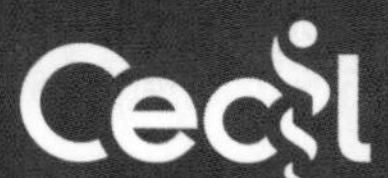

QUICK REFERENCE (QR) VIDEO ACCESS

The images below are QR codes. Each code corresponds to a video from the *Goldman's Cecil Medicine 24* collection. For fast and easy video access, right from your mobile device, follow these instructions. The videos are also available on Expertconsult.com.

What You Need

- **A mobile device, such as a smartphone or tablet, equipped with a camera and Internet access**
- **A QR code reader application (If you do not already have a reader installed on your mobile device, look for free versions in your app store.)**

How It Works

- **Open the QR code reader application on your mobile device.**
- **Point the device's camera at the code and scan.**
- **Each code opens an individual video player for instant viewing—no log-on required.**

Confusion Assessment Method (CAM)
Chapter 26, Video 1 – Sharon K. Inouye

Stress Echocardiography
Chapter 55, Video 4 – Catherine M. Otto

Interlaminar Epidural Steroid Injection
Chapter 29, Video 1 – Ali Turabi

Dilated Cardiomyopathy
Chapter 55, Video 5 – Catherine M. Otto

Standard Echocardiographic Views
Chapter 55, Video 1 – Catherine M. Otto

A Moderate Pericardial Effusion (PE)
Chapter 55, Video 6 – Catherine M. Otto

Transthoracic Versus Transesophageal Echocardiography (TEE)
Chapter 55, Video 2 – Catherine M. Otto

Secundum Atrial Septal Defect
Chapter 69, Video 1 – Ariane J. Marelli

Contrast Echocardiography
Chapter 55, Video 3 – Catherine M. Otto

Perimembranous Ventricular Septal Defect
Chapter 69, Video 2 – Ariane J. Marelli

Coronary Stent Placement
Chapter 74, Video 1 – Paul S. Teirstein

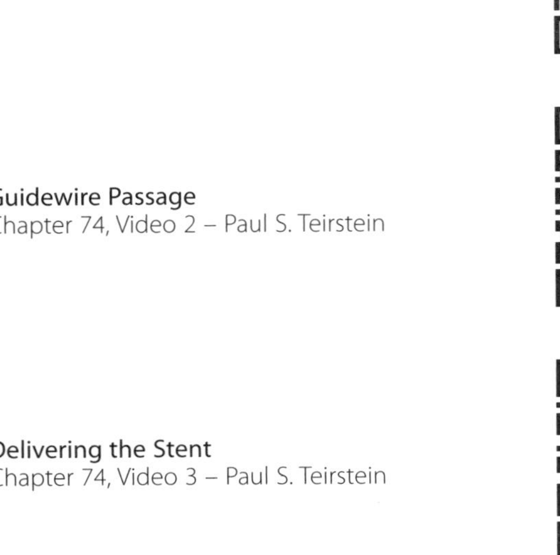

Guidewire Passage
Chapter 74, Video 2 – Paul S. Teirstein

Delivering the Stent
Chapter 74, Video 3 – Paul S. Teirstein

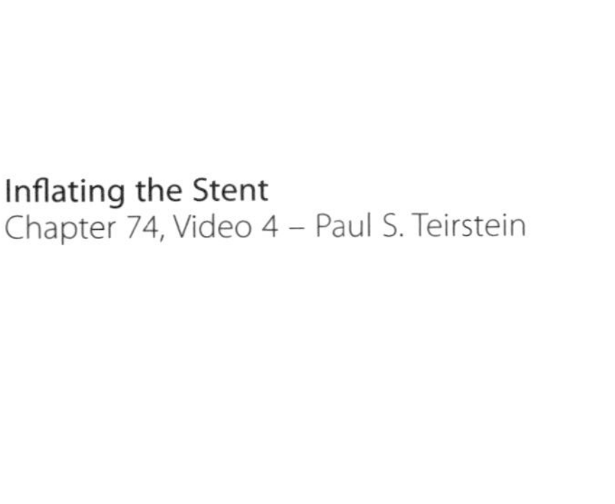

Inflating the Stent
Chapter 74, Video 4 – Paul S. Teirstein

Final Result
Chapter 74, Video 5 – Paul S. Teirstein

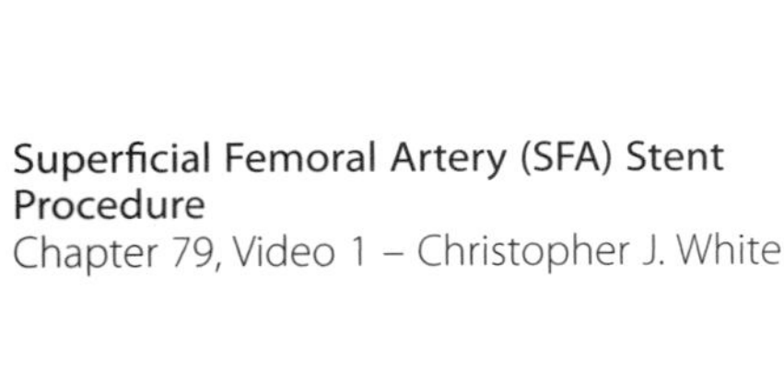

Superficial Femoral Artery (SFA) Stent Procedure
Chapter 79, Video 1 – Christopher J. White

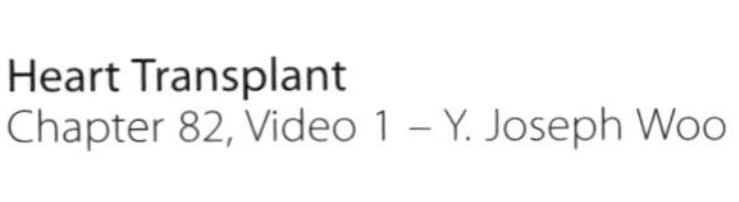

Heart Transplant
Chapter 82, Video 1 – Y. Joseph Woo

Wheezing
Chapter 87, Video 1 – Jeffrey M. Drazen

VATS Wedge Resection
Chapter 101, Video 1 – Malcolm M. DeCamp

Lung Recruitment in a Rat Lung
Chapter 105, Video 1 – Arthur S. Slutsky

Renal Artery Stent
Chapter 127, Video 1 – Thomas D. DuBose, Jr., and Renato M. Santos

Endoscopic View of Rectal Cancer
Chapter 199, Video 1 – Charles D. Blanke and Douglas O. Faigel

Endoscopic Ultrasound
Chapter 199, Video 2 – Charles D. Blanke and Douglas O. Faigel

Laparoscopic Roux-en-Y Gastric Bypass
Chapter 227, Video 1 – James M. Swain

Pituitary Surgery
Chapter 231, Video 1 – Ivan Ciric

Nasal Endoscopy
Chapter 259, Video 1 – Larry Borish

Skin Testing
Chapter 259, Video 2 – Larry Borish

Hip Arthroscopy Osteochondroplasty
Chapter 285, Video 1 – Bryan Kelly

Cervical Provocation
Chapter 407, Video 1 – Richard L. Barbano

Spurling Maneuver
Chapter 407, Video 2 – Richard L. Barbano

Cervical Distraction Test
Chapter 407, Video 3 – Richard L. Barbano

Straight Leg Raise
Chapter 407, Video 4 – Richard L. Barbano

Contralateral Straight Leg Raise
Chapter 407, Video 5 – Richard L. Barbano

Seated Straight Leg Raise
Chapter 407, Video 6 – Richard L. Barbano

Discectomy
Chapter 407, Video 7 – Jason H. Huang

Early Parkinson's Disease
Chapter 416, Video 1 – Anthony E. Lang

Freezing of Gait in Parkinson's Disease
Chapter 416, Video 2 – Anthony E. Lang

Gunslinger Gait in Progressive Supranuclear Palsy (PSP)
Chapter 416, Video 3 – Anthony E. Lang

Supranuclear Gaze Palsy in PSP
Chapter 416, Video 4 – Anthony E. Lang

Applause Sign in PSP
Chapter 416, Video 5 – Anthony E. Lang

Apraxia of Eyelid Opening (ALO) in PSP
Chapter 416, Video 6 – Anthony E. Lang

Cranial Dystonia in Multiple System Atrophy
Chapter 416, Video 7 – Anthony E. Lang

Anterocollis in Multiple System Atrophy
Chapter 416, Video 8 – Anthony E. Lang

Stridor in Multiple System Atrophy
Chapter 416, Video 9 – Anthony E. Lang

Alien Limb Phenomenon in Corticobasal Syndrome
Chapter 416, Video 10 – Anthony E. Lang

Myoclonus in Corticobasal Syndrome
Chapter 416, Video 11 – Anthony E. Lang

Levodopa-Induced Dyskinesia in Parkinson's Disease
Chapter 416, Video 12 – Anthony E. Lang

Essential Tremor
Chapter 417, Video 1 – Anthony E. Lang

Huntington's Disease
Chapter 417, Video 2 – Anthony E. Lang

Hemiballism
Chapter 417, Video 3 – Anthony E. Lang

Blepharospasm
Chapter 417, Video 4 – Anthony E. Lang

Oromandibular Dystonia
Chapter 417, Video 5 – Anthony E. Lang

Cervical Dystonia
Chapter 417, Video 6 – Anthony E. Lang

Writer's Cramp
Chapter 417, Video 7 – Anthony E. Lang

Embouchure Dystonia
Chapter 417, Video 8 – Anthony E. Lang

Sensory Trick in Cervical Dystonia
Chapter 417, Video 9 – Anthony E. Lang

Generalized Dystonia
Chapter 417, Video 10 – Anthony E. Lang

Tics
Chapter 417, Video 11 – Anthony E. Lang

Tardive Dyskinesia
Chapter 417, Video 12 – Anthony E. Lang

Hemifacial Spasm
Chapter 417, Video 13 – Anthony E. Lang

Limb Symptoms and Signs
Chapter 418, Video 1 – Pamela J. Shaw

Bulbar Symptoms and Signs
Chapter 418, Video 2 – Pamela J. Shaw

Normal Swallowing
Chapter 418, Video 3 – Pamela J. Shaw

Charcot-Marie-Tooth Disease (CMT) Exam and Walk
Chapter 428, Video 1 – Michael E. Shy

GOLDMAN'S
CECIL MEDICINE

GOLDMAN'S

CECIL MEDICINE

24TH EDITION

Volume 1

LEE GOLDMAN, MD

Dean of the Faculties of Health Sciences and Medicine
Executive Vice President for Health and Biomedical Sciences
Harold and Margaret Hatch Professor of the University
Professor of Medicine and of Epidemiology
Columbia University
New York, New York

ANDREW I. SCHAFER, MD

Chairman, Department of Medicine
The E. Hugh Luckey Distinguished Professor of Medicine
Weill Cornell Medical College
Physician-in-Chief
New York-Presbyterian Hospital/Weill Cornell Medical Center
New York, New York

ELSEVIER
SAUNDERS

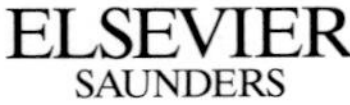

ELSEVIER
SAUNDERS

1600 John F. Kennedy Blvd.
Ste 1800
Philadelphia, PA 19103-2899

GOLDMAN'S CECIL MEDICINE, 24TH EDITION

ISBN: 978-1-4377-1604-7 (Single Volume)
978-1-4377-2788-3 (Two-Volume Set)
978-0-8089-2437-1 (International Edition)

Notices

Knowledge and best practice in this field are constantly changing. As new research and experience broaden our understanding, changes in research methods, professional practices, or medical treatment may become necessary.

Practitioners and researchers must always rely on their own experience and knowledge in evaluating and using any information, methods, compounds, or experiments described herein. In using such information or methods they should be mindful of their own safety and the safety of others, including parties for whom they have a professional responsibility.

With respect to any drug or pharmaceutical products identified, readers are advised to check the most current information provided (i) on procedures featured or (ii) by the manufacturer of each product to be administered, to verify the recommended dose or formula, the method and duration of administration, and contraindications. It is the responsibility of practitioners, relying on their own experience and knowledge of their patients, to make diagnoses, to determine dosages and the best treatment for each individual patient, and to take all appropriate safety precautions.

To the fullest extent of the law, neither the Publisher nor the authors, contributors, or editors, assume any liability for any injury and/or damage to persons or property as a matter of products liability, negligence or otherwise, or from any use or operation of any methods, products, instructions, or ideas contained in the material herein.

Library of Congress Cataloging-in-Publication Data

Goldman's Cecil medicine / [edited by] Lee Goldman, Andrew I. Schafer.—24th ed.
p. ; cm.
Cecil medicine
Rev. ed. of: Cecil medicine. 23rd ed. c2008.
Includes bibliographical references and index.
ISBN 978-1-4377-1604-7 (single v. : alk. paper)—ISBN 978-1-4377-2788-3 (two v. set : alk. paper)—ISBN 978-0-8089-2437-1 (international ed. : alk. paper)—ISBN 978-1-4377-3665-6 (e-book) 1. Internal medicine. I. Cecil, Russell L. (Russell La Fayette), 1881-1965. II. Goldman, Lee, MD. III. Schafer, Andrew I. IV. Cecil medicine. V. Title: Cecil medicine.
[DNLM: 1. Medicine. WB 100]
RC46.C423 2012
616—dc23 2011017824

Acquisitions Editor: Dolores Meloni
Developmental Editors: Catherine Carroll, Taylor Ball, Virginia Wilson
Publishing Services Manager: Patricia Tannian
Team Leader: Radhika Pallamparthy
Senior Project Manager: Linda Van Pelt
Project Manager: Anitha Sivaraj
Design Direction: Steven Stave
Marketing Manager: Helena Mutak

Printed in United States of America

Last digit is the print number: 9 8 7 6 5 4 3 2 1

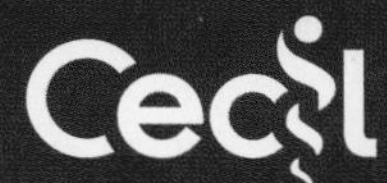

ASSOCIATE EDITORS

William P. Arend, MD
Distinguished Professor Emeritus
Arend Endowed Chair in Rheumatology
University of Colorado School of Medicine
Aurora, Colorado

James O. Armitage, MD
The Joe Shapiro Professor of Medicine
University of Nebraska College of Medicine
Section of Oncology and Hematology
University of Nebraska Medical Center
Omaha, Nebraska

David R. Clemmons, MD
Kenan Professor of Medicine
University of North Carolina at Chapel Hill School of Medicine
Chapel Hill, North Carolina

Jeffrey M. Drazen, MD
Distinguished Parker B. Francis Professor of Medicine
Harvard Medical School
Senior Physician
Division of Pulmonary and Critical Care Medicine
Brigham and Women's Hospital
Editor-in-Chief
New England Journal of Medicine
Boston, Massachusetts

Robert C. Griggs, MD, FAAN
Professor of Neurology, Medicine, Pediatrics, and Pathology and Laboratory Medicine
University of Rochester School of Medicine and Dentistry
Rochester, New York

Donald W. Landry, MD, PhD
Samuel Bard Professor and Chair, Department of Medicine
Columbia University College of Physicians and Surgeons
New York, New York

Wendy Levinson, MD
Sir John and Lady Eaton Professor and Chair
Department of Medicine
University of Toronto
Toronto, Ontario, Canada

Anil K. Rustgi, MD
T. Grier Miller Professor of Medicine and Genetics
Chief of Gastroenterology
American Cancer Society Research Professor
University of Pennsylvania School of Medicine
Philadelphia, Pennsylvania

W. Michael Scheld, MD
Bayer-Gerald L. Mandell Professor of Infectious Diseases
Director
Pfizer Initiative in International Health
Department of Medicine
University of Virginia Health System
Charlottesville, Virginia

PREFACE

The 24TH Edition of *Goldman's Cecil Medicine* symbolizes a time of extraordinary advances in medicine and in technological innovations for the dissemination of information. This textbook and its associated electronic products incorporate the latest medical knowledge in formats that are designed to appeal to learners who prefer to access information in a variety of ways.

The contents of *Cecil* have remained true to the tradition of a comprehensive textbook of medicine that carefully explains the *why* (the underlying normal physiology and pathophysiology of disease, now at the cellular and molecular as well as the organ level) and the *how* (now frequently based on Grade A evidence from randomized controlled trials). Descriptions of physiology and pathophysiology include the latest genetic advances in a practical format that strives to be useful to the nonexpert. Medicine has entered an era when the acuity of illness and the limited time available to evaluate a patient have diminished the ability of physicians to satisfy their intellectual curiosity. As a result, the acquisition of information, quite easily achieved in this era, is often confused with knowledge. We have attempted to counteract this tendency with a textbook that not only informs but also stimulates new questions and gives a glimpse of the future path to new knowledge. Grade A evidence is specifically highlighted in the text and referenced at the end of each chapter. In addition to the information provided in the textbook, the Cecil website supplies expanded content and functionality. In many cases, the full articles referenced in each chapter can be accessed from the Cecil website. The website is also continuously updated to incorporate subsequent Grade A information, other evidence, and new discoveries.

The sections for each organ system begin with a chapter that summarizes an approach to patients with key symptoms, signs, or laboratory abnormalities associated with dysfunction of that organ system. As summarized in Table 1-1, the text specifically provides clear, concise information regarding how a physician should approach more than 100 common symptoms, signs, and laboratory abnormalities, usually with a flow diagram, a table, or both for easy reference. In this way, *Cecil* remains a comprehensive text to guide diagnosis and therapy, not only for patients with suspected or known diseases but also for patients who may have undiagnosed abnormalities that require an initial evaluation.

Just as each edition brings new authors, it also reminds us of our gratitude to past editors and authors. Previous editors of *Cecil Medicine* include a short but remarkably distinguished group of leaders of American medicine: Russell Cecil, Paul Beeson, Walsh McDermott, James Wyngaarden, Lloyd H. Smith, Jr., Fred Plum, J. Claude Bennett, and Dennis Ausiello. As we welcome new associate editors—Wendy Levinson, Donald W. Landry, Anil Rustgi, and W. Michael Scheld—we also express our appreciation to Nicholas LaRusso and other associate editors from the previous editions on whose foundation we have built. Our returning associate editors—William P. Arend, James O. Armitage, David Clemmons, Jeffrey M. Drazen, and Robert C. Griggs—continue to make critical contributions to the selection of authors and the review and approval of all manuscripts. The editors, however, are fully responsible for the book as well as the integration among chapters.

The tradition of *Cecil Medicine* is that all chapters are written by distinguished experts in each field. We are also most grateful for the editorial assistance in New York of Theresa Considine and Silva Sergenian. These individuals and others in our offices have shown extraordinary dedication and equanimity in working with authors and editors to manage the unending flow of manuscripts, figures, and permissions. We also thank Faten Aberra, Reza Akari, Robert C. Brunham, Ivan Ciric, Seema Daulat, Gregory F. Erikson, Kevin Ghassemi, Jason H. Huang, Caron Jacobson, Lisa Kachnic, Bryan T. Kelly, Karen Krok, Heather Lehman, Keiron Leslie, Luis Marcos, Michael Overman, Eric Padron, Bianca Maria Piraccini, Don W. Powell, Katy Ralston, James M. Swain, Tania Thomas, Kirsten Tillisch, Ali Turabi, Mark Whiteford, and Y. Joseph Woo, who contributed to various chapters. At Elsevier, we are most indebted to Dolores Meloni and Linda McKinley, and also thank Cathy Carroll, Taylor Ball, Virginia Wilson, Linda Van Pelt, Suzanne Fannin, and Steve Stave, who have been critical to the planning and production process under the direction of Mary Gatsch. Many of the clinical photographs were supplied by Charles D. Forbes and William F. Jackson, authors of *Color Atlas and Text of Clinical Medicine*, Third Edition, published in 2003 by Elsevier Science Ltd. We thank them for graciously permitting us to include their pictures in our book. We have been exposed to remarkable physicians in our lifetimes and would like to acknowledge the mentorship and support of several of those who exemplify this paradigm—Robert H. Gifford, Lloyd H. Smith, Jr., Frank Gardner, and William Castle. Finally, we would like to thank the Goldman family—Jill, Jeff, Abigail, Mira, Daniel, and Robyn Goldman—and the Schafer family—Pauline, Eric, Pam, John, Evan, and Kate—for their understanding of the time and focus required to edit a book that attempts to sustain the tradition of our predecessors and to meet the needs of today's physician.

LEE GOLDMAN, MD
ANDREW I. SCHAFER, MD

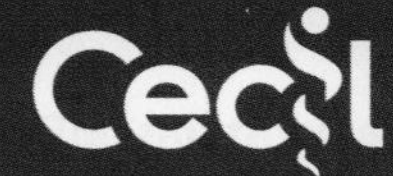

CONTRIBUTORS

Charles S. Abrams, MD
Professor of Medicine, Associate Chief, Hematology-Oncology, Department of Medicine, University of Pennsylvania School of Medicine, Philadelphia, Pennsylvania
Thrombocytopenia

Frank J. Accurso, MD
Professor of Pediatrics, University of Colorado Denver School of Medicine, Denver, Colorado
Cystic Fibrosis

Nezam H. Afdhal, MD
Associate Professor of Medicine, Harvard Medical School; Chief of Hepatology, Beth Israel Deaconess Medical Center, Boston, Massachusetts
Diseases of the Gallbladder and Bile Ducts

Cem Akin, MD, PhD
Lecturer, Harvard Medical School; Department of Internal Medicine, Division of Rheumatology, Immunology and Allergy, Brigham and Women's Hospital, Boston, Massachusetts
Mastocytosis

Allen J. Aksamit, Jr., MD
Professor, Department of Neurology, Mayo Medical School; Consultant, Department of Neurology, Mayo Clinic, Rochester, Minnesota
Acute Viral Encephalitis; Poliomyelitis

Qais Al-Awqati, MB ChB
Robert F. Loeb Professor, Department of Medicine and Department of Physiology and Cellular Biophysics, Columbia University College of Physicians and Surgeons, New York, New York
Structure and Function of the Kidneys

Ban Mishu Allos, MD
Assistant Professor of Medicine and Preventive Medicine, Vanderbilt University School of Medicine, Nashville, Tennessee
Campylobacter *Infections*

David Altshuler, MD, PhD
Professor of Genetics and Medicine, Harvard Medical School; Department of Molecular Biology and Medicine, Massachusetts General Hospital, Boston, Massachusetts; Deputy Director and Chief Academic Officer, Broad Institute of MIT and Harvard, Cambridge, Massachusetts
The Inherited Basis of Common Diseases

Michael J. Aminoff, MD, DSc
Professor, Department of Neurology, University of California, San Francisco, School of Medicine, San Francisco, California
Approach to the Patient with Neurologic Disease

Jeffrey L. Anderson, MD, MACP
Professor, Department of Internal Medicine, University of Utah School of Medicine, Salt Lake City; Associate Chief of Cardiology, Intermountain Medical Center, Murray, Utah
ST Elevation Acute Myocardial Infarction and Complications of Myocardial Infarction

Karl E. Anderson, MD
Professor of Preventive Medicine and Community Health and Internal Medicine, University of Texas Medical Branch, Galveston, Texas
The Porphyrias

Larry J. Anderson, MD
Professor and Co-Director, Division of Pediatric Infectious Diseases, Emory University School of Medicine, Atlanta, Georgia
Coronaviruses

Karen H. Antman, MD
Provost, Boston University Medical Campus, and Dean, Boston University School of Medicine, Boston, Massachusetts
Primary and Metastatic Malignant Bone Lesions

Aśok C. Antony, MD
Professor of Medicine, Indiana University School of Medicine, Indianapolis, Indiana
Megaloblastic Anemias

Gerald B. Appel, MD
Professor of Clinical Medicine, Columbia University College of Physicians and Surgeons; Director of Clinical Nephrology, Department of Medicine, Columbia University Medical Center, New York, New York
Glomerular Disorders and Nephrotic Syndromes

Frederick R. Appelbaum, MD
Professor and Head, Division of Oncology, University of Washington School of Medicine; Director, Clinical Research Division, Fred Hutchinson Cancer Research Center, Seattle, Washington
The Acute Leukemias

William P. Arend, MD
Arend Endowed Chair in Rheumatology and Distinguished Professor Emeritus, University of Colorado School of Medicine, Aurora, Colorado
Approach to the Patient with Rheumatic Disease

Paul Arguin, MD
Chief, Domestic Malaria Unit, Division of Parasitic Diseases, Centers for Disease Control and Prevention, Atlanta, Georgia
Approach to the Patient before and after Travel

James O. Armitage, MD
The Joe Shapiro Professor of Medicine, University of Nebraska College of Medicine, Section of Oncology and Hematology, University of Nebraska Medical Center, Omaha, Nebraska
Venomous Snake Bites; Approach to the Patient with Lymphadenopathy and Splenomegaly; Non-Hodgkin's Lymphomas

Cheryl A. Armstrong, MD
Professor and Chair, Department of Dermatology, University of Arkansas for Medical Sciences; Section Chief, Dermatology Section, Central Arkansas Veterans Healthcare System, Little Rock, Arkansas
Examination of the Skin and an Approach to Diagnosing Skin Diseases

M. Amin Arnaout, MD
Professor of Medicine, Harvard Medical School; Physician and Chief, Division of Nephrology, Department of Medicine, Massachusetts General Hospital, Boston, Massachusetts
Cystic Kidney Diseases

Robert Arnold, MD
Leo H. Criep Chair in Patient Care, Department of Medicine, Section of Palliative Care and Medical Ethics, University of Pittsburgh, Pittsburgh, Pennsylvania
Care of Dying Patients and Their Families

David Atkins, MD, MPH
Director, Quality Enhancement Research Initiative, Office of Research and Development, Department of Veterans Affairs, Washington, DC
The Periodic Health Examination

William L. Atkinson, MD, MPH
Medical Epidemiologist, National Center for Immunization and Respiratory Diseases, Centers for Disease Control and Prevention, Atlanta, Georgia
Immunization

Dennis Ausiello, MD
Jackson Professor of Clinical Medicine, Harvard Medical School; Physician-in-Chief, Massachusetts General Hospital, Boston, Massachusetts
Disorders of Sodium and Water Homeostasis

Bruce R. Bacon, MD
James F. King MD Endowed Chair in Gastroenterology, Professor of Internal Medicine, Division of Gastroenterology and Hepatology, Saint Louis University School of Medicine, St. Louis, Missouri
Inherited and Metabolic Disorders of the Liver; Iron Overload (Hemochromatosis)

Grover C. Bagby, MD
Professor, Department of Medicine, Department of Molecular and Medical Genetics, Oregon Health & Science University; Staff Physician, Hematology/Oncology, Portland Veterans Affairs Medical Center, Portland, Oregon
Aplastic Anemia and Related Bone Marrow Failure States

Barbara J. Bain, MB ChB
Professor in Diagnostic Haematology, Imperial College London; Consultant Haematologist, St Mary's Hospital, London, England
The Peripheral Blood Smear

Dean F. Bajorin, MD
Professor of Medicine, Department of Medicine, Weill Cornell Medical College; Attending Physician, Department of Medicine, Memorial Sloan-Kettering Cancer Center, New York, New York
Tumors of the Kidney, Bladder, Ureters, and Renal Pelvis

Mark Ballow, MD
Professor of Pediatrics, Chief, Division of Allergy and Clinical Immunology, University at Buffalo School of Medicine and Biomedical Sciences, Women & Children's Hospital of Buffalo, Buffalo, New York
Primary Immunodeficiency Diseases

Robert W. Baloh, MD
Professor of Neurology and Surgery (Head and Neck), David Geffen School of Medicine at UCLA, University of California, Los Angeles, California
Neuro-Ophthalmology; Smell and Taste; Hearing and Equilibrium

Jonathan Barasch, MD, PhD
Associate Professor of Medicine, Columbia University College of Physicians & Surgeons, New York, New York
Structure and Function of the Kidneys

Richard L. Barbano, MD, PhD
Professor of Neurology, University of Rochester; Chief of Neurology and Physical Medicine and Rehabilitation, Rochester General Hospital, Rochester, New York
Mechanical and Other Lesions of the Spine, Nerve Roots, and Spinal Cord; Videos

Murray G. Baron, MD
Professor of Radiology, Emory University School of Medicine, Atlanta, Georgia
Radiology of the Heart

Elizabeth Barrett-Connor, MD
Distinguished Professor and Chief, Division of Epidemiology, Department of Family and Preventive Medicine, University of California, San Diego, School of Medicine, La Jolla, California
Menopause

Michael J. Barry, MD
Professor of Medicine, Harvard Medical School; Medical Director, John D. Stoeckle Center for Primary Care Innovation, Massachusetts General Hospital, Boston, Massachusetts
Benign Prostatic Hyperplasia and Prostatitis

Bruce A. Barshop, MD, PhD
Professor, B. L. Maas Chair in Inherited Metabolic Disease, Department of Pediatrics, University of California, San Diego, School of Medicine, La Jolla, California
Homocystinuria and Hyperhomocysteinemia

John G. Bartlett, MD
Stanhope Bayne-Jones Professor of Medicine, Division of Infectious Diseases, Johns Hopkins University School of Medicine, Baltimore, Maryland
Bioterrorism

Mary Barton, MD, MPP
Scientific Director, U.S. Preventive Services Task Force, Center for Primary Care, Prevention and Clinical Partnerships, Agency for Healthcare Research and Quality, Rockville, Maryland
The Periodic Health Examination

Robert C. Basner, MD
Associate Professor of Clinical Medicine, Columbia University College of Physicians & Surgeons; Director, Cardiopulmonary Sleep and Ventilatory Disorders Center, Columbia University Medical Center, New York, New York
Obstructive Sleep Apnea

Stephen G. Baum, MD
Professor of Medicine and of Microbiology and Immunology, Albert Einstein College of Medicine; Senior Associate Dean for Students, Albert Einstein College of Medicine, Bronx, New York
Mycoplasma *Infections*

Daniel G. Bausch, MD, MPH&TM
Associate Professor, Department of Tropical Medicine and Section of Adult Infectious Diseases, Tulane University Health Sciences Center, New Orleans, Louisiana
Viral Hemorrhagic Fevers

Arnold S. Bayer, MD
Professor of Medicine, David Geffen School of Medicine at UCLA; Associate Chief, Adult Infectious Diseases, Senior Investigator, LA Biomedical Research Institute, Los Angeles, California
Infective Endocarditis

Hasan Bazari, MD
Associate Professor of Medicine, Harvard Medical School; Program Director, Internal Medicine Residency, Clinical Director, Nephrology Division, Massachusetts General Hospital, Boston, Massachusetts
Approach to the Patient with Renal Disease

John H. Beigel, MD
Medical Scientist, National Institute of Allergy and Infectious Diseases, National Institutes of Health, Bethesda, Maryland
Antiviral Therapy (Non-HIV)

George A. Beller, MD
Ruth C. Heede Professor of Cardiology, Division of Cardiovascular Medicine, Department of Medicine, University of Virginia Health System, Charlottesville, Virginia
Noninvasive Cardiac Imaging

Robert M. Bennett, MD
Professor of Medicine and Nursing, Oregon Health & Science University, Portland, Oregon
Fibromyalgia and Chronic Fatigue Syndrome

Joseph R. Berger, MD
Ruth L. Works Professor and Chairman, Department of Neurology, University of Kentucky, Lexington, Kentucky
Cytomegalovirus, Epstein-Barr Virus, and Other Slow Virus Infections of the Central Nervous System; Neurologic Complications of Human Immunodeficiency Virus Infection; Brain Abscess and Parameningeal Infections

Paul Berk, MD
Professor, Department of Medicine, Columbia University College of Physicians and Surgeons, New York, New York
Approach to the Patient with Jaundice or Abnormal Liver Tests

Nancy Berliner, MD
Professor of Medicine, Harvard Medical School; Chief, Division of Hematology, Department of Medicine, Brigham and Women's Hospital, Boston, Massachusetts
Leukocytosis and Leukopenia

James L. Bernat, MD
Louis and Ruth Frank Professor of Neuroscience, Professor of Neurology and Medicine, Dartmouth Medical School, Hanover, New Hampshire; Attending Neurologist, Dartmouth-Hitchcock Medical Center, Lebanon, New Hampshire
Coma, Vegetative State, and Brain Death

Philip J. Bierman, MD
Professor, Department of Internal Medicine, University of Nebraska Medical Center, Omaha, Nebraska
Non-Hodgkin's Lymphomas

Bruce R. Bistrian, MD, PhD, MPH
Professor of Medicine, Harvard Medical School; Chief, Clinical Nutrition, Beth Israel Deaconess Medical Center, Boston, Massachusetts
Nutritional Assessment

Joseph J. Biundo, MD
Clinical Professor of Medicine, Tulane Health Science Center, New Orleans, Louisiana
Bursitis, Tendinitis, and Other Periarticular Disorders and Sports Medicine

Charles D. Blanke, MD
Professor and Head, Medical Oncology, University of British Columbia; Vice President, Systemic Therapy, British Columbia Cancer Agency, Vancouver, British Columbia, Canada
Neoplasms of the Large and Small Intestine; Videos

Joel N. Blankson, MD, PhD
Associate Professor, Division of Infectious Diseases, Department of Medicine, Johns Hopkins University School of Medicine, Baltimore, Maryland
Immunopathogenesis of Human Immunodeficiency Virus Infection

Martin J. Blaser, MD
Frederick H. King Professor of Internal Medicine and Chair, Department of Medicine; Professor of Microbiology, New York University Langone Medical Center, New York, New York
Acid Peptic Disease

William A. Blattner, MD
Professor and Associate Director, Institute of Human Virology, University of Maryland School of Medicine, Baltimore, Maryland
Retroviruses Other Than Human Immunodeficiency Virus

Thomas P. Bleck, MD
Professor of Neurological Sciences, Neurosurgery, Medicine, and Anesthesiology and Assistant Dean, Rush Medical College; Associate Chief Medical Officer for Critical Care, Rush University Medical Center, Chicago, Illinois
Arboviruses Affecting the Central Nervous System

William E. Boden, MD
Clinical Chief, Division of Cardiovascular Medicine, Professor of Medicine and Preventive Medicine, University at Buffalo Schools of Medicine and Public Health; Medical Director, Cardiovascular Services, Kaleida Health, Chief of Cardiology, Buffalo General and Millard Fillmore Hospitals, Buffalo, New York
Angina Pectoris and Stable Ischemic Heart Disease

C. Richard Boland, MD
Chief, Division of Gastroenterology; Director, GI Cancer Research Laboratory, Baylor University Medical Center, Dallas, Texas
Cancer Genetics

Jean Bolognia, MD
Professor, Department of Dermatology, Yale University School of Medicine, New Haven, Connecticut
Infections, Hyper- and Hypopigmentation, Regional Dermatology, and Distinctive Lesions in Black Skin

Robert Bonomo, MD
Professor of Medicine, Pharmacology, and Molecular Biology and Microbiology, Case Western Reserve University School of Medicine; Director, VISN 10 GRECC, Louis Stokes Cleveland Veterans Affairs Medical Center, Cleveland, Ohio
Diseases Caused by Acinetobacter *and* Stenotrophomonas *Species*

Larry Borish, MD
Professor of Medicine, Asthma and Allergic Disease Center, University of Virginia, Charlottesville, Virginia
Allergic Rhinitis and Sinusitis; Videos

Patrick J. Bosque, MD
Associate Professor, Department of Neurology, University of Colorado Denver School of Medicine, Aurora, Colorado; Neurologist, Division of Neurology, Denver Health Medical Center, Denver, Colorado
Prion Diseases

Randall Brand, MD
Professor of Medicine and Academic Director, GI Division Shadyside; Director, GI Malignancy Early Detection, Diagnosis and Prevention, University of Pittsburgh Medical Center, Pittsburgh, Pennsylvania
Pancreatic Cancer

Itzhak Brook, MD, MSc
Professor, Department of Pediatrics and Medicine, Georgetown University, Washington, DC
Diseases Caused by Non–Spore-Forming Anaerobic Bacteria; Actinomycosis

Enrico Brunetti, MD
Assistant Professor of Infectious Diseases, University of Pavia; Attending Physician, Division of Infectious and Tropical Diseases, IRCCS San Matteo Hospital Foundation; Co-Director, WHO Collaborating Centre for Clinical Management of Cystic Echinococcosis, Pavia, Italy
Cestodes

David M. Buchner, MD, MPH
Professor, Department of Kinesiology and Community Health, University of Illinois at Urbana-Champaign, Champaign, Illinois
Physical Activity

Pierre A. Buffet, MD, PhD
Assistant Professor, Department of Parasitology, Pitié-Salpêtrière Hospital, Paris 6 University, Institut Pasteur, Paris, France
Leishmaniasis

H. Franklin Bunn, MD
Professor of Medicine, Harvard Medical School; Senior Physician, Brigham and Women's Hospital, Boston, Massachusetts
Approach to the Anemias

Peter A. Calabresi, MD
Professor of Neurology, Director, Johns Hopkins Multiple Sclerosis Center; Director, Division of Neuroimmunology and Neuroinfectious Diseases, Johns Hopkins University, Baltimore, Maryland
Multiple Sclerosis and Demyelinating Conditions of the Central Nervous System

David P. Calfee, MD, MSc
Associate Professor of Medicine and Public Health, Chief Hospital Epidemiologist, New York-Presbyterian Hospital/Weill Cornell Medical Center, New York, New York
Prevention and Control of Health Care–Associated Infections

Hugh Calkins, MD
Professor of Medicine, Director of Electrophysiology, Johns Hopkins Medical Institutions, Baltimore, Maryland
Principles of Electrophysiology

Douglas Cameron, MD, MBA
Emeritus Professor, Department of Ophthalmology, Mayo Medical School, Rochester, Minnesota
Diseases of the Visual System

Michael Camilleri, MD
Atherton and Winifred W. Bean Professor and Professor of Medicine and Physiology, Mayo Medical School; Consultant in Gastroenterology and Hepatology, Mayo Clinic, Rochester, Minnesota
Disorders of Gastrointestinal Motility

Grant W. Cannon, MD
Professor of Medicine, Division of Rheumatology, University of Utah School of Medicine; Associate Chief of Staff for Academic Affiliations, George E. Wahlen Veterans Affairs Medical Center, Salt Lake City, Utah
Immunosuppressing Drugs including Corticosteroids

Maria Domenica Cappellini, MD
Professor of Internal Medicine, Department of Internal Medicine, Università di Milano-Policlinico "Ca Granda" Foundation IRCCS, Milano, Italy
The Thalassemias

Blase A. Carabello, MD
Professor of Medicine, Baylor College of Medicine; Chief of Medicine, Michael E. DeBakey Veterans Affairs Medical Center, Houston, Texas
Valvular Heart Disease

Edgar M. Carvalho, MD, PhD
Professor of Clinical Medicine, Faculdade de Medicina da Bahia, Universidade Federal da Bahia, Salvador-BA, Brazil
Schistosomiasis (Bilharziasis)

Agustin Castellanos, MD
Professor of Medicine, Director, Clinical Electrophysiology, Division of Cardiovascular Medicine, University of Miami, Miller School of Medicine, Miami, Florida
Approach to Cardiac Arrest and Life-Threatening Arrhythmias

Naga P. Chalasani, MD
Professor of Medicine and Cellular and Integrative Physiology, Director, Division of Gastroenterology and Hepatology, Department of Medicine, Indiana University School of Medicine, Indianapolis, Indiana
Alcoholic and Nonalcoholic Steatohepatitis

Henry Chambers, MD
Professor of Medicine, University of California, San Francisco, School of Medicine; Chief, Division of Infectious Diseases, San Francisco General Hospital, San Francisco, California
Staphylococcal Infections

Mary Charlson, MD
William T. Foley Distinguished Professor of Medicine, Chief, Division of Epidemiology and Evaluative Sciences Research, Executive Director of Center for Integrative Medicine, Department of Medicine, Weill Cornell Medical College, New York, New York
Complementary and Alternative Medicine

William P. Cheshire, Jr., MD
Professor of Neurology, Director of Clinical Neurophysiology Laboratory, Mayo Clinic, Jacksonville, Florida
Autonomic Disorders and Their Management

Patrick F. Chinnery, MB BS
Director and Professor of Neurogenetics, Institute of Genetic Medicine, Newcastle University; Honorary Consultant Neurologist, Newcastle upon Tyne Hospitals NHS Trust, Newcastle upon Tyne, United Kingdom
Muscle Diseases

David C. Christiani, MD, MPH
Professor of Medicine, Harvard Medical School; Elkan Blout Professor of Environmental Genetics, Environmental Health, Harvard School of Public Health; Physician, Pulmonary and Critical Care Unit, Massachusetts General Hospital, Boston, Massachusetts
Physical and Chemical Injuries of the Lung

David R. Clemmons, MD
Kenan Professor of Medicine, University of North Carolina at Chapel Hill School of Medicine, Chapel Hill, North Carolina
Approach to the Patient with Endocrine Disease; Principles of Endocrinology

Jeffrey Cohen, MD
Chief, Laboratory of Infectious Diseases, National Institute of Allergy and Infectious Diseases, National Institutes of Health, Bethesda, Maryland
Varicella-Zoster Virus (Chickenpox, Shingles)

Myron S. Cohen, MD
J. Herbert Bate Distinguished Professor, Departments of Medicine, Microbiology and Public Health; Associate Vice Chancellor and Director, Institute of Global Health and Infectious Diseases, University of North Carolina at Chapel Hill School of Medicine, Chapel Hill, North Carolina
Approach to the Patient with a Sexually Transmitted Disease

Steven P. Cohen, MD
Associate Professor, Department of Anesthesiology, Johns Hopkins Medical Institutions, Baltimore, Maryland; Professor and Director of Pain Research, Department of Surgery, Walter Reed Army Medical Center, Washington, DC; Colonel, Medical Corps, U.S. Army Reserve
Pain

Steven L. Cohn, MD
Clinical Professor of Medicine, SUNY Downstate; Director, Medical Consultation Service, Kings County Hospital Center, Brooklyn, New York
Preoperative Evaluation

Robert Colebunders, MD, PhD
Professor, Department of Clinical Sciences, Institute of Tropical Medicine; Department of Epidemiology and Social Medicine, University of Antwerp, Antwerp, Belgium
Immune Reconstitution Inflammatory Syndrome in HIV/AIDS

Joseph M. Connors, MD
Clinical Professor, Division of Medical Oncology, Department of Medicine, University of British Columbia; Clinical Director, Centre for Lymphoid Cancer, British Columbia Cancer Agency, Vancouver, British Columbia, Canada
Hodgkin's Lymphoma

Deborah J. Cook, MD, MSc
Professor, Department of Medicine, Clinical Epidemiology, and Biostatistics, Academic Chair, Critical Care Medicine, McMaster University, Hamilton, Ontario, Canada
Approach to the Patient in a Critical Care Setting

C. Ralph Corey, MD
Gary Hock Distinguished Professor of Global Health, Director, Infectious Disease Research, Duke Clinical Research Institute; Director, Hubert/Yeargan Center for Global Health; Professor of Medicine and Pathology, Duke University Medical Center, Durham, North Carolina
Venomous Snake Bites

Kenneth H. Cowan, MD, PhD
Director, Eppley Cancer Center, University of Nebraska Medical Center; Director, Eppley Institute for Research in Cancer, University of Nebraska Medical Center, Omaha, Nebraska
Biology of Cancer

William A. Craig, MD
Professor Emeritus, Department of Medicine, University of Wisconsin School of Medicine and Public Health, Madison, Wisconsin
Antibacterial Chemotherapy

Simon L. Croft, PhD
Professor of Parasitology, Head, Faculty of Infectious and Tropical Diseases, London School of Hygiene and Tropical Medicine, London, England
Leishmaniasis

Mary K. Crow, MD
Joseph P. Routh Professor of Rheumatic Diseases in Medicine, Chief, Rheumatology Division, Department of Medicine, Weill Cornell Medical College; Physician-in-Chief and Chair, Rheumatology Division, Hospital for Special Surgery, New York, New York
Systemic Lupus Erythematosus

John A. Crump, MB ChB
Associate Professor of Medicine and Pathology, Division of Infectious Diseases and International Health, Duke University Medical Center; Director, Duke Tanzania Operations, Duke Global Health Institute, Duke University, Durham, North Carolina
Salmonella *Infections (including Typhoid Fever)*

Mark R. Cullen, MD
Professor of Medicine, Chief, Division of General Medical Disciplines, Stanford University School of Medicine, Stanford, California
Principles of Occupational and Environmental Medicine

Gary C. Curhan, MD, ScD
Associate Professor of Medicine, Harvard Medical School; Associate Professor of Epidemiology, Harvard School of Public Health; Physician, Renal Division and Channing Laboratory, Brigham and Women's Hospital, Boston, Massachusetts
Nephrolithiasis

Inger K. Damon, MD, PhD
Chief, Poxvirus and Rabies Branch, Centers for Disease Control and Prevention, Atlanta, Georgia
Smallpox, Monkeypox, and Other Poxvirus Infections

Troy E. Daniels, DDS, MSc
Professor, Department of Orofacial Sciences, University of California, San Francisco, School of Dentistry; Professor, Department of Pathology, University of California, San Francisco, School of Medicine, San Francisco, California
Diseases of the Mouth and Salivary Glands

Nancy Davidson, MD
Professor of Medicine and Pharmacology and Chemical Biology, University of Pittsburgh School of Medicine; Director, University of Pittsburgh Cancer Institute and UPMC Cancer Centers, Pittsburgh, Pennsylvania
Breast Cancer and Benign Breast Disorders

Lisa M. DeAngelis, MD
Professor of Neurology, Weill Cornell Medical College; Chair, Department of Neurology, Memorial Sloan-Kettering Cancer Center, New York, New York
Tumors of the Central Nervous System and Intracranial Hypertension and Hypotension

Malcolm M. DeCamp, MD
Fowler McCormick Professor of Surgery and Professor of Medicine, Northwestern University Feinberg School of Medicine; Chief, Division of Thoracic Surgery, Northwestern Memorial Hospital, Chicago, Illinois
Interventional and Surgical Approaches to Lung Disease; Video

Carlos Del Rio, MD
Hubert Professor and Chair, Hubert Department of Global Health, Rollins School of Public Health of Emory University; Professor of Medicine, Emory University School of Medicine, Atlanta, Georgia
Prevention of Human Immunodeficiency Virus Infection

George D. Demetri, MD
Associate Professor of Medicine, Harvard Medical School; Director, Ludwig Center at Dana-Farber Cancer Institute; Senior Vice President for Experimental Therapeutics, Dana-Farber Cancer Institute, Boston, Massachusetts
Sarcomas of Soft Tissue and Bone, and Other Neoplasms of Connective Tissues

Robert H. Demling, MD
Professor of Surgery, Harvard Medical School; Director of Education and Research, Department of Surgery, Brigham and Women's Hospital, Boston, Massachusetts
Medical Aspects of Trauma and Burn Care

Patricia A. Deuster, PhD, MPH
Professor and Scientific Director, Consortium for Health and Military Performance, Department of Military and Emergency Medicine, Uniformed Services University of the Health Sciences, Bethesda, Maryland
Rhabdomyolysis

Robert B. Diasio, MD
William J. and Charles H. Mayo Professor, Departments of Molecular Pharmacology and Experimental Therapeutics and Oncology, Mayo Medical School; Director, Mayo Clinic Cancer Center, Rochester, Minnesota
Principles of Drug Therapy

David J. Diemert, MD
Assistant Professor, Department of Microbiology, Immunology and Tropical Medicine, George Washington University; Director of Clinical Trials, Albert B. Sabin Vaccine Institute, Washington, DC
Intestinal Nematode Infections; Tissue Nematode Infections

Kathleen B. Digre, MD
Professor of Neurology and Ophthalmology, Adjunct Professor of Obstetrics and Gynecology, Director, Headache Clinic, University of Utah School of Medicine, Salt Lake City, Utah
Headaches and Other Head Pain

John M. Douglas, Jr., MD
Chief Medical Officer, National Center for HIV/AIDS, Viral Hepatitis, STD, and TB Prevention, Centers for Disease Control and Prevention, Atlanta, Georgia
Papillomavirus

Jeffrey M. Drazen, MD
Distinguished Parker B. Francis Professor of Medicine, Harvard Medical School; Senior Physician, Division of Pulmonary and Critical Care Medicine, Brigham and Women's Hospital; Editor-in-Chief, *New England Journal of Medicine,* Boston, Massachusetts
Asthma; Video

Stephen C. Dreskin, MD, PhD
Professor of Medicine and Immunology, Division of Allergy and Clinical Immunology, University of Colorado Denver School of Medicine, Aurora, Colorado
Urticaria and Angioedema

W. Lawrence Drew, MD, PhD
Professor, Laboratory Medicine and Medicine, University of California, San Francisco, School of Medicine, San Francisco, California
Cytomegalovirus

George L. Drusano, MD
Co-Director, Ordway Research Institute, Albany, New York
Antibacterial Chemotherapy

Thomas D. DuBose, Jr., MD
Tinsley R. Harrison Professor and Chair, Department of Internal Medicine, Wake Forest University School of Medicine, Winston-Salem, North Carolina
Vascular Disorders of the Kidney; Video

F. Daniel Duffy, MD
Steven Landgarten Professor in Medical Leadership, Dean, University of Oklahoma, School of Community Medicine, Tulsa, Oklahoma
Counseling for Behavior Change

Herbert L. DuPont, MD
H. Irving Schweppe, Jr., Chair of Internal Medicine and Vice Chairman, Department of Medicine, Baylor College of Medicine; Chief, Internal Medicine, St. Luke's Episcopal Hospital; Director, Center for Infectious Diseases, University of Texas–Houston School of Public Health, Houston, Texas
Approach to the Patient with Suspected Enteric Infection

Madeleine Duvic, MD
Professor of Dermatology and Medicine, Deputy Chairman, Department of Dermatology, The University of Texas M.D. Anderson Cancer Center, Houston, Texas
Urticaria, Drug Hypersensitivity Rashes, Nodules and Tumors, and Atrophic Diseases

Kathryn M. Edwards, MD
Sarah H. Sell Professor of Pediatrics, Vanderbilt University School of Medicine, Nashville, Tennessee
Parainfluenza Viral Disease

N. Lawrence Edwards, MD
Professor of Medicine, Vice Chairman, Department of Medicine, University of Florida College of Medicine; Chief, Section of Rheumatology, Veterans Administration Medical Center, Gainesville, Florida
Crystal Deposition Diseases

Lawrence H. Einhorn, MD
Distinguished Professor of Medicine, Lance Armstrong Foundation Professor of Oncology, Indiana University School of Medicine, Indianapolis, Indiana
Testicular Cancer

Ronald J. Elin, MD, PhD
A. J. Miller Professor and Chair, Department of Pathology and Laboratory Medicine, University of Louisville School of Medicine, Louisville, Kentucky
Reference Intervals and Laboratory Values

George M. Eliopoulos, MD
Professor of Medicine, Harvard Medical School; Division of Infectious Diseases, Beth Israel Deaconess Medical Center, Boston, Massachusetts
Principles of Anti-Infective Therapy

Perry Elliott, MBBS, MD
Reader in Inherited Cardiac Disease, The Heart Hospital, University College London, London, United Kingdom
Diseases of the Myocardium and Endocardium

Jerrold J. Ellner, MD
Professor of Medicine, Boston University; Chief, Section of Infectious Diseases, Boston Medical Center, Boston, Massachusetts
Tuberculosis

Louis J. Elsas II, MD
Professor and Chair, Department of Biochemistry and Molecular Biology, University of Miami; Professor, Department of Pediatrics, University of Miami, Miller School of Medicine, Miami, Florida
Approach to Inborn Errors of Metabolism

Dirk M. Elston, MD
Director, Department of Dermatology, Geisinger Medical Center, Danville, Pennsylvania
Arthropods and Leeches

Ezekiel J. Emanuel, MD, PhD
Chair, Department of Bioethics, The Clinical Center, National Institutes of Health, Bethesda, Maryland
Bioethics in the Practice of Medicine

Gregory F. Erickson, PhD
Professor Emeritus of Reproductive Medicine, Division of Reproductive Endocrinology, University of California, San Diego, School of Medicine, La Jolla, California
Ovaries and Development; Reproductive Endocrinology and Infertility

Armin Ernst, MD
Associate Professor of Medicine and Surgery, Harvard Medical School; Chief of Interventional Pulmonology, Beth Israel Deaconess Medical Center, Boston, Massachusetts
Interventional and Surgical Approaches to Lung Disease

Joel D. Ernst, MD
Professor, Departments of Medicine, Pathology, and Microbiology; Director, Division of Infectious Diseases, New York University School of Medicine, New York, New York
Leprosy (Hansen's Disease)

David S. Ettinger, MD
Alex Grass Professor of Oncology, Department of Oncology, The Sidney Kimmel Comprehensive Cancer Center at Johns Hopkins, Baltimore, Maryland
Lung Cancer and Other Pulmonary Neoplasms

Amelia Evoli, MD
Associate Professor, Department of Neuroscience, Catholic University, Rome, Italy
Disorders of Neuromuscular Transmission

Douglas O. Faigel, MD
Professor of Medicine, Mayo Medical School; Division of Gastroenterology and Hepatology, Mayo Clinic, Scottsdale, Arizona
Neoplasms of the Large and Small Intestine; Videos

Gary W. Falk, MD, MSc
Professor of Medicine, Division of Gastroenterology, University of Pennsylvania School of Medicine, Philadelphia, Pennsylvania
Diseases of the Esophagus

Murray J. Favus, MD
Professor of Medicine, Section of Endocrinology, Diabetes and Metabolism, University of Chicago Pritzker School of Medicine, Chicago, Illinois
Mineral and Bone Homeostasis

Gene Feder, MD
Professor of Primary Health Care, School of Social and Community Medicine, University of Bristol, Bristol, United Kingdom
Intimate Partner Violence

Stephan D. Fihn, MD, MPH
Professor, Medicine and Health Services, University of Washington School of Medicine; Director, Analytics and Business Intelligence, Department of Veterans Affairs, Seattle, Washington
Measuring Health and Health Care

Gary S. Firestein, MD
Professor of Medicine, Dean and Associate Vice Chancellor of Translational Medicine, University of California, San Diego, School of Medicine, La Jolla, California
Mechanisms of Inflammation and Tissue Repair

Neil Fishman, MD
Associate Professor of Medicine, University of Pennsylvania School of Medicine; Director, Department of Healthcare Epidemiology, Infection Prevention and Control; Director, Antimicrobial Stewardship Program, Hospital of the University of Pennsylvania, Philadelphia, Pennsylvania
Prevention and Control of Health Care–Associated Infections

Lee A. Fleisher, MD
Robert D. Dripps Professor and Chair of Anesthesiology, Professor of Medicine, University of Pennsylvania School of Medicine, Philadelphia, Pennsylvania
Overview of Anesthesia

Marsha D. Ford, MD
Adjunct Professor, Department of Emergency Medicine, University of North Carolina at Chapel Hill School of Medicine, Chapel Hill, North Carolina; Director, Carolinas Poison Center, Carolinas Medical Center, Charlotte, North Carolina
Acute Poisoning

Chris E. Forsmark, MD
Professor of Medicine, Chief, Division of Gastroenterology, Hepatology, and Nutrition, University of Florida College of Medicine, Gainesville, Florida
Pancreatitis

Vance G. Fowler, Jr., MD, MHS
Associate Professor, Department of Medicine, Division of Infectious Diseases, Duke University Medical Center, Durham, North Carolina
Infective Endocarditis

Jay W. Fox, PhD
Professor, Department of Microbiology, University of Virginia School of Medicine, Charlottesville, Virginia
Venoms and Poisons from Marine Organisms

Manuel A. Franco, MD, PhD
Director of Postgraduate Programs, School of Sciences, Pontificia Universidad Javeriana, Bogota, Colombia
Rotaviruses, Noroviruses, and Other Gastrointestinal Viruses

Martyn A. French, MD, MB ChB
Winthrop Professor in Clinical Immunology, School of Pathology and Laboratory Medicine, University of Western Australia; Consultant Clinical Immunologist, Royal Perth Hospital, Perth, Western Australia, Australia
Immune Reconstitution Inflammatory Syndrome in HIV/AIDS

Karen Freund, MD, MPH
Professor of Medicine, Director, Women's Health Interdisciplinary Research Center, Boston University School of Medicine; Professor of Epidemiology, Boston University School of Public Health, Boston, Massachusetts
Approach to Women's Health

Linda P. Fried, MD, MPH
Dean and DeLamar Professor of Public Health and of Medicine, Senior Vice President, Columbia University Medical Center; Professor of Epidemiology, Columbia University Mailman School of Public Health, New York, New York
Epidemiology of Aging: Implications of the Aging of Society

Cem Gabay, MD
Professor of Medicine, University of Geneva School of Medicine; Head, Division of Rheumatology, University Hospitals of Geneva, Geneva, Switzerland
Biologic Agents

Kenneth L. Gage, PhD
Chief, Flea-Borne Diseases Activity, Division of Vector-Borne Diseases, Centers for Disease Control and Prevention, Fort Collins, Colorado
Plague and Other Yersinia *Infections*

Robert F. Gagel, MD
Head, Division of Internal Medicine, Endocrine Neoplasia and Hormonal Disorders, The University of Texas M.D. Anderson Cancer Center, Houston, Texas
Endocrine Manifestations of Tumors: "Ectopic" Hormone Production

John N. Galgiani, MD
Professor of Medicine and Director, Valley Fever Center for Excellence, University of Arizona; Chief Medical Officer, Valley Fever Solutions Inc., Tucson, Arizona
Coccidioidomycosis

Patrick G. Gallagher, MD
Professor, Department of Pediatrics and Genetics, Yale University School of Medicine, New Haven, Connecticut
Hemolytic Anemias: Red Cell Membrane and Metabolic Defects

Eithan Galun, MD
Professor, Director, Goldyne Savad Institute of Gene Therapy, Hadassah Hebrew University Hospital, Jerusalem, Israel
Gene and Cell Therapy

Leonard Ganz, MD
Associate Professor of Medicine, University of Pittsburgh School of Medicine, UPMC-Shadyside, Pittsburgh, Pennsylvania
Electrocardiography

Guadalupe Garcia-Tsao, MD
Professor of Medicine, Section of Digestive Diseases, Yale University School of Medicine, New Haven, Connecticut; Chief, Digestive Diseases, VA-CT Healthcare System, West Haven, Connecticut
Cirrhosis and Its Sequelae

Jonathan D. Gates, MD, MBA
Assistant Professor of Surgery, Harvard Medical School; Director, Trauma Center and Vascular Surgeon, Brigham and Women's Hospital, Boston, Massachusetts
Medical Aspects of Trauma and Burn Care

William M. Geisler, MD, MPH
Associate Professor of Medicine and Epidemiology, University of Alabama at Birmingham School of Medicine, Birmingham, Alabama
Diseases Caused by Chlamydiae

Tony P. George, MD
Professor, Department of Psychiatry, Psychology and Medical Sciences, University of Toronto, Toronto, Ontario, Canada
Nicotine and Tobacco

Dale N. Gerding, MD
Professor, Department of Medicine, Loyola University Chicago Stritch School of Medicine, Maywood; Associate Chief of Staff for Research, Research Service, Hines Veterans Affairs Hospital, Hines, Illinois
Clostridial Infections

M. Eric Gershwin, MD
Distinguished Professor of Medicine, Chief, Division of Rheumatology, Allergy and Clinical Immunology, University of California, Davis, School of Medicine, Davis, California
Sjögren's Syndrome

Morie A. Gertz, MD
Professor and Chair, Department of Medicine, Mayo Medical School and Mayo Clinic, Rochester, Minnesota
Amyloidosis

Gordon D. Ginder, MD
Professor, Internal Medicine, Virginia Commonwealth University; Director, Massey Cancer Center, Virginia Commonwealth University, Richmond, Virginia
Microcytic and Hypochromic Anemias

Jeffrey Ginsberg, MD
Professor, Department of Medicine, McMaster University, Hamilton, Ontario, Canada
Peripheral Venous Disease

Geoffrey S. Ginsburg, MD, PhD
Professor of Medicine and Pathology, Duke University School of Medicine; Director, Center for Genomic Medicine, Institute for Genome Sciences and Policy; Director, Center for Personalized Medicine, Durham, North Carolina
Applications of Molecular Technologies to Clinical Medicine

Michael Glogauer, DDS, PhD
Associate Professor, Faculty of Dentistry, University of Toronto, Toronto, Ontario, Canada
Disorders of Phagocyte Function

John W. Gnann, Jr., MD
Professor of Medicine, Pediatrics, and Microbiology, University of Alabama at Birmingham School of Medicine and Birmingham Veterans Affairs Medical Center, Birmingham, Alabama
Mumps

Matthew R. Golden, MD, MPH
Associate Professor of Medicine, Director, PHSKC HIV/STD Program, University of Washington Center for AIDS and STD, Harborview Medical Center, Seattle, Washington
Neisseria Gonorrhoeae *Infections*

Lee Goldman, MD
Dean of the Faculties of Health Sciences and Medicine, Executive Vice President for Health and Biomedical Sciences, Harold and Margaret Hatch Professor of the University, Professor of Medicine and of Epidemiology, Columbia University, New York, New York
Approach to Medicine, the Patient, and the Medical Profession: Medicine as a Learned and Humane Profession; Approach to the Patient with Possible Cardiovascular Disease

Ellie J. Goldstein, MD
Clinical Professor of Medicine, David Geffen School of Medicine at UCLA, Los Angeles, California; Director, R.M. Alden Research Laboratory, Santa Monica, California
Diseases Caused by Non–Spore-Forming Anaerobic Bacteria

Lawrence T. Goodnough, MD
Professor of Pathology and Medicine, Stanford University School of Medicine; Director, Transfusion Service, Stanford University Medical Center, Stanford, California
Transfusion Medicine

Jörg J. Goronzy, MD, PhD
Professor of Medicine, Division of Immunology and Rheumatology, Stanford University School of Medicine, Stanford, California
The Innate and Adaptive Immune Systems

Eduardo Gotuzzo, MD
Principal Professor of Medicine, Universidad Peruana Cayetano Heredia; Director, Instituto de Medicina Tropical "Alexander von Humboldt," Lima, Peru
Cholera and Other Vibrio *Infections; Liver, Intestinal, and Lung Fluke Infections*

Deborah Grady, MD, MPH
Professor, Department of Medicine, University of California, San Francisco, School of Medicine; Associate Dean for Clinical and Translational Research, University of California, San Francisco, San Francisco, California
Menopause

Leslie C. Grammer, MD
Professor, Department of Medicine, Division of Allergy-Immunology, Northwestern University Feinberg School of Medicine, Chicago, Illinois
Drug Allergy

F. Anthony Greco, MD
Medical Director, Sarah Cannon Cancer Center, Nashville, Tennessee
Cancer of Unknown Primary Origin

Harry B. Greenberg, MD
Joseph D. Grant Professor of Medicine and Microbiology and Immunology; Senior Associate Dean of Research; Stanford University School of Medicine, Stanford, California
Rotaviruses, Noroviruses, and Other Gastrointestinal Viruses

Peter K. Gregersen, MD
Professor, Molecular Medicine, Director, Robert S. Boas Center for Genomics and Human Genetics, The Feinstein Institute for Medical Research, Hofstra University School of Medicine, Manhasset, New York
The Major Histocompatibility Complex

Robert C. Griggs, MD
Professor of Neurology, Medicine, Pediatrics, and Pathology and Laboratory Medicine, University of Rochester School of Medicine and Dentistry, Rochester, New York
Approach to the Patient with Neurologic Disease

Lisa M. Guay-Woodford, MD
Professor and Vice Chair, Department of Genetics; Pediatric Nephrologist, University of Alabama at Birmingham School of Medicine, Birmingham, Alabama
Hereditary Nephropathies and Developmental Abnormalities of the Urinary Tract

Richard L. Guerrant, MD
Thomas H. Hunter Professor of International Medicine, Infectious Diseases, and International Health, Director, Center for Global Health, University of Virginia School of Medicine, Charlottesville, Virginia
Escherichia Coli *Enteric Infections; Cryptosporidiosis*

Colleen Hadigan, MD, MPH
Staff Clinician, Laboratory of Immunoregulation, National Institute of Allergy and Infectious Diseases, National Institutes of Health, Bethesda, Maryland
Treatment of Human Immunodeficiency Virus Infection and Acquired Immunodeficiency Syndrome

John D. Hainsworth, MD
Chief Scientific Officer, Sarah Cannon Research Institute, Nashville, Tennessee
Cancer of Unknown Primary Origin

Anders Hamsten, MD, PhD
Professor of Cardiovascular Diseases, Department of Medicine, Center for Molecular Medicine, Karolinska University Hospital, Karolinska Institutet, Stockholm, Sweden
Atherosclerosis, Thrombosis, and Vascular Biology

Kenneth R. Hande, MD
Professor, Departments of Medicine and Pharmacology, Vanderbilt University School of Medicine, Nashville, Tennessee
Carcinoid Syndrome

H. Hunter Handsfield, MD
Clinical Professor of Medicine, Center for AIDS and STD, University of Washington School of Medicine; Senior Research Leader, Battelle Centers for Public Health Research and Evaluation, Seattle, Washington
Neisseria Gonorrhoeae *Infections*

Göran K. Hansson, MD, PhD
Professor, Center for Molecular Medicine, Department of Medicine, Karolinska University Hospital, Karolinska Institutet, Stockholm, Sweden
Atherosclerosis, Thrombosis, and Vascular Biology

Rashidul Haque, MB, PhD
Senior Scientist and Head, Parasitology Laboratory, Laboratory Sciences Division, International Centre for Diarrheal Disease Research, Bangladesh (ICDDR,B), Dhaka, Bangladesh
Amebiasis

Raymond C. Harris, MD
Anne and Roscoe R. Robinson Professor of Medicine and Chief, Division of Nephrology, Department of Medicine, Vanderbilt University School of Medicine, Nashville, Tennessee
Diabetes and the Kidney

Stephen Crane Hauser, MD
Associate Professor of Medicine, Mayo Medical School; Consultant, Division of Internal Medicine, Gastroenterology and Hepatology, Mayo Clinic, Rochester, Minnesota
Vascular Diseases of the Gastrointestinal Tract

Frederick G. Hayden, MD
Richardson Professor of Clinical Virology, Professor of Medicine, University of Virginia School of Medicine, Charlottesville, Virginia
Influenza

Letha Healey, MD
Staff Clinician, Critical Care Medicine Department, Clinical Center, National Institutes of Health, Bethesda, Maryland
Treatment of Human Immunodeficiency Virus Infection and Acquired Immunodeficiency Syndrome

Douglas C. Heimburger, MD, MS
Professor of Medicine, Associate Director for Education and Training, Vanderbilt Institute for Global Health, Vanderbilt University School of Medicine, Nashville, Tennessee
Nutrition's Interface with Health and Disease

Erik L. Hewlett, MD
Professor of Medicine and Pharmacology, Division of Infectious Diseases and International Health, University of Virginia School of Medicine, Charlottesville, Virginia
Whooping Cough and Other Bordetella *Infections*

David R. Hill, MD, DTM&H
Director, National Travel Health Network and Centre; Honorary Professor, London School of Hygiene and Tropical Medicine, London, England
Giardiasis

Nicholas S. Hill, MD
Professor of Medicine, Tufts University School of Medicine; Chief, Division of Pulmonary, Critical Care, and Sleep Medicine, Tufts Medical Center, Boston, Massachusetts
Respiratory Monitoring in Critical Care

L. David Hillis, MD
Professor and Chair, Department of Medicine, University of Texas Health Science Center at San Antonio, San Antonio, Texas
Acute Coronary Syndrome: Unstable Angina and Non-ST Elevation Myocardial Infarction

Jack Hirsh, MD, DSc
Professor Emeritus, McMaster University, Hamilton, Ontario, Canada
Antithrombotic Therapy

V. Michael Holers, MD
Scoville Professor of Rheumatology, Department of Medicine, University of Colorado Denver School of Medicine, Aurora, Colorado
Complement in Health and Disease

Steven M. Holland, MD
Chief, Laboratory of Clinical Infectious Diseases, National Institute of Allergy and Infectious Diseases, National Institutes of Health, Bethesda, Maryland
The Nontuberculous Mycobacteria

Steven Hollenberg, MD
Professor of Medicine, Robert Wood Johnson Medical School/UMDNJ; Director, Coronary Care Unit, Cooper University Hospital, Camden, New Jersey
Cardiogenic Shock

Edward W. Hook III, MD
Professor of Medicine, Epidemiology, and Microbiology, Director, Division of Infectious Diseases, University of Alabama at Birmingham School of Medicine, Birmingham, Alabama
Granuloma Inguinale (Donovanosis); Syphilis; Nonsyphilitic Treponematoses

Laurence Huang, MD
Professor of Medicine, University of California, San Francisco, School of Medicine; Chief, HIV/AIDS Chest Clinic, San Francisco General Hospital, San Francisco, California
Pulmonary Manifestations of Human Immunodeficiency Virus and Acquired Immunodeficiency Syndrome

Leonard D. Hudson, MD
Professor of Medicine, Endowed Chair in Pulmonary Disease Research, Division of Pulmonary and Critical Care Medicine, University of Washington School of Medicine, Seattle, Washington
Acute Respiratory Failure; Mechanical Ventilation

Steven E. Hyman, MD
Provost, Harvard University, Cambridge, Massachusetts; Professor, Department of Neurobiology, Harvard Medical School, Boston, Massachusetts
Biology of Addiction

Michael Iannuzzi, MD, MBA
Edward C. Reifenstein Professor and Chair, Department of Medicine, Upstate Medical University, Syracuse, New York
Sarcoidosis

Robert D. Inman, MD
Professor of Medicine and Immunology, University of Toronto; Director, Arthritis Center of Excellence, Toronto Western Hospital, Toronto, Ontario, Canada
The Spondyloarthropathies

Sharon K. Inouye, MD, MPH
Professor of Medicine, Harvard Medical School; Director, Aging Brain Center, Milton and Shirley F. Levy Family Chair, Institute for Aging Research, Hebrew SeniorLife; Faculty, Division of Gerontology, Beth Israel Deaconess Medical Center, Boston, Massachusetts
Neuropsychiatric Aspects of Aging; Delirium or Acute Mental Status Change in the Older Patient; Video

Karl L. Insogna, MD
Professor of Medicine, Section of Endocrinology, Department of Internal Medicine, Director, Yale Bone Center, Yale University School of Medicine, New Haven, Connecticut
The Parathyroid Glands, Hypercalcemia, and Hypocalcemia

Silvio E. Inzucchi, MD
Professor of Medicine, Clinical Director, Section of Endocrinology, Yale University School of Medicine; Director, Yale Diabetes Center, Yale-New Haven Hospital, New Haven, Connecticut
Type 1 Diabetes Mellitus; Type 2 Diabetes Mellitus

Eric M. Isselbacher, MD
Associate Professor of Medicine, Harvard Medical School; Associate Director, Heart Center and Co-Director, Thoracic Aortic Center, Massachusetts General Hospital, Boston, Massachusetts
Diseases of the Aorta

Ahmedin Jemal, DVM, PhD
Vice President, Surveillance Research, American Cancer Society, Inc., Atlanta, Georgia
The Epidemiology of Cancer

Joanna Jen, MD, PhD
Professor, Department of Neurology, David Geffen School of Medicine at UCLA, University of California, Los Angeles, California
Neuro-Ophthalmology; Smell and Taste; Hearing and Equilibrium

Dennis M. Jensen, MD
Professor of Medicine, David Geffen School of Medicine at UCLA, University of California, Los Angeles, CURE Digestive Diseases Research Center; Staff Physician, West Los Angeles Veterans Affairs Medical Center, Los Angeles, California
Gastrointestinal Hemorrhage and Occult Gastrointestinal Bleeding

Michael D. Jensen, MD
Professor of Medicine, Department of Endocrinology, Mayo Clinic, Rochester, Minnesota
Obesity

Robert T. Jensen, MD
Chief, Cell Biology Section, Digestive Diseases Branch, National Institute of Diabetes, Digestive and Kidney Diseases, National Institutes of Health, Bethesda, Maryland
Pancreatic Endocrine Tumors

Mariell Jessup, MD
Professor of Medicine, Department of Medicine, University of Pennsylvania School of Medicine; Medical Director, Penn Heart and Vascular Center, University of Pennsylvania Health System; Associate Chief, Clinical Affairs, Cardiovascular Division, University of Pennsylvania School of Medicine, Philadelphia, Pennsylvania
Cardiac Transplantation

Stuart Johnson, MD
Professor of Medicine, Loyola University Chicago Stritch School of Medicine, Maywood; Deputy Associate Chief of Staff for Research, Hines Veterans Affairs Hospital, Hines, Illinois
Clostridial Infections

Ralph F. Józefowicz, MD
Professor of Neurology and Medicine, Associate Chair for Education, Department of Neurology, University of Rochester School of Medicine and Dentistry, Rochester, New York
Approach to the Patient with Neurologic Disease

Stephen G. Kaler, MD
Molecular Medicine Program, Eunice Kennedy Shriver National Institute of Child Health and Human Development, Bethesda, Maryland
Wilson's Disease

Moses R. Kamya, MD, PhD
Professor of Medicine, Chair, Department of Medicine, School of Medicine, Makerere University College of Health Sciences, Kampala, Uganda
Malaria

Hagop Kantarjian, MD
Professor and Kelcie Margaret Kana Research Chair, Department of Leukemia, The University of Texas M. D. Anderson Cancer Center, Houston, Texas
The Chronic Leukemias

David R. Karp, MD, PhD
Professor and Chief, Rheumatic Diseases Division, The University of Texas Southwestern Medical Center at Dallas, Dallas, Texas
Complement in Health and Disease

Daniel L. Kastner, MD, PhD
NIH Distinguished Investigator, Scientific Director, Division of Intramural Research, National Human Genome Research Institute, National Institutes of Health, Bethesda, Maryland
The Systemic Autoinflammatory Diseases

David A. Katzka, MD
Professor of Medicine, Mayo Medical School, Rochester, Minnesota
Diseases of the Esophagus

Debra K. Katzman, MD
Professor of Pediatrics, Department of Pediatrics, University of Toronto; Head, Division of Adolescent Medicine, Senior Associate Scientist, Research Institute, The Hospital for Sick Children and University of Toronto, Toronto, Ontario, Canada
Adolescent Medicine

Carol A. Kauffman, MD
Professor, University of Michigan; Chief, Infectious Diseases Section, Veterans Affairs Ann Arbor Healthcare System, Ann Arbor, Michigan
Histoplasmosis; Blastomycosis; Paracoccidioidomycosis; Cryptococcosis; Sporotrichosis; Candidiasis

Kenneth Kaushansky, MD, MACP
Senior Vice President, Health Sciences, Dean, School of Medicine, Stony Brook University, Health Sciences Center, Stony Brook, New York
Hematopoiesis and Hematopoietic Growth Factors

Emmet B. Keeffe, MD
Professor of Medicine Emeritus, Division of Gastroenterology and Hepatology, Department of Medicine, Stanford University Medical Center, Stanford, California
Hepatic Failure and Liver Transplantation

Morton Kern, MD
Professor of Medicine, Associate Chief, Cardiology, University of California Irvine, Orange; Chief, Cardiology, Long Beach Veterans Administration Hospital, Long Beach, California
Catheterization and Angiography

Gerald T. Keusch, MD
Professor, International Health, Boston University School of Public Health; Associate Director, National Emerging Infectious Diseases Laboratory, Boston University, Boston, Massachusetts
Shigellosis

David H. Kim, MD
Associate Professor of Radiology, Section of Abdominal Imaging, University of Wisconsin School of Medicine and Public Health, Madison, Wisconsin
Diagnostic Imaging Procedures in Gastroenterology

Matthew Kim, MD
Instructor in Medicine, Harvard Medical School; Associate Physician, Division of Endocrinology, Diabetes and Hypertension, Brigham and Women's Hospital, Boston, Massachusetts
Thyroid

Louis V. Kirchhoff, MD, MPH
Professor, Departments of Internal Medicine (Infectious Diseases) and Epidemiology, University of Iowa; Staff Physician, Medical Service, Department of Veterans Affairs Medical Center, Iowa City, Iowa
Chagas' Disease

Michael J. Klag, MD, MPH
Dean, The Johns Hopkins Bloomberg School of Public Health, Baltimore, Maryland
Epidemiology of Cardiovascular Disease

Samuel Klein, MD
William H. Danforth Professor of Medicine and Nutritional Science, Director, Center for Human Nutrition, Washington University School of Medicine, St. Louis, Missouri
Protein-Energy Malnutrition

David S. Knopman, MD
Professor of Neurology and Consultant in Neurology, Mayo Clinic, Rochester, Minnesota
Regional Cerebral Dysfunction: Higher Mental Functions; Alzheimer's Disease and Other Dementias

Tamsin A. Knox, MD, MPH
Associate Professor of Medicine, Nutrition/Infection Unit, Tufts University School of Medicine, Boston, Massachusetts
Gastrointestinal Manifestions of HIV and AIDS

Albert I. Ko, MD
Associate Professor of Epidemiology and Medicine, Division Head, Epidemiology of Microbial Disease, Yale School of Public Health, New Haven, Connecticut; Collaborating Researcher, Oswaldo Cruz Foundation, Brazilian Ministry of Health, Salvador, Brazil
Leptospirosis

Rami S. Komrokji, MD
Associate Professor, Department of Oncologic Sciences, University of South Florida; Clinical Director, Department of Malignant Hematology, Associate Member, Moffitt Cancer Center and Research Institute, Tampa, Florida
Myelodysplastic Syndrome

Dimitrios P. Kontoyiannis, MD, ScD
Professor of Medicine and Deputy Chair, The University of Texas M.D. Anderson Cancer Center, Houston, Texas
Mucormycosis; Mycetoma

Barbara S. Koppel, MD
Professor of Clinical Neurology, New York Medical College, Valhalla, New York; Chief of Service, Metropolitan Hospital, New York, New York
Nutritional and Alcohol-Related Neurologic Disorders

Kevin Korenblat, MD
Associate Professor of Medicine, Washington University School of Medicine, St. Louis, Missouri
Approach to the Patient with Jaundice or Abnormal Liver Tests

Bruce R. Korf, MD, PhD
Professor and Wayne H. and Sara Crews Finley Chair in Medical Genetics, Department of Genetics; Director, Heflin Center for Genomic Sciences, University of Alabama at Birmingham, Birmingham, Alabama
Principles of Genetics

Neil J. Korman, MD, PhD
Professor, Department of Dermatology, Case Western Reserve University; Clinical Director, Murdough Family Center for Psoriasis, University Hospitals Case Medical Center, Cleveland, Ohio
Macular, Papular, Vesiculobullous, and Pustular Diseases

Joseph A. Kovacs, MD
Senior Investigator, Critical Care Medicine Department, National Institutes of Health, Bethesda, Maryland
Pneumocystis *Pneumonia*

Monica Kraft, MD
Professor of Medicine, Vice Chair for Research, Department of Medicine; Director, Duke Asthma, Allergy and Airway Center, Duke University Medical Center, Durham, North Carolina
Approach to the Patient with Respiratory Disease

Christopher M. Kramer, MD
Professor of Radiology and Medicine, Director, Cardiovascular Imaging Center, University of Virginia Health System, Charlottesville, Virginia
Noninvasive Cardiac Imaging

Donna M. Krasnewich, MD, PhD
Program Director, National Institute of General Medical Sciences, National Institutes of Health, Bethesda, Maryland
The Lysosomal Storage Diseases

Peter J. Krause, MD
Senior Research Scientist, Yale School of Public Health, Yale School of Medicine, New Haven, Connecticut
Babesiosis and Other Protozoan Diseases

Henry M. Kronenberg, MD
Professor of Medicine, Harvard Medical School; Chief, Endocrine Unit, Massachusetts General Hospital, Boston, Massachusetts
Polyglandular Disorders

Ernst J. Kuipers, MD, PhD
Professor of Medicine, Department of Gastroenterology and Hepatology, Department of Internal Medicine, Erasmus MC University Medical Center, Rotterdam, The Netherlands
Acid Peptic Disease

Paul Ladenson, MD
John Eager Howard Professor of Endocrinology; Professor of Medicine, Pathology, Oncology, Radiology and Radiological Sciences; Distinguished Service Professor, and Director, Division of Endocrinology and Metabolism, Johns Hopkins University School of Medicine, Baltimore, Maryland
Thyroid

Donald W. Landry, MD, PhD
Samuel Bard Professor of Medicine and Chair, Department of Medicine, Columbia University College of Physicians and Surgeons, New York, New York
Approach to the Patient with Renal Disease

Nancy E. Lane, MD
Professor of Medicine and Rheumatology, University of California, Davis, School of Medicine; Director, Aging Center, University of California at Davis Medical Center, Davis, California
Osteoarthritis

Anthony E. Lang, MD
Professor, Department of Medicine (Neurology), University of Toronto; Director, Movement Disorders Center, Toronto Western Hospital; Director, Division of Neurology, Jack Clark Chair for Parkinson's Disease Research, Toronto, Ontario, Canada
Parkinsonism; Other Movement Disorders; Videos

Richard A. Lange, MD, MBA
Professor and Executive Vice Chairman, Department of Medicine, University of Texas Health Science Center San Antonio, San Antonio, Texas
Acute Coronary Syndrome: Unstable Angina and Non-ST Elevation Myocardial Infarction

George V. Lawry, MD
Clinical Professor of Medicine, Chief, Division of Rheumatology, University of California Irvine, Orange, California
Approach to the Patient with Rheumatic Disease

Thomas H. Lee, MD, MSc
Professor of Medicine, Harvard Medical School; Network President, Partners Healthcare System, Boston, Massachusetts
Using Data for Clinical Decisions

William M. Lee, MD
Professor, Department of Internal Medicine, Division of Digestive and Liver Diseases, University of Texas Southwestern Medical Center, Dallas, Texas
Toxin- and Drug-Induced Liver Disease

James Leggett, MD
Associate Professor of Medicine, Oregon Health & Science University; Assistant Director of Medical Education, Providence Portland Medical Center, Portland, Oregon
Approach to Fever or Suspected Infection in the Normal Host

Adam Lerner, MD
Professor, Department of Medicine, Section of Hematology and Medical Oncology, Boston University School of Medicine, Boston, Massachusetts
Primary and Metastatic Malignant Bone Lesions

Stuart Levin, MD
The Ralph C. Brown, MD, Professor of Medicine and Chair, Department of Internal Medicine, Rush University Medical Center, Chicago, Illinois
Zoonoses

Stephanie M. Levine, MD
Professor of Medicine, Division of Pulmonary and Critical Care Diseases, University of Texas Health Science Center at San Antonio, San Antonio, Texas
Alveolar Filling Disorders

Gary R. Lichtenstein, MD
Professor of Medicine, Division of Gastroenterology, University of Pennsylvania School of Medicine; Director, Center for Inflammatory Bowel Diseases, Hospital of the University of Pennsylvania, Philadelphia, Pennsylvania
Inflammatory Bowel Disease

Henry W. Lim, MD, DSc
Chairman and C.S. Livingood Chair, Department of Dermatology, Henry Ford Hospital; Senior Vice President for Academic Affairs, Henry Ford Health System, Detroit, Michigan
Eczema, Photodermatoses, Papulosquamous (including Fungal) Diseases, and Figurate Erythemas

Aldo A. M. Lima, MD, PhD
Professor of Medicine and INCT-Biomedicine, Department of Physiology and Pharmacology, Federal University of Ceará, Fortaleza-Ceará, Brazil
Cryptosporidiosis; Schistosomiasis (Bilharziasis)

Andrew H. Limper, MD
Professor and Division Chair, Pulmonary and Critical Care Medicine, and Director, Thoracic Diseases Research Unit, Mayo Medical School; Consultant, Mayo Clinic, Rochester, Minnesota
Overview of Pneumonia

Geoffrey S. F. Ling, MD, PhD
Professor and Interim Chair, Department of Neurology, Uniformed Services University of the Health Sciences, Bethesda, Maryland; Director of Neuro Critical Care, Critical Care Medicine, Walter Reed Army Medical Center, Washington, DC
Traumatic Brain Injury and Spinal Cord Injury

Alan F. List, MD
Professor of Oncologic Sciences, University of South Florida; Executive Vice President and Physician-in-Chief, Moffitt Cancer Center; Senior Member, Malignant Hematology, Moffitt Cancer Center, Tampa, Florida
Myelodysplastic Syndrome

William C. Little, MD
McMichael Professor and Vice Chair, Department of Internal Medicine, Chief of Cardiology, Wake Forest University School of Medicine, Winston-Salem, North Carolina
Pericardial Diseases

Richard F. Loeser, MD
Professor of Internal Medicine, Section of Molecular Medicine, Wake Forest University School of Medicine, Winston-Salem, North Carolina
Connective Tissue Structure and Function

Bennett Lorber, MD
Thomas M. Durant Professor of Medicine, Professor of Microbiology and Immunology, Temple University School of Medicine, Philadelphia, Pennsylvania
Listeriosis

Donald E. Low, MD
Professor, Laboratory Medicine and Pathobiology, University of Toronto; Microbiologist-in-Chief, Mount Sinai Hospital/University Health Network; Medical Director, Public Health Laboratory–Toronto, Ontario Agency for Health Protection and Promotion, Toronto, Ontario, Canada
Nonpneumococcal Streptococcal Infections, Rheumatic Fever

Daniel R. Lucey, MD, MPH
Adjunct Professor of Microbiology and Immunology, Georgetown University Medical Center; Director, Center for Biologic Counterterrorism and Emerging Diseases, Washington Hospital Center, Washington, DC
Anthrax

James R. Lupski, MD, PhD
Cullen Professor and Vice Chair of Molecular and Human Genetics, Professor of Pediatrics, Baylor College of Medicine; Attending Medical Geneticist, Texas Children's Hospital, Ben Taub General Hospital, Houston, Texas
Gene, Genomic, and Chromosomal Disorders

Henry T. Lynch, MD
Chair, Preventive Medicine and Public Health, Professor of Medicine, Director, Creighton Hereditary Cancer Institute, Creighton University School of Medicine, Omaha, Nebraska
Cancer Genetics

Jeffrey M. Lyness, MD
Professor and Associate Chair for Education, Department of Psychiatry, University of Rochester School of Medicine and Dentistry; Medical Director for Continuing Medical Education, University of Rochester Medical Center, Rochester, New York
Psychiatric Disorders in Medical Practice

Bruce W. Lytle, MD
Chair, Heart and Vascular Institute, Department of Thoracic and Cardiovascular Surgery, The Cleveland Clinic, Cleveland, Ohio
Interventional and Surgical Treatment of Coronary Artery Disease

C. Ronald MacKenzie, MD
Associate Professor of Clinical Medicine, Department of Rheumatology, Hospital for Special Surgery and Weill Cornell Medical College, New York, New York
Surgical Treatment of Joint Disease

Harriet MacMillan, MD, MSc
Professor, Departments of Psychiatry and Behavioral Neurosciences, and Pediatrics, David R. (Dan) Offord Chair in Child Studies, Offord Centre for Child Studies, McMaster University, Hamilton, Ontario, Canada
Intimate Partner Violence

Robert D. Madoff, MD
Stanley M. Goldberg, MD, Professor of Surgery, Chief, Division of Colon and Rectal Surgery, University of Minnesota Medical School, Minneapolis, Minnesota
Diseases of the Rectum and Anus

Mark W. Mahowald, MD
Professor, Department of Neurology, University of Minnesota Medical School, Minneapolis, Minnesota
Disorders of Sleep

Atul Malhotra, MD
Associate Professor of Medicine, Harvard Medical School; Associate Physician, Brigham and Women's Hospital, Boston, Massachusetts
Disorders of Ventilatory Control

Lionel A. Mandell, MD
Professor of Medicine, Faculty of Health Sciences at McMaster University; Attending Physician, Department of Medicine, Henderson Division, Hamilton Health Sciences, Hamilton, Ontario, Canada
Streptococcus pneumoniae *Infections*

Peter Manu, MD
Professor of Medicine, Hofstra North Shore–LIJ School of Medicine at Hofstra University, Hempstead; Director of Medical Services, The Zucker Hillside Hospital, Glen Oaks, New York
Medical Consultation in Psychiatry

Marsha D. Marcus, PhD
Professor of Psychiatry and Psychology, University of Pittsburgh School of Medicine; Chief, Eating Disorders Program, Western Psychiatric Institute and Clinic, University of Pittsburgh Medical Center, Pittsburgh, Pennsylvania
Eating Disorders

Ariane J. Marelli, MD, MPH
Associate Professor, McGill University Health Center; Director, McGill Adult Unit for Congenital Heart Disease, McGill University, Montreal, Quebec, Canada
Congenital Heart Disease in Adults; Videos

Maurie Markman, MD
Vice President for Patient Oncology Services, National Director for Medical Oncology, Cancer Treatment Centers of America, Eastern Regional Medical Center, Philadelphia, Pennsylvania
Gynecologic Cancers

Andrew R. Marks, MD
Wu Professor and Chair, Department of Physiology and Cellular Biophysics and Director, Helen and Clyde Wu Center for Molecular Cardiology, Columbia University College of Physicians and Surgeons, New York, New York
Cardiac Function and Circulatory Control

Kieren A. Marr, MD
Professor of Medicine and Oncology, Director, Transplant and Oncology Infectious Disease Program, Johns Hopkins University School of Medicine, Johns Hopkins University, Baltimore, Maryland
Approach to Fever and Suspected Infection in the Compromised Host

Thomas J. Marrie, MD
Dean, Faculty of Medicine, Dalhousie University, Halifax, Nova Scotia, Canada
Legionella *Infections*

Paul Martin, MD
Professor of Medicine, Chief, Division of Hepatology, University of Miami, Miller School of Medicine, Miami, Florida
Approach to the Patient with Liver Disease

Joel B. Mason, MD
Professor of Medicine and Nutrition, Tufts University; Staff Physician, Tufts Medical Center; Director, Vitamins and Carcinogenesis Laboratory, U.S.D.A. Human Nutrition Research Center at Tufts University, Boston, Massachusetts
Vitamins, Trace Minerals, and Other Micronutrients

Barry M. Massie, MD
Professor of Medicine, University of California, San Francisco, School of Medicine; Chief, Cardiology Division, San Francisco VA Medical Center, San Francisco, California
Heart Failure: Pathophysiology and Diagnosis

Henry Masur, MD
Chief, Critical Care Medicine Department, Clinical Center, National Institutes of Health, Bethesda, Maryland
Treatment of Human Immunodeficiency Virus Infection and Acquired Immunodeficiency Syndrome

Eric L. Matteson, MD, MPH
Professor of Medicine, Division of Rheumatology and Division of Epidemiology, Mayo Medical School, Rochester, Minnesota
Infections of Bursae, Joints, and Bones

Toby Maurer, MD
Professor, Department of Dermatology, University of California, San Francisco, School of Medicine, San Francisco, California
Skin Manifestations in Patients with Human Immunodeficiency Virus Infection

Emeran A. Mayer, MD
Professor of Medicine, Physiology and Psychiatry; Director, Center for Neurobiology of Stress, Division of Digestive Diseases, David Geffen School of Medicine at UCLA, University of California, Los Angeles, California
Functional Gastrointestinal Disorders: Irritable Bowel Syndrome, Dyspepsia, and Functional Chest Pain of Presumed Esophageal Origin

Stephen A. McClave, MD
Professor of Medicine, Director of Clinical Nutrition, Division of Gastroenterology, Hepatology, and Nutrition, University of Louisville School of Medicine, Louisville, Kentucky
Enteral Nutrition

F. Dennis McCool, MD
Professor of Medicine, Alpert Medical School of Brown University, Providence, Rhode Island; Chief of Pulmonary Critical Care and Sleep Medicine, Memorial Hospital of Rhode Island, Pawtucket, Rhode Island
Diseases of the Diaphragm, Chest Wall, Pleura, and Mediastinum

Charles E. McCulloch, PhD
Professor and Head, Division of Biostatistics, Department of Epidemiology and Biostatistics, University of California, San Francisco, San Francisco, California
Statistical Interpretation of Data

Michael A. McGuigan, MDCM, MBA
Clinical Professor, Department of Emergency Medicine, State University of New York, Stony Brook; Medical Director, Long Island Regional Poison and Drug Information Center, Winthrop-University Hospital, Mineola, New York
Chronic Poisoning: Trace Metals and Others

John McHutchison, MD
Senior Vice President, Liver Disease Therapeutics, Gilead Sciences Inc., Foster City, California
Chronic Viral and Autoimmune Hepatitis

William McKenna, MD, DSc
Professor of Cardiology, Director, Institute of Cardiovascular Science, University College London, London, United Kingdom
Diseases of the Myocardium and Endocardium

Vallerie McLaughlin, MD
Professor of Medicine, Department of Internal Medicine, Division of Cardiovascular Medicine, and Director, Pulmonary Hypertension Program, University of Michigan, Ann Arbor, Michigan
Pulmonary Hypertension

John J. V. McMurray, MB, MD
Professor of Medical Cardiology, University of Glasgow; Honorary Consultant Cardiologist, Western Infirmary, Glasgow, Scotland, United Kingdom
Heart Failure: Management and Prognosis

Mary McNaughton-Collins, MD, MPH
Associate Professor of Medicine, Harvard Medical School, Boston, Massachusetts
Benign Prostatic Hyperplasia and Prostatitis

Kenneth McQuaid, MD
Professor of Clinical Medicine, University of California, San Francisco, School of Medicine; Chief, Gastroenterology Section, Veterans Affairs Medical Center, San Francisco, California
Approach to the Patient with Gastrointestinal Disease

Frederick W. Miller, MD, PhD
Chief, Environmental Autoimmunity Group, National Institute of Environmental Health Sciences, National Institutes of Health, Bethesda, Maryland
Polymyositis and Dermatomyositis

Kenneth L. Minaker, MD
Associate Professor of Medicine, Harvard Medical School; Chief, Geriatric Medicine Unit, Interim Chief, General Medicine Division, Massachusetts General Hospital, Boston, Massachusetts
Common Clinical Sequelae of Aging

Jonathan W. Mink, MD, PhD
Professor and Chief of Child Neurology, Departments of Neurology, Pediatrics, Brain and Cognitive Sciences, and Neurobiology and Anatomy, University of Rochester, Rochester, New York
Congenital, Developmental, and Neurocutaneous Disorders

Daniel R. Mishell, Jr., MD
Professor, Department of Obstetrics and Gynecology, University of Southern California, Keck School of Medicine, Los Angeles, California
Contraception

William E. Mitch, MD
Gordon Cain Chair in Nephrology and Director, Division of Nephrology, Department of Medicine, Baylor College of Medicine, Houston, Texas
Chronic Kidney Disease

Mark E. Molitch, MD
Professor of Medicine, Northwestern University Feinberg School of Medicine; Attending Physician, Northwestern Memorial Hospital, Chicago, Illinois
Neuroendocrinology and the Neuroendocrine System; Anterior Pituitary

Bruce A. Molitoris, MD
Professor of Medicine, Director of Nephrology, Director of the Indiana Center for Biological Microscopy, Indiana University School of Medicine, Indianapolis, Indiana
Acute Kidney Injury

José G. Montoya, MD
Associate Professor, Department of Medicine, Stanford University School of Medicine, Stanford, California; Director, Toxoplasma Serology Laboratory, Palo Alto Medical Foundation, Palo Alto, California
Toxoplasmosis

Fred Morady, MD
McKay Professor of Cardiovascular Diseases, Professor of Medicine, University of Michigan Health System, Ann Arbor, Michigan
Electrophysiologic Interventional Procedures and Surgery

Jeffrey A. Moscow, MD
Children's Miracle Network Professor, Chief, Hematology-Oncology, Department of Pediatrics, University of Kentucky, Lexington, Kentucky
Biology of Cancer

Andrew H. Murr, MD
Professor of Clinical Otolaryngology and Head and Neck Surgery, Roger Boles, MD, Endowed Chair in Otolaryngology Education and Vice Chair for Clinical Affairs, Department of Otolaryngology, University of California, San Francisco, School of Medicine; Chief of Service, San Francisco General Hospital, San Francisco, California
Approach to the Patient with Nose, Sinus, and Ear Disorders

Robert J. Myerburg, MD
Professor of Medicine and Physiology, Division of Cardiovascular Medicine, American Heart Association Chair in Cardiovascular Research, University of Miami, Miller School of Medicine, Miami, Florida
Approach to Cardiac Arrest and Life-Threatening Arrhythmias

Stanley Naguwa, MD
Clinical Professor, Division of Rheumatology, Allergy, Clinical Immunology, University of California, Davis, Davis, California
Sjögren's Syndrome

Stanley J. Naides, MD
Medical Director, Department of Immunology, Quest Diagnostics Nichols Institute, San Juan Capistrano, California
Arboviruses Causing Fever and Rash Syndromes

Theodore E. Nash, MD
Head, Gastrointestinal Parasites Section, Laboratory of Parasitic Diseases, National Institutes of Allergy and Infectious Diseases, National Institutes of Health, Bethesda, Maryland
Giardiasis

Avindra Nath, MD
Chief, Section of Infections of the Nervous System, National Institute of Neurological Diseases and Stroke, National Institutes of Health, Bethesda, Maryland
Cytomegalovirus, Epstein-Barr Virus, and Other Slow Virus Infections of the Central Nervous System; Neurologic Complications of Human Immunodeficiency Virus Infection; Meningitis: Bacterial, Viral, and Other; Brain Abscess and Parameningeal Infections

Eric G. Neilson, MD
Thomas Fearn Frist, Sr., Professor of Medicine and Cell Biology, Vanderbilt University School of Medicine, Vanderbilt University, Nashville, Tennessee
Tubulointerstitial Diseases

Lawrence S. Neinstein, MD
Professor of Pediatrics and Medicine, Keck School of Medicine; Executive Director, University Park Health Center, Chief, Division of College Health, Senior Associate Dean of Student Affairs, University of Southern California, Los Angeles, California
Adolescent Medicine

Thomas B. Newman, MD, MPH
Professor and Head, Division of Clinical Epidemiology, Departments of Epidemiology and Biostatistics and Pediatrics, University of California, San Francisco, School of Medicine, San Francisco, California
Statistical Interpretation of Data

William L. Nichols, MD
Associate Professor of Medicine and Laboratory Medicine, Hematology and Internal Medicine, Hematopathology and Laboratory Medicine, Mayo Medical School, Rochester, Minnesota
Von Willebrand Disease and Hemorrhagic Abnormalities of Platelet and Vascular Function

Lynnette K. Nieman, MD
Senior Investigator, Program on Reproductive and Adult Endocrinology, The Eunice Kennedy Shriver National Institute of Child Health and Human Development (NICHD), National Institutes of Health, Bethesda, Maryland
Adrenal Cortex

Dennis E. Niewoehner, MD
Professor, Department of Medicine, University of Minnesota Medical School; Chief, Pulmonary Section, Minneapolis Veterans Affairs Health Care System, Minneapolis, Minnesota
Chronic Obstructive Pulmonary Disease

S. Ragnar Norrby, MD, PhD
Director General, Swedish Institute for Infectious Disease Control, Solna, Sweden
Approach to the Patient with Urinary Tract Infection

David A. Norris, MD
Professor and Chair, Department of Dermatology, University of Colorado Denver School of Medicine, Aurora, Colorado
Structure and Function of the Skin

Susan O'Brien, MD
Professor of Medicine, Department of Leukemia, The University of Texas M.D. Anderson Cancer Center, Houston, Texas
The Chronic Leukemias

Francis G. O'Connor, MD, MPH
Associate Professor, Military and Emergency Medicine, Uniformed Services University, Bethesda, Maryland
Rhabdomyolysis

Patrick G. O'Connor, MD, MPH
Professor of Medicine, Yale University; Chief, General Internal Medicine, Yale University School of Medicine, Yale-New Haven Hospital, New Haven, Connecticut
Alcohol Abuse and Dependence

James R. O'Dell, MD
Professor and Chief of Rheumatology, Department of Internal Medicine, University of Nebraska Medical Center, Omaha, Nebraska
Rheumatoid Arthritis

Anne E. O'Donnell, MD
Professor of Medicine, Chief, Division of Pulmonary, Critical Care, and Sleep Medicine, Georgetown University Hospital, Washington, DC
Bronchiectasis, Atelectasis, Cysts, and Localized Lung Disorders

Jae K. Oh, MD
Professor, Internal Medicine, Co-Director, Echocardiography Laboratory, Division of Cardiovascular Diseases, Mayo Clinic, Rochester, Minnesota
Pericardial Diseases

Jeffrey E. Olgin, MD
Gallo-Chatterjee Distinguished Professor, Chief, Division of Cardiology, Co-Director of the Heart and Vascular Center, University of California, San Francisco, School of Medicine, San Francisco, California
Approach to the Patient with Suspected Arrhythmia

Jeffrey W. Olin, DO
Professor of Medicine, Director Vascular Medicine, Zena and Michael A. Wiener Cardiovascular Institute, Mount Sinai School of Medicine, New York, New York
Other Peripheral Arterial Diseases

Walter A. Orenstein, MD
Deputy Director for Immunization Programs, Vaccine Delivery, Global Health Program, Bill and Melinda Gates Foundation, Seattle, Washington
Immunization

Douglas R. Osmon, MD
Associate Professor of Medicine, Division of Infectious Diseases, Mayo Medical School, Rochester, Minnesota
Infections of Bursae, Joints, and Bones

Catherine M. Otto, MD
J. Ward Kennedy-Hamilton Endowed Chair of Medicine, Director, Training Programs in Cardiovascular Disease, University of Washington School of Medicine; Associate Director, Echocardiography, University of Washington Medical Center, Seattle, Washington
Echocardiography; Videos

Stephen A. Paget, MD
Professor of Medicine, Weill Cornell Medical College; Physician-in-Chief Emeritus, Hospital for Special Surgery, New York, New York
Polymyalgia Rheumatica and Temporal Arteritis

Mark Papania, MD, MPH
Medical Epidemiologist, Division of Viral Diseases, Centers for Disease Control and Prevention, Atlanta, Georgia
Measles

Peter G. Pappas, MD
Professor of Medicine, Division of Infectious Diseases, University of Alabama School of Medicine, Birmingham, Alabama
Dematiaceous Fungal Infections

Pankaj Jay Pasricha, MD
Professor of Medicine, Chief, Division of Gastroenterology and Hepatology, Stanford University School of Medicine, Stanford, California
Gastrointestinal Endoscopy

David L. Paterson, MD
Professor of Medicine, University of Queensland Centre for Clinical Research, Royal Brisbane and Women's Hospital Campus, Brisbane, Australia
Infections due to Other Members of the Enterobacteriaceae, including Management of Multidrug-Resistant Strains

Carlo Patrono, MD
Professor and Chair of Pharmacology, Catholic University School of Medicine, Rome, Italy
Prostaglandins, Aspirin, and Related Compounds

Jean-Michel Pawlotsky, MD, PhD
Professor of Medicine, University of Paris-Est; Director, National Reference Center for Viral Hepatitis B, C and Delta and Department of Virology, Henri Mondor University Hospital; Director, Department of Molecular Virology and Immunology, Institut Mondor de Recherche Biomédicale, Créteil, France
Acute Viral Hepatitis; Chronic Viral and Autoimmune Hepatitis

Richard D. Pearson, MD
Professor of Medicine and Pathology, Division of Infectious Diseases and International Health, University of Virginia School of Medicine, Charlottesville, Virginia
Antiparasitic Therapy

Eli N. Perencevich, MD, MSc
Professor of Internal Medicine, Department of Internal Medicine, University of Iowa, Carver College of Medicine; Core Investigator, Center for Research in the Implementation of Innovative Strategies in Practice, Iowa City Veterans Affairs Medical Center, Iowa City, Iowa
Enterococcal Infections

Trish M. Perl, MD, MSc
Professor, Department of Medicine, Pathology, and Epidemiology, Senior Health System Epidemiologist, Hospital Epidemiology and Infection Control, The Johns Hopkins Health System and University, Baltimore, Maryland
Enterococcal Infections

Michael C. Perry, MD, MSc
Professor of Medicine and Nellie B. Smith Chair of Oncology Emeritus, Departments of Hematology and Medical Oncology, University of Missouri, Ellis Fischel Cancer Center; Medical Director of Clinical Trials, Institute for Clinical and Translational Sciences, University of Missouri, Ellis Fischel Cancer Center, Columbia, Missouri
Approach to the Patient with Cancer

William A. Petri, Jr., MD, PhD
Professor of Medicine, Microbiology and Pathology, Wade Hampton Frost Professor of Epidemiology and Chief, Division of Infectious Diseases and International Health, University of Virginia, Charlottesville, Virginia
Relapsing Fever and Other Borrelia *Infections; African Sleeping Sickness; Amebiasis*

Marc A. Pfeffer, MD, PhD
Dzau Professor of Medicine, Harvard Medical School; Senior Physician, Cardiovascular Division, Brigham and Women's Hospital, Boston, Massachusetts
Heart Failure: Management and Prognosis

Perry J. Pickhardt, MD
Professor of Radiology and Chief, Gastrointestinal Imaging, University of Wisconsin School of Medicine and Public Health, Madison, Wisconsin
Diagnostic Imaging Procedures in Gastroenterology

Gerald B. Pier, PhD
Professor of Medicine (Microbiology and Molecular Genetics), Department of Medicine, Harvard Medical School; Microbiologist, Brigham and Women's Hospital, Boston, Massachusetts
Pseudomonas *and Related Gram-Negative Bacillary Infections*

David S. Pisetsky, MD, PhD
Professor of Medicine and Immunology, Duke University Medical Center; Chief of Rheumatology, Durham Veterans Affairs Medical Center, Durham, North Carolina
Laboratory Testing in the Rheumatic Diseases

Marshall R. Posner, MD
Professor of Medicine and of Gene and Cell Medicine, Director of Head and Neck Medical Oncology, and Director of Office of Cancer Clinical Trials, The Tisch Cancer Institute, Mount Sinai School of Medicine, New York, New York
Head and Neck Cancer

Charlene Prather, MD
Associate Professor of Internal Medicine, Saint Louis University School of Medicine, St. Louis, Missouri
Inflammatory and Anatomic Diseases of the Intestine, Peritoneum, Mesentery, and Omentum

Basil A. Pruitt, Jr., MD
Clinical Professor of Surgery and Dr. Ferdinand P. Herff Chair in Surgery, University of Texas Health Science Center at San Antonio; Consultant Surgeon, U. S. Army Institute of Surgical Research, Fort Sam Houston, San Antonio, Texas
Electric Injury

Reed E. Pyeritz, MD, PhD
Professor of Medicine and Genetics and Vice Chair for Academic Affairs, University of Pennsylvania School of Medicine, Philadelphia, Pennsylvania
Inherited Diseases of Connective Tissue

Thomas C. Quinn, MD, MSc
Professor of Medicine, Johns Hopkins University School of Medicine, Baltimore, Maryland; Associate Director for International Research, Division of Intramural Research, National Institute of Allergy and Infectious Diseases, National Institutes of Health, Bethesda, Maryland
Epidemiology of Human Immunodeficiency Virus Infection and Acquired Immunodeficiency Syndrome

Jai Radhakrishnan, MD, MSc
Associate Professor of Clinical Medicine, Department of Medicine, Division of Nephrology; Program Director, Nephrology Fellowship, Division of Nephrology, Columbia University Medical Center, New York, New York
Glomerular Disorders and Nephrotic Syndromes

Ganesh Raghu, MD
Professor of Medicine and Laboratory Medicine (Adjunct), Division of Pulmonary and Critical Care Medicine; Director, Interstitial Lung Disease, Sarcoid and Pulmonary Fibrosis Program; Medical Director, Lung Transplant Program, University of Washington, Seattle, Washington
Interstitial Lung Disease

Margaret V. Ragni, MD, MPH
Professor of Medicine and Clinical and Translational Science, Department of Medicine, Division of Hematology/Oncology, University of Pittsburgh School of Medicine; Director, Hemophilia Center of Western Pennsylvania, Pittsburgh, Pennsylvania
Hemorrhagic Disorders: Coagulation Factor Deficiencies

Srinivasa N. Raja, MD
Professor of Anesthesiology and Neurology; Director, Division of Pain Medicine, Johns Hopkins University School of Medicine, Baltimore, Maryland
Pain

S. Vincent Rajkumar, MD
Professor of Medicine and Chair, Myeloma Amyloidosis Dysproteinemia Group, Division of Hematology, Mayo Medical School and Mayo Clinic, Rochester, Minnesota
Plasma Cell Disorders

Didier Raoult, MD, PhD
Professor, Université de la Méditerranée, National Center for Scientific Research UMR 6236, Research and Development Institute 198, Université de la Méditerranée, Faculté de Médecine, Marseille, France
Bartonella *Species Infections; Rickettsial Infections*

Robert W. Rebar, MD
Volunteer Professor, Department of Obstetrics and Gynecology, Executive Director, American Society for Reproductive Medicine, University of Alabama at Birmingham School of Medicine, Birmingham, Alabama
Ovaries and Development; Reproductive Endocrinology and Infertility

Annette C. Reboli, MD
Professor of Medicine and Vice Dean, Cooper Medical School of Rowan University; Professor of Medicine, University of Medicine and Dentistry of New Jersey/Robert Wood Johnson Medical School, Department of Medicine, Division of Infectious Diseases, Cooper University Hospital, Camden, New Jersey
Erysipelothrix *Infections*

K. Rajender Reddy, MD
Professor of Medicine and of Medicine in Surgery, Director of Hepatology and Medical Director of Liver Transplantation, University of Pennsylvania School of Medicine, Philadelphia, Pennsylvania
Bacterial, Parasitic, Fungal, and Granulomatous Liver Diseases

Donald A. Redelmeier, MD, MSc
Professor of Medicine and of Health Policy Management and Evaluation, University of Toronto; Canada Research Chair, Sunnybrook Health Sciences Centre, Toronto, Ontario, Canada
Postoperative Care and Complications

Susan E. Reef, MD
Medical Epidemiologist, Global Immunization Division, Centers for Disease Control and Prevention, Atlanta, Georgia
Rubella (German Measles)

Neil M. Resnick, MD
Thomas Detre Professor of Medicine and Chief, Division of Gerontology and Geriatric Medicine; Director, University of Pittsburgh Institute on Aging, University of Pittsburgh, Pittsburgh, Pennsylvania
Incontinence

David B. Reuben, MD
Archstone Professor of Medicine; Director, Multicampus Program in Geriatric Medicine and Gerontology; Chief, Division of Geriatrics, David Geffen School of Medicine at UCLA, University of California, Los Angeles, California
Geriatric Assessment

Herbert Y. Reynolds, MD
Professor Emeritus, Department of Medicine, Penn State College of Medicine, Hershey, Pennsylvania; Adjunct Professor of Medicine, Uniformed Services University of the Health Sciences, F. Edward Hebert School of Medicine; Medical Officer, Division of Lung Diseases, National Heart, Lung, and Blood Institute, National Institutes of Health, Bethesda, Maryland
Respiratory Structure and Function: Mechanisms and Testing

Emanuel P. Rivers, MD, MPH
Clinical Professor and Senior Staff Attending, Departments of Emergency Medicine and Surgery (Critical Care), Wayne State University; Vice Chairman and Research Director, Department of Emergency Medicine, Henry Ford Hospital, Detroit, Michigan
Approach to the Patient with Shock

Robert A. Rizza, MD
Professor of Medicine, Department of Endocrinology, Mayo Clinic, Rochester, Minnesota
Hypoglycemia/Pancreatic Islet Cell Disorders

Lewis R. Roberts, MB ChB, PhD
Professor, Department of Medicine, Mayo Medical School; Consultant in Gastroenterology and Hepatology, Mayo Clinic, Rochester, Minnesota
Liver and Biliary Tract Tumors

Jean-Marc Rolain, PharmD, PhD
Professor, Université de la Méditerranée, National Center for Scientific Research UMR 6236, Research and Development Institute, Faculté de Médecine et de Pharmacie, Université de la Méditerranée, Marseille, France
Bartonella *Species Infections*

José R. Romero, MD
Professor of Pediatrics, University of Arkansas for Medical Sciences; Horace C. Cabe Professor of Pediatric Infectious Diseases, Arkansas Children's Hospital; Director, Pediatric Infectious Diseases Section; Director, Clinical Trials, Arkansas Children's Hospital Research Institute, Little Rock, Arkansas
Enteroviruses

G. David Roodman, MD, PhD
Professor of Medicine, University of Pittsburgh; Vice Chair for Research, University of Pittsburgh; Director, Center for Bone Biology, University of Pittsburgh Medical Center; University of Pittsburgh Cancer Institute, Pittsburgh, Pennsylvania
Paget's Disease of Bone

Clifford Rosen, MD
Professor, Department of Medicine, Tufts University School of Medicine, Boston, Massachusetts; Senior Scientist, Maine Medical Center Research Institute, Maine Medical Center, Portland, Maine
Osteoporosis

Karen Rosene-Montella, MD
Professor of Medicine and of Obstetrics and Gynecology, Vice Chair of Medicine for Quality and Outcomes, Alpert Medical School at Brown University; Senior Vice President, Women's Services and Clinical Integration, Lifespan; Chief of Medicine, Women and Infants Hospital, Providence, Rhode Island
Common Medical Problems in Pregnancy

Philip J. Rosenthal, MD
Professor, Department of Medicine, University of California, San Francisco, School of Medicine, San Francisco, California
Malaria

Marc E. Rothenberg, MD, PhD
Professor of Pediatrics, University of Cincinnati College of Medicine; Director, Division of Allergy and Immunology, Cincinnati Children's Hospital Medical Center, Cincinnati, Ohio
Eosinophilic Syndromes

Hope S. Rugo, MD
Clinical Professor of Medicine, Director, Breast Oncology Clinical Trials Program, University of California, San Francisco, Comprehensive Cancer Center, San Francisco, California
Paraneoplastic Syndromes and Other Non-Neoplastic Effects of Cancer

James A. Russell, MD
Professor, Department of Medicine, University of British Columbia; Principal Investigator, James Hogg Research Centre, Institute for Heart and Lung Health, St. Paul's Hospital, Vancouver, British Columbia, Canada
Shock Syndromes Related to Sepsis

Anil K. Rustgi, MD
T. Grier Miller Professor of Medicine and Genetics, Chief of Gastroenterology and American Cancer Society Research Professor, University of Pennsylvania School of Medicine, Philadelphia, Pennsylvania
Neoplasms of the Esophagus and Stomach

Robert A. Salata, MD
Professor and Vice Chair, Department of Medicine; Chief, Division of Infectious Diseases and HIV Medicine, Case Western Reserve University School of Medicine; Attending Physician and Consultant, University Hospitals Case Medical Center, Cleveland, Ohio
Brucellosis

Jane E. Salmon, MD
Professor, Department of Medicine, Weill Cornell Medical College; Collette Kean Research Chair, Divisions of Rheumatology and Research, Hospital for Special Surgery, New York, New York
Mechanisms of Immune-Mediated Tissue Injury

Renato M. Santos, MD
Assistant Professor of Internal Medicine; Associate Director, Cardiovascular Training Program, Wake Forest University School of Medicine, Winston-Salem, North Carolina
Vascular Disorders of the Kidney; Video

Michael N. Sawka, PhD
Chief, Thermal and Mountain Medicine Division, U.S. Army Research Institute of Environmental Medicine, Natick, Massachusetts
Disorders Due to Heat and Cold

Andrew I. Schafer, MD
Chairman, Department of Medicine; The E. Hugh Luckey Distinguished Professor of Medicine, Weill Cornell Medical College; Physician-in-Chief, New York-Presbyterian Hospital/Weill Cornell Medical Center, New York, New York
Approach to Medicine, the Patient, and the Medical Profession: Medicine as a Learned and Humane Profession; Approach to the Patient with Bleeding and Thrombosis; Hemorrhagic Disorders: DIC, Liver Failure, and Vitamin K Deficiency; Thrombotic Disorders: Hypercoagulable States

William Schaffner, MD
Professor and Chair, Department of Preventive Medicine; Professor of Medicine (Infectious Diseases), Vanderbilt University School of Medicine, Nashville, Tennessee
Tularemia and Other Francisella *Infections*

W. Michael Scheld, MD
Bayer-Gerald L. Mandell Professor of Infectious Diseases, Professor of Medicine, Clinical Professor of Neurosurgery, Director, Pfizer Initiative in International Health, Division of Infectious Diseases and International Health, Department of Medicine, University of Virginia Health System, Charlottesville, Virginia
Introduction to Microbial Disease: Host-Pathogen Interactions

Eileen Schneider, MD, MPH
Division of Tuberculosis Elimination, Centers for Disease Control and Prevention, Atlanta, Georgia
Coronaviruses

Thomas J. Schnitzer, MD, PhD
Professor, Physical Medicine, Rehabilitation, and Internal Medicine, Northwestern University Feinberg School of Medicine, Chicago, Illinois
Osteoarthritis

Robert T. Schooley, MD
Professor and Head, Division of Infectious Diseases, University of California, San Diego, School of Medicine, San Diego, California
Epstein-Barr Virus Infection

David L. Schriger, MD, MPH
Professor, Department of Emergency Medicine, David Geffen School of Medicine at UCLA, University of California, Los Angeles, California
Approach to the Patient with Abnormal Vital Signs

Steven A. Schroeder, MD
Distinguished Professor of Health and Healthcare, Department of Medicine, and Director, Smoking Cessation Leadership Center, University of California, San Francisco, San Francisco, California
Socioeconomic Issues in Medicine

Lynn M. Schuchter, MD
Professor of Medicine, Chief, Hematology/Oncology Division, University of Pennsylvania School of Medicine, Philadelphia, Pennsylvania
Melanoma and Nonmelanoma Skin Cancers

Sam Schulman, MD, PhD
Professor of Medicine, Department of Medicine, McMaster University, Hamilton, Ontario, Canada
Antithrombotic Therapy

Lawrence B. Schwartz, MD, PhD
Charles and Evelyn Thomas Professor of Medicine, Department of Internal Medicine, Medical College of Virginia, Virginia Commonwealth University, Richmond, Virginia
Systemic Anaphylaxis, Food Allergy, and Insect Sting Allergy

Robert S. Schwartz, MD
Distinguished Professor of Medicine, Tufts University School of Medicine, Boston, Massachusetts
Autoimmune and Intravascular Hemolytic Anemias

Carlos Seas, MD
Associate Professor of Medicine, Cayetano Heredia University; Attending Physician, Department of Tropical and Infectious Diseases, Cayetano Heredia National Hospital, Lima, Peru
Cholera and Other Vibrio *Infections*

Steven A. Seifert, MD
Professor, University of New Mexico School of Medicine; Medical Director, New Mexico Poison and Drug Information Center, Albuquerque, New Mexico
Venomous Snake Bites

Julian L. Seifter, MD
Associate Professor of Medicine, Harvard Medical School; Physician, Brigham and Women's Hospital, Boston, Massachusetts
Potassium Disorders; Acid-Base Disorders

Clay F. Semenkovich, MD
Herbert S. Gasser Professor and Chief, Division of Endocrinology, Metabolism and Lipid Research, Washington University School of Medicine, St. Louis, Missouri
Disorders of Lipid Metabolism

Carol E. Semrad, MD
Associate Professor of Medicine, Section of Gastroenterology, The University of Chicago Pritzker School of Medicine, Chicago, Illinois
Approach to the Patient with Diarrhea and Malabsorption

F. John Service, MD, PhD
Professor of Medicine, Mayo Clinic College of Medicine; Consultant in Endocrinology and Metabolism, Mayo Clinic, Rochester, Minnesota
Hypoglycemia/Pancreatic Islet Cell Disorders

George M. Shaw, MD, PhD
Professor, Division of Hematology/Oncology, Department of Medicine, University of Pennsylvania School of Medicine, Philadelphia, Pennsylvania
Biology of Human Immunodeficiency Viruses

Pamela J. Shaw, MB ChB, MD
Professor of Neurology, Academic Neurology Unit and Head of Neuroscience Department, University of Sheffield; Director, Sheffield Care and Research Centre for Motor Neuron Disorders, Sheffield, United Kingdom
Amyotrophic Lateral Sclerosis and Other Motor Neuron Diseases; Videos

Robert S. Sherwin, MD
CNH Long Professor of Medicine and Chief, Section of Endocrinology; Director, Yale Center for Clinical Investigation, Yale University School of Medicine, New Haven, Connecticut
Type 1 Diabetes Mellitus; Type 2 Diabetes Mellitus

Michael E. Shy, MD
Professor of Neurology and of Molecular Medicine and Genetics, Wayne State University School of Medicine, Detroit, Michigan
Peripheral Neuropathies; Video

Wilmer L. Sibbitt, Jr., MD
Professor of Internal Medicine, Rheumatology and Neurology, University of New Mexico Health Sciences Center, Albuquerque, New Mexico
Idiopathic Multifocal Fibrosclerosis

Ellen Sidransky, MD
Chief, Section of Molecular Neurogenetics, Medical Genetics Branch, National Human Genome Research Institute, National Institutes of Health, Bethesda, Maryland
The Lysosomal Storage Diseases

Robert F. Siliciano, MD, PhD
Professor of Medicine, Johns Hopkins University School of Medicine, Baltimore, Maryland
Immunopathogenesis of Human Immunodeficiency Virus Infection

Michael S. Simberkoff, MD
Professor of Medicine, New York University School of Medicine; Chief of Staff, Veterans Affairs New York Harbor Healthcare System, New York, New York
Haemophilus *and* Moraxella *Infections*

David L. Simel, MD, MHS
Professor and Vice Chair for Veterans Affairs, Department of Medicine, Duke University School of Medicine; Chief of Internal Medicine, Department of Medicine Service, Durham Veterans Affairs Medical Center, Durham, North Carolina
Approach to the Patient: History and Physical Examination

Karl Skorecki, MD
Annie Chutick Professor in Medicine (Nephrology) and Director, Rappaport Research Institute, Technion–Israel Institute of Technology; Director of Medical and Research Development, Rambam Health Care Campus, Haifa, Israel
Gene and Cell Therapy; Disorders of Sodium and Water Homeostasis

Arthur S. Slutsky, MD
Professor, Departments of Medicine, Surgery, and Biomedical Engineering, University of Toronto; Vice President of Research, St. Michael's Hospital, Toronto, Ontario, Canada
Acute Respiratory Failure; Mechanical Ventilation; Video

Eric J. Small, MD
Professor of Medicine and Urology, Chief, Division of Hematology and Oncology; Deputy Director and Director of Clinical Sciences, Helen Diller Family Comprehensive Cancer Center, University of California, San Francisco, California
Prostate Cancer

Gerald W. Smetana, MD
Associate Professor of Medicine, Harvard Medical School; Division of General Medicine and Primary Care, Beth Israel Deaconess Medical Center, Boston, Massachusetts
Principles of Medical Consultation

Frederick S. Southwick, MD
Professor of Medicine, Patient Quality Projects Manager, University of Florida and Shands Health System, Gainesville, Florida
Nocardiosis

Robert F. Spiera, MD
Associate Professor of Clinical Medicine, Weill Cornell Medical College; Director, Vasculitis and Scleroderma, The Hospital for Special Surgery, New York, New York
Polymyalgia Rheumatica and Temporal Arteritis

Stanley M. Spinola, MD
Professor and Chair, Department of Microbiology and Immunology; Professor of Medicine and of Pathology and Laboratory Medicine, Indiana University School of Medicine, Indianapolis, Indiana
Chancroid

Pawel Stankiewicz, MD, PhD
Associate Professor, Department of Molecular and Human Genetics, Baylor College of Medicine, Houston, Texas
Gene, Genomic, and Chromosomal Disorders

Paul Stark, MD
Professor of Clinical Radiology, University of California, San Diego, and Chief of Cardiothoracic Radiology, Radiology Service, Veterans Affairs San Diego Healthcare System, San Diego, California
Imaging in Pulmonary Disease

Lynne S. Steinbach, MD
Professor of Radiology and Orthopaedic Surgery, University of California, San Francisco, School of Medicine, San Francisco, California
Imaging Studies in the Rheumatic Diseases

Martin H. Steinberg, MD
Professor, Departments of Medicine, Pediatrics, and Pathology and Laboratory Medicine, Boston University School of Medicine; Director, Center of Excellence in Sickle Cell Disease, Boston Medical Center, Boston, Massachusetts
Sickle Cell Disease and Other Hemoglobinopathies

Theodore S. Steiner, MD
Associate Professor and Associate Head, Division of Infectious Diseases, University of British Columbia, Vancouver, British Columbia, Canada
Escherichia Coli *Enteric Infections*

David S. Stephens, MD
Stephen W. Schwarzmann Distinguished Professor of Medicine, Director, Division of Infectious Diseases, Department of Medicine, Emory University School of Medicine; Vice President for Research, Robert W. Woodruff Health Sciences Center, Emory University School of Medicine, Atlanta; Staff Physician, VA Medical Research Service (Atlanta), Decatur, Georgia
Neisseria Meningitidis *Infections; Aspergillosis*

David A. Stevens, MD
Professor, Department of Medicine, Stanford University, Stanford; Chief, Division of Infectious Diseases, Department of Medicine, Santa Clara Valley Medical Center, San Jose, California
Systemic Antifungal Agents; Aspergillosis

William G. Stevenson, MD
Professor of Medicine, Harvard Medical School; Director of Cardiac Electrophysiology, Brigham and Women's Hospital, Boston, Massachusetts
Ventricular Arrhythmias

Arthur E. Stillman, MD, PhD
William and Kay Casarella Professor, Department of Radiology, Emory University School of Medicine, Atlanta, Georgia
Radiology of the Heart

James K. Stoller, MD, MS
Jean Wall Bennett Professor of Medicine, Cleveland Clinic Lerner College of Medicine; Chair, Education Institute, Cleveland Clinic, Education Institute and Respiratory Institute, Cleveland Clinic, Cleveland, Ohio
Respiratory Monitoring in Critical Care

John H. Stone, MD, MPH
Associate Professor of Medicine, Harvard Medical School; Director, Clinical Rheumatology, Massachusetts General Hospital, Boston, Massachusetts
The Systemic Vasculitides

Edwin P. Su, MD
Assistant Professor, Clinical Orthopaedic Surgery, Weill Cornell Medical College; Assistant Attending, Department of Orthopaedic Surgery, Hospital for Special Surgery, New York, New York
Surgical Treatment of Joint Disease

Roland W. Sutter, MD, MPH&TM
Coordinator, Research and Product Development, Polio Eradication Department, World Health Organization, Geneva, Switzerland
Diphtheria and Other Corynebacteria Infections

Morton N. Swartz, MD
Professor of Medicine, Harvard Medical School; James Jackson Firm Chief of Medical Services, Massachusetts General Hospital, Boston, Massachusetts
Meningitis: Bacterial, Viral, and Other

Ronald S. Swerdloff, MD
Professor of Medicine, David Geffen School of Medicine at UCLA, Los Angeles; Chief, Division of Endocrinology and Metabolism, Harbor–UCLA Medical Center, Los Angeles Biomedical Research Institute, Torrance, California
The Testis and Male Sexual Function

Megan Sykes, MD
Michael J. Friedlander Professor of Medicine and Professor of Microbiology and Immunology and Surgical Sciences (in Surgery), Columbia University; Director, Columbia Center for Translational Immunology, Columbia University College of Physicians and Surgeons, New York, New York
Transplantation Immunology

Thomas A. Tami, MD
Medical Director, Group Health Associates; Director, Cincinnati Sinus Institute, Cincinnati, Ohio
Throat Disorders

Susan M. Tarlo, MB ChB
Professor, Department of Medicine and Dalla Lana School of Public Health, University of Toronto; Respiratory Physician, Toronto Western Hospital; Research Physician, Centre for Research Expertise in Occupational Disease, Gage Occupational and Environmental Health Unit, Toronto, Ontario, Canada
Occupational Lung Disease

Victoria M. Taylor, MD, MPH
Research Professor, Department of Health Services, University of Washington; Full Member, Cancer Prevention Program, Fred Hutchinson Cancer Research Center, Seattle, Washington
Cultural Context of Medicine

Ayalew Tefferi, MD
Professor of Medicine and Hematology, Mayo Medical School, Rochester, Minnesota
Polycythemias, Essential Thrombocythemia, and Primary Myelofibrosis

Paul S. Teirstein, MD
Visiting Professor of Medicine, Columbia University Medical Center, New York, New York; Chief of Cardiology and Director, Interventional Cardiology, Scripps Clinic, La Jolla, California
Interventional and Surgical Treatment of Coronary Artery Disease; Videos

Sam R. Telford III, ScD, MSc
Professor, Biomedical Sciences, Tufts University, North Grafton, Massachusetts
Babesiosis and Other Protozoan Diseases

Margaret Tempero, MD
Professor of Medicine, Division of Hematology and Oncology, University of California, San Francisco, School of Medicine; Leader, Pancreas Cancer Program, Director of Research Programs, Deputy Director, University of California, San Francisco, Helen Diller Family Comprehensive Cancer Center, San Francisco, California
Pancreatic Cancer

Michael J. Thun, MD, MSc
Vice President, Emeritus, Department of Epidemiology, American Cancer Society, Atlanta, Georgia
The Epidemiology of Cancer

Nina Tolkoff-Rubin, MD
Professor of Medicine, Harvard Medical School; Director of Dialysis and Renal Transplantation, Massachusetts General Hospital, Boston, Massachusetts
Treatment of Irreversible Renal Failure

Antonella Tosti, MD
Professor of Clinical Dermatology, Department of Dermatology and Cutaneous Surgery, University of Miami, Miller School of Medicine, Miami, Florida
Diseases of Hair and Nails

John J. Treanor, MD
Professor of Medicine and Chief, Infectious Diseases Division, University of Rochester Medical Center, Rochester, New York
Adenovirus Diseases

Ronald B. Turner, MD
Professor of Pediatrics, University of Virginia School of Medicine, Charlottesville, Virginia
The Common Cold

Arthur C. Upton, MD
Clinical Professor, Department of Environmental and Community Medicine, University of Medicine and Dentistry of New Jersey—Robert Wood Johnson Medical School, Piscataway, New Jersey; Professor Emeritus, Department of Environmental Medicine, New York University Medical School, New York, New York
Radiation Injury

Greet Van den Berghe, MD, PhD
Professor of Medicine, Katholieke Universiteit Leuven; Head, Department of Intensive Care Medicine, University Hospitals Leuven—Gasthuisberg, Leuven, Belgium
Parenteral Nutrition

John Varga, MD
John Hughes Professor of Medicine, Department of Medicine, Northwestern University Feinberg School of Medicine, Chicago, Illinois
Systemic Sclerosis (Scleroderma)

Adrian Vella, MD
Professor of Medicine, Division of Endocrinology and Metabolism, Mayo Clinic, Rochester, Minnesota
Hypoglycemia/Pancreatic Islet Cell Disorders

Joseph G. Verbalis, MD
Professor, Department of Medicine and Physiology, Georgetown University; Chief, Endocrinology and Metabolism, Georgetown University Hospital, Washington, DC
Posterior Pituitary

Ronald G. Victor, MD
Burns and Allen Professor of Medicine, David Geffen School of Medicine at UCLA, and Director, Hypertension Center; Co-Director, The Heart Institute, Cedars Sinai Medical Center, Los Angeles, California
Arterial Hypertension

Angela Vincent, MB ChB, MSc
Professor, Nuffield Department of Clinical Neurosciences, University of Oxford, Oxford, Oxon, United Kingdom
Disorders of Neuromuscular Transmission

Paul A. Volberding, MD
Professor and Vice Chair, Department of Medicine, University of California, San Francisco, School of Medicine; Co-Director, University of California, San Francisco–Gladstone Institute of Virology and Immunology Center for AIDS Research; Chief, Medical Service, San Francisco Veterans Affairs Medical Center, San Francisco, California
Hematology and Oncology in Patients with Human Immunodeficiency Virus Infection

Julie M. Vose, MD
Chief, Section of Hematology/Oncology, Professor of Medicine, University of Nebraska Medical Center, Omaha, Nebraska
Hematopoietic Stem Cell Transplantation

Robert M. Wachter, MD
Professor and Associate Chair, Department of Medicine, University of California, San Francisco, School of Medicine, San Francisco, California
Quality of Care and Patient Safety

Edward H. Wagner, MD, MPH
Professor of Public Health and Community Medicine, University of Washington and Director, MacColl Institute for Healthcare Innovation, Group Health Research Institute, Seattle, Washington
Comprehensive Chronic Disease Management

Edward E. Walsh, MD
Professor of Medicine, University of Rochester, Rochester, New York
Respiratory Syncytial Virus

Thomas J. Walsh, MD
Professor of Medicine, Division of Infectious Diseases, Weill Cornell Medical College, New York, New York
Aspergillosis

Christina Wang, MD
Professor of Medicine, David Geffen School of Medicine at UCLA; Program Director, General Clinical Research Center, Harbor–UCLA Medical Center, Los Angeles Biomedical Research Institute, Torrance, California
The Testis and Male Sexual Function

Christine Wanke, MD
Professor of Medicine and Public Health and Director, Division of Nutrition and Infection; Associate Chair, Department of Public Health, Tufts University School of Medicine, Boston, Massachusetts
Gastrointestinal Manifestions of HIV and AIDS

Stephen I. Wasserman, MD
Professor of Medicine, University of California, San Diego, School of Medicine, La Jolla, California
Approach to the Patient with Allergic or Immunologic Disease

Heiner Wedemeyer, MD
Professor, Department of Gastroenterology, Hepatology and Endocrinology, Hannover Medical School, Hannover, Germany
Acute Viral Hepatitis

Geoffrey A. Weinberg, MD
Professor of Pediatrics, University of Rochester School of Medicine and Dentistry; Director, Pediatric HIV Program, Golisano Children's Hospital at University of Rochester Medical Center, Rochester, New York
Parainfluenza Viral Disease

David A. Weinstein, MD, MMSc
Director, Glycogen Storage Disease Program, Division of Pediatric Endocrinology, University of Florida College of Medicine, Gainesville, Florida
Glycogen Storage Diseases

Robert S. Weinstein, MD
Professor of Medicine, University of Arkansas for Medical Sciences; Staff Physician, Department of Medicine, Central Arkansas Veterans Healthcare System, Little Rock, Arkansas
Osteomalacia and Rickets

Roger D. Weiss, MD
Professor of Psychiatry, Harvard Medical School, Boston, Massachusetts; Chief, Division of Alcohol and Drug Abuse, McLean Hospital, Belmont, Massachusetts
Drug Abuse and Dependence

Martin Weisse, MD
Professor, Department of Pediatrics, Uniformed Services University of the Health Sciences, Bethesda, Maryland; Colonel Army; Chief, Department of Pediatrics, Tripler Army Medical Center, Honolulu, Hawaii
Measles

Jeffrey I. Weitz, MD
Professor of Medicine and Biochemistry and Biomedical Sciences, McMaster University; Canada Research Chair in Thrombosis, Heart and Stroke Foundation of Ontario/J.F. Mustard Chair in Cardiovascular Research; Executive Director, Thrombosis and Atherosclerosis Research Institute, Hamilton, Ontario, Canada
Pulmonary Embolism

Samuel A. Wells, Jr., MD
Director, Thyroid Oncology Clinic, National Cancer Institute, Bethesda, Maryland
Medullary Thyroid Carcinoma and Calcitonin

Richard P. Wenzel, MD
Professor, Department of Medicine, Medical College of Virginia, Richmond, Virginia
Acute Bronchitis and Tracheitis

Victoria P. Werth, MD
Professor of Dermatology, University of Pennsylvania School of Medicine; Chief, Dermatology Section, Philadelphia Veterans Affairs Medical Center, Philadelphia, Pennsylvania
Principles of Therapy of Skin Diseases

Sterling G. West, MD
Professor of Medicine, Division of Rheumatology, University of Colorado Denver School of Medicine, Aurora, Colorado
Systemic Diseases in Which Arthritis Is a Feature

Cornelia M. Weyand, MD, PhD
Professor of Medicine, Division of Immunology and Rheumatology, Stanford University, Stanford, California
The Innate and Adaptive Immune Systems

A. Clinton White, Jr., MD
Paul R. Stalnaker, MD, Distinguished Professor and Director, Infectious Disease Division, Department of Internal Medicine, University of Texas Medical Branch, Galveston, Texas
Cestodes

Christopher J. White, MD
Professor and System Chairman for Cardiovascular Diseases, Ochsner Clinical School, University of Queensland, Ochsner Medical Institutions, New Orleans, Louisiana
Atherosclerotic Peripheral Arterial Disease; Video

Perrin C. White, MD
Professor, Department of Pediatrics, University of Texas Southwestern Medical Center; Chief, Department of Endocrinology, Children's Medical Center Dallas, Dallas, Texas
Disorders of Sexual Development

Richard J. Whitley, MD
Distinguished Professor of Pediatrics, Loeb Eminent Scholar Chair in Pediatrics, and Professor of Microbiology, Medicine and Neurosurgery, University of Alabama at Birmingham, Birmingham, Alabama
Herpes Simplex Virus Infections

Michael P. Whyte, MD
Professor of Medicine, Pediatrics, and Genetics, Division of Bone and Mineral Diseases, Washington University School of Medicine; Medical-Scientific Director, Center for Metabolic Bone Disease and Molecular Research, Shriners Hospital for Children, St. Louis, Missouri
Osteonecrosis, Osteosclerosis/Hyperostosis, and Other Disorders of Bone

Samuel Wiebe, MD, MSc
Professor and Head, Division of Neurology, Department of Clinical Neurosciences and Hotchkiss Brain Institute, University of Calgary, Calgary, Alberta, Canada
The Epilepsies

Jeanine P. Wiener-Kronish, MD
Henry Isaiah Dorr Professor of Research and Teaching in Anaesthetics, Harvard Medical School; Anesthetist-in-Chief, Department of Anesthesia, Critical Care and Pain Medicine, Massachusetts General Hospital, Boston, Massachusetts
Overview of Anesthesia

Jennifer E. Wildes, PhD
Assistant Professor of Psychiatry, University of Pittsburgh School of Medicine, Pittsburgh, Pennsylvania
Eating Disorders

Alexander Wilmer, MD, PhD
Professor of Medicine, Medical Intensive Care, Katholieke Universiteit Leuven, University Hospitals Leuven—Gasthuisberg, Belgium
Parenteral Nutrition

William Winkenwerder, Jr., MD, MBA
Chair, The Winkenwerder Company, Alexandria, Virginia
Disorders Due to Heat and Cold

Joseph I. Wolfsdorf, MB ChB
Professor of Pediatrics, Harvard Medical School; Clinical Director and Chair, Division of Endocrinology, Children's Hospital Boston, Boston, Massachusetts
Glycogen Storage Diseases

Gary P. Wormser, MD
Professor, Departments of Medicine and Pharmacology, New York Medical College; Chief of Infectious Diseases and Vice Chair of Medicine, New York Medical College; Chief of Infectious Diseases, Westchester Medical Center, Valhalla, New York
Lyme Disease

John J. Wysolmerski, MD
Professor of Internal Medicine, Section of Endocrinology and Metabolism, Department of Internal Medicine, Yale University School of Medicine, New Haven, Connecticut
The Parathyroid Glands, Hypercalcemia, and Hypocalcemia

Myron Yanoff, MD
Professor and Chair, Department of Ophthalmology, Drexel University College of Medicine; Adjunct Professor of Ophthalmology, University of Pennsylvania School of Medicine, Philadelphia, Pennsylvania
Diseases of the Visual System

Neal S. Young, MD, MACP
Chief, Hematology Branch, National Heart, Lung, and Blood Institute; Director, Center for Human Immunology, Autoimmunity, and Inflammation, National Institutes of Health, Bethesda, Maryland
Parvovirus

William F. Young, Jr., MD, MSc
Tyson Family Clinical Endocrinology Professor in Honor of Vahab Fatourechi, MD, and Professor of Medicine, Mayo Medical School; Division of Endocrinology, Diabetes, Metabolism, and Nutrition, Mayo Clinic, Rochester, Minnesota
Adrenal Medulla, Catecholamines, and Pheochromocytoma

Alan S. L. Yu, MB ChB
Solon E. Summerfield Professor of Medicine, Kansas University School of Medicine; Director of the Kidney Institute and Division of Nephrology, Kansas University Medical Center, Kansas City, Kansas
Disorders of Magnesium and Phosphorus

Mark L. Zeidel, MD
Herrman L. Blumgart Professor of Medicine, Department of Medicine, Harvard Medical School; Physician-in-Chief and Chair, Department of Medicine, Beth Israel Deaconess Medical Center, Boston, Massachusetts
Obstructive Uropathy

Peter Zimetbaum, MD
Associate Professor of Medicine, Harvard Medical School; Director, Clinical Cardiology, Beth Israel Deaconess Medical Center, Boston, Massachusetts
Cardiac Arrhythmias with Supraventricular Origin

Justin A. Zivin, MD, PhD
Professor of Neurosciences, Department of Neurosciences, University of California San Diego, La Jolla, California; Staff Neurologist, San Diego Veterans Affairs Healthcare System, San Diego, California
Approach to Cerebrovascular Diseases; Ischemic Cerebrovascular Disease; Hemorrhagic Cerebrovascular Disease

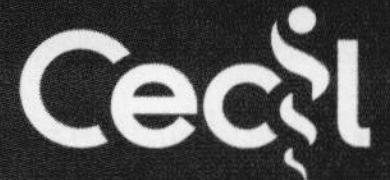

CONTENTS

SECTION VIII: CARDIOVASCULAR DISEASE

SECTION IX: RESPIRATORY DISEASES

SECTION X: CRITICAL CARE MEDICINE

SECTION XV: ONCOLOGY

VOLUME 2

SECTION XVI: METABOLIC DISEASES

SECTION XXIII: INFECTIOUS DISEASES

SECTION XXIV: HIV AND THE ACQUIRED IMMUNODEFICIENCY SYNDROME

SECTION XXV: NEUROLOGY

SECTION XXVI: EYE, EAR, NOSE, AND THROAT DISEASES

SECTION XXVII: MEDICAL CONSULTATION

SECTION XXVIII: SKIN DISEASES

APPENDIX: LABORATORY REFERENCE INTERVALS AND VALUES

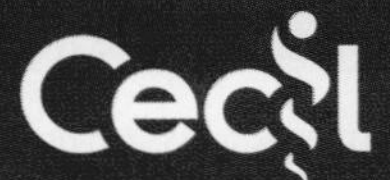

VIDEO CONTENTS

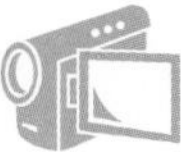

This icon appears throughout the book to indicate chapters with accompanying video available on *Expertconsult.com*. For quick viewing, use your smartphone to scan the QR codes in the front of the book.

GOLDMAN'S
CECIL MEDICINE

Cecil

I SOCIAL AND ETHICAL ISSUES IN MEDICINE

1

APPROACH TO MEDICINE, THE PATIENT, AND THE MEDICAL PROFESSION: MEDICINE AS A LEARNED AND HUMANE PROFESSION

LEE GOLDMAN AND ANDREW I. SCHAFER

APPROACH TO MEDICINE

Medicine is a profession that incorporates science and the scientific method with the art of being a physician. The art of tending to the sick is as old as humanity itself. Even in modern times, the art of caring and comforting, guided by millennia of common sense as well as a more recent, systematic approach to medical ethics (Chapter 2), remains the cornerstone of medicine. Without these humanistic qualities, the application of the modern science of medicine is suboptimal, ineffective, or even detrimental.

The caregivers of ancient times and premodern cultures tried a variety of interventions to help the afflicted. Some of their potions contained what are now known to be active ingredients that form the basis for proven medications (Chapter 28). Others (Chapter 38) have persisted into the present era despite a lack of convincing evidence. Modern medicine should not dismiss the possibility that these unproven approaches may be helpful; instead, it should adopt a guiding principle that all interventions, whether traditional or newly developed, can be tested vigorously, with the expectation that any beneficial effects can be explored further to determine their scientific basis.

When compared with its long and generally distinguished history of caring and comforting, the scientific basis of medicine is remarkably recent. Other than an understanding of human anatomy and the later description, albeit widely contested at this time, of the normal physiology of the circulatory system, almost all of modern medicine is based on discoveries made within the past 150 years. Until the late 19th century, the paucity of medical knowledge was perhaps exemplified best by hospitals and hospital care. Although hospitals provided caring that all but well-to-do people might not be able to obtain elsewhere, there is little if any evidence that hospitals improved health outcomes. The term *hospitalism* referred not to expertise in hospital care but rather to the aggregate of iatrogenic afflictions that were induced by the hospital stay itself.

The essential humanistic qualities of caring and comforting can achieve full benefit only if they are coupled with an understanding of how medical science can and should be applied to patients with known or suspected diseases. Without this knowledge, comforting may be inappropriate or misleading, and caring may be ineffective or counterproductive if it inhibits a sick person from obtaining appropriate, scientific medical care. *Goldman's Cecil Textbook of Medicine* focuses on the discipline of *internal medicine,* from which neurology and dermatology, which are also covered in substantial detail in this text, are relatively recent evolutionary branches. The term *internal medicine,* which is often misunderstood by the lay public, was developed in 19th-century Germany. *Inneren medizin* was to be distinguished from clinical medicine because it emphasized the physiology and chemistry of disease, not just the patterns or progression of clinical manifestations. *Goldman's Cecil Textbook of Medicine* follows this tradition by showing how pathophysiologic abnormalities cause symptoms and signs and by emphasizing how therapies can modify the underlying pathophysiology and improve the patient's well-being.

Modern medicine has moved rapidly past organ physiology to an increasingly detailed understanding of cellular, subcellular, and genetic mechanisms. For example, the understanding of microbial pathogenesis and many inflammatory diseases (Chapter 264) is now guided by a detailed understanding of the human immune system and its response to foreign antigens (Chapters 44 to 48).

Health, disease, and an individual's interaction with the environment are also substantially determined by genetics. In addition to many conditions that may be determined by a single gene (Chapter 40), medical science increasingly understands the complex interactions that underlie multigenic traits (Chapter 41). In the not-so-distant future, the decoding of the human genome holds the promise that personalized health care can be targeted according to an individual's genetic profile, in terms of screening and presymptomatic disease management, as well as in terms of specific medications and their adjusted dosing schedules. Currently, knowledge of the structure and physical forms of proteins helps explain abnormalities as diverse as sickle cell anemia (Chapter 166) and prion-related diseases (Chapter 424). Proteomics, which is the normal and abnormal protein expression of genes, also holds extraordinary promise for developing drug targets for more specific and effective therapies.

Concurrent with these advances in fundamental human biology has been a dramatic shift in methods for evaluating the application of scientific advances to the individual patient and to populations. The randomized controlled trial, sometimes with thousands of patients at multiple institutions, has replaced anecdote as the preferred method for measuring the benefits and optimal uses of diagnostic and therapeutic interventions (Chapter 9). As studies progress from those that show biologic effect, to those that elucidate dosing schedules and toxicity, and finally to those that assess true clinical benefit, the metrics of measuring outcome has also improved from subjective impressions of physicians or patients to reliable and valid measures of morbidity, quality of life, functional status, and other patient-oriented outcomes (Chapter 10). These marked improvements in the scientific methodology of clinical investigation have expedited extraordinary changes in clinical practice, such as recanalization therapy for acute myocardial infarction (Chapter 73), and have shown that reliance on intermediate outcomes, such as a reduction in asymptomatic ventricular arrhythmias with certain drugs, may unexpectedly increase rather than decrease mortality. Just as physicians in the 21st century must understand advances in fundamental biology, similar understanding of the fundamentals of clinical study design as it applies to diagnostic and therapeutic interventions is needed. An understanding of human genetics will also help stratify and refine the approach to clinical trials by helping researchers select fewer patients with a more homogeneous disease pattern to study the efficacy of an intervention.

This explosion in medical knowledge has led to increasing specialization and subspecialization, defined initially by organ system and more recently by locus of principal activity (inpatient vs. outpatient), reliance on manual skills (proceduralist vs. nonproceduralist), or participation in research. Nevertheless, it is becoming increasingly clear that the same fundamental molecular and genetic mechanisms are broadly applicable across all organ systems and that the scientific methodologies of randomized trials and careful clinical observation span all aspects of medicine.

The advent of modern approaches to managing data now provides the rationale for the use of health information technology. Computerized health records, oftentimes shared with patients in a portable format, can avoid duplication of tests and assure that care is coordinated among the patient's various health care providers.

APPROACH TO THE PATIENT

Patients commonly have complaints (symptoms). These symptoms may or may not be accompanied by abnormalities on examination (signs) or on laboratory testing. Conversely, asymptomatic patients may have signs or laboratory abnormalities, and laboratory abnormalities can occur in the absence of symptoms or signs.

Symptoms and signs commonly define *syndromes,* which may be the common final pathway of a wide range of pathophysiologic alterations. The fundamental basis of internal medicine is that diagnosis should elucidate the pathophysiologic explanation for symptoms and signs so that therapy may improve the underlying abnormality, not just attempt to suppress the abnormal symptoms or signs.

When patients seek care from physicians, they may have manifestations or exacerbations of known conditions, or they may have symptoms and signs that suggest malfunction of a particular organ system. Sometimes the pattern of symptoms and signs is highly suggestive or even pathognomonic for a particular disease process. In these situations, in which the physician is focusing on a particular disease, *Goldman's Cecil Textbook of Medicine* provides scholarly yet practical approaches to the epidemiology, pathobiology, clinical manifestations, diagnosis, treatment, prevention, and prognosis of entities such as acute myocardial infarction (Chapter 73), chronic obstructive lung disease (Chapter 88), obstructive uropathy (Chapter 125), inflammatory bowel disease (Chapter 143), gallstones (Chapter 158), rheumatoid arthritis (Chapter 272), hypothyroidism (Chapter 233), tuberculosis (Chapter 332), and virtually any known medical condition in adults.

Many patients, however, have undiagnosed symptoms, signs, or laboratory abnormalities that cannot be immediately ascribed to a particular disease or cause. Whether the initial manifestation is chest pain (Chapter 50), diarrhea (Chapter 142), neck or back pain (Chapter 407), or a variety of more than 100 common symptoms, signs, or laboratory abnormalities, *Goldman's Cecil Textbook of Medicine* provides tables, figures, and entire chapters to guide the approach to diagnosis and therapy (see E-Table 1-1 or table on inside back cover). By virtue of this dual approach to known disease as well as to undiagnosed abnormalities, this textbook, similar to the modern practice of medicine, applies directly to patients regardless of their mode of manifestation or degree of previous evaluation.

The patient-physician interaction proceeds through many phases of clinical reasoning and decision making. The interaction begins with an elucidation of complaints or concerns, followed by inquiries or evaluations to address these concerns in increasingly precise ways. The process commonly requires a careful history or physical examination, ordering of diagnostic tests, integration of clinical findings with test results, understanding of the risks and benefits of the possible courses of action, and careful consultation with the patient and family to develop future plans. Physicians can increasingly call on a growing literature of evidence-based medicine to guide the process so that benefit is maximized while respecting individual variations in different patients. Throughout *Goldman's Cecil Textbook of Medicine,* the best current evidence is highlighted with specific grade A references that can be accessed directly in the electronic version.

The increasing availability of evidence from randomized trials to guide the approach to diagnosis and therapy should not be equated with "cookbook" medicine. Evidence and the guidelines that are derived from it emphasize proven approaches for patients with specific characteristics. Substantial clinical judgment is required to determine whether the evidence and guidelines apply to individual patients and to recognize the occasional exceptions. Even more judgment is required in the many situations in which evidence is absent or inconclusive. Evidence must also be tempered by patients' preferences, although it is a physician's responsibility to emphasize evidence when presenting alternative options to the patient. The adherence of a patient to a specific regimen is likely to be enhanced if the patient also understands the rationale and evidence behind the recommended option.

To care for a patient as an individual, the physician must understand the patient as a person. This fundamental precept of doctoring includes an understanding of the patient's social situation, family issues, financial concerns, and preferences for different types of care and outcomes, ranging from maximum prolongation of life to the relief of pain and suffering (Chapters 2 and 3). If the physician does not appreciate and address these issues, the science of medicine cannot be applied appropriately, and even the most knowledgeable physician will fail to achieve the desired outcomes.

Even as physicians become increasingly aware of new discoveries, patients can obtain their own information from a variety of sources, some of which are of questionable reliability. The increasing use of alternative and complementary therapies (Chapter 38) is an example of patients' frequent dissatisfaction with prescribed medical therapy. Physicians should keep an open mind regarding unproven options but must advise their patients carefully if such options may carry any degree of potential risk, including the risk that they may be relied on to substitute for proven approaches. It is crucial for the physician to have an open dialogue with the patient and family regarding the full range of options that either may consider.

The physician does not exist in a vacuum, but rather as part of a complicated and extensive system of medical care and public health. In premodern times and even today in some developing countries, basic hygiene, clean water, and adequate nutrition have been the most important ways to promote health and reduce disease. In developed countries, adoption of healthy lifestyles, including better diet (Chapter 220) and appropriate exercise (Chapter 15), is the cornerstone to reducing the epidemics of obesity (Chapter 227), coronary disease (Chapter 70), and diabetes (Chapter 237). Public health interventions to provide immunizations (Chapter 17) and to reduce injuries and the use of tobacco (Chapter 31), illicit drugs (Chapter 33), and excess alcohol (Chapter 32) can collectively produce more health benefits than nearly any other imaginable health intervention.

APPROACH TO THE MEDICAL PROFESSION

In a profession, practitioners put the welfare of clients or patients above their own welfare. Professionals have a duty that may be thought of as a contract with society. The American Board of Internal Medicine and the European Federation of Internal Medicine have jointly proposed that medical professionalism should emphasize three fundamental principles: the primacy of patient welfare, patient autonomy, and social justice. As modern medicine brings a plethora of diagnostic and therapeutic options, the interactions of the physician with the patient and society become more complex and potentially fraught with ethical dilemmas (Chapter 2). To help provide a moral compass that is not only grounded in tradition but also adaptable to modern times, the primacy of patient welfare emphasizes the fundamental principle of a profession. The physician's altruism, which begets the patient's trust, must be impervious to the economic, bureaucratic, and political challenges that are faced by the physician and the patient (Chapter 5).

TABLE 1-1 PROFESSIONAL RESPONSIBILITIES

Commitment to:
Professional competence
Honesty with patients
Patient confidentiality
Maintaining appropriate relations with patients
Improving the quality of care
Improving access to care
Just distribution of finite resources
Scientific knowledge
Maintaining trust by managing conflicts of interest
Professional responsibilities

From Brennan T, Blank L, Cohen J, et al. Medical professionalism in the new millennium: a physician charter. *Ann Intern Med.* 2002;1136:243-246.

The principle of patient autonomy asserts that physicians make recommendations but patients make the final decisions. The physician is an expert advisor who must inform and empower the patient to base decisions on scientific data and how these data can and should be integrated with a patient's preferences.

The importance of social justice symbolizes that the patient-physician interaction does not exist in a vacuum. The physician has a responsibility to the individual patient and to broader society to promote access and to eliminate disparities in health and health care.

To promote these fundamental principles, a series of professional responsibilities has been suggested (Table 1-1). These specific responsibilities represent practical, daily traits that benefit the physician's own patients and society as a whole. Physicians who use these and other attributes to improve their patients' satisfaction with care are not only promoting professionalism but also reducing their own risk for liability and malpractice.

An interesting new aspect of professionalism is the increasing reliance on team approaches to medical care, as exemplified by physicians whose roles are defined by the location of their practice—historically in the intensive care unit or emergency department and more recently on the inpatient general hospital floor. Quality care requires coordination and effective communication across inpatient and outpatient sites among physicians who themselves now typically work defined hours. This transition from reliance on a single, always available physician to a team, ideally with a designated coordinator, places new challenges on physicians, the medical care system, and the medical profession.

The changing medical care environment is placing increasing emphasis on standards, outcomes, and accountability. As purchasers of insurance become more cognizant of value rather than just cost (Chapter 11), outcomes ranging from rates of screening mammography (Chapter 204) to mortality rates with coronary artery bypass graft surgery (Chapter 74) become metrics by which rational choices can be made. Clinical guidelines and critical pathways derived from randomized controlled trials and evidence-based medicine can potentially lead to more cost-effective care and better outcomes.

These major changes in many Western health care systems bring with them many major risks and concerns. If the concept of limited choice among physicians and health care providers is based on objective measures of quality and outcome, channeling of patients to better providers is one reasonable definition of better selection and enlightened competition. If the limiting of options is based overwhelmingly on cost rather than measures of quality, outcomes, and patient satisfaction, it is likely that the historic relationship between the patient and the truly professional physician will be fundamentally compromised.

Another risk is that the same genetic information that could lead to more effective, personalized medicine will be used against the very people whom it is supposed to benefit—by creating a stigma, raising health insurance costs, or even making someone uninsurable. The ethical approach to medicine

(Chapter 2), genetics, and genetic counseling (Chapter 39) provides means to protect against this adverse effect of scientific progress.

In this new environment, the physician often has a dual responsibility: to the health care system as an expert who helps create standards, measures of outcome, clinical guidelines, and mechanisms to ensure high-quality, cost-effective care and to individual patients who entrust their well-being to that physician to promote their best interests within the reasonable limits of the system. A health insurance system that emphasizes cost-effective care, that gives physicians and health care providers responsibility for the health of a population and the resources required to achieve these goals, that must exist in a competitive environment in which patients can choose alternatives if they are not satisfied with their care, and that places increasing emphasis on health education and prevention can have many positive effects. In this environment, however, physicians must beware of overt and subtle pressures that could entice them to underserve patients and abrogate their professional responsibilities by putting personal financial reward ahead of their patients' welfare. The physician's responsibility to represent the patient's best interests and avoid financial conflicts by doing too little in the newer systems of capitated care provides different specific challenges but an analogous moral dilemma to the historical American system in which the physician could be rewarded financially for doing too much.

In the current health care environment, all physicians and trainees must redouble their commitment to professionalism. At the same time, the challenge to the individual physician to retain and expand the scientific knowledge base and process the vast array of new information is daunting. In this spirit of a profession based on science and caring, *Goldman's Cecil Textbook of Medicine* seeks to be a comprehensive approach to modern internal medicine.

SUGGESTED READINGS

Ioannidis JP. Expectations, validity, and reality in omics. *J Clin Epidemiol.* 2010;63:945-949. *Perspectives on how modern biologic measurements and assays may individualize health care if appropriately validated.*

Mostaghimi A, Crotty BH. Professionalism in the digital age. *Ann Intern Med.* 2011;154:560-562. *Practical commentary.*

Qaseem A, Snow V, Gosfield A, et al. Pay for performance through the lens of medical professionalism. *Ann Intern Med.* 2010;152:366-369. *Explores how these two ideas can coexist successfully.*

Rogers W, Ballantyne A. Towards a practical definition of professional behavior. *J Med Ethics.* 2010;36:250-254. *Emphasizes the importance of responsibility; relationships with and respect for patients; probity and honesty; self awareness, and capacity for reflection.*

2

BIOETHICS IN THE PRACTICE OF MEDICINE

EZEKIEL J. EMANUEL

It commonly is argued that modern advances in medical technology, antibiotics, dialysis, transplantation, and intensive care units have created the bioethical dilemmas that confront physicians in the 21st century. In reality, however, concerns about ethical issues are as old as the practice of medicine itself. The Hippocratic Oath, composed sometime around 400 BC, attests to the need of ancient Greek physicians for advice on how to address the many bioethical dilemmas that they confronted. The Oath addresses issues of confidentiality, abortion, euthanasia, sexual relations between physician and patient, divided loyalties, and, at least implicitly, charity care and executions. Other Hippocratic works address issues such as termination of treatments to dying patients and telling the truth. Whether we agree with the advice dispensed or not, the important point is that many bioethical issues are not created by technology but are inherent in medical practice. Technology may make these issues more common and may change the context in which they arise, but there are underlying bioethical issues that seem timeless, inherent in the practice of medicine.

Many physicians have been educated that four main principles can be invoked to address bioethical dilemmas: autonomy, nonmaleficence, beneficence, and justice. Autonomy is the idea that people should have the right and freedom to choose, pursue, and revise their own life plans. Nonmaleficence is the idea that people should not be harmed or injured knowingly; this principle is encapsulated in the frequently repeated phrase that a physician has an obligation to "first do no harm"—*primum non nocere.* This phrase is not found either in the Hippocratic Oath or in other Hippocratic writing; the only related, but not identical, Hippocratic phrase is "at least, do not harm." Whereas nonmaleficence is about avoiding harm, beneficence is about the positive actions that the physician should undertake to promote the well-being of his or her patients. In clinical practice, this obligation usually arises from the implicit and explicit commitments and promises surrounding the physician-patient relationship. Finally, there is the principle of justice as the fair distribution of benefits and burdens.

Although helpful in providing an initial framework, these principles have limited value because they are broad and open to diverse and conflicting interpretations. In addition, as is clear with the principle of justice, they frequently are underdeveloped. In any difficult case, the principles are likely to conflict. Conflicting ethical principles are precisely why there are bioethical dilemmas. The principles themselves do not offer guidance on how they should be balanced or specified to resolve the dilemma. These principles, which are focused on the individual physician-patient context, are not particularly helpful when the bioethical issues are institutional and systemic, such as allocating scarce vaccines or organs for transplantation or balancing the risks and benefits of mammograms for women younger than 50 years. Finally, these four principles are not comprehensive. Other fundamental ethical principles and values, such as communal solidarity, duties to future generations, trust, and professional integrity, are important in bioethics but not encapsulated except by deformation in these four principles.

There is no formula or small set of ethical principles that mechanically or magically gives answers to bioethical dilemmas. Instead, medical practitioners should follow an orderly analytic process. First, practitioners need to obtain the facts relevant to the situation. Second, they must delineate the basic bioethical issue. Third, it is important to identify all the crucial principles and values that relate to the case and how they might conflict. Fourth, because many ethical dilemmas have been analyzed previously and subjected frequently to empirical study, practitioners should examine the relevant literature, whether it is commentaries or studies in medical journals, legal cases, or books. With these analyses, the particular dilemma should be reexamined; this process might lead to reformulation of the issue and identification of new values or new understandings of existing values. Fifth, with this information, it is important to distinguish clearly unethical practices from a range of ethically permissible actions. Finally, it is important not only to come to some resolution of the case but also to state clearly the reasons behind the decisions, that is, the interpretation of the principles used and how values were balanced. Although unanimity and consensus may be desirable ideals, reasonable people frequently disagree about how to resolve ethical dilemmas without being unethical or malevolent.

A multitude of bioethical dilemmas arise in medical practice, including issues of genetics, reproductive choices, and termination of care. In clinical practice, the most common issues revolve around informed consent, termination of life-sustaining treatments, euthanasia and physician-assisted suicide, and conflicts of interest.

PHYSICIAN-PATIENT RELATIONSHIP: INFORMED CONSENT

History

It commonly is thought that the requirement for informed consent is a relatively recent phenomenon. Suggestions about the need for a patient's informed consent can be found as far back as Plato, however. The first recorded legal case involving informed consent is the 1767 English case of *Slater v. Baker and Stapleton,* in which two surgeons refractured a patient's leg after it had healed improperly. The patient claimed they had not obtained consent. The court ruled:

> *[I]t appears from the evidence of the surgeon that it was improper to disunite the callous without consent; this is the usage and law of surgeons: then it was ignorance and unskillfulness in that very particular, to do contrary to the rule of the profession, what no surgeon ought to have done.*

Although there may be some skepticism about the extent of the information disclosed or the precise nature of the consent obtained, the notable fact is that an 18th-century court declared that obtaining prior consent of the patient is not only the usual practice but also the ethical and legal obligation of surgeons. Failure to obtain consent is incompetent and inexcusable. In contemporary times, the 1957 case of *Salgo v. Leland Stanford Junior University Board of Trustees* constitutes a landmark by stating that physicians have a positive legal obligation to disclose information about risks, benefits, and alternatives to patients; this decision popularized the term *informed consent.*

Definition and Justification

Informed consent is a person's autonomous authorization of a physician to undertake diagnostic or therapeutic interventions for himself or herself. In this view, the patient understands that he or she is taking responsibility for the decision while empowering someone else, the physician, to implement it. Not any agreement to a course of medical treatment qualifies as informed consent, however.

There are four fundamental requirements for valid informed consent: mental capacity, disclosure, understanding, and voluntariness. Informed consent assumes that people have the mental capacity to make decisions; disease, development, or medications can compromise patients' mental capacity to provide informed consent. Adults are presumed to have the legal competence to make medical decisions, and whether an adult is incompetent to make medical decisions is a legal determination. Practically, physicians usually decide whether patients are competent on the basis of whether patients can understand the information disclosed, appreciate its significance for their own situation, and use logical and consistent thought processes in decision making. Incompetence in medical decision making does not mean a person is incompetent in all types of decision making and vice versa. Crucial information relevant to the decision must be disclosed, usually by the physician, to the patient. The patient should understand the information and its implications for his or her interests and life goals. Finally, the patient must make a voluntary decision (i.e., one without coercion or manipulation by the physician). It is a mistake to view informed consent as an event, such as the signing of a form. Informed consent is viewed more accurately as a process that evolves during the course of diagnosis and treatment.

Typically, the patient's autonomy is the value invoked to justify informed consent. Other values, such as bodily integrity and beneficence, have also been cited, especially in early legal rulings.

Empirical Data

Fairly extensive research has been done on informed consent. In general, studies show that in clinical situations, physicians frequently do not communicate all relevant information for informed decision making. In a study of audiotapes from 1057 outpatient encounters, physicians mentioned alternatives in only 11.3% of cases, provided pros and cons of interventions in only 7.8% of situations, and assessed the patient's understanding of the information in only 1.5% of decisions. The more complex the medical decisions, the more likely it was that the elements of informed consent would be fulfilled. Importantly, data suggest that disclosure is better in research settings, both in the informed consent documents and in the discussions. For instance, in recorded interactions between researchers and prospective participants, the major elements of research, such as that the treatment was investigational and the risks and benefits, were disclosed in more than 80% of interactions. Greater disclosure in the research setting may be the consequence of requiring a written informed consent document. Some have suggested that for common medical interventions, such as elective surgery, standardized informed consent documents should include the risks and benefits as quantified in randomized controlled trials, as well as acceptable alternatives.

Patients frequently fail to recall crucial information disclosed, although they usually think they have sufficient information for decision making. Whether patients fail to recall key information because they are overwhelmed by the information or because they do not find much of it salient to their decision is unclear. The issue is what patients understand at the point of decision making, not what they recall later.

Studies aimed at improving informed consent in the clinical setting suggest that interactive media, such as videos, can improve understanding by patients. Conversely, data from the research setting suggest that interactive media do not improve participants' understanding, whereas more personal interaction, whether as an additional telephone call by a research nurse or as an additional face-to-face meeting, does enhance understanding.

One of the most important results of empirical research on informed consent is the gap between information and decision making. Many studies show that most patients want information, but far fewer prefer decision-making authority. One study showed that most patients wanted information, but only about one third desired decision-making authority, and patients' decision-making preferences were not correlated with their information-seeking preferences. Several investigators found that patients' preference for decision-making authority increases with higher educational levels and declines with advancing age. Most important, the more serious the illness, the more likely patients are to prefer that physicians make the decisions. Several studies suggest that patients who have less of a desire to make their own decisions generally are more satisfied with how the decisions were made.

TABLE 2-1 FUNDAMENTAL ELEMENTS FOR DISCLOSURE TO PATIENTS

Diagnosis and prognosis
Nature of proposed intervention
Reasonable alternative interventions
Risks associated with each alternative intervention
Benefits associated with each alternative intervention
Probable outcomes of each alternative intervention

Practical Considerations

Implementing informed consent raises concerns about the extent of information to be disclosed and exceptions to the general requirement. A major area of ethical and legal disagreement has been what information to disclose and how to disclose it. As a practical matter, physicians should disclose at least six fundamental elements of information to patients: (1) diagnosis and prognosis; (2) nature of the proposed intervention; (3) alternative interventions, including no treatment; (4) risks associated with each alternative; (5) benefits of each alternative; and (6) likely outcomes of these alternatives (Table 2-1). Because risk is usually the key worry of physicians, it generally is recommended that physicians disclose (1) the nature of the risks, (2) their magnitude, (3) the probability that each risk will occur, and (4) when the consequence might occur. Some argue that minor risks need not be disclosed. In general, all serious risks, such as death, paralysis, stroke, or chronic pain, even if rare, should be disclosed, as should common risks.

The central problem is that the physician should provide this detailed information within reasonable time constraints and yet not overwhelm patients with complex information in technical language. The result has been various legal standards defining how much information should be disclosed. The *physician* or *customary* standard, adapted from malpractice law, states that the physician should disclose information "which a reasonable medical practitioner would make under the same or similar circumstances." Conversely, the *reasonable person* or *lay-oriented* standard states that physicians should disclose all information that a "reasonable person in the patient's circumstances would find material to" the medical decision. The physician standard is factual and can be determined empirically, but the patient-oriented standard, which is meant to engage physicians with patients, is hypothetical. Currently, each standard is used by about half the states.

There are exceptions to the requirements of informed consent. In emergency situations, consent can be assumed because patients' interests concentrate on survival and retaining maximal mental and physical functioning; as a result, reasonable persons would want treatment. In some circumstances, physicians may believe the process of informed consent could pose a serious psychological threat. In rare cases, the "therapeutic privilege" promoting a patient's well-being trumps autonomy, but physicians should be wary of invoking this exception too readily.

If patients are deemed incompetent, family members—beginning with spouse, children, parents, siblings, then more distant relatives—usually are selected as surrogates or proxies, although there may be concerns about conflicting interests or knowledge of the patient's wishes. In the relatively rare circumstance in which a patient formally designated a proxy, that person has decision-making authority.

The *substituted judgment* standard states that the proxy should choose what the patient would choose if he or she were competent. The *best interests* standard states that the proxy should choose what is best for the patient. Frequently, it is not clear how the patient would have decided because the situation was not discussed with the patient and he or she left no living will. Similarly, what is best for a patient is controversial because there are usually tradeoffs between quality of life and survival. These problems are exacerbated because a proxy's predictions about a patient's quality of life are poor; proxies tend to underestimate patients' functional status and satisfaction. Similarly, proxy predictions are inaccurate regarding life-sustaining preferences when the patient is mentally incapacitated; families tend to agree with patients less than 70% of the time in deciding whether to provide life-sustaining treatments if the patient became demented, when chance alone would generate agreement in 50% of the cases. Such confusion about how to decide for incapacitated patients can create conflicts among family members or between the family and medical providers. In such circumstances, an ethics consultation may be helpful.

TERMINATION OF MEDICAL INTERVENTIONS

History

Since the start of medicine, it has been viewed as ethical to withhold medical treatments from the terminally ill and "let nature take its course." Hippocrates argued that physicians should "refuse to treat those [patients] who are overmastered by their disease." In the 19th century, prominent American physicians advocated withholding of cathartic and emetic "treatments" from the terminally ill and using ether to ease pain at the end of life. In 1900, editors of *The Lancet* argued that physicians should intervene to ease the pain of death but did not have an obligation to prolong a clearly terminal life. The contemporary debate on terminating care began in 1976 with the *Quinlan* case, in which the New Jersey Supreme Court ruled that patients had a right to refuse life-sustaining interventions on the basis of a right of privacy and that the family could exercise the right for a patient in a persistent vegetative state.

Definition and Justification

It generally is agreed that all patients have a right to refuse medical interventions. Ethically, this right is based on the patient's autonomy and is implied by the doctrine of informed consent. Legally, state courts have cited the right to privacy, right to bodily integrity, or common law to justify the right to refuse medical treatment. In the 1990 *Cruzan* case and in the subsequent physician-assisted suicide cases, the U.S. Supreme Court affirmed that there is a "constitutionally protected right to refuse lifesaving hydration and nutrition." The Court stated that "[A] liberty interest [based on the 14th Amendment] in refusing unwanted medical treatment may be inferred from our prior decisions." All patients have a constitutional and an ethical right to refuse medical interventions. These rulings were the basis of the consistent state and federal court rulings to permit the husband to terminate artificial nutrition and hydration in the *Schiavo* case.

Empirical Data

Data show that termination of medical treatments is now the norm. More than 85% of Americans die without cardiopulmonary resuscitation, and more than 90% of decedents in intensive care units do not receive cardiopulmonary resuscitation. Of decedents in intensive care units, 90% die after the withholding or withdrawal of medical treatments, with an average of 2.6 interventions being withheld or withdrawn per decedent. Since the 1990s, the trend has been to stop medical interventions more frequently.

Despite extensive public support for use of advance care directives and the passage of the Patient Self-Determination Act mandating that health care institutions inform patients of their right to complete such documents, only about 47% of Americans have completed one. Data suggest that over 40% of patients required active decision-making about terminating medical treatments in their final days, yet 70% lack decision-making capacity, thereby emphasizing the importance of advance directives. Efforts to improve completion of advance care directives have generated mixed results. Unfortunately, even successful pilot efforts have not been adopted or easily scaled. A persistent problem has been that even when patients complete advance care directives, the documents frequently are not available, physicians do not know they exist, or they tend to be too general or vague to guide decisions. The widespread use of electronic health records should create the possibility that advance directives will be available whenever the patient presents to a health care provider.

Just as proxies are poor at predicting patients' wishes, data show that physicians are probably even worse at determining patients' preferences for life-sustaining treatments. In many cases, life-sustaining treatments are continued even when patients or their proxies desire them to be stopped; conversely, many physicians discontinue or never begin interventions unilaterally without the knowledge or consent of patients or their surrogate decision makers. These discrepancies emphasize the importance of engaging patients early in their care about treatment preferences.

Practical Considerations

There are many practical considerations in enacting this right (Table 2-2). First, patients have a right to refuse any and all medical interventions, from blood transfusions and antibiotics to respirators, artificial hydration, and nutrition. Although initiation of cardiopulmonary resuscitation was the focus of the early court cases, this issue is viewed best as addressing just one of the many medical interventions that can be stopped or withheld. The attempt to distinguish ordinary from extraordinary or heroic treatments has been unhelpful in determining which treatments may be stopped.

Second, there is no ethical or legal difference between withholding an intervention and withdrawing it. If a respirator or other treatment is started because physicians are uncertain whether a patient would have wanted it, they always can stop it later when information clarifies the patient's wishes. Although physicians and nurses might find stopping a treatment to be more difficult psychologically, withdrawal is ethically and legally permitted—and required—when it is consonant with the patient's wishes.

Third, competent patients have the exclusive right to decide about terminating their own care. If there is a conflict between a competent patient and his or her family, the patient's wishes are to be followed. It is the patient's right to refuse treatment, not the family's right. For incompetent patients, the situation is more complex; if the patients left clear indications of their wishes, whether as explicit oral statements or as written advance care directives, these wishes should be followed. Physicians should not be overly concerned about the precise form patients use to express their wishes; because patients have a constitutional right to refuse treatment, the real concern is whether the wishes are clear and relevant to the situation. If an incompetent patient did not leave explicit indications of his or her wishes or designate a proxy decision maker, the physician should identify a surrogate decision maker and rely on the decision maker's wishes while being cognizant of the potential problems noted.

Fourth, the right to refuse medical treatment does not translate into a right to demand any treatment, especially treatments that have no pathophysiologic rationale, have already failed, or are known to be harmful. Futility has become a justification to permit physicians unilaterally to withhold or withdraw treatments despite the family's requests for treatment. Some states, such as Texas, have enacted futility laws, which prescribe procedures by which

TABLE 2-2 PRACTICAL CONSIDERATIONS IN TERMINATION OF MEDICAL TREATMENTS

PRACTICAL QUESTION	ANSWER
Is there a legal right to refuse medical interventions?	Yes. The U.S. Supreme Court declared that competent people have a constitutionally protected right to refuse unwanted medical treatments based on the 14th Amendment.
What interventions can be legally and ethically terminated?	Any and all interventions (including respirators, antibiotics, intravenous or enteral nutrition, and hydration) can be legally and ethically terminated.
Is there a difference between withholding life-sustaining interventions and withdrawing them?	No. The consensus is that there is no important legal or ethical difference between withholding and withdrawing medical interventions. Stopping a treatment once begun is just as ethical as never having started it.
Whose view about terminating life-sustaining interventions prevails if there is a conflict between the patient and family?	The views of a competent adult patient prevail. It is the patient's body and life.
Who decides about terminating life-sustaining interventions if the patient is incompetent?	If the patient appointed a proxy or surrogate decision maker when competent, that person is legally empowered to make decisions about terminating care. If no proxy was appointed, there is a legally designated hierarchy, usually (1) spouse, (2) adult children, (3) parents, (4) siblings, and (5) available relatives.
Are advance care directives legally enforceable?	Yes. As a clear expression of the patient's wishes, they are a constitutionally protected method for patients to exercise their right to refuse medical treatments. In almost all states, clear and explicit oral statements are legally and ethically sufficient for decisions about withholding or withdrawing medical interventions.

TABLE 2-3 DEFINITIONS OF ASSISTED SUICIDE AND EUTHANASIA

TERM	DEFINITION
Voluntary active euthanasia	Intentional administration of medications or other interventions to cause the patient's death with the patient's informed consent
Involuntary active euthanasia	Intentional administration of medications or other interventions to cause the patient's death when the patient was competent to consent but did not (e.g., the patient may not have been asked)
Nonvoluntary active euthanasia	Intentional administration of medications or other interventions to cause the patient's death when the patient was incompetent and was mentally incapable of consenting (e.g., the patient might have been in a coma)
Passive euthanasia	Withholding or withdrawal of life-sustaining medical treatments from a patient to let him or her die (termination of life-sustaining treatments)
Indirect euthanasia	Administration of narcotics or other medications to relieve pain with the incidental consequence of causing sufficient respiratory depression to result in the patient's death
Physician-assisted suicide	A physician provides medications or other interventions to a patient with the understanding that the patient can use them to commit suicide

physicians can invoke futility either to transfer a patient or to terminate interventions. However, the principle of futility is not easy to implement in medical practice. Initially, some commentators advocated that an intervention was futile when the probability of success was 1% or lower. Although this threshold seems to be based on empirical data, it is a covert value judgment. Because the declaration of futility is meant to justify unilateral determinations by physicians, it generally has been viewed as an inappropriate assertion that undermines physician-patient communication and violates the principle of shared decision making. Similar to the distinction between ordinary and extraordinary, futility is viewed increasingly as more obfuscating than clarifying, and it is being invoked much less often.

ASSISTED SUICIDE AND EUTHANASIA

History

Since Hippocrates, euthanasia and physician-assisted suicide have been controversial issues. In 1905, a bill was introduced into the Ohio legislature to legalize euthanasia; it was defeated. In the mid-1930s, similar bills were introduced and defeated in the British Parliament and the Nebraska legislature. As of 2010, physician-assisted suicide is legal in Oregon and Washington State, based on state-wide public referenda, and euthanasia and physician-assisted suicide are legal in the Netherlands, Belgium, Luxembourg, and Switzerland. Recently, the Montana Supreme Court did not recognize a constitutional right to physician-assisted suicide, but it ruled that the law permitting the termination of life-sustaining treatment protected physicians from prosecution if they helped hasten the death of a consenting, rational, terminally ill patient.

Definition and Justification

The terms *euthanasia* and *physician-assisted suicide* require careful definition (Table 2-3). So-called passive and indirect euthanasia are misnomers and are not instances of euthanasia, and both are deemed ethical and legal.

There are four arguments against permitting euthanasia and physician-assisted suicide. First, Kant and Mill thought that autonomy did not permit the voluntary ending of the conditions necessary for autonomy, and as a result, both philosophers were against voluntary enslavement and suicide. Consequently, the exercise of autonomy cannot include the ending of life because that would mean ending the possibility of exercising autonomy. Second, many dying patients may have pain and suffering because they are not receiving appropriate care, and it is possible that adequate care would relieve much pain and suffering (Chapter 3). Although a few patients still may experience uncontrolled pain and suffering despite optimal end-of-life care, it is unwise to use the condition of these few patients as a justification to permit euthanasia or physician-assisted suicide for any dying patient. Third, there is a clear distinction between intentional ending of a life and termination of life-sustaining treatments. The actual acts are different—injecting a life-ending medication, such as a muscle relaxant, or providing a prescription for one is not the same as removing or refraining from introducing an invasive medical intervention. Finally, adverse consequences of permitting euthanasia and physician-assisted suicide must be considered. There are disturbing reports of involuntary euthanasia in the Netherlands, and many worry about coercion of expensive or burdensome patients to accept euthanasia or physician-assisted suicide. Permitting euthanasia and physician-assisted suicide is likely to lead to further intrusions of lawyers, courts, and legislatures into the physician-patient relationship.

There are four parallel arguments for permitting euthanasia and physician-assisted suicide. First, it is argued that autonomy justifies euthanasia and physician-assisted suicide. To respect autonomy requires permitting individuals to decide when it is better to end their lives by euthanasia or physician-assisted suicide. Second, beneficence—furthering the well-being of individuals—supports permitting euthanasia and physician-assisted suicide. In some cases, living can create more pain and suffering than death; ending a painful life relieves more suffering and produces more good. Just the reassurance of having the option of euthanasia or physician-assisted suicide, even if people do not use it, can provide "psychological insurance" and be beneficial to people. Third, euthanasia and physician-assisted suicide are no different from termination of life-sustaining treatments that are recognized as ethically justified. In both cases, the patient consents to die; in both cases, the physician intends to end the patient's life and takes some action to end the patient's life; and in both cases, the final result is the same: the patient's death. With no difference in the patient's consent, the physician's intention, or the final result, there can be no difference in the ethical justification. Fourth, the supposed slippery slope that would result from permitting euthanasia and physician-assisted suicide is not likely. The idea that permitting euthanasia and physician-assisted suicide would undermine the physician-patient relationship or lead to forced euthanasia is completely speculative and not borne out by the available data.

In its 1997 decisions, the U.S. Supreme Court stated that there is no constitutional right to euthanasia and physician-assisted suicide but that there also is no constitutional prohibition against states legalizing these interventions. Consequently, the legalization of physician-assisted suicide in Oregon and Washington State was constitutional.

Empirical Data

Attitudes and practices related to euthanasia and physician-assisted suicide have been studied extensively. First, surveys indicate that about 60 to 70% of the American and British public support legalizing euthanasia and physician-assisted suicide for terminally ill patients who are suffering intractable pain. However, public support declines significantly for euthanasia and physician-assisted suicide in other circumstances. American and British physicians, however, are much less likely to support euthanasia and physician-assisted suicide, with oncologists, palliative care physicians, and geriatricians among the least supportive. Second, approximately 18 to 25% of American physicians have received requests for euthanasia or physician-assisted suicide; 43 to 63% of oncologists have received requests. Third, multiple studies indicate that less than 5% of American physicians have performed euthanasia or physician-assisted suicide. Among oncologists, 4% have performed euthanasia and 11% have performed physician-assisted suicide during their careers. Fourth, in many cases, the safeguards are violated. One study found that in 54% of euthanasia cases, it was the family who made the request; in 39% of euthanasia and 19% of physician-assisted suicide cases, the patient was depressed; in only half of the cases was the request repeated.

In the Netherlands and Belgium, where euthanasia and physician-assisted suicide are legal, less than 2% of all deaths are by these measures, with 0.4 to 1.8% of all deaths as the result of euthanasia without the patient's consent. In Oregon, about 0.2% of all deaths are by physician-assisted suicide.

Counterintuitively, data indicate that it is not pain that primarily motivates requests for euthanasia or physician-assisted suicide but rather psychological distress, especially depression and hopelessness. Interviews with physicians and with patients with amyotrophic lateral sclerosis, cancer, or infection with human immunodeficiency virus show that pain is not associated with interest in euthanasia or physician-assisted suicide; instead, depression and hopelessness are the strongest predictors of interest. Studies of patients in Australia and the Netherlands confirm the importance of depression in motivating requests for euthanasia. The desire to avoid dependence and loss of dignity are key motivations.

Finally, data from the Netherlands and the United States suggest that there are significant problems in performing euthanasia and physician-assisted suicide. Dutch researchers reported that physician-assisted suicide causes complications in 7% of cases, and in 15% of cases, the patients did not die, awoke from coma, or vomited up the medication. Ultimately, in nearly 20% of physician-assisted suicide cases, the physician ended up injecting the patient with life-ending medication, converting physician-assisted suicide to euthanasia. These data raise serious questions about how to address complications of physician-assisted suicide when euthanasia is illegal or unacceptable.

Practical Considerations

There is widespread agreement that if euthanasia and physician-assisted suicide are used, they should be considered only after all attempts at physical and psychological palliation have failed. A series of safeguards have been developed and embodied in the Oregon and the Dutch procedures, as follows: (1) the patient must be competent and must request euthanasia or physician-assisted suicide repeatedly and voluntarily; (2) the patient must have pain or other suffering that cannot be relieved by optimal palliative interventions; (3) there should be a waiting period to ensure that the patient's desire for euthanasia or physician-assisted suicide is stable and sincere; and (4) the physician should obtain a second opinion from an independent physician. Oregon and Washington State require patients to be terminally ill, whereas the Netherlands, Belgium, and Switzerland have no such requirement. Although there have been some prosecutions in the United States, there have been no convictions—except for Dr. Kevorkian—when physicians and others have participated in euthanasia and physician-assisted suicide.

FINANCIAL CONFLICTS OF INTEREST

History

Worrying about how payment and fees affect medical decisions is not new. In 1899, a physician reported that more than 60% of surgeons in Chicago were willing to provide a 50% commission to physicians for referring cases. He subsequently argued that in some cases, this fee splitting led to unnecessary surgical procedures. A 1912 study by the American Medical Association confirmed that fee splitting was a common practice. Selling patent medicines and patenting surgical instruments were other forms of financial conflicts of interest thought to discredit physicians a century ago. In the 1990s, the ethics of capitation for physician services and pharmaceutical prescriptions and payments by pharmaceutical and biotechnology companies to clinical researchers raised the issue of financial conflicts of interest.

Definition and Justification

It commonly is argued that physicians have certain primary interests: (1) to promote the well-being of their patients, (2) to advance biomedical research, (3) to educate future physicians, and, more controversially, (4) to promote public health (Table 2-4). Physicians also have other, secondary interests, such as earning income, raising a family, and pursuing avocational interests. These secondary interests are not evil; typically, they are legitimate, even admirable. A conflict of interest occurs when one of these secondary interests compromises pursuit of a primary interest, especially the patient's well-being.

Conflicts of interest are problematic because they can or appear to compromise the integrity of physicians' judgment, compromising the patient's well-being or research integrity. Conflict of interest can induce a physician to do something—perform a procedure, fail to order a test, or distort data—that would not be in a patient's best interest. These conflicts can undermine the trust of patients and the public, not only in an individual physician but also in the entire medical profession. The appearance of conflicts of interest can be damaging because it is difficult for patients and the public "to determine what motives have influenced a professional decision." The focus is on financial conflicts of interest, not because they are worse than other types of conflicts but because they are more pervasive and more easily identified and regulated compared with other conflicts. Since ancient times, the ethical norm on conflicts has been clear: the physician's primary obligation is to patients' well-being, and a physician's personal financial well-being should not compromise this duty.

TABLE 2-4 PRIMARY INTERESTS OF PHYSICIANS

Promotion of the health and well-being of their patients
Advancement of biomedical knowledge through research
Education of future physicians and health care providers
Promotion of the public health

Empirical Data

Financial conflicts are not rare. In Florida, it was estimated that nearly 40% of physicians were involved as owners of freestanding facilities to which they referred patients. Studies in the early 1990s consistently showed that self-referring physicians ordered more services, frequently charged more per service, and referred patients with less established indications. In one study, 4 to 4.5 times more imaging examinations were ordered by self-referring physicians than by physicians who referred patients to radiologists. Similarly, patients referred to joint-venture physical therapy facilities have an average of 16 visits compared with 11 at non–joint-venture facilities. Of great concern, licensed physical therapists at joint-venture facilities spent about 28 minutes per patient per visit compared with 48 minutes at non–joint-venture facilities. There are no comparable data on the influence of capitation on physicians' judgment.

Similarly, multiple studies have shown that interaction with pharmaceutical representatives can lead to prescribing of new drugs, nonrational prescribing, and decreased use of generic drugs by physicians. Industry funding for continuing medical education payment for travel to educational symposia increases prescribing of the sponsor's drug.

Regarding researcher conflicts of interest, the available data suggest that corporate funding does not compromise the design and methodology of clinical research; in fact, commercially funded research may be methodologically more rigorous than government- or foundation-supported research. Conversely, data suggest that financial interests do distort researchers' interpretation of data. The most important impact of financial interests, however, appears to be on dissemination of research studies. Growing evidence suggests the suppression or selective publication of data unfavorable to corporate sponsors but the repeated publication of favorable results.

Practical Considerations

First, financial conflicts of interest are inherent in any profession when the professional earns income from rendering a service. Second, conflicts come in many different forms, from legitimate payment for services rendered to investments in medical laboratories and facilities, drug company dinners and payment for attendance at meetings, payment for enrolling patients in clinical research trials, and consultation with companies.

Third, in considering how to manage conflicts, it is important to note that people are poor judges of their own potential conflicts. Individuals often cannot distinguish the various influences that guide their judgments, do not think of themselves as bad, and do not imagine that payment shapes their judgments. Physicians tend to be defensive about charges of conflicts of interest. In addition, conflicts tend to act insidiously, subtly changing practice patterns so that they then become what appear to be justifiable norms.

Fourth, rules—whether laws, regulations, or professional standards—to regulate conflicts of interest are based on two considerations: (1) the likelihood that payment or other secondary interests would create a conflict and (2) the magnitude of the potential harm if there is compromised judgment. Rules tend to be of three types: (1) disclosure of conflicts, (2) management of conflicts, and (3) outright prohibition. Federal law bans certain types of self-referral of physicians in the Medicare program. The American Medical Association and the Pharmaceutical Research and Manufacturers of America have established joint rules that permit physicians to accept gifts of minimal value but "refuse substantial gifts from drug companies, such as the costs of travel, lodging, or other personal expenses . . . for attending conferences or meetings."

Fifth, although there is much emphasis on disclosure of conflicts, which may be useful in publications, it is unclear whether this is a suitable safeguard in the clinical setting. Disclosure just may make patients worry more. Patients may have no context in which to place the disclosure or to evaluate the physician's clinical recommendation, and patients may have few other options in selecting a physician or getting care, especially in an acute situation. Furthermore, self-disclosure often is incomplete, even when required.

Finally, some conflicts can be avoided by a physician's own action. Physicians can refuse to engage in personal investments in medical facilities or to accept gifts from pharmaceutical companies at relatively little personal cost. In other circumstances, the conflicts may be institutionalized, and minimizing them can occur only by changing the way organizations structure reimbursement incentives. Capitation encourages physicians to limit medical services, and its potentially adverse effects are likely to be managed by institutional rules rather than by personal decisions.

FUTURE DIRECTIONS

In the near future, as genetics moves from the research to the clinical setting, practicing physicians are likely to encounter issues surrounding genetic testing, counseling, and treatment. The use of genetic tests without the extensive counseling so common in research studies would alter the nature of the bioethical issues. Because these tests have serious implications for the patient and others, scrupulous attention to informed consent must occur. The bioethical issues raised by genetic tests for somatic cell changes, such as tests that occur commonly in cancer diagnosis and risk stratification, are no different from the issues raised with the use of any laboratory or radiographic test.

In some cases, ethics consultation services may be of assistance in resolving bioethical dilemmas, although current data suggest that consultation services are used mainly for problems that arise in individual cases and are not used for more institutional or policy problems.

SUGGESTED READINGS

Brezis M, Wiist WH. Vulnerability of health to market forces. *Med Care*. 2011;49:232-239. *Explores the tension between capitalism and the goals of social justice and public health.*

Education in Palliative and End-of-life Care. http://www.epec.net; 2010. Accessed March 27, 2011. *Frequently updated website.*

Okike K, Kocher MS, Wei EX, et al. Accuracy of conflict-of-interest disclosures reported by physicians. *N Engl J Med*. 2009;361:1466-1474. *Self-disclosure often is remarkably incomplete.*

Partnership for Caring. http://www.partnershipforcaring.org; 2010. Accessed March 27, 2011. *Frequently updated website.*

3

CARE OF DYING PATIENTS AND THEIR FAMILIES

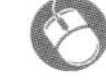

ROBERT ARNOLD

By 2030, 20% of the U.S. population will be older than 65 years. Owing to successes in public health and medicine, many of these people will live the last years of their lives with chronic medical conditions such as cirrhosis, end-stage kidney disease, heart failure, and dementia. Even human immunodeficiency virus (HIV) and many cancers, once considered terminal, have turned into chronic diseases.

The burden associated with these illnesses is high. Patients report multiple physical and psychological symptoms that lower their quality of life. The economic pressures associated with medical care may adversely affect patients' socioeconomic status and cause family stress. In addition, these chronic illnesses are incurable and often will ultimately contribute to or result in death.

The discipline of palliative care was developed to decrease the burden associated with chronic illness. The recent National Consensus Project defines palliative care as follows:

> *The goal of palliative care is to prevent and relieve suffering and to support the best possible quality of life for patients and their families. Palliative care is operationalized through effective management of pain and other distressing symptoms, while incorporating psychosocial and spiritual care with consideration of family and patient needs, preferences, values, beliefs, and culture .... Palliative care affirms life by supporting the patient and family's goals for the future, including their hopes for cure or life-prolongation, as well as their hopes for peace and dignity throughout the course of illness, the dying process, and death.*

Four points deserve special emphasis. First, palliative care can be delivered at any time during the course of an illness and is often provided concomitantly with disease-focused, life-prolonging therapy. Waiting until a patient is dying to provide palliative care is a serious error. Prognostication is an inexact science. In addition, although most elderly patients with chronic incurable illnesses are in the last 10 years of their lives, they do not consider themselves to be dying. If palliative care is to have an impact on patients' lives, it should be provided earlier in a patient's illness, in tandem with other treatments.

Second, palliative care primarily focuses on the illness's burden rather than treating the illness itself. Because these burdens can be physical, psychological, spiritual, or social, good palliative care requires a multidisciplinary approach.

Third, palliative care takes the family unit as the central focus of care. Treatment plans must be developed for both the patient and the family.

Finally, palliative care recognizes that medical treatments are not uniformly successful and that patients die. At some point in a patient's illness, the treatments may cause more burden than benefit. Palliative care recognizes this reality and starts with a discussion of the patient's goals and the development of an individualized treatment plan.

Many people confuse palliative care with hospice—an understandable confusion because hospices epitomize the palliative care philosophy. The two, however, are different. In the United States, hospice provides palliative care, primarily at home, for patients who have a life expectancy of 6 months or less and who are willing to forgo life-prolonging treatments. However, the requirement that patients must have a life expectancy of less than 6 months limits hospice's availability because this degree of prognostication is difficult to achieve for many diseases. Moreover, doctors and patients often are unwilling to cease potentially life-prolonging treatments until very late in the disease course, and thus, most patients are not enrolled in hospice until a month before death.

Palliative care, both as a philosophy of care and as a subspecialty, now includes training of medical students and residents. Although every physician should have basic knowledge about palliative care, the creation of the new subspecialty of palliative medicine allows for a growing number of physicians capable of helping with difficult patient issues, educating other physicians, and expanding the knowledge base of palliative care.

PALLIATIVE CARE DOMAINS

Palliative care is a holistic discipline with physical, psychological, spiritual, existential, social, and ethical domains. When caring for patients with chronic life-limiting illness, good palliative care requires that the following questions be addressed:

Is the Patient Physically Comfortable?

Across many chronic conditions, patients have a large number of inadequately treated physical symptoms (Table 3-1). The reasons are multifactorial and range from inadequate physician education, to societal beliefs regarding the inevitability of suffering in chronic illness, to public concerns regarding opioids.

The first step to improve symptom management is a thorough assessment. Standardized instruments such as the Brief Pain Inventory (Fig. 3-1) measure both patients' symptoms and their effect on their lives. Use of standardized instruments assures that physicians will identify overlooked or underreported symptoms and, as a result, will enhance the satisfaction of both the patient and family.

The evidence for the treatment of end-stage symptoms continues to improve. Physicians now can use proven therapies to manage pain (Chapter 29), dyspnea (Chapters 50 and 83), and depression (Chapter 404). The use of nonsteroidal anti-inflammatory agents and opioids can result in effective pain management in more than 75% of patients with cancer.■ Advances such as intrathecal pumps and neurolytic blocks are helpful in the remaining 25%. Opioids are effective in patients with unrelieved dyspnea, and oxygen is helpful for short-term relief of hypoxemia.■ Depression can be treated effectively with medications and psychotherapy.■

Is the Patient Psychologically Suffering?

Patients may be physically comfortable but still suffering. Psychological symptoms and syndromes such as depression, delirium, and anxiety are common in patients with life-limiting or chronic illnesses. It may be difficult

TABLE 3-1 APPROACHES TO THE MANAGEMENT OF PHYSICAL AND PSYCHOLOGICAL SYMPTOMS

SYMPTOM	ASSESSMENT	TREATMENT
Pain	How severe is the symptom (as assessed with the use of validated instruments) and how does it interfere with the patient's life? What is the etiology of the pain? Is the pain assumed to be neuropathic or somatic? What has the patient used in the past (calculate previous days' equal analgesic dose)?	Prescribe medications to be administered on a standing or regular basis if pain is frequent. For mild pain: use acetaminophen or a nonsteroidal anti-inflammatory agent (see Table 29-3 in Chapter 29). For moderate pain: titrate short-acting opioids (see Table 29-4 in Chapter 29). For severe pain: rapidly titrate short-acting opioids until pain is relieved or intolerable side effects develop; start long-acting opiates once pain is controlled. Rescue doses: prescribe immediate-release opioids—10% of the 24-hour total opiate every hour (orally) or every 30 minutes (parenterally) as needed. Concomitant analgesics (e.g., corticosteroids, anticonvulsants, tricyclic antidepressants, and bisphosphonates) should be used when applicable (particularly for neuropathic pain). Consider alternative medicine and interventional treatments for pain.
Constipation	Is the patient taking opioids? Does the patient have a fecal impaction?	Prescribe laxatives for all patients on opiates. If ineffective, add drugs from multiple classes (e.g., stimulant, osmotic laxatives, and enemas). Prescribe methylnaltrexone if still constipated.
Shortness of breath	Ask the patient to assess the severity of the shortness of breath. Does the symptom have reversible causes?	Prescribe oxygen to treat hypoxia-induced dyspnea, *but* not if the patient is not hypoxic. Opioids relieve breathlessness without measurable reductions in respiratory rate or oxygen saturation; effective doses are often lower than those used to treat pain. Aerosolized opiates do not work. Fans or cool air may work through a branch of the trigeminal nerve. Consider anxiolytics (e.g., low-dose benzodiazepines) and use reassurance, relaxation, distraction, and massage therapy.
Fatigue	Is the patient too tired to do activities of daily living? Is the fatigue secondary to depression? Is a disease process causing the symptom or is it secondary to reversible causes?	Provide cognitive education about conserving energy use. Treat underlying conditions appropriately.
Nausea	Which mechanism is causing the symptom (e.g., stimulation of the chemoreceptor trigger zone, gastric stimulation, delayed gastric emptying or "squashed stomach" syndrome, bowel obstruction, intracranial processes, or vestibular vertigo)? Is the patient constipated?	Prescribe an agent directed at the underlying cause (Chapter 134). If persistent, give antiemetic around the clock. Multiple agents directed at various receptors or mechanisms may be required.
Anorexia and cachexia	Is a disease process causing the symptom, or is it secondary to other symptoms (e.g., nausea and constipation) that can be treated? Is the patient troubled by the symptom or is the family worried about what not eating means?	A nutritionist may help find foods that are more appetizing (Chapter 220). Provide counseling about the prognostic implications of anorexia (Chapter 226).
Delirium	Is the confusion acute, over hours to days? Does consciousness wax and wane? Are there behavioral disturbances, marked by a reduced clarity in the patient's awareness of his environment, e.g., a problem of attention? Does the patient have disorganized thinking? Does the patient have an altered level of consciousness—either agitated or drowsy? Is there a reversible reason for the delirium? **D:** Drugs (opioids, anticholinergics, sedatives, benzodiazepines, steroids, chemotherapies and immunotherapies, some antibiotics) **E:** Eyes and ears (poor vision and hearing, isolation) **L:** Low-flow states (hypoxia, MI, CHF, COPD, shock) **I:** Infections **R:** Retention (urine/stool), Restraints **I:** Intracranial (CNS metastases, seizures, subdural, CVA, hypertensive encephalopathy) **U:** Underhydration, Undernutrition, Undersleep **M:** Metabolic disorders (sodium, glucose, thyroid, hepatic, deficiencies of vitamin B_{12}, folate, niacin, and thiamine) and toxic (lead, manganese, mercury, alcohol)	Identify underlying causes and manage symptoms (Chapter 27). Recommend behavioral therapies, including avoidance of excess stimulation, frequent reorientation, and reassurance. Ensure presence of family caregivers and explain delirium to them. Prescribe haloperidol, risperidone, or olanzapine.
Depression	Are you feeling down, depressed, or hopeless most of the time over the last 2 weeks? Do you find that little brings you pleasure or joy over the last 2 weeks? (Somatic symptoms are not reliable indicators of depression in this population.)	Recommend supportive psychotherapy, cognitive approaches, behavioral techniques, pharmacologic therapies (see Table 404-5 in Chapter 404), or a combination of these interventions; prescribe psychostimulants for rapid treatment of symptoms (within days) or selective serotonin reuptake inhibitors, which may require 3 to 4 weeks to take effect; tricyclic antidepressants are relatively contraindicated because of their side effects.
Anxiety (applicable also for family members)	Does the patient exhibit restlessness, agitation, insomnia, hyperventilation, tachycardia, or excessive worry? Is the patient depressed? Is there a spiritual or existential concern underlying the anxiety?	Recommend supportive counseling and consider prescribing benzodiazepines.
Spiritual distress	Are you at peace?	Inquire about spiritual support.

Modified from Morrison RS, Meier DE. Palliative care. *N Engl J Med.* 2004;350:2582-2590.

STUDY ID# ______________ HOSPITAL ID# ______________

DO NOT WRITE ABOVE THIS LINE

Brief Pain Inventory (Short Form)

Date: ____/____/____ Time: _____

Name: ____________________ ____________________ ____________________
Last First Middle Initial

1. Throughout our lives, most of us have had pain from time to time (such as minor headaches, sprains, and toothaches). Have you had pain other than these everyday kinds of pain today?

1. Yes 2. No

2. On the diagram, shade in the areas where you feel pain. Put an X on the area that hurts the most.

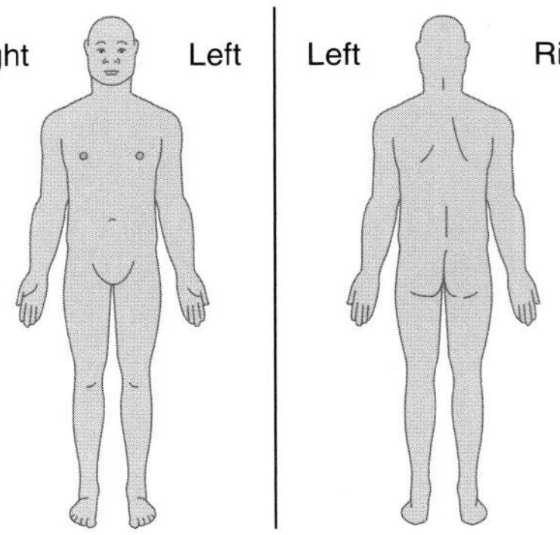

Right Left | Left Right

3. Please rate your pain by circling the one number that best describes your pain at its **worst** in the last 24 hours.

0 No pain 1 2 3 4 5 6 7 8 9 10 Pain as bad as you can imagine

4. Please rate your pain by circling the one number that best describes your pain at its **least** in the last 24 hours.

0 No pain 1 2 3 4 5 6 7 8 9 10 Pain as bad as you can imagine

5. Please rate your pain by circling the one number that best describes your pain on the **average.**

0 No pain 1 2 3 4 5 6 7 8 9 10 Pain as bad as you can imagine

6. Please rate your pain by circling the one number that tells how much pain you have **right now.**

0 No pain 1 2 3 4 5 6 7 8 9 10 Pain as bad as you can imagine

FIGURE 3-1. Brief Pain Inventory (short form). (Copyright 1991. Charles S. Cleeland, PhD, Pain Research Group. All rights reserved.)

Continued

to determine whether increased morbidity and mortality are caused by the illness's physical effects or by the psychological effects of depression and anxiety on energy, appetite, or sleep. Screening questions focusing on mood (e.g., "Have you felt down, depressed, and hopeless most of the time for the last 2 weeks?") and anhedonism (e.g., "Have you found little brings you pleasure or joy in the last 2 weeks?") have been shown to help in diagnosing depression in this population.

For patients and families facing mortality, existential and spiritual concerns are common. Progressive illness often raises questions of love, legacy, loss, and meaning. A physician's role is not to answer these questions or to provide reassurance, but rather to understand the patient's concerns, how the patient is coping, and what resources might be of help. Spirituality often is a source of comfort, and physicians can screen regarding a patient's beliefs using a brief instrument such as the FICA spiritual assessment tool (Table 3-2). A single

7. What treatments or medications are you receiving for your pain?

____

8. In the last 24 hours, how much relief have pain treatments or medications provided? Please circle the one percentage that most shows how much relief you have received.

0% No pain	10%	20%	30%	40%	50%	60%	70%	80%	90%	100% Complete relief

9. Circle one number that describes how, during the past 24 hours, pain has interfered with your:

A. General Activity

0 Does not interfere	1	2	3	4	5	6	7	8	9	10 Completely interferes

B. Mood

0 Does not interfere	1	2	3	4	5	6	7	8	9	10 Completely interferes

C. Walking Ability

0 Does not interfere	1	2	3	4	5	6	7	8	9	10 Completely interferes

D. Normal Work (includes both work outside the home and housework)

0 Does not interfere	1	2	3	4	5	6	7	8	9	10 Completely interferes

E. Relations with Other People

0 Does not interfere	1	2	3	4	5	6	7	8	9	10 Completely interferes

F. Sleep

0 Does not interfere	1	2	3	4	5	6	7	8	9	10 Completely interferes

G. Enjoyment of Life

0 Does not interfere	1	2	3	4	5	6	7	8	9	10 Completely interferes

FIGURE 3-1, cont'd.

screening question, such as "Are you at peace?," may identify patients who are in spiritual distress and facilitate referrals to hospital chaplains.

Is the Family Suffering?

Families are an important source of support for most patients. Families provide informal care-giving, often at the expense of their own physical, economic, and psychological health. Good palliative care requires an understanding of how the family is coping and a search for ways to provide family members with the social or clinical resources they need to improve their well-being. Comprehensive and individually targeted interventions can reduce caregivers' burdens, although the absolute benefits are relatively small.[1]

Because patients in palliative care often die, the palliative care team must address bereavement. A letter of condolence or a follow-up phone call to the next of kin after a patient's death is respectful and offers the opportunity to clarify questions about the patient's care. Some family members suffer from complicated grief—a recently described syndrome associated with separation and traumatic distress, with symptoms persisting for more than 6 months. Primary care physicians, who have ongoing relationships with the loved one, and hospices, which provide bereavement services for a year after the patient's death, have the opportunity to assess whether the grief symptoms persist or worsen.

Is the Patient's Care Consistent with the Patient's Goals?

The sine qua non for palliative care is ensuring that the treatment plan is consistent with the patient's values. Most elderly, seriously ill patients are not focused on living as long as possible. Instead, they want to maintain a sense

TABLE 3-2 FICA SPIRITUAL ASSESSMENT TOOL

F—What is your **faith**/religion? Do you consider yourself a religious or spiritual person? What do you believe in that gives meaning/importance to life?
I—**Importance** and **influence** of faith. Is your faith/religion important to you? How do your beliefs influence how you take care of yourself? What are your most important hopes? What role do your beliefs play in regaining your health? What makes life most worth living for you? How might your disease affect this?
C—Are you part of a religious or spiritual **community**? Is this of support to you, and how? Is there a person you really love or is very important to you? How is your family handling your illness? What are their reactions/expectations?
A—How would you like me to **address** these issues in your health care? What might be left undone if you were to die today? Given the severity or chronicity of your illness, what is most important for you to achieve? Would you like me to talk to someone about religious/spiritual matters?

From Puchalski C, Romer A. Taking a spiritual history. *J Palliat Med.* 2000;3:129-137.

of control, relieve their symptoms, improve their quality of life, avoid being a burden on their families, and have a closer relationship with their loved ones.

Ensuring that treatment is consistent with a patient's goals requires good communication skills (Table 3-3). The approaches to giving bad news, discussing goals of care, and talking about forgoing life-sustaining treatment have similar structures (Fig. 3-2). First, the patient needs to understand the basic facts about the diagnosis, possible treatments, and prognosis. The communication skill that helps physicians communicate information is *Ask-Tell-Ask*—exploring what the patient knows or wants to know, then explaining or answering questions, and then providing an opportunity for the patient to ask more. In the hospital, where discontinuity of care is common and misunderstandings frequent, it is important to determine what the patient knows before providing information so as to keep everyone well coordinated. When giving bad news, knowing what the patient knows allows the physician to anticipate the patient's reaction. Finally, information must be titrated based on the patient's preferences. Although most patients want to hear everything about their disease, a minority do not. There is no foolproof way to ascertain what any patient wants to know other than by asking.

When giving patients information, it is important to give small pieces of information, not use jargon, and check the patient's understanding. Giving information is like dosing a medication: one gives information, checks understanding, and then gives more information based on what the patient has heard.

After ensuring that the doctor and the patient have a shared understanding of the medical facts, the physician should engage in an open-ended conversation about the patient's goals as the disease progresses. This strategy requires that the patient be asked about both hopes and fears. One might ask: "What makes life worth living for you?" "If your time is limited, what are the things that are most important to achieve?" "What are your biggest fears or concerns?" "What would you consider to be a fate worse than death?" The clinician can use an understanding of these goals to make recommendations about which treatments to provide and which treatments would not be helpful. As a result, early palliative care can improve quality of life, mood, and even survival.[2]

Physicians find talking about prognosis particularly difficult for two reasons: first, it is hard to foretell the future accurately; and second, they fear this information will "take away patients' hope." Thus, they often avoid talking to patients about these issues unless specifically asked. Although some patients do not want to hear prognostic information, for many patients, this information helps them plan their lives. Given that one cannot guess how much information to provide, a physician can start these conversations by asking, "Are you the kind of person who wants to hear about what might happen in the future with your illness or would you rather take it day by day?" If the patient requests the latter, the physician can follow up by asking if there is someone else with whom he or she can talk about the prognosis. Second, before giving prognostic information, it is useful to inquire about the patient's concerns in order to provide information in the most useful manner. Finally, it is appropriate when discussing prognostic information to acknowledge uncertainty: "The course of this cancer can be quite unpredictable, and physicians don't have a crystal ball. I think you should be aware of the possibility that your health may deteriorate quickly, and you should plan accordingly. We probably are dealing with weeks to months, although some patients do better, and some do worse. Over time, the course may become clearer, and if you wish, I may be able to be a little more precise about what we are facing."

TABLE 3-3 CORE COMMUNICATION SKILLS

RECOMMENDED SKILL	EXAMPLE
A. IDENTIFYING CONCERNS AND RECOGNIZING CUES	
Elicit Concerns	
Open-ended questions	"Is there anything you wanted to talk to me about today?"
Active listening	Allowing patient to speak without interruption; allowing pauses to encourage patient to speak
Recognize Cues	
Informational concerns	Patient: "I'm not sure about the treatment options"
Emotional concerns	Patient: "I'm worried about that"
B. RESPONDING TO INFORMATIONAL CONCERNS	
"Ask-tell-ask"	Topic: communicating information about cancer stage
Ask	"Have any of the other doctors talked about what stage this cancer is?"
Tell	"That's right, this is a stage IV cancer, which is also called metastatic cancer…."
Ask	"Do you have questions about the staging?"
C. RESPONDING TO EMOTIONAL CONCERNS	
Nonverbal Empathy: S-O-L-E-R	
S	Face the patient **S**quarely
O	Adopt an **O**pen body posture
L	**L**ean toward the patient
E	Use **E**ye contact
R	Maintain a **R**elaxed body posture
Verbal Empathy: N-U-R-S-E	
N	**N**ame the emotion: "You seem worried"
U	**U**nderstand the emotion: "I see why you are concerned about this"
R	**R**espect the emotion: "You have shown a lot of strength"
S	**S**upport the patient: "I want you to know that I will still be your doctor whether you have chemotherapy or not"
E	**E**xplore the emotion: "Tell me more about what is worrying you"

From Back AL, Arnold RM, Tulsky JA. *Discussing Prognosis.* Alexandria, VA: American Society of Clinical Oncology; 2008.

The physician must discuss these topics in an empathic way. Palliative care conversations are as much about emotions as facts. Talking about disease progression or death may elicit negative emotions such as anxiety, sadness, or frustration. These emotions decrease a patient's quality of life and interfere with the ability to hear factual information. Empathic responses strengthen the patient-physician relationship, increase the patient's satisfaction, and make the patient more likely to disclose other concerns. The first step is recognizing when the patient is expressing emotions. Once the physician recognizes the emotion being expressed, he or she can respond empathically.

It is also important for physicians to recognize their own emotional reactions to these conversations. The physician's emotional reactions color impressions of the patient's prognosis, thereby making it hard to listen to the patient, and may influence the physician to hedge bad news. The physician should become aware of her or his own emotional reactions to ensure that the conversation focuses on the patient rather than the health care provider's needs.

In addition to good communication skills, palliative care requires a basic knowledge of medical ethics and the law. For example, patients have the moral and legal right to refuse any treatment, even if refusal results in their death. There is no legal difference between withholding and withdrawing life-sustaining treatment. When confronted with areas of ambiguity, the physician should know how to obtain either a palliative care or ethics consultation.

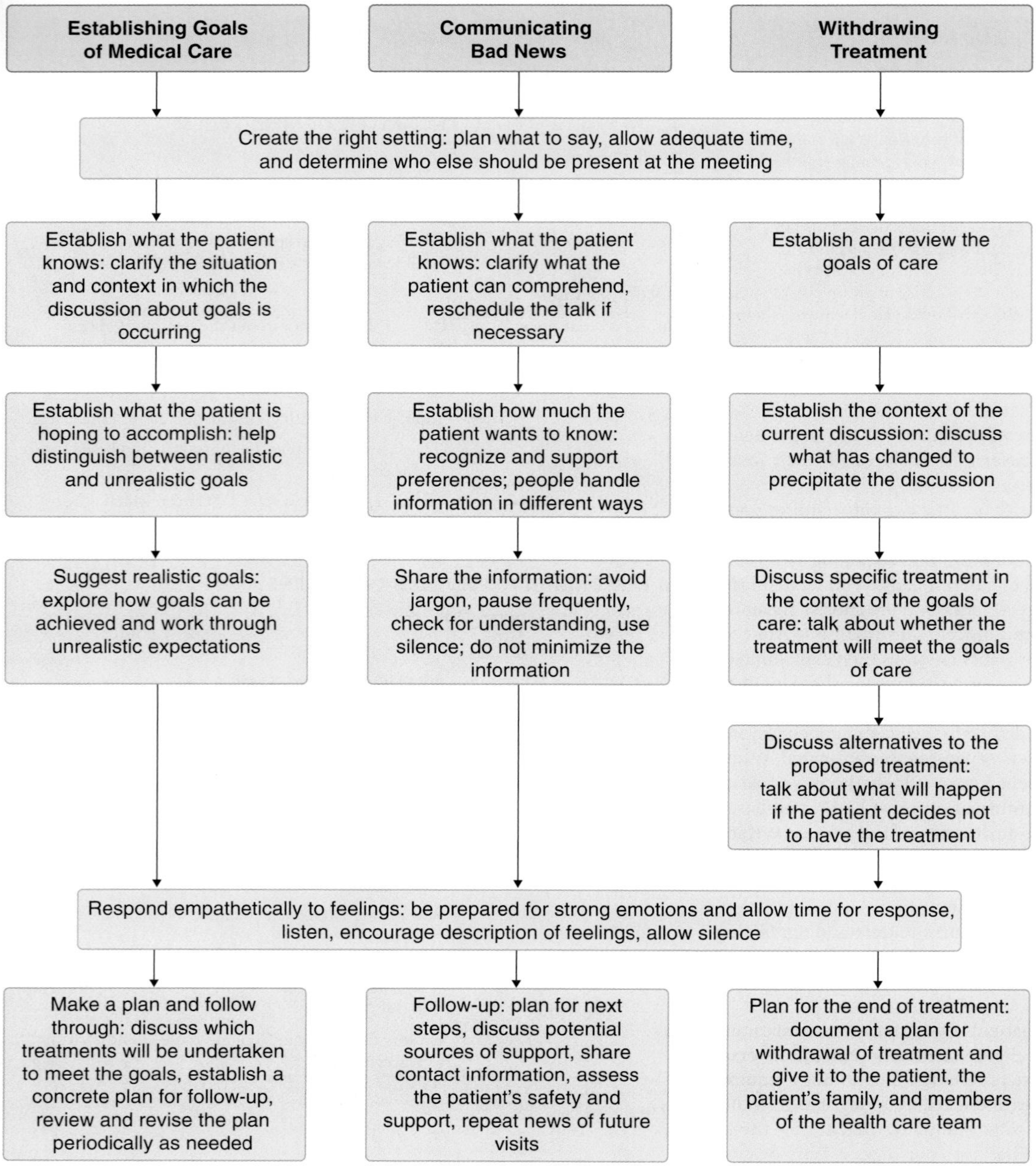

Establishing Goals of Medical Care | **Communicating Bad News** | **Withdrawing Treatment**

Create the right setting: plan what to say, allow adequate time, and determine who else should be present at the meeting

Establishing Goals of Medical Care

- Establish what the patient knows: clarify the situation and context in which the discussion about goals is occurring
- Establish what the patient is hoping to accomplish: help distinguish between realistic and unrealistic goals
- Suggest realistic goals: explore how goals can be achieved and work through unrealistic expectations

Communicating Bad News

- Establish what the patient knows: clarify what the patient can comprehend, reschedule the talk if necessary
- Establish how much the patient wants to know: recognize and support preferences; people handle information in different ways
- Share the information: avoid jargon, pause frequently, check for understanding, use silence; do not minimize the information

Withdrawing Treatment

- Establish and review the goals of care
- Establish the context of the current discussion: discuss what has changed to precipitate the discussion
- Discuss specific treatment in the context of the goals of care: talk about whether the treatment will meet the goals of care
- Discuss alternatives to the proposed treatment: talk about what will happen if the patient decides not to have the treatment

Respond empathetically to feelings: be prepared for strong emotions and allow time for response, listen, encourage description of feelings, allow silence

- **Establishing Goals of Medical Care:** Make a plan and follow through: discuss which treatments will be undertaken to meet the goals, establish a concrete plan for follow-up, review and revise the plan periodically as needed
- **Communicating Bad News:** Follow-up: plan for next steps, discuss potential sources of support, share contact information, assess the patient's safety and support, repeat news of future visits
- **Withdrawing Treatment:** Plan for the end of treatment: document a plan for withdrawal of treatment and give it to the patient, the patient's family, and members of the health care team

FIGURE 3-2. A model for discussing different palliative care topics. Protocols for Communicating with Patients about Major Topics in Palliative Care. (Adapted from the EPEC Project: Education on Palliative and End-of-Life Care. Cited in Morrison, RS, Meier DE. Palliative care. *N Engl J Med.* 2004; 350:2582-2590; accessed January 4, 2010 from http://www.epec.net.)

During the past 10 years, there has been a societal push to encourage patients to designate health care proxies and to create advance care planning documents, typified by the use of living wills. These documents are meant to protect patients against unwanted treatments and to ensure that as they are dying, their wishes are followed. Unfortunately, there are few empirical data showing that these documents actually change practice. Still, discussions of the documents with health professionals and family members generally provoke important conversations about end-of-life care decisions and may help assuage the family in that they are respecting their loved one's wishes.

Is the Patient Going to Die in the Location of Choice?

Most patients say that they want to die at home. Unfortunately, most patients die in institutions—either hospitals or nursing homes. Good palliative care requires establishing a regular system of communication to minimize transitional errors. A social worker who knows about community resources is important in the development of a dispositional plan that respects the patient's goals.

Hospice programs are an important way to allow patients to die at home. In the United States, *hospice* refers to a specific, government-regulated form of end-of-life care, available under Medicare since 1982 but subsequently adopted by Medicaid and many other third-party insurers. Hospice care typically is given at home, a nursing home, or specialized acute care unit. Care is provided by an interdisciplinary team, which usually includes a physician, nurse, social worker, chaplain, volunteers, bereavement coordinator, and home health aides, all of whom collaborate with the primary care physician, patient, and family. Bereavement services are offered to the family for a year after the death.

Hospices are paid on a per diem rate and are required to cover all the costs related to the patient's life-limiting illness. Because of this and the fact their focus is on comfort rather than life prolongation, many hospices will not cover expensive treatments such as inotropic agents in heart failure or chemotherapy in cancer, even if they have a palliative effect. This may be one of the reasons doctors are hesitant to refer patients until very late in a patient's course, and patients and families equate hospice with dying. Many hospices are experimenting with different service models in an attempt to enroll patients earlier in the course of their illness and increase access to their services.

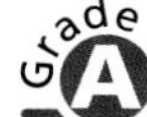

1. Lorenz KA, Lynn J, Dy SM, et al. Evidence for improving palliative care at the end of life: a systematic review. *Ann Intern Med.* 2008;148:147-159.

2. Temel JS, Greer JA, Muzikansky A, et al. Early palliative care for patients with metastatic non-small-cell lung cancer. *N Engl J Med.* 2010;363:733-742.

SUGGESTED READINGS

End of Life/Palliative Education Resource Center. http://www.eperc.mcw.edu. Accessed March 27, 2011. *Peer-reviewed instructional and evaluation materials on end-of-life care, core resources for educators, and opportunities for training and funding.*

Kane RL. Finding the right level of posthospital care: "We didn't realize there was any other option for him." *JAMA.* 2011;305:284-293. *Review.*

Pallimed. A hospice and palliative medicine blog. http://www.pallimed.org. Accessed March 27, 2011. *Reviews recent scientific articles and promotes discussion of public policy. See also http://www.eperc.mcw.edu/ for short reviews of key topics.*

Silveira MJ, Kim SY, Langa KM. Advance directives and outcomes of surrogate decision making before death. *N Engl J Med.* 2010;362:1211-1218. *Advanced directives usually result in patients' receiving desired care.*

TABLE 4-1 HEALTH INSURANCE COVERAGE AMONG ADULTS AGED 18 YEARS AND OLDER BY RACE/ETHNICITY—CALIFORNIA

RACE/ETHNICITY	CURRENTLY UNINSURED, % (95% CI)
White	9.6 (9.0-10.3)
Black	13.0 (10.9-15.5)
American Indian/Alaska Native	18.9 (14.6-24.2)
Asian American	15.0 (13.5-16.7)
Chinese	12.3 (10.1-14.7)
Filipino	11.6 (8.4-15.7)
Korean	33.6 (28.6-39.1)
South Asian	11.9 (8.0-17.4)
Vietnamese	17.9 (13.8-22.8)
Latino	28.6 (27.1-30.1)
Foreign-born	36.1 (34.1-38.0)
U.S.-born	14.3 (12.6-16.1)
Mexican	28.7 (27.1-30.3)
Central American	33.2 (28.5-38.3)
Other Latino	21.3 (17.3-26.0)

CI = confidence interval.
From Holtby S, Zahnd E, Chia YJ, et al. *Health of California's Adults, Adolescents, and Children: Findings from CHIS 2005 and CHIS 2003.* Los Angeles: UCLA Center for Health Policy Research; 2008.

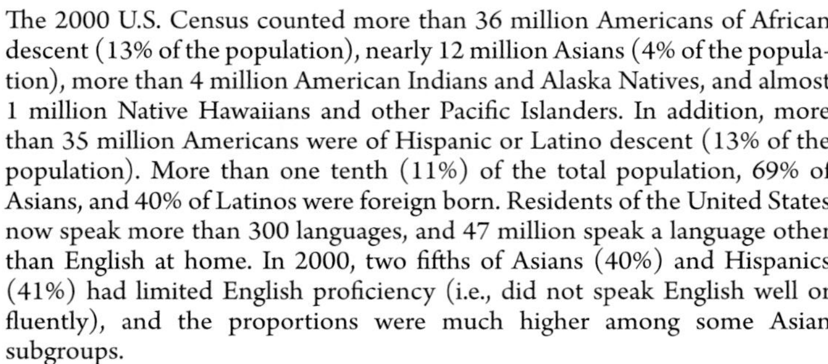

4 CULTURAL CONTEXT OF MEDICINE

VICTORIA M. TAYLOR

The 2000 U.S. Census counted more than 36 million Americans of African descent (13% of the population), nearly 12 million Asians (4% of the population), more than 4 million American Indians and Alaska Natives, and almost 1 million Native Hawaiians and other Pacific Islanders. In addition, more than 35 million Americans were of Hispanic or Latino descent (13% of the population). More than one tenth (11%) of the total population, 69% of Asians, and 40% of Latinos were foreign born. Residents of the United States now speak more than 300 languages, and 47 million speak a language other than English at home. In 2000, two fifths of Asians (40%) and Hispanics (41%) had limited English proficiency (i.e., did not speak English well or fluently), and the proportions were much higher among some Asian subgroups.

During the past two decades, a large body of literature has documented substantial disparities in health status, some based on socioeconomic status (Chapter 5), but many based on race, ethnicity, or other characteristics. For example, black men have a substantially higher age-adjusted prostate cancer incidence rate than do white men (240 per 100,000 versus 153 per 100,000). Mexican Americans and American Indians are more than twice as likely as non-Latino whites of a similar age to have diabetes. Compared with the general population, chronic hepatitis B infection is 25 to 75 times more common among Samoans and among immigrants from Cambodia, Laos, and Vietnam. Studies have documented high rates of suicidal behavior among gays and lesbians compared with heterosexuals. A major goal of Healthy People 2010 was to eliminate health differences among population subgroups for preventable and treatable conditions such as cancer, cardiovascular disease, diabetes, human immunodeficiency virus infection, and acquired immunodeficiency syndrome, among others.

Culture can be defined as a shared system of values, beliefs, and patterns of behavior, and it is not simply defined by race and ethnicity. Culture can also be shaped by factors such as country and region of origin, acculturation, language, religion, and sexual orientation. For instance, the black population of the northeastern United States includes individuals who moved from southern states decades ago as well as recent immigrants from Ethiopia. As the United States population becomes increasingly diverse and as pronounced differences in health status continue to be documented, consideration of the cultural context of medicine is becoming a national priority.

DISPARITIES IN HEALTH CARE ACCESS AND QUALITY

Components of health care access include the ability to get into the health care system as well as to obtain appropriate care once in the system. The availability of health care providers who meet an individual patient's needs is another key component of access to care. Quality care is based on scientific evidence (i.e., is effective), avoids injury to the patient (i.e., is safe), minimizes harmful delays (i.e., is timely), is responsive to the individual patient's needs (i.e., is patient centered), does not vary because of personal characteristics (i.e., is equitable), and avoids waste (i.e., is efficient) (Chapter 11).

Access and Communication

Racial and ethnic minority groups, particularly Latinos, are disproportionately represented among those with health care access problems. The proportions of Latinos who lack health insurance and have no regular source of medical care are more than twice the proportions among non-Latino whites (Table 4-1). Latinos are significantly more likely to report problems in obtaining health care for illness or injury, as well as referrals for specialist care, than are non-Latino whites, even after differences in education, income, and insurance coverage are taken into account. Black heterosexual women have significantly higher levels of health insurance coverage than do black lesbian or bisexual women.

Communication between patients and physicians is more of a problem among members of racial and ethnic minority groups than among whites. In one survey, 33% of Latinos, 27% of Asians, 23% of blacks, and 16% of whites reported one or more of the following problems with communication: the doctor did not listen to everything they said, they did not fully understand the doctor, or they had questions that they did not ask during the visit. In addition, Latinos who spoke Spanish as their primary language (43%) were more likely to have one or more communication problems than were those who spoke English as their primary language (26%).

Blacks (23%) and Latinos (26%) are far less likely than whites (82%) to have regular physicians of their own race and ethnicity. Research has shown that racial concordance between physicians and patients can improve the processes and outcomes of care. For instance, patients in race-concordant relationships with their physician rate his or her decision-making style as significantly more participatory and inclusive than do patients in race-discordant relationships. Furthermore, race-concordant office visits last significantly longer than do race-discordant visits.

Quality of Health Care

National surveys confirm population-level disparities in the quality of both preventive care and the management of chronic disease. American Indians/Alaska Natives and Latinos aged 50 years and older are far less likely to receive interval screening for colorectal cancer (Chapter 199) than are members of other racial/ethnic groups (Table 4-2). Compared with white diabetic adults, black and Latino adults with diabetes are more than 30% less likely to receive recommended preventive and screening services (Chapter 236) and are still less likely to receive them after adjustment for insurance coverage.

Racial and ethnic disparities exist in such specific clinical situations as the prescription of analgesia for pain control (blacks receive less pain medication than whites for extremity fractures), the surgical treatment of cancer (blacks are less likely than whites to receive potentially curative surgery for stage I or stage II non–small cell lung cancer), and the management of end-stage renal disease (blacks are less likely to be entered on the transplant list than are whites). Moreover, disparities in the quality of care are consistently found even when variations in such factors as insurance status, income, age, and comorbid conditions are taken into account.

Disparities in health care quality exist even in systems that are generally believed to provide equal access. For example, in Veterans Health Administration facilities, black patients who were ideal candidates to receive thrombolytic therapy (Chapter 73) on arrival were less likely to receive it than comparable white patients. Black patients were also significantly less likely to have coronary artery bypass graft surgery during their index hospitalization or within 90 days after a myocardial infarction even after adjustment for clinical characteristics and differences in patients' preferences. Similarly, of Medicare-managed care plans, black patients were less likely than white patients to receive diabetic retinal examination, post-infarction β-blockers, and post-hospitalization follow-up for mental illness after adjustment for clinical characteristics and for clustering within health plans.

TABLE 4-2 COLORECTAL CANCER SCREENING LEVELS AMONG INDIVIDUALS AGED 50 YEARS AND OLDER BY RACE/ETHNICITY—UNITED STATES, 2006

RACE/ETHNICITY	FOBT LAST YEAR OR LOWER ENDOSCOPY LAST 10 YEARS % (95% CI)
White	62.6 (62.1-63.0)
Black	59.0 (57.3-60.6)
American Indian/Alaska Native	48.4 (43.5-53.2)
Asian American/Pacific Islander	55.9 (51.0-60.7)
Latino	47.2 (44.5-49.9)

FOBT = fecal occult blood testing.
From Joseph DA, Rim SH, Seeff LC. Use of colorectal cancer tests—United States, 2002, 2004, and 2006. *MMWR Morb Mortal Wkly Rep.* 2008;57:253-258.

CULTURAL COMPETENCE IN HEALTH CARE

Health disparities can be reduced or perhaps even eliminated by maintaining culturally competent health care systems. Cultural competence may be defined as a set of congruent attitudes, behaviors, and policies that come together both among professionals and within systems to enable effective work in cross-cultural situations (Fig. 4-1). Ongoing efforts to improve cultural competence in the U.S. health care system target organizational, structural, and clinical barriers. These initiatives aim to close gaps in health status, to decrease differences in the quality of care, to enhance patients' satisfaction, and to increase patients' trust.

Organizational Barriers and Interventions

Racial and ethnic minority physicians are more likely than their white colleagues to work in medically underserved communities. Moreover, they have a better understanding of barriers to health care (such as office hours that do not match community work patterns, bureaucratic intake processes that create fear of deportation among the undocumented, and long waiting times to get an appointment and, after arrival, to keep an appointment). Finally, minority physicians bring a nuanced awareness of the needs of diverse groups of patients and share it through the critical avenues of role modeling and teaching. However, only 6% of practicing physicians are black, Native American, or Latino, and only 15% of medical school applicants are from one of these groups.

Most (approximately two thirds) patients who receive care at federally funded community health centers in medically underserved areas are members of racial and ethnic minority groups. Further, the proportion of community health center patients who have limited English proficiency is 30% and has grown rapidly since 2000. The community health center model has proved effective not only in increasing access to care but also in improving continuity of care and health outcomes. For example, one study found that medically underserved communities with federally qualifying community health centers had 5.8 fewer preventable hospitalizations per 1000 population over 3 years than did similar communities without health centers. Consequently, ongoing efforts to increase the capacity of community health centers are likely to help reduce health disparities.

Structural Barriers and Interventions

The Department of Health and Human Services has created standards on culturally and linguistically appropriate interpreter services to guide

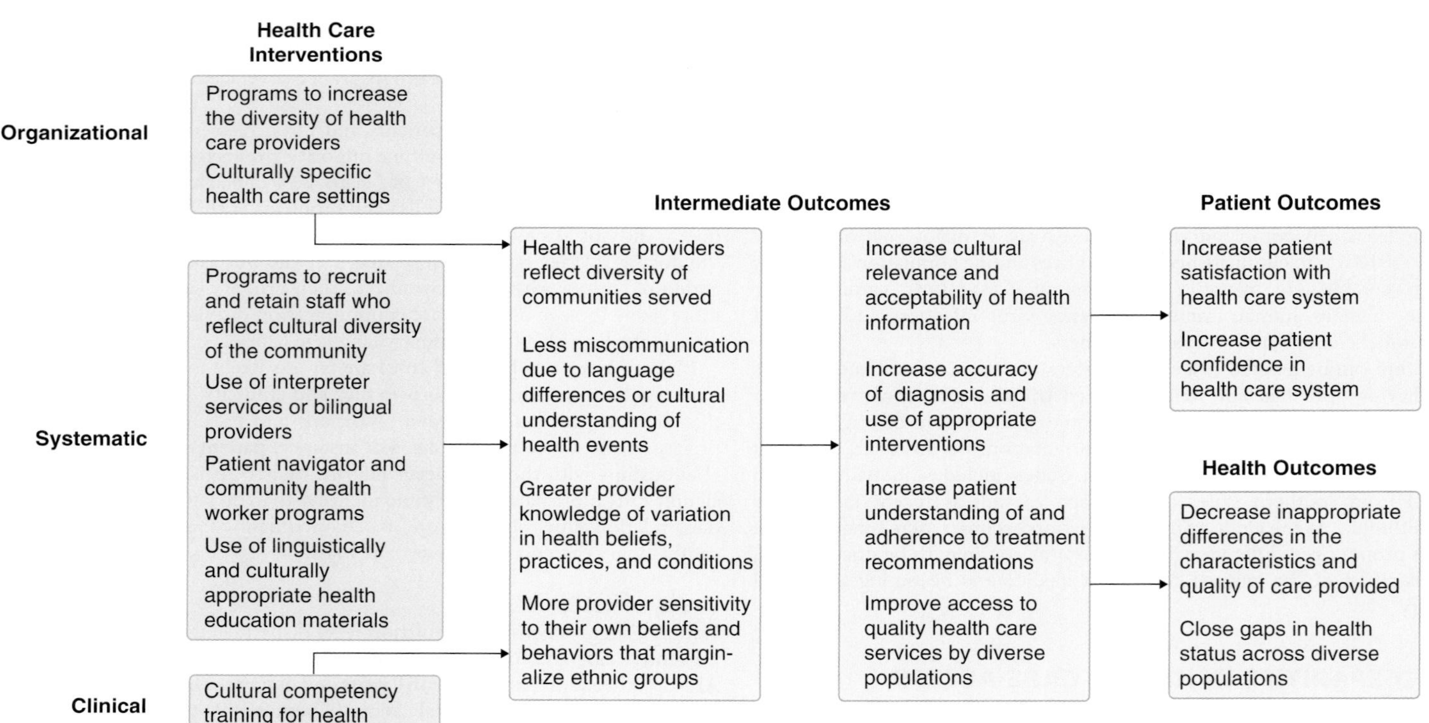

FIGURE 4-1. Analytic framework for evaluating the effectiveness of health care interventions to increase cultural competence. (From Anderson LM, Scrimshaw SC, Fullilove MT, et al, for the Task Force on Community Preventive Services. Culturally competent healthcare systems: a systemic review. *Am J Prev Med.* 2003;24[Suppl]:68-79).

providers. However, interpreter services often remain ad hoc, with family members and untrained nonclinical employees acting as interpreters. Use of ad hoc services has potentially negative clinical consequences, including breach of the patient's confidentiality and inaccurate communication. One major obstacle to the implementation of professional interpreter programs is a lack of reimbursement; Medicare and most private insurers do not pay for interpretation and related services (such as translation or telephone language lines), and only a few states currently pay for interpretation under Medicaid.

Accumulating evidence suggests that trained professional interpreters and bilingual providers can have a positive impact on the satisfaction of patients and quality of care among individuals with limited English proficiency. For example, in a health maintenance organization, the introduction of professional interpreter services for Portuguese- and Spanish-speaking patients increased their use of recommended preventive services, office visits, and number of prescriptions written and filled.

Assistance with "navigation" represents one promising model to enable racial and ethnic minority patients to move through the health system effectively and to be actively involved in decision making about their medical care. Navigator programs rely on personal guides to shepherd disadvantaged patients with chronic diseases into standard care. Guides help patients and their families navigate the treatment process, steering them around obstacles that may limit their access to quality care. For example, guides (who may be nurses, social workers, or volunteers who are familiar with the health care system) help patients choose doctors and assess treatment options. Currently, three major navigation programs (the National Cancer Institute, American Cancer Society, and Center for Medicare and Medicaid Services) are under way to address the needs of medically underserved cancer patients.

Community health workers are increasingly being used in attempts to close the gap in health care among various racial and ethnic minority populations. In general, community health workers live locally and share the language and culture of the population of patients served. Lay community health workers have several core functions; they provide cultural mediation between communities and the health care system, provide culturally appropriate and accessible health education and information, help people obtain the medical services they need, provide informal counseling and social support, and advocate for individuals within the health care system. The largest system formally to use the skills of community health workers is the Indian Health Service, which currently has about 1400 community health representatives who work with tribally managed or Indian Health Service programs in more than 550 American Indian/Alaska Native nations.

Evidence for the effectiveness of community health workers is provided by the breast and cervical cancer screening literature. For example, Vietnamese American women randomized to receive lay health worker group education are significantly more likely to obtain Papanicolaou tests than are women who do not.[1,2]

Clinical Barriers and Interventions

Patients who are members of racial and ethnic minority groups often have an understanding of health and disease (i.e., explanatory model) that differs from that of the general population. For example, many Vietnamese people believe that disease is caused by an imbalance of the humoral forces of yin and yang. When ill, they commonly use Chinese herbal medicine as well as indigenous folk practices known as Southern medicine in an effort to restore the balance of humoral forces. In addition, Vietnamese patients may think that Western medicine is too strong and will upset the internal balance. Consequently, a hypertensive patient, for example, may use Chinese herbal medicines (Chapter 38) instead of prescribed antihypertensive medication. Alternatively, the patient may take a lower dose of medication than prescribed by his or her physician.

Cultural competency training for health care providers generally includes some balance of cross-cultural knowledge and communication skills, taught while avoiding stereotypes. Examples include the effect of prejudice on gays and lesbians and how this prejudice shapes their interactions with the health care system, and common spiritual practices that might interfere with prescribed therapies (such as Ramadan fasting practices, when observed by diabetic Muslim patients). Communication skills that can be addressed in cultural competence training include approaches to eliciting patients' explanatory models and use of traditional treatments as well as methods for negotiating different styles of communication and levels of family participation in decision making. Overall, there is good evidence that cultural competency training improves the attitudes and skills of health professionals as well as patient satisfaction, but less evidence that it improves clinical outcomes.[3]

Training in cultural diversity has recently become part of medical school curricula, often by "weaving" multiculturalism into the curriculum rather than teaching it as a separate course. Program components may include home visits that allow students to hear patients' stories of illness and treatment (and learn about patient-centered care) as well as discussions of clinical cases that allow students to explore issues related to health disparities, health care access, and unequal treatment.

SUMMARY

The average life expectancy of Americans increased by more than 30 years between 1900 and 2000. However, some groups have not fully benefited from the medical and public health achievements of the last century. Although there are demonstrated correlations between racial and ethnic background and socioeconomic status (Chapter 5), poverty alone cannot explain all the gaps in health and health care that exist between minorities and whites. Although the disparities were first documented in blacks in the United States, a growing body of evidence indicates that Latinos and other racial/ethnic minority groups, as well as gays, lesbians, and bisexuals, also experience significant problems with health care access and quality, especially when their English is not proficient.

Efforts to improve cultural competence in health care, whether they are used alone or in conjunction with socioeconomic initiatives (Chapter 5), are likely to play a significant role in reducing health disparities across population subgroups. The dissemination of successful interventions through linkages with payers, policymakers, provider groups, community organizations, and the media will be critical.

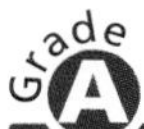

1. Mock J, McPhee SJ, Nguyen T, et al. Effective lay health worker outreach and media-based education for promoting cervical cancer screening among Vietnamese American women. *Am J Public Health.* 2007;97:1693-1700.
2. Taylor VM, Jackson JC, Yasui Y, et al. Evaluation of a cervical cancer control intervention using lay health workers for Vietnamese American women. *Am J Public Health.* 2010;100:1924-1929.
3. Sequist TD, Fitzmaurice GM, Marshall R, et al. Cultural competency training and performance reports to improve diabetes care for black patients: a cluster randomized, controlled trial. *Ann Intern Med.* 2010;152:40-46.

SUGGESTED READINGS

http://www.commonwealthfund.org/Publications/View-All.aspx?topic=Health+Care+Disparities *Website including key articles on health disparities.*

Walker R, St. Pierre-Hansen N, Cromarty H, et al. Measuring cross-cultural patient safety: identifying barriers and developing performance indicators. *Healthc Q.* 2010;13:64-71. *Review.*

5 SOCIOECONOMIC ISSUES IN MEDICINE

STEVEN A. SCHROEDER

All nations—rich and poor—struggle with how to improve the health of the public, obtain the most value from medical services, and restrain rising health care expenditures. Many developed countries also wrestle with the paradox that their citizens have never been so healthy or so unhappy with their medical care. Despite the reality that only 10% of premature deaths result from inadequate medical care, the bulk of professional and political attention focuses on how to obtain and pay for state-of-the-art medical care. By comparison, 40% of premature deaths stem from unhealthy behaviors—including smoking (about 44%; Chapter 31); excessive or unwise drinking (about 11%; Chapter 32), obesity and insufficient physical activity (about 15% but estimated to rise substantially in the years to come; Chapters 15 and 227), illicit drug use (about 2%; Chapter 33), and imprudent sexual behavior (about 3%; Chapter 293) (E-Fig. 5-1). Genetics (Chapter 39) account for an additional 30%; social factors—discussed next—account for 15%, and environmental factors (Chapter 18) account for 5%. Of the major behavioral causes of premature deaths (Fig. 5-1), tobacco use (Chapter 31) is by far the

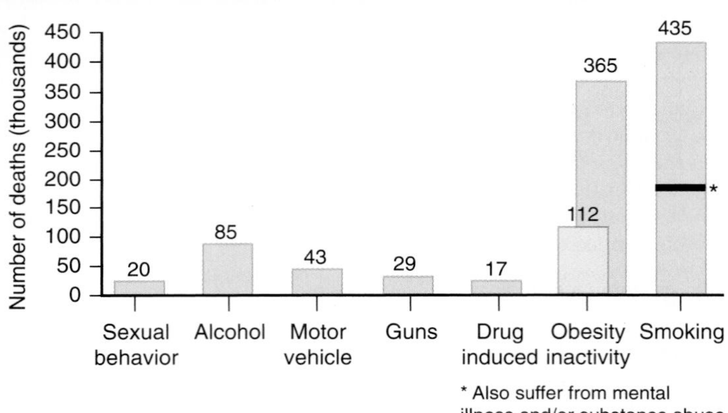

FIGURE 5-1. Number of U.S. deaths from behavioral causes. (Data from Mokdad AH, Marks JS, Stroup DF, Gerberding JL. Actual causes of death in the United States, 2000. *JAMA.* 2004;291:1238-1245; Mokdad AH, Marks JS, Stroup DF, Gerberding JL. Correction: actual causes of death in the United States, 2000. *JAMA.* 2005;293:293-294; Flegal KM, Graubard BI, Williamson DF, et al. Excess deaths associated with underweight, overweight, and obesity. *JAMA.* 2005;293:1861-1867. Adapted from Schroeder SA. Shattuck lecture: we can do better—improving the health of the American People. *N Engl J Med.* 2007;357: 1221-1228.)

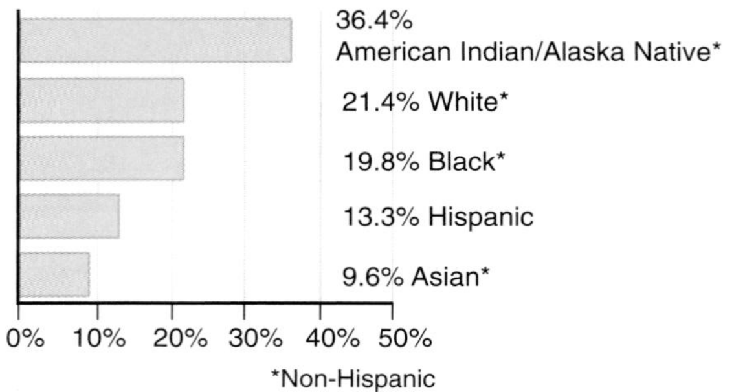

FIGURE 5-2. Prevalence of adult smoking by race/ethnicity, United States, 2007. (From Centers for Disease Control and Prevention. Cigarette smoking among adults—United States, 2007. *MMWR Morb Mortal Wkly Rep.* 2008;57:1221-1226.)

most important, although recent increases in obesity (Chapter 227) and physical inactivity (Chapter 15) are also alarming.

SOCIAL STATUS INFLUENCES HEALTH

Socioeconomic status, or class, is a composite of many different factors, including income, net wealth, education, occupation, and neighborhood. In general, people in lower classes are less healthy and die earlier than people at higher socioeconomic levels, a pattern that holds true in a stepwise fashion from the poorest to the richest. In the United States, the association between health and class is usually discussed in terms of racial and ethnic disparities; but in fact, race and class are independently associated with health status, and it can be argued that class is the more important factor. For example, U.S. racial disparities in adult smoking prevalence are relatively small among whites, blacks, and Hispanic Americans (Fig. 5-2), whereas there are huge differences among smoking rates by educational level (Fig. 5-3). U.S. physicians have reduced their smoking prevalence to a record low of only 1%.

In part, the relationship between class and health is mediated by the higher rates of unhealthy behaviors among the poor, such as the inverse relationship between educational attainment and cigarette smoking, but unhealthy behaviors do not fully explain the poor health of those in the lower socioeconomic classes. Even when behavior is held constant, people in lower socioeconomic classes are much more likely to die prematurely than are people of higher classes. Of interest is that first-generation immigrants appear to be more protected from the adverse health consequences of low socioeconomic status than are subsequent generations.

It is unclear which of the components of class—education, wealth (either absolute wealth or the extent of the gap between rich and poor), occupation, or neighborhood—makes the greatest impact on a person's health. Most likely, it is a combination of all of them. For example, the constant stress of a lower class existence—lack of control over one's life circumstances, social

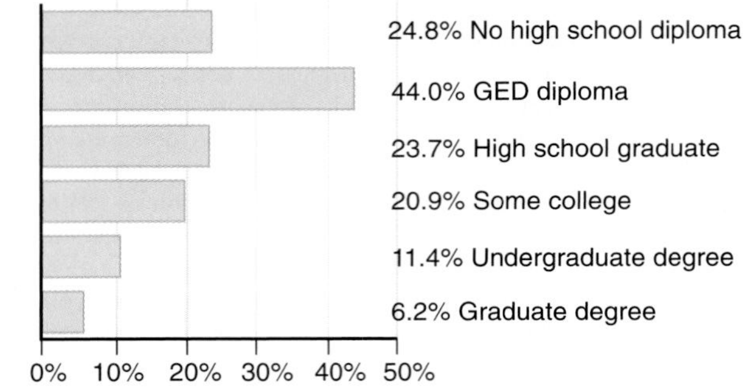

FIGURE 5-3. Age-adjusted prevalence of cigarette smoking in 2007, among persons 25 years of age or older, according to educational level. GED = General Education Development test. (From Centers for Disease Control and Prevention. Cigarette smoking among adults—United States, 2007. *MMWR Morb Mortal Wkly Rep.* 2008;57:1221-1226.)

isolation, and the anxiety derived from the feeling of having low status—is linked to poor health. This stress may trigger a variety of neuroendocrinologic responses that are useful for short-term adaptation and bring long-term adverse health consequences.

What can clinicians do with this knowledge? Clearly, it is difficult to write prescriptions for more income or for better schooling or neighborhoods or jobs, but physicians can encourage healthy behavior. At key times of transition, such as during discharge planning for hospitalized patients, clinicians should be attentive to social circumstances. For patients who are likely to be socially isolated, clinicians should encourage or arrange interactions with family, neighbors, religious organizations, or community agencies to improve the likelihood of optimal outcomes. In addition, physicians should seek to identify and to eliminate any aspects of racism in health care institutions. Finally, in their role as social advocates, physicians can promote such goals as safe neighborhoods, improved schools, and equitable taxation policies.

ECONOMIC ISSUES IN MEDICAL CARE

Medical care today is on a collision course. On the one hand, an ever-expanding science base continuously generates new technologies and drugs that promise a longer and healthier life. Add a public eager to obtain the latest breakthroughs touted in the media and over the Internet, plus a well-stocked medical industry eager to meet that demand, and it is easy to understand why expenditures continue to soar. On the other hand, payers for medical care—health insurance companies, government (federal, state, and local), and employers—increasingly bridle at medical care costs.

The United States continues to lead the world in health care expenditures (Fig. 5-4). In 2008, it spent about $2.4 trillion, amounting to 17% of its gross domestic product. It is projected that expenditures will continue to rise, exceeding 20% by 2014. Most policy analysts contend that this rate of increase in medical care expenditures is unsustainable, but the same has been said for many years. Few other countries have double-digit health care expenditures, and none comes close to 15% (see Fig. 5-4). A potent combination of supply and demand factors explains why the United States spends so much. On the supply side, it far exceeds other countries in the availability and use of expensive diagnostic technologies, such as magnetic resonance imaging and computed tomography (E-Fig. 5-2). For example, the United States has four times as many magnetic resonance imaging machines per capita as does Canada. Similar patterns exist for therapeutic technologies, whether coronary angioplasty, cancer chemotherapy, or joint prostheses. The differences are especially dramatic in older patients. For example, in the 65- to 69-year age group, the United States performed 1.95 more carotid endarterectomy procedures per capita than did Canada; but above the age of 80 years, the ratio was 8.7.

Other supply factors that drive high medical expenditures in the United States include a fee-for-service payment system that compensates physicians much more for using expensive technologies than when they do not; a medical professional work force that earns much higher incomes relative to the population than in other nations and that emphasizes specialist rather than generalist practice; accelerated development of new and costly medications that are directly marketed to consumers; much higher administrative costs; higher rates of fraud and abuse; and a high rate of defensive medicine in response to pervasive fears about medical malpractice suits. Supply factors that do not appear to be unique to the United States are the number of physicians or hospitals. Many other developed countries have a much larger

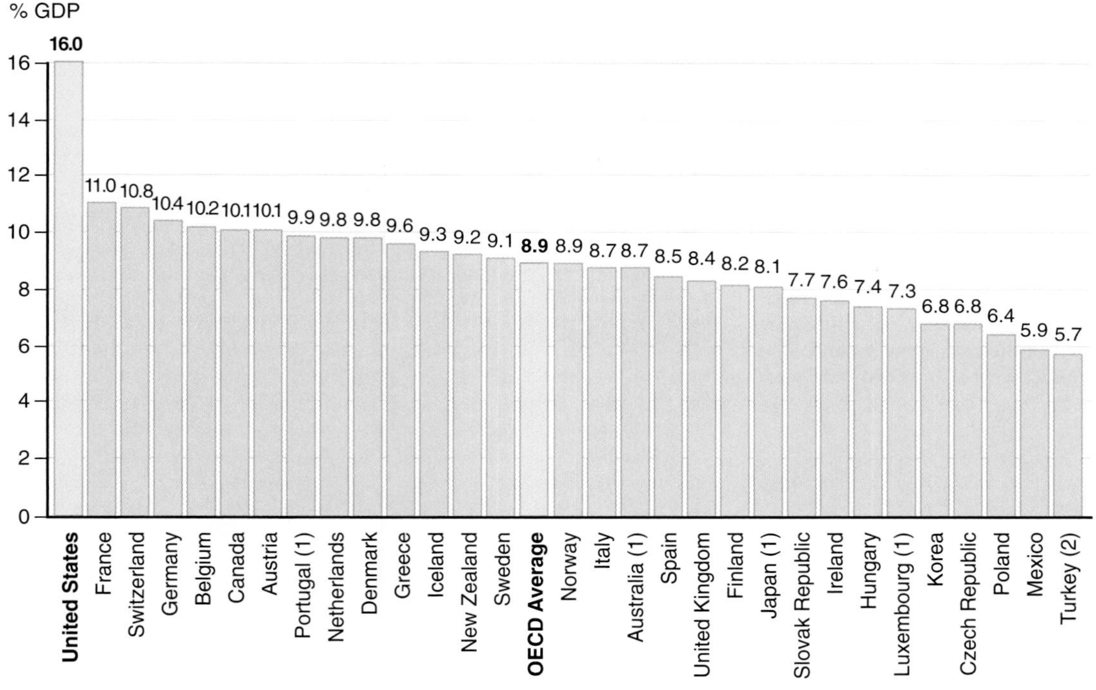

FIGURE 5-4. Health expenditure as a share of gross domestic product (GDP), 2007. OECD = Organisation for Economic Co-operation and Development. (Data from Organisation for Economic Co-operation and Development Health, 2009.)

physician work force relative to their population, as well as a much higher ratio of primary care physicians to specialists. The number of hospitals and hospital beds, the frequency of hospitalizations, and the length of hospital stay are relatively low in the United States, although it does have a much greater proportion of intensive care beds. Finally, recent analyses suggest that a principal driver of high expenditures on health care in the United States is the much greater price charged per unit of service compared with other developed countries.

Demand factors also drive medical expenditures. The extent to which the media and the medical profession feature medical "breakthroughs" is extensive and one-sided. New promising treatments merit front-page stories and commercial advertisements, whereas subsequent disappointing results are buried or ignored. The cumulative result is to whet patients' appetite for more and to leave the impression that good health depends only on finding the right treatment. This same quest explains the popularity of alternative medicine, for which patients are willing to spend $34 billion annually out of their own pockets (Chapter 38).

It could be argued that rising expenditures for medical care are not a bad thing, as what could be more important than ensuring maximal health? There are several rebuttals to that argument. First, it is not clear that money spent on medical care brings appropriate value in the United States, given that its health statistics are worse than those of virtually every other developed country. Second, there are substantial regional differences in the supply and use of medical care, such as a two-fold difference in the supply of acute hospital beds in metropolitan regions (even with adjustment for demographic variables) and a four-fold difference in the risk of being hospitalized in an intensive care unit at the end of life. Similar regional differences exist for procedures such as transurethral prostatectomy, hysterectomy, and coronary artery bypass surgery. Yet there is no evidence that "more is better" on a regional basis. In fact, geographic areas with higher consumption of medical services have been shown to have worse outcomes for some conditions, such as acute myocardial infarction.

Money spent on medical care means less to spend on other important social priorities—schools, the environment, job creation, and competition with overseas manufacturers that spend less on health care. Furthermore, many businesses are reducing their health insurance contributions to employees and retirees, passing those costs along to the beneficiaries. Consequently, health insurance coverage has emerged as the most important issue in labor contract negotiations and strikes. In addition, rising health care expenditures are stressing public programs such as Medicare, Medicaid, the Veterans Administration health system, and municipal hospitals, with budget requests outstripping the tax base to pay for them. Medical debt is by far the most important cause of bankruptcy. Finally, as health care becomes less affordable for businesses and government, the number of people without health insurance will continue to increase.

Since the mid-1970s, a variety of strategies to contain rising medical expenditures have yielded limited success. These attempts have tried to restrict the supply of costly medical technologies as well as the production of physicians, especially specialists; to promote health maintenance organizations that have incentives to spend less on medical care; to ration indirectly by limiting health insurance coverage; to institute prospective payment for hospital care; to use capitation payments or discounted fee schedules for physician reimbursement; to introduce gatekeeper mechanisms to reduce access to costly care; to put patients at more financial risk for their own medical care; to reform malpractice procedures; to reduce administrative costs; and to encourage less aggressive care at the end of life. The most recent suggestions—comparative effectiveness research to curtail unnecessary technology use, electronic medical records to avoid duplication of tests, and payment for performance—all hold the promise to improve quality, but their potential for substantial cost reduction is only theoretical at present. Fundamentally, all these strategies have failed because the political will to enforce them was missing. Americans—at least those with medical insurance—strongly resist limits on their choice of medical care, and the combined power of hospitals, medical professionals, and the pharmaceutical, medical device, and insurance industries overwhelms the meager forces pushing cost containment. Add to that the continuous production of new technologies and drugs plus the public's avidity for the latest innovations, and it is easy to see why medical costs are projected to keep rising. As a result, the costs of even modest health insurance plans are a challenge for most blue-collar and many middle-class families.

Payment for medical care varies by country. In the United States, health insurance coverage is an incomplete patchwork, consisting of government-sponsored programs for elderly people (Medicare), poor people (Medicaid), and veterans, plus employer-based coverage for workers and their families. Medicare covers acute care services in the hospital and in physicians' offices but has limited coverage for prescription drugs and long-term care. More than half of all Medicare subscribers also buy supplemental insurance. Medicaid covers more services than Medicare does, but Medicaid payments to physicians and hospitals are so low in many states that patients have restricted access to care. At any given time, more than 46 million Americans lack health insurance, and 70 million are without insurance at some point during the year. In addition, millions of immigrant workers are also uninsured. This large group must depend on charity care, often at community clinics and public hospitals, and it is well documented that lack of health insurance contributes to poor health, such as delayed diagnosis and undertreatment of asthma, diabetes, hypertension, and cancer.

The 2010 Patient Protection and Affordable Care Act (PPACA) contains insurance reform measures that took effect in 2010 and 2011, as well as coverage expansion that starts in 2014. About 32 million new people will be insured, about 50% privately and 50% in Medicaid. Revenue generating provisions are split about evenly between spending reductions and cost containment. In contrast to the passage of Medicare and Medicaid in 1965, the PPACA did not receive bipartisan support, and it is difficult to predict which of its components—if any—will survive.

Because medical care is both so valued and so expensive, physicians everywhere will inevitably become more involved in issues of medical economics. As cost-containment pressures force patients to assume more of their medical expenses, they will become more aware of costs and more demanding about the price and value of care. Informed clinical decision making will require that physicians have accurate information about the risks, benefits, and costs of medical care and better ways to communicate what is known and what is not.

SUGGESTED READINGS

Aaron HJ, Ginsburg PB. Is health care spending excessive? If so, what can we do about it? *Health Affairs.* 2009;28:1260-1276. *Analyzes the reasons the United States spends so much more on health care.*

Cubbin C, Vesely SK, Braveman PA, et al. Socioeconomic factors and health risk behaviors among adolescents. *Am J Health Behav.* 2011;35:28-39. *Shows the strong link in adolescents.*

Hajat A, Kaufman JS, Rose KM, et al. Long-term effects of wealth on mortality and self-rated health status. *Am J Epidemiol.* 2011;173:192-200. *Details the strong inverse relationship of wealth with poor health status and mortality.*

Marmot M, for the Commission on Social Determinants of Health. Achieving health equity: from root causes to fair outcomes. *Lancet.* 2007;370:1153-1163. *The quality of health and health services within and across countries corresponds with health outcomes.*

Schroeder SA. Shattuck lecture: we can do better—improving the health of the American People. *N Engl J Med.* 2007;357:1221-1228. *Reviews why, despite its high expenditures, the United States does so poorly in health outcomes.*

Seligman HK, Schillinger D. Hunger and socioeconomic disparities in chronic disease. *N Engl J Med.* 2010;363:6-9. *Perspective.*

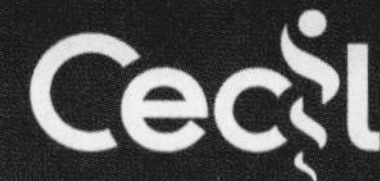

II PRINCIPLES OF EVALUATION AND MANAGEMENT

6

APPROACH TO THE PATIENT: HISTORY AND PHYSICAL EXAMINATION

DAVID L. SIMEL

OVERVIEW

Physicians may have multiple objectives with varying degrees of importance in their encounters with patients. These goals include but are not limited to the translation of symptoms and signs into diagnoses, assessment of stability or change in known conditions, provision of information and counseling for future prevention, and reaffirmation or alteration of therapeutic interventions.

The interaction between the patient and physician represents not only a scientific encounter but also a social ritual centered on locus of control and meeting each other's expectations. Patients may not be able to express their needs fully and may fear loss of control in determining their own medical fate. Conversely, physicians have expectations: a need to feel that they have not missed something important in addressing diagnostic challenges, a need to put limits on the time available for each interaction, and a need to maintain objectivity so that their evaluation and recommendations are not clouded by their emotional feelings about the patient. When the patient needs to establish the presence of health or the diagnosis for a symptom, a physician's expertise is expressed through the performance and interpretation of a rational clinical examination.

Physical Examination Begins with the History

It is almost impossible to consider the history as distinct from the physical examination because the clinical examination begins as soon as the physician sees or hears the patient. Cynics contend that physical diagnostic skills have diminished in importance because so many diagnoses are made during the history and then confirmed by a laboratory value or a radiograph. The problem may be lack of practice in detecting physical examination findings with proven accuracy. Even proponents of the clinical examination now demand proof of reasonable reproducibility and accuracy before they accept the value of specific components of the history and physical examination.

Quantitative Principles of the Clinical Examination

Data on the sensitivity, specificity, likelihood ratios (LRs), and observer variability of components of the clinical examination can be obtained by a literature search for evaluation of a disease-specific condition (e.g., melanoma) or a clinical finding (e.g., splenomegaly) (Table 6-1). For each component of the history and physical examination, there is an associated sensitivity (the percentage of patients with a disorder who have an abnormal finding), specificity (the percentage of patients without a disorder who have a normal finding), and measure of precision (the agreement beyond chance between two observers) (Chapter 9). Current research on the clinical examination uses LRs that inform clinicians how likely they are to observe a particular finding in a patient with a given condition as opposed to a patient without the condition. A patient with an abnormal glabellar tap has an LR of 4.5 for Parkinson's disease (Chapter 416), which means that the risk for parkinsonism increases 4.5-fold compared with a patient with the baseline risk. Similarly, a patient who insists that he or she does not have "shaking in the arms" has an LR of 0.25 for Parkinson's disease and is one fourth as likely (a reduced chance) to have the disease compared with the baseline risk. Evaluation of the precision of the examination uses the kappa (κ) statistic to describe the agreement beyond chance (0 = random agreement; +1 = perfect agreement).

MEDICAL HISTORY

The history begins by asking patients to describe, in their own words, the reason for seeking medical care (Table 6-2). Although patients may have many reasons for initiating a visit to the physician, they should be encouraged to select the one or two most important concerns they have. The physician should reassure the patient that he or she will not ignore other concerns but wants to understand what is most important to the patient.

History of the Present Illness

Open-ended questions facilitate descriptions of problems in the patient's own words. Subsequently, specific questions fill in gaps and help clarify important points. These questions should be asked in an order dictated by the story the patient tells and targeted to suit the individual problem. When the patient is acutely ill, the physician should limit the amount of time spent in open-ended discussion and move promptly to the most important features that allow quick evaluation and management. In general, the history of the problem under consideration includes the following:

- Description of onset and chronology
- Location of symptoms
- Character (quality) of symptoms
- Intensity
- Precipitating, aggravating, and relieving factors
- Inquiry into whether the problem or similar problems occurred before and, if so, whether a diagnosis was established at that time

It is often helpful to ask patients to express what they believe is the cause of the problem or what concerns them the most. This approach often uncovers other pertinent factors and helps establish that the physician is trying to meet the patient's needs.

Past Medical and Surgical History

An astute clinician recognizes that patients may not report all their prior problems because they may forget, may assume that previous events are unrelated to their current problem, or simply may not want to discuss past events. Open-ended statements such as "Tell me about other medical illnesses that we did not discuss" and "Tell me about any operations you had" prompt the patient to consider other items. The physician should ask the patient about unexplained surgical or traumatic scars.

A list of current medications includes prescriptions, over-the-counter medications, vitamins, and herbal preparations. Patients who do not recall the names of medications should bring all medication bottles to the next visit. Patients may not consider topical medications (e.g., skin preparations or eyedrops) as important, so they may need prompting.

Information about allergies (Chapter 262) is particularly important, but challenging, to collect. Patients may attribute adverse reactions or intolerances to allergies, but many supposed allergic reactions are not truly drug allergies. Less than 20% of patients who claim a penicillin allergy are allergic on skin testing. Eliciting the patient's actual response to medications facilitates a determination of whether the response was a true allergic reaction.

Social and Occupational History and Risk Factors

The social history not only reveals important information but also improves understanding of the patient's unique values, support systems, and social situation. The social history should be tailored to the individual patient and allow for physician-centered questioning and patient-centered expression of values and concerns.

Data that may influence risk factors for disease should be gathered, including a nonjudgmental assessment of substance abuse. The tobacco history should include the use of snuff, chewing tobacco, and cigar and cigarette smoking (Chapter 31). Alcohol use should be determined quantitatively and by the effect that it has had on the patient's life (Chapter 32). Past or present use of illicit substances, prescription pain medications or sedatives, and intravenous drugs should be assessed (Chapter 33). The sexual history should address sexual orientation as well as current and past sexual activity (including the number of partners). The employment history should include the current and past employment history, military experience, and any significant hobbies. Military veterans should be asked about their combat history, years of service, and areas of deployment.

The physician should also obtain information on socioeconomic status, insurance, the ability to afford or obtain medications, and past or current barriers to health care because of their impact on care of the patient (Chapter 5). Marital status and the living situation (i.e., whom the patient lives with, significant stressors for that patient) are important as risk factors for disease and to determine how best to care for the patient. A patient's culture (Chapter 4) and values should be known, including any prior advance directives or desire to overrule them (Chapter 3). The physician should explicitly elicit and record information regarding the next of kin; surrogate decision makers; emergency contacts; social support systems; and financial, emotional, and physical support available to the patient.

TABLE 6-1 MEDLINE SEARCH STRATEGY FOR IDENTIFYING QUANTITATIVE INFORMATION ON THE CLINICAL EXAMINATION USING THE OVID SEARCH SYSTEM*

1. exp physical examination/or physical exam$.mp
2. medical history taking.mp
3. professional competence.mp
4. (sensitivity and specificity).mp or (sensitivity and specificity).tw
5. (reproducibility of results or observer variation).mp
6. diagnostic tests, routine/
7. (decision support techniques or Bayes theorem).mp
8. 1 or 2 or 3 or 4 or 5 or 6 or 7
9. limit 8 to (Ovid full text available and human and English language)
10. exp melanoma
11. 9 and 10
12. exp splenomegaly
13. 9 and 12

*OVID Technologies, Inc. A condition and a physical finding are given as examples. Abbreviations or search term abbreviations are as follows: "exp" indicates that the topic is "exploded" to include all subheadings for the topic. The "$" is a wildcard designator, so "exam$" would include the words *examination, examining,* and *examiner.* "mp" searches for the word or phrase in the title, abstract, registry number word, or mesh subject heading. Step 9 limits the search to studies that involve humans only and where the full manuscript is available online and is written in English. If the search yields too few topics, the limitation of full text available can be removed and the search repeated. If too many results are obtained, some of the items from step 8 can be eliminated.

TABLE 6-2 PATIENT'S MEDICAL HISTORY

Description of the patient
Age, gender, ethnic background, occupation
Chief reason for seeking medical care
State the purpose of the evaluation (usually in the patient's words)
Other physicians involved in the patient's care
Include the clinician that the patient identifies as his or her primary provider or the physician who referred the patient. Record contact information for all physicians who should receive information about the visit
History of the reason for seeking medical care
In chronologic fashion, determine the evolution of the indication for the visit and then each major symptom. It is best to address the patient's reason for seeking care first rather than what the physician ultimately believes is most important
Be careful to avoid "premature closure," in which a diagnosis is assumed before all the information is collected
Past medical and surgical history
List other illnesses and previous surgeries not related to the current problem
List all prescribed and over-the-counter medications with dose
Remember to ask about vitamin and herbal supplements
Allergies and adverse reactions
List allergic reactions to medications and food. Record the specific reaction (e.g., hives). Distinguish allergies from adverse reactions or intolerance to medication (e.g., dyspepsia from nonsteroidal anti-inflammatory agents)
Social and occupational history
Describe the patient's current family and a typical day for patient. The occupational history should focus on current and past employment as it might relate to the current problem. For veterans, inquire about their military history, including combat exposure, years of service, and areas of deployment
Risk factors
Include history of tobacco use, illegal drug use, and risk factors for sexually transmitted disease (including human immunodeficiency virus and hepatitis)
Family history
History of any diseases in first-degree relatives and a listing of family members with any conditions that could be risk factors for the patient (e.g., cardiovascular disease at a young age, malignancy, known genetic disorders, longevity)
Review of systems (see Table 6-3)

Family History

The family history is never diagnostic, but it allows risk stratification, which affects the pretest probability for an increasing number of disorders (e.g., heart disease, breast cancer, or Alzheimer's disease). For common diseases such as heart disease, additional inquiry into the age of onset in first-degree relatives and death attributed to the disease should be obtained (Chapter 51). When a patient reports that a first-degree relative had a myocardial infarction, the LR is 19 that the patient has a family history of myocardial infarction. Patients may lack appropriate information about the absence of disease, however, so a reported lack of a family history of myocardial infarction reduces the likelihood only by one third. In general, the specificity of the reported family history far exceeds its sensitivity; for example, only two thirds of patients with essential tremor (Chapter 417) report a family history, but 95% of such patients have first-degree relatives with tremor. The expansion of knowledge about genetic diseases (Chapter 39) requires clinicians not only to improve their skills in eliciting the family history but also to develop methods for confirming the information. For example, patients who report that a first-degree relative had carcinoma of the colon (LR 25), breast (LR 14), ovaries (LR 34), or prostate (LR 12) are usually providing accurate information.

TABLE 6-3 REVIEW OF SYSTEMS*

FOCUS all questions on a specific time frame (e.g., within the past "month" or "now") and on items not already addressed during the clinical examination
Change in weight or appetite
Change in vision
Change in hearing
New or changing skin lesions
Chest discomfort or sensation of skipped beats
Shortness of breath, dyspnea on exertion
Abdominal discomfort, constipation, melena, hematochezia, diarrhea
Difficulty with urination
Change in menses
Joint or muscle discomfort not already mentioned
Problems with sleep
Difficulty with sexual function
Exposure to "street" drugs or medications not already mentioned
Depression (feeling "down, depressed, or hopeless"; loss of interest or pleasure in doing things)
A sensation of unsteadiness when walking, standing, or getting up from a chair

*Clinicians may start with this basic list and adapt the items to their specific patient population by considering factors such as age, gender, medications, and the problems identified during the examination. The process is facilitated by developing a routine personal approach to these questions, typically going through the systems from "head to toe."

Review of Systems

The review of systems, which is the structural assessment of each of the major organ systems, elicits symptoms or signs not covered, or overlooked, in the history of the present illness. In practice, the review of systems may be accomplished by direct questioning (Table 6-3) or by having the patient fill out a previsit questionnaire that constrains the answers to a specific time frame. When this review is directly obtained, physicians should not use open-ended questions but rather proceed with direct questions, such as "Has there been any recent change in your vision?" or "Have you recently had shortness of breath, wheezing, or coughing?" The relative value of these approaches has not been investigated fully, but restricting the symptoms to a narrower time frame prevents a complete retelling of the history. One estimate is that the review of systems yields a new important diagnosis about 10% of the time.

PHYSICAL EXAMINATION

Chaperones

Surveys suggest that most patients of either sex and all ages report a lack of preference for a chaperone; it is not clear whether this response is their true feeling or a desire to give a "correct" response. Nevertheless, many adult women (29%) and adolescent girls (46%) do express a preference for a chaperone during a breast, pelvic, or rectal examination by a male physician (especially during their first examination). Examiners should offer patients the option of a chaperone, and a chaperone should be considered when the clinician and patient are of different genders. Many examiners prefer a chaperone to allay their own anxieties attributable to gender differences or to achieve a perceived need for protection should the patient become concerned during the procedure.

Vital Signs

Vital signs include the pulse rate, blood pressure, respiratory rate, body temperature, and the patient's quantitative assessment of pain. Marked abnormalities require a rapid, focused evaluation that may take precedence over the typical structural approach to the remainder of the evaluation (Chapter 7).

The pulse should be recorded as not just the rate but also the rhythm. Physicians may prefer to initiate the examination by holding the patient's hand while palpating the pulse. This nonthreatening initial contact with the patient allows the physician to determine whether the patient has a regular or irregular rhythm.

When the blood pressure is abnormal (Chapter 67), the measurement should be repeated, assuring that the cuff size is appropriate. Many adults require a large adult cuff; using a narrow cuff can alter systolic/diastolic blood pressure by −8 to +10/+2 to +8 mm Hg. The appearance of repetitive sounds (Korotkoff sounds, phase 1) constitutes systolic pressure. (Record the value rounded upward to the nearest 2 mm Hg.) After the cuff is inflated about 20 to 30 mm Hg above the palpated pressure, the Korotkoff sounds muffle and disappear as the pressure is released (phase 5). The level at which the sounds disappear is diastolic pressure.

Respirations should be assessed with the patient unaware that the rate is being observed. The examiner should decide whether patients have tachypnea (a rapid rate of breathing) or hypopnea (a slow or shallow rate of breathing). Tachypnea is not always associated with hyperventilation, which is defined by increased alveolar ventilation resulting in a lower arterial carbon dioxide level (Chapter 103). In the evaluation of patients suspected of having pneumonia, examiners agree on the presence of tachypnea only 63% of the time. The subjective sensation of dyspnea (Chapter 83) is caused by an increased work of breathing.

The body temperature of adults is measured with an oral electric thermometer. Rectal thermometers reliably record temperatures 0.4° C higher than oral thermometers. Tympanic thermometers may vary too much in comparison to oral thermometers (−1.2° to +1.6° C vs. the oral temperature) to be reliable in hospitalized patients.

As a vital sign measure, patients should self-rate any pain on a scale of 0 to 10 (no pain to worst pain ever) (Chapter 29). However, the validity, usefulness, and value of this approach as a screening tool for clinical diagnosis are uncertain.

Head and Neck

Face

The examiner can simplify the assessment by carefully judging for facial symmetry. Asymmetrical facial features should be noted and explained. Examples of asymmetry include skin lesions (Chapter 444), cranial nerve palsies (Chapter 403), parotid enlargement (Chapter 433), or the ptosis of Horner's syndrome (Chapter 432). A variety of disorders may cause symmetrical, abnormal facies; examples include acromegaly (Chapter 231), Cushing's syndrome (Chapter 234), and Parkinson's disease (Chapter 416).

Ears

Physicians may not recognize their patient's hearing impairment (Chapter 436). The inability to appreciate the whispered voice increases the likelihood of hearing loss (LR 6). Otoscopic evaluation of the tympanic membranes should reveal a translucent membrane and an obvious cone of light reflected where the eardrum meets the malleolus (see Fig. 434-6). Cerumen impaction is an easily treated cause of diminished hearing.

Nose

Patients frequently have nasal symptoms, such as a self-diagnosis of sinusitis (Chapter 434) or snoring (Chapter 412). The nares should be examined for the presence of polyps, which can be seen as obstructing, glistening mucosal masses. Transillumination performed in a dark room is useful for diagnosing sinusitis, especially when combined with visualization of a purulent discharge, a patient's report of a poor response to decongestants or antihistamines, a maxillary toothache, and the presence of discolored rhinorrhea (Chapter 434). These patients have an LR greater than 6 for rhinosinusitis.

Mouth

The quality of the patient's dentition directly affects nutrition. Generalist physicians can be confident that the patient requires dental care if periodontal disease or dental caries are detected (LR > 4). Premalignant oral lesions (e.g., leukoplakia [see Fig. 196-1], nodules, ulcerations) found by generalist physicians are usually verified by dentists (LR > 6.5) (Chapter 433). Patients who use smokeless tobacco products are at significantly increased risk for premalignant and malignant oral lesions (Chapter 31). Bimanual palpation of the cheeks and floor of the mouth facilitates identification of potentially malignant lesions (Chapter 433).

Eyes

The eye examination begins with simple visual inspection to look for symmetry in the lids, extraocular movements, pupil size and reaction, and the presence of redness (Chapters 431 and 432). Abnormalities in extraocular movements should be grouped into nonparalytic (usually chronic with onset in childhood) or paralytic causes (third, fourth, or sixth cranial nerve palsy). Pupillary abnormalities may be symmetrical or asymmetrical (anisocoria). Red eyes should be categorized by the pattern of ciliary injection, presence of pain, effect on vision, and papillary abnormalities. When the eye examination is approached systematically, the generalist physician can evaluate the likelihood of conjunctivitis, episcleritis or scleritis, iritis, and acute glaucoma.

Routine determination of visual acuity can help confirm or refute a patient's report of diminished vision but does not replace the need for formal ophthalmologic evaluation in patients with visual complaints (Chapter 431). Cataracts can be detected with direct ophthalmoscopy, but the generalist's proficiency in this evaluation is uncertain.

After identifying the optic disc by ophthalmoscopy, the examiner should note the border of the disc for clarity, color, and the size of the central cup in relation to the total diameter (usually less than half the diameter of the disc). A careful observer usually can see spontaneous venous pulsations that indicate normal intracranial pressure, but about 10% of patients with normal intracranial pressure will not have spontaneous pulsations. Abnormalities of the optic disc include optic atrophy (a white disc), papilledema (see Fig. 431-27) (blurry margins with a pink, hyperemic disc), and glaucoma (a large, pale cup with retinal vessels that dive underneath and that may be displaced toward the nasal side). The generalist's examination inadequately detects early glaucomatous changes, so high-risk patients should undergo routine ophthalmologic examination for glaucoma.

After inspecting the disc, the examiner should examine the upper and lower nasal quadrants for the appearance of vessels and the presence of any retinal hemorrhages (see Fig. 431-24) or lesions. Proceeding from the nasal quadrants to the temporal quadrants decreases the risk of papillary constriction from the bright light focused on the fovea. Dilating the pupils leads to an improved examination. Patients with diabetes (Chapter 236) should undergo routine examination by eye care experts because the sensitivity of a generalist's examination is not adequate to exclude diabetic retinopathy or monitor it over time.

Neck

Carotid Pulses

The carotid pulses should be palpated for contour and timing in relation to the cardiac impulse. Abnormalities in the carotid pulse contour reflect underlying cardiac abnormalities (e.g., aortic stenosis) but are generally appreciated only after detecting an abnormal cardiac impulse or murmur (Chapter 50).

Many physicians listen for bruits over the carotid arteries because asymptomatic carotid bruits are associated with an increased incidence of cerebrovascular and cardiac events in older patients (Chapters 413 and 414). In asymptomatic patients, the presence of a carotid bruit increases the likelihood of a 70 to 90% stenotic lesion (LR 4 to 10), but the absence of a bruit is of uncertain value. Unfortunately, clinical data do not provide adequate data for judging the importance of detecting bruits in asymptomatic patients.

Thyroid

The thyroid gland is felt best when standing behind the patient and using both hands to palpate the thyroid gland gently (Chapter 233). The palpatory examination is enhanced by asking the patient to swallow sips of water, which allows the thyroid to glide underneath the fingers. When viewed from the side, lateral prominence of the thyroid between the cricoid cartilage and the suprasternal notch indicates thyromegaly. The generalist physician should estimate the size of the thyroid gland as normal or enlarged; the impression of an enlarged thyroid gland by a generalist physician has an LR of almost 4, whereas assessment of normal size makes thyromegaly less likely (LR 0.4).

Lymphatic System

While palpating the thyroid, the examiner may also identify enlarged cervical lymph nodes (Chapter 171). Lymph nodes can also be palpated in the supraclavicular area, axilla, epitrochlear area, and inguinofemoral region. Simple lymph node enlargement confined to one region is common and does not usually represent an important underlying disorder. Unexpected gross lymph node enlargement in a single area or diffuse lymph node enlargement is more important. Patients with febrile illnesses, underlying malignancy, or inflammatory diseases should routinely undergo an examination of each of the aforementioned areas for lymph node enlargement.

Chest

Inspection of the patient's posture may reveal lateral curves in the back (scoliosis) or kyphosis that may be associated with loss of vertebral height from osteoporosis (Chapter 251). When patients have back pain, the spine and paravertebral muscles should be palpated for spasm and tenderness (Chapter 407). The patient may be placed through maneuvers to assess loss of mobility associated with ankylosing spondylitis (Chapter 273), but a history of loss of lateral mobility may be just as efficient in the early stages of spondylitis.

Lungs

Examination of the lungs begins with inspection for chest deformities. A barrel chest, thought to be typical of obstructive airways disease, is present only in severely affected patients (Chapters 83 and 88). The incremental value of palpation and percussion of the chest to supplement the history, auscultation, and eventual chest radiograph is unknown. Medical students show more consistency than pulmonary specialists do in recording auscultatory abnormalities. The presence or absence of adventitial sounds (wheezes, crackles, or rubs) has good interobserver reliability (κ 0.30 to 0.70). The best piece of information for increasing the likelihood of chronic obstructive pulmonary disease is a history of more than 40 pack years of smoking (LR 19). The presence of wheezing or downward displacement of the larynx to within 4 cm of the sternum (distance between the top of the thyroid cartilage and the suprasternal notch) increases the likelihood of obstructive pulmonary disease (LR of 4 for either). Auscultated wheezes are continuous sounds. Crackles (formerly called rales) are discontinuous lung sounds heard in conditions that create lung stiffening (heart failure, pulmonary fibrosis, and obstructive lung disease).

Heart

The patient should be examined in the sitting and lying positions (Chapter 50). Palpation of the apical impulse in the left lateral decubitus position helps detect a displaced apical impulse and can reveal a palpable S_3 gallop. When the apical impulse is lateral to the midclavicular line, radiographic cardiomegaly (LR 3.5) and an ejection fraction of less than 50% (LR 6) are more likely. Most examiners auscultate in sequence the aortic area, pulmonic area, left sternal border, and apex. First, listen to the heart sounds and concentrate on their timing, intensity, and splitting with respiration. The first and second heart sounds are heard best with the diaphragm, as are pericardial rubs. Gallops (S_3 and S_4) are heard best with the stethoscope bell. High-pitched versus low-pitched murmurs are detected by switching from the diaphragm to the bell (see Table 50-6). The location, timing, intensity, radiation patterns, and respiratory variation of murmurs should be noted. Special maneuvers during auscultation (e.g., Valsalva, auscultation during sudden squatting or standing) do not usually need to be performed if the results of routine precordial examination are entirely normal.

There is considerable concern about the reliability and accuracy of the cardiac examination. When performed on patients (as opposed to cardiac simulators), the reliability of perceiving an S_3 or S_4 is no better than chance, and agreement on the finding among examiners does not seem to improve with the examiner's experience. Nevertheless, the presence of an S_3 on any examination is useful for detecting left ventricular systolic dysfunction (LR > 4 for identifying patients with an ejection fraction <30%). The presence of a systolic thrill (palpable murmur, LR 12) or a holosystolic murmur increases the likelihood of moderate to severe aortic stenosis or mitral regurgitation. Quiet systolic murmurs (LR 0.08) are much less likely to herald important cardiac abnormalities. A loud, early diastolic murmur (LR 4) or a diastolic murmur associated with an S_3 suggests severe aortic regurgitation.

Breast

The most important determinants of the accuracy of the breast examination are the duration of the examination; the patient's position; careful evaluation of the breast boundaries; the pattern of the examination; and the position, movement, and pressure of the examiner's fingers (Chapter 204). Interobserver variability is substantial (κ about 0.3 to 0.6) because these aspects of the examination vary among physicians. To obtain the best sensitivity, the duration of the breast examination needs to be 5 to 10 minutes' total time, but few generalist physicians perform such a lengthy examination. Clinicians should recognize that the examination may make them (or their patient) feel uncomfortable—the presence of a chaperone may give the clinician the confidence to perform an intensive examination.

The patient should be examined with the pads of the fingers while she is supine, holding her hand first on her forehead (to flatten the lateral border of the breast) and then on her shoulder (to flatten the medial border). The examiner should make small circular motions with the fingers, moving up and down in parallel rows to span the entire breast-clavicle to the bra line. Cancerous breast lumps are difficult to distinguish from benign breast lumps on examination, but the presence of a fixed mass or a mass 2 cm in diameter has an LR of about 2 to 2.5 for cancer.

Abdomen

When patients have potential abdominal symptoms and the history suggests an acute problem, the examination should focus initially on identifying patients who may require surgical evaluation. Palpation and percussion of the abdomen of patients with no symptoms or risk factors for an abdominal disorder seldom reveal important abnormalities (Chapter 134) except for asymptomatic widening of the abdominal aorta in older patients (LR of 16 for detecting aneurysms >4 cm in diameter). However, palpation misses a substantial proportion of small to medium aneurysms (Chapter 78). After specific training in palpation techniques, general internists have good agreement on the presence or absence of an aortic aneurysm ($\kappa = 0.53$).

The presence of bowel sounds in patients with acute symptoms can be falsely reassuring because bowel sounds can be present despite an ileus and may be increased early in an obstruction. For patients without gastrointestinal symptoms or abnormalities on palpation, auscultation for bruits is important primarily to detect renal bruits in patients with hypertension (Chapters 67 and 127). The presence of an abdominal bruit in a hypertensive patient, if heard in systole and diastole, strongly suggests renovascular hypertension (LR $\approx$ 40).

Liver

Detection of liver disease depends mostly on the history and laboratory evaluations (Chapter 148). By the time that signs are present on physical examination, the patient usually has advanced liver disease. The first abnormalities on physical examination associated with liver disease are extrahepatic. The clinician should assess the patient for ascites, peripheral edema, jaundice, or splenomegaly as signs of liver disease. In patients with an enlarged liver, palpation should begin at the liver edge, but palpation of the edge below the costal margin increases the likelihood of hepatomegaly only slightly (LR 1.7). The upper border of the liver may be detected by percussion, and a span of less than 12 cm reduces the likelihood of hepatomegaly. In the absence of a known diagnosis (e.g., a hepatoma, which may cause a hepatic bruit), auscultation of the liver rarely is helpful.

Spleen

Examination for splenomegaly in patients without findings suggestive of a disorder associated with splenomegaly almost always reveals nothing (Chapter 171). Approximately 3% of healthy teenagers may have a palpable spleen. The examination for an enlarged spleen begins first with percussion in the left upper quadrant to detect dullness. Percussion is performed over the lowest left anterior axillary line during inspiration and expiration while the patient is supine. In the absence of dullness, the results of palpation do not establish or exclude splenomegaly, so a radiographic image (ultrasound or nuclear scintigraphy) is required. The presence of a palpable splenic edge in patients with dullness to percussion and clinical suspicion of splenomegaly confirms enlargement. Palpation can be performed by any of the following three approaches (κ about 0.2 to 0.4): palpating with the right hand while providing counterpressure with the left hand behind the spleen, palpating with one hand without counterpressure (with the patient in the right lateral decubitus position for both techniques), or placing the patient supine with the left fist under the left costovertebral angle while the examiner tries to hook the spleen with the hands.

Musculoskeletal System

The musculoskeletal examination in adult patients is almost always driven by symptoms (Chapters 264 and 271). Most patients have back pain at some point during their lives (Chapter 407). Back pain is second only to upper respiratory illness as a reason for seeking outpatient care. Most patients' musculoskeletal discomfort will be self limited. The patient's history helps assess the likelihood of an underlying systemic disease (age, history of systemic malignancy, unexplained weight loss, duration of pain, responsiveness to previous therapy, intravenous drug use, urinary infection, or fever). The most important physical examination findings for lumbar disc herniation in patients with sciatica all have excellent reliability, including ipsilateral straight leg raising causing pain, contralateral straight leg raising causing pain, and ankle or great toe dorsiflexion weakness (all with $\kappa > 0.6$).

The generalist physician should evaluate an adult patient with knee discomfort for torn menisci or ligaments. The best maneuver for demonstrating a tear in the anterior cruciate ligament is the anterior drawer or Lachman maneuver, in which the examiner detects the lack of a discrete end point as the tibia is pulled toward the examiner while the femur is stabilized. A variety of maneuvers that assess for pain, popping, or grinding along the joint line between the femur and tibia are used to evaluate for meniscal tears. As with many musculoskeletal disorders, no single finding has the accuracy of the orthopedist's examination, which factors in the history and a variety of clinical findings.

The shoulder examination is directed toward determining range of motion, maneuvers that cause discomfort, and assessment of functional disability. Hip osteoarthritis is detected by evidence of restriction of internal rotation and abduction of the affected hip. Generalist physicians often rely on radiographs to determine the need for referral to orthopedic physicians, but routine radiographs are not needed early in the course of shoulder or hip disorders. The degree of pain and disability experienced by the patient may prompt confirmation of the diagnosis and referral.

The hands and feet may show evidence of osteoarthritis (local or as part of a systemic process) (Chapter 270), rheumatoid arthritis (Chapter 272), gout (Chapter 281), or other connective tissue diseases. In addition to regional musculoskeletal disorders, such as carpal tunnel syndrome, a variety of medical and neurologic conditions should prompt routine examination of the distal ends of the extremities to prevent complications (e.g., diabetes [neuropathy or ulcers] or hereditary sensorimotor neuropathy [claw toe deformity]).

Skin

The skin should be examined under good lighting (Chapter 444). It is best to ask the patient to point out any spots on the skin of concern. Examiner agreement on some of the most important features of melanoma (asymmetry, haphazard color, border irregularity) is fair to moderate (Chapter 210). A lesion that is symmetrical, has regular borders, is only one color, is 6 mm or smaller, or has not enlarged in size is unlikely to represent a melanoma (LR 0.07). However, an increasing number of findings greatly enhances the likelihood of melanoma (LR 2.6 for two or more findings and LR 98 for the presence of all five findings) (Chapter 210).

Basal cell carcinoma and squamous cell carcinoma occur even more frequently than melanoma (Chapter 210). These lesions can be detected during routine examination by paying careful attention to sun-exposed areas of the nose, face, forearms, and hands.

Neurologic Examination

Full details of the neurologic examination are given in Chapter 403.

Psychiatric Evaluation

During the general examination, much of the psychiatric assessment (including cognition) is accomplished while eliciting the routine history and performing the review of systems (Chapter 404). Observation of the patient's mannerisms, affect, facial expression, and behavior may suggest underlying psychiatric disturbances. When a screening survey and review of systems are obtained by a questionnaire completed by the patient, the clinician should review the responses carefully to determine whether the patient exhibits symptoms of depression. Specific questioning for symptoms of depression is appropriate for all adult patients. Military veterans should be screened for post-traumatic stress disorder and possible prior traumatic brain injuries that may affect their behaviors. Delirium (Chapter 27) is common in both medical and surgical inpatients and is recognized by fluctuating mental status.

Genitalia and Rectum

Pelvic Examination

A complete examination includes a description of the external genitalia, appearance of the vagina and cervix as seen through a speculum, and bimanual palpation of the uterus and ovaries (Chapters 205 and 245). The precision of the pelvic examination is uncertain. In the emergency setting, there is poor agreement between resident physicians and emergency physicians on the presence of cervical motion tenderness, uterine tenderness, adnexal tenderness, and adnexal masses (κ about equal to 0.2 to 0.25) (Chapter 293). Among gynecologists, assessment of uterine size by examination correlates reasonably well with measurement by pelvic ultrasound. Of asymptomatic women, 10 to 15% have some abnormality on examination, and 1.5% have abnormal ovaries. Screening for ovarian cancer is limited by the low sensitivity of the physical examination for detecting early-stage ovarian carcinoma (Chapter 205).

Male Genitalia

Examination of the male genitalia should begin with a description of whether the penis is circumcised and whether there are any visible skin lesions (e.g., ulcers or warts). Palpation should confirm the presence of bilateral testes in the scrotum. The epididymis and testes should be palpated for nodules. The low incidence of testicular carcinoma means than most nodules are benign (Chapter 206).

The prostate should be examined in all quadrants with attention focused on surface irregularities or differences in consistency throughout the prostate (Chapter 207). An estimate of prostate size may be confounded by the size of the examiner's fingers. It may be best to estimate the size of the prostate in centimeters of width and height.

Rectum

Patients can be examined while lying on their side, although this approach may place the examiner in an awkward stance (Chapters 134 and 147). The rectal examination in women can be performed as part of a bimanual examination, with the index finger in the vagina and the third finger in the rectum to permit palpation of the rectovaginal vault. Men may be asked to stand and lean over the examining table; alternatively, they may be examined while on their back with their hips and knees flexed. This latter maneuver is not used often, although it may facilitate examination of the prostate, which falls into the finger in this position.

The rectal examination begins with inspection of the perianal area for skin lesions. A well-lubricated, gloved finger is placed on the anus, and while applying gentle pressure, the examiner asks that the patient bear down as though having a bowel movement. This maneuver facilitates entry of the finger into the rectum. A normal rectal response includes tightening of the anal sphincter around the finger. The examiner should palpate circumferentially around the length of the fully inserted finger for masses. On withdrawing the gloved finger, the finger should be wiped on a stool guaiac card for fecal blood testing to assess for acute blood loss. As a screening test for colorectal carcinoma (Chapter 199), digital examination does not replace the need for testing stool samples collected by the patient (or using alternative screening strategies, such as flexible sigmoidoscopy or colonoscopy).

SUMMARIZING THE FINDINGS FOR THE PATIENT

The physician should summarize the pertinent positive and negative findings for the patient and be willing to express uncertainty to the patient, provided that it is accompanied by a plan of action (e.g., "I will reexamine you on your next visit"). The rationale for subsequent laboratory, imaging, or other tests should be explained. A plan should be established for providing further feedback and results to the patient, especially when there is a possibility that bad news may need to be delivered. Some physicians ask the patient if there is "anything else" to be covered. Patients who express additional new concerns at the end of the visit may have been fearful to address them earlier (e.g., "by the way, doctor, I'm getting a lot of chest pain"); when the problems seem non-urgent, it is acceptable to reassure the patient and offer the promise of evaluating them in a follow-up phone call or at the next visit.

FUTURE DIRECTIONS

The common assumption that physicians' diagnostic skills are deteriorating is not supported by evidence. There is considerable evidence that the scientific approach to understanding what is worthwhile and what is not worthwhile during the clinical examination identifies a core set of skills for clinical diagnosticians. Because good patient outcomes at good value are driven primarily by the quality of the information obtained during the clinical examination, continued application of scientific principles to the history and physical examination should improve diagnostic skills.

SUGGESTED READINGS

Boulware L, Marinopoulos S, Phillips K, et al. Systematic review: the value of the periodic health evaluation. *Ann Intern Med.* 2007;146:289-300. *A periodic health examination improves delivery of some recommended preventive services and may lessen patient worry.*

Society of General Internal Medicine. Website for Clinical Examination Research and Education Group. http://www.sgim.org/index.cfm?pageId=588. *Facilitates personal literature searches for topics on the clinical examination and a bibliography of the "Rational Clinical Examination Series" published in the* Journal of the American Medical Association.

7

APPROACH TO THE PATIENT WITH ABNORMAL VITAL SIGNS

DAVID L. SCHRIGER

Care of the patient is guided by integration of the chief complaint, history, vital signs, and physical examination findings (Chapter 6). Physicians should be keenly aware of a patient's vital signs but should seldom make them the centerpiece of the evaluation.

THE IMPORTANCE OF VITAL SIGNS

The importance of vital signs in medical care is a conundrum for proponents of an evidence-based approach to care of patients. No experienced physician would be willing to care for patients without them, yet a formal evaluation of the utility of vital signs for making specific diagnoses would conclude that they are not particularly useful because their likelihood ratios are too low to differentiate those who have a condition from those who do not (Chapter 6). For uncommon conditions, their predictive value is even worse. For example, the probability of tachycardia in a patient in thyroid storm is high, yet the probability of thyroid storm in a patient with isolated tachycardia is low. This application of Bayes' theorem (Chapter 9) demonstrates why there is no justification for ordering thyroid tests for every tachycardic patient and why attempts to say "When vital sign *x* is high [low], do *y*" fail. Each vital sign can be normal or abnormal in almost every acute condition (Table 7-1), and vital signs can be transiently abnormal in healthy individuals. An algorithmic approach to testing and treatment in response to abnormal vital signs would be too vague and too complex to be of use.

Predictive Value

How can it be that vital signs are poor predictors of diagnoses but central to the practice of medicine? First, although vital signs are insufficiently predictive to be of use in rigid algorithms, these algorithms are but one of several heuristics used by physicians to diagnose and to treat patients. Pattern recognition and the hypothetical-deductive model are heuristics that are based not on average tendencies of a single factor (e.g., hypotension is present in *x*% of cases of septic shock) or a small number of factors (hypotension and tachycardia are present in *y*% of cases of septic shock) but on the complex interaction of multiple factors (e.g., because this patient is an ill-appearing elderly man with an enlarged prostate and a history of urinary tract infections, is tachycardic and hypotensive, has clear lungs and an enlarged but nontender prostate, and has an oxygen saturation of 97%, he should be treated for urosepsis [Chapter 292] while awaiting results of urinalysis and urine culture).

TABLE 7-1 NORMAL AND PANIC RANGES FOR KEY VITAL SIGNS IN ADULTS*

	NORMAL	PANIC
Temperature	36°-38° C (96.8°-100.4° F)	40° C (104° F)
Pulse	60-100 beats/min	<45 beats/min, >130 beats/min
Respirations	12-20 breaths/min	<10 breaths/min, >26 breaths/min
Oxygen saturation	95-100%	<90%
Systolic blood pressure	90-130 mm Hg	<80 mm Hg, >200 mm Hg
Diastolic blood pressure	60-90 mm Hg	<55 mm Hg, >120 mm Hg

*Normal values are for healthy adults. Values outside these ranges are common in patients who are ill or are anxious about their health care encounter. Panic values demand the health care provider's attention in any adult patient. These values are specific (rarely present in healthy patients) but not sensitive (most ill patients' vital signs will not include panic values). All vital signs must be interpreted in the context of the patient's presentation (see text).

Thus, vital signs can play an important function in medical decision making even though their likelihood ratios for specific complications are unimpressive. In one study, for example, the 16% of medical and surgical ward patients with abnormal vital signs had a 20-fold higher rate of transfer to a higher level of care, cardiac arrest, or death compared with patients with persistently normal vital signs.

Vital Signs as Symptoms

Abnormal vital signs are seldom the fundamental pathophysiologic problem. In shock (Chapter 106), hypotension and tachycardia are manifestations of pathophysiologic processes occurring at cellular and molecular levels. Given the circuitous links from clinical disease to fundamental pathophysiology to abnormal vital signs, it is not surprising that the relationships between the disease states and vital signs are not strong. Until new technologies enable direct measurement of primary pathologic processes, vital signs remain an important, albeit imperfect, proxy.

The five key vital signs are temperature, pulse, blood pressure, respiratory rate, and oxygen saturation (pulse oximetry). Pulse oximetry is included because it has become widely available in acute care settings, is noninvasive and relatively inexpensive, and provides information unique from the respiratory rate. Advocates have suggested that pain, smoking status, and weight be considered routine vital signs; although a case can be made for each, they are not considered here. Clinicians should never forget that the most important vital sign is what the patient looks like; general appearance is a sign that guides the intensity and urgency of the evaluation.

MEASURING VITAL SIGNS

Although obtaining vital signs is generally straightforward, the validity and reliability of measurement depend on proper technique and, for blood pressure and pulse oximetry, well-maintained equipment. Rectal and oral temperatures are generally accurate (Chapter 288), although oral temperatures can be falsely depressed in patients who breathe through their mouths. Axillary temperature is unreliable and should not be used. There is wide variability in the validity and reliability of measurements performed with tympanic membrane thermometers. A hypothermia thermometer is preferred in patients with suspected hypothermia, and core temperature should be measured with an esophageal, bladder, or rectal temperature sensor in patients with severe hypothermia or hyperthermia (Chapter 109).

Blood pressure must be measured with an appropriately sized cuff (Chapter 67). Automated blood pressure machines occasionally provide spurious results, and questionable values should be confirmed by manual auscultation and by checking other limbs. Pulse is best obtained by palpation because this technique provides the opportunity to assess regularity and contour; the pulse should be counted for sufficient time for an accurate rate to be obtained (at least 15 seconds). High heart rates on the readout of a cardiac monitor must be confirmed by palpation because these monitors can spuriously count large P waves, T waves, or pacemaker spikes as R waves, thereby reporting a heart rate double the actual rate. Orthostatic vital signs—the comparison of blood pressure and pulse in the supine, sitting, and standing positions—are advocated by some but have proved to be insensitive and nonspecific for hypovolemia.

Because the typical respiratory rate is between 12 and 20 breaths per minute and because there is considerable breath to breath variation, the respiratory rate should be assessed for at least 30 seconds and preferably 1 minute. Oxygen saturation is dependent on technology, so an understanding of the idiosyncrasies of the device being used is critical; valid measurements are unlikely unless there is good correlation of the machine's pulse reading and the patient's pulse. The probe should be placed on a part of the body that is warm and well perfused. Pulse oximeters compare the absorption of light at two wavelengths, so readings may be spuriously high under conditions that change the color of oxygenated or deoxygenated hemoglobin, including carbon monoxide poisoning (Chapter 94), methemoglobinemia (Chapter 164), and some of the less common hemoglobinopathies.

ROLE OF VITAL SIGNS IN MANAGEMENT OF THE PATIENT

Abnormal vital signs should be remeasured. Certain abnormalities require prompt evaluation (Table 7-2). Other vital sign abnormalities should be rechecked in the future unless they have been previously noted, in which case a work-up can be initiated, guided by the patient's past history and physical examination findings. It is critical that the physician always "treat the patient, not the vital signs."

TABLE 7-2 ABNORMALITIES REQUIRING RAPID EVALUATION IN THE ASYMPTOMATIC PATIENT

An irregularly irregular rapid pulse (if it is not known to be chronic) should trigger an evaluation of the patient's rhythm so that atrial fibrillation can be identified, evaluated, and treated (Chapter 64), thereby decreasing the patient's risk of stroke.

A heart rate above 130 beats/min warrants an electrocardiogram to determine the patient's rhythm and a consideration of the differential diagnosis of tachycardia (anemia and thyroid disease in particular).

A markedly elevated diastolic blood pressure (e.g., >115 mm Hg) should stimulate an evaluation for hypertensive urgencies (Chapter 67). Note that hypertension in the absence of signs of acute end-organ damage does not require acute treatment, which can reduce intracranial perfusion pressure and cause stroke. Patients with elevated blood pressure should be offered standard evaluation and treatment for chronic hypertension (Chapter 67).

Markedly low pulse or blood pressure in patients receiving cardioactive medications should lead to a confirmation that the patient is truly asymptomatic, an inquiry into the dosing of these medications, and a reconsideration of the regimen.

Markedly low pulse in elderly patients who are not receiving rate-controlling drugs should trigger an evaluation of the patient's cardiac conduction system.

Oxygen saturation below 93% in the absence of known pulmonary problems should prompt an evaluation of the patient's pulmonary status.

Patients without Systemic Complaints

In patients presenting for a routine evaluation or nonsystemic complaint (e.g., knee pain), an abnormal vital sign will seldom be the harbinger of acute illness. Most commonly, it will be a false reading or a transient finding due to random variation or anxiety that requires no evaluation or treatment and can be rechecked in the future. On occasion, it will be the only or most apparent manifestation of a chronic condition or risk factor. The measurement of an elevated blood pressure leading to a diagnosis of hypertension is the classic example of the value of vital signs in such patients.

Patients Who Complain of Systemic Illness but Do Not Appear to Be Ill

Vital signs serve two additional roles in symptomatic patients who do not appear particularly ill. First, abnormalities in vital signs provide information that may suggest or support a diagnosis. The presence of elevated temperature in a patient with productive cough, shortness of breath, and localized rales and egophony supports a diagnosis of infectious pneumonia. Vital signs may also play a role in defining therapy and triage. For example, guidelines for patients with community-acquired pneumonia (Chapter 97) formally incorporate vital signs.

The second role of vital signs in the stable symptomatic patient is to provide warning that the patient is sicker than he or she appears. For example, the presence of hypotension in a well-appearing patient thought to have pyelonephritis may be an indication of sepsis or hypovolemia. For vital signs to be of use, the physician must be aware of them and must incorporate them explicitly into a thought process that considers the dangerous diagnoses associated with the abnormal vital sign. The physician then must decide whether the likelihood of each potentially dangerous diagnosis is high enough to warrant specific evaluation. Unfortunately, no quick or easy rules differentiate spurious abnormalities that can be ignored from those that should trigger additional testing or treatment. What can be said is that the well-trained physician who is aware of abnormal vital signs and is willing to contemplate a change in treatment or disposition in response to them is less likely to make mistakes.

A few specific points bear mention. First, for most vital signs, "normal" is relative. Blood pressure must be interpreted in the context of the patient. For example, a blood pressure of 88/64 mm Hg may be reasonable for an otherwise healthy, young 50-kg woman but should cause concern in a 90-kg middle-aged man. Similarly, a blood pressure of 128/80 mm Hg would be fine in a 60-year-old man but worrisome in a 34-week pregnant woman. Second, because vital signs are insensitive measures of disease, normal vital signs should not dissuade the physician from pursuing potentially critical diagnoses. For example, young, well-conditioned adults may maintain normal vital signs well into the course of shock.

Use of Vital Signs in Patients Who Appear to Be Ill

For some patients, abnormal vital signs are expected on the basis of their appearance and their symptoms. For patients in extremis, care should proceed according to established guidelines such as Advanced Cardiac Life Support (Chapter 63), Advanced Trauma Life Support, and algorithms for the treatment of shock (Chapters 107 and 108). For other ill-appearing patients, two processes must occur. In one, the physician, armed with knowledge of the differential diagnosis of each abnormal vital sign and the ability to take a thorough history and to perform an appropriate physical examination, narrows the list of potential diagnoses and decides which are of sufficient probability to warrant evaluation. Simultaneously, the physician considers the list of treatment options for all diagnoses associated with the abnormal vital sign and, before establishing a diagnosis, initiates those treatments for which the potential benefit of prompt administration exceeds potential harms. For example, antibiotics for febrile patients at risk for bacterial infection, hydrocortisone for hypotensive patients at risk for hypoadrenalism, and thiamine for hypothermic patients at risk for Wernicke's encephalopathy may improve outcome and are unlikely to cause harm even if the patient does not have the suspected condition. Although early presumptive treatment can be life-saving in selected patients, it should not be abused; physicians must avoid knee-jerk responses that can cause harm.

Differential Diagnosis and Treatment Options

Single Abnormal Vital Signs

Because vital signs can be abnormal in virtually any disease process, no differential diagnosis can be encyclopedic. The physician should focus initially on common diseases and diseases that require specific treatment. The thought process should begin with the chief complaint and history and then incorporate information about the vital signs and the remainder of the physical examination.

Multiple Abnormal Vital Signs

Patients who are acutely ill are likely to have several abnormal vital signs. Although certain patterns of abnormal vital signs predominate in specific conditions (e.g., hypotension, tachycardia, and hypothermia in profound sepsis), no pattern can be considered pathognomonic. The physician's goal is to work toward a diagnosis while simultaneously providing treatments whose benefits outweigh potential harms.

Fever is generally accompanied by tachycardia, with the general rule of thumb that the heart rate will increase by 10 beats per minute for every 1° C increase in temperature. The absence of tachycardia with fever is known as pulse-temperature dissociation and has been reported in typhoid fever (Chapter 316), legionnaires disease (Chapter 322), babesiosis (Chapter 361), Q fever (Chapter 335), infection with *Rickettsia* spp (Chapter 335), malaria (Chapter 353), leptospirosis (Chapter 331), pneumonia caused by *Chlamydia* spp (Chapter 326), and viral infections such as dengue fever (Chapter 390), yellow fever (Chapter 389), and viral hemorrhagic fevers (Chapter 389), although the predictive value of this finding is unknown.

Much can be learned by comparing the respiratory rate with pulse oximetry. Hyperventilation in the presence of high oxygen saturation suggests a central nervous system process or metabolic acidosis rather than a cardiopulmonary process. Low respiratory rates in the presence of low levels of oxygen saturation suggest central hypoventilation, which may respond to narcotic antagonists.

Hypertension and bradycardia in the obtunded or comatose patient are known as the Cushing reflex, a relatively late sign of elevated intracranial pressure. Physicians should strive to diagnose and treat this condition before the Cushing reflex develops.

Approach to Abnormalities of Specific Vital Signs

Elevated Temperature

Normal temperature is often cited as 37° C (98.6° F), but there is considerable diurnal variation and variation among individuals, so 38° C is the most commonly cited threshold for fever. Fever thought to be due to infection should be treated with antipyretics and appropriate antimicrobials (Chapter 288). The importance of early administration of antibiotics to potentially septic patients cannot be overstated (Chapters 108 and 288). Hyperthermia (temperature above 40° C) should be treated with cooling measures such as ice packs, cool misting in front of fans, cold gastric lavage, and, for medication-related syndromes, medications such as dantrolene (Chapter 109). Most hospital anesthesia departments will have a designated kit for the treatment of malignant hyperthermia (Chapters 440 and 442).

Low Temperature

The treatment of hypothermia is guided by its cause (Chapter 109). The body's temperature decreases when heat loss exceeds heat production. Every logically possible mechanism for this phenomenon has been observed. Decreased heat production can result from endocrine hypofunction (e.g., Addison's disease [Chapter 234], hypopituitarism [Chapter 231], hypothyroidism [Chapter 233]) and loss of the ability to shiver (e.g., drug-induced or neurologic paralysis or neuromuscular disorders). Malfunction of the hypothalamic regulatory system can be due to hypoglycemia (Chapter 236) and a variety of central nervous system disorders (Wernicke's encephalopathy [Chapter 425], stroke [Chapter 414], tumor [Chapter 195], and trauma [Chapter 406]). Resetting of the temperature set point can occur with sepsis. Increased heat loss can be due to exposure, behavioral and physical disorders that prevent the patient from sensing or responding to cold, skin disorders that decrease its ability to retain heat, and vasodilators (including ethanol). A careful history and physical examination should illuminate which of these possibilities is most likely.

Several considerations are worthy of emphasis. The spine of an obtunded hypothermic patient who is "found down" must be protected and evaluated because paralysis from a fall may have prevented the patient from seeking shelter and may have diminished the ability to produce heat. The physician should not forget to administer antibiotics to patients who may be septic (Chapter 108), thiamine to those who may have Wernicke's encephalopathy (Chapter 425), hydrocortisone to those who may be hypoadrenal (Chapter 234), and thyroid hormone to those who may have myxedema coma (Chapter 233). Severely hypothermic patients should be treated gently because any stimulation may trigger ventricular dysrhythmias (Chapter 109); even in the absence of pulses, cardiopulmonary resuscitation should be used only in patients with ventricular fibrillation or asystole.

Elevated Heart Rate

The rate, rhythm, and electrocardiogram differentiate sinus tachycardia from tachyarrhythmias (Chapters 62 to 65). Tachyarrhythmias can be instigated by conditions that may require specific treatment (e.g., sepsis [Chapter 108], electrolyte disorders [Chapters 118, 119, and 120], endocrine disorders [Chapter 233], and poisonings [Chapters 21 and 110]) before the arrhythmia is likely to resolve. For sinus tachycardia, treatment of the underlying cause is always paramount. Treatments may include antipyretics (for fever); anxiolytics; oral or intravenous fluids (for hypovolemia); nitrates, angiotensin-converting enzyme inhibitors, and diuretics (for heart failure and fluid overload [Chapter 59]); oxygen (for hypoxemia); α-blockers (for stimulant overdose); β-blockers (for acute coronary syndromes [Chapters 72 and 73] or thyroid storm [Chapter 233]); and anticoagulation (for pulmonary embolism [Chapter 98]). Tachycardia is often an appropriate response to a clinical condition and should not be treated routinely unless it is causing or is likely to cause secondary problems.

Low Pulse

Bradycardia can be physiologic (athletes and others with increased vagal tone), due to prescribed cardiac medications (e.g., β-blockers, calcium-channel blockers, digoxin), overdoses (e.g., cholinergics, negative inotropes), disease of the cardiac conducting system, electrolyte abnormalities (severe hyperkalemia), and inferior wall myocardial infarction (Chapters 64 and 73). Asymptomatic patients do not require immediate treatment. The goal of therapy is to produce a heart rate sufficient to perfuse the tissues and alleviate the symptoms (Chapter 63). Overdoses should be treated with specific antidotes (Chapter 110). Endocrine disorders should be treated with replacement therapy. In patients with acute coronary syndrome (Chapter 72), the goal is to restore perfusion and alleviate the ischemia. Patients with profound bradycardia or hypotension may require chronotropic drugs to increase perfusion even if they may increase myocardial oxygen demand. In normotensive patients with milder bradycardia, chronotropic agents should be used only if symptoms and ischemia cannot be resolved by other means. Atropine is the primary therapy for bradycardia; isoproterenol and cardiac pacing are reserved for those who do not respond (Chapter 63).

Elevated Blood Pressure

Elevated blood pressure does not require acute treatment in the absence of symptoms or signs of end-organ damage (Chapter 67). In patients whose blood pressure is markedly above their baseline, the history and physical examination should assess for the conditions that define "hypertensive emergency": evidence of encephalopathy, intracranial hemorrhage, ischemic stroke, heart failure, pulmonary edema, acute coronary syndrome, aortic dissection, renal failure, and preeclampsia. In the absence of these conditions, treatment should consist of restarting or adjusting the medications of patients with known hypertension and initiating a program of blood pressure checks and appropriate evaluation for those with no prior history of hypertension (Chapter 67).

The patient with a true hypertensive emergency should be treated with agents appropriate for the specific condition. Because rapid decreases in blood pressure can be as deleterious as the hypertensive state itself, intravenous agents with short half-lives, such as nitroprusside, labetalol, nitroglycerin, and esmolol, are preferred (Chapter 67).

Low Blood Pressure

Low blood pressure must be evaluated in the context of the patient's symptoms, general appearance, and physical examination findings. Treatment depends on context. The same blood pressure value may necessitate intravenous inotropic agents in one patient and no treatment in another.

In tachycardic hypotensive patients, the physician must rapidly integrate all available evidence to determine the patient's volume state, cardiac function, vascular capacitance, and primary etiology (Chapter 106). Not all patients with hypotension and tachycardia are in shock, and not all patients in shock will have hypotension and tachycardia. Patients in shock should be treated on the basis of the cause (Chapters 106 to 108).

Symptomatic hypotensive patients thought to be intravascularly volume depleted should receive intravenous fluid resuscitation with crystalloid or blood, depending on their hemoglobin level (Chapter 106). In patients with known heart disease, patients who are frail or elderly, and patients whose volume status is uncertain, small boluses of fluid (e.g., 250 mL of normal saline), each followed by reassessment, are preferred so that iatrogenic heart failure may be avoided. Inotropic support should be reserved for patients who do not respond to fluid resuscitation. High-output heart failure should be kept in mind in patients with possible thyroid storm or stimulant overdose.

Increased Respiratory Rate

Tachypnea is a normal response to hypoxemia (see later). Treatment of tachypnea in the absence of hypoxemia is directed at the underlying cause, which often is pain (Chapter 29). Anxiolytics (e.g., diazepam, 5 to 10 mg PO or IV; lorazepam, 1 to 2 mg PO, IM, or IV) or reassurance can calm patients with behavioral causes of hyperventilation. Breathing into a paper bag has been shown to be an ineffective treatment. Pulmonary embolism (Chapter 98) does not necessarily reduce the oxygen saturation or cause a low P_{O_2} and should always be considered in at-risk patients with unexplained tachypnea.

Decreased Respiratory Rate

Any perturbation of the respiratory center in the central nervous system can slow the respiratory drive (Chapter 86). Narcotics and other sedatives and neurologic conditions are common causes of a decreased respiratory rate. The primary treatment of apnea is mechanical ventilation (Chapter 105), but narcotic antagonists can be tried in patients with a history or physical examination findings (miosis, track marks, opiate patch) suggestive of narcotic use or abuse (Chapter 33). In nonapneic patients, mechanical ventilation is indicated for patients who are breathing too slowly to maintain an acceptable oxygen saturation and for patients who are retaining carbon dioxide in quantities sufficient to depress mental function. Patients who are unable to protect their airway should be intubated. Oxygen should be administered to all hypopneic patients who are hypoxemic (see earlier). Patients with chronic hypoventilation (Chapter 86) may have retained HCO_3^- to compensate for an elevated P_{CO_2} and so may depend on hypoxia to maintain respiratory drive; in these patients, overaggressive administration of oxygen can decrease the respiratory rate, increase the P_{CO_2}, and increase obtundation (Chapter 104).

Decreased Oxygen Saturation

In hypopneic patients, initial efforts should try to increase the respiratory rate (see earlier) and tidal volume. Regardless of etiology, oxygen, in amounts adequate to restore adequate oxygen saturation ($P_{O_2} > 60$ mm Hg, oxygen saturation >90%), is the mainstay of therapy. When oxygen alone fails, noninvasive methods for improving ventilation or tracheal intubation are required (Chapter 104). Oxygen should increase the P_{O_2} in all patients except those who have severe right-to-left shunting (Chapter 69). Treatment of conditions that cause hypoxemia includes antibiotics (pneumonia), bronchodilators (asthma, chronic obstructive pulmonary disease), diuretics and vasodilators (pulmonary edema), anticoagulants (pulmonary embolism), hyperbaric oxygen (carbon monoxide poisoning), methylene blue (methemoglobinemia, sulfhemoglobinemia), and transfusion (anemia).

SUGGESTED READINGS

Glickman SW, Cairns CB, Otero RM, et al. Disease progression in hemodynamically stable patients presenting to the emergency department with sepsis. *Acad Emerg Med.* 2010;17:383-390. *About 25% of patients with sepsis and initially normal vital signs progress to shock within 72 hours.*

Lighthall GK, Markar S, Hsiung R. Abnormal vital signs are associated with an increased risk for critical events in US veteran inpatients. *Resuscitation.* 2009;80:1264-1269. *Emphasizes that abnormal vital signs carry a 20-fold increased risk for subsequent important deterioration among general medical and surgical patients.*

8

STATISTICAL INTERPRETATION OF DATA

THOMAS B. NEWMAN AND CHARLES E. MCCULLOCH

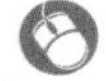

ROLE OF STATISTICS

Much of medicine is inherently probabilistic. Not everyone with hypercholesterolemia who is treated with a statin is prevented from having a myocardial infarction, and not everyone not treated does have one, but statins reduce the *probability* of a myocardial infarction in such patients. Because so much of medicine is based on probabilities, studies must be performed on *groups* of people to estimate these probabilities. Three component tasks of statistics are (1) selecting a sample of subjects for study, (2) describing the data from that sample, and (3) drawing inferences from that sample to a larger population of interest.

SAMPLING: SELECTING SUBJECTS FOR A STUDY

The goal of research is to produce generalizable knowledge, so that measurements made by researchers on samples of individuals will eventually help draw inferences to a larger group of people than was studied. The ability to draw such inferences depends on how the subjects for the study (the sample) were selected.

Sampling

The *intended sample* is the group of people who are eligible to be in the study based on meeting *inclusion criteria,* and not meeting *exclusion criteria.* For example, for a study of obesity, the intended sample (inclusion criteria) might be men and women 18 years or older who have a body mass index (BMI) of 30 kg/m^2 or higher. Exclusion criteria might include an inability to speak English or Spanish.

In some cases, the intended sample is a *simple random sample* of the target population, in which every member of the target population has an equal chance of being selected. Simple random samples are the easiest to handle statistically but are often impractical. An alternative is to take random samples of "clusters" (e.g., specific census tracts or geographic areas) and then attempt to study all of the subjects in each cluster.

Regardless of the method used to select the intended sample, the *actual sample* will almost always differ in important ways. Statistical methods address *only the effect of random variation on the inference from the intended sample to the target population.* Estimating the effects of differences between the intended sample and the actual sample depends on content knowledge about whether factors associated with being in the actual sample are related to those quantities.

DESCRIBING THE SAMPLE

Types of Variables

A key use of statistics is to describe sample data. Methods of description depend on the *type of variable. Categorical* variables consist of named characteristics, whereas *numerical* variables describe the data with numbers. Categorical variables can be further divided into *dichotomous* variables, which can take on only two possible values (e.g., alive/dead); *nominal* variables, which can take on more than two values but have no intrinsic ordering (e.g., race); and *ordinal* variables, which have more than two values and an intrinsic ordering of the values (e.g., tumor stage). *Numerical* variables include *count* variables (e.g., the number of times a woman has been pregnant), *continuous* variables (those that have a wide range of possible values), and *time-to-event* variables (e.g., the time from initial treatment to recurrence of breast cancer).

Univariate Statistics for Continuous Variables: Mean, Median, and Standard Deviation

When describing data in a sample, it is a good idea to begin with *univariate* (one variable at a time) statistics. For continuous variables, univariate statistics typically measure *central tendency* and *variability.* The most common measures of central tendency are the *mean* (or average) and the *median* (i.e., the 50th percentile).

One of the most commonly used measures of variability is the *standard deviation* (SD). A useful property of the SD is that if the distribution of the variable is the familiar bell-shaped, or "normal," distribution, about 68% of the observations will be within 1 SD of the mean, and about 95% within 2 SD. Even when the distribution is not normal, these rules are often approximately true.

For variables that are not normally distributed, the mean and SD are not as useful for summarizing the data. In that case, the median may be a better measure of central tendency because it is not influenced by observations far below or far above the center. Similarly, the range and pairs of percentiles, such as the 25th and 75th percentiles, will provide a better description of the spread of the data than the SD.

Univariate Statistics for Categorical Variables: Proportions, Rates, and Ratios

For categorical variables, the main univariate statistic is the *proportion* of subjects with each value of the variable. Ordinal variables with many categories can be summarized by using proportions or by using medians and percentiles, as with continuous data that are not normally distributed.

It is worth distinguishing between *proportions, rates,* and *ratios* because these terms are often confused. *Proportions* are unitless, always between 0 and 1 inclusive, and express what fraction of the subjects have or develop a particular characteristic or outcome. Strictly speaking, *rates* have units of inverse time; they express the proportion of subjects in whom a particular characteristic or outcome develops over a specific time period. The term is frequently misused, however. For example, the term *false-positive rate* is widely used for the proportion of subjects without a disease who test positive, even though it is a proportion, not a rate. *Ratios* are the quotients of two numbers; they can range between zero and infinity. For example, the male-to-female ratio of people with a disease might be 3:1. As a rule, if a ratio can be expressed as a proportion instead (e.g., 75% male), it is more concise and easier to understand.

Incidence and Prevalence

Two terms commonly used (and misused) in medicine and public health are *incidence* and *prevalence. Incidence* describes the number of subjects who *contract* a disease *over time* divided by the population at risk. Incidence is usually expressed as a rate (e.g., 7 per 1000 per year), but it may sometimes be a proportion if the time variable is otherwise understood or clear, as in the lifetime incidence of breast cancer or the incidence of diabetes during pregnancy. *Prevalence* describes the number of subjects who *have* a disease at *one point in time* divided by the population at risk; it is always a proportion. At any point in time, the prevalence of disease depends on how many people contract it and how long it lasts: prevalence = incidence × duration.

Bivariate Statistics

Bivariate statistics summarize the relationship between two variables. In clinical research, it is often desirable to distinguish between *predictor* and *outcome variables.* Predictor variables include treatments received, demographic variables, and test results that are thought possibly to predict or cause the *outcome variable,* which is the disease or (generally bad) event or outcome that the test should predict or treatment prevent.

Dichotomous Predictor and Outcome Variables

A common and straightforward case is when both predictor and outcome variables are dichotomous and the results can thus be summarized in a 2 × 2 table. Bivariate statistics are also called *measures of association.*

Relative Risk
The *relative risk* or *risk ratio* (RR) is the ratio of the proportion of subjects in one group in whom the outcome develops divided by the proportion in the other group in whom it develops. For example, in the Women's Health Initiative (WHI) randomized trial, estrogen use was associated with an increased risk for stroke (RR = 1.37) and decreased risk for hip fracture (RR = 0.61).

Relative Risk Reduction
The *relative risk reduction* (RRR) is 1 − RR. In the aforementioned WHI example, estrogen had an RR of 0.61 for hip fracture, so the RRR would be 1 − 0.61 = 0.39, or 39%. The RRR is commonly expressed as a percentage.

Absolute Risk Reduction
The *risk difference* or *absolute risk reduction* (ARR) is the difference in risk between the groups, as defined earlier. In the WHI, the risk for hip fracture was 0.11% per year with estrogen and 0.17% per year with placebo, so the ARR = 0.06% per year, or 6 in 10,000 per year.

Number Needed to Treat
The *number needed to treat* (NNT) is 1/ARR. To see why this is the case, consider the WHI placebo group and imagine treating 10,000 patients for a year. All but 17 would not have had a hip fracture anyway because the fracture rate in the placebo group was 0.17% per year, and 11 subjects would sustain a fracture despite treatment because the fracture rate in the estrogen group was 0.11% per year. Thus, with treatment of 10,000 patients for a year, 17 − 11 = 6 fractures prevented, or 1 fracture prevented for each 1667 patients treated.

Risk Difference
When the treatment *increases* the risk for a bad outcome, the difference in risk between treated and untreated patients should still be calculated, but it is usually just called the risk difference rather than an ARR (because the "reduction" would be negative).

Odds Ratio
Another commonly used measure of association is the *odds ratio* (OR). The OR is the ratio of the *odds* of the outcome in the two groups, where the definition of the odds of an outcome is $p/(1-p)$, with p being the probability of the outcome. From this definition it is apparent that when p is very small, $1-p$ will be close to 1, so $p/(1-p)$ will be close to p, and the OR will closely approximate the RR. When p is not small, however, the odds and probability will be quite different, and ORs and RRs will not be interchangeable.

Absolute versus Relative Measures
The choice of *absolute* versus *relative measures* of association depends on the use of the measure. RRs are more useful as summary measures of effect because they are more often generalizable across a wide variety of populations. RRs are also more helpful for understanding causality. However, absolute risks are more important for questions about clinical decision making because they relate directly to the tradeoffs between risks and benefits—specifically, the NNT, as well as the costs and side effects that need to be balanced against potential benefits. RRRs are often used in advertising because they are generally more impressive than ARRs. Unfortunately, the distinction between relative and absolute risks may not be appreciated by clinicians, thereby leading to higher estimates of the potential benefits of treatments when RRs or RRRs are used.

Risk Ratios versus Odds Ratios
The choice between RRs and ORs is easier: RRs are preferred because they are easier to understand. Because ORs that are not equal to 1 are always farther from 1 than the corresponding RR, they may falsely inflate the perceived importance of a factor. ORs are, however, typically used in two circumstances. First, in case-control studies (Chapter 10), in which subjects with and without the disease are sampled separately, the RR cannot be calculated directly. Second, in observational studies that use a type of multivariate analysis called *logistic regression* (see later), use of the OR is convenient because it is the parameter that is modeled in the analysis.

Dichotomous Predictor Variable, Continuous Outcome Variable
Many outcome variables are naturally continuous rather than dichotomous. For example, in a study of a new treatment of obesity, the outcome might be change in weight or BMI. Most measurements have units (e.g., kg, mm Hg), so differences between groups will have the same units and be meaningless without them. For measurements in unfamiliar units, such as a score on a new quality-of-life instrument, some benchmark is useful to help judge whether the difference in groups is large or small. What is typically done in that case is to express the difference in relation to the spread of values in the study, as measured by the SD. In this case, the *standardized mean difference* (SMD) is the difference between the two means divided by the SD of the measurement.

Continuous Predictor Variable
When predictor variables are continuous, the investigator can either group the values into two or more categories and calculate mean differences or SMDs between the groups as discussed earlier or use a *model* to summarize the degree to which changes in the predictor variable are associated with changes in the outcome variable. Perhaps the simplest model is to assume a linear relationship between the outcome and predictor. For example, one could assume that the relationship between systolic blood pressure (mm Hg) and salt intake (g/day) was linear over the range studied:

$$\mathrm{SBP}_i = a + (b \times \mathrm{SALT}_i) + \varepsilon_i$$

where SBP_i is the systolic blood pressure for study subject i, SALT_i is that subject's salt intake, and ε_i is an error term that the model specifies must average out to zero across all of the subjects in the study. In this model, a is a constant, the *intercept*, and the strength of the relationship between the outcome and predictor can be summarized by the slope b, which has units equal to the units of SBP divided by the units of SALT, or mm Hg per gram of salt per day in this case.

It is important to keep in mind that use of a model to summarize a relationship between two variables may not be appropriate if the model does not fit. For example, if the effect of a 1-g/day change in salt intake differed in subjects ingesting low- and high-salt diets, the model would not fit and misleading conclusions could result.

When the outcome variable is dichotomous, the relationship with the continuous predictor variable is often modeled with a *logistic* model:

$$\Pr\{Y_i = 1\} = \frac{1}{1 + e^{-(a + bx_i)}}$$

where the outcome Y_i is coded 0 or 1 for study subject i, and x_i is that subject's value of the predictor variable. Once again, a is a constant, in this case related to the probability of the disease when the predictor is equal to zero, and b summarizes the strength of the association; in this case, it is the natural logarithm of the OR rather than the slope. The OR is the OR *per unit change* in the predictor variable. For example, in a study of lung cancer, an OR of 1.06 for pack years of smoking would indicate that the odds of lung cancer increase by 6% for each pack year increase in smoking.

Multivariable Statistics
In many cases, researchers are interested in the effects of multiple predictor variables on an outcome. Particularly in observational studies, it will be of interest to estimate the effects of each predictor variable *independent* of the effects of other variables. For example, in studying whether regular exercise decreases the risk for heart disease, investigators would try to take differences in race, sex, age, cigarette smoking, blood pressure, and cholesterol into account. Trying to stratify by all of these variables would require a massive data set and raise the issue of multiple testing (see expanded chapter at www.expertconsult.com). Instead, models are used because they enable the information about individual predictors to be summarized by using the full data set. These models are similar to those described earlier but include terms for the additional variables.

INFERRING POPULATION VALUES FROM A SAMPLE
The next step after describing the data is drawing inferences from a sample to the population. Statistics mainly quantify random error. Samples that were not randomly selected from populations may be unrepresentative because of *bias*, and statistics cannot help with this type of systematic (nonrandom) error.

Inferences from Sample Means: Standard Deviation versus Standard Error
The simplest case of inference from a sample to a population involves estimating a population mean from a sample. Intuitively, the larger the sample size,

N, the more likely that the sample mean will be close to the population mean. The more variability there is within the sample, the less accurate the estimate of the population mean is likely to be. To make inferences about a population mean from a sample mean, the *standard error of the mean* (SEM), which takes both of these factors into account, is as follows:

$$\text{SEM} = \frac{\text{SD}}{\sqrt{N}}$$

Confidence Intervals

The SEM has an interpretation pertaining to means that is parallel to the SD for individual observations. Just as about 95% of *observations* in a population are expected to be within ±1.96 SD of the mean, 95% of *sample means* are expected to be within 1.96 SEM of the population mean, thereby providing the 95% confidence interval (CI), which is the range of values for the population mean consistent with what was observed from the sample.

CIs can similarly be calculated for other quantities estimated from samples, including proportions, ORs, regression coefficients, and hazard ratios. In each case, they provide a range of values consistent with what was observed in the study in the target population.

Significance Testing and *P* Values

P values start with calculation of a *test statistic* that has a known distribution under the *null hypothesis*, which states that there is no association between variables. *P* values answer the question, "If the null hypothesis were true, what would be the probability of obtaining, by chance alone, a value of the test statistic this large or larger (suggesting an association between groups of this strength or stronger)?"

There are a number of common pitfalls in interpreting *P* values. The first is that because *P* values less than .05 are customarily described as being "statistically significant," results with $P < .05$ sometimes are described as "significant" when in fact the results may not be clinically significant (i.e., important) at all. This situation may arise when studies have a large sample size.

A second pitfall is concluding that no association exists simply because the *P* value is greater than .05. This problem is particularly likely if the sample size is small. It is then helpful to look at the 95% CI to see whether a clinically significant effect may have been missed.

Finally, a common misconception about *P* values is that they indicate the probability that the null hypothesis is true (e.g., that there is no association between variables). But calculation of *P* values is *based on the assumption* that the null hypothesis is true. The probability that an association is real depends not just on the probability of its occurrence under the null hypothesis but also on the probability of another basis for the association (see later)—an assessment that depends on information from outside the study, sometimes called the *prior probability*.

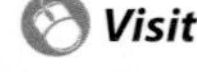

Visit expertconsult.com for e-expanded chapter

SUGGESTED READINGS

Harvey BJ, Lang TA. Hypothesis testing, study power, and sample size. *Chest*. 2010;138:734-737. *Review*.

Walker E, Nowacki AS. Understanding equivalence and noninferiority testing. *J Gen Intern Med*. 2011;26:192-196. *Review*.

9 USING DATA FOR CLINICAL DECISIONS

THOMAS H. LEE

Key functions in the professional lives of all physicians are the collection and analysis of clinical data. Decisions must be made on the basis of these data, including which therapeutic strategy is most appropriate for the patient and whether further information should be gathered before the best strategy can be chosen. This decision-making process is a blend of science and art in which the physician must synthesize a variety of concerns, including the patient's most likely outcome with various management strategies, the patient's worst possible outcome, and the patient's preferences among these strategies.

Only rarely does the physician enjoy true certainty regarding any of these issues, so a natural inclination for physicians is to seek as much information as possible before making a decision. This approach ignores the dangers inherent in the collection of information. Some of these dangers are immediate, such as the risk of cerebrovascular accident associated with coronary angiography. Other dangers are delayed, such as the risk of a malignancy due to radiation exposure from diagnostic tests.

An additional concern is the cost of information gathering, including the direct costs of the tests themselves and the indirect costs that flow from decisions made on the basis of the test results. Substantial data demonstrate marked variation in use of tests among physicians located in different regions and even within the same group practice. Standards of medical professionalism endorse the need for physicians to exert their influence to minimize inefficiency, but this challenge grows increasingly complex as medical progress leads to proliferation of alternative testing strategies.

For the physician, there are three key questions in this sequence: Should I order a test to improve my assessment of diagnosis or prognosis? Which test is best? Which therapeutic strategy is most appropriate for this patient?

SHOULD I ORDER A TEST?

The decision of whether to order a test depends on the physician's and the patient's willingness to pursue a management strategy with the current degree of uncertainty. This decision is influenced by several factors, including the patient's attitudes toward diagnostic and therapeutic interventions (e.g., a patient with claustrophobia might prefer an ultrasound to magnetic resonance imaging) and the information provided by the test itself. The personal tolerance of the patient and physician for uncertainty also frequently influences test-ordering approaches. A decision to watch and wait rather than to obtain a specific test also should be considered an information-gathering alternative because the information obtained while a patient is being observed often reduces uncertainty about the diagnosis and outcome. In other words, the "test of time" should be recognized as one of the most useful tests available when this tactic does not seem inappropriately risky.

Most tests do not provide a definitive answer about diagnosis or prognosis but instead reduce uncertainty. Accordingly, the impact of information from tests often is expressed as *probabilities* (Table 9-1). A probability of 1.0 implies that an event is certain to occur, whereas a probability of 0 implies that the event is impossible. When all the possible events for a patient are assigned probabilities, these estimates should sum to 1.0.

It is often useful to use *odds* to quantify uncertainty instead of probability. Odds of 1:2 suggest that the likelihood of an event is only half the likelihood that the event will not occur. The relationship between odds and probability is expressed in the following formula:

$$\text{Odds} = P/(1 - P)$$

where *P* is the probability of an event.

TABLE 9-1 KEY DEFINITIONS*

Probability	A number between 0 and 1 that expresses an estimate of the likelihood of an event
Odds	The ratio of [the probability of an event] to [the probability of the event not occurring]
TEST PERFORMANCE CHARACTERISTICS	
Sensitivity	Percentage of patients with disease who have an abnormal test result
Specificity	Percentage of patients without disease who have a normal test result
Positive predictive value	Percentage of patients with an abnormal test result who have disease
Negative predictive value	Percentage of patients with a normal test result who do not have disease
BAYESIAN ANALYSIS	
Pretest (or prior) probability	The probability of a disease before the information is acquired
Post-test (or posterior) probability	The probability of a disease after new information is acquired
Pretest (or prior) odds	(Pretest probability of disease)/(1 − pretest probability of disease)
Likelihood ratio	(Probability of result in diseased persons)/(probability of result in nondiseased persons)

**Disease* can mean a condition, such as coronary artery disease, or an outcome, such as postoperative cardiac complications.

Performance Characteristics

Sensitivity and *specificity* are key terms for the description of test performance. These parameters describe the test and are in theory true regardless of the population of patients to which the test is applied. Research studies that describe test performance often are based, however, on highly selected populations of patients; test performance may deteriorate when tests are applied in clinical practice. The result of a test for coronary artery disease, such as an electron beam computed tomography scan, rarely may be abnormal if it is evaluated in a low-risk population, such as high-school students. False-positive abnormal results secondary to coronary calcification in the absence of obstructive coronary disease are common when the test is performed in middle-aged and elderly people.

Although researchers are interested in the performance of tests, the true focus of medical decision making is the patient. Physicians are more interested in the implications of a test result on the probability that a patient has a specific disease or outcome, that is, the predictive values of abnormal or normal test results. These predictive values are extremely sensitive to the population from which they are derived (Table 9-2; see also Table 9-1). An abnormal lung scan result in an asymptomatic patient has a much lower positive predictive value than that same test result in a patient with dyspnea and a diminished oxygen saturation. Bayes' theorem (see later) provides a framework for analyzing the interaction between test results and a patient's pretest probability of a disease.

As useful as the performance characteristics may be, they are limited by the fact that few tests truly provide dichotomous (i.e., positive or negative) test results. Tests such as exercise tests have several parameters (e.g., ST segment deviation, exercise duration, hemodynamic response) that provide insight into the patient's condition, and the normal range for many blood tests (e.g., prostate-specific antigen) varies markedly according to the age of the tested population and one's willingness to "miss" patients with disease. Tests that require human interpretation (e.g., radiologic studies) are particularly subject to variability in the reported results.

Bayes' Theorem

The impact of a test result on a patient's probability of disease was first quantified by Bayes, an 18th-century English clergyman who developed a formula that describes the probability of disease in the presence of an abnormal test result. The classic presentation of Bayes' theorem is complex and difficult to use. A simpler form of this theorem is known as the *odds ratio* form, which describes the impact of a test result on the pretest odds (see Table 9-1) of a diagnosis or outcome for a specific patient.

To calculate the post-test odds of disease, the pretest odds are multiplied by the *likelihood ratio* (LR) for a specific test result. The mathematical presentation of this form of Bayes' theorem is as follows:

$$\text{Post-test odds} = (\text{Pretest odds}) \times (\text{LR})$$

The LR is the probability of a particular test result in patients with the disease divided by the probability of that same test result in patients without disease. In other words, the LR is the test result's sensitivity divided by the false-positive rate. A test of no value (e.g., flipping a coin and calling "heads" an abnormal result) would have an LR of 1.0 because half of patients with disease would have abnormal test results, as would half of patients without disease. This test would have no impact on a patient's odds of disease. The further an LR is above 1.0, the more that test result raises a patient's probability of disease. For LRs less than 1.0, the closer the LR is to 0, the more it lowers a patient's probability of disease.

When it is displayed graphically (Fig. 9-1), a test of no value (*dotted line*) does not change the pretest probability, whereas an abnormal or normal result from a useful test moves the probability up or down. For a patient with a high pretest probability of disease, an abnormal test result changes the patient's probability only slightly, but a normal test result leads to a marked reduction in the probability of disease. Similarly, for a patient with a low pretest probability of disease, a normal test result has little impact, but an abnormal test result markedly raises the probability of disease.

Consider how various exercise test results influence a patient's probability of coronary disease (see Table 9-2). For a patient whose clinical history, physical examination, and electrocardiographic findings suggest a 50% probability of disease, the pretest odds of disease are 1.0. LRs for various test results are developed by pooling data from published literature. The sensitivity of an exercise test with any amount of ST segment changes is the rate of such test results in patients with coronary disease, and the specificity is the percentage of patients without coronary disease who do *not* have this test result. The LR for no ST change is less than 1, whereas the LRs for patients with ST changes are greater than 1 (see Table 9-2). Therefore, when the LRs for various test results are multiplied by the pretest odds to calculate post-test odds, the odds decrease for patients without ST segment changes but increase for patients with 1 or 2 mm of ST segment change. Post-test odds can be converted to post-test probabilities according to the following formula:

$$\text{Probability} = \text{Odds}/(1 + \text{odds})$$

The calculations quantify how the absence of ST segment changes reduces a patient's probability of disease, whereas ST segment depression raises the probability of disease.

This form of Bayes' theorem is useful for showing how the post-test probability of disease is influenced by the patient's pretest probability of disease.

TABLE 9-2 EXAMPLE OF ODDS RATIO FORM OF BAYES' THEOREM

Question: What is the probability of coronary disease for a patient with a 50% pretest probability of coronary disease who undergoes an exercise test if that patient develops (a) no ST segment changes, (b) 1 mm of ST segment depression, or (c) 2 mm of ST segment depression?

Step 1. Calculate the pretest odds of disease:

$$P/(1-P) = 0.5/(1-0.5) = 0.5/0.5 = 1$$

Step 2. Calculate the likelihood ratios for the various test results, using the formula LR = sensitivity/(1 – specificity). (Data from pooled literature.)

TEST RESULT	SENSITIVITY	SPECIFICITY	LIKELIHOOD RATIO
No ST segment changes	0.34	0.15	0.4
1-mm ST segment depression	0.66	0.85	4.4
2-mm ST segment depression	0.33	0.97	11

Step 3. Calculate the post-test odds of disease and convert those odds to post-test probabilities:

TEST RESULT	PRETEST ODDS	LIKELIHOOD RATIO	POST-TEST ODDS	POST-TEST PROBABILITY
No ST segment changes	1	0.4	0.4	0.29
1-mm ST segment depression	1	4.4	4.4	0.81
2-mm ST segment depression	1	11	11	0.92

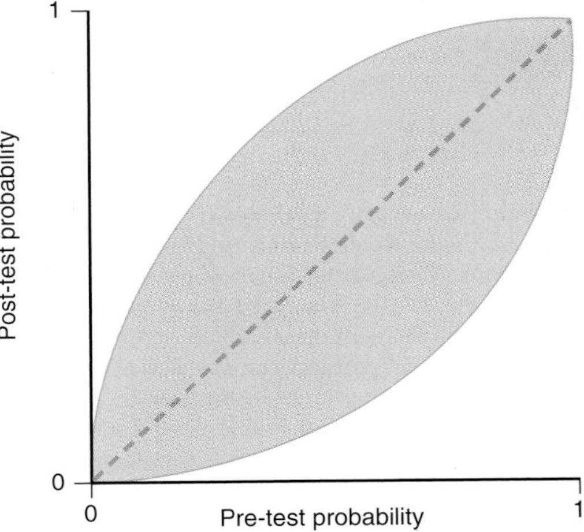

FIGURE 9-1. **Impact of various test results on the patient's probability of disease.** The x axis depicts a patient's probability of disease before a test. If the test is of no value, the post-test probability *(dotted line)* is no different from the pretest probability. An abnormal test result raises the post-test probability of disease, as depicted by the concave downward arc, whereas a normal test result lowers the probability.

TABLE 9-3 PRINCIPLES OF TEST ORDERING AND INTERPRETATION

The interpretation of test results depends on what is already known about the patient.

No test is perfect; clinicians should be familiar with their diagnostic performance (see Table 9-1) and never believe that a test "forces" them to pursue a specific management strategy.

Tests should be ordered if they may provide *additional* information beyond that already available.

Tests should be ordered if there is a reasonable chance that the data will influence the patient's care.

Two tests that provide similar information should not be ordered.

In choosing between two tests that provide similar data, use the test that has lower costs and/or causes less discomfort and inconvenience to the patient.

Clinicians should seek all of the information provided by a test, not just an abnormal or normal result.

The cost-effectiveness of strategies using noninvasive tests should be considered in a manner similar to that of therapeutic strategies.

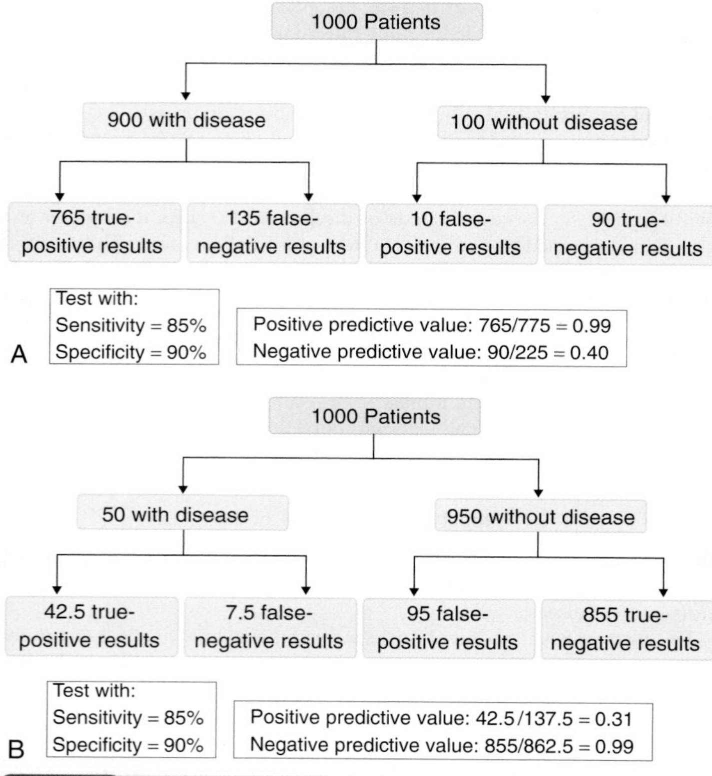

FIGURE 9-2. **Interpretation of test results in high-risk and low-risk patients. A,** High-risk population (90% prevalence of disease). **B,** Low-risk population (5% prevalence of disease).

If a patient's clinical data suggest a *probability* of coronary disease of only 0.1, the *pretest odds* of disease would be only 0.11. For such a low-risk patient, an exercise test with no ST segment changes would lead to post-test probability of coronary disease of 4%, whereas 1- or 2-mm ST segment changes would lead to a post-test probability of disease of 33 or 55%.

Even if clinicians rarely perform the calculations that are described in Bayes' theorem, there are important lessons from this theorem that are relevant to principles of test ordering (Table 9-3). The most crucial of these lessons is that the interpretation of test results must incorporate information about the patient. An abnormal test result in a low-risk patient may not be a true indicator of disease. Similarly, a normal test result in a high-risk patient should not be taken as evidence that disease is not present.

Figure 9-2 provides an example of the post-test probabilities for positive and negative results for a test with a sensitivity of 85% and a specificity of 90% (e.g., radionuclide scintigraphy for diagnosis of coronary artery disease). In a high-risk population with a 90% prevalence of disease, the positive predictive value of an abnormal result is 0.99 compared with 0.31 for the same test result obtained in a low-risk population with a 5% prevalence of disease. Similarly, the negative predictive value of a normal test result is greater in the low-risk population than in the high-risk population.

Multiple Testing

Clinicians frequently obtain more than one test aimed at addressing the same issue and at times are confronted with conflicting results. If these tests are truly independent (i.e., the tests do not have the same basis in pathophysiology), it may be appropriate to use the post-test probability obtained through performance of one test as the pretest probability for the analysis of the impact of the second test result.

If the tests are not independent, this strategy for interpretation of serial test results can be misleading. Suppose a patient with chronic obstructive pulmonary disease and a history vaguely suggestive of pulmonary embolism is found to have an abnormal lung ventilation-perfusion scan. Obtaining that same test result over and over would not raise that patient's probability of pulmonary embolism higher and higher. In this extreme case, the tests are identical; serial testing adds no information. More commonly, clinicians are faced with results from tests with related but not identical bases in pathophysiology, such as ventilation-perfusion scintigraphy and pulmonary angiography.

Regardless of whether tests are independent, the performance of multiple tests increases the likelihood that an abnormal test result will be obtained in a patient without disease. If a chemistry battery includes 20 tests and the normal range for each test has been developed to include 95% of healthy individuals, the chance that a healthy patient will have a normal result for any specific test is 0.95. However, the probability that all 20 tests will be normal is $(0.95)^{20}$, or 0.36. Most healthy people can be expected to have at least one abnormal result. Unless screening test profiles are used thoughtfully, false-positive results can subject patients to unnecessary tests and procedures.

Threshold Approach to Decision Making

Even if a test provides information, that information may not change management for an individual patient. Lumbar spine radiographs of a patient who is not willing to undergo surgery may reveal the severity of disease but expose the patient to needless radiation. Similarly, a test that merely confirms a diagnosis that already is recognized is a waste of resources (see Table 9-3).

Before ordering a test, clinicians should consider whether that test result could change the choice of management strategies. This approach is called the *threshold approach to medical decision making*, and it requires the physician to be able to estimate the threshold probability at which one strategy will be chosen over another. The management of a clinically stable patient with a high probability of coronary disease might not be changed by any of the post-test probabilities shown in Table 9-2. If that patient had no ST segment changes, the post-test probability of 0.29 still would be too high for a clinician to consider that patient free of disease. An abnormal test result that strengthened the diagnosis of coronary disease might not change management unless it suggested a greater severity of disease that might warrant another management strategy.

Testing for Peace of Mind

Physicians frequently order tests even when there is little chance that the outcomes will provide qualitatively new insights into a patient's diagnosis or prognosis or alter a patient's management. In such cases, the cited goal for testing may be to improve a patient's peace of mind. Although a decrease in uncertainty can improve quality of life for many patients, individuals with hypochondriasis and somatization disorders rarely obtain comfort from normal test results; instead, their complaints shift to a new organ system, and their demands focus on other tests. For such patients, management strategies using frequent visits and cognitive tactics are recommended.

WHICH TEST IS BEST?

If the clinician decided that more information is needed to reduce uncertainty, and if it appears possible that tests might lead to a change in management strategies, the question arises as to which test is most appropriate. Note that just because guideline-development committees have concluded that a specific test is "appropriate" in given clinical context, this does not mean that this test is the *most* appropriate option. Several factors influence the choice among diagnostic strategies, including patients' preferences, the costs and risks associated with the tests, and the diagnostic performance of alternative tests.

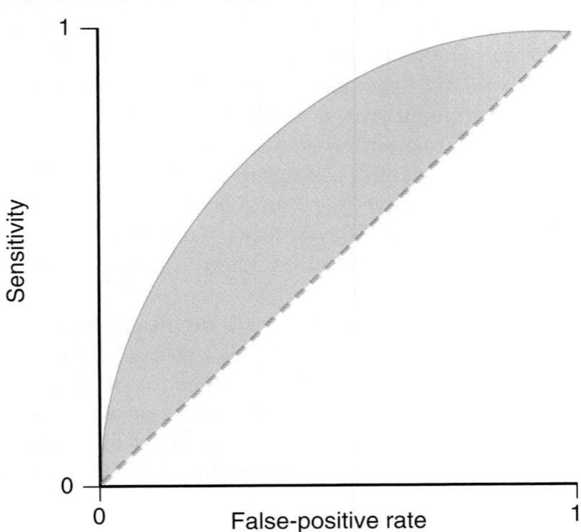

FIGURE 9-3. Receiver operating characteristic curve. The points on the curve reflect the sensitivity and false-positive (1 – specificity) rates of a test at various thresholds. As the threshold is changed to yield greater sensitivity for detecting the outcome of interest, the false-positive rate rises. The better the test, the closer the curve comes to the upper left corner. A test of no value (e.g., flipping a coin) would lead to a curve with the course of the *dotted line.* The area under the curve is used often to compare alternative testing strategies.

Diagnostic performance of a test often is summarized in terms of sensitivity and specificity, but as shown in the example in Table 9-2, these parameters depend on which threshold (e.g., 1 vs. 2 mm of ST segment change) is used. A low threshold for calling a test result abnormal might lead to excellent sensitivity for detecting disease, but at the expense of a high false-positive rate. Conversely, a threshold that led to few false-positive results might cause a clinician to miss many cases of true disease.

The receiver operating characteristic (ROC) curve is a graphic form of describing this tradeoff and providing a method for comparing test performance (Fig. 9-3). Each point on the ROC curve describes the sensitivity and the false-positive rate for a different threshold for abnormality for a test. A test of no value would lead to an ROC curve with the course of the dotted line, whereas a misleading test would be described by a curve that was concave upward (not shown).

The more accurate the test, the closer its ROC curve comes to the upper left corner of the graph, which would indicate a test threshold that has excellent sensitivity and a low false-positive rate. The closer an ROC curve comes to the upper left corner, the greater the area under the curve. The area under ROC curves can be used to compare the information provided by two tests.

Even if one test is superior to another as shown by a greater area under its ROC curve, the question still remains as to what value of that test should be considered abnormal. The choice of threshold depends on the purpose of testing and on the consequences of a false-positive or false-negative diagnosis. If the goal is to screen the population for a disease that is potentially fatal and potentially curable, a threshold with excellent sensitivity is appropriate even if it leads to frequent false-positive results. In contrast, if a test is used to confirm a diagnosis that is likely to be treated with a high-risk invasive procedure, a threshold with high specificity is preferred. Only 1 mm of ST segment depression might be the appropriate threshold when exercise electrocardiography is used to evaluate the possibility of coronary disease in a patient with chest pain. If the question is whether to perform coronary angiography in a patient with stable angina in search of severe coronary disease that might benefit from revascularization, a threshold of 2 mm or more would be more appropriate.

CHOOSING A STRATEGY

Physicians and patients ultimately must use clinical information to make decisions. These choices usually are made after consideration of a variety of factors, including information from the clinical evaluation, patients' preferences, and expected outcomes with various management strategies. Insight into the impact of these considerations can be improved through the performance of decision analysis (Table 9-4).

TABLE 9-4 STEPS IN PERFORMANCE OF DECISION ANALYSIS

Frame the question.
Create the decision tree.
- Identify the alternative strategies.
- List the possible outcomes for each of the alternative strategies.
- Describe the sequence of events as a series of decision nodes and chance nodes.

Choose a time horizon for the analysis.
Determine the probability for each chance outcome.
Assign a value to each outcome.
Calculate the expected utility for each strategy.
Perform sensitivity analysis.

The first step in a decision analysis is to define the problem clearly; this step often requires writing out a statement of the issue so that it can be scrutinized for any ambiguity. After the problem is defined, the next step is to define the alternative strategies.

Consider the question of which test is most appropriate to screen patients for breast cancer: mammography with or without breast magnetic resonance imaging—a newer technology that is highly sensitive for detecting breast cancer but is more costly and less specific. The expected outcomes for these strategies depend on each test's sensitivity and specificity for detecting breast cancer, which is influenced in turn by other factors, such as the frequency with which the test is performed. Patients' outcomes also are influenced by their underlying risk for breast cancer and the likelihood that earlier detection of tumors reduces the risk for death.

Each of these variables must be known or estimated for calculations to be made of each strategy's predicted life expectancy and direct medical costs. These outcomes differ for patients according to age, medical history, family history, and presence or absence of genetic markers such as *BRCA* mutations. Optimal strategies for an elderly patient with a short life expectancy and low clinical risk of cancer are unlikely to be the same as for a younger patient with inherited mutations of the *BRCA1* or *BRCA2* gene, indicating a cumulative lifetime risk of breast cancer of 50 to 85% (Chapter 204).

The credibility of the decision analysis depends on the credibility of these estimates. Published reports often do not provide information on the outcomes of interest for specific subsets of patients, or there may not have been sufficient statistical power within subsets of patients for the findings to be statistically significant. Randomized trial data are relevant to the populations included in the trial; the extension of the findings to other genders, races, and age groups requires assumptions by individuals performing the analysis. For many issues, expert opinion must be used to derive a reasonable estimate of the outcome.

For many diseases, the potential outcomes are more complex than perfect health or death. With chronic diseases, patients may live many years in a condition somewhere between these two, and the goal of medical interventions may be to improve quality of life rather than to extend survival. The value of life in imperfect health must be reflected in decision analyses. These values by convention are expressed on a scale of 0 to 100, where 0 indicates the worst outcome and 100 indicates the best outcome.

Life-expectancy and quality-of-life estimates are combined in many decision analyses to calculate *quality-adjusted life years.* A strategy that leads to a 10-year life expectancy with such severe disability that utility of the state of health is only half that of perfect health would have a quality-adjusted life expectancy of 5 years. With such adjustments to life-expectancy data, the impact of interventions that improve quality of life but do not extend life can be compared with interventions that extend life but do not improve its quality or perhaps even worsen it.

After the value and the probability of the various outcomes have been estimated, the expected utility of each strategy can be calculated. In comparing the different strategies available at a decision node, the analysis generally selects the option with the highest expected utility. At chance nodes, the expected utility is the weighted average of the utility of the various possible branches.

After the analysis has been performed with the baseline assumptions, *sensitivity analyses* should be performed in which these assumptions are varied over a reasonable range. These analyses can reveal which assumptions have the most influence over the conclusions and identify threshold probabilities at which the conclusions would change. For example, the threshold at which breast magnetic resonance imaging should be added to mammography is likely to be influenced by the cost of the magnetic resonance imaging and the accuracy of the radiologists who interpret the images.

Cost-Benefit and Cost-Effectiveness Analyses

For clinicians and health care policymakers, the choices that must be addressed go beyond the choices within any single decision analysis. Because resources available for health care are limited, policymakers may have to choose among many competing "investments" in health. Although such decisions frequently are made on the basis of political considerations, cost-benefit and cost-effectiveness analyses can be informative in making the choices.

The methodology of these techniques is similar to that of decision analysis except that costs for the various possible outcomes and strategies also are calculated. *Discounting* is used to adjust the value of future benefits and costs because resources saved or spent currently are worth more than resources saved or expended in the future. In *cost-benefit* analyses, all benefits are expressed in terms of economic impact. Extensions in life expectancy are translated into dollars by estimating societal worth or economic productivity.

Because of the ethical discomfort associated with expressing health benefits in financial terms, *cost-effectiveness* analyses are used more commonly than cost-benefit analyses. In these analyses, the ratio of costs to health benefits is calculated; one frequently used method for evaluating a strategy is calculation of cost per quality-adjusted life year. These estimates can be used to compare strategies and to identify settings in which strategies that may be more expensive but more effective (e.g., coronary angiography) may "purchase" quality-adjusted life years at a lower cost than less aggressive but less effective strategies (e.g., use of positron emission tomography scanning to diagnose coronary disease) (Table 9-5).

Cost-effectiveness analyses can provide important insights into the relative attractiveness of different management strategies and can help guide policymakers in decisions about which technologies to make available on a routine basis. No medical intervention can have an attractive cost-effectiveness if its effectiveness has not been proved. The cost-effectiveness of an intervention depends heavily on the population of patients in which it is applied. An

TABLE 9-5 ESTIMATED COST-EFFECTIVENESS OF COMMON HEALTH INTERVENTIONS

DISEASE CATEGORY	INTERVENTION VS. COMPARATOR IN TARGET POPULATION	COST PER QUALITY-ADJUSTED LIFE YEAR*
Circulatory	Coronary angiography vs. positron emission tomography (PET) in 55-year-old women with chest pain and risk factors that put them at intermediate pretest probability (25-75%) of coronary artery disease	Cost saving
	Angiography vs. exercise electrocardiography (ECG) in patients with no history of myocardial infarction presenting with mild chest pain (typical angina) who are able to undergo an exercise stress test	$47,000
	Exercise single-photon emission computed tomography (SPECT) vs. exercise ECG in patients with no history of myocardial infarction presenting with mild chest pain (typical angina) who are able to undergo an exercise stress test.	$52,000
	Angiography vs. exercise ECG in patients with no history of myocardial infarction presenting with mild chest pain (atypical angina) who are able to undergo an exercise stress test	$89,000
	In patients after a first stroke or transient ischemic attack, patients with heart disease receive transesophageal echocardiography and all others receive standard medical treatment vs. all receive standard medical treatment.	$240,000
	High-dose statin therapy vs. conventional-dose statin therapy in 60-year-old cohorts with acute coronary syndromes (ACS)	$14,000
	Prophylactic implantation of an implantable-cardioverter defibrillator (ICD) vs. control therapy in patients who are at risk for sudden death due to left ventricular systolic dysfunction—Sudden Cardiac Death in Heart Failure Trial (SCD HeFT) population (https://research.tufts-nemc.org/cear/search/detail.aspx?ArticleId=2005-01-01184&id=2005-01-01184-08C)	$77,000
	Cardiac resynchronization therapy (CRT-P) plus medical therapy vs. medical therapy in a 60-year-old patient with heart failure and cardiac dyssynchrony with moderate or severe symptoms (https://research.tufts-nemc.org/cear/search/detail.aspx?ArticleId=2007-01-02351&id=2007-01-02351-13C)	$9,900
Endocrine	Thyroid-stimulating hormone (TSH) screening vs. no TSH screening in women undergoing 5-year periodic health examinations, beginning at 35 years old	$13,000
	Annual diabetic retinopathy screening vs. no screening; diabetic patients receive routine medical care until they become blind in patients diagnosed with type 2 diabetes, aged 30 years or older, undergoing eye screening (https://research.tufts-nemc.org/cear/search/detail.aspx?ArticleId=2008-01-03569&id=2008-01-03569-01C)	Cost saving
	Intensive lifestyle intervention vs. usual care in 60-year-old cohort with impaired glucose tolerance	Cost saving
	Self-monitoring of blood glucose (SMBG) vs. no SMBG in patients with type 2 diabetes receiving insulin only (https://research.tufts-nemc.org/cear/search/detail.aspx?ArticleId=2006-01-02649&id=2006-01-02649-03C)	$9600
	Intensive glucose control, therapies designed to produce HbA1c (A1C) levels of 7.2% vs. conventional glucose control, therapies designed to produce HbA1c (A1C) levels of 10% in patients with new-onset type 2 diabetes at 60-65 years of age	$200,000
Digestive system	Endoscopic surveillance strategy vs. no therapy in man who has endoscopic biopsy-proven Barrett's esophagus—age 55 years	$150,000
	One-time colonoscopic screening for colorectal cancer at age 60-64 years old vs. no screening in men >40 years old	Cost saving
Infectious	One-time rapid HIV infection screening vs. no screening in U.S. communities with low to moderate HIV prevalence (0.05% to 1.0%) and annual incidence (0.0084% to 0.12%)	$35,000
	Treating patients with peginterferon alfa-2b plus ribavirin vs. no treatment in 55-year-old male naïve patients with genotypes 1, 2, and 3 chronic hepatitis C virus (HCV) infection	Cost saving
	Provision of influenza vaccine vs. no provision of service (no vaccine) in U.S. population age 50 years and older	$7,300
Injury	Driver air bag vs. no air bags in driving population (and passengers)	$36,000
	Dual air bag vs. driver air bag in driving population (and passengers)	$91,000
Obstetrics	Elective repeat cesarean section vs. vaginal birth (trial of labor) in 30-year-old patients who have had a previous low transverse cesarean delivery	$140,000
	Elective cesarean delivery vs. vaginal delivery in 25-year-old HIV-infected pregnant women with detectable HIV RNA	Cost saving
Oncology	Adjuvant chemotherapy plus trastuzumab vs. chemotherapy alone in patients with *HER2*-positive early breast cancer, from the U.S. health care system	$21,000
	MRI vs. mammography in women aged 40-49 years with *BRCA1* mutation	$16,000

*In 2008 U.S. dollars.
HIV = human immunodeficiency virus; RNA = ribonucleic acid; TSH = thyroid-stimulating hormone.
Center for the Evaluation of Value and Risk in Health. The Cost-Effectiveness Analysis Registry [Internet]. Boston: Institute for Clinical Research and Health Policy Studies, Tufts Medical Center. http://www.cearegistry.org 2009. Accessed Aug. 8, 2009.

inexpensive intervention would have a poor cost-effectiveness ratio if it were used in a low-risk population unlikely to benefit from it. In contrast, an expensive technology can have an attractive cost-effectiveness ratio if it is used in patients with a high probability of benefiting from it. Table 9-5 shows cost-effectiveness estimates from published literature for some common medical and nonmedical interventions. Such estimates should be used only with understanding of the population for which they are relevant.

SUGGESTED READINGS

Bonow RO. Should coronary calcium screening be used in cardiovascular prevention strategies? *N Engl J Med.* 2009;361:990-997. *Analysis of its potential value to improve risk stratification and management.*

CEA Registry. http://www.tufts-nemc.org/cearegistry; 2010. Accessed Nov. 11, 2010. *Through this website, the Harvard Center for Risk Analysis provides all published cost-effectiveness ratios, sorted by disease area and standardized according to 2008 dollars.*

Esserman L, Shieh Y, Thompson I. Rethinking screening for breast cancer and prostate cancer. *JAMA.* 2009;302:1685. *Assessment of the disappointing impact from breast and prostate cancer screening, with calls for new approaches.*

Kelly M, Morgan A, Ellis S, et al. Evidence based public health: a review of the experience of the National Institute of Health and Clinical Excellence (NICE) of developing public health guidance in England. *Soc Sci Med.* 2010;71:1056-1062. *Example of how data can guide health policy decisions.*

Wald NJ, Morris JK. Assessing risk factors as potential screening tests: A simple assessment tool. *Arch Intern Med.* 2011;171:286-291. *Shows when risk factors are and probably are not useful ways to screen for the probability of certain disease.*

10

MEASURING HEALTH AND HEALTH CARE

STEPHAN D. FIHN

The increasing emphasis on measuring and improving the quality of health care in the United States and elsewhere is based on several fundamental concerns. First, there is clear evidence that the health care system in the United States does not provide the highest quality of care possible. In one study, approximately 4600 randomly selected adults from 12 U.S. cities received recommended preventive, acute, or chronic care only slightly more than half the time. Second, substantial disparities in health care and outcomes persist, with women (Chapter 245), the poor (Chapter 5), and ethnic minorities (Chapter 4) typically faring less well than others. Third, there is growing concern that health care sometimes causes harm, as reflected by statistics indicating that 1 in 6.5 hospitalizations is complicated by a mistake in administering or prescribing medication, that 1 in 20 outpatient prescriptions is wrong, or that inpatient errors may cause as many as 44,000 to 98,000 deaths annually (Chapter 11). Fourth, health care is extraordinarily expensive, with an annual aggregate expenditure of more than $2 trillion (nearly $7500 per resident) that consumes nearly 17% of the U.S. gross domestic product (Chapter 5). If premiums for health insurance grow at the projected national rate of increase, the cost of family coverage will double from the 2008 average of $12,298 to $24,000 or even higher by 2020. Moreover, there is substantial evidence that the delivery system is inefficient and wasteful. Per capita expenditures for health care vary as much as 250% among communities of similar size, without any evidence that higher spending leads to better outcomes. In fact, observational data from Medicare suggest that there is actually an inverse relationship between the amount of overall health care spending at the state level and better quality.

Findings such as these have fueled demands from government, employers, and consumer groups for greater accountability and improved quality. In response, the information collected to measure health and health care has increased dramatically. Physicians and other health care providers are frequently confronted with these data in nearly every sphere of activity, including clinical care, education, and research. To interpret and apply this information correctly, health care providers should understand the basic principles of measuring the process and outcomes of health care.

MEASUREMENT OF HEALTH CARE

The basic paradigm that guides assessment of quality includes three fundamental domains: structure, process, and outcome. *Structure* refers to the stable elements that make up the health care system, such as the physical plant, administrative organizations, and qualifications of the staff. Because structural characteristics, such as whether floors are clean or doctors are board certified, are often the easiest aspects of health care to observe and measure, they were the main focus of early efforts to improve quality. Over time, however, it became clear that a clean environment and qualified providers are essential but insufficient to guarantee high quality unless the process of care is effective.

Process refers to how care is delivered, including medical interventions and interpersonal interactions. Thus it is important to know, for instance, whether the right physician has performed the right procedure on the right patient in the right way at the right time. Documenting these findings for the multitude of patients, however, can be expensive, difficult, and subjective because there may be a variety of acceptable approaches to a given clinical problem. Moreover, patients tend to be more concerned about achieving the best possible outcomes of care, such as curing disease, reducing symptoms, or improving function, than about how these outcomes are achieved.

Outcomes represent the presumptive results of care that is delivered. The concept of health outcomes encompasses a broad array of clinical indicators that include death, adverse clinical events, persistence or recurrence of disease, disability, discomfort, and pain. Outcomes from the patient's perspective include self-reported health, ability to function, burden imposed by disease, and satisfaction with care. In addition, there may be societal perspectives, such as cost-effectiveness and the cost-benefit ratio (Chapter 9). Judging care on the basis of outcomes is challenging because it may be difficult to measure outcomes reliably and because studies often fail to identify a relationship between high scores on process measures and better outcomes, such as lower in-hospital mortality. Indeed, recent studies of the quality of health care demonstrate that it is important to select measures that are adequately specified and provide a "tight" linkage between process and outcome.

STANDARDS OF MEASUREMENT

Irrespective of what aspect of health care is being evaluated, the measures used should satisfy standards that help ensure the trustworthiness of the data generated. These standards include adequate specification, reliability, validity, responsiveness, and interpretability. A measure that is *adequately specified* has a well-defined numerator that explicitly describes patients who meet the relevant criteria (e.g., patients whose blood pressure is <140/90 mm Hg or who are followed up within 2 weeks), a well-defined denominator (e.g., patients with hypertension or those discharged with heart failure), and a clear description of patients who are excluded from the calculation (e.g., patients who are younger than 18 years, who have not had an appointment within 18 months, or for whom only comfort care is being provided).

A *reliable* measure yields consistent results when repeated under similar circumstances. Although random error can never be eliminated, one would expect, for example, that two reviewers examining the same medical records would classify the outcomes in the same fashion in all but a small minority of cases. The level of reliability can be compared with common diagnostic procedures in medicine, many of which demonstrate only moderate reliability. For example, common methods of echocardiographic determination of ejection fraction vary up to 24% (Chapter 55), the intraclass coefficient for exercise treadmill tests performed a day apart is only 0.70, and the interobserver correlation for ascertaining the presence of coronary stenosis by highly trained experts is approximately 0.75 (Chapter 57).

Validity refers to the accurate measurement of an intended effect or outcome. In the case of physiologic measures, such as diagnosis of coronary artery disease with electron beam computed tomography (Chapter 56), validity would be indicated by the likelihood of coronary stenoses demonstrated angiographically. In actuality, demonstrable coronary stenoses are present in only 55 to 84% of patients who have a positive result on electron beam computed tomography, which makes it a relatively invalid outcome measure. Validity for measures of subjective outcomes, such as pain, is typically documented through correlation with other related measures, such as the use of analgesic medications or limitation of activities.

Responsiveness reflects the sensitivity of a measure to clinically meaningful changes in status. Whereas a patient with worsening osteoarthritis might record no change on an instrument assessing activities such as bathing or dressing, this patient might exhibit declining scores on a measure that addresses more vigorous activities.

These principles of measurement apply to both quality improvement and research studies, although the standards used in research are generally more rigorous. Measures are typically developed initially for use in research studies and, when shown to possess acceptable performance, are applied to routine quality improvement activities.

Additional criteria should be applied to measures that are being considered for routine use in a clinical setting (Table 10-1), including whether a measure

TABLE 10-1 CRITERIA FOR EVALUATING SUITABILITY OF A CLINICAL PERFORMANCE MEASURE

1. Are the performance characteristics of the measure well established—i.e., valid and reliable?
   The measure appears to measure what is intended (face validity).
   The measure captures most meaningful aspects of care (content validity).
   The measure is reproducible over time and in multiple organizational settings (reliability).
2. Is the measure adequately specified?
   Numerator: definition of patients meeting measure (e.g., patients with blood pressure <140/90 mm Hg or followed up within 2 wk).
   Denominator: definition of patients qualifying for measure (e.g., patients with hypertension).
   Included populations.
   Excluded populations.
3. Is the measure likely to be useful in improving patient outcomes?
   Scientific basis for the measure is well established.
   The results of the measure are interpretable by individual(s) who are responsible for relevant activity.
   The measure is actionable—i.e., addresses an activity or function that is under the control of individual(s) who are responsible and that is amenable to change.
   Implementation of the measure is anticipated to promote the adoption of interventions that have the potential to improve patient outcomes substantially.
   The clinical burden of the condition(s) related to the measure in the affected population is sufficient to warrant measurement and corresponding intervention.
   Current levels of performance related to the measure within the health system indicate substantial opportunities of performance.
4. Can the measure feasibly be implemented?
   The data required for the measure are likely to be obtained with reasonable effort, at reasonable cost, and within a reasonable time frame.
   Data for the measure can be collected automatically when possible.
   The measure has undergone adequate field testing.
5. The measure is relevant to the strategic goals of the health care system.

is *interpretable, evidence based, actionable, feasible,* and *relevant.* An interpretable measure can be understood and applied in clinical settings. For example, although most physicians understand the clinical implications of a change in arterial pH from 7.42 to 7.30, they might not have the same appreciation of a 20-point change on a 100-point scale that measures physical function or satisfaction. Moreover, a measure should be closely related to an intervention that has the potential to improve outcomes that are linked to the burden of the condition in the population.

TYPES OF MEASURES

Driven largely by efforts to compare the performance of providers and different health care systems, considerable effort has been expended to standardize measures at a national level. Examples include the Healthcare Effectiveness Data and Information Set (HEDIS), which is a set of standardized performance measures designed to assist purchasers and consumers in comparing the care and service provided by more than 90% of health plans in the United States. Another is ORYX, a set of national hospital quality measures collected by the Joint Commission on Accreditation of Healthcare Organizations (E-Table 10-1). Most of these are process measures, although some structural measures and intermediate outcome measures (see later) are included. The National Quality Forum (NQF), which is a quasi-public organization with more than 375 members from various sectors of the health care system, evaluates and issues endorsements for performance measures proposed by many different organizations.

Linkage between Process and Outcome Measures

Process measures are of greatest value when there is a close association, or tight linkage, between a process or action and an outcome. Numerous clinical trials, for example, have shown a substantial reduction in mortality when patients with hypercholesterolemia and ischemic heart disease are given a hydroxymethylglutaryl-coenzyme A reductase inhibitor (statin) to lower low-density lipoprotein cholesterol (LDL-C) levels (Chapter 213). Accordingly, the use of statins in appropriate patients is commonly used as an indicator of quality in many health care organizations. There are, however, limitations to using LDL-C measured at a single point in time; for instance, there may be a legitimate reason for LDL-C to be over the target range in as many as half of patients who would otherwise appear to have received poor-quality care. Such reasons include having only recently started taking statins, and the dosage is still being titrated; having refused therapy; having a high LDL-C level despite maximal therapy; or having experienced an adverse effect of statins.

Intermediate and Combined Outcomes

Because many outcomes of interest, such as death or the occurrence of serious adverse events, may be relatively infrequent, *intermediate* or *surrogate outcomes* are sometimes measured instead of the true outcome of interest. Intermediate outcomes are often physiologic variables such as blood pressure, cholesterol level, or hemoglobin A_{1c} concentration. For example, the primary rationale for treating diabetes is to prevent complications such as blindness, amputation, or renal failure, and the efficacy of treatment should ultimately be determined by a reduction in risk for these complications. Though important in the pathophysiology of diabetes, a change in the measured hemoglobin A_{1c} level is meaningful as an outcome measure (particularly to the patient) only insofar as it reflects a reduction in risk afforded by treatment. As opposed to standard physiologic measures, other intermediate outcomes reflect subclinical disease; for example, microalbuminuria indicates subclinical renal disease in diabetes (Chapter 236). Intermediate outcomes are attractive because they are often familiar to clinicians and can readily be measured repeatedly in most or all patients, whereas the outcome of interest (e.g., amputation) is a relatively infrequent event in patients treated for diabetes. Using intermediate outcomes may be deceptive, however, particularly when the linkage to the true outcome of interest is loose. The presence of microalbuminuria in a patient with type 2 diabetes (Chapter 237), for instance, is associated with a 2½-fold increase in the relative odds of dying over a 6-year period when compared with diabetic patients who have no protein in their urine. This sizable increase in relative risk, however, translates into a relatively small increase in absolute risk for any individual in any given year. Thus, changes in quality as measured by rates of microalbuminuria would probably not be reflected in outcome measures such as the incidence of cardiovascular events or renal failure, except in extremely large populations. Moreover, it is possible for a treatment to have a salutary effect on a surrogate outcome but a deleterious effect overall. Such was the case for short-acting dihydropyridines such as nifedipine, which effectively lowered blood pressure in hypertensive patients but doubled the incidence of myocardial infarction.

Another strategy adopted when outcome events are infrequent is the use of combined end points. An example is the incidence of cardiovascular events, including stroke, myocardial infarction, unstable angina, and sudden cardiac death. This approach can improve the statistical power of a study, but it tends to exaggerate the perceived efficacy of a particular intervention and may obscure specific effects, such as when an intervention reduces the frequency of stroke more than it does myocardial infarction.

Patient-Oriented Measures

Although physiologic and standard clinical measures are important, the assessment of outcomes from the patient's perspective has increasingly been recognized as being of equal or even greater importance, especially when evaluating treatments intended to lessen symptoms or improve function rather than improve survival. Approaches that depend on a physician's perception of a patient's condition, such as the Canadian Cardiovascular Society Classification for cardiac symptoms (Chapter 50), are limited because physicians often tend to underestimate a patient's symptoms or disability, and such assessments are difficult to standardize. Self-reporting of health and function by patients themselves via standardized questionnaires overcomes these problems. The terminology used to describe the hundreds of questionnaires now available is evolving and, at times, confusing, but the resulting scales generally address various aspects of health-related quality of life, which is a complex, multidimensional concept. Facets or subscales of quality of life may include the severity of symptoms, pain, physical functioning, social functioning, general perceptions of health, overall burden of disease, emotional well-being, and coping, among others.

General measures of health status or health-related quality of life, such as the Short-Form 36 (SF-36), do not focus on a specific disease or condition but seek to assess overall health and functioning. General measures may, however, be insensitive to a specific yet clinically meaningful change in symptoms related to a particular condition. For this reason, more than 1000 *condition-specific measures* are now available. Whereas a patient's score on a questionnaire dealing with overall health might not change in response to successful treatment of a specific condition, such as gastroesophageal reflux, the score on a questionnaire specifically addressing symptoms of heartburn would register a substantial change.

In the past, measures of self-reported health were criticized as being "soft" and overly subjective. In fact, many general and condition-specific measures demonstrate reliability and validity that equal or exceed those of many physiologic or clinical measures commonly used in research or clinical settings. For example, among patients undergoing coronary artery bypass grafting (Chapter 74), a 10-point reduction in self-reported physical functioning (on a 100-point scale) increases the risk for death by the same magnitude that the presence of diabetes or chronic obstructive pulmonary disease does.

A shortcoming of nearly all outcome measures other than death is that it is difficult or impossible to use such measures to compare alternative treatments unless they are applied in precisely the same fashion. In the case of hypertension (Chapter 67), for example, different drugs might exhibit differential effects on the risk for stroke or heart failure and also on the risk for adverse events such as fatigue, hepatotoxicity, or renal insufficiency. *Utility measures,* which are derived from economic and decision theory, seek to provide a standard method of comparing such disparate outcomes. *Utility* is the value or preference that an individual places on a given state of health or condition. Utility is scored from 0 (generally equivalent to death) to 1.0 (ideal health). Multiplication of individual utilities for different health states by their probabilities of occurrence permits computation of the overall utility of a treatment or intervention and enables comparison with therapeutic alternatives through the technique of decision analysis. When combined with probabilities of survival, utility can be used to calculate quality-adjusted life years, yet another way of comparing outcomes of different treatment strategies (Chapter 9). Outside the research setting, however, utilities have not been widely used because they are difficult to elicit from patients.

Patients' experiences with health care are commonly measured by standardized questionnaires, such as the Consumer Assessment of Healthcare Providers and Systems (CAHPS) family of surveys, which were developed through a public-private partnership and include instruments used in both ambulatory and institutional settings. Like health-related quality of life, patient experience is a broad concept that can incorporate a number of different dimensions, including satisfaction with overall health care, systems of care, hospital care, outpatient care, specific types of treatments, individual health care providers, amenities, and other aspects. Because patients' perceptions of their care may not correlate highly with other aspects of the processes and outcomes of care, results must be interpreted in the context of these other measures.

Measures of Cost and Resource Use

Given the dramatically rising expense of health care, costs are frequently measured. Because of the complexity of the health care market, including contractual arrangements and complicated formulas for reimbursement, charges (prices) rarely represent the true underlying cost of services. Therefore, careful accounting methods are necessary to accurately ascertain cost. Because these methods can be laborious and expensive, *utilization* of health care services, such as average length of stay or number of days in intensive care units, is often measured as a proxy for cost. When actual costs are measured, the costs evaluated are generally those characterized as *direct,* or the actual fixed and variable expenses for labor, materials, and equipment necessary to provide a given clinical service. Because these costs are typically the responsibility of insurers and health systems, analyses that use direct costs assume their viewpoint. When more global perspectives are incorporated, including those of patients, it is also necessary to measure *indirect costs,* such as the loss of time and the inconvenience incurred by patients or the societal burdens of disability or loss of productivity. Naturally, indirect costs are even more difficult and expensive to measure than direct costs.

From a policy or decision-making perspective, information about cost is most useful when it permits comparisons of alternatives, such as different drugs to treat hypertension. *Cost-benefit* analysis attempts to summarize all costs of treatment and all potential benefits solely in monetary terms. This approach is controversial and is not frequently applied because it necessitates assigning dollar costs to outcomes such as death or disability. *Cost-effectiveness* analysis is performed more frequently because the results are expressed in more comprehensible clinical terms, such as cost per life saved or per quality-adjusted life year (using the utilities described earlier). When a new treatment is evaluated, it is desirable to calculate its *marginal cost-effectiveness,* which describes its costs and benefits in relation to an existing standard treatment.

SOURCES OF DATA FOR THE MEASUREMENT OF HEALTH AND HEALTH CARE

Under ideal circumstances, data for measuring health care are collected prospectively with techniques and instruments specifically designed for the patient population and the problem being assessed. In reality, the time and expense required to develop or identify measures and collect primary data are often too prohibitive to address many important questions. In these situations, it can be advantageous to use information collected for administrative or billing purposes that reflects the process of health care. Such secondary sources of data have increasingly been applied to a broad range of topics, including the use and outcomes of all types of health services.

Governmental Sources of Data

Historically, federal and state governments have collected data related to public health, such as the occurrence of communicable diseases or causes of death. With the expansion of publicly funded health programs such as Medicare and Medicaid, the rise in chronic illnesses as a major cause of morbidity and mortality, and the advent of programs to promote quality and consumer awareness through public reporting of performance data, governmental agencies now maintain a broad range of databases, many of which can be accessed via the Internet (E-Table 10-2). These databases make available vast amounts of information about the incidence and prevalence of various medical conditions, characteristics of patients and health care providers, types of health care services used, burdens and cost of illness, and other important health outcomes, such as adjusted mortality.

Clinical and Quality Data

Until the latter part of the 20th century, most statistics on health care delivery and on the health of groups of patients (with the exception of individual medical records) were maintained by governmental agencies. Today, there are hundreds of public and private entities that collect, process, analyze, or disseminate this information. The consolidation of health care delivery systems within markets and the wide use of electronic health records have led to the creation of very large and rich clinical databases that can be an excellent source for monitoring and improving the quality of care. These data sources can furnish clinical details about the severity and clinical course of illnesses not obtainable from administrative databases.

Another emerging source of data is quality measurement systems developed by peer review organizations, medical care organizations, health plans, professional organizations, consumer organizations, and bodies that perform accreditation. To a greater or lesser extent, all these groups have developed systems to measure and evaluate the performance of health care providers and systems. These data may be collected through the extraction of data from secondary sources, manual abstraction of physical or electronic medical records, or primary data collection by clinical or administrative personnel. Despite the relatively low expense, ready availability, and large size of secondary data sources, there are serious potential limitations to their use (Table 10-2).

DESIGN OF MEASUREMENT STUDIES

Data used to measure the structure, process, and outcomes of health care are obtained in a variety of ways. Investigators engaged in hypothesis-driven research often apply rigorous methods of measurement and research designs, whereas those evaluating the quality of care provided within and among health care organizations tend to rely on observational studies or secondary sources of data (i.e., data initially collected for a different purpose, such as clinical care or claims processing). However, progressive overlap in the methods used and the proliferation of computerized data sources have begun to blur the boundaries between certain types of research and quality improvement studies.

Experimental Studies

Evaluation of the effects of treatments on clinical outcomes should generally be performed in randomized, controlled trials in which the intervention is randomly assigned to ensure that patients who do (subjects) and do not (controls) receive it are as similar as possible. In double-blind studies, not only the patient but also the patient's physician and certain members of the investigative team are kept uninformed about the treatment assignment. Maintenance of blinding is more difficult in studies of interventions other than drugs, but even in studies of surgery or acupuncture, for example, control patients can undergo sham procedures. In studies evaluating more

TABLE 10-2 POTENTIAL LIMITATIONS OF SECONDARY DATA

FEATURE	POTENTIAL LIMITATIONS
Accuracy and precision of data	Basic information on patient characteristics, diagnoses, and procedures may be miscoded Data generally available only for people who use services or access the health care system during the period of interest Patients may be miscounted if they have multiple sites of residence or have undergone procedures in more than one system of care
Sample size	Large sample sizes may produce statistical significance without clinical or policy significance
Characterization of patients	Patients are incompletely characterized; key clinical data on processes and outcomes may be missing
Characterization of providers	Characteristics of providers may be missing, miscoded, or inconsistently recorded
Characterization of interventions	Services or procedures may be coded imprecisely or inaccurately
Ascertainment of outcomes	Outcomes of greatest relevance may not be captured (e.g., symptom relief, quality of life, out-of-hospital events, level of satisfaction)
Completeness of follow-up	Only data about discrete episodes of care may be coded; longitudinal follow-up requires data linkage, which may not be possible

Adapted from Huston P, Naylor CD. Health services research: reporting on studies using secondary data sources. *Can Med Assoc J.* 1996;155:1697-1702.

complex interventions, such as use of a team to manage diabetes or heart failure, blinding may be impractical. To help maintain equivalence in such cases, patients serving as controls may receive a less intensive intervention to help ensure that any observed difference in health outcome between the experimental and control groups is the result of genuine treatment effects rather than nonspecific effects of increased attention.

In trials of interventions that are applied directly to patients, such as medications or procedures, allocation of the experimental treatment is generally random by patient, and results are analyzed at the level of the patient. Conversely, in trials of interventions designed to improve how care is delivered, the unit of randomization and analysis may be the patient, the health care provider, or even the entire system of care, depending on the level at which the intervention is administered. In studying the clinical effects of an educational quality improvement program targeted toward physicians, for example, participating physicians should be randomized along with their patient panels, because the effects on patients within a panel would not be independent. Similarly, in a study of a new way to organize personnel within a practice to treat depression, entire practices might be the correct unit of randomization and analysis.

Although the randomized, controlled trial is the most rigorous method of assessing treatment effects, this approach has several shortcomings. To achieve equivalence between treatment and control groups with respect to key demographic and clinical characteristics, eligibility is often restricted to a narrow range of individuals who fulfill strict criteria. Although this approach enhances the internal validity of a trial's results, applicability of the results to groups of patients who would have been deemed ineligible for the trial (often elderly or chronically ill patients) remains uncertain. Moreover, to help ensure that patients fully comply with the treatment being tested, study personnel frequently provide substantially more support and assistance to participants than similar patients would receive in ordinary clinical settings. These differences often raise concerns about the *external validity* or generalizability of results. For this reason, tightly controlled randomized trials are often considered to establish the *efficacy* of an intervention—specifically, the potential benefit of an intervention under ideal conditions. To establish whether an intervention is successful in patients more typically seen in routine practice, investigators may conduct an *effectiveness trial,* also known as a *management* or *pragmatic trial.*

Other potential drawbacks of randomized trials are the long time required for planning and execution, the high expense, and the low statistical power to assess infrequent outcomes, especially for studies in which health care providers or systems of care are randomized. To compensate in part for these drawbacks, *cluster randomized trials* are designed to permit randomization at the level of the provider or system, but they use sophisticated statistical techniques (e.g., multilevel or hierarchical regression) to perform analyses at the level of the patient so that statistical power is preserved. This approach is particularly well suited to effectiveness trials, which often involve testing of clinical strategies or programs. Other novel approaches are sequential methods, such as the *group sequential response* and *adaptive clinical trial* designs, which provide an opportunity to terminate a study, adjust the expected sample size, or modify the intervention as the trial progresses on the basis of interim analysis at predetermined points in time. These approaches, which are especially attractive when preliminary data are limited, can enhance efficiency by terminating positive or negative trials earlier than might be the case when using only initial sample size estimates.

Nonexperimental Designs

Although randomized trials remain the best approach to assess the efficacy of therapeutic interventions, other study designs, such as *observational* or *case-control* studies, are often used under certain circumstances. *Cohort* studies are a type of observational study in which one or more groups of patients are selected because they have or have not been exposed to a particular condition or intervention. Exposures can be broadly defined and can include the presence of a particular disease or condition (e.g., pneumonia or heart failure), receipt of a type of medication, provision of a certain medical service (e.g., surgical procedure) or set of services (e.g., care by a specialist physician or enrollment in a particular type of health plan), or exposure to a set of conditions (e.g., having health insurance). Cohort studies have numerous attractive features, including the ability to provide a direct estimate of the absolute risk for an outcome in exposed patients. The foremost liability of these approaches is that any observed difference in outcomes may be due to inherent differences between patients who do and do not receive the intervention because it is not randomly allocated. This dilemma can often be addressed by using statistical methods for *case mix adjustment* (described in the next section). In some circumstances, however, even extensive adjustment is inadequate, such as when there is *bias by indication.* This problem occurs in the study of a relationship between an exposure (e.g., a short-acting calcium-channel blocker) and an outcome (e.g., myocardial infarction) when one indication for the medication is treatment that is directly related to the outcome (i.e., angina pectoris). One solution to this problem is to eliminate patients for whom this bias is likely to be present. In the illustrative case, a heightened risk for myocardial infarction in patients taking short-acting calcium-channel blockers was initially demonstrated in a study restricted to persons with hypertension but no known cardiovascular disease.

In a *prospective cohort study,* participants are identified at the time of exposure and followed forward in time according to a predefined protocol and with standard measures. Prospective cohort studies often permit the enrollment of a broader cross section of patients than is possible in randomized trials and can be conducted under circumstances in which randomization is not feasible for ethical or logistic reasons. Like randomized trials, prospective cohort studies provide a means to ascertain that the exposure under study truly precedes the outcome of interest. Limitations of prospective cohort studies include the need to enroll large numbers of patients (especially when evaluating rare outcomes), the frequent loss of participants during follow-up, and the high expense, often related to the duration of follow-up.

In a *retrospective cohort study,* exposure is typically defined by using secondary data (e.g., an admitting diagnosis of acute myocardial infarction or a procedure code for spinal fusion on a hospital discharge abstract) at some point in the past, and patients are followed forward in time by using previously collected data for outcomes (e.g., death, reoperation, readmission). Formerly, retrospective cohort studies were limited in time and scope because they relied on the often tedious manual abstraction of medical charts. With the proliferation of secondary electronic data sources, this approach has become extremely popular and has several advantages—chiefly, the opportunity to study vast numbers of patients inexpensively, including those with relatively rare conditions. Standardized coding for many variables, such as diagnoses and procedures, helps reduce the variability introduced by human chart abstractors. Moreover, electronic records are far less apt to be unavailable or incomplete than paper records are. However, retrospective cohort studies are subject to a number of potentially serious flaws. Hypotheses are usually generated and studies designed well after the collection of data, which was generally done for a wholly different purpose. Thus, the reliability and validity of the data are often unknown and beyond the control of the investigator. This problem can lead to misclassification of both exposures and outcomes. For example, a diagnosis of pneumonia coded for billing purposes may not satisfy the rigorous criteria used in research. Although a patient's complete electronic record is rarely lost, missing data within records are common. Unlike with prospective studies, it may be difficult to be certain that an exposure preceded an outcome. For example, a patient might have had subclinical disease at the time of a given exposure, thereby leading to an erroneous impression of a temporal sequence when the disease was recognized clinically. Apart from methodologic limitations, the sheer volume of available data encourages investigators to conduct numerous analyses, often without prestated hypotheses. Multiple comparisons performed with very large sample sizes readily lead to erroneous conclusions that random associations are clinically meaningful because they are of marginal statistical significance.

Case-control studies differ from cohort studies in that the case and control groups are defined on the basis of whether subjects have experienced an outcome rather than on the basis of exposure. Data from existing records or gathered by interview (or both) are then used to ascertain the proportion of case and control patients who experienced the exposure of interest. As in cohort studies, exposures can be defined broadly, including a medication, a type of clinical event, or receipt of a service. Case-control studies are attractive in many settings because they require fewer patients than prospective studies do to achieve a similar level of statistical power. This attribute makes them especially useful for investigating uncommon outcomes. For example, pharmacoepidemiologists often use case-control studies to identify serious adverse effects of medications when the events are too rare to study with clinical trials or cohort studies. Case-control studies are nonetheless subject to a number of potential biases. As with cohort studies, the use of data from secondary sources can lead to misclassification of exposure or outcome. When exposure is determined by interview, differential recall by cases and controls can introduce bias. It may be even more difficult to be certain that an exposure truly occurred before the outcome than in retrospective cohort studies. Furthermore, the results of case-control studies do not yield estimates of absolute risk, as do randomized trials and cohort studies; they are expressed as the odds of an outcome in cases relative to controls. *Relative odds* only approximate the ratio of risk in cases to risk in controls.

Cross-sectional studies are performed when data on one or more groups of patients are collected at a single point in time. Although this approach is inexpensive and can provide estimates of the prevalence of a condition or outcome, it is highly subject to nearly all the biases mentioned and is the weakest method in terms of making inferences about whether a particular exposure directly causes a given outcome.

Case Mix Adjustment

Only in prospective, randomized trials is it possible to control which patients do and do not receive a specific treatment, and even then, it may not be possible to ensure the equivalence of all the characteristics that affect outcomes between subjects in the control and experimental groups. In all nonexperimental research designs, allocation of the experimental intervention is not random but is a function of a patient's personal and clinical characteristics and those of the system of care. Without consideration of such differences, it is impossible to differentiate the genuine effects of an intervention from bias related to allocation of the intervention to certain types of patients. Modern statistical techniques that can adjust for such differences are effective when many of the patient characteristics that exert an important influence on outcomes have been elucidated and relevant data are available. For example, the major factors that predict mortality after acute myocardial infarction include prolonged chest pain, tachycardia, hypotension, ST segment elevation on the admission electrocardiogram, poor left ventricular function, and initial laboratory measures that indicate a large infarct, such as a high troponin level. Thus, when comparing the outcomes of patients who are treated in different systems of care, it is essential to use multivariate statistical methods to adjust for these factors. Otherwise, differences observed between systems that are actually due to differing patient populations might erroneously be attributed to differences in quality of care. A related method is *propensity scoring*, which applies the results of modeling equations that predict how likely a person was to have received one intervention or the other based on personal and clinical characteristics. Even with sophisticated adjustments, however, studies of treatments that rely heavily on the judgment of physicians or the preference of patients are likely to have biases that cannot be addressed by statistical modeling and require randomized trials.

TABLE 10-3 EXPANDING AREAS OF STUDY FOR HEALTH CARE QUALITY AND OUTCOMES

GENERAL AREA OF STUDY	EXAMPLE OF INTERVENTION OR OUTCOME EVALUATED
Effectiveness of clinical programs	Disease management programs, specialized clinics, consultative services
Organization of care	Health maintenance organizations vs. private practice
Effects of different mechanisms of financing	Capitation vs. fee-for-service; different levels of pharmacy copayments
Outcomes of different types of providers	Generalists vs. specialists
Disparities among ethnic groups	Receipt of preventive services or sophisticated procedures
Patient safety	Occurrence of adverse drug effects or medical errors
Geographic variations in patterns of care	Use of expensive procedures

TRENDS IN OUTCOME MEASUREMENT

In recent years, the topics of studies evaluating the outcomes of health care interventions have expanded greatly. In addition to evaluating specific treatments, such as drugs or procedures, evaluations directly compare various types of clinical programs, systems of care, types of providers, mechanisms of financing, patient safety, disparities among ethnic groups, and geographic variations in patterns of care (Table 10-3). Recently, public attention has been focused on *comparative effectiveness,* which reflects the need to evaluate new and typically more expensive therapies in relation to older, well-established treatments, as opposed to the common practice of merely comparing them with placebo or clearly less effective regimens. Information from such trials is essential to identify the most cost-effective therapies.

It is safe to predict that studies on the processes and outcomes of health care will become even more ubiquitous with the expanding availability of electronic data, increasingly sophisticated statistical techniques, and growing public demand for accountability.

SUGGESTED READINGS

Fonarow GC, Peterson ED. Heart failure performance measures and outcomes: real or illusory gains. *JAMA*. 2009;302:792-794. *From 2002 to 2007, performance measures for heart failure improved 15 to 250%, but mortality, hospital readmissions, and costs remained constant.*

Nyweide DJ, Weeks WB, Gottlieb DJ, et al. Relationship of primary care physicians' patient caseload with measurement of quality and cost performance. *JAMA*. 2009;302:2444-2450. *Few primary care physicians have a sufficient number of patients to reliably detect a 10% relative difference on performance measures.*

Stulberg JJ, Delaney CP, Neuhauser DV, et al. Adherence to surgical care improvement project measures and the association with postoperative infections. *JAMA*. 2010;303:2479-2485. *Adherence was associated with fewer postoperative infections.*

11 QUALITY OF CARE AND PATIENT SAFETY

ROBERT M. WACHTER

During the past two decades, scores of studies have demonstrated that the quality and safety of modern health care leave much to be desired, despite the fact that most physicians are well trained and work very hard. Yet the evidence is undeniable, with clear documentation of stunning variations in patterns of care that are neither supported by evidence nor justified by outcomes, major gaps between evidence-based best practices and current practice, and staggering numbers of serious medical errors. The recognition of these quality and safety problems has catalyzed a major transformation in thinking and practice, with new technologies, regulations, training models, incentive systems, and more.

TABLE 11-1 THE INSTITUTE OF MEDICINE'S SIX QUALITY AIMS

Patient safety
Patient centeredness
Effectiveness
Efficiency
Timeliness
Equity

From Committee on Quality of Health Care in America, Institute of Medicine. *Crossing the Quality Chasm: A New Health System for the 21st Century*. Washington, DC: National Academy Press; 2001.

TABLE 11-2 COMPARISON OF THREE MEASURES OF CLINICAL QUALITY: THE DONABEDIAN TRIAD

MEASURE	SIMPLE DEFINITION	ADVANTAGES	DISADVANTAGES
Structure	How was care organized?	May be highly relevant in a complex health system	May fail to capture the quality of care by individual physicians Difficult to determine the "gold standard"
Process	What was done?	More easily measured and acted on than outcomes May not require case-mix adjustment No time lag—can be measured when care is provided May directly reflect quality (if carefully chosen)	A proxy for outcomes Not all may agree on "gold standard" processes May promote "cookbook" medicine, especially if physicians and health systems try to "game" their performance
Outcomes	What happened to the patient?	What we really care about	May take years to occur May not reflect quality of care Requires case-mix and other adjustment to prevent "apples-to-oranges" comparisons

Modified from Donabedian A. The quality of care. How can it be assessed? *JAMA*. 1988;270:1743-1748; and Shojania KG, Showstack J, Wachter R. Assessing hospital quality: A review for clinicians. *Eff Clin Pract*. 2001;4:82-90.

To appreciate the problem and how to address it requires an understanding of quality measurement and improvement, the safety of patients, and value, which is the confluence of safety, quality, and cost.

QUALITY

Definition

Quality of care has been defined by the Institute of Medicine as "the degree to which health services for individuals and populations increase the likelihood of desired health outcomes and are consistent with current professional knowledge." It includes six aims for a quality health care system, emphasizing that quality involves more than the delivery of evidence-based care (Table 11-1). Nevertheless, evidence-based medicine (Chapter 9) provides much of the scientific underpinning for quality measurement and improvement. Previously, the lack of clinical evidence and the apprenticeship model of medical training promoted an idiosyncratic practice style by which a senior clinician or a marquee medical center determined the standard of care—a tradition now sometimes termed *eminence-based medicine*. Without discounting the value of experience and mature clinical judgment, the modern paradigm for determining optimal practice has changed, driven by the explosion in clinical research during the past 30 years; for example, the number of randomized clinical trials grew from 350 per year in 1970 to 18,000 per year in 2008. This research has helped define "best practices" in many areas of medicine, from preventive strategies for a healthy 62-year-old outpatient (Chapters 13 and 14) to the treatment of a patient with acute myocardial infarction and cardiogenic shock (Chapters 73 and 107).

Donabedian's triad, which divides quality measures into *structure* (how care is organized), *process* (what is done), and *outcomes* (what happens to the patient), represents the most popular construct for quality measurement. Each element of the triad has important advantages and disadvantages as a quality measure (Table 11-2). Most of the widely used quality measures are process measures for which clinical research has established a link between such processes and improved outcomes. An example is the rate at which aspirin or a β-blocker is given to survivors of a myocardial infarction before hospital discharge (Chapter 73). However, when processes are less relevant and the science of case-mix adjustment is suitably advanced (e.g., cardiac bypass surgery; Chapter 74), outcome measurement is often used. In other areas involving complex processes, structural measures are used as proxies for quality; examples here include the presence of intensivists to staff critical care units, a dedicated stroke service, and computerized physician order entry (CPOE) systems.

The Epidemiology of Quality-Related Problems

It is now well established that there are large and clinically indefensible variations in care from one city to another. Furthermore, U.S. practice adheres to the best evidence only slightly more than 50% of the time, even when adherence is known to correlate with ultimate clinical outcomes.

Levers for Change

For physicians, policymakers, administrators, and patients, evidence of major problems with quality has led to the recognition of structural problems that prevent the delivery of the highest quality of care. These problems include the lack of information regarding the performance of a provider or institution, the absence of incentives for quality improvement, the challenge for practicing physicians to stay abreast of modern evidence-based medicine, and the absence of an information technology support system for quality.

The first step in quality improvement is the creation of practice standards against which to measure quality. Scores of such measures have been promulgated by a variety of organizations, including payers (such as the Centers for Medicare and Medicaid Services), accreditors (such as the Joint Commission), and medical societies. These measures have identified many opportunities for improvement among individual physicians, practices, and hospitals.

Given the volume of new literature published each year, it is impossible for an individual physician to keep up with all the evidence-based advances in his or her field. *Practice guidelines*, such as those for the treatment of community-acquired pneumonia (Chapter 97) or the prophylaxis of deep venous thrombosis (Chapter 81), aim to synthesize evidence-based best practices into a set of summary recommendations. Although concerns about "cookbook medicine" linger, there is a growing consensus that best practices should be "hardwired" if possible. The major challenges are to update guidelines as new knowledge accumulates and to recognize the complexity of guidelines when patients have multiple, potentially overlapping illnesses. *Clinical pathways* are similar to guidelines but attempt to codify a series of steps, usually temporally (on day 1, do the following; on day 2, do the following; and so forth), making them more useful for stereotypical processes such as the postoperative management of patients after hip replacement.

Although professionalism (Chapter 1) should be a sufficient incentive for physicians to provide high-quality care, reaching this goal typically depends on the existence of a system organized to translate research into practice and to deliver the right care every time. Such a system requires significant investments (in educating physicians, hiring case managers or clinical pharmacists, building information systems, and developing guidelines). The historical payment system, which compensates physicians and hospitals equally whether quality is terrific or terrible, provides no incentive to make the requisite investments.

The Changing Environment for Quality

The recent recognition of major gaps in quality and of the need for systemic change to improve quality has led to a variety of initiatives to catalyze quality improvement. Virtually all involve several steps: defining reasonable quality measures (evidence-based measures; capturing appropriate structures, process, or outcomes), measuring the performance of providers or systems, and using these results to promote change. This final imperative creates the greatest degree of uncertainty and experimentation.

Although one might hope that simply giving a physician information about prior performance would generate meaningful improvement, this strategy yields only modest change at best. Increasingly, a more aggressive and transparent strategy, such as disseminating the results of quality measurement to key stakeholders, is being adopted. In some cases, simple transparency is the main strategy—the rationale being that providers will find the exposure of their gaps in quality to be sufficiently concerning or embarrassing to motivate improvement. Although there is little evidence that patients use such data to choose among physicians or hospitals, transparency itself has frequently resulted in impressive improvements in some publicly reported quality measures.

The newest strategy in the United States is to tie payments for service to quality performance (pay for performance, or P4P). A number of P4P programs are under way, and early results indicate that differential payment leads to modest gains beyond the improvements achieved by simple transparency. P4P also raises a host of concerns, including whether presently captured quality data are accurate, whether payments should go to the best performers or those with the greatest improvements, whether existing measures adequately measure quality in patients with complex diseases, and whether P4P will create undue focus on certain measurable practices, leading to relative inattention to other important processes that are not being compensated. A recent variation on the P4P theme is Medicare's "no pay for adverse events" program, in which hospital payments are withheld for certain "preventable" adverse events. As with P4P more generally, the jury is still out regarding the impact of such programs on quality and safety.

Quality Improvement Strategies

Whether the motivation is professionalism, embarrassment, or economics, the next question is how actually to improve the quality of care. There is no simple answer; successful institutions and physicians have used a variety of strategies. In general, most use a variation of a "plan, do, study, act" (PDSA) cycle, recognizing that quality improvement activities must be carefully planned and implemented, that their impact needs to be measured, and that the results of these activities are often imperfect and require retooling.

In addition to the PDSA cycle, several other types of activities are useful. For quality improvement practices that require predictable repetition, efforts to "hardwire" the practice or to use alternative providers who focus on the activity are often beneficial. For example, the best strategy to increase the rate of pneumococcal vaccination (Chapter 17) among hospitalized patients with pneumonia is to embed it in a standard order set, either paper based or computerized. Another example is that having a nurse remove patients' shoes before the physician's entry can increase rates of diabetic foot examinations in an outpatient practice (Chapter 236).

In some areas, though, quality improvement involves much more complex and interdependent activities. In these circumstances, bringing teams together to examine their practices and to participate in a PDSA cycle is the most likely path to success. For example, a group of cardiac surgeons in the northeastern United States participated in an experiment in which they observed one another's practices, agreed on best practices, and measured one another's outcomes; the result was a 24% reduction in mortality with cardiac surgery.

PATIENT SAFETY

Epidemiology

The concept of "first, do no harm" began more than 2 millennia ago, and many hospitals host periodic forums (e.g., morbidity and mortality conferences) to discuss errors. Until recently, however, there has been little teaching about the nature of medical mistakes, investment in safety research, regulation of safety standards, or emphasis on safety improvements, despite the fact that an estimated 44,000 to 98,000 Americans die each year of medical mistakes—the equivalent of a jumbo jet crashing each day. Such deaths may be related to medication errors, gaps in the discharge process, communication problems in intensive care units, or retained sponges in surgical patients—in short, virtually every aspect of modern medical care. Moreover, detailed clinical and statistical evidence of suboptimal safety has been reinforced by several high-profile and disquieting errors, sometimes apparently related to inadequate supervision and prolonged duty hours of trainees. These errors include the wrong patient getting a major procedure, the wrong limb being operated on, chemotherapy overdoses, mistaken mastectomies, and more.

Because patients may be harmed despite receiving perfect care (i.e., from an accepted complication of surgery or a side effect of medication), it is important to separate *adverse events* from *errors*. The patient safety literature commonly defines an error as "an act or omission that leads to an unanticipated, undesirable outcome or to substantial potential for such an outcome." Adverse events, in contrast, are injuries due to medical management rather than the patient's underlying illness. This distinction is crucial. For example, when a patient who was appropriately prescribed warfarin for chronic atrial fibrillation (Chapter 64) develops a gastrointestinal bleed despite a therapeutic international normalized ratio (INR), an adverse event, not a medical error, has occurred. Conversely, if the INR was supratherapeutic because the physician prescribed a new medication without checking for possible drug interactions, a medical error would have occurred.

The Modern Approach to Patient Safety

The historical approach to medical errors often has been to blame the provider who was most proximate: whoever performed the surgery, hung the intravenous medication, or mixed the chemotherapy. It is now recognized that this approach fails to appreciate that most errors are committed by hard-working, well-trained individuals, and such errors are unlikely to be prevented by admonishing people to be more careful or by shaming and suing them. Instead, the modern approach, known as *systems thinking*, holds that humans will inevitably err and that safety depends on creating systems that anticipate errors and either prevent or catch them before they cause harm. Such an approach has been the cornerstone of safety improvements in other high-risk industries for some time.

The "Swiss cheese" model of accidents, drawn from innumerable investigations of accidents in commercial aviation and the nuclear power industry, for example, emphasizes that single errors by one individual working in an otherwise safety-conscious system rarely cause harm. Instead, such errors must penetrate multiple incomplete layers of protection ("layers of Swiss cheese") to cause terrible harm. The lesson is to focus not on the futile goal of trying to perfect human behavior but rather on creating multiple overlapping layers of protection to decrease the probability that the holes in the Swiss cheese will ever align, allowing an error to slip through.

How to Improve Patient Safety

Drawing on these models, modern thinking emphasizes efforts to design and implement systems to prevent or catch errors. For example, errors in routine behaviors can best be prevented by building in redundancies and crosschecks in the form of checklists, read-backs, and other standardized safety procedures, such as counting sponges in the operating room, signing a surgical site before an operation, or asking patients their names before administering a medication. In recent years, the use of checklists for the placement of central lines and to prepare patients for surgery has resulted in remarkable reductions in morbidity and mortality. One way to decrease errors at the person-machine interface is by the use of "forcing functions," engineering solutions that decrease the probability of human error. The classic example outside of medicine is the modification of automobile braking systems to make it impossible to place a car in reverse when the driver's foot is off the brake. In health care, forcing functions include changing the gas nozzles and connectors so that anesthesiologists cannot mistakenly hook up the wrong gas, such as nitrogen instead of oxygen, and administer it to a patient. Given the ever-increasing complexity of modern medicine, building in such forcing functions in intravenous pumps, defibrillators, mechanical ventilators, and computerized order entry systems will be crucial to safety.

In addition to better systems, communication and teamwork must be improved. All commercial pilots must take "crew resource management" courses, in which they train for emergencies with other crew members, learn to flatten hierarchies that might stifle open communication, communicate clearly with standard language, and use checklists and other systemic approaches. Recent evidence supports that such interventions in medical care can lead to fewer errors and improved outcomes. The goal is a "culture of safety"—an environment in which teamwork, clear communication, and openness about errors, both with other health care professionals and with patients, is the norm. A tailored group of discharge services, emphasizing both process improvements and better collaboration among providers, can significantly reduce hospital readmissions,[1] and a multidisciplinary fall prevention program can reduce falls in hospitalized patients.[2]

Another key principle in ensuring the safety of patients is to learn from one's mistakes. Safe systems have a culture in which errors are openly discussed, often in morbidity and mortality conferences. To be most useful, these discussions should be interdisciplinary (involving doctors and other health professionals), identify when the errors occurred, and emphasize systems thinking and solutions; they should not be punitive. In addition to open discussions during conferences, safe organizations build in mechanisms to hear about errors from frontline staff, often through "incident reporting systems"; they also perform detailed "root cause" analyses of major errors or "sentinel events" in an effort to define all the layers of Swiss cheese that need improvement. The importance of open communication extends to patients as well. Disclosure of errors is now required by the Joint Commission. Patients and families value such openness, and preliminary evidence indicates that disclosure of errors might decrease the chance of a malpractice suit.

Finally, there is increasing appreciation of the importance of a well-trained, well-staffed, and well-rested work force for the delivery of safe care. Lower nurse-to-patient ratios, long work hours for residents, and lack of board certification are all linked to poor outcomes for patients. Safer systems cannot be created if the providers are overextended or poorly trained or supervised.

In the absence of comparative evidence, and in light of the high cost of interventions such as improved staffing, computerized order entry, and teamwork training, even institutions committed to safety must often make difficult choices. Given the natural tendency to focus on practices that are measured, publicly reported, and compensated, institutions and physicians tend to focus first on areas that are subject to regulation or on initiatives with multiple potential benefits, such as computerization. Because improving culture is difficult to measure and to regulate, there is concern that it will not be as high a priority as it should be. Moreover, a safe culture depends on balancing the imperative to improve systems with the need to define and enforce accountability. The safety field is increasingly emphasizing more active enforcement of policies that address problems such as disruptive behavior by clinicians and failure to adhere to evidence-based safety practices.

VALUE: CONNECTING SAFETY AND QUALITY TO COST

Outside of health care, most purchasing decisions are based on perceived value: (quality + safety) ÷ cost. Health care decisions historically have not been made this way, in part because of the limited ability of patients and payers to make rational judgments about the quality and safety of a given provider or system, and in part because health care insurance insulates patients from the full cost of care. Much of the recent push to measure and to improve quality and safety should be seen as part of a broader effort to allow patients and payers to make rational judgments about value and to choose their providers on the basis of such judgments. Given the stakes, it is vital for physicians and other health care providers to participate in efforts to measure and improve the quality and safety of care and to do so while being mindful of the price tag.

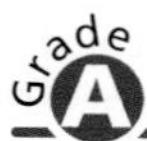

1. Jack BW, Chetty VK, Anthony D, et al. A reengineered hospital discharge program to decrease rehospitalizations: a randomized trial. *Ann Intern Med.* 2009;150:178-187.
2. Dykes PC, Carroll DL, Hurley A, et al. Fall prevention in acute care hospitals: a randomized trial. *JAMA.* 2010;304:1912-1918.

SUGGESTED READINGS

Kachalia A, Kaufman SR, Boothman R, et al. Liability claims and costs before and after implementation of a medical error disclosure program. *Ann Intern Med.* 2010;153:213-221. *A before-after demonstrating lower liability costs after implementation of a program of disclosure and, where appropriate, settlement offers.*

Neily J, Mills PD, Young-Xu Y, et al. Association between implementation of a medical team training program and surgical mortality. *JAMA.* 2010;304:1693-1700. *A team training program was associated with an 18% reduction in surgical mortality.*

Wachter RM. Why diagnostic errors don't get any respect—and what can be done about them. *Health Aff (Millwood).* 2010;29:1605-1610. *Emphasizes potentially effective strategies to address diagnostic errors.*

12

COMPREHENSIVE CHRONIC DISEASE MANAGEMENT

EDWARD H. WAGNER

Although there is no clear definition of a chronic disease, the term generally refers to long-standing degenerative conditions of noninfectious origin. However, chronic infections, such as HIV or hepatitis C, and many mental and behavioral disorders also last for months, years, or a lifetime. Regardless of cause or pathophysiology, chronic conditions require ongoing attention and adjustments by patients and their loved ones and care by professionals. Patients with a wide variety of chronic health problems have similar needs to minimize morbidity and optimize quality of life (Table 12-1). Because these needs are shared across conditions, clinical management of these seemingly disparate illnesses requires similar practice capacities and functions. For example, the design and organization of care that leads to better outcomes are remarkably similar for diseases as clinically different as diabetes, depression, and HIV.

To live effectively with their health conditions and manage their treatments, patients must have access to the necessary information, skills, and encouragement. They must also receive evidence-based therapy and preventive care to improve disease control and reduce the risk of complications and exacerbations. The severity of most chronic conditions and the effectiveness of ongoing therapy wax and wane over time. As a consequence, regular monitoring and reassessment are required by patients and clinicians alike. When chronically ill patients experience periods of increased severity and risk, they benefit from an intensification of management and support. Care for the chronically ill generally involves multiple health professionals and care settings, for which transitions must be coordinated.

THE GOALS OF CHRONIC CARE MANAGEMENT

The goals of chronic care management are to meet the aforementioned needs of patients with chronic illness routinely and efficiently by delivering care in a system organized to do so. Chronic conditions, whether medical or psychiatric, present very different challenges for patients and their caregivers than do acute illnesses or injuries. Rarely cured and often changing in severity over time, chronic illness necessitates continuous monitoring and adjustments by patients (self-management) and caregivers alike.

The decisions made and behaviors undertaken by patients to deal with their illness, generally called *self-management,* influence the course and outcomes of most chronic diseases in major ways. Patients make decisions and take action in dealing with symptoms, coping with the social and emotional impacts of illness, monitoring their condition, taking medications, adjusting lifestyle, and interacting with the health care system. Most need training and ongoing support from their clinical providers to become competent managers of their health and their illness. The competence and confidence with which patients self-manage their illness have a major impact on outcome. For example, participants in diabetes or hypertension self-management training programs generally experience clinically significant reductions in hemoglobin A_{1c} or blood pressure levels without major changes in drug therapy.[1] Self-management can be enhanced in patients of all socioeconomic

TABLE 12-1 COMMON NEEDS OF PATIENTS WITH CHRONIC ILLNESS

- Support and information that enables patients to be competent self-managers of their health and illness
- Effective clinical and behavioral treatment that keeps the disease under control and optimizes health status
- Effective preventive care to reduce the risk of complications and other morbidity
- Ongoing monitoring of the patient's condition to detect and respond to problems early in their course
- Intensification of management and support during high-risk periods
- Coordination of care to increase the efficiency and effectiveness of referrals and to prevent the mishaps that commonly occur during care transitions

groups by empowering, training, and supporting them. Modern self-management support is a collaborative rather than a didactic process that seeks concordance between providers' and patients' perspectives on the goals of treatment and the actions needed to reach those goals.

Whereas the primary goals of acute disease care are cure and recovery, cure is not an option for most chronic diseases, which are often characterized by slowly progressive deterioration, even with excellent care. Nevertheless, control of the metabolic or physiologic abnormalities or symptoms resulting from the underlying pathophysiologic processes (disease control) is now possible for many chronic conditions. Thus, a major goal for the management of many chronic illnesses is effective clinical treatment in accord with the best scientific evidence. Drugs, lifestyle modification, and other therapies attempt to minimize morbidity, limit further organ damage, reduce the risk of exacerbations and complications, and maintain quality of life and function. The metabolic or physiologic abnormalities or symptoms used to assess disease control often serve as clinical targets to guide therapy and as performance indicators to monitor the progress and quality of care for populations of patients (e.g., the percentage of diabetic patients with blood pressure <130/80 mm Hg). Disease control is best achieved through the systematic use of evidence-based treatment protocols that carefully step up or intensify treatment until clinical targets are reached.

Ongoing monitoring and assessment of chronically ill patients, including ensuring that they are not lost to follow-up, are essential to optimize therapy. Regular assessment of self-management activities reinforces their importance to the patient and to the overall management of the condition. Serious exacerbations and complications of common chronic illnesses are potentially preventable if identified early in their course and treated appropriately (e.g., recurrence of major depression, opportunistic infection in patients with HIV, lower extremity amputation among diabetic patients). The periodicity of assessments must change as the severity of illness waxes and wanes over time.

An increasingly important goal of effective chronic care management is to provide more intensive monitoring and management during periods of high risk, such as transitions from hospital to community or exacerbations. Clinical care or case management by nurses, pharmacists, or other nonphysician health professionals enables closer monitoring of patients, helps with medication adjustment, provides self-management support, and facilitates care coordination. Effective care management programs can reduce the likelihood of rehospitalization for chronically ill patients discharged from the hospital, reduce emergency room visits and hospitalizations among multiproblem ambulatory older adults, and improve disease control.

Chronically ill patients receive medical and supportive services from multiple providers with differing expertise in different settings. Without good coordination, many opportunities exist for errors, inefficiencies, and patient distress. Effective coordination of care can prevent or reduce hospital readmissions because of failures of post-discharge care, failed referrals, referrals without adequate information from the primary care provider, specialty visits without communication back to the primary care provider, duplicated testing, and so forth. Without assistance from their primary providers, patients or their loved ones must often assume responsibility for the onerous task of coordinating care.

MATCHING PATIENT NEEDS AND CARE DELIVERY

Outpatients with diseases such as diabetes, hypertension, and major depression have been estimated to receive evidence-based interventions only about half the time, and less than half achieve optimal disease control. When individual practices are audited, omissions of evidence-based care appear almost randomly across different interventions and among patients within a practice, suggesting that these omissions are related to flaws in care systems rather than cognitive gaps.

The other goals of chronic care management are met even less often, because ambulatory care systems are largely organized to react to acute problems, not to address the ongoing needs of the chronically ill. The focus on making a diagnosis and initiating treatment for the problem at hand leaves little time for addressing less urgent needs such as medication adjustment, self-management support, and preventive care. Reimbursement systems that favor multiple short encounters aggravate the problem.

Lack of attention to patient self-management and inappropriate drug management by clinicians or patients are largely responsible for the poor control of chronic illness. Abundant evidence indicates that adherence to evidence-based treatment protocols substantially increases the proportion of patients reaching therapeutic targets and reduces the risk of morbidity and mortality. The protocols for most chronic conditions include recommendations to step up or intensify therapy when clinical targets are not reached. Failure to intensify treatment in patients who have not achieved therapeutic targets, called *clinical inertia*, has been found in a large percentage of patients with uncontrolled diabetes, hypertension, depression, and other chronic illnesses. Clinicians have an understandable reluctance to increase drug doses or add new drugs, but concerns about toxicity or patient nonadherence can be mitigated if practices have organized approaches to stepping up therapy and monitoring its impact.

Deficiencies in practice infrastructure and the professional environment compound the difficulties of meeting the needs of chronically ill patients. The majority of ambulatory practices in North America still has no electronic clinical record system, performance measurement program, or access to colleagues trained to provide self-management support or clinical care management. Primary care physicians are increasingly uninvolved or even unaware when their patients are hospitalized. Specialists' communications with and support of primary care practitioners have deteriorated because of complex provider network requirements. Efforts to improve the quality of chronic care must focus on improving the infrastructure and practice systems that busy clinicians require to meet the needs of their patients.

Interventions That Improve Care and Outcomes of Chronic Diseases

A wide array of interventions can improve the care and outcomes of major chronic diseases by changing the organization and functioning of the care delivery system, regardless of the specific condition. These changes fall into four general categories. *Patient-directed interventions* try to change patient knowledge, increase their involvement in care, and alter their behavior. *Provider-directed interventions* give providers feedback about the quality of their care and aim to change providers' knowledge and behavior through education and reminders. *Organizational changes* generally focus on the composition and functioning of the care team and the organization of office visits (e.g., group visits) and other encounters (e.g., telephone management). *Information technology (IT) interventions* include the use of computer reminders and other decision support programs, as well as the use of registries for population and patient management. Growing evidence suggests that the use of registries to measure performance, identify individuals needing care, and plan individual patient care may be the IT function that contributes the most to improving the care of the chronically ill.

Provider-directed interventions, especially educational programs, generally demonstrate weak effects. Conversely, interventions that change the composition or functioning of the practice team have the most salutary effects.[2,3] Across conditions, assigning patient care responsibilities to the nonphysician members of practice teams leads to the greatest improvements in disease control and other outcomes. Better informed patients have better outcomes when they receive care from more informed providers who are supported by a well-organized clinical team and appropriate IT.

The Chronic Care Model

The chronic care model identifies features of a health care system that encourage high-quality chronic disease care: self-management support, delivery system design, decision support, clinical information systems, health care organization, and community resources. Evidence-based changes in these six areas foster productive interactions between informed patients, who take an active part in their care, and providers with resources and expertise.[4]

This approach presumes that patients with one or more chronic illnesses have a primary care clinician who assumes responsibility for managing their care and coordinating the activities of other clinicians and institutions that provide advice and services. It posits that important patient outcomes, such as the prevention of morbidity, mortality, and avoidable emergency room visits and hospitalizations, can be affected by productive medical care.

Productive interactions are more likely to occur when patients actively participate in their care. To do so, patients need to be informed—that is, they must have the relevant information and skills to manage their illness. Patients also must be empowered to take an active role in their health care. More active patients are more likely to engage in relevant self-management behaviors and to use health care more effectively. A number of group and individual interventions increase the likelihood that patients have sufficient understanding of their illness and its treatment and the skills and confidence to be competent self-managers.

The other partner in productive interactions is the primary care clinician and the practice team. Before visits with chronically ill patients, practice teams should review accessible information to determine what services are needed, have clear assignments or standing orders for the delivery of those services, and include staff trained to perform them. Although all six elements of the chronic care model contribute to a delivery system that can effectively manage chronic illness, changes in two categories—delivery system design and self-management support—are essential to improve disease control and reduce morbidity and mortality.

Self-Management Support

Didactic patient education alone has been demonstrated to have little if any impact on patient behavior or disease control. To change their lifestyle, take medications as directed, deal with symptoms and stress, and address the other challenges of living with chronic illness, patients need to participate actively in their care, understand and agree with the clinician's assessment of the problems and recommendations, learn the skills needed to carry out the recommendations, develop goals and an action plan to guide behavior change, and review their progress regularly with the primary care team.

These needs can be met in either group or individual sessions that involve skill building, discussion, and negotiation related to recommendations, goals, barriers to reaching goals, and actions to overcome barriers. Although self-management courses facilitated by peer or professional leaders improve disease control in diabetes, hypertension, and other chronic diseases, their effects diminish after termination of the program. Sustained follow-up and reinforcement are essential.

Sustained self-management support is best accomplished by the primary care team in the context of ongoing chronic illness care. Although a physician's advice and encouragement are important, most primary care clinicians have neither the time nor the training to help patients set behavioral goals and develop action plans and then follow up by telephone or e-mail. Clinical staff such as nurses or medical assistants with good communication skills and additional training in counseling methods can and should perform these functions.

Delivery System Design

Team Care

The goal of delivery system design is to match the organization of care delivery to the needs of the chronically ill. Without the help of a team, it is unlikely that, in the course of a 15- to 20-minute visit, physicians can manage intercurrent problems, review and adjust treatment, provide recommended assessments and preventive care, discuss self-management goals and plans, and plan follow-up. Designing effective team care begins with a consideration of the various tasks required to meet the needs of the chronically ill and ensure adherence to guidelines. Some of these tasks, such as self-management counseling or medication reconciliation, are generic; others are disease specific. Key tasks are allocated to the most appropriate members of the practice team. The team's routine involvement in patient visits is facilitated by protocols and/or standing orders that guide independent action by nonclinician staff. Brief meetings, often termed *huddles*, before clinic sessions allow practice teams to review key data (often from registries) on scheduled patients to identify and plan the delivery of needed services. The goal is to maximize the productivity of every patient interaction.

Planned Interactions

Much of chronic care management involves predictable preventive care or disease management activities, which are often postponed when chronically ill patients initiate care for an acute problem. The availability of key patient data gives practice teams the opportunity to update chronic illness care even during visits for more urgent problems. Practice-initiated planned visits can focus on patients who are noncompliant with guidelines, have failed to reach treatment targets, or have been lost to follow-up. The practice tries to schedule longer visits that are structured to address these patients' needs. Another format for the delivery of planned care is the group visit, in which patients receive their primary medical care together as a group. Group sessions generally include the same check-in assessments that occur during an individual visit, followed by brief individual communications between the primary care provider and each patient, opportunities for private consultations, and an educational session with ample opportunity for peer-to-peer interaction. Approximately 30 to 50% of patients offered group visits attend them, and many prefer to receive much of their care in this setting.

Follow-up and Case Management

Follow-up tailored to a patient's needs and the clinical severity of the disease is a critical component of effective chronic care management. Traditionally, follow-up consists of periodic in-person physician visits whose frequency is limited by cost and convenience. Chronically ill individuals often experience periods when more intensive monitoring would be helpful, such as during exacerbations or intercurrent illnesses, following hospital discharge, or while medications are being changed. Ample evidence indicates that follow-up by telephone, e-mail, or telemedicine can be cost-effective and far more flexible than face-to-face return visits. Nonphysician team members, guided by protocols with clear referral criteria, can effectively manage electronic follow-up. Self-monitoring by patients is an important component of the follow-up plans for many chronic illnesses and is especially useful when patients use the results to adjust their therapy[5] as well as to inform their practice team. Collecting self-monitoring data for the sole purpose of bringing them to the doctor's office appears to be far less effective. A small number of chronically ill patients at high risk of hospitalization, nursing home placement, major complication, or death need even more intensive clinical case management services. Clinical case management appears to be effective for chronically ill patients discharged from the hospital; multiproblem, high-risk older patients in community practice; high-risk patients with type 2 diabetes and other diseases; and patients with major depression and other chronic psychiatric disorders.

Disease management programs have proliferated over the past decade. These generally involve nurse case managers who have limited if any involvement with the patients' physicians or their medical care. This disconnected case management system is relatively ineffective unless the case manager collaborates closely with the primary care clinician, influences the medication regimen directly or indirectly, and reviews his or her caseload regularly with the relevant medical specialist.

Decision Support

Efforts to educate health professionals have a very limited impact on clinical performance when compared with inserting information and alerts directly into the flow of decision making. Even the most carefully developed evidence-based guidelines will have no impact on practice if they are not integrated into clinical management through computer templates, alerts, protocols, standing orders, and other efforts to standardize practice.

Many chronically ill patients who are cared for by generalists benefit from the advice and involvement of medical specialists. Communication channels between generalists and specialists (Chapter 438) can be improved by creating systems whereby consultants respond to questions in real time by secure messaging within an electronic medical record system or by reviewing the caseloads of nurse care managers.

Involving patients in decision making improves patient satisfaction with their treatment, adherence with therapy, and even some health outcomes. To support their increasing role, a wide array of decision aids has been developed for patients.

Clinical Information Systems

Well-maintained registries that are either independent or incorporated in an electronic medical record enable practices to identify patients who need additional services, produce rapid summaries of key clinical data and services for future patient encounters, and measure clinical performance. Registries allow practices to both monitor and manage their chronically ill populations. For example, individuals overdue for important preventive interventions or who fail to keep appointments can be efficiently identified and contacted.

Electronic two-way communication between patients and providers is playing an increasing role in the management of chronic disease. Telehealth and web portals enable providers to obtain and respond to clinical data from patients, and they give patients an efficient mechanism for addressing their questions and concerns.

Community Resources

Programs and organizations in patients' local communities can most effectively meet many of their needs. Such needs include transportation, homemaker services, smoking cessation (Chapter 31), exercise (Chapter 15), weight control (Chapter 227), peer support, caregiver support and respite, self-management training, and financial counseling and assistance. For commonly needed services, practices should at least be able to provide information to advise patients on their best options.

TRANSFORMING PRACTICE

Measures of disease control and other indicators of the quality of chronic care begin to improve only when practices have made system-wide changes in most of the elements of the chronic care model, such that the routine care of all their chronically ill patients has been affected. Practice routines and culture must change in ways that are initially foreign and uncomfortable for many practitioners. Team care means more meetings, new roles, and additional training for staff. To have useful registries and provide proactive care, busy practices must define their patient population and learn to manipulate software and data to get the information they need. Some of the changes may require additional financial investment. For all these reasons and more, improving chronic care management requires highly motivated physicians and practices that actively engage in continuous quality improvement. Practices must develop approaches that fit their patient population, resources, and practice style, and they must refine and adapt them using rapid cycle improvement methods.

Health Care Organization

Many practices caring for chronically ill individuals are parts of larger health care organizations that can either encourage and promote the improvement of chronic care or undermine and obstruct it. Helpful organizations promote continuous quality improvement, incorporate a trusted performance measurement system, and provide financial and/or nonfinancial incentives for high quality.

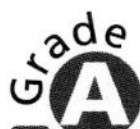

1. Chodosh J, Morton SC, Mojica W, et al. Meta-analysis: chronic disease self-management programs for older adults. *Ann Intern Med.* 2005;143:427-438.
2. Shojania KG, Ranji SR, McDonald KM, et al. Effects of quality improvement strategies for type 2 diabetes on glycemic control: a meta-regression analysis. *JAMA.* 2006;296:427-440.
3. Walsh JM, McDonald KM, Shojania KG, et al. Quality improvement strategies for hypertension management: a systematic review. *Med Care.* 2006;44:646-657.
4. Coleman K, Austin BT, Brach C, et al. Evidence on the chronic care model in the new millennium. *Health Aff (Millwood).* 2009;28:75-85.
5. Green BB, Cook AJ, Ralston JD, et al. Effectiveness of home blood pressure monitoring, web communication, and pharmacist care on hypertension control: a randomized controlled trial. *JAMA.* 2008;299:2857-2867.

SUGGESTED READINGS

Ahmed S, Gogovor A, Kosseim M, et al. Advancing the chronic care road map: a contemporary overview. *Healthc Q.* 2010;13:72-79. *Review.*

Hill MN, Miller NH, DeGeest S. American Society of Hypertension Writing Group. ASH position paper: Adherence and persistence with taking medication to control high blood pressure. *J Clin Hypertens.* 2010;12:757-764. *How to use the chronic care model to manage medications in hypertensive patients.*

Improving Chronic Care website. http://www.improvingchroniccare.org/index.php?p=Toolkit&s=244. *Advice for efficient and sustainable implementation of the chronic care model, with a downloadable copy and links to a variety of recommended tools.*

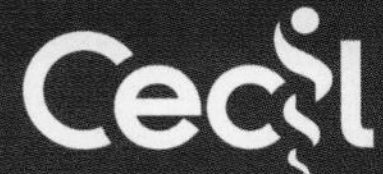

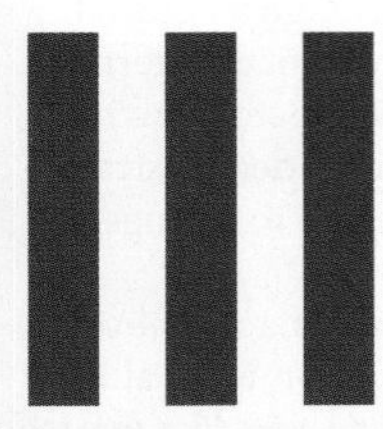

PREVENTIVE AND ENVIRONMENTAL ISSUES

13

COUNSELING FOR BEHAVIOR CHANGE

F. DANIEL DUFFY

Most office visits end with a brief conversation about diagnosis and a treatment recommendation, often including changes in long-standing behaviors. For clinicians, these conversations are routine, but for patients, these recommendations may challenge long-standing beliefs about well-being and begin repeated cycles of success and failure in replacing unhealthy habits with healthy ones. For patients with chronic illness, these habits typically include daily monitoring and medications for life.

Behavior change counseling is interpersonal therapy that changes mental models of health and internal motivational systems to reward healthy habits and extinguish unhealthy ones. The theory of behavior change counseling is grounded in cognitive behavior therapy, person-centered therapy, and social cognitive theory. Under experimental conditions and in practice, behavior change counseling delivered by trained counselors is efficacious in sustaining healthy diets, physical activity, abstinence from smoking, reduced alcohol consumption, safer sex, and daily self-care routines including adherence to medications.[1] The translation of behavior change counseling into a brief outpatient visit is challenging, owing to the long intervals between visits and the limited funding for counseling. Limited empirical evidence shows that brief office-based counseling using tailored patient-centered motivational methods and performed by trained clinicians successfully reduces smoking[2] and the hazardous use of alcohol.[3] Modest success can be achieved with brief office-based behavior change counseling for medication adherence, adopting safer sexual practices, making dietary change, and initiating physical activity.[4] The combination of direct counseling by the physician and a prepared office staff that supports patient self-care produces more effective outcomes. At a minimum, patient-centered motivational counseling improves the satisfaction of patients and physicians, forges therapeutic relationships, and influences modest changes in patients' health habits.

MODEL FOR OFFICE-BASED BEHAVIORAL CHANGE COUNSELING

Efficient behavior change counseling can be organized according to the transtheoretical model of change (Fig. 13-1), which cycles through five cognitive-experiential stages (*precontemplation*, *contemplation*, *determination*, *action*, and *maintenance*) and often through a sixth stage (*relapse*). Many patients recycle through the stages several times before establishing a new behavioral habit.

By identifying the stage of change, physicians can select efficient counseling strategies. For those who are not ready to change (precontemplation and contemplation), advice, education, and motivational counseling work best (Table 13-1). For those who are ready (determination and action), cognitive behavioral counseling based on self-determination theory works. For those who are already changing (maintenance and relapse), interventions based on social cognitive theory provides a good approach. An adaptation of the Counseling and Behavioral Interventions Work Group of the U.S. Preventive Services Task Force's "5 As" (assess, advise, agree, assist, and arrange) guides behavior change counseling in general health care settings.

Assess Risk for Unhealthy Behaviors

While taking a history of chronic illnesses (Chapter 6), physicians should ask about self-monitoring, adherence with medications, and self-care barriers and their solutions. In the personal and social history, physicians should ask about tobacco use, alcohol drinking, physical activity, diet, and sexual risks. In the family history, physicians uncover genetic and familial risks. Review of a patient's self-administered questionnaire by trained staff can help the physician obtain a health risk assessment efficiently.

Advise to Change Unhealthy Behaviors and Adopt Healthy Ones

There is strong evidence that direct, clear, nonjudgmental, and tailored advice delivered by a personal physician during a short office visit can help some patients stop smoking or reduce hazardous drinking.[4] Unfortunately, data also show that physicians rarely deliver information or advice about risky behaviors, unless behavior change is the specific agenda for an encounter or treatment for a condition.

If the patient expresses interest and time permits, physicians should give personalized advice. If time is short, the physician should arrange a counseling conversation for the near future. How advice is given influences internal motivation and self-efficacy. For example, asking permission before giving advice and postponing the conversation if the patient declines demonstrate respect for patient autonomy and acknowledge that motivation to change is entirely an internal process.

If the patient agrees, the clinician begins not by giving information about behaviors and risk, but by asking the patient to share his or her values and beliefs about the unhealthy behavior. Asking "*What do you like most about … ?*" followed by, "*What concerns you about … ?*" changes the focus of behavior change counseling from a treatment to an understanding of patients' values and beliefs. The ensuing conversation should explore the patient's perceived advantages of continuing behaviors, thoughts about changing, and confidence in the ability to do so. The physician adds information to the conversation, often by asking probing questions. This technique creates an opportunity to empathize with patients' conflict and deliberately raise their conviction that changing is important for achieving valued personal goals and enhancing self-confidence in the ability to do so.

Based on the conversation, clinicians diagnose the patient's stage of change in order to agree on goals for progressing through the cycle of change. A diagnostic tool, the *Conviction-Confidence Ruler* (Fig. 13-2), helps assess internal motivation for change. The number patients select suggests their stage of change.

Patients who select a low (0 to 2) conviction and confidence number are in the precontemplation stage. If they select low conviction and confidence scores, express ambivalence or emotional distress about advice to change, and do not intend to change soon, they are in the contemplation stage.

Patients who select a midrange conviction and confidence score (3 to 7) and state their intention to change within the next month may be in the determination stage. When they select a high conviction (8 to 10) and moderate to high confidence number (5 to 9) or report already making attempts at change, they are in the action stage.

Maintenance-stage patients select high conviction and confidence numbers. They report successful experience with the healthy behavior and effective coping in response to situations in which the unhealthy behavior appears attractive or safe to do just once more. In the relapse stage, patients reported a period of success with a new behavior but then regressed. Feelings of low self-efficacy and unrealistic expectation for positive benefits from the old behavior win over their intention to maintain the change. Disappointed and discouraged, such patients select a low confidence number. If not demoralized, they select a high conviction number; otherwise their conviction number is also low, as they recycle back into resistant precontemplation.

Agree on Appropriate Goals for the Stage of Change

In this step, physicians elicit and clarify patients' self-determined goals, articulate their own goals, and find common ground or negotiate a compromise. The result is agreement on clear, realistic, and achievable goals appropriate for the patient's stage of change (Table 13-2). Unfortunately, such agreement on goals is infrequent after usual medical encounters. Few patients are in the determination or action stages, so using only action-based behavior change counseling is often ineffective and frustrating. Patients who are in the precontemplation or contemplation stages and not ready for a change goal can agree to learn more. Most patients are in maintenance or relapse stages, with experience with both success and failure; counseling that supports self-regulation is most effective and efficient in such situations.

Assist Patient in Developing a Self-Determined and Stage-Appropriate Plan

The assist step involves stage-specific counseling, which may require training to be effective. When physicians have insufficient time or training, they can refer patients to behavior change counseling professionals, either within the practice or elsewhere in the community.

Counseling patients in the precontemplation stage raises their personal conviction that change is necessary to achieve their life and health goals. This counseling elicits the patient's commitment to seek information from family members, friends, or people who have successfully made similar changes about the behavior and what changing might be like. This cognitive, attitudinal, and emotional exploration clarifies the internal conflict between current

TABLE 13-1 STAGES OF CHANGE CHARACTERISTICS

STAGE OF CHANGE	PATIENT RESPONSE	PATIENT COPING TASKS	CLINICIAN COUNSELING TASKS	COUNSELING RESOURCES
Precontemplation	Surprise Not thinking about changing Demoralized if had relapse	Learn about risks of behavior Develop self-awareness	Reflect Advise Inform	Information media Self-assessment logs or diary
Contemplation	Ambivalence Gives reasons for concern about behavior Gives rationalization for unconcern about behavior	Emotional disturbance Self-re-evaluation Raise conviction Raise confidence	Empathize with patient's ambivalence Avoid argument Develop discrepancy Roll with resistance	Conviction-Confidence Ruler Decisional balance Feedback logs Role models Referral for group training
Determination	I must change I can do it	Raise conviction Raise confidence Develop action plan Pick start date Go public	Support self-efficacy Negotiate action plan Anticipate problems Connect to social support	Menu of options Referral for formal counseling List of role models
Action	What will I do? Who or what might help? What problems might I have?	Take action steps to change Manage withdrawal from addiction	Manage cues to old behavior Alert to consequence of new behavior Add rewards Manage withdrawal	Written plan Menu of cues Menu of consequences Menu of rewards Referral for counseling
Maintenance	Satisfied with changed self Spontaneously tells about success and difficulties	Manage cues to old behavior Manage bad effects of the new behavior Seek and use social support Become a role model to others	Discuss signs and times of relapse danger Discuss the danger of "relapse thinking" Admire new lifestyle habits	Role-model for others Frequent social support Referral for maintenance counseling
Relapse	Tells about thinking old behavior was no longer a concern Loss of control Demoralization	Learn the antecedents of relapse Recognize "relapse thinking" Keep public Call for help	Reframe relapse to be a valuable lesson Evoke self-efficiency Move quickly back into action	Referral for formal relapse counseling Contact list of recovery role models Frequent follow-up

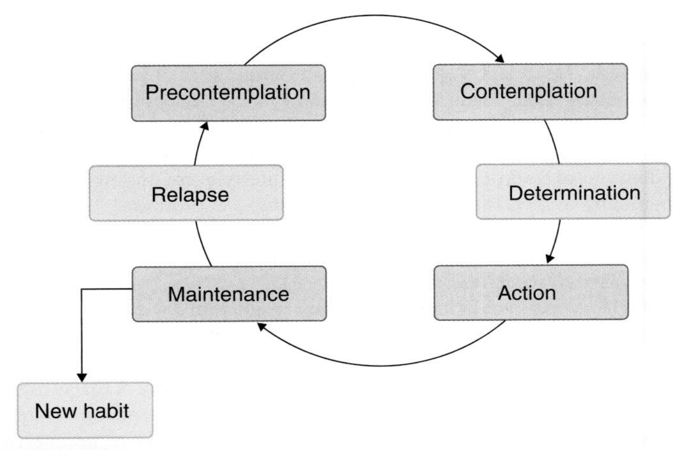

FIGURE 13-1. Cycle of change stages.

Conviction–Confidence Ruler												
On a scale of 1–10, how *convinced* are you that it is important for you to change … *(Name the behavior)* … ?"												
Not at all convinced	0	1	2	3	4	5	6	7	8	9	10	Totally convinced
On a scale of 1–10, how *confident* are you that you have the ability to change … *(Name the behavior)* … ?"												
Not at all confident	0	1	2	3	4	5	6	7	8	9	10	Totally confident

FIGURE 13-2. Motivational counseling aid.

TABLE 13-2 SUGGESTED GOALS FOR EACH STAGE OF CHANGE

STAGE OF CHANGE	EXAMPLE GOALS FOR VITAL BEHAVIORS
Precontemplation	Learn about the risk of continuing unhealthy behavior
Contemplation	Re-evaluate one's life's goals in context of unhealthy behavior
Determination/action	Commit to a start/quit date and begin vital behaviors
Maintenance	Self-monitor behavior, success, and learning
Relapse recovery	Intensify social support and self-regulating behavior

behavior and life goals or moral values. Precontemplation is not influenced by professional argument or debate.

Motivational interviewing, which is best delivered during visits specifically scheduled for behavior change counseling, is effective for patients in contemplation, especially for those with addiction. Motivational interviewing helps patients explore and resolve their ambivalence about changing. Using open-ended questions such as *"What do you like about … (the unhealthy behavior)… ?"* physicians inquire with genuine interest to reveal the patient's perceived advantages of the unhealthy habit or behavior. Turning to the healthy behavior, the physician asks with interest *"What concerns you about doing … ?"* to clarify what patients believe the risks and the benefits of adopting vital behaviors might be. A *decisional balance table* (Table 13-3) can display patients' reasons for maintaining the current behavior compared with those for adopting the healthy one. Counselors should listen to patients' statements, repeating the exact words to elicit their self-motivating statements. By guiding patients in examining both sides of their ambivalence, resistance can be reduced and readiness to change can be assessed, without attempting premature change.

By helping patients "think out loud" about their conflicting reasons for change and their rationalizations for not changing, motivational interviewing amplifies the discomfort of ambivalence and motivates change. For example,

TABLE 13-3 DECISIONAL BALANCE

BEHAVIOR	REASONS NOT TO CHANGE	REASONS TO CHANGE
Unhealthy behavior	What do you like about it?	What are your concerns about it?
Healthy behavior	What are your concerns about it?	What do you like about it?

a conviction-confidence scale can clarify a patient's values and knowledge about the behavior, thereby allowing the counselor to ask, *"Why 4 and not lower?"* Asking questions like *"What would it take to raise your conviction level?"* helps patients to voice their values and beliefs and to understand their strengths and resources.

When patients express resistance to change, motivational interviewing recommends that counselors not argue but rather make empathic statements to demonstrate their understanding of the patient's painful ambivalence, beliefs, and feelings that rationalize a low conviction about the benefits of change. Using the conviction-confidence ruler, physicians can engage a patient's self-reflection by asking, *"What makes your commitment or confidence a "2" and not "0"*? If patients report a zero for commitment or confidence, the counselor might ask, *"Zero ... that's as low as you can get....What would have to happen to make it a 1?"*

Determination/action counseling uses cognitive-behavioral methods to help patients develop a written plan to change lifestyle behaviors and to add self-monitoring and coping strategies to prevent relapse. The plan, which identifies the new behaviors patients will adopt to replace unhealthy ones, includes changing social situations that stimulate craving for the effects of the old behavior and using reminders and rewards for performing the new behavior. When the change requires an end to addictive behaviors, the plan must include treatments to manage withdrawal and craving. The plan asks partners and others who are making similar changes for support. The counseling helps patients anticipate challenges to sustaining the change and develop coping solutions for preventing and recovering from lapses. Plans work best when patients identify the people, resources, and coping strategies themselves. Exploring past experience with change may help identify strategies that were at least temporarily successful. Conversely, identifying what went wrong following a period of success clarifies how to cope with relapse situations.

Multidisciplinary teams of nurse educators, nutritionists, physical therapists, psychologists, and pharmacists can share education, counseling, and skills training. Referral is usually necessary for changing addictive behaviors and self-management of chronic illness.

The maintenance stage requires counseling in coping strategies to deal with the attraction or perceived safety of the unhealthy behavior, especially during the first months of change. Counseling aims at enhancing coping responses by self-monitoring of the positive effects of the healthy behavior, avoiding situations in which the unhealthy behavior becomes more attractive, and developing a strong social network that supports new coping responses.

Maintenance counseling conversations explore successes using questions like *"What has worked?"* and lapses using questions like *"Most people have difficulty; how has this change gone for you?"* It is useful to ask specifically about relapse thinking: *"Many people begin to think that after a while it's safe to ... (return to the old habit) just one more time; how have you handled such thoughts?"* Regarding engaging social support, counselors might ask, *"Who or what has helped you sustain your new behavior?"* Planning for lapse recovery can be initiated by asking, *"Should you slip, what will you do, or who will you call?"*

If relapse occurs, counselors should remind patients that relapse, by definition, follows success, which proves that change is possible. Relapse must become a learning opportunity to revisit pre-relapse thinking and develop a new action plan.

Arrange Follow-up and Referral for Formal Counseling

At the conclusion of counseling, counselors ask patients to rehearse the plan verbally and state their confidence in being able to execute it. Confidence ratings less than 7 may be insufficient to undertake and sustain vital behaviors. Arranging for counseling at a future date aims to identify and resolve barriers until a patient's confidence level is at least 7, or to renegotiate a goal, with a confidence level of at least 7.

The arrange step involves scheduling future office visits within an appropriate interval for the stage of change. Longer counseling visits within a few months are appropriate for the precontemplation and contemplation stages. In-person or telephone follow-up visits within a week or two are useful for counseling in the determination/action stage. For the maintenance stage, office follow-up counseling is as frequent as possible, usually monthly, and ideally combined with almost daily contact with other supporting persons or role models. When intensive counseling is necessary, counselors may arrange referral to patient education classes, behavioral counseling professionals, or self-help support groups to monitor the effectiveness of the referred behavior change counseling.

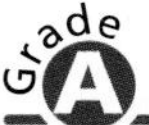

1. Schedlbauer A, Davies P, Fahey T. Interventions to improve adherence to lipid lowering medication. *Cochrane Database Syst Rev*. 2010;3:CD004371.
2. McCambridge J, Slym RL, Strang J. Randomized controlled trial of motivational interviewing compared with drug information and advice for early intervention among young cannabis users. *Addiction*. 2008;103:1809-1818.
3. Solberg LI, Maciosek MV, Edwards NM. Primary care intervention to reduce alcohol misuse ranking its health impact and cost effectiveness. *Am J Prev Med*. 2008;34:143-152.
4. Goldstein MG, Whitlock EP, DePue E. Multiple behavioral risk factor interventions in primary care: summary of research evidence. *Am J Prev Med*. 2004;27:61-79.

SUGGESTED READINGS

Gardner B, Whittington C, McAteer J, et al. Using theory to synthesize evidence from behavior change interventions: the example of audit and feedback. *Soc Sci Med*. 2010;70:1618-1625. *Emphasizes the value of audit and feedback to change behavior.*

Novack DH, Clark WD, Saizow RB, et al, eds. doc.com—An interactive learning resource for healthcare communication. [Internet]: American Academy on Communication in Healthcare/Drexel University College of Medicine; 2005. http://www.aachonline.org. Accessed Nov. 29, 2010.

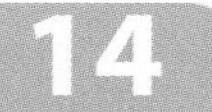

14 THE PERIODIC HEALTH EXAMINATION

DAVID ATKINS AND MARY BARTON

Primary and secondary prevention is an essential part of primary care and the patient-centered medical home (Chapter 12). The appropriate services and their frequency vary with the age, gender, and individual risk factors of each patient. A periodic health examination focusing on prevention increases the delivery of appropriate screening and lifestyle counseling. The most comprehensive prevention recommendations are produced by the U.S. Preventive Services Task Force (USPSTF), an ongoing panel of experts supported by the federal Agency for Healthcare Research and Quality (*http://www.uspreventiveservicestaskforce.org*).

USPSTF recommendations are used by major primary care subspecialty groups, many health plans, and quality organizations. The USPSTF bases its recommendations on two factors: an estimate of the *net benefits* (benefits minus harms) of a service, and an assessment of the *certainty* of that estimate, based on the rigor of supporting studies. Grade A recommendations require high certainty of a substantial net benefit, most often from large, prospective, controlled studies that measure morbidity or mortality. USPSTF recommendations are thus more conservative than those of some subspecialty organizations that may give more weight to indirect evidence, such as earlier detection of disease, and less weight to potential harms of interventions. Clinicians can draw several general conclusions from an evidence-based approach to prevention: we should be selective in our use of screening tests and involve patients in decisions about specific services for which a small chance of benefit must be balanced against possible harm.

HISTORY AND RISK ASSESSMENT

The history and risk assessment are important tools to identify individuals who may need additional screening tests or immunizations not generally recommended for their age group or who may benefit from specific counseling to address unhealthy behaviors. Formal health risk appraisals should be linked to a system to provide specific feedback and targeted interventions. Risk assessment should address the following:

- Use of tobacco, alcohol, and other drugs (especially injection drugs) (Chapters 31, 32, and 33)
- Diet (Chapter 220)
- Physical activity (Chapter 15)

- Sexual behavior that may increase the risk of sexually transmitted diseases or unintended pregnancy (Chapters 293, 392, and 395)
- Family history of cancer and heart disease
- Residence (community risk of infectious diseases)
- Presence of chronic diseases, such as diabetes, and of other cardiovascular risk factors (Chapter 51)

SCREENING FOR EARLY DISEASE OR ASYMPTOMATIC RISK FACTORS

Every year, new screening tests are introduced and marketed on the basis of their ability to detect unrecognized diseases or risk factors for disease. Other conditions need to be fulfilled for a screening test to be worthwhile for routine use, however (Table 14-1). Benefits of screening must be balanced against the potential harms, including false-positive results and the risks and costs of follow-up procedures or treatments. Even when tests have high specificity, the majority of positive results will be false-positives if the test is used to screen healthy populations for uncommon conditions such as cancer (Chapter 9). There is growing evidence that cancer screening can lead to "overdiagnosis"—detection of slow-growing cancers that would never have caused clinical symptoms in a patient's lifetime. Overdiagnosis subjects patients to the side effects of treatment with no benefits. A relatively small number of screening tests have been proved beneficial for the general population (Table 14-2), but additional tests are indicated for specific populations at risk (Table 14-3). Many commonly used tests are not recommended by the USPSTF (Table 14-4) because they provide little benefit or lack sufficient evidence to prove or disprove their value.

Depression

Depression is common and frequently undetected in primary care (Chapter 404). Simple screening instruments, including the following two questions—During the past 2 weeks, have you felt down, depressed, or hopeless? During the past 2 weeks, have you felt little interest or pleasure in doing things?—increase the detection of major depression. To improve outcomes, however, screening for depression must be linked to an organized system with staff support to ensure follow-up and treatment.[1]

High Blood Pressure, Abnormal Lipids, and Other Coronary Risk Factors

Blood pressure should be measured at least every 2 years (Chapter 67). The USPSTF recommends measuring total and high-density lipoprotein cholesterol, which can be done on fasting or nonfasting samples, beginning in middle age or earlier in the presence of other cardiovascular risk factors. The National Cholesterol Education Program guidelines recommend fasting lipoprotein analysis beginning at age 20 years (Chapter 213). Either strategy will detect the high-risk patients who need lipid-lowering therapy. Treatment decisions for elevated lipids and for blood pressure should be based on estimates of coronary heart disease risk (Chapter 51). Although factors such as C-reactive protein, homocysteine, and coronary calcification as assessed by computed tomography (CT) are associated with an increased risk of heart disease, the USPSTF found insufficient evidence to recommend their routine use.[2]

Abdominal Aortic Aneurysm

Between 5 and 9% of men older than 65 years have an abdominal aortic aneurysm (Chapter 78). The risk of aneurysm is higher in smokers and is substantially lower in women. The USPSTF recommends one-time screening with ultrasound examination in men aged 65 to 75 years who are current or former smokers, based on trials demonstrating as much as a 40% lower death rate from abdominal aortic aneurysm rupture in screened men.[3]

Colorectal Cancer

Screening can reduce both the incidence of and mortality from colorectal cancer. Options for screening men and women older than 50 years include an annual fecal occult blood test or fecal immunochemical test, flexible sigmoidoscopy every 5 to 10 years, or colonoscopy every 10 years (Chapter 199). Colonoscopy combines detection with the opportunity for biopsy and removal of lesions, so it is preferred in some guidelines. It carries higher costs and risks, however, and no single strategy has proved to be more effective or cost-effective than the alternatives.[4] In a randomized trial, a single flexible sigmoidoscopy screening between 55 and 64 years of age reduced the colorectal cancer incidence by 33% and the colorectal cancer mortality by 43% after 11 years of follow-up in people who were screened.[5] Evidence is not yet sufficient to support newer technologies such as CT colography or fecal tests for DNA markers of neoplasia. The USPSTF recommends stopping routine screening at age 75 years.

TABLE 14-1 REQUIREMENTS OF AN EFFECTIVE SCREENING TEST

The disease being screened for is an important cause of morbidity and mortality
Screening can detect disease in an early, presymptomatic phase
Screening and treatment of patients with early disease or risk factors produce better health outcomes than does treatment of patients when they present with symptoms
Screening test is acceptable to patients and clinicians—safe, convenient, acceptable false-positive rate, acceptable costs
Benefits of early detection and treatment are sufficient to justify potential harms and costs of screening

TABLE 14-2 PREVENTION RECOMMENDATIONS FOR THE GENERAL POPULATION: FROM THE U.S. PREVENTIVE SERVICES TASK FORCE AND OTHER SOURCES

SCREENING
Height, weight, and body mass index (BMI) calculation: periodically
Blood pressure: at least every 2 yr
Screen for problem drinking
Brief screen for depression*
Total blood cholesterol and HDL cholesterol: every 5 yr for men and women ≥20 yr with CHD risk factors and men ≥35 yr without CHD risk factors
Colorectal cancer screening: age ≥50 yr (see text for options)
Mammogram (± clinical breast examination): at least every 2 yr for women ≥50 yr; discuss with women 40–49
Papanicolaou (Pap) test: at least every 3 yr for sexually active women aged 21–65 yr
Chlamydia: sexually active women ≤24 yr and older women at risk
Bone mineral density test: women ≥65 yr and high-risk women <65 yr
COUNSELING
Substance use
Tobacco cessation
Reduction of risky or harmful alcohol use
Diet and exercise
Limit saturated fat; maintain calorie balance; emphasize grains, fruits, and vegetables‡
Regular physical activity†
Sexual behavior
Unintended pregnancy: contraception
STD prevention: avoid high-risk behavior, use condoms or female barrier with spermicide†
Injury prevention
Lap and shoulder belts
Motorcycle, bicycle, and ATV helmets†
Smoke detector†
Dental health
Regular visits to dental care provider†
Floss, brush with fluoride toothpaste daily†
IMMUNIZATIONS
Pneumococcal vaccine (once, age ≥65 yr)
Influenza vaccine (annual, age ≥50 yr)
Tetanus-diphtheria (Td) boosters (every 10 yr)
Measles, mumps, rubella (MMR) vaccine (susceptible adults aged 19–49 yr)§
Varicella (2 doses, susceptible adults aged 30–49 yr)§
Human papillomavirus (HPV) vaccine (3 doses, women ≤26 yr)
CHEMOPREVENTION
Multivitamin with folic acid (women planning or capable of pregnancy)
Discuss benefits and harms of aspirin to prevent vascular disease in middle-aged adults and others at increased risk of vascular disease

*Depression screening is most effective where systems exist to improve its management.
†The ability of clinician counseling to influence this behavior is uncertain.
‡Diet counseling is most effective when it targets at-risk groups.
§Immunity can be verified by serologic testing, documented history of illness, or vaccination.
Other sources for Tables 14-2 and 14-3 include U.S. Department of Health and Human Services (diet, physical activity) and Centers for Disease Control and Prevention (injury prevention, immunizations, PPD).
ATV = all-terrain vehicle; CHD = coronary heart disease; HDL = high-density lipoprotein; STD = sexually transmitted disease.

TABLE 14-3 RECOMMENDED SCREENING AND INTERVENTIONS FOR HIGH-RISK POPULATIONS

POTENTIAL INTERVENTION	POPULATION
Ultrasound examination for abdominal aortic aneurysm	Current or former male smokers aged 65–75 yr
HIV test	High-risk sexual behavior or IV drug use; consider local epidemiology*
Syphilis (RPR/VDRL)	High-risk sexual behavior; consider local epidemiology*
Gonorrhea screen	High-risk sexual behavior; consider local epidemiology*
PPD	Specific immigrant groups, prisoners, HIV patients
Hepatitis B vaccine	Exposure to blood products; IV drug use; high-risk sexual behavior; travelers to high-risk areas
Hepatitis A vaccine	Persons living in or traveling to high-risk areas; institutionalized persons and workers in these institutions; those with certain chronic medical conditions
Meningococcal vaccine	First-year college students in dormitories; military recruits; those with asplenia; travelers to high-risk areas
Varicella vaccine	Adults born after 1980 without evidence of immunity
Breast cancer chemoprevention	Women at increased risk for breast cancer and with low risk of thromboembolic complications
Diabetes screen	Persons with elevated blood pressure

*Routine screening may be indicated in communities or settings where infection is prevalent.
HIV = human immunodeficiency virus; IV = intravenous; PPD = purified protein derivative; RPR = rapid plasma reagin; VDRL = Venereal Disease Research Laboratory.

TABLE 14-4 INTERVENTIONS NOT RECOMMENDED FOR ROUTINE USE IN ASYMPTOMATIC AVERAGE-RISK ADULTS*

Resting or exercise electrocardiography or helical CT for asymptomatic coronary disease
Ultrasound examination for asymptomatic carotid artery disease
Chest radiograph
Routine blood tests for anemia
Routine urine tests
Blood tests or ultrasound examination for ovarian cancer
Whole body CT
Brief tests of mental status
Vitamin supplements
Blood test for hepatitis C infection
Blood level of C-reactive protein to predict coronary risk
Prostate-specific antigen for prostate cancer

*These tests are not recommended for routine use because there is insufficient evidence that they improve clinical outcomes or because harms exceed benefits in the general population. Any of the tests may be appropriate for selected patients on the basis of clinical judgment, and some are under investigation for more widespread use.
CT = computed tomography.

Breast Cancer

In large trials, mammography screening (at intervals of 1 to 2 years, with or without clinical breast examination) reduces breast cancer mortality by 15 to 30% (Chapter 204). Most but not all trials suggest that the benefits of screening extend to women in their 40s, but the benefits are smaller and the risks of false-positive results are higher than in women aged 50 to 70 years.[6] No studies provide data on the benefits of screening women aged 75 and older. In a collaborative study, six independent models predicted that an average of 80% of the benefit of mammography could be achieved with biennial rather than annual mammography, whereas national mammography surveillance data indicate that false-positive results and other harms of screening would be reduced by about half if women were screened every other year instead of yearly. Although many cancers are discovered by patients, teaching women to perform breast self-examination increases the likelihood that a woman will undergo further evaluation for an unimportant finding, but it does not improve outcomes. Widespread screening for *BRCA1* or *BRCA2*, inherited mutations that increase the risk for breast cancer, is not recommended, but women with a suggestive family history (multiple first-degree relatives with breast or ovarian cancer) should be referred for genetic counseling.

Cervical Cancer

Papanicolaou (Pap) screening is highly effective in preventing invasive cervical cancer, but many low-risk women in the United States are screened more often than needed. The USPSTF and American College of Obstetrics and Gynecology endorse delaying screening until age 21, screening only every 2 to 3 years instead of annually in women with previous normal test results (Chapter 205), and offering low-risk women the option of discontinuing screening after 65 years of age. Screening is not indicated in women who have undergone a hysterectomy for benign disease. Liquid-based cytology specimens do not improve clinical outcomes significantly, but they allow testing for human papillomavirus (Chapters 205 and 381), which may help in managing borderline Pap smear results, such as atypical squamous cells. Primary screening for human papillomavirus, although sensitive for cervical neoplasia, is not recommended for routine use because it identifies many younger women with transient infection. Whether women who have received the human papillomavirus vaccine (Chapter 17) need less frequent screening is not yet known.

Prostate Cancer

Screening with prostate-specific antigen (PSA) can increase the detection of organ-confined prostate cancer, but two recent large trials provided conflicting results as to whether screening lowers morbidity or mortality from prostate cancer (Chapter 207). An American trial found no benefit of annual PSA testing, but it was hampered by a high rate of screening in the control group. A European study reported that men randomized to screening every 4 years had a 20% lower risk of dying from prostate cancer after 9 years; for each prostate cancer death prevented, 48 additional men were treated for prostate cancer and 1068 men had to undergo screening. Because of the significant morbidity associated with overdiagnosis and overtreatment, including incontinence and impotence, the USPSTF does not recommend routine PSA screening, but the American Cancer Society and some specialty groups recommend discussing PSA screening with men who have a life expectancy of at least 10 years.

Osteoporosis

Tests of bone mineral density can identify men and women with a high risk of fracture due to osteoporosis and who may benefit from medications proved to lower the risk of fracture (Chapter 251). The USPSTF recommends screening for osteoporosis in women older than 65 years or earlier in the presence of risk factors for osteoporosis. The most accurate predictor of risk of hip fracture is bone mineral density of the hip assessed with dual-energy x-ray absorptiometry. A tool developed by the World Health Organization (*http://www.shef.ac.uk/FRAX/*) incorporates bone mineral density and other risk factors, such as age and fracture history, to guide treatment decisions.

Thyroid Disease

Routine thyroid testing occasionally identifies patients with symptomatic but undiagnosed hypothyroidism (Chapter 233), but it more often detects subclinical hypothyroidism, a disorder marked by elevations in thyroid-stimulating hormone with normal levels of free thyroxine. Because the benefits of treating subclinical hypothyroidism remain uncertain, the USPSTF does not recommend routine thyroid testing in the absence of symptoms. Clinicians should be alert to subtle signs of thyroid disease and have a low threshold for testing patients in high-risk groups, including postpartum and postmenopausal women.

Diabetes

Routine screening for diabetes beginning at age 45 years is recommended by some groups, but the USPSTF recommends screening only in patients with elevated blood pressure (Chapter 237). Although tight glucose control can reduce the incidence of microvascular disease, the benefit of early presymptomatic detection on retinopathy, neuropathy, and nephropathy is likely to be small. The benefits of early detection of diabetes are much greater in persons with hypertension because more aggressive treatment of blood pressure in patients with diabetes has been shown to reduce cardiovascular events within 5 years.

HIV Infection

The USPSTF recommends screening for HIV infection in all pregnant women and in adolescents and adults at increased risk. In an effort to reduce the estimated 25% of infected patients who have not yet been diagnosed, however, the Centers for Disease Control and Prevention recommends that all adolescents and adults aged 13 to 64 years have at least one HIV test and annual tests if they are at high risk.

Sexually Transmitted Disease

Screening for chlamydia (Chapter 326) is recommended for all sexually active women ages 24 years and younger and for older women at risk. Nucleic acid amplification tests can be performed on cervical or urine specimens. Early detection can reduce pelvic inflammatory disease (Chapter 293), a risk factor for infertility and ectopic pregnancy. Similar benefits are likely from screening women for gonorrhea (Chapter 307), but the risk of gonorrhea infection is more concentrated in high-risk urban and southeastern rural populations.

Vision and Hearing

Undetected but correctable vision and hearing problems are common in older adults and can be discovered by asking about problems and performing simple tests of visual acuity and hearing. Regular visual acuity testing is recommended for older adults by many organizations, but a large trial did not find any lasting benefits of screening, despite detecting many correctable causes of vision problems.

BEHAVIORAL INTERVENTIONS

Lifestyle factors contribute to a large proportion of preventable deaths in the United States. Brief interventions are effective for some behaviors such as smoking and problem drinking, but changing other behaviors usually requires more intensive approaches. The 5 *A*s framework—ask, assess, advise, assist, and arrange—which was developed from smoking cessation research, provides a useful framework for counseling (Chapter 13).

Tobacco Use

Brief interventions can produce small but clinically important increases in quit rates among smokers. Effects increase with more intensive counseling and support, including the use of medication (Chapter 31).

Problem Drinking

A variety of screening instruments can detect patients with problems due to alcohol and those with risky patterns of alcohol consumption. Brief interventions can successfully reduce alcohol consumption in at-risk drinkers (Chapter 32).

Diet

Diet counseling can reduce the intake of saturated fat and increase the consumption of fruits and vegetables. Effects are most consistent with more intensive counseling (multiple sessions with trained counselors) and in higher risk patients, such as those with elevated lipid levels (Chapter 220).

Physical Activity

Moderate physical activity reduces the risk of obesity, diabetes, and coronary heart disease, among other benefits. Studies of counseling in the primary care setting, however, have reported inconsistent effects on long-term levels of physical activity (Chapter 15).

Injury Prevention

Motor vehicle injuries are the leading cause of years of potential life lost before age 65 years. In older persons, falls are a leading cause of unintentional injury and can be reduced with targeted interventions (Chapter 24).

IMMUNIZATIONS

Recommendations regarding immunization (see Tables 14-2 and 14-3) are regularly updated by the Advisory Committee on Immunization Practices of the Centers for Disease Control and Prevention *(www.cdc.gov/vaccines)* (Chapter 17). Annual influenza immunization is effective in all adults but is most important in those older than 50 years and others at high risk because of chronic conditions or immunodeficiency. Pneumococcal immunization is recommended at least once at age 65 years or after for all adults and for younger adults with asplenia, chronic heart or lung disease, and other immune disorders. Revaccination is not generally recommended unless the initial immunization was before age 65 or the patient has immune-related risk factors. Two doses of varicella vaccine are recommended for all adults born in the United States after 1980 without other evidence of immunity, and one dose of zoster vaccine is recommended for all adults at age 60. Adults should be revaccinated once with the Tdap vaccine (tetanus, diphtheria, acellular pertussis) and every 10 years thereafter with Td, primarily to maintain levels of immunity against diphtheria.

CHEMOPREVENTION

Aspirin, postmenopausal hormone replacement therapy, and breast cancer chemopreventive drugs carry both benefits and risks. Decisions need to consider the likely benefits (which increase with the underlying risk of the disease being prevented), the probability of harm, and the individual preferences of each patient.

Aspirin

In men and women without known vascular disease, aspirin reduces the combined risk of myocardial infarction, stroke, and other serious cardiovascular events by 12%, but it also increases the risk of serious gastrointestinal bleeding and hemorrhagic stroke and does not significantly reduce cardiovascular mortality.[7] Individuals and their physicians need to assess whether the benefits, which increase with the risk of vascular disease, outweigh the bleeding risks, which increase with age (Chapter 37).

Chemoprevention of Breast Cancer

Tamoxifen and raloxifene can reduce the incidence of invasive breast cancer by nearly 50% in women at increased risk, but both agents increase risk of thromboembolic events (including stroke) and worsen menopausal symptoms; tamoxifen also increases the risk of endometrial cancer (Chapter 204). The balance of benefits and harm is most favorable in women younger than 60 years who have an increased risk of breast cancer owing to family history.

Postmenopausal Hormone Therapy

Estrogen therapy reduces the risk of fracture, but it increases the risk of thromboembolism and gallbladder disease (Chapter 248). When given with progestin, postmenopausal estrogen modestly increases the risk of heart disease and stroke (primarily in women older than 60), breast cancer, and dementia.[8] Hormone replacement therapy is a reasonable option for women with persistent, troublesome menopausal symptoms, but it should not routinely be used for preventive purposes.

Vitamin Supplementation

The USPSTF does not recommend routine vitamin supplementation because multiple large trials have failed to demonstrate the benefits of vitamins A, C, and E or folic acid against heart disease or cancer. Several studies suggested that β-carotene may increase the risk of lung cancer in smokers, and a meta-analysis suggested that folic acid supplementation could increase cancer risk.

FUTURE ISSUES

As the understanding of genetic factors that modify the risk of disease grows, clinicians may eventually be able to target screening, preventive treatments, or lifestyle interventions to those at greatest risk. The value of using currently available tests to screen average-risk individuals is limited by an incomplete understanding of the predictive value of specific genotypes in the general population, the uncertain effect of such information on clinical decisions, and concerns about the possible adverse effects of screening (e.g., anxiety or "labeling," false reassurance, discrimination).

With the current epidemic of obesity in the United States, and its attendant long-term health consequences, effective counseling tools and strategies may be more important in the coming decades than improved screening and early detection tools. Helping patients choose a healthier diet, increase their physical activity, and maintain a healthy weight is difficult, but the lessons of tobacco control over the past 30 years suggest that a combination of consistent clinical counseling and encouragement, complemented by public health messages and community strategies, can have an important health impact.

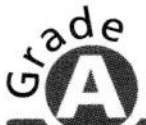

1. O'Connor EA, Whitlock EP, Beil TL, et al. Screening for depression in adult patients in primary care settings: a systematic evidence review. *Ann Intern Med*. 2009;151:793-803.

2. U.S. Preventive Services Task Force. Using nontraditional risk factors in coronary heart disease risk assessment: U.S. Preventive Services Task Force recommendation statement. *Ann Intern Med.* 2009;151:474-482.
3. Fleming C, Whitlock EP, Beil TL, et al. Screening for abdominal aortic aneurysm: a best-evidence systematic review. *Ann Intern Med.* 2005;142:203-211.
4. Whitlock EP, Lin JS, Liles E, et al. Screening for colorectal cancer: a targeted, updated systematic review for the U.S. Preventive Services Task Force. *Ann Intern Med.* 2008;149:638-658.
5. Atkin WS, Edwards R, Kralj-Hans I, et al. Once-only flexible sigmoidoscopy screening in prevention of colorectal cancer: a multicentre randomised controlled trial. *Lancet.* 2010;375:1624-1633.
6. Nelson HD, Tyne K, Naik A, et al. Screening for breast cancer: an update for the U.S. Preventive Services Task Force. *Ann Intern Med.* 2009;151:727-737.
7. Antithrombotic Trialists' Collaboration. Aspirin in the primary and secondary prevention of vascular disease: collaborative meta-analysis of individual participant data from randomized trials. *Lancet.* 2009;373:1849-1860.
8. Rossouw JE, Prentice RL, Manson JE, et al. Postmenopausal hormone therapy and risk of cardiovascular disease by age and years since menopause. *JAMA.* 2007;297:1465-1477.

SUGGESTED READINGS

Canadian Task Force on Preventive Health Care. http://www.canadiantaskforce.ca. *A Canadian counterpart to the USPSTF offers an independent perspective on preventive health interventions.*
National Guideline Clearinghouse. http://www.guidelines.gov. *Standardized descriptions of more than 1700 guidelines, with full text access to many of them. Guidelines can be searched by condition, intervention, or organization, and the site will construct a comparison of different guidelines on a given topic.*
U.S. Preventive Services Task Force. http://uspreventiveservicestaskforce.org. *This site includes all the recommendations and supporting reviews of the USPSTF.*

15

PHYSICAL ACTIVITY

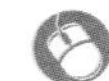

DAVID M. BUCHNER

DEFINITIONS

Physical activity can be broadly defined as body movement that is produced by skeletal muscles and expends energy. When discussing the health benefits of activity, it is useful to divide body movements into two categories. *Baseline activity* refers to light-intensity activities of daily life, such as standing, walking slowly, and lifting lightweight objects. *Health-enhancing physical activity* is activity that when added to baseline activity produces important health benefits and generally involves the large muscle groups of the body and substantial energy expenditure. Herein, *physical activity* refers to health-enhancing physical activity. *Exercise* refers to the subset of physical activity that involves a structured program to improve physical fitness.

Regular physical activity improves *health-related physical fitness*—the physiologic components of fitness that influence risk of disease, functional limitations, disability, and premature mortality. These components include cardiorespiratory endurance (aerobic capacity); skeletal muscle strength, power, and endurance; body composition and bone strength; and balance, flexibility, and reaction time.

The primary attributes of physical activity are *type* (mode), *frequency, duration,* and *intensity.* Types of physical activity (e.g., walking, swimming, lifting, stretching) are grouped according to their main physiologic effects into well-known categories: *aerobic* (or "cardio"), *muscle strengthening, flexibility,* and *balance.* Intensity is the level of effort during activity. For aerobic activity, the *absolute intensity* is measured in metabolic equivalents (METs), with 1 MET being the resting metabolic rate—an oxygen consumption of roughly 3.5 mL/kg/minute. The *relative intensity,* which is the percentage of oxygen uptake (aerobic capacity) reserve required to perform an activity, ranges from 0 to 100%. In practice, the heart rate is used to monitor relative intensity because of the generally linear relationship between heart rate and percentage of oxygen uptake. The *volume* (or amount) of activity is the product of frequency, duration, and intensity. Volume can be measured as activity-related energy expenditure (e.g., kcal/week) or as MET-minutes per week (a sum of the MET intensity of all activities multiplied by the minutes each activity is performed).

EPIDEMIOLOGY

Levels of Physical Activity

Data on long-term trends in the level of physical activity among adults are limited. Even so, it is highly likely that Americans' level of physical activity has declined since the 1950s. Levels of activity around the home, work-related activity, and transportation activity have apparently declined over the past 50 years. Trends in leisure-time physical activity are either stable or slightly improving.

In recent national surveys that track domestic, leisure-time, and transportation physical activity using questionnaires, about 45% of American adults are active at recommended levels. Using objective measurements (an accelerometer), however, less than 5% of adults meet the recommended levels of physical activity, suggesting that the lack of physical activity is a larger public health problem than previously realized.

Physical activity levels decline with age, and men report more activity than women. Higher levels of income and education are associated with greater physical activity. White Americans report higher levels of physical activity than other racial and ethnic groups do.

Preventive Health Benefits in Adults

There is strong evidence that regular moderate or vigorous physical activity (Table 15-1) reduces the risk for premature mortality and coronary artery disease (Chapter 51), stroke (Chapter 413), high blood pressure (Chapter 67), adverse lipid profile (Chapter 213), type 2 diabetes mellitus (Chapter 237), metabolic syndrome, osteoporosis (Chapter 251), colon cancer (Chapter 199), breast cancer (Chapter 204), and obesity (Chapter 227). Physical activity also reduces the risk for falls, cognitive impairment in older adults, age-related muscle loss, and depression (Chapters 24 and 404). There is moderate evidence that physical activity reduces the risk of hip fracture, lung cancer, endometrial cancer, and sleep disorders. Some evidence suggests that physical activity reduces the risk for anxiety disorders, osteoarthritis, and back pain. Observational studies consistently report that physical activity delays age-related functional limitations and loss of independence.

The benefits of physical activity are independent of other risk factors. For example, a sedentary obese smoker achieves health benefits from exercise, even if smoking and obesity persist.

Epidemiologic studies report that low levels of activity are associated with an increased risk for adverse health outcomes, including up to a 52% increase in overall mortality, a doubling of mortality from cardiovascular disease, and a 29% increase in mortality from cancer. When a healthy diet, regular activity, and abstinence from smoking are considered simultaneously, the effect of lifestyle is dramatic. For example, one study attributed 82% of coronary events in women to the lack of adherence to a healthy lifestyle.

The main determinant of the health benefits of physical activity is volume. Substantial health benefits begin to occur with a volume of 500 to 1000 MET-minutes/week. An adult can accumulate 500 MET-minutes by walking at 3.0 miles per hour (a 3.3-MET activity) on 5 days a week for 30 minutes (3.3 METs $\times$ 5 $\times$ 30 minutes = $\approx$500 MET-minutes). When measured by caloric expenditure, this volume of walking in a 75-kg (165-lb) adult expends an extra 430 kcal above the 190 kcal that would have been expended under resting conditions.

The dose-response relationship between volume and health benefits appears to be curvilinear, such that the marginal benefit of activity at lower

TABLE 15-1 EXAMPLES OF MODERATE-INTENSITY AND VIGOROUS-INTENSITY ACTIVITIES

MODERATE INTENSITY
Walking briskly (3 miles per hour or faster, but not race-walking)
Water aerobics
Bicycling slower than 10 miles per hour
Tennis (doubles)
Ballroom dancing
General gardening
VIGOROUS INTENSITY
Race-walking, jogging, or running
Swimming laps
Tennis (singles)
Bicycling 10 miles per hour or faster
Jumping rope
Heavy gardening (continuous digging or hoeing, with heart rate increases)
Hiking uphill or with a heavy backpack

From U.S. Department of Health and Human Services. *2008 Physical Activity Guidelines for Americans.* http://www.health.gov/paguidelines.

TABLE 15-2 RELATIVE RISK OF CARDIOVASCULAR DISEASE IN THE WOMEN'S HEALTH INITIATIVE OBSERVATIONAL STUDY (*N* = 73,743)

MEDIAN MET-MINUTES/WK	MULTIVARIATE ADJUSTED RELATIVE RISK OF CARDIOVASCULAR DISEASE
0	1.0
252	0.89
600	0.81
1050	0.78
1968	0.72

Data from Manson JE, Greenland P, LaCroix AZ, et al. Walking compared with vigorous exercise for the prevention of cardiovascular events in women. *N Engl J Med.* 2002;347:716-725.

levels is large, and the benefit decreases with higher activity levels. Data from the Women's Health Initiative Observational Study (Table 15-2) provide an example of the dose-response effect. Compared with the least active women, the risk for cardiovascular disease was 19% less in women who averaged 600 MET-minutes/week, yet just 28% less in women who averaged 1968 MET-minutes/week. Dose-response effects are also found in intervention studies. For example, a randomized trial of two doses of exercise (doses equivalent to jogging 12 and 20 miles/week) found that the lower volume of exercise significantly improved plasma lipoproteins, but the higher volume had greater beneficial effects.[1]

TREATMENT Rx

Therapeutic Health Benefits in Adults

Clinical practice guidelines assign a substantial therapeutic role to physical activity in patients with coronary heart disease (Chapter 51), high blood pressure (Chapter 67), type 2 diabetes (Chapter 237), obesity (Chapter 227), osteoporosis (Chapter 251), osteoarthritis (Chapter 270), claudication (Chapter 79), and chronic obstructive pulmonary disease (Chapter 88). Physical activity also plays a role in the management of depression and anxiety disorders, elevated cholesterol levels, pain, heart failure, syncope, stroke, back pain, dementia, and constipation and in the prophylaxis of venous thromboembolism.

Physical activity effectively opposes age-related loss of fitness and functional limitations. Randomized controlled trials demonstrate that exercise by sedentary older adults improves health-related physical fitness (e.g., aerobic exercise improves aerobic capacity) and has beneficial effects on functional limitations, such as a slow gait speed.[2] Generally, the benefits are most demonstrable in older adults with clinically significant functional limitations. Physical activity, especially balance training, prevents falls in older adults at increased risk for falling, such as those with impaired gait and balance.[3] It is probable that physical activity improves the ability to live independently, but evidence from randomized trials is incomplete.

Health Risks of Physical Activity

Physical activity and exercise have risks. Musculoskeletal injuries are by far the most common type of activity-related adverse event. The risk of injury depends on the type and volume of activity. Collision and contact sports have a much higher injury risk than noncontact activities such as walking, which is associated with about one musculoskeletal injury for every 1000 hours of walking for exercise. The weekly volume of activity is directly related to the risk of musculoskeletal injuries, but when following public health guidelines, which involves participating in about 500 to 1000 MET-minutes/week, the risk of injury is low. The risk of injury is directly related to the rate of increase in the dose of activity, with more rapid increases having higher risk. Previous musculoskeletal injuries and low fitness also increase the injury risk.

Overall, regular physical activity decreases the risk for sudden cardiac death and myocardial infarction; active adults have roughly a 70% lower risk of sudden death. However, relatively vigorous physical activity acutely increases the risk for these events in both active and inactive adults. About 5 to 10% of myocardial infarctions are associated with vigorous activity. Yet sudden death is a rare event during exercise, with published rates in the range of one death per year in 18,000 ostensibly healthy men and one death per 2.6 million workouts in fitness facilities.

Physical Activity Guidelines for Adults

For the first time, the U.S. Department of Health and Human Services has issued national physical activity guidelines: the *2008 Physical Activity Guidelines for Americans* (Table 15-3).

Recommended Amounts of Aerobic Activity for Prevention

To obtain substantial health benefits from physical activity, adults should do at least 150 minutes/week of moderate-intensity aerobic activity or 75 minutes/week of vigorous-intensity activity. Light-intensity activity is less than 3.0 METs, moderate-intensity activity is in the range of 3.0 to 5.9 METs, and vigorous-intensity activity is 6.0 METs or higher. There is insufficient evidence to determine whether the health benefits of 30 minutes of activity on 5 days a week differ from the health benefits of 50 minutes of activity on 3 days a week. Adults can also do an equivalent combination of both moderate- and vigorous-intensity activity, using the rule of thumb that one vigorous-intensity minute of activity counts the same as two moderate-intensity minutes.

TABLE 15-3 KEY PHYSICAL ACTIVITY GUIDELINES FOR ADULTS

All adults should avoid inactivity. Some physical activity is better than none, and adults who participate in any amount of physical activity gain some health benefits.

For substantial health benefits, adults should do at least 150 min (2.5 hr)/wk of moderate-intensity aerobic activity or 75 min (1.25 hr)/wk of vigorous-intensity aerobic activity, or an equivalent combination of moderate- and vigorous-intensity aerobic activity.

Aerobic activity should be performed in episodes lasting at least 10 min and should be spread throughout the week.

For additional and more extensive health benefits, adults should increase their aerobic physical activity to 300 min (5 hr)/wk of moderate-intensity or 150 min (2.5 hr)/wk of vigorous-intensity aerobic physical activity, or an equivalent combination of moderate- and vigorous-intensity activity. Additional health benefits are gained by engaging in physical activity beyond this amount.

Adults should also do muscle-strengthening activities that are moderate or high intensity and involve all major muscle groups on 2 or more days/wk, as these activities provide additional health benefits.

From U.S. Department of Health and Human Services. *2008 Physical Activity Guidelines for Americans.* http://www.health.gov/paguidelines.

Recommended Amounts of Muscle-Strengthening Activity for Prevention

Adults should perform activities that strengthen the major muscle groups of the body at least 2 days each week. The major muscle groups are the legs, hips, back, chest, abdomen, shoulders, and arms.

Flexibility Activity

Flexibility activities are an acceptable part of a physical activity regimen, but there is insufficient evidence that flexibility activities have any health benefits, even for preventing injuries. Flexibility training does increase flexibility, and it may facilitate the types of physical activity that do have health benefits. If so, flexibility training is more important for people with reduced flexibility, such as older adults with age- and disease-related changes in range of motion.

Balance Activity

Balance training is currently recommended only for adults at increased risk for falls, such as those older than 65 years with impaired gait or balance or frequent falls. Examples of balance exercises include sideways walking, backward walking, heel walking, and standing using a narrow base of support. Tai chi programs include exercises that improve balance. The optimal frequency, duration, and type of balance training are unknown. Preferably, adults at risk for falls should do balance training at least 3 days/week and follow an evidence-based program demonstrated to reduce the risk of falls.

Inactivity versus Sitting Time

Inactive adults engage in no activity that counts toward meeting the national guidelines. Doing some physical activity is clearly preferable to inactivity. A separate issue is whether more time spent sitting has an adverse effect on health, independent of a person's volume of moderate- to vigorous-intensity activity. It appears likely that spending more time in light-intensity baseline activity and less time sitting has an independent beneficial effect on health. Certainly, light-intensity activities expend calories and can be recommended as part of a plan to achieve and maintain a healthy weight. However, data are currently insufficient to issue guidelines on the amounts and patterns of sitting time that cause adverse health effects in adults.

Guidelines for Weight Management

The amount of activity required to maintain a healthy body weight varies widely among adults (Chapter 227). For some adults, the physical activity levels recommended in the guidelines will result in a stable, healthy body weight. Many adults, however, need higher levels of activity to achieve a healthy weight. These individuals should restrict their caloric intake and gradually increase their physical activity each week, to the point that is effective in achieving and maintaining a healthy body weight for them.

Additional Guidelines for Older Adults

In addition to balance training, the 2008 guidelines contain other recommendations specifically for older adults. Older adults who cannot do 150 minutes/week of moderate-intensity activity should be as active as their abilities and conditions allow. Progressive resistance strength training improves physical function in the elderly.[4] Older adults should determine their level of physical activity using relative intensity, not absolute intensity. This latter guideline seeks to avoid inappropriately high levels of effort in older adults with low fitness.

Recommending Physical Activity in Clinical Settings

Promoting physical activity in clinical settings involves essentially the same steps as the five As of smoking cessation: ask, advise, assess, assist, arrange. (1) Ask about the amount of physical activity a patient typically engages in each week by questionnaire or interview. (2) Advise all patients to participate in at least a moderate amount of physical activity each week. Advise patients who do not meet the recommendations to increase their physical activity gradually to a specified minimal level, and tailor the recommendations according to their medical conditions. (3) Assess the next step or steps a patient needs to take to become more active. (4) Assist the patient in taking these steps. (5) Arrange an appointment to follow up on efforts to increase activity.

Health care providers should ask and advise patients about physical activity regularly. One quality-of-care measure assesses whether asking and advising are done at least once a year in older adults. Some recommend that physical activity should be a "vital sign" that is assessed at every visit. Studies consistently report that adults (especially older adults) identify their health care providers as an important source of advice on physical activity.

The U.S. Preventive Services Task Force last reviewed the effectiveness of primary care–based counseling (i.e., assessing and assisting) in 2002. Counseling protocols vary among research studies; some have been effective, and some not. Overall, the task force concluded that the evidence was insufficient to recommend for or against counseling. In relatively healthy patients, a reasonable approach is to counsel selected patients who request information about physical activity, using a protocol that has been evaluated and shown to be effective. For example, a randomized trial demonstrated that an exercise prescription program increased physical activity and quality of life in women aged 40 to 76 over a 2-year period, although falls and injuries also increased.[5]

Exercise Prescription

For patients who want to exercise, a clinician can provide an exercise prescription. The prescription includes (1) the type, frequency, duration, and intensity of aerobic exercise; (2) the exercise movements (e.g., bench press), repetitions, and sets for resistance exercise; (3) other exercises such as stretching, balance exercises, warm-up, and cool-down; and (4) risk management strategies, such as increasing levels of activity gradually over time.

A prescription for vigorous-intensity aerobic exercise generally specifies a minimum frequency of at least 3 days/week, a minimum duration of 20 minutes, and an intensity of 70 to 85% of the maximal heart rate (HR_{max}). A prescription for moderate-intensity exercise would specify an intensity of 40 to 60% of oxygen uptake reserve (or 50 to 69% of HR_{max}) 3 or more days/week to reach an adequate volume. Training at the upper limits of vigorous intensity (85 to 89% of HR_{max}) is discouraged because of concern about injury and adherence. (Higher exercise intensities are commonly regarded as less pleasant.)

A prescription for resistance training generally specifies 8 to 10 separate exercises that train the major muscle groups, with at least one set of 8 to 12 repetitions of each exercise on 2 or 3 days/week. Some recommend that older adults do 10 to 15 repetitions in a set.

Lifestyle Prescription

A *lifestyle prescription* refers to approaches that integrate physical activity into daily life. For example, rather than walking specifically for exercise, a person walks to work or walks for pleasure as a recreational activity. Common ways to integrate physical activity into daily life are walking and biking for transportation and performing yard work and gardening.

Tailoring the Recommendation

Recommendations need to be tailored to individual abilities, individual preferences, medical conditions, and behavior techniques that improve adherence. Randomized trials show that home-based programs are superior to center-based programs in terms of long-term adherence.[6] Although center-based programs are preferred by some, in most cases they serve a short-term purpose, such as assisting adults to initiate regular exercise.

A target level of physical activity below that of preventive recommendations is appropriate for adults with very low fitness, a large burden of chronic disease (e.g., severe chronic obstructive lung disease), or major functional limitations. An assessment of the nature of the activity limitation and the individual's capabilities and preferences can determine the target activity level and other details of the activity recommendation. Often, promoting physical activity in such adults relies on health care and community resources designed for people with preexisting limitations, such as cardiac rehabilitation, pulmonary rehabilitation, and exercise classes for adults with arthritis.

Risk Management

Strategies to reduce injury include increasing physical activity gradually over time, selecting activities in which collision or contact with people or objects is unusual, increasing physical fitness, using appropriate gear and sports equipment (e.g., bike helmets), engaging in activities in safe environments, and following basic safety rules and policies. Popular activities such as walking, biking, swimming, and gardening have a low risk of injury. When increasing the level of physical activity, the guidelines recommend using relative intensity to determine the level of effort, starting with relatively moderate-intensity activity, then increasing the duration and frequency first and the intensity last. In general, adding 5 to 15 minutes of moderate-intensity activity per session, two to three times a week, to a person's usual activities carries a low risk of musculoskeletal injury and no known risk of sudden cardiac death.

There is no evidence of the protective value of a medical consultation in healthy people of any age who seek to increase their level of physical activity. The U.S. Preventive Services Task Force recommended against routine screening for coronary disease in adults at low risk for it and concluded that in adults at high risk for coronary disease, there is insufficient evidence to recommend for or against screening with resting electrocardiography, exercise treadmill test, or electron-beam computed tomography.

Coordination between Medical Care and Community

Many factors affecting physical activity levels are difficult to influence in medical care settings, such as the characteristics of the communal environment (e.g., parks and recreational facilities) and the social environment (e.g., crime and social support). Community-level interventions that address such characteristics are essential to promoting physical activity. Effective community-based interventions include school physical education, social support interventions, community-wide campaigns, enhancement of access to places where physical activity is possible, and interventions that involve community design, such as improving the connectivity of streets and the walkability of neighborhoods. Medical care and community efforts should be synergistic and mutually supportive. For example, health plans should be advocates for evidence-based community interventions. Community programs should serve as resources for evidence-based therapeutic activity for selected chronically ill adults, such as exercise classes designed to reduce the risk of falls.

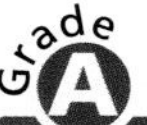

1. Kraus WE, Houmard JA, Duscha BD, et al. Effects of the amount and intensity of exercise on plasma lipoproteins. *N Engl J Med*. 2002;347:1483-1492.
2. Pahor M, Blair SN, Espeland M, et al. Effects of a physical activity intervention on measures of physical performance: results of the lifestyle interventions and independence for elders pilot (LIFE-) study. *J Gerontol Series A*. 2006;61:1157-1165.
3. Gillespie LD, Robertson MC, Gillespie WJ, et al. Interventions for preventing falls in older people living in the community. *Cochrane Database Syst Rev*. 2009;2:CD0007146.
4. Liu CJ, Latham NK. Progressive resistance strength training for improving physical function in older adults. *Cochrane Database Syst Rev*. 2009;3:CD002759.
5. Lawton BA, Rose SB, Elley CR, et al. Exercise on prescription for women age 40-74 recruited through primary care: two year randomized controlled trial. *Br J Sports Med*. 2009;43:120-123.
6. Ashworth NL, Chad KE, Harrison EL, et al. Home versus center based physical activity programs in older adults. *Cochrane Database Syst Rev*. 2005.1:CD004017.

SUGGESTED READINGS

Artinian NT, Fletcher GF, Mozaffarian D, et al. Interventions to promote physical activity and dietary lifestyle changes for cardiovascular risk factor reduction in adults: a scientific statement from the American Heart Association. *Circulation*. 2010;122:406-441. *Consensus guidelines*.

Katzmarzyk PT, Church TS, Craig CL, et al. Sitting times and mortality from all causes, cardiovascular disease, and cancer. *Med Sci Sports Exerc*. 2009;41:998-1005. *Showed a dose-response relationship between sitting time and all-cause mortality independent of the effect of moderate-to-vigorous physical activity*.

Physical Activity Guidelines Advisory Committee. Part G. Section 10. Adverse Events. In Physical Activity Guidelines Advisory Committee Report. www.health.gov/paguidelines. Accessed Dec. 4, 2010. *Reviews the determinants of activity-related adverse events and approaches to reduce injury risk*.

16

ADOLESCENT MEDICINE

DEBRA K. KATZMAN AND LAWRENCE S. NEINSTEIN

Adolescence, a period of transition between childhood and adulthood, is marked by critical biological, psychological, social, and cognitive changes. During this unique developmental period, patterns of behaviors and lifestyle choices are established that can influence current and future health, and unique medical and psychological problems can emerge. Adult-oriented health care providers play a pivotal role in engaging youth in their health and in providing health care to adolescents and young adults.

NORMAL PHYSICAL GROWTH AND DEVELOPMENT

Biologic growth and development in adolescents are signified by the onset of puberty (Chapter 243), which varies temporally among adolescents and explains why adolescents of the same chronologic age can vary greatly in physical appearance. Usually the first visible sign of puberty among females is thelarche, or the development of breast buds, which occurs on average at 10.5 years in white girls and 1 year earlier in African-American girls (Chapter 243).

Menarche occurs 2 to 4 years after the initial appearance of breast buds and pubic hair. The average age of menarche is 12.9 years for white girls and 12.2 years for African-American girls. Menstrual periods are not always regular during the first 2 years after menarche. At menarche, only 20% of cycles are ovulatory; it may take up to 4 years for 80% of cycles to be ovulatory. The average length for the completion of puberty in females is 4 years (range, 1.5 to 8.0 years).

Puberty begins about 2 years later in boys than in girls. The first physical sign of puberty in boys, testicular enlargement and thinning of the scrotum, occurs at 11.5 years. Adrenarche occurs 6 months later at an average age of 12.0 to 12.5 years (Chapter 242). Facial hair starts to grow about 3 years after pubic hair. The completion of puberty in males can take an average of 3 years (range, 2 to 5 years).

Pubertal weight gain accounts for about half of a person's ideal adult body weight. Peak weight gain follows the linear growth spurt by 3 to 6 months in adolescent girls and by about 3 months in adolescent boys. The average weight gain during puberty among adolescent females is 15 to 55 lb, or 7 to 25 kg (mean gain, 38.5 lb, or 17.5 kg). Overall, adolescent males gain 15 to 65 lb, or 7 to 30 kg, during puberty (mean gain, 52.2 lb or 23.7 kg).

Boys' body fat levels decrease during adolescence, dropping to 12% body fat by the end of puberty. On average, adolescent girls' lean body mass falls from 80 to 75%, whereas their average body fat levels increase from 16 to 27% by the end of adolescence. By the time adolescent girls are 16 years of age and adolescent boys are 18 years of age, they have accrued more than 90% of their adult skeletal mass. *Sexual maturity ratings* (SMRs), also known as Tanner staging, are used to describe the progression of secondary sexual characteristics that occur in adolescents, irrespective of chronologic age. SMR is based on the development of breasts and the appearance of pubic hair among girls (Fig. 16-1) and on testicular and penile development and the appearance of pubic hair among boys (Fig. 16-2). SMR 1 corresponds to the prepubertal stage; puberty has not begun, and no sexual development has occurred. SMR 2 to SMR 5 indicate the progression of puberty to adulthood. Once young people reach SMR 5, they have fully developed secondary sexual characteristics. Sexual maturation correlates with linear growth, changes in weight and body composition, and hormonal changes. Sexual maturation provides important assurance of the normal progression of puberty or identification of abnormal pubertal development.

NORMAL PSYCHOSOCIAL DEVELOPMENT

Adolescence is often divided into three psychosocial developmental phases: early adolescence (11 to 13 years), middle adolescence (14 to 16 years), and late adolescence (17 to 21 years). In early adolescence, adolescents begin to separate from their parents and establish an individual identity. As adolescents pull away from their parents in search of their own identity, their peer group takes on an important and special significance.

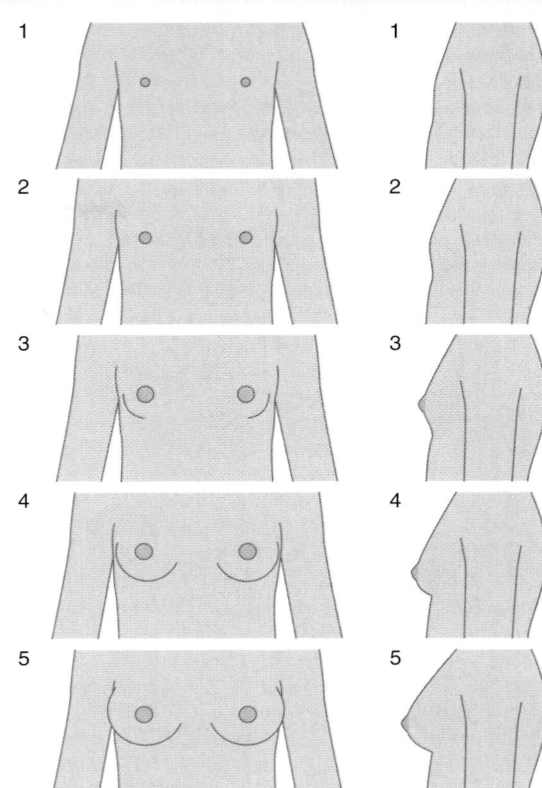

FIGURE 16-1. Female breast development. *Sexual maturity rating 1 (SMR 1)*: Preadolescent; no glandular tissue. Areola and papilla: Areola conforms to general chest line. *SMR 2:* Breast buds appear; areola is slightly widened and projects as small mound. *SMR 3:* Enlargement of the entire breast with protrusion of the papilla or of the nipple. Breast and areola enlarge with no separation of their contours. *SMR 4:* Enlargement of the breast and projection of areola and papilla as a secondary mound. *SMR 5:* Adult configuration of the breast with protrusion of the nipple; areola no longer projects separately from remainder of breast. (Redrawn from Daniel WA, Paulshock BZ. A physician's guide to sexual maturity rating. *Patient Care.* 1979;30:122. Original illustration by Paul Singh-Roy.)

At the beginning of adolescence, cognitive abilities are dominated by concrete thinking. Young adolescents lack abstract reasoning capabilities, problem-solving skills needed to overcome barriers to behavioral changes, and the ability to appreciate how their current behaviors can affect their future health status.

Middle adolescence is characterized by growth in emotional autonomy and increasing separation from family. The adolescents' peer groups play a powerful role, and adolescents are increasingly involved in partnering relationships that include dating, sexual experimentation, and adverse health behaviors such as smoking cigarettes, drinking alcohol, using street drugs, and being truant. Abstract reasoning skills emerge but often regress to concrete thinking when adolescents are faced with stressful situations. These adolescents begin to understand the relationship between health behaviors and future health status, but peer pressure makes it challenging to make health-related choices.

During late adolescence, young people become increasingly more economically and emotionally independent. Peer group values become less important, and young people spend more time in a relationship with one person. The late stage of adolescence is characterized by the development of a strong personal identity. Abstract reasoning skills expand, and older adolescents have problem-solving skills that help them overcome challenges to behavioral change.

VITAL STATISTICS

Although adolescents are generally perceived to be healthy, adolescent morbidity and mortality are the result of risky behaviors and social forces (Table 16-1). Adolescents increasingly engage in risky behaviors with each year of adolescence, especially between the ages of 11 and 16. Unintentional injury, homicide, and suicide are the leading causes of death in 15- to 24-year-olds and account for 71% of all adolescent and young adult deaths. About 75% of these causes of death and injury are preventable.

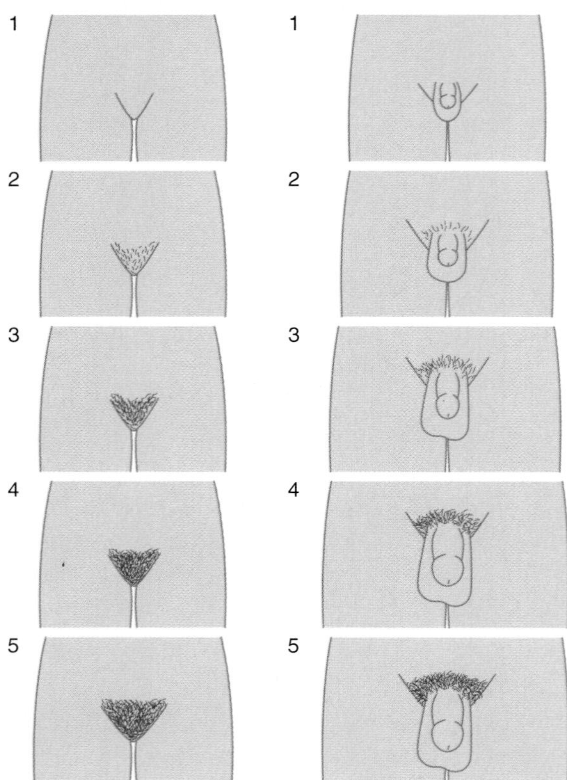

FIGURE 16-2. **Male genital development.** *SMR 1:* Penis preadolescent. Testicular volume <4 mL. *SMR 2:* Penis slight or no enlargement. Beginning enlargement of testes; testicular volume 4 to 8 mL; scrotal skin reddened, thinner. *SMR 3:* Penis increased in length. Testicular volume 10 to 15 mL. Further enlargement of scrotum. *SMR 4:* Penis larger in breadth, glans penis develops. Testes and scrotum nearly adult; testicular volume 12-20 mL. *SMR 5:* Penis adult size; testicular volume greater than 25 mL. **Female and male pubic hair development.** *Sexual maturity rating 1 (SMR 1):* Prepubertal; no pubic hair. *SMR 2:* Small amount of scanty, long, slightly pigmented, along the base of the scrotum and phallus in the male and the medial border of the labia majora in females. *SMR 3:* Darker, coarser, starts to curl, small amount, extending laterally. *SMR 4:* Coarse, curly; resembles adult type but does not extend to the medial surface of the thighs. *SMR 5:* Abundant, adult-type pattern; hair extends onto the medial aspect of the thighs. (Redrawn from Daniel WA, Palshock BZ. A physician's guide to sexual maturity rating. *Patient Care.* 1979;30:122. Original illustration by Paul Singh-Roy.)

TABLE 16-1 LEADING CAUSES OF DEATH IN U.S. ADOLESCENTS

CAUSE	PERCENTAGE OF DEATHS IN YOUTH AGED 15-24 YEARS
Unintentional injury	47
Homicide	16
Suicide	12
Malignancy	5
Heart disease	3
Congenital anomalies	1.3
Cerebrovascular disease	0.6
Human immunodeficiency virus	0.6
Influenza and pneumonia	0.5
Complicated pregnancy	0.5
All others	14

From U.S. Census Bureau, *2008 National Population Projections*, released August 2008.

Unintentional and Intentional Injuries

Unintentional injuries account for 44% of all injury deaths to children and adolescents. For every childhood death caused by injury, another 34 hospitalizations and 1000 emergency department visits occur. The major causes of unintentional injuries to adolescents are motor vehicle crashes, being struck by or against an object or person, cuts from sharp objects, and falls. Factors that contribute to adolescent injuries include socioeconomic factors (poor children are at greatest risk for injury), environmental factors (hazards such as all-terrain vehicles, backyard swimming pools, firearms, kerosene heaters, and gang activity), school environment, and developmental factors.

About 20% of all adolescents, especially adolescent girls in heterosexual relationships, report having experienced either psychological or physical violence from a dating partner. About 20 to 30% of students in grades 6 to 10 are involved in bullying, as a bully, victim, or bully-victim (those who are both aggressive to peers and victimized by peers). For younger adolescents, bullying can lead to a significantly higher risk of psychosomatic problems.

Homicide is the second leading cause of death in the 15- to 24-year-old population and the number one cause of death among African-American males 15 to 24 years of age. About 75% of homicides in older adolescents and young adults involve firearms.

Suicide (Chapter 404) is the third leading cause of death among adolescents and young adults 10 to 24 years of age. Native Americans and white youth 15 to 24 years of age have the highest suicides rates, whereas African-American youth 15 to 19 years of age and Asian youth 20 to 24 years of age have the lowest. The estimated ratio of attempted-to-completed suicides among adolescents ranges between 50:1 and 100:1. The most common methods used in suicide attempts are drugs or alcohol, whereas suffocation, hanging, or use of firearms is associated with completed suicides. Death rates caused by firearms are eight times higher in adolescent boys than in adolescent girls.

Prevention of Injuries

Clinicians should discuss the impact of alcohol and drugs on driving and stress the importance of routine use of seat belts when driving in a motor vehicle. Clinicians also should discuss safety during sports activities, such as use of bicycle helmets and sports-related protective gear.

Other Diseases

Excluding intentional and unintentional injuries, cancer is the leading cause of death in adolescents and is the leading cause of death by disease. Cancers with an increased incidence in adolescents include Hodgkin's disease (Chapter 192), germ cell tumors (Chapter 206), central nervous system tumors (Chapter 195), non-Hodgkin's lymphoma (Chapter 191), thyroid cancer (Chapter 233), malignant melanoma (Chapter 210), and acute lymphoblastic leukemia (Chapter 189). Human immunodeficiency virus (HIV) continues to be one of the ten leading causes of death among people 15 to 24 years of age.

APPROACH TO THE ADOLESCENT PATIENT

When interviewing adolescent patients, the clinician should consider the adolescents' physical, cognitive, and psychosocial developmental stage, their growing autonomy and increasing role in taking responsibility for their own health and well-being, and their individual progression from childhood to adulthood. Chronologic age is not a guarantee that all adolescents will be at the same stage of physical, cognitive, and psychosocial development. The clinician should offer adolescent health care in a sensitive, flexible, and developmentally and culturally appropriate manner.

The clinician can meet with the adolescent alone at first to give the adolescent the message that she or he is the patient and the clinician is most eager to hear what the adolescent has to say. Conversely, the clinician can meet with the adolescent and her or his parents or guardians together for the initial part of the interview and then meet with the adolescent alone; this approach permits the clinician to develop an understanding of the reason for the visit from the perspective of the adolescent and his or her parents or guardians, and to communicate that input from both the adolescent and the parents or guardians is highly valued. This approach also provides an opportunity for the clinician to observe the interaction between the adolescent and parents or guardians. The final approach to the interview is to greet the adolescent and family, and request a meeting with the parents or guardians alone. This approach allows the parents or guardians to discuss concerns about the adolescent that they may not feel comfortable raising in the presence of the adolescent. Having this information may improve the focus of the visit. Using this approach, the encounter with the parents or guardians is then followed by the clinician meeting with the adolescent alone. With this interview structure, it is important that the adolescent be present from the time he or she meets with the clinician until the end of the visit, so that the adolescent does not perceive a breach of confidentiality.

Confidentiality

Issues of consent and confidentiality are central in the physician-adolescent interaction. Adolescents appreciate clinicians whom they trust and who can assure them of confidentiality. When guaranteed confidentiality, adolescents are more likely to seek necessary medical care, disclose sensitive information, and trust their clinician. Under these circumstances, most adolescents will involve their parents in their care. Parents appreciate education about the concept of confidentiality and recognize the importance of allowing the adolescent the opportunity to speak alone with their clinician. Confidentiality is also important for clinicians. To make an accurate diagnosis and provide treatment, the clinician must obtain all relevant information from the adolescent. If the adolescent fears that such information will not be kept confidential, she or he may not provide all the necessary factual information.

Confidentiality and defining the limits of confidentiality should be discussed with the adolescent and his or her parents or guardians at the beginning of the interview. The adolescent and family need to know that the clinician will intervene if he or she believes that the adolescent's actions may cause him or her, or another person, significant harm. Examples of situations in which the clinician would not maintain confidentiality when dealing with young people include disclosure of past or current sexual abuse, current suicidal intent, and disclosure of homicidal intent.

Those who work with young people must have a clear understanding of consent and confidentiality and should make sure that adolescents are aware of confidentiality policies and practices. The duty of confidentiality does not preclude encouraging and empowering adolescents to talk to their parents or guardians about important health care issues and include them in discussions of these issues. The legal definition of confidentiality varies, depending on geographic location. It is the clinician's responsibility to familiarize himself or herself with the legal issues of confidentiality (as they relate to the adolescent patient and his or her parents or guardians) in their locality.

Another goal of the interview is to build rapport with the adolescent and his or her parents or guardians. Clinicians can establish rapport with the adolescent at the start of the interview by creating an environment that is nonjudgmental, unintimidating, and supportive. The clinician's genuine interest in the adolescent is paramount. It is helpful to encourage the adolescent to talk about himself or herself—friends, hobbies, school. The clinician should listen carefully to the adolescent's statements and feelings. Sensitivity to and understanding of the adolescent's developmental stage and cultural background are important when interviewing an adolescent and interpreting answers accurately. The clinician should be respectful of the adolescent's growing need to be independent and desire to be treated as an individual person. Taking the time to build rapport is key to engaging the adolescent in a discussion of his or her personal health concerns with the clinician.

Preventive Health Care

Preventive health care for adolescents (Chapters 14 and 17) should promote physical and mental health and healthy physical, psychological, and social growth and development. Positive behaviors such as exercise (Chapter 15) and nutritious eating (Chapter 220) should be encouraged, and health risk behaviors such as unsafe driving, use of tobacco (Chapter 31), unsafe sexual behaviors, and excess alcohol (Chapter 32) should be discouraged. Because lifelong health habits are established during adolescence, it is an important time to invest in health promotion and preventive services.

Components of the Adolescent Care Health Visit

History

Open-ended, nonjudgmental, developmentally appropriate, and gender-neutral questions help put the adolescent at ease and produce informative answers (Chapter 14). In addition to a standard medical history, the assessment should include a psychosocial history from the adolescent, either through a screening questionnaire or during the interview with the adolescent alone. The HEEADSSS assessment, which is a valuable tool for obtaining a comprehensive psychosocial history, covers the following topics:

- **Home:** Family members, living arrangements, and relationships
- **Education/Employment:** Academic or vocational success and future plans
- **Eating:** Concerns about weight or body image or disordered eating attitudes and behaviors
- **Activities**: Recreational activities, dating, and relationships
- **Drugs:** Use of tobacco, alcohol, illicit drugs, anabolic steroids, and driving while intoxicated
- **Sexuality:** Sexual orientation, sexual activity, and sexual abuse
- **Suicide** (mental health): Feelings of sadness, loneliness, depression, or suicidal thoughts
- **Safety:** Risk of unintentional injury or violence, fighting, or weapon carrying

Physical Examination

In general, the adolescent physical examination should occur without a parent or guardian present. In some situations, the adolescent is asked whether he or she would prefer to have a parent in the room during the physical examination. A male clinician should request that a female health care provider be present during the physical examination of a female patient, especially during the breast and genital examination. In theory, a female clinician should request a male health care provider be present during the genital examination of a male patient.

Care should be taken to ensure the adolescent's privacy. Providing an examination gown that covers the trunk and genital area is important. Talking with the adolescent during the examination also tends to increase comfort; explaining the procedures and commenting on the results are helpful. A comprehensive physical examination (Chapter 14) should include measuring the adolescent's weight and height, calculating his or her body mass index, plotting these measurements on standardized growth charts, and determining the adolescent's SMR.

Young women who have HIV or who are immunosuppressed (e.g., those having chemotherapy, transplantation) should have a baseline Papanicolaou smear 3 years after their first sexual intercourse. Other indications for a pelvic examination in an adolescent include symptoms of vaginal or uterine infection, menstrual irregularities (e.g., amenorrhea, dysfunctional uterine bleeding, menorrhagia, and severe dysmenorrhea), undiagnosed abdominal and pelvic pain, tenderness, mass, trauma, sexual abuse, or assault. A careful sexual history, a review of symptoms, and urine or patient-obtained specimens may be an alternative to the pelvic examination.

Conclusion of the Health Visit

At the conclusion of the adolescent health visit, the clinician should review the findings with the adolescent and talk about what happens next. This discussion should not be rushed; the adolescent should have the opportunity to ask questions, get clarification, make comments, and respond to suggestions. The clinician should discuss with the adolescent what information will remain confidential. The clinician should then meet with the adolescent and the parents or guardians (if they have accompanied the adolescent to the health visit) to review the outcomes and discuss the nonconfidential issues.

Immunizations

Adolescents should be brought up-to-date on all recommended immunizations (Chapter 17).

REPRODUCTIVE HEALTH

Reproductive health care includes issues of adolescent sexual development, adolescent sexual behaviors, adolescent pregnancy, and contraception. In the United States, nearly 50% of high school boys and girls in grades 9 to 12 have had vaginal intercourse (50% of males, 46% of females) at least once. This number increases from 27% of females and 38% of males in grade 9 to about 65% of both boys and girls by their senior year. In addition, 4% of females and 10% of males in grades 9 to 12 started having sex before they were 13 years old, 14% of adolescents have had four or more sex partners during their lives, and 38% of sexually active high school students did not used a condom when they last had sexual intercourse. About 60% of adolescent girls who are 13 years of age or younger when they first had sexual intercourse report having involuntary intercourse. Adolescents are more likely to report engaging in oral than vaginal sex because they perceive oral sex as significantly less risky (fewer health, social, and emotional consequences) than vaginal sex, but adolescents who engage in oral sex also are more likely to engage in vaginal sex.

Every year about 800,000 pregnancies occur in females 15 to 19 years of age in the United States. About 50% of these pregnancies result in a live birth, about 35% end with an abortion, and about 15% end with a miscarriage or stillbirth. The birth rate for mothers 15 to 27 years of age decreased from 38.6 in 1991 to 22.1 in 2004 because of increased use of effective contraception and decreased sexual activity. Adolescent pregnancy is more common among black and Hispanic females as well as females from low-income families.

Positive outcomes of adolescent pregnancies are enhanced with good prenatal care, adequate initial and follow-up prenatal visits, nutritional counseling, assessment of psychosocial issues, and substance abuse counseling. Adolescents younger than 15 years are at increased risk for premature and low-birthweight infants; those older than 15 years who have adequate prenatal care do not have increased adverse outcomes.

Contraception

The most commonly used contraceptive methods in adolescents are oral contraceptive pills (OCPs) and condoms, although new hormonal delivery systems such as transdermal patches, vaginal rings, and implants are convenient and effective (Chapter 246).

Sexually Transmitted Diseases

Every year, about 4 million adolescents in the United States acquire a sexually transmitted disease (Chapter 293), representing 25% of the total cases of sexually transmitted disease diagnosed annually. *Chlamydia trachomatis,* which is the most commonly reported bacterial sexually transmitted disease, is reported annually in about 2.8% of female adolescents 15 to 19 years of age and 0.5% of male adolescents of the same age. The annual incidence of gonorrhea is about 0.6% for female adolescents 15 to 19 years of age and 0.4% for adolescent males of the same age. In adolescents, HIV (Chapter 395) is contracted primarily as a sexually transmitted disease, and adolescents and young adults 15 to 24 years of age represent 14% of all new HIV diagnoses in the United States. Human papillomavirus (Chapter 381), which is the most prevalent of all sexually transmitted diseases in 15- to 24-year-olds, has a prevalence of about 20% in adolescent girls 14 to 17 years of age.

Adolescents are at greater risk of acquiring sexually transmitted diseases because they are more likely to engage in unprotected sexual intercourse with concurrent partners who have multiple other partners. Adolescent girls may have persistent vaginal columnar epithelium that is more susceptible than squamous epithelium to *Neisseria gonorrhea, C. trachomatis,* and HPV, as well lower levels of immunoglobulin A in their cervical mucus. Treatment may be delayed owing to an inability to access confidential health care services, lack of health care coverage, poverty, and drug trafficking and use.

Chlamydial infections (Chapter 326), often asymptomatic or minimally symptomatic in women, usually present with a vaginal discharge in young adolescent girls. Otherwise, clinical presentations and treatments of sexually transmitted diseases (Chapter 293) in adolescents are similar to those in adults.

About 20% of adolescents given prescriptions for a sexually transmitted disease treatment fail to fill their prescriptions. Therefore, whenever available, an observed single-dose therapy is recommended. In addition, expedited partner therapy (EPT), which is the treatment of sexual partners without requiring a prior clinical evaluation or prevention counseling, reduces the level of recurrent sexually transmitted diseases better than does standard management. Clinicians should consider the use of EPT for partners exposed within 60 days to heterosexual males and females with chlamydia or gonorrhea infections when in-person evaluation and treatment are unlikely.

ADOLESCENT EATING DISORDERS

Eating disorders (Chapter 226) commonly begin during adolescence. For adolescent-onset anorexia nervosa, bulimia nervosa, and other eating disorders, early recognition and aggressive treatment are critical to a successful outcome. The medical complications of eating disorders in adolescents include growth retardation, pubertal delay, low bone mineral density, and changes in brain structure and cognitive function. These complications, which occur early in the disease process, may not be completely reversible, thereby underscoring the need for early and aggressive treatment.

The goal of treatment is to restore physical health, normal eating-behavior patterns, and mental health and to reduce the impact of the eating disorder on the quality of life. Successful management strategies for adolescents with eating disorders include early restoration of a normal nutritional and physiologic state, involvement of the family in the treatment, and incorporation of an interdisciplinary team in the treatment. Adolescents should be treated at a facility where the health professionals understand eating disorders and have experience treating adolescents.

SUBSTANCE ABUSE

Nearly half of adolescents try an illicit drug (Chapter 33) by the time they finish high school. About 75% of adolescents consume alcohol (Chapter 32) by the end of high school, and about half report having been drunk at least once in their life. Adolescents who begin using alcohol or drugs before 15 years of age are more than five times more likely to develop an addictive disorder later in life, compared with those who first use alcohol at 21 years of age. About 45% of adolescents use marijuana, and 20% of 12th graders are current smokers.

Adolescents start using drugs or alcohol primarily because of social pressures but report continuing them to feel good or cope with difficulties. Boys tend to initiate drug and alcohol use at younger ages than girls, but once girls begin to experiment, they are just as likely as boys to use drugs. Boys are more likely to consume marijuana, steroids, and smokeless tobacco, whereas girls are more likely to abuse amphetamines and methamphetamine.

Adolescents with poor self-esteem, low motivation, and poor academic achievement have a greater propensity for alcohol and drug abuse than those with positive self-esteem. Adolescents with a family member with a history of alcohol or other drug abuse are at greater risk. Adolescents are less likely to succumb to external pressures toward drug use if they have a strong sense of attachment to parents who clearly communicate their disapproval.

Signs and symptoms suggestive of substance abuse include changes in physical appearance, poor hygiene or dress, wearing long-sleeved shirts to hide scarring at injection sites, persistent cough or bronchitis, difficulty sleeping, sudden weight loss or weight gain, sudden changes in personality, aggressive behavior, irritability, nervousness, giddiness, changes in peer group, increased isolation from peers or family, depression, loss of interest in once favorite activities, decline in performance or attendance at school or work, forgetfulness, increased secretiveness, money or objects disappearing from the household, and prescription drugs that seem to be used up too quickly.

A validated screening tool for alcohol and substance abuse (Table 16-2) should be used in adolescents. Adolescents who answer "yes" to one of the six questions should receive advice on the adverse effects of substance abuse. Those who answer "yes" to two or more questions are at high risk and require further assessment or referral (Chapters 32 and 33). Urine drug testing has low sensitivity for detecting drug use, and there is no consensus about its role for screening adolescents.

Adolescent substance use can compromise psychological and social development, cause behavioral problems, and lead to a variety of high-risk behaviors. Alcohol and drug use contributes to more than 40% of adolescent deaths from motor vehicle crashes, to suicide attempts, and to an increased risk for subsequent use and its related problems in adulthood.

Historically, substance abuse treatment has been based on abstinence. More recently, a harm-reduction approach has gained acceptance. Adolescents discontinue drug and alcohol use mainly because of concern about their negative effects, and community-based interventions can be effective.[1] To reduce alcohol abuse over time, individual interventions have a larger impact than family-based interventions.[2]

TABLE 16-2 CRAFFT SCREENING TOOL FOR DRUG AND ALCOHOL USE IN ADOLESCENTS

The adolescent is instructed, "Please answer these next questions honestly. Your answers will be kept confidential. During the past 12 months, did you ..."
- Drink any alcohol (more than a few sips)?
- Smoke any marijuana or hashish?
- Use anything else to get high?

If the adolescent answers "No" to the three opening questions, the provider only needs to ask the adolescent the first question—the CAR question. If the adolescent answers "Yes" to any one or more of the three opening questions, the provider asks all six CRAFFT questions.
- **C**—Have you ever ridden in a CAR driven by someone (including yourself) who was "high" or had been using alcohol or drugs?
- **R**—Do you ever use alcohol or drugs to RELAX, feel better about yourself, or fit in?
- **A**—Do you ever use alcohol/drugs while you are by yourself, ALONE?
- **F**—Do you ever FORGET things you did while using alcohol or drugs?
- **F**—Do your family or FRIENDS ever tell you that you should cut down on your drinking or drug use?
- **T**—Have you gotten into TROUBLE while you were using alcohol or drugs?

CRAFFT is a mnemonic acronym of first letters of key words in the six screening questions. The questions should be asked exactly as written.

CHRONIC ILLNESS AND TRANSITION

The prevalence of chronic diseases in adolescents has increased significantly because advances in medical technology and treatments have increased the survival of young people with childhood diseases formerly considered lethal. About 15% of adolescents in the United States live with a chronic illness. Chronic illness may affect the adolescent's development, or the adolescent's development may affect the illness. For example, cystic fibrosis (Chapter 89) may delay puberty and hinder normal peer development. Puberty can exacerbate diabetes mellitus (Chapter 236). Increased risk-taking by adolescents with diabetes, asthma, or chronic renal failure can hinder their compliance with their medication regimen.

Any chronic illness may limit age-appropriate activities and development. Adolescents with a chronic illness must have effective contraception and effective methods for preventing sexually transmitted diseases.

Adolescents in general, and those with special health care needs in particular, require a smooth, seamless, coordinated, and developmentally appropriate transition to the adult health care system. Barriers to a successful transition include a lack of adult physicians who can manage chronic childhood conditions (e.g., congenital heart disease; Chapter 69); patients, families, and pediatric subspecialists who are reluctant to terminate long-standing relationships; and patients and families who are poorly equipped to find their way in the adult health care system.

As adolescents move closer to the age of transfer, professionals should provide developmentally appropriate information and skills to support them and their families as they negotiate the adult health care system.

Adolescents benefit from an introductory visit with their adult-oriented care provider before leaving the pediatric health care system. This visit should give the adolescent a clearer idea about his or her new role as an adult patient, especially about expectations around decision making, giving consent, and the role of the family in his or her health care. The patient, family, and pediatric and adult health care systems should view the transition as a natural part of the developmental process of care for all adolescents.

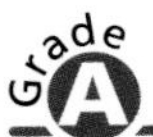

1. Oesterle S, Hawkins JD, Fagan AA, et al. Testing the universality of the effects of the communities that care prevention system for preventing adolescent drug use and delinquency. *Prev Sci.* 2010; 11:411-423.
2. Tripodi SJ, Bender K, Litschge C, et al. Interventions for reducing adolescent alcohol abuse: a meta-analytic review. *Arch Pediatr Adolesc Med.* 2010;164:85-91.

SUGGESTED READINGS

Peter NG, Forke CM, Ginsburg KR, et al. Transition from pediatric to adult care: internists' perspectives. *Pediatrics.* 2009;123:417-423. *Emphasizes how internists should be better trained regarding childhood-onset conditions.*

http://www.cdc.gov/growthcharts. *Growth charts online.*

http://brightfutures.aap.org/web. Guidelines for prevention visits for children and adolescents. *A helpful resource.*

http://www.adolescenthealth.org. Position papers from the Society for Adolescent Medicine. *A catalog of useful reports.*

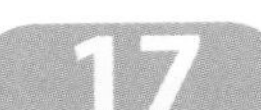

IMMUNIZATION

WALTER A. ORENSTEIN AND WILLIAM L. ATKINSON

Immunization is one of the most cost-effective means of preventing morbidity and mortality from infectious diseases. Routine immunization, particularly of children, has resulted in decreases of 90% or more in reported cases of measles, mumps, rubella, congenital rubella syndrome, poliomyelitis, tetanus, invasive *Haemophilus influenzae* and diphtheria. In many circumstances, immunization not only prevents morbidity and mortality but also, in the long run, reduces health care costs.

GENERAL CHARACTERISTICS OF IMMUNIZATIONS

Immunization protects against disease or the sequelae of disease through the administration of an immunobiologic—vaccines, toxoids, immune globulin preparations, and antitoxins. Protection induced by immunization can be active or passive.

Active Immunization

Administration of a vaccine or toxoid causes the body to produce an immune response against the infectious agent or its toxins. Vaccines consist of suspensions of live (usually attenuated) or inactivated microorganisms or fractions thereof. Toxoids are modified bacterial toxins that retain immunogenic properties but lack toxicity. Active immunization generally results in long-term immunity, although the onset of protection may be delayed because it takes time for the body to respond. With live attenuated vaccines, small quantities of living organisms multiply within the recipient until an immune response cuts off replication. In contrast, inactivated vaccines and toxoids contain large quantities of antigens. In most recipients, a single dose of a live vaccine generally induces an immune response that closely parallels natural infection and induces long-term immunity. Killed (inactivated) vaccines, in contrast, often require multiple doses.

Passive Immunization

Passive immunization with use of immune globulins or antitoxins delivers preformed antibodies to provide temporary immunity. Immune globulins obtained from human blood may contain antibodies to a variety of agents, depending on the pool of human plasma from which they are prepared. Specific immune globulins are made from the plasma of donors with high levels of antibodies to specific antigens, such as tetanus immune globulin. Most immune globulins must be injected intramuscularly, although an intravenous preparation is also available. Antitoxins are solutions of antibodies derived from animals immunized with specific antigens (e.g., diphtheria antitoxin). Passive immunization usually is indicated to protect individuals immediately before anticipated exposure or shortly after known or suspected exposure to an infectious agent (Table 17-1), when active immunization either is not possible or has not been adequate.

Route and Timing of Vaccination

Each immunobiologic has a preferred site and route of administration. In adults, vaccines containing adjuvants should be injected intramuscularly, preferably in the deltoid muscle. For most adults, intramuscular injections should be administered with a 1- to 1½-inch, 22- to 25-gauge needle. Use of the buttocks is discouraged except when large volumes are required because of the potential for damage to the sciatic nerve and because of diminished immune response to some vaccines, such as hepatitis B, probably because of injection into fat rather than into muscle. Subcutaneous vaccines also are usually administered in the triceps area. In general, inactivated vaccines and toxoids can be given at the same visit at different sites. Live and inactivated vaccines usually can be administered at the same time. For example, measles, mumps, and rubella (MMR) vaccine can be administered at the same time as inactivated poliovirus vaccine and live attenuated varicella vaccine. In general, injected and intranasally administered live vaccines not delivered on the same day should be separated by at least 4 weeks to avoid interference. Orally administered live vaccines, such as oral typhoid vaccine, can be administered at any interval before or after live injected or intranasal vaccines. Immune globulin may interfere with the replication of injected live vaccine viruses; ideally, most live vaccines should be administered at least 2 weeks before or 3 to 11 months after immune globulin. Immune globulin does not interfere with the response to yellow fever vaccine and is not believed to interfere with orally or intranasally administered live virus vaccines.

Adverse Reactions

No vaccine is completely safe or completely effective. Hypersensitivity to vaccine components, such as animal proteins, antibiotics, preservatives, and stabilizers, can lead to local and systemic reactions ranging from mild to severe. Minor reactions are common, but randomized trials caution that prophylactic antipyretic drugs at the time of vaccination reduce antibody reactions and should not be given routinely.[1] The egg protein contained in vaccines grown in chicken eggs (influenza and yellow fever vaccines) may cause reactions in persons severely allergic to eggs. In general, persons

TABLE 17-1 PASSIVE IMMUNIZATIONS FOR ADULTS

DISEASE	NAME OF MATERIAL	COMMENTS AND USE
Tetanus	Tetanus immune globulin, human	Management of tetanus-prone wounds in persons without adequate prior active immunization and treatment of tetanus
Cytomegalovirus	Cytomegalovirus immune globulin, intravenous	Prophylaxis for bone marrow and kidney transplant recipients
Diphtheria	Diphtheria antitoxin, equine	Treatment of established disease, high frequency of reactions to serum of nonhuman origin; in the United States, available only from CDC
Rabies	Rabies immune globulin, human	Postexposure prophylaxis of animal bites
Measles	Immune globulin, human	Prevention or modification of disease in contacts of cases, not for control of outbreaks
Hepatitis A	Immune globulin, human	Pre-exposure and postexposure prophylaxis for travelers and others who need protection before immunity can be achieved with hepatitis A vaccine
Hepatitis B	Hepatitis B immune globulin, human	Prophylaxis for needlestick or mucous membrane contact with HBsAg-positive persons, for sexual partners with acute hepatitis B or hepatitis B carriers, for infants born to mothers who are carriers of HBsAg, for infants whose mother or primary caregiver has acute hepatitis B
Varicella	Varicella-zoster immune globulin (VariZIG)	Persons with underlying disease and at risk for complications from chickenpox who have not had varicella or varicella vaccine and who are exposed to varicella; may be given after exposure to known susceptible adults, particularly if antibody negative. VariZIG is available under IND.
Vaccinia	Vaccinia immune globulin	Treatment of eczema vaccinatum, vaccinia necrosum, and severe inadvertent inoculations such as ocular vaccinia after vaccinia (smallpox) vaccination. Available only from the CDC.
Erythroblastosis fetalis	Rh immune globulin	Rh-negative women who give birth to Rh-positive infants or who abort
Hypogammaglobulinemia	Immune globulin, intravenous	Maintenance therapy
Idiopathic thrombocytopenic purpura	Immune globulin, intravenous	Therapy for acute episodes
Botulism	Bivalent A and B antitoxin, equine	Treatment of botulism; available through CDC
Snakebite	Antivenin, equine (North American coral snake antivenin)	Specific for North American coral snake, *Micrurus fulvius*
	Crotalidae, polyvalent	Effective for viper and pit viper bites, including rattlesnakes, copperheads, moccasins
Spider bite	Antivenin, equine	Specific for black widow spider, *Latrodectus mactans,* and other members of the genus

CDC = Centers for Disease Control and Prevention; HBsAg = hepatitis B surface antigen; IND = Investigational New Drug.

without anaphylactic-type allergies to eggs can be given these vaccines safely, but persons with anaphylactic reactions to eggs generally should not receive these vaccines except when it is absolutely necessary and then only under established protocols by physicians who are expert in such situations. Although measles and mumps vaccines are grown in chick embryo tissue culture, the risk of anaphylaxis even in persons with severe hypersensitivity to eggs is low, so they can be vaccinated without prior testing. Suspected adverse events temporally related to vaccinations should be reported to the Vaccine Adverse Events Reporting System (1-800-822-7967 or *www.vaers.hhs.gov*).

General Considerations

The major group that makes comprehensive, detailed recommendations regarding immunization of adults is the Advisory Committee on Immunization Practices of the Centers for Disease Control and Prevention (CDC), which publishes its information in *Morbidity and Mortality Weekly Report* (also available at *http://www.cdc.gov/vaccines/recs/schedules/adult-schedule.htm#print*). Immunizations for adults depend on age, lifestyle, occupation, and medical conditions. Two adult immunization schedules are available, one based on age group (Fig. 17-1 and E-Table 17-1) and one based on underlying risk (Fig. 17-2 and Table 17-2). All adults should have a primary series of tetanus and diphtheria toxoids with boosters of combined toxoids (Td) every 10 years. All adults should have a one-time dose of combined tetanus and diphtheria toxoids and acellular pertussis vaccine (Tdap) followed by Td every 10 years. Persons born in or after 1957 should have evidence of immunity to measles, mumps, and rubella (e.g., documentation of vaccination or presence of antibodies considered compatible with protection). Vaccination of susceptible adolescents and adults against varicella is desirable. Pneumococcal polysaccharide vaccine (PPSV23) is indicated for all adults 65 years and older and younger adults with certain medical conditions that place them at high risk of complications. Influenza vaccination also is recommended annually for all persons 6 months of age or older. Health care workers exposed to blood or blood products should receive hepatitis B vaccine. Health care workers likely to come in contact with persons transmitting measles, mumps, rubella, or varicella should be immune to those diseases.

Immunocompromise

Patients with conditions that compromise their immune systems generally should not receive live attenuated vaccines. Such patients include those with immunodeficiency diseases, leukemia, lymphoma, and generalized malignant disease and those who are immunosuppressed from therapy with corticosteroids, alkylating agents, antimetabolites, and radiation. An exception is infection with human immunodeficiency virus (HIV). Asymptomatic patients should receive MMR vaccine. MMR should be considered for symptomatic patients with HIV infection; however, severely immunocompromised persons should not be vaccinated. Varicella vaccination (2 doses, 3 months apart) may be considered in HIV-infected persons with $CD4^+$ T-lymphocyte counts >200 cells/μL. Patients with leukemia in remission who have not been receiving any chemotherapy for at least 3 months may receive live virus vaccines. Short-course therapy (<2 weeks) with corticosteroids, alternate-day regimens with low to moderate doses of short-acting corticosteroids, and topical applications or tendon injections are not ordinarily contraindications to the administration of live vaccines.

Immunocompromised patients can receive inactivated vaccines and toxoids, although the efficacy of such preparations may be diminished. Patients with known HIV infection should receive pneumococcal vaccine and annual influenza vaccination.

Pregnancy

In general, live vaccines should not be given to pregnant women because of the theoretical concern that the vaccines could adversely affect the fetus. No significant adverse events attributable to vaccination of pregnant women with MMR or varicella have been documented; nevertheless, pregnant women should not receive MMR or varicella vaccine, and women who do receive these vaccines should wait 1 month before becoming pregnant. Poliomyelitis and yellow fever vaccines usually should not be given to pregnant women unless the risk of disease is substantial. Td vaccination is especially

Recommended Adult Immunization Schedule
UNITED STATES–2011

Note: These recommendations *must* be read with the footnotes that follow containing number of doses, intervals between doses, and other important information.

Recommended adult immunization schedule, by vaccine and age group

Vaccine ↓ Age Group →	19–26 years	27–49 years	50–59 years	60–64 years	≥ 65 years
Influenza [1,*]	1 dose annually				
Tetanus, diphtheria, pertussis (Td/Tdap) [2,*]	Substitute 1-time dose of Tdap for Td booster; then boost with Td every 10 yrs				Td booster every 10 yrs
Varicella [3,*]	2 doses				
Human papillomavirus (HPV) [4,*]	3 doses (females)				
Zoster [5]				1 dose	
Measles, mumps, rubella (MMR) [6,*]	1 or 2 doses		1 dose		
Pneumococcal (polysaccharide) [7,8]	1 or 2 doses				1 dose
Meningococcal [9,*]	1 or more doses				
Hepatitis A [10,*]	2 doses				
Hepatitis B [11,*]	3 doses				

*Covered by the Vaccine Injury Compensation Program.

For all persons in this category who meet the age requirements and who lack evidence of immunity (e.g., lack documentation of vaccination or have no evidence of prior infection

Recommended if some other risk factor is present (e.g., based on medical, occupational, lifestyle, or other indications)

No recommendation

Report all clinically significant postvaccination reactions to the Vaccine Adverse Event Reporting System (VAERS). Reporting forms and instructions on filing a VAERS report are available at http://www.vaers.hhs.gov or by telephone, 800-822-7967.

Information on how to file a Vaccine Injury Compensation Program claim is available at htpp://www.hrsa.gov/vaccinecompensation or by telephone, 800-338-2382. Information about filing a claim for vaccine injury is available through the U.S. Court of Federal Claims, 717 Madison Place, N.W., Washington, D.C. 20005; telephone 202-357-6400.

Additional information about the vaccines in this schedule, extent of available data, and contraindications for vaccination are also available at http://www.cdc.gov/vaccines, or from the CDC-INFO Contact Center at 800-CDC-INFO (800-232-4636) in English or Spanish, 24 hours a day, 7 days a week.

FIGURE 17-1. **Recommended adult immunization schedule, by vaccine and age group, United States, 2011.** See E-Table 17-1 for footnotes. (From *http://www.cdc.gov/vaccines/recs/schedules/adult-schedule.htm#print.*)

indicated for pregnant women who are not appropriately vaccinated to prevent neonatal tetanus in their infants. Vaccination is done best after the first trimester to avoid attribution to a vaccine of an adverse outcome of pregnancy that was only coincidental. Most pregnant women should not receive TdaP. In such cases, however, TdaP should be administered postpartum. All pregnant women should be screened for hepatitis B surface antigen (HBsAg). Children born to mothers with active HBsAg infection should receive hepatitis B vaccine and hepatitis B immune globulin within 12 hours of birth. Women who will be pregnant during the influenza season should receive inactivated influenza vaccine. Pregnant women have been shown to be at particularly high risk of complications from influenza and are at high priority to receive this vaccine to protect them.

INDIVIDUAL IMMUNOBIOLOGICS

Hepatitis A

Two inactivated hepatitis A (Chapter 150) vaccines are available in the United States. Seroconversion rates after a single dose of either vaccine in persons older than 1 year exceed 95%. Antibody levels shown to be protective in animals develop in almost all persons.

Indications

The vaccine is indicated primarily for persons traveling to countries, generally the developing world, with high or intermediate endemicity for hepatitis A, but it is also recommended for other groups at high risk for infection or for development of severe hepatitis. In addition, vaccine is routinely recommended for children 12 to 23 months of age. Health care workers have not been shown to be at higher risk than the general population for hepatitis A and do not need routine immunization. Although food handlers are not at increased risk for hepatitis A compared with the general population, the consequences of infection or suspected infection in this group, which can lead to extensive public health investigations, may make vaccination cost-effective in some settings. Hepatitis A vaccine can be given to children 1 year of age or older to control outbreaks in communities with high rates of prior infection and be considered for communities with intermediate levels of prior infection (anti–hepatitis A seroprevalence of 10 to 25% by 5 years of age). Doses vary by age and product. All schedules call for a second dose at least 6 months after the first dose, with a permissible range for one of the products 18 months after the initial dose. Vaccines are not indicated for children younger than 1 year because adequate data on safety and efficacy are lacking.

Vaccines That Might Be Indicated for Adults Based on Medical and Other Indications

Vaccine ↓ Indication →	Pregnancy	Immuno-compromising conditions (excluding human immunodeficiency virus [HIV]) 3, 5, 6, 13	HIV infection 3, 6, 12, 13 CD4+ T lymphocyte count <200 cells/µL	HIV infection CD4+ T lymphocyte count ≥200 cells/µL	Diabetes, heart disease, chronic lung disease, chronic alcoholism	Asplenia 12 (including elective splenectomy) and persistent complement component deficiencies	Chronic liver disease	Kidney failure, end-stage renal disease, receipt of hemodialysis	Healthcare personnel
Influenza 1,*	1 dose TIV annually								1 dose TIV or LAIV annually
Tetanus, diphtheria, pertussis (Td/Tdap) 2,*	Td	Substitute 1-time dose of Tdap for Td booster; then boost with Td every 10 yrs							
Varicella 3,*	Contraindicated			2 doses					
Human papillomavirus (HPV) 4,*		3 doses for females through age 26 yrs							
Zoster 5	Contraindicated				1 dose				
Measles, mumps, rubella (MMR) 6,*	Contraindicated			1 or 2 doses					
Pneumococcal (polysaccharide) 7,8		1 or 2 doses							
Meningococcal 9,*	1 or more doses								
Hepatitis A 10,*	2 doses								
Hepatitis B 11,*					3 doses				

*Covered by the Vaccine Injury Compensation Program.

For all persons in this category who meet the age requirements and who lack evidence of immunity (e.g., lack documentation of vaccination or have no evidence of prior infection)

Recommended if some other risk factor is present (e.g., on the basis of medical, occupational, lifestyle, or other indications)

No recommendation

These schedules indicate the recommended age groups and medical indications for which administration of currently licensed vaccines is commonly indicated for adults ages 19 years and older, as of Febuary 4, 2011. For all vaccines being recommended on the adult immunization schedule, a vaccine series does not need to be restarted, regardless of the time that has elapsed between doses. Licensed combination vaccines may be used whenever any components of the combination are indicated and when the vaccine's other components are not contraindicated. For detailed recommendations on all vaccines, including those used primarily for travelers or that are issued during the year, consult the manufacturers' package inserts and the complete statement from the Advisory Committee on Immunization Practices (http://www.cdc.gov/vaccines/pubs/aclp-list.htm).

FIGURE 17-2. **Recommended adult immunization schedule, by vaccine and medical and other indications, United States, 2011.** See E-Table 17-1 for footnotes. (From *http://www.cdc.gov/vaccines/recs/schedules/adult-schedule.htm#print.*)

Side Effects

The most common side effect has been tenderness and soreness at the injection site. Although rare and more serious adverse events have been reported in temporal association with vaccination, a causal relationship has not been established.

Hepatitis B

Hepatitis B (Chapter 150) vaccine is the first vaccine that can prevent cancer (an estimated 800 persons per year in the United States die of hepatitis B–related liver cancer; many times more die in the developing world). It also can prevent acute and chronic complications of hepatitis B, including an estimated 4000 deaths annually from cirrhosis and 250 deaths annually from fulminant hepatic disease in the United States. Currently produced vaccines are derived from insertion of the gene for HBsAg into *Saccharomyces cerevisiae.* Hepatitis B vaccine, the first licensed vaccine made by use of recombinant techniques, produces adequate antibody responses in more than 90% of normal adults and more than 95% of normal infants, children, and adolescents when it is administered in a three-dose series. The dosage depends on the product, the age group, and the underlying clinical condition and can be determined by consulting the package insert. The duration of vaccine-conferred immunity is not known, although follow-up of vaccinees for more than 16 years indicates persistence of protection against clinically significant infections (i.e., detectable viremia and clinical disease). Booster doses are not currently recommended. Vaccine must be injected intramuscularly, preferably in the deltoid.

Indications

Hepatitis B vaccine is indicated for adults at high risk of infection (see Fig. 17-1 and E-Table 17-1). Because strategies targeting hepatitis B vaccine use only to high-risk populations have not had a significant impact on hepatitis B incidence, universal vaccination is recommended for infants and for all adolescents who have not been previously vaccinated. Universal screening for HBsAg is recommended for all pregnant women; administration of three doses of vaccine and one dose of hepatitis B immune globulin is recommended for infants of acutely or chronically infected mothers.

Side Effects

The major side effect is soreness at the injection site. Alopecia, which is usually reversible, has been reported rarely. Hepatitis B vaccine has not been shown to induce multiple sclerosis in controlled studies and has not been shown to exacerbate illness in patients with multiple sclerosis who are vaccinated.

Human Papillomavirus

Two human papillomavirus (HPV) vaccines are licensed. Both vaccines contain the L1 capsid protein of types 16 and 18, which account for about 70% of cases of cervical cancer. The quadrivalent vaccine also contains types 6 and 11, which are the most common causes of anogenital warts. Routine vaccination of 11- to 12-year-old girls is recommended in a three-dose schedule. The vaccine should be administered at 0, 1 to 2, and 6 months. Catch-up

Text continues on p. 71

TABLE 17-2 SELECTED IMMUNIZING AGENTS INDICATED FOR ADULTS*

DISEASE	IMMUNIZING AGENT	INDICATIONS	SCHEDULE	MAJOR CONTRAINDICATIONS AND PRECAUTIONS	COMMENTS
Anthrax	Anthrax vaccine, adsorbed, an inactivated vaccine	Pre-exposure prophylaxis of persons at high risk of exposure (e.g., military, certain laboratory workers) Consider with antibiotics for postexposure prophylaxis	0.5-mL dose IM at 0, 4, and 6 wk and 12 and 18 mo Manufacturer recommends booster annually thereafter If used after exposure, 3 doses at 0, 2, and 4 wk with antibiotics for at least 7-14 days after third dose	Severe allergic reaction to a vaccine component or after a prior dose Moderate or severe acute illness is a precaution to vaccination	Effectiveness against aerosol exposure inferred primarily from animal data Limited data on the benefits of postexposure use
Diphtheria	Tetanus and diphtheria toxoids combined	All adults	Two doses IM 4 wk apart, third dose 6-12 mo after second dose for primary series Booster every 10 yr No need to repeat if schedule is interrupted	History of neurologic reaction after a previous dose Severe allergic reaction to a vaccine component or after a prior dose Moderate or severe acute illness is a precaution	Tetanus and diphtheria toxoids combined with acellular pertussis vaccine (Tdap) preferred as one-time booster for all persons through 64 yr
Hepatitis A	Inactivated hepatitis A vaccine	Travelers to highly or intermediately endemic countries Men who have sex with men Illegal drug users (injection and noninjection) Persons who work with hepatitis A virus–infected primates or who do research with the virus Persons with chronic liver disease Recipients of clotting factors	Two doses at least 6 mo apart for persons aged ≥1 yr	Severe allergic reaction to a vaccine component or after a prior dose Moderate or severe acute illness is a precaution to vaccination	Recommended for all children Should be considered for outbreak control
Hepatitis B	Inactivated hepatitis B virus subunit vaccine containing HBsAg	Adolescents Health care and public safety workers potentially exposed to blood Clients and staff of institutions for the developmentally disabled Hemodialysis patients Men who have sex with men Users of illicit injectable drugs Recipients of clotting factors Household and sexual contacts of HBV carriers Inmates of long-term correctional facilities Heterosexuals treated for sexually transmitted diseases or with multiple sexual partners Travelers with close contact for ≥6 mo with populations with high prevalence of HBV carriage	Three doses IM at 0, 1, and 6 mo	Severe allergic reaction to a vaccine component or after a prior dose Moderate or severe acute illness is a precaution to vaccination	Pregnancy is not a contraindication Health care workers who have contact with patients or blood, sexual contacts of persons with chronic HBV infection, hemodialysis patients and other immunosuppressed persons, and recipients of clotting factor concentrates should be tested 1-2 mo after vaccination to determine serologic response
Human papilloma-virus	Inactivated L1 capsid proteins of types 6, 11, 16, and 18 (quadrivalent) and types 16 and 18 (bivalent)	Females at 11-12 yr; catch-up vaccination of females through 26 yr Males 9 through 26 yr for genital warts	Three 0.5-mL doses IM at 0, 1 to 2, and 6 mo	Severe allergic reaction to a vaccine component or to a prior dose Vaccine is not recommended for pregnant women	The vaccine will not protect against existing infections Because the types in the vaccine are not responsible for about 30% of infections associated with cervical cancer, screening for cancer should occur as for unvaccinated women
Influenza	Inactivated virus vaccine	All adults, with greatest priority for those ≥65 yr old, persons with underlying medical conditions, pregnant women, health care workers, and persons with close contact with children <5 years of age	Annual vaccination; see annual ACIP recommendation	Severe allergic reaction to an influenza vaccine component (including eggs) or after a prior dose Moderate or severe acute illness is a precaution to vaccination GBS within 6 wk of prior dose of influenza vaccine	Optimum timing for vaccination is October and November However, vaccination can occur in December and later, particularly for health care workers and persons at high risk for complications who were not vaccinated earlier Only one dose of influenza vaccine per season is recommended for adults

TABLE 17-2 SELECTED IMMUNIZING AGENTS INDICATED FOR ADULTS—cont'd

DISEASE	IMMUNIZING AGENT	INDICATIONS	SCHEDULE	MAJOR CONTRAINDICATIONS AND PRECAUTIONS	COMMENTS
Influenza (cont'd)	Live attenuated influenza virus	Persons 2 through 49 yr without underlying conditions that place them at high risk of complications from influenza	Annual vaccination; see annual ACIP statement Administered intranasally	Persons <2 yr or ≥50 yr Underlying disorders that place them at high risk of influenza complications History of GBS within 6 wk of prior dose of influenza vaccine Pregnant women Hypersensitivity to eggs or components of vaccine	Can be used for household contacts and health care workers caring for patients without severe immunocompromise
Japanese encephalitis	Inactivated Japanese encephalitis virus vaccine	Travelers to Asia spending at least 1 mo in endemic areas during transmission season	Two 0.5-mL doses IM on days 0 and 28 for persons 18 yr and older	Pregnancy	
Measles	Live virus vaccine	All adults born after 1956 without history of live vaccine on or after first birthday, physician-diagnosed measles, or detectable measles antibody Persons born before 1957 generally can be considered immune	One dose sufficient for most adults; 2 doses at least 1 mo apart indicated for persons entering college or medical facility employment, traveling abroad, or at risk of measles during outbreaks	Altered immunity (e.g., leukemia, lymphoma, generalized malignant disease, congenital immunodeficiency, immunosuppressive therapy) Immune globulin or other blood products within prior 3-11 mo, depending on dose of immune globulin or blood product received Untreated tuberculosis Anaphylactic hypersensitivity to neomycin or gelatin Pregnancy Thrombocytopenia	Persons with anaphylactic allergies to eggs may be vaccinated (see text) Vaccine should be administered to persons with asymptomatic HIV infection and should be considered for patients except those with severe immunocompromise
Meningococcal disease (2 vaccines)	1. Meningococcal conjugate vaccines containing polysaccharide of serogroups A, C, W135, and Y (age 2-55 yr) 2. Polysaccharide vaccine containing tetravalent A, C, W135, and Y (ages 56 yr and older)	All 11- to 18-year-old persons and all persons with persistent complement component deficiencies, anatomic or functional asplenia, persons who will travel to areas with hyperendemic or epidemic diseases; certain laboratory workers; may be useful during localized outbreaks	One dose with revaccination at age 16 yr of children who receive conjugate vaccine at 11-12 yr of age and every 5 yr for persons at high risk	1. Allergic reactions to a component of the vaccine including diphtheria toxoid and latex	Conjugate vaccine is preferred to polysaccharide alone for persons aged 2 through 55 yr
Mumps	Live virus vaccine	All adults born after 1956 without history of live vaccine on or after first birthday, physician-diagnosed mumps, or detectable mumps antibody Persons born before 1957 generally can be considered immune	One dose sufficient for most adults; 2 doses at least 1 mo apart indicated for persons entering college or medical facility employment, or traveling abroad	Altered immunity (e.g., leukemia, lymphoma, generalized malignant disease, congenital immunodeficiency, immunosuppressive therapy) Immune globulin or other blood products within prior 3-11 mo Anaphylactic hypersensitivity to neomycin or gelatin Pregnancy Thrombocytopenia if administered with measles vaccine	Although persons born after 1957 are generally immune, vaccine can be given to adults of all ages and may be particularly indicated for postpubertal males who are thought to be susceptible Persons with anaphylactic allergies to eggs may be vaccinated
Pertussis	Adult preparation of pertussis antigens combined with tetanus and diphtheria toxoids (Tdap)	All 11- to 12-year-olds Catch-up vaccination for all persons 13-64 yr of age Preferred interval of 5 yr from prior dose of Td but may be given at shorter intervals if risk of pertussis is high	One dose	Severe allergic reaction to a vaccine component or after a prior dose Moderate or severe acute illness is a precaution to vaccination	Two preparations are available, one licensed for 10- to 64-year-olds, one for 11- to 64-year-olds Administer one dose to persons 65 yr of age or older who have not previously received Td and who anticipate contact with infants younger than 1 yr of age

TABLE 17-2 SELECTED IMMUNIZING AGENTS INDICATED FOR ADULTS—cont'd

DISEASE	IMMUNIZING AGENT	INDICATIONS	SCHEDULE	MAJOR CONTRAINDICATIONS AND PRECAUTIONS	COMMENTS
Pneumococcal disease	23-Valent polysaccharide vaccine	Adults with cardiovascular disease, pulmonary disease (including asthma), diabetes mellitus, alcoholism, cirrhosis, cerebrospinal fluid leaks, splenic dysfunction or anatomic asplenia, Hodgkin's disease, lymphoma, multiple myeloma, chronic renal failure, nephrotic syndrome, immunosuppression, HIV infection, cigarette smokers 19 yr and older High-risk populations such as certain Native Americans and all adults ≥65 yr	One dose IM or SC; a second dose should be considered ≥5 yr later for adults at high risk of disease (e.g., asplenic patients) and those who lose antibody rapidly (e.g., nephrotic syndrome, renal failure, transplant recipients) Revaccinate adults who received a first dose when <65 yr who are now ≥65 yr and who received their vaccine at least 5 yr earlier	Severe allergic reaction to a vaccine component or after a prior dose Moderate or severe acute illness is a precaution to vaccination	Conjugate pneumococcal vaccine is not indicated for adults
Poliomyelitis	Inactivated poliovirus vaccine	Certain adults who are at greater risk of exposure to wild poliovirus than the general population, including travelers to countries where poliomyelitis is epidemic or endemic or specific populations with disease caused by wild poliovirus	For unvaccinated adults, two doses SC 4 wk apart and a third dose 6-12 mo after the second; if <4 wk available before protection is needed, a single dose of IPV For incompletely immunized adults, complete primary series that consists of three doses of IPV or prior OPV; no need to restart interrupted series A single dose of IPV can be given to adults who previously received a primary series but now are at high risk, such as travel to an endemic area	On theoretical grounds, pregnant women should not receive IPV, but if immediate protection is needed, IPV can be used Severe allergic reaction to a vaccine component or after a prior dose Moderate or severe acute illness is a precaution to vaccination	
Rabies	Inactivated vaccine, HDCV or PCEC	High-risk persons, including animal handlers, selected laboratory and field workers, and persons traveling for ≥1 mo to areas with high risk of rabies	Pre-exposure prophylaxis: three doses of 1 mL IM on days 0, 7, and 21 or 28	History of severe hypersensitivity reaction	Further doses needed after exposure
Rubella	Live virus vaccine	Adults, particularly women of childbearing age, who lack history of rubella vaccine and detectable rubella-specific antibodies in serum Males and females in institutions where rubella outbreaks may occur, such as hospitals, the military, and colleges Persons born before 1957, except women who can become pregnant, generally can be considered immune	One dose SC	Pregnancy, altered immunity (e.g., leukemia, lymphoma, generalized malignant disease, congenital immunodeficiency, immunosuppressive therapy) Immune globulin or other blood products within the 3-11 mo before vaccination Anaphylactic hypersensitivity to neomycin Administration of blood products should not contraindicate postpartum vaccination Thrombocytopenia if administered with measles vaccine	Women should be counseled to avoid pregnancy for 1 mo after vaccination

TABLE 17-2 SELECTED IMMUNIZING AGENTS INDICATED FOR ADULTS—cont'd

DISEASE	IMMUNIZING AGENT	INDICATIONS	SCHEDULE	MAJOR CONTRAINDICATIONS AND PRECAUTIONS	COMMENTS
Smallpox	Live vaccinia virus	Persons working with orthopox viruses Members of public health and health care response teams	One dose intracutaneously with a bifurcated needle Boosters every 10 yr and perhaps every 3 yr for persons working with virulent orthopox viruses	History or presence of eczema or other acute, chronic, or exfoliative skin condition Immunosuppression or pregnancy in patient or a close household or personal contact History of heart disease Breast-feeding Age <1 yr Allergy to a vaccine component No contraindications if exposed to smallpox	Some complications of vaccination are treatable with vaccinia immune globulin Vaccine is effective 3-4 days after exposure to variola and perhaps longer to prevent or to modify the illness Serious adverse events are rare but significant, including eczema vaccinatum, progressive vaccinia, myopericarditis, autoinoculation, and encephalitis Vaccinia is transmissible
Tetanus	Tetanus and diphtheria toxoids combined	All adults	Three doses IM needed for primary series: two doses 4 wk apart, third dose 6-12 mo after second dose Booster every 10 yr; no need to repeat if schedule is interrupted	History of neurologic or severe allergic reaction after a prior dose	Special recommendations for wound treatment (see text) Persons with GBS within the first 6 wk after immunization, particularly adults who received a prior primary series, probably should not be revaccinated in most circumstances Tetanus and diphtheria toxoids combined with acellular pertussis (Tdap) vaccine preferred for booster at age 11-12 yr One-time booster of Tdap for persons through 64 yr
Typhoid fever	Vi capsular polysaccharide vaccine Live attenuated Ty21a oral vaccine	Travelers to areas where the risk of prolonged exposure to contaminated food and water is high May be considered for family and intimate contacts of carriers and laboratory workers who work with *Salmonella typhi*	Vi polysaccharide vaccine: one dose IM 0.5 mL, boosters every 2 yr Oral vaccine: four doses on alternate days, repeat series every 5 yr if risk continues	Severe local or systemic reaction to a prior dose Ty21a vaccine should not be administered to persons with altered immunity or those receiving antimicrobial agents	Efficacy only 50-77% Food and water precautions essential
Varicella: chickenpox strain	Attenuated Oka strain of varicella virus	All persons without evidence of varicella immunity especially health care personnel, childbearing-age women, and persons with household or other contact with persons at high risk of complications of varicella (e.g., susceptible immunosuppressed persons)	Two 0.5-mL SC doses 4-8 wk apart for persons ≥13 yr A second dose is recommended for all persons who previously received one dose	Immunocompromise Pregnancy Allergy to vaccine components	Adults with a history of prior clinician-diagnosed or verified varicella can be considered immune Vaccine virus has rarely been transmitted to contacts from healthy vaccinees in whom rash developed Women who receive vaccine should not become pregnant for 1 mo
Varicella: zoster	Attenuated Oka strain of varicella virus, approximately 14 times more potent than varicella vaccine	Persons ≥60 years of age	One 0.65-mL dose SC	Immunocompromise Pregnancy Allergy to vaccine components	May be administered regardless of a prior history of shingles
Yellow fever	Live attenuated virus (17D strain)	Persons living or traveling in areas where yellow fever exists	One dose, booster every 10 yr	Immunocompromised persons History of anaphylactic allergies to eggs Pregnancy on theoretical grounds, although may be given if risk is high	Fever, jaundice, and multiple-organ system failure (viscerotropic disease) have been rarely reported in first-time recipients of 17D-derived yellow fever vaccinations Vaccinate only persons traveling to areas endemic to yellow fever

*See the text and package inserts for further details, particularly regarding indications, dosage, mode of administration, side effects, and adverse reactions and contraindications.

ACIP = Advisory Committee on Immunization Practices; GBS = Guillain-Barré syndrome; HBsAg = hepatitis B surface antigen; HBV = hepatitis B virus; HDCV = human diploid cell vaccine for rabies; HIV = human immunodeficiency virus; IM = intramuscularly; IPV = inactivated poliovirus vaccine; MMR = measles, mumps, and rubella vaccine; OPV = live trivalent oral poliovirus vaccine; PCEC = purified chick embryo cell culture rabies vaccine; SC = subcutaneously.

vaccination should be undertaken for females up through 26 years of age. Recipients of HPV vaccine should follow the same recommendations for Papanicolaou (Pap) smear screening as unvaccinated females. Persons with prior abnormal Pap smears or genital warts may be vaccinated to prevent persistent infection with types of HPV that are not in the vaccine. In 2009, the U.S. Food and Drug Administration (FDA) also licensed the quadrivalent vaccine for males, 9 through 26 years of age, for prevention of genital warts.

Side Effects

The most common reactions are local pain, swelling, and erythema, which may, in part, be explained by the aluminum-containing adjuvant rather than the L1 capsid protein. There is a slightly higher incidence of fever within 15 days of vaccination in vaccine recipients compared with placebo recipients.

Influenza

The two available influenza vaccines for seasonal influenza are the inactivated trivalent influenza vaccine (TIV) and the live attenuated influenza vaccine (LAIV). TIV, which contains split viruses of three major antigenic types, A (H3N2), A (H1N1), and B, is administered intramuscularly. LAIV, which consists of three cold-adapted, temperature-sensitive attenuated viruses, one for each of the expected circulating strains, is administered intranasally. LAIV is prepared by use of attenuated parent viruses that have been reassorted with circulating strains to contain six internal genes from the parent virus and genes for the surface hemagglutinin and neuraminidase of an A (H3N2), A (H1N1), or B strain. In 2009, a novel H1N1 virus emerged and caused a global pandemic. The 2009 H1N1 split virus vaccine is now the H1N1 component of the annual influenza vaccine.

Indications

Annual influenza (Chapter 372) vaccination with TIV is indicated for all adults but with a special emphasis on persons at high risk of complications from the disease: persons with chronic cardiopulmonary disorders, residents of nursing homes or other long-term care facilities, persons 50 years of age or older, patients with other chronic diseases (e.g., diabetes mellitus, kidney dysfunction, hemoglobinopathies, and immunosuppression) who have required regular medical follow-up or hospitalization in the prior year, adults and children who have any condition (e.g., cognitive dysfunction, spinal cord injuries, seizure disorders, or other neuromuscular disorders) that can compromise respiratory function or the handling of respiratory secretions or that can increase the risk for aspiration, and children receiving long-term aspirin therapy. Women who will be pregnant during the influenza season (usually late December through mid-March) also should be vaccinated. To reduce transmission of influenza to high-risk patients, health care workers and household contacts of high-risk patients should also be vaccinated annually, including contacts of children younger than 5 years of age. Annual vaccination is also recommended for all children 6 months through 18 years.

LAIV is licensed only for nonpregnant persons aged 2 through 49 years without underlying conditions that place them at high risk of complications from influenza. LAIV can be used for contacts of high-risk patients, if the contacts are of the appropriate age. LAIV, for theoretical concerns about live virus transmission, is not recommended for contacts of severely immunosuppressed patients such as patients with bone marrow transplants but can be given to contacts of persons with mild to moderate immunologic impairment.

The efficacy of TIV varies with the host's condition and the degree to which antigens in the vaccine match viruses in circulation the following season. Provided the match is good, the vaccine's efficacy is usually 70 to 90% in normal healthy young adults. Efficacy is substantially lower, often between 30 and 40%, in the institutionalized elderly; nevertheless, it seems to be 60 to 80% protective against pneumonia and death. LAIV has been found to be more than 85% effective in young children, even in a year when the circulating strain had antigenically drifted from the vaccine strain. Similar effects were seen in challenge studies in adults.

Ideally, seasonal vaccines should be administered as soon as they are available. If vaccine is available in December and January, vaccination should continue because it still can offer protection for many individuals. A review of influenza seasons from 1976-77 through 2008-09 documented that peak activity did not occur until January or later in more than 80% of those seasons and until February or later in more than 60%.

Side Effects

Persons with anaphylactic allergy to eggs generally should not be immunized. The most common side effect of TIV is soreness at the injection site. Fever, malaise, and myalgia may begin 6 to 12 hours after vaccination and persist for 1 to 2 days, although such reactions are most common in children exposed to vaccine for the first time. Severe allergic reactions are rare. If current influenza vaccines cause Guillain-Barré syndrome, it is likely to be rare, on the order of one case per 1 million doses. The most common adverse events after LAIV in adults are runny nose, headache, and sore throat.

Measles

Indications

Measles (Chapter 375) immunization is recommended for all persons born in or after 1957 who lack evidence of prior physician-diagnosed measles or laboratory evidence of immunity or appropriate vaccination. Before 1989, appropriate vaccination consisted of a single dose of live vaccine administered on or after the first birthday. Since then, a routine two-dose schedule has been recommended: the first dose, which is 93 to 98% effective, at 12 to 15 months of age, and the second dose at entry to primary school. All children from kindergarten through the 12th grade should have a second dose. Most adults are considered to have been appropriately vaccinated if they received one dose of vaccine administered on or after their first birthday. Some adults who are at increased risk of measles (health care workers with direct contact with patients, students in college, international travelers) should receive a second dose of vaccine, however, unless they have documentation of serologic evidence of immunity. Persons embarking on foreign travel ideally should have received two doses or have other evidence of measles immunity. Persons born before 1957 are usually immune as a result of natural infection and do not require vaccination, although vaccination is not contraindicated if they are believed to be susceptible.

During outbreaks of measles in institutions, all persons at risk who have not received two doses or who lack other evidence of measles immunity should be vaccinated. Measles vaccine is usually administered along with mumps and rubella vaccines as MMR to ensure immunity against all three diseases. Individuals already immune to one or more of the components may receive MMR without harm.

Measles vaccine is contraindicated for pregnant women on theoretical grounds, for persons with moderate to severe acute febrile illnesses, and for persons with altered immunocompetence, except those with HIV infection who are not severely immunocompromised. Patients with anaphylactic reactions to eggs can be vaccinated without prior skin testing.

Side Effects

In approximately 5 to 15% of susceptible recipients of measles vaccine, temperatures of 39.4° C or higher develop 5 to 12 days after vaccination and last 1 to 2 days. Transient rashes develop in about 5%. Thrombocytopenic purpura has been reported rarely after MMR. The overall rate of reactions after the second dose of a measles-containing vaccine is substantially lower than after the first dose. Encephalopathy or encephalitis after measles vaccination has been reported at a rate lower than the background or expected rate.

Meningococcal Vaccines

Three quadrivalent meningococcal polysaccharide vaccines against disease caused by serogroups A, C, Y, and W135 are available: meningococcal polysaccharide vaccine (MPSV4), which consists of 50 μg of polysaccharide of each of the four serogroups and is licensed for persons 2 years of age and older, and two meningococcal conjugate vaccines (MCV4). One conjugate consists of 4 μg of each polysaccharide covalently linked to 48 μg of diphtheria toxoid and licensed for persons 2 to 55 years of age. The other conjugate consists of polysaccharide linked to CRM_{197}. The four serogroups in each vaccine account for approximately two thirds of meningococcal disease in the United States and about 75% of the disease in persons 11 years of age or older (Chapter 306). Serogroup A and C polysaccharide vaccines have had 85 to 100% efficacy in epidemic settings, whereas polysaccharide vaccines for the other groups have documented good immunogenicity in adults. Meningococcal conjugate vaccine type C (MCV-C) has been associated with an estimated effectiveness of 88 to 98% in the year following vaccination in the United Kingdom, where it has been used widely. In addition, MCV-C has reduced colonization by 66% and decreased disease among unvaccinated persons by 67% in 1- to 17-year-olds and by 35% among those older than 25 years. In contrast to polysaccharide vaccines, conjugate vaccines induce immunologic memory, result in higher and more durable levels of high-avidity antibodies, and have been documented to induce herd immunity. The duration of immunity for both MPSV4 and MCV4 is thought to be about 5 years.

Indications

Routine vaccination with a single dose of MCV4 is recommended for all adolescents at 11 through 18 years of age who have not been previously vaccinated and for college freshmen who will live in dormitories. Vaccination is also recommended for very-high-risk persons, that is, those with persistent complement component deficiencies, persons with splenic dysfunction or without a spleen, microbiologists with frequent exposure to *Neisseria meningitidis* in culture, and persons who travel to or live in areas with hyperendemic or epidemic disease (e.g., the "meningitis belt" of sub-Saharan Africa, stretching from Mauritania to Ethiopia). MCV4 can be used for persons 2 to 10 years of age with high-risk conditions. It is not recommended routinely for this age group. For persons older than 55 years with an indication for vaccine, MPSV4 should be used. Meningococcal vaccination may be useful during localized epidemics of serogroups in the vaccine.

Re-vaccination is indicated at age 16 in children initially vaccinated between 11 and 12 years of age. For children initially vaccinated after age 12 years, re-vaccination recommendations are still being developed (*www.ccc.gov/vaccines*). For very high-risk persons, re-vaccination is recommended every 5 years.

Side Effects

The major side effects of MPSV4 are local reactions lasting 1 to 2 days. The incidence of local reactions and low-grade fever is slightly higher after MCV4 than with MPSV4. An excess risk of 1.25 cases of Guillain-Barré syndrome per million doses has been noted with the vaccination, although further studies have cast doubt on a causal association.

Mumps

Indications

Mumps (Chapter 377) vaccine is indicated for all persons, especially susceptible males, without evidence of immunity. For most adults, such evidence consists of a prior history of vaccination on or after the first birthday, physician-diagnosed mumps, or laboratory evidence of immunity. For adults at high risk, including health care workers, international travelers, and students at post–high school educational institutions, two doses of mumps vaccine constitute acceptable evidence of immunity. Most persons born before 1957 can be considered immune as a result of natural infection, although vaccination is not contraindicated if such persons are thought to be susceptible.

Side Effects

Adverse events after the Jeryl Lynn strain of mumps vaccine, the strain used in the United States, are uncommon—fever, parotitis, and allergic manifestations. Thrombocytopenic purpura has been reported rarely in persons administered MMR. Mumps vaccine is contraindicated for pregnant women on theoretical grounds, for persons with moderate to severe acute febrile illnesses, and for persons with altered immunocompetence. When combined with measles vaccine, it may be given to persons with asymptomatic HIV infection and considered for persons with symptomatic infection if they are not severely immunocompromised. Patients with anaphylactic reactions to eggs can be vaccinated without skin testing (see Measles earlier).

Pertussis Vaccine

In 2005, two vaccines were licensed for boosting immunity to pertussis. Both vaccines are combined with the adult preparation of tetanus and diphtheria toxoids and have a reduced content of pertussis antigens compared with the childhood pertussis-containing vaccines (Tdap). Boostrix (GlaxoSmithKline), which is licensed for adolescents and adults 10 through 64 years of age, contains three pertussis antigens—toxoid (PT), filamentous hemagglutinin (FHA), and pertactin (PRN). Adacel (Sanofi Pasteur, Inc.), which is licensed for 11- through 64-year-olds, contains five pertussis antigens, PT, FHA, PRN, and two fimbriae. Both vaccines, when administered to previously vaccinated adolescents and adults, induce serologic responses that are comparable to those induced during childhood vaccination with vaccines that have been proved effective. Adverse events, usually local reactions, are similar with the adult preparation of tetanus and diphtheria toxoids (Td) alone. A single dose of Tdap is indicated for all adolescents at 11 to 12 years of age. Older adolescents should receive Tdap instead of Td if they have not received an adolescent Td booster. Tdap can be given at any interval. All adults younger than 65 years should receive a single dose of TdaP to replace a Td booster. Persons are 65 years and older who anticipate contact with an infant should receive a single dose of Tdap.

Pneumococcal Vaccine

Pneumococcal polysaccharide vaccine consists of purified polysaccharide capsular antigens from the 23 types of *Streptococcus pneumoniae* that are responsible for 85 to 90% of the bacteremic disease in the United States (Chapter 297). Most adults, including elderly patients and those with alcoholic cirrhosis and diabetes mellitus, have a two-fold or greater rise in type-specific antibodies within 2 to 3 weeks of vaccination. Although the serologic response is generally acceptable, estimates of vaccine efficacy in preventing disease vary widely. Efficacy may be lower in some patients, such as patients with alcoholic cirrhosis or Hodgkin's disease. There is good evidence that vaccination is approximately 60% effective against bacteremic pneumococcal disease, which accounts for an estimated 50,000 cases annually. Evidence regarding efficacy against pneumonia in high-risk populations is not clear, however.

Indications

The preponderance of information supports the use of pneumococcal vaccine in high-risk populations, including all persons older than 65 years. Two groups recently added to those recommended for vaccination include persons 19 years or older who smoke cigarettes or those who have asthma. Special efforts should target hospitalized patients. Approximately two thirds of patients who are admitted later with pneumococcal disease had been hospitalized for other reasons within the preceding 5 years.

Immunity may decrease 5 years or more after initial vaccination; a single booster dose should be considered at that time for adults at highest risk of disease, such as asplenic patients, and for adults who lose antibody rapidly, such as patients with nephrotic syndrome or renal failure. Persons older than 65 years who received a dose more than 5 years earlier when they were younger than 65 years should be revaccinated.

Side Effects

Local reactions are frequent. Less than 1% of vaccinees experience severe local reactions or systemic illness, such as fever and malaise. Severe events such as anaphylaxis are rare. Because of the rarity of severe reactions in revaccinated patients, persons with indications for vaccination but with unknown histories of prior vaccination should be vaccinated.

A pneumococcal conjugate vaccine in which the polysaccharides of 13 types are covalently linked to a protein carrier was licensed and recommended for universal use in children. This vaccine, which covers substantially fewer types than the 23-valent polysaccharide vaccine, is not approved for persons 9 years of age or older. Widespread vaccination of children in the United States has led to substantial reductions of invasive pneumococcal disease in adults, suggesting that children are the source for many adult infections. Trials of conjugate vaccines in adults are ongoing.

Poliomyelitis

The last documented cases of indigenously acquired poliomyelitis (Chapters 387 and 423) caused by wild polioviruses in the United States were reported in 1979. In 2000, an all inactivated poliovirus vaccine (IPV) schedule was recommended in the United States; this vaccine replaced the live attenuated oral poliovirus vaccine (OPV), which, although it had eliminated wild poliovirus in the United States, caused about eight cases per year on average among OPV recipients or their contacts. IPV is the only vaccine available in the United States. OPV is still the vaccine used in most countries around the world, however. Between 1988, when the goal was announced to eradicate wild poliovirus from the world, and 2010, cases of poliomyelitis worldwide decreased by an estimated 99%. Four countries (Nigeria, India, Pakistan, and Afghanistan) have never interrupted endemic transmission. However, because of spread from Nigeria and India, 16 countries were reinfected in 2010. Efforts to eradicate polio globally continue.

Indications

Routine vaccination of persons 18 years of age or older is not warranted given the small risk of exposure to wild virus in the United States. The major indication for adult vaccination is travel to areas where wild poliovirus is endemic or epidemic. Previously unvaccinated adults should receive IPV. Adult travelers who have histories of partial vaccination should complete a primary series of three doses with IPV. Adults who formerly received three doses of OPV or IPV should receive a single booster of IPV. A primary series of IPV consists of three doses. A fourth dose is administered to children at school entry.

Side Effects

No serious side effects of IPV have been reported.

Rabies

Indications

Rabies (Chapter 422) vaccine is indicated for pre-exposure prophylaxis of high-risk persons, including animal handlers, selected laboratory and field workers, and persons traveling for more than 1 month to areas where rabies is a constant threat. The pre-exposure regimen consists of three 1-mL intramuscular injections on days 0, 7, and 21 or 28 for all rabies vaccines. Postexposure treatment depends on prior exposure to vaccine (Chapter 422). Persons being treated for the first time should be given four doses at days 0, 3, 7, and 14. Human rabies immune globulin is also indicated for previously unvaccinated persons who are exposed.

Rubella

Indications

Rubella (Chapter 376) vaccine is indicated for susceptible adults born in 1957 or later and for susceptible women of any age who are considering becoming pregnant. Persons without a prior history of vaccination on or after the first birthday or laboratory evidence of immunity should be considered susceptible. A single dose of vaccine is 95% or more effective. Many persons receive two doses of rubella vaccine by the two-dose schedule of MMR.

Side Effects

Follow-up of susceptible pregnant women who received rubella vaccines within 3 months of the estimated date of conception has failed to reveal any evidence of defects compatible with congenital rubella syndrome in their offspring. Nevertheless, vaccine is contraindicated in pregnant women on theoretical grounds, and conception should be delayed for 1 month after rubella vaccination.

Adverse reactions occur only in susceptible persons. Arthralgia, usually of the small peripheral joints, develops in 40% of susceptible adults, and frank arthritis develops in 10 to 20%. Joint symptoms usually begin 1 to 3 weeks after vaccination and persist for 1 day to 3 weeks. Chronic recurrent or persistent joint symptoms have developed rarely after vaccination, but controlled studies have shown that the incidence of these events in vaccinees is similar to that in nonvaccinees. Other infrequent adverse events include transient peripheral neuritis and pain in the arms and legs. Thrombocytopenic purpura has been reported rarely when rubella vaccine is administered as MMR. Rubella vaccine is contraindicated for persons with moderate to severe acute illnesses and for persons with reduced immunocompetence. When given with measles vaccine, it may be administered to persons with asymptomatic HIV infection and considered for persons with symptomatic infection without severe immunocompromise. Rubella vaccine is grown in human diploid cells and can be administered without problems to persons with allergy to eggs.

Tetanus and Diphtheria

Tetanus (Chapter 304) toxoid is one of the most effective immunizations, with more than 95% protection after a primary series. A primary series consists of three doses. In persons aged 7 years or older, it should always be used in combination with diphtheria (Chapter 300) toxoid (Td), which is more than 85% effective in preventing disease. Combinations also including pertussis antigens (Tdap) are preferred to Td for routine immunization of adolescents. Doses need not be repeated if the schedule is interrupted. A booster dose of Td is recommended every 10 years. An easy way to remember is to schedule immunization at the middle of each decade (e.g., 25 years, 35 years).

Indications

After a wound, persons of unknown immunization status or persons who have received fewer than three doses of tetanus toxoid should receive a dose of Td regardless of the severity of the wound. Td also is indicated for persons who have previously received three or more doses if more than 10 years has elapsed since the last dose, in the case of clean and minor wounds, and if more than 5 years has elapsed for all other wounds. Persons who have never received a dose of TdaP should receive it in place of Td for wound management. Tetanus immune globulin should be administered simultaneously at a separate site to persons who have not received at least three doses of toxoid and who have wounds that are not clean and minor.

Side Effects

Most reactions to Td consist of local inflammation and low-grade fever. Guillain-Barré syndrome and brachial neuritis rarely have been associated with tetanus toxoid.

Varicella: Chickenpox

A live attenuated varicella vaccine (Oka strain) was licensed in 1995. A combination measles-mumps-rubella-varicella vaccine was licensed in 2005. One dose of the vaccine protects 70 to 90% of recipients against any disease and more than 95% of recipients against severe disease. Although some studies have suggested immunity may wane with increasing time since vaccination, others have not. Use of vaccine has been associated with dramatic decreases in the incidence of varicella. Breakthrough infections in persons who have previously seroconverted have been reported. Such breakthroughs are typically mild and average fewer than 50 lesions compared with several hundred lesions in unvaccinated persons with varicella. Breakthrough illnesses do not seem to increase in incidence or severity with increasing time since vaccination, a finding compatible with long-term protection after initial vaccination. Because of persistent transmission of varicella, a two-dose schedule is recommended for all persons.

Indications

Varicella vaccine is indicated routinely for all children without a contraindication. A two-dose schedule is recommended, generally at 12 to 15 months of age and 4 to 6 years of age. For persons who previously received a single dose, catch-up vaccination with a second dose is recommended, provided at least 3 months have elapsed since the first dose. Persons who received a second dose at least 28 days after the first dose do not need a third dose. Persons 13 years or older without evidence of immunity to varicella should receive two doses at least 4 weeks apart. Persons with a clinician-diagnosed or verified history of varicella disease can be considered immune and do not need vaccination. Although a negative or unknown history of disease is predictive of susceptibility in children, many adults with such histories are immune. Serologic screening of adults in some situations may be cost-effective, provided that identified susceptible adults are vaccinated. Serologic testing is not indicated after vaccination. The vaccine is contraindicated in the immunocompromised, persons with anaphylactic allergies to vaccine components, and pregnant women. Varicella vaccine is more temperature sensitive than other vaccines used in the United States. It must be stored frozen at −15° C or colder to retain potency, and it should be discarded if it is not used within 30 minutes of reconstitution.

Side Effects

The most common side effect is soreness at the injection site, which is reported in 25 to 35% of recipients 13 years or older. Varicella-like rashes at the injection site (median of two lesions) have been reported in 3% of recipients in this age group after the first dose and in 1% after the second dose. Nonlocalized rashes with a median of five lesions have been reported in 5.5% of recipients after the first dose and in 0.9% after the second dose. Although the vaccine virus can cause herpes zoster (shingles), the incidence is substantially lower than would be expected after natural varicella (Chapter 383). More severe events occurring in temporal relation to the vaccine have been reported rarely, although a causal relationship has not been established. Transmission of vaccine virus to a contact is extremely rare and appears to take place only with vaccinees in whom a varicella-like rash has developed.

Varicella: Zoster

Clinical trials of a varicella vaccine, approximately 14 times more potent than the varicella vaccine used routinely, among persons 60 years of age or older reported a 51% reduction in the incidence of zoster and a 67% decrease in postherpetic neuralgia. The efficacy against zoster declined with increasing age from 60 to 80 years or older, but there was evidence of continuing protection against postherpetic neuralgia. The vaccine requires special freezer storage.

Indications

Zoster vaccine is recommended as a single dose for persons 60 years of age or older. Persons with a prior history of zoster may be vaccinated. It is not necessary to elicit a history of varicella or to test for varicella immunity before administration of zoster vaccine. The vaccine is not recommended for immunocompromised persons or pregnant women.

Side Effects

The most common side effect attributed to the vaccine is local reactions.

VACCINES INTENDED PRIMARILY FOR INTERNATIONAL TRAVELERS

Japanese Encephalitis Vaccine

Indications

Japanese encephalitis (Chapter 391) vaccine is indicated primarily for travelers to Asia who will spend a month or longer in endemic areas during the transmission season, especially if travel will include rural areas. In all instances, travelers should be advised to take personal precautions to reduce exposure to mosquito bites. An older vaccine was reported to be 80 to 91% effective in preventing clinical disease. The current whole virus inactivated vaccine (IXIARO, Intercell Biomedical) was licensed based on comparable immunogenicity. The primary series consists of two 0.5-mL doses given intramuscularly on days 0 and 28, with the second dose administered at least 1 week before travel (see Table 17-2). The duration of immunity is unknown. As of 2010, there were no recommendations for booster doses.

Side Effects

Headache and myalgia and local reactions (pain and tenderness) are common, occurring in more than 10% of vaccinees. However, the incidence rates of these events were similar to those in a comparison group, which received PBS and aluminum hydroxide.

Typhoid Vaccine

Indications

Two types of vaccines, a live attenuated Ty21a oral vaccine and a capsular polysaccharide vaccine (ViCPS), appear to be of comparable efficacy (50 to 77%). Typhoid (Chapter 316) vaccine is indicated primarily for travelers to areas where the risk of prolonged exposure to contaminated food and water is high. Because the vaccine is not always effective, food and water precautions are still essential. The vaccine also may be considered for family or other intimate contacts of typhoid carriers and laboratory workers who work with *Salmonella typhi*. For adults and children 6 years and older, either of the vaccines may be used. For Ty21a, one enteric-coated capsule is taken every other day for four doses. Alternatively, a single dose of the ViCPS vaccine may be given. The duration of protection with Ty21a is not known; repetition of the primary series is recommended every 5 years for persons at risk. Boosters are recommended every 2 years for the ViCPS vaccine if persons continue to be at risk. The ViCPS vaccine can be given to children as young as 2 years of age.

Side Effects

Adverse reactions are rare.

Yellow Fever Vaccine

Indications

Yellow fever (Chapter 389) occurs only in areas of South America and Africa. Vaccination with a single dose of the live attenuated 17D strain of virus confers protection to almost all recipients for at least 10 years. A booster dose is recommended every 10 years for persons at continued risk of exposure to yellow fever.

Side Effects

Side effects are uncommon. A rare syndrome of yellow fever vaccine, febrile multiple organ system failure or viscerotropic disease, has been reported, with high rates of mortality, primarily among older adults and persons who have undergone thymectomy or have severe thymic dysfunction being vaccinated for the first time. Yellow fever vaccine should be administered with caution and only after careful counseling to elderly patients who are going to spend time in yellow fever–endemic zones. Yellow fever vaccine should not be given to immunocompromised persons or persons with anaphylactic allergies to eggs. The vaccine is contraindicated in pregnant women on theoretical grounds, although if pregnant women must travel to a high-risk area, they may be vaccinated.

VACCINES FOR POSSIBLE BIOTERRORISM AGENTS

Anthrax Vaccine

Anthrax vaccine adsorbed (AVA) is prepared from a cell-free filtrate of a nonencapsulated strain of anthrax and contains many cell products including protective antigen. Protective antigen is responsible for binding to cells, allowing transport of lethal factor and edema factor into host cells. A recombinant protective antigen (rPA) vaccine is in clinical trials.

Indications

Pre-exposure prophylaxis consists of five doses intramuscularly at 0 and 4 weeks and 6, 12, and 18 months followed by annual boosters. Protective efficacy of an earlier form of the vaccine against cutaneous anthrax was 92.5%. Animal models suggest efficacy against inhalation anthrax. Pre-exposure vaccination is recommended for persons engaged in work involving exposure to high concentrations of *Bacillus anthracis* or in activities with high potential for aerosol production. Vaccine may be given with antibiotics for postexposure prophylaxis (Chapters 20 and 302); the antibiotics should be continued for 7 to 14 days after the third dose of vaccine is given.

Side Effects

The most common adverse events are local reactions, including subcutaneous nodules, which are thought to be due to the deposition of the aluminum-containing adjuvant in subcutaneous tissue.

Smallpox Vaccine

Smallpox vaccine uses vaccinia virus, an orthopox virus that is distinct from variola and cowpox viruses and that provides cross-protection from smallpox. Smallpox vaccine is close to 100% effective when it is administered properly, with a bifurcated needle. Vaccination also prevents or modifies disease when it is administered within 3 to 4 days of exposure and perhaps even after greater delays. The skin usually does not need any special preparation. If alcohol is used for cleaning, the skin should be allowed to dry before vaccination to avoid inactivation of the vaccine. The needle is held perpendicular to the skin; 3 punctures for primary vaccination and 15 punctures for revaccination are made rapidly with enough vigor to ensure that a trace of blood appears within 15 to 20 seconds. With a primary take, the vaccination site should become reddened and pruritic by 3 or 4 days after vaccination; a large vesicle with a red areola forms and becomes pustular by 7 to 11 days. The lesion scabs by the third week. Fever is the most common adverse event. Other more serious complications include eczema vaccinatum, a local or disseminated vaccinia infection in persons with a history of eczema or other exfoliative dermatitis; vaccinia necrosum, which occurs in immunocompromised persons; autoinoculation, especially of the eye, which can cause keratitis and scarring; generalized vaccinia; myopericarditis; and encephalitis. The risk for death from vaccinia has been estimated to be approximately one case per 1 million primary vaccinations.

Indications

The vaccine is indicated for persons who work with orthopox viruses. To increase preparedness for a smallpox attack, vaccination is often recommended for persons who will serve on public health or health care response teams. The duration of immunity is unclear. Revaccination is recommended at least every 10 years for persons who continue to be at risk. Contraindications include history or presence of eczema, other chronic or exfoliative skin conditions, and immunosuppression or pregnancy in the patient or a close household or other contact. Persons who are younger than 1 year, are breast-feeding, or have allergies to vaccine components should not be vaccinated. Because of reports of postvaccination cardiac events, vaccination should be deferred in persons with ischemia or other severe heart diseases or at high risk for ischemic heart disease events (*www.cdc.gov/smallpox*). In the event of exposure to variola, there are no contraindications. Should variola be introduced into a community, vaccination would be indicated for all exposed persons and their close contacts to prevent further spread, and recommendations for more widespread vaccination would have to be evaluated on a case-by-case basis.

Other Agents

Other organisms or products that have been considered potential bioterrorism threats include plague (Chapter 320) and botulinum toxin (Chapter 304). Poisoning with botulinum toxin can be treated with a trivalent antitoxin, available from the Centers for Disease Control and Prevention (see *MMWR*. 2003;52:774; *www.cdc.gov/ncidod/srp/drugs/formulary.html*). An experimental pentavalent botulinum toxoid can be obtained from the Centers for Disease Control and Prevention for laboratory workers at high risk for exposure to toxin. Pre-exposure vaccination is not warranted or feasible for the general population.

OTHER VACCINES

A protein-conjugated vaccine for *Haemophilus influenzae* type b (Hib) may be considered for some adults at high risk for invasive Hib disease (e.g., asplenia, HIV infection).

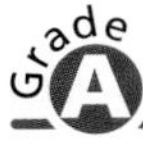

1. Prymula R, Siegrist CA, Chlibek R, et al. Effect of prophylactic paracetamol administration at time of vaccination on febrile reactions and antibody responses in children: two open-label, randomized controlled trials. *Lancet*. 2009;374:1339-1350.

SUGGESTED READINGS

Advisory Committee on Immunization Practices. Recommended adult immunization schedule: United States, 2011. *Ann Intern Med*. 2011;154:168-173. *Consensus guidelines*.

Centers for Disease Control and Prevention. Recommendations of the Advisory Committee on Immunization Practices. *Comprehensive coverage on vaccine-preventable diseases, vaccines, indications, schedules, and adverse events. Published as available in the* Morbidity and Mortality Weekly Report *as "Recommendations and Reports" supplements and available at wwwnc.cdc.gov/vaccines/recs/acip/default.htm*.

Centers for Disease Control and Prevention. Traveler's Health. www.cdc.gov/travel/default.aspx. *A complete guide for the international traveler, including required and recommended vaccinations. Revised every 1 to 2 years*.

Centers for Disease Control and Prevention. Adult Immunization Schedule—United States, 2010. www.cdc.gov/vaccines/recs/schedules/adult-schedule.htm. *The schedule is divided in two parts: (1) vaccines recommended by age group and (2) vaccines recommended by underlying medical condition*.

National Center for Immunization and Respiratory Diseases (NCIRD) Centers for Disease Control and Prevention. *The CDC has established toll-free numbers for answering questions from the general public and physicians: 1-800-232-4636. Inquiries can be made to the CDC by e-mail: cdcinfo@cdc.gov or the CDC website at www.cdc.gov/vaccine*.

18

PRINCIPLES OF OCCUPATIONAL AND ENVIRONMENTAL MEDICINE

MARK R. CULLEN

In the first several decades after World War II, when many American workers came to enjoy coverage by health insurance—for everything but workplace injuries and illnesses—the myth grew that modern work was largely free of the risks of the industrial horrors of past eras. Starting in the 1970s, however, resurgence of societal and medical interest in these consequences of work found that diseases related to work were not truly extinct, just not well observed or studied. Occupational physicians, often cut off from mainstream medical practice, had difficulty changing the perception, and most practicing internists were largely oblivious. It is now recognized that a substantial burden of ill health and disability is due to work-associated physical, chemical, and biologic hazards. Another intriguing possibility, recognized by social epidemiologists, is that work may be injurious to health in ways beyond these tangible risks.

Although tens of thousands of toxic chemicals and other hazards can potentially cause or exacerbate a wide range of acute and chronic conditions, certain basic principles and clinical approaches apply broadly to general and specialty medical practice. This chapter outlines these basics, then briefly summarizes the most common occupational disorders seen by internists in developed countries, and finally reviews the effects of the environmental exposures most likely to be encountered.

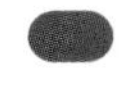

PRINCIPLES OF OCCUPATIONAL AND ENVIRONMENTAL DISEASE

It is widely imagined that the major health effects of environmental and occupational exposures are unique disorders best recognized by their failure to fit easily into other diagnostic categories (e.g., arsenic poisoning). In reality, *the major consequences of chemical and physical exposures are, without further exploration of an environmental connection, indistinguishable in clinical presentations from disorders that make up the bulk of outpatient and inpatient medical practice:* rashes, abnormal liver function studies (Chapter 149), wheezing and irritative symptoms of the upper and lower respiratory tract (Chapter 87), various cancers (Chapter 183), peripheral neuropathies (Chapter 428), dysphoria (Chapter 404), and nonspecific cognitive dysfunction (Chapter 409). Although a handful of pathologically distinct disorders still occur, such as silicosis (Chapter 93) and lead poisoning (Chapter 21), when an environmental or workplace agent causes overt disease, physiologic and radiographic studies typically reveal manifestations completely consistent with common diagnoses such as asthma (Chapter 87), contact dermatitis (Chapter 446), fatty liver (Chapter 155), and lung cancer (Chapter 197).

The underlying cause may remain obscure unless the clinician adheres to a disciplined approach designed to investigate and exclude occupational or environmental causes whenever it is appropriate. The best approach is consistent use of the occupational and environmental history, a short series of questions that can be expanded on the basis of the replies (see later). The point is that the internist cannot "wait" to consider occupational or environmental issues until other diseases have been ruled out without running the risk of missing almost every occupational and environmental effect that he or she will encounter.

Whatever the pathway or time course, exposure dose is the major determinant of the risk for development of disease. As in pharmacology (Chapter 28), it is impossible to make any meaningful statement about cause and effect without appreciation of dose. Consider, for example, the difference in health effects among aspirin at 65 mg, 650 mg, and 6500 mg (Chapter 36). Over this two-order magnitude of change, the chemical goes from having one therapeutic target organ to having many and to being potentially lethal. It is no different with lead or organophosphate pesticides or solvents, except that there is rarely as simple a way to determine dose as in the drug situation, where pill bottles are labeled and drug prescriptions are recorded. This limitation is exacerbated because, unlike with drugs, the range of toxic exposures may vary far more widely. For example, water in a contaminated drinking well or poor indoor air in an office could have toxins at a level that is two, three, or even four orders of magnitude (i.e., 10,000 times) lower than the level that may have been evaluated in an epidemiologic study of workers or tested in animals. Fortunately, it is much easier to "range find" than one might presuppose (see later discussion of history), and eagerness for precision—often unattainable—should not interfere with obtaining the great amount of information that *can* be readily gleaned and is often sufficient to act on. The key point is that no attempt to apply clinical information in relation to work or environment can be useful without some effort to characterize exposure dose.

Environmental hazards may affect preferentially vulnerable populations—those with underlying disease, those at the extremes of life, those with atopy, and those with other serious health risks such as smoking or diabetes. Genetic differences may underlie some differences, but few relevant genes have been sufficiently characterized for use in practice. Clinical studies of a host of common occupational diseases have identified behavioral and constitutional cofactors; for example, smoking dramatically increases the risk of lung cancer in asbestos-exposed workers (Chapter 197). This interaction creates a double demand on the clinician—the presence of smoking or atopy in a young woman with cough does not preclude the possibility of an occupational cause of her asthma but rather actually increases the likelihood that such a consideration may be important.

The Occupational and Environmental History and Exposure Assessment

Key to determining whether work and other environmental exposures may be causing or contributing to adverse health is the history. The approach to obtaining this information and to the use of available resources to corroborate and complement it depends on the clinical context. In primary and much specialty medical care, where it is anticipated that a patient will be observed during a long period into the future, the most important step is to establish the hazards to which the patient may be exposed at work presently, the activities that may have resulted in past harmful exposures potentially relevant to future health (because of latency), and whether the present residential environment, including air and water and food sources, is thought to be contaminated by harmful materials. The recommended approach is to use a simple questionnaire, which can be self-administered or supervised by a medical extender (E-Fig. 18-1). These instruments can then be reviewed together by the patient and physician as time permits and updated over time. When jobs or materials are noted but the actual generic exposures are unknown, the patient and available reference sources can be enlisted to "translate" the history into specifics, such as which metals are being welded or what is actually contained in a cleaning agent or plastic. This information is obligatorily maintained and supplied on request by employers in most developed countries in the form of fact sheets termed *Material Safety Data Sheets,* many of which can be easily found online as well. In this way, the ongoing and former exposures, which may have an impact on health, can be noted and, where important, incorporated into routine preventive care or clinical surveillance for sequelae.

For patients with new clinical complaints or recently diagnosed conditions, the question of an environmental cause looms more urgently, so the approach must be more focused. If symptoms or signs of acute or subacute illness are suggested, the *timing* of recent or unusual environmental exposures in relation to the symptoms is key—more important than specific chemical detail. For example, if the patient develops shortness of breath shortly after the introduction of a new chemical or process at work or after a leak or spill, that fact should drive further questions, such as Did others get sick as well? For recurrent symptoms, such as cough or rash, cyclic changes are most often the strongest clue: Do symptoms get worse on workdays and improve on days off or holidays? For more insidious symptoms, such as weakness or numbness of the extremities or new-onset hepatic dysfunction, the appropriate question would be whether the onset of the abnormality has followed by weeks or months some demonstrable change in the work or home environment. Again, the coincidence of others similarly affected may be more valuable than detailed knowledge of the constituents of that environment. When such a temporal pattern is suggested, further efforts to establish what exposure has actually occurred are warranted, often with specialty consultation when it is available.

In the elucidation of evidently more chronic conditions, such as pulmonary fibrosis, chronic renal insufficiency, or a malignant neoplasm, an alternative approach is suggested because the exposure, if relevant, is usually remote. In this situation, a detailed query about current work or ambient environments is not likely to be helpful in differential diagnosis, although knowledge of a past exposure to an important hazard (such as silica, asbestos, or cadmium) might, on the basis of the knowledge of its effects, influence the sequence of the evaluation. However, it is generally more efficient to explore past exposures *after* the pathophysiologic disturbance has been characterized, focusing inquiry exclusively on factors known to cause or suspected of causing that disorder—as is easily found in suggested texts or literature searches.

In acute or chronic cases, information about *what* the exposure has been (generically) must be augmented by an estimation of exposure dose. A brief exposure to a fume containing a small percentage of lead will not, in general, cause acute lead poisoning (although hosts may differ in their responses), nor will trace contamination of a drinking well with benzene typically cause blood dyscrasias. The patient will rarely be able to supply detailed information about past or even current "dose" but often can provide valuable clues: Did the exposure continue during many years? Were fumes or fibers grossly visible in the air? Were respirators or other protective gear necessary or offered? Have episodes of unprotected exposure ever resulted in irritation or acute discomfort? A positive reply to any of these questions would suggest "high" exposure, where the reference point is the level at which the risk for development of a health effect becomes substantial. Conversely, if exposure has occurred in an otherwise typical office or around a home renovation, the levels of exposure are more likely "low." Nevertheless, such low-level exposure does not exclude a health effect, especially one caused by idiosyncratic mechanisms or occurring in hosts who are more "sensitive" to chemical exposures, a health characteristic found in 2 to 10% of the population. Although not to be condoned because of broader public health consequences, exposures in food and drinking water are uncommon causes of perceptible clinical problems. When concern about the exposure is high, information from patients can be readily supplemented by information from employers (with the patient's consent!) and regulatory or health authorities or by consultation with specialists who should know the levels of most workplace hazards in the community. Finally, with an appropriate understanding of the limits of testing and awareness of "timing" issues in relation to exposure (as with measuring drug levels), an increasing number of hazardous chemicals can be biologically measured in blood or urine. Metals and some pesticides can be reliably tested now, and a broad array of organic chemicals should be amenable for testing in the near future. Random sampling for "unknowns" is rarely helpful and often leads to erroneous conclusions because trace chemicals are ubiquitous.

OCCUPATIONAL AND ENVIRONMENTAL HEALTH DISORDERS COMMON IN PRACTICE

Although almost any medical complaint or condition may have an occupational or environmental cause or contribution, certain conditions encountered in medical practice *commonly* do (Table 18-1). For these conditions, attention to the history is most important and most often rewarding.

Asthma

Men and women with preexisting airways disease tolerate irritants in the workplace poorly and may experience exacerbations in temporal relation to one or more exposures. More important, numerous antigens are extant in the workplace, from large proteins, such as latex and animal danders, to small molecules, such as isocyanates needed to set polyurethane. More than 250 agents have been well characterized, and many others are suspect. Virtually no profession or work is immune. Presentation is often nonspecific; timing of symptoms during or slightly staggered from exposure is the clue to diagnosis. The reward for early recognition of such causes is the likelihood that airway inflammation will abate when the noxious exposure is eliminated; otherwise lifelong, often generalized asthma is the rule (Chapter 87).

Chronic Interstitial and Parenchymal Lung Disorders

The rounded opacities of silicosis (Chapter 93) and coal workers' pneumoconiosis (Chapter 93) radiographically resemble sarcoid (Chapter 95); chronic beryllium disease (Chapter 93), a granulomatous disorder caused by sensitization to this widely used light metal, is clinically identical to sarcoid in almost all respects, but a reasonably specific test for blood and bronchoalveolar lavage fluid is now available to distinguish them. Asbestosis (Chapter 93) in every way is identical to idiopathic pulmonary fibrosis (Chapter 92) except that benign pleural changes often accompany asbestosis, which, unlike idiopathic pulmonary fibrosis, tends to run a far more indolent course and

TABLE 18-1 COMMON OCCUPATIONAL AND ENVIRONMENTAL HEALTH CONDITIONS IN GENERAL PRACTICE

CONDITION	EXPOSURE SETTINGS	COMMENT
Asthma	Virtually any indoor or outdoor workplace	New-onset, recrudescent, or exacerbated asthma
Interstitial and parenchymal lung disorders	Dusts, metals, and organic materials	All parenchymal disorders have one or more environmental causes
Cancers of the respiratory tract	Asbestos, radon, silica, mineral oils, tars, and other carcinogens	Smokers are more likely to be affected
Sensorineural hearing loss	Noise, metals, and solvents	High-frequency loss, especially in younger workers
Musculoskeletal disorders of trunk and limbs	Heavy or stereotyped activities	Cold, vibration, and work stress contribute
Upper airway irritation	Dust and fumes	More common in smokers and atopic persons
Nonspecific building-related illness	Office work	Must exclude *specific* causes
Dermatitis, allergic or irritant	Repeated exposure to unprotected skin	Work and environmental exposures should be considered in every case
Multiple chemical sensitivities	Any	Complication of adverse environmental exposure

usually stops progressing when exposure ceases or within a few years thereafter. Hypersensitivity pneumonitis (Chapter 93) is rarely suspected outside of agricultural settings but is occurring far more often; the causes are likely to be microbial contaminants of work materials, but some chemicals, such as the isocyanates, may also be causal.

Cancers of the Respiratory Tract

Although most carcinomas of the lung and upper airway occur in smokers, occupational exposures to asbestos, silica, and the polyaromatic hydrocarbons in particulate air pollution, diesel exhaust, pitch, and asphalt contribute to the burden, as do radon and carcinogenic metals such as chromium and nickel found in most alloys (Chapter 197). Some organic materials, such as formaldehyde, are also likely culprits. Until there is an established strategy for secondary prevention, patients with these exposures should be observed expectantly; at a minimum, extraordinary efforts should be made to control smoking in these exposed individuals. Asbestos-exposed workers—smokers or otherwise—are additionally at risk for malignant mesothelioma (Chapters 99 and 197), but other than primary prevention, the only clinical implication is awareness for early diagnosis and compassionate care for this still largely incurable industrial disease.

Fatty Liver

With the widespread use of abdominal imaging, fatty liver has been recognized as more common than previously thought (Chapter 155). This disorder is common among individuals exposed regularly to organic solvents, a possibility that should be considered at the same time that infectious, metabolic, and pharmaceutical causes are considered. Once it is suspected, whether or not other factors are also present, exposure should be reduced. Improvement tends to be slow, but the risk of progression is likely to have been averted or at least diminished.

Sensorineural Hearing Loss

Aside from aging, noise is the most important cause of high-frequency sensorineural hearing loss, recognizable as early as in adolescence (Chapter 436). Hobbies such as shooting and loud music may combine with industrial and agricultural noise to accelerate hearing loss. Although it is the responsibility of employers to conduct routine audiograms and to control exposure, clinicians should test noise-exposed patients periodically and reinforce whatever control strategies may be in place at work. Exposure to metals such as lead and organic solvents may compound the risk further.

Musculoskeletal Disorders of the Upper Extremity and Trunk

The most common cause of work disability, including permanent disability, is injury to the back (Chapter 407) and wrist. Repetitive, heavy, awkward, and time-pressured activities are notorious contributors, as are cold and vibration. Although an anatomically localized lesion may be identified and specifically treated in a small fraction of cases, as in carpal tunnel syndrome (Chapter 428) or thoracic outlet obstruction, the most important modalities of care in most cases are early recognition and avoidance of further insult. Physical therapy and medications may hasten recovery but cannot prevent recurrences and even progression unless the causal work and avocational activities are modified.

Upper Airway Irritation

Virtually any smoke, fume, dust, or chemical has potential to irritate the upper respiratory tract (Chapter 93), causing acute or chronic symptoms indistinguishable from common allergic manifestations (Chapter 257) or upper respiratory infections (Chapter 96). Although the mucosae of the eyes, nose, sinuses, and throat tend to be forgiving, recurrent episodes are extremely nettlesome and cause substantial disability. Atopic patients and patients with frequent infections are often the most sensitive to these ubiquitous environmental insults, which must ultimately be addressed along with the symptoms themselves and secondary infections.

Dermatitis

Erythematous rashes are a common consequence of topical exposures to workplace, avocational, and household materials, including latex, plastics, and many foods (Chapter 446). Although the keys to recognition are timing and the anatomic relation to clothing, allergenic and irritating chemicals can find their way into unlikely places, such as the groin and belt lines. Specialty consultation and patch testing are warranted in intractable cases but should not supplant careful observation and history taking in most situations.

Sick Building Syndrome and Nonspecific Building-Related Illness

The effort to reduce the influx of "fresh" air into buildings to save heating and air-conditioning costs has resulted in upper airway and dermal irritation as well as vague central nervous system symptoms such as headache and fatigue, occurring shortly after beginning work and clearing minutes to hours after leaving the affected building. Many occupants are typically affected, especially those who spend the most time in one place. The cause is unknown, but recent evidence suggests that microbial materials may be the most common culprits. In every instance, a search for a specific allergen or irritant is worth undertaking (Chapter 257), but the most remedial sources are poor overall ventilation and dampness in which molds fester. When the cause is remedied, most building occupants typically experience symptomatic improvement. From a clinical perspective, the major consideration is whether any more serious problem, such as asthma, may have also developed.

Multiple Chemical Sensitivities

An environmental illness as transient as a single noxious inhalation or as persistent as a protracted course of nonspecific building-related illness can initiate a cycle of similar symptoms after exposures to odors or irritants at very low levels so that even everyday tasks such as shopping or driving become problematic. A patient typically complains of being "allergic" to everything, although there is no evidence for allergic mechanisms (Chapter 257); the cause of this vexing complication, most prevalent in women, is unknown and may involve psychological as well as physiologic factors. Despite the severity of complaints, which often include fatigue, muscle pain, stridor, chest tightness, and palpitations, laboratory test results are normal. Coexistent anxiety and depression often prompt psychiatric referral (Chapter 404), but the disorder has proved relatively refractory to all treatment modalities. Sympathetic support, environmental modification as needed to provide some symptomatic relief, and candor regarding the unknown nature of the disorder are appropriate; extensive clinical investigations often serve only to reinforce the patient's "sick" role and are best avoided. Despite all efforts, the most severely affected individuals will often seek the care of alternative practitioners (Chapter 38) with compelling if unproven theories and expensive, potentially harmful remedies.

COMMON HAZARDOUS EXPOSURES IN THE WORKPLACE AND AMBIENT ENVIRONMENT

Tens of thousands of chemicals in the workplace, as well as important physical and biologic hazards, may be encountered in the general environment (Table 18-2). Several of these hazards are of major current concern in industrialized countries.

Metals

Exposures to lead and arsenic (Chapter 21), once commonplace in industry, are now generally controlled; concern remains highest for environmental settings, especially for children. There is now greater concern for mercury—entrained in large ocean fish worldwide—and manganese (Chapter 21), a potent neurotoxin in welding fumes and various alloys. For most metals—manganese being a notorious exception—blood or urine tests are available to quantify a patient's burden, but these tests must be mindful of timing, the form of metal, and possible "confounders," such as the largely benign form of arsenic excreted in urine for several days after even a single shellfish meal.

Organic Solvents

These petroleum derivatives remain ubiquitous in workplace and household products. All are irritating, potentially neurotoxic, and, to varying degrees, hepatotoxic (Chapter 110). A few, such as trichloroethylene and *n*-hexane, are more potent but no longer widely used. Benzene and the ethers of ethylene glycol are bone marrow toxins (Chapter 168).

Organohalides

Although these complex organic pesticides and industrial materials are no longer made and sold in developed countries, their remarkable biopersistence has resulted in entrainment into everyone's fat. Worse, the dread byproduct dioxin, once associated with herbicide manufacture, has now been recognized as a predictable consequence of combustion of any chlorine-containing materials. All are suspect carcinogens, although debate remains whether this effect is limited to soft tissue sarcomas (Chapter 209)—a relationship established for dioxin—or promotes cancers more globally.

TABLE 18-2 COMMON HAZARDS IN THE WORKPLACE AND AMBIENT ENVIRONMENT

HAZARD	HEALTH EFFECTS OF GREATEST CONCERN	COMMENTS
Metals	Neurotoxicity, cancer	Most can be measured in blood or urine to assess dose
Organic solvents	Respiratory and dermal irritation, neurotoxicity, hepatotoxicity	Benzene and a few others have unique effects
Organohalides (e.g., DDT, PCBs)	Cancer	Ubiquitous suspect carcinogens of high population concern
Herbicides and pesticides	Rare acute neurotoxicity, unknown long-term effects	Widespread hazards of high population concern
Electromagnetic radiation	Leukemia, glioblastoma	Ubiquitous exposures with unproven effects
Particulate matter	Acute and chronic atherosclerotic cardiovascular disease	Air pollution, workplace
Mold	Allergy	High population concern regarding putative chronic effects
Mineral dusts	Cancer	Old hazards still of high concern (e.g., asbestos, silica)

DDT = dichlorodiphenyltrichloroethane; PCBs = polychlorinated biphenyls.

Herbicides and Pesticides

The acute neurotoxicity and irritant properties of most herbicides and pesticides have been well studied (Chapter 110). These agents are generally well controlled, although both occupational and residential overexposures occasionally occur.

Electromagnetic Radiation

Electric wires, appliances, and, notoriously, cell phones emit low-frequency electromagnetic radiation at levels far below those that cause local thermal injuries (Chapter 19). These radiations are nonionizing, but there is some epidemiologic evidence of an increased risk of childhood leukemia with high-level exposure from household wiring and of excess brain tumors in adult workers with regular exposures. Moreover, recent reports from Europe suggest excess brain cancer in cell phone users. These data are difficult to interpret because study results differ according to how exposure is assessed; the only conclusion is that there is basis for concern and need for further study but not cause for widespread alarm or action other than precaution in the placement of new heavy power lines near schools and residences.

Particulate Matter

Evidence accumulated over the past decade points to the likelihood that ambient air pollution contributes measurably to the risk of cardiovascular disease. Focus has turned from the well-established respiratory irritants—the gases SO_2 and ozone—to the smallest particles, so-called $PM_{2.5}$. These particles are laden with polyaromatic hydrocarbons from diesel exhaust, coal burning, and industrial sources, which are proinflammatory. Unknown yet is whether this risk also accrues to more heavily exposed industrial workers, or those exposed to small particles of other composition, but it appears that controls on air quality have already resulted in reductions both of acute coronary events and overall mortality.

Mold

Molds are ubiquitous and long known for their unpleasant odors and potential for inducing allergic responses (Chapter 257), including asthma. Recently, concern has arisen over the potential for serious effects from various mycotoxins, long problems in veterinary medicine when domestic animals consume contaminated feed; however, a consensus panel concluded that there is no evidence of human risks beyond those well established from living or working in a moldy environment. Mold formation should be prevented wherever possible, especially in schools and offices, where molds contribute to problems with indoor air quality. Identification, with eradication of leaks and other sources of water accumulation, is key.

Mineral Dusts

Although asbestos has been largely abated, silica and human-made mineral fibers remain widely distributed in the environment. Silica (Chapter 93), present in virtually every form of "rock," is a potent cause of lung injury and cancer, so respiratory exposure should be carefully controlled in every setting. The evidence of serious risk from fibrous glass, mineral wool, and other human-made mineral fibers is less clear; probably only the finest fibers, such as slag wool, have cancer-causing potential, but many are potent dermal and upper respiratory irritants and should be well controlled for that reason alone.

SUMMARY

Occupational and environmental health problems remain prevalent, although their spectrum and nature have changed as rapidly as any in medicine and are likely to change even faster as technology, work, and knowledge continue to evolve. Physicians need not necessarily develop a large base of "facts"—themselves subject to revision frequently—but rather an approach that incorporates key elements and provides a foundation for efficient recognition and management of current and future clinical syndromes.

SUGGESTED READINGS

Schaafsma F, Schonstein E, Whelan KM, et al. Physical conditioning programs for improving work outcomes in workers with back pain. *Cochrane Database Syst Rev.* 2010;1:CD001822. *The effectiveness of physical conditioning programs when compared with usual care exercises in workers with back pain remains uncertain.*

Van Hee VC, Kaufman JD, Budinger GR, et al. Update in environmental and occupational medicine 2009. *Am J Respir Crit Care Med.* 2010;181:1174-1180. *Review.*

van Oostrom SH, Driessen MT, de Vet HC, et al. Workplace interventions for preventing work disability. *Cochrane Database Syst Rev.* 2009;2:CD006955. *Workplace interventions are effective to reduce sickness absence, not to improve health outcomes.*

19

RADIATION INJURY

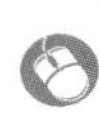

ARTHUR C. UPTON

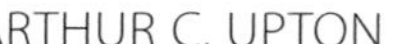

The term *radiation injury* denotes any abnormality of form or function caused by electromagnetic waves or accelerated atomic particles. The term is also often applied to the harmful effects of high-intensity ultrasound and electromagnetic fields. The different types of radiation differ markedly in their biologic effects, so each must be dealt with separately in considering the injuries it can cause.

IONIZING RADIATION INJURY

Ionizing radiation occurs as electromagnetic waves of extremely short wavelength (Fig. 19-1) and as accelerated atomic particles (e.g., electrons, protons, neutrons, α particles). The injuries they cause include mutagenic, carcinogenic, and teratogenic effects and various acute and chronic tissue reactions such as erythema, cataract of the lens, sterility, and depression of hematopoiesis.

EPIDEMIOLOGY

Precise data on the frequency of injuries caused by ionizing radiation are not available. Injuries attributable to excessive occupational exposure were prevalent among radiation workers in the era preceding modern safety standards but are seldom encountered in the United States today. The 1986 Chernobyl accident in Ukraine, however, caused radiation sickness in more than 200 emergency workers, injured 28 fatally, released enough radioactivity to require tens of thousands of inhabitants to be evacuated from the surrounding area, and resulted in a collective dose-equivalent commitment of 600,000 person-Sv for the population of the Northern Hemisphere. Less catastrophic but more numerous than reactor accidents are accidents involving medical and industrial γ-ray sources, which are occasionally serious enough to be fatal. Noteworthy in this context is the potential for terrorist attacks in which

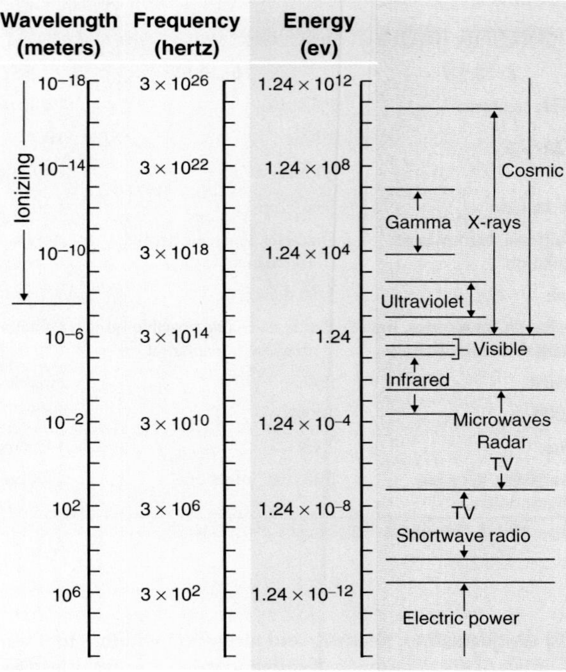

FIGURE 19-1. The electromagnetic spectrum. (From Mettler FA, Upton AC. *Effects of Ionizing Radiation*, 3rd ed. Philadelphia: WB Saunders; 2008.)

nuclear weapons, conventional explosives ("dirty bombs"), or other means may be used to disperse hazardous amounts of radioactivity.

Also of ongoing public health concern is the risk of cancer among the general population from exposure to ionizing radiation. Although no more than 3% of all cancers in the general population are thought to result from natural background ionizing irradiation, a substantially larger percentage of lung cancers are generally attributed to indoor radon. Another concern is the risk of heritable abnormalities resulting from the mutagenic and clastogenic effects of radiation, which have yet to be observed in humans but are well documented in other organisms.

Prenatal irradiation can also cause death, malformations, cataracts, mental retardation, impairment of growth, and behavioral disorders, depending on the dose and the developmental stage of the embryo at the time of exposure. Hence, special precautions are taken to avoid exposure of the embryo to irradiation.

PATHOBIOLOGY

The biologic effects of ionizing radiation result from damage to DNA and other vital molecules by locally deposited energy. Doses of ionizing radiation are therefore measured in terms of energy deposition (Table 19-1).

All humans are exposed continuously to natural background ionizing radiation from (1) cosmic rays; (2) radium and other radioactive elements in the earth's crust; (3) potassium 40, carbon 14, and other radionuclides normally present in human tissues; and (4) inhaled radon and its daughter elements (Table 19-2). In people residing at mile-high elevations, such as Denver, Colorado, the contribution from cosmic rays may be increased twofold; at jet aircraft altitudes, it may be increased more than 100-fold, exceeding 0.005 mSv/hour (1 Sv = 100 rem). Likewise, in regions where the earth's crust is rich in radium, the contribution from this radionuclide may be increased.

Among man-made sources of radiation, the largest is the use of x-rays and other radiographic procedures in medical diagnosis. Smaller amounts of radiation are also received from radioactive minerals in building materials, phosphate fertilizers, and crushed rock; radiation-emitting components of television sets, smoke detectors, and other consumer products; radioactive fallout from atomic weapons; and nuclear power.

Workers in various occupations are exposed to additional doses of ionizing radiation, depending on their job assignments and working conditions. The average annual effective dose received by monitored radiation workers in the United States is less than 1 mSv, and less than 1% of such workers approach the maximal permissible dose limit (50 mSv) in any given year.

TABLE 19-1 IONIZING RADIATION QUANTITIES AND DOSE UNITS

QUANTITY	DOSE UNIT*	DEFINITION
Radioactivity	Becquerel (Bq)	One disintegration per second
Absorbed dose	Gray (Gy)	Energy deposited in tissue (1 J/kg)
Equivalent dose	Sievert (Sv)	Absorbed dose weighted for the quality (potency) of radiation
Effective dose	Sievert (Sv)	Equivalent dose weighted for the sensitivity of exposed organs
Collective effective dose	Person-Sv	Effective dose applied to a population
Committed effective dose	Sievert (Sv)	Effective dose from a given intake of radioactivity to be received during a period extending into the future

*The units of measurement listed are those of the International System, which replaced earlier units such as the rad (1 rad = 0.01 Gy), the rem (1 rem = 0.01 Sv), and the curie (1 Ci = 3.7×10^{10} Bq).
Modified from Phillips TL. Radiation injury. In: Wyngaarden JB, Smith LH Jr, Bennett JC, eds. *Cecil Textbook of Medicine*, 19th ed. Philadelphia: WB Saunders; 1992:2351.

TABLE 19-2 AVERAGE AMOUNTS OF IONIZING RADIATION RECEIVED ANNUALLY FROM DIFFERENT SOURCES BY A U.S. RESIDENT

	*Dose**	
SOURCE	**MSV**	**%**
Natural		
Radon and thoron	2.28	37†
Cosmic	0.33	5
Terrestrial	0.21	3
Internal	0.29	5
Total natural	3.11	50
Artificial		
Computed tomography	1.47	24
X-ray diagnosis	0.33	5
Nuclear medicine	0.77	12
Interventional fluoroscopy	0.43	7
Consumer products	0.13	<0.3
Occupational	0.005	<0.3
Miscellaneous‡	<0.1	<0.3
Total artificial	3.138	50
Total natural and artificial	6.248	100

*Average effective dose.
†Average effective dose to bronchial epithelium.
‡Department of Energy, industrial, security, educational, research, and transportation facilities.
Modified from National Council on Radiation Protection and Measurements (NCRP). *Ionizing Radiation Exposure of the Population of the United States.* NCRP Report No. 160. Bethesda, MD: National Council on Radiation Protection and Measurements; 2009.

Pathogenesis

Ionizing radiation, colliding randomly with atoms and molecules in its path, gives rise to ions and free radicals, which break chemical bonds, cause other molecular alterations, and can ultimately injure the absorbing cell and its neighbors. Any molecule can be altered, but DNA is the critical biologic target because of the limited redundancy of its genetic information. A dose of radiation large enough to kill the average dividing cell (2 Sv) causes hundreds of lesions in its DNA molecules. Most such lesions are reparable, but those produced by a densely ionizing radiation (e.g., proton or α particle) are generally less reparable than those produced by a sparsely ionizing radiation (e.g., x-ray or γ-ray).

Unrepaired or misrepaired damage to DNA may be expressed in the form of mutations, the frequency of which approximates 10^{-5} to 10^{-6} per locus per sievert. Because the mutation rate tends to increase in proportion to the dose, it is inferred that a single ionizing particle traversing a genetic target may suffice to cause a mutation. Radiation damage can also cause changes in chromosome number and structure, the yields of which are characterized

TABLE 19-3 SYMPTOMS, THERAPY, AND PROGNOSIS OF WHOLE BODY IONIZING RADIATION INJURY

	0-1 SV	1-2 SV	2-6 SV	6-10 SV	10-20 SV	>50 SV
Therapeutic needs	None	Observation	Specific treatment	Possible treatment	Palliative	Palliative
Vomiting	None	5-50%	>3 Gy, 100%	100%	100%	100%
Time to nausea, vomiting	—	3 hr	2 hr	1 hr	30 min	<30 min
Main locus of injury	None	Lymphocytes	Bone marrow	Bone marrow	Small bowel	Brain
Symptoms and signs	—	Moderate leukopenia, epilation	Leukopenia, hemorrhage, epilation	Leukopenia, hemorrhage, epilation	Diarrhea, fever, electrolyte imbalance	Ataxia, coma, convulsions
Critical period	—	—	4-6 wk	4-6 wk	5-14 days	1-4 hr
Therapy	Reassurance	Observation	Transfusion of granulocytes, platelets	Transfusion, antibiotics, bone marrow transplantation	Fluids and salts, possible bone marrow transplantation	Palliative
Prognosis	Excellent	Excellent	Guarded	Guarded	Poor	Hopeless
Lethality	0	0	0-80%	80-100%	100%	100%
Time of death	—	—	2 mo	1-2 mo	2 wk	1-2 days
Cause of death	—	—	Infection, hemorrhage	Hemorrhage, infection, pneumonitis	Enteritis, infection	Cerebral edema

Modified from Phillips TL. Radiation injury. In: Wyngaarden JB, Smith LH Jr, Bennett JC, eds. *Cecil Textbook of Medicine*, 19th ed. Philadelphia: WB Saunders; 1992:2354.

well enough so that their frequency in lymphocytes can serve as a biologic dosimeter.

Radiation damage to genes, chromosomes, and other vital organelles may kill cells, especially dividing cells, which are radiosensitive as a class. Measured in terms of proliferative capacity, the survival of dividing cells tends to decrease exponentially with increasing dose; rapid exposure to 1 to 2 Sv generally reduces the surviving population of such cells by about 50%. Except for lymphocytes and oocytes, which tend to die in interphase, most cells killed by irradiation die in mitosis.

Although the killing of cells is a stochastic process, too few cells are killed by a dose less than 0.5 Sv to cause clinically detectable injury in most organs, other than the testis and organs of the embryo. The killing of dividing progenitor cells, if sufficiently extensive, can interfere with the orderly replacement of senescent cells, especially in tissues such as the epidermis, bone marrow, and intestinal epithelium, which are normally characterized by high rates of cell turnover. The timing of the resulting atrophy varies, depending on the cell population dynamics within the tissue in question; in organs such as the liver and vascular endothelium, which are characterized by slow cell turnover, expression of the injury is delayed. Also, if the volume of tissue exposed is small or if the dose is accumulated slowly enough, the effects of irradiation may be counteracted in part by adaptive responses and by compensatory regenerative hyperplasia of surviving cells.

CLINICAL MANIFESTATIONS

Ionizing radiation injuries encompass a diversity of tissue reactions that vary markedly in their dose-response relationships, manifestations, timing, and prognosis. Except for mutagenic and carcinogenic effects, the reactions generally result from the killing of sizable numbers of cells in the exposed tissues and are not detectable unless the dose of radiation exceeds a substantial threshold. For this reason, the reactions are called *nonstochastic* (or *deterministic*) effects. In contrast, the mutagenic and carcinogenic effects of radiation are presumed to have no thresholds and are considered to be *stochastic* in nature. The existing data do not exclude the possibility, however, that the latter effects may have thresholds in the millisievert dose range, and the existence of adaptive responses to radiation (e.g., DNA repair processes) has been interpreted by some observers to support the hypothesis that the net effects of small doses may be beneficial (radiation hormesis).

Tissues in which cells proliferate rapidly are generally the first to exhibit radiation injury. In such tissues, mitotic inhibition and cytologic abnormalities may be detectable immediately after irradiation, whereas ulceration, fibrosis, and other degenerative changes may not appear until months or years later.

Skin

After rapid exposure to a dose of 6 Sv or more, erythema typically appears within 1 day, lasts a few hours, and is followed 2 to 4 weeks later by one or more waves of deeper and more prolonged erythema and epilation. Brief exposure to a dose greater than 10 to 20 Sv may cause transepithelial injury, with moist desquamation, necrosis, and ulceration within 2 to 4 weeks. The ensuing fibrosis of the underlying dermis and vasculature may lead to atrophy and a second wave of ulceration months or years later.

Bone Marrow and Lymphoid Tissue

A dose of 2 to 3 Sv delivered rapidly to the whole body destroys enough lymphocytes to depress the lymphocyte count and immune response within hours. Such a dose also can damage enough hematopoietic cells to cause profound leukopenia and thrombocytopenia within 3 to 5 weeks. If the dose exceeds 5 Sv, fatal infection and hemorrhage are likely to result (Table 19-3).

Intestine

The killing of epithelial stem cells is sufficiently extensive after an acute dose of 10 Sv to cause rapid denudation of the overlying intestinal villi. If the area affected is large, death from a fatal dysentery-like syndrome may ensue within days.

Respiratory Tract

Rapid exposure of the lung to a dose of 6 to 10 Sv damages alveolar cells and the pulmonary vasculature sufficiently to result in acute pneumonitis within 1 to 3 months. If extensive, the process may lead to fatal respiratory failure within 6 months or pulmonary fibrosis and cor pulmonale months or years later.

Gonads

Spermatozoa are relatively radioresistant, but spermatogonia are highly radiosensitive; a dose of 0.15 Sv delivered rapidly to both testes causes oligospermia after a latent period of about 6 weeks, and a dose of 2 to 4 Sv may cause permanent sterility. Oocytes also are radiosensitive; a dose of 1.5 to 2 Sv delivered to both ovaries causes temporary sterility, and a larger dose causes permanent sterility, depending on the woman's age at the time of exposure.

Lens of the Eye

Acute exposure of the lens to more than 0.5 Sv may lead to a microscopic posterior polar opacity within months, and 2 to 3 Sv received in a single brief exposure or 5.5 to 14 Sv accumulated over months may result in a vision-impairing cataract.

Other Tissues and Organs

Other tissues and organs, except in the embryo, are relatively less radiosensitive. All tissues, however, are more radiosensitive when they are rapidly growing.

Whole Body Radiation Injury

Brief exposure of a major part of the body to more than 1 Sv may cause acute radiation syndrome, which is characterized by (1) an initial prodromal stage of malaise, anorexia, nausea, and vomiting; (2) an ensuing latent period; (3) a second (main) phase of illness; and (4) either recovery or death (see Table

19-3). The main phase of the illness usually takes one of four primary forms—hematologic, gastrointestinal, neurovascular, or pulmonary—depending on the size and anatomic distribution of the dose.

Localized or Regional Radiation Injury

In contrast to acute radiation syndrome, the manifestations of which are dramatic and relatively prompt, the reaction to localized irradiation in most tissues tends to evolve more slowly and does not produce symptoms or signs unless the volume of irradiated tissue or the dose is large. Injury produced by a radionuclide follows the anatomic distribution of the radionuclide and its emitted radiation, which may be influenced by the physicochemical state in which the radionuclide is encountered and its portal of entry into the body.

Heritable (Genetic) Effects of Radiation

Radiation-induced heritable mutations and chromosome abnormalities are well documented in other organisms but have yet to be observed in humans. Intensive study of more than 76,000 children of Japanese atomic bomb survivors has failed to detect definite evidence of heritable radiation effects in terms of untoward outcomes of pregnancy, neonatal death, malignant neoplasms, balanced chromosome rearrangements, sex chromosome aneuploidy, alterations in serum or erythrocyte protein phenotypes, changes in gender ratio, or disturbances in growth and development. On the basis of the existing evidence, it is inferred that a dose of at least 1 Sv is required to double the rate of heritable mutations in human germ cells and that, consequently, less than 1% of all genetically determined disease is attributable to natural background irradiation.

Carcinogenic Effects of Radiation

Many but not all types of benign and malignant growths are inducible by irradiation; however, these induced growths characteristically take years or decades to appear and possess no features distinguishing them from growths resulting from other causes. With few exceptions, such growths are detectable only after relatively large doses (>0.5 Sv) and vary in frequency based on the type of neoplasm and the age and gender of the exposed population. Because the existing data are insufficient to describe the dose-incidence relationship precisely or to define how long after irradiation the risk of cancer remains elevated in an exposed population, assessment of the risks of low-level irradiation must be based on models incorporating assumptions about these parameters (Table 19-4). Assessments depend heavily on findings in atomic bomb survivors, whose overall incidence of cancer can be inferred to increase as a linear nonthreshold function of their radiation dose. These estimates cannot be used to predict the risk of cancer attributable to a dose accumulated during weeks, months, or years, however, because experiments with laboratory animals have shown the carcinogenic potency of x-rays or γ-rays to decrease by a factor of 2 to 10 if the exposure is sufficiently prolonged. Furthermore, such estimates represent averages for a nominal population of males and females of all ages, whereas the estimates for breast cancer in women and for thyroid cancer in persons irradiated during childhood are substantially higher than those shown.

TABLE 19-4 ESTIMATED LIFETIME RISK OF VARIOUS CANCERS ATTRIBUTABLE TO 0.1-SV RAPID IRRADIATION

	Excess Cancer Deaths Per 100,000	
TYPE OR SITE OF CANCER	**No.**	**%***
Lung	205	3
Leukemia	86	14
Breast	73	2
Colon	61	3
Urinary bladder	25	5
Ovary	24	2
Stomach	22	4
Thyroid	8	16
Other	109	2
Total	613	3

*Percentage increase (rounded off) in the expected risk of death from cancer of that organ in a nonirradiated population.
Modified from National Research Council, National Academy of Sciences. *Health Risks from Exposure to Low Levels of Ionizing Radiation*. BEIR VII, phase 2. Washington, DC: National Academy Press; 2006.

Effects on Lifespan

Mortality from cardiovascular, respiratory, and other non-neoplastic diseases as well as from various forms of cancer is increased in heavily irradiated populations. In lightly irradiated populations, however, these effects are not evident, and survival appears to be enhanced in some instances. This finding has prompted some to infer that the effects of small doses may be beneficial on balance (radiation hormesis), but this hypothesis is highly controversial and has yet to be validated.

Effects of Prenatal Irradiation

The embryo is especially vulnerable to death if it is exposed before implantation; it is susceptible to malformations and other developmental disturbances if it is exposed during subsequent stages of organogenesis, and it is sensitive throughout intrauterine life to the carcinogenic effects of radiation. Among the various disturbances in growth and development, the dose-dependent increase in the frequency of severe mental retardation and the dose-dependent decrease in IQ test scores in atomic bomb survivors who were irradiated between the 8th and 15th weeks and, to a lesser extent, the 16th and 25th weeks after conception are particularly noteworthy.

DIAGNOSIS

Any facility likely to encounter radiation injuries should be able to cope with these injuries and should have personnel on call who are trained and equipped appropriately to do so. At the outset, to evaluate the dose and determine whether the patient has been contaminated with radionuclides, the nature of the exposure and any measurements by film badges or other detectors should be reviewed in detail. If exposure to radionuclides is known or suspected, radioactivity measurements of the whole body, skin, other tissue, blood, urine, and body fluid may be indicated to identify the isotope and evaluate the dose. Malaise, anorexia, nausea, and vomiting suggest a total body dose larger than 1 Sv, as do signs of erythema, hemorrhage, or infection

TREATMENT

In managing radiation injury, good medical judgment and first aid are the priorities. Even a heavily irradiated patient should be evaluated for other types of injury, such as burns, mechanical trauma, and smoke inhalation. If radioactive contamination is known or suspected, rescue and medical personnel who handle the patient should wear gloves and other protective clothing and should take precautions to isolate all contaminated objects.

Apart from symptomatic treatment, management of the hematologic form of acute radiation syndrome is similar to that of pancytopenic leukemia, including reverse isolation, antibiotics to combat infection, granulocyte and platelet transfusions as needed, and intravenous fluids as required to combat dehydration and electrolyte loss (Chapter 189). Colony-stimulating factors and interleukin may be beneficial in patients exposed to 6 to 10 Sv. Bone marrow transplantation (Chapter 181) may be life-saving after a dose of 7 to 10 Sv if a suitably matched donor is available; therefore, specimens of marrow and peripheral blood should be obtained for tissue typing as early as possible.

For localized injuries, treatment depends on the anatomic location and severity. Dry and moist desquamation of the skin, which is the most common injury requiring treatment, is usually managed adequately by simple cleansing. Large or ulcerated lesions should be covered with lanolin and closed dressings that are changed regularly. Severe injuries may require resection of necrotic tissue and skin grafting.

In the event of radioactive contamination, steps should be taken to minimize the uptake and retention of the isotope. Contaminated areas should be rinsed; the mouth, nose, and bronchial tree should be lavaged; and the gastrointestinal tract should be purged, if necessary. Additional measures to inhibit the uptake and retention of specific radionuclides may be indicated. Radioactive iodine may be released during a radiation accident or nuclear detonation and can pose a significant risk of thyroid cancer, especially in children. Stable potassium iodide should be administered to potentially exposed persons (except those who are sensitive to iodine) to inhibit the uptake of radioactive iodine by the thyroid. Its protective effect persists for about 24 hours, and the optimal effect is achieved when potassium iodide is given before exposure or concurrently with exposure. The recommended dose varies, depending on the recipient's age, expected level of thyroid exposure to radioactivity, and pregnancy or lactation status; recommendations range from 130 mg for adults to 16 mg for neonates.

in the skin, conjunctivae, or mucous membranes. The extent of lymphopenia during the first 24 hours varies with the size of the total body dose. Although the granulocyte count may be elevated temporarily during the first 24 to 48 hours, the rapidity with which it and the platelet count fall in the ensuing 2 to 4 weeks also varies with the total body dose. Cytogenetic analysis of cultured lymphocytes for chromosome aberrations can be another useful index of exposure.

PREVENTION

Because the mutagenic and carcinogenic effects of ionizing radiation may have no thresholds, unnecessary exposure should be avoided, and any doses to radiation workers and patients should be kept as low as possible, with particular care taken not to exceed the relevant maximal permissible doses. Facilities using radiation or radiation sources should be designed and equipped appropriately and should provide specialized training and supervision for all workers who may be occupationally exposed. Because indoor radon and computed tomography account for the bulk of the public's exposure to ionizing radiation, measures to limit excessive doses from these sources are warranted.

PROGNOSIS

After a total body dose of 2 Sv or less, survival is probable with little or no treatment; in the 2- to 10-Sv range, appropriate treatment can afford a high rate of survival. If the injury is localized, the prognosis depends on the nature and severity of the reaction. Although recovery is the rule after minor, acute reactions, delayed reactions tend to be irreversible and progressive.

NONIONIZING RADIATION INJURY

Ultraviolet Radiation

The ultraviolet (UV) radiation spectrum (see Fig. 19-1) is subdivided, for convenience, into three bands: UVA, or "black light," 315 to 400 nm; UVB, 280 to 315 nm; and UVC, which is germicidal, 200 to 280 nm. UV radiation does not penetrate deeply into human tissues, so the injuries it causes are confined chiefly to the skin and eyes.

EPIDEMIOLOGY

The largest source of UV radiation for the public is sunlight, which varies in intensity with latitude, elevation, and season. Important man-made sources include sun and tanning lamps, welding arcs, plasma torches, germicidal and black-light lamps, electric arc furnaces, hot-metal operations, mercury-vapor lamps, and some lasers. Low-intensity sources include fluorescent lamps and certain laboratory equipment.

Reactions of the skin to UV radiation, common among fair-skinned people, include sunburn, skin cancer (basal cell and squamous cell carcinoma and, to a lesser extent, melanoma), aging of the skin, solar elastosis, and solar keratosis. Injuries of the eye include photokeratitis, which may result from brief exposure to a high-intensity UV radiation source ("welder's flash") or more prolonged exposure to intense sunlight ("snow blindness"); cortical cataract; and pterygium.

PATHOBIOLOGY

The effects of UV radiation are primarily attributable to its absorption in DNA; pyrimidine dimers are produced and cause mutational changes in exposed cells. Sensitivity to UV radiation may be increased by DNA repair defects (as in xeroderma pigmentosum), by agents (e.g., caffeine) that inhibit repair enzymes, and by photosensitizing agents (e.g., psoralens, sulfonamides, tetracyclines, nalidixic acid, sulfonylureas, thiazides, phenothiazines, furocoumarins, and coal tar) that produce UV radiation–absorbing DNA photoproducts. The carcinogenic action of UV radiation is mediated through direct effects on the exposed cells and depression of local immunity.

CLINICAL MANIFESTATIONS

UVB in sunlight, although far less intense than UVA, plays a more important role in sunburn and skin carcinogenesis, but UVA also contributes to skin carcinogenesis, tanning, some photosensitivity reactions, and aging of the skin.

TREATMENT AND PREVENTION

Excessive exposure to sunlight or other sources of UV radiation should be avoided, especially in fair-skinned individuals. Protective clothing, UV radiation–screening lotions or creams, and UV radiation–blocking sunglasses should be used. To protect occupationally exposed workers, the American Conference of Governmental Industrial Hygienists has recommended 8-hour exposure limits for the unprotected eye that range from 3 mJ/cm^2 to 10^6 mJ/cm^2, depending on the wavelength of the radiation (note that 1 J/second = 1 W). The protective layer of ozone in the stratosphere is being depleted globally by chlorofluorocarbons and other air pollutants, and every 1% decrease in ozone is expected to increase the UV radiation reaching the earth by 1 to 2% and thus increase the rates of nonmelanotic skin cancer by 2 to 6%.

Visible Light

Visible light consists of electromagnetic waves varying in wavelength from 380 nm (violet) to 760 nm (red) (see Fig. 19-1).

PATHOBIOLOGY

Bright, continuously visible light normally elicits an aversion response to protect the eye against injury, so few sources of light other than a laser or the sun during a solar eclipse are large or bright enough to burn the retina under normal viewing conditions.

Photochemical reactions in the retina from sustained exposure to intensities exceeding 0.1 mW/cm^2, such as can result from fixing on a bright source of light, may suffice to produce photochemical blue-light injury. Brief exposure of the retina to intensities exceeding 10 W/cm^2, depending on image size, may cause a retinal burn.

CLINICAL MANIFESTATIONS

Too little illumination can cause eyestrain or seasonal affective disorder, whereas too bright a light can injure the retina (Chapter 431).

TREATMENT AND PREVENTION

Common sense usually suffices to prevent excessive exposure of the retina to light. However, in situations involving potential exposure to high-intensity sources, such as carbon arcs or lasers, appropriate training, proper design of equipment, and protective eye shields are important.

Infrared Radiation

Infrared radiation consists of electromagnetic waves ranging in wavelength from 7×10^{-5} m to 3×10^{-2} m. The injuries caused by infrared radiation are chiefly burns of the skin and cataracts of the lens of the eye.

EPIDEMIOLOGY

Potentially hazardous sources include furnaces, ovens, welding arcs, molten glass, molten metal, and heating lamps. The warning sensation of heat usually prompts aversion in time to prevent burning of the skin by infrared radiation; however, the lens of the eye is vulnerable because it lacks the ability to sense or dissipate heat.

CLINICAL MANIFESTATIONS

Glassblowers, blacksmiths, oven operators, and people working around heating and drying lamps are at increased risk of infrared radiation–induced cataracts (Chapter 431).

TREATMENT AND PREVENTION

Control of infrared radiation hazards requires appropriate shielding of its sources, training of potentially exposed persons, and use of protective clothing and goggles.

Microwave and Radio Frequency Radiation

Microwave and radio frequency radiation consists of electromagnetic waves ranging in frequency from about 3 kHz to 300 GHz.

EPIDEMIOLOGY

Sources of microwave and radio frequency radiation are used widely in radar, televisions, cellular phones, radios, other telecommunications systems, various industrial operations (e.g., heating, welding, and melting of metals; processing of wood and plastic; high-temperature plasma), household appliances (e.g., microwave ovens), and medical applications (e.g., diathermy and hyperthermia).

PATHOBIOLOGY

The biologic effects of microwave and radio frequency radiation are primarily thermal in nature, but there is growing evidence that some effects may be elicited through nonthermal mechanisms, such as DNA damage, as well. Because of the deep penetration of these types of radiation, the cutaneous burns they cause tend to involve dermal and subcutaneous tissues and to heal slowly.

CLINICAL MANIFESTATIONS

Isolated cases of skin burns, thermal injury to deeper tissues, and death from hyperthermia have been caused by industrial microwave and radio frequency radiation sources. Burns may also result from faulty or improperly used household microwave ovens and from the overexposure of patients with impaired cutaneous pain and temperature senses, which usually warn of impending injury. Other effects reported in the literature but not yet conclusively documented include cataract of the lens, impairment of fertility, developmental disturbances, neurobehavioral abnormalities, depression of immunity, and increased risk for certain cancers. Microwave and radio frequency radiation also can interfere with cardiac pacemakers (Chapter 66) and other medical devices.

TREATMENT AND PREVENTION Rx

Microwave and radio frequency radiation sources must be designed and shielded properly, and potentially exposed persons, especially those with cardiac pacemakers or other sensitive devices, must be trained and supervised properly. In general, detectable heating of tissue requires microwave and radio frequency radiation power densities greater than 10 W/cm^2; avoidance of such exposure, as prescribed by existing federal standards, suffices to prevent such injuries. Further research is needed, however, to address the potential effects of long-term exposure, such as may result from repeated use of mobile phones, especially in children.

Extremely Low Frequency Electromagnetic Fields

Extremely low frequency electromagnetic fields range in frequency from 1 to 3000 Hz, including the 50- to 60-Hz fields associated with alternating currents in electric power distribution systems and appliances. Exposure to such fields is not known to be hazardous, but data suggesting that it may cause reproductive abnormalities and carcinogenic effects have aroused public health concern.

EPIDEMIOLOGY

The earth is surrounded by a naturally occurring electromagnetic field ranging from the low end of the extremely low frequency region to radio frequencies that exist briefly as a result of lightning discharges. Localized electromagnetic fields also are generated by electric power lines, transformers, motors, household appliances, video display tubes, and various medical devices, notably nuclear magnetic resonance imaging systems. These localized fields are generally stronger than naturally existing ones; electromagnetic field flux densities near common household appliances may range up to 270 mG, compared with the average value of 0.6 mG for the earth's magnetic field.

PATHOBIOLOGY

Evaluation of epidemiologic data is complicated by the lack of any known biologic basis for the effects of extremely low frequency electromagnetic fields on tissue, especially because the currents emanating from normal nerve and muscle activity are far stronger than the currents attributable to 1- to 10-mG external 60-Hz fields. Nevertheless, such fields have been reported to influence ion transport, melatonin secretion, and tumor promotion in some model systems.

CLINICAL MANIFESTATIONS

Exceptionally strong fields may affect electrically active tissues (nerves, neuromusculature, heart) and cardiac pacemakers and may raise body temperature. Conflicting epidemiologic studies have evaluated several possibilities: that residential exposure of children to weaker electromagnetic fields may increase their risk of leukemia, that occupational exposure of male utility workers may increase their risk of brain cancer and leukemia, and that chronic exposure of pregnant women to video display tubes may increase their risk of miscarriage and of bearing children with birth defects. None of these links has been established.

TREATMENT AND PREVENTION Rx

Persons with pacemakers should avoid electromagnetic fields stronger than 0.5 mT, which exist around transformers, accelerators, nuclear magnetic resonance imaging systems, and other electrical devices; areas containing such fields should be posted with warning signs. Exposure of workers should be limited in accordance with national guidelines.

Ultrasound

Although frequently classified with nonionizing radiation, ultrasound consists of mechanical vibrations at inaudibly high frequencies (≥16 kHz) and is not a component of the electromagnetic spectrum.

EPIDEMIOLOGY

High-power, low-frequency ultrasound is used widely in science and industry for cleaning, degreasing, plastic welding, liquid extracting, atomizing, homogenizing, and emulsifying operations and in medicine for lithotripsy. Low-power, high-frequency ultrasound is used widely in analytic work and in medical diagnosis (e.g., ultrasonography).

PATHOBIOLOGY

The biologic effects of high-power ultrasound are similar in mechanism to those of mechanical vibration-localized heating, agitation, and fragmentation of tissues.

CLINICAL MANIFESTATIONS

Deleterious effects from prolonged exposure to high-power ultrasound include headache, malaise, tinnitus, vertigo, hypersensitivity to light and sound, and peripheral neuritis. Similar complaints may result from excessive exposure to high-frequency ultrasound through body contact with the source. However, adverse effects have not been shown to result from exposure to high-frequency ultrasound at the low power levels used in medical ultrasonography.

TREATMENT AND PREVENTION Rx

Protection against ultrasound injury requires appropriate isolation and insulation of generating sources and proper training and ear protective devices for persons working around such sources. Yearly audiometric and neurologic examinations of workers are advisable.

SUGGESTED READINGS

American Conference of Governmental Industrial Hygienists. 2009 Threshold Limit Values and Biological Exposure Indices. Cincinnati, OH: American Conference of Governmental Industrial Hygienists; 2009. *An authoritative listing of maximal permissible occupational exposure limits for radiation of all types.*

Einstein AJ, Weiner SD, Bernheim A, et al. Multiple testing, cumulative radiation dose, and clinical indications for patients undergoing myocardial perfusion imaging. *JAMA.* 2010;304:2137-2144. *Multiple cardiac nuclear medicine tests result in substantial radiation exposure.*

Fazel R, Krumholz HM, Wang Y, et al. Exposure to low-dose ionizing radiation from medical imaging procedures. *N Engl J Med.* 2009;361:849-857. *Imaging procedures are an important source of exposure to ionizing radiation.*

International Commission on Non-Ionizing Radiation Protection. Exposure to high frequency electromagnetic fields, biological effects and health consequences (100 kHz-300 GHz). Oberschleissheim, Germany: International Commission on Non-Ionizing Radiation Protection; 2009. *Comprehensive overview of the sources, levels, and health effects of exposure to nonionizing, high-frequency electromagnetic radiation.*

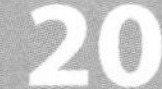

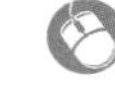

BIOTERRORISM

JOHN G. BARTLETT

BIOLOGIC WEAPONS

DEFINITION

Weapons of mass destruction are classified as biologic, chemical, or nuclear. Biologic weapons are microbes or microbial products used for bioterrorism. The potential for mass destruction is evident from a report from the U.S. Office of Technology, which predicted that the release of 100 kg of anthrax spores upwind of Washington, DC, would cause 130,000 to 3 million deaths, matching the lethal potential of a hydrogen bomb. The Centers for Disease Control and Prevention (CDC) is responsible for orchestrating the public health response to a bioterrorism threat or attack in the United States, and the FBI is responsible for the criminal aspects. The CDC has reviewed and classified various potential bioweapons based on public health impact and the properties of such weapons in terms of health consequences, ease of delivery to large populations, potential for civil disruption, and sustainability by person-to-person transmission (Table 20-1). Those with the "best" potential (category A agents) include anthrax, smallpox, plague, botulism, tularemia, and selected viruses that cause viral hemorrhagic fever (Tables 20-1 and 20-2). Of these, the two agents that stand out are anthrax and smallpox.

Despite the enormous potential for mass destruction, the actual application of bioterrorism has been quite limited. During World War II there were major bioweapons programs in the United States, the Soviet Union, Japan, and Germany, but only Japan used its program in any well-established way. The Soviet Union had the largest bioweapons program, with approximately 50 facilities and 60,000 employees. In 1972 the Biologic and Toxin Weapons Convention, which was established to eliminate the threat of bioterrorism, was signed by 140 nations, including the United States and the Soviet Union. The subsequent destiny of the enormous volume of products (e.g., smallpox virus, botulinum toxin, anthrax spores) and most of the highly skilled scientists in this area is largely unknown. Current estimates are that many nations continue to harbor bioweapons programs.

In addition to these large-scale national programs, there is the potential for individuals or dissident groups to use bioweapons. For example, in 1984 a religious cult in Oregon attempted to influence an election by contaminating restaurant salad bars with *Salmonella* to reduce voter turnout; the effort resulted in 751 cases of salmonellosis, but the election was not affected. Aum Shinrykio, a Japanese cult, was responsible for the release of sarin nerve gas, which killed 10 and injured 6000 in Tokyo.

More recently, there were 22 cases of anthrax in the United States during a 2-month period in 2001. Of the 22 cases, 20 were traced directly to six contaminated letters sent to different locations, all with the same molecular type of *Bacillus anthracis*. Some cases were cutaneous because the material in the letters was milled to a relatively large particle size that contaminated surfaces via gravity. By contrast, letters with anthrax that was milled to nearly the size of a single spore resulted in particles that were aerosolized and inhaled, causing inhalational anthrax. During this 2-month period, the CDC assigned 1000 personnel to deal with anthrax issues, prophylactic ciprofloxacin or doxycycline was delivered to 10,000 people who were exposed or possibly exposed, the New York City Health Department fielded more than 15,000 telephone calls, there were hundreds of false threats, and a hospital in Boston was closed for decontamination because of a white powder on the floor that turned out to be from a sugar donut. Ultimately, 11 cases of cutaneous anthrax and 11 of inhalational anthrax were diagnosed. Five of the 11 patients with inhalational anthrax died, despite good medical care. This experience clearly demonstrated the potential impact of a bioterrorism attack on a nation's citizenry.

The next important event was the decision to resume smallpox vaccinations in December 2002. The vaccine was mandatory for military personnel and voluntary for frontline medical personnel who were designated members of smallpox response teams. The concern was that smallpox is an ideal bioterrorism agent because vaccinations had been discontinued and the natural disease was considered to have been eradicated in 1977. The disease is contagious, highly lethal, and largely untreatable. Risk was difficult to assess, although the United States and Russia were the only countries known to have viable smallpox. The restarted vaccine program was hampered by the fact that few contemporary health care personnel knew how to deliver it and that the prior vaccine had been associated with severe complications. Despite these concerns, the experience with about 440,000 military personnel and 36,000

TABLE 20-1 CLASSIFICATION OF BIOTERRORISM AGENTS

	Public Health Impact		*Dissemination**			
Agent	**Disease**	**Death**	**Delivery Potential**	**Person To Person**	**Public Perception**[†]	**Special Preparation**[‡]
Smallpox (A)	+	++	+	+++	+++	+++
Anthrax (A)	++	+++	+++	0	+++	+++
Plague (A)	++	+++	++	+	++	+++
Botulism (A)	++	+++	++	0	++	+++
Viral hemorrhagic fever (A)	++	+++	+	++	+++	++
Tularemia (A)	++	++	+	0	+	+++
Viral encephalitis (B)	++	+	+	0	++	++
Q fever (B)	+	+	++	0	+	++
Brucellosis (B)	+	+	++	0	+	++
Glanders (B)	++	+++	++	0	0	++
Melioidosis (B)	+	+	++	0	0	++
Psittacosis (B)	+	+	++	0	0	+
Ricin toxin (B)	++	++	++	0	0	++
Typhus (B)	+	+	++	0	0	+
Cholera (B)	+	+	++	+/−	+++	+
Shigellosis (B)	+	+	++	+	+	+

*Potential for rapid large-scale dissemination.
†Need for therapeutics, surveillance, laboratory demands.
‡Media reports with +++ include more than 45 titles in a survey of 233 newspapers and 70 TV and radio sources.
+++ = death in >50%; ++ = death in 21 to 49%; + = death in <20%.
A = greatest potential for bioterrorism; B = less likely or less important for bioterrorism.

TABLE 20-2 CLINICAL FEATURES OF CATEGORY A AGENTS

	ANTHRAX (INHALATIONAL)	SMALLPOX	PLAGUE (PNEUMONIA)	BOTULISM	VIRAL HEMORRHAGIC FEVER
Cases in U.S. per year	0-1	0	8-10	200-300	0
Clinical features	Flulike, then shock	Fever, then characteristic rash	Pneumonia, hemoptysis	Descending paralysis and involvement of cranial nerves	Hemorrhage and fever
Diagnosis	Blood culture, chest CT	BSL-4 laboratory for virus	Blood and sputum culture	Toxin assay of blood, GI specimens; EMG	BSL-4 laboratory for virus
Mortality	40-50%	30%	10-20%	60%	Variable
Treatment*	Cipro, doxy, or levo + 2nd agent,† 60-100 days	None	Gent/strep (cipro/doxy), 10 days	Antitoxin, ventilator	Ribavirin (some) 7 days
Prevention*	Cipro/doxy	Vaccine	Cipro/doxy	None	None
Infection control	Not transmitted Vaccine	Contact and airborne precautions	Masks	Not transmitted	Contact precautions

*Doses: cipro 400 mg IV q8-12h or 500-750 mg PO bid; levo 500-750 mg IV qd or 500 mg PO qd; doxy 100 mg PO or IV bid; gent 5 mg/kg/day IM or IV; strep 1 g IM bid; ribavirin 16 mg/kg/day IV × 4 days, then 8 mg/kg/day × 3 days or 1000-1200 mg/day PO × 7.

†Imipenem 500 mg IV q6h, rifampin 600 mg IV or PO qd, chloramphenicol 1 g IV q6h, clarithromycin 500 mg PO bid, vancomycin 1 g IV bid, or clindamycin 600 mg IV q8h.

BSL-4 = Biologic Safety Level 4; cipro = ciprofloxacin; CT = computed tomography; doxy = doxycycline; EMG = electromyography; gent = gentamicin; GI = gastrointestinal; levo = levofloxacin; strep = streptomycin; ( ) = alternative to preferred.

civilian medical professionals showed almost none of the previously described serious reactions, but about 50 cases of myocarditis or pericarditis were reported.

More recent planning for bioterrorism has been based on extensive reviews of the anthrax experience of 2001, the 9/11 experience, and two large national simulated bioterrorism attacks: TOPOFF, which was a simulated anthrax attack carried out in Denver in 2000, and Dark Winter, which was a simulated smallpox attack in 2001. The responses have included the Biomedical Advanced Research Development Authority (BARDA), the Project BioShield Act of 2004, and the Pandemic and All-Hazards Preparedness Act of 2006. These initiatives collectively provide extensive resources, organizational structure, and preemptive planning for bioterrorism, but many of these efforts share challenges that are common to pandemics such as influenza and natural disasters such as earthquakes, as well as to bioterrorism. A major concern is surge capacity—the ability of the health system to accommodate a large number of patients in terms of demands for emergency care, medical beds, medical personnel, medications, and equipment such as ventilators.

ANTHRAX

DEFINITION

Infection is caused by *B. anthracis* (Chapter 302). The three recognized forms reflect the portal of entry: inhalation, cutaneous exposure, and ingestion.

EPIDEMIOLOGY

The greatest concern for bioterrorism is the inhaled form of anthrax, which results from the inhalation of *B. anthracis* spores and causes a devastating disease with a mortality rate of about 50%, even with optimal management. The last naturally occurring case of inhalational anthrax in the United States was in 1976. The largest epidemic followed an accidental release of anthrax in Sverdlovsk, Russia, in 1979 and resulted in an estimated 80 to 250 cases. Cutaneous anthrax is the usual naturally occurring zoonotic form. An average of less than 1 case per year now occurs in the United States, with about 2000 naturally occurring cases in the world each year.

PATHOBIOLOGY

When inhalational anthrax is associated with bioterrorism, spores must be milled to less than 5 μm to permit both aerosolization and inhalation. The spores are taken up by alveolar macrophages and migrate to the mediastinal lymph nodes, where they revert to vegetative forms and produce toxins. The protective antigen combines with lethal toxin and edema toxin; these toxins are thought to account for the clinical features.

CLINICAL MANIFESTATIONS

The incubation period is usually 4 to 5 days, but the range is 2 to 43 days after exposure. Inhalational anthrax is a two-stage disease. The initial symptoms are nonspecific and flulike. Features that distinguish this stage from influenza are the lack of coryza and the anticipated exposure history. The second stage is profound sepsis with chest pain, chest compression from large pleural effusions and mediastinal expansion, multiple organ failure, obtundation, cyanosis, hypotension, and death, which may occur within hours. Cutaneous anthrax is characterized by a vesicle that progresses to an eschar associated with substantial surrounding edema, often with regional adenopathy and systemic signs of infection.

DIAGNOSIS

The diagnosis is established by recovery of *B. anthracis* from blood or the infected site. Virtually all patients with inhalational anthrax have positive blood cultures, which frequently turn positive within 12 to 16 hours if cultures were obtained before therapy. Other highly characteristic features of the disease are a chest radiograph that shows a wide mediastinum and a computed tomography scan that shows hyperdense hilar and mediastinal lymph nodes, often with large pleural effusions. A highly characteristic feature of the disease is large, bloody pleural effusions. There may or may not be a pulmonary infiltrate.

TREATMENT

Rx

The most important facets of treatment of inhalational anthrax are supportive care, drainage of pleural effusions, and rapid administration of antibiotics. The drugs approved by the Food and Drug Administration (FDA) for B. anthracis are intravenous penicillin, doxycycline, ciprofloxacin, and levofloxacin (see Table 20-2). In reality, a bioterrorism event involving inhaled anthrax would result in specific recommendations from the CDC. In 2001 the preferred agents were doxycycline or ciprofloxacin combined with a second agent such as penicillin, imipenem, rifampin, chloramphenicol, clarithromycin, vancomycin, or clindamycin, based on sensitivity tests of the epidemic strain. After clinical improvement, the intravenous administration may be changed to oral agents such as ciprofloxacin, levofloxacin, or doxycycline; the total recommended duration of treatment is 60 to 100 days, presumably owing to the persistence of spores. For cutaneous anthrax the recommended treatment is also ciprofloxacin or doxycycline for a total of 60 to 100 days, based on the assumption that a patient with cutaneous anthrax may have inhaled organisms as well.

PREVENTION

In the event of bioterrorism, prophylaxis appears to be critical because the disease is highly lethal, even with antibiotic treatment, and prophylaxis is highly effective. The recommendation for prophylaxis has been oral doxycycline or ciprofloxacin for 60 to 100 days, although more recent animal studies suggest that shorter courses are effective. In fact, anthrax did not develop in any exposed people who received even a single dose of these drugs before the onset of symptoms. An FDA-approved anthrax vaccine administered in six doses to wool sorters and other workers in high-risk occupations is very effective, but other anthrax vaccines appear to be effective with fewer administrations and result in fewer adverse reactions.

PROGNOSIS

Data from the Sverdlovsk outbreak in Russia suggest a mortality rate of 60 to 87%, despite appropriate antibiotics. In the 2001 epidemic in the United States, 5 of 11 patients (45%) with inhalational anthrax died, despite aggressive management. In the fatal cases, the interval between the onset of symptoms and death averaged 3 to 4 days. Survivors had long-term disability.

SMALLPOX

DEFINITION

Smallpox is a systemic infection caused by the virus *Variola major* or *Variola minor* (Chapter 380). The assumption is that any attempt at bioterrorism with smallpox would use *V. major*, which is associated with a substantially higher mortality rate. The virus is viewed as ideal for bioterrorism because it is easy to culture, survives well in aerosols, and is lethal in 30% of cases. Furthermore, most humans are now susceptible because immunization was stopped in the United States and most of the world by 1973.

EPIDEMIOLOGY

The global campaign to eradicate smallpox was initiated in 1966, and the last naturally occurring case was reported in 1977. In 1980 the World Health Organization (WHO) declared smallpox eradicated and recommended that all laboratories destroy their stocks of variola or transfer them to one of two WHO reference laboratories, one in Moscow and the other at the CDC in Atlanta. These remaining isolates were to be destroyed in 1999, but the WHO agreed to retain the supplies in an effort to develop an attenuated vaccine and antiviral drugs. The number of countries that have this virus other than Russia and the United States is not known.

Smallpox is spread from person to person in droplets from the oral pharynx. The greatest risk is to persons within 6 to 8 feet of an infected individual, and prior epidemics have consistently shown that most cases occur in household members and hospital contacts. The secondary attack rate in unvaccinated household members is 37 to 88%. Because the disease has been eradicated, any confirmed case of smallpox implies bioterrorism.

CLINICAL MANIFESTATIONS

The incubation period is usually 12 to 14 days. Initial symptoms are high fever, malaise, prostration, headache, and backache. These symptoms are severe, and most patients are bedridden. The rash usually appears on day 3 as a maculopapular eruption that subsequently evolves through the vesicular and then pustular stages; at 2 to 3 weeks it forms scabs that separate and leave a characteristic pitted scar. The rash begins on the face and forearms and then spreads to the trunk and legs. Pustules have a characteristic firm, round, deep-seated appearance and measure 7 to 10 mm in diameter. Lesions are more dense on the face and extremities, all are in the same stage, and the palms and soles may be involved. An important issue in terms of disease control is that transmission takes place during the rash phase and not during the early pre-rash period of illness.

DIAGNOSIS

Laboratory diagnosis requires fluid collected from a typical vesicular or pustular lesion, preferably by a vaccinated person with appropriate protection. Laboratory testing must be done in a maximum containment facility (Biologic Safety Level 4 [BSL-4] laboratory); tissue culture is used to recover the virus, and polymerase chain reaction and restriction fragment length polymorphism are used to characterize the viral strain. For the clinician, the major issue is the distinction of smallpox from chickenpox or other illnesses characterized by a vesicular rash (Table 20-3). With chickenpox (Chapter 383), the lesions are more superficial, have a centripetal distribution with greater involvement of the trunk and face, and are not all at the same stage of evolution. Patients are also less seriously ill.

Other conditions in the differential diagnosis for a vesicular or pustular rash include disseminated herpes zoster or herpes simplex (Chapter 382), drug eruptions (Chapter 448), erythema multiforme (Chapter 446), enteroviral infection (Chapter 387), secondary syphilis (Chapter 327), monkeypox (Chapter 380), molluscum contagiosum (Chapter 446), and generalized vaccinia. With a generalized maculopapular rash, the differential diagnosis includes measles (Chapter 375), rubella (Chapter 376), drug rash, erythema multiforme, and scarlet fever (Chapter 297).

TABLE 20-3 MAJOR AND MINOR CRITERIA FOR SMALLPOX AND PRIORITY FOR REPORTING TO CENTERS FOR DISEASE CONTROL AND PREVENTION

MAJOR CRITERIA
Fever (>38.3° C) 1-4 days before the onset of rash plus one of the following: headache, prostration, chills, vomiting, abdominal pain
Typical smallpox lesions: firm, round, deep-seated vesicles or pustules with evolution to umbilicated or confluent
Lesions at same stage of development
MINOR CRITERIA
Centrifugal distribution of rash (face and extremities)
First lesions on oral mucosa, palate, face, and arms
Patient appears toxic or moribund
Slow evolution of lesions—each stage lasts at least 1-2 days
Lesions on palms and soles
REPORTING PRIORITY
Report immediately: (1) febrile prodrome, (2) classic smallpox lesions, and (3) lesions in the same stage of development (all 3 present)
Urgent assessment: (1) febrile prodrome and one other major criterion *or* (2) febrile prodrome plus ≥4 minor criteria
Manage as clinically indicated: febrile prodrome and ≥4 minor criteria

TREATMENT Rx

There is no therapy with established merit.

PREVENTION

Vaccination with vaccinia (cowpox) virus before exposure provides significant protection against smallpox. Persons in whom a vesicle or pustule develops or who have a pitted scar at a previous vaccination site have a "take" indicating an immune response. The duration of protection is not well known. Vaccination also provides some protection when given within 4 days after exposure because the immune response to vaccinia is faster than it is to smallpox. The major goal in the event of anticipated bioterrorism is to vaccinate persons with anticipated risks, such as military personnel or hospital-based smallpox response teams. In an outbreak, the highest priority would be first responders, household contacts, and others who have face-to-face contact with patients after the onset of fever.

Vaccination was associated with substantial risk when it was given routinely before 1973. The major currently recognized vaccine-associated complications (Chapter 17) include (1) postvaccinal encephalitis, which is probably an immune reaction; (2) progressive vaccinia, which is a progressive and rapidly lethal complication of disseminated vaccinia seen primarily in patients with defective cell-mediated immunity; (3) generalized vaccinia caused by dissemination of vaccinia; (4) accidental inoculation of other anatomic sites or other persons, usually bedmates; and (5) eczema vaccinatum in patients with a current or past history of eczema or atopic dermatitis. Complications that result from uncontrolled growth of vaccinia can be treated with vaccinia immune globulin. During the recent experience with smallpox vaccination in more than 500,000 U.S. military personnel and health care workers, the frequency of these adverse reactions was modest, and no deaths were recorded. However, another major complication—myopericarditis—was recognized; it was most common with primary vaccination, self-limited, and probably immune mediated.

PLAGUE

DEFINITION

Plague refers to infection by *Yersinia pestis* (Chapter 320).

EPIDEMIOLOGY

Approximately 10 cases of plague occur in the United States annually, but the pneumonic form of disease, which would be anticipated in the event of bioterrorism, is rare, with only about 7 cases in the past 50 years. Thus, any case of pneumonic plague, particularly if acquired in urban areas and outside endemic areas, should arouse suspicion of bioterrorism. An important clinical clue to the diagnosis is severe pneumonia associated with hemoptysis. It is known

TABLE 20-4 VIRAL HEMORRHAGIC FEVERS

AGENT	SOURCE	VECTOR	CLINICAL FEATURES	P-P TX	TREATMENT	MORTALITY (%)
Ebola	Africa	Not known	Fever, rash, DIC	Yes	Supportive	50-90
Marburg	Africa	Not known	Fever, rash	Yes	Supportive	20-70
Lassa fever	Africa	Rodent	Fever, conjunctivitis	Yes	Ribavirin	15-20
New World Arenaviridae	South America	Rodent	GI symptoms, conjunctivitis, adenopathy	Yes	Ribavirin	15-30
Rift Valley fever	Africa, Saudi Arabia	Mosquito	Fever, jaundice, photophobia	No	Ribavirin	<1
Yellow fever	Africa, Americas	Mosquito	Fever, jaundice, conjunctivitis	No	Supportive	20
Omsk hemorrhagic fever	Central Asia	Tick	Fever, cough, conjunctivitis, adenopathy	No	Supportive	1-10
Kyasanur	India	Tick	Biphasic encephalitis	No	Supportive	3-10

DIC = disseminated intravascular coagulation; GI = gastrointestinal; P-P Tx = person-to-person transmission.

that *Y. pestis* was produced in large quantities by Soviet scientists for bioterrorism before this program was abandoned in 1992. The WHO has estimated that a 50-kg release of *Y. pestis* over an urban area of 5 million people would result in 150,000 cases of plague pneumonia and 36,000 deaths.

CLINICAL MANIFESTATIONS

The incubation period is 1 to 6 days. The pneumonic form is associated with bloody sputum, fever, dyspnea, and frequent gastrointestinal symptoms, including nausea, vomiting, abdominal pain, and diarrhea. The course is rapidly progressive, with a sepsis syndrome at 2 to 6 days. Chest radiographs usually show consolidated infiltrates, and about 50% of patients have pleural effusions.

DIAGNOSIS

Y. pestis is a gram-negative coccobacillus that demonstrates bipolar staining and resembles a safety pin. Although the organism may be recognized by Gram stain of sputum, most laboratories require extended periods to identify it with standard methods. If this diagnosis is suspected, the laboratory should be warned so that one culture can be incubated at 28° C for rapid growth and a second at 37° C to permit identification of the capsular antigen. Rapid diagnostic tests are available in some state health departments, the CDC, and some military facilities. The differential diagnosis includes other severe forms of pneumonia or epidemic pneumonia, such as legionnaires' disease (Chapter 322), histoplasmosis (Chapter 340), anthrax (Chapter 302), tularemia (Chapter 319), and influenza (Chapter 372).

TREATMENT Rx

The preferred drugs are streptomycin or gentamicin; doxycycline and fluoroquinolones such as ciprofloxacin or levofloxacin are alternative agents. The duration of treatment is 10 days.

PREVENTION

Limited data define the efficiency of person-to-person transmission. Current recommendations are for contact and droplet precautions with the use of masks, gowns, gloves, and eye protection. Isolation may be discontinued after 48 hours of antibiotic treatment and clinical improvement. Prophylactic doxycycline or ciprofloxacin is recommended for 7 days for household members, health care workers, and other close contacts of patients. Prophylactic antibiotics are also advocated for other persons with a common-source exposure. As with anthrax, prophylaxis is virtually 100% effective, whereas treatment after the onset of symptoms is much less successful.

PROGNOSIS

The fatality rate of pneumonic plague approaches 100% without therapy. Mortality has been reduced to 5 to 14% with aminoglycoside treatment, but this experience is based largely on syndromes that are generally less severe than plague pneumonia.

BOTULISM

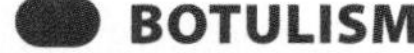

See Chapter 304.

TULAREMIA

See Chapter 319.

VIRAL HEMORRHAGIC FEVER

DEFINITION

The hemorrhagic fever viruses (Chapter 389) include diverse organisms that cause a clinical illness characterized by fever and bleeding. These agents are grouped in four families: Filoviridae, Arenaviridae, Bunyaviridae, and Flaviviridae (Table 20-4). These viruses are attractive as bioweapons for several reasons: the minimal infecting dose may be as low as 10 virions, they can be distributed by aerosols, mortality rates are virus dependent but often high, they generate great fear, many are transmitted person to person, and no good treatment is available.

EPIDEMIOLOGY

The hemorrhagic fever viruses are not normally found in the United States, Europe, or Australia. They are transmitted by contact with infected animals or arthropod vectors, although the natural reservoir for Ebola and Marburg viruses is not known. Any case of viral hemorrhagic fever in a patient who has not been in an endemic area within the previous 22 days is presumed to represent bioterrorism.

CLINICAL MANIFESTATIONS

The onset of illness is generally nonspecific and consists of fever and myalgias. Additional symptoms are virus dependent (see Table 20-4) and include rash, encephalitis, pharyngitis, adenopathy, and gastrointestinal symptoms. The syndrome progresses to thrombocytopenia with petechiae, hematuria, hematemesis, hemoptysis, and melena. Disseminated intravascular coagulation with shock, delirium, convulsions, and coma may then develop.

DIAGNOSIS

Laboratory features include thrombocytopenia, as well as leukopenia, anemia, or hemoconcentration. All specimens from patients with suspected viral hemorrhagic fever should be referred to the CDC for testing in a BSL-4 laboratory. Personnel in the referring laboratory must be warned, and only designated technicians should be assigned to processing.

TREATMENT Rx

Ribavirin has activity in vitro against Lassa fever virus, New World arenaviruses, and bunyaviruses, but clinical experience is limited. It is assumed that a limited number of cases involving these viruses would permit the use of intravenous ribavirin, but a mass casualty setting would require oral administration. Treatment of other hemorrhagic fever viruses would largely be limited to supportive care.

PREVENTION

The major concern is nosocomial and household transmission by contact with blood and other body fluids. Patients should be kept in a single-occupant negative-pressure room, and health care personnel should use N95 respirators or powered air-purifying respirators, double gloves, impermeable gowns, goggles or face shields, and leg and shoe coverings. Nonessential staff and visitors should be excluded. Dedicated medical equipment such as stethoscopes and point-of-care analyzers should be available. Laboratory specimens should not be sent in pneumonic systems, contaminated objects should be cleaned with a 1 : 100 household bleach or similar disinfectant, and contaminated cloth items should be double-bagged and incinerated or autoclaved. Particular care must be exercised in managing corpses.

SUGGESTED READINGS

Friedlander AM, Little SF. Advances in the development of next-generation anthrax vaccines. *Vaccine.* 2009;27:D28-D32. *A short course of antibiotics prevents post-exposure disease in a macaque model.*

McFadden G. Killing a killer: what next for smallpox? *PloS Pathog.* 2010;6:e1000727. *A review of the current status of variola virus and smallpox vaccines and the debate on the destruction of smallpox.*

Merkel TJ, Perera PY, Kelly VK, et al. Development of a highly efficacious vaccinia-based dual vaccine against smallpox and anthrax, two important bioterror entities. *Proc Natl Acad Sci U S A.* 2010;107:18091-18096. *A single new vaccine appears to be efficacious against both agents.*

Wright JG, Quinn CP, Shadomy S, et al. Use of anthrax vaccine in the United States: recommendations of the Advisory Committee on Immunization Practices (ACIP), 2009. *MMWR Recomm Rep.* 2010;59:1-30. *Updated consensus guideline.*

21 CHRONIC POISONING: TRACE METALS AND OTHERS

MICHAEL A. MCGUIGAN

DEFINITION

The term *chronic poisoning* refers to toxicity that develops during repeated or continuous exposure to a substance over many months or years. A *trace metal,* which by definition is present in minute quantities, usually refers to metals that are essential to an organism's function; however, this chapter includes a number of metals that are not physiologically required and does not discuss acute poisoning (Chapter 110).

EPIDEMIOLOGY

The source of most of the substances discussed in this chapter is the environment—the home, the workplace, or the outdoors—and most exposures are unintentional. Because many of these metals are essential to normal physiologic functions, another source may be dietary supplements (Chapter 225). The most common site of absorption is the gastrointestinal tract.

The medical literature on chronic low-level exposure is uneven. Although the clinical toxicology of each metal is presented individually, most if not all exposures involve a number of different metals, and the clinical impact of metal-metal interactions is poorly understood.

Lead

EPIDEMIOLOGY

Lead poisoning was recognized more than 2000 years ago. Although lead poisoning is often considered primarily a problem among children of lower socioeconomic status living in dilapidated housing with peeling lead-based paint, lead poisoning also occurs in adults exposed through occupational or nonoccupational activities (Table 21-1). In the United States, approximately 95% of cases of blood lead levels 25 μg/dL or greater in adults are attributed to occupational exposure.

PATHOBIOLOGY

Inhaled fine particulates (<5 μm in diameter) of inorganic lead reach the alveoli and are readily absorbed; larger particles come in contact with airway mucus and are eventually swallowed. Only 20 to 30% of orally ingested lead is absorbed. Organic lead compounds can also be absorbed through the skin. Absorbed lead is distributed first to blood and soft tissue and then to bone, where more than 90% of total body lead is found. Factors contributing to bone demineralization (e.g., prolonged bedrest, pregnancy, menopause) promote the release of lead from bone. Lead is excreted primarily through the kidneys at a rate of about 30 μg/day, which may increase to 200 μg/day with higher body burdens.

TABLE 21-1 COMMON SOURCES OF ADULT LEAD EXPOSURE

OCCUPATIONAL	NONOCCUPATIONAL
Manufacturing Manufacture of storage batteries Secondary smelting Manufacture of primary batteries Primary smelting Welding and cutting operations	Shooting firearms Remodeling or renovation activities Hobbies (e.g., casting, ceramics, stained glass) Retained bullets or gunshot wounds Pica Contaminated food, liquid, or nontraditional medications
Construction Special trade contractors Painting, paperhanging, decorating Lead abatement workers	
Mining Mining of lead and zinc ores	
Wholesale trades Wholesale distribution of electrical apparatus and equipment, wiring supplies, and construction materials	
Retail trades Automobile repair shops	
Transportation, communication, electric, gas, and sanitary services	

TABLE 21-2 SUMMARY OF CLINICAL LEAD TOXICITY

BLOOD LEAD LEVEL (μG/DL)	EFFECTS
<10	Aminolevulinic acid dehydrase inhibition
15–30	Elevation of erythrocyte protoporphyrin
30–39	Mild elevations in blood pressure Altered testicular function
40–49	Increased coproporphyrins and urinary aminolevulinic acid Slowed peripheral nerve conduction
50–59	Reduced hemoglobin synthesis Neurologic symptoms
60–69	Reproductive effects in women
80–90	Anemia Encephalopathic symptoms Nephropathy
100	Encephalopathic signs

CLINICAL MANIFESTATIONS

Lead binds to sulfhydryl groups and adversely affects zinc- and calcium-dependent enzyme systems. This binding interferes with heme synthesis, DNA transcription, and calcium-dependent release of neurotransmitters and of protein kinase C, which regulate cell growth, learning, and memory. In addition, lead affects membrane integrity, steroid metabolism, and vitamin D synthesis in renal tubular cells, and it produces motor axon degeneration and segmental demyelination. The clinical manifestations of lead toxicity are roughly related to the blood lead level (Table 21-2).

Cardiovascular System

A cross-sectional study of 2165 women aged 40 to 59 years found that a change in blood lead levels from the lowest quartile (mean, 1.0 μg/dL; range, 0.5 to 1.6 μg/dL) to the highest quartile (mean, 6.3 μg/dL; range, 4.0 to 31.1 μg/dL) was associated with a significant increase in systolic (by 1.7 mm Hg) and diastolic (by 1.4 mm Hg) blood pressures. At blood lead levels between 10 and 40 μg/dL, lead increases systolic blood pressure by 1 to 2 mm Hg and diastolic pressure by 1.4 mm Hg for every doubling of the blood lead level. Workers with mean blood lead levels between 40 and 70 μg/dL have an increased risk of death from renal and hypertensive cardiovascular disease. The progression, mechanisms, and effects of therapeutic intervention are unclear in lead-associated hypertension.

Reproductive System

Workplace exposure to lead is associated with decreased fertility, spontaneous abortions, stillbirths, low birthweights, and increased infant mortality. At mean blood levels above 23 μg/dL, lead has a direct toxic effect on spermatogenesis, resulting in decreased sperm counts and abnormal sperm morphology and function.

Renal System

Lead accumulates in proximal tubule cells. Reported clinical findings include Fanconi's syndrome, increased urate excretion, chronic interstitial nephritis, and interference in the renin-aldosterone system. In a population with a mean blood lead level of 8.1 μg/dL, a 10 μg/dL increase in blood lead level was associated with a decrease in creatinine clearance of 10.4 mL/minute.

Nervous System

Chronic encephalopathy is more common than acute encephalopathy (Chapter 422). Early encephalopathic manifestations include changes in cognitive function and mood, early morning sleep disturbance, headache, irritability, lassitude, and loss of libido. Abnormalities in cognition or visual-motor function may be evident on psychometric testing. These findings may occur in workers with blood levels from 18 to 30 μg/dL but are more common in those with levels in the 40- to 60-μg/dL range. The decrease in neuropsychological performance may be comparable to that expected during aging of up to 20 years, although debate continues about the predictability of the effects of blood lead levels below 70 μg/dL. Many of these manifestations respond at least partially to a reduction in the blood lead level.

Lead affects peripheral nerve conduction. Lead-induced peripheral axonal neuropathy (Chapter 428) most commonly involves the motor nerves; it tends to be more severe in the upper extremities and on the dominant side. A subclinical decrease in ulnar nerve motor conduction velocity has been demonstrated at blood lead levels as low as 30 μg/dL. Lead poisoning also predisposes to the development of carpal tunnel and tarsal tunnel syndromes (Chapter 428).

Hematologic System

Lead affects the red cell membrane and interferes with enzymes involved in the synthesis of hemoglobin. The traditional findings in severe poisoning include a hypochromic microcytic anemia and basophilic stippling (Chapter 162).

DIAGNOSIS

The initial steps in the diagnosis of lead poisoning are to identify people involved in high-risk activities (see Table 21-1) and to determine the levels of lead in the venous (not capillary) blood. The diagnosis of lead poisoning should not rely on clinical symptoms and signs because these develop late and generally correlate poorly with blood lead levels. The blood lead level that triggers intervention is not well established for adults, and no national guidelines exist for managing adults with lead poisoning. It is in the best interest of the patient to follow the most conservative standards: a confirmed venous blood lead level of 40 μg/dL or greater should trigger intervention, including improved industrial hygiene, better dust control, and increased ventilation.

TREATMENT Rx

Treatment is designed to prevent further exposure, to reduce the blood lead level to an acceptable range, and to repair any existing damage. Removal of an individual from a lead environment is recommended if the blood lead level is 50 μg/dL or greater on three tests over 6 months or if a medical condition consistent with lead poisoning has been identified. Removal from the lead source is often associated with a gradual reduction in blood lead levels. Chelation therapy is generally recommended if symptoms or signs are present or if the blood lead level is above 60 μg/dL (Table 21-3).

Calcium disodium ethylenediaminetetraacetic acid ($CaNa_2EDTA$) is the first-line drug for treating asymptomatic adults with high blood lead levels. In the treatment of symptomatic lead poisoning (with or without encephalopathy), $CaNa_2EDTA$ is used in conjunction with dimercaprol (2,3-dimercaptopropanol or BAL). Larger doses of $CaNa_2EDTA$ (50 to 75 mg/kg/day) are used for more severely poisoned patients. A third chelator, succimer (meso-2,3-dimercaptosuccinic acid, DMSA), is approved for the treatment of children with blood lead levels above 45 μg/dL; although succimer has not been approved by the Food and Drug Administration (FDA) for the treatment of adult lead poisoning, adults have been treated successfully with succimer, and it should be considered in place of $CaNa_2EDTA$ monotherapy. D-Penicillamine (3-mercapto-D-valine or penicillamine) is not recommended for the treatment of adult lead poisoning because of the high incidence of adverse drug reactions.

Chelation removes lead from the blood and soft tissues, but little is removed from bone. Redistribution of lead from deep stores after chelation may result in a rebound of blood lead levels and the redevelopment of clinical toxicity. For this reason, individuals should have their blood lead levels measured 2 weeks after the course of chelation has been completed. In general, the clinical response to chelation therapy is variable, and the data demonstrating improved outcomes are not robust. After chelation, if the blood lead level rises into the toxic range or symptoms recur, another course of chelation is indicated, with the same dose and duration used originally.

Mercury

DEFINITION

There are three chemical forms of mercury. Elemental or metallic mercury (Hg^0, quicksilver) is a silver liquid at room temperature. Inorganic mercury occurs in either a mercurous (Hg^+) or a mercuric (Hg^{++}) state. Organic mercurials are attached to short (ethyl or methyl) or long (alkyl or aryl) carbon chains. Each form of mercury can be found in a variety of occupations and products.

EPIDEMIOLOGY

The different chemical forms of mercury enter and are distributed throughout the body via different delivery systems. From a clinical perspective, the most important target organ is the central nervous system, even though the kidney accumulates the most mercury regardless of the chemical type. Chronic poisoning with any of the chemical forms of mercury results in central nervous system toxicity. Ingestion of organic mercury is the most efficient way to get mercury into the brain, followed by the inhalation of elemental mercury vapor; ingestion of inorganic mercury is the least efficient.

PATHOBIOLOGY

Mercury produces toxicity by binding to sulfhydryl groups, thereby inhibiting enzyme systems and disrupting cell membrane integrity. Mercury also binds to amide, amine, carboxyl, and phosphoryl groups. Methyl mercury inhibits choline acetyltransferase, a critical enzyme in the formation of acetylcholine.

Elemental mercury is or has been used in dental amalgams, calibration instruments, electroplating, gold extraction, manometers, and thermometers. Elemental mercury pooled under carpets or floorboards in homes has resulted in clinical toxicity. Chronic parenteral injection of elemental mercury—no longer prescribed medically, but still rarely done by individuals—may produce neurotoxicity. However, ingested elemental mercury is poorly absorbed from the gastrointestinal tract and causes virtually no toxicity. Conversely, nearly 75% of inhaled elemental mercury vapor is absorbed through the lungs. Once it is absorbed, elemental mercury is distributed to the tissues and red blood cells, where it is oxidized to the mercuric form. Some elemental mercury crosses the blood-brain barrier, and oxidation within the central nervous system leads to an accumulation of divalent mercury in the brain because ionized mercury does not readily cross the blood-brain barrier.

Inorganic mercury may be a component of disinfectants, fireworks, preservatives, and photograph developing chemicals. Application of creams or ointments containing inorganic mercury to intact or damaged skin may result in systemic absorption of mercury. Inorganic mercury solutions are corrosive to the gastrointestinal tract, but up to 15% of ingested inorganic mercury is absorbed through the gastrointestinal mucosa. After absorption, the inorganic mercury salt is ionized and penetrates the blood-brain barrier poorly. However, absorbed divalent mercury can be reduced to the metallic form, which does cross the blood-brain barrier.

Organic mercurials are used as pesticides, preservatives, and disinfectants. Coal-fired power plants are a major source of mercury

TABLE 21-3 GENERAL GUIDELINES FOR CHELATION THERAPY

DRUG	ADULT DOSE	INDICATIONS	CONTRAINDICATIONS AND CAUTIONS
Dimercaprol, British antilewisite (BAL)	3–5 mg/kg (75 mg/m^2) IM every 4 hr for 2 days; then every 6 hr for 2 days; then every 12 hr for up to an additional 7 days	Lead: symptomatic poisoning	Administration is by deep intramuscular injections, which are painful Dimercaprol is often administered with $CaNa_2EDTA$ The vehicle is peanut oil—do *not* use intravenously; use is contraindicated in those with peanut allergy
$CaNa_2EDTA$, edetate calcium disodium	20–30 mg/kg/day (1000–1500 mg/m^2/day) as a continuous infusion for 5 days	Lead: symptomatic poisoning or asymptomatic patients with high blood lead levels Manganese: symptomatic patients with blood, serum, or urine manganese levels above reference values	Do *not* use Na_2EDTA $CaNa_2EDTA$ can be given IM in two or three divided doses High doses of $CaNa_2EDTA$ increase zinc excretion and may be toxic to renal glomeruli and proximal tubules
Dimercaptopropanesulfonate (DMPS)	100 mg orally four times/day for 7 days; may repeat therapeutic course after 7 days without therapy if levels are still elevated	Arsenic: symptomatic patients with urine arsenic levels ≥50 µg/L; asymptomatic patients with urine arsenic levels >200 µg/L Manganese: symptomatic patients with blood, serum, or urine manganese levels above reference values Bismuth: symptomatic patients with bismuth blood levels >50 µg/L or urine levels >150 µg/L	
Deferoxamine	6 g as a continuous IV infusion given over 24 hr; may repeat if serum levels are still elevated	Aluminum: symptomatic patients with serum aluminum levels >100 µg/L	
Dimercaptosuccinic acid (DMSA), succimer	10 mg/kg (350 mg/m^2) orally every 8 hr for 5 days; then 10 mg/kg every12 hr for 14 days	Lead: symptomatic poisoning or asymptomatic patients with high blood lead levels Mercury: symptomatic patients with mercury whole blood levels >10 µg/L or 24-hr urine levels ≥20 µg/L	Succimer has a sulfur-like odor

in the environment. Elemental and inorganic mercurials deposited in the environment are bioconverted into organic mercury compounds that are a recognized contaminant of the food chain, particularly in fish. Consumption of fish is the source of nearly all the methyl mercury in the general population. The FDA and the Environmental Protection Agency (EPA) recommend the avoidance of fish with the highest mercury concentrations—king mackerel, shark, swordfish, and tilefish from the Gulf of Mexico. Women of childbearing age and pregnant women should limit their consumption of medium-mercury fish: fresh tuna steak, canned white or albacore tuna, grouper, orange roughy, saltwater trout, bluefish, lobster, halibut, haddock, snapper, and crab. In addition, caution is urged regarding the consumption of fish from local lakes and ponds, which may be more polluted than commercial fish sources.

Organic mercury is highly lipid soluble, well absorbed through the gastrointestinal tract, and widely distributed throughout the body. Organic mercury compounds are metabolized in the body; longer chain mercury compounds are rapidly metabolized to inorganic mercury, whereas short-chain mercury compounds (e.g., methyl mercury) are slowly metabolized to inorganic mercury. Organic mercury readily crosses the blood-brain barrier, and oxidation within the central nervous system leads to the accumulation of mercuric ions in the brain.

CLINICAL MANIFESTATIONS

The chronic inhalation of elemental mercury vapor results in two syndromes. The first syndrome consists of neuropsychiatric manifestations, gingivostomatitis, and tremor. The tremor (Chapter 417) is evident at rest or with motion and may be aggravated with purposeful movement. The second syndrome is erythism, a neuropsychiatric constellation of findings that includes fatigue, insomnia, memory impairment, nervousness, irritability, shyness, social withdrawal, loss of confidence, timidity, and depression.

Chronic occupational exposure to inorganic mercury may cause subclinical psychomotor and neuromuscular abnormalities as well as long-term behavioral impairment. Neuropsychiatric abnormalities (inattention, memory, construction, and motor performance) appear to be dose related (Chapter 409).

Methyl mercury poisoning is cumulative and develops over several years. Based on epidemics of methyl mercury poisoning in Japan and Iraq in which large quantities of organic mercury were consumed, the initial symptoms are fatigue and perioral and extremity paresthesia, followed by difficulty with hand movements and disturbances of vision. The classic picture of methyl mercury poisoning is the gradual onset of ataxia, constricted visual fields, and dysarthria. Other findings are paresthesia, deafness, incoordination, loss of voluntary movement, and mental retardation. The full picture of toxicity is that of psychological, cerebellar, sensory, and motor abnormalities. However, moderate amounts of methyl mercury in the diet have not been linked to adverse effects in adults; most concern relates to potential toxic effects on the fetus and its developing central nervous system.

DIAGNOSIS

The diagnosis of mercury poisoning requires a history of exposure, compatible clinical findings, and elevated mercury levels in blood or urine.

The mean total mercury levels in whole blood and urine in the general population are 1 to 8 µg/L and 4 to 5 µg/L, respectively. Although elevated blood or urine mercury levels are consistent with clinical toxicity, clinical signs or symptoms are poorly correlated with blood or urine mercury levels because of substantial intraindividual and interindividual variation. For example, data in urban adults (mean age, 59 years) showed no significant association between blood mercury levels (mean, 2.1 µg/L; range, 0 to 16 µg/L) and neurobehavioral performance.

A 1 : 1 ratio of red blood cell to plasma mercury suggests inorganic mercury poisoning, whereas a ratio of 10 : 1 suggests organic mercury toxicity. Red blood cell and plasma mercury levels should be requested if the source and type of mercury exposure are unknown. Methyl mercury blood levels of 3 to 5 µg/dL may be found in patients with symptoms. Determination of a methyl mercury level is recommended if the exposure is to a contaminated environmental source.

Arsenic

DEFINITION

Arsenic is a naturally occurring omnipresent element that exists in three valence states: elemental or metallic arsenic (As^0), trivalent (arsenite, As^{3+}), and pentavalent (arsenate, As^{5+}). The trivalent form of arsenic (arsenite) is the most toxic and is responsible for the worldwide public health concern about chronic arsenic poisoning. Organic alkane arsenicals are of low toxicity, and elemental arsenic is virtually nontoxic.

TREATMENT Rx

Asymptomatic patients with elevated urine mercury levels should have the analyses repeated after a 4-week period without fish consumption.

A patient with mercury poisoning should immediately be removed from the contaminated environment; the source of the mercury must then be identified and removed. Treatment is primarily symptomatic and supportive.

Chelation therapy (see Table 21-3) is used to increase the excretion of mercury, even though improved clinical outcomes have not been demonstrated; increased urinary excretion of mercury alone has become an accepted if empirical clinical goal. There is little agreement on the indications for the initiation or cessation of chelation therapy. The presence of clinical toxicity combined with elevated mercury levels is an accepted indication for chelation therapy, but its role in asymptomatic individuals with mercury levels above background values is controversial. A reasonable end point for chelation is the achievement of background levels of mercury in urine or blood (<20 μg/L or 10 μg/L, respectively). Fish eaters with elevated mercury levels should avoid eating any fish or shellfish for 1 month, after which mercury levels in blood or urine should be reanalyzed. If mercury levels have come down to reference values, low-mercury fish (shrimp, canned light tuna, salmon, pollock, catfish) can be reintroduced into the diet at a frequency of no more than two meals per week.

Succimer (see Table 21-3) is the chelator of choice because it can be given orally and has been effective in reducing brain levels of methyl mercury in animal studies. D-Penicillamine is less effective than succimer and has a higher adverse drug reaction rate. Dimercaprol is not recommended because of its potential to shift mercury from peripheral tissues into the brain. N-acetylcysteine has been proposed as a chelator of methyl mercury, and repeated oral administration may interrupt the enterohepatic recirculation of methyl mercury; however, use of the drug for this purpose has not undergone clinical trials and is not approved by the FDA.

EPIDEMIOLOGY

The major sources of human exposure to arsenic are the environment (mining, seafood, groundwater) and industry (pesticides, pigments, wood preservatives, glass or metal manufacturing, electronics, folk remedies). The arsenic content in the average North American adult diet is less than 1 μg/kg/day. Arsenic in seafood is primarily in the form of organic arsenicals, and the content is variable; freshwater fish may have up to 2 mg/kg, whereas lobster may have up to 22 mg/kg. The EPA drinking water standard is 10 μg/L.

PATHOBIOLOGY

Nearly 90% of ingested or inhaled arsenic is absorbed; little arsenic is absorbed through intact skin. Absorbed arsenic is widely distributed throughout the body, but no form of arsenic readily crosses the blood-brain barrier. Pentavalent arsenic and trivalent arsenic undergo oxidation-reduction reactions, converting one form to the other. Pentavalent arsenic is reduced by glutathione to the more toxic trivalent form. Methylation of trivalent arsenic produces the less toxic monomethylarsenate and dimethylarsenate metabolites, which are excreted in the urine. Organic arsenicals, such as those found in seafood, are essentially nontoxic; they are not metabolized to toxic forms of arsenic and are rapidly excreted in the urine, with an elimination half-life of 4 to 6 hours.

Arsenite (As^{3+}) binds to sulfhydryl groups, resulting in the inhibition of many enzyme systems (glycolysis, pyruvate dehydrogenase, Krebs cycle) and the decreased production of adenosine triphosphate. Arsenate (As^{5+}) replaces phosphate in microsomal enzyme systems, resulting in the uncoupling of oxidative phosphorylation and the decreased production of adenosine triphosphate. Pentavalent arsenate does not bind to sulfhydryl groups. Inorganic arsenic is a human carcinogen.

CLINICAL MANIFESTATIONS

Chronic poisoning develops after the ingestion or inhalation of arsenic over weeks to months, depending on the daily dose. Clinical manifestations develop gradually and are highly variable among exposed individuals. Typical initial manifestations include nonspecific complaints such as a metallic taste in the mouth, anorexia, weight loss, malaise, and weakness.

Skin lesions are some of the most common and earliest nonmalignant toxic effects. Typical dermal findings include melanosis (trunk and extremities), hyperpigmentation (tongue, oral mucosa, axilla), hyperkeratosis (palm, sole), and brittle nails. Less common or late findings include alopecia and white transverse bands (Mees' lines) in the nails (Chapter 450).

Later findings involve the nervous system and carcinogenesis. Neurologic effects are both central and peripheral. Central effects include mild dementia (Chapter 409) and headache; cranial nerves are normal. Peripheral sensory and motor neuropathies (Chapter 428) develop in a stocking-and-glove distribution and cause muscle weakness, muscle atrophy, and ataxia.

Malignant neoplasms include Bowen's disease, basal cell carcinoma, and squamous cell carcinoma (Chapter 210). Lung cancer (Chapter 197) may result from the inhalation of dust containing high levels of arsenic. Arsenic in drinking water has been associated with leukemia, bladder cancer, renal cancer, hepatic cancer, and uterine cancer (Chapter 183). The cancer risk from arsenic in drinking water may be dose related. Studies of populations outside the United States show increases in cancer only when arsenic concentrations in drinking water measure more than several hundred micrograms per liter. Studies of U.S. populations exposed to average drinking water arsenic concentrations of about 190 μg/L have not demonstrated evidence of increased cancer.

Cardiovascular disease includes atherosclerosis, coronary artery disease, and hypertension. Blackfoot disease, peculiar to the southwestern coast of Taiwan, is a form of peripheral vascular disease that results in gangrene of the lower extremities. Other manifestations of exposure to arsenic in drinking water include chronic cough, type 2 diabetes, and reproductive abnormalities such as congenital malformations, miscarriages, and low birthweights.

DIAGNOSIS

The diagnosis of chronic arsenic poisoning depends on an appropriate history of exposure (including a source), compatible clinical manifestations, and documentation of an elevated body burden of arsenic. Principal sources of arsenic are environmental (contaminated water, air, soil) and occupational or industrial. Although seafood may be a source of organic arsenic, it is not associated with clinical toxicity.

Arsenic can be measured in the hair, blood, or urine. Hair analysis is a suboptimal method of determining chronic toxicity. Environmental arsenic is adsorbed to the external surface of the hair and is difficult to remove by washing. Arsenic levels vary within a single hair and among hairs, and there is significant interindividual variability in adsorption of arsenic to hair. Nonetheless, the normal arsenic hair levels are less than 1 μg/g dry weight, and arsenic levels in hair from people with chronic toxicity range from 1 to 5 μg/g or more.

Blood levels of arsenic reflect only very recent exposure and are not reliable indicators of chronic exposure to low levels of arsenic. For example, there is no correlation between blood arsenic levels and drinking water arsenic levels of 6 to 125 μg/L.

Normal urine arsenic levels are less than 50 μg/L or less than 25 μg/24 hours in the absence of seafood consumption. Among people aged 6 years and older in the United States, the 95th percentile for total urinary arsenic is 65.4 μg/L. Urine arsenic levels above 200 μg/L are abnormal. The average urine arsenic level among people with chronic toxicity is 207 μg of

TREATMENT Rx

Treatment approaches can be stratified according to symptoms and urine levels of inorganic arsenic (Table 21-4). All patients who are symptomatic or who have urine inorganic arsenic levels of 50 μg/L or above should be removed from the source of the arsenic.

Dimercaptopropanesulfonate (DMPS) is the most widely studied chelating agent for chronic arsenic poisoning and is the drug of choice, although it is not approved by the FDA. DMPS forms a water-soluble complex with monomethyl arsenic that is excreted in the urine. In a randomized trial, DMPS therapy (100 mg orally four times/day on alternate weeks for 7 weeks) increased urine arsenic excretion and improved weakness, pigmentation, and lung disease, but it did not improve hematologic and blood chemistry abnormalities, neuropathy, hepatomegaly, keratosis, or skin histology.[1] Chelation should continue until the urine arsenic level is below 50 μg/L. Succimer has not been successful in treating chronic arsenic toxicity, and dimercaprol is not recommended because the lipid-soluble dimercaprol-arsenic complex penetrates the blood-brain barrier. The effectiveness of selenium and vitamin E supplementation in ameliorating arsenic-induced skin changes is controversial.

TABLE 21-4 ARSENIC TREATMENT STRATIFICATION

INORGANIC ARSENIC LEVELS IN URINE (μG/L)	SYMPTOMATIC	ASYMPTOMATIC
<50	Supportive care	No treatment
50–200	Chelation*	Monitor 24-hr urine levels monthly
>200	Chelation*	Chelation*

*Using DMPS (see Table 21-3).

inorganic arsenic per gram of creatinine. Because urine analysis measures total arsenic, elevated levels should be speciated to determine the fractions of inorganic and organic arsenic. If this analysis is not possible, seafood should be eliminated from the patient's diet for 1 week, and the urine analysis repeated.

A nerve conduction study is not a reliable diagnostic tool for chronic arsenic toxicity. Among patients with elevated urine arsenic levels, the results of nerve conduction tests do not correlate well with the presence or absence of clinical neuropathy.

Cadmium

EPIDEMIOLOGY

Cadmium is found as a metal and in a number of industrial chemicals. Cadmium may enter the environment through contamination, fuel combustion, or fertilizer. The majority of cadmium is used occupationally in nickel-cadmium batteries and to protect polyvinyl chloride against heat and light. Cadmium is used as a pigment in coloring the red bags used for infectious hospital waste. When they are incinerated, these bags release cadmium into the environment, so medical waste incinerators are an important environmental source of cadmium. The largest source of most human exposure to cadmium is dietary, with an average daily intake of 10 to 30 μg. Cadmium exposure is doubled in people who smoke tobacco.

PATHOBIOLOGY

Approximately 25% of inhaled cadmium is absorbed. Although normally only 5% of ingested cadmium is absorbed, gastrointestinal absorption is increased in the presence of calcium or iron deficiency or high dietary fat. Cadmium concentrates in the liver and kidneys. Cadmium is poorly excreted from the body; the geometric mean terminal half-life for elimination in creatinine-adjusted urine is estimated to be 19 years. The kidney is the primary target organ in chronic toxicity.

CLINICAL MANIFESTATIONS

The clinical picture of chronic cadmium toxicity is one of irreversible renal toxicity (Chapter 124). Proximal tubule damage results in high urine concentrations of low-molecular-weight proteins, amino acids, glucose, phosphate, and calcium. Decreased glomerular filtration rate and nephrolithiasis may occur. Renal failure is common.

The renal pathophysiologic process may result in calcium deficiency, osteoporosis, osteomalacia, and bone fractures. Other clinical manifestations of chronic cadmium poisoning include male infertility, slowing of visual-motor functioning, and peripheral neuropathies.

The EPA and the International Agency for Research on Cancer have designated cadmium a probable human carcinogen. However, this designation is controversial, and chronic exposure to cadmium may not increase cancer rates. For example, residents of a cadmium-polluted village in England had no increase in cancer rates; a study of residents of a cadmium-polluted area in Belgium found no increase in prostate, kidney, or urinary tract cancers; a retrospective comparison of Japanese residents in high, low, and no cadmium-polluted areas found no differences in cancer mortality; and a study of copper-cadmium alloy workers found no increased risk of lung cancer.

DIAGNOSIS

A tentative diagnosis of chronic cadmium poisoning can be confirmed by measuring elevated urinary cadmium levels (>5 μg/L) and elevated urinary microprotein levels, particularly β_1-microglobulin.

TREATMENT Rx

Treatment of the toxic effects of cadmium is symptomatic and supportive. There is no accepted way to reduce the body burden of cadmium. The use of $CaNa_2EDTA$ or dimercaprol may increase nephrotoxicity. Succimer and N-acetylcysteine have achieved favorable results in animal studies, but neither has been adequately evaluated in human studies.

Manganese

DEFINITION

Manganese is an increasingly important toxin, both environmentally and occupationally. Manganese exists as a metal (metallic manganese, ferromanganese), as inorganic manganese (e.g., chloride or sulfate salts), or as organic manganese.

EPIDEMIOLOGY

Metallic manganese is used in steel production. Inorganic manganese (Mn^{2+}, Mn^{3+}, and Mn^{4+}) is most commonly found in industry and in the environment. Various inorganic manganese compounds are involved in the manufacture of animal feed, batteries, fertilizers, fireworks, fungicides, matches, and potassium permanganate. Organic manganese compounds are used as a fuel oil additive, as fungicides, and as a gasoline additive (methylcyclopentadienyl manganese tricarbonyl [MMT]). Neurotoxicity seen in methcathinone (street name "Cat") abusers has been attributed to manganese.

Manganese is an essential nutrient, acting as a cofactor in enzymatic reactions involving bone mineralization as well as protein and carbohydrate metabolism. As such, it is often a component of parenteral nutrition preparations, and chronic infusion can result in manganese toxicity. Substantial exposure to manganese occurs in people who work in welding, mining, and foundry occupations. People who work with gasoline or as automobile mechanics may be exposed to MMT.

PATHOBIOLOGY

Manganese is absorbed through the gastrointestinal and respiratory tracts and is distributed widely throughout the body. Manganese accumulates in the globus pallidus of the basal ganglia. Bile is the principal route of excretion. The elimination half-life is approximately 40 days, but it is longer for manganese in the central nervous system.

The primary target organ is the central nervous system. Despite the fact that manganese adversely affects enzymes, receptors, and transport systems, the exact mechanisms of toxicity are unclear. A characteristic finding in chronic manganese poisoning is the selective destruction of dopaminergic neurons. The pathophysiologic mechanism is uncertain, but one hypothesis is that Mn^{2+} causes oxidation, the production of free radicals or reactive oxygen species, or the depletion of antioxidants.

CLINICAL MANIFESTATIONS

People who work with manganese may develop a syndrome similar to but not identical with Parkinson's disease (Chapter 416). Findings include an extrapyramidal syndrome (masklike facies, tremor of the extremities at rest or on extension, bradykinesia, stooped posture, shuffling gait, propulsion abnormalities).

Several clinical characteristics may help distinguish between Parkinson's disease and manganese-induced parkinsonism. Manganese-poisoned patients have a "cock walk" and a propensity to fall backward when pushed. These patients often exhibit psychological disturbances early in the disease process. So-called manganese madness includes aggression, irritability, nervousness, and destructive behavior. Uncontrollable spasmodic crying or laughing, singing or dancing, or unfocused running around have been described.

DIAGNOSIS

The initial diagnosis of chronic manganese poisoning relies on a history of exposure and consistent clinical findings. In patients with significant central nervous system findings, T1-weighted magnetic resonance imaging that shows bilateral, symmetrical hyperdensities in the globus pallidus lends strong support to the diagnosis of chronic manganese poisoning.

Positron emission tomography may identify reduced striatal dopamine release.

Manganese levels in body fluids are helpful in establishing a diagnosis. Reference ranges have been established: blood, 40 to 140 μg/L; serum, 1.5 to 26.5 μg/L; and urine, 9.7 to 10.7 μg/L.

TREATMENT

Treatment of chronic manganese toxicity starts with removing the source of the manganese and providing supportive care. The results of chelation with $CaNa_2EDTA$ or DMPS (see Table 21-3) have been equivocal. Although levodopa responsiveness is a hallmark of Parkinson's disease, welders with manganese-induced parkinsonism treated with levodopa showed no improvement over placebo-treated control subjects.

Nickel

EPIDEMIOLOGY

Nickel is absorbed through the lungs, gastrointestinal tract, and skin. Water-soluble nickel compounds (e.g., nickel chloride or sulfate) are absorbed better than insoluble nickel is. Approximately 25% of the nickel in drinking water is absorbed. Nickel applied to the skin is absorbed into the skin but may not reach the circulation. The urine is the primary means of excretion of nickel from the body.

PATHOBIOLOGY

Nickel is used in a large number of metal alloys and in batteries, electroplating (e.g., table cutlery and some jewelry), coins, surgical staples, and some joint prostheses. Nickel is also present in drinking water; the EPA standard is 0.02 mg/kg/day.

Nickel appears to be an essential element in the body, but its physiologic role is unclear. Nickel crosses the cell membrane through calcium channels and competes with calcium for some receptors.

CLINICAL MANIFESTATIONS

Contact dermatitis (Chapter 446) is the most common manifestation of nickel toxicity. Exposure to consumer products containing nickel, particularly jewelry, causes sensitization and contact dermatitis in as many as 30% of people. Once sensitization has occurred, the severity of subsequent reactions is related to the dose of nickel.

Chronic occupational exposure to nickel dust and fumes has been associated with respiratory tract disease, including nasal, laryngeal, and lung cancers (Chapter 183). The EPA has identified nickel dust and nickel subsulfide as class A human carcinogens. Exposure to nickel in nonindustrial settings, such as ingestion of nickel in water or food or dermal contact, has not been associated with an increased risk of cancer.

DIAGNOSIS

Nickel levels in blood or urine are not useful in establishing either excessive exposure or risk of disease.

TREATMENT

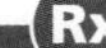

There is no specific treatment of nickel-induced dermal sensitivity.

OTHER TOXIC METALS

Aluminum

EPIDEMIOLOGY

Aluminum is the most abundant metal. It is widely available in consumer products such as food, water, cookware, food wraps, cans, antiperspirants, medications (especially antacids and phosphate binders), and dialysate fluids. North Americans consume 7 to 9 mg of aluminum in their diets each day. Industrial exposure to aluminum may result in significant toxicity.

PATHOBIOLOGY

Gastrointestinal tract absorption of aluminum ranges from 0.1 to 1%. Once it is absorbed, aluminum is bound to transferrin and distributed throughout the body, concentrating in bone and lung. The kidneys are the primary route of aluminum excretion, and a compromised ability to excrete aluminum is an important factor in the development of aluminum toxicity outside of the occupational setting. Rare individuals may accumulate significant amounts of aluminum from antiperspirants.

Aluminum blocks the incorporation of calcium into bones and inhibits osteoblastic and osteoclastic activity. In patients with renal failure, aluminum has been identified as a potential contributor to anemia, dialysis encephalopathy, and renal osteodystrophy.

CLINICAL MANIFESTATIONS

The central nervous system is a target organ for aluminum toxicity. The findings in dialysis encephalopathy (Chapters 132 and 133), which develops over months, include stuttering or stammering speech, directional disorientation, personality changes, myoclonus, motor apraxia, convulsions, and hallucinations. Industrial aluminum workers have developed cognitive defects, depression, incoordination, poor memory, and tremor. The relationship between aluminum exposure and Alzheimer's disease is controversial.

Chronic exposure to excessive aluminum may cause osteomalacia (Chapter 252), spontaneous fractures, and bone pain. Hypochromic, microcytic anemia (Chapter 162) that is unresponsive to iron therapy correlates with aluminum levels in the plasma or erythrocytes. Aluminum workers have an increased risk for the development of lung or bladder cancer (Chapter 203).

DIAGNOSIS

The background serum aluminum levels in normal individuals are less than 10 μg/L. Patients undergoing chronic dialysis may have serum aluminum levels up to 50 μg/L. Levels above 60 μg/L indicate increased absorption, serum levels above 100 μg/L are potentially toxic, and serum levels above 200 μg/L are usually associated with clinical symptoms and signs of toxicity.

TREATMENT

Elevated serum aluminum levels can be brought down with extracorporeal clearance techniques, such as hemodialysis and hemofiltration. Deferoxamine (see Table 21-3) is indicated when serum aluminum levels exceed 100 μg/L. In hemodialysis patients, 2.5 mg/kg/week is as effective as the standard dose of deferoxamine (5 mg/kg/week) for treating aluminum overload. 2

Beryllium

EPIDEMIOLOGY

Beryllium occurs naturally in rocks, coal, oil, soil, and volcanic dust. Commercially, beryllium is used in metal alloys for aerospace, aircraft, sports equipment (golf clubs, bicycle frames), and automotive manufacturing; in electronics and computers; in ceramics; and in defense weapons. Beryllium is naturally present in tobacco and may be inhaled during smoking.

PATHOBIOLOGY

Inhaled beryllium is cleared from the respiratory tract by mucociliary action and alveolar macrophages. Once it is absorbed, beryllium is distributed to the bones, liver, kidneys, lung parenchyma, and lymphatic system. The kidney is the primary route of beryllium excretion.

Repeated exposure to beryllium causes a cell-mediated immune response involving T lymphocytes and the release of T_H1 cytokines in genetically susceptible persons (Chapter 93). The cell-mediated response is persistent and results in the accumulation of immune effector cells (sensitized T lymphocytes, macrophages) that form granulomas and mononuclear cell infiltrations. A genetic predisposition to the development of chronic beryllium disease has been postulated. Dermal exposure to beryllium may cause irritative or atopic dermatitis as well as beryllium-containing foreign bodies and granulomas. The EPA considers beryllium to be a probable human carcinogen.

CLINICAL MANIFESTATIONS

Chronic beryllium disease is a progressive systemic hypersensitivity disease affecting the lungs and lymphatic system (Chapter 93). Clinical effects include progressive dyspnea, chest pain, weight loss, fatigue, anorexia, and fevers. Skin lesions, lymphadenopathy, and hepatosplenomegaly may occur. The pulmonary disease is progressive and may lead to respiratory failure within several years.

On pulmonary function testing, one third of patients have a predominantly obstructive pattern; one fourth have a predominantly restrictive pattern; one third have a reduced carbon monoxide diffusion capacity, with normal airflow and lung volumes; and some have a mix of obstruction and restriction (Chapter 85). A chest radiograph is normal early in the course, but later it shows diffuse bilateral infiltrates and hilar lymphadenopathy. Beryllium sensitivity is confirmed by the blood beryllium lymphocyte proliferation test. Tissue for histologic analysis from transbronchial or open lung biopsy may confirm the diagnosis.

TREATMENT Rx

Treatment involves removing the patient from exposure to beryllium, slowing or halting the progression of the disease with corticosteroids, and providing symptomatic and supportive care.

Bismuth

EPIDEMIOLOGY

Bismuth has been used in the treatment of gastrointestinal disorders such as ulcers, diarrhea, and *Helicobacter pylori* infection. Two forms of bismuth are toxic; lipid-soluble organic compounds (e.g., bismuth subgallate) are neurotoxic, and some water-soluble organic compounds (e.g., bismuth triglycollamate) are nephrotoxic.

PATHOBIOLOGY

Parenterally administered bismuth is distributed throughout the body but concentrates in the kidneys and liver. Elimination is through the kidneys, with a terminal elimination half-life of 3 to 10 weeks.

In the blood, bismuth binds to macroglobulins, immunoglobulins, lipoproteins, and haptoglobin. In the kidney, bismuth concentrates in the proximal tubule and causes necrosis. The mechanism of the neurologic effects is unclear.

CLINICAL MANIFESTATIONS

Chronic exposure to bismuth causes gastrointestinal, dermatologic, renal, and neurologic effects. Gastrointestinal effects include increased salivation, discoloration of the oral mucosa and gums, ulcerative stomatitis, nausea and vomiting, and diarrhea. Dermatologic effects are primarily a generalized rash after parenteral administration. Renal effects include nephritis, tubular necrosis, and renal failure.

The primary neurologic effect is an encephalopathy that develops in two distinct phases. The prodrome lasts up to several months and consists of asthenia, somnolence, depression, anxiety, and sometimes hallucinations. This prodrome is followed by the rapid onset (1 to 2 days) of encephalopathy characterized by confusion progressing to coma or dementia, dysarthria, disturbances of walking and standing, and tremor with myoclonic jerks. Chronic bismuth poisoning is associated with a distinctive electroencephalographic pattern: bilateral low-voltage diffuse beta frequencies that are maximal in the frontal and central regions and accentuated during hyperventilation.

The diagnosis of chronic bismuth toxicity is based on a history of exposure and a consistent clinical picture. Blood and urine levels of bismuth may be helpful. In chronic toxicity, the blood bismuth level is 50 to 1600 μg/L, and the urine level is 150 to 1250 μg/L. The median blood bismuth levels in patients with bismuth encephalopathy are in the range of 680 to 700 μg/L. In patients taking a bismuth product therapeutically, a blood bismuth level above 50 μg/L is a concern; a blood bismuth level above 100 μg/L is an indication to discontinue bismuth therapy.

TREATMENT 

Treatment of bismuth toxicity starts with stopping exposure to bismuth. DMPS administration (see Table 21-3) results in increased renal excretion of bismuth, but such therapy has not been shown to improve clinical outcomes.

Chromium

The most common forms of chromium in the environment are metallic chromium, trivalent chromium, and hexavalent chromium. Hexavalent chromium is the most toxic form. Trivalent chromium is essential for normal glucose tolerance; chromium picolinate is an alternative dietary supplement.

The trivalent and hexavalent chromiums are the most commonly used forms in industry. Chronic chromium toxicity is essentially an occupational disease related to tanning, metal alloys and electroplating (including surgical metals), photography, dyes, and cement.

Hexavalent chromium is absorbed primarily through the respiratory tract, with substantially smaller amounts absorbed through the gastrointestinal tract. The other valences are poorly absorbed. Hexavalent chromium is a skin and mucous membrane irritant. In dichromate compounds, hexavalent chromium binds to cellular and nuclear proteins and accumulates in red blood cells and platelets. Reduction of hexavalent to trivalent chromium creates intermediates that cause oxidative damage to DNA. Hexavalent chromium is a human carcinogen (lung cancer), but chromium and trivalent chromium are not classifiable. The EPA standard for chromium in drinking water is 100 μg/L.

Chronic occupational exposure to high levels of airborne hexavalent chromium has been associated with upper airway irritation (including nasal septum ulceration), bronchospasm, and an increased incidence of lung cancer. Repeated exposure to dichromate dust causes conjunctivitis and lacrimation. Dermal effects include irritation and chronic full-thickness ulcers. Chronic ingestion of high doses of chromium picolinate may cause renal impairment. The chronic drinking of water contaminated with hexavalent chromium may be associated with the development of stomach cancer. Reference levels of serum chromium are 0.05 to 0.16 μg/L. Treatment of chromium toxicity is symptomatic and supportive.

Cobalt

Cobalt is a naturally occurring element that exists as a metal, as a stable isotope, and as radioactive isotopes. The general public is rarely exposed to the radioactive isotopes (^{60}Co is used in radiation therapy). The metal is found in paints, enamels, and alloys used for household appliances, cutting tools, and joint replacements and surgical implants. Cobalt is a normal part of vitamin B_{12}. The average daily North American diet contains 5 to 40 μg of cobalt. Cobalt is absorbed through the gastrointestinal and respiratory tracts, distributed throughout the body, and excreted in the urine. Inhalation of cobalt is associated with obstructive and interstitial pulmonary disease. The interstitial pneumonitis is a fibrosing alveolitis, with leukocyte and multinucleated giant cell infiltration (Chapter 92). The process may be an immunoglobulin E–mediated response to cobalt reactivity. Chronic ingestion of or industrial exposure to cobalt produces a cardiomyopathy with pericardial effusions and biventricular heart failure (beer drinkers' cardiomyopathy of the 1960s). Cobalt levels are not useful in the diagnosis or management of chronic cobalt poisoning. The diagnosis is based on a history of exposure and compatible pulmonary findings. Medical evaluation should use standard methods for assessing pulmonary and cardiac function. Treatment consists of removing the patient from the source of cobalt and symptomatic and supportive care; both *N*-acetylcysteine and $CaNa_2EDTA$ have been used, but there is no definitive clinical evidence of benefit.

Selenium

Selenium is used in the vulcanization of rubber, the manufacture of some red glass, the electronics and semiconductor industries, and some pharmaceutical products and dandruff shampoos. Selenium is absorbed through the gastrointestinal and respiratory tracts and accumulates primarily in the liver and kidneys. Selenium is cleared from the body in the urine and feces. The mechanism of toxicity is not clear, but one hypothesis is that selenium inhibits sulfhydryl enzymes, resulting in a reduction in intracellular oxidative reactions.

Chronic exposure to selenium compounds in animals results in hepatotoxicity and decreased growth. In humans, dermal effects include alopecia, abnormal nail formation, and discoloration and decay of the teeth. Chronic high-dose dietary selenium can cause neurologic effects such as paresthesia and paresis. Elevated selenium levels in body fluids have been associated with clinical toxicity. The diagnosis of selenium toxicity relies on identification of a source, compatible clinical findings, and elevated whole blood selenium levels. Whole blood selenium levels vary with dietary intake; people with a normal selenium intake (90 to 168 μg/day) have levels ranging from 0.143 to 0.211 μg/L. Treatment of chronic selenium toxicity consists of removing

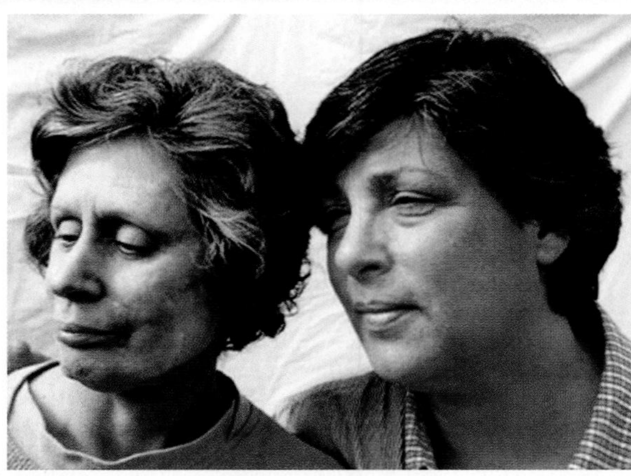

FIGURE 21-1. Fifty-six-year-old woman (left) who has had discolored skin since age 14 years. At age 11 the patient was given nose drops of unknown composition for "allergies," and 3 years later her skin turned gray. She has argyria; a skin biopsy confirmed silver deposition. A person with normal-colored skin (right) is shown for comparison. (From Bouts BA. Images in clinical medicine: Argyria. *N Engl J Med.* 1999;340:1554).

the patient from the selenium source and providing symptomatic and supportive care. Chelating agents are not useful.

Silver

Silver is used widely in photography, electronics, electrical equipment, metal alloys, and antibacterial agents. Silver is ingested in water and foods. Silver toxicity develops after the ingestion of at least 25 g of silver over 6 months.

Silver is absorbed through the gastrointestinal tract, lungs, and skin. Ingested silver undergoes a significant hepatic first-pass effect. Silver has a high affinity for sulfhydryl groups and other proteins. Inorganic silver salts precipitate intracellularly and in turn are complexed with DNA, RNA, and other proteins; alternatively, ascorbic acid or catecholamines can reduce silver salts to the metallic form. Silver is not carcinogenic. Silver is eliminated primarily in the feces; little is excreted in the urine.

The dermal picture of chronic silver poisoning is argyria, an irreversible blue-gray pigmentation of the skin (Fig. 21-1). In the kidneys, silver is deposited in the basement membrane of the glomerulus; altered renal function would be expected but has not been documented clinically. Silver levels in body fluids have not been useful in establishing the diagnosis of chronic silver intoxication. Diagnosis is based on a history of exposure and a compatible clinical picture. Reference levels of serum silver are less than 0.5 μg/L. Treatment of chronic silver intoxication consists of removing the patient from the silver source and providing symptomatic and supportive care. Chelating agents are not useful.

Uranium

Uranium causes toxicity because of its chemical effects or its radiation effects (Chapter 19). Uranium compounds are used in photography and as dyes or fixatives; depleted uranium is used in military equipment. Uranium is poorly absorbed from all exposed sites. Two percent of the uranium in drinking water and food is absorbed into the body. Two thirds of the uranium in the body is in the bones, and about 15% is in the liver.

Uranium decays into radium and then into radon, a radioactive gas that seeps into building foundations in particular geographic areas. Although radon is a respiratory carcinogen (Chapter 197), uranium itself is not carcinogenic. The chemical toxicity of uranium affects the kidneys and lungs. Uranium is nephrotoxic but has not led to increased mortality from renal disease in uranium workers. The injury to the lungs involves nonmalignant damage to alveolar type II cells, but it does not increase mortality from respiratory disease in uranium workers. Treatment of uranium toxicity consists of removing the patient from the uranium source and providing symptomatic and supportive care. Chelators are not recommended.

Although alkalinization of the urine with sodium bicarbonate enhances removal of the uranium molecule from the body, no interventions reduce the effects of chronic uranium toxicity.

Zinc

Zinc is a common element found in air, soil, water, and food. It is widely used in metal alloys, cosmetics, and medications and as an alternative dietary supplement. The oral bioavailability of zinc is variable and depends on the formulation and amount ingested. After ingestion, zinc is concentrated in the liver before being distributed throughout the body. Muscle and bone contain 90% of the total body burden of zinc. High levels of zinc stimulate the synthesis of metallothionein in the liver and in the gastrointestinal mucosal cells. Zinc is eliminated from the body primarily through the gastrointestinal tract. Chronic ingestion of zinc in doses as low as 2 mg/kg/day may lead to microcytic anemia secondary to zinc-induced copper deficiency (a result of increased gastrointestinal mucosal cell metallothionein). Chronic ingestion of high doses of zinc causes nausea, vomiting, and abdominal cramping; variable increases in low-density lipoprotein levels and decreases in high-density lipoprotein levels; and impaired white blood cell function. Treatment of chronic zinc toxicity consists of removing the patient from the zinc source and providing symptomatic and supportive care. The use of chelating agents is not recommended.

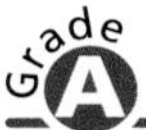

1. Mazumder DNG, De KB, Santra A, et al. Randomized placebo-controlled trial of 2,3-dimercapto-1-propanesulfonate (DMPS) in therapy of chronic arsenicosis due to drinking arsenic-contaminated water. *J Toxicol Clin Toxicol.* 2001;39:665-674.
2. Kan WC, Chien CC, Wu CC, et al. Comparison of low-dose deferoxamine versus standard-dose deferoxamine for treatment of aluminium overload among haemodialysis patients. *Nephrol Dial Transplant.* 2010;25:1604-1608.

SUGGESTED READINGS

Argos M, Kalra T, Rathouz PJ, et al. Arsenic exposure from drinking water, and all-cause and chronic-disease mortalities in Bangladesh (HEALS): a prospective cohort study. *Lancet.* 2010;376:252-258. *Chronic arsenic exposure from drinking water is associated with about a 35 to 70% increase in all-cause mortality.*

Department of Health and Human Services, Public Health Service, Agency for Toxic Substances and Disease Registry: Toxicological Profiles. http://www.atsdr.cdc.gov/toxpro2.html. *The most comprehensive review of environmental toxins available; each profile includes a public health statement for consumers.*

Kosnett MJ. Chelation for heavy metals (arsenic, lead, and mercury): protective or perilous? *Clin Pharmacol Ther.* 2010;88:412-415. *Review of risks and benefits.*

Mozaffarian D, Shi P, Morris JS, et al. Mercury exposure and risk of cardiovascular disease in two U.S. cohorts. *N Engl J Med.* 2011;364:1116-1125. *Mercury exposure did not result in increased risk of cardiovascular disease.*

IV

AGING AND GERIATRIC MEDICINE

22

EPIDEMIOLOGY OF AGING: IMPLICATIONS OF THE AGING OF SOCIETY

LINDA P. FRIED

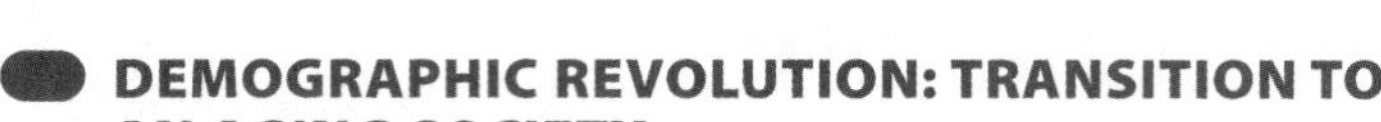

DEMOGRAPHIC REVOLUTION: TRANSITION TO AN AGING SOCIETY

There are now more than 39 million persons 65 years and older in the United States, or more than 12% of the population; in contrast, in 1900, there were 3 million persons 65 years and older, or just 4% of the population. By 2030, about 20% of the U.S. population will be older than 65. By 2050, the current population of older adults will more than double. These increases result from dramatic increases in life expectancy over the past century: in 1900, at birth, men could expect to live to 48 years, and women could expect to live to 51 years on average; by 2008, life expectancy had increased to 75 and 81 years, respectively. Substantial years are now lived after the age of 65 by a large proportion of the population.

With this significant demographic shift, older adults have become a large proportion of all persons with each of the major chronic diseases (Table 22-1). As a result of this burden of disease, people 65 years and older account for about 27% of U.S. health care expenditures, although they represent less than 13% of the U.S. population. Older adults make, on average, 11 outpatient visits per year. People age 75 years and older make almost twice as many emergency department visits as people of all younger ages combined.

HEALTH OF OLDER ADULTS

Changes in Health Status of Older Adults

By many measures, overall well-being is improving for the current generation of older adults compared with previous birth cohorts. In 2007, 39% of persons 65 years and older reported being in excellent or very good health. Educational status, a strong predictor of health behavior and health outcomes, is increasing. In 1950, 17.7% of persons 65 years and older had a high school diploma or higher, and 3.6% had a bachelor's degree or higher; by 2007, these percentages had increased to 74% and 19%. Physical disability, which is an adverse outcome of chronic diseases and aging, is reported by 37% of older adults; however, the remaining 63% are not disabled, and disability rates appear to have declined in the past 10 years.

In 1900, pneumonia and influenza, tuberculosis, diarrhea, and enteritis were the leading causes of death and accounted for 30% of all deaths in persons older than 65 years. Now, heart disease is the leading cause of death in persons 65 and older, followed by cancer, stroke, chronic lower respiratory diseases, Alzheimer's disease, diabetes mellitus, pneumonia, and influenza; the first three diseases accounted for nearly 60% of all deaths. Among persons 85 years and older, heart disease alone is responsible for about 35% of all deaths. Alzheimer's disease is the fourth leading cause of death in women 85 years and older, but it is a less common cause in men.

Death rates for people 65 years and older have declined substantially in the past three decades for heart disease, stroke, pneumonia, and influenza. The first two of these declines are due to a combination of improved medical care, risk factor reductions, and health-promoting changes in lifestyle. Conversely, mortality from chronic obstructive pulmonary disease and diabetes has increased dramatically.

Multiple Causes of Death in Older Adults

Mortality in older adults results from multiple contributing causes, even if one cause can be considered primary. One study of the predictors of 5-year mortality in older adults found that numerous types of health indices contribute: sociodemographic characteristics, health habits, cardiovascular risk factors, clinical and subclinical diseases, physical disability, and cognitive impairment (Table 22-2). After taking these risk factors and conditions into account, age itself becomes substantially less important as a predictor of mortality, up until the age of 85 years.

Disease Frequencies Rise with Increasing Age

The frequency of almost all chronic diseases increases with age, both before and after 65 years of age. For example, arthritis is reported by about 7% of adults aged 18 to 44 years, about 30% of adults aged 45 to 64 years, and about 50% of adults 65 years and older in 2007. The proportion of people who report very good or excellent health decreases with increasing age, from about 70% of persons aged 18 to 44, to about 55% of persons aged 45 to 64, to about 40% of persons 65 years and older. The prevalence of chronic diseases, especially for arthritis, diabetes, and hypertension, is higher in African Americans than in whites in the oldest age groups.

In addition to clinical diseases, subclinical disease is common in older adults. Among the 6000 men and women aged 65 years and older who participated in the Cardiovascular Health Study, 31% had evidence of clinical cardiovascular disease, whereas another 37% had subclinical disease by a variety of noninvasive measures. For example, brain infarct-like lesions, found on magnetic resonance imaging in 28% of Cardiovascular Health Study participants without a known history of stroke, are associated with falling, balance problems, and cognitive decline. Overall, subclinical cardiovascular disease is a stronger predictor of the older adults in whom clinical cardiovascular disease will develop than are other classic risk factors.

Onset of Geriatric Conditions

Health status in aging is a result of many factors, including the chronic diseases of aging and many other prevalent "geriatric" conditions that cannot be defined as classic "diseases" because they do not manifest in a single organ system or result from a single pathologic cause. Falls, which occur in one fourth of older adults, result in injuries, fractures, and high risk for disability and mortality (Chapter 24). Severe cognitive impairment, delirium (Chapters 26 and 27), and urinary incontinence (Chapter 25) have a substantial adverse impact on an older person, as does the sensory isolation resulting from hearing and visual impairment; all these conditions are frequent with aging. Frailty, occurring in 7% of community-dwelling older adults, is a geriatric syndrome that leads to heightened vulnerability to stressors and substantially increased risk for disability, falls, and mortality.

Why Geriatric Patients Are Different

Comorbid Conditions

Older patients differ from young or middle-aged adults who have the same disease in many ways. First, as a function of the high prevalences of many diseases, multimorbidity (or the co-occurrence of two or more diseases in the same individual) is common. Of people aged 65 years and older, 50% have two or more chronic diseases. The risk for becoming disabled or dependent increases with the number of diseases present, and some specific combinations of diseases synergistically increase the risk for disability. For example, arthritis and heart disease coexist in 18% of older adults; although the odds of developing disability are increased by 3-fold to 4-fold with either disease alone, the risk for disability increases 14-fold if both are present. Furthermore, one disease, such as cognitive impairment, may mask the symptoms of other important conditions, at least temporarily. Treatment of one disease may also affect another adversely, as in the use of aspirin to prevent stroke in individuals with a history of gastrointestinal bleeding.

Nonspecific Signs and Symptoms

Older adults differ also from younger adults in the greater likelihood that their diseases will have nonspecific symptoms and signs. For example, pneumonia and stroke may be associated with nonspecific changes in mentation as the primary presenting symptom. Similarly, the frequency of silent myocardial infarction increases with increasing age, as does the proportion of patients who manifest a myocardial infarction with a change in mental status, dizziness, or weakness rather than typical chest pain (Chapter 50). As a result, the diagnostic evaluation of geriatric patients must consider a wider spectrum of causes than would generally be considered in middle-aged adults.

Frailty

Another condition that is found primarily in older adults is frailty. Frailty, which is a state of decreased reserves and increased vulnerability to all kinds of stresses, from acute infection or injury to hospitalization, identifies individuals who likely will have a lower tolerance for any new medical or surgical condition. Frailty is thought to be a wasting syndrome with a characteristic clinical presentation, including weakness, poor exercise tolerance, slowed motor performance, low physical activity, and weight loss. Some estimates

TABLE 22-1 PREVALENCE OF SELECTED CONDITIONS REPORTED BY PERSONS 65 YEARS AND OLDER, UNITED STATES

	NUMBER OF PERSONS 65 YEARS AND OLDER WITH DISEASE (IN THOUSANDS)	PERCENTAGE OF PERSONS 65 YEARS AND OLDER REPORTING THE DISEASE	PERCENTAGE REPORTING THE DISEASE WHO ARE 65 YEARS AND OLDER, AMONG ALL INDIVIDUALS 18 YEARS AND OLDER REPORTING THE DISEASE, UNITED STATES
Hypertension*	19,442	54	37
Arthritis*	17,192	48	37
Disability†	13,467	37	41
Hearing impairment†	13,320	37	40
Heart disease*	11,239	31	45
Urinary incontinence†	9029[1]	25	N/A
Falls†	8379[1]	23	N/A
Malignant neoplasm*	7980	22	49
Obesity	7744	21	14
Influenza*	7744	22	N/A
Diabetes*	6748	19	39
Visual impairment†	5484	15	25
Alzheimer's disease*	4940[2]	13	96
Sinusitis*	4538	13	18
Ulcers*	4244	12	29
Stroke*	2985	8	55
Asthma*	2704	8	17
Frailty†	2528[3]	8	N/A
Emphysema*	1745	5	47
Kidney disease*	1359	4	41
Underweight	845	2	22
Liver disease*	526	2	20

*Clinical diseases.
†Geriatric conditions not associated with specific diseases.
Unless otherwise indicated, data provided by Pleis JR, Lucas JW. Summary health statistics for U.S. adults: National Health Interview Survey, 2007. National Center for Health Statistics. *Vital Health Stat.* 2009;10:240. [1]Lee PG, Cigolle C, Blaum C. The co-occurrence of chronic diseases and geriatric syndromes: the health and retirement study. *J Am Geriatr Soc.* 2009;57:511-516. [2]Hebert LE, Scherr PA, Bienias L, et al. Alzheimer's disease in the US population: prevalence estimates using the 2000 census. *Arch Neurol.* 2003;60:1119-1122. [3]Fried LP, Tangen CM, Walston J, et al. Frailty in older adults: evidence for a phenotype. *J Gerontol A Biol Sci Med Sci.* 2001;56:M146-M156.

indicate that the full syndrome is found in 7% of community-dwelling people aged 65 years and older and in 25% of community-dwelling people 85 years and older. Many institutionalized older adults are also frail. The syndrome of frailty is associated with a high risk for falls, need for hospitalization, poorer recovery after hospitalization, disability, and mortality. A core component of frailty is sarcopenia, or loss of muscle mass associated with aging, which occurs in 13 to 24% of persons aged 65 to 70 years and in 60% of persons 80 years and older. Energy dysregulation and abnormalities in multiple physiologic systems, including inflammation, immune function, hormonal status, and glucose metabolism, underlie the syndrome and decrease the ability to maintain homeostasis in the face of stress. Subclinical disease (e.g., atherosclerosis), end-stage chronic disease (e.g., heart failure, HIV/AIDS), or a combination of comorbid catabolic diseases may precipitate the clinically apparent syndrome. Evidence from randomized, controlled trials shows that resistance exercise, with (or without) nutritional supplements and home-based physical therapy, can increase lean body mass and strength in even the frailest older adults,[1,2] and that weight loss in obese, sedentary older adults has incremental benefit.[3]

Cognitive Impairment

Cognitive impairment, which increases in prevalence as people age (Fig. 22-1; Chapters 26 and 27), is a risk factor for a wide range of adverse outcomes, including falls, immobilization, dependency, institutionalization, and mortality. Cognitive impairment complicates the diagnosis of other medical conditions, necessitates targeted prevention of complications, compromises independence, and requires additional caregiving to ensure safety.

Physical Disability

A serious and common outcome of chronic diseases of aging is physical disability, defined as having difficulty or being dependent on others for the conduct of essential or personally meaningful activities of life from basic self-care (e.g., bathing or toileting) to tasks required to live independently (e.g., shopping, preparing meals, or paying bills) to a full range of activities considered to be productive or personally meaningful (Chapter 23). Among older adults, 37% report difficulty with tasks requiring mobility, and this difficulty with mobility predicts the future development of difficulty in instrumental activities of daily living (IADL; household management tasks) and activities of daily living (ADL; basic self-care tasks). In community-dwelling persons aged 65 years and older, difficulty with IADLs is reported by 20%, and difficulty with ADLs is reported by 11%; for both, the prevalence increases with age. People who have difficulty with IADLs and ADLs are at high risk of becoming dependent. Of persons older than 65 years, 3.5% reside in nursing homes, largely as a result of dependency in IADL or ADL (or both) secondary to severe disease. Generally, women live more years with disability, whereas men who become similarly disabled are more likely to die at a younger age. Although physical disability is primarily a result of chronic diseases and geriatric conditions, its onset and severity are modified by other factors, including treatments that control the underlying diseases, physical activity and rehabilitation, nutrition, smoking, and community-based services. Many intervention trials indicate that some disability can be prevented or its severity decreased.[4]

Relationships among Factors

Multimorbidity, frailty, and disability are recognized as distinct clinical entities (Fig. 22-2), although they are related in the same causal pathway. Multimorbidity may be a risk factor for frailty, and both are risk factors for disability. A vicious cycle may exist whereby inactivity resulting from disability precipitates or worsens frailty.

Thus, the health status of older adults includes a broader spectrum of issues than is found in middle-aged or younger patients, including prevalent chronic disease, recurrent disease, multimorbidity, and geriatric conditions, each of which can be an independent problem or interact with other problems

TABLE 22-2 PREDICTORS OF 5-YEAR AND LONG-TERM MORTALITY IN MEN AND WOMEN 65 YEARS AND OLDER IN THE CARDIOVASCULAR HEALTH STUDY*

RISK FACTOR CATEGORY	FIVE-YEAR MORTALITY PREDICTORS†	LONG-TERM MORTALITY PREDICTORS‡
Sociodemographic	Age (older) Gender (male) Income (<$50,000/yr)	Age (older) Gender (male) Race (black)
Anthropometric	Weight (lower)	Weight (lower)
Health habits	Physical activity (low) Smoking (pack years)	Physical activity (low) Smoking (pack years)
Cardiovascular risk factors	Brachial systolic blood pressure (elevated) Posterior tibial artery blood pressure (reduced) Diuretic use (in persons with severe CHF or liver disease) Fasting blood glucose (higher)	Fasting blood glucose (higher)
Serum measures	Albumin (lower) Creatinine (higher)	Albumin (lower) Creatinine (higher) IL-6 (greater) ApoE e4 allele
Clinically manifested disease	CHF	CHF Coronary heart disease
Subclinical disease, measured noninvasively	Forced vital capacity, mL (lower) Major ECG abnormality Ejection fraction abnormal Aortic stenosis (moderate to severe) Stenosis (maximal) of the internal carotid artery (greater)	Forced vital capacity, L (lower) Major ECG abnormality
Consequences of disease	Difficulty with instrumental activities of daily living (≥2) Cognitive impairment (greater) Poor self-assessed health	Difficulty with instrumental activities of daily living (≥2) DSST score (lower) Poor self-assessed health

ApoE = apolipoprotein E; CHF = congestive heart failure; DSST = Digit Symbol Substitution Test; ECG = electrocardiographic; IL-6, interleukin-6.
*Persons without cancer at the time of enrollment.
†Data from Fried LP, Kronmal RA, Newman AB, et al. Risk factors for 5-year mortality in older adults: the Cardiovascular Health Study. *JAMA.* 1998;279:585-592.
‡Data from Newman AB, Sachs MC, Arnold AM, et al. Total and cause-specific mortality in the Cardiovascular Health Study. *J Gerontol.* 2009;64:1251-1261.

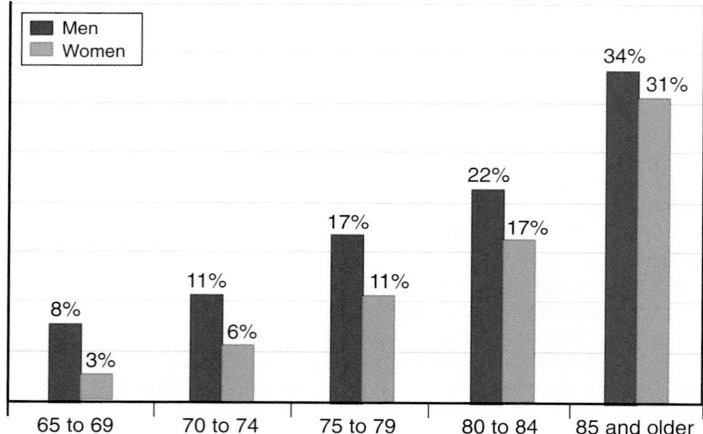

FIGURE 22-1. Percentage of persons 65 years or older with moderate or severe memory impairment (defined as ≤4 words recalled out of 20 on combined immediate and delayed recall tests). (Data from Lethbridge-Cejku M, Vickerie J. Summary health statistics for U.S. adults: National Health Interview Survey, 2003. National Center for Health Statistics. *Vital Health Stat.* 10;2005. Data also from Annual Estimates of the Population by Sex and Five-Year Age Groups for the United States April 1, 2000 to July 1, 2004 [NC-EST2004-01]. Source: Population Division, U.S. Census Bureau.)

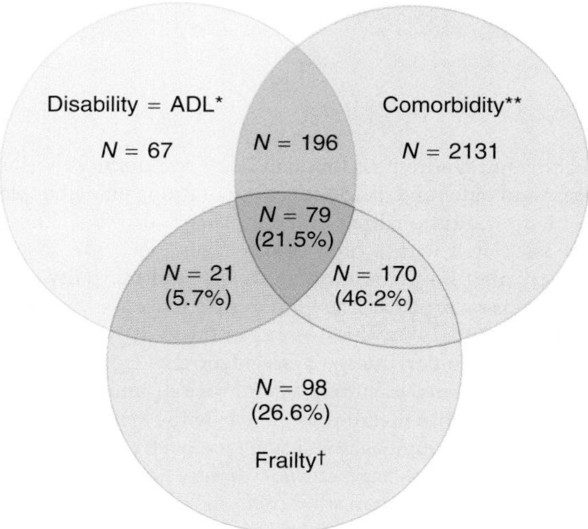

FIGURE 22-2. Overlap of frailty, disability, and comorbidity in community-dwelling older adults participating in the Cardiovascular Health Study. The total represented was 2762 subjects who had comorbidity, disability, or frailty, or any combination of these conditions. **N* = 363 with a disability in activities of daily living (ADL); of these, 100 were frail. ***N* = 2576 with comorbidity, defined as two or more of the following nine diseases: myocardial infarction, angina, heart failure, claudication, arthritis, cancer, diabetes, hypertension, and chronic obstructive pulmonary disease. Of these, 249 were also frail. †*N* = 368 frail subjects. (Adapted from Fried LP, Tangen CM, Walston J, et al. Frailty in older adults: evidence for a phenotype. *J Gerontol A Biol Sci Med Sci.* 2001;56:M146-M156.)

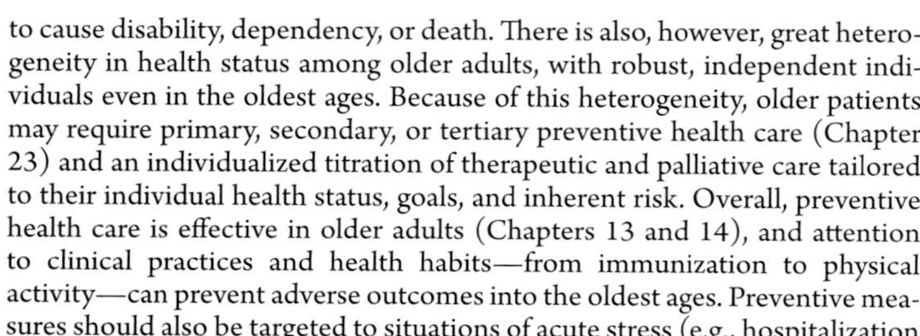

to cause disability, dependency, or death. There is also, however, great heterogeneity in health status among older adults, with robust, independent individuals even in the oldest ages. Because of this heterogeneity, older patients may require primary, secondary, or tertiary preventive health care (Chapter 23) and an individualized titration of therapeutic and palliative care tailored to their individual health status, goals, and inherent risk. Overall, preventive health care is effective in older adults (Chapters 13 and 14), and attention to clinical practices and health habits—from immunization to physical activity—can prevent adverse outcomes into the oldest ages. Preventive measures should also be targeted to situations of acute stress (e.g., hospitalization or immobilization), when the risk of decline in function is high. Health status can change rapidly as people age, so clinical care, prevention, and services must evolve in concert with the health and function of the patient. Further, there is mounting evidence that social engagement, along with physical, cognitive, and social activity, can modify key health outcomes such as cognitive function and potentially frailty and disability.

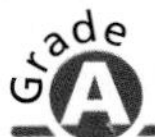

1. Liu-Ambrose T, Nagamatsu LS, Graf P, et al. Resistance training and executive functions: a 12-month randomized controlled trial. *Arch Intern Med.* 2010;170:170-178.
2. Kemmler W, von Stengel S, Engelke K, et al. Exercise effects on bone mineral density, falls, coronary risk factors, and health care costs in older women: the randomized controlled senior fitness and prevention (SEFIP) Study. *Arch Intern Med.* 2010;170:179-185.
3. Santanasto AJ, Glynn NW, Newman MA, et al. Impact of weight loss on physical function with changes in strength, muscle mass, and muscle fat infiltration in overweight to moderately obese older adults: a randomized clinical trial. *J Obes.* 2011. [Epub ahead of print.]
4. The LIFE Study Investigators. Effects of a physical activity intervention on measures of physical performance: results of the Lifestyle Intervention and Independence for Elders Pilot (LIFE-P) Study. *J Gerontol A Biol Sci Med Sci.* 2006;61A:1157-1165.

SUGGESTED READINGS

Liu L. Social connections, diabetes mellitus, and risk of mortality among white and African-American adults aged 70 and older: an eight-year follow-up study. *Ann Epidemiol.* 2010;21:26-33. *In the elderly, the lack of social connections carries a risk similar to diabetes for predicting future mortality.*

Studenski S, Perera S, Patel K, et al. Gait speed and survival in older adults. *JAMA.* 2011;305:50-58. *Better gait speed is associated with better survival.*

23 GERIATRIC ASSESSMENT

DAVID B. REUBEN

Geriatric assessment is a broad term used to describe the evaluation of older patients, a process that recognizes the diverse medical and psychosocial conditions that influence the health status of older persons. In addition to the diseases that are common in the elderly population, these influences include social, psychological, and environmental factors. Geriatric assessment can range from brief screens by individual clinicians to an intensive interdisciplinary process that includes both evaluation and management.

Three fundamental concepts guide geriatric assessment and the resulting medical management. At the core of geriatric assessment is functional status, both as a dimension to be evaluated and as an outcome to be improved or maintained. A second overarching concept guiding geriatric assessment is prognosis, particularly life expectancy. Finally, geriatric assessment must be guided by the patient's goals.

FUNCTIONAL STATUS

Functional status can be viewed as a summary measure of the overall impact of health conditions in the context of an elderly person's environment and social support network. The underlying framework of functional status is a hierarchy of increasing complexity, beginning with specific physical movements (e.g., lifting, walking) that are integrated into higher level activities (e.g., fulfilling occupational and social roles). Impairment of functional status can be triggered by the onset of disease, deconditioning, changes in social support or environment, and advanced age.

Most commonly, older adults' functional status is assessed at two levels: activities of daily living (ADLs) and instrumental activities of daily living (IADLs). ADLs refer to self-care tasks such as bathing, dressing, toileting, maintaining continence, grooming, feeding, and transferring. Dependency in these tasks, which is present in up to 10% of older persons, usually requires full-time help at home or placement in a nursing home.

IADLs refer to tasks that are integral to maintaining an independent household, such as using the telephone, doing laundry, shopping for groceries, driving or using public transportation, preparing meals, taking medications, performing housework, and handling finances. Dependency in IADLs is more common, and almost 20% of persons aged 75 years or older are impaired in at least one task. With the progressive loss of multiple IADL functions, older persons find it more difficult to remain in their homes. Accordingly, many social services (e.g., meals-on-wheels, homemaker services, transportation services) are available to compensate for these deficiencies. A move to an assisted living facility can provide most IADL functions, but many facilities do not routinely provide assistance with ADLs except at an additional cost. In the United States, the costs of assisted living facilities are not covered by Medicare.

At a higher level of function, advanced activities of daily living (AADLs) refer to the ability to fulfill societal, community, and family roles, as well as participate in recreational or occupational tasks. These advanced activities vary considerably from individual to individual but may be valuable in monitoring functional status before the development of disability.

The choice of functional assessment tool depends on the characteristics of the population being assessed. For example, nursing home residents are almost always completely dependent in IADLs, so the focus should be on assessing ADLs and other basic dimensions of health. Hospitalized older persons should be assessed with regard to their prehospitalization functional status to provide insight into what may be achievable, as well as their functional status at the time of discharge to identify any existing gap and facilitate plans to close it.

Functional status is usually measured by self-report or proxy report. However, physical and occupational therapists often add objective information using structured clinical examinations or assessments. In addition, dimensions such as mobility and balance that contribute to function can be assessed by objective measures (described later).

Functional status should be assessed periodically: at the time of an initial visit, after a major illness, and at the time of social milestones, such as the illness of a spouse or a change in living or working situation. Changes in functional status should always prompt further diagnostic evaluation and intervention unless the change is expected and reflects a trajectory that is consistent with the patient's wishes. Measurement of functional status can be valuable in monitoring response to treatment (especially of chronic diseases) and can provide prognostic information that is useful in planning short- and long-term care.

PROGNOSIS

Life expectancy affects both the assessment process and the management decisions based on that assessment. For some older patients, comorbidities can worsen prognosis, such that screening tests (e.g., mammography) and treatments (e.g., for hypertension) with demonstrated effectiveness would not be beneficial within the expected survival period.

Clinicians can estimate remaining years of life by age, gender, and race using life tables (Table 23-1). These tables, however, do not consider clinical characteristics or functional status, which can lead to wide variations in how long an individual patient will live.

PATIENT GOALS

As people age, their current and future health may become a prominent factor in determining and achieving their life goals. Among very old patients, goals may be limited to achieving a functional or health state (e.g., being able to walk independently), controlling symptoms (e.g., pain, dyspnea), maintaining their living situation (e.g., remaining at home), or short-term survival (e.g., living long enough to reach a personal milestone, such as an upcoming holiday). Sometimes the goals of patients and physicians differ. For example, a patient may want a cure, whereas the physician believes that only symptom management is possible. Conversely, the physician may believe that a better outcome is possible, but the patient declines to pursue the recommended path (e.g., hip replacement to restore mobility).

COMPONENTS OF GERIATRIC ASSESSMENT

Geriatric assessment begins with a medical evaluation. Some aspects (described later) that are rarely abnormal in younger adults (e.g., mobility, cognition) may cause substantial morbidity in older persons. In addition, some clusters of abnormal findings, such as muscle wasting, poor hygiene, bruises, pressure sores, and contractures, should raise the suspicion of elder mistreatment, neglect, or abuse. In such cases, patients should be questioned and examined without family members or caregivers present. Patients should then be queried whether anyone has threatened or hurt them, whether they have been receiving enough care, and whether anyone has taken their things. Answers to these questions may provide confirmatory information and prompt a report to adult protective services.

Nonmedical assessments are also important because they can identify problems that should be addressed and may be key to achieving the patient's goals. In addition to an assessment of functional status, older persons' environmental, financial, and nonfinancial support should be assessed. In some situations, particularly when older persons become acutely ill or experience caregiver stress or loss of a loved one, assessment of spiritual needs, with appropriate referral, may be valuable.

TABLE 23-1 LIFE EXPECTANCY (IN YEARS) FOR OLDER PERSONS BY AGE, RACE, AND SEX

	White		*Black*	
AGE	**MALE**	**FEMALE**	**MALE**	**FEMALE**
65	17.2	20	15.2	18.6
70	13.7	16.2	12.4	15.3
75	10.7	12.8	9.9	12.2
80	8.1	9.7	8.0	9.6
85	6.0	7.1	6.3	7.5
90	4.3	5.1	4.9	5.7
95	3.1	3.6	3.8	4.3
100	2.2	2.5	2.9	3.2

Advance Directives

Clinicians should discuss older patients' preferences for specific treatments while they still have the cognitive capacity to make these decisions. Patients should be asked to identify a spokesperson to make medical decisions for them if they cannot speak for themselves. This information should be conveyed through a durable power of attorney for health care, which also allows patients to specify treatments they do not want. Many states have allowed the use of Physician Orders for Life-Sustaining Treatment, a specific advance directive that documents a patient's end-of-life treatment preferences and serves as an order sheet. The standardized form is signed by both the physician and the patient and must be honored in all settings of care.

Medical Assessment

The medical assessment includes vision; hearing; cognition; mood and affect; falls, mobility, and balance; medication review; nutrition; and urinary incontinence. Numerous screening instruments have been developed that assess many of these dimensions. Other important medical components of geriatric assessment include a review of the patient's medications and a determination of whether preventive services are up-to-date.

Vision

Each of the four major eye diseases—cataract, age-related macular degeneration, diabetic retinopathy, and glaucoma (Chapter 431)—increases in prevalence with age. Moreover, presbyopia is virtually universal, and the vast majority of older persons require eyeglasses. Visual impairment has been associated with increased risk of falls, functional and cognitive decline, immobility, and depression. Corrective lenses or other treatments may restore vision or prevent further decline of visual function.

A single question can be used to screen for visual impairment: Do you have difficulty driving, watching television or reading, or doing any of your daily activities because of your eyesight, even while wearing glasses?

The Snellen eye chart is the standard method of screening for visual acuity. The patient is asked to stand 20 feet from the chart and read letters. Inability to read letters on or below the 20/40 line with their best-corrected vision (using glasses) indicates the need for further evaluation.

Hearing

Hearing loss (Chapter 436), which affects 30% of community-dwelling older adults older than 65 years and 75% of residents living in nursing home settings, is associated with reduced cognitive, social, emotional, and physical functioning. When hearing loss is detected, amplification by hearing aids or assistive listening devices can improve quality of life and functional status.

To assess hearing, the physician can administer the whisper voice test, which involves whispering three different random words in each ear at distances of 6, 12, and 24 inches from the patient's ear and then asking the patient to repeat the words. Patients who fail the screen—that is, are unable to repeat half the whispered words correctly—should be referred to an audiologist for further evaluation. Alternatively, the Hearing Handicap Inventory for the Elderly, a 10-item self-report instrument, has been used widely.

A more accurate screening tool for hearing impairment is the Welch Allyn AudioScope. This handheld otoscope has a built-in audiometer that can be set at different levels of intensity. A pretone at 60 dB is delivered to the patient, and then four tones of 500, 1000, 2000, and 4000 Hz at 40 dB are presented. The inability to hear either the 1000- or 2000-Hz frequency in both ears or both the 1000- and 2000-Hz frequencies in one ear indicates a positive screen and identifies the need for formal audiometric testing.

Cognitive Assessment

The incidence of dementia (Chapters 26 and 409) increases with age, especially among those older than 85 years. Early detection of memory problems can lead to the identification of treatable conditions that contribute to cognitive impairment and the development of a proactive management plan with the patient's full participation.

The most commonly used screen is the Mini-Mental State Examination (MMSE), a 30-item interviewer-administered assessment of several dimensions of cognitive function (see Table 26-4). However, the MMSE is too long for most practitioners to incorporate routinely into their clinical practices, and the instrument must be purchased for use. Several shorter screens have also been validated, including recall of three items at 1 minute and the Mini-Cog test (see Table 26-5), which combines three-item recall and the clock-drawing test.

Another component of cognitive assessment is decision-making capacity. In cognitively intact older persons, capacity is assumed. However, among those with cognitive impairment, decision making must be determined before many treatments are initiated. As a rule, capacity is specific to the decision the patient is being asked to make. Ask the following questions to determine a patient's decision-making capacity:

- Can the patient make and express personal preferences at all?
- Can the patient comprehend the risks and benefits?
- Does the patient comprehend the implications?
- Can the patient give reasons for the alternative selected?
- Are supporting reasons rational?

If the answer to all these questions is yes, the patient is competent to make the decision at hand. If not, then a surrogate (the durable power of attorney for health care, if the patient has identified one) should make the decision. If a durable power of attorney for health care has not been identified, the decision can be made by a family member, friend, or caregiver who knows the patient well. The order of surrogates is determined by state law. If no one is available, the health care provider should make the decision based on the patient's known value system or what the health care provider believes to be in the best interest of the patient.

Mood and Affect

Although major depression (Chapter 404) is no more common among the elderly than among the younger population, minor depression and other affective disorders are common and cause considerable morbidity. Moreover, depression may present atypically, and it may be masked in patients with cognitive impairment or other neurologic disorders such as Parkinson's disease (Chapter 416).

A two-item version of the Patient Health Questionnaire (PHQ-9) can effectively screen for depression symptoms. The screener asks the patient: Over the past 2 weeks, how often have you been bothered by any of the following problems?

- Little interest or pleasure in doing things.
- Feeling down, depressed, or hopeless.

Responses are scored as follows: 0 = not at all, 1 = several days, 2 = more than half the days, 3 = nearly every day. Persons who score a total of 3 points or higher on the two-item screen have a 75% probability of having a depressive disorder. More detailed information can be gathered using instruments such as the Geriatric Depression Scale.

Falls, Mobility, and Balance

Approximately one third of community-dwelling persons older than 65 and half of those older than 80 fall each year. Ten percent of these falls result in a serious injury. Patients who have fallen or have gait or balance problems are at higher risk of another fall. Performing a falls assessment (measuring orthostatic blood pressure; assessing vision; reviewing medications; and testing balance, gait, and lower extremity strength) and treating risk factors for falling can reduce falls by 30 to 40%.

All older patients should be asked at least annually if they have fallen, and frail older persons should be asked about falls at every visit. In addition, asking about fear of falling can identify patients at risk of future falls.

Patients who have fallen or have a fear of falling should have their balance and gait assessed by direct observation of their ability to perform specific tasks. Tests of balance include the ability to maintain a side-by-side, semitandem, and full-tandem stance for 10 seconds; resistance to a nudge; and stability during a 360-degree turn. Quadriceps strength can be assessed by observing an older person rising from a hard armless chair without using his or her hands.

In addition, direct qualitative and quantitative observation of gait to determine stability is a quick and important component of assessment. Qualitative aspects include evaluation of hesitancy; sway; step length, height, symmetry, and continuity; and path deviation. Gait speed is also a helpful marker for recurrent falls. Patients who take more than 13 seconds to walk 10 meters are more likely to have recurrent falls.

The timed "up-and-go" test combines some features of strength and gait. It is a timed test of the patient's ability to rise from a standard armchair, walk 3 meters (10 feet), turn, walk back, and sit down again. Patients who take longer than 20 seconds to complete the test should receive further evaluation.

Medication Review

Older persons often see several different health care providers who prescribe multiple medications that increase the risk for drug-drug interactions and adverse drug events. At a minimum, the clinician should review the patient's updated and accurate medication list at each visit. A good method of detecting potential problems is to have patients bring in all their medications (prescription and nonprescription) in their bottles. Entering a patient's medication list into commercially available computer drug interaction programs can help prevent adverse events.

Nutrition

Malnutrition in older adults includes obesity (Chapter 227), undernutrition (Chapter 221), and specific vitamin deficiencies (Chapter 225). Obesity in older adults is defined as a body mass index (BMI) of 30 kg/m^2 or greater. High BMI is associated with poorer function and more comorbidities, such as type 2 diabetes mellitus (Chapters 236 and 237), osteoarthritis (Chapter 270), hyperlipidemia (Chapter 213), coronary artery disease (Chapter 51), and sleep apnea (Chapter 100).

At the initial visit, patients should be weighed and asked about weight loss in the previous 12 months. They should be weighed at all follow-up visits. BMI should be calculated on the initial visit and periodically thereafter (e.g., yearly or when a change in weight suggests the need to recalculate). Serum markers, including serum albumin, prealbumin, and cholesterol levels, are nonspecific indicators of nutritional status and can be affected by inflammatory states, physiologic stress, and trauma.

Weight loss of 4% or more over 12 months predicts increased mortality and should prompt an evaluation of medical (e.g., malignancy, gastrointestinal disorders, hyperthyroidism, diabetes), psychiatric (e.g., depression, dementia), dental, and social or functional (e.g., poverty, inability to shop or prepare meals) causes.

Urinary Incontinence

Approximately one third of community-dwelling older adult women have some degree of urinary incontinence (Chapter 25), and 75% of older men have abnormal urinary tract symptoms. Complications of incontinence include skin irritation, pressure ulcers, urinary tract infections, sleep disruption, and falls. Identification of urinary incontinence is important because effective behavioral and pharmacologic treatments are available.

A simple screen for urinary incontinence asks the following question: Have you had urinary incontinence (do you "lose" your urine) to the extent that it is bothersome and you would like to know how it can be treated? This may be valuable in determining which patients want further evaluation and therapy. Patients who answer yes should be asked how much urine is leaked, how much it interferes with daily life, and when the leakage occurs. Further evaluation and treatment depend on whether the incontinence is overflow incontinence, urge incontinence, or stress incontinence (see Table 25-3).

PREVENTIVE SERVICES

Preventive services include lifestyle advice, screening tests to detect asymptomatic disease, and vaccinations. Recommended adult immunization schedules include annual influenza vaccination, one-time pneumonia vaccination, one-time pneumococcal vaccination, one-time herpes zoster vaccination (even if the patient reports a past episode of herpes zoster), and tetanus toxoid vaccination every 10 years (Chapter 17).

To help the clinician decide what is appropriate for a specific patient, the U.S. Preventive Services Task Force has created an interactive website (*http://epss.ahrq.gov/ePSS/search.jsp*) with recommendations based on the patient's age, gender, tobacco use, and current sexual activity (Chapter 14). For younger elderly persons, recommendations include screening for blood pressure, diabetes, hyperlipidemia, obesity, alcohol misuse, colorectal cancer, and osteoporosis, as well as breast cancer in women, with appropriate counseling and treatment if these disorders are detected. Aspirin may be recommended to prevent cardiovascular disease in this population. Other recommendations depend on patient-specific risk factors.

With increasing age, fewer preventive services are recommended because of limited life expectancy and greater comorbidities. Accordingly, some preventive measures (e.g., aspirin to prevent cardiovascular disease) and cancer screenings are not recommended in the very elderly. When the evidence base for preventive services is sparse, decisions should be individualized, based on the patient's personal values, goals, and preferences.

NONMEDICAL ASSESSMENTS

Environmental Assessment

Assessing a patient's environment includes evaluating three components: the person's ability to access community services (e.g., getting to the bank and stores if the patient cannot drive), the safety of the physical environment, and the appropriateness of the living situation for the person's functional ability and cognitive status. A brief screen for safety of the physical environment can be accomplished by using a checklist that is in the public domain (*http://www.cdc.gov/ncipc/pub-res/toolkit/Falls_ToolKit/DesktopPDF/English/booklet_Eng_desktop.pdf*). For home-bound older patients, a home safety evaluation by a home health agency is more appropriate.

Social Support Assessment

When older persons become frail, the adequacy of their social support network may be the determining factor in whether they can remain at home or need institutionalization. A brief screen of social support includes taking a social history, including asking who would be available to help if the patient becomes ill. For patients with functional impairment, the clinician should ascertain who can help the patient perform ADLs or IADLs. Early identification of problems with social support can help avoid crisis situations if the patient has a sudden medical or functional decline. Caregivers should be screened periodically for symptoms of depression or caregiver burnout and referred for counseling or support groups if necessary.

Financial Assessment

Although clinicians do not have the training or expertise to explore financial resources in detail, knowing the patient's insurance status may be helpful. For example, patients with Medicaid coverage may qualify for additional medical or social support benefits. Some may be eligible for other state or local benefits, depending on their income. Others may have long-term care insurance or veterans' benefits that can help pay for caregivers, obviating the need for institutionalization.

A STRATEGIC APPROACH TO GERIATRIC ASSESSMENT FOR THE PRACTICING CLINICIAN

Although assembling an interdisciplinary assessment team is beyond the capability of most practitioners, even small group practices can use teamwork and simple practice design to perform geriatric assessments efficiently and comprehensively. These assessments can lead to local implementation of or referral to comprehensive care models that can improve the outcomes of elderly individuals with a variety of chronic conditions.1,2 Because of time constraints, screening is increasingly delegated to staff and to patients and their families using standing orders, forms, and questionnaires (Table 23-2). For example, previsit questionnaires can be used to gather information about past medical and surgical history; medications and allergies; social history, including available social support resources, preventive services, ability to perform functional tasks, and need for assistance; home safety; and advance directives. In addition, the previsit questionnaire can include specific questions that assess vision, hearing, falls, urinary incontinence, and depressive symptoms. A reasonable approach is to assess these issues annually beginning at age 75 years. Persons who are younger than 75 but have multiple comorbidities should also be screened and reassessed annually. In addition, some elements of geriatrics assessment (assessing ADLs and IADLs; gait, balance, and falls; mood and affect; and cognition) should be performed after major illnesses, especially those requiring hospitalization.

TABLE 23-2 APPROACHES TO ASSESSING FUNCTION IN ELDERLY INDIVIDUALS

	Previsit Questionnaire		*Office Staff Administered*	
ASPECT BEING ASSESSED	**LENGTH OF SCREEN***	**INSTRUMENTS**	**LENGTH OF SCREEN***	**INSTRUMENTS**
Functional status	D	Activities of daily living Instrumental activities of daily living		
Advance directives	B	Specific question about advance directives		
MEDICAL ASSESSMENT				
Visual impairment	B	Single-item question	B	Snellen eye chart (see Table 431-1)
Hearing impairment	B	Hearing Handicap Inventory for the Elderly	B (if needed)	Whisper test Audioscope
Cognitive problems			B	Mini-cog 3-item recall (see Table 26-5)
Mind, affective problems	D	Geriatric depression scale (see Table 26-3)	B	
Falls, mobility, balance	B	Simple questions	B	Timed up-and-go test
Medication review			D	Inspection of medication bottles
Malnutrition	D	Single question	B	Weight
Urinary incontinence	B	Single question	B	International Consultation on Incontinence Modular Questionnaire -UI short form if single question is positive
Preventive services	D	Specific questions		
OTHER DIMENSIONS				
Environment	D	Home safety checklist		
Social support	B	Single question		
Financial status			B	Insurance status

*B = brief screen (e.g., <2 min); D = detailed evaluation (usually ≥5 min).

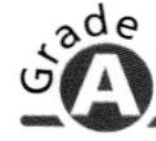

1. Boult C, Green AF, Boult LB, et al. Successful models of comprehensive care for older adults with chronic conditions: evidence for the Institute of Medicine's "Retooling for an Aging America" report. *J Am Geriatr Soc.* 2009;57:2328-2337.
2. Wenger NS, Roth CP, Shekelle PG, et al. A practice-based intervention to improve primary care for falls, urinary incontinence, and dementia. *J Am Geriatr Soc.* 2009;57:547-555.

SUGGESTED READINGS

Berry SD, Ngo L, Samelson EJ, et al. Competing risk of death: an important consideration in studies of older adults. *J Am Geriatr Soc.* 2010;58:783-787. *Emphasizes that the elderly receive less benefit from an intervention because of other adverse prognostic factors.*

Formiga F, Ferrer A, Chivite D, et al. Predictors of long-term survival in nonagenarians: the NonaSantfeliu study. *Age Ageing.* 2011;40:111-116. *Better cognitive status and lesser comorbidity are the best predictors of 5-year survival in nonagenarians.*

Reuben DB. Medical care for the final years of life: "When you're 83, it's not going to be 20 years." *JAMA.* 2009;302:2686-2694. *A practical approach to functionally impaired elderly patients.*

24

COMMON CLINICAL SEQUELAE OF AGING

KENNETH L. MINAKER

EPIDEMIOLOGY

Increased longevity throughout the world is influencing medical care dramatically as more and more older individuals survive with more complex medical conditions. Although some elderly individuals present classically with single-system disease, others have presentations and responses to treatments that are different from those in younger patients. This variation in presentation and behavior of illnesses, which is due to the combined effect of aging and comorbid disease, must be understood if elderly patients are to receive successful care.

PATHOBIOLOGY

Age-associated changes in health and disease are the result of (1) variations in the underlying physiologic changes that occur with age; (2) the presence of other diseases and medical conditions that have developed over time; (3) genetic predispositions for certain diseases; (4) lifestyle factors, including health-seeking behavior, diet, exercise, and exposure to medications and toxins; and (5) the variability intrinsic to diseases and medical conditions in general. Although no single hypothesis fully explains the process of aging at this time (Chapter 22), two major approaches have emerged (Table 24-1). The first concerns programmed causes, which are dominated by genetic theories. The second concerns stochastic causes, so-called process-of-living theories, in which genetic or environmental influences limit viability.

Spectrum of Changes Produced by Aging Processes

Perhaps the most important observation regarding normal aging is how much does not change. Most hormone levels, liver enzyme activities, electrolyte levels, body temperature, and basal glucose concentration remain constant throughout the lifespan. Long-term studies have indicated that there is no age-related anemia (Chapter 161), although the hematocrit declines slightly in men presumably because of the age-related decline in testosterone.

The passage of time results in changes that are not due to aging per se but rather may be considered "dose-time" related. For example, prolonged exposure results in the emergence of abnormalities and illnesses, such as skin cancer due to cumulative actinic injury (Chapter 210). Much of the lifetime exposure to sun is received before the age of 20 years, yet the resulting cancers follow decades later. Another example is polycystic kidney disease, which is an inheritable condition that does not appear until well into adulthood (Chapter 129); the passage of time allows the "full expression" of the genetic phenotype, but aging itself is not the key factor.

Some conditions become less likely with advancing age because of changes in the immune system. Immune disorders such as systemic lupus erythematosus (Chapter 274) and multiple sclerosis (Chapter 419) rarely appear in late life, presumably because changes in the immune system lead to less aggressive autoimmune activity. Similarly, although many cancers are more common in elderly people, many of the most aggressive tumors occur at a young age, suggesting that immune tolerance develops with advancing age.

TABLE 24-1 PATHOBIOLOGY OF AGING

THEORY	DEFINITION	CAUSE: GENETIC (G) OR ENVIRONMENTAL (E)	
PROGRAMMED THEORIES			
Programmed senescence	Aging results from gene interference with the ability of the cells to reproduce	Master clock, cancer protection	G
Hormonal	Biologic clock alters hormone secretion, resulting in tissue changes	Decrease in levels of insulin-like growth factor-I and the hormones estrogen, testosterone, DHEA, and melatonin	G
Immunologic	T-cell function declines, increasing the chances for development of infections and cancer	Alteration in the cytokines that are responsible for communication between immune cells	G
Telomere shortening	Shortening of telomeres in somatic cells lessens the ability of cells to divide	Cells cannot divide	G, E
STOCHASTIC THEORIES			
Metabolic rate	The higher the basal metabolic rate (the rate at which the body, at rest, uses energy), the shorter the lifespan	Energy demands to maintain basal metabolism	G
Glycation	Glycation (browning) causes proteins to be joined, resulting in rigidity and decreased function	Elevated glucose	G, E
Somatic mutation	Mutations in genes occur with aging, eventually causing cells to stop functioning	Errors in the transmission of genetic messages over time	G
Wear and tear	Parts of cells wear out over time	Accumulated debris mechanically disrupts cell function	E
Oxygen free radicals	Tissue damage is caused by free radicals, such as superoxide or hydroxyl radicals; this is a specific form of the wear-and-tear theory	Oxygen free radicals are unstable chemical compounds that can oxidize cell components such as DNA and proteins	E

DHEA = dehydroepiandrosterone.

Physiologic aging modulates the ways in which illnesses cause signs and symptoms. The elderly individual with hyperthyroidism often presents not with the systemic findings of agitation, irritability, hyperactivity, hyperphagia, and increased bowel movements but rather with apathy, anorexia, and atrial fibrillation (Chapter 233). The underlying pathophysiologic process may be no different, but age-related changes in physiology alter the body's sensitivity to dysfunction and influence the clinical presentation.

The most important physiologic change of aging is the predisposition to more generalized clinical syndromes and more severe disease. The lung function of a healthy 70-year-old is about 50% that of a 30-year-old (Chapters 83 and 85). Renal function commonly declines by 50% or more by the age of 70 years (Chapter 117). The resultant lack of physiologic reserve capacity does not affect day-to-day function but can affect the ability to recover from an extreme illness that exhausts the body's reserve capacity.

Geriatric syndromes emerge from these age-related changes. Many systems that maintain our upright posture are compromised by age, leading to increased postural sway. An older individual is much more likely to fall after a slip or a push. The consequences of that fall are more serious because of the age-related loss of bone mass (Chapter 251), resulting in fall-related fractures and spinal cord injuries.

Some physiologic changes imitate illness when they may be a normal part of aging. Diabetes mellitus may "appear" and "disappear" in elderly people (Chapters 236 and 237). The ability of insulin to stimulate glucose uptake declines with age and usually is manifested as postprandial hyperglycemia, but with normal fasting insulin and glucose levels. Under stress situations, older individuals can appear to be diabetic, but when the stressful situation is relieved, they no longer have chemical evidence of diabetes. Nevertheless, this loss of physiologic reserve understandably contributes to the increasing prevalence of diabetes with advancing age.

The age-related changes that make elderly people more vulnerable in daily life are often subtle. Older individuals are more likely to develop hypothermia or hyperthermia (Chapter 109) during extreme environmental exposure because of neurologic and thermoregulatory changes. The loss of brain stem neurotransmitters in older persons not only may cause a senile gait pattern but also predisposes to genetically determined conditions such as Parkinson's disease (Chapter 416). Decreases in the function of the frontal lobe inhibitory center predispose to urgency of urination.

Some age-related changes cause specific medical sequelae. Menopause (Chapter 248) is a normal aging process that produces symptoms and predisposes to future bone loss, urogenital atrophy, and atherosclerosis. Senile cataracts are caused by post-translational modifications in lens proteins combined with the inability of the lens to dispose of breakdown products associated with these processes; as a result, the lens becomes stiffer, thicker, and more opaque with age (Chapter 431).

EFFECTS OF AGING ON SPECIFIC ORGANS AND SYSTEMS

Cardiovascular System

Aging and Its Clinical Sequelae

Many important physiologic changes occur in the aging heart and help explain common age-associated cardiac disorders. Perhaps the most important physiologic change is the delay in left ventricular filling, which declines 50% between the ages of 20 and 80 years. Cardiac filling becomes more dependent on active filling late in diastole during atrial contraction (Chapter 52). This phenomenon commonly is related to thickening and stiffening of the left ventricular wall. Under normal conditions, systolic function remains unchanged, but the thickened ventricle will not produce normal output when volumes are low or be able to avoid elevated filling pressures and the resulting pulmonary congestion when volume is high. As a result, brain natriuretic peptide levels increase with age as myocardial sensors detect greater pressures in the heart.

The resting heart rate slows slightly with advancing age, and maximal and submaximal exercise-induced heart rates show an age-related decline. The loss of sinus node pacemaker cells—up to 90% at 80 years—contributes to these changes. There also are changes in central and baroreflex-mediated heart rate control (Chapter 62). Heart valves thicken and stiffen, particularly in the mitral and aortic locations (Chapter 75). The functional significance of heart valve stiffening is minimal, but 25% of older individuals have flow murmurs (Chapter 50). The aorta dilates and its walls thicken as medial walls calcify; with this loss of elasticity, there is a secondary increase in systolic blood pressure (Chapter 67). The arteriosclerosis that is due to intimal disease further causes arterial walls to thicken, calcify, and lose their elasticity, thereby predisposing aging vessels to occlude or rupture (Chapter 70).

In most industrialized countries, there is a progressive increase in blood pressure with advancing age (Chapter 67). In general, systolic blood pressure increases after the age of 30 years, continues to rise until the mid-70s, then tends to fall slightly through the 80s and 90s. Diastolic blood pressure tends to parallel the usual increase in body weight that peaks in the early 50s in men and the early 60s in women; diastolic pressures subsequently fall slightly in older age. These changes in blood pressure are not universal, suggesting varied genetic and environmental causes, such as stress, sodium and potassium intake, and obesity.

Age-Related Cardiovascular Syndromes

Although atherosclerosis is the most important cause of symptomatic cardiac disease in elderly people, age-associated vascular stiffness predisposes to left ventricular stiffness, impaired diastolic filling, and the clinical syndrome of diastolic heart failure (Chapter 58). The most common arrhythmia in older individuals is atrial fibrillation (Chapter 64), which may occur in one third of older individuals undergoing surgery and may affect 4% of community-dwelling elderly individuals. Although thyroid disease, coronary artery disease, valvular heart disease, and intrinsic conduction system disease are common causes, atrial fibrillation in elderly people is often "lone" atrial fibrillation without a detectable underlying illness.

The combination of sensitivity to filling volumes and impaired heart rate response to stress may explain the increasingly prevalent syndrome of postural hypotension that is present in 20% of older individuals (Chapter 62). Postural hypotension is also common in elderly individuals after large meals; during infections severe enough to depress salt and water intake; and during volume-depleting stresses, such as diarrhea, diuretic therapy, and bowel preparation for colonoscopy. Stiffening of vessels in which baroreceptors reside also reduces the ability to modulate blood pressure with advancing age.

Perhaps the most important principle in the approach to cardiovascular signs and symptoms with advancing age is to recognize the narrowed homeostatic capacity of elderly people. Volume status must be managed carefully, attention should be paid to standing as opposed to sitting blood pressure in patients predisposed to postural hypotension, side effects of medications must be anticipated and monitored, and cardiovascular instability must be expected during almost any major illness that an older person may experience.

Respiratory System

The most characteristic change in the chest wall with advancing age is stiffening (Chapter 85). Cartilages thicken and calcify, and spinal ligaments and joints become stiffer. The primary internal change in the lungs is the loss of the elastic recoil. The result is a modest expansion of the chest wall with the appearance of a mild barrel chest. Although resting lung mechanics do not appear to change in any major way, maximal breathing capacity declines by approximately 40%. At the alveolar level, the capacity to exchange oxygen and carbon monoxide decreases by approximately 50% between the ages of 30 and 65 years, in part as a result of ventilation-perfusion mismatching (Chapter 85). Although these changes are not noticeable at rest, individuals experience fatigue or shortness of breath when the respiratory system is under stress (e.g., during exercise or major illness). Pulmonary reflexes such as coughing and ciliary function decrease, predisposing elderly individuals to the pooling of secretions.

These changes do not produce substantial abnormalities in resting oxygen saturation, but they produce a steady decline in arterial Po_2. The arterial Po_2 of many individuals older than 80 years is about 70 to 75 mm Hg. As with other age-related physiologic findings, these changes do not interfere with function under resting conditions but dramatically affect survival during severe respiratory illness.

Age-Related Respiratory Syndromes

The major clinical impact of normal physiologic aging in the lungs is an earlier appearance of shortness of breath as a warning signal of underlying disease. Myocardial infarction and heart failure can present primarily with shortness of breath, mainly owing to age-related mechanical changes, an inability to clear blood from the lungs, and a decline in resting pulmonary function to near the threshold for clinical hypoxia. Aspiration pneumonia increases with age in association with impaired swallowing, reflux, and reduced clearance of lung secretions.

Gastrointestinal System

A broad series of changes occur in gastroenterologic tissues, but the redundancy of overall gastrointestinal function usually prevents clinical symptoms. Age-related changes in the mouth include slower production of dentine, shrinkage of the root pulp, and decreasing bone density of the jaw. Taste and smell decline progressively with advancing age, with rising thresholds for tasting salt, sweetness, and certain proteins (Chapter 435). The overall net effect is that food may taste more bitter, and more sugar is required before something tastes sweet. Salivary gland function normally does not change with age (Chapter 433). The loss of bone and tongue musculature makes the tongue appear to be enlarged.

The esophagus appears to function relatively normally. The strength of muscle contraction declines, however, and peristaltic waves slow with advancing age. There is also a tendency for the lower esophageal sphincter to become lax (Chapter 140). These changes predispose to aspiration.

The gastric mucosa secretes less acid with advancing age. Although these changes do not appear to affect digestion in most individuals, associated conditions, such as atrophic gastritis, may further decrease the absorption of nutrients to the point of producing illness. Most studies suggest that delayed gastric emptying is a feature of aging, leading to a sense of early satiety, which can impair subsequent food ingestion (Chapter 138).

Liver weight declines by one third between the ages of 30 and 90 years, primarily because of the loss of hepatocytes. The result is a decreased ability to process medications such as benzodiazepines, which require two steps for metabolism, and vitamin K–blocking agents. Doses of drugs often must be adjusted, and their blood levels should be monitored when possible.

Aging is associated with a significant reduction in small intestinal surface area with the consequence of reduced absorption of some dietary components, such as calcium. Colonic function declines with advancing age. Motility up to the rectosigmoid area, measured by passage of markers, does not appear to decline with advancing age (Chapter 138). Distal to this point, however, evacuation is characteristically slower with advancing age. Stool frequency tends to decline, and hardness of stools appears to increase with advancing age. Diverticula are present in approximately 50% of people older than 80 years and are likely to be related to reduced dietary fiber and the resulting greater intracolonic pressure (Chapter 144).

Age-Related Gastroenterologic Syndromes

The most important age-related symptom is constipation (Chapter 138), which may affect 60% of individuals in late life. Obstipation can present atypically with confusion, nausea, and vomiting or as obscure fever resulting from stercoral ulcerations. Perhaps the most common abnormality related to declining hepatic function is increased sensitivity to medications that require hepatic metabolism.

Renal and Urinary Excretory System

Overall kidney size declines by approximately one third, and blood flow through the kidney declines by about 1% per year. Beginning in the late 30s, cortical nephrons appear to drop out and sclerose at a much higher rate than medullary nephrons, creating a hyperfiltration syndrome that limits maximal concentrating capacity (Chapter 117). Resulting functional changes include decreased ability to excrete a salt load, declining glomerular filtration rate, delayed ability to regain sodium and potassium balance during deprivation states, and difficulty in conserving water under situations of dehydration. Excretion of water loads is not strikingly impaired with age, but modest and perhaps clinically significant reductions in acid secretion have been shown in older individuals.

The bladder tends to become more irritable with advancing age and may generate less power during contraction. Because of the delay in sodium excretion and orthostatic changes, nocturia is common; older individuals appear to produce more urine at night than during the day. The most important bladder change may be the slight increase in residual bladder urine volume. Atrophy of vaginal and urethral tissues due to postmenopausal estrogen deprivation predisposes women to urinary tract infections (Chapter 248).

Age-Related Renal and Urinary Tract Syndromes

The age-related increases in asymptomatic bacteriuria and urinary tract infections are almost certainly due to increased residual bladder volume and loss of protective factors in the normal anatomic structures. As the prostate gland grows with advancing age, benign prostatic hypertrophy causes urinary retention in men (Chapter 131). Urinary incontinence (Chapter 25) is more prevalent in women. The kidney is more susceptible to the effects of medications, particularly nonsteroidal anti-inflammatory drugs, which can result in sodium and fluid retention and subsequent hypertension. In elderly individuals, a slight acidemia results from impaired acid excretion and may contribute to the development of osteoporosis.

Dehydration or volume depletion, which is increasingly prevalent with advancing age, often accompanies acute infections and increases the morbidity and mortality of pneumonia or urinary tract infections. Dehydration is the most common fluid and electrolyte disorder in the frail elderly patient because of decreased fluid intake and increased fluid losses. Vomiting and diarrhea are the most common causes of isotonic dehydration. Fever associated with delirium is the leading cause of hypertonic dehydration. Hypotonic dehydration is seen most commonly with overuse of diuretics. Signs and symptoms of dehydration are notoriously vague or absent. Orthostatic tachycardia and hypotension are important clinical findings, and an acute decline in weight may be documented. Perhaps the most useful clinical parameter is a history of having missed one or more meals. A day's food contains about 1 liter of water, which may become a major water source for older individuals with impaired thirst. Laboratory tests should measure the electrolytes, osmolality, creatinine, and blood urea nitrogen; a blood urea nitrogen–to-creatinine ratio greater than or equal to 25 is suggestive of dehydration.

Anticipation and prevention of dehydration are crucial. Adequate food intake should be maintained. The total water ingested per day in persons over age 70 years ideally should be 3.7 liters for men and 2.7 liters for women. At a minimum, 30 mL of daily fluid intake per kilogram of body weight is recommended. In patients suffering from an acute medical event, it is important to review any long-term medications, particularly diuretics, that may have contributed to dehydration and to define the ethically appropriate approach to future episodes. In terminally ill patients, death from dehydration becomes a natural event in which symptom-focused care relieves discomfort from dry mucous membranes (Chapter 3).

Endocrine System

Growth hormone levels fall with advancing age, with initial loss of nocturnal growth hormone spikes (Chapter 231). These declines contribute to the decreased muscle strength, thinning of bones and skin, and increased central fat associated with aging. It is currently unclear whether replacement of growth factors can induce a permanent reversal of muscle, bone, and skin changes with advancing age.

The production rates and clearance rates of thyroxine, triiodothyronine, and calcitonin appear to be constant with advancing age despite the increased prevalence of thyroid disease in late life (Chapter 233). There is an increase in parathyroid hormone levels, particularly in women, with advancing age, perhaps in compensation for the age-related decline of the kidney's ability to maintain normal levels of phosphorus and calcium in the blood (Chapter 253).

The adrenal glands maintain their ability to secrete cortisone with advancing age (Chapter 234). Dehydroepiandrosterone declines 85 to 90% by the age of 70 years, however, perhaps contributing to impaired immune or cardiovascular function. Renin and aldosterone secretion rates decline progressively with advancing age and do not contribute to the increased rates of hypertension with advancing age.

The insulin content of the elderly pancreas is increased, but the release of insulin in response to stimulation may be blunted with advancing age (Chapters 236 and 237). There is also a concomitant decline in insulin clearance with advancing age, with the net result that plasma insulin levels in response to glucose appear to be relatively preserved. Insulin resistance may increase with advancing age, but glucagon secretion appears to be well preserved.

The ovaries show dramatic declines in estrogen and progesterone as fibrosis and scarring occur. Menopause occurs at an average age of 51 years, with subsequent hot flashes, accelerated bone loss, and atrophy of estrogen-sensitive tissues (Chapter 248). Levels of testosterone decrease in some men beginning around 50 years, but declines do not appear to affect the potency of semen. Sexual function is relatively well preserved, albeit with an increase in the refractory period, increase in the time to arousal, and a loss of tissue turgor (Chapter 242).

Age-Related Endocrine Syndromes

The most important age-related endocrine syndrome occurring with advancing age is menopause (Chapter 248). Most other endocrine changes with age may enhance the prevalence of common disorders seen with aging, especially diabetes.

Immune System

Normal aging produces an obvious decrease in the size of the thymus gland between puberty and 50 or 60 years of age, at which time the gland becomes difficult to identify anatomically. This decrease in size is accompanied by a corresponding drop in thymosin levels, which are related directly to the number of functional T cells found in older adults. T cells also appear to be less active in responding to the presence of foreign proteins, and they tend to reproduce more slowly than those in younger adults. Functional studies of immune responsiveness suggest that although antibody responses are produced by older individuals, they tend to be less robust and less long lasting than in younger individuals (Chapters 44 and 257).

Clinical Syndromes of Aging

There are increased morbidity and mortality associated with influenza and pneumonia with advancing age and reactivation of infections such as tuberculosis and herpes zoster. The decline in immune function also may make it less likely that older adults will develop autoimmune diseases, such as systemic lupus erythematosus.

Vaccine therapy, which is recommended for the prevention of herpes zoster (Chapters 17 and 383), reduces zoster-related adverse effects on functional status and quality of life.[1] It is even more critical to maintain annual immunization against influenza (Chapter 17). Pneumovax and tetanus vaccination are also important in elderly people (Chapter 17).

Hematopoietic System

The pluripotent stem cell and the erythroid and myeloid progenitor cells show no age-related reduction, indicating that there is minimal or no change in basal hematopoiesis during aging (Chapter 159). The aging hematopoietic system is less able to respond to increased demands, however, as evidenced by a slower recovery from anemia and less of a rise of hemoglobin during hypoxia. The older marrow also appears to respond less well to erythropoietin.

Neutrophils from elderly individuals show less prekilling activity and lower levels of lysozyme (Chapter 172), with a significant reduction in signal transduction and less release of inositol 1,4,5-trisphosphate and diacylglycerol during stimulation. During nutritional deprivation, there appears to be impairment in the reserve capacity to kill phagocytosed bacteria, a change that may contribute to the high prevalence of serious bacterial infections among nutritionally compromised elderly patients.

Age-Related Hematopoietic Syndromes

There are no specific syndromes of impaired hematopoiesis, aside from the clinical observation that during a comparable illness stress, hematologic abnormalities are more likely in elderly patients.

Musculoskeletal System

Bone mass and density decrease with age after reaching maximum in the 20s. In women, this loss may be about 1% per year until menopause, when it can increase to 2 to 3% per year (Chapters 248 and 251). By 5 to 10 years after menopause, bone loss returns to a rate of loss of 1% per year, but it may accelerate again in the late 80s. Because men have more bone mass than women do and lose bone mass at a similar rate of about 1% per year, the clinical effects in men are not seen until advanced age.

Tendons and ligaments become less elastic with advancing age, contributing to a higher incidence of rupture, especially of the Achilles tendon, in older individuals. Cartilage and ligaments of the ribs and spine are more likely to become calcified and less elastic.

Muscles reach their ultimate size and strength in the 20s and 30s. By 70 years of age, muscle mass declines by approximately 25% for men and women unless it is offset by exercise. By the age of 80 years, muscle size and strength in most sedentary adults decrease by 30 to 40% from the mid-30s peak. Muscle mass in late life depends on exercise earlier in life to reach a higher early mass and exercise late in life to stimulate muscle preservation.

Age-Related Musculoskeletal Syndromes

The most important age-related clinical syndrome associated with advancing age is osteoporosis (Chapter 251). Sarcopenia, or diminished muscle mass, is a clear predisposing factor for falls, which is the leading cause of accidental death at home in older individuals. Bone and muscle mass respond well to gravitational stress and resistance exercises, respectively, even in the oldest age ranges.

Falls are a major age-related syndrome involving neural, musculoskeletal, and cardiovascular systems. Most falls in older adults are due to a combination of several factors rather than a single event. Internal contributors to falls include sensory impairment from poor eyesight, hearing loss, and balance disturbances; diseases of the brain, including motor and sensory disorders, cognitive impairment that produces poor judgment or apraxia, and depression; cardiovascular, respiratory, and metabolic diseases; and musculoskeletal conditions, such as lower limb weakness, poor grip strength, osteoporosis, rheumatoid arthritis, osteoarthritis, and foot disorders. External causes of falls include medications. The risk of falling increases in patients who receive four or more prescription medications; drugs specifically shown to increase the risk of falling include hypnotics, muscle relaxants, antihypertensives, diuretics, and antidepressants. Environmental problems increase the risk of falls. Inside the home, risks include stairs (coming down is more hazardous than climbing up, as the first and last steps often have no railing or an unusable one); loose objects, such as furniture, cords, and rugs; poor lighting, particularly in areas with dark and light variability; poorly fitting shoes; surfaces with glare or patterning; and lack of bathroom safety equipment. Outdoor risks include uneven pavements and surface roads made slippery from ice, water, or fallen leaves.

For a person who has fallen, the evaluation should include a detailed history of the circumstances surrounding the fall, medications, medical problems, and mobility; an examination of vision, gait, balance, and lower extremity joint function; an examination of neurologic function, including muscle strength; and an examination of the cardiovascular system. The investigations for falls and syncope (Chapters 50 and 62) are similar. Tests are needed only if the history and physical examination do not reveal the cause of falling or if they point to a particular abnormality that requires laboratory evaluation. These tests may include the following:

- Blood tests to exclude anemia, infection, and metabolic problems such as diabetes and thyroid disease
- Electrocardiogram to evaluate heart disease
- 24-Hour electrocardiogram recording or loop monitor to evaluate arrhythmias (Chapter 62)
- Echocardiogram for patients with significant heart murmurs (Chapter 55)
- Drug levels to determine whether a patient is being undertreated or overtreated with a particular drug
- If focal neurologic signs or symptoms are present, a computed tomographic scan of the brain
- If suggestive symptoms are present, a radiograph of the neck or spine to look for spinal stenosis (Chapter 407)

The risk of falls can be reduced by exercise interventions in community-dwelling elderly persons[2] and by multifactorial interventions in elderly persons in nursing facilities and hospitals.[3]

Prevention of Fractures

The prevention of fractures has three components. First, persons with lower bone densities are more likely to fracture a bone, given the same amount of trauma, than are persons with higher bone densities. Women should be assessed for osteoporosis and treated accordingly (Chapter 251). Osteoporosis often is underdiagnosed in men, and men with fractures or repeated falls should be evaluated for possible osteoporosis; however, screening strategies for elderly men have not been defined.

Fractures can be prevented if falls can be prevented. Older people who have recurrent falls should have regular exercise and balance training after their risk factors for falling are fully addressed. The optimal type, duration, and intensity of exercise are unclear, but balance training for 10 weeks or more has the best-proven benefit. Exercise must be sustained for continued benefit. Vitamin D improves muscle strength but may not reduce falls.

When someone falls, the damage may be reduced by the intrinsic padding of fat or by devices such as mechanical hip protectors. Randomized controlled trials of hip protectors to reduce fractures in nursing home patients and in ambulatory older individuals have shown mixed results in the United States. Compliance with these cumbersome devices is only 25 to 70%.

Nervous System

Brain size decreases with advancing age; after the age of 60 years, its size declines by 5 to 10%. The decrease in size is caused primarily by a decrease in the cerebral cortex. Novel adjustments to cell loss include the formation of new connections between remaining neurons. Aging is associated with a progressive decline in the synthesis of neurotransmitters and a decline in their corresponding receptors. A major functional change is slower reaction times, which may be the result of a slower nerve conduction or trans-synaptic speed.

The farsightedness of aging is caused by the diminished ability of the lens to focus on nearby objects because of its thickening and stiffening (Chapter 431). There is reduced ability to distinguish colors, particularly blue, because of yellowing of the lens. Overall transmission of light through the lens may decline by 50 to 65% between the ages of 25 and 60 years; as a result, individuals require more ambient light. Older individuals experience more glare because light scatters through the thickened lens. Older individuals also notice more floaters as the vitreous jelly becomes slightly more liquefied and mobile with advancing age. Tear production is decreased, leading to a sense of grittiness in the older eye. Overall visual acuity tends to decrease with age; by age 65 years, 40% of men and 60% of women have a visual acuity of 20/70 or worse.

Approximately 25% of individuals older than 65 years experience hearing loss with age (Chapter 436), with men affected more than women. The degeneration of neural transmission from the ear to the brain results in difficulty in identifying a voice or understanding a spoken message when there is background noise. Presbycusis results in high-frequency sound loss and more difficulty in distinguishing high-pitched consonants and voices compared with lower-pitched vowels and sounds.

Sleep patterns change with advancing age (Chapter 412). Functionally, older adults are more wakeful during the night and spend much more time in bed. The pattern of sleep characteristically changes from the fairly regular stepwise patterns of childhood and young adulthood to a more fragmented pattern, with frequent awakenings in late life.

Defined changes in brain function also occur with age, even in persons who do not meet standardized criteria for cognitive impairment. For example, the older brain does less well with divided attentional tasks, and it processes more slowly.

Age-Related Neurologic Syndromes

Age-associated memory dysfunction is common (Chapters 26 and 409), and delirium (Chapter 27) may occur, especially during illnesses. Prevention of delirium is possible with a proactive consultation intervention, which can reduce the incidence of hospital delirium by about 40 to 50%.

Sleep-disordered breathing associated with sleep apnea appears to rise in prevalence with advancing age (Chapter 100). Anatomic changes, such as tissue laxity and diseases of the nose and sinuses, may contribute to sleep-disordered breathing. Sleep apnea may have a neurologic basis either in the sleep cycling center, leading to central sleep apnea, or in neurologic control of pharyngeal tissues.

Integumentary System

Thinning of the subcutaneous tissue begins in most people in their mid-40s, independent of the degree of sun exposure or protection from injury. The epidermis and dermis adhere less tightly, making the skin feel looser and increasing its tendency to blister and to be subject to friction burns or pressure ulceration (Chapter 443). This phenomenon also leads to senile purpura (Fig. 24-1) that results from tears in small venules when the skin is bumped or abraded (Chapter 448).

Environmental exposures, including ultraviolet sunlight, wind, and smoking, help promote the development of wrinkles by damaging the subcutaneous tissues and the epidermis, especially the elastin fibers. The process of photo injury (Chapter 446) leads to slow repair, particularly of tissues of the distal forearm and lower leg. Ultraviolet light exposure also predisposes to the development of skin cancers, the most common of which is basal cell cancer, but squamous cell cancer and melanoma are also age dependent (Chapter 210). Approximately two thirds of aging individuals experience at least one skin problem, and about 40% have two underlying skin disorders.

The most profound consequence of environmental exposure and age-related changes is that wound repair rates are significantly prolonged. In individuals older than 65 years, healing takes about 50% longer compared with individuals in their 30s; complete skin healing can take 5.5 weeks instead of 3.5 weeks.

Rates of epithelial cell regeneration decrease by about 50% from maturity to 70 years of age. A similar pattern is seen in hair, which grows more slowly.

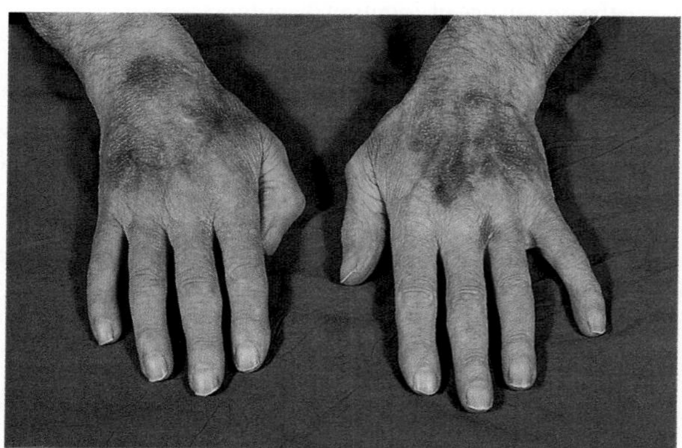

FIGURE 24-1. Senile purpura is a common and benign condition that results from impaired collagen production and capillary fragility in elderly people. In the absence of other signs of disease, no investigation is necessary. (From Forbes CD, Jackson WF. *Color Atlas and Text of Clinical Medicine,* 3rd ed. London: Mosby; 2003.)

With advancing age, graying is variable but universal because the number of melanocytes within hair bulbs declines with age (Chapter 450). Changes in skin cell size and shape cause irregular patterning and may predispose to water-induced or environment-induced cracking.

Age-Related Integumentary Syndromes

Specific illnesses affecting the skin include basal cell cancer and rosacea (Chapters 446 to 449). Aging skin syndromes also include xerosis, thermoregulatory changes, skin thinning, and hair loss. The primary therapy for xerosis is the external application of treatments to protect and moisturize the skin (Chapter 445).

Diminished sweating poses a threat during times of high ambient and environmental temperatures or in the context of fever (Chapters 109 and 289). The absence of sweating lessens heat loss by conduction and evaporation, and it diminishes the urge to move to a more protected environment. Because few elderly individuals experience thirst, dehydration may occur quickly in these settings. Environmental protection from temperature extremes is crucial (Chapter 109).

Pressure sores are necrotic areas of muscle, subcutaneous fat, and skin as a result of compression and subsequent ischemia (Fig. 24-2). Pressure sores usually occur between underlying bone and a hard surface or a soft surface during a prolonged time. Among elderly patients in acute care hospitals, the incidence rate is 8%, and the prevalence rate is 16%. Rates are even higher in patients who are in intensive care units or who have hip fractures.

A standard mattress can generate pressures as high as 150 mm Hg, well above the 30- to 35-mm Hg continuous-pressure threshold needed to cause pressure sores. In addition to pressure injury, shear injury is important. Shear injury, which occurs when local blood vessels are stretched and separated from underlying perforating vessels, is more likely when the patient is in a sloped position or is rubbing constantly against underlying surfaces. Burning injury also can result from friction of the superficial skin layers. A complicating feature of all pressure ulcers is moisture, which leads to softening of the skin, sticking to underlying surfaces, and easy access for infection.

Individuals at higher risk include those who are immobile; those who are incontinent of bowel or bladder; and those who have compromised circulation due to hypotension, dehydration, or vascular disease. Neurologic disease, particularly peripheral neuropathy that impairs sensation, can predispose to pressure ulcers, as can any neurologic condition that causes spasticity, contractures, or poor mobility.

Preventive strategies encourage safe positioning, regular turning, and avoidance of direct pressure. Judicious use of pressure-reducing beds may lower the incidence of pressure ulcers after hip fractures. Deep foam mattresses and air suspension beds are even more effective.

When pressure sores appear, they should be photographed to establish a baseline. Nutrition should be improved, all pressure on the wound should be removed, and active vigilance should be focused to prevent additional pressure ulcers. Débridement of necrotic tissue should be considered; wet-to-dry dressings and surgical or chemical débridement are often used. Infections may require topical or systemic antibiotics. Semiocclusive and occlusive dressings also can be helpful. Most pressure ulcers heal within 6 months, but operative repair is sometimes necessary.

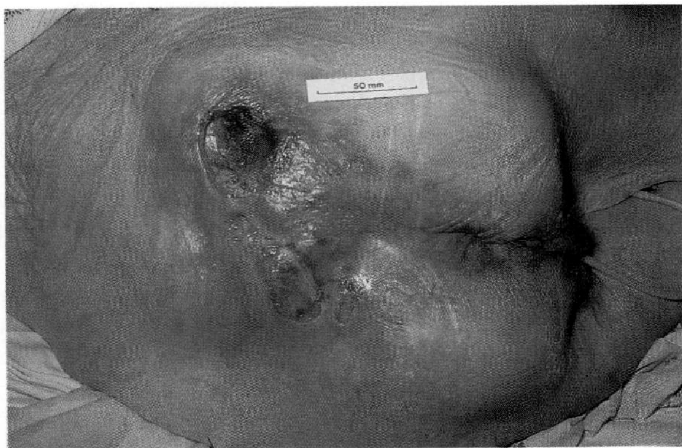

FIGURE 24-2. Severe sacral pressure sore, one of the serious but preventable complications of immobility. (From Forbes CD, Jackson WF. *Color Atlas and Text of Clinical Medicine*, 3rd ed. London: Mosby; 2003.)

Clinical Pharmacology

Of all prescription medications (Chapter 28), about 30% are taken by elderly people, even though they compose only 14% of the population. Nonprescription medications are disproportionately consumed by older individuals and are increasingly implicated in drug-drug interactions.

The gastrointestinal absorption of medications generally does not change with advancing age, despite the theoretical possibility that medications requiring acidification in the stomach may be absorbed less well because of the higher frequency of atrophic gastritis and reduced gastric acid. Drug distribution changes significantly with advancing age because medications distribute to fat or muscle. As muscle mass declines with advancing age, fat increases as a proportion of total body weight. As a result, older individuals are more sensitive to the effects of water-soluble drugs (heart) and have prolonged effects from lipophilic drugs (brain).

The decline in renal function with normal aging reduces the clearance of many drugs, especially digoxin, aminoglycosides, and cimetidine. Hepatic metabolism also may decline with age. Oxidative reactions, so-called phase 1 reactions, become impaired with normal aging, whereas phase 2 reactions (conjugation and glucuronidization) are relatively spared. A clinical example is that diazepam, which requires phase 1 and phase 2 metabolism, has a prolonged half-life with advancing age, but oxazepam, which requires only phase 2 reactions to be metabolized, does not.

The overall impact of these pharmacokinetic changes is that the half-life, which is proportional to the volume of distribution divided by drug clearance, increases for many lipophilic drugs. Poorly nourished or frail elderly persons may have a low serum albumin level. The normal age-related decline in the serum albumin level is clinically insignificant. When the albumin level is less than 3 g/dL, however, drug levels have to be interpreted on the basis of their binding to albumin; albumin levels this low are associated with an increased risk of in-hospital death and longer lengths of hospital stay.

Independent of pharmacokinetic issues, elderly people are more sensitive to many medications. The brain appears to be increasingly sensitive to many compounds, including opiates, benzodiazepines, and neuroleptics. As a result, lower doses cause effects equivalent to those seen with higher doses in younger individuals. Warfarin, which acts primarily on the liver, will maintain therapeutic anticoagulation profiles at lower doses in elderly patients because the aging liver is increasingly sensitive to blockage of vitamin K–dependent systems.

Elderly people are at higher risk for nonadherence to prescribed regimens. Factors influencing nonadherence include the number of medications and their cost, inadequate education of the patient, unacceptable side effects, and complexity of the medical regimen. Individuals who take more than three prescription drugs have lower adherence. Below three medications per day, elderly individuals in general have high adherence rates. Unfortunately, no intervention has reliably improved adherence rates in elderly people.

Perhaps the most important phenomenon in multiple-drug regimens in older individuals is the progressive accumulation of anticholinergic effects, including dry mouth, constipation, poor vision, urinary retention, balance disorders, and cognitive difficulties. Anticholinergic drugs include neuroleptics, antispasmodics, antianxiety agents, antihistamines, and medications used for urinary incontinence.

An Integrated Approach

Because elderly people commonly have many medical conditions, some of which are age-related and others exacerbated by age-related conditions, a multidisciplinary approach is often useful. For example, integrated and home-based geriatric care management improve quality of care and reduce acute care utilization among high-risk community-dwelling elderly people.[4] Collaborative care interventions are more effective for depression in older people than usual care and are also of high value.[5] Similarly, geriatric intervention improved functional abilities and mental well-being of vulnerable older people. Physicians should become aware of such community resources that can benefit these patients.

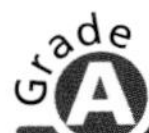

1. Schmader KE, Johnson GR, Saddier P, et al. Effect of a zoster vaccine on herpes zoster-related interference with functional status and health-related quality-of-life measures in older adults. *J Am Geriatr Soc*. 2010;58:1634-1641.
2. Gillespie LD, Robertson MC, Gillespie WJ, et al. Interventions for preventing falls in older people living in the community. *Cochrane Database Syst Rev*. 2009;2:CD007146.

3. Cameron ID, Murray GR, Gillespie LD, et al. Interventions for preventing falls in older people in nursing care facilities and hospitals. *Cochrane Database Syst Rev.* 2010;1:CD005465.
4. Melis RJ, van Eijken MI, Teerenstra S, et al. A randomized study of a multidisciplinary program to intervene on geriatric syndromes in vulnerable older people who live at home (Dutch EASYcare Study). *J Gerontol A Biol Sci Med Sci.* 2008;63:283-290.
5. Chang-Quan H, Bi-Rong D, Zhen-Chan L, et al. Collaborative care interventions for depression in the elderly: a systematic review of randomized controlled trials. *J Investig Med.* 2009;57:446-455.

SUGGESTED READINGS

Basaria S, Coviello AD, Travison TG, et al. Adverse events associated with testosterone administration. *N Engl J Med.* 2010;363:109-122. *Testosterone gel in elderly men with low testosterone levels improved strength but increased adverse cardiac events almost 5-fold.*

Delbaere K, Close JC, Heim J, et al. A multifactorial approach to understanding fall risk in older people. *J Am Geriatr Soc.* 2010;58:1679-1685. *Balance-related impairments are the critical predictors.*

Ko FC. The clinical care of frail, older adults. *Clin Geriatr Med.* 2011;27:89-100. *Review of biology and treatment.*

Steinman MA, Hanlon JT. Managing medications in clinically complex elders: "There's got to be a happy medium." *JAMA.* 2010;304:1592-1601. *Review.*

25 INCONTINENCE

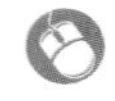

NEIL M. RESNICK

DEFINITION

Urinary incontinence is the involuntary leakage of urine sufficient to be a health or social problem.

EPIDEMIOLOGY

More than twice as common in women as in men, the prevalence of incontinence increases with age. But at no age does it affect the majority of individuals—even over age 85 years. Incontinence afflicts 15 to 30% of older adults living at home, one third of those in acute care settings, and half of those in nursing homes. It predisposes to perineal rashes, pressure ulcers, urinary tract infections, urosepsis, falls, and fractures, and it is associated with embarrassment, stigmatization, isolation, depression, anxiety, sexual dysfunction, and risk of institutionalization. Its cost in the United States exceeds $26 billion annually.

Despite these considerations, geriatric incontinence remains largely neglected, by patients and physicians alike. This is unfortunate because its increased prevalence with age relates more to age-associated diseases and functional impairments than to age itself. Most importantly, incontinence is usually treatable and often curable at all ages, even in frail elderly people, although the approach in older patients must be broader than that employed in younger patients.

PATHOBIOLOGY

At any age, continence depends not only on the integrity of lower urinary tract function but also on the presence of adequate mentation, mobility, motivation, and manual dexterity. Although incontinence in younger patients is rarely associated with deficits in these domains, such deficits occur commonly in older patients in whom they can cause or exacerbate incontinence or influence therapeutic approaches.

With age, bladder capacity does not change, but bladder sensation and contractility decrease. At the cellular level, detrusor smooth muscle develops a "dense band pattern" characterized by dense sarcolemmal bands with depleted caveolae. This depletion may mediate the age-related decline in bladder contractility. In addition, an incomplete dysjunction pattern characterized by scattered protrusion junctions develops and may underlie the high prevalence of involuntary bladder contractions (detrusor overactivity) in older adults of both sexes. Urethral length and sphincter strength decrease in women, whereas the prostate enlarges in most men and causes measurable obstruction in about half. The postvoid residual volume (PVR) in the bladder also increases but normally to less than 100 mL. In addition, elderly people often excrete most of their fluid intake at night, even in the absence of venous insufficiency, renal disease, heart failure, or prostatism. Coupled with an age-associated increase in sleep disorders, most older adults have one or two episodes of nocturia per night.

None of these changes causes incontinence, but all predispose to it. This predisposition, combined with the increased likelihood that an older person will encounter an additional pathologic, physiologic, or pharmacologic insult, explains the increased prevalence of incontinence with age. The implications are equally important. The onset or exacerbation of incontinence in an older person is likely to be due to precipitants that are outside the lower urinary tract and that are amenable to medical intervention. Furthermore, treatment of the precipitants alone may be sufficient to restore continence, even if there is coexisting urinary tract dysfunction. For example, a flare of hip arthritis in a woman with age-related detrusor overactivity may decrease mobility sufficiently to convert her urinary urgency into incontinence. Treatment of the arthritis, rather than the involuntary detrusor contractions, will not only restore continence but also lessen pain and improve mobility. Because of their frequency, reversibility, and association with morbidity beyond incontinence, the transient precipitant causes should be addressed first.

Causes of Transient Incontinence

Incontinence is transient in up to one third of community-dwelling elderly people and in up to half of acutely hospitalized patients. Although most transient causes are outside the lower urinary tract (Table 25-1), three points warrant emphasis. First, the risk of transient incontinence is increased if, in addition to physiologic changes of the lower urinary tract, there also are pathologic changes. Anticholinergic agents are more likely to cause overflow incontinence in individuals with a weak or obstructed bladder, whereas excess urine output is more likely to cause urge incontinence in people with detrusor overactivity or impaired mobility. Second, these transient causes may persist if left untreated and should not be dismissed merely because incontinence is long-standing. Third, identification of the most common cause is of little value because causes vary among individuals, and geriatric incontinence is rarely due to just one cause.

Causes of Established Incontinence Related to the Lower Urinary Tract

Detrusor overactivity, which also is called involuntary bladder contraction or *overactive bladder*, generally causes *urge incontinence* and is the most common type of lower urinary tract dysfunction in incontinent elderly people, accounting for about two thirds of cases. Histologically, detrusor overactivity is associated with the complete dysjunction pattern, with widening of the intercellular space, reduction of normal (intermediate) muscle cell junctions, and emergence of novel protrusion junctions and ultraclose abutments that connect cells together in chains. These connections may mediate a change in cell coupling from a mechanical to an electrical mechanism that results in involuntary bladder contraction. Other potential causes include ischemia, abnormalities in suburothelial myofibroblasts, and changes in central nervous system structural and functional control mechanisms.

At any age, detrusor overactivity is usually idiopathic, but it can be associated with a variety of other causes that may affect prognosis and management. Such conditions include an upper motor neuron lesion (Chapters 407 and 418), urethral obstruction, stress incontinence, bladder calculus, and bladder carcinoma (Chapter 203).

Detrusor overactivity exists as two subsets in elderly people: one in which contractile function is preserved and one in which it is impaired. The latter condition, termed *detrusor hyperactivity with impaired contractility*, has several implications. First, because the bladder is weak, these patients commonly develop urinary retention, which is also seen in patients with outlet obstruction and detrusor underactivity. Second, even in the absence of retention, detrusor hyperactivity with impaired contractility mimics other lower urinary tract causes of incontinence. For instance, if the involuntary detrusor contraction occurs coincident with a stress maneuver and if the weak contraction is not detected, detrusor hyperactivity with impaired contractility will be misdiagnosed as stress incontinence. Alternatively, because detrusor hyperactivity with impaired contractility may be associated with urinary urgency, frequency, weak flow rate, elevated residual urine, and bladder trabeculation, in men it may mimic prostatic obstruction. Third, anticholinergic therapy of detrusor hyperactivity with impaired contractility may result in urinary retention owing to bladder weakness, thereby requiring alternative therapeutic approaches.

Stress incontinence, which is the second most common cause of incontinence in older women and the dominant cause in middle-aged women, usually reflects urethral hypermobility plus some degree of sphincter

TABLE 25-1 CAUSES OF TRANSIENT INCONTINENCE: DIAPERS MNEMONIC

Delirium	Result of underlying illness or medication; incontinence is secondary and abates once the cause of delirium is corrected	
Infection—*symptomatic* UTI	Acute, symptomatic UTI causes incontinence, but the far more common asymptomatic bacteriuria does not	
Atrophic urethritis/vaginitis	Characterized by vaginal erosions, telangiectasia, petechiae, and friability; may cause or contribute to incontinence. Although oral estrogen may worsen incontinence, a 3- to 12-month course of topical estrogen can be useful	
Pharmaceuticals	*Drug type:*	*Potential effects on continence:*
	Sedative-hypnotics (e.g., long-acting benzodiazepines; alcohol)	Sedation, delirium, decreased mobility
	Anticholinergics (dicyclomine, disopyramide, sedating antihistamines, antipsychotics, tricyclic antidepressants, anti-Parkinson's, antidepressants) (*not* SSRIs)	Urinary retention, overflow incontinence, delirium, impaction; the antipsychotics also decrease mobility
	Opiates	Urinary retention, stool impaction, sedation, delirium
	α-Adrenergic antagonists	Relax sphincter; may induce stress incontinence in women
	α-Adrenergic agonists	Urinary retention in men (tighten sphincter, prostate)
	Calcium channel blockers, especially the dihydropyridines	Urinary retention; nocturnal diuresis due to fluid retention
	"Loop" diuretics (thiazide-like agents only rarely cause it)	Polyuria, frequency, urgency
	NSAIDs	Nocturnal diuresis due to fluid retention
	Thiazolidinediones	Nocturnal diuresis due to fluid retention
	Dopamine receptor agonists (e.g., ropinirole, pramipexole)	Nocturnal diuresis due to fluid retention
	Angiotensin-converting enzyme inhibitors	Drug-induced cough leads to stress incontinence in women
	Vincristine	Urinary retention due to neuropathy
Excess urine output	From large intake, diuretic agents (theophylline, caffeinated beverages, alcohol), and metabolic disorders (hyperglycemia, hypercalcemia); nocturnal incontinence may result from mobilization of peripheral edema (CHF, venous insufficiency)	
Restricted mobility	Often results from overlooked, correctable conditions such as arthritis, pain, foot problems, postprandial hypotension	
Stool impaction	May cause both fecal and urinary incontinence that remit with disimpaction	

CHF = congestive heart failure; NSAIDs = nonsteroidal anti-inflammatory drugs; SSRI = selective serotonin reuptake inhibitor; UTI = urinary tract infection.
Adapted from Resnick NM, Tadic SD, Yalla SV. Geriatric incontinence and voiding dysfunction. In: Wein AJ, Novick AC, Partin AW, et al, eds. *Campbell-Walsh Urology*, 10th ed. St. Louis: Elsevier; 2010.

weakness. Stress incontinence is rare in men but can result from sphincter damage following radical but not transurethral prostatectomy.

Urethral obstruction is the second most common cause of established incontinence in older men, although most obstructed men are not incontinent. When obstruction is associated with incontinence, it usually presents as urge incontinence owing to the associated detrusor overactivity; overflow incontinence is uncommon. Outlet obstruction is rare in women but may result from a bladder neck suspension or from urethral kinking associated with a large cystocele.

Detrusor underactivity is usually idiopathic. When it causes incontinence, it is associated with overflow incontinence (<10% of incontinence).

Damage to lower urinary tract innervation can cause several types of dysfunction. A brain lesion may cause detrusor overactivity. A spinal cord lesion (Chapters 195 and 407) above the sacral level can cause both detrusor overactivity and detrusor-sphincter dyssynergia, a condition in which the sphincter contracts rather than relaxes during detrusor contraction; the result can be severe outlet obstruction and hydronephrosis. A spinal cord lesion below the sacral level can cause detrusor underactivity, sphincter weakness, or both. Peripheral and autonomic nerve damage can cause still additional problems. Because *neurogenic bladder* is such a nonspecific term, it is preferable to refer to the dysfunction that it causes.

Causes of Incontinence Unrelated to the Lower Urinary Tract (Functional Incontinence)

"Functional" incontinence, which is often cited as a distinct type of geriatric incontinence and attributed to deficits of cognition and mobility, implies that urinary tract function is normal. However, normal urinary tract function is the exception, even in continent elderly people, and is rarely observed in incontinent elderly people. Incontinence is not inevitable, even with dementia or immobility. Among the most severely demented institutionalized residents, nearly 20% are continent; among those who can transfer from a bed to a chair, nearly half are continent. Functionally impaired individuals also are the most likely to suffer from factors that cause transient incontinence, and a diagnosis of functional incontinence may result in failure to detect these reversible causes. Finally, if functionally impaired individuals also have urethral obstruction or stress incontinence, they may benefit from targeted therapy. Nonetheless, functional impairment often contributes to incontinence, and addressing its causes and those of transient incontinence may ameliorate incontinence sufficiently to obviate the need for further investigation.

CLINICAL MANIFESTATIONS

The manifestations of transient incontinence depend on the underlying condition. For established incontinence, detrusor overactivity usually manifests as *urge incontinence,* characterized by leakage that follows the abrupt onset or intensification of a desire to void, leakage of a moderate to large amount, urinary frequency (>8 voids/day), nocturia, and nocturnal incontinence. However, some patients with detrusor overactivity may present without the urge component. *Stress incontinence* causes leakage that coincides with both the onset and cessation of a cough or other cause of increased abdominal pressure; nocturnal leakage is rare. Some patients report both types of incontinence, or *mixed incontinence,* but it is useful to determine which component is the most bothersome. Occasionally, patients present with incontinence that is more difficult to characterize clinically without further testing.

DIAGNOSIS

In addition to a targeted clinical evaluation (Table 25-2), a bladder diary can provide diagnostic clues and guide therapy (Fig. 25-1). For example, incontinence occurring only between 8 AM and noon may be caused by a morning loop diuretic. Incontinence that occurs at night in a demented man with heart failure, but not during a 4-hour nap in his wheelchair, is likely due to nocturnal diuresis associated with his heart failure and not to dementia, impaired mobility, or prostatic obstruction. A woman with volume-dependent stress incontinence may leak only on the way to void after a full night's sleep, when her bladder contains more than 400 mL—more than it ever does during her continent waking hours.

Because urinary retention is difficult to detect by examination and can affect diagnosis and therapy, the PVR volume should be determined routinely, except possibly in middle-aged women with a classic presentation of stress incontinence. Urodynamic testing is generally unnecessary unless diagnostic certainty is required, such as before surgical repair or if there is evidence of a serious underlying cause of the incontinence, such as a brain or spinal cord lesion, carcinoma of the bladder or prostate, hydronephrosis, or bladder calculus. Urodynamic evaluation comprises a battery of tests designed to assess the lower urinary tract during the filling and voiding phases of micturition. The selection among tests depends on the clinical setting and question to be answered; for instance, measuring detrusor pressure and urine flow during voiding can determine whether urethral obstruction is present, whereas monitoring bladder and urethral pressures during the filling phase and with coughing may be helpful for patients with an atypical presentation of mixed incontinence.

TABLE 25-2 CLINICAL EVALUATION OF THE INCONTINENT PATIENT

HISTORY
Type (urge, stress, overflow, or mixed) Incontinence frequency, severity, duration Pattern (diurnal, nocturnal, or both; also, e.g., after taking medications) Associated symptoms (straining to void, incomplete emptying, dysuria, hematuria, suprapubic/perineal discomfort) Alteration in bowel habit/sexual function (because of proximity to the bladder and shared innervation) Other relevant factors (cancer, acute illness, neurologic disease, pelvic or lower urinary tract surgery/radiation therapy) Medications, including nonprescription agents (see Table 25-1) Brief assessment of cognitive and physical function
PHYSICAL EXAMINATION
Identify other relevant medical conditions (e.g., congestive heart failure, peripheral edema) If stress incontinence suspected, determine whether leakage *coincides* with the onset *and* cessation of a single, forceful cough Palpate for bladder distention after voiding Pelvic examination to detect atrophic vaginitis, pelvic muscle laxity, pelvic mass Rectal examination (skin irritation, resting tone and voluntary control of anal sphincter, prostate nodule; fecal impaction (*note:* prostate size correlates poorly with presence of urethral obstruction) Neurologic examination (mental status and elemental examination, including sacral reflexes and perineal sensation)
INITIAL INVESTIGATION
Bladder diary (see Fig. 25-1) Metabolic survey (electrolytes, calcium, glucose, and urea nitrogen as appropriate) Measure postvoid residual (PVR) volume, by portable ultrasound if available Urinalysis to detect sterile hematuria or infection; culture if new-onset or worsening incontinence Renal ultrasound to detect hydronephrosis in men whose PVR urine exceeds about 200 mL Urine cytology for patients with hematuria, pain, or unexplained new-onset or worsening incontinence Uroflowmetry for men in whom urethral obstruction is suspected Cystoscopy for patients with hematuria, suspicion of lower urinary tract pathology (e.g., bladder fistula, stone, or tumor; urethral diverticulum), or need for lower urinary tract surgery

Adapted from Resnick NM, Yalla SV. Management of urinary incontinence in the elderly. *N Engl J Med.* 1985;313:800-805.

Date	Time	Volume Voided (mL)	Are You Wet or Dry?	Approximate Volume of Incontinence	Comments
4/5	3:40 pm	240	Wet	Slight	
	6:05 pm	210	Dry		
	8:15 pm	150	Dry		Running water
	10:20 pm	150	Wet	15 mL	Bowel movement
	10:30 pm	30	Dry		
4/6	3:15 am	270	Wet	Slight	
	6:05 am	300	Wet	Slight	
	7:40 am	200	Dry		
	9:50 am	?	Dry		
	11:20 am	200	Dry		
	12:50 pm	180	Dry		
	1:40 pm	240	Dry		
	3:35 pm	160	Dry		
	6:00 pm	170	Dry		
	8:20 pm	215	Wet	Slight	Running water
	10:25 pm	130	Dry		

FIGURE 25-1. Sample bladder diary. Bladder diary of an incontinent 75-year-old man. Urodynamic evaluation excluded urethral obstruction and confirmed a diagnosis of detrusor hyperactivity with impaired contractility (detrusor hyperactivity with impaired contractility). Note the 24-hour urine output of nearly 3 liters due to the belief that drinking 10 glasses of fluid per day was "good for my health." (He did not mention this until queried about the voiding record.) Given the typical voided volume of 150 to 250 mL and a measured postvoid residual of 150 mL, excess fluid intake was overwhelming his usual bladder capacity of 400 mL (150 + 250 mL). Although involuntary bladder contractions were present, the easily reversible volume component of the problem, combined with the risk of precipitating urinary retention with an anticholinergic agent, prompted treatment with volume restriction alone. After daily urinary output dropped to 1500 mL, frequency abated, and incontinence resolved. (Adapted from DuBeau CE, Resnick NM. Evaluation of the causes and severity of geriatric incontinence: a critical appraisal. *Urol Clin North Am.* 1991;18:243-256.)

TREATMENT Rx

Optimal therapy requires a multifactorial approach (Table 25-3), including treatment of transient causes, underlying medical conditions, functional impairments, and the urinary tract abnormality itself. Although pads and diapers have a role, they remain an adjunct to more specific therapy.

Behavioral Therapy

Behavioral therapy includes education, self-monitoring with a bladder diary, adjustment of fluid intake, weight loss for overweight women with stress incontinence,[1] use of aids (e.g., a bedside urinal), and various types of bladder retraining and urethral sphincter exercises (e.g., progressively increasing voiding intervals, strategies to cope with urgency, and pelvic muscle exercises).[1-3] The efficacy of behavioral therapy is equivalent to pharmacotherapy for urge incontinence and is superior to drugs for stress incontinence.[2,3] Moreover, combining behavioral and pharmacologic therapy may prove more beneficial than either treatment alone, especially for urge incontinence, because neither therapy generally abolishes involuntary bladder contractions. For institutionalized patients who are cognitively impaired but can state their name and are partly mobile, regular daytime reminders to void ("prompted voiding") have proved effective for daytime incontinence; pads and diapers are appropriate for the others.[4]

Pharmacotherapy

Currently approved drugs have generally proved ineffective for stress incontinence and overflow incontinence, but several bladder relaxants are available for urge incontinence (see Table 25-3). Each has proved superior to placebo in well-conducted trials, and most have also proved effective in trials targeting older patients.[2,3] All have antimuscarinic properties, such as dry mouth, constipation, visual blurring, and occasional confusion. Yet each is well tolerated even in cognitively impaired elderly patients when prescribed properly, although cognitive status should be monitored. These drugs also can be well tolerated in patients taking cholinesterase inhibitors. The choice among drugs often hinges on other considerations. For instance, immediate-release oxybutynin has the quickest onset of action, making it an inexpensive and effective choice for patients who need excellent control at predictable times. The other drugs, although more expensive, can be used less often and can be better tolerated for daily use.

Regardless of the agent selected, the key is to begin with a low dose and increase it slowly, realizing that the full benefit is generally not apparent for

TABLE 25-3 STEPWISE APPROACH TO TREATMENT OF URINARY INCONTINENCE*

CONDITION	CLINICAL TYPE OF INCONTINENCE[†]	TREATMENT
Detrusor overactivity with normal contractility	Urge	1. Bladder retraining or prompted voiding regimens 2. ± Bladder relaxant medication if needed and not contraindicated (see drug list below) 3. Indwelling catheterization alone is often unhelpful because detrusor spasms often increase, leading to leakage around the catheter 4. In selected cases, induce urinary retention pharmacologically and add intermittent or indwelling catheterization[‡]
Detrusor hyperactivity with impaired contractility	Urge[§]	1. If bladder empties adequately, behavioral methods (as above) ± bladder relaxant medication (low doses; especially feasible if sphincter incompetence coexists) 2. If residual urine >150 mL, augmented voiding techniques[¶] or intermittent catheterization (± bladder relaxant medication). If neither feasible, undergarment or indwelling catheter[‡] 3. In selected cases, induce urinary retention pharmacologically and add intermittent or indwelling catheterization[‡]
Stress incontinence	Stress	1. Conservative methods (weight loss if obese; treatment of cough or atrophic vaginitis; physical maneuvers to prevent leakage [e.g., tighten pelvic muscles before cough, cross legs]; occasionally, use of tampon or pessary is helpful) 2. If leakage threshold ≥150 mL identified, adjust fluid excretion and voiding intervals appropriately 3. Pelvic muscle exercises ± biofeedback/weighted intravaginal cones; must continue indefinitely 4. Surgery (sling, artificial sphincter, periurethral bulking injections)
Urethral obstruction	Urge/overflow[‖]	1. Conservative methods (including adjustment of fluid excretion, bladder retraining/prompted voiding) if hydronephrosis, recurrent symptomatic UTI, and hematuria have been excluded 2. α-Adrenergic antagonist 3. Also consider adding a bladder relaxant if detrusor overactivity coexists, PVR is small, and surgery not desired/feasible; *monitor PVR!* 4. Finasteride, if not contraindicated and the patient either prefers it or is not a surgical candidate 5. Surgery (incision, prostatectomy) is an effective alternative before or after these steps
Underactive detrusor	Overflow	1. Decompress for at least several days (the larger the PVR, the longer should be the decompression [up to a month]) and then perform a voiding trial 2. Exclude urethral obstruction if this has not already been done 3. If cannot void or PVR remains large, try augmented voiding techniques[¶] ± α-adrenergic antagonist, but only if some voiding possible; bethanechol *rarely* useful 4. If fails, or voiding is not possible, intermittent or indwelling catheterization[†]

*These treatments should be initiated only after adequate toilet access has been ensured, contributing conditions have been treated (e.g., atrophic vaginitis, UTI, fecal impaction, heart failure), fluid management has been optimized, and unnecessary or exacerbating medications have been addressed. For additional details, see text.

†*Urge:* leakage in the absence of stress maneuvers and urinary retention, usually preceded by *abrupt* onset or intensification of the need to void; *stress:* leakage that coincides *instantaneously* with stress maneuvers, in the absence of urinary retention or detrusor contraction; *overflow:* frequent leakage of small amounts associated with urinary retention.

‡UTI prophylaxis can be used for recurrent symptomatic UTIs, but only if catheter is not indwelling.

§May also mimic stress or overflow incontinence.

‖Also can cause postvoid "dribbling" alone, which is treated conservatively (e.g., by sitting to void and allowing more time, "double voiding," and in men by gently "milking" the urethra after voiding).

¶Augmented voiding techniques include Credé (application of suprapubic pressure) and Valsalva (straining) maneuvers, and double voiding. They should be performed only *after* voiding has begun.

Anticholinergic bladder relaxant agents for urge incontinence:
Oxybutynin IR, 7.5-20 mg daily (2.5-5 mg tid-qid); oxybutynin XL, 5-30 mg once daily; oxybutynin patch twice weekly; oxybutynin 10% gel (1 g topically per day)
Tolterodine, 2 mg twice daily; tolterodine LA, 4 mg once daily
Darifenacin, 7.5-15 mg once daily
Solifenacin, 5-10 mg once daily
Trospium, 20 mg daily to twice daily; XL now available
Fesoterodine, 4-8 mg once daily
PVR = postvoid residual; UTI = urinary tract infection.
Adapted and updated in 2011 from Resnick NM. Voiding dysfunction and urinary incontinence. In: Beck JC, ed. *Geriatric Review Syllabus*. New York: American Geriatrics Society, 1991:141-154.

about 2 months and that side effects may offset the benefit. With such titration, urge incontinence can be controlled in about one third of patients and substantially improved in another one third.

Surgical Procedures

Surgery for stress incontinence has proved effective for women of all ages, including elderly women, and is relatively durable. Periurethral bulking injections can help frail women or those with mild stress incontinence, but it does not generally restore continence. However, urethral sling and midurethral tape suspension procedures can cure most women for at least 5 years.[5] For women with more complex stress incontinence and for men with stress incontinence more than a year after radical prostatectomy, an artificial sphincter has proved effective and relatively durable. Experience with the "male sling" is still limited.

Surgical interventions for urge incontinence, including neuromodulation, tibial nerve stimulation, and injections of botulinum toxin are successful in selected situations. However, they have not been studied adequately in elderly people, and the limited preliminary data suggest that older patients may not fare as well as younger ones.

PREVENTION

There are scant data regarding the prevention of incontinence, but one randomized trial of an educational and behavioral modification program for women older than 55 years found that it reduced the risk of incontinence for a year.[6] A secondary analysis of the Diabetes Prevention Program found that, at the end of 3 years, an intensive lifestyle intervention was associated with reduced risk of self-reported incontinence, with most of the benefit explained by weight loss and a reduced risk of stress incontinence.[7]

PROGNOSIS

Limited data suggest that incontinence progresses in about one third of patients and remits in about 10 to 15%, although it is unclear how much of the remission reflects intervention or improvement in functional or medical status.

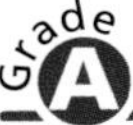

1. Subak LL, Wing R, West DS, et al. Weight loss to treat urinary incontinence in overweight and obese women. *N Engl J Med*. 2009;360:481-490.
2. Shamliyan TA, Kane RL, Wyman J, et al. Systematic review: randomized, controlled trials of nonsurgical treatments for urinary incontinence in women. *Ann Intern Med*. 2008;148:459-473.
3. Hartmann KE, McPheeters ML, Biller DH, et al. Treatment of overactive bladder in women. Evidence Report/Technology Assessment No. 187. AHRQ Publication No. 09-E017. Rockville, MD: Agency for Healthcare Research and Quality, 2009.
4. DuBeau CE, Kuchel GA, Johnson T, et al. Incontinence in the frail elderly. *Neurourol Urodyn*. 2010;29:165-179.
5. Albo ME, Richter HE, Brubaker L, et al. Burch colposuspension versus fascial sling to reduce urinary stress incontinence. *N Engl J Med*. 2007;356:2143-2155.
6. Diokno AC, Sampselle CM, Herzog AR. Prevention of urinary incontinence by behavioral modification program: a randomized controlled trial among older women in the community. *J Urol*. 2004;171:1165-1171.
7. Brown JS, Wing RA, Barrett-Connor E, et al. Lifestyle intervention is associated with lower prevalence of urinary incontinence. *Diabetes Care*. 2006;29:385-390.

SUGGESTED READINGS

Goode PS, Burgio KL, Richter HE, et al. Incontinence in older women. *JAMA*. 2010;303:2172-2181. *Evidence-based review.*

Guzzo TJ, Drach GW. Major urologic problems in geriatrics: assessment and management. *Med Clin North Am*. 2011;95:253-264. *Review.*

26 NEUROPSYCHIATRIC ASPECTS OF AGING

SHARON K. INOUYE

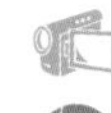

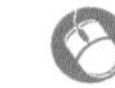

DEFINITION

The process of aging produces important physiologic changes in the central nervous system (Table 26-1), including neuroanatomic, neurotransmitter, and neurophysiologic changes. These processes result in age-related symptoms and manifestations (Table 26-2) for many older persons. These physiologic changes develop at dramatically variable rates among older persons, however, and the decline may be modified by factors such as diet, exercise, environment, lifestyle, genetic predisposition, disability, disease, and side effects of drugs. These changes can result in the common age-related symptoms of benign senescence, slowed reaction time, postural hypotension, vertigo or giddiness, presbyopia, presbycusis, stiffened gait, and sleep difficulties. In the absence of disease, these physiologic changes usually result in relatively modest symptoms and little restriction in activities of daily living. These changes decrease physiologic reserve, however, and increase the susceptibility to challenges posed by disease-related, pharmacologic, and environmental stressors.

EPIDEMIOLOGY

Neuropsychiatric disorders, the leading cause of disability in older persons, account for nearly 50% of functional incapacity. Severe neuropsychiatric conditions have been estimated to occur in 15 to 25% of older adults worldwide. These conditions are due to diseases that increase with age but are not part of the normal aging process. Alzheimer's disease and related dementias occur in approximately 10% of adults aged 65 years and older and in 40% of those older than 85 years (Chapter 409). Delirium occurs in 5 to 10% of all persons older than 65 years and in up to 80% of older persons during hospitalizations for acute illnesses (Chapter 27). Severe depression (Chapter 404) occurs in approximately 5% of older adults, with 15% having significant depressive symptoms. Anxiety disorders occur in 10% of older adults. Older individuals are also subject to substantial morbidity and functional disability from cerebrovascular disease (Chapters 413 through 415), Parkinson's disease (Chapter 416), peripheral neuropathies (Chapter 428), degenerative myelopathies (Chapters 407 and 430), spinal stenosis and disc disease (Chapter 407), seizure disorders (Chapter 410), sleep apnea (Chapter 100), visual disturbances (Chapter 431), falls (Chapter 24), incontinence (Chapter 25), and impotence (Chapter 242).

TABLE 26-1 AGE-RELATED PHYSIOLOGIC CHANGES IN THE CENTRAL NERVOUS SYSTEM

Neuroanatomic changes Brain atrophy Decreased neuron counts Increased neuritic plaques Increased lipofuscin and melanin
Neurotransmitter changes Decline in cholinergic transmission Decreased dopaminergic synthesis Decreased catecholamine synthesis
Neurophysiologic changes Decreased cerebral blood flow Electrophysiologic changes (slowing of alpha rhythm, increased latencies in evoked responses)

DIAGNOSIS

To diagnose these conditions, physicians must understand and perform a mental status examination and an assessment of functional capacity and know the uses and side effects of psychoactive drugs in geriatric patients.

Mental Status Examination

In addition to a detailed neurologic examination, evaluation of neuropsychiatric disturbances in older persons requires a careful mental status examination, including an assessment of mood, affect, and cognition. Brief screening tests are available to evaluate these domains and to assist in the detection of potential problems requiring further evaluation and treatment. For depression screening, scores of 6 or more on the 15-item short-form Geriatric Depression Scale (Table 26-3) indicate substantial depressive symptoms requiring further evaluation. Alternative depression screening instruments include the Center for Epidemiologic Studies Depression Scale (CES-D). For cognitively impaired patients, observer-rated depression scales, such as the Hamilton Depression Scale or Cornell Scale, are recommended.

TABLE 26-2 NEUROPSYCHIATRIC MANIFESTATIONS OF AGE-RELATED PHYSIOLOGIC CHANGES

SYSTEM	MANIFESTATION
Cognition	Forgetfulness Processing speed declines throughout adult life Neuropsychological declines: selective attention, verbal fluency, retrieval, complex visual perception, logical analysis
Reflexes	Stretch reflexes lose sensitivity Decreased or absent ankle reflexes Decreased autonomic and righting reflexes, postural instability
Sensory	Presbycusis (high-frequency hearing loss), tinnitus Deterioration of vestibular system, vertigo Presbyopia (decreased lens elasticity) Slowed pupil reactivity, decreased upgaze Olfactory system deterioration Decreased vibratory sensation
Gait and balance	Gait stiffer, slowed, forward flexed Increased body sway and mild unsteadiness
Sleep	Decreased sleep efficiency, fatigue Increased awakenings, insomnia Decrease in sleep stages 3 and 4 Sleep duration more variable, more naps

TABLE 26-3 GERIATRIC DEPRESSION SCALE—SHORT FORM

1. Are you basically satisfied with your life?	yes/**NO**
2. Have you dropped many of your activities and interests?	**YES**/no
3. Do you feel that your life is empty?	**YES**/no
4. Do you often get bored?	**YES**/no
5. Are you in good spirits most of the time?	yes/**NO**
6. Are you afraid that something bad is going to happen to you?	**YES**/no
7. Do you feel happy most of the time?	yes/**NO**
8. Do you feel helpless?	**YES**/no
9. Do you prefer to stay home rather than going out and doing new things?	**YES**/no
10. Do you feel you have more problems with memory than most?	**YES**/no
11. Do you think it is wonderful to be alive now?	yes/**NO**
12. Do you feel pretty worthless the way you are now?	**YES**/no
13. Do you feel full of energy?	yes/**NO**
14. Do you feel that your situation is hopeless?	**YES**/no
15. Do you think that most people are better off than you are?	**YES**/no

Scoring: Answers indicating depression are highlighted; six or more highlighted answers indicate depressive symptoms.
Modified from Yesavage J, Brink T, Rowe T, et al. Development and validation of a geriatric depression screening scale: a preliminary report. *J Psychiatr Res*. 1983;17:37-49.

MONTREAL COGNITIVE ASSESSMENT (MOCA)

NAME :
Education :
Sex :
Date of birth :
DATE :

		POINTS
VISUOSPATIAL / EXECUTIVE	(E) End, (A), (5), (B), (2), (1) Begin, (D), (4), (3), (C) [ ] · Copy cube [ ] · Draw CLOCK (Ten past eleven) (3 points) [ ] Contour [ ] Numbers [ ] Hands	___/5
NAMING	[ ] [ ] [ ]	___/3
MEMORY	Read list of words, subject must repeat them. Do 2 trials, even if 1st trial is successful. Do a recall after 5 minutes.	No points

	FACE	VELVET	CHURCH	DAISY	RED
1st trial					
2nd trial					

ATTENTION	Read list of digits (1 digit/ sec.). Subject has to repeat them in the forward order [ ] 2 1 8 5 4 · Subject has to repeat them in the backward order [ ] 7 4 2	___/2
	Read list of letters. The subject must tap with his hand at each letter A. No points if ≥ 2 errors [ ] F B A C M N A A J K L B A F A K D E A A A J A M O F A A B	___/1
	Serial 7 subtraction starting at 100 [ ] 93 [ ] 86 [ ] 79 [ ] 72 [ ] 65 · 4 or 5 correct subtractions: **3 pts**, 2 or 3 correct: **2 pts**, 1 correct: **1 pt**, 0 correct: **0 pt**	___/3
LANGUAGE	Repeat : I only know that John is the one to help today. [ ] The cat always hid under the couch when dogs were in the room. [ ]	___/2
	Fluency / Name maximum number of words in one minute that begin with the letter F [ ] _____ (N ≥ 11 words)	___/1
ABSTRACTION	Similarity between e.g. banana - orange = fruit [ ] train – bicycle [ ] watch - ruler	___/2

DELAYED RECALL	Has to recall words WITH NO CUE	FACE [ ]	VELVET [ ]	CHURCH [ ]	DAISY [ ]	RED [ ]	Points for UNCUED recall only	___/5
Optional	Category cue							
	Multiple choice cue							

ORIENTATION	[ ] Date	[ ] Month	[ ] Year	[ ] Day	[ ] Place	[ ] City	___/6

 Normal ≥ 26 / 30

TOTAL ___/30

Add 1 point if ≤ 12 yr edu

Administered by: ____________

FIGURE 26-1. Montreal Cognitive Assessment (MOCA).

Early cognitive deficits can easily be missed during conversation because intellectual impairment can be masked with intact social skills. Given the high frequency of cognitive impairment, formal cognitive screening is recommended for all older persons. Ideally, cognitive testing should evaluate at least the general domains of attention, orientation, language, memory, visuospatial ability, and conceptualization. To exclude delirium, attention should be assessed first by asking the patient to perform a task, such as repeating five digits or reciting the months backward; the remainder of cognitive testing would not be useful in an inattentive patient. For further cognitive testing, many brief, practical screening instruments are available. Historically, the most widely used instrument has been the Mini-Mental State Examination, a 19-item, 30-point scale that can be completed in 10 minutes. This copyrighted instrument now requires a per-use fee if the official version is used. A useful, brief alternative instrument is the Mini-Cog test, which can be completed in 2 to 4 minutes (Table 26-4); scores <3 suggest cognitive impairment. More detailed testing can be conducted with the Montreal Cognitive Assessment (Figure 26-1), which requires 10 to 15 minutes; scores less than 26 indicate cognitive impairment. Questions to evaluate judgment and problem-solving ability in hypothetical situations, such as in a fire or when driving, can provide crucial insight into the patient's ability to function safely and independently.

Functional Assessment

Functional impairment, defined as difficulty in performing daily activities, is common among elderly persons. Although it is not routinely evaluated in the standard medical assessment, determination of the patient's degree of functional incapacity based on medical and neuropsychiatric conditions is crucial to understanding the burden of disease and its impact on the individual's daily life. The important relationship between functional status and health in older persons is reflected by the finding that functional measures are stronger predictors of mortality after hospitalization than are admitting diagnoses. Functional measures strongly predict other important hospital outcomes in the elderly, such as length of stay, functional status at discharge, future care needs, caregiver burden, risk for institutionalization, and long-term prognosis. Functional independence is critical if patients are to remain living independently in the community, and functional decline represents a leading risk factor for nursing home placement.

The functional assessment should include an assessment of the patient's ability to perform basic self-care activities of daily living and instrumental activities of daily living, the higher level activities needed for independent living. Activities of daily living include basic self-care skills such as feeding, grooming, bathing, dressing, toileting, transferring, and walking. Instrumental activities of daily living are more complex tasks, including shopping, preparing meals, managing finances, housekeeping, using the telephone, taking medications, and driving or using public transportation. The functional assessment is conducted with the patient or the family, and the questions ascertain whether the patient can perform these activities independently. Other related domains that should be assessed include vision, hearing, continence, nutritional status, safety, falls, living situation, social support, and socioeconomic status.

The onset of acute cognitive or functional decline is often the first and sometimes the only sign of serious acute illness in older persons, and it warrants immediate medical attention. Similarly, the onset or worsening of related conditions, such as delirium, falls, incontinence, depression, frailty, or failure to thrive, heralds the need for prompt medical evaluation.

TABLE 26-4 MINI-COG TEST

1. Instruct the patient to listen carefully to and remember 3 unrelated words and then to repeat the words: BANANA, SUNRISE, CHAIR.
2. Instruct the patient to draw the face of a clock, either on a blank sheet of paper or on a sheet with a large circle already drawn on the page. After the patient puts the numbers on the clock face, ask him or her to draw the hands of the clock to read a specific time, such as 11:10. These instructions can be repeated, but no additional instructions should be given. Allow up to 3 minutes to complete the clock drawing.
3. Ask the patient to repeat the 3 previously presented words.
4. Give 1 point for each correct word and 2 points for a correctly drawn clock. Scores <3 suggest cognitive impairment.

Adapted from Borson S, Scanlan J, Watanabe J, et al. Improving identification of cognitive impairment in primary care. *Int J Geriatr Psychiatry.* 2006; 21:349-355. Reprinted by permission of the copyright holder (S. Borson).

TREATMENT Rx

Psychoactive Effects of Drugs in Older Patients

Adverse Drug Events in the Elderly

Iatrogenic complications occur in 29 to 38% of older hospitalized patients, with a three- to five-fold increased risk in older compared with younger patients. Adverse drug events, the most common type of iatrogenic complication, account for 20 to 40% of all complications. The elderly are particularly vulnerable to adverse drug reactions because of multiple-drug regimens, multiple chronic diseases, relative renal and hepatic insufficiency, decreased physiologic reserve, and altered drug metabolism with aging. Inappropriate drug use has been reported in about 40% of hospitalized older patients, with more than one quarter of these patients having absolute contraindications to the drug and the others being given a drug that was unnecessary. Because 50% of adverse drug events occur in patients receiving inappropriate drugs, the potential for reducing these adverse events is substantial.

Drugs with Psychoactive Effects

Nearly every class of drug has the potential to cause mental status changes in a vulnerable patient, but specific drugs are commonly implicated (Table 26-5) and should be used with caution in older patients. Many cases of delirium or cognitive decline in older patients may be preventable through avoidance, substitution, or dose reduction of these psychoactive drugs. Long-acting benzodiazepines (e.g., flurazepam, diazepam) are particularly problematic medications for the elderly and should be avoided whenever possible. If nonpharmacologic approaches to the management of insomnia are unsuccessful, short-term use of an intermediate-acting benzodiazepine without active metabolites (e.g., lorazepam 0.5 mg, half-life of 10 to 15 hours) is recommended. Drugs with anticholinergic effects (e.g., antihistamines, antidepressants, neuroleptics, antispasmodics) produce a panoply of poorly tolerated side effects in older patients, including delirium, postural hypotension, urinary retention, constipation, and dry mouth. Of the narcotics, meperidine causes

TABLE 26-5 DRUGS WITH PSYCHOACTIVE EFFECTS

Sedative-hypnotics Benzodiazepines (especially flurazepam, diazepam) Barbiturates Sleeping medications (chloral hydrate)
Narcotics (especially meperidine)
Anticholinergics Antihistamines (diphenhydramine, hydroxyzine) Antispasmodics (belladonna, Lomotil) Heterocyclic antidepressants (amitriptyline, imipramine, doxepin) Neuroleptics (chlorpromazine, haloperidol, thioridazine) Antiparkinson drugs (benztropine, trihexyphenidyl) Atropine, scopolamine
Cardiac drugs Digitalis glycosides Antiarrhythmics (quinidine, procainamide, lidocaine) Antihypertensives (β-blockers, methyldopa)
Gastrointestinal drugs H_2-antagonists (cimetidine, ranitidine, famotidine, nizatidine) Proton pump inhibitors (esomeprazole, lansoprazole, omeprazole, pantoprozole) Metoclopramide (Reglan)
Miscellaneous drugs Nonsteroidal anti-inflammatory drugs Corticosteroids Anticonvulsants Levodopa Lithium
Over-the-counter drugs Cold and sinus preparations (antihistamines, pseudoephedrine) Sleep aids (diphenhydramine, alcohol-containing elixirs) Stay Awake (caffeine) Nausea, gastrointestinal relief (Donnagel, meclizine, H_2-antagonists, loperamide)

delirium more frequently than other agents because of an active metabolite, normeperidine. Cardiac drugs, such as digitalis and antiarrhythmic agents, have prolonged half-lives, narrowed therapeutic windows, and decreased protein binding in older patients. The clinician should be aware that toxicity with these agents (e.g., digoxin) can occur even at therapeutic drug levels. The H_2-receptor antagonists (e.g., cimetidine, ranitidine, famotidine, nizatidine) are among the most common causes of drug-induced delirium in the elderly because of their frequent use; clinicians should strongly consider the use of less toxic alternatives (e.g., sucralfate, antacids) or dosage reductions for older patients, especially when the medication is being used for prophylaxis rather than treatment of active disease. Proton pump inhibitors have been associated with delirium in case reports; however, the overall rate of this adverse effect has not been systematically determined. The Beers list, which is updated regularly, includes drugs that are potentially inappropriate for the elderly and drugs associated with high rates of adverse events in the elderly, including mental status changes and falls.

Psychoactive drugs account for nearly 50% of preventable adverse drug events, often in patients who have been prescribed three or more psychoactive drugs, frequently at inappropriately high doses in the elderly. Delirium and cognitive impairment are the most frequent adverse outcomes of psychoactive drugs. The use of any psychoactive drug is associated with a 4-fold increased risk of delirium or cognitive decline, but the outcomes of these conditions depend on the type or class of drug administered and the total number of drugs received. Sedative-hypnotic drugs are associated with a 3- to 12-fold increased risk for delirium or cognitive decline, narcotics are associated with a 2- to 3-fold increased risk, and anticholinergic drugs are associated with a 5- to 12-fold increased risk. Each drug carries its own individual risk for adverse outcomes, and when multiple drugs are used, the overall risk is compounded by the heightened potential for drug-drug interactions. If more than three drugs are added in a 24-hour period, the risk of delirium increases 4-fold. Similarly, the risk of cognitive decline increases directly with the number of drugs prescribed, from a 3-fold increased risk with two or three drugs to a 14-fold increased risk with six or more drugs.

Principles of Drug Therapy in the Elderly

Physicians always should consider whether nonpharmacologic approaches (Chapter 38) may be used as alternatives to medications in older persons. Relaxation techniques, massage, and music are highly effective for the treatment of insomnia and anxiety; localized pain can often be managed effectively with local measures such as injection, heat, ultrasound, and transcutaneous electrical stimulation.

TABLE 26-6 GUIDELINES FOR DRUG THERAPY IN THE ELDERLY

GENERAL PRINCIPLES
Remember that the elderly are highly sensitive to the psychoactive effects of all drugs. Know the pharmacology of the drugs you prescribe. Know a few drugs well.
RECOMMENDED APPROACH
Use nonpharmacologic approaches whenever possible. Avoid *routine* use of "as needed" drugs for sleep, anxiety, pain. Choose the drug with the least toxic potential. Substitute less toxic alternatives whenever possible (antacid or sucralfate for an H_2-blocker or proton pump inhibitors, metamucil or kaopectate for imodium, or Lomotil, scheduled acetaminophen regimen for pain management). Reduce the dosage. "Start low and go slow." Start with 25-50% of the standard dose of psychoactive drugs in the elderly. Titrate the drug slowly. Set realistic end points: titrate to improvement, not elimination of symptoms. Keep the regimen simple. Regularly reassess the medication list. Have the patient bring in all bottles and review what is being taken. Re-evaluate long-time drug use because the patient is changing. Review over-the-counter medication use.

When drug therapy is required in the elderly, physicians should choose the drug with the least toxic potential and emphasize drugs that have been well tested in older populations (Table 26-6). It is often wise to start with 25 to 50% of the standard adult dosage for any psychoactive drug and increase the dose slowly. Drug regimens should be kept simple, with the fewest drugs and the fewest number of pills possible. Most important, the medication list should be reassessed frequently. Systematic interventions involving geriatricians, clinical pharmacists, and computer-based systems can significantly reduce the frequency of adverse drug reactions in older persons. [1]

Even long-standing medications should be reevaluated because the patient is changing with age and illness. Long-term use does not justify continued use. The physician should review with the patient all prescribed and over-the-counter medications on a regular basis, preferably by having the patient bring in all medication bottles and indicate how each is being taken. Patients frequently underestimate the toxic potential of over-the-counter medications and herbal remedies, and they may be using a variety of such agents that could potentiate the side effects or directly counteract the desired effects of prescription medications (Chapter 28). For example, high-risk over-the-counter medications for older persons include nonsteroidal anti-inflammatory agents, H_2-blockers, and antihistamines. In addition, herbal remedies such as gingko biloba may interact with warfarin to cause bleeding; others (such as kava kava and Chinese herbal preparations) are associated with the risk of hepatotoxicity.

FUTURE DIRECTIONS

Screening methods for cognitive and functional decline should be used for high-risk older persons. An important goal for the future is to incorporate these screening and interventional measures into the routine care of all older persons in physicians' offices, clinics, hospitals, nursing homes, and other settings.

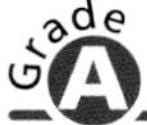

1. Schnipper JL, Hamann C, Ndumele CD, et al. Effect of an electronic medication reconciliation application and process redesign on potential adverse drug events: a cluster-randomized trial. *Arch Intern Med.* 2009;169:771-780.

SUGGESTED READINGS

Kåreholt I, Lennartsson C, Gatz M, et al. Baseline leisure time activity and cognition more than two decades later. *Int J Geriatr Psychiatry.* 2011;26:65-74. *Various forms of engagement in mid-life can protect cognition later in life.*

Ting C, Rajji TK, Ismail Z, et al. Differentiating the cognitive profile of schizophrenia from that of Alzheimer disease and depression in late life. *PLoS One.* 2010;5:e10151. *Guidance for making these important diagnostic distinctions.*

27

DELIRIUM OR ACUTE MENTAL STATUS CHANGE IN THE OLDER PATIENT

SHARON K. INOUYE

Mental status change, one of the most common presenting symptoms in acutely ill elders, is estimated to account for 30% of emergency evaluations among older patients. Mental status often serves as a barometer of the underlying health of an elderly patient and is commonly the only symptom of serious underlying disease. A broad range of medical, neurologic, and psychiatric conditions can lead to mental status changes (Chapters 404 and 409). A systematic approach aids in the evaluation of suspected mental status change in an older patient (Fig. 27-1).

The first step in evaluating suspected altered mental status in an older patient is to obtain a detailed history from a reliable informant to establish the patient's baseline level of cognitive function and the clinical course of any cognitive changes. Chronic changes (those occurring over months to years) most likely represent an underlying dementing illness and should be evaluated accordingly (Chapter 409). Acute changes (those occurring over days to weeks)—even if superimposed on an underlying dementia—should be evaluated by a detailed cognitive assessment to determine whether delirium is present. If features of delirium (e.g., inattention, disorganized thinking, altered level of consciousness, fluctuating symptoms) are not present, further evaluation for depression, acute nonorganic psychotic disorders, or other psychiatric conditions is indicated.

DELIRIUM

Delirium, a clinical syndrome characterized as an acute disorder of attention and cognitive function, is the most frequent complication of hospitalization for elders and is a potentially devastating problem. Delirium is often unrecognized despite sensitive methods for its detection, and its complications may be preventable.

DEFINITION

The definition of and diagnostic criteria for delirium are evolving. The fourth edition of the *Diagnostic and Statistical Manual of Mental Disorders* (text revision) has been used widely (Table 27-1), but the criteria in this manual were based on expert consensus, and their diagnostic sensitivity and specificity have not been determined. The Confusion Assessment Method (CAM) provides a simple, operationalized diagnostic algorithm. In studies of more than 1000 subjects, it had a sensitivity of 94%, a specificity of 89%, and a high interrater reliability.

EPIDEMIOLOGY

In persons older than 65 years, the prevalence of delirium at hospital admission is 13 to 60%. Delirium develops in 6 to 56% of patients during hospitalization. Higher rates are found when frequent surveillance is performed in older, surgical, and intensive care populations. Delirium occurs in 15 to 74% of postoperative patients, 60 to 80% of patients in medical intensive care units, up to 60% of nursing home patients, and at least 80% of patients at the end of life.

The hospital mortality rates for delirium are 25 to 33%—as high as those associated with acute myocardial infarction and sepsis. The problem of delirium in hospitalized elderly patients has assumed particular prominence because patients aged 65 years and older currently account for more than 50% of all inpatient days of hospital care. Based on U.S. vital health statistics, delirium complicates hospital stays for at least 20% of the 12.5 million older persons hospitalized each year and increases hospital costs by more than $2500 per patient, amounting to more than $6.9 billion (2004 U.S. dollars) of Medicare expenditures yearly. Substantial additional costs are incurred after hospital discharge because of the increased need for rehabilitation services, nursing home placement, home care, and rehospitalization. Health care costs associated with delirium range from $38 billion to $152 billion per year. These extrapolations highlight the extensive economic and health policy implications of delirium.

TABLE 27-1 DIAGNOSTIC CRITERIA FOR DELIRIUM

DSM-IV TR DIAGNOSTIC CRITERIA

A. Disturbance of consciousness (i.e., reduced clarity of awareness of the environment) with reduced ability to focus, sustain, or shift attention
B. A change in cognition (e.g., memory deficit, disorientation, language disturbance) or the development of a perceptual disturbance that is not better accounted for by a preexisting, established, or evolving dementia
C. The disturbance develops over a short period (usually hours to days) and tends to fluctuate during the course of the day
D. Evidence from the history, physical examination, or laboratory findings indicates that the disturbance is caused by the direct physiologic consequences of a general medical condition

CAM DIAGNOSTIC ALGORITHM*

Feature 1. Acute onset and fluctuating course. This information is usually obtained from a family member or nurse and is shown by positive responses to the following questions: Is there evidence of an acute change in mental status from the patient's baseline? Did the (abnormal) behavior fluctuate during the day—that is, tend to come and go or increase and decrease in severity?
Feature 2. Inattention. This feature is shown by a positive response to the following question: Did the patient have difficulty focusing attention—for example, was he or she easily distracted or did he or she have difficulty keeping track of what was being said?
Feature 3. Disorganized thinking. This feature is shown by a positive response to the following question: Was the patient's thinking disorganized or incoherent, such as rambling or irrelevant conversation, unclear or illogical flow of ideas, or unpredictable switching from subject to subject?
Feature 4. Altered level of consciousness. This feature is shown by any answer other than "alert" to the following question: Overall, how would you rate this patient's level of consciousness: alert (normal), vigilant (hyperalert), lethargic (drowsy, easily aroused), stupor (difficult to arouse), or coma (unable to arouse)?

*The diagnosis of delirium requires the presence of features 1 and 2 and either 3 or 4.
CAM = Confusion Assessment Method, from Inouye SK, van Dyck CH, Alessi CA, et al: Clarifying confusion: The Confusion Assessment Method. A new method for detection of delirium. *Ann Intern Med.* 1990;113:941-948. Training manual available at http://elderlife.med.yale.edu/pdf/The Confusion Assessment Method.pdf; DSM-IV = American Psychiatric Association. *Diagnostic and Statistical Manual of Mental Disorders*, 4th ed., text revision. Washington, DC: American Psychiatric Association; 2000.

PATHOBIOLOGY

Similar to other common geriatric syndromes (Chapter 24), delirium usually has multiple causes. A search for the innumerable potential underlying contributors requires clinical astuteness and a thorough medical evaluation, especially because many of these factors are treatable but may result in substantial morbidity and mortality if left untreated. The process is made more challenging by the frequently nonspecific, atypical, or muted features of the underlying illness in older persons. Delirium is commonly the only initial sign of an underlying life-threatening illness such as pneumonia (Chapter 97), urosepsis (Chapter 292), or myocardial infarction (Chapter 73) in the older population.

The development of delirium usually involves a complex interrelationship between a vulnerable patient with pertinent predisposing factors and exposure to noxious insults or precipitating factors. Delirium may develop in vulnerable patients, such as cognitively impaired or severely ill patients, after a relatively benign insult, such as a single dose of sleeping medication. Conversely, in patients who are not vulnerable, delirium may develop only after exposure to multiple noxious insults. Previous studies have shown that the effects of these risk factors may be cumulative. Recognition of this multifactorial causation is important to the clinician because the removal or treatment of one factor in isolation usually is not sufficient to resolve the delirium. The full spectrum of vulnerability and precipitating factors should be addressed.

Predisposing factors, or factors that increase vulnerability, include preexisting cognitive impairment or dementia, severe underlying illness, high levels of comorbidity, functional impairment, advanced age, chronic renal insufficiency, dehydration, malnutrition, and vision or hearing impairment. Dementia is an important and consistent risk factor for delirium; demented patients have a twofold to fivefold increased risk for delirium. Of delirious patients, 30 to 50% have underlying dementia. Delirious patients commonly have evidence of underlying chronic brain disease, particularly conditions associated with cognitive impairment such as Alzheimer's disease, Parkinson's disease, or cerebrovascular disease.

Medications, the most common remediable cause of delirium, contribute to delirium in 40% of cases (Chapter 26). Insufficiency or failure of any major

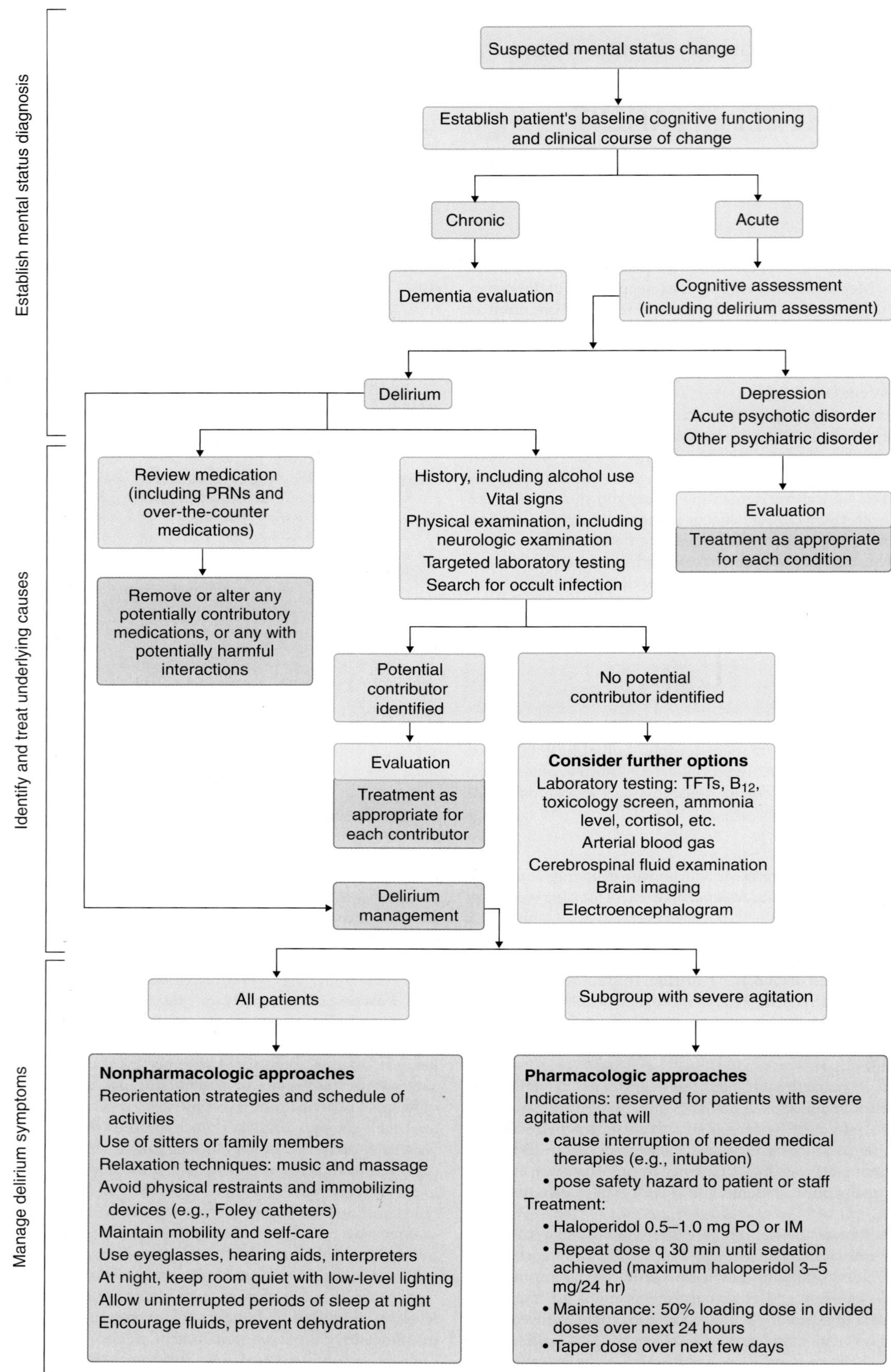

FIGURE 27-1. Algorithm for the evaluation of suspected mental status change in older patients. PRN = as needed; TFTs = thyroid function tests.

organ system, particularly renal or hepatic failure, can precipitate delirium. Hypoxemia and hypercarbia have been associated with delirium. Clinicians must be attuned to occult respiratory failure, which in the elderly often lacks the usual signs and symptoms of dyspnea and tachypnea and can be missed by the measurement of oxygen saturation alone. Acute myocardial infarction or heart failure can manifest as delirium in an elderly patient without the usual symptoms of chest pain or dyspnea. Occult infection is a particularly notable cause of delirium. Older patients frequently fail to mount the febrile or leukocytotic response to infection, and clinicians must assess them carefully for signs of pneumonia, urinary tract infection, endocarditis, abdominal abscess, or infected joints. A variety of metabolic disorders may contribute to delirium, including hypernatremia and hyponatremia, hypercalcemia, acid-base disorders, hypoglycemia and hyperglycemia, and thyroid or adrenal disorders. Immobilization and immobilizing devices (e.g., indwelling bladder catheters, physical restraints, bed alarms) are important factors in precipitating delirium. Dehydration and volume depletion and nutritional decline during hospitalization (e.g., weight loss, fall in serum albumin concentration) are well-documented factors contributing to delirium. Drug and alcohol withdrawal are important and often unsuspected causes of delirium in the elderly. Environmental factors, such as unfamiliar surroundings, sleep deprivation, deranged schedule, frequent room changes, sensory overload, and sensory deprivation, may aggravate delirium in the hospital. Psychosocial factors, such as depression, psychological stress, pain, and lack of social supports, also may precipitate delirium.

The basic pathogenesis of delirium is unclear. Most investigators agree that delirium seems to be a functional rather than a structural lesion. Electroencephalographic studies show global functional derangements in patients with delirium, characterized by generalized slowing of cortical background activity with the appearance of delta and theta activity. Neuroimaging studies coupled with cognitive testing demonstrate a generalized disruption in higher cortical function, with dysfunction in the prefrontal cortex, frontal and temporoparietal cortex, fusiform cortex, lingual gyri, subcortical structures, thalamus, and basal ganglia. The leading hypotheses for the pathogenesis of delirium focus on the roles of neurotransmission and inflammation. The most widely postulated mechanism for delirium is the failure of cholinergic transmission. Evidence supporting this hypothesis includes the frequent association of anticholinergic drugs with delirium, the reversal of delirium with procholinergic drugs such as physostigmine, the increased levels of serum anticholinergic activity in some delirious patients, and the benefit of cholinesterase inhibitors in some cases of delirium. Other neurotransmitter systems, such as dopamine, serotonin, tryptophan, norepinephrine, and γ-aminobutyric acid, may also play a role in delirium, but the evidence is less well developed. In some circumstances, such as infection or cancer, delirium may be mediated through cytokines, such as interleukin-2 and tumor necrosis factor. Although delirium has long been considered a transient syndrome, several of these basic mechanisms may not be completely reversible, particularly those resulting in hypoxic damage. Acute stress with high levels of cortisol may also contribute to delirium. The dose and duration of the noxious insult, along with the degree of vulnerability of the patient, also may exert great influence on the ultimate reversibility of the delirium.

CLINICAL MANIFESTATIONS

The cardinal features of delirium include acute onset and inattention. Establishing the acuteness of onset requires accurate knowledge of the patient's baseline cognitive function. Patients with delirium are inattentive; that is, they have difficulty focusing, maintaining, and shifting attention. They appear easily distracted and have difficulty maintaining conversation and following commands. Objectively, patients may have difficulty with simple repetitive tasks, digit spans, and recitation of months backward. Other key features include disorganized thought processes, which are usually a manifestation of underlying cognitive or perceptual disturbances; altered level of consciousness, which typically consists of lethargy with reduced awareness of the environment; and fluctuation of cognitive symptoms. Although not cardinal elements, other features that frequently occur during delirium include disorientation, cognitive deficits, psychomotor agitation or retardation, perceptual disturbances such as hallucinations and illusions, paranoid delusions, and sleep-wake cycle reversal.

DIAGNOSIS

The cornerstone of the evaluation of delirium is a comprehensive history and physical examination (Table 27-2). The first step is to establish the diagnosis of delirium through cognitive assessment and to determine whether the present condition represents an acute change from the patient's baseline cognitive function. Because cognitive impairment may not be apparent during conversation, brief cognitive screening tests, such as the Mini-Cog Test (Chapter 26) and the Confusion Assessment Method, should be used. Attention should be assessed further with other simple tests, such as a forward digit span (inattention is indicated by an inability to repeat five digits forward) or recitation of the months backward. A delirium assessment for nonverbal (e.g., intubated) patients, called the CAM-ICU, has been developed. The history, which should be obtained from a reliable informant, is targeted to establish the patient's baseline cognitive function and the time course of any mental status change and to obtain clues about potential precipitating factors, such as recent medication changes, intercurrent infection, or medical illness. Physical examination should include a detailed neurologic examination for focal deficits and a careful search for signs of occult infection or an acute abdominal process.

TABLE 27-2 EVALUATION OF DELIRIUM IN ELDERLY PATIENTS

Perform cognitive testing and determine baseline cognitive functioning: establish the diagnosis of delirium
Obtain a comprehensive history and perform a physical examination, including a careful neurologic examination for focal deficits and a search for occult infection
Review the patient's medication list: discontinue or minimize all psychoactive medications; check the side effects of all medications
Perform a laboratory evaluation (tailored to the individual): complete blood count, electrolytes, blood urea nitrogen, creatinine, glucose, calcium, phosphate, liver enzymes, oxygen saturation
Search for occult infection: physical examination, urinalysis, chest radiography, selected cultures (as indicated)
When no obvious cause is revealed after these steps, further targeted evaluation is considered in selected patients, as follows: Laboratory tests: magnesium, thyroid function, vitamin B_{12} level, drug levels, toxicology screen, ammonia level Arterial blood gas analysis: indicated in patients with dyspnea, tachypnea, any acute pulmonary process, or history of significant respiratory disease Electrocardiography: indicated in patients with chest or abdominal discomfort, shortness of breath, or cardiac history Cerebrospinal fluid examination: indicated when meningitis or encephalitis is suspected Brain imaging: indicated in patients with new focal neurologic signs or with a history or signs of head trauma Electroencephalography: useful in diagnosing occult seizure disorder and in differentiating delirium from nonorganic psychiatric disorders

Review of the patient's medication list, including over-the-counter medications, is crucial, and the use of medications with psychoactive effects should be discontinued or minimized whenever possible. In the elderly, these medications may cause psychoactive effects even at doses and measured drug levels within the "therapeutic range." Consideration should also be given to the possibility that withdrawal from alcohol or other medications is a contributor to delirium.

Laboratory Findings

Laboratory evaluation must be tailored to the individual situation (see Table 27-2). In patients with preexisting cardiac or respiratory diseases or related symptoms, electrocardiography or arterial blood gas determination may be indicated. The need for cerebrospinal fluid examination is controversial except when it is clearly indicated, such as in a febrile delirious patient. Brain imaging should be reserved for patients with new focal neurologic signs, those with a history or signs of head trauma, and those without another identifiable cause of the delirium. Electroencephalography, with a false-negative rate of 17% and a false-positive rate of 22% for distinguishing delirious from nondelirious patients, has a limited role and is most useful for detecting an occult seizure disorder and differentiating delirium from psychiatric disorders.

Differential Diagnosis

A crucial difficulty is distinguishing a long-standing confusional state (dementia) from delirium alone or delirium superimposed on dementia (see Fig. 27-1). These two conditions are differentiated by the acute onset of

TABLE 27-3 DELIRIUM RISK FACTORS AND POTENTIAL INTERVENTIONS

RISK FACTOR	INTERVENTION
Cognitive impairment	Reality orientation program (reorienting techniques, communication) Therapeutic activities program
Sleep deprivation	Noise reduction strategies Scheduling of nighttime medications, procedures, and nursing activities to allow uninterrupted period of sleep
Immobilization	Early mobilization (e.g., ambulation or bedside exercises) Minimal use of immobilizing equipment (e.g., bladder catheters)
Psychoactive medications	Restricted use of "as needed" sleep and psychoactive medications (e.g., sedative-hypnotics, narcotics, anticholinergic medications) Nonpharmacologic protocols for management of sleep and anxiety
Vision impairment	Provision of vision aids (e.g., magnifiers, special lighting) Provision of adaptive equipment (e.g., illuminated phone dials, large-print books)
Hearing impairment	Provision of amplifying devices Repair of hearing aids
Dehydration	Early recognition and volume repletion

symptoms in delirium (dementia is much more insidious) and the impaired attention and altered level of consciousness associated with delirium. The differential diagnosis also includes depression and nonorganic psychotic disorders. Although paranoia, hallucinations, and affective changes can occur with delirium, the key features of acute onset, inattention, altered level of consciousness, and global cognitive impairment assist in the recognition of delirium. At times, the differential diagnosis can be difficult, particularly with an uncooperative patient or when an accurate history is unavailable. Because of the potentially life-threatening nature of delirium, it is prudent to manage the patient as if he or she has delirium and to search for and treat underlying precipitants (e.g., intercurrent illness, metabolic derangement, drug toxicity) until further information can be obtained.

TREATMENT Rx

Prevention

The most effective strategy to reduce delirium and its associated complications is primary prevention before delirium occurs. Preventive strategies should address important risk factors and target moderate- to high-risk patients at baseline (Table 27-3). Randomized trials have shown that a geriatrics consultation or a multidisciplinary intervention aimed at the risk factors for delirium can reduce the incidence of delirium by 40%. To date, no drug treatments, including cholinesterase inhibitors, have been effective in preventing delirium.[1] On a larger scale, preventive efforts require systemwide changes to educate physicians and nurses and thus improve their recognition of delirium and heighten their awareness of its clinical implications, to provide incentives to change practice patterns that lead to delirium (e.g., immobilization, sleep medications, bladder catheters, physical restraints), and to create systems that enhance high-quality geriatric care (e.g., geriatric expertise, case management, clinical pathways, quality monitoring).

Medical Therapy

In general, nonpharmacologic approaches should be used in all delirious patients, and these are usually successful in managing symptoms. Pharmacologic approaches should be reserved for patients whose symptoms may result in the interruption of needed medical therapies (e.g., intubation, intravenous lines) or may endanger the safety of the patient or other persons. No drug is ideal for the treatment of delirium, however; any drug can cloud the patient's mental status further and obscure efforts to monitor the course of the mental status change. The drug should be given at the lowest dose and for the shortest time possible. Neuroleptics are the preferred agents. Haloperidol, the most widely used agent, causes less orthostatic hypotension and fewer anticholinergic side effects than thioridazine and is available in parenteral form; however, it has a higher rate of extrapyramidal side effects and acute dystonias. Second-generation antipsychotics have not proved superior to haloperidol.[2] If parenteral administration is required, intravenous use results in a rapid onset of action, short duration of effect, and risk of hypotension and torsades de pointes; intramuscular use has a more optimal duration of action and is preferred. The recommended starting dose is 0.25 to 0.5 mg of haloperidol orally or intramuscularly, repeated every 30 minutes after the vital signs have been rechecked, until sedation has been achieved. The end point should be an awake but manageable patient. The average elderly patient who has not been treated previously with neuroleptics should require a total loading dose of no more than 3 to 5 mg of haloperidol. Subsequently, a maintenance dose consisting of half the loading dose should be administered in divided doses during the next 24 hours, with doses tapered over the next few days as the agitation resolves.

Benzodiazepines are not recommended as the first-line treatment of delirium because of their tendency to cause oversedation and exacerbate the confusional state. They remain the drugs of choice, however, for the treatment of withdrawal syndromes from alcohol and sedative drugs (Chapters 32 and 33).

Nonpharmacologic Management

Multicomponent geriatric interventions may be effective in improving quality of life without increasing health care costs.[3] Nonpharmacologic management techniques recommended for every delirious patient include encouraging the presence of family members, using "sitters" as orienting influences, and transferring a disruptive patient to a private room or closer to the nurse's station for increased supervision. Interpersonal contact and communication, including verbal reorientation strategies, simple instructions and explanations, and frequent eye contact, are vital. Patients should be involved in their own care and allowed to participate in decision making as much as possible. Eyeglasses and hearing aids may reduce sensory deficits. Mobility, self-care, and independence should be encouraged, and physical restraints and bed alarms should be avoided, if possible, because of their tendency to increase agitation, their lack of efficacy, and their potential to cause injury. Attention must be focused on minimizing the disruptive influences of the hospital environment. Clocks and calendars should be provided to assist with orientation. Room and staff changes should be kept to a minimum. A quiet environment with low-level lighting is optimal for delirious patients. Perhaps the most important intervention is to schedule the checking of vital signs, the administration of medications, and the performance of procedures to allow the patient's uninterrupted sleep at night. Nonpharmacologic approaches to relaxation, including music, relaxation tapes, and massage, can be highly effective in managing agitation.

End-of-Life Care

Delirium occurs in at least 80% of patients at the end of life and is considered part of the dying process by many hospice care providers (Chapter 3). Establishing the goals for care in advance with the patient and family is critical to guide appropriate management. For example, some patients may prioritize the preservation of alertness and the ability to communicate with loved ones as long as possible; others may prioritize comfort above all else. Physicians must be aware that even in terminal patients, many causes of delirium are potentially reversible with simple interventions such as adjusting medications, providing oxygen, or treating dehydration; however, aggressive diagnostic evaluation is usually inappropriate in this population. Nonpharmacologic measures to treat agitation and delirium should be instituted in all patients (including massage, music, and relaxation therapies). Haloperidol remains the first-line therapy for delirium in terminally ill patients. If more sedation is indicated, a short-acting benzodiazepine such as lorazepam (starting dose, 0.5 to 1.0 mg PO, IM, or SL), which is easily titrated, is recommended in this setting. Because sedation may result in decreased interaction and communication, increased confusion, and respiratory depression, this choice should be made in conjunction with the family.

PROGNOSIS

Delirium is an important independent determinant of prolonged hospital stay, increased mortality, higher health care costs, increased rates of institutional placement, and functional and cognitive decline—even after controlling for age, gender, dementia, illness severity, and baseline functional status. Delirium was previously considered a reversible, transient condition, but more recent studies on the duration and persistence of symptoms document that delirium may be much more persistent than previously believed. Delirium typically lasts for 30 days or more, and only 20% of patients have complete resolution of all symptoms at 6-month follow-up. Delirium seems to have greater deleterious effects in patients with underlying cognitive impairment. The long-term detrimental effects are most likely related to the duration, severity, and underlying cause of the delirium and the vulnerability of the patient.

FUTURE DIRECTIONS

Because delirium is common, frequently iatrogenic, and linked to processes of care, it is considered to be a marker of the quality of care and patient safety in the hospital setting. Strategies to prevent delirium are a priority. It is hoped that future research will elucidate the pathophysiologic mechanisms of delirium by the use of neuroimaging modalities, neuropsychological testing, and genetic and laboratory markers; clarify the contribution of delirium to irreversible cognitive impairment; and improve the evidence-based management of delirium.

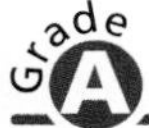

1. Overshott R, Karim S, Burns A. Cholinesterase inhibitors for delirium. Cochrane Database Syst Rev 2008, Issue 1, Art. No. CD005317.
2. Campbell N, Boustani MA, Ayub A, et al. Pharmacological management of delirium in hospitalized adults: a systemic evidence review. *J Gen Intern Med*. 2009;24:848-853.
3. Pitkala KS, Laurila JV, Strandberg TE, et al. Multicomponent geriatric intervention for elderly inpatients with delirium: effects on costs and health-related quality of life. *J Gerontol Med Sci*. 2008;63:56-61.

SUGGESTED READINGS

Clegg A, Young JB. Which medications to avoid in people at risk of delirium: a systematic review. *Age Ageing*. 2011;40:23-29. *Benzodiazepines, opioids, dihydropyridines, and antihistamine H_1 antagonists carry the highest risks.*

Witlox J, Eurelings LS, de Jonghe JF, et al. Delirium in elderly patients and the risk of postdischarge mortality, institutionalization, and dementia: a meta-analysis. *JAMA*. 2010;304:443-451. *In-hospital delirium correlates with a 2-fold increase in mortality, a 2.4-fold increase in institutionalization, and a 13-fold increase in subsequent dementia.*

Wong CL, Holroyd-Leduc J, Simel DL, et al. Does this patient have delirium?: value of bedside instruments. *JAMA*. 2010;304:779-786. *Review suggesting that the Confusion Assessment Method, which takes 5 minutes to administer, is the preferred diagnostic instrument.*

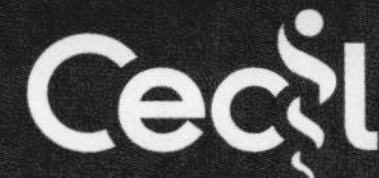

V

CLINICAL PHARMACOLOGY

PRINCIPLES OF DRUG THERAPY

ROBERT B. DIASIO

Under different conditions, a drug may produce diverse effects ranging from no effect to a desirable effect to an undesirable toxic effect. Physicians must learn how to individualize the drug dosage under different conditions to ensure effective and safe therapy. This necessitates understanding the pharmacokinetics—the movement of a drug over time through the body—and the pharmacodynamics—the relationship between drug concentration and drug effect (Fig. 28-1). This chapter reviews the basic concepts of pharmacokinetics and pharmacodynamics, followed by guidelines on how to use this information to optimize therapeutic applications. Drug interactions and adverse drug responses are briefly discussed, with advice on how both can be recognized and minimized in clinical practice.

PHARMACOKINETIC PRINCIPLES

Administration

The most efficient and straightforward means of administering a drug into the systemic circulation is by intravenous injection of the drug as a bolus. With this route, the full amount of a drug is delivered to the systemic circulation almost immediately. The same dose also may be administered as an intravenous infusion over a longer period, resulting in a decrease in the peak plasma concentration and an accompanying increase in the time the drug is present in the circulation. Many other routes of administration can be used, including sublingual, oral, transdermal, rectal, inhalational, subcutaneous, and intramuscular; each of these routes carries not only a potential delay in the time it takes the drug to enter the circulation but also the possibility that a large fraction of it will never reach the circulation.

Absorption

Absorption refers to the transfer of a drug from the site of administration to the systemic circulation. Many drugs cross a membrane barrier by passive diffusion and enter the systemic circulation. Because passive diffusion in this setting depends on the concentration of the solute at the membrane surface, the rate of drug absorption is affected by the concentration of free drug at the absorbing surface. Factors that influence the availability of free drug thus affect drug absorption from the administration site; this effect can be exploited to design medications that release a drug slowly into the circulation by prolonging drug absorption. With certain sustained-released oral preparations, the rate of dissolution of the drug in the gastrointestinal tract determines the rate at which the drug is absorbed (e.g., timed-release antihistamines). Similarly, a prolonged drug effect can be obtained by the use of transdermal medications (e.g., nitroglycerin) or intramuscular depot preparations (e.g., benzathine penicillin G).

First-Pass Effect

Some drugs that are administered orally are absorbed relatively well into the portal circulation but are metabolized by the liver before they reach the systemic circulation. Because of this "first-pass" or "presystemic" effect, the oral route may be less suitable than other routes of administration for such drugs. A good example is nitroglycerin, which is well absorbed but efficiently metabolized during the first pass through the liver. The same drug can achieve adequate systemic levels when it is given sublingually or transdermally.

Bioavailability

The extent of absorption of a drug into the systemic circulation may be incomplete. The bioavailability of a particular drug is the fraction (F) of the total drug dose that ultimately reaches the systemic circulation from the site of administration. This fraction is calculated by dividing the amount of the drug dose that reaches the circulation from the administration site by the amount of the drug dose that would enter the systemic circulation after direct intravenous injection into the circulation (essentially the total dose). Bioavailability, or F, can range from 0, in which no drug reaches the systemic circulation, to 1.0, in which essentially all the drug is absorbed. The bioavailability of a drug may vary in different formulations because the overall absorption differs. This variability has become a concern with the increasing use of generic preparations.

Distribution

After delivery of a drug into the systemic circulation either directly by intravenous injection or after absorption, the drug is transported throughout the body, initially to the well-perfused tissues and later to areas that are less perfused. The distribution phase can be assessed best by plotting the drug's plasma concentration on a log scale versus time on a linear scale (Fig. 28-2). For an intravenously administered drug, when absorption is not a factor, the initial phase—from immediately after administration through the rapid fall in concentration—represents the distribution phase, during which a drug rapidly disappears from the circulation and enters the tissues. This is followed by the elimination phase (see later), when drug in the plasma is in equilibrium with drug in the tissues. During this latter phase, the drug's plasma concentration is thought to be related to drug effect.

Volume of Distribution

The volume of distribution (VD) relates the amount of drug in the body to the concentration of drug in the plasma. It is calculated by dividing the dose that ultimately gets into the systemic circulation by the plasma concentration at time zero (C_{p0}):

$$VD = dose/C_{p0} \tag{1}$$

The C_{p0} can be calculated by extrapolating the elimination phase back to time zero (see Fig. 28-2). The VD is best considered the "apparent VD" because it represents the apparent volume needed to contain the entire amount of the drug, assuming it is distributed throughout the body at the same concentration as in the plasma. Table 28-1 lists pharmacokinetic data for commonly used drugs from several drug classes, showing the wide variation in VD. Digoxin, for example, has a large VD (>5 L), whereas glimepiride has a relatively small VD (0.18 L). As discussed later, VD is a useful pharmacokinetic tool for calculating the loading dose and appreciating how various changes can affect a drug's half-life.

Elimination

Drugs are removed from the body by two major mechanisms: hepatic elimination, in which drugs are metabolized in the liver and excreted through the biliary tract; and renal elimination, in which drugs are removed from the circulation by either glomerular filtration or tubular secretion. For most drugs, the rates of hepatic and renal elimination are proportional to the plasma concentration of the drug. This relationship is often described as a "first-order" process. Two measurements, clearance and half-life, are used to evaluate elimination.

Clearance

The efficiency of elimination can be assessed by quantifying how fast the drug is cleared from the circulation. Drug clearance is a measure of the volume of plasma cleared of drug per unit of time. It is similar to the clinical measurement used to assess renal function—creatinine clearance, which is the volume of plasma from which creatinine is removed per minute. Total drug clearance (Cl_{tot}) is the rate of elimination by all processes (El_{tot}) divided by the plasma concentration of the drug (C_p):

$$Cl_{tot} = El_{tot}/C_p \tag{2}$$

Drugs may be cleared by several organs, but as noted earlier,. renal clearance and hepatic clearance are the two major mechanisms. Total drug clearance (Cl_{tot}) can best be described as the sum of clearances by each organ. For most drugs, this is essentially the sum of renal clearance and hepatic clearance:

$$Cl_{tot} = Cl_{Ren} + Cl_{Hep} \tag{3}$$

Table 28-1 shows the wide variation in clearance values among commonly used medications; some drugs (e.g., phenobarbital) have relatively low clearances (<5 mL/minute), and other drugs (e.g., aspirin) have relatively high clearances (>500 mL/minute). Tobramycin is cleared almost entirely by the kidneys, whereas aspirin, carbamazepine, and phenytoin are cleared less than 5% by the kidneys.

Drug clearance is affected by several factors, including blood flow through the organ of clearance, protein binding to the drug, and activity of the clearance processes in the organs of elimination (e.g., glomerular filtration rate and tubular secretion in the kidney, enzyme activity in the liver). Drug clearance

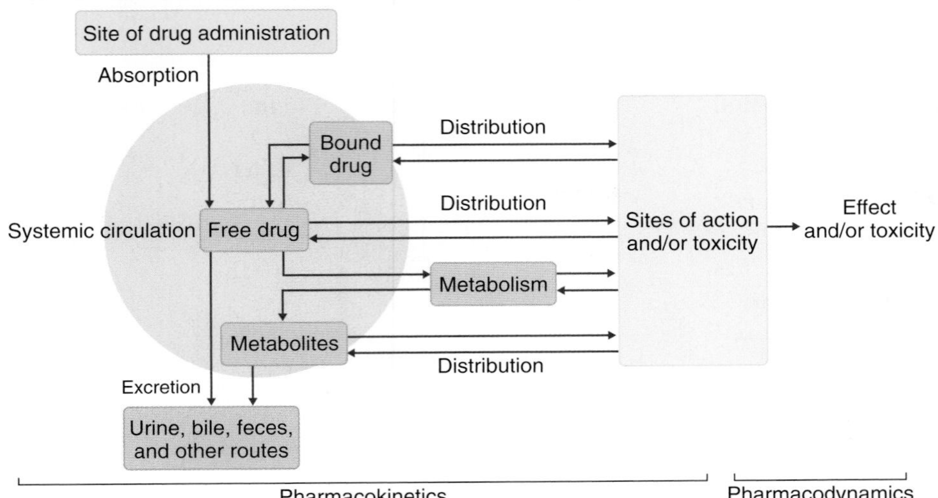

FIGURE 28-1. Schematic of a drug's movement through the body, from the site of administration to production of a drug effect. The relationship between pharmacokinetics and pharmacodynamics is shown.

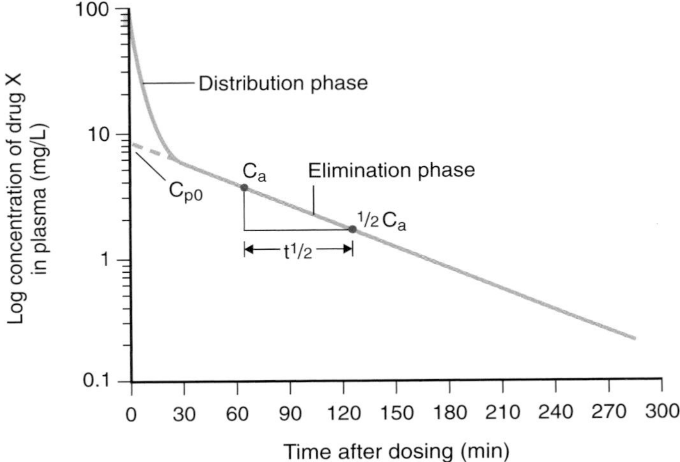

FIGURE 28-2. Representative drug concentration versus time plot used in pharmacokinetic studies. Concentration of drug is plotted with a logarithmic scale on the ordinate, and time is plotted with a linear scale on the abscissa. The resultant curve has two phases: the distribution phase, which is the initial portion of the plotted line when the concentration of drug decreases rapidly; and the later elimination phase, during which there is an exponential disappearance of drug from the plasma over time. The dotted line extrapolated from the elimination phase back to time zero is used to calculate plasma concentration at time zero (C_{p0}). During the elimination phase, the half-life ($t_{1/2}$) can be calculated as the time it takes to decrease the concentration by half (shown here as the time needed to decrease from concentration C_a to $\frac{1}{2}$ C_a).

is not affected by the distribution of drug throughout the body (VD) because clearance mechanisms act only on drug in the circulation.

Half-life

The amount of time needed to eliminate a drug from the body depends on the clearance and the VD. The first-order elimination constant (K_e) represents the proportion of the apparent VD that is cleared of drug per unit of time during the drug's exponential disappearance from the plasma over time (elimination phase):

$$K_e = \text{Cl}/\text{VD} \quad (4)$$

The value of this constant for a particular drug can be determined by plotting drug concentration versus time on a log-linear plot (see Fig. 28-2) and measuring the slope of the straight line obtained during the exponential (elimination) phase.

The time needed to eliminate the drug is best described by its half-life ($t_{1/2}$), which is the time required during the elimination phase (see Fig. 28-2) for the plasma concentration of the drug to be decreased by half. Mathematically, the half-life is equal to the natural logarithm of 2 (representing a reduction of drug concentration to half) divided by K_e. Substituting for K_e from Equation 4 and calculating the natural logarithm of 2, the half-life can be represented by the following equation:

$$t_{1/2} = 0.693\ \text{VD}/\text{Cl} \quad (5)$$

From this equation, one can predict that at a given clearance, as the VD increases, the half-life increases. Similarly, at a given VD, as the clearance increases, the half-life decreases. Clinically, many disease states (see later) can affect VD and clearance. Because disease affects VD and clearance differently, the half-life may increase, decrease, or not change much at all. Therefore, the half-life by itself is not a good indicator of the extent of abnormality in elimination.

The half-life is useful to predict how long it takes for a drug to be eliminated from the body. For any drug that has a first-order elimination, one would expect that by the end of the first half-life, the drug would be reduced to 50%; by the end of the second half-life, to 25%; by the end of the third half-life, to 12.5%; by the end of the fourth half-life, to 6.25%; and by the end of the fifth half-life, to 3.125%. In general, a drug can be considered essentially eliminated after three to five half-lives, when less than 10% of the effective concentration remains. Table 28-1 shows the wide variation in half-life for several commonly used drugs.

APPLYING PHARMACOKINETIC PRINCIPLES

Using a Loading Dose

To attain a desired therapeutic concentration rapidly, a loading dose is often used. In determining the amount of drug to be given, the physician must consider the "volume" within the body into which the drug will be distributed. This volume is best described by the apparent VD. The loading dose can be calculated by multiplying the desired concentration by the VD:

$$\text{Loading dose} = \text{desired concentration} \times \text{VD} \quad (6)$$

Rapid administration of the entire loading dose may produce an initially high peak concentration that results in toxicity. This problem can be avoided either by administering the loading dose as a divided dose or by varying the rate of access to the circulation, such as by administering the drug as an infusion (with an intravenous drug) or by taking advantage of the slower access to the circulation from various other routes (e.g., oral dosing). This approach is illustrated by phenytoin (see Table 28-1), which may need to be administered with a loading dose to achieve a therapeutic level (10 to 20 mg/L) rapidly. Because the VD for phenytoin is approximately 0.6 L/kg, the loading dose calculated from Equation 6 is 420 mg/L to attain a minimally therapeutic level of 10 mg/L in a 70-kg adult. However, administration of 420 mg of phenytoin by intravenous bolus carries the risk of cardiac arrest and death. By taking advantage of the reduced bioavailability (F = 0.8) and slow absorption of oral phenytoin, the loading dose can be administered safely as an oral dose of 500 mg.

The equation for the loading dose can also be used to calculate the dose needed to "boost" an inadequate blood level of drug to a desired therapeutic range. If therapeutic monitoring shows that the phenytoin level is 5 mg/L and the desired level is 15 mg/L, it is necessary to multiply the difference needed to achieve the desired concentration (10 mg/L) by the VD

TABLE 28-1 PHARMACOKINETIC PARAMETERS FOR SOME COMMONLY USED DRUGS

DRUG	VD (L/KG)	PROTEIN BINDING (%)	TOTAL CLEARANCE (ML/MIN)	% OF TOTAL CLEARANCE AS RENAL CLEARANCE	HALF-LIFE (HR)	THERAPEUTIC RANGE (MG/L)
Amoxicillin	0.47	17-18		86	1.2	2-8
Aspirin (acetylsalicylic acid)	0.14-0.18	80-90	575-725	<2	0.2-0.3	20-250
Carbamazepine	1.2	75-90	50-125	1-3	12-17	4-12
Digoxin	5-7.3	20-30	75	50-70	34-44	0.5-2
Glimepiride	0.18	>99.5	0.62 ± 0.26	<0.5	3.4 ± 2.0	
Lidocaine	3	60-80	700	<10	1.5-2	1-5
Lithium carbonate	0.7-1	0	20-40	95-99	20-270	0.4-1.4*
Penicillin G	0.5-0.7	45-68	—	20	0.4-0.9	Variable
Phenobarbital	0.6-0.7	20-45	4	25	2-6 days	<10-40*
Phenytoin	0.4-0.8	88-93	—	<5	7-26	10-20
Procainamide	2.2	14-23	470-600	40-70	2.5-4.7	4-8
Theophylline	0.3-0.7	60	36-50	<10	4-16	5-20
Tobramycin	0.25-0.30	<10	70	>95	2-4	0.5-2 (TR) 4-8 (PK)
Vancomycin	0.4-1	52-60	65	85	4-6	5-10 (TR) 25-35 (PK)

*Therapeutic range varies according to the indication for the drug. For example, lithium carbonate in the range of 0.4-1.3 mg/L is appropriate for affective schizophrenia disorder; a range of 1.0-1.4 mg/L is appropriate for mania. Phenobarbital concentration below 10 mg/mL is appropriate for anticonvulsant therapy; 40 mg/L is appropriate as a hypnotic.
PK = peak value; TR = trough value; VD = volume of distribution.

(0.6 L/kg) to determine the dose (in milligrams per kilogram) necessary to achieve this drug level after distribution. In a 70-kg individual, 0.6 mg/kg is multiplied by 70 kg to obtain the calculated loading dose (420 mg) that can be administered safely. A 500-mg oral dose with a bioavailability of less than 1 (e.g., F = 0.8) would deliver to the systemic circulation the approximate amount needed and avoid the risks associated with rapid intravenous administration.

Determining Drug Accumulation

Continuing to administer a drug, either as a prolonged infusion or as repeated doses, results in accumulation until a steady state occurs. Steady state is the point at which the amount of drug being administered equals the amount being eliminated so that the plasma and tissue levels remain constant. The elimination half-life determines not only the time course of drug elimination but also the time course of drug accumulation. This "mirror image" pattern of drug accumulation and elimination is illustrated in Figure 28-3. As with drug elimination, three to five half-lives determine the time it takes to reach steady state during drug accumulation. Whereas drugs with short half-lives accumulate rapidly, drugs with long half-lives require a longer time to accumulate, with a potential delay in achieving therapeutic levels. For drugs with long half-lives, a loading dose may be needed to obtain rapid drug accumulation and a more rapid therapeutic effect.

With each change in drug dose or rate of infusion, a change in steady state occurs. Although it is not obvious for drugs with short half-lives, the effects of dose adjustments for drugs with longer half-lives are delayed, and the time varies directly with the drug's half-life.

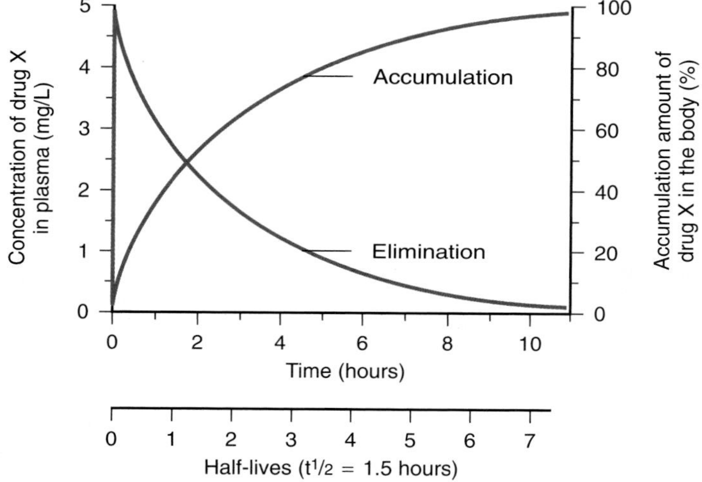

FIGURE 28-3. Representative plot of the "mirror image" relationship between the elimination of drug (after drug is discontinued) and the accumulation of drug (during infusion). The plot shows the concentration on the left *y*-axis and time on the upper *x*-axis. The lower *x*-axis shows the time in half-lives, and the *y*-axis on the right shows the percentage of drug in the body. After three to five half-lives, elimination is essentially complete, and accumulation is essentially at a steady state.

Using a Maintenance Dose

After steady state is reached in three to five half-lives with either a continuous infusion or intermittent doses, the rate of drug administered equals the rate of drug eliminated. For an intravenous drug, the administration rate is the infusion rate (I); for a drug administered by another route (e.g., orally), the administration rate is the dose per unit of time (D/t). Equation 7 shows that the rate of elimination (total) equals $Cl_{tot} \times C_p$. With an intravenously administered drug, because the infusion rate equals the elimination rate at steady state, it follows that

$$I = Cl_{tot} \times C_p \quad (7)$$

Similarly, with an orally administered drug, the dose administered per unit of time equals the elimination rate at steady state, with the result that

$$D/t = Cl_{tot} \times C_p \quad (8)$$

These equations show the direct relationship between the dose and the resultant plasma concentration at steady state. This relationship is independent of the distribution of the drug. By use of these equations, it is possible to determine the infusion rate or the interval and dose needed to achieve and maintain a specified drug concentration in the plasma.

When a drug is administered intermittently, it approaches steady-state concentration over time, with a pattern similar to that observed with continuous infusion (Fig. 28-4). With intermittent drug administration, such as with an oral dose, the drug concentration fluctuates; the magnitude of fluctuation between the peak and trough concentrations depends on the interval of administration, drug half-life, absorption characteristics, and site of administration. The effect of a change in the interval of administration for an oral drug is shown in Figure 28-4. As the intervals decrease below the half-life, the fluctuation decreases and approaches the curve produced by an intravenous infusion. Orally administered drugs may reach the blood stream more

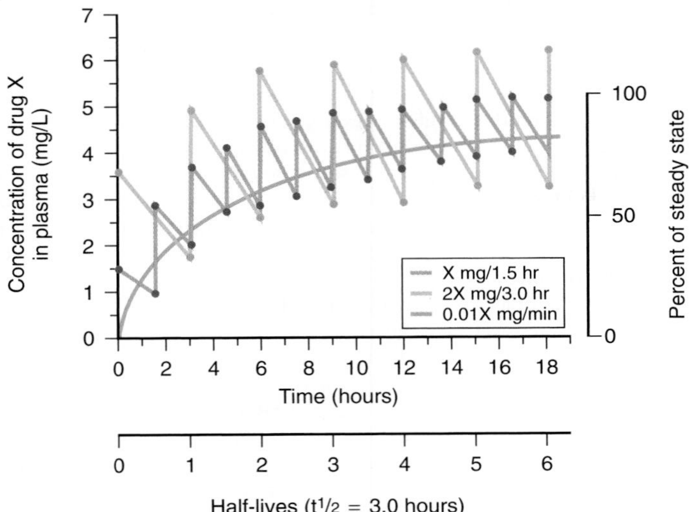

FIGURE 28-4. **Accumulation of drug over time, approaching a steady state.** Time is depicted in hours (upper *x*-axis) and half-lives (lower *x*-axis, showing that steady state is reached in three to five half-lives). The green line depicts the pattern produced by an infusion of a hypothetical drug at a dose of 0.01X. The orange line shows the pattern resulting from oral administration of a 2X dose every 3 hours, and the blue line represents the pattern produced by oral administration of dose X every 1.5 hours.

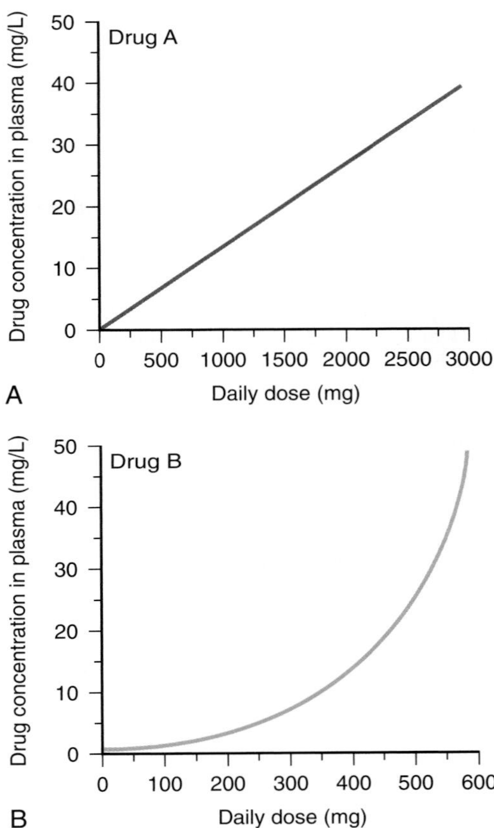

FIGURE 28-5. **Effect of increasing the dose of a drug on its serum concentration. A,** Drug A follows first-order or linear kinetics. **B,** Drug B follows zero-order or nonlinear (or saturable) kinetics.

rapidly, attaining a higher peak concentration with one formulation, whereas the same drug administered as a timed-release formulation is absorbed more slowly, with a lower peak concentration but lasting longer in the plasma. Finally, the same drug administered by different routes may have different plasma profiles not only because of differing absorption characteristics but also because of other effects, such as first-pass metabolism.

Decreasing the Drug Level

At times, it may be necessary to decrease the plasma drug level while maintaining therapy (e.g., when signs of toxicity become apparent or a potentially dangerously high concentration of drug is noted; see later). The most effective and rapid response is to discontinue the drug; the length of time for which the drug is discontinued is determined by the estimated half-life of the drug in the specific patient. After discontinuation of the drug for a time based on its half-life, the total clearance (Cl_{tot}) of the drug can be used to determine what infusion rate (I, Equation 7) or dose and interval (D/t, Equation 8) must be used to achieve the new desired concentration (C_p).

Effect of Dose Increases on Elimination Kinetics

Although the previously discussed pharmacokinetic principles can be a guide to the dose of most drugs, not all drugs behave the same when the dose is increased. The elimination of most drugs follows first-order or linear kinetics; the amount of drug eliminated is directly proportional to the concentration of drug in the plasma (Fig. 28-5A). A few drugs have a different pattern of elimination. Three of the most commonly used drugs that exhibit this different pharmacokinetic pattern are ethanol, phenytoin, and salicylate. These drugs have dose-dependent, nonlinear saturation kinetics. As the dose of drug increases and the concentration of drug in the plasma rises, the relative amount of drug being eliminated falls (i.e., the clearance decreases) until the rate of drug metabolism is at its maximum. At this point, drug elimination is said to be zero order, and the drug concentration in plasma starts to increase much more (no longer linearly) with each subsequent increase in dose (Fig. 28-5B).

MONITORING DRUG CONCENTRATION AS A GUIDE TO THERAPY

Although published pharmacokinetic data (usually population averages) such as those in Table 28-1 are useful to determine initial drug dosing, modification of the dose may be needed in an individual patient. For some drugs (e.g., certain antihypertensives or anticoagulants), the therapeutic effects (e.g., blood pressure or coagulation) can be quantified easily over a range of concentrations, permitting adequate drug adjustment. For many other drugs (e.g., some antiarrhythmics or antiseizure medications), therapeutic effects over a range of concentrations are not readily detectable. With these drugs, the plasma concentration may provide further guidance in optimizing therapy if the plasma concentration of the drug is a reflection of its concentration at the site of action and the drug effects are reversible. A third, much smaller group of drugs produces irreversible effects (e.g., aspirin inhibition of platelet aggregation). With these drugs, plasma drug concentration does not correlate with drug effect, and drug monitoring is not useful.

To use drug concentration as a guide to therapy, it is necessary to establish a range of concentrations from minimally to maximally efficacious with tolerable toxicity. This range of concentrations, or the *therapeutic window,* is usually determined from a dose-response curve generated from a population of patients who have been examined closely for therapeutic and toxic effects (Fig. 28-6). This graph also may be used to determine the *therapeutic index,* a useful measure of drug toxicity calculated by dividing the 50% value from the toxicity curve by the 50% value from the efficacy curve. Because these curves are generated from population data, the values may not be applicable to all individuals.

Table 28-1, in addition to providing useful pharmacokinetic data, lists therapeutic ranges of several common drugs for which measuring the concentration and knowing the therapeutic range may be useful in clinical management. Many of these drugs are used to treat serious or life-threatening diseases. In these cases, it is essential to avoid inadequate doses because a therapeutic effect is needed. Excessive doses must also be avoided because of the risk of toxicity with drugs that have a small therapeutic index. In contrast, it is not necessary to assay levels of drugs used to treat noncritical diseases (when inadequate treatment is not a serious problem) or for which the therapeutic index is large (when relative overtreatment is not likely to produce toxicity).

Problems with Interpreting Drug Concentration

The time of blood collection, perhaps more than any other factor, contributes to the misinterpretation of drug levels. As can be seen in Figure 28-2, if sampling is performed too early, while the drug is still in the distribution phase, the drug level may be high and not reflect drug concentration at the site of action. It is therefore important to sample after the distribution phase.

For many drugs administered intermittently, a trough level, obtained immediately before the next dose is administered, is most useful for making decisions about dose adjustments (see Table 28-1). For drugs administered by infusion or intermittently at short intervals (see Fig. 28-4), the best time to draw blood is during steady state.

Protein binding is another major factor that contributes to the misinterpretation of drug levels. Free drug (not bound to protein and able to equilibrate with tissues and to interact with the site of action) is the critical drug concentration when therapeutic decisions are being made. Many drugs are tightly bound to plasma protein, however. Table 28-1 shows that many commonly used drugs, such as aspirin, carbamazepine, phenytoin, and glimepiride, have protein binding of more than 75%. Because many of the commonly used drug assays determine total drug concentration (which includes protein-bound drug and free drug), assessment of the "true" free drug concentration may be inaccurate, particularly if the fraction of drug bound to protein varies. In addition, the drug's binding may be decreased by disease or by other drugs, leading to increased unbound drug levels that alter the interpretation of the measured drug concentrations. Kidney and liver disease can change the binding of certain drugs (e.g., phenytoin) to protein because of a decrease in protein (e.g., decreased albumin, as in nephrotic syndrome or liver disease) or as a result of competition for protein binding by endogenously produced substances (e.g., uremia in kidney disease, hyperbilirubinemia in liver disease). Similarly, other drugs may compete for binding to protein. A major problem secondary to these changes in protein binding is that free drug is not typically measured in many of the common drug assays used by clinical laboratories. Last, changes in drug binding to protein can affect the pharmacokinetics of the drug, the main effect being on the VD, which increases as protein binding decreases.

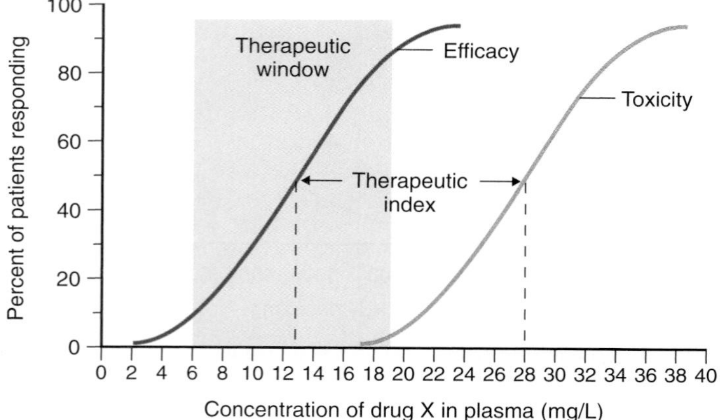

FIGURE 28-6. Pattern produced in a dose-response population study in which both effect and toxicity are measured. The therapeutic window is shown as the range of therapeutically effective concentrations, which includes most of the efficacy curve and less than 10% of the toxicity curve. The therapeutic index is calculated by dividing the 50% value on the toxicity curve by the 50% value on the efficacy curve.

The usefulness of a drug assay is also limited by physiologic changes that may alter the response at a particular drug concentration. An example of this pharmacodynamic change is the response produced by a certain level of digoxin in the presence of altered electrolyte concentrations (e.g., potassium, calcium, magnesium). Tolerance, a reduced response to a given concentration of drug with continued use, is another pharmacodynamic change that may alter how a drug concentration is interpreted. Tolerance is commonly observed with the continued use of narcotics (e.g., in terminal cancer patients); initially, adequate pain control is noted at a given drug concentration, but after long-term administration, the same drug concentration is no longer associated with pain relief.

ADJUSTING DRUG DOSE WITH DISEASE

Kidney Disease

The major questions to be answered when determining whether a drug dosage needs to be adjusted in the setting of kidney disease are the following: Is the drug primarily excreted through the kidneys? Are increased drug levels likely to be associated with toxicity? If the answer to both is yes, it is likely that with decreased renal clearance, a drug will accumulate and become toxic. With renal failure, it is necessary to adjust the dosing regimen of such drugs, particularly for a drug with a long half-life and a small therapeutic index (e.g., digoxin).

To obtain the desired concentration over time in the presence of decreased clearance, adjustments can be made by decreasing the dose while maintaining the dose interval (DD), maintaining the dose but increasing the interval between doses (II), or a combination of both (DD and II). Table 28-2 shows how these three different methods are used to adjust the dosages of several common drugs to account for renal dysfunction (see Table 28-1 for their pharmacokinetic properties with normal renal function). With these

TABLE 28-2 ADJUSTMENT OF DRUG DOSAGE IN RENAL FAILURE

		Half-Life (hr)			*Adjustment for Renal Failure*			
DRUG	TYPE OF ELIMINATION	NORMAL	END-STAGE RENAL DISEASE	METHOD*	GFR >50 ML/MIN	GFR 10-50 ML/MIN	GFR <10 ML/MIN	REMOVED BY DIALYSIS†
Amikacin	Renal	2-3	30	DD II	60-90% 12 hr	30-70% 12-18 hr	20-30% 24 hr	Yes
Aspirin	Hepatic (renal)	2-19	Unchanged	II	4 hr	4-6 hr	Avoid	Yes
Carbamazepine	Hepatic (renal)	35	?	DD	Unchanged	Unchanged	75%	No
Digoxin	Renal (nonrenal 15-40%)	36-44	80-120	DD II	Unchanged 24 hr	25-75% 36 hr	10-25% 48 hr	No
Lidocaine	Hepatic (renal <20%)	1.2-2.2	1.3-3	DD	Unchanged	Unchanged	Unchanged	No
Lithium carbonate	Renal	14-28	Prolonged	DD	Unchanged	50-75%	25-50%	Yes
Penicillin G	Renal (hepatic)	0.5	6-20	DD II	Unchanged 6-8 hr	75% 8-12 hr	25-50% 12-16 hr	Yes
Phenobarbital	Hepatic (renal 30%)	60-150	117-160	II	Unchanged	Unchanged	12-16 hr	Yes
Phenytoin	Hepatic (renal)	24	8	DD	Unchanged	Unchanged	Unchanged	No
Procainamide	Renal (hepatic 7-24%)	2.5-4.9	5.3-5.9	II	4 hr	6-12 hr	8-24 hr	Yes
Theophylline	Hepatic	3-12	?	DD	Unchanged	Unchanged	Unchanged	Yes
Tobramycin	Renal	2.5	56	DD II	60-90% 8-12 hr	30-70% 12 hr	20-30% 24 hr	Yes
Vancomycin	Renal	6-8	200-250	II	24-72 hr	72-240 hr	240 hr	No

*DD (alone) = decrease dose (maintain same interval); II (alone) = increase interval between doses (maintain dose); DD and II (together) = combination of both approaches.
†Dialysis refers to hemodialysis.
GFR = glomerular filtration rate.

adjustments, it may be possible to achieve an average concentration similar to that obtained with normal renal function; however, there may be concomitant marked changes in the magnitude of peak and trough values. In choosing the type of drug adjustment, the physician should consider not only the therapeutic index of the drug but also (1) whether an effective concentration must be achieved quickly and maintained within a narrow range (i.e., maintaining an average drug concentration and avoiding trough levels at which the drug is ineffective) and (2) whether toxicity is associated with elevated (i.e., peak) drug concentrations.

Renal drug clearance correlates with creatinine clearance (whether the drug uses glomerular filtration or tubular secretion); therefore, any adjustment of drug dose in kidney disease can use the creatinine clearance to calculate the dose needed because renal drug clearance is proportional to creatinine clearance. The creatinine clearance (Cl_{Cr}), which is used as an estimate of glomerular filtration rate, may be calculated directly from the serum creatinine concentration by the following equation:

$$Cl_{cr} = [(140 - \text{age}) \times \text{weight (kg)}]/[72 \times \text{serum creatinine (mg/dL)}] \quad (9)$$

The calculated creatinine clearance should be multiplied by 0.85 for females. (*Note:* This calculation applies only when the serum creatinine concentration is less than 5 mg/dL and renal function is not rapidly changing.)

Using Clearance for Dose Adjustment

The dose of a drug used in renal insufficiency ($\text{dose}_{D\text{-}RI}$) is proportional to the dose used with normal renal function (dose_D) in the same ratio as clearance of the drug in renal insufficiency ($Cl_{D\text{-}RI}$) to clearance with normal renal function (Cl_D). By rearranging, $\text{dose}_{D\text{-}RI}$ is defined as:

$$\text{Dose}_{D\text{-}RI} = \text{dose}_D \times [Cl_{D\text{-}RI}/Cl_D] \quad (10)$$

One can estimate the $Cl_{D\text{-}RI}$ by multiplying Cl_D by the ratio of the creatinine clearance in renal insufficiency ($Cl_{Cr\text{-}RI}$) over Cl_{Cr} with normal renal function:

$$Cl_{D\text{-}RI} = Cl_D \times [Cl_{Cr\text{-}RI}/Cl_{Cr}] \quad (11)$$

As shown in Equation 3, total clearance is the sum of clearance by renal and nonrenal (typically hepatic) mechanisms. Any nonrenal clearance is assumed to remain normal, and only the renal clearance is adjusted, with total clearance being reduced only to the extent that renal clearance is reduced. The dose may be calculated from the total (adjusted) clearance and the desired plasma concentration by either Equation 7 or Equation 8. The calculated dose is only an initial guide to the dose needed, however. By monitoring the drug response or the plasma drug concentration at various times after initial dosing, further dose adjustments can be made as necessary. From a practical perspective, most clinical dose adjustments in the presence of renal dysfunction can be guided by published tables based on changes in glomerular filtration rate (see Table 28-2) and the effectiveness of dialysis in removing the drug. Computerized decision support systems are particularly effective in guiding medication dosing for inpatients with renal insufficiency.

Loading Dose in Renal Insufficiency

For drugs typically administered with a loading dose in patients with normal renal function, the same approach can be used in those with renal insufficiency to ensure that the desired concentration is achieved rapidly. For drugs typically administered without a loading dose, the presence of a prolonged half-life resulting from renal insufficiency may delay drug accumulation to steady state. In this setting, a loading dose (equal to the amount needed to reach steady state with normal renal function) is required.

Additional Considerations in Renal Insufficiency

Because of individual differences among patients, the approaches outlined earlier should be considered only initial approximations to prevent ineffective (too low) or toxic (too high) doses. For maintenance therapy, it is desirable to monitor blood levels to guide dosing.

If a metabolite of the drug is responsible for its effect or toxicity and the metabolite accumulates in the setting of renal failure, the drug level alone may not provide sufficient guidance for planning therapy. For example, the major metabolite of procainamide is *N*-acetylprocainamide, which has a toxicity similar to that of the parent drug but only modest antiarrhythmic activity. In the setting of renal failure, *N*-acetylprocainamide may accumulate dramatically because it is more dependent on renal elimination. Measurement of procainamide levels alone does not accurately assess either the levels needed for antiarrhythmic effect or the risk of toxicity.

Liver Disease

Although many drugs are biotransformed in the liver, it is not possible to make any general recommendations for drug dose adjustments in liver disease. In contrast to renal disease, no useful laboratory test is available on which to base dose adjustments. It has been suggested that if the liver's capacity to produce protein (reflected by albumin concentration and prothrombin time) is reduced significantly, the clearance of drugs metabolized by the cytochrome P-450 enzymes is probably reduced as well.

One special situation that can develop with chronic liver disease and may require dose adjustment is the portacaval shunt. This condition produces not only a potential hemodynamic alteration, leading to decreased hepatic blood flow and accompanying decreased clearance, but also a possible bypassing of the first-pass effect, resulting in higher concentrations of drug reaching the systemic circulation. Drugs with a large hepatic extraction that are typically administered orally (e.g., propranolol) may appear in the systemic circulation at higher, potentially toxic concentrations.

Hemodynamic Diseases

Decreased cardiac output and hypotensive conditions lead to decreased perfusion of the organs, including those responsible for eliminating drugs. As noted earlier with regard to primary kidney disease, the dose can be adjusted for decreased renal perfusion by the use of creatinine clearance. The effect of decreased hepatic blood flow on pharmacokinetics is more difficult to assess. For drugs that have a high hepatic extraction (e.g., lidocaine), decreased hepatic blood flow suggests a need for dose reduction.

Altered hemodynamics also may affect the distribution of selected drugs. Drugs that have a relatively large VD (e.g., lidocaine, procainamide, quinidine) may be affected by conditions leading to hypotension, such as shock, resulting in a decrease in the apparent VD. With a reduced VD, the loading dose of a drug should be reduced to avoid potentially toxic drug levels.

In general, in the setting of severely compromised hemodynamics, it is advisable to be conservative, avoiding potentially toxic loading and maintenance doses of drugs. Drug levels and the clinical status should be monitored closely, and drug doses should be adjusted as necessary.

APPROACH TO DRUG OVERDOSE

The pharmacokinetic principles discussed earlier can be used to determine the best approach to drug removal in the setting of a drug overdose, particularly if hemodialysis or hemoperfusion is contemplated. The major goal is to increase the overall clearance of the drug, removing a substantial fraction of the total body load of drug. Examination of the VD and clearance values can provide some guidance. For drugs with a large VD (e.g., digoxin; see Table 28-1), only a small amount can be removed because clearance affects only the amount of drug present in the plasma, and a large portion of the drug is outside the plasma compartment. Similarly, for drugs with high clearance values, hemoperfusion may increase the overall clearance only minimally and is not indicated. Table 28-2 provides data for determining whether hemodialysis is likely to be useful to remove several commonly prescribed drugs.

USING DRUGS IN THE ELDERLY

Administering drugs to the elderly is perhaps the most challenging area of adult therapeutics because of several factors: the increasing likelihood of multiple illnesses, often with multisystemic involvement; the need for these patients to take multiple drugs (often prescribed by different physicians); and the increasing probability of altered pharmacokinetics and pharmacodynamics. These factors together contribute to a significantly increased frequency of drug interactions and adverse drug responses in this group of patients.

Pharmacokinetic Changes with Age

These changes can be secondary to the general physiologic effects of aging, such as alteration in body composition, or to specific changes in pharmacokinetically important organs (e.g., kidneys, liver). The distribution of drugs tends to change dramatically with age, mainly because of changes in body composition. Most typical is the increase in total body fat, with the accompanying decrease in lean body mass and total body water. The concentration of plasma proteins may also change; in particular, albumin decreases as the liver ages. Changes in drug distribution are manifested as a change in the apparent VD. For water-soluble drugs that are not bound to plasma proteins, the apparent VD is reduced; in contrast, for lipid-soluble drugs, the VD is increased. Minimal changes in metabolism accompany aging, but these alone cannot account for altered pharmacokinetics.

Excretion can be altered in the elderly, and the clearance of many drugs is decreased. Cardiac output and blood flow to the kidneys and liver also may be decreased. Glomerular filtration rate may be reduced by 50%. Hepatic elimination of drugs is less affected, except for drugs with a high hepatic clearance (e.g., lidocaine). The elimination half-life of many drugs is increased with aging as a consequence of a larger apparent VD and a decreased hepatic or renal clearance (see Equation 5).

Pharmacodynamic Changes with Age

These changes are a result of changes in the responsiveness of the target organ. They require the use of smaller drug doses in the elderly, even if the pharmacokinetics are unchanged. This affects many drugs commonly used in the elderly; for example, antianxiety drugs and drugs from the sedative-hypnotic class may produce increased central nervous system depression in the elderly at concentrations that are well tolerated in younger adults. Similarly, anticoagulants (e.g., warfarin) may produce hemorrhage in the elderly at concentrations that are well tolerated in younger adults.

General Recommendations for Drug Use in the Elderly

- Clearance of drugs eliminated by the kidneys may be reduced by 50%.
- Drugs eliminated primarily by the liver typically do not require dose adjustments for age, except for drugs with high hepatic clearances, which may be affected by the age-related decrease in hepatic blood flow.
- Because of the potential for increased target organ sensitivity in the elderly, only the lowest effective dose should be used.
- Frequent reviews of the patient's drug history should be conducted, including both prescription and over-the-counter medications, keeping in mind the increased potential risk for drug interactions and adverse drug responses.

INTERACTIONS BETWEEN DRUGS

Because patients are typically treated with multiple agents, even for a single disease, the possibilities for drug interactions are great. Most clinically important drug interactions typically involve a drug with a low therapeutic index (e.g., warfarin) and an easily detectable pharmacologic effect (e.g., bleeding), such that a small increase in the amount of drug produces a significant effect (toxicity).

It is difficult to accurately assess the prevalence of drug interactions in either the inpatient or the ambulatory setting, particularly because no formal and comprehensive surveillance mechanism is available. The risk for drug interactions seems to be increasing, particularly for critically ill, hospitalized patients, who are frequently taking more than 10 medications.

There are basically two types of drug interaction: (1) pharmacokinetic drug interactions, caused by a change in the amount of drug or active metabolite at the site of action; and (2) pharmacodynamic drug interactions (without a change in pharmacokinetics), caused by a change in drug effect.

Pharmacokinetic Drug Interactions

Less Drug at the Site of Action

Decreased Absorption

The gastrointestinal lumen is perhaps the best example of an area where drug interactions can result in decreased drug absorption. Some commonly used drugs can illustrate this type of interaction. For many drugs, a physicochemical interaction prevents the drug from being absorbed. Drugs such as colestipol and cholestyramine (resins used to lower cholesterol and bind bile acids) can also bind other drugs present in the gastrointestinal lumen, including digoxin and warfarin. Because of the potential for many other drugs to be bound, it is generally recommended that other drugs not be administered within 2 hours of colestipol or cholestyramine. Another type of interaction occurs when metal ions (e.g., aluminum, calcium, and magnesium in antacids and iron in supplements to treat iron deficiency) form insoluble complexes with tetracyclines, which can act as chelating agents. Other commonly used medications that decrease absorption include kaolin-pectin suspensions to treat diarrhea. These medications can significantly inhibit the absorption of coadministered drugs (e.g., digoxin).

Drugs that are particularly susceptible to pH changes may have decreased absorption when they are administered with other drugs that either affect gastric acidity or alter the extent of exposure to low pH. Protein pump inhibitors or H_2-receptor antagonists may elevate gastric pH, which can inhibit the dissolution and subsequent absorption of drugs that are weak bases (e.g., ketoconazole). Medications that delay gastric emptying (e.g., belladonna alkaloids) can increase the degradation of a coadministered acid-labile drug (e.g., levodopa), resulting in decreased absorption.

Altered Distribution

Drugs that use the same active transport process to reach their site of action can compete at the level of transport, resulting in lower levels of drug reaching that site. The classic example of this type of interaction is the coadministration of guanidinium-type antihypertensives with tricyclic antidepressants, phenothiazines, and certain sympathomimetic amines (e.g., ephedrine), which block the effects of the antihypertensive drug.

Increased Metabolism

Many drugs (e.g., phenobarbital, phenytoin, ethanol, glutethimide, griseofulvin, rifampin) and toxic compounds (e.g., cigarette smoke, certain chlorinated hydrocarbons) can increase the hepatic metabolism of other drugs (e.g., corticosteroids, cyclophosphamide, cyclosporine, certain β-adrenergic blockers, theophylline, warfarin) by inducing the activity of the cytochrome P-450 mixed function oxidase (CYP) system.

More Drug at the Site of Action

Increased Absorption

Any drug that increases the rate of gastric emptying (e.g., metoclopramide) can potentially increase the absorption of acid-unstable drugs. Also, drugs that decrease intestinal motility (e.g., anticholinergics) may increase the absorption of drugs that are relatively poorly absorbed (e.g., digoxin tablets) by increasing the drug's contact time with the absorbing surface.

Altered Distribution

Drugs bound to protein are limited in their distribution (particularly to the site of action) and are not available for metabolism or excretion. Drugs can compete with each other for binding to plasma proteins, resulting in drug interactions. Sulfonamides can displace barbiturates bound to serum albumin, leading to increased levels of free barbiturates and possible toxicity.

Decreased Metabolism

One of the most impressive drug interactions is produced when one drug inhibits the metabolism of another, leading to the second drug's accumulation and a significant risk of toxicity. This type of interaction results when 6-mercaptopurine, an antileukemic drug with a low therapeutic index, is used with allopurinol, often administered to control hyperuricemia. The interaction may result in potentially life-threatening toxicity.

Some drugs can inhibit the metabolism of many other drugs. For example, cimetidine can inhibit the metabolism of diazepam, imipramine, lidocaine, propranolol, quinidine, theophylline, and warfarin. Amiodarone inhibits the metabolism of calcium-channel blockers, phenytoin, quinidine, and warfarin. Of particular importance with amiodarone is its half-life of 1 to 2 months; it continues to inhibit drug metabolism for several months after it has been discontinued.

Other drugs are notable because their metabolism is inhibited by a variety of different drugs. The metabolism of the commonly used anticoagulant warfarin is inhibited not only by cimetidine and amiodarone but also by many other drugs, including alcohol, allopurinol, disulfiram, metronidazole, phenylbutazone, sulfinpyrazone, and trimethoprim-sulfamethoxazole. Similarly, the metabolism of phenytoin is inhibited by chloramphenicol, clofibrate, dicumarol, disulfiram, isoniazid (slow acetylators), phenylbutazone, and valproic acid.

Although most of these examples involve enzymes that metabolize the drug in the liver, drug-metabolizing enzymes outside the liver also may be affected by certain drugs. The best-known example is monoamine oxidase, which can be affected by nonspecific monoamine oxidase inhibitors, resulting in the accumulation of catecholamines at multiple sites after their release in response to the eating of tyramine-containing foods such as aged cheese, aged or cured meats, and any spoiled meat, poultry, or fish.

Decreased Excretion

Drugs can compete for the active transporters present in the kidney. Most of these interactions involve the acid transporters. The best-known interaction is probenecid's inhibition of penicillin transport, leading to decreased penicillin clearance and thus higher plasma levels, an interaction that was used in the past to maximize penicillin therapy. A similar inhibitory effect on the renal excretion of methotrexate can be produced by salicylates, phenylbutazone, and probenecid. The active transport of basic drugs (e.g., procainamide) can also be inhibited by other drugs (e.g., cimetidine, amiodarone).

Pharmacodynamic Drug Interactions

With pharmacodynamic interactions, drugs interact at the level of the receptor (target) or may produce additive effects by acting at separate sites on cells. An example of the first is the interaction of propranolol and epinephrine, which blocks β-adrenergic receptors; as a result, the α-adrenergic effects of epinephrine are unopposed. This undesirable interaction can result in severe hypertension.

Many examples exist of the additive effects of drugs. Aspirin, which can produce increased bleeding time by acting on platelets, can interact with warfarin, which affects clotting. The result is an increased risk of hemorrhage. Similarly, cardiac drugs, such as β-adrenergic blockers and calcium-channel blockers, have additive negative inotropic effects when they are coadministered, resulting in an increased risk of cardiac failure.

DIAGNOSIS AND PREVENTION OF DRUG INTERACTIONS

For a drug interaction to be recognized, the index of suspicion must be high whenever multiple drugs are used together. Because of the ever-increasing list of known and suspected drug interactions, it is impossible for a clinician to remember all or even many of the possible interactions.

Several clinical settings should raise concern about the possibility of drug interactions:

- The use of any drug with a low therapeutic index (Table 28-3) should be suspect.
- As the number of drugs being used concurrently increases, there is a disproportionately greater risk of drug interactions, particularly with more than 10 drugs.
- Critically ill patients who have multisystemic disease with compromised renal, hepatic, cardiac, or pulmonary function have an increased risk of drug interactions. This risk may be higher for patients with acquired immunodeficiency syndrome, who have an immunocompromised state and take a large number of drugs.
- Patients with various behavioral and psychiatric disorders (e.g., drug abusers taking a large number of prescription drugs as well as illicit drugs and alcohol) are at risk for drug interactions.

Another type of drug interaction that is becoming increasingly important is that between components of food (e.g., grapefruit juice) or natural products (e.g., herbs) and drugs. By inhibiting the intestinal cytochrome P-450 3A4 enzyme system, grapefruit juice can raise levels of drugs metabolized by this pathway (e.g., saquinavir, cyclosporine, verapamil) and result in toxicity or adverse drug effects.

Several steps can be taken to prevent drug interactions:

- When taking the medical history, it is important to document all drugs the patient is taking (and has recently taken), including prescription, over-the-counter, and other addictive drugs.
- It is desirable to minimize the number of drugs being taken by frequently reviewing the patient's drug list to ensure that each drug continues to be needed.
- There should be a high degree of suspicion when medications with a low therapeutic index known to have a high risk of drug interactions (see Table 28-3) are used.
- High-risk clinical settings, such as occur with critically ill patients, should raise the suspicion of adverse drug interactions.
- Adverse drug interactions should be considered in the differential diagnosis whenever any change occurs in a patient's course.

TABLE 28-3 DRUGS WITH LOW THERAPEUTIC INDICES AT HIGH RISK FOR ADVERSE DRUG RESPONSES AND DRUG INTERACTIONS

Anticoagulants
Antiarrhythmics
Anticonvulsants
Digoxin
Lithium carbonate
Oral hypoglycemics
Theophylline

ADVERSE REACTIONS TO DRUGS

An adverse drug response (ADR) is an undesired effect produced by a drug at standard doses, which typically necessitates reducing or stopping the suspected agent and may require treatment of the noxious effect produced. Further harm may occur with continued or future therapy with the drug.

EPIDEMIOLOGY

The financial impact of ADRs is estimated to be more than $100 billion per year. The actual incidence of ADRs is difficult to quantify because many cases are either not recognized or not reported. Several large studies have shown that the incidence may approach 20% for outpatients (even higher for patients taking more than 15 drugs) and 2 to 7% for inpatients. The incidence of ADRs increases exponentially with more than four drugs. Meta-analyses of several prospective studies suggest that ADRs are now the third leading cause of death in hospitalized patients. It is clear from more recent surveys that a relatively small group of drugs (see Table 28-3) continues to be implicated in most of the reported ADRs. Current trends suggest that the incidence of ADRs is likely to increase as a result of more prescribed and over-the-counter medications being used.

ETIOLOGY

Most ADRs are caused by an exaggerated (but predictable) pharmacologic effect of the drug or by a toxic or immunologic effect of the drug or a metabolite (not typically expected).

Predictable Toxic Responses to Drugs

Exaggerated drug responses that cause adverse drug effects may be due to any condition that causes altered pharmacokinetics or pharmacodynamics (discussed earlier). There has been increasing interest in the discipline of pharmacogenomics, which explores the role of genetic factors in altered pharmacokinetics or pharmacodynamics and the resultant increased susceptibility to ADRs. There is now ample evidence that molecular changes in the genes coding for drug-metabolizing enzymes can account for the variability in pharmacokinetics and drug effects observed in population studies. There are now many examples of the role of pharmacogenomics in altered drug response and effect. Three of the best-studied examples are genetic polymorphisms associated with debrisoquine-sparteine, *N*-acetylation, and mephenytoin. Each is associated with autosomal recessive inheritance, and together they are responsible for the metabolism of approximately 40 drugs (Table 28-4). Individuals with autosomal recessive genes are typically "poor metabolizers," with potentially altered pharmacokinetics that result in elevated plasma drug concentrations and can lead to toxicity. Recent studies have focused on genomic alterations associated with the variability in response to some commonly used drugs. Thus, the variability of response to warfarin (Chapter 37) is now understood to be due to single nucleotide polymorphisms in the cytochrome P-450 2C9 (*CYP2C9*) and vitamin K epoxide reductase (*VKOR*) genes. These single nucleotide polymorphisms have a significant effect on warfarin dose requirements. Similarly, polymorphisms in transporter genes can have profound effects on the pharmacokinetics of statins (Chapter 213). A common genetic variant of the organic anion-transporting polypeptide 1B1 can reduce the hepatic uptake of many statins, increasing the risk of statin-induced myopathy. Also, it is now appreciated that genetically impaired adenosine triphosphate–binding cassette G2 transporter efflux activity can result in an increase in systemic exposure to various statins. Of particular importance to therapeutics is that the effects of these genetic polymorphisms differ, depending on the specific statin used. This provides a rational basis for an individualized approach to the use of lipid-lowering therapeutic agents.

A particularly impressive example occurs with certain cancer chemotherapy agents that have a relatively narrow therapeutic window and the potential to produce severe cytotoxicity (e.g., deficiency in dihydropyrimidine dehydrogenase activity can result in life-threatening toxicity after the administration of 5-fluorouracil). These defects typically are not recognized until the patient is given the drug. They are often described as "pharmacogenetic" syndromes.

Other genetic alterations do not affect metabolism specifically and do not produce a range of quantitative changes. These defects can produce "qualitative" defects and are often associated with structural defects. The classic example is glucose-6-phosphate dehydrogenase. Individuals who are deficient in this enzyme cannot tolerate the oxidative stress produced by some

TABLE 28-4 GENETIC POLYMORPHISMS OF DRUG-METABOLIZING ENZYMES

TYPE	PRIMARY DRUG EXAMPLES	OTHER DRUGS THAT ARE SUBSTRATES	INCIDENCE OF "POOR METABOLIZERS" IN WHITES (%)	ENZYME INVOLVED
Debrisoquine-sparteine polymorphism	Amitriptyline, codeine, tamoxifen	Antidepressants, antiarrhythmics, β-adrenergic receptor–blocking drugs, codeine, dextromethorphan, neuroleptics	5-10	Cytochrome P-450 IID6 (CYP2D6)
Mephenytoin polymorphism	Mephenytoin	Mephobarbital, hexobarbital, diazepam, omeprazole	4 (Japanese, Chinese, 15-20)	Cytochrome P-450 IIC (CYP2C)
N-acetylation polymorphism	Isoniazid, sulfadiazine	Hydralazine, phenelzine, procainamide, dapsone, sulfamethazine, sulfapyridine, aminoglutethimide, aminosalicylic acid, sulfasalazine	40-70 (Japanese, 10-20)	*N*-acetyltransferase (NAT2)
Methyl conjugation polymorphism	Catecholamines	L-Dopa, methyldopa	25-30	Catechol-*O* methyltransferase (COMT)

drugs, leading to hemolysis (Chapter 164). Drugs that can produce this clinical picture include aspirin, nitrofurantoin, primaquine, probenecid, quinidine, quinine, sulfonamides, sulfones, and vitamin K. Another similar defect is deficiency of methemoglobin reductase, which results in an inability to maintain iron in hemoglobin in the ferrous state, causing methemoglobinemia (Chapter 161) after exposure to oxidizing drugs such as nitrites, sulfonamides, and sulfones.

Unpredictable Toxic Responses to Drugs

Other toxic or immunologic ADRs are not predictable and are not obviously due to an increase in drug concentration (pharmacokinetic) or drug effect (pharmacodynamic). Unpredictable toxic responses include direct reactions between a drug and a specific organ (e.g., platinum-containing drugs, such as cisplatin, can produce direct toxicity in the kidney and the eighth cranial nerve). With other drugs, metabolism to an active intermediate must occur first. With a standard dose of acetaminophen, no untoward effects occur because the relatively small amount of reactive metabolite formed by oxidative metabolism is detoxified rapidly by reduced glutathione. In the presence of an overdose, the glutathione is depleted, and the remaining reactive metabolite can damage the liver. Understanding the mechanism of this toxicity has provided a rationale for treating acetaminophen overdose. Sulfhydryl-containing compounds (e.g., *N*-acetylcysteine), which can complex with the reactive metabolite, can be administered to reduce the amount of free toxic metabolite present, protecting the liver.

Immunologic reactions to drugs are generally not produced by the drug alone. Similar to other low-molecular-weight compounds (<1000 D), they are typically not antigenic themselves. When a drug or reactive metabolite combines with a protein to form a drug-protein complex, it can become antigenic, capable of eliciting an immune response.

Perhaps the most impressive form of drug allergy is anaphylaxis, which is due to an immunoglobulin E–mediated hypersensitivity. Many drugs from different classes have been shown to produce this type of drug allergy. The best-known example is the anaphylactic response produced by penicillin, which can occur after its administration by any route. Skin testing with penicillin G, penicilloic acid, or penicilloyl polylysine can identify patients at risk and should be performed in those with a suspected penicillin allergy who need treatment with penicillin. If the skin test result is positive, the patient must undergo desensitization before receiving penicillin. If the skin test result is negative, penicillin can be administered with caution.

DIAGNOSIS OF ADVERSE DRUG RESPONSES

Although many of the well-known adverse drug effects are due to a relatively small group of drugs, every drug has the potential to cause an ADR. A physician should always consider the possibility of an ADR in the differential diagnosis even if none has been reported previously for the particular drug. In earlier editions of this book, we provided a table listing many diverse clinical presentations associated with ADRs. The reader is now referred to the numerous websites providing more complete and up-to-date information on ADRs than can be detailed here. For example, *www.prosoftedc.com/aers/aers.php* allows one to monitor drug safety with unlimited access to up-to-date information from the Food and Drug Administration's Adverse Event Reporting System (AERS).

In many instances, it is readily apparent that a specific drug has produced an ADR, such as the appearance of a rash in an otherwise healthy patient who was recently prescribed a single drug (e.g., penicillin). In other cases, the effect produced by the drug may be difficult to discern from other disease states. In still other cases, the adverse effect may mimic the illness being treated (e.g., development of an arrhythmia in a patient being treated with an antiarrhythmic drug).

From a public health perspective, it is highly desirable to have a mechanism available to detect, catalog, and track the incidence and severity of ADRs not only for drugs at various stages of development but also for drugs that were approved earlier. The Food and Drug Administration tracks adverse drug events through a voluntary reporting program, MedWatch. Health care professionals are encouraged to report any adverse events or product problems on a one-page form that can be sent by mail, fax, or electronically to the Food and Drug Administration. Although various methods for surveying ADRs have been proposed, ultimately, the cooperation of alert clinicians and health care professionals must be encouraged.

SUGGESTED READINGS

De Gregori M, Allegri M, De Gregori S, et al. How and why to screen for CYP2D6 interindividual variability in patients under pharmacological treatments. *Curr Drug Metab.* 2010;11:276-282. *The polymorphisms of CYP2D6 significantly affect the pharmacokinetics of about 50% of the drugs in clinical use, which are CYP2D6 substrates.*

Evans BJ. Establishing clinical utility of pharmacogenetic tests in the post-FDAAA era. *Clin Pharmacol Ther.* 2010;88:749-751. *The FDA Amendments Act, when fully implemented, will offer new sources of evidence and new regulatory mechanisms during the postmarket phase of drug life.*

Guest EJ, Rowland-Yeo K, Rostami-Hodjegan A, et al. Assessment of algorithms for predicting drug-drug interactions via inhibition mechanisms: comparison of dynamic and static models. *Br J Clin Pharmacol.* 2011;71:72-87. *Assessment of methods to predict drug-drug interactions and their clinical relevance.*

Kamali F, Wynne H. Pharmacogenetics of warfarin. *Annu Rev Med.* 2010;61:63-75. *Reviews the role of various genetic factors in warfarin therapeutics.*

Kennedy DA, Seely D. Clinically based evidence of drug-herb interactions: a systematic review. *Expert Opin Drug Saf.* 2010;9:79-124. *Overview of clinically important interactions that can result from co-exposure to commonly used herbal medicines and prescription drugs.*

Kunac DL, Tatley MV. Detecting medication errors in the New Zealand pharmacovigilance database: a retrospective analysis. *Drug Saf.* 2011;34:59-71. *The most commonly involved medications were antibacterials for systemic use and anti-inflammatory agents, with gastrointestinal and respiratory system disorders the most common adverse events reported.*

Moyer TP, O'Kane DJ, Baudhuin LM, et al. Warfarin sensitivity genotyping: a review of the literature and summary of patient experience. *Mayo Clin Proc.* 2009;84:1079-1094. *Up-to-date review of warfarin use from a pharmacogenomic perspective.*

Pai MP. Estimating the glomerular filtration rate in obese adult patients for drug dosing. *Adv Chronic Kidney Dis.* 2010;17:53-62. *Explores current approaches and controversies for estimating of GFR and creatinine clearance among obese patients in clinical practice.*

Seden K, Dickinson L, Khoo S, et al. Grapefruit-drug interactions. *Drugs.* 2010;70:2373-2407. *Review of its interactions with calcium channel blockers, immunosuppressants, antihistamines, and other drugs.*

Steinman MA, Hanlon JT. Managing medications in clinically complex elders: "there's got to be a happy medium." *JAMA.* 2010;304:1592-1601. *Systematic approach to addressing the medication regimen in the context of the clinical reality, social situation, and goals of care.*

Wang L, McLeod HL, Weinshilboum RM. Genomics and drug response. *N Engl J Med.* 2011;364:1144-1153. *Review.*

Woodcock J. Assessing the clinical utility of diagnostics used in drug therapy. *Clin Pharmacol Ther.* 2010;88:765-773. *Examination of the clinical utility and challenges of diagnostics in drug therapy.*

29 PAIN

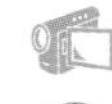

STEVEN P. COHEN AND SRINIVASA N. RAJA

Pain is ubiquitous in life, usually serving as a warning sign of impending or actual injury to the organism. As such, pain is older than humans, dating back to our most primitive ancestors. Pain is also a vital diagnostic clue for physicians. Physicians should be intimately familiar with pain because it is the most common symptom for which patients seek medical attention. According to the U.S. government's annual report on Americans' health, one in four adults suffered a day-long bout of pain within the past 30 days, and 10% suffer from pain every day. Among the various types of pain, back pain is the most common, followed by headaches and arthralgias. Spinal pain is the leading cause of disability in industrialized nations, with the economic costs exceeding $100 billion annually in the United States by some estimates. Special populations at particular risk for chronic pain include elderly people and individuals with physical and psychological morbidities. Several conditions characterized by chronic pain, such as irritable bowel syndrome, interstitial cystitis, fibromyalgia, and complex regional pain syndrome, are more prevalent in females than males.

DEFINITION

The International Association for the Study of Pain defines pain as "an unpleasant sensory and emotional experience associated with actual or potential tissue damage, or described in terms of such damage." This definition recognizes that pain may be experienced in some circumstances in the absence of ongoing tissue damage, such as phantom pain after a healed amputation. One implication of this construct is the assumption that pain is always subjective; hence, a patient's report of pain should always be accepted at face value in the absence of evidence to the contrary.

PATHOBIOLOGY

Classification of Pain States

Multiple classifications have been used to describe pain states based on duration, anatomic source, or etiology. *Acute pain* usually results from injury or inflammation, has survival value, and may play a role in the healing process by promoting behaviors that minimize reinjury. In contrast, *chronic pain* is perhaps best construed as a "disease" that serves no useful purpose. Although there is no clear threshold at which acute pain transitions to a chronic state, it is generally accepted that pain persisting beyond the expected healing period is pathologic. In most cases, this period is between 3 and 6 months. The intensity of pain can be classified as mild (1 to 3), moderate (4 to 5), or severe (≥6 on a 0 to 10 numerical rating scale).

Somatic and Visceral Pains

Pain can originate from somatic or visceral structures. *Somatic pain* is well localized and generally results from injury or disease of the skin, musculoskeletal structures, and joints. *Visceral pain* arises from internal organ dysfunction and can result from inflammation, ischemia, occlusion of flow resulting in capsular or organ distension (e.g., renal stones, bowel obstruction, cholecystitis) or from functional pathology (e.g., irritable bowel syndrome). In contrast to somatic pain, visceral pain is usually diffuse and poorly localized, is often referred to somatic regions (e.g., myocardial ischemia radiating into the arm), and tends to be associated with exaggerated autonomic reflexes and greater emotional features.

Neuropathic, Nociceptive, and Mixed Pain

Pain can be etiologically classified as neuropathic, nociceptive, or mixed (Table 29-1). *Neuropathic pain* has been defined as pain resulting from disease or injury to the peripheral or central nervous somatosensory system. Common neuropathic pain states include postherpetic neuralgia, diabetic neuropathy, and radicular pain. *Nociceptive pain* usually results from an injury or disease affecting somatic structures such as skin, muscle, tendons and ligaments, bone, and joints. Pain associated with cancer can result from the tumor itself or can be a consequence of therapy (e.g., surgery, chemotherapy, and radiation therapy). In light of the often multiple different etiologies, advanced cancer pain is a typical example of a mixed pain state.

Dysfunctional Pain

There is a group of pain syndromes that have been characterized by amplification of pain signaling in the absence of either inflammation or injury (as in nociceptive pain) or damage to the nervous system (as in neuropathic pain). These conditions include pain states such as fibromyalgia, irritable bowel syndrome, and interstitial cystitis. The precise pathophysiologic mechanisms of pain in these disorders are unclear, although they share some features of neuropathic pain. Other chronic pain states, such as primary erythromelalgia and paroxysmal extreme pain disorder, are perhaps best described as hereditary channelopathies associated with mutations of the voltage-gated sodium channel Nav1.7. These mutations lead to increased excitability of nociceptive

TABLE 29-1 CLASSIFICATION AND PREVALENCE OF COMMON PAIN CONDITIONS

Neuropathic		*Nociceptive*		
PERIPHERAL	**CENTRAL***	**SOMATIC**	**VISCERAL**	**MIXED**
Peripheral neuropathy (1-3%)	Central post-stroke pain (8%)	Arthritis (25-40% in people >40 years)	Endometriosis (10% in women of reproductive age)	Headache (15% for migraine, 20-30% for tension-type)
Postherpetic neuralgia (annual incidence 0.1-0.2%)	Spinal cord injury (30-50%)	Myofascial pain (5-10%)	Irritable bowel syndrome (5-15%)	Cancer§ (lifetime prevalence 30-40%)
Chronic postsurgical pain (2-10% after surgery)	Multiple sclerosis (25%)	Fibromyalgia† (2-4%)	Interstitial cystitis (0.2-1% of women)	Low back pain‖ (point prevalence 10-30%)
Phantom limb pain (30-60% of patients with major limb amputation)	Parkinson's disease (10%)	Connective tissue disorders (0.2-0.5%)	Ulcers/gastritis/esophagitis (3-9%)	Neck pain‖ (annual incidence 20-30%)
Trigeminal neuralgia (0.01%)	Seizure disorder (1-3%)	Burn pain‡ (annual incidence of burns requiring hospitalization 0.01%)	Cholecystitis/appendicitis	Ischemic pain¶
Radiculopathy/spinal stenosis (3-10%)				
Complex regional pain syndrome (0.03%, 3-20% after orthopedic surgery)				
Nerve entrapment syndromes (e.g., carpal tunnel, thoracic outlet, meralgia paresthetica; 2-4%)				

*Prevalence rates represent proportion of patients with condition who develop pain.
†Some cases may represent a variant of central pain.
‡Third-degree burns often associated with neuropathic pain.
§Neuropathic pain occurs in 20-50% of cases and may occur secondary to tumor invasion, surgery, chemotherapy, and radiation treatment.
‖Neuropathic pain may accompany nociceptive pain in 10-35% of cases.
¶Typically nociceptive, but long-standing pain may result in ischemic neuropathy.

afferent fibers and ongoing activity in sensory neurons, resulting in spontaneous pain.

Pain Mechanisms

Pain results from activation of specialized peripheral receptors (*nociceptors*) by a noxious event (stimulus). These stimuli fall into one of three categories: *mechanical* (e.g., pressure, tumor growth, incision), *thermal* (e.g., hot or cold), or *chemical* (e.g., ischemia or infection). The stimulus is then converted into an electrical nerve signal (*transduction*), which is conveyed along the axons of thinly myelinated (A-delta) or unmyelinated (C) nerve fibers through specific pathways (*transmission*). *Modulation* refers to the attenuation of pain signals through intrinsic inhibitory activity within the peripheral and the central nervous systems before being perceived as an unpleasant sensation (*perception*). *Pathologic pain* is the result of injury- or disease-induced changes in the peripheral or central nervous system leading to alterations in the pain signaling process. One important example of pathologic pain from injury to the nervous system is *peripheral sensitization*. This form of pain is characterized by the development of spontaneous ectopic activity in injured nerves and dorsal root ganglion cells, as well as enhanced sensitivity to mechanical, thermal, or chemical stimuli. Recent studies have shown an important role for cytokines, such as tumor necrosis factor-α (TNF-α) and interleukins, released by macrophages and other inflammatory cells, in the peripheral sensitization process.

The prolonged and repeated activation of nociceptive afferent fibers produces *central sensitization*, a state of increased sensitivity of central pain signaling neurons. Activation of *N*-methyl-D-aspartate (NMDA) receptors by glutamate is thought to be an important mechanism for central sensitization. Recent studies indicate that in addition to functional changes in neurons, microglia and astrocytes may also play an important role in the central sensitization process. Other central neuroplastic changes that may contribute to neuropathic pain states include deafferentation hyperactivity that may occur after spinal cord or avulsion injuries, loss of large fiber afferent inhibition, reorganization of central connections of primary afferent fibers, and excitatory descending modulatory mechanisms. Central and, to a lesser extent, peripheral sensitization are considered to be the prime culprits responsible for pain induced by innocuous stimuli (*allodynia*), and increased pain to normally noxious stimuli (*hyperalgesia*), that are commonly observed in neuropathic pain states.

DIAGNOSIS

History

Similar to the work-up of any symptom, the evaluation of pain begins with a thorough history. One of the primary tenets of pain assessment is that subjective complaints should always be taken seriously. There is currently no diagnostic test that can measure pain or even ascertain its existence. The most promising techniques involve functional brain imaging that reflects cerebral metabolism. Presently, these techniques are research tools that have helped us understand that the brains of chronic pain patients undergo morphologic alterations such as a diminution in gray matter in the areas involved in pain perception. A comprehensive history should include the anatomic region of pain, its quality, exacerbating and relieving factors, temporal aspects, associated symptoms and signs (e.g., numbness or weakness), interference with activities of daily living, and response to current and prior treatments. The temporal aspects of pain can provide valuable clues to etiology and help guide treatment. Most cases of acute pain develop subsequent to a specific inciting event (e.g., surgery, trauma), whereas chronic pain conditions are usually more insidious in onset. Because acute pain tends to be self-limited and the relationship to a precipitant event is more tangible, it may be better tolerated and associated with fewer psychological sequelae.

The severity of pain can be measured through a variety of different rating scales. Some of the more common instruments include categorical scales, verbal and numerical rating scales (0 to 10), and the visual analogue scale, in which a 10-cm line is anchored on each side by two points designated as "no pain" and "worst possible pain." Because there are subtle differences between different types of scales, repeat assessments and response to therapy are ideally gauged using the same instrument. For young children and mentally incapacitated patients, the use of age-appropriate substitute scales or facial expressions has been validated.

Recent guidelines from experts across multiple specialties and sectors have concluded that pain scores represent only one component of pain management. Other important aspects of treatment include assessments of functional capacity (e.g., Oswestry disability index for back pain), psychological and emotional functioning (e.g., SF-36), satisfaction ratings, adverse treatment effects, and disposition (i.e., work status). It is therefore imperative that realistic goals are established, and individually tailored treatment regimens are developed to achieve these ends.

TABLE 29-2 CATEGORIZATION OF NEUROPATHIC AND NOCICEPTIVE PAIN

CLINICAL CHARACTERISTIC	NEUROPATHIC PAIN	NOCICEPTIVE PAIN
Etiology	Nerve injury or peripheral/central sensitization	Tissue or potential tissue damage
Descriptors	Lancinating, shooting, electrical-like, stabbing	Throbbing, aching, pressure-like
Sensory deficits	Frequent (e.g., numbness, tingling, pricking)	Infrequent and, if present, in nondermatomal or non-nerve distribution
Motor deficits	Neurologic weakness may be present if motor nerve affected	May have pain-induced weakness
Hypersensitivity	Pain frequently evoked with nonpainful (allodynia) or painful (exaggerated response) stimuli	Uncommon except for hypersensitivity in the immediate area of an acute injury
Character	Distal radiation common	Distal radiation less common; proximal radiation frequent
Paroxysms	Exacerbations common and unpredictable	Exacerbations less common and associated with activity
Autonomic signs	Color changes, temperature changes, swelling, and/or sudomotor (sweating) activity occur in one third to one half of patients	Autonomic signs uncommon in chronic nociceptive pain

Distinguishing between neuropathic and nociceptive pain can have important treatment implications (Table 29-2). Neuropathic pain is characterized by positive and negative symptoms. Negative symptoms, such as a loss of sensation, are usually the result of axon and neuron loss, whereas the positive symptoms reflect abnormal excitability of the nervous system. Numbness, tingling, and other symptoms suggestive of sensory dysfunction are strongly indicative of neuropathic pain, especially when they occur in a dermatomal or solitary nerve distribution. Descriptors such as "burning," "shooting," and "electrical" are more apt to be associated with neuropathic pain, whereas adjectives such as "squeezing," "throbbing," and "aching" tend to be strongly identified with nociceptive pain states such as acute inflammatory pain or arthralgias. Other positive symptoms observed in neuropathic pain states include pain evoked by normally innocuous stimuli (allodynia) and an exaggerated or prolonged pain to noxious stimuli (hyperalgesia or hyperpathia). Although neuropathic pain tends to be more intermittent than nociceptive pain, mechanical spinal pain is classically exacerbated by movement. As alluded to earlier, some conditions such as cancer may be characterized by aspects of both nociceptive and neuropathic pain.

The proper evaluation of the patient in pain includes a psychosocial history. Between one half and two thirds of chronic pain patients exhibit varying degrees of major psychopathology, with depression being the most common comorbidity, followed by anxiety disorders, somatoform disorders, and substance abuse. Many of these coexisting psychological conditions have been associated with poor treatment prognosis. People seeking chronic pain care may also be more likely to carry a concomitant axis II diagnosis (i.e., personality disorder). Patients with axis II diagnoses are more likely to be designated as "difficult patients," which can act as an additional barrier to effective treatment. Potential social factors that can negatively affect treatment should be identified, including low job satisfaction, secondary gain, and ongoing litigation. A focused psychosocial history that includes prior psychiatric diagnoses, suicidal ideation, work history, legal history, and substance abuse, is therefore essential in the formulation of a treatment plan.

Physical Examination

Examination of the patient in pain should encompass all bodily systems because pain is a frequent manifestation of systemic disease. A physical examination finding by itself is almost never pathognomonic but usually functions to confirm suspicions garnered from the history and to select patients for imaging studies or invasive diagnostic testing. Unlike acute pain, *chronic pain is usually not associated with increased vital signs or facial grimacing.* Thorough neurologic and musculoskeletal examinations are particularly useful in evaluating pain. Sensory symptoms can precede other neurologic findings by months or weeks. The most common forms of neuropathy are associated with sensory deficits in a glove-stocking distribution, but other patterns occur as well (Chapter 428). Numbness in the distribution of a nerve root or single nerve strongly suggests neuropathic pain, but nondermatomal sensory changes can accompany nociceptive pain (e.g., fibromyalgia or arthritis) as well. Allodynia and hyperalgesia are hallmarks of neuropathic pain. Postural and gait abnormalities may be either causative factors for rheumatologic conditions (e.g., bursitis) or consequences of the underlying condition.

A careful evaluation of passive and active range of motion is useful because generalized and regional pain complaints are often accompanied by decreases in range of motion. Distinctions should be drawn between pain-induced and neurologic weakness, with the latter often occurring in conjunction with muscle atrophy or asymmetry in reflexes. Sometimes, reflex assessment is the only way to distinguish between a true neurologic condition and nonorganic etiologies; hence, deep tendon reflexes are a useful component of the pain exam.

Diagnostic Tests

Imaging has largely supplanted history and physical examination as the gold standard for diagnosing pathology, but is not without drawbacks. There is a poor correlation between findings on magnetic resonance imaging (MRI) and the intensity of spinal pain, with greater than 50% of asymptomatic individuals having abnormalities on lumbar, thoracic, and cervical films. Previous studies found that neither radiographs nor MRI studies affect treatment outcomes and are unlikely to affect decision making[1]; in fact, redundant imaging can lead to unnecessary procedures. Absolute indications for MRI in patients with back pain are (1) serious or progressive neurologic deficits, (2) new-onset bowel and bladder dysfunction, (3) suspected metastatic disease, or (4) when referring patients for procedural interventions. The presence of "red flags" suggestive of more serious pathology (e.g., extremes of age, trauma history, immunosuppressed state, persistent fever, infection, or history of intravenous drug abuse) should also alert the practitioner to seek further evaluation. Electromyography and nerve conduction studies (Chapter 428) can be used to diagnose injury to large nerve fibers. However, because these studies are associated with significant false-negative and false-positive rates and are not sensitive in detecting impairment of small fiber (nociceptive afferent fibers) function, a normal neurophysiologic study does not rule out neuropathic pain. For small fiber neuropathies, a skin biopsy demonstrating decreased density of epidermal nerve fibers is a sensitive test.

For nonspinal pain conditions, MRI is ideal for detecting inflammation and soft tissue pathology, whereas computed tomography (CT) scanning is indicated for disease processes associated with bone destruction or ossification. The main advantages of ultrasound are that it is safe, is inexpensive, does not utilize ionizing radiation, and is relatively cheap.

TREATMENT Rx

The goals of treatment should include elucidating the cause of pain and alleviating suffering. Consequently, the goal of pain treatment should not be limited to pain reduction but should encompass improving functional status, mood, and social interactions (i.e., quality of life). Chronic pain may result from diverse etiologies, including physical trauma, disease, infection, and therapies such as radiation, chemotherapy, and surgery. It has been argued that treatment should be mechanism based rather than etiology based, but at the present time, simple clinical tools to correlate symptoms and signs with mechanisms are lacking. Hence, treatment is primarily etiology based, or symptomatic. The future development and validation of diagnostic methods to identify mechanisms (e.g., intravenous infusion tests) may help develop novel target-specific pharmacologic agents.

Pain is a complex perceptual experience affected by a multitude of factors that include not only activation of nociceptors but also emotions (e.g., fear, anxiety), memory and cognition, social and cultural context, and expectations. Thus, it is not surprising that despite a paucity of studies evaluating a multidisciplinary approach to pain management, a strong consensus exists that this approach is beneficial.

Pharmacologic Therapies

Antipyretic Analgesics

Today, aspirin (Chapter 36) is the most widely used analgesic in the world. Along with its pharmacologic cousins, nonsteroidal anti-inflammatory drugs (NSAIDs) and the antipyretic drugs acetaminophen and phenacetin, this group forms the backbone of pharmacologic pain treatment. Antipyretic analgesics exert their antinociceptive effects by the inhibition of cyclooxygenase, the rate-limiting enzyme in the production of prostaglandins, which are lipid-based compounds that sensitize nociceptors and regulate inflammation. There are several pharmacologic distinctions between NSAIDs and their counterparts, phenazone and acetaminophen. Whereas NSAIDs act both centrally and peripherally, making them effective topical agents for nociceptive inflammatory conditions, the primary site of enzyme inhibition for acetaminophen is in the central nervous system. Acetaminophen is also a weaker analgesic than NSAIDs and is largely devoid of anti-inflammatory effects.

The main drawback of nonopioid antipyretic analgesics is their ceiling effect, which can render them ineffective as stand-alone agents for severe pain. For cancer pain, the World Health Organization treatment paradigm advocates adding opioids to an analgesic regimen uncontrolled by NSAIDs, not replacing them. NSAIDs may act synergistically with opioids and have proven opioid-sparing effects. It is well acknowledged that aspirin, NSAIDs, and acetaminophen are more effective in treating nociceptive than neuropathic pain, although a significant proportion of neuropathic pain sufferers regularly take NSAIDs.

The second major concern about nonopioid antipyretic agents is side effects. For NSAIDs, these include bleeding, gastrointestinal ulceration, renal toxicity, and an increased risk of cardiovascular events. Although the use of cyclooxygenase-2 selective inhibitors like celecoxib and rofecoxib may attenuate the risk of bleeding and ulcers, the risk of renal failure and cardiovascular events from these drugs remains a significant cause of morbidity and mortality. These risks are significantly increased in elderly patients and with polypharmacy. In view of its more favorable safety profile, acetaminophen is often considered a first-line therapy ahead of NSAIDs, even for pain conditions associated with inflammation.

Adjuvant Analgesics

Multiple evidence-based guidelines for the treatment of chronic pain states, particularly neuropathic pain, have been recently published. In general, these suggest that antidepressants and anticonvulsants should be the two first-line classes of medications for chronic neuropathic pain. Depending on the particular drug and condition, these medications have been demonstrated to provide significant pain relief above and beyond that observed with placebo in 20 to 40% of ideal pharmacologic candidates (i.e., number needed to treat is between 2.5 and 5 in randomized trials). Whereas opioids have shown similar efficacy for neuropathic pain, anticonvulsants and antidepressants carry a lower risk of serious adverse events (e.g., addiction) and long-term tolerance, rendering them preferable to opioids for long-standing noncancer pain (Table 29-3). In terms of efficacy, tricyclic antidepressants (TCAs) are superior to serotonin-norepinephrine reuptake inhibitors, which in turn are more effective than serotonin-specific reuptake inhibitors. Among the various TCAs, amitriptyline is the most studied but is probably comparable in efficacy to its metabolite nortriptyline and its cousin imipramine. However, the latter two drugs' more favorable side effect profiles (e.g., less sedation and anticholinergic activity) make them the preferred choices for neuropathic pain. In patients who cannot tolerate TCAs, serotonin-norepinephrine reuptake inhibitors such as duloxetine can be beneficial. In addition to neuropathic pain, antidepressants have also been shown to be effective in headache prophylaxis, chest pain, abdominal and pelvic pain, fibromyalgia, arthritis, and spinal pain.

Anticonvulsants are probably effective for neuropathic pain by virtue of their membrane-stabilizing-properties. Although anticonvulsant drugs may be slightly more effective than antidepressants for prototypical "lancinating-type" neuropathic pain, antidepressants may be more versatile in that they have proven benefit in myriad other pain conditions. Owing to their high efficacy and favorable side-effect profiles, gabapentin and its pharmacologic relative pregabalin are first-line agents for most forms of neuropathic pain. In addition to independent pain-relieving properties, these drugs may act synergistically with opioids, provide anxiolysis, and exhibit preemptive analgesic effects when administered before surgery.

When gabapentinoid drugs are ineffective or intolerable, alternative anticonvulsants that act through different cellular mechanisms such as lamotrigine and oxcarbazepine may be employed. For trigeminal neuralgia, carbamazepine remains the treatment of choice, although adverse effects, such as the risk of agranulocytosis, limit its utility for other conditions. Other classes of adjuvants that may be effective in certain contexts include topical creams (e.g., NSAIDs, capsaicin, lidocaine), *N*-methyl-D-aspartate antagonists (e.g., dextromethorphan), skeletal muscle relaxants (e.g., baclofen, cyclobenzaprine), cannabinoids, and antiarrhythmics (mexiletine). Topical lidocaine patches have been shown to reduce the pain and allodynia in patients with postherpetic neuralgia, and anecdotal evidence has suggested lidocaine may be useful in the treatment of certain types of back pain. Recently, a

TABLE 29-3 ADJUVANT ANALGESIC DRUGS FOR CHRONIC PAIN

DRUG	DOSAGE	INDICATIONS	ADVERSE EFFECTS	COMMENTS
TRICYCLIC ANTIDEPRESSANTS				
Amitriptyline, imipramine, desipramine, nortriptyline	10-150 mg/day	Peripheral neuropathy, postherpetic neuralgia, other types of peripheral neuropathic pain, central pain, facial pain, fibromyalgia, headache prophylaxis, irritable bowel syndrome, and chronic low back pain with or without radiculopathy	Sedation, dry mouth, confusion, weight gain, constipation, urinary retention, ataxia, cardiac conduction delay (QTc prolongation)	First-line agents for neuropathic pain and headache prophylaxis Secondary amine drugs (e.g., nortriptyline) have fewer side effects than tertiary amines (e.g., amitriptyline) Contraindicated in glaucoma
SEROTONIN-NOREPINEPHRINE REUPTAKE INHIBITORS				
Venlafaxine	75-225 mg/day	Peripheral neuropathy, headache prophylaxis	Sedation, dry mouth, constipation, ataxia, hypertension, hyperhidrosis	Dose adjustment in patients with renal dysfunction
Duloxetine	60-120 mg/day	Peripheral neuropathy, fibromyalgia, chronic back pain	Sedation, dry mouth, constipation, hyperhidrosis	U.S. Food and Drug Administration (FDA) approved for fibromyalgia and diabetic neuropathy Contraindicated in glaucoma
ANTICONVULSANTS				
Gabapentin	600-3600 mg/day	Peripheral neuropathy, postherpetic neuralgia, other types of peripheral neuropathic pain, central pain, pelvic pain, headache prophylaxis, radiculopathy, chronic postsurgical pain	Sedation, weight gain, dry mouth, ataxia, edema	First-line agent for neuropathic pain FDA approved for postherpetic neuralgia Effective preemptively for postoperative pain
Pregabalin	150-600 mg/day	Peripheral neuropathy, postherpetic neuralgia, central pain, fibromyalgia	Sedation, weight gain, dry mouth, ataxia, edema	First-line agent for neuropathic pain FDA approved for diabetic neuropathy, postherpetic neuralgia, fibromyalgia Effective preemptively for postoperative pain Same mechanism of action as gabapentin
Carbamazepine	200-1600 mg/day	Facial neuralgias, diabetic neuropathy	Sedation, ataxia, diplopia, hyponatremia, agranulocytosis, diarrhea, aplastic anemia, hepatotoxicity, Stevens-Johnson syndrome	First-line agent and FDA approved for trigeminal and glossopharyngeal neuralgia Contraindicated in patients with porphyria and atrioventricular conduction block
Topiramate	50-400 mg/day	Headache prophylaxis, chronic low back pain with or without radiculopathy	Sedation, ataxia, diplopia, weight loss, diarrhea, metabolic acidosis, kidney stones	First-line agent and FDA approved for migraine prophylaxis Often used as appetite suppressant
CORTICOSTEROIDS (SYSTEMIC)				
Prednisone	5-60 mg/day	Inflammatory arthritis, other inflammatory pain conditions (e.g., inflammatory bowel disease), traumatic nerve injury, complex regional pain syndrome	Myriad psychiatric, gastrointestinal, neurologic, and cardiac side effects; immunosuppression, weakness, edema, weight gain, elevated glucose, poor wound healing, others	Stronger evidence supports local (i.e., injection) administration More effective for acute pain Strong anti-inflammatory effects
MISCELLANEOUS				
Muscle relaxants	Variable depending on drug	Skeletal muscle spasm, acute spinal pain, temporomandibular disorder Baclofen effective for spasticity, dystonia, and trigeminal neuralgia	Sedation, ataxia, blurred vision, confusion, asthenia, xerostomia and other gastrointestinal effects, palpitations	First-line agents for acute back pain and skeletal muscle spasm
Lidocaine patch	1-3 patches every 12 hr	Postherpetic neuropathy, peripheral neuropathy, other types of neuropathic and possibly myofascial pain associated with allodynia	Minimal systemic side effects when applied appropriately	Second-line agent and FDA approved for postherpetic neuralgia
Capsaicin cream	0.025% applied 3 or 4 times per day	Postherpetic neuralgia, peripheral neuropathy and other types of neuropathic pain, chronic postsurgical pain, arthritis and other musculoskeletal conditions	Burning on application Minimal systemic side effects when applied appropriately	FDA approved for arthritis Second-line agent for postherpetic neuralgia and third-line agent for peripheral neuropathy Single application 8% patch providing up to 3 months of pain relief was recently approved for postherpetic neuralgia
Cannabinoids	Variable depending on drug and delivery route	Strongest evidence is for multiple sclerosis May be effective for peripheral neuropathy and other types of neuropathic pain spasticity	Myriad psychiatric, neurologic, and cardiac effects; xerostomia, abdominal pain, and other gastrointestinal effects	Fourth-line agent with narrow therapeutic index Modest analgesic effect comparable to codeine

high-concentration (8%) topical patch of capsaicin (the pungent chemical in chili pepper) has been approved for the treatment of postherpetic neuralgia. A single 1-hour application of the capsaicin patch can result in attenuation of pain for up to 12 weeks. Topical NSAIDs (e.g., diclofenac) have been shown to be effective in the short term for the treatment of osteoarthritis and other rheumatologic disorders and have been touted as having fewer adverse effects than systemic NSAIDs.

Opioid Analgesics

Opioid analgesics, such as morphine, oxycodone, hydromorphone, and methadone, are the cornerstone of treatment for cancer pain (Table 29-4). Several randomized studies have also demonstrated their usefulness in noncancer pain conditions such as chronic osteoarthritis and neuropathic pain states.2 Maximizing the therapeutic effects of opioid analgesics requires careful attention to balancing the beneficial effects with the undesirable adverse effects. Understanding the clinical pharmacology of opioids, including their relative potency, duration of action, oral bioavailability, and pharmacokinetics, is essential for rational use (see Table 29-4). Their use for chronic pain management is limited primarily by their myriad side effects that include nausea, vomiting, constipation, sedation, itch, respiratory depression, and endocrine deficiency leading to sexual dysfunction and accelerated osteoporosis. Attentive treatment to opioid-induced side effects can facilitate dose titration, maximize analgesia, and minimize adverse effects. Aggressive management with stool softeners and agents that enhance bowel motility such as docusate, lactulose, and senna, can minimize constipation. Whereas most opioids are devoid of end-organ toxicity, an exception is meperidine. A metabolite, normeperidine, can accumulate after several days of treatment, causing myoclonus and anxiety; at higher concentrations, confusion, delirium, and seizures can ensue. Opioids that are predominantly renally eliminated, such as morphine, should be used with caution in patients with renal dysfunction. Two metabolites of morphine, morphine-6-glucuronide, which contains analgesic properties, and morphine-3-glucuronide, which may amplify pain in certain contexts, can accumulate in patients with renal dysfunction and are largely responsible for the adverse effects of morphine. Alternate drugs in such patients are fentanyl and methadone.

For treatment of acute pain (e.g., postoperative pain) or an acute exacerbation of chronic pain in hospitalized patients (e.g., sickle cell crisis), patient-controlled analgesia (PCA) provides a convenient means of administering opioids. Intravenous morphine, fentanyl, or hydromorphone is commonly administered using an infusion device designed to prevent overdose. With or without a basal infusion (which can be used to replace a sustained-release opioid in a patient who is NPO), the bolus dose, lockout time interval between doses, and the maximal dose per hour can be programmed in and adjusted based on clinical circumstances. PCA devices are safe and allow patients to control their pain management with less dependence on health care providers. Studies comparing PCA with conventional administration of opioids have generally found PCAs to be associated with better pain relief and higher satisfaction rates, albeit with larger amounts of medication consumed.

The long-term use of opioids can be associated with tolerance and physical dependence. Cross-tolerance among opioids is not complete, and a strategy that is often used when tolerance to an opioid is suspected is rotation to an alternate opioid drug. Although addiction (Chapter 33) to opioids when used

TABLE 29-4 FORMULATIONS, DOSAGES, AND PHARMACOLOGIC INFORMATION ON COMMONLY PRESCRIBED OPIOIDS

DRUG	EQUIANALGESIC DOSAGE (ORAL UNLESS SPECIFIED)	READILY AVAILABLE ROUTES OF ADMINISTRATION	DURATION OF ACTION	COMMENTS
Morphine	30 mg	IV, IM, PO, PR; SR formulation	3-6 hr for short-acting, 8-12 hr for SR	Reference standard for all opioids Renally excreted active metabolite
Oxycodone	20 mg	PO, PR; SR formulation	3-6 hr for short-acting, 8-12 hr for SR	Widely available in combination form with nonopioid analgesics; SR form popular among recreational users
Hydromorphone	3-6 mg	PO, PR, IV, IM	3-6 hr	Higher PO/IV conversion ratio than other opioids
Hydrocodone	30-60 mg	PO	3-6 hr	Wide variation in morphine equivalent dose Most commonly prescribed opioid in U.S. Typically used in combination form with nonopioid analgesic Formulations containing <15 mg hydrocodone are schedule III in U.S.
Methadone	2-20 mg	PO, PR, IV	6-12 hr for pain	Morphine: methadone conversion varies according to dose and length of opioid use, ranging from 2 : 1 to >20 : 1 in patients on very high doses Any physician with a schedule II DEA license may prescribe for pain May take 5-7 days to reach steady state due to extended half-life (i.e., accumulation) Electrocardiogram monitoring recommended with higher doses Other properties such as NMDA receptor antagonism and reuptake inhibition of serotonin and norepinephrine may slow the development of tolerance and increase efficacy for neuropathic pain
Fentanyl	12.5 μg/hr (TD) 800-1000 μg (TM) 200-400 μg (B)	TD, TM, B	72 hr for TD; 1 hr-2 hr for TM and B	TD, TM, and B formulations may be useful in patients with poor bowel function TD: wide variation in conversion ratios Delivery system may be associated with fewer gastrointestinal side effects TM and B: delivery systems associated with more rapid (10-min) onset than immediate-release oral opioids. U.S. Food and Drug Administration (FDA) approved for breakthrough cancer pain in opioid-tolerant patients
Codeine	200 mg	PO, PR	3-6 hr	Often used in combination with nonopioid analgesics Efficacy and side effects may be affected by rate of metabolism to morphine Popular as cough suppressant
Propoxyphene	200 mg	PO, PR	3-6 hr	Wide variation in morphine equivalent dose Often used in combination form with nonopioid analgesic Toxic metabolite may accumulate with excessive use, especially in elderly patients Weak antagonist at NMDA receptor
Meperidine	300 mg	PO, PR, IV	2-4 hr	Toxic metabolite may accumulate with excessive use, especially in patients with renal insufficiency Associated with tachycardia and hypertension May cause more "euphoria" than other opioids
Buprenorphine	0.4 mg SL	SL, PR, IV, TD	6-8 hr	Partial opioid agonist that may precipitate withdrawal in opioid-dependent patients Lower abuse potential, and fewer psychomimetic effects, than pure agonists Not readily reversed by naloxone Schedule III drug in U.S. Primary use of SL preparation is to treat addiction

B = buccal; IV = intravenous; NMDA = *N*-methyl-D-aspartate; PO = oral; PR = rectal; SL = sublingual; SR = sustained release; TD = transdermal; TM = transmucosal.

for the treatment of chronic pain is reported to be relatively uncommon, guidelines for responsible prescribing of opioids have been published as a monograph by the Federation of State Medical Boards. The critical suggested steps in the management of chronic pain patients with opioids include appropriate patient evaluation, creating and maintaining clear and detailed documentation, creating a function-based treatment plan with well-defined patient goals that include an exit strategy, obtaining a written patient-physician agreement that includes informed consent and patient education, periodic review that focuses on progress toward functional goals, and making specialist referrals when managing difficult patients. Diversion of opioids and the increasing abuse of prescription opioids, particularly in teenagers and young adults, is another growing societal concern (Chapter 33).

Tramadol and tapentadol comprise part of a new class of analgesic drugs that have a dual mechanism of action. Tramadol is a weak agonist and inhibits the reuptake of norepinephrine and serotonin. Along with the usual side effects associated with opioids, seizures have been reported with tramadol, and adverse drug interactions can occur in patients taking warfarin sodium (Coumadin) and selective serotonin reuptake inhibitors (SSRIs). Tapentadol also has a dual mode of action as a μ–opioid agonist and a norepinephrine reuptake inhibitor. Nausea, dizziness, constipation, and sedation are reported side effects of this drug. Tramadol is presently approved for moderate to moderately severe pain, whereas tapentadol, which is currently a schedule II drug in the United States, is approved for moderate to severe acute pain.

Butorphanol, nalbuphine, and pentazocine are opioid agonist-antagonist drugs that can antagonize the actions of μ–opioid agonists and can cause psychotomimetic effects owing to their actions on the κ-opioid receptor. These drugs should be used with caution, particularly in patients receiving other μ–opioid agonists. Buprenorphine, a partial agonist at the μ–opioid receptor and an antagonist at other opioid receptors, is available as a sublingual pill that is approved for the treatment of opioid addiction. A transdermal formulation is approved in Europe for the treatment of chronic pain.

Combination Therapies

Most clinical trials have studied the effects of individual drugs in specific chronic pain states. However, no one drug is universally effective, and often the drug only provides partial pain relief. In clinical practice, two or more drugs are often used in combination to achieve an additive beneficial effect or to decrease the adverse effects associated with the use of a single drug. The rational use of polypharmacy should include drugs that act at different sites in the pain signaling process or modulate different neurotransmitter systems, or both (Fig. 29-1). Although results are conflicting, a preponderance of recent randomized trials suggest that combination therapy with opioids and either anticonvulsants or antidepressants may be more effective than using either drug class as a stand-alone treatment.[3] Similarly, combining two adjuvant medication classes (e.g., gabapentin and nortriptyline) was recently shown to be more efficacious than giving either drug alone for neuropathic pain,[4] and combination treatment with pregabalin and celecoxib was found to be superior to monotherapy in a mixed population of patients with chronic low back pain.[5] Additional studies are needed to help develop guidelines for rational polypharmacy based on pain pathophysiology, mechanisms of action, and genetic medicine.

Psychological Treatment

The relationship between pain and psychopathology is complex. The lifetime prevalence rate of coexisting psychiatric illness in chronic pain patients ranges from 50% to upward of 80%. Between 30% and 60% of chronic pain sufferers experience symptoms of depression, making it the most common comorbidity. For anxiety disorders and substance abuse, the coprevalence rates are about 30% and 10 to 15%, respectively.

Viewed from a different perspective, the relationship is even more striking. More than 60% of patients with major depression and more than half of all patients with anxiety and substance abuse disorders experience moderate to severe chronic pain. Although it is widely acknowledged that disease states and injuries that result in chronic pain can predispose patients to depression, anxiety, and even self-destructive behavior, what is less commonly appreciated is the effect preexisting psychiatric conditions have on pain perception. There is a plethora of literature demonstrating that coexisting psychopathology is a strong predictor for the development of chronic pain after an acute, traumatic event (e.g., back pain episode, surgery, motor vehicle crash).

It is necessary to screen all pain patients for psychological conditions that can adversely affect treatment (Table 29-5). Not only major psychiatric conditions such as depression and generalized anxiety but also maladaptive behaviors and secondary diagnoses such as somatization disorder and poor coping skills can negatively influence treatment. Psychological screening is mandated for pain patients being considered for neuromodulation (e.g., spinal cord stimulation), and many spine surgeons will defer surgery until major psychiatric issues are adequately addressed.

Relaxation techniques such as biofeedback, self-hypnosis, and guided imagery have proved effective in a wide array of acute and chronic pain conditions but may be especially useful in those with high levels of anxiety. Cognitive behavioral therapy is a highly structured form of psychotherapy predicated on the replacement of negative thought patterns and behaviors with more positive, constructive ones. These therapies may enhance the modulation of afferent pain signals. Ideal candidates include educated, motivated patients in whom distorted thinking (e.g., "catastrophization") and counterproductive behaviors serve to amplify pain behavior. In patients with personality disorders and ingrained maladaptive behaviors, long-term psychotherapy may be necessary.

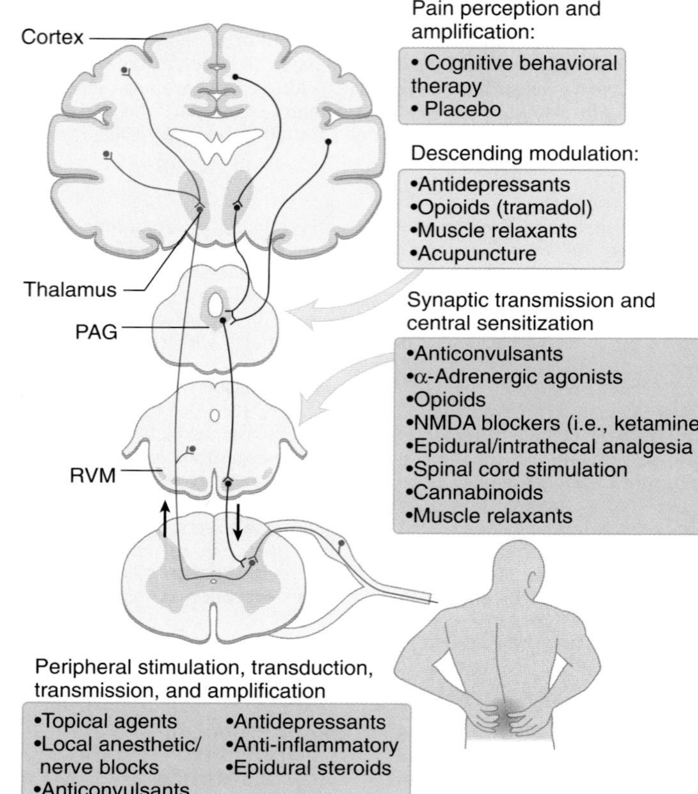

FIGURE 29-1. Rational choice of combination therapies for pain should be based on the mechanisms of drug actions. Combining drugs with disparate actions can have additive or synergistic analgesic effects and minimize adverse effects. NMDA = *N*-methyl-D-aspartate; PAG = periaqueductal gray; RVM = rostral ventromedial medulla.

TABLE 29-5 PSYCHOSOCIAL FACTORS ASSOCIATED WITH CHRONIC PAIN

Multiple pain complaints
Poor job satisfaction/low pay
Inadequate coping skills
Fear-avoidance behavior
Manual labor/physically stressful job
Obesity
Somatization
Smoking
Low baseline activity levels
Ongoing litigation
Low education level
Greater baseline disability
Anxiety
Depressed mood
Emotional distress

Interventional Therapies: Nerve Blocks, Neuromodulation, and Neurosurgery

Nerve Blocks

Nerve blocks and injections may be done for therapeutic, diagnostic, and sometimes prognostic purposes (i.e., to select candidates for surgery or radio frequency denervation). Mechanistically, injections performed with local anesthetic may work by releasing entrapped nerves, enhancing blood flow, and interrupting processes involved in central sensitization (i.e., "breaking the cycle of pain"). Additional benefits of adding corticosteroid to local anesthetic include blocking the inflammatory cascade, suppressing ectopic discharges from injured nerves, and inhibiting the synthesis of prostaglandins, some of which serve to sensitize nociceptors.

Nerve blocks are almost never a panacea for noncancer pain, but in appropriate candidates, blocks may provide intermediate-term pain relief, facilitate rehabilitative therapy, and improve quality of life for several weeks to months. Translating this relief into long-term improvement inevitably necessitates addressing the underlying etiologies and predisposing factors, which often entails physical therapy, psychotherapy, and rehabilitation. Injections that can afford benefit in well-selected individuals include trigger point injections with local anesthetic for myofascial pain and nerve blocks with corticosteroid for entrapment syndromes (e.g., carpal tunnel syndrome, occipital neuralgia). Among spinal injections, the strongest evidence is for epidural steroid injections in patients with radicular pain of less than 6 months' duration. Neurolytic procedures, such as celiac plexus neurolysis with alcohol or phenol, have been shown to provide significant pain relief lasting several months in patients with pain associated with cancer of the pancreas, liver, and gastrointestinal tract.

Spinal Cord Stimulation

Spinal cord stimulation is an effective, minimally invasive neuromodulatory technique for managing a variety of chronic pain states refractory to more conservative measures. It was developed based on the gate-control theory, which postulates that activation of peripheral sensory A-fibers can attenuate pain signaling by slower-conducting pain C-fibers. Common indications include failed back surgery syndrome, complex regional pain syndromes, and outside of the United States, ischemic pain.

Surgery

Surgical interventions are often advocated in chronic pain patients who have failed more conservative measures, but surgery is fraught with the same limitations as nerve blocks. A traumatic neuroma is an inexorable consequence of cutting or burning a nerve, formed as a result of unregulated and disorganized nerve regeneration. Neuromas have been shown to fire ectopic pain signals and are often quite painful. Hence, neurolytic procedures are rarely successful in the long-term treatment of neuropathic pain. Part of the challenge in deciding when operative therapy is indicated revolves around the difficulty involved in establishing a causative relationship between the targeted pathology and pain. Roughly 10% of women of reproductive age have endometriosis, but many patients with endometriosis have minimal symptoms, and pelvic pain is a frequent occurrence in young females with no detectable pathology. With respect to inguinal hernia repair and spinal decompression, the incidence of chronic postsurgical pain is inversely correlated with the size of the bowel and disc herniation, respectively. This illustrates that in many of these individuals, the targeted pathology may not have been the primary cause of symptoms. On a similar note, scar tissue is a predictable sequela of surgical treatment, but lysis of adhesions is only infrequently associated with long-term symptom palliation because of the high recurrence rate and absence of any means to correlate the presence of adhesions with pain. Not surprisingly, surgery done solely to remove a painful body part (e.g., hysterectomy, orchiectomy) rarely results in long-term benefit.

Back Pain

Back pain is the leading cause of disability in people younger than 45 years in the industrialized world and thus deserves separate mention when discussing interventional therapies. In patients who present with serious spinal pathology (primarily infection, tumor, and trauma), decompression, stabilization, and fusion can be highly beneficial, but outcomes are strongly dependent on the primary pathology and patient. Decompression procedures done for spinal stenosis or radiculopathy are also effective for short-term relief, but the benefits diminish with time.[6,7] With respect to fusion or disc replacement done for axial pain associated with common degenerative changes, less than 40% of patients can expect a highly functional outcome.

Physical Treatments

The use of "physical" therapies to provide pain relief and enhance function forms a cornerstone in the multimodal approach to the patient with pain. Physical therapists evaluate, educate, and provide minimally invasive and noninvasive procedural interventions to patients to help prevent and alleviate the pain and dysfunction associated with physical and mental maladies. These interventions include both addressing causative mechanisms of pain (e.g., core strengthening, correcting gait and postural abnormalities) and providing treatments (e.g., ultrasound, hot and cold packs, joint manipulation).

Exercise has been used for decades as a treatment for chronic pain and as a means to prevent injury. Exercise may work through a variety of mechanisms, including enhancing blood flow, releasing endorphins, exerting anti-inflammatory effects, activating descending inhibitory pathways, and improving sleep and mood. Whereas the largest body of research has been conducted in patients with spinal pain, benefits have also been demonstrated in those with fibromyalgia, headaches, arthritis, neuropathic pain, and cancer.

Complementary and Alternative Therapies

Physicians are referring patients for complementary and alternative medical (CAM) treatments with increasing frequency, with utilization rates exceeding one third for certain conditions. CAM therapies have been used to treat myriad pain conditions, including cancer and noncancer pain and both neuropathic and nociceptive conditions (Chapter 38). Some of the most popular and studied CAM modalities are acupuncture, chiropractic, yoga, and dietary supplements, all of which have been shown in clinical trials to reduce pain and improve functional capacity in certain contexts. However, the effect size tends to be modest for these treatments, and there is little evidence to support the superiority of any one "proven" modality over another.

Pain Management in Older Persons

Older adults often have varied and multiple pain conditions that exist with other comorbidities. Pharmacologic management of pain in this population can be challenging because of the potential for drug-drug and drug-disease interactions. The potential for drug-related adverse effects is the basis for the popular recommendation of "start low and go slow" in the titration of analgesic drugs. The potential interaction between anticoagulants, such as warfarin and aspirin, and NSAIDs can result in an increased risk for bleeding. Age-related decrease in hepatic blood flow and decreased first-pass effect can result in higher bioavailability of opioids, such as morphine. Significant interactions between analgesic drugs metabolized hepatically by CYP2D6, such as codeine, hydrocodone, oxycodone, tramadol, and antidepressants, may result in decreased metabolism and increased toxicity. Several drugs used for the management of chronic pain and their active metabolites, such as duloxetine, gabapentin, pregabalin, oxycodone, and tramadol, are primarily renally eliminated. Their dose should be adjusted accordingly. An updated guideline for the pharmacologic management of persistent pain in older persons based on a synthesis of the best available evidence has been recently published.

FUTURE DRUGS AND PREVENTION OF PAIN

Much research is being done to develop new routes of drug administration, abuse-deterrent opioids, and novel nonopioid drug treatments, which can optimize outcomes and reduce risks and side effects for pharmacotherapy. Two other areas ripe for investigation are the development of drugs that exploit the unique genetic makeup of pain patients, and refining selection criteria for various therapies. The conceptual appeal of these and other endeavors is that treatment tailored to individuals is likely to result in greater benefit and less risk than the "shotgun" approach to pain treatment that is too often used.

Regenerative therapies, which seek to facilitate the body's ability to repair, replace, restore and regenerate diseased or damaged tissue, is another frontier in pain medicine. These treatments are currently in preliminary stages of development but may someday be used to treat central, joint, and spinal pain.

Finally, identifying patients at high risk of developing pain and employing strategies to either prevent pain or minimize the disease burden represent other areas that have been henceforth underinvestigated. In patients at high risk for chronic postsurgical pain (e.g., young patients with preexisting pain and psychological comorbidities), these measures might include the use of preemptive analgesics, such as NSAIDs and anticonvulsants, and employment of surgical techniques associated with less trauma. For patients with musculoskeletal complaints, this might entail educational initiatives, extensive rehabilitation, fall-reduction classes, and increased reimbursement for walking aids and wheelchairs.

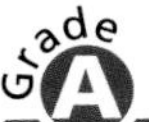

1. Modic MT, Obuchowski NA, Ross JS, et al. Acute low back pain and radiculopathy: MR imaging findings and their prognostic role and effect on outcome. *Radiology*. 2005;237:597-604.
2. Noble M, Treadwell JR, Tregear SJ, et al. Long-term opioid management for chronic noncancer pain. *Cochrane Database Syst Rev*. 2010;1:CD006605.
3. Gilron I, Bailey JM, Tu D, et al. Morphine, gabapentin, or their combination for neuropathic pain. *N Engl J Med*. 2005;352:1324-1334.
4. Gilron I, Bailey JM, Tu D, et al. Nortriptyline and gabapentin, alone and in combination for neuropathic pain: a double-blind, randomised controlled crossover trial. *Lancet*. 2009;374:1252-1261.
5. Romano CL, Romano D, Bonora C, et al. Pregabalin, celecoxib, and their combination for treatment of chronic low-back pain. *J Orthop Traumatol*. 2009;10:185-191.
6. Weinstein JN, Tosteson TD, Lurie JD, et al. Surgical vs nonoperative treatment for lumbar disk herniation. The Spine Patient Outcomes Research Trial (SPORT): a randomized trial. *JAMA*. 2006;296:2441-2450.
7. Weinstein JN, Tosteson TD, Lurie JD, et al, for the SPORT Investigators. Surgical versus nonsurgical therapy for lumbar spinal stenosis. *N Engl J Med*. 2008;358:794-810.

SUGGESTED READINGS

American Geriatrics Society Panel on the Pharmacological Management of Persistent Pain in Older Persons. Pharmacological management of persistent pain in older persons. *J Am Geriatr Soc.* 2009;57:1331-1346. *Updated guidelines developed and written by a multidisciplinary panel of the American Geriatrics Society.*

Chou R, Fanciullo GJ, Fine PG, et al, for the American Pain Society–American Academy of Pain Medicine Opioids Guidelines Panel. Clinical guidelines for the use of chronic opioid therapy in chronic noncancer pain. *J Pain.* 2009;10:113-130. *Practical guidelines on opioid use for noncancer pain by a multidisciplinary panel.*

Dunn KM, Saunders KW, Rutter CM, et al. Opioid prescriptions for chronic pain and overdose: a cohort study. *Ann Intern Med.* 2010;152:85-92. *Emphasizes the need for close supervision because higher doses of opioids increase the risk of overdose.*

Dworkin RH, O'Connor AB, Audette J, et al. Recommendations for the pharmacological management of neuropathic pain: an overview and literature update. *Mayo Clin Proc.* 2010;85(suppl):S3-S14. *A review providing an evidence-based recommendation for the pharmacological treatment of neuropathic pain.*

Morlion B. Pharmacotherapy of low back pain: targeting nociceptive and neuropathic pain components. *Curr Med Res Opin.* 2011;27:11-33. *The combination of pregabalin or antidepressants to target the neuropathic component of pain with opioids or nonsteroidal agents to target nociceptive pain may be preferable to either alone.*

30 BIOLOGY OF ADDICTION

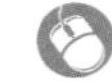

STEVEN E. HYMAN

DEFINITION

Drug addiction is defined as compulsive substance use despite serious negative consequences. Harmful drug use and addiction are significant contributors to medical morbidity and mortality both directly as a result of the toxic effects of abused drugs and indirectly through accidents, violence, nonsterile needle use, and other health hazards. By far the greatest contributors to illness and death are the widely used legal drugs, tobacco (Chapter 31) and alcohol (Chapter 32), although illegal addictive drugs and abused prescription drugs (Chapter 33) also exact a significant toll. In addition, addiction creates enormous burdens on society by impairing the function of the addicted person in multiple life roles, disrupting families and neighborhoods, and motivating crime.

Compulsive use, the cardinal feature of addiction, means that the affected person cannot control substance use for a significant period of time, despite powerful reasons to do so such as drug-related health problems, drug-associated arrest, or the threat of losing one's job or spouse. In the clinic, addiction can be remarkably frustrating to treat: drug seeking and administration are apparently voluntary behaviors that an otherwise sentient person seems unwilling to control. Even after significant efforts have been exerted to get an addicted patient into drug treatment, relapse is common, even long after the last withdrawal symptom has cleared. Relapses are often precipitated by stress or by reminders of drug use ("cues") that may range from familiar drug use contexts (such as smoking after a meal), to interactions with drug-using friends, to the smell of marijuana or tobacco smoke, to bodily feelings previously associated with drug-seeking (interoceptive cues). Cellular and molecular studies of drug action, animal models of drug use, and noninvasive human neuroimaging studies are providing significant insights into the neurobiology underlying compulsive drug taking and its persistence. Other important frontiers of research include the human genetics of addiction risk and more recently, the neurobiology of what have been called "behavioral addictions," such as compulsive gambling.

Drug users may repeatedly take drugs in order to gain pleasure or escape from negative feelings, including the aversive feelings that may occur when drugs wear off. As a result of repeated drug administration over time, drug receptors and their downstream signaling pathways (Table 30-1) are excessively stimulated and may thus undergo homeostatic adaptations. These adaptations can produce tolerance (the need for increasing drug doses to achieve desired affects) or dependence (revealed by withdrawal symptoms between drug doses or with drug cessation). Both tolerance and dependence can contribute to ongoing drug use and to dosage increases; however, neither tolerance nor dependence explains compulsive use. First, tolerance and dependence occur not only with repeated use of many addictive drugs (e.g., heroin), but also with many nonaddictive drugs (e.g., bronchodilators, nitrates, selective serotonin reuptake inhibitor [SSRI] antidepressants). Second, some highly addictive drugs such as cocaine may produce little dependence and withdrawal in some individuals who nonetheless exhibit compulsive use. Finally, if dependence and withdrawal were necessary factors in addiction, the phenomenon of late, post-detoxification relapse would not be the major clinical problem that it is. Although these forms of homeostatic adaptation play a role in addiction, as will be described, other types of plasticity within the nervous system are more significant.

The term *dependence* was selected to signify *addiction* within the *Diagnostic and Statistical Manual of Mental Disorders* of the American Psychiatric Association (DSM-IV) presumably because the term *addiction* was thought to be stigmatizing. This choice unfortunately has contributed to the confusion of physiologic dependence (the type of adaptation described previously) with addiction by physicians and patients alike. This confusion creates unnecessary obstacles to the treatment of many conditions, including cancer pain, anxiety disorders, and depression.

RISK FACTORS FOR ADDICTION

Only a minority of individuals who use drugs go on to become addicted. The best-established risk factors for addiction are male sex and family history. Across countries and cultures, males have a greater risk for both heavy drug use and addiction with risk ratios in the range of 1.4 : 1 to 2 : 1. In recent years, however, the sex ratios have narrowed in many countries, especially for tobacco use and alcohol.

Genes play the preponderant role in familial risk as evidenced by twin and adoption studies. Twin studies consistently show higher rates of concordance for heavy drug use and addiction within monozygotic twin pairs than within dizygotic twin pairs. Adoption studies that have been performed in several Scandinavian countries and in the United States have focused mostly on alcoholism. These studies demonstrate that individuals adopted early in life

TABLE 30-1 PROPERTIES OF ADDICTIVE DRUGS

DRUG	NEUROTRANSMITTER	DRUG TARGET	EFFECT AFTER BINDING
Opiates (morphine, heroin, oxycodone)	Endorphins	μ and δ opioid (agonist)	Activate G_i/G_o Activate K^+ channels
Psychostimulants (cocaine, amphetamines)	Dopamine (DA)	Dopamine transporter (DAT)* (antagonist)	Increase synaptic DA; stimulate presynaptic and postsynaptic DA receptors
Nicotine	Acetylcholine	Nicotinic acetylcholine receptors (nAChRs) (agonist)	Stimulate cation channel (may desensitize)
Alcohol	γ-Aminobutyric acid (GABA) Glutamate	$GABA_A$ receptor (agonist) *N*-methyl-D-aspartate (NMDA) receptor (antagonist)	Activate Cl^- channel Inhibit Ca^{2+} entry
Marijuana (Δ^9-tetrahydrocannabinol)	Anandamide	Cannabinoid CB_1 (agonist)	Activate G_i/G_o
Phencyclidine, ketamine		NMDA receptor channel (antagonist)	Inhibit Ca^{2+} entry

*The psychostimulants also interact with the norepinephrine and serotonin transporters, but under normal conditions, it is the DAT that is critical for rewarding and addictive properties. Unlike cocaine, amphetamines enter dopamine through the DAT and interact with a second target, the vesicular monoamine transporter (VMAT), to release DA into the cytoplasm and thence, through the DAT, to release it into the synapse.

Adapted from Hyman SE, Malenka RC, Nestler EJ. Neural mechanisms of addiction: the role of reward-related learning and memory. *Annu Rev Neurosci.* 2006;29:565-598.

tend to resemble their biologic rather than their adoptive parents with respect to patterns of alcohol use.

Although genes clearly play a significant role in vulnerability to addiction, few of the specific genetic variants that confer risk have been identified with certainty. Like all common neuropsychiatric disorders, addiction risk is highly genetically complex; there is evidence from linkage and association studies for contributions by a large number of genetic variants of relatively small effect. Large genome-wide association studies and other applications of modern genomic methods are continuing. However, the task of gene identification is also complicated by the challenges of phenotype definition. There are no objective medical tests with which to make the diagnosis, and there may be independent genetic and nongenetic risk factors for different stages of substance use disorders such as drug experimentation, addiction, and treatment responsiveness. Moreover, twin and family studies suggest that there may be both shared and unshared genetic risk factors underlying different drug preferences. As in other genetically complex disorders, it is hoped that with the identification of multiple risk-conferring variants, systems biology approaches can be brought to bear that will identify biochemical pathways involved in pathogenesis and suggest potential treatment targets.

REWARD CIRCUITRY: THE NEURAL SUBSTRATE OF ADDICTION

The survival and perpetuation of species require that animals, including humans, learn to predict threats and also learn the circumstances under which they can obtain food, water, shelter, and opportunities for mating. Neural circuits that have been highly conserved in evolution underlie these survival functions. A "fear circuit" centered on the amygdala regulates responses to threats, and a "reward circuit" centered on dopamine-releasing neurons that project from the ventral tegmental area (VTA) of the midbrain to the nucleus accumbens (NAc), prefrontal cortex, and other forebrain structures (Fig. 30-1) controls the pursuit of positive survival goals or "rewards." A simple operational definition of reward is a stimulus that elicits approach and consummatory behaviors.

Based on lesioning and physiologic studies in animals and more recently imaging in humans, the NAc (see Fig. 30-1), especially its outer region, called the *shell*, has been shown to play a necessary role in assigning motivational properties (desire, incentive salience) on rewards and to the stimuli that predict them. Thus, for example, in rat and mouse models, an intact NAc is required if the animal is to learn to work (e.g., lever pressing) to obtain natural rewards, such as palatable foods, or to learn how to self-administer drugs such as cocaine. Once an animal learns how to obtain a reward, and the relevant behaviors become ingrained, reward seeking no longer depends on the NAc and is supported by the dorsal striatum (called the *caudate* and *putamen* in humans), the brain structure that underlies well-learned behaviors and habits.

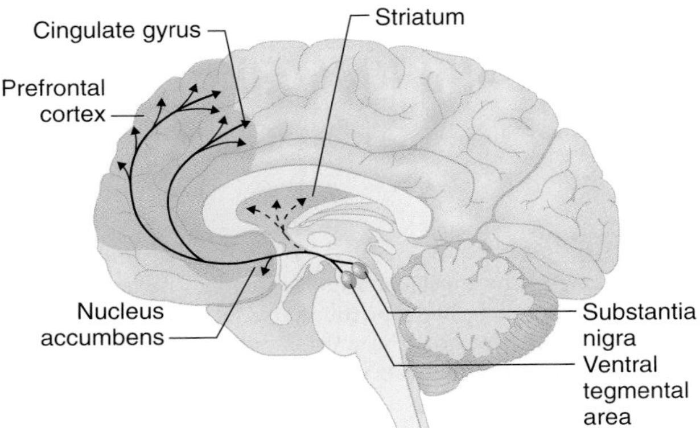

FIGURE 30-1. Brain reward circuits. The major dopaminergic projections to the forebrain that underlie brain reward are shown superimposed on a diagram of the human brain: projections from the ventral tegmental area to the nucleus accumbens, amygdala (not shown), hippocampus (not shown), and prefrontal cerebral cortex. Also shown are projections from the substantia nigra to the dorsal striatum (caudate and putamen and related structures) that play a role in habit formation and other deeply ingrained motor behaviors, including cue-dependent drug-seeking and self-administration. (From Hyman SE, Malenka RC, Nestler EJ. Neural mechanisms of addiction: the role of reward-related learning and memory. *Annu Rev Neurosci.* 2006;29:565-598.)

Under natural conditions, speed and efficiency in gaining food, water, and shelter improve the probability of survival. Thus, a critical role of reward circuitry is to facilitate the rapid learning of cues that predict the proximity of reward and of the behaviors that maximize the chances of successfully obtaining it. Once learned, predictive cues automatically activate cognitive, physiologic, and behavioral responses aimed at obtaining the predicted reward. In the laboratory, the simplest example of reward-related learning is classic (or pavlovian) conditioning in which a neutral stimulus, such as the sound of a bell, is reliably paired with a natural reward (an unconditioned stimulus) such as food. The sound of the bell quickly becomes a learned (conditioned) stimulus that henceforth activates physiologic and behavioral preparedness to obtain and consume the food.

The neurotransmitter dopamine, released from VTA neurons in the NAc, plays the key (albeit not the only) role in binding rewards and reward-associated cues to adaptive reward-seeking responses. In animals, implanted electrodes can record firing of dopamine neurons; microdialysis catheters and electrochemical methods can be used to detect dopamine that has been released from presynaptic neurons. In humans, positron emission tomography (PET) permits indirect measures of dopamine release by observing the displacement of a positron-emitting D_2 dopamine receptor ligand previously bound to receptors following a stimulus or pharmacologic challenge. Using such methods in multiple paradigms, it has been well established that natural rewards cause firing of VTA neurons and dopamine release in the NAc and other forebrain regions. When dopamine action is blocked, whether by lesioning dopamine neurons, blocking post-synaptic dopamine receptors, or inhibiting dopamine synthesis, rewards no longer motivate the behaviors necessary to obtain them.

New insights into the role of dopamine have emerged from studies of patients with Parkinson's disease (PD). PD results from the death of midbrain dopamine neurons; however, neurons within the substantia nigra (SN), which project to the caudate and putamen, are more severely affected than neurons within the VTA. Patients are generally treated with L-DOPA, a dopamine precursor, but as the disease progresses, other drugs may be needed, including selective D_2 dopamine receptor agonists. Relevant to this discussion is that a minority of patients treated with D_2 dopamine receptor agonists develop new risky, goal-directed behaviors such as compulsive gambling or compulsive shopping. These behaviors generally cease when the drug is withdrawn. It is thought that dopamine receptor agonists produce therapeutic effects on motor behavior in the more fully denervated caudate and putamen but combine with endogenous dopamine from preserved VTA neurons to overstimulate the NAc and other components of reward circuitry. These observations not only underscore the role of dopamine in motivation and reward seeking, but also suggest that what have been called *behavioral addictions* such as compulsive gambling share neural substrates with drug addiction.

Electrophysiologic recordings from nonhuman primates and functional magnetic resonance imaging (fMRI) studies in humans have converged on new views of how dopamine acts. Contrary to earlier ideas, dopamine does not appear to function as a neural representation of pleasure; rather, it serves as a learning signal in diverse forebrain circuits that are involved in responding to rewards. Dopaminergically innervated circuits underlie such functions as connecting reward-related stimuli to desire (NAc), learning and automatizing new motor behaviors (caudate and putamen), response selection, and relative valuation of experiences (orbital prefrontal cortex). Other neurotransmitters, perhaps endogenous opioid peptides, may be involved in hedonic responses (i.e., signaling pleasure). In this regard, it is noteworthy that nicotine, which is highly addictive—and causes dopamine release—does not produce significant euphoria of the sort produced by cocaine or heroin.

Much evidence suggests that the precise pattern of dopamine neuron firing, and the resulting synaptic release of dopamine in forebrain circuits, act to shape behavior so as to maximize future reward. In a basal state, dopamine neurons have a slow tonic pattern of firing. When a reward is encountered that is new, unexpected, or greater than expected, there is a phasic burst of firing of dopamine neurons causing a transient increase in synaptic dopamine. When a reward is predicted from known cues and is exactly as expected, there is no change from the tonic pattern of firing, that is, no additional dopamine release. When a predicted reward is omitted or less than expected, dopamine neurons pause their firing to levels below their tonic rate. Phasic increases in synaptic dopamine signify that the world is better than expected, facilitate learning of new predictive information, and bind the newly learned predictive cues to action.

PROPERTIES OF ADDICTIVE DRUGS

Addictive drugs are chemically diverse and interact with different molecular targets in the nervous system (see Table 30-1). They also exhibit significant differences from each other in many of their physiologic and behavioral effects. For example, cocaine and amphetamines are stimulants; they increase arousal, may cause anxiety, and at lower doses enhance cognitive performance. Alcohol is a depressant, is anxiolytic at low doses, and degrades cognitive performance. Heroin and other opiates are analgesic and cause drowsiness, constipation, and pupillary constriction. The shared behavioral effect of all addictive drugs is the liability, in vulnerable individuals, of causing compulsive use. The shared pharmacologic property that is required to cause addiction is the ability to increase levels of synaptic dopamine in the forebrain. For example, cocaine blocks the dopamine uptake transporter (DAT) that normally clears dopamine from synapses. Amphetamines cause reverse transport of dopamine into synapses through the DAT. Opiates, nicotine, alcohol, and cannabinoids cause dopamine release, acting by different initial mechanisms to release VTA neurons from resting inhibitory control.

Natural rewards, such as food or sexual opportunities, regulate the firing of dopamine neurons through highly processed sensory information, both external and interoceptive. Addictive drugs short-circuit this kind of information processing by acting directly on receptors and cells that regulate VTA dopamine neurons. Acting by such direct pharmacologic mechanisms, addictive drugs may produce greater quantities of synaptic dopamine over longer times than natural rewards. In addition, addictive drugs provide a grossly pathologic learning signal by occluding pauses in dopamine neuron firing even when drug use proves less pleasurable than expected or even aversive. For example, when the inhalation of a smoker causes painful coughing, it might seem that the brain would signal an experience that is worse than expected with a resulting decrement in VTA neuron firing rate. Because, however, nicotine causes dopamine release pharmacologically, independent of the smoker's actual experience, forebrain circuits, unavailable to conscious introspection, still receive a positive message that reinforces nicotine seeking and nicotine use. In short, addictive drugs, by virtue of their effects on dopamine, always signal "better than expected."

DRUG-INDUCED NEURAL PLASTICITY RELEVANT TO ADDICTION

In recent years, much neurobiologic research on addiction has focused on compulsive aspects of drug use, the ability of specific cues to activate drug seeking and craving, and the long persistence of stress and cue-dependent relapse risk. As described previously, compulsive drug use and the power of drug-associated cues reflect the usurpation of brain reward circuitry by drugs that directly cause dopamine release. The persistence of addiction reflects long-term changes in neurons, synapses, and circuits. Research over more than a decade has identified long-term changes in gene expression resulting from use of addictive drugs; recently, some long-lived alterations in gene expression have been attributed to drug-induced epigenetic mechanisms such as modification of chromatin.

Long-term changes in gene expression may render the addicted person susceptible to stress and may also create persistent changes in hedonic state and mood regulation that may motivate drug taking. By themselves, however, changes in gene expression do not explain the ability of exquisitely specific cues to activate drug seeking or, if seeking is impeded, intense subjective drug craving. The ability of specific cues to activate drug seeking and wanting is based on long-term associative memories consolidated under the influence of dopamine. Long-term memory formation represents perhaps the most persistent changes in brain function that may occur in adult life. The neural substrates of memory likely include alterations in synaptic weights, such as long-term potentiation (LTP) or long-term depression (LTD), and physical remodeling of dendritic spines.

The centrality of associative learning mechanisms for addiction was first recognized from clinical observation: much drug taking, and most notably late relapses, follows exposure to cues previously associated with drug use. Cues that can reinitiate drug use include environmental stimuli (e.g., persons with whom drugs have been used, drug paraphernalia) and bodily feelings. Because addictive drugs reliably increase synaptic dopamine as a result of their direct pharmacologic actions—indeed, they produce an excessive and grossly distorted dopamine signal—the brain receives a powerful impetus to connect the circumstances in which the drugs have been used with the motivation to take drugs again. Even if the drug is no longer pleasurable, the release of dopamine continues to reinforce drug wanting and seeking. Moreover, the reliability and quantity of dopamine release give drugs a marked advantage over natural rewards and other learned goals, including prosocial goals.

In the laboratory, it has been possible to study the effects of drug cues on neural circuits, physiology, and subjective responding in addicted human subjects. For example, drug-associated cues have been shown to elicit drug urges and physiologic responses (such as sympathetic activation), as well as activation of reward circuits in addicted human subjects. Using PET, cocaine-related cues have been shown to elicit dopamine release in the dorsal striatum in addicted subjects.

Investigations at the cellular and molecular levels have begun to identify the physiologic and molecular changes that underlie the effects of addictive drugs on reward-related memory processes. Among psychotropic drugs that have been examined, only those drugs that can cause addiction produce LTP in brain reward circuits including the VTA. Addictive drugs also activate transcription factors such as the cyclic adenosine monophosphate response element binding protein (CREB) and to alter the composition of activator protein 1 (AP-1) complexes in brain reward circuits. Dopamine and cocaine have been shown to regulate many genes downstream of CREB, AP-1, and other transcription factors. It has proved challenging, however, to determine which drug-regulated proteins are causally involved in addiction, as opposed to other processes such as physiologic dependence and withdrawal, or have no critical role at all. Part of the challenge is that while rodent models, including transgenic mouse models, have provided many insights into drug action and behavior, it is difficult to model human compulsion in animals, that is, to model a free-living and independent person who loses control over drug use while experiencing the negative consequences of that use. That said, a great body of detail is beginning to emerge about the neural processes that produce addiction.

SUGGESTED READINGS

Dagher A, Robbins TW. Personality, addiction, dopamine: insights from Parkinson's disease. *Neuron.* 2009;61:502-510. *Administration of dopamine agonists to patients with Parkinson's disease provides compelling new insight into the role of dopamine in addiction and into the biology of behavioral addictions.*

Haberstick BC, Zeiger JS, Corley RP, et al. Common and drug-specific genetic influences on subjective effects to alcohol, tobacco and marijuana use. *Addiction.* 2011;106:215-224. *Review.*

Hyman SE, Malenka RC, Nestler EJ. Neural mechanisms of addiction: the role of reward-related learning and memory. *Annu Rev Neurosci.* 2006;29:565-598. *Reviews behavioral and neurobiologic evidence that addictive drugs usurp normal systems underlying reward-related memory.*

Khokhar JY, Ferguson CS, Zhu AZ, et al. Pharmacogenetics of drug dependence: role of gene variations in susceptibility and treatment. *Annu Rev Pharmacol Toxicol.* 2010;50:39-61. *Reviews the genetic risk factors for drug addiction.*

Koob G. A role for brain stress systems in addiction. *Neuron.* 2008;59:11-14. *Reviews the role of stress and especially of corticotrophin releasing hormone in addictive disorders.*

31 NICOTINE AND TOBACCO

TONY P. GEORGE

DEFINITIONS

Cigarette smoking is the most common method of tobacco use (>90%), although other forms, including pipe tobacco, cigars, and smokeless tobacco, are common as well. Nicotine is the active ingredient that functions to reinforce tobacco addiction in all forms of tobacco.

EPIDEMIOLOGY

Cigarette smoking is the most preventable cause of morbidity and mortality in the Western world. In the United States, approximately 20% of the population uses tobacco, compared with 47% in 1965. Since the release of the surgeon general's report in 1965, smoking prevalence has been substantially reduced, but this reduction appears to have slowed in recent years, likely because the remaining smokers are refractory to tobacco treatment. Approximately 450,000 people die each year in the United States as a result of smoking-attributable medical illnesses such as lung cancer, chronic obstructive pulmonary disease, cardiovascular disease, and stroke; the economic and health care costs of tobacco use exceed $400 billion annually. The use of smokeless tobacco (e.g., chewing tobacco) has increased, contributing to higher rates of oral pathologies such as precancerous oral lesions and cancers of the mouth and nasopharynx. Moreover, the health risks of environmental tobacco smoke have become increasingly clear, prompting widespread tobacco bans in public settings.

Worldwide, it is estimated that approximately 1.1 billion people use tobacco on a regular basis, including approximately 65 million in the United States. Tobacco smoking is increasing rapidly throughout the developing world, and it is estimated that cigarette smoking will cause about 450 million deaths worldwide in the next 50 years. Smoking begins at a younger age in new smokers, the rates of smoking in women are increasing, and more smokers are of a lower socioeconomic status. Reducing smoking prevalence by 50% would prevent 20 million to 30 million premature deaths in the first quarter of this century and 150 million in the second quarter.

For most smokers, quitting is the single most important thing they can do to improve their health. A recent prospective cohort study in Norway suggests that even with sustained reductions (>50%) in daily smoking consumption, there is little if any reduction in cardiovascular disease and lung or other smoking-related cancer risk, further substantiating the merits of quitting versus only reducing smoking.

PATHOBIOLOGY

Nicotine is the primary reinforcer in tobacco smoke, but more than 4000 components contribute to the sensory (non-nicotinic) aspects of cigarette smoking. The primary site of action of nicotine is the $\alpha_4\beta_2$ nicotinic acetylcholine receptor, and the endogenous neurotransmitter acting on this receptor is acetylcholine. Nicotinic acetylcholine receptors in the central nervous system are pentameric ion channel complexes comprising two α and three β subunits; the eight α subunits are designated α_2 through α_9, and the three β subunits are designated β_2 through β_4. This produces considerable diversity in subunit combinations, which may explain in part the region-specific and functional selectivity of nicotine's effects in the central nervous system. Activation of nicotinic acetylcholine receptors leads to Na^+/Ca^{2+} ion channel fluxes and neuronal membrane depolarization. The receptors are located presynaptically on several neurotransmitter-secreting neuron types in the central nervous system, including mesolimbic dopaminergic (DA) neurons that project from the ventral tegmental area to the nucleus accumbens. Activation of the nicotinic acetylcholine receptors on mesolimbic DA neurons leads to dopamine secretion in the nucleus accumbens.

At low concentrations of nicotine, $\alpha_4\beta_2$ nicotinic acetylcholine receptor stimulation of afferent GABAergic projections onto mesoaccumbal DA neurons predominates, leading to reduced mesolimbic DA neuron firing and dopamine release. At higher nicotine concentrations, $\alpha_4\beta_2$ nicotinic acetylcholine receptors desensitize, and activation of α_7 nicotinic acetylcholine receptors on glutamatergic projections predominates, leading to increased mesolimbic DA neuron firing and release. Within milliseconds of activation by nicotine, nicotinic acetylcholine receptors desensitize; after overnight abstinence, they resensitize. This may explain why most smokers report that the first cigarette in the morning is the most satisfying. Interestingly, recent positron emission tomography neuroimaging studies have shown that two to three puffs on a cigarette saturate the nicotinic acetylcholine receptors in the brain reward system, suggesting that although binding to these central receptors is an important first step in the effects of nicotine, it does not fully explain continued smoking behaviors.

CLINICAL MANIFESTATIONS

Although there is a subset of cigarette smokers who do not smoke every day, most smokers are daily users and have some degree of physiologic dependence on nicotine. Smokers typically describe a "rush" and feelings of alertness, relaxation, and satisfaction when smoking, and it is well known that nicotine has both stimulating and anxiolytic effects, depending on the basal level of arousal. Airway stimulation is an important aspect of smoking behavior, and additives such as menthol enhance the experience by increasing the taste and reducing the harshness of smoked tobacco.

Interestingly, the positive effects of cigarette smoking (e.g., taste, satisfaction) appear to be mediated by non-nicotine components of tobacco such as tar. Besides positive reinforcement, withdrawal, and craving, there are several secondary effects of nicotine and tobacco use that may contribute to both the maintenance of smoking and smoking relapse, including mood modulation (e.g., reduction of negative affect), stress reduction, and weight control. In addition, conditioned cues can elicit the urge to smoke even after prolonged periods of abstinence. Specific effects might be particularly relevant to smokers wishing to lose weight and those with psychiatric disorders (mood modulation, cognitive enhancement, stress reduction). These secondary effects may present additional targets for pharmacologic intervention in certain subgroups of smokers (e.g., schizophrenic, depressed, or weight-concerned smokers).

DIAGNOSIS

Nicotine dependence is established clinically by historical documentation of daily smoking (typically 10 to 40 cigarettes/day) for several weeks, evidence of tolerance (e.g., lack of adverse effects of nicotine, such as nausea), and the presence of symptoms of nicotine withdrawal upon smoking cessation. These withdrawal symptoms, which peak within 12 to 24 hours of cessation, include dysphoria, anxiety, irritability, decreased heart rate, insomnia (waking in the middle of the night), increased appetite, and craving for cigarettes. In addition, most dependent smokers state that they smoke their first cigarette of the day within 5 minutes of awakening. Timeline follow-back procedures and smoking diaries have been used successfully to monitor smoking consumption over time. Scales such as the Fagerstrom Test for Nicotine Dependence allow an assessment of the level of nicotine dependence, with a score of 4 or greater (on a scale of 0 to 10) consistent with physiologic dependence. Nicotine craving and withdrawal can be reliably monitored with validated scales such as the Tiffany Questionnaire for Smoking Urges and the Minnesota Nicotine Withdrawal Scale. These scales have excellent test-retest reliability and internal consistency in smokers with schizophrenia when compared with nonpsychiatric control smokers, suggesting that they can be used in psychiatric populations.

TREATMENT Rx

Psychosocial Treatments

Behavioral therapies (Table 31-1) are based on the theory that learning processes operate in the development, maintenance, and cessation of smoking. Behavioral treatments for smoking can facilitate the motivation to quit, emphasize the social and contextual aspects of smoking, and enhance overall success at smoking cessation. In most reviews, 6-month quit rates with behavioral therapies are 20 to 25%, and behavioral therapy typically increases quit rates up to twofold over standard medical advice. The primary goals of behavioral therapies in the treatment of tobacco dependence are to provide smokers with the necessary skills to help them quit smoking and avoid smoking in high-risk situations.

Brief Interventions

Brief interventions can increase the rate of smoking cessation and are strongly endorsed in the latest Department of Health and Human Services Guidelines on Tobacco Dependence Treatment. It is recommended that physicians use the five As with all patients: ask patients if they smoke, advise patients to quit, assess patients' level of motivation to quit, assist with attempts to quit, and arrange follow-up contacts. Providing self-help material is a form of brief intervention used to increase the motivation to quit and impart smoking cessation skills. Several recent studies have documented that minimal behavioral interventions such as community support groups, telephone counseling, and computer-generated tailored self-help materials can augment smoking cessation rates in controlled settings.

Motivational Interventions

The goal of motivational interviewing interventions is to elicit change by addressing ambivalence, increasing the patient's intrinsic motivation for change, and creating an atmosphere of acceptance in which patients take responsibility for making change happen. Brief motivational interventions have been developed for smoking cessation, and there is some evidence of increased smoking cessation using such techniques.

Cognitive-Behavioral Therapies

In cognitive-behavioral therapy, patients learn to identify situations in which they are likely to smoke and then plan to cope with these situations using behavioral (e.g., substitution of behavior) and cognitive (e.g., challenging thoughts) techniques. Some degree of efficacy has been observed in smokers using both individual and group counseling formats.

Relapse-Prevention (Coping Skills) Therapies

A large number of smokers relapse within 6 months of quitting. Focusing on relapse-prevention skills, including recognizing high-risk situations and coping with lapses, can be included in initial smoking cessation treatment or after a quit attempt.

Pharmacologic Treatments

Three classes of smoking cessation pharmacotherapies—nicotine replacement therapies (NRTs), sustained-release bupropion, and varenicline (Table 31-2)—have been approved by the Food and Drug Administration (FDA). Other off-label and novel medications are also discussed in this section.

Nicotine Replacement Therapies

The goal of NRT is to alleviate tobacco withdrawal, which allows smokers to focus on habit and conditioning factors when attempting cessation. After smoking cessation, NRT is gradually reduced so that minimal withdrawal occurs. NRTs rely on systemic venous absorption and thus do not produce the rapid high levels of arterial nicotine achieved when cigarette smoke is inhaled. Thus, individuals are unlikely to become addicted to NRTs. NRTs should be discontinued if the person restarts smoking, although safety concerns regarding smoking while using a nicotine patch appear to be less serious than previously thought. All commercially available forms of NRT are effective and increase quit rates by approximately 1.5- to 2.5-fold compared with placebo.[1] The transdermal patch, gum, and lozenge are sold over the counter (OTC); the nasal spray and inhaler require a prescription.

TABLE 31-1 BEHAVIORAL TREATMENTS FOR TOBACCO DEPENDENCE

TREATMENT	MECHANISM OF ACTION	EFFECTIVENESS RATING*
Brief interventions	Increase motivation to quit and impart cessation skills (e.g., community support, telephone counseling)	2
Cognitive-behavioral and relapse-prevention therapies	Use behavioral strategies to manage triggers; use cognitive coping strategies to target maladaptive thoughts and prevent relapse	1
Motivational interviewing	Promote patient's self-motivational statements to gain greater awareness of the problems related to smoking and increase intention to stop smoking	2

*1 = strong evidence to support efficacy; 2= moderate evidence to support efficacy; 3= little evidence to support efficacy.

Nicotine Gum

Nicotine ingested orally is extensively metabolized on the first pass through the liver. Nicotine polacrilex gum avoids this problem through buccal absorption. Nicotine gum, which was approved as an OTC medication in the United States in 1996, contains 2 or 4 mg of nicotine that is released from a resin by chewing. Nicotine gum should be administered by scheduled dosing (e.g., 1 piece of 2-mg gum/hour). The original recommended duration of treatment was 3 months, but many experts believe longer treatment is more effective. Nicotine absorption peaks 30 minutes after beginning to chew the gum. Venous nicotine levels from 2- and 4-mg gum are about one third and two thirds, respectively, of the steady-state nicotine levels (i.e., between cigarettes) achieved with cigarette smoking. Nicotine delivered by cigarettes is absorbed directly into the pulmonary arterial circulation. Thus, arterial levels from smoking are 5 to 10 times higher than those from the 2- and 4-mg gums. Absorption of nicotine in the buccal mucosa is decreased by an acidic environment, so patients should not drink beverages (e.g., coffee, soda, juice) immediately before, during, or after nicotine gum use.

Several placebo-controlled trials established the safety and efficacy of nicotine gum for smoking cessation.[1] There appears to be some evidence to support the use of higher doses of nicotine gum (4-mg pieces) in more highly dependent cigarette smokers (≥25 cigarettes/day), which supports the idea of matching the nicotine gum dose to the smoker's dependence level. Side effects from nicotine gum are rare and include those of mechanical origin (e.g., difficulty chewing, sore jaw) or local pharmacologic origin (e.g., burning in mouth, throat irritation). Tolerance to most side effects develops over the first week, and education about proper use of the gum (e.g., not chewing too vigorously) decreases side effects.

Nicotine Lozenges

Lozenges that deliver nicotine (2- and 4-mg preparations) by buccal absorption were approved for OTC use in the United States in 2002. Lozenges offer additional nicotine replacement options for smokers and allow greater absorption of nicotine compared with nicotine gum. Mild throat and mouth irritation were reported in preliminary trials. Nicotine lozenges have shown their superiority to placebo lozenges, with a significant reduction in nicotine craving and withdrawal.[1] Furthermore, higher doses of lozenges may be more efficacious in more highly dependent smokers, suggesting that similar to nicotine gum, lozenge dose can be matched to dependence level. Interestingly, the combination of nicotine lozenge with nicotine patch may lead to the highest long-term quit rates compared with nicotine replacement monotherapies and bupropion.[2]

TABLE 31-2 PHARMACOLOGIC TREATMENTS FOR TOBACCO DEPENDENCE

TREATMENT	MECHANISM OF ACTION	EFFECTIVENESS RATING*
NICOTINE REPLACEMENT THERAPIES[†]		
Gum (OTC)	Slow nicotine absorption gradually reduces nicotine craving and withdrawal	1
TNP (OTC)	Slow nicotine absorption gradually reduces nicotine craving and withdrawal	1
Lozenge (OTC)	Slow nicotine absorption gradually reduces nicotine craving and withdrawal	1
Vapor inhaler (prescription)	Fast nicotine absorption leads to stimulation of nicotinic acetylcholine receptors, which rapidly reduces nicotine craving and withdrawal	1
Nasal spray (prescription)	Fast nicotine absorption leads to stimulation of nicotinic acetylcholine receptors, which reduces craving and withdrawal	1
NON-NICOTINE PHARMACOTHERAPIES		
Bupropion SR[†]	Blocks re-uptake of dopamine and norepinephrine; high-affinity, noncompetitive nicotinic acetylcholine receptor antagonism reduces nicotine reinforcement, withdrawal, and craving	1
Varenicline[†]	Acts as partial agonist of $\alpha_4\beta_2$ nicotinic acetylcholine receptors	1
Nortriptyline	Blocks re-uptake of norepinephrine and serotonin; probably reduces withdrawal symptoms and comorbid depressive symptoms; side effects limit utility	1-2
Clonidine	α_2-Adrenoreceptor agonist reduces nicotine withdrawal symptoms	2
Mecamylamine	Noncompetitive, high-affinity nicotinic acetylcholine receptor antagonist combined with TNP reduces nicotine reinforcement, craving, and withdrawal	2
Naltrexone	Endogenous μ-opioid peptide receptor antagonist reduces nicotine craving and withdrawal in combination with TNP; may reduce alcohol use and obviate cessation-induced weight gain	3
Monoamine oxidase inhibitors	Increased monoamine levels can reduce nicotine reinforcement, withdrawal, and craving; might be helpful for smokers with comorbid mood disorders	2
Rimonabant	Endocannabinoid receptor (CB_1) antagonist; has shown efficacy in smoking cessation trials and may be particularly useful in weight-concerned smokers	2
Nicotine vaccine	Limited evidence of efficacy for smoking cessation in early human trials; may have utility in relapse prevention	2

*1 = strong evidence to support efficacy; 2 = moderate evidence to support efficacy; 3 = little evidence to support efficacy.
[†]Approved by the Food and Drug Administration.
OTC = over the counter; SR = sustained release; TNP = transdermal nicotine patch.

Transdermal Nicotine Patch

The four transdermal nicotine patch (TNP) formulations take advantage of the ready absorption of nicotine through the skin. Three of the patches are for 24-hour use, and one is for 16-hour use. Starting doses are 21 or 22 mg/24-hour patch and 15 mg/16-hour patch. Patches are applied daily each morning. Nicotine administered by the patches is absorbed slowly, so that on the first day, venous nicotine levels peak 6 to 10 hours after application of the patch. Thereafter, nicotine levels remain fairly steady, with a decline from peak to trough of 25 to 40% with 24-hour patches. Nicotine levels obtained with the use of patches are typically half those obtained by smoking. After 4 to 6 weeks on a high-dose patch (21 or 22 mg/24 hours or 15 mg/16 hours), smokers are tapered to a medium dose (14 mg/24 hours or 10 mg/16 hours) and then, after another 2 to 4 weeks, to the lowest dose (7 mg/24 hours or 5 mg/16 hours). Most studies suggest that abrupt cessation of the use of patches causes no significant withdrawal. The recommended treatment is usually 6 to 12 weeks, but a 24-week course may be up to 50% more effective than an 8-week course.[3]

The overall efficacy of the TNP for smoking cessation has been well documented.[1] The effects are independent of patch type, treatment duration, tapering procedures, and behavioral therapy format or intensity, although it should be noted that behavioral treatment enhances outcomes compared with TNP alone. Severe adverse events have not been associated with nicotine patches. The most common minor side effects are skin reactions (50%), insomnia and increased or vivid dreams (15% with 24-hour patches), and nausea (5 to 10%). Tolerance to these side effects usually develops within a week. Rotation of patch sites decreases skin irritation. Insomnia reported in the first week after smoking cessation appears to be due to nicotine withdrawal rather than the nicotine patch itself. A 24-hour patch can be removed before bedtime to determine whether the insomnia is due to the nicotine patch. Without treatment, insomnia usually abates after 4 to 7 days. There appears to be little risk of dependence associated with patch use; only 2% of patch users continue to use it for an extended period after a cessation trial.

Nicotine Nasal Spray

Nicotine nasal spray is a nicotine solution in a nasal spray bottle similar to those used for saline sprays. This NRT was approved for the treatment of nicotine dependence in the United States in 1996. Nasal spray delivers droplets that average about 1 mg nicotine per administration, and the patient administers the spray (10 mg/mL) to each nostril every 4 to 6 hours. This formulation produces a more rapid rise in nicotine levels than does nicotine gum; the nicotine levels produced by nicotine spray fall between those produced by nicotine gum and by cigarettes. Peak nicotine levels occur within 10 minutes, and venous nicotine levels are about two thirds of between-cigarette levels. Smokers can use the nasal spray as needed up to 30 times/day for 12 weeks.

Randomized, double-blind, placebo-controlled trials of nasal spray versus placebo spray have established the safety and efficacy of nasal spray for smoking cessation.[1] These trials employed treatment for 3 to 6 months, and nicotine nasal spray led to a doubling of quit rates during active use. Differences were reduced or absent with extended follow-up, suggesting the need to continue using this agent. However, such long-term studies have not been published. Major side effects from nicotine nasal spray are nasal and throat irritation, rhinitis, sneezing, coughing, and watering eyes. Nicotine nasal spray may have some risk of dependence; prolonged use occurs in about 10% of smokers using the nasal spray, so follow-up is recommended.

Nicotine Inhaler

Cartridges (plugs) of nicotine (containing about 1 mg of nicotine each) are placed inside hollow cigarette-like plastic rods. The cartridges produce a nicotine vapor when warm air is passed through them. Absorption from a nicotine inhaler is primarily buccal rather than respiratory. More recent versions of inhalers produce a more rapid rise in venous nicotine levels compared with nicotine gum but a less rapid rise compared with nicotine nasal spray, with nicotine blood levels of about one third that of between-cigarette levels. Smokers are instructed to puff continually on the inhaler (0.013 mg/puff) during the day, and the recommended dosing is 6 to 16 cartridges daily. The inhaler is used as needed for about 12 weeks. No serious medical side effects have been reported with nicotine inhalers. Fifty percent of subjects report throat irritation or coughing. Randomized, double-blind, placebo-controlled trials have demonstrated the superiority of the nicotine inhaler to placebo inhalers for smoking cessation.[1] Results revealed a two- to threefold increase in quit rates (17 to 26%) at trial end point compared with placebo inhalers, and smaller differences at follow-up periods of 1 year or longer. These data support the short-term efficacy of inhalers in cigarette smokers, but longer-term trials are needed. There is also some modest concern about the risk of abuse, based on long-term use of the product in less than 10% of smokers.

Sustained-Release Bupropion

Bupropion, a phenylaminoketone atypical antidepressant agent, in the sustained-release (SR) formulation (Zyban), is a non-nicotine first-line pharmacologic treatment for nicotine-dependent smokers who want to quit. The mechanism of action in the treatment of nicotine dependence likely involves dopamine and norepinephrine reuptake blockade, as well as antagonism of high-affinity nicotinic acetylcholine receptors. The exact mechanism by which bupropion exerts antismoking effects is unclear. The goals of bupropion therapy are smoking cessation, reduction of nicotine craving and withdrawal symptoms, and prevention of cessation-induced weight gain.

The target dose of this agent in nicotine-dependent patients is 300 mg daily (150 mg twice a day). It is typically started 7 days before the target quit date (TQD) at 150 mg daily, then increased to 150 mg twice a day after 3 to 4 days. Unlike NRTs, there is no absolute requirement that smokers completely cease smoking by the TQD, although many smokers report a significant reduction in the urge to smoke and cravings, which facilitates cessation at the TQD when drug levels reach steady-state plasma levels. Some smokers gradually reduce their cigarette smoking over several weeks before quitting completely.

A pivotal multicenter study established the efficacy and safety of bupropion SR for the treatment of nicotine dependence, which led to its FDA approval in 1998. In a 7-week double-blind, placebo-controlled multicenter trial, four doses of bupropion SR (0, 100, 150, and 300 mg/day in twice-a-day dosing), in combination with weekly individual cessation counseling, were prescribed to 615 cigarette smokers using at least 15 cigarettes/day. At 1-year follow-up, cessation rates were 12.4%, 19.6%, 22.9%, and 23.1%, respectively. Bupropion SR treatment dose-dependently reduced weight gain associated with smoking cessation and significantly reduced nicotine withdrawal symptoms at doses of 150 and 300 mg/day.

Subsequently, the efficacy of combined bupropion SR and TNP was studied in a double-blind, placebo-controlled, randomized multicenter trial. A total of 893 cigarette smokers, using at least 15 cigarettes/day, were randomized to one of four experimental groups: (1) placebo bupropion + placebo patch; (2) placebo bupropion + TNP; (3) bupropion (300 mg/day) + placebo patch; or (4) bupropion + TNP. Cessation rates at the 1-year follow-up assessment were 15.6%, 16.4%, 30.3%, and 35.5% respectively. The bupropion groups did significantly better than the placebo and TNP alone groups, but the combination of bupropion and TNP was not significantly better than bupropion alone. Weight suppression after cessation was most robust in the combination therapy group.

Finally, a randomized, controlled trial demonstrated the efficacy of bupropion SR in relapse prevention after smoking cessation.[4] In individuals who had quit smoking with 7 weeks of bupropion (300 mg/day) treatment, bupropion SR versus placebo for 12 months delayed smoking relapse and resulted in weight gain.

Common side effects reported with bupropion administration in cigarette smokers are headache, nausea and vomiting, dry mouth, insomnia, and activation, most of which occur during the first week of treatment. The main contraindication for the use of bupropion is a past history of seizures of any cause. The rates of de novo seizures are low with this agent (<0.5%) at doses of 300 mg/day or less, but they have been observed when daily dosing exceeds 450 mg/day.

Varenicline

Varenicline tartrate (Chantix in the United States; Champix in Europe and Canada), a partial $\alpha_4\beta_2$ nicotinic acetylcholine receptor agonist, was approved as a first-line smoking cessation agent in the United States in 2006 and in Canada and Europe in 2007. The initial phase II trials of varenicline established its safety and efficacy in comparison to placebo and suggested an optimal dose of 2 mg/day.[5] Two independent but identical 12-week phase III trials comparing varenicline (2 mg/day) to bupropion SR (300 mg/day) were then conducted.[6,7] The quit rates for both studies were similar for continuous abstinence over the last 4 weeks (weeks 9 to 12) of the study. For study 1, the quit rates were as follows: varenicline, 43.9%; bupropion SR, 29.8%; and placebo, 17.6%.[6] For study 2, they were varenicline, 44.0%; bupropion SR, 29.5%; and placebo, 17.7%.[7] Quit rates were significantly higher for participants taking varenicline compared with bupropion SR, and both drugs resulted in significantly higher quit rates than placebo. Continuous abstinence over the follow-up period (weeks 9 to 52) was lower, but participants taking varenicline continued to show a higher rate of abstinence than those taking bupropion and placebo. Varenicline is also more effective in smoking relapse prevention compared with placebo.[8]

Varenicline reduces tobacco cravings and smoking satisfaction and is generally well tolerated. The most common adverse events reported in the initial studies were nausea and insomnia. Since the drug's approval, however, concerns have arisen over treatment-emergent neuropsychiatric events, including agitation, suicidal and homicidal ideation, mania, and psychosis. Thus, close monitoring of smokers, especially those with a history of psychiatric illness, is strongly advised when prescribing this agent.

Off-Label Medications

Other medications (see Table 31-2) have demonstrated some efficacy for tobacco treatment but are not approved for this indication and should be considered second-line treatments.

Novel Medications on the Horizon: Cannabinoid Antagonists and Nicotine Vaccines

Two novel pharmacologic strategies not yet approved in the United States may offer some additional strategies for smoking cessation and smoking relapse prevention. The cannabinoid receptor (CB_1) antagonist rimonabant demonstrated promising results in clinical trials in the United States and Europe; at the 20 mg/day dose, it doubled the chance of quitting compared with placebo. Most notably, it potently suppresses smoking cessation–related weight gain. Side effects, which include nausea, vomiting, and tremors, are dose dependent. Unfortunately, rimonabant was not approved for smoking cessation by the FDA and was recently withdrawn as a pharmacologic treatment for obesity by the European Medications Agency owing to safety concerns related to the emergence of clinical depression. Trials with other CB_1 antagonists are in progress.

Nicotine vaccines are being developed by a number of companies. They appear to be well tolerated and enhance smoking cessation rates. Higher abstinence rates are observed as a function of higher serum antibody titers. The nicotine vaccine also shows promise for the prevention of smoking initiation or relapse and will likely be tested for these indications. Side effects include soreness at the injection site and hypersensitivity reactions to vaccine components.

PREVENTION

Tobacco dependence remains one of the leading preventable causes of morbidity and mortality in the Western world. Although smoking cessation therapies are among the most cost-effective and proven therapies in medicine, most health care providers do not identify tobacco use in their patients. The U.S. Public Health Service recently published updated clinical practice guidelines for nicotine dependence that provide standards for the treatment of tobacco dependence. In addition, effective tobacco policies such as state taxes and prevention efforts targeted at reducing the initiation of tobacco use by youths and adults are critical elements in the overall strategy to reduce the burden of tobacco-related disease and related social and health care costs.

PROGNOSIS

The prognosis for tobacco smokers who quit is excellent in terms of years of life and quality of life gained. Bans on smoking in public places can reduce local rates of acute myocardial infarction by about 17%.

Although medications and behavioral treatments have documented efficacy in treating tobacco dependence, these therapies must be used in combination to achieve the best overall results and ensure adequate skill acquisition and treatment adherence. Novel treatment and prevention interventions, such as the nicotine vaccine and the employment of personalized medicine—matching the right medications to smokers with preferential responses using pharmacogenetic approaches—are generating considerable excitement in the tobacco treatment field and may be available within the next decade. Further, given the high rates of tobacco use and dependence in psychiatric populations and the lower rates of quitting in this subset of smokers compared with the general population, the specific adaptation of tobacco treatments to mentally ill smokers will be of paramount importance in improving prognosis and outcome in these hard-to-treat smokers. Additional future challenges include developing safer and more effective smoking cessation therapies and making these therapies available to all smokers who wish to quit.

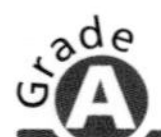

1. Silagy C, Lancaster T, Stead L, et al. Nicotine replacement therapies for smoking cessation. *Cochrane Database Syst Rev.* 2004;3:CD000146.
2. Piper ME, Smith SS, Schlam TR, et al. A randomized placebo-controlled clinical trial of 5 smoking cessation pharmacotherapies. *Arch Gen Psychiatry.* 2009;66:1253-1262.
3. Schnoll RA, Patterson F, Wileyto EP, et al. Effectiveness of extended-duration transdermal nicotine therapy: a randomized trial. *Ann Intern Med.* 2010;152:144-151.
4. Hays JT, Hurt RD, Rigotti NA, et al. Sustained-release bupropion for pharmacologic relapse-prevention after smoking cessation: a randomized, controlled trial. *Ann Intern Med.* 2001;135:423-433.
5. Oncken C, Gonzales D, Nides M, et al. Efficacy and safety of the novel selective nicotinic acetylcholine receptor partial agonist, varenicline, for smoking cessation. *Arch Intern Med.* 2006;166:1571-1577.
6. Gonzales D, Rennard SI, Nides M, et al. Varenicline, an $alpha_4$ $beta_2$ nicotinic acetylcholine receptor partial agonist, vs. sustained release bupropion and placebo for smoking cessation. *JAMA.* 2006;296:47-55.
7. Jorenby DE, Hays JT, Rigotti NA, et al. Efficacy of varenicline, an $alpha_4$ $beta_2$ nicotinic acetylcholine receptor partial agonist, vs. placebo or sustained release bupropion for smoking cessation. *JAMA.* 2006;296:56-63.
8. Tonstad S, Tonnesen P, Hajek P, et al. Effect of maintenance therapy with varenicline on smoking cessation. *JAMA.* 2006;296:64-71.

SUGGESTED READINGS

Hamer M, Stamatakis E, Kivimaki M, et al. Objectively measured secondhand smoke exposure and risk of cardiovascular disease: what is the mediating role of inflammatory and hemostatic factors? *J Am Coll Cardiol.* 2010;56:18-23. *Secondhand smoke elevates the CRP level, which accounts for about 50% of its effect on increasing the risk of cardiovascular disease.*

Piano MR, Benowitz NL, Fitzgerald GA, et al. Impact of smokeless tobacco products on cardiovascular disease: implications for policy, prevention, and treatment: a policy statement from the American Heart Association. *Circulation.* 2010;122:1520-1544. *Policy statement emphasizing their risks.*

Strand BH, Mishra G, Kuh D, et al. Smoking history and physical performance in midlife: results from the British 1946 birth cohort. *J Gerontol A Biol Sci Med Sci.* 2010;66:142-149. *Lifetime cigarette pack years are strongly related to poorer midlife physical performance.*

32 ALCOHOL ABUSE AND DEPENDENCE

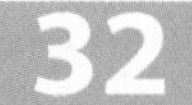

PATRICK G. O'CONNOR

DEFINITION

A variety of terms have been used to describe the spectrum of medical, psychological, behavioral, and social problems associated with excessive consumption of alcohol (*alcohol problems*). *Alcoholism* is perhaps the most widely used term to describe patients with alcohol problems. In an attempt to define *alcoholism* more precisely, a panel of 23 experts convened by the National Council on Alcoholism and Drug Dependence and the American Society of Addiction Medicine developed a definition of alcoholism that included "a primary chronic disease with genetic, psychosocial and environmental factors . . . often progressive and fatal . . . characterized by impaired control over drinking, preoccupation with the drug alcohol, use of alcohol despite future consequences, and distortions of thinking, most notably denial." Because the term *alcoholism* is so broad, it also can be imprecise in defining the entire spectrum of alcohol problems.

Abstainers are individuals who consume no alcohol. *Moderate drinking* is defined by the National Institute on Alcohol Abuse and Alcoholism as the average number of drinks consumed daily that places an adult at low risk for alcohol problems. There is some epidemiologic evidence to suggest that moderate drinking may have some health benefits by reducing the risk of cardiovascular disease (Chapter 51). The scope of alcohol consumption that imparts this benefit may be low, however (e.g., less than one drink per day).

At-risk drinking is a level of alcohol consumption that imparts health risks (Table 32-1). This category of drinking behavior has been identified on the

TABLE 32-1 TERMS AND CRITERIA FOR PATTERNS OF ALCOHOL USE

AT-RISK DRINKING
Men: >14/week or >4 drinks/day Women: >7/week or >3 drinks/day
ALCOHOL ABUSE
Maladaptive pattern of alcohol use leading to clinically significant impairment or distress, manifested within a 12-month period by one or more of the following: Failure to fulfill role obligations at work, school, or home Recurrent use in hazardous situations Legal problems related to alcohol Continued use despite alcohol-related social or interpersonal problems Symptoms have never met criteria for alcohol dependence
ALCOHOL DEPENDENCE
Maladaptive pattern of alcohol use leading to clinically significant impairment or distress, manifested within a 12-month period by three or more of the following: Tolerance (either increasing amounts used or diminished effects with the same amount) Withdrawal (withdrawal symptoms or use to relieve or avoid symptoms) Use of larger amounts for a longer period than intended Persistent desire or unsuccessful attempts to cut down or control use Great deal of time spent obtaining, using, or recovering from use Important social relationships, occupations, or recreational activities given up or reduced Use despite knowledge of alcohol-related physical or psychological problems

basis of epidemiologic evidence that certain threshold levels of alcohol consumption are associated with increased risk of specific health problems. At-risk drinking is defined differently for men younger than 65 years than for women of all ages because of generally lower body weights and lower rates of metabolism of alcohol in women; the definition in men older than 65 years is the same as in women because of the age-related increased risk of alcohol problems, in part due to changes in alcohol metabolism in older individuals. *Binge drinking* or *heavy drinking* is the episodic consumption of large amounts of alcohol, usually five or more drinks per occasion for men and four or more drinks per occasion for women. One standard drink contains 12 g of pure alcohol, an amount equivalent to that contained in 5 ounces of wine, 12 ounces of beer, or 1.5 ounces of 80-proof spirits. *Problem drinking* refers to a level of alcohol consumption that causes any problems for the patient (medical, psychiatric, behavioral, or social—*alcohol problems*).

Alcohol abuse and *alcohol dependence,* which are alcohol use disorders defined in the *Diagnostic and Statistical Manual of Mental Disorders,* 4th edition, require the presence of specific social or clinical phenomena (see Table 32-1). *Alcohol abuse* includes criteria that indicate social dysfunction or use in high-risk situations (e.g., driving). *Alcohol dependence* includes social consequences along with criteria related to physiologic aspects of dependence (e.g., tolerance, loss of control) and use despite physical or psychological problems. The distinction between *alcohol abuse* and *alcohol dependence* is important given the general need for more intensive treatment services for patients who are alcohol dependent.

EPIDEMIOLOGY

In national surveys, 64% of American adults reported that they use alcoholic beverages (liquor, wine, or beer), whereas 36% reported that they were abstinent. Among individuals who use alcohol, many experience problems because of their drinking. It has been estimated that more than $100 billion is spent by American society each year to treat alcohol use disorders and to recover the costs of alcohol-related economic losses. Excessive alcohol consumption ranks as the third leading preventable cause of death in the United States after cigarette smoking and obesity. More than 100,000 deaths per year in the United States are attributed to alcohol use disorders.

Population-based epidemiologic studies have shown that alcohol use disorders are among the most prevalent medical, behavioral, or psychiatric disorders in the general population. An epidemiologic survey of the general population in the United States documented a prevalence of alcohol abuse and dependence estimated to be between 7.4 and 9.7%. The lifetime prevalence of abuse and dependence is estimated to be even higher. Despite higher thresholds and tolerance, men are at least twice as likely as women to meet criteria for alcohol abuse and dependence by standard diagnostic survey techniques. Although sociodemographic features, such as young age, low income, and low education level, have been associated with an increased risk for problem drinking, alcohol use disorders are prevalent throughout all sociodemographic groups, and all individuals should be screened carefully. The "skid row" stereotype of the alcohol-dependent patient is much more the exception than the rule.

The prevalence of alcohol use disorders is higher in most health care settings than it is in the general population because alcohol problems often result in treatment-seeking behaviors. The prevalence of problem drinking in general outpatient and inpatient medical settings has been estimated between 15 and 40%. These data strongly support the need for physicians to screen all patients for alcohol use disorders.

PATHOBIOLOGY

Beverage alcohol contains ethanol, which acts as a sedative-hypnotic drug. Alcohol is absorbed rapidly into the blood stream from the stomach and intestinal tract. Because women have lower levels of gastric alcohol dehydrogenase, the enzyme primarily responsible for metabolizing alcohol, they experience higher blood alcohol concentrations than do men who consume similar amounts of ethanol per kilogram of body weight. The absorption of alcohol can be affected by other factors, including the presence of food in the stomach and the rate of alcohol consumption. By means of metabolism in the liver, alcohol is converted to acetaldehyde and acetate (Fig. 32-1). Metabolism is proportional to an individual's body weight, but a variety of other factors can affect how alcohol is metabolized. A genetic variation in a significant proportion of the Asian population alters the structure of an aldehyde hydrogenase isoenzyme, resulting in the development of an alcohol flush reaction, which includes facial flushing, hot sensations, tachycardia, and hypotension.

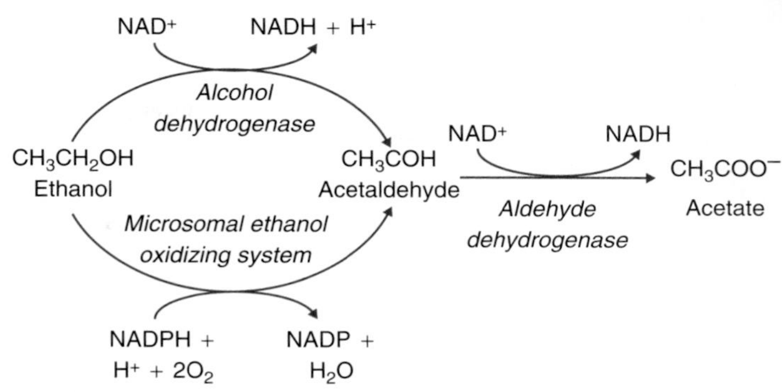

FIGURE 32-1. Ethanol metabolism. Alcohol dehydrogenase predominates at low to moderate ethanol doses. The microsomal ethanol-oxidizing system is induced at high ethanol levels of chronic exposure and by certain drugs. Aldehyde dehydrogenase inhibition (genetic or drug induced) leads to acetaldehyde accumulation.

In the brain, alcohol seems to affect a variety of receptors, including γ-aminobutyric acid (GABA), *N*-methyl-D-aspartate, and opioid receptors. Glycinuric and serotoninergic receptors also are thought to be involved in the interaction between alcohol and the brain. The phenomena of reinforcement and cellular adaptation are thought, at least in part, to influence alcohol-dependent behaviors. Alcohol is known to be reinforcing because withdrawal from ethanol and ingestion of ethanol itself are known to promote further alcohol consumption. After chronic exposure to alcohol, some brain neurons seem to adapt to this exposure by adjusting their response to normal stimuli. This adaptation is thought to be responsible for the phenomenon of tolerance, whereby increasing amounts of alcohol are needed over time to achieve desired effects. Although much has been learned about the variety of effects alcohol can have on various brain receptors, no single receptor site has been identified. A variety of neuropsychological disorders are seen in association with chronic ethanol use, including impaired short-term memory, cognitive dysfunction, and perceptual difficulties.

Although the brain is the primary target of alcohol's actions, a variety of other tissues have a major role in how alcohol affects the human body. Direct liver toxicity may be among the most important consequences of acute and chronic alcohol use (Chapter 155). A variety of histologic abnormalities ranging from inflammation to scarring and cirrhosis have been described. The pathophysiologic mechanism of these effects is thought to include the direct release of toxins and the formation of free radicals, which can interact negatively with liver proteins, lipids, and DNA. Alcohol also has substantial negative effects on the heart and cardiovascular system. Direct toxicity to myocardial cells frequently results in heart failure (Chapter 58), and chronic heavy alcohol consumption is considered to be a major contributor to hypertension (Chapter 67). Other organ systems that experience significant direct toxicity from alcohol include the gastrointestinal tract (esophagus, stomach), immune system (bone marrow, immune cell function), and endocrine system (pancreas, gonads).

CLINICAL MANIFESTATIONS

Alcohol has a variety of specific acute and chronic effects. The acute effects seen most commonly are alcohol intoxication and alcohol withdrawal. Chronic clinical effects of alcohol include almost every organ system.

Acute Effects

Alcohol Intoxication

After entering the blood stream, alcohol rapidly passes through the blood-brain barrier. The clinical manifestations of alcohol intoxication are related directly to the blood level of alcohol. Because of tolerance, individuals chronically exposed to alcohol generally experience less severe effects at a given blood alcohol level than do individuals who are not chronically exposed to alcohol.

The symptoms of mild alcohol intoxication in nontolerant individuals typically occur at blood alcohol levels of 20 to 100 mg/dL and include euphoria, mild muscle incoordination, and mild cognitive impairment. At higher blood alcohol levels (100 to 200 mg/dL), more substantial neurologic dysfunction occurs, including more severe mental impairment, ataxia, and prolonged reaction time. Individuals with blood alcohol levels in these ranges can be obviously intoxicated with slurred speech and lack of coordination.

These effects progress as the blood alcohol level rises to higher levels, to the point at which stupor, coma, and death can occur at levels equal to or greater than 300 to 400 mg/dL, especially in individuals who are nontolerant to the effects of alcohol. The usual cause of death in individuals with very high blood levels of alcohol is respiratory depression and hypotension.

Alcohol Withdrawal Syndrome

Alcohol withdrawal can occur when individuals decrease their alcohol use or stop using alcohol altogether. The severity of symptoms can vary greatly. Many individuals experience alcohol withdrawal without seeking medical attention, whereas others require hospitalization for severe illness. Because ethanol is a central nervous system depressant, the body's natural response to withdrawal of the substance is a hyperexcitable neurologic state. This state is thought to be the result of adaptive neurologic mechanisms being unrestrained by alcohol, with an ensuing release of a variety of neurohumoral substances, including norepinephrine. In addition, chronic exposure to alcohol results in a decrease in the number of GABA receptors and impairs their function.

The clinical manifestations of alcohol withdrawal include hyperactivity resulting in tachycardia and diaphoresis. Patients also experience tremulousness, anxiety, and insomnia. More severe alcohol withdrawal can result in nausea and vomiting, which can exacerbate metabolic disturbances. Perceptual abnormalities, including visual and auditory hallucinations and psychomotor agitation, are common manifestations of more moderate to severe alcohol withdrawal. Grand mal seizures commonly occur during alcohol withdrawal, although they do not generally require treatment beyond the acute withdrawal phase.

The time course of the alcohol withdrawal syndrome can vary within an individual and by symptom complex, and the overall duration of symptoms can be a few to several days (Fig. 32-2). Tremor is typically among the earliest symptoms and can occur within 8 hours of the last drink. Symptoms of tremulousness and motor hyperactivity typically peak within 24 to 48 hours. Although mild tremor typically involves the hands, more severe tremors can involve the entire body and greatly impair a variety of basic motor functions. Perceptual abnormalities typically begin within 24 to 36 hours after the last drink and resolve within a few days. When withdrawal seizures occur, they are typically generalized tonic-clonic seizures and most often occur within 12 to 24 hours after reduction of alcohol intake. Seizures can occur, however, at later time periods as well.

The most severe manifestation of the alcohol withdrawal syndrome is delirium tremens. This symptom complex includes disorientation, confusion, hallucination, diaphoresis, fever, and tachycardia. Delirium tremens typically begins after 2 to 4 days of abstinence, and the most severe form can result in death.

Chronic Effects

Acute manifestations, including intoxication and withdrawal, are generally stereotypical in their appearance and time course, but chronic manifestations tend to be more varied. Many patients with alcohol dependence may be without evidence of any chronic medical manifestations for many years. As time goes on, however, the likelihood that one or more of these manifestations will occur increases considerably. All major organ systems can be affected, but the primary organ systems involved are the nervous system, cardiovascular system, liver, gastrointestinal system, pancreas, hematopoietic system, and endocrine system (Table 32-2). Patients who drink are at risk for a variety of malignant neoplasms, such as head and neck, esophageal, and liver cancers (Chapters 196, 198, and 202). Excessive alcohol use often causes significant psychiatric and social morbidity that can be more common and more severe than the direct medical effects, especially earlier in the course of problem drinking.

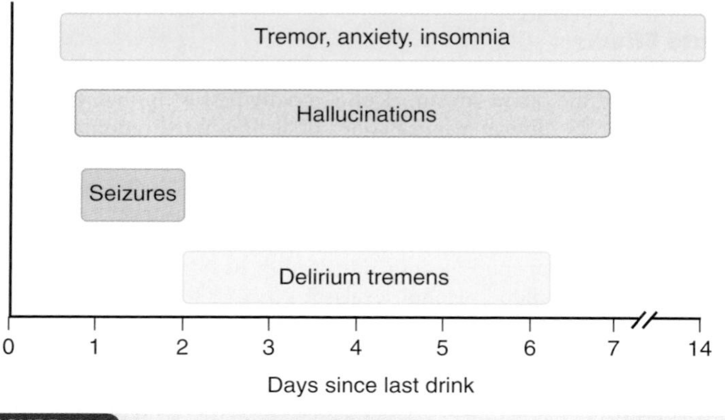

FIGURE 32-2. Time course of alcohol withdrawal.

Nervous System

In addition to the acute neurologic manifestations of intoxication and withdrawal, alcohol has major chronic neurologic effects. About 10 million Americans have identifiable nervous system impairment from chronic alcohol use. Individual predisposition to these disorders is highly variable and is related to genetics, environment, sociodemographic features, and gender; the relative contribution of these factors is unclear.

In the central nervous system, the major effect is cognitive impairment. Patients may present with mild to moderate short-term or long-term memory problems or may have severe dementia resembling Alzheimer's disease (Chapter 409). The degree to which the direct toxic effect of alcohol is responsible for these problems or the impact of alcohol-related nutritional deficiencies is uncertain (Chapter 425). The deficiency of vitamins such as thiamine may play a major role in promoting alcoholic dementia and severe cognitive dysfunction, as is seen in Korsakoff's syndrome. Alcohol also causes a polyneuropathy that can present with paresthesias, numbness, weakness, and chronic pain (Chapters 425 and 428). As with the central nervous system, peripheral nervous system effects are thought to be caused by a combination of the direct toxicity of alcohol and nutritional deficiencies. A small proportion (<1%) of patients with alcohol dependence may develop midline cerebellar degeneration, which presents as an unsteady gait.

Cardiovascular System

The most common cardiovascular complications of chronic alcohol consumption are cardiomyopathy, hypertension, and supraventricular arrhythmias. Alcoholic cardiomyopathy can present clinically in a manner similar to

TABLE 32-2 ALCOHOL-RELATED COMPLICATIONS

SYSTEM/REALM OF PROBLEM	COMPLICATIONS
Nervous system	Intoxication Withdrawal Cognitive impairment Cerebellar degeneration Peripheral neuropathy
Cardiovascular system	Cardiac arrhythmias Chronic cardiomyopathy Hypertension
Liver	Fatty liver Alcoholic hepatitis Cirrhosis
Gastrointestinal tract	
Esophagus	Chronic inflammation Malignant neoplasms Mallory-Weiss tears Esophageal varices
Stomach	Gastritis Peptic ulcer disease
Pancreas	Acute pancreatitis Chronic pancreatitis
Other medical problems	Cancers: mouth, oropharynx, esophagus Hepatoma Pneumonia Tuberculosis
Psychiatric	Depression Anxiety Suicide
Behavioral and psychosocial	Injuries Violence Crime Child or partner abuse Tobacco, other drug abuse Unemployment Legal problems

other causes of heart failure (Chapter 58). It is the most common cause of nonischemic cardiomyopathy in Western countries, accounting for about 45% of cases. Like these other causes, alcoholic cardiomyopathy also responds to conventional treatments of heart failure (Chapter 59). Abstinence from alcohol can result in significant improvement in cardiomyopathy in some patients. Increasing levels of alcohol consumption also are associated with increasing levels of systolic and diastolic hypertension (Chapter 67).

The most common arrhythmias associated with chronic alcohol use include atrial fibrillation and supraventricular tachycardia; these are seen commonly in the setting of acute intoxication and withdrawal (Chapter 64). The prevalence of alcohol-induced arrhythmias is unclear. Alcoholic cardiomyopathy also is associated with arrhythmias, in particular, ventricular arrhythmias (Chapter 65).

Liver

Alcohol abuse is the major cause of morbidity and mortality from liver disease in the United States. It has been estimated that there are more than 2 million people with known alcoholic liver disease in the United States. Factors that predispose to early liver disease include the quantity and duration of alcohol exposure, female gender, and malnutrition. The range of clinical manifestations includes acute fatty liver, alcoholic hepatitis, and cirrhosis (Chapter 156). Fatty liver associated with alcohol ingestion can be asymptomatic or associated with nonspecific abdominal discomfort; it generally improves with abstinence from alcohol. Alcoholic hepatitis can present as an asymptomatic condition identified through abnormalities in liver enzymes or as an acute episode with abdominal pain, nausea, vomiting, and fever. Patients with alcoholic hepatitis have particularly high levels of aspartate aminotransferase in the blood and elevated levels of γ-glutamyltransferase. Alcoholic hepatitis typically improves with abstinence from alcohol.

Alcohol-related cirrhosis is a major cause of death in the United States (Chapter 157). Although patients are often asymptomatic, patients with more advanced cirrhosis may present with a variety of symptoms and signs, including jaundice, ascites, and coagulopathy. Cirrhosis also is associated with gastrointestinal bleeding from esophageal varices (Chapter 140). Although there is some controversy about the use of liver transplantation to treat patients with alcoholic cirrhosis, many believe that patients in established recovery are good candidates for liver transplantation (Chapter 157).

Gastrointestinal Disease

Chronic alcohol use is associated with a variety of esophageal problems, including esophageal varices, Mallory-Weiss tears, and squamous cell carcinoma of the esophagus. The risk of squamous cell carcinoma is increased further in patients who smoke tobacco and drink alcohol. Patients with these problems can present with difficulty swallowing, chest pain, gastrointestinal blood loss, and weight loss. Acute alcoholic gastritis typically presents with abdominal discomfort, nausea, and vomiting (Chapter 137).

Pancreas

The risk of pancreatitis in individuals with alcohol dependence is approximately four times that in the general population. Quantity and duration of alcohol exposure and a history of pancreatitis are predictive of future episodes. Acute alcoholic pancreatitis, which may present with severe abdominal pain, nausea, vomiting, fever, and hypotension, can be life-threatening (Chapter 146). Individuals who have recurrent acute pancreatitis may develop chronic pancreatitis, which typically presents with chronic abdominal pain, malabsorption, weight loss, and malnutrition.

Hematopoietic System

The anemia that commonly is seen in patients with chronic alcohol problems can be multifactorial (e.g., blood loss, nutrient deficiency, secondary to liver disease and hypersplenism). Studies of selected inpatients with alcohol dependence showed the prevalence of anemia to range from about 10 to 60%. Gastrointestinal blood loss due to Mallory-Weiss tears (Chapter 137), alcoholic gastritis (Chapter 134), or esophageal varices (Chapters 137 and 156) may be a key factor, and many patients develop subsequent iron deficiency. Dietary folate deficiency can be associated with megaloblastic anemias (Chapter 167). Alcohol also has a direct toxic effect on the bone marrow, which can lead to sideroblastic anemia that resolves after abstinence. Alcohol can suppress megakaryocyte production and cause thrombocytopenia, which may manifest as petechiae or bleeding (Chapter 175); the thrombocytopenia is particularly sensitive to abstinence, with platelet counts usually rebounding or returning to normal within 5 to 7 days after cessation of alcohol intake. Alcohol also appears to interfere directly with platelet function. Alcohol-related immune dysfunction, as evidenced by decreased production and function of white blood cells and derangement in humoral and cell-mediated immunity, partly explains why alcohol-dependent individuals are at higher risk for infectious diseases, such as pneumonia and tuberculosis.

Malignant Neoplasms

Alcohol intake has been associated with upper digestive, respiratory, and liver malignant neoplasms. Alcohol use is associated with squamous cell carcinomas of the esophagus (Chapter 198) and of the head and neck (Chapter 196). The co-occurrence of alcohol and tobacco abuse seems to be synergistic. Either heavy alcohol use or smoking individually increases the rate of oropharyngeal cancer by about six or seven times that of the general population, whereas the rate for people with both risk factors is about 40 times that of the general population. Patients with alcohol-induced liver disease who also have a history of hepatitis B or C are at particularly increased risk for hepatocellular carcinoma (Chapter 202).

Chronic alcohol use also has been associated with malignant neoplasms of the breast (Chapter 204), prostate (Chapter 207), pancreas (Chapter 200), cervix (Chapter 205), lung (Chapter 197), and colon (Chapter 199). Women who have more than one or two alcoholic drinks per day may increase their breast cancer risk 1.5-fold or more. Hormonal mechanisms and direct carcinogenic effects of alcohol have been postulated as causes of this association. The association of cervical cancer with alcohol dependence may be due to alcohol-associated high-risk sexual behaviors that are thought to increase the risk of cervical cancer.

Other Medical Issues

Gout has been associated with alcohol abuse, and flares can occur at lower serum urate levels than in nonalcoholic patients (Chapter 281). Alcoholic ketoacidosis (Chapter 120), which usually follows an alcoholic binge, presents as nausea, vomiting, abdominal pain, and volume depletion. Typically, ketoacidosis is seen with low or normal glucose readings. Mild or nonspecific abnormalities in thyroid function, especially in patients with underlying liver disease, may reflect abnormalities in the clearance of thyroid-stimulating hormone or the impact of elevated circulating estrogens. Infertility and menstrual irregularities have been associated with chronic alcohol consumption, presumably due to alcohol-induced hypothalamic-pituitary dysfunction, gonadal toxicity, and impaired hepatic metabolism of circulating hormones. Hypogonadism is highly prevalent in male alcoholics with cirrhosis. Alcohol dependence also is associated with higher rates of dental and periodontal disease (Chapter 433) and with a variety of dermatologic problems, including spider angiomas and, in patients with poor hygiene, skin infestations. Both at-risk drinking and alcohol dependence have been shown to be associated with an increased risk of hospital-acquired infections, sepsis, and mortality, especially in intensive care patients.

Psychiatric Issues

Psychiatric symptoms and illnesses are exceedingly common among individuals with alcohol problems. The prevalence of anxiety disorders is about 40%, and the prevalence of affective disorders is about 30%. Antisocial personality disorder is also more common in individuals with alcohol problems than in the general population. These psychiatric problems are more prevalent during periods of heavy drinking and withdrawal. All patients with alcohol use disorders require careful screening for psychiatric illnesses. Effective treatment of underlying psychiatric disorders may result in improved drinking behaviors.

Other Behavioral and Psychosocial Issues

Alcohol commonly is the underlying cause of domestic abuse, injuries, trauma, motor vehicle crashes, and burns. Patients presenting with injuries should be questioned carefully about their alcohol use. Tobacco (Chapter 31) and other drug abuse (Chapter 33) is more prevalent in people with alcohol problems than in the general population.

DIAGNOSIS

Data from the history, physical examination, and laboratory generally are needed to provide a complete picture of the extent of alcohol problems in affected patients (Table 32-3).

TABLE 32-3 DIAGNOSIS OF ALCOHOL PROBLEMS

HISTORY
Step 1: Ask all patients about current and past use.
Do you drink alcohol (ever or currently)?
Do you have a family history of alcohol problems?
Step 2: Obtain detailed history regarding quantity and frequency of alcohol use.
What types of alcohol do you consume?
How often do you drink?
How much do you usually drink?
Do you ever drink more, and if so, how much?
Step 3: Standardized questionnaire
CAGE questions:
Have you ever felt that you should *c*ut down on your drinking?
Have people *a*nnoyed you by criticizing your drinking?
Have you ever felt bad or *g*uilty about drinking?
Have you ever taken a drink first thing in the morning (*e*ye opener) to steady your nerves or get rid of a hangover?
Step 4: Assess specific areas in suspected or known problem drinkers.
Criteria for alcohol abuse and dependence
Evidence of medical and psychiatric problems
Evidence of behavioral or social problems
Use of other substances
Tobacco
Mood-altering prescription drugs
Illicit drugs (e.g., heroin, cocaine)
Prior alcohol or substance abuse treatment
PHYSICAL EXAMINATION
Thorough and complete examination important in all patients
Focus attention to system with identified problems
In all patients, carefully examine
Central and peripheral nervous systems
Cardiovascular system
Liver
Gastrointestinal tract
LABORATORY STUDIES (IN SELECTED PATIENTS)
Liver enzymes
Coagulation studies
Complete blood count
Carbohydrate-deficient transferrin

Discussing the Diagnosis with Patients

In discussing alcohol problems, it is crucial that physicians be sensitive to the stigma and shame that may be felt by patients with alcohol problems and by their families. Alcohol-related diagnoses or problems should be discussed in a nonjudgmental manner, which forges a partnership and indicates commitment to helping with whatever problems the patients might have. Setting the stage for the discussion should include educating patients about the various levels of alcohol problems (e.g., at-risk drinking, alcohol abuse, alcohol dependence) so that patients have an understanding of the spectrum of alcohol problems. Many patients may have a skewed view of what qualifies as problem drinking and may believe that only individuals with severe alcohol problems are truly problem drinkers. The history, physical examination, and laboratory studies should be provided as "proof" that a problem may or does exist.

History

A four-step approach to the alcohol history includes comprehensive questions about alcohol use and a thorough evaluation for alcohol-related problems.

Step 1: Ask All Patients about Current and Past Alcohol Use

A single question—Do you currently or have you ever used alcohol?—can identify quickly patients who are not lifetime abstainers and require further screening. Patients who answer yes to this question should proceed through the subsequent three steps. Patients who answer no can be classified as lifetime abstainers from alcohol and require no further questioning unless their answer changes over time. It is crucial to ask about current and past alcohol use because many patients who meet lifetime criteria for alcohol dependence but who are currently in recovery answer no to the question about current use; unless it is specifically asked about, important past use information may be missed.

Step 2: Obtain Detailed History Regarding Quantity and Frequency of Alcohol Use

A question to be asked routinely is, What type or types of alcoholic drinks (beer, wine, spirits) do you consume? Many patients do not consider the use of beer or wine "drinking." Quantity should be determined for typical use—How much do you usually drink on a typical drinking day?—and for range of use—Do you ever drink more than your usual amount, and if so, how much? This second question can be particularly important for identifying binge drinking. Quantity questions offer easy identification of at-risk drinking. Asking about the frequency of alcohol consumption—How often do you drink?—helps distinguish daily from nondaily alcohol users. Binge drinkers who drink only on weekends tend to have significant alcohol problems yet not be daily drinkers. A major goal of step 2 is to acquire a complete characterization of current alcohol use behaviors and the pattern of quantity and frequency of alcohol use during the patient's lifetime.

Step 3: Use Standardized Screening Instruments

Many standardized questionnaires have been developed to detect alcohol abuse and dependence. The two questionnaires that have been evaluated most extensively in medical settings are the CAGE (Cut down, Annoyed, Guilty, and Eye opener) questionnaire (see Table 32-3) and the Alcohol Use Disorder Identification Test (AUDIT). The CAGE questionnaire includes four questions and is scored by giving 1 point for each positive response. Given that the word *ever* is used in the CAGE questions, by definition this instrument is designed to detect lifetime alcohol problems and does not distinguish between lifetime problems and current problems. To screen for alcohol abuse and dependence, the CAGE has a sensitivity of 43 to 94% and a specificity of 70 to 97% when a cutoff score of 2 is used to indicate a "positive" result.

The AUDIT's ten questions cover the quantity and frequency of alcohol use, drinking behaviors, adverse psychological symptoms, and alcohol-related problems. It was developed by the World Health Organization to identify hazardous (e.g., at-risk) drinking and harmful (e.g., alcohol use that results in physical or psychological harm) drinking. In contrast to the CAGE questionnaire, the AUDIT focuses on recent (current to past year) drinking behaviors. Each question is scored 0 to 4 (range for total score is 0 to 40), and a total score of 8 is considered to be a positive result.

Step 4: Assess Specific Areas in Suspected or Known Problem Drinkers

Questions asked in step 4 are based on the results of the questions asked in steps 2 and 3 to obtain more detailed information in patients with potential alcohol problems. Even patients who do not screen positive on the CAGE questionnaire may warrant detailed questioning about alcohol abuse and dependence (see Table 32-1), especially if they are drinking at or above at-risk levels or there is other evidence of possible alcohol problems. A detailed review for evidence of alcohol-related medical and psychiatric problems should occur, and the need for further medical and psychiatric evaluation should be determined. The physician should look for evidence of behavioral and social problems commonly associated with alcohol use and screen for family and occupational dysfunction and other problems, such as domestic violence. Patients should be asked about their use of tobacco, mood-altering prescription medications, and illicit drugs such as heroine and cocaine.

Finally, many patients with alcohol problems have prior treatment episodes that should be detailed. The inquiry should include questions not only about formal alcohol treatment (including number of episodes, duration of treatment, and inpatient versus outpatient treatment) but also about more informal treatments, such as attendance at self-help groups like Alcoholics Anonymous (AA). For patients who require a referral for treatment, knowledge of prior treatment experience is a crucial determinant of future referral recommendations.

The National Institute on Alcohol Abuse and Alcoholism has published *Helping Patients Who Drink Too Much: A Clinician's Guide,* which provides a similar approach to screening and evaluating patients for alcohol-related problems and includes an appendix of useful supporting materials.

Physical Examination

Patients with potential alcohol use disorders require a detailed physical examination to complement the history. In addition, attention should be focused on detecting common alcohol-related problems, including the nervous system, cardiovascular system, liver, and gastrointestinal system (see Table 32-2).

Laboratory Findings

A variety of laboratory tests have been proposed to aid screening for alcoholic abuse and dependence. Aminotransferase levels, red blood cells, mean corpuscular volume, and carbohydrate-deficient transferrin, alone or in combination, are not as effective as screening questionnaires, such as the CAGE and the AUDIT.

Laboratory tests do have a role in diagnosis and assessment of patients with potential alcohol problems. Routine laboratory testing including liver enzymes (Chapter 149), bilirubin, complete blood count, and prothrombin time should be obtained in all patients with alcohol problems on a regular basis so that an appropriate and complete picture of the effects of alcohol on the individual can be obtained.

PROGNOSIS

Alcohol abuse and dependence are chronic disorders that are characterized by exacerbations and remissions. The prognosis is better for patients who seek treatment and receive it in a systematic way (Table 32-6), but it can be poor for patients with advanced liver disease and continued alcohol use. In addition, the use of combinations of medications (e.g., naltrexone plus acamprosate) is under investigation.

PREVENTION AND TREATMENT

The relationship of change in alcohol use with prevention of subsequent problems has been well established. Treatment of alcohol use disorders should be based on the severity of potential or actual alcohol problems and tailored to meet the needs of individual patients. Separate advice and management approaches are suggested for nondependent at-risk or problem drinkers compared with individuals who are alcohol dependent (Table 32-4).

Treatment of At-Risk Drinkers

Evidence confirms that generalist physicians, in a cost-effective manner, can help patients reduce their alcohol intake and prevent subsequent alcohol-related problems by using brief (5 to 20 minutes), focused counseling techniques (brief interventions) that are well suited for primary care and other medical settings. The brief counseling strategy includes four main components: motivational techniques, feedback about the problems with alcohol use, discussion of the adverse effects of alcohol, and setting recommended drinking limits. Motivational techniques are designed to motivate patients to change their alcohol use behavior by identifying potential or actual problems with which their alcohol use is associated. Feedback about these problems can make it clear to the patient that the problems exist. For at-risk and problem drinkers who do not meet criteria for alcohol dependence, setting recommended drinking limits below at-risk levels (e.g., less than one drink per day for women and less than two drinks per day for men) is a realistic and suitable goal. Epidemiologic evidence suggests that drinking below these levels is less likely to be associated with problems. Several randomized clinical trials confirm that patients who receive brief interventions significantly decrease their alcohol intake, often to "safe" levels, and can decrease health care use as well.

Treatment of Alcohol Dependence

Patients who meet criteria for alcohol dependence typically require more intensive services than do patients who meet criteria for at-risk drinking. Most patients can be managed in outpatient treatment settings, whereas patients with more severe alcohol dependence or comorbid problems initially may require inpatient management, specific counseling programs, and pharmacologic therapy. Before entering a formal program to maintain remission, many patients first require medical management of alcohol withdrawal. Professional organizations have published practice guidelines that provide useful recommendations for how to select among treatment options for patients with alcohol dependence.

Management of Alcohol Withdrawal

Many patients may not present for medical management of alcohol withdrawal and deal with it on their own. However, a substantial subset do present for alcohol withdrawal treatment. Patients with mild to moderate withdrawal generally can be managed safely as outpatients with close follow-up. Patients with moderate to severe withdrawal, as manifested by hypertension, tremor, and any mental status changes, especially patients with significant comorbid medical or psychiatric illnesses, generally are treated best as inpatients. Patients who have a history of severe withdrawal in the past (e.g., delirium tremens) or who have a history of alcohol withdrawal seizures also generally should be managed as inpatients. The three major goals of medical management of alcohol withdrawal are to minimize the severity of withdrawal-related symptoms; to prevent specific withdrawal-related complications, such as seizures and delirium tremens; and to provide referral to relapse prevention treatment.

A wide variety of medications have been evaluated for their effectiveness in managing the alcohol withdrawal syndrome (Table 32-5). Longer-acting benzodiazepines are preferred because they provide a smoother withdrawal. Shorter-acting benzodiazepines, such as oxazepam, may be indicated in individuals with severe liver disease. The most common approach is to administer a standing dose of a benzodiazepine, with additional medication being given "as needed" on the basis of withdrawal symptoms. The specific benzodiazepine and dose often depend on the experience of the prescribing physician and the characteristics of the patient, including the severity of withdrawal (higher doses are used if withdrawal is more severe), the presence of liver disease (patients with severe liver disease should receive lower doses or shorter-acting medications), and the response to prior doses of medication (higher doses are given if symptom control is inadequate; lower doses are given if adverse effects, such as oversedation, have occurred). In general, the amount of medication per dosing period is decreased gradually as the withdrawal syndrome abates. An individualized "symptom-triggered" dosing approach, in which benzodiazepines are administered on a dose-by-dose basis as guided by withdrawal symptoms, is safe and effective in certain patients and can reduce the total doses of benzodiazepines needed to treat withdrawal. β-Blockers (atenolol and propranolol), α-agonists (clonidine), and antiepileptics (carbamazepine) improve signs and symptoms of alcohol withdrawal but are viewed best as adjunctive medications to be used in addition to benzodiazepines.

Prevention of Relapse

Counseling Strategies Used by Alcohol Treatment Programs

Three commonly used psychotherapeutic techniques are motivational enhancement therapy, 12-step facilitation, and cognitive-behavioral coping skills. Two of these techniques are designed to give patients specific tools to help them avoid relapse to alcohol use. In motivational enhancement therapy, patients identify reasons for staying away from alcohol. The 12-step facilitation therapy uses the principles of AA to help patients focus their attention on abstinence. In cognitive-behavioral coping skills therapy, the patient identifies triggers to alcohol use and develops strategies to help deal with the triggers when they are present.

Project MATCH (Matching Alcohol Treatments to Client Heterogenicity) showed equivalence among three counseling approaches (cognitive-behavioral coping skills therapy, motivational enhancement therapy, or 12-step facilitation therapy) to treat alcohol dependence. At 1-year follow-up, most enrolled patients either remained abstinent or significantly decreased their alcohol use.

Self-Help Groups

Self-help groups such as AA and Rational Recovery are an important source of support and treatment for many patients with alcohol dependence. AA has

TABLE 32-4 ADVICE FOR PATIENTS WITH ALCOHOL PROBLEMS

State your medical concern:
Be specific about your patient's drinking patterns and related health risks.
Ask: How do you feel about your drinking?

Agree on a plan of action:
Ask: Are you ready to try to cut down or abstain?
Talk with patients who are ready to make a change in their drinking about a specific plan of action.

For patients who are not alcohol dependent:
Advise the patient to cut down if drinking is at or above at-risk drinking amounts (see Table 32-1) and there is no evidence of alcohol dependence.
Ask the patient to set a specific drinking goal: Are you ready to set a drinking goal? Some patients choose to abstain for a period of time or for good; others prefer to limit the amount they drink. What do you think will work best for you?
Provide patient education materials and tell the patient: It helps to think about your reasons for wanting to cut down and examine what situations trigger unhealthy drinking patterns. These materials will give you some useful tips on how to maintain your drinking goal.

For patients with evidence of alcohol dependence:
Advise to abstain if:
- Evidence of alcohol dependence
- History of repeated failed attempts to cut down
- Pregnant or trying to conceive
- Contraindicated medical condition or medication

Refer for additional diagnostic evaluation or treatment.
Procedures for patient in making referral decisions:
- Involve your patient in making referral decisions.
- Discuss available alcohol treatment services.
- Schedule a referral appointment while the patient is in the office.

TABLE 32-5 MEDICATIONS FOR THE TREATMENT OF ALCOHOL DEPENDENCE*

MEDICATION	DOSE AND ROUTE	FREQUENCY	EFFECTS	MAJOR COMMON ADVERSE EFFECTS
ALCOHOL WITHDRAWAL				
Benzodiazepines[‡]				
Chlordiazepoxide* Diazepam[†] Oxazepam[†] Lorazepam[†]	25-100 mg, PO/IV/IM[‡] 5-10 mg, PO/IV/IM[‡] 15-30 mg, PO[‡] 1-4 mg, PO/IV/IM[‡]	Every 4-6 hr Every 6-8 hr Every 6-8 hr Every 4-8 hr	Decreased severity of withdrawal; stabilization of vital signs; prevention of seizures and delirium tremens	Confusion, oversedation, respiratory depression
β-Blockers				
Atenolol Propranolol	25-50 mg, PO 10-40 mg, PO	Once a day Every 6-8 hr	Improvement in vital signs Reduction in craving	Bradycardia, hypotension
α-Agonists				
Clonidine	0.1-0.2 mg, PO	Every 6 hr	Decreased withdrawal symptoms	Hypotension, fatigue
Antiepileptics				
Carbamazepine	200 mg, PO	Every 6-8 hr	Decreased severity of withdrawal; prevention of seizures	Dizziness, fatigue, red blood cell abnormalities
PREVENTION OF RELAPSE				
Disulfiram[†]	125-500 mg, PO	Daily	Decreased alcohol use among those who relapse	Disulfiram-alcohol reaction, rash, drowsiness, peripheral neuropathy
Naltrexone[†]	50 mg, PO 380 mg, IM	Daily Every 4 wk	Increased abstinence, decreased drinking days	Nausea, abdominal pain, myalgias-arthralgias
Acamprosate[†]	666 mg, PO	Three times a day	Increased abstinence	Diarrhea

*Most commonly used medications listed.
[†]Currently approved by U.S. Food and Drug Administration for the indication noted.
[‡]Dose and routes given for standard fixed-dose regimens, which include dose tapers over time.

TABLE 32-6 OVERVIEW OF TREATMENT APPROACH FOR PATIENTS WITH ALCOHOL PROBLEMS

Evaluate all patients
- For patterns of problem alcohol use (Table 32-1)
- For alcohol-related complications, if indicated (Table 32-2)
- With use of data collected from history, physical examination, and laboratory testing (Table 32-3)

For at-risk and nondependent problem drinkers
- Advise to decrease alcohol use to below at-risk levels (Table 32-4)
- Advise patients who cannot decrease use to below at-risk levels to abstain

For patients who are alcohol dependent
- Assess for need for withdrawal management medications (Table 32-5)
- Refer to an alcohol treatment program
- Consider medication to prevent relapse (Table 32-5)

the advantage of being widely available throughout the United States and is free of charge. The overall approach to treatment is based on the 12 steps for maintaining abstinence and dealing with the various effects of alcohol. AA meetings can be either "open" to anybody in the community or "closed" for active members only. The meetings vary in format, size, location, and demographic makeup. In counseling patients about attending AA, it is important for physicians to make them aware that variations in the nature of specific meetings, especially location and demographics of participants, require patients to be willing to attend more than one meeting site on a trial basis so that they find a comfortable setting.

Research of the effectiveness of AA has been limited, and there are no large controlled studies. Indirect evidence suggests, however, a significant improvement in alcohol use behaviors.

Pharmacotherapy to Prevent Relapse to Alcohol Use

The addition of medication to enhance the effectiveness of counseling therapies has been the subject of research for the past 40 years. As the neurobiology of alcohol use disorders has become more clearly understood, the potential to develop medications that may promote abstinence or decreased alcohol use has grown. Three medications—disulfiram, naltrexone, and acamprosate—are approved for the treatment of alcohol dependence in the United States[1] (see Table 32-5).

Disulfiram

Disulfiram is designed to prevent alcohol use by causing a severe adverse reaction when patients use alcohol. The disulfiram reaction, which includes flushing, nausea, vomiting, and diarrhea, is mediated by the inhibition of alcohol dehydrogenase and the resulting increase in serum levels of acetaldehyde and acetate after ingestion of alcohol. Disulfiram also affects monoamine metabolism, and the alcohol-disulfiram reaction may be related to changes in central monoamine functioning. Although disulfiram offers little benefit to most patients, it is effective in reducing alcohol intake in highly motivated patients who are supervised in an alcohol treatment program.

Naltrexone

Naltrexone is thought to decrease alcohol use by diminishing the euphorigenic effects of alcohol and by decreasing craving in alcohol-dependent patients. Randomized, placebo-controlled trials generally have shown that alcohol-dependent patients who receive naltrexone (50 mg/day) are more likely to decrease their alcohol use or remain abstinent compared with patients who receive placebo,[2] and the effects persist after discontinuation of treatment, although one randomized trial did not show benefit in male veterans with severe alcohol dependence. Although most studies of naltrexone were performed in a specialty alcohol treatment setting and observed subjects for only 10 to 12 weeks, one study demonstrated that naltrexone can be effective in primary care settings in patients who were observed for up to 34 weeks.[3] Side effects of naltrexone are infrequent, most notably self-limited nausea in about 10% of patients. Dose-related hepatotoxicity has been reported in patients treated for obesity with high-dose naltrexone (300 mg/day). Mild liver enzyme abnormalities are not a contraindication to naltrexone, but patients should be followed with repeated liver enzyme studies. Patients with acute hepatitis or liver failure should not use naltrexone. In addition to the oral naltrexone, a newer long-acting injectable form of naltrexone was approved by the U.S. Food and Drug Administration (FDA) in 2006.[4] Injectable naltrexone is typically administered at a dose of 380 mg intramuscularly every 4 weeks. Before beginning naltrexone, it is important to be sure that the patient is not opioid dependent in order to avoid a potentially severe opioid withdrawal reaction. Complete opioid abstinence for at least 7 to 10 days is recommended. Adverse reactions seen most commonly in patients who receive injectable naltrexone include injection site reactions (e.g., induration, itching) and symptoms such as nausea and headache, which are generally self-limited.

Acamprosate

Approved by the FDA in 2004, acamprosate (calcium acetylhomotaurinate) has been identified as an effective agent for treatment of alcohol dependence. The precise mechanism of action of acamprosate is uncertain, but it may be related to its effects on neuroexcitatory amino acids and the inhibitory GABA system. In a randomized, placebo-controlled clinical trial, subjects who received acamprosate were more likely to remain abstinent compared with subjects who received placebo.[5] Side effects are minimal and typically include diarrhea. Like naltrexone, acamprosate is given as an adjunctive therapy to psychological treatments for alcohol dependence.

Other Pharmacologic Approaches to Prevent Relapse

There has been much interest in evaluation of the effectiveness of combinations of drug therapies to treat alcohol dependence. One study of 160 patients suggested that the combination of naltrexone and acamprosate was more effective than either medication alone. A larger federally funded study that enrolled 1383 subjects, Project COMBINE, examined naltrexone and acamprosate alone and in combination with two different psychological therapies to see which combination of pharmacologic and behavioral therapies is most effective.[6] The behavioral therapies were medical management, which was designed to approximate counseling that can be provided in primary care and other medical settings, and combined behavioral intervention, which incorporated counseling techniques that are provided in alcohol treatment specialty settings. Results from this study demonstrated that patients receiving medical management with naltrexone, combined behavioral intervention, or both fared best, lending further support to the idea that alcohol-dependent patients can be effectively treated in primary care and other medical settings. Interestingly, acamprosate was not shown to be effective in this study.

Topiramate, a fructopyranose derivative, has been shown to be an effective treatment of alcohol dependence in randomized clinical trials at a dose of up to 300 mg/day.[7] Other medications that have shown promise include ondansetron, bromocriptine, and sodium valproate. Other drugs have shown possible benefits in patients with concurrent depression (e.g., fluoxetine) or anxiety (e.g., buspirone) or no effect (e.g., lithium).

FUTURE DIRECTIONS

To date, most studies have focused on shorter-term outcomes, from a few months to a year. It is important to understand more clearly what happens to these patients over time, especially the need for "booster sessions" to sustain improvements provided by brief interventions. Newer pharmacologic therapies may help many patients.

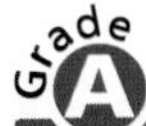

1. Laaksonen E, Koski-Jannes A, Salaspuro M, et al. A randomized, multicentre, open-label, comparative trial of disulfiram, naltrexone and acamprosate in the treatment of alcohol dependence. *Alcohol Alcohol.* 2008;43:53-61.
2. Rösner S, Hackl-Herrwerth A, Leucht S, et al. Opioid antagonists for alcohol dependence. *Cochrane Database Syst Rev.* 2010;12:CD001867.
3. O'Malley SS, Rounsaville BJ, Farren C, et al. Initial and maintenance naltrexone treatment for alcohol dependence using primary care vs specialty care: a nested sequence of 3 randomized trials. *Arch Intern Med.* 2003;163:1695-1704.
4. Garbutt JC, Kranzler HR, O'Malley SS, et al, for the Vivitrex Study Group. Efficacy and tolerability of long-acting injectable naltrexone for alcohol dependence: a randomized controlled trial. *JAMA.* 2005;293:1617-1625.
5. Rösner S, Hackl-Herrwerth A, Leucht S, et al. Acamprosate for alcohol dependence. *Cochrane Database Syst Rev.* 2010;9:CD004332.
6. Anton RF, O'Malley SS, Ciraulo, DA, et al, for the COMBINE Study Research Group. Combined pharmacotherapies and behavioral interventions for alcohol dependence. The COMBINE study: a randomized controlled trial. *JAMA.* 2006;295:2003-2017.
7. Flórez G, Saiz PA, Garcia-Portilla P, et al. Topiramate for the treatment of alcohol dependence: comparison with naltrexone. *Eur Addict Res.* 2011;17:29-36.

SUGGESTED READINGS

Amato L, Minozzi S, Vecchi S, et al. Benzodiazepines for alcohol withdrawal. *Cochrane Database Syst Rev.* 2010;3:CD005063. *Benzodiazepines protect against alcohol withdrawal symptoms, especially seizure.*

Johnson BA. Medication treatment of different types of alcoholism. *Am J Psychiatry.* 2010;6:630-639. *Review.*

Minozzi S, Amato L, Vecchi S, et al. Anticonvulsants for alcohol withdrawal. *Cochrane Database Syst Rev.* 2010;3:CD005064. *Anticonvulsants have no obvious benefit for treating alcohol withdrawal.*

Saitz R. Alcohol screening and brief intervention in primary care: absence of evidence for efficacy in people with dependence or very heavy drinking. *Drug Alcohol Rev.* 2010;29:631-640. *These interventions are disappointingly ineffective.*

Schuckit MA. Alcohol-use disorders. *Lancet.* 2009;373:492-501. *Review of diagnosis and treatment, emphasizing importance of clinicians routinely screening for alcohol disorders.*

Zarkin GA, Bray JW, Aldridge A, et al. The effect of alcohol treatment on social costs of alcohol dependence: results from the COMBINE study. *Med Care.* 2010;48:396-401. *Combined pharmacotherapies and behavioral intervention are a cost-savings strategy for patients who are alcohol dependent.*

33 DRUG ABUSE AND DEPENDENCE

ROGER D. WEISS

DEFINITION

The terms *drug abuse* and *drug dependence* refer to a clinical syndrome characterized by the following statement from the fourth edition of the American Psychiatric Association's *Diagnostic and Statistical Manual of Mental Disorders*: "The essential feature of dependence is a cluster of cognitive, behavioral, and physiological symptoms indicating that the individual continues substance use despite significant substance-related problems." There is no single pathognomonic symptom that is diagnostic of drug dependence. Rather, the syndrome of drug dependence as described in the text above is a series of seven symptoms, of which the individual needs to meet three in the same 12-month period to warrant a diagnosis of dependence (Table 33-1). Several points are important to keep in mind when considering the diagnosis of drug dependence.

The criteria for the diagnosis are the same regardless of the substance used. Thus, the criteria for opioid dependence are the same as those for nicotine dependence and cocaine dependence, although different drugs are more likely to produce different symptoms.

The diagnostic term *drug dependence* should only be used with people whose drug use is problematic; tolerance and physical dependence are neither necessary nor sufficient for a diagnosis of drug dependence. If someone is using legitimately prescribed medications as intended (e.g., opioids for chronic pain or benzodiazepines for panic disorder), and those medications are helping the person to function better, that person will not meet criteria for drug dependence, even if the person is tolerant to the medication and is physically dependent.

Finally, the 5th edition of the American Psychiatric Association's *Diagnostic and Statistical Manual of Mental Disorders* may no longer distinguish between abuse and dependence, using the term *substance abuse disorder* instead. However, that decision has not yet been finalized.

EPIDEMIOLOGY

Use of illicit drugs and nonmedical use of prescribed drugs is quite common. In 2009, approximately 22 million Americans reported using an illicit drug in

TABLE 33-1 DIAGNOSTIC CRITERIA FOR DRUG DEPENDENCE AND DRUG ABUSE

"A maladaptive pattern of substance use, leading to clinically significant impairment or distress."

DEPENDENCE (≥3 IN 12-MONTH PERIOD)

1. Tolerance
2. Withdrawal
3. The substance is often taken in larger amounts for a longer period than intended
4. Unsuccessful efforts or a persistent desire to cut down or to control substance use
5. A great deal of time is spent in activities necessary to obtain the substance or to recover from its effects
6. Important social, occupational, or recreational activities given up or reduced because of substance use
7. Continued substance use despite knowledge of having had persistent or recurrent physical or psychological problems that are likely to be caused or exacerbated by the substance

ABUSE (≥1 IN A 12-MONTH PERIOD)

1. Recurrent substance use resulting in failure to fulfill major role obligations at work, school, or home
2. Recurrent substance use in situations in which it is physically hazardous
3. Recurrent substance-related legal problems
4. Continued substance use despite having persistent or recurrent social or interpersonal problems caused or exacerbated by the effects of the substance

and

Never met criteria for dependence

From American Psychiatric Association. *Diagnostic and Statistical Manual of Mental Disorders*, 4th ed. Washington DC: American Psychiatric Association; 1994.

the previous month, representing approximately 9% of the population: when asked about their substance use in the past month, 17 million people reported using marijuana, 7 million reported using potentially psychoactive prescription drugs nonmedically, 2 million people used cocaine, and 1 million people used hallucinogens; in fact, 10% of youths aged 12 to 17 years reported using an illicit drug in the past month. Drug abuse produces substantial medical morbidity and mortality as well as tremendous social and economic costs.

PATHOBIOLOGY

Drug abuse and dependence are complex disorders involving the interaction between the pharmacology of a specific drug, an individual's genetic makeup, psychological strengths and weaknesses, environmental circumstances, and societal influences such as physical and perceived drug availability, legal status and cost of the drug, religious and cultural mores, and presence of alternative rewarding activities. Thus, one can conceptualize the etiology of drug abuse by employing the public health model frequently cited when studying infectious disease, that is, as an interaction among the host (i.e., the potential drug user), the agent (a specific drug in this case, as opposed to an infectious microorganism), and the environment (the person's family life, peer group, and the social, cultural, and religious attitudes toward use of that substance).

The Host

A host factor that is well known to heighten vulnerability to drug abuse problems is a positive family history of a substance use disorder, which has been shown to increase the likelihood of development of both alcohol and drug dependence. Twin studies and adoption studies have shown that both genetic and environmental factors contribute to this vulnerability, although the precise nature by which this occurs is still unknown and a subject of active research. One area of great research interest relates to whether people can be vulnerable to drug dependence in general (e.g., as a result of a risk-taking temperament or poor decision making) or whether they are at high risk to abuse particular substances (perhaps because of a highly reinforcing response to a specific drug).

Psychiatric illness and personality disorders have been shown to influence the likelihood of developing drug abuse problems. For example, the presence of conduct disorder in childhood and adolescence and antisocial personality disorder in adulthood have both been shown to predispose to subsequent drug abuse problems. Psychiatric disorders such as mood disorders are frequently found in people with drug abuse problems. However, it is important to note that the presence of these two disorders in the same person does not necessarily imply causation, even if one of the disorders manifests first.

In addition to the risk factors mentioned previously, certain individual protective factors may reduce the likelihood of an addictive disorder. Individuals who have positive familial relationships, success in academic activities, and meaningful religious affiliation have a lower likelihood of developing drug abuse problems. The fact that many people have a mixture of risk and protective factors speaks to the complex etiologic nature of drug abuse problems.

The Agent

Most drugs of abuse are inherently reinforcing; animals typically will self-administer most of the commonly abused drugs. Not all drugs are equally reinforcing in general, however, and there is a great deal of individual variation in drug preference. Some people like the stimulating effects of drugs such as cocaine and amphetamine, whereas others experience that level of stimulation as extremely uncomfortable. Some people like the relaxation induced by drugs such as marijuana and sedative-hypnotics, whereas others feel deadened and overly slowed down by these drugs. Although some people gravitate toward particular drugs of abuse because of their specific pharmacologic properties, other will use a variety of drugs indiscriminately, based on level of availability; some of these people are primarily seeking to alter their current emotional state, regardless of the direction in which it is changed. The reinforcing properties of many drugs of abuse appear to be mediated through dopaminergic pathways, although other neurotransmitters, including γ-aminobutyric acid (GABA), serotonin, and norepinephrine are also involved in mediating drug-induced reinforcement.

The Environment

The third critical factor in the development, maintenance, and (perhaps) cessation of drug abuse is the environment in which the use occurs. Drug use does not occur in a vacuum. Rather, many societal factors, including legal status, availability, price, perception of dangerousness, social desirability, peer group, and religious beliefs influence behavior relating to substance use. Drug availability is known to be a substantial influence on likelihood of substance use. For example, alcohol consumption has been shown to increase when the hours during which alcohol can be sold are extended. The restriction of alcohol availability by restricting hours of sale or by increasing its cost through taxation, in turn, reduces consumption. Illicit drugs are, of course, by definition less available than alcohol or tobacco. A major factor that influences use of these agents is the potential user's perception of the drug's safety, social cachet (or lack thereof), likelihood of incurring legal consequences, and peer group behavior. Treatment research has shown that environmental influences can have a powerful effect on drug use: studies have shown, for example, that offering an alternative positive reward (e.g., a voucher that can be exchanged for desired goods and services such as movie tickets or clothes) in response to abstaining from drugs may help drug-dependent individuals overcome their severe craving and reduce their substance use. In fact, this type of treatment approach, based on the use of motivational incentives for abstinence, has been shown to be one of the most powerful treatment interventions available for the treatment of drug dependence. The responsiveness of drug-dependent individuals to environmental contingencies demonstrates the importance of appreciating the complexity of the interaction among the individual, the drug, and the environment in the determination of drug use.

CLINICAL MANIFESTATIONS

Medical Complications Related to Drug Abuse and Dependence

Drug abuse is associated with significant medical morbidity and sometimes with mortality. Medical complications related to drug abuse are often directly related to the pharmacology of the abused agent, for example, the vasoconstrictor properties of cocaine; drug-specific complications are described later in the sections focusing on particular drugs of abuse.

In addition to these drug-specific sequelae, however, many medical complications incurred by drug-dependent patients occur not as a result of the particular drug being abused. Rather, serious complications may occur as a result of three factors that cut across many of the drugs of abuse: (1) paraphernalia, particularly unsterile needles; (2) adulterants; and (3) lifestyle issues.

Paraphernalia

Some of the most serious medical problems that occur in individuals with drug abuse and dependence occur as a result of the route of administration rather than from the actual drug being used. The use of unsterile needles, particularly if shared with other drug users, can lead to a variety of localized and systemic infections, some of which can be life-threatening. Skin infections and cellulitis are relatively common among injection drug users. Systemic infections related to needle use are often quite serious; individuals who inject drugs may develop infective endocarditis (Chapter 76). Other relatively common infections among injection drug users include hepatitis B, hepatitis C, and HIV infection.

Adulterants

Drugs that are purchased and sold illicitly are often adulterated or "cut" with other similar-looking products, with the intention of increasing the dealer's profit margin. For example, other white powdery substances are typically added to cocaine and heroin during the dealing process, to dilute their purity. Some of these adulterants can, in turn, cause medical problems. At times, these complications occur because of the combined toxicity of the adulterant and the route of administration. Thus, for example, a patient may have a granuloma in the lung or liver as a result of talc use; talc is commonly added to street heroin and can also cause difficulties in users who crush talc-containing pharmaceutical tablets (e.g., opioids) and then inject them. Other common adulterants in street drugs include quinine (frequently used with heroin) and lidocaine (often added to cocaine), but such toxic materials as strychnine and ground glass have been found in samples of street drugs, leading to serious medical sequelae.

Lifestyle Issues

Many drug-dependent patients expose themselves to multiple risks due to intoxication, participating in dangerous illegal activities, and associating with potentially violent people. As a result, these individuals experience a high rate of traumatic injuries and are at greater risk of being victims of assault, homicide, or suicide. Suicide is far more common among people with substance abuse problems than among the general population; this may be related to a combination of the effects of acute intoxication, the high prevalence of depression among drug-dependent patients, and the higher rate of antisocial personality disorder in this population, which is associated with a propensity toward impulsiveness, risk taking, and violence. Although it is well known that intoxication can lead to motor vehicle crashes, intoxication can also serve as a risk factor for becoming a victim of someone else's vehicle; one study reported that one third of pedestrians who are killed by motor vehicles have alcohol in their blood, perhaps a reflection of the combination of risk taking, poor judgment, and impaired motor coordination that can occur during periods of intoxication.

TREATMENT Rx

General Treatment Principles

Drug abuse and dependence represent a relatively heterogeneous group of disorders, based on type of drug or drugs used, frequency and amount of use, severity of medical, behavioral, and social consequences, presence and severity of comorbid medical and psychiatric illness, and motivation to change. Treatment thus requires a careful medical and psychiatric assessment, including a detailed substance use history and laboratory testing. It is often helpful to enlist the help of a family member or significant other (with the patient's permission) in obtaining historical information. Intoxication and withdrawal syndromes need to be treated acutely; longer-term treatment involves helping the patient to reduce or (ideally) abstain from substances of abuse and thus improve overall functioning.

Among the common drugs of abuse, medications with approval by the U.S. Food and Drug Administration (FDA) are only available for opioids. However, researchers are actively studying a number of compounds for the treatment of other drugs of abuse, particularly stimulants and marijuana. Behavioral treatments are critically important in the treatment of substance use disorders. A number of behavioral treatments have a substantial evidence base supporting their efficacy; these include cognitive-behavioral therapy, motivational enhancement therapy, contingency management (also referred to as *motivational incentive*) therapy, 12-step facilitation therapy, and behavioral couples therapy. In addition to professional treatment, peer support groups such as the 12-step-oriented Alcoholics or Narcotics Anonymous and non-12-step groups such as SMART Recovery can be extremely helpful in facilitating recovery from drug abuse problems.

MAJOR DRUGS OF ABUSE

Opioids

For centuries, opioids have been a core part of the medical pharmacopoeia, primarily because of their capacity to treat pain, but also because of their antitussive and antidiarrheal properties. Unfortunately, opioids are also powerful euphoriants and thus have substantial abuse liability. Although opium itself has been used for centuries, the isolation of morphine and codeine from opium in the 19th century, along with the introduction of the hypodermic needle, led to the increased prevalence of intravenous opioid use. Ironically, heroin was introduced near the end of the 19th century as a treatment for morphine addiction.

Opioids can be divided into four categories: (1) natural opium alkaloids, including opium, morphine, and codeine; (2) semisynthetic derivatives of morphine, including heroin and oxycodone; (3) synthetic opioids that are not derived from morphine, including methadone and meperidine; and (4) opioid-containing preparations such as elixir of terpin hydrate.

EPIDEMIOLOGY

Opioid dependence represents a significant public health problem and accounts for more admissions for substance use disorder treatment than any substance other than alcohol. In the past decade, there has been a shift in the epidemiology of opioid abuse, however, with a reduction in heroin use and an increase in the abuse of opioid analgesic drugs; the latter has occurred as a result of either misuse of prescription opioids or illicit use of these agents. Approximately 600,000 people reported using heroin in 2009, with 180,000 trying the drug for the first time. During the same year, over 12 million people either misused prescription opioids or used them illicitly, with 2 million doing so for the first time; opioids are currently the most commonly misused prescription drugs. Most people who use opioid analgesics in this way report that they obtained them from a friend or relative. It is thus likely that a portion of these people might, for example, have used a relative's opioid for the treatment of a temporary painful condition such as a migraine headache. However, the number of people seeking treatment for dependence on opioid analgesics has increased dramatically in the past decade.

PATHOBIOLOGY

Opioids are readily absorbed when taken orally, intranasally, or by smoking or injection. Heroin, which is almost immediately converted to morphine in the liver, is most commonly injected but may be smoked or used intranasally.

Opioids work by binding to specific opioid receptors and then exerting their activity. Three major subtypes of opioid receptors have been identified and well described for many years. Most of the commonly abused opioids bind as agonists to the μ-receptor and typically produce the effects most commonly associated with opioids: miosis, respiratory depression, analgesia, euphoria, and drowsiness. Opioids that bind to the κ-receptor, unlike μ-receptor agonists, often produce dysphoria rather than euphoria. The other two receptors, δ- and N/OFQ-receptors, do not appear to play a known significant role in opioid dependence.

Opioid analgesics are ordinarily taken by the oral route, but they may be altered to be used through a different route of administration. This is particularly common with the extended release preparations, which may be altered by chewing the pill (facilitating a rapid release of the opioid medication) or by crushing the pill, dissolving it in water, and then injecting it or using it intranasally.

CLINICAL MANIFESTATIONS

The initial response to the administration of heroin, particularly when used intravenously, is a "rush," often described as orgasmic, lasting 30 to 60 seconds. This sensation is generally followed by a profound sense of relaxation that is sometimes referred to as being "wrapped in warm cotton." During this period, the user generally feels drowsy and may be seen to be "nodding," with mental clouding and a sense of tranquility. A reduction in respiratory rate occurs, along with miosis, reduced contractility of smooth muscle, and reduced secretions in the stomach, pancreas, and biliary tract. Thus, constipation and urinary hesitancy may occur. Itching is commonly seen during opioid intoxication. Many people experience nausea and vomiting in their initial use of opioids, although tolerance tends to develop to this effect over time. Tolerance also occurs to some other effects rather quickly, particularly the analgesic, respiratory depressant, and euphoriant properties of opioids. In contrast, relatively little tolerance occurs to constipation or to pupillary constriction. It is important to be aware, then, that miosis is a manifestation of opioid use, but it is not diagnostic of opiate overuse or intoxication.

Physical Dependence

Physical dependence on opioids leads to a characteristic withdrawal syndrome, the key signs of which include elevated heart rate and blood pressure, mydriasis, abdominal cramps, sweating, gooseflesh, rhinorrhea, lacrimation, and gastrointestinal distress, particularly diarrhea, nausea, and vomiting. Insomnia is common, particularly difficulty falling asleep; this is often the most long-lasting complaint among people who experience opioid withdrawal. Yawning, muscle twitches, and difficulty with body temperature regulation are also commonly seen. The severity of withdrawal can be highly variable, depending on the dose of opioids taken, the length of time that they have been taken, and individual factors. For short-acting opioids such as heroin and hydrocodone, the earliest stages of withdrawal typically occur approximately 6 to 12 hours after the last use. Peak symptoms tend to occur 48 to 72 hours after the last dose, and most clinical symptoms usually resolve within 7 to 10 days. For longer-acting opioids such as methadone, each of these time periods associated with withdrawal from short-acting opioids should be approximately doubled or tripled.

Other Medical Complications

The most common serious medical complications that occur from opioid use are typically related to factors other than the opioids themselves, particularly needle use and adulterants; these were discussed previously. Common medical problems among those dependent on heroin include hepatitis B, hepatitis C, infective endocarditis, talc granulomatosis, HIV infection, cellulitis, and abscesses, all typically related to needle use.

An important noninfectious complication that has been reported with opioid abuse is alteration of the cardiac conduction system, with a prolongation of the QT interval; this can lead to potentially serious arrhythmias, including torsades de pointes. This complication has been particularly noted with the long-acting opioid L-α-acetylmethadol (LAAM) and with methadone.

Chronic pain is commonly seen among opioid-dependent individuals, not just those who have received opioids for the treatment of pain. Pain can occur in opioid-dependent individuals for numerous reasons. In addition to the possibility that a chronic painful condition led to the use of opioids in the first place, those dependent on opioids are more likely to experience accidents, violence, and other forms of physical trauma that could produce chronic pain. There is also some evidence that chronic opioid use may lead to hyperalgesia, although there is some controversy regarding this issue. As with all substance use disorders, psychiatric illnesses (particularly mood disorders) are more common in opioid-dependent patients than in the general population. Moreover, it is important to note that the use of multiple drugs is extremely common in patients with opioid dependence, particularly among those using heroin. Indeed, the use of more than one drug is typically the rule rather than the exception in most substance use disorders.

TREATMENT Rx

Opioid Withdrawal

Opioid detoxification can be accomplished by switching patients from their current drug of abuse (e.g., heroin, hydrocodone) to methadone or buprenorphine and then tapering that medication. Although the details of accomplishing this vary, one method commonly used in hospital settings is to administer methadone 10 mg orally whenever a patient experiences objective signs of opioid withdrawal (e.g., mydriasis, tachycardia, hypertension, and sweating). This process can be repeated every 2 to 4 hours for 24 hours after the initial dose; the total amount of methadone given in that 24-hour period is the "stabilization dose," which should not ordinarily exceed 40 mg. The stabilization dose is then reduced by 5 mg a day until the detoxification is completed.

Buprenorphine can also be used successfully for opioid detoxification[1]; patients who demonstrate objective signs of opioid withdrawal (often measured with a standardized withdrawal severity scale) can be stabilized on buprenorphine over a 1- to 2-day period; the subsequent taper from buprenorphine may occur either right away or after a period of stabilization on buprenorphine. The dose of buprenorphine will depend on whether the medication will be used for a brief, several-day detoxification or for longer-term stabilization or maintenance treatment.

Longer-Term Opioid Dependence Treatment

There are three effective medications that are approved by the FDA for the treatment of opioid dependence: methadone (a full opioid agonist), buprenorphine (a partial agonist), and naltrexone (an opioid antagonist). Methadone has been used successfully for both detoxification from opioids and maintenance treatment for many years.[2] Unlike buprenorphine and naltrexone, which can be prescribed by physicians in their offices (although physicians wishing to prescribe buprenorphine for the treatment of opioid dependence must receive specialized training and certification to do so), methadone is available for the treatment of opioid dependence only in specially licensed treatment programs. Methadone is a long-acting μ-receptor agonist with a slow onset of peak effects (typically approximately 2 to 6 hours) and a slow offset of action, allowing for once-a-day administration. Methadone reduces opioid craving and induces cross-tolerance, thus blocking or attenuating the effects of other opioid use. Although the therapeutic dose of methadone for a particular individual may vary, doses of 60 mg or higher have typically been shown to be more effective than lower doses; there is some evidence that even higher doses (e.g., 80 mg a day or more) may be more effective than 60 mg. Methadone treatment has been shown to reduce opioid use, increase employment, decrease criminal behavior, and reduce the rate of development of HIV infection.

When a patient enrolled in a methadone treatment program experiences pain (e.g., postoperatively) requiring opioid analgesia, the patient should continue to receive the baseline methadone maintenance treatment dose for the addiction and should receive a different opioid for treatment of the pain (Chapter 29); before administering methadone, it is a good idea to confirm the methadone dose with the patient's treatment program whenever possible. The fact that the patient is receiving methadone every day does not obviate the need for opioid analgesia, however. In fact, many patients receiving methadone treatment for opioid dependence will require a dose of opioids that is relatively high as a result of cross-tolerance to other opioid drugs.

The Drug Addiction Act of 2000 revolutionized the treatment of opioid dependence by enabling the approval of the partial opioid agonist buprenorphine for the treatment of opioid dependence and allowing treatment with buprenorphine to be administered in physicians' offices rather than only in specialized opioid treatment programs. To prescribe buprenorphine, physicians must apply to the Substance Abuse and Mental Health Services Administration (SAMHSA) for a waiver that allows them to prescribe buprenorphine, after taking an 8-hour training course on buprenorphine. At the time of this writing, physicians may treat up to 100 patients with buprenorphine in their office practice. Buprenorphine, a partial μ-agonist and κ-antagonist, has a more favorable safety profile than methadone because of its partial agonist properties. Respiratory depression, which can be induced by full agonists, and which is responsible for some overdose deaths, is far less likely to occur with buprenorphine because its partial agonist properties cause a plateau of opioid effects as the dose increases. Buprenorphine is administered sublingually for the treatment of opioid dependence either as buprenorphine alone (sometimes referred to as the "mono" product) or (more commonly, in the United States) as a combination product of buprenorphine and naloxone; the naloxone is added to discourage users from dissolving the tablet and injecting the medication because the naloxone in the combination product will precipitate withdrawal when injected. Buprenorphine has been shown to be effective for both opioid detoxification and for maintenance treatment. A randomized trial has shown that extended treatment with buprenorphine-naloxone for 12 weeks improved outcome compared with short-term detoxification in opioid-addicted youth (aged 15 to 21 years).[3] Typical doses of 12 to 16 mg of sublingual buprenorphine per day appear to be as effective as methadone in doses up to approximately 60 mg a day. However, individuals who require much higher doses of methadone may respond better to that agent than to buprenorphine.[4]

Naltrexone, a pure opioid antagonist, blocks the effects (including euphoria) of opioids. As a result, individuals taking naltrexone should have a reduced desire to use opioids because the latter drug will have no desired effect. When used orally (50 mg/day) or in its long-acting form (380 mg intravenously every 4 weeks), naltrexone is highly effective at suppressing illicit opioid use. However, naltrexone suffers from very low acceptability; few patients are interested in being treated with naltrexone. Moreover, among those who initially accept this treatment, the dropout rate is extremely high. Nevertheless, naltrexone can be a useful medication for patients who are willing (either as the result of external pressure or for internal motivation) to use it.

Methadone, buprenorphine, and naltrexone are not designed to be delivered alone but should be given along with counseling to be effective. It has been well demonstrated that the administration of methadone in the absence of counseling is an inadequate treatment approach; less is known about the optimal combination of buprenorphine and counseling. One study demonstrated that counseling delivered within a medical office setting can be quite effective in conjunction with buprenorphine treatment, suggesting that general physicians who are trained to use buprenorphine can effectively treat at least a portion of patients with opioid dependence in their offices with a combination of buprenorphine and counseling.

Central Nervous System Stimulants: Cocaine and Amphetamines

The two most important central nervous system stimulants, cocaine and amphetamine (including methamphetamine), are derived from different sources; the former is extracted from coca leaves, whereas the latter is a synthetic compound. However, both induce similar psychoactive activity when taken illicitly and can produce similar adverse consequences. Amphetamine has been used over the years to treat obesity and to combat fatigue and depression. Cocaine is still used as a topical anesthetic for otolaryngologic surgery. Ironically, its vasoconstrictor action, which is responsible for many of the cocaine-related medical complications described later, can be valuable for surgeons because of the resultant reduction of blood flow in the operating field. Although cocaine was not extracted from the coca leaf until the 19th century, coca leaves have been chewed for more than 1500 years for medicinal and religious purposes, as well as to combat work-related fatigue. Sigmund Freud was one of the foremost advocates of cocaine, both extolling its psychoactive properties and discovering its ability to relieve pain, thus eventually leading to its discovery as the first local anesthetic. Cocaine was seen in the late 19th century as a "cure-all" and was included in numerous patent medicines as well as in Coca-Cola. The Harrison Narcotic Act of 1914 restricted the use of cocaine, and the drug was not widely used until the late 1970s, when there was a resurgence in cocaine use in the United States.

Like cocaine, amphetamine was synthesized for the first time in the late 19th century. It was used for clinical purposes for the first time in the 1920s. Reports of amphetamine abuse first occurred in the 1930s, with intermittent epidemics since that time. In recent years, methamphetamine abuse has been particularly prevalent and worrisome in the United States, with particularly high concentration of its use in the Midwestern and Western states, including Hawaii.

Cocaine can be used either intranasally, by intravenous injection, or by smoking. Cocaine hydrochloride, which is the form of the drug used in medical therapeutics, is a water-soluble compound that can be used intranasally ("snorted") or injected. Adding an alkaline compound such as baking soda to an aqueous solution of cocaine hydrochloride produces a rocklike compound known as *crack*, which can be smoked. Smoking cocaine produces the most rapid onset of intoxication (6 to 10 seconds) and the shortest period of drug effect (10 to 15 minutes). Methamphetamine can also be used in multiple ways—either orally, by smoking, or intravenously. Methamphetamine effects last much longer than those produced by cocaine; psychiatric symptoms such as paranoia that typically last only a matter of hours in cocaine users may persist for days to weeks after methamphetamine use and occasionally may result in a chronic psychotic state.

EPIDEMIOLOGY

Approximately 37 million Americans have used cocaine during their lifetime. In 2009, just under 5 million people used cocaine; 1.6 million people, or 0.7% of the population, reported using cocaine in the past month. Of these past-month cocaine users, 30% (492,000) used crack, an increase from 2008. There were 600,000 new users in 2009, a number that has been in decline since 2002. Cocaine had the third highest rate of drug abuse or dependence in 2009 and was the second most common drug associated with a recent treatment episode; cocaine use is also associated with 28% of emergency room visits associated with drug abuse.

Other stimulant use is less common; approximately 22 million Americans have used stimulants nonmedically during their lifetime, with 12.8 million lifetime methamphetamine users. Methamphetamine use in the past month was reported by 500,000 people in the United States in 2009, a number comparable to the number of past-month crack cocaine users.

PATHOBIOLOGY

Both cocaine and amphetamine increase the accumulation and activity of specific neurotransmitters in the synaptic cleft, including dopamine, norepinephrine, and serotonin. Cocaine is believed to exert this effect by binding to the dopamine transporter. Increased dopaminergic activity, particularly in the nucleus accumbens, is thought to be responsible for the reinforcing effects of cocaine. Amphetamines appear to increase the level of dopamine in the synaptic cleft primarily by stimulating presynaptic dopamine release as opposed to reuptake blockade.

CLINICAL MANIFESTATIONS

Both cocaine and amphetamines reliably produce euphoria, wakefulness, a sense of initiative, increased self-confidence (sometimes to the point of grandiosity), and in some instances, sexual stimulation. With higher doses, users may feel "wired," a syndrome characterized by anxiety, irritability, and perhaps paranoia. Withdrawal from either of these agents leads to opposite effects from those of intoxication: increased appetite, hypersomnia, and depression, which can occasionally be serious. Medical complications related to cocaine use are related to a combination of cocaine's stimulant activity (increased heart rate and blood pressure) and its vasoconstrictor properties. Local complications that result from the drug's vasoconstrictor activity include ulcerations of the nasal mucosa, perforation of the nasal septum, and decreased pulmonary diffusion capacity. Systemic complications include myocardial infarction, intracranial hemorrhage, grand mal seizures (as a result of intoxication, not withdrawal), and ventricular tachyarrhythmias, which may be responsible for sudden death. Physicians seeing a patient in an emergency room for an unexplained seizure should consider drug abuse as a potential cause (not only cocaine, but also phencyclidine and meperidine intoxication may lead to seizures, as can sedative-hypnotic or alcohol withdrawal). A serum or urine toxicology screen may thus be an important diagnostic tool in such a situation.

TREATMENT (Rx)

The treatment of central nervous system stimulant abuse and dependence primarily consists of behavioral therapies, including individual and group therapy, and self-help groups. Specific forms of treatment, such as cognitive-behavioral therapy, individual drug counseling using a 12-step-oriented disease model, and a behavioral treatment in which patients are reinforced for positive outcomes (e.g., drug-free urine screens), have been found to be successful. A great deal of research has been conducted in search of an effective pharmacotherapeutic treatment for stimulant dependence, but there is as yet no medication that has consistently been found to be effective enough to warrant approval by the FDA for this purpose.

Sedative-Hypnotic and Anxiolytic Drugs

Benzodiazepines and other sedative-hypnotic and anxiolytic medications such as barbiturates and zolpidem are frequently prescribed for the treatment of anxiety and sleep difficulties. Although different classifications of these drugs have very different chemical structures, they are grouped together according to their therapeutic applications. Most of these drugs act at the γ-aminobutyric acid type A ($GABA_A$) receptor and can cause physical dependence and both dispositional and pharmacodynamic tolerance. According to epidemiologic studies, approximately 9 million people, or 3.6% of the population aged 12 years and over, have used a sedative-hypnotic drug nonmedically.

Because the benzodiazepines are far and away the most commonly prescribed sedative-hypnotics, they are also the most widely abused. There are two major patterns of benzodiazepine abuse. Many people who ultimately abuse these medications have initially received a legitimate benzodiazepine prescription for the treatment of anxiety or insomnia. However, a combination of tolerance and decreased effectiveness of the agent over time may lead some people to increase their dose on their own. In such circumstances, attempts by the physician to taper the person off of the medication can be very difficult.

A second pattern of benzodiazepine abuse occurs among individuals who are using other drugs of abuse, most commonly opioids or stimulants. For example, many individuals who are dependent on heroin or other opioids may use benzodiazepines as a means of either enhancing the opioid effect or buffering symptoms of opioid withdrawal. Such individuals typically use relatively large doses of benzodiazepines intermittently, and therefore many of these patients do not develop physical dependence on benzodiazepines, unlike the first category of patients described previously, for whom physical dependence is common.

TREATMENT (Rx)

The treatment of people who are abusing benzodiazepines depends to some extent on the pattern of abuse. For individuals who have an anxiety disorder and have been misusing a legitimately prescribed medication, a common approach would be to taper the benzodiazepine and to institute a different type of treatment, such as an antidepressant along with cognitive-behavioral therapy. Tapering a benzodiazepine that a person has been taking for an extended period of time (sometimes many years) often requires a slow process, with careful monitoring of withdrawal symptoms (anxiety, agitation, insomnia, tachycardia, palpitations). Because benzodiazepine withdrawal, like alcohol withdrawal, can precipitate a seizure, gradual withdrawal is preferred. Most patients tolerate a benzodiazepine dose reduction initially with relatively little difficulty. However, as with most drug withdrawal regimens, people experience their greatest difficulty toward the end of the taper. One reason for this is that the percent dose reduction at the low end of a taper regimen continues to increase over time; a reduction from 2 mg to 1.5 mg of clonazepam, for instance, is a 25% reduction, whereas the same half-milligram dose reduction from 1 mg to 0.5 mg represents a 50% drop.

For patients who are abusing benzodiazepines as part of a pattern of multiple substance use, medical detoxification from the benzodiazepine itself will often not be necessary; for this population, psychosocial approaches that advocate abstinence from all substances of abuse, in conjunction with appropriate pharmacotherapy as needed (e.g., in the case of opioid dependence), is the preferred approach. It is important to note, however, that some deaths have been reported in France and elsewhere as a result of combinations of buprenorphine and benzodiazepines, usually used parenterally. Thus, physicians who are treating patients who are abusing both opioids and benzodiazepines need to be mindful of this issue when considering the use of buprenorphine.

Marijuana

Marijuana, which refers to the dried leaves and flowers of the plant *Cannabis sativa*, has been used for its psychoactive and medicinal properties for centuries. The major psychoactive substance in marijuana is δ-9-tetrahydrocannabinol (THC); the concentration of THC has increased from 1 to 3% in 1970 to nearly 8% in 2005; more potent varieties such as sinsemilla may contain nearly twice as much THC.

EPIDEMIOLOGY

Marijuana is the most commonly used illicit drug worldwide; it is estimated that approximately 160 million people have used marijuana. More than 16 million Americans state that they have used marijuana in the past month, with 104 million people in the United States having used marijuana during their lifetime.

PATHOBIOLOGY

Marijuana and other cannabinoids such as hashish (dried cannabis resin) exert their effects by binding to the cannabinoid receptors, of which two are currently known. Binding to the CB1 receptor, which is located primarily in the brain, appears to be responsible for the psychoactive effects of THC, whereas the CB2 receptor may be associated with immune system responses.

CLINICAL MANIFESTATIONS

When marijuana is smoked, its psychoactive effects occur almost immediately, with peak intensity approximately 30 minutes later; effects tend to disappear within 3 hours. Oral administration of marijuana leads to a delayed onset of action, but the effects of the drug persist for a longer period of time. Because THC is highly soluble in lipids, it can be stored in fat depots of regular users for several weeks, sometimes longer, with resultant positive urine tests for THC. Physiologic effects of marijuana intoxication include increased heart rate and conjunctival injection. Psychological effects include a sense of euphoria and well-being, friendliness, increased appetite, a distorted sense of time, impaired short-term memory, and sometimes a feeling of having achieved special insights. Cannabis has the capacity to cause tolerance in regular users, and some regular heavy users experience withdrawal symptoms on cessation of use, including irritability, difficulty sleeping, and anxiety.

TREATMENT Rx

The most common acute adverse event that occurs in marijuana smokers is a sense of acute panic, most common in inexperienced smokers, when the user's level of intoxication is greater than expected and the individual feels out of control. This can be best managed with reassurance that the effects will go away as the drug wears off. Recent evidence has shown that cannabis use, particularly during adolescence, may increase the likelihood of development of a psychotic disorder such as schizophrenia later in life.

Compared with alcohol, opioids, and stimulants, it is relatively uncommon for people to seek treatment of cannabis dependence itself. However, that situation has gradually changed in recent years, and an increasing number of people have sought treatment because of difficulty stopping marijuana use. There are no medications approved by the FDA for the treatment of cannabis dependence. Psychosocial approaches similar to the treatment of other substance use disorders are currently the treatment of choice.

Hallucinogens

Hallucinogens are a group of plant-based and synthetic drugs that lead to (primarily visual) perceptual alterations such as illusions and hallucinations, along with an alteration in the experience of external stimuli; ordinary events can appear quite profound to people while they are under the influence of these agents. The most common hallucinogens are lysergic acid diethylamide (LSD), mescaline, and psilocybin. Methylene dioxymethamphetamine (MDMA), also known as *ecstasy,* has both mild stimulant and potentially hallucinogenic properties and is thus sometimes categorized with the hallucinogens and sometimes as a stimulant.

EPIDEMIOLOGY

Approximately 1.3 million people in the United States report having used a hallucinogen in the previous month; approximately 37 million people have used these drugs during their lifetime. LSD is the most commonly used hallucinogen, with 24 million lifetime users in the United States; approximately 60% of that number have used MDMA.

PATHOBIOLOGY

LSD is thought to exert its action through serotonin agonist activity, particularly at the 5-HT_{2A} receptor. Other neurotransmitters may be involved in hallucinogenic activity as well. Hallucinogens can produce tolerance in a matter of days, but they do not produce physical dependence.

CLINICAL MANIFESTATIONS

In addition to their effects on perception and behavior, hallucinogens can produce sympathomimetic effects such as tachycardia, increased blood pressure and body temperature, and pupillary dilatation. Hyperreflexia and muscle weakness can also be seen. The most commonly seen medical consequence of hallucinogen use is hyperthermia, which can occur most commonly in users of MDMA.

The most common acute psychological adverse event, similar to marijuana, is a feeling of panic over the sense of loss of control that a person may feel as a result of intoxication; as is the case with marijuana, this is most likely to occur in inexperienced users. Some hallucinogen users will develop psychotic symptoms that fail to remit after the drug has worn off. Some hallucinogen use can also lead to longer-term perceptual difficulties. When these occur, a spontaneous return of very brief hallucinogen-induced symptoms long after the drug has worn off is known as a *flashback.* People who have perceptual difficulties that are much more pervasive may be said to have *hallucinogen persisting perception disorder,* which can at times be quite disabling.

TREATMENT 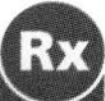

Symptomatic treatment is focused on the specific adverse medical and psychiatric sequelae described previously. If a psychotic episode that occurs after use of a hallucinogen persisted over time, it would be treated like any other psychotic disorder. There is no specific treatment for abuse of or dependence on hallucinogens per se, and it is very uncommon for people to seek treatment specifically because they want to stop using hallucinogens.

Phencyclidine

Phencyclidine (PCP) was originally developed as a human general anesthetic, but its use for that purpose was stopped in the 1960s because it frequently led to psychosis and hallucinations in the postoperative period. Approximately 120,000 individuals report that they used PCP during 2009, which represents more than a 40% decline from 5 years previous to that. Low doses of PCP can lead to symptoms that resemble alcohol intoxication, with slurred speech, ataxia, and a subjective feeling sometimes described as "feeling dead." PCP intoxication typically is accompanied by increased muscle tone, hyperreflexia, nystagmus, and ataxia.

When taken in high doses, PCP can have serious medical and psychiatric consequences. High-dose users may experience psychosis, catatonia, and extremely violent behavior. Medical sequelae of PCP intoxication can include muscle rigidity, seizures, hyperthermia, coma, and occasionally death.

Anabolic-Androgenic Steroids

Anabolic-androgenic steroids differ from other drugs described in this chapter because the motivation for use is typically related to the drug's physical rather than behavioral effects. Anabolic-androgenic steroids such as testosterone and its synthetic analogues have traditionally been used primarily to enhance strength and thus athletic performance, although in recent years, an increasing number of people have used these drugs primarily in an attempt to improve their physical appearance. Anabolic-androgenic steroids can have a legitimate medical purpose; they have most commonly been used to treat testosterone deficiency in men and more recently have been used to treat wasting syndromes in patients with AIDS.

Abuse of anabolic-androgenic steroids can cause a number of medical and psychiatric problems, including hypertension, elevated low-density lipoprotein cholesterol, cardiomyopathy, hepatotoxicity, acne, feminization (gynecomastia and reduced testicular size) in men, and masculinization (hirsutism, reduction in breast tissue, deeper voice) in women. Behavioral effects include aggressiveness (sometimes leading to violence) and an increased prevalence of mood disorders. There is no specific treatment to help people abusing anabolic steroids to stop. Rather, behavioral treatment approaches that are commonly used to treat other substance use disorders should be employed with this population.

CONCLUSION AND FUTURE DIRECTIONS

The ever-changing epidemiology of drug abuse means that the next decade will likely present new challenges as new drugs of abuse become increasingly popular. Recent research has focused on developing and testing effective pharmacologic and behavioral treatments for drug abuse and dependence. Screening for these disorders in general medical practice and combining office-based interventions with referrals to specialty drug abuse treatment as indicated can lead to successful outcomes for many of these patients.

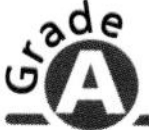

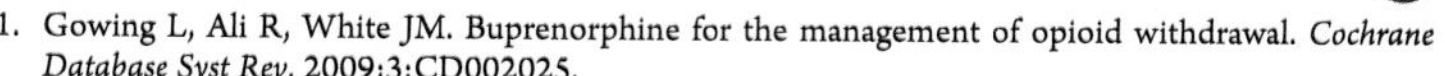

1. Gowing L, Ali R, White JM. Buprenorphine for the management of opioid withdrawal. *Cochrane Database Syst Rev.* 2009;3:CD002025.
2. Mattick RP, Breen C, Kimber J, et al. Methadone maintenance therapy versus no opioid replacement therapy for opioid dependence. *Cochrane Database Syst Rev.* 2009;3:CD002209.
3. Woody GE, Poole SA, Subramaniam GA, et al. Extended vs. short-term buprenorphine-naloxone for treatment of opioid-addicted youth: a randomized trial. *JAMA.* 2008;300:2003-2011.

4. Mattick RP, Kimber J, Breen C, et al. Buprenorphine maintenance versus placebo or methadone maintenance for opioid dependence. *Cochrane Database Syst Rev.* 2008;2:CD002207.

SUGGESTED READINGS

Benotsch EG, Koester S, Luckman D, et al. Non-medical use of prescription drugs and sexual risk behavior in young adults. *Addict Behav.* 2011;36:152-155. *Young adults who use prescription medication recreationally also use marijuana, ecstasy, cocaine, methamphetamine, and poppers and tend to engage in risky sexual behaviors.*

Haber PS, Demirkol A, Lange K, et al. Management of injecting drug users admitted to hospital. *Lancet.* 2009;374:1284-1293. *Review.*

Ling W, Casadonte P, Bigelow G, et al. Buprenorphine implants for treatment of opioid dependence: a randomized controlled trial. *JAMA.* 2010;304:1576-1583. *Buprenorphine implants (4 implants of 80 mg each) reduce opioid use, with about twice as many patients (40% vs. 20%) drug free for 16 weeks.*

Meader N. A comparison of methadone, buprenorphine and alpha(2) adrenergic agonists for opioid detoxification: a mixed treatment comparison meta-analysis. *Drug Alcohol Depend.* 2010;108:110-114. *Buprenorphine and methadone appear to be the most effective detoxification treatments.*

Oviedo-Joekes E, Brissette S, Marsh DC, et al. Diacetylmorphine versus methadone for the treatment of opioid addiction. *N Engl J Med.* 2009;361:777-786. *In a randomized trial, diacetylmorphine treatment resulted in a 40% greater decrease in the rate of illicit-drug use or other illegal activity as compared with methadone.*

Strang J, Metrebian N, Lintzeris N, et al. Supervised injectable heroin or injectable methadone versus optimised oral methadone as treatment for chronic heroin addicts in England after persistent failure in orthodox treatment (RIOTT): a randomised trial. *Lancet.* 2010;375:1885-1895. *Injectable heroin is more effective than oral methadone for lowering street heroin use.*

34 IMMUNOSUPPRESSING DRUGS INCLUDING CORTICOSTEROIDS

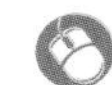

GRANT W. CANNON

IMMUNOSUPPRESSIVE DRUGS

The immune response is an essential host defense mechanism to control and fight infection. The ability to suppress immune reactions is a critical component in autoimmune disease treatment and transplantation management. During autoimmune diseases, the basic immune physiology is altered, and one or more components of this process do not function properly. Current challenges related to the selection, dosing, monitoring, and development of immunosuppressive drugs involve identifying the component of the immune system to be altered by the immunosuppressive therapy while maintaining a competent immune response to fight infection and perform other important immunoregulatory functions. After organ transplantation, most patients have an immune response to reject the implanted organ. Thus, immunosuppression during transplantation management involves the suppression of normal immune reactions rather than a pathologic process, as in the treatment of autoimmune disease. Suppression of natural host immune responses inevitably affects the ability of these protective mechanisms to fight infection. The general principles for selecting immunosuppressive therapy in transplantation patients involve specific monitoring for organ rejection and the selection of immunosuppressive therapy proportionate to the degree of rejection or to maintain tolerance of the implanted organ. Selection of the most effective therapy requires an individualized treatment program. These decisions require an understanding of the underlying pathophysiologic process, prognosis, and potential adverse events associated with the agents selected.

This chapter describes the mechanism of action—including the components of the immune response affected by the therapy—indications, and adverse events associated with commonly used immunosuppressive agents in autoimmune diseases and transplantation. Although each of these agents is discussed individually, these drugs are frequently used in combination to take advantage of their complementary effects. An understanding of the principles and adverse events associated with immunosuppressive therapy is important for all physicians as the use of these drugs becomes more widespread; however, the initiation and management of immunosuppressive therapy, particularly in patients with organ transplants and severe autoimmune diseases, should generally be limited to specialists with specific training in its use.

Corticosteroids

Historically, the initial enthusiasm related to the marked clinical benefit of corticosteroids in the treatment of rheumatoid arthritis was dampened by the significant adverse effects that developed after prolonged use. As opposed to allergic and idiosyncratic reactions to medications, the majority of adverse effects related to corticosteroid therapy are a direct consequence of the physiologic effects of the drug. This observation sparked a determined effort to understand the mechanisms of action of corticosteroids at physiologic levels and therapeutic doses. The objectives of these investigations have been to modify the naturally occurring hormones to exploit their clinical benefits while avoiding the associated adverse effects.

Mechanism of Action

Corticosteroids affect multiple physiologic functions at the molecular, cellular, and organ levels. The final result of corticosteroid treatment represents the composite effects of the drug on these multiple functions, which vary with the particular agent, dose, route, and duration of treatment (Table 34-1).

Molecular Action

Genomic Effects

Corticosteroids are lipophilic and rapidly cross cell membranes into the cytosol, where they bind to the glucocorticoid receptor. The complex of glucocorticoid and its receptor then enters the nucleus and affects gene transcription by binding to glucocorticoid response elements. The complex may either stimulate or suppress gene transcription and subsequent protein production. This mechanism may have an impact on the function of 1% of all genes and suppresses the production of cytokines and other important inflammatory proteins. In addition to binding to glucocorticoid response elements, the glucocorticoid–glucocorticoid receptor complex suppresses signal transduction pathways such as transcription factor activator protein-1, nuclear factor-κB, and nuclear factor of activator of T cells. Corticosteroids may also affect post-transcription and post-translation steps of protein synthesis. The anti-inflammatory actions of corticosteroids may be related to

TABLE 34-1 MECHANISM OF ACTION OF IMMUNOSUPPRESSIVE AGENTS

CORTICOSTEROIDS
Binding to cytosol glucocorticoid receptor results in suppression of pro-inflammatory cytokines (genomic effects)
Inhibition of arachidonic acid release and binding to surface receptor (nongenomic effects)
Results of corticosteroid actions:
Leukocyte numbers
Increase in circulating neutrophils
Decrease in circulating lymphocytes, monocytes, eosinophils, and basophils
Leukocyte function
Decreased trafficking of neutrophils
Decrease in leukocytes' cellular immune functions and immunoglobulin production
Cytokines
Decrease in pro-inflammatory cytokines: IL-1, IL-2, IL-6, and tumor necrosis factor-α
Increase in anti-inflammatory cytokines: IL-4, IL-10, and IL-13
Decreased production of prostaglandins and leukotrienes
PURINE PATHWAY INHIBITORS
Azathioprine: inhibition of DNA synthesis and purine synthesis
Mycophenolate mofetil: inhibition of purine synthesis
PYRIMIDINE PATHWAY INHIBITORS
Leflunomide: inhibition of pyrimidine synthesis by inhibiting dihydroorotate dehydrogenase
IMMUNOPHILIN-BINDING AGENTS
Calcineurin inhibition
Cyclosporine: binds with cyclophilin to inhibit calcineurin, resulting in decreased T-cell activation
Tacrolimus: binds with FKBP12 to inhibit calcineurin, resulting in decreased T-cell activation
Mammalian target of rapamycin (mTOR) inhibition
Sirolimus: binds to FKBP12 to inhibit mTOR, resulting in decreased T-cell activation
ALKYLATING AGENTS
Cyclophosphamide: alkylation of nucleic acids with cytotoxic action

FKBP12 = 12-kD FK-binding protein; IL = interleukin.

their action on the nuclear factor-κB and activator protein-1 pathways; the adverse events produced are related more to the activation or suppression of gene transcription.

Nongenomic Effects

The genomic effects of corticosteroids require the diffusion of the drug into the cell, binding to the receptor, entry into the nucleus, and alteration of transcription. The ultimate effect on protein synthesis is not immediate, and it generally takes at least 30 minutes before any response is seen. The observation that some actions of corticosteroids are seen immediately has directed a search for nongenomic effects of these drugs. The glucocorticoid–glucocorticoid receptor complex can inhibit arachidonic acid release. In addition to the cytosol glucocorticoid receptor, a membrane-bound receptor may be present that mediates nongenomic functions.

Systemic Effects

Impact on Leukocytes

Corticosteroids affect the activation, production, circulation, function, and survival of leukocytes. Whereas these impacts appear to be modulated principally by the genomic effects of corticosteroids on cytokines, corticosteroids act on adhesion molecules and other mechanisms as well. The effects are on neutrophils, monocytes, macrophages, lymphocytes, eosinophils, and basophils. With corticosteroid therapy, neutrophils increase in the peripheral circulation, primarily because of demargination; in contrast, there is a decrease in monocytes, lymphocytes, eosinophils, and basophils. Although the number of circulating neutrophils may increase, trafficking appears to be impaired. The impact on T cells is more pronounced than the effects on B cells, with the induction of apoptosis particularly in immature and activated T cells. Although the function of B cells and neutrophils is not affected as strongly as that of T cells, prolonged use of high-dose corticosteroids can lead to suppression of antibody production.

Changes in Inflammatory Mediators

Corticosteroids result in a decrease in multiple pro-inflammatory cytokines and interleukins (ILs), including IL-1, IL-2, IL-6, and tumor necrosis factor-α, at the same time that there is an increase in anti-inflammatory cytokines such as IL-4, IL-10, and IL-13. Corticosteroids have been associated with a reduction in the production of prostaglandins, leukotrienes, and other arachidonic acid metabolites, probably related to the reduced production of cyclooxygenase 2 and phospholipase A_2–related pro-inflammatory compounds (Chapter 36).

TREATMENT Rx

Specific Issues with Corticosteroid Therapy

Multiple corticosteroid compounds and preparations are available (Table 34-2). These compounds have differences in potency, half-life, and sodium-retaining properties. In many conditions, the local administration of corticosteroids provides clinical benefit without the systemic toxicity associated with oral therapy. Local therapies include topical, ophthalmic, inhaled, and local injection, such as soft tissue and intra-articular injections. Although the potential for adverse events is generally reduced with local therapy, local toxicities as well as systemic effects can develop if large doses of topical corticosteroids are used.

Whereas most conditions can be treated with local or oral corticosteroids, intravenous administration can provide pulse doses if desired. Intravenous therapy can also be used when the patient cannot take oral medication or the absorption of oral agents is impaired. Pulse therapy generally consists of high-dose intravenous treatment that is often administered as divided doses over 3 to 5 days. High-dose pulse therapy has been advocated in acute organ transplantation rejection, severe systemic lupus erythematosus (SLE), aggressive vasculitis, and other acute and severe autoimmune disorders. The use of high-dose corticosteroid pulse therapy has been associated with the development of sudden cardiac arrhythmias and sudden death. However, many of these patients had serious concurrent diseases that could have been partly responsible for electrolyte abnormalities and other associated morbidities contributing to these complications. Because of this possible association, close monitoring of patients receiving high-dose corticosteroid pulse therapy is warranted.

Indications

Corticosteroids are employed in a wide range of autoimmune disorders and transplantation procedures. A listing of each indication for which corticosteroids have been used and proved effective is beyond the scope of this chapter, but indications range from multiple rheumatologic disorders and many other inflammatory conditions to transplantation. For example, the demonstration that inflammation plays a significant role in reactive airway disease has dramatically increased the use of systemic and inhaled corticosteroids in asthma and chronic obstructive pulmonary disorders. The challenge is to determine the appropriate dose, route, and duration of therapy. For severe autoimmune disorders, high doses of corticosteroids are indicated. In many cases, oral prednisone, 60 to 80 mg/day as single or divided doses, can be employed. If patients cannot take oral medication or higher doses of corticosteroids are indicated, they can be administered intravenously. Comparative data on the most appropriate doses and routes of administration are generally not available. Clinical judgment and empirical literature form the basis of these treatment regimens.

Adverse Effects

With most medications, adverse events are the result of allergic and idiosyncratic reactions. The adverse events associated with corticosteroids, however, are generally caused by the drug's physiologic action. Investigations are ongoing to determine whether separate mechanisms might account for the therapeutic benefits of corticosteroids, whereas other pathways are involved in the adverse events related to these drugs. Currently available forms of corticosteroids do not allow the separation of adverse events from therapeutic effects. For example, the increase in infection associated with corticosteroids is a result of the drug's impact on leukocyte function and antibody production; it is not an allergic reaction. The prevalence and severity of these adverse effects increase in proportion to the dose and duration of therapy. The key to reducing adverse events is to use the lowest dose needed for the shortest possible duration. Data also suggest that intermittent and every-other-day dosing may be associated with less toxicity than daily or divided daily doses.

Despite these limitations, corticosteroids are the only viable treatment option in many conditions, and efforts must be made to prevent, detect the development of, and monitor these adverse events. In most situations, education of the patient coupled with vigilant surveillance can detect these adverse events and often reduce their serious impact.

The following discussion is not a comprehensive list of all reported adverse events associated with corticosteroids. Infection, osteoporosis, metabolic abnormalities, and cardiovascular effects are highlighted because specific interventions can have an impact on these problems through proper education of the patient, monitoring, or prophylactic therapy.

Infection

Infections are increased in patients taking corticosteroids, particularly bacterial, fungal, and mycobacterial infections. These opportunistic infections are seen much less frequently in healthy individuals with normal immune function. The increased incidence and general severity of these infections are complicated by the anti-inflammatory actions of corticosteroids, which can mask many of the cardinal signs of infection such as fever, inflammation, and local discomfort. Patients taking corticosteroids should be alerted to the possibility of these "subclinical" infections, and the provider must be vigilant in investigating signs and symptoms that might be less concerning in patients not taking corticosteroids. Management of infections in patients receiving corticosteroids requires close monitoring. Appropriate diagnostic procedures, antimicrobial therapy, and supportive measures are key to the successful management of infections in immunocompromised hosts. Patients with adrenal suppression may require "stress doses" of corticosteroids during the initial treatment. However, when a reduction in corticosteroid dose is possible, this may help restore the host immune response to the infection, particularly with chronic infections.

Preventive measures to reduce infections include proper immunizations. For example, in a patient being evaluated for future transplantation, immunizations should be given before the immunosuppressive therapy, if possible. In many cases, however, a delay of immunosuppressive therapy is not possible to allow immunizations to be updated. In patients receiving chronic immunosuppressive therapy, routine immunizations should be offered when the disease is stable. Prophylactic antibiotics are generally not recommended to prevent infections in patients receiving corticosteroid therapy. However, two notable exceptions are the use of antituberculosis therapy in purified protein derivative (PPD)–positive patients and trimethoprim-sulfamethoxazole therapy in patients receiving high-dose corticosteroid therapy for *Pneumocystis jirovecii* (previously *Pneumocystis carinii*) prophylaxis.

TABLE 34-2 GLUCOCORTICOID PREPARATIONS

	ANTI-INFLAMMATORY POTENCY	EQUIVALENT DOSE (MG)	SODIUM-RETAINING POTENCY	PLASMA HALF-LIFE (MIN)	BIOLOGIC HALF-LIFE (HR)
Hydrocortisone	1	20	2+	90	8-12
Cortisone	0.8	25	2+	30	8-12
Prednisone	4	5	1+	60	12-36
Prednisolone	4	5	1+	200	12-36
Methylprednisolone	5	4	0	180	12-36
Triamcinolone	5	4	0	300	12-36
Betamethasone	20-30	0.6	0	100-300	36-54
Dexamethasone	20-30	0.75	0	100-300	36-54

From Garber EK, Targoff C, Paulus HE. Glucocorticoid preparations. In: Paulus HE, Furst DE, Droomgoole SH, eds. *Drugs for Rheumatic Diseases*. New York: Churchill Livingstone; 1987:446.

Osteoporosis

Bone loss associated with corticosteroids affects multiple sites and has a greater impact on trabecular bone than cortical bone. Common sites of involvement are the spine and femur; associated fracture rates may be as high as 20%, depending on the dose and duration of therapy. On initiation of long-term corticosteroid therapy, all patients should be evaluated for osteoporosis prophylactic therapy (Chapter 251). Unless it is contraindicated, patients should be receiving adequate calcium and vitamin D through diet or supplements. In many patients, bisphosphonates provide significant protection. Postmenopausal women may be evaluated for potential estrogen replacement therapy, which may be helpful if the benefits of therapy with corticosteroids outweigh the risks for cardiovascular disease and malignancy. If osteoporosis develops in a patient receiving corticosteroids, efforts should be made to discontinue therapy or reduce the dose. Agents used for the treatment of osteoporosis should also be administered (Chapter 251). Effective therapies include bisphosphonates and anabolic agents such as parathyroid hormone preparations. These agents are generally used in association with calcium and vitamin D supplementation. An algorithm for the prevention and treatment of glucocorticoid-induced osteoporosis is provided in Figure 34-1.

Metabolic Effects

The metabolic effects of corticosteroids may influence glucose metabolism, with results ranging from mild glucose intolerance to frank diabetes. Patients beginning corticosteroid therapy should be monitored for glucose intolerance and treated if significant hyperglycemia develops. The management of patients with existing diabetes is particularly challenging during corticosteroid therapy; they require close monitoring and adjustments to their diabetes management programs.

Exogenous corticosteroids suppress the hypothalamic-pituitary-adrenal (HPA) axis (Chapters 230 and 234). The likelihood of adrenal suppression increases with the dose and duration of therapy. HPA axis suppression should be considered in patients receiving doses of 20 mg/day or more for 3 weeks or longer, although suppression can occur with lower doses. Formal evaluations can be performed to test the integrity of the HPA axis, but in most cases, a scheduled tapering of corticosteroid dose over several weeks allows the return of HPA axis function without signs of adrenal insufficiency. The ideal rate for the tapering of corticosteroids has not been evaluated by clinical trials. The rate of reduction in corticosteroid dose is often limited more by the relapse of disease activity than by the development of adrenal insufficiency. In general, a rapid reduction in dose (about 10 mg prednisone-equivalent/day), as tolerated by the patient's clinical disease, can be undertaken until a dose reflecting the normal physiologic production of cortisol is achieved. After this point, reductions of 1 to 2.5 mg/day every 1 to 2 weeks are generally well tolerated and can be accomplished by decreasing the dose of alternate-day treatment over 6 to 8 weeks. However, with an acute medical illness, patients who received corticosteroid doses in the past sufficient to cause HPA suppression should receive stress doses of steroids for up to 1 year after steroid treatment. Other metabolic complications of corticosteroid treatment include weight gain with truncal obesity; electrolyte abnormalities, including hypokalemia; and fluid retention.

Cardiovascular Effects

Corticosteroids may induce or exacerbate cardiovascular risk factors, including hypertension, hyperlipidemia, and diabetes. Multiple mechanisms have been proposed for these effects, but the end result is that patients taking corticosteroids have an increased prevalence of atherosclerotic diseases and their associated complications. This problem is complicated by the recent observation that many patients with inflammatory conditions, including rheumatoid arthritis and SLE, may have an increased risk for cardiovascular disease above that predicted by traditional risk factors. These observations emphasize the need to monitor corticosteroid-treated patients closely for cardiovascular risk factors (Chapter 51) and to treat detected abnormalities aggressively.

Other Adverse Effects

Many other adverse events have been reported with corticosteroid therapy and are listed in Table 34-3. Osteonecrosis (avascular necrosis) is common during corticosteroid therapy and often involves the femoral head. Peptic ulcer disease is increased independent of concurrent nonsteroidal anti-inflammatory therapy. Cataracts and a variety of dermatologic abnormalities are more common. Muscle weakness or steroid myopathy, alteration of mood and behavior, and psychosis may develop. This broad spectrum of clinical complications requires the prescriber of corticosteroids to be aware of and alert to the development of these adverse events.

Purine Inhibition

Purines are critical components of nucleic acids and are particularly important in proliferating cells as part of cell growth and division. The inhibition of purines by competitive inhibitors (azathioprine and 6-mercaptopurine) and the blocking of critical enzymes (mycophenolate mofetil) in the purine pathway are effective methods of immunosuppression.

Azathioprine and 6-Mercaptopurine

Mechanism of Action

Azathioprine is an inactive compound that is metabolized to the active compound 6-mercaptopurine (6-MP). The exact mechanisms of action of 6-MP and its metabolites have not been fully established. At high doses, 6-MP may be incorporated into RNA and DNA, resulting in a cytotoxic effect; however, this effect is probably not the drug's major action at the usual doses employed. Most likely through the feedback inhibition of de novo purine synthesis, 6-MP and its metabolites may reduce cell proliferation and thus produce immunosuppression. Genetically controlled differences in the activity of enzymes involved in the metabolism of 6-MP have been identified. The enzyme thiopurine *S*-methyltransferase is responsible for the metabolism of 6-MP to the metabolite methyl-6-MP. A rare homozygous (0.3%) and heterozygous (10%) defect in thiopurine *S*-methyltransferase is associated with increased toxicity, with severe hematologic toxicity in homozygous patients.

The drug is eventually metabolized by xanthine oxidase. Because xanthine oxidase is inhibited by allopurinol, the concurrent use of allopurinol and azathioprine or 6-MP can result in a significant reduction in the metabolism of the active compounds and a significant increase in drug toxicity. For this reason, the combination of allopurinol and azathioprine should be avoided.

Indications

Azathioprine is approved by the Food and Drug Administration (FDA) for the prevention of renal transplant rejection and for the treatment of rheumatoid arthritis. Clinical trials and reports suggest that azathioprine also has efficacy in other types of organ transplantation and autoimmune diseases. Azathioprine has been particularly effective as an adjunct to corticosteroid

TABLE 34-3 MAJOR ADVERSE EVENTS ASSOCIATED WITH IMMUNOSUPPRESSIVE THERAPIES*

CORTICOSTEROIDS
Serious and opportunistic infections Osteoporosis Metabolic disorders: hyperglycemia, adrenal suppression, hyperlipidemia, electrolyte abnormalities, fluid retention, hypertension, truncal obesity Cardiovascular Miscellaneous: osteonecrosis, peptic ulcer disease, cataracts, dermatologic abnormalities, steroid myopathy, psychosis, growth retardation, altered mood and behavior
AZATHIOPRINE
Serious and opportunistic infections Hematologic abnormalities: leukopenia, thrombocytopenia, anemia Gastrointestinal: nausea, vomiting, rare hepatitis Reproductive: pregnancy class D Miscellaneous: pancreatitis, interstitial pneumonitis, rashes
MYCOPHENOLATE MOFETIL
Serious and opportunistic infections Leukopenia Gastrointestinal: diarrhea, nausea, dyspepsia, elevated transaminases Reproductive: pregnancy class C
CYCLOSPORINE
Serious and opportunistic infections Renal disease and hypertension Potential for increased malignant neoplasms Reproductive: pregnancy class C Miscellaneous: hirsutism, gingival hyperplasia, hyperuricemia, electrolyte abnormalities
TACROLIMUS
Serious and opportunistic infections Renal disease and hypertension (perhaps lower than with cyclosporine) Potential for increased malignant neoplasms Post-transplantation diabetes mellitus Neurotoxicity: tremor, headaches, motor function abnormalities, mental status alteration, sensory changes Reproductive: pregnancy class C Miscellaneous: hirsutism, gingival hyperplasia, myocardial hypertrophy
SIROLIMUS
Serious and opportunistic infections Renal disease and hypertension Potential for increased malignant neoplasms Reproductive: pregnancy class C Miscellaneous: hyperlipidemia, pneumonitis, interstitial lung disease
CYCLOPHOSPHAMIDE
Serious and opportunistic infections Increased incidence of malignant neoplasms Hematologic toxicity: leukopenia, thrombocytopenia, anemia Reproductive: pregnancy class D, premature ovarian failure, oligospermia, fetal abnormalities Urologic: hemorrhagic cystitis, bladder cancer Miscellaneous: nausea, vomiting, diarrhea, pulmonary fibrosis

*This list highlights the most serious and common adverse events but does not include all reported adverse events with these agents.

therapy, allowing a reduction in corticosteroid dose and avoiding the associated adverse events.

Adverse Effects

Serious infection has been reported during treatment with azathioprine, similar to that seen with other immunosuppressive drugs. Opportunistic infections are a particular concern. Hematologic abnormalities include leukopenia, thrombocytopenia, and anemia. A complete blood count (CBC) is recommended on a regular basis, with greater frequency at the initiation of therapy. Current guidelines recommend a CBC weekly during the first month of azathioprine therapy, every 2 weeks during the second and third months, and monthly thereafter. Genotyping of the enzyme thiopurine S-methyltransferase may identify subjects at the highest risk for hematologic toxicity, but it does not substitute for monitoring of the CBC. Gastrointestinal toxicity is usually minor, but patients may have significant symptomatic complaints of nausea, vomiting, diarrhea, and epigastric pain; these are often self limited and reversible. Severe hepatic toxicity has been rarely reported, leading to a recommendation for regular monitoring of serum transaminases, alkaline phosphatase, and bilirubin, particularly during the first 6 months of therapy. Rare complications of azathioprine treatment include fever, arthralgia, rash, pancreatitis, and interstitial pneumonitis.

Azathioprine use in pregnancy is classified as category D and has been associated with fetal abnormalities in animals. The use of azathioprine should be avoided, if possible, in pregnant women and nursing mothers, although patients with organ transplants and autoimmune disease have had successful pregnancies while receiving azathioprine.

The association between azathioprine treatment and the development of malignant neoplasms is controversial. In most clinical situations, azathioprine is used in conditions and in combination or temporal sequence with other drugs that are associated with the development of malignancies. For example, patients with systemic vasculitis or SLE may initially be treated with cyclophosphamide and then with azathioprine. An increase in malignant neoplasms in this population could be related to azathioprine treatment, but the prior cyclophosphamide therapy may be a greater risk factor. In addition, patients with solid organ transplantation, another circumstance in which azathioprine is frequently used, appear to have a higher rate of malignant neoplasms unrelated to the use of immunosuppressive drugs. Extensive efforts to identify an independent increased risk for malignant neoplasms with azathioprine have not produced consistent results. These results suggest that the risk for malignant transformation with azathioprine is very low, if it exists at all.

Azathioprine is an important and effective therapy in organ transplantation and autoimmune disease. It is often used in combination with other agents and as a corticosteroid-sparing drug. Surveillance for infection and monitoring for hematologic toxicity are important. Concurrent treatment with allopurinol should be avoided to prevent serious toxicity from an interaction of the two drugs.

Mycophenolate Mofetil

Mechanism of Action

Mycophenolate mofetil is a prodrug that is converted in vivo to the active compound mycophenolic acid. Mycophenolic acid acts through inhibition of the enzyme inosine monophosphate dehydrogenase, resulting in an increase in 6-thionosinic acid, which is normally metabolized by this enzyme. The accumulation of 6-thionosinic acid acts via a negative feedback loop to suppress the de novo synthesis of purines and associated DNA production. Although it is not a cytotoxic agent, the actions of mycophenolic acid are most pronounced on proliferating cells, such as lymphocytes, reducing cell division and associated functions of these critical cells in the immune response.

Indications

Mycophenolate mofetil is approved by the FDA for the prevention of allograft rejection in renal, hepatic, and cardiac transplantation. In addition to these approved indications, mycophenolate mofetil has been evaluated in SLE; its principal use is in patients with lupus nephritis, although the drug has been used for other manifestations. Current studies are seeking to determine whether this agent can replace cytotoxic agents, such as cyclophosphamide, in the treatment of SLE, particularly as initial and maintenance therapy for lupus nephritis. Limited use has been reported in other autoimmune diseases such as rheumatoid arthritis, vasculitis, and polymyositis.

Adverse Effects and Monitoring

Common adverse events with mycophenolate mofetil include hematologic and gastrointestinal complications. Leukopenia is reported in 20 to 35% of patients receiving this drug for organ transplantation; however, severe neutropenia is seen in only 2 to 3% of subjects. Patients receiving mycophenolate mofetil have a higher susceptibility to infections, including opportunistic infections, similar to that seen with other immunosuppressive agents. Diarrhea, nausea, and dyspepsia are frequent. Abnormalities of liver enzymes are commonly noted and appear to be dose dependent. Rare complications include pulmonary fibrosis and malignant neoplasms. Mycophenolate mofetil is classified as category C by the FDA for use in pregnant women. Although the agent should be avoided in patients who are pregnant or not practicing adequate contraception, this drug appears to have less impact on the reproductive system than does cyclophosphamide. Patients with SLE who are concerned about cyclophosphamide's potential

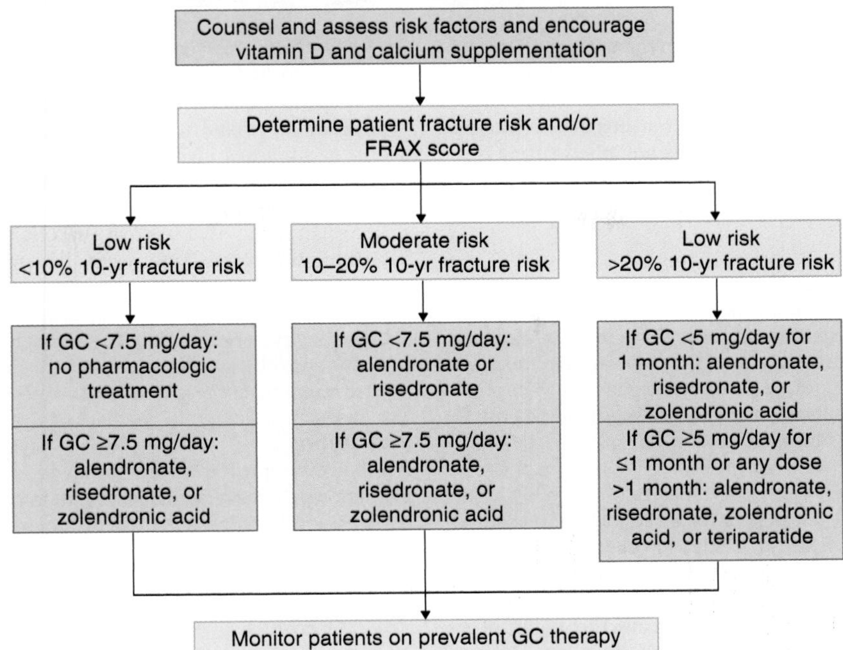

FIGURE 34-1. Algorithm for the prevention of steroid-induced osteoporosis on initiation of glucocorticoid (GC) therapy. FRAX = World Health Organization Fracture Assessment Tool. (Modified from American College of Rheumatology 2010 recommendations for the prevention and treatment of glucocorticoid-induced osteoporosis. *Arthritis Rheum.* 2010;62:1515-1526.)

severe impact on reproductive organs may elect to use mycophenolate mofetil instead.

Monitoring of patients receiving mycophenolate mofetil should include a monthly CBC and hepatic enzyme activities. Monitoring for gastrointestinal and infectious complications should be conducted during regular clinical follow-up.

Mycophenolate mofetil is an important and effective agent in the management of transplant patients. Ongoing studies are evaluating the role of this drug in other autoimmune diseases. It is hoped that mycophenolate mofetil can provide effective therapy for rheumatic and autoimmune disorders with less toxicity than that associated with currently available agents. It has particular potential for use in lupus nephritis.

Immunophilin-Binding Agents

The development of immunophilin inhibitors has significantly advanced organ transplantation. Each of these drugs—cyclosporine, tacrolimus (also known as FK506), and sirolimus (also known as rapamycin)—has significant immunosuppressive activity on T-cell–mediated functions. Although the mechanism of action for each drug differs, they all bind to a cytosolic protein. This binding results in a decrease in T-cell cytokine production and T-cell proliferation. These separate sites of action allow these agents to be used in combination in transplantation management. In addition, because of these differences in action and binding, each drug has a unique adverse event profile.

Cyclosporine

Mechanism of Action

Cyclosporine acts by binding to the cytosolic protein cyclophilin to form a cyclosporine-cyclophilin complex. The cyclosporine-cyclophilin complex inhibits the enzyme calcineurin, which is involved in multiple T-cell functions and is of particular importance in enhancing the transcription of genes for pro-inflammatory cytokines. The use of cyclosporine inhibits the production of IL-2, resulting in a decrease in T-cell activation. Cyclosporine also inhibits the production of other cytokines, including IL-3, IL-4, granulocyte-macrophage colony-simulating factor, tumor necrosis factor-α, and interferon-γ. The overall impact of these actions is to reduce immune function and inflammation.

Indications

The use of cyclosporine and other calcineurin inhibitors has revolutionized treatment after solid organ transplantation. The specific FDA-approved indications include renal, liver, and heart transplantation. Most often the drug is used in conjunction with other immunosuppressive agents, including corticosteroids and azathioprine. The critical clinical challenge is to balance the potent immunosuppressive effects of the drug against its adverse effects, with particular attention to the avoidance of infectious complications and monitoring for hypertension and renal toxicity. Because of these critical issues, prescription of this drug is limited to physicians experienced in the use of immunosuppressive agents.

Oral cyclosporine is also approved for the treatment of rheumatoid arthritis as a disease-modifying antirheumatic drug (DMARD), either alone or in combination with methotrexate. Although it is effective in the treatment of rheumatoid arthritis and other rheumatic diseases, cyclosporine does not have substantially greater efficacy than the other DMARDs. Cyclosporine is also approved for the treatment of psoriasis. Because of its significant adverse event profile, cyclosporine is generally reserved for patients with autoimmune diseases who have failed therapy with more traditional and less toxic agents.

Topical cyclosporine is effective and is approved to increase tear production, presumed to be suppressed secondary to inflammation, in patients with keratoconjunctivitis sicca syndrome. Topical treatment is associated with a much lower frequency of adverse drug events than is systemic cyclosporine therapy.

Adverse Effects

Close monitoring is required during cyclosporine therapy. Blood levels can be measured, which is useful to ensure that the drug remains within the therapeutic range and below levels associated with increased toxicity. Because many potential drug and food interactions can either raise or lower cyclosporine levels, such as increased levels seen with the ingestion of grapefruit and grapefruit juice, patients should be constantly monitored, and blood levels should be obtained when indicated. These evaluations should ensure that when medical therapy is added, changed, or deleted, these adjustments do not have an impact on the effects of the cyclosporine.

Infection

Patients receiving cyclosporine and other calcineurin inhibitors have an increased risk of developing infections. Opportunistic infections associated with impaired cell-mediated immunity are particularly increased in these patients.

Renal Disease and Hypertension

Renal disease and hypertension are common adverse events during cyclosporine therapy and increase in prevalence with increased doses and duration of therapy. Close monitoring of blood pressure and serum creatinine concentration is critical during treatment with cyclosporine. In many cases, these conditions are reversible if they are detected early and appropriate dose adjustments are implemented. In many patients, a mild increase in serum creatinine concentration may be tolerated if the level remains stable. Although renal abnormalities and hypertension are commonly identified during treatment with cyclosporine, most patients can continue taking the drug if adjustments in dose or other interventions are implemented to avoid these complications.

Malignant Neoplasia

Malignant neoplasms, particularly lymphomas, are more common in patients receiving solid organ transplants and immunosuppressive therapy. However, the exact cause of these malignant neoplasms has not been determined. In vitro mutagenesis assays with cyclosporine have been negative. In vivo animal studies have yielded equivocal results, with some data suggesting a possible increased rate of malignant neoplasms in rats and mice.

Reproductive Issues

Cyclosporine is a pregnancy class C drug. Data in animals have demonstrated toxicity to both the embryo and the fetus. Patients should practice effective contraception while receiving this drug. Data from pregnant transplant patients are difficult to interpret because cyclosporine is generally not the only medical therapy being given to these women, and the impact of the disease associated with organ transplantation may be difficult to separate from the impact of therapy. Despite these limitations, normal pregnancies and early childhood development have been reported in many women receiving cyclosporine and their children. Premature birth and low birthweight are more common among women receiving cyclosporine. Therefore, although the use of cyclosporine during pregnancy and breast-feeding should be avoided if possible, in patients who become pregnant, an assessment can determine whether the immunosuppressive therapy should be continued. In some cases, the risk of organ rejection with the discontinuation of cyclosporine therapy may exceed the risk of exposure to the fetus during pregnancy.

Other Adverse Effects

Cyclosporine has also been associated with the development of hirsutism, gingival hyperplasia, hyperuricemia, and electrolyte abnormalities.

Tacrolimus

Mechanism of Action

Whereas cyclosporine binds to cyclophilin, tacrolimus binds to a different protein, the 12-kD FK-binding protein (FKBP12). The binding of FKBP12 and tacrolimus forms a complex that inhibits calcineurin in a fashion similar to cyclosporine. Through this mechanism, tacrolimus has similar inhibitory effects on T-cell function and cytokine production.

Indications

Tacrolimus is approved for the prophylactic treatment of organ rejection after kidney and liver transplantation. Its efficacy and safety in rheumatoid arthritis are limited but encouraging. Experience with this agent is less extensive than that with cyclosporine.

Adverse Effects

The major adverse events associated with tacrolimus are similar to those associated with cyclosporine and include increased susceptibility to infection, renal disease, and hypertension. An increase in malignant neoplasia is also reported, with a pattern similar to that in patients receiving cyclosporine.

In addition to the adverse events similar to those reported with other calcineurin inhibitors, some specific complications have been reported with tacrolimus, including the development of post-transplantation diabetes mellitus. This was seen in 20% of subjects in phase III clinical trials of tacrolimus, with the onset generally occurring within the first 3 months of therapy. In many patients, post-transplantation diabetes mellitus resolves after the drug is discontinued. Neurotoxicity has been reported, including tremor, headache, motor function abnormalities, mental status alterations, and sensory changes. Myocardial hypertrophy has also been reported. Tacrolimus, like cyclosporine, is pregnancy class C; patients receiving this drug should practice effective contraception.

Sirolimus

Mechanism of Action

Sirolimus (or rapamycin) in not a calcineurin inhibitor, but it has many actions and mechanisms similar to that class of drug. The mechanism of action of sirolimus involves binding to FKBP12, the binding protein for tacrolimus, but the effect of this binding is different. Instead of acting on calcineurin, the sirolimus-FKBP12 complex binds to another protein, the mammalian target of rapamycin (mTOR), which is a key regulatory kinase. The inhibition of mTOR results in significant immunosuppression by decreasing T-cell proliferation and the progression from G_1 phase to S phase in the cell cycle. Because sirolimus works through a different mechanism of action from cyclosporine, the two drugs have been studied in combination. In renal transplantation patients, these two agents in combination have a greater immunosuppressive effect than that of cyclosporine alone.

Indications

Sirolimus is approved for the prophylaxis of organ rejection in renal transplantation patients older than 12 years, in combination with cyclosporine and corticosteroids. Data on the use of sirolimus in other populations, including subjects with autoimmune diseases, are limited and are generally derived from animal models.

Adverse Effects

The adverse event profile of sirolimus in terms of infections and malignant neoplasms is similar to that of the calcineurin inhibitors. Renal disease in patients taking cyclosporine and sirolimus in combination has been reported more frequently than in those receiving cyclosporine alone. Adverse reactions specific for sirolimus include hyperlipidemia, interstitial lung disease, and the syndrome of calcineurin-induced hemolytic-uremic syndrome, thrombotic thrombocytopenic purpura, and thrombotic microangiopathy.

Alkylating Agents

Alkylating agents are an important component of immunosuppressive therapy in autoimmune diseases. The use of these agents is limited by their toxicity, particularly the potential for the development of malignant neoplasia, reproductive toxicity, and an increased incidence of infection. Patients considered candidates for alkylating therapy should be fully informed of the potential risks and benefits of these drugs and should concur with the decision to use them. Regular monitoring of the CBC and urinalysis is important in patients receiving these drugs.

Cyclophosphamide

Cyclophosphamide has been used primarily as a cytotoxic drug for the treatment of malignant neoplasms; it is currently approved for this indication as well as for biopsy-proven minimal change nephrotic disease in children. Several severe autoimmune diseases are also responsive to cyclophosphamide, which is often given in conjunction with initial high-dose corticosteroid therapy. Because of the significant toxicities associated with these drugs, a benefit-to-risk assessment and discussion should be undertaken with each patient for whom cyclophosphamide is being considered. In most cases, the diseases warranting cyclophosphamide therapy are life-threatening conditions with a poor prognosis, justifying the use of such a toxic agent.

Mechanism of Action

Cyclophosphamide is an inactive compound that can be administered either orally or intravenously. It is metabolized to the active drug by the cytochrome P-450 mixed-function oxidase system. This process produces the active compounds phosphoramide mustard and the toxic metabolite acrolein. The cytotoxic effect of this drug results from the alkylation of various cellular constituents, especially nucleic acids. Changes in immune function with cyclophosphamide include depletion of lymphoid tissues, with decreases in both B and T cells, suppression of cellular immune function, and decreased antibody production.

Indications

The use of cyclophosphamide in the treatment of rheumatic diseases is most common and well studied in lupus nephritis and severe systemic vasculitis. Controlled clinical trials have demonstrated improved outcomes in these conditions, with reduced progression to end-stage renal disease in patients with SLE and improved survival in those with systemic vasculitides such as Wegener's granulomatosis. The evaluation of cyclophosphamide in patients with SLE has demonstrated the benefit of intermittent, usually monthly, intravenous pulse therapy as a method to avoid some of the most severe toxic side effects while maintaining therapeutic efficacy. However, pulse intravenous cyclophosphamide is not as effective as continuous oral cyclophosphamide in all conditions, particularly Wegener's granulomatosis. Patients with other conditions, such as polyarteritis nodosa, Takayasu's arteritis, and Churg-Strauss syndrome, reportedly benefit from cyclophosphamide therapy; however, the low prevalence of these diseases has prohibited the conduct of controlled clinical trials to prove its efficacy. Cyclophosphamide is also effective in the treatment of rheumatoid arthritis, but it is generally not used in this condition because of its toxicity and the availability of other effective agents. Although the advent of cyclophosphamide has been a tremendous advance in the treatment of these life-threatening diseases, the use of less toxic medications with similar clinical efficacy is currently under investigation.

Adverse Effects

Before the initiation of cyclophosphamide therapy, a frank discussion with the patient about potential serious and even life-threatening adverse events should be undertaken and documented.

MALIGNANT NEOPLASIA. Malignant neoplasms may develop in patients receiving cyclophosphamide for the treatment of both malignant and nonmalignant diseases. The risk of malignant change appears to increase with the duration and dose of cyclophosphamide. The most common malignant neoplasms are bladder, myeloproliferative, and lymphoproliferative disorders. The use of intravenous pulse cyclophosphamide may reduce but not eliminate the risk of bladder cancer. These malignant neoplasms may develop years after discontinuation of the drug.

REPRODUCTIVE ISSUES. Cyclophosphamide can be teratogenic, affect female reproduction, and reduce male fertility. Cyclophosphamide is pregnancy category D and should not be used in pregnant women unless life-threatening disease is present that warrants this treatment. Although successful pregnancies have been reported in patients receiving cyclophosphamide during pregnancy, fetal abnormalities are well documented secondary to chromosome damage. The use of cyclophosphamide in premenopausal women can induce premature ovarian failure. The use of gonadotropin-releasing hormone analogues during intravenous pulse cyclophosphamide therapy may reduce but not eliminate the risk of premature ovarian failure in patients with SLE. In males, a temporary or permanent decrease in sperm count may occur with cyclophosphamide. Because the recovery of fertility after cyclophosphamide therapy is variable, sperm banking should be considered before treatment is begun.

OTHER ADVERSE EFFECTS. As with other immunosuppressive agents, infections are more frequent and potentially more serious in patients receiving cyclophosphamide. Opportunistic infections are more likely to be seen in these subjects. Hematologic abnormalities can involve all cell lines. The CBC should be monitored regularly, and cyclophosphamide should be discontinued or the dose reduced when cytopenias develop. Cyclophosphamide treatment may be complicated by hemorrhagic cystitis and bladder cancer, which are probably related to the toxic metabolite acrolein. Efforts to reduce the potential for hemorrhagic cystitis and malignant bladder neoplasms include the use of intravenous pulse therapy, hydration, frequent voiding, and treatment with agents containing sulfhydryl groups to scavenge acrolein. Regular urinalysis for blood is indicated to monitor for bladder toxicity. Patients may develop severe nausea, vomiting, and diarrhea with cyclophosphamide therapy.

Chlorambucil

Chlorambucil has not been evaluated as extensively as cyclophosphamide, but this agent appears to have similar properties and a similar adverse event profile. Like cyclophosphamide, chlorambucil is associated with the development of malignant neoplasms and should be avoided during pregnancy.

Miscellaneous Agents

Although principally prescribed for other indications, methotrexate and leflunomide have been evaluated and used for their potential immunosuppressive effects. Leflunomide blocks the enzyme dihydroorotate dehydrogenase, resulting in the inhibition of pyrimidine synthesis and a reduction in T-cell activation. Methotrexate has multiple mechanisms of action, but its major effect in autoimmune diseases is mediated by inhibition of the enzyme aminoimidazole-4-carboxamide ribonucleotide transformylase. This inhibition affects purine synthesis, increasing the intracellular concentration of aminoimidazole-4-carboxamide ribonucleotide, which stimulates the release of adenosine, a potent anti-inflammatory compound. Methotrexate has principally been advocated for its corticosteroid-sparing effects. Both methotrexate and leflunomide are effective DMARDs in the treatment of rheumatoid arthritis.

SUGGESTED READINGS

Grossman JM, Gordon R, Ranganath VK, et al. American College of Rheumatology 2010 recommendations for the prevention and treatment of glucocorticoid-induced osteoporosis. *Arthritis Care Res*. 2010;62:1515-1526. *Consensus guidelines.*

Kuypers DR. Immunotherapy in elderly transplant recipients: a guide to clinically significant drug interactions. *Drugs Aging*. 2009;26:715-737. *A detailed review of medications that interact with immunosuppressive medications.*

Lui JC, Baron J. Effects of glucocorticoids on the growth plate. *Endocr Dev*. 2011;20:187-193. *Glucocorticoids inhibit chondrocyte proliferation, hypertrophy, and cartilage matrix synthesis, but after their discontinuation, the growth plate grows more rapidly than normal for age.*

35

BIOLOGIC AGENTS

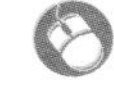

CEM GABAY

Biologic agents are a new class of therapeutic agents that target different mediators involved in the pathogenesis of human diseases. The development of these therapies has markedly improved the management of many diseases. In addition, their use has greatly increased our understanding of the pathophysiology of these diseases. One of the most compelling examples is the efficacy of tumor necrosis factor (TNF)-α inhibitors in rheumatoid arthritis and inflammatory bowel disease.

Classification systems for the different biologic therapies have been established (Table 35-1). The pharmaceutical company usually provides the prefix of the name, and the suffix defines whether this is a monoclonal antibody (mab), a soluble receptor (cept), or a kinase inhibitor (inib). Monoclonal antibodies, by far the largest group of biologic agents today, also include in their names the type of target (immune system, cancer, cardiovascular system, bone), as well as their origin (chimeric, humanized, human). Rather than providing an exhaustive review of all tested approaches, this chapter reviews the currently approved treatments.

TUMOR NECROSIS FACTOR-α INHIBITORS

The cytokine TNF-α binds to two different receptors, TNF-R55 and TNF-R75, and exerts important functions in the control of host responses against infection. However, uncontrolled TNF-α production may lead to chronic inflammation and subsequent tissue damage.

Types of TNF Inhibitors

Different agents have been developed to inhibit the biologic activity of TNF-α, including monoclonal antibodies and soluble receptors. Monoclonal antibodies include infliximab (Remicade), adalimumab (Humira), and golimumab (Simponi). Infliximab is a chimeric antibody, whereas the other two are fully human antibodies. Certolizumab-pegol (Cimzia) is a pegylated humanized anti–TNF-α antibody Fab′ fragment. Etanercept (Enbrel) is a fusion protein that contains the extracellular portion of TNF-R75 coupled to the Fc domain of human immunoglobulin (Ig) G1. All these agents bind to TNF-α and block its biologic activity. Etanercept also binds to lymphotoxin-α (previously termed TNF-β). Infliximab has been shown to exert cytotoxic effects on macrophages and T lymphocytes expressing TNF-α on their surface.

Indications

TNF-α antagonists are approved for the treatment of rheumatoid arthritis (Chapter 272). They exert marked anti-inflammatory effects and prevent the progression of structural joint damage. TNF-α inhibitors are efficacious in

TABLE 35-1 NOMENCLATURE OF MONOCLONAL ANTIBODIES

Nomenclature for monoclonal antibodies (mAbs) are composed of a prefix, a substem A, a substem B, and a suffix.
The common stem for all mAbs is *–mab*, placed as a suffix.
Substems B and A preceding *–mab* represent source identifiers of the antibody, as follows:

TARGET (MOLECULE, CELL, ORGAN)	SUBSTEM A
Immunomodulating	*-l(i)-*
Cardiovascular	*-c(i)-*
Bone	*-o(s)-*
Interleukin	*-k(i)-*
Tumor	*-t(u)-*
SOURCE	**SUBSTEM B**
Human	*-u-*
Humanized	*-zu-*
Chimeric	*-xi-*
Rat	*-a-*
EXAMPLE	**INDICATES**
Ri***tux***imab	**Tumor, chimeric**
Den***osu***mab	**Bone, human**
Tras***tuzu***mab	**Tumor, humanized**
Beva***cizu***mab	**Cardiovascular, humanized**

From the International Nonproprietary Names (INN) Program of the World Health Organization, 2009: www.who.int/medicines/services/inn/Generalpoliciesformonoclonalantibodies2009.pdf.

early rheumatoid arthritis and in long-standing disease refractory to conventional disease-modifying antirheumatic drugs (DMARDs) such as methotrexate. TNF-α inhibitors are also approved for the treatment of ankylosing spondylitis refractory to nonsteroidal anti-inflammatory drugs (NSAIDs) and psoriatic arthritis refractory to DMARDs (Chapter 273). Anti–TNF-α antibodies, but not etanercept, have proven efficacy in severe Crohn's disease (Chapter 143) by reducing the disease activity score, inducing closure of draining fistulas, and allowing a decrease in the dose of chronic glucocorticoid medication. Infliximab is approved for the treatment of ulcerative colitis refractory to conventional therapy. Infliximab, adalimumab, and etanercept are also approved for the treatment of chronic plaque psoriasis (Chapter 446) refractory to phototherapy or systemic therapy.

Adverse Effects

TNF-α inhibitors can cause allergic reactions. Postmarketing data have shown that TNF-α inhibitors are associated with an increased risk of infections, including all types of bacterial and opportunistic infections. In particular, the use of TNF-α inhibitors has been associated with an increased risk of reactivation of latent tuberculosis. The results of cohort studies do not support an increased risk of cancer. Rare cases of demyelinating disorders, lupus-like manifestations, and cytopenia have also been reported.

INTERLEUKIN-1 INHIBITORS

Interleukin (IL)-1 (both IL-1α and IL-1β) binds to IL-1 receptors (type I IL-1R and IL-1R accessory protein) to induce a vast array of inflammatory signals. IL-1 receptor antagonist (IL-1Ra) competitively inhibits the interaction of IL-1 with its receptors.

Types of IL-1 Inhibitors

Anakinra (Kineret), recombinant human IL-1Ra, was the first IL-1 inhibitor used in clinical trials. Rilonacept (Arcalyst) is a fusion protein including the IL-1 binding motifs of IL-1 receptors coupled to the Fc domain of human IgG1. Canakinumab (Ilaris) is a fully human monoclonal antibody against IL-1β.

Indications

Anakinra is approved for the treatment of rheumatoid arthritis refractory to conventional DMARDs, but it has relatively modest efficacy. Anakinra, canakinumab, and rilonacept exert marked anti-inflammatory effects in hereditary systemic autoinflammatory diseases (Chapter 269) characterized by enhanced IL-1β production, leading to their approval for this indication. Anakinra is effective in some patients with systemic inflammatory diseases, including systemic-onset juvenile idiopathic arthritis, adult-onset Still's disease, and other autoinflammatory conditions. Clinical trials have reported encouraging results in crystal-induced arthritis such as gout and chondrocalcinosis. Promising results have also been reported from the use of anakinra in type 2 diabetes mellitus and smoldering/indolent multiple myeloma.

Adverse Effects

Anakinra is frequently associated with injection site reactions. A modest increase in serious infections has been reported with anakinra. The combination of anakinra and etanercept (and probably other TNF-α antagonists as well) increases the risk of infections and is not recommended.

INTERLEUKIN-6 INHIBITORS

IL-6 is a pro-inflammatory cytokine that binds to a heterodimeric receptor, including IL-6Rα and gp130. Tocilizumab (Actemra) is a humanized monoclonal antibody against IL-6Rα that inhibits its interaction with IL-6.

Indications

Tocilizumab is approved for the treatment of rheumatoid arthritis refractory to conventional DMARDs and TNF-α antagonists.[1] In clinical trials, tocilizumab prevented the progression of radiographic damage. Tocilizumab is also effective in controlling the inflammatory manifestations of systemic-onset juvenile idiopathic arthritis. Clinical trials are in progress in other inflammatory rheumatic diseases.

Adverse Effects

Tocilizumab has been associated with an increased risk of serious infections. A transient increase in transaminase levels has been reported. Hypercholesterolemia and cytopenia may appear in some patients.

ANTIBODY AGAINST INTERLEUKIN-12 AND INTERLEUKIN-23

IL-12 and IL-23 are heterodimeric cytokines, including a common p40 subunit and a specific subunit—p35 for IL-12, and p19 for IL-23. IL-23 participates in the differentiation of T_H17 cells that produce IL-17. Recent experimental findings indicate that IL-23 and IL-17 are critical for the development of autoimmune pathologies. Ustekinumab (Stelara) is a human monoclonal antibody against p40 that targets both IL-12 and IL-23 and blocks their biologic activities.

Indications

Ustekinumab is approved for the treatment of psoriasis in patients who have had prior exposure to phototherapy or other systemic therapies. In clinical trials, ustekinumab was associated with the successful treatment of Crohn's disease. In addition, ustekinumab was effective in patients with psoriatic arthritis refractory to conventional DMARDs. Anti–IL-17 antibodies are also in clinical trials for the treatment of psoriasis and rheumatoid arthritis.

Adverse Effects

Ustekinumab has been well tolerated in clinical trials.

INHIBITORS OF ANGIOGENESIS

Vascular endothelial growth factor (VEGF) is a family of growth factors involved in vasculogenesis and angiogenesis. VEGF-A binds to the tyrosine kinase receptors VEGFR1 and VEGFR2. VEGF has been implicated in tumor growth and metastasis, in diabetic retinopathy, and in age-related macular retinopathy.

Types of Angiogenesis Inhibitors

Bevacizumab (Avastin) is a humanized monoclonal antibody against VEGF that acts as an angiogenesis inhibitor. VEGF Trap is a fusion protein containing extracellular immunoglobulin motifs of VEGFR1 and VEGFR2 coupled to human IgG1. Sunitinib (Sutent) and sorafenib (Nexavar) are two orally available tyrosine kinase inhibitors that block not only VEGFR2 but also platelet-derived growth factor receptor β, C-kit, and Flt3 receptor.

Indications

Bevacizumab is approved for the treatment of glioblastoma (Chapter 195) and also for some patients with non–small cell lung cancer (Chapter 197) and metastatic colorectal cancer (Chapter 199). The absence of clear benefit on survival in patients with metastatic breast cancer led to the removal of the indication by the FDA. Bevacizumab is still approved in Europe in combination with placitaxel for this indication. Intraocular injections of ranibizumab (Lucentis), an antibody fragment derived from bevacizumab, are effective in maintaining vision in the vast majority of patients with wet macular degeneration (Chapter 431) and are approved for this indication.

Sunitinib is approved for the treatment of metastatic renal cell carcinoma (Chapter 203) and gastrointestinal stromal tumor refractory to imatinib (Chapter 209). Sorafenib is approved for advanced renal cell carcinoma and some cases of hepatocarcinoma (Chapter 202).

Adverse Effects

Bevacizumab has been associated with a heightened risk of bleeding and gastrointestinal tract perforation. Delayed wound healing and hypertension have also been reported. Sunitinib and sorafenib are generally well tolerated. Reported adverse events include hypertension, fatigue, asthenia, diarrhea, and some abnormal laboratory tests, including lipase, amylase, leukocytes, and platelets.

INHIBITORS OF TUMOR GROWTH FACTORS

Epidermal growth factor receptor (EGFR), a member of the ErbB-1 (HER-1) family of receptors, is a cell surface receptor for EGF and transforming growth factor-α. Binding of EGFR tyrosine kinase activity leads to increased gene transcription, cell proliferation, and inhibition of apoptosis. Human epithelial growth factor receptor (HER)-2 (also known as ErbB-2) is a receptor with tyrosine kinase activity that is expressed at high levels in 20 to 30% of breast cancers and other types of cancers and may cause uncontrolled tumor cell proliferation.

Types of Tumor Growth Factor Inhibitors

Two types of strategies target the EGFR pathway: monoclonal antibodies to the extracellular domain of EGFR, and orally available tyrosine kinase inhibitors. Cetuximab (Erbitux) is a chimeric monoclonal IgG1 anti-EGFR antibody that inhibits EGFR signaling and may also induce tumor cell death by antibody-dependent cellular cytotoxicity. Panitumumab (Vectibix) is a fully human monoclonal IgG2 antibody directed against EGFR. Erlotinib (Tarceva) and gefitinib (Iressa) are the two most commonly studied EGFR tyrosine kinase inhibitors.

Trastuzumab (Herceptin) is a humanized monoclonal IgG1 antibody that binds to the extracellular domain of HER-2. Lapatinib (Tykerb) is a small molecule with inhibitory activity on EGFR and HER-2 tyrosine kinases.

Indications

Cetuximab is an approved second- and third-line treatment for colorectal cancer and squamous cell carcinoma of the head and neck.[2] Positive results were also reported in clinical trials of cetuximab as first- or second-line treatment in patients with non–small cell lung cancer. Panitumumab is approved for the treatment of metastatic colorectal cancer. Erlotinib is approved for the treatment of metastatic non–small cell lung carcinoma and advanced pancreatic cancer, and gefitinib is approved for the treatment of advanced non–small cell lung carcinoma. Trastuzumab and lapatinib are approved for the treatment of metastatic breast cancer expressing HER-2.

Adverse Effects

Cetuximab is sometimes associated with severe allergic reactions during infusion. Acne-like skin rash is commonly reported. Erlotinib and gefitinib are associated with acne-like rash and mild gastrointestinal symptoms. Cardiotoxicity is a major problem in patients treated with trastuzumab. Approximately 10% of patients are unable to tolerate this drug because of preexisting heart problems. The risk of cardiomyopathy is increased when combined with anthracycline (which itself is associated with cardiac toxicity). Lapatinib is generally well tolerated, but some cases of hepatotoxicity have been reported.

OTHER TYROSINE KINASE INHIBITORS

Imatinib mesylate (Gleevec, Glivec) works by binding to the adenosine triphosphate (ATP) binding site of Bcr-abl, resulting in competitive inhibition of its enzymatic activity. Imatinib also inhibits the tyrosine kinase activity of C-kit and platelet-derived growth factor receptor.

Indications

Imatinib represents a major advance over conventional treatments for chronic myelogenous leukemia (Chapter 190), with more than 90% of patients obtaining a complete hematologic response and 70 to 80% achieving a complete cytogenetic response. Resistance to imatinib is often a result of point mutations causing a conformation change in Bcr-abl, which impairs imatinib binding. Dasatinib (Sprycel) and nilotinib (Tasigna), two other tyrosine kinase inhibitors, are approved for the treatment of chronic myelogenous leukemia that is not responsive or is intolerant to imatinib, and dasatinib can provide more rapid and possibly durable responses than does imatinib.[3]

Imatinib is also approved for the treatment of patients with C-kit–positive advanced gastrointestinal stromal tumor (Chapter 209). Early clinical trials also showed imatinib's potential beneficial effects in systemic mastocytosis, hypereosinophilic syndrome, and dermatofibrosarcoma protuberans. Imatinib is in clinical trials for systemic sclerosis.

Adverse Effects

Imatinib has been associated with cytopenia, edema, nausea, and rash, as well as rare cases of congestive heart failure. Cytopenia and congestive heart failure are also reported with dasatinib, and cytopenia can occur with nilotinib. The latter drug also carries a potential risk of severe cardiac arrhythmias.

BIOLOGIC AGENTS TARGETING T LYMPHOCYTES

T cells play a central role in immune responses and are thus important targets for therapies against graft rejection and autoimmune diseases.

Types of Agents Modulating T-Cell Activity

The agents targeting T cells include antibodies against T cells, soluble receptors inhibiting costimulation signals, and antibodies blocking T-cell migration. Therapies targeting CD3 were developed more than 30 years ago with a mouse monoclonal IgG2 antibody called OKT3. These antibodies were used in the treatment of kidney transplant rejection but were associated with limiting side effects due to the occurrence of a "cytokine release syndrome." A series of non-Fc binding humanized anti-CD3 monoclonal antibodies was developed to overcome this problem, along with the development of antimurine immunoglobulin antibodies.

Abatacept (Orencia) is a fusion protein containing the extracellular portion of cytotoxic T-lymphocyte antigen-4 coupled to the Fc portion of human IgG1; it inhibits costimulatory signals between CD28 and CD80/86. Alefacept (Amevive) is a recombinant fully human fusion protein in which the extracellular domain of CD2 has been linked to the Fc portion of IgG1; it inhibits costimulatory signals between CD2 and LFA-3.

Natalizumab (Tysabri), a humanized monoclonal antibody against α_4-integrin, inhibits the migration of T cells by blocking the interaction between α_4-integrin and adhesion molecules expressed on endothelial cells.

Indications

Different monoclonal anti-CD3 antibodies are used in clinical trials for the prevention of transplant rejection (Chapter 48), as well as for the treatment of acute graft-versus-host disease and type 1 diabetes mellitus.

Abatacept is approved for the treatment of rheumatoid arthritis refractory to conventional DMARDs and TNF-α inhibitors. Positive results have been reported in psoriasis and psoriatic arthritis. Alefacept is approved for the treatment of chronic plaque psoriasis. Natalizumab is approved for the treatment of patients with highly active remitting-relapsing multiple sclerosis on monotherapy (Chapter 419) and for severe Crohn's disease.

Adverse Effects

Abatacept is generally well tolerated, but serious infections may occur. Lymphopenia may occur with alefacept, and infections, malignancies, and hepatotoxicity have been reported in clinical trials. Natalizumab can be associated with allergic reactions and hepatotoxicity. Some cases of multifocal progressive leukoencephalopathy (Chapter 378), a fatal neurologic complication of JC virus reactivation in immunosuppressed individuals, have been reported, thus limiting the use of natalizumab.

BIOLOGIC AGENTS TARGETING B LYMPHOCYTES

The B-cell lineage plays a critical role in immune responses through the production of immunoglobulins, the presentation of antigen to T cells, and the production of cytokines. Therapies targeting B cells are used in B-cell lymphoma and autoimmune diseases.

Mode of Action

B cells can be targeted either by the use of monoclonal antibodies depleting B cells or by the inhibition of cytokines essential for their maturation and survival, such as B-cell activating factor of the TNF family (BAFF) and a proliferation-inducing ligand (APRIL). Rituximab (Rituxan, MabThera), ofatumumab (Arzerra), and ocrelizumab are B-cell–depleting monoclonal antibodies binding to CD20. Belimumab is a fully human monoclonal antibody against BAFF. Atacicept is a fusion protein containing the extracellular domain of TACI (BAFF and APRIL receptor), which inhibits BAFF and APRIL biologic activities.

Indications

Rituximab is approved for the treatment of non-Hodgkin's B-cell lymphoma (Chapter 191). More recently, rituximab has also been approved for rheumatoid arthritis patients with an inadequate response to TNF-α inhibitors. Ofatumumab is approved for the treatment of chronic lymphocytic leukemia (Chapter 190). Ocrelizumab is currently in clinical trials in multiple sclerosis and systemic lupus erythematosus. Epratuzumab, a humanized monoclonal anti-CD22 B-cell–depleting antibody, is in clinical trials for non-Hodgkin's B-cell lymphoma and systemic lupus erythematosus.

The administration of belimumab in patients with systemic lupus erythematosus has led to positive results regarding the number of flares and disease activity. Atacicept is in clinical trials for rheumatoid arthritis and systemic lupus erythematosus.

Adverse Effects

Rituximab is associated with an allergic reaction during infusions, a systemic reaction due to tumoral B-cell lysis, and an increased risk of infections. Rare cases of multifocal progressive leukoencephalopathy have been reported. Hypogammaglobulinemia may occur, particularly after several series of infusions.

CONCLUSIONS

The use of biologic agents has led to major advances in the management of many severe diseases refractory to conventional therapies. These agents have also provided a unique way to confirm the role of basic mechanisms in human diseases. New developments in this field will take different directions, including the refinement of existing strategies (using more selective inhibitors or human rather than chimeric antibodies), the extension to indications other than those for which the agents were primarily designed, and the selection of novel targets.

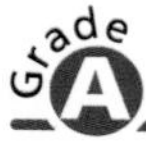

1. Singh JA, Beg S, Lopez-Olivo MA. Tocilizumab for rheumatoid arthritis. *Cochrane Database Syst Rev.* 2010;7:CD008331.
2. Liu L, Cao Y, Tan A, et al. Cetuximab-based therapy versus non-cetuximab therapy for advanced cancer: a meta-analysis of 17 randomized controlled trials. *Cancer Chemother Pharmacol.* 2010;65:849-861.
3. Kantarjian H, Shah NP, Hochhaus A, et al. Dasatinib versus imatinib in newly diagnosed chronic-phase chronic myeloid leukemia. *N Engl J Med.* 2010;362:2260-2270.

SUGGESTED READINGS

Devine EB, Alfonso-Christancho R, Sullivan SD. Effectiveness of biologic therapies for rheumatoid arthritis: an indirect comparisons approach. *Pharmacotherapy.* 2011;31:39-51. *All approved biologic agents are significantly better than placebo, with the TNFα inhibitor certolizumab perhaps the most efficacious.*

Gabay C, Lamacchia C, Palmer G. IL-1 pathways in inflammation and human diseases. *Nat Rev Rheumatol.* 2010;6:232-241. *Describes some basic findings on IL-1 biology and their implications for the use of IL-1 inhibitors in the management of different inflammatory diseases.*

Graudal N, Jürgens G. Similar effects of disease-modifying antirheumatic drugs, glucocorticoids, and biologic agents on radiographic progression in rheumatoid arthritis: meta-analysis of 70 randomized placebo-controlled or drug-controlled studies, including 112 comparisons. *Arthritis Rheum.* 2010;62:2852-2863. *All agents were beneficial, thereby suggesting that biologic agents should be reserved for patients resistant to DMARD therapy.*

Grothey A, Galanis E. Targeting angiogenesis: progress with anti-VEGF treatment with large molecules. *Nat Rev Clin Oncol.* 2009;6:507-518. *Discusses the rationale for using antiangiogenic compounds in the treatment of cancer, with a focus on antibodies that target the VEGF system.*

36

PROSTANOIDS, ASPIRIN, AND RELATED COMPOUNDS

CARLO PATRONO

Arachidonic acid, or 5,8,11,14-eicosatetraenoic acid, is a 20-carbon polyunsaturated fatty acid esterified in the phospholipid domain of cell membranes. In response to chemical, physical, and hormonal stimuli, arachidonic acid is released from the glycerol backbone sn-2 position by the action of various phospholipases A_2, and can be subjected to rapid enzymatic conversion to a series of oxygenated derivatives collectively called *eicosanoids*. The enzymes catalyzing various structural modifications of free arachidonic acid include prostaglandin H synthases (commonly known as *cyclooxygenases* [COX]), *lipoxygenases*, and *cytochrome P-450 isozymes*. The resulting eicosanoids include prostanoids (prostaglandins and thromboxane A_2), leukotrienes, lipoxins, and epoxylins. Esterified arachidonic acid can also be subjected to in situ peroxidation, catalyzed by oxygen radicals, to form a series of corresponding isomers called *isoeicosanoids*.

Eicosanoids are not stored but are produced in response to diverse stimuli, with a pattern that reflects the cell-specific distribution of arachidonic acid–metabolizing enzymes and downstream isomerases and synthases. Eicosanoids are not circulating hormones but rather ubiquitous autacoids that modulate the intensity and duration of many important cellular responses in an autocrine (acting on the same cells that produced them) or paracrine (acting on nearby cells) fashion.

BIOSYNTHESIS AND ACTION OF PROSTANOIDS

Prostanoids include prostaglandins D_2, E_2, $F_{2\alpha}$, and I_2 (prostacyclin) and thromboxane A_2. They are formed through the sequential actions of phospholipase A_2 to release arachidonic acid from membrane phospholipids, prostaglandin H synthase to catalyze the cyclooxygenation of arachidonic acid to form the unstable intermediate prostaglandin G_2 and its reduction to prostaglandin H_2, and specific isomerases and synthases to catalyze the conversion of prostaglandin H_2 to different prostanoids (Fig. 36-1). Once formed, prostanoids interact with specific G protein–coupled receptors to evoke a variety of cellular responses, depending on the site of their biosynthesis (see Fig. 36-1).

Two prostaglandin H synthases have been identified: prostaglandin H synthase-1 is expressed constitutively in all cells; prostaglandin H synthase-2 is constitutively expressed in some cells (e.g., neurons and renal cells) and is induced in other cell types in response to cytokines (e.g., in monocytes), tumor promoters (e.g., in intestinal epithelial cells), growth factors (e.g., in bone marrow–derived stem cells), and laminar shear stress (e.g., in endothelial cells). Because nonsteroidal anti-inflammatory drugs (NSAIDs) target the COX activity of these enzymes, they have become known colloquially as COX-1 and COX-2. Both enzymes are homodimers that convert arachidonic acid, two O_2 molecules, and two electrons from one or more unknown reductants to prostaglandin H_2. COX-1 and COX-2 are found predominantly in the same cellular organelles, at the luminal surface of the endoplasmic reticulum and nuclear envelope of cells. Only one monomer of a dimer catalyzes arachidonic acid oxygenation at any given time. The cross-talk between monomers serves as a way for COX-2 to exhibit selectivity toward arachidonic acid, even when it is a minor component of the available fatty acid pool, and to sustain a "late phase" of prostanoid production. In contrast, COX-1 may efficiently oxygenate arachidonic acid in the early phase of prostanoid production, when this substrate represents a large fraction of free fatty acids, but may be inhibited by other competing fatty acids in the late phase.

Phenotypical analyses of COX-1-deficient and COX-2-deficient mice, as well as studies with isoform-selective inhibitors, suggest that there are processes in which each isozyme is uniquely involved (e.g., platelet aggregation for COX-1, ovulation and neonatal development for COX-2) and others in which both isozymes function coordinately (e.g., inflammation and its resolution, gastrointestinal ulceration and healing, and carcinogenesis). A way in which the two biosynthetic pathways may be dissociated metabolically is by a preferential coupling of the COX isozymes to various upstream phospholipases and downstream synthases, conditioning preferential formation of a particular prostanoid by a given cell type (e.g., COX-2-dependent prostacyclin by vascular endothelial cells).

Moreover, COX-2 oxygenation may play a unique role in a novel signaling pathway dependent on agonist-induced release of endocannabinoids. Among the products of COX-2 oxygenation of endocannabinoids are glyceryl prostaglandins, some of which (e.g., glyceryl prostaglandin E_2 and glyceryl prostaglandin I_2) exhibit interesting biologic activities in inflammatory, neurologic, and vascular systems.

MEASUREMENTS OF THE PROSTAGLANDIN H SYNTHASE PATHWAY

Prostanoids are formed in vivo at a relatively low rate (e.g., 0.1 ng/kg per minute for both prostacyclin and thromboxane A_2) and are metabolized extensively by lung and liver enzymes to form chemically stable, but biologically inactive, derivatives that are excreted primarily through the kidney. Given the chemical instability and extremely low concentrations (1 to 2 pg/

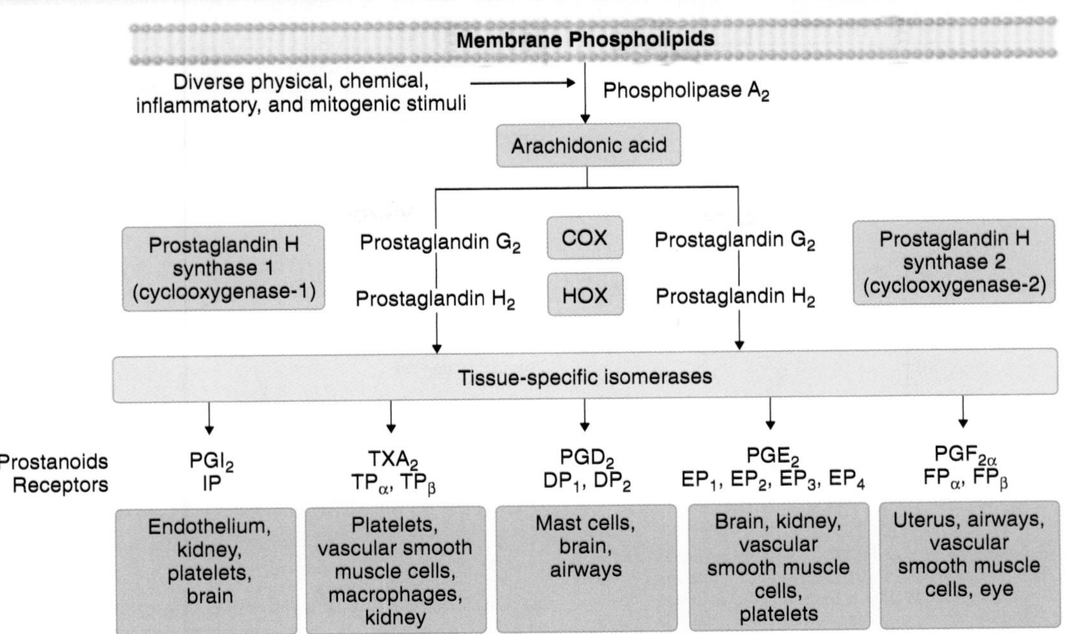

FIGURE 36-1. Production and actions of prostaglandins and thromboxane. Arachidonic acid, a 20-carbon fatty acid containing four double bonds, is liberated from the *sn*2 position in membrane phospholipids by phospholipase A_2, which is activated by diverse stimuli. Arachidonic acid is converted by prostaglandin H synthases, which have both cyclooxygenase (COX) and hydroperoxidase (HOX) activity, to the unstable intermediate prostaglandin H_2. The synthases are colloquially termed *cyclooxygenases* and exist in two forms, cyclooxygenase-1 and cyclooxygenase-2. Prostaglandin H_2 is converted by tissue-specific isomerases to multiple prostanoids. These bioactive lipids activate specific cell membrane receptors of the superfamily of G protein–coupled receptors. Some of the tissues in which individual prostanoids exert prominent effects are indicated. IP denotes prostacyclin receptor, TP thromboxane receptor, DP prostaglandin D_2 receptor, EP prostaglandin E_2 receptor, and FP prostaglandin $F_{2\alpha}$ receptor.

mL) of prostanoids in the systemic circulation, assessment of their production in humans is largely based on measurements of stable urinary metabolites (e.g., 11-dehydro-thromboxane B_2, a major enzymatic derivative of thromboxane A_2, and 2,3-dinor-6-keto-$PGF_{1\alpha}$, a major enzymatic derivative of prostacyclin). These analytical measurements have established that thromboxane metabolite excretion is primarily derived from platelet thromboxane biosynthesis and largely reflects the rate of platelet activation in vivo. Similarly, prostacyclin metabolite excretion largely reflects the rate of vascular prostacyclin biosynthesis in vivo. Thromboxane biosynthesis is persistently enhanced in association with the major cardiovascular risk factors (e.g., diabetes mellitus). Both thromboxane and prostacyclin biosynthesis are episodically increased in patients with acute coronary syndromes, perhaps reflecting a homeostatic response to accelerated platelet-vascular interactions.

Studies of the human pharmacology of COX inhibitors have largely relied on the development of whole blood assays of platelet COX-1 (based on serum thromboxane B_2 measurements) and monocyte COX-2 (based on lipopolysaccharide-induced prostaglandin E_2 production) activities. These assays have been useful in characterizing the variable potency of NSAIDs in inhibiting COX-1 and COX-2 in vitro (a measure of isozyme selectivity) and in determining ex vivo the dose- and time-dependence of their inhibitory effects in health and disease.

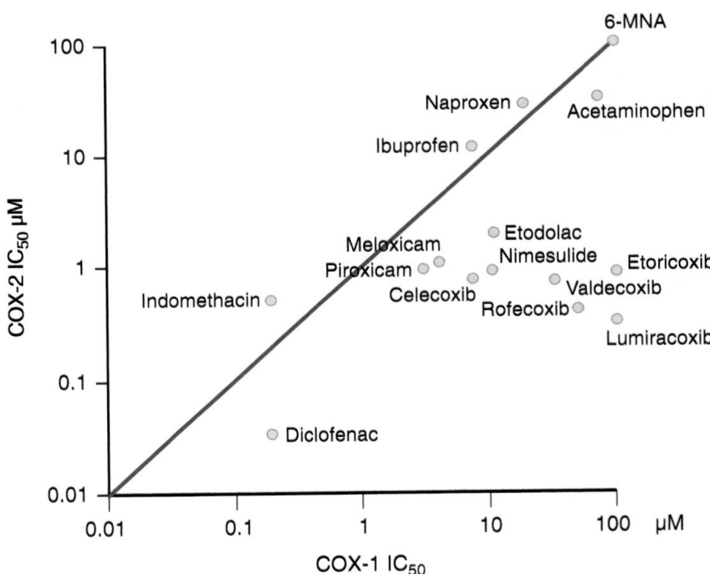

FIGURE 36-2. COX-2 selectivity as a continuous variable. Concentrations of various COX-2 inhibitors to inhibit the activity of platelet COX-1 and monocyte COX-2 by 50% (IC_{50}) are plotted on the abscissa and ordinate scales, respectively. The *solid line* describes equipotent inhibition of both COX-1 and COX-2. Symbols to the left of this line denote greater inhibition of COX-1 than COX-2. Symbols to the right of this line indicate progressively greater inhibition of COX-2 than COX-1, that is, increasing degrees of COX-2 selectivity. Aspirin is not shown on the figure because the long-term incubation required for monocyte COX-2 expression in human whole blood affects the chemical stability of the drug and underestimates its inhibitory potency. 6-MNA denotes 6-methoxy-2-naphthylacetic acid, the active metabolite of nabumetone.

CLINICAL PHARMACOLOGY OF PROSTAGLANDIN H SYNTHASE INHIBITION

Most traditional NSAIDs inhibit COX-1 and COX-2 with similar potency (Fig. 36-2). Some traditional NSAIDs (e.g., nimesulide and diclofenac) and a class of COX-2 inhibitors called coxibs (e.g., celecoxib and etoricoxib) are more potent in inhibiting COX-2 than COX-1 (see Fig. 36-2). These drugs fall into three general categories based on their mechanism of action. One category of inhibitors includes freely reversible competitive inhibitors, such as ibuprofen and mefenamic acid. Binding of these inhibitors to the COX sites of both monomers comprising a dimer is required for inhibition of COX-2 oxygenation of the substrate. A second group of inhibitors, including flurbiprofen, meclofenamate, diclofenac, and indomethacin, comprises time-dependent, noncovalent inhibitors. These NSAIDs are allosteric inhibitors that bind to one monomer of COX to inhibit its activity. Aspirin is unique to a third group of inhibitors that cause a time-dependent, covalent inhibition. Binding of aspirin to COX-1 or COX-2 leads to irreversible acetylation of a highly conserved serine residue (Ser-529 and Ser-516 in human COX-1 and COX-2, respectively). Aspirin acetylates only one monomer of a COX-1 dimer to cause complete loss of COX activity. Aspirin also maximally acetylates one monomer of human COX-2. The acetylated monomer of aspirin-treated COX-2 forms 15-hydroperoxyeicosatetraenoic acid from arachidonic acid, whereas the nonacetylated partner monomer forms mainly prostaglandin H_2 but only at 15 to 20% of the rate of native COX-2. Thus, the effect of

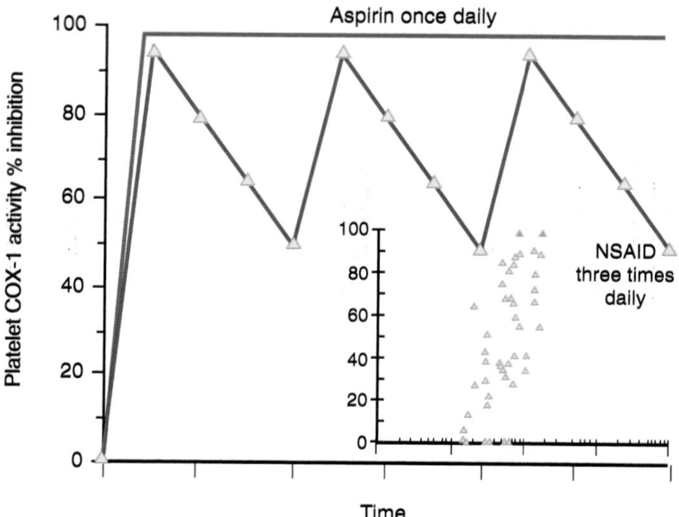

FIGURE 36-3. Time-dependent inhibition of platelet COX-1 activity by aspirin and a traditional nonsteroidal anti-inflammatory drug (NSAID). The average time course of inhibition of serum TXB_2, an ex vivo index of platelet COX-1 activity, is depicted over 24 hours following the administration of low-dose aspirin once daily and a traditional NSAID with short half-life given every 8 hours. The *inset* depicts the interindividual variability in the relationship between NSAID plasma levels plotted on the abscissa log scale and the corresponding level of inhibition of platelet COX-1 plotted on the ordinate.

TABLE 36-1 VASCULAR DISORDERS FOR WHICH ASPIRIN HAS BEEN SHOWN TO BE EFFECTIVE AND THE LOWEST EFFECTIVE DOSE

DISORDER	LOWEST EFFECTIVE DAILY DOSE (MG)
TIA and ischemic stroke*	50
Men at high cardiovascular risk	75
Essential hypertension	75
Chronic stable angina	75
Unstable angina or NSTEMI*	75
Severe carotid artery stenosis*	75
Polycythemia vera	100
Acute ischemic stroke*	160
Acute STEMI	162

*Higher doses were tested and not found to confer any greater risk reduction.
NSTEMI = non–ST elevation myocardial infarction; STEMI = ST elevation myocardial infarction; TIA = transient ischemic attack.

aspirin on COX-2 is an incomplete allosteric inhibition compared with that seen with COX-1.

Traditional NSAIDs typically inhibit platelet COX-1 and monocyte COX-2 by 50 to 90%, depending on dose; this effect is usually transient, depending on dose and half-life (Fig. 36-3). Coxibs inhibit monocyte COX-2 to the same extent as other NSAIDs, while substantially sparing platelet (and presumably other cells) COX-1 in most patients exposed to therapeutic doses. In contrast, aspirin achieves virtually complete (i.e., >97%) and persistent (i.e., ≥ 24 hour) inactivation of platelet COX-1 by virtue of its irreversible mechanism of action and inability of anucleate platelets to resynthesize the enzyme. Aspirin is equally potent in acetylating COX-1 and COX-2 in vitro. However, its unique mechanism of action and unusual pharmacokinetic features (20-minute half-life; presystemic encounter with the platelet target in the portal blood before first-pass liver metabolism) allow selective, cumulative inhibition of platelet COX-1 at low doses while substantially sparing vascular COX-2. The effect of aspirin on COX-1-dependent TXA_2 production is saturable at daily doses as low as 30 to 50 mg; in contrast, its inhibitory effect on COX-2-dependent prostaglandin I_2 biosynthesis is dose dependent up to daily doses of 650 to 1300 mg.

The relationships among inhibition of COX isozyme activity, reduced prostanoid formation, and changes in prostanoid-dependent cell function in vivo are not necessarily linear. The strikingly nonlinear relationship between inactivation of platelet COX-1 and inhibition of thromboxane-dependent platelet activation in vivo has important clinical implications for the cardiovascular effects of low-dose aspirin versus traditional NSAIDs (see later). In addition, interindividual variability in drug plasma levels as well as in the corresponding level of COX isozyme inhibition contributes to substantial unpredictability of the individual clinical response to COX inhibitors (E-Fig. 36-1).

Low-Dose Aspirin as an Antithrombotic and Anti-cancer Agent

The efficacy and safety of aspirin as an antithrombotic agent have been evaluated in several populations, ranging from apparently healthy persons at low risk of vascular complications (so-called primary prevention) to high-risk patients presenting with or surviving an acute myocardial infarction or an acute ischemic stroke (so-called secondary prevention). The clinical efficacy of aspirin was demonstrated at doses ranging from 50 to 162 mg given once daily (Table 36-1), consistent with the irreversible nature of its mechanism of action. Furthermore, higher doses (e.g., 300 to 325 mg) were not found to confer additional benefits, consistent with saturability of platelet COX-1 acetylation at low doses.[1]

In the six primary prevention trials among 95,000 low-risk individuals, aspirin allocation yielded a 12% relative risk reduction in serious vascular events (myocardial infarction, stroke, or vascular death).[2] This protective effect was mainly due to a reduction in nonfatal myocardial infarction. The net effect on stroke was not significant, reflecting a small reduction in presumed ischemic stroke and counterbalancing effects on hemorrhagic stroke and other (probably ischemic) stroke. There was no significant reduction in vascular mortality. Aspirin increased gastrointestinal (or other extracranial) bleeds by approximately 50%.[2]

In 16 secondary prevention trials in 17,000 high-risk patients with prior myocardial infarction, or prior stroke or transient cerebral ischemia, aspirin allocation yielded 19% fewer serious vascular events, with similar proportional reductions in coronary events (20% relative risk reduction) and ischemic stroke (22% relative risk reduction) but a nonsignificant increase in hemorrhagic stroke.[2] The absolute benefit of aspirin was about 25 times larger in secondary than in primary prevention (15 vs. 0.6 fewer vascular events per 1000 per year). In both primary and secondary prevention trials, the proportional reductions in serious vascular events appeared similar for men and women and for older and younger people. The risks of serious vascular events and of major extracranial bleeds were predicted by the same independent risk factors (age, male gender, diabetes mellitus, current smoking, blood pressure, and body mass index), so those with high risk of vascular complications also had a high risk of bleeding.

For secondary prevention of cardiovascular disease, the net benefits of adding aspirin to other preventive measures (e.g., statins) substantially exceed the bleeding hazards, irrespective of age and gender. In addition, aspirin, 75 mg daily or more for at least several years, reduces the incidence and mortality of colorectal cancer.[3]

Traditional Nonsteroidal Anti-inflammatory Drugs and Coxibs

NSAIDs constitute a chemically heterogeneous group of compounds that provide symptomatic relief of pain and inflammation associated with a variety of human disorders, including the rheumatic diseases. Their shared therapeutic actions (i.e., analgesic, anti-inflammatory, and antipyretic) are usually accompanied by mechanism-based adverse effects on gastrointestinal, cardiovascular, and renal functions. Prostanoids reproduce the main signs and symptoms of the inflammatory response and cause hyperalgesia and fever. Because of the redundancy of mediators of these responses, it is not surprising that NSAIDs only exert a moderate anti-inflammatory effect, are effective only against pain of low to moderate intensity and reduce fever, but do not interfere with the physiologic control of body temperature. The analgesic, anti-inflammatory, and antipyretic actions of traditional NSAIDs are largely reproduced by coxibs, a class of selective inhibitors of COX-2.

COX-2 selectivity is a continuous variable (see Fig. 36-2). Thus, one can pragmatically characterize three levels of COX-2 selectivity in terms of the probability of sparing COX-1 at therapeutic plasma levels: low (e.g., acetaminophen), intermediate (e.g., celecoxib, nimesulide, and diclofenac), and high (e.g., rofecoxib, etoricoxib, and lumiracoxib).

NSAIDs can modify the pharmacokinetics or pharmacodynamics of other drugs given concurrently, resulting in clinically important drug interactions. A pharmacodynamic interaction may occur between most NSAIDs and several classes of antihypertensive drugs. Reduced production of vasodilator prostacyclin and natriuretic prostaglandin E_2, as a consequence of renal

COX-2 inhibition, results in vasoconstriction and sodium and water retention that in turn tend to elevate blood pressure, regardless of the mechanism of action of antihypertensive drugs. This pharmacodynamic interaction has been described with most traditional NSAIDs (including acetaminophen) and coxibs, but not with low-dose aspirin.

Some NSAIDs favoring COX-1 over COX-2 inhibition, such as ibuprofen and naproxen, may interfere with the antiplatelet effect of low-dose aspirin by competing with acetylsalicylic acid for a common docking site (arginine-120) within the COX-1 channel. Drugs favoring COX-2 versus COX-1 inhibition, such as acetaminophen and diclofenac, do not interfere with the pharmacodynamic effect of low-dose aspirin, similarly to celecoxib and rofecoxib.

Upper gastrointestinal complications (bleeds, perforations, and obstructions) occur in 1 to 2% of NSAID-treated patients (Chapter 141). The mortality rate associated with hospitalization due to major gastrointestinal events is 5 to 6% in recent studies. Mortality rates associated with upper or lower gastrointestinal complications due to NSAIDs are similar. The major risk factors for upper gastrointestinal bleeding are represented by age and a prior history of gastrointestinal disorders (E-Fig. 36-1). Male gender, cigarette smoking, and heavy alcohol intake increase this risk by less than two-fold, as do oral glucocorticoids. Oral anticoagulants, thienopyridines, and low-dose aspirin increase the risk of NSAID-induced bleeding complications by two- to three-fold. The excess of these complications due to traditional NSAIDs has been estimated to range between 3 and 30 events per 1000 patients treated per year depending on the absence or presence of risk factors (E-Fig. 36-1).

Highly selective COX-2 inhibitors are associated with a statistically significant 50 to 66% relative risk reduction in ulcer complications compared with naproxen or ibuprofen.[4] However, no such agent is available on the U.S. market.

A meta-analysis of tabular data from 138 randomized trials of five different coxibs in approximately 145,000 patients has revealed that, in placebo comparisons, allocation to a coxib was associated with a 42% increased incidence of vascular events with no statistically significant heterogeneity among the different coxibs.[5] This excess risk of vascular events was derived primarily from a two-fold increased risk of myocardial infarction. Overall, there was no significant difference in the incidence of vascular events between a coxib and any traditional NSAID, but there was evidence of significant heterogeneity between naproxen and the other traditional NSAIDs (largely represented by ibuprofen and diclofenac).[5]

Current evidence suggests that the risk of myocardial infarction depends on the extent of COX-2 inhibition and not on the variable COX-2 selectivity of the inhibitor. This risk appears to be modulated by concomitant high-grade and persistent inhibition of platelet COX-1 activity, as suggested by the neutral cardiovascular phenotype associated with a high-dose regimen of naproxen. However, in patients at high cardiovascular risk, whose platelet COX-1 is completely and persistently inactivated by low-dose aspirin, the administration of any COX-2 inhibitor (including naproxen) is likely to produce detrimental cardiovascular consequences.

Given the nonlinear relationship between inhibition of platelet COX-1 activity and inhibition of platelet activation in vivo, it is perhaps not surprising that the cardiovascular safety profiles of coxibs and some traditional NSAIDs appear similar because they both fail to inhibit platelet activation adequately irrespective of their COX-2 selectivity. Early appearance, dose dependence, and slow dissipation of risk are important features of COX-2-related cardiotoxicity.

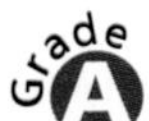

1. CURRENT-OASIS 7 Investigators, Mehta SR, Bassand JP, et al. Dose comparisons of clopidogrel and aspirin in acute coronary syndromes. *N Engl J Med.* 2010;363:930-942.
2. Baigent C, Blackwell L, Collins R, et al, for the Antithrombotic Trialists' (ATT) Collaboration. Aspirin in the primary and secondary prevention of vascular disease: collaborative meta-analysis of individual participant data from randomised trials. *Lancet.* 2009;373:1849-1860.
3. Rothwell PM, Wilson M, Elwin CE, et al. Long-term effect of aspirin on colorectal cancer incidence and mortality: 20-year follow-up of five randomised trials. *Lancet.* 2010;376:1741-1750.
4. Schnitzer TJ, Burmester GR, Mysler E, et al, for the TARGET Study Group. Comparison of lumiracoxib with naproxen and ibuprofen in the Therapeutic Arthritis Research and Gastrointestinal Event Trial (TARGET), reduction in ulcer complications: randomised controlled trial. *Lancet.* 2004;364:665-674.
5. Kearney PM, Baigent C, Godwin J, et al. Do selective cyclooxygenase-2 inhibitors and traditional non-steroidal anti-inflammatory drugs increase the risk of atherothrombosis? Meta-analysis of randomized trials. *BMJ.* 2006;332:1302-1308.

SUGGESTED READINGS

Patrono C, Baigent C. Low-dose aspirin, coxibs, and other NSAIDs: a clinical mosaic emerges. *Mol Interv.* 2009;9:31-39. *This review discusses the mechanisms underlying the cardiovascular effects of low-dose aspirin, traditional NSAIDs, and coxibs.*

Patrono C, Rocca B. The future of antiplatelet therapy in cardiovascular disease. *Annu Rev Med.* 2010;61:49-61. *This review discusses different mechanisms of platelet inhibition with emphasis on the pharmacokinetic and pharmacodynamic determinants of clinical efficacy and safety of antiplatelet drugs.*

Stavrakis S, Stoner JA, Azar M, et al. Low-dose aspirin for primary prevention of cardiovascular events in patients with diabetes: a meta-analysis. *Am J Med Sci.* 2011;341:1-9. *Argues against low-dose aspirin for primary prevention of cardiovascular events in patients with diabetes.*

Sung JJ, Lau JY, Ching JY, et al. Continuation of low-dose aspirin therapy in peptic ulcer bleeding: a randomized trial. *Ann Intern Med.* 2010;152:1-9. *In a small randomized trial, low-dose aspirin therapy increased the risk of recurrent bleeding from 5.4 to 10.3%, but reduced mortality by 11.6%.*

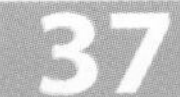

ANTITHROMBOTIC THERAPY

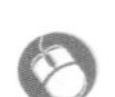

SAM SCHULMAN AND JACK HIRSH

Antithrombotic therapy suppresses the natural hemostatic mechanisms (Chapter 174) and is effective for preventing and treating venous, cardiac, and arterial thromboembolism. A variety of medications are now available that interfere with different steps in coagulation and platelet activation, sometimes with synergistic effects. In recent years, randomized clinical trials have produced a substantial body of evidence-based literature to guide the use of antithrombotic therapy for a wide range of clinical conditions.

PHARMACOLOGIC AGENTS

Vitamin K Antagonists

For more than 60 years, vitamin K antagonists have been the only oral anticoagulants available for clinical use. Now, with the development of novel oral agents that target single coagulation enzymes (see later), the situation is changing. Coumarins are vitamin K antagonists, of which warfarin is the most widely used. Coumarins inhibit a vitamin K reductase that catalyzes the reduction of 2,3-epoxide (vitamin K epoxide), thereby leading to the depletion of vitamin KH_2, which is required for the production of functionally active (γ-carboxylated) coagulation proteins (factors II [prothrombin], VII, IX, and X) and anticoagulant proteins (protein C and protein S) (Chapter 178). Vitamin K_1 in food sources can reverse these effects of coumarins because it is reduced to vitamin KH_2 by a warfarin-insensitive vitamin K reductase (Fig. 37-1).

Warfarin is rapidly and almost completely absorbed from the gastrointestinal tract. It has a half-life of about 40 hours, a delayed onset of action (2 to 7 days, depending on dose), and a residual anticoagulant effect for up to 5 days after treatment is discontinued. The dose-response relationship of warfarin varies widely among individuals and is influenced by many factors, including age, body weight, liver disease, dietary vitamin K_1, genetic factors, concomitant drug use, compliance of the patient, and inappropriate dosage adjustments.[1] Of these factors, inappropriate dosage adjustment and improved compliance through patient education are the most readily correctable.

The effect of warfarin must be monitored closely to prevent overdosing or underdosing. Laboratory monitoring is performed by measuring the prothrombin time and is reported as an international normalized ratio (INR). During initiation of warfarin therapy, the INR reflects primarily the depression of factor VII, which has a half-life of only 6 hours. There is evidence that the reliability of warfarin monitoring is improved by having the dosage controlled by an anticoagulation management service and by using computer-assisted algorithms. The convenience of monitoring is increased with a portable point-of-care instrument. Pharmacogenetic-guided dosing of warfarin has been evaluated in four randomized trials without producing evidence that the rate of major hemorrhage or thromboembolic complications is reduced, and the current cost is \$100 to \$200 per patient.

Indications for Warfarin

Warfarin is effective in the primary and secondary prevention of systemic embolism in patients with atrial fibrillation (Chapter 64); in the prevention of systemic arterial embolism in patients with valvular heart disease

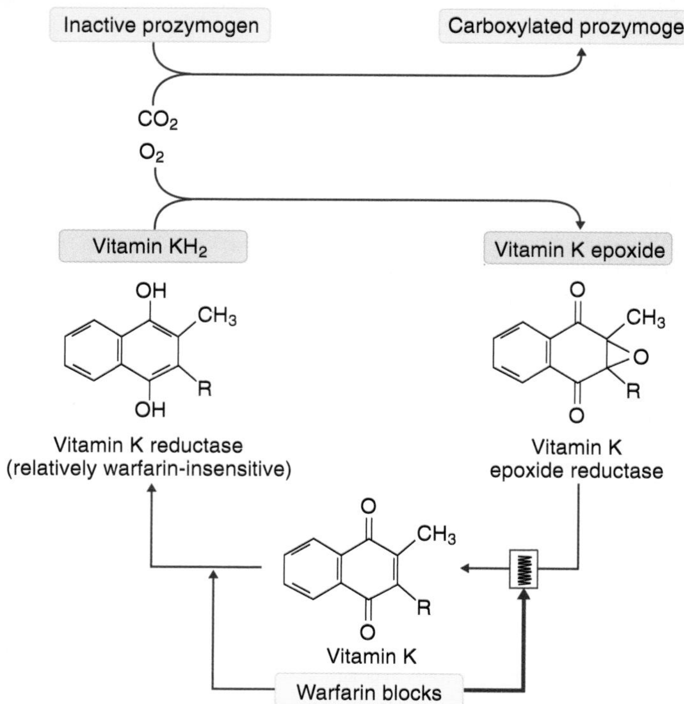

FIGURE 37-1. Warfarin inhibits vitamin K epoxide reductase and leads to the intracellular depletion (in the hepatocyte) of vitamin KH_2. Vitamin KH_2 is required for the conversion (by γ-carboxylation) of functionally inactive to active coagulation proteins. The anticoagulant effect of warfarin can be reversed by vitamin K_1 in food because it is reduced to vitamin KH_2 by a warfarin-insensitive vitamin K reductase.

(bioprosthetic and mechanical heart valves [Chapter 75]); in the primary and secondary prevention of venous thromboembolism (Chapters 81 and 98); in the prevention of acute myocardial infarction in high-risk patients (Chapters 72 and 73); and in the prevention of stroke (Chapter 414), recurrent infarction, and death in patients with acute myocardial infarction (Chapter 73).[2] A target INR of 2.5 (range, 2.0 to 3.0) is recommended for almost all indications. Exceptions are mechanical prosthetic heart valve in the mitral position or caged-ball or caged-disk valve in the aortic position or any mechanical aortic valve in combination with atrial fibrillation, anterior myocardial infarction, left atrial enlargement, or low ejection fraction, when an INR of 3.0 (range, 2.5 to 3.5) is recommended.

Dosing and Monitoring

If a rapid anticoagulant effect is required, heparin and warfarin should be started at the same time and overlapped for at least 5 days. Warfarin is started with the estimated maintenance dose of about 5 mg/day, with the first INR measurement after 2 to 3 days, and patients usually reach an INR of 2.0 in 4 or 5 days. If there is no increase of the INR after two or three doses, the daily dose should be progressively increased until an INR response is observed. In patients with a low risk of bleeding, warfarin may be started at a dose of 10 mg and then adjusted according to daily INR results. Heparin treatment is discontinued when the INR has been in the therapeutic range for 2 days. The INR is then performed two or three times weekly for 1 to 2 weeks and then weekly up to a maximal interval of 4 weeks, depending on the stability of INR results, and more frequently when a new drug is added to the treatment.

Adjustments to the dose when the INR drifts out of the therapeutic range should be gradual and based on the weekly dose (e.g., a 10 to 20% change in weekly dose). Patients should be encouraged to keep a log of their dose and their INR response.

Adverse Effects

Warfarin-related bleeding is increased by the level of the INR. The risk of bleeding is also increased with concomitant aspirin use, in persons older than 65 years, in those with a history of stroke or gastrointestinal bleeding, and in those with serious comorbid conditions. Elderly patients are more sensitive to warfarin, requiring lower doses to reach the therapeutic range, and have an increased tendency to bleed, including intracranially, even when their INR is in the therapeutic range (Chapter 23).

TABLE 37-1 RECOMMENDED MANAGEMENT OF ELEVATED INR WITH OR WITHOUT BLEEDING IN PATIENTS TREATED WITH WARFARIN

INR	BLEEDING	WARFARIN	VITAMIN K_1	FFP/PCC/rFVIIa
<5.0	Negligible	Hold 1 dose or reduce dose	No	No
5.0-9.9	Negligible	Hold 1-2 doses	1-2.5 mg PO*	No
≥10	Negligible	Hold	2.5-5 mg PO	No
Any	Serious or life-threatening	Hold	10 mg IV[†] and repeat PRN	Yes

*Only for patients at increased risk of bleeding.[26]
[†]Intravenous (IV) infusion should be given slowly.
FFP = fresh-frozen plasma; INR = International Normalized Ratio; PCC = prothrombin complex concentrate; PO = orally; PRN = as needed; rFVIIa, recombinant factor VIIa.

Warfarin-induced skin necrosis occurs in 1 in 5000 patients, more frequently in women, and affects mainly breasts, buttocks, and thighs. An imbalance between moderately reduced procoagulant factors and severely depressed natural inhibitors may cause this hypercoagulable state in patients with congenital deficiency of protein C or protein S (Chapter 179), dietary deficiency of vitamin K, cancer, or heparin-induced thrombocytopenia with premature start of vitamin K antagonists (Chapter 175).

Reversing the Effect of Warfarin

The anticoagulant effect of warfarin can be reversed in one of three ways: by discontinuation of therapy, with the expectation that the INR will return to baseline in about 5 days; by administration of vitamin K_1, with the expectation that the anticoagulant effect will be reduced in 6 hours and reversed in 24 hours; and by infusion of fresh-frozen plasma (FFP), prothrombin complex concentrate (PCC), or recombinant coagulation factor VIIa (rFVIIa), which produce immediate reversal (Table 37-1).

Heparin and Low-Molecular-Weight Heparins

Heparin

Heparin binds to antithrombin (AT), thereby increasing the rate at which AT inactivates thrombin, activated factor X (factor Xa), and other coagulation enzymes. Heparin accelerates the inactivation of thrombin by AT by providing a template to which both the enzyme and the inhibitor bind to form a ternary complex (Fig. 37-2). In contrast, the inactivation of factor Xa by the AT-heparin complex does not require ternary complex formation and is achieved by binding of the heparin-bound AT to factor Xa. Heparin binds to a number of plasma, platelet, and endothelial cell–derived proteins that compete with AT for heparin binding. Binding of heparin to plasma proteins contributes to the variability of its anticoagulant response, whereas binding to hepatic macrophages is responsible for its dose-dependent clearance. Both properties contribute to the unpredictable anticoagulant effect of heparin and the need for laboratory monitoring.

Heparin is effective for the prevention and treatment of venous thromboembolism,[3-5] for the early treatment of patients with unstable angina and acute myocardial infarction,[6,7] for patients who have cardiac surgery under cardiopulmonary bypass,[8] for patients undergoing vascular surgery,[9] and during and after coronary angioplasty and coronary stent placement.[8]

The anticoagulant effects of heparin are usually monitored by the activated partial thromboplastin time (aPTT). A therapeutic effect is achieved when the aPTT ratio is equivalent to a heparin level of 0.3 to 0.7 anti–factor Xa units, which for many reagents is an aPTT ratio of 1.5 to 2.5.[4] The risk of bleeding complications is increased with increasing heparin dosage, which in turn is related to the anticoagulant response. However, other clinical factors, such as recent surgery, trauma, and invasive procedures, are also important as predictors of bleeding during heparin treatment.

For the treatment of venous thromboembolism, heparin is given in doses of 80 U/kg followed by 18 U/kg per hour by continuous infusion; the dose is adjusted according to the aPTT result at 6 hours by use of a validated nomogram. Lower doses (70 U/kg or 5000 U followed by 15 U/kg/h or 1000 U/hour) of heparin are used in patients with acute myocardial ischemia, who also receive aspirin and platelet glycoprotein IIb/IIIa complex (GPIIb-IIIa) antagonists or thrombolytic therapy.

The main complications of heparin are bleeding and heparin-induced thrombocytopenia. Less common complications are heparin-induced osteoporosis and hyperkalemia. Heparin-related bleeding is dose related, and the risk is increased in patients who undergo an invasive procedure and if heparin is used in combination with a platelet GPIIb-IIIa antagonist or a thrombolytic agent.

If heparin-induced thrombocytopenia (Chapter 175) is suspected on clinical grounds and anticoagulant treatment is indicated, heparin should be stopped and replaced with a thrombin inhibitor, either hirudin (lepirudin) or argatroban. Warfarin should not be used alone to treat acute heparin-induced thrombocytopenia because it can aggravate the thrombotic process, but it is safe in combination with a thrombin inhibitor after the platelet count has risen above 100×10^9/L.

Low-Molecular-Weight Heparins

LMWHs are fragments produced by either chemical or enzymatic depolymerization of heparin. LMWHs are approximately one third the size of heparin (Table 37-2). Depolymerization of heparin changes the anticoagulant profile. As a result, LMWHs have less protein and cellular binding and, as a consequence, have a more predictable dose response, better bioavailability, and a longer plasma half-life than regular heparin. LMWHs can therefore be administered subcutaneously once daily without laboratory monitoring.

Compared with heparin, which has a ratio of anti–factor Xa to anti–factor IIa activity of approximately 1:1, the various commercial LMWHs have ratios of anti–factor Xa to anti–factor IIa varying between 4:1 and 2:1, depending on their molecular size distribution. LMWHs are cleared principally by the renal route. LMWHs are associated with a lower incidence of heparin-induced thrombocytopenia and heparin-induced osteoporosis than is heparin.

LMWHs are effective in the prevention and treatment of venous thromboembolism (VTE) (Chapter 81),[3-5] in the treatment of patients with unstable angina and non–ST elevation myocardial infarction (Chapters 72 and 73),[7] and as an adjunct to fibrinolytic therapy in patients with acute ST elevation myocardial infarction (Chapter 73).[6]

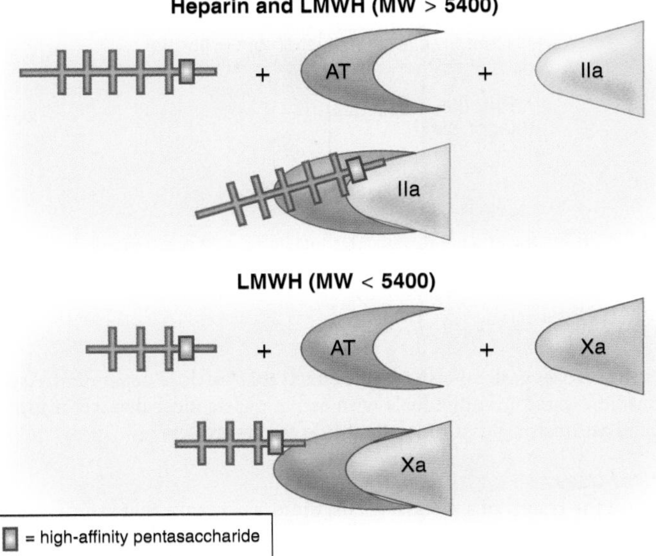

FIGURE 37-2. Only one third of high-affinity pentasaccharide-containing heparin molecules and one fifth of pentasaccharide-containing low-molecular-weight heparin (LMWH) molecules activate antithrombin (AT). Virtually all of the high-affinity heparin molecules are large enough to bridge between AT and factor IIa (thrombin). In contrast, only 25 to 50% of LMWH molecules have a molecular weight (MW) of 5400 or more, and although these smaller molecules inactivate factor Xa, they do not inactivate factor IIa. Although heparin has equal anti–factor IIa and anti–factor Xa activities, LMWH has reduced anti–factor IIa activity.

Pentasaccharides

On the basis of knowledge of the AT-binding sequence on heparin, a pentasaccharide, fondaparinux, with high affinity for AT has been synthesized. The structure of fondaparinux has been modified to increase its affinity to AT. Fondaparinux inactivates factor Xa through an AT-mediated mechanism. Because it is too short to bridge AT to thrombin, fondaparinux has no activity against thrombin.

After subcutaneous injection, fondaparinux is rapidly and completely absorbed and exhibits a bioavailability of 100%. The volume of distribution is similar to the blood volume. The drug is mainly excreted unchanged in the urine, with a terminal half-life of 17 hours in young volunteers and 21 hours in elderly volunteers.[4]

Fondaparinux circulates extensively bound to AT with minimal binding to other plasma proteins. Limited experimental and clinical studies suggest that fondaparinux has a lower risk of heparin-induced thrombocytopenia than that of heparin or LMWH as well as a lower risk of bone loss and of local skin reactions.

Fondaparinux is effective in the prevention and treatment of VTE[3,5] and is also effective in the treatment of acute coronary syndromes.[6,7]

New Anticoagulants

The limitations of established anticoagulants have prompted the development of a variety of new anticoagulant agents that target various specific steps in the coagulation mechanism.

Direct Thrombin Inhibitors

Direct thrombin inhibitors act independently of AT to inactivate both free thrombin and thrombin bound to fibrin. The direct thrombin inhibitors include hirudin, synthetic hirudin fragments (hirugen, lepirudin, and

TABLE 37-2 ANTICOAGULANT PROFILES, MOLECULAR WEIGHTS, PLASMA HALF-LIVES, AND RECOMMENDED DOSES OF COMMERCIAL LOW-MOLECULAR-WEIGHT HEPARINS

				Recommended Dose (International Anti-Xa Units)		
AGENT	ANTI-X_a/ANTI-II_a RATIO	MOLECULAR WEIGHT	PLASMA HALF-LIFE (MIN)	GENERAL SURGERY PROPHYLAXIS	ORTHOPEDIC SURGERY PROPHYLAXIS	ACUTE TREATMENT
Enoxaparin	2.7:1	4500	129-180	4000 U SC daily	4000 U SC daily or 3000 U SC bid	7000 U SC bid*† or 10,500 U SC daily*
Dalteparin	2:1	5000	119-139	2500 U SC daily	2500 U SC bid or 5000 U SC daily	8400 U SC bid*† or 14,000 U SC daily*
Nadroparin	3.2:1	4500	132-162	2850 U SC daily	2700 U SC daily,* 4000 U SC daily* from day 4	13,300 U SC daily*
Tinzaparin (Innohep)	1.9:1	4500	111	3500 U SC daily	3500 U SC daily* or 4500 U SC daily*	12,250 U daily*
Ardeparin	2:1	6000	200		50 U/kg SC bid	
Danaparoid‡	20:1	6500	1100	750 U SC daily	750 U SC bid	2500 U IV, then 4 hr each of 400 U/hr and 300 U/hr, then 200 U/hr; or 2000 U SC bid

*Weight-adjusted dose; stated dose for 70-kg patient.
†The higher daily dose is for acute coronary syndromes; the lower dose is for deep vein thrombosis.
‡Danaparoid sodium is a heparinoid.
IV = intravenously; SC = subcutaneously.

bivalirudin [Hirulog]), and low-molecular-weight inhibitors that react with the active site of thrombin (dabigatran and argatroban).[10]

Bivalirudin is approved for use in coronary angioplasty (Chapter 73),[11] and both argatroban and lepirudin are approved in patients with heparin-induced thrombocytopenia (Chapter 175). Data comparing argatroban with hirudin in heparin-induced thrombocytopenia are too limited for conclusions to be drawn about their relative efficacy and safety. Argatroban is metabolized in the liver and can be used in patients with renal failure, whereas the other direct thrombin inhibitors depend on elimination through renal excretion, and they may be used in patients with liver disease.

Dabigatran etexilate is metabolized by ubiquitous esterases to dabigatran, a reversible, active-site thrombin inhibitor. The bioavailability after oral administration is 6%; the half-life is 12 to 17 hours with substantial prolongation in case of renal failure, owing to predominant elimination through the kidneys. Dabigatran etexilate has been approved in Europe and several other countries for prophylaxis against VTE after hip or knee arthroplasty (first dose, 110 mg; then 220 mg once daily; for patients over 70 years of age or with creatinine clearance, 30 to 50 mL/minute, first dose 75 mg and then 150 mg daily). The effect is similar to that of enoxaparin (40 mg subcutaneously daily).[12] Dabigatran (150 mg twice daily) is more effective than warfarin for stroke prophylaxis in atrial fibrillation, whereas a lower dose (110 mg twice daily) is equally effective with lower risk for major bleeding. Both doses resulted in fewer intracranial hemorrhages than warfarin.[13] Dabigatran has been approved for this use in the United States and Canada. In the treatment of VTE, dabigatran (150 mg twice daily) has comparable effect to warfarin and is at least as safe regarding bleeding.[14]

Direct Factor Xa Inhibitors

A number of orally available low-molecular-weight active site-directed factor Xa inhibitors have been designed and are in various stages of clinical development (rivaroxaban, apixaban, betrixaban, edoxaban). Unlike heparins and pentasaccharides, direct inhibitors inactivate factor Xa without the need for AT as a cofactor.[10]

Rivaroxaban, an oxazolidinone derivative, has a bioavailability of 80%, reaches maximal plasma concentration 1 to 4 hours after oral administration, and has a half-life of 5 to 9 hours in young volunteers and 11 to 13 hours in elderly volunteers. Elimination occurs to one third each through the hepatofecal route, intact through the kidneys, and as a metabolite through the kidneys. Rivaroxaban (10 mg daily for 30-39 days) is more effective than enoxaparin in patients undergoing hip or knee arthroplasty but with a trend to more bleeding.[15]

Apixaban has also a high bioavailability, mixed pathway elimination, and a half-life of 12 hours. Given for prophylaxis against VTE after knee arthroplasty, apixaban (2.5 mg twice daily) has similar or better efficacy than LMWH and similar or lower risk of bleeding.[16,17]

Platelet-Active Drugs

The platelet-active drugs inhibit different steps in either platelet activation (aspirin, ticlopidine, clopidogrel, prasugrel, cilostazol, and dipyridamole) or platelet recruitment (GPIIb-IIIa antagonists abciximab, tirofiban, and eptifibatide) (Fig. 37-3).[10,18]

Aspirin and Other Cyclooxygenase Inhibitors

Mechanism of Action and Pharmacology

Aspirin permanently inactivates cyclooxygenase isoenzymes (COX-1 and COX-2) that catalyze the conversion of arachidonic acid to prostaglandin H_2, a precursor of a variety of eicosanoids including thromboxane A_2 in platelets and prostacyclin (prostaglandin I_2) in vascular endothelial cells.

Aspirin is rapidly absorbed in the stomach and upper intestine, attaining peak plasma levels about 30 minutes after ingestion; it has a half-life of about 15 minutes. Inhibition of platelet function is evident by 1 hour with uncoated aspirin but can be delayed after administration of enteric-coated aspirin. Therefore, if only enteric-coated tablets are available when a rapid effect is required, the tablets should be chewed.

Aspirin potentiates the antithrombotic effects of warfarin (in high-risk subjects), dipyridamole (in those with ischemic stroke), clopidogrel (in those with coronary stents or acute myocardial ischemia), and heparin (in the prevention of recurrent miscarriages in pregnant women with antiphospholipid antibody syndrome and in patients with acute coronary ischemia). Aspirin produces a small increase in major bleeding and a very small increase in the risk of cerebral hemorrhage. It also potentiates bleeding when it is added to another antithrombotic agent.

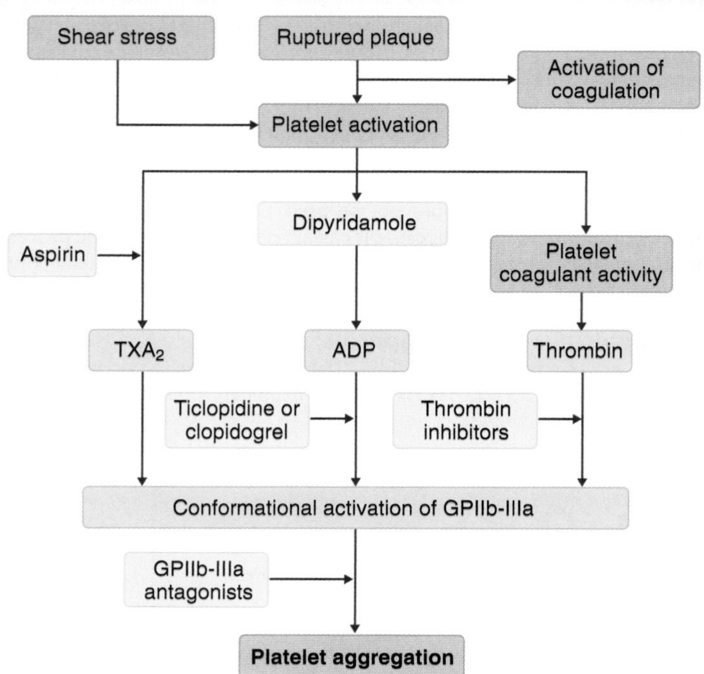

FIGURE 37-3. **Sites of action of platelet inhibitors.** ADP = adenosine diphosphate; GPIIb-IIIa = glycoprotein IIb/IIIa complex; TXA_2 = thromboxane A_2.

Aspirin causes gastrointestinal side effects that are dose dependent. Aspirin is contraindicated in individuals with active peptic ulcer disease or aspirin-induced asthma or if gastrointestinal side effects are severe.

Clinical Uses

Based on the results of a meta-analysis, there is evidence that aspirin reduces vascular death by approximately 15% and nonfatal vascular events by about 30% in patients with cardiovascular disease (Table 37-3).[18] These effects are achieved in patients with silent myocardial ischemia or stable angina, unstable angina, non–ST elevation myocardial infarction, ST elevation myocardial infarction, and ischemic cerebrovascular disease.[6-8,19] Aspirin is also effective in patients after coronary angioplasty or coronary artery bypass surgery[8] and in preventing symptomatic coronary events in asymptomatic men and women older than 50 years.[8,18] Aspirin has a favorable risk-to-benefit ratio for secondary prevention in patients with overt vascular disease, but the risk-to-benefit ratio is marginal when aspirin is used as primary prevention in asymptomatic individuals, even individuals with type 2 diabetes.[20] Aspirin is less effective than oral anticoagulants in the prevention of recurrent stroke in atrial fibrillation[21] and less effective than LMWH or warfarin in preventing venous thromboembolism.[3]

Phosphodiesterase Inhibitors

Dipyridamole and cilostazol are phosphodiesterase inhibitors, which elevate platelet cyclic adenosine and guanine monophosphate (cAMP and cGMP) levels. They block platelet reactivity and also inhibit vasoconstriction. The most common side effect is headache.

Dipyridamole is a pyrimidopyrimidine derivative with a terminal half-life of 10 hours and elimination primarily by biliary excretion. Favorable results were obtained with a modified-release preparation in patients with prior stroke or transient ischemic attack, in whom the risk of stroke was reduced by 16% with dipyridamole alone and by 37% with aspirin and dipyridamole in combination, compared with placebo.[18,19]

In a meta-analysis, cilostazol (100 mg twice daily) was shown to improve maximal and pain-free walking distance in patients with intermittent claudication.[22] Cilostazol is contraindicated in patients with congestive heart failure, owing to reports of fatal events with similar drugs.

Thienopyridines

Ticlopidine, clopidogrel, and prasugrel are thienopyridines that inhibit adenosine diphosphate–induced platelet aggregation through the action of their active metabolites at the $P2Y_{12}$ receptor level. The drugs are administered orally, but their onset of action is delayed until their active metabolites are formed. Similarly, recovery of platelet function is delayed until the circulating affected platelets are replaced by newly formed, unaffected platelets.

Based on a better safety profile and equal efficacy, clopidogrel has replaced ticlopidine. Clopidogrel is rapidly absorbed and metabolized, producing inhibition of platelet aggregation as soon as 90 minutes after an oral loading dosing of 300 mg. With repeated daily administration of low doses (75 mg), there is cumulative inhibition of platelet function with a return to normal 7 days after the last dose of clopidogrel.

Clopidogrel is more effective than aspirin in patients who have experienced a recent stroke or recent myocardial infarction and in patients presenting with symptomatic peripheral arterial disease.[6,9,19] The additional benefit over aspirin is modest and similar to that observed with ticlopidine (about 10% relative risk reduction). The combination of clopidogrel and aspirin is also more effective than aspirin alone in patients with unstable angina and non–ST elevation myocardial infarction (20% risk reduction)[7] and in patients with atrial fibrillation,[23] but at a cost of a modest increase in bleeding. The combination of clopidogrel and aspirin is also more effective than

TABLE 37-3 SUMMARY OF GRADE A RECOMMENDATIONS FOR ANTITHROMBOTIC THERAPY

Grade 1A indicates that experts are certain that benefits do or do not outweigh risks, burdens, and costs. Grade 2A indicates that they are less certain, resulting in a weaker recommendation.

PREVENTION OF VENOUS THROMBOEMBOLISM (Chapters 81 and 98)[3]

General Recommendations

Every general hospital should develop a formal, active strategy to prevent venous thromboembolism, such as computer decision support systems (grade 1A).
Patients at high risk for or with active bleeding: mechanical methods—elastic stockings or intermittent pneumatic compression (grade 1A)

General Surgery

Moderate-risk general surgery: LMWH, low-dose unfractionated heparin or fondaparinux (grade 1A)
Higher-risk general surgery: LMWH, low-dose unfractionated heparin or fondaparinux; for major procedures until discharge from hospital (grade 1A)
Major gynecologic surgery for benign disease: LMWH, or low-dose unfractionated heparin every 12 hours (grade 1A)
Extensive gynecologic surgery for malignant disease: low-dose unfractionated heparin every 8 hours, higher doses of LMWH, or intermittent pneumatic compression as long as patient is not ambulating (grade 1A)

Major Orthopedic Surgery

Elective total hip replacement surgery: subcutaneous LMWH, started either 12 hours before or 12-24 hours after surgery or 4-6 hours after surgery at half dose; fondaparinux, started 6-24 hours after surgery; or adjusted-dose warfarin (INR target of 2.5; range, 2.0 to 3.0), started preoperatively or immediately after surgery (grade 1A)
Elective total knee replacement surgery: LMWH, fondaparinux, or adjusted-dose warfarin (grade 1A)
Hip fracture surgery: fondaparinux (grade 1A)
Anticoagulant prophylaxis should be continued for at least 10 days (grade 1A). Extended prophylaxis should be given for up to 35 days with LMWH after total hip replacement and with fondaparinux after hip fracture surgery (grade 1A). Routine duplex ultrasonography screening at the time of hospital discharge or during outpatient follow-up is not recommended in asymptomatic patients after total hip replacement or total knee replacement (grade 1A).
Isolated distal lower-extremity injuries: routine thromboprophylaxis is not recommended (grade 2A)

Neurosurgery, Burns, Trauma, and Acute Spinal Cord Injury

Neurosurgery: intermittent pneumatic compression (grade 1A) or LMWH started after surgery (grade 2A)
Trauma or burn patients: all burn patients with at least one risk factor for VTE and all patients with major trauma or acute spinal cord injury should receive thromboprophylaxis, if it is not contraindicated (grade 1A). LMWH is started as soon as it is considered safe (grade 1A).

Medical Conditions

Acutely ill medical patients, confined to bed and with at least one additional risk factor for VTE: low-dose unfractionated heparin, LMWH or fondaparinux (grade 1A)

Critical Care

Most patients should, after appropriate assessment of the risk for VTE, receive thromboprophylaxis: if medically ill or postoperative—with unfractionated heparin or LMWH; with major trauma or orthopedic surgery—with LMWH (grade 1A).

TREATMENT OF VENOUS THROMBOEMBOLIC DISEASE (Chapters 81 and 98)[5]

Acute Treatment

Acute treatment: LMWH, or unfractionated heparin IV, adjusted dose SC or fixed dose SC, or fondaparinux (grade 1A)
Start treatment with vitamin K antagonists on the first day (grade 1A).
Patients with DVT: early ambulation when feasible (grade 1A)

Long-Term Anticoagulation

Patients with VTE and cancer: treat with LMWH for the first 3-6 months (grade 1A).
Patients with a first episode of VTE and reversible or time-limited risk factors: treat with vitamin K antagonists for 3 months (grade 1A).
Patients with a first episode of unprovoked VTE: treat for at least 3 months and extend long-term if risk factors for bleeding are absent and good anticoagulation monitoring is achievable (grade 1A).
After two or more episodes: treat long-term (grade 1A).
Adjust the dose of vitamin K antagonist to maintain a target INR of 2.5 with a range of 2.0 to 3.0 for all treatment durations (grade 1A). In patients with a strong preference for less frequent INR testing after the first 3 months, continue with INR range 1.5 to 1.9 (grade 1A).
Prescribe an elastic compression stocking with an ankle pressure of 30 to 40 mm Hg for 2 years after a proximal DVT (grade 1A).
Women treated with warfarin after VTE and who become pregnant: substitute with unfractionated heparin or LMWH (grade 1A).
Women using warfarin or unfractionated heparin and who wish to breast-feed: continue the medication (grade 1A).

ATRIAL FIBRILLATION (Chapter 64)[21]

Patients with Previous Ischemic Stroke, TIA, Systemic Embolism, or at Least One Other Risk Factor for Stroke

Standard approach: warfarin anticoagulation (INR of 2.5; range, 2.0 to 3.0) (grade 1A)
Warfarin contraindicated or declined by patient: aspirin, 75 to 325 mg daily
Aspirin plus low-, fixed-dose warfarin should not be used.

VALVULAR AND STRUCTURAL HEART DISEASE (Chapter 75)[27]

Mitral Valve Disease

Rheumatic mitral valve disease with atrial fibrillation, previous systemic embolism, or left atrial thrombus: warfarin anticoagulation (INR of 2.5; range, 2.0 to 3.0) (grade 1A)
Mitral valve prolapse with documented but unexplained TIA: long-term aspirin, 50 to 162 mg daily (grade 1A)

Mechanical Heart Valves

Warfarin anticoagulation (grade 1A)

Patent Foramen Ovale

Patent foramen ovale and stroke: platelet-active drug

ACUTE ST SEGMENT ELEVATION MYOCARDIAL INFARCTION AND CORONARY THROMBOLYSIS (Chapter 73)[6,7]

All patients with acute myocardial infarction should receive aspirin (160 to 325 mg), chewed and swallowed, at initial evaluation by health care personnel (grade 1A).
Maintenance dose of 75 to 162 mg daily should be continued indefinitely (grade 1A).
All patients should also receive clopidogrel, 300 mg for patients less than 75 years old and 75 mg for older patients without reperfusion therapy, followed by 75 mg daily for up to 28 days (grade 1A).
All patients should also receive anticoagulation (grade 1A), with fondaparinux for patients with no reperfusion therapy (first dose 2.5 mg IV, then SC daily for up to 9 days) (grade 1A), or with enoxaparin for patients with fibrinolytic therapy and preserved renal function (grade 2A).
Anticoagulation should be extended for at least 3 months, using warfarin (INR 2.0 to 3.0), for patients with large anterior myocardial infarction, significant heart failure, intracardiac thrombus, or atrial fibrillation (grade 2A).
Patients with ischemic symptoms characteristic of myocardial infarction of less than 12 hours' duration and persistent ST segment elevation should be rapidly evaluated for reperfusion therapy with primary percutaneous coronary intervention or thrombolysis (grade 1A).
Thrombolytic therapy should be given before arrival to the hospital, when feasible (grade A), and otherwise ideally within 30 minutes from arrival (grade 1A).
Choice of fibrinolytic agent for patients with symptom duration <12 hours: streptokinase, anistreplase, reteplase, tenecteplase, or alteplase (grade 1A).
Choice of fibrinolytic agent for patients with symptom duration <6 hours: alteplase and tenecteplase are superior to streptokinase (grade 1A).

TABLE 37-3 SUMMARY OF GRADE A RECOMMENDATIONS FOR ANTITHROMBOTIC THERAPY—cont'd

NON–ST SEGMENT ELEVATION ACUTE CORONARY SYNDROMES AND PERCUTANEOUS CORONARY INTERVENTIONS (Chapters 72 and 74)[7,8]

Platelet-Active Drugs

Aspirin, non–enteric-coated, at an initial dose of 162 to 325 mg to chew and swallow as soon as possible after the clinical impression of unstable angina is formed (grade 1A). Aspirin by mouth, 75 to 100 mg, should be continued indefinitely (grade 1A).
In cases of aspirin allergy or intolerance: clopidogrel at a bolus dose of 300 mg orally and then 75 mg indefinitely (grade 1A).
Patients at a moderate to high risk for an ischemic event and planned for early invasive strategy: "upstream" clopidogrel (300-mg bolus orally, followed by 75 mg daily) or a GPIIb-IIIa antagonist IV (eptifibatide or tirofiban) (grade 1A) or both (grade 2A).
Clopidogrel should be continued, in addition to aspirin, for 12 months (grade 1A).

Anticoagulants

Unfractionated heparin, LMWH, bivalirudin or fondaparinux (grade 1A). For patients with early conservative strategy: fondaparinux (grade 1A)

CHRONIC CORONARY ARTERY DISEASE (Chapter 71)[8]

Primary Prevention

Moderate or high risk for a coronary event: aspirin, 75 to 100 mg daily (grade 2A)
Very high risk with easily monitored INR: warfarin targeted at INR of approximately 1.5 (grade 2A)

CORONARY ARTERY BYPASS GRAFTS (Chapter 74)[8]

Aspirin, 75 to 100 mg (75 to 162 mg for internal mammary bypass grafting) indefinitely (grade 1A), starting after surgery (grade 2A)
Discontinue clopidogrel 5 days before the operation (grade 2A).

ANTITHROMBOTIC THERAPY IN PATIENTS UNDERGOING PERCUTANEOUS CORONARY INTERVENTION (Chapters 72 and 74)[8]

Platelet-Active Drugs

Aspirin, 162 to 325 mg, should be administered before PCI (grade 1A).
Aspirin, 75 to 100 mg daily, should be used for secondary prevention of cardiovascular events (grade 1A).

Thienopyridines

Clopidogrel should be combined with aspirin for 12 months after bare metal stent placement (grade 1A) and for at least 12 months after drug-eluting stent (grade 1A).

Platelet Glycoprotein IIb/IIIa Antagonists

Abciximab (0.25 mg/kg bolus and 12-hour infusion at 10 μg/min) or eptifibatide (two bolus doses of 180 μg/kg 10 minutes apart) should be considered in all patients undergoing percutaneous coronary intervention, particularly patients with refractory unstable angina or with other high-risk features (grade 1A).

ANTITHROMBOTIC THERAPY IN PERIPHERAL ARTERIAL OCCLUSIVE DISEASE (Chapter 79)[9]

Patients should be treated indefinitely with a platelet-active agent (grade 1A).
Moderate to severe disabling intermittent claudication, not responding to exercise and not candidate for invasive procedures: cilostazol (grade 1A)
Patients with carotid endarterectomy should be treated preoperatively and continued indefinitely with aspirin, 75 to 100 mg daily (grade 1A).
Adding warfarin to aspirin for peripheral arterial disease is not more effective but increases life-threatening bleeding.[28]

Peripheral Vascular Reconstructive Surgery

Patients having infrainguinal bypass operations: aspirin, 75 to 100 mg/day, begun preoperatively (grade 1A)

Intraoperative Anticoagulation Therapy

Patients undergoing major vascular reconstructive operations should be systemically anticoagulated with heparin at the time of application of cross-clamps (grade 1A).

ANTITHROMBOTIC AND THROMBOLYTIC THERAPY FOR ISCHEMIC STROKE (Chapter 414)[19]

Acute ischemic stroke treatment within 3 hours of onset of symptoms:
Thrombolytic therapy: in eligible patients, IV t-PA in a dose of 0.9 mg/kg (maximum of 90 mg), with 10% of the total dose given as an initial bolus and the remainder infused during 60 minutes (grade 1A).
Streptokinase is not recommended (grade 1A).
Acute ischemic stroke patients not receiving thrombolysis:
Aspirin, 150 to 325 mg/day, started early (grade 1A)

DVT or Pulmonary Embolism Prophylaxis

For acute stroke patients with restricted mobility: low-dose subcutaneous heparin or LMWH, provided there are no contraindications to anticoagulation (grade 1A)

Stroke Prevention

Noncardioembolic cerebral ischemic events (stroke or TIA; atherothrombotic, lacunar, or cryptogenic): platelet-active drugs (grade 1A); preferably the combination of aspirin and extended-release dipyridamole (25/200 mg bid) (grade 1A) or otherwise aspirin, 50 to 100 mg/day or clopidogrel (75 mg daily) are acceptable options for initial therapy.
Patients with recent acute coronary syndrome: clopidogrel plus aspirin (75 to 100 mg daily) (grade 1A)
Stroke and aortic atherosclerotic lesions: platelet-active drugs
Cardioembolic ischemic events: long-term warfarin (target INR of 2.5; range, 2.0 to 3.0) for atrial fibrillation (grade 1A)
Carotid endarterectomy: aspirin, 50 to 100 mg/day, before carotid endarterectomy and continued long-term after the procedure

aPTT = activated partial thromboplastin time; DVT = deep vein thrombosis; ECG = electrocardiogram; FFP = fresh-frozen plasma; INR = International Normalized Ratio; IV = intravenous; LMWH = low-molecular-weight heparin; PCC = prothrombin complex concentrate; PCI = percutaneous coronary intervention; rFVIIa = recombinant factor VIIa; SC = subcutaneously; TIA = transient ischemic attack; t-PA = tissue plasminogen activator; VTE = venous thromboembolism.

aspirin alone in patients who have percutaneous coronary intervention procedures. Clopidogrel appears to be as well tolerated as aspirin.[18]

Prasugrel is more potent and has a more rapid onset of action than clopidogrel.[10] Given as a bolus dose of 60 mg, followed by 10 mg daily, when compared with clopidogrel, prasugrel reduces the absolute risk of cardiovascular death or nonfatal myocardial infarction or stroke by 2.2%, which is partly offset by an absolute increase of serious bleeding of 0.5%.[24]

Ticagrelor, an oral direct and reversible $P2Y_{12}$ receptor inhibitor, provides a faster response than the thienopyridines.[10] In a randomized trial in patients with acute coronary syndromes, ticagrelor was more effective than clopidogrel, providing an absolute risk reduction for cardiovascular death, myocardial infarction, or stroke of 1.9% without any significant increase of major bleeding.[25]

Integrin $\alpha_{IIb}\beta_3$ (GPIIb-IIIa) Receptor Antagonists

The final common pathway of platelet aggregation is mediated by the binding of fibrinogen to the functionally active integrin $\alpha_{IIb}\beta_3$ (GPIIb-IIIa) on the platelet surface. Inhibitors of this process include monoclonal antibodies, synthetic peptides containing Arg-Gly-Asp (RGD) or Lys-Gly-Asp (KGD), and peptidomimetic and nonpeptide RGD mimetics. These compounds are administered intravenously and inhibit platelet function by competing with fibrinogen (and von Willebrand factor) for occupancy on the platelet integrin receptor.[18] Abciximab (ReoPro), a mouse-human chimeric 7E3 Fab antibody, inhibits platelet aggregation in a concentration-dependent manner. Platelet function is impaired rapidly after an intravenous bolus of abciximab and gradually recovers over 24 to 48 hours. Tirofiban (MK-383, Aggrastat) is a nonpeptide derivative of tyrosine. It has a plasma half-life of 1.6 hours, and its effect on hemostasis is reversed within 4 hours of stopping treatment. Eptifibatide (Integrilin) is a synthetic disulfide-linked cyclic heptapeptide. It has a rapid onset and offset of action, and its effect on platelet function is reduced by more than 50% after 4 hours.

All three GPIIb-IIIa receptor antagonists are effective intravenous agents in patients undergoing percutaneous coronary interventions[8] (Chapter 74), and tirofiban and eptifibatide are effective in patients with unstable angina or non–ST elevation myocardial infarction.[7] The GPIIb-IIIa receptor antagonists are administered in combination with heparin and aspirin. Orally active nonpeptide GPIIb-IIIa inhibitors have been developed for long-term use, but the results of clinical trials have been disappointing.

Fibrinolytic Agents

Fibrinolytic agents convert plasminogen to the enzyme plasmin, which then degrades fibrin to soluble fragments, thereby lysing the thrombus. Of the available fibrinolytic agents, streptokinase and urokinase are not fibrin specific; in contrast, recombinant tissue-type plasminogen activator (rt-PA, alteplase) and the rt-PA variant tenecteplase are relatively fibrin specific (Chapter 73).

Streptokinase is an indirect fibrinolytic agent. It binds to plasminogen, converting it into a plasmin-like molecule that in turn converts plasminogen to plasmin. Streptokinase has a number of disadvantages. It is antigenic, rendering its repeated use problematic, and allergenic, producing chills, fever, and rigors in some patients and, in rare instances, anaphylaxis. Anistreplase (APSAC) is an acylated complex of streptokinase and Lys-plasminogen. Compared with streptokinase, it is more fibrin specific, has a longer plasma half-life, and is inactive until it is selectively activated by deacylation on the fibrin surface. Its side-effect profile, antigenicity, and efficacy are similar to those of streptokinase.

Urokinase is a naturally occurring plasminogen activator that differs from streptokinase in that it directly activates plasminogen and is not antigenic. Urokinase was used extensively to treat peripheral vascular occlusions, but production problems have curtailed its availability.

In its natural state, tissue plasminogen activator is produced by vascular endothelium; rt-PA (alteplase) is produced by recombinant DNA technology. Alteplase is not antigenic or allergenic, and it has greater fibrin specificity than does streptokinase. It has a short half-life of about 3.5 minutes and therefore is given as a continuous intravenous infusion.

Truncated forms of rt-PA have been developed; the first was reteplase (r-PA), a single-chain deletion mutant that lacks certain domains. As a result, its half-life is about twice that of rt-PA, permitting double-bolus therapy 30 minutes apart. r-PA has lower affinity for fibrin than does rt-PA, but fibrinogen depletion with r-PA is less than that with streptokinase. No antigenicity has been reported with this compound.

Tenecteplase (TNK-tPA) is a mutant tissue plasminogen activator with amino acid substitution at three sites. Compared with rt-PA, it has a longer half-life, allowing single-bolus administration, increased fibrin specificity, and increased resistance to inhibition by plasminogen activator inhibitor 1.

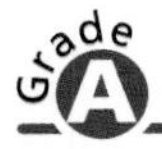

1. Ansell J, Hirsh J, Hylek E, et al. Pharmacology and management of the vitamin K antagonists. *Chest.* 2008;133:160S-198S.
2. Schulman S. Care of patients receiving long-term anticoagulant therapy. *N Engl J Med.* 2003; 349:675-683.
3. Geerts WH, Bergqvist D, Pineo GF, et al. Prevention of venous thromboembolism: American College of Chest Physicians Evidence-Based Clinical Practice Guidelines, 8th ed. *Chest.* 2008;133:381S-453S.
4. Hirsh J, Bauer KA, Donati MB, et al. Parenteral anticoagulants: American College of Chest Physicians Evidence-Based Clinical Practice Guidelines. 8th ed. *Chest.* 2008;133:141S-159S.
5. Kearon C, Kahn SR, Agnelli G, et al. Antithrombotic therapy for venous thromboembolic disease: American College of Chest Physicians Evidence-Based Clinical Practice Guidelines, 8th ed. *Chest.* 2008;133:454S-545S.
6. Goodman SG, Menon V, Cannon CP, et al. Acute ST-segment elevation myocardial infarction: American College of Chest Physicians Evidence-Based Clinical Practice Guidelines. 8th ed. *Chest.* 2008;133:708S-775S.
7. Harrington RA, Becker RC, Cannon CP, et al. Antithrombotic therapy for non-ST-segment elevation acute coronary syndromes: American College of Chest Physicians Evidence-Based Clinical Practice Guidelines. 8th ed. *Chest.* 2008;133:670S-707S.
8. Becker RC, Meade TW, Berger PB, et al. The primary and secondary prevention of coronary artery disease: American College of Chest Physicians Evidence-Based Clinical Practice Guidelines. 8th ed. *Chest.* 2008;133:776S-814S.
9. Sobel M, Verhaeghe R. Antithrombotic therapy for peripheral artery occlusive disease: American College of Chest Physicians Evidence-Based Clinical Practice Guidelines. 8th ed. *Chest.* 2008;133:815S-843S.
10. Weitz JI, Hirsh J, Samama MM. New antithrombotic drugs: American College of Chest Physicians Evidence-Based Clinical Practice Guidelines. 8th ed. *Chest.* 2008;133:234S-256S.
11. Stone GW, Witzenbichler B, Guagliumi G, et al. Bivalirudin during primary PCI in acute myocardial infarction. *N Engl J Med.* 2008;358:2218-2230.
12. Wolowacz SE, Roskell NS, Plumb JM, et al. Efficacy and safety of dabigatran etexilate for the prevention of venous thromboembolism following total hip or knee arthroplasty: a meta-analysis. *Thromb Haemost.* 2009;101:77-85.
13. Connolly SJ, Ezekowitz MD, Yusuf S, et al. Dabigatran versus warfarin in patients with atrial fibrillation. *N Engl J Med.* 2009;361:1139-1151.
14. Schulman S, Kearon C, Kakkar AK, et al. Dabigatran versus warfarin in the treatment of acute venous thromboembolism. *N Engl J Med.* 2009;361:2342-2352.
15. Eriksson BI, Kakkar AK, Turpie AG, et al. Oral rivaroxaban for the prevention of symptomatic venous thromboembolism after elective hip and knee replacement. *J Bone Joint Surg Br.* 2009;91: 636-644.
16. Lassen MR, Raskob GE, Gallus A, et al. Apixaban or enoxaparin for thromboprophylaxis after knee replacement. *N Engl J Med.* 2009;361:594-604.
17. Lassen MR, Raskob GE, Gallus A, et al. Apixaban versus enoxaparin for thromboprophylaxis after knee replacement (ADVANCE-2): a randomized double-blind trial. *Lancet.* 2010;375:807-815.
18. Patrono C, Baigent C, Hirsh J, et al. Antiplatelet drugs: American College of Chest Physicians Evidence-Based Clinical Practice Guidelines. 8th ed. *Chest.* 2008;133:199S-233S.
19. Albers GW, Amarenco P, Easton JD, et al. Antithrombotic and thrombolytic therapy for ischemic stroke: American College of Chest Physicians Evidence-Based Clinical Practice Guidelines. 8th ed. *Chest.* 2008;133:630S-669S.
20. De Berardis G, Sacco M, Strippoli GF, et al. Aspirin for primary prevention of cardiovascular events in people with diabetes: meta-analysis of randomised controlled trials. *BMJ.* 2009;339:b4531.
21. Singer DE, Albers GW, Dalen JE, et al. Antithrombotic therapy in atrial fibrillation. *Chest.* 2008;133:546S-592S.
22. Robless P, Mikhailidis DP, Stansby GP. Cilostazol for peripheral arterial disease. *Cochrane Database Syst Rev.* 2008;1:CD003748.
23. Connolly SJ, Pogue J, Hart RG, et al. Effect of clopidogrel added to aspirin in patients with atrial fibrillation. *N Engl J Med.* 2009;360:2066-2078.
24. Wiviott SD, Braunwald E, McCabe CH, et al. Prasugrel versus clopidogrel in patients with acute coronary syndromes. *N Engl J Med.* 2007;357:2001-2015.
25. Wallentin L, Becker RC, Budaj A, et al. Ticagrelor versus clopidogrel in patients with acute coronary syndromes. *N Engl J Med.* 2009;361:1045-1057.
26. Crowther MA, Ageno W, Garcia D, et al. Oral vitamin K versus placebo to correct excessive anticoagulation in patients receiving warfarin: a randomized trial. *Ann Intern Med.* 2009;150:293-300.
27. Salem DN, O'Gara PT, Madias C, et al. Valvular and structural heart disease: American College of Chest Physicians Evidence-Based Clinical Practice Guidelines. 8th ed. *Chest.* 2008;133: 593S-629S.
28. Anand S, Yusuf S, Xie C, et al. Oral anticoagulant and antiplatelet therapy and peripheral arterial disease. *N Engl J Med.* 2007;357:217-227.

SUGGESTED READINGS

Baigent C, Blackwell L, Collins R, et al. Aspirin in the primary and secondary prevention of vascular disease: collaborative meta-analysis of individual participant data from randomised trials. *Lancet.* 2009;373:1849-1860. *The net benefit of aspirin is more convincing in secondary than in primary prevention of vascular disease.*

Gurbel PA, Tantry US. Combination antithrombotic therapies. *Circulation.* 2010;121:569-583. *Review.*

Krishnaswamy A, Lincoff AM, Cannon CP. Bleeding complications of unfractionated heparin. *Expert Opin Drug Saf.* 2011;10:77-84. *Practical approaches to dosing and monitoring.*

Matchar DB, Jacobson A, Dolor R, et al. Effect of home testing of international normalized ratio on clinical events. *N Engl Med.* 2010;363:1608-1620. *In a randomized trial, weekly INR self-testing was not effective for delaying the time until first stroke, major bleed, or death compared with monthly high-quality standard testing.*

38

COMPLEMENTARY AND ALTERNATIVE MEDICINE

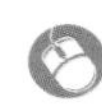

MARY CHARLSON

COMPLEMENTARY AND INTEGRATIVE INTERVENTIONS

Despite tremendous strides by modern medicine in understanding the mechanisms of disease and improving treatments, many patients faced with illness find that conventional therapies do not completely alleviate their suffering. As a result, many patients, particularly those who have experienced life-threatening illnesses, turn to alternative or complementary therapies that they believe will make them feel better.

Most complementary therapies are provided in community settings, not in health institutions. In 2007 a nationally representative sample showed that almost 40% of adults and 11% of children in the United States had used complementary or alternative medical (CAM) therapies in the prior year. CAM modalities include biologically based therapies, body-based practices, mind-body therapies, energy medicine, and whole medical systems; the proportion of U.S. adults using these CAM modalities in 2007 is shown in Table 38-1. Of note, adults had more visits with CAM practitioners, including acupuncturists, massage therapists, and herbalists, than they had with primary care physicians. Most people who use CAM modalities do not disclose this to their physicians because they are concerned that their physicians may not understand or support the use of such approaches.

The use of CAM modalities is particularly high in cancer patients. Eighty percent of patients who are undergoing treatment for cancer use one or more CAM modalities, and about half tell their oncologists. The use of CAM modalities does not stop when treatment is over; in fact, patients may seek such modalities even more aggressively after treatment is completed, much to the surprise of their physicians. When oncologists tell patients that their treatment is over and that they have an excellent prognosis or that the critical time frame for recurrence has passed, they expect the patients to be enormously relieved. All too often, patients experience distress when told that they can go back to their usual lives, asking, "What life?" The growing field

TABLE 38-1 USE OF COMPLEMENTARY OR ALTERNATIVE MEDICINE BY U.S. ADULTS IN 2007

MODALITY	% OF ADULTS WHO USED IT
BIOLOGICALLY BASED THERAPIES	
Herbal or natural products	17.7
Dietary supplements	N/A
Diet-based therapy	3.5
BODY-BASED PRACTICES	
Chiropractic or osteopathic manipulation	8.6
Massage	8.3
Movement therapies*	1.5
MIND-BODY THERAPIES	
Biofeedback	0.2
Hypnosis	0.2
Meditation	9.4
Guided imagery	2.2
Progressive relaxation	2.9
Deep breathing	12.7
Yoga	6.1
Tai chi	1.0
Qi gong	0.3
ENERGY MEDICINE†	
Reiki, biofield, and other therapies	0.5
WHOLE MEDICAL SYSTEMS	
Naturopathy	0.3
Homeopathy	1.8
Ayurveda	0.1
Traditional Chinese medicine (acupuncture)	1.4
Traditional healers	0.4

*Pilates, Trager, Feldenkrais, and Alexander.
†Energy medicine is based on the theory that there are energy fields surrounding and penetrating the human body. Energy therapies are intended to manipulate these energy fields.

of survivorship medicine recognizes that patients who have had cancer may face ongoing physical, psychological, and spiritual challenges.

Most often, patients who are feeling distressed are referred to support groups. Surprisingly, support groups were not shown to improve quality of life in breast cancer survivors in randomized trials. Cognitive-behavioral therapy may also be recommended for patients who experience anxiety after treatment for cancer. Randomized trials have shown that cognitive-behavioral therapy may be effective in improving mood in cancer patients. More and more, cancer survivors reach for complementary or integrative approaches to healing and health to address their psychological, physical, and spiritual needs.

Integrative health is a broad framework that encompasses complex biologic, psychological, cultural, and social pathways to health and disease. *Complementary medicine* encompasses adjunctive approaches to conventional medicine for preventing or treating illness or distress. These alternative approaches are embraced in many different communities and cultures.

THE IMPORTANCE OF PATIENT BELIEFS, EXPECTATIONS, AND CULTURES

Beliefs about illness and health and about the risks and benefits of treatment are deeply rooted at a cultural and social network level. Americans rely on family and social networks for advice about how to handle most illnesses and see physicians for only 10 to 20% of illness episodes. Social networks in many communities help determine many individuals' beliefs and expectations with regard to health and the use of different treatment modalities. Emerging data suggest that apart from determining expectations about disease and treatment, social networks can have a profound impact on health and affect. A recent analysis of the Framingham data showed that obesity spreads through social networks. The chance of becoming obese increased by 171% if a friend became obese or 40% if a sibling became obese. Obesity was not higher in neighbors, suggesting that the findings were not due to environmental confounding. Instead, obesity appears to be propagated through social networks. A similar analysis of the Framingham data suggested that happiness is also spread through social networks. Such social network influences are rarely considered in modern medicine, except in approaches to HIV and drug addiction.

TABLE 38-2 QUESTIONS PHYSICIANS CAN ASK TO EXPLORE PATIENTS' BELIEFS

What do you think this illness does?
What worries you with this illness?
Why did you think you got this illness?
How do you think it should be treated?
Who do you ask for advice about illness?

Physicians are often not aware that their patients have beliefs about the cause of their illness (i.e., their explanatory model). As a result, it is common for patient-doctor discussions to involve major discrepancies in understanding, expectations, and goals. For example, Hmong parents in Minnesota who placed heated cups on their children's skin to relieve chest congestion (a traditional practice) were mistakenly reported for child abuse because the cups caused erythematous patches. Puerto Rican women who reported having visions during religious ceremonies (as was expected) were incorrectly diagnosed as having schizophrenia. Understanding and addressing patients' beliefs is critical to overcoming otherwise hidden barriers to adopting effective treatments and preventing unintended consequences. Questions that can be employed to elucidate patients' beliefs are shown in Table 38-2. Explanatory models of illness are deeply rooted in culture and embedded in indigenous medical systems and healing practices.

INDIGENOUS MEDICAL SYSTEMS AND TRADITIONAL HEALING PRACTICES

Having evolved over thousands of years, most indigenous medical systems frame health as balance or harmony and illness as imbalance. To treat illness, indigenous systems seek to restore balance using a combination of foods, herbs, physical manipulation, movement, prayer, and social interventions. Each has its own methods of diagnosis, using the patient's symptoms and often his or her family or social situation.

For Native Americans, health means staying strong in spirit, mind, and body and staying in harmony with oneself, one's community, and the earth. Efforts to restore health focus on healing the spirit of the person who is ill and healing the community and the environment. Ceremonies and rituals such as the sweat lodge as well as herbal remedies may be used. Ayurvedic (ancient Indian) medicine focuses on achieving a balance of three elements—vata (air), pita (bile), and kapha (phlegm)—through the use of foods, herbs, yoga, meditation, and massage. Traditional Chinese medicine draws on ancient theory to achieve a balance of yin and yang (opposites) and the five elements (water, wood, fire, earth, and metal) through acupuncture, herbs, foods, and massage. The life force or energy, called *Qi*, is believed to flow through meridians; acupuncture, tai chi, and qi gong are all thought to balance the flow of energy. Tibetan medicine combines elements from Ayurvedic, Greek, and Chinese medical systems with the Buddhist philosophy that all illness and suffering come from the mind; it emphasizes guided meditation as central to harmony and healing. African traditional medicine frames illness as a physical or mental problem caused by a disruption of a person's own balance or his or her social relationships. Diagnosis involves identifying the spiritual cause of the illness; treatments are designed to restore spiritual and social balance and may involve herbals, prayers to ancestors, and family interventions, as well as rituals and ceremonies. Obviously, these descriptions are too short to do justice to any of these traditions, but they emphasize that each of these indigenous medical systems has specific theories about the cause of, susceptibility to, and treatment for certain conditions and specific strategies for diagnosis. These traditional systems are currently being used to treat millions of people worldwide. In Asia and Africa, the World Health Organization estimates that 80% of people currently depend primarily on traditional medicine.

There is limited research about the effectiveness of indigenous medical systems as a whole because these systems are deeply intertwined with culture. Most Western research has taken one element or tool from a traditional system and tested its use to treat a specific condition or disease. For example, acupuncture has been shown to reduce nausea and vomiting induced by chemotherapy. Iyengar yoga improves function and reduces pain in patients with chronic back pain. Tai chi reduces pain and improves function among patients with osteoarthritis of the knee. Our knowledge is limited about the effectiveness of specific practices across diverse communities; specifically, we do not know whether responses to therapies differ between populations that have used "alternative" approaches for many years as part of their healing traditions and those that have only recently begun to incorporate them.

TRADITIONAL VERSUS MODERN MEDICINE: THE MIND AND THE BODY

In traditional medical systems, the mind and spirit were not viewed as separate from the body; the health of the mind and spirit was viewed as central to physical health. Many traditional systems held that physical illness is caused by disturbances of the mind or spirit. As a result, many interventions were designed to improve the health of the mind and spirit.

In the Indo-Tibetan Buddhist tradition, healing focuses on building the discipline of attention through healing visualization, recitation, and deep breathing. The Tibetans developed a comprehensive system of self-healing and learning called the *gradual path*, which deals with the causes of suffering and the approaches to end suffering. Self-healing is taught through meditation guided by a mentor. Recently, guided meditation in this tradition has been shown to improve quality of life in breast cancer survivors.

African traditional medicine focuses on the spiritual causes of illness and then on the physical manifestations. The traditional healer understands the beliefs and normative values of the community and interprets what the patient has done wrong to cause the illness. The intervention may involve prayer, dancing, singing, drumming, ritual, or community ceremonies. Recently, traditional healers have developed rituals for the rehabilitation of children who were abducted and forced to become soldiers. Reconciliation with their dead ancestors and with those who died is a central part of the ritual. These rituals were adapted from those used for centuries to peacefully reintegrate returning warriors into the community.

Native American healing focuses on restoring health and harmony with the community and with nature. Illness is believed to stem from spiritual imbalances. Purifying and cleansing the body and spirit through sweat lodge ceremonies is an important healing tradition. Other rituals may include the whole community and involve drumming, singing, chanting, and prayers. Sweat lodge rituals have improved the success of interventions designed to change addictive behaviors.

For the most part, Western medicine does not have equivalent approaches. The focus of Western medicine has been medical and surgical treatments for the physical body. Most interventions target the individual patient. Community-based rituals or interventions for improving health are still largely the province of religious institutions. The difference between modern medicine and indigenous systems grew out of the mind-body dichotomy. Introduced by Descartes in the West, the philosophy that the mind and the body are separate and distinct provided the foundation for modern medicine. The physical body became the focus of Western medicine, while the mind and the spirit were exclusively the domain of the church.

THE MIND-BODY CONNECTION

For some time it has been clear that psychosocial states such as stress, social isolation, and depression alter the risk of developing chronic illness and increase the risk of adverse outcomes. For example, depression increases the risk of developing heart disease. Depressive symptoms also increase the risk of morbidity and mortality among patients who have heart disease. Lack of emotional support increases mortality in patients who have had a myocardial infarction. Sudden emotional stress can precipitate heart failure in patients without coronary artery disease.

Psychosocial stress may be caused by a discrete life event such as the death of a family member, chronic situations related to social role or work, or small day-to-day hassles. The impact of a given event depends on how the individual perceives it: is the event a threat, and if so, how severe? An individual's interpretation of events as physical or psychological threats is based on his or her own experience and that of the individual's social network. Once an event is perceived as a potential threat, an individual may experience negative emotions, such as anger or anxiety. Such emotions activate emotional memory and trigger reaction patterns learned in response to prior stresses, initiating the neuroendocrine stress response. People react to stress with their own patterned behavioral responses, and most resultant behaviors tend to increase the negative impact of stress (e.g., eating unhealthy food, gaining weight, smoking, living a sedentary life, not taking medications). The impact of negative psychosocial states on health has been clear for several decades; however, we have recently gained a greater understanding of the potential mechanisms.

How Does Psychosocial Stress Impact Health?

The repeated triggering of the stress cascade can adversely affect multiple aspects of health and adaptation. There is emerging evidence that psychosocial stress is one of the most salient, potentially modifiable mechanisms linking illness and health.

Allostatic Load

An approach has been defined to measure the cumulative toll exacted by adverse behavioral, psychological, social, physiologic, and environmental stressors. Stress causes specific neural and endocrine responses, with sympathetic activation resulting in the release of catecholamines from the adrenal medulla and cortisol from the adrenal cortex. The acute stress response is designed to protect against threats to survival. However, chronic stress, especially psychosocial stress, can have a negative impact on health. Chronic stress interferes with biologic regulatory processes central to homeostasis. Chronic stress disrupts the hypothalamic-pituitary-adrenal (HPA) axis, resulting in abnormal circadian cortisol rhythms, with elevated and flattened diurnal cortisol levels and elevated overnight urinary cortisol. Stress also disrupts the autonomic balance, resulting in an increase in sympathetic versus parasympathetic function and elevated levels of urinary catecholamines. There are multiple biologic markers of the stress response that indicate cumulative stress-related wear and tear, which is called *allostatic load*. The potential adverse consequences of allostatic load were evaluated in the MacArthur Studies of Successful Aging, which followed 736 healthy men and women between 70 and 79 years of age. Among patients without cardiovascular disease at baseline, patients with a higher allostatic load had a higher mortality and greater functional decline that those with a lower allostatic load. Of note, older men with more social network ties and greater social integration had lower allostatic load scores. Therefore, individuals under chronic stress had greater neuroendocrine and cardiovascular responses and subsequent adverse health outcomes.

Stress Reactivity

Efforts to measure sympathetic-parasympathetic balance have focused on measures of stress reactivity, including heart rate variability and blood pressure. Studies measuring cardiovascular reactivity in the context of daily life have yielded valuable insights. For example, day-to-day social interactions may be associated with changes in cardiovascular reactivity; the changes depend on the relationships involved. Negative social relationships may cause activation of the sympathetic nervous system, leading to increased cardiovascular reactivity. People who have increased reactivity to stress have a larger, longer-lasting increase in negative affect. In contrast, during positive social interaction with one's partner, blood pressure levels are lower than during interactions with other people.

In some studies, the health impact of heightened cardiovascular reactivity depended on socioeconomic status. Thus, social context and social support may alter stress reactivity. Increased cardiovascular reactivity to stressors may predict cardiovascular disease.

Chronic work stress has significant health consequences. The Whitehall study showed that workers with higher chronic work-related stress had a higher incidence of coronary heart disease and higher death rates from heart disease. Higher work stress was associated with four components of the metabolic syndrome (higher fasting glucose, higher triglycerides, greater waist circumference, and lower high-density lipoprotein cholesterol), as well as worse health behaviors (lower physical activity, poor diet) and the development of obesity.

Importantly, higher work stress was also associated with lower heart rate variability. Lower heart rate variability indicates lower vagal tone—that is, reduced parasympathetic and increased sympathetic activity. Lower heart rate variability predicts increased all-cause mortality and increased risk of coronary heart disease. There is a correlation between heart rate variability (the high-frequency component reflecting vagal activity) and emotion-specific changes in blood flow in the medial prefrontal cortex.

The Cholinergic Inflammatory Pathway

The vagus nerve, which controls parasympathetic tone and heart rate variability, also mediates the release of pro- and anti-inflammatory cytokines. Through the vagus nerve, the nervous system has the ability to sense and suppress inflammation through the cholinergic anti-inflammatory pathway. Stimulation of the vagus nerve leads to the release of acetylcholine, which in turn inhibits the inflammatory response by inhibiting the release of pro-inflammatory cytokines (interleukin-6 and tumor necrosis factor). When pro-inflammatory cytokines are released to defend against pathogens, the release is a rapid and localized reflex; however, if pro-inflammatory cytokines are released over a prolonged period, they can create a systemic humoral response, leading to or exacerbating diseases such as rheumatoid arthritis, inflammatory bowel disease, and atherosclerosis.

Stress and the Brain

A large body of literature highlights the effects of chronic stress on the structure and function of the hippocampus and amygdala. The hippocampus is important for both contextual and declarative memory. Severe stress and elevated steroid levels impair memory reversibly and may affect the reliability of contextual memories, which are important in evaluating a potential threat. High levels of stress hormones also impair declarative memory reversibly. Chronic stress can cause a reduction in the size of the hippocampus (which provides negative feedback to the HPA axis). However, there is some evidence of plasticity at least in the dentate gyrus in the hippocampus: in primates, new cells are increased by exercise and enriched environments. A study showed that older patients who are socially disengaged experience cognitive decline, leading to speculation that social engagement may buffer against stress-related damage to the hippocampus.

The amygdala and the prefrontal cortex are also involved in the affective and attentional response to stress. The amygdala is important to threat recognition and fear, as well as emotional learning. Chronic stress causes increases in the amygdala (which provides positive feedback to the HPA axis). The prefrontal cortex likely exerts a major inhibitory influence on the amygdala. Chronic stress interferes with the prefrontal cortex and results in decreased working memory and impaired problem solving. It has been shown that among medical students experiencing the same examination stress, those with higher perceived stress levels also had more impairment in attentional control compared with those whose perceived stress levels were lower. Importantly, after 1 month of vacation, the impairment in prefrontal cortex function was reversible. Thus, stress results in both reversible and irreversible changes in the hippocampus, amygdala, and prefrontal cortex that are involved in multiple aspects of cognition, attention, and emotion.

Stress and Telomere Length

Chronic stress is also associated with telomere length, a marker of cellular age. When telomeres shorten sufficiently, the cell becomes senescent. An important study evaluated mothers of healthy children versus mothers of chronically ill children; the hypothesis was that mothers of ill children would have greater perceived stress than mothers of healthy children and thus shorter telomeres. Instead, the investigators found no difference in telomere length, telomerase activity, or oxidative stress. However, in both groups of mothers, telomere length was correlated with perceived stress; specifically, the higher the mother's perceived stress, the shorter her telomeres were. High-stress mothers had the equivalent of 1 decade of aging in telomere length in contrast to the low-stress mothers. Because the study was cross-sectional, it could not establish whether the correlation represented causation.

Thus, if the stress response, which is designed to protect against acute events, becomes a chronic response, it can have an adverse impact on cellular aging and multiple aspects of regulatory systems, including the HPA axis, parasympathetic-sympathetic tone, the vagus nerve, and the central nervous system.

How Do Integrative Interventions Reduce the Impact of Stress?

Reducing the impact of stress is likely a key mechanism through which many integrative interventions work. It is important to realize that it is not the actual magnitude of the stressor that has the adverse health impact; it is the individual's perception of the stressor. Thus, in two mothers with chronically ill children, telomeres are shortened in the mother with high perceived stress but not in the mother with a low level of perceived stress. Medical students with high levels of perceived stress about an upcoming examination have attentional shifts and impairment in prefrontal cortex function, whereas those with low perceived stress do not.

Integrative interventions are almost uniformly designed to increase confidence in one's own control and in one's ability to self-regulate emotion and mood. Many of these interventions focus on the individual's being present in the moment and achieving nonjudgmental awareness. They are also designed, using different theories, to create greater harmony between the mind and the body.

Cognitive neuroscience has begun to understand meditation as a discipline of attention; stress reduction is achieved through learning. This model is consistent with the view of traditional medical systems that use meditation, prayer, guided imagery, recitation, singing, drumming, and chanting to build present awareness, attention, and harmony. Yoga, tai chi, and qi gong are examples of practices that involve movement and meditation.

Studies of clinically stressed populations indicate that interventions aimed at reducing stress by promoting the cognitive regulation of attention and affective behavior yield enhancements in neuroendocrine and immune function and clinically significant improvements in quality of life. A few small studies have reported changes in heart rate variability in response to an intervention. Transcendental meditation[1] and biofeedback can increase heart rate variability in cardiac patients; acupuncture may also increase heart rate variability. It has been suggested that interventions designed to increase heart rate variability should target patients whose conditions are associated with high levels of pro-inflammatory cytokines, such as inflammatory bowel disease or rheumatoid arthritis. Meditation may also improve blood pressure and insulin resistance.[1] With regard to brain plasticity and telomere shortening, studies have only begun to evaluate interventions' potential to effect changes.

WHY DO PATIENTS SEEK INTEGRATIVE INTERVENTIONS?

First, patients want to play an active role in their recovery and return to health—that is, self-healing. Self-healing is a concept that may seem strange to physicians, yet we know that self-healing (i.e., regeneration) allows repair to occur after injury.

Patient empowerment and active engagement are major determinants of health outcomes. An overwhelming body of literature has shown that confidence in one's ability to do something—that is, self-efficacy—is a powerful predictor of success. More and more studies have shown the importance of whether patients believe they can influence their own health outcomes. People who think they can influence their own outcomes (those with an internal locus of control) fare better than those who believe that what they do does not matter (those with an external locus of control). Of note, it has been known for more than 20 years that locus of control can predict health outcomes and behaviors. Ten-year-olds who believed they could influence events by their own actions had a reduced risk of obesity and psychological distress than those with a greater external locus of control.

Self-efficacy can be enhanced; that is, patients can learn strategies to increase confidence in their ability to cope with illness and thereby improve their health outcomes, at least over the short term.[2] A self-management course, including action planning, modeling of behaviors, problem solving, and a decision-making model, may increase self-efficacy and reduce hospitalizations. Many disease management courses cite this model but miss the critical ingredients of improving self-efficacy, decision making, and problem solving, focusing instead on specific things the patient should monitor and report to the nurse or doctor, potentially undermining self-efficacy and reinforcing the external locus of control.

To date, only a few complementary approaches have achieved widespread use in medical centers. Among commonly used complementary and alternative medical therapies, acupuncture is beneficial for tension-type headache[3]; can improve nausea, vomiting, and other symptoms in cancer patients[4]; can lower blood pressure by about 5.4/2.0 mm Hg during treatment but not after it is stopped[5]; has some benefit for chronic lower back pain,[6] but has small and probably not clinically relevant benefits for peripheral joint osteoarthritis.[7] Tai Chi may be an effective treatment for fibromyalgia.[8] By comparison, Echinacea is not effective for the common cold,[9] hypnotherapy is not effective for smoking cessations,[10] and glucosamine and chondroitin are not beneficial for osteoarthritis of the hip or knee.[11]

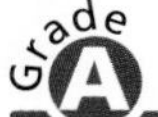

1. Paul-Labrador M, Pol D, Dwyer JH, et al. Effects of a randomized controlled trial of transcendental meditation on components of the metabolic syndrome in subjects with coronary heart disease. *Arch Intern Med*. 2006;166:1218-1224.
2. Foster G, Taylor SJ, Eldridge SE, et al. Self-management education programmes by lay leaders for people with chronic conditions. *Cochrane Database Syst Rev*. 2007;4:CD005108.
3. Linde K, Allais G, Brinkhaus B, et al. Acupuncture for tension-type headache. *Cochrane Database Syst Rev*. 2009;1:CD007587.
4. Capodice JL. Acupuncture in the oncology setting: clinical trial update. *Curr Treat Options Oncol*. 2010;11:87-94.
5. Flachskampf FA, Gallasch J, Gefeller OY, et al: Randomized trial of acupuncture to lower blood pressure. *Circulation*. 2007;115:3121-3129.
6. Berman BM, Langevin HH, Witt CM, et al. Acupuncture for chronic low back pain. *N Engl J Med*. 2010;363:454-461.
7. Manheimer E, Cheng K, Linde K, et al. Acupuncture for peripheral joint osteoarthritis. *Cochrane Database Syst Rev*. 2010;1:CD001977.
8. Wang C, Schmid CH, Rones R, et al. A randomized trial of tai chi for fibromyalgia. *N Engl J Med*. 2010;363:743-754.
9. Barrett B, Brown R, Rakel D, et al. Echinacea for treating the common cold: a randomized trial. *Ann Intern Med*. 2010;153:769-777.
10. Barnes J, Dong CY, McRobbie H, et al. Hypnotherapy for smoking cessation. *Cochrane Database Syst Rev*. 2010;10:CD001008.
11. Wandel S, Jüni P, Tendal B, et al. Effects of glucosamine, chondroitin, or placebo in patients with osteoarthritis of hip or knee: network meta-analysis. *BMJ*. 2010;341:c4675.

SUGGESTED READINGS

Kennedy DA, Seely D. Clinically based evidence of drug-herb interactions: a systemic review. *Expert Opin Drug Saf*. 2010;9:79-124. *Review*.

Liston C, McEwen BS, Casey BJ. Psychosocial stress reversibly disrupts prefrontal processing and attentional control. *Proc Natl Acad Sci U S A*. 2009;106:912-917. *Documents the effect of stress on mental function*.

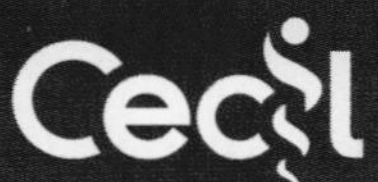

VI GENETICS

39

PRINCIPLES OF GENETICS

BRUCE R. KORF

The elucidation of the structure and function of the genome is one of the great scientific triumphs of the 20th century. The relevance of inheritance to health and disease probably has been recognized throughout history, but it is only during the last century that the rules governing inheritance and the mechanisms whereby genetic information is stored and used have come to light. The application of this knowledge to medical practice so far has focused on relatively rare monogenic and chromosomal disorders. Major contributions have been made in these areas in the form of approaches to genetic counseling, genetic testing, prenatal diagnosis, newborn screening, carrier screening, and, to a limited extent, treatment. As important as these contributions are, however, their impact has been limited by the rarity of these disorders. Powerful tools resulting from the Human Genome Project are changing this situation (Chapter 42). Genetic factors that contribute to common and rare disorders are being identified, leading to new approaches to diagnosis, prevention, and treatment. Genetics and genomics are increasingly occupying center stage in medical practice, guiding treatment decisions and preventive strategies. This chapter reviews the paradigm whereby genetics is being integrated into the routine practice of medicine.

GENETIC CONTRIBUTION TO DISEASE

It may be argued that no disorder is either completely determined genetically or completely determined by nongenetic factors. Even monogenic conditions, such as phenylketonuria, are modified by the environment, in this case by dietary intake of phenylalanine. Genetically determined host factors are known to modify susceptibility to infection or other environmental agents. Even individuals who are victims of trauma may find themselves at risk in part because of genetic traits that affect behavior or ability to perceive or escape from danger.

Multifactorial Inheritance

Complex traits that are important for both health and disease are the result of an interaction of multiple genes with one another and with the environment (Fig. 39-1). In some cases, individual genes or environmental factors contribute overwhelmingly to the cause of a disorder, as with a genetic condition, such as neurofibromatosis or Marfan syndrome, or an acquired disorder, such as bacterial infection or trauma. Other times, there may be interplay among many factors, making it difficult to dissect out the specific genes or environmental exposures.

From a medical perspective, it is helpful to divide the genetic contribution to disease into three categories: high-penetrance monogenic or chromosomal disorders, monogenic versions of common disorders, and complex, multifactorial disorders. Each of these has an impact on medical practice in distinctive ways.

High-Penetrance Monogenic or Chromosomal Disorders

High-penetrance monogenic or chromosomal disorders are the disorders that most clinicians think of as "genetic conditions." They include rare but familiar single-gene disorders, such as neurofibromatosis, Marfan syndrome, and cystic fibrosis, and chromosomal abnormalities, such as trisomy 21 (Down syndrome). Several thousand distinct human genetic disorders have been described and cataloged in *Mendelian Inheritance in Man* (available at www.ncbi.nlm.nih.gov/Omim/). These include mendelian dominant or recessive disorders, sex-linked disorders, and conditions that are due to mutations within the 16.6-kilobase mitochondrial genome. They also include major chromosomal aneuploidy syndromes and syndromes associated with duplication or deletion of small regions of the genome that result in either reproducible syndromes, such as Williams syndrome (deletion of contiguous loci from a region of chromosome 7), or nonspecific mental retardation.

Role of the Nonspecialist

Because of the rarity of many of these conditions, most practitioners have limited experience with a given disorder and are likely to need to refer the patient to an appropriate specialist for assistance with diagnosis and management. Nevertheless, the nonspecialist has many distinct roles in the care of these patients. These roles begin with the recognition of the fact that the patient may have a disorder and arrangement for appropriate diagnostic evaluation. Many genetic disorders produce obvious signs or symptoms that at least prompt referral even if they are not immediately suggestive of a diagnosis. Others can be more subtle, with nevertheless significant consequences if the diagnosis is missed. An example is Marfan syndrome (Chapter 268). The physician needs to be alert to the physical characteristics of patients with Marfan syndrome because life-threatening aortic dissection can be avoided with appropriate monitoring and treatment. Table 39-1 lists examples of some adult-onset monogenic conditions with which the internist should be familiar.

Treatment of Patients with Genetic Disorders

The treatment of patients with genetic disorders may require the assistance of a specialist, but the nonspecialist is likely to be the first contact when an affected individual is ill. The primary care physician needs to be familiar with the disorder and major potential complications. For example, the patient with neurofibromatosis who experiences chronic back pain may be presenting with a malignant peripheral nerve sheath tumor, requiring more aggressive evaluation than would be typical for an unaffected individual with back pain. Formation of a good working relationship between the specialist and nonspecialist is crucial to ensure effective care.

The nonspecialist also has an important role in supporting the patient and helping to explain the difficult choices that may be offered for management. This includes providing support for patients who have disorders that cannot be treated and for the emotional impact that accompanies knowledge that a disorder may be transmitted to one's offspring or shared with other relatives. Most patients have little understanding of the mechanisms of genetics and genetic disease. Although the responsibility to explain these issues may reside with specialists and counselors, the primary care provider has an important supportive role.

Advances in Genetics

Many of the disorders in this group have been known for a long time, but more recent advances in genetics have had a substantial impact on approaches to diagnosis and management. Genetic testing has been refined with the advent of molecular diagnostic tests that detect mutations within individual genes. Even rare disorders may be amenable to diagnostic testing; a database of testing laboratories can be found on the Internet (available at www.genetests.org). Whole-genome scanning for small deletions or duplications is revealing mutations in patients with disorders such autism, for which standard chromosomal analysis had previously been unrevealing. Population screening for carrier status of some disorders now is offered routinely. Some tests are targeted to particular ethnic groups, such as Ashkenazi Jews (Tay-Sachs disease, Canavan disease, cystic fibrosis, Gaucher's disease) or individuals of African, Mediterranean, or Asian ancestry (hemoglobinopathies) (Table 39-2). Pan-ethnic screening is now being made available for cystic fibrosis, although risks differ in different ethnic groups. Newborn screening is being expanded beyond inborn errors of metabolism such as phenylketonuria and galactosemia, with the advent of tandem mass spectrometry and the availability of a standardized panel of tests. Finally, treatment of some monogenic disorders is becoming feasible. Life expectancy for patients with cystic fibrosis has been increasing gradually with better treatments for chronic lung disease; dietary therapy is available for many inborn errors of metabolism; novel therapies that use either pharmaceuticals or gene or enzyme replacement strategies are in use or being tested for many conditions. The principles of management of genetic disorders are evolving rapidly so that care of patients increasingly requires active partnership of specialists and primary care providers. Moreover, individuals with congenital disorders such as Down syndrome are routinely surviving to adulthood and require primary care providers who are familiar with their special needs.

Monogenic Versions of Common Disorders

Not all monogenic disorders produce obscure phenotypes, and not all common disorders are due to complex multifactorial causes. Some common disorders occur in some families as single-gene traits (Table 39-3). This is usually true for only a proportion of affected individuals, but in some cases it is a significant proportion and represents an important group of patients to be recognized.

Breast Cancer

An example is breast cancer (Chapter 204). About 10% of cases of this common form of cancer can be attributed to mutation in one of two genes, *BRCA1* or *BRCA2*. Women who inherit a mutation in one of these genes face a high risk of eventually developing breast or ovarian cancer—more than 80% by age 70 years for breast cancer. Women at risk because of mutation do not look different from women with sporadic breast cancer but can be distinguished by many features, including family history of breast or ovarian cancer in multiple relatives, early age at onset of cancer, and multifocality of the cancer (e.g., bilateral breast cancer or breast and ovarian cancer).

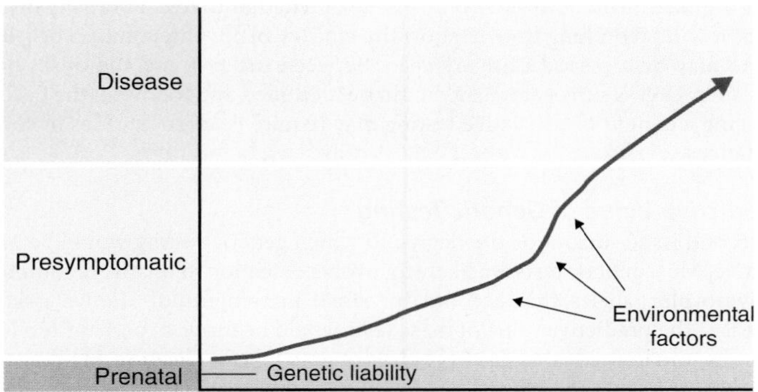

FIGURE 39-1. Multifactorial etiology of disease. An individual is born with a genetic liability but remains in a presymptomatic state for some time until additional events occur, including exposure to environmental factors, that result in crossing a threshold that is identified as *disease.* In instances of high-penetrance monogenic disorders, the genetic liability may be overwhelming. In other instances, genetic factors may contribute only slightly to disease risk.

TABLE 39-1 HIGH-PENETRANCE SINGLE-GENE DISORDERS THAT MAY PRESENT IN ADULTHOOD, WITH SOME MAJOR MEDICAL IMPLICATIONS*

DISORDER	INHERITANCE	MAJOR MEDICAL IMPLICATIONS
CARDIOVASCULAR		
Marfan syndrome	AD	Risk of aortic dissection; lens dislocation
Long QT syndrome	AD, AR	Arrhythmia, sudden death
RENAL		
Adult polycystic kidney disease	AD	Renal failure
PULMONARY		
α_1-Antitrypsin deficiency	AR	Emphysema, cirrhosis
NEUROLOGIC		
NF1	AD	Benign and malignant nerve sheath tumors, gliomas
NF2	AD	Schwannomas (especially vestibular), meningiomas
Von Hippel-Lindau	AD	Hemangioblastoma of cerebellum, brain stem, eye; pheochromocytoma; renal cell carcinoma
Huntington disease	AD	Movement disorder, psychiatric disorder, dementia
HEMATOLOGIC		
Globin disorders	AR	Stroke, iron overload
ENDOCRINE		
MEN syndromes	AD	Tumors of thyroid and parathyroid, pheochromocytoma

*See Table 39-3 for examples of lower penetrance disorders.
AD = autosomal dominant; AR = autosomal recessive; MEN = multiple endocrine neoplasia; NF = neurofibromatosis.

Colon Cancer and Other Common Disorders

Another example from cancer genetics is colon cancer (Chapter 199). Two syndromes, familial adenomatous polyposis and hereditary nonpolyposis colon cancer, are autosomal dominantly inherited and convey a high risk of colon cancer. Other noncancer examples are hemochromatosis (Chapter 219), in which cirrhosis, cardiomyopathy, diabetes, joint disease, and other problems ensue from excessive iron absorption; 10% of whites carry an allele that predisposes to this recessive disorder. Mutations in the factor V gene or the prothrombin gene occur commonly and predispose to deep venous thrombosis (Chapter 179). Rarer examples include inherited forms of cardiomyopathy, hypertension, and familial hypercholesterolemia.

Management

The physician may be called on to address these disorders in many ways. There is a compelling reason to make an early diagnosis of hemochromatosis because the complications can be prevented, but not reversed, by phlebotomy and subsequent monitoring of iron stores. Individuals at risk of colon cancer can be offered surveillance with colonoscopy or surgical resection of the colon to reduce the risk of cancer. Individuals at risk of breast and ovarian cancer likewise can be offered surveillance, chemoprevention, or surgery. The benefits of knowledge of genetic risks are less clear in some instances. Carriers of the factor V Leiden mutation would not be treated with anticoagulation until after an event of thrombosis, and the treatment may not be different for a carrier versus a noncarrier. In some cases, however, knowledge of carrier status might help ensure prompt diagnosis or avoid situations of high risk.

TABLE 39-2 MAJOR RECESSIVE DISORDERS FOR WHICH CARRIER SCREENING COMMONLY IS OFFERED IN THE UNITED STATES

DISORDER	MAJOR AT-RISK POPULATION	CARRIER FREQUENCY
Cystic fibrosis	White Ashkenazi Jewish	1:25 1:29
Sickle cell anemia	African American	1:10
β-Thalassemia	Mediterranean	1:30
α-Thalassemia	Southeast Asian, Chinese	1:30
Tay-Sachs disease	Ashkenazi Jewish French Canadian	1:30 1:30
Canavan's disease	Ashkenazi Jewish	1:40
Familial dysautonomia	Ashkenazi Jewish	1:30

TABLE 39-3 SINGLE-GENE DISORDERS WITH INCOMPLETE PENETRANCE THAT MAY ACCOUNT FOR INHERITED FORMS OF SELECTED COMMON DISORDERS

DISORDER	INHERITANCE: GENES	MAJOR MEDICAL IMPLICATIONS
Hemochromatosis	AR: *HFE*	Cirrhosis, cardiomyopathy, diabetes mellitus
Thrombophilia	AD, AR: multiple genes	Deep venous thrombosis
Breast and ovarian cancers	AD: *BRCA1, BRCA2*	Breast and ovarian cancers
Familial adenomatous polyposis	AD: *APC*	Multiple colonic polyps, colon cancer
Hereditary nonpolyposis colorectal cancer	AD: DNA mismatch repair genes	Colorectal cancer, endometrial cancer
Maturity-onset diabetes of the young	AD: multiple genes	Diabetes mellitus
Cardiomyopathy	AD: genes involved in cardiac contractile apparatus	Arrhythmia, heart failure

AD = autosomal dominant; AR = autosomal recessive.

Genetic Testing

As with other medical tests, the physician should carefully consider risks, benefits, and clinical utility in deciding to use a genetic test. Some distinct ethical and legal risks may apply to some genetic tests. These may include anxiety, stigmatization, guilt, and possibly discrimination for insurance or employment. Some of these risks may be addressed by legislation to maintain privacy of genetic information, such as the Genetic Information Nondiscrimination Act, but the risks of anxiety, guilt, and stigmatization cannot be legislated away. To some extent, further research may improve the basis for surveillance or lead to effective treatments. For now, many of these disorders present a double-edged sword of potentially useful knowledge and potentially harmful information.

Role of the Physician

The role of the physician in dealing with monogenic disorders includes recognition of individuals at risk and participation in formulation of a care plan. Individuals at risk cannot be identified by physical appearance and usually are not evident from medical history or physical examination findings. The most valuable screening tool is the family history. Directed questioning about a family history of major monogenic disorders, especially breast, ovarian, and colon cancer, as well as hypercholesterolemia, hypertension, deep venous thrombosis, cirrhosis, and diabetes, can identify the occasional patient with mendelian segregation of these common disorders. Even if the information is of uncertain reliability, eliciting a family history can prompt referral for further evaluation, documentation of the family history, and consideration for genetic testing. The physician's job is not simply to identify individuals at risk; some people believe they are at high risk even in the absence of well-documented risk factors. Addressing these misconceptions can bring peace of mind and usually does not require genetic testing.

Complex, Multifactorial Disorders

Understanding the genetics of common disorders is one of the great challenges of modern medicine, with the promise of major returns in terms of prevention, diagnosis, and treatment. The etiology of these disorders is complex in that they result from an interaction of multiple genes with one another and with environmental factors. The specific genes that are relevant may be different from one person to the next. Identification of these genes is difficult given this heterogeneity and the relatively small impact that any particular gene may have in a particular person.

Population Studies

Dissection of the genetic contribution to common disease cannot be accomplished by the standard genetic approaches involving study of rare variants or family-based linkage studies. Most recent efforts have focused on study of large groups of patients, comparing the prevalence of particular genetic markers in case patients and control subjects. The availability of markers has been boosted by the identification of single-nucleotide polymorphisms (SNPs) (Chapter 42). These are differences in single DNA bases between individuals that occur every several hundred bases. Some of these account for common genetic differences between people, including differences that may contribute to disease. The catalog of SNPs currently includes several million variants; it has been found that the genome has evolved as blocks of clusters of genes, making it possible to use only a limited number of SNPs within a given region to determine whether there is a gene in that region that is associated with a disease. Since completion of the HapMap Project, there has been a dramatic increase in the number of SNPs found to be associated with common disorders. As genetic risk factors for common disorders come to light, it is likely that there will be advances in risk assessment, disease stratification, and developing new approaches to treatment.

Genetic Risk Assessment

The goal of genetic risk assessment is the identification of individuals at risk of disease before the onset of signs or symptoms. In principle, the genetic factors could be identified at birth, or any time in life, by testing a DNA sample. Individuals found to be at risk might be offered treatment in advance of onset of the disease to avoid complications or might be advised to modify their lifestyle to avoid exposure to environmental factors that might increase their risk of disease. Several companies have begun to offer "personalized genomic testing." Tests are usually accessed through an Internet site without intervention of a health professional and involve analysis of hundreds of thousands of SNPs in a clinical laboratory. Results are provided through a secure Internet site, sometimes with an option for genetic counseling.

Although the concept of genomic risk assessment would appear to be an attractive paradigm, many questions may be raised about its practicality and implementation. First, predictive testing is useful only insofar as it guides further management. This is likely to be a moving target because ability to test for risk can be developed more quickly than ability to modify that risk. The utility of interventions may be valued differently by different people. This already has been the case for testing of disorders such as breast cancer. Some women at risk choose not to know their *BRCA* status because the options, including surveillance or prophylactic surgery, are unacceptable to them. If there were a low-cost, safe, and effective treatment that would neutralize any risk the decision to test would be simple, but short of that, there are reasonable arguments on both sides of the issue of whether to test. For many disorders, it will take a long time to show the efficacy of any intervention because there may be a period of many years between the test and the onset of a disorder. Unless surrogate markers can be identified and followed, the task of proving a benefit to predictive testing may require years to decades in some instances.

Predictive Value of Genetic Testing

A second issue surrounds the degree to which genetic testing would be predictive. Most genetic tests are likely to involve detection of relatively common polymorphic alleles that account for small increments of relative risk of disease. The predictive value of these tests would be modest, perhaps too low to induce an individual to modify behavior or to take medication. Here, again, much depends on the efficacy of any intervention that can be offered. There may be some disorders for which testing would have substantial predictive value and clinical utility and others for which testing would not be justified.

Social and Ethical Issues

A third concern relates to social and ethical issues. Will people use test results as an excuse to pursue self-destructive behaviors, having received what may be false reassurance of "immunity"? Will genetic testing further exacerbate the divide between individuals who can afford to pay for their care and those who cannot? Will people misinterpret results of testing in terms of a simplistic notion of genetic determinism, erroneously believing that their futures have been written, leaving them no recourse but to meet their fate? The rapid pace of technologic change is going to challenge the ability of the social and legal systems to keep pace.

Service Models

Finally, there are questions of the ideal context in which to offer such testing. The personal genomics companies provide their services directly to the consumer in most cases. This creates the obvious risk for incorrect interpretation of results by the patient, although it is not clear that the health care work force is otherwise prepared to deal with the challenges of interpretation of genome-wide studies. The challenges will only increase if whole-genome sequencing at modest cost (e.g., <$1,000) becomes available, as is widely anticipated.

Disease Stratification

A second application of genomics in medical practice entails stratification of disease. Even if genetic testing is not used to predict individuals at risk, it may well be used to determine the most appropriate treatment for a clinically diagnosed disorder. Most common disorders, such as hypertension and diabetes, are symptom complexes that probably result from a variety of causes. The particular combination of causes may differ in different individuals and may respond to different types of treatments. Choice of antihypertensive drug may come to depend on genetic testing to determine the specific cause of hypertension in a patient. There are already examples of genotypes that predict response to drugs, for example, in lung cancer. It is possible that genetic tests eventually will accompany many if not most treatment decisions.

Effects and Identification of Drugs

Aside from helping to choose the most efficacious drug, genetic testing may play a role in avoidance of side effects and in appropriate dosing. Many drugs are known to be associated with rare side effects, some of which are sufficiently severe as to lead the drug to be withdrawn from use. Some of these side effects may occur only in individuals who are susceptible on the basis of having a particular allele at a polymorphic locus. An example is the

TABLE 39-4 GENES IN WHICH COMMON POLYMORPHISMS AFFECT RATES OF DRUG METABOLISM OR ACTION

GENE	MEDICATIONS (EXAMPLES)
CYP2C9	Phenytoin, warfarin
CYP2D6	Debrisoquin, β-blockers, antidepressants
VKORC1	Warfarin
UGT1A1	Irinotecan
Thiopurine methyltransferase	Mercaptopurine, azathioprine
N-acetyltransferase	Isoniazid, hydralazine
CYP2C19	Clopidogrel

association of polymorphisms in certain sodium or potassium channel genes with risk of arrhythmia on exposure to specific drugs.

Absorption and metabolism of drugs are largely under genetic control. Several polymorphisms are known to lead to particularly rapid or slow metabolism, accounting for individuals who experience dose-related side effects or lack of efficacy at standard dosages (Table 39-4). Detection of these polymorphisms would allow customization of drug dosage to an individual's pattern of metabolism, increasing the likelihood of efficacy without a prolonged period of trial-and-error dosing. There has been a major interest in applying this paradigm to warfarin dosing, although questions remain about the cost-effectiveness and practicality of genetic testing in routine use of this drug.

The greatest gift of genetics and genomics to medicine may be in the ability to identify new drug targets and develop new approaches to treatment. Identification of genes that contribute to common disorders is revealing the cellular mechanisms that lead to disease. This knowledge offers the opportunity to develop new pharmaceutical agents that would target the physiologic mechanisms more precisely, leading to drugs that work better and cause fewer side effects. New approaches to gene replacement or insertion of genes into cells as localized drug delivery systems also may be developed. The treatment of common disorders likely would entail the use of approaches developed as a result of genomics even in cases in which genetic testing is not used to predict individuals who are at risk.

CONCLUSION

The Human Genome Project began after most practicing physicians completed their medical training, and few are familiar with the methods and approaches of medical genetics and genomics. Nevertheless, physicians will be using the products of the genome project increasingly in their day-to-day practice during the coming years. Whether they are providing care for a patient with a rare genetic disorder or for a patient with a common condition not usually regarded as genetic, management choices increasingly will be informed by tests and treatments that in some way are based on information from the genome sequence.

The essence of the encounter between a physician and a patient can be distilled to two questions: Why this person? Why this time? A person who seeks medical care is doing so as the product of human evolution, having an ancestry associated with certain genetic vulnerabilities, because of inheritance of certain familial risk factors, because of exposure to some environmental factors, because of a particular physiologic process gone awry, because of behavioral traits that lead the person to seek medical care, because of prompting by family or friends to go to the doctor, because society makes medical services available, and because the person can afford to seek care. Genetics cannot answer all of these questions, but it is providing the key to addressing many of the biologic questions that underlie the medical mysteries that have puzzled humankind for generations.

SUGGESTED READINGS

Ginsburg GS, Willard HF. Genomic and personalized medicine: foundations and applications. *Transl Res.* 2009;154:277-278. *Overview of the role genetics and genomics increasingly will play in medical practice.*

Guttmacher AE, McGuire AL, Ponder B, et al. Personalized genomic information: preparing for the future of genetic medicine. *Nat Rev Gen.* 2010; 11:161-165. *Four experts with different insights into the field of genomic medicine.*

Khoury MJ, McBride CM, Schully SD, et al. The Scientific Foundation for personal genomics: recommendations from a National Institutes of Health-Centers for Disease Control and Prevention multidisciplinary workshop. *Genet Med.* 2009;11:559-567. *Report of a workshop on issues related to personal genomic testing.*

Limdi NA, Veenstra DL. Expectations, validity, and reality in pharmacogenetics. *J Clin Epidemiol.* 2009;63:960-969. *Review of the use of pharmacogenetics in medicine.*

Rotimi CN, Jorde LB. Ancestry and disease in the age of genetic medicine. *N Engl J Med.* 2010;363:1551-1558. *Review.*

40 GENE, GENOMIC, AND CHROMOSOMAL DISORDERS

PAWEŁ STANKIEWICZ AND JAMES R. LUPSKI

THE HUMAN GENOME

Unprecedented technologic advances in molecular biology during the past two decades have enabled the determination of the entire DNA (deoxyribonucleic acid) sequence content of the human genome (Human Genome Project, HGP; *www.ornl.gov/sci/techresources/Human_Genome/home.shtml*) and establishment of a reference haploid genome. To date, a few other personal diploid human genomes have been sequenced, and the enormous amount of available DNA sequence data has expanded our view of the genetic bases of disease.

Human genomic DNA is packaged within the nucleus in 23 chromosome pairs, 22 autosomes, and two sex chromosomes, XX in females and XY in males. The diploid genome (2n) in each cell consists of two identical haploid copies of about 3×10^9 base pairs (bp), thus equaling in total 6 billion nucleotides. Most of the human genome consists of repetitive elements: tandem repeats (e.g., satellite sequences in centromeres), telomeric repeats, microsatellites, minisatellites, and short and long interspersed retrotransposable elements (e.g., *Alu* elements and LINE elements, respectively) (Table 40-1). These elements form heterochromatin; however, their functional role remains largely unknown. The unique DNA sequences constituting euchromatin compose the minority of our genome and include 20,000 to 25,000 genes, 700 micro-RNA genes, pseudogenes, gene fragments, nongenic sequences, and regulatory elements. Although protein coding sequences occupy only about 2% of the human genome, it has been demonstrated recently that the majority of our DNA may be transcribed into RNA.

Approximately 4 to 5% of the human genome, including both repetitive and unique sequences, is present in two or more copies in the haploid genome. DNA fragments larger than 1 kb in size and of DNA sequence identity greater than 90% have been termed *low-copy repeats* (LCRs) or segmental duplications (SDs). Most LCRs have arisen during primate speciation. A subset of LCRs with DNA sequence identity greater than 95 to 97% and longer than 10 kb can lead to local genome instability during both meiotic (constitutional) and mitotic (somatic) cell divisions, resulting in genomic rearrangements.

GENE

The concept of a gene can be traced back to 1865 when Gregor Mendel observed the inheritance of phenotypic traits in the garden pea, *Pisum sativum*. Mendel noted that two *factors*, which we now know to be corresponding DNA loci (alleles) located on homologous chromosomes, separate from each other during meiosis and segregate to two different gametes. This phenomenon of independent segregation is now known as *Mendel's First Law*. *Mendel's Second Law* described the independent segregation of two different (nonallelic) loci during gamete formation. The *inheritance factors* or *units of heredity* encoding the genetic information were later defined as *genes*. We now define *gene* as a fragment of DNA that carries the information used to transcribe it into a functional RNA (ribonucleic acid).

The DNA double helix is composed of four nucleotides: two purine bases, adenine (A) and guanine (G), and two pyrimidine bases, thymine (T) and cytosine (C), all connected to deoxyribose sugars and linked by phosphodiester bonds at the 5′ and 3′ carbons of the sugar (in RNA, thymine is replaced by uracil, U). Three consecutive nucleotides (triplet codon) of the coding DNA encode an amino acid. There are 64 possible different codons (4^3 combinations) but only 20 amino acids; therefore, the genetic code has been termed *degenerate*. Most of the genes in our genome comprise several coding

TABLE 40-1 STRUCTURE OF THE HUMAN GENOME

CHROMATIN FEATURE	SEQUENCE TYPE	HUMAN GENOME (HAPLOID)	SIZE (% OF 3 MILLION BASE PAIRS)*
Euchromatin	Protein coding	20,000-25,000 genes	~2
	Noncoding	RNA genes	
		Regulatory elements	
		Pseudogenes	~38
		Gene fragments	
		Conserved sequences	
Heterochromatin	Repetitive		~60
		Tandem: Satellite DNA, minisatellites, microsatellites	~14
		Interspersed (transposons):	~45
		Retro-transposons	~8
		LTR	
		Non-LTR	
		SINE (*Alu*)	~13
		LINE	~21
		DNA transposons	~3

*Estimated.
LTR = Long-terminal repeat.

regions or exons that are separated by noncoding introns. The entire gene (exons and introns) is transcribed into messenger RNA (mRNA) by RNA polymerase II starting from its 5′ end and continuing beyond the polyA recognition signal at the 3′ end. Typically, mRNA begins with a cap and terminates with a polyadenylated (polyA) tail at the 3′ end. In the subsequent process of splicing, the intervening noncoding introns are deleted, and the spliced, mature mRNA is translated into a polypeptide. The polypeptides start at the 5′ end (NH_2) with a methionine encoded by the AUG triplet. At the 3′ end (COOH), the polypeptides are terminated by one of three termination codons: UAA, UAG, or UGA (Fig. 40-1).

Micro-RNAs are single-stranded, 21- to 24-bp RNA molecules encoded by their own genes or introns of other genes but not translated into protein (i.e., they are noncoding RNAs). Micro-RNAs are thought to regulate (usually downregulate) gene expression of more than half of all human protein-coding genes. The phenotypic consequences of micro-RNAs are mainly unknown; they are believed to prevent the development of cancer and other diseases.

GENETIC VARIATION

In addition to the HGP, the International HapMap (*http://hapmap.ncbi.nlm.nih.gov*), Human Genome Diversity (*www.stanford.edu/group/morrinst/hgdp.html*), ENCODE (*www.genome.gov/10005107*), and ongoing personal genome sequencing projects have revealed the tremendous and underappreciated extent of variation in our genome. Genetic variation consists of two major types: (1) nucleotide sequence changes, or single nucleotide variation (SNV), and (2) genome structural changes, or copy-number variation (CNV) (Fig. 40-2).

Single Nucleotide Variation

A genetic polymorphism is defined as a heterozygous DNA variation present in greater than 1% of the population. Genome-wide nucleotide variation has been uncovered in the early phase of DNA sequencing analyses, which showed that human genomes differ mainly by single nucleotide changes. These differences have been termed *single nucleotide polymorphisms* (SNPs) and defined as a nucleotide change at a given position generated by substitution (usually there are two alleles per SNP). Only a minority of SNPs map to exons; however, SNPs located outside of the protein-coding regions can still exert phenotypic effects, such as by modifying gene regulatory elements or transcription factor binding sites, generating splicing mutations, or affecting noncoding RNAs. Any two humans differ on average by about 3.5 million SNVs or SNPs, about 0.1% of the 3.0×10^9 reference haploid genome (phase 3 of the International HapMap project).

A set of consecutive SNPs (or other markers) is defined as a *haplotype*. A nonrandom association of markers in a population not interrupted by meiotic recombination (*crossing-over*) is described as *linkage disequilibrium*. (Note that linkage disequilibrium exemplifies the exception to Mendel's Second Law.)

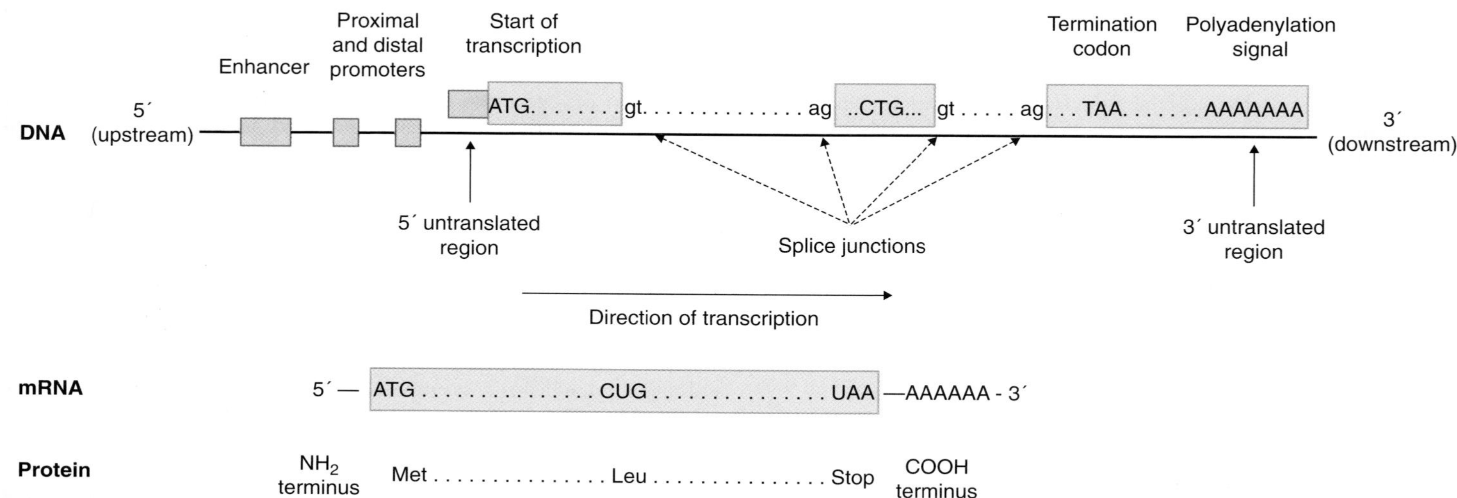

FIGURE 40-1. Gene structure. Schematic representation of the general structure of a typical human gene. Three exons are depicted as *orange open rectangles*. Note that the transcription usually starts with an ATG triplet encoding methionine. The 5′ (upstream) portion of a gene corresponds to the NH_2 terminus, and the 3′ (downstream) segment encodes the COOH terminus of the polypeptide. Enhancers and promoters are shown as *blue rectangles*.

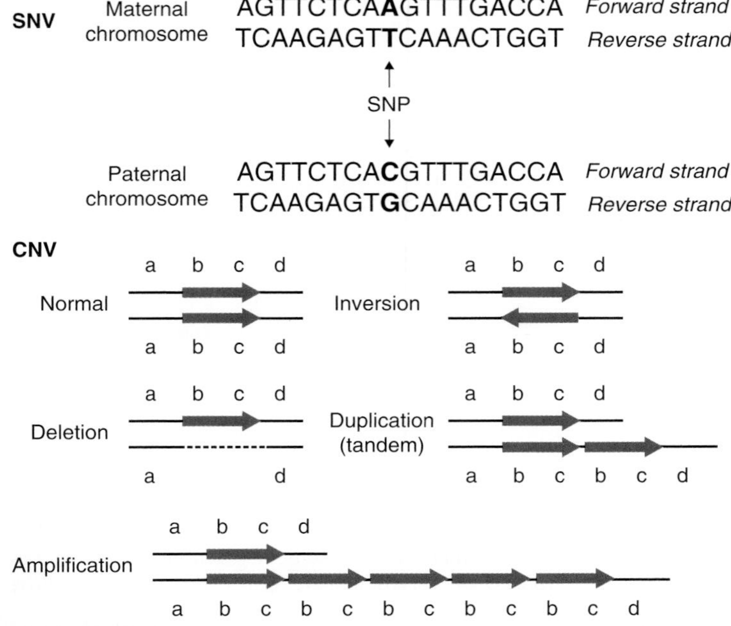

FIGURE 40-2. **Genetic variation.** *Top,* Heterozygous single nucleotide polymorphism (SNP, or single nucleotide variation SNV) representing the most common transition C→T is shown. *Bottom,* Structural genomic changes: a balanced inversion and the unbalanced copy-number variations (CNVs), deletion, duplication, and amplification are shown with *black arrows* on two homologous chromosomes (*black lines*). The *dashed line* represents a deleted fragment of one chromosome.

Tandem Repeats

Variable number of tandem repeats (VNTRs), or *minisatellites,* and short tandem repeats (STRs) such as unstable dinucleotides, trinucleotides, and tetranucleotides, $(GT)_n$, $(CAA)_n$, or $(GATA)_n$, referred to as *microsatellites,* are highly variable. Both minisatellites and microsatellites have been successfully used in linkage and association studies that enable the mapping of traits and the identification of genes and loci responsible for both mendelian disorders and complex traits. These highly polymorphic sequence repeats are extremely variable in the copy number of their repeating subunits; this property enables the use of a number of such markers to derive a unique pattern of marker genotypes for each human individual. Thus, such markers have been useful for identity testing and DNA forensics.

Repetitive Elements

The other group of polymorphic elements in the human genome is represented by retrotransposons, long and short interspersed nuclear elements (LINEs and SINEs) (see Table 40-1). The most common *Alu* and L1 elements introduce recombinogenic genomic instability and insertional mutagenic activity; their positions within an individual human personal diploid genome can vary tremendously.

Copy-Number Variation

A more recently characterized group of major polymorphic genetic variation in the human genome is represented by structural changes. In this postgenomic era, high-resolution genome-wide analysis of human genome sequences has revealed higher-order architectural features, with a potential to cause genomic instability and extensive submicroscopic structural variations. These structural variations consist of unbalanced CNVs, including deletions, duplications, triplications, insertions, and translocations, that differ from the normal diploid state, as well as balanced rearrangements, such as genomic inversions. Both CNVs and SNVs have been shown to play a major role in human genetic diversity, evolution, and susceptibility to diseases. Surprisingly, it has been found that any two human genomes contain more base pair differences due to CNVs than SNVs.

Recent analyses have revealed over 38,000 CNVs (greater than 100 bp) that occupy more than 29% of the reference human genome. A validated subset of these CNVs overlaps 13% of the Reference Sequence (*www.ncbi.nlm.nih.gov/projects/RefSeq/RSG*) genes and 12% of the Online Mendelian Inheritance in Man (OMIM) (*www.ncbi.nlm.nih.gov/sites/entrez?db=omim*) genes and was predicted by conceptual translation to alter the structure of 12.5% gene transcripts and 5.5% mRNAs. Despite all these recent achievements, the total number, position, size, gene content, and population distribution of CNVs remain obscure because we still do not have accurate and reliable molecular methods to study smaller CNVs on a genome-wide scale in different populations, particularly when copy-number changes are greater than 4 or 5.

CNVs have been shown to be responsible for mendelian diseases, nonmendelian traits such as complex diseases, and common traits (including neurobehavioral traits) or to represent benign polymorphic variation. CNVs can lead to an abnormal phenotype by disrupting the gene structure or changing the copy number of dosage-sensitive genes. However, long-range effects of CNVs involving nongenic sequences, leaving a gene intact, have been also demonstrated. Furthermore, evidence suggests that a combination of two or more CNVs at the same or different loci may be responsible for phenotypic variation. The genome-wide scale of phenotypic effects exerted by CNVs (genomic load) are unknown and await further studies.

Any two individuals differ by about 1000 CNVs ranging in size from about 500 bp to 1 Mb. An updated summary of CNVs can be found in the Toronto Database of Genomic Variants (*http://projects.tcag.ca/variation*). Many clinically relevant CNVs can be found in the Database of Chromosomal Imbalance and Phenotype in Humans using Ensembl Resources (DECIPHER) (*https://decipher.sanger.ac.uk/information*).

CHROMOSOMES

The recombined haploid (1n) human genome formed during meiosis is stored as chromosomes in female and male gametes. They merge at conception, and this diploid genome instructs the development of a zygote; the diploid human genome is subsequently transmitted to the mitotically dividing daughter cells. Human chromosomes can be distinguished from each other in a light microscope by differences in size and characteristic banding patterns after specific chemical staining (e.g., G-banding with Giemsa) when the chromosomes are arrested in a condensed phase (metaphase) of mitotic divisions.

Each human metaphase chromosome is composed of two chromatids that form short (p) and long (q) arms connected by a centromere built with α-satellite DNA. Based on the relative position of the centromere along the chromosome, chromosomes have been described as metacentric (similarly sized p and q arms), submetacentric (q arm significantly longer than p), and acrocentric (chromosomes 13, 14, 15, 21, and 22, with centromeres located close to the end of a chromosome) (Fig. 40-3).

Telomeres consist of repetitive DNA sequences (thousands of copies of TTAGGG repeats) located at the ends of both chromosome arms that are stabilized by a reverse transcriptase enzyme, telomerase, which adds TTAGGG sequence to the 3′ end of DNA strands. In contrast to germline and cancer cells, human somatic cells lacking telomerase gradually lose the telomeric sequences. As a result, cells reach the limit of their replicative capacity and fall into senescence.

Chromosomal Aberrations

Numerical Aberrations

Microscopically visible chromosomal aberrations have been divided into numerical and structural aberrations and are found in 1 in about 160 live births. The numerical aberrations are usually lethal. Polyploidies (multiplication of a haploid set of 23 chromosomes), such as triploidies (3n), 69,XXX, 69,XXY, and 69,XYY, and tetraploidies (4n), 92,XXYY or 92,XXXX, are caused by abnormal egg fertilization by two sperms or by a failure in zygote division, respectively.

The most commonly detected viable chromosomal aneuploidies, trisomies and monosomies, involve chromosomes X, Y, 21, 18, and 13 and arise as a result of meiotic nondisjunctions. Sex chromosome aneuploidies are more common and are found in 1 in 440 newborns. Monosomy X (45,X cell line) in female patients with Turner's syndrome is identified in every 4000 female newborns. However, this birth rate represents only 1% of all fetuses with 45,X because more than 99% are spontaneously aborted (this is similar to the most frequent fetal aneuploidy, trisomy 16, that results in 100% miscarriages). In most cases, the 45,X cell line is found as a mosaic along with another cell line that has either a normal karyotype or a structural rearrangement of the X chromosome (e.g., deletion of the short arm, ring chromosome, or isochromosome of the long or short arms). One in every 1000 males has a 47,XXY chromosome complement that is responsible for Klinefelter's syndrome.

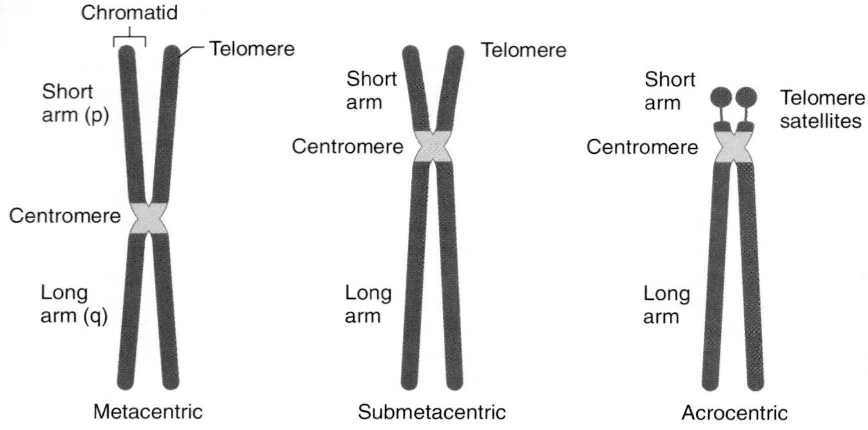

FIGURE 40-3. Types of metaphase chromosomes. Metacentric, submetacentric, and acrocentric chromosomes are composed of two arms connected by a centromere. Each chromosome arm consists of two chromatids.

In contrast to gonosomes, monosomies of all autosomes are lethal. The only trisomies compatible with life are found in patients with Down syndrome (trisomy 21 in every 670 newborns), Edwards' syndrome (trisomy 18 in 1 in 5000 newborns), and Patau's syndrome (trisomy 13 in every 10,000 newborns).

Incomplete supernumerary chromosomes are termed *marker chromosomes*. They usually originate from acrocentric autosomes (~ 50% from chromosome 15) and are found in every 4000 newborns. The severity of the abnormal phenotype in carriers of marker chromosomes varies among different chromosomes and is estimated as 28% in de novo cases.

Structural Aberrations

Chromosomal deletions and duplications have been categorized as microscopically visible or submicroscopic, terminal or interstitial, recurrent or nonrecurrent. The most frequent are recurrent common-sized rearrangements flanked by directly oriented LCRs or SDs that mediate nonallelic homologous recombination (NAHR). For example, an about 3 Mb microdeletion in chromosome 22q11.2 occurs in patients with DiGeorge velocardiofacial syndrome and is found in 1:4000 newborns. The 1.4-Mb Charcot-Marie-Tooth disease type 1A (CMT1A) duplication causes greater than half of all adult-onset inherited Charcot-Marie-Tooth neuropathy, and de novo events account for up to 90% of sporadic cases. The phenotypic consequences of deletion/duplication CNVs depend on whether the CNVs harbor a dosage-sensitive (e.g., haploinsufficient for deletion) gene.

Balanced reciprocal translocations result from an exchange of the DNA material between two chromosomes and are found in 1 in about 600 individuals. During meiosis, the translocation chromosomes form a pachytene tetrad structure and, depending on the segregation type (alternate or adjacent, symmetric or asymmetric), either balanced or unbalanced products are transmitted to progeny. The unbalanced products often lead to either spontaneous abortions or births of clinically affected children. Recently, it has been shown by high-resolution genome analyses that up to 40% of apparently balanced translocations found in subjects with abnormal phenotypes are associated with additional imbalances at or near the translocation breakpoint or somewhere else in the genome.

Translocations involving short arms (or centromeres) of acrocentric chromosomes are described as robertsonian translocations. Balanced robertsonian translocations (45-chromosome complement) are present in 1 in 900 newborns; thus, these are the most common chromosome rearrangements in humans. The most frequent robertsonian translocation, t(13;14), is found in 1 in 1300 individuals. The carriers of balanced robertsonian translocations have a significantly increased risk for an unbalanced karyotype in progeny (e.g., trisomy 21 or trisomy 13) or uniparental disomy for chromosomes 14 and 15 that are known to contain imprinted genes.

Constitutional nonrobertsonian chromosomal translocations are nonrecurrent, with the exception of five recurrent translocations: t(11;22)(q11.2;q23.3) and t(8;22)(q24.13;q11.21), that use AT-rich cruciforms, and translocations t(4;8)(p16;p23), t(8;12)(p23.1p13.31), and t(4;11)(p16;p15.2) that are mediated by LCR gene clusters.

When a fragment of one chromosome is translocated into another chromosome's arm, the aberration is termed an *insertion* or *insertional translocation*. Insertional translocations have been recently shown by high-resolution human genome analyses to occur more than 100 times more frequently than recognized previously. The carrier of a balanced insertion has up to a 50% chance of an unbalanced offspring.

An inversion is defined when a chromosome fragment is reversed end to end. Inversions harboring the centromere are termed *pericentric,* and those with breakpoints mapping in the same chromosome arm are termed *paracentric*. Usually, only the products of pericentric inversions (unbalanced terminal deletion of one chromosome arm accompanied by a terminal duplication of the second arm) are found in a progeny. The acentric or dicentric products of paracentric inversions are unstable and thus not transmitted.

Other, less common structural chromosomal abnormalities include ring chromosomes, isochromosomes, complex chromosome rearrangements, and heterochromatin variants. Rings arise when two broken ends of the same chromosome fuse. Usually, chromosome material telomeric to the breakpoints is lost and leads to an abnormal phenotype. Rings are commonly unstable mitotically and often form double ring structures. Isochromosomes arise when one part of the chromosome is duplicated and separated from the other. Isochromosomes can be monocentric (breakpoint in the centromere) or dicentric and thus unstable, unless one of the centromeres becomes inactivated (pseudoisodicentric). Chromosome aberrations with more than two breakpoints on two or more chromosomes are termed *complex chromosome rearrangements* and often result in an unbalanced product of meiotic division.

Mosaicism and Chimeras

The presence of two or more cell lines with different chromosome complements in one individual is termed *mosaicism* when they originate from the same zygote or *chimeras* when the cells originate from different zygotes. Chromosomal mosaicism is a common phenomenon, observed in about 50% of embryos at the eight-cell stage and in up to 75% of blastocysts. Somatic chromosomal mosaicism is found, for example, in patients with hypomelanosis of Ito and Pallister-Killian syndrome (tetrasomy 12p).

MUTATION

Mutation is defined as a change in nucleotide sequence due to errors of DNA replication, recombination, or repair or to radiation, chemical mutagens, viruses, or transposons. Gene mutations can be inherited from a parent (hereditary, germline, or constitutional) and thus present in every cell. Alternatively, mutations can be acquired in some tissues at some time either during an individual's development or at any time throughout a person's life (somatic) (Fig. 40-4). Recent whole genome sequencing of lung cancer tissue suggests one new point mutation for every pack of cigarettes smoked. Point mutations, usually involving only one or a few nucleotides, have been divided into substitutions, insertions, and deletions. Mutations mapping in protein-coding sequences and changing the protein structure have been termed *nonsynonymous,* whereas those that do not lead to protein change are known as *synonymous* or silent mutations. The latter mutations can still have functional consequences (e.g., by generating a cryptic splice site, an exon splice enhancer, or affecting the regulatory elements).

Based on the functional consequences, mutations have been divided into loss-of-function and gain-of-function mutations. The former, also known as *hypomorphic* (partial loss) or *amorphic* or *null* (complete *loss*), affect the dosage-sensitive or haploinsufficient genes, in which a decreased amount of protein is not sufficient for normal function. Gain-of-function mutations

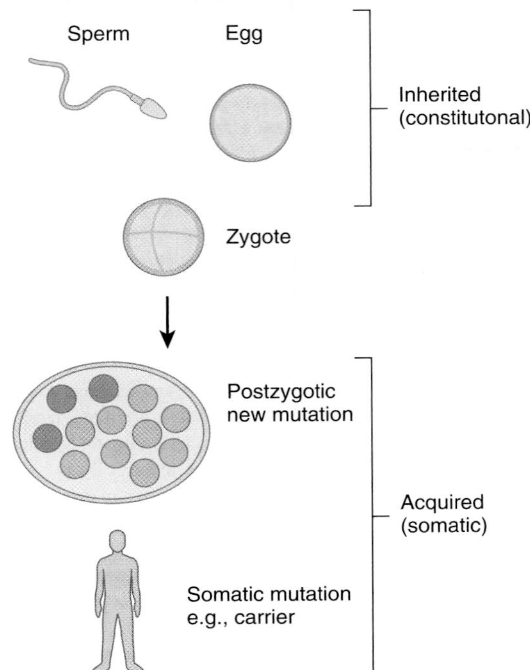

FIGURE 40-4. Mutation. Constitutional mutations are inherited from one of the parents. They can be present in the somatic cells of a parent (carrier) or can arise during gametogenesis (de novo). Mutations that occur postzygotically (acquired, somatic) are usually found in a mosaic state.

increase or add a new function for the protein (*neomorphic*), and dominant negative mutations are translated into a protein that interacts antagonistically with the normal product from the other allele (*antimorphic*).

The situation in which one allele is mutated and the second is normal (wild-type) is referred to as *heterozygous*. A combination of the same two mutations in each of the alleles of the same locus (e.g., in consanguineous families) is defined as *homozygous* mutations, or compound heterozygotes when the two mutant alleles are distinct. Two mutant alleles at different loci are described as *double heterozygote*. When one of the autosomal alleles is absent (e.g., because of a deletion CNV and for most of the X chromosome genes in males), the locus is referred to as *hemizygous*.

Different mutations in one gene can manifest with the same or distinct phenotypes, phenomena called *allelic heterogeneity* or *allelic affinity*, respectively. By contrast, the same abnormal clinical phenotype can be caused by mutations in different genes (genetic or locus heterogeneity).

Single Nucleotide Variation

Nonsynonymous mutations can lead to a single amino acid change (*missense*), modify the downstream protein structure (*frameshift*), introduce a stop codon (*premature termination codon [PTC]*) that truncates the protein prematurely (*nonsense*), or abolish the specific site at which splicing of an intron takes place during the processing of precursor mRNA into mature mRNA (*splice site*). The PTC-mutated mRNAs are inactivated and removed from cells by a surveillance mechanism called *nonsense mediated decay* that is initiated by a premature termination codon in any exon, except the last and a 50- to 55-bp portion of the second to last (i.e., penultimate) exon that usually escape nonsense mediated decay.

Transition mutations refer to changes from pyrimidine to pyrimidine (e.g., C to T) or purine to purine (e.g., A to G), and are more frequent than exchanges from purine to pyrimidine (e.g., A to C) or pyrimidine to purine (e.g., T to G), that is, transversions. The most common C-to-T transition (about ten-fold relative to other bases) occurs in the methylated CpG dinucleotide because methylated C is subject to deamination and becomes T.

Mutations that are unstable have been termed *dynamic*. Pathogenic dynamic expansion of trinucleotide, tetranucleotide, and pentanucleotide repeat sequences can be located in coding (e.g., CAG triplet in Huntington's disease) or noncoding regions such as introns (e.g., GAA in Friedreich's ataxia) or untranslated regions, either 5′ (e.g., CGG in fragile X syndrome, OMIM 300624) or 3′ (e.g., CTG in myotonic dystrophy). The mutations convey phenotypes that can be inherited as autosomal dominant (e.g., myotonic dystrophy), autosomal recessive (e.g., Friedreich's ataxia), or X-linked (e.g., fragile X syndrome) traits due to gain- or loss-of-function mutations. For each of the dynamic mutation diseases, there is a specific repeat number limit, above which the disease is manifested. The number of repeats below that threshold but greater than in normals is referred to as a *premutation*. However, in some "disease genes," premutations are also associated with a milder, nonspecific phenotype (e.g., ovarian failure in females and late-onset neurologic disorders in males with premutations in the fragile X *FMR1* gene). The number of repeats tends to expand in the next generations, a phenomenon called *anticipation*; this typically occurs in a sex-specific manner.

Copy-Number Variation

It has now become apparent that the Watson-Crick DNA base pair changes are not the only mutational mechanism responsible for mendelian monogenic diseases and complex traits. Higher-order genomic architectural features can lead to a regional instability and susceptibility to DNA rearrangements or CNVs, which can be a frequent cause of diseases in humans. Such conditions due to structural genome changes or CNV have been referred to as *genomic disorders*.

A major mechanism by which rearrangements convey phenotypes is gene dosage due to a variation in gene copy number. CNVs can lead to deletion, duplication, or disruption of the dosage-sensitive gene, generate gene fusions, exert position effects, or unmask mutations in the coding region or other functional SNPs in the second allele, as when a deletion CNV results in a hemizygous state.

Different calculations have shown that the de novo locus-specific mutation rates for genomic rearrangements are between 10^{-4} and 10^{-5}, at least 1000 to 10,000 fold more frequent than de novo point mutations. Thus, new mutation CNV can contribute significantly to sporadic disease.

Many genomic disorders occur sporadically and are often caused by de novo rearrangements. Recurrent rearrangements (deletions, duplications, or inversions) are caused by NAHR between LCR that are located less than 5 to 10 Mb from each other and have greater than 97% DNA sequence identity. The fixed position of these LCRs and SDs in the human genome result in recurrent rearrangements having a common size for a given region. NAHR between directly oriented LCRs leads to deletions or reciprocal duplications of the genomic region located between them, and NAHR between the oppositely oriented LCRs results in an inversion of the intervening genomic segment. Interestingly, the strand exchanges for NAHR sites are not scattered throughout the entire length of homology within LCRs, but instead cluster in recombination hot spots.

Most nonrecurrent CNVs appear to occur by nonhomologous recombination mechanisms, and one often observes microhomology at the breakpoints. One prominent mechanism, particularly for complex (e.g., deletion/normal/duplication) rearrangements is the microhomology-mediated break-induced replication mechanism. The remainder of nonrecurrent different-sized rearrangements likely result from a nonhomologous end-joining recombination mechanism.

Microduplication and Microdeletion Syndromes

Some of the microduplication and microdeletion syndromes are caused by a copy-number change of the dosage-sensitive or haploinsufficient gene. Among the best characterized genomic disorders are common autosomal dominant peripheral neuropathies, CMT1A and hereditary neuropathy with liability (HNPP) to pressure palsies, that in more than 99% of cases are caused by duplication and deletion CNV, respectively, of an about 1.4-Mb genomic interval within 17p12 harboring a dosage-sensitive myelin gene *PMP22*. This genomic segment is flanked by two about 24-kb and about 98.7% identical LCRs, called the *proximal CMT1A-REP* and the *distal CMT1A-REP*, which serve as substrates for NAHR. Another example of common predominantly monogenic reciprocal microdeletion and microduplication syndromes include Potocki-Lupski syndrome due to dup(17)(p11.2p11.2), reciprocal to del(17)(p11.2p11.2) found in patients with Smith-Magenis syndrome. When two or more dosage-sensitive genes that are usually functionally unrelated are involved, these are referred to as *contiguous gene deletion* or *duplication syndromes*, for example, Potocki-Shaffer syndrome resulting from deletion del(11)(p11.2p11.2).

LCR-mediated recurrent microdeletion and microduplication syndromes usually have similar prevalence in different populations; however, for a few genomic disorders, significant differences in incidences in different world populations have been observed, likely demonstrating that variation of genomic architecture is a significant factor for disease susceptibility (e.g.,

17q21.31 microdeletion syndrome, Sotos' syndrome, 5q35). Examples of well-known and characterized microdeletion syndromes include Williams-Beuren syndrome (7q11.23), Prader-Willi and Angelman syndromes (15q11.2q12), DiGeorge velocardiofacial syndrome (22q11.2), microdeletion 17q21.31 syndrome, and Sotos' syndrome. For all these microdeletions, the reciprocal microduplications predicted by the NAHR model have been reported with phenotypes typically being milder. Recent studies revealed that some fraction of patients with autism and of patients with schizophrenia have deletion or duplication CNV involving specific loci (e.g., 1q21.1, 15q13.3, and 16p11.2); for 16p11.2, deletion CNV is more frequently associated with an autism phenotype, whereas duplication CNV can cause schizophrenia.

PATTERNS OF INHERITANCE

Mendelian Inheritance

Most characterized disease-associated mutations in humans can be assigned to a single gene (monogenic) or locus and segregate as a mendelian trait in an autosomal dominant, autosomal recessive, or X-linked fashion.

Autosomal dominant mutation is present in only one allele and thus is transmitted in meiosis to 50% of the gametes and is expected to manifest in half the offspring unless the trait is incompletely penetrant (e.g., in Marfan syndrome), represents variable expressivity (e.g., in cystic fibrosis), is age dependent (e.g., in Huntington disease), or lethal (e.g., alveolar capillary dysplasia). In pedigree analysis, autosomal dominant inheritance is revealed as a vertical transmission of the trait.

In an autosomal recessive trait, the affected individuals carry two mutant alleles at a specific locus that are either the same (usually in consanguineous families) or different. In general, both mutations are inherited from unaffected carrier parents (note that occasionally heterozygous carriers of the mutated allele may manifest a mild phenotype or have an increased susceptibility to complex or multifactorial traits). Theoretically, affected probands represent 25% of the progeny; two thirds of the unaffected siblings carry one mutated allele, and the remaining one fourth of all progeny (one third of unaffected) have two wild-type alleles. In pedigree analysis, autosomal recessive inheritance is observed as horizontal transmission of the trait.

In X-linked (both dominant and recessive) diseases, no male-to-male transmission is observed, and all daughters of affected fathers are obligate carriers of the mutated allele. X-linked dominant diseases are more rare than X-linked recessive disorders and present both in males and in females. Usually, there are twice as many affected females as males; however, if the disease is lethal in males, only females are affected (e.g., Rett's syndrome). Because of X-inactivation, the phenotype in females is milder than in males. In an X-linked recessive trait, only males are affected; in female carriers, the X chromosome harboring a mutated recessive allele is preferentially inactivated by nonrandom X-inactivation. However, females with an incomplete or skewed X inactivation, females with only one X chromosome (Turner's syndrome), or females carrying a balanced translocation between the X chromosome and an autosome (X material on the derivative chromosomes is not inactivated) can manifest the X-linked recessive disease.

Nonmendelian Inheritance

The occurrence of sporadic cases of the disease can be explained by a classic mendelian inheritance, such as de novo autosomal dominant, autosomal recessive, or X-linked mutation; however, one has to consider other possibilities, including nonmendelian inheritance—genomic imprinting, uniparental disomy, mosaicism, mitochondrial DNA mutations, and digenic or triallelic inheritance.

Some genes acquire different activity status (usually methylation) after passage through spermatogenesis compared with oogenesis. As a result, a gene can be silenced (imprinted), depending on the parent of origin. This parent-of-origin effect is observed for the *UBE3A* gene on chromosome 15q12 that is imprinted during spermatogenesis, and only the maternal copy is active. When the active maternal copy of *UBE3A* is mutated, deleted, or inactivated in a different way, the offspring is affected with Angelman's syndrome.

Sporadically, a chromosome pair may not be inherited from both parents. This distortion from biparental inheritance, termed *uniparental disomy* (UPD), may have clinical consequences when the uniparental chromosomes contain an autosomal recessive mutation or an imprinted gene. When both homologues are inherited from one parent, it is referred as *heterodisomy*. In isodisomy, both homologues in an offspring originate from only one of the parental homologues. The most common mechanism for UPD is trisomy rescue, in which an early postzygotic embryo is trisomic, as a result of chromosome nondisjunction in meiosis I, and the extra chromosome is then lost during further development to restore disomy. Because this is a random event, in one third of cases, the disomic chromosomes remaining after trisomy to disomy rescue will represent UPD. Consequently, UPD is associated with advanced maternal age.

In some diseases, pathogenic mutations have been found in single alleles of two different genes with the other alleles at each given locus being normal. This double heterozygous phenomenon of two interacting genes has been reported, for example, for *ROM1* and *RDS* in retinitis pigmentosa and *GJB6* and *GJB2* in deafness.

In some patients, three abnormal alleles in two different genes have been identified. The phenomenon of triallelic (or oligogenic) inheritance has been observed, for example, in Bardet-Biedl syndrome, familial hypercholesterolemia, and cortisone reductase deficiency. Monogenic chromosomal microduplication syndromes (e.g., CMT1A) can also be categorized as triallelic given the presence of three alleles at a given locus owing to duplication CNV.

Another distortion from mendelian inheritance can be caused by mosaicism. Two or more cell lines can be present either in the gonads only (germline mosaicism) or in somatic cells. Mosaicism should be suspected when healthy parents have two or more children with a dominant disease. Mosaicism can be particularly relevant when mutational processes involve DNA replication errors and occur mitotically (e.g., point mutation and microhomology-mediated break-induced replication).

Very rarely, a disease trait is transmitted to daughters and sons only from mothers. In such cases, one should consider a mitochondrial disease. Mitochondrial DNA (mtDNA) is present in multiple copies in the cell cytoplasm and is transmitted to progeny only through the oocytes. Initial clinical signs and symptoms typically originate from the most energy-dependent tissues (e.g., eyes, brain, skeletal muscle, and heart), and the phenotypic expression among family members varies and depends mainly on the proportion of mtDNA in the cytoplasm that carries the mutation, that is, heteroplasmy.

ASSAYING GENETIC VARIATION

Chromosome aberrations larger than about 5 Mb can be detected by light microscopy after specific staining that reveals characteristic banding patterns (e.g., G-banded karyotype analysis). Submicroscopic rearrangements, such as microdeletions or microduplications (30 kb to 5 Mb), have been analyzed for the past two decades using molecular cytogenetic techniques such as fluorescence in situ hybridization. In these routine clinical cytogenetic techniques, usually a subpopulation of peripheral blood phytohemagglutinin-stimulated T lymphocytes is analyzed. Rearrangements of similar size (i.e., 30 kb to 5 Mb in size) can be analyzed also using pulsed-field gel electrophoresis. However, both these technologies are limited to the analysis of specific genomic regions, that is, locus-specific testing.

The recent development of array-based comparative genomic hybridization (array CGH) has enabled screening of the entire human genome for imbalances, with the level of genome resolution depending only on the number, size, and distance between the arrayed interrogating probes. These genome-wide imaging techniques are analogous to digital photography wherein the resolution observed is dependent on the pixels used. Initial clinical array CGH used large genomic clones, BACs and PACs (bacterial or P1 artificial chromosomes), as interrogating probes. Recently, they have been replaced by oligonucleotides, of which millions can be synthesized on one glass slide. Oligonucleotide probes are also used on SNP arrays that, in contrast to microarray-based CGH, enable association studies or detection of uniparental disomies.

For detection of genomic imbalances, an alternative quantitative polymerase chain reaction–based technique, multiplex ligation-dependent probe amplification (MLPA) has been developed. MLPA is an inexpensive, simple, rapid, and sensitive tool to detect dosage alterations in selected genomic regions.

Most recently, several next-generation sequencing (NGS) technologies have been developed that enable massively parallel DNA sequencing reactions simultaneously and thus whole genome sequencing, or sequencing of the entire genome of an individual, to enable the determination of a Personal Genome Sequence (Fig. 40-5). In NGS, DNA sequencing uses chemistries other than the traditional Sanger dideoxy chain termination method. NGS methods generate far larger quantities of data at less expense; however, the individual raw sequence reads that are generated from individual amplified DNA template sequences have shorter read lengths and lower quality. Nevertheless, massive redundant sequencing of a personal diploid human genome (e.g., 30-fold coverage with respect to the haploid human reference genome sequence) can provide a robust and accurate Personal Genome Sequence.

CONCLUSION

Mutations in humans are caused by SNVs and CNVs. New mutations can contribute to sporadic disease. The total genomic load can be important to a clinical phenotype. Individual genetic variation is extensive. It is a sobering thought that for more than 90% of the annotated genes in the reference human genome, a function remains to be elucidated for the potential clinical consequences of mutations. Furthermore, 98% of the human genome is noncoding, and the functional consequences of variation within it cannot be assisted using the genetic code.

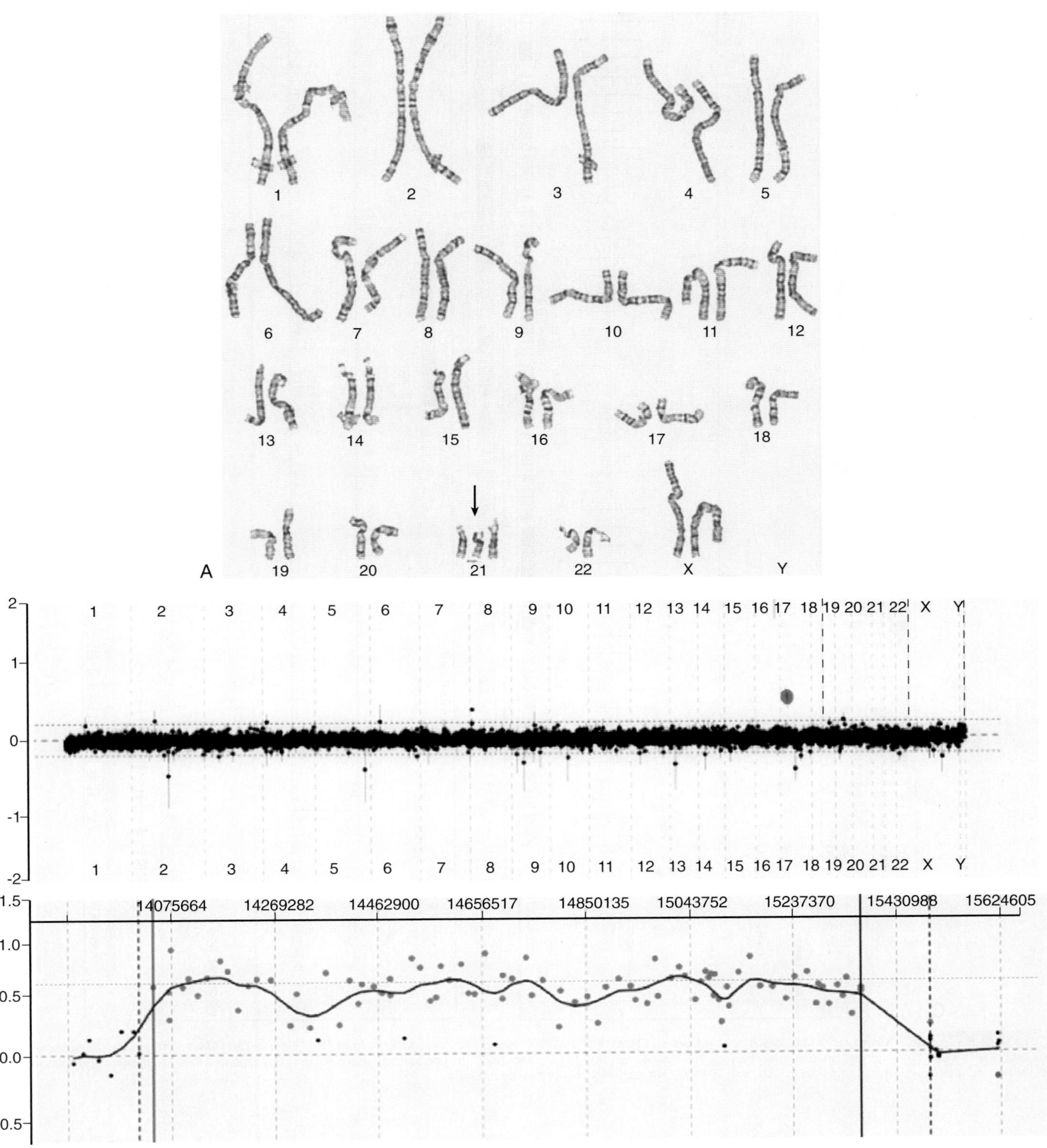

FIGURE 40-5. Assaying copy-number variation (CNV). A, G-banded metaphase chromosomes (karyogram) in a female (two X chromosomes) with trisomy 21 (Down syndrome). **B,** The genome-wide (*upper*) and region-specific (*bottom*) plots of the oligonucleotide-based array comparative genomic hybridization (array CGH) showing a 1.4-Mb CMT1A duplication (*green*) on chromosome 17p12. Oligonucleotides presented with *green color* and displaced upward, indicating a gain of chromosome material in the patient versus the reference DNA.

Continued

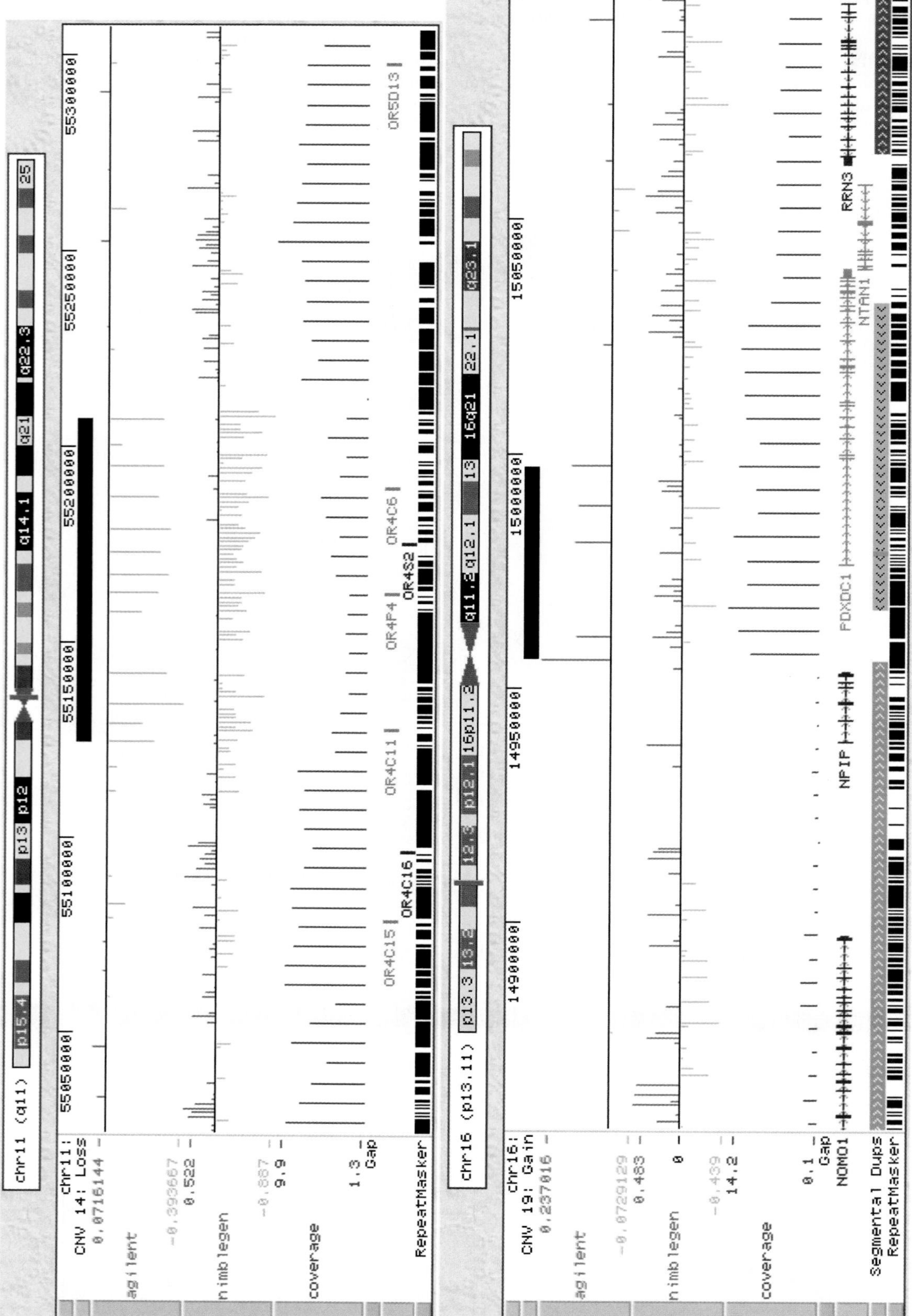

FIGURE 40-5, cont'd. **C,** Heterozygous CNV loss (*black bar* from 55,124,00 to 55,207,000) (*upper*) and gain (*black bar* from 73,071,000 to 73,114,000) (*bottom*) identified using oligonucleotide array CGH (Agilent Technology and Roche-NimbleGen) and next-generation sequencing (NGS) 454 Life Sciences (Roche). Low-copy repeats (LCRs) are shown at the bottom as *orange, dark yellow*, and *gray* bars representing >99%, >98%, and 90-98% DNA sequence identity, respectively.

SUGGESTED READINGS

Conrad DF, Pinto D, Redon R, et al. Origins and functional impact of copy number variation in the human genome. *Nature.* 2010;464:704-712. *Describes the most updated set of CNVs greater than 443 base pairs detected using tiling oligonucleotide microarrays with 42 million probes.*

Dietz HC. New therapeutic approaches to Mendelian disorders. *N Engl J Med.* 2010;363:852-863. *Review.*

Lupski JR, Reid JG, Gonzaga-Jauregui C, et al. Complete genome sequencing reveals *SH3TC2* mutations causing CMT1 neuropathy. *N Engl J Med.* 2010;362:1181-1191. *First use of personal whole genome sequencing to identify the genetic basis of disease in a single patient.*

Sheehan NA, Meng S, Didelez V. Mendelian randomization: a tool for assessing causality in observational epidemiology. *Methods Mol Biol.* 2011;713:153-166. *Methods for determining independent importance of a genetic variant based on epidemiologic data.*

Stankiewicz P, Lupski JR. Structural variation in the human genome and its role in disease. *Annu Rev Med.* 2010;61:437-455. *Reviews the role of CNV in disease.*

41

THE INHERITED BASIS OF COMMON DISEASES

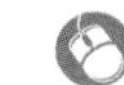

DAVID ALTSHULER

A central question in medicine is to understand why some people get sick and others do not. We seek these answers for multiple reasons: to provide explanations to our patients, to improve our ability to predict disease risk, and most importantly, to understand pathophysiology as a foundation for designing rational approaches to prevention and therapy. In some cases, a single environmental exposure is found to play a major role in disease (e.g., smoking and lung cancer, or human immunodeficiency virus infection [HIV] and acquired immunodeficiency syndrome [AIDS]). In others, such as Huntington's disease or cystic fibrosis, mutation of a single gene is necessary and can be sufficient to cause illness. Such singular answers are the exception; in most cases, disease is attributable neither to a single environmental factor nor to mutation of a single gene. Rather, most cases of disease result from the combined action of inborn and somatically acquired alterations in gene sequence, environmental and behavioral exposures, and bad luck. Such disorders, which make up most of the morbidity and mortality in the population, are termed *complex traits.*

Human genetics is a unique tool for generating new hypotheses about the root causes of disease, based on genome-wide searches in the human population that are unlimited by prior assumptions about underlying pathophysiologic processes. Because the sequence of the human genome and much of its common variation is now known, and given emerging tools and methods to directly determine genome sequences of individuals, we are entering an era in which medicine can be informed by knowledge of the specific genes and variants that contribute to risk for common human diseases.

HERITABILITY: INHERITED VARIATION IN DISEASE RISK

Susceptibility to disease varies within and across human populations. Studies of *familial aggregation* can determine the extent to which inheritance contributes to these patterns. These studies are simple in concept and ask whether members of the same family display more similar rates of disease than do individuals chosen at random from the population. Of course, familial clustering can reflect not only shared genes but also shared environment. The contribution of shared genotype can be dissected further by comparing rates of disease within families as a function of the extent of genetic relatedness. The cleanest such design involves the comparison of disease concordance among dizygotic and monozygotic twin pairs. For common diseases such as types 1 and 2 diabetes mellitus, obesity, hypertension, coronary artery disease, autoimmune diseases, common cancers, schizophrenia, and bipolar disease, twin studies have documented that rates of concordance are significantly higher in monozygotic than in dizygotic twin pairs. For many other traits of clinical interest (e.g., most drug responses), formal tests of heritability have not yet been performed, and the role of inheritance in these characteristics is less well documented.

Data about familial aggregation allow the calculation of *heritability,* or the fraction of interindividual variability in disease risk attributable to additive genetic influences. The remaining variability among individuals is due to all other contributions: environmental influences on disease, nonadditive (*epistatic*) genetic effects (e.g., gene-gene interactions or gene-environment interactions), error in the measurement of relatedness or disease, and random chance. For most clinically important traits (diseases and risk factors), empirical estimates of heritability range from 20 to 80% (see Online Mendelian Inheritance in Man, available at *www.ncbi.nlm.nih.gov:80/entrez/query.fcgi?db=OMIM,* for comprehensive information).

When interpreting estimates of heritability, it is important to consider two crucial factors: the effect of measurement errors and the environmental context. *Measurement errors* can decrease the estimate of the heritability of a trait. A single measurement of blood pressure is much less heritable than a composite score based on serial measures of blood pressure over time. That is, day-to-day variability and imprecision in clinical measures can obscure an underlying biologic susceptibility that is entrained by inheritance. For the patient and physician, this means that although the blood pressure on a given day may not be particularly heritable, the blood pressure over time (which is presumably the relevant risk factor for vascular disease) is heritable to a much greater extent.

Second, estimates of heritability must be interpreted in the context of the environment in which the study was performed. In the case in which environmental triggers of disease are relatively constant across a study population, inherited factors may explain much of the variation in rates of disease. In contrast, in the case in which exposure to environmental causes of disease is highly varied across the study population, nongenetic factors may outweigh the contribution of inborn susceptibility. For example, the rate and diversity of smoking behavior will have a major impact on how much of the variability in rates of lung cancer (in any given study or patient cohort) may be explained by inheritance. If nobody smoked (or everyone smoked), little of the variation in lung cancer risk would be due to smoking behavior; if, in contrast, half the population smoked multiple packs a day, and the other half not at all, this behavior would no doubt dominate over inborn susceptibility.

For these reasons, heritability is not a fixed characteristic of a given disease, but an assessment of a given population, set of measurements, and the extent to which variability in genetic and environmental exposure explains disease risk. This sheds light on what is sometimes thought to be a contradiction between rates of disease being highly heritable (in a given population) and yet varying dramatically across populations separated by time, geography, or socioeconomic status. In broad comparisons across groups, environmental exposure and methods of clinical ascertainment can vary substantially and contribute to secular changes in patterns of disease. Conversely, within a group exposed to a relatively uniform environment and studied in a standardized manner, genetic susceptibility may play a major role in determining individual risk.

HETEROZYGOSITY: INHERITED VARIATION IN GENOME SEQUENCE

Heritability expresses the patterns of inherited variation in rates of disease; *heterozygosity* expresses the rate of inherited variation in genome sequences (Table 41-1). Heterozygosity is defined as the proportion of sites on the chromosome at which two randomly chosen copies differ in DNA sequence. Because cells are *diploid* (carry two copies of the genome sequence) and because these two copies were selected in a semirandom manner from the population, heterozygosity is equivalent to the fraction of base pairs that vary between the two copies each of us inherited from our mother and our father. That is, heterozygosity is the rate of genetic variation in the individual.

Single-nucleotide polymorphisms (SNPs) are sites at which a single letter in the DNA code has been swapped for a single alternate letter. Such variants are observed at approximately 1 in 1000 positions in the human genome sequence. In the protein coding regions of genes, rates of genetic variation are lower—less than 1 in every 2000 bases; the rate of variation that substantially alters the sequence of the encoded protein is lower still (see Table 41-1). These rates can be understood in light of darwinian selection against changes that alter the amino acid sequence of encoded proteins.

Genomes also contain larger scale variation: insertions and deletions of nucleotides, alteration in the number of copies of particular genes and sequences, and larger-scale alterations such as inversions and translocations. Both SNPs and larger-scale alterations can influence gene function and contribute to disease.

TABLE 41-1 CHARACTERISTICS OF HUMAN GENOME SEQUENCE VARIATION

Length of the human genome sequence (base pairs)	3,000,000,000
Number of human genes (estimated)	20,000
Fraction of base pairs that differ between the genome sequence of a human and a chimpanzee	1.3% (1 in 80)
Fraction of base pairs that vary between the genome sequence of any two humans	0.1% (1 in 1000)
Fraction of coding region base pairs that vary in a manner that substantially alters the sequence of the encoded protein	0.2% (1 in 5000)
Number of sequence variants present in each individual as heterozygous sites	3,000,000
Number of amino acid–altering variants present in each individual as heterozygous sites	12,000
Number of sequence variants in any given human population with frequency of >1%	10,000,000
Number of amino acid polymorphisms present in the human genome with a population frequency of >1%	75,000
Fraction of all human heterozygosity attributable to variants with a frequency of >1%	98%

The genetic variation in each of us is due largely to common variants. Empirically, more than 98% of the heterozygous sites in each individual display frequency of greater than 1% in the worldwide human population. Because most human heterozygosity is due to common variants, a database containing all common (>1% frequency) sequence variants in the human population can be constructed by sequencing the genomes of only hundreds of individuals, and yet would capture most of the genetic variation in any individual.

Built on the foundation of the human genome project, a catalogue of common DNA variants has been created by a series of public-private projects, including the SNP Consortium, International HapMap, and 1000 Genomes Projects. At the time of this writing, the public database contains more than 17 million human genetic variants (*www.ncbi.nlm.nih.gov:80/SNP/index.html*). Not all these entries represent common variants (some are rare), and some may represent technical false-positive findings. Nonetheless, the existing collection represents most of the common variants in each individual and has fueled efforts to systematically measure genetic variants for their contribution to disease.

The major role of common variation in human sequence diversity is explained by the unique demographic history of the human population. Despite the global distribution of the current human population, it is now clear that all people on the planet are the descendants of a single population that lived in Africa only 10,000 to 40,000 years ago. The ancestral population was small (with an effective size of perhaps 10,000 individuals), lived a hunter-gatherer existence at low population densities (relative to other humans and later domesticated animals), and had evolved in Africa over millions of years. Most human genetic variation arose in this phase of human history, before the more recent migrations, expansions, and invention of technologies (e.g., farming) that resulted in widespread population of the globe. Most common human genetic variation predates the Diaspora and is shared by all populations on earth.

A second factor is the slow rate of change in human DNA. Mutation and recombination occur at very low rates: on the order of 10^{-8} per base pair per generation. And yet, any pair of human genes traces a lineage back to a shared ancestor who lived on the order of 10^3 to 10^4 generations ago (if a generation is 20 years, then 10^4 generations is 200,000 years). In other words, considering the typical nucleotide in two unrelated humans, it is more likely that they trace back to a shared ancestor without any mutation having occurred than it is that a mutation has arisen in the intervening time. This explains why 99.9% of base pairs are identical when any two copies of the human genome are compared.

Another aspect of human variation is explained by these simple mathematical and population genetic relationships: the extent of human DNA sequence diversity attributable to rare and common variants. Each of us inherits from our parents some 3 million common polymorphisms (classically defined as those with frequency of >1%). We inherit common variants that are shared by apparently unrelated individuals but do not reach a frequency of 1% or higher. Finally, we inherit thousands of variants that are unique to each individual and their closest relatives. The question of how these different classes of variants influence disease is of central interest and importance to medical genetics.

The shared ancestry of human populations explains another aspect of human genetic variation: the correlations among nearby variants known as *linkage disequilibrium*, or *haplotypes*. Empirically, individuals who carry a particular variant at one site in the genome are observed to be more likely than chance to carry a particular set of variants at nearby positions along the chromosome. That is, not all combinations of nearby variants are observed in the population, but rather only a small subset of the possible combinations. These correlations reflect the fact discussed earlier that most variants in our genomes arose once in human history (typically long ago) and did so on an arbitrary but unique copy carried by some individual in the population. The ancestral copy of the genome on which the mutation occurred can be recognized in the current population as a stretch of particular alleles (known as a *haplotype*) that track together in the population. That is, although most variations in our genome arose before written human history, the DNA sequence in each of us carries a record of the evolution and demographic history of the human population.

These ancestral haplotypes, passed down from shared prehistoric ancestors in Africa, can be recognized in the current human population. The haplotype structure of the human genome offers a practical tool in association studies of human disease because it is not necessary to measure directly each nucleotide in order to capture much of the information. Such haplotype-based methods are the foundation for genome-wide association studies, discussed later.

THE SEARCH FOR GENES UNDERLYING MONOGENIC DISEASES

The *genetic architecture* of a disease refers to the number and magnitude of genetic risk factors that exist in each patient and in the population and their frequencies and interactions. Diseases can be due to a single gene *(monogenic)* in each family or to multiple genes *(polygenic)*. It is easiest to identify genetic risk factors when only a single gene is involved and this gene has a large impact on disease in that family. In cases in which a single gene is necessary and sufficient to cause disease, the condition is termed a *mendelian* disorder because the disease tracks perfectly with a mutation (in the family) that obeys Mendel's simple laws of inheritance.

Some single-gene disorders are caused by the same gene in all affected families; for example, cystic fibrosis is always caused by mutations in *CFTR*. Although many individuals with cystic fibrosis carry the same founder mutation (δ-508), others carry any pair of a wide variety of different mutations in *CFTR*. The existence of many different mutations at a given disease gene is known as *allelic heterogeneity*.

A mendelian disorder can be due to a single genetic lesion in any given family, but in different families can be due to mutations in a variety of genes. This phenomenon, termed *locus heterogeneity*, is illustrated by retinitis pigmentosa. Although mutation in a single gene is typically necessary and sufficient to cause retinitis pigmentosa, there are dozens of different genes in which retinitis pigmentosa mutations have been found (Online Mendelian Inheritance in Man #268000). In each family, however, only one such gene is mutated to cause disease.

Most single-gene disorders are rare (present in <1% of the population) and are manifested early in life. Many are severe and cause death before reproduction in the absence of modern medical care. The fact that most monogenic disorders are severe in childhood and rare in the population is probably not a coincidence, but reflects the impact of *natural selection*. The deleterious effect of these mutations results in a decrease in reproductive fitness (in individuals unlucky enough to inherit them), and the mutations and the disease are therefore unlikely to drift to high frequency in the population.

There are exceptions to this general idea: cases in which the mutation causing a severe monogenic disease (such as *HbS*, the cause of sickle cell anemia) is common in the population at large. Such cases appear to be the result of a different kind of selection, known as *balancing selection*—situations in which a gene mutation is beneficial in one circumstance (a genotype or environment) but deleterious in another. Heterozygous carriers for *HbS* are relatively protected against malaria, and this benefit balances the deleterious effect of sickle cell disease in homozygotes.

Starting in the 1980s, the advent of genome-wide linkage analysis led to rapid success at identifying the specific genetic mutations that cause mendelian disorders, with hundreds of genes identified for clinically important conditions (for comprehensive information, see *www.ncbi.nlm.nih.gov:80/entrez/query.fcgi?db=OMIM*). Progress was sparked by the development of a suite of powerful research techniques—*family-based linkage analysis* followed by *positional cloning*—in which a genome-wide search is undertaken for the causal gene, which is first localized to a chromosomal region. (The initial idea of genetic linkage mapping traces to Sturtevant in fruit flies in 1913 but did not become practical in humans until the 1980s.)

Once the search has been focused by the discovery of linkage between a chromosomal region and a disease, that chromosomal neighborhood is scoured for the genetic culprit, which is recognized based on the observation of mutations that alter the protein coding sequence, and are enriched in cases of disease compared with unaffected relatives and population-based controls. The power of these approaches prompted and was fuelled by the Human Genome Project, which provided the foundation of information on DNA structure, sequence, and genetic variation required to undertake such searches.

GENETIC INVESTIGATION OF COMMON DISEASES

Similar to mendelian disorders, most common diseases are influenced by inheritance. In contrast to mendelian disorders, however, the genetic contribution to common diseases appears to be due to the action of many genes rather than a single gene in each family. Empirical evidence in favor of this model comes from efforts to use the same approach (positional cloning) for complex traits that was applied successfully to monogenic disorders.

In the 1990s, the tools of family-based linkage analysis were applied to nearly all common disorders. Much of this work was done in isolated founder populations (such as Finland and Iceland) with the goal of simplifying the genetic architecture and accessing extended pedigrees. Excepting a few notable successes, however, these studies revealed few strong signals that localized the genes responsible for disease. In most of the hundreds of such studies that have been published, there are many weak statistical signals (few if any are statistically significant given the large number of hypotheses tested) and little agreement between different studies of the same disease.

In view of the well-understood statistical power of family-based linkage methods (based on their extensive use for monogenic disorders) and their relatively limited success despite extensive efforts in common diseases, it was concluded by most investigators that rare variants in single genes do not explain a large fraction of the risk for common diseases. If a single gene contained rare mutations of large effect that explained 20% or more of the inherited risk for type 2 diabetes, hypertension, or schizophrenia, it is likely that its location would long since have been found based on linkage analysis.

A next potential shortcut to understanding the genetic determinants of common diseases is to identify and study rare, early-onset forms of diseases that clearly demonstrate mendelian patterns of inheritance. Because these families display patterns of inheritance consistent with a major gene of large effect, the powerful tools of positional cloning can be and have been used successfully to identify the genes responsible. Important examples include the role of *BRCA1* and *BRCA2* in early-onset breast cancer, maturity-onset diabetes of the young as a form of type 2 diabetes, many monogenic disorders of blood pressure and electrolyte regulation, early-onset Alzheimer's disease, and many others.

These successes provide diagnostic information for families burdened with severe, early-onset forms of disease and insight into the underlying pathways responsible for disease. For example, more than 20 genes have been identified that, when mutated, cause rare mendelian disorders of blood pressure and electrolyte regulation. So far, every one of these genes is active in the kidney, and most are involved in the renin-angiotensin-aldosterone pathway. This result is a compelling demonstration of the central importance of the kidney in human blood pressure regulation and has suggested new therapeutic targets of substantial promise.

It was hoped that the genes found to be responsible for early-onset, monogenic forms of common diseases would contribute to the more common forms of disease in the population. In this scenario, severe mutations might cause early-onset forms, and more prevalent but subtle alterations in the same genes might contribute to common forms of disease. A comprehensive test of this hypothesis awaited tools from the human genome project and improved methods of genetic epidemiologic analysis.

ASSOCIATION STUDIES: FROM CANDIDATE GENES TO GENOME-WIDE ASSOCIATION STUDIES

Genome-wide association studies (GWAS) are simple in concept. A genetic variant is identified, its frequency is measured in individuals with the disease of interest, and it is compared with well-matched controls (drawn from the population at large or unaffected family members). This process can be repeated for as many genetic variants as exist—up to and including a genome-wide collection. Appropriate analyses need be performed to rule out alternative explanations for an association to disease, such as mismatching of cases and controls, or technical artifacts. Because the null distribution is well described (under the hypothesis of no association between genotype and phenotype), it is possible to calibrate such analyses and to identify reproducible associations from out of the large sea of benign polymorphisms.

Genetic association studies were pioneered in the context of the *HLA* locus on chromosome 6. The *HLA* was discovered based on its role in transplantation tolerance and is characterized by diverse allelic variation that can be measured based on interactions of antibodies and antigens. By measuring these protein-based (immunologic) readouts of the underlying genetic variation, *HLA* alleles were found to be a major determinant of susceptibility to infectious and autoimmune diseases. Starting in the 1960s, empirical data on human population genetics and genetic association studies were developed in the context of the *HLA*.

By the 1980s, tools of molecular biology made it possible to directly measure DNA variation (rather than using protein or phenotype measurements as surrogates for the underlying genetic variation), ushering in the modern era of human genetic research. In this pregenomic era, it was only practical to measure one or a small number of genetic variations in each study, limiting association studies to incomplete assessments of individual "candidate" genes selected based on biologic criteria.

The study of candidate genes led to a modest number of robust and reproducible associations, such as the contribution of Apo-ε4 to Alzheimer's disease; factor V Leiden to deep venous thrombosis; a 32-base deletion in the chemokine receptor CCR5 to HIV infection; common variants in the insulin gene to type 1 diabetes; SNPs in the peroxisome proliferator-activated receptor γ (PPAR-γ) and the β-cell potassium channel Kir6.2 to the risk for type 2 diabetes.

By early in the 2000s, comprehensive surveys of published genetic association studies showed that valid associations were few and far between, with many initial claims of association proving irreproducible, likely representing false-positive claims. One such analysis estimated that, in the pre-GWAS era, only 10 to 20 bona fide associations had been documented of common genetic variants with common diseases.

A major reason for the state of this literature was the intrinsically low likelihood of finding a gene and variant contributing to any given disease. Each genome contains millions of genetic variants, and presumably only a small fraction of these influence disease. This is often described as a problem of "multiple hypothesis testing," with the investigative community searching for associations between multiple genes, multiple variants in each gene, and multiple diseases. An alternative (bayesian) statistical framework frames this issue based on low prior probabilities of association. Regardless, it is conceptually clear that much more stringent statistical thresholds (than the traditional $P < .05$) are required for declaring association of genetic variants and disease.

As in linkage analysis for mendelian traits, a key to success in association studies was the advent of genome-wide search, unbiased by prior hypotheses about biologic mechanisms. With the sequencing of the human genome, development of large-scale SNP databases, and tools for genotyping up to 1M SNPs per individual, by 2005 it became practical to perform GWAS to identify genomic loci harboring allelic variation. With a recognition that any given variant had a very low likelihood of truly being associated with disease, much more stringent statistical thresholds were deployed (typically requiring a P value of 10^{-7} or lower to declare "genome-wide significance").

Age-related macular degeneration (AMD) provided an early success of GWAS. AMD is a typical common, polygenic disease (Chapter 431); siblings of affected patients are perhaps three to six times as likely as unrelated individuals to become afflicted, and yet family-based linkage analysis revealed only modestly significant (and modestly reproducible) linkage results. The pathophysiologic defects that underlie AMD were largely unknown until it was found that a common coding polymorphism in the gene for complement factor H is a major risk factor for AMD. The variant *(Y402H)* has a high population frequency (approximately 35% in European populations) and increases risk by 2.5- to 3-fold in heterozygotes and by 5- to 7-fold in homozygotes. Multiple other complement factors have since been found to harbor common genetic variation that influences the risk for AMD in a highly reproducible manner, providing unambiguous information about the primary role of complement in this common disease.

Since 2005, GWAS has been used to identify literally hundreds of novel genetic variants that show reproducible associations to a large variety of common human diseases. The field evolved a set of criteria and standards that largely eliminated the previous difficulties with irreproducible claims of association, making association studies a reliable method to identify genomic loci related to human diseases. The National Human Genome Research Institute of the National Institutes of Health maintains a catalogue of GWAS findings (www.genome.gov/26525384) that, at the time of this writing, included 904 such associations for 165 traits. This represents rapid progress compared with the two dozen or so such findings known at the start of the decade.

The results of GWAS support a number of conclusions about the role of common genetic variants in common disease. First, most diseases investigated by GWAS have yielded novel findings, suggesting that the approach has general utility. Second, only a small fraction of these findings were previously known, indicating that new clues can be obtained by genetic mapping of common diseases. Third, most of the associations demonstrate extremely modest odds ratios (on the order of 1.1-fold to 1.5-fold), indicating that natural selection has purged alleles of large effect from the pool of common variants. Fourth, most of the associated SNPs lie in noncoding regions, suggesting that they act through effects on gene regulation rather than directly altering protein-coding sequences. Fifth, only a modest fraction of the estimated heritability of each disease has yet been explained, indicating a role for other common variants of more modest effect, rare variants, genetic interactions, or other (as yet unanticipated) influences.

Because GWAS are genome-wide (not limited to "candidate" genes), they provide a test of the hypothesis that prior investigations had identified sets of genes relevant to each disease (relevant, that is, through the lens of genetic variation and inheritance). In the case of autoimmune diseases, many (perhaps half) of the 100 or more findings from GWAS lie near a gene previously known to play a role in the immune system. Similarly, a substantial fraction of the genetic variants found to influence lipid levels lie near genes that were previously known to play a role in lipid biology (because they were known already either through rare mutations that contribute to mendelian forms of hyperlipidemia or through biologic investigations). These findings confirm that the basic pathophysiologic mechanisms already known can be "validated" through the lens of inherited risk factors and encourage investigation of the new findings offered by GWAS.

In contrast, for some diseases, most of the genetic variants found are novel and do not lie near genes previously studied. One such case is type 2 diabetes, for which 35 independent genomic loci have been found to influence risk for disease, and yet only a handful were previously implicated by other methods. This may indicate and illuminate gaps in our previous knowledge of the pathophysiology of type 2 diabetes.

Although tantalizing, the results of GWAS have raised many more questions than they have answered. These discoveries implicate particular genomic regions, but to date in only a few cases have the causal genes been proved. This is challenging in large part because so many of these common variants are noncoding, and it remains difficult to connect noncoding variation to the genes thereby regulated. To the extent that truly novel genes are identified, much work is needed to discover their biologic and physiologic functions. Finally, GWAS findings explain only a modest fraction of the estimated heritability of most diseases, leaving open the question of which genes, and which types of variants and genetic effects, explain the remainder.

FROM COMMON VARIANTS TO INDIVIDUAL GENOMES

Although much of human genetic variation is due to common DNA variants (such as those tested through GWAS), each of us also inherits many thousands of variants that arose more recently and that tend to be lower in frequency and more population specific. To the extent that such variants have very large effects on phenotype, they may have been previously identified based on family-based linkage studies of mendelian disorders. However, there almost certainly exists a large universe of lower-frequency variations that are too rare to have been captured by the first generation of GWAS and that have effects too modest to have been recognized and identified in family-based linkage analyses.

The study of such lower-frequency and rare variants is now becoming practical owing to advances in technology for DNA sequencing. With dramatic drops in price and increases in throughput, it is increasingly practical to sequence individual genomes in the context of medical research (and, in the future, clinical practice). Such an approach will provide a much more complete assessment of genetic variation than was previously obtainable and will incorporate common as well as rare variants.

The first task will be to develop methods to interpret the millions of variants in each genome. Variants of high frequency have already been well studied by GWAS, and each is increasingly annotated with information about disease association. For variants that are lower in frequency, but still observed in a substantial number of unrelated individuals, the basic association methodology can be applied. That is, the frequencies of each specific variant can be measured in affected cases and in unaffected controls and compared with an appropriately constructed null distribution and statistical threshold. Moreover, the availability of a much more complete database of DNA variation (as is being created by the 1000 Genomes Project) will lead to a second generation of GWAS that is more complete for lower-frequency variation.

Many DNA variants will be unique to individuals (and their close relatives), however, and will require different approaches. If the analysis includes a large pedigree, with multiple affected and unaffected relatives, it may be possible to perform the association analysis in single families. More typically, however, it will be necessary to analyze large sets of samples, measure the rate of different (individually rare) variants in each gene, and compare these rates between cases and controls.

In the distant future, we may learn to "read" genome sequences and predict the effect of a variant never before observed. For the foreseeable future, however, interpretation will require statistical analysis of genomes, documenting that variation in particular genes is robustly and reproducibly associated with each particular disease.

IMPLICATIONS AND FUTURE DIRECTIONS

Inherited factors contribute substantially to common as well as rare diseases. Mendelian disorders are typically caused by rare mutations in the protein-coding regions of genes. Common variants, investigated through GWAS, have typically modest effects and often act through noncoding effects on gene regulation. Each of us carries a deep reservoir of less common variation that will soon be tested for a role in disease using methods of next-generation DNA sequencing. It seems reasonable to expect that an integrative analysis of this information will result in a defined list of genes and variants in those genes (both common and rare) that contribute to each human disease.

Success identifying genes and mutations will only prove of value if it leads to improved prediction, diagnosis, understanding, and treatment. Prediction and personalized medicine require a foundation of evidence that demonstrates clinical benefit. This will involve incorporating DNA variation in epidemiologically valid cohorts and testing particular approaches to genetic prediction in clinical trials. The fact that some genetic tests may prove predictive in no way means that routine genome sequencing will be useful to patients, and much work will be needed to offer the public and physicians guidance in interpreting such data.

Biologic understanding requires bedside-to-bench research, in which genes found as mutated in patients are studied in the laboratory. It will be necessary to place these new genes into known (and as yet unrecognized) biologic pathways and to understand how dysfunction and dysregulation lead to disease. In some cases, such as the role of complement in AMD (see earlier), initial answers may come quickly; in others, in which the relevant pathobiology is as yet unknown, the information to be gleaned from following these clues is unpredictable. Presumably, in the fullness of time, the genetic insights gleaned from patients will lead to a new generation of therapies that more directly target the underlying root causes of risk in the population. What is most certain is that genetic and genomic information is accumulating at a staggering rate and holds both much potential and much challenge for the future of medicine.

SUGGESTED READINGS

Altshuler D, Daly MJ, Lander ES. Genetic mapping in human disease. *Science.* 2008;322:881-888. *A review of genetic mapping of human disease.*

Lifton RP. Individual genomes on the horizon. *N Engl J Med.* 2010;362:1235-1236. *A commentary previewing the use of individualized genome sequences in clinical medicine.*

Manolio TA. Genomewide association studies and assessment of the risk of disease. *N Engl J Med.* 2010;363:166-176. *Review.*

Fark YJ, Claus R, Weichenhan D, et al. Genome-wide epigenetic modifications in cancer. *Prog Drug Res.* 2011;67:25-49. *Review.*

42

APPLICATION OF MOLECULAR TECHNOLOGIES TO CLINICAL MEDICINE

GEOFFREY S. GINSBURG

MOLECULAR TECHNOLOGIES ALONG THE CONTINUUM FROM HEALTH TO DISEASE

Along the continuum from health to disease (as shown in Fig. 42-1), there are now several important points in clinical decision making for which molecular technologies are being applied to health care (Table 42-1). Using DNA-based approaches, risk estimates for developing some diseases can now be quantified during health and possibly even at birth. Molecular signatures from technology platforms that measure the expressed genome (RNA, proteins, metabolites) now allow interventions at the level of the individual by defining physiologic states in response to our environment that predict future clinical outcomes. These methods can also provide more precise ways to screen for and to detect disease at its earliest molecular manifestations. Similarly, they are the basis for a new molecular classification of disease and diagnosis that foretells prognosis. The selection of certain drugs now may be guided by a patient's underlying genetic makeup as well as the molecular makeup of the disease. Given that a disease's evolution from baseline risk often occurs over many years, molecular profiling over time defines a novel form of health care that focuses on disease prevention and proactive management rather that the current paradigm of acute intervention and crisis management.

GENES, GENOMES, DISEASE, AND TREATMENT

A key question in medicine is to what extent genetic variation influences the likelihood of disease onset, affects the natural history of disease in combination with the environment, or provides clues relevant to the management of disease. And it is not just the human genome that is relevant to an individual's state of health—the genomes of thousands of microorganisms are relevant to human phenotypes, and insights from their genomes are providing new approaches for the diagnosis, study, and treatment of disease (see Microbiome).

Variation in the Human Genome

It is now estimated that any two randomly selected individuals have sequences that are 99.5% identical, or that an individual genome would be heterozygous at approximately 15 to 25 million positions. Most of the differences involve a single base in the DNA code, referred to as single nucleotide polymorphisms (SNPs). The remaining variation consists of insertions or deletions of short sequence stretches, and copy-number variation (CNV) in the number of repeated elements at a particular locus in the genome. These types of variation can influence disease, and this must be accounted for in any attempt to understand the contribution of genetics to human health.

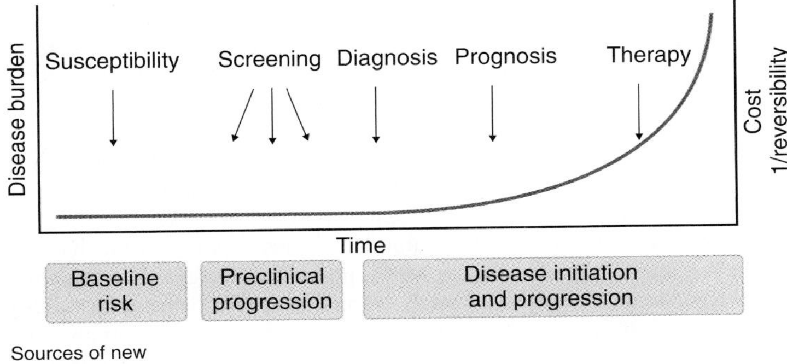

FIGURE 42-1. Use of molecular technologies across the continuum from health to disease. Various molecular technologies may be used to complement the traditional approach to evaluating at the time points indicated. SNP = single nucleotide polymorphism. (Adapted from Snyderman R. The role of genomics in enabling prospective health care. In: Willard H, Ginsburg G, eds. *Genomic and Personalized Medicine*. Burlington, Mass: Elsevier; 2009:378-385.)

Genome-wide Association Studies

The "common allele, common disease" hypothesis has been explored with notable success in a number of conditions, using large cohorts of well-phenotyped patients and high-throughput methods to genotype up to 1 million variants in the genome. Genome-wide association studies (GWAS) report the statistical association of one or more variants in a narrow genomic region with the presence or absence of the clinical condition. The reported SNPs define risk factors for that condition, at least in the populations under study, and can provide novel insights into the biology of the disease. As of December 2010, more than 3500 SNPs have been reported to be associated with more than 50 phenotypes in published studies (www.genome.gov/gwastudies/). It should be stressed that in most instances, *causality* of the reported SNP and the increased risk has not been proved; it may be that the actual causal variant is not the SNP itself but is a currently undetected variant that lies in linkage disequilibrium with the SNP. In most instances, the functional impact of the associated SNP is obscure, and it will require integrated genomic and functional studies to elucidate the precise basis for the roles of genome variation in disease.

Medical Resequencing

Resequencing specific genes in a cohort of affected individuals with disease is an alternative or complementary approach to GWAS to uncover rare variants responsible for the disease in question. It may indeed be that these more rare variants are responsible for most genetic risk, but there are insufficient data to draw conclusions. Most efforts have focused on one or several genes that are believed to be strong candidates for the phenotype under study. Using this approach, rare variants in relevant candidate genes have been detected at a statistically significant higher frequency in the genomes of patients with common clinical conditions. These early successes suggest a strategy of resequencing relevant genes in individuals at the extremes of the population distribution for measurable traits.

Somatic Mutations

It has been of interest to use medical resequencing to search for somatic mutations in tumor tissue in order to identify genes potentially relevant to cancer progression. The Cancer Genome Atlas (http://cancergenome.nih.gov/index.asp), started in 2006, has begun to explore systematically the entire spectrum of genomic changes in human cancers and has already published its first results for glioblastoma. The genes implicated in these studies tend to be different from those identified as inherited risk factors in previous genetic studies and provide novel insights into the biology of human cancer and suggest candidates for exploring mechanisms of tumorigenesis or metastasis or for developing therapeutic approaches.

Copy-Number Variation

There has been an unanticipated prevalence of structural variants in the genome that collectively account for more variation in genome sequence than do SNPs. The most common types of structural variations are CNVs. A dedicated effort is under way to catalogue CNVs in the human genome and to associate these with clinical phenotypes. Although most CNVs are inherited, some occur de novo or even in somatic cells; in these cases, an individual will have different repeat lengths from either of his or her parents. CNVs can contribute to human diseases in at least two ways:

1. *Pathogenic* CNVs are certain genomic imbalances that appear to cause neurodevelopmental diseases directly. Pathogenic CNVs are usually de novo in nature and have associated specific genomic imbalances with as many as 50 genetic syndromes (*www.sanger.ac.uk/PostGenomics/decipher/*).
2. *Benign* CNVs have been identified in healthy individuals and may have more subtle consequences on human health.

Epigenetics and the Epigenome

Epigenetic changes, in DNA methylation or in histone modification over time, in the genome may result in aberrant gene expression and human

TABLE 42-1 APPLICATION OF MOLECULAR DIAGNOSTICS ALONG THE CONTINUUM FROM HEALTH TO DISEASE: EXAMPLES

TIME POINT IN CLINICAL DECISION MAKING	Cancer		Cardiovascular Disease	
	Test	**Indication**	**Test**	**Indication**
Risk/susceptibility	*BRCA1, BRCA2* *HNPCC* *TP53, PTEN*	Breast Colon Sarcomas	*KIF6, 9p21* Familion 5-gene profile	CAD LQTS
Screening	HPV genotypes	Cervical	Corus CAD	CAD
Diagnosis	Pathwork Tissue of Origin	Cancer of unknown primary	Corus CAD	CAD
Prognosis	Oncotype DX (21-gene assay) MammaPrint (70-gene assay) HER2/neu, ER, PR	Breast	TnI, BNP, CRP	ACS
Pharmacogenomics	HER2/neu *UGT1A1* *KRAS* *EGFR* AmpliChip; DMET *CYP2D6/ CYP2C19*	Herceptin Irinotecan Cetuximab Erlotinib, gefitinib Various (see Table 42-2)	*KIF6, SLCO1B1* AmpliChip; DMET *CYP2D6/CYP2C19* *VKORC1*	Statins Various (see Table 42-2) Warfarin
Monitoring	CTCs	Tumor recurrence or progression	AlloMap gene profile	Transplant rejection

ACS = acute coronary syndromes; BNP = brain natriuretic peptide; CAD = coronary artery disease; CRP = C-reactive protein; CTCs = circulating tumor cells; ER = estrogen receptor; HPV = human papillomavirus; LQTS = long QT syndrome; PR = progesterone receptor; TnI = troponin I.

disease in response to environmental influences. It has become clear during the past two decades that epigenetic changes (methylation) play a crucial role in carcinogenesis. Similar research is emerging on DNA methylation in other diseases, especially autoimmune and cardiovascular disorders. For example, aberrantly hypomethylated DNA in circulation in systemic lupus erythematosus (SLE) (Chapter 274) might induce an immune response because of its similarity to unmethylated microbial DNAs. Further contributions of defective methylation to SLE pathogenesis could be due to the transcription of endogenous retroviruses or the increase in the expression of certain genes related to autoreactivity. In cardiovascular disease, global DNA hypomethylation and coexisting hyperhomocystinemia have been observed. Taken together, these data reinforce the notion that methylation profiles can be highly valuable to study the pathogenesis of a variety of conditions. The National Institutes of Health have initiated the Human Epigenome Project, whose goal is to indentify, catalogue, and interpret widespread DNA methylation patterns of all human genes in all major tissues; this effort has now been expanded internationally.

Microbiome

The genome sequences of thousands of microorganisms have been determined and are being used to provide rapid diagnostic tests in clinical settings; to predict antibiotic or antifungal efficacy; to identify the source of airborne, water, or soil contaminants; to monitor hospital or community environments; and to understand better the contribution of microbial ecosystems and various environmental exposures to diverse human phenotypes. For example, the human colon contains more than 400 bacterial species comprising some 10^{13} to 10^{14} microorganisms. The gastrointestinal tract (as well as other body cavities and the skin) provides a unique environment for microorganisms, the microbiome, whose impact on human health and disease is just being explored. The genomes of the microbiota are significantly different from the human genome and have the capacity to alter the metabolic profile of different individuals or different populations, with clinically meaningful effects on drug metabolism, toxicity, and efficacy. The applications to microbiomes of approaches in genomics are revolutionizing clinical diagnostics, for example, to identify unknown viral infections or to diagnose antibiotic resistance in infections such as methicillin-resistant *Staphylococcus aureus* (MRSA). A number of diseases have been associated with large-scale imbalances in the gut microbiome, including inflammatory bowel disease, antibiotic-resistant diarrhea, and obesity.

Personal Genomics

The delivery of information from individual genomes is a fast-moving area of technology development that is spawning a social and information revolution among consumers. Dramatic improvements in sequencing technology have reduced the cost and time of resequencing projects to approach the long awaited personal "$1000 genome." What remains unsettled for now is what degree of genome surveillance will be most useful, either for research or for clinical practice. The push for incorporation of genome information into clinical practice may come as much or more from consumers as from professionals. Several companies offer genome-wide SNP profiles to the public, some with associated risk estimates for relevant clinical conditions. There is a clear and important research agenda that needs to be developed in concert with these technologic breakthroughs that allows health providers and the public to understand the information and, more importantly, to believe that it is accurate, informative, and actionable. With the vast amount of information contained in the human genome sequence, it will be critically important that the proper reading, interpretation, and communication of the information are carried out. This may be a "disruptive technology" in health care delivery, providing health and disease risk information to consumers without physician intervention and guidance. Patients are already bringing reports from these analyses to their health providers and requesting guidance. What are providers, armed with a paucity of genomic training, telling them?

Pharmacogenetics

DNA variation that is associated with response to drugs is referred to as *pharmacogenetics,* and there are now numerous examples of molecularly guided therapies that use DNA assays (E-Table 42-1). To assist clinicians in the practice of pharmacogenetics across a broad number of medications, the first microarray-based gene chip, approved both in the United States and European Union, was released in 2003 as the AmpliChip CYP450. The product was designed to identify key genetic polymorphisms in two CYP450 enzymes, *CYP2D6* and *CYP2C19*, cumulatively responsible for much of the first-pass metabolism of many currently prescribed drugs. The regulatory agencies cleared this test based solely on analytic performance and validity information, but indicated that its utility specifically for clinical application needed to be proved. Thus, clinicians remain unclear about the impact of these tests on clinical decision-making guidelines.

Perhaps the best example of a pharmacogenetic association for which the clinical relevance is clear features management of treatment with warfarin. The oral anticoagulant warfarin (Chapter 37) is prescribed for the long-term treatment and prevention of thromboembolic events, with more than 31 million prescriptions annually in the United States alone. However, because of the drug's narrow therapeutic index, a variety of complications are associated with its treatment, even after dose adjustment according to age, gender, weight, disease state, diet, and concomitant medications. Investigation of pharmacokinetic and pharmacodynamic drug properties indicated the additive involvement of two genes in determination of warfarin maintenance dose. One of these genes encodes CYP2C9, which is responsible for most of the metabolic clearance (~80%) of the more pharmacologically potent S-enantiomer of warfarin. Both *CYP2C9*2* and *3 cause a reduction in S-warfarin clearance, with ten-fold variation seen from the genotype linked with the highest (*CYP2C9*1/*1*) to lowest (*CYP2C9*3/*3*) activity. It is estimated that *CYP2C9* variants account for 10 to 20% of the total variation in warfarin dose, with additional genetic and environmental factors playing larger roles in dose determination. The second gene is the vitamin K epoxide reductase complex protein 1 (*VKORC1*), targeted by warfarin. Consideration of *VKORC1* genotype, together with *CYP2C9* genotype and factors such as age and body size, is estimated to account for 35 to 60% of the variability in warfarin dosing requirements. Although further studies are under way, the clinical pharmacology advisory panel to the U.S. Food and Drug Administration (FDA) acknowledged the importance and potential for genotyping of *CYP2C9* and *VKORC1* during the early phase of warfarin therapy, and the drug label was amended accordingly in August 2007; however, the Center for Medicare and Medicaid Services announced in 2009 that it would not reimburse for testing until there was more evidence of a clinical benefit.

THE EXPRESSED GENOME

Gene Expression

Information from (RNA, protein, or metabolite) expression informs three areas relevant to clinical decision making:

- Disease diagnosis and classification
- Disease prognosis
- Pharmacogenomics

Disease Diagnosis and Classification

Whole-genome RNA expression data can be used to identify subtypes of cancer not previously recognized by traditional methods of analysis (Table 42-2). Among many examples, patterns of RNA expression have identified subclasses of tumors that define the acute leukemias or Burkitt's lymphoma from diffuse large B-cell lymphomas (DLBCL). Breast cancer profiling has defined four different gene expression subtypes; these molecularly defined subtypes have important prognostic relevance. Outside of cancer, complementary DNA microarray technology has proved useful for classifying a broad range of diseases, such as rheumatoid arthritis, Crohn's disease, schizophrenia, and multiple sclerosis, and for differentiating between ischemic and nonischemic cardiomyopathy.

Disease Prognosis

The first prognostic application of gene expression signatures described two molecularly distinct forms of DLBCL previously not appreciated using traditional histopathology techniques: germinal center B-like DLBCL and activated B-like DLBCL. Their clinical significance is that patients with germinal center B-like DLBCL have significantly better overall survival when treated with standard chemotherapy. Similarly, microarray studies of breast cancer have proved more powerful than traditional methods for predicting a patient's outcome, such as tumor size, lymph node status, and estrogen receptor status; for example, a 70-gene expression signature was found to be a strong predictor of metastasis, outperforming all currently used clinical predictors.

In 2009, oncologists used RNA expression signatures (Oncotype DX) for risk stratification and prognosis in more than 40,000 breast cancer patients and had cumulatively ordered more than 135,000. A prospective cooperative group clinical trial in Europe (MINDACT) aims to measure the effectiveness of a gene expression predictor of breast cancer prognosis in guiding adjuvant chemotherapy when compared with predictions based solely on the traditional clinical parameters for prognoses. A current study sponsored by the National Cancer Institute aims to use the Oncotype DX test from Genomic Health, Inc., to identify low-risk breast cancer patients unlikely to benefit from chemotherapy. For lung cancer, a similar opportunity now exists to refine prognosis and redirect treatment in early-stage disease and a clinical trial has been developed that uses this signature to randomize patients to surgical treatment with or without adjuvant chemotherapy.

Pharmacogenomics

The use of complex molecular information from the genome (as opposed to DNA variation) is often referred to as *pharmacogenomics.* (As described earlier, *pharmacogenetics* refers to individual responses to drugs as a function of DNA variation.) The expressed genome has provided several important

TABLE 42-2 PERIPHERAL BLOOD GENE EXPRESSION SIGNATURES TO CLASSIFY DISEASE STATES

	TARGET CELL	RESULTS	CHAPTER
Autoimmune	Whole blood RNA	A 41-gene signature differentiates **infliximab** responders from nonresponders.	35
	Whole blood RNA	A 29-gene signature best differentiates active from inactive **systemic lupus erythematosus.**	274
Inflammatory	Peripheral monocytes	A 53-gene signature distinguishes between patients with active **multiple sclerosis** and healthy controls.	419
	Peripheral monocytes	A 136-gene signature distinguishes active **multiple sclerosis** patients on TNF-α therapy from treatment-naïve patients.	419
	Whole blood RNA	A 10-gene-based composite score for diagnosing **atopy** and **asthma** performs better than the total IgE count, with a sensitivity and specificity of 96% and 92%, respectively.	257
Neoplasm	$CD27^+$ and $CD19^+$ B cells; $CD4^+$ T cells	A 2984-gene signature can distinguish subtypes of **diffuse large B-cell lymphoma**.	191
	Bone marrow mononuclear cell RNA	A 50-gene signature is highly correlated with **AML-ALL distinction** and is used to develop a classification scheme.	189
	$CD34^+$ blast cells RNA	A 2856-gene signature allows **classification of AML** into 16 distinct groups.	189
Transplant	$CD4^+$ and $CD8^+$ T-cell RNA	A 17-gene signature identifies donor samples **likely to cause GVHD** with 80% accuracy.	181
	Whole blood RNA	A 91-gene signature distinguishes between **transplant rejection** (grade 3A) and controls (grade 0).	48
Environmental Exposure	Whole blood RNA	A 216-gene profile differentiates **oxidative damage** from active oxidative damage in active and passive smokers.	31
	Whole blood RNA	A 62-gene profile correlates with severity of **arsenic poisoning.**	21
	Whole blood RNA	A 25-gene signature identifies **exposure to ionizing radiation** with overall accuracy of 90%.	19
Cardiovascular Disease	Platelet RNA	A 54-gene signature classifies **STEMI and stable CAD**. Moreover, MRP8/14 predicts risk for a future cardiovascular event.	71, 73
	Whole blood RNA	A 160-gene signature correlates with extent of **coronary stenosis** and is associated with atherosclerotic vascular disease.	70
	Whole blood RNA	A 14-gene signature confirmed by PCR is associated with the **presence and extent of CAD.**	71

ALL = acute lymphoblastic leukemia; AML = acute myelogenous leukemia; CAD = coronary artery disease; GVHD = graft-versus-host disease; IgE = immunoglobulin E; PCR = polymerase chain reaction; STEMI = ST elevation myocardial infarction; TNF = tumor necrosis factor.

Adapted from Aziz H, Zaas A, Ginsburg G. Peripheral blood gene expression profiling for cardiovascular disease assessment. *Genomic Med.* 2007;1:105-112.

TABLE 42-3 MOLECULAR MARKER INFORMED CANCER THERAPIES (TARGETED THERAPEUTICS)

BIOMARKER	DRUG	CANCER TYPE	DRUG EFFECT	FDA DRUG LABELING RECOMMENDED OR REQUIRED
Estrogen receptor	Tamoxifen	Breast	Response	Yes
HER2/neu	Trastuzumab	Breast	Response	Yes
EGFR	Cetuximab	Colorectal	Response	Yes
Kras	Cetuximab	Colorectal	Response	Yes
EGFR	Panitumumab	Colorectal	Response	Yes
Kras	Panitumumab	Colorectal	Response	Yes
DPYD	5-FU	Breast/colorectal	Response	No
EGFR	Erlotinib	Lung	Response	No
EGFR	Gefitinib	Lung	Response	No
BCR-ABL	Imatinib	CML	Response	Yes
C-KIT	Imatinib	CML/ALL	Response	Yes

5-FU, 5-fluorouracil; ALL = acute lymphocytic leukemia; CML = chronic myelogenous leukemia; DPD = dihydropyrimidine dehydrogenase; EGFR = epidermal growth factor receptor.
Adapted from Freedman A, Sansbury L, Figg W, et al. Cancer pharmacogenomics and pharmacoepidemiology: setting a research agenda to accelerate translation. *J Natl Cancer Inst*. 2010;102:1698-1705.

examples of novel biomarkers that can be used to guide therapy selection. An iconic form of pharmacogenomics is "targeted therapy," of which there are now several examples in clinical practice (E-Table 42-1 and Table 42-3). Trastuzumab therapy (a monoclonal antibody specifically targeting *HER2/neu*-overexpressing breast tumors) is an example of a protein therapeutic for which an obligatory biomarker assay and diagnostic test have been developed to identify the patients most likely to benefit from this drug. Trastuzumab is marketed solely for the subset of patients (~10%) who overexpress *HER2/neu* (Chapter 204). Given the low prevalence of marker-positive breast cancers, it has been suggested that if it were not for the use of the diagnostic marker the drug would not have been successfully developed. In cardiovascular medicine, a targeted approach to acute coronary syndromes has been practiced for more than a decade with the use of cardiac troponin I (cTnI) measurements to dictate the beneficial use of glycoprotein IIb/IIIa inhibitors.

Recently, a series of gene expression signatures have been developed to predict the activation state of various oncogenic signaling pathways, thereby portending the advent of personalized cancer treatment based on a tumor's gene expression pattern. When evaluated in several large collections of human cancers, these gene expression signatures identify patterns of pathway deregulation in tumors and clinically relevant associations with disease outcomes, including prognosis. Linking pathway deregulation with sensitivity to therapeutics that target components of the pathway provides an opportunity to make use of these "oncogenic signatures" to guide the use of target therapeutics.

Proteomics

Proteomics is the large-scale study of proteins. The *proteome* often refers to the full complement of proteins and their various derivatives (e.g., splice variants or post-translational modification). In the context of health and disease, proteomics seeks to define the full set of proteins associated with a particular physiologic state. The capabilities and direction of proteomics is evolving in terms of both protein identification and differential expression between two physiologic states (such as health and a specific disease). Quantitative proteomics, in which global differences in protein abundances are measured, continues to be a priority area for biomarker discovery and molecular medicine. This area has been dominated by stable isotope approaches, but recent label-free quantitative methods have been developed that rely on the measured intensity of a peptide ion and compares this to its intensity in other samples. Label-free methods have the advantage of higher throughput and fewer sample manipulation steps. Multiple-reaction monitoring of specific peptides within biofluids allows quantitation of absolute abundance of proteins in clinical samples. Although this technology is relatively immature in its applications to human health and disease compared with RNA and metabolic profiling, it is anticipated that these methods, combined with the development of mass spectroscopy (MS) technology, will advance proteomics to more routine use in disease classification and diagnosis, prognosis, and pharmacogenomics within the next several years.

Metabolic Profiling

A metabolic profile is very similar to some of the traditional targeted profiles, such as a lipid profile, although it is more comprehensive. Metabolomics measures changes in the metabolic or chemical milieu that are downstream of genomic and proteomic alterations. It is estimated that humans contain approximately 5000 discrete small molecule metabolites, and the identification of metabolic fingerprints for specific diseases may have particular practical utility for the development of therapies because metabolic changes immediately suggest enzymatic drug targets. Similar to genomics and proteomics, metabolomics may be useful in disease diagnosis, prognosis, and drug development. In particular, metabolomics will likely be a valuable tool in assessing drug toxicity. Targeted MS-based metabolic profiling has also been increasingly applied to studies of human diseases and conditions. These tools are being applied to diverse areas, such as diabetes, obesity, cardiovascular disease, cancer, and mental disorders.

ASSEMBLING MOLECULAR INFORMATION FOR CLINICAL DECISION MAKING

Despite the potential for molecular information to transform health care, past experience indicates that new molecular interventions, like any new medical intervention, will remain substantially underused for many years unless a robust infrastructure is established for supporting their appropriate use. Moreover, molecular interventions may face even greater barriers to clinical adoption compared with more traditional medical interventions, owing to such factors as limited clinician familiarity with molecular technologies, the volume and complexity of the underlying data that may need to be considered, and financial coverage of additional testing in an already financially challenged health care system.

Of the many strategies that have been evaluated for promoting evidence-based care, one strategy has been found to be particularly effective: clinical decision support (CDS), which entails providing clinicians, patients, and other health care stakeholders with pertinent knowledge or person-specific information, intelligently filtered or presented at appropriate times, to enhance health and health care. Clinician-directed CDS interventions evaluated in randomized controlled trials have significantly improved patient care, provided that the CDS was delivered automatically as a part of clinician workflow, offered at the time and location of decision making, recommended a specific course of action, and used a computer to generate the recommendations.

Extended to molecular medicine, CDS supports its consistent and evidence-based application in health care. For example, when initiating warfarin therapy using an electronic prescribing system, a clinician could be provided with recommendations on dosing and monitoring that account for the patient's *CYP2C9* and *VKORC1* genotypes. As another example, to

TABLE 42-4 CLINICAL DECISION SUPPORT REQUIREMENTS TO APPLY MOLECULAR TECHNOLOGIES TO CLINICAL MEDICINE

NEED	AVAILABLE RESOURCES
Centrally managed repositories of medical knowledge	Authoritative knowledge on how molecular interventions should be used in clinical practice (e.g., U.S. Preventive Services Task Force, U.S. Evaluation of Genomic Applications in Practice and Prevention initiative) Repositories of structured experimental genomic and molecular data (e.g., PharmGKB for pharmacogenetic and pharmacogenomic experimental data and curated knowledge; NCBI dbGaP for data from studies evaluating the interaction between genotypes and phenotypes; and NCBI GEO for gene expression data) Large-scale efforts at managing medical information in health systems (Intermountain Healthcare, Partners HealthCare)
Standardized representation of molecular and patient data	Standardized information terminologies for both molecular and traditional patient data (e.g., HL7 data standards, including HL7 Clinical Genomics data standards and emerging HL7 virtual medical record standard; openEHR Archetypes; SNOMED CT; LOINC; BSML; MAGE-ML; National Cancer Institute/caBIG Common Data Elements)
Standard approaches for locating and retrieving patient and molecular data	Approaches for locating and retrieving patient data across systems (e.g., HL7 Retrieve, Locate, and Update Service draft standard and corresponding OMG technical specification) Regional and national initiatives for secure health data exchange (e.g., U.K. National Health Service Connecting for Health, U.S. Nationwide Health Information Network prototypes, caBIG, Indiana Health Information Exchange)
Sharing and coordination of information	Initiatives to share medical knowledge (e.g., Morningside Initiative, U.S. Federal CDS Collaboratory) Efforts to specify functional requirements of EHR systems (e.g., HL7 EHR System Functional Model standard) Coordinated use of available health information technology standards (e.g., U.S. Health Information Technology Standards Panel, Integrating the Healthcare Enterprise)

BSML = Bioinformatic Sequence Markup Language; caBIG = cancer Biomedical Informatics Grid; dbGaP = database of Genotype and Phenotype; EHR = electronic health record; GEO = Gene Expression Omnibus; LOINC = Logical Observation Identifiers Names and Codes; MAGE-ML = microarray and gene expression markup language; NCBI = National Center for Biotechnology Information; PharmGKB = Pharmacogenomics and Pharmacogenetics Knowledge Base; SNOMED CT = Systematized Nomenclature of Medicine, Clinical Terms.
Adapted from Kawamoto K, Lobach D, Willard H, Ginsburg G. National clinical decision support infrastructure to enable the widespread and consistent application of genetics and genomics in healthcare. PMCID: PMC2666673 2009;9:17.

support a clinician in his or her treatment of a patient with breast cancer, an electronic health record (EHR) system could consider the gene expression profile of the patient's cancer biopsy and provide an individually tailored prediction of how the patient is likely to respond to various therapeutic options. Critical to the vision of molecular medicine supported by information technologies will be a national CDS infrastructure (Table 42-4) that enables authoritative, centrally curated knowledge of molecular information that can be consistently leveraged in clinical practices across the nation. The true application of molecular technologies will require robust CDS systems that (1) access molecular and other patient data located within the EHR, (2) evaluate and integrate this information in relation to rule sets, and (3) deliver the information in a fashion that allows real-time actionable recommendations for the individual patient.

SUGGESTED READINGS

Chadwick R. Personal genomes: no bad news? *Bioethics.* 2011;25:62-65. *Thoughtful review of whole genome sequencing's potential effects on people and their lives.*

Ginsburg GS, Willard HF, eds. *Genomic and Personalized Medicine.* 2nd ed. Philadelphia: Elsevier; 2011. *A comprehensive work on the discovery, translational, clinical, and policy research and evidence to guide molecular information and technologies from bench to bedside.*

43

CELL AND GENE THERAPY

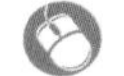

KARL SKORECKI AND EITHAN GALUN

CELL THERAPY

Cell therapy refers to the provision of living cells to patients for the prevention or treatment of human disease. The best established and most widely practiced form of cell therapy is the administration of blood and blood products in transfusion medicine. Other emerging applications of cell therapy involve the use of cells as vehicles for the delivery of genes or gene products, as discussed in the section on gene therapy.

In regenerative medicine, cells from various sources are administered to augment, repair, or replace tissues or organs damaged by disease, injury, or congenital anomaly. In this regard, solid organ transplantation can be considered a form of cell therapy. Like blood and blood product transfusion (Chapter 180), solid organ transplantation provides fully differentiated, functioning replacement cells of the transplanted organ (Chapter 48). One of the most important practical limitations of solid organ transplantation is the shortage of available organs relative to the growing demand. In certain forms of irreversible organ system failure, such as neurodegenerative disease, organ transplantation is not a therapeutic option. For these reasons, the development of safe and effective cell therapies is progressing rapidly.

Stem Cells of Human Origin

Stem cells possess two defining properties: (1) the capacity for self-renewal, and (2) the capacity to differentiate into cell types with specialized cellular functions. This may occur at the individual stem cell level through the process of asymmetrical cell division (Fig. 43-1) or at the cell population level wherein a subset of cells differentiate and the remaining stem cells remain dormant or replicate themselves as stem cells. After asymmetrical cell division, non–stem cell derivatives may either generate a pool of organ system–restricted, transit-amplifying cells with enhanced proliferative capacity or differentiate by epigenetic and gene expression profile changes until reaching the terminally differentiated state. This framework was developed after the discovery of bone marrow cells that were capable of reconstituting the adult hematopoietic system. These hematopoietic stem cells constitute the basis for hematopoietic stem cell transplantation, the only form of stem cell therapy currently well established in clinical practice (Chapter 181). Besides these two cardinal properties of self-renewal and differentiation capacity, stem cells can also be classified according to three additional attributes. These are replicative capacity (limited versus unlimited), the scope or potency of differentiation (e.g., pluripotent, multipotent, oligopotent, unipotent), and their place in the life history of the organism (developmental or postdevelopmental). Thus, more recent terminology has broadened use of the term *stem cells* to cover a wider array of cell types that contribute to organ development or have the capacity to repopulate tissues and organ systems. The term *stem cell*, together with the formulations noted previously, has also recently been extrapolated to describe certain cellular subpopulations that may be principally responsible for the growth of malignant tumors. However, because cancer stem cells (Chapter 185) have no role in tissue regeneration, they are not considered further in this chapter.

Embryonic and Induced Pluripotent Stem Cells

The fertilized egg, or zygote, develops first into a blastocyst, then an embryo, and then a fetus. The blastocyst is evident on day 5 after fertilization and consists of 200 to 250 cells, 30 to 34 of which consist of the inner cell mass, or epiblast. The remaining cells are the outer cell mass (Fig. 43-2). After the entire blastocyst attaches to the lining of the uterus, embryonic and extraembryonic development begins. At the blastocyst stage, each cell in the inner cell mass has the capacity to differentiate into derivatives of all three germline layers (ectoderm, mesoderm, and endoderm). In normal development, these cells do not persist beyond the blastocyst stage. Unused preimplantation

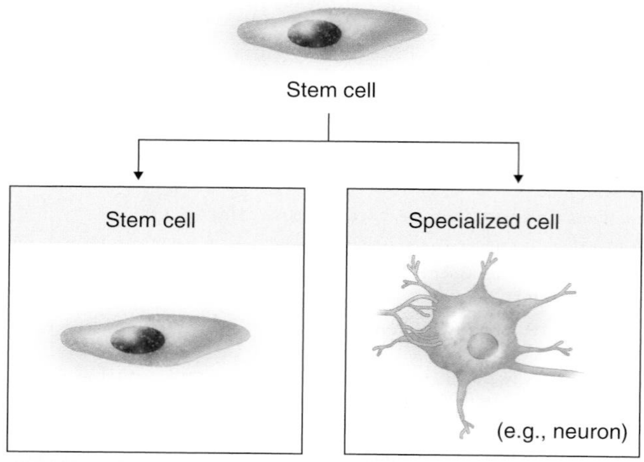

FIGURE 43-1. Asymmetrical cell division. Although this first characteristic was considered a *required characteristic* for stem cells based on their original description in the adult hematopoietic system, not all cell types currently named as stem cells necessarily display this property. For instance, human embryonic stem cells divide by symmetrical cell division.

blastocysts generated for in vitro fertilization can be used to generate human embryonic stem cells (hESCs) from the microdissected inner cell mass. Under appropriate culture conditions, these hESCs exhibit unlimited self-renewal in cell culture in the undifferentiated state without undergoing replicative senescence (i.e., losing the ability to divide). This occurs by virtue of the expression of high levels of the telomerase enzyme, which protects against senescence-associated attrition of the telomeric ends of linear chromosomes during repeated rounds of cell division. Under appropriate cell culture conditions, hESCs are pluripotent; they can differentiate into any of the known cell types of the body.

A major goal of embryonic stem cell research is to direct the differentiation process to enable enrichment to homogeneity of a replacement cell type by adding growth factors that activate cell signaling pathways used in normal embryonic development. This approach has yielded partial enrichment of cells with properties similar to those of authentic fetal pancreatic β cells, vascular endothelial cells, and cardiomyocytes, as well as more mature cells with properties similar to those of bone, connective tissue, and retinal, neuronal, and hepatic cells.

More recently, methods have been developed to reprogram differentiated adult somatic cells into a state of pluripotency, thereby generating induced pluripotent stem cells (iPSCs; Fig. 43-3). The methods to achieve this were enabled by identifying the various cell signaling and gene regulatory pathways that confer pluripotency on hESCs—including the transcription factors Nanog, Oct-4, and Sox-2. The availability of iPSCs from a given patient in need of replacement cells potentially avoids problems of immune rejection because the iPSCs will be recognized as autologous or self rather than allogeneic in origin. In addition, the use of iPSCs appears to invoke fewer ethical concerns, as outlined later. iPSCs derived from patients with certain genetic diseases also provide a unique experimental platform for studying the cellular and molecular pathways that go awry during the development of the affected cell types and tissues.

During the later stages of prenatal human development, cells of fetal origin often show enhanced proliferative capacity as well as the ability to differentiate into more than one type of mature or specialized cell. Thus, these cells have also been used as sources of cell therapy in regenerative medicine and can also be considered stem or progenitor cells—but with more restricted replicative capacity and differentiation potential than is the case for hESCs and iPSCs. To date, the only fetal-derived stem cells that have been used with documented success in human clinical applications are the dopaminergic cells derived from the developing fetal nervous system for the treatment of Parkinson's disease (Chapter 416).

Translating hESCs and iPSCs into a therapeutic platform has the potential for the development of teratomas and malignant tumors from residual undifferentiated cells, following administration of what appears to be a homogeneous population of fully differentiated replacement cells. Progress to clinical trials requires definitive clarification of this concern.

Adult (Postnatal) Stem Cells

After birth, many tissues are thought to contain a subpopulation of cells with the capacity for extended self-renewal, combined with the ability to differentiate into more mature cell types with specialized functions. Adult stem cells generate an intermediate state characterized by enhanced proliferation (transit-amplifying cells or progenitor cells), before reaching full terminal differentiation (Fig. 43-4).

Adult stem cells, thought to represent less than 0.01% of the total number of cells, are located in specialized supportive niche compartments at various sites within the hematopoietic system and elsewhere, and respond to cues in their local microenvironment. As a result of the success of hematopoietic stem cell transplantation in the treatment of bone marrow failure or in conjunction with myeloablative therapy in malignancy, scientists have been motivated to find adult stem cells in other organs and other organ systems. Adult tissues and organ systems reported to contain stem cells include bone marrow (hematopoietic and mesenchymal compartments) and peripheral blood, the central nervous system, blood vessel endothelium, dental pulp, epithelia of the skin, adipose tissue, digestive system, cornea, retina, testis, and liver. Controversy exists regarding the existence of adult stem cells in the kidney, pancreas, and heart. Whether adult stem cells represent remnants of developmental stem cells that persist into adulthood for purposes of organ maintenance and repair or represent a distinct cell type dedicated for this latter purpose is not clear.

Given their low percentage, dispersed tissue distribution, and markers that are not fully defined, isolation of adult stem cells for therapeutic use has been technically challenging, with the greatest successes to date reported for mesenchymal stem cells. Mesenchymal stem cells represent a type of multipotential adult progenitor cell found in the bone marrow niche that supports hematopoiesis. Mesenchymal stem cells have also been isolated from adipose tissue, blood, umbilical cord, and muscle. Although mesenchymal and other multipotential adult progenitor cells have been shown in some experimental animal models to differentiate into a wide variety of cell types representing all three germ layers, they do not possess the capacity to develop into every cell type, as do hESCs and iPSCs.

There is some evidence that beyond the therapeutic value to hematopoietic reconstitution, bone marrow transplantation may also make some contribution to restoration of organ system function after certain forms of solid organ transplantation. Although adult stem cells are classically thought to be committed to a narrow spectrum of differentiation within the organ system, some studies have suggested the possibility that certain adult stem cells may display unexpected degrees of plasticity. *Plasticity* refers to the ability of differentiated cells to undergo transdifferentiation into mature cell derivatives of another germline origin. Such plasticity would allow bone marrow-derived hematopoietic or mesenchymal stem cells to transdifferentiate into cardiac, vascular endothelial, connective tissue, neuronal, or other cells that show promise in clinical trials of regenerative medicine.

Like iPSCs, postnatal or adult stem cells have the potential to circumvent two of the obstacles in developmental stem cell therapy: ethical concerns regarding the use of cells of developmental origin, and alloimmunologic rejection. Adult stem cells may have the additional advantage of being less prone to teratoma and tumor development. hESCs and their derivatives generally emanate from a source not related to the potential recipient and can therefore be considered an allogeneic graft. Research studies have confirmed the immunogenicity of hESCs despite their very early developmental origin. Adult stem cells and iPSCs of autologous origin should not elicit an alloimmunologic response and therefore offer a potential solution. On the other hand, when the underlying disease is an active autoimmune destructive process (e.g., type 1 diabetes mellitus), it can be expected that replacement cells of autologous origin might also be targets of the immune-mediated pathophysiologic process.

Specific Disease Applications in Cell Therapy

Except for hematopoietic stem cell and solid organ transplantation, experimental cell therapies have been implemented in a limited number of patient trials.

Neurodegenerative Disease and Neuronal Injury

Parkinson's disease (Chapter 416) involves loss of melanin-containing dopaminergic neurons within the substantia nigra pars compacta of the midbrain, coupled with accompanying depletion of striatal dopamine. This cellular loss is responsible for the major motor features of the disease. Although

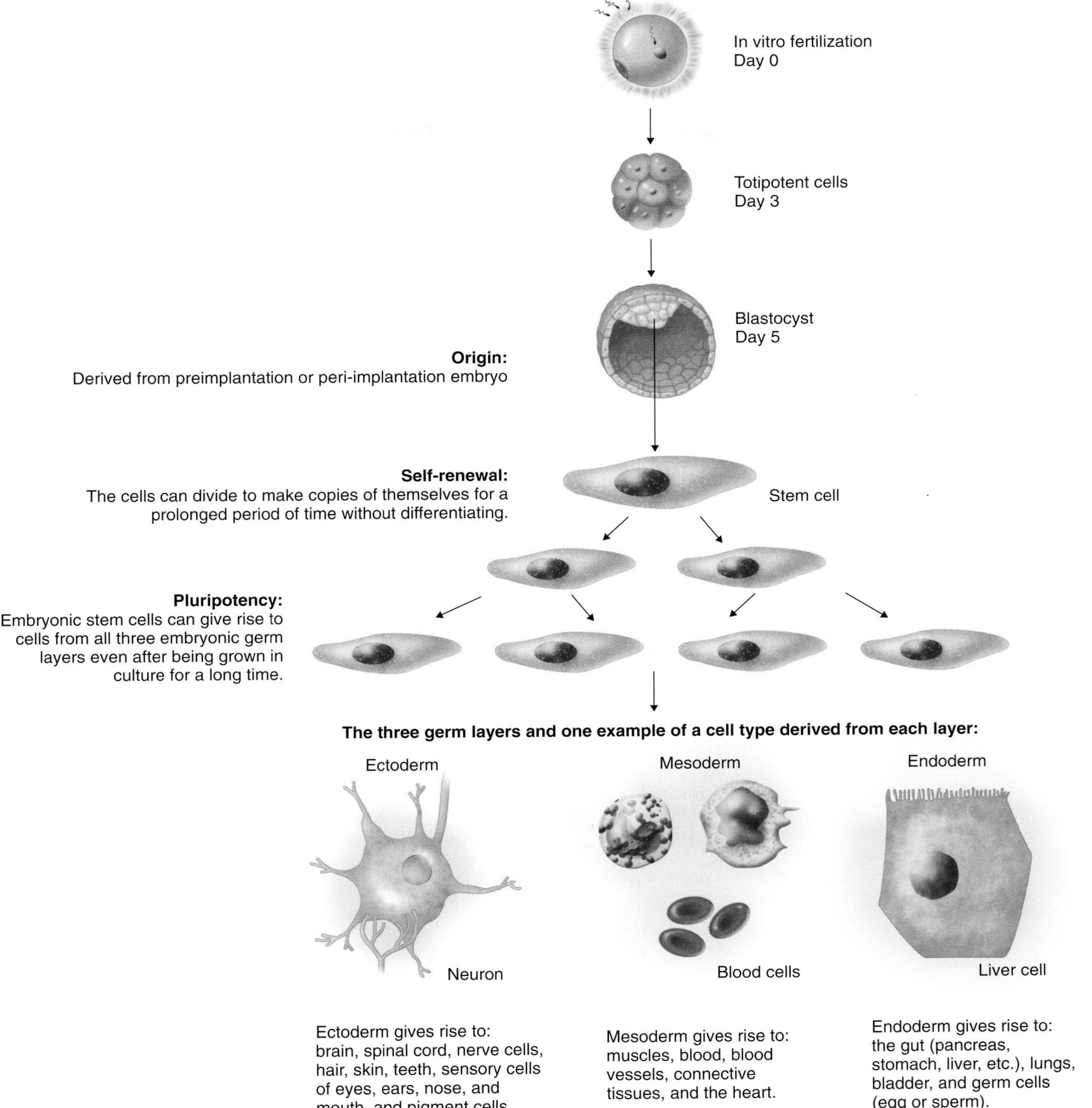
In vitro fertilization
Day 0
Totipotent cells
Day 3
Blastocyst
Day 5
Origin:
Derived from preimplantation or peri-implantation embryo
Self-renewal:
The cells can divide to make copies of themselves for a prolonged period of time without differentiating.
Stem cell
Pluripotency:
Embryonic stem cells can give rise to cells from all three embryonic germ layers even after being grown in culture for a long time.
The three germ layers and one example of a cell type derived from each layer:
Ectoderm
Mesoderm
Endoderm
Neuron
Blood cells
Liver cell
Ectoderm gives rise to: brain, spinal cord, nerve cells, hair, skin, teeth, sensory cells of eyes, ears, nose, and mouth, and pigment cells.
Mesoderm gives rise to: muscles, blood, blood vessels, connective tissues, and the heart.
Endoderm gives rise to: the gut (pancreas, stomach, liver, etc.), lungs, bladder, and germ cells (egg or sperm).

FIGURE 43-2. Embryonic stem cells. *Totipotency* refers to the capacity to differentiate into all cell types in an organism, including extraembryonic tissues, placenta, and umbilical cord, a property confined to the fertilized egg itself, including the cells derived from the first few cell divisions after fertilization. *Pluripotency* refers to the capacity to differentiate into all the specialized cell types derived from the three germ layers (ectoderm, mesoderm, endoderm) of the developing embryo and is a hallmark feature of embryonic stem and germ cells.

pharmacologic dopaminergic replacement therapy is effective in the early stages of illness, prolonged treatment with pharmacologic agents alone is associated with refractoriness and complications and fails to halt the underlying neurodegeneration. In the search for more definitive therapy, early reports of cell replacement suggested significant improvement in motor function after intrastriatal implantation of mesencephalic tissue, obtained from aborted human fetuses aged 6 to 9 weeks after conception. Long-term immunosuppressive treatment is essential to allow transplanted dopaminergic neurons to develop into their full functional potential despite the notion of an immunologic sanctuary within the brain. Clinical assessment standards have provided evidence of long-lived graft survival and clinical benefit after therapy with cells of fetal origin that has now lasted up to 10 years or longer in some patients. Further progress is limited by lack of sufficient source tissue to treat a large number of affected patients, prohibitive variability in functional outcome, reports of serious dyskinesias in a subset of treated patients, and ethical considerations.

Investigations of stem cell–based approaches for the treatment of other neurodegenerative diseases, including Alzheimer's disease, Batten's disease, amyotrophic lateral sclerosis, stroke, and brain and spinal cord injury, are now moving between experimental animal model studies to planning of clinical trials. Recent reports have shown a major clinical benefit in animal models on directed differentiation and transplantation of hESCs toward a retinal pigment epithelium. Human studies with these cells may be soon initiated for patients suffering from age-related macular degeneration.

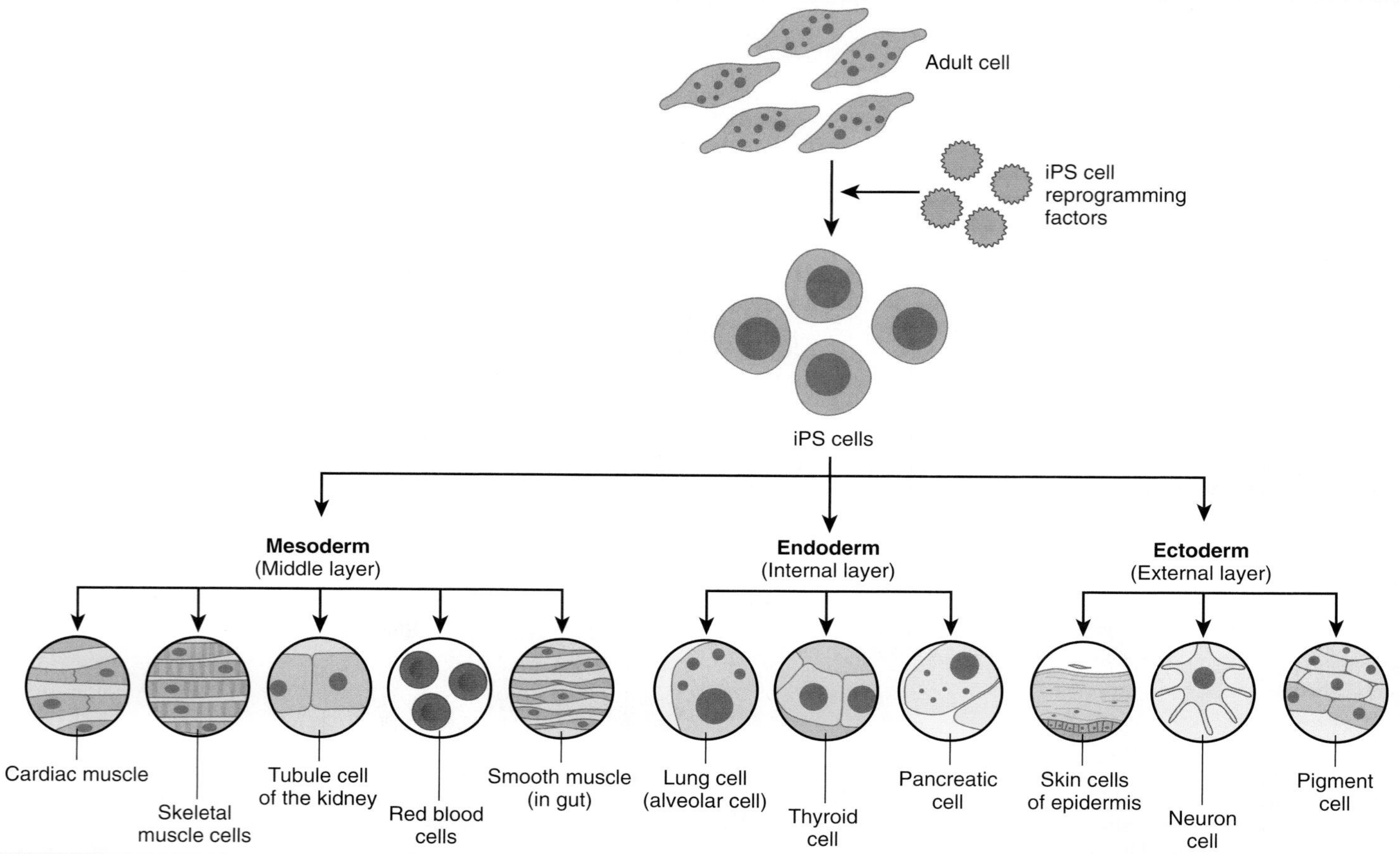

Adult cell
iPS cell reprogramming factors
iPS cells
Mesoderm (Middle layer)
Endoderm (Internal layer)
Ectoderm (External layer)
Cardiac muscle
Skeletal muscle cells
Tubule cell of the kidney
Red blood cells
Smooth muscle (in gut)
Lung cell (alveolar cell)
Thyroid cell
Pancreatic cell
Skin cells of epidermis
Neuron cell
Pigment cell

FIGURE 43-3. Induced pluripotent stem (iPS) cells. Introduction of three growth factors and a chemical agent that modifies gene expression is sufficient to restore pluripotency to adult somatic cells. (Adapted from http://www.sigmaaldrich.com/life-science/stem-cell-biology/ipsc.html.)

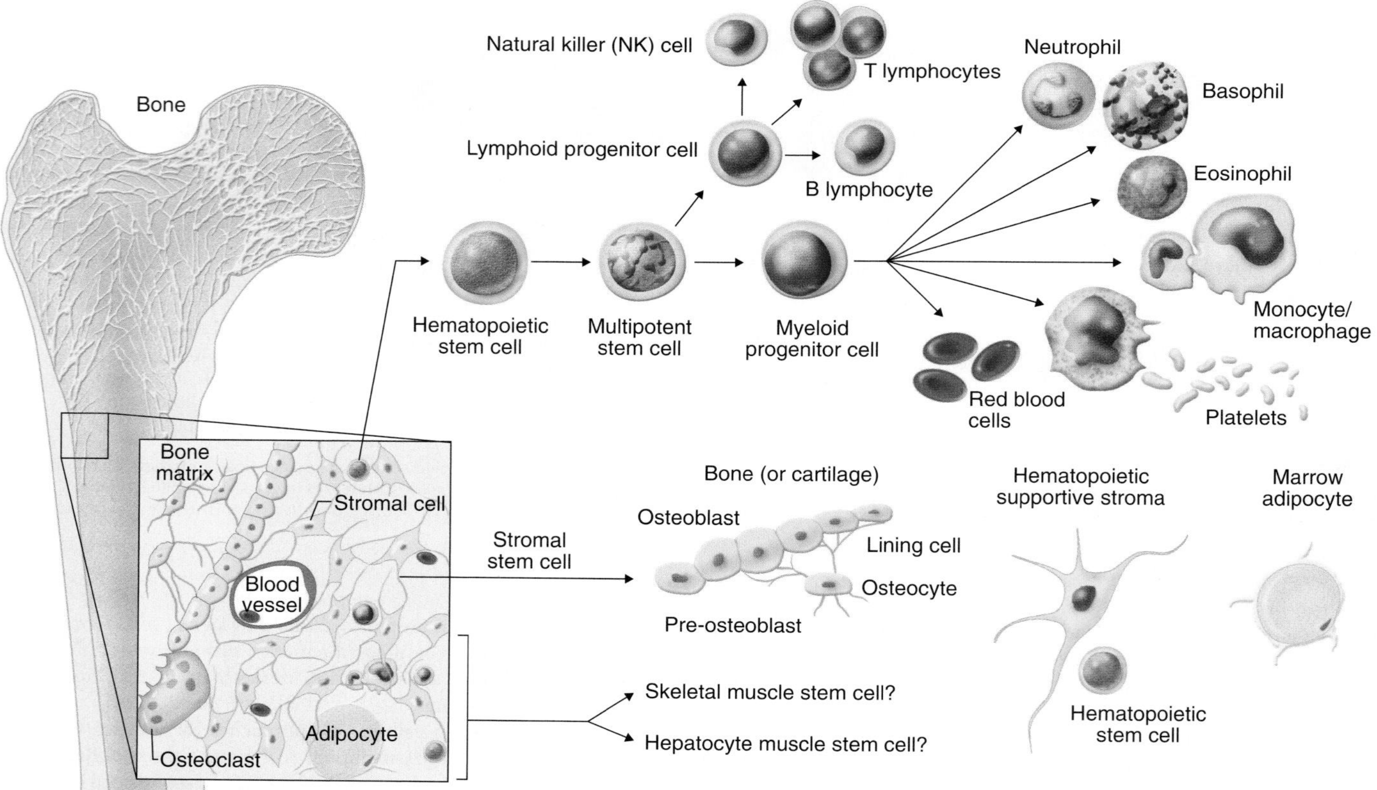

FIGURE 43-4. Adult stem cells. Adult stem cells can be multipotent and have the capacity to differentiate into a limited number of different cell types, often restricted to a given tissue or organ system, as in the case of adult hematopoietic or epidermal stem cells. Two stem cell types have been isolated from adult bone marrow—the hematopoietic stem cell and the mesenchymal stem cell. Adult mesenchymal stem cells of bone marrow origin, although their range of differentiation has been shown to be broader than that of any other adult stem cell type, do not reach pluripotency. It is thought that in some organ systems, such as the gastrointestinal epithelium, a unipotent pool of progenitors exists for repopulating a rapid population turnover of only one type of cell—although it is difficult to be certain whether such progenitors can be distinguished from the overall population of fully differentiated cells in tissues with high cellular turnover.

Muscular Dystrophies and Other Disorders of the Musculoskeletal System

In the major genetic forms of muscular dystrophy (Chapter 429), a range of approaches have been developed that aim to correct the genetic defect, restore functional expression of the missing gene product (e.g., dystrophin), and thereby slow disease progression. Implantation of myoblast muscle precursor cells might enable the improved repopulation of degenerating dystrophic muscles in these disease states. Although initial success in harvesting myoblasts was reported, clinical benefit did not ensue because of an inflammatory response that destroys most injected myoblasts. Furthermore, failure of myoblasts to migrate meaningful distances from the injection site renders implantation by direct needle injection impractical in acute muscular dystrophy disorders.

Protocols have been devised for the development of mixed biomechanical substitutes for bone, tendon, cartilage, and other connective tissues that incorporate or produce relevant surrounding matrix. For these forms of cell therapy, connective tissue scaffold can be produced in vitro and then repopulated with endogenous recipient cells in the patient, thus potentially preempting immune rejection and other problems related to the presence of cells of allogeneic origin.

Heart Disease

In heart failure (Chapters 58 and 59), limitations of clinical therapy have motivated the search for cell-based therapies to restore or augment myocardial contractile function or reestablish functional cardiomyocytes in damaged cardiac regions.

Autologous skeletal myoblasts have been shown in clinical trials to grow in scarred cardiac tissue after direct intracardiac injection. However, histologic or functional evidence of electrical or mechanical coupling has not been demonstrated. Currently, most experimental work selects a specific preparation of bone marrow and peripheral stem cells and progenitors. In some cases, the apparent differentiation of bone marrow cells into cardiac myocyte phenotypes has been subsequently refuted. In cell culture, hESCs are easily induced into a cardiomyocyte phenotype, including the following features: rhythmic contraction, gene and protein expression markers for cardiomyocyte differentiation, electrical coupling through gap junctions, responsiveness to chronotropic and inotropic agents, and electromechanical coupling with heterotypic cardiomyocytes derived from other sources. Cardiomyocytes of human embryonic stem cell origin have been shown to serve as a biologic pacemaker after conduction system ablation in experimental animals. They have also been shown to enhance cardiac contractility after myocardial infarction induced by coronary ligation in experimental animals. For the treatment of refractory cardiac rhythm disturbances, a combination of cell and gene therapy involves the stable expression of potassium conductance or other ion channels in skin fibroblasts derived from patients suffering from refractory rhythm disturbances, followed by their implantation into electrically unstable regions of the heart by guided endomyocardial injection. A major experimental effort in the use of bone marrow–derived cells through intracoronary administration aims to improve left ventricular function after acute myocardial infarction. Clinical experience with more than 1000 patients who received stem cell therapy indicates a favorable safety profile with a modest improvement in cardiac function and structural remodeling in the setting of acute myocardial infarction or chronic heart failure. Direct intracardiac muscle administration was more frequently associated with lesser degrees of improvement and sometimes with arrhythmias.

Diabetes Mellitus

Successful pancreatic transplantation and improved glucocorticoid-free protocols for transplantation of islets of Langerhans have been shown not only to restore glucose control in patients with diabetes mellitus but also to prevent or even reverse some of the disease's complications (Chapters 236 and 237). However, whole organ or islet-based transplantation approaches are limited both by immunologic rejection and by limitation of an available source of transplantable tissues. This has motivated the search for cell types that can replace (type 1 diabetes mellitus) or augment (type 2 diabetes mellitus) deficient β-cell function. Although no clinical applications have been reported, significant progress has been made with cells of human origin tested in cell culture and in animal models. Strategies that have been pursued include the developmental reprogramming of hepatic cells along the endocrine pancreatic lineage differentiation to provide these cells with the appropriate machinery for glucose-mediated insulin release. Protocols have also been established for differentiation of hESCs to either a precursor or mature β-cell phenotype. Because the pathogenesis of type 1 diabetes mellitus involves autoimmune destruction of pancreatic islet cells, the β cells derived from autologous sources, such as the patient's own iPSCs, might also become a target for autoimmune destructive processes unless preemptive measures are taken. In addition, because glucose monitoring and insulin delivery systems are constantly improving, any cell therapy–based approach must provide a clear advantage over existing therapeutic modalities while meeting the most rigorous standards of patient safety.

Stem Cell–Derived Platforms in Gene and Drug Discovery

In addition to the generation of cells for regenerative applications, the ability to grow a wide variety of different specialized cell types of human origin in culture provides unparalleled opportunities for gene and drug discovery and testing. For example, the ability to grow human cardiomyocytes in culture provides a preclinical human cellular-based experimental platform for screening newly developed drugs in terms of their potential to cause QT-interval prolongation and hence the risk for arrhythmia in the clinical setting. Other examples include the creation of an experimental tissue microenvironment of human origin for studying the stromal response to tumor growth and testing anticancer drugs that target tumorigenic responses such as angiogenesis. By combining technologies such as RNA interference (RNAi) with human stem cell growth and technology (E-Fig. 43-1), it will also be possible to uncover the role of certain gene products in the biochemical pathways and cellular responses in gene therapy.

Societal, Ethical, and Legal Considerations in Stem Cell Research and Therapy

Societal, ethical, and legal concerns about defining the concept of personhood status before birth have emerged among countries and political or religious constituencies in the field of stem cell research and therapy. Although there is a broad consensus that full personhood sanctity and associated rights should be accorded to each individual from at least the moment of birth, similar consensus does not apply to the status of an individual before birth. Various guidelines for research have been developed worldwide based on milestones in embryonic development. Bioethicists and legislators are often concerned about the possibility that research scientists and clinicians will move beyond allowable activities into prohibited domains. Previous concerns about therapeutic cloning, in which the first step is oocyte somatic nuclear transfer, or replacement of the haploid nucleus of a harvested oocyte with the diploid nucleus derived from the somatic cell of a potential cell therapy recipient were based mostly on the fear of a slippery slope to reproductive cloning. However, the successful generation of human iPSCs has for the most part supplanted the incentive for oocyte somatic nuclear transfer. Continued civil discourse and strict regulatory guidelines to ensure patient safety in clinical trials will remain key in resolving the bioethical dilemmas and societal concerns raised by stem cell and related emerging biomedical technologies.

GENE THERAPY

The use of genes as therapeutic platforms emerged during the mid-20th century, and in the 1990s, the first regulated registered studies were performed in the United States. Since then, more than 10,000 patients have been treated in more than 1000 studies in 15 countries across all continents with various modalities of gene therapy for a variety of diseases. About 50 studies have been performed for tracking gene delivery and more than 1000 for therapeutic assessment. One hundred studies involved monogenic diseases, and 1000 involved cancer patients, which is also the most common disease category for gene therapy studies worldwide. Two gene therapy agents are currently available on the market. Fomivirsen (Vitravene) is used for the treatment of cytomegalovirus retinitis (Chapter 384) in patients with acquired immunodeficiency syndrome (AIDS). The *p53* tumor suppressor coding sequence in an adenovirus vector is used for the treatment of head and neck cancer patients and is registered only in China. Most patients who participated in the first gene therapy clinical trials were administered marker or reporter genes rather than actual therapeutic genes. Of the thousands treated, two deaths have been attributed directly to gene therapy. The mortality statistics attributed to gene therapy are very low when compared with those associated with chemotherapy and transplantation, two therapeutic modalities frequently used today in clinical practice for disease targets of gene therapy.

Genetic Material

The therapeutic payload in most cases, the core of every gene therapy drug, is composed of an expression cassette. Essential clinical objectives of gene therapy are based on controlling gene expression through regulation of a tissue-specific promoter for expression. Although a few systems have been developed in the experimental setting, none has yet received approval for clinical use by the U.S. Food and Drug Administration or any other regulatory authority, other than the expression of *p53* in head and neck tumors by regulatory authorities in China.

Gene Therapy Delivery Methods

Gene therapy agents are often composed of two elements: the genetic material and the delivery system. The latter is usually the more complex and limiting component, and it is important to select the most efficient delivery method for any genetic therapy. Unfortunately, many gene therapy delivery methods are associated with potential adverse effects, thus necessitating tailoring of therapy to specific clinical considerations. The most commonly used delivery systems have used retrovirus- and adenovirus-based approaches. Virus-based approaches take advantage of the fact that viruses have been designed through evolution to serve as genetic material delivery systems. However, for each specific virus-based gene therapy vector, there have been major disadvantages that should be balanced against potential therapeutic benefits. Nonviral methods have also been used in many studies. The most commonly used nonviral delivery methods involve the use of naked/plasmid DNA and liposome-mediated delivery. In cancer gene therapy, the immune response to the delivery vehicle carrying the anticancer genetic material can be used to advantage by serving as an adjuvant. However, the system for delivery of a gene to be expressed for a prolonged period to replace or supplement a missing gene product in monogenic disease states should preferably be ignored by the immune system.

Naked/Plasmid DNA

In theory, the most straightforward approach to gene therapy would be the introduction of genetic material, such as an antisense molecule, short interfering RNA (siRNA), or an expression cassette, directly into the targeted cellular compartment (i.e., DNA into the nucleus or RNA into the cytoplasm). However, in clinical practice, this turns out not to be efficient. Systemic administration of naked DNA into the blood stream generally results in loss of the delivered genetic material, nonspecific interactions with serum proteins, and active degradation mediated by the innate immune system (e.g., tissue macrophages). Direct administration or application to target organs or tissues may circumvent some of these problems, but certain barriers must also be overcome. When the payload is a DNA expression cassette, it will need to interact with the cellular membrane and penetrate it, escape the endosomal compartment and cytosolic degradation by nucleases, and traverse the nuclear pores to reach the nucleus of the cell. This is a long process that is prone to failure unless supported by additional means that allow the DNA to pass the cellular barriers. Electroporation is an approach that has been applied to well-circumscribed body compartments or masses, such as muscle, skin, and tumors. Patients treated with electroporation have experienced tissue damage and associated pain. Additional methods have also been developed for the administration of naked DNA, including the different types of gene guns used for DNA vaccination and ultrasound energy for the transduction of endothelial cells, which could be used for cardiovascular applications and against tumor angiogenesis.

Naked DNA has also been formulated as part of DNA vaccination approaches to the treatment of cancer and immune and infectious diseases. Although preclinical studies have been promising, successful extrapolation to the clinic has not yet been achieved.

Nonviral Vectors

Nonviral vectors have been designed to overcome the cell membrane barrier and, in some cases, intracytoplasmic compartmentalization of the administered genetic material. These nonviral vectors are efficient at enhancing membrane penetration in vitro; however, their efficiency in vivo is significantly reduced. There are additional advantages to nonviral delivery systems: they are inexpensive and can carry large DNA molecules, and their structure can be modified to comply with specific needs, such as conjugation to short peptides for targeting. After systemic and, in some cases, local administration, these nonviral vectors stimulate the innate immune response by serving as adjuvants. They interact with serum proteins as well as cells that were not meant to be targeted, and with extracellular matrix. Once the DNA reaches the nucleus, it is subject to silencing. After cell division, expression is significantly reduced. Currently, nonviral vectors are used in specific selected cases. Local and systemic delivery of nonviral delivery systems could induce reciprocal immune effects with an undesirable inflammatory clinical response.

Adenovirus as a Viral Vector

Adenovirus is a nonenveloped DNA virus with the capacity to carry a large genetic payload. Adenoviruses, as well as adenovectors (the virally based vector), transduce nondividing cells, a property that is important for gene therapy for many cell types, such as hepatocytes (<0.1% of hepatocytes are replicating in humans at any given time). These vectors have been modified to prevent their replication in healthy tissues. Replication-defective (RD) adenovectors are used for short-term expression. Additional modifications of the viral genome and the cellular system supporting production of the viral particles have enabled deletion of all the viral coding sequences, thereby converting it into a "gutted" vector (helper-dependent [HD] adenovector). It is possible to clone the therapeutic genes into the RD adenovirus and generate recombinant adenovectors in a relatively short time. An additional advantage of adenovectors is that the relatively simple production system enables the generation of a very high titer. High viral titers are essential when administration is parenteral or when production of a large amount of a given protein is needed, such as in disease states in which secretion of a protein is impaired and each cell needs to encode its own normal protein. The HD adenovectors, which do not harbor virus-encoded genes, are able to support the transgene expression for months and possibly for more than a year. RD adenovector-transduced cells express viral proteins and induce an immune response. They are thus used in clinical cases in which the therapeutic gene needs to be expressed at high levels for a short period. High-titer systemic administration of adenovectors could be associated with severe adverse effects, such as disseminated intravascular coagulopathy (Chapter 178).

Retroviral Vectors

Retroviral vectors are an RNA group of viruses that harbor two RNA genomic copies in each viral particle, which is composed of a capsid and surrounded by an envelope. For gene therapy applications, two groups of viruses have been modified for clinical assessment and use: the oncoretroviruses and the lentiviruses. Vectors generated from both groups have already entered clinical testing.

Gammaretroviral Vectors

Gammaretroviral vectors are derived from different gammaretroviruses, including the murine leukemia virus and the Moloney murine leukemia virus. RD viruses are produced in special packaging cells that supply all the essential components in *trans* for viral replication and structural proteins. The viral gene therapy vector is composed of (1) a genome without any encoded viral sequences that is responsible for the production of viral proteins; (2) the therapeutic genetic payload and the structural components; and (3) the capsid and envelope. These viral vectors can carry transgenic payloads up to 8 kilobases (kb) in length. Retroviral vectors are capable of transducing only dividing cells. If the DNA reaches the nucleus, integration of the viral genome into the host cell chromosome can occur and lead to stable, long-term transgene expression. At its peak, a multiplicity of infection (MOI) integration occurs at numerous sites. Therefore, if long-term correction of a genetic disorder is required, the target cells must first be induced to replicate. The integration is a random event, with preference within an approximately 5-kb nucleotide window around the transcription initiation site. Thus, there is concern that interference with normal cell function could occur, including the activation of oncogenes or the disruption of tumor suppressor genes. Such events have occurred and have led to the development of malignant transformation both in animal models (rodents and primates) and in humans. There is evidence that "young" cells of the hematopoietic system and hepatocytes are more susceptible to malignant transformation than are terminally differentiated cells. On the other hand, the selectivity for dividing cells is advantageous if one aims to deliver a toxin gene to a growing tumor surrounded by quiescent normal parenchyma. The production of retroviral vectors is less efficient than that of adenovectors. As a result, the application of retroviruses is, in most cases, not by systemic administration but by ex vivo or direct injection into normal or tumor tissue.

Lentiviral Vectors

This group of viruses has been developed more recently for gene therapy applications. Human immunodeficiency virus (HIV) and the feline, simian, and equine immunodeficiency virus (FIV, SIV, and EIV, respectively) lentivirus family members were converted to become lentivectors for gene therapy. These vectors are deprived of the structural and most nonstructural and accessory genomic sequences that are supplied in *trans* in the packaging cell line for vector production. In addition, the envelope glycoprotein is of nonlentivirus origin, and for safety measures, the origin of replication is inactivated to generate a self-inactivating vector. All these genomic manipulations have been introduced to improve the safety of the lentivector and to enable a large cloning capacity of up to 8 kb. The lentivectors have been applied in only a few gene therapy studies, mainly for the treatment of AIDS patients. However, additional studies using lentivirus-based delivery systems are under way in patients with hemoglobinopathies, Parkinson's disease, X-linked adrenoleukodystrophy, and other genetic and degenerative diseases, with promising results. The long-term risk of using retroviral vectors, including gammaretroviral and lentiviral vectors, is not known. The possible development of clonal dominance, transformation, and cancer in the case of retroviral stem cell transduction is judiciously monitored in all appropriately registered studies.

Adenovirus-Associated Virus

Adenovirus-associated virus (AAV) is a single-strand DNA, nonenveloped, nonpathogenic human parvovirus. Viral vectors were derived from several serotypes, which exhibit different tissue and cell tropism. The capacity of AAV vectors is smaller, which is a limitation for certain AAV vector gene therapy approaches. The capacity for high titers (10^{12} transducing units per milliliter) of AAV serotypes enables systemic injections with reasonable MOI in targeted cells and tissues. Additional advantages of AAV vectors are that they transduce nondividing cells and do not integrate into the target cell genome. The innate immune system detects the AAV and responds to it, and antibodies generated against the viral capsid after a single injection attenuate the effect of a second administration of AAV vector. Long-term expression is detected with the use of AAV vectors. Phase I to III clinical studies have assessed the AAV vector for genetic, viral, inflammatory, degenerative, and malignant diseases. A study with AAV coagulation factor IX showed short-term efficacy owing to the development of an immune attack against the transduced hepatocytes. Studies both in Europe and the United States have shown a long-term benefit for patients with Leber's congenital amaurosis treated by subretinal administration of AAV to express retinal pigment epithelium-specific 65-kD protein (RPE65). Success was also reported in Parkinson's disease. Furthermore, more than 2 years of follow-up showed no significant side effects.

Special Virus-Derived Vectors

In addition to the adenoviral, retroviral, and AAV vectors, numerous, more specialized virus-based vectors with interesting properties and clinical objectives have been developed during the past 10 years.

Herpes simplex virus type 1 (HSV-1) is a DNA virus that can be manipulated to become RD and accommodate a large amount of foreign DNA for gene delivery. Expression of the transgene payload is transient. The HSV-1 amplicon has been used in numerous clinical trials of gene therapy for neurologic diseases.

Virus-like particles (VLPs) were recently developed for vaccination or gene therapy. VLPs of human papillomavirus were recently used as empty particles for vaccination against cervical cancer with significant success. Viruses of the same group, including SV40, which is also a DNA virus, are used for the generation of VLPs to carry gene therapy payloads. One advantage of SV40 is the low immune response against the virus. Again, similar barriers will slow the development of these vehicles, such as limitation of titers and production capacity.

Recombinant vaccinia virus (rVV) was initially developed for the expression of proteins in transduced tissues. Clinical studies in this avenue have encountered limited success. However, recent development of rVV for the treatment of malignant diseases through the expression of antigens might yield clinical benefit.

Oncolytic Viruses

Oncolytic viruses replicate in tumor cells and induce a cytopathic effect or kill tumor cells through other means, such as induction of apoptosis. The major obstacle facing the current development of antitumor drugs is not their potency, but rather their low selectivity for tumor cells. High therapeutic selectivity is essential to enable a safe therapeutic window. Virotherapy has such properties, but these viruses are still waiting to be proved clinically effective. Tumor-targeted oncolytic viruses are composed of two groups. Genetically engineered viruses are designed to replicate in tumor cells preferentially. This group includes adenoviruses that can replicate only in the presence of a nonfunctioning tumor suppressor gene, such as *p53* or *Rb*. The latter viruses will selectively replicate in tumor cells and induce their killing. The engineered HSV-1 and rVV viruses can also be included in this group. The second group consists of inherently antitumor-selective viruses found to possess antitumor effects through specific protein expression (reovirus) or viruses that activate the innate or adaptive immune response against the tumor, such as the Newcastle disease virus, measles virus strains, Sindbis virus, poliovirus, and vesicular stomatitis virus. The rationale for the use of reovirus in a virotherapeutic approach against cancer is based on the observation that reovirus infection activates host protein kinases to shut down protein production, an essential protection against the infection. Activated Ras signaling is known to interfere with protein kinase activation and with its signaling after reovirus infection. This allows the reovirus to continue to replicate in tumor cells and spare normal tissues. Such replication induces a specific cytopathic effect in malignant cells. Genetically engineered viruses and inherently antitumor-selective viruses have been tested in early clinical trials and are awaiting studies to determine their effectiveness in specific types of cancer. Virotherapy, in combination with standard chemotherapy, has the potential to further increase the antitumor activity of oncolytic virotherapy in a synergistic manner.

Diseases Treated by Gene Therapy

Inherited Immunodeficiency

More than 30 patients reported to date worldwide have undergone treatment with different retroviral vectors for inherited immunodeficiencies (Chapter 258). Patients with one of the following three diseases are included in this group: two types of severe combined immunodeficiency (SCID), both of which are characterized by dysregulation of lymphocyte development, and X-linked chronic granulomatous disease (X-CGD), an inherited immune deficiency with absent phagocyte reduced nicotinamide adenine diphosphate (NADPH) oxidase activity caused by mutations in the *gp91* (*phox*) gene. Individuals with adenosine deaminase (ADA) SCID suffer from premature death of T, B, and natural killer (NK) cells as a result of the accumulation of purine metabolites; patients with this condition have been treated with vectors expressing the *ADA* gene. In the first patients with ADA SCID, transduced T cells expressing transgenic *ADA* have been shown to persist for longer than 10 years; however, the therapeutic effect of gene therapy resulted in incomplete correction of the metabolic defect. More recently, an improved gene transfer protocol of bone marrow CD34-positive cells, combined with low-dose busulfan, resulted in multilineage, stable engraftment of transduced progenitors at substantial levels, restoration of immune function, correction of the *ADA* metabolic defect, and proven clinical benefit. Overall, no adverse effect or toxicity has been observed in patients treated with *ADA* gene transfer in mature lymphocytes or hematopoietic progenitors.

The X-linked type (X-SCID group), in which there is defective cytokine-dependent survival signaling in T and NK cells, was shown to be corrected by introduction of the wild-type sequence of the common γ-C chain, which is an essential component of five cytokine receptors. In one clinical study, hematologic malignancies developed in four patients. One of the four died of this complication. A group of ten patients treated with a different viral transduction protocol were successfully treated, with one reported malignancy in up to 8 years of follow-up. Two adult X-CGD patients who suffered recurrent bacterial infections have been treated with CD34-positive cells transduced with a gammaretroviral vector expressing *gp91 phox*, with significant clinical improvement in the short term. However, in both of these patients, there was an expansion of gene-transduced cells caused by the transcriptional activation of growth-promoting genes leading to myelodysplasia and gradual loss of efficacy.

In summary, of the close to 30 patients worldwide treated with gene therapy for immunodeficiency disorders, significant clinical improvement has been observed in many. However, severe and even life-endangering adverse consequences have been encountered with certain viral vectors and protocols. Additional clinical information from long-term observation and new clinical studies will be important for a clearer assessment of clinical benefit.

Hematologic Disorders

Additional inherited diseases treated in recent years with gene therapy have included mostly hematologic conditions in which a low amount of a secreted protein could reverse the clinical phenotype, and partial success has been achieved in various inherited bleeding disorders. However, the response has not usually been sustained or has been accompanied by adverse reactions, such as increases in hepatic enzymes in the case of hepatic artery administration.

Cardiovascular and Pulmonary Conditions

The most common cardiovascular-related syndromes are related to atherosclerotic arterial occlusive disease. To overcome arterial occlusions, especially when conventional treatments fail to improve blood supply to the ischemic organs, therapeutic angiogenesis has been advocated as a therapeutic option. Transfer of genes encoding angiogenic growth factors (vascular endothelial growth factor and fibroblast growth factor), delivered by nonviral and viral vectors, has been tested in phase II and III studies in patients with coronary and peripheral arterial disease.

Cystic Fibrosis

Experimental protocols for gene therapy for cystic fibrosis (CF) (Chapter 89) have been implemented since 1990. The cystic fibrosis transmembrane conductance regulator (CFTR) protein is mutated in patients with CF. Transducing the epithelium of the nasal and bronchial tree is potentially feasible through nonsystemic approaches. Nonviral gene therapy methods that deliver a copy of the *CFTR* gene to the airway of CF patients have been developed. Several placebo-controlled clinical trials of liposome-mediated *CFTR* gene transfer to the nasal epithelium have confirmed its safety and demonstrated variable degrees of functional correction.[1] In addition, several clinical studies have assessed the potential of retrovectors, adenovectors, and AAV vectors for gene therapy for CF.[2,3] With both nonviral and viral delivery systems, there were only mild side effects. However, the long-term clinical benefit has been marginal. Improved vectors are being assessed in preclinical studies.

Cancer

Gene therapy approaches to treatment of cancer have been based on perturbation of pathways in the tumorigenesis process (Chapter 185), which has led to diverse anticancer gene therapy approaches.

Tumor-Specific Expression of Anticancer Proteins

Certain promoters are activated in many types of tumors (e.g., human telomerase or survivin), whereas others are activated in specific types of tumors (probasin in prostate cancer, ceruloplasmin in ovarian cancer, HER2 in breast cancer, carcinoembryonic antigen in colon cancer). Targeting of tumor-specific promoters constitutes a rational basis for anticancer therapeutics, which may fall into different categories, including cellular proteins that are involved in apoptosis or antiproliferation, or both (e.g., p53, Fas, p202, E1A, and BAX). Their expression induces tumor-specific killing. The most clinically advanced gene therapy drug against cancer is the RD adenovector expressing the human *p53* gene. This therapy (Gendicine) is approved in China for the treatment of patients with head and neck squamous cell carcinoma by direct administration into the tumor bed. According to the results emanating from China[4] and clinical phase III studies in the United States, this treatment has therapeutic benefits. Additionally, the use of suicide genes is one of the most promising approaches for cancer gene therapy.

DNA Vaccines

Human clinical trials using DNA vaccines against cancer (as well as infectious diseases) have been conducted in the past several years. Although these studies have consistently demonstrated the safety of such DNA vaccines, the resultant immunologic responses have not been encouraging, including lack of or low antibody response detected in most cases and somewhat weak cellular response in some trials. Disappointing results were also reported with the use of DNA vaccines against HIV and other infectious agents. However, new methods are currently being assessed for DNA vaccination, such as electroporation and new generations of gene guns. Tumor gene knockdown has been used in many different clinical studies. This approach involves the use of antisense oligonucleotides (ASOs) to target genes involved in cancer progression. ASOs inhibit translation through a mechanism that involves the formation of an mRNA-ASO duplex, which leads to RNase-H-mediated cleavage of the target mRNA. The disappointing lack of clinical efficacy for some first-generation ASOs indicates that challenges remain to be confronted and overcome.

RNA Interference

RNA interference regulates gene expression by a highly precise mechanism of sequence-directed gene silencing at the stage of translation by degrading specific messenger RNAs or by blocking its translation into protein. Research into the use of RNAi for therapeutic applications has gained considerable momentum. It has been suggested that many of the novel disease-associated targets that have been identified are amenable to conventional small molecule drug blockade and can potentially be targeted with RNAi. In the coming years, the concept of RNAi will be actively translated into a therapeutic option, with numerous phase I and II trials currently being conducted. Local and systemic approaches of delivery are under development.

Gene Therapy Ethics and Regulation

There are major differences in the ethical issues pertaining to somatic as opposed to germline gene therapy. In most countries, germline gene therapy, because of its potential effect on future generations, is appropriately outlawed. Our limited understanding of the complex interactions that have shaped human evolution, together with societal and cultural considerations, precludes the possibility of conceiving of responsible programs for germline genetic modifications in humans, as well as germline gene therapy approaches. However, somatic gene therapy is encouraged and performed worldwide under strict regulatory authority with remarkable congruency of guidelines in different countries and global constituencies. The concept that gene therapies constitute novel biologic drugs provides an appropriate framework for regulatory oversight.

Future Directions

In recent years, the genetic payload/transgene and delivery systems have experienced significant improvements. Rapid advances in understanding the molecular underpinnings of pathogenetic processes have facilitated translation to novel biologically based therapeutics, including gene therapy approaches. The major developments in recent years have been in the design of new types of transgenes. The discovery of RNAi (see E-Fig. 43-1) and the biogenesis and potential role of siRNA, including their apparent efficiency in the knockdown of gene expression, suggests that these developments will revolutionize gene therapy in the coming years. Viral infections still pose a major threat to humanity. Because viruses are developing resistance to the current available therapies, there is an ongoing battle between the viruses and our ability to develop novel strategies to fight them. In vitro and in vivo experiments demonstrate the effectiveness of RNAi in inhibiting many viruses that cause severe health and economic problems, including respiratory syncytial, hepatitis C, and influenza viruses.

The tragic occurrence of tumors in patients after retroviral vector-based treatment of X-SCID has motivated researchers to direct the integration of transgenes to specific human genomic sites. It is hoped that assessment of these transgene insertion navigation tools will reduce the random occurrence of insertional mutagenic events. In addition to the development of novel transgenes, there is progress with viral and nonviral vectors. The AAV vector has experienced significant improvement as a delivery system in recent years because of its capacity for targeting with different capsid serotypes and more efficient production, and this has resulted in high-level AAV transgene expression early after transduction. The lentivectors are safer now than in earlier generations and will be the subject of newly planned clinical trials.

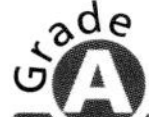

1. Lee T, Southern KW. Topical cystic fibrosis transmembrane conductance regulator gene replacement for cystic fibrosis-related lung disease. *Cochrane Database Syst Rev*. 2007;18:CD005599.
2. Moss RB, Milla C, Colombo J, et al. Repeated aerosolized AAV-CFTR for treatment of cystic fibrosis: a randomized placebo-controlled phase 2B trial. *Hum Gene Ther*. 2007;18:726-732.
3. Moss RB, Rodman D, Spencer LT, et al. Repeated adeno-associated virus serotype 2 aerosol-mediated cystic fibrosis transmembrane regulator gene transfer to the lungs of patients with cystic fibrosis: a multicenter, double-blind, placebo-controlled trial. *Chest*. 2004;125:509-521.
4. Zhang SW, Xiao SW, Liu CQ. Recombinant adenovirus-p53 gene therapy combined with radiotherapy for head and neck squamous-cell carcinoma. *Zhonghua Zhong Liu Za Zhi*. 2005;27:426-428.

SUGGESTED READINGS

Aiuti A, Cattaneo F, Galimberti S, et al. Gene therapy for immunodeficiency due to adenosine deaminase deficiency. *N Engl J Med*. 2009;360:447-458. *Gene therapy, combined with reduced-intensity conditioning, can be a safe and effective treatment for SCID in patients with ADA deficiency.*

Castanotto D, Rossi JJ. The promises and pitfalls of RNA-interference-based therapeutics. *Nature*. 2009;457:426-433. *The ability of short RNA sequences to modulate gene expression has provided a powerful tool with which to study gene function and is set to revolutionize the treatment of disease.*

Daley GQ. Stem cells: roadmap to the clinic. *J Clin Invest*. 2010;120:8-10. *Introduces a series of articles providing a balanced and realistic perspective on some of the major advances that might lead to clinical applications of stem cells in regenerative medicine.*

Davies JC, Alton EW. Gene therapy for cystic fibrosis. *Proc Am Thorac Soc*. 2010;7:408-414. *Review.*

Hyun I. The bioethics of stem cell research and therapy. *J Clin Invest*. 2010;120:71-75. *Consideration of the bioethics of human stem cell research taking into account recent scientific developments.*

Katz MG, Swain JD, Tomasulo CE, et al. Current strategies for myocardial gene delivery. *J Mol Cell Cardiol*. 2011;50:766-776. *Review.*

Kitchen SG, Zack JA. Stem cell-based approaches to treating HIV infection. *Curr Opin HIV AIDS*. 2011;6:68-73. *Review of recent trials.*

Maguire AM, High KA, Auricchio A, et al. Age-dependent effects of RPE65 gene therapy for Leber's congenital amaurosis: a phase 1 dose-escalation trial. *Lancet*. 2009;374:1597-1605. *Gene therapy has the potential to reverse disease or prevent further deterioration of vision in patients with otherwise incurable inherited retinal degeneration.*

Parmacek MS, Epstein JA. Cardiomyocyte renewal. *N Engl J Med*. 2009;361:86-88. *Thoughtful review indicating that progress toward regenerative therapy for heart disease should be based on a sound formulation of cardiac cell and developmental biology.*

VII

PRINCIPLES OF IMMUNOLOGY AND INFLAMMATION

44

THE INNATE AND ADAPTIVE IMMUNE SYSTEMS

JÖRG J. GORONZY AND CORNELIA M. WEYAND

GENERAL PRINCIPLES OF THE IMMUNE SYSTEM

The immune system has evolved as a complex network of molecules, cells, and organs to defend against pathogenic microorganisms and noninfectious foreign substances. Beyond its role in host protection, it regulates tissue homeostasis and tissue repair. Cells of the immune system identify and remove injured, dead, and malignant cells. Immune system cells derive from hematopoietic stem cells in the bone marrow, circulate in the blood and lymph, form complex microstructures in specialized lymphoid organs, and infiltrate virtually every tissue. These cells express characteristic profiles of surface molecules, also referred to as *cluster of differentiation* (CD) molecules, with which they sense soluble or cell-bound ligands in their microenvironment. Molecular structure, ligands, and main functions of more than 300 molecules have been defined; a selected list is given in E-Table 44-1. The anatomic organization of immune system cells in lymphoid organs and their ability to circulate throughout the body and to migrate between blood and lymphoid tissues are crucial components of host defense. On activation, these cells transcribe and release cytokines, small soluble proteins that communicate between cells within the immune system or between immune system cells and cells in other tissues (Table 44-1).

Innate and Adaptive Immunity

Principally, host protection is accomplished by two types of immunity: innate and adaptive. The *innate immune system* is present in all vertebrates and is widely conserved among species. It provides the first line of defense and functions through immediate responses that use preformed proteins and preexisting cells. *Innate immunity,* broadly defined, includes physical barriers, such as epithelial layers, and chemical impediments, such as antimicrobial substances at these surfaces. Using a narrower definition, the innate immune system mediates nonspecific protection through a diverse set of cells, including monocytes, macrophages, dendritic cells, natural killer (NK) cells, eosinophils, basophils, neutrophils, and mast cells. A variety of chemical mediators, such as members of the complement system, acute phase reactants, and cytokines, contribute to inflammatory responses that develop to prevent tissue invasion by pathogens. The need for immediacy is irreconcilable with selectivity and adaptivity. Response patterns of the innate immune system are broad, and collateral tissue damage is often unavoidable. Despite the lack of specificity, innate immunity is highly effective; microbial invasion is frequently controlled, and pathogens are often eliminated. The pathogenicity of microorganisms is largely related to their ability to resist and overcome the first line of defense mounted by the innate immune system.

If invading microorganisms succeed in escaping the host's nonspecific defense mechanisms, a second line of defense, *adaptive immunity,* secures host survival. Adaptive immune responses depend on innate immunity for supplementation and augmentation and to provide crucial information about the nature of the attacker. The term *adaptive* relates to the ability of the system to adapt to the microbial challenge; it is also called *acquired* or *specific immunity*. The adaptive immune system has unique attributes, such as specificity, diversity, memory, specialization, tolerance, and homeostasis.

Immune specificity relies on two major cell types: B lymphocytes and T lymphocytes. These cells possess receptors that specifically recognize antigenic determinants and that distinguish subtle differences. To contend with the gamut of possible antigens, the adaptive immune system requires an enormous spectrum of specific receptors. An extremely high degree of discriminatory specificity is achieved by clonal distribution of the recognition structures; each individual T cell and B cell expresses a unique receptor.

The diversity of the adaptive immune system is not inherited; it is acquired somatically and is called the *lymphocyte repertoire*. The frequency of T or B cells in the naïve repertoire specific for a particular antigenic determinant is less than 1 in 10^5 and is therefore extremely low. On recognition of an antigen, the adaptive immune system reacts with clonal expansion of these infrequent antigen-responsive cells to build up a line of defense. Proliferating antigen-specific cells acquire new properties, including effector functions and the ability to function as memory cells. Specificity and memory are prerequisites for heightened reactivity to recurrent or persistent infections and also provide the basis for vaccination. Another example of the adaptive power of the specific immune system lies in specialized responses to different classes of microbes (e.g., parasites vs. viral infections). Specialization is a consequence of differentiation during the evolution of the immune response; it results in selection of the most appropriate effector pathway for a particular microbial challenge.

Molding the responding lymphocyte population to the antigenic profile of the invading pathogen inevitably involves the risk of generating cells that respond to self-antigens. To prevent injury to the host, the adaptive immune system discriminates between self and nonself. Nonreactivity to self is actively acquired and is maintained by several mechanisms, collectively called *self-tolerance*. Distinguishing self and nonself is individualized for each host and requires the selection of an individual set of nonself-reactive receptors. Consequently, the outcome of self/nonself discrimination is not transferred from generation to generation and is devoid of evolutionary pressure. In contrast, innate immunity relies on genetically programmed recognition structures and receptors that have been evolutionarily selected to recognize pathogens but not self.

Together with the capability of generating tremendous diversity and specificity, the adaptive immune system has a built-in ability to self-limit responses and to regain homeostasis. This mechanism is crucial in preventing excessive immune responses and in providing space for emerging lymphocytes that are required for a new specific immune response.

Leukocyte Migration and Homing

Mobility of the cellular constituents is fundamental to innate and adaptive immunity. To home to the site of tissue injury or to enter lymphoid organs, cells use a multistep process of adherence and activation. Initially, leukocytes roll on activated endothelial cells, activate chemokine receptors, increase adhesiveness, and eventually migrate through the endothelial layer across a chemokine gradient. The selectin family of proteins mediates the first steps of leukocyte migration. Selectins have a lectin domain and bind to carbohydrate ligands. L-selectin is present on virtually all leukocytes; P-selectin and E-selectin are expressed on activated endothelial cells, and P-selectin is also stored in platelets. Selectins capture floating leukocytes and initiate their attachment and rolling on activated endothelial cells. To transform attachment and rolling into firm adhesion, the concerted action of chemokines, chemokine receptors, and integrins is necessary. Integrins are heterodimers formed of many different α chains and β chains; different α/β combinations are expressed on different cell subsets. Only after activation can integrins interact with ligands on endothelial cells. Activation involves modification of the cytoplasmic domain of the β chain, which leads to a structural change of the extracellular domains. This process is termed *inside-out signaling*. The last step of homing is transendothelial migration. Here, the firmly attached leukocytes migrate through the endothelial cell monolayer and the basement membrane.

INNATE IMMUNE SYSTEM

Principles of Innate Immune System Activation

Activation by Pattern Recognition Receptors

The strategy of the innate immune system is to focus on the recognition of a few highly conserved structures that are preserved in large groups of microorganisms shared by entire classes of pathogens and essential for their survival and pathogenicity. The system uses a few hundred receptor structures to identify microbial invaders. This set of receptors is insufficient to cover the entire spectrum of antigens expressed on infectious agents. Structures recognized by pattern recognition receptors (PRRs) are collectively referred to as *pathogen-associated molecular patterns* (PAMPs). Examples of PAMPs are bacterial lipopolysaccharides, peptidoglycans, mannans, bacterial DNA, double-stranded RNA, and glucans.

PAMP-binding receptor families share structural characteristics, such as leucine-rich repeated domains, calcium-dependent lectin domains, and scavenger-receptor protein domains. They can be secreted to act as opsonins; the best-characterized receptor of this class is the mannose-binding lectin that binds to microbial carbohydrates and activates the lectin pathway of complement activation. Another functional class of PRRs is expressed on the

TABLE 44-1 CYTOKINES AND CYTOKINE FUNCTION

CYTOKINES	MAJOR PRODUCER CELLS	PRINCIPAL ACTION
HEMATOPOIETIN FAMILY		
IL-2	T cells	Proliferation of T cells, B cells, and NK cells
IL-3	T cells	Early hematopoiesis
IL-4	T cells, mast cells	B-cell activation, IgE switch, inhibition of T_H1 cells
IL-5	T cells, mast cells	Eosinophil growth and differentiation
IL-6	Macrophages, endothelial cells	T-cell and B-cell growth and differentiation, induction of acute phase proteins
IL-7	Bone marrow, thymic epithelium	Growth of pre-B cells and pre-T cells
IL-9	T cells	Stimulation of mast cells and T_H2 cells
IL-11	Stromal fibroblasts	Hematopoiesis
IL-13	T cells	B-cell growth and differentiation, inhibition of T_H1 cells and macrophages
G-CSF	Fibroblasts and monocytes	Neutrophil development and differentiation
IL-15	Non-T cells	Growth of T cells and NK cells
GM-CSF	Macrophages, T cells	Growth and differentiation of myelomonocytic lineage cells
INTERFERON FAMILY		
IFN-α	Leukocytes	Antiviral; increases MHC class I expression
IFN-β	Fibroblasts	Antiviral; increases MHC class I expression
IFN-γ	T cells, NK cells	Macrophage activation; increases expression of MHC molecules, Ig class switching, inhibition of T_H2 cells
TNF FAMILY		
TNF-α	Macrophages, NK cells, T cells	Induction of pro-inflammatory cytokines, endothelial cell activation, apoptosis
TNF-β (LT-α)	T cells, B cells	Cell death, endothelial activation, lymphoid organ development
LT-β	T cells, B cells	Cell death, lymphoid organ development
OTHERS		
TGF-β	Monocytes, T cells	Anti-inflammatory; inhibits cell growth, induces IgA secretion
IL-1α, IL-1β	Macrophages, endothelial cells	Acute phase response, fever, macrophage activation, costimulation
IL-10	T cells, macrophages	Suppression of macrophage functions
IL-12	Macrophages, dendritic cells	NK cell activation, T_H1 cell differentiation
IL-16	T cells, mast cells, eosinophils	Chemoattractant for CD4 T cells, monocytes, and eosinophils
IL-17	CD4 memory cells	Cytokine production by epithelia, endothelia, and fibroblasts
IL-18	Macrophages	IFN-γ production by T cells and NK cells
IL-23	Macrophages, dendritic cells	T_H17 cell differentiation

CD = cluster of differentiation; G-CSF = granulocyte colony-stimulating factor; GM-CSF = granulocyte-macrophage colony-stimulating factor; IFN = interferon; Ig = immunoglobulin; IL = interleukin; LT = lymphotoxin; MHC = major histocompatibility complex; NK = natural killer; TGF = transforming growth factor; T_H = helper T lymphocyte; TNF = tumor necrosis factor.

surface of phagocytes and facilitates endocytosis. The macrophage mannose receptor and the macrophage scavenger receptor are the best-known examples. These receptors are essential for the clearance of microbes from the circulation. A third class of PRRs controls cell activation (Fig. 44-1); the most important members are toll-like receptors (TLRs). TLRs are expressed on either the cell membrane or the endosome to sense extra- or intracellular pathogens. They function by regulating the activity of nuclear factor-κB (NF-κB) and interferon signaling pathways and control the expression of many inflammatory cytokines and cell surface molecules. Prominent members of the TLR family are TLR4, which, in conjunction with other cell surface molecules, binds bacterial lipopolysaccharides; TLR2, which recognizes bacterial peptidoglycans and lipoproteins; and TLR9, which binds to bacterial DNA motifs.

PRRs used by the innate immune system are fundamentally different from the antigen-specific receptors generated in the adaptive immune system. The receptors of the innate immune system are encoded in the germline and are under evolutionary pressure. They are shared by many different cells, including macrophages and dendritic cells, and are not clonally distributed (i.e., different cell types display identical specificity). Finally, PRRs do not recognize self, so they do not carry the risk for autoimmune injury, although exceptions to this rule (e.g., recognition of heat shock proteins) have been described.

Regulation by Major Histocompatibility Complex Class I–Recognizing Receptors

Several cells of the innate immune system require reversal of inhibition to enter the activation cycle. Loss of inhibitory signals in constitutively activated cells is particularly important for NK cells. NK cells are poised to attack, but they are held in check by inhibitory receptors that recognize major histocompatibility complex (MHC) class I or MHC class I–like molecules. The observation that NK cells kill target cells lacking MHC class I molecules led to the *missing-self hypothesis*. The principle that immune cells are kept in check by recognizing self-determinants is appreciated now as fundamental in the immune system.

Provision of negative signals is closely linked to the recognition of MHC class I molecules. Currently, three types of MHC class I–recognizing receptors are known. C-type lectin receptors (CD159) recognizing human leukocyte antigen E (HLA-E) and killer immunoglobulin-like receptors (CD158) specific for HLA-C and, to a lesser extent, HLA-A and HLA-B are expressed predominantly on NK cells. Immunoglobulin-like transcript receptors (CD85) are more widely expressed. Immunoglobulin-like transcript receptor 2 is expressed on NK cells, B cells, monocytes, dendritic cells, and macrophages. Immunoglobulin-like transcript receptors 3 and 4 are encountered on monocytes, dendritic cells, and macrophages. By screening cell surfaces for the expression of MHC class I molecules, the innate immune system collects information about the intactness of tissues, emphasizing the crucial role of MHC class I molecules as markers of tissue integrity. Recognition of MHC class I molecules provides a negative signal that suppresses cell activity. However, all receptor families also include stimulatory isoforms that mediate an activating signal. The balance between these opposing signals is finely tuned, ultimately determining whether innate immunity is initiated.

Activation by Fc Receptors

Most cells of the innate immune system possess immunoglobulin crystallizable fragment (Fc) receptors (FcRs) and can bind antibodies attached to antigens (see Fig. 44-1). FcRs specifically interact with the constant region (Fc portion) of immunoglobulins. Each member of the FcR family displays specificity for one or a few immunoglobulin isotypes. The isotype of the antibody determines which cell type is activated in a given response. Triggering of most FcRs transmits activating signals; however, inhibitory FcRs do exist. Phagocytic cells, such as neutrophils and macrophages, are equipped with FcγRs that are activated by immunoglobulin G (IgG) antibodies,

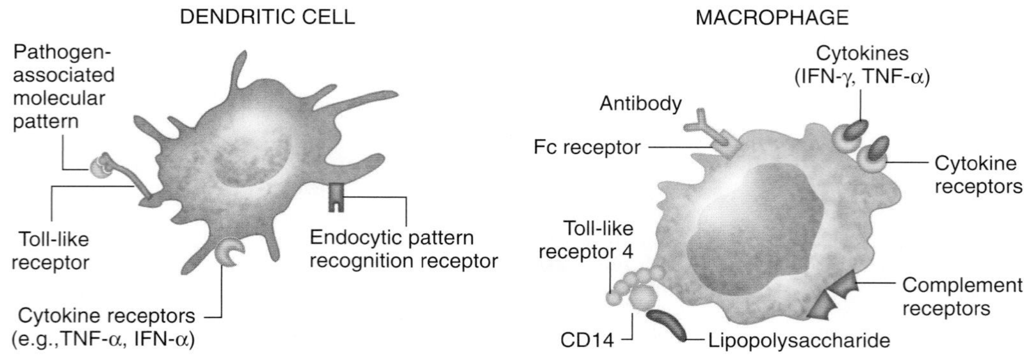

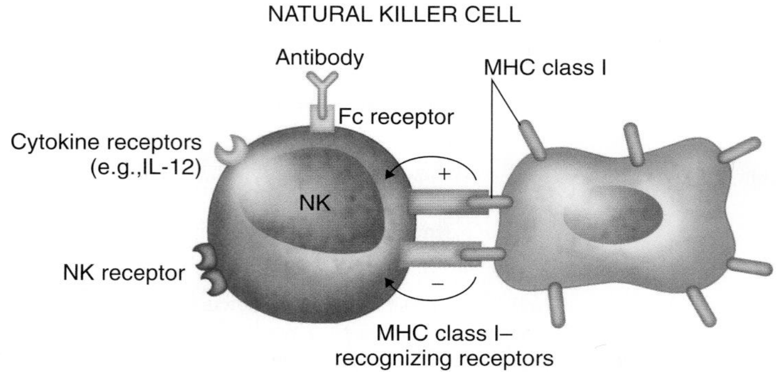

FIGURE 44-1. Activation pathways in the innate immune system. Cells of the innate immune system recognize microorganisms and tissue damage caused by either infection or malignancy. Dendritic cells and monocytes/macrophages use a multitude of receptors to sense constituents of pathogens—often bacterial molecules common to many classes of microorganisms—and respond to cytokines and endogenous stimulators released from injured cells. Binding of complement factors can also trigger cell activation. Self-recognition of major histocompatibility complex (MHC) class I molecules by natural killer (NK) cells can deliver positive or negative signals. Lack of MHC class I molecules on the target cell surface activates NK cells to kill the target. IFN = interferon; IL = interleukin; TNF = tumor necrosis factor.

particularly IgG1. Ligation of an FcγR triggers phagocytosis of the antigen, activation of respiratory burst, and induction of cytotoxicity. On NK cells, FcγRs initiate antibody-dependent cell-mediated cytotoxicity. In this process, the cytolytic machinery of NK cells is triggered by the binding of IgG1-coated or IgG3-coated target cells. FcRs on mast cells, basophils, and activated eosinophils are specific for IgE. In contrast to other FcRs, they bind monomeric antibody molecules with extremely high affinity. Cross-linking of the constitutively cell surface–bound IgE induces cell activation and the release of cytoplasmic granules.

Activation by Cytokines

Generally, cells of the innate immune system are exquisitely sensitive to the action of cytokines. Cytokines are soluble, low-molecular-weight glycoproteins that derive from many tissue sources. They are chemical messengers that convey information between cells, regulate the differentiation of effector cells, and modulate immune responses. Important examples of cytokine-mediated signals in the innate immune system are interferon-γ (IFN-γ), produced by NK cells, which is the most potent activator of macrophages; interleukin-6 (IL-6), which induces acute phase reactants; IL-12, IL-23, and IL-27, derived from macrophages and dendritic cells, which coordinate the development of adaptive immune responses; IL-15, which regulates the activity and proliferation of NK cells; and type I IFN secreted at the time of injury, which activates NK cells and dendritic cells (see Fig. 44-1).

Cellular Elements of the Innate Immune System

Monocytes and Macrophages

Monocytes circulate in the peripheral blood with a half-life of 1 to 3 days. Macrophages arise from monocytes that have migrated out of the circulation and have proliferated and differentiated in tissue. Tissue macrophages are common in lymphoid organs, but they are also present in connective tissues, such as the perivascular space, and in the lining of serous cavities (pleura and peritoneum). Specialized macrophages include alveolar macrophages in the lung, Kupffer cells in the liver, osteoblasts in bone, microglia in the central nervous system, and type A synoviocytes in the synovial membrane. Macrophages are activated through the triggering of PRRs or FcRs, and they respond vigorously to IFN-γ (see Fig. 44-1). They secrete myriad products, including hydrolytic enzymes, reactive oxygen species, cytokines (tumor necrosis factor-α [TNF-α], IL-1, IL-6, IL-10, IL-12, IL-15, and IL-18), and chemokines. They phagocytose and expose the engulfed microorganism to a wide range of toxic intracellular molecules, including reactive oxygen species, nitric oxide, antimicrobial cationic proteins and peptides, and lysosomal enzymes. In addition to attacking microbial organisms, macrophages remove dying and dead host cells. They recognize molecules expressed on apoptotic cells and eliminate them without initiating an inflammatory response. Finally, they play a crucial role in the recruitment of adaptive immune responses. After capturing antigen, they function as antigen-presenting cells for T lymphocytes. In this function, however, they are less important than dendritic cells.

Dendritic Cells/Langerhans Cells

Dendritic cells represent the major cell type linking the innate and adaptive immune systems. Their primary function is the presentation of antigens to T cells. They are the only cell type that can activate naïve T cells and initiate adaptive immune responses. Two major lineages of dendritic cells exist: myeloid and plasmacytoid dendritic cells. When positioned in the skin, myeloid dendritic cells are referred to as *Langerhans cells.* They constantly endocytose and digest extracellular molecules but usually do not display these molecules at a sufficient density to activate T cells. On receiving a stimulatory signal, they convert into highly efficient antigen-presenting cells. Activation signals can derive from PAMPs or from host cells that react to injury and secrete mediators such as TNF-α or heat shock proteins (see Fig. 44-1). Activation causes dendritic cells to change their expression profile of chemokine receptors and to migrate from the local tissue to lymph nodes. In parallel, they begin expressing accessory molecules on their cell surface, a prerequisite for T-cell activation, and to secrete cytokines (e.g., IFN-α by plasmacytoid dendritic cells, or IL-12 and IL-23 by myeloid dendritic cells) that orchestrate T-cell differentiation. When they arrive in the T-cell zone of the lymph node, they display MHC–peptide complexes with peptides derived from endocytosed and digested antigens. With high surface expression of MHC and accessory molecules, dendritic cells optimize the process of antigen presentation and T-cell priming (Fig. 44-2).

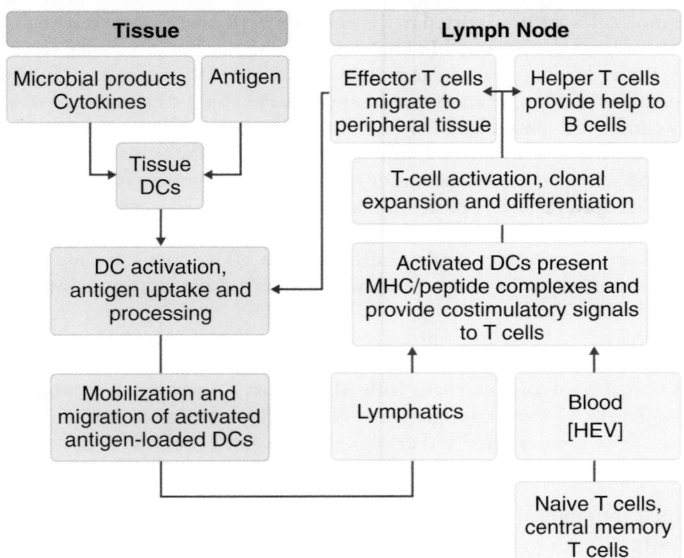

FIGURE 44-2. Interface between the innate and adaptive immune systems. Dendritic cells (DCs) reside in the tissue, where they recognize and ingest antigens. If they also receive an activating signal (e.g., by binding pathogen-associated molecular patterns or cytokines), they enter lymph vessels and travel to regional lymph nodes. In parallel, they mature into efficient antigen-presenting cells that express high levels of cell surface major histocompatibility complex (MHC) and costimulatory molecules. In the T-cell zones, DCs present the antigen engulfed in the peripheral tissue to prime naïve T cells. By capturing and transporting antigens and priming naïve T cells, DCs integrate responses of the innate and adaptive immune systems. HEV = high endothelial venules.

Natural Killer Cells

NK cells provide the first line of defense against viral infections and other intracellular pathogens while adaptive responses are generated. NK cells are sensitized by cytokines released from macrophages and dendritic cells. They function by secreting cytokines, mainly IFN-γ, which activate macrophages and other cells. They also are poised to kill virus-infected cells. NK cells induce apoptosis of the target cells by injecting pore-forming enzymes and granzymes. One of the interesting features of NK biology is the activation of these lymphocytes when MHC class I molecules on target cells are lost (see Fig. 44-1). NK cells are important in tumor surveillance because they are able to kill MHC class I–deficient tumor cells that are no longer susceptible to adaptive immune responses.

Neutrophils, Eosinophils, and Basophils

Neutrophils

Neutrophils are the most abundant circulating white blood cells. They are recruited rapidly to inflammatory sites and are capable of phagocytosing and digesting microbes. Activation of neutrophils and phagocytosis is facilitated through the triggering of FcRs or complement receptors. During phagocytosis, the pathogen is first surrounded by the phagocyte membrane, and then internalized in membrane-bound vesicles known as *phagosomes*. Phagosomes fuse with lysosomes, which contain enzymes, proteins, and peptides that inactivate and digest microbes. Beyond their phagocytic capability, neutrophils produce a variety of toxic products. The release of toxic products is known as the *respiratory burst* because it is accompanied by an increase in oxygen consumption. During the respiratory burst, oxygen radicals are generated by lysosomal reduced nicotinamide adenine dinucleotide phosphate (NADPH) oxidases. Neutrophils are short-lived cells, dying soon after they have been activated. Secretion of their granule products, in particular enzymes (myeloperoxidase, elastase, collagenase, and lysozyme), causes direct cellular injury and damages macromolecules at inflamed sites.

Eosinophils

In contrast to macrophages and neutrophils, eosinophils (Chapter 173) are only weakly phagocytic. They are potent cytotoxic effector cells against parasites. Their major effector mechanism is the secretion of various cationic proteins (major basic protein, eosinophil cationic protein, and eosinophil-derived neurotoxin). These proteins are released into the extracellular space, where they directly destroy the invading microorganism, but they can also damage host tissue.

Basophils

Basophils and tissue mast cells are important reservoirs of inflammatory mediators such as histamines, prostaglandins, leukotrienes, and selected cytokines. Basophils and tissue mast cells have high-affinity receptors for monomeric IgE. They play a role in atopic allergies, in which allergens bind immunoglobulin (IgE) and cross-link FcεRs. Their function in normal immune responses is incompletely understood.

Soluble Factors in Innate Defenses

Effector functions of the cells of the innate immune system are enhanced by many circulating proteins. A particularly important contribution derives from the complement system, a group of plasma enzymes and regulatory proteins that are converted from inactive pro-enzymes to active enzymes in a controlled and systematic cascade, which is crucial in linking microbial recognition to cellular effector function (Chapter 47). Mannose-binding lectin circulates in the plasma, functioning as an opsonin, and is involved in activation of the complement pathway. C-reactive protein, an acute phase protein, participates in opsonization by binding to bacterial phospholipids. Finally, the innate immune system could not work without the cytokines that regulate the recruitment and activation of leukocytes (see Table 44-1). Cells of the innate immune system are not only the principal producers of such cytokines but also their targets.

ADAPTIVE IMMUNE SYSTEM

Principles of Adaptive Immune System Activation: Recognition of Antigen

Structure of Antigen-Specific Receptors

The innate immune system recognizes structural patterns that are common in the microbial world, whereas the adaptive immune system is designed to respond to the entire continuum of antigens. This goal is achieved through two principal types of antigen recognition receptors: antibodies and T-cell receptors (TCRs). Antibodies are expressed as cell surface receptors on B cells or are secreted. They recognize conformational structures formed by the tertiary configuration of proteins. In contrast, α/β TCRs fit specifically to epitopes formed by a small linear peptide embedded into MHC molecules on the surface of antigen-presenting cells.

Antibodies consist of two identical heavy chains and two identical light chains, which are covalently linked by disulfide bonds. The amino (N)-terminal domain of each chain is variable and represents the recognition structure that interacts with the antigen. Each antibody has two binding arms of identical specificity. The carboxy (C)-terminal ends of the heavy and light chains form the constant region, which defines the subclass of the antibody (κ or λ for light chains; IgM, IgA, IgD, IgE, or IgG for heavy chains). Additional subclasses can be distinguished for IgG and IgA. The constant region of antibodies includes the Fc region. Fc regions can polymerize (IgA) or pentamerize in the presence of a J (joining) chain (IgM). Fc regions are also the ligand for the FcRs on cells of the innate immune system.

TCRs are dimers of α chains and β chains or of γ chains and δ chains, each of which contains three complementary-determining binding sites in the N-terminal domain. These complementary-determining sites define the specificity. α/β TCRs exclusively recognize peptide fragments in the context of MHC molecules. γ/δ TCRs are more variable and can recognize certain glycolipid antigens in the context of MHC-like molecules or even unprocessed antigens, functioning similar to antibodies. The repertoires of antibodies and TCRs are extremely diverse and have been estimated in the human to account for 10^8 to 10^9 unique (of 10^{15} possible) combinations. This enormous diversity cannot be genetically encoded; it must be acquired. Its foundation consists of fewer than 400 genes that are recombined and modified. Immunoglobulin heavy chains are formed from four gene segments encoded on chromosome 14—the variable, diversity, joining, and constant region gene segments. Also, TCR β chains and δ chains are assembled by the recombination of variable, diversity, joining, and constant region segments of TCR genes. Immunoglobulin light chains and TCR α chains and γ chains lack the diversity segment and are composed of three gene segments. During antibody or TCR rearrangement, gene segments are cut out by nucleases and spliced together at the DNA level to form linear coding units for each receptor gene. Through the combination of several different mechanisms, an enormous diversity of receptors is generated. First, the genome contains multiple forms of gene segments; each receptor or antibody uses a different combination of these gene segments. Second, the splicing process is imprecise, introducing nucleotide variations at the variable-diversity, diversity-joining, and variable-joining junctions. These inaccuracies lead to frame shifts and result in completely different amino acid sequences. Finally, random nucleotides can be inserted at the junctional region by an enzyme, deoxyribonucleotidyl transferase.

Once generated, TCR sequences remain unchanged. This rule does not apply to immunoglobulins, which can undergo editing. Immunoglobulin editing includes replacement of an entire variable region (receptor editing); class switching during immune responses, in which the variable-diversity-joining unit combines with different constant region genes (isotype switching); or somatic hypermutation, in which the antigen contact areas of the antibody undergo mutations during an immune response to improve the affinity (affinity maturation).

Antigen Processing

T cells do not recognize native antigens but rather peptide fragments that are displayed in the context of MHC class I and class II molecules. The two classes of MHC molecules are used as restriction elements by two different subsets of T cells. $CD4^+$ T cells recognize antigen peptides embedded into MHC class II molecules, whereas $CD8^+$ T cells are directed against peptides complexed with MHC class I molecules. Generally, MHC class II molecules are expressed only on specialized antigen-presenting cells, such as dendritic cells, monocytes, macrophages, and B cells. Peptides bound to MHC class II molecules derive from extracellular antigens that are captured and internalized into endosomes to be digested by proteinases, notably cathepsin. Occasionally, intracellular proteins or membrane proteins are also funneled into this pathway. MHC class II molecules are assembled in the endoplasmic reticulum in association with a protein called the *invariant chain* (Fig. 44-3). The molecules are transported to the endosome, where the invariant chain is removed from the peptide-binding cleft, making the cleft accessible to peptides derived from extracellular proteins. MHC class II molecules, stabilized by peptides of 10 to 30 amino acids, are displayed on the cell surface, where they can be recognized by $CD4^+$ T cells.

MHC class I–associated peptides are produced in the cytosol by the proteosome, a large cytoplasmic multiprotein enzyme complex (see Fig. 44-3). Specialized transporter proteins, called *transporter in antigen processing* (TAP), facilitate translocation from the cytosol to the endoplasmic reticulum. There, the peptides bind to newly formed MHC class I molecules and are transported to the cell surface, where they are recognized by antigen-specific $CD8^+$ T cells.

The nature of the antigen-processing pathway determines the sequence of events in immune responses. Extracellular antigens, in general, enter the endosomal pool and associate with MHC class II molecules to stimulate $CD4^+$ T cells. Cytosolic antigens, including antigens from intracellular infectious agents, are degraded and displayed in the context of MHC class I molecules to initiate $CD8^+$ T-cell responses.

Cellular Elements of the Adaptive Immune System

T Cells

T-Cell Development

T precursor cells are derived from hematopoietic stem cells seeded into the thymus, where all the subsequent stages of T-cell maturation occur (Fig. 44-4). Pre-T cells express two enzymes, recombinase and terminal

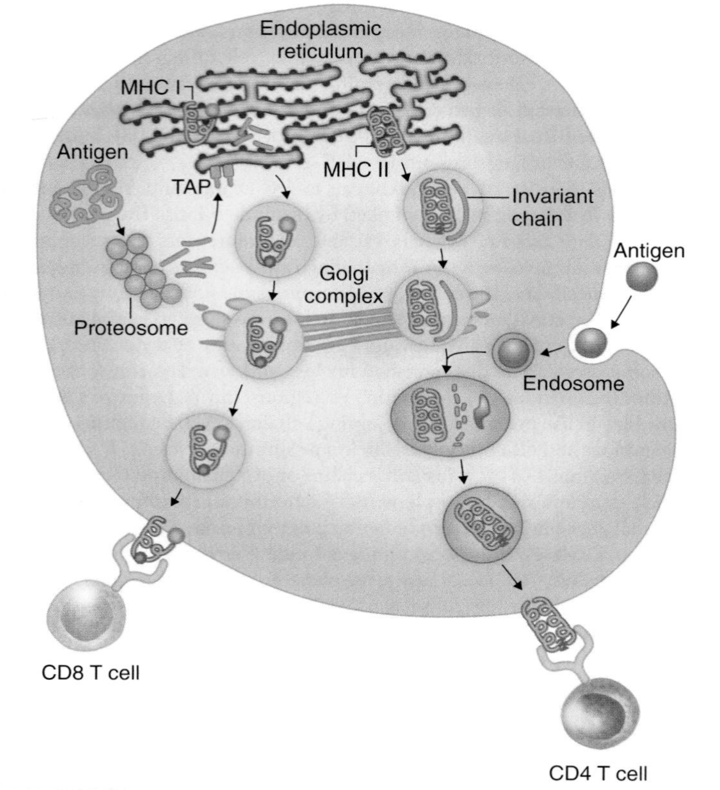

FIGURE 44-3. Pathways of antigen processing and delivery to major histocompatibility complex (MHC) molecules. Cytosolic proteins are broken down by the proteosome to generate peptide fragments, which are transported into the endoplasmic reticulum by specialized peptide transporters (TAP). After peptides are bound to MHC class I molecules, MHC-peptide complexes are released from the endoplasmic reticulum and travel to the cell surface, where they are ligands for $CD8^+$ T-cell receptors (TCRs). Extracellular foreign antigens are taken into intracellular vesicles, called *endosomes*. As the pH in the endosomes gradually decreases, proteases are activated that digest antigens into peptide fragments. After fusing with vesicles that contain MHC class II molecules, antigenic peptides are placed in the antigen-binding groove. Loaded MHC class II–peptide complexes are transported to the cell surface, where they are recognized by the TCRs of $CD4^+$ T cells.

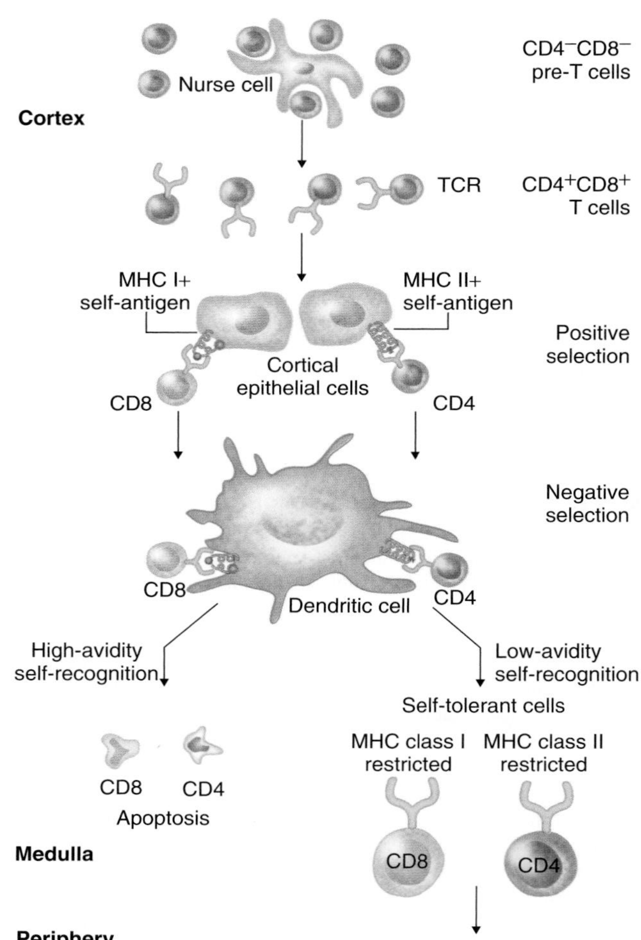

FIGURE 44-4. Maturation of T cells in the thymus. Precursors committed to the T-cell lineage arrive in the thymus and begin to rearrange their T-cell receptor (TCR) genes. Immature T cells with receptors binding to self–major histocompatibility complex (MHC) on cortical epithelial cells receive signals for survival (positive selection). At the corticomedullary junction, surviving T cells probe self-antigens presented by dendritic cells and macrophages. T cells reacting strongly to self-antigens are deleted by apoptosis (negative selection). T cells released into the periphery are tolerant toward self and recognize foreign antigens in the context of self-MHC.

deoxynucleotidyl transferase, enabling them to recombine TCR genes. The β chain of the TCR is rearranged first and is expressed together with a pre-TCR α chain. Signals from the immature TCR complex inhibit rearrangement of the second β-chain allele and induce T-cell proliferation and expression of the CD4 and CD8 molecules. Subsequently, the TCR α chain is recombined. From here, the T cell undergoes many differentiation and selection steps modulated by the thymic microenvironment. Early stages of thymocytes reside in the thymic cortex, where they mostly interact with epithelial cells. They then migrate toward the medulla, encountering dendritic cells and macrophages at the corticomedullary junction. Thymic stromal cells regulate T-cell proliferation by secreting lymphopoietic growth factors, such as IL-7. Interactions of the TCR with MHC molecules expressed on epithelial cells and on dendritic cells or macrophages determine the fate of the thymocyte. Low-avidity recognition of peptide-MHC complexes on thymic epithelial cells by the TCR results in positive selection. This recognition event rescues cells from apoptotic cell death and ensures that only T cells with functional receptors survive. Thymocytes that express a receptor not fitting any MHC antigen complex die by neglect. High-affinity interaction between the TCR and peptide-MHC complex induces apoptotic death of the recognizing T cell. This process of negative selection eliminates T cells with specificity for self-antigens and is responsible for central tolerance to many autoantigens. It has been estimated that approximately 1% of thymocytes survive the stringent selection process. While undergoing selection, T cells continue to differentiate, with orderly expression of cell surface molecules. Thymocytes expressing CD4 and CD8 molecules develop into single-positive $CD4^+$ helper T cells that have been selected on MHC class II complexes or $CD8^+$ cytotoxic T cells that are restricted to MHC class I complexes.

T-Cell Stimulation and Accessory Molecules

T-cell activation is initiated when TCR complexes recognize antigenic peptides in the context of the appropriate MHC molecule on the surface of an antigen-presenting cell. Antigen recognition by T cells results in proliferation and differentiation and triggers various effector functions. Stimulation of the TCR is not sufficient and needs to be complemented by the interaction of accessory molecules on the T cell and their ligands on the antigen-presenting cell. A spectrum of accessory molecules is known (see E-Table 44-1). The coreceptors CD4 and CD8 interact with MHC class II and class I molecules and support activation signals through the TCR. Adhesion molecules (integrins) stabilize the interactions between T cells and antigen-presenting cells. Finally, specialized costimulatory molecules provide a second signal in addition to the TCR signal. In the absence of such a second signal, T cells undergo apoptosis or are rendered nonresponsive and anergic.

The best-known and best-studied costimulatory molecule expressed on T cells is the CD28 molecule, which binds to the CD80/CD86 ligands expressed on activated antigen-presenting cells. CD28-mediated signals are mandatory for the expression of many activation markers on the responding T cells and, in particular, for the secretion of IL-2.

Signals from the TCR result in the activation of many genes and entry of the T cell into the cell cycle. The signals are transmitted by a cascade of cytoplasmic events. Cross-linking of the TCR and associated CD3 molecules results in the recruitment and activation of phosphotyrosine kinases and the phosphorylation of molecular constituents of the TCR and various adapter molecules; signals mediated through the TCR activate several biochemical pathways, which collectively lead to the activation of transcription factors that regulate gene expression.

Three major variables determine the outcome of TCR stimulation: the duration and affinity of the TCR-antigen interaction, the maturation stage of the responding T cell, and the nature of the antigen-presenting cell. Antigen-presenting cells are gatekeepers in the initiation of T-cell responses. They can upregulate the expression of accessory molecules that provide costimulatory signals. MHC-peptide complexes are particularly dense on dendritic cells, enabling them to activate naïve T cells. In contrast, memory and effector cells have a lower threshold for activation and can react to antigens presented on peripheral tissue cells.

T-Cell Differentiation and Effector Functions

T-cell activation induces T-cell proliferation, with the goal of clonally selecting and expanding antigen-specific T cells. The extent of clonal proliferation is impressive. Antigen-specific $CD8^+$ T cells expand by a factor of 50,000; $CD4^+$ T cells expand slightly less. During the phase of rapid growth, T cells differentiate from naïve T cells that are essentially devoid of effector functions into effector T cells. The transition into effector cells is associated with a fundamental shift in functional profiles. First, effector T cells have a lower activation threshold; they do not require costimulation and can scan tissues that lack professional antigen-presenting cells. Second, they switch the expression of chemokine receptors and adhesion molecules to gain access to peripheral tissues. Finally, they gain effector functions. The principal effector function of $CD8^+$ T cells is to lyse antigen-bearing target cells. $CD4^+$ T cells produce many cytokines and express cell surface molecules that are important in the activation of phagocytes and other lymphocytes. $CD8^+$ T cells are committed to differentiating into cytotoxic T cells as they emerge from the thymus; the spectrum of options for $CD4^+$ T cells is larger. Different subsets of $CD4^+$ effector T cells can be distinguished based on the preferential production of certain cytokines (see Table 44-1). T_H1 T cells produce predominantly IFN-γ and TNF-α and are involved in cell-mediated immunity, such as delayed-type hypersensitivity reactions. T_H2 T cells preferentially produce IL-4, IL-5, and IL-13, cytokines that regulate B-cell responses and the activation of eosinophils. T_H17 T cells producing IL-17 and IL-22 induce an intense inflammatory response to eliminate difficult to clear pathogens. Follicular T helper cells home to lymphoid follicles, where they express CD40 ligand (CD154) and secrete IL-21 and other cytokines to provide B-cell help. The decision as to which differentiation pathway to take is made during the early stages of T-cell activation and depends on many factors, including the cytokines produced by cells of the innate immune system in the microenvironment, the nature of costimulatory signals, and the avidity of the TCR–MHC antigen interaction. Lineage development is generally correlated with the expression of specific transcription factors (T-bet for T_H1 cells, GATA3 for T_H2 cells, or RORγt for T_H17 cells). Lineage commitment is not absolute and is not terminal, and transition between different effector types is possible.

Cytotoxic T-cell effector functions are also triggered by antigen recognition by the TCR. On recognizing the appropriate MHC class I–peptide complex, $CD8^+$ T cells induce apoptosis in target cells. The T cell polarizes toward the area of antigen contact; specialized lytic granules are clustered in the contact area. A pore-forming protein, perforin, is released from the lytic granules and inserted into the target cell membrane. Proteases (granzymes) are injected into the target cells to initiate the apoptotic process by activating enzyme cascades. Mechanisms deployed by $CD8^+$ T cells are essentially identical to those of NK cells. $CD4^+$ T cells can also induce apoptosis, but by a different mechanism from $CD8^+$ T cells. Upon activation, they express cell surface molecules such as Fas ligand (CD178) and TRAIL, which initiate the apoptotic cascade selectively in cells expressing the respective ligands Fas (CD95) or the death receptors DR4 and DR5.

Regulatory T Cells

Depending on their cytokine profile, $CD4^+$ T cells have the ability to cross-regulate each other, influence T-cell differentiation, and suppress T-cell effector activity. Classic examples of T cells with regulatory activity cells generated during the normal immune response are IL-10– and transforming growth factor-β (TGF-β)–producing cells. In addition, specialized subsets of regulatory T (Treg) cells are characterized by expression of the transcription factor forkhead box P3 (Foxp3). Naturally occurring $Foxp3^+$ Treg cells are generated during T-cell development in the thymus and recognize self-antigens. $Foxp3^+$ Treg cells can also arise from conventional $CD4^+$ T cells in the periphery. Phenotypically and functionally, natural and inducible Treg cells are indistinguishable; their development and function depend on Foxp3, and they are able to suppress T-cell expansion and constitutively express several cell surface markers. However, none of these markers is specific for Treg, as activated T cells can also express them. Treg cells are important in peripheral tolerance, controlling the expansion of autoreactive T cells, and they also play a role in immune responses to pathogens by virtue of their ability to suppress T-cell effector function. Despite extensive studies in various models, the mechanism by which Treg cells functions in vivo remains poorly understood.

T-Cell Homeostasis

Effective immunity depends on the ability of the immune system to generate large numbers of antigen-specific T cells rapidly, yet the space in the T-cell compartment is limited. To avoid competition for space and resources and to prevent perturbation of T-cell diversity by lifelong exposure to antigens, the adaptive immune system employs several counterbalancing mechanisms. In the later stages of the activation process, a strong negative signal derives from interaction of the T-cell molecule cytotoxic T-lymphocyte antigen (CTLA)-4 (CD152) with CD80/CD86 on antigen-presenting cells. In addition, T cells undergo activation-induced cell death. Activated CD4$^+$ T cells begin to secrete Fas ligand and acquire sensitivity to Fas-mediated death, inducing apoptotic suicide and fratricide in neighboring T cells. These mechanisms impose constraints in the early stages of the T-cell antigen response. Other mechanisms control the rapid decline of expanded antigen-specific T cells when elimination of the antigen has been achieved. Removal of the driving antigen causes a deprivation of cytokines and costimulatory molecules, and growth factor–deprived T cells die from apoptosis. It has been estimated that only 5% of the antigen-expanded population survives after antigen clearance.

B Lymphocytes

B-Cell Development

B cells are generated in the bone marrow. Supported by a specialized microenvironment of nonlymphoid stromal cells, lymphoid stem cells differentiate into distinctive B-lineage cells. Driven by chemokines (stromal cell–derived factor 1) and cytokines (IL-7), precursor B cells enter a process of tightly controlled sequential rearrangements of heavy chain and light chain immunoglobulin genes. On pre-B cells, the membrane μ chain is associated with a surrogate light chain to form a pre-B-cell receptor (BCR). Signals provided through this receptor induce proliferation of a progeny that subsequently rearranges different light chain gene segments.

It is estimated that only 10% of B cells generated in the bone marrow reach the circulating pool. Losses are mostly due to negative selection and clonal deletion of immature B cells that express receptors directed against self-antigens. Cross-linking of surface IgM by multivalent self-antigens causes immature B cells to die. Such self-reactive B cells can be rescued from death by replacing the light chain with a newly rearranged light chain that is no longer self-reactive (receptor editing). On maturation, B cells begin to express surface IgD. B cells positive for IgD and IgM are exported from the bone marrow and seed peripheral lymphoid tissues (Fig. 44-5).

B-Cell Stimulation

Mature B cells are activated by soluble and cell-bound antigens to develop into antibody-secreting effector cells. B cells respond to a large variety of antigens, including proteins, polysaccharides, and lipids. Binding of antigen to cell surface IgM molecules induces BCR clustering. In addition to the antigen-binding immunoglobulin, the BCR comprises two proteins, Ig-α and Ig-β. The Ig-α/Ig-β heterodimer functions to transduce a signal and initiates the intracellular signaling cascade. The composition of the BCR, with a ligand-binding and a signal-transducing unit, and the signaling events that lead to gene induction are similar to those of the TCR. BCR triggering can be enhanced by coreceptors. The coreceptor complex is composed of CD81, CD19, and CD21; CD21 binds to complement fragments on opsonized antigens.

Naïve B cells require accessory signals in addition to triggering of the immunoglobulin receptor. They receive second signals either from helper T cells or from microbial components. Microbial constituents, such as bacterial polysaccharides, can induce antibody production in the absence of helper T cells (thymus-independent antigens). In the case of protein antigens (thymus-dependent antigens), the initial BCR stimulation prepares the cell for subsequent interaction with helper T cells. These activated B cells start to enter the cell cycle; upregulate cell surface molecules, such as CD80 and CD86, that provide costimulatory signals to T cells; and upregulate certain cytokine receptors. These B cells are prepared to activate helper T cells and to respond to cytokines secreted by those T cells, but they cannot differentiate into antibody-producing cells in the absence of T-cell help.

B-Cell Differentiation

Differentiation of antigen-activated B cells depends on interaction with helper T cells. B cells use their antigen receptor not only to recognize antigens but also to internalize them. After processing endocytosed antigens, MHC class II–peptide complexes appear on the cell surface, where antigen-specific CD4$^+$ T cells detect them. Also, B cells express costimulatory molecules and provide optimal conditions for T-cell activation. On activation, CD4$^+$ T cells express CD154 on their surface and are able to stimulate the CD40 molecule on their B-cell partner. CD40-CD154 interaction is essential for subsequent B-cell proliferation and differentiation. Cytokines secreted by the helper T cells act in concert with CD154 to amplify B-cell differentiation and to determine the antibody type by controlling isotype switching. Isotypes greatly influence the versatility of antibodies as effector molecules, and cytokines drive isotype switching by stimulating the transcriptional activation of heavy chain constant region genes. T-cell–dependent B-cell differentiation and maturation take place in germinal centers, specialized structures in secondary lymphoid tissues (see Fig. 44-5). There, the variable regions of B cells are altered by somatic hypermutation, leading to the production of large amounts of high-affinity antibodies. Subsequently, B cells that possess immunoglobulin receptors with high affinity for antigens in the germinal center are selected for survival (affinity maturation).

Lymphocytes and Lymphoid Tissue

The initiation of adaptive immune responses depends on rare antigen-specific T cells and B cells meeting antigen-presenting cells and their relevant antigen. The recognition of a specific antigen in the tissue by uncommon T

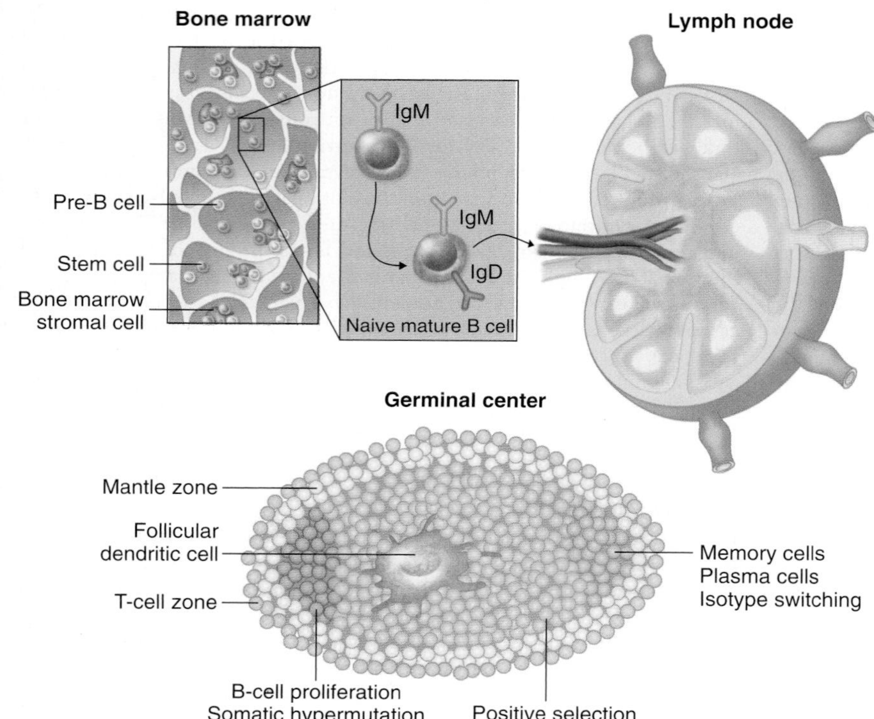

FIGURE 44-5. B-cell development and differentiation. The early stages of B-cell development occur in the bone marrow, with cells progressing through a developmental program determined by the rearrangement and expression of immunoglobulin (Ig) genes. Immature B cells with receptors for multivalent self-antigens die in the bone marrow. Surviving B cells coexpress IgD and IgM surface receptors. They are seeded into peripheral lymphoid organs, where they home to selected locations and receive signals to survive and become longer-lived naïve B cells. Antigen-binding B cells and antigen-presenting B cells that receive help from antigen-specific T cells are activated through membrane-bound and secreted molecules. Activated B cells migrate into the follicles, leading to the formation of germinal centers. B cells in germinal centers undergo somatic hypermutation of immunoglobulin genes; cells with high affinity for antigens presented on the surface of follicular dendritic cells are selected to differentiate into either memory B cells or plasma cells.

cells has a low probability, and it is unlikely that sufficient numbers of antigen-presenting cells and lymphocytes can be brought together to provide crucial momentum. The immune system uses specialized lymphoid microstructures to bring antigens to the site of lymphocyte traffic and accumulation. Secondary lymphoid organs include the spleen for blood-borne antigens, the lymph nodes for antigens encountered in peripheral tissues, and the mucosa-associated, bronchial-associated, and gut-associated lymphoid tissues, where antigens from epithelial surfaces are collected. Lymphocytes circulate through secondary lymphoid organs, constantly searching for their antigen. Their homing to secondary lymphoid organs is facilitated by specialized microvessels, called *high endothelial venules*. Secondary lymphoid tissues have developed several strategies to sequester the relevant antigen. Antigens in peripheral tissue are encountered first by dendritic cells that, after activation, are mobilized to transport antigens into the local lymph nodes by the draining lymph. These antigen-bearing dendritic cells enter the lymph nodes through the afferent lymphatic vessel and settle in the T-cell–rich zones to present processed antigens to T cells. The net result of this process is an accumulation and concentration of the antigen in an environment that can be readily screened by infrequent antigen-specific T cells (see Fig. 44-2).

B cells are segregated from T cells in the lymph nodes and are localized in follicles. If B cells find their cooperating T cells, they enter germinal centers. Germinal centers contain a network of follicular dendritic cells that capture particulate antigen or immune complexes on the cell surface. This unprocessed antigen is taken up by antigen-specific B cells, processed and presented, and recognized by antigen-specific T cells. These T cells provide cytokines and cell-cell contact signals to support the germinal center reaction, a process that includes somatic hypermutation, affinity selection, and isotype switching (see Fig. 44-5). Germinal centers are essential for generating antibody-secreting plasma cells and memory B cells.

Lymphoid organ development is highly dependent on environmental cues. The symbiotic relationship between the host immune system and microorganisms is best exemplified in the gastrointestinal tract. Development of gut-associated lymphoid tissue is absolutely dependent on bacterial colonization. Increasing evidence suggests that host-symbiont interactions regulate adaptive immune functions throughout life. Disturbances in the bacterial microbiota and failure to maintain intestinal homeostasis are important in diverse diseases, including inflammatory bowel disease (Chapter 143) and HIV-associated immune defects.

Memory

An important consequence of adaptive immunity is the generation of immunologic memory, the basis for long-lived protection after a primary infection. Memory induction by vaccination is one of the landmark successes in medicine. Immunologic memory is defined as the ability to respond more rapidly and effectively to pathogens that have been encountered previously. The bases of immunologic memory are qualitative and quantitative changes in antigen-specific T cells and B cells. As a direct result of clonal expansion and selection in antigen-driven responses, the frequencies of antigen-specific memory B cells and memory T cells are increased 10-fold to 1000-fold compared with the naïve repertoires. The mechanisms through which memory T cells and B cells escape clonal downsizing in the terminal stages of the primary immune response are not clear. The enrichment of antigen-specific B cells and T cells enhances the sensitivity of the system to renewed challenges and provides a head start of 4 to 10 cell divisions. In addition to increased frequencies, memory T cells and B cells are functionally different from their naïve counterparts. Memory cells are long-lived and survive in the presence of certain cytokines without the need for continuous antigenic stimulation, guaranteeing immunologic memory for the life expectancy of the individual cell. Memory B cells produce predominantly IgG and IgA antibodies with evidence of somatic hypermutation and high affinity for the antigen. Cell surface expression of high-affinity antibodies allows more efficient antigen uptake, which enhances the crucial interaction with T cells. High affinity also gives memory B cells a competitive advantage over naïve B cells in antigen binding, leading to progressive affinity maturation of somatically mutated antibody molecules.

Because the TCR does not undergo isotype switching or affinity maturation, memory T cells are more difficult to distinguish from naïve or effector T cells. In contrast to effector cells, memory T cells lack activation markers and need antigen stimulation to resume effector functions. In contrast to naïve T cells, memory T cells have a lower activation threshold and are less dependent on costimulatory signals. In essence, their requirements for antigen stimulation are fewer, and their clonal size is larger, permitting fast, efficient responses to secondary antigen encounters. Also, memory T cells resume effector functions without having to undergo cell divisions.

Immunologic Tolerance and Autoimmunity

Unresponsiveness to self is a fundamental property of the immune system and is a condition, sine qua non, to maintain tissue integrity of the host. Self/nonself distinction is relatively straightforward for the innate immune system, in which receptors to nonself molecules are genetically encoded and evolutionarily selected. Self/nonself discrimination is much more complex for the adaptive immune system, in which antigen-specific receptors are generated randomly and the entire spectrum of antigens can be recognized. The adaptive immune system must acquire the ability to distinguish between self and nonself. Several different mechanisms are used, collectively called *tolerance*. Tolerance is antigen specific; its induction requires the recognition of antigen by lymphocytes in a defined setting. Failure of self-tolerance results in immune responses against self-antigens. Such reactions are called *autoimmunity* and may give rise to chronic inflammatory autoimmune disease.

Central and peripheral tolerance mechanisms can be distinguished. In central tolerance, self-reactive lymphocytes are deleted during development. This process of negative selection is particularly important for T cells. During thymic development, T cells that recognize antigen with high affinity, in particular antigens that are constitutively expressed on antigen-presenting cells, are deleted. Central tolerance for B cells follows the same principles. Recognition of antigen by developing B cells in the bone marrow induces apoptosis. Negative selection is particularly important for B cells that recognize multivalent antigens because they do not depend on T-cell help and cannot be controlled peripherally.

Not all self-reactive T cells are centrally purged from the repertoire; certain antigens are not encountered at sufficient densities in the thymus. Also, all T cells have some degree of self-reactivity, which is necessary for positive selection in the thymus and for peripheral survival. Mechanisms of peripheral T-cell tolerance include anergy, peripheral deletion, clonal ignorance, and suppression of immune responses by regulatory T cells. T-cell anergy is transient and is actively maintained. It is induced if $CD4^+$ T cells recognize antigens without receiving costimulatory signals. In general, costimulatory molecules are restricted to antigen-presenting cells, and their expression is activation dependent. Antigen recognition on immature or resting antigen-presenting cells or on any cell other than peripheral antigen-presenting cells results in anergy. Tissue-residing immature dendritic cells need to be activated by cytokines or recognition of PAMPs to stimulate and not to anergize T cells. Peripheral deletion is induced as a consequence of hyperstimulation. Hyperstimulation of T cells (e.g., by high doses of antigen and high concentrations of IL-2) preferentially activates pro-apoptotic pathways and causes elimination of the responding T-cell specificity. This mechanism may be responsible for the elimination of T cells specific for plentiful peripheral self-antigens and for foreign antigens abundantly present during infection. Whereas induction of anergy and activation-induced cell death are active consequences of antigen recognition, the third tolerance mechanism, clonal ignorance, is less well understood. Clonal ignorance is defined as the presence of self-reactive lymphocytes that fail to recognize or to respond to peripheral antigens. These cells remain responsive to antigenic challenge if given in the right setting. An example of clonal ignorance is nonresponsiveness to sequestered antigens that are not accessible to the immune system. Other mechanisms must exist, however, because clonal ignorance has also been shown for accessible antigens. Treg cells play a pivotal role in maintaining peripheral tolerance. During an immune response, T cells can acquire the ability to produce regulatory cytokines, such as TGF-β, IL-10, or IL-4, that dampen or suppress immune responses. A dedicated subset of Treg cells, Foxp3 $CD4^+$ T cells, has been identified and characterized. Harnessing the frequencies and function of these cells may offer a promising approach to restoring peripheral tolerance in treating autoimmune diseases or facilitating transplantation tolerance; their elimination or functional suppression may potentiate cancer immunotherapy.

Peripheral tolerance of B cells is maintained through the absence of T-cell help. B cells require signals from T cells to differentiate into effector cells. B lymphocytes that recognize self-antigens in the periphery in the absence of T-cell help are rendered anergic or are unable to enter lymphoid follicles, where they could receive T-cell help, effectively excluding them from immune responses.

Generation and maintenance of self-tolerance can fail, in which case autoimmune responses are generated. Overall, chronic inflammatory diseases induced by tolerance failure occur in about 5% of the general population. Given the complexity of regulation, it is surprising that autoimmune diseases are not more frequent. It is thought that most autoimmune diseases result from dysfunction of the adaptive immune system. Many models of autoimmunity rely on the hypothesis that peripheral anergy is broken. Aberrant expression of costimulatory molecules on nonprofessional antigen-presenting cells or inappropriate activation of tissue-residing dendritic cells sets the stage for the induction of "forbidden" T-cell responses. Also, autoreactive B cells that recognize self-antigen complexed with foreign antigen may engulf this complex and receive help from T cells specific for the foreign antigen. Autoimmunity also may emerge if antigen ignorance is broken. This could happen if tissue barriers break down and antigens that are usually sequestered from the immune system, such as antigens from the central nervous system or the eye, become accessible. Tolerance mechanisms of anergy or clonal ignorance can also fail if a foreign antigen is sufficiently different from a self-antigen to initiate an immune response but sufficiently similar for activated T cells to elicit T-cell and B-cell effector functions (molecular mimicry).

SUGGESTED READINGS

Bonilla FA, Oettgen HC. Adaptive immunity. *J Allergy Clin Immunol.* 2010;125:S33-S40. *Concise review of the current understanding of the mechanisms of adaptive immunity.*

Delano MJ, Thayer T, Gabrilovich S, et al. Sepsis induces early alterations in innate immunity that impact mortality to secondary infection. *J Immunol.* 2011;186:195-202. *Sepsis impairs innate immunity and increases susceptibility to secondary infections.*

Iwasaki A, Medzhitov R. Regulation of adaptive immunity by the innate immune system. *Science.* 2010;327:291-295. *Review of mechanisms by which pathogen-specific innate immune recognition activates antigen-specific adaptive immune responses.*

Littman DR, Rudensky AY. Th17 and regulatory T cells in mediating and restraining inflammation. *Cell.* 2010;140:845-858. *Discussion of how immune balance is achieved by interactions of different T-lymphocyte classes with pro- or anti-inflammatory activities in the context of genetic and environmental factors.*

Von Boehmer H, Melchers F. Checkpoints in lymphocyte development and autoimmune disease. *Nat Immunol.* 2010;11:14-20. *Discussion of how failures at B-cell and T-cell developmental checkpoints result in autoimmunity.*

45 THE MAJOR HISTOCOMPATIBILITY COMPLEX

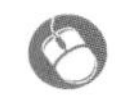

PETER K. GREGERSEN

HUMAN LEUKOCYTE ANTIGENS

The major histocompatibility complex (MHC) occupies a unique position in the nexus of clinical medicine, immunology, and genetics. Hundreds of diseases and clinical phenotypes have been associated with genes located within the MHC. The most important of these genes encode the human leukocyte antigens (HLAs), a family of cell surface proteins that are essential for normal immune function. HLA genes display a remarkably high degree of genetic variation among individuals in the population, and this variability is largely responsible for individual differences in immune responsiveness. These effects on immune responsiveness are in turn related to individual differences in susceptibility to a variety of autoimmune, inflammatory, and infectious disorders. Thus, the structural variability of the HLA molecules themselves underlies most but not all of the HLA disease associations reported over the past 3 decades.

Structure of HLA Molecules

Discovery of the x-ray crystallographic structure of an HLA molecule had a major impact on understanding the molecular basis of immune recognition by T cells. A ribbon diagram of the structure of an HLA class I molecule is shown in Figure 45-1. The "business end" of the molecule contains a peptide-binding cleft formed by the two membrane distal domains (α_1 and α_2) of the HLA class I heavy chain, as seen in the side view in Figure 45-1A. A view from the top of this cleft is shown in Figure 45-1B, which can be thought of as the "T-cell view" of the HLA molecule. It illustrates that the base of the peptide-binding cleft is formed by β-pleated sheets, with two α-helical structures forming the sides of the cleft. It is now known that the T-cell receptor physically interacts with both the HLA molecule and the peptide bound within the cleft to form a "trimolecular complex" (E-Fig. 45-1). Thus, it is not surprising that structural differences in HLA molecules, particularly in amino acids surrounding the peptide-binding cleft, have a major role in many immunologically mediated diseases.

Properties of HLA Class I and Class II Isoforms

There are two major isoforms of HLA molecules, termed *class I* and *class II.* Both isoforms are anchored in the cell membrane and contain a peptide-binding cleft similar to that shown in Figure 45-1. However, their specific structural and functional features differ, as summarized in Table 45-1 (E-Fig. 45-2). In the case of class I molecules, a highly variable α chain (45 kD) forms a noncovalent heterodimer with an invariant β_2-microglobulin (12 kD) and is anchored to the cell by a single transmembrane segment on the α chain. In contrast, HLA class II molecules are formed by α chain (32 kD) and β chain (28 kD) heterodimers, and in many cases both chains exhibit structural variability among individuals. HLA class I molecules are expressed on nearly all nucleated cells. HLA class II molecules are found on more restricted cell populations, including B cells, monocytes, macrophages, dendritic cells, and other "professional" antigen-presenting cells such as Langerhans cells in the skin. Certain subsets of T cells also express class II molecules. In addition, HLA class II molecules are expressed on thymic epithelium, where they are involved in thymic selection of the T-cell receptor repertoire (see later). The size of the peptides bound to HLA class I molecules is

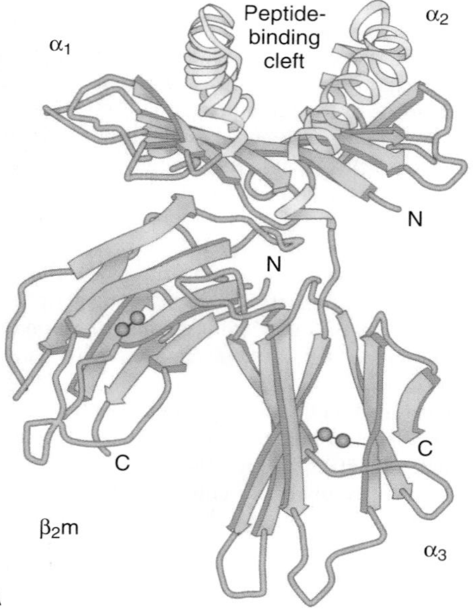

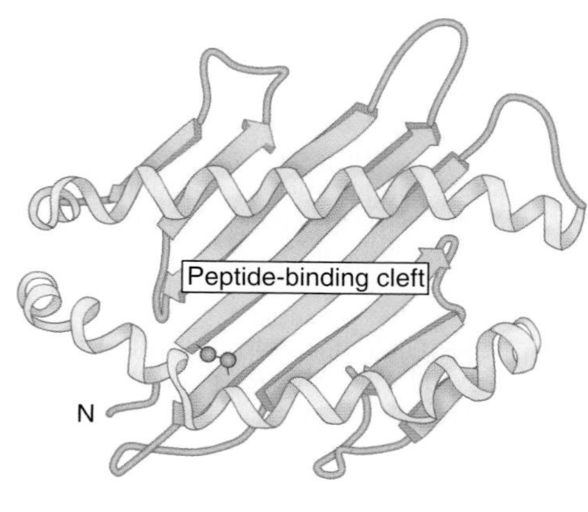

FIGURE 45-1. Two views of an HLA class I molecule. A, Ribbon diagram showing the x-ray crystallographic structure of an HLA class I molecule (side view). The β-strand structures are indicated by *thick green arrows* (oriented in an amino to carboxy direction), whereas connecting loops are indicated as *thin lines.* The α-helices are shown flanking a peptide-binding cleft at the top (membrane distal portion) of the molecule. The base (membrane proximal portion) of the molecule is formed by the noncovalent association between the α_3 domain of the class I α chain and β_2-microglobulin (β_2m). **B,** View from the top of the molecule emphasizing that the base of the peptide-binding cleft consists of β-pleated sheets flanked by α-helical structures. C = C terminal; N = N terminal. (Adapted from Bjorkman PJ, Saper MA, Samraoi B, et al. Structure of the class I histocompatibility antigen HLA-A2. *Nature.* 1987;329:506-512.)

circumscribed to 8 or 9 amino acids in length, whereas the peptides presented by HLA class II molecules are longer and more variable in size, with lengths usually ranging from 10 to 20 amino acids. HLA class I molecules generally present peptides for recognition by $CD8^+$ T cells, such as in cytotoxic $CD8^+$ T-cell responses against virally infected tissues. In contrast, HLA class II molecules are primarily involved in presenting antigenic peptides to $CD4^+$ T cells.

TABLE 45-1 COMPARISON OF STRUCTURAL AND FUNCTIONAL FEATURES OF HLA CLASS I AND CLASS II ISOTYPES

FEATURE	HLA CLASS I	HLA CLASS II
Chain structure of heterodimer	45-kD α chain 12-kD β_2-microglobulin	34-kD α chain 28-kD β chain
Tissue distribution	All nucleated cells	Antigen-presenting cells (monocytes, B cells, dendritic cells, Langerhans cells), thymic epithelium, and some T cells; inducible on other cell types by interferon-γ
Size of bound peptides	8-9 amino acids	10-20 amino acids
Source peptides	Cytosolic	Endosomal
Functions	Presentation of antigenic peptides to $CD8^+$ T cells; ligands for natural killer cell receptors	Presentation of antigenic peptides to $CD4^+$ T cells

Sources of the peptide antigens presented by class I and class II molecules are quite distinct. In the case of class I molecules, the bound peptides are derived from cytosol and are loaded onto the class I molecules during their synthesis in the endoplasmic reticulum. Thus, either host or virally derived peptides may be present in the peptide cleft, and a peptide is required for proper folding and surface expression of class I molecules. In contrast, HLA class II molecules present peptides that are present in endosomes, and peptide loading onto class II molecules occurs in endocytic vesicles. These peptides are derived from sources exogenous to the cell, such as soluble proteins, particles, cell debris, or whole organisms. In the case of B cells, surface immunoglobulin can facilitate the internalization of highly specific antigens, whereas in macrophages and other antigen-presenting cells, endocytosis and phagocytosis mediate less specific cellular internalization of antigens. Mycobacteria and intracellular parasites such as *Leishmania* replicate inside vesicular compartments of the cell; therefore, peptides from these agents are generally presented on class II molecules.

Organization of HLA Molecules

Genetic Map of HLA Genes

The MHC is contained within a 3.6 million–base pair region located at chromosome 6p21 and encodes more than 200 different genes, approximately 40% of which appear to have some role in immune function. Figure 45-2 shows a simplified map of the major HLA loci. The HLA class I and class II regions are separated by a gene-dense region often referred to as the *central* MHC. This central region encodes a number of genes of immunologic importance, including several complement components and tumor necrosis factor-α and -β, to name only a few. The class I heavy chains for HLA-A, HLA-B, and HLA-C are encoded on the telomeric side of the MHC, along with a number of other class I–like molecules, as shown in Figure 45-2. The HLA class II region is considerably more complicated, with multiple α and

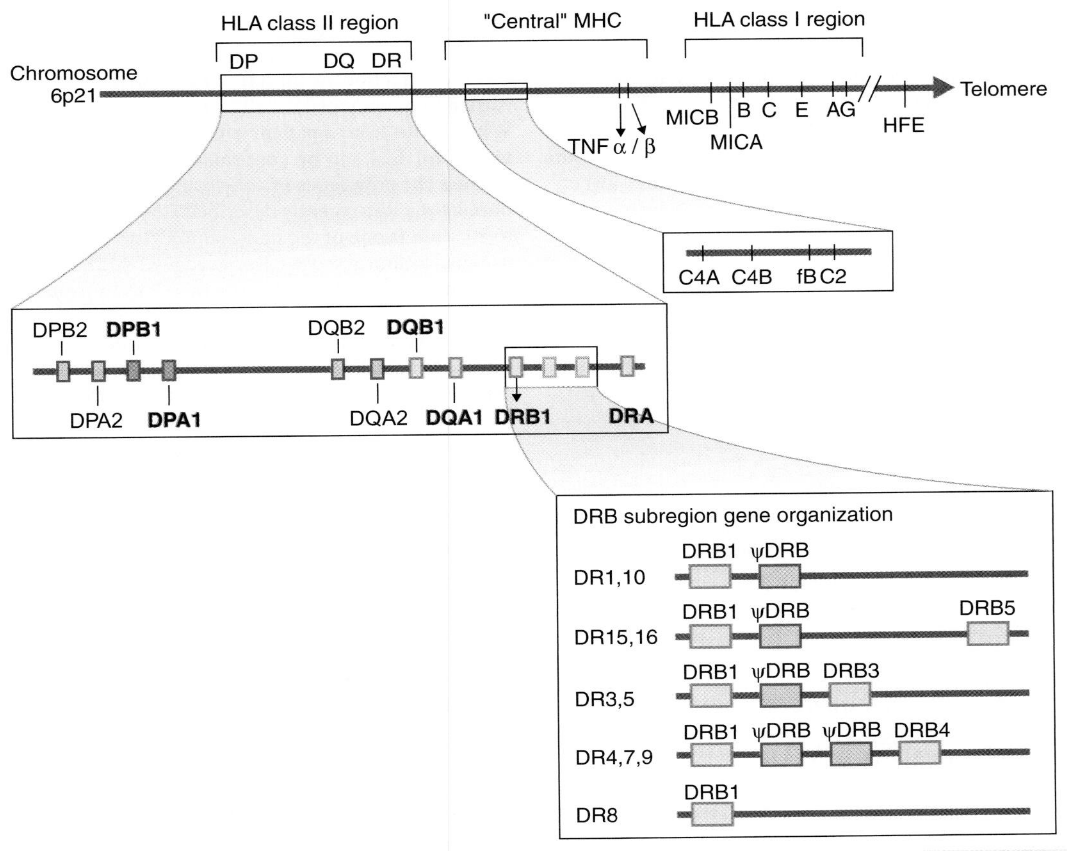

FIGURE 45-2. Map of the human major histocompatibility complex (MHC) spanning approximately 3.5 million base pairs on the short arm of chromosome 6. The HLA class I and class II molecules are encoded in distinct regions of the MHC. The HLA class II region contains three subregions: DR, DQ, and DP. Each of these subregions contains a variable number of α- and β-chain genes. HLA class II loci with known functional protein products are labeled in bold. In the case of DR, different numbers of DRB genes are present in different haplotypes, some of which are nonfunctional pseudogenes (ψ). A summary of the most common of these is shown in the *box*. The DQ and DP subregions each contain one pair of functional α- and β-chain genes. The HLA class I region contains the three "classic" class I genes—HLA-A, HLA-B, and HLA-C—as well as other related "nonclassic" class I molecules such as MICA, MICB, HLA-E, and HLA-G. The gene for familial hemochromatosis (HFE) is found just telomeric to the HLA class I region, about 3 million base pairs distant from HLA-A. The "central" MHC also contains a number of genes related to immune function, including the complement components (C4A, C4B, C2, and factor B), as well as tumor necrosis factor (TNF)-α and -β. Not shown in the figure are more than 100 additional genes, many of which are located in the central MHC. A complete listing of MHC-encoded genes can be found in Horton R, Wilming L, Rand V, et al. Gene map of the extended human MHC. *Nat Rev Genet*. 2004;5:889-899.

β chains encoded for each of the major HLA class II isotypes: HLA-DR, HLA-DQ, and HLA-DP. Of these, HLA-DR exhibits additional complexity, in that a different gene organization of β chains is seen, depending on the particular DR haplotype.

HLA Typing Nomenclature and Patterns of Allelic Sequence Variation

In addition to the organizational complexity of the HLA region, the nomenclature for HLA typing of different alleles at each locus presents some challenges for the nonexpert. In the past decade, hundreds of HLA alleles have been sequenced, and each HLA allelic variant is defined by its locus and sequence. For example, B*2701 indicates allele 2701 at the HLA-B locus, and DRB1*0401 indicates allele 0401 at the DRB1 locus. This nomenclature is, in principle, quite straightforward. However, there are many different alleles at each of these loci; for example, more than 100 alleles have been identified at the HLA-B locus, and similar allelic diversity is seen at HLA-A and HLA-C, as well as in many of the HLA class II loci. The sequence relationships between alleles are both complex and informative for understanding HLA associations with disease, and the nomenclature reflects this to some degree. It is therefore worth understanding the origins of these naming conventions.

The current HLA nomenclature contains traces of the early history of HLA typing. A serologic approach was initially used for HLA typing. HLA protein variation is highly immunogenic between individuals; therefore, typing alloantisera can be derived either from multiply transfused individuals (who make an antibody response to HLA molecules on the donor white cells) or from multiparous women (who commonly form antibodies to the paternal HLA antigens expressed by the fetus). Thus, by screening large numbers of individuals, panels of alloantisera were developed as the first HLA typing reagents. These original HLA typing sera did not distinguish all the variation at a particular locus, and it is now apparent that serologic typing actually detects rather large groups of structurally related alleles. For example, the serologically defined allele HLA-DR4 contains well over 30 different alleles at the DRB1 locus, although only a few of these alleles are common in the population. Table 45-2 summarizes the major allelic groups at the DRB1 locus and shows the relationship between the original serologic typing and the various groups of alleles defined at the sequence level. For some allelic groups, such as HLA-DR3, there is little sequence diversity within the group, depending on the population; thus, almost all white Europeans carry just one type of DR3 allele, DRB1*0301. As a result, the term *DR3* is often used in conversation to refer to the DRB1*0301 allele and is reasonably precise when talking about a white population. In contrast, *DR4* could refer to any one of several different alleles (see Table 45-2).

TABLE 45-2 SUMMARY OF MAJOR ALLELIC GROUPS AT THE DRB1 LOCUS AND THEIR RELATIONSHIP TO COMMON DRB1 ALLELES DEFINED AT THE SEQUENCE LEVEL

Allelic Groups (Serologic Typing)		
MAJOR GROUPS	**SEROLOGIC "SPLITS"**	**EXAMPLES OF COMMON ALLELES (NORTHERN EUROPEAN WHITE INDIVIDUALS) DEFINED BY SEQUENCE***
DR1		DRB1***0101**, 0102, 0103
DR2	DR15 DR16	DRB1***1501**, 1502 DRB1*1601
DR3		DRB1***0301**
DR4		DRB1***0401**, 0402, 0403, 0404, 0405, 0406, 0407, 0408
DR5	DR11 DR12	DRB1*1101, 1102, 1103, 1104 DRB1*1201
DR6	DR13 DR14	DRB1*1301, 1302, 1303 DRB1*1401
DR7		DRB1***0701**
DR8		DRB1*0801, 0802, 0803, 0804, 0806
DR9		DRB1*0901
DR10		DRB1*1001

*Alleles in bold are found in at least 10% of individuals in the population.
From Williams F, Meenagh A, Single R, et al. High resolution HLA-DRB1 identification of a Caucasian population. *Hum Immunol.* 2004;65:66-77.

In addition to having large numbers of alleles at each locus, the frequency distribution of these alleles is highly variable in human populations. As shown in Table 45-2, five DRB1 alleles predominate in the northern European white population (shown in bold), with frequencies ranging from 10 to 30%. This frequency distribution would be quite different in a different population group, even among white subgroups, such as a comparison of northern and southern European populations. The population differences emphasize the importance of matching controls to cases by ethnic origin when comparing allele frequencies between them.

HLA Associations with Disease: The Concept of Disease Susceptibility

Table 45-3 provides a representative sample of some well-established HLA associations with human disease. The overwhelming majority of these studies were conducted with a case-control design in which the frequency of alleles was compared in subjects with appropriately matched controls. Matching of controls is a critical part of the study design because HLA alleles can differ greatly between different populations; as a result, many early reports in the literature turned out to be false positives. Nevertheless, hundreds of diseases and medically relevant phenotypes have confirmed associations with HLA alleles.

As shown in Table 45-3, the strength of many of these disease associations is rather modest, with an estimated relative risk of 10 or less. Therefore, HLA alleles confer a state of susceptibility, or risk, for disease. Because the HLA risk alleles are usually quite common in the population, and the diseases are relatively uncommon, many individuals who carry these risk alleles do not contract the disease. Conversely, a substantial number of individuals with the disease do not carry the known HLA risk-conferring alleles. Thus, in a practical sense, HLA typing alone is not very useful in a clinical setting for most diagnostic purposes. Even for a disease such as ankylosing spondylitis (Chapter 273), where the relative risk approaches 100, the disease develops in only a fraction of the HLA-B27 carriers in the population because the carrier frequency of HLA-B27 in a white population is approximately 8%. When confronting a patient with typical symptoms of ankylosing spondylitis, testing for B27 can be confirmatory; however, it is not diagnostic by itself because the prevalence of ankylosing spondylitis is very low (≈0.12%) in the population. The recently described association of B57 with adverse reactions to abacavir is one of the first examples in which HLA testing may be directly useful in a clinical setting. Knowledge of this association has now been shown to reduce the incidence of drug reactions in treated populations.

This pattern of association, in which HLA alleles confer a state of risk or susceptibility to disease, implies that other factors must be involved for a disease to actually manifest. In general, these other factors can include other genes, environmental factors, and nongenetic factors such as stochastic or "epigenetic" events that may occur at any time during development. Somatic rearrangements of T-cell and B-cell receptor genes are one example of such a stochastic process. These factors explain why concordance rates for many autoimmune disorders in monozygotic twins are only in the 30% range, even though these diseases all exhibit significant genetic associations with particular HLA alleles and have a strong genetic component. The genetic predisposition conferred by the MHC is only part of the overall genetic contribution to most autoimmune disorders, and the MHC component varies in importance, depending on the particular disease.

Linkage Disequilibrium

An understanding of the concept of linkage disequilibrium is critical to the proper interpretation of HLA associations or, indeed, any genetic associations with human diseases. The term *linkage disequilibrium* is used to describe the fact that alleles at adjacent loci are often found together on the same chromosomal segment, or haplotype, more frequently than would be predicted by chance. This phenomenon occurs throughout the genome, and the MHC is no exception. Indeed, because of the high degree of allelic diversity at HLA loci, the pattern of linkage disequilibrium between HLA alleles can be quite complicated and, like the alleles themselves, often varies among different population groups. For example, in most white populations, the DRB1*0301 allele is almost always found on the same haplotype with the DQB1*0201 allele at the DQB1 locus. (Note that the DQB1 locus is situated several hundred thousand base pairs away from the DRB1 locus; see Fig. 45-2.) Likewise, DR4 alleles (at DRB1) are often found to be in linkage

TABLE 45-3 SELECTED HLA ASSOCIATIONS WITH HUMAN DISEASES

DISEASE	MAJOR HLA ASSOCIATION (ALLELIC GROUP OR HAPLOTYPE)	EFFECT/APPROXIMATE RELATIVE RISK/RELATIVE HAZARD
AUTOIMMUNE DISEASES		
Type 1 diabetes	DR3-DQ2 DR4-DQ3	10
Multiple sclerosis	DR2-DQ1	3-5
Celiac disease	DR3-DQ2 DR4-DQ3	30
Rheumatoid arthritis	DR1, DR4	2-5
Systemic lupus erythematosus	DR2, DR3, DR8	2-10
Ankylosing spondylitis	B27	100
Psoriasis	Cw6	10
INFECTIOUS DISEASES		
Progression to AIDS	B35	2-3
Severe malaria	B53	0.5 (protective)
Transient vs persistent hepatitis C infection	DR11-DQ3	5-10
OTHER		
Hemochromatosis	A3	10
Adverse drug reaction (allopurinol)	B58	>100
Cervical cancer	DR11-DQ3	2-3

AIDS = acquired immunodeficiency syndrome; HFE = hereditary hemochromatosis gene.

disequilibrium with DQB1*0302. These two haplotypes are both associated with type 1 diabetes (see Table 45-3).

Occasionally, linkage disequilibrium can extend to very long chromosomal segments. For example, a common haplotype in northern European white populations extends to several million base pairs and contains the HLA alleles A*0101-B*0801-DRB1*0301-DQB1*0201, often referred to as the *A1-B8-DR3* or *8.1 haplotype*. This particular haplotype accounts for about a third of all DR3 haplotypes in a U.S. white population and is of particular interest because it is associated with a variety of diseases, some of which are listed in Table 45-4. Because haplotypes such as these are inherited as a unit, it can be difficult to determine which specific genes on the haplotype are actually responsible for the disease association in a population.

There are a number of possible explanations for linkage disequilibrium. In part, it reflects the fact that meiotic recombination in the genome is discontinuous, and some loci have very low recombination rates between them—such as between the DRB1 and DQB1 loci. In addition, population migrations can introduce haplotypes into new population groups and thereby generate common "founder" haplotypes. Finally, some haplotypes may be kept intact because of selection. For example, it may be that the combination of genes found on the A1-B8-DR3 haplotype confers a survival advantage. Whatever the underlying reason, it is important to keep in mind that any HLA association may reflect the presence of linkage disequilibrium with another allele at another locus on the same haplotype.

TABLE 45-4 DISEASES AND PHENOTYPES ASSOCIATED WITH THE A1-B8-DR3 (8.1) HAPLOTYPE

IgA deficiency
Common variable immunodeficiency
Myasthenia gravis
Dermatitis herpetiformis
Rheumatoid arthritis (central portion of the 8.1 haplotype only)
Rapid loss of CD4⁺ T cells in HIV infection
Low antibody response to hepatitis B immunization
Increases (tumor necrosis factor) or decreases (interleukin-5) in cytokine production in vitro

HLA Associations with Autoimmune and Infectious Diseases

The majority of autoimmune disorders exhibit some association with HLA class II alleles, although because of linkage disequilibrium, it is not always clear which locus is actually responsible for the association. In the case of type 1 diabetes, the bulk of evidence suggests that alleles at the HLA-DQ locus play a predominant role by virtue of specific amino acid substitutions that are present on multiple different DQB1 alleles; aspartic acid at amino acid position 57 of the DQβ chain is thought to be of particular importance. Rheumatoid arthritis is another autoimmune disorder in which the molecular basis of HLA class II associations has been partially worked out. In this case, a series of DRB1 alleles, including DRB1*0101, *0401, *0404, *0405, all share a common amino acid sequence (Q-K or R-R-A-A) at positions 70 to 74 of the DRβ1 chain, located on the rim of the peptide-binding cleft (see Fig. 45-1). This sequence is known as the *shared epitope* and provides an appealing unifying explanation for the complex patterns of HLA-DR associations with rheumatoid arthritis. However, for both type 1 diabetes and rheumatoid arthritis, there are exceptions to these observations, and certain combinations of HLA alleles can confer very high degrees of risk. For most of the HLA-associated diseases, the exact molecular basis of the association has not been definitively established, and in some cases, even the causative locus is uncertain (see Table 45-3). For ankylosing spondylitis, it appears that most allelic variants of HLA-B27 are associated with disease. Recent genetic data provide support for the C*0601 allele being causative for psoriasis. However, in the case of systemic lupus erythematosus and multiple sclerosis, the relative importance of DRB1 versus DQB1 alleles is not clear.

For infectious diseases, such as the role of HLA-B35 in the progression of acquired immunodeficiency syndrome (AIDS), there is evidence that particular amino acid residues on the HLA-B molecule are especially important. The amino acids that distinguish risk alleles (B*3502, B*3503) from nonrisk alleles (B*3501) alter the structure of a "pocket" within the peptide-binding cleft on the various HLA-B35 proteins and therefore can affect the kinds of human immunodeficiency virus (HIV) antigenic peptides that are bound by these alleles. Other HLA-B alleles, such as B27 and B58, protect against progression of HIV, apparently by similar mechanisms. Aside from HLA-B associations with HIV outcome, specific structural explanations have not yet been defined for most HLA associations with infectious diseases.

Mechanisms Explaining HLA Associations with Disease

It is fair to say that the mechanisms underlying HLA disease associations are still not fully explained for any disorder, and the mechanisms clearly differ for different diseases. However, there are two general categories of mechanisms that are likely to be important. First, a pattern of immune responsiveness, or lack of immune responsiveness, can be related to the ability of an individual's HLA molecules to bind and present antigenic peptides (either foreign or self) to T cells. This mechanism is often referred to as *determinant selection*, which means that HLA molecules are involved in selecting which antigenic determinants are selected for presentation to responding T cells. As mentioned earlier, this probably underlies the contrasting HLA-B allelic associations with AIDS progression.

An alternative mechanism invokes the role of HLA molecules in regulating thymic selection of the mature T-cell repertoire. During thymic development, thymocytes either survive or die of apoptosis, depending in large part on their ability to recognize "self" HLA molecules (and associated "self" peptides) on thymic epithelium or on other antigen-presenting cells in the thymus. This recognition is mediated through the α/β T-cell receptor. Thus, the structural repertoire of T-cell receptors in the mature circulating T-cell population is shaped by the structural variation of the selecting HLA molecules. This may lead to "holes" in the T-cell repertoire or, alternatively, enrichment for particular T-cell specificities. In this view, the presence of particular sets of potentially responding T cells provides a risk factor for response, or lack of response, to autoantigens or foreign antigens. It implies the need for an environmental trigger to actually cause this risk to manifest as overt clinical disease.

In addition to these two basic models, it has been proposed that HLA molecules can themselves serve as a source of antigenic peptides and may predispose to disease by means of molecular mimicry or other more complex mechanisms. However, none of these proposed mechanisms has been definitively proved for any disorder.

HLA Associations with Disease May Reflect Linkage Disequilibrium with Non-HLA Genes

In most cases, HLA associations such as those listed in Table 45-3 probably reflect the mechanistic involvement of the HLA molecules themselves in the disease or phenotype under study. However, the MHC is one of the most gene-dense segments in the human genome, and other genes in the region may in fact be responsible for the observed disease association. A good example of this is hemochromatosis (Chapter 219). Early studies showed that certain HLA class I alleles, such as HLA-A3, were highly associated with this disorder. However, it is now clear that the causative gene, *HFE*, is actually more than 3 million base pairs distant from the HLA-A locus (see Fig. 45-2). The HLA-A3 association is observed because the *HFE* C282Y allele (causative for hemochromatosis) is frequently found on the same haplotype as HLA-A3 in many white populations.

Some of the associations with the A1-B8-DR3 haplotype almost certainly reflect linkage disequilibrium with genes other than HLA class I and class II genes (see Table 45-3). Although the HLA genes may contribute to some of these disorders, it is likely that other genes on the 8.1 haplotype also contribute to risk. The central portion of the MHC in particular (see Fig. 45-2) is very dense with many genes of uncertain function, as well as genes for important inflammatory cytokines such as tumor necrosis factor and complement components C2 and C4. Indeed, the combination of several different genes may well explain why this haplotype is associated with so many different immunologic disorders.

HLA Typing and Bone Marrow Transplantation

As the term *histocompatibility* implies, the ability of the MHC to control graft rejection in experimental animals led to the realization that HLA matching is important for transplant survival. For solid organ transplantation, treatment with immunosuppressive agents often prevents the rejection of HLA-mismatched transplants. However, for bone marrow transplantation (Chapter 181), careful matching of the major HLA class I and class II loci is important for a successful outcome, regardless of whether the donor is related or unrelated to the recipient. Because of the extensive sequence diversity of HLA alleles, very large numbers of unrelated donors are required to ensure a reasonable probability of a match for any given recipient who does not have a living related donor. This has led to the development of international bone marrow donor registries that now contain more than 10 million potential donors who have been screened for HLA type. If transplantation is performed in the presence of a significant mismatch at either class I or class II loci, T cells from the recipient may recognize the donor HLA molecules or their bound peptides as foreign and initiate an immune response, leading to graft rejection. Interestingly, even when HLA molecules are completely matched, T cells still occasionally initiate rejection because of individual differences in "minor" histocompatibility antigens that are not encoded within the MHC but are processed and presented as antigenic peptides that appear foreign to the host.

HLA Class I: Alternative Forms and Functions

The HLA class I region of the MHC contains a number of genes that encode so-called nonclassic class I genes, including HLA-E, HLA-G, MICA, and MICB (see Fig. 45-2). These molecules do not present peptides to α/β T cells but rather interact with a variety of other ligands that are generally found on natural killer cells and some other types of T cells. In addition, certain allelic subsets of the "classic" class I molecules (e.g., HLA-A, -B, and -C) can interact with some of these other ligands. Among these ligands, the killer cell immunoglobulin-like receptor (KIR) family displays a large degree of genetic variation in both gene structure and gene number and has been associated with human disease. For example, certain combinations of HLA class I alleles and KIR alleles have been associated with risk for rheumatoid vasculitis as well as outcome of HIV infection. These genetic relationships are complex, and this aspect of HLA class I function in disease has been relatively understudied.

HLA and Clinical Medicine

The identification of risk genes within the MHC may hold the key to understanding a large number of immunologically related disorders. However, we are far from identifying all of these genes, and in the few cases in which the actual risk alleles are known with confidence, their mechanism of action is not clear. Moreover, most HLA-associated disorders are complex, and additional genetic or environmental factors (or both) are likely to be involved, most of which have not yet been identified. Therefore, in most cases, HLA typing alone has limited diagnostic utility. HLA typing may be diagnostically important in the future if used in combination with other biomarkers, and HLA typing remains critical to successful bone marrow transplantation. Thus, it is likely that future advances in immunology and genetics will lead to greater clinical use of genetic typing of HLA genes, as well as other genes, within the MHC.

SUGGESTED READINGS

Claas FH. Clinical relevance of circulating donor-specific HLA antibodies. *Curr Opin Organ Transplant.* 2010;15:462-466. *Which HLA antibodies are the direct cause of graft failure remains uncertain.*

Howell WM, Carter V, Clark B. The HLA system: immunobiology, HLA typing, antibody screening and crossmatching techniques. *J Clin Pathol.* 2010;63:387-390. *Overview of biology and methodologies.*

Shiina T, Hosomichi K, Inoko H, et al. The HLA genomic loci map: expression, interaction, diversity and disease. *J Hum Genet.* 2009;54:15-39. *A detailed review of the genetics and disease associations within the HLA region.*

Zachary AA, Eng HS. Desensitization: achieving immune détente. *Tissue Antigens.* 2011;77:3-8. *Desensitization can increase the rate of transplantation among sensitized patients.*

46

MECHANISMS OF IMMUNE-MEDIATED TISSUE INJURY

JANE E. SALMON

THE ADAPTIVE IMMUNE RESPONSE

Definition

The adaptive immune response is a crucial component of host defense against infection. Its distinguishing and unique feature is the ability to recognize pathogens specifically, based on clonal selection of lymphocytes bearing antigen-specific receptors. Antigens unassociated with infectious agents also may elicit adaptive immune responses. Many clinically important diseases are characterized by normal immune responses directed against an inappropriate antigen, typically in the absence of infection. Immune responses directed at noninfectious antigens occur in allergy, in which the antigen is an innocuous foreign substance, and in autoimmunity, in which the response is to a self-antigen.

Effector mechanisms that eliminate pathogens in adaptive immune responses are essentially identical to those of innate immunity. The specific antigen recognition feature of the adaptive immune response seems to have been appended to the preexisting innate defense system. As a result, the inflammatory cells and molecules of the innate immune system are essential for the effector functions of B and T lymphocytes. In addition to initiating protective responses, they mediate tissue injury in allergy, hypersensitivity, and autoimmunity.

Effector Mechanisms

Effector actions of antibodies depend on recruiting cells and molecules of the innate immune system. Antibodies are adapters that bind antigens to nonspecific inflammatory cells and direct their destructive effector responses. Antibodies also activate the complement system, which enhances opsonization of antigens, recruits phagocytic cells, and amplifies (or "complements") antibody-triggered damage. The isotype or class of antibodies produced determines which effector mechanisms are engaged.

Cell-bound receptors for immunoglobulin (Ig) constitute the link between humoral and cellular aspects of the immune cascade and play an integral part in the process by which foreign and endogenous opsonized material is identified and destroyed. These cell-based binding sites for antibodies, termed *Fc receptors,* interact with the constant region (Fc portion) of the immunoglobulin heavy chain of a particular antibody class regardless of its antigen specificity. Accessory cells that lack intrinsic specificity, such as neutrophils, macrophages, and mast cells, are recruited to participate in inflammatory responses through the interaction of their Fc receptors with antigen-specific antibodies. Distinct receptors for different immunoglobulin isotypes are expressed on different effector cells.

Receptors for IgG (FcγRs) are a diverse group of receptors expressed as hematopoietic cell surface molecules on phagocytes (macrophages, monocytes, neutrophils), platelets, mast cells, eosinophils, and natural killer (NK) cells. FcγRs often are expressed as stimulatory and inhibitory pairs. Triggering of stimulatory FcγRs initiates a series of events, including phagocytosis; antibody-dependent, cell-mediated cytotoxicity; secretion of granules; and release of inflammatory mediators, such as cytokines, reactive oxidants, and proteases. Extensive structural diversity among FcγR family members leads to differences in binding capacity, signal transduction pathways, and cell type–specific expression patterns. This diversity allows IgG complexes to activate a broad program of cell functions relevant to inflammation, host defense, and autoimmunity. Phagocyte activation is triggered by stimulatory FcγRs, facilitating the recognition, uptake, and destruction of antibody-coated targets, whereas multivalent IgG binding to FcγRs on platelets leads to platelet aggregation and thrombosis, and binding to FcγRs on NK cells mediates cytotoxicity of antibody-coated targets.

IgE binds to high-affinity FcεRs on mast cells, basophils, and activated eosinophils. In contrast to FcγRs, which are low affinity and bind to multivalent IgG rather than circulating individual IgG molecules, FcεRs can bind monomeric IgE. A single mast cell may be armed with IgE molecules specific for different antigens, all bound to surface FcεRs. Mast cells, localized beneath the mucosa of the gastrointestinal and respiratory tracts and the dermis of the skin, await exposure to multivalent antigens, which cross-link surface IgE bound to FcεRs and cause release of histamine-containing granules and generation of cytokines and other inflammatory mediators. IgE-mediated activation of eosinophils, cells normally present in the connective tissue of underlying respiratory, urogenital, and gut epithelium, leads to the release of highly toxic granule proteins, free radicals, and chemical mediators such as prostaglandins, cytokines, and chemokines. These amplify local inflammatory responses by activating endothelial cells and recruiting and activating more eosinophils and leukocytes. Prepackaged granules and high-affinity FcεRs that bind to free monomeric IgE enable an immediate response to pathogens or allergens at the first site of entry, a location where FcεR-bearing cells reside.

Inhibitory FcγRs, which modulate activation thresholds and terminate stimulating signals, are key elements in the regulation of effector function. Given that inhibitory and stimulatory Fc receptors are often coexpressed on the same cells, the effector response to a specific stimulus in a particular cell represents the balance between stimulatory and inhibitory signals. Inhibitory FcγRs can dampen responses triggered by FcεRs on mast cells and FcγR-mediated inflammation at sites of immune complex deposition.

Effector activities targeted by IgG and IgM also may be mediated by components of the complement system (Chapter 49). Antigen-bound multimeric immunoglobulin can initiate activation of the classical pathway of complement, causing enhanced phagocytosis of antigen-antibody complexes, increased local vascular permeability, and recruitment and activation of inflammatory cells. The target of injury is specified by the antibody, and the extent of damage is determined by the synergistic activities of immunoglobulin and complement.

Antigen-specific effector T cells also may initiate tissue injury. On exposure to an appropriate antigen, memory T cells are stimulated to release cytokines and chemokines that activate local endothelial cells and recruit and activate macrophages and other inflammatory cells. The effector cells directed by T-cell–derived cytokines, or cytolytic T cells themselves, mediate tissue damage. T_H1 cells produce interferon-γ (IFN-γ) and activate macrophages to cause injury, whereas T_H2 cells produce interleukin-4 (IL-4), IL-5, and eotaxin (an eosinophil-specific chemokine) and trigger inflammatory responses in which eosinophils predominate.

HYPERSENSITIVITY REACTIONS

In predisposed individuals, innocuous environmental antigens may stimulate an adaptive immune response, immunologic memory, and, on subsequent exposure to the antigen, inflammation. These "overreactions" of the immune system to harmless environmental antigens (allergens), called *hypersensitivity* or *allergic reactions,* produce tissue injury and can cause serious disease. Hypersensitivity reactions are grouped into four types according to the effector mechanisms by which they are produced (Table 46-1). The effectors for types I, II, and III hypersensitivity reactions are antibody molecules, whereas type IV reactions are mediated by antigen-specific effector T cells.

Autoimmune disease is characterized by the presence of antibodies and T cells specific for self-antigens expressed on target tissues. The mechanisms of antigen recognition and effector function that lead to tissue damage in autoimmune disease are similar to the mechanisms elicited in response to pathogens and environmental antigens. These mechanisms resemble certain hypersensitivity reactions and may be classified accordingly (Table 46-2). Autoimmune disease caused by antibodies directed against cell surface or extracellular matrix antigens corresponds to type II hypersensitivity reactions; disease caused by formation of soluble immune complexes that subsequently are deposited in tissue corresponds to type III hypersensitivity; and disease caused by effector T cells corresponds to type IV hypersensitivity. Typically, several of these pathogenic mechanisms are operative in autoimmune disease. However, IgE responses are not associated with damage in autoimmunity.

Type I Hypersensitivity Reactions

Type I hypersensitivity reactions (Fig. 46-1) are triggered by the interaction of antigen with antigen-specific IgE bound to FcεRs on mast cells, which causes mast cell activation. Proteolytic enzymes and toxic mediators, such as histamine, are released immediately from preformed granules, and chemokines, cytokines, and leukotrienes are synthesized after activation. Together, these mediators increase vascular permeability, break down tissue matrix proteins, promote eosinophil production and activation (IL-3, IL-5, and granulocyte-macrophage colony-stimulating factor [GM-CSF]), and cause influx of effector leukocytes (tumor necrosis factor-α [TNF-α], platelet-activating factor, and macrophage inflammatory protein [MIP-1]), constriction of smooth muscle, stimulation of mucus secretion, and amplification of T_H2 cell responses (IL-4 and IL-13). Eosinophils and basophils, activated through cell surface FcεRs, rapidly release highly toxic granular proteins (major basic protein, eosinophil peroxidase, and collagenase) and, over a longer period, produce cytokines (IL-3, IL-5, and GM-CSF), chemokines (IL-8), prostaglandins, and leukotrienes that activate epithelial cells, leukocytes, and eosinophils to augment local inflammation and tissue damage.

FcεR-bearing effectors act in a coordinated fashion. The immediate allergic inflammatory reaction initiated by mast cell products is followed by a late-phase response that involves recruitment and activation of eosinophils, basophils, and T_H2 lymphocytes. The manifestations of IgE-mediated reactions depend on the site of mast cell activation. Mast cells reside in vascular and epithelial tissue throughout the body. In a sensitized host (an individual with IgE responses to antigens), re-exposure to antigen leads to type I hypersensitivity responses only in the mast cells exposed to the antigen. Inhalation of antigens produces bronchoconstriction and increased mucus secretion

TABLE 46-1 FOUR MAJOR TYPES OF IMMUNOLOGICALLY MEDIATED HYPERSENSITIVITY REACTIONS*

IMMUNOLOGIC SPECIFICITY	TYPE I (IgE ANTIBODY)	TYPE II (IgG ANTIBODY)	TYPE III (IgG ANTIBODY)	Type IV (T Cells)			
				T_H1 CELLS	T_H2 CELLS	T_H17 CELLS	T CELLS
Antigen	Soluble antigen allergen	Cell- or matrix-associated antigen	Soluble antigen	Soluble antigen	Soluble antigen	Soluble antigen	Cell-associated antigen
Effector mechanism	FcεRI- or FcγRIII-dependent mast cell activation, with release of mediators/cytokines	FcγR$^+$ cells (phagocytes, NK cells), complement	FcγR$^+$ cells, complement	Macrophage activation	Eosinophil activation	Macrophage activation Neutrophil activation	Direct cytotoxicity
Examples	Systemic anaphylaxis, asthma, allergic rhinitis, urticaria, angioedema	Certain drug reactions and reactions to incompatible blood transfusions	Arthus reaction and other immune complex–mediated reactions (e.g., serum sickness, subacute bacterial endocarditis)	Contact dermatitis, tuberculin reaction	Chronic allergic inflammation (e.g., chronic asthma, chronic allergic rhinitis)	Contact dermatitis, atopic dermatitis, asthma, rheumatoid arthritis	Contact dermatitis (e.g., poison ivy), reactions to certain virus-infected cells, some instances of graft rejection

*Hypersensitivity reactions were classified into four types by Coombs and Gell (1963) and modified by Janeway and colleagues (2001).
FcγR = Fc receptor for immunoglobulin G; FcεR = Fc receptor for immunoglobulin E; NK = natural killer.
(From Coombs RRA, Gell PGH: Classification of allergic reactions responsible for clinical hypersensitivity and disease. In Gell PGH, Coombs RA [eds]: *Clinical Aspects of Immunology.* Oxford, UK: Blackwell; 1963; and Janeway C, Travers P, Walport M, Shlomchick M: *Immunobiology: The Immune System in Health and Disease.* 5th ed. New York: Garland Publishing; 2001.)

TABLE 46-2 CLASSIFICATION OF AUTOIMMUNE DISEASES ACCORDING TO MECHANISM OF TISSUE INJURY

HYPERSENSITIVITY REACTION	AUTOIMMUNE DISEASE	AUTOANTIGEN
TYPE II		
Antibody against cell-surface antigens	Autoimmune hemolytic anemia	Rh blood group antigens, I antigen
	Autoimmune thrombocytopenic purpura	Platelet integrin glycoprotein IIb:IIIa
Antibody against receptors	Graves' disease	Thyroid-stimulating hormone receptor (agonistic antibodies)
	Myasthenia gravis	Acetylcholine receptor (antagonistic antibodies)
Antibody against matrix antigens	Goodpasture's syndrome	Basement membrane collagen (α_3-chain of type IV collagen)
	Pemphigus vulgaris	Epidermal cadherin (desmoglein)
TYPE III		
Immune complex diseases	Mixed essential cryoglobulinemia	Rheumatoid factor IgG complexes (with or without hepatitis C antigens)
	Systemic lupus erythematosus	DNA, histones, ribosomes, binuclear proteins
TYPE IV		
T-cell-mediated diseases	Insulin-dependent diabetes mellitus	Pancreatic B-cell antigen
	Rheumatoid arthritis	Unknown synovial joint antigen
	Multiple sclerosis	Myelin basic protein, proteolipid protein

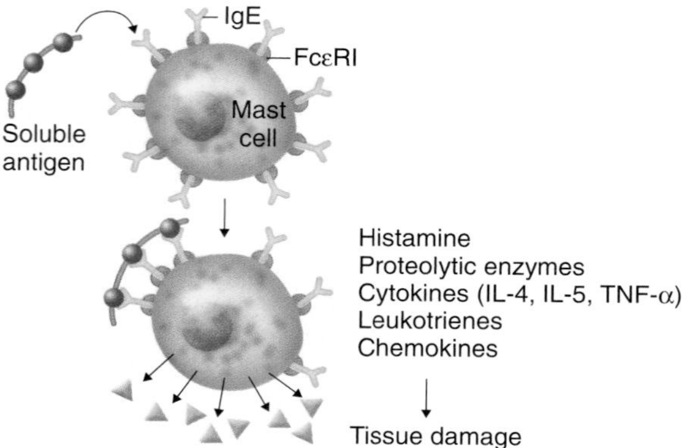

FIGURE 46-1. Type I hypersensitivity. Type I responses are mediated by immunoglobulin E (IgE), which induces mast cell activation. Cross-linking of the Fc receptor for IgE (FcεR) on mast cells, triggered by the interaction of multivalent antigen with antigen-specific IgE bound to FcεR, causes the release of preformed granules containing histamine and proteases. Cytokines, chemokines, and lipid mediators are synthesized after cell activation. IL = interleukin; TNF = tumor necrosis factor.

(asthma and allergic rhinitis); ingestion of antigens causes increased peristalsis and secretion (diarrhea and vomiting); and the presence of subcutaneous antigens initiates increased vascular permeability and swelling (urticaria and angioedema). Blood-borne antigens cause systemic mast cell activation, increased capillary permeability, hypotension, tissue swelling, and smooth muscle contraction—the characteristics of systemic anaphylaxis.

Type II Hypersensitivity Reactions

Type II hypersensitivity reactions (Fig. 46-2) are caused by chemical modification of cell surface or matrix-associated antigens that generates "foreign" epitopes to which the immune system is not tolerant. B cells respond to this antigenic challenge by producing IgG, which binds to these modified cells and renders them susceptible to destruction through complement activation, phagocytosis, and antibody-dependent cytotoxicity.

This phenomenon is seen clinically when drugs interact with blood constituents and alter their cellular antigens. Hemolytic anemia caused by immune-mediated destruction of erythrocytes (Chapter 163) and thrombocytopenia caused by destruction of platelets (Chapter 175), both type II hypersensitivity reactions, are adverse effects of certain drugs. Chemically reactive drug molecules bind covalently to the surface of red cells or platelets creating new epitopes that in a small subset of individuals are recognized as foreign antigens by the immune system and stimulate production of IgM and IgG antibodies reactive with the conjugate of drug and cell surface protein. Penicillin-specific IgG binds to penicillin-modified proteins on red blood cells and triggers activation of the complement cascade. Activation of complement components C1 through C3 results in covalent binding of C3b to the red cell membrane and renders circulating red cells susceptible to phagocytosis by FcγR and complement receptor–bearing macrophages in the spleen or liver. Activation of complement components C1 through C9 and formation of the membrane attack complex cause intravascular lysis of red cells. The factors that predispose only some people to drug-induced type II hypersensitivity reactions are unknown. Penicillin, quinidine, and methyldopa have been associated with hemolytic anemia and thrombocytopenia through this mechanism. Another example is heparin-induced

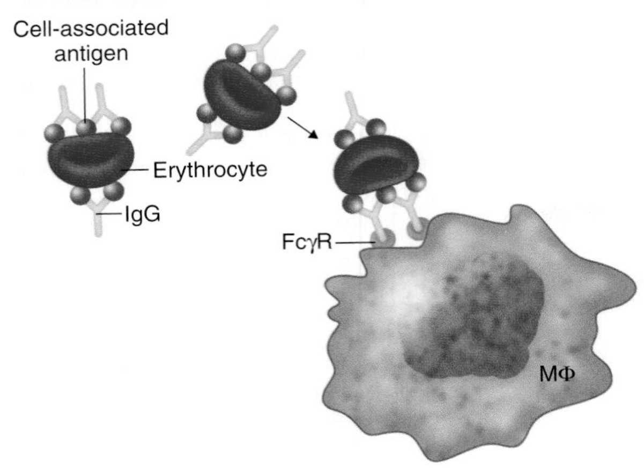

FIGURE 46-2. Type II hypersensitivity. Type II responses are mediated by immunoglobulin G (IgG) directed against cell surface or matrix antigens, which initiates effector responses through the Fc receptor for IgG (FcγR) and complement. The relative contributions of these pathways vary with the IgG subclass and the nature of the antigen. Only FcγR-mediated phagocytosis by macrophages (MΦ) is depicted in this figure. Activation of complement components would result in binding of C3b to the red blood cell membrane, rendering red blood cells susceptible to phagocytosis and leading to formation of the membrane attack complex and cell lysis.

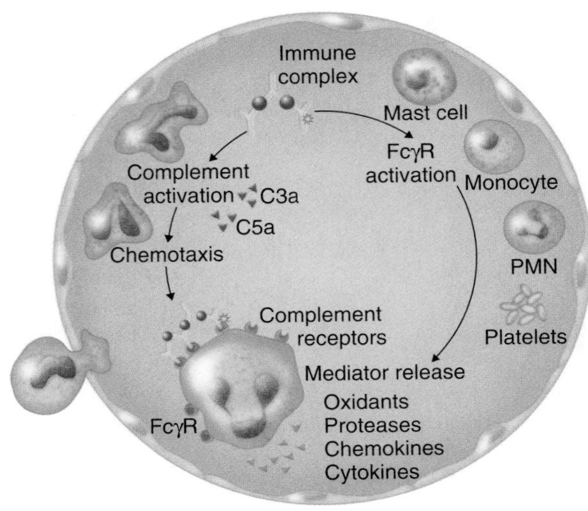

FIGURE 46-3. Type III hypersensitivity. Type III responses are mediated by immunoglobulin G (IgG) directed against soluble antigens. Localized deposition of immune complexes activates mast cells, monocytes, neutrophils, and platelets bearing the Fc receptor for IgG (FcγR), and initiates the complement cascade, all effectors of tissue damage. Generation of complement components C3a and C5a recruits and stimulates inflammatory cells and amplifies effector functions. PMN = polymorphonuclear leukocyte (also called *neutrophil*).

thrombocytopenia or thrombosis, a severe, life-threatening complication that occurs in 1 to 3% of patients exposed to heparin (Chapter 175). Interactions among heparin, human platelet factor 4, antibodies to the human platelet factor 4–heparin complex, platelet FcγRIIA, and splenic FcγRs (which remove opsonized platelets) are involved in the pathogenesis of this disease.

Autoantibodies directed at antigens on the cell surface or extracellular matrix cause tissue damage by mechanisms similar to type II hypersensitivity reactions. IgG or IgM antibodies against erythrocytes lead to cell destruction in autoimmune hemolytic anemia because opsonized cells (coated with IgG or IgM and complement) are removed from the circulation by phagocytes in the liver and spleen or are lysed by formation of the membrane attack complex. Platelet destruction in autoimmune thrombocytopenic purpura occurs through a similar process. Because nucleated cells express membrane-bound complement regulatory proteins, they are less sensitive to lysis through the membrane attack complex, but when coated with antibody, they become targets for phagocytosis or antibody-dependent cytotoxicity. This mechanism is responsible for autoimmune and alloimmune neutropenia (Chapter 170).

IgM and IgG antibodies recognizing antigens within tissue or binding to extracellular antigens cause local inflammatory damage through FcγR and complement mechanisms. Pemphigus vulgaris (Chapter 447) is a serious blistering disease that results from a loss of adhesion between keratinocytes caused by autoantibodies against the extracellular portions of desmoglein 3, an intercellular adhesion structure of epidermal keratinocytes. Another example of a type II hypersensitivity reaction is Goodpasture's disease (Chapter 123), in which antibodies against the α_3-chain of type IV collagen (the collagen in basement membranes) are deposited in glomerular and lung basement membrane. Tissue-bound autoantibodies activate monocytes, neutrophils, and basophils through FcγRs, initiating release of proteases, reactive oxidants, cytokines, and prostaglandins. Local activation of complement, particularly C5a, recruits and activates inflammatory cells and amplifies tissue injury. Neighboring cells are lysed by assembly of the membrane attack complex or by FcγR-initiated, antibody-dependent cytotoxicity.

Autoantibodies against cell surface receptors produce disease by stimulating or blocking receptor function. In myasthenia gravis (Chapter 430), autoantibodies against the acetylcholine receptors on skeletal muscle cells bind the receptor and induce its internalization and degradation in lysosomes, reducing the efficiency of neuromuscular transmission and causing progressive muscle weakness. In contrast, Graves' disease (Chapter 233) is characterized by autoantibodies that act as agonists. Autoantibodies to thyroid-stimulating hormone receptors bind the receptor, mimicking the natural ligand, inducing thyroid hormone overproduction, disrupting feedback regulation, and causing hyperthyroidism.

Type III Hypersensitivity Reactions

Type III hypersensitivity reactions (Fig. 46-3) are caused by tissue deposition of small soluble immune complexes that contain antigens and high-affinity IgG antibodies directed at these antigens. Localized deposition of immune complexes activates FcγR-bearing mast cells and phagocytes and initiates the complement cascade, all effectors of tissue damage.

Immune complexes are generated in all antibody responses. The formation and the fate of immune complexes depend on the biophysical and immunologic properties of the antigen and the antibody. These properties include the size, net charge, and valence of the antigen; the class and subclass of the antibody; the affinity of the antibody-antigen interaction; the net charge and concentration of antibody; the molar ratio of available antigen and antibody; and the ability of the immune complex to interact with the proteins of the complement system. The lattice size of the immune complex is influenced strongly by the physical size and valence of the antigen, the association constant of antibody for that antigen, the molar ratio of antigen and antibody, and the absolute concentrations of the reactants. Larger aggregates fix complement more efficiently, present a broader multivalent array of ligands for complement and FcγRs to bind, and are taken up more readily by mononuclear phagocytes in the liver and spleen and thereby removed from the circulation. Smaller immune complexes, which form in antigen excess—as occurs early in an immune response—circulate in the blood and are deposited in blood vessels, where they initiate inflammatory reactions and tissue damage through interactions with FcγRs and complement receptors.

Serum sickness is a systemic type III hypersensitivity reaction, historically described in patients injected with therapeutic horse antiserum for the treatment of bacterial infections. In general, serum sickness occurs after the injection of large quantities of a soluble antigen. Clinical features include chills, fever, rash, urticaria, arthritis, and glomerulonephritis. Disease manifestations become evident 7 to 10 days after exposure to the antigen, when antibodies are generated against the foreign protein and form immune complexes with these circulating antigens. Immune complexes are deposited in blood vessels, where they activate phagocytes and complement, producing widespread tissue injury and clinical symptoms. The effects are transient, however, and resolve after the antigen is cleared.

A syndrome similar to serum sickness occurs in chronic infections in which pathogens persist in the face of continued immune response. In subacute bacterial endocarditis (Chapter 76), antibody production continues but fails to eliminate the infecting microbes. As the pathogens multiply, generating new antigens, immune complexes form in the circulation and are deposited in small blood vessels, where they lead to inflammatory damage of skin, kidney, and nerve. Hepatitis B virus infection (Chapters 150 and 151) may be associated with immune complex deposition early in its course,

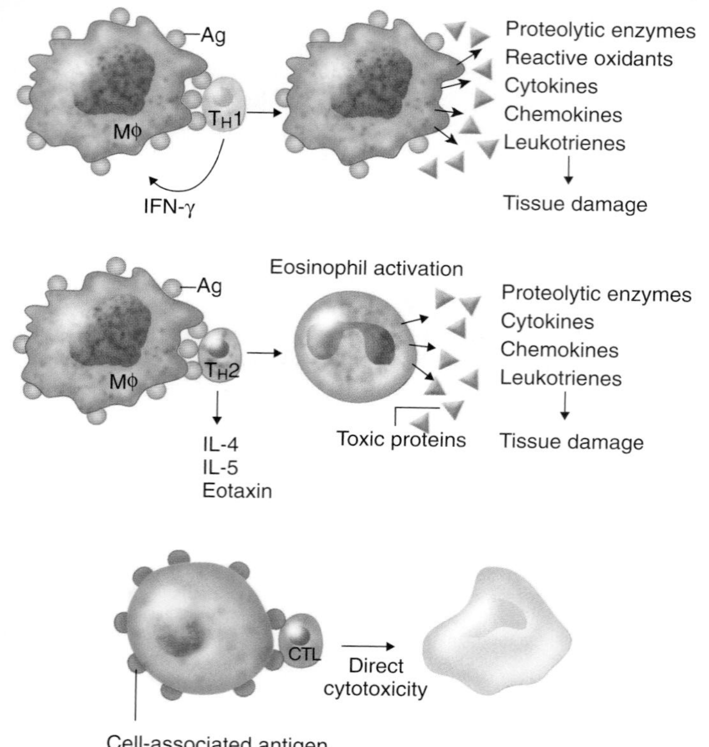

FIGURE 46-4. **Type IV hypersensitivity.** Type IV responses are mediated by T cells through three different pathways. In the first, type 1 helper T (T_H1) cells recognize soluble antigens (Ag) and release interferon-γ (IFN-γ) to activate effector cells, in this case macrophages (MΦ), and cause tissue injury. In T_H2-mediated responses, eosinophils predominate. T_H2 cells produce cytokines to recruit and activate eosinophils, leading to their degranulation and tissue injury lymphocytes (CTLs). In the third pathway, damage is caused directly by cytolytic T cells. IL = interleukin.

during a period of antigen excess, because antibody production in response to hepatitis B surface antigen is as yet relatively insufficient; some anicteric patients may present with acute arthritis. Mixed essential cryoglobulinemia, which may be associated with hepatitis C viral infection, is an immune complex–mediated vasculitis in which deposition of complexes containing IgG, IgM, and hepatitis C antigens causes inflammation in peripheral nerves, kidneys, and skin. Serum sickness also can develop in transplant recipients who are treated with mouse monoclonal antibodies specific for human T cells to prevent rejection, and in patients with myocardial infarction who are treated with the bacterial enzyme streptokinase to effect thrombolysis.

Systemic lupus erythematosus (Chapter 274), the prototypical immune complex–mediated autoimmune disease, is characterized by circulating IgG directed against common cellular constituents, typically DNA and DNA-binding proteins. Small immune complexes are deposited in skin, joints, and glomeruli and initiate local tissue damage.

Type IV Hypersensitivity Reactions

Type IV hypersensitivity reactions (Fig. 46-4), also known as *delayed-type hypersensitivity reactions,* are mediated by antigen-specific effector T cells. They are distinguished from other hypersensitivity reactions by the lag time from exposure to the antigen until the response is evident (1 to 3 days). Antigen is taken up, processed, and presented by macrophages or dendritic cells. Type 1 helper T (T_H1) effector cells that recognize the specific antigen (these are scarce and take time to arrive) are stimulated to release chemokines, which recruit macrophages to the site and release cytokines that mediate tissue injury. IFN-γ activates macrophages and enhances their release of inflammatory mediators, whereas TNF-α and TNF-β activate endothelial cells, enhance vascular permeability, and damage local tissue. The prototypical type IV hypersensitivity reaction is the tuberculin test, but similar reactions can occur after contact with sensitizing antigens (e.g., poison ivy, certain metals) and lead to epidermal reactions characterized by erythema, cellular infiltration, and vesicles. $CD8^+$ T cells also may mediate damage by direct toxicity.

In contrast to T_H1-mediated hypersensitivity reactions, in which the effectors are macrophages, eosinophils predominate in T_H2-mediated responses. T_H2 effector T cells are associated with tissue damage in chronic asthma (Chapter 87). T_H2 cells produce cytokines to recruit and activate eosinophils (IL-5 and eotaxin), leading to degranulation, further tissue injury, and chronic, irreversible airway damage.

T_H17 cells, members of the helper T-cell lineage, produce IL-17 family cytokines that regulate innate effectors and orchestrate local inflammation by inducing release of proinflammatory cytokines and chemokines, recruiting neutrophils, and enhancing T_H2 cytokine production to amplify allergic and autoimmune responses. T_H17 cells have been implicated in contact dermatitis, atopic dermatitis, asthma, and rheumatoid arthritis.

In some autoimmune diseases, effector T cells specifically recognize self-antigens to cause tissue damage, either by direct cytotoxicity or by inflammatory responses mediated by activated macrophages. In type 1 insulin-dependent diabetes mellitus, T cells mediate destruction of B cells of the pancreatic islets. IFN-γ–producing T cells specific for myelin basic proteins have been implicated in multiple sclerosis. Rheumatoid arthritis is another autoimmune disease caused, at least in part, by activated T_H1 cells.

SUGGESTED READINGS

Khosroshahi A, Stone JH. Treatment approaches to IgG4-related systemic disease. *Curr Opin Rheumatol.* 2011;23:67-71. *Review of this systemic fibroinflammatory condition.*

Klareskog L, Gregersen PK, Huizinga TW. Prevention of autoimmune rheumatic disease: state of the art and future perspectives. *Ann Rheum Dis.* 2010;69:2062-2066. *Review of suspected inciting antigens.*

Mauri C. Regulation of immunity and autoimmunity by B cells. *Curr Opin Immunol.* 2010;22:761-767. *Review.*

47

MECHANISMS OF INFLAMMATION AND TISSUE REPAIR

GARY S. FIRESTEIN

THE INFLAMMATORY RESPONSE

Host defense mechanisms have evolved to recognize pathogens rapidly, render them harmless, and repair the damaged tissue. This complex and highly regulated sequence of events can also be triggered by environmental stimuli such as noxious mechanical and chemical agents. Under normal circumstances, tightly controlled responses protect against further injury and clear damaged tissue. In disease states, however, pathologic inflammation can lead to marked destruction of the extracellular matrix (ECM) and organ dysfunction.

Initiation of the Inflammatory Response

When normal tissue encounters a pathogen, resident cells are stimulated by engagement of pattern recognition receptors that activate an ancient arm of host defense known as *innate immunity.* In contrast to *adaptive immunity,* which provides exquisite antigen specificity, innate immune responses recognize common motifs on pathogens (Chapter 44). Additional cytoplasmic receptors can sense "danger" signals from a toxic environment or cellular stress, such as urate or adenosine triphosphate (ATP). Innate mechanisms are designed for rapid responses (minutes to hours) compared with the more leisurely adaptive system that can take days to weeks to develop. In addition to orchestrating early events that are critical to host defense, cells of the innate system like dendritic cells orchestrate the subsequent adaptive cascade through the generation of chemokines that organize lymphoid tissue and presentation of antigens to lymphocytes. Innate immunity provides intergenerational continuity in that the receptors are encoded in the germline and are passed unchanged to progeny to protect the species. In contrast, each individual must generate his or her own adaptive immune system through complex somatic mutations and gene rearrangements. This provides defense tailored for each member of the species; its complexity and beauty permit specificity but also provide opportunities for error such as responses against self-antigens in autoimmunity.

Pattern Recognition Receptors and Innate Immunity

The toll-like receptor (TLR) family of proteins, which bind molecular structures on microbial pathogens that normally are not found in mammalian cells, are critical members of the innate immune system. Some are expressed on the cell surface, such as TLR2, which is activated primarily by bacterial peptidoglycan and lipoproteins, and TLR4, which is activated by lipopolysaccharide (LPS, or endotoxin). Others are expressed mainly on the inner leaflet of cytoplasmic vesicles, like TLR9, which is activated by unmethylated bacterial sequences that are enriched for CpG motifs, or TLR3 and TLR7, which are important for antiviral defense because they bind double-stranded and single-stranded viral RNA, respectively. In addition to exogenous molecules, some endogenous structures can bind to TLRs, including heat shock proteins and oxidized low-density lipoproteins (oxLDLs). The latter might be especially important in the pathogenesis of atherosclerosis, where LDL activates TLR4 within vascular plaques. Local endothelial cell– and macrophage-derived chemotactic factors can then recruit activated T cells into the atheroma.

Signaling by TLR2 and TLR4 progresses through adaptor proteins and often converges on a kinase known as MyD88, which orchestrates several downstream cascades. By directing the phosphorylation of IκB kinase-β (IKKβ), MyD88 activates nuclear factor-κB (NF-κB), a master switch for inflammatory genes. Translocation of NF-κB to the cell nucleus stimulates the production of cytokines (e.g., interleukin-6 [IL-6], IL-8, and tumor necrosis factor [TNF]), the machinery for prostaglandin release (e.g., cyclo-oxygenase 2 [COX2]), and genes that regulate the ECM (e.g., metalloproteinases). This rapid response is normally transient, although it can persist in pathogenic states. MyD88-independent pathways that stimulate innate immunity also exist. For instance, TLR3 stimulation by RNA viruses uses a separate pathway involving IKKβ and interferon regulating factor-3 (IRF-3). IRF-3, in combination with several other transcription factors, induces the expression of genes such as interferon-β (IFN-β) to establish an antiviral state.

These genes primarily offer protection against pathogens by initiating key defense mechanisms. However, these same pathways can create a hazardous milieu that is toxic to normal cells through the production of oxygen radicals, nitric oxide, and other reactive intermediaries. These molecules can damage DNA and harm bystander cells, or even lead to neoplasia (E-Table 47-1). For instance, long-standing inflammation in the colon, as in ulcerative colitis, is associated with adenocarcinoma. Increased COX2 expression as a result of NF-κB translocation is another mechanism that contributes to the development of tumors at inflammatory sites. An unanticipated finding is that NF-κB itself can also directly augment carcinogenesis by serving as a survival signal for damaged cells that would normally be deleted by apoptosis.

The TLR signal transduction mechanisms, initiated by broad categories of nonmammalian structures, integrate the environmental stimuli and generate a broadly antipathogenic response. Fine-tuning of host defenses against unique pathogen structures to provide long-lived immunity requires the slower, more precise adaptive immune system. Although it is more cumbersome and primitive, innate immunity provides signals that activate adaptive responses. For instance, TLRs can stimulate dendritic cells (Chapter 44), which have internalized and processed antigen, to migrate from peripheral tissues to central lymphoid organs. The dendritic cells can also produce cytokines and, after maturation, present antigens to T cells in the context of class II major histocompatibility molecules and surface costimulatory proteins. The activated T cells can then migrate to the tissue to enhance and amplify the host response. T cells also provide help to B cells, thereby stimulating antibody production and activating other components of innate immunity (e.g., the complement system).

The Inflammasome and Innate Immune Responses

Receptors that can recognize "danger" signals and potential pathogens are present in the cell cytoplasm. The inflammasome is among the best characterized systems and includes the 22-family-member human Nod-like receptor (NLR) family of cytoplasmic proteins. The activated NLR proteins recruit additional proteins to form a complex with caspase-1 and adaptor molecule apoptosis-associated specklike protein (ASC). Activation of caspase-1 is one of the critical functions of inflammasomes, with resultant cleavage and activation of IL-1, IL-18, and IL-33.

Disorders of the inflammasome can lead to autoinflammatory diseases. The prototypic syndromes known as familial cold autoinflammatory disease, Muckle-Wells disease, and neonatal-onset multisystem inflammatory disease (NOMID) are due to nonconserved mutations in the NLR gene that encodes cryopyrin (also known as NALP3). These three rare diseases are characterized by abnormal inflammasome activation with aberrant release of processed IL-1β. The clinical manifestations, including fever, rash, hearing impairment, and arthritis, depend on the specific amino acid substitution as well as other less well-defined genetic influences. The critical role of IL-1 has been proved by studies using treatment with IL-1 inhibitors, which prevent flares and, in some cases, appear to reverse end-organ disease. The inflammasome also appears to play a key role in other more common diseases, such as gout, in which urate crystals can activate the inflammasome. IL-1 inhibitors also appear to be effective in some patients, although long-term controlled studies are needed.

Immune Complexes and Complement

The complement system (Chapter 49) is another ancient defense mechanism that links innate immunity and the humoral arm of adaptive immunity. Both the classical complement pathway, activated by immunoglobulin G (IgG)– and IgM-containing immune complexes, and the alternative pathway, activated by bacterial products, converge at the third component of complement, C3, with proteolytic release of fragments that amplify the inflammatory response and mediate tissue injury. The anaphylotoxins C3a and C5a directly increase vascular permeability and contraction of smooth muscle. C3a and C3a desArg also induce TNF and IL-1β production by peripheral blood mononuclear cells. C5a induces mast cell release of histamine, thereby indirectly mediating increased vascular permeability. C5a also activates leukocytes and enhances their chemotaxis, adhesion, and degranulation, with release of proteases and toxic metabolites. C5b attaches to the surface of cells and microorganisms and is the first component in the assembly of the C5b-9 membrane attack complex.

Individuals with abnormalities of the early complement components, especially C1q, C2, and C4, usually have a minimally increased incidence of infection but demonstrate an enhanced risk of developing autoimmune diseases such as systemic lupus erythematosus (SLE) (Chapter 274). The mechanism of increased disease susceptibility is probably related to inefficient clearance of immune complexes. Enhanced activation and consumption of complement proteins can also occur in SLE accompanied by low plasma C3 and C4 levels, especially in association with disease exacerbations. C3 or C5 deficiency causes increased susceptibility to bacterial infections, whereas defects in the late components that form the membrane attack complex result in an increased incidence of *Neisseria* sp bacteremia.

Environmental Stress and Tissue Damage

Tissue injury due to direct trauma or noxious stimulus also initiates an inflammatory response and is associated with microvascular damage, extravasation of leukocytes through vascular walls, and leakage of plasma and proteins into the tissue. As noted previously, the inflammasome acts as a sensor that can initiate this program in some cases. In other cases, such as ischemia, acid-sensitive ion channels on the cell surface can detect the environmental stress due to a decrease in tissue pH. Thrombus formation at the site of vascular damage begins the inflammatory cascade through the release of vasoactive amines (e.g., serotonin), release of lysosomal proteases, and formation of eicosanoid products. The platelets can also later regulate healing with release of growth factors such as platelet-derived growth factor (PDGF) and transforming growth factor-β (TGF-β).

Second Wave of the Inflammatory Response

Activation of innate immunity quickly leads to the robust influx of inflammatory cells. Resident cells, such as vascular endothelial cells, mast cells, dendritic cells, and interstitial fibroblasts, respond by releasing soluble mediators, including eicosanoids and pro-inflammatory cytokines (E-Table 47-2). These mediators amplify the inflammatory response and recruit additional leukocytes. Locally stimulated cells, along with the newly arrived inflammatory cells, release toxic reactive intermediates of nitrogen and oxygen as well as a myriad of proteases, principally matrix metalloproteinases (MMPs), serine proteases, and cysteine proteases. These molecules are designed to help destroy infectious agents and remove damaged cells, thus clearing the injured site for tissue repair. Prolonged stimulation of acute inflammatory mechanisms can cause severe tissue destruction. However, in most situations, the normal physiologic response is an exquisitely coordinated program that uses proteolytic enzymes to remodel the ECM and promote a supportive environment for wound healing rather than tissue damage.

Cellular Response

Inflammatory cell infiltration at the site of initial tissue damage typically progresses in an orderly fashion. The process begins with release of chemokines and soluble mediators from resident cells, including interstitial fibroblasts, mast cells, and vascular endothelial cells. Signaling from these events alters the local adhesion molecule profile and creates a chemotactic gradient that recruits cells from the blood stream. Mast cells, in particular, act as sentinels and can degranulate within seconds to release vasoactive amines. In most acute responses, polymorphonuclear leukocytes (PMNs) are the first inflammatory cells to extravasate from the circulation and arrive at the site of injury, followed later by mononuclear cells under the influence of separate signals.

Most tissue fibroblasts and vascular endothelial cells are quiescent before migration of PMNs into the tissue. However, these resident cells can be triggered to proliferate and migrate toward the site of injury as well as to synthesize cytokines, proteases, and ECM components. Growth factors are released, such as basic fibroblast growth factor (bFGF) and vascular endothelial growth factor (VEGF), stimulating new blood vessel formation. Together with granulocyte-macrophage colony-stimulating factor (GM-CSF), these locally released growth factors contribute to cellular proliferation and amplification of the inflammatory response and also induce maturation of dendritic cells that process antigens. In addition, fibroblasts and endothelial cells secrete new ECM proteins, MMPs, and other ECM-digesting enzymes. The balance of protease and ECM production varies as tissue is remodeled during the course of inflammation. Initially, the response favors proteolytic activity to clear damaged infrastructure. This is followed by a shift to increased production of new ECM to allow tissue repair and wound healing.

Increased vascular permeability, caused by disruption of endothelial cell tight junctions, allows blood-borne proteins such as fibrinogen, fibronectin, and vitronectin to extravasate into the perivascular ECM. Interaction with preexisting ECM allows the assembly of new ligands for a subset of adhesion molecules (e.g., integrins $\alpha5\beta1$ and $\alpha v\beta3$). This increased vascular permeability and change in the profiles of adhesion molecules and ligands, in conjunction with release of chemoattractant molecules, lead to the recruitment of leukocytes to sites of inflammation. Some of the chemokines involved are IL-8 (for neutrophils), macrophage chemoattractant protein-1 (MCP-1) for monocytes, RANTES (regulated on activation, T-cell expressed and secreted) for monocytes and eosinophils, and IL-16 (for $CD4^+$ T cells). In addition, chemokines recruit specific subsets of cells by binding to chemokine receptors.

The precise combination of chemokines and vascular adhesion molecules present in an inflammatory lesion determines the specificity of time and event for the recruitment of subsets of inflammatory cells. Ligation of integrins on leukocytes also prolongs cell survival once they have moved into the tissue, by preventing apoptosis. The central role of certain specific adhesion molecule-ligand pairs has been confirmed in human diseases. For instance, $\alpha4\beta1$ plays a key role in the recruitment of lymphocytes to the central nervous system in multiple sclerosis, and blocking this interaction suppresses disease activity (Chapter 419). Eosinophils also use the same adhesion receptors to migrate into the lung in allergen-induced asthma (Chapter 87).

Increased expression of intracellular adhesion molecule 1 (ICAM-1) and vascular cell adhesion molecule 1 (VCAM-1), as well as increased chemokine expression, is also evident in other cell types, such as the airway epithelium after allergen challenge in asthma. Rapid and transient influx of neutrophils occurs in allergic airway disease, along with activation of the local T cells and mast cells. These neutrophils produce lipid mediators, reactive oxygen intermediates, and proteases such as elastase, which may contribute to airflow obstruction, epithelial damage, and remodeling. Neutrophil elastase, together with chemokines released by both recruited and allergen-activated T cells and mast cells, serves to recruit eosinophils.

Soluble Mediators

Pro-inflammatory Cytokines

Pro-inflammatory cytokines, often derived from macrophages and fibroblasts, are mediators that activate the immune system. The pro-inflammatory members of the IL-1 family (IL-α, IL-1β, IL-18, and IL-33) and TNF have pleiotropic activities and can enhance adhesion molecule expression on endothelial cells, induce proliferation of endogenous cells, and stimulate antigen presentation. IL-1 and TNF also increase expression of matrix-degrading enzymes, such as collagenase and stromelysin. In addition, they stimulate synthesis of other inflammatory mediators such as prostaglandin E_2 (PGE_2) from fibroblasts. Inhibitors of TNF are effective therapeutic agents in inflammatory diseases such as psoriasis, rheumatoid arthritis, and inflammatory bowel disease, and IL-1 inhibitors are beneficial in genetic diseases such as Muckle-Wells syndrome and familial cold autoinflammatory syndrome.

IL-1 and TNF comprise only a small fraction of the acute cytokine response. Many other factors also participate, including IL-6 and its related cytokines (IL-11, osteopontin, and leukemia inhibitory factor), which can both induce acute phase reactants and bias an immune response toward a helper T type 1 (T_H1) or T_H2 phenotype (Chapter 46). GM-CSF can regulate dendritic cell maturation, increase expression of human leukocyte antigen (HLA-DR) on these cells, and enhance antigen presentation. The T_H1 lymphokine IFN-γ, although often considered part of the secondary wave that ensues after T-cell activation, can also induce expression of HLA-DR, increase expression of endothelial cell adhesion molecules, and inhibit collagen production. IL-1, IL-6, and IL-23 coordinate differentiation toward Th17 cells, a phenotype that is thought to play a major role in inflammation and autoimmunity owing to the production of IL-17 family members (IL-17A through F). Of these, IL-17A and perhaps IL-17F are especially important because they can synergize with IL-1 and TNF. The growth factor TGF-β biases cells toward the regulatory T cell (Treg) phenotype, which can suppress antigen-specific responses of other T cells (see later).

Cytokines play a key role in the establishment and perpetuation of inflammatory diseases. In rheumatoid arthritis (Chapter 272), autocrine and paracrine cytokine networks play a critical role in the perpetuation of inflammation. Effects of IL-1 and TNF are often central to continued synovitis, and there is increasing evidence that IL-15 participates by enhancing TNF production. IL-17A contributes to synoviocyte activation, and IL-18 can trigger T-cell differentiation toward a T_H1 phenotype. Factors such as MCP-1 recruit and activate macrophages into atheromas containing oxLDLs and foam cells. In allergic asthma (Chapter 87), IL-13 is emerging as a central inflammatory cytokine. IL-13 functions through binding to cell surface IL-4 receptors, and IL-4R–deficient mice are relatively resistant to the development of asthma. An IL-23 inhibitor, ustekinemab, has shown dramatic efficacy in psoriasis, indicating a major role for this pathway in inflammatory skin disease.

Eicosanoids

In addition to cytokines and immune complexes, local inflammatory responses lead to the release of eicosanoids, which are lipid-derived molecules. Because lipids are present in the cell membrane, they are readily available substrates for the synthesis of mediators. These molecules are functional immediately adjacent to sites of synthesis, and their half-lives range from seconds to minutes. Eicosanoids are not stored but are produced de novo from membrane lipids when cell activation by mechanical trauma, cytokines, growth factors, or other stimuli leads to release of arachidonic acid. Cytosolic phospholipase A_2 ($cPLA_2$) is the key enzyme in eicosanoid production. Cell-specific and agonist-dependent events coordinate the translocation of $cPLA_2$ to the nuclear envelope, endoplasmic reticulum, and Golgi apparatus, where interaction with cyclooxygenase (COX) (in the case of prostaglandin synthesis) or 5-lipoxygenase (in the case of leukotriene synthesis) can occur.

Prostaglandins

Prostanoids are produced when arachidonic acid is released from the plasma membrane of injured cells by phospholipases and metabolized by cyclooxygenases and specific isomerases (Chapter 36). These molecules act both at peripheral sensory neurons and at central sites within the spinal cord and brain to evoke pain and hyperalgesia. Their production is increased in most acute inflammatory conditions, including arthritis and inflammatory bowel disease. In response to exogenous and endogenous pyrogens, PGE_2 derived from COX2 mediates a central febrile response. In addition, prostaglandins synergize with bradykinin and histamine to enhance vascular permeability and edema. The levels of prostaglandins are usually very low in normal tissues and increase rapidly with acute inflammation, well before leukocyte recruitment. COX2 induction with inflammatory stimuli most likely accounts for the high levels of prostanoids in chronic inflammation.

COX2 also plays a key role in platelet-endothelial cell interactions by increasing the production of prostacyclin (PGI_2) in endothelial cells (Chapter 36). Increased risk of myocardial infarction associated with the use of selective COX2 inhibitors might be related to unopposed production of thromboxane A_2 by COX1 in platelets. Prostacyclin production also protects against atherosclerosis in female mice, and COX2 blockade abrogates this beneficial effect. Thus, COX inhibitors can potentially increase thrombotic events.

Leukotrienes

In addition to prostaglandins, a distinct set of enzymes direct arachidonic acid metabolites toward the synthesis of leukotrienes (Chapter 87). Their relative importance depends on the specific target organ of an inflammatory response. For instance, leukotriene receptor antagonists have demonstrated efficacy in asthma, whereas similar approaches have been less impressive in rheumatoid arthritis. Unlike prostaglandins, leukotrienes are primarily produced by inflammatory cells such as neutrophils, macrophages, and mast cells. 5-Lipoxygenase is the key enzyme in this cascade, transforming released arachidonic acid to the epoxide leukotriene A_4 (LTA_4) in concert with 5-lipoxygenase-activating protein (FLAP). LTA_4 can be hydrolyzed by cytosolic LTA_4 hydrolase to LTB_4, a potent neutrophil chemoattractant and stimulator of leukocyte adhesion to endothelial cells. LTA_4 can also conjugate with glutathione to form LTC_4 by LTC_4 synthase at the nuclear envelope. LTC_4 migrates out of the cell, using transporters such as the multidrug resistance–associated protein, and can be metabolized extracellularly to LTD_4 and LTE_4. These three cysteinyl leukotrienes comprise the "slow-reacting substance of anaphylaxis" for their slow and sustained smooth muscle–contracting abilities. They promote plasma leakage from postcapillary venules, upregulation of expression of cell surface adhesion molecules, and bronchoconstriction.

Histamine

Histamine is a vasoactive amine produced by basophils and mast cells that markedly increases capillary leakage. In basophils, histamine is released in response to bacterial formylmethionyl-leucyl-phenylalanine (f-MLP) sequences, complement fragments C3a and C5a, and IgE. The resultant edema can be readily observed clinically in urticaria (Chapters 260 and 448) and allergic rhinitis (Chapter 259). Despite the production of histamine in asthma and in acute synovitis, histamine blockers have minimal therapeutic effect in these conditions. The stimulus for release of histamine from mast cell granules is the same as in basophils, except for the absence of f-MLP receptors in this cell type. Histamine can also synergize with locally produced LTB_4 and LTC_4. In addition, histamine enhances leukocyte rolling and firm adhesion, and induces gaps in the endothelial cell lining, enhancing leukocyte extravasation.

Kinins

Kinins induce vasodilation, edema, and smooth muscle contraction, as well as pain and hyperalgesia, through stimulation of C fibers. They are formed from high- and low-molecular-weight kininogens by the action of serine protease kallikreins in plasma and peripheral tissues. The primary products of kininogen digestion are bradykinin and lysyl-bradykinin. These products have high affinity for the B2 receptor, which is widely expressed and is responsible for the most common effects of kinins. The peptides desArg-BK and Lys-desArg-BK are generated by carboxypeptidases and bind the kinin B1 receptor subtype, which is not expressed in normal tissues but is rapidly upregulated by TLR ligands and cytokines. The kinin B2 receptor is internalized rapidly and desensitized, whereas the B1 receptor remains highly responsive. Kinin actions are associated with the secondary production of other mediators of inflammation, including nitric oxide, mast cell–derived products, and the pro-inflammatory cytokines IL-6 and IL-8. In addition, kinins can increase IL-1 production through initial stimulation of TNF and can increase prostanoid production through activation of phospholipase A_2 and release of arachidonic acid.

Mechanisms of Tissue Damage in Inflammation

Reactive Oxygen and Nitrogen

Macrophages, neutrophils, and other phagocytic cells can generate large amounts of toxic reactive oxygen intermediates (ROIs) and reactive nitrogen intermediates (RNIs) that can directly kill pathogens. ROIs and RNIs also serve as critical signal transduction molecules that regulate expression of inflammatory genes.

These molecules can have deleterious effects on normal tissue by damaging DNA, oxidizing membrane lipids, and nitrosylating proteins. Release of reactive intermediates can be initiated by microbial products such as LPS and lipoproteins, by cytokines such as IFN-γ and IL-8, and by engagement of Fc receptors by IgG. These events cause translocation of several cytosolic proteins, including Rac2 and Rho-family guanosine triphosphatase (GTPase) to the membrane-bound complex carrying cytochrome *c*, with subsequent activation of reduced nicotinamide adenine dinucleotide phosphate (NADPH) oxidase. The reaction catalyzed by NADPH oxidase leads to superoxide production, which, in turn, increases hydrogen peroxide, hydroxyl radicals and anions, hypochlorous acid, and chloramines.

In some cases, ROIs can contribute directly to the initiation of chronic disease. Lipid oxidation produces aldehydes that substitute lysine residues in apolipoprotein B-100. This altered moiety either binds to TLR2 to induce cytokine production or is internalized by macrophages, leading to the production of foam cells and fatty streaks, the primary lesions of atherosclerosis (Chapter 70). Subsequently, altered epitopes in damaged host proteins can be presented to T cells to initiate an adaptive immune response that amplifies the inflammatory vascular lesion.

Nitric oxide synthases (NOS) convert L-arginine and molecular oxygen to L-citrulline and nitric oxide (NO). There are three known isoforms of NOS: neuronal NOS (ncNOS or NOS1) and endothelial cell NOS (ecNOS or NOS3) are both constitutively expressed, whereas macrophage NOS (macNOS, iNOS, or NOS2) is induced by inflammatory cytokines such as TNF-α and IFN-γ, as well as by products of viruses, bacteria, protozoa, and fungi and by low oxygen tension and low environmental pH.

Together with prostaglandins, the production of NO by NOS2 and ROIs by NADPH oxidase is a key mechanism by which macrophages paradoxically impair T-cell proliferation. This might control inflammatory processes or delete autoreactive T cells and partially accounts for the immunosuppression observed in certain infections and malignancies.

Proteases

Production of enzymes that degrade the ECM represents a key mechanism of tissue turnover in inflammation. Reconfiguring of the matrix remodels damaged tissue, releases matrix-bound growth factors and cytokines, prepares the tissue for the ingrowth of new blood vessels, and alters the local milieu to permit adherence and retention of newly recruited cells.

The MMPs are a family of more than 20 extracellular endopeptidases that participate in degradation and remodeling of the ECM matrix (Table 47-1). They are produced as pro-enzymes and require limited proteolysis or partial denaturation to expose the catalytic site. Their name is derived from their dependence on metal ions (zinc/metzincin superfamily) for activity and from their potent ability to degrade structural ECM proteins. MMPs can also cleave cell surface molecules and other pericellular nonmatrix proteins, thereby regulating cell behavior. For instance, MMPs can alter cell growth by digesting matrix proteins associated with growth factors. FGF and TGF-β

TABLE 47-1 COMMON MATRIX METALLOPROTEINASES (MMPS) AND THEIR SUBSTRATES

MMP FAMILY	MATRIX SUBSTRATES	OTHER SUBSTRATES
Collagenases	Collagen I, II, III, VII, and X Aggrecan	Pro-MMP-1, -2, -8, -9, and -13 Pro-TNF-α
Entactin	α_1-Proteinase inhibitors Gelatin Tenascin	
Gelatinases	Aggrecan Denatured collagen Elastin Fibronectin Laminin Vitronectin	Pro-MMP-1, -2, and -13 Pro-TNF-α Pro-IL-1β Latent TGF-β
Matrilysins	Proteoglycans Denatured collagens Entactin Fibrin, fibrinogen Fibronectin Gelatin Laminin Tenascin Vitronectin	Pro-MMP-2 and -7 Pro-TNF-α Membrane-bound Fas ligand (FasL) Plasminogen β4 Integrins
Stromelysins	Proteoglycans Aggrecan Collagen III, IV, V, IX, X, and XI Entactin Fibrin, fibrinogen Fibronectin Gelatin Laminin Tenascin Vitronectin	Pro-MMP-1, -3, -7, -8, -9, -10, and -13 Pro-TNF-α Pro-IL-1β Plasminogen α_1-Proteinase inhibitors

IL = interleukin; MMP = matrix metalloproteinase; TGF = transforming growth factor; TNF = tumor necrosis factor.

have high affinities for matrix molecules that serve as depots for storage of these cytokines in their activation state. Matrix proteolysis releases some growth factors and can make them available to cell surface receptors. In addition, MMPs can directly cleave and activate growth factors. MMPs affect cell migration by altering cell-matrix or cell-cell receptor sites. For instance, the adhesion molecule β4 integrin is cleaved by MMP-7. MMP-3 and MMP-7 digest E-cadherin and not only disrupt endothelial cell junctions but also stimulate cell migration.

Degradation of the ECM is usually initiated by collagenases, which cleave native collagen. Denatured collagen is then recognized and further degraded by gelatinases and stromelysins. Unlike the collagenases, stromelysins demonstrate broad substrate specificity and act on many ECM proteins, such as proteoglycan, fibronectin, laminin, and many cartilage proteins. Stromelysins can also amplify the remodeling process by activating collagenase through limited proteolysis. MMP gene expression can be induced by many pro-inflammatory cytokines, including TNF, IL-1, IL-17, and IL-18, through MAP kinase signal transduction pathways.

Several other classes of proteases remodel the matrix, including serine proteases and cysteine proteases. High levels of active serine proteases, such as trypsin, chymotrypsin, and elastase, are released by infiltrating PMNs at sites of inflammation and can directly digest the ECM or activate the pro-enzyme forms of secreted MMPs. The ADAM (a disintegrin and metalloproteinase) family can cleave the extracellular domain of cytokine receptors. These ECM proteases include two members of the aggrecanase family. One of the aggrecanases (aggrecanase 2, or ADAMTS5) has been implicated in osteoarthritis because mice deficient in this enzyme have decreased cartilage destruction in models of osteoarthritis.

Tissue Repair and Resolution of Inflammation

Inflammation is a normal physiologic response, but it can cause serious host injury if it is allowed to persist. Hence, additional mechanisms are required to reestablish homeostasis once this response is initiated. Suppression of acute inflammation by removal or deactivation of mediators and effector cells permits the host to repair damaged tissues through elaboration of appropriate growth factors and cytokines (Fig. 47-1). As in the initial generation of an inflammatory response, components of resolution include a cellular response (apoptosis and necrosis), formation of soluble mediators (such as anti-inflammatory cytokines and antioxidants), and production of direct effectors (such as protease inhibitors).

Deletion of Inflammatory Cells

Cells can be removed from an inflammatory site by several mechanisms. First, the influx of cells can be decreased by suppressing chemotactic factor production and vascular adhesion molecule expression. Second, cells, especially lymphocytes, can be released from the tissue and return to the circulation through lymphatics. Third, stressed cells can undergo necrosis with the release of their contents into the local environment. Perhaps the most critical mechanism for clearing cells from an inflammatory site is programmed cell death, or apoptosis.

Apoptosis is a highly regulated process in eukaryotic cells that leads to cell death and marks the surface membrane for rapid removal by phagocytes. This clearance process does not elicit an inflammatory response, in contrast to cell death by necrosis. PMN phagocytes have a very short half-life in the tissue, and the persistence or release of their contents into the microenvironment after death can be deleterious. In some pathologic conditions, such as leukocytoclastic vasculitis (Chapter 278), abundant neutrophil apoptosis is readily apparent on histopathologic examination; in fact, it is one of the pathologic criteria for this diagnosis. Other cells, including T lymphocytes, undergo postactivation apoptosis to prevent their overwhelming of host responses. Defective apoptosis or even persistence of apoptotic cells that escape clearance may contribute to chronic inflammatory and autoimmune diseases. For instance, loss of tolerance to self-antigens might participate in autoimmune responses in SLE.

Commitment of a cell to apoptosis can be initiated by a number of factors, including the ROIs in the cellular microenvironment as well as signaling through several death receptor pathways (e.g., FasL/Fas and TNF-related apoptosis-inducing ligand [TRAIL]). The former can damage DNA, which is a common byproduct of the genotoxic environment created by inflammation. If DNA damage is excessive, repair by tightly regulated mismatch repair mechanisms is terminated, and programmed cell death begins. The burden of mutations induced by ROIs or RNIs in chronic inflammation can potentially accumulate over time and eventually lead to amino acid substitutions in key regulatory proteins. Ultimately, as has been observed in ulcerative colitis, neoplastic disease can ensue.

Removal of apoptotic bodies, or the remnants of packaged apoptotic cells, is rapid and can be accomplished by macrophages, fibroblasts, epithelial and endothelial cells, muscle cells, and dendritic cells. The surface receptors used in recognition and engulfment of apoptotic cells include integrins (e.g., αvβ3), lectins, scavenger receptors, adenosine triphosphate (ATP)-binding cassette transporter 1, LPS receptor, CD14, and complement receptors CR3 and CR4. However, some of these membrane molecules can be used in both pro-inflammatory and apoptotic pathways, the divergence of which may be based on differing ligands and accessory molecules. Apoptotic cells display a series of membrane-associated molecular patterns that interact with receptors on phagocytes. The details of interactions between apoptotic cells and phagocytes are only partially understood. A general feature of apoptotic cells is loss of phospholipid asymmetry, with external presentation of phosphatidylserine. Externalized phosphatidylserine may be sufficient to trigger phagocytosis, but other apoptotic cell surface structures exist.

Although some inflammatory and immune cells are being deleted, other cell lineages expand during the resolution phase. Mesenchymal cells, especially fibroblasts, proliferate and produce new matrix that can contract to form

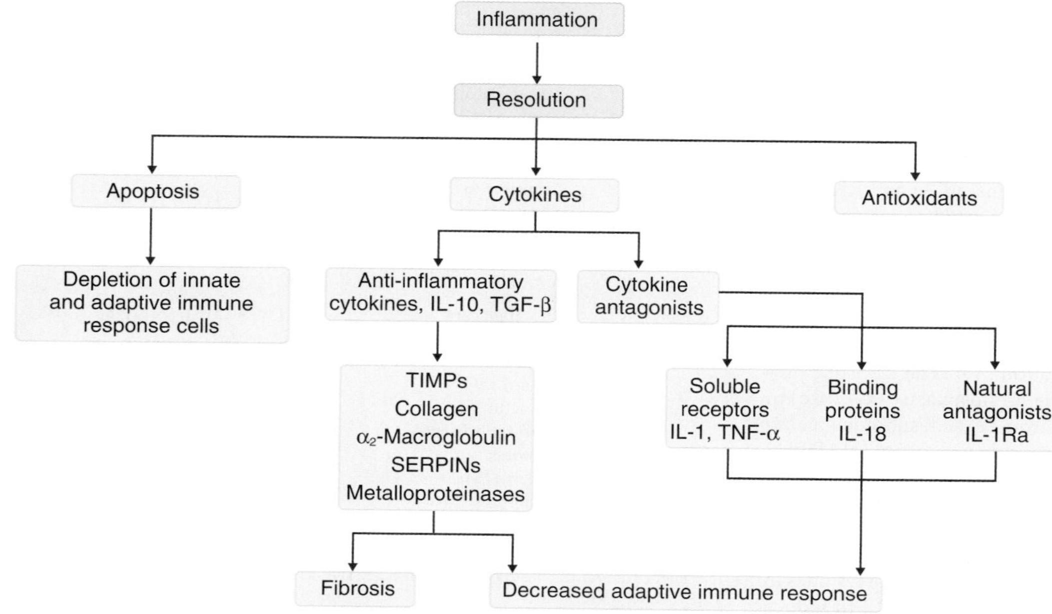

FIGURE 47-1. Anti-inflammatory mechanisms that resolve inflammation and lead to repair of the extracellular matrix. IL = interleukin; SERPINs = serine protease inhibitors; TGF = transforming growth factor; TIMPs = tissue inhibitor of metalloproteinases; TNF = tumor necrosis factor.

a fibrotic scar. Locally produced growth factors such as PDGF and TGF-β induce DNA synthesis of these stromal cells. In addition, mesenchymal stem cells that either reside in the tissue or migrate from the peripheral blood can differentiate into the appropriate organ-specific lineage. The pluripotential cells, in the presence of the appropriate milieu, can become adipocytes, chondrocytes, bone cells, or other terminally differentiated stromal cells.

Soluble Mediators

Anti-inflammatory Cytokines

A variety of anti-inflammatory cytokines are released by resident and infiltrating cells. TGF-β and IL-10 are examples that are produced by macrophages, interstitial fibroblasts, or T cells. Some T-cell cytokines, including IL-4, IL-10, and IL-13, suppress the expression of MMP by cells stimulated by IL-1 or TNF. In addition to increasing fibroblast proliferation, TGF-β suppresses collagenase production, increases collagen deposition, and decreases MMP activity by inducing production of the tissue inhibitors of metalloproteinases (TIMPs). The repair phase is abnormal in diseases in which tissue fibrosis represents a major pathologic manifestation. For example, scleroderma (Chapter 275) is marked by diffuse fibrosis and is accompanied by high levels of TGF-β and increased production of ECM.

Cytokine decoy receptors can also downregulate the inflammatory response. Receptors can also be shed from the cell surface after proteolytic cleavage and can absorb cytokines, thereby preventing them from ligating functional receptors on cell membranes. These cytokine inhibitors can be released as a coordinated attempt to prevent unregulated inflammation, as in septic shock (Chapter 108), in which endotoxin induces production of soluble receptors after initial massive production of TNF and IL-1. Other types of cytokine-binding proteins are also produced as counter-regulatory mechanisms, including IL-18-binding protein (IL-18BP), which is an Ig superfamily-related receptor that captures IL-18. In bone remodeling (Chapter 251), interactions of receptor activator of NF-κB (RANK) with RANK ligand are required for osteoclast-mediated resorption. The competitive antagonist osteoprotegerin is a member of the TNF receptor family that binds to RANK ligand and inhibits osteoclast activation.

The need for tight control of the pro-inflammatory cytokine IL-1 is demonstrated by the existence of two separate mechanisms. An IL-1 decoy receptor, known as the type II IL-1R, has both cell membrane and soluble forms that neutralize IL-1 activity. In addition, a natural IL-1 antagonist, IL-1Ra, can bind to functional IL-1 receptors and compete with IL-1α or IL-1β. However, IL-1Ra does not transduce a signal to the cell and blocks the biologic functions of ambient IL-1. The balance of IL-1 and IL-1Ra production depends on many influences. For instance, monocytes produce more IL-1, whereas mature macrophages produce IL-1Ra.

Prostanoids and Cyclooxygenase

COX2 induced by pro-inflammatory mediators appears early and can contribute to inflammatory responses. However, COX2 expression late in the process has led to speculation that it also functions in the resolution of inflammation. This regulation might occur through formation of the cyclopentenone prostaglandins (CyPG). The prostanoids can serve as ligands for peroxisome proliferator-activated receptors (PPARs) (Chapter 213). There are three main classes of PPAR receptors—PPARα, PPARβ/δ, and PPARγ—all of which bind to DNA as heterodimers in association with the retinoid X receptor. Activation of PPARγ by CyPG is associated with the suppression of activator protein 1 (AP-1) and signal transducer and activator of transcription (STAT) transcriptional pathways in macrophages. A variety of natural and synthetic PPAR agonists have demonstrated efficacy in models of ischemia-reperfusion injury, arthritis, and inflammatory airway disease.

Inhibitors of Direct Effectors

Antioxidants

Antioxidant enzymes that can inactivate the toxic intermediates and protect normal tissues include catalase and superoxide dismutase. Catalase is a peroxisomal enzyme that catalyzes the conversion of hydrogen peroxide to water and oxygen. Superoxide dismutases (SOD) catalyze the dismutation of superoxide to hydrogen peroxide, which is then removed by catalase or glutathione peroxidase. Glutathione peroxidases and glutathione reductase are additional mechanisms for maintaining redox balance and removal of toxic metabolites. Insufficient production of intracellular antioxidants such as glutathione can suppress lymphocyte responses and could account for defective T-cell receptor signaling and blunted immunity in T cells derived from rheumatoid arthritis synovium (Chapter 272).

Interactions of free radicals with surrounding molecules can generate secondary radical species in a self-propagating chain reaction. Chain-breaking antioxidants are small molecules that can receive or donate an electron and thereby form a stable byproduct with a radical. These antioxidant molecules are categorized as either aqueous phase (vitamin C, albumin, reduced glutathione) or lipid phase (vitamin E, ubiquinol-10, carotenoids, and flavonoids). In addition, transition metal-binding proteins (ceruloplasmin, ferritin, transferrin, and lactoferrin) can serve as antioxidants by sequestering cationic iron and copper and thereby inhibiting the propagation of hydroxyl radicals.

Protease Inhibitors

Protease inhibitors regulate the function of endogenous proteases and reduce the likelihood of collateral damage to tissues. These proteins form two functional classes, active site inhibitors and α_2-macroglobulin (α2M). The latter class of protease inhibitors acts by covalently linking the protease to the α2M chain and thereby blocking access to substrates. α2M binds to all classes of proteases and, after forming a covalent bond, conveys them to cells through receptor-mediated endocytosis with subsequent enzymatic inactivation. The family of inhibitors of serine proteases (SERPINs) are the most abundant members of the former class of protease inhibitors and play a major role in regulation of blood clot resolution and inflammation, as indicated by many of their names: antithrombin III, plasminogen activator inhibitors 1 and 2, α_2-antiplasmin, α_1-antitrypsin, and kallistatin.

The tissue inhibitor of metalloproteinases (TIMP) family blocks the function of most MMPs. The TIMPs bind to activated MMPs and irreversibly block their catalytic sites. Examples of disease states with an unfavorable balance between TIMPs and MMPs include loss of cartilage in arthritis and regulation of tumor metastasis. TIMP-MMP imbalance in destructive forms of arthritis appears be caused by the limited production capacity for protease inhibitors, which is overwhelmed by the prodigious expression of MMPs. Whereas IL-1 and TNF-α induce MMPs, IL-6, TGF-β, and several other growth factors suppress production of MMPs and increase levels TIMPs. Therefore, the cytokine profile has a pivotal influence on the status of remodeling. When pro-inflammatory cytokines predominate, the balance favors matrix destruction; in the presence of pro-inflammatory cytokine inhibitors and growth factors, matrix protein production increases, and MMPs are inhibited by TIMPs.

SUGGESTED READINGS

Davis DM. Mechanisms and functions for the duration of intercellular contacts made by lymphocytes. *Nat Rev Immunol.* 2009;9:543-555. *Detailed discussion of structure and function relationships in key adhesion molecules as they relate to cell-cell communication.*

Karin M. The IκB kinase: a bridge between inflammation and cancer. *Cell Res.* 2008;18:334-342. *Discusses mechanisms that link inflammation and cancer, with an emphasis on NF-κB.*

Lee SB, Kaluri R. Mechanistic connection between inflammation and fibrosis. *Kidney Int.* 2010;78:S22-S26. *Review.*

Martinon F, Mayor A, Tschopp J. The inflammasomes: guardians of the body. *Annu Rev Immunol.* 2009;27:229-265. *Review of how the inflammasome regulates innate immunity and host defense.*

Wang J, Hori K, Ding J, et al. Toll-like receptors expressed by dermal fibroblasts contribute to hypertrophic scarring. *J Cell Physiol.* 2011;226:1265-1273. *Rationale for manipulating these receptors to ameliorate scarring.*

48 TRANSPLANTATION IMMUNOLOGY

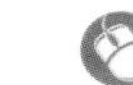

MEGAN SYKES

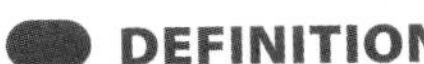

DEFINITION

Clinical transplantation encompasses the transplantation of organs and islets of Langerhans, in which it is necessary to overcome the host-versus-graft (HVG) immune response to avoid rejection, as well as hematopoietic cell transplantation (HCT; Chapter 181), in which not only the HVG but also the graft-versus-host (GVH) immune response must be contended with. Because preparations of marrow or mobilized peripheral blood stem cells contain mature T cells, their administration to conditioned, and consequently immunoincompetent, recipients is associated with the risk of GVH disease. Organs transplanted include the cornea, kidney, liver, heart, lung,

TABLE 48-1 LYMPHOCYTES INVOLVED IN GRAFT REJECTION

CELL TYPE	ANTIGENS RECOGNIZED	FUNCTION	ROLE IN TRANSPLANTATION
$CD4^+$ T cells	Allogeneic MHC class II (± peptide) Self–MHC class II + donor peptide	1. Assistance (cytokines and costimulation) in $CD8^+$ T-cell activation, expansion, and CTL differentiation; B-cell Ig class switching, expansion, and effector differentiation 2. Cytotoxicity 3. Regulatory function	Organ allografts Cellular allografts Xenografts GVHD
$CD8^+$ T cells	Allogeneic MHC class I (± peptide) Self–MHC class I + donor peptide	1. Cytotoxicity 2. Cytokine production 3. Regulatory function	Organ allografts Cellular allografts Xenografts GVHD
NK cells	MHC class I (activates or inhibits NK cell function) Other activating ligands	1. Cytotoxicity 2. Cytokine production	? Organ allografts Cellular allografts Xenografts
B cells	MHC class I and II Blood group antigens Xenogeneic carbohydrates	1. Antibody-mediated rejection (hyperacute, acute humoral, and chronic rejection)	Organ allografts Cellular allografts Xenografts

CTL = cytotoxic T lymphocyte; GVHD = graft-versus-host disease; Ig = immunoglobulin; MHC = major histocompatibility complex; NK = natural killer.

small intestine, and pancreas, and even the hand and face. The list of transplanted allogeneic cells is likely to expand in the future to include other cell types such as hepatocytes, myoblasts, and stem cell–derived replacement cells. Transplants originating from a member of the same species are referred to as *allotransplants.* However, many believe that transplants from other species, termed *xenografts,* represent a promising solution to the severely inadequate supply of allogeneic organs and tissues, and such grafts may be used in the future.

ANTIGENS IN TRANSPLANTATION

The major antigens recognized during graft rejection and the cell types targeting them are summarized in Table 48-1.

Major Histocompatibility Antigens

The major histocompatibility complex (MHC; Chapter 45)—consisting of human leukocyte antigens (HLAs) in humans—presents the strongest immunologic obstacle to all types of allografts. Because of its uniquely extensive polymorphism, truly MHC-identical, unrelated donors are difficult to find in an outbred species such as humans. The strong immunogenicity of allogeneic MHC molecules relates to the manner in which T cells are selected in the thymus; developing thymocytes do not survive unless they can weakly recognize a self-MHC/peptide complex on a thymic stromal cell. This process is termed *positive selection.* However, because thymocytes whose receptors have high affinity for self-MHC complexes are deleted, strongly autoreactive T cells rarely make it into the peripheral T-cell pool. Allogeneic antigens are not part of this *negative selection* process. The net result of these two selection steps is that the human T-cell "repertoire" is strongly biased to have cross-reactivity to allogeneic MHC molecules, providing a barrier to organ and hematopoietic cell transplantation. In the case of organ transplantation, in which long-term pharmacotherapy with powerful immunosuppressive drugs is used in an effort to prevent graft rejection, this can translate into improved results with matched organs in some situations. However, for unrelated, cadaveric donor transplantation, the benefits of HLA matching may be counterbalanced by the disadvantages associated with prolonged graft ischemia when attempts are made to transport organs to the most closely matched recipient. For HCT, the risks of GVH disease and marrow graft failure are so greatly amplified in the presence of extensive HLA mismatches that such transplants are generally avoided; if a sufficiently matched, related donor cannot be found, a search is conducted through large registries containing millions of volunteer unrelated donors.

Minor Histocompatibility Antigens

Minor histocompatibility antigens are peptides derived from polymorphic peptides presented by an MHC molecule. Even genotypically HLA-identical siblings have different minor histocompatibility antigens. These are sufficient to induce graft rejection if immunosuppressive pharmacotherapy is not used. In the case of HCT, significant GVH disease frequently (about 30 to 50% of the time) complicates transplantation between HLA-identical siblings, even with the use of pharmacologic immunoprophylaxis.

Other Antigens

The major blood group (ABO) antigens can be the target of a dramatic "hyperacute" rejection process that occurs when mismatched vascularized grafts are transplanted. Recognition of blood group antigens on the endothelial surface of the graft vessels by recipient "natural" antibodies (antibodies without known sensitization to the antigens) activates the complement and coagulation cascades, resulting in rapid graft thrombosis and ischemia. A similar outcome can occur after transplantation to an individual with preformed antidonor HLA antibodies resulting from presensitization by prior transplantation, transfusion, or pregnancy. Antibodies against other polymorphic antigens, such as MHC class I–related chain A, have been associated with graft rejection. Until recently, successful transplantation was not possible in the presence of a positive antidonor crossmatch. However, considerable success has now been achieved in the transplantation of ABO-mismatched kidneys, livers, and hearts (the last in the neonatal period only) and in the transplantation of kidneys to highly presensitized patients. In the case of kidney and liver transplantation, initial removal of the antibody and sometimes depletion of B cells, as well as the infusion of intravenous immunoglobulin, have led to success. ABO-mismatched neonatal heart transplantation has been successful because the transplant is performed before the recipient has developed high levels of anti–blood group antigen antibodies, and the B cells seem to be rendered tolerant to the donor blood group antigen by the grafting process. Recognition of blood group antigens can also be of significance in HCT, in which ABO barriers are routinely crossed in both directions. This can cause hemolysis of recipient erythrocytes if the mismatch is in the GVH direction, but this complication can be avoided by washing the cellular product before infusion. Mismatches in the HVG direction can cause more persistent problems due to ongoing destruction of donor erythropoietic cells, resulting in pure red cell aplasia. More often, however, donor erythropoiesis is established, and antidonor isohemagglutinins disappear from the circulation.

A and B blood group antigens are caused by the presence or absence of specific glycosylation enzymes in different individuals. Likewise, an antigenic specificity of the utmost importance in xenotransplantation is a carbohydrate epitope, Galα1-3Galα1-4GlcNAc (αGal), which is produced by a specific galactosyl transferase. Humans and Old World monkeys lack a functional αGal transferase and produce high levels of natural antibodies against the ubiquitous αGal epitope. Because animals of interest as xenograft sources (e.g., pigs) express αGal at high levels on their vascular endothelium, transplantation of vascularized organs from pigs results in hyperacute rejection unless something is done to absorb the antibodies or inactivate complement. The recent development of αGal-knockout pigs is therefore an important milestone, and encouraging results have been obtained in initial studies of pig-to-primate transplantation.

In another type of transplant reaction, recognition as foreign results not from the presence of an antigen but, paradoxically, from the absence of a self-MHC molecule. Natural killer (NK) cells express a series of surface inhibitory and activating receptors that determine, collectively, whether the NK cell does or does not kill a potential target cell. The ligands for the inhibitory receptors are MHC class I molecules, and the receptors recognize specific groups of alleles. An NK cell may kill an allogeneic target that lacks a self-MHC inhibitory ligand. In animal models, this phenomenon results in rapid bone marrow rejection when the donor marrow cells are not given in excess numbers or when a fraction of them is destroyed by an incompletely suppressed T-cell response. A similar phenomenon has not been clearly demonstrated in clinical HCT. The possibility that NK cells play a role in organ allograft rejection has long been an area of controversy. NK cells may be of particular importance in xenotransplantation, where they appear early in infiltrates of organ xenografts undergoing acute vascular rejection. NK cells clearly play a strong role in the rejection of xenogeneic bone marrow, an observation that is relevant in one approach to inducing tolerance (see the later discussion).

MECHANISMS OF REJECTION AND GRAFT-VERSUS-HOST DISEASE

Cellular Mediators

Many different cell types participate in rejection responses, and there is considerable redundancy. T cells are key players in most forms of rejection, with the exception of rejection that can be induced by antibodies in the absence of T-cell help. These include hyperacute and acute vascular rejection processes that may be induced by natural antibodies, as described earlier, or by antibodies that are present due to presensitization. The possible role of NK cells has already been discussed.

Direct and Indirect Allorecognition

T-cell responses are induced by antigen-presenting cells (APCs) that present alloantigens. There are two forms of alloantigen recognition—direct and indirect (Fig. 48-1). Direct allorecognition denotes recognition of donor antigens on donor APCs provided by the graft. The extraordinarily high frequency of T cells with alloreactivity is caused by direct recognition of allogeneic MHC. Indirect recognition is the recognition of donor antigens that are picked up and presented on recipient MHC molecules on recipient APCs. The indirect response is more similar to "normal" T-cell responses, in which professional APCs present peptide antigens to T cells that are present at relatively low frequency in the naïve repertoire.

Direct alloreactivity is particularly important in the early post-transplantation period, when APCs within the transplanted organ are still present; many of these cells migrate to the lymphoid tissues, where they initiate the alloresponse. However, the APC supply that comes with the donor graft is not renewable; therefore, if the direct response is not maintained by the recognition of donor antigens on endothelial cells or other cells in the graft, it recedes in importance. The indirect response, in contrast, can be maintained by the constantly renewed pool of recipient APCs. The indirect response is of particular importance in inducing antibody responses.

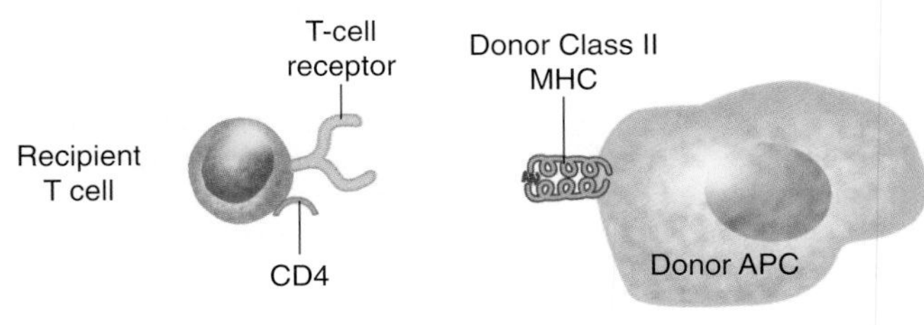

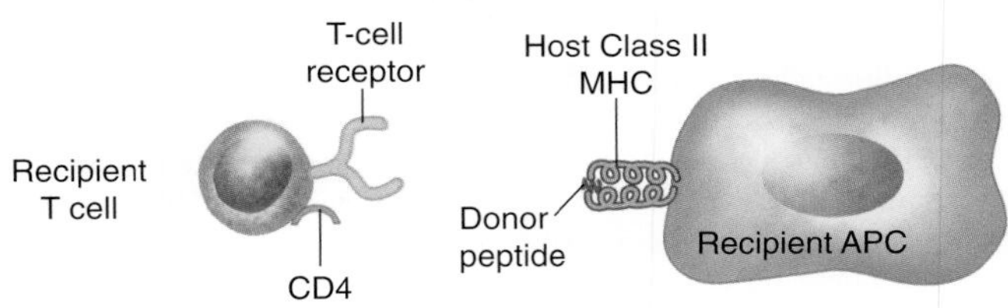

FIGURE 48-1. Direct and indirect allorecognition. Direct allorecognition involves the recognition by a T-cell receptor of major histocompatibility complex (MHC) molecules (with or without a peptide) on a donor antigen-presenting cell (APC). Indirect allorecognition involves recognition by the T-cell receptor of a donor peptide presented on a recipient APC that has picked up and processed donor antigens.

Effector Mechanisms of Rejection

T cells can promote graft rejection through several effector mechanisms. One is the antibody-dependent processes that have already been discussed, which can be induced by $CD4^+$ helper T cells that promote the differentiation and immunoglobulin (Ig) class switching of B cells that recognize other specificities on the same alloantigens. T cells provide cognate help to B cells when they recognize complexes of self-MHC with donor MHC-derived peptide antigens (produced by B cells whose surface Ig receptors recognize and pick up the donor MHC antigen). If antidonor antibody is not present before transplantation but is induced afterward, the response can lead to the pathologic picture of acute humoral rejection. Antibodies may also participate in a slower, poorly understood process of chronic rejection, which, in the case of kidney and heart transplantation, is characterized by unique vascular lesions with intimal thickening and loss of the vessel space and, in the case of lung transplantation, by obliterative bronchiolitis. The mechanisms underlying these chronic rejection lesions are not well understood, and several different immune processes may in fact lead to similar lesions.

Another major effector pathway leading to graft rejection involves cytotoxic T lymphocytes (CTLs), which are predominantly members of the $CD8^+$ T-cell subset but also include $CD4^+$ T cells. Several effector mechanisms lead to the killing of target cells by CTLs; these include the granzyme/perforin-mediated pathway and the pathways involving Fas/Fas ligand (FasL) and other members of the tumor necrosis factor (TNF) receptor family and their ligands (Chapter 46). Because $CD8^+$ cells recognize MHC class I molecules, which are widely expressed, it is not difficult to envision graft destruction by $CD8^+$ CTLs. $CD8^+$ CTLs may be activated via an APC that is initially stimulated through contact with an alloreactive $CD4^+$ cell. This is one form of CD4 "help" for $CD8^+$ cells. In addition, $CD8^+$ cells may be dependent on cytokines such as interleukin-2 (IL-2) from $CD4^+$ cells for their expansion and cytotoxic differentiation. However, there are also many examples of $CD8^+$ cell-mediated rejection that is independent of "help" from $CD4^+$ cells. MHC class II, which is recognized by $CD4^+$ T cells, is less widely expressed on graft tissues than is MHC class I, although it may be induced on endothelial cells and graft parenchymal cells in the presence of inflammatory cytokines such as interferon-γ (IFN-γ).

In addition to cytotoxic mechanisms resulting from direct allorecognition, $CD4^+$ and $CD8^+$ T cells with indirect specificity seem to be capable of causing graft destruction under some circumstances. Cytokines such as IFN-γ have been implicated in some instances, but the pathways of indirect graft destruction are not well understood. A $CD8^+$ cell-mediated form of skin graft rejection dependent on donor antigens cross-presented on recipient MHC molecules (a form of indirect allorecognition for $CD8^+$ cells) has been described in an animal model. This form of graft rejection may be directed at antigen presented on the endothelial cells of recipient vessels that revascularize the graft. This mechanism would not apply to primarily vascularized organ allografts.

The Role of T-Cell Trafficking

All the rejection processes described require trafficking of T cells into the graft. This process is made possible after the initial activation of naïve T cells in the lymphoid tissues. Naïve T cells can migrate into lymph nodes because of their expression of the CCR7 chemokine receptor and the adhesion molecule L-selectin. These T cells are activated by migratory graft APCs that also enter the lymph nodes. T-cell activation is associated with the loss of CCR7 and L-selectin expression and the acquisition of a new set of chemokine receptors and adhesion molecules that allow rolling and adhesion on the graft endothelium and entry into the graft parenchyma (Chapter 46). Inflammation in the graft, such as that induced by ischemia-reperfusion injury and the transplantation procedure itself, as well as that induced by initially responding T cells, is associated with the upregulation of chemokines and adhesion ligands that promote the entry of lymphocytes into the graft. Nevertheless, well-healed grafts can be slowly rejected by adoptively transferred memory T cells, demonstrating that acute graft injury and inflammation are not essential for rejection in the presence of an established memory T-cell response. Rejection of hematopoietic cell grafts may involve many of the same mechanisms involved in solid organ rejection, although less work has been done in this area.

Mechanisms of Graft-versus-Host Disease

Initiation of GVH disease (Chapter 181) requires that donor T cells recognize host alloantigens. The disease attacks a variety of recipient epithelial

TABLE 48-2 EXPERIMENTAL STRATEGIES TO PREVENT GRAFT-VERSUS-HOST DISEASE

STRATEGY	ADVANTAGES	LIMITATIONS
Donor T-cell T_H2 polarization (e.g., conditioning with ATG and TLI, in vitro stimulation with cytokine exposure)	May preserve GVL	May limit GVL; T_H2 can contribute to acute and chronic GVHD
Tolerance induction of donor T cells (e.g., costimulatory blockade, regulatory cells)	Some strategies may selectively tolerize GVH-reactive T cells (e.g., in vitro antigen exposure with costimulatory blockade)	Global immunosuppression may limit GVL and anti-infectious immunity; tolerance (i.e., GVH protection) may be incomplete
Donor T-cell depletion plus NK-cell infusion with class I mismatched transplantation	NK cells do not cause GVHD but may mediate antitumor effects; donor NK cells may eliminate host APCs that trigger GVHD	May require very large numbers of donor NK cells; antitumor effect may not apply to all tumors; requires appropriate MHC disparity and expression of polymorphic NK cell receptors; insufficient T-cell immunity to infection
Donor T-cell depletion followed by delayed DLI	Preserves high level of GVL due to GVH reactivity; GVHD does not occur if host inflammation from conditioning has subsided and initial HCT was devoid of donor T cells	Antitumor effect delayed until time of DLI; most applicable for indolent lymphohematopoietic tumors; GVHD more difficult to control in humans than in animal models
Depletion of donor T cells recognizing host alloantigens by in vitro activation/depletion (i.e., "allodepletion")	Preserves anti-infectious immunity and tumor antigen-specific responses	Loss of GVH reactivity limits GVL; highly efficient allodepletion methods not yet available; residual T cells may cause GVHD
Donor T-cell depletion with infusion of expanded infection-specific T cells (e.g., CMV or EBV-specific)	Reduced GVHD potential while protecting against significant infectious organisms	Lack of GVL effect; lack of broad anti-infectious immunity; expense and inefficiency of in vitro T-cell expansion; loss of survival/homing potential of cultured T cells
Donor T-cell depletion with infusion of expanded tumor antigen-specific T cells	GVL without GVHD	Lack of anti-infectious immunity; expense and inefficiency of in vitro expansion of tumor-specific T cells; loss of survival/homing potential of cultured T cells
Insertion of suicide gene (e.g., thymidine kinase) into donor T cells	Drugs targeting inserted gene (e.g., gancyclovir) kill donor T cells to treat GVHD after GVL initiated	Expense and inefficiency of in vitro transduction of T cells; loss of function/survival/homing potential of cultured T cells; risk of GVHD if transduction incomplete; curtailment of GVL when donor T cells killed in vivo
Block T-cell trafficking to epithelial GVHD target tissues (e.g., blockade of adhesion molecules or chemokines, sphingosine 1 phosphate agonists)	Permits lymphohematopoietic GVH reactions to occur, with associated GVL effects	Redundancy of trafficking pathways in inflammatory environment may limit efficacy; tumors outside of lymphohematopoietic system not targeted
Block injury/promote repair in epithelial target tissues (e.g., keratinocyte growth factor)	Permits lymphohematopoietic GVH reactions to occur, with associated GVL effects	Efficacy may be limited

APC = antigen-presenting cell; ATG = antithymocyte globulin; CMV = cytomegalovirus; DLI = donor lymphocyte infusion; EBV = Epstein-Barr virus; GVH = graft versus host; GVHD = graft-versus-host disease; GVL = graft-versus-leukemia effects; HCT = hematopoietic cell transplantation; MHC = major histocompatibility complex; NK = natural killer; T_H2 = helper T lymphocytes type 2; TLI = total lymphoid irradiation.

tissues, including the skin, intestine, and liver. Animal models have demonstrated clear roles for both $CD4^+$ and $CD8^+$ cells in initiating GVH disease, and each subset can do so independently of the other. The mechanisms of GVH disease include activation of alloreactive donor T cells by recipient APCs, leading to the differentiation of effector cells with direct cytotoxic activity and cytokine production in response to host antigens. A prominent role is played by TNF-α, whose production is induced in part by the translocation of bacteria across the intestinal wall, promoting activation of the innate immune system via toll-like receptors (Chapter 44). An intensely proinflammatory environment is produced by the combination of conditioning-induced tissue injury and disruption of mucosal barriers, bacterial activation of the innate immune system, and the GVH alloresponse. It is now appreciated that the inflamed microenvironment in target tissues plays an important role in promoting the trafficking of GVH-reactive T cells into these tissues.

STRATEGIES TO PREVENT GRAFT-VERSUS-HOST DISEASE

In view of the critical role of donor T cells in inducing GVH disease (Chapter 181), an obvious strategy to prevent this complication is to remove mature T cells from the marrow graft. In both animal models and clinical studies, this approach has been effective in preventing GVH disease; however, it has several disadvantages. One is that adult humans, particularly those who have undergone prior chemotherapy and radiotherapy, have little remaining thymic tissue and therefore demonstrate sluggish T-cell recovery, leading to serious opportunistic infections.

The second disadvantage applies to the most common indication for allogeneic HCT—the treatment of hematologic malignancies (Chapter 181). In this setting, T-cell depletion is often associated with an increased relapse rate due to the loss of a graft-versus-tumor effect, which is in large part mediated by GVH alloreactivity. Separation of GVH disease from graft-versus-tumor effects is a major goal of research in HCT, and some promising strategies are being explored (Table 48-2). These include the control of T-cell trafficking so that the GVH alloresponse is confined to the lymphohematopoietic tissues where the tumor resides, as well as host conditioning with total lymphoid irradiation in combination with antithymocyte globulin in an attempt to enrich NKT cells, which may inhibit GVH disease without impeding graft-versus-tumor effects.

The third disadvantage of donor T-cell depletion in HCT is that it increases the rate of engraftment failure. GVH alloreactivity and a "veto" effect of donor T cells help overcome host resistance to donor engraftment. A "veto" cell, which may be a T cell or an NK cell, kills a CTL that recognizes it. Although this phenomenon has been well established in animal models, its mechanisms have not been clearly determined, and its potential role in humans is uncertain. NK-cell recognition in the GVH direction, resulting from the absence in the recipient of an MHC class I ligand (E-Fig. 48-1) that can trigger a donor NK-cell inhibitory receptor (KIR), may promote donor marrow engraftment and antitumor effects in the setting of T-cell–depleted, HLA-mismatched HCT.

Clinically, pharmacologic immunosuppressive prophylaxis is usually used for at least 6 months after HCT to minimize the complication of GVH disease. Additionally, HLA-matched or closely matched donors are chosen whenever possible, because GVH disease increases in frequency and severity as more HLA barriers are transgressed. These measures are insufficient, however, and GVH disease remains a major complication of HCT. Therefore, many of the new strategies being explored in organ transplantation and other fields are also being examined for the prevention of GVH disease in experimental models. It should be borne in mind, however, that donor T cells' tolerance to recipient alloantigens (see the later discussion) might not be entirely beneficial in the setting of HCT for the treatment of malignant disease, because the loss of GVH alloreactivity is likely to come with a loss of antitumor effects.

STRATEGIES TO PREVENT ALLOGRAFT REJECTION

Nonspecific Immunosuppression

Immunosuppressive drugs are the mainstay of clinical organ transplantation, and improvements in these drugs have allowed the transplantation of hearts, lungs, pancreatic islets, and livers. The mechanisms of action of these agents are discussed in Chapter 34. However, it is noteworthy that despite these improvements and their enormous impact on early graft survival, these agents have been less effective in attenuating late graft loss. Because chronic immunologic rejection processes and the side effects of immunosuppressive drugs themselves are responsible for much of this late graft loss, better immunosuppressive agents and the induction of immune tolerance (see the later discussion) are major research goals.

Costimulatory Blockade

As our understanding of immune responses has increased, efforts to improve allograft survival have focused on numerous biologic agents, including antibodies and small molecules that target receptors of the immune system, as well as cell-based therapies. Because of the central role played by T cells in the immune response, considerable attention has been paid to blockers of T-cell costimulation. When a naïve T cell recognizes antigen through its unique T-cell receptor, additional costimulatory signals are required to allow full activation, expansion, and differentiation to occur. These signals are often provided by APCs in the form of ligands (e.g., B7-1, B7-2) for costimulatory receptors (e.g., CD28) on the T cell. Cross-talk between the T cell and the APC (e.g., due to CD40 activation by CD154 upregulation on the activated T cell) further amplifies the costimulatory activity of the APC, allowing it to effectively activate other T cells as well. The CD154 (T cell)–CD40 (B cell) interaction also promotes Ig class switching and the functioning of B cells as APCs. Blockade of these processes (e.g., by CTLA4Ig and anti-CD154 monoclonal antibodies) has led to marked prolongation of allograft survival in stringent rodent and large-animal models. Robust, systemic tolerance to donor antigens has been achieved in rodents receiving bone marrow transplants with costimulatory blockade and little or no additional conditioning. Some of these agents have been or are currently being evaluated in clinical trials of transplantation and autoimmune diseases. Anti-CD154 antibodies have been associated with thromboembolic complications, however, and their evaluation in transplantation trials is currently on hold. Numerous additional costimulatory and inhibitory pathways that affect T-cell responses have been described, and these are all potential targets for further manipulation of the alloresponse.

Immune Tolerance

Immune tolerance denotes a state in which the immune system is specifically unreactive to the donor graft (or recipient, in the case of GVH reactivity), while remaining normally responsive to other antigens. Tolerance is distinct from the state produced by nonspecific immunosuppressive agents, which increases the risk of infection and malignancy. Numerous approaches to tolerance induction have been described in rodent models, largely owing to the strong tolerogenicity of primarily vascularized heart, liver, and kidney grafts in these animals. Because such grafts are less tolerogenic in humans, none of these strategies has been applied clinically to date. Therefore, tolerance strategies that are appropriate for clinical evaluation must first be tested in stringent models, including relatively nontolerogenic grafts such as MHC-mismatched skin in rodents and vascularized organ graft models in large animals. In most of the models, only a superficial understanding of the mechanisms leading to tolerance has been achieved.

The three major mechanisms of T-cell tolerance are deletion, anergy, and suppression (often referred to as *regulation*). *Deletion* denotes the destruction of T cells with receptors that recognize donor antigens; it can be achieved during T-cell development in the thymus, for example, by the induction of mixed chimerism in T-cell–depleted hosts. Deletion can also be applied to mature T cells in the periphery, for example, by transplantation of a tolerogenic organ or marrow graft in combination with blockade of costimulatory molecules. *Anergy* denotes the inability of T cells to respond fully to antigens they recognize, and it can be induced by antigen presentation without costimulation. *Suppression* has attracted considerable interest since the discovery that constitutively $CD25^+$ T cells of the $CD4^+$ subset have suppressive activity that is dependent on expression of the transcription factor forkhead box protein 3 (Foxp3). These and other types of suppressive T cells (e.g., NKT cells) have been implicated in rodent transplantation tolerance models and in the prevention of autoimmunity. However, it seems likely that large numbers of regulatory cells recognizing the relevant antigens would be needed to apply this type of cellular therapy clinically, and the ultimate practicality of the approach remains to be determined. Nevertheless, an improved understanding of this type of immune regulation may lead to effective strategies for activating or expanding regulatory T cells in vivo, thereby favoring the suppressive immune response over destructive alloimmunity.

These developments in animal models and in the understanding of immune mechanisms have encouraged efforts to achieve immune tolerance in the setting of clinical transplantation. Every transplantation center has anecdotal cases of patients who have removed themselves from chronic immunosuppression without experiencing graft rejection. However, for every such patient, there are dozens more who have experienced rejection episodes with dose reductions or discontinuation of immunosuppressive drugs. Although trials of minimization and slow withdrawal of nonspecific immunosuppressive therapy are under way in organ transplant recipients, a major limitation is the absence of good predictors of success. It remains to be seen whether recently identified molecular "tolerance signatures" will provide markers with sufficient predictive value to allow such withdrawal to be undertaken safely.

One approach developed in animal models has been successfully applied to the induction of immune tolerance in a small group of patients receiving renal allografts. This approach involves bone marrow transplantation after nonmyeloablative conditioning, which is much less toxic than standard HCT conditioning. It was shown to be effective in the most stringent rodent and large-animal models before being evaluated clinically. Initial success using combined kidney and bone marrow transplantation in patients with renal failure due to multiple myeloma led to pilot studies in patients with renal failure without malignant disease, with encouraging preliminary results. This approach and others that have emerged from ongoing investigations provide hope that, in the future, transplant recipients might not need chronic immunosuppressive therapy, with its attendant complications and its limited ability to control chronic rejection. Because autoimmune diseases are major contributors to end-stage renal disease, diabetes, and other types of organ failure, the potential of tolerance strategies to reverse autoimmunity while inducing allograft tolerance is a source of hope for those patients as well. All these approaches must be undertaken with the caution, however, because successful regimens could lead to immune tolerance to active infectious organisms as well.

SUGGESTED READINGS

Gooley TA, Chien JW, Pergam SA, et al. Reduced mortality after allogeneic hematopoietic-cell transplantation. *N Engl J Med*. 2010;363:2091-2101. *Mortality from allogeneic hematopoietic stem cell transplantation decreased from 63% in 1993-1997 to 47% in 2003-2007, but the risk of relapse or progression of the underlying disease did not change.*

Locascio SA, Morokata T, Chittenden M, et al. Mixed chimerism, lymphocyte recovery, and evidence for early donor-specific unresponsiveness in patients receiving combined kidney and bone marrow transplantation to induce tolerance. *Transplantation*. 2010;90:1607-1615. *Potential role of chimerism to induce tolerance.*

Sánchez-Fueyo A, Strom TB. Immunologic basis of graft rejection and tolerance following transplantation of liver or other solid organs. *Gastroenterology*. 2011;140:51-64. *Review.*

Sarwal MM. Deconvoluting the "omics" for organ transplantation. *Curr Opin Organ Transplant*. 2009;14:544-551. *An overview of the role of genomics, proteomics, and the like in transplantation medicine.*

Sykes M. Hematopoietic cell transplantation for tolerance induction: animal models to clinical trials. *Transplantation*. 2009;87:309-316. *A review of animal studies and recent clinical studies of tolerance induction using hematopoietic cell transplantation.*

49 COMPLEMENT IN HEALTH AND DISEASE

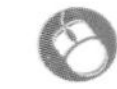

DAVID R. KARP AND V. MICHAEL HOLERS

The complement system consists of more than 30 serum and membrane proteins that participate in both host defense and a wide variety of pathologic states. This system serves many protective functions ascribed to the innate immune system (Chapter 44). It helps to maintain blood sterility by depositing the membrane attack complex (MAC) in bacterial cell walls and lysing them. It also participates in the opsonization of pathogens for phagocytic removal. The peptide *anaphylatoxins* produced during complement activation promote inflammatory responses with microbicidal effects. The deposition of complement on immune complexes helps to keep them soluble and remove them from the circulation.

There also is increasing evidence that complement can shape the adaptive immune response (Chapter 44). Antigens decorated by complement proteins are taken up by B cells and other antigen-presenting cells, resulting in T-cell activation. Complement activation is needed for optimal antibody production by B cells. Lastly, humans and experimental animals that are deficient in early complement components are often predisposed to autoimmune diseases, particularly systemic lupus erythematosus (SLE) (Chapter 274). This observation suggests that complement is required in some way to identify soluble self-antigens and eliminate self-reactive B cells.

Complement is activated immediately on exposure to immune complexes, but it lacks the immunologic memory of T or B cells with clonotypic receptors that discriminate between self and non-self. Activated complement can be deposited on host and pathogenic surfaces. This potentially dangerous situation is controlled by a series of genetically, structurally, and functionally similar proteins termed the *regulators of complement activation* (RCA). These proteins provide species-specific downregulation of complement activation on host tissues.

Inappropriate complement action occurs when the nondiscriminating activating proteins function in excess of the regulatory proteins that limit damage on self-tissues. This can be seen in almost any inflammatory disease. Some conditions are obvious, such as autoimmune hemolytic anemia, lupus nephritis, and immune complex vasculitis. In other diseases, the role of complement may be contributory but is less clear. These include myocardial infarction, stroke, cardiopulmonary bypass, and hemodialysis. Table 49-1 lists conditions in which complement activation is associated with pathology rather than protection.

In each of these conditions, inhibition of complement activation potentially would limit tissue damage. Many strategies have been developed to discover inhibitors that can work at various sites in the complement activation cascades for use as possible therapeutic agents in human diseases. These potential complement inhibitors include small molecules designed similarly to traditional drugs and newer biologic agents, particularly antibodies that inhibit complement activation.

Although the complement system plays important roles in infection and inflammatory responses, it also has many deleterious effects that must be controlled in conditions ranging from immune complex injury to reproduction. The critical feature of complement-mediated pathology is the alternative pathway amplification loop. As shown in Figure 49-1, failure to control this response results in the generation of potent inflammatory signals and the recruitment of tissue-damaging neutrophils, monocytes, and mast cells. Because more than half of the proteins associated with the complement system are dedicated to the control of activation or effector functions, it is clear that discrimination between "self" and "non-self" must occur even in the innate immune system.

Knowledge of how complement is activated and how it can be controlled offers new opportunities for the development of therapeutic agents for human diseases. Recently, anti-C5 monoclonal antibody therapy has been approved for treatment of paroxysmal nocturnal hemoglobinuria (Chapter 163), and it is anticipated that within the next few years, many additional complement-targeted drugs will be approved for clinical use. The diseases most likely to be improved by complement inhibition are autoimmune and inflammatory injuries to retina and the kidney.

ACTIVATION OF COMPLEMENT

As an essential component of the innate immune system, complement is endowed with redundant yet carefully controlled activation pathways. The molecular events that occur during activation not only are responsible for the pathology of complement-associated disease states but also offer opportunities for the rational design of inhibitors. For simplicity, it is convenient to think of the different parts of the complement activation pathways as involving *recognition, convertase/amplification,* and *effector* mechanisms.

Classical Pathway

Although traditionally thought of as activated only by immune complexes containing immunoglobulin M (IgM) or IgG, the classical pathway has been shown to be activated by targets other than immune complexes (Fig. 49-2). Notably, apoptotic cells bind C1q and activate the C1 proteases. C1 also is

TABLE 49-1 PATHOLOGIC CONDITIONS PRIMARILY ASSOCIATED WITH COMPLEMENT ACTIVATION

Allotransplantation	Macular degeneration
Alzheimer's disease	Meconium pneumonitis
ARDS	Multiple sclerosis
Arthus reaction	Multisystem organ failure
Asthma	Myasthenia gravis
Bullous pemphigoid	Post–cardiopulmonary bypass
Burns	Psoriasis
Crohn's disease	Recurrent spontaneous abortion
Glomerulonephritis (many causes)	Rheumatoid arthritis
Hemodialysis	Septic shock
Hemolytic anemia	Stroke
Hereditary angioedema	Systemic lupus erythematosus
Immune complex vasculitis	Traumatic brain injury
Ischemia-reperfusion injury	Xenotransplantation

ARDS = adult respiratory distress syndrome.

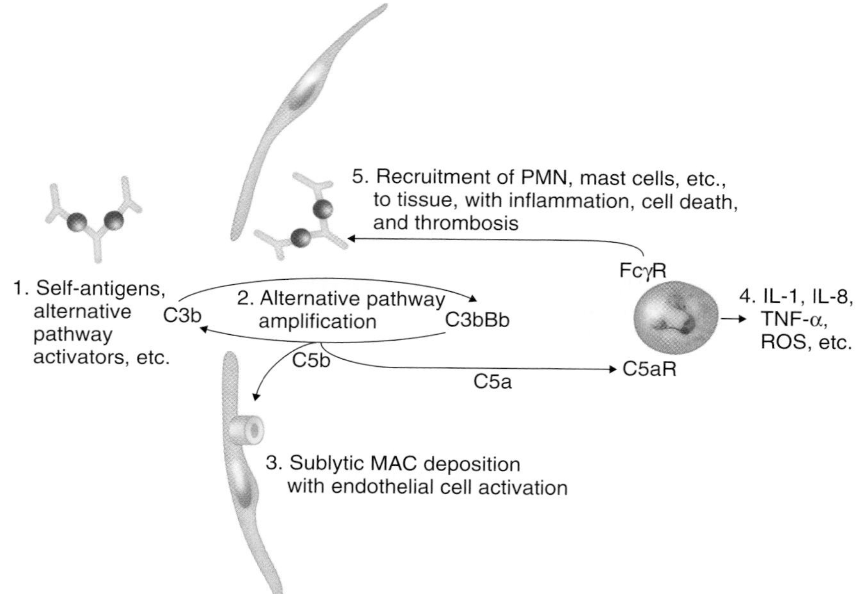

FIGURE 49-1. Pathogenic effect of complement. 1, Complement is activated by immune complexes or the exposure of surfaces that lack regulatory proteins. **2,** In the absence of effective regulation, the alternative pathway activation loop produces large amounts of both C5a and C5b. **3,** C5b initiates the deposition of sublytic amounts of the membrane attack complex (MAC), leading to cellular activation and proliferation. **4,** C5a is a potent chemoattractant and activator of polymorphonuclear neutrophils (PMN), mast cells, and other leukocytes, resulting in production of inflammatory cytokines and chemokines. **5,** Leukocytes also express Fc receptors (e.g., FcγR) that interact with immunoglobulin G bound to damaged tissue, further amplifying the generation of inflammatory mediators and activating coagulation pathways. IL = interleukin; ROS = reactive oxygen species; TNF-α = tumor necrosis factor-α.

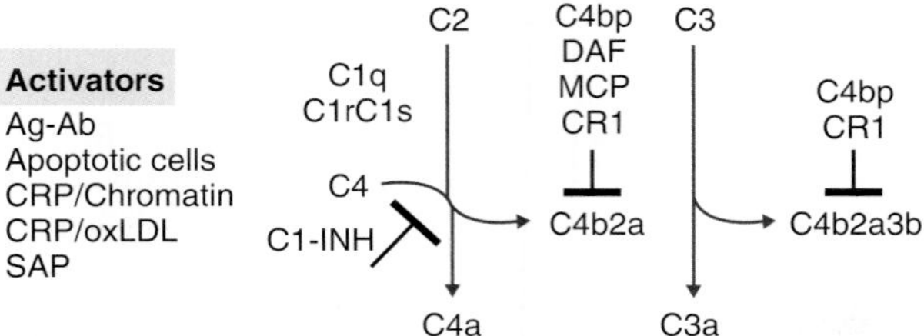

FIGURE 49-2. Schematic representation of the activation of the classical pathway and generation of its C3 convertase. Included are naturally occurring regulators (inhibitors) of this pathway. Ag-Ab = antigen-antibody complex; C1-INH = C1 inhibitor; C4bp = C4-binding protein; CR = complement receptor; CRP = C-reactive protein; DAF = decay-accelerating factor; MCP = membrane cofactor protein; oxLDL = oxidized low-density lipoprotein; SAP = serum amyloid protein.

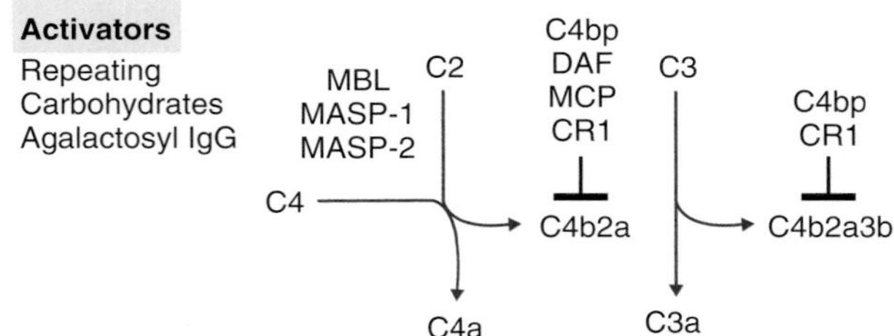

FIGURE 49-3. Schematic representation of the activation of the lectin pathway and generation in concert with the classical pathway of a C3 convertase. Included are naturally occurring regulators (inhibitors) of this pathway. CR = complement receptor; C4bp = C4-binding protein; DAF = decay-accelerating factor; IgG = immunoglobulin G; MASP = MBL-associated serine protease; MBL = mannose-binding lectin; MCP = membrane cofactor protein.

activated by the accumulated Aβ protein found in the neuritic plaques of patients with Alzheimer's disease. C-reactive protein (CRP) and serum amyloid protein bind to chromatin and other ribonucleoprotein complexes released from apoptotic cells. The CRP–nuclear antigen complexes bind and activate C1. C1q and the classical pathway appear to play a role in the opsonization and removal of nuclear materials that frequently contain autoantigens. The few patients with hereditary C1q deficiency all eventually develop SLE. The addition of CRP and enzymatically modified low-density lipoprotein to human serum causes the activation of complement, as determined by the almost quantitative conversion of C3 to C3b. Finally, deposits of CRP and activated C1 have been shown in infarcted human myocardium. Together, these observations suggest that activation through the antibody-independent classical pathway is important in protective immune responses and in pathogenic inflammatory reactions.

Regulation of the classical pathway activation occurs at several levels. First is the serine protease inhibitor (serpin), C1-inhibitor (C1-INH). C1-INH blocks the activity of many proteases, including factor XIIa, kallikrein, and factor XIa of the clotting system and C1r and C1s in the complement system. The importance of C1-INH is seen in hereditary angioedema (Chapter 260). In this instance, the heterozygous deficiency of C1-INH allows uncontrolled proteolysis of C2 and C4 after minor trauma. A vasoactive peptide is released from C2 and leads to painless (but occasionally life-threatening) soft tissue swelling. Treatment of acute attacks of hereditary angioedema includes purified C1-INH and antifibrinolytic drugs such as ε-aminocaproic acid.

Classical pathway activation also is regulated by RCA proteins. These proteins form the basis for the ability of the complement system to discriminate self from nonself targets. They are discussed in depth later in this chapter. The RCA proteins C4-binding protein (C4-bp) and complement receptor 1 (CR1) provide classical pathway regulation.

Lectin Pathway

The most recently described complement recognition and activation pathway is the lectin pathway (Fig. 49-3). The protein mannose-binding lectin (MBL) is a member of the collectin family that includes pulmonary surfactants A and D. MBL has a structure similar to C1q, in that it consists of several subunits, each having a globular recognition domain and a collagen-like portion that interacts with serine proteases. In the case of MBL, the globular domain is a lectin that binds to repeating carbohydrates (mannose and *N*-acetylglucosamine) on the surface of pathogens. Many microorganisms are recognized by MBL, including gram-positive and gram-negative bacteria, mycobacteria, fungi, parasites, and viruses, including human immunodeficiency virus 1 (HIV-1). In general, mammalian glycoproteins and glycolipids are not recognized by MBL. One notable exception is agalactosyl IgG. The levels of this modified immunoglobulin are increased in inflammatory conditions such as rheumatoid arthritis, raising the possibility that excessive activation of the lectin pathway is clinically relevant.

Three serine proteases, MASP-1, MASP-2, and MASP-3, associate with MBL, presumably through the collagen-like domain. Although not formally proved, this is analogous to the association of C1r and C1s with C1q. Activation of MASP-1 and MASP-2 results in cleavage of C2 and C4, with the subsequent formation of the classical pathway C3 convertase (C4b2a).

Variation in the structural and regulatory portions of the MBL gene leads to wide individual differences in serum levels. Low levels of MBL have been associated with recurrent infections in children and adults and have been shown to be a minor risk factor for the development of SLE. More striking is the association of low levels of MBL with infection in SLE. In a study of Danish lupus patients, heterozygous MBL deficiency was associated with a fourfold increase in the risk of bacterial pneumonia, and homozygous deficiency with a more than 100-fold increase.

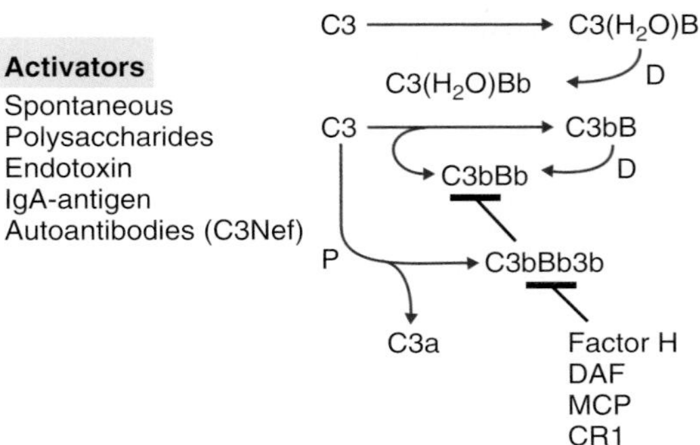

FIGURE 49-4. Schematic representation of the activation of the alternative pathway and generation of its C3 convertase. Included are naturally occurring regulators (inhibitors) of this pathway. C3Nef = C3-nephritic factor; CR = complement receptor; DAF = decay-accelerating factor; IgA = immunoglobulin A; MCP = membrane cofactor protein.

Alternative Pathway

The alternative pathway is much less stringent in its recognition requirements. It takes advantage of the fact that C3 undergoes spontaneous low-grade activation in the fluid phase (Fig. 49-4). This allows the covalent attachment of C3 to the polysaccharides of fungi and bacteria and to other appropriately charged targets, such as endotoxin and virally infected cells. Other alternative pathway activators include IgA immune complexes and biomaterials, such as cardiopulmonary bypass and hemodialysis membranes.

During spontaneous activation, called *tickover*, C3 acquires a C3b-like conformation and binds factor B, which is cleaved by the serine protease factor D to form the alternative pathway C3 convertase C3bBb. This complex has a short half-life. It is stabilized by properdin (factor P) during physiologic complement activation. This convertase cleaves more C3, which leads to additional C3bBb production. In fact, the C3b can also come from either the classical or alternative pathway. Thus, the activation of complement from any of the three pathways is greatly amplified. The alternative pathway C3 convertase is negatively regulated by the RCA proteins factor H, decay-accelerating factor (DAF), and CR1.

The central role of the alternative pathway as an essential amplifier of complement activation is borne out in its association with a number of clinicopathologic states. For example, membranoproliferative glomerulonephritis type II (Chapter 123) is associated with excessive C3 deposition in the kidney due either to the presence of autoantibodies (C3 nephritic factor) that stabilize the alternative C3 convertase or to genetic deficiencies in the complement regulatory proteins factor H and factor I. Likewise, the atypical form of hemolytic-uremic syndrome (i.e., not associated with shiga-like toxin) (Chapter 175) is found in families that harbor heterozygous mutations in factor H or I or have activating mutations in factor B or C3. Strong genetic associations have linked age-related macular degeneration (Chapter 431) to functional mutations in factor H as well as factor B and C3. Finally, rodent models of many of the complement-associated diseases listed in Table 49-1 are ameliorated when the alternative pathway is genetically disrupted.

C3 and C5 Convertases

The three activation pathways converge at C3. C3 (and C4) contains a reactive glutamic acid residue buried within the three-dimensional structure of the protein. Normally the γ-carboxy group of the reactive glutamic acid in C3 (and C4) is linked to a nearby cysteine in an "internal thioester." On activation, the thioester is exposed to the surface of the protein, where it can react with amino or hydroxyl groups. Most of the thioesters are hydrolyzed by water to form inactive C3 or C4. Some of the thioesters form amide or ester bonds to proteins or carbohydrates, covalently attaching C3b (and C4b) to target surfaces. This enables cells bearing CR1 to bind these targets and opsonize them, representing one of the effector mechanisms of complement.

The covalently bound C3b associates with C4b2a (classical or lectin pathway) or with C3bBb (alternative pathway) to form a convertase for C5. C3b is part of the alternative-pathway C3 convertase, and its product generates an amplification loop that can deposit thousands of C3b molecules on a target, regardless of the initial activation step.

Regulators of Complement Activation

The major function of the protein regulators of complement activation (RCA) (E-Fig. 49-1) as a group is to limit the production of C3b by either the classical or the alternative C3 convertases. Because the addition of C3b to a C3 convertase makes it a C5 convertase, regulation of the two enzyme complexes is linked. Modulation of their activity on host cells limits tissue destruction and the production of inflammatory mediators.

There are six RCA proteins that control the C3/C5 convertases, listed in Table 49-2. The genes for all of these proteins are found in a cluster on human chromosome 1.q32. Structurally, they are composed of repeating subunits termed *short consensus repeats* (SCRs), sometimes referred to as *complement control protein* modules. Each SCR has about 60 amino acids with four invariant cysteine residues. The pairing of the disulfides leads to a four- to five-β pleated sheet structure, causing the SCRs to appear like beads on a string.

Although the SCRs are structurally related, the individual RCA proteins may recognize different parts of the C3 molecule. They do so using specific combinations of SCRs. The RCA proteins function to control complement activation by two processes. First is *decay acceleration*. This refers to the process whereby the RCA protein binds to C3b or C4b in the convertase and dissociates the other members of the complex, rendering it enzymatically inactive. The second effect is *cofactor* activity. Some of the RCA proteins facilitate the recognition of C3b or C4b by a serum protease, factor I. Cleavage of C3b or C4b by factor I renders the convertase irreversibly inactive.

Despite their relatedness, the RCA proteins exhibit differences in their overall structure, distribution, and function (see Table 49-2). All of the RCA

TABLE 49-2 DISTRIBUTION AND FUNCTION OF REGULATORS OF COMPLEMENT ACTIVATION (RCA) PROTEINS

RCA PROTEIN	DISTRIBUTION	FUNCTION
C4-binding protein	Serum	Cofactor for C4b; decay of classical C3/C5 convertases
Factor H	Serum	Cofactor for C3b; decay of alternative C3/C5 convertases
Decay-accelerating factor	Widely distributed on most cell types	Decay of classical and alternative C3/C5 convertases
Membrane cofactor protein	Widely distributed on most cell types	Cofactor for C3b and C4b (not RBCs)
Complement receptor 1	Most blood cells; mast cells	Cofactor for C3b and C4b; decay of C3/C5 convertases; receptor for C3b/C4b
Complement receptor 2	B cells; follicular dendritic cells	Receptor for C3b fragments; regulation of B cells

RBCs = red blood cells.

proteins except MCP and CR2 have decay acceleration activity; it is the only function of DAF. This glycosyl phosphatidylinositol-linked protein is widely expressed and causes the removal of C2a or Bb from the C3 and C5 convertases. DAF lacks the cofactor activity seen with the other RCA proteins (except CR2). Factor H and C4bp are serum proteins. MCP and DAF are ubiquitously expressed membrane proteins. CR1 and CR2 are membrane proteins expressed primarily on hematopoietic cells.

RCA proteins have been linked to several disease states. DAF is missing from the abnormal erythrocytes of patients with paroxysmal nocturnal hemoglobinuria (Chapter 163). Although the hemolysis of these cells is ultimately due to the fact that the cells also lack CD59 (see later discussion), the DAF deficiency promotes complement activation on these cells. The association between genetic factor H deficiency and type II membranoproliferative glomerulonephritis and familial hemolytic-uremic syndrome has been mentioned. Lastly, low levels of CR1 and/or CR2 have been seen in patients with SLE. CR1 has cofactor and decay activity, and its major role is in the removal of immune complexes from the circulation. CR2 is necessary for optimal B-cell regulation, including the downmodulation of autoreactive B cells.

Membrane Attack Complex

The cleavage of C5 by either convertase generates C5a, the most potent of the complement anaphylatoxins, and C5b. C5b associates with C6 and C7 to create a lipophilic trimer as part of the MAC (E-Fig. 49-2). On the surface of a target cell, fewer than 1% of the C5b67 trimers that are formed insert into the lipid bilayer and serve as binding sites for C8. This attracts C9 to the membrane, and C9 has the capacity to self-polymerize. A total of 12 to 18 C9 molecules form a ring structure, completing the MAC. In its complete form, the MAC appears like a doughnut with a 10-nm pore running through the center. This pore can allow water and ions to enter the cells, ultimately leading to cell lysis. A MAC with only one or two C9 molecules also can cause lysis, however, suggesting that the MAC disrupts the lipid integrity in its general vicinity, rather than creating holes in the membrane.

The MAC itself appears to be largely redundant in terms of protection against infection. It appears to be essential only for efficient elimination of *Neisseria* species. Individuals who are homozygous deficient for C6, C7, or C8 are at risk for meningococcal and gonococcal infection (Chapters 306 and 307). C9 deficiency is the most common immunodeficiency in Japan, with a heterozygote frequency of 3 to 5%, which notably is not associated with an increased risk of *Neisseria* infection. Absence of an efficient MAC is not deleterious to the population in general and may have some selective advantage.

Extensive complement activation during an inflammatory response can result in sufficient MAC deposition to cause host cell lysis. Most nucleated cells have mechanisms to resist the osmotic changes caused by the MAC, however, and they may "disassemble" the MAC as it is formed. Rather, the nonlethal effects of sublytic MAC deposition are more likely to contribute to pathology. In most cells, this occurs through a general activation of multiple cell signaling pathways. Calcium enters the cell, activating protein kinases and phospholipase C, and upregulates the production of cyclic adenosine monophosphate (cAMP). G proteins and their associated factors are concentrated at the cell membrane, perhaps localized to C9 directly. The mitogen-activated protein kinase pathways (extracellular signal-regulated kinase [ERK], c-Jun N-terminal kinase [JNK], and p38) are activated, resulting in the induction of transcription factors such as c-jun and c-fos, cell proliferation, and inhibition of apoptosis.

The response to MAC deposition depends on the cell type (E-Table 49-1). In phagocytic cells, such as polymorphonuclear neutrophils or macrophages, sublytic MAC activation leads to the production of reactive oxygen species (e.g., superoxide, hydrogen peroxide), as well as prostaglandins and leukotrienes. Platelets undergo the exposure of phosphatidylserine on their outer membrane, facilitating formation of blood coagulation enzyme complexes with a potentially procoagulant effect. On endothelial cells, MAC deposition induces the synthesis of interleukin-1α (IL-1α), which leads to further autocrine and paracrine endothelial cell activation; stimulates a procoagulant state by altering the phospholipid composition of the endothelial membrane, inducing the synthesis of tissue factor and upregulating the synthesis of plasminogen activator inhibitor; induces the expression of adhesion molecules, including intercellular adhesion molecule 1 (ICAM-1) and E-selectin; and stimulates endothelial cells to proliferate through growth factor production. Despite the fact that cell death does not occur, deposition of the sublytic levels of MAC leads to a potentially more dangerous situation, with increased inflammation, coagulation, and cellular proliferation.

Regulation of MAC formation is important clinically and has become an area of therapeutic research. Two fluid-phase proteins, clusterin and S-protein (vitronectin), bind the C5b-7 complex and prevent its association with the lipid membrane. C8 and usually two to four C9 molecules bind to this soluble complex, termed *sC5b-9*, which is lytically inactive. CD59 is a membrane-bound inhibitor of MAC formation. This small glycoprotein is attached to the cell membrane through a glycosyl phosphatidylinositol tail. It binds tightly to C5b-8, preventing the binding and polymerization of C9. CD59 shows strong species restriction, being most effective in the inhibition of MAC formation by the same or closely related species. The expression of CD59 is defective in patients with paroxysmal nocturnal hemoglobinuria, owing to the failure to synthesize the glycosyl phosphatidylinositol tail on this and many other cell surface proteins, including DAF. The clinical features of paroxysmal nocturnal hemoglobinuria are protean. The hemolysis is believed to be caused by low-grade complement activation on red blood cells due to the lack of DAF; without CD59, MAC formation then proceeds and allows hemolysis (Chapter 163).

Anaphylatoxins

In addition to the MAC, the other major source of pathologic damage resulting from complement activation comes from the action of the anaphylatoxins. These are the peptides C3a, C4a, and C5a, which are cleaved from their respective proteins during activation. They were named by Friedberger in 1910 to describe toxic effects after the transfer of complement-activated serum into laboratory animals. They are 77 (C3a and C4a) or 74 (C5a) amino acids long and contain a carboxy (C)-terminal arginine. The structures of C3a and C5a have been determined by x-ray crystallography and nuclear magnetic resonance; they exhibit a compact amino (N)-terminal region that is held together by conserved disulfide bonds. This part of the molecule contains cationic amino acids that are believed to interact with the anaphylatoxin receptors. The C-terminal regions of the anaphylatoxins are extended sequences. Only the last five amino acids are required for activity. In plasma, the C-terminal arginine is removed rapidly by carboxypeptidase N from anaphylatoxins not bound to their receptors. Depending on the response studied, this removal totally inactivates the anaphylatoxin or reduces its potency by 1000-fold.

The C5a receptor (C5aR [CD88]) was the first anaphylatoxin receptor to be characterized. It is a seven-transmembrane-spanning protein that couples ligand binding to G-protein signaling. Expressed on myeloid cells, particularly neutrophils and eosinophils, it mediates the potent chemoattractant property of C5a for both of these cell types. Signaling through CD88 leads to rapid secretion of all granule contents. These include proteases, peroxidases, and lactoferrin from neutrophils, and peroxidase, major basic protein, and eosinophil cationic protein from eosinophils. C5a also induces the release of cytokines, such as tumor necrosis factor (TNF), IL-1, IL-6, and IL-8, and adhesion molecules, promoting the inflammatory response. The C5aR also has been found on numerous other tissues (E-Table 49-2). These include hepatocytes, bronchial and alveolar epithelium, vascular endothelium, renal mesangial and tubular epithelial cells, and brain neuronal cells. The function of C5a in these tissues is not clear. In vitro experiments have shown that these cells are activated by exposure to the anaphylatoxins, leading to production of cytokines, chemokines, and prostaglandins, and to cell proliferation.

The C3a receptor is also a seven-transmembrane-domain protein. It is expressed on almost all myeloid cells, including mast cells, where it mediates the release of allergic mediators. The C3aR also has been detected on many tissues, including in the brain.

The anaphylatoxins have many biologic effects. In general, they cause smooth muscle contraction and recruitment of granulocytes, monocytes, and mast cells. In theory, they can contribute to the pathophysiology of any inflammatory condition. C3a and C5a have been shown to play a role in diseases such as adult respiratory distress syndrome, multisystem organ failure, septic shock, myocardial ischemia-reperfusion injury, asthma, rheumatoid arthritis, SLE, and inflammatory bowel disease. The anaphylatoxin peptides also are responsible for the "postpump" syndrome seen in patients undergoing cardiopulmonary bypass or hemodialysis. Exposure of blood to dialysis or perfusion membranes leads to complement activation. Within minutes of starting bypass, there is a sharp increase in the levels of C3a and C5a in the extracorporeal circuit being returned to the patient. This increase can be associated with respiratory distress, pulmonary hypertension, and pulmonary edema. It has been shown that the length of time that patients stay on the ventilator after bypass surgery depends on the level of C3a generated during reperfusion.

C3a and C5a have been implicated in the initiation and prolongation of adult respiratory distress syndrome (Chapter 104) and multisystem organ failure (Chapter 106). After severe trauma (Chapter 112), levels of C3a have been measured that suggest activation of the entire circulating C3 pool. This activation leads to bronchoconstriction, increased vascular permeability, and vascular plugging with leukocytes. The activation of white blood cells continues the cycle of tissue damage with further complement activation. Continued elevation of C3a in shock or adult respiratory distress syndrome is a poor prognostic sign. C3a also appears to play a major role in the pathogenesis of asthma (Chapter 87).

COMPLEMENT INHIBITORS

Given the many disease states in which complement is one of the central mediators of pathology, it is no surprise that several complement inhibitors are in preclinical or clinical development for treatment of human diseases. These inhibitors take several different forms. Some are variations of physiologic inhibitors, whereas others are the products of molecular biologic searches for novel compounds.

It is important to consider where in the complement pathway to design an inhibitor to act. Inhibition of the activation pathways limits the production of biologically active peptides. All three pathways need to be inhibited, however, for this approach to be effective. Inhibiting the activation of C3 not only prevents the generation of the C3a anaphylatoxin but also may leave the patient susceptible to infection by limiting the deposition of C3b on targets as an opsonin. Inhibition of C3b deposition also theoretically would decrease the patient's ability to clear immune complexes, resulting in renal, pulmonary, and vascular damage. It also might promote the development of antibodies to self-antigens.

Inhibition of the C5 convertases is an attractive goal because it would prevent the generation of the C5a anaphylatoxin and the MAC. This strategy would inhibit complement activation from any cause without the potentially immunosuppressive effects of limiting C3b deposition. Inhibitors based on this concept are the farthest along in clinical treatment.

Other concerns about complement inhibition include whether it is short-term or long-term and whether it is systemic or localized. Long-term inhibition of complement, particularly at early steps, is likely to predispose the patient to infection. Short-term (hours to days) inhibition at any step is unlikely to cause problems. Given that inflammation is usually a local phenomenon, there are several mechanisms being tested to target complement inhibitors to these sites. In this way, higher levels of inhibition can be achieved where needed with lower doses of inhibitor.

Natural Complement Inhibitors

Naturally occurring compounds that control complement activation include products or extracts of plants, fungi, insects, venoms, and cell lines. The mechanism of complement inhibition by some of these natural products is known and is of clinical and experimental importance. Cobra venom factor isolated from *Naja naja* is a 144,000-D glycoprotein that forms an alternative pathway convertase in association with Bb; this leads to massive activation of complement that causes pulmonary microvascular injury in experimental animals. Perhaps the most widely used natural inhibitor of complement activation is heparin. It decreases activation of the classical and the alternative pathways. In clinical practice, the anticomplementary effect of heparin has been used to prevent complement activation during cardiopulmonary bypass. Measurement of complement activation products such as C3a or soluble C5b-9 after bypass showed decreases of 35 to 70% for adult and pediatric patients when heparin-coated extracorporeal circuits (e.g., Duraflo II) were used. Although numerous studies have looked at the decrease in complement activation by heparin-coated bypass circuits, there have been few attempts to correlate this with clinical outcome.

Anti-C5

The complement inhibitor that has achieved the widest attention as a therapeutic agent is a monoclonal antibody to C5. The advantage to this strategy is that it prevents the generation of C5a, the most potent of the anaphylatoxins, and of the MAC. The generation of C3b and C4b opsonins still would occur, allowing proper clearance of pathogens and immune complexes even if C5 conversion were inhibited chronically. Because there is evidence that activation of early complement components is important for the maintenance of tolerance to self-antigens, inhibition of C5 activation may be less worrisome than inhibition of C3 activation. Lastly, there appears to be little detrimental effect of genetic C5 deficiency. The only consequence of C5 deficiency in humans seems to be an increased risk of *Neisseria* infection.

The anti-C5 monoclonal antibody eculizumab has been approved for use in patients with paroxysmal nocturnal hemoglobinuria to block intravascular hemolysis and stabilize hemoglobin levels.[1] Several groups have also reported the favorable use of an anti-C5 monoclonal antibody in animal model systems of arthritis and lupus nephritis.

Soluble CR1

Soluble CR1 (sCR1) was the first rationally designed complement inhibitor to undergo extensive testing. The idea behind the use of this RCA protein was that it had multiple mechanisms of action. It has two separate binding sites for C3b and one for C4b. It not only serves as a cofactor for the enzymatic degradation of C3b and C4b but also can dissociate the classical (C3b4b) and the alternative (C3b2) C5 convertases. It is produced by recombinant methodology in animal cells. A modified version, produced in a manner that decorates the protein with the carbohydrate sialyl Lewis^x, the ligand for P-selectin and E-selectin, targets sCR1 directly to activated (inflamed) endothelium. Another modified form of sCR1 targets the protein to the lipid membrane of cells. This technique has been shown to be experimentally effective in situations in which sCR1 can be delivered locally, such as intra-articular injections or the perfusion of donor organs before transplantation.

Soluble CR1 blocks activation of complement in many experimental animal models of disease, including myocardial ischemia-reperfusion injury, intestinal ischemia, and middle cerebral artery ligation in rodents. In each case, the administration of sCR1 was associated with decreased tissue injury, less neutrophil accumulation, and lower concentrations of inflammatory mediators such as leukotriene B_4. In allograft transplantation, the donor organ undergoes significant ischemia-reperfusion injury. Animal models of allogeneic renal and lung transplantation have shown that sCR1 prolongs graft survival, which may prevent early rejection episodes. In pig-to-primate cardiac xenotransplantation, sCR1 prolonged graft survival remarkably. In one study of human lung transplantation, patients were randomly assigned to receive or not receive a single infusion of 10 mg/kg of sCR1 before restoration of blood flow in the graft. Complement activation was suppressed for 2 days after surgery. There were trends for all patients toward decreased time on the ventilator and in the intensive care unit that did not reach statistical significance. For patients who had been receiving cardiopulmonary bypass during surgery (and may have had more complement activation), however, there was a 56% decrease in time spent on the ventilator postoperatively if they were treated with sCR1.

sCR1 has also been found to have salutary effects in animal models of autoimmune disease, including collagen-induced arthritis, experimental autoimmune neuritis, a model for Guillain-Barré syndrome, and models of myasthenia gravis, multiple sclerosis, and glomerulonephritis.

Transgenic Animals

Xenotransplantation offers a solution to the chronic lack of solid organs for transplantation. The most studied donor animal is the pig because swine have many desirable experimental and practical characteristics, such as size and ease of production. Although immunosuppression and other strategies may be able to overcome cellular immune barriers, the most pressing current problem facing xenotransplantation is hyperacute rejection. This is the immediate (within minutes) cessation of graft function owing to natural IgM antibodies that react with the vascular endothelium of the xenograft. The target of these antibodies is mainly the carbohydrate moiety galactose-(α1,3)-galactose present on the graft. These antibodies quickly activate complement, leading to intravascular coagulation, tissue edema, hemorrhage, and endothelial activation. Prevention of hyperacute rejection would require reducing the levels of antibodies or of their antigens, inhibiting complement activation, or a combination of all three. Because complement regulatory proteins display species specificity, the approach to limit complement activation in xenografts has been to make transgenic pigs that express one or more membrane proteins of human origin. In one study, kidneys from the triple-transgenic pigs were transplanted into bilaterally nephrectomized baboons. No immunosuppression or pretreatment of the recipients was given. Under these circumstances, the function of a nontransgenic pig kidney ceases within 3 minutes, and the graft rapidly becomes nonviable. The function of transgenic kidneys was maintained with good urine output for 3 to 5 days in the six baboons that received these grafts.

C3a and C5a Receptor Antagonists

The profound biologic effects of the anaphylatoxins and the many conditions in which C3a and C5a are believed to play a pathologic role make the development of specific inhibitors of these proteins attractive. Because the active portion of the anaphylatoxins is contained in the C-terminal part of the protein, it is possible that small-molecule antagonists could be developed that are orally available, easy to synthesize, and inexpensive. These are all advantages over the use of biologics such as monoclonal antibodies or recombinant RCA proteins. To date, several synthetic C5a antagonists have been described. C5a inhibitors are in early human clinical trials. Finally, a potent small-molecule inhibitor of C3a has been found to be active in vitro as an inhibitor of C3a-mediated cellular activation, chemotaxis, and smooth muscle contraction.

Anti–Factor B

Inactivation of the factor B gene in mice prevents a number of autoimmune or inflammatory diseases. Presumably, this represents the necessity for an intact alternative pathway to amplify subclinical complement activation. Inhibition of the alternative pathway activation loop is an attractive target for therapy because it would allow for protective immunity against pathogens through the classical pathway. The efficacy of this approach has been demonstrated using a monoclonal antibody to factor B that inhibits its function. This antibody blocks activation of the alternative pathway in the serum of a number of species, including mice, rats, nonhuman primates, and humans. In a mouse model of complement-mediated pregnancy loss, administration of the anti–factor B antibody resulted in a 50% decrease in fetal death. In models of asthma and renal ischemia-reperfusion injury, this antibody ameliorated disease. This strategy could have wide applicability in a number of disease states.

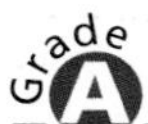

1. Hillmen P, Young NS, Schubert J, et al. The complement inhibitor eculizumab in paroxysmal nocturnal hemoglobinuria. *N Engl J Med*. 2006;355:1233-1243.

SUGGESTED READINGS

Dunkelberger JR, Song WC. Complement and its role in innate and adaptive immune responses. *Cell Res*. 2010;20:34-50. *Review*.

Lynch AM, Gibbs RS, Murphy JR, et al. Early elevations of the complement activation fragment C3a and adverse pregnancy outcomes. *Obstet Gynecol*. 2011;117:75-83. *Elevated C3a as early as the first trimester of pregnancy is an independent predictor of adverse pregnancy outcomes*.

Ram S, Lewis LA, Rice PA. Infections of people with complement deficiencies and patients who have undergone splenectomy. *Clin Microbiol Rev*. 2010:23:740-780. *Practical review*.

Rutkowski MJ, Sughrue ME, Kane AJ, et al. Cancer and the complement cascade. *Mol Cancer Res*. 2010;8:1453-1465. *Complement proteins can promote carcinogenesis by a variety of mechanisms via dysregulation of mitogenic signaling pathways*.

VIII

CARDIOVASCULAR DISEASE

50

APPROACH TO THE PATIENT WITH POSSIBLE CARDIOVASCULAR DISEASE

LEE GOLDMAN

Patients with cardiovascular disease may present with a wide range of symptoms and signs, each of which may be caused by noncardiovascular conditions. Conversely, patients with substantial cardiovascular disease may be asymptomatic. Because cardiovascular disease is a leading cause of death in the United States and other developed countries, it is crucial that patients be evaluated carefully to detect early cardiovascular disease, that symptoms or signs of cardiovascular disease be evaluated in detail, and that appropriate therapy be instituted. Improvements in diagnosis, therapy, and prevention have contributed to a 70% or so decline in age-adjusted cardiovascular death rates in the United States since the 1960s. However, the absolute number of deaths from cardiovascular disease in the United States has not declined proportionately because of the increase in the population older than 40 years as well as the aging of the population in general.

In evaluating a patient with known or suspected heart disease, the physician must determine quickly whether a potentially life-threatening condition exists. In these situations, the evaluation must focus on the specific issue at hand and be accompanied by the rapid performance of appropriately directed additional tests. Examples of potentially life-threatening conditions include acute myocardial infarction (Chapter 73), unstable angina (Chapter 72), suspected aortic dissection (Chapter 78), pulmonary edema (Chapter 59), and pulmonary embolism (Chapter 98).

USING THE HISTORY TO DETECT CARDIOVASCULAR SYMPTOMS

Patients may complain spontaneously of a variety of cardiovascular symptoms (Table 50-1), but sometimes these symptoms are elicited only by obtaining a careful, complete medical history. In patients with known or suspected cardiovascular disease, questions about cardiovascular symptoms are key components of the history of present illness; in other patients, these issues are a fundamental part of the review of systems.

Chest Pain

Chest discomfort or pain is the cardinal manifestation of myocardial ischemia resulting from coronary artery disease or any condition that causes myocardial ischemia by an imbalance of myocardial oxygen demand compared with myocardial oxygen supply (Chapter 71). New, acute, often ongoing pain may indicate an acute myocardial infarction, unstable angina, or aortic dissection; a pulmonary cause, such as acute pulmonary embolism or pleural irritation; a musculoskeletal condition of the chest wall, thorax, or shoulder; or a gastrointestinal abnormality, such as esophageal reflux or spasm, peptic ulcer disease, or cholecystitis (Table 50-2). The chest discomfort of myocardial infarction commonly occurs without an immediate or obvious precipitating clinical cause and builds in intensity for at least several minutes; the sensation can range from annoying discomfort to severe pain (Chapter 73). Although a variety of adjectives may be used by patients to describe the sensation, physicians must be suspicious of any discomfort, especially if it radiates to the neck, shoulder, or arms. The probability of an acute myocardial infarction can be estimated by integrating information from the history, physical examination, and electrocardiogram (Fig. 50-1).

The chest discomfort of unstable angina is clinically indistinguishable from that of myocardial infarction except that the former may be precipitated more clearly by activity and may be more rapidly responsive to antianginal therapy (Chapter 72). Aortic dissection (Chapter 78) classically presents with the sudden onset of severe pain in the chest and radiating to the back; the location of the pain often provides clues to the location of the dissection. Ascending aortic dissections commonly present with chest discomfort radiating to the back, whereas dissections of the descending aorta commonly present with back pain radiating to the abdomen. The presence of back pain or a history of hypertension or other predisposing factors, such as Marfan syndrome, should prompt a careful assessment of peripheral pulses to determine whether the great vessels are affected by the dissection and of the chest radiograph to evaluate the size of the aorta. If this initial evaluation is suggestive, further testing with transesophageal echocardiography, computed tomography (CT), or magnetic resonance imaging (MRI) is indicated. The pain of pericarditis (Chapter 77) may simulate that of an acute myocardial infarction, may be primarily pleuritic, or may be continuous; a key physical finding is a pericardial rub. The pain of pulmonary embolism (Chapter 98) is commonly pleuritic in nature and is associated with dyspnea; hemoptysis also may be present. Pulmonary hypertension (Chapter 68) of any cause may be associated with chest discomfort with exertion; it commonly is associated with severe dyspnea and often is associated with cyanosis.

Recurrent, episodic chest discomfort may be noted with angina pectoris and with many cardiac and noncardiac causes (Chapter 71). A variety of stress tests (Table 50-3) can be used to provoke reversible myocardial ischemia in susceptible individuals and to help determine whether ischemia is the pathophysiologic explanation for the chest discomfort (Chapter 71).

Dyspnea

Dyspnea, which is an uncomfortable awareness of breathing, is commonly due to cardiovascular or pulmonary disease. A systematic approach (see Fig. 83-3 in Chapter 83) with selected tests nearly always reveals the cause. Acute dyspnea can be caused by myocardial ischemia, heart failure, severe hypertension, pericardial tamponade, pulmonary embolism, pneumothorax, upper airway obstruction, acute bronchitis or pneumonia, or some drug overdoses (e.g., salicylates). Subacute or chronic dyspnea is also a common presenting or accompanying symptom in patients with pulmonary disease (Chapter 83). Dyspnea also can be caused by severe anemia (Chapter 161) and can be confused with the fatigue that often is noted in patients with systemic and neurologic diseases (Chapters 264 and 403).

In heart failure, dyspnea typically is noted as a hunger for air and a need or an urge to breathe. The feeling that breathing requires increased work or effort is more typical of airway obstruction or neuromuscular disease. A feeling of chest tightness or constriction during breathing is typical of bronchoconstriction, which is commonly caused by obstructive airway disease (Chapters 87 and 88) but also may be seen in pulmonary edema. A feeling of heavy breathing, a feeling of rapid breathing, or a need to breathe more is classically associated with deconditioning.

In cardiovascular conditions, chronic dyspnea usually is caused by increases in pulmonary venous pressure as a result of left ventricular failure (Chapters 58 and 59) or valvular heart disease (Chapter 75). Orthopnea, which is an exacerbation of dyspnea when the patient is recumbent, is due to increased work of breathing because of either increased venous return to the pulmonary vasculature or loss of gravitational assistance in diaphragmatic effort. Paroxysmal nocturnal dyspnea is severe dyspnea that awakens a patient at night and forces the assumption of a sitting or standing position to achieve gravitational redistribution of fluid.

Palpitations

Palpitations (Chapter 62) describe a subjective sensation of an irregular or abnormal heartbeat. Palpitations may be caused by any arrhythmia (Chapters 64 and 65) with or without important underlying structural heart disease. Palpitations should be defined in terms of the duration and frequency of the episodes; the precipitating and related factors; and any associated symptoms of chest pain, dyspnea, lightheadedness, or syncope. It is crucial to use the history to determine whether the palpitations are caused by an irregular or a regular heartbeat. The feeling associated with a premature atrial or ventricular contraction, often described as a "skipped beat" or a "flip-flopping of the heart," must be distinguished from the irregularly irregular rhythm of atrial fibrillation and the rapid but regular rhythm of supraventricular tachycardia. Associated symptoms of chest pain, dyspnea, lightheadedness, dizziness, or diaphoresis suggest an important effect on cardiac output and mandate further evaluation. In general, evaluation begins with ambulatory electrocardiography (ECG) (Table 50-4), which is indicated in patients who have palpitations in the presence of structural heart disease or substantial accompanying symptoms. Depending on the series, 9 to 43% of patients have important underlying heart disease. In such patients, more detailed evaluation is warranted (see Fig. 62-1).

Lightheadedness or *syncope* (Chapter 62) can be caused by any condition that decreases cardiac output (e.g., bradyarrhythmia, tachyarrhythmia, obstruction of the left ventricular or right ventricular inflow or outflow, cardiac tamponade, aortic dissection, or severe pump failure), by

TABLE 50-1 CARDINAL SYMPTOMS OF CARDIOVASCULAR DISEASE

Chest pain or discomfort
Dyspnea, orthopnea, paroxysmal nocturnal dyspnea, wheezing
Palpitations, dizziness, syncope
Cough, hemoptysis
Fatigue, weakness
Pain in extremities with exertion (claudication)

reflex-mediated vasomotor instability (e.g., vasovagal, situational, or carotid sinus syncope), or by orthostatic hypotension (see Table 62-1 in Chapter 62). Neurologic diseases (e.g., migraine headaches, transient ischemic attacks, or seizures) also can cause transient loss of consciousness. The history, physical examination, and ECG are often diagnostic of the cause of syncope (see Table 62-2 in Chapter 62). Syncope caused by a cardiac arrhythmia usually occurs with little warning. Syncope with exertion or just after conclusion of exertion is typical of aortic stenosis and hypertrophic obstructive cardiomyopathy. In many patients, additional testing is required to document central nervous system disease, the cause of reduced cardiac output, or carotid sinus

TABLE 50-2 CAUSES OF CHEST PAIN

CONDITION	LOCATION	QUALITY	DURATION	AGGRAVATING OR RELIEVING FACTORS	ASSOCIATED SYMPTOMS OR SIGNS
CARDIOVASCULAR CAUSES					
Angina	Retrosternal region; radiates to or occasionally isolated to neck, jaw, epigastrium, shoulder, or arms (left common)	Pressure, burning, squeezing, heaviness, indigestion	<2-10 min	Precipitated by exercise, cold weather, or emotional stress; relieved by rest or nitroglycerin; atypical (Prinzmetal's) angina may be unrelated to activity, often early morning	S_3 or murmur of papillary muscle dysfunction during pain
Rest or unstable angina	Same as angina	Same as angina but may be more severe	Usually <20 min	Same as angina, with decreasing tolerance for exertion or at rest	Similar to stable angina but may be pronounced; transient heart failure can occur
Myocardial infarction	Substernal and may radiate like angina	Heaviness, pressure, burning, constriction	≥30 min but variable	Unrelieved by rest or nitroglycerin	Shortness of breath, sweating, weakness, nausea, vomiting
Pericarditis	Usually begins over sternum or toward cardiac apex and may radiate to neck or left shoulder; often more localized than the pain of myocardial ischemia	Sharp, stabbing, knifelike	Lasts many hours to days; may wax and wane	Aggravated by deep breathing, rotating chest, or supine position; relieved by sitting up and leaning forward	Pericardial friction rub
Aortic dissection	Anterior chest; may radiate to back	Excruciating, tearing, knifelike	Sudden onset, unrelenting	Usually occurs in setting of hypertension or predisposition, such as Marfan syndrome	Murmur of aortic insufficiency, pulse or blood pressure asymmetry; neurologic deficit
Pulmonary embolism (chest pain often not present)	Substernal or over region of pulmonary infarction	Pleuritic (with pulmonary infarction) or angina-like	Sudden onset; minutes to <1 hr	May be aggravated by breathing	Dyspnea, tachypnea, tachycardia; hypotension, signs of acute right ventricular failure, and pulmonary hypertension with large emboli; rales, pleural rub, hemoptysis with pulmonary infarction
Pulmonary hypertension	Substernal	Pressure; oppressive	Similar to angina	Aggravated by effort	Pain usually associated with dyspnea; signs of pulmonary hypertension
NONCARDIAC CAUSES					
Pneumonia with pleurisy	Localized over involved area	Pleuritic, localized	Brief or prolonged	Painful breathing	Dyspnea, cough, fever, dull to percussion, bronchial breath sounds, rales, occasional pleural rub
Spontaneous pneumothorax	Unilateral	Sharp, well localized	Sudden onset, lasts many hours	Painful breathing	Dyspnea; hyperresonance and decreased breath and voice sounds over involved lung
Musculoskeletal disorders	Variable	Aching	Short or long duration	Aggravated by movement; history of muscle exertion or injury	Tender to pressure or movement
Herpes zoster	Dermatomal in distribution	Burning, itching	Prolonged	None	Vesicular rash appears in area of discomfort
Esophageal reflux	Substernal, epigastric	Burning, visceral discomfort	10-60 min	Aggravated by large meal, postprandial recumbency; relief with antacid	Water brash
Peptic ulcer	Epigastric, substernal	Visceral burning, aching	Prolonged	Relief with food, antacid	
Gallbladder disease	Epigastric, right upper quadrant	Visceral	Prolonged	May be unprovoked or follow meals	Right upper quadrant tenderness may be present
Anxiety states	Often localized over precordium	Variable; location often moves from place to place	Varies; often fleeting	Situational	Sighing respirations, often chest wall tenderness

Modified from Andreoli TE, Carpenter CCJ, Griggs RC, et al. Evaluation of the patient with cardiovascular disease. In: *Cecil Essentials of Medicine*, 6th ed. Philadelphia: WB Saunders; 2004:34-35.

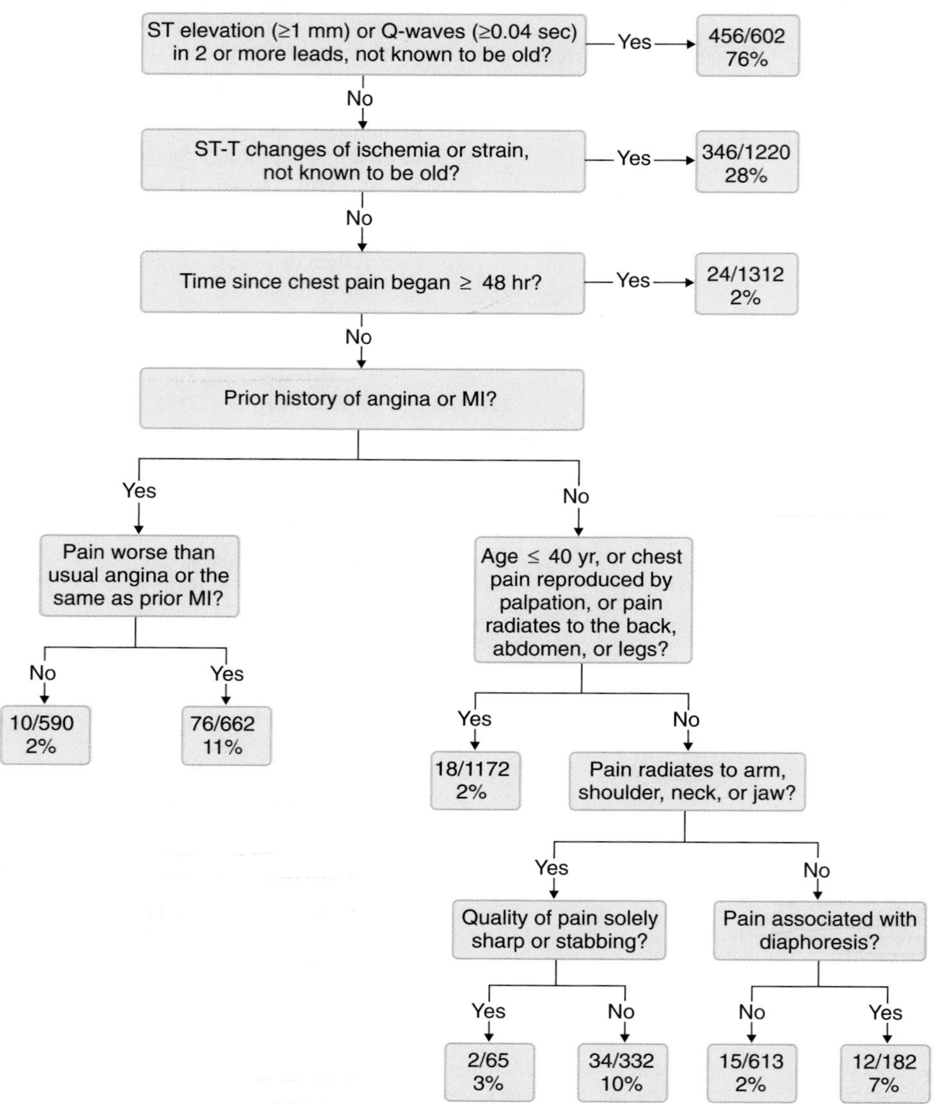

FIGURE 50-1. Flow diagram to estimate the risk for acute myocardial infarction in emergency departments in patients with acute chest pain. For each clinical subset, the numerator is the number of patients with the set of presenting characteristics who had a myocardial infarction; the denominator is the total number of patients presenting with that characteristic or set of characteristics. CHF = congestive heart failure; DVT = deep vein thrombosis. (Modified from Pearson SD, Goldman L, Garcia TB, et al. Physician response to a prediction rule for the triage of emergency department patients with chest pain. *J Gen Intern Med*. 1994;9:241-247.)

TABLE 50-3 COMMON EXERCISE TEST PROTOCOLS*

PROTOCOL	STAGE	DURATION (min)	GRADE (%)	RATE (mph)	METABOLIC EQUIVALENTS AT COMPLETION	FUNCTIONAL CLASS
Modified Bruce protocol†	1	3	0	1.7	2.5	III
	2	3	10	1.7	5	II
	3	3	12	2.5	7	I
	4	3	14	3.4	10	I
	5	3	16	4.2	13	I
Naughton protocol‡	0	2	0	2	2	III
	1	2	3.5	2	3	III
	2	2	7	2	4	III
	3	2	10.5	2	5	II
	4	2	14	2	6	II
	5	2	17.5	2	7	I

*Ramp protocols in which the workload is gradually increased on the basis of the patient's estimated functional capacity to achieve maximal effort in approximately 10 minutes are also useful.
†Commonly used in ambulatory patients.
‡Commonly used in patients with recent myocardial infarction, unstable angina, or other conditions that are expected to limit exercise.
Modified from Braunwald E, Goldman L, eds. *Primary Cardiology*, 2nd ed. Philadelphia: WB Saunders; 2003.

TABLE 50-4 AMERICAN HEART ASSOCIATION/AMERICAN COLLEGE OF CARDIOLOGY GUIDELINES FOR USE OF DIAGNOSTIC TESTS IN PATIENTS WITH PALPITATIONS*

AMBULATORY ELECTROCARDIOGRAPHY	
Class I	Palpitations, syncope, dizziness
Class II	Shortness of breath, chest pain, or fatigue (not otherwise explained, episodic, and strongly suggestive of an arrhythmia as the cause because of a relation of the symptom with palpitation)
Class III	Symptoms not reasonably expected to be due to arrhythmia
ELECTROPHYSIOLOGIC STUDY	
Class I	Patients with palpitations who have a pulse rate documented by medical personnel as inappropriately rapid and in whom electrocardiographic recordings fail to document the cause of the palpitations Patients with palpitations preceding a syncopal episode
Class II	Patients with clinically significant palpitations, suspected to be of cardiac origin, in whom symptoms are sporadic and cannot be documented; studies are performed to determine the mechanisms of arrhythmias, to direct or provide therapy or to assess prognosis
Class III	Patients with palpitations documented to be due to extracardiac causes (e.g., hyperthyroidism)
ECHOCARDIOGRAPHY	
Class I	Arrhythmias with evidence of heart disease Family history of genetic disorder associated with arrhythmias
Class II	Arrhythmias commonly associated with, but without evidence of, heart disease Atrial fibrillation or flutter
Class III	Palpitations without evidence of arrhythmias Minor arrhythmias without evidence of heart disease

*Class I, general agreement the test is useful and indicated; class II, frequently used, but there is a divergence of opinion with respect to its utility; class III, general agreement the test is not useful.
From Braunwald E, Goldman L, eds. *Primary Cardiology*, 2nd ed. Philadelphia: WB Saunders; 2003:132.

TABLE 50-5 A COMPARISON OF THREE METHODS OF ASSESSING CARDIOVASCULAR DISABILITY

CLASS	NEW YORK HEART ASSOCIATION FUNCTIONAL CLASSIFICATION	CANADIAN CARDIOVASCULAR SOCIETY FUNCTIONAL CLASSIFICATION	SPECIFIC ACTIVITY SCALE
I	Patients with cardiac disease but without resulting limitations of physical activity Ordinary physical activity does not cause undue fatigue, palpitation, dyspnea, or anginal pain.	Ordinary physical activity, such as walking and climbing stairs, does not cause angina. Angina with strenuous or rapid or prolonged exertion at work or recreation	Patients can perform to completion any activity requiring ≥7 metabolic equivalents, e.g., can carry 24 lb up 8 steps; carry objects that weigh 80 lb; do outdoor work (shovel snow, spade soil); do recreational activities (skiing, basketball, squash, handball, jog or walk 5 mph)
II	Patients with cardiac disease resulting in slight limitation of physical activity They are comfortable at rest. Ordinary physical activity results in fatigue, palpitations, dyspnea, or anginal pain.	Slight limitation of ordinary activity Walking or climbing stairs rapidly, walking uphill, walking or stair climbing after meals, in cold, in wind, or when under emotional stress, or only during the few hours after awakening Walking >2 blocks on the level and climbing >1 flight of ordinary stairs at a normal pace and in normal conditions	Patient can perform to completion any activity requiring ≥5 metabolic equivalents but cannot and does not perform to completion activities requiring ≥7 metabolic equivalents, e.g., have sexual intercourse without stopping, garden, rake, weed, roller skate, dance foxtrot, walk at 4 mph on level ground
III	Patients with cardiac disease resulting in marked limitation of physical activity They are comfortable at rest. Less than ordinary physical activity causes fatigue, palpitations, dyspnea, or anginal pain.	Marked limitation of ordinary physical activity Walking 1 or 2 blocks on the level and climbing >1 flight in normal conditions	Patient can perform to completion any activity requiring ≥2 metabolic equivalents but cannot and does not perform to completion any activities requiring ≥5 metabolic equivalents, e.g., shower without stopping, strip and make bed, clean windows, walk 2.5 mph, bowl, play golf, dress without stopping
IV	Patients with cardiac disease resulting in inability to carry on any physical activity without discomfort Symptoms of cardiac insufficiency or of the anginal syndrome may be present even at rest. If any physical activity is undertaken, discomfort is increased.	Inability to carry on any physical activity without discomfort—anginal syndrome may be present at rest	Patient cannot or does not perform to completion activities requiring ≥2 metabolic equivalents; cannot carry out activities listed above (Specific Activity Scale, class III)

From Goldman L, Hashimoto B, Cook EF, et al. Comparative reproducibility and validity of systems for assessing cardiovascular functional class: advantages of a new specific activity scale. *Circulation.* 1981;64:1227-1234. Reproduced by permission of the American Heart Association.

syncope. When the history, physical examination, and ECG do not provide helpful diagnostic information that points toward a specific cause of syncope, it is imperative that patients with heart disease or an abnormal ECG be tested with continuous ambulatory ECG monitoring to diagnose a possible arrhythmia (see Fig. 62-1 in Chapter 62); in selected patients, formal electrophysiologic testing may be indicated (Chapter 62). In patients with no evident heart disease, tilt testing (Chapter 62) can help detect reflex-mediated vasomotor instability.

Other Symptoms

Nonproductive *cough* (Chapter 83), especially a persistent cough (see Fig. 83-1 in Chapter 83), can be an early manifestation of elevated pulmonary venous pressure and otherwise unsuspected heart failure. *Fatigue* and *weakness* are common accompaniments of advanced cardiac disease and reflect an inability to perform normal activities. A variety of approaches have been used to classify the severity of cardiac limitations, ranging from class I (little or no limitation) to class IV (severe limitation) (Table 50-5). *Hemoptysis*

(Chapter 83) is a classic presenting finding in patients with pulmonary embolism, but it is also common in patients with mitral stenosis, pulmonary edema, pulmonary infections, and malignant neoplasms (see Table 83-5 in Chapter 83). *Claudication,* which is pain in the extremities with exertion, should alert the physician to possible peripheral arterial disease (Chapters 79 and 80).

Complete Medical History

The complete medical history should include a thorough review of systems, family history, social history, and past medical history (Chapter 14). The review of systems may reveal other symptoms that suggest a systemic disease as the cause of any cardiovascular problems. The family history should focus on premature atherosclerosis or evidence of familial abnormalities, such as may be found with various causes of the long QT syndrome (Chapter 65) or hypertrophic cardiomyopathy (Chapter 60).

The social history should include specific questioning about cigarette smoking, alcohol intake, and use of illicit drugs. The past medical history may reveal prior conditions or medications that suggest systemic diseases, ranging from chronic obstructive pulmonary disease, which may explain a complaint of dyspnea, to hemochromatosis, which may be a cause of restrictive cardiomyopathy. A careful history to inquire about recent dental work or other procedures is crucial if bacterial endocarditis is part of the differential diagnosis.

PHYSICAL EXAMINATION FOR DETECTION OF SIGNS OF CARDIOVASCULAR DISEASE

The cardiovascular physical examination, which is a subset of the complete physical examination, provides important clues to the diagnosis of asymptomatic and symptomatic cardiac disease and may reveal cardiovascular manifestations of noncardiovascular diseases. The cardiovascular physical examination begins with careful measurement of the pulse and blood pressure (Chapter 7). If aortic dissection (Chapter 78) is a consideration, blood pressure should be measured in both arms and, preferably, in at least one leg. When coarctation of the aorta is suspected (Chapter 69), blood pressure must be measured in at least one leg and in the arms. Discrepancies in blood pressure between the two arms also can be caused by atherosclerotic disease of the great vessels. Pulsus paradoxus, which is more than the usual 10 mm Hg drop in systolic blood pressure during inspiration, is typical of pericardial tamponade (Chapter 77).

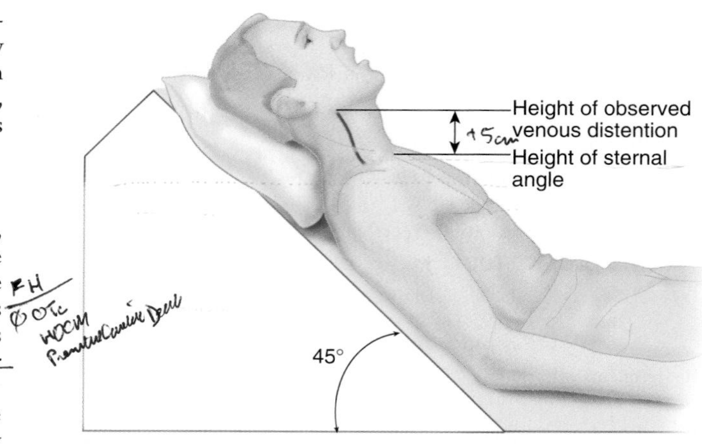

FIGURE 50-2. Jugular venous distention is defined by engorgement of the internal jugular vein more than 5 cm above the sternal angle at 45 degrees. The central venous pressure is the observed venous distention above the sternal angle plus 5 cm. (From American Academy of Family Physicians Online. http://www.aafp.org/afp/20000301/1319.html. Accessed June 9, 2010.)

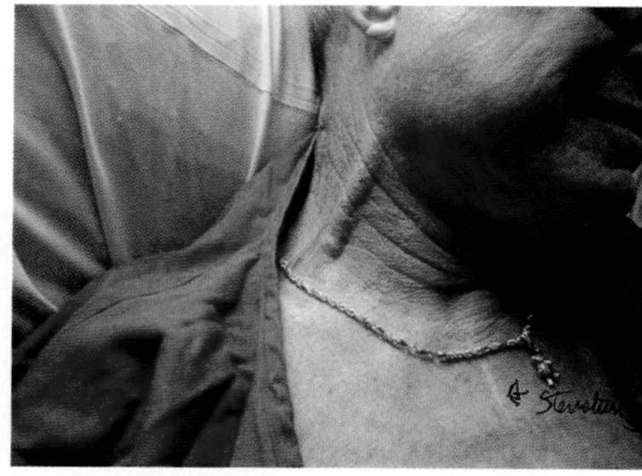

FIGURE 50-3. Typical distention of the internal jugular vein. (From http://courses.cvcc.vccs.edu/WisemanD/jugular_vein_distention.htm.)

General Appearance

The respiratory rate may be increased in patients with heart failure. Patients with pulmonary edema are usually markedly tachypneic and may have labored breathing. Patients with advanced heart failure may have Cheyne-Stokes respirations.

Systemic diseases, such as hyperthyroidism (Chapter 233), hypothyroidism (Chapter 233), rheumatoid arthritis (Chapter 272), scleroderma (Chapter 275), and hemochromatosis (Chapter 219), may be suspected from the patient's general appearance. Marfan syndrome (Chapter 268), Turner's syndrome (Chapter 243), Down syndrome (Chapter 40), and a variety of congenital anomalies also may be readily apparent.

Ophthalmologic Examination

Examination of the fundi may show diabetic (see Fig. 431-24 in Chapter 431) or hypertensive retinopathy (see Fig. 67-11 in Chapter 67) or Roth's spots (see Fig. 431-28 in Chapter 431) typical of infectious endocarditis. Beading of the retinal arteries is typical of severe hypercholesterolemia. Osteogenesis imperfecta, which is associated with blue sclerae, also is associated with aortic dilation and mitral valve prolapse. Retinal artery occlusion (see Fig. 431-29 in Chapter 431) may be caused by an embolus from clot in the left atrium or left ventricle, a left atrial myxoma, or atherosclerotic debris from the great vessels. Hyperthyroidism may present with exophthalmos and typical stare (see Fig. 431-6 in Chapter 431), whereas myotonic dystrophy, which is associated with atrioventricular block and arrhythmia, often is associated with ptosis and an expressionless face (see Fig. 429-2 in Chapter 429).

Jugular Veins

The external jugular veins help in assessment of mean right atrial pressure, which normally varies between 5 and 10 cm H_2O; the height (in centimeters) of the central venous pressure is measured by adding 5 cm to the height of the observed jugular venous distention above the sternal angle of Louis (Fig. 50-2). The normal jugular venous pulse, best seen in the internal jugular vein (and not seen in the external jugular vein unless insufficiency of the jugular venous valves is present), includes an *a* wave, caused by right atrial contraction; a *c* wave, reflecting carotid artery pulsation; an *x* descent; a *v* wave, which corresponds to isovolumetric right ventricular contraction and is more marked in the presence of tricuspid insufficiency; and a *y* descent, which occurs as the tricuspid valve opens and ventricular filling begins (Fig. 50-3). Abnormalities of the jugular venous pressure (Fig. 50-4) and arterial pulse are useful in detecting conditions such as heart failure, pericardial disease, tricuspid valve disease, and pulmonary hypertension (Table 50-6).

Carotid Pulse

The carotid pulse should be examined in terms of its volume and contour. The carotid pulse (Fig. 50-5) may be increased in frequency and may be more intense than normal in patients with a higher stroke volume secondary to aortic regurgitation, arteriovenous fistula, hyperthyroidism, fever, or anemia. In aortic regurgitation or arteriovenous fistula, the pulse may have a bisferious quality. The carotid upstroke is delayed in patients with valvular aortic stenosis (Chapter 75) and has a normal contour but diminished amplitude in any cause of reduced stroke volume.

Cardiac Inspection and Palpation

Inspection of the precordium may reveal the hyperinflation of obstructive lung disease or unilateral asymmetry of the left side of the chest because of right ventricular hypertrophy before puberty. Palpation may be performed with the patient either supine or in the left lateral decubitus position; the latter position moves the left ventricular apex closer to the chest wall and increases the ability to palpate the point of maximal impulse and other phenomena. Low-frequency phenomena, such as systolic heaves or lifts from the left ventricle (at the cardiac apex) or right ventricle (parasternal in the third or fourth intercostal space), are felt best with the heel of the palm. With the patient in the left lateral decubitus position, this technique also may allow palpation of an S_3 gallop in cases of advanced heart failure or an S_4 gallop in cases of poor left ventricular distensibility during diastole. The left ventricular apex is more diffuse and sometimes may be frankly dyskinetic in patients with advanced heart disease. The distal palm is best for feeling thrills, which are the tactile equivalent of cardiac murmurs. By definition, a thrill denotes a murmur of grade 4/6 or louder. Higher-frequency events may be felt best with the fingertips; examples include the opening snap of mitral stenosis or the loud pulmonic second sound of pulmonary hypertension.

Auscultation

The first heart sound (Fig. 50-6), which is largely produced by closure of the mitral and—to a lesser extent—the tricuspid valves, may be louder in patients with mitral valve stenosis and intact valve leaflet movement and less audible in patients with poor closure due to mitral regurgitation (Chapter 75). The second heart sound is caused primarily by closure of the aortic valve, but closure of the pulmonic valve is also commonly audible. In normal individuals, the louder aortic closure sound occurs first, followed by pulmonic closure. With expiration, the two sounds are virtually superimposed. With inspiration, by comparison, the increased stroke volume of the right ventricle commonly leads to a discernible splitting of the second sound. This splitting may be fixed in patients with an atrial septal defect (Chapter 69) or a right bundle

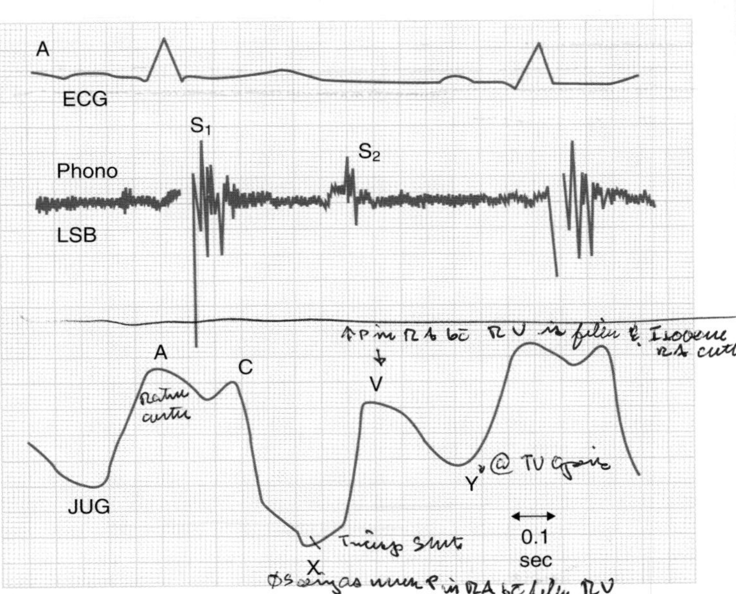

FIGURE 50-4. Normal jugular venous pulse. ECG = electrocardiogram; JUG = jugular vein; LSB = left sternal border; phono = phonocardiogram; S_1 = first heart sound; S_2 = second heart sound.

TABLE 50-6 ABNORMALITIES OF VENOUS PRESSURE AND PULSE AND THEIR CLINICAL SIGNIFICANCE

Positive hepatojugular reflux	Suspect heart failure, particularly left ventricular systolic dysfunction (echocardiography recommended)
Elevated systemic venous pressure without obvious *x* or *y* descent, quiet precordium, and pulsus paradoxus	Suspect cardiac tamponade (echocardiography recommended)
Elevated systemic venous pressure with sharp *y* descent, Kussmaul's sign, and quiet precordium	Suspect constrictive pericarditis (cardiac catheterization and MRI or CT recommended)
Elevated systemic venous pressure with a sharp brief *y* descent, Kussmaul's sign, and evidence of pulmonary hypertension and tricuspid regurgitation	Suspect restrictive cardiomyopathy (cardiac catheterization and MRI or CT recommended)
A prominent *a* wave with or without elevation of mean systemic venous pressure	Exclude tricuspid stenosis, right ventricular hypertrophy due to pulmonary stenosis, and pulmonary hypertension (echo-Doppler study recommended)
A prominent *v* wave with a sharp *y* descent	Suspect tricuspid regurgitation (echo-Doppler or cardiac catheterization to determine etiology)

CT = computed tomography; MRI = magnetic resonance imaging.
From Braunwald E, ed. *Heart Disease: A Textbook of Cardiovascular Medicine*, 5th ed. Philadelphia: WB Saunders; 1997.

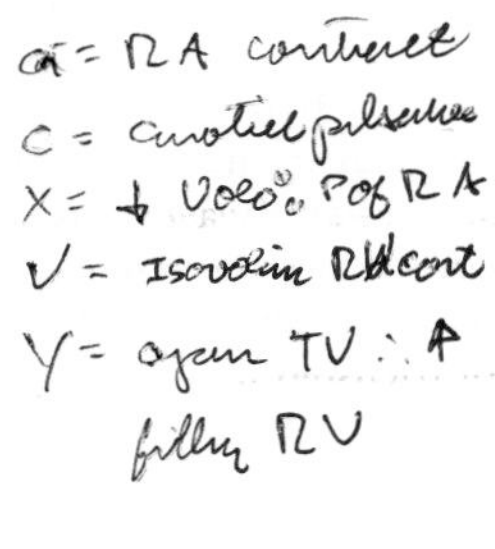

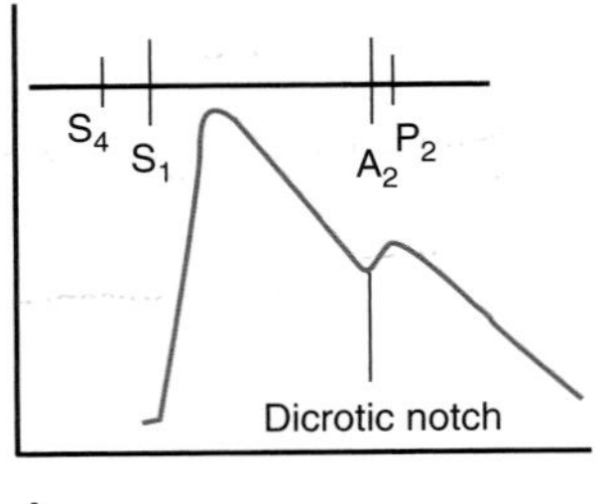

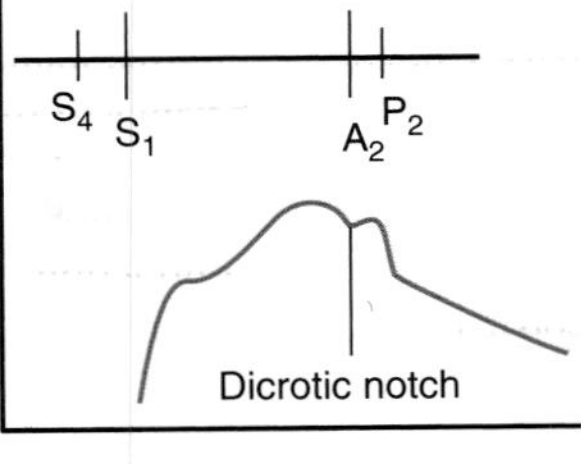

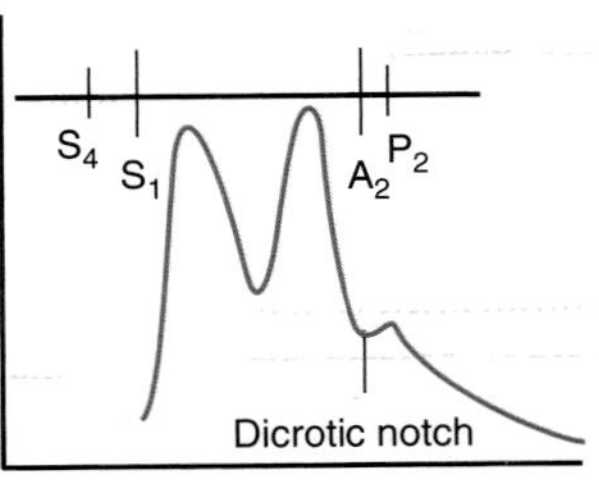

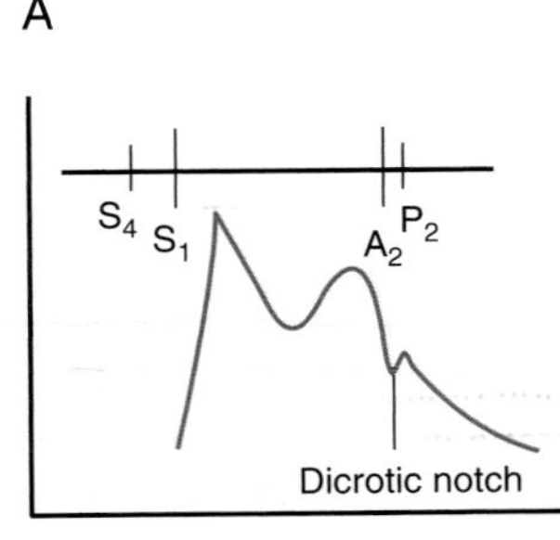

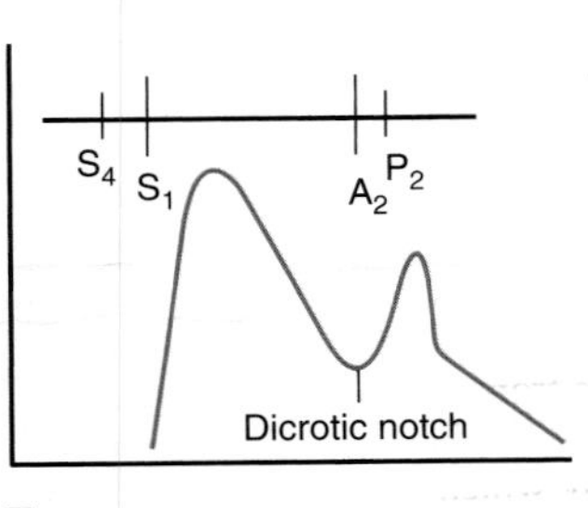

FIGURE 50-5. Schematic diagrams of the configurational changes in the carotid pulse and their differential diagnosis. Heart sounds also are illustrated. **A,** Normal. **B,** Anacrotic pulse with slow initial upstroke. The peak is close to the second heart sound. These features suggest fixed left ventricular outflow obstruction, such as valvular aortic stenosis. **C,** Pulsus bisferiens, with percussion and tidal waves occurring during systole. This type of carotid pulse contour is observed most frequently in patients with hemodynamically significant aortic regurgitation or combined aortic stenosis and regurgitation with dominant regurgitation. It rarely is observed in patients with mitral valve prolapse or in normal individuals. **D,** Pulsus bisferiens in hypertrophic obstructive cardiomyopathy. This finding rarely is appreciated at the bedside by palpation. **E,** Dicrotic pulse results from an accentuated dicrotic wave and tends to occur in sepsis, severe heart failure, hypovolemic shock, and cardiac tamponade and after aortic valve replacement. A_2 = aortic component of the second heart sound; P_2 = pulmonary component of the second heart sound); S_1 = first heart sound; S_4 = atrial sounds. (From Chatterjee K. Bedside evaluation of the heart: the physical examination. In: Chatterjee K, Chetlin MD, Karliner J, et al, eds. *Cardiology: An Illustrated Text/Reference.* Philadelphia: JB Lippincott; 1991:3.11-3.51.)

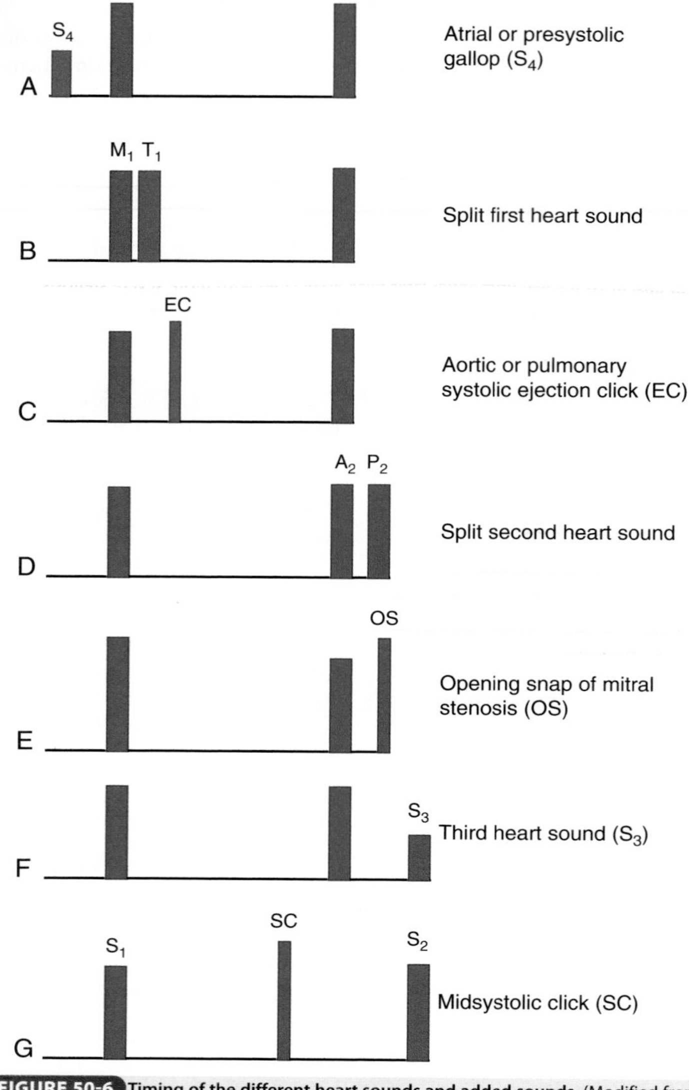

FIGURE 50-6. Timing of the different heart sounds and added sounds. (Modified from Wood P. *Diseases of the Heart and Circulation*, 3rd ed. Philadelphia: JB Lippincott; 1968.)

branch block. The split may be paradoxical in patients with left bundle branch block or other causes of delayed left ventricular emptying. The aortic component of the second sound is increased in intensity in the presence of systemic hypertension and decreased in intensity in patients with aortic stenosis. The pulmonic second sound is increased in the presence of pulmonary hypertension.

Early systolic ejection sounds are related to forceful opening of the aortic or pulmonic valve. These sounds are common in congenital aortic stenosis, with a mobile valve; in hypertension, with forceful opening of the aortic valve; and in healthy young individuals, especially when cardiac output is increased. Midsystolic or late systolic clicks are caused most commonly by mitral valve prolapse (Chapter 75). Clicks are relatively high-frequency sounds that are heard best with the diaphragm of the stethoscope.

An S_3 corresponds to rapid ventricular filling during early diastole. It may occur in normal children and young adults, especially if stroke volume is increased. After about 40 years of age, however, an S_3 should be considered abnormal; it is caused by conditions that increase the volume of ventricular filling during early diastole (e.g., mitral regurgitation) or that increase pressure in early diastole (e.g., advanced heart failure). A left ventricular S_3 gallop is heard best at the apex, whereas the right ventricular S_3 gallop is heard best at the fourth intercostal space at the left parasternal border; both are heard best with the bell of the stethoscope. An S_4 is heard rarely in young individuals but is common in adults older than 40 or 50 years because of reduced ventricular compliance during atrial contraction; it is a nearly ubiquitous finding in patients with hypertension, heart failure, or ischemic heart disease.

The opening snap of mitral and, less commonly, tricuspid stenosis (Chapter 75) occurs at the beginning of mechanical diastole, before the onset of the rapid phase of ventricular filling. An opening snap is high pitched and is heard best with the diaphragm; this differential frequency should help distinguish an opening snap from an S_3 on physical examination. An opening snap commonly can be distinguished from a loud pulmonic component of the second heart sound by the differential location (mitral opening snap at the apex, tricuspid opening snap at the left third or fourth intercostal space, pulmonic second sound at the left second intercostal space) and by the longer interval between S_2 and the opening snap.

Heart murmurs may be classified as systolic, diastolic, or continuous (Table 50-7). Murmurs are graded by intensity on a scale of 1 to 6. Grade 1 is faint and appreciated only by careful auscultation; grade 2, readily audible; grade 3, moderately loud; grade 4, loud and associated with a palpable thrill; grade 5, loud and audible with the stethoscope only partially placed on the chest; and grade 6, loud enough to be heard without the stethoscope on the chest. Systolic ejection murmurs usually peak in early to mid systole when left ventricular ejection is maximal; examples include fixed valvular, supravalvular, or infravalvular aortic stenosis and pulmonic stenosis. The murmur of hypertrophic obstructive cardiomyopathy has a similar ejection quality, although its peak may be later in systole when dynamic obstruction is maximal (Chapter 60). Pansystolic murmurs are characteristic of mitral or tricuspid regurgitation or with a left-to-right shunt from conditions such as a ventricular septal defect (left ventricle to right ventricle). A late systolic murmur is characteristic of mitral valve prolapse (Chapter 75) or ischemic papillary muscle dysfunction. Ejection quality murmurs also may be heard in patients with normal valves but increased flow, such as occurs with marked anemia, fever, or bradycardia secondary to congenital complete heart block; they also may be heard across a valve that is downstream from increased flow because of an intracardiac shunt. Maneuvers such as inspiration, expiration, standing, squatting, and hand gripping can be especially useful in the differential diagnosis of a murmur; however, echocardiography commonly is required to make a definitive diagnosis of cause and severity (Table 50-8).

High-frequency, early diastolic murmurs are typical of aortic regurgitation and pulmonic regurgitation from a variety of causes. The murmurs of mitral and tricuspid stenosis begin in early to mid-diastole and tend to diminish in intensity later in diastole in the absence of effective atrial contraction, but they tend to increase in intensity in later diastole if effective atrial contraction is present.

Continuous murmurs may be caused by any abnormality that is associated with a pressure gradient in systole and diastole. Examples include a patent ductus arteriosus, ruptured sinus of Valsalva aneurysm, arteriovenous fistula (of the coronary artery, pulmonary artery, or thoracic artery), and a mammary soufflé. In some situations, murmurs of two coexistent conditions (e.g., aortic stenosis and regurgitation; atrial septal defect with a large shunt and resulting flow murmurs of relative mitral and pulmonic stenosis) may mimic a continuous murmur.

Abdomen

The most common cause of hepatomegaly in patients with heart disease is hepatic engorgement from elevated right-sided pressures associated with right ventricular failure of any cause. Hepatojugular reflux is elicited by pressing on the liver and showing an increase in the jugular venous pressure; it indicates advanced right ventricular failure or obstruction to right ventricular filling. Evaluation of the abdomen also may reveal an enlarged liver caused by a systemic disease, such as hemochromatosis (Chapter 219) or sarcoidosis (Chapter 95), which also may affect the heart. In more severe cases, splenomegaly and ascites also may be noted. Large, palpable, polycystic kidneys (Chapter 129) commonly are associated with hypertension. A systolic bruit suggestive of renal artery stenosis (Chapter 127) or an enlarged abdominal aorta (Chapter 78) is a clue of atherosclerosis.

Extremities

Extremities should be evaluated for peripheral pulses, edema, cyanosis, and clubbing. Diminished peripheral pulses suggest peripheral arterial disease (Chapters 79 and 80). Delayed pulses in the legs are consistent with coarctation of the aorta and are seen after aortic dissection.

TABLE 50-7 SOME COMMON CAUSES OF HEART MURMURS*

	USUAL LOCATION	COMMON ASSOCIATED FINDINGS
SYSTOLIC		
Holosystolic		
Mitral regurgitation	Apex → axilla	↑ with handgrip; S_3 if marked mitral regurgitation; left ventricular dilation common
Tricuspid regurgitation	LLSB	↑ with inspiration; right ventricular dilation common
Ventricular septal defect	LLSB → RLSB	Often with thrill
Early–mid systolic		
Aortic valvular stenosis	RUSB	
Fixed supravalvular or subvalvular	RUSB	Ejection click if mobile valve; soft or absent A_2 if valve immobile; later peak associated with more severe stenosis
Dynamic infravalvular	LLSB → apex + axilla	Hypertrophic obstructive cardiomyopathy; murmur louder if left ventricular volume lower or contractility increased, softer if left ventricular volume increased†; can be later in systole if obstruction delayed
Pulmonic valvular stenosis	LUSB	↑ with inspiration
Infravalvular (infundibular)	LUSB	↑ with inspiration
Supravalvular	LUSB	↑ with inspiration
"Flow murmurs"	LUSB	Anemia, fever, increased flow of any cause‡
Mid–late systolic		
Mitral valve prolapse	LLSB or apex → axilla	Preceded by click; murmur lengthens with maneuvers that decrease left ventricular volume†
Papillary muscle dysfunction	Apex → axilla	Ischemic heart disease
DIASTOLIC		
Early diastolic		
Aortic regurgitation	RUSB, LUSB	High-pitched, blowing quality; endocarditis, diseases of the aorta, associated aortic valvular stenosis; signs of low peripheral vascular resistance
Pulmonic valve regurgitation	LUSB	Pulmonary hypertension as a causative factor
Mid–late diastolic		
Mitral stenosis, tricuspid stenosis	Apex, LLSB	Low pitched; in rheumatic heart disease, opening snap commonly precedes murmur; can be due to increased flow across normal valve‡
Atrial myxomas	Apex (L), LLSB (R)	"Tumor plop"
Continuous		
Venous hum	Over jugular or hepatic vein or breast	Disappears with compression of vein or pressure of stethoscope
Patent ductus arteriosus	LUSB	
Arteriovenous fistula		
Coronary	LUSB	
Pulmonary, bronchial, chest wall	Over fistula	
Ruptured sinus of Valsalva aneurysm	RUSB	Sudden onset

*See also Chapters 69 and 75.
†Left ventricular volume is decreased by standing or during prolonged, forced expiration against a closed glottis (Valsalva maneuver); it is increased by squatting or by elevation of the legs; contractility is increased by adrenergic stimulation or in the beat after an extrasystolic beat.
‡Including a left-to-right shunt through an atrial septal defect for tricuspid or pulmonic flow murmurs, and a ventricular septal defect for pulmonic or mitral flow murmurs.
LLSB = left lower sternal border (4th intercostal space); LUSB = left upper sternal border (2nd-3rd intercostal spaces); RLSB = right lower sternal border (4th intercostal space); RUSB = right upper sternal border (2nd-3rd intercostal spaces).

Edema (Fig. 50-7) is a cardinal manifestation of right-sided heart failure. When it is caused by heart failure, pericardial disease, or pulmonary hypertension, the edema is usually symmetrical and progresses upward from the ankles; each of these causes of cardiac edema commonly is associated with jugular venous distention and often with hepatic congestion. Unilateral edema suggests thrombophlebitis or proximal venous or lymphatic obstruction (Fig. 50-8). Edema in the absence of evidence of right-sided or left-sided heart failure suggests renal disease, hypoalbuminemia, myxedema, or other noncardiac causes. Among unselected patients with bilateral edema, about 40% have an underlying cardiac disease, about 40% have an elevated pulmonary blood pressure, about 20% have bilateral venous disease, about 20% have renal disease, and about 25% have idiopathic edema.

Cyanosis (Fig. 50-9) is a bluish discoloration caused by reduced hemoglobin exceeding about 5 g/dL in the capillary bed. Central cyanosis is seen in patients with poor oxygen saturation resulting from a reduced inspired oxygen concentration or inability to oxygenate the blood in the lungs (e.g., as a result of advanced pulmonary disease, pulmonary edema, pulmonary arteriovenous fistula, or right-to-left shunting); it also may be seen in patients with marked erythrocytosis. Methemoglobinemia (Chapter 161) also can present with cyanosis. Peripheral cyanosis may be caused by reduced blood flow to the extremities secondary to vasoconstriction, heart failure, or shock.

Clubbing (Fig. 50-10), which is loss of the normal concave configuration of the nail as it emerges from the distal phalanx, is seen in patients with pulmonary abnormalities such as lung cancer (Chapter 197) and in patients with cyanotic congenital heart disease (Chapter 69).

Examination of the Skin

Examination of the skin may reveal bronze pigmentation typical of hemochromatosis (Chapter 219); jaundice (see Fig. 149-2 in Chapter 149) characteristic of severe right-sided heart failure or hemochromatosis; or capillary hemangiomas typical of Osler-Weber-Rendu disease (see Fig. 176-1 in Chapter 176), which also is associated with pulmonary arteriovenous fistulas and cyanosis. Infectious endocarditis may be associated with Osler's nodes (see Fig. 76-2 in Chapter 76), Janeway's lesions, or splinter hemorrhages (Fig. 50-11) (Chapter 76). Xanthomas (Fig. 50-12) are subcutaneous deposits of cholesterol seen on the extensor surfaces of the extremities or on the palms and digital creases; they are found in patients with severe hypercholesterolemia.

Laboratory Studies

All patients with known or suspected cardiac disease should have an ECG and chest radiograph. The ECG (Chapter 54) helps identify rate, rhythm,

TABLE 50-8 SENSITIVITY AND SPECIFICITY OF BEDSIDE MANEUVERS IN THE IDENTIFICATION OF SYSTOLIC MURMURS

MANEUVER	RESPONSE	MURMUR	SENSITIVITY (%)	SPECIFICITY (%)
Inspiration	↑	RS	100	88
Expiration	↓	RS	100	88
Valsalva maneuver	↑	HC	65	96
Squat to stand	↑	HC	95	84
Stand to squat	↓	HC	95	85
Leg elevation	↓	HC	85	91
Handgrip	↓	HC	85	75
Handgrip	↑	MR and VSD	68	92
Transient arterial occlusion	↑	MR and VSD	78	100

HC = hypertrophic cardiomyopathy; MR = mitral regurgitation; RS = right sided; VSD = ventricular septal defect.

Modified with permission from Lembo NJ, Dell'Italia IJ, Crawford MH, et al. Bedside diagnosis of systolic murmurs. *N Engl J Med.* 1988;318:1572-1578.

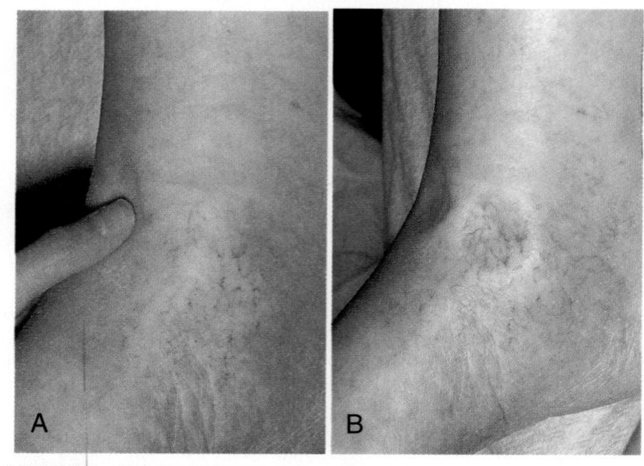

FIGURE 50-7. Pitting edema in a patient with cardiac failure. A depression ("pit") remains in the edema for some minutes after firm fingertip pressure is applied. (From Forbes CD, Jackson WD. *Color Atlas and Text of Clinical Medicine*, 3rd ed. London: Mosby; 2003.)

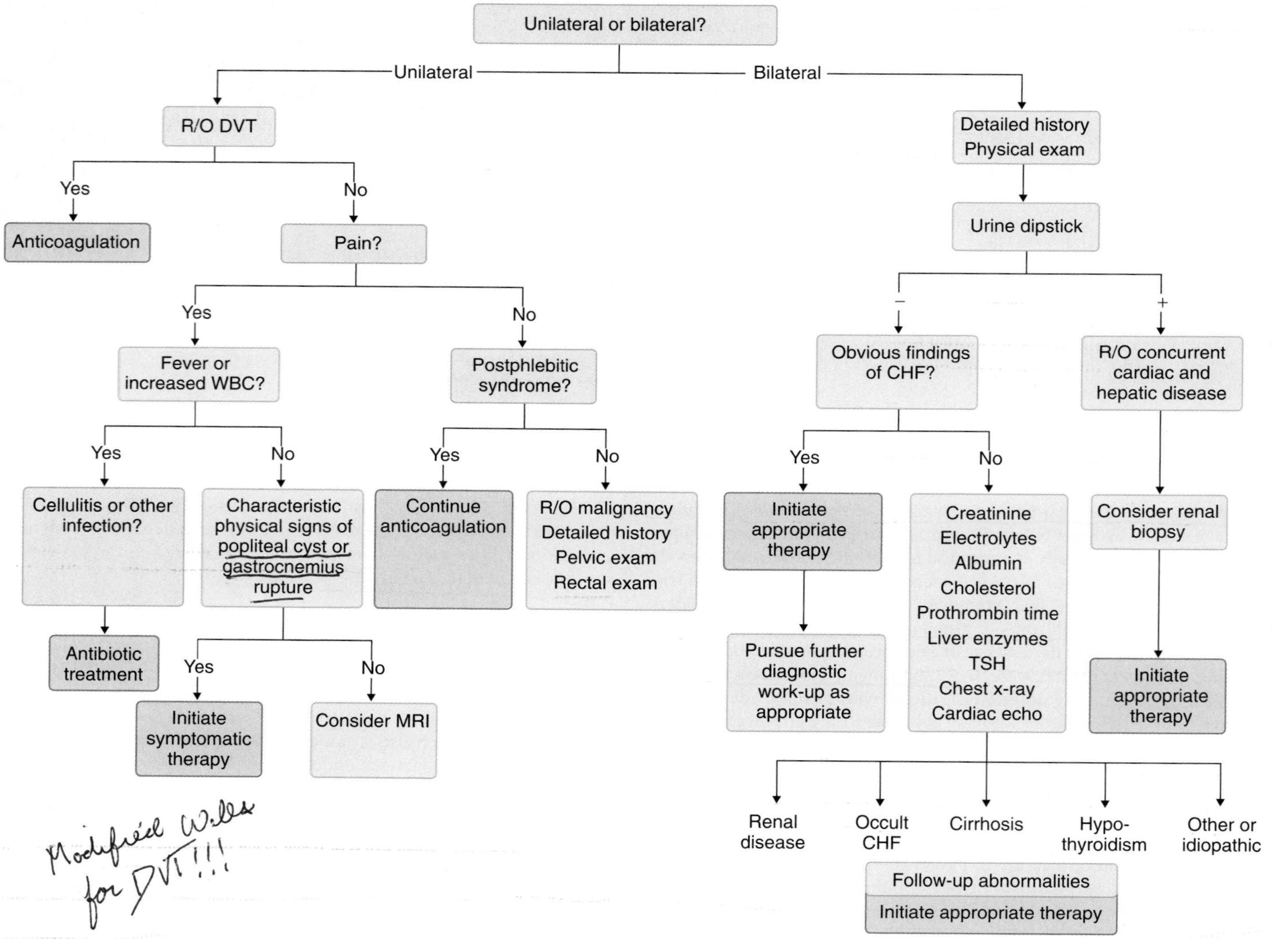

Unilateral or bilateral?

- Unilateral → R/O DVT
  - Yes → Anticoagulation
  - No → Pain?
    - Yes → Fever or increased WBC?
      - Yes → Cellulitis or other infection? → Antibiotic treatment
      - No → Characteristic physical signs of popliteal cyst or gastrocnemius rupture
        - Yes → Initiate symptomatic therapy
        - No → Consider MRI
    - No → Postphlebitic syndrome?
      - Yes → Continue anticoagulation
      - No → R/O malignancy; Detailed history; Pelvic exam; Rectal exam
- Bilateral → Detailed history; Physical exam → Urine dipstick
  - – → Obvious findings of CHF?
    - Yes → Initiate appropriate therapy → Pursue further diagnostic work-up as appropriate
    - No → Creatinine; Electrolytes; Albumin; Cholesterol; Prothrombin time; Liver enzymes; TSH; Chest x-ray; Cardiac echo
      - Renal disease; Occult CHF; Cirrhosis; Hypo-thyroidism; Other or idiopathic
      - Follow-up abnormalities; Initiate appropriate therapy
  - + → R/O concurrent cardiac and hepatic disease → Consider renal biopsy → Initiate appropriate therapy

FIGURE 50-8. Diagnostic approach to patients with edema. CHF = congestive heart failure; DVT = deep venous thrombosis; MRI = magnetic resonance imaging; R/O = rule out; TSH = thyroid-stimulating hormone; WBC = white blood cell count. (From Chertow G. Approach to the patient with edema. In: Braunwald E, Goldman L, eds. *Primary Cardiology*, 2nd ed. Philadelphia: WB Saunders; 2003.)

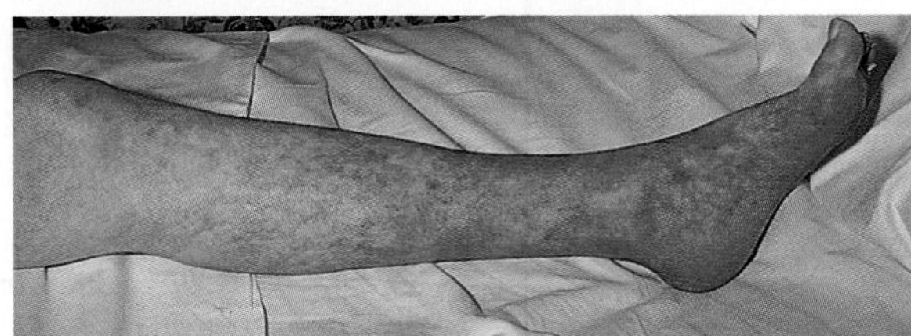

FIGURE 50-9. **Arterial embolism causing acute ischemia and cyanosis of the leg. Initial pallor of the leg and foot was followed by cyanosis.** (From Forbes CD, Jackson WD. *Color Atlas and Text of Clinical Medicine*, 3rd ed. London: Mosby; 2003.)

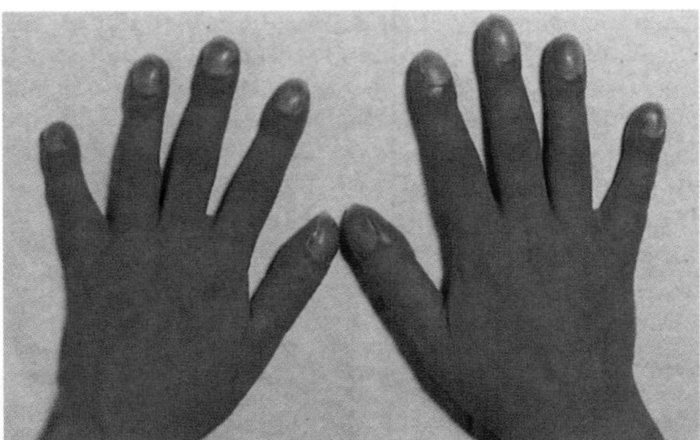

FIGURE 50-10. **Severe finger clubbing in a patient with cyanotic congenital heart disease.** (From Forbes CD, Jackson WD. *Color Atlas and Text of Clinical Medicine*, 3rd ed. London: Mosby; 2003.)

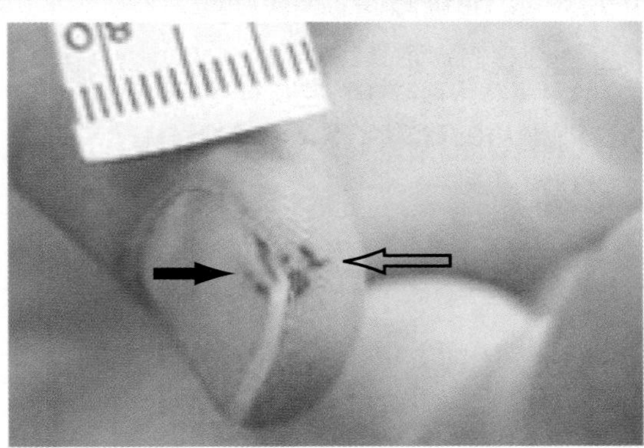

FIGURE 50-11. **Splinter hemorrhage (*solid arrow*) and Janeway's lesions (*open arrow*).** These findings should stimulate a work-up for endocarditis. (From American Academy of Family Physicians Online. http://www.aafp.org/afp/20040315/1417.html. Accessed June 9, 2010.)

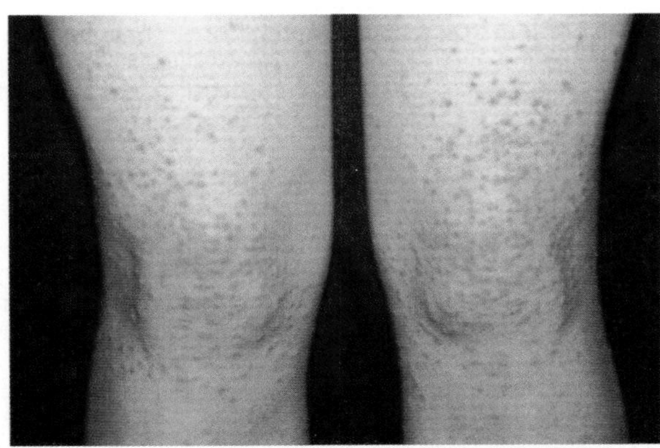

FIGURE 50-12. **Eruptive xanthomas of the extensor surfaces of the lower extremities.** This patient had marked hypertriglyceridemia. (From Massengale WT, Nesbitt LT Jr. Xanthomas. In: Bolognia JL, Jorizzo JL, Rapini RP, eds. *Dermatology*. Philadelphia: Mosby; 2003:1449.)

conduction abnormalities, and possible myocardial ischemia. The chest radiograph (Chapter 53) yields important information on chamber enlargement, pulmonary vasculature, and the great vessels.

Blood testing in patients with known or suspected cardiac disease should be targeted to the conditions in question. In general, a complete blood cell count, thyroid indices, and lipid levels are part of the standard evaluation. Point-of-care biomarker measurements in the emergency department can decrease unnecessary admissions and reduce median length-of-stay.

Echocardiography (Chapter 55) is the most useful test to analyze valvular and ventricular function. By use of Doppler flow methods, stenotic and regurgitant lesions can be quantified. Hand-held ultrasonography performed by generalists can improve the assessment of left ventricular function, cardiomegaly, and pericardial effusion. Transesophageal echocardiography is the preferred method to evaluate possible aortic dissection and to identify clot in the cardiac chambers. Radionuclide studies (Chapter 56) can measure left ventricular function, assess myocardial ischemia, and determine whether ischemic myocardium is viable. CT can detect coronary calcium, which is a risk factor for symptomatic coronary disease (Chapter 56). In the setting of acute chest pain, multislice CT is effective in diagnosing coronary disease, but it currently cannot adequately determine the physiologic significance.[1]

Stress testing by exercise or pharmacologic stress is useful to precipitate myocardial ischemia that may be detected by ECG abnormalities, perfusion abnormalities on radionuclide studies, or transient wall motion abnormalities on echocardiography. These tests are often crucial in diagnosis of possible myocardial ischemia (Chapter 71) and in establishment of prognosis in patients with known ischemic heart disease.

Cardiac catheterization (Chapter 57) can measure precise gradients across stenotic cardiac valves, judge the severity of intracardiac shunts, and determine intracardiac pressures. Coronary angiography provides a definitive diagnosis of coronary disease and is a necessary prelude to coronary revascularization with a percutaneous coronary intervention (Chapter 74) or coronary artery bypass graft surgery (Chapter 74).

Continuous ambulatory ECG monitoring can help diagnose arrhythmias. A variety of newer technologies allow longer-term monitoring in patients with important but infrequently occurring symptoms (Chapter 62). Formal invasive electrophysiologic testing can be useful in the diagnosis of ventricular or supraventricular wide-complex tachycardia, and it is crucial for guiding a wide array of new invasive electrophysiologic therapies (Chapter 66).

SUMMARY

The history, physical examination, and laboratory evaluation should help the physician establish the cause of any cardiovascular problem; identify and quantify any anatomic abnormalities; determine the physiologic status of the valves, myocardium, and conduction system; determine functional capacity; estimate prognosis; and provide primary or secondary prevention. Key preventive strategies, including diet modification, recognition and treatment of hyperlipidemia, cessation of cigarette smoking, and adequate physical exercise, should be part of the approach to every patient, with or without heart disease.

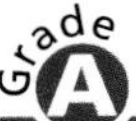

1. Goodacre SW, Bradburn M, Cross E, et al. The randomised Assessment of Treatment using Panel Assay of Cardiac Markers (RATPAC) trial: a randomised controlled trial of point-of-care cardiac markers in the emergency department. *Heart.* 2011;97:190-196.

SUGGESTED READINGS

Amsterdam EA, Kirk JD, Bluemke DA, et al. Testing of low-risk patients presenting to the emergency department with chest pain: a scientific statement from the American Heart Association. *Circulation.* 2010;122:175-1776. *Guidelines.*

Brown AF, Cullen L, Than M. Future developments in chest pain diagnosis and management. *Med Clin North Am.* 2010;94:375-400. *Review.*

Martin LD, Howell EE, Ziegelstein RC, et al. Hand-carried ultrasound performed by hospitalists: does it improve the cardiac physical examination? *Am J Med.* 2009;122:35-41. *It improves the accuracy of the assessment of left ventricular dysfunction, cardiomegaly, and pericardial effusion.*

51 EPIDEMIOLOGY OF CARDIOVASCULAR DISEASE

MICHAEL J. KLAG

DEFINITION OF CARDIOVASCULAR DISEASES

Cardiovascular diseases, which encompass congenital malformations (Chapter 69) and acquired diseases of the circulatory system, include coronary heart disease (Chapters 70 to 74), arrhythmias (Chapters 62 to 65), valvular heart disease (Chapter 75), cardiomyopathy (Chapter 60), pericardial disease (Chapter 77), heart failure (Chapter 59), stroke (Chapter 413), peripheral arterial disease (Chapter 79), aortic diseases (Chapter 78), venous diseases (Chapter 81), and pulmonary vascular diseases (Chapter 68). However, because of their incidence and prevalence, their impact on survival and quality of life, and their shared pathogenesis (Chapter 70), this chapter mainly focuses on the epidemiology of coronary heart disease, stroke, and heart failure.

BURDEN OF CARDIOVASCULAR DISEASE

Impact in the United States

The age-adjusted mortality rate for cardiovascular disease has decreased substantially in the past few decades, with a 69% decline for coronary heart disease and a 76% decline for stroke in 2006 compared with 1950 (Fig. 51-1). This decline is considered to be about equally attributable to reductions in major risk factors and to evidence-based medical therapies.

Despite this decline in the cardiovascular disease mortality rate, heart disease (about 620,000 out of about 2.4 million deaths total) and stroke (about 135,000 deaths) are still the first and third leading causes of deaths in the United States. Because of a growing and aging population, the total number of cardiovascular disease deaths has decreased only modestly, by about 16% since 1979. Cardiovascular disease, including congenital defects, still accounts for more than one of every three deaths in the United States.

An estimated 17.6 million American adults currently have coronary heart disease, about 6.4 million have had a stroke, and 5.8 million have heart failure. The prevalence of peripheral arterial disease is estimated to be 8 million, and about 2.2 million people are estimated to have atrial fibrillation.

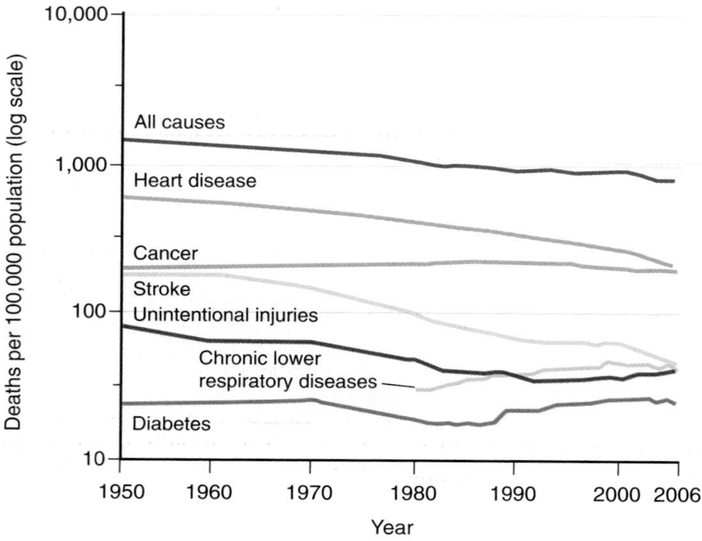

FIGURE 51-1. Age-adjusted death rates for selected leading causes of death: United States, 1958-2006. (From CDC/NCHS, Health United States, 2009. Figure 18. Data from the National Vital Statistics System.)

The annual estimated incidence in the United States is 785,000 for coronary heart disease, 610,000 for stroke, and 670,000 for heart failure. Importantly, heart disease and stroke are the 3rd and 12th leading chronic conditions that limit activity, and stroke is the leading cause of serious long-term disability.

Hospitalization rates for myocardial infarction and stroke have been relatively steady in the United States over the past few decades. However, diagnostic measures have improved substantially during this time period, likely leading to hospitalization of milder cases. Improved survival of patients with severe disease, who are at greater risk for recurrence, may also have contributed to this constant hospitalization rate. In contrast, hospitalization rates for heart failure and atrial fibrillation have substantially increased (two- to three-fold) in the past few decades.

In 2010, cardiovascular diseases are projected to cost $324 billion in health care expenditures (direct costs) and $189 billion in lost productivity (indirect costs). Direct and indirect costs are estimated to be $96 billion and $81 billion for coronary heart disease, $48 billion and $26 billion for stroke, and $35 billion and $4 billion for heart failure, respectively.

Worldwide Impact

Coronary heart disease and stroke are the leading causes of death in both economically developed and developing countries. Each year, more than 17 million people die from cardiovascular disease worldwide. Currently, 80% of deaths due to coronary heart disease or stroke take place in developing countries. Cardiovascular disease occurs at a younger age in developing countries than in developed countries, thereby resulting in serious loss of productivity. For example, 50% of cardiovascular disease deaths in India occur before 70 years of age, whereas only about 25% of cardiovascular disease deaths in developed countries occur before age 70 years. Traditional risk factors play an important role in the excess risk for cardiovascular disease in developing countries, thereby emphasizing the urgent need to develop cost-effective programs to control these risk factors in settings with limited resources.

PRIMARY AND SECONDARY PREVENTION

Primary prevention is defined as preventing cardiovascular disease among persons without clinically apparent cardiovascular disease. *Secondary prevention* denotes preventing the recurrence of cardiovascular disease among those who already have it. Preventive interventions are largely the same for primary and secondary intervention, except that the targeted levels of low-density lipoprotein cholesterol (LDL-C) are lower when cardiovascular disease is present (Chapter 213), and some medications, such as aspirin, are recommended for every patient with coronary heart disease.[1] Cardiovascular disease is also an indication for influenza vaccination.

The absolute risk of a future cardiovascular disease event is substantially higher in persons who already have cardiovascular disease. Because the reduction in absolute risk is greater for secondary than primary prevention, secondary prevention is more cost-effective than primary prevention. Nevertheless, the control of blood pressure (Chapter 67) and the use of statins (Chapter 213) can markedly lower the risk of cardiovascular disease in apparently healthy individuals, with low rates of adverse effects.[2]

RISK FACTORS FOR CARDIOVASCULAR DISEASE

Atherosclerotic disease in the arteries of the heart and brain is the most common cause of clinically apparent coronary heart disease and stroke. Heart failure most commonly occurs as a result of coronary heart disease or hypertension, although valvular heart disease (Chapter 75) and cardiomyopathy (Chapter 60) also can lead to heart failure.

Risk factors for cardiovascular disease can be categorized as traditional (i.e., those identified in the Framingham Heart Study) or novel (Table 51-1). Risk factors can also be grouped as modifiable or nonmodifiable.

Individual Risk Factors

Age

Older age is one of the strongest risk factors for coronary heart disease, stroke, and heart failure. An age over 45 years in men and 55 years in women is considered a risk factor for coronary heart disease, and every 10 years of older age imparts a risk of coronary heart disease equivalent to the presence of hypertension or diabetes. In general, traditional risk factors are more strongly associated with the risk of cardiovascular disease at younger compared with older ages.

TABLE 51-1 RISK FACTORS FOR CORONARY HEART DISEASE AND/OR STROKE

	TRADITIONAL (OR ESTABLISHED)*	NOVEL (OR LESS ESTABLISHED)
Modifiable	Hypertension Diabetes Dyslipidemia† Smoking Obesity Physical inactivity Kidney dysfunction/damage Left ventricular hypertrophy Alcohol Atrial fibrillation‡	Socioeconomic status Psychological factors Inflammatory markers Infection Homocysteine Thrombotic factors Natriuretic peptide Troponin†
Nonmodifiable	Age Gender Ethnicity Family history	Genetic polymorphism Coronary artery calcification†

*Factors incorporated in multiple risk scoring systems or dealt with in clinical guidelines and potentially affecting clinical decisions for cardiovascular disease prevention.
†Risk factor mainly for coronary heart disease.
‡Risk factor mainly for stroke.

Gender

Before age 60, men have a 1.5- to 2-fold higher risk of coronary heart disease and stroke than do women. After 60 years of age, however, the risk of coronary heart disease and stroke in women increases at a faster rate than men, and the risk becomes equivalent in both sexes at 80 years of age. This gender difference at younger ages is thought to be primarily due to differences in levels of estrogen and other endogenous sex hormones. Clinical trials of hormone replacement therapy in postmenopausal women, however, have not reduced the risk of cardiovascular disease.[3]

Race and Ethnicity

The incidence and prevalence of cardiovascular disease vary substantially across ethnic groups. For example, the incidence of stroke and heart failure in the United States is 1.5- to 2-fold higher in blacks compared with whites, whereas the incidence of coronary heart disease is relatively comparable between these groups. Asians are less prone to developing coronary heart disease than whites or blacks. These differences in the incidence of cardiovascular disease among ethnic groups are largely attributable to differences in risk factor profiles. Numerous studies demonstrate that migrants assume the cardiovascular disease risk of their new environment within two generations. Thus, lifestyle and other environmental factors appear to be more important than ethnicity in influencing the risk of cardiovascular disease. There are also ethnic differences in awareness of traditional modifiable risk factors. Individual ancestry, as estimated by genetic markers, may provide better information for differentiating the genetic and environmental contributions to ethnic differences.

Hypertension

Hypertension (Chapter 67), defined as systolic/diastolic blood pressure of 140/90 mm Hg or higher, is the most prevalent modifiable risk factor for coronary heart disease, stroke, and heart failure. Hypertension affects one third of U.S. adults. Systolic pressure is a stronger risk predictor than diastolic blood pressure, and each 20-mm Hg increase in systolic blood pressure is associated with two-fold increased risk of coronary heart disease in middle-aged populations. Numerous studies have demonstrated that blood pressure control by antihypertensive drug therapy decreases cardiovascular disease risk when used in either primary or secondary prevention.[4] Adoption of a diet that is rich in potassium, magnesium, calcium, protein, and fiber can reduce blood pressure to a degree equivalent to using one antihypertensive medication, and substituting additional protein or unsaturated fats leads to additional improvement in blood pressure and the lipid profile.[5]

Diabetes Mellitus

Diabetes mellitus (Chapters 236 and 237), which is defined as fasting plasma glucose of 126 mg/dL or higher, a nonfasting plasma glucose or a plasma glucose 2 hours after an oral glucose tolerance test of 200 mg/dL or higher, or a hemoglobin A_{1c} level of 6.5% or higher, is associated with a two-fold increased risk for cardiovascular disease. Diabetes is often considered as equivalent to a history of coronary heart disease in terms of predicting the risk for coronary heart disease events. Intensive glucose control among diabetic patients has been associated with a reduction in the incidence or progression of microvascular disease, such as retinopathy or nephropathy, but not necessarily with that of macrovascular disease.[6] By comparison, aggressive blood pressure reduction in persons with diabetes prevents both microvascular and macrovascular disease.[7]

Dyslipidemia

Elevated LDL-C is a strong risk factor, particularly for coronary heart disease (Chapter 213). Each 1-mg/dL increase in the LDL-C level is associated with approximately a 1% higher risk of coronary heart disease. Decreased HDL-C levels and elevated triglyceride levels are also associated with the risk of coronary heart disease. Current clinical guidelines for treatment of hyperlipidemia (Chapter 213) are based mainly on LDL-C levels, but the nonfasting non-HDL cholesterol level (total cholesterol minus HDL-C) and the HDL cholesterol level are sufficient to estimate the risk of coronary heart disease.

The effectiveness of statins to reduce coronary heart disease risk is established in both primary and secondary prevention.[8] In contrast, drugs that specifically increase HDL-C and reduce triglycerides have not demonstrated consistent benefits for reducing cardiovascular events.[9,10]

Serum total cholesterol and triglyceride levels are inversely associated with the risk of hemorrhagic stroke in many, but not all, studies. Persons with the highest blood pressures and lowest serum cholesterol levels are at the greatest risk. Several studies have reported neutral or weak associations of dyslipidemia with ischemic stroke. Nevertheless, statin treatment reduces the incidence of stroke.[8]

Smoking

Current smokers have an approximately two-fold higher risk of cardiovascular disease compared with former and never smokers. Second-hand smoke is also associated with a 30% or greater increase in the risk of coronary heart disease. Bans on smoking in public places have been associated with a 20% reduction in incident coronary heart disease.

In patients with coronary heart disease, the risk for recurrent coronary heart disease events is substantially reduced by smoking cessation, and the risk in former smokers returns to the level of nonsmokers within 3 years. Smoking cessation is associated with increased risk of incident diabetes, in part due to weight gain. Thus, body weight and glucose metabolism should be carefully monitored among persons who attempt to quit smoking.

Obesity

Obesity (Chapter 227) is closely associated with hypertension, dyslipidemia, and diabetes. Even accounting for these traditional cardiovascular risk factors, obesity may be an independent predictor of coronary heart disease, stroke, and heart failure. Each 5-kg/m^2 higher body mass index (BMI) is associated with 40% increased risk for cardiovascular mortality in middle-aged populations. Among individuals with morbid obesity (BMI $\geq$ 35 kg/m^2), weight reduction through bariatric surgery may reduce the risk of coronary heart disease by more than 50%.

Among patients with established coronary heart disease or heart failure, higher adiposity is paradoxically associated with better prognosis, probably because of weight loss in persons with severe illness, especially heart failure, who also experience high mortality. In addition, persons with severe heart disease who are very obese probably die earlier than persons who weigh less. Thus, prevalent patients with heart disease and obesity likely have less severe disease, thereby imparting a survival advantage.

Physical Inactivity

Physical inactivity and sedentary lifestyle (Chapter 15) are associated with increased risk for cardiovascular disease. Exercise is an important adjunct to diet for achieving and maintaining weight loss, and exercise improves lipid and glucose metabolism and decreases blood pressure. In patients who have survived an acute myocardial infarction, exercise-based cardiac rehabilitation is associated with reduction of mortality but not of recurrent myocardial infarction. 11

Kidney Dysfunction or Damage

Chronic kidney disease (Chapter 132), defined as a persistently reduced glomerular filtration rate of less than 60 mL/minute/1.73 m^2 or kidney damage, usually detected by albuminuria, raises the risk of incident cardiovascular disease. Cardiovascular mortality increases exponentially with lower glomerular filtration rate and increases linearly on a log-log scale at higher levels of albuminuria. Cardiovascular mortality is two-fold higher at a glomerular filtration rate of 30 to 45 mL/minute/1.73 m^2 or albuminuria of more than 100 mg/day, compared with normal levels of about 90 mL/minute/1.73 m^2 and about 5 mg/day, respectively, independently of each other and of traditional risk factors.

Left Ventricular Hypertrophy

Left ventricular hypertrophy usually represents target-organ damage from hypertension, although multiple factors play a role in its development. The regression of left ventricular hypertrophy by antihypertensive treatment may be associated with more favorable outcomes.

Socioeconomic Status

Most of the evidence for the link between socioeconomic status, an individual's social position relative to other members of a society, and cardiovascular disease comes from economically developed countries. In general, low socioeconomic status is associated with increased risk of cardiovascular disease. The mechanism for this association is multifactorial, perhaps mediated through in utero and childhood exposures and lack of educational opportunities that result in deleterious health behaviors and risk factor patterns (Chapter 4). In addition, a reduced accessibility to health care (Chapter 5) and greater exposure to residential and occupational harmful exposures almost certainly play a role. For example, neighborhood characteristics, such as accessibility to healthy food and walkability, are associated with higher prevalence of obesity, and air pollution predicts incident coronary heart disease.

Psychological Factors

Acute and chronic stress, in daily life or due to a natural disaster, is associated with an increased risk for cardiovascular disease. Acute or chronic stress may raise blood pressure, alter glucose or lipid metabolism, and increased blood viscosity.

Inflammation

Higher levels of inflammatory markers are associated with a higher risk of cardiovascular disease, consistent with the concept that atherosclerosis is an inflammatory process (Chapter 70). C-reactive protein, which is the most studied inflammatory marker, is undoubtedly associated with the future risk for cardiovascular disease, although this association is considerably attenuated by the adjustment for conventional risk factors. Genotypes associated with elevated levels of C-reactive protein are not associated with the risk of coronary heart disease, suggesting that C-reactive protein itself is not a cause of cardiovascular disease. Nevertheless, the C-reactive protein can be used for risk stratification beyond traditional risk factors.

Infection

Infection with microorganisms such as *Chlamydophila pneumoniae* (Chapter 326), *Helicobacter pylori* (Chapter 141), cytomegalovirus (Chapter 384), hepatitis A virus (Chapter 150), and influenza virus (Chapter 372) has been reported to be associated with the risk of coronary heart disease. However, antibiotic treatment of these pathogens has not reduced risk. 12 In contrast, vaccination for influenza virus may help prevent recurrent coronary heart disease and is currently recommended for secondary prevention.

Homocysteine

Blood homocysteine levels are associated with the risk of cardiovascular disease, but reducing blood homocysteine levels using folic acid alone or in combination with other B vitamins is not effective for either primary or secondary prevention. 13

Alcohol

A J-shaped association between alcohol consumption (Chapter 32) and the risk of incident coronary heart disease has been noted in both primary and secondary prevention settings, with the lowest risk at light (<3 drinks per week) to moderate (3 to 7 [for female] or 14 [for male] per week) alcohol consumption. Alcohol use, however, is also associated with injuries and other harmful outcomes, including hypertension and atrial fibrillation. Thus, persons who do not drink should not be encouraged to initiate regular alcohol consumption.

Family History

Premature coronary heart disease in a first-degree relative (male relative <55 years and female <65 years or <60 years in both genders) is associated with increased risk of coronary heart disease. Family history of premature coronary heart disease likely integrates genetic predisposition to cardiovascular disease or cardiovascular risk factors, lifestyle preferences, and environmental factors.

Genetic Factors

Numerous single nucleotide polymorphisms have been associated with cardiovascular disease risk factors or the incidence of cardiovascular disease. Nevertheless, current genetic risk scoring using 101 single nucleotide polymorphisms has not yet improved the prediction of incident cardiovascular disease after accounting for traditional risk factors. However, single nucleotide polymorphisms have been associated with differing response to specific antihypertensive and antiplatelet drugs.

Thrombotic and Fibrinolytic Factors

Various thrombotic and fibrinolytic factors, such as fibrinogen and plasminogen activator inhibitor, have been associated with incident cardiovascular disease. Whether such information improves the prediction of prognosis over prediction based on traditional risk factors alone and, if so, whether such factors provide targets for prevention, are not yet clear.

Risk Prediction

Although clinical interventions to prevent cardiovascular disease usually target individual risk factors, methods to predict the risk of cardiovascular disease use information on multiple risk factors, including age, gender, smoking, hypertension, diabetes, and lipids. Of these, the Framingham Risk Score is most commonly used in the United States. Some clinical guidelines use an individual's probability of coronary heart disease within 10 years to make clinical decisions about treatment with statins and aspirin. Although the original Framingham Risk Score estimated coronary heart disease risk, a new score predicting global cardiovascular disease risk (coronary heart disease, stroke, heart failure, and peripheral artery disease) has recently been published (Tables 51-2 and 51-3).

New Aspects of Traditional Risk Factors

Global risk prediction and the management of traditional risk factors in clinical practice are generally based on the most recent assessments of risk factors or the average of multiple measurements over a short period of time. However, change over time or the duration of an abnormal risk factor level may be associated with future risk independent of baseline values. The association of traditional risk factors with cardiovascular disease risk is generally graded and continuous, such that higher levels of the risk factors impart greater risk; as a result, cutoffs to define elevated levels of risk factors are somewhat arbitrary. In general, the definition of normal is becoming stricter with increasing recognition that "borderline" levels of risk factors are associated with cardiovascular risk, that the greatest population burden may be in persons with lower elevations of risk because they are much more numerous than persons with very high levels of risk, and because interventions are becoming safer and more effective. For example, diabetes is now defined as a fasting glucose level of 126 mg/dL rather than 140 mg/dL.

NEW BIOMARKERS OF SUBCLINICAL DAMAGE OR DISEASE

New biomarkers of subclinical cardiovascular disease include the coronary artery calcium score (Chapter 56), troponin level, and natriuretic peptide levels. Because these biomarkers are related to ongoing pathophysiologic processes, it is not surprising that they may be better predictors of future events than are traditional risk factors.

TABLE 51-2 POINTS OF FRAMINGHAM RISK SCORE FOR CARDIOVASCULAR DISEASE PREDICTION ACCORDING TO TRADITIONAL RISK FACTORS

POINTS	AGE (YR)	HDL-C (MG/DL)	TOTAL CHOLESTEROL (MG/DL)	SBP NOT TREATED	SBP TREATED	SMOKER	DIABETES
WOMEN							
−3				<120			
−2		60+					
−1		50-59			<120		
0	30-34	45-49	<160	120-129		No	No
1		35-44	160-199	130-139			
2	35-39	<35		140-149	120-129		
3			200-239		130-139	Yes	
4	40-44		240-279	150-159			Yes
5	45-49		280+	160+	140-149		
6					150-159		
7	50-54				160+		
8	55-59						
9	60-64						
10	65-69						
11	70-74						
12	75+						
MEN							
−2		60+		<120			
−1		50-59					
0	30-34	45-49	<160	120-129	<120	No	No
1		35-44	160-199	130-139			
2	35-39	<35	200-239	140-159	120-129		
3			240-279	160+	130-139		Yes
4			280+		140-159	Yes	
5	40-44				160+		
6	45-49						
7							
8	50-54						
9							
10	55-59						
11	60-64						
12	65-69						
13							
14	70-74						
15	75+						

HDL-C = high-density lipoprotein cholesterol; SBP = systolic blood pressure.

TABLE 51-3 CARDIOVASCULAR RISK ACCORDING TO TOTAL POINTS OF FRAMINGHAM RISK SCORE

Women		Men	
POINTS	10-YEAR RISK, %	POINTS	10-YEAR RISK, %
		≤−3	<1
≤−2	<1	−2	1.1
−1	1.0	−1	1.4
0	1.2	0	1.6
1	1.5	1	1.9
2	1.7	2	2.3
3	2	3	2.8
4	2.4	4	3.3
5	2.8	5	3.9
6	3.3	6	4.7
7	3.9	7	5.6
8	4.5	8	6.7
9	5.3	9	7.9
10	6.3	10	9.4
11	7.3	11	11.2
12	8.6	12	13.2
13	10.0	13	15.6
14	11.7	14	18.4
15	13.7	15	21.6
16	15.9	16	25.3
17	18.5	17	29.4
18	21.5	18+	>30
19	24.8	—	—
20	28.5	—	—
21+	>30	—	—

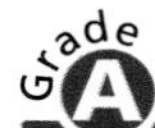

1. Smith SC Jr, Allen J, Blair SN, et al. AHA/ACC guidelines for secondary prevention for patients with coronary and other atherosclerotic vascular disease: 2006 Update. Endorsed by the National Heart, Lung, and Blood Institute. *Circulation.* 2006;113:2363-2372.
2. Ridker PM, Danielson E, Fonseca FA, et al. Rosuvastatin to prevent vascular events in men and women with elevated C-reactive protein. *N Engl J Med.* 2008;359:2195-2207.
3. Sare GM, Gray LJ, Bath PMW. Association between hormone replacement therapy and subsequent arterial and venous vascular events: a meta-analysis. *Eur Heart J.* 2008;29:2031-2041.
4. Turnbull F. Effects of different blood-pressure-lowering regimens on major cardiovascular events: results of prospectively-designed overviews of randomised trials. *Lancet.* 2003;362:1527-1535.
5. Appel LJ, Giles TD, Black HR, and American Society of Hypertension Writing Group. ASH position paper: dietary approaches to lower blood pressure. *J Am Soc Hypertens.* 2009;5:321-331.
6. Ray KK, Seshasai SRK, Wijesuriya S, et al. Effect of intensive control of glucose on cardiovascular outcomes and death in patients with diabetes mellitus: a meta-analysis of randomised controlled trials. *Lancet.* 2009;373:1765-1772.
7. UK Prospective Diabetes Study Group. Tight blood pressure control and risk of macrovascular and microvascular complications in type 2 diabetes: UKPDS 38. *BMJ.* 1998;317:703-713.
8. Baigent C, Keech A, Kearney PM, et al. Efficacy and safety of cholesterol-lowering treatment: prospective meta-analysis of data from 90,056 participants in 14 randomized trials of statins. *Lancet.* 2005;366:1267-1278.
9. The ACCORD Study Group. Effects of combination lipid therapy in type 2 diabetes mellitus. *N Engl J Med.* 2010;362:1563-1574.
10. Barter PJ, Caulfield M, Eriksson M, et al, for the ILLUMINATE Investigators. Effects of torcetrapib in patients at high risk for coronary events. *N Engl J Med.* 2007;357:2109-2122.
11. Lavie CJ, Thomas RJ, Squires RW, et al. Exercise training and cardiac rehabilitation in primary and secondary prevention of coronary heart disease. *Mayo Clin Proc.* 2009;84:373-383.
12. Andraws R, Berger JS, Brown DL. Effects of antibiotic therapy on outcomes of patients with coronary artery disease: a meta-analysis of randomized controlled trials. *JAMA* 2005;293:2641-2647.
13. Clarke R, Halsey J, Lewington S, et al. Effects of lowering homocysteine levels with B vitamins on cardiovascular disease, cancer, and cause-specific mortality: meta-analysis of 8 randomized trials involving 37,485 individuals. *Arch Intern Med.* 2010;170:1622-1631.

SUGGESTED READINGS

Bui AL, Horwich TB, Fonarow GC. Epidemiology and risk profile of heart failure. *Nat Rev Cardiol.* 2011;8:30-41. *Review.*

Greenland P, Alpert JS, Beller GA, et al. 2010 ACCF/AHA guideline for assessment of cardiovascular risk in asymptomatic adults: executive summary: a report of the American College of Cardiology Foundation/American Heart Association Task Force on practice guidelines. *Circulation.* 2010;122:2748-2764. *Guidelines.*

Lloyd-Jones D, Adams RJ, Brown TM, et al. Heart disease and stroke statistics—2010 update: a report from the American Heart Association. *Circulation.* 2010;121:e46-e215. *Updated U.S. statistics.*

Wijeysundera HC, Machado M, Farahati F, et al. Association of temporal trends in risk factors and treatment uptake with coronary heart disease mortality, 1994-2005. *JAMA.* 2010;303:1841-1847. *The decline in CHD mortality in 1994 and 2005 in Ontario, Canada, was about equally attributable to reductions in risk factors and to improvements in treatment.*

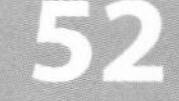

52 CARDIAC FUNCTION AND CIRCULATORY CONTROL

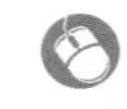

ANDREW R. MARKS

The heart has the daunting task of pumping sufficient amounts of blood to meet both its own metabolic demands and those of the other organs. Uniquely among all the organs, the heart's failure to perform its task for even a few minutes causes death. The heart continuously fulfills this physiologic role with a variety of electrical, contractile, and structural functions that control the flow of blood to the organs.

STRUCTURE OF THE HEART

Cardiac Development

In humans, the formation of a linear heart tube from the primary cardiac crescent occurs between days 21 and 23 of gestation. Looping of the heart tube and trabecular formation of the ventricle occurs at 26 days of gestation (E-Fig. 52-1). At 6 weeks, the embryonic interventricular communication closes, followed by thickening and remodeling of the ventricular walls in the first trimester. By the end of week 7, heart development is essentially finished, although the heart continues to enlarge throughout gestation.

Electrical Cells

The heart is a muscular pump controlled by regular electrical discharges from specialized muscle cells in the conduction system (Chapter 61). The molecular basis for the electrical activity of the heart is the activation of specific ion-conducting channels (Fig. 52-1). Coordinated activation and inactivation of cardiac ion channels regulate the membrane potential of the cardiac cells, thereby resulting in a rapid sequence of depolarization followed by repolarization. This electrical activity, which is manifested on the body surface as the electrocardiogram (ECG), is known as the action potential, and it is responsible for activating the contraction of the cardiac muscle. At a typical heart rate of 70 beats per minute, the heart beats about 100,000 times per day, or 37 million beats a year, corresponding to 3 billion beats over a lifespan of 80 years. Failure to propagate the signal throughout the heart (e.g., heart block), or abnormal rhythms (arrhythmias) that are either too slow (bradycardia) or too fast (tachycardia), can result in death (Chapter 63).

Ion Channels

Sodium, potassium, and calcium channels determine the electrical activity of the heart by opening and closing in a highly choreographed pattern that determines the action potential of the heart. The electrical regulation of the heart, which is reflected in the relative concentrations of ions inside and outside the heart muscle cells, determines the five phases of the action potential. The action potential is initiated when the opening of sodium channels results in a rapid influx of sodium (phase 0) down its concentration gradient (~145 mmol outside the heart muscle cell, ~10 mmol inside). After a brief early repolarization owing to activation of potassium channels (phase 1), the rapid sodium influx depolarizes the cell, thereby activating calcium channels that allow calcium influx (phase 2) down its concentration gradient (~3 mmol outside, ~100 nmol inside). This calcium influx triggers excitation-contraction coupling that results in pumping by the heart. Potassium channels then open and cause repolarization (phase 3) as potassium fluxes out of the cell down its concentration gradient (~4 mmol outside, ~135 mmol inside). The membrane potential returns to the resting level of about −90 mV (phase 4).

Conduction System

Specialized pacemaker cells in the sinoatrial (SA) node (Fig. 52-2) have slightly higher (less negative) resting potentials and gradually depolarize

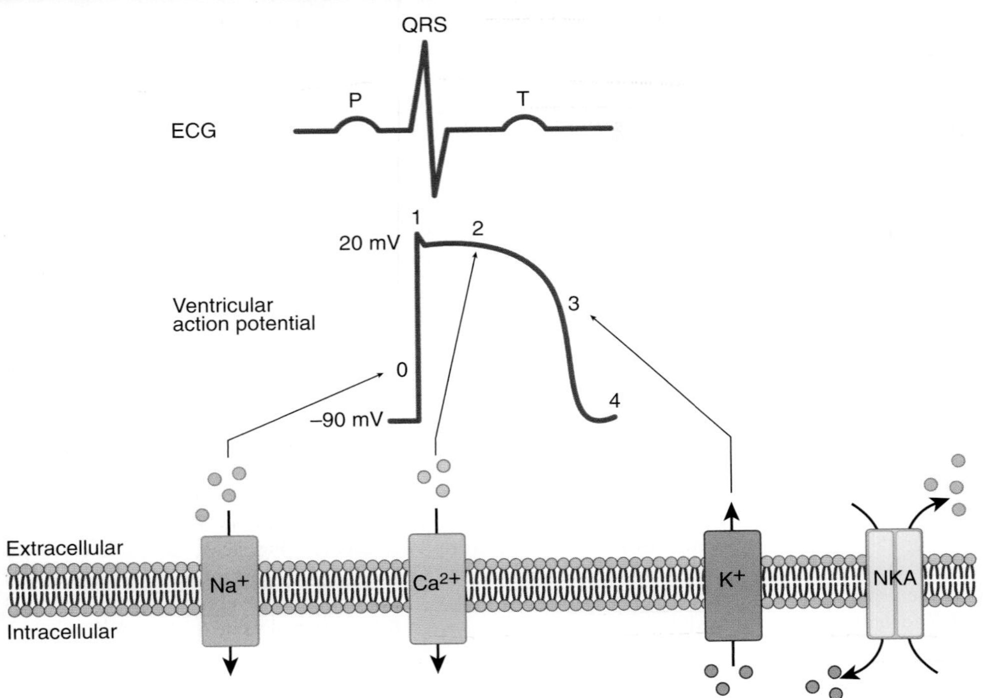

FIGURE 52-1. Cardiac action potential and ion channels. Myocardial contraction begins when sodium channels open and positively charged sodium ions flow into the cell and cause membrane depolarization (phase 0). During phases 1, 2, and 3, calcium ions flow into the cell through L-type calcium channels, while potassium flows out of the cell through voltage-gated potassium channels. These three phases correspond to the myocardial contraction, which corresponds to the QRS complex on the surface electrocardiogram (ECG). The sodium-potassium adenosine triphosphatase (NKA) helps return the system to its resting state.

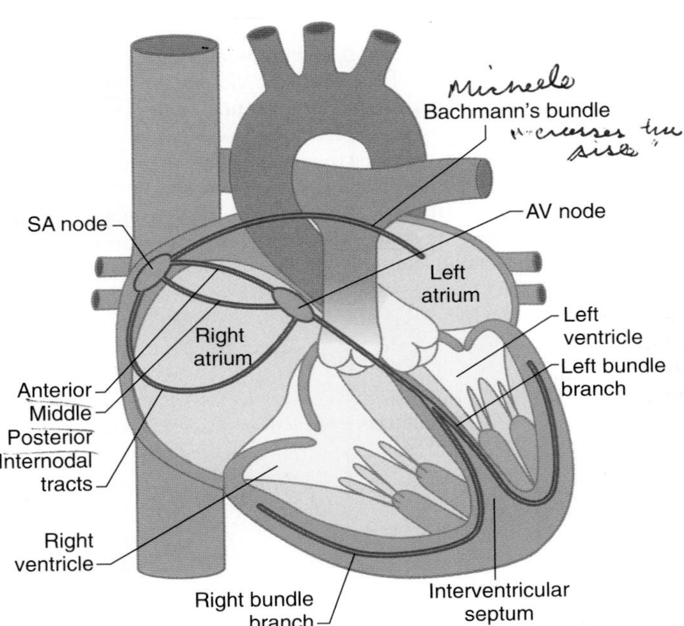

FIGURE 52-2 Cardiac anatomy. Cardiac anatomy comprises electrical and structural components. The electrical impulse that directs cardiac contraction originates in the sinoatrial (SA) node and is rapidly conducted through the atria by specialized conduction tracts. The impulses merge at the atrioventricular (AV) node where, after a brief pause, they are rapidly conducted into the ventricles through the bundle of His, which is composed of specialized Purkinje cells. Blood moves from the atria into the ventricles through the tricuspid and mitral valves during diastole. During systole, blood from the ventricles is pumped into the pulmonary artery and aorta through the pulmonic and aortic valves.

during phase 5 owing to the activity of the potassium and calcium channels and the hyperpolarization-activated cyclic nucleotide gated (HCN) channels that are responsible for a small inward (depolarizing) current. In the normal heart, pacemaker cells are the first cells to depolarize, and they trigger the subsequent depolarization of the cells in specialized conducting fibers that propagate the electrical signal throughout the heart muscle in a highly regular and integrated fashion. Electrical activation (depolarization) spreading through the atria to the atrioventricular (AV) node is reflected as the P wave on the ECG (Chapter 54). The slowing of conduction in the AV node accounts for the PR interval on the ECG. After passing through the AV node, the depolarizing signal enters the bundle of His, where conduction is rapid. The bundle of His divides into the right and left bundle branches, which conduct the depolarizing signals into the ventricles and account for the QRS complex on the ECG. Repolarization is represented by the ST segment and the T and U waves of the ECG.

Contractile Cells

Heart muscle is composed of millions of individual cells, which are known as *cardiomyocytes* and which contain an elaborate machinery required for coordinated contraction that pumps blood. Each cardiomyocyte is connected to its neighbors through specialized junctions that enable them to work as a single contractile unit.

Ultrastructure

The basic unit of the contractile system is the sarcomere, which is defined anatomically as the distance between two Z lines that anchor thin filaments composed of actin, tropomyosin, and troponin. Thin filaments slide past thick filaments (composed of myosin and titin) in a calcium-dependent manner to shorten the sarcomere length. The contractile proteins are surrounded by a calcium-filled membrane called the *sarcoplasmic reticulum.* The sarcoplasmic reticulum forms specialized associations with the transverse tubules, which are invaginations of the plasma membrane and contain voltage-gated calcium channels. When the muscle is activated by depolarization of its membrane, this electrical signal travels deep into the muscle through the transverse tubules. Inside the muscle, the electrical depolarizing signal activates the voltage-gated channels, which open to allow a small amount of calcium to enter the muscle cells. This influx of calcium in turn activates the type 2 ryanodine receptor (RyR2)–calcium release channels on the sarcoplasmic reticulum. The RyR channels open and release enough calcium from the sarcoplasmic reticulum to raise the calcium concentration in the myoplasm about ten-fold. As a result, calcium binds to troponin C in the thin filaments and causes a conformational change that enables cross-bridging between actin and myosin, thereby leading to sliding of the filaments, shortening of the sarcomere, and muscle contraction. Hydrolysis of adenosine triphosphate (ATP) provides the energy required for the generation of force by the actin-myosin interaction. The conversion of electrical energy (depolarization of the cell membrane) to mechanical energy is known as excitation-contraction coupling. Relaxation of the heart muscle occurs when calcium is pumped back into the sarcoplasmic reticulum through the sarcoendoplasmic reticulum ATPase. Contractile force can be enhanced during stress by activation of the β-adrenergic pathway, which increases both the amount of calcium released and the rate of calcium uptake in the sarcoplasmic reticulum (E-Fig. 52-3).

Although the heart is a muscular pump, 60 to 70% of its cells are cardiac fibroblasts, not muscle cells. These fibroblasts provide critical components of the extracellular matrix that determine the structure of the heart.

ANATOMY OF THE HEART

The primary pumping chamber of the heart is the thick-walled left ventricle, which is composed of billions of cardiomyocytes connected end to end through gap junctions. The right ventricle is a thinner-walled chamber, divided from the left ventricle by the *interventricular septum*. Above the ventricles are the right and left atria, which are thin-walled chambers that receive low-pressure venous blood; they are separated from the ventricles by the *tricuspid valve* on the right side and the *mitral valve* on the left side. These valves are attached to *papillary muscles* that emerge from the ventricular walls through *chordae tendineae*. The pressure gradient between the ventricles and the atria opens the AV valves. The papillary muscles help establish the positions of the valve leaflets and prevent regurgitant flow during contraction. The *aortic and pulmonary valves* separate the left and right ventricles from their arterial connections and enable blood flow out of the ventricles.

Coronary Blood Flow

The coronary arteries receive blood from the aorta, directly above the aortic valve, and travel through the epicardium that surrounds the heart to supply blood to the heart muscle (see Fig. 57-3 in Chapter 57). The diastolic blood pressure in the ascending aorta just above the aortic valve determines most of the flow of blood into the normal (nonstenosed) coronary arteries while the heart is relaxed. During systole, coronary flow is determined by the left ventricular intracavitary pressure, which equals the pressure within the inner myocardial wall, where coronary arteries are compressed during systole. Coronary blood flows to the epicardium during both systole and diastole but flows to the endocardium predominantly during diastole.

Metabolic Regulation of the Cardiovascular System

Cardiac muscle requires constant coronary perfusion to supply oxygen and other metabolites. Increased energy consumption owing to enhanced contractility necessitated by increased pressures or higher heart rates (e.g., during exercise) can be met only by increased coronary blood flow. Signals that augment coronary blood flow (by up to six-fold) include nitric oxide, adenosine, bradykinins, prostaglandins, and carbon dioxide. The breakdown of ATP is the source of adenosine, whereas nitric oxide is produced by the action of nitric oxide synthases that metabolize the amino acid L-arginine. Autoregulatory mechanisms, including constriction in response to increased luminal pressures and dilation in response to reduced pressure, also play a role in determining coronary artery blood flow. Other metabolic factors that cause vasoconstriction include endothelin peptides, serotonin, 5-hydroxytryptamine, thromboxane, angiotensin II, and β-adrenergic stimulation.

Sympathetic and parasympathetic pathways of the autonomic nervous system and the renin-angiotensin system exert potent regulatory effects on cardiovascular function. The sympathetic nervous system plays the key role in the response to stress (e.g., the fight-or-flight response) by increasing heart rate and myocardial contractility and decreasing vascular tone. Regulation of cardiovascular function by the sympathetic nervous system is mediated by norepinephrine that is released at the nerve endings and by epinephrine from the adrenal gland. β-Adrenergic signaling is mediated by epinephrine, which increases the heart rate and vasodilates the central arterial bed, thereby resulting in reduced afterload, which in turn helps augment cardiac output.

PHYSIOLOGY OF THE HEART AND CIRCULATORY CONTROL

Cardiac Energetics

The major immediate source of energy in the heart is the oxidation of fatty acids and glucose. When oxygen supply is limited, glucose metabolism is favored because it generates more ATP per oxygen consumed. The heart has virtually no ability to conduct anaerobic metabolism (i.e., glycolysis) and therefore is dependent on oxygen for its function. For example, heart function deteriorates immediately under conditions of hypoxia, ischemia, and carbon monoxide poisoning.

Basal metabolism, total mechanical work performed by the heart, contractility, and heart rate determine the oxygen and energy consumption of the heart. During excitation-contraction coupling, two key steps require energy consumption (ATP hydrolysis): release of the myosin head–actin interaction, and reuptake of calcium into the sarcoplasmic reticulum.

The mechanical work of the heart is determined by the total *pressure-volume area* (E-Fig. 52-4), which is related to the number of actin-myosin cross-bridges formed during the contraction. It is the sum of the external work performed by the heart in pumping blood from the ventricle to the aorta (represented by the area inside the pressure-volume loop) plus energy stored in the myocardium at the end of contraction. Enhanced contractility requires increased oxygen consumption because an increased amount of calcium released from the sarcoplasmic reticulum requires increased ATP and oxygen consumption to pump the released calcium back into the sarcoplasmic reticulum through the sarcoplasmic reticular ATPase. Based on these principles, increasing the heart rate requires increased oxygen consumption. If the heart rate increases from 70 to 140 beats per minute during exercise or stress, oxygen consumption increases almost two-fold over the basal value.

Contractility and Relaxation

The Cardiac Cycle

In resting humans, the heart beats approximately once per second. With each beat, the heart cycles through a series of four hemodynamic events represented by changes in pressures and volumes (Fig. 52-3) as well as electrical activity as represented by the ECG. When the heart muscle is relaxed at end diastole, the ventricular pressure is at its resting level (*end-diastolic pressure*) and the ventricular volumes are at their maximal value (*end-diastolic volume*). Aortic pressure declines as the blood ejected into the aorta during the previous ventricular contraction flows to the peripheral circulation. Atrial contraction provides a final boost to ventricular volume immediately before ventricular systole. Ventricular contraction increases the pressure in the ventricle; when this pressure exceeds the pressure in the atrium, the mitral valve closes. However, because ventricular pressure remains less than aortic pressure, the aortic valve remains closed, and no blood enters or leaves the ventricle during this first phase of the cardiac cycle, the *isovolumic contraction* phase. During systole, ventricular pressure eventually exceeds aortic pressure, at which time the aortic valve opens, blood is ejected into the aorta, and ventricular volume decreases during the *ejection* phase of the cycle. At the end of systole when contraction is maximum, ejection ends, and the ventricular volumes are at their lowest (*end-systolic volume*). The volume of the ejected blood, which is termed the *stroke volume* (SV), is defined as the difference between the end-diastolic and end-systolic volumes. The ejection fraction

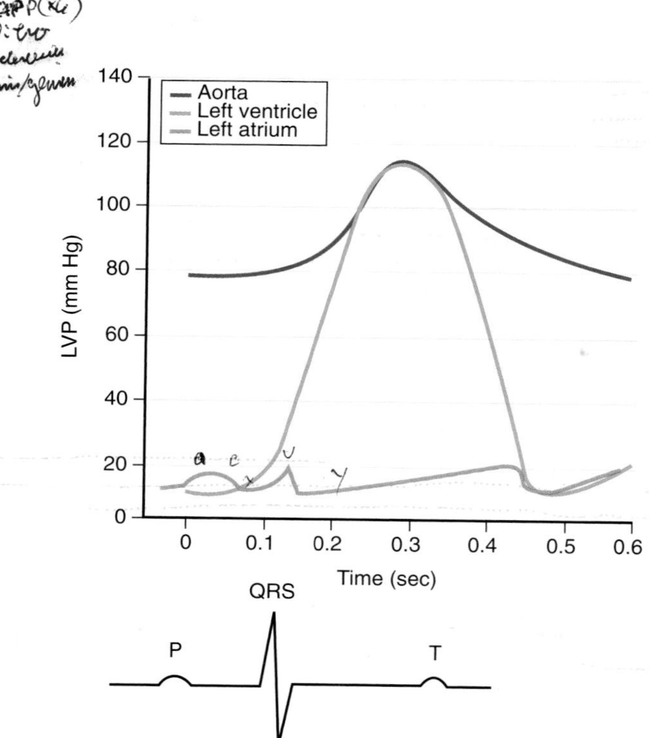

FIGURE 52-3. Wigger's diagram. Changes in aortic, left ventricular, and left atrial pressures represented graphically as a function of time, with the corresponding electrocardiogram signal for each. LVP = left ventricular pressure.

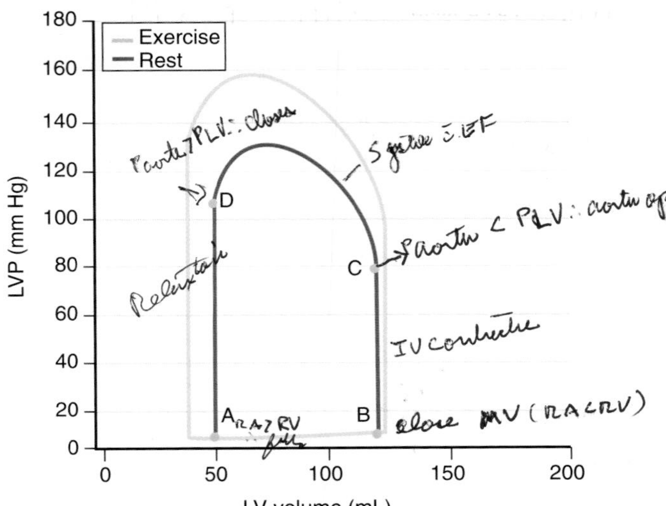

FIGURE 52-4. **Pressure-volume loop.** The left ventricle (LV) begins to fill when pressure in the chamber falls below that of the left atrium, and the mitral valve opens (point A). Pressure in the ventricle slowly rises as the muscle fibers are stretched by the increasing volume. When the myocardium contracts (point B), pressure in the left ventricle rises, causing the mitral valve to close and trapping the blood inside the chamber (isovolumic contraction). When the pressure in the left ventricle is higher than in the aorta, the aortic valve opens (point C), and blood is ejected out of the left ventricle. As the left ventricle stops contracting, pressure in the aorta becomes higher than that in the left ventricle, and the aortic valve closes (point D). During this period of isovolumic relaxation, the ventricle rapidly relaxes until it starts filling again. During exercise, the release of norepinephrine from sympathetic nerve terminals leads to enhanced myocardial contractility. As a result, the left ventricle generates higher pressures and ejects a greater volume of blood during each beat. LVP = left ventricular pressure.

(EF), defined as the percentage of end-diastolic volume (EDV) ejected during a contraction (EF = 100 × SV/EDV), is an index of heart function. The next phase in the cycle occurs when the heart muscle relaxes, ventricular pressures are less than the aorta pressure, and the aortic valve closes. During this *isovolumic relaxation* phase, ventricular volumes remain constant because, once again, both the mitral and aortic valves are closed. When ventricular pressures fall below atrial pressures, the mitral and tricuspid valves open, and blood flows from the atria into the ventricles during the *filling* phase.

These four phases of the cardiac cycle can be represented by a *pressure-volume diagram* (Fig. 52-4), which plots the instantaneous ventricular pressure versus volume to calculate the *pressure-volume loop*. Similar effects occur on the left and right sides of the heart, but with higher pressures on the left side (Table 52-1).

Pressure-Volume Relationships

The volume of a ventricular chamber correlates with length of its muscles and sarcomeres. In the left ventricle, with its circular cross section, Laplace's law defines the relationship among pressure in the chamber (P), muscle tension (T, force/unit cross-sectional area of the muscle), chamber wall thickness (h), and the internal radius of the chamber (R): $P \approx 2 \cdot T \cdot h/R$. Both calcium and the length of the heart muscle determine force (Fig. 52-5). Each muscle is composed of a linear array of sarcomere bundles. Maximal force is achieved at a sarcomere length of about 2.2 to 2.3 mm, which results in the optimal overlap of thick and thin filaments. When the sarcomere length is less than 2.0 mm, the ends of the thin filaments contact each other, thereby resulting in a reduction in force. Conversely, when sarcomeres are stretched beyond 2.3 mm, force decreases owing to reduced overlap between myosin heads and actin.

Force-length relationships, which are determined by measuring the force developed at different muscle lengths while preventing the muscle from shortening (isometric contractions), characterize the systolic and diastolic contractile properties of cardiac muscle. With increasing muscle length, end-systolic force increases to a greater degree than does end-diastolic force. The difference in force at end diastole versus end systole increases as muscle length increases as a result of the greater developed force of the stretched muscle. This relationship of force to length is referred to as the Frank-Starling law of the heart.

TABLE 52-1 RANGE OF NORMAL RESTING HEMODYNAMIC VALUES

PRESSURE
Central venous (mean): 0-5 mm Hg
Right atrial (mean): 0-5 mm Hg
Right ventricular (systolic/diastolic): 20-30/0-5 mm Hg
Pulmonary artery (systolic/diastolic): 20-30/8-12 mm Hg
Left atrial (mean): 8-12 mm Hg
Left ventricular (systolic/diastolic): 100-150/8-12 mm Hg
Aortic (systolic/diastolic): 100-150/70-90 mm Hg
VOLUME-RELATED MEASURES
Right ventricular end-diastolic volume: 70-100 mL
Left ventricular end-diastolic volume: 70-100 mL
Stroke volume: 40-70 mL
Cardiac index: 2.5-4 L/min/m^2
Ejection fraction: 55-70%
ARTERIAL RESISTANCE
Systemic vascular resistance: 10-20 mm Hg · min/L
Pulmonary vascular resistance: 0.5-1.5 mm Hg · min/L

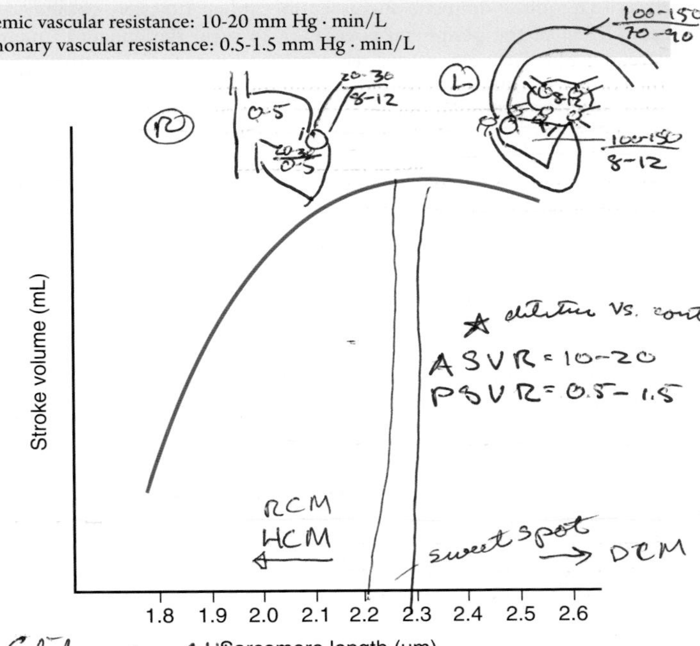

FIGURE 52-5. **Starling's law.** Cardiac output, represented as stroke volume (end-systolic volume minus end-diastolic volume), as a function of initial sarcomere stretch. The greater the initial stretch on the fibers during diastole, referred to as *preload*, the more force is generated during systole.

Work of the Heart

Cardiovascular performance is reflected in the arterial blood pressure and cardiac output (mean arterial blood flow), which in turn are dependent on four factors: preload, afterload, ventricular contractility, and heart rate.

Preload, which refers to the degree to which sarcomeres are stretched just before systole, is defined as the end-diastolic pressure or volume. The Frank-Starling law of the heart dictates that ventricular pressure and output vary with preload, so a decrease in preload decreases end-diastolic volume and pressure, peak pressure, and stroke volume. Conversely, increased preload increases ventricular pressure and output, subject to the limits to which preload pressures can be increased. Left ventricular end-diastolic pressures of 20 to 25 mm Hg and greater cause exudation of fluid into the alveoli and pulmonary edema (Chapter 58).

Afterload refers to the stress that the ventricle must overcome to eject blood. Peak arterial pressure reflects the peak stress imposed on cardiomyocytes according to Laplace's law (described previously as $P \approx 2 \cdot T \cdot h/R$). As long as there is no left ventricular outflow obstruction, arterial pressure reflects myocyte afterload, as does *total peripheral resistance* (TPR), which corresponds to the tone of the resistance vessels. TPR is the ratio between the mean pressure decrease across the arterial system (mean arterial pressure [MAP] minus mean central venous pressure [CVP]) and cardiac output (CO): TPR = (MAP − CVP)/CO. When TPR is increased, the pressure-volume relationship shifts such that peak pressure is increased whereas stroke volume and ejection fraction are decreased.

Contractility of cardiac muscle (*myocardial contractility*) or a ventricle (*ventricular contractility*) is the intrinsic ability to generate force independent of preload or afterload. When contractility is increased, the pressure-volume relationship shifts so that pressure, stroke volume, and ejection fraction are increased at constant preload volume and arterial resistance.

Cardiac output is measured in liters per minute and is equal to the amount of blood ejected at each heartbeat (stroke volume in liters per beat) multiplied by the number of beats per minute. As a result, *heart rate* is a powerful determinant of cardiac performance. Cardiac output and mean arterial pressure can be related to preload, afterload, contractility, and heart rate through the Frank-Starling curves, which plot end-diastolic pressure versus cardiac output or mean arterial pressure, to yield an overall picture of left ventricular function.

CARDIOVASCULAR RESPONSES TO STRESSORS

Exercise

Exercise requires dramatic increases in cardiac function combined with remodeling of the peripheral circulation to meet the enhanced metabolic demands of critical organs and redirect blood flow to those organs. Indeed, the oxygen consumption during exercise can increase as much as 18-fold. About one third of the requirement for increased oxygen consumption is met by improved extraction of oxygen from the blood in the muscles (reducing venous saturation from about 75% to about 25%) and the remainder by increasing cardiac output as much as 6-fold. Increased cardiac function is achieved largely through sympathetic stimulation and reduction in vagal tone, which combine to increase the heart rate, contractility, ejection fraction, filling rates, and systolic blood pressure and to decrease aortic impedance. In young healthy individuals, heart rate can increase from a baseline of 60 to 70 beats per minute at rest to as much as 170 to 200 beats per minute with exercise. To increase rather than decrease cardiac output at these high heart rates, which can limit ventricular filling and stroke volume, contractility must also increase, through a phenomenon known as the positive force frequency relationship or Bowditch phenomenon. Along with increased cardiac contractility, arterial vasodilation in the aorta and other major arteries reduces the resistance to cardiac outflow. Both enhanced cardiac contractility and arterial vasodilation are triggered by the same sympathetic nervous system signals. With increased cardiac outflow, venous return also must increase, so preload can be maintained as well as possible to enhance cardiac function by the Frank-Starling mechanism.

Heart Failure

Heart failure can be defined as the inability of the heart to provide sufficient blood flow to meet the metabolic demands of the organs (Chapter 58). Heart failure can be due to systolic dysfunction with volume overload, most often as the consequence of ischemic heart disease (myocardial infarction) or as the end-stage consequence of hypertension. Systolic heart failure is characterized by increases in the size of the various cardiac chambers (rightward shift of the end-diastolic pressure-volume relationship). In another form of heart failure, known as *diastolic heart failure*, the heart is not necessarily increased in size, and systolic function is preserved.

Aging

Prolongation of contraction and relaxation times, which are common abnormalities in older individuals, may be related to cardiac hypertrophy as a consequence of the high prevalence of hypertension with advancing age (Chapter 67). A progressive "stiffening" of the large arteries with advancing age increases resistance, although the mechanism underlying this change is not understood. The heart rate and contractile responses to sympathetic signals are reduced and lead to a diminished ability to respond to conditions of acute overload, such as increased blood pressure or an acute myocardial infarction.

Visit expertconsult.com for e-expanded chapter

SUGGESTED READINGS

Burkhoff D, Dickstein ML, Ferber P. The Heart Simulator. http://www.columbia.edu/itc/hs/medical/heartsim. Accessed Sept. 22, 2010. *A useful web-based learning tool for cardiac physiology.*

Gandhi MS, Kamalov G, Shahbaz AU, et al. Cellular and molecular pathways to myocardial necrosis and replacement fibrosis. *Heart Fail Rev.* 2011;16:23-34. *Review.*

Rawlins J, Carre F, Kervio G, et al. Ethnic differences in physiological cardiac adaptation to intense physical exercise in highly trained female athletes. *Circulation.* 2010;121:1078-1085. *Addresses the question of "what is normal" cardiac physiology.*

TPR = (MAP - CVP) / CO   ↑ TPR

53

RADIOLOGY OF THE HEART

MURRAY G. BARON

The heart casts a homogeneous shadow on the chest film. No internal detail can be seen within its contours because the radiodensities of blood, myocardium, and other cardiac tissues are so similar that one cannot be distinguished from the others. Only two borders of the heart, where it contacts the radiolucent, air-containing lung, can be discerned in any one projection. Changes in the size or shape (or both) of the chambers of the heart and the great vessels usually alter the shape of the cardiac silhouette. However, because the heart is a three-dimensional structure, multiple views are required for complete radiographic evaluation. With the advent of echocardiography, the need for this "cardiac series" has disappeared. However, a remarkable amount of information regarding the heart is contained on standard frontal and lateral chest films, which remain a useful tool for detecting disease, evaluating the severity of known disease, documenting the progress of disease, and assessing the efficacy of treatment.

RADIOLOGIC ANATOMY

Except for the more complex cardiac anomalies, which are rare, especially in adults, the positions and spatial relationships of the cardiac chambers and the great vessels are the same from one patient to the next and are not significantly affected by disease. On a frontal chest film, the right cardiac border is composed of a straight vertical upper half formed by the superior vena cava and a gently convex lower half representing the lateral wall of the right atrium (Fig. 53-1). The break in the contour of this border of the heart indicates the

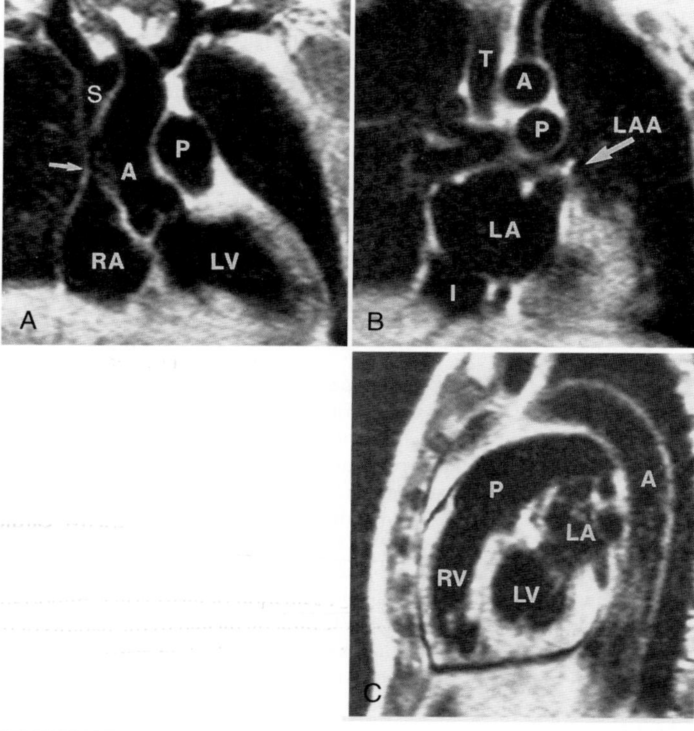

FIGURE 53-1. Normal radiographic anatomy, magnetic resonance images. A, Coronal section at the level of the aortic valve. The right border of the cardiac silhouette is formed by the superior vena cava (S) and the right atrium (RA). The *arrow* indicates the caval-atrial junction. The lower portion of the left cardiac border is formed by the left ventricle (LV). A = ascending aorta; P = main pulmonary artery. **B,** Coronal section at the level of the left atrium. The upper portion of the left cardiac border is formed by the aorta (A), main pulmonary artery (P), and left atrial appendage (LAA), see *arrow*. I = inferior vena cava; LA = left atrium; T = trachea. **C,** Sagittal section near the midline. The right ventricle (RV) forms the anterior surface of the heart, which abuts the sternum. The pulmonary artery (P) extends upward and posteriorly from the ventricle. The posterior border of the heart is formed by the left atrium (LA) and left ventricle (LV). The aorta (A) is behind the heart.

caval-atrial junction. Some patients are able to inhale deeply enough to uncover a small, straight segment of the inferior vena cava between the diaphragm and the right atrium.

Abnormalities of the caval segment are usually due to dilation of the ascending aorta. A localized bulge in its midportion usually indicates poststenotic dilation secondary to aortic valve stenosis, whereas aortic insufficiency is commonly associated with a more generalized dilation of the aorta. A bulge in the region of the caval-atrial junction may be due to an aneurysm of either the right coronary artery or the noncoronary sinus of Valsalva or to a markedly enlarged left atrium. Dilation of either atrium tends to extend the cardiac silhouette to the right, whereas dilation of either ventricle enlarges the silhouette to the left.

The left cardiac border is composed of four distinct segments. The uppermost bulge represents the aortic knob, the most distal portion of the aortic arch where it turns downward to become the descending aorta. The prominence below the knob is formed by the main pulmonary artery and the subvalvular portion of the outflow tract of the right ventricle. The lowermost third of this border represents the anterolateral wall of the left ventricle. Between this bulge and that of the pulmonary artery is a short, flat, or slightly concave segment where the left atrial appendage reaches the border of the heart.

Aneurysms of the descending thoracic aorta commonly involve its most proximal portion in the region of the ligamentum arteriosum and appear as a dilated aortic knob. Prominence of the pulmonary artery segment is common in younger individuals, but after the age of 35 to 40 years, such dilation is almost always an indicator of pulmonary arterial hypertension.

In the lateral view (see Fig. 53-1C), the anterior border of the cardiac silhouette is formed by the body and the outflow tract of the right ventricle. The heart lies in the anterior portion of the chest, and the right ventricle abuts the lower third of the sternum. Both the outflow tract and the pulmonary artery slope posteriorly. Air-containing lung interposed between this portion of the heart and the anterior chest wall forms the "retrosternal clear space." The posterior border of the heart extends from the level of the pulmonary carina to the diaphragm. Its upper half is formed by the back of the left atrium, and the lower half represents the posterior wall of the left ventricle. The shadow of the inferior vena cava is usually seen in the lateral projection extending obliquely upward and anteriorly from the diaphragm to enter the posterior aspect of the right atrium. The lowermost contour of the normal left ventricle curves anteriorly and crosses the inferior vena cava about 2 cm above the left side of the diaphragm.

Alterations in the contour of the heart usually reflect dilation or hypertrophy of the chambers, or both. Many times the pattern of these changes, together with the appearance of the pulmonary vasculature, points to a specific underlying cardiac abnormality. Chest films are most sensitive for detecting chamber dilation. Cardiac hypertrophy is more difficult to recognize because the thickened myocardium tends to encroach on the ventricular lumen more than extending outward and enlarging the cardiac silhouette. With severe hypertrophy, as in hypertrophic cardiomyopathy, the heart enlarges to the left and the apex becomes blunted, but this appearance is not pathognomonic.

HEART SIZE

A normal-sized heart does not guarantee the absence of cardiac disease. Angina, for example, no matter how severe, does not affect heart size until the left ventricle decompensates. Similarly, patients with restrictive cardiomyopathy may be in severe heart failure with a normal-appearing heart. Conversely, an enlarged heart always indicates the presence of cardiac or pericardial disease. Therefore, accurate evaluation of heart size is important.

Heart size, in the absence of disease, is directly related to the habitus of the patient. The cardiothoracic ratio, which compares the transverse diameter of the heart with the width of the chest, gives a readily obtainable, rough estimate of heart size. This ratio is measured by dropping a vertical line through the heart and summing the greatest distance to the right and left cardiac borders (Fig. 53-2) to give the transverse cardiac diameter. The transverse thoracic diameter, the greatest width of the chest, is measured from the inner surfaces of the ribs. Dividing the cardiac diameter by the chest diameter gives the cardiothoracic ratio. A value of less than 0.6 can be considered within the limits of normal. Setting this value at 0.5, as is often done, produces too many false-positive results.

In most cases, exact measurement of the cardiac silhouette is not necessary, and a reasonably experienced observer can achieve an acceptable degree of accuracy by visual estimation. With either method, several cautions must be observed. The single greatest effect on apparent cardiac size is the degree of inspiration. The volume of the heart is essentially constant throughout the cardiac cycle. As the diaphragm moves up with expiration, the vertical diameter of the heart is shortened, and its transverse diameter increases. Because heart size is estimated primarily from its width, the heart appears larger on expiratory films. The degree of inspiration can be determined from the relationship of the diaphragm to the ribs. On a properly positioned frontal chest film, a reasonable degree of inspiration is indicated if the diaphragm is lowered to at least the level of the posterior portion of the ninth rib.

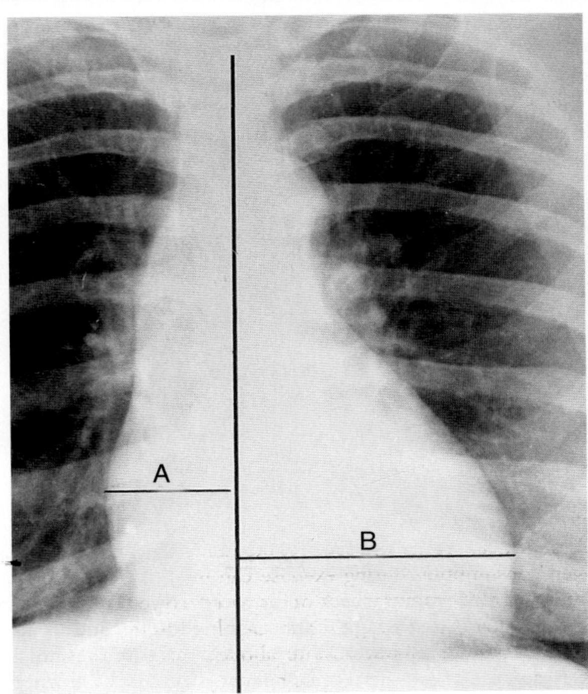

FIGURE 53-2. Measurement of the transverse cardiac diameter. Severe aortic stenosis with a 95-mm systolic gradient across the valve is present. The heart, though considerably hypertrophied, is normal in size and configuration. A *vertical line* is drawn through the heart. The greatest distances to the right cardiac border (A) and to the left cardiac border (B) are then measured. Transverse cardiac diameter = A + B.

When the anteroposterior diameter of the chest is small, the heart may be compressed between the sternum and the spine so that it splays to one or both sides. For this reason, the heart often appears enlarged in patients with the straight back syndrome or with a pectus excavatum deformity of the sternum. An epicardial fat pad (actually it is extrapleural fat outside the pericardium) can occur in one or both cardiophrenic angles and make the heart appear larger than it actually is. The fat pad can be recognized because the cardiophrenic angle appears obtuse or the cardiac apex is indistinct. In addition, the slightly greater density of the heart can usually be distinguished from the more radiolucent image of the fat.

A change in size of the cardiac silhouette can also occur between systole and diastole. This point is important because chest films are exposed at random with reference to the cardiac cycle, so a change in heart size between two examinations may be solely due to the timing of filming. In most cases, the difference in the transverse cardiac diameter between systole and diastole is small, no more than several millimeters. However, in younger patients, especially the more athletic with a slow heart rate and a large stroke volume, phasic change in the normal cardiac diameter can be as large as 2 cm.

CHAMBER ENLARGEMENT

Left Atrium

Dilation of the left atrium alone, in the absence of a left-to-right shunt, is most often due to disease of the mitral valve, although it can also result simply from atrial fibrillation. The two "popular" radiologic signs of left atrial enlargement—a double contour within the right cardiac border and elevation of the left main bronchus—are accurate when present, but they are insensitive and seen in only about half the cases of mitral valve disease. To produce a discernible margin within the cardiac silhouette in the frontal projection, the thickness of the heart must increase sharply at some point. This increase in thickness occurs in mitral disease when the left atrium enlarges and

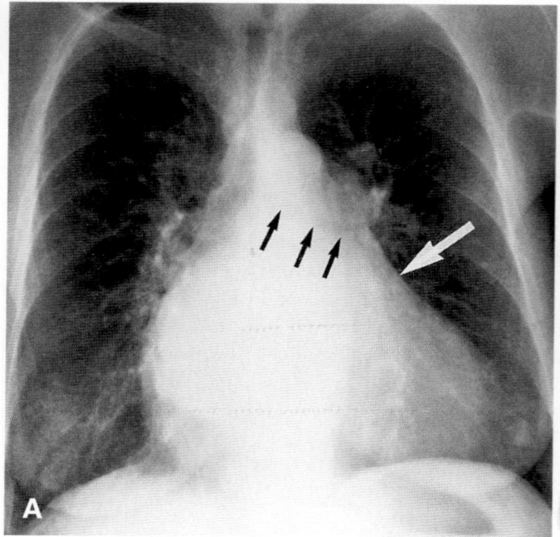

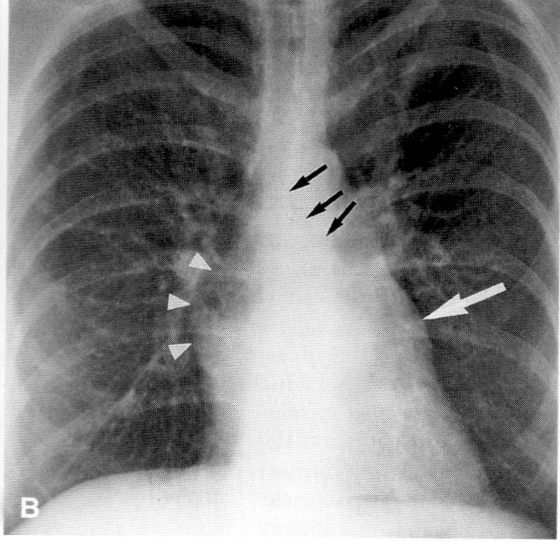

FIGURE 53-3. Left atrial enlargement in mitral valve disease. A, Patient 1: The enlarged left atrium is causing the central portion of the cardiac silhouette to be abnormally dense. The right border of the atrium is seen within the right side of the cardiac silhouette. The left main bronchus *(black arrows)* is elevated. The region of the left atrial appendage *(white arrow)* is slightly concave because this structure was resected at a previous mitral commissurotomy. **B,** Patient 2: The enlarged left atrial appendage bulges from the left side of the heart *(white arrow),* whereas the body of the atrium *(arrowheads)* extends beyond the right atrium to form a part of the right heart border. No double density is seen within the heart, and the left main bronchus *(black arrows)* is not elevated.

protrudes posteriorly from the back of the heart. The right border of the left atrium is then silhouetted where it abuts the right lung, and its contour is seen within the cardiac silhouette (Fig. 53-3A). This pattern is not apparent with lesser degrees of left atrial enlargement. Conversely, when the right atrium also enlarges, as is common in long-standing mitral valve disease, it forms a continuous curve on the posterior cardiac border with the enlarged left atrium. Thus, the double contour is not seen with mild left atrial enlargement or in severe cases of mitral valve disease. Furthermore, because the radiologic technique used for chest films is chosen to provide optimal images of the lungs, the enlarged heart is underexposed and the double contour may be hidden within its opaque silhouette. For the same reason, the position of the left main bronchus often cannot be clearly visualized through the mediastinal shadow.

A more sensitive sign of left atrial enlargement in the frontal projection is dilation of the left atrial appendage. The appendage extends anteriorly from the atrium along the left side of the heart, below the level of the pulmonary artery (see Fig. 53-1B). It forms the part of the left heart border between the pulmonary artery segment and the left ventricular segment. Normally, the border of the appendage is flat or slightly concave. Any convexity is abnormal and usually indicates left atrial enlargement.

Left Ventricle

The shape of the dilated left ventricle depends to a large extent on the underlying cause. When it is due to insufficiency of the aortic or mitral valve, the ventricle elongates and its apex is displaced downward, to the left, and posteriorly (Fig. 53-4). When the dilation is due to coronary artery disease or primary myocardial disease, the ventricle tends to assume a more globular shape. In the lateral view, the downward extension of the enlarged left ventricle covers more of the vena cava shadow than normal, and the crossing point of their posterior borders occurs nearer to the diaphragm than normal. Unfortunately, the usefulness of this sign is limited because of the distortion produced by even slight rotation of the patient from the true lateral position.

Enlargement of the left ventricle produces a smoothly curved dilation of the lower portion of the cardiac silhouette. A localized bulge in this contour most often represents a ventricular aneurysm (Fig. 53-5). Dilation of the left ventricle is usually associated with elevated left ventricular end-diastolic pressure. The latter increases resistance to left atrial emptying and can result in dilation of the atrium. Therefore, left atrial enlargement in the presence of a large left ventricle does not necessarily indicate the presence of mitral valve disease.

Right Atrium

Enlargement of only the right chambers of the heart is seen in severe pulmonary hypertension without coexisting left heart failure, in bacterial endocarditis of the tricuspid or pulmonic valve (or both), and in carcinoid syndrome. Dilation of the right atrium causes an accentuation and outward bowing of the curvature on the lower half of the right cardiac contour in the frontal view. With greater degrees of dilation, the cardiac silhouette enlarges to the right (Fig. 53-6).

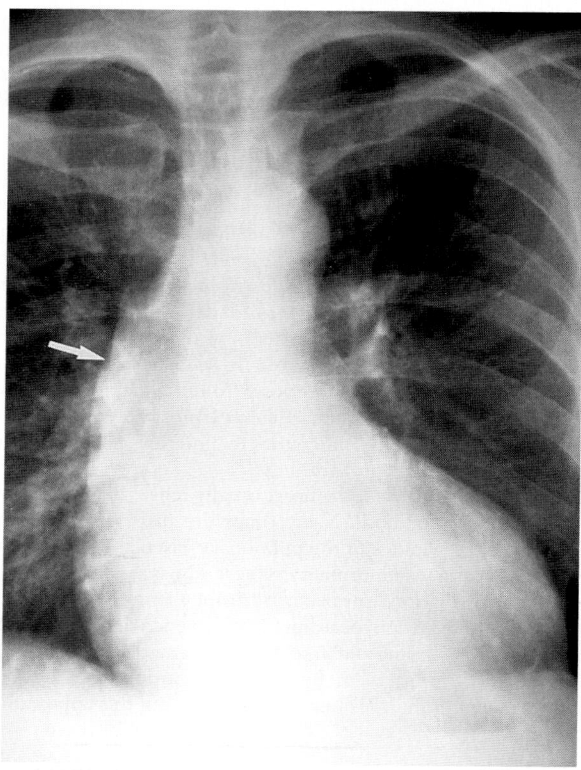

FIGURE 53-4. Left ventricular dilation, aortic insufficiency. The apex of the heart is displaced downward and to the left. The ascending aorta *(arrow)* is diffusely dilated. The pulmonary vasculature is normal.

Right Ventricle

The right ventricle is the most difficult of the four cardiac chambers to evaluate on chest films. Except for a small area in the subpulmonic region, the chamber is not border-forming in the frontal projection. Even moderate right ventricular enlargement may produce no abnormality in this view other than some prominence of the main pulmonary artery. As right ventricular size increases, the transverse diameter of the heart enlarges to the left, and the cardiac apex becomes blunted and elevated (see Fig. 53-6). Enlargement of either or both ventricles displaces the apex of the heart to the left. It is not often possible to distinguish between biventricular enlargement and dilation of one or the other ventricle.

As the right ventricle enlarges, its area of contact with the sternum increases and tends to obliterate the retrosternal clear space in the lateral view. This sign is nonspecific inasmuch as it also depends on the shape of the chest and the size of the left ventricle, as well as the size of the right ventricle.

CALCIFICATION

Most calcifications involving the heart occur in cardiac structures as a result of inflammatory or necrotic processes (or both) or degenerative disease. Because the calcific deposits have greater radiodensity than cardiac tissues, they can often be seen within the cardiac silhouette.

The aortic and mitral valves abut each other, both inserting on the central fibrous tendon of the heart. On a frontal chest film, the two valves lie next to each other in the midportion of the cardiac silhouette, to the left of the spine (Fig. 53-7A), the aortic valve being slightly higher. It is often difficult to determine which valve is calcified in this view. They can be separated by fluoroscopy because the aortic valve tends to move in a vertical direction as the heart beats, whereas the motion of the mitral valve approximates the horizontal. This distinction can also be made accurately from the lateral chest film. If a line is drawn from the left main bronchus, seen as a dark circular shadow over the lower end of the trachea, to the anterior costophrenic angle, the mitral valve lies below the line and the aortic valve above it (Fig. 53-7B).

In the United States, calcification of only the aortic valve is most likely to represent degenerative disease of the cusps (a process in older patients akin to coronary artery calcification) or deterioration of a congenitally bicuspid valve (Chapter 75). In developing countries, calcification of the aortic or mitral valves, or both, is usually a late sequela of rheumatic fever. Calcification of the mitral annulus, which is seen in patients older than 70 years and is about four times more frequent in women than in men, is only rarely of clinical significance. The pattern of calcification is characteristic and should not be confused with that of the mitral valve. Calcium is deposited mainly between the base of the posterior mitral leaflet and the posterior wall of the left ventricle. It is seen as a broad, curvilinear band of calcium in a C shape, open superiorly and to the right on the frontal film and anteriorly on the lateral. In severe cases, the calcific deposits may also extend across the base of the anterior mitral leaflet and then form an O encircling the mitral orifice.

Calcification of the myocardium almost always indicates a previous transmural infarction and, frequently, a ventricular aneurysm. The calcified scar appears as a fine, curvilinear density, most commonly on the anterolateral

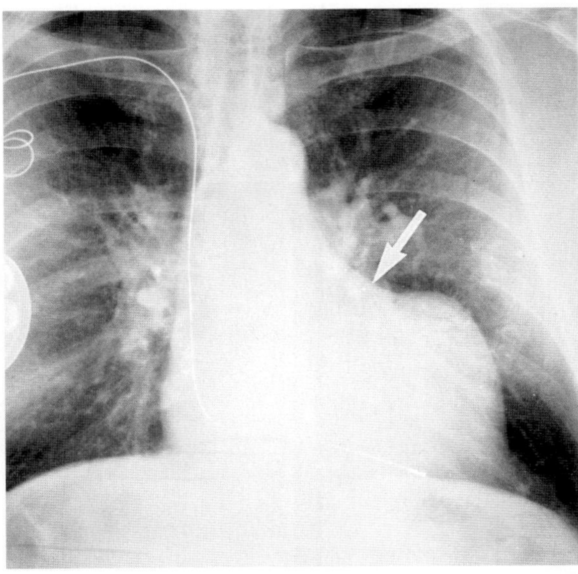

FIGURE 53-5. Left ventricular aneurysm. A bulge on the lower portion of the left cardiac border, formed by the anterolateral wall of the left ventricle, represents a ventricular aneurysm. The patient had suffered a myocardial infarction 1 year previously. The left atrial appendage segment *(arrow)* is normal. A transvenous pacemaker has been inserted through the right subclavian vein. The electrode tip is situated in the apex of the right ventricle.

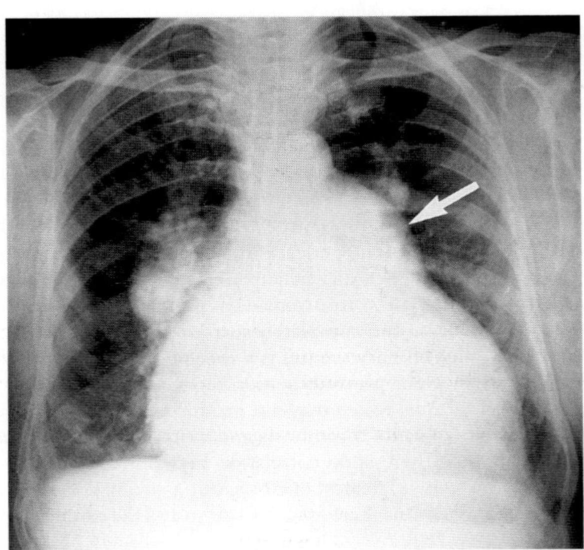

FIGURE 53-6. Right ventricular enlargement seen in a patient with resistive pulmonary hypertension secondary to an atrial septal defect. The main pulmonary artery *(arrow)* and the right pulmonary artery are markedly dilated. The left pulmonary artery was also dilated but is hidden by the heart in this view. The sudden "cutoff" of the vascular shadows just beyond the hila is characteristic of resistive pulmonary hypertension. Enlargement of the right ventricle is elevating the cardiac apex and displacing it to the left. Accentuation of the curvature of the lower right cardiac border and enlargement of the cardiac silhouette to the right are caused by dilation of the right atrium.

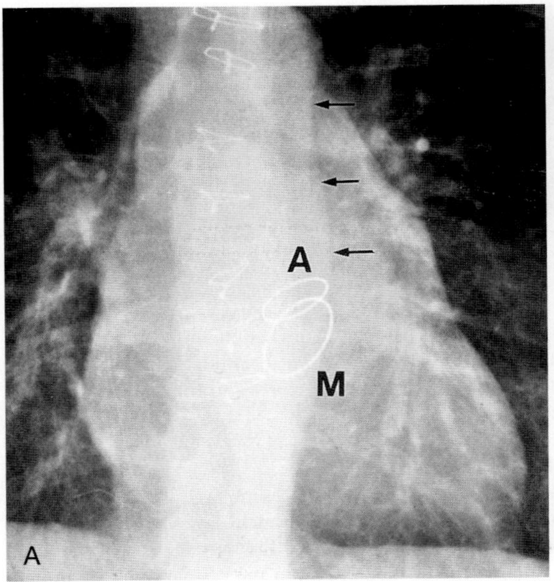

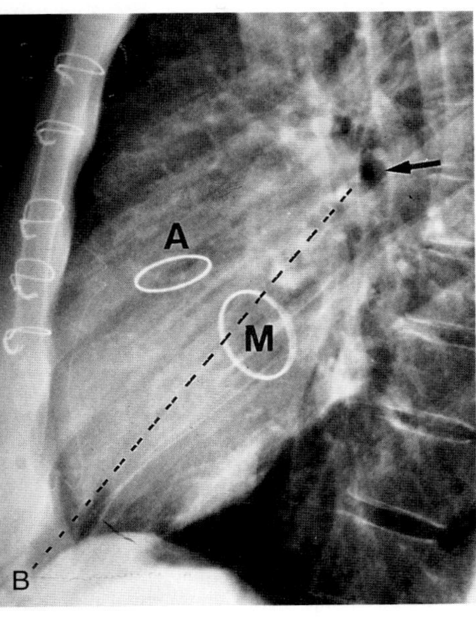

FIGURE 53-7. Location of the mitral and aortic valves. Both the mitral (M) and aortic (A) valves have been replaced by porcine heterografts. The circular stents indicate the location and tilt of each valve. **A,** Frontal projection. The two valves are normally in contact with each other, and it is difficult to separate them in the frontal projection. Furthermore, on a routinely exposed film, calcific deposits are not easily seen because of the overlapping shadows of the descending aorta *(arrows)* and the spine. **B,** Lateral projection. The valves can be differentiated on the lateral view by drawing a line from the left main bronchus *(arrow)* to the anterior costophrenic sulcus. The aortic valve lies above this line and the mitral valve below it.

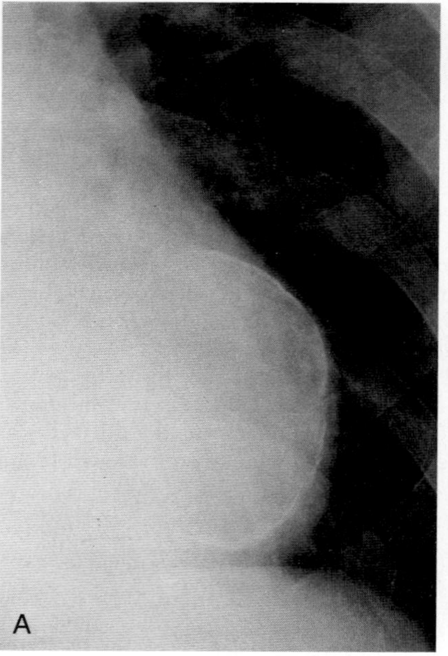

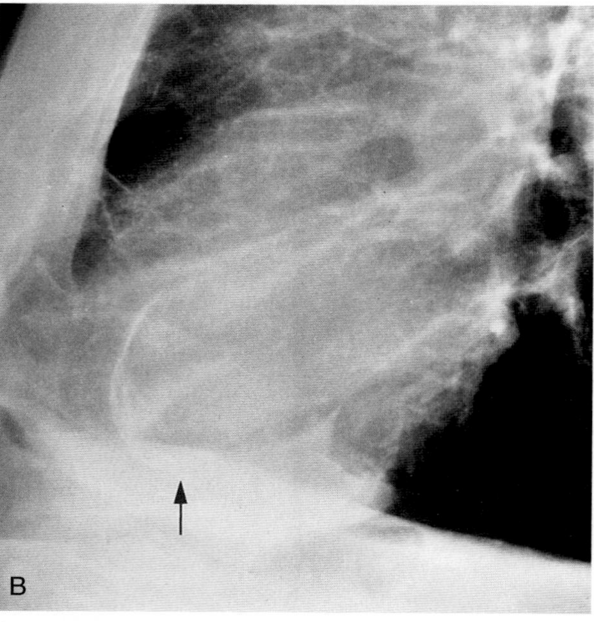

FIGURE 53-8. Calcified myocardial infarctions. **A,** Patient 1: frontal projection of an anterolateral left ventricular aneurysm. The fine calcific line outlines an anterolateral aneurysm of the left ventricle. The calcific deposit is much finer than that seen with pericardial calcification. The patient had suffered a myocardial infarction several years earlier. **B,** Patient 2: lateral projection of a septal infarction. The curvilinear calcific deposit is within the scarred lower portion of the ventricular septum. The infarction extended posteriorly along the base of the heart to involve the diaphragmatic wall of the left ventricle *(arrow).*

aspect of the heart, best seen on the frontal view (Fig. 53-8A), or in the lower portion of the interventricular septum, best seen on the lateral projection (see Fig. 53-8B). Calcification of the pericardium is usually coarser and tends to occur in clumps. Often, pericardial calcium is distributed primarily over the interventricular sulcus and the atrioventricular grooves, but when extensive, the deposits may coalesce and completely surround the heart (Fig. 53-9).

Calcification of the coronary arteries is a specific sign of complicated atheromatous plaques in which previous hemorrhage has occurred. Not uncommonly, this type of plaque, which may not produce significant narrowing of the vessel, is the site of acute thrombosis and vascular occlusion leading to myocardial infarction. There is no correlation between the sites of calcium deposition and the sites of greatest stenosis, but a strong correlation exists between the extent of coronary artery calcification and the extent of coronary arterial sclerosis.

Calcification of the coronary arteries is difficult to visualize on chest films because the deposits are thin and their shadows are blurred by the motion of the heart. Ultrafast computed tomography (CT) scanning using either electron beam or helical CT is very sensitive and accurate for detecting and quantifying the extent of coronary arterial calcification (Chapter 56). However, the data accumulated to date have not clearly shown a correlation between the volume of coronary calcification and the clinical status of the patient. Although high calcium scores indicate extensive atherosclerosis, acute events, such as myocardial infarction or sudden death, can occur in patients with little or no calcification of their coronary arteries.

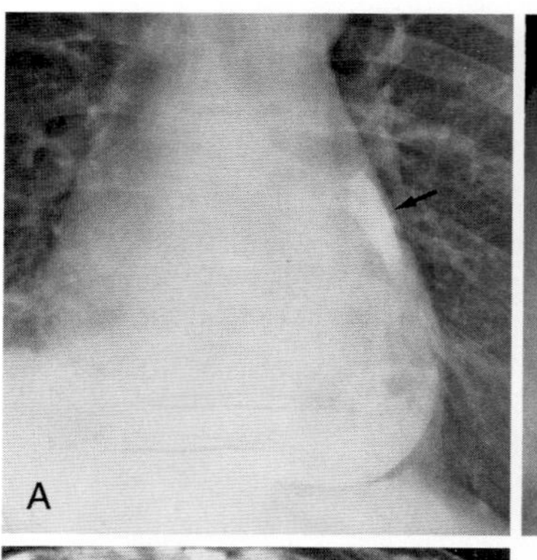

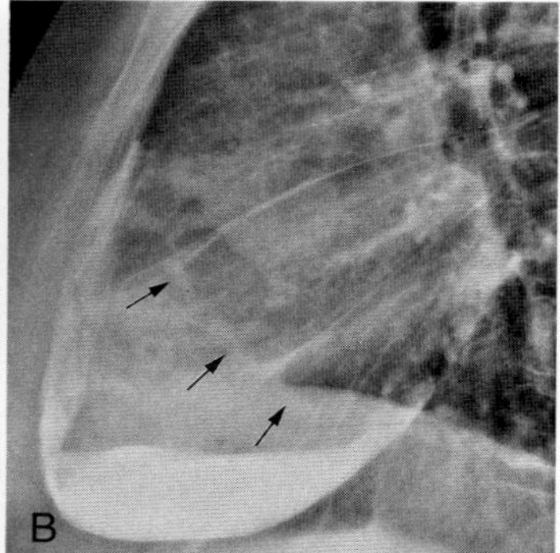

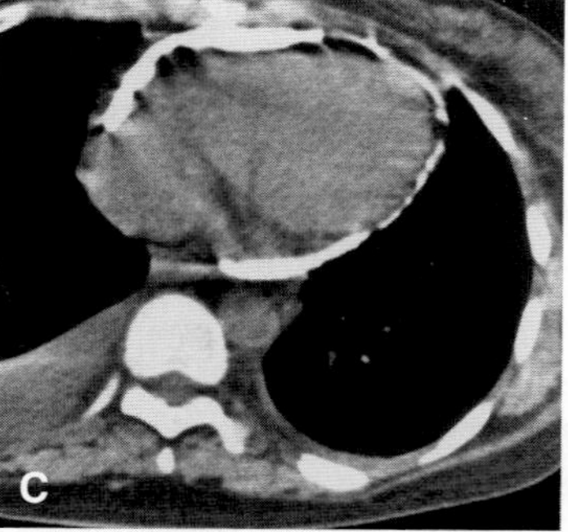

FIGURE 53-9. Calcific pericarditis. **A,** Frontal projection. A large, thick, calcific plaque *(arrow)* lies just below the level of the left upper lobe bronchus. More caudad, the calcific deposits become confluent and cover the diaphragmatic surface of the heart. **B,** The dense calcific peel around the cardiac apex and the diaphragmatic aspect of the heart is better seen. Linear calcific deposits *(arrows)* lie within the atrioventricular sulcus. **C,** Nonenhanced computed tomography shows the irregular, thick, calcific peel almost encircling the heart.

PERICARDIAL EFFUSION

The pericardium completely invests the heart, except for a small area on its posterior surface between the entrances of the pulmonary veins and the superior and inferior venae cavae. When fluid accumulates in the pericardium, the sac distends smoothly to enlarge the cardiac silhouette and give it a flask-shaped appearance. A similar shape can occur with a dilated, failing heart.

The two conditions are readily differentiated by the appearance of the pulmonary hila on a frontal chest film. The pericardial sac extends onto the great vessels and up to or slightly above the level of the bifurcation of the main pulmonary artery (Fig. 53-10). As the sac distends with fluid, it tends to overlap and obscure the hilar vessels. Conversely, when the heart fails, the vessels become congested and appear more prominent than normal (Fig. 53-11).

Posterior displacement of the epicardial fat line is a second reliable sign of pericardial effusion (Chapter 77). In adults, fat is often insinuated between the myocardium and the visceral pericardium (the epicardium) and is sometimes seen on the lateral projection as a curvilinear, radiolucent shadow paralleling the anterior aspect of the heart. The anterior surface of the parietal pericardium borders the retrosternal mediastinal fat. The soft tissue density between these two fat lines therefore represents the pericardium, the epicardium, and the fluid between them. When normal, this stripe is no more than 2 to 4 mm thick. As fluid accumulates in the pericardial sac, the epicardial fat line is displaced posteriorly and the pericardial stripe widens (Fig. 53-12).

PULMONARY VASCULATURE

Almost all of the linear shadows in the lung represent large and medium-sized pulmonary arteries and veins. The terminal branches of the vessels are too small to be visualized as individual structures. The same is true of the interstitial tissues that support the alveoli and form the primary and secondary interlobular septa. However, summation of the minimal densities cast by these structures gives the pulmonary fields an overall grayish cast. The large vessels are seen because their soft tissue density is contrasted against the surrounding air-containing alveoli.

The caliber of the pulmonary vessels reflects the volume of blood flowing through the lungs. When this volume is diminished because of a right-to-left shunt, venous blood bypasses the pulmonary vessels, and, as a result, these vessels are smaller in caliber and the lungs appear abnormally radiolucent. Increased size and prominence of the pulmonary vessels, both central and peripheral, usually indicate an increase in pulmonary blood flow secondary to a left-to-right shunt (Fig. 53-13A). The vessels in the lower as well as the upper lung fields are dilated. Although pulmonary arteries and veins also become abnormally prominent in patients with heart failure, the vessels are not usually sharply outlined, and additional signs of pulmonary venous hypertension or interstitial edema are present (Chapter 58).

The vessels to the lower lobes carry about 60 to 70% of the pulmonary blood flow and are normally of greater caliber than the vessels to the upper lobes. As pulmonary venous pressure increases, the lower lobe vessels become constricted, so more blood is distributed to the upper lobes, which makes their vessels more prominent. This redistribution of the pulmonary vasculature is a reliable sign of pulmonary venous hypertension (see Fig. 53-13B), although it is often difficult to recognize unless quite marked. With a sufficient further increase in venous pressure, pulmonary edema develops.

Pulmonary Edema

Normally, extravascular circulation of fluid in the lungs from the capillaries through the interstitium and back to the blood stream by way of the lymphatics is constant. When pulmonary venous pressure increases, more and more fluid leaks from the capillary bed, the capacity of the lymphatics to remove the fluid is exceeded, and the interstitium becomes waterlogged. Because the interlobular septa in the outer portions of the lung bases are oriented parallel to the x-ray beam on an erect film, when thickened, they are seen as parallel, short horizontal lines extending to the pleural surfaces (Kerley B lines). Kerley A lines also represent thickened interlobular septa, but they are longer and are seen in the upper lung fields. These lines are within the depth of the lung and do not usually reach the pleural surface. Most of the other septa, even when thickened, are too fine to be identified as individual structures. However, the summation pattern creates random "noise" on the film that obscures the shadows of the pulmonary vessels (Fig. 53-14). A ground-glass appearance of the lung fields without identifiable vascular markings within them is characteristic of interstitial pulmonary edema (Chapter 58). The patient is generally severely tachypneic at this stage, but rales may not be

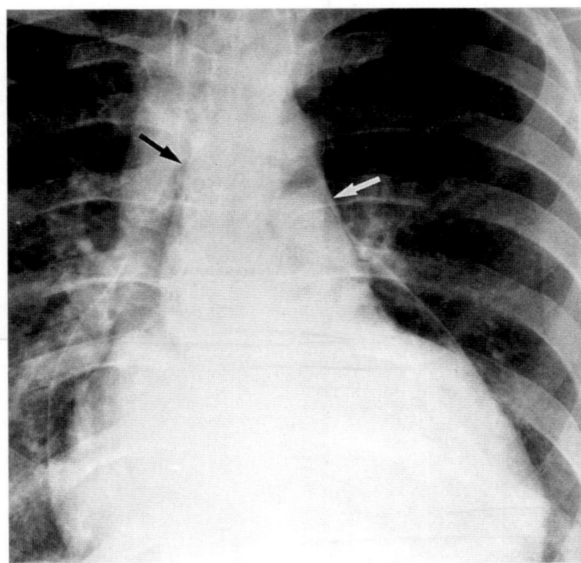

FIGURE 53-10. Superior pericardial reflection with effusion after a tap. During pericardiocentesis, some of the fluid withdrawn was replaced with air. The normal pericardium is now outlined between the intrapericardial air and the air in the lungs and is seen as a thin linear shadow along the outer border of the cardiac silhouette. The film is made in the erect position, and the air has risen to the highest point of the pericardial cavity *(arrows)*, above the level of the pulmonary hila and almost reaching the aortic arch.

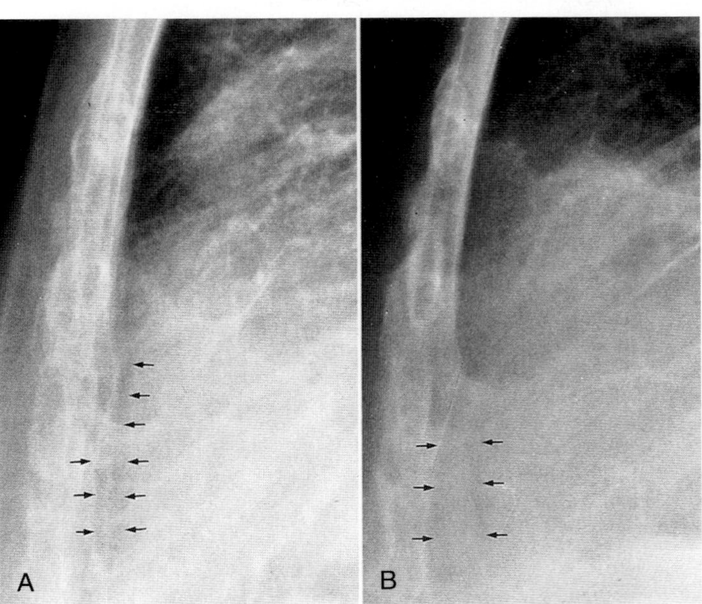

FIGURE 53-12. Pericardial effusion with posterior displacement of the epicardial fat line. The *two lines of arrows* point to the substernal fat and the subepicardial fat layers. **A,** Normal. The fine line of soft tissue density between the fat layers represents the epicardium, the pericardium, and the fluid between them. **B,** Same patient with a pericardial effusion. The epicardial fat line is displaced posteriorly, and the pericardial stripe is abnormally wide.

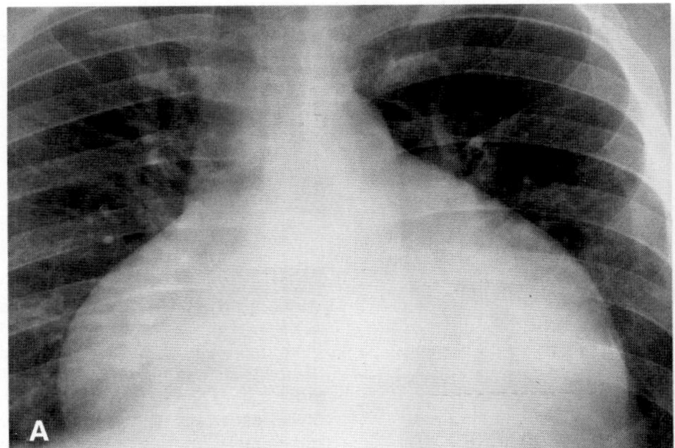

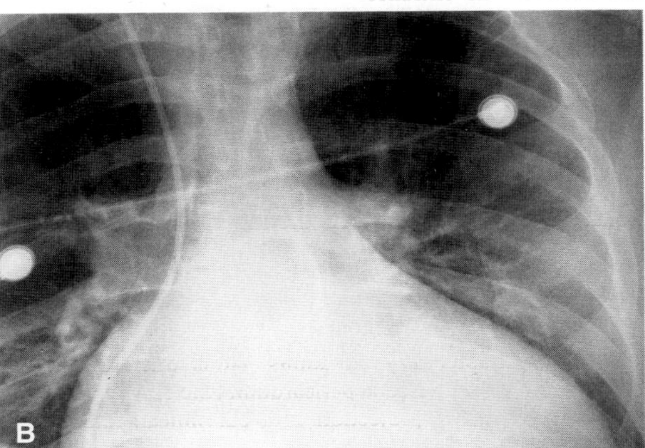

FIGURE 53-11. Hilum overlay sign. A, Pericardial effusion. The heart is diffusely enlarged. Its silhouette extends outward and is obscuring the hilar shadows in each lung. **B,** Dilated cardiomyopathy. The heart is diffusely enlarged. The failing left ventricle has caused congestion of the hilar vessels, and they are more prominent than normal.

present. Interstitial edema also causes thickening of the bronchial walls and peribronchial connective tissue, best seen when they are projected on end. This "peribronchial cuffing" is best visualized in the superior portion of the pulmonary hila, where the anterior segmental bronchus of the upper lobes is viewed on end. When the interstitium can no longer accommodate the excess fluid, it spills into the alveoli (Fig. 53-15). At this point, as air bubbles through the fluid, the typical auscultatory findings of pulmonary edema appear.

Pulmonary Arterial Hypertension

Resistive pulmonary hypertension can result from a left-to-right intracardiac shunt, mitral valve disease, or extracardiac disease, such as repeated episodes of pulmonary embolization (Chapter 98). The central pulmonary arteries become grossly dilated. Instead of gradually tapering as they bifurcate, a sudden, sharp change in the caliber of the vessels is noted. The size and number of the smaller arterial branches decrease, and they take on the appearance of a "pruned tree" (see Fig. 53-6). With severe pulmonary hypertension, the right heart chambers may dilate. The radiographic appearance of pulmonary hypertension is relatively specific but not sensitive, and clinically significant pulmonary hypertension can be present with a normal-appearing pulmonary vascular bed.

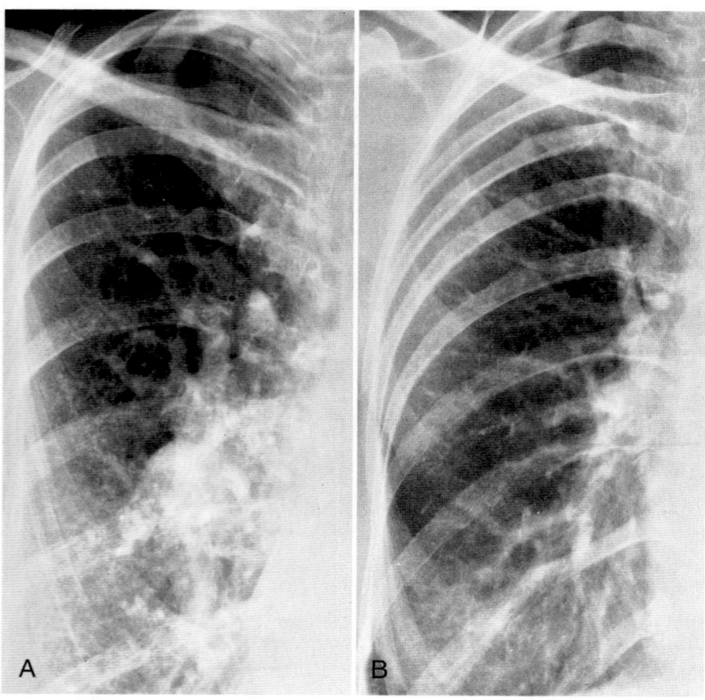

FIGURE 53-13. **Pulmonary vasculature. A,** Atrial septal defect, left-to-right shunt. All pulmonary vessels, to the lower lobes as well as to the upper lobes, are dilated, which is indicative of increased blood flow. **B,** Mitral stenosis, pulmonary venous hypertension with redistribution of the pulmonary vasculature. The lower lobe vessels are constricted and the upper vessels, which now carry more blood, are of greater caliber.

The Cardiac Veins

Almost all coronary blood returns to the heart through the coronary sinus. The orifice of the coronary sinus is in the base of the right atrium just above the entrance of the inferior vena cava and behind the tricuspid valve. Three major cardiac veins drain through the coronary sinus. The great cardiac vein runs upward in the anterior portion of the interventricular sulcus to the atrioventricular sulcus, where it turns to the right (Fig. 53-16) and is joined by the posterior vein of the left ventricle. The drainage area of the latter vein roughly corresponds to the distribution of the circumflex coronary artery. These combined veins continue in the atrioventricular sulcus around the back of the heart as the coronary sinus, which empties into the right atrium. The third vein, the middle cardiac vein, courses in the posterior portion of the interventricular sulcus together with the posterior descending branch of the right coronary artery and joins the coronary sinus near its entrance into the right atrium.

Although percutaneous ventricular pacing initially was limited to the right ventricle, an electrode can now be safely placed percutaneously into a cardiac vein. If a venous catheter in the right atrium curves anteriorly in the lateral view, it extends into the right ventricle. However, if it curves posteriorly, it almost certainly enters the coronary sinus. In the frontal projection, the courses of a catheter in the coronary sinus and a catheter in the right ventricle are almost identical, although one is located on the back of the heart and the

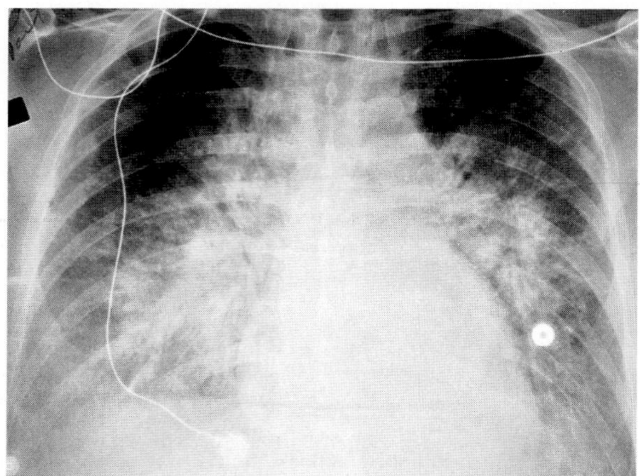

FIGURE 53-15. **Alveolar pulmonary edema, acute myocardial infarction.** Patchy areas of consolidation can be seen in the perihilar regions of both lungs. Dilation of the heart after a massive myocardial infarction may not be seen for the first 24 to 48 hours.

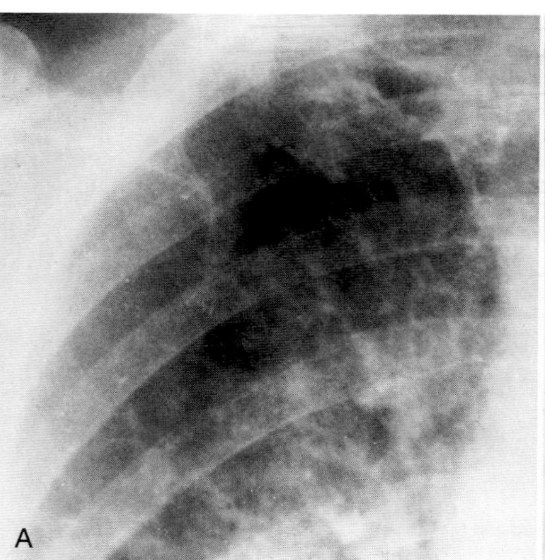

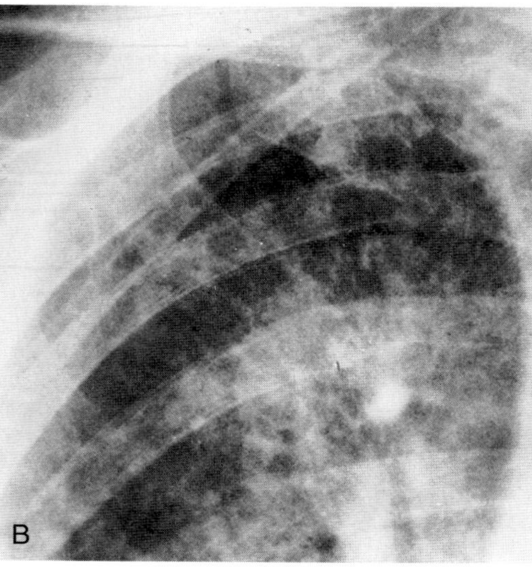

FIGURE 53-14. **Interstitial pulmonary edema.** **A,** Close-up of the right upper lobe; portable film of a patient with an acute myocardial infarction. The pulmonary vessels are well outlined. **B,** Two days later, the patient became tachypneic. No abnormal auscultatory findings were present in the lungs. Radiographically, the lung fields are noisy, with numerous random shadows obscuring the outline of the pulmonary vessels. The appearance and the time sequence of the changes are characteristic of interstitial pulmonary edema.

other is more anterior in the right ventricular cavity. Because the coronary sinus courses directly above the attachment of the posterior leaflet of the mitral valve (Fig. 53-17), it can be used for the percutaneous placement of a device to constrict the mitral orifice, thereby producing the same effect as a surgical mitral annuloplasty (Chapter 75).

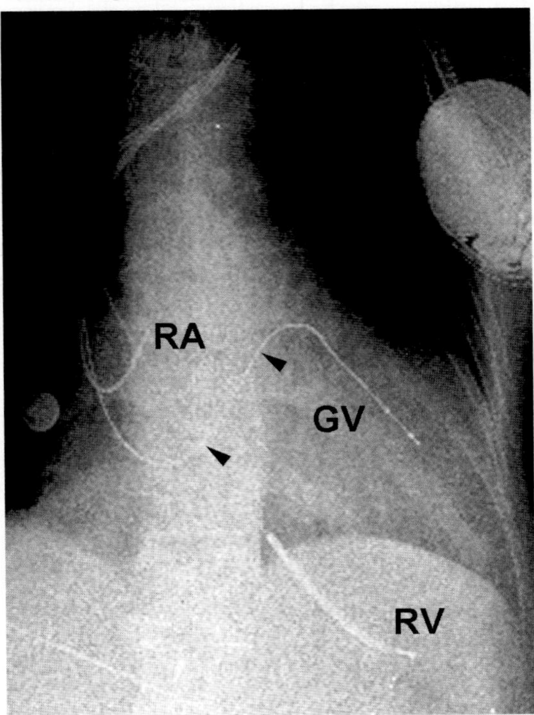

FIGURE 53-16. Biventricular pacemaker, frontal view. The left ventricular lead extends retrograde through the coronary sinus into the great cardiac vein (GV), running in the anterior interventricular sulcus. The section of the coronary sinus between the *arrowheads* is the portion adjacent to the insertion of the posterior mitral leaflet. RA = right atrial lead; RV = right ventricular lead.

THE HEART AND PORTABLE FILMS

Not uncommonly, cardiac patients are too ill to be transported, so their studies must be performed with portable equipment at the bedside. The resulting images are less sharp and have less contrast, and the degree of magnification of the intrathoracic structures can vary considerably. Portable images can also vary from one to the next because the positioning of the patient and the film and the distance between the patient and the x-ray tube are all dependent, in practice, on visual estimation of the technologist. Despite these differences, the same principles of interpretation also apply to portable images, with a few important caveats:

1. The size of the heart, especially relative to the width of the chest, is magnified on a portable image, so the cardiothoracic ratio is not particularly useful. Furthermore, small changes in cardiac size from one portable film to the next have little significance because of the likelihood of variations in technique. Conversely, if the heart appears smaller on a portable than on an erect film, the decrease in size is almost certainly real.
2. If the technologist tilts the x-ray tube even slightly toward the patient's head, the heart will appear even larger and will be projected over the hilar vessels, thereby mimicking the "hilum overlay" sign of a pericardial effusion. Thus, this sign is not useful with portable images.
3. Free pleural fluid collects in the dependent portions of the pleural space, at first in the costophrenic sulci. With fixed equipment in which the x-ray beam is horizontal, the lateral costophrenic sulci are usually obliterated by the fluid, and the upper level of the fluid can be seen. When the patient is supine or slightly tilted, the fluid flows out of the costophrenic sulci and layers along the posterior chest wall. The x-ray beam, although still at right angles to the patient, is no longer horizontal, so the fluid, now viewed en face, appears as an ill-defined haze.
4. Portable films are frequently used to confirm the position of various inserted devices. Without any sense of depth, however, all that is really known is that the object is "projected over" the region of interest; it could actually be some distance away.

SUGGESTED READINGS

Kasznia-Brown J. Cardiac disease on chest x-ray: a pictorial view. *Br J Hosp Med (Lond)*. 2010;71:182-184. *Practical clinical pearls.*

Miller RR, Ely EW. Radiographic measures of intravascular volume status: the role of vascular pedicle width. *Curr Opin Crit Care*. 2006;12:255-262. *Assessment of the value of radiographic markers of volume status.*

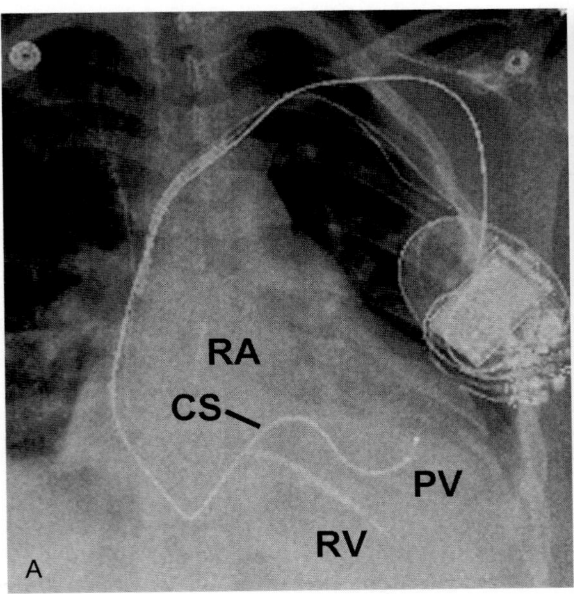

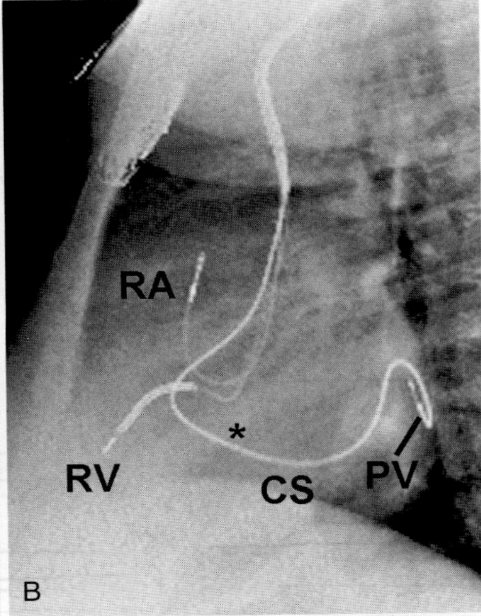

FIGURE 53-17. Left subclavian biventricular pacemaker. Frontal **(A)** and lateral **(B)** images. The right ventricular lead (RV) is seen in the lateral view to curve anteriorly through the tricuspid valve. Its tip is in the apex of the right ventricle. The left ventricular lead curves posteriorly in the atrium and enters the coronary sinus (CS), continuing to the posterior vein of the left ventricle (PV). Note how the right ventricular lead and coronary sinus are superimposed in the frontal projection (RA) right atrial lead.

54

ELECTROCARDIOGRAPHY

LEONARD GANZ

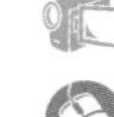

Electrocardiography, which has changed surprisingly little since it was initially introduced by Einthoven in the early 1900s, allows recording of myocardial activation from several vantage points on the body's surface, thereby permitting analysis of electrical activation in different myocardial regions. Surface electrocardiography may be supplemented with intracardiac recordings, which are particularly helpful in the diagnosis and management of cardiac arrhythmias (Chapter 62).

NORMAL FUNCTION AND ELECTROCARDIOGRAM

Normal Cardiac Activation

Electrical activation of the heart depends on the spread of a depolarizing wave front from pacemaker cells through cardiac muscle, as well as specialized conducting tissues (Fig. 54-1). Under normal circumstances, cells in the sinoatrial (SA) nodal complex in the high lateral aspect of the right atrium have the highest spontaneous depolarization rate and are therefore the dominant cardiac pacemaker (Chapter 61). This electrical wave front spreads throughout the right and left atria; specialized conducting tracts called *Bachmann's* bundle speed the depolarizing wave front to the left atrium. Electrical atrial activation triggers atrial muscular contraction, which pumps blood through the tricuspid and mitral valves into the right and left ventricles. Normally, the atrioventricular (AV) node, where conduction delay is physiologic, serves as the only electrical connection linking the atria and ventricles; the AV valve rings are insulated. The depolarizing wave front exits the AV node into the bundle of His, a specialized conducting tissue capable of rapid conduction. The bundle of His bifurcates into right and left bundle branches; the left bundle branch divides into the left anterior and left posterior fascicles. The bundle branches, as well as their more distal ramifications of specialized conducting tissue, are called the *Purkinje system*. From these specialized conducting tissues, the depolarizing wave front enters into and then moves through ventricular muscle. As in the atria, ventricular electrical activation begets muscular contraction, which pumps blood through the semilunar valves into the pulmonary and systemic circulations. After electrical activation, or depolarization, a period of electrical recovery, or repolarization, is necessary before repeated activation.

At the cellular level, a complex orchestration of ion channels opening and closing determines the membrane potential throughout this process. The flow of ions into and out of the myocardial cells inscribes an action potential, which reflects depolarization and repolarization, as well as spontaneous depolarization of pacemaker cells (Chapter 61).

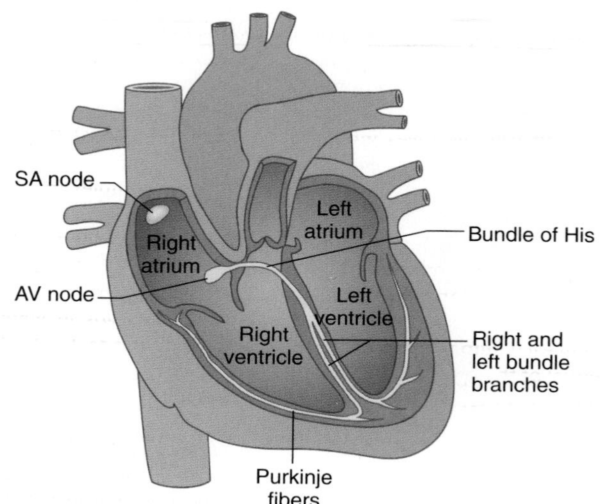

FIGURE 54-1. Cardiac conduction system. The normal conducting system consists of pacemaker cells in the sinoatrial (SA) nodal complex, specialized intra-atrial conducting tracts (including Bachmann's bundle), the atrioventricular (AV) node, the His-Purkinje system, and working atrial and ventricular myocardium.

The Electrocardiographic Waves

Labeled alphabetically, beginning with the P wave, the basic waves of the electrocardiogram (ECG) correspond to these electrical events (Fig. 54-2). The P wave represents atrial muscular depolarization; in severe hyperkalemia, atrial electrical activation may be unaccompanied by atrial muscular activation, and no P wave is inscribed. The QRS complex represents ventricular muscular depolarization; because of the disparity between ventricular and atrial muscle mass, the QRS complex is typically much larger in voltage amplitude than the P wave is. Recorded from multiple vantage points, the QRS complex harbors tremendous information about the structure and function of ventricular tissue. Under normal circumstances, the PR interval, which is the segment from the onset of the P wave to the onset of the QRS complex, represents the delay between atrial and ventricular depolarization. The ST segment and T wave (and occasionally the U wave) reflect ventricular repolarization, a process of electrical recovery that must take place before the ventricle can be depolarized again. Atrial muscle also requires repolarization before the next depolarizing wave front. Because ventricular mass far exceeds atrial muscular mass, the low-amplitude atrial repolarization wave is buried underneath the QRS complex and is rarely manifested on the ECG.

Electrocardiography Standards

A standard ECG is recorded on paper with 1-mm ("small" boxes) as well as 5-mm ("big" boxes) gridlines. Voltage amplitude is measured on the vertical axis (typically 10 mm equaling 1 mV) and time on the horizontal axis. Because the usual ECG recording speed is 25 mm per second, each 1-mm gridline ("small" box) represents 0.04 second (40 msec), and each 5-mm gridline ("big" box) equals 0.2 second (200 msec). These parameters are the usual calibration or standardization. Necessary for proper interpretation, the standardization parameters are typically printed on the ECG.

A standard ECG is recorded over a 10-second period, although a rhythm or monitor strip can be recorded for substantially longer if necessary. Multiple leads are typically recorded simultaneously from the top to the bottom of the page. The usual groupings of leads include I, II, and III; aVR, aVL, and aVF; V_1, V_2, and V_3; and V_4, V_5, and V_6 (see later). Each group of leads is recorded for 2.5 seconds. A single lead (or multilead) rhythm strip is recorded below for the entire 10 seconds. Thus, as the ECG is scanned from left to right, one sees 10 seconds of cardiac activity, with each complex recorded simultaneously in multiple leads.

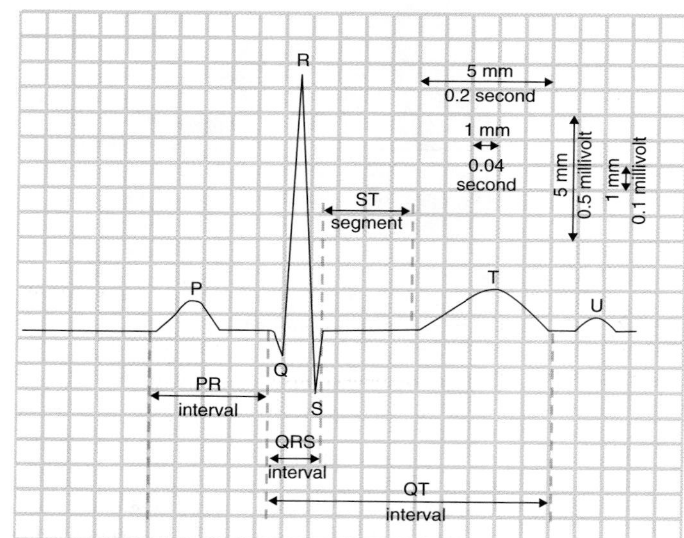

FIGURE 54-2. Inscription of a normal electrocardiogram (ECG). Sinoatrial nodal depolarization is not visible on the surface ECG; the P wave corresponds to atrial mechanical contraction. The PR interval denotes conduction through the atrial muscle, atrioventricular node, and His-Purkinje system. The QRS complex reflects ventricular muscle depolarization. The ST segment and T wave correspond to ventricular repolarization. Atrial repolarization also occurs, but the signal is of low amplitude and buried underneath the QRS complex. Note the gridlines. On the horizontal axis, each 1-mm line ("small" box) denotes 0.04 second (40 msec); a "big" box denotes 0.2 second (200 msec). On the vertical axis, 1 mm ("small" box) corresponds to 0.1 mV; 10 mm (two "big" boxes) therefore denotes 1 mV.

TABLE 54-1 NORMAL ELECTROCARDIOGRAPHIC INTERVALS

Heart rate	50-100 beats per minute
P wave duration	<0.12 sec (120 msec)
PR interval	0.09 (90 msec) to 0.20 sec (200 msec)
QRS duration	0.075 (75 msec) to 0.11 sec (110 msec)
QTc	0.45 sec (450 msec) males, 0.46 sec (460 msec) females
QRS axis	−30 to + 90 degrees

Normal Intervals

Each of the various ECG waves and intervals has normal ranges, defined from large numbers of electrocardiographic recordings in (presumably) healthy subjects (Table 54-1; see Fig. 54-2).

The RR interval (or PP interval), which is the measurement from R wave to R wave (or P wave to P wave), allows calculation of the heart rate. Because there are 60,000 msec in a minute, the heart rate (HR) in beats per minute can be easily calculated from the RR or PP interval in milliseconds:

$$HR = \frac{60{,}000}{RR}$$

Although traditionally the normal resting heart rate has been defined as 60 to 100 beats per minute, a range of 50 to 90 at rest may actually be more reflective of normal physiology. When the heart rate is grossly irregular, as in atrial fibrillation (Chapter 64), the RR interval can be averaged over a number of cardiac cycles to estimate the heart rate. Because a standard ECG records 10 seconds in time, the heart rate (beats per minute) will equal the number of QRS complexes recorded on a standard ECG multiplied by 6.

P Wave Duration

The P wave duration, from the beginning to the end of a P wave, is typically less than 0.12 second (120 msec, three small boxes) in length. A broader P wave reflects an intra-atrial or interatrial conduction delay, or both. Abnormalities in P wave amplitude, morphology, and axis may reflect atrial enlargement.

PR Interval

The PR interval, which is measured from the onset of the P wave to the onset of the QRS complex, is normally between 0.09 and 0.2 second (90 to 200 msec). One-to-one AV conduction with a PR interval greater than 0.2 second has traditionally been called first-degree AV block, but *delayed AV conduction* may be a more appropriate term. Conduction through the atrial tissue, the AV node, and the His-Purkinje system contributes to the PR interval. When the PR interval is prolonged, delay is usually present in the AV node, although other sites of delay are possible. Prolongation of the PR interval is associated with an increased risk of atrial fibrillation, need for a pacemaker, and higher overall mortality. A short PR interval may reflect ventricular preexcitation (Wolff-Parkinson-White syndrome), a junctional rhythm, or other conditions.

QRS Complex

The QRS complex, which reflects ventricular muscular electrical activation, carries important information in patients with coronary artery disease, cardiomyopathy, metabolic abnormalities, and other conditions. Capital letters (Q, R, S) denote large-amplitude deflections (≥5 mm or 0.5 mV), whereas lowercase letters (q, r, s) signify low-amplitude deflections (<5 mm or 0.5 mV). Q, q, S, and s waves are negative excursions from the isoelectric baseline, whereas R and r waves are positive deflections. Q and q waves are initial negative deflections, and S and s waves are negative deflections that follow a positive deflection (R or r wave); a QS complex is an entirely negative deflection. An R′ or r′ wave refers to a second positive deflection after an S (or s) wave. The duration of the QRS complex reflects the time required for ventricular depolarization. Ventricular activation usually requires at least 0.075 second (75 msec, nearly two small boxes). There is some debate regarding the upper limit of the normal range for QRS duration; a recent consensus document specified 0.11 second (110 msec, nearly three small boxes). If the QRS duration is prolonged, an intraventricular or interventricular conduction delay (IVCD), or both, is present. Particular patterns of IVCD have been termed *bundle branch block* (see later).

QT Interval

The QT interval, which reflects ventricular repolarization, is measured from the onset of the QRS complex to the end of the T wave. Accurate assessment of the repolarization interval is important inasmuch as patients with prolonged repolarization, either congenital or acquired, may be at risk for torsades de pointes ventricular tachycardia (Chapter 65). The QT interval must be corrected to allow comparison of this interval at differing heart rates. Bazett's formula defines a corrected QT interval (QTc):

$$QTc = \frac{QT}{\sqrt{RR}}$$

Bazett's formula works reasonably well at heart rates in the normal range but overcorrects at high rates and undercorrects at low rates. Although more complex regression formulas have been developed to correct the QT interval at different heart rates, none has achieved widespread clinical use. Irregular rhythms (notably atrial fibrillation) complicate calculation of the QTc. Calculating multiple QTc intervals and then taking the average is reasonable; alternatively, the QTc after the longest RR interval can be considered the "worst-case scenario" of the repolarization interval.

The presence of a U wave complicates measurement of the QT (and therefore QTc) interval because it is not always clear where the T wave ends and whether the U wave should be included in a QTU interval. If the isoelectric baseline is reached between the T and U waves, the U wave is not generally included in the QT interval. If the T wave "merges" into the U wave without reaching the isoelectric baseline, the U wave is included in the QT (or QTU) interval. Short QTc intervals are unusual. The QTc in a given patient may vary somewhat over the course of the day and tends to be slightly longer in young and middle-aged women than in men. The upper limit of a normal QTc is somewhat debatable, but a cutoff of 0.45 second (450 msec) in men and 0.46 second (460 msec) in women was proposed recently in a consensus document. The QT interval is quite sensitive to drug effects, as well as to electrolyte and metabolic derangements.

Electrocardiographic Leads

Recording a single ECG lead allows calculation of the heart rate and, frequently, accurate diagnosis of the heart rhythm. When the ECG is recorded from multiple skin leads simultaneously, the direction (or vector) of activation as the electrical wave front moves through the heart can be inferred. Although a number of different lead systems are possible (and some are actually used in research settings), standard electrocardiography uses 12 leads from 12 vantage points, recorded with 10 electrodes, 6 on the chest wall and 4 on the limbs. In reality, only three limb leads are actually used to generate recordings; the right leg lead serves as an electrical ground. The limb leads, called the *frontal plane leads,* generate bipolar and augmented unipolar lead recordings. The chest or precordial electrodes record unipolar recordings. Bipolar leads record the potential difference between two skin electrodes. In unipolar recordings, the lead of interest, the exploring electrode, is compared with a reference electrode. By convention, a positive deflection is recorded if the electrical wave front is moving toward the positive electrode in a bipolar pair or toward the exploring electrode in a unipolar lead.

The bipolar limb leads measure potential differences between electrodes on pairs of limb electrodes. Lead I compares the right arm (negative) and left arm (positive), lead II the right arm (negative) and left leg (positive), and lead III the left arm (negative) and left leg (positive) (Fig. 54-3). Because the direction of both atrial and ventricular depolarization is away from the right arm and toward the left arm, a positive P wave and QRS complex are generally recorded in lead I. Similarly, the P wave and QRS complexes are positive in leads II and III in normal SA to AV conduction because atrial and ventricular activation proceeds in a craniocaudal direction. The bipolar limb leads closely resemble Einthoven's original string galvanometer recordings.

Leads aVR, aVL, and aVF are augmented unipolar leads in which the potential in each limb is compared with a reference electrode. For lead aVR, the potential of the right arm is compared with a reference composed of the left arm and left leg electrodes. Lead aVL compares the left arm potential with a reference combining the right arm and left leg; aVF compares the left leg with a right and left arm reference. Because atrial and ventricular activation normally moves from right to left and in a craniocaudal direction, the P wave and QRS complex are negative in lead aVR but positive in lead aVF. In lead aVL, P waves and QRS complexes are generally upright, although an rS complex may be recorded, particularly in young patients.

The precordial electrodes are positioned at specific points on the chest wall (Fig. 54-4A). These unipolar leads compare electrical potential between the

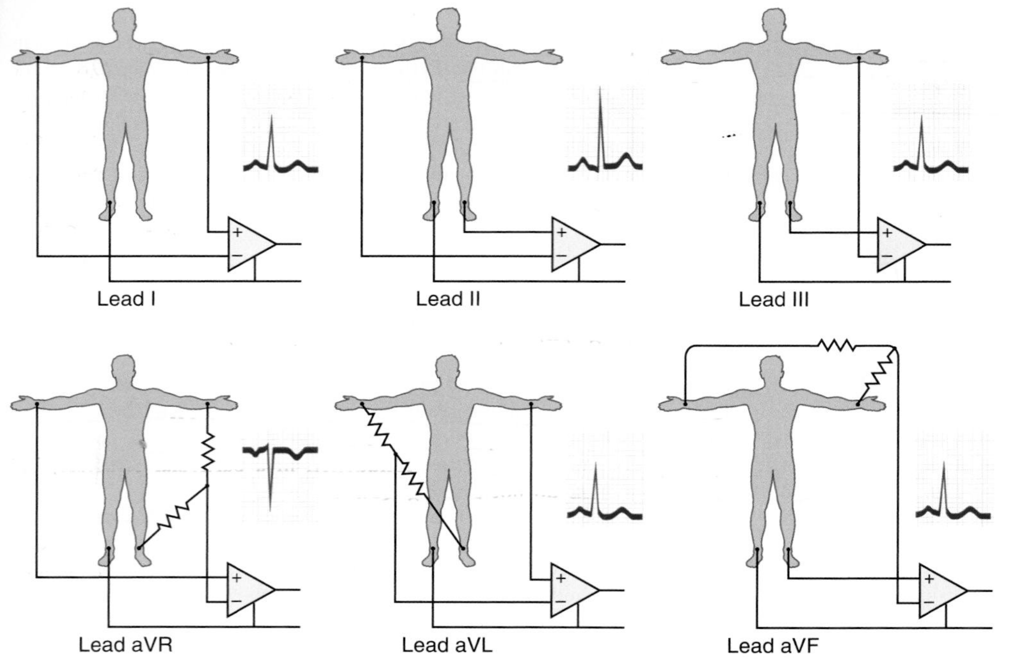

FIGURE 54-3. Normal cardiac activation as manifested in the limb leads. Under normal circumstances, P waves and QRS complex are typically upright in leads I, II, III, and aVF and inverted in aVR. In lead aVL, P waves are usually upright, although QRS complexes may be either upright or inverted. The right leg electrode serves to ground the system.

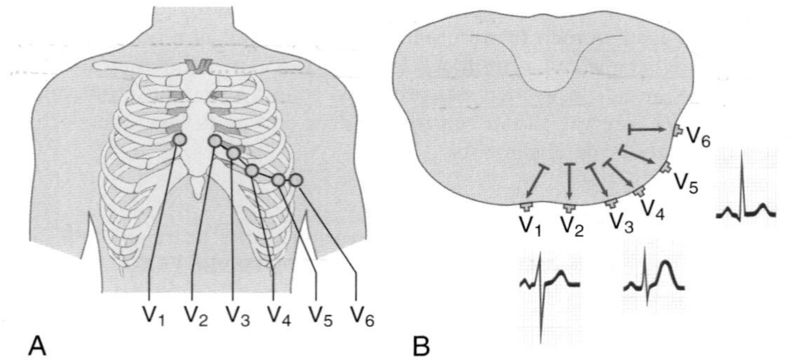

FIGURE 54-4. Precordial leads. A, Positioning of the precordial leads on the chest wall. **B,** Normal cardiac activation as manifested in the precordial leads. Note the small r wave and deep S wave in lead V_1, the transition at around V_3 or V_4, and the "septal" q wave and large R wave in lead V_6.

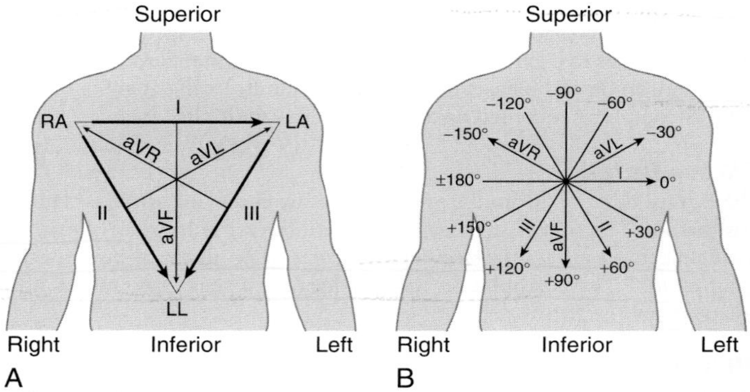

FIGURE 54-5. Axis of electrical activation. A, Vectors for the limb leads (LL) in the frontal plane. **B,** Hexaxial reference for determining the frontal plane axis. Note that the vectors for leads I, II, and III are in the same direction as in **A,** but now, like the augmented limb leads, these standard limb lead vectors have been moved so that they emanate from the center of the figure. LA = left atrium; RA = right atrium.

chest electrode and a reference electrode called the *Wilson central terminal.* The Wilson central terminal combines the right arm, left arm, and left leg potentials through 5000-Ω resistors. The six precordial leads define atrial and ventricular activation with respect to a somewhat transverse plane through the chest wall (see Fig. 54-4B). In this plane, atrial activation moves from right to left. Initial ventricular activation involving the septum is directed from left to right; left ventricular depolarization, which dominates right ventricular depolarization because of the differential in myocardial mass, then moves apically and laterally. In lead V_1, to the right of the sternum, the P wave is biphasic (reflecting right and then left atrial activation). Initial ventricular activation of the septum inscribes an r wave, whereas subsequent activation away from lead V_1 records a dominant S wave. In lead V_6, the P wave is positive. Initial septal depolarization inscribes a tiny "septal" q wave (usually ≤0.02 second), and subsequent ventricular depolarization records a dominant R wave.

Right-sided chest leads should be recorded when right ventricular abnormalities are suspected. RV_3, the mirror image of lead V_3, is routinely recorded in pediatric patients because of the possibility of congenital heart disease. In adults, ST elevation in lead RV_3 is quite specific for acute right ventricular infarction in those being evaluated for an acute inferior wall myocardial infarction.

Axis

An axis of electrical activation can be defined in the frontal plane axis by combining the bipolar and augmented unipolar limb leads (Fig. 54-5A). By convention, the axis parallel to lead I, toward the left arm, is called 0 degrees. A frontal plane axis between −30 and +90 degrees is normal; other axes are abnormal (Fig. 54-6). Right axis deviation is a normal variant in children and

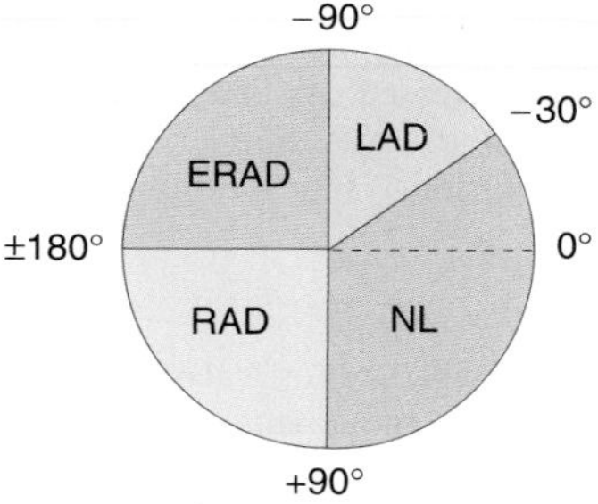

FIGURE 54-6. Chart of frontal plane axes. Normal (NL) = −30 to +90 degrees; left axis deviation (LAD) = −30 to −90 degrees (moderate, −30 to −45 degrees; marked, −45 to −90 degrees); right axis deviation (RAD) = +90 to +180 degrees (moderate, +90 to +120 degrees; marked, +120 to +180 degrees); extreme right axis deviation (ERAD) = −90 to ±180 degrees. Mild RAD is considered normal in children, adolescents, and young adults.

adolescents. The frontal plane axis can be estimated by identifying the limb lead in which the QRS complex is most nearly isoelectric (similar positive and negative deflections); the axis is perpendicular to this lead (see Fig. 54-5B). Because two lines pointing 180 degrees apart can be drawn perpendicular to any given line, examination of the other limb leads defines the direction in which the axis points. If the QRS complex is positive in any given limb lead, the axis will be oriented toward that limb lead, not away from it. Alternatively, the axis is in the normal range if the QRS complexes are primarily positive in both leads I and II.

An axis per se is not defined in the precordial leads. Rather, because the typical progression from leads V_1 to V_6 is from a predominantly negative to a positive QRS complex, the transition point is usually defined as the point at which the amplitude of the R wave begins to exceed the amplitude of the S wave.

APPROACH TO INTERPRETING THE ELECTROCARDIOGRAM

A stepwise approach to interpreting the ECG ensures that no features of the tracing will be overlooked (Table 54-2).

Normal Electrocardiogram

Figure 54-7 is an example of a normal ECG. Sinus rhythm occurs at about 78 beats per minute, with minor variations in the RR intervals (sinus arrhythmia). The PR interval, QRS duration, and QTc are all normal. The QRS complex is most nearly isoelectric in lead aVL, so the QRS axis will be perpendicular to lead aVL. Because aVL points to −30 degrees, the QRS axis must be approximately −120 or +60 degrees. Because the QRS complex is positive in leads I and II (large R waves), the QRS axis is approximately +60 degrees. The transition in the precordial leads is between leads V_3 and V_4. The P wave is biphasic in lead V_1 and then positive in the other precordial leads. "Septal" q waves, reflecting not lateral infarction but rather normal early septal depolarization, are present in leads V_5 and V_6. Tiny q waves, a normal variant, are seen in the inferior leads.

TABLE 54-2 STEPWISE APPROACH TO INTERPRETING THE ELECTROCARDIOGRAM

- Estimate the heart rate
- Define the heart rhythm (regular vs. irregular; relationship of P waves to QRS complexes)
- Measure intervals (PR, QRS duration, QT)
- Calculate/estimate QTc
- Estimate QRS axis
- Examine P wave morphology, duration, and axis
- Examine QRS progression and transition in precordial leads
- Examine QRS complexes in regional groupings (septal leads [V_1,V_2], anterior leads [V_2, V_3, V_4], lateral leads [I, aVL, V_5, V_6], inferior and posterior leads [II, III, aVF, V_1, V_2])
- Examine ST segments in regional groupings
- Examine T waves in regional groupings

Abnormal Electrocardiogram

Electrocardiography in patients with coronary artery disease is reviewed in Chapters 71 to 73 and arrhythmias in Chapters 61 to 66.

Conduction Abnormalities and Axis Deviation

Abnormalities of the specialized conduction system (i.e., His-Purkinje system) reflect slow or absent conduction in a particular structure, but fascicular blocks do not prolong QRS duration beyond 120 msec (Table 54-3). An IVCD is generally defined as a QRS duration of more than 0.11 second (110 msec). When the QRS has a duration of at least 0.12 second (120 msec), it often has the configuration of a specific bundle branch block (Fig. 54-8).

Chamber Hypertrophy

A number of criteria for defining left ventricular hypertrophy (LVH; Fig. 54-9) and right ventricular hypertrophy (RVH) have been proposed. All of the LVH criteria suffer from poor sensitivity (ranging from 30 to 50%), although the specificity is good (85 to 95%). The Cornell voltage criterion, developed with an echocardiographic standard for LVH, simply adds the S wave amplitude in V_3 and the R wave amplitude in aVL; a total greater than

TABLE 54-3 FASCICULAR AND BUNDLE BRANCH BLOCKS

	QRS DURATION	AXIS	QRS MORPHOLOGY	ST SEGMENTS AND T WAVES
LAFB	<0.12 sec (120 msec)	−45 to −90 degrees	Delayed transition across the precordium qR aVL	Normal
LPFB	<0.12 sec (120 msec)	+90 to +180 degrees	Delayed transition across the precordium rS in I, aVL qR in III, aVF	Normal
RBBB	≥0.12 sec (120 msec)	Normal	rsr′, rsR′, rSR′ in V_1 (and usually V_2); wide S in V_6 and I	Discordant in V_1 and V_2
RBBB with LAFB	≥0.12 sec (120 msec)	−45 to 90 degrees	rsr′, rsR′, rSR′ in V_1 (and usually V_2); wide S in V_6 and I	Discordant in V_1 and V_2
RBBB with LPFB	≥0.12 sec (120 msec)	+ 90 to +180 degrees	rsr′, rsR′, rSR′ in V_1 (and usually V_2); wide S in V_6 and I	Discordant in V_1 and V_2
LBBB	≥0.12 sec (120 msec)	Variable	rS or QS in V_1 (S wide and notched); wide notched R without q in V_5, V_6, and I Wide notched R with or without small q in aVL	Discordant in V_1 to V_6

LAD = left axis deviation; LAFB = left anterior fascicular block; LBBB = left bundle branch block; LPFB = left posterior fascicular block; RBBB = right bundle branch block.

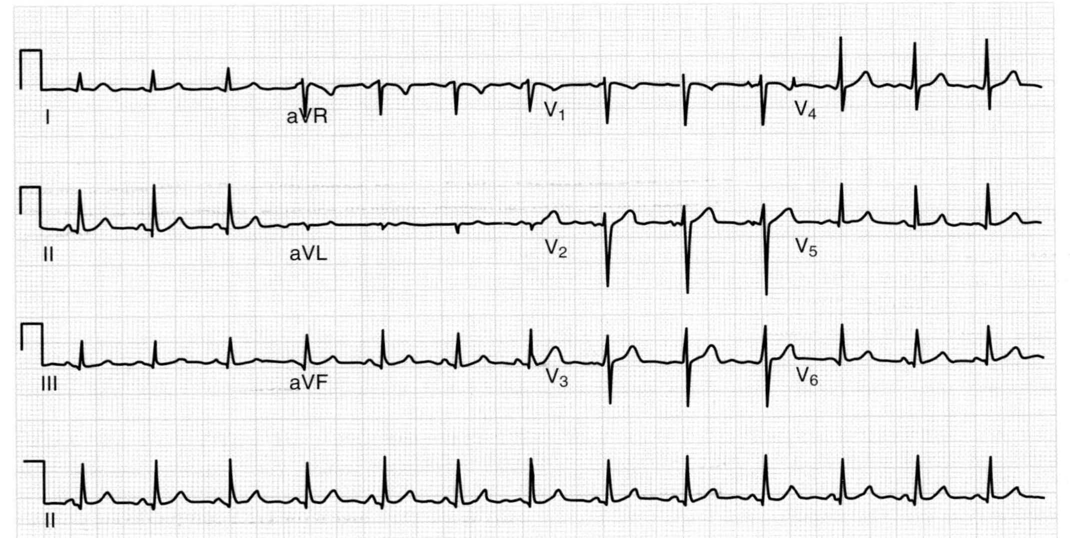

FIGURE 54-7. **Normal electrocardiogram.** The heart rate is approximately 78 beats per minute, with minor irregularity. Sinus arrhythmia is present. The axis is approximately +60 degrees. The PR, QRS, and QT intervals are approximately 140, 90, and 360 msec, respectively. P wave morphology, duration, and axis are normal. The transition is between leads V_3 and V_4. No abnormal Q waves are present. ST segments are isoelectric, and T waves are concordant with QRS complexes.

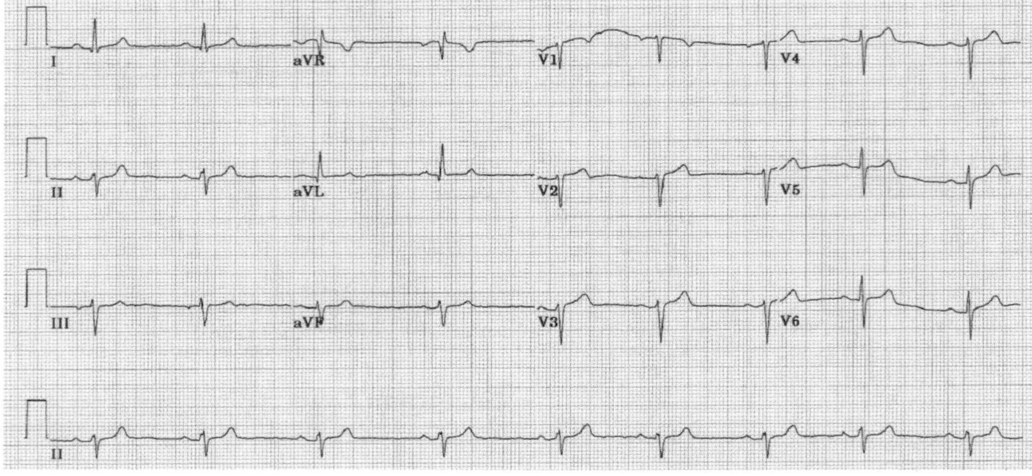

A

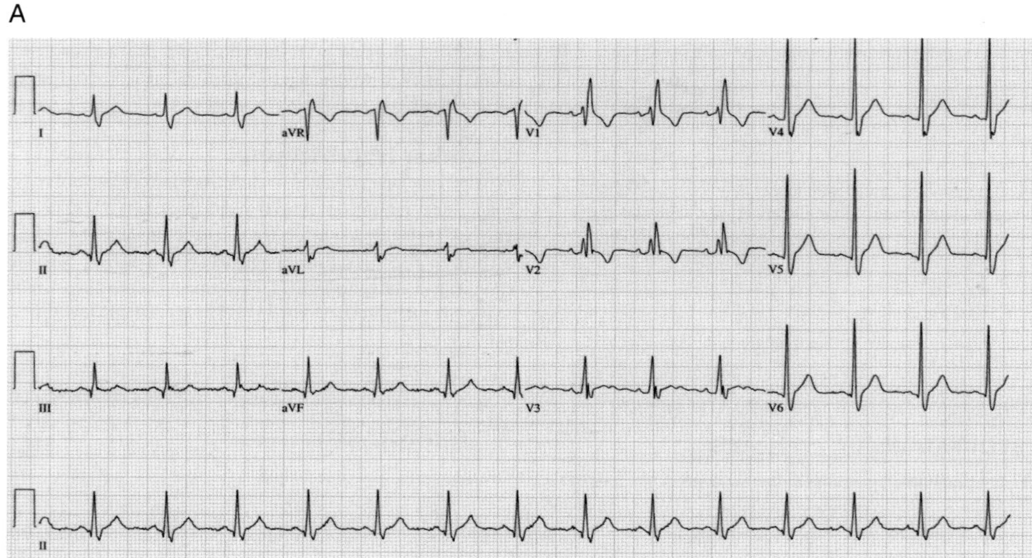

B

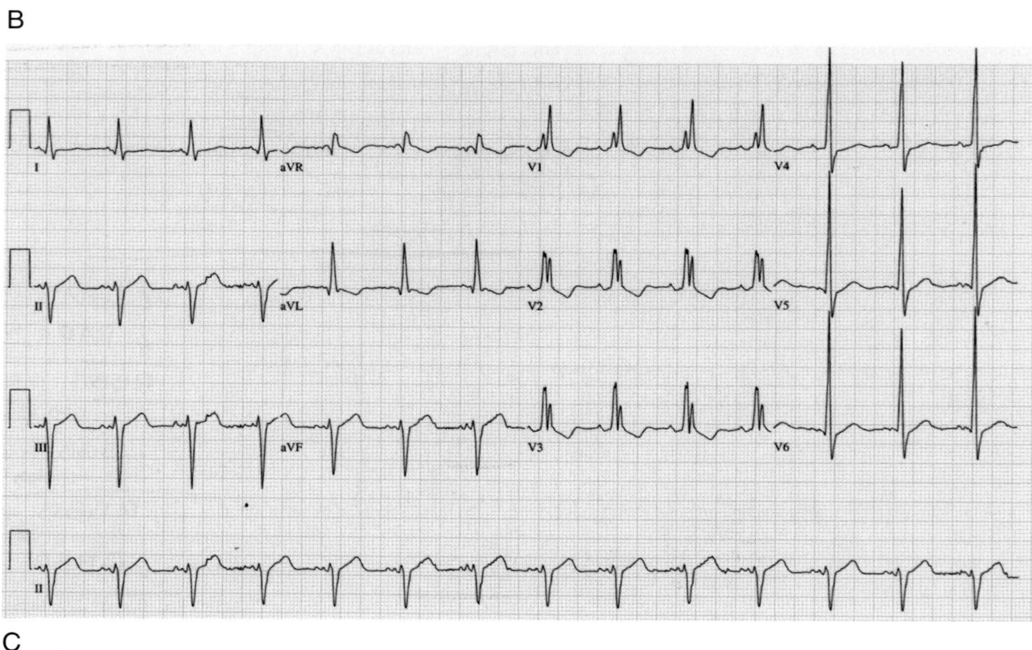

C

FIGURE 54-8. **Fascicular and bundle branch blocks. A,** Left anterior fascicular block (LAFB). Left axis deviation is present; the axis is approximately −60 degrees. The QRS duration is normal, and there is a delay in R wave progression across the precordial leads (late transition). Small q waves are present in leads I and aVL and small r waves in leads II, III, and aVF. **B,** Right bundle branch block (RBBB). The QRS is widened, with an rsR′ pattern in lead V_1 and a wide terminal S wave in lead V_6. ST segments are downsloping, and T waves are discordant with the QRS complex in the right precordial leads. The axis is normal, and signs of normal septal activation (q waves in lead V_6) are present. **C,** RBBB and LAFB. In addition to features diagnostic of RBBB, an axis of −60 degrees is present.

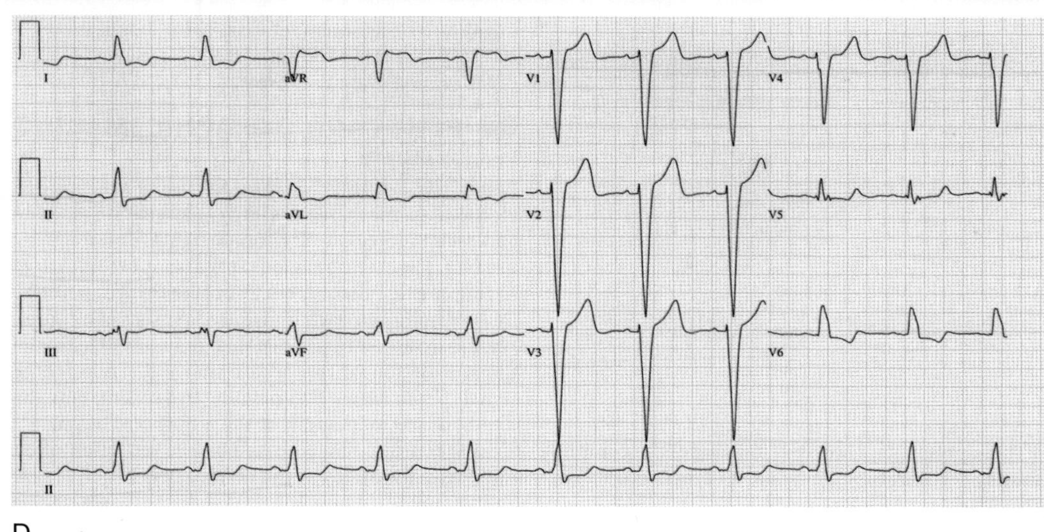

D

FIGURE 54-8, cont'd. D, Left bundle branch block (LBBB). The QRS is widened, with a broad, notched complex in leads I, aVL, and the left precordial leads. Small r waves and broad, deep S waves are present in the right precordial leads. With LBBB, the axis is usually normal or deviated to the left. ST segments and T waves are discordant with the QRS complex throughout the precordium.

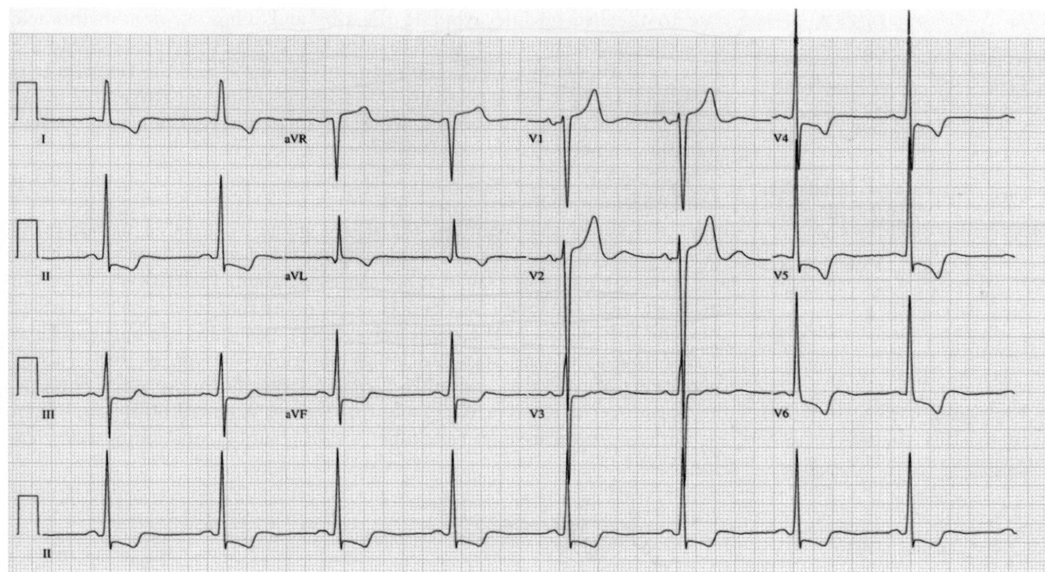

FIGURE 54-9. Left ventricular hypertrophy. Note the striking S wave amplitude in the right precordial leads and R wave amplitude in the left precordial leads. Repolarization abnormalities are present in the left precordial leads, as well as the limb leads. The S wave amplitude in V_3 (2.4 mV) plus the R wave amplitude in aVL (1.0 mV) total 3.4 mV, easily satisfying the Cornell voltage criteria in this 76-year-old hypertensive man. Sinus bradycardia (50 beats per minute) is present as well.

2.0 mV in women and 2.8 mV in men implies LVH. In many clinical settings, the Cornell criterion has replaced the more complicated Romhilt-Estes criteria, which assign points for QRS amplitude, repolarization abnormalities ("strain" pattern), left axis deviation, and other electrocardiographic features. RVH is much less common than LVH. Electrocardiographic criteria for diagnosing RVH have even lower sensitivity (10 to 20%) than for LVH, although the specificity is similar. The Sokolow-Lyon criterion for RVH adds the R wave amplitude in lead V_1 to the S wave amplitude in lead V_5 or V_6; a sum of 1.05 mV or greater implies RVH.

Low QRS Voltage

Low QRS voltage is defined as limb lead voltage less than 5 mm (0.5 mV) in all leads or precordial voltage less than 10 mm (1 mV) in all leads. The differential diagnosis is broad (Table 54-4), and no underlying explanation is defined in many cases.

TABLE 54-4 CAUSES OF LOW QRS VOLTAGE
Normal variant
Pericardial effusion
Myocardial infarction
Cardiomyopathy
Hypothyroidism
Obesity
Sarcoidosis
Amyloidosis
Chronic obstructive pulmonary disease
Anasarca

Repolarization Abnormalities

Abnormalities of the ST segment or T waves, or both, are extremely common (Table 54-5). Electrolyte and other metabolic abnormalities, drug effects (particularly digoxin and antiarrhythmic drugs), and secondary effects caused by LVH or bundle branch block are all commonly encountered. Early repolarization, a relatively common pattern of ST segment elevation previously thought to be benign, occurs more commonly in patients with idiopathic ventricular fibrillation than in controls and has also been associated with an increased risk of cardiac mortality.

Pitfalls of Automated Computerized Electrocardiographic Readings

Automatic interpretations of ECG tracings are generally quite accurate for calculating heart rates, axes, and intervals. Interpretation of the significance of repolarization abnormalities may be less accurate, and diagnosis of rhythms

TABLE 54-5 CAUSES OF REPOLARIZATION ABNORMALITIES
Athlete's heart
Early repolarization (normal variant)
Myocardial ischemia/injury
Pericarditis
Electrolyte abnormalities
Left ventricular hypertrophy
Intraventricular conduction delay/bundle branch block
Drug effects (digitalis, antiarrhythmic drugs, etc.)
Long QT syndrome
Stroke/neurologic catastrophe

is the striking weakness of these programs. Thus, over-reading of the computerized interpretation by the physician and comparison with previous tracings, when available, remain mandatory.

SUGGESTED READINGS

Cheng S, Keyes MJ, Larson MG, et al. Long-term outcomes in individuals with prolonged PR interval or first-degree atrioventricular block. *JAMA*. 2009;301:2571-2585. *Prolongation of the PR interval increases the risk of atrial fibrillation, need of a pacemaker, and overall mortality by 10 to 20%.*

Steinvil A, Chundadze T, Zeltser D, et al. Mandatory electrocardiographic screening of athletes to reduce their risk for sudden death: proven fact or wishful thinking? *J Am Coll Cardiol*. 2011;57:1291-1296. *Mandatory ECG does not change risk of sudden death.*

Tikkanen JT, Anttonen O, Junttila MJ, et al. Long-term outcome associated with early repolarization on electrocardiography. *N Engl J Med*. 2009;361:2529-2537. *In Finnish men and women with mean follow-up of 30 ± 11 years, an early repolarization pattern in the inferior leads was associated with a significantly increased risk of cardiac death.*

55

ECHOCARDIOGRAPHY

CATHERINE M. OTTO

Echocardiography is the clinical standard for evaluating cardiac function in patients with known or suspected heart disease. This chapter reviews the basic principles of echocardiography, echocardiographic approaches, quantitative measurements, and clinical indications. The specific use of echocardiography and additional images is shown in other chapters on individual types of cardiovascular diseases.

ECHOCARDIOGRAPHIC IMAGING

Principles

Echocardiography is based on the use of a piezoelectric crystal that converts electrical to mechanical energy, and vice versa, allowing both transmission and reception of an ultrasound signal. The frequency of ultrasound waves used for diagnostic imaging ranges from 2 to 10 MHz, with lower frequencies having greater tissue penetration and higher frequencies providing better image resolution. Each transducer consists of a complex array of piezoelectric crystals arranged to provide images in a fanlike two-dimensional image, with the narrow top of this sector scan indicating the origin of the ultrasound signal. Transducers also include an acoustic lens that determines the focal depth, height, and width of the ultrasound beam.

Images are generated based on the reflection of ultrasound from acoustic interfaces: for example, the boundary between the blood in the left ventricle and the myocardium. The time delay between transmission and reception is used to determine the depth of origin of the ultrasound reflection. The depths of the reflected signals from multiple ultrasound beams are combined to generate a two-dimensional image. The speed of signal analysis allows acquisition of two-dimensional ultrasound images at frame rates of 30 to 60 per second. Ultrasound is strongly attenuated by bone and air, so echocardiography relies on acoustic "windows" where, for example, ultrasound can penetrate to the heart while avoiding the ribs and lungs. With transthoracic imaging, the patient is positioned to bring the cardiac structures close to the chest wall, usually in a left lateral decubitus position, and the transducer is placed on the chest, using gel to provide acoustic coupling between the transducer and skin. Standard acoustic windows are parasternal, apical, subcostal, and suprasternal notch.

Standard Image Planes

From the parasternal window, the image plane is adjusted manually by an experienced physician or sonographer to provide long and short axis views. Standard cardiac imaging planes are aligned relative to the axis of the heart, with the long axis defined as the plane that intersects the cardiac apex and the middle of the aortic valve. Short axis views are perpendicular to this long axis, with standard image planes at the cardiac base (aortic valve level), mitral valve, and midventricular levels. From the apical window, the transducer is rotated to provide three views oriented 60 degrees from each other, producing a four-chamber, a two-chamber, and a long axis view (Fig. 55-1).

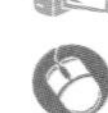

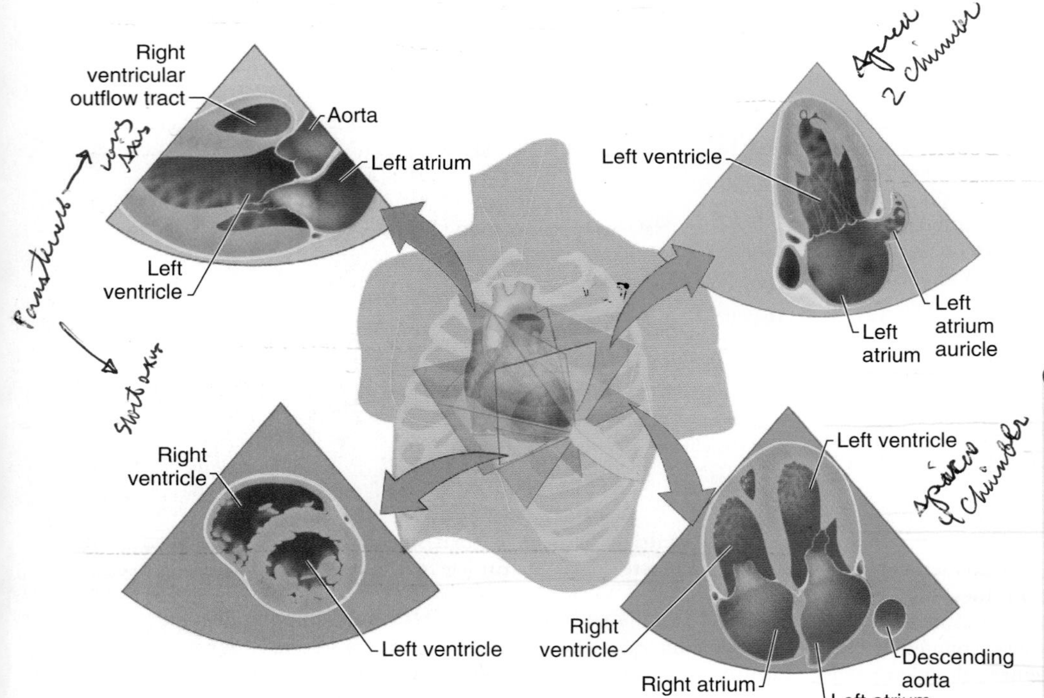

FIGURE 55-1. The four basic image planes used in transthoracic echocardiography. A parasternal transducer position or "window" is used to obtain long and short axis views. The long axis view *(purple outline)* extends from the left ventricular apex through the aortic valve plane. The short axis view is perpendicular to the long axis view, resulting in a circular view of the left ventricle *(red outline)*. The transducer is placed at the ventricular apex to obtain the two-chamber *(blue outline)* and four-chamber *(green outline)* views, each of which is about a 60-degree rotation from the long axis view and perpendicular to the short axis view. The four-chamber view includes both ventricles and both atria. The two-chamber view includes the left ventricle and left atrium; sometimes the atrial appendage is visualized. (From Otto CM. *Textbook of Clinical Echocardiography*, 4th ed. Philadelphia: Elsevier Saunders; 2009:32, Fig. 2-1.)

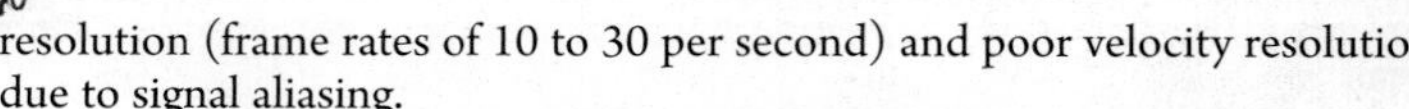

Measurements

Echocardiography provides accurate cardiac dimensions from two-dimensional or two-dimensional-guided linear depth (M-mode) recordings. The measurements typically provided include left ventricular (LV) end-diastolic and end-systolic internal dimensions, LV wall thickness, left atrial anterior-posterior diameter, and aortic sinus dimension. LV ejection fraction (EF) is determined by visual estimation or, more accurately, by tracing the endocardial borders at end diastole and end systole in two orthogonal views. End-diastolic and end-systolic ventricular volumes (EDV and ESV, respectively) are calculated using validated formulas, and the EF is determined as follows:

$$EF = (EDV - ESV)/EDV$$

Limitations

Echocardiography is a very accurate, widely available, and widely used imaging approach. However, the quality of images can be suboptimal because of poor tissue penetration (e.g., excessive adipose tissue, position of the lungs relative to the heart), although images are nondiagnostic in fewer than 5% of patients with current instrumentation. Reflections are stronger when the interface is perpendicular to the ultrasound beam, so structures that are parallel to the beam may not be visible, an artifact called *echo dropout*. This potential limitation may be avoided by the use of appropriate imaging planes and the integration of data from multiple transducer positions. Ultrasound artifacts, such as beam width, shadowing, and reverberations, may be misinterpreted by inexperienced observers.

DOPPLER ECHOCARDIOGRAPHY

Principles

Ultrasound energy that is backscattered from moving red blood cells is shifted to a higher frequency when the blood is moving toward the transducer and a lower frequency when it is moving away. The magnitude of this Doppler shift corresponds to the velocity of blood flow.

Modalities

Pulsed Doppler allows measurement of flow velocity at a specific intracardiac site with the advantages of high spatial and temporal resolution. However, spatial localization is based on intermittent sampling at a time interval corresponding to the depth of interest. The sampling frequency, which is depth dependent, limits the maximum detectable velocity because of a phenomenon called *signal aliasing*. Normal intracardiac flow velocities are about 1 m/second, which can usually be recorded with pulsed Doppler.

Continuous-wave Doppler allows measurement of high velocities along the entire length of the ultrasound beam, but the origin of the high-velocity signal must be inferred from the two-dimensional images. With stenotic and regurgitant valves, blood flow velocities may be as high as 5 to 6 m/second, requiring the use of the continuous-wave Doppler mode. Both pulsed and continuous-wave Doppler velocities are displayed as a graph of velocity versus time, with the density of the spectral display corresponding to signal strength.

Color flow Doppler imaging is a modification of pulsed Doppler in which the flow velocity is displayed across a two-dimensional image using a color scale to indicate direction and velocity. The advantage is a visually appealing display of intracardiac flow patterns. Disadvantages are low temporal resolution (frame rates of 10 to 30 per second) and poor velocity resolution due to signal aliasing.

Tissue Doppler uses the Doppler principle to record the velocity of motion of the myocardial wall. Tissue Doppler recordings of the myocardium adjacent to the mitral annulus are used to evaluate diastolic ventricular function.

Measurements

A standard echocardiographic study includes pulsed Doppler measurement of antegrade flow velocities (transmitral and transaortic) and evaluation for valve regurgitation using continuous-wave and color Doppler modalities. Other Doppler measurements depend on the specific clinical indication.

Quantitative measurements using Doppler data are derived from two basic concepts: volume flow rate and the pressure-velocity relationship. Stroke volume (in cubic centimeters) can be calculated as the volume of a cylinder, where the base is the spatial cross-sectional area (CSA, in square centimeters) of flow, determined as the area of a circle from a two-dimensional diameter measurement. The height of the cylinder is the distance the average blood cell travels in one cardiac cycle, which is the velocity time integral (VTI, in centimeters) of flow. Therefore,

$$SV\,(cm^3) = CSA\,(cm^2) \times VTI\,(cm)$$

This approach has been validated for measurement of transaortic, transmitral, and transpulmonic flow. Measurement of volume flow rate at two different intracardiac sites allows quantitation of intracardiac shunts and valvular regurgitation.

The relationship between the pressure gradient (ΔP) across a narrowing and the velocity (v) of blood flow is described by the simplified Bernoulli equation:

$$\Delta P = 4v^2$$

This equation allows calculation of maximum and mean gradients across stenotic valves, estimation of pulmonary systolic pressure, and detailed evaluation of intracardiac hemodynamics with regurgitant valves.

ECHOCARDIOGRAPHIC APPROACHES

Several echocardiographic modalities are in clinical use. If it is unclear which modality is optimum in a specific clinical setting, consultation with the echocardiographer is appropriate.

Transthoracic echocardiography (TTE) is the standard clinical approach in most patients with suspected or known cardiac disease. Advantages are that it is noninvasive, has no known adverse effects, and provides detailed data on cardiac anatomy and physiology. Limitations include poor image quality in some patients, limited visualization of structures distant from the transducer (e.g., atrial septum, left atrial appendage), and the inability to visualize structures immediately distal to prosthetic heart valves (acoustic shadowing).

Transesophageal echocardiography (TEE) offers superior image quality because of a shorter distance between the transducer and the heart, the absence of interposed bone or lung, and the use of a higher-frequency transducer. TEE usually is well tolerated, but intubation of the esophagus entails some risk, and most clinicians do this procedure with the patient under conscious sedation. TEE is much more sensitive than TTE for detection of left atrial thrombus (95% vs. 50%), valvular vegetations (99% vs. 60%), and prosthetic mitral valve regurgitation (Fig. 55-2).

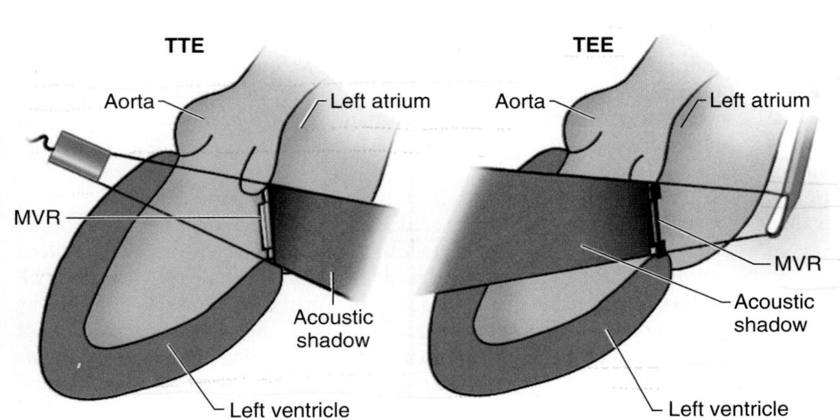

FIGURE 55-2. The problem of acoustic shadowing from a prosthetic mitral valve replacement (MVR). On the left, with transthoracic echocardiography (TTE), the acoustic shadow distal to the prosthetic valve obscures the left atrium, limiting assessment of valve regurgitation by Doppler techniques. On the right, with transesophageal echocardiography (TEE), the left atrium now can be evaluated for valvular regurgitation. However, the acoustic shadow now obscures the left ventricle. (From Otto CM. *Textbook of Clinical Echocardiography,* 4th ed. Philadelphia: Elsevier Saunders; 2009:117, Fig. 5-9.)

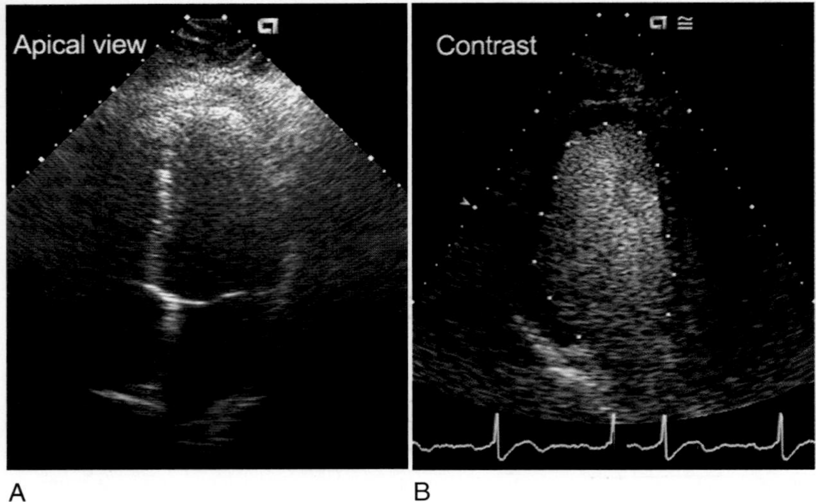

FIGURE 55-3. Poor-quality apical view (A) with marked improvement in definition of the left ventricular cavity after opacification using contrast echocardiography (B). The *dots* indicate the left ventricular endocardial tracing for calculation of ejection fraction.

Handheld echocardiography refers to the use of smaller, less expensive ultrasound systems that can be carried by the physician, who can perform quick, limited examinations in the office or at the bedside. These laptop-sized echocardiography units range from the very simple, with only two-dimensional imaging and limited controls, to systems with high-quality imaging and all Doppler modalities. Handheld echocardiography does not replace a complete imaging study but can serve as an adjunct to the physical examination, particularly in the acute care setting, such as to distinguish ventricular dilation from a pericardial effusion or to estimate ventricular systolic performance.

Contrast echocardiography may be performed using intravenous injection of agitated saline to opacify the right-sided heart chambers. These microbubbles are relatively large and do not pass through pulmonary capillaries. Therefore, appearance of contrast in the left side of the heart within one or two beats after right heart opacification is consistent with an intracardiac shunt. Although most atrial-level shunts are predominantly left-to-right shunts, a small amount of right-to-left shunting occurs, which is the basis of this approach.

Contrast echocardiography also may be performed with commercially available microbubbles in the range of 1 to 5 μm. Because these microbubbles are smaller than the pulmonary capillaries, right heart opacification is followed by left heart opacification, which can enhance the evaluation of systolic function when image quality is suboptimal, especially during stress echocardiography (Fig. 55-3).

Three-dimensional echocardiography is increasingly available and is useful in some clinical settings, particularly for the evaluation of complex structural heart disease and for transcatheter interventions (Fig. 55-4).

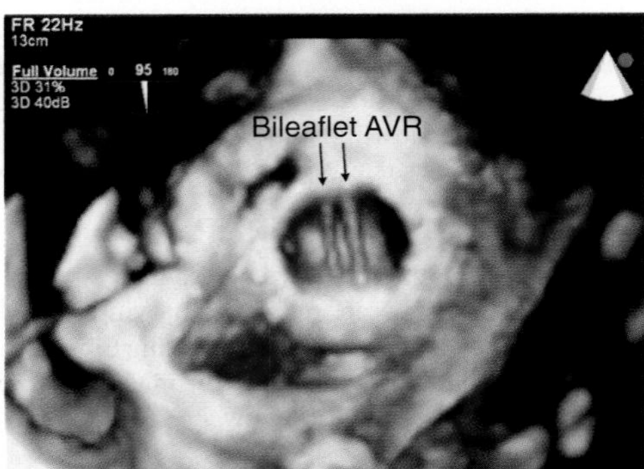

FIGURE 55-4. Real-time three-dimensional transesophageal echocardiographic imaging of a bileaflet aortic valve replacement (AVR) with the leaflets open during systole. The three-dimensional data set was cropped and rotated so that the viewer is looking at the valve from the aortic side. (From Otto CM. *Textbook of Clinical Echocardiography,* 4th ed. Philadelphia: Elsevier Saunders; 2009:91, Fig. 4-3.)

Stress echocardiography is a standard approach for evaluating patients with known or suspected coronary artery disease; it has a sensitivity (85 to 95%) and a specificity (80 to 90%) similar to those of radionuclide stress imaging (Chapters 56 and 71). Myocardial infarction results in thinning and akinesis of the affected wall. However, in the absence of infarction, resting myocardial function is normal, even when severe epicardial coronary disease is present. The increased myocardial demand associated with exercise or pharmacologic stress leads to myocardial ischemia, which results in a regional wall motion abnormality, often before the onset of chest pain or electrocardiographic changes (Fig. 55-5).

In patients who can exercise, standard views of the left ventricle are recorded at baseline and immediately after maximal treadmill or bicycle exercise. If endocardial definition is suboptimal, left-sided contrast is used. The rest and exercise images are compared in a side-by-side cine loop format. Myocardial ischemia is present if resting wall motion is normal but hypokinesis or akinesis is seen after exercise. The pattern of regional wall motion accurately identifies the area of myocardium at risk and is reasonably reliable for identification of the affected coronary artery. With three-vessel coronary disease, rather than a regional wall motion abnormality, the only clue on imaging may be an absence of the expected decrease in chamber size at peak exercise, caused by diffuse ischemia. Interpretation of an exercise echocardiogram includes exercise duration, hemodynamic response, symptoms, and electrocardiographic changes, in addition to the echocardiographic images (see Fig. 55-5).

In patients who are unable to exercise, stress testing is performed using a graded intravenous infusion of dobutamine, beginning at 5 to 10 μg/kg/minute and increasing every 3 minutes to a maximum dose of 40 μg/kg/minute. If needed, atropine is used to achieve 85% of the maximum predicted heart rate. In addition to evaluation for myocardial ischemia, dobutamine stress echocardiography can assess myocardial viability in areas of stunning or hibernation, based on an improvement in endocardial motion from baseline to low-dose dobutamine, with subsequent worsening of function at higher doses—the "biphasic" response.

Intracardiac echocardiography (ICE) is performed using an ultrasound probe on a catheter that is inserted into the right side of the heart through the femoral vein. ICE is used in the cardiac catheterization laboratory to guide percutaneous closure of a patent foramen ovale (PFO) and other procedures. In the electrophysiology laboratory, ICE helps guide catheter positioning and identify complications.

CARDIAC FUNCTION MEASUREMENTS

In addition to qualitative descriptions of cardiac anatomy and physiology, echocardiography provides precise and accurate quantitation of cardiac function, including ventricular systolic and diastolic function, an estimate of the severity of valve stenosis and regurgitation, and a noninvasive estimate of pulmonary pressures.

Systolic Ventricular Function

Overall LV systolic function is graded by visual estimation, with an approximate correspondence to EF as follows: normal (EF > 55%), mildly reduced (EF, 40 to 55%), moderately reduced (EF, 20 to 40%), severely reduced (EF < 20%). More precise quantitation is performed when clinically indicated by calculation of a biplane ejection fraction. Cardiac output calculations are not routine but may be helpful for noninvasive monitoring of therapy in patients with heart failure. Because EF measurements are affected by preload and afterload, measures that are less dependent on loading conditions, including

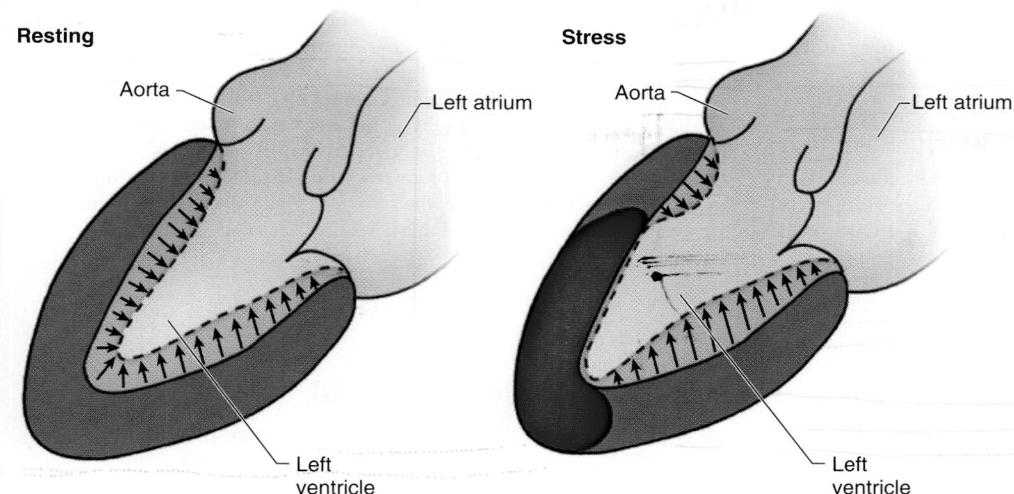

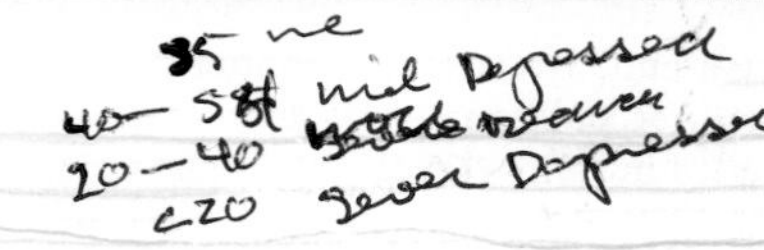

FIGURE 55-5. The concept of stress echocardiography in a patient with 70% stenosis in the proximal third of the left anterior descending (LAD) coronary artery. At rest *(left)*, endocardial motion and wall thickening are normal. After stress *(right)*, either exercise or pharmacologic, the middle and apical segments of the anterior wall become ischemic, showing reduced endocardial wall motion and wall thickening. If the LAD extends around the apex, the apical segment of the posterior wall also will be affected, as shown here. The normal segment of the posterior wall shows compensatory hyperkinesis. (From Otto CM. *Textbook of Clinical Echocardiography,* 4th ed. Philadelphia: Elsevier Saunders; 2009:191, Fig. 8-9.)

the end-systolic dimension or volume, are generally preferred for clinical decision making in situations such as the timing of surgery for chronic valvular regurgitation.

Diastolic Ventricular Function

Evaluation of diastolic ventricular function is challenging because the patterns of ventricular filling are affected by preload, heart rate, and coexisting valvular regurgitation in addition to the diastolic properties of the ventricle. However, echocardiography can classify diastolic function based on the combination of LV inflow, pulmonary vein flow, tissue Doppler velocities, and the isovolumic relaxation time. An estimate of LV filling pressure (e.g., LV end-diastolic pressure) also can be inferred using these approaches.

Valvular Stenosis

Echocardiography is the clinical standard for evaluation of aortic valvular heart disease (see Fig. 75-1). Cardiac catheterization can be reserved for cases in which echocardiography is nondiagnostic, clinical data are discrepant with echocardiographic findings, or coronary anatomy needs to be assessed (Chapter 75).

In patients with aortic stenosis, the most direct measure of stenosis severity is the antegrade velocity across the valve, indicating mild (<3 m/second), moderate (3 to 4 m/second), or severe (>4 m/second) valve obstruction. The maximum and mean transaortic pressure gradients also can be calculated using the Bernoulli equation. Accurate evaluation depends on a careful examination by an experienced echocardiographer.

Aortic valve area (AVA) is calculated using the continuity equation, based on the concept that volume flow rates proximal to and within the narrowed orifice are equal:

$$AVA \times VTI_{AS} = CSA_{LVOT} \times VTI_{LVOT}$$

or

$$AVA = (CSA_{LVOT} \times VTI_{LVOT})/VTI_{AS}$$

where LVOT = left ventricular outflow tract, VTI = velocity time integral, CSA = cross-sectional area, and AS = aortic stenosis (Fig. 55-6). It is especially important to calculate the AVA when LV systolic dysfunction accompanies aortic valve disease. In some patients, dobutamine stress echocardiography is helpful in distinguishing ventricular dysfunction caused by severe aortic stenosis from primary myocardial disease with concurrent moderate stenosis.

The evaluation of mitral stenosis (see Fig. 75-3) includes measurement of the mean transmitral gradient from the velocity curve and calculation of the valve area, both from two-dimensional planimetry of a short-axis image of the orifice and from the deceleration slope of the Doppler curve (pressure half-time method).

Valvular Regurgitation

The current approach to evaluating valvular regurgitation is based on the proximal geometry of the regurgitant jet, with measurement of the narrowest jet width (vena contracta; see Fig. 75-5). When further quantitation is

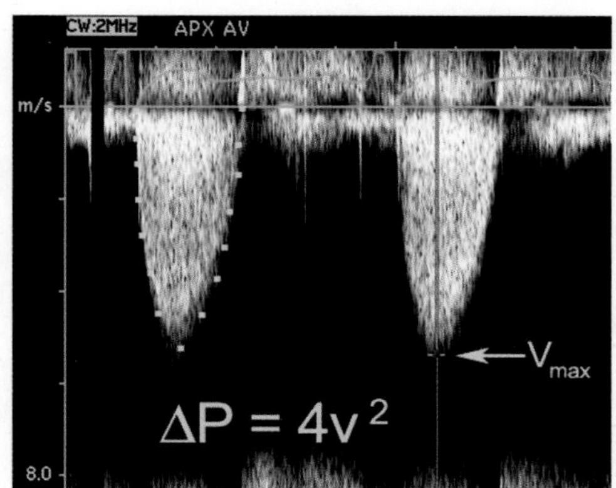

FIGURE 55-6. In a patient with aortic stenosis, the aortic jet velocity is recorded with continuous wave Doppler from the window that yields the highest velocity signal. Maximum velocity (V_{max}) is used to calculate the maximum systolic gradient. The Doppler curve is traced, as shown, to calculate the mean systolic gradient, using the Bernoulli equation, by which the pressure gradient (ΔP) equals four times the square of the velocity.

needed, regurgitant volume (RV), regurgitant fraction (RF), and regurgitant orifice area (ROA) are calculated. Although color flow visualization of the flow disturbance may be helpful for detection of regurgitation and for understanding the mechanism of valve dysfunction, this approach should no longer be used to evaluate severity.

For aortic regurgitation, a narrow vena contracta (<3 mm) indicates mild regurgitation, whereas a wide vena contracta (>6 mm) indicates severe regurgitation. Additional evaluation of the severity of aortic regurgitation is based on the presence of holodiastolic flow reversal in the abdominal aorta and the density and slope of the continuous wave Doppler velocity curve. The approach to evaluating mitral regurgitation (see Fig. 75-5) is similar, beginning with measurement of the vena contracta. In addition to calculation based on transmitral versus transaortic volume flow rates, the proximal acceleration of flow into the regurgitant orifice allows evaluation with central regurgitant jets. Color flow shows a proximal isovelocity surface area (PISA).

Pulmonary Pressures

Estimation of pulmonary artery systolic pressure (PAP) is a standard component of a complete examination. The systolic pressure difference between the right ventricle and right atrium is calculated from the peak velocity in the tricuspid regurgitant (V_{TR}) jet, using the Bernoulli equation. Then, the right atrial pressure (RAP) is estimated from the size and appearance of the inferior vena cava. Because right ventricular and pulmonary artery systolic pressures are equal (in the absence of pulmonic stenosis),

$$PAP = 4(V_{TR})^2 + RAP$$

A small amount of tricuspid regurgitation is present in most patients, so pulmonary pressures can be estimated with this approach in more than 90%

of patients. Because this approach measures only pulmonary systolic pressure, not pulmonary vascular resistance, invasive evaluation may still be needed in some clinical situations (Chapter 68).

THE ECHOCARDIOGRAPHIC EXAMINATION

Clinical Indications

Echocardiography is an effective approach to the initial evaluation of many cardiac signs and symptoms (Table 55-1). Even when transesophageal imaging might be helpful, most clinicians begin with a transthoracic examination; exceptions are for the patient with a possible acute aortic dissection (Chapter 78), in whom TEE should be performed as quickly as possible, and in the evaluation of possible left atrial thrombosis before cardioversion without anticoagulation (Chapter 64). It is important to remember that resting echocardiography is not helpful for diagnosis of coronary artery disease; stress imaging is needed if this diagnosis is suspected (Chapter 71). In patients with known cardiac disease, echocardiography is used to evaluate severity, assess the results of medical and surgical interventions, and guide procedures (Table 55-2).

TABLE 55-1 COMMON SYMPTOMS AND SIGNS EVALUATED BY ECHOCARDIOGRAPHY

REASON FOR ECHOCARDIOGRAPHY	POSSIBLE ECHOCARDIOGRAPHIC FINDINGS OR DIAGNOSIS
Chest pain	Coronary artery disease Acute myocardial infarction on resting echocardiography Stress echocardiography needed to detect coronary disease Aortic dissection Pericarditis Valvular aortic stenosis Hypertrophic cardiomyopathy
Heart failure	Left ventricular systolic dysfunction (global or segmental) Valvular heart disease Left ventricular diastolic dysfunction Pericardial disease Right ventricular dysfunction
Palpitations	Left ventricular systolic dysfunction Mitral valve disease Congenital heart disease (e.g., ASD, Ebstein's anomaly) Pericarditis No structural cardiac disease
Cardiac murmur Systolic	Flow murmur (no valve abnormality) Aortic stenosis—valvular or subaortic Hypertrophic cardiomyopathy Mitral regurgitation Ventricular septal defect Pulmonic stenosis Tricuspid regurgitation
Diastolic	Mitral stenosis Aortic regurgitation Pulmonic regurgitation Tricuspid stenosis
Cardiomegaly on chest radiography	Pericardial effusion Dilated cardiomyopathy Specific chamber enlargement (e.g., left ventricle in chronic aortic regurgitation)
Systemic embolic event	Left ventricular systolic function and segmental wall motion abnormalities (aneurysms) Left ventricular thrombus Aortic valve disease Mitral valve disease Left atrial thrombus (TTE has low sensitivity, TEE required) Atrial septal defect or patent foramen ovale

ASD = atrial septal defect; TEE = transesophageal echocardiography; TTE = transthoracic echocardiography.
From Otto CM. *Textbook of Clinical Echocardiography*, 4th ed. Philadelphia: Elsevier Saunders; 2009:114-115, Tables 5-1 and 5-2.

TABLE 55-2 INDICATIONS FOR ECHOCARDIOGRAPHY BY KNOWN DIAGNOSIS

CLINICAL DIAGNOSIS	KEY ECHOCARDIOGRAPHIC FINDINGS	LIMITATIONS OF ECHOCARDIOGRAPHY	ALTERNATIVE APPROACHES
VALVULAR HEART DISEASE (CHAPTER 75)			
Valve stenosis	Etiology of stenosis, valve anatomy Transvalvular ΔP, valve area Chamber enlargement and hypertrophy LV and RV systolic function Associated valvular regurgitation	Possible underestimation of the severity of stenosis Possible coexisting coronary artery disease	Cardiac catheterization; MRI
Valve regurgitation	Mechanism and etiology of regurgitation Severity of regurgitation Chamber enlargement LV and RV systolic function PA pressure estimate	TEE may be needed to evaluate mitral regurgitant severity and valve anatomy (especially before MV repair)	Cardiac catheterization; MRI
Prosthetic valve function	Evidence for stenosis Detection of regurgitation Chamber enlargement Ventricular function PA pressure estimate	Imaging of prosthetic valves is limited by shadowing and reverberations TEE is needed for suspected prosthetic MR due to "masking" of the LA on TTE	Cardiac catheterization
Endocarditis (Chapter 76)	Detection of vegetations (TTE sensitivity 70-85%) Presence and degree of valve dysfunction Chamber enlargement and function Detection of abscess Possible prognostic implications	TEE more sensitive for detection of vegetations (>90%) A definite diagnosis of endocarditis also depends on bacteriologic criteria TEE more sensitive for detecting an abscess	Blood cultures and clinical findings also are diagnostic criteria for endocarditis

TABLE 55-2 INDICATIONS FOR ECHOCARDIOGRAPHY BY KNOWN DIAGNOSIS—cont'd

CLINICAL DIAGNOSIS	KEY ECHOCARDIOGRAPHIC FINDINGS	LIMITATIONS OF ECHOCARDIOGRAPHY	ALTERNATIVE APPROACHES
CORONARY ARTERY DISEASE			
Acute myocardial infarction (Chapters 72 and 73)	Segmental wall motion abnormality reflects "myocardium at risk" Global LV function (EF) Complications: Acute MR vs. VSD Pericarditis LV thrombus, aneurysm RV infarct	Coronary artery anatomy itself is not directly visualized	Coronary angiography Radionuclide LV angiography Cardiac catheterization
Angina (Chapter 71)	Global and segmental LV systolic function Exclude other causes of angina (e.g., AS, HOCM)	Resting wall motion may be normal despite significant CAD Stress echocardiography is needed to induce ischemia and wall motion abnormality	Coronary angiography Stress thallium ETT
Pre-revascularization/ post-revascularization	Assess wall thickening and endocardial motion at baseline Improvement in segmental function after procedure	Dobutamine stress and/or contrast echocardiography is needed to detect viable but nonfunctioning myocardium	MRI PET Thallium ETT Contrast echocardiography
End-stage ischemic disease	Overall LV systolic function (EF) PA pressures Associated MR LV thrombus RV systolic function	—	Coronary angiography Radionuclide EF
CARDIOMYOPATHY (CHAPTERS 58-60)			
Dilated	Chamber dilation (all four) LV and RV systolic function (qualitative and EF) Coexisting atrioventricular valve regurgitation PA systolic pressure LV thrombus	Indirect measures of LVEDP Accurate EF may be difficult if image quality is poor	Radionuclide EF LV and RV angiography
Restrictive	LV wall thickness LV systolic function LV diastolic function PA systolic pressure	Must be distinguished from constrictive pericarditis	Cardiac catheterization with direct, simultaneous RV and LV pressure measurement after volume loading
Hypertrophic	Pattern and extent of LV hypertrophy Dynamic LVOT obstruction (imaging and Doppler) Coexisting MR Diastolic LV dysfunction	—	—
Hypertension (Chapter 67)	LV wall thickness and chamber dimensions LV mass LV systolic function Aortic root dilation	—	—
PERICARDIAL DISEASE (CHAPTER 77)			
	Pericardial thickening Detection, size, and location of PE 2D signs of tamponade physiology Doppler signs of tamponade physiology	Diagnosis of tamponade is a hemodynamic and clinical diagnosis Constrictive pericarditis is a difficult diagnosis Not all patients with pericarditis have an effusion	Intracardiac pressure measurements for tamponade or constriction MRI or CT to detect pericardial thickening
DISEASES OF THE AORTA (CHAPTER 78)			
Aortic root dilation	Etiology of aortic dilation Accurate aortic root diameter measurements Anatomy of sinuses of Valsalva (especially Marfan syndrome) Associated aortic regurgitation	—	CT, MRI, aortography
Aortic dissection	2D images of ascending aorta, aortic arch, descending thoracic and proximal abdominal aorta Imaging of dissection "flap" Associated aortic regurgitation Ventricular function	TEE more sensitive (97%) and more specific (100%) Cannot assess distal vascular beds	Aortography CT MRI TEE
CARDIAC MASSES (CHAPTER 60)			
LV thrombus	High sensitivity and specificity for diagnosis of LV thrombus Suspect with apical wall motion abnormality or diffuse LV systolic dysfunction	Technical artifacts can be misleading 5-MHz or higher frequency transducer and angulated apical views needed TEE is needed to detect LA thrombus reliably	LV thrombus may not be recognized on radionuclide or contrast angiography
LA thrombus	Low sensitivity for detection of LA thrombus, although specificity is high Suspect with LA enlargement, MV disease	—	TEE

TABLE 55-2 INDICATIONS FOR ECHOCARDIOGRAPHY BY KNOWN DIAGNOSIS—cont'd

CLINICAL DIAGNOSIS	KEY ECHOCARDIOGRAPHIC FINDINGS	LIMITATIONS OF ECHOCARDIOGRAPHY	ALTERNATIVE APPROACHES
Cardiac tumors	Size, location, and physiologic consequences of tumor mass	Extracardiac involvement is not well seen Cannot distinguish benign from malignant tumor or tumor from thrombus	TEE CT MRI (with cardiac gating) Intracardiac echocardiography
PULMONARY HYPERTENSION (CHAPTER 68)			
	Estimate of PA pressure Evidence of left-sided heart disease to account for increased PA pressures RV size and systolic function (cor pulmonale) Associated TR	Indirect PA pressure measurement Cannot determine pulmonary vascular resistance accurately	Cardiac catheterization
CONGENITAL HEART DISEASE (CHAPTER 69)			
	Detection and assessment of anatomic abnormalities Quantitation of physiologic abnormalities Chamber enlargement Ventricular function	No direct intracardiac pressure measurements Complicated anatomy may be difficult to evaluate if image quality is poor (TEE is helpful)	MRI with 3D reconstruction Cardiac catheterization TEE

2D = two-dimensional; 3D = three-dimensional; AS = aortic stenosis; CAD = coronary artery disease; CT = computed tomography; EF = ejection fraction; ETT = exercise treadmill test; HCM = hypertrophic cardiomyopathy; LA = left atrial; LV = left ventricular; LVEDP = left ventricular end-diastolic pressure; LVOT = left ventricular outflow tract; MR = mitral regurgitation; MRI = magnetic resonance imaging; MV = mitral valve; ΔP = pressure gradient; PA = pulmonary artery; PE = pericardial effusion; PET = positron emission tomography; RV = right ventricular; TEE = transesophageal echocardiography; TR = tricuspid regurgitation; TTE = transthoracic echocardiography; VSD = ventricular septal defect.
From Otto CM. *Textbook of Clinical Echocardiography*, 4th ed. Philadelphia: Elsevier Saunders; 2009:475-478.

Normal Findings

Trace to mild regurgitation is considered "physiologic" and is seen with 70 to 80% of mitral valves, 80 to 90% of tricuspid valves, and 70 to 80% of pulmonic valves in normal individuals. The prevalence of aortic regurgitation increases with age, but it is found in only 5% of young normal adults; the presence of aortic regurgitation raises the possibility of subtle aortic valve or root abnormalities.

A PFO (Chapter 69) is present in 25 to 35% of normal individuals and may be identified by color Doppler or by contrast echocardiography. Use of the Valsalva maneuver enhances identification of a PFO because the slight elevation in right atrial pressure may lead to a brief right-to-left shunt. The significance of a PFO in patients without clinical events is unclear. Other common anatomic variants seen on echocardiography include aberrant chords (or "webs") in the left ventricle; small, linear, mobile echoes associated with the valves (Lambl's excrescences); and normal ridges in the left and right atrium.

Unexpected abnormal findings also may be found on studies requested for other indications. A bicuspid aortic valve is present in 1 to 2% of the population; most of these patients are asymptomatic until late in life, so many cases are diagnosed "incidentally" by echocardiography. Aortic valve sclerosis, which is a frequent unexpected echocardiographic diagnosis, is a marker of cardiovascular disease and an increased risk of myocardial infarction even if valve function is normal.

INTEGRATING THE ECHOCARDIOGRAPHIC AND CLINICAL FINDINGS

The echocardiographic request should indicate the specific reason for the study and any relevant symptoms or signs. The echocardiographic examination then can be tailored to answer the clinical question. The echocardiographic results should be interpreted in conjunction with other clinical data. If the echocardiographic data seem discrepant with the clinical data, the requesting physician should review the images with the echocardiographer to identify areas of uncertainty and to determine the next best diagnostic step.

SUGGESTED READINGS

Melamed R, Sprenkle MD, Ulstad VK, et al. Assessment of left ventricular function by intensivists using hand-held echocardiography. *Chest.* 2009;135:1416-1420. *A small bedside diagnostic ultrasound imaging system can allow intensivists, after a short training period, to estimate left ventricular systolic function.*

Mitiku TY, Heidenreich PA. A small pericardial effusion is a marker of increased mortality. *Am Heart J.* 2011;161:152-157. *Even a small asymptomatic pericardial effusion is associated with a 17% increased mortality after adjustment for other clinical factors.*

Pepi M, Evangelista A, Nihoyannopoulos P, et al. Recommendations for echocardiography use in the diagnosis and management of cardiac sources of embolism: European Association of Echocardiography (EAE) (a registered branch of the ESC). *Eur J Echocardiogr.* 2010;11:461-476. *Consensus guidelines.*

56

NONINVASIVE CARDIAC IMAGING

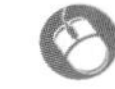

CHRISTOPHER M. KRAMER AND GEORGE A. BELLER

NUCLEAR CARDIOLOGY

The techniques of nuclear cardiology permit the noninvasive imaging of myocardial perfusion under stress and resting conditions and of resting regional and global function by use of radionuclide imaging agents and gamma or positron cameras with associated computer processing. All these techniques are based on acquiring images of radioactivity emanating from tracers localized in heart muscle or in the blood pools of the left and right ventricles. Myocardial perfusion imaging is the most commonly performed nuclear cardiology technique, most often in conjunction with either exercise or pharmacologic stress intended to produce flow heterogeneity between relatively hypoperfused and normally perfused myocardial regions. Radionuclide angiography, in which technetium-99m (^{99m}Tc)-labeled red blood cells or other ^{99m}Tc-labeled agents are injected intravenously, is used for measurement of left ventricular ejection fraction and assessment of regional wall motion, especially to monitor changes in global left ventricular function in patients undergoing chemotherapy with cardiac toxic drugs. Positron emission tomography (PET) can assess regional myocardial metabolism to estimate myocardial viability, most often with fluorine-18–labeled 2-deoxyglucose (FDG), as well as myocardial perfusion by use of rubidium-82 (^{82}Rb). Hybrid cameras with computed tomography (CT) permit multimodality imaging of coronary anatomy and physiologic perturbations in flow or myocardial function.

Myocardial Perfusion Imaging

Imaging Agents

For the assessment of myocardial perfusion, ^{99m}Tc-labeled perfusion agents, which provide higher-quality images more quickly, are used more commonly than thallium-201 (^{201}Tl) for exercise or pharmacologic stress perfusion imaging to evaluate patients with suspected or known coronary heart disease (CHD). Of the various ^{99m}Tc-labeled agents, ^{99m}Tc-sestamibi and ^{99m}Tc-tetrofosmin are the most common. These ^{99m}Tc agents permit simultaneous assessment of regional and global left ventricular function and volumes with gated single-photon emission computed tomography (SPECT) technology.

Some laboratories use dual-isotope rest ^{201}Tl/stress ^{99m}Tc-sestamibi imaging, in which patients undergo ^{201}Tl imaging at rest and then, immediately

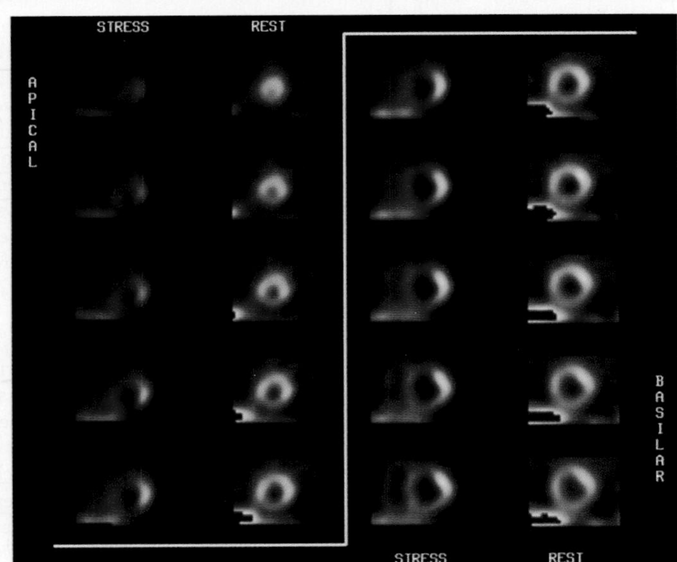

FIGURE 56-1. **Short-axis images showing a moderately large, reversible defect of the apex, anterior wall, and septum.** This defect is consistent with disease of the proximal left anterior descending coronary artery.

afterward, undergo ^{99m}Tc-sestamibi imaging during stress. Reversibility is identified by comparing the perfusion pattern on the stress ^{99m}Tc-sestamibi images with the pattern on the baseline resting ^{201}Tl images. The major advantage of this technique is the marked decrease in total imaging time, but the disadvantage is a substantially higher radiation dose. In patients with a low to intermediate pretest probability of CHD, a normal stress myocardial perfusion study obviates the need for a resting study, reducing both cost and radiation.

Detection of Coronary Heart Disease

The major indications for stress and rest myocardial perfusion imaging are to diagnose CHD, to assess prognosis, and to detect myocardial viability. Exercise or pharmacologic stress myocardial perfusion imaging in patients with chest pain yields a sensitivity for detecting CHD in the 85 to 90% range (Fig. 56-1). The specificity for excluding CHD is in the 85% range for ^{99m}Tc-sestamibi SPECT imaging and increases to 90% with gated SPECT. Exercise or pharmacologic stress SPECT perfusion imaging have sensitivities and specificities that are superior to those of exercise electrocardiogram (ECG) testing alone. The specificity of gated SPECT for detecting CHD with use of one of the ^{99m}Tc-labeled perfusion agents is 20 to 30% higher than that of ^{201}Tl SPECT in women.

Radionuclide stress perfusion imaging is of particular value compared with exercise ECG testing alone in (1) patients with resting ECG abnormalities, such as those seen with left ventricular hypertrophy, digitalis effect, Wolff-Parkinson-White syndrome, and intraventricular conduction abnormalities; and (2) patients who fail to achieve more than 85% of maximal predicted heart rate. Approximately 40% of patients with a low to intermediate pretest likelihood of CHD who manifest 1.0 mm or more of horizontal or downsloping ST segment depression have no evidence of CHD (false-positive findings). The addition of stress perfusion imaging can assist in differentiating true-positive from false-positive ST depression. Detection of proximal left anterior descending stenoses and proximal multivessel CHD is enhanced by identifying regional systolic thickening or wall motion abnormalities on the gated SPECT images compared with assessment based on perfusion alone. If possible, drugs such as long-acting nitrates, β-blockers, and rate-lowering calcium blockers should be discontinued for 24 hours before exercise stress testing that is performed to diagnose or to exclude CHD as the cause of chest pain.

Pharmacologic Stress Imaging

In patients who are unable to exercise to adequate heart rates and workloads on exercise stress testing protocols, pharmacologic stress testing with use of vasodilators (e.g., dipyridamole), adenosine, regadenoson, or inotropic agents (e.g., dobutamine) is an alternative to exercise for detecting physiologically significant coronary artery stenoses. Sensitivity and specificity for CHD detection are comparable for dipyridamole and adenosine. The addition of limited exercise to dipyridamole or adenosine imaging can prevent the vasodilator-induced hypotension, improve the ECG detection of ischemia, and enhance image quality by increasing the heart-to-liver ratio of tracer uptake. Dobutamine stress is preferred in patients who have bronchospasm or a history of asthma or who have consumed caffeine, which is an adenosine receptor antagonist, within 12 hours before testing. Patients who experience side effects such as hypotension and chest pain during dipyridamole or adenosine infusion should be treated with intravenous aminophylline, an adenosine antagonist that immediately reverses these side effects. Regadenoson has fewer side effects than adenosine. PET myocardial perfusion imaging, which is performed only with vasodilator stress, has a higher specificity and better ability to detect multivessel disease than SPECT.

Assessment of Prognosis

The extent of hypoperfusion on post-stress SPECT perfusion images provides important incremental prognostic information when added to clinical characteristics, the resting left ventricular ejection fraction, exercise ECG stress test variables, and even coronary artery anatomy. Nondiabetic patients with chest pain and a normal myocardial perfusion scan at peak exercise or under vasodilator stress have a subsequent cardiac death or infarction rate of less than 1% per year and are generally appropriate candidates for medical therapy (Chapter 71) or require further diagnostic evaluation for a noncardiac cause of chest pain (Chapters 50 and 139). Conversely, patients with high-risk imaging results may benefit from early referral for invasive strategies, including coronary revascularization (Chapter 74), even if symptoms are mild. Patients who show inducible ischemia involving more than 20% of the left ventricular myocardium may have a better outcome with coronary revascularization compared with medical therapy.

Transient ischemic left ventricular cavity dilation, by which the left ventricular cavity appears more dilated on stress images compared with rest images, is a particularly high-risk finding on SPECT. This finding occurs when subendocardial ischemia after stress causes a decrease in tracer uptake in the subendocardium, thereby yielding what appears to be a larger left ventricular cavity than was observed on the resting images.

Patients with abnormal pharmacologic stress studies have a worse prognosis than patients with comparable defect patterns seen on exercise scans, perhaps because their inability to exercise is also a prognostic factor. Assessment of regional left ventricular function on post-stress gated SPECT images enhances the detection of three-vessel CHD. Exercise or pharmacologic stress perfusion imaging also provides useful prognostic information for predischarge risk stratification in clinically low- to intermediate-risk patients who have experienced an uncomplicated myocardial infarction or unstable angina. Demonstration of defects remote from the zone of infarction (which indicate underlying multivessel disease), evidence for residual ischemia within the infarct zone, or both identify patients with an increased risk of reinfarction and subsequent cardiac death.

Exercise or pharmacologic stress perfusion imaging is superior to exercise ECG testing alone for detection of coronary restenosis in patients presenting with recurrence of symptoms after a percutaneous coronary intervention (Chapter 74). Stress perfusion imaging also has proved useful for identifying high-risk asymptomatic patients who have undergone previous coronary artery bypass graft surgery (Chapter 74) and patients who have intermediate or nonevaluable stenoses on coronary angiography.

Determination of Myocardial Viability with Single-Photon Emission Computed Tomography or Positron Emission Tomography

SPECT perfusion imaging is performed in the resting state to identify residual myocardial viability in zones corresponding to severe regional wall motion abnormalities in patients with CHD and depressed left ventricular function. When severe left ventricular dysfunction is caused by "hibernation" (a state of chronic reduced contractility because of substantial ischemia), and not by irreversible myocardial necrosis, areas of resting hypoperfusion that are viable and contributing to hibernation show initial defects on early images but no or less severe defects on 3-hour delayed images. If uptake ultimately exceeds 50 or 60% of peak uptake in these regions, there is a high probability (65 to 75%) that regional myocardial function will improve after successful revascularization, compared with only a 10 to 20% probability for myocardial zones showing less than 50% of peak uptake on resting images.

Regional myocardial metabolism can be assessed noninvasively by PET with FDG and a flow tracer such as [^{13}N]ammonia or ^{82}Rb. FDG is a glucose analogue that is taken up initially in myocardial cells and is trapped by conversion to FDG-6-phosphate. FDG is cell membrane impermeable and remains within viable cells at high concentrations for more than 40 to 60 minutes. Increased FDG activity on clinical PET images in areas of diminished regional blood flow, as determined by [^{13}N]ammonia imaging, is characteristic of myocardial viability. These areas of blood flow/FDG mismatch usually show improved regional function after coronary revascularization. Regions of the heart that show both diminished perfusion and FDG uptake (a "match" pattern) represent predominantly nonviable myocardium, with only a 10 to 15% probability of showing improved systolic function after revascularization. Patients who have an ischemic cardiomyopathy with poor viability on either resting SPECT or PET have a worse outcome after coronary revascularization compared with patients with predominantly viable myocardium.

Imaging of Ventricular Function

Global and segmental left and right ventricular function can be evaluated accurately by gated cardiac blood pool imaging to provide a radionuclide angiogram or ventriculogram. The equilibrium radionuclide angiographic approach is performed after thorough mixing of ^{99m}Tc-labeled blood cells within the intravascular compartment. Because ^{99m}Tc remains within the blood pool, serial imaging studies can be acquired during several hours. Acquisition of the images is synchronized with the QRS complex on the ECG through a multigated approach by which each cardiac cycle is divided into multiple frames. A uniform diminution of left ventricular systolic function without segmental wall motion abnormalities suggests nonischemic dilated cardiomyopathy (Chapter 60), whereas depressed global left ventricular function associated with segmental wall motion abnormalities suggests ischemic heart disease.

CARDIAC COMPUTED TOMOGRAPHY

For CT, imaging with high spatial and temporal resolution and ECG gating during a breath-hold yields snapshots of the heart reconstructed from the same phase of the cardiac cycle. Multidetector computed tomography (MDCT), which has almost entirely replaced electron beam CT, can capture a three-dimensional image of the heart in one to two heartbeats on the latest generation scanners as well as provide coronary artery calcium scoring without the use of contrast and with only 1 to 3 millisievert (mSv) of radiation. MDCT coronary arteriography requires 60 to 100 mL of iodinated contrast and average radiation doses less than 5 mSv. However, without careful planning of the imaging approach, radiation doses on the order of 10 to 25 mSv have been reported on 64-detector scanners. β-Blockade is often used to achieve a heart rate of less than 60 beats per minute to optimize imaging, and irregular rhythms such as atrial fibrillation may diminish image quality.

Coronary Artery Calcium Scoring

Coronary calcium is an indicator of the burden of atherosclerotic plaque, and very high levels confer an increased risk of future cardiac events (Fig. 56-2). Calcium scores are generally calculated as an Agatston score, which corresponds to each coronary lesion's calcium area multiplied by the maximal CT attenuation value of that lesion, and then summed for the entire coronary tree. Calcium scores are age, gender, and race dependent and must be normalized by these factors. In a large prospective, population-based study, the coronary calcium score predicted coronary events independently of either standard risk factors or C-reactive protein and was a better predictor than the Framingham risk score. Calcium scores above 300 were associated with an increased risk of myocardial infarction and cardiac death at every risk level. The utility of calcium scoring is highest in intermediate-risk patients on the basis of Framingham risk data, and there is no evidence that a calcium score in otherwise low- or high-risk groups would change risk factor management. Importantly, there is no correlation between coronary calcium and the physiologic or anatomic significance of a stenosis. Consensus guidelines suggest that stress testing may be indicated in patients with high calcium scores (>300 to 400).

Computed Tomographic Coronary Angiography

MDCT is an excellent technique to diagnose anomalous coronary arterial anatomy in adults (Fig. 56-3). For detection of coronary artery disease, 64-detector scanners have consistently demonstrated sensitivities on a per-segment basis in the 95% range, specificities of 85 to 98%, positive-predictive values of 64 to 91%, and negative-predictive values of 99%. Thus, the technique appears to be an excellent way to exclude significant coronary artery disease (Fig. 56-4). Initial studies with 256- and 320-detector row scanners are even more promising. A limitation of the technique, however, is its lower specificity in heavily calcified vessels, which are more common in elderly patients. MDCT tends to overestimate the percentage of stenosis when compared with intravascular ultrasound. The accuracy for detecting stenoses in bypass grafts is quite high, although evaluation of native vessel coronary artery disease is limited in postbypass patients owing to extensive calcification and smaller size vessels. Stents less than 3 mm in diameter cannot be

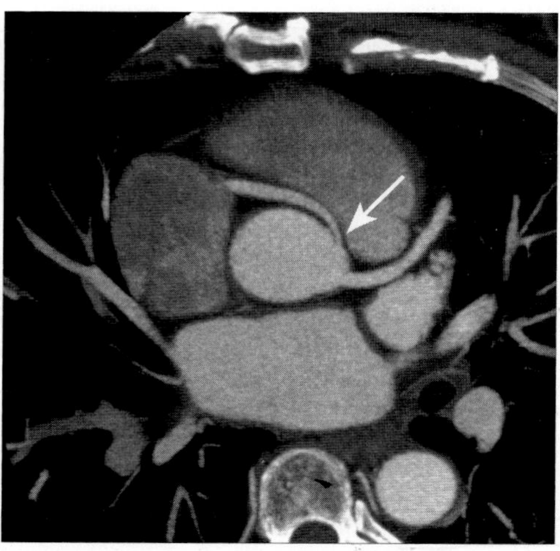

FIGURE 56-3. **Contrast-enhanced computed tomographic angiogram in a young patient with chest pain and an anomalous right coronary artery (RCA).** The RCA originates with a slit-like origin from the left coronary cusp *(arrow)* and passes anteriorly between the aorta and right ventricular outflow tract. The left main coronary artery originates normally from the left cusp.

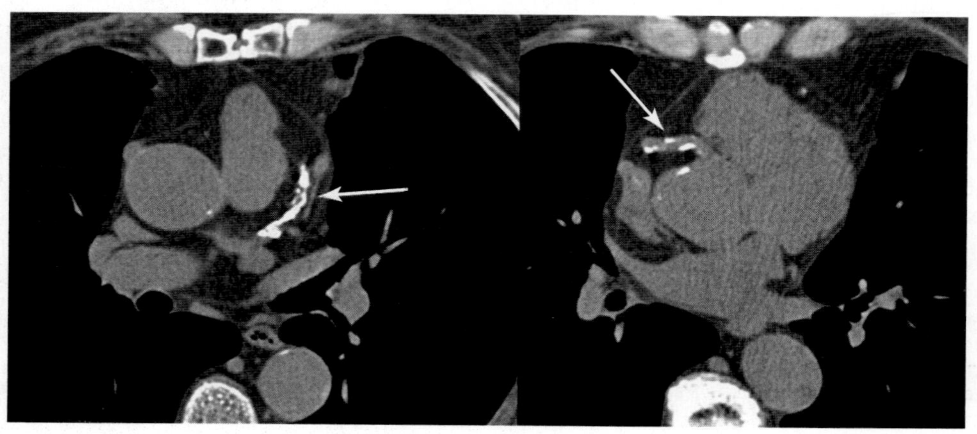

FIGURE 56-2. **Non–contrast-enhanced computed tomography axial slices through the heart at two locations for coronary calcium scoring as risk assessment in an asymptomatic patient.** On the *left,* the slice includes the left anterior descending artery with extensive calcification in its proximal portion *(arrow).* On the *right,* the slice includes the right coronary artery with proximal spotty calcification *(arrow).* This patient's calcium score was 457, putting him in a higher risk group regardless of his Framingham risk score.

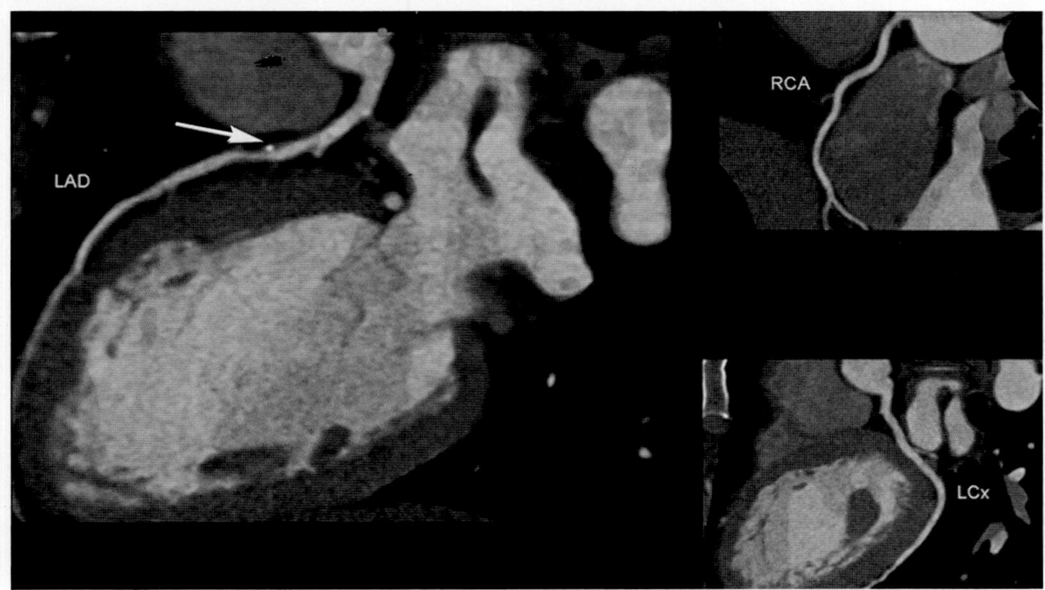

FIGURE 56-4. Contrast-enhanced computed tomographic coronary angiogram obtained on a dual source 64-detector scanner in a patient with atypical chest pain. The left anterior descending (LAD) artery has a nonobstructive lesion *(arrow)* containing both noncalcified (soft) plaque, which appears dark, and a focal area of calcification. The right coronary artery (RCA) and left circumflex coronary artery (LCx) are normal.

adequately evaluated by MDCT, although accuracy in larger stents is improving with the use of advanced postprocessing techniques.

MDCT coronary angiography is not recommended as a routine screening test, but it can be useful in selected situations, such as in low- or low-intermediate-risk patients who present to emergency departments with chest pain but without ECG changes or elevations of cardiac biomarkers (Chapter 50). The high negative-predictive value of MDCT often can exclude important CHD and avoid the need for other testing in this patient group. MDCT also may be useful in patients with equivocal or nondiagnostic stress testing or new-onset heart failure. The extent and severity of coronary disease found at CT coronary angiography correlate with subsequent all-cause mortality in a similar fashion to catheter-based coronary angiography.

Other Cardiac Applications

The same data acquired by MDCT for coronary artery imaging can be reformatted and used for functional cardiac imaging, including measurement of left ventricular volumes, ejection fraction, wall thickness, and global and segmental wall motion. In acute and chronic myocardial infarction, contrast-enhanced MDCT can demonstrate late enhancement in a manner similar to cardiovascular magnetic resonance imaging (CMR), albeit with a lower signal and contrast-to-noise ratio. MDCT also can complement echocardiography to evaluate cardiac anatomy in patients with congenital heart disease, especially in patients with contraindications to CMR. MDCT can evaluate pericardial thickness and calcification in patients with suspected constrictive pericarditis (see Fig. 77-10 in Chapter 77) and can evaluate native and prosthetic valvular structures and cardiac masses when imaging with other modalities is inadequate.

Cardiac CT is often used to image the left atrium and pulmonary venous anatomy for preprocedural planning for pulmonary vein ablations for atrial fibrillation (Chapter 66). Cardiac venous anatomy may be imaged to aid in the implantation of left ventricular pacemakers in the cardiac venous system for biventricular pacing for heart failure (Chapters 59 and 66).

CARDIOVASCULAR MAGNETIC RESONANCE IMAGING

Indications, Contraindications, and Pulse Sequences

CMR is a tremendously versatile and flexible imaging modality. CMR is typically performed on 1.5-Tesla (T) scanners, although problems with ECG gating and off-resonance effects previously encountered at higher field strength (3 T) have largely been overcome. Advantages of CMR include the lack of ionizing radiation, the variety of tissues that can be characterized, and the ability to image the heart in any arbitrary plane. Images typically are obtained using ECG gating and breath-hold techniques.

In addition to general restrictions regarding magnetic resonance (e.g., certain intracranial aneurysm clips, transcutaneous electrical nerve stimulation units, intra-auricular implants), patients with cardiac pacemakers and implantable cardioverter-defibrillators generally should *not* undergo CMR because of concern regarding reprogramming of the device, direct stimulation of the heart during gradient switching, or localized heating in the lead system. Newer pacemaker systems and defibrillator models may not be susceptible, but even in these cases, careful precautions must be taken, including close monitoring and device testing and reprogramming after the procedure. CMR is safe for all prosthetic heart valves, although image distortions immediately around the prosthesis will obscure nearby pathology. CMR is safe for patients with intracoronary stents, including at 3 T. Gadolinium-based contrast agents are now contraindicated in patients with a glomerular filtration rate of less than 30 mL/minute/1.83 m^2, owing to the recently identified complication of nephrogenic systemic fibrosis (Chapter 275) in a small subset of patients with severe chronic kidney disease, especially those on dialysis.

A comprehensive CMR study includes evaluation of cardiac structure, function, tissue characteristics, perfusion, and scarring or fibrosis. The components of the examination are tailored to the particular diagnostic question at hand.

Specific Clinical Applications

Coronary Disease

For detection of myocardial ischemia, gadolinium perfusion imaging during vasodilator stress with adenosine or regadenoson shows defects, generally in the subendocardium, that persist for at least 5 heartbeats during the first pass of contrast. Imaging is often repeated at rest after approximately 10 minutes to be sure any defect seen with stress was not either artifactual or due to an infarct (the latter is excluded in combination with late gadolinium enhancement). Head-to-head comparisons of vasodilator stress perfusion CMR and dobutamine stress CMR suggest a higher sensitivity for contrast-enhanced perfusion imaging and higher specificity for dobutamine wall motion imaging. MDCT has superior spatial resolution and accuracy compared with CMR for imaging of the coronary arteries. However, CMR coronary imaging is ideal for the diagnosis of anomalous coronary arteries.

CMR with late gadolinium enhancement is the gold standard technique for assessment of myocardial scar owing to myocardial infarction, with a better accuracy than nuclear imaging approaches, especially for smaller non–Q wave infarctions (Fig. 56-5). In acute myocardial infarction, CMR techniques assess the myocardium at risk and estimate the amount of salvaged myocardium owing to reperfusion. Areas of low signal in the subendocardial core of the infarction represent regions of microvascular obstruction with severe capillary destruction and are a marker of subsequent adverse left ventricular remodeling and poorer outcome.

Cardiomyopathies

CMR is increasingly used to identify the underlying etiology of cardiomyopathies and is the best test to diagnose arrhythmogenic right ventricular

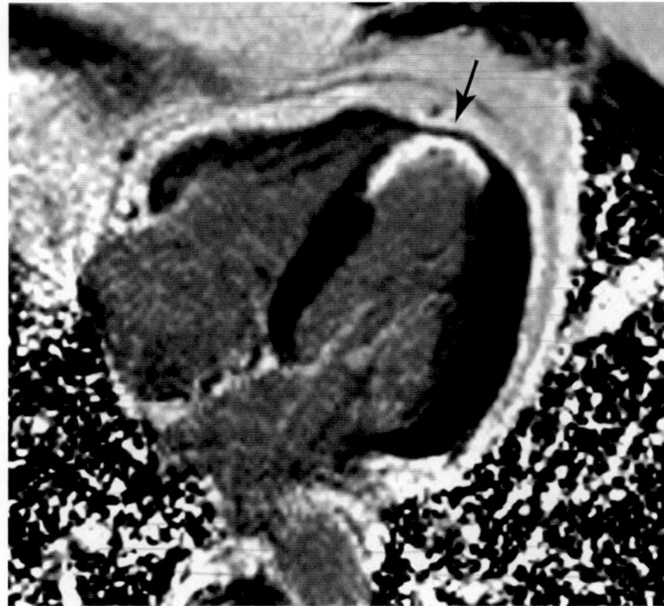

FIGURE 56-5. Late gadolinium-enhanced four-chamber long-axis image in a patient with a scar *(arrow)* from a prior anterior myocardial infarction.

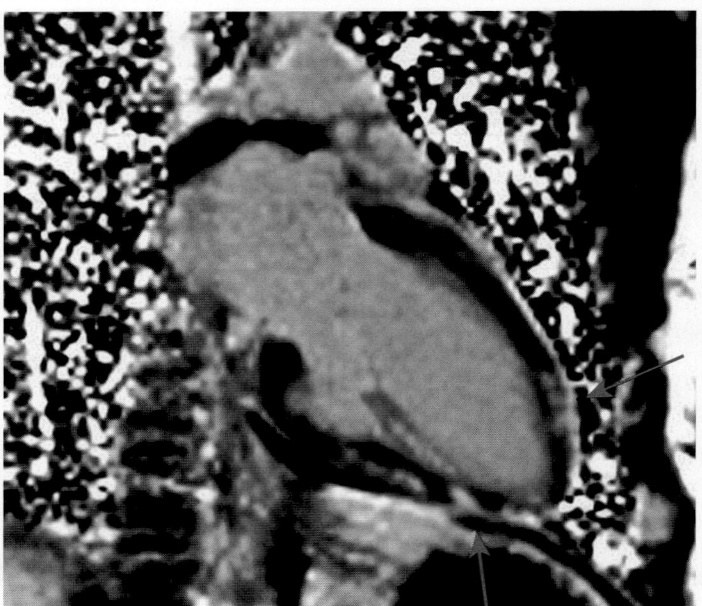

FIGURE 56-7. Gadolinium-enhanced image in a 22-year-old man shows patchy subepicardial enhancement *(arrows)*, characteristic of acute myocarditis.

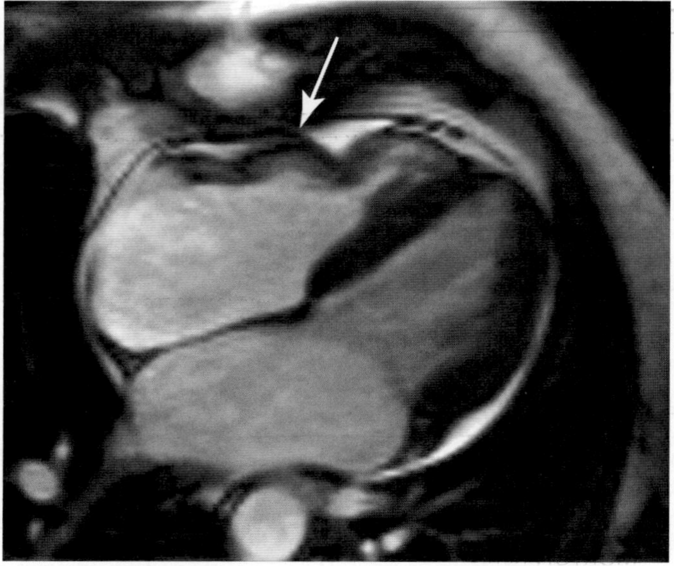

FIGURE 56-6. Magnetic resonance image in a 27-year-old woman with arrhythmogenic right ventricular cardiomyopathy demonstrates regional right ventricular (RV) systolic dysfunction, which is the hallmark of the disease. The *arrow* points to a region of RV dyskinesis at end systole, and the RV appears like an accordion at end systole.

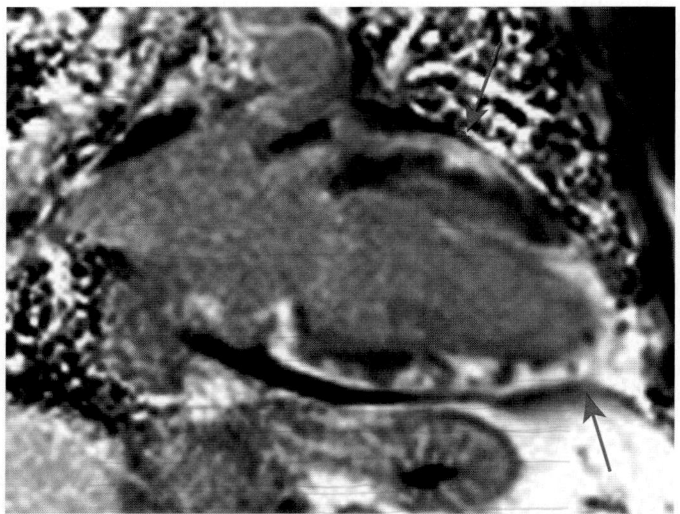

FIGURE 56-8. Late gadolinium-enhanced magnetic resonance image in a 47-year-old man with heart failure, heart block, and hilar lymphadenopathy shows patchy late gadolinium enhancement in a noncoronary distribution, including subepicardial anterior wall enhancement *(upper arrow)* and near transmural apical enhancement *(lower arrow)* consistent with myocardial sarcoidosis.

dysplasia (Fig. 56-6), which is associated with an increased risk of sudden death (Chapters 60 and 65). Arrhythmogenic right ventricular cardiomyopathy is characterized by regional or global right ventricular dilation and dysfunction. Late gadolinium enhancement may be seen but can be difficult to identify in the thin-walled right ventricle in this disease. Fat is a nonspecific finding.

In patients who present in acute heart failure or with chest pain, elevated troponins, but a negative coronary arteriogram, CMR is ideally suited to identify myocarditis (Chapter 60) noninvasively (Fig. 56-7), with changes most often in the basal lateral wall pattern seen as chronic midwall enhancement, which is a poor prognostic marker in the setting of dilated cardiomyopathy. CMR is more sensitive than echocardiography to measure regional wall thickness and left ventricular outflow tract gradients in patients with hypertrophic cardiomyopathy (Chapter 60). Cardiac amyloidosis (Chapters 60 and 194) can be seen as diffuse subendocardial enhancement, patchy enhancement, or simply difficulty in nulling normal myocardium. Patchy fibrosis is readily identified in cardiac sarcoidosis (Chapters 60 and 95) (Fig. 56-8) and may be more sensitive than endomyocardial biopsy. In iron overload conditions such as thalassemia (Chapter 165), multi-echo T1-weighted imaging of T2* can identify the extent of iron overload. Rarer causes of cardiomyopathy, such as ventricular noncompaction, Chagas' disease (Chapters 60 and 355), and takotsubo cardiomyopathy (Chapter 60), also have characteristic CMR findings. CMR is highly accurate for the noninvasive quantitative assessment of left and right ventricular volumes and ejection fraction but is rarely needed clinically for this purpose unless adequate echocardiography (Chapter 55) cannot be obtained.

Aortic Dissection, Pericardial Disease, and Masses

CMR is an excellent test to detect aortic dissection (see Fig. 78-5 in Chapter 78) or intraluminal aortic hematoma (see Fig. 78-6 in Chapter 78) in patients who are stable enough for it and have no contraindications. CMR is also an excellent test for the evaluation of chronic pericardial disease (Fig. 56-9) because it accurately identifies pericardial thickness as well as adherence of the pericardium to the epicardium in constrictive pericarditis. Real-time

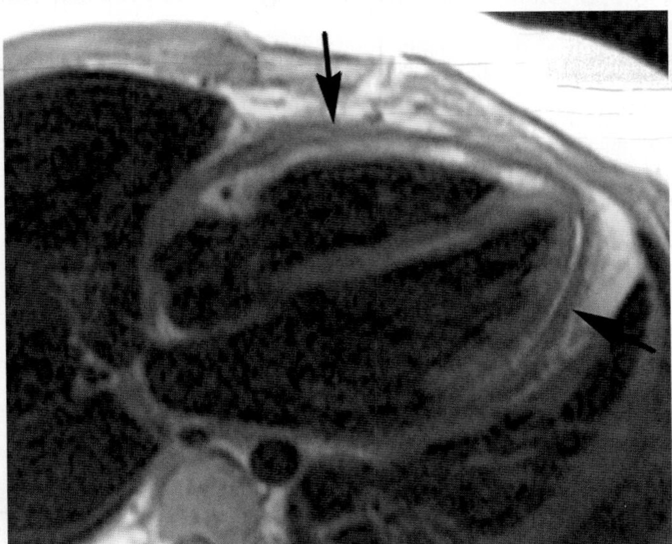

FIGURE 56-9. Magnetic resonance image of a 35-year-old man with dyspnea many years after mantle radiation for Hodgkin's lymphoma shows a thickened pericardium *(arrows)* circumferentially around the left and right ventricles.

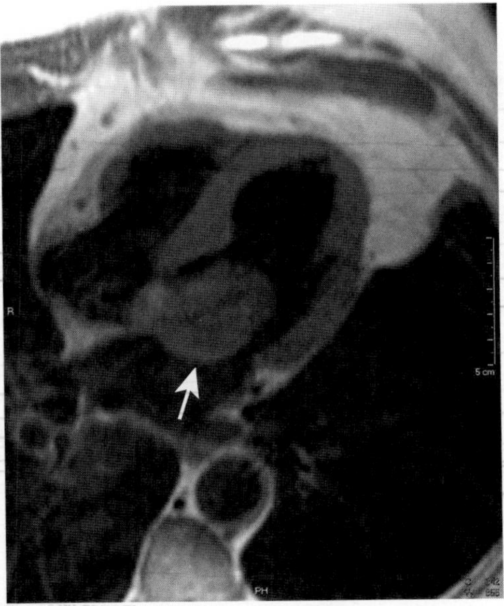

FIGURE 56-10. Diastolic magnetic resonance image of a large left atrial myxoma *(arrow)* showing that it is attached to the atrial septum and is prolapsing across the mitral valve.

imaging can demonstrate ventricular interdependence, a hallmark of this disease.

CMR is also an ideal tool to diagnose intracardiac (Fig. 56-10) and extracardiac masses such as myxomas, thrombus, and tumors, owing to its high spatial resolution and ability to perform tissue characterization.

Congenital Heart Disease

CMR is useful for the assessment of both simple and complex congenital heart disease (Chapter 69). Although atrial septal defects and ventricular septal defects in adults are generally well appreciated by echocardiography, phase velocity CMR readily quantifies blood flow through the major blood vessels, thereby facilitating accurate assessment of the ratio of pulmonary to systemic blood flow. CMR is particularly valuable for assessing abnormalities of the great vessels, such as aortic coarctation (Fig. 56-11), extracardiac anatomy, or anomalous pulmonary venous drainage, and in patients with complex congenital heart disease who have undergone prior corrective or palliative shunt surgery, such as in tetralogy of Fallot. CMR is uniquely able to measure right ventricular volumes accurately, an often important determination in this setting.

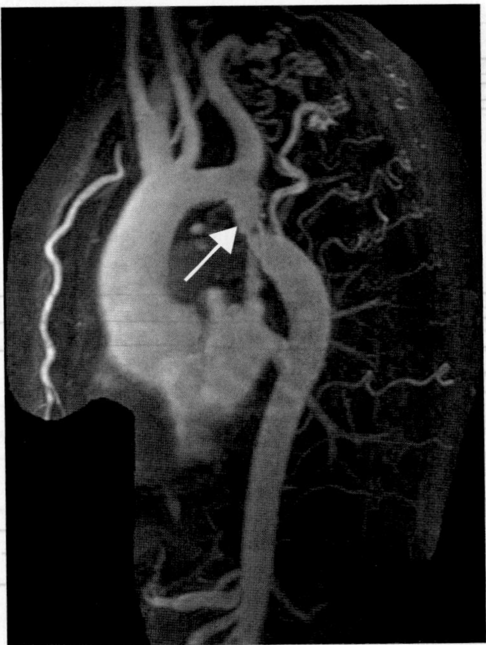

FIGURE 56-11. Three-dimensional contrast-enhanced magnetic resonance angiogram in a patient with an aortic coarctation *(arrow)*.

SUGGESTED READINGS

Flotats A, Knuuti J, Gutberlet M, et al. Hybrid cardiac imaging: SPECT/CT and PET/CT. A joint position statement by the European Association of Nuclear Medicine (EANM), the European Society of Cardiac Radiology (ESCR) and the European Council of Nuclear Cardiology (ECNC). *Eur J Nucl Med Mol Imaging.* 2011;38:201-212. *Consensus guidelines.*

Harrington RA, Bates ER, Bridges CR, et al. ACCF/ACR/AHA/NASCI/SAIP/SCAI/SCCT 2010 expert consensus document on coronary computed tomographic angiography: a report of the American College of Cardiology Foundation Task Force on Expert Consensus Documents. *Circulation.* 2010;121:2509-2543. *Consensus guidelines.*

Hundley WG, Bluemke DA, Finn JP, et al. ACCF/ACR/AHA/NASCI/SCMR 2010 expert consensus document on cardiovascular magnetic resonance: a report on the American College of Cardiology Foundation Task Force on Expert Consensus Documents. *Circulation.* 2010;121:2462-2508. *Consensus guidelines.*

Pennell DJ. Cardiovascular magnetic resonance. *Circulation.* 2010;121:692-705. *A comprehensive review.*

57 CATHETERIZATION AND ANGIOGRAPHY

MORTON KERN

Cardiac catheterization is insertion and passage of small plastic tubes (catheters) into arteries and veins to the heart to obtain radiographic images of coronary arteries and cardiac chambers (angiography and ventriculography) and to measure pressures in the heart (hemodynamics). Coronary angiography defines the site, severity, and morphology of atherosclerotic lesions, and it identifies collateral blood supply beyond occluded vessel segments. Cardiac catheterization is used not only to diagnose coronary artery, valvular (Chapter 75), and myocardial diseases (Chapter 60), but also to perform therapeutic (interventional) procedures to relieve obstructing arterial stenoses (Chapter 74), open narrowed valves, or close intracardiac defects (Chapter 69) through catheter-based, minimally invasive percutaneous techniques. These same diagnostic and therapeutic techniques are also used in the peripheral arterial circulation in a modified fashion to address carotid, renal, and peripheral vascular disease (Chapter 80), aortic aneurysms (Chapter 78), and vascular shunts (Table 57-1).

INDICATIONS AND CONTRAINDICATIONS FOR CARDIAC CATHETERIZATION

The indications to perform cardiac catheterization include the need to diagnose atherosclerotic coronary artery disease, abnormalities of cardiac muscle

TABLE 57-1 PROCEDURES THAT MAY ACCOMPANY CORONARY ANGIOGRAPHY

PROCEDURE	COMMENTS
Central venous access: femoral, internal jugular, subclavian	Uses IV access for emergency medications or fluids, temporary pacemaker; pacemaker not mandatory for most coronary angiography
Hemodynamic assessment, left heart pressures, aorta, and left ventricle	Routine for all studies
Right and left heart combined pressures	Not routine for coronary artery disease but mandatory for valvular heart disease and routine for heart failure, right ventricular dysfunction, pericardial disease, cardiomyopathy, intracardiac shunts, congenital abnormalities
Left ventriculography	Routine for all studies; may be excluded with high-risk patients and those with left main coronary or aortic stenosis, severe congestive heart failure, or renal failure
Internal mammary selective angiography	Routine for coronary bypass conduit
Pharmacologic studies: Complication of coronary spasm, use of ergonovine or acetylcholine conducted in specialized centers Use of vasodilators	Conducted routinely for coronary angiography with nitroglycerin and commonly nitric oxide used for pulmonary hypertension
Aortography	Routine for aortic insufficiency, aortic dissection, and aneurysm and may be performed with or without aortic stenosis; routine to locate bypass graft conduits not visualized by selective angiography
Cardiac pacing electrophysiologic studies	Arrhythmia evaluation routine
Interventional and special techniques	Percutaneous coronary angioplasty including balloon stenting, Rotablator, and coronary atherectomy Intracoronary pressure flow assessment of lesion severity routine Balloon catheter valvuloplasty, myocardial biopsy, atrial septal defect or patent foramen ovale defect closure, transseptal or direct left ventricular function to assess valvular heart disease and invasive interventional electrophysiologic catheter ablation
Vascular closure devices	Routinely available for patients prone to femoral artery access bleeding

From Kern MJ, ed. *The Cardiac Catheterization Handbook*, 5th ed. St. Louis: Mosby; 2010.

TABLE 57-2 INDICATIONS AND CONTRAINDICATIONS FOR CARDIAC CATHETERIZATION

INDICATIONS

1. Identification of the extent and severity of coronary artery disease and evaluation of left ventricular function
2. Assessment of the severity of valvular or myocardial disorders such as aortic stenosis and/or insufficiency, mitral stenosis and/or insufficiency, and various cardiomyopathies to determine the need for surgical correction
3. Collection of data to confirm and complement noninvasive studies
4. Determination of the presence of coronary artery disease in patients with confusing clinical presentations or chest pain of uncertain origin

ABSOLUTE CONTRAINDICATIONS

1. Inadequate facilities
2. Patient refusal

RELATIVE CONTRAINDICATIONS

1. Severe uncontrolled hypertension
2. Ventricular arrhythmias
3. Recent acute stroke
4. Severe anemia
5. Active gastrointestinal bleeding
6. Allergy to radiographic contrast
7. Acute renal failure
8. Uncompensated congestive failure (patient cannot lie flat)
9. Unexplained febrile illness and/or untreated active infection
10. Electrolyte abnormalities (e.g., hypokalemia)
11. Severe coagulopathy
12. Pregnancy
13. Uncontrolled arrhythmias, hypertension
14. Uncooperative patient or patient refusal

function, valvular abnormalities, and congenital heart disease (Table 57-2). Contraindications to cardiac catheterization are few. Absolute contraindications involve only inadequate facilities or equipment for catheterization. Relative contraindications depend on the urgency of the procedure and conditions.

TECHNIQUE OF CATHETERIZATION

After the procedure and its indications, risks, and benefits are explained to the patient, the patient is placed on the cardiac catheterization table and centered under the C-arm of the radiographic gantry (E-Fig. 57-1). After sterile preparation and draping, local anesthetic is administered over the vascular access site (most commonly the femoral but, alternatively, the radial artery). The artery is punctured, and a vascular sheath is inserted, through which the angiographic catheter is advanced over a soft spring-tipped 0.035-inch guidewire that permits safe, atraumatic passage of the catheter to the heart. The specially shaped catheters are seated and connected to a manifold to measure pressure and inject radiographic contrast media.

Coronary arteriography records the images from multiple angles by rotating the C-arm. The images are displayed and preserved on digital imaging systems.

After coronary angiography, the catheter is exchanged for a ventriculography catheter that is inserted into the left ventricle. After left ventricular (LV) pressure is measured, radiographic contrast media (approximately 35 to 45 mL) is injected under high pressure (1000 psi) to assess LV wall motion, chamber size, presence of mitral valve regurgitation, and the shape of the aortic root. The LV ejection fraction (normal is 50 to 70%), a measure of the heart function, is computed as a percentage of the diastolic volume ejected.

After the diagnostic angiograms are completed, the need for coronary revascularization (Chapter 74) is assessed. If suitable symptomatic coronary artery obstructions are present, percutaneous coronary intervention (PCI) may be performed at the same time, if discussed and consented to in advance. Alternatively, the patient may be referred for later PCI or for coronary artery bypass graft (CABG) surgery.

At the conclusion of the catheterization procedure, the catheters are removed. For the femoral artery, hemostasis is achieved either by manual compression, which requires the patient to remain stationary in bed for 4 hours, or by use of a vascular closure device while the patient remains in bed for 1 to 2 hours. For the radial approach, the arterial sheath is removed with the simple application of a specialized compression wrist band; the patient can ambulate immediately.

COMPLICATIONS OF CARDIAC CATHETERIZATION

For the diagnostic cardiac catheterization, risks are less than 0.2% for death, less than 0.5% for myocardial infarction, less than 0.07% for stroke, less than 0.5% for serious arrhythmia, and less than 1% for major vascular complications, including thrombosis and bleeding requiring transfusion or pseudoaneurysm (Table 57-3). Vascular complications occur more frequently with the femoral artery approach than with the radial artery approach; the brachial artery approach, which is used only when neither femoral nor radial access is possible, has the highest rate of vascular complications, and the radial artery has the lowest.

Patients are not routinely anticoagulated for a diagnostic catheterization, and special preparations must be made for patients who are receiving anticoagulants, patients who have diabetes or renal insufficiency, and patients who may have a potential allergy to radiographic contrast media. For the anticoagulated patient, provisions to withhold warfarin or heparin must be made

TABLE 57-3 COMPLICATIONS OF CARDIAC CATHETERIZATION

MAJOR COMPLICATIONS

1. Death
2. Cerebrovascular accident
3. Myocardial infarction, shock
4. Ventricular tachycardia/fibrillation

RARE BUT SERIOUS COMPLICATIONS

1. Aortic dissection
2. Cardiac perforation
3. Tamponade
4. Congestive heart failure
5. Contrast reaction/anaphylaxis
6. Nephrotoxicity
7. Arrhythmias, including heart block, asystole, supraventricular tachyarrhythmias
8. Hemorrhage, including local or retroperitoneal
9. Infection
10. Protamine reaction
11. Vascular complications, including thrombosis, embolus, vascular injury, pseudoaneurysm

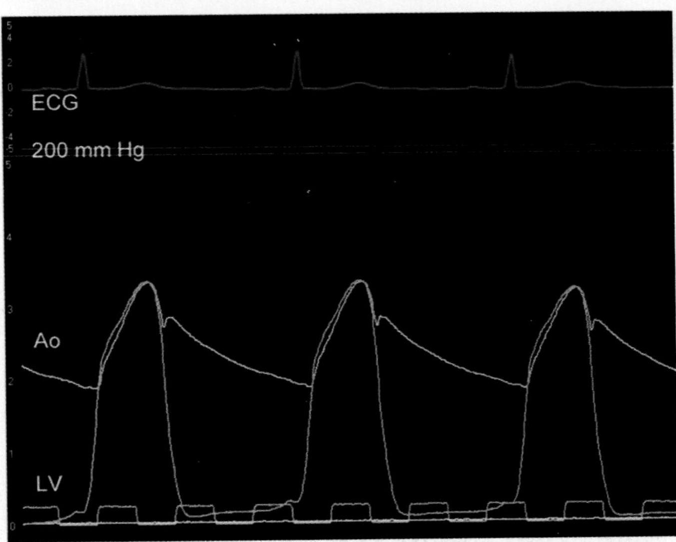

FIGURE 57-1. Normal left ventricular (LV) and aortic (Ao) pressures measured with high-fidelity pressure transducers.

to reduce the potential for femoral puncture site bleeding complications (e.g., retroperitoneal hematoma or pseudoaneurysm). For example, a patient taking warfarin after an aortic valve replacement would have the warfarin withheld for about 3 days before the catheterization, the international normalized ratio would be monitored, and the patient might be administered bridging heparin to the time of the procedure; warfarin would be restarted after the procedure.

For elective catheterizations in patients with insulin-dependent diabetes, half of the usual morning dose of insulin generally is given the morning of the procedure to provide reasonable diabetic coverage and to avoid hypoglycemia. Metformin should be withheld before study. Medications for hypertension and other medical conditions are continued up to and including the morning of the procedure.

Contrast-induced nephropathy, which generally becomes clinically apparent 2 to 3 days after the catheterization, is uncommon. Patients with diabetes or renal insufficiency and patients who are dehydrated from any cause are at a three- to five-fold increased risk for contrast-induced renal failure. For patients with renal insufficiency and those at high risk for contrast-induced renal failure because of diabetes or dehydration, hydration and treatment with *N*-acetylcysteine (Mucomyst, 600 mg evening and morning of procedure) are used routinely in most catheterization laboratories in an attempt to reduce the risk for contrast-induced renal failure.

Contrast media reactions are rare, with an overall incidence of 5% or less, but potentially serious. Adverse reactions occur in 10 to 12% of patients with a history of allergy and in 15% of patients with reported reaction on a previous contrast radiographic examination. There are three types of contrast allergies: cutaneous and mucosal manifestations, smooth muscle and minor anaphylactoid responses, and cardiovascular and major anaphylactoid responses involving laryngeal or pulmonary edema. Pretreatment with corticosteroids is helpful in reducing all types of reactions except urticaria. Patients reporting previous allergic reactions to contrast media should be premedicated with prednisone (60 mg orally the evening before and morning of the procedure) and diphenhydramine (25 to 50 mg orally the morning of the procedure). Patients with known prior anaphylactoid reactions should be pretreated with steroids in the same dose as above. Routine treatment with a histamine-2 blocker (e.g., cimetidine) does not appear to have any benefit.

Hypotension during and after cardiac catheterization may occur from a vasovagal response, bleeding (often occult), myocardial ischemia or infarction, or cardiac tamponade. Vasovagal hypotension is treated with volume and atropine (0.5 to 1.0 mg intravenously). Hypotension due to cardiac tamponade, which may occur during or after PCI, requires reversal of anticoagulation and urgent pericardiocentesis (Chapter 77).

Pulmonary congestion may develop in patients with marginal LV function or critical valvular heart disease. Congestion compromising respiratory and hemodynamic function is an emergency treated with oxygen, diuretics, nitroglycerin, inotropic agents, and intraaortic balloon pumping as indicated (Chapter 107).

Chest pain during coronary angiography is unusual, but myocardial ischemia with pain and ST segment changes may occur during PCI (Chapter 74). Treatment with nitroglycerin, heparin, and antiplatelet medications usually controls myocardial ischemia before revascularization (Chapter 72). Minor arrhythmias (e.g., atrial or ventricular premature beats, brief episodes of supraventricular tachycardia) are common and usually resolve without treatment. Ventricular tachycardia or fibrillation is a rare occurrence but requires prompt defibrillation (Chapter 63).

HEMODYNAMIC DATA OBTAINED DURING CARDIAC CATHETERIZATION

Hemodynamic data are the pressure and flow measurements generated by the heart and recorded during the catheterization procedure. A pressure wave is created by cardiac muscular contraction and is transmitted from the cardiac chamber through the arterial circuit (Fig. 57-1). The pressure waves are measured using the fluid-filled catheters with a pressure transducer, which converts the mechanical pressure to an electrical signal that is displayed on a video monitor.

Simultaneous pressure measurements across the heart valves are used to diagnose valve function. Hemodynamic data also include sampling multiple blood oxygen saturations throughout the right and left sides of the heart for intracardiac shunt identification. Cardiac output is commonly measured by a thermodilution technique. Hemodynamic data permit calculation of vascular and pulmonary resistances and cardiac valve areas (see Table 52-1 in Chapter 52). Complete hemodynamic data requiring right and left heart catheterization are indicated to evaluate dyspnea of any cause; to confirm echocardiographic findings when data are not concordant with clinical or other testing results; and to determine the status of valvular heart disease, cardiomyopathy, and constrictive or restrictive coronary physiology.

Complications of right heart catheterization are rare. The most common problem is transient arrhythmia resulting from mechanical stimulation by the catheter as it passes through the right ventricular outflow tract. In patients with left bundle branch block, a temporary pacemaker may be needed if right bundle branch block occurs during right-sided heart catheterization.

Examples of Hemodynamics for Valvular Heart Disease

The severity of a valvular stenosis is based on the pressure gradient and flow across the valve. In patients with suspected aortic stenosis, a transvalvular pressure gradient should be obtained whenever there is conflicting clinical or echocardiographic data. The pressure recordings most commonly used to assess the aortic valve gradients are the left ventricle and the femoral artery through a side arm of the femoral artery sheath (Fig. 57-2). The normal aortic valve area is 2.5 to 3.5 cm^2 in adults. Severe aortic valve stenosis is associated with valve areas smaller than 1.0 cm^2.

In patients with mitral stenosis, the valve gradient usually is measured using the LV and pulmonary capillary wedge pressures (Fig. 57-3). The most accurate method to compute the mitral stenosis gradient uses the left atrial (obtained by transseptal puncture) and LV pressures. The normal mitral valve area is 4 to 6 cm^2. Valve areas smaller than 1.0 to 1.2 cm^2 are considered severe mitral stenosis.

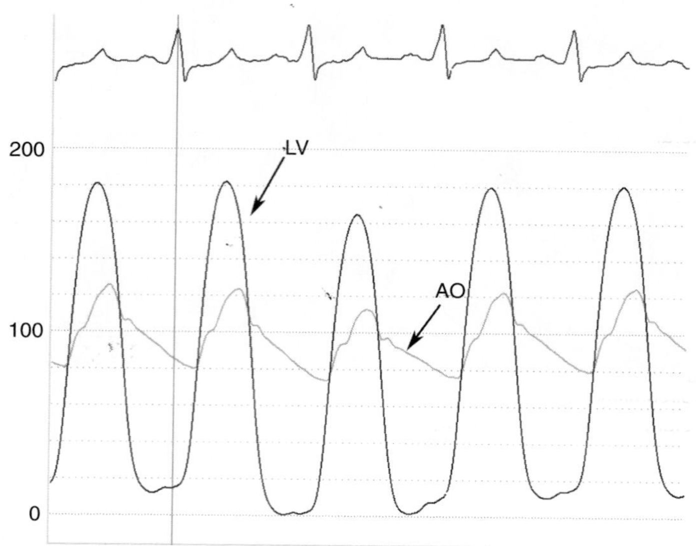

FIGURE 57-2. Hemodynamics of aortic stenosis. Left ventricular (LV) and aortic (AO) pressures are measured simultaneously. Aortic pressure is measured from a central position.

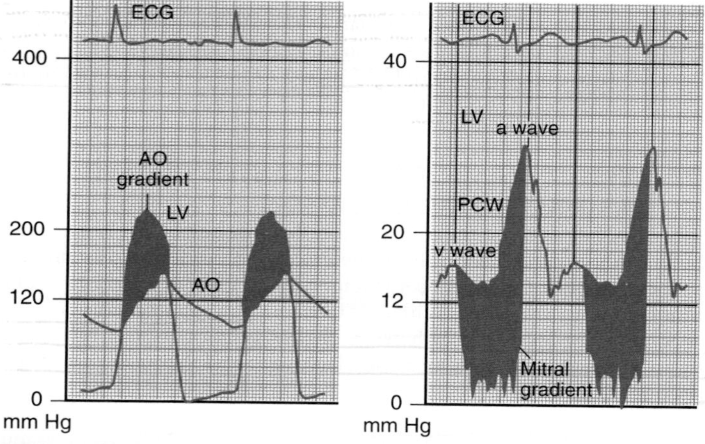

FIGURE 57-3. Examples of the hemodynamic findings in aortic and mitral stenosis. *Left panel,* Simultaneous recording of aortic (AO) and left ventricular (LV) pressure shows a 50-mm Hg systolic pressure gradient. *Right panel,* There is a 15-mm Hg diastolic gradient between the pulmonary capillary wedge pressure (PCW) and the LV pressure. The a wave in the PCW tracing is larger than the v wave, indicating increased resistance to LV filling in this patient. ECG = electrocardiogram.

In patients with mitral regurgitation, the hemodynamics often show a characteristic large v wave on the pulmonary capillary wedge (PCW) tracing (Fig. 57-4). The grading of mitral regurgitation is on a semiquantitative 1 to 4 severity scale based on the amount of contrast seen passing backward from the left ventricle through the incompetent mitral valve into the left atrium. Grade 1 angiographic mitral regurgitation demonstrates a brief puff of contrast filling the left atrium and emptying immediately; grade 2 shows contrast filling the left atrium on 3 beats with moderate density; grade 3 shows contrast filling immediately and moderate density persisting for 2 to 3 beats; and grade 4 shows contrast filling the entire left atrium, often including the appendage, with a density equal to that of the left ventricle for several beats after injection.

CORONARY ANGIOGRAPHY

Coronary angiography visualizes the epicardial arteries, branches, collaterals, and anomalies to diagnose and treat in patients with coronary artery disease (Fig. 57-5). In anticipation of PCI, the angiogram documents not only the presence and location of stenoses but also proximity to major and minor side branches, luminal abnormalities (e.g., thrombi), areas of calcification, and collateral supply, which will influence the decision and techniques used for revascularization. For the two-dimensional radiographic images to depict the three-dimensional coronary tree, multiple angulations of the radiographic imaging system are required.

Assessment of Coronary Stenoses

The degree of a stenosis is most often reported as the estimated percentage diameter luminal reduction of the most severely narrowed segment compared with the adjacent angiographically normal vessel segment, seen in the worst radiographic projection (Fig. 57-6). Because the operator uses visual estimations, an exact evaluation is impossible with less than 20% variation between readings of two or more experienced angiographers. The severity of a stenosis alone should not always be assumed to be associated with abnormal physiology (flow) and ischemia. Moreover, coronary artery disease is a diffuse process, so minimal luminal irregularities on angiography may represent significant, albeit nonobstructive, coronary artery disease at the time of angiography. The precise physiologic impact or morphologic detail of stenosis can be made with specialized catheters and sensor-tipped guidewires. For example, intermediately severe lesions (40 to 70% narrowed) without prior evidence of ischemia can be assessed using a pressure sensor guidewire to measure the translesional pressure during maximal blood flow (e.g., hyperemia induced by adenosine). This pressure measurement, which is called the *fractional flow reserve* (FFR), represents the percentage of normal flow across the stenosis. FFR values higher than 0.80 are considered nonischemic and do not require revascularization. Conversely, if the FFR is lower than 0.80, PCI may be undertaken. The lesion's length, true diameter, eccentricity, and degree of calcium involvement can be determined by intravascular ultrasound catheter-based imaging (IVUS); such information can help guide subsequent PCI (Fig. 57-7).

Coronary Artery Anomalies

Coronary artery anomalies may be present in patients with chest pain syndromes or in young individuals who have survived sudden death. The

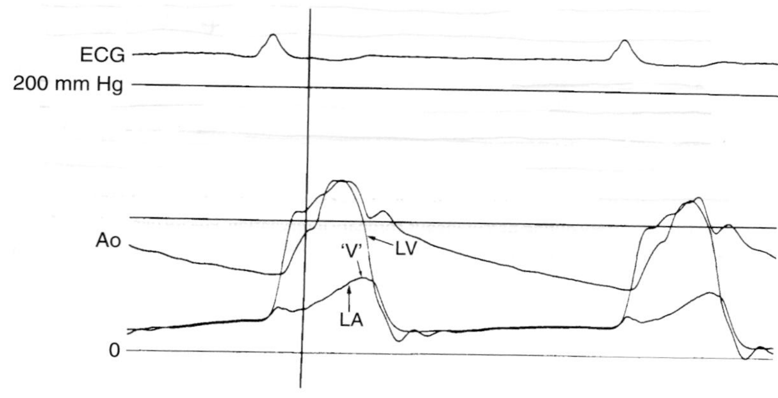

FIGURE 57-4. Hemodynamic tracings in a patient with mitral regurgitation characterized by giant v wave ('V') in the left atrial pressure (LA). This v wave corresponds to marked increase in flow and volume into the left atrium. Ao = aortic pressure; LV = left ventricular pressure.

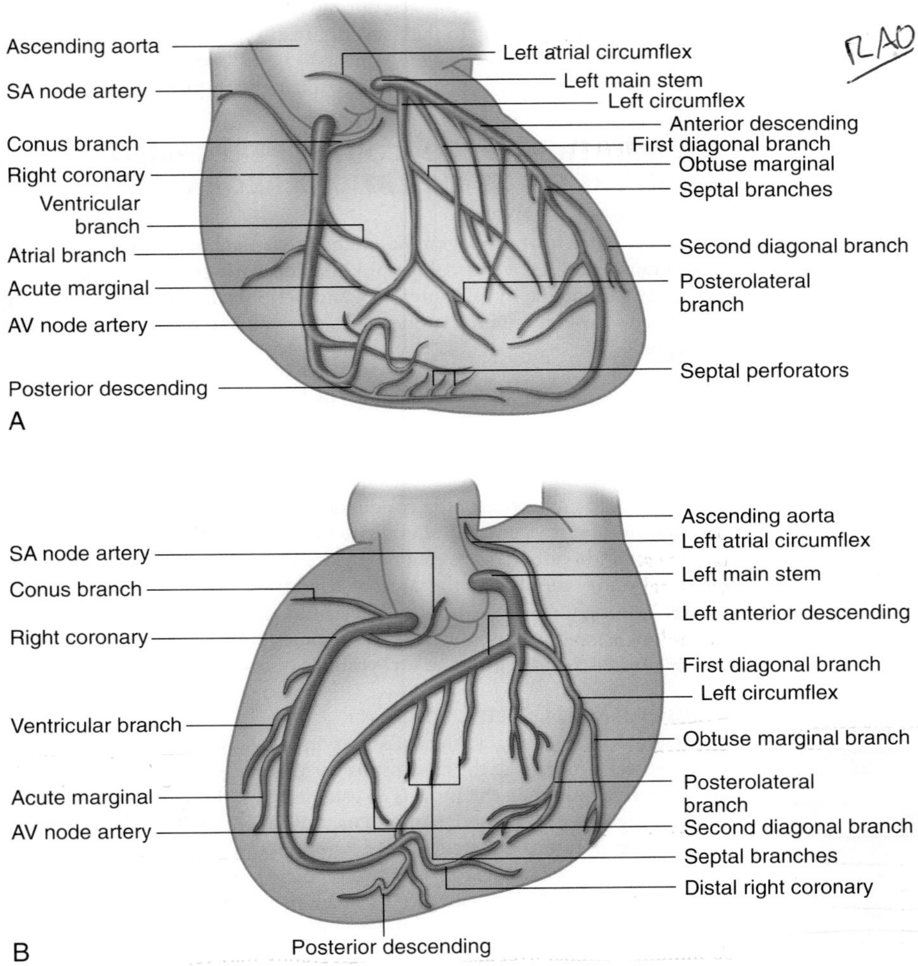

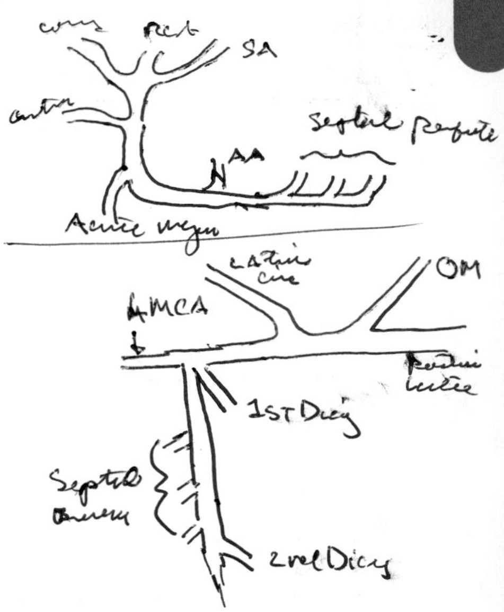

Ascending aorta
SA node artery
Conus branch
Right coronary
Ventricular branch
Atrial branch
Acute marginal
AV node artery
Posterior descending
Left atrial circumflex
Left main stem
Left circumflex
Anterior descending
First diagonal branch
Obtuse marginal
Septal branches
Second diagonal branch
Posterolateral branch
Septal perforators
A
RAO
Ascending aorta
Left atrial circumflex
Left main stem
Left anterior descending
First diagonal branch
Left circumflex
Obtuse marginal branch
Posterolateral branch
Second diagonal branch
Septal branches
Distal right coronary
Posterior descending
SA node artery
Conus branch
Right coronary
Ventricular branch
Acute marginal
AV node artery
B
LAO

SA
OM
1st Diag
2nd Diag

FIGURE 57-5. **Coronary vessels.** The right anterior oblique (**A**) and left anterior oblique (**B**) views are shown. The major arteries are the left main, left anterior descending, circumflex, and right coronary arteries. AV = atrioventricular; SA = sinoatrial. (Modified from Yang SS, Bentivoglio LG, Maranhao V, et al, eds. *From Cardiac Catheterization Data to Hemodynamic Parameters.* Philadelphia: Oxford University Press; 1988.)

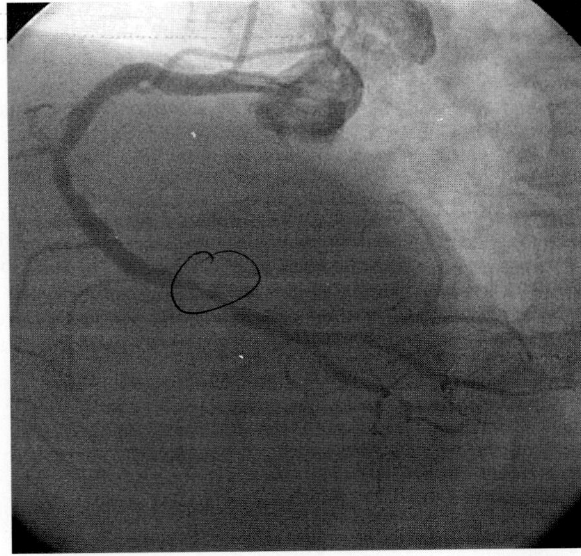

FIGURE 57-6. **Example of a significant stenosis in the right coronary artery.**

VOLCANO IVUS
KIM NGUYEN
20041382812
VL1: (PAUSED)
Diameters
1 0.0mm
2 1.9mm
Live
Diameter
Draw
Dots
Delete
Patient
Home
VH
End Case
Archive
Retrieve
Press Measure for Autoborders or Select from Measurement Toolbar

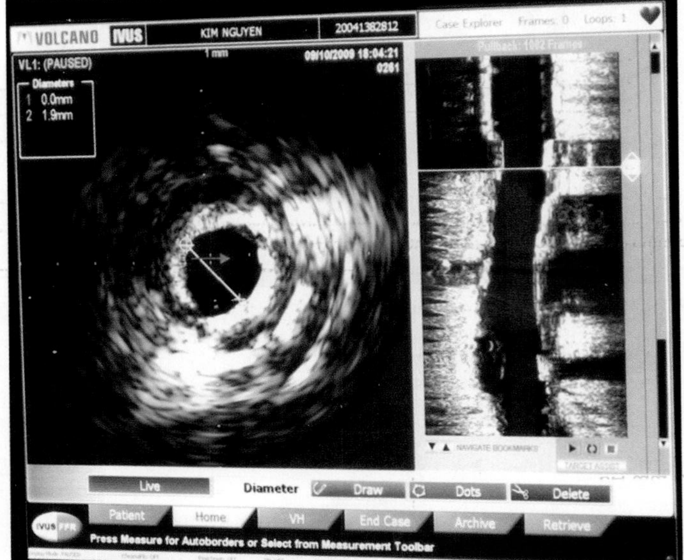

FIGURE 57-7. **Angiographic monitor display of intravascular ultrasound (IVUS) image of coronary artery during percutaneous coronary intervention.** Precise dimensions of the artery and lumen are provided.

angiographic appearance of coronary anomalies is not always straightforward, and computed tomographic angiography (Chapter 56) has become the diagnostic modality best suited to delineate the origin and course of the anomaly (Fig. 57-8).

At the time of coronary angiography, the misdiagnosis of an unsuspected anomalous origin of a coronary artery is a potential problem. Because the natural history of a patient with an anomalous origin of a coronary artery may depend on the anatomic pathway of the anomalous vessel, it is important to define accurately the origin and course of the vessel. Even experienced angiographers have difficulty delineating the true course of the anomalous vessel.

The most critical coronary anomaly is when the left main coronary artery arises from the right cusp and traverses a course between the aorta and pulmonary artery. The artery's initial course through the aortic wall creates a narrow oval opening; with aortic stretch during exercise, coronary blood flow is limited.

Ventriculography

The left ventriculogram, an integral part of nearly every coronary angiographic study, provides information on the motion of the walls of the heart (Fig. 57-9), LV volumes during systole and diastole, the LV ejection fraction, the rate of ejection, the quality of contractility, the presence of hypertrophic myopathy, and valvular regurgitation. The normal pattern of LV contraction is a coordinated, uniform, almost concentric inward motion of all points along the ventricular inner surface during systole. Uncoordinated contractions are named according to their severity (e.g., moderate or severe hypokinesis, akinesis, and aneurysm-dyskinesis). Focal abnormal wall motion indicates the presence of ischemia, infarction, or aneurysm.

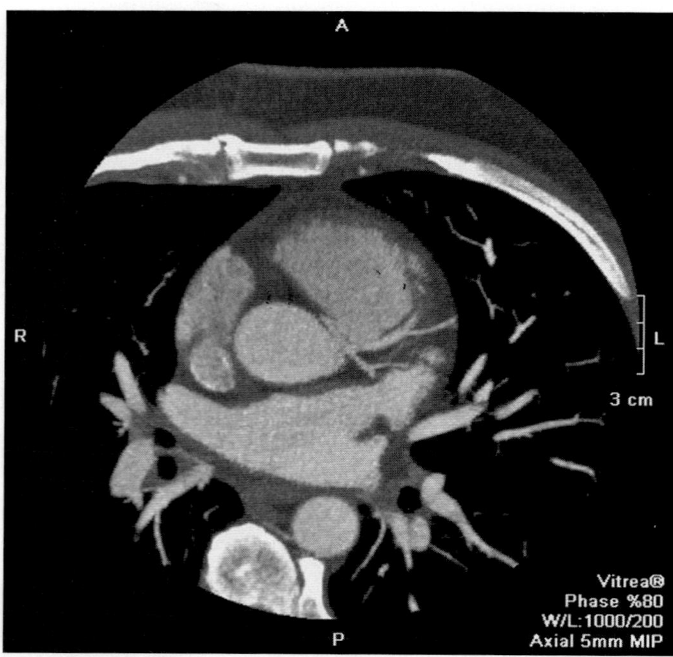

FIGURE 57-8. Frame from a computed tomographic angiographic study showing the origin of the left main coronary artery arising from the right sinus of Valsalva and coursing anteriorly between the aorta and pulmonary artery.

ADDITIONAL PROCEDURES PERFORMED IN THE CATHETERIZATION LABORATORY

Noncardiac Angiography

Other cardiovascular angiographic studies that may accompany coronary angiography and left ventriculography include aortography (Chapter 78), pulmonary angiography (Chapter 98), and peripheral vascular angiography of iliac and lower extremity arteries (Chapters 80 and 81) or renal arteries (Chapter 127).

Electrophysiologic Studies and Ablation Techniques

An electrophysiologic study (EPS) is an invasive procedure that involves the placement of multipolar catheter electrodes at various intracardiac sites (Chapter 62). The general purposes of an EPS are to characterize the electrophysiologic properties of the conduction system, induce and analyze the mechanism of arrhythmias, and evaluate the effects of therapeutic interventions. Electrode catheters are routinely placed in the right atrium, across the tricuspid valve annulus in the area of the atrioventricular node and His bundle, the right ventricle, the coronary sinus, and sometimes the left ventricle. EPS is routinely used in the clinical management of patients who have supraventricular and ventricular arrhythmias (Chapters 64 and 65).

Transseptal Heart Catheterization

Transseptal access using a long catheter with a needle to puncture the thin atrial septal membrane at the fossa ovalis permits placement of a catheter into the left atrium and then the LV. It is an established technique used to acquire precise, high-quality hemodynamic data for patients with aortic stenosis, mitral valve disease (both stenosis and regurgitation), and hypertrophic cardiomyopathy (outflow tract obstructive gradient) and to provide access for valvuloplasty techniques (Chapter 75). The risks of transseptal catheterization, which include punctures of the aortic root, the coronary sinus, or the posterior free wall of the atrium, are potentially lethal problems.

Endomyocardial Biopsy

Endomyocardial biopsy procedures use venous access from the internal jugular vein or femoral vein to insert a flexible metal bioptome to obtain four to six 1-mm^3 pieces of right ventricular myocardium. There are two definitive indications for endomyocardial biopsy: monitoring for cardiac transplant rejection (Chapter 82) and detection of anthracycline cardiotoxicity (Chapter 60). Other indications in selected patients include diagnosis of cardiomyopathy and myocarditis and differentiation between restrictive and constrictive cardiomyopathies.

Other Procedures

Pericardiocentesis (Chapter 77) and PCI (Chapter 74) are performed in the catheterization laboratory for specific indications. Other procedures include balloon valvuloplasty for stenotic heart valves (Chapter 75) and closure of an atrial septal defect or patent foramen ovale (Chapter 69), which is confirmed by typical oxygen saturations detected at catheterization. Percutaneous implantation of prosthetic heart valves is a newer procedure that may become routine for many laboratories in the future.

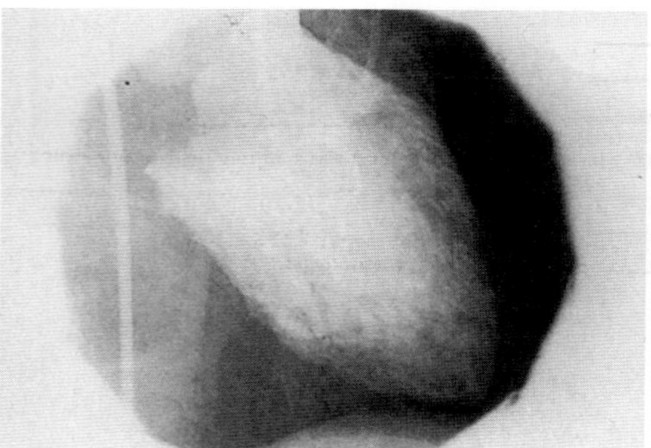

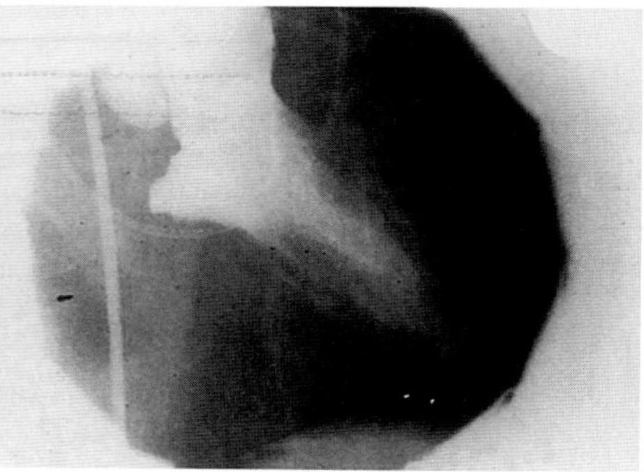

FIGURE 57-9. **Example of left ventriculography.** The ventricular contour is seen in diastole *(left panel)* and in systole *(right panel)*.

SUGGESTED READINGS

Kern MJ, Samady H. Current concepts of integrated coronary physiology in the cath lab. *J Am Coll Cardiol.* 2010;55:173-185. *How to use coronary pressure and flow measurements to achieve optimal outcomes.*

Patel MR, Peterson ED, Dai D, et al. Low diagnostic yield of elective coronary angiography. *N Engl J Med.* 2010;362:886-895. *Among patients who do not have known coronary disease but undergo elective coronary angiography for suspected coronary disease, only about one third have obstructive coronary disease.*

58

HEART FAILURE: PATHOPHYSIOLOGY AND DIAGNOSIS

BARRY M. MASSIE

HEART FAILURE

DEFINITION

Heart failure is a heterogeneous syndrome in which abnormalities of cardiac function are responsible for the inability of the heart to pump blood at an output sufficient to meet the requirements of metabolizing tissues or the ability to do so only at abnormally elevated diastolic pressures or volumes. The heart failure syndrome is characterized by signs and symptoms of intravascular and interstitial volume overload (shortness of breath, rales, elevated jugular venous pressure, and edema) or manifestations of inadequate tissue perfusion (impaired exercise tolerance, fatigue, signs of hypoperfusion, renal dysfunction), or both. Heart failure may occur as a result of (1) impaired myocardial contractility (systolic dysfunction, commonly characterized as reduced left ventricular [LV] ejection fraction [EF]); (2) increased ventricular stiffness or impaired myocardial relaxation in the absence of systolic dysfunction (diastolic dysfunction, which is commonly associated with a relatively normal LVEF and is often termed *heart failure with preserved EF*); (3) a variety of other cardiac abnormalities, including obstructive or regurgitant valvular disease, intracardiac shunting, or disorders of heart rate or rhythm; or (4) states in which the heart is unable to compensate for increased peripheral blood flow or metabolic requirements. In adults, LV involvement is almost always present even if the manifestations are primarily those of right ventricular (RV) dysfunction (fluid retention without dyspnea or rales). Heart failure may result from an acute insult to cardiac function, such as a large myocardial infarction (MI), or, more commonly, from a chronic process. The focus in this chapter is on the syndrome of *chronic* heart failure, including its presentation in an acutely decompensated state. The most common causes of de novo acute heart failure, such as MI (Chapter 73), valvular disease (Chapter 75), myocarditis (Chapter 60), and cardiogenic shock (Chapter 107), are discussed elsewhere.

EPIDEMIOLOGY

Both the incidence and the prevalence of heart failure are growing, as is the resulting burden of deaths and hospitalizations. Although these trends primarily reflect the strong association between heart failure and advancing age, they also are influenced by the rising prevalence of precursors such as hypertension, diabetes, dyslipidemia, and obesity in industrialized societies and the improved long-term survival of patients with ischemic and other forms of heart disease. The annual incidence of heart failure rises from less than 1 per 1000 patient years among those younger than 45 years, to 10 per 1000 patient years for those older than 65 years, to 30 per 1000 patient years (3%) for those older than 85 years. Prevalence figures follow a similar exponential pattern, increasing from 0.1% before 50 to 55 years of age to almost 10% after age 80 years. About 20% of U.S. adults will develop heart failure in their lifetimes. Overall in the United States, the estimated prevalence of heart failure is 5.8 million patients, with an annual incidence of 670,000 new cases per year. Heart failure results in 1.1 million hospital discharges and causes or contributes to 280,000 deaths per year. Although the relative incidence and prevalence of heart failure are lower in women than men, women constitute at least half of the cases because of their longer life expectancy. Any condition that causes myocardial necrosis or produces chronic pressure or volume overload can induce myocardial dysfunction and heart failure. In developed countries, the causes of heart failure have changed greatly over several decades. Valvular heart disease, with the exception of calcific aortic stenosis, has declined markedly, whereas coronary heart disease has become the predominant cause in men and women, being responsible for 60 to 75% of cases. Hypertension, although less frequently the primary cause of heart failure than in the past, continues to be a major factor in 75%, including most of the patients with coronary disease.

Prevention of Heart Failure

Treatment of hypertension, with a focus on the systolic pressure, reduces the incidence of heart failure by 50%. This intervention remains effective even in patients older than 75 years (Chapter 67). Any intervention that reduces the risk of a first or recurrent MI (Chapter 51) will also reduce the incidence of heart failure. In patients with reduced LVEF, angiotensin-converting enzyme (ACE) inhibitors, aldosterone blockers, and β-blockers prevent or delay progressive LV dysfunction and dilation and the onset or worsening of heart failure. Well-timed intervention for progressive valvular disease affords another opportunity to prevent eventual heart failure (Chapter 75).

Stages of Heart Failure

The recognition that most patients who develop heart failure have underlying risk factors or predisposing clinical conditions that precede its development, usually by many years, has led to a greater emphasis on early detection and treatment of predisposing factors, on the staging of heart failure (Fig. 58-1), and on early intervention. *Stage A* heart failure includes patients who are at risk for development of heart failure but do not as yet have either symptoms or apparent structural abnormalities of the heart; this includes patients with hypertension, atherosclerotic disease, diabetes, obesity, or the

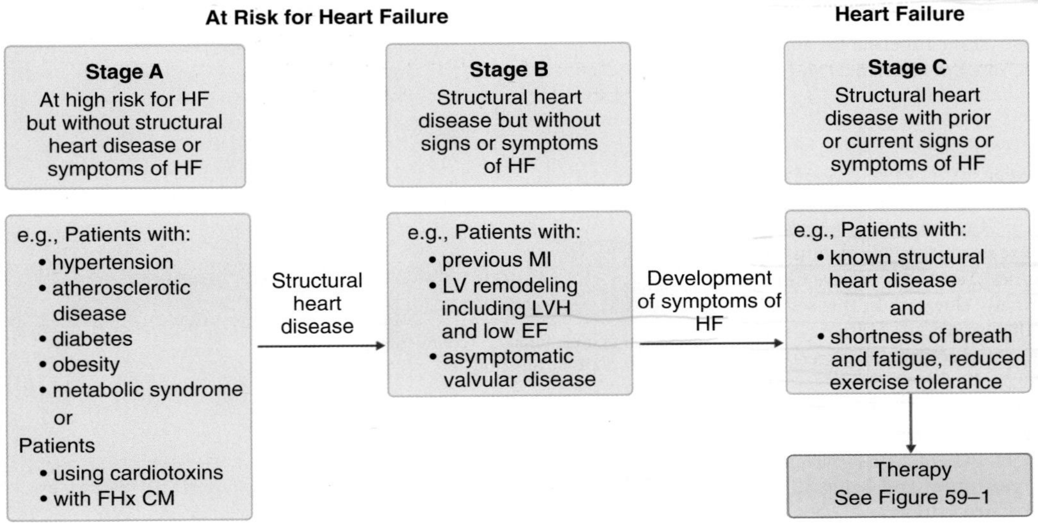

FIGURE 58-1. **Stages of heart failure.** EF = ejection fraction; FHx CM = family history of cardiomyopathy; HF = heart failure; LV = left ventricle; LVH = left ventricular hypertrophy; MI = myocardial infarction. (Modified from Hunt SA. ACC/AHA 2005 guideline update for the diagnosis and management of chronic heart failure in the adult: a report of the American College of Cardiology/American Heart Association Task Force on Practice Guidelines [Writing Committee to Update the 2001 Guidelines for the Evaluation and Management of Heart Failure]. *J Am Coll Cardiol.* 2005;46:e1-e82.)

metabolic syndrome and individuals with ongoing excessive alcohol intake, use of cardiotoxic drugs, a familial history of cardiomyopathy, or a known genetic abnormality associated with cardiomyopathy (Chapter 60). *Stage B* encompasses asymptomatic patients who have demonstrable structural abnormalities that predispose to heart failure, such as prior MI, LV hypertrophy diagnosed by electrocardiography or echocardiography, reduced LVEF or LV dilation, or asymptomatic but hemodynamically significant valvular heart disease. *Stage C* heart failure includes patients who have exhibited symptoms or signs of heart failure. These patients may have improved to the point of being relatively asymptomatic, but they still are classified as stage C and usually continue to receive treatment with agents that are known to improve their natural history, such as β-blockers and inhibitors of the renin-angiotensin-aldosterone system.

PATHOBIOLOGY

Differing Mechanisms of Heart Failure

Heart failure is a syndrome that may result from many cardiac and systemic disorders (Table 58-1). Some of these disorders, at least initially, do not involve the heart, and the term *heart failure* may be confusing. Even in high-output states, however, the patient may present with the classic findings of exertional dyspnea and edema *(high-output heart failure)* that resolve if the underlying disorder is eliminated. If they persist, these conditions may impair myocardial performance secondarily as a result of chronic volume overload or direct deleterious effects on the myocardium. Other conditions, including mechanical abnormalities, disorders of rate and rhythm, and pulmonary abnormalities, do not primarily affect myocardial function but are frequent causes of heart failure.

Abnormalities of Cardiac Function

Systolic Function

In the normal left ventricle, stroke volume increases over a wide range of end-diastolic volumes (the Frank-Starling effect). If contractility (or the inotropic state of the myocardium) is enhanced, such as during exercise or catecholamine stimulation, this increase is correspondingly greater (Table 58-2). In the failing heart with depressed contractility, there is relatively little increment in systolic function with further increases in LV volume, and the ventricular function curve is shifted downward and flattened (Chapter 52). In the clinical setting, systolic dysfunction is characterized by depressed stroke volume despite elevated ventricular filling pressures. The resulting symptoms are those of pulmonary or systemic congestion, activity intolerance, and organ dysfunction.

Assessment of systolic function clinically is more problematic. The most useful measure is the LVEF (stroke volume/end-diastolic volume, usually expressed as a percentage), which reflects a single point on the ventricular function curve. The EF is *load dependent*, however, meaning that alterations in afterload (see later discussion) can affect it independently of contractility. In addition, mitral regurgitation, which facilitates ejection into the low-pressure left atrium, may lead to an overestimation of systolic function by the EF. Nonetheless, with the exceptions indicated earlier, when the EF is normal (>50 to 55% in most laboratories), systolic function is usually adequate. LVEFs that are mildly (40 to 50%), moderately (30 to 40%), or severely (<30%) depressed are associated with reduced survival and, in the severe range, with reduced functional reserve, if not overt symptoms of heart failure. Cardiac output, in contrast, is a poor measure of systolic function because it can be affected markedly by heart rate, systemic vascular resistance, and the degree of LV dilation.

Diastolic Function

Diastole is the portion of the cardiac cycle between aortic valve closure and mitral valve closure. Diastole consists of three phases: (1) active relaxation, (2) the conduit phase, and (3) atrial contraction. If relaxation is delayed or if the myocardium is abnormally stiff (e.g., an excessively steep relationship between change in pressure and change in volume [$\Delta P/\Delta V$]), passive filling may be impaired and atrial pressures are abnormally elevated. In this setting of a noncompliant ventricle (compliance is the inverse of stiffness—the change in volume for a given change in pressure), atrial contraction is responsible for a disproportionately large amount of diastolic filling.

The importance of abnormalities of diastolic function in the pathogenesis of heart failure is increasingly appreciated. Because relaxation is energy dependent, it frequently is impaired in the presence of ischemia or hypoxemia. Recurring myocardial ischemia, myocardial hypertrophy, and aging all are associated with interstitial fibrosis and impaired diastolic function.

TABLE 58-1 PATHOGENESIS OF HEART FAILURE

IMPAIRED SYSTOLIC (CONTRACTILE) FUNCTION
Ischemic damage or dysfunction
Myocardial infarction
Persistent or intermittent myocardial ischemia
Hypoperfusion (shock)
Chronic pressure overloading
Hypertension
Obstructive valvular disease
Chronic volume overload
Regurgitant valvular disease
Intracardiac left-to-right shunting
Extracardiac shunting
Nonischemic dilated cardiomyopathy
Familial/genetic disorders
Toxic/drug-induced damage
Immunologically mediated necrosis
Infectious agents
Metabolic disorders
Infiltrative processes
Idiopathic conditions
IMPAIRED DIASTOLIC FUNCTION (RESTRICTED FILLING, INCREASED STIFFNESS)
Pathologic myocardial hypertrophy
Primary (hypertrophic cardiomyopathies)
Secondary (hypertension)
Aging
Ischemic fibrosis
Restrictive cardiomyopathy
Infiltrative disorders (amyloidosis, sarcoidosis)
Storage diseases (hemochromatosis, genetic abnormalities)
Endomyocardial disorders
MECHANICAL ABNORMALITIES
Intracardiac
Obstructive valvular disease
Regurgitant valvular disease
Intracardiac shunts
Other congenital abnormalities
Extracardiac
Obstructive (coarctation, supravalvular aortic stenosis)
Left-to-right shunting (patent ductus arteriosus)
DISORDERS OF RATE AND RHYTHM
Bradyarrhythmias (sinus node dysfunction, conduction abnormalities)
Tachyarrhythmias (ineffective rhythms, chronic tachycardia)
PULMONARY HEART DISEASE
Cor pulmonale
Pulmonary vascular disorders
HIGH-OUTPUT STATES
Metabolic disorders
Thyrotoxicosis
Nutritional disorders (beriberi)
Excessive blood flow requirements
Chronic anemia
Systemic arteriovenous shunting

TABLE 58-2 MAJOR DETERMINANTS OF CARDIAC PERFORMANCE

Ventricular systolic function (contractility)
Ventricular diastolic function
Relaxation
Stiffness
Ventricular preload
Ventricular afterload
Cardiac rate and conduction
Myocardial blood flow

Ventricular Preload

In the intact heart, preload is best characterized by the end-diastolic volume or pressure, which are indirect indicators of end-diastolic fiber length (Chapter 52). The performance of the normal left ventricle is highly preload dependent, but the failing heart operates at high preloads and on the flat part of the LV function curve (see Fig. 52-3 in Chapter 52). In contrast to the normal ventricle, an increase in preload does not improve systolic function but worsens pulmonary congestion further. Preload reduction by diuresis or by reduction of venous return with venodilating agents generally has a beneficial effect on symptoms of heart failure.

Ventricular Afterload

LV afterload frequently is equated with arterial pressure or systemic vascular resistance, but a more accurate measurement of afterload is systolic wall stress (Chapter 52), defined as follows:

$$\text{Systolic wall stress} = (\text{Pressure} \times \text{radius of left ventricle}) \div (2 \times \text{thickness of left ventricle})$$

At any given arterial pressure, afterload is increased with a dilated, thin-walled ventricle and decreased with a smaller or thicker ventricle. Increased afterload has an effect similar to that of depressed contractility, so afterload reduction can improve cardiac performance.

Heart Rate and Rhythm

Heart rate affects cardiac performance by two mechanisms. First, increasing the heart rate enhances the inotropic state by upregulating cytosolic calcium concentrations. Second, heart rate is an important determinant of cardiac output and is the primary mechanism by which cardiac output is matched to demand in situations such as exercise. Because stroke volume is relatively fixed in the failing heart, heart rate becomes a major determinant of cardiac output. Chronic tachycardia impairs ventricular performance, however, and cardiac function can decline rapidly with sustained tachyarrhythmias (as seen in atrial fibrillation, atrial flutter, chronic atrial tachycardia, and even inappropriate sinus tachycardia).

Optimal cardiac performance depends on a well-coordinated sequence of contraction. Normal atrioventricular conduction times (0.16 to 0.20 second) enhance the contribution of atrial contraction to LV filling, which is particularly important in the noncompliant ventricle. Patients with heart failure frequently have intraventricular conduction abnormalities, which result in dyssynchronous contractions, such that the septum and parts of the anterior wall begin contracting only after systole has ended in other regions. Cardiac resynchronization therapy can prevent the onset of heart failure in patients with significant ventricular dyssynchrony, usually manifest electrically as a left bundle branch block.

Myocardial Blood Flow and Oxygen Requirements

In the normal heart, myocardial blood flow is closely coupled to oxygen requirements, and it is not ordinarily considered a determinant of cardiac performance. However, myocardial ischemia is associated with a rapid decline in contractile function that may persist long beyond the episode (myocardial stunning). Chronically inadequate blood flow may lead to a reduction in contractility, which reestablishes the balance between oxygen delivery and demands (hibernation). Low arterial diastolic pressures may interfere with the autoregulatory reserve of the coronary circulation, which is limited at diastolic pressures of less than 60 mm Hg. Endothelial dysfunction, which is common in patients with heart failure, also may limit blood flow. At the same time, tachycardia, increased afterload, and substantial LV hypertrophy increase myocardial oxygen requirements. Inadequate myocardial blood flow plays an important role in the pathogenesis of cardiac dysfunction, sometimes even in patients without obstructive coronary disease.

Genetic Causes of Dilated Cardiomyopathy

Although much less is known about the genetics of dilated cardiomyopathy than that of hypertrophic cardiomyopathy (Chapter 60), several forms of familial cardiomyopathy have been recognized, most of which are inherited in an autosomal dominant pattern. Mutations of genes encoding for nuclear membrane proteins (emerin, lamin) or for contractile or cytoskeletal proteins (desmin, a cardiac myosin, vinculin) have been identified. Cardiomyopathy also is associated with muscular dystrophies (Duchenne's, Becker's, and limb-girdle dystrophies; Chapter 429) and other forms of myopathy. As research in this area burgeons, it is estimated that genetic abnormalities may be involved in 20 to 30% of cases of idiopathic dilated cardiomyopathy.

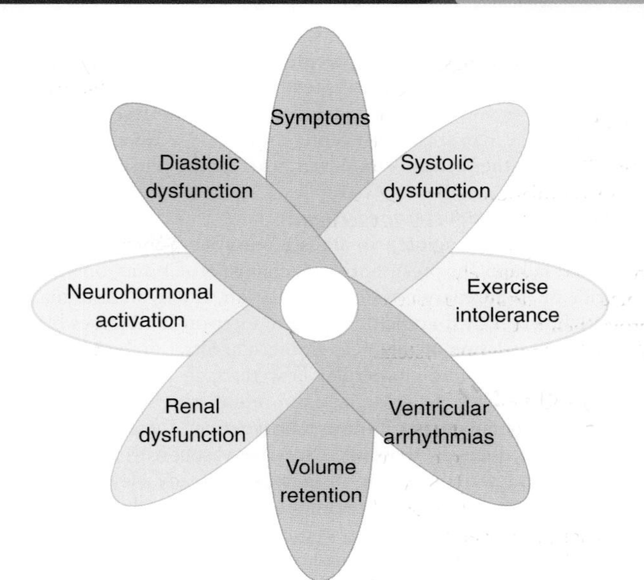

FIGURE 58-2. Pathophysiology of heart failure, illustrated by Venn diagram.

TABLE 58-3 NEUROHORMONES THAT MAY BE INCREASED IN CHRONIC HEART FAILURE

Norepinephrine	Natriuretic peptides
Epinephrine	Endothelin
Plasma renin activity	Endorphins
Angiotensin II	Calcitonin gene–related peptide
Aldosterone	Growth hormone
Prostaglandins	Cortisol
Vasopressin	Proinflammatory cytokines
Neuropeptide Y	Neurokinin A
Vasoactive intestinal peptides	Substance P

Heart Failure Syndrome

Chronic heart failure is a multifaceted syndrome with diverse presentations (Fig. 58-2). The initial manifestations of hemodynamic dysfunction are a reduction in stroke volume and a rise in ventricular filling pressures, perhaps in the basal state but consistently under conditions of increased systemic demand for blood flow. These changes have downstream effects on cardiovascular reflexes and systemic organ perfusion and function, which in turn stimulate a variety of interdependent compensatory responses involving the cardiovascular system, neurohormonal systems, and alterations in renal physiology. It is this constellation of responses that leads to the characteristic pathophysiology of the heart failure syndrome. Recognition of the role of neurohormonal activation in heart failure has grown with the increasing understanding of its pathophysiology and with evidence that blockade of some of these responses can have a profound effect on the natural history of the disease (Table 58-3). The number of hormonal systems that are known to be activated in heart failure continues to grow.

Neurohormonal Responses

Sympathetic Nervous System

Initial activation of the sympathetic nervous system probably results from reduced pulse pressures, which activate arterial baroreceptors, and renal hypoperfusion. Evidence for its activation comes from elevated levels of circulating norepinephrine, direct sympathetic nerve recordings showing increased activity, and increased release of norepinephrine by several organs, including the heart. As cardiac function deteriorates, responsivity to norepinephrine diminishes, as evidenced by baroreceptor desensitization and downregulation of cardiac adrenergic receptors and signal transduction. This desensitization may further stimulate sympathetic responses.

The adaptive role of norepinephrine is to stimulate heart rate and myocardial contractility and to produce vasoconstriction. These actions reverse the depression of cardiac output and blood pressure. Increased levels of plasma norepinephrine are associated with a worse prognosis, although it is unclear whether this is a cause-and-effect relationship. There is also convincing, albeit circumstantial, evidence that norepinephrine has adverse effects on the myocardium. In this regard, β-adrenoceptor blockade, which once was considered dangerous in heart failure because it would interfere with important compensatory mechanisms, consistently improves LV function and prognosis. The roles of other catecholamines in heart failure remain undefined.

Renin-Angiotensin-Aldosterone System

Elements of the renin-angiotensin-aldosterone system are activated relatively early in heart failure. The presumptive mechanisms of induction include renal hypoperfusion, β-adrenergic system stimulation, and hyponatremia. All may be activated further by diuretic therapy. Angiotensin II increases blood pressure by vasoconstriction; it enhances glomerular filtration by increasing renal pressure and maintaining glomerular flow through its intrarenal hemodynamic effects. Aldosterone causes sodium retention, which restores normal cardiac output by enhancing intravascular volume. These adaptations have deleterious consequences, however. Excessive vasoconstriction can depress LV function, and sodium retention increases already elevated ventricular filling pressures. There also is experimental evidence indicating that angiotensin II may have pathologic effects on the myocardium and may induce vascular hypertrophy, whereas aldosterone induces myocardial fibrosis. The striking success of ACE inhibitors and aldosterone blockers in improving the natural history of heart failure suggests that the adverse effects of renin-angiotensin-aldosterone activation may outweigh the benefit in patients with or at risk of heart failure.

Other Neurohormonal Systems

Levels of several natriuretic peptides are elevated consistently in heart failure, and they may counterbalance the vasoconstricting and sodium-retaining actions of the renin-angiotensin-aldosterone and sympathetic nervous systems. However, the renal responses to these natriuretic hormones are often downregulated in patients with heart failure, so they do not have the same natriuretic effects in patients with chronic heart failure that they manifest in normal individuals. Elevated circulating and tissue levels of vasodilating prostaglandins may improve glomerular hemodynamics, and inhibitors of prostaglandin synthesis (including aspirin and other nonsteroidal anti-inflammatory agents) interfere with the hemodynamic and renal actions of ACE inhibitors.

Endothelin and arginine vasopressin are elevated in many patients with heart failure, and interference with their actions may promote vasodilation and aquaresis. Arginine vasopressin induces vasoconstriction through a vascular (V-1) receptor and reduces free water clearance through a renal tubular (V-2) receptor. Endothelin causes prolonged vasoconstriction, reductions in glomerular filtration, and pulmonary arteriolar constriction. Although endothelin is a theoretically attractive target for therapy, clinical trials with endothelin antagonists have been negative or even shown harm, thereby indicating that interdiction of neurohormonal activation is not uniformly beneficial.

Cytokine Activation

Circulating levels of many proinflammatory cytokines, including tumor necrosis factor-α (TNF-α), interleukin-1β, and interleukin-6, are elevated in patients with relatively severe heart failure and may be involved in the syndrome of cardiac cachexia. These cytokines also may induce contractile dysfunction, myocardial fibrosis, and myocyte necrosis, perhaps by mediating some of the deleterious responses to catecholamines and angiotensin II. Nonetheless, trials using antagonists of TNF-α have not shown clinical benefit.

Altered Renal Physiology

In most patients with chronic heart failure, the kidneys are anatomically and structurally normal. Reduced blood pressure, diminished stroke volume, and reduced renal perfusion pressure and flow are sensed as reduced blood volume by the high-pressure baroreceptors and the juxtaglomerular apparatus, which maintain cardiovascular homeostasis. In chronic heart failure, these receptors become desensitized, generating reduced afferent responses. The low-pressure intracardiac pressure and volume receptors also are desensitized. Thirst and fluid intake may be increased as a result of activation of the cerebral thirst center. Although heart failure usually is associated with a normal or increased blood volume, it paradoxically is characterized by activation of the same homeostatic responses as those that act in hemorrhage and shock; the result is abnormal retention of sodium and water. In advanced heart failure, which is usually characterized by low cardiac output or hypotension (or coexisting renal vascular disease), the glomerular filtration rate may become so severely reduced that sodium and fluid retention becomes refractory to diuretic therapy.

Left Ventricular Remodeling and Progression of Heart Failure

After an initial insult precipitates heart failure, progressive alterations occur in myocardial structure and function owing to continuing damage by the underlying process and responses to hemodynamic stresses and neurohormonal activation. The left ventricle progressively dilates and changes from the normal ellipsoid shape to a more spherical geometry. This "remodeling" is accompanied by changes in the cardiac interstitium that lead to altered orientation of the myofibrils and progressive fibrosis. The result is more discoordinate and less effective contraction. Inhibitors of the renin-angiotensin-aldosterone system and β-blockers slow, halt, or reverse this remodeling process, preventing LV dilation, geometric distortion, and deterioration in contractile function.

CLINICAL MANIFESTATIONS

Heart failure may manifest acutely in a de novo manner, chronically, or as recurring exacerbations of chronic heart failure.

Acute Decompensation of Heart Failure

Most episodes of acute worsening of heart failure occur in patients with previously recognized symptoms of chronic heart failure. Patients with such decompensations usually present with shortness of breath, generally after a period of fluid retention or signs of congestion, as manifested by worsening edema and some degree of worsening dyspnea (Fig. 58-3).

Occasionally, the initial presentation may be more acute, with rapid progression to resting dyspnea or pulmonary edema, or both. The acute presentation is often associated with severe hypertension and is particularly characteristic of patients who have diastolic dysfunction and whose stiff left ventricle tolerates fluid retention poorly. In patients without a preceding history of heart failure, other precipitating factors, such as acute MI (Chapter 73), tachyarrhythmias (Chapters 64 and 65), previously unrecognized or new valvular abnormalities (Chapter 75), toxic damage (including alcohol excess), or acute myocarditis (Chapter 60), should be considered. Rapid diagnosis by noninvasive testing and early cardiac catheterization is essential. In patients whom myocarditis is suspected, particularly when the clinical presentation suggests giant cell myocarditis, early endomyocardial biopsy is recommended. Treatment is cause specific and may include early coronary revascularization, valve repair or replacement, or supportive care (e.g., inotropic support, intra-aortic balloon pumping, ventricular assist devices). If the condition does not improve, cardiac transplantation (Chapter 82) may be the best option for appropriate candidates.

Chronic Heart Failure

Left-Sided and Right-Sided Heart Failure

Most adult patients with heart failure have abnormalities of the left ventricle as the underlying cause. Nonetheless, the clinical presentation may be

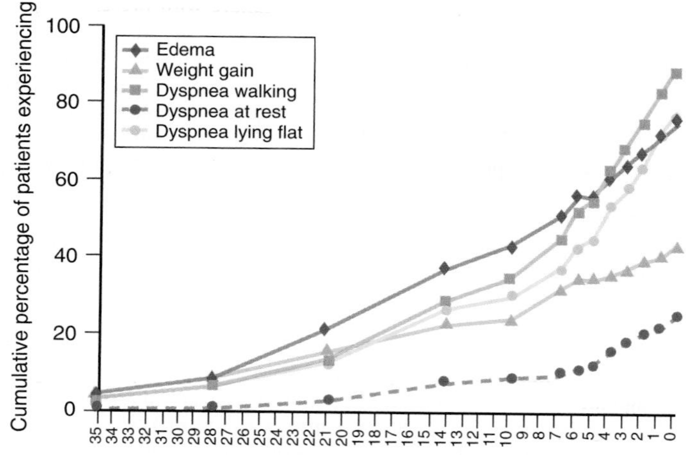

FIGURE 58-3. **Number of days from onset of worsening of selected symptoms of heart failure to admission to hospital: cumulative percentage of patients.** (Reprinted with permission from Schiff GD, Fung S, Speroff T, et al. Decompensated heart failure: symptoms, patterns of onset, and contributing factors. *Am J Med.* 2003;114:625-630.)

variable, sometimes suggesting predominantly or even exclusively RV dysfunction. The manifestations of LV dysfunction are related to elevated filling (diastolic) pressures, which are transmitted backward to the left atrium and pulmonary veins, or inadequate cardiac output. The former results in dyspnea (sometimes at rest but usually with activity) and, when severe, pulmonary edema (classically associated with rales and possibly pleural effusions). The cardiac output may be insufficient to support peripheral organ function, causing exertional muscle fatigue, impaired renal function and salt excretion, or depressed mentation.

Right-sided heart failure results from either chronic RV pressure overload (e.g., pulmonary hypertension resulting from cor pulmonale, pulmonary vascular disease or pulmonary embolism) or intrinsic dysfunction of the right ventricle or its valves. However, the most common cause of RV pressure overload is left-sided heart dysfunction, which results in pulmonary hypertension. If the symptoms and signs of left-sided heart failure are absent or difficult to elicit, the physician inappropriately may seek a primarily right-sided pathology. The primary manifestations of right-sided failure are related to chronically elevated right atrial and systemic venous pressures: jugular venous distention, peripheral edema, ascites, hepatic and bowel edema, and varied gastrointestinal complaints. These patients are especially vulnerable to renal dysfunction because elevated venous pressures may cause renal medullary ischemia and depress renal function.

Heart Failure with Preserved Ejection Fraction

Myocardial mechanisms that lead to the syndrome of heart failure can be differentiated into conditions that depress LV systolic function and conditions that occur despite normal or relatively preserved contractility. Although it is arbitrary, an LVEF threshold of 45 to 50% often is used for this distinction

Until the widespread use of noninvasive assessments of LV function, heart failure with preserved EF was considered unusual in the absence of valvular abnormalities or other specific and uncommon causes. It is now recognized that at least 40-50% of patients with heart failure have relatively normal EFs. In the ongoing Cardiovascular Health Study, a population-based study of more than 5000 patients aged 65 years and older, more than 70% of the patients developing heart failure had normal or only mildly impaired EFs. As the population ages and as interventional and pharmacologic approaches reduce infarct sizes and prevent LV remodeling, it is likely that heart failure with preserved EF will become increasingly common.

Although there are many potential causes of heart failure with preserved EF, most patients have current hypertension or a history of treated hypertension; the resulting LV hypertrophy and fibrosis are probably responsible for increased chamber stiffness. Ischemic heart disease also may contribute to heart failure with preserved systolic function, probably by virtue of subendocardial fibrosis or as a result of acute, intermittent ischemic dysfunction. Diabetes mellitus is often present, especially in women. Age itself is a crucial predisposing factor because it causes loss of myocytes (apoptosis), increased fibrosis with shifts to more rigid forms of collagen, and loss of vascular compliance.

The mortality rate of patients with heart failure with preserved systolic function is somewhat lower than the rate for those with low EFs but still is high, often owing to the significant comorbid conditions that are common in these older-aged individuals. Hospitalization and rehospitalization rates for these patients are comparable to those for patients with reduced EFs. Unfortunately, clinical trials have yet to identify any therapeutic interventions that improve the outcomes of the patients with heart failure with preserved systolic function.

Although patients who have heart failure with preserved systolic function are often considered to have *diastolic dysfunction,* other explanations for this presentation must be considered, some of which are reversible or warrant specific therapy (Table 58-4). The first two questions to consider are whether the patient's symptoms are caused by heart failure of any type and whether important valvular abnormalities are present. LVEF measurements may be inaccurate, particularly if their technical quality is suboptimal. Regurgitant valve disease may lead to a dissociation between the LVEF and underlying myocardial dysfunction because afterload may be low in this setting. There also are many conditions in which LV function is impaired transiently, but subsequently measured EFs may be normal. Intermittent ischemia, presenting as episodic heart failure *(flash pulmonary edema)*, is the most important of these conditions because revascularization may be indicated. Severe hypertension with subsequent control and transient tachyarrhythmias also may have temporary effects on EF. Some patients with alcoholic cardiomyopathy exhibit rapid recovery in EF when they cease drinking.

The remaining patients most likely have diastolic dysfunction as the underlying disorder. The noninvasive measurement of diastolic function remains problematic. The most commonly used test, Doppler echocardiography, is neither sensitive nor specific for diastolic dysfunction. Particularly in elderly patients, Doppler mitral valve filling patterns show impaired early diastolic filling in most subjects, whether or not they have evidence of heart failure. Diastolic dysfunction is basically a diagnosis of exclusion based on accompanying conditions and circumstantial evidence.

TABLE 58-4 CAUSES OF (AND ALTERNATIVE EXPLANATIONS FOR) HEART FAILURE WITH PRESERVED LEFT VENTRICULAR EJECTION FRACTION (>45-50%)

Inaccurate diagnosis of heart failure (e.g., pulmonary disease, obesity)
Inaccurate measurements of ejection fraction
Systolic function overestimated by ejection fraction (e.g., mitral regurgitation)
Episodic, unrecognized systolic dysfunction
Intermittent ischemia
Arrhythmia
Severe hypertension
Alcohol abuse
Diastolic dysfunction
Abnormalities of myocardial relaxation Ischemia Hypertrophy
Abnormalities of myocardial compliance Hypertrophy Aging Fibrosis Diabetes Infiltrative disease (amyloidosis, sarcoidosis) Storage disease (hemochromatosis) Endomyocardial disease (endomyocardial fibrosis, radiation, anthracyclines)
Pericardial disease (constriction, tamponade)

TABLE 58-5 FACTORS THAT MAY PRECIPITATE ACUTE DECOMPENSATION OF CHRONIC HEART FAILURE

Discontinuation of therapy (patient noncompliance or physician initiated)
Initiation of medications that worsen heart failure (calcium antagonists, β-blockers, nonsteroidal anti-inflammatory drugs, antiarrhythmic agents)
Iatrogenic volume overload (transfusion, fluid administration)
Dietary indiscretion
Alcohol consumption
Increased activity
Pregnancy
Exposure to high altitude
Arrhythmias
Myocardial ischemia or infarction
Worsening hypertension
Worsening mitral or tricuspid regurgitation
Fever or infection
Anemia

Factors Precipitating Acute Decompensation of Chronic Heart Failure

Many patients with chronic heart failure maintain a stable course, and then abruptly present with acutely or subacutely worsening symptoms. Although this decompensation may reflect unrecognized gradual progression of the underlying disorder, many precipitating events must be considered and, if present, addressed (Table 58-5). An important focus is on changes in medications (by patient or physician), diet, or activity. Superimposed new or altered cardiovascular conditions, such as arrhythmias, ischemic events, hypertension, or valvular abnormalities, should be considered. Systemic processes, such as fever, infection, declining renal function, or anemia, also can cause cardiac decompensation.

DIAGNOSIS

The diagnosis of heart failure is straightforward when a patient presents with classic symptoms and accompanying physical findings. In patients with chronic heart failure, however, the diagnosis is often delayed or missed entirely because no single sign or symptom is diagnostic.

CLINICAL EVALUATION

The most frequent symptoms, dyspnea and fatigue, are not specific for heart failure, especially in older individuals, but their presence always should lead to a more complete evaluation. The more specific symptoms of orthopnea, paroxysmal nocturnal dyspnea, and severe edema are much less common. Although the physical examination may be helpful, characteristic physical findings may be absent. The chest radiograph (Chapter 53), on which many physicians rely, adds relatively little to the clinical evaluation except when pulmonary edema is present (see Fig. 53-15 in Chapter 53).

The key to making the timely diagnosis of chronic heart failure is to maintain a high degree of suspicion, particularly in high-risk patients with coronary artery disease, chronic hypertension, diabetes, a history of heavy alcohol use, or advanced age. If such patients present with any of the symptoms or physical findings suggestive of heart failure, additional testing (see later discussion) should be undertaken, typically beginning with echocardiography (Chapter 55).

The common symptoms of heart failure are well known but are frequently absent and variably specific for this condition. The symptoms generally reflect, but may be dissociated from, the hemodynamic derangements of elevated left-sided and right-sided pressures and impaired cardiac output or cardiac output reserve.

Dyspnea

Dyspnea (Chapter 83), or perceived shortness of breath, is the most common symptom of heart failure. In most patients, dyspnea is present only with activity or exertion. The underlying mechanisms are multifactorial. The most important is pulmonary congestion with increased interstitial or intra-alveolar fluid, which activates juxtacapillary J receptors, stimulating a rapid and shallow pattern of breathing. Increased lung stiffness may enhance the work of breathing, leading to a perception of dyspnea. Central regulation of respiration may be disturbed in those with more severe heart failure, resulting in disordered sleep patterns and sleep apnea. Cheyne-Stokes respiration, or periodic breathing, is common in advanced heart failure, is usually associated with low-output states, and may be perceived by the patient (and the patient's family) as either severe dyspnea or transient cessation of breathing. Hypoxia, which is uncommon in heart failure unless there is accompanying pulmonary disease, suggests the presence of pulmonary edema. Dyspnea is a relatively sensitive symptom of heart failure when patients maintain or attempt a moderate level of activity. However, in patients who are inactive, dyspnea may not be prominent, and the diagnosis of heart failure is often delayed or overlooked. In addition, dyspnea may become less prominent with the onset of RV failure and tricuspid regurgitation, which may lead to lower pulmonary venous pressures. Dyspnea, moreover, is also a common symptom of patients with pulmonary disease (Chapter 83), obesity, or anemia and of sedentary individuals.

Orthopnea and Paroxysmal Nocturnal Dyspnea

Orthopnea is dyspnea that is positional, occurring in the recumbent or semirecumbent position. It occurs as a result of the increase in venous return from the extremities and splanchnic circulation to the central circulation with changes in posture, with resultant increases in pulmonary venous pressures and pulmonary capillary hydrostatic pressure. Nocturnal cough may be a manifestation of this process and is an under-recognized symptom of heart failure. Orthopnea is a relatively specific symptom of heart failure, although it may occur in patients with pulmonary disease who breathe more effectively in an upright posture and in individuals with significant abdominal obesity or ascites. Most patients with mild or moderate heart failure do not experience orthopnea if they are treated adequately.

Paroxysmal nocturnal dyspnea is an attack of acute, severe shortness of breath that awakens the patient from sleep, usually 1 to 3 hours after the patient retires. Symptoms usually resolve over 10 to 30 minutes after the patient arises, often gasping for fresh air from an open window. Paroxysmal nocturnal dyspnea results from increased venous return and mobilization of interstitial fluid from the extremities and elsewhere, with accumulation of alveolar edema. Paroxysmal nocturnal dyspnea almost always represents heart failure, but it is a relatively uncommon finding.

Acute Pulmonary Edema

Pulmonary edema results from transudation of fluid into the alveolar spaces due to acute rises in capillary hydrostatic pressures caused by an acute depression of cardiac function or an acute rise in intravascular volume. The initial symptoms may be cough or progressive dyspnea. Because alveolar edema may precipitate bronchospasm, wheezing is common. If the edema is not treated, the patient may begin coughing up pink (or blood-tinged), frothy fluid and become cyanotic and acidotic.

Exercise Intolerance

Activity or exercise intolerance is, together with dyspnea, the most characteristic symptom of chronic heart failure. Intuitively, it might be assumed that exercise would be limited by shortness of breath because of rising pulmonary venous pressures and pulmonary congestion. Although this mechanism may contribute, it is only one of many operating. Blood flow to exercising muscles is impaired as a result of reduced cardiac output reserve and impaired peripheral vasodilation; oxygen delivery is limited, and early fatigue ensues. Heart failure is associated with additional abnormalities of skeletal muscle itself, including biochemical changes and alterations in fiber types, which increase muscle fatigue and impair muscle function. Finally, heart failure may affect adversely respiratory muscle function and ventilatory control.

Fatigue

Fatigue is a common, if nonspecific, complaint of patients with heart failure. Perhaps the most common origin of this complaint is muscle fatigue. Fatigue also may be a nonspecific response to the systemic manifestations of heart failure, such as chronic increases in catecholamines and circulating levels of cytokines, sleep disorders, and anxiety.

Edema and Fluid Retention (Ascites, Pleural Effusion, Pericardial Effusion)

Elevated right atrial pressures increase the capillary hydrostatic pressures in the systemic circulation, with resultant transudation. The location of edema fluid is determined by position (e.g., dependent) and by the accompanying pathology. Most commonly, edema accumulates in the extremities and resolves at night, when the legs are not dependent. Edema may occur only in the feet and ankles, but if it is more severe, it may accumulate in the thighs, scrotum, and abdominal wall. Edema is more likely and more severe in patients with accompanying venous disease, in those who have had veins harvested for coronary bypass surgery, and in patients taking calcium channel blockers, which themselves cause edema. Fluid retention associated with thiazolidinediones (Chapter 237) and nonsteroidal anti-inflammatory drugs may precipitate heart failure or mimic it.

Fluid also may accumulate in the peritoneal cavity and in the pleural or pericardial spaces. Ascites occurs as a result of elevated pressures in the hepatic, portal, and systemic veins draining the peritoneum. Ascites is unusual in heart failure and almost always is associated with peripheral edema. Most commonly, there is severe tricuspid regurgitation, with potential damage to the liver. Otherwise, significant primary liver disease should be suspected as an exacerbating factor or cause of ascites. Pleural effusions are fairly common in chronic heart failure, especially when they are accompanied by left-sided and right-sided manifestations. The effusions result from an increase in transudation of fluid into the pleural space and from impaired lymphatic drainage caused by elevated systemic venous pressures. Pericardial effusions are far less frequent but may occur.

Abdominal and Gastrointestinal Symptoms

Passive congestion of the liver may lead to right upper quadrant pain and tenderness and mild jaundice. Usually only mild elevations of transaminase levels and modest increases in bilirubin levels are observed. With severe, acute rises in central venous pressures, especially if associated with systemic hypotension, a severe congestive and ischemic hepatopathy may occur, with striking elevations in liver function markers and hypoglycemia. Recovery is usually rapid and complete if the hemodynamic abnormalities are corrected.

Bowel wall edema may lead to early satiety (a common symptom in heart failure), nausea, diffuse abdominal discomfort, malabsorption, and a rare form of protein-losing enteropathy. The potential role of heart failure in producing these nonspecific gastrointestinal symptoms is often overlooked, leading to extensive diagnostic testing or unnecessary discontinuation of medications.

Sleep Disorders and Central Nervous System Manifestations

Periods of nocturnal oxygen desaturation to less than 80 to 85% are relatively common in patients with heart failure; they coincide with episodes of apnea (Chapter 100) and often are preceded or followed by episodes of hyperventilation. These are similar to, and may represent truncated forms of, Cheyne-Stokes respiration. These episodes reflect altered central nervous system ventilatory control and have been associated with diminished heart rate variability. Supplemental oxygen appears to reverse some of the ventilatory disorders, and the apneic spells respond to nasal positive-pressure ventilation. In some patients, these interventions have a striking beneficial effect on fatigue and other symptoms of heart failure.

Aside from the common complaint of fatigue, which originates in part in the central nervous system, brain function is not affected in most patients with heart failure. In advanced heart failure, cerebral hypoperfusion can cause impairment of memory, irritability, limited attention span, and altered mentation.

Cardiac Cachexia

In chronic, severe heart failure, unintentional chronic weight loss may occur, leading to a syndrome of cardiac cachexia. The mechanisms underlying this syndrome are unclear, but it may result from many factors, including increased levels of pro-inflammatory cytokines (e.g., TNF), elevated metabolic rates, loss of appetite, and malabsorption. Cardiac cachexia carries a poor prognosis.

PHYSICAL EXAMINATION

The physical findings associated with heart failure generally reflect elevated ventricular filling pressures and, to a lesser extent, reduced cardiac output. In chronic heart failure, many of these findings are absent, often obscuring the correct diagnosis.

Appearance and Vital Signs

Compensated patients may be comfortable, but patients with more severe symptoms are often restless, dyspneic, and pale or diaphoretic. Although the heart rate is usually at the high end of the normal range or higher (>80 beats per minute), it may be lower in patients with chronic, stable heart failure. Premature beats and arrhythmias are common. Pulsus alternans (alternating amplitude of successive beats) is a sign of advanced heart failure (or of a large pericardial effusion). The blood pressure may be normal or high, but in advanced low-output heart failure, it is usually on the low end of normal or lower.

Jugular Veins and Neck Examination

Examination of the jugular veins is one of the most useful aspects of the evaluation of patients with heart failure. The jugular venous pressure should be quantified in centimeters of water (normal = 8 cm H_2O) (see Figs. 50-2 and 50-3 in Chapter 50), estimating the level of pulsations above the sternal angle (and arbitrarily adding 5 cm H_2O in any posture). The presence of abdominal-jugular reflux should be assessed by putting pressure on the right upper quadrant of the abdomen for 30 seconds and avoiding an induced Valsalva maneuver; a positive finding is a rise in the jugular pressure of at least 1 cm. Either an elevated jugular venous pressure or an abnormal abdominal-jugular reflux has been reported in 80% of patients with advanced heart failure. No other simple sign is nearly as sensitive.

An additional important finding in the neck is evidence of tricuspid regurgitation—a large "cv" wave, usually associated with a high jugular venous pressure. This finding is confirmed by hepatic pulsations, which can be detected during the abdominal-jugular reflux determination. The carotid pulses should be evaluated for evidence of aortic stenosis, and thyroid abnormalities should be sought.

Pulmonary Examination

Although dyspnea is the most common symptom of patients with heart failure, the pulmonary examination is usually unremarkable. Rales, representing alveolar fluid, are a hallmark of heart failure; when they are present in patients without accompanying pulmonary disease, they are highly specific for the diagnosis. In chronic heart failure, they are often absent, however, even in patients known to have pulmonary capillary wedge pressures greater than 20 mm Hg (normal, <12 mm Hg). LV failure cannot be excluded by the absence of rales. Pleural effusions, which tend to lateralize on the right side because of the greater surface area of the lungs, are not uncommon, but large effusions are relatively rare in chronic heart failure.

Cardiac Examination

The cardiac examination is a crucial part of the evaluation of the patient with heart failure, but it is more useful for identification of associated cardiac abnormalities than for assessment of the severity of the heart failure (Chapter 50). Assessment of the point of maximal impulse may provide information concerning the size of the heart (enlarged if displaced below the fifth intercostal space or lateral to the midclavicular line) and its function (if sustained beyond one third of systole or palpable over two interspaces). Additional precordial pulsations may indicate an LV aneurysm. A parasternal lift is valuable evidence of pulmonary hypertension.

The first heart sound (S_1) may be diminished in amplitude when LV function is poor, and the pulmonic component of the second heart sound (P_2) may be accentuated when pulmonary hypertension is present. An apical third heart sound (S_3) is a strong indicator of significant LV systolic dysfunction, but it is present only in a minority of patients with low EFs and elevated LV filling pressures. A fourth heart sound (S_4) is not a specific indicator of heart failure, but it is usually present in patients with diastolic dysfunction. An S_3 at the lower left or right sternal border or below the xiphoid indicates RV dysfunction. Murmurs may indicate the presence of significant valvular disease as the cause of heart failure, but mitral and tricuspid regurgitation also are common secondary manifestations of severe ventricular dilation and dysfunction.

Examination of the Abdomen and Extremities

The size, pulsatility, and tenderness of the liver should be evaluated as evidence of passive congestion and tricuspid regurgitation. Ascites and edema should be sought and quantified.

Characterization: Essential and Contingent Tests

Essential Tests

Chest Radiography

Although the standard posteroanterior and lateral chest radiographs provide limited information about chamber size, the presence of overall cardiomegaly (a cardiothoracic ratio of >0.50, especially if >0.60) is a strong indicator of heart failure or another cause of cardiomegaly (especially valvular insufficiency) (see Fig. 53-4 in Chapter 53). However, almost 50% of patients with heart failure do not have this high a cardiothoracic ratio.

Most patients with acute heart failure, but only a minority of those with chronic heart failure, have clear evidence of pulmonary venous hypertension (upper lobe redistribution, enlarged pulmonary veins), interstitial edema (haziness of the central vascular shadows or increased central interstitial lung markings), or pulmonary edema (perihilar or patchy peripheral infiltrates). The absence of these findings reflects the subjectivity of interpretation and the increased capacity of the lymphatics to remove interstitial and alveolar fluid in chronic heart failure. This absence of radiographic findings is consistent with the absence of rales in most patients with chronic heart failure despite markedly elevated pulmonary venous pressures. Pleural effusions are important adjunctive evidence of heart failure. Characteristically, these are more common and larger on the right than on the left side, reflecting the greater pleural surface area of the right lung.

Electrocardiography

The major importance of the electrocardiogram is to evaluate cardiac rhythm, identify prior MI, and detect evidence of LV hypertrophy (Chapter 54). Prior MI suggests that the cause is ischemic cardiomyopathy with systolic dysfunction. LV hypertrophy is a nonspecific finding but may point toward LV diastolic dysfunction if the EF is not depressed.

Echocardiography

Noninvasive cardiac imaging is a crucial part of the diagnosis and evaluation of heart failure. The most useful procedure is transthoracic echocardiography (Chapter 55), which provides a quantitative assessment of LV function; in the presence of appropriate symptoms and signs, it can confirm the presence of heart failure resulting from systolic dysfunction or indicate whether the patient has heart failure with preserved systolic function. The echocardiogram also provides a wealth of additional valuable information, including assessment of LV and RV size and regional wall motion (as an indicator of prior MI), evaluation of the heart valves, and diagnosis of LV hypertrophy. Particularly valuable are quantitative measurements of pulmonary artery and central venous pressures. The echocardiogram generally has replaced the chest radiograph in the diagnostic assessment of heart failure, and it can provide useful hemodynamic measurements without cardiac catheterization.

Measurements of Natriuretic Peptides

Serum levels of natriuretic peptides can be measured quickly and accurately, including point-of-care testing at the bedside. B-type natriuretic peptide (BNP) and amino (N)-terminal pro-BNP are relatively sensitive and specific markers for clinically confirmed heart failure These peptides have been found to be useful adjuncts in the diagnosis of patients presenting in the acute care setting with possible heart failure, particularly when the diagnosis remains uncertain.[1] However, levels of both BNP and N-terminal pro-BNP increase with age in the absence of clinical heart failure, especially in women, probably reflecting increased ventricular stiffness associated with aging and hypertension. BNP levels may also be increased slightly in patients with chronic obstructive pulmonary disease, in whom elevations may reflect diastolic dysfunction or RV dysfunction but nonetheless may lead to a false-positive clinical diagnosis of heart failure. Elevated natriuretic peptide measurements are associated with a worse prognosis and may be helpful in assessing the response to therapy. Randomized clinical trials that have assessed the clinical value of serial measurements in guiding therapy suggest a reduction in all-cause mortality compared with usual clinical practice.[2]

Contingent Tests

After the diagnosis of heart failure is made, the goal of additional testing is to identify potentially correctable or specifically treatable causes and to obtain further information that is necessary for future management.

Laboratory Testing

An extensive battery of laboratory tests is not required for most patients with heart failure. Routine testing should include a complete blood cell count (to detect anemia and systemic diseases with hematologic manifestations); measurement of renal function and electrolytes, including magnesium (to exclude renal failure and to provide a baseline for subsequent therapy); liver function tests (to exclude accompanying liver pathology and provide a baseline); and blood glucose and lipid testing (to diagnose diabetes and dyslipidemia, both of which should be managed aggressively in patients with heart failure).

A few additional tests may be indicated. Thyrotoxicosis, and to a lesser extent hypothyroidism, may cause heart failure and may be difficult to diagnose clinically, especially in older patients (Chapter 233). Many guidelines recommend thyroid function tests for all patients, or at least all elderly patients and those with atrial fibrillation. Hemochromatosis (Chapter 219) is a potentially treatable cause of heart failure; particularly if there is accompanying diabetes or hepatic disease, measurement of serum ferritin levels is indicated. Sarcoidosis (Chapter 95) is another potentially treatable cause, although it would be unusual not to have evidence of accompanying lung disease. Amyloidosis (Chapter 194) should be considered in patients with other manifestations, but treatment of the cardiac manifestations is rarely successful except with heart transplantation.

Assessment of Left Ventricular Function

Although heart failure is a syndrome with many pathogenic mechanisms, the most common are LV systolic dysfunction and LV diastolic dysfunction. In some patients, it is almost impossible to distinguish between these two forms of heart failure by clinical evaluation because both may present with the same symptoms and with only subtle differences on physical examination. However, it is important to distinguish between these two entities because they may require different diagnostic evaluations and different therapeutic approaches (Chapter 59). The most useful and practical test is the echocardiogram (Chapter 55); alternative approaches include radionuclide measurements of LVEF (Chapter 56) and left ventriculography if cardiac catheterization (Chapter 57) is being performed. All these tests allow the detection of significant systolic dysfunction; diastolic dysfunction sometimes can be documented (Chapter 55) but often is identified primarily as a process of exclusion in patients with preserved systolic function. Randomized trials have found no benefit, in terms of days alive and out of hospital or in a number of other relevant end points, among patients who were monitored with pulmonary artery catheterization compared with those who were not.[3]

DIAGNOSTIC EVALUATION

Assessment for Coronary Artery Disease

Coronary artery disease is the most common cause of heart failure in industrialized societies, particularly in men. Often it is known that a patient has coronary disease based on a prior history of MI or positive results on an angiogram or noninvasive test, but in some patients, MI can be silent. There are two reasons to identify the coexistence of heart failure and coronary disease: first, to treat symptoms that may be caused by ischemia and, second, to improve prognosis (Chapters 71, 72, and 73). A prudent approach is to divide patients with heart failure into three groups: (1) those with clinical evidence of ongoing ischemia (active angina or a possible ischemic equivalent), (2) those who have had a prior MI but do not currently have angina, and (3) those who may or may not have underlying coronary disease. The first group of patients may be evaluated most expeditiously by coronary angiography because they stand to benefit in terms of symptoms and probably have more extensive ischemia. In the second group are patients with heart failure and prior MI who by other criteria (age, absence of other major comorbid conditions) are good candidates for coronary revascularization; they generally should undergo noninvasive stress testing in conjunction with nuclear myocardial perfusion imaging or echocardiography to assess regional function and myocardial viability (Chapter 71). CT angiography is a useful screening test to evaluate coronary anatomy (Chapter 56), but it provides little physiologic information. These procedures identify individuals with extensive ischemic but viable myocardium, whose prognosis and symptoms also may be improved with revascularization. The third group, patients without either angina or prior MI, are much less likely to benefit from an evaluation for asymptomatic coronary disease.

Myocardial Biopsy

There is no rationale for routine myocardial biopsy in patients with heart failure, even in the subgroup without apparent coronary disease. Few entities that might be detected are amenable to specific therapy, and those that are (hemochromatosis, sarcoidosis) usually can be detected by their other manifestations or other procedures. A possible exception is acute fulminant myocarditis (Chapter 60), particularly eosinophilic and giant cell myocarditis, which may respond to immunosuppressive therapy. Another exception is in the patient being evaluated for cardiac transplantation (Chapter 82) because the presence of some entities may preclude this procedure.

Assessment of Exercise Capacity

Quantitative assessment of exercise capacity provides additional insight into prognosis beyond the clinical evaluation and measurements of cardiac function, particularly when a detailed history of activity tolerance cannot be obtained. Exercise testing with measurements of peak oxygen uptake by respiratory gas exchange has become a routine part of the evaluation for transplantation (Chapter 82) because it provides an indication of need for early intervention and an additional method for follow-up. In most patients, testing is not necessary, however. Emphasis should be placed on eliciting each patient's maximum tolerated activity and the minimum activity associated with symptoms; both can be monitored from visit to visit as a guide to management.

Assessment of Arrhythmias

Ventricular arrhythmias are extremely common in patients with chronic heart failure, with 50 to 80% of patients exhibiting nonsustained ventricular tachycardia during 24-hour monitoring. Because approximately 50% of cardiac deaths in these patients are sudden, these arrhythmias have been viewed with concern. In multivariate analyses, asymptomatic ventricular arrhythmias carry little independent prognostic significance when the severity of symptoms, EF, and presence of concurrent coronary disease are taken into account. Arrhythmias are no more predictive of sudden death than of total mortality. Ventricular arrhythmias associated with syncope or hemodynamic compromise must be taken seriously and require further evaluation and treatment (Chapter 65). Selected patients with advanced heart failure will benefit from implantable cardioverter defibrillators (Chapters 59 and 66).

Differential Diagnosis

Although it is not difficult to make the definitive diagnosis of heart failure in a patient who presents with the classic symptoms and signs, several alternative diagnoses need to be considered in less clear-cut situations, such as in the patient with normal LV function and less definitive clinical evidence. The most common alternative diagnosis is pulmonary disease, for which pulmonary function testing is usually helpful (Chapter 85). If LV systolic function is normal, it may be difficult to make a conclusive determination of the relative role of diastolic heart failure compared with other concomitant conditions, such as severe obesity, chronic anemia, or other systemic illnesses; in some patients, a therapeutic trial of treatment for heart failure (Chapter 59) may be diagnostic.

Follow-Up Testing

After the diagnosis of heart failure is confirmed and the initial evaluation is complete, there is little need for further testing beyond the laboratory tests necessary to monitor therapy (primarily renal function and electrolytes). If the status of ventricular function is known, there are few indications for retesting. Exceptions are monitoring for transplantation and important changes in clinical status, such as marked deterioration in a patient previously known to have preserved LV function or the occurrence of new murmurs in conjunction with declining status.

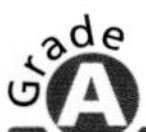

1. Lam LL, Cameron PA, Schneider HG, et al. Meta-analysis: effect of B-type natriuretic peptide testing on clinical outcomes in patients with acute dyspnea in the emergency setting. *Ann Intern Med.* 2010;153:728-735.
2. Porapakkham P, Zimmet H, Billah B, et al. B-type natriuretic peptide-guided heart failure therapy: a meta-analysis. *Arch Intern Med.* 2010;170:507-514.
3. The ESCAPE Investigators. Evaluation study of congestive heart failure and pulmonary artery catheterization effectiveness. The ESCAPE trial. *JAMA.* 2005;294:1625-1633.

SUGGESTED READINGS

Al-Mohammad A, Mant J. The diagnosis and management of chronic heart failure: review following the publication of the NICE guidelines. *Heart.* 2011;97:411-416. *Review.*

Heart Failure Society of America. 2010 Comprehensive guideline: executive summary. *J Cardiac Failure.* 2010;16:475-539. *Consensus guidelines.*

Hunt SA. Focused update incorporated into the ACC/AHA 2005 guidelines for the diagnosis and management of heart failure in adults. *Circulation.* 2009;119:e391-479. *Consensus guideline update.*

McMurray JJ. Clinical practice: systolic heart failure. *N Engl J Med* 2010;362:228-238. *Practical overview.*

59 HEART FAILURE: MANAGEMENT AND PROGNOSIS

JOHN J. V. MCMURRAY AND MARC A. PFEFFER

EVALUATION AND MANAGEMENT OF HEART FAILURE

Heart failure is an overarching term for a syndrome (i.e., a constellation of signs and symptoms) that encompasses a vast spectrum of cardiovascular disorders and is associated with a greatly heightened risk for death and nonfatal adverse cardiovascular events (Chapter 58). Treatment is initially directed toward prevention of cardiac injury (e.g., due to hypertension or myocardial infarction) or toward limiting structural progression if cardiac damage has already occurred (e.g., left ventricular remodeling with declining left ventricular ejection fraction) and delaying the development of symptomatic heart failure. Once symptoms develop, treatments are also directed at improving functional status as well as prognosis.

Approximately one in five adults will develop heart failure. In the United States, 5.8 million people have heart failure, and U.S. hospitals annually admit 1.1 million patients with a primary diagnosis of heart failure. The estimated cost of heart failure in the United States is about $39 billion per year. Randomized controlled clinical trials (RCTs) supply the framework for quantifying what different therapeutic approaches can offer. Even when they are definitive, RCTs only generate data about average risks and benefits of the tested therapeutic option in a selected cohort. Because an individual patient's responses can only be implied from the overall estimated group responses, RCTs cannot definitively direct the approach of every patient or answer the myriad questions that confront the practitioner regarding the specific circumstances of the patient. Another major limitation of RCTs is the relatively narrow time frame of observation, generally only months to several years, compared with epidemiologic experiences during decades. Despite these limitations, RCTs are the premier tool of evidence-based medicine, and the field of heart failure has fortunately been the focus of relatively high-quality RCTs that have provided robust evidence to improve clinical care and prognosis (Table 59-1). Indeed, the implementation of evidence from RCTs into clinical practice has resulted in impressive temporal improvements in survival after discharge from a first hospital admission for heart failure. Moreover, the age at which symptomatic heart failure first becomes evident has increased. Despite these tangible advances, heart failure continues to be a leading cause of morbidity and mortality in elderly people.

STAGES OF HEART FAILURE

The American Heart Association/American College of Cardiology Guidelines for the Evaluation and Management of Chronic Heart Failure in the Adult use a staging classification to underscore the evolution and progression of heart failure severity (Fig. 59-1). This classification emphasizes the use of different strategies and therapeutic options across the full spectrum of the syndrome, from prevention of heart failure to palliation of patients with end-stage disease.

Stage A: Individuals at Risk for Development of Heart Failure

Stage A designates patients at risk for development of heart failure based on concomitant cardiovascular diseases such as hypertension, coronary artery disease, and diabetes mellitus. Also included in stage A are individuals with prior exposure to cardiotoxic agents such as doxorubicin (Chapter 182) and those with a family history of a cardiomyopathy (Chapter 60). Although these predisposing factors do not by themselves technically constitute the syndrome of heart failure, the guidelines stress the importance of identifying individuals with modifiable factors because this represents an important opportunity to reduce the reservoir of patients at risk.

Population-based preventive approaches can reduce the incidence of heart failure. For example, public health programs targeting the eradication of the insect vector for *Trypanosoma cruzi* (Chapter 355) have reduced the incidence of Chagas' cardiomyopathy (Chapter 60) in endemic regions of South and Central America.

Other population-based approaches to reduce the incidence of heart failure require specific screening efforts to identify individuals with modifiable risk factors. The most important, although unfortunately nonmodifiable, risk factor for the development of heart failure is advanced age; the incidence of heart failure rises sharply per decade after the age of 45 years (Chapter 58). For each decade of age after 45 years, the incidence of heart failure doubles, and heart failure is the leading hospital diagnosis for patients older than 65 years in the United States.

Hypertension

Of the modifiable factors, hypertension (Chapter 67) undoubtedly contributes the greatest population-attributable risk for heart failure. In other words, even though the increased risk of heart failure in an individual with hypertension is modest, the high prevalence of hypertension in the general population means that at a population level, hypertension is the major cause of heart failure.

The contribution of hypertension to the risk of heart failure was a consistent finding from all major cardiovascular epidemiologic studies, and the earliest RCTs of antihypertensive therapy showed unambiguous reductions in the risk of heart failure. Of the components of blood pressure, elevated systolic pressure has a greater influence on the incidence of heart failure than does diastolic pressure. In fact, aging is associated with a progressive rise in systolic blood pressure and fall in diastolic pressure as the compliance of the arterial tree diminishes (Chapter 67). In community-based studies, isolated systolic hypertension and elevated pulse pressure have been the most predictive blood pressure measurements for development of heart failure. In the Systolic Hypertension in the Elderly Program, antihypertensive treatment with chlorthalidone followed by atenolol reduced the incidence of new heart failure by about 50%, a treatment effect size recently exceeded (relative risk reduction, 64%) with indapamide followed by perindopril in the Hypertension in Very Elderly Trial, probably the last placebo-controlled

TABLE 59-1 CONTROLLED TRIALS* IN SYMPTOMATIC HEART FAILURE WITH REDUCED SYSTOLIC FUNCTION

TRIAL, TREATMENT, AND YEAR PUBLISHED	*N*	SEVERITY OF HEART FAILURE	ESTIMATED FIRST-YEAR PLACEBO/CONTROL GROUP MORTALITY	BACKGROUND TREATMENT†	TREATMENT ADDED	TRIAL DURATION (YR)	PRIMARY END POINT	RELATIVE RISK REDUCTION (%)‡	*Events Prevented Per 1000 Patients Treated*§‖		
									DEATH	HF HOSP.	DEATH OR HF HOSP.
ACE INHIBITORS											
CONSENSUS, 1987[5]	253	End stage	52	Spironolactone	Enalapril, 20 mg bid	0.54‡	Death	40	146	—	—
SOLVD-T, 1991[6]	2569	Mild-severe	15.7	—	Enalapril, 20 mg bid	3.5	Death	16	45	96	108
β-BLOCKERS											
CIBIS-2, 1999[a]	2647	Moderate-severe	13.2	ACE-I	Bisoprolol, 10 mg qd	1.3‡	Death	34	55	56	—
MERIT-HF, 1999[b]	3991	Mild-severe	11.0	ACE-I	Metoprolol CR/XL, 200 mg qd	1.0‡	Death	34	36	46	63
COPERNICUS, 2001[10]	2289	Severe	19.7	ACE-I	Carvedilol, 25 mg bid	0.87‡	Death	35	55	65	81
SENIORS, 2005[c]	2128	Mild-severe	10.4	ACE-I + spironolactone	Nebivolol, 10 mg qd	1.75	Death or CV hosp.	14	23	0	—
ANGIOTENSIN RECEPTOR BLOCKERS											
Val-HeFT, 2001[8]	5010	Mild-severe	~8.0	ACE-I	Valsartan, 160 mg bid	1.9	CV death or morbidity	13	0	35	33¶
CHARM-Alternative, 2003[7]	2028	Mild-severe	12.6	BB	Candesartan, 32 mg qd	2.8	CV death or HF hosp.	23	30	31	60
CHARM-Added, 2003[9]	2548	Moderate-severe	10.6	ACE-I + BB	Candesartan, 32 mg qd	3.4	CV death or HF hosp.	15	28	47	39
ALDOSTERONE BLOCKADE											
RALES, 1999[11]	1663	Severe	~25	ACE-I	Spirolactone, 25-50 mg qd	2.0‡	Death	30	113	95	—
EMPHASIS-HF, 2011[13]	2737	Mild	8.1	ACE-I + BB	Eplerenone, 50 mg qd	1.75	Death or HF hosp.	37	30	64	66
HYDRALAZINE-ISDN											
V-HeFT-1, 1986[d]	459	Mild-severe	26.4	—	Hydralazine, 75 mg tid-qid ISDN, 40 mg qid	2.3	Death	34	52	0	—
A-HeFT, 2004[15]	1050	Moderate-severe	~9.0	ACE-I + BB + spironolactone	Hydralazine, 75 mg tid ISDN, 40 mg tid	0.83‡	Composite	—	40	80	—

DIGITALIS GLYCOSIDES											
DIG, 1997[14]	6800	Mild-severe	~11.0	ACE-I	Digoxin	3.1	Death	0	0	79	73
SHIFT, 2010	6558	Mild-severe	~7.5	ACE-I + BB + spironolactone	Ivabradine 7.5 mg bid	1.9	CV death or HF hosp.	18	14	47	—
CRT											
COMPANION, 2004[20]	925	Moderate-severe	19.0	ACE-I + BB + spironolactone	CRT	1.35[‡]	Death or any hospital admission	19	38	—	87
CARE-HF, 2005[21]	813	Moderate-severe	12.6	ACE-I + BB + spironolactone	CRT	2.45	Death or CV hospital admission	37	97	151	184
CRT-D											
COMPANION, 2004[20]	903	Moderate-severe	19.0	ACE-I + BB + spironolactone	CRT-ICD	1.35[‡]	Death or any hospital admission	20	74	—	114
MADIT-CRT, 2009[23]	1820	Mild	~3.0%	ACE-I + BB + spironolactone + ICD	CRT-ICD	2.4[‡]	Death or HF event**	34	5	—	—
RAFT, 2010[22]	1798	Mild-moderate	~6.5	ACE-I + BB + spironolactone + ICD	CRT-ICD	3.3	Death or HF hosp.	25	53	66	70
IMPLANTABLE CARDIOVERTER-DEFIBRILLATOR											
SCD-HeFT, 2005[19]	1676	Mild-severe	~7.0	ACE-I + BB	ICD	3.8	Death	23	—	—	—
VENTRICULAR ASSIST DEVICE											
REMATCH, 2001[e]	129	End stage	75	ACE-I + spironolactone	LVAD	1.8	Death	48	282	—	—
EXERCISE TRAINING											
HF-ACTION, 2009[17]	2231	Mild-severe	~6.0	ACE-I + BB+ spironolactone	Exercise training	2.5	Death or any hosp.	7	6	—	—

*Excluding active-controlled trials.

[†]In more than one third of patients, ACE-I + BB means that ACE inhibitors were used in almost all patients and BB in the majority; most patients were also taking diuretics, and many digoxin (except in DIG). Spironolactone was used at baseline in 5% Val-HeFT, 8% MERIT-HF, 17% CHARM-Added, 19% SCD-HeFT, 20% COPERNICUS, and 24% CHARM-Alternative.

[‡]Relative risk reduction in primary end point.

[§]Stopped early for benefit.

[||]Individual trials may not have been designed or powered to evaluate effect of treatment on these outcomes.

[¶]Primary end point that also included treatment of heart failure with intravenous drugs for 4 hours or more without admission and resuscitated cardiac arrest (both added small numbers).

[a]The Cardiac Insufficiency Bisoprolol Study II (CIBIS-II): a randomised trial. *Lancet.* 1999;353:9-13.

[b]Effect of metoprolol CR/XL in chronic heart failure: metoprolol CR/XL Randomised Intervention Trial in Congestive Heart Failure (MERIT-HF). *Lancet.* 1999;353:2001-2007.

[c]Cohn JN, Archibald DG, Ziesche S, et al. Effect of vasodilator therapy on mortality in chronic congestive heart failure: results of a Veterans Administration Cooperative Study. *N Engl J Med.* 1986;314:1547-1552.

[d]Rose EA, Gelijns AC, Moskowitz AJ, et al. Long-term mechanical left ventricular assistance for end-stage heart failure. *N Engl J Med.* 2001;345:1435-1443.

[e]Flather MD, Shibata MC, Coats AJ, et al. Randomized trial to determine the effect of nebivolol on mortality and cardiovascular hospital admission in elderly patients with heart failure (SENIORS). *Eur Heart J.* 2005;26:215-225.

ACE-I = ACE inhibitor; BB = β-blocker; CRT = cardiac resynchronization therapy (biventricular pacing); CRT-D = CRT device that also defibrillates; CV = cardiovascular; HF hosp. = patients with at least one hospital admission for worsening heart failure—some patients had multiple admissions; ICD = implantable cardioverter-defibrillator; ISDN = isosorbide dinitrate; LVAD = left ventricular assist device.

Modified from McMurray JJ, Pfeffer MA. Heart failure. *Lancet.* 2005;365:1877-1889.

Trials

Therapy	Stage A	Stage B	Stage C	Stage D
Antihypertensives	VA Study I and II SHEP HOT ALLHAT	→	→	
Statins	HPS WOSCOPS ASCOT-LLA AFCAPS-Texcaps	HPS 4S CARE	→	→
β-Blockers		BHAT Norwegian β-blocker trial CAPRICORN	CIBIS II MERIT HF COPERNICUS COMET SENIORS	
ACE inhibitors	HOPE EUROPA (PEACE)	SAVE AIRE TRACE SOLVD-P	SOLVD-T CONSENSUS	
Angiotensin II receptor blockers (ARBs)		VALIANT	CHARM alternative CHARM added → Val-HeFT	→
Hydralazine/ nitrates			V-HeFT I and II A-HeFT →	→
Digoxin			DIG	
Aldosterone antagonists		EPHESUS →	→ RALES →	→
Implantable cardioverter-defibrillator (ICD)		MADIT II	SCD-HeFT →	→
Cardiac resynchronization therapy (CRT)			COMPANION CARE HF MADIT-CRT →	→
Left ventricle assist device (LVAD)				REMATCH

Stage A	Stage B	Stage C	Stage D
High risk for HF without structural heart disease or symptoms of HF	Structural heart disease but without signs or symptoms of HF	Structural heart disease with prior or current symptoms of HF	Refractory HF requiring specialized interventions
Patients with • Hypertension • Artherosclerotic disease • Diabetes • Obesity • Metabolic syndrome or Patients using • Cardiotoxins with family history of cardiomyopathy (FHx CM)	Patients with • Previous MI • LV remodeling including LVH and low EF • Asymptomatic valvular disease	Patients with • Known structural heart disease • Shortness of breath and fatigue, reduced exercise tolerance	Patients with marked symptoms at rest despite maximal medical therapy (e.g., those who are recurrently hospitalized or cannot be safely discharged from the hospital without specialized interventions)
↓	↓	↓	↓

THERAPY
Goals
• Treat hypertension
• Encourage smoking cessation
• Treat lipid disorders
• Encourage regular exercise
• Discourage alcohol intake, illicit drug use
• Control metabolic syndrome
Drugs
• ACEI or ARB as appropriate patients for vascular or diabetes
	THERAPY
	Goals
	• Treat hypertension
	• Encourage smoking cessation
	• Treat lipid disorders
	• Encourage regular exercise
	• Discourage alcohol intake, illicit drug use
	• Control metabolic syndrome
	Drugs
	• ACEI or ARB as appropriate patients for vascular or diabetes
	• β-Blockers in appropriate patients
	Devices in selected patients
	• Implantable defibrillators
		THERAPY
		Goals
		• Treat hypertension
		• Encourage smoking cessation
		• Treat lipid disorders
		• Encourage regular exercise
		• Discourage alcohol intake, illicit drug use
		• Control metabolic syndrome
		• Dietary salt restriction
		Drugs for routine use
		• Diuretics for fluid retention
		• ACEI
		• β-Blockers in appropriate patients
		Drugs in selected patients
		• Aldosterone antagonist
		• ARBs
		• Digitalis
		• Hydralazine/nitrates
		Devices in selected patients
		• Biventricular pacing
		• Implantable defibrillators
			THERAPY
			Goals
			• Appropriate measures under stages A, B, C
			• Decision re: appropriate level of care
			Options
			• Compassionate end-of-life care/hospice
			• Extraordinary measures
			  • Heart transplantation
			  • Chronic inotropes
			  • Permanent mechanical support
			  • Experimental surgery or drugs

antihypertensive trial. In general, the actual extent of blood pressure lowering achieved, not the agent used, is the most important factor in reducing overall rates of major cardiovascular events. However, the greatest reduction in risk of heart failure seems to be seen when initial therapy is based on a diuretic and angiotensin-converting enzyme (ACE) inhibitor. By comparison, treatment with α-blockers increases the risk of heart failure compared with other antihypertensive drugs. Most important, it is estimated that effective treatment of hypertension (Chapter 67) will substantially reduce the age-adjusted incidence of heart failure by approximately 60% in women and 50% in men.

Other Risk Factors

Treatment of atherosclerotic risk factors, such as hypercholesterolemia (Chapter 213), and promotion of measures that encourage healthier lifestyles, such as smoking cessation (Chapter 31), weight control (Chapter 227), and aerobic exercise (Chapter 15), should also reduce the number of individuals who progress from stage A to stage B (structural heart disease but without symptoms of heart failure). ACE inhibitors protect against the development of heart failure in patients with diabetes mellitus or with evidence of atherosclerosis. Although obesity is correlated with hypertension, lipid abnormalities, and glucose intolerance, an elevated body mass index is also an independent risk factor for the development of heart failure.

Stage B: Asymptomatic Structural or Functional Heart Disease

Stage B identifies asymptomatic (class I; Chapter 58) patients who have a structural or functional cardiac disorder (e.g., left ventricular hypertrophy, enlargement, or dysfunction and valvar abnormalities) but do not have the signs and symptoms, such as dyspnea and fatigue, of the heart failure syndrome. In addition to history, physical examination, and electrocardiography (Chapter 54), more extensive screening with echocardiography (Chapter 55) or other imaging modalities (Chapter 56) is often required to detect patients with asymptomatic cardiac structural abnormalities.

A patient who has an acute myocardial infarction not complicated by early heart failure is an obvious example of someone who transitions from stage A to stage B. Rapid pharmacologic or mechanical coronary reperfusion is one of the immediate goals of therapy, with the aim of limiting the extent of myocardial injury and reducing the risk for death and future development of heart failure (Chapters 72 and 73). Survivors of the acute phase of myocardial infarction, a well-studied stage B cohort, are at particularly high risk for the future development of heart failure, with an overall annual incidence of 2% per year—but higher in patients who are older, have a lower left ventricular ejection fraction (LVEF), do not routinely perform at least moderate exercise, or have concomitant hypertension or diabetes mellitus. For example, a clinically stable asymptomatic patient who has recovered from a myocardial infarction but who is older than 60 years with an LVEF of less than 50% and a history of diabetes and hypertension has an estimated 30% 5-year likelihood of experiencing death or heart failure; without diabetes or hypertension, the 5-year estimated rate becomes 12%. By comparison, a younger myocardial infarction survivor who has an LVEF over 50% and does not have hypertension or diabetes would be anticipated to have a 5-year rate for heart failure or death of only 3%. Data also suggest that an assessment of right ventricular function provides further independent incremental prediction for the risk of developing heart failure. With the continued improvements in care of patients with acute myocardial infarction (Chapters 72 and 73) and the use of implantable cardioverter-defibrillators (ICDs) after myocardial infarction in patients with reduced LVEF, this pool of stage B patients, who represent a reservoir for new-onset heart failure, has been expanding.

The impaired left ventricle, often due to a prior myocardial infarction, can undergo progressive chamber enlargement. This process, also termed *left ventricular remodeling*, describes the time-dependent and often insidious structural alterations of the impaired left ventricle, whereby the relationship of the left ventricular cavity volume increases out of proportion to mass, so the overall ventricular geometry becomes more distorted, usually more spherical. This distortion of left ventricular geometry often leads to mitral regurgitation. These structural changes produce regional and global increases in myocardial wall stress, which can promote further remodeling and contribute to the progressive deterioration of cardiac function and structure often associated with the later stages of symptomatic heart failure.

TREATMENT Rx

ACE Inhibitors and Angiotensin Receptor Blockers

Mechanistic studies confirm that ACE inhibitors inhibit progressive left ventricular enlargement by reducing wall stress during the entire cardiac cycle as well as by more direct inhibition of the intracellular signaling pathways involved in myocardial hypertrophy and interstitial fibrosis. This attenuation of ventricular remodeling by ACE inhibitors reduces the development of symptomatic heart failure and death in stage B asymptomatic patients with left ventricular dysfunction by about 20%.[1,2] In addition, deaths, often sudden and unexpected, attributed to cardiovascular causes, are reduced in stage B patients by ACE inhibitor therapy.

Several ACE inhibitors are effective as prophylactic therapy for high-risk stage B patients (see Fig. 59-1), and the target dose of each agent is established (Table 59-2). The angiotensin receptor blocker (ARB) valsartan (Table 59-3) is as effective as captopril in reducing risk for cardiovascular death and other nonfatal cardiovascular outcomes,[3] thereby providing an alternative pharmacologic class of agents. Importantly, in patients with left ventricular dysfunction or acute heart failure in the context of a myocardial infarction, the combination of an ACE inhibitor and ARB is not better than either alone, so combination therapy is not recommended in this setting.

β-Blockers

β-Adrenergic receptor blockers (β-blockers) have long been known to reduce death and recurrent myocardial infarction when they are administered during the acute phase of myocardial infarction in patients without pulmonary congestion (Chapter 73). However, carvedilol (Table 59-4) also improves survival, reduces subsequent nonfatal myocardial infarctions, and has a favorable trend for reduced hospitalizations for heart failure in patients with a recent myocardial infarction and reduced LVEF (≤40%) when it is added to an ACE inhibitor.[4] For stage B patients whose left ventricular dysfunction does not have an ischemic etiology, the evidence for β-blockers is less firm.

Treatment of Arrhythmias

Functional as well as structural problems may lead to the development of heart failure. For example, a persistently rapid ventricular rate in patients with atrial fibrillation can cause a rate-related (tachycardia-induced) cardiomyopathy (Chapter 64). Adequate pharmacologic control of the ventricular rate or interventions to restore sinus rhythm or to ablate re-entry pathways (Chapter 66) may reduce the risk for heart failure.

Other Therapies

Any treatments that control hypertension or reduce the risk of myocardial infarction will benefit stage B patients. Examples include statins, antiplatelet agents, and smoking cessation.

FIGURE 59-1. Stages of heart failure (HF). 4S = Scandinavian Simvastatin Survival Study; AFCAPS-Texcaps = Air Force/Texas Coronary Atherosclerosis Prevention Study; A-HeFT = African American Heart Failure Trial; AIRE = Acute Infarction Ramipril Efficacy study; ALLHAT = Antihypertensive and Lipid Lowering to Prevent Heart Attack Trial; ASCOT-LLA = Anglo-Scandinavian Cardiac Outcomes Trial—Lipid Lowering Arm; BHAT = The Beta-Blocker Heart Attack Trial; CAPRICORN = Carvedilol Post-Infarct Survival Control in LV Dysfunction; CARE HF = Cardiac Resynchronization in Heart Failure; CHARM added = Candesartan in Heart Failure—Added Trial; CHARM alternative = Candesartan in Heart Failure—Alternative Trial; CIBIS II = Cardiac Insufficiency Bisoprolol Study II; COMET = Carvedilol or Metoprolol European Trial; COMPANION = Comparison of Medical Therapy, Pacing, and Defibrillation in Heart Failure; CONSENSUS = Cooperative North Scandinavian Enalapril Survival Study; COPERNICUS = Carvedilol Prospective Randomized Cumulative Survival Trial; DIG = Digitalis Investigation Group; EPHESUS = Eplerenone Post-Acute Myocardial Infarction Heart Failure Efficacy and Survival Study; EUROPA = European Trial on Reduction of Cardiac Events with Perindopril in Stable Coronary Artery Disease; HOPE = Heart Outcomes Prevention Evaluation; HOT = Hypertension Optimal Treatment; HPS = Heart Protection Study; MADIT II = Multicenter Automatic Defibrillator Implantation Trial II; MERIT-HF = Metoprolol CR/XL Randomized Intervention Trial in Congestive Heart Failure; PEACE = Prevention of Events with ACE inhibition; RALES = Randomised Aldactone Evaluation Study; REMATCH = Randomized Evaluation of Mechanical Assistance for the Treatment of Congestive Heart Failure; SAVE = Survival and Ventricular Enlargement trial; SCD-HeFT = Sudden Cardiac Death in Heart Failure Trial; SHEP = Systolic Hypertension in the Elderly Program; SOLVD-P = Studies of Left Ventricular Dysfunction-Prevention; SOLVD-T = Studies of Left Ventricular Dysfunction-Treatment; TRACE = Trandolapril Cardiac Evaluation; VALIANT = Valsartan in Acute Myocardial Infarction Trial; VHeFT = Vasodilator-Heart Failure Trials; WOSCOPS = West of Scotland Coronary Prevention Study.

TABLE 59-2 PRACTICAL GUIDANCE ON THE USE OF ANGIOTENSIN-CONVERTING ENZYME INHIBITORS IN PATIENTS WITH HEART FAILURE DUE TO LEFT VENTRICULAR SYSTOLIC DYSFUNCTION

WHY?

Two major randomized trials (CONSENSUS I and SOLVD-T) and a meta-analysis of smaller trials have conclusively shown that angiotensin-converting enzyme (ACE) inhibitors increase survival, reduce hospital admissions, and improve NYHA class and quality of life in patients with *all* grades of symptomatic heart failure. Other major randomized trials in patients with systolic dysfunction after acute myocardial infarction (SAVE, AIRE, TRACE) have shown that ACE inhibitors increase survival. In patients with heart failure (ATLAS), the composite end point of death or hospital admission was reduced by higher doses of ACE inhibitor compared with lower doses. ACE inhibitors have also been shown to delay or to prevent the development of symptomatic heart failure in patients with *asymptomatic* left ventricular systolic dysfunction.

IN WHOM AND WHEN?

Indications:
- Potentially *all* patients with heart failure and a low ejection fraction
- First-line treatment (along with β-blockers) in patients with NYHA class II-IV heart failure; start as early as possible in course of disease. ACE inhibitors are also of benefit in patients with asymptomatic left ventricular systolic dysfunction (NYHA class I).

Contraindications:
- History of angioedema
- Known bilateral renal artery stenosis

Cautions/seek specialist advice:
- Significant hyperkalemia ($K^+ > 5.0$ mmol/L)
- Significant renal dysfunction (creatinine >221 μmol/L or >2.5 mg/dL)
- Symptomatic or severe asymptomatic hypotension (systolic blood pressure <90 mm Hg)

Drug interactions to look out for:
- K^+ supplements/K^+-sparing diuretics, e.g., amiloride and triamterene (beware combination preparations with furosemide)
- Aldosterone antagonists (spironolactone, eplerenone), angiotensin receptor blockers, NSAIDs*
- "Low-salt" substitutes with a high K^+ content

WHERE?

In the community for most patients
Exceptions—see *Cautions/seek specialist advice*

WHICH ACE INHIBITOR AND WHAT DOSE?

	Starting Dose	Target Dose
Captopril	6.25 mg thrice daily	50 mg thrice daily
Enalapril	2.5 mg twice daily	10-20 mg twice daily
Lisinopril	2.5-5.0 mg once daily	20-35 mg once daily
Ramipril	2.5 mg once daily	5 mg twice daily or 10 mg once daily
Trandolapril	0.5 mg once daily	4 mg once daily

HOW TO USE?

- Start with a low dose (see above).
- Double dose at not less than 2-week intervals.
- Aim for target dose (see above) or, failing that, the highest tolerated dose.
- Remember: some ACE inhibitor is better than no ACE inhibitor.
- Monitor blood pressure and blood chemistry (urea/blood urea nitrogen, creatinine, K^+).
- Check blood chemistry 1-2 weeks after initiation and 1-2 weeks after final dose titration.
- When to stop up-titration, reduce dose, stop treatment—see Problem Solving.
- A specialist heart failure nurse may assist with education of the patient, follow-up (in person or by telephone), biochemical monitoring, and dose up-titration.

ADVICE TO PATIENT

- Explain expected benefits (see Why?).
- Treatment is given to improve symptoms, to prevent worsening of heart failure leading to hospital admission, and to increase survival.
- Symptoms improve within a few weeks to a few months of starting treatment.
- Advise patients to report principal adverse effects, (i.e., dizziness/symptomatic hypotension, cough)—see Problem Solving.
- Advise patients to avoid NSAIDs* not prescribed by a physician (self-purchased over-the-counter) and salt substitutes high in K^+—see Problem Solving.

PROBLEM SOLVING

Asymptomatic low blood pressure
- Does not usually require any change in therapy

Symptomatic hypotension
- If dizziness, lightheadedness, or confusion and a low blood pressure, reconsider need for nitrates, calcium-channel blockers,† and other vasodilators.
- If no signs or symptoms of congestion, consider reducing diuretic dose.
- If these measures do not solve problem, seek specialist advice.

Cough
- Cough is common in patients with heart failure, many of whom have smoking-related lung disease.
- Cough is also a symptom of pulmonary edema, which should be excluded when a new or worsening cough develops.
- ACE inhibitor–induced cough rarely requires treatment discontinuation.
- When a troublesome cough does develop (e.g., one stopping the patient from sleeping) and can be proved to be due to ACE inhibition (i.e., recurs after ACE inhibitor withdrawal and rechallenge), substitution of an angiotensin receptor blocker can be considered (see Table 59-3).

Worsening renal function
- Some rise in urea (blood urea nitrogen), creatinine, and potassium is to be expected after initiation of an ACE inhibitor; if an increase is small and asymptomatic, no action is necessary.
- An increase in creatinine of up to 50% above baseline, or ≤266 μmol/L (3 mg/dL), whichever is the smaller, is acceptable.
- An increase in potassium to ≤5.5 mmol/L is acceptable.
- If urea, creatinine, or potassium does rise excessively, consider stopping concomitant nephrotoxic drugs (e.g., NSAIDs*) and other potassium supplements or retaining agents (triamterene, amiloride, spironolactone-eplerenone‡) and, if no signs of congestion, reducing the dose of diuretic.
- If greater rises in creatinine or potassium than those outlined above persist despite adjustment of concomitant medications, the dose of the ACE inhibitor should be halved and blood chemistry rechecked within 1-2 weeks; if there is still an unsatisfactory response, specialist advice should be sought.
- If potassium rises to >5.5 mmol/L or creatinine increases by >100% or to above 310 μmol/L (3.5 mg/dL), the ACE inhibitor should be stopped and specialist advice sought.
- Blood chemistry should be monitored frequently and serially until potassium and creatinine have plateaued.

Note: It is very rarely necessary to stop an ACE inhibitor, and clinical deterioration is likely if treatment is withdrawn. Ideally, specialist advice should be sought before treatment discontinuation.
*Avoid nonsteroidal anti-inflammatory drugs (NSAIDs) unless essential.
†Calcium-channel blockers should be discontinued unless absolutely essential (e.g., for angina or hypertension).
‡The safety and efficacy of an ACE inhibitor used with an angiotensin receptor blocker and spironolactone (as well as β-blocker) are uncertain, and the use of all three inhibitors of the renin-angiotensin-aldosterone system together is not recommended.
Modified from McMurray J, Cohen-Solal A, Dietz R, et al. Practical recommendations for the use of ACE inhibitors, β-blockers, aldosterone antagonists and angiotensin receptor blockers in heart failure: putting guidelines into practice. *Eur J Heart Fail.* 2005;7:710-721.

Stages C and D: Symptomatic Heart Failure

The development of symptoms and signs of the heart failure syndrome defines the transition from patients in the asymptomatic "at-risk" stages (A and B) to those who fulfill the clinical diagnosis of symptomatic heart failure (Chapter 58). This transition to the symptomatic phase underscores the progressive nature of heart failure and heralds a marked decline in prognosis. In one study, for example, the 2-year mortality rate was 27% in symptomatic patients compared with 10% in asymptomatic patients despite similarly reduced LVEFs and comorbidities.

TABLE 59-3 PRACTICAL GUIDANCE ON THE USE OF ANGIOTENSIN RECEPTOR BLOCKERS IN PATIENTS WITH HEART FAILURE DUE TO LEFT VENTRICULAR SYSTOLIC DYSFUNCTION

WHY?

Added to standard therapy, including an angiotensin-converting enzyme (ACE) inhibitor, in patients with all grades of symptomatic heart failure, the angiotensin receptor blockers (ARBs) valsartan and candesartan have been shown, in two major randomized trials (Val-HeFT and CHARM), to reduce heart failure hospital admissions, to improve NYHA class, and to maintain quality of life. The two CHARM low-left ventricular ejection fraction trials (CHARM-Alternative and CHARM-Added) also showed that candesartan reduced all-cause mortality. In patients previously intolerant of an ACE inhibitor, candesartan has been shown to reduce the risk of the composite outcome of cardiovascular death or heart failure hospitalization, to reduce the risk of heart failure hospital admission, and to improve NYHA class. These findings in heart failure are supported by another randomized trial in patients with left ventricular systolic dysfunction, heart failure, or both complicating acute myocardial infarction (VALIANT) in which valsartan was as effective as the ACE inhibitor captopril in reducing mortality and cardiovascular morbidity.

IN WHOM AND WHEN?

Indications:
- Potentially *all* patients with heart failure
- First-line treatment (along with β-blockers) in patients with NYHA class II-IV heart failure intolerant of an ACE inhibitor
- Second-line treatment (after optimization of ACE inhibitor and β-blocker*) in patients with NYHA class II-IV heart failure

Contraindications:
- Known bilateral renal artery stenosis

Cautions/seek specialist advice:
- Significant hyperkalemia ($K^+ > 5.0$ mmol/L)
- Significant renal dysfunction (creatinine, >221 μmol/L or >2.5 mg/dL)
- Symptomatic or severe asymptomatic hypotension (systolic blood pressure < 90 mm Hg)

Drug interactions to look out for:
- K^+ supplements/K^+-sparing diuretics, e.g., amiloride and triamterene (beware combination preparations with furosemide)
- Aldosterone antagonists (spironolactone, eplerenone), ACE inhibitors, NSAIDs†
- "Low-salt" substitutes with a high K^+ content

WHERE?

In the community for most patients
Exceptions—see *Cautions/seek specialist advice*

WHICH ARB AND WHAT DOSE?

	Starting Dose	Target Dose
Candesartan	4 or 8 mg once daily	32 mg once daily
Valsartan	40 mg twice daily	160 mg twice daily
Losartan	50 mg once daily	150 mg daily

HOW TO USE?

Start with a low dose (see above).
Double dose at not less than 2-week intervals.
Aim for target dose (see above) or, failing that, the highest tolerated dose.
Remember: some ARB is better than no ARB.
Monitor blood pressure and blood chemistry (urea/blood urea nitrogen, creatinine, K^+).
Check blood chemistry 1-2 weeks after initiation and 1-2 weeks after final dose titration.
When to stop up-titration, reduce dose, stop treatment—see Problem Solving.
A specialist heart failure nurse may assist with education of the patient, follow-up (in person or by telephone), biochemical monitoring, and dose up-titration.

ADVICE TO PATIENT

Explain expected benefits (see Why?).
Treatment is given to improve symptoms, to prevent worsening of heart failure leading to hospital admission, and to increase survival.
Symptoms improve within a few weeks to a few months of starting treatment.
Advise patients to report principal adverse effect (i.e., report dizziness/symptomatic hypotension)—see Problem Solving.
Advise patients to avoid NSAIDs† not prescribed by a physician (self-purchased over-the-counter) and salt substitutes high in K^+—see Problem Solving.

PROBLEM SOLVING

Asymptomatic low blood pressure
- Does not usually require any change in therapy

Symptomatic hypotension
- If dizziness, lightheadedness, or confusion and a low blood pressure, reconsider need for nitrates, calcium-channel blockers,‡ and other vasodilators.
- If no signs or symptoms of congestion, consider reducing diuretic dose.
- If these measures do not solve problem, seek specialist advice.

Worsening renal function
- Some rise in urea (blood urea nitrogen), creatinine, and potassium is to be expected after initiation of an ARB; if the increase is small and asymptomatic, no action is necessary.
- An increase in creatinine of up to 50% above baseline, or ≤266 μmol/L (3 mg/dL), whichever is the smaller, is acceptable.
- An increase in potassium to ≤5.5 mmol/L is acceptable.
- If urea, creatinine, or potassium does rise excessively, consider stopping concomitant nephrotoxic drugs (e.g., NSAIDs†) and potassium supplements or retaining agents (triamterene, amiloride, spironolactone-eplerenone*) and, if no signs of congestion, reducing the dose of diuretic.
- If greater rises in creatinine or potassium than those outlined above persist despite adjustment of concomitant medications, the dose of the ARB should be halved and blood chemistry rechecked within 1-2 weeks; if there is still an unsatisfactory response, specialist advice should be sought.
- If potassium rises to >5.5 mmol/L or creatinine increases by >100% or to above 310 μmol/L (3.5 mg/dL), the ARB should be stopped and specialist advice sought.
- Blood chemistry should be monitored frequently and serially until potassium and creatinine have plateaued.

Note: It is very rarely necessary to stop an ARB, and clinical deterioration is likely if treatment is withdrawn. Ideally, specialist advice should be sought before treatment discontinuation.
*The safety and efficacy of an ARB used with an ACE inhibitor and spironolactone (as well as a β-blocker) are uncertain, and the use of all three inhibitors of the renin-angiotensin-aldosterone system together is not recommended.
†Avoid nonsteroidal anti-inflammatory drugs (NSAIDs) unless essential.
‡Calcium-channel blockers should be discontinued unless absolutely essential (e.g., for angina or hypertension).
Modified from McMurray J, Cohen-Solal A, Dietz R, et al. Practical recommendations for the use of ACE inhibitors, β-blockers, aldosterone antagonists and angiotensin receptor blockers in heart failure: putting guidelines into practice. *Eur J Heart Fail.* 2005;7:710-721.

TREATMENT Rx

The goals of treatment for patients with stage C and stage D heart failure are relief of symptoms, avoidance of hospital admission, and prevention of premature death. In general, the preventive measures that are of value during stages A and B should be sustained in patients with stages C and D heart failure.

Heart Failure with Reduced Left Ventricular Ejection Fraction

Pharmacologic Treatment

Drugs are the mainstay of the treatment of patients with symptomatic heart failure on the basis of the cumulative experiences from RCTs (see Table 59-1), particularly for patients with reduced LVEF. However, devices and surgery have an important and increasing role in patients with advanced symptomatic heart failure (stages C and D; see Fig. 59-1). Exercise clearly improves well-being and clinical outcomes (see Table 59-1), but the evidence base for other lifestyle interventions is less robust. The organization and delivery of care can also have a substantial impact on outcomes.

Diuretics

Mechanism of Action. Diuretics act by blocking sodium reabsorption at specific sites in the renal tubule, thereby enhancing urinary excretion of sodium and water.

Clinical Benefits. Although not proven to improve mortality and morbidity in large trials, diuretics are required in nearly all patients with symptomatic heart failure (stages C and D) to relieve dyspnea and the signs of sodium and water retention ("congestion"), that is, peripheral and pulmonary edema. No other treatment relieves symptoms and the signs of sodium and water overload as rapidly and effectively. Once a patient needs a diuretic, treatment is usually necessary for the rest of the patient's life, although the dose and type of diuretic may vary.

TABLE 59-4 PRACTICAL GUIDANCE ON THE USE OF β-BLOCKERS IN PATIENTS WITH HEART FAILURE DUE TO LEFT VENTRICULAR SYSTOLIC DYSFUNCTION

WHY?

Several major randomized controlled trials (i.e., USCP, CIBIS II, MERIT-HF, COPERNICUS) have shown, conclusively, that certain β-blockers increase survival, reduce hospital admissions, and improve NYHA class and quality of life when added to standard therapy (diuretics, digoxin, and angiotensin-converting enzyme [ACE] inhibitors) in patients with *stable* mild and moderate heart failure and in some patients with severe heart failure. In the SENIORS trial, which differed substantially in design from the aforementioned studies (older patients, some patients with preserved left ventricular systolic function, longer follow-up), nebivolol appeared to have a smaller treatment effect, although direct comparison is difficult. One other trial (BEST) did not show a reduction in all-cause mortality but did report a reduction in cardiovascular mortality and is otherwise broadly consistent with the aforementioned studies. The COMET trial showed that carvedilol was substantially more effective than a low dose of short-acting metoprolol tartrate* (long-acting metoprolol succinate was used in MERIT-HF).

IN WHOM AND WHEN?

Indications:
- Potentially *all* patients with *stable* mild and moderate heart failure; patients with severe heart failure should be referred for specialist advice
- First-line treatment (along with ACE inhibitors) in patients with *stable* NYHA class II-III heart failure; start as early as possible in course of disease

Contraindications:
- Asthma
- Second- or third-degree atrioventricular block

Cautions/seek specialist advice:
- Severe (NYHA class IV) heart failure
- Current or recent (<4 wk) exacerbation of heart failure (e.g., hospital admission with worsening heart failure, heart block, or heart rate <60/min)
- Persisting signs of congestion, hypotension/low blood pressure (systolic <90 mm Hg), raised jugular venous pressure, ascites, marked peripheral edema

Drug interactions to look out for:
- Verapamil, diltiazem (should be discontinued)†
- Digoxin, amiodarone

WHERE?

In the community in stable patients (NYHA class IV/severe heart failure patients should be referred for specialist advice)
Not in unstable patients hospitalized with worsening heart failure
Other exceptions—see *Cautions/seek specialist advice*

WHICH β-BLOCKER AND WHAT DOSE?

	Starting Dose	Target Dose
Bisoprolol	1.25 mg once daily	10 mg once daily
Carvedilol	3.125 mg twice daily	25-50 mg twice daily
Metoprolol CR/XL	12.5-25 mg once daily	200 mg once daily*
Nebivolol	1.25 mg once daily	10 mg once daily

HOW TO USE?

Start with a low dose (see above).
Double dose at not less than 2-week intervals.
Aim for target dose (see above) or, failing that, the highest tolerated dose.
Remember: some β-blocker is better than no β-blocker.
Monitor heart rate, blood pressure, and clinical status (symptoms, signs—especially signs of congestion, body weight).
Check blood chemistry 1-2 weeks after initiation and 1-2 weeks after final dose titration.
When to stop up-titration, reduce dose, stop treatment—see Problem Solving.
A specialist heart failure nurse may assist with education of the patient, follow-up (in person or by telephone), and dose up-titration.

ADVICE TO PATIENT

Explain expected benefits (see Why?).
Treatment is given to improve symptoms, to prevent worsening of heart failure leading to hospital admission, and to increase survival.
Symptomatic improvement may develop slowly after starting treatment, taking 3-6 months or longer.
Temporary symptomatic deterioration may occur during initiation or up-titration phase; in the long term, β-blockers improve well-being.
Advise patient to report deterioration (see Problem Solving) and that deterioration (tiredness, fatigue, breathlessness) can usually be easily managed by adjustment of other medication; patients should be advised not to stop β-blocker therapy without consulting the physician.
To detect and to treat deterioration early, patients should be encouraged to weigh themselves daily (after waking, before dressing, after voiding, before eating) and to increase their diuretic dose should their weight increase, persistently (>2 days), by >1.5-2.0 kg.‡

PROBLEM SOLVING

Worsening symptoms or signs (e.g., increasing dyspnea, fatigue, edema, weight gain)
- If increasing congestion, increase dose of diuretic or halve dose of β-blocker (if increasing diuretic does not work).
- If marked fatigue (or bradycardia—see below), halve dose of β-blocker (rarely necessary); review patient in 1-2 weeks; if not improved, seek specialist advice.
- If serious deterioration, halve dose of β-blocker or stop this treatment (rarely necessary); seek specialist advice.

Low heart rate
- If <50 beats/min and worsening symptoms, halve dose of β-blocker or, if severe deterioration, stop β-blocker (rarely necessary).
- Review need for other heart rate–slowing drugs (e.g., digoxin, amiodarone, diltiazem, or verapamil†).
- Arrange electrocardiogram to exclude heart block.
- Seek specialist advice.

Asymptomatic low blood pressure
- Does not usually require any change in therapy

Symptomatic hypotension
- If dizziness, lightheadedness, or confusion and a low blood pressure, reconsider need for nitrates, calcium-channel blockers,† and other vasodilators.
- If no signs or symptoms of congestion, consider reducing diuretic dose or ACE inhibitor.
- If these measures do not solve problem, seek specialist advice.

Note: β-Blockers should not be stopped suddenly unless absolutely necessary (there is a risk for a "rebound" increase in myocardial ischemia or infarction and arrhythmias). Ideally, specialist advice should be sought before treatment discontinuation.
*Metoprolol tartrate should not be used in preference to an evidence-based β-blocker in heart failure.
†Calcium-channel blockers should be discontinued unless absolutely necessary, and diltiazem and verapamil are generally contraindicated in heart failure.
‡This is generally good advice for all patients with heart failure.
Modified from McMurray J, Cohen-Solal A, Dietz R, et al. Practical recommendations for the use of ACE inhibitors, β-blockers, aldosterone antagonists and angiotensin receptor blockers in heart failure: putting guidelines into practice. *Eur J Heart Fail.* 2005;7:710-721.

Practical Use. The key principle is to prescribe the minimum dose of diuretic needed to maintain an edema-free state ("dry weight"). Excessive use can lead to electrolyte imbalances, such as hyponatremia, hypokalemia (and risk of digitalis toxicity), hyperuricemia (and risk of gout), and uremia. The risk of renal dysfunction is increased by concomitant use of nonsteroidal anti-inflammatory drugs (NSAIDs). Diuretic-induced hypovolemia may also cause symptomatic hypotension and prerenal azotemia. Restriction of dietary sodium intake may help reduce but does not eliminate the requirement for diuretics. Diuretic dosing should be flexible, with temporary increases for evidence of fluid retention (e.g., increasing symptoms, weight gain, edema) and decreases for evidence of hypovolemia (e.g., as a consequence of increased electrolyte loss due to gastroenteritis, decreased fluid intake, or both).

In some patients with milder symptoms of heart failure and preserved renal function (stage C), a thiazide diuretic such as chlorthalidone may suffice. In more advanced heart failure (stage D) or in patients with concomitant renal dysfunction, a loop diuretic such as furosemide is often needed. Loop diuretics cause a rapid onset of an intense but relatively short-lived diuresis compared with the longer-lasting but gentler effect of a thiazide diuretic. The timing of administration of a loop diuretic, which need not be taken first thing every morning, can be adjusted according to the patient's social activities. The dose may be postponed or even temporarily omitted if the patient has to travel or has another activity that might be compromised by the prompt action of the diuretic. In severe heart failure (stage D), the effects of long-term administration of a loop diuretic may be diminished by increased sodium reabsorption at the distal tubule. This problem can be offset by use of the combination of a loop diuretic and a thiazide or thiazide-like diuretic (e.g., hydrochlorothiazide or metolazone), which act in synergy with a loop diuretic by blocking sodium reabsorption in different segments of the nephron. This combination requires more frequent monitoring of electrolytes and renal function for diuretic-induced hyponatremia, abnormalities of the serum potassium level, and prerenal azotemia.

A period of intravenous loop diuretic, given either as bolus injections or by continuous infusion, may be required in patients who become resistant to the action of oral diuretics. Why this resistance develops is uncertain, but factors thought to be important include impaired absorption of oral diuretics due to gut edema, hypotension, reduced renal blood flow, and adaptive changes in the nephron.

In patients with advanced heart failure (stage D), an aldosterone antagonist, such as spironolactone, which increases excretion of sodium but not of potassium, usually should be added. Patients receiving a combination of diuretics require careful monitoring of blood chemistry and clinical status. The use of an aldosterone antagonist (or, rarely, a potassium-sparing diuretic) along with an ACE inhibitor or ARB (treatment with all three is not recommended) requires particular care and surveillance for hyperkalemia.

Although they are highly effective in relieving symptoms and signs, diuretics alone are not sufficient for treatment of heart failure. In cases of severe resistant volume overload, mechanical removal of fluid by ultrafiltration may be considered. The addition of other treatments will better maintain clinical stability, slow structural progression, and reduce the risk of hospital admission and premature death.

ACE Inhibitors

Mechanism of Action. These drugs act by inhibiting the enzyme that converts the inactive decapeptide angiotensin I to the active octapeptide angiotensin II (and that also breaks down bradykinin). In patients with heart failure, excessive angiotensin II is thought to exert myriad harmful actions mediated through stimulation of the angiotensin II type 1 receptor subtype (AT_1R), including vasoconstriction (which increases ventricular afterload), excessive growth of myocytes and the extracellular matrix (contributing to maladaptive left ventricular remodeling), activation of the sympathetic nervous system, prothrombotic actions, and augmentation of the release of arginine vasopressin and the retention of sodium (both directly and through stimulation of aldosterone secretion).

ACE inhibitors also reduce the breakdown of bradykinin (as ACE is identical to kininase II), and the resultant accumulation of bradykinin is directly or indirectly responsible for two of the specific adverse effects of ACE inhibitors, cough and angioedema. Bradykinin may, however, also have beneficial effects (vasodilation, inhibition of adverse cardiovascular remodeling, and antithrombotic actions), although the importance of these bradykinin-mediated actions to the clinical benefits of ACE inhibition is uncertain.

Clinical Benefits. Clinical trials have shown that treatment with an ACE inhibitor, when it is used alone or added to diuretics and digoxin, decreases left ventricular size, improves systolic function, reduces symptoms and hospital admissions, and prolongs survival (see Table 59-1).[5,6] These agents also reduce the risk for development of myocardial infarction, diabetes, and atrial fibrillation. Consequently, treatment with an ACE inhibitor is recommended for all patients with systolic dysfunction, irrespective of symptoms or etiology. ACE inhibitors are not a substitute for a diuretic but mitigate diuretic-induced hypokalemia.

Practical Use. ACE inhibitors should be introduced as early as possible in a patient's treatment. The only contraindications are current symptomatic hypotension and bilateral renal artery stenosis (Chapter 127); the latter is often associated with a prompt and marked increase in serum levels of blood urea nitrogen and creatinine when renal perfusion is reduced precipitously by inhibiting the production and actions of angiotensin. Treatment should be started in a low dose (see Table 59-2), with the dose gradually increased toward a target dose proven of benefit in a clinical trial. The patient should be evaluated for symptomatic hypotension, uremia, and hyperkalemia after each dose increment; these adverse effects are uncommon and can usually be resolved by reduction in the dose of diuretic (if the patient is edema free) or concomitant hypotensive or nephrotoxic medications (e.g., nitrates, calcium-channel blockers, or NSAIDs). A dry, nonproductive cough occurs in approximately 15% of patients treated with an ACE inhibitor, and if it is troublesome, substitution of an ARB is recommended. In the rare cases of angioedema (Chapter 260), the ACE inhibitor should be stopped and not used again; an ARB can be cautiously substituted.

Angiotensin Receptor Blockers

Mechanism of Action. Instead of inhibiting the production of angiotensin II through ACE, ARBs block the binding of angiotensin II to the AT_1R. This pharmacologically distinct mechanism of action may be important because angiotensin II is also believed to be produced by other enzymes, such as chymase. ARBs do not inhibit kininase II or the breakdown of bradykinin, so they do not cause cough and cause less angioedema than do ACE inhibitors.

Clinical Benefits. When they are used as the sole agent in heart failure, ARBs produce benefits similar to those of ACE inhibitors and can be substituted for them in patients who have cough or angioedema with ACE inhibitors.[7,8] When they are used in clinically effective doses, other adverse effects such as hypotension, renal dysfunction, and hyperkalemia are encountered as frequently as with an ACE inhibitor. As with an ACE inhibitor, the specific agents, dosing regimens, and target doses that were of demonstrable benefit in clinical trials are recommended (see Table 59-1).

In the broader population of patients with symptomatic (stage C or stage D, functional class II to class IV) heart failure that can be treated with an ACE inhibitor, an ARB *in combination with* an ACE inhibitor (and β-blocker) further improves LVEF, relieves symptoms, reduces the risk of hospital admission for worsening heart failure, and can also reduce the risk for cardiovascular death (see Table 59-3).[8,9] Consequently, the addition of an ARB to both an ACE inhibitor and a β-blocker may be considered in any patient with persisting symptoms (stages C and D). There is, however, also strong evidence that addition of an aldosterone antagonist to an ACE inhibitor is of benefit in patients with advanced (classes III to IV) heart failure (see later), but the efficacy and safety of the four-drug combination of an ACE inhibitor, β-blocker, ARB, and aldosterone antagonist are uncertain. Consequently, either an ARB or an aldosterone antagonist, but not both, should be added to an ACE inhibitor and a β-blocker in such patients.

The approach to initiation, titration, and monitoring of an ARB is similar to that of an ACE inhibitor (see Table 59-3). The adverse effects, with the exception of cough and angioedema, are similar. Use of multiple inhibitors of the renin-angiotensin-aldosterone system requires even more diligent monitoring, especially in patients at higher risk for uremia, hypotension, or hyperkalemia (i.e., patients 75 years of age and older or with a systolic blood pressure below 100 mm Hg, diabetes, or renal impairment) because combined treatment with an ACE inhibitor and an ARB significantly increases the risks of worsening renal function, hyperkalemia, and symptomatic hypotension.

As with ACE inhibitors, β-blockers, and aldosterone antagonists, treatment with ARBs should be indefinite unless there is intolerance.

β-Blockers

Mechanism of Action. Heart failure is characterized by excessive activation of the sympathetic nervous system, which causes vasoconstriction and sodium retention, thereby increasing cardiac preload and afterload and often inducing myocardial ischemia or arrhythmias. In addition, norepinephrine can cause hypertrophy of myocytes and augment their apoptosis. β-Blockers counteract many of these harmful effects of the hyperactivity of the sympathetic nervous system.

Clinical Benefits. The long-term addition of a β-blocker to an ACE inhibitor (and diuretic and digoxin) further improves left ventricular function and symptoms, reduces hospital admissions, and strikingly improves survival.[10] Consequently, a β-blocker is recommended for all patients with symptomatic systolic dysfunction, irrespective of etiology and severity, and the combination of a β-blocker with an ACE inhibitor is now the cornerstone of the treatment of symptomatic heart failure (see Fig. 59-1).

Practical Use. The major contraindications to use of a β-blocker in heart failure are asthma (although it is important to note that the dyspnea caused by pulmonary congestion can be confused with reactive airway disease) and second- or third-degree atrioventricular block. Initiation of treatment during an episode of acute decompensated heart failure should also generally be avoided. In addition, caution is advised in patients with a heart rate below 60 beats per minute or a systolic blood pressure below 90 mm Hg. It is recommended that a β-blocker shown to produce benefits in a randomized trial be used (see Table 59-1).

Like ACE inhibitors, β-blockers should be introduced as early as possible in a patient's treatment, started in a low dose (see Table 59-4), and increased gradually toward a target dose used in a clinical trial (the "start low–go slow" approach). The patient should be checked for symptomatic hypotension and excessive bradycardia after each dose increment, but both of these side effects are uncommon, and hypotension can often be resolved by reduction in the dose of other nonessential blood pressure–lowering medications (e.g., nitrates and calcium-channel blockers). Bradycardia is more likely in patients who are also taking digoxin or amiodarone, and the simultaneous use of these agents should be reviewed if excessive bradycardia occurs. On occasion, symptomatic worsening and fluid retention (e.g., weight gain or edema) may occur after initiation of a β-blocker or during dose up-titration; these side effects usually can be resolved by a temporary increase in the diuretic dose without necessitating discontinuation of the β-blocker.

Treatment with a β-blocker should be given for life, although the dose may need to be decreased (or, rarely, treatment discontinued) during episodes of acute decompensation if the patient shows signs of circulatory underperfusion or refractory congestion.

Aldosterone Antagonists

Mechanism of Action. Aldosterone, which is the second effector hormone in the renin-angiotensin-aldosterone cascade, has detrimental vascular, renal, autonomic, and cardiac actions when it is produced in excess in patients with heart failure. Excessive aldosterone promotes sodium retention and hypokalemia, and it is believed to contribute to myocardial fibrosis, all of which predispose to arrhythmias. Aldosterone antagonists block these undesirable actions and act as potassium-sparing diuretics.

Clinical Benefits. The aldosterone antagonist spironolactone (Table 59-5) improves symptoms, reduces hospital admissions, and increases survival when it is added to an ACE inhibitor (and diuretics and digoxin) in patients with a reduced LVEF and severely symptomatic heart failure. 11 Eplerenone, another aldosterone antagonist, reduces mortality and morbidity when it is added to both an ACE inhibitor and β-blocker in patients with a reduced LVEF and heart failure or diabetes after a recent myocardial infarction (see Table 59-5) 12 and when added to an ACE inhibitor/ARB and β-blockers in class II heart failure. 13 Consequently, an aldosterone antagonist should be considered in patients who remain in severe heart failure (class III or IV) despite treatment with a diuretic, ACE inhibitor (or ARB), and β-blocker. When begun, it should be given indefinitely. The combination of an ACE inhibitor, an ARB, and an aldosterone antagonist has not been adequately evaluated and is not recommended.

Treatment with an aldosterone antagonist should be initiated with a low dose (see Table 59-5) with careful monitoring of serum electrolytes and renal function. Hyperkalemia and uremia are the adverse effects of greatest concern (as with ACE inhibitors and ARBs), and an aldosterone antagonist should not be given to patients with a serum potassium concentration of more than 5.0 mmol/L, serum creatinine concentration above 2.5 mg/dL (>221 μmol/L) or other evidence of markedly impaired renal function. The importance of selection of patients and dose is underscored by reports of a worrisome incidence of serious hyperkalemia in community practice settings. Spironolactone can have antiandrogenic effects, especially painful gynecomastia, in men; because eplerenone has less of an action on the androgen receptor, it is a reasonable substitute in patients who experience this adverse effect.

Digoxin

Mechanism of Action. Digitalis glycosides inhibit the cell membrane Na^+,K^+-ATPase pump, thereby increasing intracellular calcium and myocardial contractility. In addition, digoxin is thought to enhance parasympathetic and reduce sympathetic nervous activity as well as to inhibit renin release.

TABLE 59-5 PRACTICAL GUIDANCE ON THE USE OF SPIRONOLACTONE IN PATIENTS WITH HEART FAILURE DUE TO LEFT VENTRICULAR SYSTOLIC DYSFUNCTION

WHY?

The RALES study showed that low-dose spironolactone increased survival, reduced hospital admissions, and improved NYHA class when added to standard therapy (diuretic, digoxin, angiotensin-converting enzyme [ACE] inhibitor, and, in a minority of cases, β-blocker) in patients with severe (NYHA class III or IV) heart failure. In patients with left ventricular systolic dysfunction and heart failure (or diabetes) complicating *acute* myocardial infarction (EPHESUS) and in patients with NYHA class II symptoms on an ACE inhibitor/ARB and β-blocker (EMPHASIS-HF), another aldosterone antagonist, eplerenone, increased survival and reduced hospital admissions for cardiac causes.

IN WHOM AND WHEN?

Indications:
- Potentially all patients with symptomatic heart failure (class II-IV NYHA)
- Second-line therapy (after ACE inhibitors and β-blockers*) in patients with NYHA class II-IV heart failure

Cautions/seek specialist advice:
- Significant hyperkalemia ($K^+ > 5.0$ mmol/L)†
- Significant renal dysfunction (creatinine > 221 μmol/L or 2.5 mg/dL)†

Drug interactions to look out for:
- K^+ supplements/K^+-sparing diuretics (e.g., amiloride and triamterene; beware combination preparations with furosemide)
- ACE inhibitors, angiotensin receptor blockers, NSAIDs‡
- "Low-salt" substitutes with a high K^+ content

WHERE?

In the community or in the hospital
Exceptions—see *Cautions/seek specialist advice*

WHICH DOSE?†

	Starting Dose	Target Dose
Spironolactone	25 mg once daily or on alternate days	25-50 mg once daily
Eplerenone	25 mg once daily	50 mg once daily

HOW TO USE?

Start with a low dose (see above).
Check blood chemistry at 1, 4, 8, and 12 weeks; 6, 9, and 12 months; every 6 months thereafter.
If K^+ rises above 5.5 mmol/L or creatinine rises to ≥221 μmol/L (2.5 mg/dL), reduce dose to 25 mg on alternate days and monitor blood chemistry closely.
If K^+ rises to ≥6.0 mmol/L or creatinine to ≥310 μmol/L (3.5 mg/dL), stop spironolactone immediately and seek specialist advice.
A specialist heart failure nurse may assist with education of the patient, follow-up (in person or by telephone), biochemical monitoring, and dose up-titration.

ADVICE TO PATIENT

Explain expected benefits (see Why?).
Treatment is given to improve symptoms, to prevent worsening of heart failure leading to hospital admission, and to increase survival.
Symptom improvement occurs within a few weeks to a few months of starting treatment.
Avoid NSAIDs‡ not prescribed by a physician (self-purchased over-the-counter) and salt substitutes high in K^+.
If diarrhea or vomiting occurs, patients should stop spironolactone and contact the physician.

PROBLEM SOLVING

Worsening renal function/hyperkalemia
- See How to Use?

Major concern is hyperkalemia (>6.0 mmol/L); although this was uncommon in RALES, it has been seen more commonly in clinical practice.
- Conversely, a high-normal potassium level may be desirable in patients with heart failure, especially if they are taking digoxin.
- It is important to avoid other K^+-retaining drugs (e.g., K^+-sparing diuretics such as amiloride and triamterene) and nephrotoxic agents (e.g., NSAIDs‡).
- The risk for hyperkalemia and renal dysfunction when an aldosterone antagonist is given to patients already taking an ACE inhibitor and angiotensin receptor blocker is higher than when an aldosterone antagonist is added to just an ACE inhibitor or angiotensin receptor blocker given singly; close and careful monitoring is mandatory.*
- Some "low-salt" substitutes have a high K^+ content.
- Male patients treated with spironolactone may develop breast discomfort or gynecomastia (these problems are significantly less common with eplerenone).

*The safety and efficacy of spironolactone used with an ACE inhibitor *and* an angiotensin receptor blocker (as well as a β-blocker) are uncertain, and the use of all three inhibitors of the renin-angiotensin-aldosterone system together is not recommended.
†It is extremely important to adhere to these cautions and doses in light of recent evidence of serious hyperkalemia with spironolactone in usual clinical practice in Ontario.
‡Avoid nonsteroidal anti-inflammatory drugs (NSAIDs) unless essential.
Modified from McMurray J, Cohen-Solal A, Dietz R, et al. Practical recommendations for the use of ACE inhibitors, β-blockers, aldosterone antagonists and angiotensin receptor blockers in heart failure: putting guidelines into practice. *Eur J Heart Fail.* 2005;7:710-721.

Clinical Benefits. Only one large RCT has examined the effects of starting (as opposed to withdrawing) digoxin on mortality and morbidity in patients with heart failure in sinus rhythm. In that trial, digoxin did not reduce mortality but did decrease the risk for admission to hospital for worsening heart failure when it was added to a diuretic and an ACE inhibitor.[14] In patients in sinus rhythm, addition of digoxin is recommended only for those whose heart failure remains symptomatic despite standard three-drug treatment with a diuretic, ACE inhibitor, and β-blocker plus an ARB or aldosterone antagonist. In patients with atrial fibrillation, digoxin may be used at an earlier stage if a β-blocker fails to control the ventricular rate (ideally less than 70 beats per minute at rest and less than 100 beats per minute during exercise; Chapter 64). Digoxin can also be used to control the ventricular rate when β-blocker treatment is being initiated or up-titrated.

If the effect of digoxin is needed urgently, loading with 10 to 15 μg/kg *lean* body weight, given in three divided doses 6 hours apart, may be used. The maintenance dose should be one third of the loading dose. Smaller maintenance doses (e.g., one fourth of the loading dose and not more than 62.5 μg/day) should be used in elderly patients and in patients with reduced renal function as well as in patients with a low body mass. Monitoring of the serum digoxin concentration is recommended because of the narrow therapeutic window. A steady state is reached 7 to 10 days after treatment is started; blood should be collected at least 6 hours (and ideally 8 to 24 hours) after the last dose. The currently recommended therapeutic range is 0.5 to 1.0 ng/mL.

Digoxin can cause anorexia, nausea, arrhythmias, confusion, and visual disturbances, especially if the serum concentration is above 2.0 ng/mL. Hypokalemia increases susceptibility to the adverse effects. The dose of digoxin should be reduced in elderly patients and patients with renal dysfunction. Certain drugs increase serum digoxin concentration, including amiodarone.

Hydralazine and Isosorbide Dinitrate

Mechanism of Action. Hydralazine is a powerful direct-acting arterial vasodilator. Its mechanism of action is not understood, although it may inhibit enzymatic production of superoxide, which neutralizes nitric oxide and may induce nitrate tolerance. Nitrates dilate both veins and arteries, thereby reducing preload and afterload by stimulating the nitric oxide pathway and increasing cyclic guanosine monophosphate in vascular smooth muscle. Neither drug on its own nor any other direct-acting vasodilator has been demonstrated to be beneficial in heart failure.

Clinical Benefits. Although this combination has been known for some time to improve systolic function and probably to reduce death in classes II to IV heart failure compared with placebo, head-to-head comparison showed that an ACE inhibitor is superior for improving survival. Nevertheless, on the basis of subgroup analyses suggesting that African Americans responded better to hydralazine and isosorbide dinitrate, a subsequent RCT showed that the addition of hydralazine and isosorbide dinitrate in African Americans, most of whom were receiving an ACE inhibitor and β-blocker and many of whom were taking spironolactone, further reduced mortality and hospital admissions for heart failure and improved quality of life.[15]

A fixed combination of 37.5 mg of hydralazine and 20 mg of isosorbide dinitrate was used in the trial; one tablet was given and if tolerated, a second was given 12 hours later. One tablet was then prescribed three times daily for 3 to 5 days, at which point the dose was increased to the target maintenance of two tablets three times daily, that is, a daily dose of 225 mg hydralazine and 120 mg isosorbide dinitrate. Because of the limited inclusion criteria of this RCT, however, it is uncertain whether this combination of vasodilators is an effective addition in other populations of patients.

Practical Use. Other than for African Americans, the main indication for hydralazine and isosorbide dinitrate is in patients with intolerance to an ACE inhibitor and an ARB. Hydralazine and isosorbide dinitrate should be used as additional treatment in African Americans and considered for other patients who remain symptomatic with other proven therapies. The main dose-limiting adverse effects are headache and dizziness. A rare adverse effect of higher doses of hydralazine, especially in slow acetylators, is a systemic lupus erythematosus–like syndrome (Chapter 274).

Omega-3 Polyunsaturated Fatty Acids (n-3 PUFA)

A trial of 1 g of n-3 PUFA (850 to 852 mg eicosapentaenoic acid and docosahexaenoic acid as ethyl esters in the average ratio of 1 : 1.2) per day led to a small reduction in cardiovascular morbidity and mortality in patients with heart failure. However, in light of negative trials in post-MI patients and for the prevention of AF, the role of these agents remains uncertain.

Other Pharmacologic Issues

Ivabradine, a specific inhibitor of the sinus node (at 7.5 mg twice daily), reduces mean heart rate from 75 to 64 beats per minute and reduced subsequent hospital admission in patients with chronic heart failure by about 25%. However, this agent has not reduced mortality, and the risks of symptomatic bradycardia and other side effects offset much of its benefits. Some therapies that are of proven value for cardiovascular conditions that underlie or are associated with heart failure are of uncertain benefit (antiplatelet treatment, Chapter 37) or do not improve outcomes (statins, Chapter 213) in patients with persistent, symptomatic heart failure. Warfarin is indicated in patients with atrial fibrillation, provided there is no contraindication to its use (Chapter 64). Warfarin may also be used in patients with evidence of intracardiac thrombus (e.g., detected during echocardiographic examination) or systemic thromboembolism. The many interactions of warfarin with other drugs, including some statins and amiodarone (Chapter 37), must always be considered when warfarin or another drug in a patient taking warfarin is initiated. Heparin prophylaxis (Chapter 37) against deep venous thrombosis is indicated when patients with heart failure are bed bound, such as during hospital admission.

Vaccination against influenza and pneumococcal infection is advised (Chapter 17) in all patients with heart failure because infection can lead to clinical deterioration.

The aforementioned treatments are the only pharmacologic therapies shown to be of benefit in patients with heart failure and a reduced LVEF. Other treatments have been tested in randomized trials and shown to have a neutral (e.g., amlodipine) or uncertain (e.g., bosentan and etanercept) effect on mortality and morbidity or to increase mortality (e.g., milrinone, flosequinan, vesnarinone, and moxonidine).

Drugs to Use with Caution in Heart Failure

Patients with heart failure, especially if it is severe, often have renal and hepatic dysfunction, so any drug excreted predominantly by the kidneys or metabolized by the liver may accumulate (Chapter 28). Similarly, because of their extensive comorbidity, patients with heart failure are inevitably treated with multiple drugs, thereby increasing the risk of drug interactions.

Drugs that should be avoided, if possible, in heart failure include thiazolidinediones (because of the risk of fluid retention), most antiarrhythmic drugs (including dronedarone, although amiodarone and dofetilide may be used), most calcium-channel blockers (with the exception of amlodipine), corticosteroids, NSAIDs, cyclooxygenase 2 inhibitors, many antipsychotics (e.g., clozapine), and antihistamines. Metformin (because of the risk of lactic acidosis) should be used with caution. Some salt substitutes contain substantial amounts of potassium and must be used cautiously. Other dietary constituents (e.g., grapefruit and cranberry juice) and supplements such as St. John's wort can interact with drugs taken by patients with heart failure, especially warfarin and digoxin.

Organization of Care

Several studies have shown that organized, nurse-led, multidisciplinary care can improve outcomes in patients with heart failure, particularly by reducing recurrent hospital admissions. The most successful approach seems to involve education of the patients, their families, and caregivers about heart failure and its treatment (including flexible diuretic dosing and reinforcing the importance of adherence), recognizing (and acting on) early deterioration (dyspnea, sudden weight gain, edema), and optimizing proven pharmacologic treatments.[16] A home-based rather than clinic-based approach may be best, although trials are needed to compare these types of interventions directly. Even telephone follow-up is of value. New technology enabling noninvasive home telemonitoring of physiologic measures (e.g., heart rate and rhythm, blood pressure, temperature, respiratory rate, weight, and estimated body water content) and implanted devices, which collect similar data and may be interrogated remotely, are also being tested as aids to monitoring and management. Despite the usefulness of B-type natriuretic peptide (BNP) in the diagnosis of heart failure and as a prognostic measure, treatment guided by BNP levels has not been shown in randomized trials to be any better than standard, evidence-based care.

Education

Education of the patient, family, and caregivers is invaluable (Table 59-6). Self-detection of early signs and symptoms of deterioration provides for earlier intervention. Counseling on the proper use of therapies, with an emphasis on adherence, is critical.

Useful patient-oriented material is available from several reliable sources the Heart Failure Society of America (*www.abouthf.org/education_modules.htm*), American Heart Association (*www.americanheart.org/presenter.jhtml?identifier=1486*), National Heart, Lung, and Blood Institute (*www.nhlbi.nih.gov/health/dci/Diseases/Hf/HF_WhatIs.html*), the Heart Failure Association of the European Society of Cardiology (*www.heartfailurematters.org/EN/Pages/index.aspx*), and other organizations.

Medication Use Counseling. When appropriate, a patient should be taught how to adjust the dose of diuretic within individualized limits. The dose should be increased (or a supplementary diuretic added) if there is evidence of fluid retention (symptoms of congestion) and decreased if there is evidence of hypovolemia (e.g., increased thirst associated with weight loss or postural dizziness, especially during hot weather or an illness causing decreased fluid intake or sodium and water loss). If hypovolemia is more marked, the doses of other medications also will have to be reduced.

The expected effects, beneficial and adverse, of other drugs should also be explained in detail (e.g., possible association of cough with ACE inhibitor). It is useful to inform patients that improvement with many drugs is gradual and may become fully apparent only after several weeks or even months of

TABLE 59-6 TOPICS THAT SHOULD BE DISCUSSED WITH A PATIENT WITH HEART FAILURE AND WITH HIS OR HER FAMILY AND CAREGIVERS

General advice
- Explain what heart failure is and why symptoms occur
  - Causes of heart failure
  - How to recognize symptoms
  - What to do if symptoms occur
  - Self-weighing (to identify fluid retention)
- Rationale for treatments
- Importance of adhering to pharmacologic and nonpharmacologic (e.g., dietary) treatments
- Smoking advice
- Prognosis

Drug counseling
- Rationale (i.e., benefits of individual drugs)
- Dose and time of administration
- Potential adverse effects (and what, if any, action to take)
- What to do in case of missed or skipped doses
- Self-management (e.g., flexible diuretic dosing)

Rest and exercise
- Rest
- Exercise and activities related to work
- Daily physical activity
- Sexual activity
- Rehabilitation

Vaccinations and immunizations

Travel

Driving

Dietary and social habits
- Control sodium intake when necessary (e.g., some patients with severe heart failure)
- Avoid excessive fluids in severe heart failure
- Avoid excessive alcohol intake

Modified from Swedberg K, Cleland J, Dargie H, et al, for the Task Force for the Diagnosis and Treatment of Chronic Heart Failure of the European Society of Cardiology. Guidelines for the diagnosis and treatment of chronic heart failure: executive summary (update 2005). *Eur Heart J.* 2005;26:1115-1140.

treatment. It is also important to explain the need for gradual titration with ACE inhibitors, ARBs, and β-blocking drugs to a desired dose level, which again may take weeks or even months to achieve. Patients should be advised not to use NSAIDs without consultation and to be cautious about using herbal or other nonproprietary preparations (Chapter 38).

Adherence. Education and counseling of the patient, caregiver, and family promote adherence, which is associated with better outcomes. Drug adherence can also be helped by certain pharmacy aids, such as dose allocation (dosette) boxes.

Exercise. Tailored, structured, supervised aerobic exercise is safe and improves functional capacity and quality of life in patients with heart failure (see Table 59-1). 17 An appropriate exercise prescription may also reduce hospitalizations and mortality in patients with heart failure.

Diet, Nutrition, Alcohol. Most guidelines advocate avoidance of foods containing relatively high salt content in the belief that doing so may reduce the need for diuretic therapy. This recommendation is based on clinical experience, which suggests that excess sodium intake can be a precipitant of clinical decompensation. Some salt substitutes have a high potassium content, which can lead to hyperkalemia.

Restriction of fluid intake is indicated only during episodes of decompensation associated with peripheral edema or hyponatremia. In these situations, daily intake should be restricted to 1.5 to 2.0 L to help facilitate reduction in extracellular fluid volume and to avoid hyponatremia.

Reducing excessive weight will reduce the work of the heart and may lower blood pressure (Chapter 67). Conversely, malnutrition is common in severe heart failure, and the development of cardiac cachexia is an ominous sign. Reduced food intake is sometimes caused by nausea (e.g., related to digoxin use or hepatosplenic congestion) or abdominal bloating (e.g., due to ascites). In these cases, small frequent meals and high-protein and high-calorie liquids may be helpful. In severe decompensated heart failure, eating may be difficult because of dyspnea.

Moderate alcohol intake is not thought to be harmful in heart failure, although excessive intake can cause cardiomyopathy and atrial arrhythmias in susceptible individuals. In patients with suspected alcoholic cardiomyopathy, abstinence from alcohol may improve cardiac function.

Smoking. Smoking causes peripheral vasoconstriction, which is detrimental in heart failure. Nicotine replacement therapy (Chapter 31) is believed to be safe in heart failure. The safety of bupropion in heart failure is uncertain, especially as it is known to increase blood pressure.

Sexual Activity. Sexual activity need not be restricted in patients with compensated heart failure, although dyspnea may be limiting. In men with erectile dysfunction (Chapter 242), treatment with a cyclic guanine monophosphate phosphodiesterase type 5 inhibitor can be useful, but these drugs must not be taken within 24 hours of prior nitrate use, and nitrates must not be restarted for at least 24 hours afterward.

Driving. Patients with heart failure can continue to drive, provided their condition does not induce undue dyspnea, fatigue, or other incapacitating symptoms. Patients with recent syncope, cardiac surgery, percutaneous coronary intervention, or device placement may be restricted from driving, at least temporarily, according to local regulations. Patients holding an occupational or commercial license may also be subject to additional restrictions.

Traveling. Short flights are unlikely to cause problems for a patient with compensated heart failure. Cabin pressure is generally maintained to provide an oxygen level no lower than equivalent to 6000 feet above sea level, which should be well tolerated in patients without severe pulmonary disease or pulmonary hypertension. Longer journeys may cause limb edema and dehydration, thereby predisposing to venous thrombosis. Adjustment of the dose of diuretics and other treatments should be discussed with the patient wishing to travel to a warm climate or a country where the risk of gastroenteritis is high. It is also advisable for heart failure patients to carry a list of medications and contact information for their health care provider.

Comorbidity

Comorbid conditions, which are common and important in patients with heart failure, may be due to the underlying cardiovascular disease that caused or contributed to heart failure (e.g., hypertension, coronary artery disease, diabetes mellitus), may arise as a complication of heart failure (e.g., arrhythmias), or can result from an adverse effect of treatment given for heart failure (e.g., gout). The exact causes of other comorbidities in heart failure, such as diabetes (Chapters 236 and 237), depression (Chapter 404), sleep apnea (Chapter 100), renal dysfunction (Chapter 132), and anemia (Chapter 161), are complex and uncertain. These and other comorbid conditions, such as chronic obstructive pulmonary disease and asthma, are important because they are a major determinant of prognosis and may limit the use of certain treatments for heart failure (e.g., renal dysfunction limiting use of ACE inhibitors or asthma limiting β-blockers) and because treatment of comorbidities may affect the stability of heart failure (e.g., NSAIDs needed for rheumatic conditions can cause salt and water retention and renal dysfunction). Both prevention (e.g., diabetes mellitus) and treatment (e.g., anemia) of comorbidities are being evaluated as a potential new therapeutic goal in heart failure.

Angina. β-Blockers are of benefit in both angina (Chapter 71) and heart failure. Ivabradine, which is an inhibitor of the I_f current in the sinus node, reduces heart rate, is an effective antianginal agent at 2.5 to 7.5 mg twice daily, and is safe in patients with left ventricular systolic dysfunction. Nitrates relieve angina but on their own are not of proven value in chronic heart failure. Calcium-channel blockers should generally be avoided in heart failure because they have a negative inotropic action and cause peripheral edema; only amlodipine has been shown to have no adverse effect on survival. Trimetazidine, ranolazine, and nicorandil are antianginal drugs that are available in certain countries; their safety in patients with heart failure is uncertain. Percutaneous and surgical (Chapter 74) revascularization is also of value in relieving angina in selected patients with heart failure (see below).

Atrial Fibrillation. Atrial fibrillation (Chapter 64) may be the cause of or a consequence of heart failure in a patient presenting with atrial fibrillation and a rapid ventricular rate, and the distinction can be difficult, especially because prolonged atrial fibrillation may lead to a rate-related cardiomyopathy. Thyrotoxicosis (Chapter 233) and mitral valve disease (Chapter 75), especially stenosis, must be excluded. Alcohol abuse should also be considered. β-Blockers and digoxin are given to control the ventricular rate. The patient should be supervised closely after the initiation of these treatments because underlying sinus node dysfunction may raise the risk of bradycardia. Unless the patient presents emergently with symptoms or signs of heart failure, myocardial ischemia, or hypertension, there is little or no evidence to support a strategy of restoring sinus rhythm rather than controlling the ventricular rate in most patients with heart failure (Chapter 64). 18 Atrioventricular node ablation and pacing may be required to control ventricular rate (Chapter 66). The use of catheter ablation to cure atrial fibrillation in patients with heart failure is promising but is not currently recommended routinely (Chapter 66). There is a strong indication for thromboembolism prophylaxis with warfarin in patients with heart failure and atrial fibrillation (Chapter 64).

Asthma and Reversible Airways Obstruction. Asthma is a contraindication for use of a β-blocker, but most patients with chronic obstructive pulmonary disease (Chapter 88) can tolerate a β-blocker. Pulmonary congestion can mimic chronic obstructive pulmonary disease. Systemic administration of a corticosteroid to treat reversible airways obstruction may cause sodium and water retention and exacerbate heart failure, whereas inhalation therapy is better tolerated.

Diabetes Mellitus. Diabetes mellitus is discussed in detail elsewhere (Chapters 236 and 237). The prevalence and incidence of diabetes mellitus are high in heart failure, and the risk for development of type 2 diabetes may be reduced by ACE inhibitors and ARBs. β-Blocker treatment is not contraindicated and is of benefit in patients with diabetes and heart failure. Thiazolidinediones cause sodium and water retention, may lead to decompensation, and are not recommended in patients with or at risk of heart failure. Metformin may cause lactic acidosis and is not recommended in patients with severe heart failure.

Abnormal Thyroid Function. Both thyrotoxicosis and hypothyroidism can cause heart failure (and thyrotoxicosis can cause atrial fibrillation, which may precipitate heart failure). Amiodarone can also induce both hypothyroidism and hyperthyroidism, the latter being particularly difficult to diagnose. The risk of thyroid dysfunction may be less with the related antiarrhythmic agent dronedarone, but dronedarone increases mortality in severe heart failure and should be avoided in patients with stage C or D heart failure or recently decompensated heart failure.

Gout. Hyperuricemia and gout (Chapter 281) are common in heart failure and can be caused or aggravated by diuretic treatment. Allopurinol may prevent gout, and acute attacks are better treated with colchicine, oral steroids, or intra-articular steroids rather than by an NSAID.

Renal Dysfunction. Most patients with heart failure have a reduced glomerular filtration rate. ACE inhibitors, ARBs, and aldosterone antagonists often cause a further small reduction in glomerular filtration rate and rise in serum blood urea nitrogen and creatinine levels, which, if limited, should not lead to discontinuation of treatment. Marked increases in blood urea nitrogen and creatinine, however, should prompt consideration of underlying renal artery stenosis (Chapter 127). Renal dysfunction may also be caused by sodium and water depletion, leading to relative hypovolemia (e.g., due to excessive diuresis, diarrhea, and vomiting) or hypotension. Nephrotoxic agents such as NSAIDs are also a common cause of renal dysfunction in heart failure.

Prostatic Obstruction. For prostatic disease (Chapter 131), a 5α-reductase inhibitor may be preferable to an α-adrenoceptor antagonist, which can cause hypotension and salt and water retention. Prostatic obstruction should also be considered in male patients with deteriorating renal function.

Anemia. A normocytic, normochromic anemia (Chapter 161) is also common in heart failure, in part because of the high prevalence of renal dysfunction. Malnutrition and blood loss may also contribute. Intravenous iron treatment with 200 mg of ferric carboxymaltose improves quality of life and reduces symptoms in patients with class II or III heart failure and iron deficiency without adverse effects.[19]

Depression. Depression (Chapter 404) is common in patients with heart failure, perhaps partly owing to disturbance of the hypothalamic-pituitary axis and other neurochemical pathways but also as a result of social isolation and the adjustment to chronic disease. Depression is associated with worse functional status, reduced adherence to treatment, and poor clinical outcomes. Both psychosocial interventions and pharmacologic treatment are helpful. Selective serotonin reuptake inhibitors are believed to be the best tolerated pharmacologic agents, whereas tricyclic antidepressants should be avoided because of their anticholinergic actions and potential to cause arrhythmias.

Cancer. Many anticancer drugs, particularly anthracyclines, cyclophosphamide, and trastuzumab (Herceptin), can cause myocardial damage and heart failure, as can mediastinal radiotherapy. Pericardial constriction can be a result of previous radiotherapy, and malignant pericardial involvement can cause effusion and tamponade (Chapter 77).

Devices and Surgery

Implantable Cardioverter-Defibrillators

About half of patients with heart failure die suddenly, mainly as the result of a ventricular arrhythmia. The relative risk of sudden death, as opposed to death from progressive heart failure, is greatest in patients with milder heart failure. In patients with more advanced heart failure, progressive pump failure deaths are relatively more common. Antiarrhythmic drugs have not been shown to improve survival in heart failure, but ICDs (Chapter 66) reduce the risk of death in selected patients after myocardial infarction (Chapter 73) and improve survival in patients with class II or III heart failure and systolic dysfunction who were otherwise treated with optimal medical therapy.[20,21] All patients with class II or class III heart failure, irrespective of etiology, and an LVEF of 35% or less should be considered for an ICD provided they have no other conditions greatly limiting life expectancy (i.e., have an anticipated survival of at least a year) or quality of life.

Cardiac Resynchronization Therapy

About 30% of patients with heart failure have substantial prolongation of the QRS duration on the surface electrocardiogram, which is a marker of abnormal electrical activation of the left ventricle causing dyssynchronous contraction, less efficient ventricular emptying, and, often, mitral regurgitation. Atrioventricular coupling may also be abnormal, as reflected by a prolonged PR interval, as may interventricular synchrony. Cardiac resynchronization therapy (CRT) with atrial-biventricular or multisite pacing optimizes atrioventricular timing and improves synchronization of cardiac contraction. In selected patients with marked systolic dysfunction (LVEF ≤ 35%), severe symptoms (functional class III or IV), and a wide QRS (120 milliseconds or more, usually manifest with left bundle branch block morphology), CRT improves pump function, reduces mitral regurgitation, relieves symptoms, and significantly prolongs exercise capacity. CRT reduces the composite of death or hospital admission in such patients (see Table 59-1) by more than 35%,[21] and in one trial, it also reduced the risk of death from any cause by 36%.[21] Many other outcome measures, including quality of life, were also improved. The combination of CRT plus an ICD also reduces all-cause mortality by 25% in patients with an LVEF <30%, a QRS >120 milliseconds, and functional class II or III heart failure.[22] In patients with New York Heart Association (NYHA) class I and II symptoms, an LVEF of 30% or less, and a QRS duration of 130 milliseconds or more, CRT (plus an ICD) improved ventricular function and reduced the risk of worsening heart failure, compared with an ICD alone (see Table 59-1); these effects were most pronounced in individuals with a QRS 150 milliseconds or more. CRT did not reduce the risk of death in this population with a relatively low mortality.[23]

The current debate focuses on whether additional patients will benefit from CRT. CRT appears to be beneficial in patients in sinus rhythm, class I or II symptoms, LVEF of 30% or less, a left bundle branch block morphology, and a QRS duration of at least 130 milliseconds. The combination of a CRT plus an ICD improves ventricular function and reduces the risk of worsening heart failure compared with an ICD alone (see Table 59-1), especially in patients with a QRS ≥150 milliseconds.[23] CRT has not been shown to help patients with echocardiographic dyssynchrony but a narrow QRS (<120 milliseconds).

Whether patients with right bundle branch block and atrial fibrillation are helped by CRT is still uncertain. There is no consensus yet about whether (or in whom) CRT alone or a CRT with implantable cardioverter-defibrillator capabilities should be used.

Surgery

With the exception of cardiac transplantation and ventricular assist devices, there are no generally accepted criteria for surgical intervention. Use of operative procedures is variable among centers and greatly dependent on local experience and expertise. Expert imaging and detailed hemodynamic and functional assessments are usually required when any patient with heart failure is considered for surgery, and close liaison between the relevant experts in these fields is essential. The collective expertise in surgical centers is often used to make highly individualized decisions about whether to operate and what procedures will be attempted. "Established" operative treatments for patients with heart failure include coronary artery bypass grafting, surgery for mitral valve incompetence, left ventricular remodeling surgery (including aneurysmectomy), implantation of ventricular assist devices, and heart transplantation. "Experimental" approaches include ventricular constraint devices and intramyocardial cell transplantation.

A recent trial showed no benefit (in symptoms or rates of death or hospitalization for cardiac causes) of surgical ventricular reconstruction. Cardiomyoplasty and partial left ventriculectomy are other recently developed operations for heart failure now thought to be without benefit.

Percutaneous Coronary Intervention or Coronary Artery Bypass Grafting. Percutaneous coronary intervention or coronary artery bypass grafting (Chapter 74), as appropriate, is indicated for relief of angina. The extent of ischemia and residual myocardial viability can be determined by noninvasive assessments such as dobutamine echocardiography (Chapter 55), magnetic resonance imaging (Chapter 56), and positron emission tomographic scanning (Chapter 56) in patients with impaired LVEF. In patients with coronary artery disease and an ejection fraction ≤35%, coronary artery bypass surgery plus optimal medical therapy can significantly reduce cardiovascular mortality but not overall mortality compared with optimal medical therapy alone.[24] As a result, the role of surgery in such patients should be individualized.

Cardiac Transplantation. Cardiac transplantation (Chapter 82) remains the most accepted surgical intervention in end-stage heart failure. Selection criteria usually focus on patients with refractory heart failure, that is, those with severe symptoms and functional limitations (peak oxygen consumption of less than 10 mL/kg/min), as well as a particularly worrisome clinical course and prognosis attributed to their cardiac condition. These patients are often dependent on intravenous inotropic agents and mechanical support.

Left Ventricular Assist Devices. Given the scarcity of organ donors, left ventricular assist devices are used as a "bridge to transplantation" or even as a permanent, definitive, procedure ("destination therapy") for some patients with advanced heart failure. A pulsatile volume-displacement left ventricular assist device can provide a short but significant prolongation of survival in patients who have end-stage heart failure and are ineligible for transplantation (see Table 59-1), but the rates of bleeding, infective and thrombotic complications, and mechanical dysfunction necessitating repeat surgery were high with this older device. In patients with end-stage heart failure ineligible for transplantation, a new continuous-flow device is significantly better than this older device in terms of 2-year survival without repeat device surgery or disabling stroke (46% versus 11%).[25]

A recent trial showed no benefit (in symptoms or rates of death or hospitalization for cardiac causes) of surgical ventricular reconstruction. Cardiomyoplasty and partial left ventriculectomy are other recently developed operations for heart failure now thought to be without benefit.

Heart Failure with Preserved Left Ventricular Ejection Fraction (Diastolic Dysfunction)

Although all patients with symptomatic heart failure share a constellation of signs and symptoms, impaired physical capacity, and reduced quality of life, some have a preserved LVEF (generally above 40 or 50%) and many are thought to have diastolic dysfunction (Chapter 58). Diastolic heart failure often has a cause different from that of systolic heart failure and a better survival rate (Chapters 52, 58, and 60), but sometimes it is an early manifestation of what will evolve into heart failure with a reduced LVEF. The distinction is important, however, because most of the RCTs that generated the evidence for treatment of heart failure included only patients with reduced LVEFs (see Table 59-1). Treatment of the underlying cardiovascular and other disorders that contribute to symptomatic stage C and stage D of heart failure with preserved LVEF, such as hypertension, myocardial ischemia, and diabetes, is critical and is as for stages A and B (see earlier). In patients with atrial fibrillation, control of the ventricular rate with a β-blocker or a rate-limiting calcium-channel blocker (or restoration of sinus rhythm) is particularly important (Chapter 64). Diuretics are used empirically to treat sodium and water retention, according to the same principles as in heart failure with reduced LVEF. In one trial of patients with an LVEF higher than 40% (mean, 54%), treatment with the ARB candesartan decreased the risk of hospital admission for heart failure but did not improve survival or the composite outcome of cardiovascular death or hospital admission for worsening heart failure. In a more recent study of patients with an LVEF of 45% or higher (mean, 60%), the ARB irbesartan had no beneficial effect, raising the possibility that the benefit of candesartan in the earlier trial was largely in patients with borderline systolic dysfunction (i.e., LVEF of 40-50%).[26] Smaller studies in patients in sinus rhythm have shown that the calcium-channel blocker verapamil or the nonselective β-adrenergic blocker propranolol can improve symptoms and exercise capacity in patients with heart failure and preserved LVEF, possibly by reducing heart rate and thereby increasing the duration of diastolic left ventricular filling as well as by directly enhancing myocardial relaxation. There are, however, no current RCTs in which these drugs decisively reduced mortality or morbidity in patients with heart failure and preserved LVEF, so treatment currently is aimed to relieve symptoms.

Heart Failure Due to Valvular Heart Disease

Heart failure also can arise as a result of regurgitant and stenotic valve disease (Chapter 75). It can sometimes be difficult to determine whether mitral regurgitation is primary or secondary in a patient with heart failure and left ventricular dilation, although a prior history of known valve disease or rheumatic fever may suggest a primary valve problem. The objective of treatment of primary valve disease is the prevention of heart failure by surgical repair or replacement of the diseased valve or valves (Chapter 75). The development of overt heart failure is an ominous sign, sometimes requiring emergent valve replacement (e.g., aortic stenosis) but sometimes indicating that valve replacement may not be possible (e.g., because of severe pulmonary hypertension).

Aortic Stenosis

Evaluation of the aortic valve (Chapter 75) can be difficult in patients with poor left ventricular systolic function. Such patients may have insufficient cardiac output to generate a high gradient across even a severely stenotic valve. Conversely, a calcified and degenerate but nonstenotic aortic valve may appear stenosed simply because it does not open normally in patients with very low cardiac output. A calculated valve area provides a better assessment of the severity of aortic stenosis in these patients. Stress echocardiography (Chapter 55) may help assess the potential for ventricular recovery after relief of aortic stenosis. Consideration should be given as to whether concomitant myocardial ischemia from coronary artery disease may also be contributing to a reversible depression of systolic function. Transcatheter valve replacement is a promising new technique for patients who have aortic stenosis but are at very high risk for open valve replacement.

Mitral Regurgitation

Mitral regurgitation can be a primary cause or a secondary manifestation in a patient with heart failure and left ventricular dilation (Chapter 75). Surgery sometimes will result in clinical improvement, but some patients with advanced left ventricular dysfunction will not achieve substantial benefit (e.g., mitral valve surgery in a patient with long-standing severe mitral regurgitation). Valve repair or annuloplasty may, however, be beneficial in carefully selected patients with secondary mitral regurgitation caused by or exacerbated by left ventricular dilation. Valve repair is generally preferable to valve replacement.

Heart Failure Due to Nonischemic Dilated Cardiomyopathy

Patients with heart failure and normal coronary arteries should be evaluated for possible reversible causes. Untreated hypertension is now an unusual cause of dilated cardiomyopathy in the United States, but hypertension was once a leading cause in the United States and remains a major consideration in many parts of the world. Infiltrative cardiomyopathies (e.g., hemochromatosis, amyloid, sarcoid) and arteritides sometimes have specific recommended therapies (Chapters 60, 95, 194, and 219). Chagas' disease (Chapter 355) must be considered in patients from endemic areas. Alcohol and other toxins (e.g., chemotherapeutic agents) are other recognized causes of dilated cardiomyopathy. Dilated cardiomyopathy can also develop in the peripartum period. Most cases of nonischemic dilated cardiomyopathy are usually labeled idiopathic (i.e., no specific etiology can be determined), although many may have a genetic origin, especially if there is a positive family history. Irrespective of etiology, patients with nonischemic dilated cardiomyopathy should be treated in the same way as patients whose dilated, poorly contracting left ventricle is a result of coronary artery disease.

Heart Failure Due to Hypertrophic Cardiomyopathy

Heart failure can arise in patients with hypertrophic cardiomyopathy because of predominant diastolic dysfunction, associated mitral incompetence, or the development of systolic dysfunction. The management of hypertrophic cardiomyopathy and its complications is often very different from the management of dilated cardiomyopathy (Chapter 60), thereby underscoring the value of echocardiography in the evaluation of the patient with heart failure.

Acute Decompensated Heart Failure and Pulmonary Edema

Patients presenting with acute heart failure include those who develop heart failure de novo as a consequence of another cardiac event, usually a myocardial infarction, and those who present for the first time with decompensation of previously asymptomatic and often unrecognized cardiac dysfunction (patients previously in stage B, a transition with profound prognostic implications). However, because of frequent recurrences, most episodes of acute decompensation occur in patients with established, chronic heart failure that has worsened as a result of the unavoidable natural progression of the syndrome, with an intercurrent cardiac (e.g., arrhythmia) or noncardiac (e.g., pneumonia) event, or as a consequence of an avoidable reason, such as nonadherence with treatment or use of an agent that can alter renal function. Although it is not always identified, searching for a reversible precipitant is an important aspect of the initial therapy plan (Table 59-7).

Most patients with acute heart failure require admission to the hospital, especially if pulmonary edema is present. In contrast to chronic heart failure, data from RCTs generally are not available to guide effective therapy for patients with acute decompensated heart failure. The principal goals of management of this heterogeneous group of patients are to relieve symptoms, the most important of which is extreme dyspnea, and to maintain or restore vital organ perfusion. An intravenous bolus or infusion of a loop diuretic (e.g., furosemide, 50 to 100 mg intravenous bolus twice daily, or 10 mg per hour continuous intravenous infusion, titrated according to the symptom response,[27] the reduction in edema, and renal function) and, in hypoxemic patients, oxygen are the key first-line treatments. An intravenous opiate may also be given to relieve anxiety and distress. Noninvasive ventilation using a tight-fitting mask to provide positive-pressure ventilation reduces respiratory distress and metabolic disturbances more rapidly than does standard oxygen therapy but has not reduced short-term mortality.[28] Intravenous infusion of a nitrate (e.g., continuous intravenous infusion of 20 to 200 μg/mm of nitroglycerin, titrated according to the symptomatic response and hemodynamic measurements, particularly arterial blood pressure) is also valuable in patients with a systolic blood pressure of 100 mm Hg or higher (Fig. 59-2). Intravenous nesiritide (human BNP as a 2.0 μg/kg intravenous bolus followed by a continuous intravenous infusion of 0.01 to 0.03 μg/kg/mm titrated according to the symptomatic response and hemodynamic measurements, particularly arterial blood pressure) can reduce the pulmonary capillary wedge pressure more promptly than intravenous nitroglycerin, but the effect of this short-term

TABLE 59-7 SOME COMMON PRECIPITATING CAUSES OF HEART FAILURE

Myocardial ischemia or infarction
Atrial fibrillation or other supraventricular tachycardias
Uncontrolled hypertension
Valvular disease
Ventricular tachycardia
Pulmonary embolism
Pericardial disease
Sepsis
Anemia
Nutritional and medical noncompliance
Adverse drug effects
Hyperthyroidism or hypothyroidism

From Kimmelstiel CD, DeNofrio D, Konstam MA. Heart failure. In: Wachter RM, Goldman L, Hollander H, eds. *Hospital Medicine,* 2nd ed. Philadelphia: Lippincott Williams & Wilkins; 2005:360.

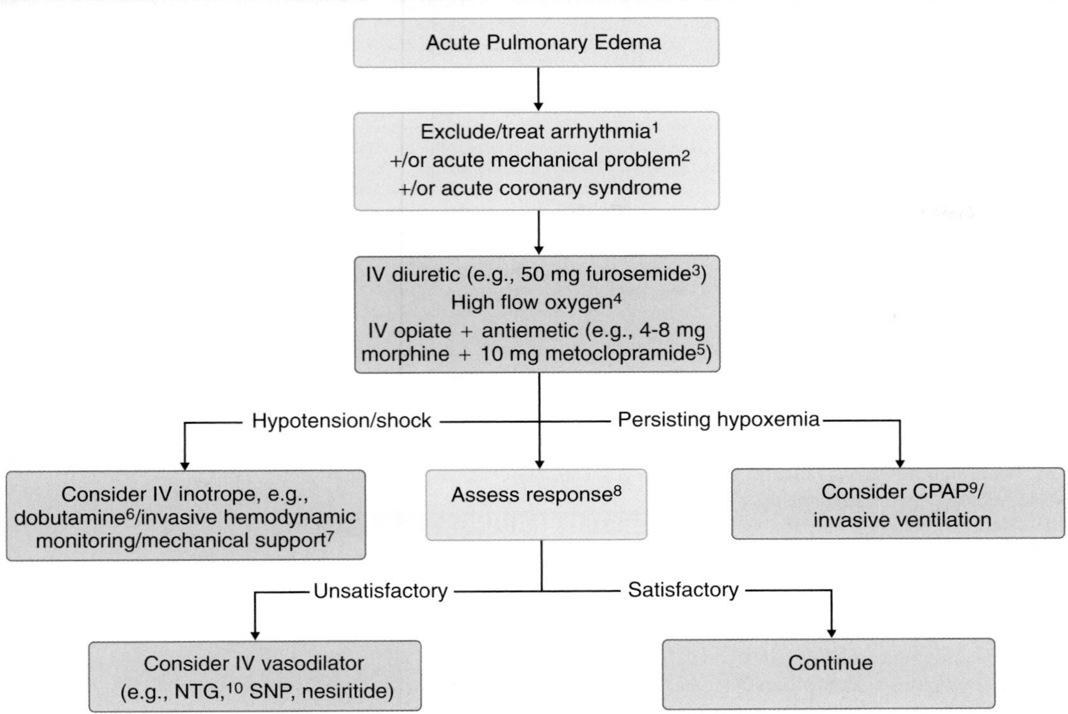

1 Causal arrhythmia (e.g., ventricular tachycardia). It can be difficult to determine whether atrial fibrillation is a primary cause of acute pulmonary edema or secondary to it. An ECG is an essential investigation.

2 Acute mechanical problems include ventricular septal rupture and mitral valve papillary muscle rupture. Mechanical support (e.g., an intra-aortic balloon pump) and urgent surgery should be considered. An echocardiogram should be performed as soon as possible, especially in a patient without a prior diagnosis of heart failure/other relevant heart disease (e.g., prior myocardial infarction or valve disease).

3 Dose of diuretic depends on prior diuretic use and renal function—a lower dose may suffice if preserved renal function and no prior diuretic use.

4 Oxygen causes an increase in systemic vascular resistance and a reduction in heart rate and cardiac output and should only be administered to patients with hypoxemia.

5 Consider if patient agitated/distressed/in pain; may cause respiratory depression and dose should be reduced in very elderly.

6 An intravenous infusion of dobutamine may be started at a dose of 2.5 μg/kg/min, doubling every 15 minutes according to response and tolerability (dose titration usually limited by excessive tachycardia, arrhythmias, or ischemia). A dose above 20 μg/kg/min is rarely needed.

7 E.g., an intra-aortic balloon pump

8 Improvement in symptoms and peripheral perfusion and adequate urine output—patient should be monitored closely, and usually a response will occur within 30 minutes. Bladder catheterization may help in monitoring urine output.

9 Continuous positive airways pressure (CPAP) is valuable in severe pulmonary edema, especially if associated with hypoxemia. Endotracheal intubation and invasive mechanical ventilation should be considered in patients with persisting hypoxemia and physical ventilatory exhaustion.

10 An intravenous infusion of nitroglycerin (NTG) should be started at a dose of 10 μg/min and doubled every 10 minutes according to response and tolerability (usually dose up-titration is limited by hypotension). A dose of more than 100 μg/min is rarely needed.

FIGURE 59-2. Approach to the patient with acute pulmonary edema. ECG = electrocardiogram.

therapy on other clinical outcomes is controversial. In volume-overloaded patients with severe heart failure unresponsive to diuretics, ultrafiltration is an option at specialized centers.

In patients with marked hypotension or other evidence of organ hypoperfusion, an inotropic agent such as dobutamine (continuous intravenous infusion of 2.5 to 25 μg/kg/mm, titrated according to hemodynamic and heart rate response and induction of arrhythmias or myocardial ischemia) or a phosphodiesterase inhibitor (e.g., milrinone) should be considered, although neither treatment has ever been shown to reduce in-hospital deaths. In some countries, the calcium sensitizer levosimendan is also available for use in these patients. In general, potent inotropic agents should be used in a cardiac-monitored setting at the lowest clinically effective dose and for the shortest duration possible (Chapter 107). Although there are limited data supporting a benefit, low-dose dopamine (intravenous infusion of 2.5 μg/kg/mm) may be administered in an attempt to improve renal function. Patients with severe hyponatremia may benefit from the arginine vasopressin antagonist tolvaptan (15 to 60 mg orally once daily).

In more critically ill patients, mechanical support (e.g., with an intra-aortic balloon pump) may also be considered (Chapter 107). The aim of treatment is to support the patient's circulation and vital organ function until either the patient's heart recovers or a definitive operative procedure can be performed (e.g., transplantation or permanent implantation of a ventricular-assist device).

In patients admitted to the hospital, discharge planning and subsequent management to reduce the risk of readmission are important. Ideally, an effective oral diuretic regimen should have been identified, and fluid-volume and biochemical stability should have been achieved. This optimization of volume status and development of a stable oral regimen before discharge is thought to reduce the risk of early readmission. Treatment with an ACE inhibitor, β-blocker, and ARB or aldosterone antagonist, as appropriate, should also be started and titrated in the stabilized patient before discharge. Outpatient follow-up should be arranged to ensure that any of those treatments that have not been started before discharge are initiated after discharge and that the dose of each drug is increased, as tolerated, to the appropriate target.

Outpatient Follow-Up

The key to successful follow-up is the careful tracking of clinical symptoms and the patient's weight, which often involves interviewing not only the patient but also family members, who may be more aware of changes in status than the patient (see Organization of Care, earlier). Continuity of care and seamless transitions from the inpatient to the outpatient setting are crucial aspects of optimal management. Patients with advanced heart failure and patients requiring frequent hospitalization require special handling. Programs that provide telephone-based tracking of daily weights and symptoms can detect deterioration in time to intervene before the need for hospitalization. Although these programs may be costly, several evaluations have found them to be cost-effective. Because the management of these patients requires considerable experience and expertise, specialized heart failure programs and clinics have been developed and may provide additional benefit compared with traditional care.

PROGNOSIS

The prognosis of patients with heart failure is poor despite advances in therapy. Of patients who survive the acute onset of heart failure, only 35% of men and 50% of women are alive after 5 years. Although it is difficult to predict prognosis in individual patients, patients with symptoms at rest (class IV) have a 30 to 50% annual mortality rate, patients who are symptomatic with mild activity (class III) have mortality rates of 10 to 20% annually, and patients with symptoms only with moderate activity (class II) have a 5 to 10% annual mortality rate. Mortality rates are higher in older patients, men, and patients with a reduced LVEF or underlying coronary heart disease.

END-OF-LIFE CONSIDERATIONS

Although predicting the trajectory of illness in patients with advanced heart failure is notoriously difficult, it is often apparent when a patient has progressed to end-stage heart failure, commonly associated with concomitant renal failure. In these circumstances, the expertise of the palliative care team may be especially helpful (Chapter 3). Useful websites providing information on palliative care relevant to heart failure are available (*www.goldstandardsframework.nhs.uk/* and *www.palliativecarescotland.org.uk/assets/files/AR%2031%20March%202009.pdf*). Medications such as parenteral opiates (with an antiemetic) and benzodiazepines may be particularly helpful in relieving dyspnea, anxiety, and pain that arises from ascites, hepatic congestion, lower limb edema, and pressure points. At this stage in the patient's illness, it may be appropriate to discuss withdrawal of conventional treatment, deactivation of an ICD to avoid undesired and unpleasant electrical discharges, and a do-not-resuscitate order if the patient and others involved in the patient's care agree that "comfort care" is appropriate. Hospice care may be chosen by some at this point.

FUTURE DIRECTIONS

The discovery of primitive pluripotent stem cells that have the potential to differentiate into contractile tissue has generated considerable optimism about their transplantation into patients with impaired systolic function. Stimulation of the small population of resident stem cells in adult myocardium may also be possible.

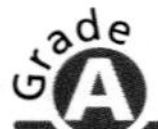

1. Pfeffer MA, Braunwald E, Moyé LA, et al. Effect of captopril on mortality and morbidity in patients with left ventricular dysfunction after myocardial infarction: results of the survival and ventricular enlargement trial. The SAVE Investigators. *N Engl J Med.* 1992;327:669-677.
2. The SOLVD Investigators. Effect of enalapril on mortality and the development of heart failure in asymptomatic patients with reduced left ventricular ejection fractions. *N Engl J Med.* 1992;327:685-691.
3. Pfeffer MA, McMurray JJ, Velazquez EJ, et al. Valsartan, captopril, or both in myocardial infarction complicated by heart failure, left ventricular dysfunction, or both. *N Engl J Med.* 2003;349:1893-1906.
4. Dargie HJ. Effect of carvedilol on outcome after myocardial infarction in patients with left-ventricular dysfunction: the CAPRICORN randomised trial. *Lancet.* 2001;357:1385-1390.
5. The CONSENSUS Trial Study Group. Effects of enalapril on mortality in severe congestive heart failure: results of the Cooperative North Scandinavian Enalapril Survival Study (CONSENSUS). *N Engl J Med.* 1987;316:1429-1435.
6. The SOLVD Investigators. Effect of enalapril on survival in patients with reduced left ventricular ejection fractions and congestive heart failure. *N Engl J Med.* 1991;325:293-302.
7. Granger CB, McMurray JJ, Yusuf S, et al. Effects of candesartan in patients with chronic heart failure and reduced left-ventricular systolic function intolerant to angiotensin-converting-enzyme inhibitors: the CHARM-Alternative trial. *Lancet* 2003;362:772-776.
8. Cohn JN, Tognoni G: A randomized trial of the angiotensin-receptor blocker valsartan in chronic heart failure. *N Engl J Med.* 2001;345:1667-1675.
9. McMurray JJ, Östergren J, Swedberg K, et al. Effects of candesartan in patients with chronic heart failure and reduced left-ventricular systolic function taking angiotensin-converting-enzyme inhibitors: the CHARM-Added trial. *Lancet.* 2003;362:767-771.
10. Packer M, Coats AJ, Fowler MB, et al. Effect of carvedilol on survival in severe chronic heart failure. *N Engl J Med.* 2001;344:1651-1658.
11. Pitt B, Zannad F, Remme WJ, et al. The effect of spironolactone on morbidity and mortality in patients with severe heart failure: randomized Aldactone Evaluation Study Investigators. *N Engl J Med.* 1999;341:709-717.
12. Pitt B, Remme W, Zannad F, et al. Eplerenone, a selective aldosterone blocker, in patients with left ventricular dysfunction after myocardial infarction. *N Engl J Med.* 2003;348:1309-1321.
13. Zannad F, McMurray JJ, Krum H, et al. Eplerenone in patients with systolic heart failure and mild symptoms. *N Engl J Med.* 2011;364:11-21.
14. The Digitalis Investigation Group. The effects of digoxin on mortality and morbidity in patients with heart failure. *N Engl J Med.* 1997;336:525-533.
15. Taylor AL, Ziesche S, Yancy C, et al. Combination of isosorbide dinitrate and hydralazine in blacks with heart failure. *N Engl J Med.* 2004;351:2049-2057.
16. Sochalski J, Jaarsma T, Krumholz HM, et al. What works in chronic care management: the case of heart failure. *Health Aff (Millwood).* 2009;28:179-189.
17. O'Connor CM, Whellan DJ, Lee KL, et al. HF-ACTION Investigators. Efficacy and safety of exercise training in patients with chronic heart failure: HF-ACTION randomized controlled trial. *JAMA.* 2009;301:1439-1450.
18. Roy D, Talajic M, Nattel S, et al. Atrial Fibrillation and Congestive Heart Failure Investigators. Rhythm control versus rate control for atrial fibrillation and heart failure. *N Engl J Med.* 2008;358:2667-2677.
19. Anker SD, Comin Colet J, Filippatos G, et al. Ferric carboxymaltose in patients with heart failure and iron deficiency. *N Engl J Med.* 2009;361:2436-2448.
20. Bardy GH, Lee KL, Mark DB, et al. Amiodarone or an implantable cardioverter-defibrillator for congestive heart failure. *N Engl J Med.* 2005;352:225-237.
21. Cleland JG, Daubert JC, Erdmann E, et al. The effect of cardiac resynchronization on morbidity and mortality in heart failure. *N Engl J Med.* 2005;352:1539-1549.
22. Tang AS, Wells GA, Talajic M, et al. Cardiac-resynchronization therapy for mild-to-moderate heart failure. *N Engl J Med.* 2010;363:2385-2395.
23. Moss AJ, Hall WJ, Cannom DS, et al. Cardiac-resynchronization therapy for the prevention of heart-failure events. *N Engl J Med.* 2009;361:1329-1338.
24. Velazquez EJ, Lee KL, Deja MA, et al, for the STICH Investigators. Coronary-artery bypass surgery in patients with left ventricular dysfunction. *N Engl J Med.* 2011;364:1607-1616.
25. Slaughter MS, Rogers JG, Milano CA, et al. Advanced heart failure treated with continuous-flow left ventricular assist device. *N Engl J Med.* 2009;361:2241-2251.
26. Massie BM, Carson PE, McMurray JJ, et al. I-PRESERVE Investigators. Irbesartan in patients with heart failure and preserved ejection fraction. *N Engl J Med.* 2008;359:2456-2467.
27. Felker GM, Lee KL, Bull DA, et al. Diuretic strategies in patients with acute decompensated heart failure. *N Engl J Med.* 2011;364:797-805.
28. Weng CL, Zhao YT, Liu Qh, et al. Meta-analysis: noninvasive ventilation in acute cardiogenic pulmonary edema. *Ann Intern Med.* 2010;152:590-600.

SUGGESTED READINGS

Joynt KE, Orav EJ, Jha AK. The association between hospital volume and processes, outcomes, and costs of care for congestive heart failure. *Ann Intern Med.* 2011;154:94-102. *Experience is associated with better outcomes but a higher cost.*

McMurray JJV. Systolic heart failure. *N Engl J Med.* 2010;362:32-42. *Concise review.*

Weintraub NL, Collins SP, Pang PS, et al. Acute heart failure syndromes: emergency department presentation, treatment, and disposition: current approaches and future aims: a scientific statement from the American Heart Association. *Circulation.* 2010;122:1975-1996. *Guidelines.*

60

DISEASES OF THE MYOCARDIUM AND ENDOCARDIUM

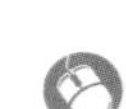

WILLIAM MCKENNA AND PERRY ELLIOTT

MYOCARDIAL DISEASE

A substantial minority of cases of heart failure result from familial (genetic) or nonfamilial (acquired) disorders, which can be confined to the heart or be multisystem disorders. The term *cardiomyopathy* refers to myocardial disorders in which the heart muscle is structurally and functionally abnormal in the absence of coronary artery disease (Chapter 73), hypertension (Chapter 67), valvular disease (Chapter 75), or congenital heart disease (Chapter 69) sufficient to cause the observed myocardial abnormality. Cardiomyopathies are classified according to ventricular morphology and pathophysiology into four major types: dilated cardiomyopathy, hypertrophic cardiomyopathy, restrictive cardiomyopathy, and arrhythmogenic right ventricular cardiomyopathy (ARVC) (Table 60-1; Fig. 60-1). Diseases that do not fit into these groups (such as endocardial fibroelastosis and left ventricular noncompaction) are termed *unclassified cardiomyopathies.* Mixed phenotypes can exist; for example, patients with hypertrophic and dilated cardiomyopathies frequently have a restrictive left ventricular physiology or develop ventricular dilation.

Hypertrophic Cardiomyopathy

DEFINITION AND EPIDEMIOLOGY

Hypertrophic cardiomyopathy is defined as unexplained left ventricular hypertrophy in the absence of abnormal loading conditions (valve disease, hypertension, congenital heart defects) sufficient to explain the degree of hypertrophy. The disease occurs in all racial groups, with a prevalence of between 0.2 and 0.5%.

PATHOBIOLOGY

Hypertrophic cardiomyopathy is usually familial with autosomal dominant inheritance. Mutations in sarcomeric contractile protein genes (Table 60-2) account for approximately 50 to 60% of cases. More than 400 different

TABLE 60-1 PROFILES OF MYOCARDIAL DISEASE

	HYPERTROPHIC	DILATED	RESTRICTIVE	ARVC
Causes	Genetic (see Table 60-2)	Myocarditis (see Table 60-4) Metabolic/endocrine Genetic (see Table 60-2)	Infiltrative or storage diseases (see Table 60-8) Endomyocardial (e.g., Löffler's, carcinoid) Genetic (see Table 60-2)	Genetic (see Table 60-2)
Ejection fraction	Increased	Reduced	25-50%	Normal until end stage 30% regional LV disease
Left ventricular End-diastolic dimension	Usually decreased	Increased	Normal	Normal until end stage Right ventricle dilated
Left ventricular wall thickness	Increased	Normal	Normal or mildly increased	Normal
Atrial size	Increased	Increased	Increased; may be massive	Left atrium normal; right dilated in severe disease
Valvular disease	Mitral regurgitation (SAM)	Mitral (functional); tricuspid regurgitation in late stages	Mitral and tricuspid regurgitation, rarely severe	Tricuspid regurgitation in severe disease
Common symptoms	Dyspnea; chest pain, syncope Late: orthopnea, PND	Dyspnea, fatigue Late: orthopnea, PND	Dyspnea Late: orthopnea, PND, right heart failure	Palpitations, syncope Late: right heart failure
Arrhythmia	Atrial fibrillation, ventricular tachycardia; conduction block in PRKAG2, mitochondrial; Fabry's disease	Ventricular tachyarrhythmias; heart block in Chagas' disease, giant cell myocarditis, laminopathies	Atrial fibrillation; conduction block in sarcoid, amyloidosis, desminopathy	Ventricular ectopy and tachycardia

ARVC = arrhythmogenic right ventricular cardiomyopathy; LV = left ventricular; SAM = systolic anterior motion of mitral valve; PND = paroxysmal nocturnal dyspnea.

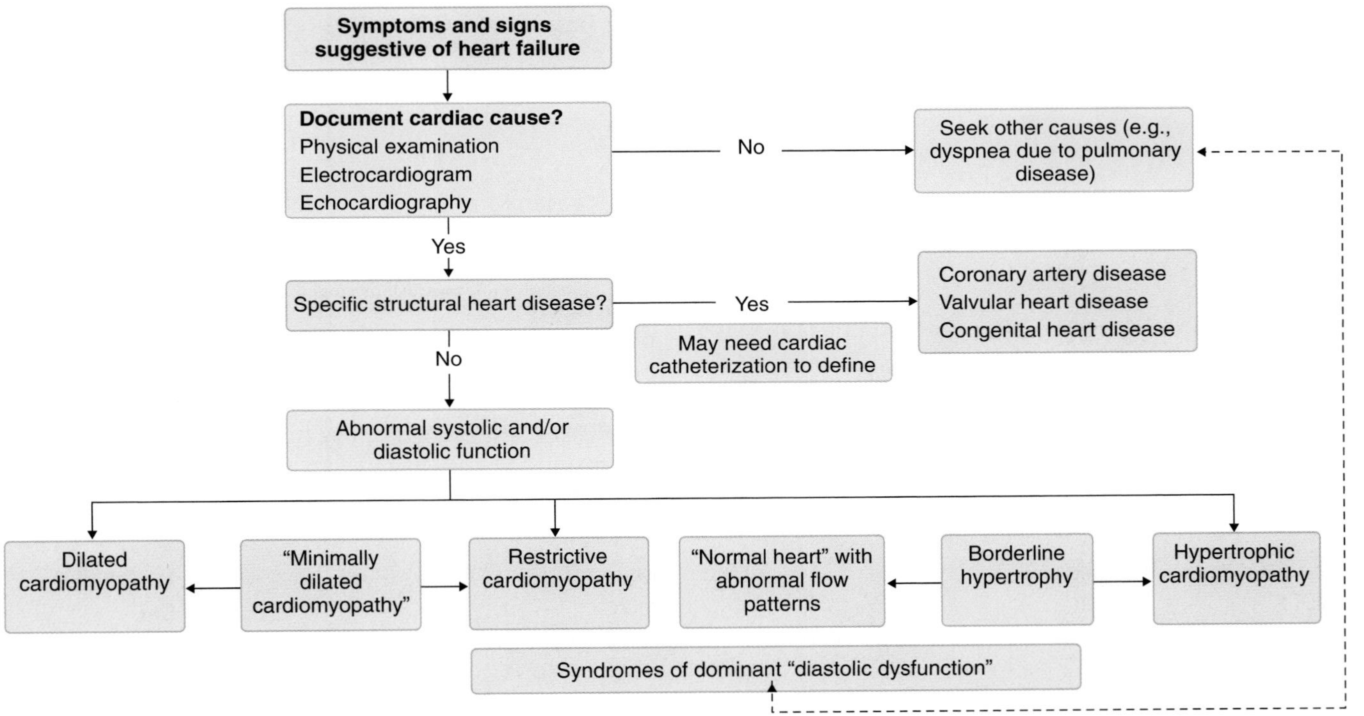

FIGURE 60-1. Initial approach to classification of cardiomyopathy. The evaluation of symptoms or signs consistent with heart failure first includes confirmation that they can be attributed to a cardiac cause. Although this conclusion is often apparent from routine physical examination and electrocardiography, echocardiography serves to confirm cardiac disease and provides clues to the presence of other cardiac diseases, such as focal abnormalities, suggesting primary valve disease or congenital heart disease. Having excluded these conditions, cardiomyopathy is generally considered to be dilated, restrictive, or hypertrophic, as shown in Table 60-1. Patients with apparently normal cardiac structure and contraction are occasionally found to demonstrate abnormal intracardiac flow patterns consistent with diastolic dysfunction but should also be evaluated carefully for other causes of their symptoms. Most patients with so-called diastolic dysfunction also demonstrate at least borderline criteria for left ventricular hypertrophy, frequently in the setting of chronic hypertension and diabetes. A moderately decreased ejection fraction without marked dilation or a pattern of restrictive cardiomyopathy is sometimes referred to as *minimally dilated cardiomyopathy*, which may represent either a distinct entity or a transition between acute and chronic disease.

mutations have been identified, with marked variation in disease penetrance and clinical expression. A similar clinical phenotype is seen in association with other uncommon genetic disorders, including Noonan's syndrome (Chapter 69), Friedreich's ataxia (Chapter 429), neurofibromatosis (Chapter 426), hereditary spherocytosis (Chapter 164), respiratory chain disorders, glycogen storage diseases (Chapter 214), and lysosomal storage disorders (Chapter 215) (see Table 60-2).

PATHOLOGY

In the common form of autosomal dominant hypertrophic cardiomyopathy, myocardial hypertrophy usually affects the interventricular septum more than other regions of the left ventricle. Other patterns, including concentric, mid-ventricular (sometimes associated with a left ventricular apical diverticulum), and apical also occur. Coexistent right ventricular hypertrophy is

TABLE 60-2 GENETIC CAUSES OF CARDIOMYOPATHY

GENE	SYMBOL	INHERITANCE	PHENOTYPES	FREQUENCY
SARCOMERIC PROTEINS				
Cardiac β-myosin heavy chain	MYH7	AD	Variable: moderate to severe prognosis; HCM; LVNC; DCM; Laing distal myopathy	HCM 30-40%; DCM 4-6%
Cardiac troponin T	TNNT2	AD	HCM: possible high incidence of sudden death; DCM	HCM 5%; DCM 3%
Cardiac troponin I	TNNI3	HCM, AD; DCM, AR	Can present with restrictive physiology/ cardiomyopathy; HCM; DCM	HCM 5%, DCM <1%
Cardiac troponin C	TNNC	AD	DCM	<1%
Cardiac myosin binding protein C	MYBPC3	AD	Late onset of the disease described; cases of children with a severe hypertrophy also reported; DCM	HCM 30-40%; DCM (?)
Cardiac α-myosin heavy chain	MYH6	AD	DCM, HCM	DCM (?) 2-3%; HCM <1%
Titin	TTN	AD	DCM, HCM	DCM (?); HCM rare
Cardiac actin	ACTC	DCM and HCM AD	DCM, LVNC, HCM	DCM <1%; HCM ≈1%
Essential myosin light chain	MYL3	AD	HCM	(?)
Regulatory myosin light chain	MYL2	AD	HCM	≈1%
α-Tropomyosin	TPM1	AD	HCM, DCM	HCM ≈1-2%; DCM <1%
Z-DISC PROTEINS				
Cypher/ZASP	LDB3		LVNC	
Metavinculin	VCL	AD	DCM, HCM	DCM <1-1%; HCM rare
LIM binding domain 3	LDB3	AD	DCM, HCM	DCM <1-1%; HCM rare
Titin-cap or telethonin	TCAP	AD	DCM, HCM	DCM <1-1%; HCM <1%
Myozenin 2	MYOZ2	AD	HCM	<1%
Muscle LIM protein	CSRP3	AD	DCM, HCM	DCM <1%; HCM rare
CYTOSKELETAL PROTEINS				
Desmin	DES	AD	DCM	<1-1%
α- and β-dystroglycans	DAG1	NA	DCM	NA
α-, β-, γ-, and δ-sarcoglycans	SGCA, SGCB, SGCG, SGCD	SGCD AD	DCM	SGCD <1%
Caveolin-3	CAV3	AD	DCM, HCM	HCM rare
Lamin A/C	LMNA	DCM, AD; EMD2, AD; EMD3, AR; LGMD1B, AD	LVNC, DCM, DCM in Emery-Dreifuss muscular dystrophy types 2 and 3 (EMD2 and EMD3), DCM in limb girdle muscular dystrophy (LGMD) 1B	DCM 4-8%
Syntrophin	SNT	NA	DCM	NA
Dystrobrevin	DTN	NA	DCM	NA
Dystrophin	DMD	XL	DCM in Duchenne muscular dystrophy (DMD), Becker muscular dystrophy (BMD)	(?)
DESMOSOMAL PROTEINS				
Plakoglobin	JUP	Naxos disease, AR	ARVC, ARVC in Naxos disease	Rare
Desmoplakin	DSP	Carvajal syndrome, AR; ARVC, AD	ARVC, DCM in Carvajal syndrome	ARVC 6-16%
Desmoglein 2	DSG2	AD	ARVC	12-40%
Desmocollin 2	DSC2	AD	ARVC	Rare
Plakophilin-2	PKP2	AD, AR	ARVC	AD 11-43%, AR rare
SARCOPLASMIC RETICULUM				
Phospholamban	PLN	AD	DCM, HCM	DCM (?); HCM rare
METABOLIC PROTEINS				
Protein kinase, AMP-activated, γ_2 noncatalytic subunit	PRKAG2	AD	HCM in Wolff-Parkinson-White syndrome	NA
α-Galactosidase A	GLA	XL	HCM in Anderson-Fabry disease	NA
Lysosomal-associated membrane protein 2	LAMP2	XL	HCM in Danon disease	NA
OTHERS				
Hereditary hemochromatosis	HFE	AR	DCM and RCM in hereditary hemochromatosis	NA
Hereditary amyloidosis	TTR	AD	HCM and RCM in hereditary amyloidosis	NA
RAS-MAPK pathway genes	PTPN11/RAF1/ SOS1/KRAS/ HRAS/ BRAF/MEK1-2	AD	HCM in Noonan syndrome and LEOPARD syndrome	NA
Frataxin	FRDA	AR	HCM in Friedreich ataxia	NA

AD = autosomal dominant; AR = autosomal recessive; ARVC = arrhythmogenic right ventricular cardiomyopathy; DCM = dilated cardiomyopathy; HCM = hypertrophic cardiomyopathy; NA = not available; RCM = restrictive cardiomyopathy; XL = X-linked.

present in up to 17% of cases. The papillary muscles are often displaced anteriorly, thereby contributing to systolic anterior motion of the anterior mitral valve leaflet in 25% of patients and of the posterior leaflets in 10% of cases in the resting state. Often, the mitral valve is structurally abnormal, with elongation of the anterior leaflet and occasional direct insertion of the papillary muscle into the anterior leaflet. The histologic hallmark of hypertrophic cardiomyopathy is a triad of myocyte hypertrophy, myocyte disarray, and interstitial fibrosis. Myocyte disarray refers to architectural disorganization of the myocardium, with adjacent myocytes aligned obliquely or perpendicular to each other in association with increased interstitial collagen. The myofibrillar architecture within the myocyte is also disorganized. Although myocyte disarray occurs in aortic stenosis, long-standing hypertension, and some forms of congenital heart disease, the presence of extensive disarray (more than 10% of ventricular septal myocytes) is thought to be a highly specific marker for hypertrophic cardiomyopathy. Small intramural coronary arteries are often dysplastic and narrowed owing to wall thickening by smooth muscle cell hyperplasia.

PATHOPHYSIOLOGY

Abnormal ventricular geometry, wall thickening, myocyte hypertrophy, myocyte and myofibrillar disarray, and myocardial fibrosis all contribute to impairment of left ventricular diastolic function. The net result is elevation of left ventricular end-diastolic pressures, symptoms of heart failure, and reduced exercise tolerance. Global measures of left ventricular systolic function are often normal, but regional myocardial dysfunction and progressive systolic impairment are relatively common.

Approximately 25% of patients have left ventricular outflow tract obstruction at rest caused by contact between the anterior leaflet of the mitral valve and the interventricular septum during ventricular systole. Many patients without outflow obstruction at rest develop it during physiologic and pharmacologic interventions that reduce left ventricular end-diastolic volume or increase left ventricular contractility (e.g., amyl nitrate inhalation, Valsalva maneuver, and administration of intravenous inotropic agents).

CLINICAL MANIFESTATIONS

Most patients are asymptomatic or have only mild or intermittent symptoms. Symptomatic progression is usually slow, age related, and associated with a gradual deterioration in left ventricular function over decades. Fewer than 5% of patients may have rapid, symptomatic deterioration. Symptoms can develop at any age, even many years after the appearance of electrocardiographic (ECG) or echocardiographic manifestations of left ventricular hypertrophy. Occasionally, sudden death may be the initial presentation. However, most individuals with hypertrophic cardiomyopathy have few if any symptoms, and the diagnosis is often made as a result of family screening or the incidental detection of a heart murmur or an abnormal ECG.

Approximately 20 to 30% of adults develop chest pain (Chapters 50 and 71), which may occur on exertion, at rest, or nocturnally. Postprandial angina associated with mild exertion is typical. Mild to moderate dyspnea on exertion is relatively common, and some patients develop paroxysmal nocturnal dyspnea that may be caused by transient myocardial ischemia or arrhythmia. Approximately 20% of patients experience syncope (Chapters 50 and 62), and a similar proportion complain of presyncope. Palpitations (Chapter 62) are frequent and are usually attributable to supraventricular or ventricular ectopy or to forceful cardiac contraction. Sustained palpitations are usually caused by supraventricular tachyarrhythmias, but initial presentation with a symptomatic arrhythmia is uncommon. Patients with distal or apical hypertrophy have fewer symptoms, better exercise capacity, no arrhythmias, and good prognosis. Occasionally, however, patients with distal or apical hypertrophy may have severe refractory chest pain or may present with troublesome supraventricular arrhythmias.

DIAGNOSIS

A three- to four-generation family history, which should be obtained in all patients with a new diagnosis of cardiomyopathy, helps to determine the probability of familial disease and its mode of inheritance. The initial diagnostic evaluation includes a family history focusing on premature cardiac disease or death, a comprehensive medical history focusing on cardiovascular symptoms, a careful physical examination, a 12-lead ECG, and a two-dimensional echocardiogram.

The general evaluation may provide diagnostic clues in patients whose hypertrophic cardiomyopathy is associated with syndromes or metabolic disorders. For example, Noonan's syndrome (Chapter 69) is characterized by short stature, developmental delay, cutaneous abnormalities (café au lait spots), hypertelorism, ptosis, low-set posteriorly rotated ears, and a webbed neck. These features are shared with the less common LEOPARD syndrome. Angiokeratomas, anhidrosis, Raynaud's-like symptoms with neuropathy, cornea verticillata, retinal vascular dilation, tinnitus, diarrhea, and proteinuria are typical features of Fabry's disease (Chapter 215).

Clinical examination of the cardiovascular system is often normal. In the presence of left ventricular outflow tract obstruction, the arterial pulse has a rapid upstroke and downstroke (sometimes with a bisferiens character), the apex beat is sustained or double (reflecting a palpable atrial impulse followed by left ventricular contraction), and auscultation will demonstrate a systolic ejection murmur that is heard loudest at the left sternal edge and that radiates to the right upper sternal edge and apex (Chapter 50). Most patients with left ventricular outflow tract obstruction also have the murmur of mitral regurgitation, which results from failure of the mitral valve leaflets to coapt owing to the systolic anterior motion of the mitral valve. Physiologic and pharmacologic maneuvers that decrease afterload or venous return (e.g., standing, Valsalva maneuver, inhalation of amyl nitrite) or increase contractility (e.g., a post-extrasystole beat) will increase the intensity of the murmur, whereas interventions that increase afterload and venous return (e.g., squatting or handgrip) will reduce it (see Table 50-2 in Chapter 50). In contrast, physical signs in most patients who do not have left ventricular outflow tract obstruction are subtle and are limited to features that reflect the hyperdynamic contraction (rapid upstroke pulse) and poorly compliant right (prominent a wave in jugular venous pressure) and left (S_4 gallop, double-apex beat) ventricles (Chapter 50).

Diagnostic Testing

More than 90% of patients have abnormal ECG findings, but no changes are disease specific. The most common abnormalities are increased QRS voltage consistent with left ventricular hypertrophy, left axis deviation (15 to 20%), abnormal Q waves (25 to 30%, most commonly in inferolateral leads), and ST segment or T wave changes (>50%). An isolated increase in the QRS voltage without ST segment changes or T wave inversion is rare in hypertrophic cardiomyopathy. The presence of predominantly distal or apical thickening is associated with giant negative T wave inversion on the ECG tracing.

Two-dimensional echocardiography (Chapter 55) is the mainstay of diagnostic imaging, but magnetic resonance imaging (Chapter 56) and computed tomography (Chapter 56) provide alternatives if the echocardiogram is of poor quality. In most patients, the hypertrophy is asymmetrical and involves the anterior and posterior intraventricular septum (Fig. 60-2). The hypertrophy, however, may be more generalized and involve the free wall of the left ventricle, or it may be localized and confined to areas other than the septum, such as the lateral or posterior wall of the left ventricle. The echocardiogram can measure left ventricular outflow tract obstruction, both at rest and after provocative maneuvers. Patients with an outflow tract gradient of 30 mm Hg or more typically have systolic anterior motion of the mitral valve, with contact of either the anterior or (less commonly) the posterior mitral leaflet with the intraventricular septum during systole, in association with a posteriorly directed jet of mitral regurgitation, the severity of which is proportionate to the severity of the obstruction. Most patients with hypertrophic cardiomyopathy have left atrial enlargement as well as echocardiographic evidence of diastolic dysfunction.

When available, cardiopulmonary exercise testing with metabolic gas exchange measurements provides an accurate and reproducible assessment of exercise capacity, which can be followed serially. Cardiac catheterization is rarely required for diagnosis or management, but it may be indicated when measurement of intracardiac pressures is required to guide therapeutic decisions (e.g., in patients with severe mitral regurgitation) and for the exclusion of coexistent coronary artery disease in patients with chest pain.

Diagnostic Criteria

A wall thickness of more than 2 standard deviations above the mean, corrected for age, gender, and height, is generally accepted as diagnostic. In adults, this value is typically 1.5 cm or greater in men and 1.3 cm or greater in women. In the presence of other causes of left ventricular hypertrophy such as long-standing systemic hypertension or aortic stenosis, the diagnosis of hypertrophic cardiomyopathy may be problematic. However, secondary hypertrophy from other causes rarely exceeds 1.8 cm. Hypertrophy in the

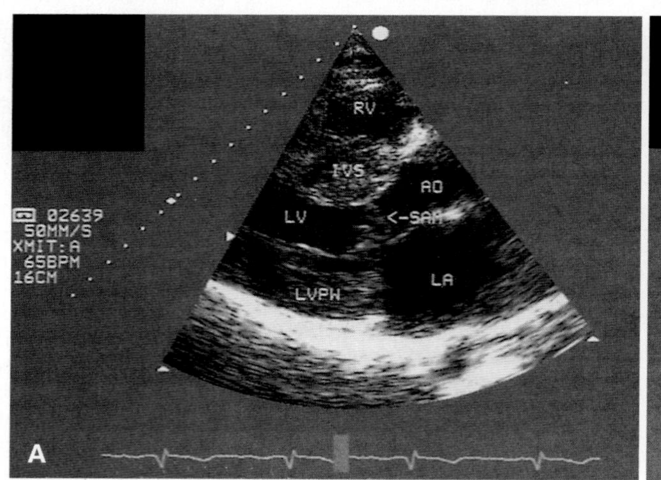

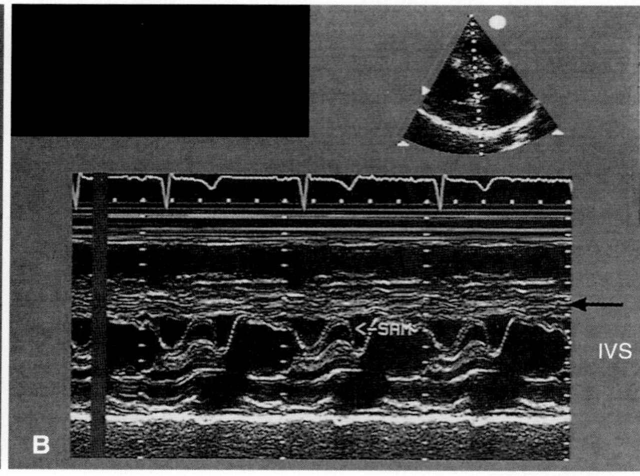

FIGURE 60-2. Hypertrophic obstructive cardiomyopathy. A, The two-dimensional long-axis parasternal view shows the chambers of the heart. The left ventricle posterior wall (LVPW) is thickened, and the most striking abnormality is the hypertrophy of the interventricular septum (IVS). Another characteristic feature is a Venturi effect: as blood leaves the left ventricle (LV), it sucks the anterior leaflet of the mitral valve forward, a phenomenon called *systolic anterior motion* (SAM). **B,** This phenomenon is more clearly shown in the parasternal long-axis M-mode echocardiogram. The massive thickening of the septum is also obvious in the M-mode image (IVS). AO = aorta; LA = left atrium; RV = right ventricle. (From Forbes CD, Jackson WF. *Color Atlas and Text of Clinical Medicine,* 3rd ed. London: Mosby; 2003.)

TABLE 60-3 DIAGNOSTIC CRITERIA FOR HYPERTROPHIC CARDIOMYOPATHY IN FIRST-DEGREE RELATIVES OF AFFECTED PATIENTS*

MAJOR CRITERIA	MINOR CRITERIA
ECHOCARDIOGRAPHY	
Left ventricular wall thickness ≥13 mm in the anterior septum or posterior wall or ≥15 mm in the posterior septum or free wall	Left ventricular wall thickness of 12 mm in the anterior septum or posterior wall or of 14 mm in the posterior septum or free wall
Severe SAM of the mitral valve (septal-leaflet contact)	Moderate SAM of the mitral valve (no mitral leaflet-septal contact)
	Redundant mitral valve leaflets
ELECTROCARDIOGRAPHY	
Left ventricular hypertrophy with repolarization changes (Romhilt and Estes)	Complete bundle branch block or (minor) interventricular conduction defects (in left ventricular leads)
T wave inversion in leads I and aVL (≥3 mm with QRS-T wave axis difference ≥30 degrees), V_3-V_6 (≥3 mm) or II and III and aVF (≥5 mm)	Minor repolarization changes in left ventricular leads
	Deep S wave in lead V_2 (>25 mm)
Abnormal Q waves (>40 msec or >25% R wave) in at least two leads from II, III, aVF (in absence of left anterior hemiblock), and V_1-V_4; or I, aVL, V_5-V_6	Unexplained chest pain, dyspnea, or syncope

*The diagnosis of hypertrophic cardiomyopathy in first-degree relatives of patients with the disease is based on the presence of one major criterion or two minor echocardiographic criteria or one minor echocardiographic and two minor electrocardiographic criteria.
aVF = augmented voltage unipolar left foot lead; aVL = augmented voltage unipolar left arm lead; SAM = systolic anterior motion.
Adapted from McKenna WJ, Spirito P, Desnos M, et al. Experience in clinical genetics in hypertrophic cardiomyopathy. *Heart.* 1997;77:130-132.

highly trained athlete is usually less than 1.6 cm in males and 1.4 cm in females, and typically occurs in association with an increased left ventricular end-diastolic dimension and stroke volume. An ECG tracing showing Q waves or inferolateral repolarization changes in an athlete favors the diagnosis of hypertrophic cardiomyopathy.

Given the 50% probability of disease in a first-degree relative of a patient with hypertrophic cardiomyopathy, modified diagnostic criteria (Table 60-3) consider the high probability that their otherwise unexplained ECG and echocardiographic findings reflect incomplete disease expression, with the corresponding risks for complications and for passing the gene to their children.

TREATMENT Rx

Clinical management is based mainly on symptoms (Fig. 60-3). Exceptions include specific therapies for lysosomal storage diseases, such as Pompe's (Chapter 214) and Fabry's disease (Chapter 215), and for Friedreich's ataxia (Chapter 429). The treatment of the remaining patients with hypertrophic cardiomyopathy focuses on the counseling of family members, the management of symptoms, and the prevention of disease-related complications.

Family Evaluation

All patients with hypertrophic cardiomyopathy should be counseled on the implications of the diagnosis for their families. Careful pedigree analysis can reassure relatives who are not at risk for inheriting the disease. For those who are at risk, current guidelines recommend screening with a 12-lead ECG and echocardiogram at intervals of 12 to 18 months, usually starting at the age of 12 years (unless there is a "malignant" family history of premature sudden death, the child is symptomatic or a competitive athlete, or there is a clinical suspicion of left ventricular hypertrophy) until full growth and maturation are achieved (usually by the age of 18 to 21 years). Thereafter, if there are no signs of disease expression, screening approximately every 5 years is advised because the onset of left ventricular hypertrophy may be delayed until well into adulthood in some families. Modified diagnostic criteria (see Table 60-3) consider the high probability that otherwise unexplained ECG and echocardiographic findings in first-degree relatives reflect incomplete disease expression.

When available, genetic testing can identify a disease-causing mutation in an index case and thereby provide presymptomatic diagnosis of family members. Whenever genetic testing is considered, individuals should be informed about the purpose of the test, the most probable mode of inheritance, and the potential hazards and limitations of genetic testing.

Symptom Management

Medical Therapy

Therapeutic options in patients *without* left ventricular outflow gradients are limited predominantly to pharmacologic therapy. β-Blockade may improve chest pain and dyspnea. The dose (starting at a dose equivalent to propranolol, 120 mg/day) should be titrated to achieve a target heart rate of 50 to 70 beats per minute at rest and 130 to 140 beats per minute at peak exercise. Calcium antagonists such as verapamil (starting at a dose of 120 mg/day) and diltiazem (starting at a dose of 180 mg/day) are useful alternatives, particularly in patients with refractory chest pain, but high doses (e.g., verapamil >480 mg/day, diltiazem >360 mg/day) may be required. In patients with paroxysmal nocturnal dyspnea and no evidence of ventricular outflow obstruction, a transient mechanism such as myocardial ischemia or arrhythmia may be the cause, although investigations usually fail to identify the precise cause. Such patients, as well as those with chronically raised pulmonary pressures, may require diuretics (e.g., furosemide, 20 to 40 mg orally as needed, followed by 20 mg/day if required). The dose and duration of diuretic therapy should be minimized because injudicious use of these drugs can be dangerous, particularly in patients with severe diastolic impairment or labile obstruction.

In patients with symptoms caused by left ventricular outflow tract obstruction, the main aim of treatment is to reduce the outflow tract gradient. Options include negative inotropic drugs, surgery, atrioventricular sequential pacing, and percutaneous alcohol ablation of the interventricular septum. Approximately 60 to 70% of patients improve with β-blockers, although high doses (equivalent to propranolol at 480 mg/day) are frequently required, and side effects are often limiting. When β-blockade alone is ineffective, disopyramide, titrated to the maximal tolerated dose (usually between 400 and 600 mg/day), may be effective in up to two thirds of patients, but side effects related to the anticholinergic effects (e.g., dry eyes and mouth) limit its use. Disopyramide should be given concomitantly with a small to medium dose of a β-blocker (e.g., propranolol, 120 to 240 mg/day), which will slow the heart rate and also blunt rapid atrioventricular nodal conduction should supraventricular arrhythmias develop. In patients who have left ventricular outflow tract obstruction and are taking a β-blocker and disopyramide, other antiarrhythmic drugs that alter repolarization (e.g., sotalol or amiodarone) must be avoided because of the potential proarrhythmic effect. In patients with outflow tract gradients, verapamil can be effective, but caution is required in patients with severe obstruction or elevated pulmonary pressures.

Interventional Therapy

Surgery should be considered for significant outflow obstruction (gradient >50 mm Hg) in patients who have symptoms refractory to medical therapy. The most commonly performed surgical procedure, ventricular septal myectomy, either abolishes or substantially reduces the gradient in 95% of cases, reduces mitral regurgitation, and improves exercise capacity and symptoms. Surgery should be performed in an experienced center, where mortality rates should be less than 1% for isolated myomectomy. The main complications (atrioventricular block, ventricular septal defects) are rare. In some patients, concomitant mitral valve repair or replacement may be required.

In experienced centers, the selective injection of alcohol into a septal perforator branch of the left anterior descending coronary artery to create a localized septal scar yields outcomes similar to surgery. The main nonfatal complication is atrioventricular block requiring a pacemaker in 5 to 20% of patients.

Dual-chamber pacing using a short-programmed atrial ventricular delay to produce maximal pre-excitation while maintaining effective atrial transport can reduce the outflow gradient by 30 to 50% but provides little objective improvement in exercise capacity in most patients.

Supraventricular Arrhythmia

Atrial fibrillation in hypertrophic cardiomyopathy is associated with a high risk for systemic embolization, so anticoagulation (international normalized ratio in the range of 2.0 to 3.0) should be considered in all patients with sustained or paroxysmal atrial fibrillation (Chapter 64). Treatment with low-dose amiodarone, 1000 to 1400 mg/week, is effective in maintaining sinus rhythm and in controlling the ventricular response during breakthrough episodes. The addition of a low-dose β-blocker, verapamil, or diltiazem may be required for rate control. Serious side effects on low-dose amiodarone are uncommon. β-blockers, particularly those with class III action (e.g., sotalol), are less effective alternatives. In general, the principles of managing atrial fibrillation in patients with hypertrophic cardiomyopathy are similar to those in other conditions (Chapter 64), with the provision that the threshold to use anticoagulation should be low because of the significant embolic risk.

Prevention of Sudden Death

The overall risk for sudden death in children and adults with hypertrophic cardiomyopathy is approximately 1% per year, but a minority of individuals have a much greater risk for ventricular arrhythmia and sudden death. The most powerful predictor of sudden cardiac death in hypertrophic cardiomyopathy is a history of previous cardiac arrest. In patients without such a history, the most useful markers of risk are a family history of premature (<40 years of age) sudden cardiac death; unexplained syncope (unrelated to neurocardiogenic mechanisms); a flat or hypotensive blood pressure response to upright exercise; nonsustained ventricular tachycardia on ambulatory electrocardiographic monitoring or during exercise; and severe left ventricular hypertrophy on echocardiography (defined as a maximal left ventricular wall thickness of 30 mm or more). Patients with two or more of these markers have an annual mortality rate of 3 to 6% and should receive an implantable cardioverter-defibrillator (ICD) (Chapter 66). All patients with hypertrophic cardiomyopathy should be advised to avoid competitive sports and intense physical exertion. Patients without any risk factors do not warrant an ICD. For patients with one risk factor, decisions regarding an ICD should be individualized based on the patient's age and severity of disease.

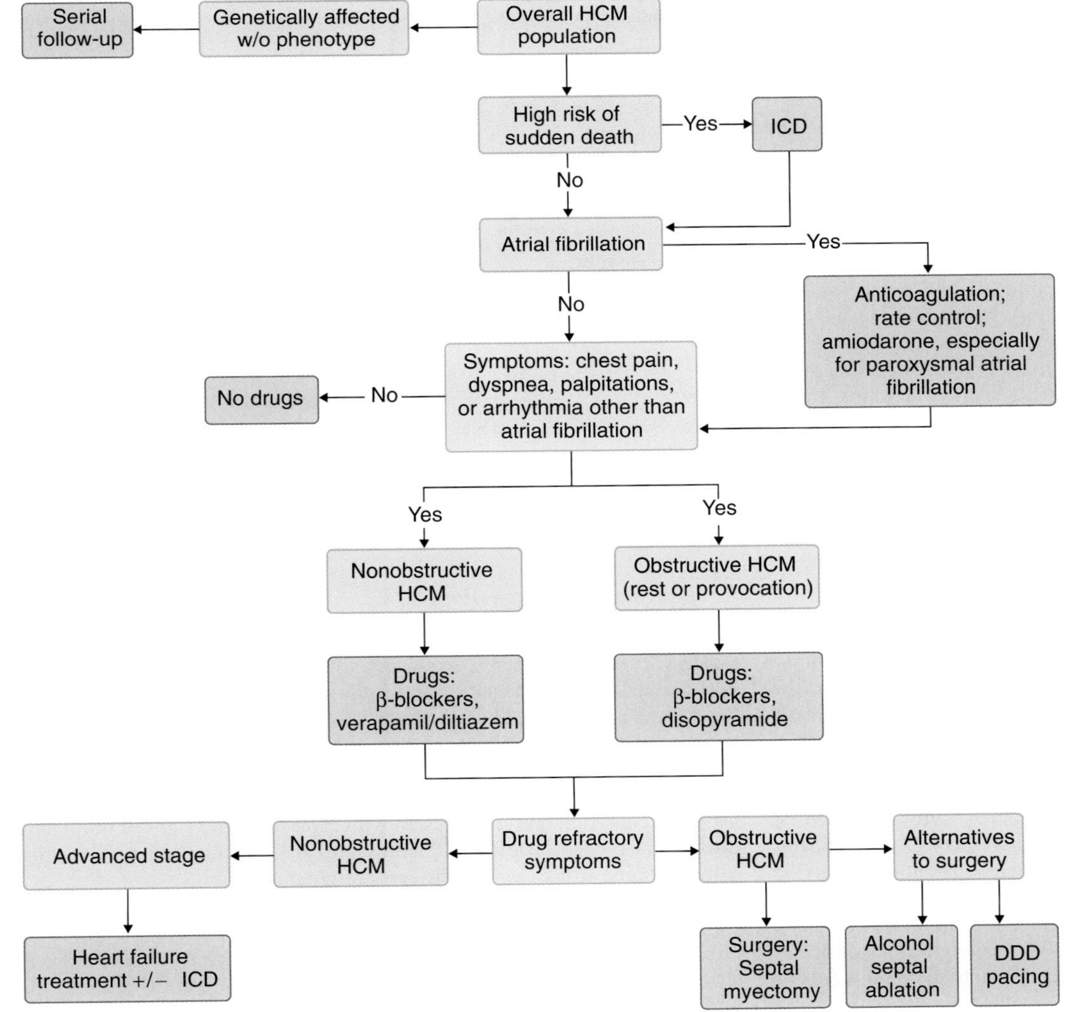

FIGURE 60-3. Approach to the management of hypertrophic cardiomyopathy (HCM). ICD = implantable cardioverter-defibrillator. (Adapted from Maron BJ, McKenna WJ, Danielson GK, et al. American College of Cardiology/European Society of Cardiology clinical expert consensus document on hypertrophic cardiomyopathy. *J Am Coll Cardiol.* 2003;42:1687-1713.)

PROGNOSIS

Most patients with hypertrophic cardiomyopathy follow a stable and benign course with a low risk for adverse events and a survival similar to that of age- and gender-matched normal populations, but many experience progressive symptoms caused by atrial arrhythmia and gradual deterioration in left ventricular systolic and diastolic function. About 1% of affected individuals die suddenly each year. The annual incidence of stroke varies from 0.56 to 0.8%/year, rising to 1.9% in patients older than 60 years, and 23% of strokes are fatal. The development of severe systolic heart failure is associated with a poor prognosis, with an overall mortality rate of up to 11% per year. The incidence of infective endocarditis is 1.4 per 1000 person-years overall but 3.8 per 1000 person-years in patients with obstruction.

Myocarditis

DEFINITION AND EPIDEMIOLOGY

Myocarditis, which is an inflammatory process involving the myocardium, can be caused by infections, immune-mediated damage, or toxins (Table 60-4). The incidence and prevalence of myocarditis are difficult to estimate because the clinical presentation varies from asymptomatic ECG abnormalities to hemodynamic collapse and sudden death. Population estimates of the prevalence of myocarditis range from 1 in 100,000 to 1 in 10,000, whereas postmortem studies report myocarditis in up to 12% of young victims of sudden cardiac death.

Worldwide, the most common infective myocarditis is Chagas' disease, caused by *Trypanosoma cruzi,* a protozoan organism endemic in rural areas of South and Central America (Chapter 355). In the Western world, viral myocarditis is the most common cause of inflammatory heart disease. Human immunodeficiency virus (HIV) infection (Chapter 392) is associated with lymphocytic monocarditis and is a strong predictor of poor prognosis. Smallpox vaccination (Chapter 17) causes myopericarditis, with a reported incidence of 7.8 cases per 100,000 vaccine administrations. Other rare myocarditises include giant cell myocarditis, myocarditis complicating autoimmune disorders such as systemic lupus erythematosus (Chapter 274), and cocaine abuse (Chapter 33).

PATHOBIOLOGY

Myocarditis is defined histologically by the presence of myocyte injury, with degeneration or necrosis, and an inflammatory infiltrate not due to ischemia. Four patterns are recognized: *active myocarditis,* with myocyte degeneration or necrosis and definite cellular infiltrate with or without fibrosis; *borderline myocarditis,* with a definite cellular infiltrate without evidence of myocardial cellular injury; *persistent myocarditis,* with continued active myocarditis on repeat biopsy; and *resolving or resolved myocarditis,* characterized by a diminished or absent infiltrate with evidence of connective tissue healing on repeat biopsy. Despite their widespread use, these criteria have low specificity and sensitivity, with a diagnostic yield as low as 10 to 20% in some series. Therefore, newer virology techniques used in conjunction with conventional light microscopy include nested polymerase chain reaction (PCR) or reverse transcription PCR on RNA and DNA extracted from endomyocardial biopsy specimens, as well as immunohistochemical staining for subtypes of infiltrating lymphocytes and abnormal expression of cellular adhesion molecules on interstitial or endothelial cells.

Viral Myocarditis

Most data on the pathology of viral myocarditis come from murine models. Initially, there is direct invasion of the myocardium by cardiotropic viruses, which enter the cardiomyocyte through receptor-mediated endocytosis. The viral genome, which translated intracellularly to produce viral protein or is incorporated into the host cell genome, may contribute to myocyte dysfunction by cleaving dystrophin. In the second phase, activation of the host immune system, including recruitment of natural killer cells and macrophages, increases the expression of proinflammatory cytokines such as interleukin-1 and tumor necrosis factor. Activation of $CD4^+$ T lymphocytes promotes clonal expansion of B lymphocytes, thereby resulting in further myocardial cell damage, inflammation, and the production of circulating antiheart antibodies directed against contractile, structural, and mitochondrial proteins. This autoimmune response may result in long-term ventricular remodeling owing to direct effects on myocardial structural components or alterations in the extracellular matrix.

TABLE 60-4 CAUSES OF MYOCARDITIS

INFECTION
Viral
Coxsackievirus, human immunodeficiency virus, echovirus, adenovirus, influenza, measles, mumps, parvovirus, poliovirus, rubella, varicella-zoster virus, herpes simplex virus, cytomegalovirus, hepatitis C virus, rabies virus, respiratory syncytial virus, vaccine virus, dengue virus, yellow fever virus
Protozoal
Trypanosoma cruzi, Toxoplasma gondii
Bacterial
Brucella, Corynebacterium diphtheriae, Salmonella, Haemophilus influenzae, Mycoplasma pneumoniae, Neisseria meningitidis (meningococcus), *Streptococcus pneumoniae, Staphylococcus, Mycobacterium, Neisseria gonorrhoeae* (gonococcus), *Vibrio cholerae*
Spirochetal
Treponema pallidum, Borrelia, Leptospira
Fungal
Aspergillus, Candida, Cryptococcus, Actinomyces, Blastomyces, Histoplasma, Coccidioides
Rickettsial
Coxiella burnetii, Rickettsia rickettsii, Rickettsia tsutsugamushi
Parasitic
Trichinella spiralis, Echinococcus granulosus, Taenia solium
IMMUNE-MEDIATED DISORDERS
Alloantigens
Heart transplant rejection
Autoantigens
Churg-Strauss syndrome, celiac disease, Whipple's disease, giant cell myocarditis, Kawasaki disease, systemic lupus erythematosus, systemic sclerosis, sarcoidosis, scleroderma, polymyositis, thrombocytopenic purpura
Allergens (Drugs)
Penicillin, sulfonamides, tetracycline, methyldopa, streptomycin, tricyclic antidepressants, thiazide diuretics, dobutamine, indomethacin
TOXIC CAUSES
Drugs
Anthracyclines, catecholamines, amphetamines, cocaine, cyclophosphamide, 5-fluorouracil, Herceptin, interferon, interleukin-2
Physical Agents
Electric shock, radiation, hyperpyrexia
Heavy Metals
Copper, iron, lead
Others
Arsenic, snake bite, scorpion bite, wasp and spider stings, phosphorus, carbon monoxide
GENETIC DISORDERS
Inherited cardiomyopathies with immune-mediated pathogenesis (dilated and right ventricular cardiomyopathy)

CLINICAL MANIFESTATIONS

Some patients report prodromal symptoms of viremia, including fever, myalgia, coryzal symptoms, or gastroenteritis, but many individuals with myocarditis are asymptomatic and manifest only transient ECG abnormalities such as nonspecific ST segment and T wave abnormalities, pathologic Q waves, and low QRS voltages. Less common ECG presentations include acute myocardial infarction (Chapter 73), atrioventricular block (Chapter 64), and ventricular arrhythmias (Chapter 65). Patients with impairment of left ventricular function may present with symptoms and signs of fulminant cardiogenic shock (Chapter 107) with acute cardiovascular collapse. In some cases, sudden cardiac death is the first presentation.

DIAGNOSIS

The diagnosis of myocarditis requires a high index of suspicion because it may mimic other common conditions. On echocardiography, evidence of impaired left ventricular systolic performance, often without significant left ventricular dilatation, is typical. Regional wall motion abnormalities are common, and left (or right) ventricular thrombus may be present. Evidence of left ventricular diastolic impairment and pericardial effusions is common. Cardiac magnetic resonance imaging can detect myocardial inflammation and myocyte injury, with pericellular and cellular edema.

Routine blood tests such as full blood count and erythrocyte sedimentation rate are usually unhelpful, but serum markers of myocardial injury such as troponin T and I may be elevated. Creatine kinase and its cardiac isoform CK-MB are less sensitive and specific than troponin and are not useful as screening tests. Increased levels of autoantibodies against myocardial proteins (such as myosin and the adenine nucleotide translocator protein) correlate with progressive worsening of ventricular function.

Cardiac catheterization with right ventricular endomyocardial biopsy remains the gold standard diagnostic test for myocarditis. However, it is generally reserved for patients with heart failure refractory to standard management, features suggestive of systemic disease (e.g., connective tissue disease [Chapter 268], amyloidosis [Chapter 193], hemochromatosis [Chapter 219], sarcoidosis [Chapter 95]), or suspicion of giant cell myocarditis because of new-onset heart failure associated with tachyarrhythmias or conduction disease.

Specific Causes

Viral myocarditis may be suspected from the clinical picture of recent febrile illness, often with prominent myalgias, followed by angina-like chest pain, dyspnea, or arrhythmias. Elevated troponin levels support the diagnosis, and increasing viral titers (to coxsackievirus, echovirus, adenovirus, or influenza virus) confirm recent infection. Clinical cardiomyopathy occurs in 10 to 40% of patients infected with HIV, owing to the HIV itself or to coinfection with cytomegalovirus.

Giant cell myocarditis, which accounts for 10 to 20% of biopsy-positive cases of myocarditis, presents with the rapid onset of chest pain, fever, and hemodynamic compromise, often with ventricular tachycardia or atrioventricular block. When ventricular tachyarrhythmias are a major feature of myocarditis, particularly in a young person, endomyocardial biopsy is generally recommended to determine whether giant cell myocarditis is present, even though the diagnosis is statistically unlikely.

Toxoplasmosis (Chapter 357) *myocarditis,* owing to intermittent rupture of cysts in the myocardium, can cause atypical chest pain, arrhythmias, pericarditis, and symptomatic heart failure. Diagnosis is made from antibody titers. Lyme carditis (Chapter 329) classically presents with conduction system abnormalities resulting from infection with *Borrelia burgdorferi,* which is diagnosed serologically.

Immune-mediated myocarditis can be associated with polymyositis (Chapter 277) or systemic lupus erythematosus (Chapter 274), although pericarditis and coronary artery vasculitis are more common. Hypersensitivity reactions, especially to drugs (Chapter 262), can cause myocarditis that is often associated with peripheral eosinophilia and can be confirmed by endomyocardial biopsy.

TREATMENT (Rx)

The first-line treatment of myocarditis is supportive with afterload reduction and diuresis (Chapter 59). Patients with fulminant acute myocarditis may require inotropic support, mechanical assist devices, or extracorporeal membrane oxygenation (Chapter 107). Following initial stabilization, patients with symptoms and signs of heart failure should receive angiotensin-converting enzyme inhibitors, diuretics, β-blockers, and anticoagulants in accordance with standard guidelines (Chapter 59). Patients with intractable and deteriorating heart failure may require cardiac transplantation (Chapter 82).

The role of immunosuppression is uncertain. In one randomized, placebo-controlled trial of 111 adults with biopsy-proven myocarditis, there was no difference in mortality or improvement in left ventricular function in patients treated with prednisolone plus either cyclosporine or azathioprine.[1] Conversely, in a randomized trial of patients who had major histocompatibility complex expression on endomyocardial biopsy samples and who were randomized to prednisolone (1 mg/kg/day tapering to a maintenance dose of 0.2 mg/kg/day for a total of 90 days) and azathioprine (1 mg/kg/day for a total of 100 days) versus placebo, left ventricular ejection fraction improved in the immunosuppressed group, but no difference was observed in mortality or rates of transplantation or rehospitalization over a 2-year follow-up period.[2] At present, immunosuppression is generally reserved for patients with giant cell myocarditis, in whom there is some benefit,[3] although the optimal regimen is yet to be determined. Intravenous immunoglobulin therapy is not helpful.[4]

PROGNOSIS

Patients with acute myocarditis with mild heart failure or symptoms suggestive of myocardial ischemia or infarction typically improve within weeks without sequelae. An acute presentation of myocarditis with advanced heart failure (ejection fraction <35%) may resolve but can lead to chronic left ventricular dysfunction (dilated cardiomyopathy) or progress to death or cardiac transplantation. Patients who present with acute fulminant myocarditis, however, have an excellent prognosis, with survival rates of more than 90%. Giant cell myocarditis is usually fatal without heart transplantation.

Dilated Cardiomyopathy

DEFINITION AND EPIDEMIOLOGY

Dilated cardiomyopathy is a heart muscle disorder defined by dilation and impaired systolic function of the left or both ventricles, in the absence of coronary artery disease, valvular abnormalities, or pericardial disease. In adults, prevalence estimates range from 14 to 36 per 100,000. In children, dilated cardiomyopathy is the most common cardiomyopathy, accounting for up to 58% of cases. Overall, males and females are approximately equally affected, except for dilated cardiomyopathy associated with neuromuscular disorders or inborn errors of metabolism, for which there is male predominance, because some of these conditions have an X-linked inheritance.

PATHOBIOLOGY

A number of conditions are associated with dilated cardiomyopathy, including neuromuscular disorders, inborn errors of metabolism, and malformation syndromes. In most patients, no identifiable cause is found, and the disease is termed *idiopathic dilated cardiomyopathy*.

Genetic Dilated Cardiomyopathy

Between 20 and 50% of individuals with dilated cardiomyopathy have evidence of familial disease (see Table 60-2). Autosomal dominant inheritance, which accounts for 68% of familial cases, has two major forms: isolated dilated cardiomyopathy and dilated cardiomyopathy associated with conduction system disease. The latter patients may also have an associated skeletal myopathy. Genes implicated in isolated dilated cardiomyopathy include cytoskeletal and sarcomeric protein genes. Mutations in the lamin A/C gene, which encodes a nuclear envelope protein, cause atrial arrhythmia and progressive atrioventricular conduction disease, which precede the development of dilated cardiomyopathy by several years.

X-linked inheritance accounts for between 2 and 5% of familial cases of dilated cardiomyopathy Neuromuscular disorders account for 26% of cases, 90% of which are Duchenne, Becker's, and Emery-Driefuss muscular dystrophies (Chapter 429). Isolated X-linked dilated cardiomyopathy, also caused by mutations in the dystrophin gene, is characterized by raised serum creatine kinase muscle isoforms but does not result in clinical signs or symptoms of skeletal muscular dystrophy.

Acquired Dilated Cardiomyopathy

Common acquired causes of dilated cardiomyopathy include infectious myocarditis, chemotherapy (Chapter 182), radiotherapy (Chapter 19), alcohol (Chapter 32), cocaine (Chapter 33), nutritional deficiencies (Chapter 222), iron overload (Chapter 219), inflammatory and autoimmune disorders (Chapters 274 and 278), endocrinopathies (Chapter 233), and pregnancy (Chapter 247). Tachycardia-mediated cardiomyopathy (tachycardiomyopathy) is rare and usually reverses once the tachycardia is controlled.

CLINICAL MANIFESTATIONS

The symptoms and signs associated with dilated cardiomyopathy depend on the age of the patient and the degree of left ventricular dysfunction. Although the first presentation may be with sudden death or a thromboembolic event, most patients present with symptoms of high pulmonary venous pressure or low cardiac output (Chapter 58), which can be acute, sometimes precipitated by intercurrent illness or arrhythmia, or chronic. Increasingly, dilated cardiomyopathy is diagnosed incidentally in asymptomatic individuals during family screening.

Adults initially present with reduced exercise tolerance and dyspnea on exertion. With worsening left ventricular function, patients may develop dyspnea at rest, orthopnea, paroxysmal nocturnal dyspnea, peripheral edema, and ascites. Symptoms related to mesenteric ischemia, such as abdominal pain after meals, nausea, vomiting, and anorexia, may dominate, especially in children. Arrhythmia symptoms, such as palpitations, presyncope, and syncope, can occur at any age.

In advanced disease, features of low cardiac output include sinus tachycardia, weak peripheral pulses, and hypotension. The jugular venous pressure may be elevated, and the apical impulse is displaced. Peripheral edema, hepatomegaly, and ascites are common in patients with heart failure. Auscultation of the chest typically reveals basal crackles. Auscultation of the heart may reveal the presence of a third (and sometimes also a fourth) heart sound. In patients with functional mitral regurgitation, a pansystolic murmur may be heard at the apex and radiate to the axilla, but frequently no murmurs are heard, even in the presence of mitral incompetence, especially if cardiac output is very low.

DIAGNOSIS

The ECG may be normal but more typically shows sinus tachycardia, nonspecific ST segment and T wave changes (most commonly in the inferior and lateral leads), atrial enlargement, and voltage criteria for ventricular hypertrophy. Atrioventricular block raises the possibility of mutations in the lamin A/C gene. Supraventricular and ventricular arrhythmias are common. The chest radiograph is usually abnormal, with an increased cardiothoracic ratio (greater than 0.5) reflecting left ventricular and left atrial dilation. Patients with pulmonary edema have increased pulmonary vascular markings and pleural effusion.

On echocardiography, the presence of ventricular end-diastolic dimensions greater than 2 standard deviations above body surface area–corrected means (or greater than 112% of predicted dimension) and fractional shortening less than 25% are sufficient to make the diagnosis. Other common features include functional mitral and tricuspid regurgitation and abnormalities of diastolic left ventricular function. Cardiac magnetic resonance imaging may show areas of myocardial fibrosis.

Other recommended tests (Table 60-5) include a complete blood count and tests of renal, thyroid, and hepatic function. Levels of serum creatine kinase should be measured in all patients with dilated cardiomyopathy because this may provide important clues to the etiology. Other cardiac biomarkers, such as troponin I and troponin T, can be elevated. Plasma B-type natriuretic peptide levels predict survival, hospitalization rates, and listing for cardiac transplantation. Symptom-limited exercise testing, combined with respiratory gas analysis, is a useful technique to assess functional limitation and disease progression in patients with stable dilated cardiomyopathy.

Cardiac catheterization is rarely needed except perhaps to exclude severe coronary artery disease or to provide more precise information about possible valvular heart disease. Endomyocardial biopsy may be diagnostic for myocarditis and for some metabolic or mitochondrial disorders but is rarely advised. Hemodynamic assessment of left ventricular end-diastolic and pulmonary artery pressures may be necessary before transplantation.

TABLE 60-5 LABORATORY EVALUATION OF CARDIOMYOPATHY

CLINICAL EVALUATION
History and physical examination to identify cardiac and noncardiac disorders*
Assessment of ability to perform routine and desired activities*
Assessment of volume status*
LABORATORY EVALUATION
Electrocardiogram*
Chest radiograph*
Two-dimensional and Doppler echocardiogram*
Chemistry
Serum sodium,* potassium,* glucose, creatinine,* blood urea nitrogen,* calcium,* magnesium*
Albumin,* total protein,* liver function tests,* serum iron, ferritin
Urinalysis
Creatine kinase
Thyroid-stimulating hormone*
Hematology
Hemoglobin/hematocrit*
White blood cell count with differential,* including eosinophils
Erythrocyte sedimentation rate
INITIAL EVALUATION IN SELECTED PATIENTS ONLY
Titers for suspected infection
Acute viral (coxsackievirus, echovirus, influenza virus)
Human immunodeficiency virus, Epstein-Barr virus
Lyme disease, toxoplasmosis
Chagas' disease
Catheterization with coronary angiography in patients with angina who are candidates for intervention*
Serologic studies for active rheumatologic disease
Endomyocardial biopsy

*Level I recommendations from Hunt SA, Abraham WT, Chin MH, et al. ACC/AHA 2005 Guideline Update for the Diagnosis and Management of Chronic Heart Failure in the Adult. *Circulation.* 2005;112:e154-e235.

TREATMENT Rx

Supportive therapy includes sodium and fluid restriction, avoidance of alcohol and other toxins, and use of established heart failure medications (Chapter 59). Although older recommendations emphasized rest and avoidance of exercise, this advice should be limited to patients with myocarditis or peripartum cardiomyopathy; for other patients, a submaximal exercise regimen is desirable to sustain mobility, to avoid deconditioning, and to maintain physical and psychological health. Patients with atrial fibrillation or with echocardiographic evidence of a left atrial or left ventricular mural thrombosis should be anticoagulated to an international normalized ratio of 2.0 to 3.0. An ICD is preferred over medication for ventricular arrhythmias,[5] and some patients require management for advanced heart failure (Chapter 59) with biventricular pacing, inotropic medications, ventricular assist devices, and cardiac transplantation (Chapter 82).

Family Screening

Familial evaluation of first-degree relatives by history and physical examination and with 12-lead ECG and two-dimensional echocardiographic studies is warranted at the time of diagnosis and serially thereafter. Precise algorithms to guide the interval of evaluation remain to be determined; because disease progression is usually slow, evaluation about every 5 years until age 50 years appears appropriate. The detection of early disease in a family member offers an opportunity to initiate treatment, usually with an angiotensin-converting enzyme inhibitor or β-blocker, but the efficacy of such therapy remains to be proved.

PROGNOSIS

The prognosis of idiopathic and genetically determined dilated cardiomyopathy is related to the severity of disease at the time of presentation and the response to treatment. Most patients improve with treatment, but 5-year survival is less than 50% in patients who present with severe disease (e.g., ejection fraction <25%, left ventricular end-diastolic dimension >65 mm, peak oxygen consumption <12 mL/kg/minute).

Specific Causes of Dilated Cardiomyopathy

Alcoholic Cardiomyopathy

In the United States, excess alcohol consumption (Chapter 32) contributes to more than 10% of cases of heart failure. Alcohol and its metabolite, acetaldehyde, are cardiotoxins. Myocardial depression is initially reversible but, if alcohol consumption is sustained, can lead to myocyte vacuolization, mitochondrial abnormalities, and myocardial fibrosis. Even in chronic stages, however, the heart failure represents a sum of both reversible and irreversible myocardial dysfunction. The amount of alcohol necessary to produce symptomatic cardiomyopathy in susceptible individuals is not known but has been estimated to be six drinks (~4 oz of pure ethanol) a day for 5 to 10 years. Frequent binging without heavy daily consumption may also be sufficient. Alcoholic cardiomyopathy can develop in patients without social evidence of an alcohol problem. Abstinence leads to improvement in at least 50% of patients with severe symptoms, some of whom normalize their left ventricular ejection fractions. Patients with other causes of heart failure also should limit alcohol consumption.

Chemotherapy

Anthracycline (doxorubicin, daunorubicin, epirubicin) cardiotoxicity (Chapter 182) causes characteristic histologic changes on endomyocardial biopsy with overt heart failure in 5 to 10% of patients who receive doses greater than or equal to 450 mg/m^2 of body surface area. Patients who have received anthracyclines in the prepubertal period without apparent cardiotoxicity may develop cardiac failure in young adulthood. The risk is higher in patients who have lower baseline ejection fractions, concomitant radiation therapy, or higher doses of anthracycline. *Cyclophosphamide* and *ifosfamide* can cause acute severe heart failure and malignant ventricular arrhythmias. Some *tyrosine kinase inhibitors* (e.g., sunitinib) cause a reduction in systolic function, especially in the presence of coronary artery disease, but there is good response to withdrawal and conventional medical therapy (Chapter 190). *5-Fluorouracil* can cause coronary artery spasm and depressed left ventricular contractility. Up to 11% of patients who receive *trastuzumab* (Chapter 204), a recombinant monoclonal antibody that binds to human epidermal growth factor type 2, develop dilated cardiomyopathy, which is reversible after withdrawal and conventional drug treatment. The risk for cardiotoxicity increases with previous anthracycline and radiation treatment. *Interferon-α* may be associated with hypotension and arrhythmias in up to 10% of patients, and *interleukin-2* rarely has been associated with cardiotoxicity.

Metabolic and Endocrine Disease

Excess catecholamines, as in *pheochromocytoma* (Chapter 235), may injure the heart by compromising the coronary microcirculation or by direct toxic effects on myocytes. *Cocaine* (Chapter 33) increases synaptic concentrations of catecholamines by inhibiting reuptake at nerve terminals; the result may be an acute coronary syndrome or chronic cardiomyopathy.

Thiamine deficiency from poor nutrition or alcoholism (Chapter 225) can cause beriberi heart disease, with vasodilation and high cardiac output followed by low output. *Calcium deficiency* resulting from hypoparathyroidism, gastrointestinal abnormalities, or chelation directly compromises myocardial contractility.

Hypophosphatemia (Chapter 121), which may occur in alcoholism, during recovery from malnutrition, and in hyperalimentation, also reduces myocardial contractility. Patients with *magnesium depletion* owing to impaired absorption or increased renal excretion (Chapter 121) also may present with left ventricular dysfunction.

Hypothyroidism (Chapter 233) depresses contractility and conduction and may cause pericardial effusions, whereas *hyperthyroidism* increases cardiac output, can worsen underlying heart failure, and may rarely be the sole cause of heart failure.

The presenting sign of *diabetes* (Chapter 236) can be cardiomyopathy, especially with diastolic dysfunction, independent of epicardial coronary atherosclerosis, for which it is a major risk factor.

Obesity (Chapter 227) can cause cardiomyopathy with increased ventricular mass and decreased contractility, which improve after weight loss, or it can aggravate underlying heart failure from other causes.

Peripartum Cardiomyopathy

Peripartum cardiomyopathy appears in the last month of pregnancy or in the first 5 months after delivery in the absence of preexisting cardiac disease (Chapter 247). The incidence is between 1 in 3000 and 1 in 15,000 deliveries, with increased risk in older mothers or in the setting of twins, malnutrition, tocolytic therapy, toxemia, or hypertension. Lymphocytic myocarditis, found in 30 to 50% of biopsy specimens, suggests an immune component, perhaps cross-reactivity between uterine and cardiac myocyte proteins or an enhanced susceptibility to viral myocarditis. More recently, it has been suggested that enhanced oxidative stress triggers activation of cathepsin D, a ubiquitous lysosomal enzyme, which cleaves serum prolactin in its antiangiogenic and proapoptotic 16-kD form. The latter appears to promote endothelial inflammation and impair cardiomyocyte metabolism and contraction. Presentation is usually with orthopnea and dyspnea on minimal exertion, most often within the first weeks after delivery when the excess volume of pregnancy would normally be mobilized. Preexisting cardiac disease must be excluded. Diuretics facilitate postpartum diuresis, and angiotensin-converting enzyme inhibitors improve symptoms (Chapter 59). In a small randomized trial, oral bromocriptine (2.5 mg twice daily for 2 weeks, then daily for 6 weeks) significantly improved recovery of left ventricular function and may reduce deaths.[6] The prognosis is improvement to normal or near-normal ejection fraction during the next 6 months in more than 50% of patients. About 4% require heart transplantation, and about 9% die suddenly or from complications of heart transplantation.

Overlap with Restrictive Cardiomyopathy

Diseases causing primarily restrictive cardiomyopathies can occasionally overlap to cause a picture consistent with dilated cardiomyopathy. For example, *hemochromatosis* (Chapter 219) and *sarcoidosis* (Chapter 95) should be considered when evaluating any patient with a cardiomyopathy, although these conditions are more often considered with the restrictive diseases. *Amyloidosis* (Chapter 194) is less commonly confused with dilated than with hypertrophic cardiomyopathy but should be considered in a patient with a thick-walled ventricle with moderately depressed contractile function.

Arrhythmogenic Right Ventricular Cardiomyopathy

DEFINITION AND EPIDEMIOLOGY

ARVC (Chapter 65) is a genetically determined heart muscle disorder characterized histologically by loss of cardiomyocytes with replacement by fibrous or fibrofatty tissue in the right ventricular myocardium; clinically by ventricular arrhythmias, heart failure, and sudden death; and histologically by cardiomyocyte loss and replacement. It is associated with arrhythmia, heart failure, and premature sudden death. The disease is seen in patients of European, African, and Asian descent, with an estimated prevalence between 1 in 1000 and 1 in 5000 adults.

PATHOBIOLOGY

ARVC is inherited as an autosomal dominant disease, with incomplete penetrance, although recessive forms with cutaneous manifestations are recognized (see Table 60-2). Most cases are caused by heterozygous mutations in genes encoding components of the desmosome and adherens junction of cardiomyocytes. The most common occur in plakophilin-2, desmocollin-2, desmoplakin, and desmoglein-2. Homozygous mutations in plakoglobin are responsible for the rare autosomal recessive form, Naxos disease. Recently, a mutation in the transmembrane cytoplasmic protein 43 (TNEM43) has been described. Two other nondesmosomal genes, the cardiac ryanodine receptor and transforming growth factor-β3 (TGF-β3), have been linked with ARVC but are probably not important in most patients.

Pathology

The main pathologic feature is progressive loss of right ventricular myocardium, which is replaced by adipose and fibrous tissue. These changes begin in the inflow, outflow, and apical regions of the right ventricle. Aneurysm formation in these areas is typical. Progressive myocardial involvement may lead to global right ventricular dilation. Severe right ventricular disease is often associated with fibrofatty substitution of the left ventricular myocardium, with the posterolateral wall preferentially affected.

Mutations in desmosomal protein genes may increase the susceptibility of the myocardium to the damaging effects of mechanical stress, thereby predisposing to cardiomyocyte detachment, death, and eventual replacement with fibrofatty tissue. The acute phase of myocardial injury may be accompanied by inflammation. The predilection for the right ventricle has been explained by its thin wall and greater distensibility. As desmosomal proteins interact with many other proteins, including components of the cellular cytoskeleton and intermediate filaments, it is possible that ventricular dysfunction occurs as the result of reduced cytoskeletal integrity and impaired force transduction. Some desmosomal proteins, in particular plakoglobin, are also important signaling molecules that regulate the transcription of many other genes. Finally, a reduction in the number and size of gap junctions may result in a electrical coupling defect, thereby increasing the propensity to arrhythmia without significant morphologic changes.

CLINICAL MANIFESTATIONS

By convention, the natural history of ARVC is divided into four phases, but it is not inevitable that patients will progress through all phases. In the early phase, patients are usually asymptomatic, but resuscitated cardiac arrest and sudden death may be the initial manifestations, particularly in adolescents and young adults. The overt arrhythmic phase usually begins in adolescents and young adults, when patients note palpitations or syncope. Symptomatic sustained arrhythmias are usually accompanied by morphologic and functional abnormalities of the right ventricle. The third phase, characterized by diffuse right ventricular disease, occurs in the middle and later decades; patients may present with right-sided heart failure despite relatively preserved left ventricular function. In the advanced stage, left ventricular involvement and biventricular heart failure are seen.

DIAGNOSIS

Clinical evaluation includes inquiry for symptoms of arrhythmia (syncope, presyncope, sustained palpitation); a family history of premature cardiac symptoms or sudden death; 12-lead, 24-hour, and maximal exercise ECG testing; and two-dimensional echocardiography with specific right ventricular views. Contrast echocardiography may be required to obtain better endocardial definition of the right ventricular myocardium and apex of the left ventricle. Magnetic resonance imaging may provide accurate assessment of ventricular volumes as well as noninvasive characterization of fibrous tissue and fat.

Ventricular arrhythmias with a left bundle branch block morphology, consistent with a right ventricular origin, are characteristic. However, the ECG and arrhythmic manifestations are not specific to ARVC and overlap with many other disease states, so standard criteria are recommended for diagnosis (Table 60-6). Because these criteria are highly specific but lack sensitivity for detecting early disease, more sensitive criteria are recommended for first-degree relatives of known cases (Table 60-7). The diagnosis of ARVC in a proband also raises the possibility of mutation analysis in the family to identify those at risk and in need of serial evaluation as well as those who need no specific follow-up.

Differential Diagnosis

The differential diagnosis includes other inherited cardiomyopathies, the inherited arrhythmia syndromes (long QT syndrome, Brugada's syndrome, and catecholaminergic polymorphic ventricular tachycardia; Chapter 65), and causes of right ventricular dilation such as intracardiac or extracardiac shunts (Chapter 69). The differentiation from so-called benign right ventricular outflow tract tachycardia may be problematic, although in the latter the 12-lead ECG and right ventricular imaging studies are typically normal, and no familial disease is present. Some patients with desmosomal protein

TABLE 60-6 REVISED TASK FORCE CRITERIA FOR ARRHYTHMOGENIC RIGHT VENTRICULAR CARDIOMYOPATHY IN PROBANDS*

Criteria	
MAJOR	**MINOR**
I. GLOBAL OR REGIONAL DYSFUNCTION AND STRUCTURAL ALTERATIONS*	
By two-dimensional echo: • Regional RV akinesia, dyskinesia, or aneurysm • *and* 1 of the following (end diastole): PLAX RVOT ≥32 mm (corrected for body size [PLAX/BSA] ≥19 mm/m^2) PSAX RVOT ≥36 mm (corrected for body size [PLAX/BSA] ≥21 mm/m^2) *or* fractional area change ≤33%	**By two-dimensional echo:** • Regional RV akinesia or dyskinesia • *and* 1 of the following (end diastole): PLAX RVOT ≥29 to <32 mm (corrected for body size [PLAX/BSA] ≥16 to <19 mm/m^2) PSAX RVOT ≥32 to <36 mm (corrected for body size [PSAX/BSA] ≥18 to <21 mm/m^2) *or* fractional area change >33% to ≤40%
By MRI: • Regional RV akinesia or dyskinesia or dyssynchronous RV contraction • *and* 1 of the following: RV end-diastolic volume indexed to BSA ≥110 mL/m^2 (male) or ≥100 mL/m^2 (female) or RV ejection fraction ≤40%	**By MRI:** • Regional RV akinesia or dyskinesia or dyssynchronous RV contraction • *and* 1 of the following: RV end-diastolic volume indexed to BSA ≥100 to <110 mL/m^2 (male) or ≥90 to <100 mL/m^2 (female) or RV ejection fraction >40% to ≤45%
By RV angiography: • Regional RV akinesia, dyskinesia, or aneurysm	
II. TISSUE CHARACTERIZATION OF WALL	
• Residual myocytes <60% by morphometric analysis (or <50% if estimated), with fibrous replacement of the RV free wall myocardium in ≥1 sample, with or without fatty replacement of tissue on endomyocardial biopsy	• Residual myocytes 60% to 75% by morphometric analysis (or 50% to 65% if estimated), with fibrous replacement of the RV free wall myocardium in ≥1 sample, with or without fatty replacement of tissue on endomyocardial biopsy
III. REPOLARIZATION ABNORMALITIES	
• Inverted T waves in right precordial leads (V_1,V_2, and V_3) or beyond in individuals >14 years of age (in the absence of complete right bundle-branch block QRS ≥120 msec)	• Inverted T waves in leads V_1 and V_2 in individuals >14 years of age (in the absence of complete right bundle branch block) or in V_4, V_5, or V_6 • Inverted T waves in leads V_1, V_2, V_3, and V_4 in individuals >14 years
IV. DEPOLARIZATION/CONDUCTION ABNORMALITIES	
• Epsilon wave (reproducible low-amplitude signals between end of QRS complex to onset of the T wave) in the right precordial leads (V_1 to V_3)	• Late potentials by SAECG in ≥1 of 3 parameters in the absence of a QRS duration ≥110 msec on the standard ECG • Filtered QRS duration (fQRS) ≥114 msec • Duration of terminal QRS <40 µV (low-amplitude signal duration) ≥38 msec • Root-mean-square voltage of terminal 40 msec ≤20 µV • Terminal activation duration of QRS ≥55 msec measured to the end of the QRS, including R′, in V_1, V_2, or V_3, in the absence of complete right bundle-branch block
V. ARRHYTHMIAS	
• Nonsustained or sustained ventricular tachycardia of left bundle branch morphology with superior axis (negative or indeterminate QRS in leads II, III, and aVF and positive in lead aVL)	• Nonsustained or sustained ventricular tachycardia of RV outflow configuration, left bundle branch block morphology with inferior axis (positive QRS in leads II, III, and aVF and negative in lead aVL) or of unknown axis • >500 ventricular extrasystoles per 24 hours (Holter)
VI. FAMILY HISTORY	
• ARVC confirmed in a first-degree relative who meets current Task Force criteria • ARVC confirmed pathologically at autopsy or surgery in a first-degree relative • Identification of a pathogenic mutation[†] categorized as associated or probably associated with ARVC in the patient under evaluation	• History of ARVC in a first-degree relative in whom it is not possible or practical to determine whether the family member meets current Task Force criteria • Premature sudden death (<35 years of age) due to suspected ARVC in a first-degree relative

*Hypokinesis is not included in this or subsequent definitions of right ventricular (RV) regional wall motion abnormalities for the proposed modified criteria.
†A pathogenic mutation is a DNA alteration associated with ARVC that alters or is expected to alter the encoded protein, is unobserved or rare in a large non-ARVC control population, and either alters or is predicted to alter the structure or function of the protein or has demonstrated linkage to the disease phenotype in a conclusive pedigree.
ARVC = arrhythmogenic right ventricular cardiomyopathy; aVF = augmented voltage unipolar left foot lead; aVL = augmented voltage unipolar left arm lead; BSA = body surface area; PLAX = parasternal long-axis view; PSAX = parasternal short-axis view; RVOT = right ventricular outflow tract.
Diagnostic terminology for original criteria: this diagnosis is fulfilled by the presence of 2 major, 1 major plus 2 minor, or 4 minor criteria from different groups.
Diagnostic terminology for revised criteria: definite diagnosis: 2 major, 1 major and 2 minor, or 4 minor criteria from different categories; borderline: 1 major and 1 minor or 3 minor criteria from different categories; possible: 1 major or 2 minor criteria from different categories.
From Marcus FI, McKenna WJ, Sherrill D, et al. Diagnosis of arrhythmogenic right ventricular cardiomyopathy/dysplasia: proposed modification of the task force criteria. *Circulation.* 2010;121:1533-1541.

TABLE 60-7 ARRHYTHMOGENIC RIGHT VENTRICULAR CARDIOMYOPATHY: CRITERIA FOR DIAGNOSIS OF FIRST-DEGREE RELATIVES WHO DO NOT FULFILL CRITERIA AS PROBANDS*

ARVC in a first-degree relative plus one of the following:

ECG	T wave inversion in right precordial leads (V_2 and V_3)
Signal-averaged ECG	Late potentials seen on signal-averaged ECG
Arrhythmia	Left bundle branch block–type ventricular tachycardia on ECG, Holter monitoring, or during exercise testing; >200 extrasystoles over a 24-hour period
Structural or functional abnormality of the right ventricle	Mild global right ventricular dilation or reduction in ejection fraction with normal left ventricle; mild segmental dilation of the right ventricle; regional right ventricular hypokinesia

*Any one criterion is adequate for the diagnosis.
ARVC = arrhythmogenic right ventricular cardiomyopathy; ECG = electrocardiogram.
From Hamid MS, Norman M, Quraishi A, et al: Prospective evaluation of relatives for familial arrhythmogenic right ventricular cardiomyopathy reveals a need to broaden diagnostic criteria. *J Am Coll Cardiol* 2002;40:1445-1450.

gene mutations demonstrate left ventricular involvement early in the disease may have a predominant left ventricular dilated cardiomyopathy phenotype.

TREATMENT

Rx

Pharmacologic treatment is the first-line therapy for patients with well-tolerated, non–life-threatening ventricular arrhythmias, such as frequent ventricular extrasystoles. Treatment of patients with symptomatic ventricular arrhythmias is with an ICD, with supplemental sotalol (160 to 240 mg/day) or even amiodarone (maintenance dose of 200 mg/day). Catheter ablation (Chapter 66) is indicated in patients with drug-refractory incessant ventricular arrhythmia or frequent recurrences of ventricular tachycardia after implantation of an ICD, although recurrence is common.

Retrospective analyses of clinical and pathologic series have identified a number of possible predictors of adverse outcome in probands, including an early age of onset of symptoms; competitive sporting activity; a malignant family background; severe right ventricular dilation; left ventricular involvement; syncope; episodes of complex ventricular arrhythmias or VT; and increased QRS dispersion on 12-lead ECG. ICD implantation is recommended for the prevention of sudden cardiac death in patients with documented sustained ventricular tachycardia or ventricular fibrillation and a reasonable expectation of survival with a good functional status for longer than 1 year. ICD implantation may also be appropriate in patients with extensive disease, including those with left ventricular involvement, or undiagnosed syncope when ventricular tachycardia or ventricular fibrillation has not been excluded as the cause.

Standard heart failure therapy, including diuretics, angiotensin-converting enzyme inhibitors, and β-blockers is indicated in patients in whom ARVC has progressed to severe heart failure or biventricular systolic dysfunction (Chapter 59). Anticoagulation should be considered in the presence of atrial fibrillation (Chapter 64), marked ventricular dilation, or ventricular aneurysms. In patients in whom heart failure is refractory, cardiac transplantation (Chapter 82) should be considered.

PROGNOSIS

Most data on prognosis in ARVC are derived from small, high-risk populations. By the age of 40 years, event-free survival is 50 to 60% in patients with Naxos disease and some autosomal dominant forms. In patients who have syncope or sustained ventricular arrhythmias and are treated with an ICD, freedom from appropriate shock therapy is about 75% at 48 months after implantation, with 96% of patients alive. Risk factors for sudden cardiac death include severe right ventricular disease, left ventricular involvement, and a history of unexplained syncope.

Restrictive Cardiomyopathy

DEFINITION AND EPIDEMIOLOGY

The incidence and prevalence of restrictive cardiomyopathy in adults are unknown. Restrictive cardiomyopathies (Table 60-8) are characterized by

TABLE 60-8 CAUSES OF RESTRICTIVE CARDIOMYOPATHIES

INFILTRATIVE DISORDERS
Amyloidosis Sarcoidosis
STORAGE DISORDERS
Hemochromatosis Fabry's disease Glycogen storage diseases
FIBROTIC DISORDERS
Radiation Scleroderma Drugs (e.g., doxorubicin, serotonin, ergotamine)
METABOLIC DISORDERS
Carnitine deficiency Defects in fatty acid metabolism
ENDOMYOCARDIAL DISORDERS
Endomyocardial fibrosis Hypereosinophilic syndrome (Löffler's endocarditis)
MISCELLANEOUS CAUSES
Carcinoid syndrome

stiffness, impaired filling, elevated left ventricular diastolic pressures, and reduced diastolic volume of the left or right ventricle despite normal or near-normal systolic function and wall thickness. Primary forms are uncommon, whereas secondary forms, in which the heart is affected as a part of a multisystem disorder, usually present at the advanced stage of an infiltrative disease (e.g., amyloidosis or sarcoidosis) or a systemic storage disease (e.g., hemochromatosis). Idiopathic restrictive cardiomyopathy affects both male and female patients and may manifest in children and young adults.

PATHOBIOLOGY

Approximately 30% of patients with idiopathic restrictive cardiomyopathy have familial disease. Mutations in the gene encoding desmin (an intermediate filament) cause restrictive cardiomyopathy associated with skeletal myopathy and cardiac conduction system abnormalities. Mutations in the cardiac sarcomere protein genes also cause restrictive cardiomyopathy.

The macroscopic features of restrictive cardiomyopathy include biatrial dilation and small ventricular cavities. In many hearts, there is thrombus in the atrial appendages and patchy endocardial fibrosis. The histologic features of idiopathic restrictive cardiomyopathy are typically nonspecific with patchy interstitial fibrosis, but myocyte disarray is not uncommon in patients with pure restrictive cardiomyopathy. Amyloidosis, hemochromatosis, and sarcoidosis are among the systemic diseases that cause restrictive cardiomyopathy (see later).

CLINICAL MANIFESTATIONS

Most patients present with symptoms and signs of heart failure and arrhythmia. Common symptoms include dyspnea on exertion, recurrent respiratory tract infections, general fatigue, and weakness. Symptoms may progress rapidly to dyspnea at rest, orthopnea, and paroxysmal nocturnal dyspnea. Many patients complain of chest pain and palpitation. Syncope is a presenting symptom in 10% of children. Rarely, sudden death is the initial manifestation of the disease.

Physical examination typically reveals an elevated jugular venous pressure, which has a prominent y descent and fails to fall (or rises) during inspiration (Kussmaul's sign). On cardiac auscultation, the pulmonary component of the second heart sound may be loud if pulmonary vascular resistance is high. A third heart sound and occasionally a fourth heart sound commonly produce a gallop rhythm. Peripheral edema, ascites, and hepatomegaly are common.

DIAGNOSIS

The most frequent ECG abnormalities include p-mitrale and p-pulmonale, nonspecific ST segment and T wave abnormalities, ST segment depression, and T wave inversion, usually in the inferolateral leads. Voltage criteria for left and right ventricular hypertrophy may be present, although patients with amyloidosis have low-voltage QRS complexes. Conduction abnormalities include intraventricular conduction delay and abnormal Q waves.

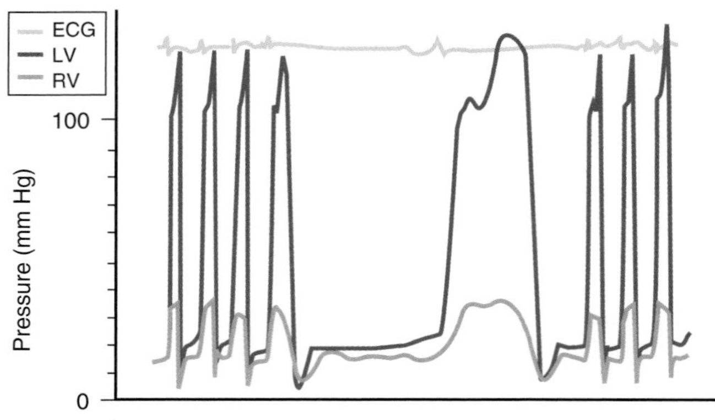

FIGURE 60-4. Idiopathic restrictive cardiomyopathy. Right ventricular (RV) and left ventricular (LV) pressure electrocardiographic (ECG) tracings in a patient with idiopathic restrictive cardiomyopathy. A dip-and-plateau pattern is seen in both ventricles, and diastolic filling pressures are elevated. The plateaus occur at different pressures, approximately 16 mm Hg for the RV tracing compared with 20 mm Hg for the LV tracing. The diagnosis of restrictive disease was confirmed by thoracotomy. (Redrawn from Benofti JR, Grossman W, Cohn PF. The clinical profile of restrictive cardiomyopathy. *Circulation.* 1980;61:1206.)

On cardiac imaging, both atria are markedly dilated and can dwarf the size of the ventricles in patients with normal global systolic function and a nonhypertrophied, nondilated left ventricle. Pulsed-wave Doppler velocities typically show increased early diastolic filling velocity, decreased atrial filling velocity, an increased ratio of early diastolic filling to atrial filling, decreased E wave deceleration time, and decreased isovolumic relaxation time. Pulmonary vein and hepatic vein pulsed-wave Doppler velocities demonstrate higher diastolic than systolic velocities, increased atrial reversal velocities, and an atrial reversal duration greater than mitral atrial filling duration. Tissue Doppler imaging usually shows reduced diastolic annular velocities and an increased ratio of early diastolic tissue Doppler annular velocity to mitral early diastolic filling velocity, reflecting elevated left ventricular end-diastolic pressures.

The characteristic hemodynamic feature on cardiac catheterization is a deep and rapid early decline in ventricular pressure at the onset of diastole, with a rapid rise to a plateau in early diastole ("dip-and-plateau" or "square root sign") (Fig. 60-4). Left ventricular end-diastolic, left atrial, and pulmonary capillary wedge pressures are markedly elevated, usually 5 mm Hg or more above right atrial and right ventricular end-diastolic pressures. Volume loading and exercise accentuate the difference between left-sided and right-sided pressures.

The diagnostic evaluation aims to exclude potentially reversible conditions. In such cases, the cardiac manifestations may provide the clues, but definitive diagnosis relies on the demonstration of disease-specific features, such as amyloid protein in amyloidosis (Chapter 194), noncaseating granulomas in sarcoidosis (Chapter 95), abnormal iron studies in hemochromatosis (Chapter 219), or reduced α-galactosidase A levels in Fabry's disease (Chapter 215). Endomyocardial biopsy is rarely required to make these diagnoses.

TREATMENT (Rx)

Diuretics are the main therapy for heart failure symptoms (Chapter 59), but they must be carefully administered so as not to reduce left ventricular filling pressures to the point of hypotension. Angiotensin-converting enzyme inhibitors and β-blockers are commonly recommended despite few data on their benefit. In patients with secondary restrictive cardiomyopathies, specific treatment of the underlying systemic disease is often appropriate (see later). Referral for transplant assessment should be considered early because pulmonary hypertension may develop and necessitate heart and lung transplantation.

PROGNOSIS

In adults with restrictive cardiomyopathy, the clinical course is usually slow and protracted. Survival from the time of diagnosis is often 10 years or more, except for amyloidosis, which progresses much more rapidly. Symptoms of heart failure are generally progressive and respond poorly to treatments for heart failure.

Specific Clinical Syndromes

SARCOIDOSIS

The frequency of myocardial involvement in patients with sarcoidosis (Chapter 95) is difficult to determine because it is frequently subclinical and patchy in nature. Postmortem studies suggest that the heart is involved in at least 25% of patients, but clinical cardiac involvement occurs in fewer than 10% of patients. Clinical manifestations of sarcoid include heart failure, conduction abnormalities, atrial and ventricular arrhythmias, pericardial effusion, valvular dysfunction, and, rarely, sudden cardiac death. Right heart failure secondary to pulmonary hypertension may occur in patients with extensive fibrotic lung disease. Myocardial infiltration by sarcoid granulomas results in restrictive or dilated cardiomyopathy. The most common site is in the lateral wall of the left ventricle. Papillary muscle involvement is responsible for the most common valvulopathy, mitral regurgitation. Granuloma formation in the basal interventricular septum may cause conduction abnormalities. Ventricular arrhythmias are also frequent. Biopsy of extracardiac sites is usually adequate for the diagnosis, but a gallium scan often demonstrates cardiac inflammation. A myocardial biopsy may show granulomas but, because of the focal distribution of the lesions, may be nondiagnostic. Corticosteroid therapy may improve arrhythmias, but heart failure may worsen despite such therapy. An ICD is generally indicated for ventricular arrhythmias.

AMYLOIDOSIS

EPIDEMIOLOGY AND PATHOBIOLOGY

Amyloidosis can result in deposition of amyloid protein in the atria, ventricles, coronary vessels, conduction system, and valves. The degree of cardiac involvement varies among subtypes. Hematologic disorders (Chapter 193) associated with excessive light chain (AL) immunoglobulin production are the most common cause of cardiac amyloid. Familial forms caused by the accumulation of mutant proteins (transthyretin or A-apolipoprotein) (Chapter 194) have variable cardiac involvement. Secondary amyloidosis, due to deposition of serum amyloid A protein in chronic inflammatory diseases, rarely affects the heart. In senile systemic amyloidosis, cardiomyopathy is by caused deposition of normal wild-type transthyretin; this disease nearly always affects elderly persons (>70 years), with a clinical course that is considerably slower than other types of amyloid.

DIAGNOSIS

The ECG tracing in most forms of cardiac amyloid characteristically shows decreased voltage despite increased wall thickness on echocardiography. Characteristic two-dimensional echocardiographic findings in advanced cardiac amyloidosis are biventricular hypertrophy, thickened valves and interatrial septum, dilated atria, and a small pericardial effusion. The myocardium has a hyperreflective granular texture (Fig. 60-5), best seen on digital image

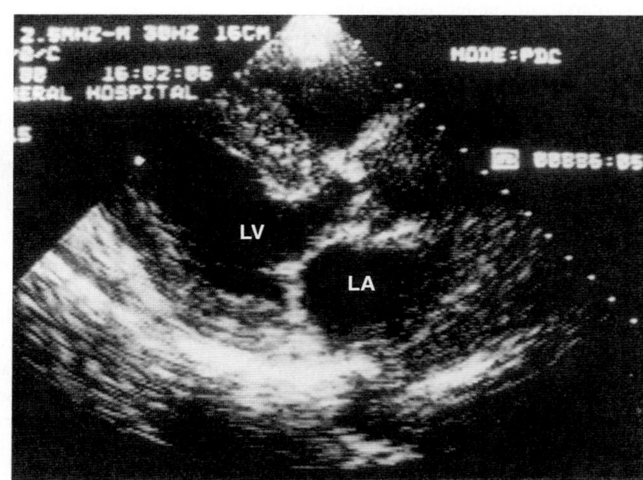

FIGURE 60-5. Amyloidosis. An apical four-chamber echocardiographic image demonstrates biventricular hypertrophy in a patient with biopsy-proved amyloidosis. RA = right atrium; RV = right ventricle. (From Levine RA. Echocardiographic assessment of the cardiomyopathies. In: Weyman AE, ed. *Principles and Practice of Echocardiography,* 2nd ed. Philadelphia: Lea & Febiger; 1994:810.)

analysis. Echo Doppler in advanced disease demonstrates a restrictive left ventricular filling pattern. Cardiac magnetic resonance imaging may show subendocardial late gadolinium enhancement with abnormal gadolinium kinetics. Nuclear scans with ^{123}I-labeled serum amyloid P component are highly specific.

A definitive diagnosis of amyloidosis requires a tissue biopsy, which can be obtained from other sites. For example, fine-needle aspiration of abdominal fat is positive for amyloid deposits in more than 70% of patients with AL amyloidosis. If negative, endomyocardial biopsy has a very high sensitivity.

TREATMENT AND PROGNOSIS (Rx)

Specific therapies to impede precursor protein production and fibril formation should be implemented whenever possible (Chapter 194). Diuretics, often in high doses (e.g., furosemide 40 to 80 mg daily), are the mainstay of the palliative heart failure regimen. Angiotensin-enzyme converting or angiotensin II inhibitors should be used very cautiously because they are often poorly tolerated and of unproven efficacy in cardiac amyloid. Aldosterone inhibitors might be helpful in advanced cases. Patients may be hypersensitive to digoxin because of enhanced drug binding with amyloid fibrils. Patients with atrial fibrillation in AL amyloidosis should receive anticoagulation with warfarin (Chapter 37) because of a very high rate of thromboembolism. Cardiac transplantation remains controversial, but heart transplantation (Chapter 82) with high-dose chemotherapy and with stem cell transplantation (Chapter 181) has been used in patients with AL amyloidosis.

Patients with amyloidosis with heart failure have a median survival time of less than 1 year and a 5-year survival rate of less than 5%. Most deaths occur suddenly. Patients with familial amyloidosis have a slower course than do patients with a monoclonal gammopathy.

HEREDITARY HEMOCHROMATOSIS

Hereditary hemochromatosis (Chapter 219) is an autosomal recessive disorder caused by excessive iron deposition in various organs, including the liver, spleen, pancreas, endocrine glands, and heart. In whites, its prevalence is between 1 in 200 and 1 in 500, with an even higher prevalence in the Irish population. The most common form is caused by mutations in the *HFE* gene, with two missense mutations accounting for most cases (C282Y and H63D).

Most patients with classical disease present between the ages of 40 and 60 years with hyperpigmentation, diabetes mellitus, and hepatomegaly. Up to 35% of patients with hemochromatosis experience heart failure, and 36% develop arrhythmias. Restrictive physiologic features dominate early in the disease, followed by ventricular dilation. The diagnosis is generally made from the clinical picture, an elevated serum iron level, and a high transferrin saturation. Genetic testing is helpful, and the diagnosis can be confirmed by endomyocardial biopsy. Phlebotomy and iron chelation therapy with deferoxamine (Chapter 219) may improve cardiac function before cell injury becomes irreversible. Standard heart failure treatment (Chapter 59) is generally recommended. Death from hemochromatosis results more often from cirrhosis and liver carcinoma than from cardiac disease.

Unclassified Cardiomyopathies

LEFT VENTRICULAR NONCOMPACTION

Failure of the trabecular or spongiform layer of the myocardium to compact may occur with congenital heart disease, including atrial and ventricular septal defects and coarctation of the aorta (Chapter 69), and with the rare X-linked multisystem disorder, Barth's syndrome. With recent improvements in imaging technology, it has also been recognized in patients with hypertrophic and dilated cardiomyopathy. The prevalence of localized areas of noncompaction is unknown, but clinically significant isolated left ventricular noncompaction in the absence of other cardiac abnormalities is uncommon.

Areas of noncompacted myocardium may be best delineated from normal myocardium by the demonstration of flow within the myocardium by Doppler or contrast echocardiography. When extensive areas are involved, systolic performance may be impaired, and there is a risk of ventricular arrhythmias and systemic emboli. Treatment, when necessary, is for associated heart failure (Chapter 59), arrhythmias (Chapters 64 and 65), and the risk of emboli (Chapter 59). Natural history and prognosis are not well established.

TAKOTSUBO CARDIOMYOPATHY

Takotsubo cardiomyopathy is a syndrome of transient apical left ventricular dysfunction that mimics myocardial infarction (Chapter 73). Postulated mechanisms include coronary artery spasm, myocarditis, and dynamic mid-cavity obstruction.

The clinical syndrome classically includes chest pain, ST segment elevation, and raised cardiac biomarkers in association with emotional or physical stress. Coronary arteriography reveals normal epicardial vessels. Conservative treatment with rehydration and removal of the determinants of stress usually results in rapid resolution within hours of the symptoms, ECG changes, and wall motion abnormalities.

DISEASES OF THE ENDOCARDIUM

Endocardial fibrosis, fibroelastosis, and thrombosis are subclassified into endomyocardial diseases with hypereosinophilia (hypereosinophilic syndromes) and endomyocardial disease without hypereosinophilia (e.g., endomyocardial fibrosis) (see Table 60-8).

Hypereosinophilic Syndrome

Hypereosinophilic syndromes are a rare and heterogeneous group of disorders defined as persistent blood eosinophilia ($>1.5 \times 10^9$/L) for more than 6 consecutive months, associated with evidence of eosinophil-induced organ damage in the absence of causes of hypereosinophilia, such as allergic, parasitic, and malignant disorders (Chapter 173). Pathogenic mechanisms include stem cell mutations that lead to expression of PDGFRA-containing fusion genes, mainly the *FIP1L1-PDGFRA* fusion gene, with constitutive tyrosine kinase activity and sustained overproduction of interleukin-5 by activated T-cell subsets. Clinically, hypereosinophilic syndrome can be classified into chronic eosinophilic leukemia, lymphocytic hypereosinophilic syndrome, myeloproliferative hypereosinophilic syndrome, and idiopathic hypereosinophilic syndrome. The term *organ-restricted eosinophilic disease*, such as eosinophilic gastroenteritis, dermatitis, or pneumonia, is used when a specific organ or tissue is the exclusive target of eosinophilic infiltration and damage. The term *Löffler's fibroplastic endocarditis* with eosinophilia has been used to describe cardiac damage caused by direct toxicity of circulating eosinophils in patients with persistent hypereosinophilia, but its use is now discouraged.

CLINICAL MANIFESTATIONS AND DIAGNOSIS

Hypereosinophilic syndrome is a rare disorder that tends to occur in patients 20 to 50 years of age, but all age groups are affected. Cardiac involvement generally evolves in three phases: an early necrotic stage that involves the endomyocardium, which is usually asymptomatic but can present as acute heart failure; a thrombotic stage, in which thrombi develop on the ventricular endocardium, sometimes causing peripheral emboli; and the final fibrotic stage, endomyocardial fibrosis, which causes restrictive cardiomyopathy and damage to atrioventricular valves. Chest pain, cough, dyspnea or orthopnea, and edema of the lower extremities are typical symptoms. Some patients may develop arrhythmias.

The characteristic two-dimensional echocardiographic findings include endocardial thickening, apical obliteration of one or both ventricles by an echogenic material, hyperdynamic contraction of the spared ventricular walls with bilateral atrial enlargement, and a restrictive pattern on echo Doppler.

TREATMENT (Rx)

Patients with the F/P fusion gene chromosomal rearrangement should be treated with the tyrosine kinase inhibitor, imatinib (100 mg daily for 1 week, increasing by 100 mg each week to 400 mg as guided by toxicity and hematologic response); the duration of therapy is still under investigation. Because some patients develop severe congestive heart failure within days after initiation of therapy, pretreatment with corticosteroids is recommended by some authorities. For patients without the F/P fusion gene, corticosteroids (median maximal daily dose of prednisone 40 mg, range 5 to 625 mg; duration 2 months to 20 years; median maintenance dose of 10 mg daily, range 1 to 40 mg/day) are the most common first-line therapy. Steroid-sparing and second-line drugs include hydroxyurea (median maximal daily dose of 1000 mg, range 500 to 2000 mg, adjusted to response), interferon-α (median maximal dose of 14 million units per week, range 3 to 40 million units per week, adjusted to response), and imatinib (as above).

Tropical Endomyocardial Fibrosis

Tropical endomyocardial fibrosis is probably the most common type of restrictive cardiomyopathy worldwide. The disease occurs predominantly within the tropics and affects mostly children and adolescents, usually from low socioeconomic backgrounds. Its cause is unknown, but potential contributors include infection, autoimmunity, genetic predisposition, ethnicity, diet, climate, and poverty.

Severe hypereosinophilia is found in some patients early in the initial stage of the illness, which is characterized by febrile illness, pancarditis, facial and periorbital swelling, pruritus, urticaria, and neurologic symptoms. This phase is followed by ventricular thrombosis that affects the apices and the subvalvular apparatus and then evolves to endocardial fibrosis. The final stage is characterized by restrictive physiology, atrioventricular valve regurgitation, and marked atrial dilation. Death results from complications of chronic heart failure but can occur suddenly owing to thromboembolism or arrhythmia.

Atrial fibrillation is common at presentation. In advanced disease, the ECG shows low-voltage QRS complexes, nonspecific ST-T wave changes, and conduction abnormalities. Echocardiography demonstrates apical obliteration, reduction of ventricular cavity size, and tethering or retraction of mitral or tricuspid leaflets, or both. There is no specific laboratory test, and hypereosinophilia is present only early in the disease.

There is no specific treatment for endomyocardial fibrosis. Medical treatment is used to control the heart failure (Chapter 59) and arrhythmias (Chapters 64 and 65). Surgical endocardial resection, combined with valve repair or replacement, has an early postoperative mortality between 15 and 30%. The overall prognosis is poor, with a 44% mortality rate at 1 year, increasing to nearly 90% at 3 years.

Carcinoid Syndrome

EPIDEMIOLOGY AND PATHOBIOLOGY

Carcinoid tumors are rare (1 in 100,000) neuroendocrine malignancies originating mostly from enterochromaffin cells in the gastrointestinal tract (Chapter 240). Carcinoid syndrome, with flushing, diarrhea, and bronchospasm, occurs after tumor cells metastasize to the liver and the vasoactive substances produced by the tumors enters the systemic circulation through the hepatic vein. Carcinoid heart disease occurs in up to 70% of cases of carcinoid syndrome.

The typical cardiac lesion is the carcinoid plaque, which is composed of smooth muscle cells, myofibroblasts, and elastic tissue that forms a fibrous layer on the endocardial surface of the right ventricle and atrium, the valve leaflets, and the subvalvular apparatus, including the chordae and papillary muscles. The tricuspid valve plaques tend to develop on the ventricular side of the leaflets, where they adhere to the mural endocardium and cause valvular regurgitation. On the pulmonary valve, the predominant lesion is stenosis. In patients with a patent foramen ovale, left-sided valvular involvement can occur. Occasional patients may have concomitant myocardial metastases and pericardial effusions from direct tumor invasion.

The most common presentation is dyspnea with signs and symptoms of right-sided heart failure. The ECG and radiograph are nonspecific. Echocardiography shows thickening of the tricuspid valve, the subvalvular apparatus, and the pulmonary valve. In severe disease, the tricuspid leaflets are retracted and fixed, with loss of normal coaptation. Similar findings can be seen on cardiac magnetic resonance imaging.

TREATMENT AND PROGNOSIS Rx

Treatment of the underlying carcinoid with a somatostatin analogue can improve systemic symptoms (Chapter 240). Valve replacement now has an operative mortality of less than 10% (Chapter 240). Without treatment, patients with carcinoid heart disease have a mean life expectancy of 1.6 years. In one series, cardiac surgery for valve disease was associated with about a 50% risk reduction.

Nonbacterial Thrombotic (Marantic) Endocarditis

EPIDEMIOLOGY AND PATHOBIOLOGY

Platelet-fiber masses that are adherent to the mitral or aortic valves are seen in about 20% of patients with malignant tumors, especially mucin-producing adenocarcinomas, melanomas, leukemias, and lymphomas. The lesions are sterile, commonly verruciform, and without accompanying inflammation.

CLINICAL MANIFESTATIONS AND DIAGNOSIS

Nonbacterial thrombotic endocarditis is virtually always asymptomatic but occasionally is a source of systemic emboli. Because of the small size of many of the emboli, the first presentation is often with cerebral symptoms. Larger lesions are detectable by echocardiography, but even transesophageal echocardiography is not sufficiently sensitive to identify lesions that may be found at autopsy and that may have been the source of systemic emboli.

TREATMENT

No treatment has been proved efficacious. However, systemic anticoagulation similar to that used in patients with tumor-associated deep vein thrombosis is often tried (Chapters 81 and 187).

CARDIAC TUMORS

Myocardial Tumors

Most primary cardiac tumors (Table 60-9) are benign. However, all tumors that extend from other tissues into the heart are malignant, as are metastatic lesions.

EPIDEMIOLOGY AND PATHOBIOLOGY

Primary tumors of the heart are unusual, with a prevalence of 1 in 2000 to 1 in 4000 in autopsy series. Nearly all these primary tumors are benign myxomas, although fibromas, lipomas, and fibroelastomas also occur. Rhabdomyomas are seen in children, especially with tuberous sclerosis (Chapter 426). The rare primary malignant tumors include sarcomas, especially angiosarcomas (see Table 60-9). Rarely, a primary mesothelioma or lymphoma may originate in the heart.

Up to 20% of advanced cancers may involve the pericardium, epicardium, or cardiac chambers either by direct extension of the primary tumor or by metastatic disease. Direct extension occurs principally from cancers of the lung, breast, esophagus, and mediastinum. Extension through the inferior vena cava to the right atrium and even to the right ventricle occurs with cancers of the kidney, adrenal gland, and liver. Metastatic spread is most common with melanomas or lymphomas.

TABLE 60-9 CARDIAC TUMORS

PRIMARY
Benign
Myxoma
Lipoma
Fibroma
Rhabdomyoma
Fibroelastoma
Malignant
Sarcoma
Mesothelioma
Lymphoma
SECONDARY
Direct Extension
Lung cancer
Breast cancer
Mediastinal tumors
Metastatic Tumors
Malignant melanoma
Leukemia
Lymphoma
Venous Extension
Renal cell cancer
Adrenal cancer
Liver cancer

Pericardial Tumors

CLINICAL MANIFESTATIONS

Pericardial tumors almost always result from direct extension of tumors, principally lung and breast, which produce a pericardial effusion that can progress to cardiac tamponade (Chapter 77). Patients typically are asymptomatic or minimally symptomatic in terms of the cardiac involvement until the effusion is very large, although they often may be very ill owing to progressive tumor elsewhere.

DIAGNOSIS

The diagnosis is often suspected in a patient with advanced malignant disease based on evidence of heart failure, hypertension, or arrhythmia and is confirmed by echocardiography. The differentiation between pericardial involvement by tumor and postradiation pericarditis depends on pericardiocentesis, often guided by echocardiography, and cytologic examination.

TREATMENT (Rx)

Cardiac tamponade must be treated with urgent pericardiocentesis, preferably under echocardiographic or radiologic guidance (Chapter 77). Although such a procedure can be life-saving and provide short-term to immediate-term palliation, control of the effusion often requires prolonged drainage, administration of intrapericardial chemotherapeutic agents, or limited or full pericardiectomy (Chapter 77). Some patients with pericardial tumors may respond to aggressive systemic chemotherapy, but recurrent accumulation of fluid is sufficiently likely that creation of a pericardial window should be considered before hospital discharge.

PROGNOSIS

In many cases, a tumor that is causing pericarditis has extended or will eventually extend through the pericardial space and into the myocardium, so no therapy is likely to be successful. The prognosis is very poor, except in unusual cases in which the tumor responds dramatically to systemic therapy.

Intracavitary Tumors

MYXOMA

DEFINITION AND EPIDEMIOLOGY

A *myxoma* is a benign polypoid neoplasm that originates from endocardial cells and is attached to the interatrial septum, usually protruding into the left atrium but occasionally into the right atrium and rarely into the ventricles. Myxomas are more common in women, especially between the ages of 30 and 60 years, than in men. These tumors can be familial and are rarely associated with other systemic abnormalities.

CLINICAL MANIFESTATIONS

Myxomas are slow growing and usually do not produce symptoms or signs until they enlarge. The typical presentation is with a tumor embolus, whereby usually small portions of the myxoma break loose and cause a single embolism or a shower of emboli. However, a large embolism from a myxoma can be of sufficient size to obstruct a medium-sized artery. Some patients have systemic symptoms, including fever, malaise, and arthralgias, as part of a clinical syndrome that may be confused with bacterial endocarditis (Chapter 76) or a collagen vascular disease. Large myxomas can prolapse into the mitral valve orifice during diastole, or they may obstruct blood flow from the left atrium to the left ventricle and mimic rheumatic mitral stenosis.

DIAGNOSIS

A myxoma large enough to obstruct the mitral orifice can produce an audible "tumor plop" when the myxoma prolapses and obstructs blood flow during diastole, at the same time that the opening snap of mitral stenosis would typically be heard. If obstruction is incomplete, the tumor plop may be followed by a diastolic rumble. As obstruction becomes more severe, cardiac output may fall precipitously. Echocardiography (Chapter 53) is usually definitive; transesophageal echocardiography provides a higher sensitivity than does transthoracic echocardiography, and magnetic resonance imaging can be helpful.

TREATMENT (Rx)

Surgical removal is generally curative, although myxomas can be multiple or recur in about 5% of cases. Follow-up postoperative echocardiography is generally recommended. However, the optimal frequency and duration for follow-up screening are uncertain.

OTHER PRIMARY INTRACAVITARY TUMORS

Papillary fibroelastomas are rare, typically frondlike tumors that may arise from a cardiac valve, often the mitral valve, and are generally detected incidentally by echocardiography. However, like myxomas, they can manifest with systemic or even coronary emboli. Surgical excision is usually successful.

Angiosarcomas, which are more frequent in men than in women, typically involve the pericardium and right atrium. They cause obstruction with clinical signs and symptoms of right-sided heart failure. These sarcomas are generally not amenable to therapy.

EXTENSION OF TUMOR INTO THE CARDIAC CAVITIES

Direct extension of tumor up the inferior vena cava into the right atrium can be seen with renal cell carcinomas and less commonly with liver and adrenal cancers. In some cases, tumor extension is accompanied by adherent clot, and either the tumor or the clot may cause obstruction or pulmonary emboli (Chapter 98). No treatments are generally successful, and the prognosis is grim.

Intramyocardial Tumors

Benign tumors in the myocardium include lipomas, fibromas, and rhabdomyomas. Primary malignant tumors include sarcomas, lymphomas, and mesotheliomas. Metastatic tumors include melanomas, lymphomas, and leukemias. The tumors may be clinically silent, or they may produce arrhythmias or even impinge on coronary arteries, thereby causing ischemic syndromes. Large tumors may protrude into the cardiac chamber and cause obstruction. Therapies are not successful, except for occasional patients whose metastatic tumors may respond to systemic chemotherapy or whose primary tumors have been cured by heart transplantation.

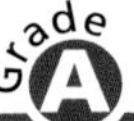

1. Mason JW, O'Connell JB, Herskowitz A, et al. A clinical trial of immunosuppressive therapy for myocarditis: the Myocarditis Treatment Trial Investigators. *N Engl J Med.* 1995;333:269-275.
2. Wojnicz R, Nowalany-Kozielska E, Wojciechowska C, et al. Randomized, placebo-controlled study for immunosuppressive treatment of inflammatory dilated cardiomyopathy: two-year follow-up results. *Circulation* 2001;104:39-45.
3. Cooper LT Jr, Hare JM, Tazelaar HD, et al. Usefulness of immunosuppression for giant cell myocarditis. *Am J Cardiol.* 2008;102:1535-1539.
4. Robinson J, Hartling L, Vandermeer B, et al. Intravenous immunoglobulin for presumed viral myocarditis in children and adults. *Cochrane Database Syst Rev.* 2005;25:CD004370.
5. Kadish A, Dyer A, Daubert JP, et al. Prophylactic defibrillator implantation in patients with nonischemic dilated cardiomyopathy. *N Engl J Med.* 2004;350:2151-2158.
6. Sliwa K, Blauwet L, Tibazarwa K, et al. Evaluation of bromocriptine in the treatment of acute severe peripartum cardiomyopathy: a proof-of-concept pilot study. *Circulation.* 2010;121:1465-1473.

SUGGESTED READINGS

Basso C, Corrado D, Marcus FI, et al. Arrhythmogenic right ventricular cardiomyopathy. *Lancet.* 2009;373:1289-1300. *Review of the genetics, pathology, and clinical manifestations of ARVC.*

Blauwet LA, Cooper LT. Myocarditis. *Prog Cardiovasc Dis.* 2010;52:274-288. *Review.*

Cardinale D, Colombo A, Lamantia G, et al. Anthracycline-induced cardiomyopathy: clinical relevance and response to pharmacologic therapy. *J Am Coll Cardiol.* 2010;55:213-220. *Prompt treatment can reduce the risk of major cardiac events.*

Gujja P, Rosing DR, Tripodi DJ, et al. Iron overload cardiomyopathy: better understanding of an increasing disorder. *J Am Coll Cardiol.* 2010;56:1001-1012. *Review.*

Jeffries JL, Towbin JA. Dilated cardiomyopathy. *Lancet.* 2010;375:752-762. *Review.*

Seward JB, Casaclang-Verzosa G. Infiltrative cardiovascular diseases. *J Am Coll Cardiol.* 2010;55:1769-1779. *Review.*

Sorajja P, Nishimura RA, Gersh BJ, et al. Outcome of mildly symptomatic or asymptomatic obstructive hypertrophic cardiomyopathy: a long-term follow-up study. *J Am Coll Cardiol.* 2009;5:234-241. *Patients with obstructive HCM and with mild or no symptoms are at a very small increased risk for mortality unless they have very elevated resting gradients.*

van Spaendonck-Zwarts KY, van Tintelen JP, van Veldhuisen DJ, et al. Peripartum cardiomyopathy as a part of familial dilated cardiomyopathy. *Circulation.* 2010;121:2169-2175. *Some cases of peripartum cardiomyopathy represent the first presentation of a familial dilated cardiomyopathy.*

61

PRINCIPLES OF ELECTROPHYSIOLOGY

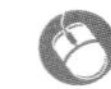

HUGH CALKINS

The function of the human heart requires rhythmic beatings occurring on the average 70 times a minute, 24 hours a day, for 80 or more years. The close to 3 billion contractions of the cardiac musculature that must occur without fail are coordinated by an intricate network of specialized electrically active cells that are integrated with the myocytes that comprise the predominant mass of the heart. Any loss of electrical activity, even for a few seconds, results in syncope (Chapters 50 and 62); loss of electrical activity for a few minutes may end in death.

CARDIAC ELECTROPHYSIOLOGY

Ion channels are integral membrane-spanning proteins, which allow the rapid movement of specific ions, most importantly Na^+, K^+, Cl^-, and Ca^{2+}, across the cell membrane at rates of 10^8 ions per second (E-Fig. 61-1). The opening and closing of the channels occur through a process of gating, whereby changes in the voltage, ligand, or receptor associated with the channel lead to alterations in the conformation of the proteins that activate or inactivate the channel pore. Voltage gating is the predominant method of regulating ion channels in the heart and is found in sodium and various potassium channels. Ligand-gated ion channels use ligands such as neurotransmitters, ions such as intracellular calcium, and metabolic products such as adenosine triphosphate (ATP) to activate a variety of channels, including those for potassium. Receptor-gated channels use changes in the physical environment, such as stretch, to activate channels, including those for chloride, which regulate intracellular volume.

The coordinated activity of numerous ion channels contributes to the creation of the cardiac action potential (Fig. 61-1). There are five phases to the cardiac action potential. At rest, the transmembrane potential of the cell exists close to −90 mV (the inside of the cell is positive with respect to the outside). With depolarization of the cell either from depolarization of adjacent cells or from an external change in voltage, sodium channels change from a closed to an open state and rapidly move sodium ions down a gradient into the interior of the cell, creating the sodium current I_{Na} and the rapid upstroke of phase 0 of the action potential. At the peak of depolarization, approximately +40 mV, the sodium current is inactivated, and the transient outward current I_{to} is activated with the opening of various voltage-gated potassium channels, resulting in the rapid decrease in voltage and phase 1 of the action potential. The plateau of the action potential, phase 2, follows and is an amalgamation of multiple currents representing inward and outward movement of ions. Contributors to this phase include the rapid component of the delayed rectifier potassium current I_{Kr}, the slow component of the delayed rectifier potassium current I_{Ks}, the L-type calcium channel, and the Na^+-Ca^{2+} exchanger. As the outward potassium currents increase and the calcium current decreases at the end of phase 2, the action potential progresses to phase 3, the phase of rapid repolarization. The inward rectifier potassium current I_{K1} contributes significantly to this final phase of repolarization and brings the action potential to its resting membrane potential. During phase 4, the heart is in diastole, with most cells at −85 to −90 mV. Specialized cells located in the sinoatrial and atrioventricular nodes repolarize to approximately −60 mV and contain currents that contribute to spontaneous depolarization during phase 4. These pacemaker cells contain the inward activation, or funny, current I_f activated by hyperpolarization and carried by sodium, and the background sodium current $I_{Na\text{-}B}$. The calcium currents $I_{Ca,L}$ and $I_{Ca,T}$, the sodium-potassium pump $I_{Na,K}$, and the sodium calcium exchanger $I_{Na,Ca}$ additionally may contribute to diastolic depolarization.

Variations in the duration and shape of the cardiac action potential depend on its location in the heart (Fig. 61-2). Likewise, alterations of ion channel expression and activity in disease states contribute to prolongation of the action potential. The atrial action potential has a typical duration of 100 to 200 msec, whereas the ventricular action potential typically lasts 250 to 300 msec. Different layers of the ventricle exhibit marked changes in the action potential. Epicardial cells have a prominent phase 1 compared with endocardial cells, in which phase 1 is blunted. The phase 2 plateau is decreased in epicardial cells, leading to less activation of the delayed rectifier currents

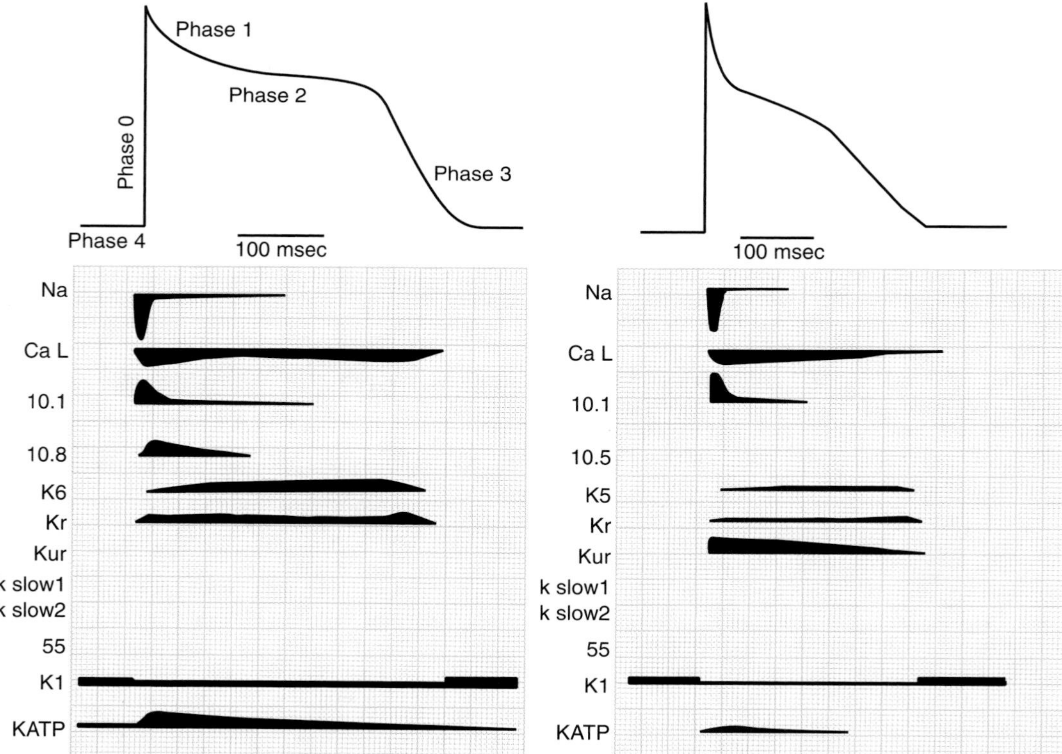

FIGURE 61-1. The cardiac action potential waveforms and underlying ionic currents in adult human and ventricular *(left)* and atrial *(right)* myocytes. The time- and voltage-dependent properties of the voltage-gated inward Na^+ (Nav) and Ca^{2+} (Cav) currents expressed in human atrial and ventricular myocytes are similar. In contrast, multiple types of K^+ currents, particularly Kv currents, contribute to atrial and ventricular action potential repolarization. The properties of the various Kv currents are distinct, and, in contrast to the inward currents, there are multiple Kv currents expressed in individual myocytes throughout the myocardium. (From Kass R. Molecular physiology of cardiac repolarization. *Physiol Rev.* 2005;85:1207.)

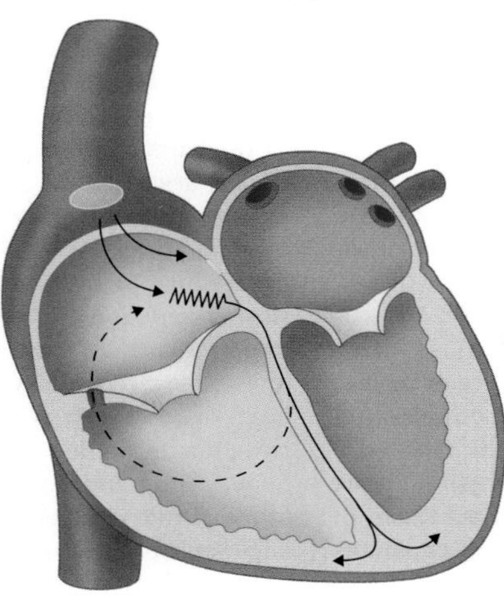

FIGURE 61-2. Accessory pathway in sinus rhythm and in orthodromic re-entrant tachycardia. (From Bassam CT. A molecular basis for Wolff-Parkinson-White syndrome. *N Engl J Med.* 2001;344:1861. Copyright © 2001 Massachusetts Medical Society. All rights reserved.)

and a prolonged action potential in epicardial cells. M cells found in the midmyocardium have the longest action potential duration and may contribute to the U wave seen on the surface electrocardiogram (ECG). The J (Osborne) wave seen on the ECG in cases of hypothermia (see Fig. 109-2 in Chapter 109) may be due to the increased prominence of I_{to} in the epicardial cells. Prolongation of the action potential is seen in cardiac hypertrophy or failure. At the molecular level, downregulation of the transient outward current I_{to} plays a prominent role in these disease states.

In a normal heart, the source of initial depolarizations occurs in the pacemaker cells of the sinus node (E-Fig. 61-2). The sinoatrial (SA) node is found at the lateral border of the superior vena cava and right atrial junction in the sulcus terminalis. It is an ovoid structure measuring up to 2 cm long by 0.5 cm wide. The sinus node artery, branching from either the right coronary artery (55 to 60%) or the left coronary artery (40 to 45%), runs through the middle of the sinus node. Pacemaker cells, seen as spider-shaped and spindle-shaped cells in the node, spontaneously depolarize during diastole. The wave of depolarization spreads through the sinus node and into the surrounding myocardium. The sympathetic and parasympathetic nervous systems affect the sinus rate. Adrenergic stimulation increases the rate by increasing $I_{Ca,L}$ and I_f activity. Cholinergic stimulation decreases the rate by decreasing $I_{Ca,L}$ and I_f activity. Stretch mediators found in the node and coupled to chloride channels also may increase the atrial rate with increasing atrial pressure. The SA node is the predominant pacemaker in the heart owing to its rapid rates of depolarization and overdrive suppression of secondary pacemakers.

Depolarization occurs through the atria to the atrioventricular (AV) node and from the right atrium to the left atrium. Three intra-atrial pathways—anterior, middle, and posterior—connect the right and left atria. Three intranodal pathways—superior, middle, and inferior tracts—also may connect the SA node to the AV node, although various investigators have disputed their presence. The P wave on the ECG is formed by atrial depolarization. The AV node is found at the apex of the triangle of Koch, formed by the tendon of Todaro on one side and the tricuspid annulus on the other, on the right side of the heart and anterior to the os of the coronary sinus. The arterial supply of the AV node arises from the right coronary artery in 85 to 90% of cases. The AV node itself is complex and can be divided into three general regions, with further subdivisions possible. A transitional zone contains multiple atrial inputs that extend to the compact AV node, which penetrates the central fibrous body and becomes the bundle of His. The compact AV node ranges from 5 to 7 mm by 2 to 5 mm in size. At least two distinct populations of AV node cells, rod-shaped and ovoid, have been described. These cells spontaneously depolarize because of a strong I_f current. Most ovoid cells lack I_{Na} and I_{to}, leading to slower depolarization. Conduction is relatively slow through the AV node compared with atrial and ventricular tissue, in part because of the decreased density of gap junction proteins, such as connexin 43, which is 33 times less prevalent in the AV node compared with ventricular cells. This reduction in gap junctions and intercalated discs leads to slower depolarization of neighboring cells. On the surface ECG, most of the PR interval depends on this slow AV node conduction.

The bundle of His arises from the compact AV node as it enters the central fibrous body. Conduction through the His bundle is rapid, on the order of 35 to 55 msec to the ventricles, owing to the presence of rapidly acting sodium channels. The arterial supply of the bundle of His originates from the left anterior descending artery in 90% of cases, with 10% emanating from the right coronary artery. The right and left bundle branches originate from the bundle of His. The left bundle branch further subdivides into the left anterior fascicle and left posterior fascicle before supplying the ventricular endocardium with Purkinje fibers. The right bundle branch trifurcates distally into a network that supplies the anterolateral papillary muscle, the low right septum, and the parietal band. Activation of the His-Purkinje system can be seen as the later portion of the PR interval on the surface ECG.

Ventricular activation occurs first from the left to right septum, followed by the synchronized depolarization of both ventricles from apex to base and endocardium to epicardium. The rapid activation of myocardial cells is due in part to the strong presence of the gap junction protein connexin 43. Knockout mice homozygous for connexin 43 deletions die with conotruncus malformations early in life, whereas mice heterozygous for connexin 43 deletion (Cx43+/−) have significant decreases in ventricular conduction in otherwise normal ventricles. Ventricular depolarization can be seen as the QRS complex on the surface ECG and is followed by repolarization seen as the ST, T, and U waves.

Normally the only connection between the atria and the ventricles is through the AV node and His bundle because the fibrous rings surrounding the tricuspid valve and mitral valve are electrically insulating. In a small percentage of the population (0.15 to 0.25%), anomalous myocardial bypass tracts join atrium to ventricle (Kent bundle) or, less frequently, atrium to AV node (James fiber), atrium to His bundle (Brechenmacher fiber), or AV node or His to Purkinje fiber or ventricle (Mahaim fiber). The classic AV bypass tract involved in the Wolff-Parkinson-White syndrome is composed of fibers containing I_{Na} and conducts rapidly in a nondecremental manner similar to that seen in the atria, His-Purkinje, or ventricular tissue (Fig. 61-2). A missense mutation in the $\gamma 2$ regulatory subunit of adenosine monophosphate (AMP)-activated protein kinase gene *PRKAG2* can cause the Wolff-Parkinson-White syndrome, with a possible effect of interfering with muscle fiber regression during embryogenesis. The surface ECG often shows a δ wave (see Fig. 64-19 in Chapter 64), the hallmark of ventricular preexcitation, preceding the QRS complex.

The heart is innervated by the sympathetic and the parasympathetic nervous systems, with their influence on ion channels manifested as changes in the heart rate, refractoriness, and contractility. Sympathetic stimulation causes the release of norepinephrine at the postganglionic nerve terminal, leading to β_1-adrenergic and β_2-adrenergic receptor activation, followed by G protein–mediated adenylyl cyclase production, which increases production of cyclic AMP (cAMP), which leads to the activation of protein kinase A, ultimately resulting in the phosphorylation of ion channels, which alter their gating and function. Parasympathetic activity leads to release of acetylcholine at the nerve terminal, which stimulates muscarinic cholinergic receptors, followed by direct G protein–mediated activation of channels, or indirect G protein–mediated secondary messenger activation using cAMP. Multiple membrane currents are influenced by sympathetic or parasympathetic activity. The L-type calcium channel current $I_{Ca,L}$ is increased four times with β-adrenergic stimulation, leading to increased conduction of the SA and AV nodes. β-Adrenergic stimulation also leads to a cAMP-mediated change in the activation of I_f, with the result being increased activity of cardiac pacemaker cells and higher heart rates. Parasympathetic stimulation leads to activation of the acetylcholine-activated potassium current I_{KACh}, which results in decreased pacemaker activity and slowing of conduction over the AV node. Purinergic receptors are a third family of G protein–coupled receptors that are activated by adenosine. Exposure to adenosine leads to activation of I_{KACh} and inhibition of $I_{Ca,L}$, resulting in slowing of the pacemaker activity for SA and AV nodes and conduction delay through the AV node.

Mechanisms of Cardiac Tachyarrhythmias

A cardiac arrhythmia is an abnormality in the timing or sequence of cardiac depolarization. There are two predominant types of cardiac arrhythmias: (1) tachyarrhythmia—an abnormally rapid cardiac rhythm (heart rate >100 beats per minute) and (2) bradyarrhythmia—a slow cardiac rhythm (heart rate <60 beats per minute) (Chapters 62, 64, and 65). The mechanism of cardiac tachyarrhythmias can be grouped into two general categories, abnormalities of impulse formation and re-entry (E-Fig. 61-3). Abnormalities of impulse formation can be subdivided further into abnormal automaticity and triggered activity. In the normal heart, the sinus node is the predominant pacemaker, with secondary pacemakers located in the atria, AV node, and His-Purkinje system, which function in the event that normal initiation or propagation is affected by disease or drugs. Automaticity is the ability to initiate spontaneous impulses. Under normal circumstances, there is a hierarchical sequence in the rate of firing of the heart cells that have the capacity for automaticity. Normally, spontaneous firing is fastest in the sinus node (70 to 80 beats per minute under resting conditions), and the sinus node is the predominant pacemaker. The AV node and His bundle fire at 50 to 60 beats per minute, and the Purkinje fibers fire at 30 to 40 beats per minute. The lower pacemaker may take over the pacemaking function of the heart if the faster pacemaker fails or slows. Variations in autonomic tone may have a major effect on normal automaticity. In general, activation of the sympathetic nervous system increases automaticity, whereas activation of the parasympathetic nervous system decreases automaticity. Under pathologic conditions that depolarize cells, myocardial cells outside the specialized conduction system also may acquire automaticity, a phenomenon termed *abnormal automaticity*.

Triggered activity is an uncommon mechanism of cardiac arrhythmias. Triggered activity occurs when a preceding depolarization does not repolarize completely before depolarizing again. *Early afterdepolarizations* (EADs) occur during phase 2 and phase 3 of the action potential. The basis for EADs appears to involve the L-type calcium channel. EADs are facilitated by increased repolarization times, as seen in either congenital or acquired long QT syndromes. With drugs that prolong the QT interval, such as erythromycin, quinidine, sotalol, and procainamide, the block of potassium channels involved in repolarization leads to prolongation of the action potential. The ultimate effect of EADs may be in initiating polymorphic ventricular tachycardia or torsades de pointes (Chapter 65). *Delayed afterdepolarizations* (DADs) arise during phase 4 of the action potential, when the cell membrane is completely repolarized. Transient inward currents, which are not normally present, may be initiated by the action of elevated intracellular calcium on the sodium-calcium exchanger or by release of calcium from the sarcoplasmic reticulum, and they may form the basis for DADs. Rapid heart rates, increased extracellular calcium, and adrenergic stimulation all may contribute to DADs. DADs are thought to form the basis of arrhythmias resulting from digitalis, idiopathic ventricular tachyarrhythmias, and idioventricular rhythms, and they may be reduced by drugs that block the uptake of calcium by the sarcoplasmic reticulum. Multifocal atrial tachycardia is another example of an arrhythmia that results from DAD-mediated triggered activity. The third type of automaticity, *depolarization-induced automaticity*, has been reproduced in cardiac tissues but may not lead to clinically relevant arrhythmias. Depolarization-induced automaticity arises from the constant application of current to muscle, a process that leads to spontaneous firing of the muscle.

Re-entry is the most common mechanism of cardiac arrhythmias. Re-entry generally occurs in the setting of abnormalities in impulse conduction. The abnormalities in impulse conduction may result from an anomalous electrical connection in the heart (i.e., an accessory pathway) or from poor impulse propagation. The basis for poor propagation of the depolarizing wave front in the heart may be attributed to pathology, drugs, or hormonal modulation of the conduction system. Fibrosis or calcification of the AV node, His bundle, or right and left bundle branches may lead to AV block or right and left bundle-branch blocks. AV nodal block may be a result of high vagal tone, as seen during sleep or in a well-conditioned athlete, or may be due to agents that act on the AV node, such as digitalis, β-adrenergic blockers, or calcium-channel blockers. Slowing of conduction in the atrium and ventricles also may be affected directly by hyperkalemia or ischemia.

The basis for poor propagation of the depolarizing wave front in the heart usually results from pathologic changes in patients with structural heart disease, including coronary artery disease, left ventricular hypertrophy, and heart failure. Fibrotic changes in the heart, with increases in collagen and intracellular matrix as seen in hypertrophy or infarction, can lead to areas of slow conduction and provide portals for re-entry. Changes in the gap junction proteins have been noted in hypertrophy with increases of connexin 43. These changes typically result from advanced age or the presence of structural heart disease, such as a prior myocardial infarction or a cardiomyopathy. In ischemia, the action potential is abbreviated owing to activation of I_{KACh}; in hypertrophy and failure, action potential prolongation from loss of I_{to} is found. Other influences on remodeling include catecholamines, free radicals, angiotensin-converting enzyme, angiotensin II, aldosterone, cytokines, and nitric oxide. Re-entry occurs when there is continuation of a propagating wave front, which reactivates areas of the heart that previously have depolarized and are not refractory. The refractory period, which is the time interval in which the cells are unable to depolarize after a second stimulus, often persists until the transmembrane voltage is +60mV at the activation threshold of I_{Na}.

Three types of re-entry have been described: circus movement re-entry, reflection, and phase 2 re-entry. The simplest model of circus movement tachycardia, the ring model, requires the presence of unidirectional block, in which the wave front can travel only in one direction, and a long enough circuit, in which recovery from refractoriness occurs before the approach of the leading edge of depolarization (Fig. 61-3). The length of the circuit must be equal to or greater than the wavelength (conduction velocity × refractory period) of the tachycardia. Three criteria for circus movement tachycardia include the presence of unidirectional block, the presence of a distinct path of recurrent propagation, and the fact that disrupting the circuit at any point along the path terminates the tachycardia. AV reciprocating tachycardia is an example of a re-entrant tachycardia (see Fig. 64-20 in Chapter 64). During sinus rhythm, the cardiac impulse activates the ventricle through the AV node and the accessory pathway. The tachycardia is initiated when a premature atrial impulse blocks the accessory pathway and conducts down the AV node (owing to differences in refractoriness). The impulse then returns to the atria by conduction through the accessory pathway, resulting in a re-entrant or circus movement tachycardia. Atrial fibrillation is the most common type of arrhythmia that results from re-entry. In contrast to arrhythmias with an accessory pathway in which there is only a single fixed re-entrant circuit, however, atrial fibrillation results from the presence of many functional re-entrant wavelets that propagate throughout the atria simultaneously. It has been estimated that at least three re-entrant wavelets must coexist for atrial fibrillation to be sustained. *Re-entry resulting from reflection* occurs when an

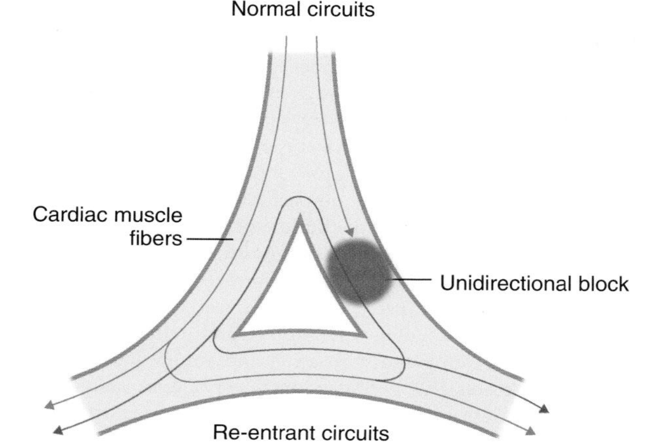

FIGURE 61-3. Unidirectional block as a result of abnormal repolarization, conduction, or intracellular calcium homeostasis. *Red arrows* show normal conduction, and *blue arrows* show re-entry through previously refractory tissue. (From Keating MT, Sanguinetti MC. Molecular and cellular mechanisms of cardiac arrhythmias. *Cell.* 2001;104:569.)

impulse proceeds back and forth over a functionally unexcitable pathway, depolarizing proximal tissue on each return cycle. *Phase 2 re-entry* occurs when an action potential dome during phase 2 is propagated from normal myocytes to myocytes lacking the dome, followed by local reexcitation, extrasystolic beats, and circus movement re-entry. Phase 2 re-entry notably is found in Brugada's syndrome (Chapter 65). Brugada's syndrome is the result of a sodium channel mutation in the α-subunit SCN5A. The hallmark of Brugada's syndrome is ST segment elevation and a right bundle branch pattern in V_1 to V_3 on the ECG. The ECG abnormalities can be explained by the loss of a phase 2 action potential dome in the epicardium but not in the endocardium owing to a failure of I_{Na} to reach a more positive voltage before phase 1. Endocardium-to-epicardium phase 2 re-entry occurs, leading to the ventricular tachycardia or ventricular fibrillation that is seen in Brugada's syndrome.

Multiple intrinsic and extrinsic factors can affect the initiation and propagation of cardiac arrhythmias (E-Fig. 61-4). At the molecular level, multiple mutations contribute to the inherited long QT syndrome and to idiopathic ventricular fibrillation (Brugada's syndrome). Twelve different subtypes of long QT syndrome have been described, and the genetic mutations of each have been identified. Genetic testing now can find a mutation in approximately two thirds of patients with long QT syndrome. The three most common types are LQT1 and LQT2, which account for approximately 90% of genotyped cases, and LQT3, which accounts for an additional 5% to 8% of cases. The mutations in long QT syndrome affect the sodium channel and potassium channels involved in repolarization with either gain of function for the sodium channel or loss of function for the potassium channels, resulting in a prolonged phase 2. The most common subtype, LQT1, is a disorder of the potassium channel α-subunit KVLQT1 responsible in part for I_{Ks}. LQT2 is due to mutations in HERG, a component of I_{Kr}. LQT3 affects the sodium channel SCN5A at a site leading to incomplete inactivation, and a continuing inward current Brugada's syndrome has been shown to be due to mutations in SCN5A, causing faster inactivation of the sodium channel. Familial polymorphic ventricular tachycardia has been linked to mutations in the cardiac ryanodine receptor (*RyR2*) gene of the cardiac sarcoplasmic reticulum, mutations that may lead to changes in calcium-induced activation.

Mechanism of Bradyarrhythmias

Cardiac bradyarrhythmias may result from either abnormalities in impulse formation or abnormalities in impulse conduction. Sinus bradycardia is the most common type of bradyarrhythmia. Sinus bradycardia results from a decreased rate of firing of the sinus node, which may be physiologic and result from increased parasympathetic tone (i.e., during sleep) or pathologic and result from a fibrosis of the sinus node, such as occurs with aging. Bradyarrhythmias also occur when abnormalities of conduction interrupt the normal sequence of cardiac depolarization. Depending on the site of block, subsidiary pacemakers begin to fire, creating an "escape" rhythm. Conduction block usually is due to fibrosis or calcification of the AV node, His bundle, or right and left bundle branches. Conduction block also may result from increased parasympathetic tone, however, as seen during sleep or in a well-conditioned athlete, or may be due to agents that act on the AV node, such as digitalis, β-adrenergic blockers, or calcium channel blockers.

SUGGESTED READINGS

Boyett MR. 'And the beat goes on.' The cardiac conduction system: the wiring system of the heart. *Exp Physiol.* 2009;94:1035-1049. *Detailed overview.*

Park DS, Fishman GI. The cardiac conduction system. *Circulation.* 2011;123:904-915. *Review.*

Trayanova NA. Whole-heart modeling: application to cardiac electrophysiology and electromechanics. *Circ Res.* 2011;108:113-128. *Review.*

62

APPROACH TO THE PATIENT WITH SUSPECTED ARRHYTHMIA

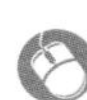

JEFFREY E. OLGIN

CLINICAL MANIFESTATIONS

Patients with suspected arrhythmias can present in a variety of ways. Typical symptoms include palpitations, syncope, and presyncope (dizziness). On occasion, arrhythmias can manifest more subtly as exercise intolerance, lethargy, and vague complaints of malaise or without any symptoms at all. Conversely, arrhythmias occasionally manifest as aborted sudden cardiac death (cardiac arrest) (Chapter 63). The specific differential diagnosis, prognosis, and treatment of these symptoms are determined by the severity of the symptom (i.e., whether it results in syncope) and whether the patient has underlying structural heart disease. In general, the likelihood of a life-threatening arrhythmia, such as ventricular tachycardia or ventricular fibrillation, in a patient with symptoms of palpitations or syncope is significantly greater in a patient who has structural heart disease. Therefore, the determination of whether structural heart disease is present is a key step in the diagnosis and prognosis of patients with suspected arrhythmias.

Palpitations

Palpitations, defined as an awareness of an irregular or rapid heartbeat, are most commonly due to ectopic beats—namely, premature atrial contractions (PACs; Chapter 64) and premature ventricular contractions (PVCs; Chapter 65)—or to tachyarrhythmias. A careful history can often distinguish benign palpitations from those that need further evaluation. It can be useful to have the patient tap out with a finger what the palpitations feel like. An irregularly irregular pattern suggests atrial fibrillation, whereas a more regular, rapid pattern suggests a sustained tachycardia. A reliable symptom suggesting that palpitations are caused by a tachyarrhythmia, particularly a supraventricular tachycardia, is the sensation of a regular, rapid-pounding sensation in the neck. Conversely, most patients who complain of symptoms from PACs or PVCs are often more aware of the post-extrasystolic pause or the accentuated output of the post-extrasystolic beat than of the actual premature beat itself. The majority of patients who have symptoms suggestive of premature beats but not of sustained tachycardia do not require further evaluation if they have no other symptoms and no evidence of structural heart disease—that is, an otherwise normal cardiac history, physical examination, and electrocardiogram (ECG) (see Table 50-4 in Chapter 50). If, however, the symptoms are not due to a single occasional extrasystole or are accompanied by presyncope or syncope, further evaluation is required (Fig. 62-1). Antiarrhythmic therapy is usually not necessary to treat PACs or PVCs unless the symptoms are frequent or severe. β-Blockers (e.g., metoprolol 25 mg/day or atenolol 25 mg/day) are first-line therapy in highly symptomatic patients with documented PACs or PVCs.

Palpitations are the most common presentation of tachyarrhythmias. The majority of tachyarrhythmias in patients without structural heart disease are due to supraventricular tachycardias (Chapter 64) that resolve spontaneously within several seconds. When the tachyarrhythmia is more prolonged, it often resolves with simple interventions. Patients themselves can cough several times, perform the Valsalva maneuver, exhale forcefully against a closed glottis for several seconds, or even rub gently on their eyeballs. A physician can use carotid sinus massage (Chapter 64), performed by pressing and rubbing the carotid pulse just below the angle of the mandible for 5 to 15 seconds. This maneuver should be avoided in elderly patients and in patients with a history of cerebrovascular accident, known carotid artery stenosis, or carotid bruit on auscultation. In patients with structural heart disease, palpitations may signify ventricular tachycardia (Chapter 65), particularly if they occur with syncope or presyncope. Rarely do bradyarrhythmias manifest as palpitations.

Presyncope and Syncope

Syncope, defined as a sudden loss of consciousness, and presyncope, or lightheadedness, are caused by global impairment of blood flow to the brain

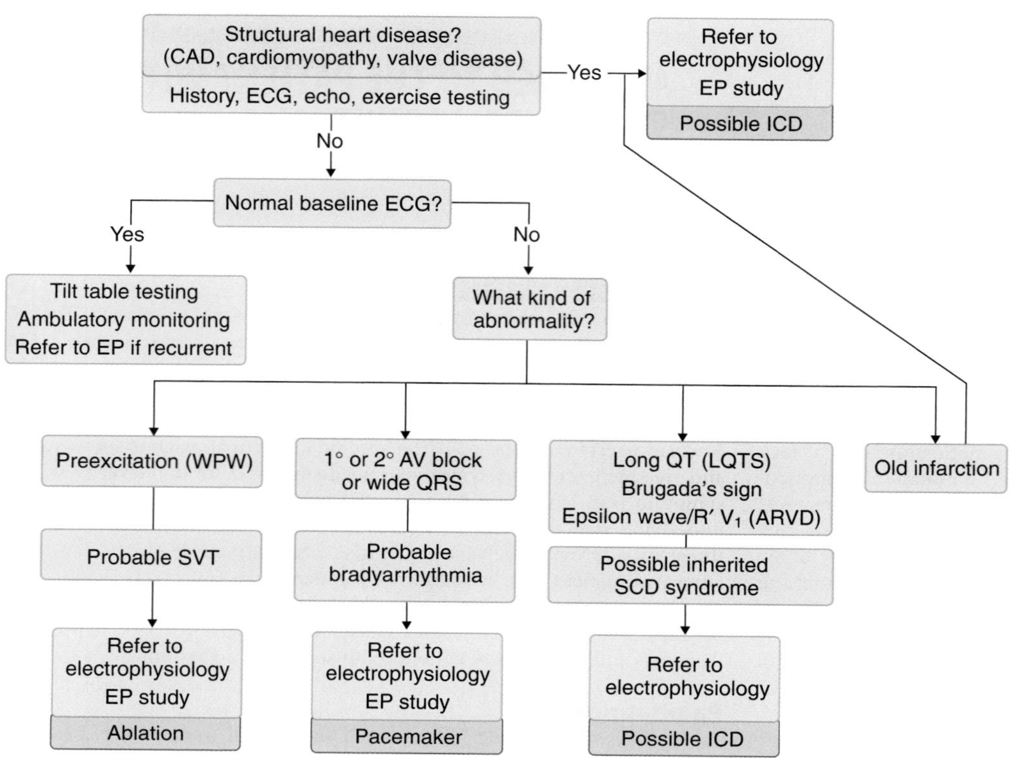

FIGURE 62-1. **Algorithm for evaluating patients with symptoms of palpitation, dizziness, or syncope.** ARVD = arrhythmogenic right ventricular dysplasia; AV = atrioventricular; CAD = coronary artery disease; ECG = electrocardiogram; echo = echocardiogram; EP = electrophysiology; ICD = implantable cardioverter-defibrillator; LQTS = long QT syndrome; SCD = sudden cardiac death; SVT = supraventricular tachycardia; WPW = Wolff-Parkinson-White syndrome.

(Table 62-1). Syncope can be a manifestation of tachyarrhythmias, bradyarrhythmias, or neurocardiogenic syncope, or it can be unrelated to any arrhythmia. A careful history and physical examination are necessary to exclude other cardiac causes (e.g., acute ischemia, aortic stenosis) or neurologic causes. Important historical features that suggest an arrhythmic cause are an association with palpitations and the lack of any neurologic deficits preceding or following the event. Important differential diagnoses include conditions other than lightheadedness that may be termed dizziness by the patient. Vertigo (Chapter 436), a sense of imbalance or of the “room spinning,” and ataxia (Chapter 417) can usually be distinguished by the history and physical examination. The possibility of seizures (Chapter 410) must also be evaluated; syncope from an arrhythmia or neurocardiogenic syncope occasionally results in seizure-like activity, and seizures can sometimes be confused with syncope. The most important distinguishing feature is that postictal symptoms, a key feature of seizure disorders, are absent when syncope is the result of an arrhythmia. Patients with syncope from an arrhythmia usually awaken without any neurologic residual, unless the patient experienced a cardiac arrest with prolonged hypoxia and required resuscitation.

Because most spells of episodic loss of consciousness occur outside medical observation, the history is the most critical part of the evaluation (Table 62-2). Each syncopal episode should be reviewed in detail, with special attention to symptoms preceding the episode, events during unconsciousness, and the symptoms and time course of regaining orientation after consciousness is restored. Information from a witness can be essential to the evaluation.

The patient's presymptomatic activity and positioning, as well as symptoms when the syncopal episode began, are important clues to diagnosis. Seizures or cardiac arrhythmias can occur in any body position, but recumbent patients rarely develop neurocardiogenic (vasovagal) syncope and never have orthostatic hypotension. Prodromal lightheadedness, dizziness (but uncommonly vertigo), bilateral tinnitus, nausea, diffuse weakness, and dimming of vision are symptoms of cerebral hypoperfusion and support the diagnosis of syncope, which may be from a cardiac, orthostatic, or neurocardiogenic cause. Loss of consciousness so rapid that a prodrome is absent may occur with seizures and with some cardiac arrhythmias such as asystole, which typically causes loss of consciousness within 4 to 8 seconds in the

TABLE 62-1 CAUSES OF SYNCOPE AND THEIR PREVALENCE

NEUROCARDIOGENIC CAUSES
Vasovagal (8–41% of patients)
Situational (1–8% of patients)
Micturition
Defecation
Swallow
Cough
Carotid sinus syncope (0.4% of patients)
Neuralgias
Psychiatric disorders
Medications, exercise
ORTHOSTATIC HYPOTENSION (4–10% OF PATIENTS)
DECREASED CARDIAC OUTPUT
Obstruction to flow (1–8% of patients)
Obstruction to left ventricular outflow or inflow: aortic stenosis, hypertrophic obstructive cardiomyopathy, mitral stenosis, myxoma
Obstruction to right ventricular outflow or inflow: pulmonic stenosis, pulmonary embolism, pulmonary hypertension, myxoma
Other heart disease
Pump failure, myocardial infarction, coronary artery disease, coronary spasm, tamponade, aortic dissection
ARRHYTHMIAS (4–38% OF PATIENTS)
Bradyarrhythmias: sinus node disease, second- and third-degree atrioventricular block, pacemaker malfunction, drug-induced bradyarrhythmias
Tachyarrhythmias: ventricular tachycardia, torsades de pointes (e.g., associated with congenital long QT syndrome or acquired QT prolongation), supraventricular tachycardia
NEUROLOGIC AND PSYCHIATRIC DISEASES (3–32% OF PATIENTS)
Migraine
Transient ischemic attacks
UNKNOWN (13–41% OF PATIENTS)

Adapted from Kapoor W. Approach to the patient with syncope. In: Braunwald E, Goldman L, eds. *Primary Cardiology*, 2nd ed. Philadelphia: Saunders; 2003.

TABLE 62-2 CLINICAL FEATURES SUGGESTING SPECIFIC CAUSES

SYMPTOM OR FINDING	DIAGNOSTIC CONSIDERATION
After sudden unexpected pain, fear, or unpleasant sight, sound, or smell	Vasovagal
Prolonged motionless standing	Vasovagal
Well-trained athlete after exertion (without heart disease)	Vasovagal
During or immediately after micturition, cough, swallowing, or defecation	Situational syncope
Syncope with throat or facial pain (glossopharyngeal or trigeminal neuralgia)	Neurocardiogenic syncope with neuralgia
With head rotation, pressure on the carotid sinus (as in tumors, shaving, tight collars)	Carotid sinus syncope
Immediately on standing	Orthostatic hypotension
Medication that may lead to long QT syndrome, orthostasis, or bradycardia	Drug induced
Associated with headaches	Migraine, seizures
Associated with vertigo, dysarthria, diplopia	Transient ischemic attack, subclavian steal, basilar migraine
With arm exercise	Subclavian steal
Confusion after a spell or loss of consciousness for >5 min	Seizure
Differences in blood pressure or pulse in the two arms	Subclavian steal or aortic dissection
Syncope and murmur with changing position (from sitting to lying, bending, turning over in bed)	Atrial myxoma or thrombus
Syncope with exertion	Aortic stenosis, pulmonary hypertension, mitral stenosis, obstructive hypertrophic cardiomyopathy, coronary artery disease
Family history of sudden death	Long QT syndrome, Brugada's syndrome
Brief loss of consciousness, no prodrome, with heart disease	Arrhythmias
Frequent syncope, somatic complaints, no heart disease	Psychiatric illness

From Kapoor WN. Syncope. *N Engl J Med.* 2000;343:1856-1862.

upright position but usually requires 12 to 15 seconds in the recumbent position. Palpitations during the prodrome suggest a tachyarrhythmia. The activity of the patient immediately before the onset of symptoms may also provide clues. Syncope associated with the cessation of exertion or with anxiety or pain suggests neurocardiogenic syncope, whereas symptoms during exertion suggest an arrhythmia. Syncope associated with a change in posture suggests orthostatic causes, whereas syncope while straining at urination suggests situational neurocardiogenic syncope.

A witness's description of the events during the episode of unconsciousness is very helpful. Although body stiffening and limb jerking occur with generalized seizures, similar movements can result from cerebral hypoperfusion, especially if perfusion is not restored rapidly. Such muscle jerking is often multifocal and can be synchronous or asynchronous. In contrast to epileptic seizures, which generally produce tonic-clonic activity for at least 1 to 2 minutes, muscle jerking in syncope rarely persists for longer than 30 seconds. If an arrhythmia continues or the patient is physically maintained upright, tonic stiffening of the body followed by jerking movements of the limbs can occur. Occasionally, motor movements identical to a tonic-clonic seizure occur, and a mistaken diagnosis of epilepsy can be made. Urinary incontinence during the spell is frequently used to support or refute a diagnosis of epilepsy; however, fainting with a full bladder can result in incontinence, whereas seizures with an empty bladder will not. Tongue biting favors seizures.

The time frame over which consciousness and orientation are regained is perhaps the most important clue in differentiating seizures from syncope. Recovery of orientation after neurocardiogenic syncope occurs within seconds of regaining consciousness. Recovery of orientation after self-reversible arrhythmia-associated syncope is usually proportional to the duration of the unconsciousness and is usually rapid (0 to 10 seconds). Life-threatening arrhythmias (e.g., prolonged asystole or ventricular fibrillation) usually do not resolve without resuscitation, and the confusion after regaining consciousness may be permanent owing to ischemic brain injury (Chapter 63). By comparison, the period of confusion after seizures, often accompanied by agitation, continues for 2 to 20 minutes after recovery of consciousness.

DIAGNOSIS

Arrhythmias are generally categorized as bradyarrhythmias (slow heart rates), tachyarrhythmias (fast heart rates), or premature beats (single extrasystoles from the atrium or the ventricle—PACs [see Fig. 64-12 in Chapter 64] or PVCs [see Fig. 65-3 in Chapter 65], respectively) (see Table 62-1). Although not a primary arrhythmia, neurocardiogenic syncope is a related diagnostic and management issue because its symptoms are frequently similar to those of arrhythmias and because neurocardiogenic syncope secondarily results in bradycardia (see later).

Bradyarrhythmias

Bradyarrhythmias (Chapter 64) can be due to dysfunction in the sinoatrial node, atrioventricular (AV) node, or His-Purkinje system (below the AV node). Sinus bradycardia manifests as a slow atrial (sinus) rate and can occur at rest or as an inappropriately slow rate during exercise (chronotropic incompetence). Sinus arrest can be intermittent, when transient loss of sinus activity (loss of the P wave on the ECG) causes brief sinus pauses, or persistent, with prolonged loss of atrial activation. The sinus rate and even the presence of sinus pauses are influenced by autonomic tone. Therefore, healthy individuals—particularly younger patients and well-trained athletes (with high vagal tone)— have occasional sinus slowing, often during sleep. A sinus pause of more than 3 seconds is considered pathologic when it is associated with symptoms. Sinus bradycardia and sinus arrest can also be the result of medications, typically β-blockers and calcium-channel blockers. When not "physiologic" or due to medications, sinus bradycardia and sinus arrest are the result of intrinsic conduction system disease. Sinus bradycardia, especially if it is intermittent, can also signify disease of the right coronary artery.

Bradyarrhythmias from AV nodal disease result from the failure of impulse conduction from the atrium to the ventricle. Like the sinus node, the AV node is dramatically affected by autonomic tone. Mobitz type I second-degree AV block (Wenckebach block; see Fig. 64-8 in Chapter 64) can be seen during periods of high vagal tone and is not necessarily pathologic; for example, it does not progress to complete heart block and is not associated with a widened QRS. Many drugs, such as β-blockers and calcium-channel blockers, commonly cause first-degree AV block and should be considered a potential cause of any degree of AV block. Mobitz type II block (see Fig. 64-9 in Chapter 64) signifies that the level of AV block is below the AV node in the His-Purkinje system, which is not sensitive to autonomic tone; the resulting QRS is widened, and there is a high likelihood of progression to complete heart block (third-degree AV block; see Figs. 64-10 and 64-11 in Chapter 64). Intermittent complete heart block, which can result in drop attacks or Stokes-Adams attacks, is usually preceded by abnormal baseline findings on the ECG, such as a bundle branch block or second-degree AV block. The treatment of choice for symptomatic bradyarrhythmias or those likely to progress to complete heart block is implantation of a permanent pacemaker (Chapter 66).

Tachyarrhythmias

Tachyarrhythmias can arise from the atrium or AV node (supraventricular tachycardia) or from the ventricle (ventricular tachycardia). Supraventricular tachyarrhythmias that may be associated with palpitations, presyncope, or syncope include atrial tachycardia (see Fig. 64-18 in Chapter 64), AV nodal re-entrant tachycardia (see Fig. 64-19 in Chapter 64), AV junctional tachycardia (see Fig. 64-20 in Chapter 64), atrial flutter (see Fig. 64-23 in Chapter 64), and atrial fibrillation (see Fig. 64-24 in Chapter 64), sometimes in association with accessory conduction pathways that facilitate the re-entry needed to sustain the arrhythmia. Ventricular tachyarrhythmias include the various forms of ventricular tachycardia (see Fig. 65-3 in Chapter 65). Treatment is guided by the specific tachyarrhythmia and its underlying cause (see Table 62-3 and Tables 64-6 and 64-7 in Chapters 62 and 64, respectively) (Chapters 63 through 66).

Neurocardiogenic Syncope and Related Syndromes

Neurocardiogenic syncope is the sudden onset of lightheadedness or loss of consciousness as a result of autonomic reflexes and is more common in

TABLE 62-3 ARRHYTHMIC CAUSES OF PALPITATIONS AND SYNCOPE

ETIOLOGY	SPECIFIC ARRHYTHMIA	*Symptoms* PALPITATIONS	DIZZINESS	SYNCOPE	TREATMENT	COMMENTS
BRADYARRHYTHMIAS						
Sinus node dysfunction	Sinus bradycardia	No	Occasional	Rare	Pacemaker (if symptoms)	Can be seen in association with neurocardiogenic syncope
	Sinus arrest	Occasional	Yes	Occasional	Pacemaker	Pause >3 sec
	Sick sinus syndrome	Occasional	Yes	Occasional	Pacemaker	
AV nodal disease	First-degree AV block	No	No	No	None	
	Type I second-degree AV block	Occasional	No	No	None	Can be seen in association with neurocardiogenic syncope
	Type II second-degree AV block	Occasional	Rare	No	Pacemaker if severe	Can progress to complete heart block
	Third-degree AV block	Yes	Yes	Yes	Pacemaker	
Tachy-brady syndrome		Yes	Yes	Occasional	Treat tachycardia if possible Pacemaker	Can also be manifestation of sick sinus syndrome
TACHYARRHYTHMIAS						
SVT	Atrial tachycardia	Yes	Occasional	Rare	Ablation β-Blockers (e.g., metoprolol, atenolol)* Calcium-channel blockers (e.g., diltiazem)*	
	Atrial flutter	Yes	Occasional	Rare	Ablation Antiarrhythmic drugs (e.g., amiodarone)* Cardioversion (acute episode)	Often difficult to control rate
	Atrial fibrillation	Yes	Occasional	Rare	Ventricular rate control Warfarin Antiarrhythmic drugs (e.g., amiodarone)* Cardioversion (acute episode) Ablation	
	AV nodal re-entrant tachycardia	Yes	Yes	Rare	Ablation β-Blockers (e.g., metoprolol, atenolol)* Calcium-channel blockers (e.g., diltiazem)*	
	AV re-entrant tachycardia (WPW)	Yes	Yes	Rare	Ablation Antiarrhythmic drugs*	
VT	Idiopathic (RV outflow tract, fascicular)	Yes	Yes	Occasional	Ablation	Absence of structural heart disease Low risk of sudden death
	VT secondary to CAD, cardiomyopathy	Yes	Yes	Yes	ICD Amiodarone (400 mg qd)* Ablation	Increased incidence of sudden death
	Bundle branch re-entry	Yes	Yes	Yes	Ablation	Usually in the setting of LV dysfunction and baseline intraventricular conduction delay
	Genetic syndromes (e.g., long QT syndrome, Brugada's, arrhythmic right ventricular dysplasia)	Occasional	Yes	Yes	ICD	Not always a clear family history Increased incidence of sudden death
Ectopy	PACs	Occasional	No	No	None β-Blockers (e.g., atenolol, metoprolol) if symptomatic*	
	PVCs	Occasional	No	No	None β-Blockers (e.g., atenolol, metoprolol) if symptomatic*	Benign in absence of structural heart disease
NEUROCARDIOGENIC SYNCOPE		No	Yes	Yes	Behavioral (hydration, avoid triggers, abort episodes) Midodrine (10 mg tid)	

*See Table 64-7 in Chapter 64 for drug doses.
AV = atrioventricular; CAD = coronary artery disease; ICD = implantable cardioverter-defibrillator; LV = left ventricle; PACs = premature atrial contractions; PVCs = premature ventricular contractions; RV = right ventricle; SVT = supraventricular tachycardia; VT = ventricular tachycardia; WPW = Wolff-Parkinson-White syndrome.

younger patients (teenage to third decade of life). It is sometimes called a vasovagal episode, a common faint, or situational syncope if it is clearly induced by a particular activity (e.g., micturition syncope). In this form of neurocardiogenic syncope, heightened parasympathetic output, either due to direct stimulation (e.g., micturition, defecation, abdominal pain or other gastrointestinal conditions) or as a reflex in response to sympathetic stimulation (e.g., seeing blood, abrupt cessation of exercise), results in arterial dilation (called the vasodilatory response) and an inhibition of sinus and AV node activity (the cardioinhibitory response). The result is a transient decrease in blood pressure, often manifested as lightheadedness or syncope. Because they are associated with parasympathetic (vagal) output, episodes are frequently accompanied by nausea, diaphoresis, and salivation.

Treatment of this form of syncope can be challenging. The most effective therapies are behavioral (avoidance of triggers), wearing of compression stockings, and maintenance of adequate hydration and salt intake. Lying down with the feet elevated and performing isometric hand exercises may abort an acute episode. Medical therapy, including β-blockers (pindolol 5 to 15 mg twice daily), mineralocorticoids (fludrocortisone 0.1 mg/day), paroxetine (10 to 20 mg/day), and midodrine (an α-adrenergic agonist and vasoconstrictor; 2.5 to 5 mg three times daily), has shown some efficacy in reducing recurrence rates, although the efficacy of β-blockers for reducing syncopal episodes has been inconsistent. Even though bradycardia is a dominant feature of neurocardiogenic syncope, a pacemaker is not effective for the prevention of episodes because most patients also have a major vasodilatory component.

Rarely, situational syncope is associated with swallowing or coughing. Swallowing can trigger brain stem reflexes that lead to vagally induced bradyarrhythmias, with resultant syncope. This phenomenon may or may not be associated with severe pain in the tonsillar pillar, which may radiate to the ear (i.e., glossopharyngeal neuralgia; Chapter 405). The pain can usually be prevented by carbamazepine (400 to 1000 mg/day orally); in refractory cases, 300 mg/day of phenytoin can be added. Cough-related syncope can occur with severe, repeated coughing, which may increase thoracic pressure and result in increased vagal tone or a transient reduction in outflow from the intracranial veins, followed by a transient increase in intracranial pressure and impaired blood flow.

A related cause of syncope is carotid body hypersensitivity, in which vagal tone is increased by direct stimulation of the carotid body. This condition is frequently seen in older patients (particularly men older than 60 years), in whom episodes are associated with mechanical stimulation of the neck (e.g., turning the head, shaving, wearing a tight collar or necktie). Use of β-blockers, calcium-channel blockers, and digitalis can exacerbate or predispose to this condition. This form of syncope is diagnosed by documenting pauses longer than 3 seconds in response to carotid sinus massage and is curable with a pacemaker because carotid body stimulation does not cause significant vasodilation.

Postural or orthostatic hypotension can result in recurrent syncope. The history confirms that the patient is in the upright posture during spells, that the prodromal symptoms are those of cerebral hypoperfusion, and that the symptoms are relieved with recumbency. The diagnosis is supported by detecting a decrease of 30 mm Hg or greater in systolic blood pressure or a decrease of 10 mm Hg or greater in diastolic blood pressure between recumbent and upright postures. The many causes include drugs, polyneuropathies (Chapter 428), and neurodegenerative disorders (Chapter 416).

Cerebrovascular syncope results from cerebral hypoperfusion due to vascular phenomena, as opposed to generalized hypotension caused by arrhythmias or neurocardiogenic reflexes. Loss of consciousness can be a component of a basilar artery transient ischemic attack, but other brain stem symptoms nearly always precede or accompany the unconsciousness. Vertigo is most frequent, but diplopia or visual field disturbances, hemifacial or perioral numbness, and dysarthria or ataxia are also common. Recovery of consciousness may require 30 to 60 minutes. Although the diagnosis is suggested by the history and clinical presentation, imaging studies can be useful to confirm the diagnosis. Carotid Doppler studies may show various degrees of stenosis, especially in older patients. However, unconsciousness requires bihemispheric dysfunction; thus, unilateral carotid stenosis alone does not cause syncope. Transcranial Doppler studies or magnetic resonance angiography of the basilar artery is indicated only if brain stem ischemic symptoms are present in addition to loss of consciousness; false-positive tests are common, especially with increasing age. These patients, who are at risk for basilar artery stroke, should be treated with aspirin and should be considered for other treatments (e.g., surgery, stent placement) appropriate for their symptoms and anatomy (Chapter 414).

Other syndromes that can cause syncope include subclavian artery stenosis, which may result in retrograde blood flow from the vertebral artery to one arm, with resultant brain stem hypoperfusion (i.e., subclavian steal syndrome). Asymmetry in upper extremity systolic blood pressure, typically averaging 45 mm Hg, is nearly always present. Brain stem symptoms are similar to those in basilar transient ischemic attacks, including loss of consciousness, but a subsequent stroke from subclavian steal is rare. Repair of the stenosis is the treatment of choice. Syncope may also occur in up to 10% of patients with basilar artery migraine (Chapter 405). It can have a postural (orthostatic) manifestation or be associated with other basilar artery symptoms.

Neuropsychiatric syncope is a diagnosis of exclusion but is suggested by young age, frequent spells, multiple symptoms (e.g., dizziness, vertigo, lightheadedness, numbness), and duplication of the patient's symptoms by hyperventilation with the mouth open for 2 to 3 minutes. Whereas syncope and seizures occur with the eyes open, often with gaze deviation, psychogenic events frequently begin with eye closing.

Seizures (Chapter 410) can cause loss of consciousness and occasionally present clinically as syncope. However, seizures usually have a characteristic presentation and include a postictal phase, whereas most patients experiencing a syncopal episode quickly regain consciousness, except when cerebral perfusion is so compromised as to cause a secondary seizure or persistent anoxia and brain damage.

Diagnostic Tests

Electrocardiography

The baseline ECG is critical in the evaluation of a patient with palpitations or syncope. The presence of ventricular preexcitation, as manifested by a short PR interval and a delta wave (see Fig. 64-21 in Chapter 64), establishes the likely diagnosis of Wolff-Parkinson-White syndrome in a patient with palpitations and AV reciprocating tachycardia (Chapter 64); it can also be used to determine the location of the responsible accessory pathway. The baseline ECG provides useful predictive information about the likelihood of conduction system abnormalities being responsible for bradyarrhythmias (e.g., sinus bradycardia suggests sinus node dysfunction, a prolonged PR interval suggests AV nodal disease, and a widened QRS suggests disease below the AV node). The ECG is also useful in diagnosing prior myocardial infarction (i.e., pathologic Q waves), which raises the likelihood of ventricular tachycardia as a potential cause of syncope or palpitations. Abnormalities such as a prolonged QT interval in a patient with syncope and a family history of syncope or sudden death suggest one of the congenital long QT syndromes (Chapter 65). An incomplete right bundle branch block with coved ST segment elevation in ECG lead V_1 or V_2 in a patient with syncope or palpitations suggests Brugada's syndrome, whereas an epsilon wave, incomplete right bundle branch block, and inverted T waves in V_1 are suggestive of right ventricular dysplasia (Chapter 65). All these syndromes carry an increased risk of recurrent syncope and sudden death if untreated (Chapters 63 through 65).

Performing an ECG during an episode of palpitations is extremely useful in making a definitive diagnosis. For narrow–QRS complex tachycardias, the specific supraventricular tachycardia can often be surmised from the 12-lead ECG obtained during symptoms (Fig. 62-2). Moreover, for wide–QRS complex tachycardias, the 12-lead ECG is useful in distinguishing a supraventricular tachycardia (with aberrancy) from a ventricular tachycardia (Fig. 62-3). The presence of fusion beats or AV dissociation during a wide–QRS complex tachycardia leads to the diagnosis of ventricular tachycardia. For ventricular tachycardias, the morphology of the QRS complex is useful in determining the location of the ventricular tachycardia focus and in identifying idiopathic ventricular tachycardia (right ventricular outflow tract or fascicular), which has a much more benign course than ventricular tachycardia in the setting of coronary disease (Chapter 65).

The effect of carotid sinus massage, vagal maneuvers, or adenosine (given as a rapid intravenous bolus of 6 mg and repeated at a dose of 12 mg if the initial dose is ineffective) is also useful in narrowing the differential diagnosis of a tachycardia. These maneuvers slow conduction through the AV node. Therefore, tachycardias that terminate with either maneuver are likely to involve the AV node as a critical component of the re-entrant circuit (AV nodal re-entrant tachycardia or AV re-entrant tachycardia). If the maneuver induces AV block but does not terminate the arrhythmia, likely causes are atrial fibrillation, atrial flutter, and atrial tachycardias (or occasionally ventricular tachycardia if the QRS is wide). On rare occasions, atrial tachycardias and some idiopathic ventricular tachycardias terminate in response to

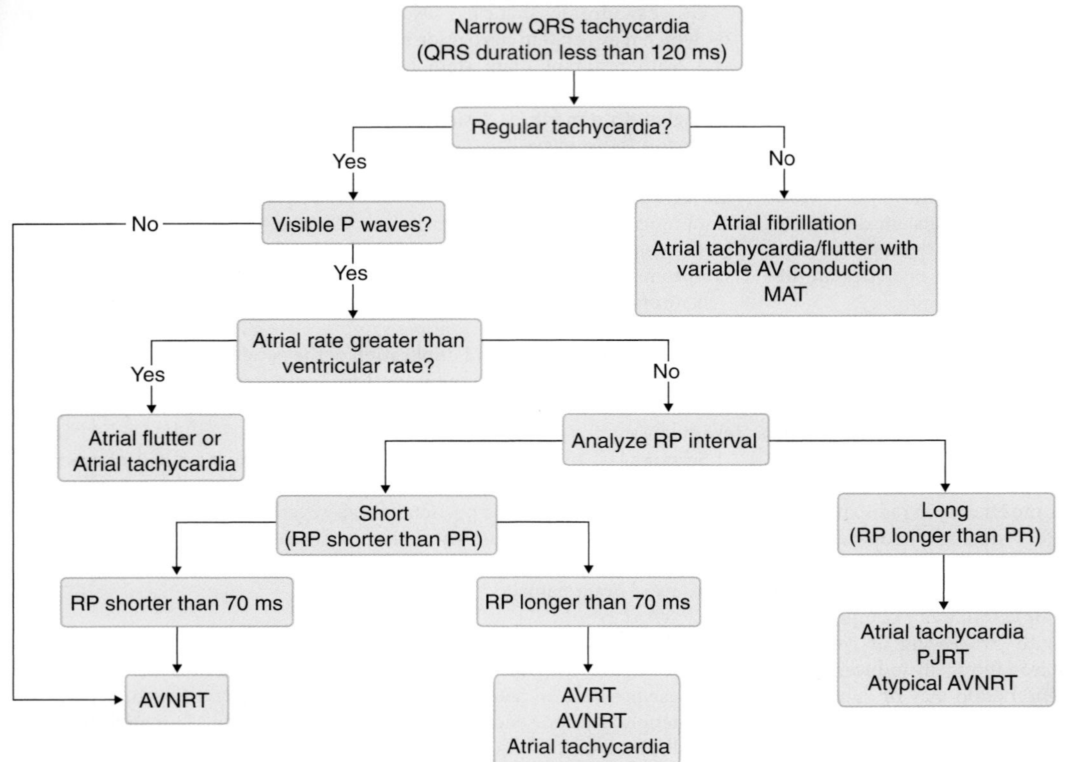

FIGURE 62-2. ECG algorithm for diagnosis of narrow-complex tachycardias. AVNRT = atrioventricular nodal reciprocating tachycardia; AVRT = atrioventricular reciprocating tachycardia; MAT = multifocal atrial tachycardia; PJRT = permanent form of junctional reciprocating tachycardia. (From Blomstrom-Lundqvist C, Scheinman MM, Aliot EM, et al. ACC/AHA/ESC guidelines for the management of patients with supraventricular arrhythmias—executive summary. *Circulation.* 2003;108:1871-1909.)

adenosine. Important clues to the specific mechanism can be obtained at the onset or termination of tachycardia, so obtaining a continuous 12-lead ECG during carotid sinus massage or the administration of adenosine is useful.

During bradycardias, the ECG is useful in determining the level of the conduction system (sinus node, AV node, or His bundle) responsible for the bradycardia. Sinus bradycardia is diagnosed when a slow (<50/minute at rest) atrial rate (P wave) conducts to the ventricle. Sinus arrest or sinus pauses (see Fig. 64-6 in Chapter 64) are diagnosed by absent or dropped P waves. First-degree AV block (see Fig. 64-7 in Chapter 64) is defined as a prolonged PR interval (>200 msec), and second-degree AV block is defined by P waves that occasionally do not conduct to the ventricle (P wave without an ensuing QRS); Mobitz type I second-degree AV block (also known as Wenckebach block; see Fig. 64-8 in Chapter 64) is characterized by progressive lengthening of the PR interval until one P wave does not conduct to the ventricle. This form of AV block is often seen in younger patients, is usually benign, and rarely progresses to complete AV (third-degree) block. Mobitz type II second-degree AV block (see Fig. 64-9 in Chapter 64), which is characterized by the sudden, unexpected loss of conduction of a P wave to the ventricle (dropped QRS), signifies disease of the His-Purkinje system and often progresses to complete heart block. Complete heart block or third-degree AV block (see Figs. 64-10 and 64-11 in Chapter 64) is diagnosed by the dissociation of P waves from QRS complexes, with an atrial rate faster than the ventricular rate.

Ambulatory Monitoring

For intermittent symptoms such as palpitations, dizziness, or syncope, it is often difficult to obtain a 12-lead ECG while the symptoms are occurring. Therefore, ambulatory monitoring, which allows ECG monitoring over long periods, is a vital diagnostic tool. There are currently three types of ambulatory monitors: Holter monitors, which continuously record the ECG for 24 to 48 hours; event recorders, which are wearable loop recorders that record only during specific events (when the patient activates the recorder because of symptoms or the recorder detects a heart rate above or below a specified threshold) and can be worn for 1 month or more; and implantable loop recorders, which function similarly to event recorders but can be used for up to 14 months. More recently, home telemetry units have been developed, allowing patients to undergo prolonged continuous remote monitoring by wireless or Internet connections. The choice of ambulatory monitoring method is largely determined by the frequency of the symptoms and the likelihood of capturing an episode during a given monitoring period.

Ambulatory monitoring is diagnostic only if abnormalities occur during symptoms or if the patient has typical symptoms without any concurrent abnormalities. A "normal" monitoring record is nondiagnostic if the patient does not have symptoms during the period.

Holter Monitors

Holter monitors use either a tape (in older devices) or digital media (in newer devices) to record a 3-, 5-, or 12-lead surface ECG continuously for 24 to 48 hours. Processing, printing, and analysis of the recordings are performed offline with commercial systems. In addition to recording the rhythm, analyses of heart rate variability and ST segment changes and accurate counts of PACs and PVCs can be automated. Some systems allow extrapolation to produce a "virtual" 12-lead recording at any time during the monitoring period. Holter monitoring is useful for detecting symptoms that are frequent (multiple times daily) and for diagnosing sinus node dysfunction (sinus node arrest, sick sinus syndrome) or intermittent AV block. It can also be useful to assess the adequacy of control of the ventricular rate in a patient with atrial fibrillation.

Event Monitors

Event monitors, also known as loop recorders, are designed to record intermittent episodes during long periods (weeks to months) and are thus useful for patients with less frequent symptoms. The system records the ECG into a loop buffer that is continuously updated and overwritten. The duration of memory varies from a few seconds to a few minutes and is usually programmable. When activated, the information is "locked" into memory and continues to record forward for a preprogrammed amount of time. Newer systems allow both patient-activated (when symptoms occur) and event-triggered (when the heart rate is above or below a preset threshold) recording. Some recorders have algorithms to detect and record atrial fibrillation automatically, regardless of the heart rate. After episodes have been recorded, the patient transmits the recording over the telephone to centralized receivers. Some event monitors require leads similar to Holter monitors, whereas others are worn on the wrist or are put into small credit card–sized devices that are placed on the chest during symptoms. The latter type is useful only in patients whose symptoms last for several minutes and who do not have syncope.

IMPLANTABLE LOOP RECORDERS. Implantable loop recorders are small devices with integrated leads that are implanted in a small subcutaneous pocket during a simple surgery, usually performed in the electrophysiology

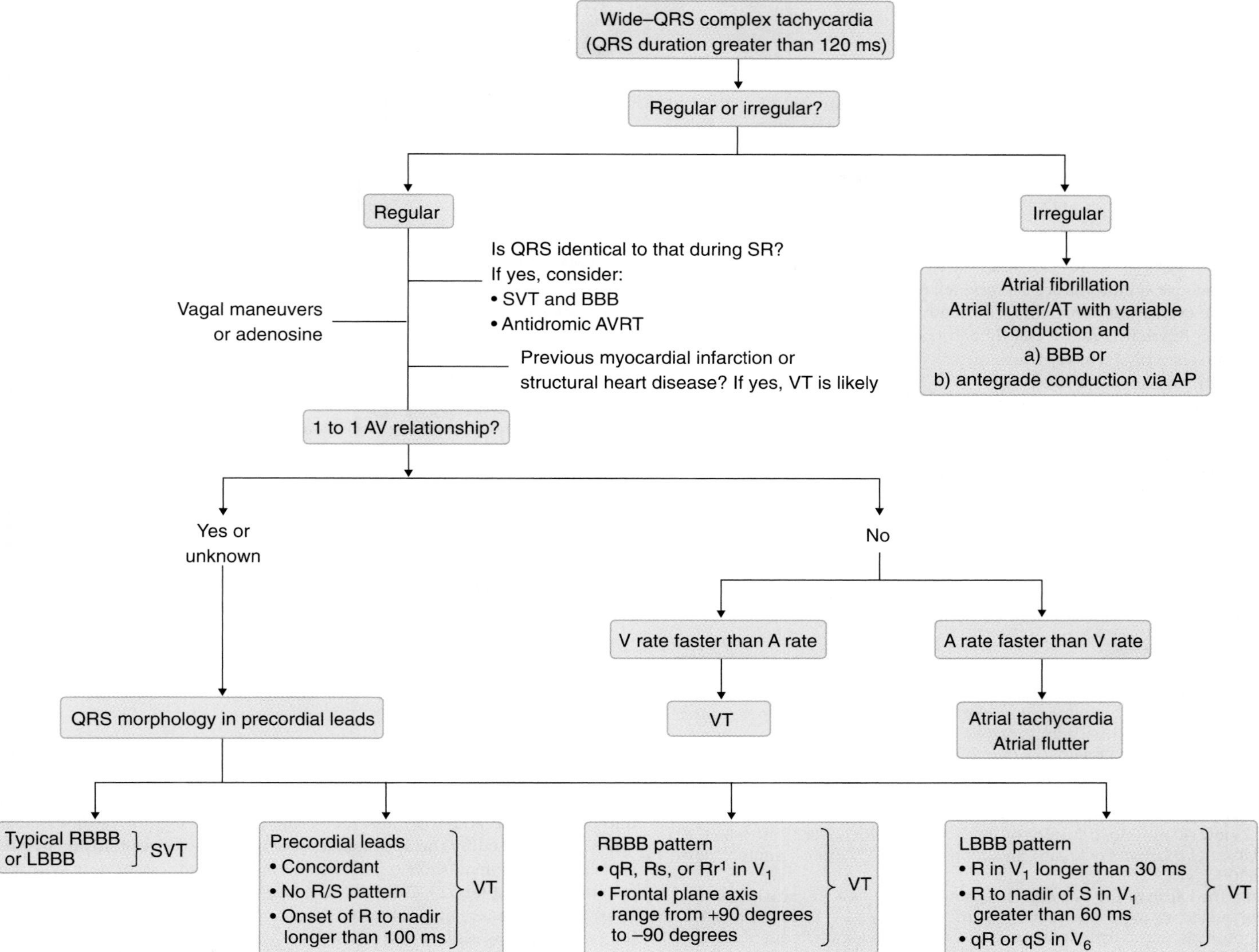

FIGURE 62-3. ECG algorithm for diagnosis of wide-complex tachycardias. A = atrial; AP = accessory pathway; AT = atrial tachycardia; AV = atrioventricular; AVRT = atrioventricular reciprocating tachycardia; BBB = bundle branch block; LBBB = left bundle branch block; RBBB = right bundle branch block; SR = sinus rhythm; SVT = supraventricular tachycardia; V = ventricular; VT = ventricular tachycardia. (From Blomstrom-Lundqvist C, Scheinman MM, Aliot EM, et al. ACC/AHA/ESC guidelines for the management of patients with supraventricular arrhythmias—executive summary. *Circulation.* 2003;108:1871-1909.)

laboratory. They function similarly to event recorders in terms of recording ECGs. Patients can activate the device with a small transmitter, or the device can be autotriggered on the basis of preprogrammed heart rates. The device can be interrogated by a computer, similar to the way pacemakers are interrogated to program the device's parameters and to retrieve ECGs that have been recorded. In patients with recurrent, difficult-to-diagnose syncope, an implantable loop recorder is better than the combination of tilt testing, an external loop recorder, and electrophysiologic testing.

Tilt Table Testing

Tilt table testing is used to confirm the diagnosis of neurocardiogenic syncope. The test involves continuous heart rate and blood pressure monitoring during head-up tilting. After baseline measurements in the supine position, the patient is tilted head-up at 60 to 80 degrees for 60 minutes. Some laboratories use isoproterenol or nitroglycerin as additional provocation. A positive result is a sudden and precipitous fall in blood pressure and heart rate, with concurrent reproducibility of symptoms (syncope). Because there is an appreciable false-positive rate, the test is best used as a confirmatory test in patients with a history suggestive of neurocardiogenic syncope or in patients with syncope in whom structural heart disease and other causes of syncope have been excluded.

Electrophysiologic Studies

Electrophysiologic studies involve the placement of several transvenous catheters in the heart to make temporary measurements of intracardiac electrograms and to perform pacing. Electrophysiologic studies are useful to identify the precise mechanism of tachyarrhythmias and are a necessary prelude to curative ablation (Chapter 66). Most arrhythmias, especially those with re-entrant mechanisms, can be readily induced during electrophysiologic studies. In addition, the existence and characteristics of accessory AV pathways (i.e., those responsible for Wolff-Parkinson-White syndrome or other re-entrant tachyarrhythmias) can be readily assessed by an electrophysiologic study. In patients with previous myocardial infarction, electrophysiologic studies are useful in determining the existence of a substrate for ventricular arrhythmias (Chapter 65), which may be treated with ablation or implantable defibrillators (Chapter 66). Electrophysiologic studies are also useful to determine the integrity of the conduction system and the precise mechanism of bradyarrhythmias that may be causing syncope. Therefore, electrophysiologic studies are indicated in patients with documented or suspected tachyarrhythmias as a prelude to curative ablation; in patients with a previous myocardial infarction and syncope, presyncope, or palpitations to exclude ventricular tachycardia; and in patients with severe or prolonged symptoms and no apparent diagnosis by history or ambulatory monitoring, especially in the setting of an abnormal ECG.

Other Tests

Echocardiography

Echocardiography (Chapter 55) can be useful to ensure that a patient does not have underlying structural heart disease, which can be an important prognostic factor in patients with ventricular tachycardia or syncope. Echocardiography should be performed in patients who present with syncope that is not obviously neurocardiogenic to ensure that there is no valvular or myocardial cause.

Exercise Testing

Exercise testing (Chapter 50) can be useful to assess arrhythmias, particularly in patients whose symptoms are exercise related. Exercise testing can also be useful in the evaluation of patients with bradyarrhythmias to diagnose chronotropic incompetence, and it can differentiate AV block due to autonomic tone (improves with exercise) from intrinsic conduction disease (generally worsens with an increasing rate).

Neurologic Testing

Routine electroencephalography (Chapter 403) is not helpful because a single study may be normal, even in epileptic patients. Structural brain diseases rarely cause episodic loss of consciousness, and routine brain imaging studies are indicated only in patients with focal neurologic findings. Carotid Doppler (Chapter 414) studies can document stenosis, but unconsciousness requires bihemispheric dysfunction. Transcranial Doppler or magnetic resonance angiography of the basilar artery is indicated only in patients with symptoms suggestive of brain stem ischemia.

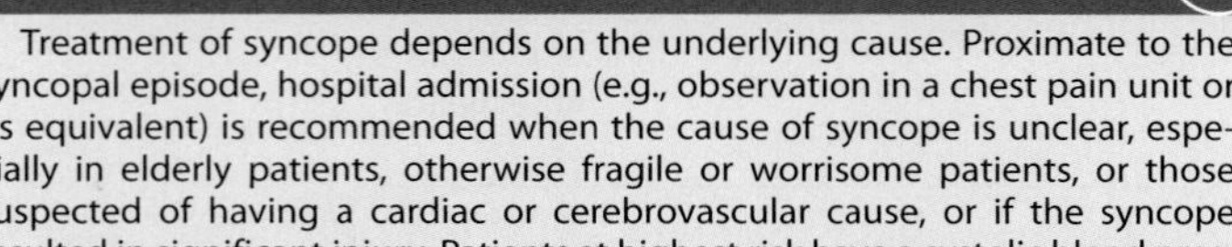

TREATMENT Rx

Treatment of syncope depends on the underlying cause. Proximate to the syncopal episode, hospital admission (e.g., observation in a chest pain unit or its equivalent) is recommended when the cause of syncope is unclear, especially in elderly patients, otherwise fragile or worrisome patients, or those suspected of having a cardiac or cerebrovascular cause, or if the syncope resulted in significant injury. Patients at highest risk have a systolic blood pressure below 90 mm Hg, a history of myocardial infarction or heart failure, a complaint of shortness of breath, an abnormal initial ECG, or a hematocrit less than 30%.

Until the cause of the syncope is determined and treated, patients should be instructed to avoid situations that may cause injury as a result of the syncope, especially if there is no prodrome and episodes are frequent. Careful consideration should be given to driving restrictions, which may be mandatory depending on local laws, and restrictions on dangerous work-related activity (e.g., for pilots, heavy machine operators, bus drivers) until definitive therapy is given.

In patients with a cardiac cause of syncope, targeted treatments include valve replacement for aortic stenosis (Chapter 75); medications for hypertrophic cardiomyopathy (Chapter 60); cardioversion, a pacemaker, an implantable cardioverter-defibrillator, ablation, or medications for tachyarrhythmias (Table 62-3; Chapters 63 through 65); and fluid repletion for orthostatic hypotension.

In patients with neurocardiogenic syncope, behavioral guidance should encourage an increased intake of fluid and salt, as well as the avoidance of situations that precipitate symptoms. Patients should also be taught how to tense their arms and legs and grip their hands during prodromal symptoms to increase peripheral resistance and systemic blood pressure.[2] If neurocardiogenic syncope recurs despite education and lifestyle changes, fludrocortisone (0.1 mg/day, starting dose) can expand intravascular volume but has not been proved to prevent syncope. Midodrine (usually 10 mg three times daily), an α_1-receptor agonist and vasoconstrictor, has shown potential benefit,[3] but other α-agonists have not. Paroxetine (20 mg/day), a selective serotonin re-uptake inhibitor, reduced recurrent neurocardiogenic syncope in one trial of very symptomatic patients but otherwise has been disappointing.[3] In randomized trials, β-blockers have not been useful. Pacemakers do not reduce recurrent neurocardiogenic syncope,[4] but they are very effective in patients with cardioinhibitory syncope as a result of severe bradycardia.[3]

PROGNOSIS

One syncopal event predicts a substantial risk for recurrent syncope. Although syncope itself does not appear to increase the risk of death, patients with cardiac or cerebrovascular causes have higher mortality rates than patients with definable noncardiac causes or those without a definable cause. Among patients who come to an emergency department, the overall death rate of about 7.5% at 1 year reflects patients' underlying abnormalities.

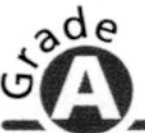

1. Krahn AD, Klein GJ, Yee R, et al. Randomized assessment of syncope trial: conventional diagnostic testing versus a prolonged monitoring strategy. *Circulation.* 2001;104:46-54.
2. van Dijk N, Quartieri F, Blanc JJ, et al. Effectiveness of physical counterpressure maneuvers in preventing vasovagal syncope: the Physical Counterpressure Manoeuvres Trial (PC-Trial). *J Am Coll Cardiol.* 2006;48:1652-1657.
3. Moya A, Sutton R, Ammirati F, et al. Guidelines for the diagnosis and management of syncope (version 2009): the Task Force for the Diagnosis and Management of Syncope of the European Society of Cardiology (ESC). *Eur Heart J.* 2009;30:2631-2671.
4. Connelly SJ, Sheldon R, Thorpe KE, et al. Pacemaker therapy for prevention of syncope in patients with recurrent severe vasovagal syncope: Second Vasovagal Pacemaker Study (VPS II): a randomized trial. *JAMA.* 2003;289:2224-2229.

SUGGESTED READINGS

Duncan GW, Tan MP, Newton JL, et al. Vasovagal syncope in the older person: differences in presentation between older and younger patients. *Age Ageing.* 2010;39:465-470. *Older patients were more likely to fall and less likely to report palpitations or to lose consciousness totally.*

Thavendiranathan P, Bagai A, Khoo C, et al. Does this patient with palpitations have a cardiac arrhythmia? *JAMA.* 2009;302:2135-2143. *Review.*

Zimetbaum P, Goldman A. Ambulatory arrhythmia monitoring: choosing the right device. *Circulation.* 2010;122:1629-1636. *Review emphasizing the role of loop recorders and post-event recorders.*

63

APPROACH TO CARDIAC ARREST AND LIFE-THREATENING ARRHYTHMIAS

ROBERT J. MYERBURG AND AGUSTIN CASTELLANOS

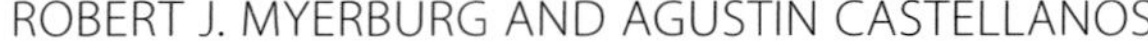

Cardiac arrest is characterized by an abrupt loss of consciousness because of absence of blood flow owing to loss of cardiac pumping action. If not treated promptly, it will lead to central nervous system injury or death within minutes. Cardiac arrest is often forewarned by a change in cardiovascular status, as indicated by the appearance or worsening of symptoms related to transient arrhythmias, such as palpitations, lightheadedness, or near-syncope or syncope (Chapter 62). Other forewarnings may include new or worsening chest pain, dyspnea, or weakness. These warning symptoms, however, are limited by their sensitivity and predictive power in individual patients. Moreover, cardiac arrest may occur unexpectedly as a first cardiac event in an apparently healthy individual, in a patient with known previous cardiac disease, or as the final event in any fatal disease.

The most common electrical mechanisms of cardiac arrest are the ventricular tachyarrhythmias (Chapter 65)—ventricular fibrillation (VF) or pulseless ventricular tachycardia (VT). In a substantial minority of cardiac arrests, severe bradyarrhythmia, asystole, or pulseless electrical activity is the first rhythm abnormality noted. The latter may be the primary mechanism of the cardiac arrest or a result of deterioration of VT/VF. Pulseless electrical activity or asystole may also be seen after termination of VT/VF by electrical cardioversion. Pulseless electrical activity is defined as secondary when it occurs in the setting of predisposing factors, such as hypoxia or other metabolic disorders, and primary when it is the initial rhythm noted in patients with predisposing cardiac disorders. The probability of survival after intervention is far better for ventricular tachyarrhythmias than for bradyarrhythmic or asystolic mechanisms. The interval between cardiac arrest and the initiation of resuscitation and cardioversion is the major determinant of survival.

PREDISPOSING WIDE-QRS COMPLEX TACHYCARDIAS

Sustained tachycardias with wide QRS complexes should be considered of ventricular origin and potentially high risk until determined otherwise. Most wide-QRS tachycardias are initially approached as a medical urgency or emergency, whereas most narrow-QRS tachycardias of supraventricular origin are approached with less urgency (Chapters 64 and 65).

Management of Sustained Ventricular Tachycardia

Sustained VT occurs most commonly in the presence of structural heart disease and must be interpreted as a forewarning of fatal arrhythmia in that setting. It is characterized by QRS complexes that are usually longer than 0.12

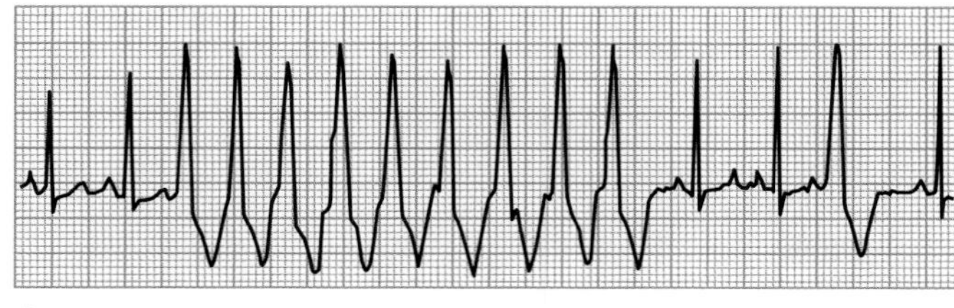

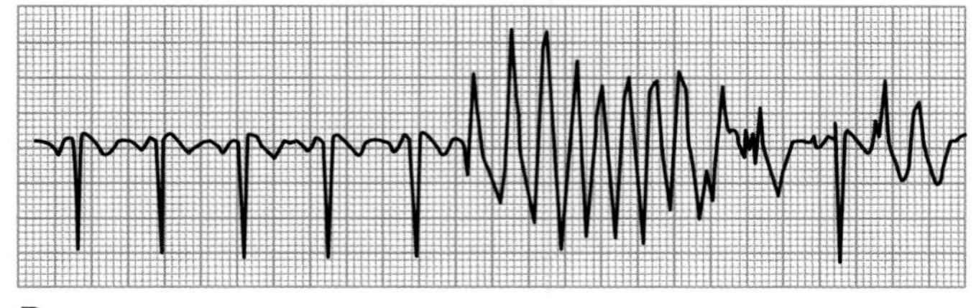

FIGURE 63-1. Nonsustained ventricular tachycardia. Monomorphic patterns **(A)** are characterized by a slower and more stable electrical pattern than polymorphic patterns **(B)**. Both have long-term prognostic implications in patients with advanced structural heart disease, but monomorphic patterns tend to be more stable over the short term.

second, with a mean vector that is markedly different from the QRS vector of normally conducted impulses. The rate of most VTs is between 140 and 200 impulses per minute, but rates may be slower or faster. VT may be electrically stable (such as monomorphic VT patterns at relatively slow rates; Fig. 63-1A) or unstable (such as polymorphic VTs or monomorphic VTs at rates exceeding 190 to 200 per minute; see Fig. 63-1B) (Chapter 65). Slower monomorphic VT may be better tolerated, whereas rapid VT is often associated with hemodynamic instability. In the latter circumstance, VT must be managed as a life-threatening or imminently fatal event, analogous to a VT/VF cardiac arrest (see later) that is usually treated with electrical cardioversion as initial therapy. Long-term management strategies, often involving consideration of implantable cardioverter-defibrillator therapy, are based on consideration of the likelihood of recurrent tachycardias and the extent of underlying disease (Chapter 65). Some well-tolerated, slow monomorphic VTs, especially in the absence of structural heart disease, may be more benign and treated with less urgency, usually with antiarrhythmic drugs or β-adrenergic blocking agents (see Table 64-5 in Chapter 64).

Distinguishing Supraventricular from Ventricular Tachycardias

It is important to distinguish between supraventricular tachycardia (SVT) (Chapter 64) and VT for both risk prediction and therapy. Although it is generally assumed that narrow-QRS tachycardias are supraventricular in origin, VT occasionally has a narrow QRS complex on a one- or two-lead rhythm strip, thereby mimicking SVT. Whenever possible, the diagnosis of tachycardia should be based on a 12-lead electrocardiogram (ECG). However, a standard ECG will not always suffice because patients with intraventricular conduction abnormalities (such as a left or right bundle branch block) will have wide-complex tachycardias during SVTs, usually with a QRS vector similar to that seen in normal sinus rhythm. In addition, when an SVT is very rapid, a functional bundle branch block may generate a widened QRS duration and shift the axis transiently. In both these examples, the wide QRS may mimic VT, and it may be necessary to perform an electrophysiologic study to determine the diagnosis (Chapter 62).

When wide-complex SVT is suspected clinically, transient vagal stimulation by carotid sinus massage or an atrioventricular nodal blocking agent, such as intravenous adenosine (see Table 64-5 in Chapter 64), may be useful for slowing the rate or terminating an SVT. Intravenous calcium-blocking agents generally should not be used for the diagnosis or treatment of wide-QRS tachycardias, especially in the presence of structural heart disease, because of their myocardial depressant effects. The exception is when it is known with certainty that the tachycardia is an SVT in a patient with normal or near-normal left ventricular function.

SVTs can result in a risk for generating life-threatening ventricular arrhythmias in two circumstances. One is in patients with high-grade coronary artery stenoses, in whom rapid heart rates can cause myocardial ischemia because of the dependence of coronary blood flow on the diastolic interval; the arrhythmia should be treated urgently, usually by electrical direct current (DC) cardioversion (Chapter 66), unless specific medical therapy is available and controls the rate promptly (Chapter 64). The second is in patients with Wolff-Parkinson-White syndrome, who may have ventricular rates greater than 300 beats per minute during atrial fibrillation when the accessory pathway has a short refractory period (see Fig. 64-19 in Chapter 64). This arrhythmia, which can cause hypotensive VT or VF, requires prompt therapy (Chapter 64).

GENERAL MANAGEMENT OF CARDIAC ARREST

Basic life-support (BLS) and advanced cardiac life support (ACLS) strategies for initial and definitive responses to cardiac arrest have improved survival in victims of cardiac arrest. The principles of BLS and ACLS apply to both in-hospital and out-of-hospital cardiac arrest, but their applications and outcomes depend on the setting. In the hospital, the probability of survival is determined by the specific patient category (acute syndromes better than end-stage diseases), the mechanism of cardiac arrest (better for tachyarrhythmias than for bradyarrhythmias, asystole, or pulseless electrical activity), and the hospital site (better in intensive care units or other monitored settings than on an unmonitored general care unit). In many acute care settings, including patients with acute coronary syndromes (Chapters 72 and 73), outcomes can be excellent. For other in-hospital settings and most out-of-hospital settings, the absolute number and proportion of survivors remain low, except in unique out-of-hospital settings that can provide an extraordinarily rapid response time to victims in VF or VT. When immediate defibrillation in highly protected environments is available, such as monitored intensive care units and electrophysiology laboratories, where response times of less than 60 seconds are the norm, the survival rate after VF is greater than 90% in the absence of pathophysiologic conditions that favor persistence of the potentially fatal arrhythmia.

Once 2 to 3 minutes have elapsed from the onset of cardiac arrest to attempted defibrillation, the survival probability falls below 50% in most in-hospital and out-of-hospital circumstances. Survival rates continue to fall rapidly thereafter, decreasing to 25% or less by 4 to 6 minutes and less than 10% by 10 minutes. Although immediate defibrillation is the preferred method within the first few minutes after the onset of cardiac arrest, a brief period of cardiopulmonary resuscitation (CPR) to provide oxygenation of the victim improves survivability when the time to defibrillation exceeds 4 to 5 minutes.

Basic Life Support

The activities included within BLS encompass the initial responses for diagnostic evaluation, followed by a seamless flow into establishing ventilation and perfusion through the techniques of CPR or the newly proposed concept of cardiocerebral resuscitation (see later). The first action is to confirm that the collapse is the result of a cardiac arrest. After an initial evaluation for response to voice or tactile stimulation, observation for respiratory movements and skin color, and simultaneous palpation of major arteries for the presence of a pulse, the determination that a life-threatening incident is in progress should immediately prompt a call to an emergency medical rescue system (911).

The absence of respiratory efforts, or the presence of only gasping agonal respirations in conjunction with an absent pulse, is diagnostic of cardiac arrest. Although the absence of a carotid or femoral pulse is a primary diagnostic criterion for the health care professional, palpation for a pulse is no longer recommended for lay responders. The absence of respiratory efforts or severe stridor with *persistence of a pulse* suggests a primary respiratory arrest that may lead to cardiac arrest in a short time; skin color may be pale or intensely cyanotic. In the latter circumstance, initial efforts should include oropharyngeal exploration in search of a foreign body and the Heimlich maneuver, which entails wrapping the arms around the victim from the back and delivering a sharp thrust to the upper part of the abdomen with a closed fist, particularly in a setting in which aspiration is likely (e.g., collapse in a restaurant).

Once a pulseless cardiac arrest is established, a blow to the chest (precordial thump) may be attempted by a properly trained rescuer as part of an initial response when monitoring and a defibrillator are not immediately available. A precordial thump should not be used in an unmonitored patient with a perceptible rapid tachycardia or without complete loss of consciousness because of concern about converting organized electrical activity into VF. The technique involves one or two blows delivered firmly to the junction of the middle and lower thirds of the sternum from a height of 8 to 10 inches, but the effort should be abandoned if a spontaneous pulse does not immediately occur or if the patient begins to breathe.

The precordial thump should be followed immediately by the initiation of CPR so as to maintain viability of the central nervous system, heart, and other vital organs until a definitive intervention can be carried out. CPR can be performed by professional and paraprofessional personnel, by experienced emergency medical technicians, and by trained laypersons. Time is the key element for success, and there should be minimal delay between the diagnosis and preparatory efforts in the initial response and institution of CPR. If only one witness is present, the only activity that should precede BLS is telephone contact (911) of emergency personnel.

Clearing the airway, which is a critical step in preparing for successful resuscitation, includes tilting the head backward and lifting the chin, in addition to exploring the airway for foreign bodies—including dentures—and removing them. The Heimlich maneuver should be performed if there is reason to suspect a foreign body lodged in the oropharynx, as suggested by severe respiratory stridor rather than by slow agonal respirations or apnea. When the person at the scene has insufficient physical strength to perform the maneuver, mechanical dislodgement of a foreign body can sometimes be achieved by abdominal thrusts with the unconscious patient in a supine position. If there is suspicion that respiratory arrest precipitated the cardiac arrest, particularly in the presence of a mechanical airway obstruction, a second precordial thump should be delivered after the airway has been cleared.

With the head properly placed and the oropharynx clear, mouth-to-mouth respiration can be initiated, but bystander compression-only CPR is as good as, if not better than, compression plus mouth-to-mouth respiration.[1] A variety of devices are available for establishing ventilation, including plastic oropharyngeal airways, esophageal obturators for establishing ventilation, a masked Ambu bag, and endotracheal tubes. Intubation is the preferred procedure, but time should not be sacrificed, even in the in-hospital setting, while awaiting an endotracheal tube or a person trained to insert it quickly and properly. Temporary support with Ambu bag ventilation is the usual method in the hospital until endotracheal intubation can be accomplished; in the out-of-hospital setting, mouth-to-mouth resuscitation is performed while awaiting emergency rescue personnel. The lungs should be inflated twice in succession after every 30 chest compressions.

The third element of BLS, circulation, is intended to maintain blood flow until definitive steps can be taken. The rationale is based on the hypothesis that chest compression maintains an externally driven pump function by sequential emptying and filling of its chambers, with competent valves favoring the forward direction of flow. The palm of one hand is placed over the lower part of the sternum while the heel of the other rests on the dorsum of the lower hand. The sternum is then depressed with the resuscitator's arms straight at the elbows to provide a less tiring and more forceful fulcrum at the junction of the shoulders and back. With this technique, sufficient force is applied to depress the sternum about 4 to 5 cm, with abrupt relaxation. The cycle is carried out at a rate of about 100 compressions per minute. In the 2005 modification of guidelines for emergency cardiac care, the integration of respiratory and compression actions was changed to a compression-ventilation ratio of 30 : 2 for single responders to victims from infancy (excluding newborns) through adulthood, and two responders for adults. For two-rescuer CPR for infants and children, the former compression-ventilation ratio of 15 : 2 was retained. Another recently suggested modification, which is intended to encourage more bystander CPR by untrained or remotely trained bystanders who lack confidence, is the "hands-only" (cardiac-only, compression-only) technique, which uses 200 successive compressions without interruption. This variation, which may be more effective than compression-ventilation sequences, also allays concerns about bystander mouth-to-mouth ventilation of unknown victims in the absence of mechanical airway devices.

Automated External Defibrillators—Intermediate Life Support

Because time to defibrillation is the major determinant of survival, despite any temporizing benefit of BLS, and because ACLS strategies are generally implemented by in-hospital personnel or out-of-hospital emergency medical rescue system responders, an intermediate strategy has emerged that is based on the availability of automated external defibrillators (AEDs) for use by nonconventional first responders. Referred to as public access defibrillation or lay first-responder systems, the strategy relies on devices that prompt the user to deliver a defibrillation shock when deemed appropriate by a computerized rhythm detection system in the device. The operators can be trained police officers, security guards, airline personnel, or trained (or even untrained) lay responders (Table 63-1). A number of studies have suggested improved survival rates when such strategies are deployed in public sites, but an initial study of a home deployment strategy was disappointing.[2] Further study is warranted because most out-of-hospital cardiac arrests occur at home. AED programs are not a replacement for ACLS (see later), but rather an intermediate supplement to the BLS-ACLS sequence that is intended to attempt earlier defibrillation while awaiting the arrival of ACLS-trained emergency rescue personnel.

Advanced Cardiac Life Support

ACLS methods, other than those directly related to control of tachyarrhythmias, have led to the generation of comprehensive protocols to guide responders over a broad expanse of clinical circumstances and mechanisms of cardiac arrest ranging from transient clinical events to end-stage multisystem disease. The general goals of ACLS are to restore a hemodynamically effective cardiac rhythm, optimize ventilation, and maintain and support the restored circulation. During ACLS, the patient's cardiac rhythm is promptly cardioverted or defibrillated as the first priority, if appropriate equipment is immediately available. If cardiac arrest has lasted for 4 to 5 minutes before the availability of a defibrillator, a short period of closed-chest cardiac compression immediately before defibrillation increases the probability of survival.[3] Additional survival benefit has not been observed for delays greater than 10 minutes.

After the initial attempt to restore a hemodynamically effective rhythm, the patient is intubated and oxygenated, if needed, and the heart is paced if a bradyarrhythmia or asystole occurs. An intravenous line is established to deliver medications. After intubation, the goal of ventilation is to reverse hypoxemia and not merely to achieve a high alveolar Po_2. When available, oxygen rather than room air should be used to ventilate the patient, and arterial O_2 saturation should be monitored, when possible. In the out-of-hospital setting, a face mask or an Ambu bag by means of an endotracheal tube is generally used.

TABLE 63-1 AUTOMATED EXTERNAL DEFIBRILLATOR STRATEGIES FOR RAPID RESPONSE TO CARDIAC ARRESTS CAUSED BY VENTRICULAR FIBRILLATION

DEPLOYMENT	EXAMPLES	RESCUERS	ADVANTAGES	LIMITATIONS
Emergency vehicles	Police cars Fire engines Ambulances	Trained emergency personnel	Experienced users Broad deployment Objectivity	Deployment time Arrival delays Community variations
Public access sites	Public buildings Stadiums, malls Airports Airliners	Security personnel Designated rescuers Random laypersons	Population density Shorter delays Lay and emergency personnel access	Low event rates Inexperienced users Panic and confusion
Multifamily dwellings	Apartments Condominiums Hotels	Security personnel Designated rescuers Family members	Familiar locations Defined personnel Shorter delays	Infrequent use Low event rates Geographic factors
Single-family dwellings	Private homes Apartments Neighborhood "Heart Watch"	Family members	Immediate access Familiar setting	Acceptance Victim may be alone One-time user; panic

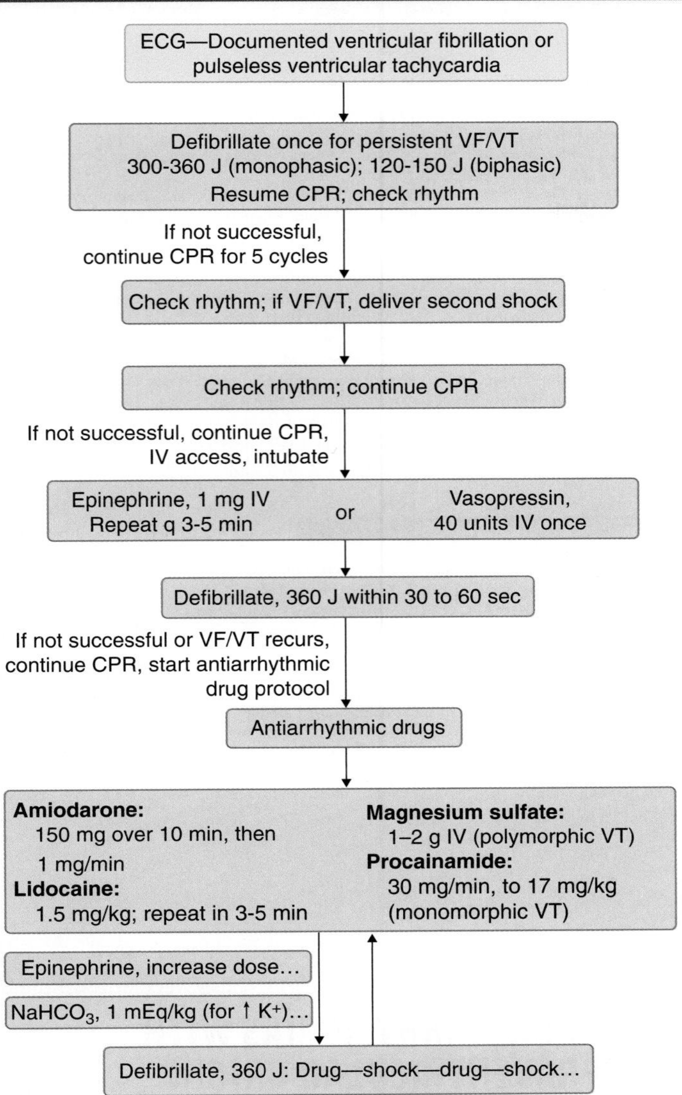

FIGURE 63-2. General algorithm for advanced cardiac life support (ACLS) response to ventricular fibrillation (VF) or pulseless ventricular tachycardia (VT). For more detail, see the ACLS guidelines in Suggested Readings. *Note:* In a 2008 advisory, 200 compression-only sequences were suggested as an alternative to standard CPR cycles between shocks, and this approach is under consideration for future guidelines. CPR = cardiopulmonary resuscitation; ECG = electrocardiogram.

MANAGEMENT OF TACHYARRHYTHMIC CARDIAC ARRESTS

Direct Current Cardioversion

When VF or a rapid VT is identified on a monitor or by telemetry, defibrillation should be performed immediately (Fig. 63-2). When a reversible cause, such as an acute ischemic syndrome or electrolyte disturbance, is the mechanism, normal rhythm can be successfully restored in up to 90% of VF victims weighing up to 90 kg with a DC monophasic shock of up to 360 J, or a with a biphasic shock of up to 200 J, delivered within 2 to 3 minutes. Failure of the initial shock to restore an effective rhythm is a poor prognostic sign. Although some algorithms suggest a succession of monophasic shock energies from 200 to 360 J, or biphasic waveforms from 100 to 200 Joules, during a sequence of attempts to defibrillate, there is little to be gained from beginning with energies less than 300 J monophasic or less than 150 J biphasic during a cardiac arrest response.

After a single shock at 300 or 360 J of monophasic energy, or 150 or 200 J biphasic, the patient should be checked for restoration of a spontaneous pulse; CPR should be continued for five cycles if a pulse remains absent. Subsequently, a second shock should be delivered, followed by epinephrine, 1 mg intravenously (IV). If a pulse is still absent, CPR is repeated for five cycles before the next shock. Epinephrine may be repeated at 3- to 5-minute intervals with defibrillator shocks in between, but high-dose epinephrine does not appear to provide added benefit. Vasopressin, 40 U given IV once, is an equally good alternative to epinephrine,[4] but the combination does not appear to be better than either one alone.[5]

This algorithm is based on the 2005 update. In a 2008 advisory, use of 200 compression-only sequences was suggested as an alternative to standard CPR cycles between shocks.

Pharmacotherapy for Resistant Arrhythmias

For a patient who continues in VF or pulseless VT despite multiple attempts at DC cardioversion after epinephrine, or who has recurrent episodes of VF or VT after cardioversion, electrical stability may be achieved by administering intravenous antiarrhythmic agents while continuing resuscitative efforts (see Fig. 63-2). Amiodarone (150 mg IV over a 10-minute period, followed by 1 mg/minute for up to 6 hours and 0.5 mg/minute thereafter) is the initial treatment of choice.[6] Additional bolus dosing, to a maximum of 500 mg, can be tried if the initial bolus is unsuccessful. Amiodarone need not be given as a routine to individuals who respond to initial defibrillation with a persistently stable rhythm, but it is preferred for those who have recurrent episodes of VT or VF after initial defibrillation and oxygenation.

If there is sufficient clinical evidence that the cardiac arrest was heralded by the onset of an acute coronary syndrome, lidocaine (1.0- to 1.5-mg/kg bolus given IV, with the dose repeated in 2 minutes) may be used instead of amiodarone, or if amiodarone has failed. When acute or intermittent ischemia is not thought to be the mechanism, intravenous amiodarone is the preferred initial drug, but lidocaine may be tried if amiodarone fails. Intravenous procainamide (loading infusion of 100 mg/5 minutes to a total dose of 500 to 800 mg, followed by a continuous infusion at 2 to 5 mg/minute) is now rarely used but may be tried in those with persisting, hemodynamically unstable arrhythmias.

In patients with acute hyperkalemia as the triggering event for resistant VF, hypocalcemia, or arrest potentially caused by excess doses of calcium-blocking drugs, 10% calcium gluconate (5 to 20 mL infused at a rate of 2 to 4 mL/minute) may be helpful. Otherwise, calcium should not be used routinely during resuscitation, even though ionized Ca^{2+} levels may be low during resuscitation from cardiac arrest.

Some resistant forms of polymorphic VT (*torsades de pointes*), rapid monomorphic VT, ventricular flutter (rate > 260/minute), or resistant VF respond to $MgSO_4$ (1 to 2 g IV given over a 1- to 2-minute period) or to β-blocker therapy (propranolol, 1-mg boluses IV to a total dose of up to 15 to 20 mg; or metoprolol, 5 mg IV, up to 20 mg). $MgSO_4$ is specifically indicated for polymorphic VTs due to inherited or acquired (drug-induced) long QT patterns (Chapter 65). This VT pattern also occurs with marked hypokalemia, so 20 mEq/hour of intravenous potassium chloride should be included in the treatment of patients who have a serum K^+ of less than 3 mEq/L and whose polymorphic VT is resistant to other therapies. However, hypokalemia also may follow the acid-base and electrolyte shifts associated with prolonged arrests and should not be considered a primary cause of the cardiac arrest in that circumstance.

MANAGEMENT OF CARDIAC ARREST CAUSED BY ASYSTOLE, BRADYARRHYTHMIAS, OR PULSELESS ELECTRICAL ACTIVITY

The approach to a patient with bradyarrhythmic or asystolic arrest or with pulseless electrical activity differs from the approach to patients with tachyarrhythmic events (VT/VF). Once this form of cardiac arrest is recognized, efforts should focus on first establishing control of the patient's cardiorespiratory status (i.e., continue CPR, intubate, and establish intravenous access), then reconfirming the rhythm (in two leads if possible), and finally taking actions that favor the emergence of a stable spontaneous rhythm or attempt to pace the heart. Possible reversible causes, particularly for bradyarrhythmia and asystole, should be considered and excluded (or treated) promptly (Fig. 63-3), including hypovolemia, hypoxia, cardiac tamponade, tension pneumothorax, preexisting acidosis, drug overdose, hypothermia, and hyperkalemia. Epinephrine (1.0 mg IV every 3 to 5 minutes) and atropine (1.0 to 2.0 mg IV) or isoproterenol (up to 15 to 20 μg/minute IV), which are commonly used in an attempt to elicit spontaneous electrical activity or increase the rate of a bradycardia, have only limited success. In the absence of an intravenous line, epinephrine (1 mg, i.e., 10 mL of a 1 : 10,000 solution) may be given by the intracardiac route, but there is danger of coronary or myocardial laceration. Sodium bicarbonate, 1 mEq/kg, may be tried for known or

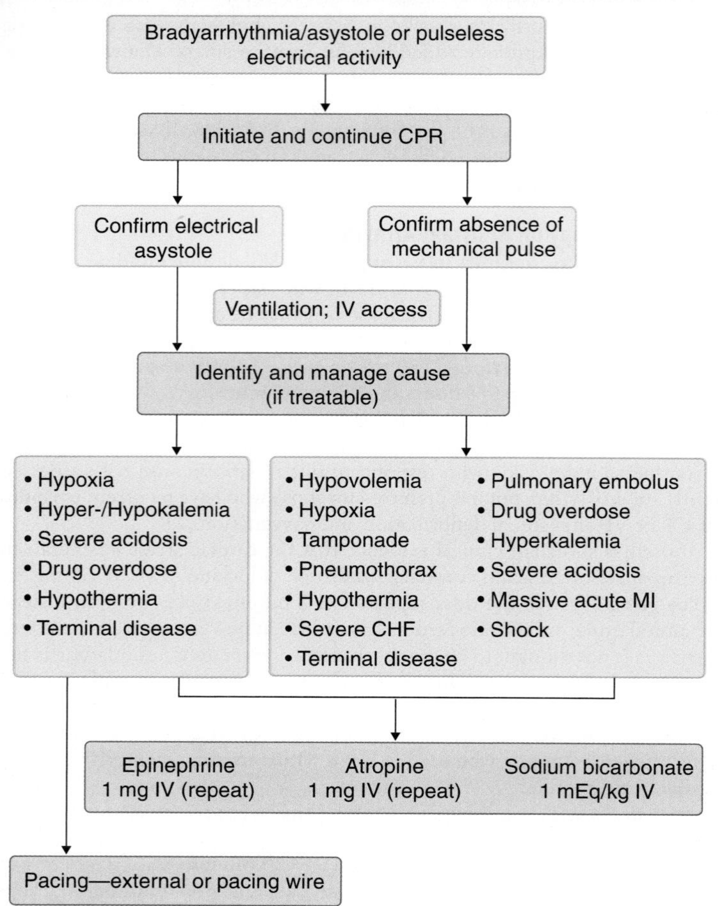

FIGURE 63-3. General algorithm for advanced cardiac life support response to bradycardic or asystolic cardiac arrest or pulseless electrical activity. For more detail, see Suggested Readings. CHF = congestive heart failure; CPR = cardiopulmonary resuscitation; MI = myocardial infarction.

strongly suspected preexisting hyperkalemia or bicarbonate-responsive acidosis.

External pacing systems (Chapter 66) should be used for out-of-hospital bradycardic or asystolic arrest, although its influence on outcome is not well documented. In the hospital setting, external pacing is generally used during the initial response to a bradycardic or asystolic arrest, but it should be superseded by transvenous pacing if the arrest is prolonged, if continuous pacing is needed, or if the external device fails to pace. Unfortunately, an *asystolic* patient continues to have a very poor prognosis despite available techniques.

ADJUNCTIVE THERAPEUTIC ACTIONS

During or after therapy targeted to restoration of an electrically stable cardiac rhythm, the patient's general metabolic state should be addressed by improving oxygenation and reversing acidosis. Intravenous sodium bicarbonate (1 mEq/kg), with up to 50% of this dose repeated every 10 to 15 minutes during the course of CPR, is recommended for patients with known or suspected preexisting bicarbonate-responsive causes of acidosis, for certain drug overdoses (Chapter 110), and after prolonged and unsuccessful attempts at resuscitation. Caution must be exercised, however, because excessive quantities of sodium bicarbonate can be deleterious by causing alkalosis, hypernatremia, and hyperosmolality. When possible, arterial pH, Po_2, and Pco_2 should be monitored during the resuscitation. In addition, moderate therapeutic hypothermia (32° to 34° C) is now recommended for post–cardiac arrest improvement of cerebral function and of survival[7] as part of the concept of "cardiocerebral resuscitation."

LONG-TERM MANAGEMENT

Survivors of a cardiac arrest that is not due to transient factors remain at high risk for recurrent cardiac arrest and sudden cardiac death. An implantable defibrillator improves outcomes in survivors of cardiac arrest.[8]

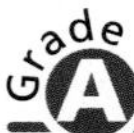

1. Hüpfl M, Selig HF, Nagele P. Chest-compression-only versus standard cardiopulmonary resuscitation: a meta-analysis. *Lancet.* 2010;376:1552-1557.
2. Bardy GH, Lee KL, Mark DB, et al. Home use of automated external defibrillators for sudden cardiac arrest. *N Engl J Med.* 2008;358:1793-1804.
3. Wik L, Hansen TB, Fylling F, et al. Delaying defibrillation to give basic cardiopulmonary resuscitation to patients with out-of-hospital ventricular fibrillation: a randomized trial. *JAMA.* 2003;289:1389-1395.
4. Aung K, Htay T. Vasopressin for cardiac arrest: a systematic review and meta-analysis. *Arch Intern Med.* 2005;165:17-24.
5. Gueugniaud PY, David JS, Chanzy E, et al. Vasopressin and epinephrine vs. epinephrine alone in cardiopulmonary resuscitation. *N Engl J Med.* 2008;359:21-30.
6. Dorian P, Cass D, Schwartz B, et al. Amiodarone as compared with lidocaine for shock-resistant ventricular fibrillation. *N Engl J Med.* 2002;346:884-890.
7. Arrich J, Holzer M, Herkner H, et al. Hypothermia for neuroprotection in adults after cardiopulmonary resuscitation. *Cochrane Database Syst Rev.* 2009;4:CD004128.
8. Connolly SJ, Hallstrom AP, Cappato R, et al. Meta-analysis of the implantable cardioverter defibrillator secondary prevention trials. AVID, CASH and CIDS studies. Antiarrhythmics vs Implantable Defibrillator study. Cardiac Arrest Study Hamburg. Canadian Implantable Defibrillator study. *Eur Heart J.* 2000;21:2071-2078.

SUGGESTED READINGS

Brooks SC, Bigham BL, Morrison LJ. Mechanical versus manual chest compressions for cardiac arrest. *Cochrane Database Syst Rev.* 2011;1:CD007260. *Review finding no benefit from mechanical devices.*

Field JM, Hazinski MF, Sayre MR, et al. Executive summary: 2010 American Heart Association Guidelines for Cardiopulmonary Resuscitation and Emergency Cardiovascular Care. *Circulation.* 2010;122:S640-S656. *Review.*

Kong MH, Fonarow GC, Peterson ED, et al. Systematic review of the incidence of sudden cardiac death in the United States. *J Am Coll Cardiol.* 2011;57:794-801. *Review.*

Maron BJ, Estes NA 3rd. Commotio cordis. *N Engl J Med.* 2010;362:917-927. *Review.*

Nichol G, Aufderheide TP, Eigel B, et al. Regional systems of care for out-of-hospital cardiac arrest: a policy statement from the American Heart Association. *Circulation.* 2010;121:709-729. *Advocates national implementation of systems known to be effective.*

Stub D, Bernard S, Duffy SJ, et al. Post cardiac arrest syndrome: a review of therapeutic strategies. *Circulation.* 2011;123:1428-1435. *Review.*

64

CARDIAC ARRHYTHMIAS WITH SUPRAVENTRICULAR ORIGIN

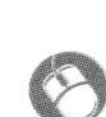

PETER ZIMETBAUM

Supraventricular arrhythmias are divided into bradyarrhythmias and tachyarrhythmias. Any rhythm that originates above where the His bundle bifurcates into the right and left bundle branches is considered to be supraventricular in origin.

ANATOMY AND NORMAL ELECTROPHYSIOLOGY

The normal cardiac impulse begins in the sinus node complex, which is located at the junction of the right atrium and the superior vena cava. It then travels through the right atrium and primarily activates the left atrium through the coronary sinus. The time it takes to activate the atria is represented by the P wave on the electrocardiogram (ECG). After depolarizing the atria, the impulse enters the atrioventricular (AV) node, which is located in the inferior septal region of the right atrium, where a delay occurs. This delay allows time for the atria to contract and fill the ventricles. In most individuals, the impulse travels through the AV node over a uniform functional pathway or route. Some people have two or more functional pathways called dual AV nodal pathways (fast and slow pathways). The delay in the AV node represents most of the isoelectric portion of the PR interval on the ECG (E-Fig. 64-1). The usual duration of atrial activation including delay in the AV node is up to 140 msec and can be measured directly as the atrial-His interval. The impulse then travels into the specialized infranodal conducting system, i.e., through the His bundle, then right and left bundle branches, and into the Purkinje network. The Purkinje network extends or fans out throughout the ventricular endocardium. Impulses conduct rapidly through the Purkinje network, thereby allowing nearly simultaneous activation of the ventricles. A small portion of the isoelectric segment of the PR interval represents infranodal conduction. This infranodal conduction through the His-Purkinje system can also be measured directly (His-ventricle interval) and should take between 40 and 60 msec. Once out of the Purkinje network, the impulse proceeds relatively slowly from the endocardial to epicardial surface of the ventricles. The QRS complex on ECG represents depolarization of the bundle branches and ventricular myocardium. Patients who have ventricular preexcitation activate the ventricles through an alternative route to the normal ventricular conduction system. These patients have bypass tracts or accessory pathways over which the ventricular myocardium can be activated directly rather than traveling over the AV node and His-Purkinje network. These pathways, which develop as a failure of the normal fibrous separation of the atria and ventricles, are located in proximity to the tricuspid and mitral valves. Direct activation of the ventricular myocardium without the usual delay in the AV node results in a slurred upstroke of the QRS complex called a delta (δ) wave (E-Fig. 64-2).

The normal heart rate is generated by tissues or pacemaker cells with intrinsic automaticity. The sinus node cells produce the greatest rate (60 to 100 beats/minute) of automaticity and suppress other potentially automatic (AV junctional, 40 to 55 beats/minute; His-Purkinje cells, 15 to 40 beats/minute) tissues with slower rates of depolarization. The sinus node and AV node are heavily influenced by the parasympathetic (vagal) and sympathetic (adrenergic) nervous system. At rest, the parasympathetic system controls sinus node automaticity. With exertion or emotional or physical stress, a withdrawal of parasympathetic tone and an increase in heart rate, which is then perpetuated by sympathetic tone, further increase heart rate. Sinus arrhythmia refers to the normal variation in heart rate with inspiration and expiration. With inspiration, a withdrawal of vagal tone increases heart rate; by comparison, expiration is associated with a drop in heart rate (Fig. 64-1). During sleep, a dominance of vagal tone slows heart rate.

BRADYARRHYTHMIAS

Bradyarrhythmias may be caused by sinus node, AV node, or His-Purkinje dysfunction (Table 64-1).

Sinus Bradycardia and Sinus Node Dysfunction

Sinus bradycardia (Fig. 64-2) is generally defined as a sinus rate of less than 60 beats per minute. It should be noted, however, that sinus rates as low as 45 to 50 beats per minute, particularly at rest, can be physiologically normal. Sinus node dysfunction encompasses a group of disorders including sinus bradycardia, sinoatrial (SA) exit block, sinus arrest (pause of >2 to 3 seconds) during sinus rhythm, chronotropic incompetence, and tachycardia-bradycardia (tachy-brady) syndrome. Sinus node dysfunction in combination with symptoms such as fatigue, dizziness, near or complete syncope (Chapters 50 and 62), or worsening of heart failure (Chapter 58) is called sick sinus syndrome. The tachy-brady syndrome is often identified by a prolonged delay in sinus node recovery following the termination of atrial fibrillation (AF) (Fig. 64-3). SA exit block refers to the electrophysiologic phenomenon of sinus node firing with delay or block of the impulse as it travels from the sinus node to the surrounding atrial tissue (Fig. 64-4). SA exit block can be first degree, second degree (type 1 or 2), and third degree. First-degree SA block is difficult to diagnose from the surface ECG. Second-degree SA exit block type 1 is manifest by progressive PP shortening preceding the sinus pause. The PP interval following the pause must be greater than twice the PP interval that preceded the pause. Second-degree SA exit block type 2 is characterized by a pause equaling an exact multiple of the sinus rate (i.e., constant PP interval before and after the pause). High-degree SA exit block refers to the absence of multiple P waves with a pause still corresponding to an absolute multiple of the underlying PP intervals, and third-degree AV block results in a complete absence of sinus P waves.

Chronotropic incompetence refers to the inability to increase the sinus rate appropriately in response to exercise or other physiologic demand. In most patients, chronotropic incompetence is manifest by a maximal heart rate of less than 100 beats per minute.

TABLE 64-1 BRADYCARDIAS

SINUS NODE DYSFUNCTION
Sinus bradycardia < 45 beats/min
Sinoatrial exit block
First-degree
Second-degree
Third-degree
Sinus arrest
Bradycardia-tachycardia syndrome
ATRIOVENTRICULAR BLOCK
First-degree
Second-degree
Mobitz type I (Wenckebach phenomenon)
Mobitz type II
Higher degree (e.g., 2:1, 3:1)
Third-degree
Atrioventricular node
His-Purkinje system

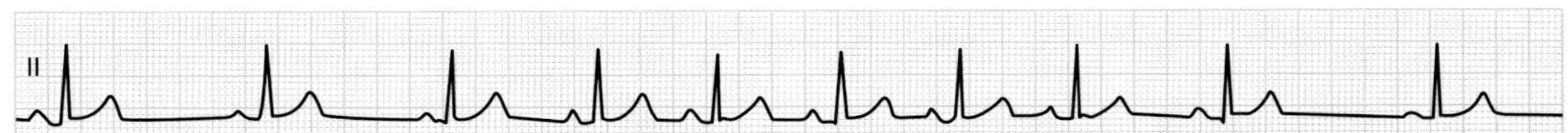

FIGURE 64-1. Sinus arrhythmia. Note the variation in sinus rates, which fluctuate with normal variations in autonomic tone.

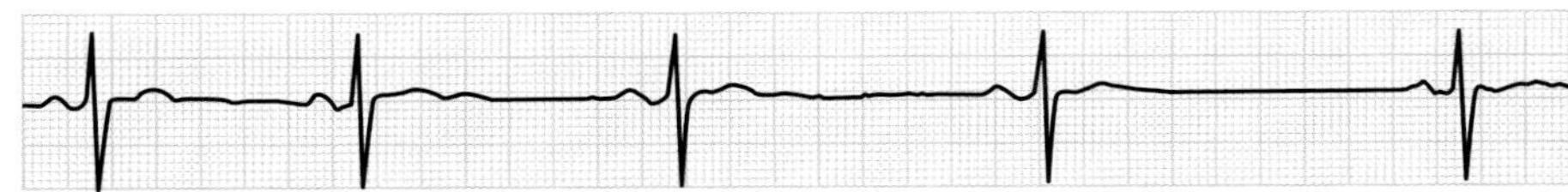

FIGURE 64-2. Sinus bradycardia. Progressive sinus bradycardia—in this case related to heightened vagal tone while sleeping.

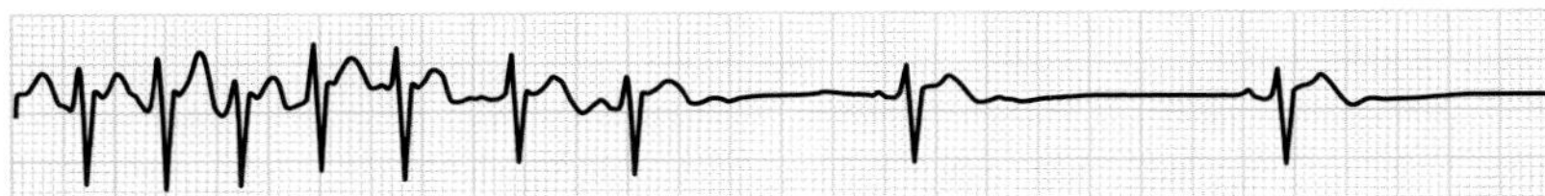

FIGURE 64-3. Electrocardiographic evidence of tachy-brady syndrome. Atrial fibrillation with a tachycardic ventricular response followed by conversion to sinus bradycardia.

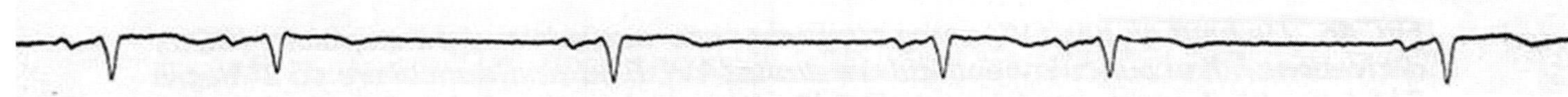

FIGURE 64-4. Sinoatrial block. Sinoatrial exit block, probably type 2, is characterized by a pause equaling an exact multiple of the sinus rate.

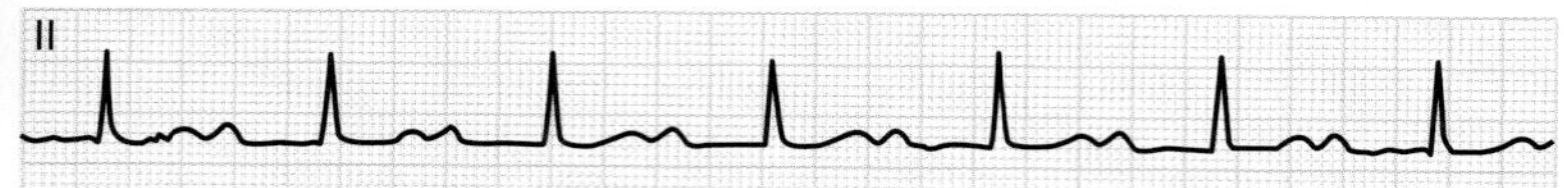

FIGURE 64-5. **First-degree atrioventricular (AV) block.** Note the prolonged (>200 msec) AV conduction.

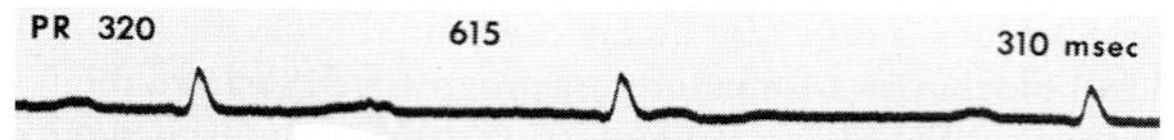

FIGURE 64-6. **Mobitz I block.** Progressive PR prolongation from 320 to 615 msec, followed by a blocked P wave. The subsequent conducted PR interval is less than the PR interval before the dropped P wave.

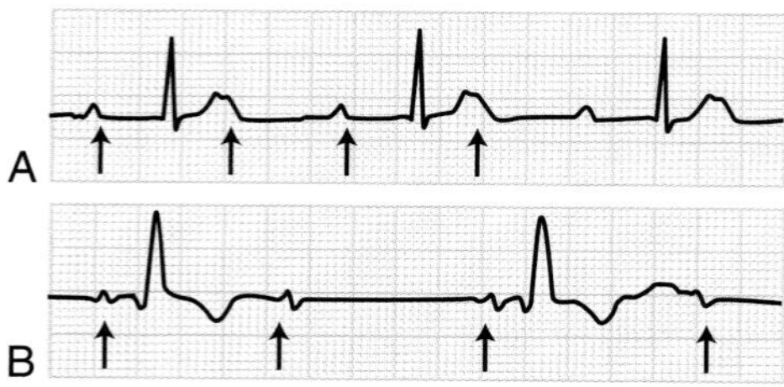

FIGURE 64-7. **Two-to-one conduction in the atrioventricular (AV) node and below the AV node. A,** Two-to-one conduction, with the conducted beats demonstrating a prolonged PR interval (>300 msec) and a narrow QRS, indicating Mobitz I block in the AV node. **B,** Normal-duration conducted PR interval and a wide QRS duration favoring Mobitz II block into an infranodal site of block.

Atrioventricular Conduction Disturbances

AV conduction disturbances refer to abnormal conduction in the AV node or in the His-Purkinje system (HPS) below the AV node. Electrical transmission through the AV conduction system is primarily limited by the AV node, which conducts in a decremental fashion to prevent excessively rapid conduction to the ventricles. The normal AV node rarely conducts faster than 200 beats per minute and slows with aging. The AV node is heavily influenced by autonomic tone and may conduct more than 200 beats per minute in the presence of heightened sympathetic and withdrawal of parasympathetic tone. Conduction through the HPS system is faster and nondecremental.

The AV blocks are classified as first, second, high, and third degree. First-degree AV block is a misnomer because nothing is actually blocked—rather, there is delay, usually in the AV node, manifest by a prolonged PR interval (Fig. 64-5). Second-degree AV block is divided into Mobitz type I (Wenckebach) or Mobitz type II. Mobitz type I is defined by progressive PR prolongation with eventual block after a P wave (Fig. 64-6). The initial PR prolongation is longest, the subsequent RR intervals shorten, and the PR interval following the blocked P wave is shorter than the last conducted PR interval before the blocked P wave. Mobitz type I usually occurs in the AV node. Mobitz type II, which is characterized by the abrupt failure of conduction after a P wave without preceding PR prolongation, usually represents conduction disease below the AV node. In patients with 2 : 1 block (two P waves for every QRS), it can be difficult to determine whether the block is Mobitz I in the AV node or Mobitz II below the AV node. Clues to conduction disease in the AV node include a prolonged PR interval (i.e., more than 300 msec) and a narrow QRS duration. Clues to conduction disease below the node include a normal PR interval but with bundle branch block (Fig. 64-7).

High-degree or advanced AV block, which is a form of second-degree block with multiple or successive nonconducted P waves, or both (Fig. 64-8), frequently recurs or persists. Third-degree block (or complete heart block) refers to a rhythm in which the atrial and ventricular activity occur independently, and the atrial rate usually exceeds the ventricular rate. Third-degree heart block can be seen with sinus rhythm or any atrial tachyarrhythmia with a regular escape rhythm in the AV junction or below (Fig. 64-9). Sometimes there is no escape rhythm, and heart block results in asystole. Complete heart block, particularly when it is acute and accompanied by an escape rhythm, can be associated with marked QT prolongation, which signifies a risk of torsades de pointes (Chapter 65). For this reason, patients who undergo AV node ablation have their pacemakers set at 80 beats per minute for at least 6 weeks after the procedure to prevent QT prolongation and torsades de pointes. Eventually, the pacing rate can be reduced to more physiologic levels without the ongoing risk of ventricular arrhythmia. Complete heart block and other types of severe bradyarrhythmia may present with syncope if there is a prolonged pause before an escape rhythm develops. More often, these rhythms present with fatigue and dyspnea. The blood pressure is often elevated owing to peripheral vasoconstriction, and there may be renal insufficiency secondary to reduced cardiac output.

The term AV dissociation refers to any rhythm in which the atria and ventricles beat independently of one another. If the atrial rate is faster than the ventricular rate, it is called complete heart block or third-degree AV block. AV dissociation with an atrial rate slower than the subsidiary pacemaker is usually seen with junctional or ventricular tachycardias.

CLINICAL MANIFESTATIONS

Sinus bradycardia and various degrees of AV nodal blocks can occur asymptomatically during sleep in healthy individuals. Asymptomatic first- and second-degree AV block, particularly when partially or completely reversed by exercise, is usually benign. Persistent second-degree and third-degree AV nodal block is abnormal and is often associated with dizziness, fatigue, exertional dyspnea, worsening of heart failure, near-syncope, or syncope. Third-degree AV block with a good junctional escape mechanism that accelerates during exercise, as often noted in patients with congenital AV block, may remain asymptomatic. Patients with congenital heart block may not appreciate their potential for a more active lifestyle because of the lack of a reference point but often feel much better when an appropriate heart rate acceleration can be achieved after pacemaker therapy.

DIAGNOSIS

Bradycardias are typically diagnosed by the ECG. In symptomatic patients with symptoms suggestive of bradyarrhythmia, 24-hour Holter monitoring or prolonged loop monitoring usually can make the diagnosis, but some patients may require formal electrophysiologic testing (Chapter 62). Any bradycardias, including sinus node dysfunction (Table 64-2) and AV nodal block (Table 64-3), can be caused at least in part by vagal influences, such as vasovagal episodes, vomiting, abdominal surgery, and upper and lower gastrointestinal invasive procedures. Syncope, sometimes caused by the bradycardia and sometimes by vasodepression with hypotension, may result (Chapters 50 and 62). Medications, infiltrative diseases, fibrocalcific degeneration, and a variety of other causes must be considered.

TREATMENT Rx

The treatment of sinus node dysfunction and AV blocks consists of first removing any medications that may precipitate dysfunction (see Table 64-2). Although some patients will recover normal conduction, the susceptibility to medications usually indicates an underlying conduction abnormality that may worsen over time.

Asymptomatic sinus node dysfunction requires no therapy. Asymptomatic atrioventricular nodal block can also be managed without intervention unless the QT interval is markedly prolonged, in which case a pacemaker should be considered. For symptomatic sinus node dysfunction and second- and third-degree AV block, acute management includes intravenous atropine (1 mg) or isoproterenol (usually 1 to 2 μ/minute infusion) to increase the heart rate. Temporary cardiac pacing (Chapter 66) may be required. If sinus node dysfunction or AV block is due to transient abnormalities, such as drug-induced or acute ischemic syndromes, temporary pacing is usually sufficient; however, when infra-His or intra-His block is suspected (e.g., exercise-induced AV block or asymptomatic Mobitz type II block) and the site can be documented with His bundle recording, permanent pacing (see Tables 66-1 and 66-2 in Chapter 66) is the only effective chronic therapy, and consensus recommendations for pacemaker implantation should guide its use. For all forms of persistent symptomatic sinus node dysfunction or second- or third-degree AV block, permanent pacing is the therapy of choice (Chapter 66).

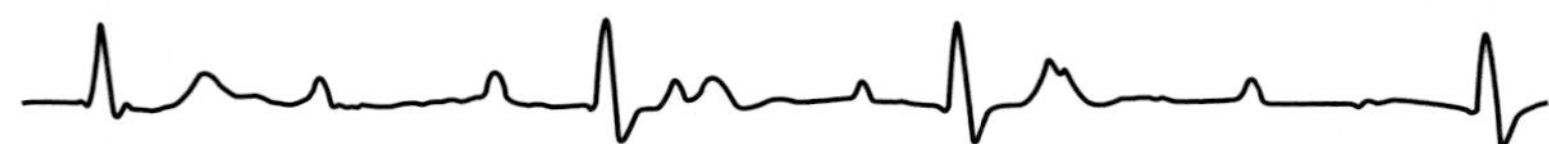

FIGURE 64-8. High-degree atrioventricular block. Periods of complete heart block with three nonconducted P waves (the first of which is buried in the first QRS complex) followed by two P waves, the second of which is conducted to the ventricle with a long PR interval. The subsequent three P waves are once again nonconducted, with the last P wave buried in the last QRS complex.

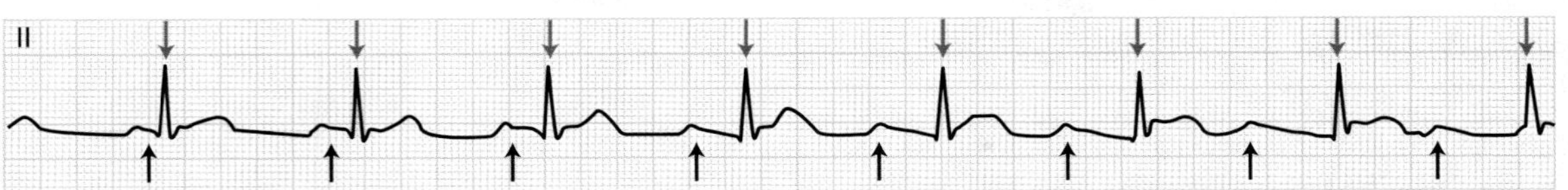

FIGURE 64-9. Complete heart block with the atrial beats *(black arrows)* dissociated from the ventricular beats *(red arrows)*. Note the ST elevation in leads III and aVF indicating acute inferior myocardial infarction as the cause of complete heart block.

TABLE 64-2 CAUSES OF SINUS NODE DYSFUNCTION
INTRINSIC
Hypothyroidism Fibrocalcific degeneration Increased vagal tone, especially in sleep apnea Congenital mutations Scleroderma Amyloidosis Chagas' disease
EXTRINSIC

Trauma, including cardiac surgery
Drugs
  Calcium-channel blockers
  β-Blockers
  Digoxin
  Antiarrhythmic medications (amiodarone, dronedarone, sotalol, flecainide, propafenone)
  Lithium

TABLE 64-3 CAUSES OF ATRIOVENTRICULAR BLOCK

All causes of sinus node dysfunction and
  Lyme disease
  Bacterial endocarditis with abscess formation
  Cardiac sarcoidosis with granuloma
  Inferior myocardial infarction
  Anterior myocardial infarction (less common and often associated with cardiogenic shock)
  Congenital mutations (possibly associated with maternal lupus erythematosus and transmission of anti-Ro and La antibodies)

Corrected transposition of the great vessels
Chagas' disease
Some neurologic conditions (especially myotonic dystrophy)
Drugs as in Table 64-2

Supraventricular Rhythms with a Normal Rate

Atrial premature beats (APBs) can arise from the right or left atrium or the pulmonary veins. The P wave, which differs from the P wave of sinus rhythm unless the APB originates near the sinus node, always precedes the QRS complex (Fig. 64-10). If the P wave is blocked, however, it is not followed by a QRS complex. A blocked premature atrial contraction may be confused with second-degree AV block, unless its prematurity is recognized, or with sinus node dysfunction, if it is inconspicuous. Altered appearance of the ST-T segment is often a clue to the presence of a P wave. A premature QRS complex with the morphology of the underlying sinus rhythm in the absence of a premature P wave represents an AV junctional beat (Fig. 64-11).

An ectopic atrial rhythm refers to a nonsinus atrial rhythm from a single focus with a single P wave morphology (Fig. 64-12). Wandering atrial pacemaker refers to an ectopic atrial rhythm with at least three distinct P wave morphologies at rates between 50 and 100 beats per minute (Fig. 64-13).

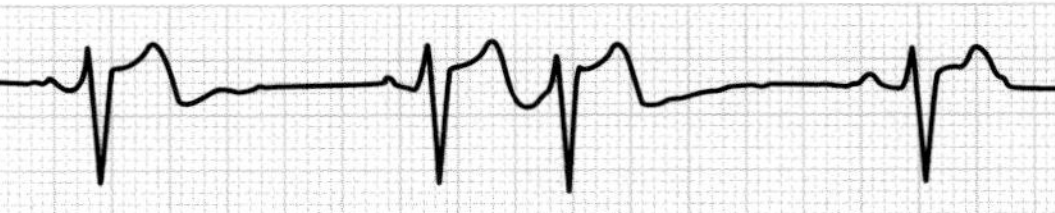

FIGURE 64-10. Atrial premature beat. Sinus rhythm with an atrial premature beat as the third complex in the rhythm strip. The P wave is buried in the preceding T wave.

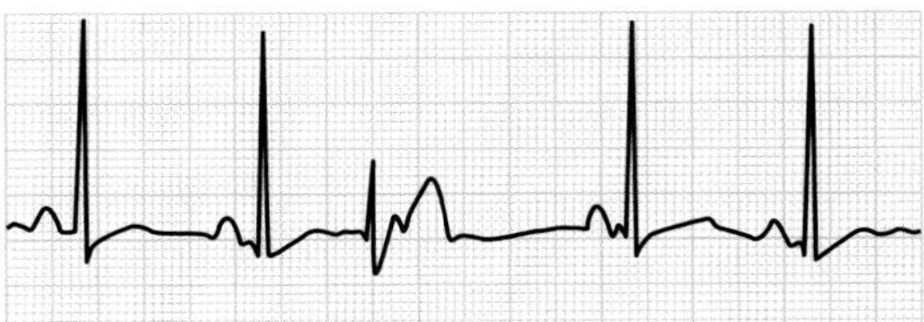

FIGURE 64-11. Junctional premature beat. The premature beat is narrow but slightly different in morphology compared with the surrounding sinus beats. This premature beat is from the atrioventricular junction or slightly more distal in the fascicles. The inverted P wave following the QRS represents retrograde activation of the atria.

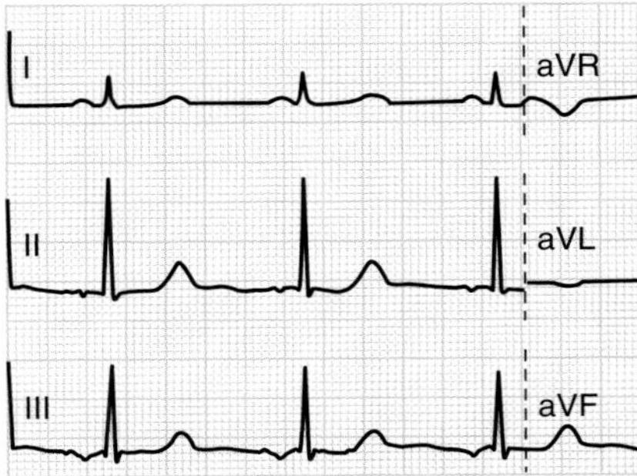

FIGURE 64-12. Ectopic atrial rhythm. The inverted P waves in leads II, III, and aVF indicate a nonsinus P wave originating in the low right atrium.

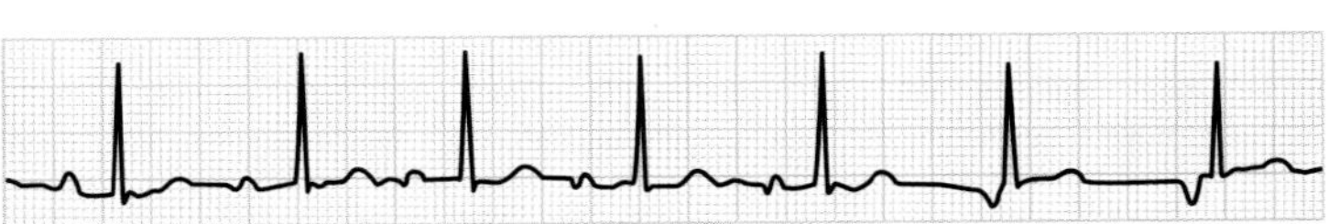

FIGURE 64-13. Wandering atrial pacemaker. Rhythm with three distinct P wave morphologies.

CLINICAL MANIFESTATIONS

APBs are most often asymptomatic but can occasionally be experienced as palpitations (Chapter 62). Similarly, ectopic atrial rhythms, including a wandering atrial pacemaker, are virtually always asymptomatic. Rarely, ectopic atrial rhythm can be very slow and associated with symptoms of fatigue.

DIAGNOSIS

The diagnosis of atrial premature beats, ectopic atrial rhythms, and wandering atrial pacemakers are all made by ECG or on an ambulatory Holter monitor or loop event recorder (Chapter 62).

TREATMENT Rx

Premature atrial contractions do not generally require treatment unless they are associated with significant symptoms. Treatment consists primarily of β-blockers (e.g., atenolol, 25 to 100 mg daily) or calcium-channel blockers (e.g., long-acting diltiazem, 180 to 300 mg daily). Ectopic atrial rhythms and wandering atrial pacemakers are rarely symptomatic and are not treated with medications. Rarely, a slow ectopic rhythm associated with fatigue can be treated with atrial pacing at a rate faster than the ectopic atrial rhythm.

Supraventricular Tachyarrhythmias

The supraventricular tachycardias (SVTs) are defined as arrhythmias with three or more beats at a rate of greater than 100 beats per minute (Table 64-4). The beats, which can be regular or irregular, are usually narrow complex but can be wide complex when associated with bundle branch block (aberration) or conduction over an accessory pathway. Atrial dilation, acute myocardial infarction, pulmonary embolism, acute or chronic inflammatory states, or scars from prior surgery involving atrial myocardium or pericardium are among the causes of atrial tachyarrhythmias.

TABLE 64-4 SUPRAVENTRICULAR TACHYCARDIAS

	R-R REGULARITY	P WAVE MORPHOLOGY
ATRIAL TACHYCARDIAS		
Sinus tachycardia	Regular	Positive in II, III, aVF; negative in aVR
Sinus node re-entry	Regular	Positive in II, III, aVF; negative in aVR
Atrial tachycardia, unifocal	Regular	P different from sinus
Atrial tachycardia, multifocal	Irregular	Three or more different P wave morphologies
Atrial flutter, common, counterclockwise	Regular; irregular if variable AV block	Sawtooth flutter waves; regular waveform; negative in II, III, aVF, positive in V_1, negative in V_6
Clockwise		Positive in II, III, aVF; negative in V_1; positive in V_6
Atrial flutter, uncommon	Regular; irregular if variable AV block	Pattern different than common atrial flutter (counterclockwise or clockwise)
Atrial fibrillation	Irregularly irregular	Irregular fibrillation waves
AV JUNCTIONAL TACHYCARDIAS		
AV re-entry (using accessory pathways)		
Orthodromic	Regular	Retrograde P in ST-T wave
Antidromic	Regular preexcited	Retrograde P, short RP
Slow conducting	Regular	Retrograde P at end of T wave or later (long RP)
Atriofascicular (antidromic)	Regular preexcited	Retrograde P, short RP
AV nodal re-entry		
Common (slow-fast)	Regular	Retrograde P obscured by QRS or alters the end of QRS (short RP)
Uncommon (fast-slow)	Regular	Retrograde P at end of T wave or later (long RP)
Others (slow-slow)	Regular	PR-RP approximately equal
Nonparoxysmal junctional tachycardia*	Regular, slow rate	AV dissociation
Automatic junctional tachycardia*	Regular	AV dissociation

*Site of origin usually infranodal.
AV = atrioventricular.

Sinus Tachycardia

Sinus tachycardia (Fig. 64-14) is an arrhythmia that is almost always a physiologic response to an emotional or physical stress such as anxiety, exercise, anemia, hypotension, hypoxemia, fever, thyrotoxicosis, or heart failure. It is characterized by a gradual increase and decrease in heart rate and rarely exceeds 180 beats per minute. In rare cases, it may be a nonphysiologic condition called inappropriate sinus tachycardia, which is characterized by sinus tachycardia that develops in response to minimal stress and that continues beyond the time when the normal response would have slowed. This disorder is difficult to manage but is sometimes responsive to β-blockade.

Sinus node re-entry is a rare form of SVT caused by re-entry in the sinus node. As opposed to physiologic ST, it begins abruptly, is often triggered by a premature atrial beat, and ends abruptly. The P wave morphology is identical to sinus rhythm, and β-blockers are the treatment of choice if required for symptoms.

Atrial Tachycardia

The term atrial tachycardia refers to a group of SVTs that originate from focal anatomic locations in the atria and propagate in a centrifugal pattern (Fig. 64-15). These locations include the pulmonary veins, crista terminalis in the right atrium, tricuspid or mitral annulus, coronary sinus, or regions of scar tissue from previous cardiac surgery. Atrial tachycardias, which are usually regular rhythms that rarely exceed 200 beats per minute, may present in young age but more often develop later in life. Atrial tachycardias can be re-entrant, triggered, or automatic in mechanism. Some forms of atrial tachycardia are incessant and can predispose to a tachycardia-related cardiomyopathy (Chapter 60). Other forms of atrial tachycardia are paroxysmal and may remit spontaneously without treatment. When persistent, atrial tachycardias can be managed with medications (calcium-channel or β-blockers or other antiarrhythmic drugs). Electrical mapping and ablation (Chapter 66) of atrial

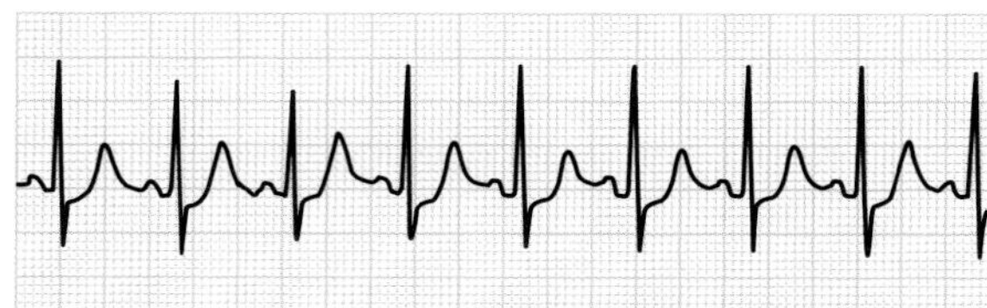

FIGURE 64-14. Sinus tachycardia at 120 beats/min.

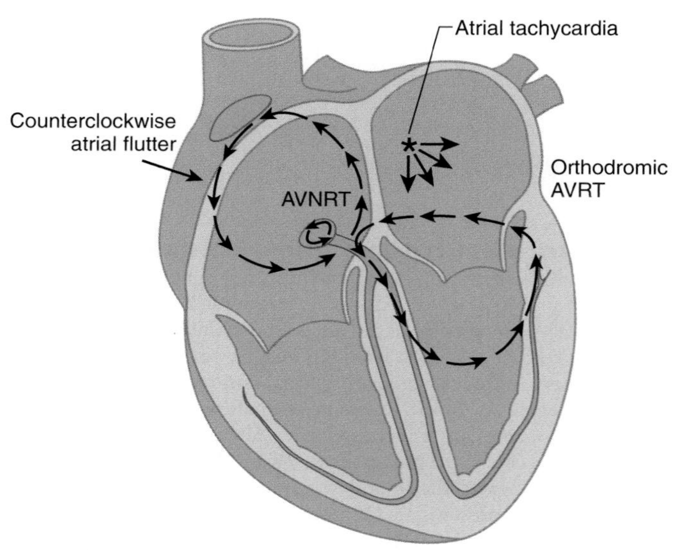

FIGURE 64-15. **Diagram of the site and mechanism of common forms of supraventricular tachycardia.** AVNRT = atrioventricular nodal re-entrant tachycardia; AVRT = atrioventricular re-entrant tachycardia.

tachycardia are highly effective and are increasingly offered as first-line therapy. Multifocal atrial tachycardia (Fig. 64-16), which is a unique form of atrial tachycardia characterized by three or more P wave morphologies, is distinguished from wandering atrial pacemaker when the rate is 100 beats per minute or more rather than less than 100 beats per minute. It is an irregular rhythm and occurs almost exclusively in patients with advanced pulmonary disease.

Atrioventricular Nodal Re-entrant Tachycardia

Atrioventricular nodal re-entrant tachycardia (AVNRT), which is a common form of SVT in all age groups, presents most often in young adulthood and frequently occurs after a change in position. It is more common in women than men and may develop or be exacerbated by pregnancy or certain phases of the menstrual cycle. Patients with AVNRT have two functional AV nodal pathways (dual pathways). Typically, an atrial premature beat blocks in one pathway (fast pathway) and conducts slowly over the other pathway (slow pathway). If this beat conducts back up the fast pathway and then re-enters the slow pathway, AV nodal re-entry occurs (Fig. 64-17). This re-entrant circuit is confined to the AV node, and the result is that both the atria and ventricles are activated nearly simultaneously. P waves may not be visible on the ECG because they are buried in the QRS complex. When P waves are present, they usually are seen just after the QRS and have a negative or superior axis (negative in leads II, III, and aVF; short RP tachycardia) (see Fig. 64-15). Atypical AVNRT is rare and occurs with conduction down the fast pathway and up the slow pathway, with a long interval between the preceding R wave and subsequent negative P wave (e.g., long RP tachycardia).

Junctional Tachycardia

Junctional tachycardia refers to a focal (non-re-entrant) tachycardia originating in the AV junction (Fig. 64-18). A number of different forms of junctional tachycardia have differing clinical patterns. Nonparoxysmal junctional tachycardia is a benign arrhythmia that rarely exceeds 120 beats per minute and typically exhibits a "warm-up" and "cool-down" pattern. A more rapid paroxysmal form of junctional tachycardia occurs in young adults and is often associated with exercise. Congenital junctional ectopic tachycardia, which occurs in the pediatric population, is associated with very rapid rates and a risk of tachycardia-related cardiomyopathy.

Accessory Pathway Tachycardias

Tachycardias associated with an accessory pathway or bypass tract are called atrioventricular re-entrant tachycardia (AVRT). These tachycardias most often conduct down the normal AV conducting system and back up the accessory pathway (orthodromic AVRT) (see Fig. 64-15). Antidromic tachycardia is rare and represents conduction down the accessory pathway and back up the normal conducting system or less commonly, a second accessory pathway. Wolff-Parkinson-White syndrome is defined by the presence of delta waves or preexcitation on the ECG in sinus rhythm (Fig. 64-19), often with a

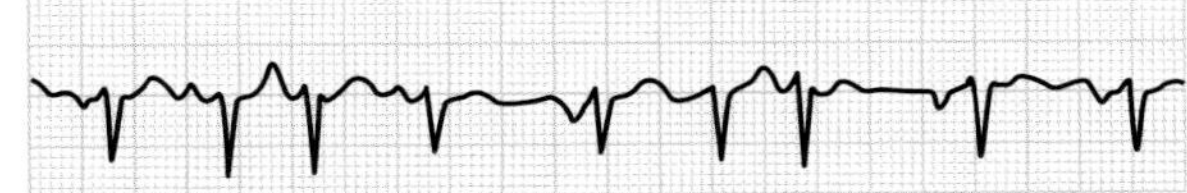

FIGURE 64-16. Multifocal atrial tachycardia. An atrial tachycardia with three different P wave morphologies.

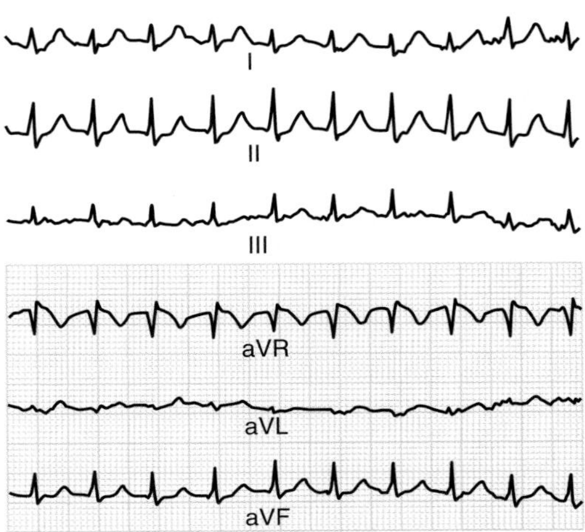

FIGURE 64-18. Junctional tachycardia. A tachycardia without evident P waves. The negative deflections at the end of leads II, III, and aVF represent retrograde P waves. This rhythm is impossible to distinguish from atrioventricular nodal re-entrant tachycardia on the surface electrocardiogram.

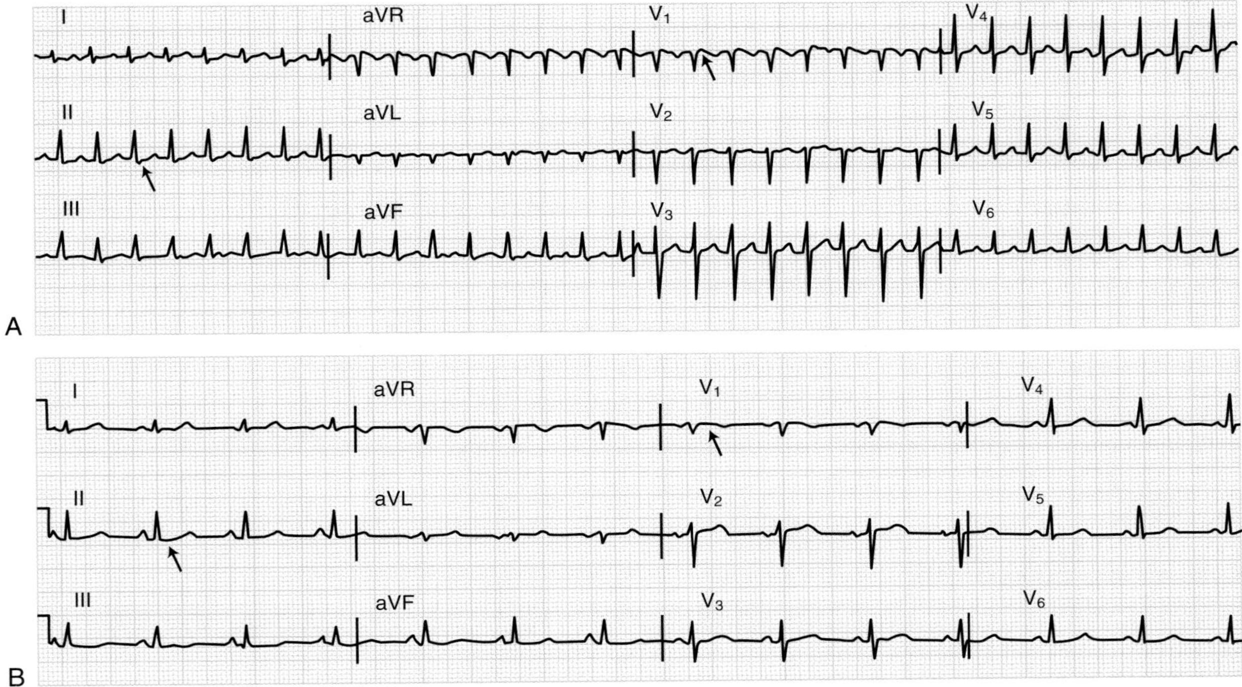

FIGURE 64-17. Electrocardiograms demonstrating different rhythms in the same patient. A, Atrioventricular nodal re-entrant tachycardia, with *arrows* indicating retrograde P waves (negative in lead II, positive in V_1). **B,** Same patient in sinus rhythm. The absence of a negative deflection at the end of the QRS in lead II and positive deflection in V_1 confirms that those findings in panel **A** were retrograde P waves.

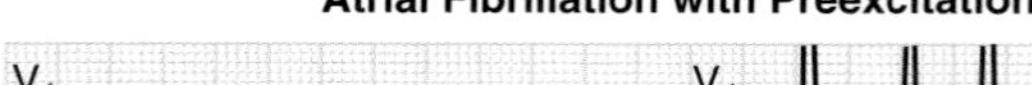

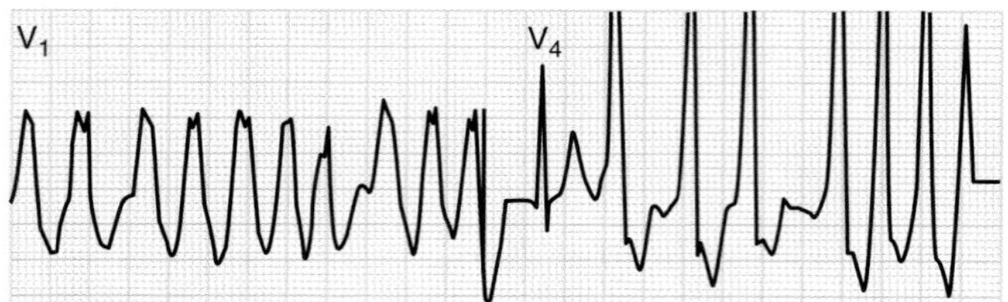

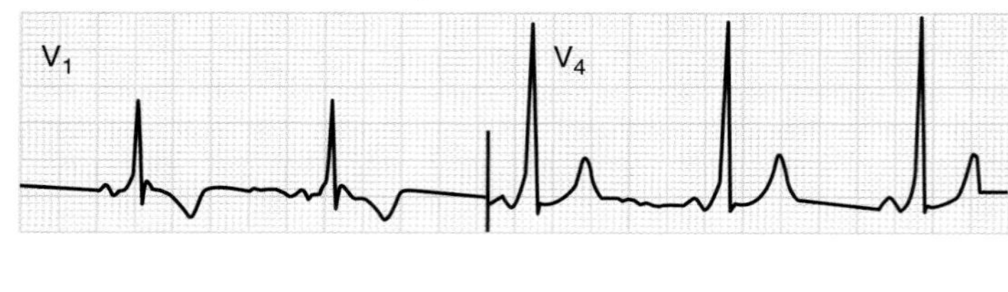

FIGURE 64-19. Two panels of the same patient with ventricular preexcitation. The rhythm on the left is fast, broad, and irregular, indicating atrial fibrillation with conduction over an accessory pathway. The rhythm on the right is sinus with conduction over an accessory pathway.

history of AVRT, but many patients with ventricular preexcitation never get AVRT. Up to 40% of patients with accessory pathways have AF. Because accessory pathway tissue, unlike the AV node, is usually nondecremental, a rapidly conducting accessory pathway may allow AF to conduct to the ventricles at excessive rates and precipitate ventricular fibrillation. Drugs like digoxin, which accelerate accessory pathway conduction, should be avoided in these patients.

The ECG during orthodromic AVRT can have a narrow complex, but a wide QRS complex will be seen if there is aberration from a bundle branch block, especially at more rapid rates. The retrograde P wave is negative in leads I and aVL if it conducts over a left lateral accessory pathway and negative in leads II, III, and aVF if it conducts over a septal or postural septal accessory pathway (Fig. 64-20). The P wave occurs later (after the preceding R wave) compared with AVNRT because in AVRT, the impulse must conduct beyond the AV node and into the ventricle before returning to the atria over an accessory pathway. In antidromic AVRT, the QRS complex is wide with a slurred upstroke and resembles that seen with ventricular tachycardia as opposed to a bundle branch block. Antidromic conduction with AF is often fast, broad, and irregular (see Fig. 64-19).

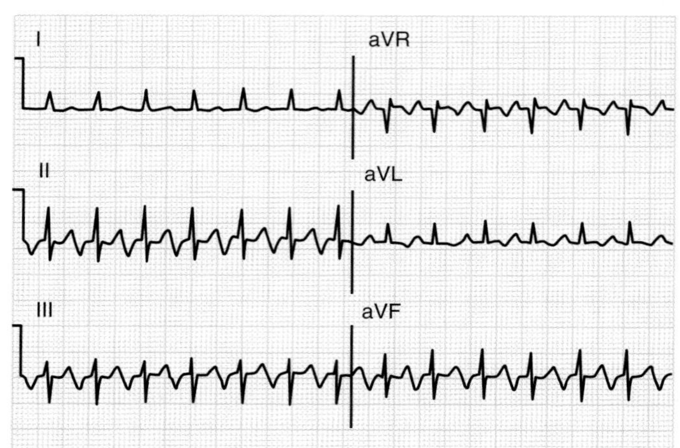

FIGURE 64-20. Atrioventricular re-entrant tachycardia. Negative P waves are seen in leads II, III, and aVF indicative of retrograde conduction to the atria over a septal accessory pathway.

Atrial Flutter

Atrial flutter is an arrhythmia with an atrial rate of approximately 300 beats per minute and a ventricular response of 150 (2 : 1), 100 (3 : 1), or slower multiples. Typical atrial flutter is a macro-re-entrant circuit that circulates in the right atrium in a clockwise or counterclockwise loop (Fig. 64-21). The inferior portion of typical flutter uses the narrow region between the inferior vena cava and tricuspid annulus as a critical isthmus of conduction. Typical atrial flutter almost always occurs in patients with underlying cardiovascular or pulmonary disease. It can also develop in patients who receive anti-arrhythmic drugs (e.g., sodium-channel blocking drugs) for AF. Atypical atrial flutter refers to macro-re-entrant atrial circuits that do not use this critical cavotricuspid isthmus of tissue. These atypical forms of atrial flutter often occur in the left atrium after mitral valve surgery or catheter ablation of AF. Typical atrial flutter can be recognized by a "sawtooth" P wave morphology, which is predominantly negative in leads II, III, and aVF and positive in V_1 (counterclockwise atrial flutter) or positive in leads II, III, and aVF and negative in V_1 (clockwise atrial flutter).

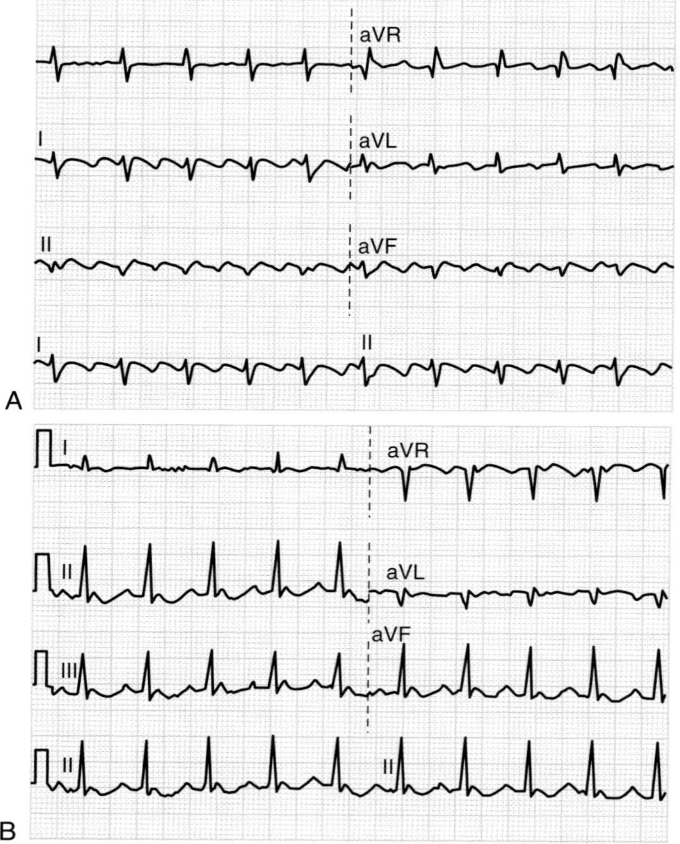

FIGURE 64-21. Two examples of atrial flutter. A, Typical counterclockwise right atrial flutter with classic sawtooth flutter waves seen in leads II, III, and aVF. **B,** Clockwise right atrial flutter.

Atrial Fibrillation

AF is identified by the absence of P waves and the presence of an irregularly irregular ventricular rate. Coarse AF, which describes the presence of residual atrial activity on the ECG, is generally best seen in lead V_1 with the absence of P wave–like activity in other leads (Fig. 64-22). AF can be present with a regular ventricular rate when there is concomitant AV dissociation (e.g., complete heart block or ventricular tachycardia).

AF, which is the most common arrhythmia in clinical practice, afflicts over two million Americans. The likelihood of developing AF increases with aging, with an anticipated three-fold increase in prevalence as the U.S. population ages in the next 20 years. AF is almost always a recurrent disorder with the possible exception of AF that develops in association with hyperthyroidism (Chapter 233) and surgery (Chapter 441). AF can be paroxysmal (terminates spontaneously) or persistent (persists for at least 7 days or until cardioverted). Paroxysmal AF can occur as self-remitting arrhythmia for decades or can progress to permanent AF. Patients with persistent AF generally progress to permanent AF unless sinus rhythm is restored with cardioversion.

In addition to its association with aging, AF frequently occurs in association with hypertension (Chapter 67) or other comorbid conditions such as

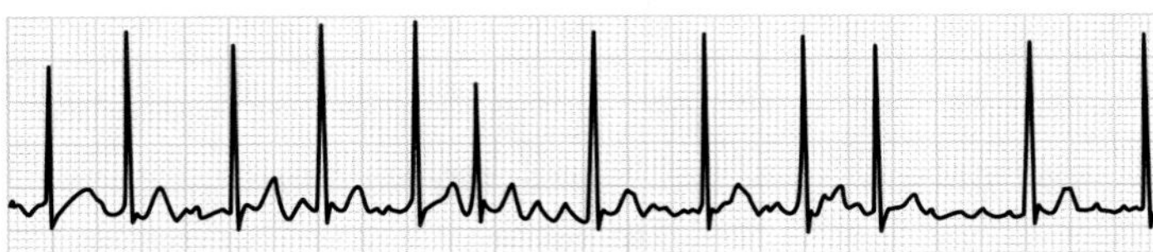

FIGURE 64-22. **Coarse atrial fibrillation.** The wavy baseline is suggestive of atrial activity and can be misinterpreted as P waves or flutter waves. The irregularity of the QRS complexes indicates that this is atrial fibrillation.

diabetes mellitus, thyrotoxicosis, heart failure, coronary artery disease, valvular heart disease, or lung disease such as chronic obstructive pulmonary disease or obstructive sleep apnea. About 20% of patients have no associated comorbidity and have what may be termed *lone AF*. Some patients develop AF after binges of alcohol use ("holiday heart") or after parasympathetic surges such as after vigorous exercise or a large meal (vagally induced AF). Excessive caffeine intake is an often cited but very rare cause of AF. AF requires a trigger in the form of atrial premature depolarizations, which often originate in the pulmonary veins and which, in the susceptible individual, result in AF. The susceptibility to AF may relate to changes in the electrical function of the left atrium. Prolonged periods of AF can lead to electrical and structural remodeling of the atria and promote the further perpetuation of AF ("AF begets AF").

AF results in the loss of the atrial contribution to ventricular filling. This so-called loss of atrial kick is generally well tolerated in normal individuals, in whom only about 15% of ventricular filling is the result of atrial contraction. In patients who have stiff, noncompliant ventricles (e.g., patients with aortic stenosis, hypertrophic or restrictive cardiomyopathy, or long-standing hypertension), however, up to 40% of ventricular filling may be related to atrial contraction, so stroke volume may fall noticeably in such patients.

The primary morbidity associated with AF is thromboembolism. Thromboembolism in patients with nonvalvular AF typically results from thrombus formation in and dislodgement from the left atrial appendage. The risk of thromboembolism is unrelated to the pattern of AF (paroxysmal or persistent) but is increased in the first 3 to 4 weeks after cardioversion, when the gradual return of atrial mechanical function can result in a particularly high risk of thromboembolism. The risk of thromboembolism in AF increases with age, diabetes mellitus, hypertension, previous embolic episodes, and heart failure. The lowest incidence (<1% annually) is in patients younger than 65 years with lone AF.

CLINICAL MANIFESTATIONS

SVTs can produce symptoms specifically related to the rhythm itself, including fatigue, palpitations (Chapter 62), dizziness, shortness of breath, chest discomfort, presyncope, and syncope. These symptoms are mostly related to the rapidity of the ventricular response and are most prevalent at the onset of the arrhythmia. In contrast to other forms of SVT, asymptomatic episodes of AF are common in patients who also have symptomatic AF.

Incessant SVT and uncontrolled ventricular rates can cause tachycardia-related cardiomyopathy, which is reversible with control of these arrhythmias. In some situations, however, the clinical presentation may be dominated by the underlying condition that precipitates the arrhythmia, such as fever, physical stress, hypovolemia, heart failure (Chapter 58), hypoxia, sympathomimetic or parasympatholytic medications, thyrotoxicosis (Chapter 233), and pheochromocytoma (Chapter 235).

Re-entrant tachycardias begin and end abruptly, whether without treatment or when terminated with vagal maneuvers or intravenous medications. An accessory pathway with ventricular preexcitation can be undiagnosed into adulthood, when it can mimic myocardial infarction or right ventricular hypertrophy on the electrocardiogram.

DIAGNOSIS

The key to diagnosis is the 12-lead ECG if the symptoms are very frequent. A Holter monitor is useful if the arrhythmia is likely to be detected by 24 to 48 hours of monitoring, whereas a continuous loop event recorder, which can be worn for up to a month and activated by the patient for symptoms, is preferred if the arrhythmia is less frequent (Chapter 62). Another alternative is a device that records data continuously and transmits to a central station, capturing both symptomatic and asymptomatic arrhythmias over a period of up to a month.

On physical examination, patients with a blocked atrial beat or AVNRT may have large (cannon) "a" waves detected in their jugular veins (see Fig. 50-4 in Chapter 50). Carotid sinus massage, which has a vagal effect on the AV node, can terminate SVTs that depend on the AV node as part of the circuit (AVNRT and AVRT). Carotid sinus massage also can occasionally terminate atrial tachycardia but more often will slow the pulse by reducing the number of atrial inputs conducted through the AV node. Similarly, carotid sinus massage will slow but not terminate atrial flutter and AF.

Electrophysiologic testing (Chapter 66) is the definitive way to distinguish SVT from VT (see Table 65-2 in Chapter 65). The SVT can often be initiated by paced premature beats, after which the mechanism and location of the arrhythmia can be determined.

TREATMENT Rx

Acute Therapy

Sinus, Atrial, Atrioventricular Nodal Re-entrant, and Junctional Tachycardias

Sinus tachycardia rarely should be treated directly. Instead, treatment should focus on identifying and treating any precipitating underlying conditions, especially heart failure, pulmonary disease, fever, and thyroid disease. Multifocal atrial tachycardia is relatively unresponsive to medical therapy, is very difficult to ablate, and is best treated by management of the underlying pulmonary disorder. Nondihydropyridine calcium-channel blocking drugs (diltiazem, verapamil; Table 64-5) are most often used if a therapy is absolutely required.

Sustained or repeated episodes of nonsustained SVT, however, generally require effective therapy. If rapid control is desired (e.g., in patients with myocardial ischemia or hypotension), cardioversion is the best solution (Chapter 66). Atrial tachycardias, including atrial flutter or AF, may also convert spontaneously or convert after treatment of an underlying cause, such as hypoxia or heart failure, or after cessation of precipitating medications.

An acute episode of either AVNRT or junctional tachycardia can often be terminated with vagal maneuvers, such as carotid massage. In most atrial tachycardias, adenosine or vagal stimulation (or both) produces enough AV block to unmask the atrial origin of the tachycardia. However, some atrial tachycardias and most episodes of AVNRT terminate after administration of adenosine. Intravenous β-blockers or calcium-channel blockers (see Table 64-5) can be used for the same purpose. For sustained control of the ventricular rate during atrial tachycardia, intravenous esmolol and diltiazem are effective.

Accessory Pathway Tachycardia

The acute management of SVTs that use an accessory pathway (AVRT) depends on the mechanism of the rhythm. If the tachycardia uses the AV node as one limb of the circuit, it may terminate with vagal maneuvers such as carotid sinus massage. If the tachycardia uses an accessory pathway as the antegrade limb (antidromic AVRT), it is important to avoid measures that may accelerate the conduction properties of the accessory pathway. For example, digoxin and epinephrine will increase conduction over the accessory pathway and potentially accelerate the tachycardia. Patients may have an adrenergic response to a drop in blood pressure induced by the vasodilating properties of β-blockers and calcium-channel blockers, particularly when AF conducts over an accessory pathway. As a result of these potential complications, adenosine (see Table 64-5) is the drug of choice for the acute termination of antidromic AVRT, but a true antiarrhythmic drug, such as intravenous amiodarone, or cardioversion should be considered for antidromically conducted AF. In orthodromic AVRT, in which the AV node is the antegrade limb of the tachycardia, β-blockers or calcium-channel blockers can be used as well as adenosine.

Atrial Flutter

It can be very difficult to control the rate of acute atrial flutter, which generally must be treated by restoring sinus rhythm. Intravenous ibutilide is approximately 60% effective for converting atrial flutter to sinus rhythm. Direct current electrical cardioversion, which is highly (>95%) effective for restoring sinus rhythm, should not be performed unless the episode of atrial flutter is believed to be less than 48 hours in duration, or transesophageal echocardiogram has excluded clot in the left atrial appendage, or until the risk of stroke has been minimized by achieving a therapeutic international normalized ration (INR) of 2 to 3 for the prior 4 weeks.

Atrial Fibrillation

For acute AF without hypotension, rate control is crucial and can be accomplished with esmolol, metoprolol, verapamil, or diltiazem (see Table 64-5); digoxin is usually a third-line agent (Fig. 64-23). All patients with new-onset AF should receive anticoagulation acutely with heparin (Chapter 37). The decision of whether to restore and maintain sinus rhythm or allow recurrences or progression to permanent AF is a fundamental component of AF management. Trials of a strategy of rate control compared with a

TABLE 64-5 ANTIARRHYTHMIC DRUGS: DOSES AND SIDE EFFECTS

ANTIARRHYTHMIC DRUG AND COMMON USE	DOSE/METABOLISM	SIDE EFFECTS AND REQUIRED MONITORING	SELECTED DRUG INTERACTIONS
Quinidine	Hepatic CYP 3A4 (70%), renal (30%) Dose: sulfate—600 mg tid, gluconate—324 to 648 mg q8h Dose reduced for renal failure	Thrombocytopenia Cinchonism Pruritus, rash QT prolongation/torsades de pointes	↑ Digoxin and amiodarone concentrations Quinidine inhibits CYP 2D6 and may increase drugs metabolized by this enzyme, e.g., ↑ effect of tricyclic antidepressants, haloperidol, some β-blockers, fluoxetine, narcotics Quinidine metabolism inhibited by cimetidine Quinidine metabolism increased by phenobarbital, phenytoin, and rifampicin
Procainamide	Mostly hepatic—rapid acetylators produce more NAPA; NAPA renally cleared PO dose: 50 mg/kg/24 hr IV dose: 1 g over 25 min, then 20-60 μg/kg/min infusion Reduce dose for renal dysfunction or low cardiac output	Rash, fever, arthralgias, drug-induced lupus, particularly in slow acetylators Agranulocytosis QT prolongation/torsades de pointes	Procainamide clearance reduced by trimethoprim, cimetidine, and ranitidine
Disopyramide	Renal, hepatic (CYP 3A4) Dose: 100-400 mg q8-12h; max dose, 800 mg/24 hr Reduce dose for renal or hepatic dysfunction	Anticholinergic (contraindicated for narrow-angle glaucoma): dry mouth, urinary retention, constipation, blurry vision QT prolongation/torsades de pointes	None
Propafenone	Hepatic: 150-300 mg q8h or sustained release 225-425 mg bid	Metallic taste, dizziness, SIADH Atrial flutter, ventricular tachycardia	May decrease the metabolism of warfarin Increase digoxin levels
Flecainide	Renal, hepatic CYP 2D6 50-100 mg bid; max dose, 300-400 mg/day	Dizziness, headache, visual blurring Atrial flutter, ventricular tachycardia	May increase digoxin levels Flecainide levels increased by amiodarone, haloperidol, quinidine, cimetidine, and fluoxetine
β-Blockers (selected)	Hepatic, renal Only renal (atenolol, nadolol) IV esmolol: 250-500 μg over 1 min, then 50-300 μg/kg/min over 4 min Acebutolol, 200-600 mg bid; atenolol, 25-100 mg qd; carvedilol, 3.125-50 mg bid; metoprolol, 25-150 mg bid; nadolol, 20-120 mg qd; nebivolol, 5-40 mg qd; propranolol, 10-120 mg bid	Fatigue, depression, bronchospasm, impotence	Minimal, except for carvedilol and metoprolol, whose levels may be increased by amiodarone, propafenone, quinidine, fluoxetine, haloperidol, paroxetine, and cimetidine
Sotalol	Renal: 80-120 mg bid Max dose, 240 mg bid	Bronchospasm QT prolongation/torsades de pointes	No significant interactions
Dofetilide	Renal, hepatic CYP 3A4 CrCl > 60 (500 μg bid), CrCl 40-60 (250 μg bid), CrCl 20-39 (125 μg bid)	QT prolongation and torsades de pointes Three days of in-hospital monitoring is required during drug initiation	Contraindicated with verapamil, ketoconazole, cimetidine, megestrol, prochlorperazine, and trimethoprim Hydrochlorothiazide increases dofetilide levels Must discontinue amiodarone at least 3 mo before dofetilide initiation
Ibutilide	Hepatic CYP 3A4 1 mg IV over 10 min, repeat after 10 min if necessary	Nausea QT prolongation and torsades de pointes Must monitor for 4 hr after drug initiation	None
Amiodarone	Hepatic half-life 50 days PO load 10 g over 7-10 days, then 400 mg for 3 wk, then 200 mg/day for atrial fibrillation Maintenance dose of 400 mg/day for VT Dose reduce load for bradycardia or QT prolongation IV: 150-300 mg bolus, then 1 mg/min infusion for 6 hr, followed by 0.5 mg/min thereafter	Pulmonary (acute hypersensitivity pneumonitis, chronic interstitial infiltrates), hepatitis Thyroid (hypo- or hyperthyroidism) Photosensitivity, blue-gray discoloration with chronic high dose, nausea, ataxia, tremor, alopecia Avoid if identified thyroid nodule LFTs two to three times a year, TFTs twice yearly, PFTs and CXR at initiation and CXR yearly thereafter. QT prolongation expected; reduce dose if exceeds 500 msec	Inhibits CYP 450 enzymes—increases concentrations of warfarin, digoxin, cyclosporine, alprazolam, carbamazepine, HMG-CoA inhibitors, phenytoin, and quinidine
Dronedarone	Hepatic CYP 3A4 half-life 30 hr PO 400 mg bid Improved absorption with food	Reduces the secretion of creatinine without a reduction in GFR Hepatic failure Avoid in heart failure	Increases digoxin levels (dose reduce digoxin by half) May increase myositis with simvastatin Avoid grapefruit
Calcium-channel blocker (nondihydropyridine)	Hepatic Inhibit CYP 3A4 IV diltiazem, 20 mg bolus over 2 min, then 5-15 mg per hour maintenance infusion Verapamil long-acting 120-480 mg qd Diltiazem long-acting 180-300 mg qd	Constipation, rash, peripheral edema	Inhibits CYP 3A4—will increase levels of alprazolam, carbamazepine, dihydropyridine, cyclosporine, HMG-CoA inhibitors. Verapamil (but not diltiazem) increases digoxin levels

TABLE 64-5 ANTIARRHYTHMIC DRUGS: DOSES AND SIDE EFFECTS—cont'd

ANTIARRHYTHMIC DRUG AND COMMON USE	DOSE/METABOLISM	SIDE EFFECTS AND REQUIRED MONITORING	SELECTED DRUG INTERACTIONS
Adenosine	Erythrocyte, endothelial cell 6-mg IV push, followed if necessary by 12 mg after 1-2 min	Nausea, headache, flushing, chest pain, bronchospasm (contraindicated if asthma)	Methylxanthines compete for adenosine receptors with adenosine Dipyridamole decreases the metabolism of adenosine
Digoxin	Renal, hepatic, gastrointestinal, 0.125-375 mg/day	Anorexia, nausea, fatigue, confusion, altered vision with green-yellow halos	Levels of or sensitivity to digoxin increased by hypokalemia, quinidine, verapamil, amiodarone, propafenone, renal failure, hypoxia, decreased muscle mass Levels of or sensitivity to digoxin decreased by malabsorption, hyperkalemia, hypocalcemia

CXR = chest x-ray; CYP = cytochrome P-450; GFR = glomerular filtration rate; HMG-CoA = 3-hydroxy-3-methylglutaryl coenzyme A; IV = intravenous administration; LFT = liver function test; NAPA = *N*-acetyl procainamide; PFT = pulmonary function test; PO = oral administration; SIADH = syndrome of inappropriate diuretic hormone; TFT = thyroid function test; VT = ventricular tachycardia.

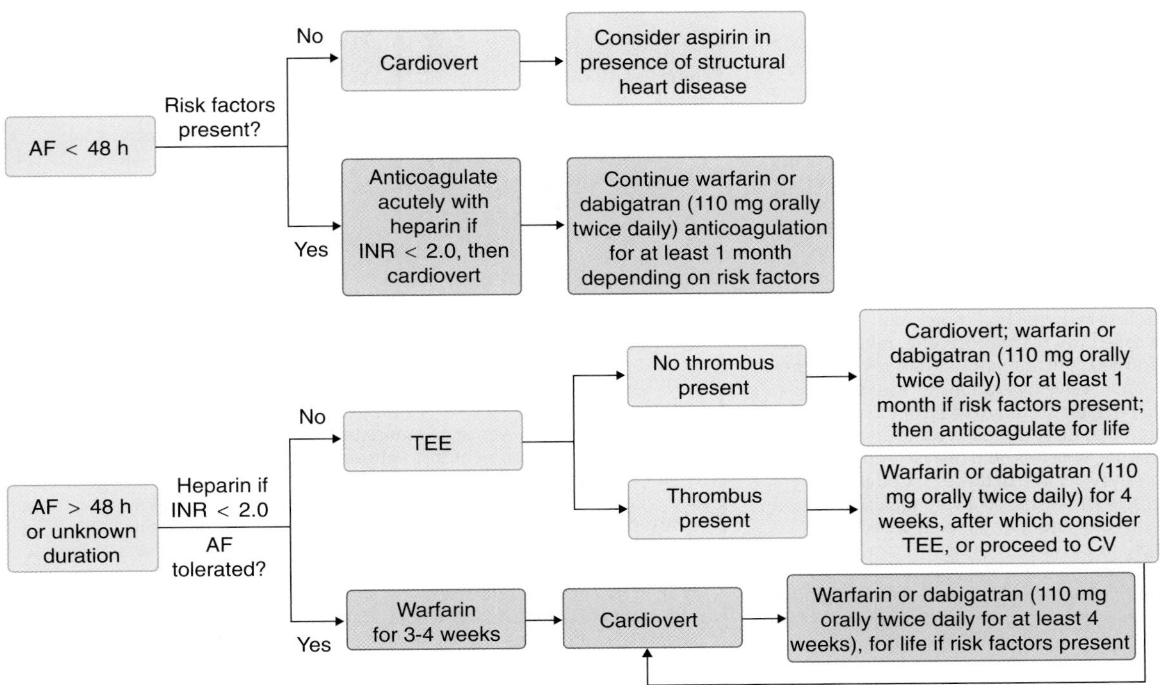

FIGURE 64-23. Management of recent-onset atrial fibrillation (AF). CV = Cardioversion; INR = International Normalized Ratio; TEE = Transesophageal echocardiography.

strategy of rhythm control with antiarrhythmic drugs have demonstrated no difference in total or arrhythmic mortality associated with these two approaches,[1-3] even in patients with a reduced ejection fraction.[4] Because a significant component of the adverse events experienced in the rhythm control arms of these studies was due to stroke in un-anticoagulated patients and toxicity from antiarrhythmic drugs, advances in antiarrhythmic and anticoagulant medications as well as the advent of reliable ablative therapies for AF may necessitate a reevaluation of this question.

If a strategy of rate control is chosen, it is important to confirm a heart rate of 80 to 110 beats per minute at rest and less than 140 beats per minute with exercise, preferably by monitoring the heart rate during exercise on an exercise treadmill test or with an ambulatory monitor. More strict rate control is not beneficial.[5] Failure to confirm rate control can result in the development of tachycardia-induced cardiomyopathy. First-line therapy for rate control includes β-blockers or calcium-channel blockers; digoxin can also be used but is generally less effective. Patients commonly require a combination of mediations to achieve goal heart rates.

If a strategy of rhythm control is chosen, many patients will first require cardioversion, either pharmacologic or electrical (Chapter 66). The risk of clot formation must be mitigated before cardioversion in all patients with AF of more than 48 hours' duration. The first step generally is to perform transesophageal echocardiography (TEE) (Chapter 55). If TEE shows no evidence of a left atrial clot, cardioversion can be undertaken without systemic anticoagulation; if the patient has risk factors for stroke in association with AF, however, most clinicians administer anticoagulation during the cardioversion and for the subsequent 4 weeks. If the TEE shows evidence of clot, 4 consecutive weeks of anticoagulation with an INR of at least 2 is required, and anticoagulation must be maintained for at least 3 to 4 weeks after cardioversion. Electrical cardioversion, which should be performed with a minimum of 200 joules, is successful in more than 90% of cases. Pharmacologic cardioversion can be performed with intravenous drugs such as ibutilide, which is more successful for atrial flutter (60% efficacy) than AF (50%). Oral medications can also be used as a "pill in the pocket" strategy. Patients can take a single dose of propafenone (600 mg) or flecainide (300 mg) with a conversion rate for recent-onset AF (<48 hours' duration) of approximately 50% without the need for a screening TEE. Oral amiodarone (typically loaded with 10 g over the first week, followed by 400 to 600 mg a day for the next 3 weeks) can also be used for cardioversion and is successful in approximately 50% of patients with both recent and more prolonged AF.

Long-Term Management

AVNRT, AVRT, Atrial Tachycardias, and Atrial Flutter

Chronic therapy for AVNRT is guided by the frequency and severity of symptoms. Many patients are able to live with this rhythm with infrequent recurrences, which terminate spontaneously or with adenosine. If chronic therapy is required, β-blockers or calcium-channel blockers and less commonly digoxin are used. Ablation of AVNRT (Chapter 66) is highly effective and should be considered before using sodium- or potassium-channel blocking drugs.

Most patients with symptomatic AVRT are treated with catheter ablation (Chapter 66). Ablation of an accessory pathway located near the AV node or His bundle carries a 1% risk of complete heart block, whereas ablation of accessory pathways on the left side of the heart and distant from the AV node and His bundle region is not associated with a risk of heart block but carries a small risk of stroke. At present, it is not standard of care to ablate accessory pathways in patients without symptomatic arrhythmias.

The long-term management of atrial tachycardia depends on symptoms. If the rhythm is highly symptomatic, it is generally managed with a β-blocker or calcium-channel blocker. If these medications are unsuccessful or not tolerated, ablation is frequently recommended, but antiarrhythmic medications are an alternative.

In patients with atrial flutter, ventricular rate control is possible by achieving AV nodal block with β-blockers, calcium-channel blockers, and digitalis. However, radio frequency ablation, which is curative, is now the preferred choice for most patients with atrial flutter (Chapter 66), especially recurrent atrial flutter. Because atrial flutter carries a 3% per year risk of thromboembolism, patients with atrial flutter should also receive long-term anticoagulation similar to what is recommended for AF (see later). If atrial flutter is successful, the risk of recurrence is very small, and long-term anticoagulation is not necessary.

Atrial Fibrillation

Therapies for the chronic maintenance of sinus rhythm in patients with AF include pharmacologic and procedural approaches. The procedural approaches include catheter-based ablation inside the left atrium with the goal of electrically isolating the pulmonary veins from the left atrium. Similarly, a minimally invasive surgical approach can electrically isolate the pulmonary veins from the external surface of the heart with the additional resection of the left atrial appendage. Both these procedures have become standard options for AF, especially in patients who have recurrent AF despite at least one antiarrhythmic drug.[6,7] The catheter approach carries a small risk of cardiac perforation, including pericardial tamponade and atrioesophageal fistula formation, and a 1% risk of stroke. There is also a small risk of pulmonary vein stenosis, which has been reduced by newer technologies. The surgical approach carries a higher risk of cardiac bleeding, particularly during the resection of the left atrial appendage, and is associated with a significantly longer recovery time than the percutaneous approach. However, there should be no stroke risk associated with the surgical procedure because it is performed completely from the epicardial surface of the heart. In addition, the exclusion of the left atrial appendage may prove protective in regard to future thromboembolic risk.[8] Both procedures appear to be equally effective, with approximately 60 to 70% of patients experiencing a significant reduction or absence of AF following either procedure. It is typical to offer a second procedure to patients who have recurrent AF following a first catheter-based procedure. Finally, a more extensive surgical operation, called the maze procedure, requires a full thoracotomy and is most often performed concomitantly as part of open coronary artery bypass surgery or an open valve operation. In this procedure, electrical lines of block are created in the left atrium to interrupt the perpetuation of AF, the pulmonary veins are isolated, and the left atrial appendage is resected. Success rates for this procedure, which should be reserved for refractory, symptomatic AF, exceed 80%. However, none of these procedures has yet been demonstrated to reduce the risk of stroke risk, so anticoagulation should be maintained for 6 months after the procedure in patients without clinical risk factors for stroke and chronically in patients with risk factors. Catheter-based procedures directed at excluding the left atrial appendage from the systemic blood stream may become options in patients who have a high risk of stroke and who cannot tolerate systemic anticoagulation owing to an excessive risk of bleeding.

The pharmacologic options for the treatment of AF work by blocking sodium, potassium, or a combination of cardiac channels. Blockade of these channels results in slowing of cardiac conduction (sodium channels) and prolongation in cardiac repolarization (potassium channels) as well as additional effects from modulation of the autonomic nervous system. The choice of antiarrhythmic drug is based on the patient's underlying clinical condition (Table 64-6).

Amiodarone is the most widely used medication for AF with an efficacy of 60 to 70% at 1 year. It is associated with a number of drug interactions, most notably with warfarin and digoxin. Its associated risk of thyroid, liver, and lung toxicities, related in part to the iodine moieties on this compound, necessitate careful follow-up. For prevention of recurrent AF, oral amiodarone is significantly more effective than propafenone and sotalol, which are the recommended alternatives. Another alternative is 400 mg twice daily of dronedarone, which is related to amiodarone but has no iodine and a 24-hour half-life, significantly reduced cardiovascular hospitalizations by 16% and death from 3.9% to 2.7% at 21 months in patients with AF.[9] Dronedarone is currently thought to be safe, however, only in patients with an ejection fraction greater than 35% and no evidence of advanced heart failure.

Quinidine, procainamide, and disopyramide are predominantly sodium-channel blocking drugs that also block potassium channels at slow heart rates. Each of these drugs is moderately successful in AF, with about 50% of treated patients in sinus rhythm at 1 year, but each also has idiosyncratic noncardiovascular toxicities that can significantly limit their utility (see Table 64-5). Propafenone and flecainide are also sodium-channel blockers that are widely used for the maintenance of sinus rhythm. These drugs are moderately effective, with a 50% rate of sinus rhythm at 1 year, and are generally well tolerated but must be avoided in patients with structural heart disease, particularly with a history of prior myocardial infarction and impaired left ventricular function, because of a risk for drug-induced ventricular arrhythmia. Dofetilide is a potassium-channel blocking medication that is moderately effective for suppressing AF but carries a dose-dependent risk of QT prolongation and torsades de pointes.

TABLE 64-6 SELECTION OF ANTIARRHYTHMIC DRUGS

PATIENT CHARACTERISTICS	ANTIARRHYTHMIC DRUG CHOICES
No structural heart disease	*First line:* flecainide, propafenone, dronedarone, sotalol *Second line:* amiodarone, dofetilide
Depressed left ventricular ejection fraction with heart failure	*First line:* amiodarone, dofetilide *Avoid:* dronedarone, flecainide, propafenone
Coronary artery disease without congestive heart failure	*First line:* sotalol, dronedarone, dofetilide, amiodarone *Avoid:* flecainide, propafenone
Hypertrophic cardiomyopathy	*First line:* amiodarone, sotalol, dronedarone *Second line:* disopyramide

TABLE 64-7 CURRENT RECOMMENDATIONS FOR THROMBOEMBOLIC PROPHYLAXIS FOR PATIENTS WITH ATRIAL FIBRILLATION BASED ON RISK FACTORS FOR STROKE

No risk	Aspirin (81 to 325 mg/day) or nothing
One moderate risk factor (age ≥ 75 yr, hypertension, heart failure, left ventricular ejection fraction ≤ 35%, diabetes mellitus)	Warfarin (INR 2-3) or dabigatran (110 mg orally twice daily) preferred in patients age ≥ 65 yr with heart failure or age 65-74 yr with diabetes or coronary disease; otherwise aspirin (81 or 325 mg)
At least two moderate risk factors or one high risk factor (prior stroke or transient ischemic attack, mitral stenosis, prosthetic valve)	Warfarin (INR 2-3, or 2.5-3.5 with prosthetic valve) or dabigatran (110 mg orally twice daily)

Anticoagulation

The presence or absence of associated conditions help determine which patients with AF require chronic anticoagulation with warfarin or other systematic coagulants (Table 64-7). Long-term anticoagulation therapy with warfarin or dabigatran is generally recommended in all patients who have persistent or paroxysmal AF, who are older than 65 years, and who have no contraindications to anticoagulation.[10] Warfarin alone is superior to aspirin[11] or the combination of clopidogrel and aspirin, with meta-analysis showing that adjusted-dose warfarin and antiplatelet agents reduce stroke by approximately 60% and 20%, respectively.[12] Although there is some protective effect at an INR as low as 1.8, the target INR for chronic anticoagulation with warfarin should be 2 to 3 to avoid INRs less than 1.8. For patients who do not require or cannot tolerate warfarin, aspirin is a reasonable alternative. Clopidogrel (75 mg/day), in addition to aspirin, reduces the risk of major vascular events from 7.6% per year to 6.8% per year compared with aspirin alone, but increases the risk of major bleeding from 1.3% per year to 2% per year.[13] Dabigatran at 110 mg twice daily is as effective as warfarin but causes less bleeding.[14] Newer alternatives include direct thrombin inhibitors and factor Xa inhibitors. For example, in a randomized study of patients unable to tolerate warfarin, the factor Xa inhibitor apixaban (5 mg daily) reduced stroke and systemic embolism without major increases in bleeding.[15] These new classes of anticoagulants do not require monitoring with blood tests and do not interact with food or medications. Aspirin may be better than no treatment for patients who cannot tolerate warfarin. The addition of aspirin to moderate-intensity warfarin in anticoagulation (INR 2 to 3) can decrease vascular events and is recommended in high-risk patients.[16]

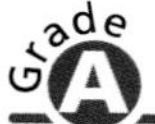

1. Hohnloser SH, Kuck K-H, Lilienthal J. Rhythm or rate control in atrial fibrillation. Pharmacological Intervention in Atrial Fibrillation (PIAF): a randomized trial. *Lancet.* 2000;356:1789-1794.
2. Wyse DG, Waldo AL, DiMarco JP, et al. A comparison of rate control and rhythm control in patients with atrial fibrillation. *N Engl J Med.* 2002;347:1825-1833.
3. Van Gelder IC, Hagens VE, Bosker HA, et al. A comparison of rate control and rhythm control in patients with recurrent persistent atrial fibrillation. *N Engl J Med.* 2002;347:1834-1840.
4. Roy D, Talajic M, Nattel S, et al. Rhythm control versus rate control for atrial fibrillation and heart failure. *N Engl J Med.* 2008;358:2667-2677.
5. Van Gelder I, Groenveld H, Crijns H. Lenient versus strict rate control in patients with atrial fibrillation. *N Engl J Med.* 2010;362:1363-1373.
6. Wilber DJ, Pappone C, Neuzil P, et al. Comparison of antiarrhythmic drug therapy and radiofrequency catheter ablation in patients with paroxysmal atrial fibrillation: a randomized controlled trial. *JAMA.* 2010;303:333-340.
7. Terasawa T, Balk EM, Chung M, et al. Systematic review: comparative effectiveness of radiofrequency catheter ablation for atrial fibrillation. *Ann Intern Med.* 2009;151:191-202.

8. Holmes DR, Reddy VY, Turi ZG, et al. Percutaneous closure of the left atrial appendage versus warfarin therapy for prevention of stroke in patients with atrial fibrillation: a randomized non-inferiority trial. *Lancet.* 2009;374:534-542.
9. Hohnloser SH, Crijns HJ, van Eickels M, et al. Effect of dronedarone on cardiovascular events in atrial fibrillation. *N Engl J Med.* 2009;360:668-678.
10. Perez-Gomez F, Alegria E, Berjon J, et al. Comparative effects of antiplatelet, anticoagulant, or combined therapy in patients with valvular and nonvalvular atrial fibrillation: a randomized multi-center study. *J Am Coll Cardiol.* 2004;44:1557-1566.
11. Mant J, Richard FD, Fletcher K, et al. Warfarin versus aspirin for stroke prevention in an elderly community population with atrial fibrillation (the Birmingham atrial fibrillation treatment of the aged study, BAFTA). *Lancet.* 2007;370:493-503.
12. Hart RG, Pearce LA, Aguilar MI, et al. Meta-analysis: antithrombotic therapy to prevent stroke in patients who have nonvalvular atrial fibrillation. *Ann Intern Med.* 2007;146:857-867.
13. Connolly SJ, Pogue J, Hart RG, et al, for the ACTIVE Investigators. Effect of clopidogrel added to aspirin in patients with atrial fibrillation. *N Engl J Med.* 2009;360:2066-2078.
14. Connolly SJ, Ezekowitz MD, Yusuf S, et al. Dabigatran versus warfarin in patients with atrial fibrillation. *N Engl J Med.* 2009;361:1139-1151.
15. Connolly SJ, Eikelboom J, Joyner C, et al. Apixaban in patients with atrial fibrillation. *N Engl J Med.* 2011;364:806-817.
16. Taylor FC, Cohen H, Ebrahim S. Systematic review of long term anticoagulation or antiplatelet treatment in patients with non-rheumatic atrial fibrillation. *BMJ.* 2001;322:321-326.

SUGGESTED READINGS

Dobrev D, Nattel S. New antiarrhythmic drugs for treatment of atrial fibrillation. *Lancet.* 2010;375:1212-1223. *Review.*

Wann LS, Curtis AB, January CT, et al. 2011 ACCF/AHA/HRS focused update on the management of patients with atrial fibrillation (updating the 2006 guideline). A report of the American College of Cardiology Foundation/American Heart Association Task Force on Practice Guidelines. *Circulation.* 2011;123:104-123. *Consensus guidelines.*

Zimetbaum P, Goldman A. Ambulatory arrhythmia monitoring: choosing the right device. *Circulation.* 2010;122:1629-1636. *Comprehensive review.*

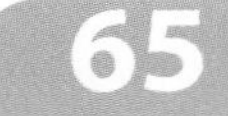

VENTRICULAR ARRHYTHMIAS

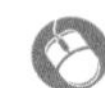

WILLIAM G. STEVENSON

Ventricular arrhythmias originate below the atrioventricular (AV) node in the ventricular myocardium or His-Purkinje system. These include premature ventricular beats, ventricular couplets, nonsustained and sustained ventricular tachycardias (VTs), and ventricular fibrillation (VF). These arrhythmias occur in all forms of heart disease and can be the initial presentation of disease. Sustained arrhythmias are an important cause of sudden death. Arrhythmias associated with genetic abnormalities of cardiac ion channels can cause sudden death despite the absence of identifiable structural heart disease. Ventricular arrhythmias that occur in the absence of structural heart disease or a defined ion channel abnormality are referred to as *idiopathic* and are usually benign. Evaluation and management are guided by the risk of arrhythmic death, which is determined by the presenting symptoms, type of arrhythmia, and associated underlying heart disease.

EPIDEMIOLOGY

Premature ventricular contractions (PVCs) are encountered on a standard electrocardiogram (ECG) in fewer than 1% of subjects younger than 20 years of age. The prevalence increases with age to greater than 2% of patients older than 50 years. Premature ventricular beats can be a sign of increased sympathetic tone, myocardial ischemia, hypoxia, and electrolyte abnormalities, particularly hypokalemia (Table 65-1), or underlying heart disease.

Sustained ventricular arrhythmias are usually caused by underlying structural heart disease, and the prevalence of arrhythmias increases with the severity of the heart disease. Ventricular arrhythmias are responsible for most of the 150,000 to 350,000 sudden deaths (Chapter 63) that occur annually in the United States and account for approximately 13% of all mortality. VF due to acute myocardial ischemia (Chapter 73) in the setting of coronary artery disease is the most common cause. The annual incidence of out-of-hospital VF is approximately 8 per 100,000. A 24-hour ECG recording will show premature ventricular beats and nonsustained VT in more than half of patients with advanced heart failure (Chapter 59). In the heart failure population, sustained VT or VF develops at a rate of approximately 2% per year or less when the left ventricular ejection fraction is above about 30%, but the rate doubles for patients with worse ventricular function.

TABLE 65-1 POTENTIAL FACTORS AGGRAVATING VENTRICULAR ARRHYTHMIAS

Elevated sympathetic tone
Acute illness
Central nervous system injury
Hypovolemia
Exertion/emotion
Fever
Myocardial ischemia/infarction
Tachycardia
Atrial fibrillation
Sinus tachycardia
Bradycardia
Electrolyte abnormalities
Hypokalemia, hypomagnesemia, hypocalcemia
Hypoxia
Hyperthyroidism
Sleep apnea
Toxins
Amphetamines, caffeine, ephedrine, pseudoephedrine
QT prolonging drugs/toxins (see Table 65-3)
Digitalis glycosides

PATHOBIOLOGY

Ventricular arrhythmia can be caused by automaticity or re-entry. Purkinje fibers have the capability for spontaneous automaticity that emerges normally at rates slower than 50 beats per minute. Abnormal automaticity occurs in partially depolarized ventricular or Purkinje myocytes. Triggered automaticity results from afterdepolarizations, which may be early or delayed in relation to the completion of ventricular repolarization. Delayed afterdepolarizations, which are membrane depolarizations that follow the completion of repolarization (i.e., usually after the completion of the T wave on the ECG), can occur when intracellular calcium overload increases the activity of the sodium-calcium exchanger, thereby producing a depolarizing inward flux of sodium. This mechanism is implicated in the ventricular arrhythmias seen in digitalis toxicity, familial catecholaminergic polymorphic VT, and some idiopathic right ventricular outflow tract arrhythmias. Rapid pacing and β-adrenergic stimulation promote delayed afterdepolarizations, so these arrhythmias are often exercise induced. Early afterdepolarizations occur before the completion of repolarization, that is, before the end of the T wave on the ECG, because a prolonged time to repolarization allows recovery of ion channels before the end of repolarization. Early afterdepolarizations are involved in the genesis of polymorphic VT associated with QT prolongation in the long QT syndromes and possibly during myocardial ischemia.

Re-entry in regions of myocardial scar is the most common cause of sustained VT associated with structural heart disease. The scar contains areas of fibrous tissue as well as surviving myocyte bundles that can create channels for propagation through the scar. Separation of myocyte bundles by fibrous tissue and uncoupling of adjacent bundles leads to slow conduction through these regions, thereby promoting re-entry (Fig. 65-1).

Re-entry can also occur in the absence of a fixed structural abnormality in the tissue. Spiral wave re-entry is one such formation that can be provoked in normal tissue by electrical stimulation (Fig. 65-2). The core of the spiral wave may wander through the tissue, thereby changing the ventricular activation sequence and producing polymorphic VT (see later). Alternatively, the spiral wave may anchor on anatomic discontinuities to produce a consistent beat-to-beat ventricular activation. Spiral waves that encounter refractory tissue can break into daughter waves and disorganize to VF.

CLINICAL MANIFESTATIONS AND DIAGNOSES

Ventricular arrhythmias can be asymptomatic and be detected by an irregular pulse, on a routine ECG, on routine monitoring in the hospital, or on an exercise test. Ventricular arrhythmias also can present symptomatically as palpitations (Chapters 50 and 62), dizziness, exercise intolerance, syncope (Chapters 50 and 62), or sudden cardiac arrest (Chapter 63). The diagnosis should be confirmed with an ECG. Individuals often have substantial hour-to-hour and day-to-day variation in the frequency of ventricular arrhythmias, so ambulatory monitoring is useful to record the cardiac rhythm at the time of symptoms (Chapter 62) if the arrhythmia is not present on the resting ECG. Exercise testing should be considered in patients with exercise-induced symptoms.

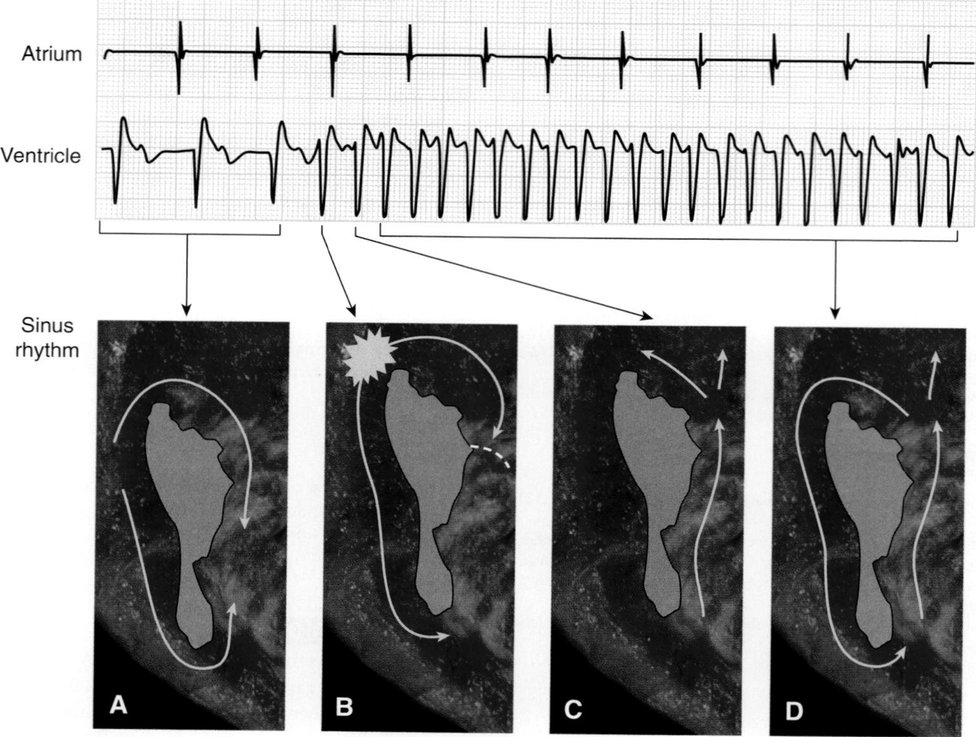

FIGURE 65-1. Initiation of scar-related re-entry. At the *top* are cardiac electrograms recorded by an implanted cardioverter-defibrillator. The *top tracing* is an atrial electrogram. The *bottom tracing* is the electrogram recorded from the lead in the right ventricular apex. Three beats of sinus rhythm are followed by a premature beat, which initiates ventricular tachycardia. The schematics below the tracings illustrate a potential mechanism of initiation of scar-related re-entry. In each panel, a cross section through the myocardium includes a region of scar *(white and gray regions)* that contains surviving myocyte bundles. A dense region of fibrosis *(solid gray region)* causes conduction block that creates a channel for conduction along the right-hand side of the fibrosis region. **A,** During sinus rhythm, wave fronts *(yellow arrows)* enter the channel from both sides and collide within the channel, thereby preventing re-entry. **B,** A premature beat *(star)* produces a wave front that reaches the superior end of the channel and finds it refractory, where it blocks *(dashed white line)*. The wave front that reaches the lower end of the channel enters the channel. **C,** Conduction through the channel is slow, allowing time for the initial region of block to recover. The wave front emerges from the exit of this channel, where it produces the first beat of ventricular tachycardia. **D,** The complete re-entry circuit.

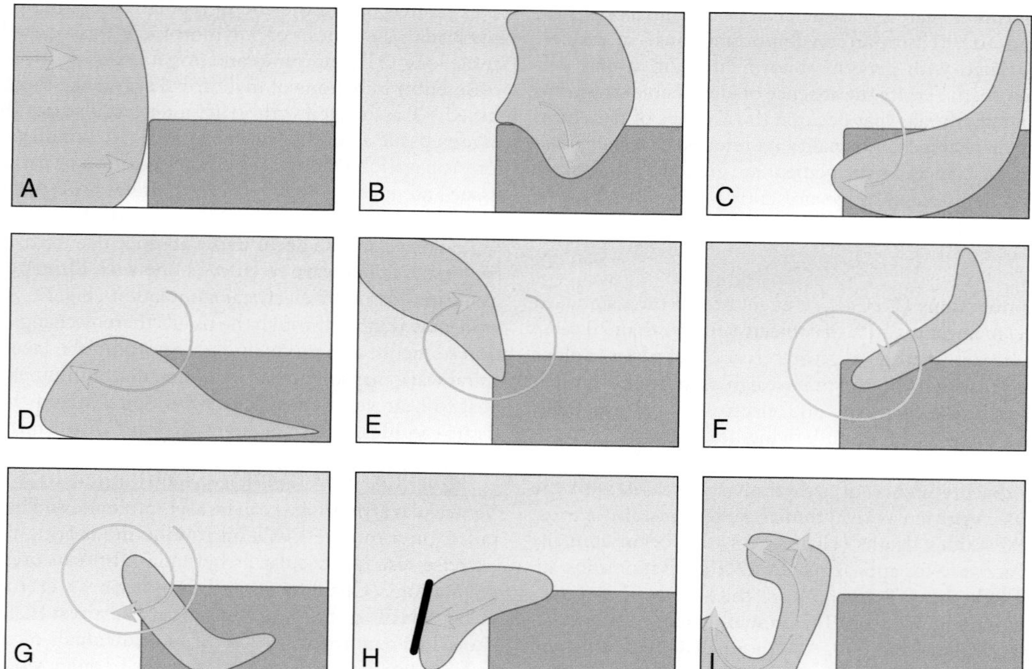

FIGURE 65-2. Spiral wave re-entry. The area of *blue* represents an excitation wave of depolarization. **A,** A wave front propagates from left to right and encounters a region of incompletely recovered tissue *(dark red region)*. **B,** The wave front propagates along the margin of refractory tissue until it reaches recovered tissue and propagates inferiorly (**C**). **D** to **G,** The wave front continues re-entering and establishing a circuit that continues to spiral through the tissue *(yellow arrow)*. **H,** The spiral wave encounters a region of block *(black line)*, which splits the wave front (**I**). Multiple potential wave fronts can be generated, thereby leading to fibrillation.

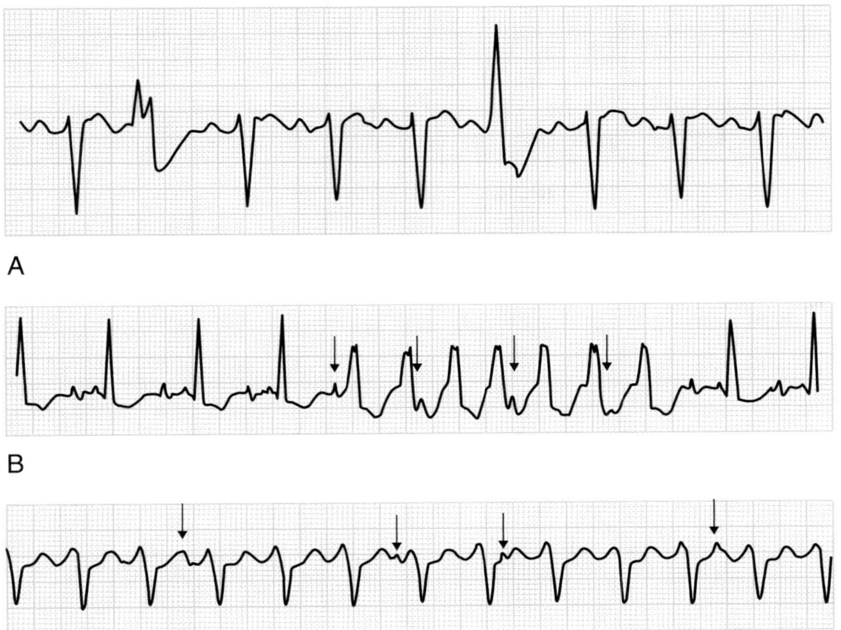

FIGURE 65-3. **Ventricular arrhythmias. A,** Multifocal premature ventricular beats. **B,** Nonsustained monomorphic ventricular tachycardia. Note dissociated P waves indicated by *arrows*. **C,** Sustained monomorphic ventricular tachycardia. Dissociated P waves are indicated by *arrows*.

TYPES OF VENTRICULAR ARRHYTHMIAS

A single beat is referred to as a *premature ventricular* beat (Fig. 65-3). Two consecutive beats are *ventricular couplets.* Three or more consecutive beats at a rate faster than 100 beats per minute are *VT* (see Fig. 65-3B and C). Three or more consecutive beats at slower rates are designated *idioventricular rhythms.* VT that terminates spontaneously within 30 seconds is *nonsustained* (see Fig. 65-3B), whereas *sustained VT* persists longer than 30 seconds.

The QRS morphology of the arrhythmia is determined by the sequence of ventricular activation. Conduction through the ventricular myocardium is slower than activation of the ventricles over the Purkinje system, so the QRS complex will be wide, typically more than 0.12 second. When VT is caused by repetitive activation from the same source, the QRS complexes are the same from beat to beat, and VT is monomorphic (see Fig. 65-3B and C). A continually changing activation sequence produces polymorphic VT with a changing QRS morphology (Fig. 65-4A). VF has continuous irregular activation with no discrete QRS complexes (see Fig. 65-4D). Although underlying structural heart disease is usually present, these arrhythmias do not require a fixed structural substrate.

The QRS morphology of an individual beat is determined largely by the site of initial ventricular activation. Arrhythmias that originate from the right ventricle or septum result in late activation of much of the left ventricle, thereby producing a prominent S wave in V_1, referred to as a *left bundle branch block–like configuration* (Fig. 65-5). Arrhythmias that originate from the free wall of the left ventricle have a prominent positive deflection in V_1, thereby producing a right bundle branch block–like morphology (Fig. 65-6). The axis of the QRS is also useful. A frontal plane axis that is directed inferiorly, as indicated by dominant R waves in leads II, III, and aVF, suggests initial activation of the cranial portion of the ventricle, whereas a frontal plane axis that is directed superiorly (dominant S waves in II, III, and aVF) suggests initial activation at the inferior wall.

Very rapid monomorphic VT has a sinusoidal appearance, also called *ventricular flutter,* because it is not possible to distinguish the QRS complex from the T wave (see Fig. 65-4B). Relatively slow sinusoidal VTs have a wide QRS indicative of slowed ventricular conduction (see Fig. 65-4C). Hyperkalemia, toxicity from excessive effects of drugs that block sodium channels (e.g., flecainide, propafenone, or tricyclic antidepressants), and severe global myocardial ischemia are causes.

PREMATURE VENTRICULAR CONTRACTIONS AND NONSUSTAINED VENTRICULAR TACHYCARDIA

PVCs can be due to automaticity or re-entry. PVCs that have the same QRS morphology, which indicates that they have the same origin, are unifocal PVCs (see Fig. 65-5). PVCs from more than one focus give rise to PVCs with different QRS morphologies and are known as *multifocal premature ventricular beats* (see Fig. 65-3A).

During myocardial ischemia or in association with other heart disease, PVCs can be a harbinger of sustained VT or VF. When encountered during acute illness or as a new finding, the possibility of myocardial ischemia and other aggravating factors (Table 65-1) should be considered, and evaluation for underlying heart disease is warranted.

Three or more consecutive ventricular beats that occur at a rate faster than 100 beats per minute and that terminate spontaneously are nonsustained VT (see Fig. 65-3B). In patients with heart disease, nonsustained VT is associated with more severe disease and increased mortality. However, suppression of nonsustained VT with antiarrhythmic drugs does not improve survival. In ambulatory patients, nonsustained VT is usually monomorphic, with rates of less than 200 beats per minute and a duration of less than 8 beats. Nonsustained VT that is rapid, polymorphic, or with a first beat that occurs before the peak of the T wave ("short coupled") (see Fig. 65-4A) is uncommon and should prompt careful evaluation for causes of sustained VT and diseases associated with a high risk of sudden death (Table 65-3).

Idiopathic PVCs and nonsustained VT occur in the absence of structural or genetic heart disease. Most frequently, these PVCs originate from the right ventricular outflow tract and have a left bundle branch block configuration, with an inferiorly directed frontal plane axis (see Fig. 65-5). Less common sites of origin are the aortic and mitral valve annuli, the left ventricular papillary muscles, and the Purkinje system.

Once the diagnosis is established, further evaluation assesses the possible presence and severity of underlying heart disease. A family history of sudden death should prompt evaluation for genetic syndromes associated with sudden death, including cardiomyopathy (Chapter 60), long QT syndrome (see later), and arrhythmogenic right ventricular cardiomyopathy (Chapter 60). Any abnormality on the 12-lead ECG warrants further evaluation. Repolarization abnormalities are seen in a number of genetically determined syndromes associated with sudden death, including the long QT syndrome, Brugada's syndrome, arrhythmogenic right ventricular cardiomyopathy, and hypertrophic cardiomyopathy (Chapter 60). An echocardiogram (Chapter 55) is often warranted to assess ventricular function, wall motion abnormalities, and valvular heart disease. Cardiac magnetic resonance imaging is also useful for this purpose and for the detection of ventricular scarring that is the substrate for sustained VT. Exercise stress testing should be performed in patients who have exertional symptoms and for those who are at risk for coronary artery disease.

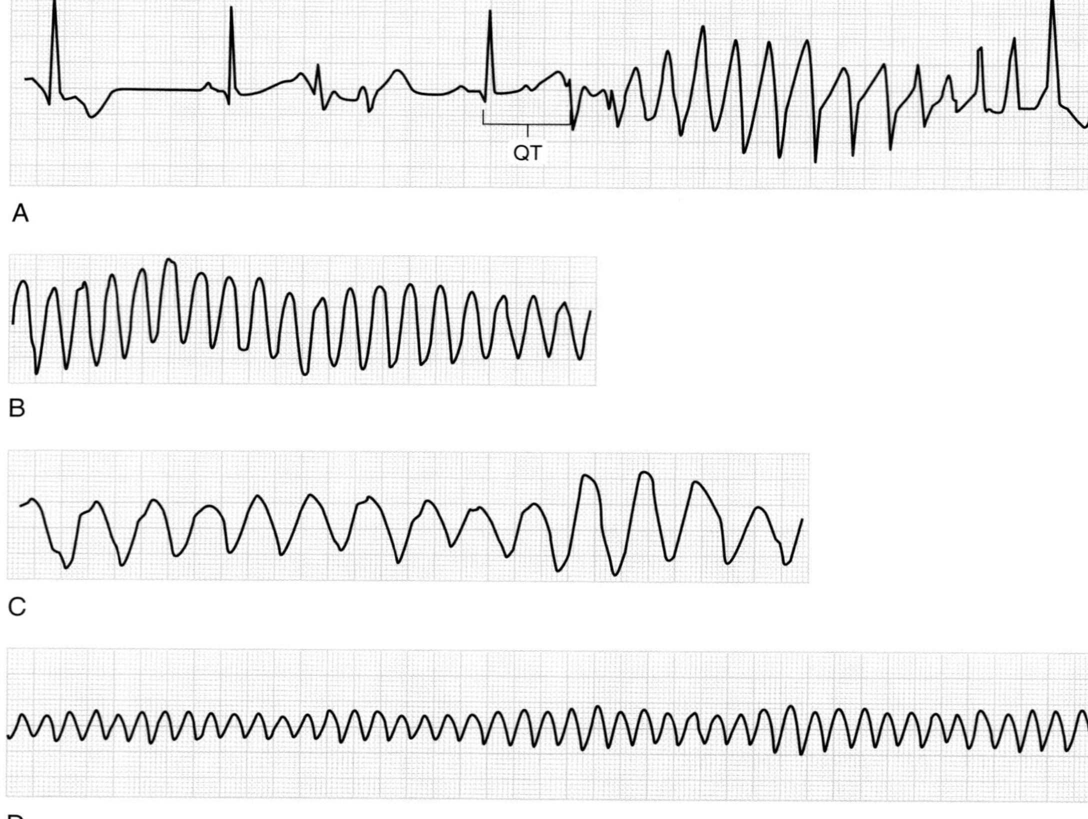

FIGURE 65-4. **A,** Polymorphic ventricular tachycardia associated with QT prolongation. Sinus rhythm, with a couplet of premature ventricular contractions, is followed by a sinus beat, and then by a polymorphic ventricular tachycardia. The QT interval of the sinus beats is markedly prolonged, exceeding 0.56 second. **B,** Rapid sinusoidal ventricular tachycardia with a rate approximating 250 beats/minute. **C,** Sinusoidal ventricular tachycardia owing to hyperkalemia. The rate is slower than 150 beats/minute, but the QRS duration exceeds 200 msec, thereby creating the sinusoidal appearance. **D,** Ventricular fibrillation.

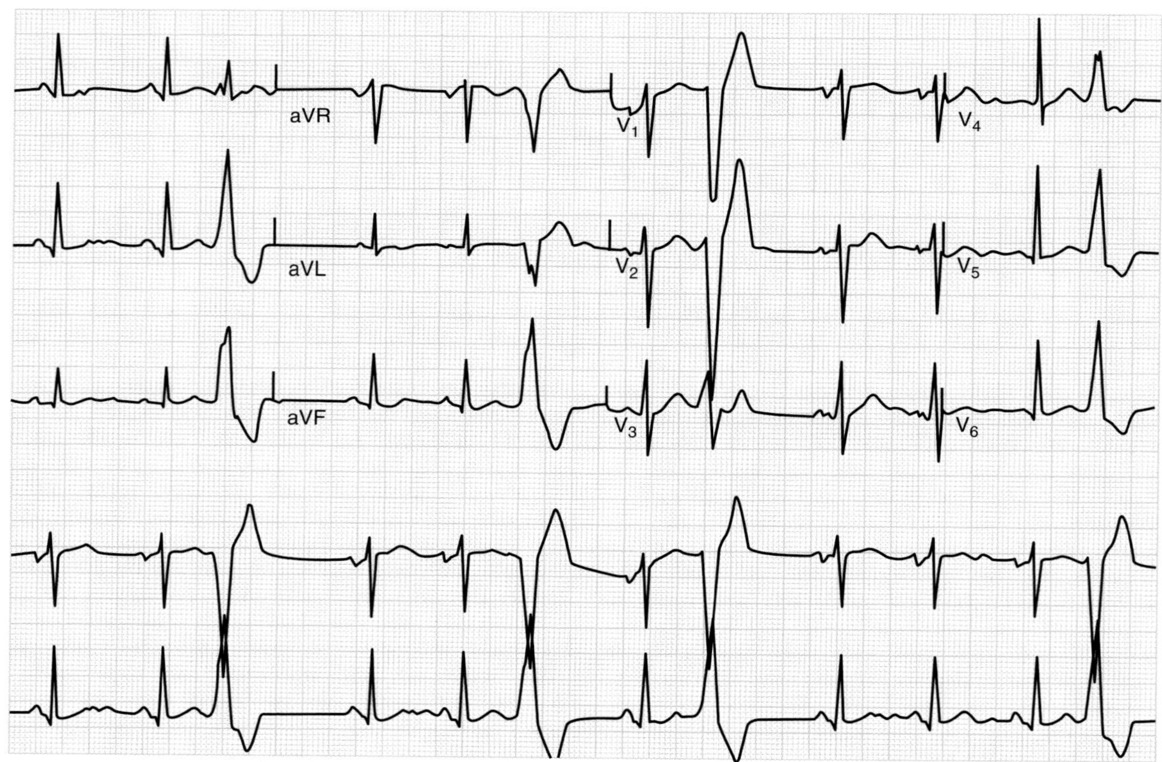

FIGURE 65-5. **Twelve-lead electrocardiogram with simultaneous two-lead rhythm strip (V_2 and V_5) showing premature ventricular beats that originated from the right ventricular outflow tract.** Sinus rhythm and frequent premature ventricular beats are present. The premature ventricular contractions all have the same morphology, best appreciated in the bottom two continuous leads, with a left bundle branch block–like configuration in V_1 consistent with an origin in the right ventricle or septum. The frontal plane axis is directed inferiorly, indicating initial depolarization from the cranial aspect of the ventricle.

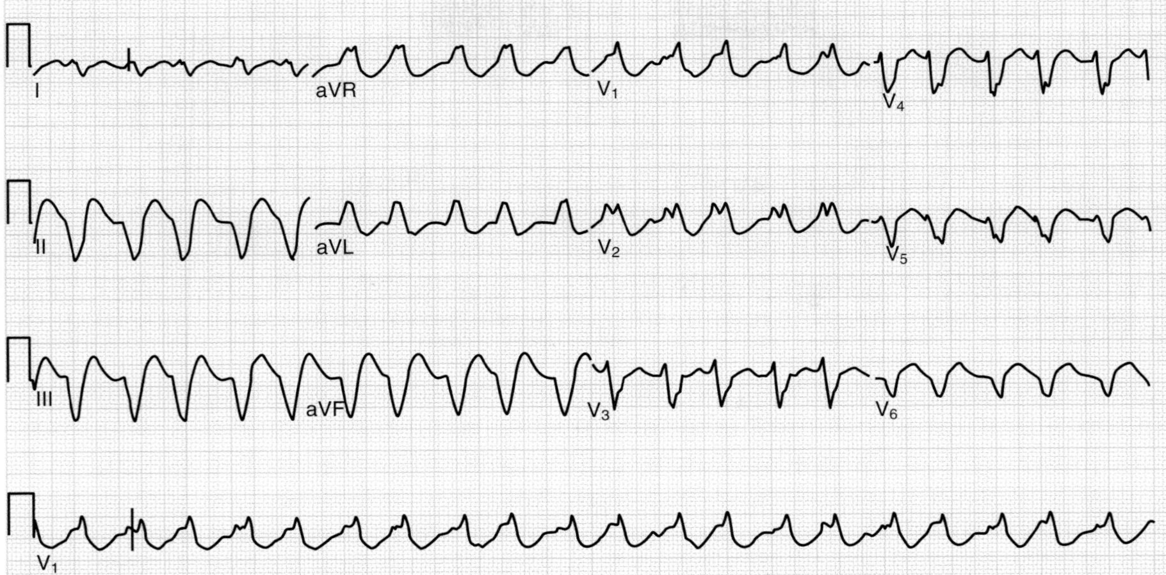

FIGURE 65-6. Sustained monomorphic ventricular tachycardia (VT) originating from an inferior left ventricular infarct region. VT has a right bundle branch block–like configuration in V_1, consistent with an origin in the left ventricle. The frontal plane axis is directed superiorly, consistent with initial depolarization of the inferior wall of the left ventricle.

TABLE 65-2 DISTINGUISHING VENTRICULAR TACHYCARDIA FROM SUPRAVENTRICULAR TACHYCARDIA WITH ABERRANT CONDUCTION

VENTRICULAR TACHYCARDIA	SUPRAVENTRICULAR TACHYCARDIA
AV dissociation AVR: initial R > S or initial r or q > 40 msec V_1 to V_6: absence of rs V_1 to V_6: onset of R to S > 100 msec in any lead V_6: QS or QR	Same QRS morphology as preexisting bundle branch block in sinus rhythm V_1: rsR′

TREATMENT Rx

Idiopathic Ventricular Tachycardia

For idiopathic PVCs and nonsustained VT in the absence of underlying heart disease, no specific therapy is needed unless the patient has significant symptoms or evidence that ectopy is depressing ventricular function. Reassurance that the arrhythmia is benign is often sufficient to allow the patient to cope with the symptoms, which will often wax and wane in frequency over years. Avoiding stimulants, such as caffeine, is helpful in some patients. If symptoms require treatment, β-adrenergic blockers and nondihydropyridine calcium-channel blockers (verapamil and diltiazem) are sometimes helpful (see Table 64-7 in Chapter 64). Suppression with more potent antiarrhythmic drugs can be effective but warrants careful consideration of the risks. Catheter ablation can be considered, particularly if unifocal PVCs are causing significant symptoms or contributing to depressed ventricular function, but the potential benefit must be carefully weighed against the procedure risks (Chapter 66).

For PVCs and nonsustained VT that have an impact on quality of life or are extremely frequent such that they may be contributing to ventricular dysfunction, chronic therapy with β-adrenergic blockers (Table 64-7) should be considered. Amiodarone and catheter ablation may be considered if β-adrenergic blockers are ineffective (see later).

Acute Coronary Syndromes

During and early after acute myocardial infarction (MI) (Chapter 73), PVCs and nonsustained VT are common and can be an early manifestation of ischemia and a harbinger of subsequent VF. Treatment with β-adrenergic blockers and correction of hypokalemia and hypomagnesemia reduce the risk of VF. Routine administration of the antiarrhythmic drug lidocaine does not reduce mortality.

Following recovery from acute MI, frequent PVCs (typically more than 10 PVCs per hour), repetitive PVCs with couplets, and nonsustained VT are markers for depressed ventricular function and increased mortality, but suppression of the arrhythmias with antiarrhythmic drug therapy does not improve survival and is not recommended. For survivors of an acute MI, an implantable cardioverter-defibrillator (ICD) reduces mortality in certain high-risk groups: patients who have survived more than 40 days after the acute MI and have a left ventricular ejection fraction of 30% or less or who have an ejection fraction of less than 0.35% and have symptomatic heart failure (functional class II or III); and patients more than 5 days after MI who have a reduced left ventricular ejection fraction, nonsustained VT, and inducible sustained VT or VF on electrophysiologic testing.[1] ICDs do not reduce mortality when routinely implanted soon after MI or in patients after recent coronary artery revascularization surgery.[2]

Depressed Ventricular Function and Heart Failure

Premature ventricular beats and nonsustained VT are common in patients with depressed ventricular function and heart failure, in whom they are markers for disease severity and increased mortality. Suppression of PVCs with antiarrhythmic drug therapy does not improve survival and is not routinely warranted. For example, in patients with prior MI and a depressed left ventricular ejection fraction, chronic antiarrhythmic drug therapy with the sodium-channel blocking antiarrhythmic drugs flecainide or moricizine increases mortality despite suppression of ventricular ectopy, apparently because of their proarrhythmic and negative inotropic effects. Therefore, antiarrhythmic drugs whose major action is blockade of the cardiac sodium channel (flecainide, propafenone, mexiletine, quinidine, disopyramide) are avoided in patients with structural heart disease. Therapy with dofetilide (see Table 64-7 in Chapter 64), which blocks the repolarizing current IKr, does not improve survival. In patients with heart failure and depressed left ventricular function, amiodarone suppresses ventricular ectopy and reduces sudden death but does not appear to improve survival,[3,4] whereas insertion of an ICD reduces the mortality rate by 20%, from 36% to 29%, over 5 years.[4]

Other Cardiac Disease

Ventricular ectopy is associated with increased mortality in patients with *hypertrophic cardiomyopathy* (Chapter 60) or with *congenital heart disease* (Chapter 69) associated with right or left ventricular dysfunction. In these patients, management is similar to what is recommended in patients with ventricular dysfunction. Pharmacologic suppression of the arrhythmia does not improve mortality, and ICDs are warranted for high-risk patients.

Premature Ventricular Contraction–Induced Ventricular Dysfunction

Very frequent ventricular ectopy can depress ventricular function, probably by a mechanism similar to that by which any chronic tachycardia causes tachycardia-induced cardiomyopathy. PVCs rarely contribute to depressed ventricular function unless they account for more than 10% of beats. The PVCs that cause ventricular depression typically are unifocal, most commonly originating from the left ventricular papillary muscles or outflow tract regions. The distinction between PVC-induced ventricular dysfunction compared with a cardiomyopathy that causes ventricular dysfunction independent of the ventricular arrhythmia is difficult and often can be made only retrospectively by observing an improvement in ventricular function after the arrhythmia is suppressed with amiodarone or catheter ablation.

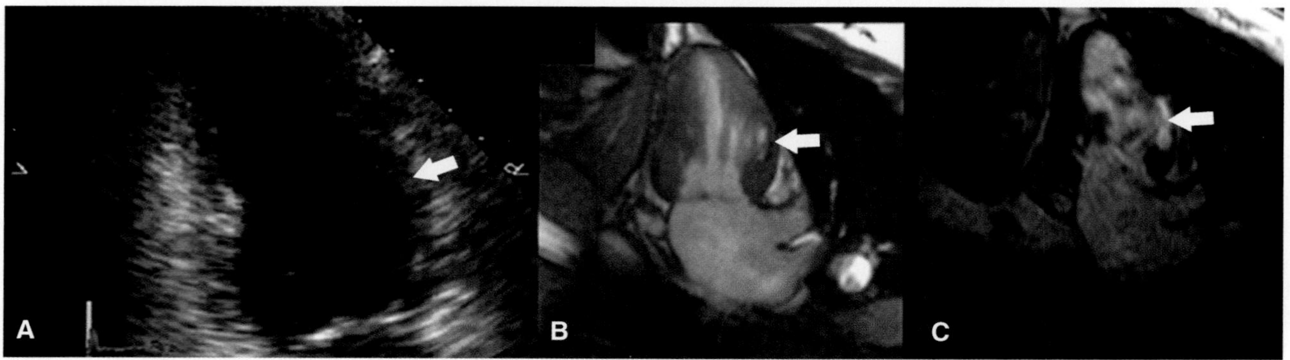

FIGURE 65-7. Images from a patient with an area of scar in the anterior left ventricular wall. **A,** Echocardiography shows a region of akinesis *(arrow)*. **B,** Cardiac magnetic resonance imaging shows the same area of akinesis *(arrow)*. **C,** Magnetic resonance imaging after administration of gadolinium contrast shows a region of delayed enhancement *(arrow)* consistent with scar.

IDIOVENTRICULAR RHYTHMS

Three or more ventricular beats at a rate slower than 100 beats/minute is an *idioventricular rhythm*. Automaticity is the likely mechanism. Idioventricular rhythms are common during acute MI (Chapter 73), when atropine therapy is occasionally indicated, and are seen as an escape rhythm during bradycardias. This rhythm is more common in patients with cardiomyopathies or sleep apnea, and it also can be idiopathic, often emerging when the sinus rate slows during sleep. Therapy targets any underlying cause and correction of bradycardia (Chapter 64).

SUSTAINED MONOMORPHIC VENTRICULAR TACHYCARDIA

CLINICAL MANIFESTATIONS

Sustained monomorphic VT presents as a wide QRS tachycardia. Presentations include palpitations, dyspnea, lightheadedness, syncope (Chapters 50 and 62), cardiac arrest, and sudden death (Chapter 63). During cardiac arrest, VT often deteriorates to VF, which may be the initial cardiac rhythm recorded. Structural heart disease with ventricular scarring that allows re-entry is the most common cause. Scars can be due to prior MI (Chapter 73), cardiomyopathies (Chapter 60), sarcoidosis (Chapter 95), and prior ventricular surgery, such as repair of tetralogy of Fallot (Chapter 69). Less commonly, VT is related to re-entry or automaticity in a diseased Purkinje system. Idiopathic VT occurs in the absence of structural heart disease. Management is determined by the underlying heart disease and the frequency and severity of symptoms.

DIAGNOSIS

All patients with monomorphic VT must be evaluated for possible underlying heart disease. When left ventricular function is depressed or there is evidence of structural myocardial disease, scar-related re-entry is the most likely diagnosis. Scars are suggested by pathologic Q waves on the ECG (see Fig. 73-1 in Chapter 73), segmental left or right ventricular wall motion abnormalities on echocardiogram (Fig. 65-7) or nuclear imaging, and areas of delayed gadolinium enhancement during magnetic resonance imaging (see Fig. 65-7). Patients who present with sustained VT associated with coronary artery disease typically have had large MIs and may present years after the acute infarct with a remodeled ventricle and markedly depressed left ventricular function.

TREATMENT AND PROGNOSIS Rx

Initial management is according to advanced cardiac life support (ACLS) guidelines (Chapters 7 and 63). Following restoration of sinus rhythm, hospitalization and evaluation to define underlying heart disease are required. Sustained monomorphic VT must be distinguished from supraventricular tachycardia with aberrancy (Chapter 64) to guide further therapy. The presence of AV dissociation is the most reliable maker for VT (see Fig. 65-3C), but P waves can be difficult to define, and 1:1 conduction from ventricle to atrium occurs in some VTs, so a 1:1 relationship of P waves to the QRS does not exclude the diagnosis of VT. A number of QRS morphologic criteria for distinguishing VT from supraventricular tachycardia with aberrancy (Table 65-2) have been described but are less reliable in patients with severe heart disease. The presence of underlying structural heart disease, particularly a history of prior MI, favors a diagnosis of VT rather than supraventricular tachycardia with aberrancy. An electrophysiologic study (Chapter 62) is sometimes required for definitive diagnosis.

Following restoration of sinus rhythm, assessment of cardiac biomarkers for evidence of MI (Chapter 72) is appropriate, but acute MI is rarely a cause of sustained monomorphic VT, and elevations in troponin or CK-MB are more likely to indicate MI that is secondary to hypotension and ischemia from the VT. Even when there is evidence of acute MI, a preexisting scar from previous MI should be suspected as the cause of the VT. Scar-related re-entry is not dependent on recurrent acute myocardial ischemia, so coronary revascularization cannot be anticipated to prevent recurrent VT, even when it may be appropriate for other indications (Chapter 74).

Scars provide a durable substrate for sustained VT, and up to 70% of patients have a recurrence of the arrhythmia within 2 years. Most patients with sustained monomorphic VT have depressed ventricular function, which is a risk factor for sudden death. ICDs reduce annual mortality from 12.3% to 8.8% and reduce arrhythmic deaths by 50% in patients with hemodynamically significant sustained VT or a history of cardiac arrest compared with pharmacologic therapy,[5] and they are usually warranted in such patients, provided that there is a reasonable expectation of survival with acceptable functional status for the next year after recovery from the VT episode. Chronic amiodarone therapy may be considered for patients who are not candidates for or who decline ICD placement.[3] Patients with frequent symptomatic VT require antiarrhythmic drug therapy or catheter ablation[5,6] to reduce recurrences.

Following ICD implantation, patients remain at risk for heart failure, recurrent ischemic events, and recurrent VT, with a 5-year mortality rate that exceeds 30%. Attention to therapies with survival benefit, including β-adrenergic blocking agents, angiotensin-converting enzyme inhibitors, and statins (Chapter 73) is critical.

Nonischemic Dilated Cardiomyopathy

Sustained monomorphic VT associated with cardiomyopathy is usually due to areas of ventricular scar. The etiology of scar is often unclear, but progressive fibrosis is a potential cause. On magnetic resonance imaging, scars are detectable as areas of delayed gadolinium enhancement and are more often intramural or subepicardial in location compared with those in patients with prior MI. Scars that cause VT are often located adjacent to a valve annulus and can occur in either ventricle. Any cardiomyopathic process can cause scars and VT, but cardiac sarcoidosis (Chapters 60 and 95) and Chagas' disease (Chapter 355) are particularly associated with monomorphic VT. An ICD is usually warranted.[7] Antiarrhythmic drugs and catheter ablation are used to control recurrent episodes in patients with an ICD.

Arrhythmogenic Right Ventricular Cardiomyopathy

Arrhythmogenic right ventricular cardiomyopathy (ARVC) (Chapter 60) is a rare genetic disorder with an estimated prevalence of 1 in 5000. Patients typically present between the second and fifth decades with palpitations, syncope, or cardiac arrest owing to sustained monomorphic VT, although polymorphic VT can also occur. Most cases are due to genetic mutations involving desmosomal proteins, including plakoglobin, plakophilin-2, desmin, desmocollin, and desmoglein-2. Inheritance is usually autosomal dominant with variable penetrance. Fibrosis and fibrofatty replacement of right ventricular myocardium, and less often the left ventricle, provide the substrate for reentrant VT that usually has a left bundle branch block–like configuration, consistent with a right ventricular origin.

The sinus rhythm ECG suggests the disease in more than 90% of patients, most often showing T wave inversions in V_1 to V_3 (Fig. 65-8C). Delayed activation of the right ventricle may cause a widened QRS (≥110 msec) in the right precordial leads and a prolonged S wave upstroke in those leads. Cardiac imaging may show right ventricular enlargement or areas of abnormal motion, or reveal areas of scar on magnetic resonance imaging with gadolinium. Distinction from idiopathic right ventricular outflow tract VT can be difficult.

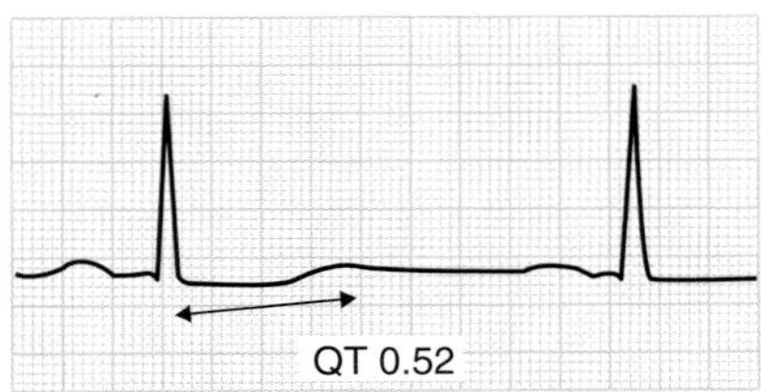

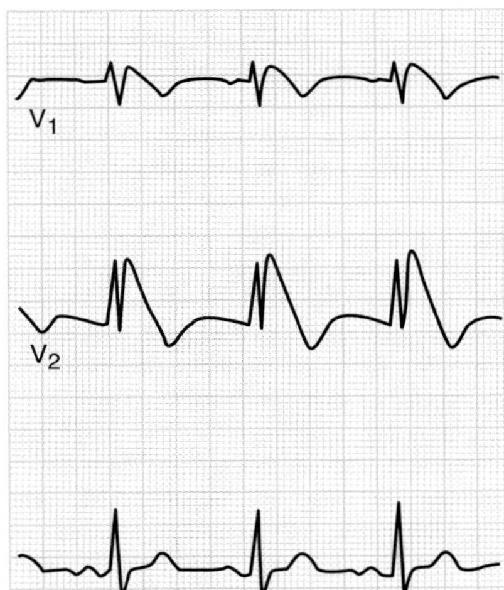

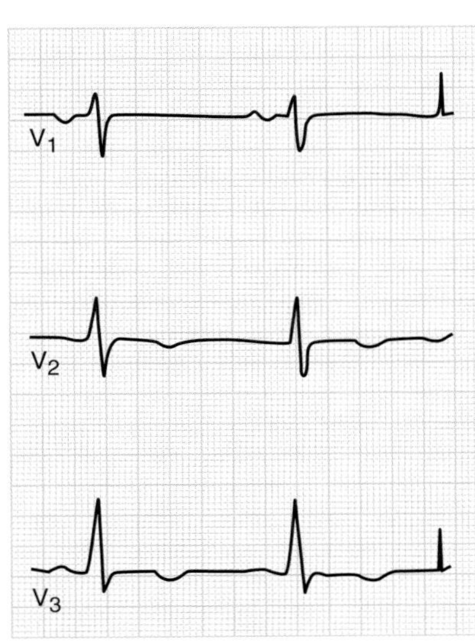

FIGURE 65-8. Sinus rhythm electrocardiogram findings in three genetic sudden death syndromes. A, QT prolongation during sinus rhythm in a patient with long QT syndrome. **B,** ST elevation in V_1 and V_2 in a patient with Brugada's syndrome. **C,** T wave inversion in V_1-V_3 in a patient with arrhythmogenic right ventricular dysplasia.

Left ventricular function is usually preserved, heart failure is rare, and survival to advanced age can be anticipated provided that VT can be controlled. An ICD is routinely recommended. When VT is exercise induced, it may respond to β-adrenergic blockers and prohibition of exercise. Sotalol, amiodarone, and catheter ablation have been used to reduce recurrences.

Tetralogy of Fallot

Ventricular tachycardia occurs in approximately 3 to 14% of patients late after repair of tetralogy of Fallot (Chapter 69) and contribute to a 2% per decade risk of sudden death. Factors associated with VT risk include age more than 5 years at repair, high-grade ventricular ectopy, inducible VT on an electrophysiologic study, abnormal right ventricular hemodynamics, and sinus rhythm QRS duration of more than 180 msec. An ICD is usually warranted for patients who have a spontaneous episode of VT, but criteria for a prophylactic ICD in other patients has not been established.

Bundle Branch Re-entry Ventricular Tachycardia

Re-entry through the Purkinje system occurs in approximately 5% of patients with monomorphic VT in the presence of structural heart disease. The re-entry circuit typically revolves retrograde up the left bundle and anterograde down the right bundle, thereby producing VT that has a left bundle branch block configuration. Catheter ablation of the right bundle branch abolishes this VT. Other scar-related VTs are often present and may require additional therapy.

IDIOPATHIC MONOMORPHIC VENTRICULAR TACHYCARDIA

CLINICAL MANIFESTATIONS AND DIAGNOSIS

Idiopathic VT in patients without structural heart disease usually presents with palpitations, lightheadedness, and occasionally syncope, often provoked by sympathetic stimulation during exercise or emotional upset. The QRS morphology of the arrhythmia suggests the diagnosis (see later). The sinus rhythm ECG is normal. Cardiac imaging shows normal ventricular function and no evidence of ventricular scar. Occasionally, a patient with structural heart disease is found to have concomitant idiopathic VT, unrelated to the structural disease. Sudden death is rare.

TREATMENT Rx

Treatment is required for symptoms or when frequent or incessant arrhythmias depress ventricular function. β-Adrenergic blockers are first-line therapy. Nondihydropyridine calcium-channel blockers (diltiazem and verapamil) are sometimes effective. Catheter ablation is warranted for severe symptoms or when β-blockers or calcium-channel blockers are not effective or not desired. Efficacy and risks of catheter ablation vary with the specific site of origin of the VT, being most favorable for arrhythmias originating in the right ventricular outflow tract.

Outflow tract VTs originate from a focus, usually with features consistent with triggered automaticity. The arrhythmia may present with sustained VT, nonsustained VT or PVCs, often provoked by exercise or emotional upset. Repeated bursts of nonsustained VT, which may occur incessantly, are known as repetitive monomorphic VT and can cause tachycardia-induced cardiomyopathy with depressed ventricular function that recovers after suppression of the arrhythmia.

Origin in the right ventricular outflow tract, which is the most common site of origin, gives rise to VT that has a left bundle branch block configuration in V_1 and an axis that is directed inferiorly, with tall R waves in leads II, III, and aVF (see Fig. 65-5). The arrhythmia can also arise in the left ventricular outflow tract or in sleeves of myocardium that extend along the aortic root. Left ventricular origin should be suspected when lead V_1 or V_2 has prominent R waves. Although the typical outflow tract QRS morphology favors idiopathic VT, cardiomyopathies can also cause PVCs or VT from this region; in such cases, management is the same as for arrhythmias in patients with structural heart disease (see earlier).

Left ventricular intrafascicular verapamil-sensitive VT arrhythmia presents with sustained VT that has a right bundle branch block–like configuration. It is often exercise induced and occurs more often in men than women. The mechanism is re-entry in or near the septal ramifications of the left ventricular Purkinje system. VT can be terminated by intravenous administration of verapamil, although chronic therapy with oral verapamil is not always effective. Catheter ablation is recommended if β-adrenergic blockers or calcium-channel blockers are ineffective or not desired.

TABLE 65-3 POLYMORPHIC VENTRICULAR TACHYCARDIA

ETIOLOGY	MECHANISM/CAUSES	CLINICAL FEATURES
Acute myocardial infarction/ischemia	Re-entry through the ischemic border zone	VT degenerating to VF, greatest risk during the first hour of infarction Common cause of sudden death
Ventricular hypertrophy, cardiomyopathy, heart failure, myocarditis	Multiple factors likely contribute (ion channel remodeling, abnormal calcium handling, ischemia)	Sudden death
Idiopathic VF		PVCs from the Purkinje system or RVOT initiating VF
Idiopathic VT with acquired QT prolongation	Early afterdepolarizations Bradycardia Hypokalemia, hypomagnesemia, hypocalcemia Antiarrhythmic drugs: disopyramide, dofetilide, ibutilide, procainamide, quinidine, sotalol, amiodarone (rare) Psychotropic drugs: haloperidol, droperidol, phenothiazines, pimozide, mesoridazine, tricyclic antidepressants Antibiotics: chloroquine, erythromycin, pentamidine, halofantrine, sparfloxacin, trimethoprim-sulfamethoxazole Other drugs: arsenic, methadone, others	Torsades de pointes causing syncope or cardiac arrest
GENETIC SUDDEN DEATH SYNDROMES		
Congenital long QT syndrome LQTS-1 LQTS-2 LQTS-3	Abnormal gene and ion current *KCNQ1* Iks *KCNQ2* Ikr *SCN5A* Ina	Sudden death or syncope due to torsades de pointes Events during swimming, exertion Events with emotional or auditory stimuli Events at rest and sleep
Short QT syndrome	Mutations affecting IKr, IKs, IK1	QTc < 320 msec
Brugada's syndrome	*SCN5A* mutations affecting INa account for approximately 25% of cases	J-point elevation in leads V_1-V_3 Events at night, during fever
Catecholaminergic polymorphic VT	Mutations affecting the ryanodine receptor or calsequestrin	Events during exertion or emotional upset

LQTS = long QT syndrome; PVC = premature ventricular contraction; RVOT = right ventricular outflow tract; VF = ventricular fibrillation; VT = ventricular tachycardia.

POLYMORPHIC VENTRICULAR TACHYCARDIA

Sustained polymorphic VT (see Fig. 65-4A) can be seen with any form of structural heart disease. However, unlike sustained monomorphic VT, polymorphic VT does not always indicate a structural abnormality or focus of automaticity. Re-entry with multiple or moving wave fronts, spiral wave re-entry (see Fig. 65-2), and multiple automatic foci are potential mechanisms. Sustained polymorphic VT usually degenerates rapidly into VF. Causes include acute MI or ischemia, ventricular hypertrophy, and a number of gene mutations that affect cardiac ion channels (Table 65-3).

Acute Myocardial Infarction and Ischemia

Acute MI or ischemia is a common cause of polymorphic VT and always should be considered immediately. Approximately 10% of patients with acute MI develop VT that degenerates to VF, related to re-entry through the infarct border zone. The risk is greatest in the first hour of acute MI. Following resuscitation (Chapter 63), management is as for acute MI (Chapter 73). β-Adrenergic blockers, intravenous amiodarone, and correction of hypokalemia and hypomagnesemia are warranted. Repeated episodes of polymorphic VT suggest ongoing myocardial ischemia and warrant assessment of whether coronary reperfusion has been re-established. Episodes that occur within the first 48 hours of acute MI do not necessarily confer a long-term risk, and long-term therapy usually is not required after recovery from the MI.

Acquired Long QT Syndrome

QT prolongation is associated with polymorphic VT that often has a characteristic waxing and waning QRS amplitude (see Fig. 65-4A) and is called *torsades de pointes* (twisting about the points). The VT often has a characteristic initiation sequence of PVCs that induces a pause, followed by a sinus beat that has a longer QT interval and interruption of the T wave by the PVC that is the first beat of the polymorphic VT. This characteristic initiation is called *pause dependent.* Causes of QT prolongation include electrolyte abnormalities, chronic bradycardia, and a large number of medications that block repolarizing potassium currents, notably the antiarrhythmic drugs sotalol, dofetilide, and ibutilide, but also a number of other medications used for noncardiac diseases, including erythromycin, pentamidine, haloperidol, phenothiazines, and methadone (see Table 65-3). Individual susceptibility may be related to genetic polymorphisms or mutations that influence repolarization.

Patients present with near-syncope, syncope, or cardiac arrest. Sustained episodes degenerate to VF requiring defibrillation. PVCs and nonsustained VT often precede episodes of sustained VT. Prevention of further episodes can usually be achieved by administration of 1 to 2 g of $MgSO_4$ intravenously. If bradycardia is present, the heart rate should be increased sufficiently to suppress PVCs, often to 100 beats per minute, with temporary pacing or administration of isoproterenol (starting at 1 μg/minute and titrating to the desired heart rate, up to 10 μg/minute). Rapid pacing in addition to $MgSO_4$ (1 to 2 g) administration is sometimes required. Potential contributing factors should be corrected, including removal of all medications that prolong the QT interval and correction of electrolyte abnormalities. Drug interactions that elevate levels of the offending agent are an important cause. Patients who experience a polymorphic VT induced by QT prolongation should be considered to have a susceptibility to the arrhythmia, and medications known to prolong the QT interval are contraindicated.

Congenital Long QT Syndrome

The congenital long QT syndrome (LQTS) is caused by mutations that interfere with ventricular repolarization, prolong the QT interval, and predispose to polymorphic VT. The syndrome is rare, with a prevalence of approximately 1 in 7000. The most frequently encountered mutations, LQTS-1 and -2 (see Table 65-3), cause abnormalities of potassium channels, but mutations affecting the sodium channel (LQTS-3) and calcium channels have also been described.

Patients present with syncope or cardiac arrest, often in childhood. In LQTS-1, episodes tend to occur during exertion, particularly swimming. In LQTS-2, sudden auditory stimuli or emotional upset predispose to events. Asymptomatic patients may be discovered in the course of family screening or on a routine ECG. Penetrance is variable, such that the QT interval is usually, but not always, prolonged to more than 0.44 second (see Fig. 65-8A). LQTS-1 responds well to chronic therapy with β-adrenergic blockers (e.g., nadolol, 0.5 to 3.5 mg/kg daily). ICDs are recommended for patients with arrhythmias despite β-adrenergic blocker therapy or other high-risk disease features, including a (QTc > 0.5 second). Family members of the proband should be screened with an ECG. The type of LQTS identified by genetic testing can help guide management decisions and family screening, but the clinical utility of genotype-phenotype correlations are still being defined. All mutations have not been identified, and failure to identify a known mutation does not exclude the syndrome.

Brugada's Syndrome and Other Repolarization Syndromes

Brugada's syndrome is a rare familial syndrome characterized on the ECG by more than 0.2 mV of ST segment elevation with a coved ST segment and negative T wave in more than one anterior precordial lead (V_1 to V_3) (see Fig. 65-8B) and clinically by episodes of polymorphic VT that present as syncope or cardiac arrest in the absence of structural heart disease. Cardiac arrest may occur during sleep or be provoked by febrile illness. Males are more commonly affected than females. Mutations involving cardiac sodium channels are identified in approximately 25% of cases. Distinction from patients with similar ST elevation owing to left ventricular hypertrophy, pericarditis (Chapter 77), myocardial ischemia or MI (Chapter 72), hyperkalemia (Chapter 119), hypothermia (Chapter 109), right bundle branch block (see Fig. 54-8B in Chapter 54), and ARVC is often difficult. Furthermore, the characteristic ST segment elevation can wax and wane over time. Administration of sodium-channel blocking drugs, such as flecainide, causes further ST elevation in affected individuals. An ICD is recommended. Quinidine has been used successfully to suppress frequent VT.

The short QT syndrome is a very rare familial disorder characterized by a short QTc interval (<0.32) and susceptibility to polymorphic VT and sudden death due to mutations involving cardiac potassium channels. Rare patients with idiopathic polymorphic VT and VF associated with ST elevation in inferior and lateral ECG leads have been reported. This type of ECG pattern, known as *early repolarization,* can also be a normal variant.

Catecholaminergic Polymorphic Ventricular Tachycardia

This rare familial syndrome causes exercise-induced PVCs, a characteristic VT with alternating QRS morphologies termed *bidirectional tachycardia,* polymorphic VT, and VF. Mutations involving the cardiac ryanodine receptor and calsequestrin are identified causes. Patients usually present during childhood with exercise- or emotion-induced palpitations, syncope, or cardiac arrest. β-Adrenergic blockers (e.g., nadolol, 1 to 2 mg/kg/day, or propranolol, 2.5 to 3.5 mg/kg/day) and an implantable defibrillator are recommended. Verapamil (240 to 480 mg daily), or flecainide (50 to 100 mg twice daily), or surgical left cardiac sympathetic denervation reduces or prevents recurrent VT in some patients.

VENTRICULAR FIBRILLATION

VF is characterized by disordered electrical ventricular activation without identifiable QRS complexes (see Fig. 65-4C). Spiral wave re-entry (see Fig. 65-2) and multiple circulating re-entry wave fronts are possible mechanisms. Sustained polymorphic or monomorphic VT that degenerates to VF is a common cause of out-of-hospital cardiac arrest. Treatment follows ACLS guidelines (Chapters 7 and 63), with defibrillation to restore sinus rhythm. If resuscitation is successful, further evaluation is performed to identify and treat underlying heart disease and potential causes of the arrhythmia, including the possibility that VF was initiated by monomorphic or polymorphic VT. If a transient reversible cause, such as acute MI, is not identified, therapy to reduce the risk of sudden death is often warranted. An ICD is often warranted provided the patient has reasonable expectation for survival over the following year with acceptable functional capacity. Chronic amiodarone therapy may be considered for individuals who are not ICD candidates.[3]

INCESSANT VENTRICULAR TACHYCARDIA AND ELECTRICAL STORM

VT is incessant when it continues to recur shortly after electrical, pharmacologic, or spontaneous conversion to sinus rhythm. "VT storm" or "electrical storm" refers to three or more separate episodes of VT within 24 hours. Slow incessant VT is sometimes asymptomatic, but it can cause heart failure or tachycardia-induced cardiomyopathy. More commonly, these presentations are life-threatening and require emergent therapy. Measures to reduce sympathetic tone, including β-adrenergic blockade, sedation, and general anesthesia, have been used effectively. Intravenous administration of amiodarone can be effective. Urgent catheter ablation can be life-saving. Rare patients with idiopathic VF due to rapid polymorphic VT from the Purkinje system or outflow tract in the absence of heart disease benefit from catheter ablation of the initiating focus.

VENTRICULAR ARRHYTHMIAS IN PATIENTS WITH IMPLANTABLE DEFIBRILLATORS

ICDs effectively terminate VT when it occurs and markedly reduce the risk of death from arrhythmias. ICDs do not, however, prevent the arrhythmia. ICDs can be programmed to provide antitachycardia pacing in an attempt to terminate VT by rapid pacing (Fig. 65-9B), which is painless and often asymptomatic. If antitachycardia pacing fails or is not a programmed treatment for rapid VT or VF, an ICD shock is administered. Interrogation of the ICD, which commonly can be performed remotely and communicated by the Internet, allows assessment of any arrhythmias detected by the ICD and of therapies delivered (Fig. 65-9).

Despite effective termination of VT by the ICD, the occurrence of VT predicts an increased risk of mortality and heart failure. VT episodes can be evidence of deteriorating heart failure or myocardial ischemia. Evaluation for progression of heart disease and optimization of medical therapy are warranted.

ICD shocks are painful, reduce quality of life, and can cause post-traumatic stress syndrome. Patients with recurrent episodes of symptomatic VT warrant therapy to prevent episodes. Amiodarone is more effective than β-adrenergic blockers or sotalol.[5] Changes in antiarrhythmic drug therapy can alter the VT rate and the energy required for defibrillation, thereby necessitating programming changes in the ICD algorithms for detection and therapy. Catheter ablation reduces episodes of VT in more than 70% of patients with monomorphic VT.[6]

ANTIARRHYTHMIC DRUGS FOR VENTRICULAR ARRHYTHMIAS

Use of antiarrhythmic drugs (see Table 64-5 in Chapter 64 for dosing) is based on consideration of the risks and potential benefit for individual patients. Many drugs have the potential to induce "proarrhythmia," thereby increasing the frequency of the arrhythmia or causing a new arrhythmia, such as torsades de pointes for QT interval–prolonging drugs.

β-Adrenergic Blockers

Many ventricular arrhythmias are sensitive to sympathetic stimulation, and β-adrenergic stimulation also diminishes the electrophysiologic effects of many antiarrhythmic drugs. The safety of β-blocking agents makes them the first choice of therapy for most ventricular arrhythmias. They are particularly effective for exercise-induced arrhythmias and idiopathic arrhythmias. Bradyarrhythmias are the major cardiac toxicity.

Calcium-Channel Blockers

The nondihydropyridine calcium-channel blockers diltiazem and verapamil can be effective for ventricular arrhythmias and for some idiopathic ventricular arrhythmias.

Sodium-Channel Blockers

Antiarrhythmic drugs with prominent sodium-channel blocking effects can suppress ventricular arrhythmias. Mexiletine, quinidine, disopyramide, flecainide, and propafenone are available for chronic oral therapy. Quinidine, disopyramide, and procainamide also have potassium-channel blocking effects that prolong the QT interval. These agents have potential proarrhythmic effects and, with the possible exception of quinidine, also have negative inotropic effects that may contribute to the increased mortality observed in patients with prior MI. Long-term therapy is generally avoided in patients with structural heart disease but may be used to reduce symptomatic arrhythmias in some patients with ICDs. Lidocaine and procainamide can be used for acute intravenous therapy.

Potassium-Channel Blockers

Sotalol and dofetilide block the delayed rectifier potassium channel IKr, thereby prolonging the QT interval. Sotalol also has nonselective β-adrenergic blocking activity. Sotalol has been shown to reduce ICD shocks, but it is less effective than amiodarone for this purpose.[5] Proarrhythmia with torsades de pointes occurs in 3% of patients. These drugs are excreted by the kidney, so dose adjustment is required according to renal function. These drugs must be avoided in patients with other risk factors for torsades de pointes, including QT prolongation and hypokalemia.

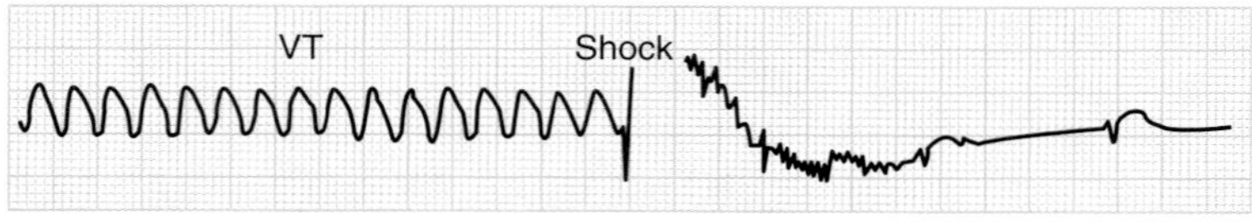

A

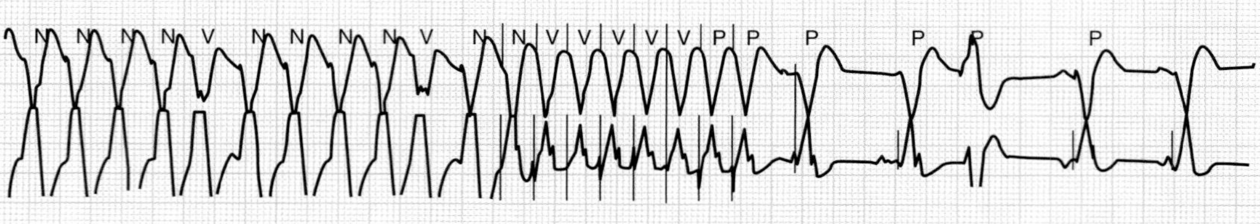

B VT Antitachycardia pacing A–V pacing

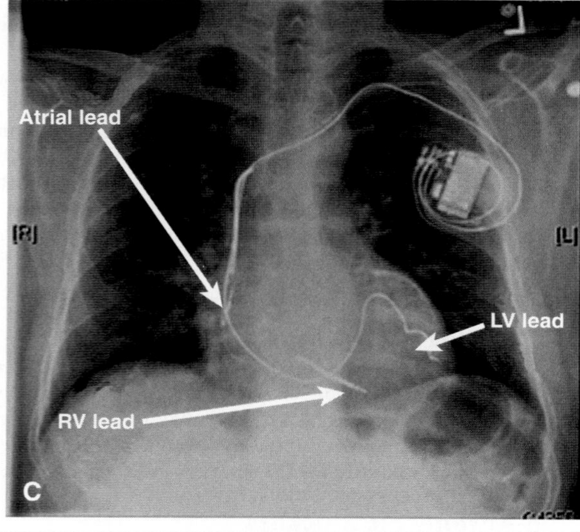

FIGURE 65-9. **Implantable cardioverter-defibrillator (ICD). A,** An electrocardiogram (ECG) tracing of sustained monomorphic ventricular tachycardia (VT) terminated by a shock from an ICD. **B,** Two-lead ECG tracing showing sustained monomorphic VT that is detected by the implanted ICD. A burst of rapid pacing terminates VT. The ICD then provides atrioventricular (A-V) pacing to prevent bradyarrhythmia. **C,** Anterior-posterior radiograph showing an ICD that incorporates a lead to the right atrium, right ventricular (RV) apex, and through the coronary sinus to an epicardial vein over the lateral left ventricle (LV). The pulse generator is evident in the left infraclavicular region.

Amiodarone and Dronedarone

Amiodarone, which blocks multiple cardiac ionic currents and has sympatholytic activity, suppresses a variety of ventricular arrhythmias. It is administered intravenously for life-threatening arrhythmias. During chronic oral therapy, electrophysiologic effects develop over several days, depending on dosing. It is more effective than sotalol in reducing ICD shocks and is the preferred drug in patients who are not candidates for an ICD.[3,5] Bradyarrhythmia is the major cardiac adverse effect. Ventricular proarrhythmia can occur, but torsades de pointes is uncommon. Noncardiac toxicities contribute to drug discontinuation in approximately one third of patients during long-term therapy. Pneumonitis or pulmonary fibrosis occurs in approximately 1% of patients. Photosensitivity is common, and neuropathy and ocular toxicity can occur. Systematic monitoring is recommended during chronic therapy: assessment for thyroid and liver toxicity with thyroid-stimulating hormone and aminotransferase levels every 6 months, and lung toxicity with a chest radiograph and determination of lung diffusing capacity annually. In a randomized study, dronedarone, which is related to amiodarone but without iodine in it, resulted in a 2.13-fold increase in mortality in patients with heart failure.[8]

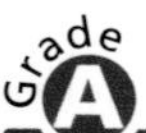

1. Goldenberg I, Gillespie J, Moss AJ, et al. Long-term benefit of primary prevention with an implantable cardioverter-defibrillator: an extended 8-year follow-up study of the Multicenter Automatic Defibrillator Implantation Trial II. *Circulation*. 2010;122:1265-1271.
2. Steinbeck G, Andresen D, Seidl K, et al. Defibrillator implantation early after myocardial infarction. *N Engl J Med*. 2009;361:1427-1436.
3. Piccini JP, Berger JS, O'Connor CM. Amiodarone for the prevention of sudden cardiac death: a meta-analysis of randomized controlled trials. *Eur Heart J*. 2009;30:1245-1253.
4. Bardy GH, Lee KL, Mark DB, et al. Amiodarone or an implantable cardioverter-defibrillator for congestive heart failure. *N Engl J Med*. 2005;352:225-237.
5. Connolly SJ, Dorian P, Roberts RS, et al. Comparison of beta-blockers, amiodarone plus beta-blockers, or sotalol for prevention of shocks from implantable cardioverter defibrillators. The OPTIC Study: a randomized trial. *JAMA*. 2006;295:165-171.
6. Kuck KH, Schaumann A, Eckardt L, et al. Catheter ablation of stable ventricular tachycardia before defibrillator implantation in patients with coronary heart disease (VTACH): a multicentre randomized controlled trial. *Lancet*. 2010;375:4-6.
7. Kadish A, Dyer A, Daubert JP, et al. Prophylactic defibrillator implantation in patients with nonischemic dilated cardiomyopathy. *N Engl J Med*. 2004;350:2151-2158.
8. Kober L, Torp-Pedersen C, McMurray JJ, et al. Increased mortality after dronedarone therapy for severe heart failure. *N Engl J Med*. 2008;358:2678-2687.

SUGGESTED READINGS

Aliot EM, Stevenson WG, Almendral-Garrote JM, et al. EHRA/HRS Expert consensus on catheter ablation of ventricular arrhythmias. *Heart Rhythm*. 2009;6:886-933. *Consensus statement on outcomes and risks.*

Heist EK, Ruskin JN. Drug-induced arrhythmia. *Circulation*. 2010;122:1426-1435. *Review.*

Jacobson JT, Weiner JB. Management of ventricular tachycardia in patients with structural heart disease. *Cardiovasc Ther*. 2010;28:225-263. *Review.*

Manuchehry A, Agusala K, Montevecchi M, et al. Ventricular tachyarrhythmias in patients receiving an implantable cardioverter-defibrillator for primary versus secondary prophylaxis indications. *Pacing Clin Electrophysiol*. 2011. [Epub ahead of print.] *Monomorphic VT is the most common cause of appropriate ICD therapy regardless of implant indication thereby suggesting it is the most common trigger of SCD.*

Probst V, Veltmann C, Eckardt L, et al. Long-term prognosis of patients diagnosed with Brugada syndrome: results from the FINGER Brugada Syndrome Registry. *Circulation*. 2010;121:635-643. *The rate of cardiac events at 32-month follow-up was 7.7% in patients with aborted SCD, 1.9% in patients with syncope, and 0.5% in patients with no symptoms.*

Vest RN 3rd, Gold MR. Risk stratification of ventricular arrhythmias in patients with systolic heart failure. *Curr Opin Cardiol*. 2010;25:268-275. *Emphasizes that symptomatic heart failure is the most powerful predictor of sudden cardiac death from ventricular arrhythmias.*

66

ELECTROPHYSIOLOGIC INTERVENTIONAL PROCEDURES AND SURGERY

FRED MORADY

PACEMAKERS

Pacemaker Generators and Leads

Pacemaker batteries, which are lithium iodide cells that typically have a lifespan of 7 to 8 years, now often weigh less than 30 g. They are usually implanted subcutaneously in the infraclavicular area (Fig. 66-1). The programmability of many different variables has become standard, as has the ability of the pacemaker to provide diagnostic and telemetric data.

Pacemaker leads are generally bipolar, with the distal electrode serving as the cathode. Unipolar leads are less commonly used because of the potential for pacing chest wall muscles and for inhibition of pacing by skeletal muscle myopotentials. The leads are inserted into the heart either percutaneously through a subclavian vein or by cutdown into a cephalic vein. Atrial leads are usually positioned in the right atrial appendage, and ventricular leads are placed in the right ventricular apex. Fixation to the myocardium is achieved either passively with tines or actively with a screw mechanism. Newer lead and electrode designs, such as high-impedance leads and carbon-tipped electrodes, have resulted in lower acute and chronic pacing thresholds.

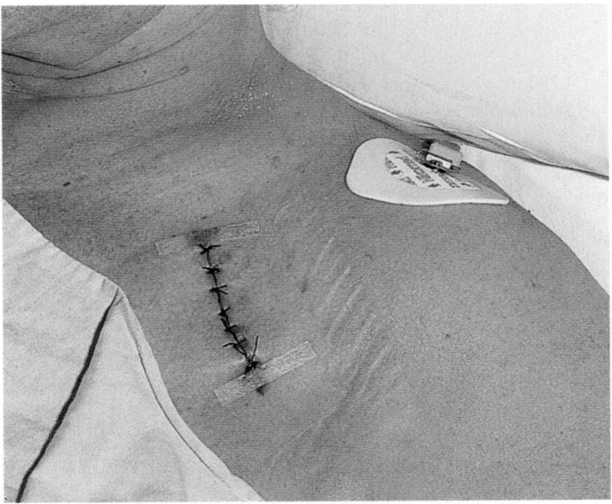

FIGURE 66-1. Site of implantation of a permanent pacemaker or automatic implantable cardioverter-defibrillator. The pacemaker is usually implanted in the left pectoral region, but it may be placed elsewhere if necessary. (From Forbes CD, Jackson WF. *Color Atlas and Text of Clinical Medicine,* 3rd ed. London: Mosby; 2003.)

Pacing Modes

The mode of pacing is described in shorthand fashion by a three- to five-letter code. The first letter designates the chamber being paced (A for atrium, V for ventricle, D for dual chamber); the second letter designates the chamber in which the depolarizations are sensed by the pacemaker (A, V, D, or O for no sensing); the third letter designates whether the pacemaker functions in an inhibited (I) or tracking mode (T), in both modes (D), or asynchronously (O); and the fourth letter indicates whether the pacemaker is capable of rate modulation independent of atrial activity. An additional fifth letter may be used to designate the capability for antitachycardia pacing (P), delivery of shocks (S), or both (D). The most commonly used pacing modes are VVI (pacing and sensing within the ventricle in inhibited fashion), VVIR (VVI plus rate responsiveness), and DDD (pacing and sensing of the atrium and ventricle in both inhibited and tracking fashion).

The most appropriate pacing mode must always be determined on an individual basis, the goal being to meet the patient's physiologic needs with the simplest system possible. For example, in a patient with chronic atrial fibrillation who has symptomatic pauses but not chronotropic incompetence, a VVI pacemaker is sufficient. However, if the patient also has chronotropic incompetence, a VVIR pacemaker is necessary to restore a normal rate response to exercise. In a patient with a high-degree atrioventricular (AV) block and normal sinus node function, DDD pacing is optimal. However, if a patient with a high-degree AV block also has sinus node dysfunction, the ideal pacing mode is DDDR.

In patients who have paroxysmal atrial fibrillation and a high-degree AV block, no single pacing mode is optimal. DDD pacing is ideal when the patient is in sinus rhythm, but during atrial fibrillation, DDD pacing may result in tracking of the atrium at the upper rate limit of the pacemaker. Conversely, VVIR pacing, which is ideal during atrial fibrillation, will not provide AV synchrony during periods of sinus rhythm. The development of mode-switching pacemakers has solved this dilemma. Mode-switching pacemakers are capable of pacing in the DDD mode during sinus rhythm and automatically switching to rate-responsive ventricular pacing during atrial fibrillation or other supraventricular arrhythmias (Fig. 66-2).

The choice between ventricular (VVIR) and atrial (AAIR) or dual-chamber (DDDR) pacing remains controversial. Although a randomized trial of 225 patients with sinus node dysfunction reported a significant reduction in cardiovascular death at 8 years with AAIR versus VVIR pacing,[1] studies of nearly 5000 patients have shown no survival differences when patients were randomized to DDDR or VVIR pacing. Dual-chamber pacing, like atrial pacing, reduces the incidence of atrial fibrillation and appears to result in slightly better quality of life.[2] In these randomized trials, 5 to 25% of patients who initially received VVIR pacemakers "crossed over" to DDDR pacing because of physician-diagnosed pacemaker syndrome (see Complications of Pacemakers).

Several studies have demonstrated that the ventricular dyssynchrony induced by right ventricular pacing may have deleterious effects on ventricular function and functional capacity and may also predispose to the development of atrial fibrillation. Therefore, pacemakers should always be programmed to minimize the amount of ventricular pacing.

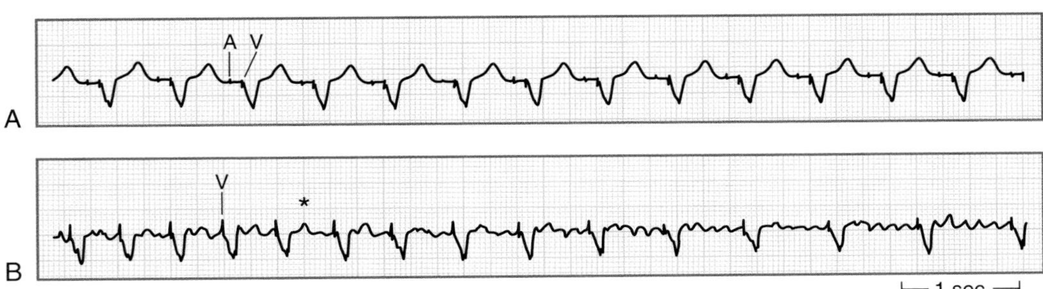

FIGURE 66-2. Rhythm strips from a Holter monitor in a patient with complete atrioventricular block, sinus bradycardia, paroxysmal atrial fibrillation, and a rate-responsive dual-chamber pacemaker with mode-switching capability. A, When the patient is in sinus rhythm, the pacemaker functions in a DDDR mode, with synchronized atrial and ventricular pacing at 105 beats per minute while the patient is walking. **B,** At the onset of an episode of atrial fibrillation, there is tracking of the atrium that results in ventricular pacing at 140 beats per minute, which is the upper rate limit of the pacemaker. Within 2 seconds *(asterisk),* the mode-switch feature results in VVIR pacing, and the ventricular pacing rate gradually falls to 70 beats per minute, which is the lowest rate limit of the pacemaker. A = atrial stimulus; V = ventricular stimulus.

TABLE 66-1 CLASS I INDICATIONS* FOR IMPLANTATION OF A PERMANENT PACEMAKER

SINUS NODE DYSFUNCTION

1. Symptomatic sinus bradycardia
2. Symptomatic chronotropic incompetence
3. Symptomatic sinus bradycardia resulting from required drug therapy

ATRIOVENTRICULAR (AV) BLOCK

1. Third-degree and advanced second-degree AV block associated with symptomatic bradycardia
2. Third-degree and advanced second-degree AV block in an awake patient with asystole of >3 seconds or an escape rate of <40 beats per minute or with an infranodal escape rhythm
3. Atrial fibrillation with a pause of ≥5 seconds
4. Third-degree and advanced second-degree AV block due to postoperative AV block that is not expected to resolve
5. Third-degree and advanced second-degree AV block with neuromuscular diseases such as myotonic muscular dystrophy, Kearns-Sayre syndrome, and Erb dystrophy
6. Asymptomatic third-degree AV block if cardiomegaly or left ventricular dysfunction is present, or if the block is below the AV node

CHRONIC BIFASCICULAR BLOCK

1. Advanced second-degree or intermittent third-degree AV block
2. Type II second-degree AV block
3. Alternating bundle branch block

AFTER ACUTE PHASE OF MYOCARDIAL INFARCTION

1. Second-degree infranodal AV block with alternating bundle branch block
2. Third-degree infranodal AV block
3. Transient advanced second-degree or third-degree infranodal AV block and associated bundle branch block
4. Persistent symptomatic second-degree or third-degree AV block

CAROTID SINUS SYNDROME

1. Recurrent syncope caused by spontaneous carotid sinus stimulation or carotid sinus pressure that induces asystole of >3 seconds in duration

*Class I indications are conditions for which a pacemaker is indicated.
Adapted from Epstein AE, DiMarco JP, Ellenbogen KA, et al. ACC/AHA/HRS 2008 guidelines for device-based therapy of cardiac rhythm abnormalities: executive summary. *J Am Coll Cardiol.* 2008;51:2085-2105.

TABLE 66-2 CLASS IIA INDICATIONS* FOR IMPLANTATION OF A PERMANENT PACEMAKER

SINUS NODE DYSFUNCTION

1. Heart rate of <40 beats per minute when a clear association between symptoms consistent with bradycardia and the actual presence of bradycardia has not been demonstrated
2. Syncope of unclear etiology when sinus node dysfunction is demonstrated by electrophysiologic testing

ATRIOVENTRICULAR (AV) BLOCK

1. Persistent third-degree AV block with an escape rate of >40 beats per minute in an asymptomatic adult without cardiomegaly
2. Asymptomatic second-degree infranodal AV block
3. First-degree or second-degree AV block associated with symptoms similar to pacemaker syndrome
4. Asymptomatic type II second-degree AV block with a narrow QRS

CHRONIC BIFASCICULAR BLOCK

1. Syncope, when other potential causes of syncope have been excluded
2. An HV interval of ≥100 msec
3. Pathologic pacing-induced infranodal AV block during electrophysiologic testing

CAROTID SINUS SYNDROME

1. Syncope without clear provocative events and with asystole of >3 seconds during carotid sinus pressure

*Class IIA indications are conditions for which a pacemaker is reasonable.
Adapted from Epstein AE, DiMarco JP, Ellenbogen KA, et al. ACC/AHA/HRS 2008 guidelines for device-based therapy of cardiac rhythm abnormalities: executive summary. *J Am Coll Cardiol.* 2008;51:2085-2105.

Indications for a Permanent Pacemaker

In general, pacemakers are implanted either to alleviate symptoms caused by bradycardia or to prevent severe symptoms in patients in whom symptomatic bradycardia is likely to develop (Tables 66-1 and 66-2). The most common bradycardia-induced symptoms are dizziness or lightheadedness, syncope or near-syncope (Chapters 50 and 62), exercise intolerance, and symptoms of heart failure. Because these symptoms are nonspecific, documentation of an association between symptoms and bradycardia should be obtained before pacemaker implantation. If the bradycardia is persistent, such as in a patient with a complete AV block, a simple electrocardiogram may be sufficient to document the need for a pacemaker. If the bradycardia is intermittent, other diagnostic testing, such as 24-hour ambulatory monitoring, a continuous loop recorder, an implantable event monitor, or an electrophysiology test (Chapter 62), may be needed to document a relationship between symptoms and bradycardia.

After a symptomatic bradycardia has been documented, a correctable cause for the bradycardia should be excluded before a pacemaker is implanted. Correctable causes of symptomatic bradycardia include hypothyroidism, an overdose with drugs such as digitalis, electrolyte disturbances, and several categories of medications, most commonly β-adrenergic blocking agents (administered either orally or in the form of eyedrops for glaucoma), calcium-channel blocking agents, and antiarrhythmic medications (Chapter 64). At times, a pacemaker is necessary to allow continued treatment with a medication that is responsible for the bradycardia, such as in a patient in whom symptomatic sinus bradycardia develops after initiation of therapy with a β-adrenergic blocking agent for paroxysmal atrial fibrillation associated with a rapid ventricular response.

Complications of Pacemakers

Complications related to the implantation procedure occur in less than 2% of patients and include pneumothorax, perforation of the atrium or ventricle, lead dislodgement, infection, and erosion of the pacemaker pocket. Thrombosis of the subclavian vein occurs in 10 to 20% of patients and is more likely in the presence of multiple leads; it rarely causes symptoms.

Pacemaker-mediated tachycardia is a possible complication of DDD pacing when the atrial lead senses retrograde depolarizations because of ventriculoatrial conduction. The resulting tachycardia often has a rate equal to the upper rate limit of the pacemaker. Pacemaker-mediated tachycardia can be eliminated by various reprogramming maneuvers, such as lengthening of the postventriculoatrial refractory period. Patients with dual-chamber pacemakers for sinus node disease are at risk for future atrial fibrillation. In a randomized study, minimizing dual-chamber ventricular pacing reduced the risk of atrial fibrillation by 40%. 3

The pacemaker syndrome consists of symptoms of weakness, lightheadedness, exercise intolerance, or palpitations caused by the absence of AV synchrony during ventricular pacing. It is treated by restoring AV synchrony with DDD pacing or, if AV conduction is intact, with AAI pacing. During long-term follow-up after pacemaker implantation, potential problems include failure to pace, failure to capture, and changes in the pacing rate. These problems may be a manifestation of suboptimal programming, fracture of a lead or a break in the insulation, generator malfunction, or battery depletion.

Temporary Pacemakers

Temporary pacemaker leads are generally inserted percutaneously into an internal jugular or subclavian vein or by cutdown into a brachial vein and then positioned under fluoroscopic guidance in the right ventricular apex and attached to an external generator. Temporary pacing is used to stabilize patients awaiting permanent pacemaker implantation, to correct a transient symptomatic bradycardia caused by drug toxicity or a metabolic defect, or to suppress torsades de pointes by maintaining a rate of 85 to 100 beats per minute until the causative factor has been eliminated. Temporary pacing may also be used in prophylactic fashion in patients at risk for symptomatic bradycardia during a surgical procedure or high-degree AV block in the setting of an acute myocardial infarction. The most common complication of temporary pacemakers is infection; this risk is minimized by limiting the use of a pacemaker lead to 48 hours. In emergency situations, ventricular pacing can be instituted immediately by transcutaneous pacing with electrode pads applied to the chest wall.

TRANSTHORACIC CARDIOVERSION AND DEFIBRILLATION

Mechanism of Action

Direct current defibrillators store an electrical charge and discharge it across two paddle electrodes in a damped, sinusoidal waveform. The shock terminates arrhythmias caused by re-entry by simultaneously depolarizing large portions of the atria or ventricles, thereby causing the re-entry circuits to extinguish (Chapters 61, 64, and 65).

A nonsynchronized shock that is delivered coincident with the T wave during supraventricular tachycardia (SVT) or ventricular tachycardia (VT) may precipitate ventricular fibrillation (VF). *Cardioversion* refers to the termination of SVT or VT by delivery of a shock in synchrony with the QRS complex. When shocks are delivered to terminate VF, synchronization to the QRS complex is not necessary, and this process is referred to as *defibrillation.*

Technique

Whenever cardioversion or defibrillation is performed on an elective basis, the patient should be in a fasting state. Intravenous access to a peripheral vein should be established, and oxygen, suction, and equipment needed for airway management should be readily available. Transthoracic shocks are painful, and drugs commonly used for anesthesia or amnesia include short-acting barbiturates such as methohexital or a short-acting amnestic agent such as midazolam. In the anteroapical configuration, one electrode is positioned to the right of the sternum at the level of the second intercostal space, and the second electrode is positioned at the midaxillary line, lateral to the apical impulse. In the anteroposterior configuration, an electrode is placed to the left of the sternum at the fourth intercostal space, and the second electrode is positioned posteriorly, to the left of the spine, at the same level as the anterior electrode. These two-electrode configurations result in similar success rates of cardioversion and defibrillation.

Important variables affecting the success of cardioversion or defibrillation are the shock waveform and shock strength. Defibrillators that deliver biphasic shocks are now clinically available and have a significantly higher success rate than conventional defibrillators. Other technique-dependent variables that maximize delivery of energy to the heart include firm paddle pressure, delivery of the shock during expiration, and repetitive shocks. Patient-related variables that may decrease the probability of successful cardioversion and defibrillation include metabolic disturbances, long arrhythmia duration, some antiarrhythmic drugs such as amiodarone, and body weight in excess of 80 kg.

Because cardioversion of atrial fibrillation (Chapter 64) may be complicated by thromboembolism, anticoagulation with warfarin is generally necessary for 3 weeks before cardioversion and for 1 month after cardioversion whenever atrial fibrillation has been present for 48 hours or longer. The 3-week period of anticoagulation before cardioversion can be eliminated if no atrial thrombi are seen on a transesophageal echocardiogram, but anticoagulation for 1 month after cardioversion is still necessary to prevent thrombus formation secondary to transient, postconversion atrial stunning.

Indications

The most common arrhythmias treated by cardioversion and defibrillation are VF, VT, atrial fibrillation, and atrial flutter (Chapters 63, 64, and 65). Treatment of VF is always an emergency, and a 200-J shock should be delivered as quickly as possible, followed by one or more 360-J shocks if necessary. Depending on the patient's hemodynamic status, cardioversion of VT may be performed electively or on an emergency basis; if elective, an initial shock strength of 50 J is appropriate, followed by higher energy levels if additional shocks are needed. An initial energy level of 50 J is appropriate for cardioversion of atrial flutter. In atrial fibrillation, in which cardioversion is generally performed on an elective basis, an initial shock of 100 to 200 J is appropriate, depending on the patient's body weight. Shocks of 300 to 360 J are then used if necessary. If atrial fibrillation must be treated on an urgent basis, for example, in a patient with Wolff-Parkinson-White syndrome who has a very rapid ventricular rate and hemodynamic compromise, an initial shock of 200 J should be followed by 360-J shocks, as needed. Because the defibrillation energy requirement is a probability function and not a discrete value, subsequent shocks may be effective for cardioversion and defibrillation even when the first 360-J shock is ineffective.

Complications

Asynchronous shocks may precipitate VF. Rarely, VF may occur even when shocks are synchronized to the QRS complex. The risk for post-shock ventricular arrhythmias is increased in the presence of a supratherapeutic plasma concentration of digitalis, so cardioversion in patients with digitalis toxicity should be avoided.

Transient ST segment elevation may occur after cardioversion and is usually of no clinical consequence. Mild myocardial necrosis may occasionally occur if a total energy exceeding 425 J is delivered in a short period. Another rare complication of cardioversion is pulmonary edema, which may be due to transient left ventricular dysfunction.

Post-shock bradycardia or asystole may occur because of vagal discharge or an underlying sick sinus syndrome. At times, atropine or emergency transcutaneous pacing may be necessary. In patients who have a pacemaker or implantable cardioverter-defibrillator (ICD), the shocking electrodes should be positioned as far away from the generator as possible, and the generator and pacing threshold should be checked afterward.

IMPLANTABLE CARDIOVERTER-DEFIBRILLATORS

ICD Pulse Generators and Leads

ICDs now weigh as little as 60 g, are multiprogrammable, have improved detection algorithms, are capable of antitachycardia and antibradycardia (including dual-chamber) pacing, can deliver biphasic shocks at strengths of less than 1 to 42 J, and provide a record of the electrograms recorded during arrhythmic episodes. With the development of pulse generators small enough to implant in the infraclavicular area and endocardial leads that are inserted transvenously, the implantation procedure has been greatly simplified and is now very similar to that for permanent pacemakers.

ICDs that deliver shocks to terminate atrial fibrillation, as well as VT and VF, are clinically available. Biventricular ICDs are available for patients who need an ICD and have advanced (class III or IV) heart failure and a bundle branch block.

A single lead that contains a pacing-sensing electrode and two defibrillating coils can be used. If adequate defibrillation is not achieved with a single-lead configuration, a subcutaneous patch electrode or subcutaneous array can be added. In another commonly used configuration, the pulse generator itself functions as an electrode, and a lead that has a pacing-sensing electrode at its tip and a distal defibrillating coil electrode is positioned at the right ventricular apex. Multiple other combinations of a chest wall patch electrode and defibrillating electrodes in the right ventricular apex, superior vena cava, or coronary sinus can also be used. When a biventricular ICD is implanted, a lead is inserted into a branch of the coronary sinus for left ventricular pacing.

Indications

ICDs have become first-line therapy in patients who have survived an episode of VF not associated with acute myocardial infarction or who have had an episode of hemodynamically significant, sustained VT (Chapter 65).[4] ICDs are also implanted in individuals at high risk for cardiac arrest, including patients with idiopathic, dilated cardiomyopathy and unexplained syncope or patients with coronary artery disease (CAD), an ejection fraction of less than 35%, spontaneous episodes of nonsustained VT, and inducible sustained VT in the electrophysiology laboratory (Chapter 65).[5] Based on the results of large-scale clinical trials, the indications for implantation of an ICD include patients with a previous myocardial infarction and an ejection fraction of 30% or less, as well as patients with dilated cardiomyopathy (ischemic or nonischemic), an ejection fraction of 35% or less, and class II or III heart failure.[6-8]

Programming of ICDs

Testing is performed at the time of implantation to determine the energy requirement for defibrillation. A safety margin of at least 10 J should be present; for example, if the maximum output of the pulse generator is 32 J, successful defibrillation should be achieved with shocks of 22 J or less in strength. If the patient has had episodes of VT, antitachycardia pacing can be evaluated and programmed as needed to terminate the VT. Appropriate programming of the device is performed during predischarge testing.

With ICDs that are tiered-therapy devices, as many as two VT zones and one VF zone are available to provide individualized therapy for ventricular arrhythmias that have different rates. The rate threshold and various sequences of antitachycardia pacing and low- or high-energy shocks can be programmed for each of the two VT zones. The VF zone is a high-rate zone in which high-energy shocks are delivered. Optimal programming is important for many reasons, including minimizing patient discomfort, reducing the chance of

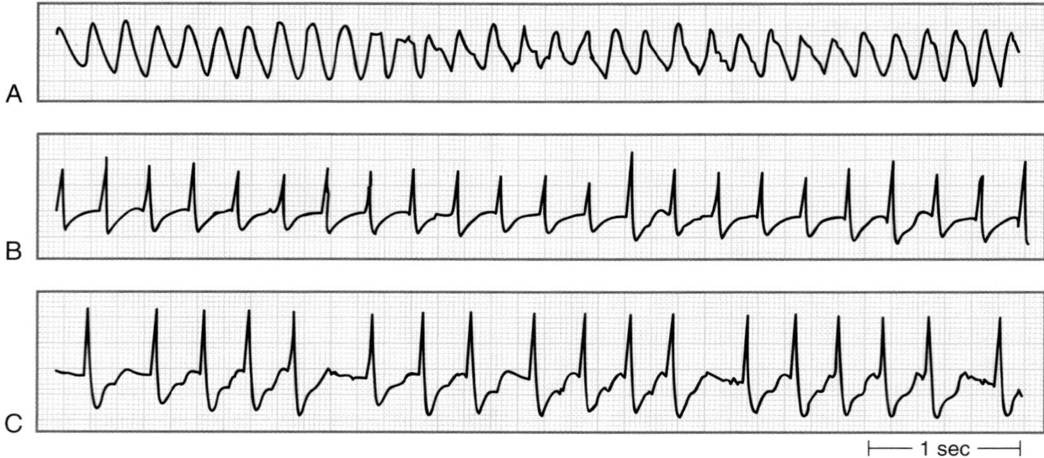

FIGURE 66-3. **Examples of stored electrograms obtained several hours after three different patients had experienced a flurry of shocks from an implantable cardioverter-defibrillator and showing the rhythm recorded by the device immediately before a shock was delivered.** **A,** In this patient, the stored electrogram demonstrates ventricular tachycardia at a rate of 300 beats per minute, thus indicating that the shock was appropriate. He was treated with amiodarone to reduce the frequency of episodes of ventricular tachycardia. **B,** This patient received shocks because of paroxysmal supraventricular tachycardia at a rate of 206 beats per minute, which exceeded the programmed rate cutoff of 170 beats per minute. He underwent radio frequency ablation of the paroxysmal supraventricular tachycardia and received no further inappropriate shocks. **C,** The stored electrograms in this patient indicate that the patient received inappropriate shocks that were triggered by atrial fibrillation at a rate of 180 beats per minute. The rate cutoff of the device in this patient was 150 beats per minute. This patient was treated with a β-blocker to keep the ventricular rate less than 150 beats per minute during atrial fibrillation.

syncope with an arrhythmia episode, maximizing the battery life of the pulse generator, and preventing inappropriate shocks.

Complications

Complications related to the implantation procedure include pneumothorax, myocardial perforation, and infection, all of which should have an incidence of less than 1%. Complications associated with the subcutaneous or submuscular pocket into which the device is placed include hematoma formation and erosion of the pocket. The endocardial leads that are used in the ICD system occasionally become dislodged shortly after implantation, thus necessitating a second procedure to reposition the leads. Other lead complications include fracture or breakdown of the insulation, either of which may result in failure to defibrillate. Fracture of a lead may also result in an artifact that mimics VF and triggers inappropriate shocks.

Patients who have an ICD do not require evaluation every time that they experience a device discharge. However, urgent evaluation is necessary if the patient experiences flurries of discharges. Analysis of stored electrograms often reveals the underlying problem (Fig. 66-3). The frequent shocks may be appropriate shocks triggered by flurries of VT or VF; if a correctable cause such as a metabolic defect or proarrhythmic drug cannot be identified, antiarrhythmic drug therapy or catheter ablation, or both, should be used to eliminate these arrhythmia flurries. Flurries of shocks may be triggered by atrial fibrillation with a rapid ventricular response, in which case aggressive management of the atrial fibrillation is indicated. In addition, flurries of shocks may be a manifestation of a lead fracture, in which case lead replacement is necessary.

RADIO FREQUENCY CATHETER ABLATION

Tissue Effects of Radio Frequency Energy

Radio frequency ablation is a percutaneous catheter technique that can permanently eliminate a variety of SVTs and VTs that previously required either chronic pharmacologic treatment for suppression or surgery for cure. Radio frequency energy is delivered through an electrode catheter whose tip is in contact with tissue that is critical to maintenance of the tachycardia. The radio frequency energy results in resistive heating of the tissue and irreversible tissue destruction when the tissue temperature exceeds 50° C. Depending on the type of catheter and the power settings, the lesions that are created are up to 7 to 8 mm in diameter and up to 6 to 8 mm deep. Chronic lesions demonstrate coagulation necrosis and are well demarcated.

Procedural Aspects

Diagnostic electrophysiologic testing (Chapter 62) and radio frequency ablation are often performed during the same procedure, sometimes on an outpatient basis, such as in patients with paroxysmal SVT. Various pacing techniques or infusions of isoproterenol (or both) are used to induce the patient's arrhythmia and allow the specific mechanism of the tachycardia to be determined. Depending on the type of tachycardia, the sites in the heart targeted for ablation are determined by the results of mapping or as guided by specific anatomic landmarks. Radio frequency energy is delivered, typically in applications of 1 minute, at a power setting sufficient to result in adequate tissue heating of 60° to 70° C.

Radio Frequency Ablation of Supraventricular Arrhythmias

AV nodal re-entrant tachycardia (Chapter 64), the most common type of paroxysmal SVT, is eliminated by radio frequency ablation of the "slow" limb of the re-entry circuit. Target sites for ablation are located in the posteroseptal aspect of the right atrium, near the ostium of the coronary sinus. In experienced hands, slow-pathway ablation has a success rate of 98% and is associated with a less than 1% risk of high-degree AV block.

Cryoablation, which is an alternative to radio frequency ablation, is associated with a lower risk for AV block but a lower long-term success rate. Cryoablation is useful in patients at higher risk for AV block, such as small children.

Left-sided accessory pathways are ablated by using either a retrograde aortic or a transseptal approach, and those that are right sided or septal are ablated with a venous approach. Detailed mapping of the accessory pathway is essential for identification of an appropriate ablation site, and the ablation catheter is positioned on either the atrial or the ventricular aspect of the mitral or tricuspid annulus. The success rate of accessory pathway ablation is 90 to 98%, and the complication rate is 2 to 3%. A fatal complication occurs in less than 0.1% of patients. The most common nonfatal but serious complications are cardiac tamponade as a result of mechanical perforation of the heart by an electrode catheter and high-degree AV block in patients with a septal accessory pathway. Cryoablation is associated with a lower risk for AV block and is useful for ablation of accessory pathways located near the AV node.

Detailed mapping is also needed to identify sites for ablation of atrial tachycardias. Most atrial tachycardias arise in the right atrium and are mapped by using a venous approach, but left atrial tachycardias are mapped via a transseptal approach. Assuming that the atrial tachycardia is arising only at one site, the success rate of ablation is approximately 90%, and complications are rare.

Type I atrial flutter (Chapter 64) arises in the right atrium and can be eliminated by radio frequency ablation directed at a critical isthmus in the low right atrium, between the tricuspid annulus and the inferior vena cava. The success rate of this type of ablation is greater than 90%, and the risk for a serious complication is less than 1%.

Catheter ablation aimed at the elimination of atrial fibrillation is useful in patients with symptomatic, drug-refractory atrial fibrillation.[9] The 1-year efficacy of catheter ablation appears to be in the range of 75 to 85% for paroxysmal atrial fibrillation and 65 to 75% for chronic atrial fibrillation. The most serious complications are myocardial perforation, thromboembolism, and atrioesophageal fistula, with an overall risk of 1 to 2%. Pulmonary vein stenosis is a potentially serious complication that can be avoided by not delivering radio frequency energy applications within the tubular portion of the pulmonary veins.

In patients with refractory atrial fibrillation (Chapter 64) associated with an uncontrolled ventricular rate, radio frequency ablation of the AV node can improve symptoms, functional capacity, and left ventricular function. In AV node ablation, a third-degree AV block is intentionally induced; the success rate is 100%, and all patients require a permanent pacemaker.

Inappropriate sinus tachycardia can also be managed with radio frequency ablation, but this approach should be recommended only as a last resort. The sinus node, located in the high lateral portion of the right atrium, is targeted for ablation. The success rate is 80%, and 10% of patients require a pacemaker because of an inadequate atrial escape rate.

Because of a very favorable risk-benefit ratio, radio frequency ablation is appropriate first-line therapy for any patient with paroxysmal SVT, Wolff-Parkinson-White syndrome, or type I atrial flutter that is symptomatic enough to warrant therapy (Chapter 64). For atrial flutter other than type I and inappropriate sinus tachycardia, an ablation procedure is appropriate only in patients with severe symptoms who are refractory to medication.

Ablation techniques and new technologies for ablation of atrial fibrillation are still evolving, and their long-term efficacy is not yet established. After 1 year, rates of recurrent atrial fibrillation have been reduced by catheter ablation, but rates of stroke and mortality have not.[10]

Radio Frequency Ablation of Ventricular Tachycardia

Radio frequency ablation has been used as first-line treatment of idiopathic VT. The most common type of idiopathic VT arises in the outflow tract of the right ventricle and has a left bundle branch block configuration and superior axis. Another type of idiopathic VT has a right bundle branch block configuration and a superior axis and arises in the inferoapical aspect of the left ventricle (Chapter 65). The success rate of radio frequency ablation of these types of VT has been 85 to 100%, and complications have been rare.

In patients with CAD, VT usually arises in diseased tissue adjacent to an area of previous infarction in the left ventricle. Because the disease process is diffuse instead of focal and because VT may originate at multiple sites, radio frequency ablation of VT is not usually curative in patients with CAD. More often, radio frequency ablation is used as adjunctive therapy with an ICD or with antiarrhythmic drug therapy. In the setting of CAD, the success rate of radio frequency ablation of VT has been 65 to 95%, with serious complications occurring in approximately 5% of patients.

ARRHYTHMIA SURGERY

Wolff-Parkinson-White Syndrome

At present, surgical ablation of an accessory pathway may be indicated for the rare patient with Wolff-Parkinson-White syndrome who has potentially dangerous arrhythmias and in whom catheter ablation is unsuccessful. When performed by an experienced surgeon, the success rate of surgical ablation of an accessory pathway approaches 100%, and the risk for a serious complication is low. Intraoperative mapping is necessary to establish the location of the accessory pathway, which then can be ablated either cryosurgically using an epicardial approach or by direct dissection using an endocardial approach.

Ventricular Tachycardia in Patients with Coronary Artery Disease

The substrate for monomorphic VT in patients with CAD usually lies within visually apparent scar tissue surrounding an area of previous myocardial infarction (Chapter 65). Subendocardial resection has been successful in eliminating VT when performed either on a visual basis, with resection or cryoablation of all visually apparent scar tissue, or on a map-guided basis, with resection or cryoablation limited to the areas found to be participating in generation of the VT. At centers experienced in this type of surgery, the success rate of subendocardial resection has been 85 to 90%, and the operative mortality rate has been in the range of 5 to 10%. Although subendocardial resection has the potential advantage of preventing recurrences of VT, the relatively high operative mortality rate and the widespread availability of ICDs have discouraged its use.

Atrial Fibrillation

In the maze procedure, a series of incisions or linear lesions or both (created by cryoablation or radio frequency ablation) are made in specific regions of the left and right atria to subdivide the atria into parts too small to sustain atrial fibrillation. The operative mortality rate associated with the maze procedure is less than 2%, and more than 90% of patients have had no recurrences of atrial fibrillation during long-term follow-up. However, because it requires extensive surgery, the maze procedure is performed by only a small number of surgeons.

A variety of simpler operative procedures for atrial fibrillation have been developed, some of which can be performed with minimally invasive surgery. The long-term efficacy of these simpler "mini-maze" procedures is lower than that of the maze procedure, but because of their ease and low risk, their use has become widespread, mostly as an adjunct to valve or coronary bypass surgery.

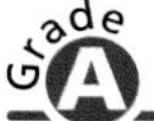

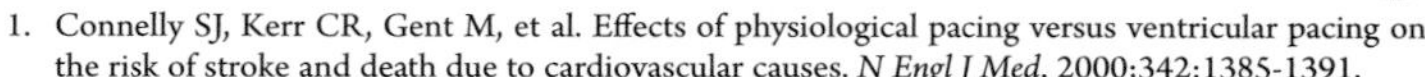

1. Connelly SJ, Kerr CR, Gent M, et al. Effects of physiological pacing versus ventricular pacing on the risk of stroke and death due to cardiovascular causes. *N Engl J Med.* 2000;342:1385-1391.
2. Lamas GA, Lee KL, Sweeney MO, et al. Ventricular pacing or dual-chamber pacing for sinus-node dysfunction. *N Engl J Med.* 2002;346:1854-1862.
3. Sweeney MO, Bank AJ, Nsah E, et al. Minimizing ventricular pacing to reduce atrial fibrillation in sinus-node disease. *N Engl J Med.* 2007;357:1000-1008.
4. The Antiarrhythmics versus Implantable Defibrillators (AVID) Investigators. A comparison of antiarrhythmic-drug therapy with implantable defibrillators in patients resuscitated from near-fatal ventricular arrhythmias. *N Engl J Med.* 1997;337:1576-1583.
5. Buxton AE, Lee KL, Fisher JD, et al. A randomized study of the prevention of sudden death in patients with coronary artery disease. Multicenter Unsustained Tachycardia Trial Investigators. *N Engl J Med.* 1999;341:1882-1890.
6. Goldenberg I, Gillespie J, Moss AJ, et al. Long-term benefit of primary prevention with an implantable cardioverter-defibrillator: an extended 8-year follow-up study of the Multicenter Automatic Defibrillator Implantation Trial II. *Circulation.* 2010;122:1265-1271.
7. Bardy GH, Lee KL, Mark DB, et al. Amiodarone or an implantable cardioverter-defibrillator for congestive heart failure. *N Engl J Med.* 2005;352:225-237.
8. Bristow MR, Saxon LA, Boehmer J, et al. Cardiac-resynchronization therapy with or without an implantable defibrillator in advanced chronic heart failure. *N Engl J Med.* 2004;350:2140-2150.
9. Jaïs P, Cauchemez B, Macle L, et al. Catheter ablation versus antiarrhythmic drugs for atrial fibrillation: the A4 study. *Circulation.* 2008;118:2498-2505.
10. Wilber DJ, Pappone C, Neuzil P, et al. Comparison of antiarrhythmic drug therapy and radiofrequency catheter ablation in patients with paroxysmal atrial fibrillation: a randomized controlled trial. *JAMA.* 2010;303:333-340.

SUGGESTED READINGS

Bardy GH, Smith WM, Hood MA, et al. An entirely subcutaneous implantable cardioverter-defibrillator. *N Eng J Med.* 2010;363:36-44. *In a non-randomized study, an entirely subcutaneous ICD detected and treated tachyarrhythmias.*

Weerasooriya R, Khairy P, Litalien J, et al. Catheter ablation for atrial fibrillation: are results maintained at 5 years of follow-up? *J Am Coll Cardiol.* 2011;57:160-166. *Arrhythmia-free survival rates after a single ablation were 40%, 37%, and 29% at 1, 2, and 5 years.*

67 ARTERIAL HYPERTENSION

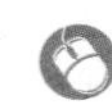

RONALD G. VICTOR

DEFINITION

Hypertension has been defined as a usual blood pressure of 140/90 mm Hg or higher (Table 67-1), blood pressure levels for which the benefits of drug treatment have been shown in randomized controlled trials. This conservative definition has been called into question by epidemiologic data showing continuous positive relationships between the risk for death from coronary artery disease (CAD) and stroke with systolic or diastolic blood pressure values as low as 115/75 mm Hg (Fig. 67-1). Thus, an artificial dichotomy between "hypertension" and "normotension" may delay medical treatment until vascular health has been irreversibly compromised by elevated blood pressure values previously considered normal. For certain high-risk patients, such as those with CAD, the recommended medical treatment threshold recently has been lowered to 130/80 mm Hg.

EPIDEMIOLOGY

Affecting one fourth of the adult population (70 million people in the United States and 1 billion people worldwide), arterial hypertension is the leading cause of death in the world and the most common cause for an outpatient visit to a physician; it is the most easily recognized treatable risk factor for

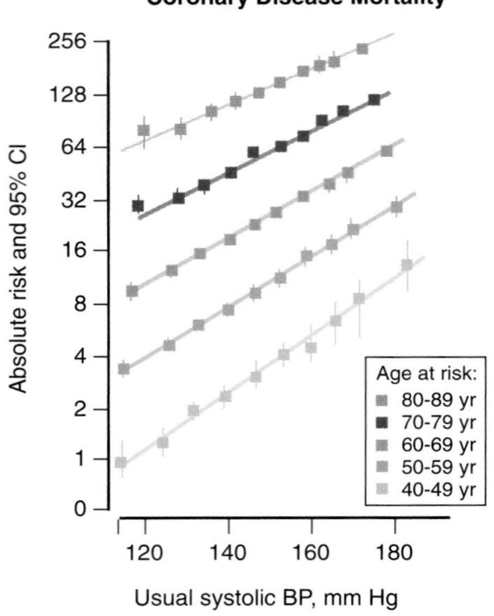

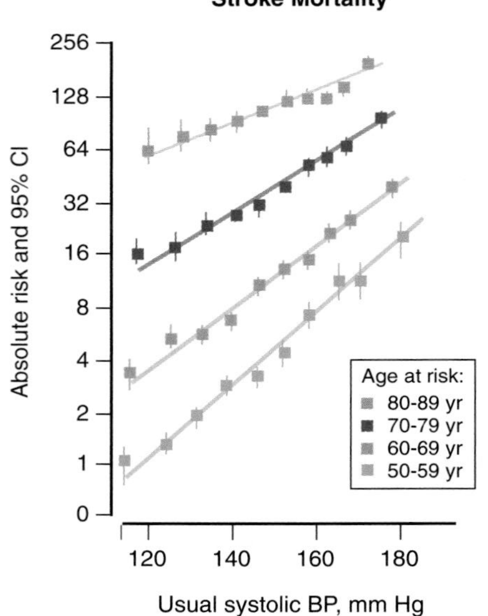

FIGURE 67-1. Absolute risk of coronary artery disease and stroke mortality by usual systolic blood pressure (BP) levels. (From Lewington S, Clarke R, Qizilbash N, et al, for the Prospective Studies Collaboration. Age-specific relevance of usual blood pressure to vascular mortality: a meta-analysis of individual data for one million adults in 61 prospective studies. *Lancet.* 2002;360:1903-1913.)

TABLE 67-1 STAGING OF OFFICE BLOOD PRESSURE*

BLOOD PRESSURE STAGE	SYSTOLIC BLOOD PRESSURE (mm Hg)	DIASTOLIC BLOOD PRESSURE (mm Hg)
Normal	<120	<80
Prehypertension	120-139	80-89
Stage 1 hypertension	140-159	90-99
Stage 2 hypertension	≥160	≥100

*Calculation of seated blood pressure is based on the mean of two or more readings on two separate office visits.
From Chobanian A, Bakris G, Black H, et al. The Seventh Report of the Joint National Committee on the Prevention, Evaluation, and Treatment of High Blood Pressure: the JNC 7 report. *JAMA.* 2003;289:2560-2572.

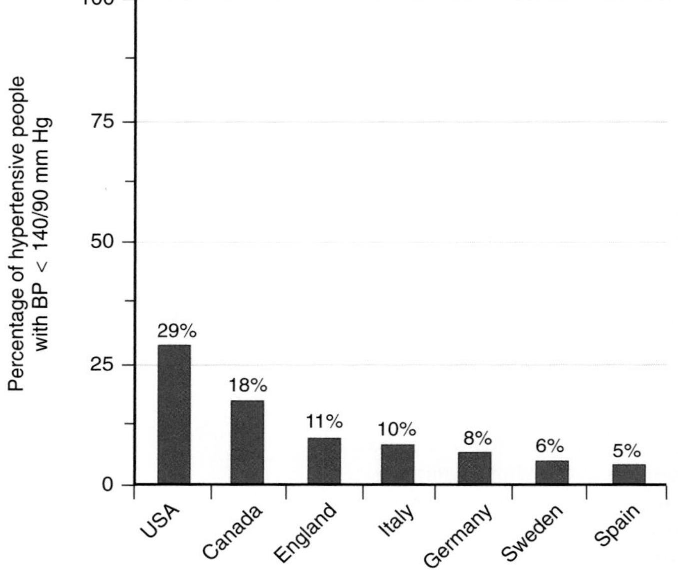

FIGURE 67-2. Hypertension control rates in North America and Europe. (From Wolf-Maier K, Cooper RS, Kramer H, et al. Hypertension treatment and control in five European countries, Canada, and the United States. *Hypertension.* 2004;43:10-17.)

stroke (Chapters 413, 414, and 415), myocardial infarction (Chapters 72 and 73), heart failure (Chapters 58 and 59), peripheral vascular disease (Chapter 79), aortic dissection (Chapter 78), atrial fibrillation (Chapter 64), and end-stage kidney disease (Chapter 132). Because of increasing rates of obesity and aging of the population, hypertension is projected to affect 1.5 billion persons, one third of the world's population, by the year 2025. Presently, about 54% of strokes and 47% of ischemic heart disease worldwide is attributable to high blood pressure. Half of this disease burden is in people who meet the definition of hypertension, and the remainder is in people with lesser degrees of high blood pressure (*prehypertension*).

The asymptomatic nature of most cases of hypertension and the inherent variability in blood pressure can delay diagnosis and treatment. Most cases of hypertension are multifactorial. Blood pressure control typically requires empirical treatment with several classes of prescription medication. Pill burden, prescription drug costs, medication side effects, and insufficient time for patient education contribute to nonadherence to medications. Physicians can be too slow to initiate and intensify blood pressure medication. Lifestyle modification (particularly diet and exercise) can lower blood pressure somewhat, but the reduction rarely is enough to eliminate the need for medication. For all these reasons, blood pressure is controlled to a value below 140/90 mm Hg in less than one third of affected individuals, even in higher-income countries with the most advanced systems of health care (Fig. 67-2). Effective management requires continuity of care by a knowledgeable physician and continued active involvement by an educated patient.

Aging and Pulse Pressure

Patients often ask: Is systolic or diastolic blood pressure more important? Both are (Fig. 67-3). In industrialized societies, systolic pressure rises progressively with age; if individuals live long enough, almost all (>90%) will develop hypertension. This age-dependent rise in blood pressure is not an essential part of human biology. In less developed countries where consumption of calories and salt is low, blood pressures remain low and do not rise with age. In developed countries, diastolic pressure rises until the age of 50 years and decreases thereafter, producing a progressive rise in pulse pressure (systolic pressure minus diastolic pressure) (Fig. 67-4).

Different hemodynamic faults underlie hypertension in younger and older persons. Patients who develop hypertension before the age of 50 years typically have *combined systolic and diastolic hypertension:* systolic pressure above 140 mm Hg *and* diastolic pressure above 90 mm Hg. The main hemodynamic fault is vasoconstriction at the level of the resistance arterioles. In contrast, most patients who develop hypertension after the age of 50 years have *isolated systolic hypertension:* systolic pressure above 140 mm Hg but diastolic pressure below 90 mm Hg (often below 80 mm Hg). In isolated systolic hypertension, the primary hemodynamic fault is decreased distensibility of the large conduit arteries. Collagen replaces elastin in the elastic lamina of the aorta, a process that is accelerated by both aging and hypertension. When pulse wave velocity increases sufficiently, the rapid return of the arterial pulse wave from the periphery augments central systolic (rather than diastolic) pressure. The augmented systolic load on the left ventricle increases myocardial oxygen demands, whereas the rapid diastolic runoff compromises myocardial perfusion. As the population ages, most uncontrolled hypertension occurs in older patients with isolated systolic hypertension.

Gender and Race/Ethnicity

Before the age of 50 years, hypertension is less common in women than men, suggesting a protective effect of estrogen. After menopause, hypertension is more common in women than men.

One in three African American individuals has hypertension, compared with one in four or five white and Mexican American individuals. In African Americans, hypertension also starts at a younger age, is more severe, and causes more target organ damage, leading to premature disability and death. In the Bogalusa Heart Study, African American children already had higher blood pressures than white children by grade school. However, hypertension is more prevalent in the white populations of several European countries (e.g., Finland, Germany, Spain) than in African Americans and is rare among Africans living in Africa (Fig. 67-5). These international data emphasize the importance of environmental factors.

PATHOBIOLOGY

In 90 to 95% of hypertensive patients, a single reversible cause of the elevated blood pressure cannot be identified, hence the term *primary hypertension*. However, in most patients with primary hypertension, readily identifiable behaviors—habitually excessive consumption of calories, salt, or alcohol—contribute to the elevated blood pressure. In the remaining 5 to 10%, a more discrete mechanism can be identified, and the condition is termed *secondary or identifiable hypertension*. At the organ-system level, hypertension results from a gain in function of pathways that promote vasoconstriction and renal sodium retention or a loss in function of pathways that promote vasodilation and renal sodium excretion. Neural, hormonal, renal, and vascular mechanisms are involved. There is increasing evidence that neurohormonal activation contributes to the early pathogenesis by compromising vascular function (e.g., endothelium-dependent vasodilation) and structure (e.g., inward remodeling) that precede hypertension.

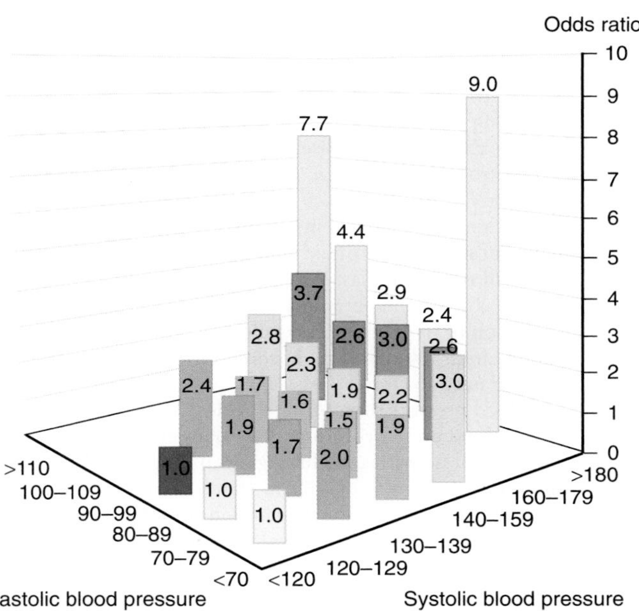

FIGURE 67-3. Joint influences of systolic blood pressure and diastolic blood pressure on the risk (odds ratio) of a cardiovascular event. (Modified from Franklin SS, Lopez VA, Wong ND, et al. Single versus combined blood pressure component and risk for cardiovascular disease: the Framingham Heart Study. *Circulation.* 2009;119:243-250.)

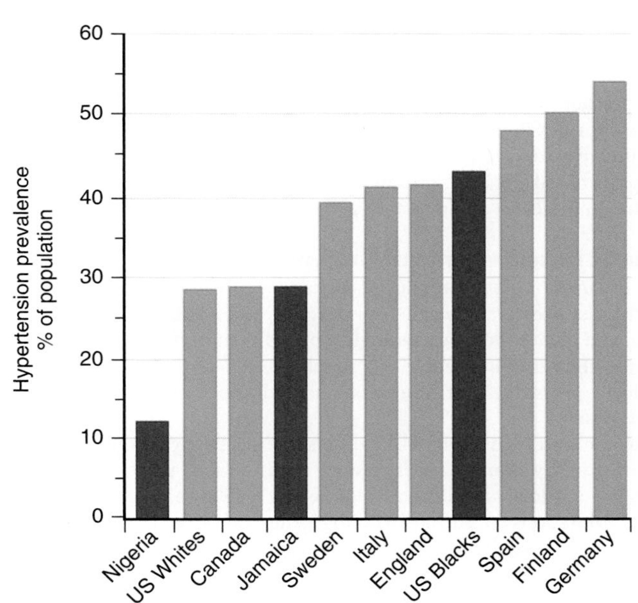

FIGURE 67-5. Geographic variation in hypertension prevalence in populations of African and European ancestries. (From Cooper RS, Wolf-Maier K, Luke A, et al. An international comparative study of blood pressure in populations of European vs. African descent. *BMC Med.* 2005;3:1-8.)

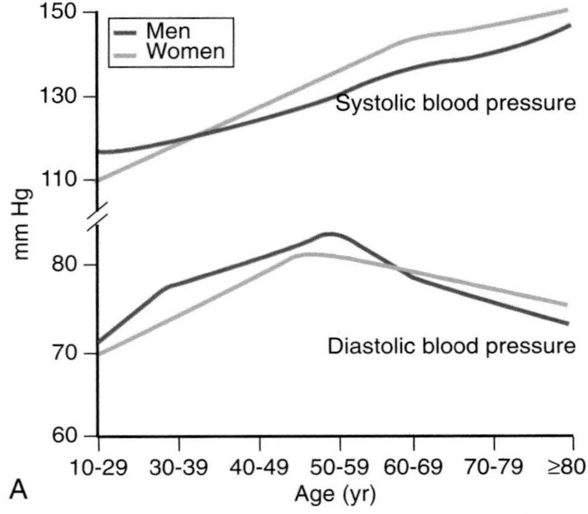

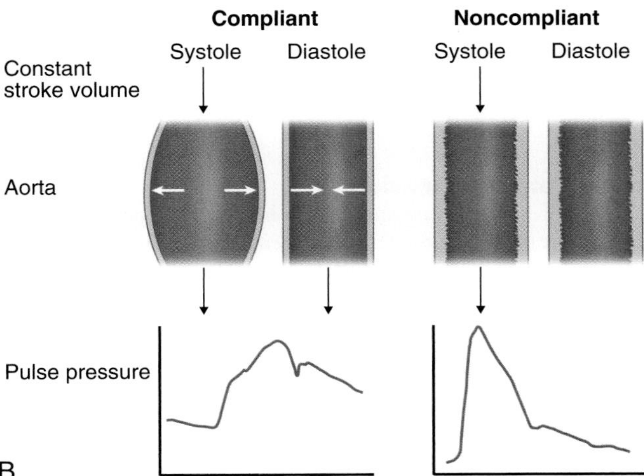

FIGURE 67-4. Aging and pulse pressure. A, Age-dependent changes in systolic and diastolic blood pressure in the United States. **B,** Schematic diagram showing the relation between aortic compliance and pulse pressure. (**A,** From Burt V, Whelton P, Rocella EJ, et al. Prevalence of hypertension in the U.S. adult population: results from the Third National Health and Nutrition Examination Survey, 1988-1991. *Hypertension.* 1995;25:305-313; **B,** Courtesy of Dr. Stanley Franklin, University of California at Irvine.)

Behavioral Determinants of Human Blood Pressure Variation

The most important behavioral determinants of blood pressure are related to dietary consumption of calories and salt. Across populations, the prevalence of hypertension increases linearly with average body mass index. With the unrelenting obesity epidemic in both developed and developing societies, increasing attention is being paid to the *metabolic syndrome* (Chapter 237) that often accompanies hypertension. The metabolic syndrome refers to the frequent clustering of elevated blood pressure with abdominal ("male pattern") adiposity, insulin resistance with glucose intolerance, and a dyslipidemic pattern consisting typically of elevated plasma triglyceride and low high-density lipoprotein cholesterol levels. In the Framingham Heart Study, obesity has been estimated to account for as much as 60% of the new cases of hypertension. The underlying mechanisms by which weight gain leads to hypertension are incompletely understood, but there is mounting evidence for an expanded plasma volume plus sympathetic overactivity. The sympathetic overactivity is thought to be a compensatory attempt to burn fat but at the expense of peripheral vasoconstriction, renal salt and water retention, and hypertension. In some obese individuals, sleep apnea (Chapter 100) is an important cause of hypertension. Repeated arterial desaturation sensitizes the carotid body chemoreceptors, causing sustained sympathetic overactivity even during waking hours.

Dietary sodium intake is another key behavioral determinant of human hypertension. In the INTERSALT study of 52 locations around the world, the risk for development of hypertension during three decades of adult life was linearly and tightly related to dietary sodium intake. Interindividual variability in blood pressure responses to dietary sodium loading and sodium restriction indicates an important genetic underpinning.

Genetic Determinants of Human Blood Pressure Variation

Concordance of blood pressures is greater within families than in unrelated individuals, greater between monozygotic twins than between dizygotic twins, and greater between biologic siblings than between adoptive siblings living in the same household. As much as 70% of the familial aggregation of blood pressure is attributed to shared genes rather than to shared environment.

The complex regulation of blood pressure has thwarted the genetic dissection of primary human hypertension, with the first positive genome-wide association studies suggesting multiple risk alleles, each having very small effects. Mutations in 20 salt-handling genes cause ultra-rare syndromes of severe, early-onset hypotension (salt-wasting syndromes) or hypertension (all inherited as mendelian traits). The clinical relevance of these mutations to common primary hypertension has been limited, although recent data indicate that heterozygous mutations in genes underlying the pediatric salt-wasting syndromes (Bartter's and Gitelman's) are present in 1 to 2% of the general adult population and confer resistance against primary hypertension.

CLINICAL MANIFESTATIONS

Hypertension has been called the silent killer, an asymptomatic chronic disorder that silently damages the blood vessels, heart, brain, and kidneys if it is undetected and untreated. Although headaches (Chapter 405) are common in patients with mild to moderate hypertension, episodes of headaches do not correlate with fluctuations in blood pressure. Rather, they correlate with a person's awareness of his or her diagnosis.

DIAGNOSIS

Initial Evaluation for Hypertension

The initial evaluation for hypertension should accomplish three goals: (1) stage the blood pressure, (2) assess the patient's overall cardiovascular risk, and (3) detect clues of secondary hypertension that require further evaluation.

Goal 1: Accurate Assessment of Blood Pressure

Office Blood Pressure

Traditionally, blood pressure has been staged as normal, prehypertension, or hypertension based on the average of two or more readings taken at two or more office visits (see Table 67-1). The blood pressure should be measured at least twice after 5 minutes of rest with the patient seated, the back supported, and the arm bare and at heart level. A large adult-sized cuff should be used to measure blood pressure in overweight adults because the standard-sized cuff will cause falsely elevated readings. Tobacco and caffeine should be avoided for at least 30 minutes. Blood pressure should be measured in both arms, to exclude coarctation of the aorta, and after 5 minutes of standing, to exclude a significant postural fall, particularly in older persons and persons with diabetes or other conditions (e.g., Parkinson's disease) that predispose to autonomic insufficiency.

Home and Ambulatory Blood Pressure Monitoring

A person's blood pressure varies so much throughout a 24-hour period that it is impossible to characterize it accurately except by repeated measurements under various conditions. Out-of-office readings are the only way to obtain a clear picture of a person's usual blood pressure for accurate diagnosis and management. These readings are more predictive of cardiovascular events than office readings and overcome many of the pitfalls of office measurement, including physician errors and "white coat" reactions. Home blood pressure monitoring also improves medication adherence by actively involving patients in their own medical care.

New recommendations include the following: (1) home blood pressure monitoring should become a routine part of the clinical management of patients with known or suspected hypertension the same way that home blood glucose monitoring is essential to the management of patients with diabetes; (2) two (or three) readings should be taken in the morning and at night for 1 week, with a total of at least 12 readings being averaged before making clinical decisions; and (3) the target treatment goal is an average home blood pressure of less than 135/85 mm Hg for most patients and less than 130/80 mm Hg for high-risk patients, such as those with CAD, heart failure, diabetes, or chronic kidney disease.

A validated electronic oscillometric monitor with an arm cuff should be chosen from the dabl Educational Web site (*www.dableducational.org*). Each patient's monitor should be checked in the physician's office for its accuracy and appropriate cuff size. Patients must be taught correct measurement techniques and to avoid reporting bias. Wrist monitors are inaccurate and thus not recommended. The oscillometric method may not work well in patients with atrial fibrillation or frequent extrasystoles, for whom manual sphygmomanometry is required. Rare patients become obsessed about taking their blood pressure and need to stop.

Ambulatory blood pressure monitoring (Table 67-2) provides automated measurements of blood pressure during a 24-hour period while patients are engaged in their usual activities, including sleep (Fig. 67-6). Ambulatory blood pressure measurement is superior to standard office measurement in predicting fatal and nonfatal myocardial infarction and stroke. Recommended normal values are an average daytime blood pressure below 135/85 mm Hg, nighttime blood pressure below 120/70 mm Hg, and 24-hour blood pressure below 130/80 mm Hg. Some experts have recommended a lower cutoff value of 130/80 mm Hg as a more stringent definition of normal daytime blood pressure.

About 20% of patients with elevated office blood pressures have normal home or ambulatory blood pressures. If the daytime blood pressure is below 135/85 mm Hg (or preferably below 130/80 mm Hg) and there is no target organ damage despite consistently elevated office readings, the patient has

TABLE 67-2 RECOMMENDED INDICATIONS FOR AMBULATORY BLOOD PRESSURE MONITORING

Suspected "white coat hypertension" (high office blood pressure readings in patients with otherwise low total cardiovascular risk)*
Considerable variability of clinic blood pressure readings
Marked discrepancy between home and office blood pressure readings (e.g., suspected masked hypertension)
Suspected nocturnal hypertension
Suspected resistance to drug treatment
Suspected orthostatic hypotension or autonomic failure, particularly in elderly or diabetic patients
Elevated office blood pressure in pregnant women or suspected preeclampsia

*Medicare currently reimburses for ambulatory monitoring only to confirm the diagnosis of white coat hypertension that is suspected on the basis of three normal home readings in patients with no evidence of target organ damage despite repeatedly elevated office blood pressure readings (ICD 796.2).

Modified from Mancia G, DeBacker G, Dominickak A, et al. 2007 Guidelines for the management of arterial hypertension of the European Society of Hypertension (ESH) and the European Society of Cardiology (ESC). *Eur Heart J.* 2007;23:1462-1536.

"office-only" or "white coat" hypertension, caused by a transient adrenergic response to the measurement of blood pressure in the physician's office. The cardiovascular risk is intermediate to that in persons with consistently normal blood pressure and those with consistently high blood pressure. Many patients do not have pure white coat hypertension but rather white coat aggravation, a white coat reaction superimposed on a milder level of out-of-office hypertension that nevertheless needs treatment. For example, up to 30% of treated patients who have persistently elevated office blood pressure readings will be shown by ambulatory monitoring to have adequate or even excessive control of their hypertension, thereby eliminating overtreatment (see Fig. 67-6). In other patients, office readings underestimate ambulatory blood pressures, presumably because of sympathetic overactivity (e.g., owing to job stress, home stress, or tobacco smoke) that dissipates when the patient comes to the office. Such "masked hypertension," present in up to 10% of patients, increases cardiovascular risk.

Ambulatory monitoring is the only way to detect hypertension during sleep. Blood pressure normally dips during sleep and increases sharply when a person awakens and becomes active (see Fig. 67-6). Nocturnal hypertension increases the aggregate blood pressure burden on the cardiovascular system and is a stronger predictor of cardiovascular outcomes than daytime ambulatory blood pressure or office measurements. Nocturnal hypertension is particularly common in patients with chronic kidney disease (Chapter 132), presumably because of their sustained sympathetic overactivity, which does not shut down during sleep, and centralization of blood volume with nocturnal recumbence.

Goal 2: Cardiovascular Risk Stratification

Although cardiovascular risk increases with increasing blood pressure, it also increases if the patient has hypertensive target organ damage or additional cardiovascular risk factors. More than 75% of hypertensive patients meet current U.S. criteria for initiation of lipid-lowering medication (low-density lipoprotein cholesterol more than 130 mm Hg), and 25% have diabetes. Thus, the minimal laboratory testing required for the initial evaluation of hypertension is determination of blood electrolyte, fasting glucose, and serum creatinine levels (with calculated glomerular filtration rate [GFR]), a fasting lipid panel, hematocrit, spot urinalysis (including urine albumin-to-creatinine ratio), and a resting 12-lead electrocardiogram (ECG).

The gradient of increasing levels of blood pressure with cardiovascular risk steepens as additional risk factors are added (Fig. 67-7). As the overall risks multiply, blood pressure control becomes more important. Current U.S. guidelines recommended a usual blood pressure of 140/90 mm Hg as the threshold for initiating antihypertensive medication in most patients, with a lower threshold of 130/80 mm Hg for high-risk patients with diabetes or chronic kidney disease. Based on more recent data, the operational definition of high-risk patients has been expanded to include most patients with established CAD, carotid artery disease, peripheral artery disease, abdominal aortic aneurysm, heart failure, or high risk for CAD (10-year Framingham risk score of >10%) (Table 67-3). Because cardiovascular risk increases so steeply with age (see Fig. 67-1), most hypertensive men older than 55 years and most hypertensive women older than 65 years will have a Framingham risk score higher than 10% (*http://hp2010.nhlbihin.net/atpiii/calculator.asp*).

Goal 3: Identification and Treatment of Secondary (Identifiable) Causes of Hypertension

The third goal of the initial evaluation is to screen for identifiable causes of hypertension (Table 67-4), in the hope of finding a cure. A thorough search for secondary causes, which is not cost-effective in most patients with hypertension, becomes critically important in two circumstances: (1) when there is a compelling finding on the initial evaluation and (2) when the hypertensive process is so severe that it either is refractory to intensive multiple-drug therapy or requires hospitalization.

Renal Parenchymal Hypertension

Chronic kidney disease (Chapter 132) is the most common cause of secondary hypertension. Hypertension is present in more than 85% of patients with

TABLE 67-3 RECOMMENDED (TARGET) BLOOD PRESSURE VALUES*

BP < 150/80 mm Hg
Very elderly persons (80+ years of age)
BP < 140/90 mm Hg
Uncomplicated hypertension
BP < 130/80 mm Hg
Diabetes mellitus
Chronic kidney disease
GFR <60 mL/min/1.73 m^2
Urine albumin-to-creatinine ratio ≥30 mg/g (consider <120/80 mm Hg if >1 g of proteinuria per day)
Other patients at high risk for coronary artery disease (primary prevention)
Coronary artery disease risk equivalents
Carotid artery disease
Peripheral arterial disease
Abdominal aortic aneurysm
10-year Framingham risk score > 10% (most men over age 55, most women over age 65)
Established coronary artery disease: stable or unstable (secondary prevention)
Secondary prevention of stroke or TIA
Heart failure or left ventricular systolic dysfunction (consider BP < 120/80 mm Hg)

*Values are for office readings; target values for home or daytime ambulatory monitoring are generally set 5 mm Hg lower.
BP = blood pressure; GFR = glomerular filtration rate; TIA = transient ischemic attack.
Adapted from Rosendorff C, Black HR, Cannon CP, et al. Treatment of hypertension in the prevention and management of ischemic heart disease: a scientific statement from the American Heart Association Council for High Blood Pressure Research and the Councils on Clinical Cardiology and Epidemiology and Prevention. *Circulation.* 2007;115:2761-2788.

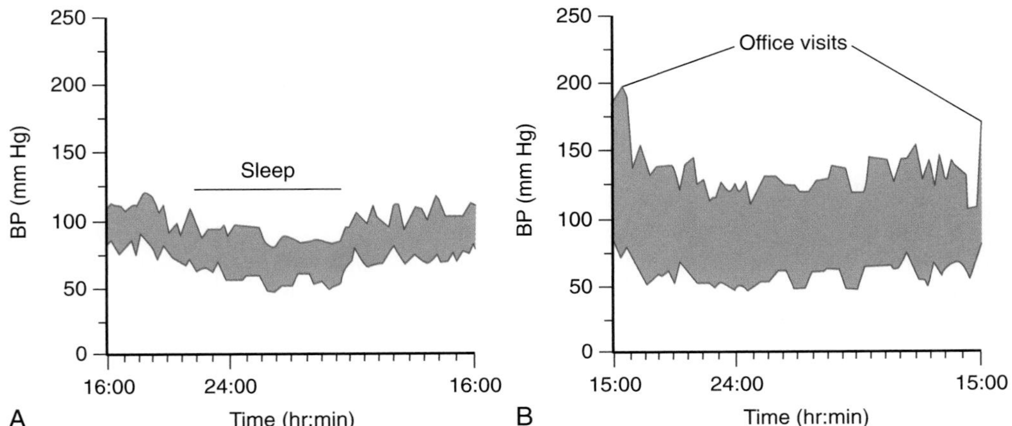

FIGURE 67-6. The 24-hour ambulatory blood pressure (BP) monitor tracings of two different patients. A, Optimal blood pressure in a healthy 37-year-old woman. Note the normal variability in blood pressure, the nocturnal dip in blood pressure during sleep, and the sharp increase in blood pressure on awakening. **B,** Pronounced white coat effect in an 80-year-old woman referred for evaluation of medically refractory hypertension. Documentation of the white coat effect prevented overtreatment of the patient's isolated systolic hypertension. (**A,** Courtesy of Ronald G. Victor, MD, Hypertension Division, Department of Internal Medicine, University of Texas Southwestern Medical Center, Dallas, Texas; **B,** Courtesy of Wanpen Vongpatanasin, MD, Hypertension Division, Department of Internal Medicine, University of Texas Southwestern Medical Center, Dallas, Texas.)

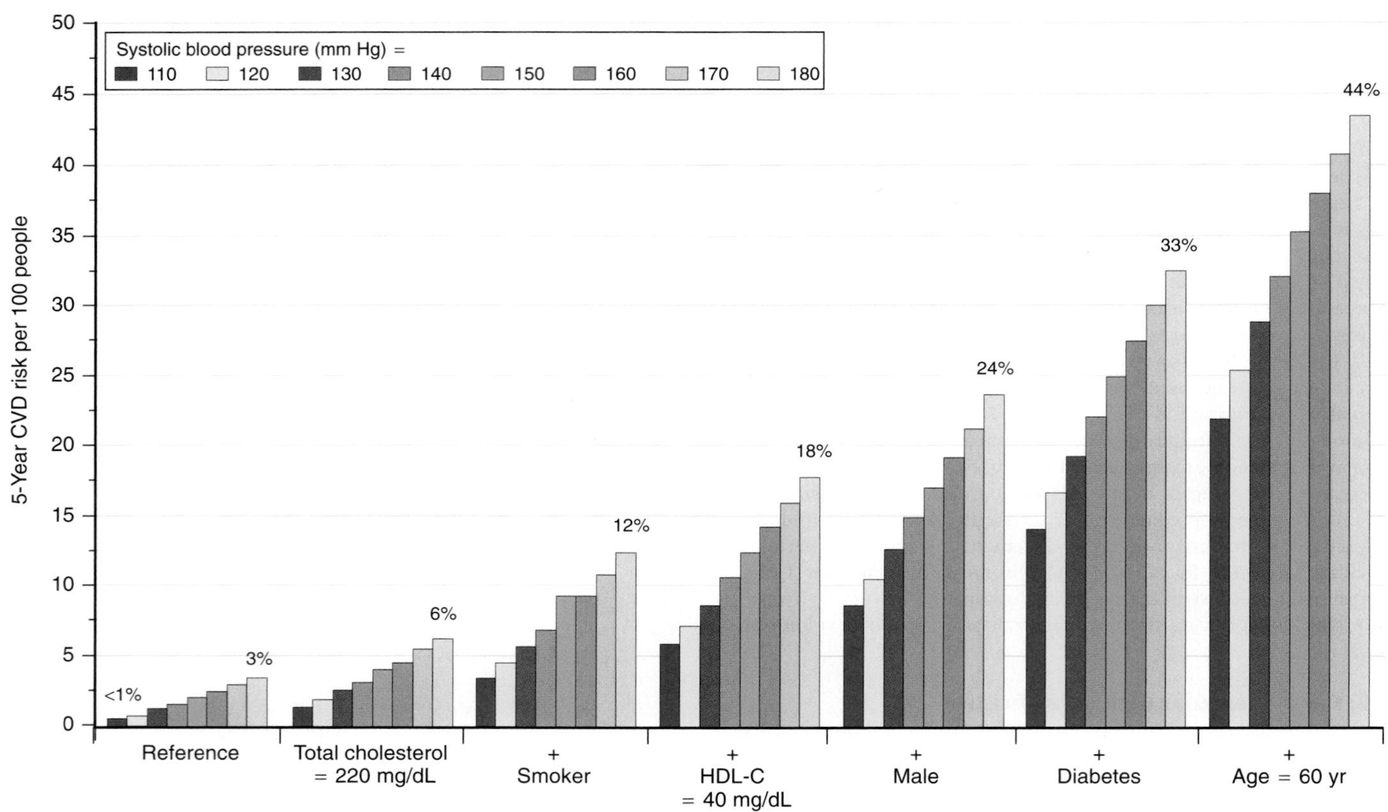

FIGURE 67-7. Absolute risk of cardiovascular disease (CVD) during 5 years in patients by systolic blood pressure at specified levels of other risk factors. The reference category is a nondiabetic, nonsmoking woman aged 50 years with a total cholesterol value of 190 mg/dL and a high-density lipoprotein cholesterol (HDL-C) value of 60 mg/dL. Risks are given for systolic pressures of 110, 120, 130, 140, 150, 160, 170, and 180 mm Hg. In the other categories, additional risk factors are added consecutively. (From Jackson R, Lawes CMM, Benett DA, et al. Treatment with drugs to lower blood pressure and blood cholesterol based on an individual's absolute cardiovascular risk. *Lancet.* 2005;365:434-441.)

TABLE 67-4 GUIDE TO EVALUATION OF IDENTIFIABLE CAUSES OF HYPERTENSION

SUSPECTED DIAGNOSIS	CLINICAL CLUES	DIAGNOSTIC TESTING
Chronic kidney disease	Estimated GFR <60 mL/min/1.73 m^2 Urine albumin-to-creatinine ratio ≥30 mg/g	Renal sonography
Renovascular disease	New elevation in serum creatinine, marked elevation in serum creatinine with ACEI or ARB, drug-resistant hypertension, flash pulmonary edema, abdominal or flank bruit	Renal sonography (atrophic kidney), CT or MR angiography, invasive angiography
Coarctation of the aorta	Arm pulses > leg pulses, arm BP > leg BP, chest bruits, rib notching on chest radiography	MR angiography, TEE, invasive angiography
Primary aldosteronism	Hypokalemia, drug-resistant hypertension	Plasma renin and aldosterone, 24-hour urine aldosterone and potassium after oral salt loading, adrenal vein sampling
Cushing's syndrome	Truncal obesity, wide and blanching purple striae, muscle weakness	1 mg dexamethasone-suppression test, urinary cortisol after dexamethasone, adrenal CT
Pheochromocytoma	Paroxysms of hypertension, palpitations, perspiration, and pallor; diabetes	Plasma metanephrines, 24-hour urinary metanephrines and catecholamines, abdominal CT or MR imaging
Obstructive sleep apnea	Loud snoring, large neck, obesity, somnolence	Polysonography

ACEI = angiotensin-converting enzyme inhibitor; ARB = angiotensin receptor blocker; BP = blood pressure; CT = computed tomography; GFR = glomerular filtration rate; MR, magnetic resonance; TEE = transesophageal echocardiography.

chronic kidney disease and is a major factor causing their increased cardiovascular morbidity and mortality. The mechanisms causing the hypertension include an expanded plasma volume and peripheral vasoconstriction; the peripheral vasoconstriction is caused by both activation of vasoconstrictor pathways (renin-angiotensin and sympathetic nervous systems) and inhibition of vasodilator pathways (nitric oxide).

Measurement of serum creatinine alone is an inadequate screening test for renal insufficiency. A spot urine specimen should be obtained to screen for microalbuminuria, which is defined as a urine albumin-to-urine creatinine ratio of 30 to 300 mg/g (equivalent to excretion of 30 to 300 mg of albumin per 24 hours); higher levels of albuminuria indicate more advanced kidney disease. Using the spot urine specimen, creatinine clearance should be calculated (*www.nephron.com; www.newtech.kidney.org*) (Chapter 116) to screen for an estimated GFR below 60 mL/min/1.73 m^2.

In patients with mild (stage 2: GFR of 60 to 90 mL/min/1.73 m^2) or moderate (stage 3: GFR of 30 to 60 mL/min/1.73 m^2) proteinuric chronic kidney disease, stringent blood pressure control is imperative both to slow the progression to end-stage renal disease and to reduce the excessive cardiovascular risk. In patients with severe chronic kidney disease, hypertension often becomes difficult to treat and may require either (1) intensive medical treatment with loop diuretics, potent vasodilators (e.g., minoxidil), high-dose β-adrenergic blockers, and central sympatholytics; or (2) initiation of chronic hemodialysis as the only effective way to reduce plasma volume. In chronic hemodialysis patients, the challenge is to control interdialytic hypertension without exacerbating dialysis-induced hypotension. The annual mortality rate in the hemodialysis population is 25%; half of this excessive mortality is caused by cardiovascular events that are related, at least in part, to hypertension.

Renovascular Hypertension

PATHOBIOLOGY AND CLINICAL MANIFESTATIONS

The two main causes of renal artery stenosis (Chapter 127) are atherosclerosis (85% of cases), typically in older persons with other clinical manifestations of systemic atherosclerosis, and fibromuscular dysplasia (15% of cases), typically in young women who are otherwise healthy. Although renal artery stenosis and hypertension frequently coexist, the presence of a renal artery stenosis does not prove that the patient's hypertension is renovascular in origin or that revascularization will improve renal perfusion and blood pressure.

Unilateral renal artery stenosis can lead to underperfusion of the juxtaglomerular cells, thereby causing renin-dependent hypertension even though the contralateral kidney is able to maintain normal blood volume. In contrast, bilateral renal artery stenosis (or unilateral stenosis with a solitary kidney) constitutes a potentially reversible cause of progressive renal failure and volume-dependent hypertension. The following clinical clues increase the suspicion of renovascular hypertension: any hospitalization for urgent or emergent hypertension; recurrent "flash" pulmonary edema; recent worsening of long-standing, previously well-controlled hypertension; severe hypertension in a young adult or after the age of 50 years; precipitous and progressive worsening of renal function in response to angiotensin-converting enzyme (ACE) inhibition or angiotensin II receptor blockade; unilateral small kidney by any radiographic study; extensive peripheral arteriosclerosis; and a flank bruit.

DIAGNOSIS

Contrast-enhanced computed tomography (CT) and magnetic resonance angiography are the preferred screening tests for renal artery stenosis, but gadolinium-enhanced magnetic resonance imaging (MRI) is contraindicated in patients with advanced chronic kidney disease to avoid potentially fatal gadolinium-induced nephrogenic systemic fibrosis (Chapter 275). Fibromuscular dysplasia classically causes a "string of beads" lesion in the midportion of a renal artery (Fig. 67-8A), whereas atherosclerotic renal artery lesions are proximal and discrete (see Fig. 67-8B). Invasive renal angiography is the "gold standard" for confirming the diagnosis of renal artery stenosis.

TREATMENT Rx

Balloon angioplasty is the treatment of choice for fibromuscular dysplasia, with overall favorable outcomes. In contrast, medical management of hypertension and the associated atherosclerotic risk factors is first-line treatment for atherosclerotic renal artery stenosis. Truly drug-resistant hypertension and a progressive decline in renal function (ischemic nephropathy) currently are the only two firm indications for balloon angioplasty. Most atherosclerotic renal artery lesions do not cause hypertension or progressive renal failure, and most patients will not benefit from revascularization (balloon angioplasty or stenting), which carries substantial risks of serious complications.[1] About 15% of patients undergoing cardiac catheterization will have a renal artery lesion when coronary angiography is followed by routine ("drive-by") renal angiography, but evidence does not support this diagnostic practice or therapy based on it.

Mineralocorticoid-Induced Hypertension Due to Primary Aldosteronism

PATHOBIOLOGY

The most common causes of primary aldosteronism (Chapter 234) are a unilateral aldosterone-producing adenoma and bilateral adrenal hyperplasia. Because aldosterone is the principal ligand for the mineralocorticoid receptor in the distal nephron, excessive aldosterone production causes excessive renal Na^+-K^+ exchange, often resulting in hypokalemia.

CLINICAL MANIFESTATIONS AND DIAGNOSIS

The diagnosis should always be suspected when hypertension is accompanied by either unprovoked hypokalemia (serum potassium concentration below 3.5 mmol/L in the absence of diuretic therapy) or a tendency to develop excessive hypokalemia during diuretic therapy (serum potassium concentration below 3.0 mmol/L). However, more than one third of patients do not have hypokalemia on initial presentation, and the diagnosis should also be considered in any patient with resistant hypertension.

Screening for hyperaldosteronism should be restricted to the small fraction of hypertensive patients with hypokalemia or severe drug-resistant hypertension. If such patients have a positive screening test—a high serum aldosterone level and a suppressed plasma renin activity level— and want to consider laparoscopic adrenalectomy, the patient should be referred to an experienced center for further evaluation: salt-loading to test for nonsuppressible aldosteronism and, if present, adrenal vein sampling to test for lateralization.

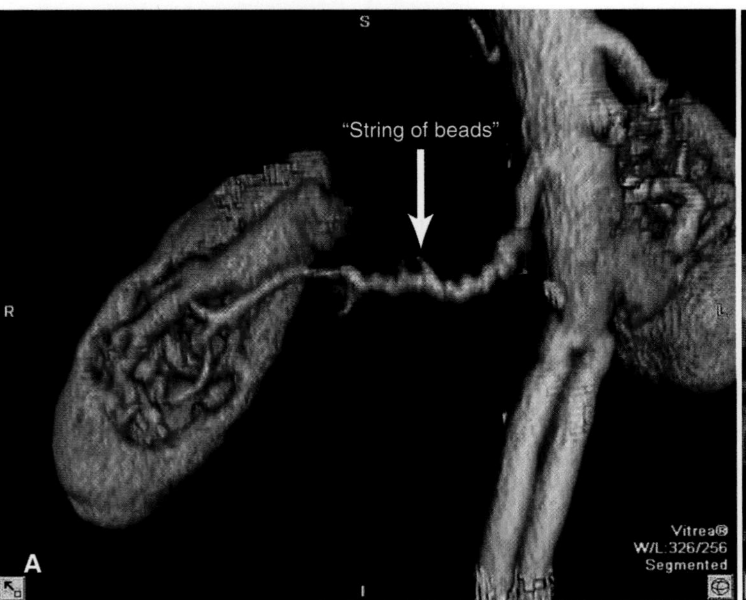

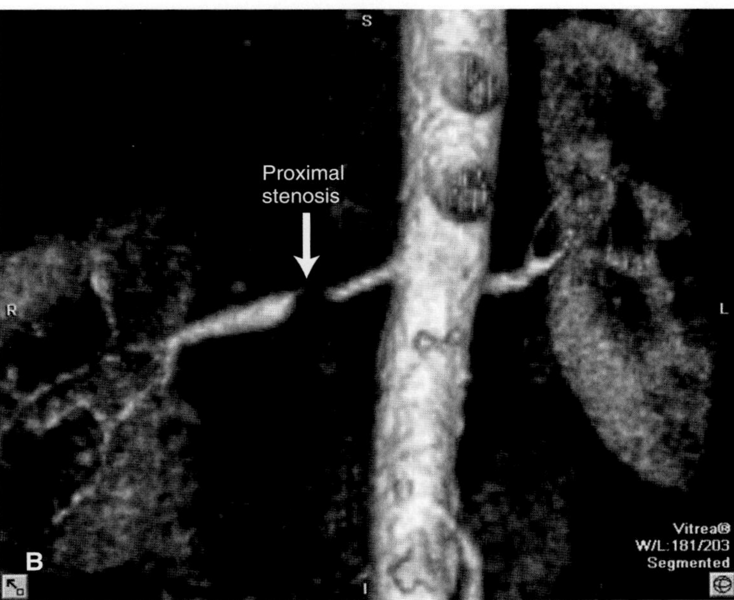

FIGURE 67-8. Computed tomographic angiogram with three-dimensional reconstruction. A, The classic "string of beads" lesion of fibromuscular dysplasia (bilateral in this patient). **B,** A severe proximal atherosclerotic stenosis of the right renal artery and mild stenosis of the left renal artery. (Images courtesy of Bart Domatch, MD, Radiology Department, University of Texas Southwestern Medical Center, Dallas, Texas.)

TREATMENT

Rx

CT has too many false-positive and false-negative results to be used as a noninvasive alternative to invasive adrenal vein sampling. Laparoscopic adrenalectomy and mineralocorticoid receptor blockade with eplerenone (50 to 100 mg per day) constitute highly effective therapeutic options that target the disease-causing mechanism with a favorable risk-to-benefit ratio.

Mendelian Forms of Mineralocorticoid-Induced Hypertension

Almost all the rare mendelian forms of hypertension are mineralocorticoid induced and involve excessive activation of the epithelial Na^+ channel (ENaC), the final common pathway for reabsorption of sodium from the distal nephron (Fig. 67-9). Thus, salt-dependent hypertension can be caused both by gain-of-function mutations of ENaC or the mineralocorticoid receptor and by increased production or decreased clearance of mineralocorticoid receptor ligands, which are aldosterone, deoxycorticosterone, and cortisol.

Pheochromocytomas and Paragangliomas

Pheochromocytomas are rare catecholamine-producing tumors of the adrenal chromaffin cells, whereas paragangliomas are even rarer tumors of the extra-adrenal chromaffin cells (Chapter 235). The diagnosis should be suspected when hypertension is drug resistant or paroxysmal, particularly when accompanied by paroxysms of headache, palpitations, pallor, or diaphoresis. In some patients, pheochromocytoma is misdiagnosed as panic disorder. A family history of early-onset hypertension may suggest pheochromocytoma as part of the multiple endocrine neoplasia syndromes (Chapter 239). An increasing number of pheochromocytomas are being detected incidentally on abdominal imaging studies for nonadrenal indications. If the diagnosis is missed, outpouring of catecholamines from the tumor can cause unsuspected hypertensive crisis during unrelated surgical procedures, in which case mortality rates exceed 80%.

Other Neurogenic Causes

Other causes of neurogenic hypertension that can be confused with pheochromocytoma include sympathomimetic agents (cocaine, methamphetamine; Chapter 33), baroreflex failure, and obstructive sleep apnea (Chapter 100). A history of surgery and radiation therapy for head and neck tumors (Chapter 196) raises suspicion of baroreceptor damage. Snoring and somnolence suggest sleep apnea, but continuous positive airway pressure to treat the sleep apnea rarely improves blood pressure substantially (Chapter 100).

Other Causes of Secondary Hypertension

Coarctation of the aorta typically occurs just distal to the origin of the left subclavian artery, so the blood pressure is lower in the legs than in the arms (opposite of the normal situation) (see Fig. 69-7 in Chapter 69). The clue is that the pulses are weaker in the lower than in the upper extremities, indicating the need to measure blood pressure in the legs as well as in both arms. Intercostal collaterals can produce bruits on examination and rib notching on the chest radiograph. Coarctations can be cured with surgery or angioplasty.

Hyperthyroidism tends to cause systolic hypertension with a wide pulse pressure, whereas hypothyroidism tends to cause mainly diastolic hypertension. Treatment is for the underlying disease. Hyperparathyroidism (Chapter 253) also has been associated with hypertension. Cyclosporine and tacrolimus are important causes of secondary hypertension in transplant recipients, apparently by inhibition of calcineurin, the calcium-dependent phosphatase that is expressed not only in lymphoid tissue but also in neural, vascular, and renal tissue. In the absence of outcomes data, nondihydropyridine calcium-channel blockers (CCBs) have become the drugs of first choice, but they increase cyclosporine blood levels. Combination therapy with diuretics, CCBs, and central sympatholytics often is required.

PREVENTION AND TREATMENT OF HYPERTENSION

Rx

At the population level, the primary prevention of hypertension requires large-scale societal changes, including further efforts to influence the food industry to reduce salt in processed foods, efforts to increase exercise, and the availability of fresh fruits and vegetables. Once a person's blood pressure rises to prehypertensive levels, lifestyle modifications alone are almost never enough to return blood pressure to normal, and recidivism is almost universal.

Although short-term pharmacologic therapy with a low-dose angiotensin receptor blocker (ARB) has been advocated to prevent conversion from prehypertension to full-blown hypertension, blood pressure quickly rises again once the ARB is discontinued.[2] Thus, lifelong prescription medication is the cornerstone of effective therapy for primary hypertension, with lifestyle modification serving as an adjunct but not as an alternative. The objective is to reduce the blood pressure and associated metabolic abnormalities sufficiently to reduce the risk for cardiovascular events and end-stage renal disease without compromising the patient's quality of life.

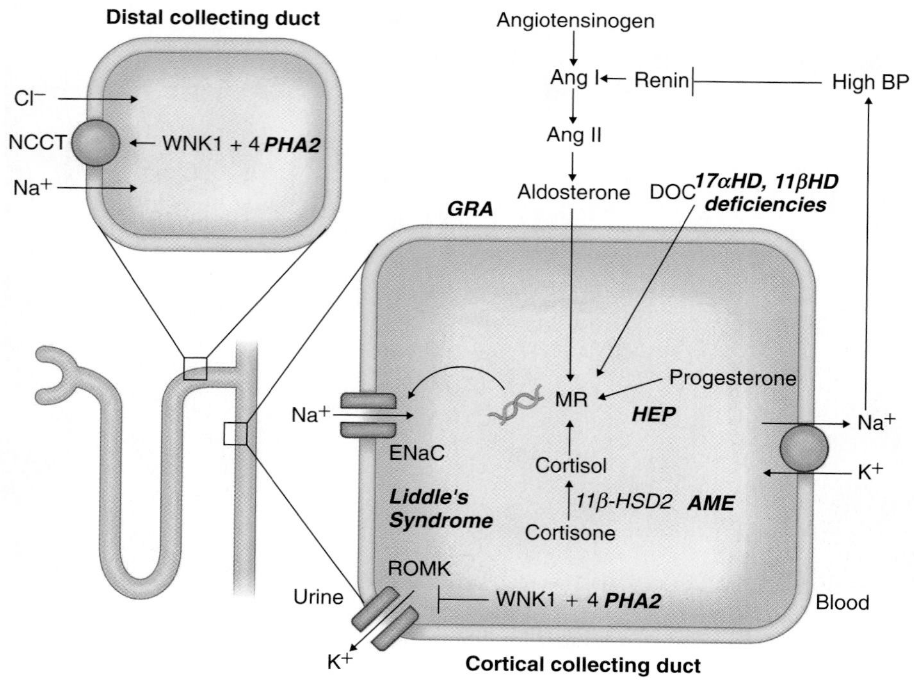

FIGURE 67-9. Mendelian forms of hypertension that cause mineralocorticoid-induced hypertension. AME = apparent mineralocorticoid excess; Ang = angiotensin; BP = blood pressure; GRA = glucocorticoid-remediable aldosteronism; 17αHD and 11βHD = 17α- and 11β-hydroxylase deficiency; 11β-HSD2 = 11β-hydroxysteroid dehydrogenase type 2; DOC = deoxycorticosterone; ENaC = epithelial Na^+ channel; HEP = hypertension exacerbated by pregnancy; MR = mineralocorticoid receptor; NCCT = sodium-chloride cotransporter; PHA2 = pseudohypoaldosteronism type 2; ROMK = rectifying outer medullary K^+ channel; WNK = with no lysine kinases. See text for explanation. (Modified from Lifton RP, Gharavi AG, Geller DS. Molecular mechanisms of human hypertension. *Cell.* 2001;104:545-556.)

Randomized trials have proved beyond any doubt that antihypertensive drug therapy reduces cardiovascular risk, with benefits that are proportional to the reduction in blood pressure achieved.[3] However, in practice, most treated patients do not achieve the same low risk levels of truly normotensive persons because their blood pressures remain higher than optimal owing to the threshold levels of guidelines, the hesitation of practicing physicians to start and intensify drug treatment, the costs of medications, and nonadherence despite the generally declining costs of medications as they become generic.

Multidrug regimens with two, three, or even more medications of different drug classes are almost always required to achieve currently recommended blood pressure goals, particularly for high-risk patients. Low-dose drug combinations exert synergistic effects on blood pressure while minimizing dose-dependent side effects. For most patients with hypertension, lipid-lowering therapy and antiplatelet therapy are indicated as part of a comprehensive cardiovascular risk-reduction strategy (Chapter 51).

Lifestyle Modification

Every antihypertensive regimen should include lifestyle modification. The Seventh Report of the Joint National Committee on Prevention, Detection, Evaluation, and Treatment of High Blood Pressure (JNC 7) recommended a trial of lifestyle modification alone for an unspecified time (6 to 12 months in prior guidelines) before antihypertensive medication is prescribed, even for high-risk patients. This is wishful thinking and may be a cause of therapeutic inertia. More recent data, however, support greater urgency in achieving pharmacologic control of high blood pressure to reduce cardiovascular risk, at least in patients with multiple risk factors. In sufficiently motivated individuals, lifestyle modification can decrease medication requirements, have a favorable impact on associated cardiovascular risk factors, and emphasize the active role patients can play in controlling their blood pressure.

Moderate dietary sodium reduction (Chapter 220) reduces renal potassium wasting during diuretic therapy and lowers blood pressure by 2/2 mm Hg on average. Most dietary sodium comes from processed foods rather than from the salt shaker. Without draconian measures, daily salt consumption can be reduced from 10 to 6 g by teaching patients to read food labels (6 g of NaCl = 2.4 g of sodium = 100 mmol of sodium). The Dietary Approaches to Stop Hypertension (DASH) study showed that individuals with prehypertension or stage 1 hypertension can lower their blood pressures, at least over the short term, by as much as 11/6 mm Hg even without restricting calorie or sodium intake if they adhere to a diet rich in fresh fruits and vegetables (for high potassium content) and low-fat dairy products.[4] This diet (*www.nhlbi.nih.gov/health/public/heart/hbp/dash/*) is strongly recommended because the blood pressure–lowering effects can approach the magnitude of drug monotherapy, can be enhanced by an additional 2/1 mm Hg by dietary sodium restriction, and are seen in all ethnic groups, especially African Americans.

Smokers should be counseled to quit because tobacco (Chapter 31) is such a potent risk factor for coronary heart disease, stroke, and progression of hypertensive nephrosclerosis to end-stage renal disease. Because blood pressure increases transiently by 10 to 15 mm Hg after each cigarette, smokers of more than 20 cigarettes per day often have higher blood pressures out of the office than in the smoke-free medical office. Blood pressure increases similarly with the first morning cup of coffee, but the pressor response to caffeine usually (but not always) habituates throughout the day. Thus, caffeine consumption need not be eliminated.

Moderate alcohol (Chapter 32) consumption (one or two drinks per day) does not increase the risk for hypertension in Western populations; but in Japanese populations, hypertension is more common in men who are moderate drinkers than in men who cannot drink because of a loss-of-function mutation in the alcohol dehydrogenase gene. In all populations, heavy drinking (three or more standard-sized drinks per day) and especially binge drinking activate the sympathetic nervous system the next day during withdrawal and are associated with an increased incidence and severity of hypertension, which is reversible if alcohol consumption decreases.

After a bout of aerobic exercise (Chapter 15), a small reduction in blood pressure can persist for several hours. Relaxation techniques (e.g., meditation, biofeedback, breathing exercises) can decrease blood pressure transiently but generally produce little if any demonstrable effect on ambulatory blood pressure (Chapter 38). However, in some individuals in whom overwhelming home or job strain or anger is a major determinant of high blood pressure, cognitive behavior therapy and anxiolytics (Chapter 404) may be beneficial. Patients often associate hypertension directly with life stress, but stress management alone rarely is sufficient to control their hypertension.

Pharmacologic Therapy

More than 100 antihypertensive medications are marketed (Table 67-5). Lowering blood pressure with medication reduces but does not eliminate cardiorenal risks.

Classes of Oral Antihypertensive Drugs

The various classes of oral antihypertensive drugs have different mechanisms of actions, which explain the therapeutic principles of their use as well as their major contraindications and side effects (Table 67-6).

Diuretics

Mechanism of Action. With initiation of diuretic therapy, contraction of blood volume causes the initial fall in blood pressure. With continued therapy, blood volume is partially restored, and vasodilator mechanisms (e.g., opening of adenosine triphosphate [ATP]-sensitive K^+ channels) sustain the antihypertensive action. Loop diuretics block Na^+-K^+-$2Cl^-$ transport in the thick ascending loop of Henle, where a large portion of the filtered sodium is reabsorbed. Thiazide diuretics and the indoline derivative indapamide block Na^+-Cl^- cotransporter in the distal convoluted tubule, where a smaller portion of the filtered sodium is reabsorbed. Spironolactone and eplerenone prevent aldosterone from activating the mineralocorticoid receptor, thereby inhibiting the downstream activation of ENaC, whereas triamterene and amiloride block ENaC directly; because less sodium is presented to the Na^+,K^+-ATPase on the vascular side of the collecting duct cells, less potassium is excreted in the urine.

Therapeutic Principles. Diuretics are the oldest, least expensive, and still among the most effective antihypertensive medications. In the Antihypertensive and Lipid-Lowering Treatment to Prevent Heart Attack Trial (ALLHAT), the thiazide-type diuretic chlorthalidone was at least as effective as (and in some instances more effective than) newer and more expensive agents (the ACE inhibitor lisinopril or the dihydropyridine CCB amlodipine) in lowering blood pressure and preventing the attendant cardiovascular complications in all subgroups of patients.[5] Combined with other classes of antihypertensive medications, diuretics exert a synergistic effect on blood pressure. The most common cause of apparently drug-resistant hypertension is the failure to include a diuretic in the therapeutic regimen or to dose it correctly.

Because of their long half-lives, thiazides are more effective than short-acting loop diuretics for most patients with hypertension. Chlorthalidone, the thiazide-type diuretic used in the ALLHAT and many other trials, is more potent and has a much longer duration of action than hydrochlorothiazide, which for decades has replaced chlorthalidone as the main thiazide-type diuretic in clinical practice. Low-dose hydrochlorothiazide (12.5 mg/day), often in fixed-dose combination with an ACE inhibitor or ARB, is recommended for mild uncomplicated hypertension, whereas chlorthalidone (typically 25 mg/day, which has a potency equivalent to about 40 mg of hydrochlorothiazide [HCTZ]) is recommended for more severe or more difficult hypertension.

When the GFR falls below 50 mL/min/1.73 m^2, standard doses of hydrochlorothiazide become ineffective, although chlorthalidone or much higher doses of HCTZ can be effective. Loop diuretics are the diuretics of choice for treating hypertension in patients with chronic kidney disease or heart failure. Because the duration of action of furosemide is less than 6 hours, torsemide is a better choice owing to its longer half-life. The addition of chlorthalidone to a loop diuretic can sometimes restore blood pressure responsiveness in patients with resistant hypertension due to volume expansion in the setting of advanced chronic kidney disease.

Thiazides can aggravate glucose intolerance (especially when used in combination with a β-blocker), cause hypokalemia and hyponatremia (especially in older persons), precipitate gout, elevate serum lipids, and rarely cause severe photosensitive dermatitis. They are more likely than any other antihypertensive drugs to cause erectile dysfunction.

With its more favorable side-effect profile, eplerenone (50-100 mg/day) has replaced spironolactone as the drug of choice for primary aldosteronism. Low-dose eplerenone (12.5 to 50 mg/day) and low-dose spironolactone (6.25 to 50 mg/day) have been understudied and underused in primary hypertension. Both drugs are powerful antihypertensives and avoid hypokalemia. Either drug can be remarkably effective as add-on therapy for otherwise drug-resistant hypertension. Hyperkalemia must be avoided when using these agents in patients with kidney disease.

Angiotensin-Converting Enzyme Inhibitors and Angiotensin Receptor Blockers

Mechanism of Action. The renin-angiotensin-aldosterone system is one of the most important targets for antihypertensive drugs. The interaction of angiotensin II with G protein–coupled receptors, termed *AT_1 receptors*, accelerates numerous cellular processes that contribute not only to hypertension but also to its end-organ damage. The ACE inhibitors block the conversion of angiotensin I to angiotensin II, initially leading to a dramatic fall in plasma angiotensin II levels; with continued treatment, however, plasma angiotensin II levels return to normal (the phenomenon of "ACE escape") because ACE inhibitors do not block alternative pathways that generate angiotensin II. The sustained antihypertensive action of ACE inhibitors is explained in part by their ability to block the metabolism of bradykinin, a potent endothelium-dependent vasodilator. These agents slow the deterioration of renal function in patients with chronic kidney disease by causing greater dilation of the efferent renal arteriole, thereby reducing intraglomerular pressure.

By comparison, ARBs lower blood pressure specifically by blocking the interaction of angiotensin II on the AT_1 receptors. Thus, ARBs do not increase bradykinin, which has been implicated in both the therapeutic benefits and the side effects of ACE inhibitors (i.e., cough, angioedema).

Therapeutic Principles. Because of their favorable side-effect profiles and putative ancillary benefits on vascular health, ACE inhibitors and ARBs have gained popularity for the general treatment of hypertension. As monotherapy,

TABLE 67-5 ORAL ANTIHYPERTENSIVE AGENTS

DRUG	DOSE RANGE, TOTAL, MG/DAY (DOSES PER DAY)	USUAL STARTING DOSE, MG/DAY (DOSES PER DAY)
DIURETICS		
Thiazide Diuretics		
Chlorthalidone	6.25-50 (1)	12.5 (1)
HCTZ	6.25-50 (1)	12.5 (1)
Indapamide	1.25-5 (1)	1.25 (1)
Metolazone	2.5-5 (1)	2.5 (1)
Loop Diuretics		
Bumetanide	0.5-2 (2)	1 (2)
Ethacrynic acid	25-100 (2)	25 (2)
Furosemide	20-160 (2)	20 (2)
Torsemide	2.5-20 (1-2)	5 (2)
Potassium Sparing		
Amiloride	5-20 (1)	10 (2)
Eplerenone	25-100 (1-2)	25 (1)
Spironolactone	6.25-400 (1-2)	6.25 (1)
Triamterene	25-100 (1)	37.5 (1)
β-BLOCKERS		
Acebutolol	200-800 (2)	200 (2)
Atenolol	25-100 (1)	25 (1)
Betaxolol	5-20 (1)	5 (1)
Bisoprolol	2.5-20 (1)	2.5 (1)
Carteolol	2.5-10 (1)	2.5 (1)
Metoprolol	50-450 (2)	50 (2)
Metoprolol XL	50-200 (1-2)	50 (1)
Nadolol	20-320 (1)	40 (1)
Penbutolol	10-80 (1)	10 (1)
Pindolol	10-60 (2)	10 (1)
Propranolol	40-180 (2)	40 (2)
Propranolol LA	60-180 (1-2)	60 (1)
Timolol	20-60 (2)	20 (2)
α-/β-BLOCKERS/VASODILATING β-BLOCKERS		
Carvedilol	6.25-50 (2)	6.25 (2)
Carvedilol CR	20-80 (1)	20 (1)
Labetalol	200-2400 (2)	200 (2)
Nebivolol	5-40 (1)	5 (1)
CALCIUM-CHANNEL BLOCKERS		
Dihydropyridines		
Amlodipine	2.5-10 (1)	2.5 (1)
Felodipine	2.5-20 (1-2)	2.5 (2)
Isradipine CR	2.5-20 (2)	2.5 (2)
Nicardipine SR	30-120 (2)	30 (2)
Nifedipine XL	30-120 (1)	30 (1)
Nisoldipine	10-40 (1-2)	10 (2)
Nondihydropyridines		
Diltiazem CD	120-540 (1)	180 (1)
Verapamil HS	120-480 (1)	180 (1)
ANGIOTENSIN-CONVERTING ENZYME INHIBITORS		
Benazepril	10-80 (1-2)	20 (1)
Captopril	25-150 (2)	25 (2)
Enalapril	2.5-40 (2)	5 (2)
Fosinopril	10-80 (1-2)	20 (2)
Lisinopril	5-80 (1-2)	40 (2)
Moexipril	7.5-30 (1)	7.5 (1)
Perindopril	4-16 (1)	4 (1)
Quinapril	5-80 (1-2)	40 (2)
Ramipril	2.5-20 (1)	2.5 (1)
Trandolapril	1-8 (1)	2 (1)
ANGIOTENSIN RECEPTOR BLOCKERS		
Candesartan	8-32 (1)	16 (1)
Eprosartan	400-800 (1-2)	400 (1)
Irbesartan	150-300 (1)	150 (1)
Losartan	25-100 (2)	50 (1)
Olmesartan	5-40 (1)	20 (1)
Telmisartan	20-80 (1)	40 (1)
Valsartan	80-320 (1-2)	160 (2)
DIRECT RENIN INHIBITOR		
Aliskiren	150-300 (1)	150 (1)
α-BLOCKERS		
Doxazosin	1-16 (1)	1 (1)
Prazosin	1-40 (2-3)	1 (2)
Terazosin	1-20 (1)	1 (1)
Phenoxybenzamine for pheochromocytoma	20-120 (2)	20 (2)
CENTRAL SYMPATHOLYTICS		
Clonidine	0.2-1.2 (2-3)	0.2 (2)
Clonidine patch	0.1-0.6 (weekly)	0.1 (weekly)
Guanabenz	2-32 (2)	2 (2)
Guanfacine	1-3 (1) (qhs)	1 (1)
Methyldopa	250-1000 (2)	250 (2)
Reserpine	0.05-0.25 (1)	0.05 (1)
DIRECT VASODILATORS		
Hydralazine	10-200 (2)	20 (2)
Minoxidil	2.5-100 (1)	2.5 (1)
FIXED-DOSE COMBINATIONS		
Aliskiren/HCTZ	150/12.5-300/25 (1)	150/12.5 (1)
Amiloride/HCTZ	5/50 (1)	5/50 (1)
Amlodipine/benazepril	2.5-5/10-20 (1)	2.5/10 (1)
Amlodipine/olmesartan	5/20-10/40 (1)	5/20 (1)
Amlodipine/telmisartan	5/20-10/80 (1)	5/20 (1)
Amlodipine/valsartan	5/160-10/320 (1)	5/160 (1)
Atenolol/chlorthalidone	50-100/25 (1)	50/25 (1)
Benazepril/HCTZ	5-20/6.25-25 (1)	20/6.25 (1)
Bisoprolol/HCTZ	2.5-10/6.25 (1)	2.5/6.25 (1)
Candesartan/HCTZ	16-32/12.5-25 (1)	16/12.5 (1)
Enalapril/HCTZ	5-10/25 (1-2)	5/25 (1)
Eprosartan/HCTZ	600/12.5-25 (1)	600/12.5 (1)
Fosinopril/HCTZ	10-20/12.5 (1)	10/12.5 (1)
Irbesartan/HCTZ	150-300/12.5-25 (1)	150/12.5 (1)
Losartan/HCTZ	50-100/12.5-25 (1)	50/12.5 (1)
Olmesartan/HCTZ	20-40/12.5 (1)	20/12.5 (1)
Spironolactone/HCTZ	25/25 ($^1/_2$-1)	25/25 (1/2)
Telmisartan/HCTZ	40-80/12.5-25 (1)	40/12.5 (1)
Trandolapril/verapamil	2-4/180-240 (1)	2/180 (1)
Triamterene/HCTZ	37.5/25 ($^1/_2$-1)	37.5/25 (1/2)
Valsartan/HCTZ	80-160/12.5-25 (1)	160/12.5 (1)

HCTZ = hydrochlorothiazide.

TABLE 67-6 MAJOR CONTRAINDICATIONS AND SIDE EFFECTS OF ANTIHYPERTENSIVE DRUGS

DRUG CLASS	MAJOR CONTRAINDICATIONS	SIDE EFFECTS
Diuretics		
Thiazides	Gout	Insulin resistance, new-onset type 2 diabetes Hypokalemia, hyponatremia Hypertriglyceridemia Hyperuricemia, precipitation of gout Erectile dysfunction (more than other drug classes) Potentiate nondepolarizing muscle relaxants Photosensitivity dermatitis
Loop diuretics	Hepatic coma	Interstitial nephritis Hypokalemia Potentiate succinylcholine Potentiate aminoglycoside ototoxicity
Potassium-sparing diuretics	Serum potassium concentration > 5.5 mEq/L GFR < 30 mg/mL/1.73 m^2	Hyperkalemia
ACEIs	Pregnancy Bilateral renal artery stenosis Hyperkalemia	Cough Hyperkalemia Angioedema Leukopenia Fetal toxicity Cholestatic jaundice (rare fulminant hepatic necrosis if the drug is not discontinued)
Dihydropyridine CCBs	As monotherapy in chronic kidney disease with proteinuria	Headaches Flushing Ankle edema CHF Gingival hyperplasia Esophageal reflux
Nondihydropyridine CCBs	Heart block Systolic heart failure	Bradycardia, AV block (especially with verapamil) Constipation (often severe with verapamil) Worsening of systolic function, CHF Gingival edema or hypertrophy Increase cyclosporine blood levels Esophageal reflux
ARBs, DRI	Pregnancy Bilateral renal artery stenosis Hyperkalemia	Hyperkalemia Angioedema (very rare) Fetal toxicity
β-Adrenergic blockers	Heart block Asthma Depression Cocaine and methamphetamine abuse	New-onset type 2 diabetes (especially in combination with a thiazide) Heart block, acute decompensated CHF Bronchospasm Depression, nightmares, fatigue Cold extremities, claudication (β_2 effect) Stevens-Johnson syndrome Agranulocytosis
α-Adrenergic blockers	Orthostatic hypotension Systolic heart failure Left ventricular dysfunction	Orthostatic hypotension Drug tolerance (in the absence of diuretic therapy) Ankle edema CHF First-dose effect (acute hypotension) Potentiate hypotension with PDE-5 inhibitors (e.g., sildenafil)
Central sympatholytics	Orthostatic hypotension	Depression, dry mouth, lethargy Erectile dysfunction (dose dependent) Rebound hypertension with clonidine withdrawal Coombs' test–positive hemolytic anemia and elevated liver enzymes with α-methyldopa
Direct vasodilators	Orthostatic hypotension	Reflex tachycardia Fluid retention Hirsutism, pericardial effusion with minoxidil Lupus with hydralazine

ACE = angiotensin-converting enzyme; ARBs = angiotensin receptor blockers; AV = atrioventricular; CCBs = calcium-channel blockers; CHF = congestive heart failure; DRI = direct renin inhibitor; GFR = glomerular filtration rate; NSAIDs = nonsteroidal anti-inflammatory drugs; PDE-5 = phosphodiesterase-5.

they generally are less potent than diuretics or CCBs, particularly in African Americans, but they amplify the effects of these other drug classes when they are used in combination. An ACE inhibitor or an ARB is considered the basis for antihypertensive drug therapy in mild or moderate chronic kidney disease (Chapter 116) because they rarely precipitate hyperkalemia or acute renal failure and appear to provide renoprotection. Serum creatinine and potassium concentrations must be monitored in all patients receiving an ACE inhibitor or ARB. In patients with chronic kidney disease, initiation of an ACE inhibitor or ARB often causes small and transient increases in serum creatinine concentration that do not necessitate discontinuation. ACE inhibitors and ARBs can precipitate acute renal failure in patients with bilateral renal artery stenosis (Chapter 127) or hypovolemia. After correction of hypovolemia, the ACE inhibitor or ARB usually can be restarted safely at a lower dose.

The most common side effect of ACE inhibitors is a dry cough. Patients may complain not of a cough but rather of having to clear the throat or loss of voice later in the day. These symptoms occur in 3 to 39% of patients, resolve in a few days after the drug is discontinued, and can be eliminated by switching the patient to an ARB. The incidence is higher in African Americans than in whites and is highest in Asians.

The ARBs are less effective than dihydropyridine CCBs in controlling hypertension but are increasingly popular because they have a more favorable side-effect profile than ACE inhibitors. Their efficacy is enhanced by addition of low-dose HCTZ or a dihydropyridine CCB. An increasing number of fixed-dose combinations are available (see Table 67-5). Losartan, the prototype, differs from the other ARBs in two ways: a shorter duration of action, requiring twice-daily dosing if it is used as monotherapy; and a uricosuric effect, which may be beneficial in patients with hyperuricemia. Newer ARBs vary in potency and duration of action. The putative special metabolic benefit of telmisartan, which shares structural homology with the insulin sensitizer pioglitazone, remains unproved.

Direct Renin Inhibitors

Aliskiren is the first in a new class of orally effective, nonpeptide, low-molecular-weight renin inhibitors. Direct renin inhibitors block the renin-angiotensin-aldosterone system at its origin without increasing bradykinin. By eliminating the reactive rise in plasma renin activity seen with ACE inhibitors and ARBs, direct renin inhibition may prevent more hypertensive complications, particularly renal complications. Short-term studies in patients with mild or moderate hypertension suggest that once-daily low-dose (150 mg) or high-dose (300 mg) aliskiren is equivalent to an ARB in terms of both blood pressure–lowering effect and favorable side-effect profile. The contraindications are the same. Randomized trials of cardiovascular outcomes compared with other drugs are pending.

Calcium-Channel Blockers

Mechanism of Action. The CCBs are antiarrhythmic, antianginal, and antihypertensive because they block the opening of voltage-gated (L-type) Ca^{2+} channels in cardiac myocytes and vascular smooth muscle cells. The resultant decrease in the cytosolic Ca^{2+} signal decreases heart rate and ventricular contractility and relaxes vascular smooth muscle. Blood pressure lowering is related mainly to peripheral arterial vasodilation, with the rank order of potency being dihydropyridines > diltiazem >> verapamil. In contrast, for negative chronotropic and inotropic effects, the rank order of potency is verapamil >> diltiazem > dihydropyridines.

Therapeutic Principles. *Short-acting dihydropyridines should not be used to treat hypertension.* By triggering an abrupt fall in blood pressure with reflex sympathetic activation, these rapidly acting arterial vasodilators can precipitate myocardial ischemia, infarction, stroke, and death. By comparison, the safety and efficacy of long-acting dihydropyridine CCBs was confirmed by ALLHAT and the VALUE (Valsartan Antihypertensive Long-term Use Evaluation) trial.[6] For most hypertensive patients, these are among the most potent, best tolerated, and safest antihypertensive medications available, but there are some caveats. For comparable degrees of blood pressure lowering, dihydropyridine CCBs exert protection against myocardial infarction and stroke equivalent to that of diuretics, but their use is associated with a greater risk for heart failure. For patients with renal insufficiency and proteinuria, dihydropyridine CCB-based therapy is less renoprotective than ARB- or ACE inhibitor–based therapy. However, in most patients with renal disease, multiple classes of medications, including dihydropyridines, are required to achieve blood pressure goals. Thus, dihydropyridine CCBs should not be used as first-line therapy for hypertension in patients with proteinuria, but they may be used as adjunctive therapy once the dose of the ACE inhibitor or ARB has been maximized in combination with an appropriate diuretic.

Verapamil is a weak antihypertensive and of limited utility because of dose-dependent constipation. Diltiazem is intermediate in potency between verapamil and the dihydropyridines; it is usually well tolerated. Verapamil and diltiazem can cause heart block, especially in older patients and in patients taking digoxin.

Adrenergic Receptor Blockers and Central Sympatholytics

Sympathetic drive to the sinus node increases heart rate and cardiac output through β-adrenergic receptors, whereas sympathetic drive to the peripheral vasculature causes neurogenic vasoconstriction through α-adrenergic receptors. Sustained activation of the sympathetic nervous system is thought to contribute to chronic hypertension by vascular remodeling, renin release, and attenuation of renal sodium excretion by an action on the distal tubules.

β-Adrenergic Blockers

Mechanism of Action. Interaction of epinephrine or norepinephrine with β_1-adrenoreceptors in the heart causes G protein–linked activation of adenylate cyclase, resulting in positive chronotropic and inotropic effects. Interaction of catecholamines with β_2-adrenoreceptors relaxes bronchiolar and arteriolar smooth muscle. With the initiation of β-blocker therapy, blood pressure at first is little affected because the fall in cardiac output is offset by a compensatory increase in peripheral resistance. Over time, blood pressure falls progressively as the peripheral vasculature relaxes. Thus, the antihypertensive effect of β-blockade involves decreases in cardiac output (β_1-receptors), renin release (β_1-receptors), and norepinephrine release (prejunctional β_2-receptors).

The prototype β-blocker, propranolol, nonselectively blocks both β_1- and β_2-receptors. Other standard β-blockers (metoprolol, atenolol, acebutolol, and bisoprolol) are *relatively* cardioselective. In low doses, they exert a greater inhibitory effect on β_1- than on β_2-receptors, but selectivity is lost at high doses. In contrast, combined α- and β-blockers (labetalol, carvedilol, nebivolol) cause vasodilation by blocking α_1-adrenoreceptors on vascular smooth muscle and possibly by increasing the bioavailability of nitric oxide.

Therapeutic Principles. Although standard β-blockers are first-line medical therapy for ischemic heart disease (Chapters 72 and 73) and heart failure (Chapter 59), they are no longer first-line or even second-line agents for uncomplicated hypertension. They predispose to diabetes, particularly when combined with a thiazide, and offer less stroke protection than other antihypertensive drugs.[7] In addition to being rather weak antihypertensives, they are less effective than other agents in lowering central aortic blood pressure because bradycardia allows more time for wave reflection and thus central pressure augmentation. β-blockers can cause fatigue, limit exercise tolerance, and worsen depression.

Compared with standard β-blockers, combined α-/β-blockers are better antihypertensives. They lower blood pressure more and have a more favorable metabolic profile. Generic carvedilol is now widely affordable ($10 for a 90-day supply), but its patent has expired, and no outcomes trials have been performed. Labetalol, which rarely causes severe hepatotoxicity, should be reserved for hypertensive urgencies, perioperative management, or very difficult hypertension. All β-blockers can precipitate heart block, and they can aggravate preexisting asthma.

α-Adrenergic Blockers

Mechanism of Action. By blocking the interaction of norepinephrine on vascular α-adrenergic receptors, these drugs cause peripheral vasodilation, thereby lowering blood pressure. By increasing skeletal muscle blood flow, they increase insulin sensitivity. By dilating urethral smooth muscle, they improve symptoms of prostatism. Prazosin, doxazosin, terazosin, and intravenous phentolamine selectively block α_1-adrenoreceptors; phenoxybenzamine blocks both α_1- and α_2-receptors.

Therapeutic Principles. Phenoxybenzamine remains the drug of choice for preoperative management of pheochromocytoma (Chapter 235); after α-blockade is achieved, a β-blocker should be added to block an otherwise excessive reflex tachycardia. The selective α_1-blockers are not first-line agents and should not be used as monotherapy because their propensity to cause fluid retention can lead to tachyphylaxis and unmask or exacerbate heart failure. However, when they are prescribed as part of a combination regimen that includes a diuretic, they are effective fourth- or fifth-line therapy for difficult hypertension and are particularly useful in older men with prostatism. Although marketed specifically for prostatism and not as an antihypertensive agent, the selective α_{1A}-blocker tamsulosin lowers blood pressure in some men.

Central Sympatholytics

Mechanism of Action. Stimulation of postsynaptic α_2-adrenergic receptors and imidazoline receptors in the central nervous system lowers central sympathetic outflow, whereas stimulation of presynaptic α_2-receptors causes feedback inhibition of norepinephrine release from peripheral sympathetic nerve terminals. The combined effect is reduced sympathetic drive to the heart and peripheral circulation, thereby leading to decreased heart rate, cardiac output, and peripheral vascular resistance.

Therapeutic Principles. The central sympatholytics are best reserved for short-term oral treatment of severe uncontrolled hypertension. They are potent antihypertensive agents that may be needed as fourth- or fifth-line therapy for very difficult hypertension, but their troublesome central nervous system side effects often reduce quality of life. To avoid rebound hypertension between doses, short-acting clonidine must be given every 6 to 8 hours or, whenever possible, discontinued using a gradual tapering schedule. Rebound hypertension is less of a problem with longer-acting preparations (guanfacine, clonidine patch). α-Methyldopa remains the drug of choice for chronic hypertension in pregnancy (Chapter 247).

Direct Vasodilators

Mechanism of Action. Minoxidil and hydralazine are potent hyperpolarizing arterial vasodilators that work by opening vascular ATP-sensitive K^+ channels.

Therapeutic Principles. By causing selective and rapid arterial dilation, both drugs cause profound reflex sympathetic activation and tachycardia as well as ankle edema. For this reason, hydralazine has largely been replaced by the longer-acting dihydropyridine CCBs. However, hydralazine remains the treatment of choice for acute severe hypertension in pregnancy (Chapter 247). A combination of hydralazine plus nitroglycerin now is recommended for the treatment of heart failure specifically in African Americans, in whom hypertensive heart disease is the most common cause of heart failure (Chapter 58). Severe hypertension accompanying advanced chronic kidney disease (Chapter 132) is the main indication for minoxidil, which must be combined with a β-blocker to prevent excessive reflex tachycardia and with a loop diuretic to prevent excessive fluid retention. Institution of hemodialysis is usually a more effective means of controlling hypertension.

Antihypertensive Drug Interactions

By inhibiting the kidney's ability to excrete sodium, nonsteroidal anti-inflammatory drugs (including aspirin in daily doses above 81 mg), can negate the antihypertensive action of diuretics and renin-angiotensin system inhibitors, but they do not interfere with CCBs. However, even a single glass of grapefruit juice increases the bioavailability of dihydropyridine CCBs by inhibiting the intestinal cytochrome P-450 3A4 system, which is responsible for the first-pass metabolism of many oral medications. Acetaminophen per se does not appear to cause salt retention, but in Great Britain, and not in the United States, each acetaminophen tablet contains 1000 mg of sodium. A high-fat meal will impair aliskiren absorption. Verapamil and diltiazem will increase blood levels of cyclosporine and digoxin.

Which Drugs for Which Patients?

Choosing the best drugs to treat hypertension in a given patient is based primarily on effective lowering of blood pressure and prevention of hypertensive complications with minimal side effects (see Table 67-6) and cost. A secondary consideration is concomitant treatment of comorbid cardiovascular diseases (e.g., angina, heart failure). According to a strict evidence-based approach, a "compelling indication" is defined as a comorbid condition for which the use of a specific antihypertensive drug has been shown to improve disease outcomes in a randomized controlled trial (Table 67-7).

Choice of Therapy for the Patient with "Uncomplicated" Primary Hypertension

To date, a few DNA sequence variations have been proposed to identify individual patients whose blood pressure is particularly sensitive to a specific drug class. However, pharmacogenetic research has yet to affect the clinical treatment of hypertension.

In the absence of such ideal scientific information, the now outdated 2003 JNC 7 guidelines recommended a thiazide-type diuretic as cost-effective first-line therapy for most patients with hypertension. They also recommended initiation of therapy with two drugs (one being a thiazide) for stage 2 hypertension. In contrast, the European Society of Hypertension–European Society of Cardiology makes no specific drug class recommendation, arguing that the most effective drugs are those that the patient will tolerate and take. The revised guidelines of the British Hypertension Society previously advocated initiation of therapy with an ACE inhibitor or ARB ("A" drug) for young white patients (<55 years), who often have high-renin hypertension, but a CCB or diuretic ("C" or "D" drug) for older and black patients, who often have low-renin hypertension.

In contrast, there is growing evidence and consensus about the overriding importance of lowering blood pressure with combinations of drugs with different mechanisms of action (see Table 67-5), rather than belaboring the choice of the single best initial agent, to reach currently recommended blood pressure treatment targets (see Table 67-3). For example, tight control (goal systolic pressure of <130 mm Hg) of systolic blood pressure in nondiabetic patients is significantly more effective than usual control (goal systolic pressure of <140 mm Hg) in reducing subsequent left ventricular hypertrophy by electrocardiography, and it can reduce important cardiovascular events by 50%.[8] Systolic blood pressure targets are achieved in only 50 to 60% of hypertensive patients, even when they receive an average of three drugs in the idealized setting of a randomized trial.

Low-dose combination drug therapy is not only the best way to control blood pressure but also the best way to minimize side effects because the dose-response relationship for blood pressure is rather flat, occurring at the lower end of the dose range for most medications, whereas many of the side effects are steeply dose dependent. Synergistic combinations achieve blood pressure control at lower doses.

The question is: Which drug combinations are best?

Dual therapy with an ACE inhibitor plus amlodipine (the longest-acting, best studied, and now generic dihydropyridine CCB) was found in recent trials to offer more cardiovascular protection, particularly against stroke, than dual therapy with either a β-blocker plus a thiazide[9] or an ACE inhibitor plus thiazide.[10] Other recent data indicate that ACE inhibitors or ARBs offer similar cardiovascular protection[11] and thus are interchangeable, except for higher cost of ARBs and almost no cough. All the ACE inhibitors and ARBs are available as fixed-dose combinations with a low dose of hydrochlorothiazide (see Table 67-5). Lotrel is the prototype ACE inhibitor–amlodipine fixed-dose combination, and several new (branded) ARB-CCB combinations recently have been marketed (see Table 67-5).

Amlodipine and other dihydropyridine CCBs cause dose-dependent ankle edema because they preferentially dilate arteries rather than veins, thereby elevating hydrostatic pressure; the resulting ankle edema often can be relieved by the addition of an ACE inhibitor, ARB, or aliskiren, which dilate the veins as well as the arteries. Standard β-blockers are no longer recommended to treat uncomplicated hypertension. In contrast, generic carvedilol is being used increasingly as third- or fourth-line therapy. Central sympatholytic agents should be reserved as fifth-line therapy for patients with difficult hypertension.

Despite much compelling basic research on ancillary (pleiotropic) benefits of ACE inhibitors or ARBs to block multiple adverse effects of angiotensin II, in clinical trials most of the cardiovascular benefit derived from these and all other classes of antihypertensive agents comes directly from lowering blood pressure (Fig. 67-10). Dual therapy with an ACE inhibitor and ARB provides no more cardiovascular protection than either alone and is associated with more hypotension and renal failure.[11]

Along with antihypertensive medication and lifestyle modification, additional cardiovascular risk reduction with low-dose aspirin (81 mg) (Chapter 37) and lipid-lowering medication (Chapter 213) should be strongly considered as an integral part of cardiovascular risk reduction. In treated hypertensive

TABLE 67-7 "COMPELLING" INDICATIONS AND PUBLISHED EVIDENCE

COMPELLING INDICATION	DRUG CLASS (RELEVANT CLINICAL TRIALS*)
Systolic heart failure	ACEI (CONSENSUS, SAVE) ARB (Val-HeFT, CHARM) β-Blocker (MERIT-HFCOMET) Aldosterone antagonist (RALES)
Recent MI	β-Blockers (ISIS)
Reduced left ventricular function after MI	ACEI (SAVE, TRACE) Aldosterone antagonist (EPHESUS) β-Blocker (CAPRICORN)
Type 1 diabetes	ACEI (CCSG)
Type 2 diabetes	ACEI (MICRO-HOPE)
Type 2 diabetic nephropathy	ARB (IDNT, RENAAL, IRMA-2, MOSES, ONTARGET)
Nondiabetic chronic kidney disease	ACEI (REIN, AIPRI, AASK, ONTARGET)
CV disease	ACEI (HOPE, EUROPA) ARB (ONTARGET)
Prior stroke or TIA	ACEI + thiazide (PROGRESS)
Isolated systolic hypertension in older persons	DHP-CCB (Syst-Eur, Syst-China, STOP-2) Thiazide (SHEP) ACEI (STOP-2) ARB (SCOPE, second-line)
Hypertension in the very elderly	ACEI + thiazide (HYVET)
Left ventricular hypertrophy by electrocardiography	ARB plus thiazide (LIFE)

*CONSENSUS, Cooperative North Scandinavian Enalapril Survival Study (*N Engl J Med.* 1987;316:1429-1435); SAVE, Survival and Ventricular Enlargement study (*N Engl J Med.* 1992;327:669-677); Val-HeFT, Valsartan Heart Failure Trial (*N Engl J Med.* 2001;345:1667-1675); CHARM, Candesartan in Heart Failure: Assessment of Reduction in Morbidity and Mortality (*Lancet.* 2003;362:759-766); MERIT-HF, Metoprolol Randomized Intervention Trial in Congestive Heart Failure (*JAMA.* 2000;283:1295-1302); COMET, comparison of carvedilol and metoprolol on clinical outcomes in patients with chronic heart failure in the Carvedilol Or Metoprolol European Trial (*Lancet.* 2003;362:7-13); RALES, Randomized Aldactone Evaluation Study (*N Engl J Med.* 1999;341:709-717); ISIS, International Study of Infarct Survival (*Lancet.* 1986;2:57-66); TRACE, Trandolapril Cardiac Evaluation (*N Engl J Med.* 1995;333:1670-1676); EPHESUS, Eplerenone Post-Myocardial Infarction Heart Failure Efficacy and Survival Study (*N Engl J Med.* 2003;348:1309-1321); CAPRICORN, effect of carvedilol on outcome after myocardial infarction in patients with left-ventricular dysfunction (*Lancet.* 2001;357:1385-1390); CCSG, Captopril Cooperative Study Group (*N Engl J Med.* 1993;323:1456-1462); MICRO-HOPE, Microalbuminuria, Cardiovascular and Renal Outcomes substudy of the Heart Outcomes Prevention Evaluation (*Lancet.* 2000;355:253-259); IDNT, Irbesartan Diabetic Nephropathy Trial (*N Engl J Med.* 2001;345:841-860); RENAAL, Reduction of Endpoints in NIDDM with the Angiotensin II Antagonist Losartan (*N Engl J Med.* 2001;345:861-869); IRMA-2, Irbesartan Microalbuminuria study 2 (*N Engl J Med.* 2001;345:870-878); REIN, Ramipril Evaluation in Nephropathy trial (*Lancet.* 1998;352:1252-1256); AIPRI, ACE Inhibition in Progressive Renal Insufficiency (*Kidney Int.* 1997;63[Suppl]:S63-S67); AASK, African American Study of Kidney Disease and Hypertension (*JAMA.* 2002;288:2421-2431); ONTARGET, Ongoing Telmisartan Alone and in combination with Ramipril Global Endpoint Trial (*N Engl J Med.* 2008;358:1547-1559; *Lancet.* 2008;372:547-553); HOPE, Heart Outcomes Prevention Evaluation (*N Engl J Med.* 2000;342:145-153); EUROPA, European Reduction of Cardiac Events with Perindopril in Stable Coronary Artery Disease (*Lancet.* 2003;362:782-788); PROGRESS, Perindopril Protection Against Recurrent Stroke Study (*Lancet.* 2001;358:1033-1041); Syst-Eur, Systolic Hypertension in Europe trial (*Lancet.* 1997;360:757-764); Syst-China, Systolic Hypertension in China trial (*J Hypertens.* 1998;16:1823-1829); STOP-2, Swedish Trial in Old Patients with Hypertension 2 (*Lancet.* 1999;354:1751-1756); SHEP, Systolic Hypertension in the Elderly Program (*JAMA.* 1991;265:3255-3264); SCOPE, Study on Cognition and Prognosis in the Elderly (*J Hypertens.* 2003;21:875-886); HYVET, Hypertension in the Very Elderly Trial (*N Engl J Med.* 2008;358:1887-1898); LIFE, Losartan Intervention for Endpoint Reduction (*Lancet.* 2002;359:995-1003).

ACE = angiotensin-converting enzyme; ACEI = angiotensin-converting enzyme inhibitor; ARB = angiotensin receptor blocker; CHF = congestive heart failure; CV = cardiovascular; DHP-CCB = dihydropyridine calcium-channel blocker; MI = myocardial infarction; TIA = transient ischemic attack.

Modified and updated from Elliott WJ. *Compelling Indications for Antihypertensive Drugs.* ASH Clinical Hypertension Review Course. New York: American Society of Hypertension; 2005:333-351.

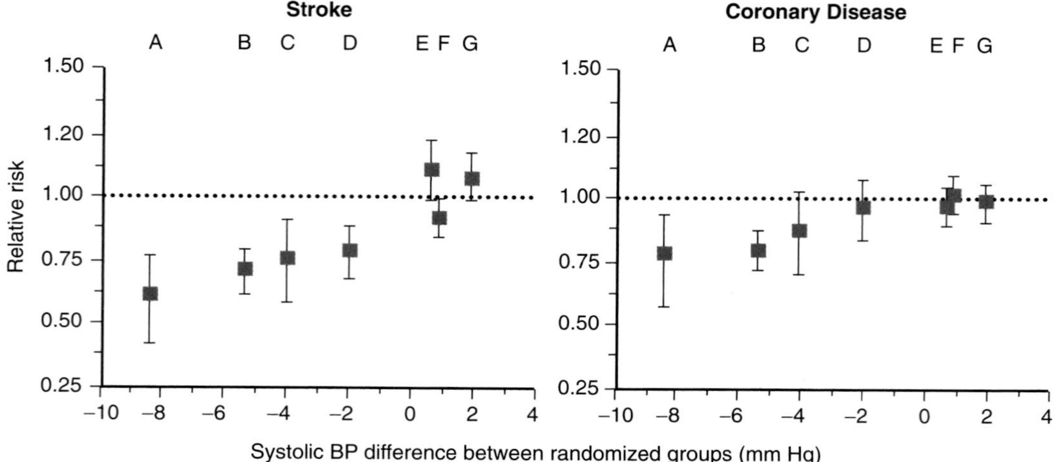

FIGURE 67-10. Meta regression analysis of randomized controlled intervention trials. (12 trials, $N = 94{,}338$ patients with hypertension, coronary artery disease, or diabetic nephropathy who were assigned to treatment with amlodipine or an angiotensin receptor blocker.) Systolic blood pressure (BP) differences were obtained by subtracting the mean change in the amlodipine or ARB group from the corresponding mean change in the reference group. Regardless of drug class, most of the protection against stroke and myocardial infarction was related to lowering of systolic BP. (From Wang J-G, Li Y, Franklin SS, et al. Prevention of stroke and myocardial infarction by amlodipine and angiotensin receptor blockers: a quantitative review. *Hypertension.* 2007;50:181-188.)

patients, low-dose aspirin reduces the risk for myocardial infarction by 36% without increasing the risk for intracerebral hemorrhage. In patients with moderate hypertension, additional cardiovascular risk factors, and an average low-density lipoprotein cholesterol level of 130 mg/dL, the addition of 10 mg of atorvastatin to the antihypertensive regimen results in a 36% reduction in fatal and nonfatal myocardial infarction and a 27% reduction in fatal and nonfatal stroke.[12] Thus, statin therapy should be used in such patients with the goal of reducing the low-density lipoprotein cholesterol level to below 100 mg/dL or even lower (Chapter 213).

Hypertension in Minority Populations

Mexican Americans have the lowest rate of control of hypertension of all U.S. race/ethnic groups but also have the highest risk for diabetes. Thus, antihypertensive regimens should be tailored to avoid causing more new cases of diabetes. In African Americans, hypertension not only is more prevalent than in the general population but also starts at a younger age, is less well controlled, and causes disproportionate and premature disability and death. African Americans commonly have lower plasma renin levels and have less response to monotherapy with an ACE inhibitor, ARB, or β-blocker than do white hypertensive patients. In one randomized trial, African American participants in the ALLHAT had a 40% higher risk for fatal stroke when taking an ACE inhibitor than when taking a diuretic, probably because blood pressure remained higher on the ACE inhibitor. However, when high doses of an ACE inhibitor or ARB are used in combination with a diuretic, antihypertensive efficacy is amplified, and racial/ethnic differences disappear. ACE inhibitors or ARBs can help achieve excellent control of hypertension in African American patients when used as part of an appropriate multidrug regimen.

Hypertensive Nephrosclerosis: A Misnomer?

Second only to diabetes, hypertension is thought to be the next most common cause of end-stage renal disease (ESRD; Chapter 132). Because African Americans are at increased risk for both hypertension and chronic kidney disease, most cases of nondiabetic kidney disease in African Americans have been attributed to *hypertensive nephrosclerosis*—small shrunken kidneys caused by chronic glomerular ischemia owing to severe constriction of the afferent renal arteriole. However, most cases of presumed hypertensive nephrosclerosis are due primarily to a West African ancestral gene locus on chromosome 21 (ApoL1), which both confers resistance against trypanosomiasis and is a powerful risk factor for non-diabetic chronic kidney disease. This risk allele, which is present in 30% of African Americans, may explain why intensive lowering of blood pressure failed to prevent ESRD in the African American Study of Kidney Disease trial.[13]

Mild to moderate nondiabetic chronic kidney disease has been considered a compelling indication for ACE inhibitors, but the renal benefit of an ACE inhibitor–based regimen in nondiabetic chronic kidney disease has been confined to short-term trials and was not demonstrated during long-term follow-up.[13] A recommended multidrug regimen for hypertension in patients with stage II or stage III chronic kidney disease is a loop diuretic (for effective control of obligatory sodium retention), a low-dose ACE inhibitor or ARB (to reduce intraglomerular hypertension), and a central sympatholytic (to reduce sympathetic overactivity from a pressor reflex arising in the failing kidneys). If proteinuria is present, the blood pressure should be lowered gradually to 130/80 mm Hg, if possible, without causing a progressive rise in serum creatinine levels. The ACE inhibitor and loop diuretic will need to be held temporarily if the rise in serum creatinine concentration exceeds 30% of the baseline value or the serum potassium concentration increases to more than 5.6 mmol/L; they often can be restarted at lower doses once the acute deterioration in renal function has resolved.

Hypertension in Patients with Diabetes

Compared with its 25% prevalence in the general adult population, hypertension is present in 75% of diabetic patients and is a major factor contributing to an excessive risk for myocardial infarction, stroke, heart failure, microvascular complications, and diabetic nephropathy progressing to ESRD (Chapter 237). Compared with less intensive treatment, more intensive reduction of blood pressure has been proved to reduce stroke and microvascular end points dramatically in patients with diabetes. To reduce these risks, blood pressures should be lowered to 130/80 mm Hg, a goal that typically requires three to five drugs.[14] On the basis of data from randomized trials, type 1 diabetes (Chapter 236) with renal insufficiency is a compelling indication for ACE inhibitor–based antihypertensive therapy, whereas type 2 diabetes (Chapter 237) with renal insufficiency is now considered to be a compelling indication for ARB-based antihypertensive therapy because similar data do not exist for ACE inhibitor–based regimens in type 2 diabetic patients (see Table 67-7). However, an ACE inhibitor or ARB alone rarely achieves the stringent blood pressure goals; a loop diuretic is usually needed to shrink the expanded plasma volume, and a dihydropyridine CCB is usually needed for antihypertensive synergy. To optimize renal protection, the CCB should not be started until antihypertensive therapy has been initiated with an ACE inhibitor or ARB. A β-blocker should be added if the patient has coronary disease, which is prevalent in diabetes or heart failure. The α- and β-blocker carvedilol has a better metabolic profile than the pure β-blockers.

Systolic Hypertension in Older Persons

In older persons with isolated systolic hypertension, lowering systolic pressure from above 160 to below 150 mm Hg has been shown to reduce the risk for stroke by 30%, myocardial infarction by 23%, and overall cardiovascular mortality by 18%; it also reduces heart failure admissions and slows the progression of dementia. Even hypertensive patients older than 80 years have benefited from treatment with an ACE inhibitor and thiazide regimen (perindopril plus indapamide) compared with placebo.[15]

However, because of slower drug metabolism and reduced postural autonomic reflexes in older persons, it is important to start with low doses of antihypertensive medication and titrate slowly. If orthostatic hypotension is present, medication should be titrated to standing blood pressure. The same triple combination therapy for systolic and diastolic hypertension should be used for isolated systolic hypertension: an ACE inhibitor (or ARB), a dihydropyridine CCB, and thiazide. In some older patients, even low-dose thiazides cause unacceptable degrees of hyponatremia. β-blockers should be restricted to patients with coronary disease or heart failure and should be used with caution because they are more likely to precipitate heart block, to impair exercise tolerance, and to cause depression.

Blood Pressure Lowering for Secondary Prevention of Stroke

Most neurologists recommend minimal or no blood pressure reduction during an acute ischemic stroke unless the patient is a candidate for thrombolytic therapy (Chapters 414 and 415). Once the patient's condition has stabilized, however, lowering blood pressure by 12/5 mm Hg with a combination of the thiazide diuretic indapamide plus the ACE inhibitor perindopril reduces the risk for recurrent stroke by 43%.[16]

Hypertension in Patients with Ischemic Heart Disease

In patients with stable coronary disease, 130/80 mm Hg is an appropriate threshold for starting an antihypertensive regimen. Blood pressure should be lowered slowly, and caution is advised in lowering diastolic blood pressure below 60 mm Hg to avoid the potential risk for subendocardial ischemia. To lower myocardial oxygen demands in patients with coronary disease, the antihypertensive regimen should reduce blood pressure without causing reflex tachycardia. Thus, a β-blocker is often prescribed in conjunction with a dihydropyridine CCB. β-Blockers are indicated for hypertensive patients who have sustained a myocardial infarction (Chapters 72 and 73) and for most patients with chronic heart failure (Chapter 59), and they are typically first-line therapy in patients with angina (Chapter 71). ACE inhibitors are indicated for almost all patients with left ventricular systolic dysfunction (Chapters 59 and 60) and may be considered for post–myocardial infarction patients even in the absence of ventricular dysfunction (Chapters 72 and 73). In patients with very high cardiovascular risk profiles but without known left ventricular dysfunction, the ACE inhibitor ramipril (10 mg/day) reduces cardiovascular events, an effect that may or may not be beyond what can be explained by blood pressure reduction alone. In normotensive patients with stable coronary artery disease, data are conflicting as to whether the addition of an ACE inhibitor reduces the risk for subsequent cardiovascular events.

The CCBs, including amlodipine, and the α-blockers have a greater propensity than other antihypertensive drugs to precipitate heart failure and should be avoided in hypertensive patients with known heart failure and those with asymptomatic left ventricular systolic dysfunction. Optimal control of hypertension is perhaps the best way to prevent diastolic heart failure.

Hypertension Associated with Oral Contraceptives and Estrogen Replacement

Oral contraceptives, particularly current low-dose estrogen preparations, cause a small increase in blood pressure in most women but rarely cause a large increase into the hypertensive range. The mechanism is unknown, but women older than 35 years and those who smoke or are overweight appear to be at increased risk. Drospirenone, a progestin with structural homology to spironolactone, is claimed to have neutral or beneficial effects on blood pressure from mineralocorticoid reception antagonism. If hypertension develops, oral contraceptive therapy should be discontinued in favor of other methods of contraception. Oral estrogen replacement therapy after menopause appears to cause a small increase in blood pressure, whereas transdermal estrogen (which bypasses first-pass hepatic metabolism) appears to cause a small decrease in blood pressure.

Hypertension in Pregnancy

Hypertension, the most common nonobstetric complication of pregnancy, is present in about 10% of all pregnancies (Chapter 247). About one third is caused by chronic hypertension and two thirds by preeclampsia, defined as an increase in blood pressure to 140/90 mm Hg or more after the 20th week of gestation, accompanied by proteinuria (>300 mg/24 hours) and pathologic edema. Preeclampsia sometimes also is accompanied by seizures (eclampsia) and the multisystem HELLP syndrome (Chapters 153 and 247) of hemolysis, elevated liver enzymes, and low platelets. Preeclampsia is the most common cause of maternal mortality and perinatal mortality. Given the current trend of childbearing in women older than 35 years, the prevalence of chronic hypertension in pregnancy is rising. In the absence of randomized trials, α-methyldopa remains the drug of choice for chronic hypertension in pregnancy, and hydralazine (plus bedrest) for preeclampsia. In preeclampsia, magnesium sulfate is predictably effective in preventing seizures but, despite being a vasodilator, has inconsistent effects on blood pressure.

Resistant Hypertension

One in five hypertensive patients has drug-resistant hypertension, in which blood pressure remains above goal values despite concurrent treatment with three antihypertensive drugs of different classes. Most such patients actually have *pseudoresistance* from (1) improper blood pressure measurement technique, (2) white coat reactions, (3) medication nonadherence, (4) ingestion of pressor substances (e.g., nonsteroidal anti-inflammatory drugs, excessive alcohol, psychiatric drugs), or (5) an inadequate blood pressure regimen. Common correctable issues are clonidine rebound (especially with as-needed dosing), inadequate diuretic therapy, inappropriate use of a loop diuretic in a patient with normal renal function, infrequent dosing with a short-acting loop diuretic (e.g., once-a-day furosemide), and low-dose thiazide in a patient with impaired renal function. Significant impairment in renal function can be present with serum creatinine concentrations in the range of 1.2 to 1.4 mg/dL or even lower, particularly in older patients with little muscle mass. GFR should be estimated by standard equations (Chapter 116), and urinary albumin-to-creatinine ratio from a spot urine specimen should be obtained.

Truly drug-resistant patients should be screened for secondary hypertension, especially unrecognized chronic kidney disease, obstructive sleep apnea, and primary aldosteronism. In the absence of an identifiable cause for the hypertension, a mineralocorticoid receptor antagonist and an α-/β-blocker are recommended as highly effective fourth- and fifth-line therapy. Low-dose eplerenone or spironolactone can be remarkably effective for resistant hypertension—even when serum aldosterone is within the normal range. An implantable carotid baroreceptor pacemaker and radio frequency ablation of the renal nerves are potentially useful device-based treatments currently undergoing evaluation for drug-resistant hypertension.

Acute Severe Hypertension

Twenty-five percent of all emergency department patients present with an elevated blood pressure (Chapter 7). *Hypertensive emergencies* are acute, often severe, elevations in blood pressure, accompanied by rapidly progressive target organ dysfunction, such as myocardial or cerebral ischemia or infarction, pulmonary edema, or renal failure. *Hypertensive urgencies* are severe elevations in blood pressure without severe symptoms and without evidence of acute or progressive target organ dysfunction. The key distinction depends on the state of the patient and the assessment of target organ damage, not just the absolute level of blood pressure.

The full-blown clinical picture of a hypertensive emergency is a critically ill patient who presents with a blood pressure above 220/140 mm Hg, headaches, confusion, blurred vision, nausea and vomiting, seizures, pulmonary edema, oliguria, and grade 3 or grade 4 hypertensive retinopathy (Fig. 67-11). Hypertensive emergencies require immediate intensive care unit (ICU) admission for intravenous therapy and continuous blood pressure monitoring. Hypertensive emergencies often can be managed with oral medications and appropriate outpatient follow-up in 24 to 72 hours. The most common hypertensive cardiac emergencies include acute aortic dissection (Chapter 78), hypertension after cardiac surgery (Chapter 74), acute myocardial infarction (Chapter 73), and unstable angina (Chapter 72). Other hypertensive emergencies include cocaine-induced sympathetic crisis, eclampsia (Chapter 247), head trauma (Chapter 406), severe body burns (Chapter 112), postoperative bleeding from vascular suture lines, and epistaxis that cannot be controlled with anterior and posterior nasal packing. Neurologic emergencies—acute ischemic stroke, hemorrhagic stroke, subarachnoid hemorrhage, and hypertensive encephalopathy—can be difficult to distinguish from one another (Chapters 413 to 415). Hypertensive encephalopathy (Chapter 415) is characterized by severe hypertensive retinopathy (retinal hemorrhages and exudates, with or without papilledema) and a posterior leukoencephalopathy (affecting mainly the white matter of the parieto-occipital regions) seen on cerebral MRI or CT. A new focal neurologic deficit suggests a stroke in

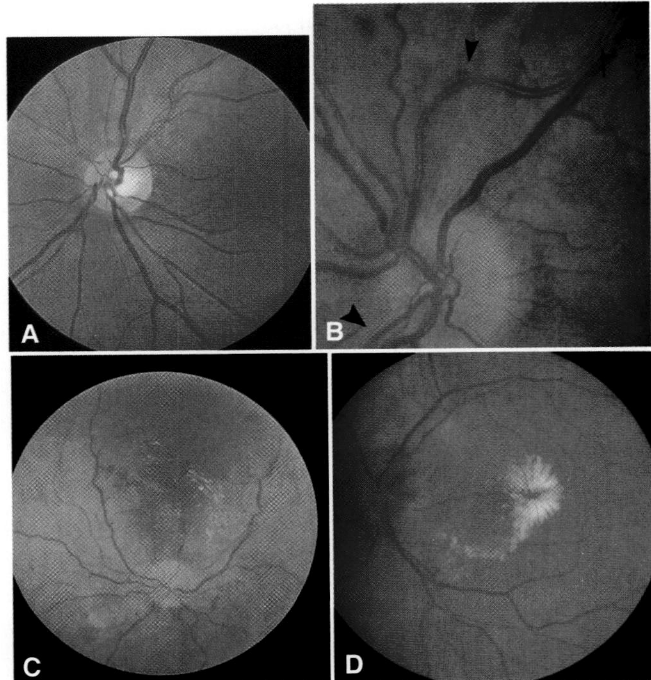

FIGURE 67-11. Hypertensive retinopathy is traditionally divided into four grades. **A,** Grade 1 shows early and minor changes in a young patient. Increased tortuosity of a retinal vessel and increased reflectiveness (silver wiring) of a retinal artery are seen at 1 o'clock in this view. Otherwise, the fundus is completely normal. **B,** Grade 2 also shows increased tortuosity and silver wiring *(arrowheads)*. In addition, there is "nipping" of the venules at arteriovenous crossings. **C,** Grade 3 shows the same changes as grade 2 plus flame-shaped retinal hemorrhages and soft "cotton-wool" exudates. **D,** In grade 4, there is swelling of the optic disc (papilledema), retinal edema is present, and hard exudates may collect around the fovea, producing a typical "macular star." (From Forbes CD, Jackson WF. *Color Atlas and Text of Clinical Medicine,* 3rd ed. London: Mosby; 2003.)

evolution, which demands a much more conservative approach to the elevated blood pressure (Chapter 414).

In most other hypertensive emergencies, the goal of parenteral therapy is to achieve a controlled and gradual lowering of blood pressure. A good rule of thumb is to lower the initially elevated arterial pressure by 10% in the first hour and by an additional 15% during the next 3 to 12 hours to a blood pressure of no less than 160/110 mm Hg. Blood pressure can be reduced further during the next 48 hours. Exceptions to this rule are aortic dissection (Chapter 78) and postoperative bleeding from vascular suture lines, two situations that demand much more rapid normalization of blood pressure. In most other cases, unnecessarily rapid correction of the elevated blood pressure to completely normal values places the patient at high risk for worsening cerebral, cardiac, and renal ischemia. In chronic hypertension, cerebral autoregulation is reset to higher than normal blood pressures. This compensatory adjustment prevents tissue overperfusion (increased intracranial pressure) at very high blood pressures, but it also predisposes to tissue underperfusion (cerebral ischemia) when an elevated blood pressure is lowered too quickly (Chapter 414). In patients with coronary disease, overly rapid or excessive reduction in diastolic blood pressure in the ICU can precipitate an acute myocardial ischemia or infarction.

Intravenous Drugs for Hypertensive Emergencies. Among parenteral agents for hypertensive emergencies (Table 67-8), no definitive comparisons of efficacy and safety exist. Sodium nitroprusside, which is a nitric oxide donor that causes both venous and arterial dilation, has been the most widely used agent for hypertensive emergencies because it can be titrated rapidly to control blood pressure. Disadvantages are reflex tachycardia, rebound hypertension after discontinuation, and thiocyanate toxicity in patients with renal insufficiency. Intravenous nitroglycerin, another nitric oxide donor, is a potent coronary vasodilator and therefore the drug of choice for hypertension in the setting of acute coronary syndromes, when it typically is combined with intravenous β-blockade (metoprolol) to reduce the double product (systolic blood pressure times heart rate) and thus myocardial oxygen demands. Nitroglycerin also is a potent venodilator that lowers preload in patients with hypertension in the setting of exacerbated heart failure. However, nitroprusside may be necessary if pulmonary edema results from severe hypertension (increased afterload). Compared with nitroprusside, the fall in blood pressure is less predictable with nitroglycerin. Intravenous labetalol is an effective treatment of hypertensive crisis, particularly in the setting of myocardial ischemia with preserved ventricular function. Nicardipine is a parenteral dihydropyridine CCB that is used most often in the postoperative cardiac surgery patient. Clevidipine, a new dihydropyridine CCB with an ultrafast onset and offset of action of 1 minute, is a pure arterial vasodilator that does not depress cardiac output and appears safe for patients with heart failure. Fenoldopam mesylate is a selective dopamine-1 receptor agonist that causes both systemic and renal vasodilation as well as increased glomerular filtration, natriuresis, and diuresis; it is a good choice for hypertensive emergencies in the setting of acute renal failure. Hydralazine (intravenous or intramuscular) is recommended only for hypertension during pregnancy because of the marked reflex tachycardia it precipitates.

After the blood pressure has been brought under acute control, oral labetalol and dihydropyridine CCBs are particularly useful agents in weaning patients from parenteral therapy so they can be transferred from the ICU. A few doses of intravenous furosemide are often needed to overcome drug resistance due to secondary volume expansion resulting from parenteral vasodilator therapy.

Secondary hypertension should be suspected in patients admitted to the ICU with hypertensive crisis. Normal 24-hour urinary catecholamine values or normal plasma normetanephrine and metanephrine values collected when the blood pressure is the highest (first 24 hours in ICU) effectively rule out pheochromocytoma (Chapter 235). Bilateral renal artery stenosis (Chapter 127) and other secondary causes should be excluded after the patient has been transferred out of the ICU but before discharge from the hospital.

Oral Medications for Hypertensive Urgencies. Most patients who present to the emergency department with hypertensive urgencies either are not adhering to their medical regimen or are being treated with an inadequate regimen. To expedite medication changes, outpatient follow-up should be arranged within 72 hours. Uncontrolled severe chronic hypertension may not require acute treatment in the emergency department if the patient clearly has adequate outpatient follow-up. Otherwise, for management of the patient during the short interim period, labetalol is effective in a dose of 200 to 300 mg, which can be repeated in 2 to 3 hours and then prescribed in twice-daily dosing. If a β-blocker is contraindicated, clonidine is effective in an initial dose of 0.1 or 0.2 mg followed by additional hourly doses of 0.1 mg. Captopril, a short-acting ACE inhibitor, lowers blood pressure within 15 to 30 minutes of oral dosing. A small test dose of 6.25 mg should be used to avoid an excessive fall in blood pressure in hypovolemic patients; then, the full oral dose is 25 mg, which can be repeated in 1 to 2 hours and prescribed as 25 to 75 mg twice daily.

Incidental Blood Pressure Elevation in the Emergency Department

Blood pressures above 160/110 mm Hg are a common incidental finding among patients who present to emergency departments and other acute care settings for urgent medical or surgical care of symptoms that are unrelated to blood pressure (e.g., musculoskeletal pain, orthopedic injury). The elevated blood pressure more often is the first indication of chronic hypertension than a simple physiologic stress reaction, so there is an important opportunity to initiate primary care referral for formal evaluation of possible chronic hypertension. Home or ambulatory blood pressure monitoring is indicated to determine whether the patient's blood pressure normalizes completely once the acute illness has resolved.

PROGNOSIS

An important prognostic factor in hypertension is electrocardiographic or echocardiographic left ventricular hypertrophy (LVH), with the latter already present in as many as 30% of patients with newly diagnosed hypertension and

TABLE 67-8 PARENTERAL AGENTS FOR MANAGEMENT OF HYPERTENSIVE EMERGENCIES

AGENT	DOSE	ONSET OF ACTION	PRECAUTIONS
PARENTERAL VASODILATORS			
Sodium nitroprusside	0.25-10 μg/kg/min IV infusion	Immediate	Thiocyanate toxicity, rebound hypertension
Nitroglycerin	5-100 μg/min IV infusion	2-5 min	Headache, tachycardia, tolerance
Nicardipine	5-15 mg/hr IV infusion	5-10 min	Protracted hypotension after prolonged use
Clevidipine	1-2 mg as rapid IV infusion, rapidly increase dose to 16 mg	2-4 min	Minimal
Fenoldopam mesylate	0.1-0.3 μg/kg/min IV infusion	1-5 min	Headache, tachycardia, increased intraocular pressure
Hydralazine	5-10 mg as IV bolus or 10-40 mg IM; repeat q4-6h	10 min IV; 20 min IM	Unpredictable and excessive falls in pressure; reflex tachycardia, angina exacerbation
Enalaprilat	0.625-1.25 mg q6h IV bolus	15-60 min	Unpredictable and excessive falls in pressure; acute renal failure (in bilateral renal stenosis)
PARENTERAL ADRENERGIC INHIBITORS			
Labetalol	20-80 mg as slow IV injection q10min, or 0.5-2 mg/min IV as infusion hypotension	5-10 min	Bronchospasm, heart block, orthostatic hypotension
Metoprolol	5 mg IV q10min × 3 doses	5-10 min	Bronchospasm, heart block, heart failure, exacerbation of cocaine-induced MI
Esmolol	500 μg/kg IV during 3 min, then 25-100 mg/kg/min as IV infusion	1-5 min	Bronchospasm, heart block, heart failure
Phentolamine	5-10 mg IV bolus q5-15min	1-2 min	Tachycardia, orthostatic hypotension

90% of patients with severe hypertension. LVH is associated with an increased risk for heart failure, stroke, and kidney failure. All drugs that lower blood pressure will reduce left ventricular mass, but the reduction averages only 12% or less and is less with β-blockers. With regression of LVH, the associated risks are reduced but not eliminated.

Because of their relatively short duration (typically <5 years), randomized trials may underestimate the lifetime protection against disability and death afforded by several decades of antihypertensive therapy in clinical practice. In the Framingham Heart Study, treatment of hypertension for 20 years in middle-aged adults reduced total cardiovascular mortality by 60%, which is considerably greater than the results of most randomized controlled trials despite the less intense treatment guidelines when therapy was initiated in the 1950s to 1970s. Further benefits may be seen with lower blood pressure treatment thresholds and goals than those presently endorsed, along with better control of associated cardiovascular risk factors.

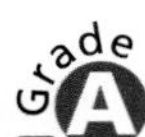

1. The ASTRAL Investigators. Revascularization versus medical therapy for renal-artery stenosis. *N Engl J Med.* 2009;361:1953-1962.
2. Julius S, Nesbitt SD, Egan BM, et al. Feasibility of treating prehypertension with an angiotensin-receptor blocker. *N Engl J Med.* 2006;354:1685-1697.
3. Law MR, Morris JK, Wald NJ. Use of blood pressure lowering drugs in the prevention of cardiovascular disease: meta-analysis of 147 randomized trials in the context of expectations from prospective epidemiological studies. *BMJ.* 2009;338:1665-1684.
4. Elmer PJ, Obarzanek E, Vollmer WM, et al. Effects of comprehensive lifestyle modification on diet, weight, physical fitness, and blood pressure control: 18-month results of a randomized trial. *Ann Intern Med.* 2006;144:485-495.
5. The ALLHAT Officers and Coordinators for the ALLHAT Collaborative Research Group. The major outcomes in high-risk hypertensive patients randomized to angiotensin-converting enzyme inhibitor or calcium channel blocker vs. diuretic: the Antihypertensive and Lipid-Lowering Treatment to Prevent Heart Attack Trial (ALLHAT). *JAMA.* 2002;288:2981-2997.
6. Julius S, Kjeldsen SE, Weber M, et al. Outcomes in hypertensive patients at high cardiovascular risk treated with regimens based on valsartan or amlodipine: the VALUE randomised trial. *Lancet.* 2004;363:2022-2031.
7. Lindholm LH, Carlberg B, Samuelsson O. Should beta blockers remain first choice in the treatment of primary hypertension? A meta-analysis. *Lancet.* 2005;366:1545-1553.
8. Verdecchia P, Staessen JA, Angeli F, et al. Usual versus tight control of systolic blood pressure in non-diabetic patients with hypertension (Cardio-Sis): an open-label randomized trial. *Lancet.* 2009;374:525-533.
9. Dahlof B, Sever PS, Poulter NR, et al. Prevention of cardiovascular events with antihypertensive regimen of amlodipine adding perindopril as required versus atenolol adding bendroflumethiazide as required, in the Anglo-Scandinavian Cardiac Outcomes Trial—Blood Pressure Lowering Arm (ASCOT-BPLA): a multicentre randomised controlled trial. *Lancet.* 2005;366:895-906.
10. Jamerson K, Weber MA, Bakris GL, et al. Benazepril plus amlodipine or hydrochlorothiazide for hypertension in high-risk patients. *N Engl J Med.* 2008;359:2417-2428.
11. The ONTARGET Investigators. Telmisartan, ramipril, or both in patients at high risk for vascular events. *N Engl J Med.* 2008;358:1547-1559.
12. Sever PS, Dahlof B, Poulter NR, et al. Prevention of coronary and stroke events with atorvastatin in hypertension patients who have average or lower-than-average cholesterol concentrations, in the Anglo-Scandinavian Cardiac Outcomes Trial—Lipid Lowering Arm (ASCOT-LLA): a multicentre randomized controlled trial. *Lancet.* 2003;361:1149-1158.
13. Appel LJ, Wright JT, Greene T, et al. Long-term effects of renin-angiotensin system-blocking therapy and a low blood pressure goal on progression of hypertensive chronic kidney disease in African Americans. *Arch Intern Med.* 2008;168:832-839.
14. The ACCORD Study Group. Effects of intensive blood-pressure control in type 2 diabetes mellitus. *N Engl J Med.* 2010;362:1575-1585.
15. Beckett NS, Peters R, Fletcher AE, et al. Treatment of hypertension in patients 80 years of age or older. *N Engl J Med.* 2008;358:1887-1898.
16. PROGRESS Collaborative Group. Randomised trial of a perindopril-based blood-pressure-lowering regimen among 6,105 individuals with previous stroke or transient ischaemic attack. *Lancet.* 2001;358:1033-1041.

SUGGESTED READINGS

Appel LJ, Frohlich ED, Hall JE, et al. The importance of population-wide sodium reduction as a means to prevent cardiovascular disease and stroke: a call to action from the American Heart Association. *Circulation.* 2011;123:1138-1143. *Recommendation for primordial prevention of hypertension by population-wide reduction in the sodium content of processed food.*

Drazner MH. The progression of hypertensive heart disease. *Circulation.* 2011;123:327-334. *Review.*

Rothwell PM, Howard SC, Dolan E, et al. Prognostic significance of visit-to-visit variability, maximum systolic blood pressure, and episodic hypertension. *Lancet.* 2010;375:895-905. *High visit-to-visit variability in systolic blood pressure is associated with an increased risk of stroke.*

68

PULMONARY HYPERTENSION

VALLERIE MCLAUGHLIN

DEFINITION

The normal pulmonary vasculature is a low-pressure system, with less than one tenth the resistance to flow observed in the systemic vasculature. Pulmonary hypertension refers to the hemodynamic state in which the pressure in the pulmonary artery is elevated above a mean of 25 mm Hg. A specific type of pulmonary hypertension, pulmonary arterial hypertension, also requires that the left heart filling pressure (pulmonary capillary wedge pressure, left ventricular end-diastolic pressure, or left atrial pressure) be 15 mm Hg or less. The syndrome of pulmonary arterial hypertension results when blood flow through the pulmonary circulation is restricted, thereby leading to pathologic increases in pulmonary vascular resistance and, ultimately, to right ventricular failure. Pulmonary hypertension may also be a consequence of many other chronic diseases, including left heart failure (Chapter 58), a variety of parenchymal lung diseases, and thromboembolic disease (Chapter 98) (Table 68-1).

EPIDEMIOLOGY

Normal pulmonary blood pressure is 20/10 (mean 15) mm Hg at rest at sea level, rising to 30/13 (mean 20) mm Hg with mild exercise. Pressures rise with altitude, and at an altitude of about 15,000 feet, normal resting pulmonary artery pressures are about 38/14 (mean 20) mm Hg. Pulmonary arterial systolic pressure rises gradually with age, and each 10-mm Hg increase is associated with a 2.7-fold greater risk for mortality.

Idiopathic pulmonary arterial hypertension, formerly called primary pulmonary hypertension, is the prototype of group 1 pulmonary arterial hypertension. This disease affects women more than men in a 2 : 1 ratio. It may present at any age, with a mean age of onset of 37 years. The prevalence of pulmonary arterial hypertension is between 15 and 26 per million persons. Heritable pulmonary arterial hypertension occurs in a familial context, most often (70%) owing to a mutation in the bone morphogenic protein receptor type 2. Less commonly, mutations in activin receptor–like kinase type 1, or endoglin, have been identified in patients with pulmonary arterial hypertension, predominately with coexistent hereditary hemorrhagic telangiectasia (Chapter 176). Drug- and toxin-induced pulmonary arterial hypertension has been most clearly linked to anorexigens, including aminorex, fenfluramine, and dexfenfluramine. Although these agents are no longer used, observational studies suggest that amphetamines, methamphetamines, and L-tryptophan are likely related to the development of pulmonary arterial hypertension.

One of the most common types of group 1 pulmonary arterial hypertension occurs in the setting of connective tissue diseases. For example, the prevalence of pulmonary arterial hypertension in patients with scleroderma (Chapter 275) is in the range of 7 to 12%. It is less common in systemic lupus erythematosus (Chapter 274), rheumatoid arthritis (Chapter 272), and other systemic vasculitides (Chapter 278). Pulmonary arterial hypertension is a rare but well established complication of human immunodeficiency virus (HIV) infection, with a prevalence of 0.5%. Prospective hemodynamic studies show that 2 to 6% of patients with portal hypertension (Chapter 148) develop pulmonary arterial hypertension, although the reason for the association is not clear.

A significant proportion of patients with untreated systemic-to-pulmonary shunts, commonly owing to congenital heart disease (Chapter 69), develop pulmonary arterial hypertension. Persistent exposure of the pulmonary vasculature to increased blood flow and pressure leads to an elevated pulmonary vascular resistance. In some cases, Eisenmenger's syndrome (Chapter 69), with a reversal of flow across the defect, results in right-to-left shunting. Pulmonary veno-occlusive (Chapter 98) disease and pulmonary capillary hemangiomatosis are rare disorders that directly affect the pulmonary vasculature. The presentation of each is often similar to pulmonary arterial hypertension, but the prognosis is particularly poor.

Pulmonary hypertension owing to left heart disease probably represents the most frequent cause of pulmonary hypertension seen in practice (group 2 patients). Left-sided ventricular (Chapter 58) or valvular disease

TABLE 68-1 UPDATED CLINICAL CLASSIFICATION OF PULMONARY HYPERTENSION

GROUP 1
Pulmonary arterial hypertension (PAH)
Idiopathic PAH
Heritable
BMPR2
ALK1, endoglin (with or without hereditary hemorrhagic telangiectasia)
Unknown
Drug and toxin induced
Associated with
Connective tissue diseases
HIV infection
Portal hypertension
Congenital heart diseases
Schistosomiasis
Chronic hemolytic anemia
Persistent pulmonary hypertension of the newborn
Pulmonary veno-occlusive disease with left to right shunts and/or pulmonary capillary hemangiomatosis
GROUP 2
Pulmonary hypertension owing to left heart disease
Systolic dysfunction
Diastolic dysfunction
Valvular disease
GROUP 3
Pulmonary hypertension owing to lung diseases and/or hypoxia
Chronic obstructive pulmonary disease
Interstitial lung disease
Other pulmonary diseases with mixed restrictive and obstructive pattern
Sleep-disordered breathing
Alveolar hypoventilation disorders
Chronic exposure to high altitude
Developmental abnormalities
GROUP 4
Chronic thromboembolic pulmonary hypertension
GROUP 5
Pulmonary hypertension with unclear multifactorial mechanisms
Hematologic disorders: myeloproliferative disorders, splenectomy
Systemic disorders: sarcoidosis, pulmonary Langerhans cell histiocytosis: lymphangioleiomyomatosis, neurofibromatosis, vasculitis
Metabolic disorders: glycogen storage disease, Gaucher's disease, thyroid disorders
Others: tumoral obstruction, fibrosing mediastinitis, chronic renal failure on dialysis

ALK1 = activin receptor-like kinase type 1; BMPR2 = bone morphogenetic protein receptor type 2; HIV = human immunodeficiency virus.

Reprinted from Simonneau G, Robbins IM, Beghetti M, et al. Updated clinical classification of pulmonary hypertension. *J Am Coll Cardiol.* 2009;54:S43-S54.

(Chapter 75) may increase left atrial pressure, which then is transmitted back to the pulmonary vasculature. Often, the transpulmonary gradient and pulmonary vascular resistance are normal. In such cases, optimal treatment of the left heart disease results in reduction of the left heart filling pressures and, consequently, a reduction in the pulmonary artery pressures. On occasion, patients with left heart disease have an elevation of pulmonary artery pressure greater than expected based on the elevation of left heart filling pressures, with a transpulmonary gradient of more than 12 mm Hg and a pulmonary vascular resistance of more than 3 Wood units (Wood units = [pulmonary artery pressure minus mean pulmonary capillary wedge pressure] divided by cardiac output). This difference may be due to an increase in pulmonary artery vasomotor tone or pulmonary vascular remodeling in the setting of persistently elevated left heart filling pressures.

Group 3 patients have pulmonary hypertension owing to lung diseases or hypoxia. Any disorder that results in hypoxemia (e.g., chronic obstructive lung disease [Chapter 88], interstitial lung disease [Chapter 92], sleep-disordered breathing [Chapter 100]) may result in pulmonary hypertension, although the pressure elevation tends to be modest, with a mean pulmonary artery pressure of 25 to 35 mm Hg. Echocardiography-based observations have suggested that up to 80% of patients with chronic obstructive lung disease and idiopathic pulmonary fibrosis have elevated pulmonary artery pressures. In patients who have more advanced parenchymal lung disease and undergo evaluation for lung volume reduction surgery or lung transplantation, 40 to 50% have pulmonary hypertension at the time of right heart catheterization. Most often, the elevations in pulmonary artery pressures are modest, but a small proportion of patients have more substantial elevations.

Group 4 patients have chronic thromboembolic pulmonary hypertension (Chapter 98), which must be differentiated from the other groups because the treatment is quite different. Approximately 4% of patients who have suffered an acute pulmonary embolism progress to develop chronic thromboembolic pulmonary hypertension. Approximately half of those ultimately diagnosed with chronic thromboembolic pulmonary hypertension do not have a known history of an acute pulmonary embolism. Patients with a significant clot burden can be candidates for a pulmonary thromboendarterectomy, which is a potentially curative procedure for this disorder.

Group 5 pulmonary arterial hypertension consists of several forms for which the etiology is unclear or multifactorial. Among these conditions are a number of hematologic, systemic, and metabolic disorders.

PATHOBIOLOGY

The pathobiology of pulmonary arterial hypertension is complex and incompletely elucidated (Fig. 68-1). The pulmonary arterial hypertension phenotype is characterized by endothelial dysfunction, a decreased ratio of apoptosis to proliferation in pulmonary artery smooth muscle cells, and a thickened, disordered adventitia in which adventitial metalloproteases are excessively activated. The evolution of pulmonary vascular disease frequently originates with the interaction of a predisposing state and one or more inciting stimuli, a concept referred to as the "multiple-hit hypothesis."

In group 1 pulmonary arterial hypertension, patients have a panvasculopathy predominantly affecting the small pulmonary arterioles. It is characterized by a variety of arterial abnormalities, including intimal hyperplasia, medial hypertrophy, adventitial proliferation, thrombosis in situ, varying degrees of inflammation, and plexiform lesions. An individual patient may manifest all or some of these lesions, and the distribution of the lesions may be diffuse or focal.

The genetic defect best characterized in heritable pulmonary arterial hypertension is that of the bone morphogenetic protein receptor type 2, a member of the transforming growth factor-β signaling family. This defect accounts for 70% of heritable pulmonary arterial hypertension cases, although it has also been detected in 11 to 40% of patients with apparently idiopathic pulmonary arterial hypertension and no family history. Characteristics of this gene include incomplete penetrance (20%) and genetic anticipation. Less commonly, mutations in activin receptor–like kinase type 1, or endoglin, have been identified, usually in families with coexistent hereditary hemorrhagic telangiectasia.

The imbalance in the production or metabolism of vasoactive mediators in the pulmonary vasculature includes a reduction in prostacyclin and nitric oxide, which have vasodilator and antiproliferative properties, and an increase in thromboxane and endothelin, which are vasoconstrictors as well as mitogens. The reduction in nitric oxide synthase in pulmonary arterial hypertension diminishes nitric oxide and, subsequently, cyclic guanosine monophosphate production. Endothelin-1 is a potent vasoconstrictor and smooth muscle mitogen that may contribute to the development of pulmonary arterial hypertension. Prostacyclin synthase is reduced in pulmonary arterial hypertension, resulting in an inadequate production of prostacyclin I_2, which is a vasodilator with potent antiproliferative effects. Other aberrations include those of the voltage-dependent potassium channels and serotonin pathways. Disorders of inflammatory and coagulation pathways have also been described.

Chronic changes in the pulmonary vasculature also occur as a result of other types of pulmonary hypertension. Chronic elevation of left heart filling pressures causes a backward transmission of pressure to the pulmonary venous system and triggers vasoconstriction in the pulmonary arterial bed. Histologically, the veins thicken abnormally, and a neointima is formed. As secondary features, medial hypertrophy and thickening of the neointima on the arterial side of the pulmonary circulation occur. These changes can be reversed with therapies that result in chronic reduction of left heart filling pressures.

In parenchymal lung disease, changes in the distal pulmonary arterial vessels are related to hypoxia. Hypoxia induces muscularization of the distal

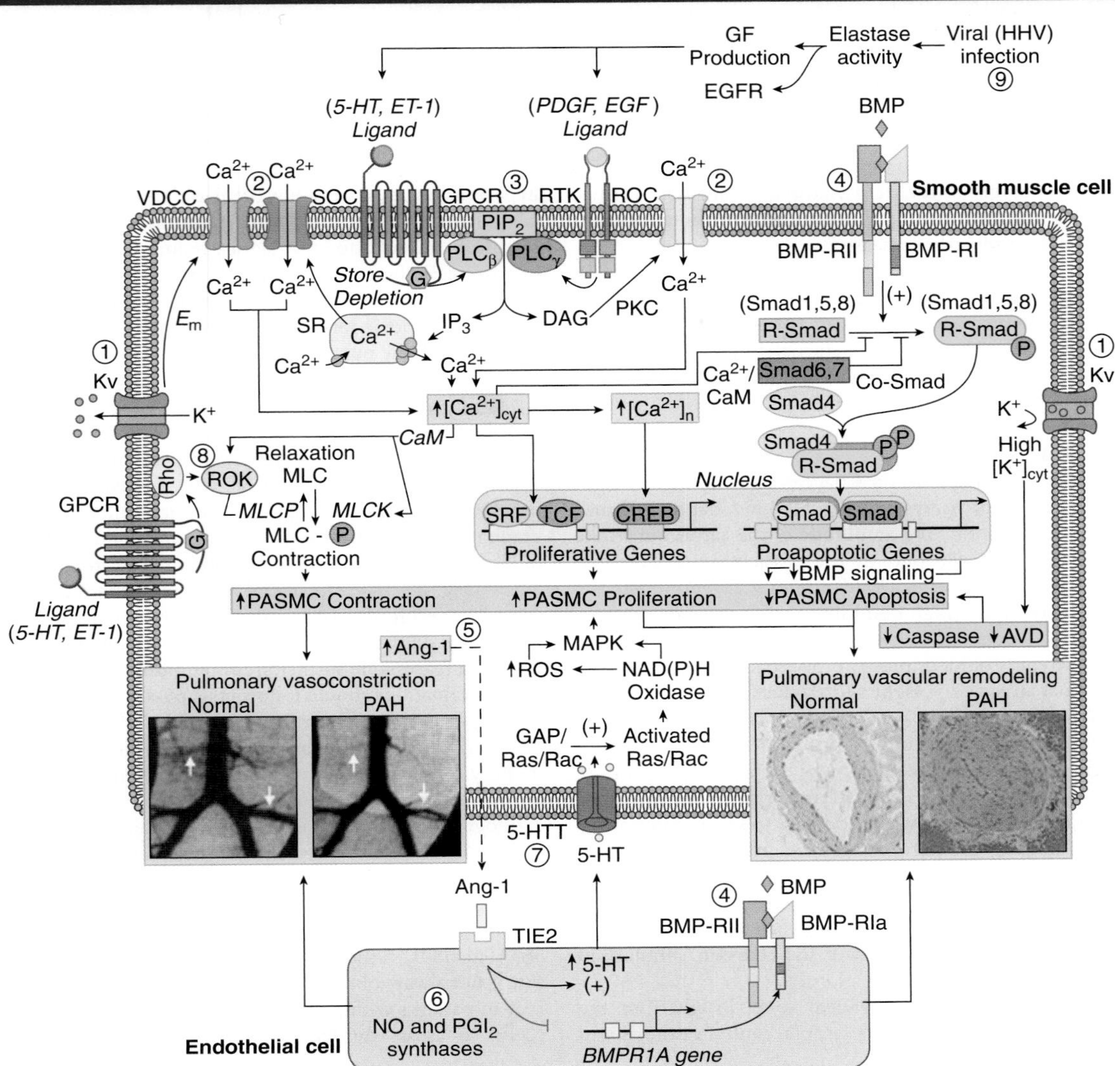

FIGURE 68-1. Potential mechanisms involved in the development of pulmonary arterial hypertension (PAH). Ang = angiopoietin; AVD = apoptotic volume decrease; BMP = bone morphogenetic protein; BMPR = bone morphogenetic protein receptor; CaM = calmodulin; CREB = cAMP-response element binding protein; DAG = diacylglycerol; E_m = membrane potential; EGF = epidermal growth factor; EGFR = epidermal growth factor receptor; ET = endothelin; GAP = GTPase-activating protein; GPCR = G protein–coupled receptor; HHV = human herpesvirus; HT = hydroxytryptamine (serotonin); HTT = hydroxytryptamine (serotonin) transporter; IP_3 = inositol 1,4,5-trisphosphate; Kv = voltage-gated K^+; MAPK = mitogen-activated protein kinase; MLC = myosin light chain; MLCK = myosin light chain kinase; NA(D)PH = nicotinamide adenine dinucleotide phosphate; NO = nitric oxide; PASMC = pulmonary artery smooth muscle cell; PDGF = platelet-derived growth factor; PGI_2 = prostacyclin; PKC = protein kinase C; PLC = phospholipase C; ROC = receptor-operated Ca^{2+} channels; ROS = reactive oxygen species; RTK = receptor tyrosine kinase; SR = sarcoplasmic reticulum; SRF = serum response factor; TCF = T-cell factor; TIE = endothelial-specific tyrosine kinase; VDCC = voltage-dependent calcium channel. (Modified from Morrell NW, Adnot S, Archer SL, et al. Cellular and molecular basis of pulmonary hypertension. *J Am Coll Cardiol.* 2009;54:S20-S31.)

vessels and medial hypertrophy of the more proximal vessels. Neither neointima formation nor the development of plexiform lesions is observed.

The pathology of chronic thromboembolic pulmonary hypertension is often distinct from idiopathic pulmonary arterial hypertension. The lesions are frequently more variable, with some arterial pathways that appear relatively unaffected and others that show recanalized vascular thromboses. However, the involvement of distal microvessels, particularly when thromboses have occurred in subsegmental arteries, can resemble idiopathic pulmonary arterial hypertension with the formation of plexiform lesions.

Pathophysiology

The normal pulmonary vasculature bed has a remarkable capacity to dilate and recruit unused vasculature to accommodate increases in pulmonary blood flow. In pulmonary hypertension, the pulmonary artery pressure and pulmonary vascular resistance are increased at rest and further increase with exertion. In response to this increased afterload, the normally very thin right ventricle hypertrophies and eventually dilates. Early on in the process, the right ventricle may be capable of maintaining normal cardiac output at rest, although it may fail to augment cardiac output with exercise, thereby leading to exertional dyspnea. As the disease progresses, the right ventricular dysfunction may progress to the point that resting cardiac output is impaired. Right ventricular function is a major determinant of functional capacity and prognosis in pulmonary arterial hypertension. Although the left ventricle is not affected by pulmonary vascular disease itself, progressive right ventricular dilation can impair left ventricular filling and lead to mildly increased left heart filling pressure. The pathophysiology of pulmonary hypertension related to left heart and lung disease is further complicated by those underlying disorders.

The two most frequent mechanisms of death are progressive right ventricular failure and sudden death. Right ventricular failure, as evidence by elevated jugular venous pressure, lower extremity edema, and occasionally ascites, may also be accompanied by evidence of poor forward flow owing to inadequate filling of the left ventricle. Hypotension, hypoperfusion, and renal insufficiency may result. Other potential causes of death include pneumonia, sepsis, and pulmonary embolism.

CLINICAL MANIFESTATIONS

History

Dyspnea, which is the most common symptom of pulmonary hypertension, initially may be attributed to underlying disorders such as heart failure or obstructive lung disease, but the dyspnea of pulmonary hypertension typically is insidious in progression and reproducible. Dyspnea is classified by the

World Health Organization (WHO) system, which is similar to the New York Heart Association classification system for angina and heart failure (see Table 50-5 in Chapter 50), and may progress to dyspnea at rest.

Other common symptoms of pulmonary hypertension include fatigue, lightheadedness, chest pain (Chapter 50), and palpitations (Chapters 50 and 62). Syncope (Chapter 62), which is an ominous finding, is often exertional in nature; it signifies the inability of the right ventricle to augment cardiac output as needed for physical activity. Symptoms of right heart failure, including edema and ascites, signify advanced disease.

Patients often have symptoms associated with their underlying disease, which typically is far advanced by the time pulmonary arterial hypertension develops. For example, patients with pulmonary hypertension associated with left heart disease often have paroxysmal nocturnal dyspnea and orthopnea. Patients with pulmonary hypertension related to hypoxic lung disease may have cough, sputum production, or wheezing.

Physical Examination

Distention of jugular veins (see Fig. 50-3 in Chapter 50) may signify right ventricular failure, and prominent v ways (see Fig. 50-4 in Chapter 50) may be a result of tricuspid regurgitation. The amplitude of the carotid upstroke may give some insight into the cardiac output. The classic physical examination finding in pulmonary hypertension is a loud pulmonic component to the second heart sound, which reflects high pulmonary pressures that increase the force of the pulmonic valve closure. Palpation of the sternum often reveals a parasternal lift as the hypertrophied, pressure-overloaded right ventricle obliterates the retrosternal air space. A right ventricular fourth heart sound reflects diastolic filling of the hypertrophied, noncompliant right ventricle, akin to the left-sided fourth heart sound in a patient with systemic hypertension and left ventricular hypertrophy. The murmur of tricuspid regurgitation, which is holosystolic, located at the left lower sternal border, and augments with inspiration, is common in patients with moderate to severe pulmonary hypertension. Other findings on auscultation may include an early systolic click and the murmur of pulmonic regurgitation. A right ventricular third heart sound often signifies advanced disease and right heart failure. Other signs consistent with right ventricular failure include hepatomegaly, peripheral edema (see Fig. 50-7 in Chapter 50), ascites, hypotension, diminished pulse pressure, and cool extremities.

Other physical examination findings may give some insight into the etiology of the pulmonary hypertension. For example, central cyanosis and clubbing may suggest an intracardiac shunt and Eisenmenger's physiology. Sclerodactyly, telangiectasias (see Fig. 275-3 in Chapter 275), arthritis, Raynaud's phenomenon (see Fig. 80-5 in Chapter 80), and skin rashes may increase the suspicion of an underlying connective tissue disease. Splenomegaly, spider angioma, palmar erythema (see Fig. 148-2 in Chapter 148), icterus (see Fig. 148-1 in Chapter 148), and caput medusa may suggest portal hypertension as an etiology. Signs of left heart disease, such as pulmonary congestion, a left-sided third heart sound, or findings of mitral or aortic valve disease on auscultation may signify pulmonary hypertension as a result of left heart disease. Fine rales, accessory muscle use, wheezing, protracted expiration, and productive cough may denote group 3 pulmonary hypertension as a result of hypoxic lung disease. Pulmonary vascular bruits suggest chronic thromboembolic pulmonary hypertension.

DIAGNOSIS

Initial assessments include an electrocardiogram (ECG) and chest radiograph. The ECG may show right axis deviation, right ventricular enlargement, right atrial enlargement, and ST and T wave changes across the anterior precordium that reflect right ventricular strain (Fig. 68-2). The chest radiograph may demonstrate enlarged proximal pulmonary arteries (see Fig. 53-6 in Chapter 53) with peripheral tapering or pruning of the pulmonary vasculature (Fig. 68-3A). The lateral may reveal the reduction in retrosternal air space as a result of right ventricular enlargement (see Fig. 68-3B).

If, based on the history, physical examination, ECG, and chest radiograph, there is a reasonable suspicion for pulmonary hypertension, a series of diagnostic evaluations should follow (Fig. 68-4), usually beginning with an echocardiogram, and with further testing guided by the patient subtype (Table 68-2). The echocardiogram gives insight not only into the presence of pulmonary hypertension but also into the presence of common disorders of the left heart that may result in pulmonary hypertension. Two-dimensional echocardiographic findings reflective of elevated pulmonary artery pressures include right atrial enlargement, right ventricular enlargement, flattening of the intraventricular septum, and an underfilled left ventricle (Fig. 68-5). The right ventricular systolic pressure may be estimated based on the velocity of the tricuspid regurgitant jet using the modified Bernoulli equation (Chapter 55) (Fig. 68-6), although a reliable estimate of right ventricular systolic pressure is not always obtainable, and this measurement is prone to error, particularly in patients with parenchymal lung disease, The echocardiogram is also useful to assess for left heart causes of pulmonary hypertension, such

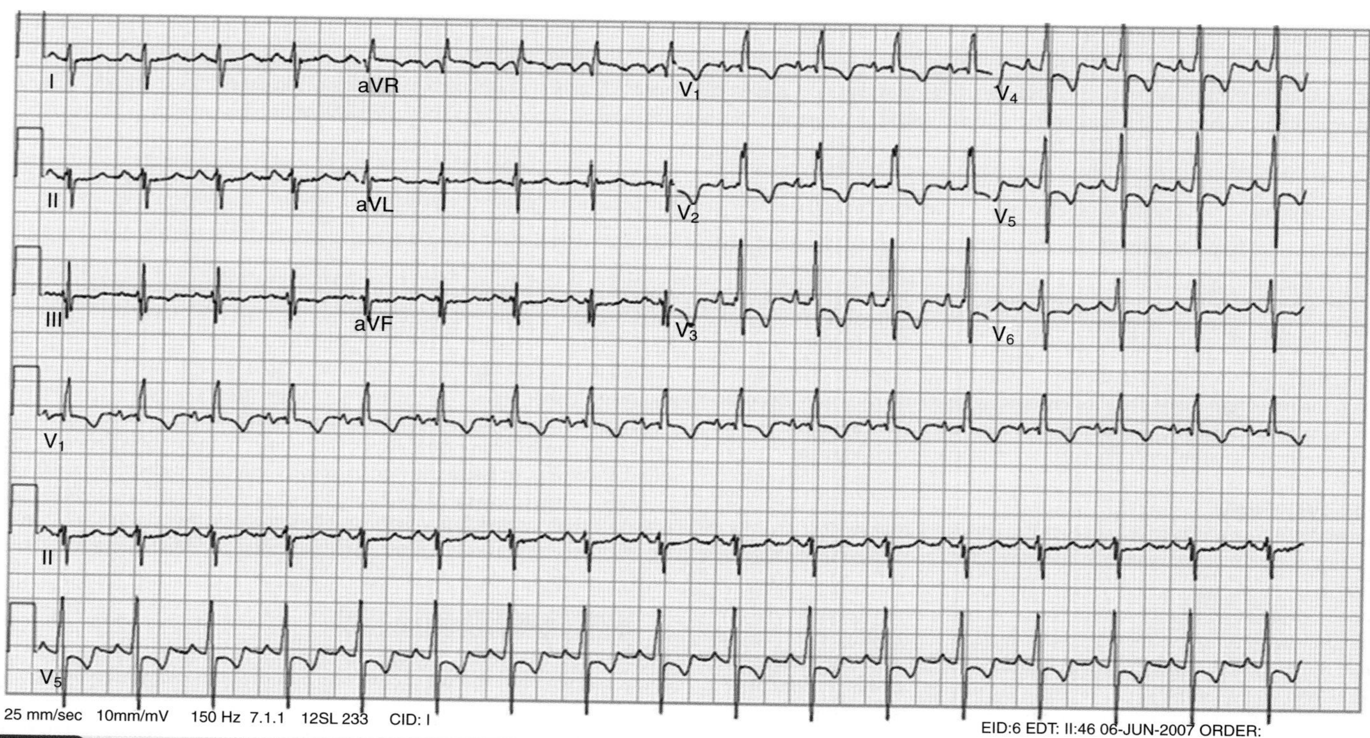

FIGURE 68-2. Electrocardiogram demonstrating sinus rhythm, right axis deviation, and right ventricular hypertrophy with a strain pattern.

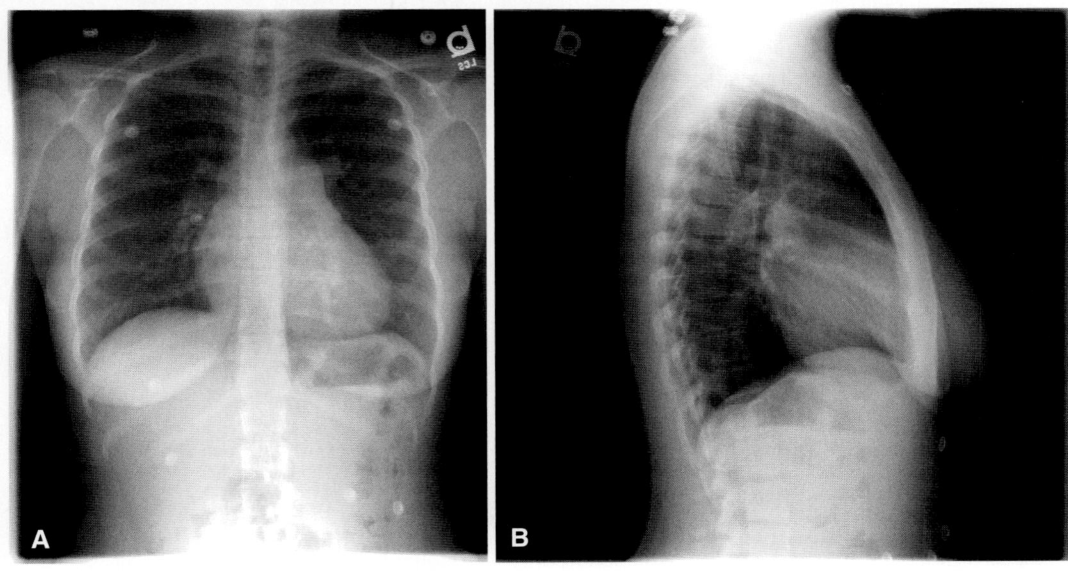

FIGURE 68-3. Posterior-anterior **(A)** and Lateral **(B)** chest radiographs demonstrating enlarged proximal pulmonary arteries and right ventricular enlargement.

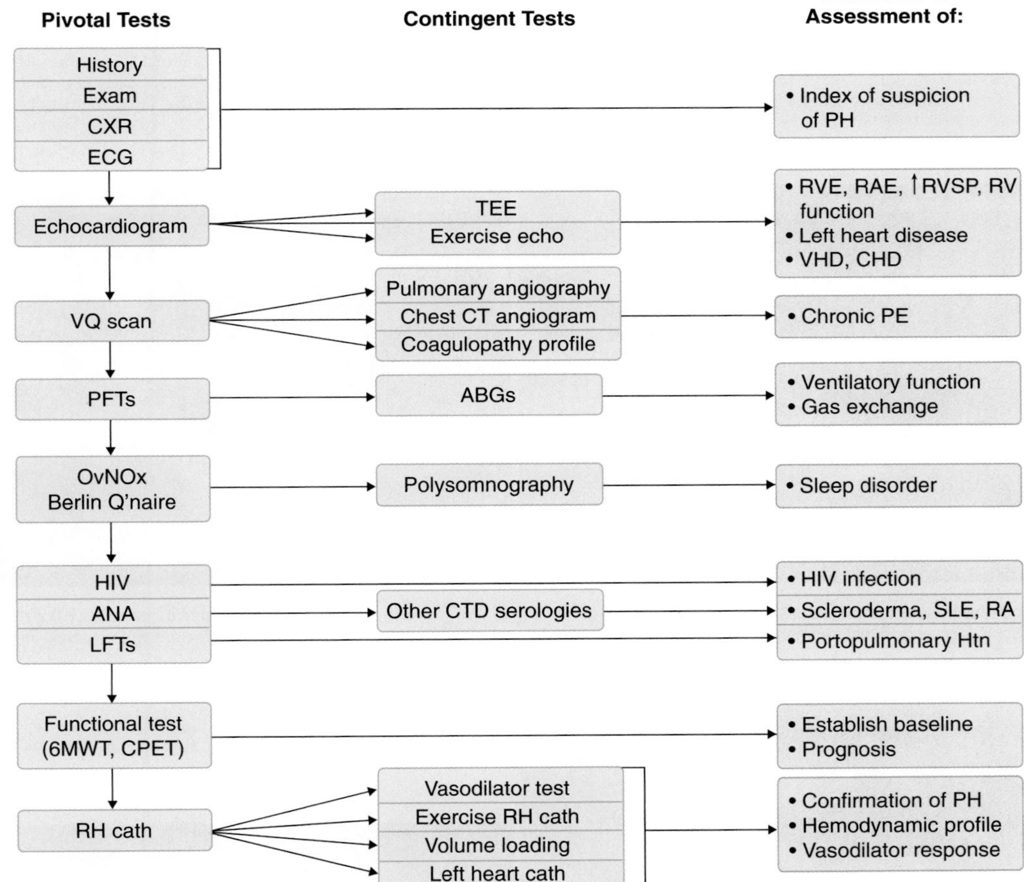

FIGURE 68-4. Diagnostic approach to pulmonary arterial hypertension (PH). Because the suspicion of PH may arise in various ways, the sequence of tests may vary. However, the diagnosis of PH requires that certain data support a specific diagnosis. In addition, the diagnosis of idiopathic pulmonary arterial hypertension (IPAH) is one of excluding all other reasonable possibilities. *Pivotal tests* are those that are essential to establishing a diagnosis of any type of PH by either identification of criteria of associated disease or exclusion of diagnoses other than IPAH. All pivotal tests are required for a definitive diagnosis and baseline characterization. An abnormality of one assessment (such as obstructive pulmonary disease on pulmonary function tests [PFTs]) does not preclude that another abnormality (chronic thromboembolic disease on VQ scan and pulmonary angiogram) is contributing or predominant. *Contingent tests* are recommended to elucidate or confirm results of the pivotal tests and need only be performed in the appropriate clinical context. The *combination* of pivotal and appropriate contingent tests contributes to assessment of the differential diagnoses in the right-hand column. It should be recognized that definitive diagnosis may require additional specific evaluations not necessarily included in this general guideline. 6MWT = 6-minute walk test; ABGs = arterial blood gases; ANA = antinuclear antibody serology; CHD = congenital heart disease; CPET = cardiopulmonary exercise test; CT = computed tomography; CTD = connective tissue disease; CXR = chest X-ray; ECG = electrocardiogram; HIV = human immunodeficiency virus screening; Htn = hypertension; LFTs = liver function tests; PE = pulmonary embolism; RA = rheumatoid arthritis; RAE = right atrial enlargement; RH cath = right heart cath; RVE = right ventricular enlargement; RVSP = right ventricular systolic pressure; SLE = systemic lupus erythematosus; TEE = transesophageal echocardiography; VHD = valvular heart disease; VQ scan = lung ventilation-perfusion scintigram. (From McLaughlin VV, Archer SL, Badesch DB, et al. ACCF/AHA 2009 expert consensus document on pulmonary hypertension: a report of the American College of Cardiology Foundation Task Force on Expert Consensus Documents and the American Heart Association developed in collaboration with the American College of Chest Physicians; American Thoracic Society, Inc.; and the Pulmonary Hypertension Association. *J Am Coll Cardiol.* 2009;53:1573-1619.)

TABLE 68-2 APPROACH TO SPECIFIC PATIENT SUBGROUPS

	FURTHER ASSESSMENT	RATIONALE
BMPR2 mutation	Echocardiogram yearly; RHC if echocardiogram demonstrates evidence of PAH (high right ventricular systolic pressure or right heart chamber enlargement)	Early detection of PAH; 20% chance of developing PAH
First-degree relative of patient with BMPR2 mutation or within pedigree of two or more patients with a diagnosis of PAH	Genetic counseling and recommendation for BMPR2 genotyping; proceed as above if positive	Autosomal dominant transmission
Systemic sclerosis	Echocardiogram yearly; RHC if echocardiogram demonstrates evidence of PAH (high right ventricular systolic pressure or right heart chamber enlargement)	About 8% (by RHC): 27% (by echo screening) prevalence of PAH in systemic sclerosis
HIV infection	Echocardiogram if symptoms or signs suggestive of PAH; RHC if echo demonstrates evidence of PAH (high right ventricular systolic pressure or right heart chamber enlargement)	0.5% prevalence of PAH
Portal hypertension	Echocardiogram if OLT considered; RHC if echocardiogram demonstrates evidence of PAH (high right ventricular systolic pressure or right heart chamber enlargement)	4% prevalence of PAH in candidates for OLT; PAH is predictive of poor OLT outcome
Prior appetite suppressant use (fenfluramine)	Echocardiogram only if symptomatic	Incidence of PAH is approximately 0.005% if agent used >3 mo
Congenital heart disease with shunt	Echocardiogram and RHC at time of diagnosis; consider repair of defect if significant left-to-right shunt present	High probability of PAH developing in unrepaired shunt (Eisenmenger's syndrome)
Recent acute pulmonary embolism	Ventilation-perfusion (V/Q) scintigraphy 3 mo after event if symptomatic; pulmonary angiogram if positive	3% risk of chronic thromboembolic PH; negative V/Q scan excludes chronic thromboembolism
Sickle cell disease	Echocardiogram yearly; RHC if echocardiogram demonstrates evidence of PAH (high right ventricular systolic pressure or right heart chamber enlargement)	Increased mortality if PH present, early detection of PH, 30% develop PH, about 10% develop PAH

BMPR2 = bone morphogenic protein receptor 2; HIV = human immunodeficiency virus; OLT = orthotopic liver transplantation; PAH = pulmonary arterial hypertension; RHC = right heart catheterization. From McLaughlin VV, Archer SL, Badesch DB, et al. ACCF/AHA 2009 expert consensus document on pulmonary hypertension: a report of the American College of Cardiology Foundation Task Force on Expert Consensus Documents and the American Heart Association developed in collaboration with the American College of Chest Physicians; American Thoracic Society, Inc.; and the Pulmonary Hypertension Association. *J Am Coll Cardiol.* 2009;53:1573-1619.

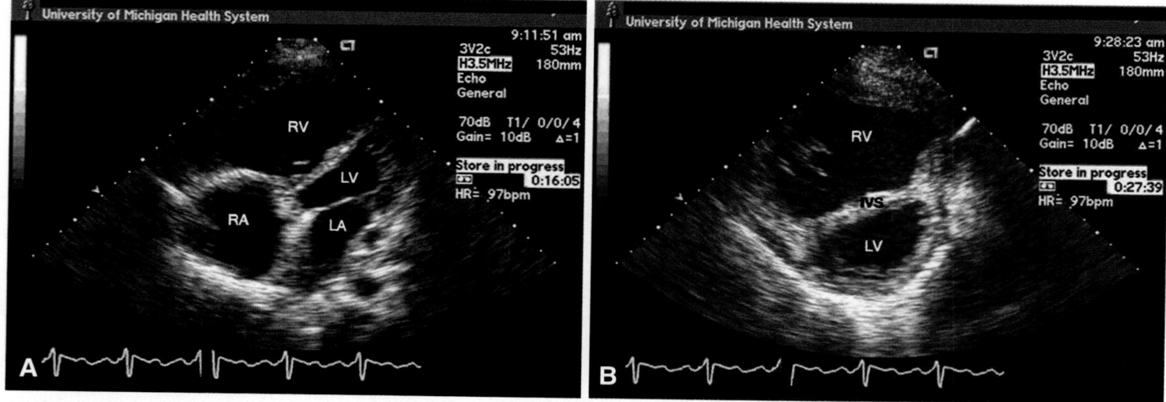

FIGURE 68-5. **Echocardiographic images of the heart. A,** Four-chamber view. Right atrial (RA) enlargement, right ventricular (RV) enlargement. The left atrium (LA) and left ventricle (LV) are small and underfilled. **B,** Short axis view. RV enlargement is present. Flattening of the intraventricular septum (IVS) results from pressure and volume overload of the RV.

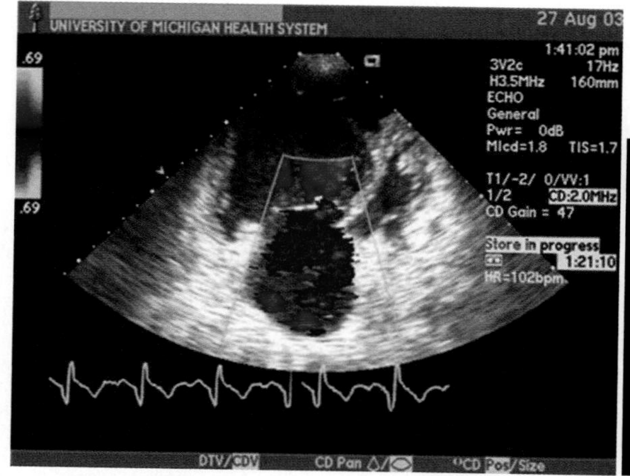

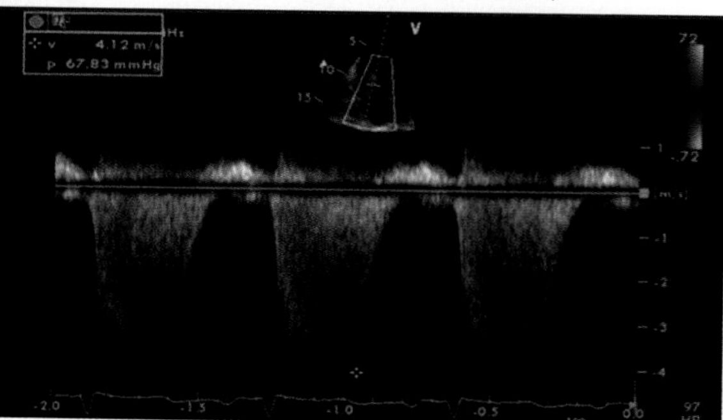

FIGURE 68-6. **Calculation of estimated pulmonary artery pressure based on the velocity of the tricuspid regurgitant jet.** RAP = right atrial pressure; RVSP = right ventricular systolic pressure; PASP = pulmonary artery systolic pressure; V = tricuspid jet velocity (m/sec).

as systolic dysfunction, diastolic dysfunction, and valvular heart disease. Occasionally, a previously unknown congenital heart defect is discovered during this evaluation. In approximately 25% of patients, a previously trivial patent foramen ovale may shunt blood from the right atrium to the left atrium, owing to the high pulmonary vascular resistance, and thereby worsen systemic oxygenation.

In a patient with unexplained dyspnea and evidence of pulmonary hypertension on echocardiogram, chronic thromboembolic pulmonary hypertension must be excluded. The study of choice for this assessment is the ventilation-perfusion scan (see Fig. 98-4 in Chapter 98), which often shows multiple perfusion defects that are not matched on ventilation. Although spiral computed tomography (CT) is excellent for the assessment of acute pulmonary embolus, it sometimes fails to detect surgically accessible chronic thromboembolic disease. If either of these studies is abnormal, further evaluation with a pulmonary angiogram may be required to determine whether chronic thrombolic disease is the diagnosis and, if so, whether it is surgically accessible.

Pulmonary function tests in patients with pulmonary arterial hypertension may show mild restrictive disease and a mildly reduced diffusing capacity for carbon monoxide. Patients with the scleroderma spectrum of diseases tend to have more substantial reductions in the diffusing capacity for carbon monoxide, which may even precede the development of pulmonary hypertension. Pulmonary function tests may disclose evidence of obstructive or restrictive lung disease; further evaluation with chest CT may be necessary. Overnight oximetry is useful to screen for obstructive sleep apnea (Chapter 100). If indicated, formal polysomnography may be required.

Recommended serologic testing, given the known associations, includes an antinuclear antibody test and HIV serology, in addition to liver function tests to assess for chronic liver disease. A study of functional capacity, most commonly the 6-minute walk test, is useful to assess the severity of disease, to determine the potential need for oxygen, and to establish a baseline against which to assess subsequent changes in exercise capacity as a result of medical interventions.

If pulmonary arterial hypertension is suspected based on the noninvasive evaluation, the diagnosis must be confirmed with a right heart catheterization that measures right atrial pressure, right ventricular pressure, pulmonary artery (systolic, diastolic, and mean) pressures, pulmonary arterial wedge pressure (reflective of left ventricular end-diastolic pressure or left atrial pressure), cardiac output and index, heart rate, systemic blood pressure, and oxygen saturations in the superior vena cava, inferior vena cava, pulmonary artery, and a systemic artery. From this information, pulmonary vascular resistance and systemic vascular resistance may be calculated, right ventricular performance can be assured, and an intracardiac or intrapulmonary shunt can be confirmed or excluded.

In patients with left heart or parenchymal lung disease, however, optimal management of the underlying condition is often undertaken before considering right heart catheterization. Patients with suspected chronic thromboembolic disease often undergo both right heart catheterization and pulmonary angiography (Chapter 98) to assess surgical candidacy and operative risk.

Measurement of the wedge pressure, a surrogate for left atrial pressure in the absence of pulmonary vein obstruction, is useful to exclude pulmonary hypertension caused by left heart disease or, in rare cases, pulmonary veno-occlusive disease. If an optimal wedge pressure tracing cannot be obtained, or if there is any question about the accuracy of the wedge pressure tracing, a left ventricular end-diastolic pressure should be obtained.

Acute vasodilator testing is often performed at the time of the initial right heart catheterization, not only for its prognostic implications but also to identify patients who might be candidates for therapy with calcium-channel blockers. Although the data regarding vasodilator testing and treatment with calcium-channel blockers are largely restricted to patients with idiopathic pulmonary arterial hypertension, vasodilator testing is often performed in patients with other types of pulmonary arterial hypertension. However, acute vasodilator testing is not indicated and may be harmful in patients with significantly elevated left heart filling pressures because pulmonary edema may ensue.

The three agents most commonly used for acute vasodilator testing in the cardiac catheterization laboratory are inhaled nitric oxide, intravenous epoprostenol, and intravenous adenosine. A positive response to an acute vasodilator is a decrease in mean pulmonary artery pressure by at least 10 mm Hg, to a mean pulmonary artery pressure of less than 40 mm Hg, without a decrease in cardiac output. If a patient meets these criteria, it is reasonable to administer a trial of oral calcium-channel blockers.

TREATMENT Rx

General Measures

Important goals of therapy in patients with pulmonary arterial hypertension include alleviation of symptoms, particularly dyspnea; improvement of functional capacity, which is often measured by the 6-minute walk test; and improvement of hemodynamics by lowering pulmonary artery pressure and increasing cardiac output. Another important goal of therapy is to reverse, or at least prevent, disease progression, often measured in clinical trials as hospitalization, escalation of therapy, and lung transplantation.

Patients are encouraged to engage in low-level graded aerobic exercise, such as walking, as tolerated. Patients are advised to avoid heavy physical exertion or isometric exercise because this may provoke exertional syncope. Exposure to high altitudes may contribute to hypoxic pulmonary vasoconstriction and may not be well tolerated. A sodium-restricted diet (<2400 mg/day) is advised and is particularly important to manage volume status in patients with right ventricular failure. Routine immunizations, such as those against influenza and pneumococcal pneumonia, are advised. Because hypoxia is a potent pulmonary vasoconstrictor, supplemental oxygen is recommended to maintain saturations above 90% at rest, with exertion, and during sleep. In patients with intracardiac shunting and Eisenmenger's physiology (Chapter 69), this goal may not be possible.

Patients with pulmonary arterial hypertension are advised against pregnancy because the hemodynamic fluctuations of pregnancy, labor, delivery, and the postpartum period are potentially life-threatening, with a 30 to 50% mortality rate in some series. Current guidelines recommend that pregnancy be avoided or terminated early in women with pulmonary arterial hypertension. Women of childbearing potential should be counseled on contraception options at the time of diagnosis.

For patients with idiopathic, heritable, anorexigen-induced, and connective tissue disease–associated pulmonary arterial hypertension (group 1 pulmonary arterial hypertension), clinical trial data can guide effective therapy (Fig. 68-7). For all other types of pulmonary hypertension, the safety and efficacy of pulmonary arterial hypertension–specific therapies have not been demonstrated, so treatment should instead be targeted at the underlying disease.

Treatment of the Underlying Conditions

The initial treatment should be directed at any underlying or associated conditions, especially lung disease, that also directly affect exercise tolerance and systemic diseases that have effective therapies. After these disorders have been optimally treated, specific therapy of the pulmonary arterial hypertension itself should be considered.

Background Therapy

In three uncontrolled observational series in patients with primarily idiopathic pulmonary arterial hypertension, warfarin coagulation improved survival. Consensus recommendations advocate the use of warfarin titrated to an INR of 1.5 to 2.5 in patients with idiopathic pulmonary arterial hypertension. Although no data are available to guide recommendations in patients with other types of pulmonary arterial hypertension, warfarin is generally recommended in patients with advanced disease and severe right heart failure, in the absence of contraindications. Diuretics (e.g., furosemide, initiated at 20 mg and titrated as needed) are indicated to manage right ventricular volume overload; in some patients, intravenous diuretics may be necessary. Serum electrolytes and renal function must be closely monitored. Digoxin, 0.125 to 0.25 mg/day, is sometimes used in patients with right ventricular failure and a low cardiac output and in patients with atrial arrhythmias, despite the paucity of data; if the patient experiences any evidence of digoxin toxicity, the drug should be discontinued because of the unfavorable risk-to-benefit ratio.

Vasodilator Therapy

Calcium-Channel Blockers

Approximately 7% of adult patients with idiopathic pulmonary arterial hypertension have a favorable response to acute vasodilator testing and excellent prognosis with calcium-channel blockers. Long-acting nifedipine, diltiazem, and amlodipine are the most commonly used calcium-channel blockers. Because of its potential negative inotropic effects, verapamil should be avoided. Patients must be followed closely for both the safety and efficacy of this therapy. If a patient who meets the definition of an acute response does not improve to WHO class I or II on calcium-channel blocker therapy, the patient should not be considered a chronic responder; alternative or additional pulmonary arterial hypertension specific therapy should be instituted.

Targeted Therapies

In clinical trials, intravenous epoprostenol improves functional class, exercise endurance, hemodynamics, and survival in patients with idiopathic pulmonary arterial hypertension,[1] and it also improves exercise tolerance and hemodynamics in patients with pulmonary arterial hypertension related to

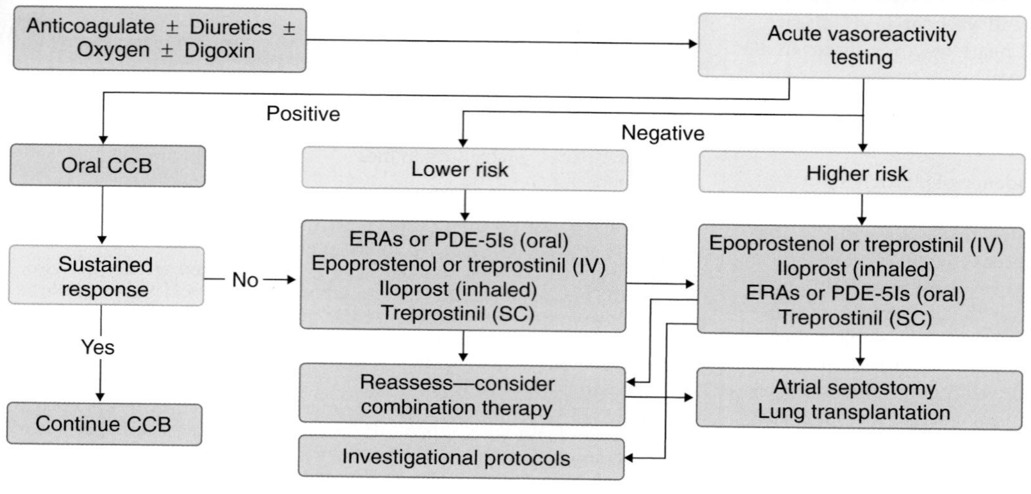

FIGURE 68-7. Pulmonary hypertension treatment algorithm. CCB = calcium-channel blocker; ERA = endothelin receptor antagonist; IV = intravenous; PDE-5I = phosphodiesterase type 5 inhibitor; SC = subcutaneous. (From McLaughlin VV, Archer SL, Badesch DB, et al. ACCF/AHA 2009 expert consensus document on pulmonary hypertension: a report of the American College of Cardiology Foundation Task Force on Expert Consensus Documents and the American Heart Association developed in collaboration with the American College of Chest Physicians; American Thoracic Society, Inc.; and the Pulmonary Hypertension Association. *J Am Coll Cardiol.* 2009; 53:1573-1619.)

the scleroderma spectrum of diseases.[2] Uncontrolled studies have also reported favorable effects with intravenous epoprostenol in patients with numerous forms of associated pulmonary arterial hypertension. Observational series suggest a long-term survival benefit with intravenous epoprostenol compared with historical controls. Epoprostenol must be delivered by continuous intravenous infusion, commonly initiated in the hospital at a dose of 2 ng/kg/minute, with the dose titrated up based on symptoms of pulmonary arterial hypertension and side effects of the therapy. Each patient must learn the techniques of sterile preparation of the medication, operation of the ambulatory infusion pump, and care of the central venous catheter. Although dosing must be highly individualized, maintenance doses in the range of 25 to 40 ng/kg/minute are typically needed for patients on monotherapy. Common side effects include headache, jaw pain, flushing, nausea, diarrhea, skin rash, and musculoskeletal pain. Infections and infusion interruption can be life-threatening.

Subcutaneous treprostinil can provide a modest but statistically significant improvement in exercise tolerance.[3] The main limitation of this therapy is pain and erythema at the site of the subcutaneous infusion, a complication that occurs in 85% of patients. Other prostanoid-type side effects, including headache, diarrhea, rash, and nausea, also occur. Subcutaneous treprostinil is often started in the home, with the dose titrated up based on symptoms of pulmonary arterial hypertension and drug side effects. Treprostinil is less potent than epoprostenol, and higher doses are required to achieve the desired efficacy. Inhaled treprostinil four times daily[4] and inhaled iloprost six to nine times daily[5] also are effective for improving exercise capacity. However, cough is an additional side effect with this method of administration.

The endothelin receptor antagonist bosentan (initiated orally at 62.5 mg twice daily and titrated up to 125 mg twice daily after 1 month) improves hemodynamics and exercise capacity and the clinical course of pulmonary arterial hypertension.[6,7] Ambrisentan (administered orally at doses of either 5 mg or 10 mg once daily) has similar benefits.[8] Liver enzymes must be monitored on a monthly basis; the dose should be reduced if liver enzymes rise to greater than three to five times the upper limits of normal and discontinued if they rise to five times the upper limit of normal. Other side effects include lower extremity edema, headache, and nasal congestion.

The chronic administration of inhaled nitric oxide is cumbersome and not clinically useful. However, the phosphodiesterase type 5 antagonists sildenafil and tadalafil are effective and useful for pulmonary arterial hypertension.[9,10] Sildenafil is approved at a dose of 20 mg three times daily and tadalafil at a dose of 40 mg once daily. The most common side effects of the phosphodiesterase inhibitors are headache, flushing, dyspepsia, and epistaxis.

Given the availability of therapies that target different pathologic processes, combination therapy is an attractive theoretical option in pulmonary arterial hypertension. Emerging data support the incremental benefit of combining more than one targeted therapy[4,11-12] under careful observation, usually in a specialized center.

Invasive Therapies

Despite advances in medical therapies for pulmonary arterial hypertension, many patients experience progressive functional decline, largely related to worsening right heart failure. In carefully selected patients, atrial septostomy may improve symptoms. Atrial septostomy creates a right-to-left interatrial shunt, thereby decreasing right heart filling pressures and improving right heart function and left heart filling. Although the right-to-left shunting decreases systemic arterial oxygen saturation, it is anticipated that the improvement in cardiac output will result in overall augmentation in systemic oxygen delivery. Contraindications to performing atrial septostomy include severe right ventricular failure on cardiorespiratory support, mean right atrial pressure of more than 20 mm Hg, pulmonary vascular resistance index of more than 55 U/m^2, resting oxygen saturation of less than 90% on room air, and left ventricular end-diastolic pressure of more than 18 mm Hg. Because of the high morbidity and mortality associated with this procedure, it should be performed only by experienced operators in specialized centers.

Bilateral lung (Chapter 101) or heart-lung transplantation (Chapter 82) is the final option for selected patients with pulmonary arterial hypertension when medical therapy fails. The 1-, 3-, 5-, and 10-year survival rates are 66%, 57%, 47%, and 27%, respectively, in patients with idiopathic pulmonary arterial hypertension who undergo transplantation. Transplantation as a potential therapeutic option should be discussed with selected patients at the time of diagnosis, although timing of referral is challenging. Patients who are otherwise good transplant candidates should be referred when they have an unacceptable response to medical therapies.

Assessing Response to Therapy

Given the complexity of the disease, the variable response to therapy, and the goal of optimizing and individualizing care, patients with pulmonary arterial hypertension must be followed closely. The usual recommendation is every 3 to 6 months in stable patients and every 1 to 3 months in patients with worsening or unstable symptoms or signs.

PROGNOSIS

Several clinical factors are correlated with prognosis (Table 68-3). The natural history of idiopathic pulmonary arterial hypertension is a median survival of 2.8 years with 1-, 3-, and 5-year survival rates of 68%, 48%, and 34%, respectively. Patients with pulmonary arterial hypertension related to the scleroderma spectrum of diseases tend to have a poorer prognosis than those with idiopathic pulmonary arterial hypertension, whereas patients with pulmonary arterial hypertension related to congenital heart disease tend to have a better prognosis, perhaps because they have better right ventricular function. Observational series suggest survival benefits for modern treatments, including epoprostenol, treprostinil, bosentan, and ambrisentan, but data are limited. Nevertheless, studies have demonstrated the 1-year survival on current medical therapy to be in the 85 to 88% range.

The natural history of patients with groups 2 and 3 pulmonary hypertension are influenced by their left heart and lung disease. In most cases, the presence of pulmonary hypertension in addition to the underlying disease portends a poor prognosis.

TABLE 68-3 PULMONARY ARTERIAL HYPERTENSION: DETERMINANTS OF PROGNOSIS*

DETERMINANTS OF RISK	LOWER RISK (GOOD PROGNOSIS)	HIGHER RISK (POOR PROGNOSIS)
Clinical evidence of RV failure	No	Yes
Progression of symptoms	Gradual	Rapid
WHO class†	II, III	IV
6-MW test‡	Longer (>400 m)	Shorter (<300 m)
CPET	Peak Vo_2 > 10.4 mL/kg/min	Peak Vo_2 < 10.4 mL/kg/min
Echocardiography	Minimal RV dysfunction	Pericardial effusion, significant RV enlargement or dysfunction, right atrial enlargement
Hemodynamics	RAP < 10 mm Hg, CI > 2.5 L/min/m^2	RAP > 20 mm Hg, CI < 2.0 L/min/m^2
BNP§	Minimally elevated	Significantly elevated

*Most data available pertain to idiopathic pulmonary arterial hypertension. Few data are available for other forms of PAH. One should not rely on any single factor to make risk predictions.
†WHO class is the functional classification for PAH and is a modification of the New York Heart Association functional class.
‡6-MW test is also influenced by age, gender, and height.
§Because there are currently limited data regarding the influence of BNP on prognosis, and many factors including renal function, weight, age, and gender may influence BNP, absolute numbers are not given for this variable.
6-MW = 6-minute walk; BNP = brain natriuretic peptide; CI = cardiac index; CPET = cardiopulmonary exercise testing; peak Vo_2 = average peak oxygen uptake during exercise; RAP = right atrial pressure; RV = right ventricle; WHO = World Health Organization.
From McLaughlin VV, Archer SL, Badesch DB, et al. ACCF/AHA 2009 expert consensus document on pulmonary hypertension: a report of the American College of Cardiology Foundation Task Force on Expert Consensus Documents and the American Heart Association developed in collaboration with the American College of Chest Physicians; American Thoracic Society, Inc.; and the Pulmonary Hypertension Association. *J Am Coll Cardiol.* 2009;53:1573-1619.

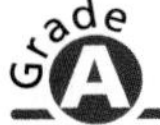

1. Barst RJ, Rubin LJ, Long WA, et al. A comparison of continuous intravenous epoprostenol (prostacyclin) with conventional therapy for primary pulmonary hypertension. *N Engl J Med.* 1996;334:296-301.
2. Badesch DB, Tapson VF, McGoon MD, et al. Continuous intravenous epoprostenol for pulmonary hypertension due to the scleroderma spectrum of disease: a randomized, controlled trial. *Ann Intern Med.* 2000;132:425-434.
3. Simonneau G, Barst RJ, Galiè N, et al. Continuous subcutaneous infusion of treprostinil, a prostacyclin analogue, in patients with pulmonary arterial hypertension. *Am J Respir Crit Care Med.* 2002;165:800-804.
4. McLaughlin VV, Benza RL, Rubin LJ, et al. Addition of inhaled treprostinil to oral therapy for pulmonary arterial hypertension: a randomized controlled clinical trial. *J Am Coll Cardiol.* 2010; 55:1915-1922.
5. Olschewski H, Simonneau G, Galiè N, et al. Inhaled iloprost for severe pulmonary hypertension. *N Engl J Med.* 2002;347:322-329.
6. Channick RN, Simonneau G, Sitbon O, et al. Effects of the dual endothelin-receptor antagonist bosentan in patients with pulmonary hypertension: a randomised placebo-controlled study. *Lancet.* 2001;358:1119-1123.
7. Rubin LJ, Badesch DB, Barst RJ, et al. Bosentan therapy for pulmonary arterial hypertension. *N Engl J Med.* 2002;346:896-903.
8. Galiè N, Olschewski H, Oudiz R, et al. Ambrisentan for the treatment of pulmonary arterial hypertension: results of the ambrisentan in pulmonary arterial hypertension, randomized, double-blind, placebo-controlled, multicenter, efficacy (ARIES) study 1 and 2. *Circulation.* 2008;117:3010-3019.
9. Galiè N, Ghofrani HA, Torbicki A, et al. Sildenafil citrate therapy for pulmonary arterial hypertension. *N Engl J Med.* 2005;353:2148-2157.
10. Galiè N, Brundage BH, Ghofrani HA, et al. Tadalafil therapy for pulmonary arterial hypertension. *Circulation.* 2009;119:2894-2903.
11. McLaughlin VV, Oudiz RJ, Adaani F, et al. Randomized study of adding inhaled iloprost to existing bosentan in pulmonary arterial hypertension. *Am J Respir Crit Care Med.* 2006;174:1257-1263.
12. Simonneau G, Rubin LJ, Galiè N, et al. Addition of sildenafil to long-term intravenous epoprostenol therapy in patients with pulmonary arterial hypertension: a randomized trial. *Ann Intern Med.* 2008;149:521-530.

SUGGESTED READINGS

Humbert M, Sitbon O, Chaouat A, et al. Survival in patients with idiopathic, familial, and anorexigen-associated pulmonary arterial hypertension in the modern management era. *Circulation.* 2010;122:156-163. *Estimated survivals are 86% at 1 year, 70% at 2 years, and 55% at 3 years.*

Kaw R, Pasupuleti V, Deshpande A, et al. Pulmonary hypertension: an important predictor of outcomes in patients undergoing non-cardiac surgery. *Respir Med.* 2011;105:619-624. *Mean pulmonary arterial pressure is an independent predictor of post-operative morbidity.*

McLaughlin VV, Archer SL, Badesch DB, et al. ACCF/AHA 2009 expert consensus document on pulmonary hypertension: a report of the American College of Cardiology Foundation Task Force on Expert Consensus Documents and the American Heart Association developed in collaboration with the American College of Chest Physicians; American Thoracic Society, Inc.; and the Pulmonary Hypertension Association. *J Am Coll Cardiol.* 2009;53:1573-1619. *Expert consensus document.*

Nef HM, Möllmann H, Hamm C, et al. Pulmonary hypertension: updated classification and management of pulmonary hypertension. *Heart.* 2010;96:552-559. *Review.*

69

CONGENITAL HEART DISEASE IN ADULTS

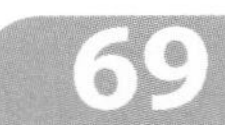

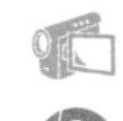

ARIANE J. MARELLI

The convergence of major progress in medicine, pediatrics, and cardiovascular surgery has resulted in the survival of an increasingly large number of adult patients with congenital heart disease. Adult physicians are becoming increasingly responsible for these patients, commonly in concert with a cardiologist and a tertiary care facility.

DEFINITIONS

Patients can be divided into three categories according to the surgical status: unoperated, surgically palliated, or physiologically repaired. Congenital heart lesions can be classified as *acyanotic* or *cyanotic*. *Cyanosis* refers to a blue discoloration of the mucous membranes resulting from an increased amount of reduced hemoglobin. Central cyanosis occurs when the circulation is mixed because of a right-to-left shunt.

A *native lesion* refers to an anatomic lesion present at birth. Acquired lesions, naturally occurring or as a result of surgery, are superimposed on the native anatomy. *Palliative* interventions are performed in patients with cyanotic lesions and are defined as operations that either increase or decrease pulmonary blood flow while allowing a mixed circulation and cyanosis to persist (Table 69-1). *Physiologic* repair applies to procedures that provide total or nearly total anatomic and physiologic separation of the pulmonary and systemic circulations in complex cyanotic lesions and result in patients who are acyanotic.

Eisenmenger's complex refers to flow reversal across a ventricular septal defect (VSD) when pulmonary vascular resistance exceeds systemic levels. *Eisenmenger's physiology* designates the physiologic response in a broader category of shunt lesions in which a right-to-left shunt occurs in response to an elevation in pulmonary vascular resistance. *Eisenmenger's syndrome* is a term applied to common clinical features shared by patients with Eisenmenger's physiology.

Each congenital lesion can influence the course of another. For example, the physiologic consequences of a VSD are different if it occurs in isolation or in combination with pulmonary stenosis. A *simple lesion* is defined as either a shunt lesion or an obstructive lesion of the right or left heart occurring in isolation. A *complex lesion* is a combination of two or more abnormalities.

EPIDEMIOLOGY

Genetic Determinants

In 90% of patients, congenital heart disease is attributable to multifactorial inheritance; only 5 to 10% of malformations are due to primary genetic factors, either chromosomal or related to a single mutant gene. The most common defect observed in patients with chromosomal aberrations is a VSD, which occurs in 90% of patients with trisomy 13 and trisomy 18. Defects of the endocardial cushions and the ventricular septum are found in 50% of patients with Down syndrome (trisomy 21). The most frequently observed defects in patients with Turner's syndrome (45,X) are aortic coarctation, aortic stenosis, and atrial septal defect (ASD). About 15% of patients with tetralogy of Fallot have a deletion on chromosome 22q11; prevalence is higher in those with a right aortic arch. Abnormalities involving the chromosomal band 22q11 can also result in a group of syndromes, the most common of which is DiGeorge syndrome. The shared phenotypic features are designated CATCH-22 syndromes, that is, a combination of cardiac defects, abnormal facies, thymic hypoplasia, cleft palate, and hypocalcemia. The

TABLE 69-1 PALLIATIVE SURGICAL SHUNTS FOR CONGENITAL HEART LESIONS

PALLIATIVE SHUNT	ANASTOMOSIS
SYSTEMIC ARTERIAL TO PULMONARY ARTERY SHUNTS	
Classic Blalock-Taussig	Subclavian artery to PA
Modified Blalock-Taussig	Subclavian artery to PA (prosthetic graft)
Potts anastomosis	Descending aorta to left PA
Waterston shunt	Ascending aorta to right PA
SYSTEMIC VENOUS TO PULMONARY ARTERY SHUNTS	
Classic Glenn	SVC to right PA
Bidirectional Glenn	SVC to right and left PA
Bilateral Glenn	Right and left SVC to right and left PA

PA = pulmonary artery; SVC = superior vena cava.
From Marelli A, Mullen M. Palliative surgical shunts for congenital heart lesions. *Clin Paediatr.* 1996;4:189.

recurrence risk for families with a child who carries a congenital cardiac malformation due to a chromosomal anomaly is related to the recurrence risk of the chromosomal anomaly itself.

Typically, single mutant genes are also associated with syndromes of cardiovascular malformations, although not every patient with the syndrome has the characteristic cardiac anomaly. Examples include osteogenesis imperfecta (autosomal recessive), associated with aortic valve disease; Jervell and Lange-Nielsen syndrome (autosomal recessive) and Romano-Ward syndrome (autosomal dominant), associated with a prolonged QT interval and sudden death; and Holt-Oram syndrome (autosomal dominant), in which an ASD occurs with a range of other skeletal anomalies. Osler-Weber-Rendu telangiectasias are associated with pulmonary arteriovenous fistulas. Williams syndrome occurs with supravalvular aortic stenosis in most cases. Noonan's syndrome is associated with pulmonary stenosis, ASD, and hypertrophic cardiomyopathy. Although autosomal dominant inheritance has been implicated for both, most cases are sporadic. Deletion at chromosome 7q11.23 has been identified in patients with Williams syndrome, and a gene defect has been mapped to 12q22-qter in patients with Noonan's syndrome.

The risk for recurrence when the mother carries a sporadically occurring congenital lesion varies from 2.5 to 18%, depending on the lesion. Obstructive lesions of the left ventricular outflow tract have the highest recurrence rates in offspring. When the father carries the lesion, 1.5 to 3% of the offspring are affected. When a sibling has a congenital cardiac anomaly, the risk for recurrence in another sibling varies from 1 to 3%.

Incidence and Prevalence

Cardiac malformations occur at a rate of 8 per 1000 live births, or 32,000 infants with new diagnoses yearly in the United States. The prevalence of congenital heart disease has increased in the general population, with the steepest rise observed in adults with severe or complex lesions. An estimated 20% die in the first year of life—a substantial decrease from the late 1960s. An overall prevalence of 4 per 1000 adults has been documented. The median age of patients with severe lesions has increased from childhood to late adolescence. Currently, more than 1 million patients are thought to be alive in the United States with congenital heart disease.

Bicuspid aortic valve occurs in about 2% of the general population, is the most common congenital cardiac anomaly encountered in adult populations, and accounts for up to half of surgical cases of aortic stenosis in adults (Chapter 75). ASDs constitute 30 to 40% of cases of congenital heart disease in adults, with ostium secundum ASD accounting for 7% of all congenital lesions. A solitary VSD represents 15 to 20% of all congenital lesions and is the most common congenital cardiac lesion observed in children; its high spontaneous closure rates explain the lesser prevalence in adults. Patent ductus arteriosus (PDA) accounts for 5 to 10% of all congenital cardiac lesions in infants with a normal birthweight. Pulmonary stenosis and coarctation of the aorta represent 3 to 10% of all congenital lesions.

Tetralogy of Fallot is the most common cyanotic congenital anomaly observed in adults. Together with complete transposition of the great arteries, these lesions account for 5 to 12% of congenital heart disease in infants. More complex lesions such as tricuspid atresia, univentricular heart, congenitally corrected transposition of the great arteries, Ebstein's anomaly, and double-outlet right ventricle account for 2.5% or less of all congenital heart disease.

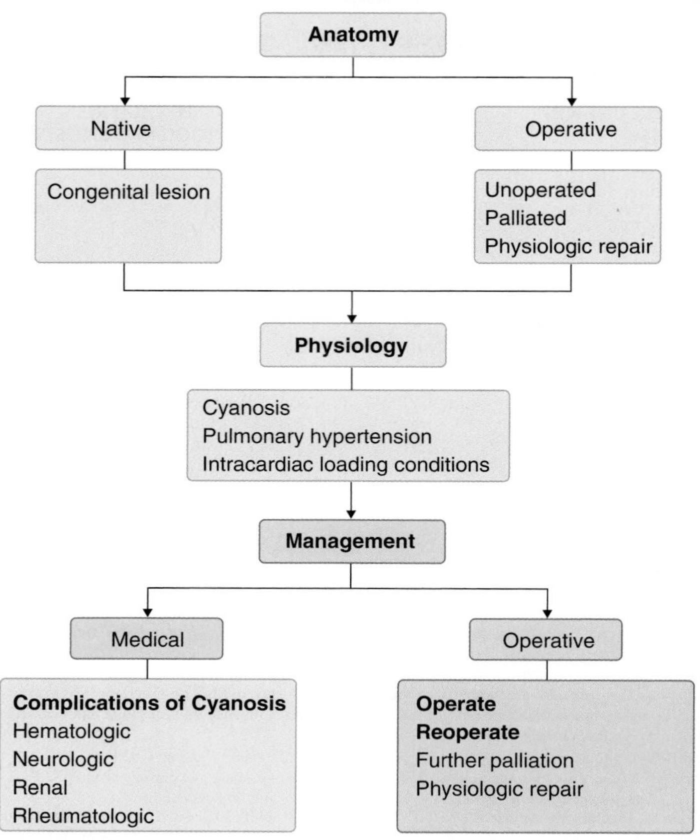

FIGURE 69-1. The goals of complete clinical assessment in congenital heart disease are to define the anatomy and physiology to determine appropriate management.

CLINICAL MANIFESTATIONS

Congenital heart disease is a lifelong condition during which the patient and the lesion evolve concurrently. A patient may have been monitored for many years because of an erroneous diagnosis made in infancy or childhood when diagnostic techniques were more limited. The differential diagnosis of native and surgical anatomy in the adult with an unknown diagnosis depends on whether the patient is cyanotic or acyanotic. On completion of the evaluation, the following questions should be answered (Fig. 69-1): What is the native anatomy? Has this patient undergone surgery for the condition? What is the physiology? What can and should be done for this patient both medically and surgically, and importantly, who should do it?

If the patient has not undergone surgery, the question is, Why not? If the patient is palliated, has the degree of cyanosis progressed as evidenced by a drop in systemic saturation or a rise in hemoglobin? If the patient has undergone a physiologic repair, what procedure was performed? Are residual lesions present, and have new lesions developed as a consequence of surgery? The patient's physiology is determined by the presence or absence of cyanosis, pulmonary hypertension, adequate filling of the cardiac chambers, and any resulting medical complications.

A clinical assessment, 12-lead electrocardiogram (ECG), chest radiograph, and baseline oxygen saturation should be part of every initial assessment. Two-dimensional transthoracic echocardiography (Chapter 55) and Doppler and color flow imaging are used to establish the diagnosis and to monitor the evolution of documented hemodynamic complications. Transesophageal echocardiographic examination is particularly useful in adults and is increasingly important during interventional catheter-guided therapy and surgery. Magnetic resonance imaging (Chapter 56) and computed tomography (Chapter 56) are useful adjuncts. Cardiac catheterization for congenital heart disease has shifted from pure diagnosis to include intervention. Coronary arteriography is recommended for adults older than 40 years in whom surgical intervention is contemplated.

Pulmonary Hypertension and Its Complications

Pulmonary hypertension secondary to structural disease of the heart or circulation can occur with or without an increase in pulmonary vascular resistance. Pulmonary vascular obstructive disease occurs when pulmonary vascular resistance rises and becomes fixed and irreversible. In the most common congenital anomalies, pulmonary hypertension is a result of increased pulmonary blood flow because of a native left-to-right shunt. Examples include ASD, a moderately sized VSD, PDA, and a variety of complex lesions. The rate at which pulmonary hypertension progresses to become pulmonary vascular obstructive disease varies from one lesion to another and depends at least in part on the source of pulmonary blood flow. Pulmonary hypertension typically develops in patients with an ASD after the fourth decade; Eisenmenger's syndrome is a late complication seen in only 5 to 10% of cases. In contrast, in patients with a large VSD or persistent PDA, progressive elevation in pulmonary vascular resistance occurs rapidly because the pulmonary vascular bed is exposed not only to the excess volume of the left-to-right shunt but also to systemic arterial pressures. As a result, Eisenmenger's complex develops in approximately 10% of patients with a large VSD during the first decade. Surgical pulmonary artery banding is a palliative measure aimed at decreasing pulmonary blood flow and protecting the pulmonary vascular bed against the development of early pulmonary vascular obstructive disease.

If forward flow from the right side of the heart is insufficient, native collaterals or surgical shunts provide an alternative source of pulmonary blood flow (see Table 69-1). With large surgical shunts, however, direct exposure of the pulmonary vascular bed to the high pressures of the systemic circulation causes pulmonary vascular obstructive disease. As a result, systemic to pulmonary arterial shunts are currently less favored in neonates and infants, in whom systemic venous to pulmonary arterial shunts are now preferred.

The term *Eisenmenger's syndrome* should be reserved for patients in whom pulmonary vascular obstructive disease is present and pulmonary vascular resistance is fixed and irreversible. These findings, in combination with the absence of left-to-right shunting, render the patient inoperable.

The clinical manifestations of Eisenmenger's syndrome include dyspnea on exertion, syncope, chest pain, congestive heart failure, and symptoms related to erythrocytosis and hyperviscosity. On physical examination, central cyanosis and digital clubbing are hallmark findings. Systemic oxygen saturations typically vary between 75 and 85%. The pulse pressure narrows as the cardiac output falls. Examination of jugular venous pressure can reveal a dominant a wave reflecting a noncompliant right ventricle until tricuspid insufficiency is severe enough to generate a large v wave. A prominent right ventricular impulse is felt in the left parasternal border in end expiration or in the subcostal area in end inspiration. A palpable pulmonary artery is commonly felt. The pulmonary component of the second heart sound is increased and can be felt in most cases. Pulmonary ejection sounds are common when the pulmonary artery is dilated with a structurally normal valve. Right atrial gallop is heard more frequently when the a wave is dominant. A murmur of tricuspid insufficiency is common, but the inspiratory increase in the murmur (Carvallo's sign) disappears when right ventricular failure occurs. In diastole, a pulmonary insufficiency murmur is often heard. The 12-lead ECG shows evidence of right atrial enlargement, right ventricular hypertrophy, and right axis deviation. Chest radiographic findings include a dilated pulmonary artery segment, cardiac enlargement, and diminished pulmonary vascular markings. Echocardiography confirms the right-sided pressure overload and pulmonary artery enlargement as well as the tricuspid and pulmonary insufficiency. Cardiac catheterization is indicated if doubt exists about the potential reversibility of the elevated pulmonary vascular resistance in a patient who might otherwise benefit from surgery.

Cyanosis occurs when persistent venous to arterial mixing results in hypoxemia. Adaptive mechanisms to increase oxygen delivery include an increase in oxygen content, a rightward shift in the oxyhemoglobin dissociation curve, a higher hematocrit, and an increase in cardiac output. When cyanosis is not relieved, chronic hypoxemia and erythrocytosis result in hematologic, neurologic, renal, and rheumatic complications.

Hematologic complications of chronic hypoxemia include erythrocytosis, iron deficiency, and bleeding diathesis. Hemoglobin and hematocrit levels, as well as red blood cell indices, should be checked regularly and correlated with systemic oxygen saturation levels. Symptoms of hyperviscosity include headaches, faintness, dizziness, fatigue, altered mentation, visual disturbances, paresthesias, tinnitus, and myalgia. Symptoms are classified as mild to moderate when they interfere with only some activities, or they can be marked to severe and interfere with most or all activities. Patients with compensated erythrocytosis establish an equilibrium hematocrit at higher levels in an iron-replete state with minimal symptoms. Patients with decompensated erythrocytosis manifest unstable, rising hematocrit levels and experience severe hyperviscosity symptoms.

Hemostatic abnormalities can occur in up to 20% of cyanotic patients with erythrocytosis. Bleeding is usually mild and superficial and leads to easy bruising, skin petechiae, or mucosal bleeding, but epistaxis, hemoptysis, or even life-threatening postoperative bleeding can occur. A variety of clotting factor deficiencies and qualitative and quantitative platelet disorders have been described.

Neurologic complications, including cerebral hemorrhage, can be caused by hemostatic defects and are most often seen after inappropriate use of anticoagulant therapy. Patients with right-to-left shunts may be at risk for paradoxical cerebral emboli. Focal brain injury may provide a nidus for brain abscess if bacteremia supervenes. Attention should be paid to the use of air filters in peripheral intravenous lines to avoid paradoxical emboli through a right-to-left shunt.

Prophylactic phlebotomy has no place in the prevention of cerebral arterial thrombosis. Indications for phlebotomy are the occurrence of symptomatic hyperviscosity in an iron-repleted patient and prevention of excessive bleeding perioperatively.

Pulmonary complications include massive pulmonary hemorrhage and in situ arterial thrombosis. A rapid clinical deterioration associated with progressive hypoxemia often marks the terminal stage of disease. No clear benefits are observed with the use of anticoagulants (systemic or intrapulmonary) because of the risk for prolonged bleeding due to the underlying coagulopathy. The chronic disease process and high mortality prohibit pulmonary endarterectomy.

Renal dysfunction can be manifested as proteinuria, hyperuricemia, or renal failure. Focal interstitial fibrosis, tubular atrophy, and hyalinization of afferent and efferent arterioles can be seen on renal biopsy. Increased blood viscosity and arteriolar vasoconstriction can lead to renal hypoperfusion with progressive glomerulosclerosis. Hyperuricemia is commonly seen in patients with cyanotic congenital heart disease and is thought to be due mainly to the decreased reabsorption of uric acid rather than overproduction from erythrocytosis. Asymptomatic hyperuricemia need not be treated because lowering of uric acid levels has not been shown to prevent renal disease or gout.

Rheumatologic complications include gout and hypertrophic osteoarthropathy, which is thought to be responsible for the arthralgias affecting up to one third of patients with cyanotic congenital heart disease. In patients with right-to-left shunting, megakaryocytes released from the bone marrow bypass the lung and are entrapped in systemic arterioles and capillaries, where they release platelet-derived growth factor, which promotes local cell proliferation. Digital clubbing and new osseous formation with periostitis occur and cause the symptoms of arthralgia. Symptomatic hyperuricemia and gouty arthritis can be treated as necessary with colchicine, probenecid, or allopurinol; nonsteroidal anti-inflammatory drugs are best avoided, given the baseline hemostatic anomalies in these patients.

TREATMENT Rx

In patients with Eisenmenger's syndrome, bosentan (62.5 mg twice daily for 4 weeks, then 125 mg twice daily) improves hemodynamics and exercise capacity for at least 40 weeks. 1 Chronic oxygen therapy is unlikely to benefit hypoxemia secondary to right-to-left shunting in the setting of a fixed pulmonary vascular resistance. Chronic oxygen therapy results in mucosal dehydration with an increased incidence of epistaxis and is therefore not recommended.

In the iron-replete state, moderate to severe hyperviscosity symptoms typically occur when hematocrit levels exceed 65%. If no evidence of dehydration is present, removal of 500 mL of blood during a 30- to 45-minute period should be followed by quantitative volume replacement with normal saline or dextran (Fig. 69-2). The procedure may be repeated every 24 hours until symptomatic improvement occurs.

Treatment of spontaneous bleeding is dictated by its severity and the abnormal hemostatic parameters (Fig. 69-3). For severe bleeding, platelet transfusions, fresh-frozen plasma, vitamin K, cryoprecipitate, and desmopressin have been used. Reduction in erythrocyte mass also improves hemostasis, so cyanotic patients undergoing surgery should have prophylactic phlebotomy if the hematocrit is greater than 65%.

Iron deficiency is common in cyanotic adult patients because of excessive bleeding or phlebotomy. In contrast to normocytic erythrocytosis, which is rarely symptomatic at hematocrit levels less than 65%, iron deficiency may manifest with hyperviscosity symptoms at hematocrit levels well below 65%. The treatment of choice is not phlebotomy but oral iron repletion until a rise in hematocrit is detected, typically within 1 week.

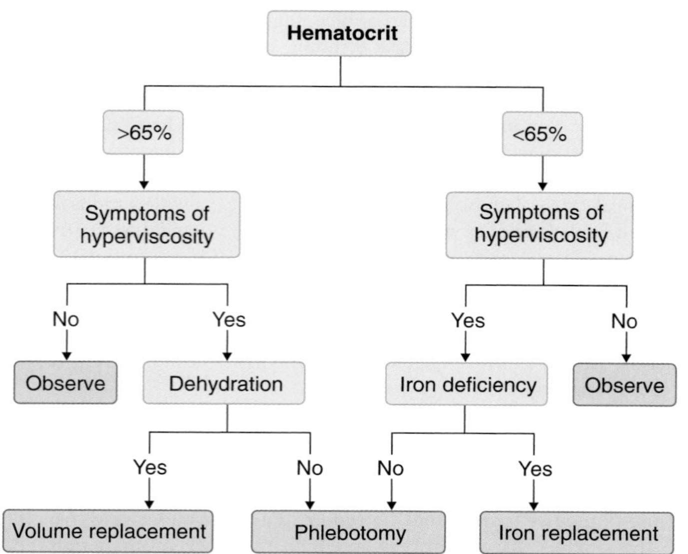

FIGURE 69-2. Treatment algorithm for erythrocytosis of cyanotic congenital heart disease.

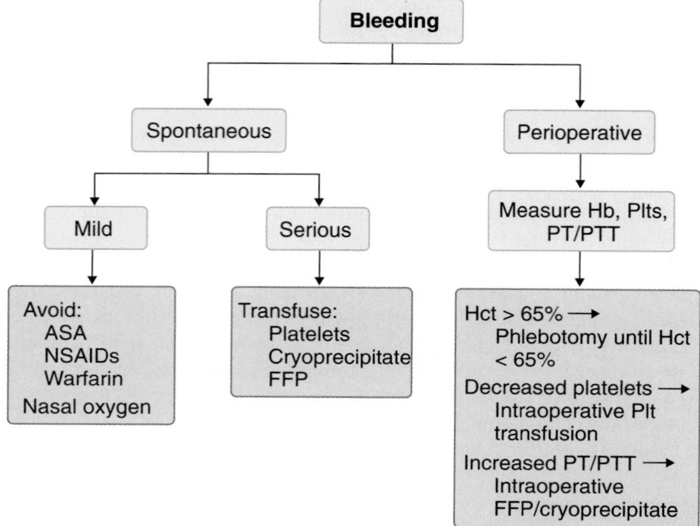

FIGURE 69-3. Treatment algorithm for bleeding diathesis of cyanotic congenital heart disease. ASA = acetylsalicylic acid; FFP = fresh-frozen plasma; Hb = hemoglobin; Hct = hematocrit; NSAIDs = nonsteroidal anti-inflammatory drugs; Plts = platelets; PT = prothrombin time; PTT = partial thromboplastin time.

SIMPLE LESIONS

Isolated Shunt Lesions

Hemodynamic complications of significant shunts relate to volume overload and chamber dilation of the primary chamber receiving the excess left-to-right shunt and to secondary complications of valvular dysfunction and damage to the pulmonary vascular bed. The size and duration of the shunt determine the clinical course and therefore the indications for closure. The degree of shunting is a function of both the size of the communication and, depending on its location, biventricular compliance or pulmonary and systemic vascular resistance. Clinically apparent hemodynamic sequelae of shunts are typically apparent or can be expected to occur when pulmonary to systemic flow ratios exceed 1.5:1.

Shunt size can be inferred and measured with cardiac ultrasonography. Secondary enlargement of the cardiac chambers receiving excess shunt flow in diastole occurs as the shunt size becomes hemodynamically significant; in addition, the pulmonary artery becomes enlarged as pulmonary pressure rises. When tricuspid insufficiency occurs primarily from right ventricular dilation or secondary to pulmonary hypertension, the regurgitant jet can be used to estimate the pulmonary pressure as another indicator of shunt significance. When the pulmonary to systemic flow ($\dot{Q}:\dot{Q}$) exceeds 2:1, the volume of blood in both circulations can be estimated by comparing the stroke volume at the pulmonary and aortic valves. Shunt detection and quantification can also be obtained by a first-pass radionuclide study. As a bolus of radioactive substance is injected into the systemic circulation, the rise and fall of radionuclide activity can be measured in the lungs. When a shunt is significant, the rate of persistent activity in the lungs over time can be used to calculate the shunt fraction. For both echocardiographic and radionuclide quantification of shunt size, sources of error are multiple. The most predictable results are obtained only in experienced laboratories. Uncertainty about the physiologic significance of a borderline shunt can be minimized by integrating serial determinations from multiple clinical and relevant diagnostic sources rather than basing management decisions on a single calculated shunt value.

Atrial Septal Defect

Classification of ASDs is based on anatomic location. Most commonly, an ostium secundum ASD occurs in the central portion of the interatrial septum as a result of an enlarged foramen ovale or excessive resorption of the septum primum. The combination of a secundum ASD and acquired mitral stenosis is known as *Lutembacher's syndrome,* the pathophysiology of which is determined by the relative severity of each. Abnormal development of the embryologic endocardial cushions results in a variety of atrioventricular canal defects, the most common of which consists of a defect in the lower part of the atrial septum in the ostium primum location, typically accompanied by a cleft mitral valve and mitral regurgitation. The sinus venosus defect, which accounts for 2 to 3% of all interatrial communications, is located superiorly at the junction of the superior vena cava and right atrium and is generally associated with anomalous drainage of the right-sided pulmonary veins into the superior vena cava or right atrium. Less commonly, interatrial communications can be seen at the site of the coronary sinus, typically associated with an anomalous left superior vena cava.

The pathophysiology is determined by the effects of the shunt on the heart and pulmonary circulation. Right atrial and right ventricular dilation occurs as shunt size increases with pulmonary to systemic flow ratios greater than 1.5:1. Superimposed systemic hypertension and coronary artery disease modify left ventricular compliance and favor left-to-right shunting. Mitral valve disease can occur in up to 15% of patients older than 50 years. Right-sided heart failure, atrial fibrillation, or atrial flutter can occur as a result of chronic right-sided volume overload and progressive ventricular and atrial dilation. Stroke can result from paradoxical emboli, atrial arrhythmias, or both. A rise in pulmonary pressure occurs because of the increased pulmonary blood flow. Pulmonary hypertension is unusual before 20 years of age but is seen in 50% of patients older than 40 years. The overall incidence of pulmonary vascular obstructive disease is 15 to 20% in patients with ASD. Eisenmenger's disease with reverse shunting, a late and rare complication of isolated secundum ASD, is reported in 5 to 10% of patients.

DIAGNOSIS

Although most patients are minimally symptomatic in the first three decades, more than 70% become impaired by the fifth decade. Initial symptoms include exercise intolerance, dyspnea on exertion, and fatigue caused most commonly by right-sided heart failure and pulmonary hypertension. Palpitations, syncope, and stroke can occur with the development of atrial arrhythmias.

On physical examination, most adults have a normal general physical appearance. When Holt-Oram syndrome is present, the thumb may have a third phalanx or may be rudimentary or absent. With an uncomplicated nonrestrictive communication between both atria, the a and v waves are equal in amplitude. Precordial palpation typically discloses a normal left ventricular impulse unless mitral valve disease occurs. Characteristically, if the shunt is significant, a right ventricular impulse can be felt in the left parasternal area in end expiration or in the subxiphoid area in end inspiration. A dilated pulmonary artery can sometimes be felt in the second left intercostal space. On auscultation, the hallmark of an ASD is the wide and fixed splitting of the second heart sound. Pulmonary valve closure, as reflected by P_2, is delayed because of right ventricular overload and the increased capacitance of the pulmonary vascular bed. The A_2-P_2 interval is fixed because the increase in venous return elevates the right atrial pressure during inspiration, thereby decreasing the degree of left-to-right shunting and offsetting the usual phasic respiratory changes. In addition, compliance of the pulmonary circulation is reduced from the high flow, thus making the vascular compartment less susceptible to any further increase in blood flow. A soft midsystolic murmur generated by the increased flow across the pulmonary valve is usually heard in the second left interspace. In the presence of a high left-to-right shunt volume, increased flow across the tricuspid valve is heard as a mid-diastolic murmur at the lower left sternal border. With advanced right-sided heart failure, evidence of systemic venous congestion is present.

The ECG characteristically shows an incomplete right bundle branch block pattern (Fig. 69-4). Right axis deviation and atrial abnormalities, including a prolonged PR interval, atrial fibrillation, and flutter, are also seen. Typically, the chest radiograph shows pulmonary vascular plethora with increased markings in both lung fields consistent with increased pulmonary blood flow (see Fig. 53-13 in Chapter 53). The main pulmonary artery and both its branches are dilated. Right atrial and right ventricular dilation can be seen. Cardiac ultrasonography is diagnostic and provides important prognostic information (Fig. 69-5). Ostium primum and secundum ASDs are easily identifiable with transthoracic imaging, but a sinus venosus ASD can be missed unless it is specifically sought. For more accurate visualization of the superior interatrial septum and localization of the pulmonary veins, transesophageal echocardiography is useful. With Doppler study, pulmonary artery pressures can be quantified, and the $\dot{Q}:\dot{Q}$ can be measured.

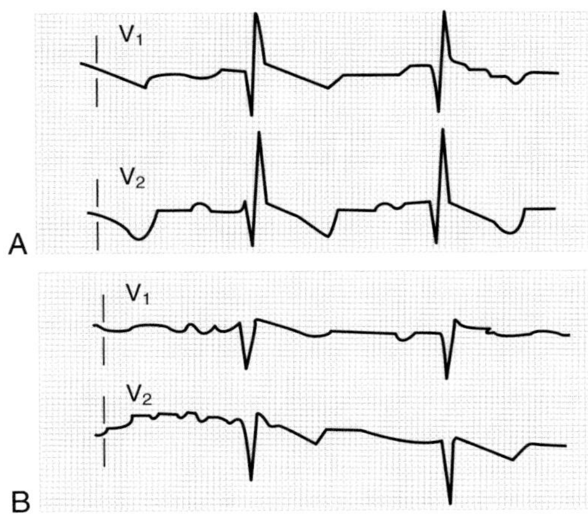

FIGURE 69-4. Electrocardiographic hallmark in atrial septal defect. Right precordial leads V_1 and V_2 illustrate two variants of an incomplete right bundle branch block pattern, the rSrT pattern (**A**) and the rsR′ pattern (**B**).

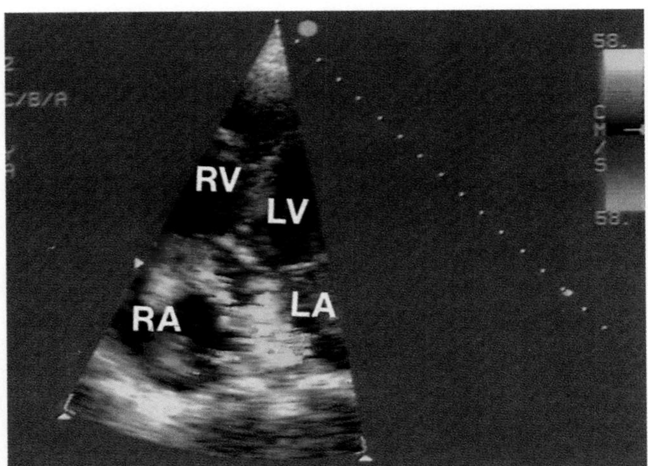

FIGURE 69-5. Color flow Doppler apical four-chamber view showing blood flow from the left atrium (LA) to the right atrium (RA) through a moderately sized atrial septal defect. LV = left ventricle; RV = right ventricle. (From Forbes CD, Jackson WF. *Color Atlas and Text of Clinical Medicine,* 3rd ed. London: Mosby; 2003.)

TREATMENT Rx

Closure of an ASD either percutaneously or surgically is indicated in the presence of right heart enlargement, with or without symptoms. Centrally located defects measuring up to 3.5 cm can be occluded by transcatheter techniques in a cardiac catheterization laboratory. Advantages of this approach include the avoidance of sternotomy and cardiopulmonary bypass. Uncomplicated secundum ASDs may be closed surgically in children and adults with minimal operative mortality, although surgical closure is usually reserved for patients in whom concomitant repair of associated valvular anomalies is required, anomalous pulmonary veins are present, or device closure is not technically feasible.

In patients older than 40 years with symptoms and significant shunts, closure improves functional status and survival. [2] In the presence of a significant shunt, closure of an ASD before 25 years of age without evidence of pulmonary hypertension results in a long-term outcome that is similar to that of age- and sex-matched controls. Advanced age (60 years) is not a contraindication to ASD closure in the presence of a significant shunt because a significant number of patients will show evidence of symptomatic improvement. Preoperative pulmonary artery pressure and the presence or absence of pulmonary vascular disease are important predictors of successful interventional outcome.

Patent Foramen Ovale

Integrity of the fetal circulation depends on the patency of the foramen ovale. In most cases, the fall in pulmonary vascular resistance at birth induces the foramen to become sealed. Necropsy studies have revealed that the foramen ovale remains patent beyond the first year of life in about 30% of individuals, and clinical studies have demonstrated that the prevalence of patent foramen ovale is three times greater in patients with cryptogenic stroke (Chapter 414), particularly before the age of 55 years, because of right-to-left shunting and paradoxical embolization of material from the venous circulation. Cardiac investigation of the patient with cryptogenic stroke includes transesophageal echocardiography with agitated saline injection to visualize the presence of a right-to-left shunt (Chapter 55). Patent foramen ovale most likely to result in future paradoxical embolization is found in patients younger than 55 years with a prior cryptogenic stroke, in association with a hypermobile septum with aneurysm formation, and when a significant amount of right-to-left shunting is present at rest without provocative maneuvers. Some data suggest that a patent foramen ovale also may be associated with migraine headaches.

TREATMENT Rx

Currently there are no data to support closure of a patent foramen ovale for primary stroke prevention in a patient in whom it is fortuitously diagnosed on routine echocardiography. Ongoing randomized trials are addressing the benefit of closure versus medical therapy after a stroke; in the meantime, warfarin to an international normalized ratio of 2.0 to 3.0 is usually recommended over aspirin for secondary stroke prevention. Primary closure of a patent foramen ovale is indicated when a patient has contraindications to medical therapy, if medical therapy has failed, or in the presence of a hypercoagulable state not treatable by medical therapy. Device closure in experienced centers is usually preferred to surgical closure, although surgical closure is performed if the patient undergoes cardiac surgery for other reasons. Device closure appears to be associated with a low incidence of yearly recurrence rates. Despite the potential link with migraine headaches, closure of a patent foramen ovale does not result in symptomatic improvement. [3]

Ventricular Septal Defect

For anatomic classification of VSDs, the interventricular septum can be divided into four regions. Defects of the membranous septum, or infracristal VSDs, are located in a small translucent area beneath the aortic valve and account for up to 80% of VSDs. These VSDs typically show a variable degree of extension into the inlet or outlet septum, hence their designation as perimembranous. Infundibular defects or supracristal outlet VSDs occur in the conal septum above the crista supraventricularis and below the pulmonary valve. Inlet defects are identified at the crux of the heart between the tricuspid and mitral valves and are usually associated with other anomalies of the atrioventricular canal. Defects of the trabecular or muscular septum can be multiple and occur distal to the septal attachment of the tricuspid valve and toward the apex.

The pathophysiology and clinical course of VSDs depend on the size of the defect, the status of the pulmonary vascular bed, and the effects of shunt size on intracardiac hemodynamics. Unlike ASDs, a VSD may decrease in size with time. Approximately half of all native VSDs are small, and more than half of them close spontaneously; moderate or even large VSDs may also close in 10% or less of cases. The highest closure rates are observed in the first decade of life; spontaneous closure in adult life is unusual.

Patients who have a small defect with trivial or mild shunts are defined as those with a $\dot{Q}:\dot{Q}$ of less than 1.5 and normal pulmonary artery pressure and vascular resistance. Patients with moderate defects have a $\dot{Q}:\dot{Q}$ ratio of greater than 1.2 and elevated pulmonary artery pressure but not elevated pulmonary vascular resistance. Patients with a large and severe defect have an elevated $\dot{Q}:\dot{Q}$ ratio with high pulmonary pressure and elevated pulmonary vascular resistance. Eisenmenger's complex develops in about 10% of patients with VSDs, usually when there is no resistance to flow at the level of the defect, which can be as large as the aorta. When a systolic pressure gradient is present between the ventricles, the physiologic severity may be trivial or mild but can also be moderate or severe.

Minimal or mild defects usually cause no significant hemodynamic or physiologic abnormality. A moderate or severe defect causes left atrial and ventricular dilation consistent with the degree of left-to-right shunting. Shunting across the ventricular septum occurs predominantly during systole when left ventricular pressure exceeds that on the right; diastolic filling abnormalities occur in the left atrium. With moderate or severe defects, the right side of the heart becomes affected as a function of the rise in pulmonary pressure and pulmonary blood flow.

DIAGNOSIS

An adult with a VSD most commonly has a small restrictive lesion that either was small at birth or has undergone some degree of spontaneous closure. A second group of patients consists of those with large, nonrestrictive VSDs that have not been operated on; these patients have had Eisenmenger's complex for most of their lives. Patients with a moderately sized defect are typically symptomatic as children and are therefore more likely to have repair at a young age.

Patients with a trivial or mild shunt across a small, restrictive VSD are usually asymptomatic. Physical examination discloses no evidence of systemic or pulmonary venous congestion, and jugular venous pressure is normal. A thrill may be palpable at the left sternal border. Auscultation reveals normal S_1 and S_2 without gallops. A grade 4 or louder, widely radiating, high-frequency, pansystolic murmur is heard maximally in the third or fourth intercostal space and reflects the high-pressure gradient between the left and right ventricles throughout systole. The striking contrast between a loud murmur and an otherwise normal cardiac examination is an important diagnostic clue. The ECG and chest radiograph are also normal in patients with small VSDs.

At the other end of the spectrum are patients with Eisenmenger's complex (see earlier). Between these two extremes are patients with a moderate defect, whose pathology reflects a combination of pulmonary hypertension and left-sided volume overload resulting from a significant left-to-right shunt. In adults, shortness of breath on exertion can be the result of both pulmonary venous congestion and elevated pulmonary pressure. On physical examination, a diffuse palpable left ventricular impulse occurs with a variable degree of right ventricular hypertrophy and an accentuated second heart sound. A systolic murmur persists as long as pulmonary vascular resistance is below systemic resistance. The ECG commonly shows left atrial enlargement and left ventricular hypertrophy. The chest radiograph shows shunt vascularity with an enlarged left atrium and ventricle. The degree of pulmonary hypertension determines the size of the pulmonary artery trunk.

Echocardiography can identify the defect and determine the significance of the shunt by assessing left atrial and ventricular size, pulmonary artery pressure, and the presence or absence of right ventricular hypertrophy. Cardiac catheterization is reserved for those in whom surgery is considered. Adults with a small defect of no physiologic significance need not be studied invasively. Those with Eisenmenger's complex have severe pulmonary vascular disease and are not surgical candidates. Patients who have a moderately sized shunt that appears hemodynamically significant and in whom pulmonary pressures are elevated are most likely to benefit from direct measurements of pulmonary vascular resistance and reactivity.

TREATMENT

Patients with Eisenmenger's complex have pulmonary vascular resistance that is prohibitive to surgery. For this group of patients, management centers on the medical complications of cyanosis (see earlier). In a few patients with small defects, complications can relate to progressive tricuspid insufficiency caused by septal aneurysm formation or to acquired aortic insufficiency when an aortic cusp becomes engaged in the high-velocity jet flow generated by the defect. The intermediate group of patients with a defect of moderate physiologic significance should have surgical closure unless it is contraindicated by high pulmonary vascular resistance.

Late results after operative closure of isolated VSDs include residual patency in up to 20% of patients, only about 5% of whom need a reoperation. Rhythm disturbances after surgical closure of VSDs include tachyarrhythmias and conduction disturbances. Right bundle branch block occurs in one third to two thirds of patients, whereas first-degree atrioventricular block and complete heart block occur in less than 10%. Sudden cardiac death after surgical repair of VSD occurs in 2% of patients.

Patent Ductus Arteriosus

The ductus arteriosus connects the descending aorta to the main pulmonary trunk near the origin of the left subclavian artery (Fig. 69-6). Normal postnatal closure results in fibrosis and degenerative changes in the ductal lumen, leaving in its place the residual ligamentum arteriosum, which rarely can become part of an abnormal vascular ring. When the duct persists, significant calcification of the aortic ductal end is observed.

The physiologic consequences of a PDA are determined by its size and length as well as by the ratio of pressure and resistance of the pulmonary and aortic circulations on either end of the duct. If systolic and diastolic pressure in the aorta exceeds that in the pulmonary artery, aortic blood flows continuously down a pressure gradient into the pulmonary artery and then returns to the left atrium. The left atrium and subsequently the left ventricle dilate, whereas the right side of the heart becomes progressively affected as pulmonary hypertension develops.

A small PDA has continuous flow throughout the entire cardiac cycle without left-sided heart dilation, pulmonary hypertension, or symptoms. Patients with a small PDA, although protected from hemodynamic complications of a significant left-to-right shunt, remain at risk for infectious endarteritis, which usually develops on the pulmonary side of the duct and occurs at a rate of about 0.45% per year after the second decade. Because endarteritis accounts for up to one third of the total mortality in patients with PDA, ductal closure should be considered even when the PDA is small.

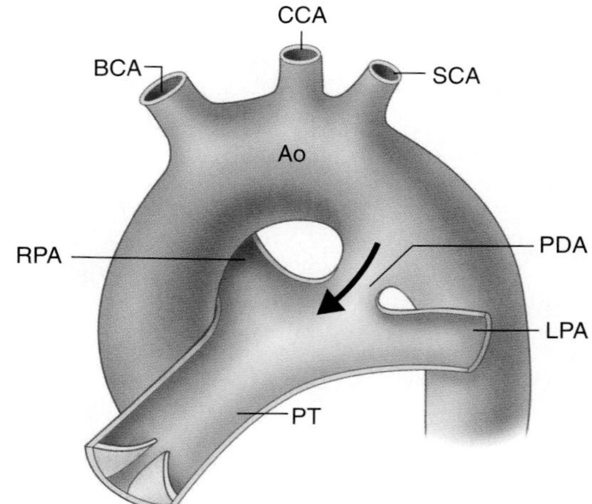

FIGURE 69-6. Anatomy of a patent ductus arteriosus. Note the relationships among the position of the ductus, left subclavian artery, and pulmonary artery bifurcation. Ao = aorta; BCA = brachiocephalic; CCA = common carotid artery; LPA = left pulmonary artery; PDA = patent ductus arteriosus; PT = pulmonary trunk; RPA = right pulmonary artery; SCA = subclavian artery. (From Perloff JK, ed. *Clinical Recognition of Congenital Heart Disease*, 4th ed. Philadelphia: WB Saunders; 1994:510.)

A PDA is of moderate or large size but still restrictive when a left-to-right shunt occurs throughout systole and diastole is of variable duration. Left atrial or ventricular dilation and pulmonary hypertension will vary with the quantity of left-to-right shunting as well as with the secondary effects on the pulmonary vascular bed. Symptoms generally increase by the second and third decades and include dyspnea, palpitations, and exercise intolerance. As heart failure, pulmonary hypertension, or endarteritis develops, mortality rises to 3 to 4% per year by the fourth decade, and two thirds of patients die by 60 years of age. Eisenmenger's physiology with systemic or suprasystemic pulmonary pressure and a right-to-left shunt develops in 5% of patients with an isolated PDA.

DIAGNOSIS

In patients with Eisenmenger's physiology, a right-to-left shunt from the pulmonary artery to the descending aorta results in decreased oxygen saturation in the lower extremities compared with the upper extremities. This difference in cyanosis and clubbing is most prominent in the toes; the left arm is variably affected through the left subclavian artery, and the right arm is typically spared. With a large left-to-right shunt, the pulse pressure widens as diastolic flow into the pulmonary artery lowers systemic diastolic pressure. The arterial pulse becomes bounding as a result of increased stroke volume. Precordial palpation discloses variable left and right ventricular impulses as determined by the relative degree of left-sided volume overload and pulmonary hypertension. In the presence of a continuous aortopulmonary gradient, the classic "machinery" murmur of a PDA can be heard at the first or second left intercostal space below the left clavicle. As the pulmonary pressure rises, the diastolic component of the murmur becomes progressively shorter. With the development of Eisenmenger's physiology and equalization of aortic and pulmonary pressure, the entire murmur may disappear, and the clinical findings are dominated by pulmonary hypertension.

In adult patients with a significant left-to-right shunt, the ECG shows a bifid P wave in at least one limb lead consistent with left atrial enlargement and a variable degree of left ventricular hypertrophy. The PR interval is prolonged in about 20% of patients. In older patients, the chest radiograph shows calcification at the location of the PDA. Characteristically, the ascending aorta and pulmonary artery are dilated, and the left-sided chambers are enlarged. Echocardiography may not directly visualize the PDA but can accurately identify it by a Doppler signal that often parallels the length of the murmur. Left-sided heart dilation and pulmonary hypertension can be quantified and monitored. Cardiac catheterization to assess pulmonary vascular resistance is commonly indicated before closure.

TREATMENT Rx

After ligation of a PDA in infancy or early childhood, cardiac function is commonly normal, and no special follow-up is required. If pulmonary artery pressure and pulmonary vascular resistance are substantially elevated, preoperative evaluation should assess the degree of reversibility. With Eisenmenger's disease, closure is contraindicated. Closure of a PDA either percutaneously or surgically is indicated in the presence of left heart enlargement or if prior endarteritis has occurred. Reported operative mortality rates vary from less than 1 to 8%, depending on the presence of calcification and the degree of pulmonary hypertension. Transcatheter or coil occlusion is an accepted procedure in adults. Residual shunt rates vary from 0.5 to 8%, depending on the device used. Small residual defects that are detected by echocardiography but are not associated with an audible murmur or hemodynamic findings do not appear to carry a significant risk for endarteritis.

Aortopulmonary Window

An aortopulmonary window is typically a large defect across the adjacent segments of both great vessels above their respective valves and below the pulmonary artery bifurcation. The pathophysiology is similar to that of a PDA. The shunt is usually large, so pulmonary vascular resistance rises rapidly and abolishes the aortopulmonary gradient in diastole. The murmur is usually best heard at the third left intercostal space. With a right-to-left shunt, differential cyanosis never occurs because the shunt is proximal to the brachiocephalic vessels. Differentiation of an aortopulmonary window from a PDA can usually be confirmed with echocardiography; the left-to-right shunt is seen in the main pulmonary artery in the aortopulmonary window compared with the left pulmonary artery bifurcation in PDA. Cardiac catheterization confirms the diagnosis and hemodynamics. Surgical repair is necessary unless pulmonary vascular obstructive disease precludes closure.

Pulmonary Arteriovenous Fistulas

Pulmonary arteriovenous fistulas can occur as isolated congenital disorders or as part of generalized hereditary hemorrhagic telangiectasia (Osler-Weber-Rendu syndrome). These fistulas typically occur in the lower lobes or the right middle lobe and can be small or large, single or multiple. The arterial supply usually comes from a dilated, tortuous branch of the pulmonary artery.

The most common finding is that of abnormal opacity on a chest radiograph in a patient with buccal ruby patches or in an otherwise healthy adult who has mild cyanosis. Shunting between deoxygenated pulmonary arterial blood and the oxygenated pulmonary venous blood results in a physiologic right-to-left shunt. The degree of shunting is typically small and not significant enough to result in dilation of the left atrium and ventricle. Heart failure is unusual. Hemoptysis can result if a fistula ruptures into a bronchus. In patients with hereditary hemorrhagic telangiectasia, angiomas occur on the lips and mouth as well as in the gastrointestinal tract and on pleural, liver, and vaginal surfaces. Epistaxis is most common, but cerebrovascular accidents can also occur. Patients with hereditary hemorrhagic telangiectasia can have symptoms that resemble those of a transient ischemic attack even in the absence of right-to-left shunting. On physical examination, cyanosis and clubbing can be notable or barely detectable. Auscultation can disclose soft systolic or continuous noncardiac murmurs on the chest wall adjacent to the fistula. The murmur typically increases with inspiration. The ECG is usually normal. The chest radiograph shows one or more densities, typically in the lower lobes or in the right middle lobe. An echocardiogram can confirm the presence of the fistula by showing early opacification of the left atrium in the absence of any other intracardiac communication when saline is injected into a peripheral vein. The absence of a hemodynamically significant shunt can be confirmed by documenting normal cardiac chamber size.

If the hypoxemia is progressive or if a neurologic complication is documented to have occurred because of paradoxical emboli, fistula closure should be considered. Options include percutaneous catheter techniques if the fistula is small and accessible or a pulmonary wedge resection or lobectomy if the fistula is large. Multiple or recurrent fistulas create a major therapeutic challenge.

Isolated Obstructive Lesions of the Right and Left Ventricular Outflow Tract

Complications of obstructive lesions of the outflow tract relate to the secondary effects of exposure to pressure overload in the chamber proximal to the obstruction. The inability to increase systemic or pulmonary blood flow in the face of a fixed obstruction can cause exercise intolerance, inadequate myocardial perfusion, ventricular arrhythmias, and sudden death.

RIGHT VENTRICULAR OUTFLOW TRACT OBSTRUCTION

Obstruction of the right ventricular outflow tract can occur at the level of the pulmonary valve (see later), above it in the main pulmonary artery or its branches, or below it in the right ventricle itself. Supravalvular and branch pulmonary artery stenoses are important and common complications in patients with tetralogy of Fallot (see later). Residual supravalvar pulmonary stenosis is sometimes seen after palliative pulmonary artery banding to decrease pulmonary blood flow in patients with large left-to-right shunts. Congenital branch pulmonary artery stenosis can occur in isolation or with valvar pulmonary stenosis, shunt lesions, or a variety of syndromes. Patients with Noonan's syndrome have a characteristic phenotypic facial appearance, short stature, and webbed neck; cardiac lesions may include a dysplastic pulmonary valve, left ventricular hypertrophic cardiomyopathy, and peripheral pulmonary artery stenosis. Supravalvular pulmonary stenosis can be seen with supravalvular aortic stenosis in Williams (elfin facies) syndrome.

Pulmonary atresia refers to an absent, imperforate, or closed pulmonary valve, which typically occurs in conjunction with other malformations. Pulmonary atresia with a nonrestrictive VSD is a complex cyanotic malformation that is discussed later.

Primary infundibular stenosis with an intact ventricular septum can result from a fibrous band just below the infundibulum. In a double-chambered right ventricle, obstruction is caused by anomalous muscle bundles that divide the right ventricle into a high-pressure chamber below the hypertrophied muscle bundles and a low-pressure chamber above the bundles and below the valve. The clinical features vary according to the presence or absence of other lesions, such as pulmonary valvular stenosis or VSD.

VALVULAR PULMONARY STENOSIS

Isolated congenital valvular pulmonary stenosis (Chapter 75) is a common lesion due to a bicuspid valve in 20% of cases, a dysplastic valve caused by myxomatous changes and severe thickening in 10% of cases, and an abnormal trileaflet valve in most of the remaining cases. Fusion of the leaflets results in a variable degree of thickening and calcification in older patients.

The 25-year survival of patients with valvular pulmonary stenosis is greater than 95% but is worse in those with severe stenosis and peak systolic gradients greater than 80 mm Hg. For patients with mild (<50 mm Hg gradients) and moderate (50 to 80 mm Hg gradients) pulmonary stenosis, bacterial endocarditis, complex ventricular arrhythmias, and progression of the stenosis are uncommon.

DIAGNOSIS

A patient with moderate or even severe pulmonary stenosis may be asymptomatic. With severe stenosis, exercise intolerance can be associated with presyncope and ventricular arrhythmias. Progressive right-sided heart failure is the most common cause of death. On physical examination of patients with significant pulmonary stenosis, jugular venous pressure has a dominant a wave, reflecting a noncompliant right ventricle. Palpation discloses a sustained parasternal lift of right ventricular hypertrophy. An expiratory systolic ejection click is characteristic if the leaflets are still mobile. In moderate or severe stenosis, a grade 3 or louder systolic murmur can be heard and felt in the second left interspace. The length of the murmur increases as it peaks progressively later in systole with an increasing degree of obstruction. If right-sided heart failure occurs, tricuspid insufficiency and systemic venous congestion develop. The ECG can show right axis deviation and tall, peaked right atrial P waves in lead II. With more than mild stenosis, the R wave exceeds the S wave in lead V_1. On chest radiography, the main pulmonary artery can be dilated even if the stenosis is mild. Characteristically, the left pulmonary artery is more dilated than the right because of the leftward direction of the high-velocity jet. A variable degree of right ventricular hypertrophy is manifested as right-sided chamber enlargement. Echocardiography can establish the diagnosis and determine the severity by Doppler ultrasound examination. Patients with valvar pulmonary stenosis do not require cardiac catheterization. The mean gradient at echocardiography correlates well with the gradient measured at cardiac catheterization and should be used for therapeutic decisions because peak instantaneous Doppler gradients tend to overestimate the severity of disease.

TREATMENT Rx

Depending on symptoms, percutaneous balloon valvotomy should be considered for patients with isolated valvar pulmonary stenosis and mean Doppler gradients of 30 mm Hg or greater unless there is moderate or severe pulmonary regurgitation. In the presence of a doming valve, pulmonary angioplasty is the procedure of choice for adults, who achieve persistently good results at 10-year follow-up. For patients with hypoplastic pulmonary arteries or subvalvular stenosis (double-chambered right ventricle), surgical resection of right ventricular muscle bands can be performed.

LEFT VENTRICULAR OUTFLOW TRACT OBSTRUCTION

Stenosis of the left ventricular outflow tract can occur at, below, or above the aortic valve. Discrete subaortic stenosis, most commonly caused by a fibromuscular ring just below the valve, accounts for 15 to 20% of all cases of congenital obstruction of the left ventricular outflow tract. Concomitant aortic insufficiency occurs in 50% of cases. Supravalvular aortic stenosis results from thickened media and intima above the aortic sinuses; early coronary atherosclerosis or even ostial coronary obstruction can occur.

CONGENITAL VALVULAR AORTIC STENOSIS

The normal aortic valve has three cusps and commissures. A unicuspid aortic valve accounts for most cases of severe aortic stenosis in infants (Chapter 75). A bicuspid aortic valve, which is the most common congenital cardiac malformation, functions normally at birth but often becomes gradually obstructed as calcific and fibrous changes occur; prolapse of one or both cusps can cause aortic insufficiency.

The pathophysiology of aortic stenosis depends not only on its severity but also on the age at diagnosis. When a bicuspid aortic valve becomes stenotic in adulthood because of degenerative changes, criteria for diagnosis and intervention parallel those for other forms of acquired aortic stenosis (Chapter 75). The estimated overall 25-year survival rate for patients with congenital valvular aortic stenosis diagnosed in childhood is 85%. Children with initial peak cardiac catheterization gradients of less than 50 mm Hg have long-term survival rates of higher than 90%, as opposed to survival rates of 80% in those with gradients of 50 mm Hg or greater.

DIAGNOSIS

Symptoms include angina, exertional dyspnea, presyncope, and syncope and may progress to heart failure. The auscultatory hallmark of a bicuspid aortic valve is an audible systolic ejection click that is typically of a higher pitch than the first heart sound and is best heard not at the cardiac base but at the apex. The sound is caused by sudden movement of the stenotic valve as it moves superiorly in systole and is followed by the typical aortic stenosis murmur (Chapter 75). When significant calcification of the valve results in reduced mobility, the ejection sound is no longer heard. The diagnosis is easily confirmed by two-dimensional echocardiography, with which the number and orientation of aortic cusps can readily be identified.

TREATMENT Rx

Conservative management is generally indicated for mild stenosis with a peak gradient of less than 25 mm Hg, but close supervision is required because 20% of these patients require an intervention during long-term follow-up. Unlimited athletic participation is allowed only for asymptomatic patients with peak gradients of less than 20 to 25 mm Hg, a normal ECG, and a normal exercise test. For children who are symptomatic or have gradients greater than 30 mm Hg but do not have significant aortic insufficiency, transcatheter aortic valvotomy is preferred. Aortic valvuloplasty can be considered in young adults, but calcification limits its success, and valve replacement is usually required (Chapter 75). For adults, treatment decisions are similar to those for aortic stenosis from other causes. For patients with subvalvular aortic stenosis, surgical intervention is indicated in the presence of peak gradients above 50 mm Hg, symptoms, or progressive aortic insufficiency.

COARCTATION OF THE AORTA

Aortic coarctation typically occurs just distal to the left subclavian artery at the site of the aortic ductal attachment or its residual ligamentum arteriosum. Less commonly, the coarctation ridge lies proximal to the left subclavian. A bicuspid aortic valve is the most common coexisting anomaly, but VSDs and PDAs are also seen. Pseudocoarctation refers to buckling or kinking of the aortic arch without the presence of a significant gradient.

The most common complications of aortic coarctation are systemic hypertension (Chapter 67) and secondary left ventricular hypertrophy with heart failure. Systemic hypertension is caused by decreased vascular compliance in the proximal aorta and activation of the renin-angiotensin system in response to renal artery hypoperfusion below the obstruction. Left ventricular hypertrophy occurs in response to chronic pressure overload. Congestive heart failure occurs most commonly in infants and then after 40 years of age. The high pressure proximal to the obstruction stimulates the growth of collateral vessels from the internal mammary, scapular, and superior intercostal arteries to the intercostals of the descending aorta. Collateral circulation increases with age and contributes to perfusion of the lower extremities and the spinal cord. This mechanism, although adaptive in a patient who has not undergone surgery, accounts for significant morbidity during surgery when the motor impairment results from inadequate protection of spinal perfusion. Aneurysms occur most notably in the ascending aorta and in the circle of Willis. Premature coronary disease is thought to be related to the resulting hypertension. Complications, including bacterial endarteritis at the coarctation site or, more commonly, endocarditis at the site of a bicuspid aortic valve, cerebrovascular complications, myocardial infarction, heart failure, and aortic dissection, occur in 2 to 6% of patients, more frequently in those with advancing age who have not undergone surgery.

DIAGNOSIS

Young adults may be asymptomatic with incidental systemic hypertension and decreased lower extremity pulses. Coarctation should always be considered in adolescents and young adult men with unexplained upper extremity hypertension. The pressure differential can cause epistaxis, headaches, leg fatigue, or claudication. Older patients have angina, symptoms of heart failure, and vascular complications.

On physical examination, the lower half of the body is typically slightly less developed than the upper half. The hips are narrow and the legs are short, in contrast to broad shoulders and long arms. Blood pressure measurements

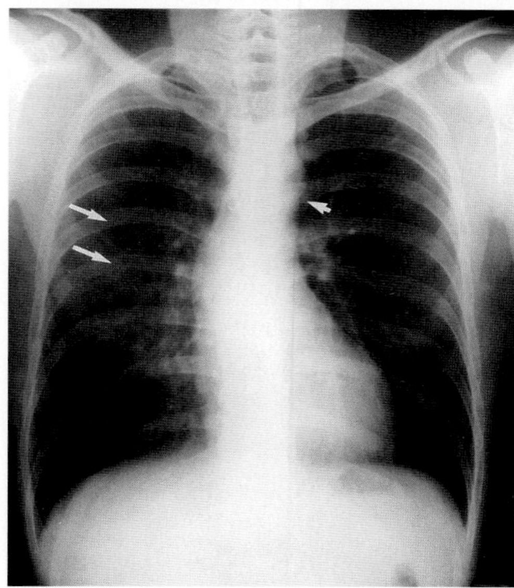

FIGURE 69-7. Chest radiograph of a patient with coarctation of the aorta. The radiographic *3* formed by the dilated subclavian artery above and the dilated aorta below *(short arrow)* is shown. Note the notching, best seen at the level of the seventh and eighth ribs *(long arrows)*. The dilated ascending aortic segment can also be seen.

should be obtained in each arm and one leg; an abnormal measurement is an increase of less than 10 mm Hg in popliteal systolic blood pressure compared with arm systolic blood pressure. The diastolic pressure should be the same in the upper and lower extremities. A pressure differential of more than 30 mm Hg between the right and the left arms is consistent with compromised flow in the left subclavian artery. Right brachial palpation characteristically reveals a strong or even bounding pulse compared with a slowly rising or absent femoral, popliteal, or pedal pulse. Examination of the eyegrounds can reveal tortuous or corkscrew retinal arteries. Precordial palpation is consistent with left ventricular pressure overload. On auscultation, a systolic ejection sound reflecting the presence of a bicuspid aortic valve should be sought. The coarctation itself generates a systolic murmur heard posteriorly, in the midthoracic region, the length of which correlates with the severity of the coarctation. Over the anterior of the chest, systolic murmurs reflecting increased collateral flow can be heard in the infraclavicular areas and the sternal edge or in the axillae.

In adult coarctation, the most common finding on the ECG is left ventricular hypertrophy. Chest radiographic findings are diagnostic. Location of the coarctation segment between the dilated left subclavian artery above and the leftward convexity of the descending aorta below results in the "3 sign" (Fig. 69-7). Bilateral rib notching as a result of dilation of the posterior intercostal arteries is seen on the posterior of the third to eighth ribs when the coarctation is below the left subclavian. Unilateral rib notching sparing the left ribs is observed when the coarctation occurs proximal to the left subclavian artery. Transthoracic echocardiography documents the gradient in the descending aorta and determines the presence of left ventricular hypertrophy. Magnetic resonance imaging (Chapter 56) is the best modality for visualizing the anatomy of the descending aorta. Cardiac catheterization should measure pressures and assess collaterals when surgery is contemplated.

TREATMENT Rx

Intervention is recommended in patients who have gradients of 20 mm Hg or more on cardiac catheterization (Chapter 57) or who have evidence of significant collateral flow on imaging studies. The choice between catheter interventional and surgical intervention, which should be made in conjunction with a specialist, depends on the associated anomalies and the anatomy of the coarctation segment. Fifty percent of patients repaired when they are older than 40 years have residual hypertension, whereas those who have undergone surgery between the ages of 1 and 5 years have a less than 10% prevalence of hypertension on long-term follow-up. Balloon angioplasty is the treatment of choice for focal recoarctation in patients who have previously been operated on. The incidence of incomplete relief and restenosis is decreased in adults by endovascular stent placement. Focal complications include aortic aneurysms and, rarely, aortic rupture.

Anomalies of the Sinuses of Valsalva and Coronary Arteries

SINUS OF VALSALVA ANEURYSMS

At the base of the aortic root, the aortic valve cusps are attached to the aortic wall, above which three small pouches, or sinuses, are seated. The right coronary artery originates from one sinus and the left main coronary artery from a second; the third is called the *noncoronary sinus.* A weakness in the wall of the sinus can result in aneurysm formation with or without rupture. In more than 90% of cases, the aneurysm involves the right or noncoronary cusp. Rupture typically occurs into the right side of the heart at the right atrial or ventricular level with a resulting large left-to-right shunt driven by the high aortic pressure.

A previously asymptomatic young man typically has chest pain and rapidly progressing shortness of breath sometimes after physical strain. The physical examination is consistent with significant heart failure. Even if the communication is between the aorta and the right side of the heart, biventricular failure is not unusual. The classic murmur is loud and continuous, often with a thrill. A murmur of aortic insufficiency secondary to damage to the adjacent aortic valve may be superimposed. The chest radiograph shows volume overload of both ventricles with evidence of shunt vascularity and pulmonary venous congestion. The echocardiogram is diagnostic. Cardiac catheterization can verify the integrity of the coronary artery adjacent to the ruptured aneurysm.

Even though symptoms may abate as the heart dilates, progressive cardiac decompensation typically results in death within 1 year of the rupture. A ruptured sinus of Valsalva aneurysm therefore requires urgent surgical repair.

CORONARY ARTERY FISTULAS

Fistulas arise from the right or left coronary arteries and in 90% of cases drain into the right ventricle, the right atrium, or the pulmonary artery in order of decreasing frequency. Typically, young patients are asymptomatic, but supraventricular arrhythmias are seen with progressive dilation of the intracardiac chambers. Angina can occur as the fistula creates a coronary steal by diverting blood away from the myocardium. Heart failure is seen with large fistulas. A continuous murmur heard in a young, otherwise normal acyanotic, asymptomatic patient should suggest the diagnosis. Most fistulas are associated with a small shunt, and hence the murmur is often less than grade 3 and is heard in the precordial area. Unless the shunt is large, the ECG is normal, as is the chest radiograph. The echocardiogram, especially the transesophageal echocardiogram, is diagnostic. Percutaneous transcatheter closure with coil embolization is preferred, but surgical ligation is also an alternative.

ANOMALOUS ORIGIN OF THE CORONARY ARTERIES

The left main coronary artery normally arises from the left sinus of Valsalva and courses leftward, posterior to the right ventricular outflow tract. The right coronary artery arises from the right sinus of Valsalva and courses rightward to the right ventricle. Isolated ectopic or anomalous origins of the coronary arteries (see Fig. 57-8 in Chapter 57) are seen in 0.6 to 1.5% of patients undergoing coronary angiography.

The most common anomaly is ectopic origin of the left circumflex artery from the right sinus of Valsalva, followed by anomalous origin of the right coronary artery from the left sinus and anomalous origin of the left main coronary artery from the right sinus. If the anomalous coronary artery does not course between the pulmonary artery and aorta, the prognosis is favorable. Risks of ischemia, myocardial infarction, and death are greatest when the left main coronary artery courses between both great vessels.

Coronary arteries can also originate from the pulmonary trunk. If both the right and left arteries originate from the pulmonary trunk, death usually occurs in the neonatal period. If only the left anterior descending coronary artery originates from the pulmonary trunk, the rate of survival to adulthood is approximately 10%, depending on the development of collateral retrograde flow to the anomalous artery from a normal coronary artery. This collateral flow may cause a continuous murmur along the left sternal border, congestive heart failure from the large shunt, and a coronary steal syndrome as blood is diverted away from the normal artery.

A single coronary ostium can provide a single coronary artery that branches into right and left coronary arteries, the left then giving rise to the circumflex and the anterior descending arteries. The ostium can originate from the right or left aortic sinus. The coronary circulation is functionally normal unless one of the branches passes between the aorta and the pulmonary artery.

Diagnostic procedures include angiography, magnetic resonance imaging, and transesophageal echocardiography. For an anomalous coronary artery that originates from the pulmonary artery, surgical reimplantation into the aorta is preferred. For an anomalous artery that courses between the pulmonary artery and aorta, a bypass graft to the distal vessel is preferred.

SPECIFIC COMPLEX LESIONS

Tetralogy of Fallot

Tetralogy of Fallot, the most common cyanotic malformation, is characterized by superior and anterior displacement of the subpulmonary infundibular septum, which causes the tetrad of pulmonary stenosis, VSD, aortic override, and right ventricular hypertrophy. The VSD is perimembranous in 80% of cases. Additional cardiac anomalies include a right-sided aortic arch in up to 25% of patients. An anomalous left anterior descending artery originating from the right coronary cusp and crossing over the right ventricular outflow tract is seen in 10% of cases. Other associated anomalies include ASD, left superior vena cava, defects of the atrioventricular canal, and aortic insufficiency. With pulmonary atresia, pulmonary blood flow occurs through aortic to pulmonary collaterals. Life expectancy is limited unless staged reconstructive surgery is performed.

The physiology in unrepaired tetralogy of Fallot is determined by the severity and location of the pulmonic outflow obstruction and by the interaction of pulmonary and systemic vascular resistance across a nonrestrictive VSD. Because the pulmonary stenosis results in a relatively fixed pulmonary resistance, a drop in systemic vascular resistance as occurs with exercise is associated with increased right-to-left shunting and increasing cyanosis. A child who squats after running is attempting to reverse the process by increasing systemic vascular resistance by crouching with bent knees. Native pulmonary blood flow is typically insufficient. Unless a PDA has remained open, a cyanotic adult will typically have undergone a palliative procedure to increase pulmonary blood flow.

Examination of unrepaired patients reveals central cyanosis and clubbing. The right ventricular impulse is prominent. The second heart sound is single and represents the aortic closure sound with an absent or inconspicuous P_2. Typically, little or no systolic murmur is heard across the pulmonary valve because the more severe the obstruction, the more right-to-left shunting occurs and the less blood flows across a diminutive right ventricular outflow tract. A diastolic murmur of aortic insufficiency is often heard in adults. In the presence of a palliative systemic arterial to pulmonary artery shunt, the high-pressure gradient generates a loud continuous murmur. In a patient who has not undergone surgery, progressive infundibular stenosis and cyanosis occur. Before the advent of palliative surgery, mortality rates were 50% in the first few years of life, and survival past the third decade was unusual.

Complete surgical repair consists of patch closure of the VSD and relief of the right ventricular outflow tract obstruction. Adequate pulmonary blood flow is ensured by reconstruction of the distal pulmonary artery bed. Previous palliative shunts are usually taken down. Complete repair in childhood yields a 90 to 95% 10-year survival rate with good functional results, and 30-year survival rates may be as high as 85%. Total correction with low mortality and a favorable long-term follow-up is possible even in adulthood.

After repair, residual pulmonary stenosis, proximal or distal, with a right ventricular pressure greater than 50% of systemic occurs in up to 25% of patients. Some degree of pulmonary insufficiency is common, particularly if a patch has been inserted at the level of the pulmonary valve or if a pulmonary valvotomy has been performed. Residual VSDs can be found in up to 20% of patients. Patients may be asymptomatic or may have symptoms related to long-term complications after surgical repair. Symptoms can reflect residual right ventricular pressure or volume overload or arrhythmias at rest or with exercise. Angina can occur in a young patient if surgical repair has damaged an anomalous left anterior descending artery as it courses across the right ventricular outflow tract. In acyanotic adults, clubbing commonly regresses. A right ventricular impulse is often felt as a result of residual pulmonary insufficiency or stenosis. Typically, no functioning pulmonary valve is present, and hence the second heart sound is still single. A systolic murmur can represent residual pulmonary stenosis, residual VSD, or tricuspid insufficiency. A diastolic murmur can reflect aortic or pulmonary insufficiency. Ventricular arrhythmias are common after repair, with an incidence of sudden death as high as 5%.

The ECG in unrepaired tetralogy of Fallot shows right axis deviation, right atrial enlargement, and dominant right ventricular forces over the precordial leads. The most common finding after repair is complete right bundle branch block, which is seen in 80 to 90% of patients. The chest radiograph typically shows an upturned apex with a concave pulmonary artery segment giving the classic appearance of a boot-shaped heart. Figure 69-8 demonstrates the findings in an adult after repair. The apex is persistently upturned, although the pulmonary artery segment is no longer concave. Echocardiography can confirm the diagnosis and document intracardiac complications in repaired and unrepaired patients. Shunt patency can be determined by Doppler examination. Magnetic resonance imaging can accurately document stenosis in the distal pulmonary artery bed. Cardiac catheterization is reserved for patients in whom operative or reoperative treatment is contemplated or in whom the integrity of the coronary circulation needs to be verified.

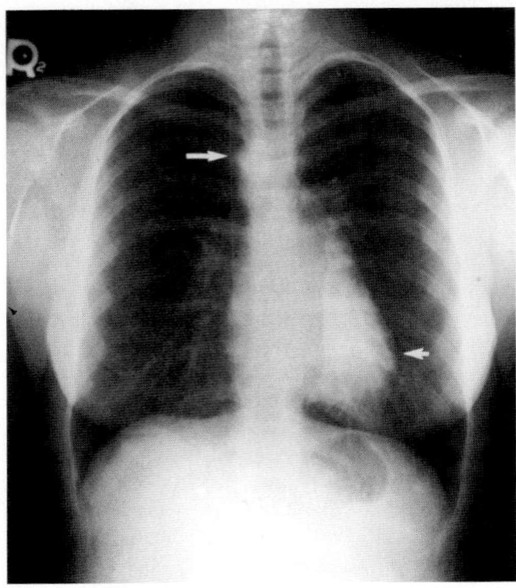

FIGURE 69-8. Chest radiograph of an adult after tetralogy of Fallot repair. A right aortic arch with rightward indentation of the trachea *(long arrow)* can be seen. The right ventricular apex remains upturned *(short arrow)*. Note the sternal wires consistent with intracardiac repair, clarifying the fullness of the pulmonary artery segment often seen after extensive enlargement of the right ventricular outflow tract.

Patients with a change in exercise tolerance, angina, or evidence of heart failure and those with symptomatic arrhythmias or syncope should be referred for complete evaluation. Surgical reintervention is generally considered when right ventricular pressure is more than two thirds as high as systemic pressure because of residual right ventricular outflow tract obstruction, free pulmonary regurgitation occurs with right ventricular dysfunction or sustained arrhythmias, or a residual VSD causes a significant shunt.

Complete Transposition of the Great Arteries

Complete transposition of the great arteries is the second most common cyanotic lesion, and surgically corrected adults are increasingly common. In simple transposition of the great arteries, the atria and ventricles are in their normal positions, but the aorta arises from the right ventricle, and the pulmonary artery arises from the left ventricle. When the aorta is anterior and rightward with respect to the pulmonary artery, as is most common, D-transposition is present. The native anatomy has the pulmonary and systemic circulations in parallel, with deoxygenated blood recirculating between the right side of the heart and the systemic circulation, whereas oxygenated blood recirculates from the left side of the heart to the lungs. The condition is incompatible with life unless a VSD, PDA, or ASD is present or an ASD is created; a hemodynamically significant VSD is present in 15% of cases. Subpulmonary obstruction of the left ventricular outflow tract occurs in 10 to 25% of cases.

The Senning or Mustard atrial baffle repairs, which were the first corrective procedures, redirect oxygenated blood from the left atrium to the right ventricle so that it may be ejected into the aorta while deoxygenated blood detours the right atrium and heads for the left ventricle and into the pulmonary artery. Although this operation results in acyanotic physiology, the right ventricle assumes a permanent position under the aorta and pumps against systemic pressures, a lifelong task for which it was not designed. When the subpulmonary obstruction is significant, the Rastelli procedure reroutes blood at the ventricular level by tunneling the left ventricle to the aorta inside the heart through a VSD. A conduit is then inserted outside the heart between the left ventricle and aorta. More recently, the arterial switch operation transects the aorta and pulmonary artery above their respective valves and switches them to become realigned with their physiologic outflow tracts and appropriate ventricles. The proximal coronary arteries are translocated from the sinuses of the native aorta to the neoaorta (native pulmonary artery). In this operation, each ventricle reassumes the role that it was embryologically destined to fulfill.

If an adult patient is cyanotic and has a native intracardiac shunt or a palliative shunt, referral to an appropriate facility should be undertaken to explore the possibility of intracardiac repair. At present, adults with transposition of the great arteries most commonly have undergone an atrial baffle repair, with an expected 15-year survival rate of 75% and a 20-year survival rate of 70%. For patients with an atrial baffle procedure, symptoms include exercise intolerance, palpitations caused by bradyarrhythmias or atrial flutter, and right ventricular failure. The patient is typically acyanotic unless a baffle leak exists. The clinical findings are determined by the presence or absence of systemic right ventricular failure. On auscultation, the second heart sound is classically single. The ECG reveals sinus bradycardia, but nodal rhythms and heart block occur as the patient ages. The chest radiograph shows a variable degree of right ventricular enlargement. Echocardiography can be used to confirm the diagnosis and to explore related abnormalities. Cardiac catheterization is performed when an operation or reoperation is contemplated. Reoperation is performed in approximately 20% of patients for baffle-related complications, progressive left ventricular outflow tract stenosis, or severe tricuspid regurgitation.

Congenitally Corrected Transposition of the Great Arteries

In congenitally corrected transposition of the great arteries, the great arteries are transposed, the ventricles are inverted, but the atria remain in their normal position. The systemic circulation (left atrium, morphologic right ventricle, and aorta) and pulmonary circulation (right atrium, morphologic left ventricle, and pulmonary artery) are in series. The patient is therefore acyanotic unless an intracardiac shunt is also present. The right ventricle is aligned with the aorta and performs lifelong systemic work, which accounts in part for its eventual failure. Associated lesions include a VSD, pulmonary stenosis, and Ebstein's malformation of the left-sided tricuspid valve. Complete heart block develops at a rate of 2% per year. Patients with congenitally corrected transposition of the great arteries and no other associated defects can remain free of symptoms until the sixth decade, at which time significant atrioventricular valve regurgitation, failure of the right (systemic) ventricle, supraventricular arrhythmias, and heart block occur.

Right-Sided Ebstein's Anomaly

The septal and posterior cusps of the tricuspid valve are largely derived from the right ventricle as it liberates a layer of muscle that skirts away from the cavity to become valve tissue. When this process occurs abnormally, the posterior and septal cusps of the tricuspid valve remain tethered to the muscle and adhere to the right ventricular surface—hence the diagnostic hallmark of Ebstein's anomaly, apical displacement of the septal tricuspid leaflet.

In right-sided Ebstein's anomaly of the tricuspid valve, the right side of the heart consists of three anatomic components: the right atrium proper, the true right ventricle, and the atrialized portion of the right ventricle between the two. The displaced septal and posterior tricuspid leaflets lie between the atrialized right ventricle and the true right ventricle. In mild Ebstein's anomaly, the degree of tricuspid leaflet tethering is only mild, the anterior leaflet retains mobility, and the size of the true right ventricle is only mildly reduced. Severe Ebstein's anomaly is associated with severe tethering of the tricuspid leaflet tissue and a diminutive, hypocontractile true right ventricle. Functionally, the valve is regurgitant because it is unable to appose its three leaflets during ventricular contraction. Valvular regurgitation and asynchronous, abnormal right ventricular function cause the dilation and right-sided heart failure observed in the more severe forms of the lesion. The wide spectrum of severity of the anomaly is based on the degree of tricuspid leaflet tethering and the relative proportion of atrialized and true right ventricle. The most common associated cardiac defect, a secundum ASD or patent foramen ovale, is reported in more than 50% of patients. On physical examination, a clicking "sail sound" is heard as the second component of S_1 when tricuspid valve closure becomes loud and delayed.

The 12-lead ECG typically shows highly peaked P waves with a wide, often bizarre-looking QRS complex. Preexcitation occurs in 20% of patients; supraventricular tachyarrhythmias, atrial fibrillation, and atrial flutter occur in 30 to 40% of patients and constitute the most common findings in adolescents and adults with right-sided Ebstein's anomaly.

When patients of all ages are taken together, the predicted mortality is approximately 50% by the fourth or fifth decade. Complications include atrial arrhythmias due to severe right atrial enlargement and cyanosis caused by a right-to-left atrial shunt as tricuspid insufficiency increases and the right ventricle fails. Atrial arrhythmias, cyanosis, and the presence of an intra-atrial communication also increase the risk for stroke.

Intervention is considered when functional status or cyanosis worsens, significant atrial arrhythmias are documented, or a cerebrovascular accident occurs. Surgical options include replacement or repair of the tricuspid valve and closure of the ASD. The feasibility of tricuspid valvuloplasty depends on the size and mobility of the anterior tricuspid leaflet, which is used to construct a unicuspid right-sided valve.

Atrioventricular Canal Defect

Embryologic septation of the atrioventricular canal results in closure of the inferior portion of the interatrial septum and the superior portion of the interventricular septum. Septation is achieved with the growth of endocardial cushions, which also contribute to development of the mitral and tricuspid valves. Hence, the nomenclature *atrioventricular canal defect* or *endocardial cushion defect* is used to designate this group of anomalies.

A partial atrioventricular canal defect refers to an ostium primum ASD with a cleft mitral valve. The anomaly is manifested as a hemodynamic combination of an ASD with a variable degree of mitral regurgitation. The 12-lead ECG shows the typical findings of left axis deviation with a Q wave in leads I and aVL and a prolonged PR interval. The echocardiogram shows a defect in the inferior portion of the interatrial septum and a cleft mitral valve.

A complete atrioventricular canal defect is an uncommon defect consisting of a primum ASD, an inlet VSD that usually extends to the membranous interventricular septum, and a common atrioventricular valve. Adults who have not been operated on usually have Eisenmenger's syndrome unless concomitant pulmonary stenosis has protected the pulmonary vascular bed or the VSD has undergone spontaneous closure, in which case the physiologic consequences are similar to those of a partial atrioventricular canal.

Surgical repair of an atrioventricular defect consists of closing the interatrial or interventricular communication with reconstruction of the common atrioventricular valve or closure of the cleft in the mitral valve. An adult who has undergone repair may have significant residual regurgitation of the mitral or tricuspid valve. Even after surgery, acquired subaortic obstruction can occur in the long left ventricular outflow tract, which has a classic gooseneck deformity on cardiac angiography.

Univentricular Heart and Tricuspid Atresia

The terms *single ventricle, common ventricle,* and *univentricular heart* have been used interchangeably to describe the double-inlet ventricle, in which one ventricular chamber receives flow from both the tricuspid and mitral valves. In 75 to 90% of cases, the single ventricle is a morphologic left ventricle. Obstruction of one of the great arteries is common, and life expectancy is short without an operation. The patients most likely to survive to adulthood palliated or, rarely, without surgery have a single ventricle of the left morphologic type, with pulmonary stenosis protecting the pulmonary vascular bed.

In tricuspid atresia, no orifice is found between the right atrium and right ventricle, and an underdeveloped or hypoplastic right ventricle is present. The morphologic left ventricle is consistently normally developed and therefore becomes the single functional ventricle. Typically, blood flows into the right atrium, then through an obligatory ASD and to the left atrium, where it then proceeds to the left ventricle. Variable features include a VSD, the abnormal position of the great arteries, and the relative degree of pulmonary stenosis, all of which are used to classify tricuspid atresia. Without surgery, 50% of patients die in the first 6 months and 90% in the first decade.

Adult patients rarely have not been operated on. They may be acyanotic after the Fontan operation; if cyanotic and palliated, the patient may benefit from further palliation or may be eligible for the Fontan operation. With the Glenn shunt or the Fontan operation, a direct anastomosis is created between the systemic venous and pulmonary circulations. Venous blood flows passively from the systemic veins to the pulmonary circulation and returns oxygenated to a left-sided atrium and into the single functional ventricle, which then pumps oxygenated blood into the systemic circulation. The Glenn anastomosis diverts part of the systemic venous return to the lungs, whereas the Fontan procedure makes the patient acyanotic by diverting the entire systemic venous circulation to the pulmonary vascular bed. For optimal results, a successful Fontan operation requires low pulmonary vascular resistance, preserved single ventricular function, and unobstructed anastomosis between the systemic veins and the pulmonary arteries. At 5-year follow-up, 80% or more of Fontan survivors are in New York Heart Association functional class I or II, with successful pregnancy reported in a small number of patients. When patients of all ages are considered together, 10-year survival rates vary from 60 to 70%. Late deaths are due to reoperation, arrhythmia, ventricular failure, and protein-losing enteropathy.

Vascular Malformations

AORTIC ARCH ANOMALIES

Vascular Rings and Other Arch Anomalies

One of the most frequent developmental errors of the aortic arch is an aberrant right subclavian artery originating distal to the left subclavian and coursing rightward behind the esophagus at the level of the third thoracic vertebrae. Although the finding is frequent, symptoms are uncommon. When symptoms occur, the term *dysphagia lusoria* has been used in reference to swallowing difficulties that result from esophageal compression. Abnormal development of the brachial arches and dorsal aorta can result in a variety of anomalies that lead to the formation of vascular rings around the trachea and esophagus. The outcome is often benign, but symptoms of respiratory compromise or dysphagia warrant surgery. When the left pulmonary artery arises from the right and passes leftward between the trachea and esophagus, a pulmonary artery sling occurs. Symptoms of tracheal compression warrant correction.

A right aortic arch occurs when the aortic arch courses toward the right instead of the left. Mirror-image branching is the most common anatomic variant. In most cases, this anomaly coexists with other congenital lesions, notably tetralogy of Fallot.

ANOMALOUS VENOUS CONNECTIONS

Anomalies of Systemic Venous Return

A persistent left superior vena cava can be fortuitously diagnosed on chest radiography or on echocardiography. Its clinical relevance depends on development of the coronary sinus. If the coronary sinus is normally formed, typically the left superior vena cava drains into the right atrium through the coronary sinus. If the coronary sinus is not normally developed, the persistent left superior vena cava drains into the left atrium, and cyanosis results from the obligatory right-to-left shunt. The latter commonly occurs with an ASD or a complex cardiac anomaly.

Venous return above the renal veins can be abnormal with inferior vena cava interruption and azygos or hemiazygos continuation. In the former, inferior vena cava flow above the renal veins continues into the azygos vein, which courses normally up the right of the spine to empty into the junction between the superior vena cava and right atrium. In a less common anatomic arrangement, the caval flow empties into a hemiazygos vein, which empties into a persistent left superior vena cava. The finding rarely occurs in isolation but can be seen in patients with associated simple or complex malformations.

Anomalies of Pulmonary Venous Return

In partial anomalous pulmonary venous return, one or more, but not all four, pulmonary veins are not connected to the left atrium. The most common pattern has the right pulmonary veins connected to the superior vena cava, usually with a sinus venosus ASD. Anomalous connection of the right pulmonary veins to the inferior vena cava results in a chest radiographic shadow that resembles a Turkish sword, hence the designation *scimitar syndrome*. Associated anomalies include hypoplasia of the right lung, anomalies of the bronchial system, hypoplasia of the right pulmonary artery, and dextroposition of the heart. Partial anomalous pulmonary venous return results in a left-to-right shunt physiology similar to that of an ASD.

In total anomalous pulmonary venous return, all the pulmonary veins connect abnormally to either the right atrium or one of the systemic veins above or below the diaphragm. Concurrent obstruction of the pulmonary veins is present when drainage occurs below the diaphragm and variable when drainage occurs above it. An ASD is essential to sustain life. One third of cases occur with major complex cardiac malformations.

In cor triatriatum, the pulmonary veins drain into an accessory chamber that is usually connected to the left atrium through an opening of variable size. The hemodynamic consequences are determined by the size of this opening and are similar to those of mitral stenosis. If symptoms of pulmonary venous hypertension occur, surgical treatment is indicated.

CARDIAC MALPOSITIONS

The normal heart is left sided and hence the designation *levocardia*. Cardiac malpositions are defined in terms of the intrathoracic position of the heart in relation to the position of the viscera (visceral situs), which are usually concordant with the position of the atria. That is, when the liver is on the right and the stomach is on the left, the atrium receiving systemic venous blood (right atrium) is right sided and the atrium receiving pulmonary venous blood (left atrium) is left sided. Asplenia and polysplenia syndromes are associated with a variety of complex cardiovascular malformations.

Dextrocardia and Mesocardia

In dextrocardia, the heart is on the right side of the thorax with or without situs inversus. When the heart is right sided with inverted atria, the stomach is right sided, and the liver is left sided, the combination is dextrocardia with situs inversus. In this arrangement, also called *mirror-image dextrocardia*, the ventricles are inverted, but so are the viscera and therefore the atria. The heart usually functions normally, and the diagnosis is often fortuitous. The heart sounds are louder on the right side of the chest, and the liver is palpable on the left. The chest radiograph shows a right-sided cardiac apex with a lower left hemidiaphragm and a right-sided stomach bubble. The ECG shows an inverted P and T wave in lead I with a negative QRS deflection and a reverse pattern between aVR and aVL. A mirror-image progression is seen from V_1 to a right-sided V_6 lead. An echocardiogram should be performed to ensure that intracardiac anatomy is normal.

When dextrocardia with situs solitus occurs, the ventricles are inverted but not the viscera and therefore not the atria. Associated severe cardiac malformations are typical.

In mesocardia, the heart is centrally located in the chest with normal atrial and visceral anatomy. The apex is central or rightward displaced on the chest radiograph. Typically, no associated cardiac malformations are present.

SPECIALIZED ISSUES

Endocarditis Prophylaxis

Prolonged survival of patients with complex congenital heart disease has resulted in a population at increased risk for infective endocarditis (Chapter 76). Adults with congenital heart disease should be informed about the risks of endocarditis. Any unexplained fever requires blood cultures to be drawn before antibiotics are initiated. Thorough transthoracic and transesophageal echocardiograms should be performed to assess the presence of vegetations. If infection of prosthetic material is suspected, early consultation with a specialist who has access to a congenital heart surgeon should be initiated because of the potential for rapid deterioration.

Antibiotic prophylaxis before dental procedures that involve manipulation of the gingiva, periapical regions of the teeth, or mucosal tissue is indicated in patients with previous infective endocarditis; unrepaired cyanotic lesions; palliative shunts or conduits; prosthetic valves or prosthetic materials used for valve repair; repaired congenital heart disease with prosthetic material or transcatheter device within 6 months of intervention; and repaired congenital heart disease with residual lesions at or adjacent to the site of a prosthetic patch or device (Chapter 76). It is also reasonable to consider prophylaxis against endocarditis before vaginal delivery at the time of membrane rupture in such patients. Prophylaxis is not indicated for nondental procedures in the absence of active infection.

Exercise

The goal of exercise evaluation is to assess the functional results of therapeutic interventions and to provide guidelines for exercise prescriptions. Patients with residual hemodynamic lesions or unrepaired congenital cardiac anomalies should be evaluated on an annual basis with a physical examination, an ECG, and a cardiac ultrasonographic examination if indicated. Pertinent additional tests may include Holter monitoring and exercise testing. Attention should be directed to the detection of pulmonary hypertension, arrhythmias, myocardial dysfunction, and symptoms such as exercise-induced dizziness, syncope, dyspnea, or chest pain.

A series of exercise guidelines have been proposed for major groups of congenital heart defects (Table 69-2). Patients beyond 6 months after repair of a single shunt lesion without pulmonary hypertension, arrhythmias, or evidence of myocardial dysfunction can participate in all sports. With

TABLE 69-2 EXERCISE RECOMMENDATIONS IN ADULTS WITH CONGENITAL HEART DISEASE

CONDITION	UNRESTRICTED	LOW-MODERATE INTENSITY*	PROHIBITED
ASD†	No PHT; no arrhythmia; normal ventricular function	PA pressure >40 mm Hg *with* normal ETT; no arrhythmia	Eisenmenger's
VSD†	Small; no PHT; no arrhythmia; normal ventricular function	Moderate VSD	Eisenmenger's
PDA†	Small; no PHT; no arrhythmia; normal ventricular function	PA pressure >40 mm Hg *with* normal ETT; no arrhythmia	Eisenmenger's
Coarctation‡	Gradient ≤20 mm Hg arm to leg; normal BP at rest and exercise	Gradient ≥20 mm Hg arm to leg *with* normal BP and normal ETT	Gradient ≥50 mm Hg arm to leg *or* aortic aneurysm
PS	Gradient <50 mm Hg; no arrhythmia; normal ventricular function	Gradient ≥50 mm Hg	Gradient ≥70 mm Hg *or* ventricular arrhythmia
AS	Gradient ≤20 mm Hg; normal ECG; normal ETT; asymptomatic	Gradient >20 mm Hg *with* normal ECG, normal ETT; asymptomatic	Gradient ≥50 mm Hg *or* ventricular arrhythmia
TOF after repair	Normal RV pressure; no shunt; no arrhythmia	Increased RV pressure *or* moderate PR *or* SVT	RV pressure ≥65% systemic *or* ventricular arrhythmia on ETT *or* severe PR
Mustard or Senning		No cardiomegaly, arrhythmia, or syncope; normal ETT	Cardiomegaly *or* arrhythmia at rest or exercise
c-TGA unoperated	No cardiomegaly; mild TR; no arrhythmia; normal ETT	Moderate RV dysfunction, moderate TR; no arrhythmia	Severe TR *or* uncontrolled arrhythmia
Ebstein's	Mild Ebstein's; no arrhythmia; operated with mild TR	Moderate TR *with* no arrhythmia	Severe Ebstein's *or* uncontrolled arrhythmia
Fontan		Normal O_2 saturation *with* near-normal ETT and ventricular function	Moderate-severe MR or TR *or* uncontrolled arrhythmia

*Based on peak dynamic and static components of exercise during competition for individual sports (see credit line).
†Unoperated or 6 months after surgery.
‡Unoperated or 1 year after surgery.
AS = aortic stenosis; ASD = atrial septal defect; BP = blood pressure; c-TGA = corrected transposition of the great arteries; ECG = electrocardiogram; ETT = exercise tolerance test; MR = mitral regurgitation; PA = pulmonary artery; PDA = patent ductus arteriosus; PHT = pulmonary hypertension; PR = pulmonary regurgitation; PS = pulmonary stenosis; RV = right ventricle; SVT = supraventricular tachyarrhythmia; TOF = tetralogy of Fallot; TR = tricuspid regurgitation; VSD = ventricular septal defect.
Based on guidelines recommended in Graham TP, Bricker TJ, James FW, et al. 26th Bethesda conference: recommendations for determining eligibility for competition in athletes with cardiovascular abnormalities. Task Force 1: Congenital heart disease. *J Am Coll Cardiol.* 1994;24:867. Reprinted with permission of the American College of Cardiology.

residual shunts, if the peak pulmonary artery pressure is less than 40 mm Hg in the absence of ventricular dysfunction or significant arrhythmias, patients can enjoy a free range of activity. Patients with elevated pulmonary vascular resistance are at risk of sudden death during intense exercise; although most self-limit their activity, participation in competitive sports is contraindicated. Patients with aortic and pulmonary stenosis should be counseled as recommended earlier, according to gradient severity. For patients with uncomplicated aortic coarctation, athletic participation is permitted if the arm-leg blood pressure gradient is 20 mm Hg or less at rest and the peak systolic blood pressure during exercise is normal. For patients after tetralogy of Fallot repair, repair of transposition of the great arteries, and the Fontan operation, exercise recommendations vary according to residual ventricular function and the presence or absence of arrhythmias.

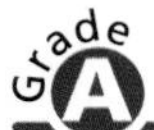

1. Gatzoulis MA, Beghetti M, Galiè N, et al. Longer-term bosentan therapy improves functional capacity in Eisenmenger syndrome: results of the BREATHE-5 open-label extension study. *Int J Cardiol.* 2008;127:27-32.
2. Attie F, Rosas M, Granados N, et al. Surgical treatment for secundum atrial septal defects in patients >40 years old: a randomized clinical trial. *J Am Coll Cardiol.* 2001;38:2035-2042.
3. Dowson A, Mullen MJ, Peatfield R, et al. Migraine intervention with STARFlex Technology (MIST) trial: a prospective, multicenter, double-blind, sham-controlled trial to evaluate the effectiveness of patent foramen ovale closure with STARFlex septal repair implant to resolve refractory migraine headache. *Circulation.* 2008;117:1397-1404.

SUGGESTED READINGS

Penny DJ, Vick GW 3rd. Ventricular septal defect. *Lancet.* 2011;377:1103-1112. *Review.*

Silversides CK, Marelli A, Beauchesne L, et al. Canadian Cardiovascular Society 2009 Consensus Conference on the Management of Adults with Congenital Heart Disease: executive summary. *Can J Cardiol.* 2010;26:143-150. *Practical guidelines.*

Thaler DE, Kent DM. Rethinking trial strategies for stroke and patent foramen ovale. *Curr Opin Neurol.* 2010;23:73-78. *Review of potential risks and benefits.*

Warnes CA, Williams RG, Bashore TM, et al. ACC/AHA 2008 Guidelines for the Management of Adults with Congenital Heart Disease: a report of the American College of Cardiology/American Heart Association Task Force on Practice Guidelines (writing committee to develop guidelines on the management of adults with congenital heart disease). *Circulation.* 2008;118:e714-833. *Consensus guidelines.*

70

ATHEROSCLEROSIS, THROMBOSIS, AND VASCULAR BIOLOGY

GÖRAN K. HANSSON AND ANDERS HAMSTEN

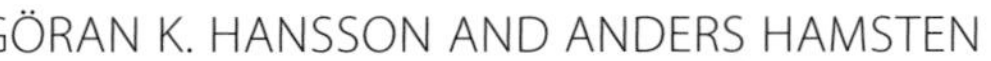

Atherosclerosis is the underlying cause of most cases of myocardial infarction, ischemic stroke, and peripheral arterial disease. It is also a major cause of chronic heart failure and vascular dementia. Atherosclerosis, which is a chronic inflammatory response to the accumulation of lipid in the artery wall, initially is typically characterized by clinically silent intimal plaques in arteries for years and even decades. Fissuring or erosion of atherosclerotic plaques triggers the formation of a thrombus that accumulates over seconds to minutes to cause acute ischemia of the end organ. This ischemia, in turn, results in the dramatic clinical manifestations. It is estimated that approximately 90% of cases of myocardial infarction (Chapter 73), 60% of strokes (Chapter 414), most cases of heart failure (Chapter 58), and up to one third of all cases of dementia (Chapter 409) are due to atherosclerosis.

RISK FACTORS FOR ATHEROSCLEROSIS

The major risk factors that promote the development of atherosclerosis are an elevated low-density lipoprotein (LDL) cholesterol level, a low high-density lipoprotein (HDL) level (Chapter 213), cigarette smoking, type 2 diabetes (Chapter 237), hypertension (Chapter 67), and a family history of coronary heart disease, ischemic stroke, or peripheral arterial disease. Other conditions thought to increase the risk of atherosclerotic disease include abdominal obesity, hypertriglyceridemia, high plasma levels of lipoprotein (a) [Lp(a)], hyperfibrinogenemia, the inflammatory marker C-reactive protein (CRP), and physical inactivity. Other emerging risk factors, including uric acid, psychosocial stress, encompassing external stressors (e.g., job stress, life events, and financial problems), and reactions to stress (e.g., depression [Chapter 404], anxiety, psychosocial distress, and sleep disturbances [Chapter 100]), also appear to contribute. Elevation of plasma total homocysteine is also associated with increased cardiovascular risk, but it is possible that chronic renal dysfunction accounts for at least some of the vascular pathology seen in hyperhomocysteinemia.

An atherogenic lipoprotein phenotype has been defined as the presence of a predominance of small, dense LDL particles, hypertriglyceridemia, and low plasma HDL cholesterol concentration. This lipoprotein phenotype, which is strongly linked to obesity, insulin resistance, hypertension, and abnormalities in postprandial lipoprotein metabolism, is similar to the so-called metabolic syndrome, in that both are associated with a cluster of atherogenic and thrombotic risk factors—raised plasma levels of fibrinogen, plasminogen activator inhibitor-1 (PAI-1), and coagulation factor VII, as well as platelet hyperactivity.

FORMATION OF ATHEROSCLEROTIC LESIONS

Atherosclerosis is thought to be initiated when apolipoprotein B (apoB100)-containing lipoproteins, predominantly LDL, accumulate in the vascular intima, the innermost layer of the artery (Fig. 70-1). Small dense LDL particles are particularly prone to accumulate in the intima, where they associate with proteoglycans of the extracellular matrix. Lipoprotein lipase produced locally in the artery can bridge LDL to the extracellular matrix, and phospholipase and sphingomyelinase actions may contribute to the entrapment of LDL. Once trapped in the artery wall, LDL particles can be attacked by enzymes such as myeloperoxidase and NADPH oxidases; they may also be modified by nonenzymatic oxidation. During oxidative modification of LDL, certain biologically active oxidized phospholipid species are released and activate endothelial cells and macrophages. Such activation leads to production of chemokines and expression of leukocyte adhesion molecules that together instigate recruitment of monocytes and T cells to the intima. Local growth factors induce recruited monocytes to develop into macrophages.

In the intima, macrophages take up oxidized LDL through their scavenger receptors, start to accumulate cholesterol, and are gradually transformed into cholesterol-laden foam cells. Some macrophages in the intima produce proinflammatory mediators, including tumor necrosis factor (TNF), interleukin-1 (IL-1), proinflammatory eicosanoids, radical oxygen and nitrogen species, and prothrombotic factors.

T cells that are stimulated to enter the intima may recognize antigens presented by macrophages. These antigens include components of LDL, other endogenous proteins, and possibly microbial antigens. Activated intimal T cells produce T_H1-type cytokines, such as interferon-γ, TNF, and lymphotoxin, all of which are strongly proatherogenic. With the entry and activation of T cells and macrophages, the accumulation of lipid in the intima leads to the chronic inflammatory disease process of atherosclerosis.

Although adaptive immunity is believed to exert a net proatherogenic effect, antiatherogenic immune responses against LDL involve activation of regulatory T cells, secretion of the anti-inflammatory cytokines IL-10 and transforming growth factor-β, and production of anti-LDL antibodies. In addition to T cells and macrophages, atheroma formation is also stimulated by dendritic cells that take up and present antigen and by mast cells that secrete enzymes and bioactive mediators.

Triglyceride-rich lipoprotein remnant particles, which have adverse effects on endothelial function, penetrate into the subendothelial space of normal intima and atherosclerotic plaques, where they are retained. The LDL-like Lp(a) lipoprotein particle exerts both proatherogenic and prothrombotic actions.

Conversely, antiatherogenic HDL particles counteract the formation of atherosclerotic lesions. These particles mediate cholesterol efflux from cells by acting as acceptors of cholesterol delivered from specific transport proteins termed adenosine triphosphate–binding cassette (ABC) A1 and G1. In addition, HDL particles carry anti-inflammatory and antioxidant proteins.

GROWTH, DEATH, AND THE PROGRESSION OF DISEASE

Early atherosclerotic lesions grow by the accumulation of cholesterol; infiltration of inflammatory cells; the activation, proliferation, and death of such cells; and the gradual development of a core that contains cellular debris and lipids. As a tissue response to this process, smooth muscle cells form a

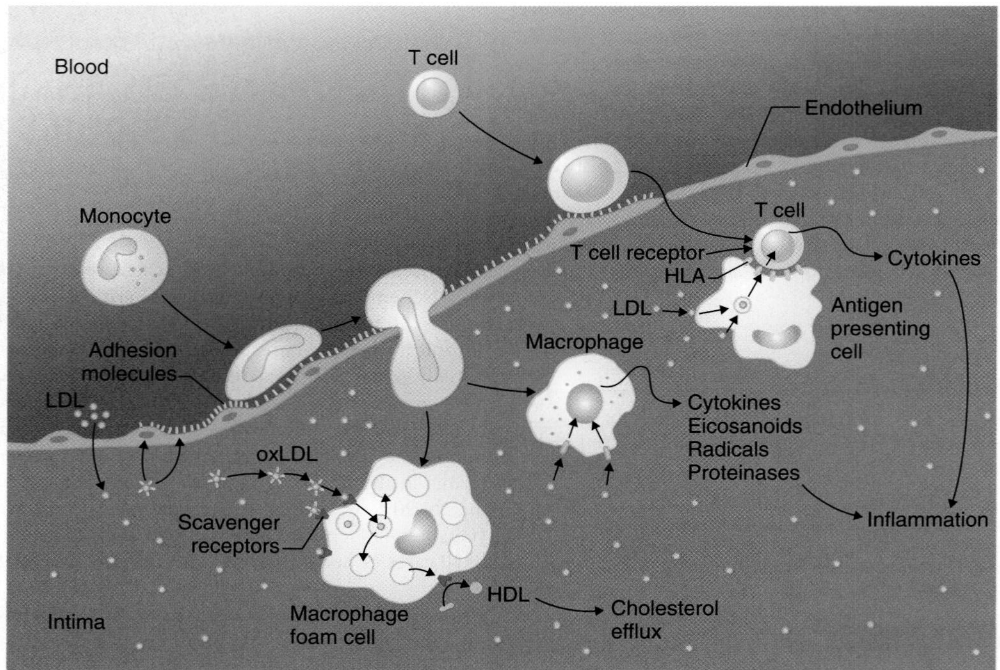

FIGURE 70-1. Formation of atherosclerotic plaques. Low-density lipoproteins (LDL) transit from the blood stream to the arterial intima and accumulate under the endothelial cell layer. LDL particles undergo oxidative modification in the intima (denoted by spikes on LDL particles), thereby leading to their binding to scavenger receptors and uptake by macrophages, which accumulate cholesterol and develop into foam cells. Cholesterol efflux to high-density lipoprotein (HDL) counteracts the tendency to foam cell formation. Molecules released from oxidatively modified LDL activate endothelial cells to express leukocyte adhesion molecules that promote binding of monocytes and T cells to the surface of the artery. Chemokines stimulate monocytes and T cells to migrate into the intima, where the monocytes differentiate into macrophages. Although many macrophages develop into foam cells, some are activated, thereby leading to release of proinflammatory cytokines, eicosanoids, radicals, and proteases. T cells entering through similar mechanisms as monocytes can recognize local antigens, such as LDL components, which are presented to them by antigen-presenting cells (dendritic cells and macrophages) that express HLA molecules. T cells whose receptors can recognize local antigens are activated, thereby leading to release of a host of cytokines that can activate macrophages and enhance vascular inflammation. (Modified from Hansson GK. Inflammation, atherosclerosis, and coronary artery disease. *N Engl J Med.* 2005;352:1685-1695.)

subendothelial cap structure dominated by collagen fibers that are produced by these cells. The collagen cap mechanically stabilizes the plaque and creates a barrier between the hemostatic components of the blood and the thrombogenic material of the plaque. Until the plaque is far advanced, compensatory enlargement ("remodeling") of the arterial wall prevents it from significantly protruding into the arterial lumen. However, after the plaque enlarges to a sufficient size, the lumen narrows as the plaque grows, and the artery remodels inward, often accompanied by exaggerated or paradoxical vasoconstriction.

PLAQUE ACTIVATION, THROMBOSIS, AND INFARCTION

The atherosclerotic process typically is silent for months, years, and even decades, and it may never result in clinical manifestations. However, if and when the plaque's surface is damaged, thrombotic occlusion of the artery may ensue. Surface continuity may be damaged by fissuring (so-called plaque rupture, observed in 60 to 80% of cases of acute coronary syndrome) or surface erosion (present in 20 to 40% of cases with coronary thrombosis, especially women and young victims of sudden coronary death). Fissures and erosions stimulate atherothrombosis by exposing thrombogenic material inside the plaque, such as phospholipids, tissue factor, and matrix molecules, to platelets and coagulation factors (Fig. 70-2). Platelet aggregates formed on exposed surfaces are stabilized by a fibrin network. Tissue factor, expressed in vascular smooth muscle cells and macrophages of the atherosclerotic plaque, is the primary cellular initiator of the blood coagulation cascade that leads to fibrin formation. Atherothrombi expand rapidly and can fill the lumen within minutes, thereby leading to ischemia and infarction.

The cause of plaque rupture remains unclear. Clinical studies have associated ischemic atherothrombotic events such as myocardial infarction (Chapter 73) and stroke (Chapter 414) with infections and stressful events. Histopathologic analysis shows increased inflammation with infiltration of macrophages, activated T cells, dendritic cells, and mast cells, as well as reduced thickness of the fibrous cap and increased neovascularity at sites of plaque rupture and thrombosis. Ruptured plaques also tend to have a large necrotic lipid core. In contrast, plaques underlying erosions do not have a large lipid core and show less inflammation compared with ruptured plaques.

Several members of the matrix metalloproteinase and cysteine proteinase families are found at sites of plaque rupture and have been implicated in plaque rupture, but their effects on the composition and size of lesions are complex. Apoptosis of inflammatory cells and smooth muscle cells, which are contained in the plaque and are likely to contribute to plaque rupture, may be initiated by activation of the death receptor group of the TNF receptor superfamily. Apoptotic macrophages release tissue factor, and a reduced number of smooth muscle cells leads to matrix depletion and destabilizes the plaque. In addition, activated T cells inhibit matrix synthesis by production of interferon-γ, a cytokine that inhibits collagen fiber formation as well as proliferation of smooth muscle cells.

Although a range of factors contribute to atherothrombosis, the precise sequence of events is not yet known. Similarly, the precise role of the activation of coagulation pathways and platelets, combined with the inhibition of fibrinolysis, remains to be defined. Importantly, plaque rupture frequently occurs without clinical manifestations, possibly reflecting variation in the thrombotic response depending on the thrombogenicity of exposed plaque constituents, local hemorrheology, shear-induced platelet activation, systemic clotting activity, fibrinolytic function, and the sensitivity of the end organ to ischemia.

PRINCIPLES OF ANTIATHEROSCLEROTIC THERAPY

Current treatment of atherosclerosis aims at controlling risk factors and maintaining perfusion in affected arteries. However, progress in understanding the pathogenesis of atherosclerosis is expected to result in more direct approaches. To date, firmly established interventions include smoking cessation, dietary and pharmacologic reduction of LDL cholesterol (Chapter 213), and management of blood pressure (Chapter 67). Available data also strongly support intervention directed toward hyperglycemia (Chapter 237), low HDL cholesterol levels (Chapter 213), hypertriglyceridemia (Chapter 213), obesity (Chapter 227), and physical inactivity (Chapter 15). Statins clearly reduce atherosclerotic lesions and inhibit their progression.[1,2] Statins also can prevent nitroglycerin-induced endothelial dysfunction and nitrate tolerance.[3] Aspirin and other inhibitors of platelet aggregation, β-adrenergic receptor blockers, and angiotensin-converting enzyme inhibitors[4] or angiotensin II antagonists are also part of the routine secondary prevention of coronary heart disease (Chapter 71). Inhibitors of platelet aggregation are widely used for secondary prevention of atherosclerotic cardiovascular disease. Aspirin inhibits formation of proaggregatory prostaglandins, whereas other inhibitors of platelet aggregation modulate

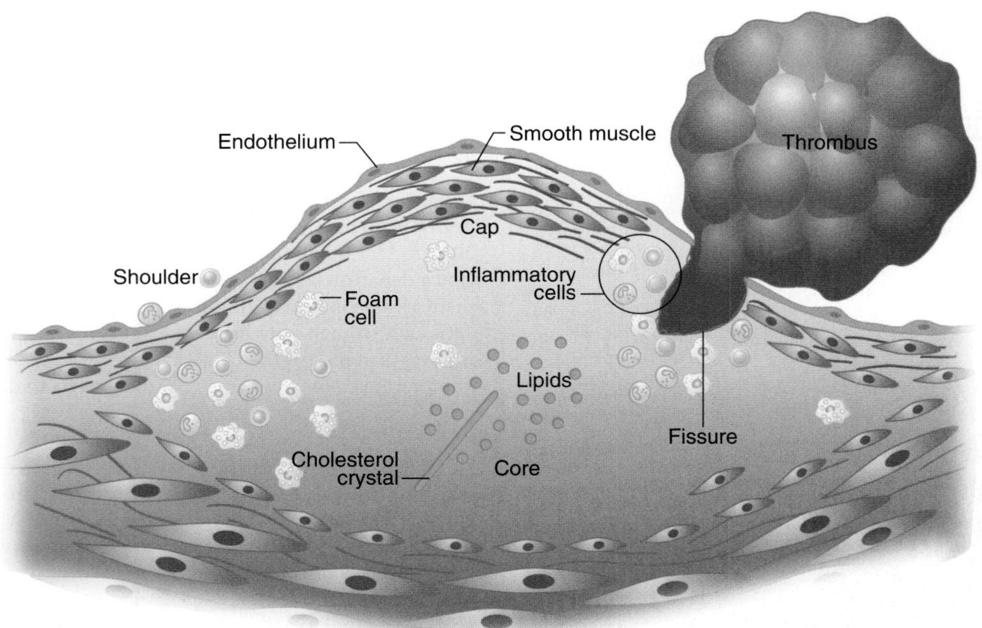

FIGURE 70-2. Plaque rupture and atherothrombosis. The advanced atherosclerotic plaque has a central core with lipids, especially cholesterol, live and dead cells, necrotic material from dead foam cells, and calcium salts. The plaque is overlaid by a fibrous cap that consists of smooth muscle cells and collagen (produced by the muscle cells) and covered by an intact layer of endothelial cells. Inflammatory cells (macrophages, T cells, mast cells, dendritic cells, and occasional B cells) are interspersed with these components and are particularly abundant in the shoulder regions of plaques, where fissures (also called ruptures) may expose thrombogenic core material (e.g., lipids, collagen, tissue factor) to blood components. This event triggers platelet aggregation and humoral coagulation, thereby leading to thrombus formation at the site of fissuring. Thrombi may expand locally to obstruct blood flow or they may detach to cause embolization. (Modified from Hansson GK. Inflammation, atherosclerosis, and coronary artery disease. *N Engl J Med.* 2005;352:1685-1695.)

expression of platelet adhesion molecules. Nitroglycerin and similar compounds that mimic the action of endogenous nitric oxide remain the most important vasodilators used in secondary prevention (Chapter 71). In one preliminary trial, eicosapentaenoic acid reduced coronary events for 4 to 6 years after treatment.5

FUTURE DIRECTIONS

Novel therapeutic opportunities that are currently being considered include new targets for lipid-lowering treatment, use of new immunosuppressing and anti-inflammatory compounds, and vaccination with disease-related antigens. Investigational agents targeting atherogenic lipoproteins include inhibitors of squalene synthase, microsomal triglyceride transfer protein, proprotein convertase subtilisin kexin type 9 (PCSK9), and antisense oligonucleotides to apoB. Compounds targeting HDL include liver X receptor (LXR) agonists, inhibitors of endothelial lipase, and apoA-I mimetic peptides. Statins (Chapter 213) have an array of beneficial actions that are independent of LDL cholesterol reduction, including attenuation of inflammation and inhibition of antigen presentation. Besides their beneficial effects on lipid and blood glucose levels, peroxisome proliferator-activated receptor (PPAR) agonists (Chapter 237) exhibit direct antiatherosclerotic effects in experimental studies.

Members of the TNF superfamily of proinflammatory proteins, eicosanoids, and cell surface proteins promoting antigen-specific T-cell activation are particularly promising targets of anti-inflammatory therapy, whereas stimulation of anti-inflammatory signaling pathways represents a different potential antiatherosclerotic therapy. Inhibition of secreted and lipoprotein-associated phospholipase A_2 is already being examined in clinical trials. Similarly, vaccination against immunogenic epitopes in the protein and lipid moieties of LDL may induce anti-inflammatory regulatory immunity and reduce LDL uptake in cells of the atherosclerotic lesion.

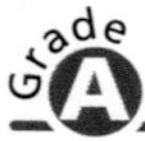

1. Corti R, Fuster V, Fayad ZA. Effects of aggressive versus conventional lipid-lowering therapy by simvastatin on human atherosclerotic lesions: a prospective, randomized, double-blind trial with high-resolution magnetic resonance imaging. *J Am Coll Cardiol.* 2005;46:106-112.
2. Crouse JR 3rd, Raichlen JS, Riley WA, et al. Effect of rosuvastatin on progression of carotid intima-media thickness in low-risk individuals with subclinical atherosclerosis: the METEOR trial. *JAMA.* 2007;297:1344-1353.
3. Liuni A, Luca MC, Di Stolfo G, et al. Coadministration of atorvastatin prevents nitroglycerin-induced endothelial dysfunction and nitrate tolerance in healthy humans. *J Am Coll Cardiol.* 2011;57:93-98.
4. Dagenais GR, Pogue J, Fox K, et al. Angiotensin-converting-enzyme inhibitors in stable vascular disease without left ventricular systolic dysfunction or heart failure: a combined analysis of three trials. *Lancet.* 2006;368:581-588.
5. Yokoyama M, Origasa H, Matsuzaki M, et al. Effects of eicosapentaenoic acid on major coronary events in hypercholesterolaemic patients (JELIS): a randomised open-label, blinded endpoint analysis. *Lancet.* 2007;369:1090-1098.

SUGGESTED READINGS

Alsheikh-Ali AA, Kitsios GD, Balk EM, et al. The vulnerable atherosclerotic plaque: scope of the literature. *Ann Intern Med.* 2010;153:387-395. *Review.*

Bäck M, Ketelhuth DF, Agewall S. Matrix metalloproteinases in atherothrombosis. *Prog Cardiovasc Dis.* 2010;52:410-428. *Proteolytic enzymes may play a key role in plaque rupture and myocardial infarction.*

Khera AV, Cuchel M, de la Llera-Moya M, et al. Cholesterol efflux capacity, high-density lipoprotein function, and atherosclerosis. *N Engl J Med.* 2011;364:127-135. *Cholesterol efflux capacity is negatively associated with carotid intima-media thickness and the likelihood of angiographic coronary artery disease.*

71

ANGINA PECTORIS AND STABLE ISCHEMIC HEART DISEASE

WILLIAM E. BODEN

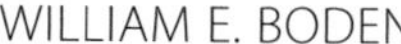

DEFINITION

Ischemic heart disease is most commonly caused by obstruction or stenosis of one or more of the coronary arteries by atheromatous plaque (Chapter 70). Obstruction can result in myocardial ischemia and infarction (Chapters 72 and 73) with associated symptoms of angina, ischemia, myocardial remodeling, heart failure (Chapter 58), arrhythmic complications (Chapters 63, 64, 65), and ultimately death.

Angina pectoris is generally a consequence of a supply-demand imbalance between an activity that increases cardiac workload or "demand," thereby resulting in an increase in heart rate, blood pressure, or both, and the inability of the narrowed epicardial coronary arteries (Chapter 57) to augment antegrade flow or "supply" in response to this increase in demand. Such an imbalance classically results in chest discomfort (Chapter 50) of varying intensity and duration. Angina pectoris is generally defined as a discomfort in the chest or adjacent areas caused by myocardial ischemia. Often, angina is described incorrectly as "chest pain." The term *angina*, however, derives from a neologism of two Latin words, "angor animi," which literally translates into "fear of life being extinguished ('from the breast')," according to Heberden's original description in 1768. Had Heberden been trying to convey the term for chest pain, he would more likely have used the Latin term *dolor pectoris*.

Grading of Angina Pectoris

The Canadian Cardiovascular Society (CCS) angina grading scale is a widely used four-point ordinal scale that classifies angina pectoris from mild (class I: angina occurring only during strenuous or prolonged physical activity) to severe (class IV: inability to perform any activity without angina, or angina at rest) and includes the full spectrum of angina from chronic stable to unstable (see Table 50-5 in Chapter 50). Operationally, the CCS angina scale permits clinicians to categorize patients as mild or stable (generally CCS classes I and II) versus severe or unstable (typically CCS classes III and IV). Other grading systems include a specific activity scale, which is based on the metabolic cost of specific activities, and an anginal score, which integrates the clinical features and tempo of angina with electrocardiographic (ECG) changes and offers independent prognostic information beyond that provided by age, gender, ventricular function, and coronary anatomy.

EPIDEMIOLOGY

It is currently estimated that 17,600,000 adults in the United States have heart disease, 10,200,000 of whom have angina pectoris and 8,500,000 of whom have had acute myocardial infarction (MI). Approximately 785,000 Americans will experience a new ischemic heart disease event annually, and about 470,000 will have a recurrent event. In 2006, ischemic heart disease accounted for 52% of all deaths caused by cardiovascular disease and was the single most frequent cause of death in American men and women, resulting in more than one in every six deaths. The economic burden of ischemic heart disease in the United States in 2010 has been estimated at $177.1 billion. Despite the sustained decline in age-specific case-fatality rates from coronary artery disease over the past several decades, ischemic heart disease is now the leading cause of death worldwide, and it is expected that this rate of rise will continue to accelerate over the coming decade as a consequence of the epidemic rise in obesity (Chapter 227), type 2 diabetes (Chapter 237), and the metabolic syndrome, which may give rise to an increasing risk of developing premature coronary artery disease in younger generations. The World Health Organization has projected that, over the next decade, the global number of deaths from coronary artery disease will increase by 46% from 7.6 million in 2005 to 11.1 million in 2020. An estimated 8 million patients come to emergency departments annually for chest pain, and approximately 1.5 million of them are hospitalized with the acute coronary syndrome (ACS; Chapter 72). Although women may have typical angina less frequently than men, more women than men in the United States die annually of ischemic heart disease or its complications, and, overall, ischemic heart disease is the most common cause of death in women.

PATHOBIOLOGY

Angina is the most frequent clinical expression of myocardial ischemia. Ischemia, which rapidly develops when a mismatch arises between myocardial oxygen needs and myocardial oxygen supply, can manifest clinically in many different ways besides angina, from no symptoms (e.g., silent ischemia) to unstable angina, MI, or sudden cardiac death. It may remain stable for many years in selected patients or may be rapidly progressive with an abrupt change in frequency and tempo over days to weeks. Conversely, atherosclerosis, which is the most common cause of myocardial ischemia, may evolve for years without any manifestations of ischemia.

In contrast to the inherent pathogenetic complexity mediated by differing mechanisms associated with abrupt plaque rupture, fissuring, or erosion in patients with ACS (Chapters 70 and 72), the pathogenesis of chronic stable angina is, by comparison, seemingly less complicated and heterogeneous because it fundamentally involves a myocardial supply-demand mismatch. In most patients with stable ischemic heart disease, the process of atherosclerosis involves a fundamentally different histopathology (small lipid core with a thick or very thick fibrous cap and a low proclivity to rupture) compared with ACS or unstable angina, in which the principal histopathologic picture is that of a large lipid core subtended by a thinned, inflamed cap, which harbors the high-risk or vulnerable plaque with a high proclivity for rupture (Chapter 70).

Two major pathogenetic mechanisms may result in myocardial ischemia and angina in the chronic setting: so-called demand angina, which is caused by an increase in myocardial oxygen requirements and workload, and supply angina, which is caused by diminished oxygen delivery to myocardial tissue. Demand angina is a consequence of the increased myocardial oxygen (O_2) requirements that occur with increased physical activity, emotion, or stress. In a patient with chronic, restricted O_2 delivery owing to atherosclerotic narrowing of a coronary artery, this increased demand may precipitate angina. Other extracardiac precipitants of angina include the excessive metabolic demands imposed by fever, thyrotoxicosis (Chapter 233), severe anemia (Chapter 161) from blood loss, tachycardia from any cause (Chapters 62, 63, 64), and hypoglycemia (Chapter 238).

By contrast, supply angina may occur in patients with either unstable angina (Chapter 72) or chronic stable angina by transient reductions in myocardial O_2 delivery as a consequence of coronary vasoconstriction with resulting dynamic coronary stenosis. In the presence of coronary luminal narrowing due to atherosclerosis, superimposed platelet thrombi and leukocytes may elaborate vasoconstrictor substances, such as serotonin and thromboxane A_2, whereas endothelial damage in diseased coronary arteries may decrease production of vasodilator substances such as nitric oxide and adenosine. The result is an abnormal vasoconstrictor response to exercise and other stimuli, such as exogenously administered adenosine or the paradoxical vasoconstrictor response to the typical flow-mediated reactive hyperemia associated with brachial artery compression. In some clinical settings, patients who have normal coronary arteries or non-flow-limiting stenoses may exhibit dynamic obstruction alone, which can cause myocardial ischemia and result in angina at rest (Prinzmetal's [variant] angina). Conversely, in patients with severe fixed obstruction to coronary blood flow, only a minor increase in dynamic obstruction can reduce blood flow below a critical level and cause myocardial ischemia.

The pathophysiologic basis for angina and ischemia in patients with stable ischemic heart disease has important implications for the selection of anti-ischemic agents. The greater the contribution from increased myocardial O_2 requirements to the imbalance between supply and demand, the greater the likelihood that agents such as β-blockers or heart rate–lowering calcium antagonists will provide clinical benefit, whereas nitrates and calcium antagonists with more potent vasodilatory properties (particularly the dihydropyridines) will be more beneficial to alleviate angina and ischemia mediated by coronary vasoconstriction.

Although the most common cause of ischemic heart disease is atherosclerotic narrowing of the epicardial coronary arteries resulting in flow-limiting obstruction to blood flow, obstructive coronary artery disease may also have nonatherosclerotic causes, such as congenital abnormalities of the coronary arteries (Chapter 69), vasospasm, myocardial bridging, coronary arteritis in association with systemic vasculitides (Chapter 278), and radiation-induced coronary disease (Chapter 19). Myocardial ischemia and angina pectoris may also occur in the absence of obstructive coronary artery disease, as in the case of aortic valve disease (Chapter 75), hypertrophic cardiomyopathy (Chapter 60), and idiopathic dilated cardiomyopathy. Moreover, ischemic heart disease may coexist with these other forms of heart disease.

TABLE 71-1 PROBABILITY (%) OF CORONARY ARTERY DISEASE BY AGE, GENDER, AND SYMPTOMS

GENDER	AGE (yr)	DEFINITE ANGINA	ATYPICAL ANGINA	NONCARDIAC CHEST PAIN
Men	30-39	83	46	3
	40-49	88	57	12
	50-59	94	71	18
	60-69	95	78	31
	≥70	97	94	63
Women	30-39	—	20	4
	40-49	56	31	4
	50-59	68	30	6
	60-69	81	48	10
	≥70	96	56	—

From Chaitman BR, Bourassa MG, Davis K, et al. Angiographic prevalence of high-risk coronary artery disease in patient subsets (CASS). *Circulation*. 1981;64:360-367.

TABLE 71-2 NON–CHEST PAIN SYMPTOMS OF CHRONIC ISCHEMIC HEART DISEASE

DYSPNEA

Dyspnea on exertion
Dyspnea at rest
Paroxysmal nocturnal dyspnea
Temporal change of increasing exertional dyspnea with declining effort tolerance

NON–CHEST LOCATIONS OF DISCOMFORT (EITHER EXERTIONAL OR AT REST)

Neck or mandibular discomfort or pain
Throat tightness
Shoulder discomfort
Upper arm or forearm discomfort (more often left-sided)
Interscapular or infrascapular discomfort

MID-EPIGASTRIC OR ABDOMINAL

Mid-epigastric burning, often postprandially
Sharp abdominal pain (atypical, but more common in women)
Right-upper quadrant discomfort (may mimic gallbladder disease or pancreatitis)
Nausea and/or vomiting (often associated with increased vagal tone secondary to inferior myocardial ischemia or infarction)

DIAPHORESIS

EXCESSIVE FATIGUE AND WEAKNESS

Often a discernible prodrome of increasing fatigue with declining effort tolerance

DIZZINESS AND SYNCOPE

Uncommon, unless precipitated or exacerbated by alterations in heart rate or rhythm (e.g., bradyarrhythmia, tachyarrhythmia, heart block), blood pressure (e.g., hypotension), or cardiac output (e.g., decreased cerebral perfusion)

CLINICAL MANIFESTATIONS

History

It is important to recognize that there are many causes of chest pain (see Table 50-2 in Chapter 50), that angina-like chest pain may not represent ischemic heart disease (Table 71-1), that ischemic heart disease causes symptoms other than anginal pain (Table 71-2), and that nonatherosclerotic coronary artery abnormalities may cause ischemic chest pain (Table 71-3).

Angina pectoris has four cardinal clinical features: the character of the discomfort, its site and distribution, its provocation, and its duration. The character of anginal discomfort is typically described as a pressure sensation that conveys a feeling of strangling and anxiety (Chapter 50). Other adjectives frequently used to describe this discomfort include heavy, squeezing, constricting, viselike, suffocating, and, at times, crushing. In some patients, the quality of the sensation is more vague and atypical (often in women and elderly patients), and these patients may describe the discomfort as a burning sensation in the mid-epigastrium or as an uncomfortable, numb sensation. Anginal equivalents (i.e., symptoms of myocardial ischemia other than angina), such as dyspnea, fatigue, lightheadedness or dizziness, and gastric eructations, may likewise be described.

The site and distribution of anginal discomfort are predominantly midsternal or retrosternal but can be precordial. Radiation is common, usually to the left neck and shoulder and down the ulnar surface of the left arm; the right arm and the outer surfaces of both arms may also be involved. Discomfort that radiates to the jaw may be confused with dental pain. Epigastric discomfort alone or in association with chest pressure may occur. Provocation of angina is classically caused by physical exertion or activity, emotional stress, exposure to the cold, sexual intercourse, or eating a large meal. Angina that occurs at rest or nocturnally often heralds a change in the pattern from stable to unstable and may indicate that there is an incipient plaque rupture leading

TABLE 71-3 NONATHEROSCLEROTIC CAUSES OF ISCHEMIC CHEST PAIN

PRIMARY CARDIAC CAUSE
Coronary artery abnormalities
Coronary spasm
Coronary arteritis
Coronary dissection
Coronary artery anomalies
Radiation-induced coronary disease
Myocardial bridging
Aortic stenosis
Hypertrophic cardiomyopathy
Dilated cardiomyopathy
Tachycardia
PRIMARY NONCARDIAC CAUSE
Anemia
Sickle cell disease
Hypoxemia
Carbon monoxide poisoning
Hyperviscosity (e.g., polycythemia)
Hyperthyroidism
Pheochromocytoma

to ACS. Vasospastic (or Prinzmetal's) angina may occur spontaneously at rest or nocturnally without provocation.

The typical duration of an episode of angina pectoris is brief. An episode usually begins gradually and reaches its maximal intensity over a period of minutes before abating. It is unusual for angina pectoris to peak and trough in less than a minute, and it is common that patients with exertional angina usually prefer to rest, sit, or stop walking during episodes that may be precipitated by the offending activity. Chest discomfort that persists for more than 15 to 20 minutes, especially at rest or nocturnally, is likely to represent ACS or MI. By contrast, features that suggest a noncardiac etiology of angina pectoris include pleuritic pain, pain reproduced by movement or palpation of the chest wall or arms, sharp or constant pain lasting for many hours, pain or discomfort that a patient can localize to the chest wall with the tip of one finger, or very brief episodes of pain lasting seconds (Chapter 50). Typical angina pectoris is generally relieved within minutes by rest or the use of sublingual, oral, or cutaneous nitroglycerin. The response to sublingual nitroglycerin is often a helpful diagnostic tool, although it should be emphasized that some noncardiac pain (e.g., esophageal spasm) may also respond to nitroglycerin.

Although chest discomfort is usually the predominant symptom in chronic (stable) angina, unstable angina, Prinzmetal's (variant) angina, microvascular angina, and acute MI, chest discomfort is absent, atypical, or not prominent in some patients. Patients with chronic ischemic heart disease may complain predominantly or exclusively of dyspnea, diminishing exercise tolerance or weakness. Others will first present with an abnormal exercise test result or other evidence of myocardial ischemia without any symptoms. Some patients will present with cardiac arrhythmias or even sudden cardiac death.

Physical Examination

Many patients with stable ischemic heart disease present with normal physical findings, but a diligent physical examination may reveal findings that represent either the consequences of myocardial ischemia or evidence of risk factors for coronary artery disease. Inspection of the eyes may reveal a corneal arcus, and examination of the skin may show xanthomas (see Fig. 50-12 in Chapter 50). Retinal arteriolar changes are common in patients with coronary artery disease who have hypertension or diabetes mellitus (see Figs. 431-26 and 431-24 in Chapter 431).

The cardiac examination is generally of limited benefit in evaluating patients with chest pain or establishing a diagnosis of ischemic heart disease. During an episode of chest discomfort, myocardial ischemia may produce either a third or fourth heart sound.

Myocardial ischemia also can cause a transient holosystolic or mid-late systolic apical murmur owing to reversible papillary muscle dysfunction that results in mitral regurgitation. These murmurs are more prevalent in patients with extensive coronary artery disease, especially with inferior or inferoposterior ischemia owing to right coronary artery disease. It is important to distinguish such a murmur from the murmur of aortic stenosis or obstructive hypertrophic cardiomyopathy (see Tables 50-7 and 50-8 in Chapter 50). A displaced left ventricular (LV) apical impulse, particularly if dyskinetic, is a sign of significant LV systolic dysfunction.

If patients have coexisting heart failure, an elevated jugular venous pressure, pulmonary rales, and peripheral edema may be present (Chapter 58). The physical examination may reveal other implicating or contributing conditions, such as thyroid enlargement (Chapter 233) or severe anemia (Chapter 161).

DIAGNOSIS AND EVALUATION

In addition to a careful history and physical examination, assessment of patients with stable ischemic heart disease includes the 12-lead ECG, measurement of biochemical and inflammatory markers, and noninvasive diagnostic testing. The first goal is to assess the patient's probability of ischemia so that an appropriate evaluation can expedite effective therapy (Fig. 71-1).

Resting Electrocardiogram

Although there may be focal, diagnostic findings of ST segment depression and T wave inversions (Fig. 71-2) on the resting ECG in chronic ischemic heart disease, even patients with extensive anatomic coronary artery disease may have a normal tracing at rest. In addition to myocardial ischemia, other conditions that can produce ST-T wave abnormalities include LV hypertrophy and dilation due to long-standing hypertension and valvular heart disease (e.g., aortic stenosis, hypertrophic cardiomyopathy), electrolyte abnormalities, neurogenic effects, and antiarrhythmic drugs. The presence of new ST-T wave abnormalities on the resting ECG, however, can be helpful in the diagnosis of coronary artery disease and may correlate with the severity of the underlying heart disease.

In addition to focal ST-T wave abnormalities, the ECG may reveal various conduction disturbances, most frequently left bundle branch block and left anterior fascicular block (Chapter 54). The finding of abnormal Q waves is relatively specific for the presence of previous MI but may not help to determine when such an event occurred. Arrhythmias, especially ventricular premature beats (Chapter 65), may be present on the ECG but have a low sensitivity and specificity for coronary artery disease.

During a spontaneous episode of angina pectoris or during exertion or stress, the ECG becomes abnormal in 50% or more of patients with normal resting ECGs. The most common abnormality observed is focal ST segment depression, usually in one or more ECG lead groups, which signifies the presence of subendocardial ischemia. On occasion, transient, but diminutive, ST segment elevation and normalization of previous resting ST-T wave depression or inversion (pseudonormalization) may develop during chronic angina and ischemia, although ST segment elevation is far more commonly observed in ACS patients with plaque rupture.

Laboratory Testing

In patients with new-onset or worsening symptoms, a troponin level can distinguish MI and ACS from stable ischemic heart disease (Chapters 72 and 73). An elevated plasma concentration of brain natriuretic peptide does not help diagnose stable ischemic heart disease but is suggestive of heart failure (Chapter 58) and is associated with a higher risk of future cardiovascular events. High-sensitivity C-reactive protein, an acute phase reactant of inflammation, has a strong and consistent relationship to the risk of future cardiovascular events, and an elevated level may warrant more aggressive diagnostic evaluation and therapy.

All patients with chronic angina should have biochemical evaluation of total cholesterol, low-density lipoprotein (LDL) cholesterol, high-density lipoprotein (HDL) cholesterol, triglyceride, serum creatinine (estimated glomerular filtration), and fasting blood glucose levels (Table 71-4). Other biochemical markers that are not routinely recommended but are associated with higher risk of future cardiovascular events include lipoprotein (a), apoprotein B, small dense LDL cholesterol, and lipoprotein-associated phospholipase A_2 (Lp-PLA_2). Homocysteine levels correlate with the risk of developing coronary heart disease, but randomized trials have failed to demonstrate a reduction of clinical events when elevated homocysteine levels are reduced; as a result, screening for an elevated homocysteine level is not recommended.

Noninvasive Testing

Noninvasive stress testing with a standard ECG treadmill or bicycle exercise, radionuclide imaging (Chapter 56), stress echocardiography (Chapter 55), or newer diagnostic modalities such as cardiac magnetic resonance (CMR;

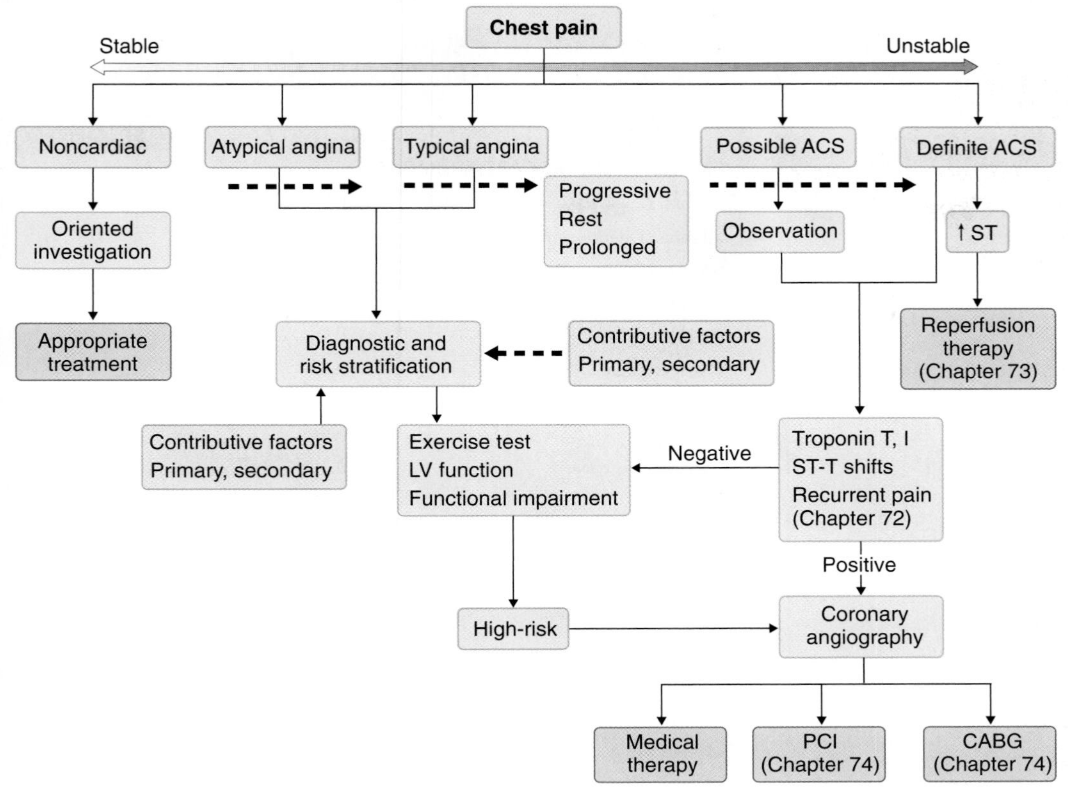

FIGURE 71-1. **Evaluation of chest pain.** ACS = acute coronary syndrome; CABG = coronary artery bypass graft; LV = left ventricular; PCI = percutaneous coronary intervention. (Adapted from Théroux P. Angina pectoris. In: Goldman L, Ausiello DA, eds. *Cecil Textbook of Medicine,* 23rd ed. Philadelphia: Saunders Elsevier; 2008.)

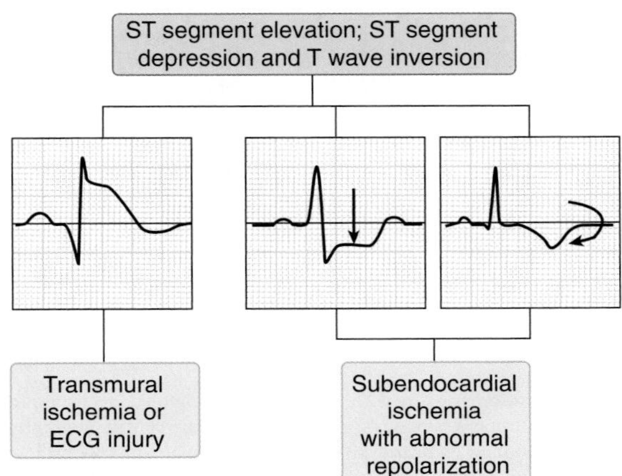

FIGURE 71-2. **Ischemic ST segment shifts and repolarization changes on electrocardiogram (ECG).**

TABLE 71-4 BLOOD TESTS TO OBTAIN ROUTINELY (OR SELECTIVELY*) IN PATIENTS WITH CHRONIC STABLE ISCHEMIC HEART DISEASE

LIPID LEVELS
Low-density lipoprotein (LDL) and high-density lipoprotein (HDL) cholesterol Triglyceride level *LDL electrophoresis (especially apoprotein B and small dense LDL) *Lipoprotein (a) *Lipoprotein-associated phospholipase (Lp-PLA2)
METABOLIC EVALUATION
Fasting plasma glucose Serum creatinine Thyroxine level *Hemoglobin A_{1c} in patients with known or suspected diabetes
MARKERS OF INFLAMMATION OR CARDIAC FUNCTION
*High-sensitivity C-reactive protein (hs-CRP) *Brain natriuretic peptide (BNP)
PROTHROMBOTIC ASSESSMENT
Plasma fibrinogen Platelet count *Factor V Leiden *D-dimer *Plasminogen activator inhibitor (PAI) type 1
TO ASSESS OTHER POTENTIAL CARDIAC RISK FACTORS
*Serum homocysteine

Chapter 56) or positron-emission tomography (PET; Chapter 56) (Fig. 71-3) is a useful and clinically important approach to establishing the diagnosis and prognosis in patients with stable ischemic heart disease. The predictive accuracy of these tests is defined not only by their sensitivity and specificity but also by the prevalence of disease (or pretest probability) in the population under study. Noninvasive testing should be performed only if the incremental information is likely to alter the planned management strategy. Thus, the value of noninvasive stress testing is greatest when the pretest likelihood is intermediate because the test result is likely to have the greatest effect on the post-test probability of coronary artery disease and, hence, on clinical decision making.

Each noninvasive test has a sensitivity and specificity (Table 71-5), which, when combined with a patient's pretest probability (see Table 71-1), can yield a post-test probability for coronary artery disease (Fig. 71-4). The choice among tests depends on the patient's characteristics (Table 71-6).

Exercise Electrocardiography

An exercise ECG is the preferred test in patients who have suspected angina pectoris and are considered to have a moderate probability of coronary artery disease if the resting ECG is normal (i.e., ST segments are not obscured by structural heart disease or medication), provided that subjects are capable of achieving an adequate workload. Interpretation of the exercise ECG should include the exercise capacity achieved (duration and metabolic equivalents of the external workload; see Table 50-3 in Chapter 50), the magnitude and extent of ST segment deviation, and clinical and hemodynamic responses to exercise.

The exercise test protocol is usually adjusted to a patient's tolerance, aiming for 6 to 12 minutes of exercise time (i.e., Bruce protocol stages II to

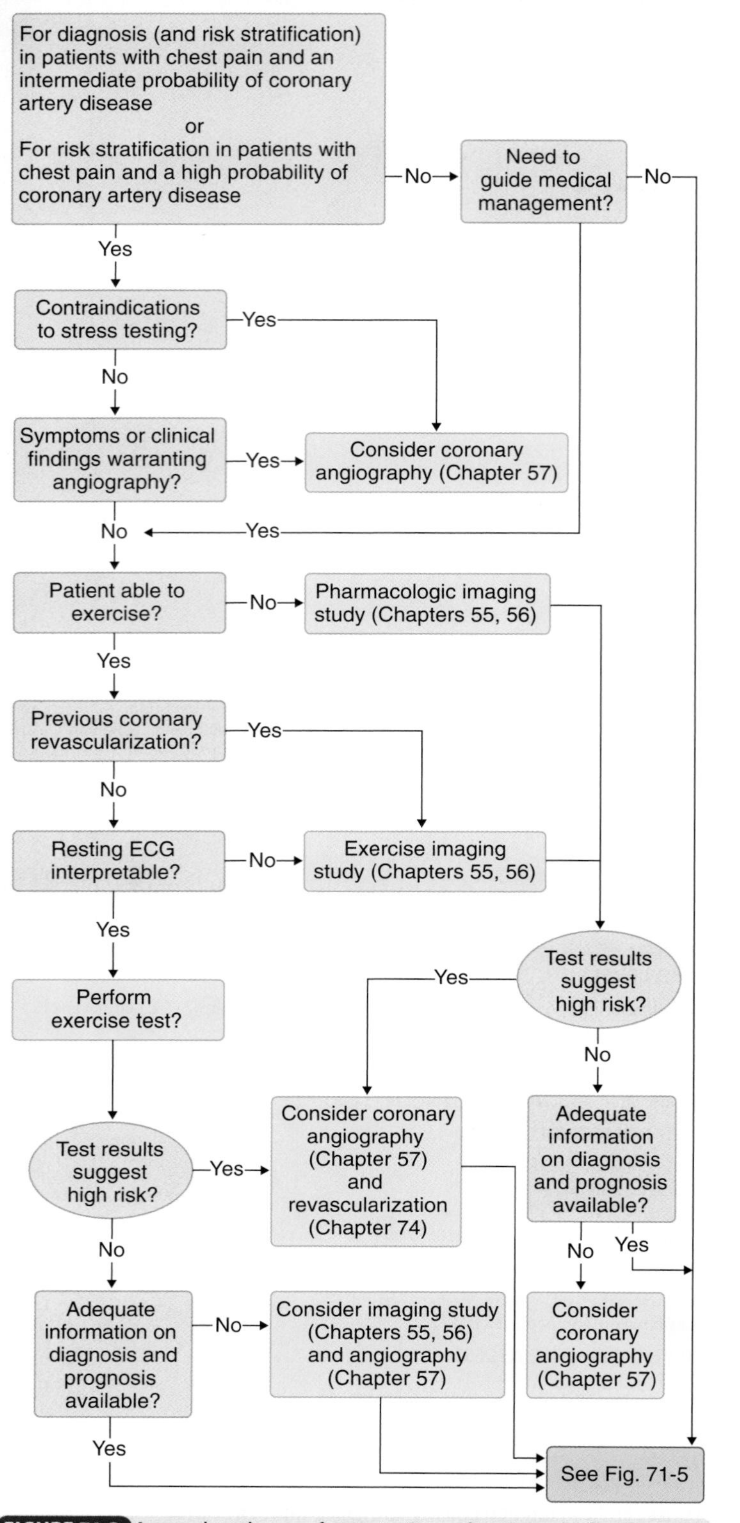

FIGURE 71-3. Approach to the use of stress testing and angiography for the evaluation of chronic stable angina. ECG = electrocardiogram. (Modified from American College of Cardiology/American Heart Association Task Force on Practice Guidelines. *Management of Patients with Chronic Stable Angina. ACC/AHA/ACP-ASIM Pocket Guidelines.* Philadelphia: Elsevier Science; 2000.)

TABLE 71-5 APPROXIMATE SENSITIVITY AND SPECIFICITY OF COMMON TESTS TO DIAGNOSE CORONARY ARTERY DISEASE

	SENSITIVITY	SPECIFICITY
EXERCISE ELECTROCARDIOGRAPHY		
>1 mm ST depression	0.70	0.75
>2 mm ST depression	0.33	0.97
>3 mm ST depression	0.20	0.99
PERFUSION SCINTIGRAPHY		
Exercise SPECT	0.88	0.72
Pharmacologic SPECT	0.90	0.82
ECHOCARDIOGRAPHY		
Exercise	0.85	0.81
Pharmacologic stress	0.81	0.79
PET	0.95	0.95

PET = positron emission tomography; SPECT = single-photon emission computed tomography.
From Gibbons RJ, Abrams J, Chatterjee K, et al. ACC/AHA 2002 guideline update for the management of patients with chronic stable angina—summary article: a report of the American College of Cardiology/American Heart Association Task Force on Practice Guidelines (Committee on Management of Patients with Chronic Stable Angina). *Circulation.* 2003;107:149-158.

TABLE 71-6 SUGGESTED NONINVASIVE TESTS IN DIFFERENT TYPES OF PATIENTS WITH STABLE ANGINA

Exertional angina, mixed angina, walk-through angina, postprandial angina with or without prior myocardial infarction	
Normal resting ECG	Treadmill exercise ECG test
Abnormal, uninterpretable resting ECG	Exercise myocardial perfusion scintigraphy (^{201}Tl, ^{99m}Tc-sestamibi) or exercise echocardiography
Unsuitable for exercise	Dipyridamole, adenosine, or regadenoson myocardial perfusion scintigraphy, dobutamine stress echocardiography
Atypical chest pain with normal or borderline abnormal resting ECG or with nondiagnostic stress ECG, particularly in women	Exercise myocardial perfusion scintigraphy, exercise echocardiography
Vasospastic angina	ECG during chest pain, ST segment ambulatory ECG, exercise test
Dilated ischemic cardiomyopathy with typical angina or for assessment of hibernating or stunned myocardium	Regional and global ejection fraction by radionuclide ventriculography or two-dimensional echocardiography, radionuclide myocardial perfusion scintigraphy; in selected patients, flow and metabolic studies with positron emission tomography
Syndrome X	Treadmill exercise stress ECG, coronary blood flow by positron emission tomography, Doppler probe
Known severe aortic stenosis or severe hypertrophic cardiomyopathy with stable angina	Exercise stress tests contraindicated; dipyridamole, adenosine, or regadenoson myocardial perfusion scintigraphy in selected patients; coronary angiography preferred
Mild aortic valvar disease or hypertrophic cardiomyopathy with typical exertional angina	"Prudent" treadmill myocardial perfusion scintigraphy, dipyridamole or adenosine or regadenoson myocardial perfusion scintigraphy

ECG = 12-lead electrocardiogram.
Modified from Braunwald E, Goldman L, eds. *Primary Care Cardiology*, 2nd ed. Philadelphia: WB Saunders; 2003.

IV) to achieve maximal oxygen consumption and to elicit objective evidence of inducible ischemia, if present. Exercise stress testing is generally very safe, with death or MI occurring in less than one case per 2500 tests, when such provocative testing is avoided in patients with severe aortic stenosis, severe hypertension, or uncontrolled heart failure. Other contraindications are acute MI, symptomatic arrhythmias, acute pulmonary embolism, and suspected acute aortic dissection. Relative contraindications are hypertension greater than 200 mm Hg systolic or 110 mm Hg diastolic, hypertrophic cardiomyopathy, and high-degree atrioventricular block.

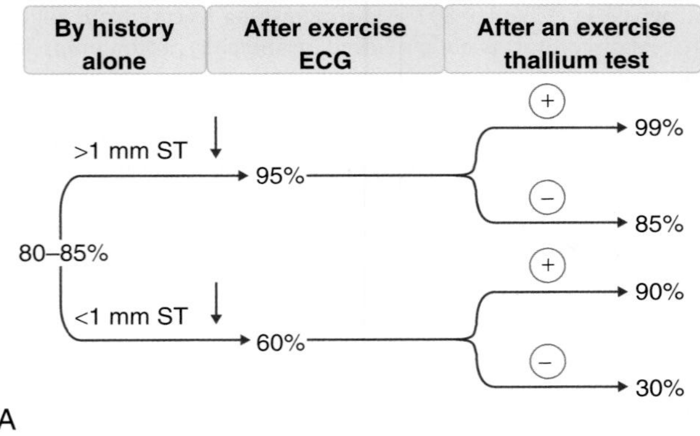

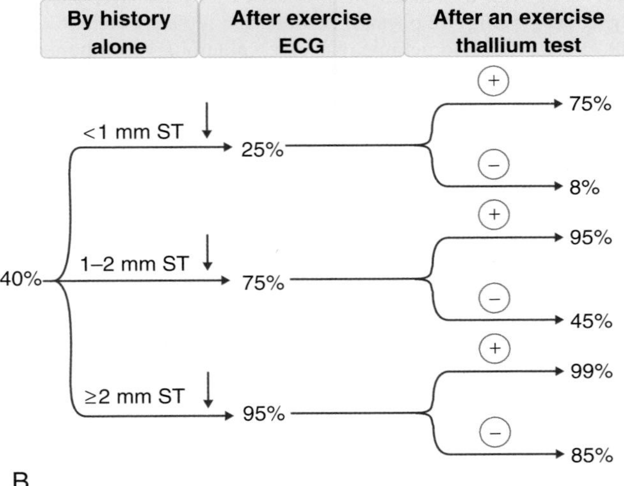

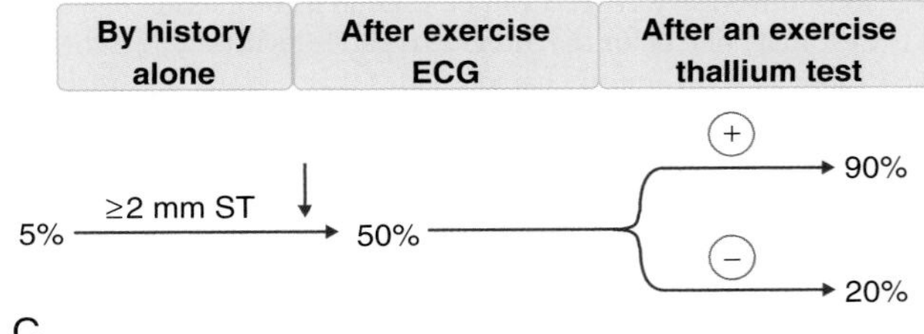

FIGURE 71-4. Approximate probabilities of coronary artery disease in different patient groups. A, Approximate probability of coronary artery disease before and after noninvasive testing in a patient with typical angina pectoris. These percentages demonstrate how the sequential use of an electrocardiogram (ECG) and an exercise thallium test may affect the probability of coronary artery disease in a patient with typical angina pectoris. **B,** Approximate probability of coronary artery disease before and after noninvasive testing in a patient with atypical angina symptoms. **C,** Approximate probability of coronary artery disease before and after noninvasive testing in an asymptomatic subject in the coronary artery disease age range. (Redrawn from Branch WB Jr, ed. *Office Practice of Medicine*, 3rd ed. Philadelphia: WB Saunders; 1994:45.)

Concomitant antianginal therapy (notably the use of β-blockers) reduces the sensitivity of exercise testing as a screening tool. If the purpose of the exercise test is to diagnose ischemia, it should be performed, whenever possible, before initiating β-blockers, or 2 to 3 days after their discontinuation.

Nuclear Cardiology Imaging

Stress myocardial perfusion imaging (Chapter 56) using single-photon emission computed tomography (SPECT) with simultaneous electrocardiographic testing (see Fig. 56-1 in Chapter 56) is particularly helpful in the diagnosis of coronary artery disease in patients with abnormal resting ECGs and among those in whom ST segment responses cannot be interpreted accurately, such as patients with repolarization abnormalities caused by LV hypertrophy, those with left bundle branch block, and those receiving digitalis. Its sensitivity and specificity are superior to exercise electrocardiography alone in detecting coronary artery disease, especially multivessel disease, in identifying regional perfusion defects that may localize to and correlate with diseased vessels, and in delineating the magnitude and extent of ischemic and infarcted myocardium. Treadmill testing is preferred for patients who are capable of performing such physical activity because of the additional diagnostic and prognostic information achieved with graded exercise. In the 40 to 50% of patients who are unable to exercise adequately, however, pharmacologic vasodilator stress with dipyridamole, adenosine, or regadenoson may be the preferred approach to noninvasive testing.

Stress Echocardiography

Stress two-dimensional echocardiography using exercise or pharmacologic stress can detect regional ischemia by identifying new wall motion abnormalities (see Fig. 55-5 in Chapter 55). Additional clinical information regarding associated structural heart disease, chamber dimensions, and valve function can be readily obtained. Exercise echocardiography can detect the presence of coronary artery disease with a similar accuracy as achieved with stress myocardial perfusion imaging and is useful for localizing and quantifying ischemic myocardial segments. Pharmacologic stress is usually performed with dobutamine in patients who are unable to exercise and in those unable to achieve adequate heart rates with exercise.

Ambulatory Ischemic Monitoring

Patients with symptomatic myocardial ischemia have episodes of silent ischemia that occur with the activities of daily living and are detectable on ambulatory monitoring but go unrecognized clinically because of the absence of angina or anginal equivalents. Although such "silent myocardial ischemia" may be detected during 24-hour ambulatory ECG recordings and may provide a quantitative estimate of the frequency and duration of ischemic episodes, its sensitivity for detecting coronary artery disease is much less reliable than that of exercise ECG.

Stress Cardiac Magnetic Resonance Imaging

Pharmacologic stress perfusion with CMR imaging is becoming increasingly available in many centers and may provide additional diagnostic capability in detecting the presence of structural heart disease, in addition to suspected coronary artery disease. CMR with gadolinium enhancement is the most accurate way to diagnose a scar from a prior MI (see Fig. 56-7 in Chapter 56).

Chest Roentgenography

Unless there is no history of prior MI, heart failure, or structural heart disease, the chest radiograph (Chapter 53) is usually normal in patients with chronic angina or stable ischemic heart disease. If an enlarged cardiac silhouette is present, it is generally indicative of a previous MI with LV dilation and cardiac remodeling. Other causes of cardiomegaly include long-standing hypertension, concomitant valvular heart disease, pericardial effusion, or nonischemic cardiomyopathy.

Cardiac Computed Tomographic Angiography

Cardiac computed tomographic angiography (CCTA; Chapter 56) is a highly sensitive method to detect coronary calcification (see Fig. 56-2 in Chapter 56), which is strongly associated with coronary atherosclerosis and can also provide noninvasive angiography of the proximal coronary arteries. Although coronary calcification is a highly sensitive (approximately 90%) finding in patients with coronary artery disease, the specificity for identifying patients with obstructive coronary artery disease is much lower (approximately 50%). Because of the potential unnecessary testing from false-positive results, CCTA is currently not recommended as a routine screening approach for suspected obstructive coronary artery disease in individuals at low risk (<10% 10-year estimated risk of coronary events). CCTA can be coupled with PET imaging in a hybrid PET and computed tomography scanner, which can provide a quantitative assessment of coronary anatomy along with regional myocardial blood flow and cardiac metabolism.

Diagnostic Coronary Angiography

Despite the continued evolution of noninvasive diagnostic testing, invasive coronary angiography (Chapter 57) remains the gold standard for anatomic definition of coronary artery disease. Among patients with the clinical diagnosis of stable ischemic heart disease referred for coronary angiography, a 70% or more luminal diameter narrowing is found in one (about 25%), two (about 25%), or all three (about 25%) epicardial coronary arteries, in about 75% of cases; another 5 to 10% of patients have obstruction of the left main

TABLE 71-7 CORONARY ANGIOGRAPHY FOR DIAGNOSIS AND RISK STRATIFICATION IN PATIENTS WITH CHRONIC ANGINA AND STABLE ISCHEMIC HEART DISEASE

FOR INITIAL DIAGNOSTIC INDICATION
Recommended on the basis of evidence or general consensus
Patients with suspected angina and evidence of intermediate-high risk, moderate-severe ischemia on noninvasive testing, or a changing angina pattern who have survived sudden cardiac death or serious ventricular arrhythmia
Weight of evidence or opinion is in favor
Uncertain diagnosis after noninvasive testing, and the benefit of a more certain diagnosis outweighs the risk and cost of coronary angiography
Inability to undergo noninvasive testing because of disability, illness, or morbid obesity
Occupational requirement for a definitive diagnosis
Suspected nonatherosclerotic cause of myocardial ischemia
Suspicion of a coronary spasm
High pretest probability of left main or three-vessel disease
Recurrent hospitalization for chest pain in the absence of definitive diagnosis
Overriding desire for a definitive diagnosis and a greater than low probability of CAD
Not recommended
Significant comorbidity in patients in whom the risk of coronary arteriography outweighs the benefit of the procedure
Overriding personal desire for a definitive diagnosis and a low probability of CAD
FOR INITIAL RISK STRATIFICATION OR TREATMENT INDICATION
Recommended on the basis of evidence or general consensus
With disabling (CCS class III and class IV) chronic stable angina despite medical therapy
With high-risk criteria on noninvasive testing regardless of anginal severity
Patients with angina who have survived sudden cardiac death or serious ventricular arrhythmia
Angina and symptoms and signs of congestive heart failure
Clinical characteristics that indicate a high likelihood of severe CAD
Weight of evidence or opinion is in favor
Significant left ventricular dysfunction (EF < 45%), CCS class I or class II angina, and demonstrable ischemia but less than high-risk criteria on noninvasive testing
High-risk criteria suggesting ischemia on noninvasive testing
Inadequate prognostic information after noninvasive testing
Clinical characteristics that indicate a high likelihood of severe CAD
CCS class I or class II angina, preserved left ventricular function (EF > 45%), and less than high-risk criteria on noninvasive testing
CCS class III or class IV angina that improves to class I or class II with medical therapy
CCS class I or class II angina but intolerance (unacceptable side effects) to adequate medical therapy
Not recommended
CCS class I or class II angina in patients who respond to medical therapy and who have no evidence of ischemia on noninvasive testing
Patients who prefer to avoid revascularization after adequate explanation

CAD = coronary artery disease; CCS = Canadian Cardiovascular Society; CHD = coronary heart disease; EF = ejection fraction.

Modified from Gibbons RJ, Abrams J, Chatterjee K, et al. ACC/AHA 2002 guideline update for the management of patients with chronic stable angina—summary article: a report of the American College of Cardiology/American Heart Association Task Force on Practice Guidelines (Committee on Management of Patients with Chronic Stable Angina). *Circulation.* 2003;107:149-158.

coronary artery; and the remaining 15 to 20% have no flow-limiting coronary obstructions. These data emphasize the persisting role of coronary angiography for diagnostic purposes (Table 71-7), but angiography is also helpful for risk stratification in patients with clear-cut angina and ischemic heart disease. In patients with less severe coronary stenoses (i.e., 50 to 70% on angiography), coronary intravascular ultrasonography (see Fig. 57-7 in Chapter 57) can substantially enhance the quantification of obstruction and vulnerability of the coronary atheroma to future instability. A pressure wire positioned proximal and distal to a coronary stenosis can measure the severity of the stenosis and determine whether functionally significant flow reduction may be ameliorated by myocardial revascularization.

Differential Diagnosis of Angina

Many common noncardiac disorders may present with clinical features that can be confused with angina pectoris (see Table 50-2 in Chapter 50). In some instances, symptoms may be indistinguishable from ischemic heart disease. For example, many patients with angina have coexisting esophageal disorders (Chapter 140), and both angina and esophageal discomfort may be relieved by nitroglycerin (Chapter 50). A distinguishing feature from angina is that esophageal discomfort is often relieved by antacids, proton pump inhibitors, or food.

Costochondritis can mimic angina but can typically be distinguished by the presence of well-localized pain on palpation. However, pressure, if applied too firmly to the anterior chest wall during examination of a patient with suspected angina pectoris, may elicit symptoms of discomfort even in normal subjects. Cervical radiculopathy may cause pain radiating to the shoulders, neck, or upper arms and can be confused with angina. However, this condition typically causes a constant ache that is often exacerbated by neck movement or rotation and may be accompanied by a focal sensory deficit or radiculopathy.

Pulmonary hypertension (Chapter 68) can cause exertional chest discomfort that may share many of the characteristics of angina pectoris. It is believed that right ventricular ischemia during physical exertion may cause this discomfort along with associated symptoms of exertional dyspnea, dizziness, and syncope. Findings on physical examination typically include a parasternal lift, a loud (and sometimes palpable) pulmonary component of the second heart sound, and findings of right ventricular hypertrophy on ECG.

Chest pain may also be an important presenting clinical feature of pulmonary embolism (Chapter 98). Physical findings typically include tachycardia and tachypnea, an accentuated pulmonic component of the second heart sound, and occasionally a right-sided S_4 gallop. Pleuritic discomfort suggests pulmonary infarction, whereas a history of pain exacerbated by inspiration or deep breathing, along with a pleural friction rub, usually helps distinguish it from angina pectoris.

Acute pericarditis (Chapter 77) may be confused with the discomfort of angina pectoris, but pericarditis tends to cause chest pain that is generally sharp, is not relieved by rest or nitroglycerin, is exacerbated by movement or deep breathing, and is associated with a pericardial friction rub that may be evanescent. Aortic dissection (Chapter 78), which may present with acute, severe chest pain, may be confused with an acute MI but generally not with angina.

Risk Stratification

Clinical and noninvasive criteria can be used in a complementary fashion to refine the estimate of risk for the individual patient with stable ischemic heart disease (Table 71-8). Clinical characteristics that include age, male sex, diabetes mellitus, previous MI, and the presence of symptoms typical of angina are predictive of the presence of coronary artery disease. Heart failure and LV dysfunction (generally defined by an ejection fraction < 50%), the severity and extent of angina, and associated symptoms such as dyspnea are also important predictors of outcome in patients with stable ischemic heart disease.

The simple classification of disease into single-, double-, or triple-vessel or left main coronary artery disease remains the most widely used approach (Table 71-9). Additional prognostic information is provided by the severity and extent of coronary luminal narrowing and its location. For example, high-grade lesions of the left main coronary artery or its equivalent, as defined by severe proximal left anterior descending and proximal left circumflex coronary artery disease, are particularly life-threatening. The SYNTAX trial has permitted the identification of subsets of coronary artery disease patients into three tertiles of low-, moderate-, and high-risk anatomic findings, based on multiple lesional characteristics (see Tables 71-8 and 71-9). It should be kept in mind, however, that the plaque causing the most severe chronic stenosis is not necessarily the one that will subsequently rupture to cause acute coronary syndrome or acute MI.

TREATMENT Rx

Comprehensive management of angina and stable ischemic heart disease (Fig. 71-5) entails multiple therapeutic approaches to the identification and treatment of associated diseases that can precipitate or worsen angina and ischemia (Table 71-10): cardiac risk factor identification and intervention; application of pharmacologic and nonpharmacologic interventions for secondary prevention; pharmacologic and symptomatic management of angina and ischemia; and myocardial revascularization with percutaneous coronary intervention (PCI) or coronary artery bypass graft (CABG) surgery, when indicated (Table 71-11). A multidimensional management approach integrates all of these considerations, often simultaneously, in each patient. Among pharmacotherapies, three drug classes are classified as being "disease modifying" in that they have been demonstrated to reduce mortality and morbidity in patients with stable ischemic heart disease and preserved LV function: aspirin,

TABLE 71-8 USING THE RESULTS OF NONINVASIVE RISK STRATIFICATION TO GUIDE CLINICAL DECISION MAKING

HIGH RISK (>3% ANNUAL MORTALITY RATE)

Severe resting left ventricular dysfunction (LVEF < 35%)
High-risk treadmill score (≤ −11)*
Severe exercise left ventricular dysfunction (exercise LVEF < 35%)
Stress-induced large perfusion defect (particularly if anterior)
Stress-induced multiple perfusion defects of moderate size
Large, fixed perfusion defect with left ventricular dilation or increased lung uptake (^{201}Tl)
Stress-induced moderate perfusion defect with left ventricular dilation or increased lung uptake (^{201}Tl)
Echocardiographic wall motion abnormality (involving more than two segments) developing at low dose of dobutamine or at a low heart rate (<120 beats/min)
Stress echocardiographic evidence of extensive ischemia

INTERMEDIATE RISK (1-3% ANNUAL MORTALITY RATE)

Mild to moderate resting left ventricular dysfunction (LVEF = 35-49%)
Intermediate-risk treadmill score (−11 < score < 5)*
Stress-induced moderate perfusion defect without left ventricular dilation or increased lung intake (^{201}Tl)
Limited stress echocardiographic ischemia with a wall motion abnormality only at higher doses of dobutamine involving two segments or less

LOW RISK (<1% ANNUAL MORTALITY RATE)

Low-risk treadmill score (≥ 5)*
Normal or small myocardial perfusion defect at rest or with stress†
Normal stress echocardiographic wall motion or no change of limited resting wall motion abnormalities during stress†

*Score = (duration of exercise in minutes) − (5 × mm of ST segment depression) − (4 × angina score), where 0 = no angina, 1 = nonlimiting angina, and 2 = angina that causes discontinuation of the test.
†Although the published data are limited, patients with these findings will probably not be at low risk in the presence of either a high-risk treadmill score or severe resting left ventricular dysfunction (LVEF < 35%).
LVEF = left ventricular ejection fraction.
From Gibbons RJ, Abrams J, Chatterjee K, et al. ACC/AHA 2002 guideline update for the management of patients with chronic stable angina—summary article: a report of the American College of Cardiology/American Heart Association Task Force on practice guidelines (Committee on the Management of Patients with Chronic Stable Angina). *J Am Coll Cardiol.* 2003;41:159-168.

TABLE 71-9 CORONARY ARTERY DISEASE PROGNOSTIC INDEX

EXTENT OF CORONARY ARTERY DISEASE	5-YEAR MORTALITY RATE (%)*
1-vessel disease, 75%	7
>1-vessel disease, 50-74%	7
1-vessel disease, ≥95%	9
2-vessel disease	12
2-vessel disease, both ≥95%	14
1-vessel disease, ≥95% proximal LAD	17
2-vessel disease, ≥95% LAD	17
2-vessel disease, ≥95% proximal LAD	21
3-vessel disease	21
3-vessel disease, ≥95% in at least 1	27
3-vessel disease, 75% proximal LAD	33
3-vessel disease, ≥95% proximal LAD	41

*Assuming medical treatment only.
LAD = left anterior descending coronary artery.
From Califf RM, Armstrong PW, Carver JR, et al. Task Force 5: stratification of patients into high, medium and low risk subgroups for purposes of risk factor management. *J Am Coll Cardiol.* 1996;27:1007-1019.

angiotensin-converting enzyme (ACE) inhibition, and effective lipid lowering. Other therapies such as nitrates, β-blockers, calcium antagonists, and ranolazine have been shown to improve angina, exercise performance, and reduce ischemia, but have not been proved to reduce mortality in patients with stable ischemic heart disease.

Disease-Modifying Therapies

Careful attention to lifestyle and the management of coronary risk factors is essential (Fig. 71-6). Such secondary prevention strategies can reduce the risk of progressive coronary disease, morbidity, and mortality.

Drugs That Alter Lipid Metabolism

Each 1% increase in the LDL cholesterol level results in a 2 to 3% increase in risk for coronary events (Chapter 51). Large, randomized clinical trials in patients with ischemic heart disease have shown a consistent and significant reduction in mortality and cardiac events with statin therapy (Chapter 213). Patients with stable angina should routinely be treated with statins to a target of less than 70 mg/dL,[1] using any of a variety of specific statin drugs (see Table 213-5 in Chapter 213).

Gemfibrozil, a fibrate at 1200 mg daily, can reduce fatal and nonfatal MI in men who have coronary heart disease and normal levels of LDL cholesterol but who also have low levels of HDL cholesterol and elevated triglycerides,[2] but fibrates have not been shown to reduce overall mortality despite about a 10% reduction in major cardiovascular events.[3] Other cholesterol-lowering agents such as ezetimibe or bile acid sequestrants can be used instead of statins in those who are intolerant or can be added to high-dose statins in those in whom the LDL goal has not been achieved, but there are no studies to indicate whether these agents reduce cardiac events or mortality.

Each 1-mg/dL decline in HDL cholesterol is associated with a 2 to 3% increase in the risk of MI and death from cardiac causes. Nicotinic acid raises HDL cholesterol by about 25 to 30% on an average at doses of 1 to 2 g/day, but its use has been limited by side effects, notably flushing. Nicotinic acid reduces carotid artery intimal media thickness, a surrogate for atherosclerotic progression, but clinical outcomes data are lacking. Cholesteryl ester transfer protein inhibitors may be quite effective in raising HDL levels but have had no benefit in clinical trials to date.

Angiotensin-Converting Enzyme Inhibitors

ACE inhibitor administration (see Table 67-5 in Chapter 67) reduces cardiac events, cardiovascular mortality, and all-cause mortality in patients with risk factors for or with previously diagnosed coronary artery disease,[1,4] including high-risk patients with vascular disease or diabetes and patients with stable coronary artery disease and no clinical evidence of heart failure. By contrast, ACE inhibitors do not appear to prevent future cardiac events in post-MI patients with preserved LV function. Whether angiotensin receptor blockers have similar benefits in patients with chronic angina and stable ischemic heart disease is not yet known.

Antiplatelet Agents and Anticoagulants

Aspirin reduces the risk of adverse cardiovascular events by 33% in patients with stable angina. The reduction in vascular events is comparable for doses of 75 to 150 mg daily and 160 to 325 mg daily, but daily doses of less than 75 mg have less benefit.[5] Therefore, in the absence of contraindications, aspirin, 75 to 325 mg once daily, should be administered routinely in all patients with angina and stable ischemic heart disease.

Clopidogrel (Chapter 37), which is the most widely used thienopyridine in the treatment of patients with coronary artery disease, is of proven benefit when combined with aspirin to reduce the composite end point of death, MI, or stroke in patients after an acute coronary event. The standard regimen is an initial loading dose of 300 to 600 mg orally, followed by a maintenance dose of 75 mg daily. In patients with angina and stable ischemic heart disease, however, adding clopidogrel to low-dose (75 to 162 mg/day) aspirin does not reduce the primary composite end point of MI, stroke, or death from cardiovascular causes,[6] so clopidogrel should be reserved for patients who cannot tolerate aspirin or who have had an acute coronary event (Chapter 72) or a stent implantation (Chapter 74). Prasugrel is a new thienopyridine that is approved in patients with ACS and in those who undergo PCI with stent placement, but it has not yet been studied in the medical management of patients with chronic angina and stable coronary artery disease.

Warfarin is generally as effective as aspirin for preventing coronary events in patients with angina and is preferred over aspirin for patients with concomitant atrial fibrillation (Chapter 66), but it is associated with a higher risk of bleeding. Combination therapy with warfarin plus aspirin is superior to aspirin alone if the international normalized ratio is maintained above 2.0, but the benefit of the combination must be weighed against a 1 per 100 patient years risk of bleeding.[7] Anticoagulants are more commonly used in Europe than in America.

Therapeutic Agents to Reduce Angina and Ischemia

The goal of antianginal therapy is to reduce symptoms of cardiac ischemia and to improve quality of life. β-Blockers, which prevent the binding of catecholamines to the β-adrenergic receptor, lower heart rate and myocardial contractility, thereby reducing myocardial workload, myocardial oxygen demand, and ischemia and anginal symptoms. β-Blockers raise the ischemic threshold and delay or prevent the onset of angina with exercise. β-Blockers also reduce the rate of secondary cardiac events and sudden cardiac death in post-MI patients, but there have been no placebo-controlled outcome trials in angina patients. All β-blockers appear to be equally effective in patients with chronic stable angina (Table 71-12). The β-blocker dose should be titrated to a target resting heart rate of 50 to 60 beats per minute as tolerated by the patient.

Calcium-channel blockers (Table 71-13) reduce afterload owing to their peripheral vasodilatory effects and thus lower myocardial workload and myocardial oxygen demand. Calcium-channel blockers also reduce coronary vascular resistance and inhibit coronary vasospasm by preventing coronary arterial smooth muscle contraction. This favorable reduction in myocardial oxygen demand, coupled with an increase in myocardial oxygen supply, results in a reduction in angina and ischemia. Nondihydropyridine calcium-channel blockers, such as verapamil and diltiazem, also reduce heart rate. Conversely, dihydropyridine calcium channel antagonists, such as amlodipine, have greater effect on vascular smooth muscle, are better peripheral and coronary vasodilators, and hence may have advantages for use in the hypertensive patient with angina. In randomized clinical trials, calcium-channel blockers and β-blockers are generally equally effective in relieving angina, improving time to onset of angina, and improving time to ischemic ST depression during exercise. Because calcium-channel blockers have not been shown to reduce death or MI in patients with stable or previously unstable ischemic heart disease, these agents are usually used in patients who cannot tolerate β-blockers or who require additional pharmacotherapy to control their symptoms. When used with β-blockers, care must be taken not to cause symptomatic bradycardia with verapamil and diltiazem. When used alone, diltiazem is

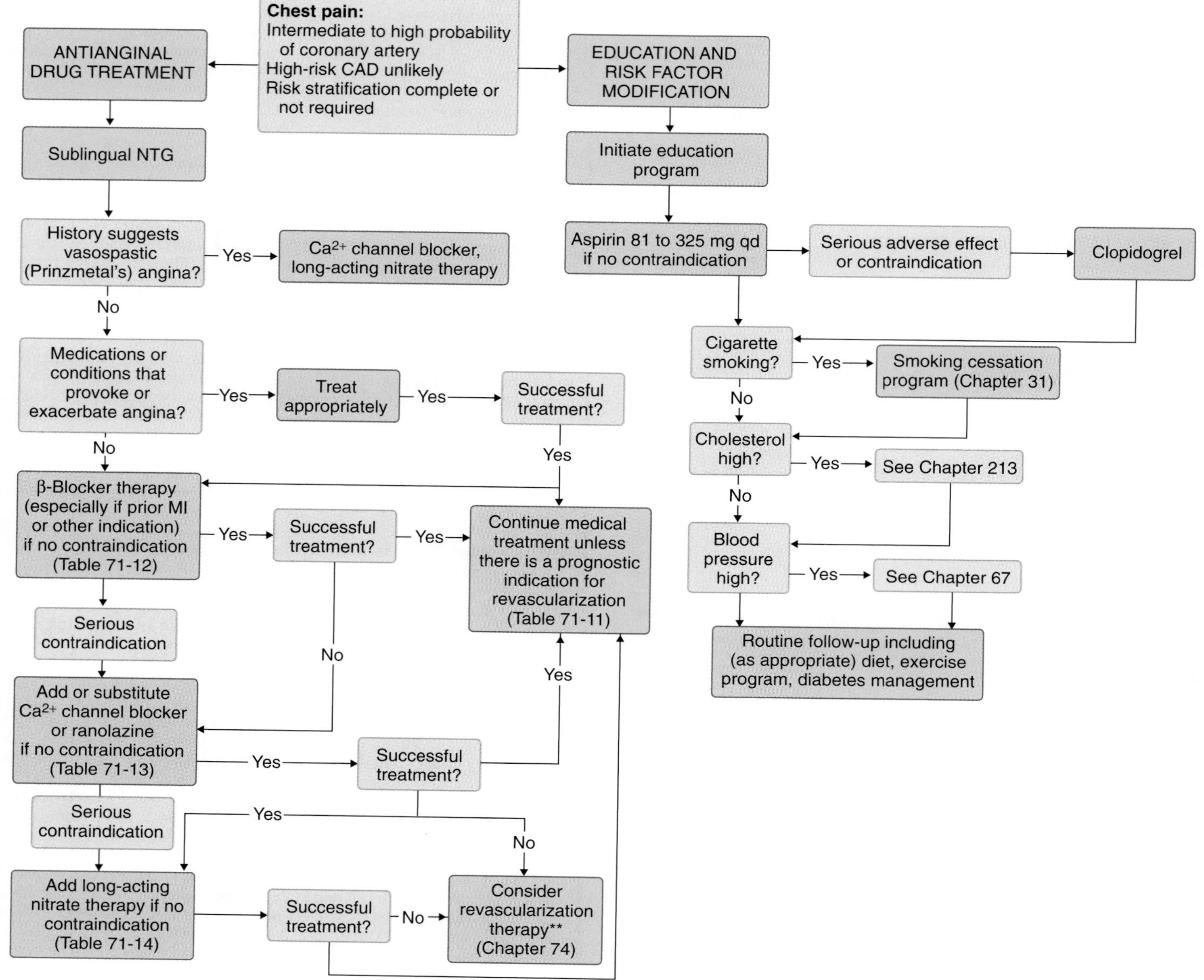

*Conditions that exacerbate or provoke angina:

Medications:
Vasodilators
Excessive thyroid replacement
Vasoconstrictors

Other medical problems:
Profound anemia
Uncontrolled hypertension
Hyperthyroidism
Hypoxemia

Other cardiac problems:
Tachyarrythmias
Bradyarrythmias
Valvular heart disease (espec. AS)
Hypertrophic cardiomyopathy

**At any point in this process, based on coronary anatomy, severity of anginal symptoms, and patient preferences, it is reasonable to consider evaluation for coronary revascularization. Unless a patient is documented to have left main, three-vessel, or two-vessel CAD with significant stenosis of the proximal left anterior descending coronary artery, there is no demonstrated survival advantage associated with revascularization in low-risk patients with chronic stable angina; thus, medical therapy should be attempted in most patients before considering PTCA or CABG.

FIGURE 71-5. Algorithm for the treatment of stable angina. AS = aortic stenosis; CABG = coronary artery bypass graft; CAD = coronary artery disease; MI = myocardial infarction; NTG = nitroglycerin; PTCA = percutaneous transluminal coronary angioplasty. (Modified from American College of Cardiology/American Heart Association Task Force on Practice Guidelines. *Management of Patients with Chronic Stable Angina. ACC/AHA/ACP-ASIM Pocket Guidelines.* Philadelphia: Elsevier Science; 2000.)

TABLE 71-10 TREATMENT OF PATIENTS WITH STABLE ANGINA

GENERAL MEASURES

Rule out and control aggravating conditions
- Associated noncardiac diseases
- Associated cardiac disease
- Use of drugs aggravating angina

Smoking cessation
Dietary counseling for body weight and lipid control
Exercise prescription
Treat to targets
- Hypertension
- Blood lipids
- Diabetes

PHARMACOLOGIC THERAPY: RECOMMENDATIONS FOR PHARMACOTHERAPY TO PREVENT MI AND DEATH AND TO REDUCE SYMPTOMS

Recommended on the basis of evidence or general consensus
Aspirin in the absence of contraindications
β-Blockers as initial therapy in the absence of contraindications in patients with prior MI or without prior MI
Angiotensin-converting enzyme inhibitor in all patients with CAD who also have diabetes or left ventricular systolic dysfunction
Low-density lipoprotein-lowering therapy in patients with documented or suspected CAD and LDL cholesterol greater than 130 mg/dL, with a target LDL of less than 100 mg/dL
Sublingual nitroglycerin or nitroglycerin spray for the immediate relief of angina
Calcium-channel antagonists or long-acting nitrates as initial therapy for reduction of symptoms when β-blockers are contraindicated
Calcium-channel antagonists or long-acting nitrates in combination with β-blockers when initial treatment with β-blockers is not successful
Calcium-channel antagonists and long-acting nitrates as a substitute for β-blockers if initial treatment with β-blockers leads to unacceptable side effects
Weight of evidence or opinion is in favor
Clopidogrel when aspirin is contraindicated
Long-acting nondihydropyridine calcium-channel antagonists instead of β-blockers as initial therapy
In patients with documented or suspected CAD and LDL cholesterol level of 100 to 129 mg/dL, several therapeutic options are available (Level of Evidence: B)
Lifestyle and/or drug therapies to lower LDL to less than 100 mg/dL
Weight reduction and increased physical activity in persons with the metabolic syndrome
Institution of treatment of other lipid or nonlipid risk factors; consider use of nicotinic acid or fibric acid for elevated triglycerides or low HDL cholesterol
Angiotensin-converting enzyme inhibitor in patients with CAD or other vascular disease
Usefulness unclear
Low-intensity anticoagulation with warfarin in addition to aspirin
Not recommended
Dipyridamole
Chelation therapy

CAD = coronary artery disease; HDL = high-density lipoprotein; LDL = low-density lipoprotein; MI = myocardial infarction.
From Gibbons RJ, Abrams J, Chatterjee K, et al. ACC/AHA 2002 guideline update for the management of patients with chronic stable angina—summary article: a report of the American College of Cardiology/American Heart Association Task Force on practice guidelines (Committee on the Management of Patients with Chronic Stable Angina). *J Am Coll Cardiol.* 2003;41:159-168.

often preferred because the dihydropyridine calcium-channel blockers can increase the heart rate.

Nitrates (Table 71-14) continue to be widely prescribed for antianginal treatment and are effective when administered sublingually, orally, or topically. They act as vasodilators by entering vascular smooth muscle, where they are metabolized to nitric oxide, which relaxes vascular smooth muscle, including in coronary arteries. These effects reduce angina by improving coronary blood flow. Nitrates also lower preload owing to their venodilator effects, with a resulting reduction in LV end-diastolic pressure and wall tension, which, in turn, lowers subendocardial oxygen demand. When used in patients with stable angina, nitrates improve exercise tolerance, time to onset of angina, and ST segment depression during treadmill exercise testing. Long-acting nitrates, which are frequently combined with β-blockers and calcium-channel blockers, have additive antianginal and anti-ischemic effects in patients with stable ischemic heart disease. Sublingual nitroglycerin or oral spray can terminate an angina attack and can be used as prophylaxis to prevent exertional angina. Long-acting nitrates administered orally or transdermally are used to prevent angina and to improve exercise tolerance. For avoidance of nitrate tolerance

TABLE 71-11 CURRENT RECOMMENDATIONS FOR MYOCARDIAL REVASCULARIZATION IN PATIENTS WITH CHRONIC STABLE ANGINA

CABG SURGERY VERSUS MEDICAL THERAPY

Among patients with medically refractory angina pectoris, CABG surgery is indicated for symptom improvement.

Among patients with medically stable angina pectoris, CABG surgery is indicated to prolong life in left main coronary artery disease or three-vessel disease (regardless of left ventricular function) and, possibly, to help symptoms.

CABG surgery may be indicated for prolongation of life if the proximal left anterior descending coronary artery is involved (regardless of the number of diseased vessels).

CABG surgery may reduce the composite end point of death, myocardial infarction, or stroke in diabetic patients with extensive multivessel (two- to three-vessel) coronary artery disease compared with medical therapy.

PCI VERSUS MEDICAL THERAPY

For the initial management of patients with stable ischemic heart disease, PCI does not reduce the risk of death, myocardial infarction, or other major cardiovascular events when added to optimal medical therapy.

Among patients with medically refractory angina pectoris, PCI is indicated for symptom improvement.

PCI may be indicated in the presence of severe myocardial ischemia, regardless of symptoms. PCI does not appear to improve survival compared with medical treatment among patients with one- or two-vessel disease.

In the absence of symptoms or myocardial ischemia, PCI is not indicated (merely for the presence of an anatomic stenosis).

PCI VERSUS CABG SURGERY

For single-vessel disease, PCI and CABG surgery provide excellent symptom relief, but repeated revascularization procedures are required more frequently after PCI. Intracoronary stenting is preferred to regular PCI, but direct comparison with CABG surgery is limited.

For treated diabetic patients with two- or three-vessel disease, CABG surgery is the treatment of choice.

For nondiabetic patients, multivessel PCI and CABG surgery are acceptable alternatives. The choice of PCI or CABG surgery for initial treatment depends primarily on local expertise and the patient's and physician's preferences.

In general, PCI is preferred for patients at low risk and CABG surgery for patients at high risk.

CABG = coronary artery bypass graft; PCI = percutaneous coronary intervention.

or tachyphylaxis, an 8- to 12-hour nitrate-free interval daily is recommended. Nitroglycerin and nitrates can cause vasodilation-induced headache, a decrease in blood pressure, and, more rarely, severe hypotension with bradycardia due to activation of the vagal Bezold-Jarisch reflex. Because the vasodilation by nitroglycerin is markedly exaggerated and prolonged in the presence of the phosphodiesterase inhibitors sildenafil (Viagra), vardenafil (Levitra), and tadalafil (Cialis), these agents and nitrates should not be used concurrently.

Ranolazine (initiated at a dose of 500 mg twice daily and titrated up to a maximal dose of 1000 mg twice daily) is the newest U.S. Food and Drug Administration–approved antianginal agent and the first new drug class for angina since calcium-channel blockers were introduced clinically 30 years ago. Ranolazine acts by reducing intracellular calcium overload in ischemic myocytes by inhibiting late inward sodium current entry. The net effect of reduced late inward sodium current is a reduction in LV wall tension and myocardial oxygen demand, thereby reducing angina and ischemia. Ranolazine increases exercise tolerance in patients with stable angina, reduces episodes of recurrent ischemia, and provides additional antianginal benefit in patients who are already on intensive antianginal therapy with β-blockers and calcium-channel blockers. In patients with ACS, ranolazine also reduces hemoglobin A_{1c} concentrations in diabetic patients, and it is associated with a reduction in arrhythmic events, in particular, episodes of ventricular tachycardia and atrial fibrillation.[8] Although ranolazine can minimally prolong the QT interval (on average, 6 to 8 msec), it has not been shown to increase the risk of torsades de pointes. Its precise role in the management of stable angina remains to be determined.

Nonpharmacologic Treatment

Enhanced external counterpulsation (EECP) is an alternative treatment for patients with refractory angina. EECP is generally administered as 35 sequential treatments (1 hour daily; 5 days/week) over 7 weeks. EECP does not reduce ischemia on myocardial perfusion imaging, and the mechanisms underlying

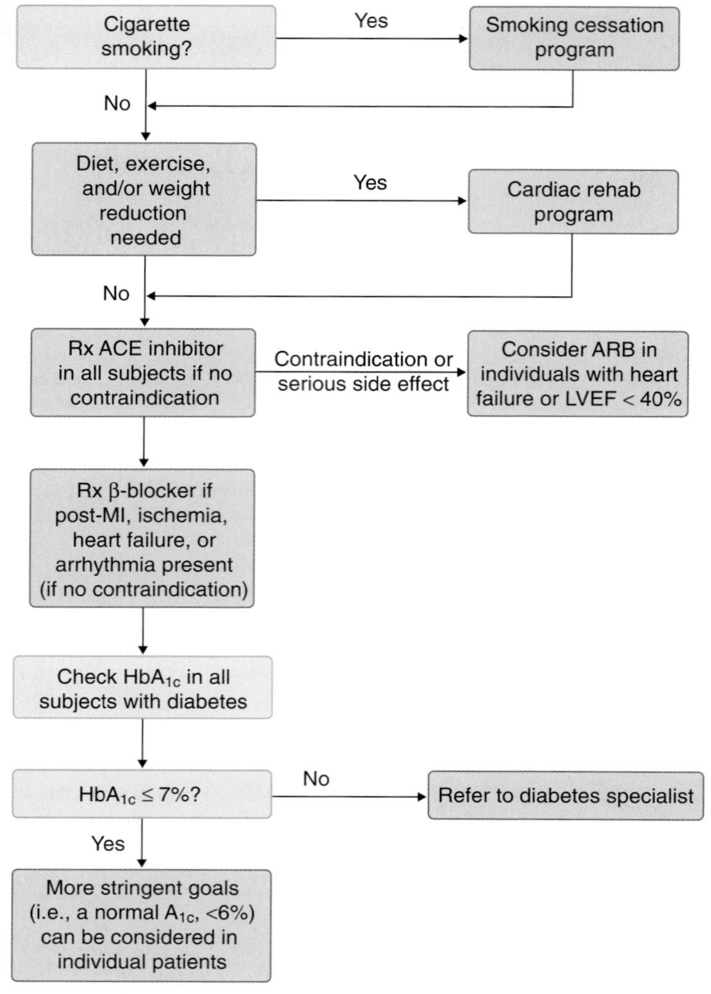

FIGURE 71-6. Approach to lifestyle interventions and pharmacotherapy. ACE = angiotensin-converting enzyme; ARB = angiotensin receptor blocker; HbA_{1c} = hemoglobin A_{1c}; LVEF = left ventricular ejection fraction; MI = myocardial infarction; Rx = prescribe.

its effects are poorly understood. Possible mechanisms include durable hemodynamic changes that reduce myocardial O_2 demand, improvement in myocardial perfusion by diastolic augmentation of retrograde coronary flow, and improved endothelial function. Although EECP increased the time to ST segment depression during exercise testing, reduced angina, and improved health-related quality of life for at least 1 year in one randomized, double-blind study of patients with chronic stable angina, its role in the treatment of angina remains unclear.[9]

Myocardial Revascularization

Coronary revascularization with either PCI or CABG (Chapter 74) can prolong life, reduce major cardiovascular events, and improve health status, quality of life, and functional capacity in selected patients with chronic, stable ischemic heart disease.

Comparisons of PCI with Optimal Medical Therapy

Randomized clinical trials comparing PCI with medical therapy in patients with stable coronary heart disease are few in number, and many recruited patients predominantly with single-vessel disease and were completed before the routine use of coronary stenting and contemporary aggressive preventive medical therapy. In general, these studies showed benefits of PCI in terms of symptoms[10] but not in terms of subsequent MI or death.[11] In the most recent trial of modern PCI (the Clinical Outcomes Utilizing Revascularization and Aggressive druG Evaluation [COURAGE] trial), including stents, versus aggressive medical therapy, there were no significant differences in the composite primary outcome of all-cause mortality or nonfatal MI or in stroke or hospitalization for ACS between the two strategies during a 2.5- to 7.0-year (median, 4.6-year) follow-up period.[12] PCI improved symptoms for 2 years, especially in patients with more severe angina, but differences were no longer present at 36 months, at which time both PCI and intensive medical therapy led to better symptom control than was noted at baseline. Because PCI as an initial management strategy in patients with stable coronary artery disease does not reduce death, MI, or other major cardiovascular events when added to optimal medical therapy, the importance of preventive pharmacotherapy and lifestyle modification for secondary prevention of major cardiovascular events in patients with stable CHD must be paramount.

Comparisons of CABG with Medical Therapy

Randomized trials comparing CABG with medical therapy indicate that a greater severity of ischemia, a greater extent of disease, and the presence of LV dysfunction favor a greater magnitude of benefit of CABG over medical therapy on survival. CABG prolongs survival in patients with significant left main coronary artery disease irrespective of symptoms, in patients with multivessel coronary artery disease and impaired LV function (ejection fraction < 50%), and in patients with three-vessel coronary artery disease that includes the proximal left anterior descending coronary artery. Patients with extensive multivessel coronary artery disease appear to benefit more from CABG surgery, particularly if they also have diabetes, whereas PCI is most appropriate for patients with one- or two-vessel coronary artery disease. Of note is that these randomized trials found little difference in mortality between CABG surgery and medical therapy at 1 year, but the benefits of CABG surgery over medical therapy steadily emerged over the next 3 to 5 years. Thereafter, the benefits of CABG surgery diminished, perhaps as a result of late occlusion of saphenous vein grafts, progression of disease in the nonbypassed native coronary arteries, and increasing rates of CABG surgery in the medical group among those with high-risk anatomy and severe symptoms ("crossovers"). It is important to emphasize that very few patients in these early trials received arterial grafts (which would likely improve the long-term results of CABG surgery), aspirin to prevent graft occlusion, lipid-lowering drugs to mitigate late graft disease progression, or inhibitors of the renin-angiotensin-aldosterone system. With improvements in operative techniques, more common use of antiplatelet-agents, more intensive use of disease-modifying therapies, and more aggressive risk factor management over the past decade, the benefits of modern-day CABG surgery compared with contemporary medical therapy may have changed.

Comparisons of PCI with CABG Surgery for Multivessel Coronary Artery Disease

Of the randomized outcomes trials that have compared PCI with CABG in patients with multivessel coronary artery disease, most excluded patients with significant left main coronary artery disease and were conducted in an era before the advent of stents and other advances in PCI technology, including newer adjunctive medical therapies that are increasingly in widespread clinical use. The Bypass Angioplasty Revascularization Investigation (BARI) trial found no overall difference in survival or MI rates between percutaneous balloon angioplasty and CABG surgery at 10 years, but CABG provided a significantly better survival advantage in patients with diabetes.[13] CABG also was associated with a greater initial improvement in angina and with a diminished frequency of repeat revascularization procedures compared with balloon angioplasty. A significant survival advantage was observed in patients with previously treated diabetes who underwent CABG rather than angioplasty.

More recently, the BARI-2D trial of 2368 diabetic patients with coronary artery disease who were randomized to prompt revascularization with PCI or CABG versus delayed or no revascularization with optimal medical therapy found no significant difference for the primary end point of total mortality.[14] Thus, the BARI-2D results replicate the principal finding of the COURAGE trial[10]—namely, that an initial strategy of PCI provides no incremental clinical benefit over intensive medical therapy and lifestyle intervention alone, and that an "optimal medical therapy first" instead of a "PCI first" strategy seems justifiable in many diabetic patients with coronary disease.

In a randomized trial of CABG or PCI patients with three-vessel or left main coronary artery disease, rates of major adverse cardiac or cerebrovascular events (i.e., death from any cause, stroke, MI, or repeat revascularization) at 12 months were significantly higher in the PCI group (18% vs. 12% for CABG), in large part because of an increased rate of repeat revascularization (14% vs. 6%).[15] At 12 months, the rates of death and MI were similar between the two groups, although stroke was significantly more likely to occur with CABG (2.2% vs. 0.6% with PCI). Thus, based on these 1-year findings, CABG still is generally considered the preferred option for patients with three-vessel or left main coronary artery disease.

In summary, among those who remain symptomatic despite intensive treatment, or who have substantial ischemia or extensive coronary artery disease, revascularization with either PCI or CABG is appropriate, depending on the anatomic complexity of disease (see Table 71-11; Chapter 73). CABG surgery appears to be preferable to PCI in symptomatic patients with three-vessel or

TABLE 71-12 CLINICAL USE OF β-BLOCKERS

COMPOUND BY RECEPTOR ACTIVITY	INTRINSIC SYMPATHOMIMETIC ACTIVITY*	MEMBRANE STABILITY EFFECT	HALF-LIFE (hr)	EXCRETION	USE
β_1 AND β_2					
Propranolol	–	++	1-6	Hepatic	20-80 mg bid-tid
Propranolol long-acting	–	++	8-11	Hepatic	80-360 mg/day
Nadolol	–	–	40-80	Renal	40-80 mg/day
Pindolol	+	+	3-4	Renal	2.5-7.5 mg tid
Sotalol	–	–	7-18	Renal	40-160 mg bid
Timolol	–	–	4-5	Hepatic-renal	10-15 mg bid
β_1 SELECTIVE					
Acebutolol	+	+	3-4	Hepatic	200-600 mg bid
Atenolol	–	–	6-9	Renal	50-200 mg/day
Bisoprolol	–	–	9-12	50% renal	5-20 mg/day
Metoprolol	–	–	3-7	Hepatic	50-200 mg bid
Metoprolol long-acting	–	–	14-25	Hepatic	100-400 mg
Esmolol	–	–	4.5 min	Esterases in red cells	Bolus 500 μg/kg 50-300 μg/kg/min IV
β_1, β_2, α_2					
Labetalol	+	–	6	Hepatic	200-600 mg bid
Carvedilol	–	+	6-10	Hepatic	2.5-25 mg bid

*Presence commonly associated with maintenance of or increase in heart rate; absence associated with decrease in heart rate.
From Théroux P. Angina pectoris. In: Goldman L, Ausiello DA, eds. *Cecil Textbook of Medicine*, 23rd ed. Philadelphia: Saunders Elsevier; 2008.

TABLE 71-13 PROPERTIES OF CALCIUM-CHANNEL BLOCKING DRUGS IN CLINICAL USE

DRUGS	USUAL DOSE	ELIMINATION HALF-LIFE (HR)	*Hemodynamic Effect* HR	PVR	SIDE EFFECTS
DIHYDROPYRIDINES					
Nifedipine PA*	10-40 mg bid	10	↑↑	↓↓↓	Hypotension, dizziness, flushing, edema, constipation
Nifedipine XL*	30-120 mg/day	24	↑	↓↓	
Amlodipine	2.5-10 mg/day	30-50	=	↓↓↓	Headache, edema
Felodipine	2.5-10 mg/day	11-16	↑	↓↓↓	Headache, dizziness
Isradipine	2.5-10 mg bid	8	=	↓↓↓	Headache, fatigue
Nicardipine	20-40 mg tid	2-4	↑	↓↓↓	
Nicardipine SR*	30-60 mg bid	8-10	↑	↓↓	Headache, dizziness, flushing, edema
Nisoldipine	10-40 mg/day	7-12	=	↓↓↓	As for nifedipine
Nitrendipine	20 mg/day or bid	5-12	↑	↓↓↓	As for nifedipine
OTHERS					
Bepridil	200-400 mg/day	24-40	↓	↓	Arrhythmias, dizziness, nausea
Diltiazem	30-90 mg tid	4-6	↓	↓	Hypotension, dizziness, bradycardia, edema
Diltiazem CD*	120-540 mg/day	—	↓	↓	
Verapamil	80-160 mg tid	3-8	↓	↓↓	
Verapamil SR*	120-480 mg/day	—	↓	↓↓	Hypotension, heart failure, edema, bradycardia

*PA, XL, SR, CD: long acting.
HR = heart rate; PVR = peripheral vascular resistance.
From Théroux P. Angina pectoris. In: Goldman L, Ausiello DA, eds. *Cecil Textbook of Medicine*, 23rd ed. Philadelphia: Saunders Elsevier; 2008.

TABLE 71-14 CLINICAL USE OF NITROGLYCERIN AND NITRATES

	DOSE	DURATION OF ACTION	INDICATION
NITROGLYCERIN			
Sublingual or buccal spray	0.15-1.5 mg	Relief of angina	Before or at onset of pain
Ointment	7.5-40 mg	8-12 hr	Prophylaxis of angina
Transdermal	0.2-0.8 mg/hr	8-16 hr	Prophylaxis of angina
Intravenous	5-400 μg/hr	Ongoing; increasing doses as needed	Recurrent chest pain, systemic hypertension, left-sided heart failure
ISOSORBIDE DINITRATE			
Oral	5-40 mg tid	6-8 hr	Prophylaxis of angina
ISOSORBIDE-5-MONONITRATE			
Oral	20 mg bid	8-12 hr	Prophylaxis of angina
Oral, slow release	30-240 mg/day	12-20 hr	Prophylaxis of angina

From Théroux P. Angina pectoris. In: Goldman L, Ausiello DA, eds. *Cecil Textbook of Medicine*, 23rd ed. Philadelphia: Saunders Elsevier; 2008.

left main coronary artery disease and in diabetic patients with stable ischemic heart disease. PCI provides equivalent survival outcomes, but repeat procedures are more often needed, and symptomatic outcomes are generally not as good as after CABG. 16 Whether newer stent technologies will alter these findings remains unclear.

Other Anginal Syndromes

Variant Angina or Prinzmetal's Angina

The diagnosis of variant or Prinzmetal's angina is based on the documentation of transient ST segment elevation during an episode of chest pain in the absence of a severe, fixed coronary stenosis. Prinzmetal's variant angina typically is caused by an occlusive spasm superimposed on a nonsevere coronary artery stenosis. In some patients, however, no underlying stenoses are seen, or the underlying stenosis may be severe. Associated Raynaud's phenomenon and migraine headache have been described in some patients, suggesting that the syndrome may be part of a more generalized vasospastic disorder.

The chest pain occurs predominantly at rest, although approximately one third of patients may also experience pain during exercise. There is a predilection for the pain to wake the patient in the early morning hours when sympathetic activity is increasing. The syndrome is often cyclical, with periods of exacerbation with repetitive episodes of chest pain that may persist only for seconds or be more prolonged and severe, alternating with periods with few or no symptoms. The pain is typically relieved by nitroglycerin. The ST segment elevation accompanying the pain signifies transmural ischemia owing to total abrupt occlusion of a nonsignificant stenosis in the absence of adequate collateral circulation. The subsequent rapid reperfusion may explain the high prevalence of severe life-threatening arrhythmias.

Coronary angiography, with a provocative test for spasm such as injection of acetylcholine into the affected coronary artery, usually precipitates the syndrome. Such testing is useful to establish the diagnosis and to assess the response to therapy, especially in patients with normal or nearly normal coronary angiograms, in whom the diagnosis is otherwise unclear. Dihydropyridine calcium-channel blockers (e.g., amlodipine, 5 to 10 mg orally per day) are preferred in patients with Prinzmetal's angina.

Microvascular Angina with Normal Coronary Angiography

Angina can occur despite normal coronary arteries, even after an acetylcholine challenge. More detailed testing may reveal increased coronary resistance and an inability to increase coronary resistance and increase coronary flow in response to stimuli such as exercise, adenosine, dipyridamole, and atrial pacing.

Symptoms occur most frequently at rest and often in relation to emotional stress. Periods of exacerbation commonly alternate with symptom-free periods. The syndrome is more frequent in women, and some patients have an altered perception of pain or hypersensitivity to certain stimuli.

The diagnosis requires objective documentation of ischemia based on ST-T segment changes, a metabolic abnormality, a transient regional perfusion defect or new wall motion abnormality on echocardiography, or endothelial dysfunction that limits blood flow reserve. Abnormal endothelium-dependent vasoreactivity can be associated with regional myocardial perfusion defects on SPECT and PET imaging.

β-blockers may be useful, particularly when a relative tachycardia, hypertension, or decreased heart rate variability on Holter monitoring is present. Nitroglycerin can relieve symptoms in approximately 50% of patients, and long-acting nitrates or calcium antagonists are sometimes helpful.

The prognosis in general is favorable and not different from that of a general age-matched population in the absence of coronary artery disease. However, some studies have indicated that an ischemic response to exercise is associated with increased mortality.

Silent Myocardial Ischemia

Up to 20% of patients with ischemic heart disease may not present with angina. Such patients are often described as having silent myocardial ischemia. Some patients are totally asymptomatic despite obstructive coronary artery disease, which may be severe. Others have silent ischemia after a prior documented MI. The third and most common form occurs in patients who may also exhibit the usual forms of chronic stable angina, unstable angina, and Prinzmetal's angina. When monitored, these patients, who typically have silent ischemia episodes in addition to symptomatic ischemia, are sometimes referred to as having *mixed angina*. This mixed angina is estimated to be present in approximately one third of all treated patients with angina, although an even higher prevalence has been reported in diabetic patients. In these patients, about 85% of ambulant ischemic episodes occur without chest pain, and 66% of angina episodes are not accompanied by ST segment depression, suggesting that overt angina pectoris is merely the "tip of the ischemic iceberg." Pharmacologic agents that reduce or abolish episodes of symptomatic ischemia also reduce or abolish episodes of silent ischemia.

PROGNOSIS WITH OPTIMAL MANAGEMENT

Modern treatments have improved the prognosis of patients with stable ischemic heart disease to an annual mortality rate of 1 to 3% and a 1 to 2% rate of major ischemic events. The 1-year rate of cardiovascular death is now 1.9% (95% confidence interval [CI], 1.7 to 2.1), with a 2.9% (95% CI, 2.6 to 3.2) rate of all-cause mortality, and a 4.5% (95% CI, 4.2 to 4.8) rate of the combined outcome of cardiovascular death, MI, or stroke.

Recurrent angina is a common subsequent complaint in many patients with stable ischemic heart disease—even those who were initially treated successfully with PCI. About 30% of patients continue to experience angina one or more times per week, with associated greater physical limitation and worse quality of life, and almost 80% of patients who underwent initially successful PCI for chronic angina still take one or more antianginal agents at 1 year.

Selection of optimal treatment requires a full understanding of the potential risks and benefits of each treatment approach. In patients with stable symptoms who have not had an adequate trial of medical therapy (e.g., 8 to 12 weeks of multifaceted medical therapy and lifestyle intervention), such an initial approach of aggressive medical therapy is recommended. For patients whose angina or quality of life is not adequately controlled with optimal medical therapy, revascularization with either PCI or CABG surgery should be considered. Although the results of randomized trials must be individualized for specific patients, a multidisciplinary approach to clinical decision making can ensure that all therapeutic options are fully and transparently discussed so that patients are offered the most appropriate evidence-based treatment recommendations.

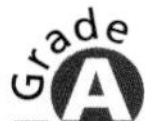

1. Cannon CP, Braunwald E, McCabe CH, et al. Intensive versus moderate lipid lowering with statins after acute coronary syndromes. *N Engl J Med.* 2004;350:1495-1504.
2. Tenkanen L, Mänttäri M, Kovanen PT, et al. Gemfibrozil in the treatment of dyslipidemia: an 18-year mortality follow-up of the Helsinki Heart Study. *Arch Intern Med.* 2006;166:743-748.
3. Jun M, Foote C, Lv J, et al. Effects of fibrates on cardiovascular outcomes: a systematic review and meta-analysis. *Lancet.* 2010;375:1875-1884.
4. Dagenais GR, Pogue J, Fox K, et al. Angiotensin-converting enzyme inhibitors in stable vascular disease without left ventricular systolic dysfunction or heart failure: a combined analysis of three trials. *Lancet.* 2006;368:581-588.
5. Lièvre M, Cucherat M. Aspirin in the secondary prevention of cardiovascular disease: an update of the APTC meta-analysis. *Fundam Clin Pharmacol.* 2010;24:385-391.
6. Bhatt DC, Fox KA, Hacke W, et al. Clopidogrel and aspirin versus aspirin alone for the prevention of atherothrombotic events. *N Engl J Med.* 2006;354:1706-1717.
7. Anand SS, Yusuf S. Oral anticoagulants in patients with coronary artery disease. *J Am Coll Cardiol.* 2003;41:62S-69S.
8. Morrow DA, Scirica BM, Karwatowska-Prokupczok E, et al. Effects of ranolazine on recurrent cardiovascular events in patients with non-ST-segment elevation acute coronary syndromes: the MERLIM TIMI-36 randomized trial. *JAMA.* 2007;297:1775-1784.
9. McKenna C, McDaid C, Suekarran S, et al. Enhanced external counterpulsation for the treatment of stable angina and heart failure: a systematic review and economic analysis. *Health Technol Assess.* 2009;13:1-90.
10. Weintraub WS, Spertus JA, Kolm P, et al. Effect of PCI on quality of life in patients with stable coronary disease. *N Engl J Med.* 2008;359:677-687.
11. Trikalinos TA, Alsheikh-Ali AA, Tatsioni A, et al. Percutaneous coronary interventions for non-acute coronary artery disease: a quantitative 20-year synopsis and a network meta-analysis. *Lancet.* 2009;373:911-918.
12. Boden WE, O'Rourke RA, Teo KK, et al. Optimal medical therapy with or without PCI for stable coronary disease. *N Engl J Med.* 2007;356:1503-1516.
13. BARI Investigators. The final 10-year follow-up results from the BARI randomized trial. *J Am Coll Cardiol.* 2007;49:1600-1606.
14. Frye R, August P, Brooks M, et al. BARI 2D: a randomized clinical trial of treatment strategies for type 2 diabetes and coronary artery disease. *N Engl J Med.* 2009;360:2503-2515.
15. Serruys PW, Morice MC, Kappetein AP, et al. Percutaneous coronary intervention versus coronary artery bypass grafting for severe coronary artery disease. *N Engl J Med.* 2009;360:961-972.
16. Hlatky MA, Boothroyd DB, Bravata DM, et al. Coronary artery bypass surgery compared with percutaneous coronary interventions for multivessel disease: a collaborative analysis of individual patient data from 10 randomised trials. *Lancet.* 2009;373:1190-1197.

SUGGESTED READINGS

Patel MR, Peterson ED, Dai D, et al. Low diagnostic yield of elective coronary angiography. *N Engl J Med.* 2010;362:886-895. *Only about one third of patients had significant coronary disease.*

Pfister ME, Zellweger MJ, Gersh BJ. Management of stable coronary artery disease. *Lancet.* 2010;375:763-772. *Review.*

Wijeysundera HC, Nallamothu BK, Krumholz HM, et al. Meta-analysis: effects of percutaneous coronary intervention versus medical therapy on angina relief. *Ann Intern Med.* 2010;152:370-379. *In a meta-analysis, PCI was associated with better relief of angina than was medical therapy, although the benefit is attenuated in contemporary studies with better use of evidence-based medical therapies.*

72

ACUTE CORONARY SYNDROME: UNSTABLE ANGINA AND NON–ST ELEVATION MYOCARDIAL INFARCTION

RICHARD A. LANGE AND L. DAVID HILLIS

DEFINITION

The term *acute coronary syndrome* (ACS) is used to describe the continuum of myocardial ischemia (unstable angina pectoris) or infarction (with or without concomitant ST segment elevation). The patient with *unstable angina* has cardiac chest pain that is new, worsening (i.e., more severe, prolonged, or frequent than previous episodes of angina), or occurring at rest, *without* serologic evidence of myocyte necrosis (i.e., no elevation of serum concentrations of troponin or the MB isoenzyme of creatine kinase [CK-MB]). The patient with cardiac chest pain *with* serologic evidence of myonecrosis and without ST segment elevation is said to have a *non–ST segment elevation myocardial infarction* (MI). Because unstable angina and non–ST segment elevation MI are characterized by the absence of ST segment elevation, they are collectively termed *non–ST segment elevation ACS*, or NSTE-ACS (Fig. 72-1). The patient with acute-onset cardiac chest pain, serologic evidence of myonecrosis, and persistent (>20 minutes) ST segment elevation is said to have an *ST segment elevation MI* (Chapter 73).

EPIDEMIOLOGY

More than 1.4 million individuals in the United States are hospitalized annually with ACS, of whom approximately two thirds have NSTE-ACS. More than half of those with NSTE-ACS are older than 65 years, and almost half are women. NSTE-ACS is more common in individuals with one or more risk factors for atherosclerosis (Chapter 51), peripheral vascular disease, or a chronic inflammatory disorder, such as rheumatoid arthritis, psoriasis, or infection.

Most subjects with ACS have so-called *primary* ACS, which is precipitated by rupture of a coronary arterial atherosclerotic plaque, with subsequent platelet aggregation and thrombus formation, leading, in turn, to compromised blood flow in the involved artery. An occasional individual has so-called *secondary* ACS, which is caused by a transient or sustained marked imbalance between myocardial oxygen supply and demand. Substantial reductions in oxygen supply, for example, can be caused by severe systemic arterial hypotension, anemia, or hypoxemia; dramatic increases in oxygen demand can be caused by fever, tachycardia, severe systemic arterial hypertension, or thyrotoxicosis. In the subject thought to have secondary ACS, therapy should be directed at correcting the underlying cause.

PATHOBIOLOGY

The precipitating event in almost all subjects with NSTE-ACS is atherosclerotic coronary arterial plaque rupture or erosion, with subsequent platelet aggregation and thrombus formation, leading to subtotal occlusion of the involved artery. In an occasional patient with extensive collateral blood supply to the region of myocardium that is perfused by an occluded artery, total thrombotic occlusion of the artery leads to NSTE-ACS rather than to ST segment elevation MI.

Rarely, intense vasospasm of a segment of an epicardial coronary artery, due to focal endothelial dysfunction (i.e., Prinzmetal's angina) or drug ingestion (caused, for example, by cocaine, chemotherapeutic agents, or one of the serotonin receptor agonist "triptans"), causes a transient or sustained compromise of coronary arterial blood flow, with resultant NSTE-ACS. Spontaneous coronary arterial dissection, which occurs most often in peripartum women and patients with vasculitis, may result in NSTE-ACS.

Plaque Rupture

Atherosclerotic coronary arterial plaque rupture (Chapter 70) or erosion is the initiating event in most patients with NSTE-ACS. Several factors may play a role in the deterioration of the protective fibrous cap that separates the atheroma in the vessel wall from the coronary arterial lumen. Local and systemic inflammation, mechanical features, and anatomic changes contribute to the transformation of a stable atherosclerotic plaque to a so-called "vulnerable" plaque, the rupture of which triggers platelet adherence, activation, and aggregation, with subsequent thrombus formation.

The deposition of oxidized low-density lipoprotein (LDL) in the coronary arterial wall stimulates an inflammatory response, which results in the accumulation of macrophages and T lymphocytes at the plaque border. These inflammatory cells secrete cytokines (e.g., interferon-γ), which inhibit collagen synthesis and deposition, as well as enzymes (e.g., matrix metalloproteinases and cathepsins), which promote collagen and elastin degradation, thereby rendering the overlying fibrous cap vulnerable to rupture.

Systemic inflammation may play a role in plaque rupture as evidenced by the predisposition of individuals with chronic gingivitis, rheumatoid arthritis, and chronic or acute infection to develop ACS. Angiographic and angioscopic studies of the coronary arteries of ACS patients often demonstrate plaque ulceration and thrombosis at more than one site, thereby suggesting that a systemic and diffuse inflammatory process is present.

The mechanical characteristics and location of coronary arterial plaques appear to influence their stability. For example, thin fibrous caps are more likely to erode or rupture than are thick ones. Sites of low shear stress, such as vessel bifurcations, have reduced production of endothelial vasodilator substances (i.e., nitric oxide and prostacyclin), accelerated accumulation of lipids and inflammatory cells, increased degradation of the extracellular matrix, and thinning of the fibrous cap, all of which contribute to plaque instability.

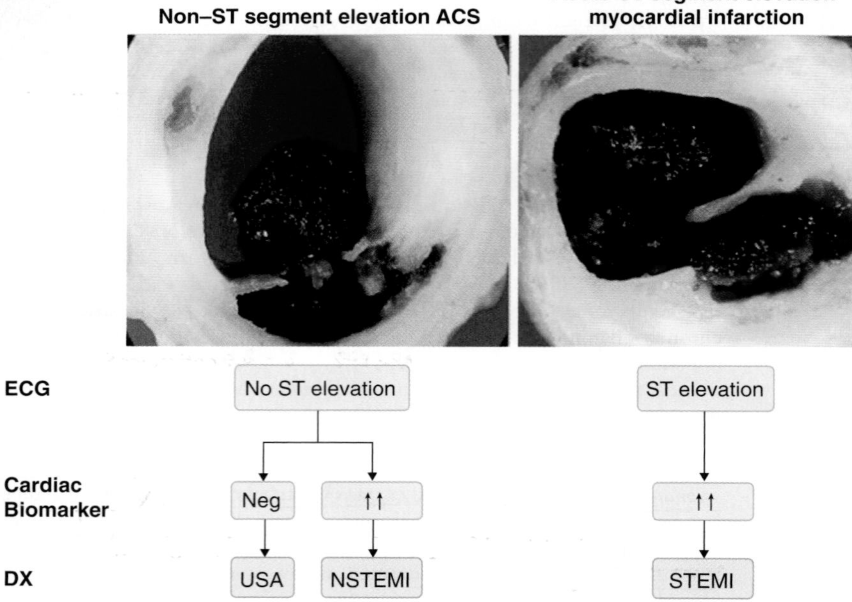

FIGURE 72-1. **Acute coronary syndrome (ACS).** Symptomatic, morphologic, electrocardiographic (ECG), and serologic findings in patients with various kinds of ACS. Subjects with ACS usually complain of chest pain. If the involved coronary artery is totally occluded by fresh thrombus (shown on the *right*), the patient's ECG reveals ST segment elevation; cardiac biomarkers subsequently are elevated; and he or she is diagnosed with an ST segment elevation myocardial infarction (STEMI). If the involved coronary artery is partially occluded by fresh thrombus (shown on the *left*), the patient's ECG does not show ST segment elevation. If cardiac biomarkers are not elevated, he or she is diagnosed with unstable angina (USA). If cardiac biomarkers are elevated, the patient is diagnosed with a non–ST segment elevation MI (NSTEMI). Dx = diagnosis.

Detailed histologic examination of evolving atherosclerotic plaques reveals a rich neovascularization that is the result of angiogenic peptides, such as fibroblast growth factors, vascular endothelial growth factor, placental growth factor, oncostatin M, and hypoxia-inducible factor, which are secreted by smooth muscle cells, inflammatory cells, and platelets. This neovascularization contributes to the growth of atheroma and to leukocyte trafficking, plaque hemorrhage, and destabilization.

Thrombus Formation

Platelets play a pivotal role in the pathobiology of ACS. Following erosion or rupture of a "vulnerable" plaque, circulating platelets *adhere* to the exposed subendothelial proteins, after which they are *activated*. With activation, the platelets change shape from discoid to stellate, thereby increasing the surface area on which thrombin formation can occur. The platelets then release the contents of their intracellular granules (i.e., thromboxane, serotonin, adenosine diphosphate, von Willebrand factor, fibrinogen) into the immediate environment and promote focal vasoconstriction of the adjacent arterial segment and activation of nearby platelets. Platelets also augment their number of surface glycoprotein IIb/IIIa receptors and the affinity of these receptors to bind circulating fibrinogen. The result is platelet *aggregation*, which occurs as fibrinogen binds to the glycoprotein IIb/IIIa receptors of adjacent platelets, thereby creating a "platelet plug."

Simultaneously with formation of the platelet plug, activation of the coagulation system with the generation of thrombin is a powerful stimulator of platelet activation and aggregation. In addition, thrombin converts fibrinogen to fibrin, which is incorporated into the thrombus. Subtotal coronary arterial occlusion by this platelet-rich thrombus compromises blood flow in the involved artery, thereby resulting in an imbalance of oxygen supply and demand of the myocytes perfused by the artery. Distal embolization of platelet-rich thrombi from the site of a ruptured plaque contributes to the compromise in blood flow. If the supply-demand imbalance is transient, the involved myocytes become ischemic but do not die because the ischemia is of insufficient duration to cause necrosis. The patient typically complains of cardiac chest pain at rest, but serologic evidence of myonecrosis, as evidenced by elevated serum concentrations of troponin or CK-MB, is absent; a diagnosis of *unstable angina* is made. In contrast, if the supply-demand imbalance is sustained, ischemic myocytes begin to die, and infarction occurs. The patient typically complains of cardiac chest pain at rest, and serologic evidence of myonecrosis confirms the diagnosis of *non–ST segment elevation MI.*

CLINICAL MANIFESTATIONS

Symptoms

The patient with NSTE-ACS typically complains of retrosternal pressure, squeezing, or heaviness that may be intermittent and recurrent or persistent (Chapter 50). If the episodes are intermittent and recurrent, the duration of each episode may range from only a few minutes to several hours. The chest pain may radiate to the left arm, neck, or jaw, and it may be accompanied by diaphoresis, nausea, abdominal pain, dyspnea, or syncope.

Atypical presentations of NSTE-ACS are not uncommon and may include aching or vague chest discomfort, epigastric pain, acute-onset indigestion, unexplained fatigue, or dyspnea. Such atypical complaints are often observed in younger (25 to 40 years of age) and older (>75 years of age) patients, women, and patients with diabetes mellitus, chronic renal insufficiency, or dementia.

Women with NSTE-ACS are more likely to have diabetes mellitus, hypertension, hyperlipidemia, and heart failure and to be older than men. They are less likely to be smokers or to have had a previous MI or coronary revascularization.

Physical Examination

The patient with NSTE-ACS often has a normal physical examination. On occasion, evidence of left ventricular dysfunction (Chapter 58), such as basilar rales or a ventricular gallop, hypotension, or peripheral hypoperfusion, may accompany an episode of NSTE-ACS or appear shortly thereafter. An important goal of the physical examination is to exclude noncardiac causes of the subject's symptoms (i.e., costochondritis, pneumothorax, pulmonary embolism, pneumonia) and nonischemic cardiac disorders (i.e., aortic dissection, pericarditis, severe systemic arterial hypertension) that can cause chest pain, other symptoms, or an elevation of cardiac biomarkers (Chapter 50). Accordingly, differences in blood pressure between the upper and lower limbs, decreased lung sounds, friction rubs, and pain on sternal palpation suggest a diagnosis other than NSTE-ACS. Other findings on physical examination—such as an elevated blood pressure, pallor, or increased sweating or tremor—point toward precipitating conditions, such as uncontrolled hypertension (Chapter 67), anemia (Chapter 161), or thyrotoxicosis (Chapter 233), respectively.

DIAGNOSIS

The patient with suspected ACS should be evaluated promptly because an expedient and accurate diagnosis permits the timely initiation of appropriate therapy, which can reduce the rate of complications. The initial assessment should be directed at determining whether the subject's symptoms are likely caused by myocardial ischemia, MI, or some other disorder. The likelihood of ACS can be estimated from the history, physical examination, and electrocardiogram (ECG) (Table 72-1).

In the acute setting, the presence or absence of traditional risk factors for atherosclerosis is far less important for determining the presence or absence of ACS than are the patient's symptoms, ECG findings, and serologic evidence of myonecrosis. As a result, these long-term risk factors are not the key factors that should be used to determine whether an individual should be evaluated, hospitalized, or treated for ACS.

TABLE 72-1 LIKELIHOOD THAT SYMPTOMS AND SIGNS REPRESENT AN ACUTE CORONARY SYNDROME CAUSED BY CORONARY ARTERIAL PLAQUE RUPTURE

HIGH LIKELIHOOD
Any of the following features:
Chest or left arm pain as the main symptom, similar in nature to previously noted angina
Known coronary artery disease
Evidence on physical exam of transient mitral regurgitation murmur, hypotension, diaphoresis, or pulmonary edema
New or transient ST segment deviation (≥1 mm) or T wave inversion in multiple precordial leads
Elevated serum troponin or CK-MB concentration
INTERMEDIATE LIKELIHOOD
Absence of high-likelihood features and any of the following:
Chest or left arm discomfort as main symptom
Age > 70 yr
Male gender
Diabetes mellitus
Extracardiac vascular disease
Q waves, ST segment depression (0.5-1 mm), or T wave inversion (>1 mm) in leads with dominant R waves
Normal cardiac troponin or CK-MB
LOW LIKELIHOOD
Absence of high- or intermediate-likelihood features, but may have:
Probable ischemic symptoms in the absence of any of the intermediate likelihood characteristics
Recent cocaine use
Chest discomfort reproduced by palpation
T wave flattening or inversion < 1 mm in leads with dominant R waves
Normal electrocardiogram
Normal serum troponin or CK-MB concentration

Modified from Anderson JL, Adams CD, Antman EM, et al. ACC/AHA 2007 Guidelines for the management of patients with unstable angina/non-ST-elevation myocardial infarction. *Circulation.* 2007;116:e148-e304.

Conditions that increase the likelihood that the symptomatic patient is experiencing myocardial ischemia or MI include older age, male gender, diabetes mellitus, extracardiac vascular disease, and chest pain radiating to the left arm, neck, or jaw as the presenting symptom. Myocardial ischemia is highly likely if anginal symptoms are accompanied by ECG abnormalities (i.e., ST segment depression or elevation ≥1 mm in magnitude or T wave inversion in multiple precordial leads), elevated serum concentration of troponin or CK-MB, or evidence of left ventricular dysfunction.

In a patient with known coronary artery disease, typical symptoms are likely to be caused by myocardial ischemia or MI rather than by another condition, particularly if the patient confirms that his or her symptoms are similar to previous anginal episodes. Conversely, a young individual who has a normal ECG and no risk factors for atherosclerosis is unlikely to be having ACS even when complaining of chest pain with features consistent with ischemia or infarction.

It is important to inquire about the use of cocaine and methamphetamines in the patient with suspected ACS, especially patients who are less than 40 years of age or have few traditional risk factors for atherosclerosis. These drugs can increase myocardial oxygen demand and concomitantly decrease oxygen supply by causing vasospasm and thrombosis. A urine toxicologic analysis should be considered when substance abuse is suspected as a cause of or contributor to ACS.

Electrocardiogram

An ECG should be obtained and examined promptly in the patient with suspected ACS. An ECG obtained during a symptomatic episode is particularly valuable. If the patient has persistent (>20 minutes) ST segment elevation, prompt reperfusion therapy should be initiated (Chapter 73). Transient ST segment abnormalities that develop during a symptomatic episode at rest and resolve when the patient is asymptomatic strongly suggest NSTE-ACS. ST segment depression (or transient ST segment elevation) and T wave abnormalities occur in up to 50% of NSTE-ACS patients.

A completely normal ECG does not exclude the possibility of NSTE-ACS; in fact, about 5% of patients who are discharged from the emergency department and ultimately diagnosed with ACS have a normal ECG. Ischemia or infarction in the territory of the left circumflex coronary artery often escapes detection with a standard 12-lead ECG, but it may be detected with right-sided leads (V_{4R} and V_{3R}) or posterior leads (V_7 to V_9). In the patient whose initial ECG is normal, subsequent ECGs should be obtained in the first 24 hours and during symptomatic episodes, and they should be compared with previous tracings to identify new ST segment or T wave abnormalities. Deep (>2 mm), symmetrical T wave inversion in the anterior chest leads is often associated with a hemodynamically significant stenosis of the left main or proximal left anterior descending coronary artery.

More than half of all episodes of myocardial ischemia are asymptomatic. On-line continuous computer-assisted 12-lead ST segment monitoring is a valuable diagnostic tool for detecting such episodes. Continuous ST segment monitoring also adds independent prognostic information to the resting ECG, serum cardiac enzymes, and other variables.

Serum Biomarkers

Troponin (Chapter 73) is detectable in the blood with conventional assays within 3 to 4 hours of the onset of myonecrosis, but in some individuals, its detection may be delayed for up to 8 hours. As a result, single negative assessment of serum troponin is insufficient to exclude MI in a patient with recent symptoms. To demonstrate or to exclude myonecrosis, repetitive blood sampling and troponin measurements should be performed 6 to 12 hours after the initial evaluation of the patient and following any additional episodes of chest pain. High sensitivity troponin assays can detect extremely small amounts of troponin in the blood, thereby improving the early (i.e., within 2 hours of symptom onset) diagnosis of MI. Troponin levels can be measured in the hospital's central chemistry laboratory or with point-of-care instruments at the patient's bedside using desktop devices or handheld bedside rapid qualitative assays. The advantage of point-of-care systems for avoiding delays must be weighed against their higher costs and the need for stringent quality control. In addition, point-of-care assays are qualitative or semiquantitative and observer dependent, whereas the central laboratory provides more accurate quantitative information concerning biomarker concentrations.

Up to one third of ACS patients whose serum CK-MB concentrations are normal have detectable serum concentrations of troponin T and I, indicating that myonecrosis has occurred and establishing the diagnosis of NSTE-MI. Current recommendations call for the use of the serum troponin concentration for acute risk stratification at the time of the patient's arrival to hospital.

Noninvasive Testing

The patient considered to have a low likelihood for ACS (based on the history, physical examination, ECG, and serum biomarkers) should undergo timely stress testing (Chapter 50), which does not absolutely establish or exclude the presence of coronary artery disease but has a high enough predictive value to guide acute decision making. Alternatively, multidetector computed tomographic (CT) coronary angiography has a high (>98%) negative predictive value to exclude coronary artery disease when performed and interpreted at centers experienced in its use. Conversely, the patient who is believed to be at intermediate or high risk for ACS and who continues to have typical ischemic chest pain with ECG abnormalities or elevated cardiac biomarkers should not undergo urgent diagnostic stress testing or CT coronary angiography; when such patients become symptom free with medical therapy and otherwise do not have indications for coronary angiography (see later), stress testing, often with myocardial perfusion imaging, should be performed before hospital discharge.

An echocardiogram may be helpful in the patient with chest pain if the ECG is nondiagnostic (i.e., minimal ST segment or T wave abnormalities). If left ventricular hypokinesis or akinesis is observed during an episode of chest pain and then improves when symptoms resolve, myocardial ischemia is likely. In the patient with T wave inversion in the anterior leads of uncertain etiology, hypokinesis of the left ventricular anterior wall suggests that the observed T wave abnormality is due to a severe stenosis of the left anterior descending coronary artery. Because echocardiography can help evaluate and identify alternative causes for the patient's chest pain, such as myocarditis (Chapter 60), aortic dissection (Chapter 78), or pulmonary embolism (Chapter 98), it is recommended in patients whose diagnosis is uncertain.

Coronary Angiography

Coronary angiography (Chapter 57) should be performed in patients who are thought to be at high risk for a cardiac ischemic event (death, MI, or recurrent ischemia) in the ensuing days, weeks, and months (see later); have spontaneous or inducible myocardial ischemia despite appropriate medical therapy; or have a confusing or difficult clinical presentation and a subsequent inconclusive noninvasive evaluation. The results of angiography help determine whether revascularization is appropriate and, if so, whether it should be attempted surgically (through coronary artery bypass grafting [CABG]) or percutaneously (through percutaneous coronary intervention [PCI]) (Chapter 74).

In patients with NSTE-ACS, coronary angiography demonstrates more than 50% luminal diameter narrowing of the left main coronary artery in about 15% of patients, of all three major epicardial coronary arteries in about 30 to 35% of patients, of two of the three epicardial arteries in about 20 to 30% of patients, and of one major epicardial artery in 20 to 30% of patients. About 15% of patients have no coronary arterial narrowing of hemodynamic significance. Women with NSTE-ACS are likely to have less extensive coronary artery disease than men, and patients with non–ST segment elevation MI on average have more extensive disease than those with unstable angina.

The coronary arterial lesion responsible for NSTE-ACS (the so-called culprit lesion) typically is asymmetrical or eccentric, with scalloped or overhanging edges and a narrow base or neck. These angiographic features reflect underlying plaque disruption and thrombus formation. Although obvious thrombus is visible angiographically in only one third of patients with NSTE-ACS, coronary angioscopy shows plaque rupture with overlying thrombus in most.

If the patient had previous coronary angiography, the culprit lesion usually can be seen to have progressed substantially. Interestingly, the lesion that is the nidus for ACS often is not severely stenotic when assessed on the previous angiogram; in fact, two thirds of culprit lesions previously had less than 50% luminal diameter narrowing (and, therefore, would not have been considered appropriate for surgical or percutaneous revascularization).

During the months after a NSTE-ACS, the culprit coronary arterial lesion is more likely to progress and to precipitate another ACS than are other lesions in the same patient. Lesions with irregular borders, overhanging edges, or obvious thrombus at angiography are more likely to precipitate another ACS in the ensuing months when compared with those that do not display these morphologic characteristics.

Risk Assessment and Triage

The initial evaluation of the patient with possible or suspected ACS should focus on an assessment of his or her risk of acutely sustaining a cardiac ischemic event (death, MI, or recurrent ischemia). Patients may be admitted immediately to a coronary intensive care unit or to an intermediate care unit, watched carefully in a monitored chest pain evaluation unit, or discharged home based on their risk of an MI (Fig. 72-2; see Fig. 50-1 in Chapter 50). Patients considered to be at low risk for a cardiac ischemic event should be discharged home, with further evaluation performed as an outpatient. Conversely, patients not at low risk should be hospitalized for further evaluation and treatment.

After the initial triage decision is made, urgent therapeutic interventions are based on the risk of adverse events in the coming hours, days, weeks, and months—estimated by using either the Thrombolysis in Myocardial Infarction (TIMI) or Global Registry of Acute Coronary Events (GRACE) risk algorithm—balanced against the risk of a bleeding complication from intensive medical therapy (Table 72-2) or an adverse event from an invasive cardiac procedure. Based on this initial assessment, the patient's therapy can be tailored, thereby reducing the likelihood of adverse events.

Although serum markers of myonecrosis comprise only one of the TIMI or GRACE risk variables, the presence of this variable alone appears to identify the patient as being "high risk." However, although elevated serum markers indicate myonecrosis, they provide no insight into its cause: in some subjects, myonecrosis occurs with disease entities other than coronary artery disease (e.g., pulmonary embolism, decompensated heart failure, severe hypertension or tachycardia, anemia, sepsis). Thus, when evaluating the patient with possible ACS, the presence of elevated serum markers should be assessed in conjunction with other variables.

Increasing age is associated with a higher incidence of both ACS-related cardiac ischemic events and complications from intensive medical therapy and invasive cardiac procedures. Even though elderly people are at increased risk of such treatment-related complications, they nonetheless derive a greater absolute and relative benefit from such intensive therapy when compared with younger individuals. Apart from this initial risk assessment, the ACS patient's general medical and cognitive status, anticipated life expectancy, risk of treatment-related complications, and, most importantly, personal preferences should be evaluated and considered.

TABLE 72-2 RISK VARIABLES FOR ISCHEMIC EVENTS AND BLEEDING COMPLICATIONS

1. RISK VARIABLES PREDICTIVE OF DEATH, MYOCARDIAL INFARCTION, OR RECURRENT ISCHEMIA
A. Thrombolysis in Myocardial Infarction (TIMI) Score*
Age > 65 yrs
Three or more risk factors for atherosclerosis
Known coronary artery disease (previous coronary arteriography or myocardial infarction)
Two or more episodes of anginal chest pain in the 24 hr before hospitalization
Use of aspirin in the 7 days before hospitalization
ST segment deviation ≥ 0.5 mV
Elevated serum concentrations of troponin or CK-MB
B. Global Registry of Acute Coronary Events (GRACE)†
Age
Heart failure class
Heart rate
Systolic blood pressure
ST segment deviation
Cardiac arrest during presentation
Serum creatinine concentration
Elevated serum markers of myonecrosis
2. RISK FACTORS FOR BLEEDING COMPLICATIONS WITH INTENSIVE THERAPY‡
Female gender
Older age
Renal insufficiency
Low body weight
Tachycardia
Systolic arterial pressure (high or low)
Anemia
Diabetes mellitus

*Individuals with three or more of these variables are considered to be "high risk," whereas those with 0, 1, or 2 are considered to be "low risk." (From Diez JG, Cohen M. Balancing myocardial ischemic and bleeding risks in patients with non-ST-segment elevation myocardial infarction. *Am J Cardiol.* 2009;103:1396-1402.)

†Each variable is assigned a numerical score based on its specific value, and the eight scores are summed to yield a total score, which is applied to a reference nomogram to determine the patient's risk. The GRACE application tool is available online at *www.outcomes-umassmed.org/grace.* (From Brieger D, Fox KA, Fitzgerald G, et al. Predicting freedom from clinical events in non-ST-elevation acute coronary syndromes: the Global Registry of Acute Coronary Events. *Heart.* 2009;95:888-894.)

‡The patient's bleeding risk can be estimated with the tool available at *www.crusadebleedingscore.org.* (From Subherwal S, Bach RG, Chen AY, et al. Baseline risk of major bleeding in non-ST-segment-elevation myocardial infarction: the CRUSADE [Can Rapid risk stratification of Unstable angina patients Suppress ADverse outcomes with Early implementation of the ACC/AHA Guidelines] Bleeding Score. *Circulation.* 2009;119:1873-1882.)

Once the risk status of the ACS patient is established, management is initiated and tailored to the patient's risk of sustaining a subsequent ischemic cardiac event or a treatment-related complication (Table 72-3). For example, the patient considered to be at low risk of a subsequent ischemic event does not benefit from intensive antithrombotic therapy or routine coronary angiography and revascularization. 1 Conversely, in patients considered to be at high risk of sustaining an ischemic event, optimal therapy—including coronary angiography and revascularization (if appropriate)—results in a substantial 20 to 40% decrease in the risk of recurrent ischemia and MI and an approximately 10% reduction in mortality. 2,3 In short, the magnitude of benefit of intensive therapy correlates with the patient's level of risk.

Differential Diagnoses

Several cardiac and noncardiac conditions, some of which are potentially life-threatening, may mimic NSTE-ACS. The patient with a pulmonary

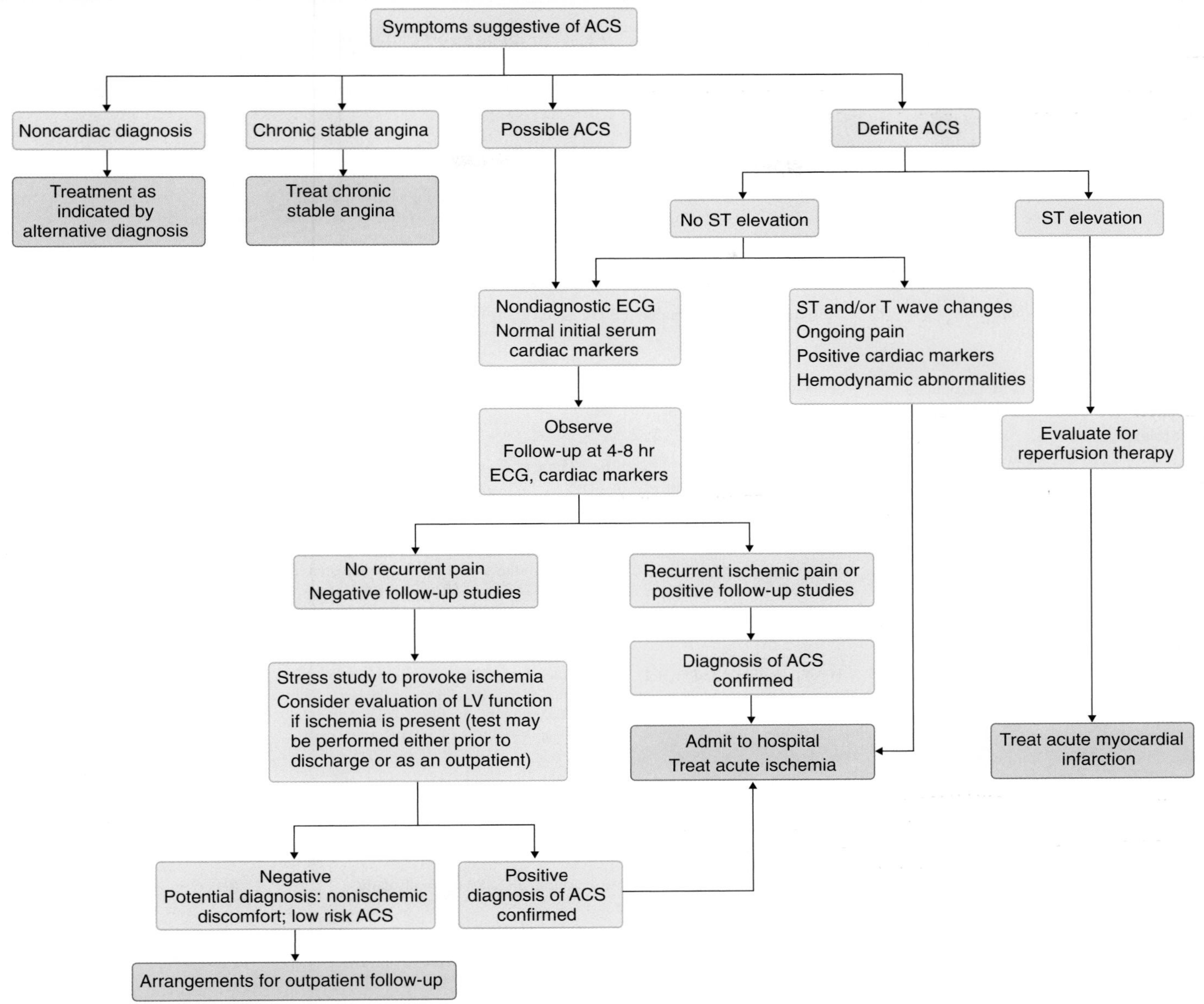

FIGURE 72-2. Initial triage for patients with symptoms suggestive of an acute coronary syndrome (ACS). ECG = electrocardiogram; LV = left ventricular. (Modified from Anderson JL, Adams CD, Antman EM, et al. ACC/AHA 2007 guidelines for the management of patients with unstable angina and non-ST-segment elevation myocardial infarction. A report of the American College of Cardiology/American Heart Association Task Force on Practice Guidelines. *Circulation.* 2007;116:e148-e304.)

embolism (Chapter 98) often complains of dyspnea and chest pain and may have ECG abnormalities and elevated serum concentrations of troponin and CK-MB. Aortic dissection (Chapter 78) should be considered and excluded because the therapies for NSTE-ACS are contraindicated in patients with this condition. Stroke (Chapter 414) and subarachnoid hemorrhage (Chapter 415) may be accompanied by ECG abnormalities, segmental wall motion abnormalities, and elevated serum biomarker concentrations. Underlying chronic cardiac conditions, such as valvular heart disease (i.e., aortic stenosis, aortic regurgitation) and hypertrophic cardiomyopathy (Chapter 60), may be associated with symptoms similar to those of NSTE-ACS, elevated serum biomarker concentrations, and ECG abnormalities. Myocarditis (Chapter 60), pericarditis (Chapter 77), and myopericarditis often cause chest pain that resembles angina, ECG abnormalities, and elevated serum biomarker concentrations. A flu-like or upper respiratory tract infection often precedes or accompanies these conditions. Patients with "stress cardiomyopathy" (takotsubo syndrome) typically have chest pain, ST segment abnormalities and deeply inverted T waves, and mildly elevated serum biomarker concentrations (Chapter 60).

PREVENTION AND TREATMENT Rx

The goals of treatment of the patient with NSTE-ACS are to prevent recurrent ischemia by correcting the imbalance between myocardial oxygen supply and demand; to prevent thrombus propagation; and to stabilize the "vulnerable" plaque. Antianginal medications, such as nitroglycerin, β-adrenergic blockers, and calcium-channel blockers, favorably affect myocardial oxygen supply and demand, thereby preventing recurrent ischemia. Antiplatelet and antithrombotic agents retard thrombus propagation, and statins promote plaque stabilization. Once the risk status of the ACS patient is established, treatment is initiated (see Table 72-3).

Every NSTE-ACS patient, regardless of the level of risk, should promptly receive antianginal medications, antiplatelet therapy (aspirin and clopidogrel), and a statin, unless contraindicated. A "low-risk" patient should also receive unfractionated heparin but not more intensive antiplatelet or anticoagulant therapy because anticoagulation beyond aspirin, clopidogrel, and heparin increases the risk of bleeding without further reducing the risk of an ischemic cardiac event. Routine coronary angiography and revascularization are not beneficial and should be reserved for the patient with recurrent ischemia despite intensive medical therapy.

TABLE 72-3 MANAGEMENT STRATEGIES FOR PATIENTS WITH ACUTE CORONARY SYNDROME

THERAPY	INITIATION	DURATION	DOSE, ROUTE, AND DURATION	BENEFIT VS. PLACEBO (REDUCED INCIDENCE OF …)
LOW-RISK PATIENT				
Antianginal				
β-Blocker*	Immediately	Hospitalization ± indefinitely	Metoprolol, 5 mg IV boluses (three given 2 to 5 minutes apart) then 50 mg orally twice daily titrated up to 100 mg twice daily or atenolol, 5-10 mg IV bolus then 100 mg orally daily	Recurrent ischemia
Nitroglycerin	Immediately	Hospitalization ± indefinitely	0.3 to 0.6 mg sublingually or 5 to 10 μg/min IV initially and increased by 10 μg/min every 5 min	Not studied
Diltiazem or verapamil*	Immediately	Hospitalization ± indefinitely	30 to 90 mg orally four times daily or up to 360 mg of long-acting preparation orally daily	MI, recurrent ischemia
Lipid Lowering				
Statin	Before hospital discharge	Indefinitely	Atorvastatin, up to 80 mg orally daily	Recurrent ischemia
Antiplatelet				
Aspirin	Immediately	Indefinitely	162-325 mg orally initial dose then 81 mg orally daily	Death, MI
Clopidogrel	Immediately	1-12 mo	300 mg orally initial dose then 75 mg orally daily	MI, recurrent ischemia
Anticoagulant				
Unfractionated heparin	Immediately	2 to 5 days	60 U/kg IV bolus then 12 U/kg IV adjusted to achieve an aPTT of 50 to 70 sec	Death or MI (combined)
HIGH-RISK PATIENT				
Antianginal				
β-Blocker*	Immediately	Hospitalization ± indefinitely	Metoprolol, 5 mg IV boluses (three given 2 to 5 minutes apart) then 50 mg orally twice daily titrated up to 100 mg twice daily or atenolol, 5-10 mg IV bolus then 100 mg orally daily	Death, MI, recurrent ischemia
Nitroglycerin	Immediately	Hospitalization ± indefinitely	0.3 to 0.6 mg sublingually or 5 to 10 μg/min IV initially and increased by 10 μg/min every 5 min	Not studied
Diltiazem or verapamil*	Immediately	Hospitalization ± indefinitely	30 to 90 mg orally four times daily or up to 360 mg of long-acting preparation orally daily	MI, recurrent ischemia
Lipid Lowering				
Statin	Before hospital discharge	Indefinitely	Atorvastatin, up to 80 mg orally daily	Recurrent ischemia
Antiplatelet				
Aspirin	Immediately	Indefinitely	162-325 mg orally initial dose then 81 mg orally	Death, MI
Clopidogrel	Immediately	≥12 mo	300 mg orally initial dose then 75 mg orally daily	MI, recurrent ischemia
Glycoprotein IIb/IIIa inhibitor (eptifibatide, tirofiban, or abciximab)	At time of PCI	12-24 hr post-PCI	Abciximab, 0.25 mg/kg IV bolus then 0.125 μg/kg/min IV (max 10 μg/min) for 12 hr or eptifibatide, 180 μg/kg IV bolus then 2.0 μg/kg/min IV for 18-24 hr or tirofiban, 0.4 μg/kg/min IV for 30 min then 0.1 μg/kg/min IV for 12 to 24 hr	MI
Anticoagulants				
Unfractionated heparin or	Immediately	2 to 5 days; discontinue after successful PCI	60 U/kg IV bolus then 12 U/kg IV adjusted to achieve an aPTT of 50 to 70 sec	Death or MI (combined)
Enoxaparin or	Immediately	Duration of hospitalization (up to 8 days); discontinue after successful PCI	1 mg/kg subcutaneously twice daily	MI, recurrent ischemia[†]
Bivalirudin	Immediately	Up to 72 hr; discontinue 4 hr after PCI	0.1 mg/kg IV bolus then 1.75 mg/kg/hr IV	Bleeding[‡]
Invasive Management				
Coronary angiography followed by revascularization (if appropriate)	Up to 36-80 hr after hospitalization; within 24 hr in "very high risk" patients			MI, recurrent ischemia

*Avoid in the patient with decompensated heart failure, hypotension, or hemodynamic instability.
[†]As compared with unfractionated heparin.
[‡]As monotherapy compared with heparin and glycoprotein IIb/IIIa inhibitor combination.
aPTT = activated partial thromboplastin time; IV = intravenous; MI = myocardial infarction; PCI = percutaneous coronary intervention.
Modified from Lange RA, Hillis LD. Optimal management of acute coronary syndromes. *N Engl J Med.* 2009;260:2237-2240.

Conversely, the high-risk patient should receive antianginal medications, antiplatelet therapy (aspirin and clopidogrel), a statin, more intensive anticoagulant therapy, and coronary angiography followed by revascularization (if indicated). In the patient whose coronary anatomy is suitable, revascularization reduces the incidence of ischemia and recurrent MI, and in certain patients (see later), it improves survival.

Antianginal Therapy

Nitroglycerin

Nitroglycerin (Chapter 71), which is a venodilator at low doses and an arteriolar dilator at higher doses, may prevent recurrent ischemia in patients with unstable angina, but no studies of sufficient statistical power have determined whether it reduces the risk of MI in this patient population. In patients who complain of recurrent symptoms, nitroglycerin should be given sublingually or by buccal spray (0.3 to 0.6 mg). Patients with ongoing or recurrent chest pain should receive intravenous nitroglycerin (5 to 10 μg/minute using nonabsorbable tubing), with escalation of the dose in increments of 10 μg/minute until symptoms resolve or adverse effects develop. Nitroglycerin's most common adverse effects are headache, nausea, dizziness, hypotension, and reflex tachycardia.

Nitrate tolerance can be avoided by providing the patient with a "nitrate-free" period (i.e., a brief cessation of drug administration). Nitroglycerin should not be given to the patient who has received a phosphodiesterase-5 inhibitor (i.e., sildenafil, tadalafil, or vardenafil) within the previous 24 to 48 hours, as severe hypotension may ensue.

β-Adrenergic Blockers

β-Adrenergic blockers diminish symptoms and the risk of MI in patients who are not already taking a β-blocker at the time of hospital admission. In the normotensive patient without ongoing chest pain or tachycardia, metoprolol should be initiated at 50 mg orally every 6 to 8 hours, with the dose increased (to 100 mg twice daily) as necessary to control heart rate, blood pressure, and symptoms. In high-risk patients and in patients with tachycardia or elevated systemic arterial pressure, metoprolol should be administered intravenously (3 boluses of 5 mg each given 5 minutes apart) initially, after which an oral dose should be initiated. A reasonable target heart rate is 50 to 60 beats per minute at rest.

β-Blockers should not be administered to patients with decompensated heart failure, hypotension, hemodynamic instability, or advanced atrioventricular block. Because most patients with chronic obstructive pulmonary disease or peripheral vascular disease tolerate β-blockers without difficulty, these conditions should not preclude their use.

Calcium-Channel Blockers

Calcium-channel blockers, which cause coronary and systemic arterial vasodilation, increase coronary arterial blood flow and lower systemic arterial pressure. The nondihydropyridine calcium-channel blockers, diltiazem and verapamil, slow heart rate and are recommended for the patient with a contraindication to a β-adrenergic blocker or persistent or recurrent symptoms despite treatment with nitroglycerin or a β-blocker. Oral diltiazem (30 to 90 mg four times daily of the short-acting preparation or up to 360 mg once daily of the long-acting preparation) is the preferred agent because studies have shown that it reduces the incidence of myocardial ischemia and recurrent MI in patients with NSTE-ACS.[4] Diltiazem is contraindicated in patients with left ventricular dysfunction or pulmonary vascular congestion. Caution should be exercised when combining a β-blocker with diltiazem because the two drugs may act synergistically to depress left ventricular systolic function as well as sinus and atrioventricular nodal conduction. Short-acting nifedipine should not be administered to the patient with ACS unless the patient is already receiving a β-blocker because it may increase the risk of death. The risks and benefits of long-acting dihydropyridines in patients with NSTE-ACS are undefined.

Antiplatelet Agents

In patients with NSTE-ACS, *aspirin* (Chapter 36), 75 to 1300 mg daily, reduces the risk of death or MI by roughly 50%.[5] Because high-dose aspirin increases the risk of gastrointestinal bleeding but is no more efficacious than low-dose aspirin, the patient should be treated with 75 to 162 mg daily, unless contraindicated (i.e., the patient has an aspirin allergy or active bleeding). Once initiated, aspirin therapy should be continued indefinitely.

Clopidogrel (Chapter 37) is a thienopyridine that blocks the $P2Y_{12}$ adenosine diphosphate (ADP) receptor, thereby diminishing ADP-mediated platelet activation. Its antiplatelet activity is synergistic with aspirin because the two agents inhibit different platelet-activating pathways. Clopidogrel is a prodrug that must be metabolized by the cytochrome P-450 system to the active form. Polymorphisms in the cytochrome P-450 isoform CYP2C19, present in 15 to 20% of individuals, slow metabolism of the prodrug to the active form, thereby reducing the magnitude of platelet inhibition.

In patients with NSTE-ACS, the addition of clopidogrel to aspirin reduces the composite end point of cardiovascular death, nonfatal MI, or stroke by 20% (2.1% reduction in absolute risk) compared with treatment with aspirin alone.[6] The benefit of an aspirin-clopidogrel combination is seen as early as 24 hours after drug initiation and persists for the 12 months of the study; an increase in minor bleeding is observed in those receiving both agents.

Dual antiplatelet therapy (aspirin and clopidogrel) should be administered routinely to the ACS patient, unless contraindicated. The patient who is allergic to or intolerant of aspirin should receive clopidogrel alone. Because maximal platelet inhibition occurs 3 to 5 days after clopidogrel is initiated unless a large dose is given initially, the patient should receive a loading dose of 300 to 600 mg, then 75 mg daily for at least 1 year.

Clopidogrel treatment increases the risk of bleeding in the patient undergoing CABG. Clopidogrel should not be initiated in likely candidates for CABG; if already begun, it should be discontinued 5 days before the planned surgery. Drugs that are potent inhibitors of the CYP2C19 enzyme should not be administered with clopidogrel because they affect the metabolism to its active form and reduce its antiplatelet effects. Such drugs include omeprazole, esomeprazole, cimetidine, fluconazole, ketoconazole, voriconazole, etravirine, felbamate, fluoxetine, and fluvoxamine. For clopidogrel-treated patients who need antacid therapy, treatment with ranitidine or pantoprazole is recommended.

Prasugrel (Chapter 37) is another thienopyridine with a greater antiplatelet effect and a more rapid onset of action than clopidogrel. In patients with ACS who are referred for PCI, prasugrel in combination with aspirin reduces ischemic events (i.e., a combination of cardiovascular death, nonfatal MI, and stroke) by 20% compared with concomitant clopidogrel and aspirin (2.2% absolute risk reduction) therapy.[7] However, this benefit is obtained at a 0.5% increased risk of life-threatening bleeding and a 0.3% increased risk of fatal bleeding. At present, prasugrel is approved for use in the ACS patient who is referred for PCI. In combination with aspirin, it is administered as a 60 mg oral loading dose followed by a 10 mg daily maintenance dose. Because prasugrel-associated bleeding complications are highest in patients with a previous stroke or transient ischemic attack, age older than 75 years, or a body weight of less than 60 kg, its use should be avoided in the patient with any of these features.

Glycoprotein IIb/IIIa inhibitors (Chapter 37) block platelet aggregation in response to all potential agonists and are the most potent antiplatelet agents available. Three glycoprotein IIb/IIIa inhibitors, each of which must be administered parenterally, are available: abciximab is the Fab fragment of a monoclonal antibody to the receptor; eptifibatide is a peptide; and tirofiban is a peptidomimetic molecule.

Glycoprotein IIb/IIIa inhibitors reduce the incidence of recurrent ischemic events in patients with NSTE-ACS who undergo PCI, but not in patients who are managed with medical therapy alone. If a glycoprotein IIb/IIIa inhibitor is administered, it should be initiated at the time of angiography because previously published studies have shown that its routine administration beforehand carries an increased bleeding risk and no improvement in outcomes.[8] The glycoprotein IIb/IIIa inhibitor infusion (see Table 72-3) typically is continued for 12 to 24 hours following PCI.

Anticoagulants

Anticoagulant therapy should be administered to all patients with ACS unless a contraindication, such as active bleeding, is present. For the patient in whom a noninvasive, ischemia-guided management strategy is selected, treatment with unfractionated heparin, low-molecular-weight heparin (LMWH), or fondaparinux is appropriate, with fondaparinux recommended for the patient at increased risk of bleeding. For the patient in whom an invasive management strategy is selected, unfractionated heparin and LMWH are the agents of choice. Bivalirudin may be preferred in the individual undergoing PCI, but it should not be used in the initial management of the patient with ACS.

Heparin

Unfractionated heparin (Chapter 37) exerts its anticoagulant effect by accelerating the action of circulating antithrombin and prevents thrombus propagation but does not lyse existing thrombi. In the patient with NSTE-ACS, the addition of heparin to aspirin reduces the rate of in-hospital ischemic events (i.e., death or MI) by 33%.[9]

Unfractionated heparin should be initiated with an intravenous bolus of 60 U/kg, followed by a continuous infusion of approximately 12 U/kg/hour (maximum, 1000 U/hour), adjusted to maintain the activated partial thromboplastin time (aPTT) at 1.5 to 2.5 times control (i.e., 50 to 70 seconds) or a heparin concentration at 0.3 to 0.7 U/mL (by anti–factor Xa determinations). The infusion should be continued for 48 hours or until revascularization is performed, whichever occurs sooner. Frequent monitoring of the aPTT or heparin concentration is necessary because the anticoagulant response to a standard dose of unfractionated heparin varies widely among individuals; even when a weight-based nomogram (see Table 81-4 in Chapter 81) is followed, the aPTT is outside the therapeutic range more than one third of the time.

Mild thrombocytopenia occurs in 10 to 20% of patients treated with unfractionated heparin. In 1 to 5% of patients, a more severe form of thrombocytopenia develops. This antibody-mediated response usually occurs 4 to 14 days after the initiation of treatment, although it may become manifest far more quickly in the subject who received heparin within the preceding 6 months. Such antibody-mediated thrombocytopenia is associated with thromboembolic sequelae in 30 to 80% of subjects.

Low-Molecular-Weight Heparin

LMWHs (Chapter 37), which are fragments of unfractionated heparin, exert a more predictable anticoagulant effect, have a longer half-life, and are less likely to cause thrombocytopenia compared with unfractionated heparin. Because they provide predictable and sustained anticoagulation with once- or twice-daily subcutaneous administration, monitoring of their anticoagulant effect is not required.

LMWH is superior to unfractionated heparin in preventing MI or death during hospitalization in patients with NSTE-ACS who have elevated serum cardiac biomarkers as well as in those considered to be at high risk for recurrent ischemia (i.e., the subject with three or more TIMI risk factors).[10] In the low-risk subject, unfractionated heparin and LMWH have similar efficacy.[10] In the patient who is likely to undergo CABG surgery during the hospitalization, unfractionated heparin is preferred over LMWH because its anticoagulant effects can be more readily reversed with protamine.

Two LMWHs are approved for the treatment of the patient with NSTE-ACS, enoxaparin and dalteparin. The dose of enoxaparin is 1 mg/kg subcutaneously twice daily, and the dose of dalteparin is 120 IU/kg (maximum, 10,000 IU) subcutaneously twice daily. Therapy should be continued for the duration of the hospitalization, up to 8 days, or until revascularization is performed (whichever occurs first). In obese (>120 kg), thin (<60 kg), or renally impaired (creatinine clearance < 30 mL/minute) patients, the LMWH dose should be adjusted to achieve an anti–factor Xa concentration of 0.5 to 1.5 IU/mL 4 to 6 hours after drug administration.

LMWH should be avoided in the patient with a history of heparin-induced thrombocytopenia. In the patient with renal failure, treatment with LMWH has been associated with the development of hyperkalemia.

Fondaparinux

Fondaparinux (Chapter 37), which is a selective factor Xa inhibitor, does not require dose adjustment and monitoring. Fondaparinux does not cause thrombocytopenia. Fondaparinux is as effective as enoxaparin in preventing ischemic cardiac events but with 50% fewer major bleeding episodes (from 4.1% to 2.2%).[11] An increased incidence of catheter-related thrombosis has been reported following fondaparinux treatment, so it is not recommended for the patient who is likely to undergo coronary angiography. Thus, fondaparinux is a desirable anticoagulant for the patient with ACS who is managed with a noninvasive approach, especially if he or she is at higher risk of a bleeding complication with anticoagulant therapy, but not for other patients.

For the patient with ACS, fondaparinux is administered as a 2.5-mg subcutaneous injection once daily for up to 5 days or until hospital discharge. Its use is contraindicated in patients with severe renal impairment and in those who weigh 50 kg or less, and it should not be used as the sole anticoagulant during a PCI.

Bivalirudin

Bivalirudin, a direct thrombin inhibitor, is currently recommended as an alternative anticoagulant for patients undergoing PCI. It has not been tested in the patient with ACS who is managed with an ischemia-guided strategy. Hence, the administration of bivalirudin in a setting other than the cardiac catheterization laboratory is not recommended. In the patient undergoing PCI, bivalirudin (0.75 mg/kg intravenous bolus followed by an infusion of 1.75 mg/kg/hr for up to 4 hours after the PCI) is as effective as combination heparin and glycoprotein IIb/IIIa inhibitor therapy in preventing ischemic events, but it causes fewer major bleeding episodes.[12] Bivalirudin is the anticoagulant of choice for the patient with ACS who has heparin-induced thrombocytopenia.

Statins

Prompt initiation of statin therapy is recommended in all patients with NSTE-ACS to promote plaque stabilization and to restore endothelial function. Moreover, when statin therapy is initiated during the patient's hospitalization (rather than at hospital discharge), long-term medical compliance is substantially improved. In the absence of contraindications, high-dose atorvastatin (80 mg daily) should be given orally to the patient with NSTE-ACS, regardless of the baseline serum LDL cholesterol concentration; a lower dose is not as effective in reducing ischemic events.[13]

Recurrent or Refractory Unstable Angina

In most patients hospitalized with NSTE-ACS, symptoms do not recur after the institution of appropriate antianginal therapy. The occasional patient with continued or recurrent chest pain despite optimal medical therapy is at high risk for an MI. For the patient with refractory myocardial ischemia or hemodynamic instability despite optimal medical therapy, intraaortic balloon counterpulsation can reduce the ischemic episodes until revascularization can be performed. Intra-aortic balloon function is synchronized with the patient's ECG so that it inflates during diastole and deflates during systole, thereby augmenting coronary arterial blood flow and reducing myocardial oxygen demand by decreasing afterload. Intra-aortic balloon counterpulsation causes lower limb ischemia in approximately 3% of patients in whom the device is placed, but this complication usually resolves with its removal.

Coronary Revascularization

Coronary revascularization is performed to relieve angina that is persistent or recurrent despite optimal medical therapy, to prevent recurrent ischemia or MI in patients at high risk for a subsequent ischemic event, and to improve survival in patients with suitable anatomy.

Coronary revascularization is successful in relieving symptoms in 90% of the patients with angina refractory to medical therapy. Whether coronary bypass surgery or PCI is the more appropriate method of revascularization is determined by the location and severity of coronary arterial stenoses and the presence of comorbid medical conditions that may affect the performance or safety of the revascularization procedure.

The patient who has been rendered symptom free with optimal medical therapy should undergo an assessment to determine whether he or she is at high risk or relatively low risk of sustaining a cardiac ischemic event (death, MI, or recurrent ischemia) in the ensuing days, weeks, and months and a bleeding complication from intensive medical therapy or an invasive cardiac procedure. Patients who are at low risk of having an ischemic event (those with a normal serum troponin concentration, age less than 75 years, and zero, one, or two TIMI risk variables) should be evaluated noninvasively for inducible ischemia before hospital discharge. If the patient has spontaneous or provocable ischemia, coronary angiography and, if appropriate, revascularization should be performed.

The ACS patient with a detectable serum troponin concentration, age more than 75 years, or three or more TIMI risk variables is considered to be high risk and should be referred for routine coronary angiography and revascularization (if appropriate) during the hospitalization because this management strategy reduces the incidence of subsequent ischemic cardiac events.[3,14] In most subjects, early (within 24 hours of hospitalization) invasive therapy is no better at preventing death, MI, or stroke than somewhat delayed (median, 50 hours) invasive management, although it is associated with a modest decrease in the occurrence of recurrent ischemia.[2] In contrast, in the one third of subjects considered to be very high risk (GRACE risk score of >140, corresponding to an incidence of in-hospital death or MI of >20%), an early invasive management strategy is superior to a delayed strategy in reducing the incidence of death, MI, or stroke.[2]

The patient with clinical features or noninvasive test results suggestive of severe coronary artery disease (i.e., left ventricular dysfunction, hemodynamic instability, life-threatening ventricular arrhythmias, or extensive inducible ischemia) should be referred for coronary angiography to determine whether left main or three-vessel coronary arterial disease is present because patients with these coronary anatomic findings derive a survival benefit with coronary revascularization compared with medical therapy (Chapter 74).

Complications

Patients with NSTE-ACS can develop recurrent ischemic events or any of the complications associated with ST segment elevation MI, including arrhythmias, heart failure, and mechanical complications (Chapter 73). However, the acute complications other than recurrent ischemia occur less often in subjects with NSTE-ACS because the amount of myocardial damage usually is less.

Because intensive medical therapy in conjunction with invasive management can lead to life-threatening bleeding complications, the patient's risk of such should be assessed before these therapies are instituted. Female gender, older age, renal insufficiency, low body weight, tachycardia, systolic arterial pressure, hematocrit, and diabetes mellitus predict an increased risk of major bleeding, often due to excessive dosing of antiplatelet or anticoagulant agents. The bleeding risk can be estimated with the tool available at *www.crusadebleedingscore.org*.

Integrated Approach to Treatment

Although the treatment of the subject with NSTE-ACS should be individualized, taking into account the specific features of the disease and the particular circumstances of the patient, algorithms nonetheless provide a useful framework (Fig. 72-3).

NSTE-ACS is an acute episode related to one active culprit lesion, but the patient often has diffuse atherosclerosis. Smoking cessation (Chapter 31), cholesterol lowering (Chapter 213), control of blood pressure (Chapter 67), and diabetes mellitus (Chapters 236 and 237) are important long-term prevention strategies. Maintaining compliance long-term with medical therapy appears to reduce the risk of a future ischemic event by up to 80%.

PROGNOSIS

Because the number of ECG leads demonstrating ST segment depression and the magnitude of such depression are indicative of the extent and severity of myocardial ischemia and MI, it is not surprising that ST segment depression correlates with the patient's prognosis. Compared with subjects without

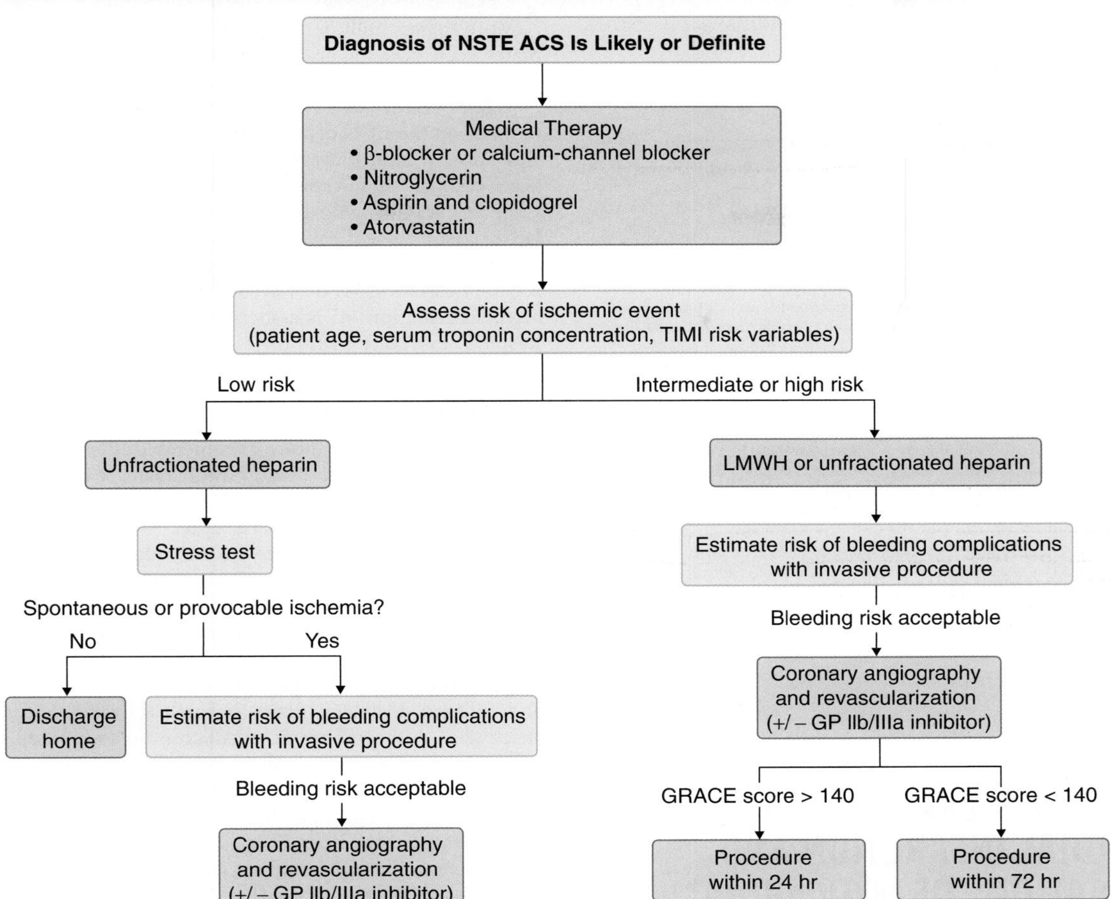

FIGURE 72-3. Approach to the patient with acute coronary syndrome (ACS). Low-risk patients have age < 75 years, no elevation in serum troponin concentration, and two or fewer Thrombolysis in Myocardial Infarction (TIMI) risk variables. Intermediate- or high-risk patients are those with age > 75 years, elevated serum troponin concentration, or three or more TIMI risk variables. The Global Registry of Acute Coronary Events (GRACE) score is available at *www.outcomes-umassmed.org/grace*. GP = glycoprotein; LMWH = low-molecular-weight heparin; NSTE = non–ST segment elevation.

ST segment depression, the patient with NSTE-ACS who has ST segment depression of 1 mm or greater in two or more leads is almost four times as likely to die within 1 year, and the patient with ST segment depression of 2 mm or greater in magnitude is almost six times as likely to die within 1 year. If ST segment depression of 2 mm or greater is present in more than one region of the ECG, the mortality is increased ten-fold. Even the 20% of patients with ACS who have only 0.5 to 1 mm of ST segment depression have an adverse prognosis. Patients with ST segment depression also have a higher risk for subsequent cardiac events compared with patients with only T wave inversion (>1 mm).

The magnitude of the serum troponin concentration predicts short-term (30 days) and long-term (1 year) risks of recurrent MI and death, independent of ECG abnormalities or markers of inflammatory activity. C-reactive protein measured with a highly sensitive assay, which is a widely used marker of inflammation, has no role in the diagnosis of ACS but is predictive of long-term (6 months) mortality among patients with troponin-negative NSTE-ACS. Elevated levels of natriuretic peptides (B-type natriuretic peptide [BNP] or its N-terminal prohormone [NT-proBNP]) are associated with a three- to five-fold increased mortality in patients with NSTE-ACS, although they have limited value for diagnosis, initial risk stratification, and selection of an initial management strategy. Natriuretic peptide concentrations measured a few days after the onset of symptoms have better predictive value than those measured at the time of hospitalization. In patients with NSTE-ACS, a simultaneous assessment of troponin, hsCRP, and BNP is superior to a single biomarker assessment at predicting short-term (in-hospital and 30-day) outcome.

During the past two decades, the prognosis of patients with ACS has improved dramatically with the introduction of more effective medical therapy and revascularization techniques. In contrast to individuals with ST segment elevation MI, in whom most events occur before or shortly after presentation to the hospital, patients with NSTE-ACS continue to have these events during the ensuing days, weeks, and months. Although in-hospital mortality is higher in patients with ST segment elevation MI than among those with NSTE-ACS (7 vs. 5%, respectively), the mortality rates at 6 months are similar for the two conditions (12 vs. 13%, respectively). During long-term follow-up of patients hospitalized with ACS, rates of death are actually higher in those with NSTE-ACS than in those with ST segment elevation MI, with a two-fold difference after 4 years. As a result, treatment strategies for NSTE-ACS should address the issues related to both the acute event and longer-term treatment.

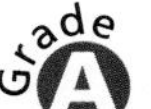

1. Morrow DA, Cannon CP, Rifai N, et al. Ability of minor elevations of troponins I and T to predict benefit from an early invasive strategy in patients with unstable angina and non-ST elevation myocardial infarction: results from a randomized trial. *JAMA*. 2001;286:2405-2412.
2. Mehta SR, Granger CB, Boden WE, et al. Early versus delayed invasive intervention in acute coronary syndromes. *N Engl J Med*. 2009;360:2165-2175.
3. O'Donoghue M, Boden WE, Braunwald E, et al. Early invasive vs conservative treatment strategies in women and men with unstable angina and non-ST-segment elevation myocardial infarction: a meta-analysis. *JAMA*. 2008;300:71-80.
4. Gibson RS, Boden WE, Theroux P, et al. Diltiazem and reinfarction in patients with non-Q-wave myocardial infarction: results of a double-blind, randomized, multicenter trial. *N Engl J Med*. 1986;315:423-429.
5. Collaborative meta-analysis of randomised trials of antiplatelet therapy for prevention of death, myocardial infarction, and stroke in high risk patients. *BMJ*. 2002;324:71-86.
6. Yusuf S, Mehta SR, Zhao F, et al. Early and late effects of clopidogrel in patients with acute coronary syndromes. *Circulation*. 2003;107:966-972.
7. Wiviott SD, Braunwald E, McCabe CH, et al. Prasugrel versus clopidogrel in patients with acute coronary syndromes. *N Engl J Med*. 2007;357:2001-2015.
8. Giugliano RP, White JA, Bode C, et al. Early versus delayed, provisional eptifibatide in acute coronary syndromes. *N Engl J Med*. 2009;360:2176-2190.
9. Eikelboom JW, Anand SS, Malmberg K, et al. Unfractionated heparin and low-molecular-weight heparin in acute coronary syndrome without ST elevation: a meta-analysis. *Lancet*. 2000;355:1936-1942.
10. Antman EM, Cohen M, Bernink PJ, et al. The TIMI risk score for unstable angina/non-ST elevation MI: a method for prognostication and therapeutic decision making. *JAMA*. 2000;284:835-842.

11. Yusuf S, Mehta SR, Chrolavicius S, et al. Comparison of fondaparinux and enoxaparin in acute coronary syndromes. *N Engl J Med.* 2006;354:1464-1476.
12. Stone GW, McLaurin BT, Cox DA, et al. Bivalirudin for patients with acute coronary syndromes. *N Engl J Med.* 2006;355:2203-2216.
13. Cannon CP, Braunwald E, McCabe CH, et al. Intensive versus moderate lipid lowering with statins after acute coronary syndromes. *N Engl J Med.* 2004;350:1495-1504.
14. Cannon CP, Weintraub WS, Demopoulos LA, et al. Comparison of early invasive and conservative strategies in patients with unstable coronary syndromes treated with the glycoprotein IIb/IIIa inhibitor tirofiban. *N Engl J Med.* 2001;344:1879-1887.

SUGGESTED READINGS

Anderson JL, Adams CD, Antman EM, et al. ACC/AHA 2007 guidelines for the management of patients with unstable angina/non ST-elevation myocardial infarction: a report of the American College of Cardiology/American Heart Association Task Force on Practice Guidelines (Writing Committee to Revise the 2002 Guidelines for the Management of Patients With Unstable Angina/Non ST-Elevation Myocardial Infarction): developed in collaboration with the American College of Emergency Physicians, the Society for Cardiovascular Angiography and Interventions, and the Society of Thoracic Surgeons: endorsed by the American Association of Cardiovascular and Pulmonary Rehabilitation and the Society for Academic Emergency Medicine. *Circulation.* 2007;116:e148-304. *Comprehensive guidelines.*

Chew DP, Anderson FA, Avezum A, et al. Six month survival benefits associated with clinical guideline recommendations in acute coronary syndromes. *Heart.* 2010;96:1201-1206. *PCI, CABG, statins, and clopidogrel were the major contributors to better outcomes with guideline-driven care.*

Hillis LD, Lange RA. Optimal management of acute coronary syndromes. *N Engl J Med.* 2009;360:2237-2240. *Review.*

Stone GW, Maehara A, Lansky A, et al. A prospective natural-history study of coronary atherosclerosis. *N Engl J Med.* 2011;364:226-235. *Coronary lesions responsible for ACS are often initially angiographically mild (~30% stenosis) with a thin-cap fibroatheroma, large plaque burden, small luminal area, or some combination of these.*

73 ST SEGMENT ELEVATION ACUTE MYOCARDIAL INFARCTION AND COMPLICATIONS OF MYOCARDIAL INFARCTION

JEFFREY L. ANDERSON

DEFINITION

Conceptually, myocardial infarction (MI) is myocardial necrosis caused by ischemia. Practically, MI can be diagnosed and evaluated by clinical, electrocardiographic, biochemical, radiologic, and pathologic methods. Technologic advances in detecting much smaller amounts of myocardial necrosis than previously possible (e.g., by troponin determinations) have required a redefinition of MI. Given these developments, the term *MI* now should be qualified with regard to size, precipitating circumstance, and timing. This chapter focuses on acute MI associated with ST segment elevation on the electrocardiogram (ECG). This category of acute MI is characterized by profound ("transmural") acute myocardial ischemia affecting relatively large areas of myocardium. The underlying cause essentially always is *complete* interruption of regional myocardial blood flow (resulting from coronary occlusion, usually atherothrombotic) (Chapter 70). This clinical syndrome should be distinguished from non–ST segment elevation MI, in which the blockage of coronary flow is incomplete and for which different acute therapies are appropriate (Chapter 72).

EPIDEMIOLOGY

Cardiovascular disease is responsible for almost one half of all deaths in the United States and other developed countries and for one fourth of deaths in the developing world (Chapter 51). By 2020, cardiovascular disease will cause one of every three deaths worldwide. Cardiovascular disease causes almost 1 million deaths in the United States each year; it accounts for 37% of all deaths and contributes to 58% of deaths. Annually, an estimated 1.2 million U.S. residents suffer a fatal or nonfatal acute MI. Coronary heart disease, the leading cause of cardiovascular death, underlies or is a contributing cause of 650,000 deaths annually. Half of coronary heart disease deaths (250,000/year) are directly related to acute MI, and at least half of these acute MI–related deaths occur within 1 hour of onset of symptoms and before patients reach a hospital emergency department.

More than 5 million people visit emergency departments in the United States each year for evaluation of chest pain and related symptoms, and almost 1.5 million are hospitalized for an acute coronary syndrome (Chapter 50). The presence of ST segment elevation or new left bundle branch block (LBBB) on the ECG distinguishes patients with acute MI who require consideration of immediate recanalization therapy from other patients with an acute coronary syndrome (non–ST segment elevation MI/unstable angina; Chapter 72). Changing demographics, lifestyles, and medical therapies have led to a decrease in the ratio of ST segment elevation MI to non–ST segment elevation acute coronary syndromes over the past 10 to 15 years, so ST segment elevation MI now accounts for about 30% of all MIs. However, ST segment elevation MI is associated with greater in-hospital (but not post-hospital) mortality than non–ST segment elevation MI, and it remains an important contributor to total population mortality.

PATHOBIOLOGY

Erosion, fissuring, or rupture of vulnerable atherosclerotic plaques has been determined to be the initiating mechanism of coronary thrombotic occlusion, thereby precipitating intraplaque hemorrhage, coronary spasm, and occlusive luminal thrombosis (Chapter 70). Plaque rupture most frequently occurs in lipid-laden plaques with an endothelial cap weakened by internal collagenase (metalloproteinase) activity derived primarily from macrophages. These macrophages are recruited to the plaque from blood monocytes responding to inflammatory mediators and adhesion molecules.

With plaque rupture, elements of the blood stream are exposed to the highly thrombogenic plaque core and matrix containing lipid, tissue factor, and collagen. Platelets adhere, become activated, and aggregate; vasoconstrictive and thrombogenic mediators are secreted; vasospasm occurs; thrombin is generated and fibrin formed; and a partially or totally occlusive platelet- and fibrin-rich thrombus is generated. When coronary flow is occluded, electrocardiographic ST segment elevation occurs (ST segment elevation acute MI). Partial occlusion, occlusion in the presence of collateral circulation, and distal coronary embolization result in unstable angina or non–ST segment elevation MI (Chapter 72). Ischemia from impaired myocardial perfusion causes myocardial cell injury or death, ventricular dysfunction, and cardiac arrhythmias.

Although most MIs are caused by atherosclerosis, occasional patients can develop complete coronary occlusions owing to coronary emboli, in situ thrombosis, vasculitis, primary vasospasm, infiltrative or degenerative diseases, diseases of the aorta, congenital anomalies of a coronary artery, or trauma (Table 73-1). In a canine model of coronary occlusion and recanalization, myocardial cell death begins within 15 minutes of occlusion and proceeds rapidly in a wave front from endocardium to epicardium. Partial myocardial salvage can be achieved by releasing the occlusion within 3 to 6 hours; the degree of salvage is inversely proportional to the duration of ischemia and occurs in a reverse wave front from epicardium to endocardium. The extent of myocardial necrosis can also be altered by modification of metabolic demands and collateral blood supply. The temporal dynamic of infarction in human disease, although more complex, is generally similar.

CLINICAL MANIFESTATIONS

Traditionally, the diagnosis of acute MI has rested on the triad of ischemic-type chest discomfort, ECG abnormalities, and elevated serum cardiac markers. Acute MI was considered present when at least two of the three were present. With their increasing sensitivity and specificity, serum cardiac markers (e.g., troponin I [TnI] or troponin T [TnT]) have assumed a dominant role in confirming the diagnosis of acute MI in patients with suggestive clinical or ECG features.

History

Ischemic-type chest discomfort is the most prominent clinical symptom in most patients with acute MI (see Table 50-1 in Chapter 50). The discomfort is characterized by its quality, location, duration, radiation, and precipitating and relieving factors. The discomfort associated with acute MI is qualitatively similar to that of angina pectoris but more severe. It often is perceived as heavy, pressing, crushing, squeezing, bandlike, viselike, strangling, constricting, aching, or burning; it rarely is perceived as sharp pain and generally not as stabbing pain (Chapters 50 and 71).

The primary location of typical ischemic pain is most consistently retrosternal, but it also can present left parasternally, left precordially, or across the anterior chest (Chapter 50). Occasionally, discomfort is

TABLE 73-1 CONDITIONS OTHER THAN CORONARY ATHEROSCLEROSIS THAT CAN CAUSE ACUTE MYOCARDIAL INFARCTION

Coronary emboli	Causes include aortic or mitral valve lesions, left atrial or ventricular thrombi, prosthetic valves, fat emboli, intracardiac neoplasms, infective endocarditis, and paradoxical emboli
Thrombotic coronary artery disease	Can occur with oral contraceptive use, sickle cell anemia and other hemoglobinopathies, polycythemia vera, thrombocytosis, thrombotic thrombocytopenic purpura, disseminated intravascular coagulation, antithrombin III deficiency and other hypercoagulable states, macroglobulinemia and other hyperviscosity states, multiple myeloma, leukemia, malaria, and fibrinolytic system shutdown secondary to impaired plasminogen activation or excessive inhibition
Coronary vasculitis	Seen with Takayasu's disease, Kawasaki disease, polyarteritis nodosa, lupus erythematosus, scleroderma, rheumatoid arthritis, and immune-mediated vascular degeneration in cardiac allografts
Coronary vasospasm	Can be associated with variant angina, nitrate withdrawal, cocaine or amphetamine abuse, and angina with "normal" coronary arteries
Infiltrative and degenerative coronary vascular disease	Can result from amyloidosis, connective tissue disorders (e.g., pseudoxanthoma elasticum), lipid storage disorders and mucopolysaccharidoses, homocystinuria, diabetes mellitus, collagen vascular disease, muscular dystrophies, and Friedreich's ataxia
Coronary ostial occlusion	Associated with aortic dissection, luetic aortitis, aortic stenosis, and ankylosing spondylitis syndromes
Congenital coronary anomalies	Including Bland-White-Garland syndrome of anomalous origin of the left coronary artery from the pulmonary artery, left coronary artery origin from the anterior sinus of Valsalva, coronary arteriovenous fistula or aneurysms, and myocardial bridging with secondary vascular degeneration
Trauma	Associated with and responsible for coronary dissection, laceration, or thrombosis (with endothelial cell secondary to trauma such as angioplasty) and with radiation and cardiac contusion
Augmented myocardial oxygen requirements exceeding oxygen delivery	Encountered with aortic stenosis, aortic insufficiency, hypertension with severe left ventricular hypertrophy, pheochromocytoma, thyrotoxicosis, methemoglobinemia, carbon monoxide poisoning, shock, and hyperviscosity syndromes

predominantly perceived in the anterior neck, jaw, arms, or epigastrium. It generally is somewhat diffuse; highly localized pain (finger point) is rarely angina or acute MI. The most characteristic pattern of radiation is to the left arm, but the right arm or both arms can be involved. The shoulders, neck, jaw, teeth, epigastrium, and interscapular areas also are sites of radiation. Discomfort above the jaws or below the umbilicus is not typical of acute MI. Associated symptoms often include nausea, vomiting, diaphoresis, weakness, dyspnea, restlessness, and apprehension.

The discomfort of acute MI is more severe and lasts longer (typically 20 minutes to several hours) than angina, and it is not reliably relieved by rest or nitroglycerin. The onset of acute MI usually is unrelated to exercise or other apparent precipitating factors. Nevertheless, acute MI begins during physical or emotional stress and within a few hours of arising more frequently than explained by chance.

It is estimated that at least 20% of acute MIs are painless ("silent") or atypical (unrecognized). Elderly patients and patients with diabetes are particularly prone to painless or atypical MI, which occurs in as many as one third to one half of such patients. Because the prognosis is worse in elderly patients and in those patients with diabetes, diagnostic vigilance is required. In these patients, acute MI can present as sudden dyspnea (which can progress to pulmonary edema), weakness, lightheadedness, nausea, and vomiting. Confusional states, sudden loss of consciousness, a new rhythm disorder, and an unexplained fall in blood pressure are other uncommon presentations. The differential diagnosis of ischemic chest discomfort also should include gastrointestinal disorders (e.g., reflux esophagitis; Chapter 140), musculoskeletal pain (e.g., costochondritis), anxiety or panic attacks, pleurisy or pulmonary embolism (Chapter 98), and acute aortic dissection (see Table 50-2 in Chapter 50 and Chapter 78).

Physical Examination

No physical findings are diagnostic or pathognomonic of acute MI. The physical examination can be entirely normal or may reveal only nonspecific abnormalities. An S_4 gallop frequently is found if carefully sought. Blood pressure often is initially elevated, but it may be normal or low. Signs of sympathetic hyperactivity (tachycardia, hypertension, or both) often accompany anterior wall MI, whereas parasympathetic hyperactivity (bradycardia, hypotension, or both) is more common with inferior wall MI.

The examination is best focused on an overall assessment of cardiac function. Adequacy of vital signs and peripheral perfusion should be noted. Signs of cardiac failure, both left and right sided (e.g., S_3 gallop, pulmonary congestion, elevated neck veins) should be sought, and observation for arrhythmias and mechanical complications (e.g., new murmurs) is essential. If hypoperfusion is present, determination of its primary cause (e.g., hypovolemia, right heart failure, left heart failure) is critical to management.

DIAGNOSIS

Electrocardiogram

In patients with a possible acute MI, an ECG must be obtained immediately. Although the initial ECG is neither perfectly specific nor perfectly sensitive in all patients who develop acute ST segment elevation myocardial infarction (STEMI), it plays a critical role in initial stratification, triage, and management (Chapter 50). In an appropriate clinical setting, a pattern of regional ECG ST segment elevation suggests coronary occlusion causing marked myocardial ischemia; hospital admission is indicated with triage to the coronary care unit (CCU). An emergency recanalization strategy (primary angioplasty or fibrinolysis) should be used unless it is contraindicated. Other ECG patterns (ST segment depression, T wave inversion, nonspecific changes, normal ECG) in association with ischemic chest discomfort are consistent with a non–ST segment elevation acute coronary syndrome (non–ST segment elevation MI or unstable angina) and are treated with different triage and initial management strategies (Chapter 72).

Electrocardiographic Evolution

Serial ECG tracings improve the sensitivity and specificity of the ECG for the diagnosis of acute MI and assist in assessing the outcomes of therapy. When typical ST segment elevation persists for hours and is followed within hours to days by T wave inversions and Q waves, the diagnosis of acute MI can be made with virtual certainty. The ECG changes in ST segment elevation acute MI evolve through three overlapping phases: (1) hyperacute or early acute, (2) evolved acute, and (3) chronic (stabilized).

Early Acute Phase

This earliest phase begins within minutes, persists, and evolves over hours. T waves increase in amplitude and widen over the area of injury (hyperacute pattern). ST segments evolve from concave to a straightened to a convex upward pattern (acute pattern). When prominent, the acute injury pattern of blended ST-T waves can take on a tombstone appearance (Figs. 73-1 and 73-2). ST segment depressions that occur in leads opposite those with ST segment elevation are known as *reciprocal changes* and are associated with larger areas of injury and a worse prognosis but also with greater benefits from recanalization therapy.

Other causes of ST segment elevation must be considered and excluded. These conditions include pericarditis (Chapter 77), left ventricular (LV) hypertrophy with J point elevation, and normal variant early repolarization (Chapter 54). Pericarditis (or perimyocarditis) is of particular concern because it can mimic acute MI clinically, but fibrinolytic therapy is *not* indicated and can be hazardous.

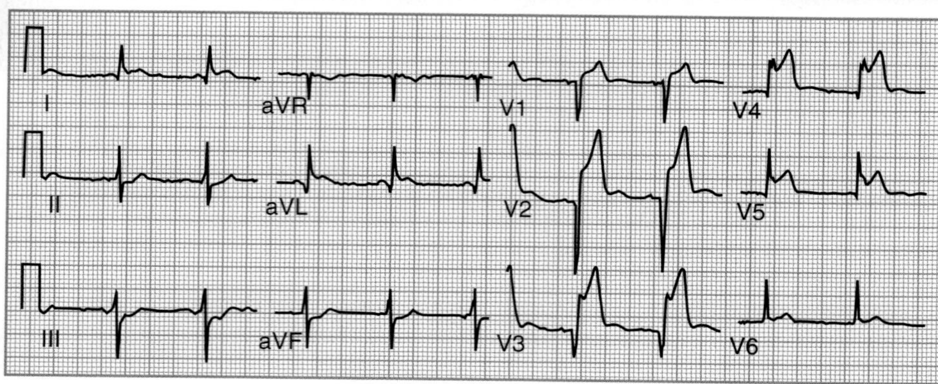

FIGURE 73-1. **Electrocardiographic tracing shows an acute anterolateral myocardial infarction.** Note ST segment elevation in leads I, L, and V_1 to V_6 with Q waves in V_1 to V_4.

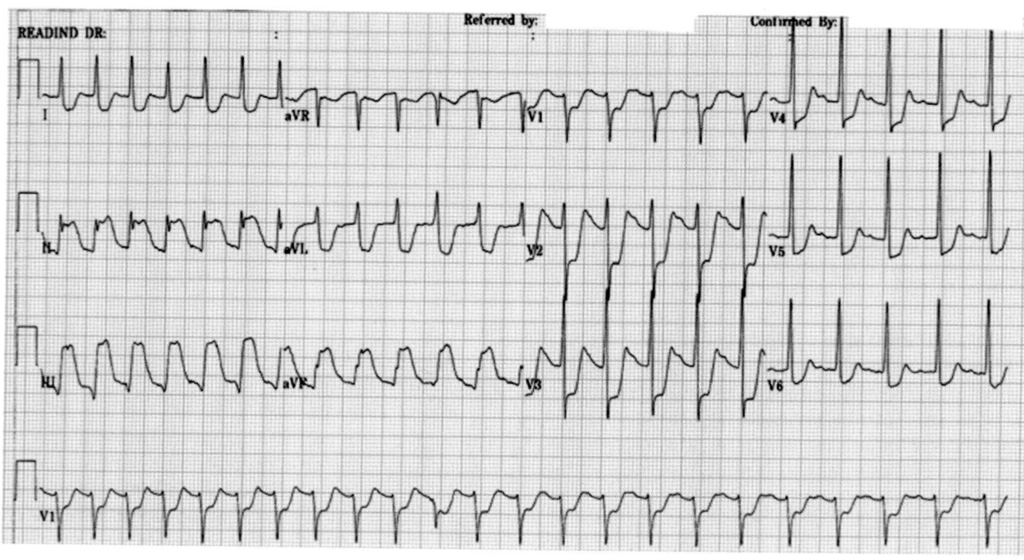

FIGURE 73-2. **Electrocardiographic tracing shows an acute inferoposterior myocardial infarction.**

Evolved Acute Phase

During the second phase, ST segment elevation begins to regress, T waves in leads with ST segment elevation become inverted, and pathologic Q or QS waves become fully developed (>0.03-second duration or depth >30% of R wave amplitude, or both).

Chronic Phase

Resolution of ST segment elevation is quite variable. It is usually complete within 2 weeks of inferior MI, but it can be delayed further after anterior MI. Persistent ST segment elevation, often seen with a large anterior MI, is indicative of a large area of akinesis, dyskinesis, or ventricular aneurysm. Symmetrical T wave inversions can resolve over weeks to months or can persist for an indefinite period; hence, the age of an MI in the presence of T wave inversions is often termed *indeterminate.* Q waves usually do not resolve after anterior MI but often disappear after inferior wall MI.

Early recanalization therapy accelerates the time course of ECG changes so that, on coronary recanalization, the pattern can evolve from acute to chronic over minutes to hours instead of days to weeks. ST segments recede rapidly, T wave inversions and losses of R wave occur earlier, and Q waves may not develop or progress and occasionally may regress. Indeed, failure of ST segment elevation to resolve by more than 50 to 70% within 1 to 2 hours suggests failure of fibrinolysis and should prompt urgent angiography for "rescue angioplasty."

True Posterior Myocardial Infarction and Left Circumflex Myocardial Infarction Patterns

"True posterior" MI presents a mirror-image pattern of ECG injury in leads V_1 to V_2 to V_4 (Fig. 73-2). Anatomically, the location of injury of "true posterior MI" by magnetic resonance imaging actually involves portions of the *lateral* left ventricular wall and is typically caused by occlusion of a nondominant left circumflex artery. The acute phase is characterized by ST segment depression, rather than ST segment elevation. The evolved and chronic phases show increased R wave amplitude and widening instead of Q waves. Recognition of a true posterior acute MI pattern is challenging but important because the diagnosis should lead to an immediate recanalization strategy. Extending the ECG to measure left posterior leads V_7 to V_9 increases sensitivity for detecting acute left circumflex–related injury patterns (i.e., ST segment elevation) with excellent specificity (Chapter 54). Other causes of prominent upright anteroseptal forces include right ventricular (RV) hypertrophy, ventricular preexcitation variants (Wolff-Parkinson-White syndrome; Chapter 64), and normal variants with early R wave progression. New appearance of these changes or the association with an acute or evolving inferior MI usually allows the diagnosis to be made.

Right Ventricular Infarction

Proximal occlusion of the right coronary artery before the acute marginal branch can cause RV as well as acute inferior MI in about 30% of cases. Because the prognosis and treatment of acute inferior MI differ in the presence of RV infarction, it is important to make this diagnosis. The diagnosis is assisted by obtaining right precordial ECG leads, which are routinely indicated for inferior acute MI (Chapter 54). Acute ST segment elevation of at least 1 mm (0.1 mV) in one or more of leads V_{4R} to V_{6R} is both sensitive and specific (>90%) for identifying acute RV injury, and Q or QS waves effectively identify RV infarction.

Diagnosis in the Presence of Bundle Branch Block

The presence of LBBB often obscures ST segment analysis in patients with suspected acute MI. The presence of a new (or presumed new) LBBB in association with clinical (and laboratory) findings suggesting acute MI is associated with high mortality; patients with new-onset LBBB benefit substantially from recanalization therapy and should undergo triage and treatment in the same way as patients with ST segment elevation MI. Certain ECG patterns, although relatively insensitive, suggest acute MI if present in

TABLE 73-2 CONDITIONS THAT CAN MIMIC ST SEGMENT ELEVATION MYOCARDIAL INFARCTION

Early repolarization with non-coronary chest pain
Myocarditis
Pericarditis
Takotsubo cardiomyopathy

the setting of LBBB: Q waves in two of leads I, aVL, V_5, V_6; R wave regression from V_1 to V_4; ST segment elevation of 1 mm or more in leads with a positive QRS complex; ST segment depression of 1 mm or more in leads V_1, V_2, or V_3; and ST segment elevation of 5 mm or more associated with a negative QRS complex. The presence of right bundle branch block (RBBB) usually does not mask typical ST-T wave or Q wave changes, except for rare cases of isolated true posterior acute MI, characterized by tall right precordial R waves and ST segment depressions.

Differential Diagnosis

Although ST-segment elevation MI is often an easy diagnosis to make based on the presentation and test results (see later), other considerations include acute pericarditis (Chapter 77), acute myocarditis (Chapter 60), stress-induced takotsubo syndrome (Chapter 60), and early repolarization (Table 73-2). All but early repolarization can be associated with abnormal biomarkers, but none is associated with a coronary occlusion. Early coronary angiography is advised when any of these conditions is suggested or when MI may be related to a cause other than atherosclerosis (see Table 73-1).

Serum Cardiac Markers

Ideal markers are not normally present in serum, become rapidly and markedly elevated during acute MI, and are not released from other injured tissues (see Table 73-2). The increasing sensitivity and specificity of serum cardiac markers, which are macromolecules (proteins) released from myocytes undergoing necrosis, have made them the "gold standard" for detection of myocardial necrosis. However, because of the 1- to 12-hour delay after the onset of symptoms before markers become detectable or diagnostic, and given laboratory delays even when markers are positive, the decision to proceed with an urgent recanalization strategy (primary angioplasty or fibrinolysis) must be based on the patient's clinical history and initial ECG (Chapter 50).

Troponins I and T

Troponins have replaced other markers because they are more specific in the setting of injuries to skeletal muscle or other organs and also are more sensitive in the setting of minimal myocardial injury. Cardiac-derived TnI (cTnI) and TnT (cTnT), proteins of the sarcomere, are not normally present in the blood with standard sensitivity assays and have amino acid sequences distinct from their skeletal muscle isoforms. With even small acute MIs, troponins increase to 20-fold or more above the lower limits of the assay, and elevations persist for several days.

The troponins generally are first detectable 2 to 4 hours after the onset of acute MI, are maximally sensitive at 8 to 12 hours, peak at 10 to 24 hours, and persist for 5 to 14 days. Their long persistence has allowed them to replace other markers for the diagnosis of acute MI in patients presenting late (>1 to 2 days) after symptoms. However, this persistence can obscure the diagnosis of an early recurrent MI, for which more rapidly cleared markers (i.e., CK-MB) are more useful. Clinically, cTnI and cTnT appear to be of approximately equivalent utility, except renal failure is more likely to be associated with false-positive elevations of cTnT than of cTnI.

Ultrasensitive troponin assays increase assay sensitivity and enable even earlier diagnosis. However, because troponins also may be present in low concentration in a number of nonischemic cardiovascular conditions, specificity for MI remains an issue.

Other Laboratory Tests

On admission, routine assessment of complete blood count and platelet count, standard blood chemistry studies, a lipid panel, and coagulation tests (prothrombin time, partial thromboplastin time) are useful. Results assist in assessing comorbid conditions and prognosis and in guiding therapy. Hematologic tests provide a useful baseline before initiation of antiplatelet, antithrombin, and fibrinolytic therapy or coronary angiography or angioplasty. Myocardial injury precipitates polymorphonuclear leukocytosis, commonly resulting in an elevation of white blood cell count of up to 12,000 to 15,000/μL, which appears within a few hours and peaks at 2 to 4 days. The metabolic panel provides a useful check on electrolytes, glucose, and renal function. On hospital admission or the next morning, a fasting lipid panel is recommended to assist in decision making for inpatient lipid lowering (e.g., statin therapy if low-density lipoprotein is greater than 70 mg/dL (Chapter 213). Unless carbon dioxide retention is suspected, finger oximetry is adequate to titrate oxygen therapy. The C-reactive protein level increases with acute MI, but its incremental prognostic value in the acute setting is unknown. B-type natriuretic peptide, which increases with ventricular wall stress and relative circulatory fluid overload, may provide useful incremental prognostic information in the setting of acute MI.

Imaging

A chest radiograph is the only imaging test *routinely* obtained on admission for acute MI. Although the chest radiograph is often normal, findings of pulmonary venous congestion, cardiomegaly, or widened mediastinum can contribute importantly to diagnosis and management decisions. For example, a history of severe, "tearing" chest and back pain in association with a widened mediastinum should raise the question of a dissecting aortic aneurysm (Chapter 78). In such cases, fibrinolytic therapy must be withheld pending more definitive diagnostic imaging of the aorta. Other noninvasive imaging (e.g., echocardiography [Chapter 55], cardiac nuclear scanning [Chapter 56], and other testing) is performed for evaluation of specific clinical issues, including suspected complications of acute MI. Coronary angiography (Chapter 57) is performed urgently as part of an interventional strategy for acute MI or later for risk stratification in higher-risk patients who are managed medically.

Echocardiography

Two-dimensional transthoracic echocardiography with color-flow Doppler imaging is the most generally useful noninvasive test obtained on admission or early in the hospital course (Chapter 55). Echocardiography efficiently assesses global and regional cardiac function and enables the clinician to evaluate suspected complications of acute MI. The sensitivity and specificity of echocardiography for regional wall motion assessment are high (>90%), although the age of the abnormality (new versus old) must be distinguished clinically or by ECG. Echocardiography is helpful in determining the cause of circulatory failure with hypotension (relative hypovolemia, LV failure, RV failure, or mechanical complication of acute MI). Echocardiography also can assist in differentiating pericarditis and perimyocarditis from acute MI. Doppler echocardiography is indicated to evaluate a new murmur and other suspected mechanical complications of acute MI (papillary muscle dysfunction or rupture, acute ventricular septal defect, LV free wall rupture with tamponade or pseudoaneurysm). Later in the course of acute MI, echocardiography may be used to assess the degree of recovery of stunned myocardium after recanalization therapy, the degree of residual cardiac dysfunction and indications for angiotensin-converting enzyme (ACE) inhibitors and other therapies for heart failure, and the presence of LV aneurysm and mural thrombus (requiring oral anticoagulants).

Radionuclide, Magnetic Resonance, and Other Imaging Studies

Radionuclide techniques generally are too time consuming and cumbersome for routine use in the acute setting. More commonly, they are used in risk stratification before or after hospital discharge to augment exercise or pharmacologic stress testing (Chapter 56). Thallium-201 and, increasingly, technetium-99m sestamibi (alone or together—dual isotope imaging) remain the most frequently used "cold spot" tracers to assess myocardial perfusion and viability, as well as infarct size, although additional tracers are becoming available. Infarct-avid tracers to identify, locate, and size recent myocardial necrosis are available but are rarely required for ST segment elevation MI. Computed tomography (Chapter 56) and magnetic resonance imaging (Chapter 56) can be useful to evaluate patients with a suspected dissecting aortic aneurysm and, together with positron emission tomography, for research purposes and in selected clinical applications such as for assessment of myocardial viability (infarct sizing). When the issue of a nonatherosclerotic cause of myocardial necrosis is raised (e.g., perimyocarditis simulating acute MI), contemporary multislice (e.g., 64-slice) coronary computed tomography (Chapter 56) can assess coronary artery disease qualitatively and semiquantitatively, and it can also distinguish other causes of chest pain syndromes (Chapters 50 and 56).

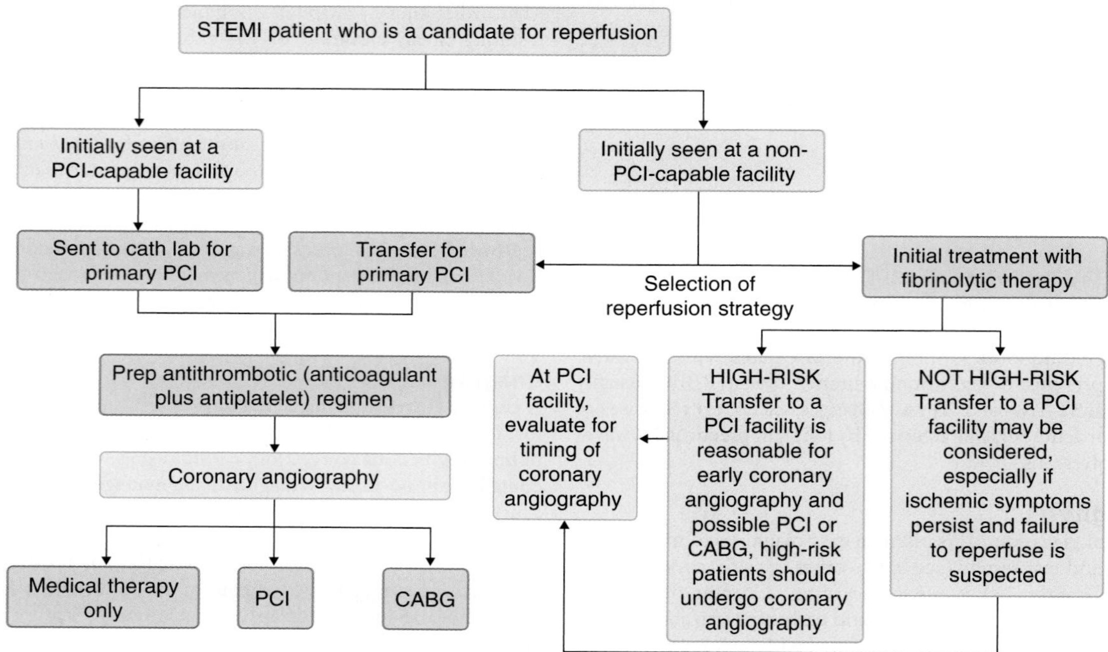

FIGURE 73-3. **Evidence-based approach to percutaneous coronary intervention (PCI) and coronary artery bypass grafting (CABG) after ST segment elevation myocardial infarction (STEMI).** (Adapted from Kushner FG, Hand M, Smith SC Jr, et al. 2009 Focused updates: ACC/AHA guidelines for the management of patients with ST-elevation myocardial infarction and the ACC/AHA/SCAI guidelines on percutaneous coronary intervention. *J Am Coll Cardiol.* 2009;54:2205-2241.)

TREATMENT Rx

Assessment and Management

Prehospital Phase

More than one half of deaths related to acute MI occur within 1 hour of onset of symptoms and before the patient reaches a hospital emergency department. Most of these deaths are caused by ischemia-related ventricular fibrillation (VF) and can be reversed by defibrillation (Chapters 63 and 66). Rapid defibrillation allows resuscitation in 60% of patients when treatment is delivered by a bystander using an on-site automatic external defibrillator or by a first-responding medical rescuer (Chapter 63). Moreover, the first hour represents the best opportunity for myocardial salvage with recanalization therapy. Thus, the three goals of prehospital care are as follows: (1) to recognize symptoms promptly and seek medical attention; (2) to deploy an emergency medical system team capable of cardiac monitoring, defibrillation and resuscitation, and emergency medical therapy (e.g., nitroglycerin, lidocaine, atropine); and (3) to transport the patient expeditiously to a medical care facility staffed with personnel capable of providing expert coronary care, including recanalization therapy (primary angioplasty or fibrinolysis).

The greatest time lag to recanalization therapy is the patient's delay in calling for help. Public education efforts have yielded mixed results, and innovative approaches are needed. The feasibility of initiating fibrinolytic therapy by highly trained ambulance personnel in coordinated ambulance and emergency department systems has been shown. More recently, data indicate that high-dose prehospital tirofiban (25 μg/kg bolus, then 0.15 μg/kg/minute for 18 hours) can improve intermediate outcomes in patients with acute ST elevation MI who undergo percutaneous coronary intervention and is equivalent to abciximab.[1] In coordinated systems and when transportation delays are substantial, initiation of fibrinolytic or other antithrombotic therapy in the field may be considered, thereby shortening the time to recanalization.

Hospital Phases

Emergency Department

The goals of emergency department care are to identify patients with acute myocardial ischemia rapidly, to stratify them into acute ST segment elevation MI as compared with other acute coronary syndromes (see Fig. 72-1 in Chapter 72 and Fig. 73-1), to initiate a recanalization strategy and other appropriate medical care in qualifying patients with acute ST segment elevation MI, and to prioritize by triage rapidly to inpatient care (CCU, step-down unit, observation unit) or outpatient care (patients without suspected ischemia) (see Fig. 72-2 in Chapter 72).

The evaluation of patients with chest pain and other suspected acute coronary syndromes begins with a 12-lead ECG even as the physician is beginning a focused history, including contraindications to fibrinolysis, and a targeted physical examination. Continuous ECG monitoring should be started, an intravenous line should be established, and admission blood tests should be drawn (including cardiac markers such as cTnI or cTnT). As rapidly as possible, the patient should be stratified as having a probable ST segment elevation acute MI, a non–ST segment elevation acute MI, probable or possible unstable angina, or likely noncardiac chest pain.

In patients with ST segment elevation acute MI by clinical and ECG criteria, a recanalization strategy must be selected: alternative choices are primary percutaneous coronary intervention (primary PCI; the patient is transferred directly to the cardiac catheterization laboratory with a goal of door-to-balloon time of less than 90 minutes) or fibrinolysis (begun immediately in the emergency department with a goal of door-to-needle time of less than 30 minutes) (Fig. 73-3).

Aspirin (162 to 325 mg) should be given to all patients unless it is contraindicated (see Fig. 73-3). A loading dose of a thienopyridine (e.g., clopidogrel, 600 mg, or prasugrel, 60 mg) also is recommended for STEMI patients for whom PCI is planned. In addition, it is reasonable to start treatment with a glycoprotein IIb/IIIa (GPIIb-IIIa) receptor antagonist (abciximab, 0.25 mg/kg IV bolus, then 0.125 μg/kg/minute [maximum, 10 μg/minute] for up to 12 hours), tirofiban (25 μg/kg IV bolus, then 0.15 μg/kg/minute for 12 to 18 hours; reduce infusion rate by 50% for estimated creatinine clearance less than 30 mL/minute) or eptifibatide (180 μg/kg IV bolus, second bolus after 10 minutes, then 2.0 μg/kg/minute for up to 18 hours; reduce infusion by 50% for estimated creatinine clearance less than 50 mL/minute) at the time of primary PCI for STEMI in selected patients, such as those with a large burden of thrombus or those who have not received adequate thienopyridine loading. It is uncertain whether there is any incremental usefulness of starting GPIIb-IIIa receptor antagonists "upstream," before arrival in the catheterization laboratory.

Intravenous heparin (initial bolus 60 IU/kg, maximum, 4000 IU, then 12 IU/kg/hour, maximum 1000 IU/hour, for patients >70 kg, adjusted to maintain activated partial thromboplastin time 1.5 to 2 times the control value) or low-molecular-weight heparin (LMWH; e.g., enoxaparin, 30 mg intravenous bolus, then 1 mg/kg subcutaneously twice daily, for patients <75 years old without renal insufficiency) or bivalirudin (for those undergoing a primary PCI strategy—0.75 mg/kg bolus, then 1.75 mg/kg/hour infusion) is appropriate in most patients. In STEMI patients who are undergoing PCI who are at higher risk for bleeding, evidence supports using bivalirudin anticoagulation with a thienopyridine but without a GPIIb-IIIa receptor antagonist.[2]

Patients with chest pain should be given sublingual nitroglycerin (0.4 mg every 5 minutes for up to three doses), after which an assessment should be made of the need for intravenous nitroglycerin. Persistent ischemic pain may be treated with titrated intravenous doses of morphine (i.e., 2 to 4 mg intravenously [IV], repeated every 5 to 15 minutes to relieve pain). Initiation of β-blocker therapy is usually indicated, especially in patients with hypertension, tachycardia, and ongoing pain; however, decompensated heart failure is a contraindication to the acute initiation of β-blocker therapy, particularly by the intravenous route. Oxygen should be used in doses sufficient to avoid hypoxemia (e.g., initially at 2 to 4 L/minute by nasal cannula; fingertip oximetry may be used to monitor effect). The ideal systolic blood pressure is 100 to 140 mm Hg. Excessive hypertension usually responds to titrated nitroglycerin, β-blocker therapy, and morphine (also given for pain). Relative hypotension could require discontinuation of these medications, fluid administration, or other measures as appropriate to the hemodynamic subset (Table 73-3). Atropine (0.5 to 1.5 mg IV) should be available to treat symptomatic bradycardia and hypotension related to excessive vagotonia. Direct transfer to the catheterization laboratory or fibrinolysis followed by transfer to the CCU should occur as expeditiously as possible.

Early Hospital Phase: Coronary Care

Coronary care for early hospital management of acute MI has reduced in-hospital mortality by more than 50%. The goals of CCU care include (1) continuous ECG monitoring and antiarrhythmic therapy for serious arrhythmias (i.e., rapid defibrillation of VF), (2) initiation or continuation of a coronary recanalization strategy to achieve myocardial reperfusion, (3) initiation or continuation of other acute medical therapies, (4) hemodynamic monitoring and appropriate medical interventions for different hemodynamic subsets of patients, and (5) diagnosis and treatment of mechanical and physiologic complications of acute MI. General care and comfort measures also are instituted. A sample of CCU admission orders is given in Table 73-4.

General care measures include attention to activity, diet, and bowels, education, reassurance, and sedation. Bedrest is encouraged for the first 12 hours. In the absence of complications, dangling, bed to chair, and self-care activities can begin within 24 hours. When stabilization has occurred, usually within 1 to 3 days, patients may be transferred to a step-down unit where progressive reambulation occurs. The risk for emesis and aspiration or the anticipation of angiography or other procedures usually dictates nothing by mouth or clear liquids for the first 4 to 12 hours. Thereafter, a heart-healthy diet in small portions is recommended. In patients at high risk for bleeding gastric stress ulcers, a proton pump inhibitor or an H_2-antagonist is recommended for prophylaxis in patients receiving antithrombotic therapy. Many patients benefit from an analgesic (e.g., morphine sulfate, in 2- to 4-mg increments) to relieve ongoing pain and an anxiolytic or sedative during the CCU phase. A benzodiazepine is frequently selected. Sedatives should not be substituted for education and reassurance from concerned caregivers to relieve emotional distress and improve behavior; routine use of anxiolytics is neither necessary nor recommended. Constipation often occurs with bedrest and narcotics; stool softeners and a bedside commode are advised.

The ECG should be monitored continuously in the CCU (and usually in the step-down unit) to detect serious arrhythmias and to guide therapy. Measures to limit infarct size (i.e., coronary recanalization) and to optimize hemodynamics also stabilize the heart electrically. Routine antiarrhythmic prophylaxis (e.g., with lidocaine or amiodarone) is not indicated, but specific arrhythmias require treatment (see later text).

Hemodynamic evaluation is helpful in assessing prognosis and in guiding therapy (see Table 73-3). Clinical and noninvasive evaluation of vital signs is adequate for normotensive patients without pulmonary congestion. Patients with pulmonary venous congestion alone can usually be managed conservatively. Invasive monitoring is appropriate when the cause of circulatory failure is uncertain and when titration of intravenous therapies depends on hemodynamic measurements (e.g., pulmonary capillary wedge pressure and cardiac output). Similarly, an arterial line is not necessary in all patients and may be associated with local bleeding after fibrinolysis or potent antiplatelet and antithrombin therapy. Arterial catheters are appropriate and useful in clinically unstable, hypotensive patients who do not respond to intravenous fluids to replete or expand intravascular volume (see the later discussion of complications).

Later Hospital Phase

Transfer from the CCU to the step-down unit usually occurs within 1 to 3 days, when the cardiac rhythm and hemodynamics are stable. The duration of this late phase of hospital care is usually an additional 2 to 3 days in uncomplicated cases. Activity levels should be increased progressively under continuous ECG monitoring. Medical therapy should progress from parenteral and short-acting agents to oral medications appropriate and convenient for long-term outpatient use.

Risk stratification and functional evaluations are critical to assess prognosis and to guide therapy as the time for discharge approaches. Functional evaluation also can be extended to the early period after hospital discharge. Education must be provided about diet, activity, smoking, and other risk factors (e.g., lipids, hypertension, diabetes).

Specific Therapeutic Measures

Recanalization Therapy

Early reperfusion of ischemic, infarcting myocardium represents the most important conceptual and practical advance for ST segment elevation acute MI and is the primary therapeutic goal. Coronary recanalization is accomplished by using primary PCI with angioplasty and, commonly, stenting or with fibrinolytic (thrombolytic) therapy. With broad application of recanalization therapy, 30-day mortality rates from ST segment elevation acute MI have progressively declined over the past 3 decades (from 20 to 30% to 5 to 10%). Each community should develop and follow a multidisciplinary STEMI system of care that provides consistently optimal STEMI care within the resources available.

Fibrinolytic Therapy

Various fibrinolytic agents (Table 73-5) are useful in patients with ST segment elevation or new or presumed-new LBBB who present for treatment within 12 hours of the onset of symptoms and who have no contraindications to the use of these agents (Table 73-6). Compared with no recanalization therapy, older fibrinolytics such as streptokinase reduced mortality by 18% (from 11.5 to 9.8%) at 5 weeks. Patients with anterior ST segment elevation benefit more (37 lives saved per 1000) than those with inferior ST segment elevation only (8 lives saved per 1000), and younger patients benefit more than elderly (>75 years) patients. No benefit or a slight adverse effect is seen in patients presenting with normal ECGs or ST depression alone. Benefit is time dependent; it declines from about 40 lives or more saved per 1000 within the first hour, to 20 to 30 lives saved per 1000 for hours 2 to 12, to a nonsignificant 7 lives saved per 1000 for hours 13 to 24. An accelerated regimen of tissue plasminogen activator (t-PA plus intravenous heparin) further reduces mortality at 30 days (by 14%, from 7.3 to 6.3%), compared with streptokinase because the patency rate of the infarct-related artery at 90 minutes is higher with t-PA (81%) than with streptokinase (53 to 60%). Longer-acting variants of t-PA, given by single-bolus (tenecteplase) or double-bolus (reteplase) injections are now in widespread clinical use because they are more convenient to give, but they have not improved survival further.

The major risk of fibrinolytic therapy is bleeding. Intracerebral hemorrhage is the most serious and frequently fatal complication; its incidence rate is 0.5 to 1% with currently approved regimens. Older age (>70 to 75 years), female gender, hypertension, and higher relative doses of t-PA and heparin increase

TABLE 73-3 HEMODYNAMIC SUBSETS OF ACUTE MYOCARDIAL INFARCTION

	BLOOD PRESSURE (RELATIVE)	TYPICAL PHYSICAL FINDINGS	CARDIAC INDEX (L/min/m²)	PA WEDGE PRESSURE (mm Hg)	SUGGESTED INTERVENTIONS
Normal	Normal	±S_4	>2.5	≤12	None required
Hyperdynamic	Normal or high	Anxious	>3	<12	Control pain, anxiety; β-blocker; treat SBP to <140 mm Hg
Hypovolemia	Low	Dry	≤2.7	≤9	Add fluids to maintain normal pressure; can develop pulmonary edema if hypotension caused by unrecognized LV failure
Mild LV failure	Low to high	Rales, ±S_3	2-2.5	>15	Diuresis; nitrates, ACE inhibitor; consider low-dose β-blocker
Severe LV failure	Low to normal	Above +S_3, ± ↑ JVP, ± edema	<2	>20	Diuresis; nitrates; low-dose ACE inhibitor; avoid β-blockers; consider inotropes, urgent revascularization
Cardiogenic shock	Very low	Above + cool, clammy; ↓ mental or renal function	≤1.5	>25	Avoid hypotensive agents; place intra-aortic balloon pump; urgent revascularization if possible
RV infarct	Very low	↑ JVP with clear lungs	<2.5	≤12	Give IV fluids; avoid nitrates and hypotensive agents; dobutamine if refractory to fluids

↑ = increased; ↓ = decreased; ACE = angiotensin-converting enzyme; IV = intravenous; JVP = jugular venous pressure; LV = left ventricle; PA = pulmonary artery; RV = right ventricle; SBP = systolic blood pressure.

Adapted from Forrester JS, Diamond G, Chatterjee K, et al. Medical therapy of acute myocardial infarction by application of hemodynamic subsets (second of two parts). *N Engl J Med*. 1976;295:1404-1413.

TABLE 73-4 SAMPLE ADMISSION ORDERS FOR ST SEGMENT ELEVATION ACUTE MYOCARDIAL INFARCTION

Diagnosis:	Acute ST segment elevation myocardial infarction
Admit:	Coronary care unit with telemetry
Condition:	Serious
Vital signs:	q½h until stable, then q1-4h and PRN; pulse oximetry × 24 hr; notify if heart rate <50 or >100; respiratory rate <8 or >20; SBP <90 or >150 mm Hg; O_2 saturation <90%
Activity:	Bedrest × 12 hr with bedside commode; thereafter, light activity if stable
Diet:	NPO except for sips of water until pain free and stable; then 2 g sodium, heart-healthy diet as tolerated, unless on call for catheterization (or other test requiring NPO)
Laboratory tests:*	Troponin I or T and CK/CK-MB q8h × 3; comprehensive blood chemistry, magnesium, CBC with platelets; PT/INR, aPTT; BNP; lipid profile (fasting in morning); portable CXR
IV therapy:	D_5W or NS to keep vein open (increase fluids for relative hypovolemia); second IV if IV medication given
Recanalization therapy:*	Emergency primary coronary angioplasty, or fibrinolysis (if appropriate) 1. Primary angioplasty (preferred if available within 90 min) 2. Tenecteplase, alteplase, reteplase, or streptokinase (see Table 73-5 for doses)
Medications:	1. Nasal O_2 at 2 L/min × 6 hr, then by order (titrate to keep O_2 saturation >90%) 2. Aspirin 162-325 mg chewed on admission, then 81-162 mg PO daily 3. IV heparin, 60 U/kg bolus (maximum, 4000 U) and 12 U/kg/hr (maximum, 1000 U/hr), titrate to target aPTT 1.5-2.0 × control (about 50-70 sec), OR enoxaparin (preferred with fibrinolytic), 30 mg IV, then 1 mg/kg SC q12h (maximum SC doses, 100 mg on day 1; reduce to 0.75 mg/kg for age ≥75, increase interval to q24h for CrCl <30 mL/min), OR bivalirudin (with primary PCI), 0.75 mg/kg IV bolus, then 1.75 mg/kg/hr (delay 30 min if heparin given) 4. Metoprolol, 12.5 PO q6h, incremented to 25-50 mg q6h as tolerated (hold for SBP < 100 mm Hg, pulse < 50 beats/min, asthma, heart failure); may consider IV metoprolol if immediate effect required (tachyarrhythmia, severe hypertension, unrelieved pain) in the absence of heart failure 5. Consider IV nitroglycerin drip × 24-48 hr (titrated to SBP 100-140 mm Hg) 6. Morphine sulfate, 2-4 mg IV and increment at 5-15 min PRN for unrelieved pain 7. Stool softener 8. Anxiolytic or hypnotic if needed 9. ACE inhibitor for hypertension, anterior acute MI, or LV dysfunction, in low oral dose (e.g., captopril, 6.25 mg q8h), begun within 24 hours or when stable (SBP > 100 mm Hg) and adjusted upward 10. Lipid-lowering therapy (i.e., statin) regardless of LDL: target LDL at least <100 mg/dL (<70 mg/dL reasonable); clopidogrel, 300-600 mg PO, then 75 mg PO daily, or prasugrel 60 mg PO, then 10 mg PO daily (with PCI strategy), begun immediately after PCI (if CABG not planned) 11. Specific treatments for hemodynamic subgroups (see Table 73-3)

*If not ordered in the emergency department.
ACE = angiotensin-converting enzyme; aPTT = activated partial thromboplastin time; BNP = brain natriuretic peptide; CABG = coronary artery bypass graft surgery; CBC = complete blood count; CK = creatine kinase; CrCI = creatinine clearance; CXR = chest radiograph; D_5W = 5% dextrose in water; GP = glycoprotein; INR = International Normalized Ratio; IV = intravenous; LDL = low-density lipoprotein; LV = left ventricle; MI = myocardial infarction; NPO = nothing by mouth; NS = normal saline; PCI = percutaneous coronary intervention; PO = orally; PRN = as needed; PT = prothrombin time; daily = once daily; SBP = systolic blood pressure; SC = subcutaneous.
Adapted from Kushner FG, Hand M, Smith SC Jr, et al. 2009 Focused updates: ACC/AHA guidelines for the management of patients with ST-elevation myocardial infarction and the ACC/AHA/SCAI guidelines on percutaneous coronary intervention. *Circulation.* 2009;120:2271-306.

TABLE 73-5 CHARACTERISTICS OF INTRAVENOUS FIBRINOLYTIC AGENTS APPROVED BY THE FOOD AND DRUG ADMINISTRATION

	STREPTOKINASE (SK)	ALTEPLASE (T-PA)	RETEPLASE (R-PA)	TENECTEPLASE (TNK-T-PA)
Dose	1.5 MU in 30-60 min	100 mg in 90 min*	10 U + 10 U, 30 min apart	30-50 mg† over 5 sec
Circulating half-life (min)	≅20	≅4	≅18	≅20
Antigenic	Yes	No	No	No
Allergic reactions	Yes	No	No	No
Systemic fibrinogen depletion	Severe	Mild to moderate	Moderate	Minimal
Intracerebral hemorrhage	≅0.4%	≅0.7%	≅0.8%	≅0.7%
Patency (TIMI-2/3) rate, 90 min‡	≅51%	≅73-84%	≅83%	≅77-88%
Lives saved per 100 treated	≅3§	≅4¶	≅4	≅4
Cost per dose (approximate U.S. dollars)	300	1800	2200	2200

*Accelerated t-PA given as follows: 15-mg bolus, then 0.75 mg/kg over 30 min (maximum, 50 mg), then 0.50 mg/kg over 60 min (maximum, 35 mg).
†TNK-t-PA is dosed by weight (supplied in 5-mg/mL vials): <60 kg = 6 mL; 61-70 kg = 7 mL; 71-80 kg = 8 mL; 81-90 kg = 9 mL; >90 kg = 10 mL.
‡TIMI = Thrombolysis in Myocardial Infarction. Data from Granger CB, Califf RM, Topol EJ. Thrombolytic therapy for acute myocardial infarction: a review. *Drugs.* 1992;44:293-325; and Bode C, Smalling RW, Berg G, et al. Randomized comparison of coronary thrombolysis achieved with double-bolus reteplase (recombinant plasminogen activator) and front-loaded, accelerated alteplase (recombinant tissue plasminogen activator) in patients with acute myocardial infarction: the RAPID[II] Investigators. *Circulation.* 1996;94:891-898.
§Patients with ST segment elevation or bundle branch block, treated <6 hr.
¶Based on the finding from the GUSTO trial that t-PA saves one more additional life per 100 treated than does SK. Data from The GUSTO Investigators. An international randomized trial comparing four thrombolytic strategies for acute myocardial infarction. *N Engl J Med.* 1993;329:673-682; and Simes RJ, Topol EJ, Holmes DR Jr, et al. Link between the angiographic substudy and mortality outcomes in a large randomized trial of myocardial reperfusion: importance of early and complete infarct artery reperfusion. GUSTO-I Investigators. *Circulation.* 1995;91:1923-1928.

TABLE 73-6 INDICATIONS AND CONTRAINDICATIONS TO FIBRINOLYTIC THERAPY

INDICATIONS

Ischemic-type chest discomfort or equivalent for 30 min-12 hr with new or presumed new ST segment elevation in two contiguous leads of ≥2 mm (≥0.2 mV) in leads V_1, V_2, or V_3 or ≥1 mm in other leads
New or presumed-new left bundle branch block with symptoms consistent with myocardial infarction
Absence of contraindications

CONTRAINDICATIONS, ABSOLUTE

Active bleeding or bleeding diathesis (menses excluded)
Prior hemorrhagic stroke, ischemic stroke within 3 months, except acute ischemic stroke within 3-4.5 hours
Intracranial or spinal cord neoplasm or arteriovenous malformation
Suspected or known aortic dissection
Closed head or facial trauma within 3 months

CONTRAINDICATIONS, RELATIVE

Severe, uncontrolled hypertension by history or on presentation (>180/110 mm Hg)
Anticoagulation with therapeutic or elevated international normalized ratio (>2-3)
Old ischemic stroke (>3 mo ago); intracerebral disease other than above
Recent (<3 wk) major trauma/surgery or prolonged (>10 min) cardiopulmonary resuscitation or internal bleeding
Active peptic ulcer
Recent noncompressible vascular punctures
Pregnancy
For streptokinase/anistreplase: prior exposure (especially if >5 days ago) or allergic reaction

Adapted from Kushner FG, Hand M, Smith SC Jr, et al. 2009 Focused updates: ACC/AHA guidelines for the management of patients with ST-elevation myocardial infarction and the ACC/AHA/SCAI guidelines on percutaneous coronary intervention. *Circulation.* 2009;120:2271-2306.

TABLE 73-7 INDICATIONS FOR PRIMARY ANGIOPLASTY AND COMPARISON WITH FIBRINOLYTIC THERAPY

INDICATIONS

Alternative recanalization strategy for ST segment elevation or LBBB acute MI within 12 hr of symptom onset (or >12 hr if symptoms persist)
Cardiogenic shock developing within 36 hr of ST segment elevation/Q wave acute MI or LBBB acute MI in patients <75 yr old who can be revascularized within 18 hr of shock onset
Recommended only at centers performing >200 PCI/yr with backup cardiac surgery and for operators performing >75 PCI/yr

ADVANTAGES OF PRIMARY PCI

Higher initial recanalization rates
Reduced risk of intracerebral hemorrhage
Less residual stenosis; less recurrent ischemia or infarction
Usefulness when fibrinolysis contraindicated
Improvement in outcomes with cardiogenic shock

DISADVANTAGES OF PRIMARY PCI (COMPARED WITH FIBRINOLYTIC THERAPY)

Access, advantages restricted to high-volume centers, operators
Longer average time to treatment
Greater dependence on operators for results
Higher system complexity, costs

LBBB = left bundle branch block; MI = myocardial infarction; PCI = percutaneous coronary intervention (includes balloon angioplasty, stenting).

the risk for intracranial hemorrhage. The risk-to-benefit ratio should be assessed in each patient when fibrinolysis is considered and specific regimens are selected.

For failed fibrinolysis, rescue PCI is more effective than repeat fibrinolysis.[3] After fibrinolysis, regardless of its apparent success, the best strategy is to transfer all STEMI patients with high-risk features rapidly to a hospital with PCI facilities to undergo angiography, rather than to transfer only selected patients in whom fibrinolysis failed or recurrent ischemia developed.[4,5] This early transfer and angiography strategy at a median of 3 hours after fibrinolysis reduces the risk for recurrent ischemia, reinfarction, heart failure, cardiogenic shock or death by 36%.

Primary Percutaneous Coronary Intervention

Prompt PCI is the preferred recanalization strategy (Table 73-7).[6,7] PCI achieves mechanical recanalization by inflation of a catheter-based balloon centered within the thrombotic occlusion. Percutaneous transluminal coronary angioplasty (PTCA) is generally augmented by placing a stent at the site of occlusion as a scaffold to enlarge the lumen and to retain optimal postangioplasty expansion. Preference is often given to drug-eluting stents (e.g., sirolimus, paclitaxel), which markedly reduce the rates of restenosis but can increase the risk of late thrombosis (Chapter 74). Factors favoring a bare metal stent include inability to maintain at least 1 year of dual antiplatelet therapy because of an increased risk for bleeding, need for concomitant anticoagulation, risk for poor adherence or anticipated need for surgery requiring interruption of thienopyridine.

The relative benefits of primary PTCA or PCI over fibrinolysis are confirmed by a meta-analysis that found a significantly lower mortality rate (4.4 versus 6.5%; odds ratio, 0.66) and lower rates of nonfatal reinfarction (2.9 versus 5.3%; odds ratio, 0.53) and intracerebral hemorrhage with primary PTCA compared with fibrinolysis. PCI yields better outcomes than fibrinolysis across all age groups when it is performed within 1 to 2 hours of presentation to a health care facility.

Currently, a primary PCI strategy begins with initiation of a thienopyridine in the emergency department, together with aspirin and an anticoagulant (e.g., heparin or bivalirudin), followed by rapid application of coronary angioplasty with stenting. Augmented antiplatelet therapy with a GPIIb-IIIa inhibitor may be added in selected patients, generally at the time of catheterization. The addition of a reduced dose of a plasminogen activator to GPIIb-IIIa therapy in the field or emergency department may further improve outcomes only in selected patients who undergo early PCI, but this approach is generally not recommended.[8] Facilitated PCI, whereby patients at hospitals without PCI capabilities are given adjusted doses of fibrinolytic or GPIIb-IIIa inhibitors, or both, and then are transferred to other hospitals for emergent (i.e., within 1 to 2 hours) PCI, overall appears to be no better than rapid transfer for primary PCI within 1 to 2 hours.[8,9]

Operator and institutional experience is an issue more important to outcomes with primary PCI than fibrinolysis and has been incorporated into current recommendations (see Table 73-7). Primary PCI is feasible in community hospitals without surgical capability, but concerns about timing and safety remain. Current guidelines allow that primary PCI "might be considered" in hospitals without on-site cardiac surgery, provided (1) there is a proven plan for rapid and safe transport to a nearby hospital with cardiac surgery capability and availability, and (2) the PCI is done by a skilled operator (≥75 PCIs/year) in a hospital with adequate experience (≥36 primary PCIs/year).

Mechanical reperfusion, primarily with stenting and a GPIIb-IIIa receptor antagonist, for patients presenting more than 12 hours but less than 48 hours after the onset of symptoms, also can reduce infarct size and perhaps adverse events.[10] Extending PCI to ST segment elevation MI beyond 12 hours deserves further testing in larger studies.

An additional important indication is cardiogenic shock occurring within 36 hours of the onset of acute MI and treated within 18 hours of the onset of shock (Chapter 107). However, benefit was not established for patients older than 75 years, and benefit was greater with earlier PCI.

Increasing positive experience with PCI of the left main coronary artery with stents, especially drug-eluting stents, suggests that it may be an alternative to coronary artery bypass grafting (CABG) in patients with an amenable anatomy, a low risk of PCI procedural complications, and an increased risk of adverse surgical outcomes.

Mechanical thrombus aspiration at the time of angiography may improve outcomes of patients with STEMI undergoing primary PCI.[11] To reduce the risk for contrast-induced nephropathy, an isosmolar or a low-molecular-weight contrast medium together with preprocedure hydration is recommended in patients undergoing angiography.

Selecting a Recanalization Regimen

Whether to use PCI or fibrinolytic therapy depends on local resources and experience as well as on patient factors. Outcomes appear to be determined both by timing and by institutional and operator experience. In general, in experienced facilities (≥200 PCIs/center; surgical capability; ≥75 PCIs/operator annually; frequent primary PCI, e.g., ≥36/year/center; ≥4/operator/year) that are able to mobilize and treat patients quickly (<90 minutes to balloon inflation), primary PCI is considered the preferred strategy, with stenting preferred over balloon PTCA. PCI is particularly preferred for patients at higher risk for mortality (including shock), for later presentations (>3 hours), and for patients with greater risk of intracerebral hemorrhage (age >70 years, female gender, therapy with hypertensive agents). Ancillary antithrombotic therapy with primary PCI includes aspirin, unfractionated heparin or LMWH or bivalirudin, and a GPIIb-IIIa inhibitor (preferably initiated on admission before catheterization). Clopidogrel is begun directly after PCI and is continued after discharge.

For other situations, fibrinolytic therapy becomes the recommended recanalization strategy. If time since the onset of symptoms is within 3 hours and the difference between expected time to PCI and fibrinolytic administration is more than 1 hour, fibrinolysis is often the preferred strategy. Fibrinolysis also is preferred in centers without sufficient PCI experience or capability. In hospitals with long ambulance transport times (>60 to 90 minutes), a strategy for initiating prehospital fibrinolysis may be considered. Very early or prehospital fibrinolysis followed by a routine emergent (i.e., within 1 to 2 hours) invasive strategy on hospital arrival, that is, "pharmacoinvasive therapy," although an appealing concept, appears to cause a *higher* rate of in-hospital mortality, cardiac ischemic events, and strokes compared with primary PCI alone or by a more delayed invasive approach after fibrinolysis in stabilized patients,4,5,12 and its use cannot be recommended as a primary recanalization strategy. Whether fibrinolysis before PCI will be beneficial in selected subgroups with MI, such as patients seen within the first hour of symptoms and with an expected delay to PCI of 2 hours or more, deserves further testing. Currently, however, efforts should be made to provide primary PCI to a larger percentage of patients with acute MI.

The selection of a specific fibrinolytic regimen is based on the risk of complications of the acute MI, the risk of intracerebral hemorrhage, and a consideration of economic constraints. Using these factors, longer-acting variants of t-PA (i.e., tenecteplase and reteplase) have become dominant in the United States and other affluent medical markets; in other countries, less costly streptokinase is still widely used. A nonimmunogenic fibrinolytic agent is preferred for patients with a history of prior streptokinase use. Streptokinase is associated with a lower risk for intracerebral hemorrhage than other regimens if excessive heparin is avoided. Tenecteplase combined with enoxaparin was more effective than tenecteplase with standard heparin or with a GPIIb-IIIa inhibitor (abciximab) and heparin in one but not another trial. Reteplase with abciximab showed no mortality advantage when combined (in half-dose) with abciximab than with heparin alone; ischemic events decreased, but intracerebral hemorrhage increased, especially in elderly patients. Over the past decade, the application of recanalization therapy has remained relatively constant in the United States and other Western countries at 70 to 75% of "eligible" patients with acute MI. Primary PCI use has increased substantially over time, although fibrinolytic therapy continues to be more commonly applied, particularly in developing countries.

Ancillary and Other Therapies

Antiplatelet Therapy

Aspirin

Platelets form a critical component of coronary thrombi. Aspirin inhibits platelet aggregation by irreversibly blocking cyclooxygenase 1 activity by selective acetylation of serine at position 530. Cyclooxygenase 1 catalyzes the conversion of arachidonic acid to thromboxane-A_2, a potent platelet aggregator (Chapter 36).

Aspirin has been extensively tested to prevent coronary heart disease (Chapter 37). Aspirin trials in ST segment elevation acute MI have been more limited but positive. The most important trial of aspirin in ST segment elevation acute MI randomized more than 17,000 patients with "suspected acute MI" (representing mostly, but not entirely, ST segment elevation acute MI) to aspirin or control and to intravenous streptokinase or control. At 5 weeks, the relative risk for vascular death was reduced 21% by aspirin alone, 25% by streptokinase alone, and 40% by aspirin in combination with streptokinase. Since that time, aspirin has been included as standard therapy in most treatment regimens for ST segment elevation acute MI.

Current guidelines strongly recommend aspirin (class I indication) on admission in a dose of 162 to 325 mg, preferably chewed. Aspirin administration is continued throughout hospitalization and then indefinitely in a maintenance dose of 75 to 162 mg/day on an outpatient basis (enteric-coated forms are popular).

Adenosine Diphosphate Receptor Antagonists

The thienopyridine clopidogrel exerts potent antiplatelet effects by blocking the platelet membrane adenosine diphosphate receptor (Chapter 37). For patients allergic to aspirin, clopidogrel has become the alternative of choice for short- and long-term therapy of ST segment elevation acute MI. A single loading dose is given, usually 300 mg with fibrinolytic therapy but 600 mg with PCI. The maintenance dose is 75 mg/day.

In patients who can take aspirin, the addition of clopidogrel (300 mg followed by 75 mg/day) to aspirin and fibrinolytic therapy in patients 75 years or younger reduces predischarge occlusion rates of infarct-related arteries (by 41%) and reduces ischemic complications at 30 days (by 20%) without increasing rates of intracerebral hemorrhage.13 When given without a loading dose but also without an upper age restriction, clopidogrel reduces 15-day ischemic complications by 9% and death from any cause by 7%.14 Hence, clopidogrel appears to represent a beneficial initial adjunctive therapy in patients with STEMI who are treated with fibrinolytic agents. However, clopidogrel increases the risk for bleeding with CABG, so it is commonly initiated only after coronary angiography has been performed and early surgery has been excluded as a therapeutic choice; if CABG is planned, clopidogrel should be withheld for 5 to 7 days unless the urgency of surgery outweighs the risk of excessive bleeding.

Prasugrel, a new and more potent thienopyridine, may reduce ischemic events at the cost of a small increase in bleeding compared with clopidogrel after PCI in patients with acute STEMI.15 Prasugrel is contraindicated in patients with a prior history of stroke or transient ischemia attack and should be used with caution (or in reduced doses) in older (≥75 years) and smaller (<60 kg) patients.

Clopidogrel added to aspirin on admission for patients with non–ST segment elevation acute MI or unstable angina (Chapter 72) or after a PCI reduces vascular events (by 22%) at 3 to 12 months compared with aspirin alone. Extrapolation of these findings led to the recommendations that clopidogrel be used for 3 to 12 months as an alternative antiplatelet agent in patients with ST segment elevation acute MI when aspirin is contraindicated and that it be considered routinely (in addition to aspirin) in patients after primary PCI.

Glycoprotein IIB/IIIA Inhibitors

Inhibitors of the platelet membrane GPIIb-IIIa receptor, a fibrinogen receptor, have been shown to benefit high-risk patients with non–ST segment elevation acute coronary syndrome (Chapters 37 and 72) on admission or after PCI. The benefit in STEMI is smaller when routine stenting is used and when GPIIb-IIIa therapy is administered only in the catheterization laboratory. Earlier ("upstream") glycoprotein inhibition before hospital admission or in the emergency department (precatheterization) is effective in improving coronary patency by the time of emergency angiography, but incremental benefit on clinical outcomes has not been established. If early CABG is a possibility after angiography, a shorter-acting inhibitor (eptifibatide, tirofiban) may impart a lower perioperative risk for bleeding than abciximab.

Antithrombin Therapy

Low-Molecular-Weight Heparins

Compared with unfractionated heparins, LMWHs have enhanced inhibitory activity for factor Xa (Chapter 37). They also have more reliable bioavailability and longer durations of action, thus permitting subcutaneous administration once or twice daily in fixed (weight-adjusted) doses. Evidence suggests that in patients with ST segment elevation acute MI who are treated with fibrinolytic therapy, LMWH can improve angiographic outcomes and can reduce reinfarction rates by 25% and mortality by about 10% compared with unfractionated heparin.16 Enoxaparin may thus be preferred over unfractionated heparin as an antithrombotic agent for ST segment elevation acute MI in most patients treated with a fibrinolysis strategy. When used as ancillary therapy with a fibrinolytic agent, enoxaparin may be given to patients younger than 75 years who do not have renal insufficiency as a 30-mg intravenous bolus, followed by 1 mg/kg subcutaneously twice daily until hospital discharge, and to those 75 years and older as 0.75 mg/kg subcutaneously twice daily without a bolus.

Unfractionated Heparin

Unfractionated heparin can be used in patients undergoing primary PCI and in those receiving fibrin-specific lytic agents (i.e., alteplase, reteplase, or tenecteplase; see Fig. 73-3 and Table 73-4). It also can be used with intravenous streptokinase or anistreplase for patients at high risk for systemic emboli (e.g., large or anterior acute MI with LV thrombus, atrial fibrillation [AF]). Excessive bleeding when heparin is used in combination with antithrombotic regimens has led to reductions in heparin doses, with improved safety. When given with a fibrinolytic agent, intravenous heparin is begun concurrently and is given for 48 hours. Currently recommended doses include a 60 U/kg bolus (maximum, 4000 U), followed initially by a 12 U/kg/hour infusion (maximum, 1000 U/hour), with adjustment after 3 hours based on activated partial thromboplastin time (target of 50 to 70 seconds, 1.5 to 2 times control). Experimental regimens including a GPIIb-IIIa inhibitor and a fibrinolytic agent have used even lower heparin doses. During primary PCI, high-dose heparin is used (activated clotting time, 300 to 350 seconds). Given together with a GPIIb-IIIa inhibitor during PCI, the dose of heparin is adjusted to a lower activated clotting time range (150 to 300 seconds).

Factor Xa Inhibitors

Selective factor Xa inhibitors (e.g., fondaparinux, 2.5 mg subcutaneously once daily for up to 8 days during index hospitalization) reduce the end point of death or reinfarction at 30 days by 18 to 23% independent of heparin use in patients who receive fibrinolysis or no recanalization therapy but have no benefit in patients who have undergone PCI.18 These results suggest that fondaparinux may be a preferred alternative to unfractionated heparin or no heparin (e.g., in patients who present later, in patients treated with streptokinase) in patients with STEMI who are not undergoing a primary PCI strategy.

Direct Antithrombins

Bivalirudin, a synthetic hirudin analogue with direct antithrombin activity (Chapter 37), compares favorably with heparin and a glycoprotein IIb/IIIa inhibitor for ST segment elevation acute MI managed by primary PCI, with better survival rates at 1 year.18 However, an increased risk of ischemic events and stent thrombosis occurs in bivalirudin patients who do not receive upstream therapy with a 600-mg loading dose of clopidogrel. As a result, bivalirudin, together with early administration of clopidogrel, has become a

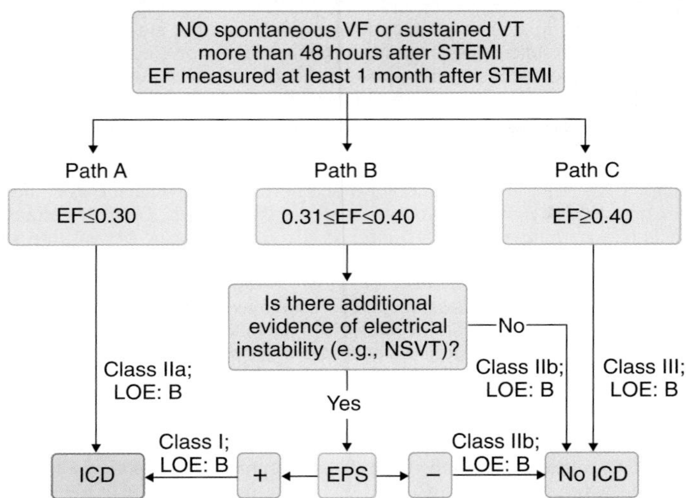

FIGURE 73-4. Algorithm to aid in selection of implantable cardioverter-defibrillator (ICD) in patients with ST segment elevation myocardial infarction (STEMI) and diminished ejection fraction (EF). The appropriate management path is selected based on left ventricular EF measured at least 1 month after STEMI. All patients, whether an ICD is implanted or not, should receive medical therapy. EPS = electrophysiologic studies; LOE = level of evidence; NSVT = nonsustained ventricular tachycardia; VF = ventricular fibrillation; VT = ventricular tachycardia. (Adapted from Antman EM, Anbe DT, Armstrong PW, et al. 2004 Update: ACC/AHA guidelines for the management of patients with ST-elevation myocardial infarction—executive summary. A Report of the American College of Cardiology/American Heart Association Task Force on Practice Guidelines. *Circulation*. 2004;110:588-536.)

widely used antithrombotic regimen in primary PCI for ST segment elevation acute MI.

Other Pharmacologic Therapies

Nitrates

Nitroglycerin and other organic nitrates (isosorbide dinitrate and isosorbide mononitrate) induce vascular smooth muscle relaxation by generating vascular endothelial nitric oxide. The resulting vasodilation of veins and peripheral and coronary arteries can beneficially reduce excessive cardiac preload and afterload, increase coronary caliber in responsive areas of stenosis, reverse distal small coronary arterial vasoconstriction, improve coronary collateral flow to ischemic myocardium, and inhibit platelet aggregation in acute MI (Chapter 71). The results are improved oxygen delivery and reduced oxygen consumption. Potential clinical benefits include relief of ischemia, limitation of infarct size, prevention of dilative remodeling, control of hypertension (afterload), and relief of congestion (preload).

In the era before reperfusion, nitrates appeared to confer a mortality benefit in acute MI. In the context of fibrinolytic therapy and aspirin, however, mortality benefits are modest, with a relative survival benefit of about 4 lives saved per 1000 patients treated. Nitroglycerin is definitely recommended for the first 24 to 48 hours for patients with acute MI and pulmonary congestion, large anterior MI, persistent ischemia, or hypertension. For other patients without contraindications, nitrates are possibly useful.

When nitrates are clearly indicated early in acute MI, intravenous nitroglycerin is preferred. Intravenous nitroglycerin may begin with a bolus injection of 12.5 to 25 μg followed by an infusion of 10 to 20 μg/minute. The infusion rate is increased by 5 to 10 μg every 5 to 10 minutes up to about 200 μg/minute during hemodynamic monitoring until clinical symptoms are controlled or blood pressure targets are reached (blood pressure decreased by 10% in normotensive patients or by 30% in hypertensive patients but not less than 80 mm Hg mean or 90 mm Hg systolic).

β-Blockers

β-Adrenoceptor blockers reduce heart rate, blood pressure, and myocardial contractility, and they stabilize the heart electrically. These actions provide clinical benefit to most patients with acute MI by limiting myocardial oxygen consumption, relieving ischemia, reducing infarct size, and preventing serious arrhythmias.

In the era before fibrinolysis, a meta-analysis of 28 randomized trials involving 27,500 patients found a modest early benefit on mortality (14% odds reduction), cardiac arrest (16% reduction), and nonfatal reinfarction (19% reduction). In patients with acute MI who are receiving fibrinolytic therapy, immediate (intravenous then oral) metoprolol reduces recurrent ischemic events and reinfarction compared with deferred oral therapy. Further experience has shown that moderate to severe heart failure should preclude the early use of intravenous β-blockers, but not predischarge and outpatient oral therapy initiated in small doses and carefully adjusted once stability is achieved.

Early (first-day) initiation of oral β-blockade is generally recommended for patients with acute MI who have ongoing or recurrent ischemic pain or tachyarrhythmias if they do not have heart failure or other contraindications (asthma, hypotension, severe bradycardia), regardless of concomitant fibrinolysis or PCI. Intravenous initiation (e.g., metoprolol, 5 mg over 2 minutes to a total of 15 mg over 10 to 15 minutes, or atenolol, 2.5 to 5 mg over 2 minutes to a total of 10 mg over 10 to 15 minutes) is reasonable in the absence of contraindications if an indication for immediate therapy is present, such as a tachyarrhythmia or hypertension. However, the routine, short-term initiation of intravenous β-blockade should be avoided because it is not associated with benefit and, indeed, causes a small excess of early death from cardiogenic shock, primarily in patients with preexisting heart failure.[14] All patients without contraindications or intolerance to β-blocker therapy should receive oral doses, titrated to tolerance or goal (e.g., metoprolol, 25 to 100 mg twice daily; atenolol, 50 to 100 mg/day; or carvedilol, 6.25 to 25 mg twice daily). β-Blocker therapy should begin promptly, in the absence of heart failure and if not otherwise contraindicated, and should be continued during the in-hospital convalescent phase of STEMI and beyond.

Renin-Angiotensin-Aldosterone System Inhibitors

The renin-angiotensin-aldosterone system is activated in acute MI and heart failure. Use of an ACE inhibitor has been shown to improve remodeling after acute MI (especially after large anterior MI). ACE inhibitors also have demonstrated efficacy in heart failure, wherein they prevent disease progression, hospitalization, and death (Chapter 59). A meta-analysis of three major trials and 11 smaller ones involving more than 100,000 patients showed an overall mortality reduction of 6.5%, representing about 5 lives saved per 1000 patients treated. Benefit is concentrated and greater in higher-risk patients with large or anterior MI and with LV dysfunction or heart failure, although patients with lesser degrees of LV dysfunction and only moderate cardiovascular risk can also benefit in the long term.

Oral *ACE inhibitor therapy* should begin within the first 24 hours in patients with anterior infarction, pulmonary congestion, or low ejection fraction (<0.40) in the absence of hypotension (systolic pressure <100 mm Hg or >30 mm Hg less than usual baseline) or known contraindications. An *angiotensin receptor blocker* (ARB) should be given to otherwise qualifying patients who are intolerant of ACE inhibitors. An ACE inhibitor or an ARB also should be considered for other patients with STEMI, especially those with a relative indication (e.g., hypertension, diabetes, or mild renal insufficiency), with the expectation of a smaller but worthwhile benefit. All patients without contraindications or intolerance to initial ACE inhibitor or ARB therapy also should receive these drugs during the in-hospital convalescent phase. ACE inhibitor therapy should begin with low oral doses and should be progressively adjusted to full dose as tolerated. For example, the short-acting agent captopril may be started in a dose of 6.25 mg or less and adjusted over 1 to 2 days to 50 mg twice daily. Before discharge, a transition may be made in graded dose schedules to longer-acting agents such as ramipril (2.5 mg titrated to 10 mg/day), lisinopril (2.5 to 5 mg titrated to 10 mg/day), or enalapril (2.5 mg, titrated to up to 20 mg twice daily). In patients who cannot tolerate ACE inhibitors (e.g., because of cough), graded doses of an ARB may be substituted (e.g., valsartan, 80 to 160 mg twice daily, or losartan, 50 to 100 mg/day).

Selective *aldosterone receptor blockade* with eplerenone (25 to 50 mg/day) reduces total and cardiovascular mortality (including sudden death) as well as cardiovascular hospitalizations in post-MI patients who have an ejection fraction of 0.40 or less and heart failure or diabetes and who are already receiving other optimal therapies, including ACE inhibitors.[19] Spironolactone also benefits patients with advanced heart failure, including those in whom it is caused by a remote MI. Hence, aldosterone receptor blockade should be added to other standard therapies during convalescence in patients with these characteristics. Hyperkalemia, which is the most common side effect, requires monitoring (Chapter 59).

Antiarrhythmic Agents

Antiarrhythmic therapy is reserved for treatment of, or short-term prevention after, symptomatic or life-threatening ventricular arrhythmias, together with other appropriate measures (cardioversion, treatment of ischemia and metabolic disturbances). An implantable cardioverter-defibrillator (ICD) is indicated in patients with VF or hemodynamically significant sustained ventricular tachycardia (VT) occurring more than 2 days after STEMI or in patients with inducible VT or VF at electrophysiologic study and a depressed ejection fraction (≤0.40) at least 1 month after STEMI (Chapter 65). An ICD also may be considered for patients with severe LV dysfunction (ejection fraction ≤0.30) at least 1 month after STEMI and 3 months after CABG without spontaneous or induced VT or VF.[20] These differences reflect an apparent time dependence, in which the benefit of an ICD appears to be delayed until the early post-MI and post-revascularization periods (Chapter 66). By comparison, early ICD implantation is not beneficial in a broader group of patients because its usefulness in preventing similar deaths is offset by the high rate of nonsudden deaths.[21]

Inotropes

Digitalis and intravenous inotropes can increase oxygen demand, provoke serious arrhythmias, and extend infarction. Current recommendations support the use of digoxin in selected patients recovering from acute MI who develop supraventricular tachyarrhythmias (e.g., AF) or heart failure refractory to ACE inhibitors and diuretics. Intravenous inotropes (e.g., dobutamine, dopamine, milrinone, and norepinephrine) are reserved for temporary support of patients with hypotension and circulatory failure that is unresponsive to volume replacement (Chapters 59 and 107). Other treatment measures for these patients (e.g., intra-aortic balloon pump, early revascularization) are discussed herein.

Lipid-Lowering Therapy

Lipid lowering, particularly with hydroxymethylglutaryl–coenzyme A reductase inhibitors (statins), reduces event rates in patients with coronary disease, and a more aggressive approach appears to provide superior benefits (Chapter 213).[22] A fasting lipid profile should be obtained on admission, so a statin can be started promptly in the hospital with a low-density lipoprotein cholesterol goal of less than 70 mg/dL.

Other Medical Therapies

Calcium channel blockers, although anti-ischemic, also are negatively inotropic and have not been shown to reduce mortality after ST segment elevation acute MI. With certain agents and in specific groups of patients, harm has been suggested. For example, short-acting nifedipine has been reported to cause reflex sympathetic activation, tachycardia, hypotension, and increased mortality. Verapamil or diltiazem (heart rate–slowing drugs) may be given to patients in whom β-blockers are ineffective or contraindicated for control of rapid ventricular response with AF or relief of ongoing ischemia *in the absence of heart failure, LV dysfunction, or atrioventricular (AV) block.*

Magnesium is of no benefit in patients with acute MI who are treated with fibrinolysis. Supplementation is recommended if the magnesium level is lower than normal or in patients with torsades de pointes–type VT associated with a prolonged QT interval.

Glucose-insulin-potassium affords no benefit on mortality, cardiac arrest, or cardiogenic shock when this combination is added to usual care in patients with acute STEMI. However, *glucose control,* using an insulin-based regimen to achieve and maintain glucose levels less than 180 mg/dL while avoiding hypoglycemia, is recommended in the acute phase of STEMI. After the acute phase, individualized treatment is indicated using agents or combinations of agents that best achieve glycemic control and are well tolerated (Chapters 236 and 237).

Management of Complications

Recurrent Chest Pain

When chest pain recurs after acute MI, the diagnostic possibilities include post-infarction ischemia, pericarditis, infarct extension, and infarct expansion. Characterization of the pain, physical examination, ECG, echocardiography, and cardiac marker determinations assist in the differential diagnosis. CK-MB often discriminates reinfarction better than cTnI or cTnT.

Post-infarction angina developing spontaneously during hospitalization for acute MI despite medical therapy usually merits coronary angiography. β-blockers (IV, then orally) and nitroglycerin (IV, then orally or topically) are recommended medical therapies. Pain with recurrent ST segment elevation or recurrent elevation of cardiac markers may be treated with (re)administration of t-PA or, possibly, a GPIIb-IIIa inhibitor, together with nitroglycerin, β-blockade, and heparin. Streptokinase, which induces neutralizing antibodies, generally should not be readministered after the first few days. If facilities for angiography, PCI, and surgery are available, an invasive approach is recommended to relieve discomfort occurring hours to days after an acute MI that is associated with objective signs of ischemia. Radionuclide perfusion stress testing can be helpful in patients with discomfort that is transient or of uncertain ischemic origin. For lesions with questionable degrees of stenosis at angiography, coronary pressure (fractional flow reserve) or Doppler velocimetry can determine whether PCI is warranted.

Infarct expansion implies circumferential slippage with thinning of the infarcted myocardium. Infarct expansion can be associated with chest pain but without recurrent elevation of cardiac markers. Expansive remodeling can lead to an LV aneurysm. The risk for remodeling is reduced with early recanalization therapy and administration of ACE inhibitors.

Acute pericarditis most commonly manifests on days 2 to 4 in association with large, "transmural" infarctions causing pericardial inflammation. Occasionally, hemorrhagic effusion with tamponade develops; thus, excessive anticoagulation should be avoided. Pericarditis developing later (2 to 10 weeks) after acute MI could represent Dressler's syndrome, which is believed to be immune mediated. The incidence of this post-MI syndrome has decreased dramatically in the modern reperfusion era. Pericardial pain is treated with aspirin (preferred, especially in the acute setting) or other nonsteroidal agents (e.g., indomethacin); patients with severe symptoms could require corticosteroids.

Rhythm Disturbances

Ventricular Arrhythmias

Acute MI is associated with a proarrhythmic environment that includes heterogeneous myocardial ischemia, heightened adrenergic tone, intracellular electrolyte disturbance, lipolysis and free fatty acid production, and oxygen free radical production on recanalization. Arrhythmias thus are common early during acute MI. Micro-re-entry is likely the most common electrophysiologic mechanism of early-phase arrhythmias, although enhanced automaticity and triggered activity also are observed in experimental models.

Primary VF, the most serious MI-related arrhythmia, contributes importantly to mortality within the first 24 hours. It occurs with an incidence of 3 to 5% during the first 4 hours and then declines rapidly over 24 to 48 hours. Polymorphic VT and, less commonly, monomorphic VT are associated life-threatening arrhythmias that can occur in this setting. Clinical features (including warning arrhythmias) are not adequately specific or sensitive to identify patients at risk for sustained ventricular tachyarrhythmias, so all patients should be continuously monitored. Prophylactic lidocaine, which reduces primary VF but does not decrease (and may increase) mortality, is not recommended. Primary VF is associated with a higher rate of in-hospital mortality, but long-term prognosis is unaffected in survivors.

Accelerated idioventricular rhythm (60 to 100 beats per minute) frequently occurs within the first 12 hours and is generally benign (i.e., is not a risk factor for VF). Indeed, accelerated idioventricular rhythm frequently heralds recanalization after fibrinolytic therapy. Antiarrhythmic therapy is not indicated except for sustained, hemodynamically compromising accelerated idioventricular rhythm.

Late VF, which is defined as VF developing more than 48 hours after the onset of acute MI, often occurs in patients with larger MIs or heart failure, portends a worse prognosis for survival, and is an indication for aggressive measures (e.g., consideration of an ICD). Monomorphic VT resulting from re-entry in the context of a recent or old MI also can appear late after MI, and patients may require long-term therapy (e.g., an ICD).

Electrical cardioversion is required for VF and sustained polymorphic VT (unsynchronized shock) and for sustained monomorphic VT that causes hemodynamic compromise (synchronized shock) (Chapters 65 and 66). Brief intravenous sedation is given to conscious, "stable" patients. For slower, stable VT and nonsustained VT requiring therapy, intravenous amiodarone or intravenous lidocaine is commonly recommended. After episodes of VT or VF, infusions of antiarrhythmic drugs may be given for 6 to 24 hours; the ongoing risk for arrhythmia then is reassessed. Electrolyte and acid-base imbalance and hypoxia should be corrected. β-Blockade is useful in patients with frequent polymorphic VT associated with adrenergic activation ("electrical storm"). Additional, aggressive measures should be considered to reduce cardiac ischemia (e.g., emergency PCI or CABG) and LV dysfunction (intra-aortic balloon pump) in patients with recurrent polymorphic VT despite the use of β-blockers or amiodarone, or both.

Patients with sustained VT or VF occurring late in the hospital course should be considered for long-term prevention and therapy. An ICD provides greater survival benefit than antiarrhythmic drugs in patients with ventricular arrhythmias and can improve survival after acute MI for patients with an ejection fraction of 30% or less, regardless of their rhythm status.[20]

Atrial Fibrillation and Other Supraventricular Tachyarrhythmias

AF occurs in up to 10 to 15% of patients after an acute MI, usually within the first 24 hours (Chapter 64). The incidence of atrial flutter or another supraventricular tachycardia is much lower. The risk for AF increases with age, larger MIs, heart failure, pericarditis, atrial infarction, hypokalemia, hypomagnesemia, hypoxia, pulmonary disease, and hyperadrenergic states. The incidence of AF is reduced by effective early recanalization. Hemodynamic compromise with rapid rates and systemic embolism (in ~2%) are adverse consequences of AF. Systemic embolism can occur on the first day, so prompt anticoagulation with heparin is indicated.

Recommendations for management of AF include the following: electrical cardioversion for patients with severe hemodynamic compromise or ischemia; rate control with intravenous digoxin for patients with ventricular dysfunction (i.e., give 1.0 mg, one half initially and one half in 4 hours), with an intravenous β-blocker (e.g., metoprolol, 5 mg over 2 minutes to a total of 15 mg over 10 to 15 minutes) in those without clinical ventricular dysfunction, or with intravenous diltiazem or verapamil in hemodynamically compensated patients with a contraindication to β-blockers; and anticoagulation with heparin (or LMWH). Amiodarone, which is generally reserved for patients with or at high risk for recurrence, may be continued for 6 weeks if sinus rhythm is restored and maintained.

Bradycardias, Conduction Delays, and Heart Block

Sinus and AV nodal dysfunction is common during acute MI. Sinus bradycardia, a result of increased parasympathetic tone often in association with inferior acute MI, occurs in 30 to 40% of patients. Sinus bradycardia is particularly common during the first hour of acute MI and with recanalization of the right coronary artery (Bezold-Jarisch reflex). Vagally mediated AV block also can occur in this setting. Anticholinergic therapy (atropine, 0.5 to 1.5 mg IV) is indicated for *symptomatic* sinus bradycardia (heart rate generally <50 beats per minute associated with hypotension, ischemia, or escape ventricular arrhythmia), including ventricular asystole, and *symptomatic* second-degree (Wenckebach) or third-degree block at the AV nodal level (narrow QRS complex escape rhythm). Atropine is not indicated and can worsen infranodal AV block (anterior MI, wide complex escape rhythm).

New-onset infranodal AV block and intraventricular conduction delays or bundle branch blocks (BBBs) predict substantially increased in-hospital mortality. Fortunately, their incidence has declined in the recanalization era (from 10 to 20% to ~4%). Mortality is related more to extensive myocardial damage than to heart block itself, so cardiac pacing only modestly improves survival. Prophylactic placement of multifunctional patch electrodes, which allow for immediate transcutaneous pacing (and defibrillation) if needed, is indicated for symptomatic sinus bradycardia refractory to drug therapy, infranodal second-degree (Mobitz II) or third-degree AV block, and new or indeterminate-age bifascicular (LBBB; RBBB with left anterior or left posterior fascicular block) or trifascicular block (bilateral or alternating BBB [any age], BBB with first-degree AV block). Transcutaneous pacing is uncomfortable and is intended for prophylactic and temporary use only. In patients who require a pacemaker to maintain a rhythm or who are at very high risk (>30%) of requiring pacing (including patients with alternating, bilateral BBB, with new or indeterminate-age bifascicular block with first-degree AV block, and with infranodal second-degree AV block) should have a transvenous pacing electrode inserted as soon as possible.

Indications for permanent pacing after acute MI depend on the prognosis of the AV block and not solely on symptoms. Class I indications include even transient second- or third-degree AV block in association with BBB and symptomatic AV block at any level. Advanced block at the AV nodal level (Wenckebach) rarely is persistent or symptomatic enough to warrant permanent pacing.

Heart Failure and Other Low-Output States

Cardiac pump failure is the leading cause of circulatory failure and in-hospital death from acute MI. Manifestations of circulatory failure can include a weak pulse, low blood pressure, cool extremities, a third heart sound, pulmonary congestion, oliguria, and obtundation. However, several distinct mechanisms, hemodynamic patterns, and clinical syndromes characterize the spectrum of circulatory failure in acute MI. Each requires a specific approach to diagnosis, monitoring, and therapy (see Table 73-3).

Left Ventricular Dysfunction

The degree of LV dysfunction correlates well with the extent of acute ischemia or infarction. Hemodynamic compromise becomes evident when impairment involves 20 to 25% of the left ventricle, and cardiogenic shock or death occurs with involvement of 40% or more (Chapter 107). Pulmonary congestion and S_3 and S_4 gallops are the most common physical findings. Early recanalization (with fibrinolytic agents, PCI, or CABG) is the most effective therapy to reduce infarct size, ventricular dysfunction, and associated heart failure. Medical treatment of heart failure related to the ventricular dysfunction of acute MI is otherwise generally similar to that of heart failure in other settings (Chapter 59) and includes adequate oxygenation and diuresis (begun early, blood pressure permitting, and continued on a long-term basis if needed). Morphine sulfate (i.e., 2 to 4 mg IV, with increments as needed after 5 to 15 minutes or more) is useful for patients with pulmonary congestion. Nitroglycerin also reduces preload and effectively relieves congestive symptoms. Titrated oral ACE inhibitor therapy (e.g., captopril, incremented from 3.125 to 6.25 mg three times daily to 50 mg twice daily as tolerated) also is indicated for heart failure and pulmonary edema unless excessive hypotension (systolic blood pressure <100 mm Hg) is present. Treatment can be begun sublingually (0.4 mg every 5 minutes three times), and then the transition can be made to intravenous therapy (initially 5 to 10 μg/minute, incrementing by 5 to 20 μg/minute until symptoms are relieved or until mean arterial pressure falls by 10% in normotensive or 30% in hypertensive patients but not <90 mm Hg or >30 mm Hg lower than baseline). Intravenous vasodilator therapy to reduce preload and afterload, inotropic support, and intra-aortic balloon counterpulsation (IABP), together with urgent recanalization, are indicated in cardiogenic shock (Chapter 107).

Volume Depletion

Relative or absolute hypovolemia is a frequent cause of hypotension and circulatory failure and is easily corrected if it is recognized and treated promptly. Poor hydration, vomiting, diuresis, and disease- or drug-induced peripheral vasodilation can contribute to this condition. Hypovolemia should be identified and corrected with intravenous fluids before more aggressive therapies are considered. An empirical fluid challenge may be tried in the appropriate clinical setting (e.g., for hypotension in the absence of congestion, for inferior or RV infarction, and for hypervagotonia). If filling pressures are measured, cautious fluid administration to a pulmonary capillary wedge pressure of up to about 18 mm Hg may optimize cardiac output and blood pressure without impairing oxygenation.

Right Ventricular Infarction

RV ischemia and infarction occur with proximal occlusion of the right coronary artery (before the take-off of the RV branches). Ten to 15% of inferior acute STEMIs show classic hemodynamic features, and these patients form the highest-risk subgroup for morbidity and mortality (25 to 30% versus <6% hospital mortality). Improvement in RV function commonly occurs over time, a finding suggesting reversal of ischemic stunning and other favorable accommodations, if short-term management is successful.

Hypotension in patients with clear lung fields and elevated jugular venous pressure in the setting of inferior or inferoposterior acute MI should raise the suspicion of RV infarction. Kussmaul's sign (distention of the jugular vein on inspiration) is relatively specific and sensitive in this setting. Right-sided ECG leads show ST segment elevation, particularly in V_{4R} (Chapter 54), in the first 24 hours of RV infarction. Echocardiography is helpful in confirming the diagnosis (RV dilation and dysfunction are observed). When right-sided heart pressures are measured, a right atrial pressure of 10 mm Hg or greater and 80% or more of the pulmonary capillary wedge pressure are relatively sensitive and specific for RV ischemic dysfunction.

Management of RV infarction consists of early maintenance of RV preload with intravenous fluids, reduction of RV afterload (i.e., afterload-only reducing drugs as for LV dysfunction; consider intra-aortic balloon pump), early recanalization, short-term inotropic support if needed, and avoidance of venodilators (e.g., nitrates) and diuretics used for LV failure (they may cause marked hypotension). Volume loading with normal saline solution alone is often effective. If the cardiac output fails to improve after 0.5 to 1 L fluid, inotropic support with intravenous dobutamine (starting at 2 μg/kg/minute and titrating to hemodynamic effect or tolerance, up to 20 μg/kg/minute) is recommended. High-grade AV block is common, and restoration of AV synchrony with temporary AV sequential pacing can lead to substantial improvement in cardiac output. The onset of AF (in up to one third of RV infarcts) can cause severe hemodynamic compromise requiring prompt cardioversion. Early coronary recanalization with fibrinolysis or PCI markedly improves outcomes.

Cardiogenic Shock

Cardiogenic shock (Chapter 107) is a form of severe LV failure characterized by marked hypotension (systolic pressures <80 mm Hg) and reductions in cardiac index (to <1.8 L/minute/m^2) despite high LV filling pressure (pulmonary capillary wedge pressure >18 mm Hg). The cause is loss of a critical functional mass (>40%) of the left ventricle. Cardiogenic shock is associated with mortality rates of more than 70 to 80% despite aggressive medical therapy. Risk factors include age, large (usually anterior) acute MI, previous MI, and diabetes. In patients with suspected shock, hemodynamic monitoring and IABP are indicated. Intubation often is necessary. Vasopressors are often needed. Early urgent mechanical revascularization (PCI or CABG), if feasible, affords the best chance for survival, especially in patients younger than 75 years (Chapter 107).

IABP remains useful for patients with medically refractory unstable ischemic syndromes and for cardiogenic shock. The deflated balloon catheter is introduced into the femoral artery and is advanced into the aorta. The ECG triggers balloon inflation during early diastole, thereby augmenting coronary blood flow; deflation then occurs in early systole, thereby reducing LV afterload. Primary IABP therapy for cardiogenic shock associated with acute MI provides temporary stabilization but does not reduce mortality (>80%). IABP is currently recommended in the setting of acute MI as a stabilizing measure for patients undergoing angiography and subsequent PCI or surgery for (1) cardiogenic shock, (2) mechanical complications (acute mitral regurgitation, acute ventricular septal defect), (3) refractory post-MI ischemia, or (4) recurrent intractable VT or VF associated with hemodynamic instability. IABP is not useful in patients with significant aortic insufficiency or severe peripheral vascular disease.

Mechanical Complications

Mechanical complications usually occur within the first weeks and account for approximately 15% of MI-related deaths. Such complications include acute mitral valve regurgitation, ventricular septal defect, free wall rupture, and LV aneurysm. Suspicion and investigation of a mechanical defect should be prompted by a new murmur or sudden, progressive hemodynamic deterioration with pulmonary edema or a low output state. Transthoracic or transesophageal Doppler echocardiography usually establishes the diagnosis. A balloon flotation catheter can be helpful in confirming the diagnosis. Arteriography to identify correctable coronary artery disease is warranted in most cases. Surgical consultation should be requested promptly, and urgent repair is usually indicated.

Acute mitral valve regurgitation (Chapter 75) results from infarct-related rupture or dysfunction of a papillary muscle. Total rupture leads to death in 75% of patients within 24 hours. Medical therapy is initiated with nitroprusside (beginning with 0.1 μg/kg/minute and titrating upward every 3 to 5 minutes to the desired effect, as tolerated by blood pressure response, up to 5 μg/kg/minute), to lower preload and to improve peripheral perfusion, and inotropic support (e.g., dobutamine, titrated from 2 up to 20 μg/kg/minute in normotensive patients; dopamine, titrated from 2 up to 20 μg/kg/minute in hypotensive patients; or combined dobutamine and dopamine). An IABP is used to maintain hemodynamic stability. Emergency surgical repair (if possible) or replacement is then undertaken. Surgery is associated with high mortality (≥25 to 50%), but it leads to better functional and survival outcomes than medical therapy alone.

Post-infarction septal rupture with *ventricular septal defect,* which occurs with increased frequency in elderly patients, in patients with hypertension, and possibly after fibrinolysis, also warrants urgent surgical repair. Because a small post-MI ventricular septal defect can suddenly enlarge and cause rapid hemodynamic collapse, all septal perforations should be repaired. On diagnosis, invasive monitoring is recommended, together with vasodilators (e.g., nitroprusside, initially 0.1 μg/kg/minute, titrated upward every 3 to 5 minutes to desired effect, as tolerated by blood pressure response, up to 5 μg/kg/minute) and, if needed, judicious use of inotropic agents (e.g., dobutamine, titrated from 2 up to 20 μg/kg/minute in normotensive patients; dopamine, titrated from 2 up to 20 μg/kg/minute in hypotensive patients; or combined dobutamine and dopamine). An IABP should be inserted, a surgical consultation promptly obtained, and surgical repair undertaken as soon as feasible.

LV free wall rupture usually causes acute cardiac tamponade with sudden death. In a small percentage of cases, however, resealing or localized containment ("pseudoaneurysm") can allow medical stabilization, usually with inotropic support or an IABP, followed by emergency surgical repair.

An *LV aneurysm* can develop after a large, usually anterior, acute MI. If refractory heart failure, VT, or systemic embolization occurs despite medical therapy and PCI, aneurysmectomy with CABG is indicated.

Thromboembolic Complications

Thromboembolism has been described in approximately 10% of clinical series and 20% of autopsy series, a finding suggesting a high rate of undiagnosed events. Thromboembolism contributed to up to 25% of hospital deaths from acute MI in the past, but the incidence has declined in the recanalization era in association with greater use of antithrombotics, reductions of infarct size, and earlier ambulation. Systemic arterial emboli (including cerebrovascular emboli) typically arise from an LV mural thrombus, whereas pulmonary emboli commonly arise from thrombi in leg veins. Arterial embolism can cause dramatic clinical events, such as hemiparesis, loss of a pulse, ischemic bowel, or sudden hypertension, depending on the regional circulation involved.

Mural thrombosis with embolism typically occurs in the setting of a large (especially anterior) ST segment elevation acute MI and heart failure. The risk for embolism is particularly high when a mural thrombus is detected by echocardiography. Thus, in patients with anterior ST segment elevation acute MI and in other high-risk patients, echocardiography should be performed during hospitalization; if results are positive, anticoagulation should be started (with an antithrombin), if not already initiated, and continued (with warfarin) for 6 months.

Deep vein thrombosis can be prevented by lower extremity compression therapy, by limiting the duration of bedrest, and by the use of subcutaneous unfractionated heparin or LMWH (in patients at risk not receiving intravenous heparin) until patients are fully ambulatory (Chapter 81). Patients with pulmonary embolism are treated with intravenous heparin, then oral anticoagulation for 6 months (Chapter 98).

Risk Stratification after Myocardial Infarction

The goal of risk stratification before and early after discharge for acute MI is to assess ventricular and clinical function, latent ischemia, and arrhythmic risk, to use this information for patient education and prognostic assessment, and to guide therapeutic strategies (see Fig. 73-3).

Cardiac Catheterization and Noninvasive Stress Testing

Risk stratification generally involves functional assessment by one of three strategies: cardiac catheterization, submaximal exercise stress ECG before discharge (at 4 to 6 days), or symptom-limited stress testing at 2 to 6 weeks after discharge. Many or most patients with ST segment elevation acute MI undergo invasive evaluation for primary PCI or after fibrinolytic therapy. Catheterization generally is performed during hospitalization for patients at high risk. In others, predischarge submaximal exercise testing (to peak heart rate of 120 to 130 beats per minute or 70% of the predicted maximum) appears safe when it is performed in patients who are ambulating without symptoms; it should be avoided within 2 to 3 days of acute MI and in patients with unstable post-MI angina, uncompensated heart failure, or serious cardiac arrhythmias. Alternatively or in addition, patients may undergo symptom-limited stress testing at 2 to 6 weeks before they return to work or resume other increased physical activities. Abnormal test results include not only ST segment depression but also low functional capacity, exertional hypotension, and serious arrhythmias. Patients with positive test results should be considered for coronary angiography.

The sensitivity of stress testing can be augmented with radionuclide perfusion imaging (thallium-201 or technetium-99m sestamibi, or both; Chapter 56) or echocardiography (Chapter 55). Supplemental imaging also can quantify the LV ejection fraction and size the area of infarction or ischemia (e.g., by cardiac magnetic resonance imaging; Chapter 56). For patients taking digoxin or for those with ST segment changes that preclude accurate ECG interpretation (e.g., baseline LBBB or LV hypertrophy), an imaging study is recommended with initial stress testing. In others, an imaging study may be performed selectively for those in whom the exercise ECG test result is positive or equivocal. For patients unable to exercise, pharmacologic stress testing can be performed using adenosine, a long-acting bolus analogue of adenosine (e.g., regadenoson) or dipyridamole scintigraphy or using dobutamine echocardiography.

Electrocardiographic Monitoring

Modern telemetry systems capture complete rhythm information during hospital observations and allow for identification of patients with serious arrhythmias, so routine 24- to 48-hour ambulatory ECG (Holter) monitoring before or after hospital discharge is not recommended. Patients with sustained VT or VF occurring late during hospitalization or provoked during electrophysiologic study with nonsustained VT on monitoring are candidates for an ICD, especially if the ejection fraction is less than 40% (Fig. 73-4) (Chapters 65 and 66). Prophylactic ICD placement at least 1 month after acute MI prevents sudden death for patients with severely depressed function (ejection fraction ≤ 0.30) regardless of the rhythm status. [22]

Secondary Prevention, Patient Education, and Rehabilitation

Secondary Prevention

Advances in secondary prevention have resulted in increasingly effective measures to reduce recurrent MI and cardiovascular death. Secondary prevention should be conscientiously applied after acute MI (Table 73-8).

A fasting *lipid profile* is recommended on admission, and *lipid-lowering therapy,* typically with a statin, is begun in the hospital, generally with an LDL cholesterol goal of less than 70 mg/dL (Chapter 213). Continued smoking doubles the subsequent mortality risk after acute MI, and *smoking cessation* reduces the risk for reinfarction and death within 1 year (Chapter 31). An individualized smoking cessation plan should be formulated, including pharmacologic aids (nicotine gum and patches, bupropion, or varenicline).

Antiplatelet therapy (Chapter 37; Fig. 73-5) should consist of aspirin, given on a long-term basis to all patients without contraindications (maintenance dose, 75 to 162 mg/day). Clopidogrel (75 mg/day) or prasugrel (10 mg/day) is given to patients who received PCI with stenting, and clopidogrel is also appropriate for others at higher risk for recurrent vascular events. Therapy is recommended for a minimum of 1 month after a bare metal stent, for at least 3 months for sirolimus-eluting stents, and for at least 6 months for paclitaxel-eluting stents. If patients are not at high risk for bleeding, therapy is continued for up to 1 year or more.

Anticoagulant therapy (i.e., warfarin, with an international normalized ratio goal of 2.0 to 3.0) is indicated after acute MI for patients unable to take antiplatelet therapy (aspirin or clopidogrel), for those with persistent or paroxysmal AF, for those with LV thrombus, and for those who have suffered a systemic or pulmonary embolism. Anticoagulants also may be considered for patients with extensive wall motion abnormalities and markedly depressed ejection fraction with or without heart failure. Data on the benefits and risks of warfarin added to antiplatelet therapy (Fig. 73-5) are sparse.

ACE inhibitor therapy can prevent adverse myocardial remodeling after acute MI and can reduce heart failure and death; it is clearly indicated for long-term use in patients with anterior acute MI or an LV ejection fraction of less than 40%. ACE inhibitors also reduce recurrent MI in higher-risk patients with an ejection fraction greater than 40%. In contrast, ACE inhibition, when added to other contemporary therapies, provides little additional benefit in reducing cardiovascular events in patients who have stable coronary disease and a low risk (<5%/year) for a coronary event. These data suggest a rationale for the long-term use of ACE inhibitors (e.g., ramipril, 2.5 mg titrated to 10 mg/day, or lisinopril, 2.5 to 5 mg titrated to 10 mg/day) in all patients after MI, except perhaps those at lowest risk (i.e., without heart failure, hypertension, glucose intolerance, or reduced ejection fraction). An ARB (e.g., valsartan, 80 to 160 mg twice daily, or losartan, 50 to 100 mg/day) should be substituted in patients who cannot tolerate an ACE inhibitor; in patients with advanced heart failure, both an ACE inhibitor and an ARB may be complementary (Chapter 59). An aldosterone receptor blocker (e.g., eplerenone, 25 mg/day orally, increased to 50 mg/day after 4 weeks if tolerated, with monitoring of serum potassium levels) also should be added to the ACE inhibitor or ARB (but not both) regimen on a long-term basis in patients with depressed ejection fraction (≤0.40) and clinical heart failure or diabetes, unless this approach is contraindicated.

Long-term β-blocker therapy is strongly recommended for all MI survivors without uncompensated heart failure or other contraindications. Options include metoprolol, 20 to 200 mg per day, or carvedilol, 6.25 to 25 mg twice daily. Long-term therapy in patients at low risk (normal ventricular function, successful recanalization, absence of arrhythmias) is reasonable but not mandatory.

Nitroglycerin (0.4 mg) is prescribed routinely for sublingual or buccal administration for acute anginal attacks. Longer-acting oral therapy (isosorbide mononitrate, 30 to 60 mg orally every morning, or dinitrate, 10 to 40 mg orally two to three times daily) or topical nitroglycerin (e.g., start 0.5 inch, can titrate up to 2 inches, every 6 hours for 2 days) may be added to treatment regimens for angina or heart failure in selected patients.

Calcium-channel blockers are negatively inotropic and are *not* routinely given on a long-term basis; however, they may be given to selected patients without LV dysfunction (ejection fraction > 0.40) who are intolerant of β-blockers and who require these drugs for antianginal therapy (e.g., amlodipine, 5 to 10 mg/day orally, or diltiazem, 120 to 480 mg/day orally as sustained release or divided doses) or for control of heart rate in AF (e.g., diltiazem, 120 to 480 mg/day orally, or verapamil, 180 to 480 mg/day orally, as sustained release or in divided doses). Short-acting nifedipine should be avoided.

Hormone therapy with estrogen with or without progestin is not begun after an acute MI because it increases thromboembolic risk and does not prevent reinfarction. For women already receiving hormone replacement, therapy

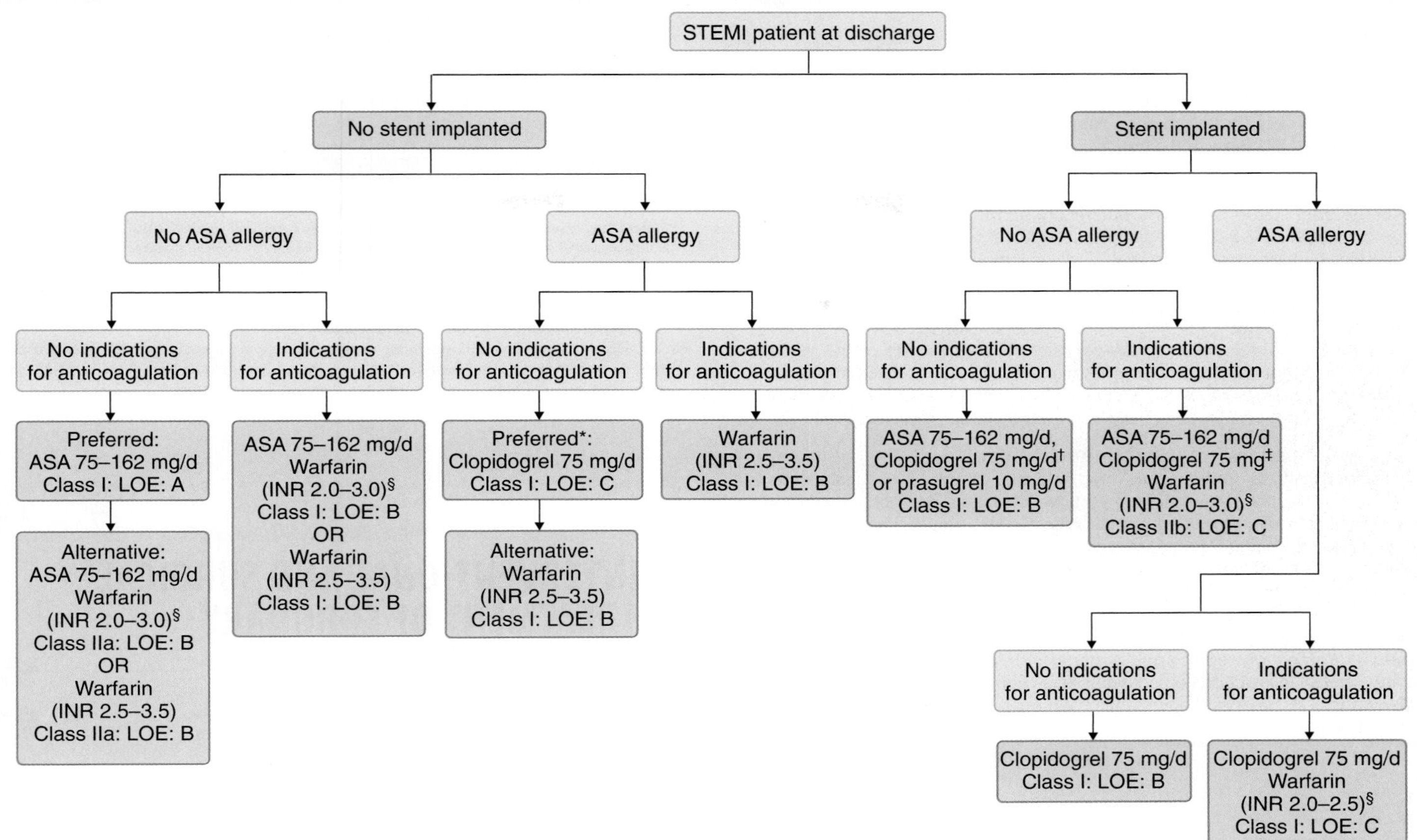

FIGURE 73-5. Long-term antithrombotic therapy at hospital discharge after ST segment elevation myocardial infarction (STEMI). *Clopidogrel is preferred over warfarin because of increased risk of bleeding and low patient compliance in warfarin trials. †For 12 months. ‡Discontinue clopidogrel 1 month after implantation of a bare metal stent or several months after implantation of a drug-eluting stent (3 months after sirolimus and 6 months after paclitaxel) because of the potentially increased risk of bleeding with warfarin and two antiplatelet agents. Continue aspirin (ASA) and warfarin on a long-term basis if warfarin is indicated for other reasons such as atrial fibrillation, left ventricular thrombus, cerebral emboli, or extensive regional wall motion abnormality. §An International Normalized Ratio (INR) of 2.0 to 3.0 is acceptable with tight control, but the lower end of this range is preferable. The combination of antiplatelet therapy and warfarin may be considered in patients younger than 75 years who have a low bleeding risk and who can be monitored reliably. LOE = level of evidence. (Adapted from Antman EM, Anbe DT, Armstrong PW, et al. ACC/AHA guidelines for the management of patients with ST-elevation myocardial infarction—executive summary. A report of the American College of Cardiology/American Heart Association Task Force on Practice Guidelines [Writing Committee to Revise the 1999 Guidelines for the Management of Patients with Acute Myocardial Infarction]. *Circulation*. 2004;110:588-636.)

TABLE 73-8 DISCHARGE MEDICATION CHECKLIST AFTER MYOCARDIAL INFARCTION*

MEDICATION	DOSES	REASONS NOT TO USE	COMMENTS
Aspirin	Initial: 162-325 mg Maintenance: 75-162 mg daily	High bleeding risk	Reduces mortality, reinfarction, and stroke
Clopidogrel	Initial dose: 300-600 mg (75-150 mg after fibrinolysis in patients >75 years old) Maintenance: 75 mg daily	High bleeding risk; suboptimal antiplatelet response	Indicated after PCI for at least 1 yr (shorter time for BMS if high bleeding risk); also reduces vascular events when added to aspirin in non–ST segment elevation acute MI (also useful based on recent clinical trials after ST segment elevation acute MI) Genetic variants (CYP2C19) may reduce response Controversial interaction with PPIs (e.g., omeprazole)
Prasugrel	Initial dose: 60 mg Maintenance: 10 mg daily	High bleeding risk	Avoid with history of prior stroke/TIA Consider 5 mg daily in patients >75 years old or <60 kg
β-Blocker (e.g., metoprolol, carvedilol)	Metoprolol: 25-200 mg daily Carvedilol: 6.25-25 mg bid	Asthma, bradycardia, heart failure	Reduces mortality, reinfarction, sudden death, arrhythmia, hypertension, angina, atherosclerosis progression
ACE inhibitor (e.g., ramipril, lisinopril) or ARB (e.g., valsartan, losartan)	Ramipril: 2.5-10 mg daily Lisinopril: 5-10 mg daily Valsartan: 80-160 mg daily-bid Losartan: 50-100 mg daily	Hypotension, allergy, hyperkalemia	Reduces mortality, reinfarction, stroke, heart failure, diabetes, atherosclerosis progression
Lipid-lowering agent (e.g., a statin) (e.g., atorvastatin, simvastatin)	Atorvastatin: 10-80 mg daily Simvastatin: 20-40 mg daily	Myopathy, rhabdomyolysis, hepatitis	Goal = LDL <100 and preferably <70 (statins also can benefit patients with lower LDL†); consider addition of niacin or fibrate for high non-HDL cholesterol, low HDL
Nitroglycerin sublingual	0.4 mg SL PRN for angina	Aortic stenosis; sildenafil (Viagra) use	Instruct on PRN use and appropriate need for medical attention

*Medications given at hospital discharge improve long-term compliance.
†Heart Protection Study (*Lancet*. 2002;360:7); and PROVE-IT Study (*N Engl J Med*. 2004;350:1495).
ACE, angiotensin-converting enzyme; ARB = angiotensin receptor blocker; bid = twice daily; BMS = bare metal stent; HDL = high-density lipoprotein; LDL = low-density lipoprotein; MI = myocardial infarction; PCI = percutaneous coronary intervention; PRN = as needed; daily = once daily, SL = sublingual; TIA, transient ischemic attack.
Adapted from Kushner FG, Hand M, Antman EM, et al. 2009 Focused updates: ACC/AHA guidelines for the management of patients with ST-elevation myocardial infarction and the ACC/AHA/SCAI guidelines on percutaneous coronary intervention. *Circulation*. 2009;120:2271-2306.

should be discontinued unless it is being given for another compelling indication.

Hypertension (Chapter 67) and diabetes mellitus (Chapter 236) must be assessed and tightly controlled in patients after acute MI. ACE inhibitors or β-blockers as described earlier are usually the first-choice therapies for hypertension, with ARBs indicated when ACE inhibitors are not tolerated. ACE inhibitors and ARBs also can reduce the long-term complications of diabetes.

Antioxidant supplementation (e.g., vitamin E, vitamin C) does not benefit patients after acute MI and is *not* recommended. Folate therapy reduces homocyst(e)ine levels, but it has not been effective in reducing clinical events in large secondary prevention trials. Fish oil supplements showed no benefit in the best randomized trial.

Antiarrhythmic drugs are *not* generally recommended after acute MI, and class I antiarrhythmic agents can increase the risk for sudden death. Class III drugs (amiodarone, sotalol, dofetilide) may be used as part of the management strategy for specific arrhythmias (e.g., AF, VT) (Chapters 64 and 65).

The intracoronary infusion of stem cells has been proposed as a mechanism to reduce infarct size. To date, however, trials have been inconclusive.

Patient Education and Rehabilitation

The hospital stay provides an important opportunity to educate patients about their MI and its treatment, coronary risk factors, and behavioral modification. Education should begin on admission and should continue after discharge. However, the time before hospital discharge is particularly opportune. Many hospitals use case managers and prevention specialists to augment physicians and nurses, to provide educational materials, to review important concepts, to assist in formulating and actualizing individual risk-reduction plans, and to ensure proper and timely outpatient follow-up. This follow-up should include early return appointments with the patient's physician (within a few weeks). Instructions on activities also should be given before discharge. Many hospitals have cardiac rehabilitation programs that provide supervised, progressive exercise.

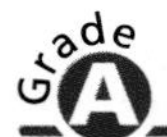

1. Van't Hof AW, Ten Berg J, Heestermans T, et al. Prehospital initiation of tirofiban in patients with ST-elevation myocardial infarction undergoing primary angioplasty (On-TIME 2): a multicentre, double-blind, randomised controlled trial. *Lancet.* 2008;372:537-546.
2. Stone GW, Witzenbichler B, Guagliumi G, et al. Bivalirudin during primary percutaneous coronary intervention in acute myocardial infarction. *N Engl J Med.* 2008;358:2218-2230.
3. Wijeysundere HC, Vijayaraghavan R, Nallamothu BK, et al. Rescue angioplasty or repeat fibrinolysis after failed therapy for ST-segment myocardial infarction: a meta-analysis of randomized trials. *J Am Coll Cardiol.* 2007;49:422-430.
4. Cantor WJ, Fitchett D, Borgundvaag G, et al. Routine early angioplasty after fibrinolysis for acute myocardial infarction. *N Engl J Med.* 2009;360:2705-2718.
5. DiMario C, Dudek D, Piscione F, et al. Immediate angioplasty versus standard therapy with rescue angioplasty after thrombolysis in the Combined Abciximab REteplase Stent study in acute myocardial infarction (CARESS-in-AMI): an open, prospective, randomised, multicentre trial. *Lancet.* 2008;371:559-568.
6. Keeley EC, Boura JA, Grines CL. Primary angioplasty versus intravenous thrombolytic therapy for acute myocardial infarction: a quantitative review of 23 randomised trials. *Lancet.* 2003;361:13-20.
7. Andersen HR, Nielsen TT, Rasmussen K, et al. A comparison of coronary angioplasty with fibrinolytic therapy in acute myocardial infarction. *N Engl J Med.* 2003;349:733-742.
8. Kushner FG, Hand M, Antman EM, et al. 2009 focused updates: ACC/AHA guidelines for the management of patients with ST-elevation myocardial infarction and the ACC/AHA/SCAI guidelines on percutaneous coronary intervention. *Circulation.* 2009;120:2271-2306.
9. Ellis SG, Tendera M, de Belder MA, et al. Facilitated PCI in patients with ST-elevation myocardial infarction. *N Engl J Med.* 2008;358:2205-2217.
10. Schomig A, Mehilli J, Antoniucci D, et al. Mechanical reperfusion in patients with acute myocardial infarction presenting more than 12 hours from symptom onset: a randomized controlled trial. *JAMA.* 2005;293:2865-2872.
11. Svilass T, Vlaar PJ, vander Horst I, et al. Thrombus aspiration during primary percutaneous coronary intervention. *N Engl J Med.* 2008;358:557-567.
12. Keeley EC, Boura JA, Grines CL. Comparison of primary and facilitated percutaneous interventions for ST-elevation myocardial infarction: quantitative review of randomized trials. *Lancet.* 2006;367:579-588.
13. Sabatine MS, Cannon CP, Gibson M, et al. Addition of clopidogrel to aspirin and fibrinolytic therapy for myocardial infarction with ST-segment elevation. *N Engl J Med.* 2005;352:1179-1189.
14. COMMIT (Clopidogrel and Metoprolol in Myocardial Infarction Trial) Collaborative Group. Early intravenous then oral metoprolol in 45 of 852 patients with acute myocardial infarction: randomised placebo-controlled trial. *Lancet.* 2005;366:1622-1632.
15. Montalescot G, Wiviott SD, Braunwald E, et al. Prasugrel compared with clopidogrel in patients undergoing percutaneous coronary intervention for ST-elevation myocardial infarction (TRITON-TIMI 38): double-blind, randomised controlled trial. *Lancet.* 2009;373:723-731.
16. Antman EM, Morrow DA, McCabe CH, et al. Enoxaparin versus unfractionated heparin with fibrinolysis for ST-elevation myocardial infarction. *N Engl J Med.* 2006;354:1477-1488.
17. Yusuf S, Mehta SR, Chrolavicius S, et al. Effects of fondaparinux on mortality and reinfarction in patients with acute ST-segment elevation myocardial infarction: the OASIS-6 randomized trial. *JAMA.* 2006;295:1519-1530.
18. Mehran R, Lansky AJ, Witzenbichler B, et al. Bivalirudin in patients undergoing primary angioplasty for acute myocardial infarction (HORIZONS-AMI): 1-year results of a randomised controlled trial. *Lancet.* 2009;374:1149-1159.
19. Pitt B, Remme W, Zannad F, et al. Eplerenone, a selective aldosterone blocker, in patients with left ventricular dysfunction after myocardial infarction. *N Engl J Med.* 2003;348:1309-1321.
20. Moss AJ, Zareba W, Hall J, et al. Prophylactic implantation of a defibrillator in patients with myocardial infarction and reduced ejection fraction. *N Engl J Med.* 2002;346:877-883.
21. Steinbeck G, Andresen D, Seidl K, et al. Defibrillator implantation early after myocardial infarction. *N Engl J Med.* 2009;361:1427-1436
22. Cannon CP, Steinberg BA, Murphy SA, et al. Meta-analysis of cardiovascular outcomes trials comparing intensive versus moderate statin therapy. *J Am Coll Cardiol.* 2006;48:438-445.

SUGGESTED READINGS

Cohen M, Boiangiu C, Abidi M. Therapy for ST-segment elevation myocardial infarction patients who present late or are ineligible for reperfusion therapy. *J Am Coll Cardiol.* 2010;55:1895-1906. *Low-molecular-weight heparin is recommended for patients who have ST segment elevation myocardial infarction but who present late or are ineligible for reperfusion therapy.*

Lambert L, Brown K, Segal E, et al. Association between timeliness of reperfusion therapy and clinical outcomes in ST-elevation myocardial infarction. *JAMA.* 2010;303:2148-2155. *Prompt reperfusion improves outcomes compared with delayed reperfusion.*

Suh HS, Song HJ, Choi JE, et al. Drug-eluting stents versus bare-metal stents in acute myocardial infarction: a systematic review and meta-analysis. *Int J Technol Assess Heatlh Care.* 2011;27:11-22. *Drug-eluting stents provided better 1-year outcomes but equivalent 2-year outcomes.*

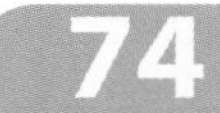

INTERVENTIONAL AND SURGICAL TREATMENT OF CORONARY ARTERY DISEASE

PAUL S. TEIRSTEIN AND BRUCE W. LYTLE

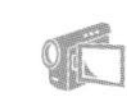
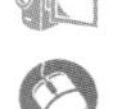

Percutaneous coronary intervention (PCI) and coronary artery bypass graft (CABG) surgery represent alternative and sometimes complementary approaches to coronary revascularization. Each has its relative indications, advantages, disadvantages, and contraindications.

PERCUTANEOUS CORONARY INTERVENTION

PCI is applicable to most forms of coronary artery disease, including multivessel disease, total occlusions, saphenous vein graft disease, unstable angina (Chapter 72), and acute myocardial infarction (MI) (Chapter 73). An estimated 2 million PCIs are performed worldwide each year, making it one of the most widely used medical procedures. Its popularity is based largely on its simplicity, the need for only local anesthesia, a short (approximately 1 day) hospitalization, and negligible postprocedure recovery time.

Mechanisms and Technical Considerations

Under local anesthesia, a hollow-bore needle is inserted percutaneously into a peripheral artery (usually the femoral or radial artery). A guidewire (approximately 0.038 inch) is placed through this needle and advanced into the aorta. The needle is removed, leaving the guidewire, over which a small-caliber (approximately 3 mm), specially shaped catheter (called a guiding catheter) is advanced under fluoroscope guidance into the ostium of the obstructed coronary artery. By use of radiographic contrast injections that provide fluoroscopic visualization of the coronary artery lumen, a thin (approximately 0.014 inch), highly steerable guidewire is directed down the coronary artery and across the stenotic lesion. This guidewire becomes a "rail" over which therapeutic tools such as inflatable balloons, stents, and atherectomy catheters are passed to the diseased segment (Fig. 74-1).

Balloon catheters (Fig. 74-2) typically have two lumens, one to allow passage over the guidewire and another to carry a mixture of saline and radiographic contrast material to inflate a balloon at the distal catheter tip. Under fluoroscopy, the balloon is centered across the lesion and inflated to 3 to 20 atmospheres of pressure. Balloon inflation widens the narrowed lumen by stretching the vessel and, in most cases, causing a tear (a therapeutic dissection) at the edges of the plaque, where the atheroma meets the nondiseased media. Atherectomy catheters, which also are passed over a guidewire to the diseased segment, remove plaque by a shaving, grinding, slicing, or suction mechanism. Coronary stents are metallic scaffolding devices that are crimped onto a deflated balloon catheter before insertion into the diseased vessel. During balloon inflation, the collapsed stent expands to support the vessel lumen (Fig. 74-3). Whereas balloons and atherectomy devices create an adequate, albeit rough channel through diseased arteries, the supporting structure of the stent can widen the lumen to near its predisease dimensions.

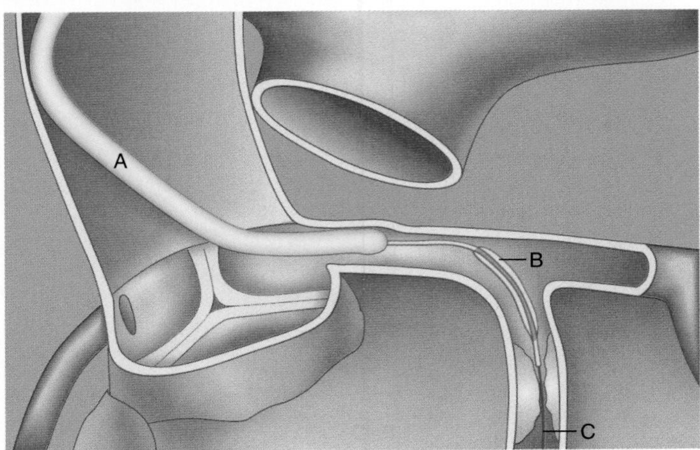

FIGURE 74-1. **Schematic view of coronary angioplasty technique.** A guide catheter (A) is inserted into the orifice of the coronary artery (in this figure, the left main); a balloon catheter (B) is advanced over a thin guidewire (C) into the lesion. Balloon inflation dilates the stenotic region. (Modified from Baim DS. Percutaneous balloon angioplasty and general coronary intervention. In: Baim DS, ed. *Grossman's Cardiac Catheterization, Angiography, and Intervention,* 7th ed. Philadelphia: Lippincott Williams & Wilkins; 2005.)

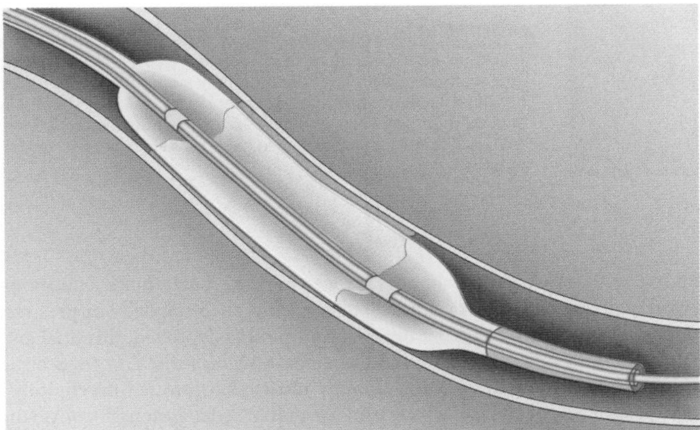

FIGURE 74-2. **Balloon angioplasty catheter.** The catheter consists of two lumens, an inflation lumen and a guidewire lumen. Two radiopaque markers, indicating the lateral balloon margins, aid in positioning of the balloon before inflation.

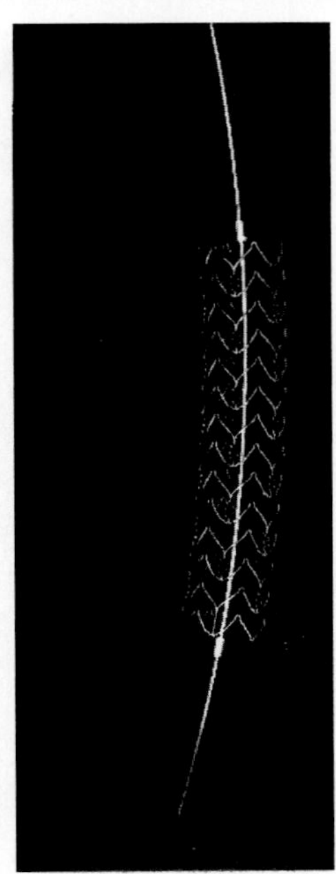

FIGURE 74-3. **Balloon-expandable coronary stent.** The stainless steel stent is crimped onto a balloon catheter to allow low-profile passage through the coronary artery. When it is positioned across the lesion, the balloon is inflated, expanding the stent. After balloon deflation and removal, the stent remains, providing a scaffold that supports the vessel lumen.

With a stent, tissue flaps are "pinned" against the wall, and recoil is limited. Most stents are designed so that the metallic struts compose only about 20% of the surface area to allow a rapid endothelialization (during about 2 weeks) and a reduced risk of thrombosis. Because coronary stents are able to obtain a larger and more secure lumen, some resist restenosis, and some elute beneficial medications, they are now used in more than 95% of PCIs.

During the PCI procedure, the interventional cardiologist is able to assess the target vessel fluoroscopically by injections of contrast material through the guiding catheter (Fig. 74-4). When the coronary artery has been opened successfully, all catheters are withdrawn, and the arterial access site is sealed by mechanical pressure, an absorbable plug, or a remote suturing device. Patients without comorbidity ambulate in 3 to 6 hours. Discharge from the hospital usually occurs on the morning after the procedure, after stability of the arterial access site, cardiac biomarkers, and electrocardiogram is confirmed. Selected patients in some medical centers are treated as outpatients and released 6 to 12 hours after the procedure without an overnight stay.

Selection of Patients

Any decision to perform PCI must include a review of the coronary angiogram (Chapter 57) by an experienced interventional cardiologist to assess the lesion's technical suitability for the procedure. The disease must narrow the coronary artery lumen by at least 60%, and the quantity of myocardium subtended by the vessel should not be trivial. High-risk lesion characteristics, such as longer lesion length, vessel tortuosity, lesion calcification, or the presence of thrombus, must be taken into consideration. Subtle angiographic findings, such as the presence of collateral vessels that supply a different myocardial territory and that originate distal to the target, should be appreciated. For each patient, the benefits of PCI must be weighed against the procedural risk. Characteristics of the patient conveying increased risk include advanced age (i.e., >75 years), diabetes, smaller vessels that are often found in women, prior MI, significant impairment of left ventricular function, and renal insufficiency.

Procedural Success and Complications

With use of modern techniques in appropriately selected patients, most PCI procedures have a greater than 95% success rate. The single exception is a chronic total coronary occlusion (100% obstruction of the lumen), in which the interventional cardiologist's ability to negotiate a guidewire through the blockage is only about 50 to 80%. With the increased use of coronary stents and adjunctive antiplatelet agents (thienopyridines and platelet glycoprotein IIb/IIIa inhibitors), abrupt coronary artery closure is rarely encountered. When PCI is performed by an experienced interventional cardiologist in appropriately selected patients, the risk of in-hospital death is less than 1%; MI (usually small, non–ST segment elevation MI) is approximately 5%; the need for urgent or emergent CABG surgery is less than 1%; the risk of stroke is less than 0.1%; the chance of coronary perforation is less than 1%; and morbidity at the arterial access site (i.e., hematoma, pseudoaneurysm, or arteriovenous fistula) occurs in less than 5%. Balloons and filters deployed within a coronary vessel beyond the target lesion to limit distal embolization of plaque, platelet aggregates, and other "debris" can further reduce ischemic complications in selected, high-risk patients.

Restenosis and Thrombosis

Restenosis is a renarrowing of an artery after a PCI procedure, usually resulting from one of two general mechanisms. The first mechanism, unfavorable remodeling and elastic recoil, is a mechanical renarrowing caused by adventitial constriction and shrinkage of the vessel lumen. The second mechanism, neointimal hyperplasia, is due to the proliferation of smooth muscle cells and matrix in response to the injury caused by balloons, stents, or atherectomy devices. Restenosis occurs in 10 to 50% of PCI patients after balloon angioplasty without stenting, usually within the first 6 months after the procedure. Characteristics associated with higher risk of restenosis include longer lesions, small-diameter vessels, diabetes, and multivessel disease. Treatment with either balloon angioplasty or atherectomy devices results in similar rates of restenosis. Coronary stents provide a semirigid scaffolding within the lumen and reduce restenosis by eliminating the mechanical renarrowing

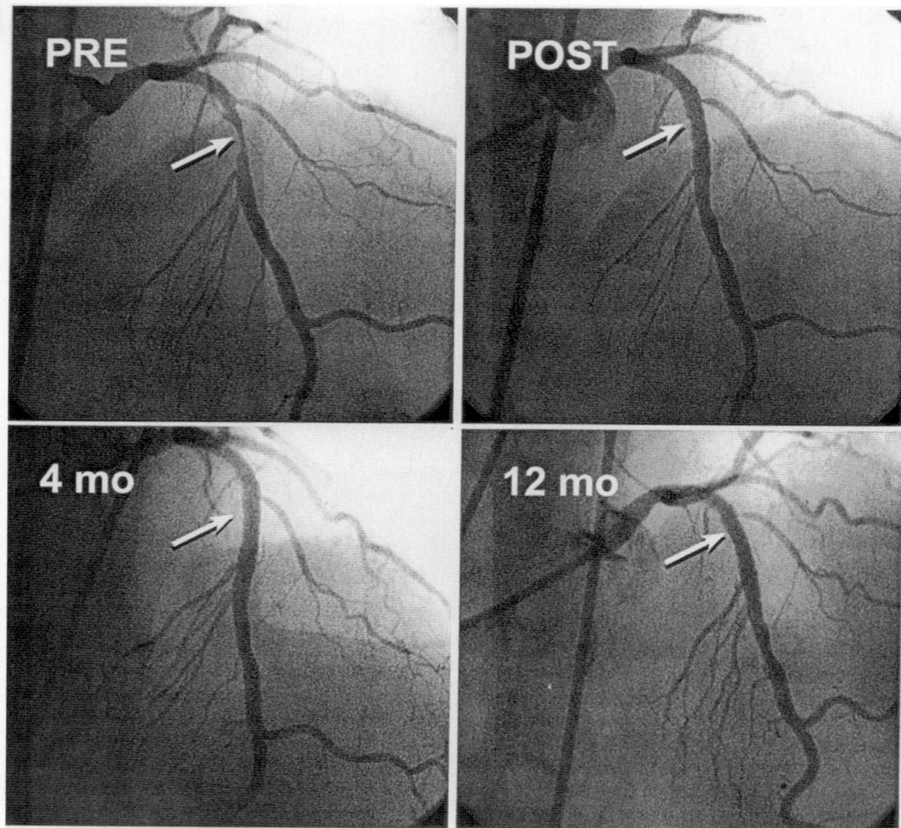

FIGURE 74-4. Angiographic images before, after, and at late follow-up after placement of a sirolimus-eluting stent. The left anterior descending artery contains a tight stenosis *(arrow, upper left panel)*. After stent implantation *(upper right panel)*, the stenosis is abolished *(arrow)*. Follow-up at 4 and 12 months *(bottom panels)* reveals a completely open lumen, with no evidence of restenosis *(arrows)*.

caused by unfavorable remodeling and elastic recoil. In randomized trials, bare metal stents reduce restenosis by about one third, from approximately 30 to 40% in patients randomized to balloon angioplasty to 20 to 30% in patients receiving stents.[1]

Although bare metal stents reduce restenosis, they do not eliminate restenosis because the stent struts that embed into the vessel wall increase the intimal proliferative response to injury. With bare metal stents, the mechanical component of restenosis is eliminated, but the proliferative component is enhanced. Smooth muscle cell division and matrix formation can migrate through the stent struts to renarrow the vessel lumen. Antiproliferative drugs that are embedded into a polymer stent coating are extremely effective for the control of restenosis. However, drug-eluting stents carry a slightly higher risk of thrombosis later (>1 year), especially if patients cannot or do not continue with aspirin plus a thienopyridine. As a result, trials of stents that release the cell cycle inhibitors sirolimus, everolimus, zotarolimus, and paclitaxel have demonstrated a reduced need for early repeated procedures,[2] but have not always found improved long-term outcome compared with bare metal stents.[3,4] Among the drug-eluting stents, the most favorable current data are for everolimus and sirolimus.[5,6]

Choices Related to Stenting

Based on long-term follow-up data, the choice between a bare metal stent and a drug-eluting stent remains controversial. Patients receiving drug-eluting stents must continue dual antiplatelet therapy with aspirin and a thienopyridine for a minimum of 12 months. If a patient is unlikely to be able to adhere to such therapy because of bleeding risks or the need for an invasive or surgical procedure, a bare metal stent is preferable. Atherectomy is rarely used, with the exception of the Rotablator (Boston Scientific, Maple Grove, MN), which pulverizes plaque into microparticles that pass through the coronary microcirculation and is particularly helpful for the treatment of heavily calcified lesions. After plaque debulking with the Rotablator, a drug-eluting stent is usually implanted.

Discharge Issues

Discharge planning after PCI represents an important opportunity to emphasize evidence-based medical treatment of atherothrombotic disease and coronary risk factor modification. All patients should receive aspirin (81 to 325 mg/day) indefinitely. For patients receiving bare metal stents, a minimum 2-week course of a thienopyridine (i.e., clopidogrel 75 mg daily or prasugrel 10 mg daily) is mandatory. If a drug-eluting stent is deployed, this dual antiplatelet therapy must be extended for at least 12 months, and then either aspirin alone or dual antiplatelet therapy must be continued indefinitely if possible.[7] Prolonged use of aspirin, clopidogrel, angiotensin-converting enzyme inhibitors, β-blockers, and lipid-lowering agents should be considered on the basis of randomized trials showing improved long-term outcome, particularly in patients who present with unstable angina syndromes (Chapters 71, 72, and 73). Smoking cessation (Chapter 31), blood pressure control (Chapter 67), stress management, exercise, weight loss, changes in dietary habits, and strict blood glucose control for diabetic patients (Chapter 237) also are important elements of the discharge plan.

Activity restrictions after PCI are modest. If the femoral artery was instrumented, heavy lifting is discouraged for several days. Intense aerobic exercise is usually discouraged for 2 to 4 weeks (especially after stent implantation) because exercise can activate platelets and lead to formation of thrombus at the angioplasty site. Patients may return to work 1 or 2 days after the procedure if their occupation does not include heavy lifting or excessive physical exercise. There is usually no restriction on driving an automobile.

CORONARY ANGIOPLASTY VERSUS MEDICAL THERAPY

PCI reduces angina and commonly leads to better treadmill exercise performance and improved quality-of-life measurements. However, PCI has not been shown to reduce the risks of death, MI, or other major cardiovascular events compared with modern optimal medical therapy in patients with stable angina (Chapter 71).[8] PCI reduces symptoms for the first 24 months, especially in patients with more severe angina, but symptoms were similarly improved over baseline with both intensive medical therapy and PCI at 36 months.[9] In truly asymptomatic patients, significant ischemia first should be documented by functional testing, or a large quantity of myocardium should be supplied by the stenotic coronary artery. Patients experiencing acute ST elevation MI (Chapter 73) represent an important subgroup in whom PCI has proved beneficial compared with medical therapy (Fig. 74-5). In ST elevation MI, randomized trials consistently have reported a reduction in

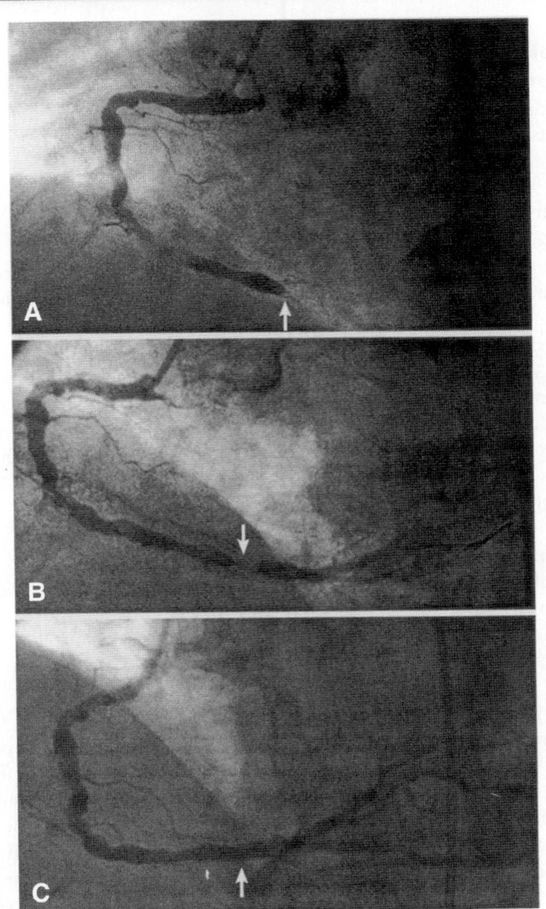

FIGURE 74-5. Primary coronary angioplasty for acute myocardial infarction. This 50-year-old man presented at midnight with 70 minutes of crushing substernal chest pressure accompanied by inferior ST segment elevation. Emergency angiography performed 45 minutes after arrival found 100% occlusion of the right coronary artery (**A**, *arrow*). Within 10 minutes, a guidewire was negotiated through the obstruction (presumably caused by fresh thrombus), allowing perfusion into the distal vessel and uncovering a high-grade stenotic lesion (**B**, *arrow*). After deployment of a coronary stent (**C**, *arrow*), the stenosis was abolished and significant myocardial damage aborted.

mortality, stroke, subsequent MI, and recurrent ischemia with immediate PCI compared with thrombolytic therapy[10] or with initial thrombolytic therapy followed by rescue PCI as needed,[11] even if immediate PCI requires transfer to another hospital. For non–ST elevation MI and many patients with unstable angina, an early aggressive approach that includes either PCI or CABG in angiographically suitable patients is generally preferable to a conservative strategy,[12,13] except in lower-risk patients (Chapter 72).

CORONARY ARTERY SURGERY

CABG is based on the premise that the morbidity and mortality associated with coronary atherosclerosis are largely related to atherosclerotic coronary stenoses that can be demonstrated by coronary angiography (Chapter 57) and that if grafts are constructed to route blood flow around these stenoses, myocardial blood supply can be improved or preserved, cardiac symptoms relieved, cardiac events diminished, and survival prolonged. Over time, the fundamentals of that concept have been shown to be correct.

The most common types of grafts for coronary artery bypass have been reversed segments of saphenous vein and the internal thoracic arteries. Saphenous vein grafts are anastomosed to the aorta (proximal anastomosis) and to the coronary artery distal to the major obstruction (Fig. 74-6). Saphenous vein grafts have the advantages of availability, larger size than most coronary arteries, and favorable handling characteristics. However, with time, saphenous vein grafts may develop intrinsic pathologic changes, intimal fibroplasia, and vein graft atherosclerosis, each of which may lead to narrowing or occlusions. By 10 years after surgery, approximately 30% of saphenous vein grafts become occluded, and 30 to 35% of those remaining exhibit angiographic evidence of vein graft atherosclerosis. Treatment with platelet inhibitors and statins (Chapter 213) decreases the risk of vein graft failure but does not eliminate it.

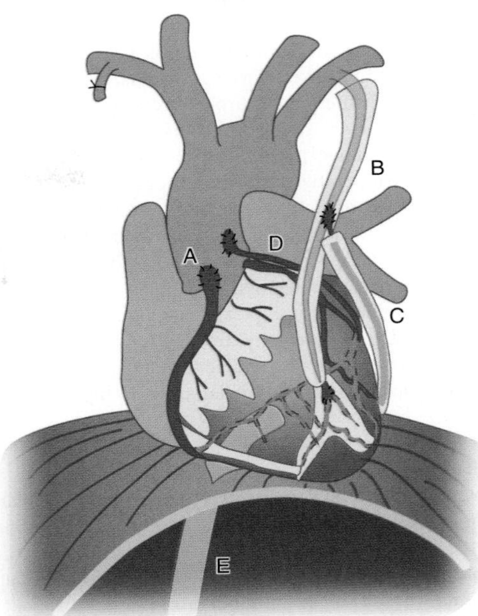

FIGURE 74-6. Types of bypass grafts. Bypass grafts include reversed saphenous vein graft from aorta to right coronary artery (A), in situ left internal mammary artery graft to anterior descending coronary artery (B), Y graft of right internal mammary artery from left internal mammary artery to circumflex coronary artery (C), radial artery graft from aorta to circumflex coronary artery (D), and in situ gastroepiploic graft to posterior descending branch of the right coronary artery (E).

Internal thoracic artery grafts, on the other hand, are resistant to the development of late atherosclerosis. When it is used as an in situ (subclavian origin intact) graft to the left anterior descending (LAD) coronary artery, the left internal thoracic artery graft has a more than 90% patency rate up to 20 years after operation. Because the LAD coronary artery has a strong prognostic influence, the left internal thoracic artery to LAD graft is a clinically important part of myocardial revascularization. Patients who receive a left internal thoracic artery to LAD graft with or without saphenous vein grafts have a better long-term survival rate, fewer reoperations, and fewer cardiac events compared with patients receiving only saphenous vein grafts. The right internal thoracic artery may also be used for revascularization as an in situ graft, as an aorta to coronary artery graft, or as a composite arterial graft from the left internal thoracic artery to a coronary artery. Use of both internal thoracic arteries as grafts provides incremental benefit over a single internal thoracic artery graft strategy and produces an improved survival with a lower risk for reoperation. By comparison, radial artery grafts provide outcomes that are essentially equivalent to those with saphenous vein grafts.[14]

Most CABG operations have been performed with a full median sternotomy incision, historically with the aid of cardiopulmonary bypass, aortic cross-clamping, and cardioplegic solution—techniques that allow exposure and arrest of the heart such that detailed microsurgical anastomoses can be constructed while myocardial function is effectively protected. By comparison, strategies for performing operations through smaller incisions (minimally invasive surgery) have had limited application for coronary revascularizations. Although beating heart ("off-pump") surgery without cardiopulmonary bypass has been widely advocated to avoid neurologic complications, it apparently does not provide such protection and leads to lower rates of graft patency compared with traditional on-pump CABG.[15]

Perioperative Risks

The risk of mortality associated with CABG correlates with ischemia at the time of operation, left ventricular function, extent of coronary stenoses, noncardiac atherosclerosis, and comorbid conditions and with the experience, skill, and judgment of the surgeon. Effective myocardial protection has diminished much of the incremental risk based on the severity of cardiac disease. For patients younger than 70 years without serious comorbid conditions, the mortality risk of primary CABG surgery is less than 1% in experienced hands regardless of the number of coronary arteries that are stenotic, and left ventricular dysfunction only slightly increases risk. Nevertheless, CABG surgery in the presence of ongoing myocardial ischemia due to acute myocardial infarction, unstable angina, or acute vessel closure after PCI is still associated with increased risk. National data on primary CABG operations show a 1.7% mortality rate for elective operations, a 2.6% rate for "urgent" operations, a 6% rate for "emergency" procedures, and a 23% rate for "salvage" operations. Noncardiac comorbid conditions (aortic atherosclerosis, renal function, chronic obstructive pulmonary disease, and coagulation system disorders) increase perioperative risk when these conditions are severe.

The most serious postoperative morbidity after CABG is stroke, often related to aortic or cerebrovascular atherosclerosis and atherosclerotic embolization. Heightened awareness of the importance of aortic and carotid atherosclerosis and improved management strategies appear to have decreased the risk of focal stroke in patients previously at high risk. Serious wound complications of median sternotomy are uncommon (1 to 2%). Obesity, diabetes, and bilateral internal thoracic artery grafting (particularly in combination with diabetes) are associated with higher rates of wound complications.

Late Outcomes

The late outcomes after CABG are related to age, severity of cardiac disease before operation, noncardiac comorbid conditions, progression of atherosclerosis, and the operation itself. Many of these factors can be influenced by treatment choices. CABG tends to diminish but not to eliminate long-term survival differences based on the number of diseased coronary vessels, left main stenosis, and different levels of left ventricular function. The achievement of complete revascularization (bypass grafts to all stenotic coronary vessels) and the use of internal thoracic artery grafts improve long-term survival rates and symptomatic status.

Patients often have prolonged survival after CABG; more than 80% of patients are alive more than 10 years after operation. Over the long term, control of the progression of atherosclerosis by lifestyle modifications, pharmacologic treatment of hypertension (Chapter 67) and lipids (Chapter 213), and platelet inhibitors (Chapter 37) appears to extend the benefits of CABG.

INDICATIONS FOR BYPASS SURGERY

The goals of CABG are to relieve symptoms and to prolong life expectancy. On the basis of randomized trials and the emergence of alternative medical treatments and PCI, the surgical population has evolved toward patients with complex conditions, often involving left main or triple-vessel disease, diffuse coronary stenoses, totally obstructed vessels, abnormal left ventricular function, and diabetes. Surgically treated patients with single-vessel disease usually have LAD stenoses or have failed alternative treatments.

Symptom Relief

If patients who experience angina have severe stenoses in graftable coronary arteries that supply areas of myocardium ischemic at rest or with stress, CABG will reliably relieve angina. Randomized trials have shown that the relief of angina after CABG is more consistent than that achieved with alternative treatments. When intermittent heart failure symptoms represent an "anginal equivalent" that is also caused by ischemia, such symptoms also respond well to relief of that ischemia by CABG. Patients with symptoms of heart failure at rest are more complex, but dobutamine echocardiography (Chapter 55) and positron emission tomography (Chapter 56) can identify segments of viable but hibernating myocardium (ischemic at rest) that may improve with bypass grafting, thus reducing symptoms of heart failure.

Survival

Chronic Stable Angina

In randomized trials of patients with mild to moderate chronic stable angina, an improved survival rate has been documented for patients treated with initial CABG compared with initial medical treatment in the presence of a left main stenosis of more than 50% of the diameter, triple-vessel disease, double-vessel disease with a proximal LAD lesion, abnormal left ventricular function, or a strongly positive exercise test result (Chapter 71). Meta-analysis of these randomized trials also suggests a survival benefit of CABG for any patient with a proximal LAD lesion and myocardial ischemia. These are subgroups of patients for whom bypass surgery should be strongly considered even in the absence of severe symptoms. During these trials, patients with severe angina were not randomized but were included in observational studies that noted improved survival rates with CABG for patients with double- and triple-vessel disease and normal or abnormal left ventricular function. Medical, interventional, and surgical treatments have all advanced substantially since these trials were completed.

Unstable Angina or Non–ST Elevation Myocardial Infarction

Current data suggest an aggressive strategy, including CABG when indicated, in patients with unstable angina or non–ST elevation acute myocardial infarction (Chapter 72).[12]

Ischemic Syndromes without Randomized Trials

ST Elevation Acute Myocardial Infarction

For patients with ST segment elevation acute myocardial infarction, CABG may be indicated in the acute setting when thrombolytic therapy or PCI has not been effective, ischemia is ongoing, and large areas of myocardium remain jeopardized. CABG after a completed MI may be indicated in patients in whom persistent ischemia in noninfarcted areas of myocardium produces post-infarction angina or hemodynamic instability. Mechanical complications of myocardial necrosis, including papillary muscle rupture, ventricular septal rupture, and myocardial free wall rupture, are acute life-threatening situations that usually require urgent operation for repair of the defect, often combined with CABG (Chapter 73).

Failed Percutaneous Coronary Intervention

The availability of intracoronary stents has decreased the need for emergency CABG to treat acute failure of PCIs. Current indications for emergency CABG include closure or threatened closure of a vessel supplying a significant amount of myocardium.

Coronary Bypass Reoperations

Patients in whom new stenoses develop in native arteries or in bypass grafts may have recurrent ischemic syndromes. Observational study of patients with severe vein graft atherosclerosis indicate that this is an unstable lesion often leading to serious cardiac events, particularly if the LAD or multiple vessels are jeopardized; reoperation appears to improve the survival rate of these patients. Reoperations are more difficult and dangerous than primary procedures, but the risk now approaches that for primary procedures in institutions performing a large number of reoperations. PCI is sometimes an alternative for the treatment of vein graft disease.

Coexisting Cardiac Disease

During cardiac operations performed for valvular (Chapter 75) or aortic (Chapter 78) disease, the standard treatment is to perform bypass grafts to major coronary arteries with angiographic stenoses of more than 50% of the luminal diameter. No randomized trials have addressed this issue, and these indications, although logical given the natural history of atherosclerosis, remain practice patterns based on consensus but not on definitive data.

PERCUTANEOUS CORONARY INTERVENTION VERSUS CORONARY ARTERY BYPASS GRAFTING

The decision between PCI and CABG surgery is largely determined by clinical status and anatomic features but remains controversial. For patients with acute coronary syndromes, PCI is the preferred initial approach and is known to improve the survival rate of patients with ST elevation M. CABG is reserved for patients with failed acute PCI or residual myocardial ischemia. For patients with chronic coronary syndromes, there are currently no data to confirm that PCI prolongs life regardless of anatomy, whereas randomized trials, albeit older trials, demonstrate that CABG prolongs the life expectancy of patients with severe coronary artery disease, particularly patients with left ventricular dysfunction or severe ischemia. Surgery, therefore, is often the initial approach to these patient subsets.

For patients in whom the survival benefit of revascularization is less clear, the decision is often related to anatomic features. For low-risk patients followed for 1 year after revascularization, repeat revascularization is more frequent after PCI (14%) than CABG (6%), stroke is more common after CABG (2.2%) than PCI (0.6%), and the rates of death and MI are similar (Fig. 74-7). Patients with extensive and diffuse coronary stenoses appear to benefit most from surgery, whereas patients with more limited coronary stenoses, including some with left main stenosis, have equivalent outcomes with PCI.[16]

The need for repeated revascularization procedures is consistently higher in patients randomized to PCI.[17] In several randomized trials, diabetic patients with multivessel coronary disease have better outcomes with CABG surgery.[18,19]

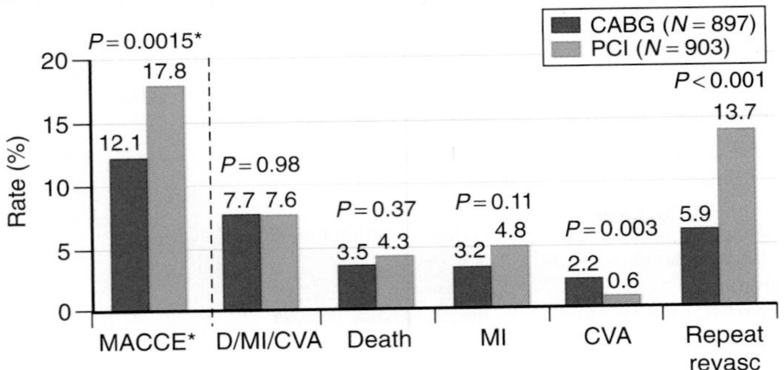

FIGURE 74-7. The SYNTAX trial randomized patients with left main vessel or three-vessel coronary artery disease to coronary artery bypass grafting (CABG) versus percutaneous coronary intervention (PCI). At 12 months, rates of death and myocardial infarction were similar, CABG increased stroke risk (2.2% vs. 0.6%), and PCI resulted in more repeat revascularizations. CVA = cerebrovascular accident, or stroke; MACCE = death, MI, CVA, and repeat revascularization; MI = myocardial infarction; repeat revasc = repeat revascularization. (Data from Serruys PW, Morice MC, Kappetein AP, et al. Percutaneous coronary intervention versus coronary-artery bypass grafting for severe coronary artery disease. *N Engl J Med.* 2009;360:961-972.)

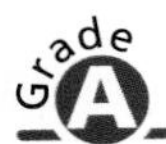

1. Fischman DL, Leon MB, Baim DS, et al. A randomized comparison of coronary-stent placement and balloon angioplasty in the treatment of coronary artery disease. *N Engl J Med.* 1994;331:496-501.
2. Moses JW, Leon MB, Popma JJ, et al. Sirolimus-eluting stents versus standard stents in patients with stenosis in a native coronary artery. *N Engl J Med.* 2003;349:1315-1323.
3. Kastrati A, Mehilli J, Pache J, et al. Analysis of 14 trials comparing sirolimus-eluting stents with bare-metal stents. *N Engl J Med.* 2007;356:1030-1039.
4. Spaulding C, Daemen J, Boersma E, et al. A pooled analysis of data comparing sirolimus-eluting stents with bare-metal stents. *N Engl J Med.* 2007;356:989-997.
5. Stone GW, Rizvi, Newman W, et al. Everolimus-eluting versus paclitaxel-eluting stents in coronary artery disease. *N Engl J Med.* 2010;362:1663-1674.
6. Rasmussen K, Maeng M, Kaltoft A, et al. Efficacy and safety of zotarolimus-eluting and sirolimus-eluting coronary stents in routine clinical care (SORT OUT III): a randomized controlled superiority trial. *Lancet.* 2010:375:1090-1099.
7. Park SJ, Park DW, Kim YH, et al. Duration of dual antiplatelet therapy after implantation of drug-eluting stents. *N Engl J Med.* 2010;362:1374-1382.
8. Boden WE, O'Rourke RA, Teo KK, et al. Optimal medical therapy with or without PCI for stable coronary disease. *N Engl J Med.* 2007;356:1503-1516.
9. Weintraub WS, Spertus JA, Kolm P, et al. Effect of PCI on quality of life in patients with stable coronary artery disease. *N Engl J Med.* 2008;359:677-687.
10. Keeley EC, Boura JA, Grines CL. Primary angioplasty versus intravenous thrombolytic therapy for acute myocardial infarction: a quantitative review of 23 randomised trials. *Lancet.* 2003;361:13-20.
11. Di Mario C, Dudek D, Piscione F, et al. Immediate angioplasty versus standard therapy with rescue angioplasty after thrombolysis in the Combined Abciximab REteplase Stent Study in Acute Myocardial Infarction (CARESS-in-AMI): an open, prospective, randomised, multicentre trial. *Lancet.* 2008;371:559-568.
12. Mehta SR, Granger CB, Boden WE, et al, for the TIMACS Investigators. Early versus delayed invasive intervention in acute coronary syndromes. *N Engl J Med.* 2009;360:2165-2175.
13. O'Donoghue M, Boden WE, Braunwald E, et al. Early invasive vs. conservative treatment strategies in women and men with unstable angina and non-ST-segment elevation myocardial infarction: a meta-analysis. *JAMA.* 2008;300:71-80.
14. Goldman S, Sethi GK, Holman W, et al. Radial artery grafts vs saphenous vein grafts in coronary artery bypass surgery: a randomized trial. *JAMA.* 2011;305:167-174.
15. Shroyer AL, Grover FL, Brack H, et al. On-pump versus off-pump coronary artery bypass surgery. *N Engl J Med.* 2009;361:1827-1837.
16. Serruys PW, Morice MC, Kappetein AP, et al. Percutaneous coronary intervention versus coronary-artery bypass grafting for severe coronary artery disease. *N Engl J Med.* 2009;360:961-972.
17. Hlatky Ma, Boothroyd DB, Bravata DM, et al. Coronary artery bypass surgery compared with percutaneous coronary interventions for multivessel disease: a collaborative analysis of individual patient data from ten randomised trials. *Lancet.* 2009;373;1190-1197.
18. The BARI Investigators. The final 10-year follow-up results from the BARI randomized trial. *J Am Coll Cardiol.* 2007;49:1600-1606.
19. Frye RL, August P, Brooks MM, et al, for the BARI 2D Study Group. A randomized trial of therapies for type 2 diabetes and coronary artery disease. *N Engl J Med.* 2009;360:2503-2515.

SUGGESTED READING

Garg S, Serruys PW. Coronary stents: current status. *J Am Coll Cardiol.* 2010;56:S1-S42. *Review.*

Magro M, Garg S, Serruys PW. Revascularization treatment of stable coronary artery disease. *Expert Opin Pharmacother.* 2011;12:195-212. *Review.*

75

VALVULAR HEART DISEASE

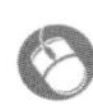

BLASE A. CARABELLO

The cardiac valves permit unobstructed forward blood flow through the heart when they are open while preventing backward flow when they are closed. Most valvular heart diseases cause either valvular stenosis with obstruction to forward flow or valvular regurgitation with backward flow. Valvular stenosis imparts a pressure overload on the left or right ventricle because these chambers must generate higher than normal pressure to overcome the obstruction to pump blood forward. Valvular regurgitation imparts a volume overload on the heart, which now must pump additional volume to compensate for what is regurgitated. When valve disease is severe, these hemodynamic burdens can lead to ventricular dysfunction, heart failure, and sudden death (Table 75-1). In almost every instance, definitive therapy for severe valvular heart disease is mechanical restoration of valve function.

AORTIC STENOSIS

EPIDEMIOLOGY

Bicuspid and Other Congenitally Abnormal Aortic Valves

Approximately 1% of the population is born with a bicuspid aortic valve, with a male preponderance (Chapter 69). Although this abnormality does not usually cause a hemodynamic disturbance at birth, bicuspid aortic valves tend to deteriorate with age. Approximately one third of these valves become stenotic, another third become regurgitant, and the remainder cause only minor hemodynamic abnormalities. When stenosis develops, it usually occurs when patients are in their 40s, 50s, and 60s.

Sometimes, congenital aortic stenosis from a unicuspid, bicuspid, or even abnormal tricuspid valve causes symptoms during childhood and requires correction by adolescence. Occasionally, these congenitally stenotic aortic valves escape detection until adulthood.

Tricuspid Aortic Valve Stenosis

In some patients born with apparently normal tricuspid aortic valves, thickening and calcification develop similar to what occurs in bicuspid valves. When aortic stenosis develops in previously normal tricuspid aortic valves, it usually does so in the 60s to 80s. Although stenosis and calcifications of bicuspid and tricuspid aortic valves were formerly considered to be degenerative processes, it is clear that this type of aortic stenosis arises from an active inflammatory process similar to that of coronary heart disease. This concept is supported by many pieces of evidence. First, the initial lesion of aortic stenosis is similar to the plaque of coronary disease. Second, both diseases have hypertension and hyperlipidemia as risk factors. Third, there is excellent correlation between calcification of the aortic valve and calcification of the coronary arteries. Fourth, patients with the most severe aortic stenosis have the highest levels of C-reactive protein. However, statins, which are so effective in treating coronary disease, have been ineffective in retarding the progression of moderately advanced aortic stenosis.

Rheumatic Valvular Heart Disease

Rheumatic valve disease is now a rare cause of aortic stenosis in developed countries. In virtually every case, the mitral valve is also detectably abnormal.

PATHOBIOLOGY

The normal aortic valve area is 3 to 4 cm^2, and little hemodynamic disturbance occurs until the orifice is reduced to about one third of normal, at which point a systolic gradient develops between the left ventricle and aorta. Left ventricular (LV) and aortic pressures are normally nearly equal during systole. In aortic stenosis, intracavitary LV pressure must increase above aortic pressure, however, to produce forward flow across the stenotic valve and to achieve acceptable downstream pressure (see Fig. 57-2 in Chapter 57). There is a geometric progression in the magnitude of the gradient as the valve area narrows. Given a normal cardiac output, the gradient rises rapidly from 10 to 15 mm Hg at valve areas of 1.5 to 1.3 cm^2 to about 25 mm Hg at 1.0 cm^2, 50 mm Hg at 0.8 cm^2, 70 mm Hg at 0.6 cm^2, and 100 mm Hg at

TABLE 75-1 SUMMARY OF SEVERE VALVAR HEART DISEASE

	AORTIC STENOSIS	MITRAL STENOSIS	MITRAL REGURGITATION	AORTIC REGURGITATION
Etiology	Idiopathic calcification of a bicuspid or tricuspid valve Congenital Rheumatic	Rheumatic fever Annular calcification	Mitral valve prolapse Ruptured chordae Endocarditis Ischemic papillary muscle dysfunction or rupture Collagen vascular diseases and syndromes Secondary to LV myocardial diseases	Annuloaortic ectasia Hypertension Endocarditis Marfan syndrome Ankylosing spondylitis Aortic dissection Syphilis Collagen vascular disease
Pathophysiology	Pressure overload on the LV with compensation by LV hypertrophy As disease advances, reduced coronary flow reserve causes angina. Hypertrophy and afterload excess lead to systolic and diastolic LV dysfunction.	Obstruction to LV inflow increases left atrial pressure and limits cardiac output, thus mimicking LV failure. Mitral valve obstruction increases the pressure work of the right ventricle Right ventricular pressure overload is augmented further when pulmonary hypertension develops.	Places volume overload on the LV. Ventricle responds with eccentric hypertrophy and dilation, which allow increased ventricular stroke volume. Eventually, however, LV dysfunction develops if volume overload is uncorrected.	*Chronic:* Total stroke volume causes hyperdynamic circulation, induces systolic hypertension and causes pressure and volume overload. Compensation is by concentric and eccentric hypertrophy. *Acute:* Because cardiac dilation has not developed, hyperdynamic findings are absent. High diastolic LV pressure causes mitral valve preclosure and potentiates LV ischemia and failure.
Symptoms	Angina Syncope Heart failure	Dyspnea Orthopnea PND Hemoptysis Hoarseness Edema Ascites	Dyspnea Orthopnea PND	Dyspnea Orthopnea PND Angina Syncope
Signs	Systolic ejection murmur radiating to the neck Delayed carotid upstroke S_4, soft or paradoxical S_2	Diastolic rumble after an opening snap Loud S_1 Right ventricular lift Loud P_2	Holosystolic apical murmur radiating to the axilla, S_3 Displaced PMI	*Chronic:* Diastolic blowing murmur Hyperdynamic circulation Displaced PMI Quincke pulse de Musset's sign *Acute:* Short diastolic blowing murmur Soft S_1
Electrocardiogram	LAA LVH	LAA RVH	LAA LVH	LAA LVH
Chest radiograph	Boot-shaped heart Aortic valve calcification on lateral view	Straightening of left heart border Double density at right heart border Kerley B lines Enlarged pulmonary arteries	Cardiac enlargement	*Chronic:* Cardiac enlargement Uncoiling of the aorta *Acute:* Pulmonary congestion with normal heart size
Echocardiographic findings	Concentric LVH Reduced aortic valve cusp separation Doppler shows mean gradient ≥40 mm Hg in most severe cases	Restricted mitral leaflet motion Valve area ≤1 cm^2 in most severe cases Tricuspid Doppler may reveal pulmonary hypertension	LV and LAA in chronic severe disease Doppler: large regurgitant jet	*Chronic:* LV enlargement Large Doppler jet PHT <400 msec *Acute:* Small LV Mitral valve preclosure
Catheterization findings	Increased LVEDP Transaortic gradient 50 mm Hg AVA ≤0.7 in most severe cases	Elevated pulmonary capillary wedge pressure Transmitral gradient usually >10 mm Hg in severe cases MVA <1 cm^2	Elevated pulmonary capillary wedge pressure Ventriculography shows regurgitation of dye into LV	Wide pulse pressure Aortography shows regurgitation of dye into LV Usually unnecessary
Medical therapy	Avoid vasodilators Digitalis, diuretics, and nitroglycerin in inoperable cases	Diuretics for mild symptoms Anticoagulation in atrial fibrillation Digitalis, β-blockers, verapamil, or diltiazem for rate control	Vasodilators in acute disease No proven therapy in chronic disease	*Chronic:* Vasodilators may help in chronic asymptomatic disease with normal left ventricular function. *Acute:* Vasodilators
Indications for surgery	Appearance of symptoms in patients with severe disease (see text)	Appearance of more than mild symptoms Development of pulmonary hypertension Appearance of persistent atrial fibrillation	Appearance of symptoms EF <0.60 ESD ≥40 mm	*Chronic:* Appearance of symptoms EF <0.55 ESD ≥55 mm *Acute:* Even mild heart failure Mitral valve preclosure

AVA = aortic valve area; EF = ejection fraction; ESD = end-systolic diameter; LAA = left atrial enlargement; LV = left ventricle; LVEDP = left ventricular end-diastolic pressure; LVH = left ventricular hypertrophy; MVA = mitral valve area; PHT = pressure half-time; PMI = point of maximal impulse; PND = paroxysmal nocturnal dyspnea; RVH = right ventricular hypertrophy.

0.5 cm^2. The rate of progression of aortic stenosis varies widely from patient to patient; it may remain stable for many years or increase by more than 15 mm Hg per year.

A major compensatory response to the increased LV pressure associated with aortic stenosis is the development of concentric LV hypertrophy. The Laplace equation—stress (s) = pressure (p) × radius (r)/2 × thickness (th)—indicates that the force on any unit of LV myocardium (afterload) varies directly with ventricular pressure and radius and inversely with wall thickness. As pressure increases, it can be offset by increased LV wall thickness (concentric hypertrophy). The determinants of LV ejection fraction are contractility, preload, and afterload. By normalizing afterload, the development of concentric hypertrophy helps preserve ejection fraction and cardiac output despite the pressure overload. Although hypertrophy clearly serves a compensatory function, it also has a pathologic role and is in part responsible for the classic symptoms of aortic stenosis.

Angina

In general, angina (Chapter 71) results from myocardial ischemia when LV oxygen (and other nutrient) demand exceeds supply, which is predicated on coronary blood flow. In normal subjects, coronary blood flow can increase five- to eight-fold under maximum metabolic demand, but in patients with aortic stenosis, this reserve is limited. Reduced coronary blood flow reserve may be caused by a relative diminution in capillary ingrowth to serve the needs of the hypertrophied left ventricle or by a reduced transcoronary gradient for coronary blood flow because of the elevated LV end-diastolic pressure. Restricted coronary blood flow reserve appears to be responsible for angina in many patients who have aortic stenosis despite normal epicardial coronary arteries. In other patients, angina is due to increased oxygen demand when inadequate hypertrophy allows wall stress, a key determinant of myocardial oxygen consumption, to increase.

Syncope

Syncope (Chapters 50 and 62) generally occurs because of inadequate cerebral perfusion. In aortic stenosis, syncope is usually related to exertion. It may result when exertion causes a fall in total peripheral resistance that cannot be compensated by increased cardiac output because output is limited by the obstruction to LV outflow; this combination reduces systemic blood pressure and cerebral perfusion. In addition, high LV pressure during exercise may trigger a systemic vasodepressor response that lowers blood pressure and produces syncope. Cardiac arrhythmias, possibly caused by exertional ischemia, also cause hypotension and syncope.

Heart Failure

In aortic stenosis, contractile dysfunction (systolic failure) and failure of normal relaxation (diastolic failure) occur and cause symptoms (Chapter 58). The extent of ventricular contraction is governed by contractility and afterload. In aortic stenosis, contractility (the ability to generate force) is often reduced. The mechanisms of contractile dysfunction may include abnormal calcium handling, microtubular hyperpolymerization causing an internal viscous load on the myocyte, and myocardial ischemia. In some cases, contractile function is normal, but the hypertrophy is inadequate to normalize wall stress and excessive afterload results. Excessive afterload inhibits ejection, reduces forward output, and leads to heart failure.

The increased wall thickness that helps normalize stress increases diastolic stiffness. Even if muscle properties remain normal, higher filling pressure is required to distend a thicker ventricle. As aortic stenosis advances, collagen deposition also stiffens the myocardium and adds to the diastolic dysfunction.

CLINICAL MANIFESTATIONS

The diagnosis of aortic stenosis is usually first suspected when the classic systolic ejection murmur is heard during physical examination (Chapter 50). The murmur is loudest in the aortic area and radiates to the neck. In some cases, the murmur may disappear over the sternum and reappear over the LV apex, thereby giving the false impression that a murmur of mitral regurgitation is also present (Gallavardin's phenomenon). The intensity of the murmur increases with cycle length because longer cycles are associated with greater aortic flow. In mild disease, the murmur peaks in intensity in early systole or mid-systole. As the severity of stenosis worsens, the murmur peaks progressively later in systole. Perhaps the most helpful clue to the severity of aortic stenosis by physical examination is the characteristic delay in the carotid pulse with a diminution in its volume (see Fig. 50-5 in Chapter 50); in elderly patients, however, increasing carotid stiffness may pseudonormalize the carotid upstrokes. The LV apical impulse in aortic stenosis is not displaced but is enlarged and forceful. The simultaneous palpation of a forceful LV apex beat and a delayed and weakened carotid pulse is a persuasive clue that severe aortic stenosis is present. S_1 in aortic stenosis is generally normal. In congenital aortic stenosis when the valve is not calcified, S_1 may be followed by a systolic ejection click. In calcific disease, S_2 may be single and soft when the aortic component is lost because the valve neither opens nor closes well. In some cases, delayed LV emptying secondary to LV dysfunction may create paradoxical splitting of S_2. An S_4 gallop is common. In advanced disease, pulmonary hypertension and signs of right-sided failure are common.

Because of the dire consequences of missing the diagnosis of aortic stenosis, the physician must have a low threshold for obtaining an echocardiogram whenever aortic stenosis cannot be excluded by physical examination, especially in patients with a history of angina, syncope, or heart failure. In asymptomatic patients with suspicious murmurs, early diagnosis allows the patient and physician to be more vigilant regarding possible early signs and symptoms.

DIAGNOSIS

The electrocardiogram (ECG) in patients with aortic stenosis usually shows LV hypertrophy (Chapter 54). In some cases of even severe aortic stenosis, however, LV hypertrophy is absent on the ECG, possibly because of the lack of LV dilation. Left atrial abnormality is common because the stiff left ventricle increases left atrial afterload and causes the left atrium to dilate.

The chest radiograph in aortic stenosis is generally nondiagnostic. The cardiac silhouette is not usually enlarged but may assume a boot-shaped configuration. In advanced cases, there may be signs of cardiomegaly and pulmonary congestion; aortic valve calcification may be seen in the lateral view.

Echocardiography (Chapter 55) is indispensable to assess the extent of LV hypertrophy, systolic ejection performance, and aortic valve anatomy (Fig. 75-1). Doppler interrogation of the aortic valve makes use of the modified Bernoulli equation (gradient = 4 × $velocity^2$) to assess the severity of the stenosis (Chapter 55). As blood flows from the body of the left ventricle across the stenotic valve, the flow rate must accelerate for the volume to remain constant. Doppler interrogation of the valve can be performed to detect this increase in velocity for estimation of the valve gradient. The peak aortic flow velocity in patients with preserved LV systolic function is a useful clinical guide to prognosis. In patients with a flow velocity of 3.0 mL/second or less, symptoms are unlikely to develop in the next 5 years; by comparison, in patients with a flow velocity of 4.0 mL/second or greater, symptoms usually develop within 2 years.

Although exercise testing is contraindicated in symptomatic patients with aortic stenosis because of the high risk for complications, cautious exercise

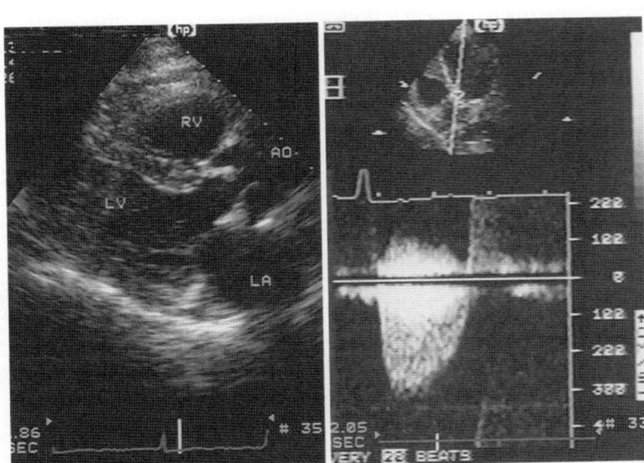

FIGURE 75-1. Doppler echocardiogram from a patient with aortic stenosis. The *left panel* shows thickened aortic valve leaflets that dome into the aorta with restricted opening in systole. The *top right panel* shows a miniaturized apical four-chamber view at the top with a Doppler cursor through the aorta, whereas the *bottom right panel* shows a continuous-wave spectral Doppler signal with a peak velocity of 3 m/sec. The peak valve gradient can be calculated as 4 × 3^2, or 36 mm Hg. AO = aorta; LA = left atrium; LV = left ventricle; RV = right ventricle. (Courtesy of Dr. Anthony DeMaria.)

testing is gaining favor in asymptomatic patients. Such testing often reveals latent symptoms or hemodynamic instability that have gone unrecognized during the patient's normal daily activities. Exercise-induced hypotension or symptoms are indications for aortic valve replacement in patients with severe aortic stenosis; in patients with mild to moderate aortic stenosis, another source of exercise limitation should be sought.

Brain natriuretic peptide levels may be higher in patients who will become symptomatic in a short time span. Levels exceeding 550 pg/mL portend a poor prognosis, but use of this biomarker to indicate the need for valve replacement is still premature.

Cardiac catheterization for performance of coronary arteriography is usually undertaken before surgery because most patients with aortic stenosis are of the age at which coronary disease is common. When echocardiography shows severe aortic stenosis and the patient has one or more of the classic symptoms of the disease, formal invasive documentation of the severity of the stenosis is not necessary, and coronary angiography need not be performed in young adults. When the hemodynamic diagnosis is unclear, however, right-sided and left-sided heart catheterization should be performed to determine the transaortic valvular pressure gradient and cardiac output, which are used to calculate the aortic valve area by the Gorlin formula:

$$A = \frac{CO/SEP \times HR}{44.3\sqrt{h}}$$

where CO is cardiac output (mL/min), SEP is the systolic ejection period (seconds), HR is the heart rate, and h is the mean gradient.

TREATMENT

Rx

Medical Therapy

In asymptomatic patients, no treatment is indicated, nor is any known to be beneficial. Even statins are not useful, despite the similar pathobiology between aortic stenosis and coronary disease.

There also is no accepted effective medical therapy for symptomatic aortic stenosis. In patients with heart failure awaiting surgery, diuretics can be used cautiously to relieve pulmonary congestion. Nitrates may also be used cautiously to treat angina pectoris. Although vasodilators, especially angiotensin-converting enzyme inhibitors, have become a cornerstone of therapy for heart failure, they are not recommended for aortic stenosis. With fixed valvular obstruction to outflow, vasodilation reduces pressure distal to the obstruction without increasing cardiac output and may cause syncope. Statins do not slow the progression of calcific aortic stenosis. When surgery and valvoplasty are unsuccessful or impossible, digitalis and diuretics can be used to improve symptoms with the understanding that they will not improve life expectancy.

Invasive Therapy

Valve Replacement Surgery

The only proven effective therapy for aortic stenosis is aortic valve replacement. Even octogenarians benefit from valve replacement unless other comorbid factors preclude surgery, so aortic valve replacement should not be denied simply on the basis of age. Valve replacement should also not be denied because the ejection fraction is reduced; the excess afterload imposed by the stenotic valve is relieved with valve replacement, and a depressed ejection fraction usually improves dramatically after surgery. The exception to this rule is a severely reduced ejection fraction in the face of only a small aortic valve gradient; in this case, the severity of the aortic stenosis may be overestimated because the failing left ventricle has difficulty opening a mildly to moderately stenotic valve. In such patients, LV muscle dysfunction either has another cause or is often so severe that it does not recover after valve replacement. Evidence indicates, however, that even some well-selected patients in this category, such as patients who demonstrate increased cardiac output during dobutamine infusion, may benefit from aortic valve replacement.

Percutaneous Aortic Valve Replacement

Percutaneous transcatheter aortic valve implantation reduces 1-year mortality by 45% (from 51 to 31%) in patients who have severe aortic stenosis and are too ill to undergo surgery.[1] It also is not inferior to standard valve replacement in high-risk adults.[2] In this procedure, the native valve is dilated, and then a stented valve is inserted over a balloon into the aortic annulus (Fig. 75-2). The balloon is expanded to secure the valve and its stent, which is intended to help prevent restenosis. Two such valves have been approved in Europe, where thousands of patients have already received successful implants.

Balloon Aortic Valvotomy

In acquired calcific aortic stenosis, leaflet restriction results from heavy calcium deposition in the leaflets themselves and is not due to commissural fusion. Balloon aortic valvotomy is relatively ineffective in improving aortic stenosis; it generally results in a residual gradient of 30 to 50 mm Hg and a valve area of 1.0 cm^2. Mortality after this procedure is similar to that in untreated patients. The only occasional indication for balloon aortic valvotomy is palliative in cases in which aortic valve replacement is impossible because of comorbidity or is impractical when immediate temporary relief is required because of the demands of other noncardiac conditions.

PROGNOSIS

In asymptomatic patients with normally functioning or minimally dysfunctional bicuspid aortic valves, survival is similar to age-matched controls, and sudden death is rare, occurring in less than 1% of asymptomatic patients. However, 27% of patients require surgery by 20 years after diagnosis. In adults with asymptomatic but hemodynamically significant aortic stenosis, symptoms typically develop within 5 years. A higher peak aortic-jet velocity and high β-type natriuretic peptide levels predict a worse prognosis.

The progression of mild to moderate aortic stenosis to severe disease is the key to the natural history of the disease and is quite variable. Aortic stenosis may remain mild for a decade or more in some patients, whereas in others, it may progress to severe disease in as little as 5 years.

When symptoms develop, survival declines precipitously. Approximately 35% of patients with aortic stenosis are initially evaluated for angina. Of these, 50% are dead in 5 years unless aortic valve replacement is performed. Approximately 15% have syncope; of these, 50% are dead in only 3 years unless the aortic valve is replaced. Of the 50% with symptoms of heart failure, 50% are dead in 2 years without aortic valve replacement. In all, only 25% of patients with symptomatic aortic stenosis survive 3 years in the absence of valve replacement, and the annual risk for sudden death ranges from 10% in patients with angina to 15% with syncope to 25% with heart failure.

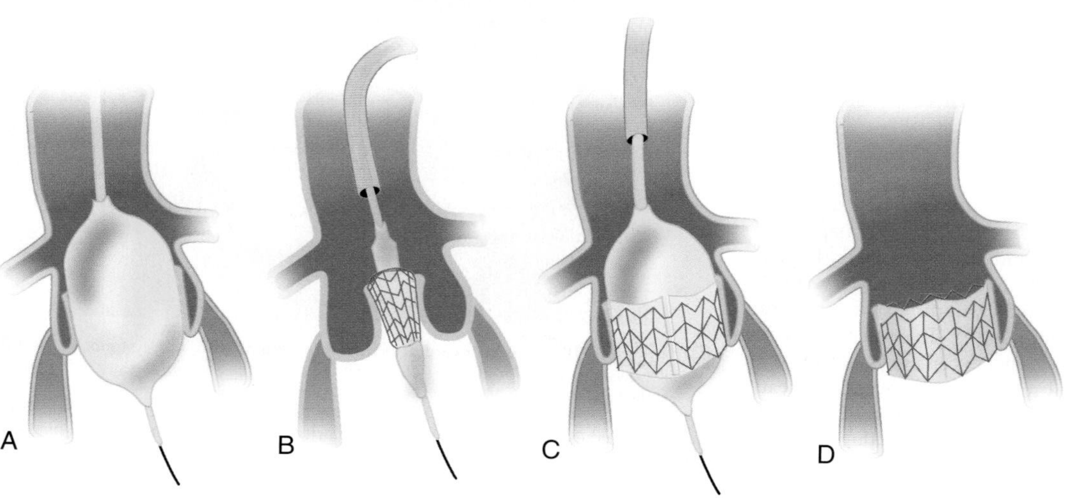

FIGURE 75-2. Steps for percutaneous balloon valvotomy. A, Dilation of the native stenotic valve. **B,** A crimped stented valve has been inserted over a guidewire into the aortic annulus. **C,** Inflation of the balloon deploys the valve. **D,** The balloon is deflated and removed with the aortic valve replaced. (Modified from http://my.clevelandclinic.org/heart/percutaneous/percutaneousValve.aspx.)

After valve replacement surgery, prognosis improves to near normal, especially for patients older than 65 years at the time of valve implantation, presumably because older patients have fewer years at risk for valve-related complications.

MITRAL STENOSIS

EPIDEMIOLOGY

In almost all cases of acquired mitral stenosis, the cause is rheumatic heart disease. Occasionally, severe calcification of the mitral annulus can lead to mitral stenosis in the absence of rheumatic involvement. Mitral stenosis is three times more common in women and usually develops in the 40s and 50s. Although the disease has become rare in developed countries because of the waning incidence of rheumatic fever, mitral stenosis is still prevalent in developing nations, where rheumatic fever is common.

PATHOBIOLOGY

At the beginning of diastole, a transient gradient between the left atrium and left ventricle normally initiates LV filling. After early filling, left atrial and LV pressures equilibrate. In mitral stenosis, obstruction to LV filling increases left atrial pressure and produces a persistent gradient between the left atrium and the left ventricle (see Fig. 57-2 in Chapter 57). The combination of elevated left atrial pressure (and pulmonary venous pressure) and restriction of inflow into the left ventricle limits cardiac output. Although myocardial involvement from the rheumatic process occasionally affects LV muscle function, the muscle itself is normal in most patients with mitral stenosis. However, in approximately one third of patients with mitral stenosis, LV ejection performance is reduced despite normal muscle function because of reduced preload (from inflow obstruction) and increased afterload as a result of reflex vasoconstriction caused by reduced cardiac output.

Because the right ventricle generates most of the force that propels blood across the mitral valve, the right ventricle incurs the pressure overload of the transmitral gradient. In addition, secondary but reversible pulmonary vasoconstriction develops, thus further increasing pulmonary artery pressure and the burden on the right ventricle. As mitral stenosis worsens, right ventricular (RV) failure develops.

CLINICAL MANIFESTATIONS

Patients with mitral stenosis usually remain asymptomatic until the valve area is reduced to about one third its normal size of 4 to 5 cm^2. Then the symptoms typical of left-sided failure—dyspnea on exertion, orthopnea, and paroxysmal nocturnal dyspnea—develop. As the disease progresses and RV failure occurs, ascites and edema are common. Hemoptysis, which is common in mitral stenosis but uncommon in other causes of left atrial hypertension, develops when high left atrial pressure ruptures the anastomoses of small bronchial veins. In some cases, a large left atrium may impinge on the left recurrent laryngeal nerve and cause hoarseness (Ortner's syndrome) or may impinge on the esophagus and cause dysphagia.

Physical Examination

Although mitral stenosis produces typical and diagnostic findings on physical examination, the diagnosis is missed frequently because the auscultatory findings may be subtle. Palpation of the precordium finds a quiet apical impulse. If pulmonary hypertension and RV hypertrophy have developed, the examiner notes a parasternal lift. S_1 is typically loud and may be the most prominent physical finding of the disease. A loud S_1 is present because the transmitral gradient holds the mitral valve open throughout diastole until ventricular systole closes the fully opened valve with a loud closing sound. In far-advanced disease, the mitral valve may be so damaged, however, that it neither opens nor closes well, so S_1 may become soft. S_2 is normally split; the pulmonic component is increased in intensity if pulmonary hypertension has developed. Left-sided S_3 and S_4 gallop sounds, which represent the ventricular and atrial components of rapid LV filling, are exceedingly rare in mitral stenosis because obstruction at the mitral valve prevents rapid filling. S_2 is usually followed by an opening snap. The distance between S_2 and the opening snap provides a reasonable estimation of left atrial pressure and the severity of the mitral stenosis. The higher the left atrial pressure, the sooner the left atrial pressure and the falling LV pressure of early ventricular relaxation equilibrate. At this equilibration point, the mitral valve opens, and the opening snap occurs. When left atrial pressure is high, the opening snap closely (0.06 second) follows S_2. Conversely, when left atrial pressure is relatively normal, the snap occurs later (0.12 second) and may mimic the cadence of an S_3 gallop. The opening snap is followed by the classic low-pitched early diastolic mitral stenosis rumble, which increases in length as the mitral stenosis worsens. This murmur may be inaudible if the patient has a relatively low resting cardiac output. Modest exercise, such as isometric handgrip, may accentuate the murmur's intensity. If the patient is in sinus rhythm, atrial systole may produce a presystolic accentuation of the murmur. If pulmonary hypertension has developed, the pulmonic component of S_2 increases in intensity to become as loud or louder than the aortic component. With pulmonary hypertension, a diastolic blowing murmur of pulmonary insufficiency (Graham Steell's murmur) is often heard, although in many cases, a coexistent murmur of mild aortic insufficiency is mistaken for this murmur. Neck vein elevation, ascites, and edema are present if RV failure has developed.

DIAGNOSIS

If the patient is in sinus rhythm, left atrial abnormality is generally present on the ECG. Atrial fibrillation is common, however. If pulmonary hypertension has developed, there is often evidence of RV hypertrophy.

On the chest radiograph, left atrial enlargement produces straightening of the left heart border and a double density at the right heart border as a result of the combined silhouettes of the right atrium and left atrium. Pulmonary venous hypertension produces increased vascularity. Kerley B lines, which represent thickening of the pulmonary septa secondary to chronic venous engorgement, may also be seen.

The echocardiogram produces excellent images of the mitral valve and is the most important diagnostic tool in confirming the diagnosis (Fig. 75-3). Transthoracic echocardiography or, if necessary, transesophageal echocardiography makes the diagnosis in nearly 100% of cases and accurately assesses severity. Mitral stenosis, similar to aortic stenosis, can be quantified by assessing the transvalvular gradient with the modified Bernoulli principle. The stenosis is considered mild when the calculated or planimetered valve area is more than 1.75 cm^2, moderate at 1.25 to 1.75 cm^2, moderately severe at 1.0 to 1.25 cm^2, and severe at less than 1.0 cm^2.

During echocardiography, the suitability of the valve for balloon valvotomy can also be assessed (see later). If even mild tricuspid regurgitation is present, the systolic gradient across the tricuspid valve can be used to gauge pulmonary artery pressure, which is an important prognostic factor in mitral stenosis because the prognosis worsens as pulmonary pressure increases.

Invasive Evaluation

Cardiac Catheterization

Cardiac catheterization is usually unnecessary to assess the severity of mitral stenosis. Because many patients with mitral stenosis are of an age when coronary disease might be present, however, coronary arteriography is generally performed if cardiac surgery is anticipated or if the patient has coexistent angina. In these cases, it is common to perform left-sided and right-sided heart catheterization to confirm the transmitral gradient and to calculate the valve area from the Gorlin formula (see earlier).

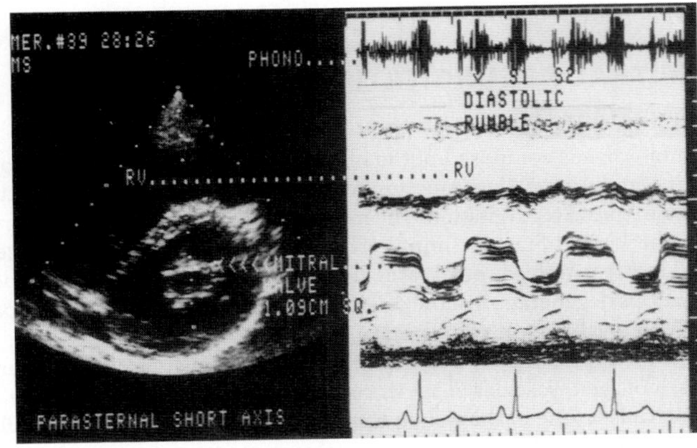

FIGURE 75-3. Mitral stenosis. An en face view of a stenotic mitral valve in the short-axis view of the left ventricle is shown on the *left*. Planimetry for the mitral valve orifice yielded an area of 1.09 cm^2. The M-mode echocardiogram on the *right* has been aligned with the appropriate structures on the *left*. It shows the restricted opening of the mitral valve in diastole associated with the classic diastolic rumbling murmur. RV = right ventricle. (From Assey ME, Usher BW, Carabello BA. The patient with valvular heart disease. In: Pepine CJ, Hill JA, Lambert CR, eds. *Diagnostic and Therapeutic Cardiac Catheterization,* 3rd ed. Baltimore: Williams & Wilkins; 1998:709.)

PREVENTION, TREATMENT, AND PROGNOSIS (Rx)

Mitral stenosis can be prevented by appropriate antibiotic treatment of β-hemolytic streptococcal infections (Chapter 298).

Medical Therapy

Asymptomatic patients with mitral stenosis and sinus rhythm require no therapy. Symptoms of mild dyspnea and orthopnea can be treated with diuretics alone. When symptoms worsen to more than mild or if pulmonary hypertension develops, mechanical correction of the stenosis is preferable to medical therapy because it improves longevity in severely symptomatic patients.

Patients with mitral stenosis in whom atrial fibrillation develops usually decompensate because the rapid heart rate reduces diastolic filling time, increases left atrial pressure, and decreases cardiac output. The heart rate must be controlled promptly, preferably with an infusion of diltiazem or esmolol for acute atrial fibrillation or with a β-blocker, a calcium-channel blocker, or oral digoxin in chronic atrial fibrillation (Chapter 64).

Conversion to sinus rhythm is routinely recommended either pharmacologically or with direct-current countershock (Chapter 64) after anticoagulation is therapeutic. It should be noted that patients with rheumatic atrial fibrillation have been excluded from trials of echocardiogram-guided cardioversion without anticoagulation and trials of rate control versus rhythm control for the chronic management of atrial fibrillation. If sinus rhythm cannot be maintained, mechanical therapy for the mitral stenosis is generally recommended in the hope that sinus rhythm can be restored after the obstruction to atrial outflow is corrected. However, the cause of atrial fibrillation in patients with mitral stenosis probably includes atrial rheumatic inflammation, so restoration of sinus rhythm is unpredictable even after mechanical intervention.

Because patients with concomitant mitral stenosis and atrial fibrillation have an extraordinarily high risk for systemic embolism, they should undergo chronic anticoagulation with warfarin at an international normalized ratio (INR) target of 2.5 to 3.5. Anticoagulation is warranted in all patients unless there is a serious contraindication to its use.

Mechanical Therapy

When symptoms progress past early functional class II, that is, symptoms with more than ordinary activity, or if pulmonary hypertension develops, the prognosis is worse unless the mitral stenosis is relieved. In most instances, an excellent result can be achieved with percutaneous balloon valvotomy. In contrast to aortic stenosis, in mitral stenosis there is fusion of the valve leaflets at the commissures. Balloon dilation produces a commissurotomy and a substantial increase in valve area that appears to persist for at least a decade and provides improvement comparable to that of closed or open commissurotomy in suitable patients. Suitability for balloon valvotomy is determined partially during echocardiography. Patients with pliable valves, little valvular calcification, little involvement of the subvalvular apparatus, and less than moderate mitral regurgitation are ideal candidates. Even when valve anatomy is not ideal, however, valvotomy may be attempted in patients with advanced age or in situations in which comorbid risk factors increase surgical risk. In otherwise healthy patients with unfavorable valve anatomy, surgery to perform an open commissurotomy or valve replacement is undertaken.

MITRAL REGURGITATION

EPIDEMIOLOGY

The mitral valve is composed of the mitral annulus, the leaflets, the chordae tendineae, and the papillary muscles. Abnormalities in any of these structures may lead to mitral regurgitation. The most common cause of mitral regurgitation in the United States is mitral valve prolapse, which is responsible for approximately two thirds of all cases and comprises many diseases, including myxomatous degeneration of the valve. Myocardial ischemia leading to papillary muscle dysfunction or infarction is the next most common cause and accounts for approximately a fourth of all cases. Annular calcification, endocarditis, collagen vascular disease, and rheumatic heart disease are less common causes. Use of the weight loss agents dexfenfluramine and fenfluramine has been implicated in causing valve damage in a few patients who received these drugs.

Mitral regurgitation can be subdivided on the basis of chronicity. Common causes of severe acute mitral regurgitation include ruptured chordae tendineae, ischemic papillary muscle dysfunction or rupture, and infective endocarditis. Chronic severe mitral regurgitation is more likely to be due to myxomatous degeneration of the valve, rheumatic heart disease, or annular calcification.

PATHOBIOLOGY

The pathophysiology of mitral regurgitation can be divided into three phases (Fig. 75-4). In acute mitral regurgitation of any cause, the sudden option for ejection of blood into the left atrium "wastes" a portion of the LV stroke volume as backward rather than forward flow. The combined regurgitant and forward flow causes volume overload of the left ventricle and stretches the existing sarcomeres toward their maximum length. Use of the Frank-Starling mechanism is maximized, and end-diastolic volume increases concomitantly. The regurgitant pathway unloads the left ventricle in systole because it allows ejection into the relatively low-impedance left atrium and thereby reduces end-systolic volume. Although increased end-diastolic volume and decreased

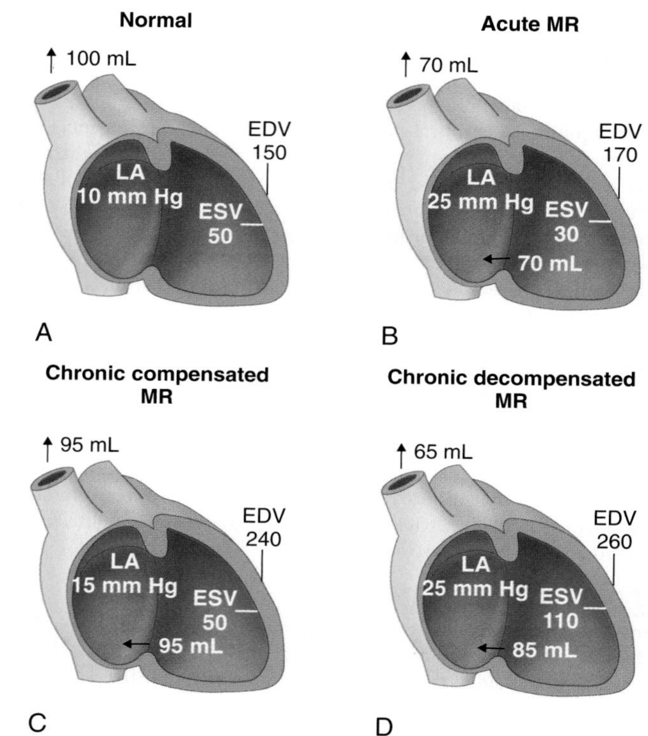

	Preload SL (μ)	Afterload ESS (kdyne/cm^2)	CF	EF	RF	FSV (mL)
N	2.07	90	N	.67	.0	100
AMR	2.25	60	N	.82	.50	70
CCMR	2.19	90	N	.79	.5	95
CDMR	2.19	120	↓	.58	.57	65

FIGURE 75-4. Mitral regurgitation. A and **B,** Normal physiology (N) **(A)** is compared with the physiology of acute mitral regurgitation (AMR) **(B).** Acutely, the volume overload increases preload (sarcomere length [SL]), and end-diastolic volume (EDV) increases from 150 to 170 mL. Unloading of the left ventricle by the presence of the regurgitant pathway decreases afterload (end-systolic stress [ESS]), and end-systolic volume (ESV) falls from 50 to 30 mL. These changes result in an increase in the ejection fraction (EF). Because 50% of the total left ventricular (LV) stroke volume (regurgitant fraction [RF]) is ejected into the left atrium (LA), however, forward stroke volume (FSV) falls from 100 to 70 mL. At this stage, contractile function (CF) is normal. **C,** Chronic compensated mitral regurgitation (CCMR). In CCMR, eccentric cardiac hypertrophy has developed, and EDV has increased substantially. Increased EDV, combined with normal contractile function, permits ejection of a larger total stroke volume and a larger forward stroke volume than in the acute phase. Left atrial enlargement permits lower left atrial pressure. Because the radius term in the Laplace equation has increased with increasing LV volume, afterload and ESV return to normal. **D,** Chronic decompensated mitral regurgitation (CDMR). In this stage, contractile dysfunction causes a large increase in ESV with a fall in total and forward stroke volume. Additional LV enlargement leads to worsening mitral regurgitation. The relatively favorable loading conditions in this phase still permit a normal EF, however, despite contractile dysfunction. (From Carabello BA. Mitral regurgitation: basic pathophysiologic principles. *Mod Concepts Cardiovasc Dis.* 1988;57:53-57.)

end-systolic volume act in concert to increase total stroke volume, forward stroke volume is subnormal because a large portion of the total stroke volume is regurgitated into the left atrium. This regurgitant volume increases left atrial pressure, so the patient experiences heart failure with low cardiac output and pulmonary congestion despite normal LV contractile function.

In many cases, severe acute mitral regurgitation necessitates emergency surgical correction. Patients who can be managed through the acute phase may enter the phase of compensation. In this phase, eccentric LV hypertrophy and increased end-diastolic volume, combined with normal contractile function, allow ejection of a sufficiently large total stroke volume to permit forward stroke volume to return toward normal. Left atrial enlargement allows accommodation of the regurgitant volume at a lower filling pressure. In this phase, the patient may be relatively asymptomatic even during strenuous exercise.

Although severe mitral regurgitation may be tolerated for many years, the lesion often causes LV dysfunction, atrial fibrillation, or heart failure within 5 years of the detection of severe mitral regurgitation. The now damaged ventricle has impaired ejection performance, and end-systolic volume increases. Greater LV residual volume at end systole increases end-diastolic volume and end-diastolic pressure, and the symptoms of pulmonary congestion may reappear. Additional LV dilation may worsen the amount of regurgitation by causing further enlargement of the mitral annulus and malalignment of the papillary muscles. Although there is substantial contractile dysfunction, the increased preload and the presence of the regurgitant pathway, which tends to normalize afterload despite ventricular enlargement, augment the ejection fraction and may maintain it in a relatively normal range.

The causes of LV contractile dysfunction in patients with mitral regurgitation may relate to loss of contractile proteins and abnormalities in calcium handling. In at least some cases, contractile dysfunction is reversible by timely mitral valve replacement.

CLINICAL MANIFESTATIONS

In the medical history, the standard symptoms of left-sided heart failure should be sought (Chapter 58). An attempt to discover potential causes should be made by questioning for a prior history of a heart murmur or abnormal findings on cardiac examination (Chapter 50), rheumatic heart disease, endocarditis (Chapter 76), myocardial infarction (Chapter 73), or the use of anorexigenic drugs.

Volume overload of the left ventricle displaces the apical impulse downward and to the left. S_1 may be reduced in intensity, whereas S_2 is usually physiologically split. In severe mitral regurgitation, S_2 is followed by S_3, which does not indicate heart failure but reflects rapid filling of the left ventricle by the large volume of blood stored in the left atrium during systole. The typical murmur of mitral regurgitation is a holosystolic apical murmur that often radiates toward the axilla (Chapter 50). There is a rough correlation between the intensity of the murmur and the severity of the disease, but this correlation is too weak to use in clinical decision making because the murmur may be soft when cardiac output is low. In contrast to aortic stenosis, murmur intensity does not usually vary with the RR interval. In acute mitral regurgitation, the presence of a large v wave may produce rapid equilibration of left atrial and LV pressure, thereby reducing the driving gradient and shortening the murmur. Pulmonary hypertension may develop and produce right-sided signs, including an RV lift, an increased P_2, and if RV dysfunction has developed, signs of right-sided heart failure.

DIAGNOSIS

The ECG usually shows LV hypertrophy and left atrial abnormality. The chest radiograph typically shows cardiomegaly; the absence of cardiomegaly indicates either that the mitral regurgitation is mild or that it has not been chronic enough to allow cardiac dilation to occur.

Echocardiography shows the extent of left atrial and LV enlargement (Chapter 55). Ultrasonic imaging of the mitral valve is excellent and offers clues to the mitral valve abnormalities responsible for the regurgitation. In some patients, three-dimensional echocardiography can add pathoanatomic information of potential use in aiding surgical repair of the valve. Color flow Doppler interrogation of the valve (Fig. 75-5) helps assess the severity of regurgitation, but because this technique images flow velocity rather than actual flow, it is subject to errors in interpretation. The Doppler technique is excellent for excluding the presence of mitral regurgitation and for distinguishing between mild and severe degrees. Although newer techniques may quantify regurgitation more precisely, they are not yet in widespread use, and standard color flow Doppler examination may not be sufficient for exact quantification of mitral regurgitation or to determine whether the severity of the lesion is sufficient to cause eventual LV dysfunction. When the severity of mitral regurgitation is in doubt or if mitral valve surgery is being contemplated, cardiac catheterization (Chapter 57) is helpful in resolving the severity of the lesion; coronary arteriography should be included in patients older than 40 years or with symptoms suggesting coronary disease (Chapter 71).

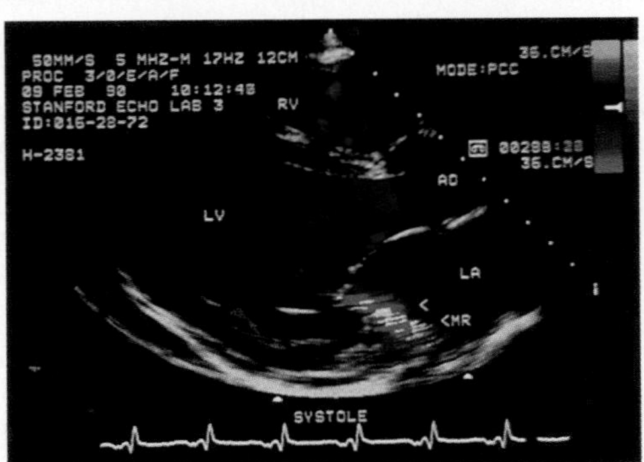

FIGURE 75-5. Two-dimensional echocardiogram of mitral regurgitation with Doppler flow mapping superimposed on a portion of the image. The color information is represented in the sector of the imaging plane extending from the apex of the triangular plane to the *two small arrows* at the *bottom* of the image plane. Mitral regurgitation (MR) is indicated (*open arrows*) and extends from the mitral valve leaflets toward the posterior aspect of the left atrium (LA) during systole. The mosaic of colors representing the mitral regurgitant signal is typical of high-velocity turbulent flow. The low-intensity *orange-brown* signal represents flow directed away from the transducer on the chest wall, and the *blue* shades represent blood in the left ventricular outflow tract moving toward the transducer. AO = aorta; LV = left ventricle; RV = right ventricle.

TREATMENT AND PROGNOSIS

Rx

Medical Therapy

Severe Acute Mitral Regurgitation

In severe acute mitral regurgitation, the patient is usually symptomatic with heart failure or even shock. The goal of medical therapy is to increase forward cardiac output while concomitantly reducing regurgitant volume (Chapter 59). Arterial vasodilators reduce systemic resistance to flow and preferentially increase aortic outflow and simultaneously decrease the amount of mitral regurgitation and left atrial hypertension. If hypotension already exists, vasodilators such as nitroprusside lower blood pressure further and cannot be used. In these cases, intra-aortic balloon counterpulsation (Chapter 107) is preferred if the aortic valve is competent. Counterpulsation increases forward cardiac output by lowering ventricular afterload while augmenting systemic diastolic pressure.

Chronic Symptomatic Mitral Regurgitation

In patients with *symptomatic* mitral regurgitation, angiotensin-converting enzyme inhibitors (such as lisinopril, 20 mg per day) reduce LV volume and improve symptoms. Mitral valve surgery rather than medical therapy is generally preferred, however, in most symptomatic patients with mitral regurgitation. When atrial fibrillation is present, long-term anticoagulation should achieve the same INR goal as for mitral stenosis.

Chronic Asymptomatic Mitral Regurgitation

Vasodilators have had little effect in reducing LV volume or improving normal exercise tolerance in patients with mitral regurgitation, perhaps because afterload is not usually increased in those with chronic asymptomatic mitral regurgitation. There is no definitive indication to begin afterload reduction before symptoms appear because no large randomized trials have been performed, and smaller trials have generally shown no benefit from these therapies.

Surgical Therapy

The timing of mitral valve surgery must weigh the risks of the operation and placement of a prosthesis, if one is inserted, against the risk for irreversible LV dysfunction if surgery is delayed unwisely. For most other types of valve diseases, surgical correction usually requires placement of a prosthetic valve, but in patients with mitral regurgitation, the native valve can often be repaired. Because conservation of the native valve obviates the risks associated with a prosthesis, the option of mitral valve repair should influence the patient and physician toward earlier surgery.

Types of Mitral Valve Surgery

Mitral Valve Repair

When feasible, mitral valve repair (Fig. 75-6) is the preferred operation. Repair restores valve competence, maintains the functional aspects of the apparatus, and avoids the insertion of a prosthesis. Repair is most applicable in cases of posterior chordal rupture; anterior involvement and rheumatic involvement make repair more difficult. Currently, the percentage of mitral valve surgeries that are valve repair varies from 0 to 95% at different hospital centers, averaging about 60% across the United States overall. Percutaneous mitral valve repair with implantation of a clip device is less effective than conventional mitral valve repair for reducing the amount of mitral regurgitation but is safer and provides equivalent clinical benefit.[3] In all cases, the feasibility of repair depends on the pathoanatomy that is causing the mitral regurgitation and the skill and experience of the operating surgeon.

Mitral Valve Replacement with Preservation of the Mitral Apparatus

In this procedure, a prosthetic valve is inserted, but continuity between the native leaflets and the papillary muscles is maintained. This procedure has the advantage of ensuring mitral valve competence while preserving the LV functional aspects of the mitral apparatus. Even if only the posterior leaflets and chordae are preserved, the patient benefits from improved postoperative ventricular function and better survival. In many cases, it is possible to preserve the anterior and posterior chordal attachments, although anterior continuity can be associated with LV outflow tract obstruction. Although the patient benefits from restored mitral valve competence and maintenance of LV function, insertion of a prosthesis still carries all prosthesis-associated risks.

Mitral Valve Replacement without Preservation of the Mitral Apparatus

When the native valve cannot be repaired or the chordae preserved, such as in severe rheumatic deformity, the mitral valve leaflets and its apparatus are removed, and a prosthetic valve is inserted. Although this operation almost guarantees mitral valve competence, the mitral valve apparatus is responsible for coordinating LV contraction and for helping maintain the efficient prolate ellipsoid shape of the left ventricle. Destruction of the apparatus leads to a sudden fall in LV function and a decline in postoperative ejection fraction that is often permanent.

Timing of Surgery

Symptomatic Patients

Most patients with symptoms of dyspnea, orthopnea, or fatigue should undergo surgery regardless of which operation is performed because they already have lifestyle limitations from their disease. The mere presence of symptoms may worsen the prognosis despite relatively well-preserved LV function. The onset or worsening of symptoms is a summary of the patient's pathophysiology and may give a broader view of cardiovascular integrity than possible with any single measurement of pressure or function.

Asymptomatic Patients with Normal Left Ventricular Function

Surgery has increasingly been considered in asymptomatic patients who have normal LV function but echocardiographic findings indicating that valve *repair* is likely to be successful. Although these patients are at low risk without surgery, the risk associated with valve repair is less than 1%, and this approach avoids the risks of later valve *replacement*, which may be required if the valvular disease progresses. Valve repair obviates the need for protracted, expensive follow-up and provides a durable correction of the lesion. This approach is sensible, however, only if it is certain that valve repair can be performed because insertion of a prosthesis carries unacceptable risk in this low-risk group.

Asymptomatic Patients with Left Ventricular Dysfunction

The onset of LV dysfunction in patients with mitral regurgitation may occur without causing symptoms. Early surgery is warranted to prevent the muscle dysfunction from becoming severe or irreversible. Regardless of whether valve repair or replacement is eventually performed, survival is prolonged to or toward normal if surgery is performed before the ejection fraction declines to less than 0.60 or before the left ventricle is unable to contract to an end-systolic dimension of 40 mm. Patients with severe mitral regurgitation should be monitored yearly with a history, physical examination, and echocardiographic evaluation of LV function. When the patient reports symptoms or echocardiography shows the onset of LV dysfunction, surgery should be undertaken.

Asymptomatic Elderly Patients

Patients older than 75 years may have poorer surgical results than younger patients, especially if coronary disease is present or if mitral valve replacement rather than repair must be performed. However, results of surgery in older patients with mitral regurgitation have steadily improved during the past decade, and elderly patients with symptoms refractory to medical therapy may benefit from surgery. Nevertheless, there is little compelling reason to commit elderly *asymptomatic* patients to a mitral valve operation.

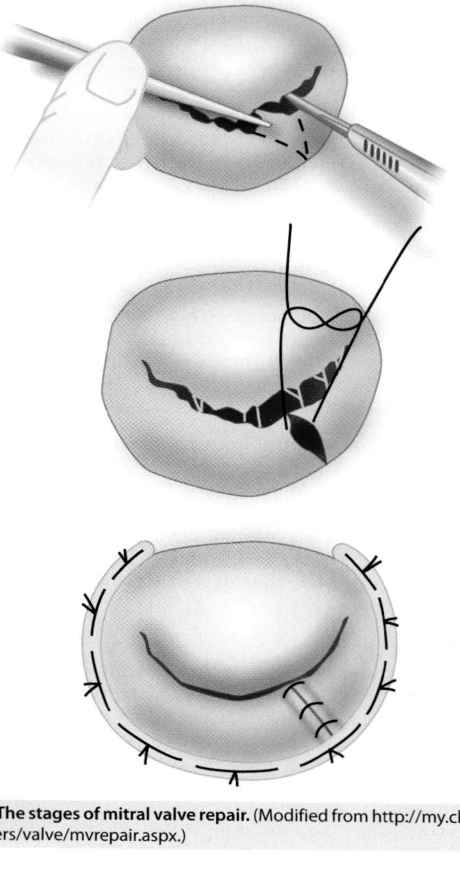

FIGURE 75-6. The stages of mitral valve repair. (Modified from http://my.clevelandclinic.org/heart/disorders/valve/mvrepair.aspx.)

MITRAL VALVE PROLAPSE

DEFINITION

Mitral valve prolapse occurs when one or both of the mitral valve leaflets prolapse into the left atrium superior to the mitral valve annular plane during systole. The importance of mitral valve prolapse varies from patient to patient. In some cases, prolapse is simply a consequence of normal LV physiology without significant medical impact, such as in situations that produce a small left ventricle (e.g., the Valsalva maneuver or an atrial septal defect), in which reduction of ventricular volume causes relative lengthening of the chordae tendineae and subsequent mitral valve prolapse. At the other end of the spectrum, severe redundancy and deformity of the valve, which occurs in myxomatous valve degeneration, increases the risk for stroke, arrhythmia, endocarditis, and progression to severe mitral regurgitation.

DIAGNOSIS

History

Most patients with mitral valve prolapse are asymptomatic. In some cases, however, mitral valve prolapse is associated with symptoms, including palpitations, syncope, and chest pain. In some cases, chest pain is associated with a positive thallium scintigram indicating the presence of true ischemia despite normal epicardial coronary arteries, perhaps because excessive tension on the papillary muscles increases oxygen consumption and causes ischemia. Palpitations, syncope, and presyncope, when present, are linked to autonomic dysfunction (Chapters 50, 62, and 427), which appears to be more prevalent in patients with mitral valve prolapse.

Physical Examination

On physical examination, the mitral valve prolapse syndrome produces the characteristic findings of a midsystolic click and a late systolic murmur. The click occurs when the chordae tendineae are stretched taut by the prolapsing mitral valve in mid-systole. As this occurs, the mitral leaflets move past their coaptation point, permit mitral regurgitation, and cause the late systolic murmur (see Table 50-7 in Chapter 50). Maneuvers that make the left ventricle smaller, such as the Valsalva maneuver, cause the click to appear earlier and the murmur to be more holosystolic and often louder (see Table 50-8 in Chapter 50). In some cases of echocardiographically proven mitral valve prolapse, neither the click nor the murmur is present; in other cases, only one of these findings is present.

Noninvasive Evaluation

Echocardiography is useful to prove that prolapse is present, to image the amount of regurgitation and its physiologic effects, and to discern the pathoanatomy of the mitral valve. Although an echocardiogram is not necessary to diagnose prolapse in patients with the classic physical findings, the echocardiogram adds significant prognostic information because it can detect patients who have specifically abnormal valve morphology and in whom most of the complications of the disease occur.

In the 1990s, it became clear that the mitral annulus did not exist in a single plane but had a saddleback shape. Prolapse shown in the four-chamber echocardiographic view should be confirmed in the parasternal long-axis view. Echocardiographic diagnoses made before the understanding that the mitral valve plane was multidimensional (circa 1987) may have been made in error.

TREATMENT Rx

Because most cases of mitral valve prolapse are asymptomatic, therapy is unnecessary. Although prophylaxis against infective endocarditis was previously recommended in these patients, guidelines no longer recommend antibiotic prophylaxis based on available data (Chapter 76). In patients with palpitations and autonomic dysfunction, β-blockers are often effective in relieving symptoms. Low-dose aspirin therapy has been recommended for patients with redundant leaflets because these patients have a slightly increased risk for stroke. No data from large studies are available to support this contention, however. If severe mitral regurgitation develops, the therapy is the same as for other causes of mitral regurgitation.

PROGNOSIS

Most patients with mitral valve prolapse have a benign clinical course; even for complication-prone patients with redundant and misshapen mitral leaflets, complications are relatively rare. Approximately 10% of patients with thickened leaflets experience infective endocarditis, stroke, progression to severe mitral regurgitation, or sudden death. The progression to severe mitral regurgitation varies with gender and age, and men are approximately twice as likely to progress as women. By 50 years of age, only approximately 1 in 200 men requires surgery to correct mitral regurgitation. By the age of 70 years, the risk increases to approximately 3%.

AORTIC REGURGITATION

DEFINITION

Aortic regurgitation is caused either by abnormalities of the aortic leaflets or by abnormalities of the proximal aortic root. Leaflet abnormalities causing aortic regurgitation include a bicuspid aortic valve, infective endocarditis, and rheumatic heart disease; anorexigenic drugs have also been implicated. Common aortic root abnormalities that cause aortic regurgitation include Marfan syndrome (Chapter 268), hypertension-induced annuloaortic ectasia, aortic dissection (Chapter 78), syphilis (Chapter 327), ankylosing spondylitis (Chapter 273), and psoriatic arthritis (Chapter 273). Acute aortic regurgitation is usually caused by infective endocarditis (Chapter 76) or aortic dissection.

PATHOBIOLOGY

As with mitral regurgitation, aortic regurgitation imparts a volume overload on the left ventricle because the left ventricle must pump the forward flow entering from the left atrium and the regurgitant volume returning through the incompetent aortic valve. Also as with mitral regurgitation, the volume overload is compensated for by the development of eccentric cardiac hypertrophy, which increases chamber size and allows the ventricle to pump a greater total stroke volume and a greater forward stroke volume. Ventricular enlargement also allows the left ventricle to accommodate the volume overload at a lower filling pressure. In contrast to mitral regurgitation, the entire stroke volume is ejected into the aorta in aortic regurgitation. Because pulse pressure is proportional to stroke volume and elastance of the aorta, the increased stroke volume increases systolic pressure. Systolic hypertension leads to afterload excess, which does not generally occur in mitral regurgitation. Ventricular geometry also differs between mitral and aortic regurgitation because the afterload excess in aortic regurgitation causes a modest element of concentric hypertrophy, as well as severe eccentric hypertrophy.

In acute aortic insufficiency, such as might occur in infective endocarditis, severe volume overload of the previously unprepared left ventricle results in a sudden fall in forward output while precipitously increasing LV filling pressure. It is probably this combination of pathophysiologic factors that leads to rapid decompensation, presumably because the severely diminished gradient for coronary blood flow causes ischemia and progressive deterioration in LV function. In acute aortic insufficiency, reflex vasoconstriction increases peripheral vascular resistance. In compensated chronic aortic insufficiency, vasoconstriction is absent, and vascular resistance may be reduced and contribute to the hyperdynamic circulation observed in these patients.

CLINICAL MANIFESTATIONS

The most common symptoms from chronic aortic regurgitation are those of left-sided heart failure, that is, dyspnea on exertion, orthopnea, and fatigue. In acute aortic regurgitation, cardiac output and shock may develop rapidly. The onset of symptoms in patients with chronic aortic regurgitation usually heralds the onset of LV systolic dysfunction. Some patients with symptoms have apparently normal systolic function, however, and the symptoms may be attributed to diastolic dysfunction. Other patients may have ventricular dysfunction yet remain asymptomatic.

Angina may also occur in patients with aortic insufficiency but less commonly than in those with aortic stenosis. The cause of angina in aortic regurgitation is probably multifactorial. Coronary blood flow reserve is reduced in some patients because diastolic runoff into the left ventricle lowers aortic diastolic pressure while increasing LV diastolic pressure—these two influences lower the driving pressure gradient for flow across the coronary bed. When angina occurs in aortic regurgitation, it may be accompanied by flushing. Other symptoms include carotid artery pain and an unpleasant awareness of the heartbeat.

DIAGNOSIS

Physical Examination

Aortic regurgitation produces a myriad of signs because a hyperdynamic, enlarged left ventricle ejects a large stroke volume at high pressure into the systemic circulation. Palpation of the precordium finds a hyperactive apical impulse displaced downward and to the left. S_1 and S_2 are usually normal. S_2 is followed by a diastolic blowing murmur heard best along the left sternal border with the patient sitting upright. In mild disease, the murmur may be short and heard only in the beginning of diastole when the gradient between the aorta and the left ventricle is highest. As the disease worsens, the murmur may persist throughout diastole. A second murmur, a mitral valve rumble, is heard at the LV apex in patients with severe aortic insufficiency. Although the cause is still debated, this Austin Flint murmur is probably produced as the regurgitant jet impinges on the mitral valve and causes it to vibrate.

In chronic aortic regurgitation, the high stroke volume and reduced systemic arterial resistance result in a wide pulse pressure, which may generate a number of signs, including Corrigan's pulse (sharp upstroke and rapid decline of the carotid pulse), de Musset's sign (head bobbing), Duroziez's sign (combined systolic and diastolic bruits created by compression of the femoral artery with the stethoscope), and Quincke's pulse (systolic plethora and diastolic blanching in the nail bed when gentle traction is placed on the nail). Perhaps the most reliable of physical signs indicating severe aortic regurgitation is Hill's sign, an increase in femoral systolic pressure of 40 mm Hg or more compared with systolic pressure in the brachial artery.

In contrast to chronic aortic insufficiency with its myriad clinical signs, acute aortic insufficiency may have a subtle manifestation. The eccentric hypertrophy, which compensates for chronic aortic insufficiency, has not yet had time to develop, and the large total stroke volume responsible for most of the signs of chronic aortic insufficiency is absent. The only clues to the presence of acute aortic insufficiency may be a short diastolic blowing murmur and reduced intensity of S_1. This latter sign occurs because high diastolic LV pressure closes the mitral valve early in diastole (mitral valve preclosure) so that when ventricular systole occurs, only the tricuspid component of S_1 is heard.

Noninvasive Evaluation

The ECG in patients with aortic insufficiency is nonspecific but almost always demonstrates LV hypertrophy. The chest radiograph shows an enlarged heart, often with uncoiling and enlargement of the aortic root.

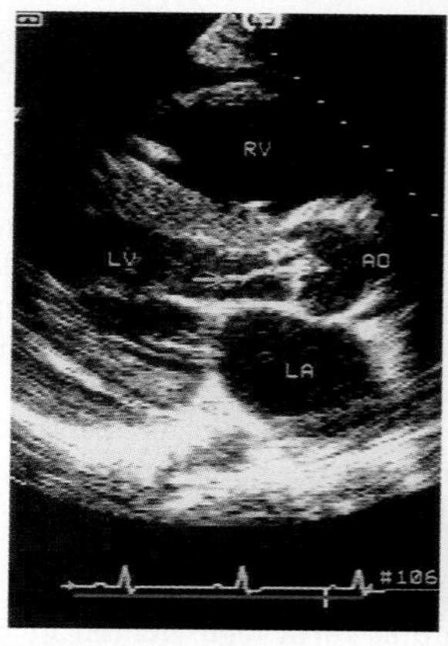

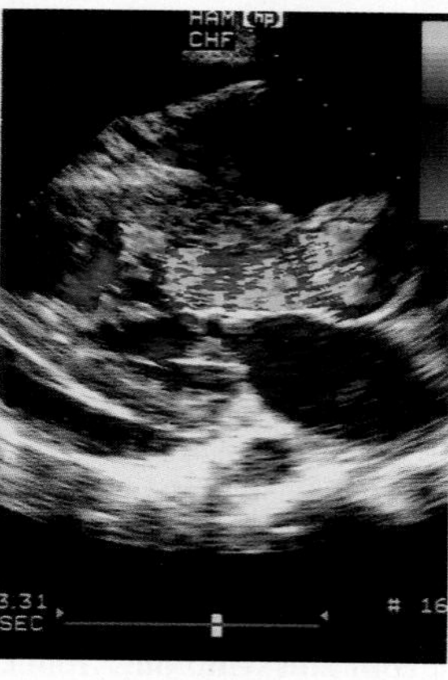

FIGURE 75-7. **Echocardiogram of a patient with aortic regurgitation caused by infective endocarditis.** The *left panel* shows a linear vegetation (*arrow*) prolapsing into the left ventricular outflow tract from the aortic valve leaflet in diastole. The *right panel* is a color flow Doppler image exhibiting turbulent blood flow filling the left ventricular tract during diastole. AO = aorta; LA = left atrium; LV = left ventricle; RV = right ventricle. (Courtesy of Dr. Anthony DeMaria.)

Echocardiography (Chapter 55) is the most important noninvasive tool for assessing the severity of aortic insufficiency and its impact on LV geometry and function (Fig. 75-7). During echocardiography, the LV end-diastolic dimension, end-systolic dimension, and fractional shortening are determined. Aortic valve anatomy and aortic root anatomy can be assessed and the cause of the aortic regurgitation can often be determined. Color flow Doppler examination of the aortic valve helps quantify the severity of aortic regurgitation by assessing the depth and width to which the diastolic jet penetrates the left ventricle. Another way to assess the severity of aortic regurgitation is the pressure half-time method: continuous-wave Doppler interrogation of the aortic valve displays the decay of the velocity of retrograde flow across the valve. In mild aortic insufficiency, the gradient across the valve is high throughout diastole, and its rate of decay is slow, with production of a long Doppler half-time (the time that it takes the velocity to decay from its peak to that value divided by the square root of 2). In severe aortic regurgitation, there is rapid equilibration between pressure in the aorta and pressure in the left ventricle, and the Doppler half-time is short. If mitral valve preclosure is detected in acute aortic insufficiency, urgent surgery is necessary. In cases in which the severity of aortic insufficiency is in doubt, catheterization to perform aortography is useful in resolving the issue.

TREATMENT AND PROGNOSIS Rx

Medical Therapy

Asymptomatic Patients with Normal Left Ventricular Function

Because aortic regurgitation increases LV afterload, which decreases cardiac efficiency, afterload reduction with nifedipine and other vasodilators, including angiotensin-converting enzyme inhibitors and hydralazine, improves hemodynamics in the short term. Although initial data suggested that such therapy could delay or reduce the need for aortic valve surgery without any adverse effects when surgery is finally performed, more recent data suggest no benefit from such therapy. These discrepant results from relatively small trials preclude firm recommendations.

Symptomatic Patients or Patients with Left Ventricular Dysfunction

Patients who have symptoms or manifest LV dysfunction should not be treated medically, except for short-term stabilization, but should undergo aortic valve surgery as soon as feasible.

Surgical Therapy

Acute Aortic Regurgitation

When any of the symptoms or signs of heart failure develop, even if mild, medical mortality is high and approaches 75%. Therapy with vasodilators, such as nitroprusside, may temporarily improve the patient's condition before surgery but is never a substitute for surgery. In patients with acute aortic regurgitation caused by bacterial endocarditis (Chapter 76), surgery may be delayed to permit a full or partial course of antibiotics, but persistent, severe aortic regurgitation requires emergency valve replacement. Even when blood cultures have been positive recently and antibiotic therapy has been of brief duration, the valve reinfection rate is low, 0 to 10%, with valve replacement or valve repair. Emergency surgery should not be withheld simply because the duration of antibiotic therapy has been brief.

Chronic Aortic Regurgitation

Asymptomatic patients who manifest evidence of LV dysfunction benefit from surgery. Because loading conditions differ between aortic and mitral regurgitation, the objective markers for the presence of LV dysfunction also differ. In aortic regurgitation, when the ejection fraction is less than 0.55 or the end-systolic dimension is greater than 55 mm, postoperative outcome is impaired, presumably because these markers indicate that LV dysfunction has developed. Surgery should be performed before these benchmarks are reached. A calculated regurgitant orifice above 40 mm^2 portends a poorer prognosis and also may warrant surgery.

Patients with advanced symptoms are at increased risk for a suboptimal surgical outcome regardless of whether they have evidence of LV dysfunction. Patients should undergo aortic valve replacement before symptoms impair lifestyle.

Although some patients may be able to undergo successful aortic valve repair to restore aortic valve competence, most patients require insertion of an aortic valve prosthesis.

TRICUSPID REGURGITATION

DEFINITION

Tricuspid regurgitation is usually secondary to a hemodynamic load on the right ventricle rather than a structural valve deformity. Diseases that cause pulmonary hypertension, such as chronic obstructive airway disease or intracardiac shunts, lead to RV dilation and subsequent tricuspid regurgitation. Because most of the force that is needed to fill the left ventricle is provided by the right ventricle, LV dysfunction leading to elevated LV filling pressure also places the right ventricle under a hemodynamic load and can eventually lead to RV failure and tricuspid regurgitation. In some instances, tricuspid regurgitation may be caused by pathology of the valve itself. The most common cause of primary tricuspid regurgitation is infective endocarditis, usually stemming from drug abuse and unsterile injections. Other causes include carcinoid syndrome, rheumatic involvement of the tricuspid valve, myxomatous degeneration, RV infarction, and mishaps during endomyocardial biopsy.

DIAGNOSIS

The symptoms of tricuspid regurgitation are those of right-sided heart failure and include ascites, edema, and occasionally right upper quadrant pain. On physical examination, tricuspid regurgitation produces jugular venous distention accentuated by a large v wave as blood is regurgitated into the right atrium during systole. Regurgitation into the hepatic veins causes hepatic enlargement and liver pulsation. RV enlargement is detected as a parasternal lift. Ascites and edema are common.

The definitive diagnosis of tricuspid regurgitation is made during echocardiography. Doppler interrogation of the tricuspid valve shows systolic disturbance of the right atrial blood pool. Echocardiography (Chapter 55) can also be used to determine the severity of pulmonary hypertension, measure RV dilation, and assess whether the valve itself is intrinsically normal or abnormal.

TREATMENT AND PROGNOSIS Rx

Therapy for secondary tricuspid regurgitation is generally aimed at the cause of the lesion. If LV failure has been responsible for RV failure and tricuspid regurgitation, the standard therapy for improving LV failure (Chapter 59) lowers LV filling pressure, reduces secondary pulmonary hypertension, relieves some of the hemodynamic burden of the right ventricle, and partially restores tricuspid valve competence. If pulmonary disease is the primary cause, therapy is directed toward improving lung function. Vasodilators, so useful in the treatment of left-sided heart failure, are often ineffective in treating pulmonary hypertension itself. Medical therapy directed at tricuspid regurgitation is usually limited to diuretic use.

Surgical intervention for the tricuspid valve is rarely entertained in isolation. However, if other cardiac surgery is planned in a patient with severe tricuspid regurgitation, concomitant ring annuloplasty or tricuspid valve repair is frequently attempted to ensure postoperative tricuspid competence. Since a second operation to address residual tricuspid regurgitation after successful left-sided valve surgery carries an unacceptably high mortality rate, concomitant tricuspid annuloplasty is now entertained for even mild to moderate tricuspid regurgitation during left-sided valve surgery. Tricuspid valve replacement is often not well tolerated and is rarely performed except when severe deformity, as is often seen in endocarditis or carcinoid disease, precludes valve repair.

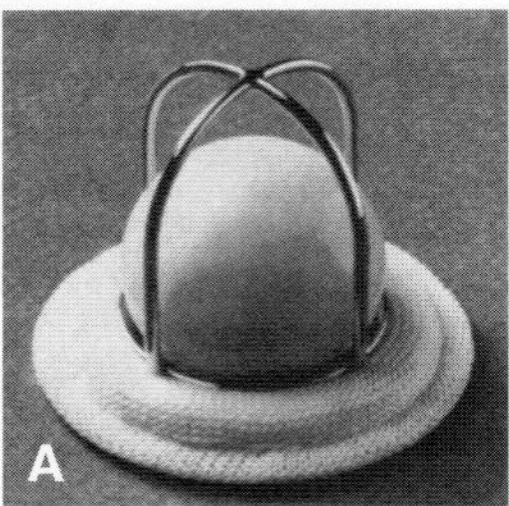
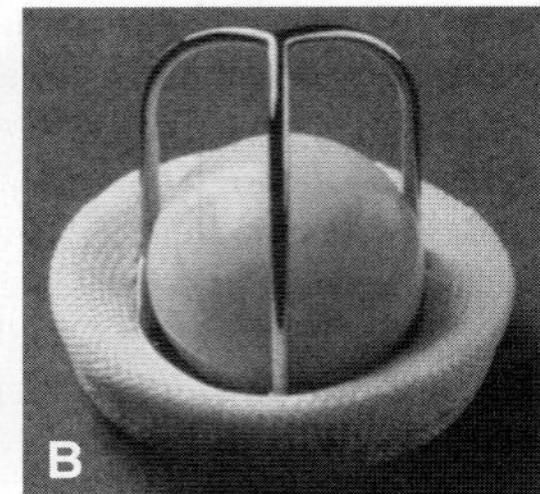
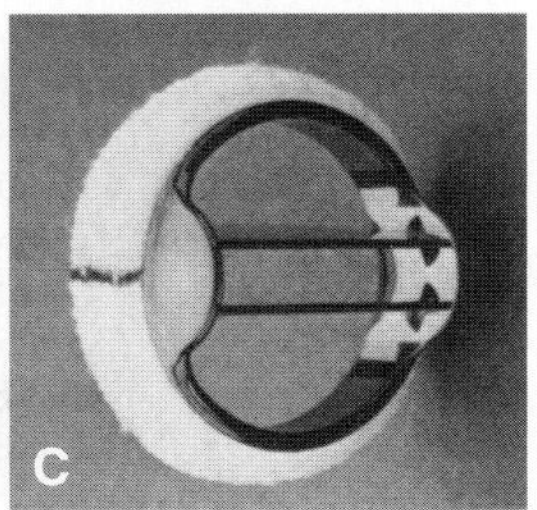
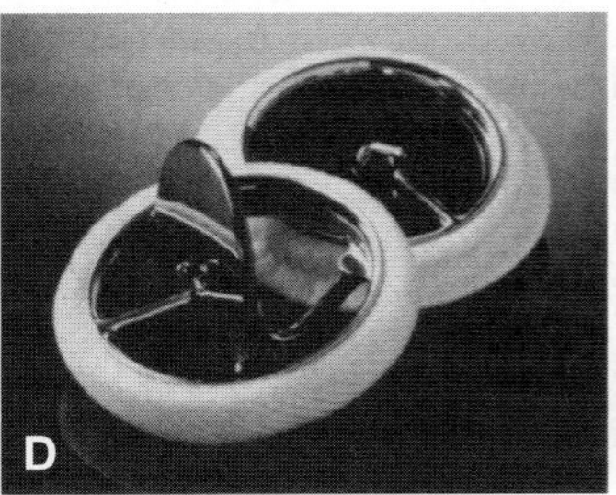
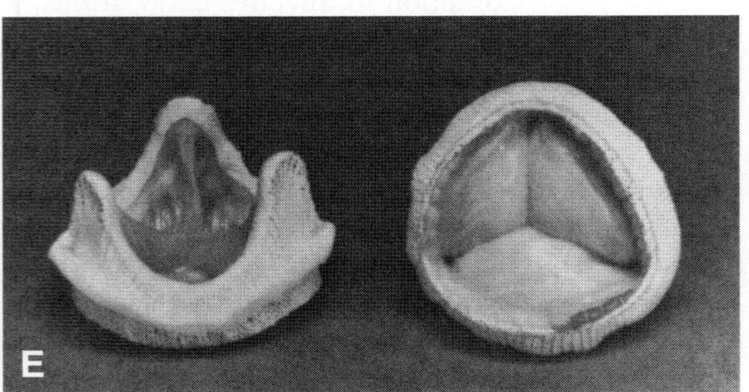

FIGURE 75-8. Different types of commonly used prosthetic valves. **A,** Starr-Edwards caged ball mitral prosthesis. **B,** Starr-Edwards aortic prosthesis. **C,** St. Jude Medical bileaflet prosthesis. **D,** Medtronic-Hall tilting disc valve. **E,** Carpentier-Edwards bioprosthesis. (From Wernly JA, Crawford MH. Choosing a prosthetic heart valve. *Cardiol Clin.* 1991;9:329-338.)

PULMONIC STENOSIS

DEFINITION

Pulmonic stenosis is a congenital disease resulting from fusion of the pulmonic valve cusps (Chapter 69). It is usually detected and corrected during childhood, but occasionally cases are diagnosed for the first time in adulthood. Symptoms of pulmonic stenosis include angina and syncope. Occasionally, symptoms of right-sided heart failure develop. During physical examination, the uncalcified valve in pulmonic stenosis produces an early systolic ejection click on opening. During inspiration, the click diminishes or disappears because increased flow into the right side of the heart during inspiration partially opens the pulmonic valve in diastole so that systole causes less of an opening sound. The click is followed by a systolic ejection murmur that radiates to the base of the heart. If the transvalvular gradient is severe, RV hypertrophy develops and produces a parasternal lift.

The diagnosis of pulmonic stenosis is confirmed by echocardiography, which quantifies the transvalvular gradient and the degree of RV hypertrophy and dysfunction.

TREATMENT AND PROGNOSIS Rx

In asymptomatic patients with a gradient less than 25 mm Hg, no therapy is required. If symptoms develop or the gradient exceeds 50 mm Hg, balloon commissurotomy is effective in reducing the gradient and relieving symptoms. Although long-term prognosis is not yet established, 90% of patients do not require reintervention 10 years after balloon therapy.

Postoperative Care of Patients with Substitute Heart Valves

After a prosthetic valve has been inserted, a baseline echocardiogram should be obtained to provide a reference point in the event that valve dysfunction is suspected at a later date. Echocardiography does not need to be repeated unless there is a change in clinical status or physical findings. The major causes of valve dysfunction are infective endocarditis, clot, and valve degeneration. Dysfunction is manifested most commonly by valvular regurgitation, but valvular stenosis can also occur with a clot, vegetations, or degeneration, especially degeneration of a bioprosthesis.

Whenever a patient with a prosthetic heart valve has a temperature higher than 100° F, endocarditis must be excluded by blood culture; for fever with signs of sepsis, broad-spectrum antibiotics must be begun while awaiting culture results. For patients with bioprosthetic valves, mechanical prostheses, and homografts, endocarditis prophylaxis should be instituted at the time of procedures that are associated with a high risk for bacteremia (Chapter 76). Whether prophylaxis is necessary for pulmonary autografts is currently unclear, but physicians usually prescribe prophylaxis for these patients.

All patients with a mechanical heart valve require anticoagulation. Recommended INR values range from 2.0 for a young normotensive patient in sinus rhythm with an aortic valve prosthesis to 3.5 for a patient with atrial fibrillation and a mitral valve prosthesis. Aspirin, 325 mg, is recommended in addition to warfarin to reduce the risk for valve thrombosis in patients who have mechanical prosthetic valves that are at higher risk for thromboembolic complications. When thrombosis occurs on a prosthetic valve, about 60% of patients can have restored valve function after intravenous infusion of a thrombolytic agent.

TABLE 75-2 ADVANTAGES AND DISADVANTAGES OF SUBSTITUTE CARDIAC VALVES

TYPE OF VALVE	ADVANTAGES	DISADVANTAGES
Bioprosthesis (Carpentier-Edwards, Hancock)	Avoids anticoagulation in patients with sinus rhythm	Durability limited to 10-15 yr Relatively stenotic
Mechanical valves (St. Jude, Medtronic-Hall, Starr-Edwards)	Good flow characteristics in small sizes Durable	Require anticoagulation
Homografts and autografts	Anticoagulation not required Durability increased over that of bioprostheses	Surgical implantation technically demanding

Choices among Prosthetic Valves

Different types of prosthetic valves (Fig. 75-8) have different advantages and disadvantages (Table 75-2). At long-term follow-up, primary valve failure with resulting need for reoperation is much more common with bioprosthetic valves,[4,5] and bleeding is generally more common with mechanical valves. For mitral valves, long-term survival is similar with bioprosthetic and mechanical valves.[4] Survival after aortic valve replacement is probably better with mechanical valves. Another alternative is to use the patient's own pulmonic valve to replace the diseased aortic valve and then to implant a prosthetic pulmonic valve (the Ross procedure). In a randomized trial, this procedure was superior to homograft valve and root replacement, with a 10-year survival of 97% compared with 83%.[6]

In general, a tissue valve is recommended in patients who have a life expectancy of less than 15 years or who are unable or unwilling to maintain warfarin anticoagulation. A mechanical valve is preferred in patients who already have another indication for anticoagulation or who have a longer life expectancy and want to minimize the risk of reoperation. Because many patients prefer the risk of reoperation to that of anticoagulation, the age at which bioprostheses are implanted has steadily declined, and many 60-year-old patients now request and receive a bioprosthetic valve.

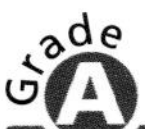

1. Leon MB, Smith CR, Mack M, et al. Transcatheter aortic-valve implantation for aortic stenosis in patients who cannot undergo surgery. *N Engl J Med.* 2010;363:1597-1607.
2. Smith CR, Leon MB, Mack MJ, et al, for the PARTNER Trial Investigators. Comparison of transcatheter and surgical aortic valve replacement for aortic stenosis in patients at high risk for operation. *N Engl J Med.* 2011. [Epub ahead of print.]
3. Feldman T, Foster E, Glower DG, et al. Percutaneous repair or surgery for mitral regurgitation. *N Engl J Med.* 2011;364:1395-1406.
4. Hammermeister K, Sethi GK, Henderson WG, et al. Outcomes 15 years after valve replacement with a mechanical versus a bioprosthetic valve: final report of the Veterans Affairs randomized trial. *J Am Coll Cardiol.* 2000;36:1152-1158.
5. Stassano P, Di Tommaso L, Monaco M, et al. Aortic valve replacement: a prospective randomized evaluation of mechanical versus biological valves in patients ages 55 to 70 years. *J Am Coll Cardiol.* 2009;54:1862-1868.

6. El-Hamamsy I, Eryigit Z, Stevens LM, et al. Long-term outcomes after autograft versus homograft aortic root replacement in adults with aortic valve disease: a randomised controlled trial. *Lancet.* 2010;376:524-531.

SUGGESTED READINGS

Foster E. Clinical practice. Mitral regurgitation due to degenerative mitral-valve disease. *N Engl J Med.* 2010;363:156-165. *Review.*

Rahimtoola SH. Choice of prosthetic heart valve in adults an update. *J Am Coll Cardiol.* 2010;55:2413-2426. *Review.*

Siu SC, Silversides CK. Bicuspid aortic valve disease. *J Am Coll Cardiol.* 2010;55:2789-2800. *Review.*

Vaishnava P, Fuster V, Goldman M, et al. Surgery for asymptomatic degenerative aortic and mitral valve disease. *Nat Rev Cardiol.* 2011;8:173-177. *Review suggesting a targeted role for pre-emptive intervention in selected, asymptomatic individuals with AS or MR.*

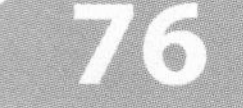

INFECTIVE ENDOCARDITIS

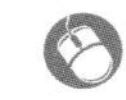

VANCE G. FOWLER JR. AND ARNOLD S. BAYER

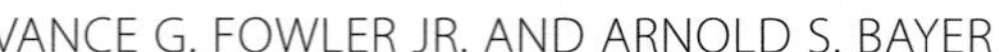

DEFINITION

Infective endocarditis is defined as an infection, usually bacterial, of the endocardial surface of the heart. Infective endocarditis affects primarily the cardiac valves, although in some cases the septa between the chambers or the mural endocardium may be involved. Traditionally, infective endocarditis has been categorized as acute or subacute, depending on the duration of symptoms before presentation; however, this distinction is somewhat arbitrary. A classification that considers the causative organism and the valve involved is more clinically relevant.

EPIDEMIOLOGY

The incidence of infective endocarditis is difficult to determine because of the different criteria for diagnosis and methods of reporting. An analysis based on strict case definitions reveals that only a relatively small proportion (about 20%) of clinically diagnosed cases are categorized as definite. Nevertheless, in 10 large surveys, infective endocarditis accounted for approximately 1 case per 1000 U.S. hospital admissions, with a range of 0.16 to 5.4 cases per 1000 admissions. This incidence has not changed appreciably over the past 30 years. Estimates from the American Heart Association place the annual incidence of infective endocarditis in the United States at 10,000 to 20,000 new cases.

Men are more commonly affected than women (mean male-female ratio of 1.7 : 1 in 18 large series). However, in patients younger than 35 years, more cases occur in women. More than 50% of patients with infective endocarditis in the United States are now older than 50 years owing to the low incidence of acute rheumatic fever (Chapter 298) and the low subsequent prevalence of rheumatic heart disease compared with prior eras and with developing countries, as well as a simultaneous rise in the prevalence of degenerative heart disease as the population lives longer.

Although some patients have no clearly definable risk factor for endocarditis, cardiac conditions that cause turbulent flow at the endocardial surface or across a valve (Chapter 75) predispose patients to infective endocarditis (Table 76-1). Historically, rheumatic heart disease with valvular dysfunction was the most common underlying condition, although its contribution has diminished in the antibiotic era, especially in developed countries.

TABLE 76-1 PREDISPOSING CONDITIONS ASSOCIATED WITH INCREASED RISK OF ENDOCARDITIS

MORE COMMON	LESS COMMON
Mitral valve prolapse	Rheumatic heart disease
Degenerative valvular disease	Idiopathic hypertrophic subaortic stenosis
Intravenous drug use*	Pulmonary-systemic shunts*
Prosthetic valve*	Coarctation of the aorta
Congenital abnormalities (valvular or septal defect)	Previous endocarditis*
	Complex cyanotic congenital heart disease*

*Indicates conditions with highest risk for endocarditis.

Degenerative valvular disease is also associated with infective endocarditis, particularly in elderly patients; the increasing relevance of senile calcification as a risk factor is reflected in the increasing proportion of aortic valve involvement in infective endocarditis. Most significant congenital heart defects (Chapter 69) confer an increased risk of infective endocarditis, particularly complex cyanotic disease such as single-ventricle states, transposition of the great vessels, and tetralogy of Fallot. Similarly, surgically constructed pulmonary-systemic shunts and ventricular septal defects place patients at high risk for infective endocarditis.

Mitral valve prolapse is currently the most common underlying cardiac condition in infective endocarditis, a statistic that reflects its prevalence in the general population (4%). Notably, mitral valve prolapse is a risk only in patients with thickened mitral leaflets and/or regurgitation, in which case the risk of endocarditis increases by about 10-fold over that of the general population. In addition, patients with hypertrophic cardiomyopathy are at increased risk of infective endocarditis, particularly in the presence of outflow obstruction. Finally, previous endocarditis is among the highest risk factors for infective endocarditis.

Prosthetic cardiac valves represent an important risk factor for infective endocarditis. More than 150,000 heart valves are implanted annually worldwide, and prosthetic valve infective endocarditis develops in 1 to 4% of prosthetic valve recipients in the first year after valve replacement and in approximately 0.8% of recipients annually thereafter. Mechanical prosthetic valves may initially be more susceptible to infective endocarditis, but bioprosthetic valves are more likely to develop infective endocarditis after 1 year; overall, the rate is similar with either type of valve.

The incidence of infective endocarditis in injection drug users (Chapter 33) may be 30 times higher than in the general population and 4 times higher than in adults with rheumatic heart disease. In some areas of the United States, injection drug use is the most common predisposing cause of infective endocarditis in patients younger than 40 years. *Staphylococcus aureus* is the predominant organism, and tricuspid valve involvement is noted in 78% of cases, mitral involvement in 24%, and aortic involvement in 8%. More than one valve is infected in approximately 20% of cases, and some of these infections are polymicrobial.

Health care–associated infective endocarditis arises primarily as a consequence of invasive therapies, including intravenous catheters, hyperalimentation lines, pacemakers, and dialysis shunts. In a recent prospective multinational cohort study of more than 1600 patients with native valve endocarditis and no injection drug use, more than one third of patients had health care–associated endocarditis, and many of these cases were community acquired (e.g., in patients on outpatient hemodialysis). The emerging importance of health care–associated infective endocarditis in industrialized nations has also influenced the microbiology of the disease, with an increasing prevalence of *S. aureus* and a decreasing prevalence of viridans streptococci in much of the industrialized world.

Systemic medical conditions predispose patients to the development of infective endocarditis. For example, HIV infection is an independent risk factor for the development of infective endocarditis in injection drug users, with the risk increasing as the CD4 count decreases. Catheter-related bacteremia is an important risk factor for nosocomial infective endocarditis. Patients with end-stage renal disease—particularly those receiving long-term hemodialysis—and patients with diabetes mellitus are also at increased risk, presumably because of the recurrent vascular access associated with the former and the low-level immunosuppression associated with both conditions.

The mitral valve has classically been the most commonly affected valve, followed by the aortic valve. Although mitral valve relapse remains the most common underlying condition, the decreasing frequency of rheumatic mitral disease and the increasing senescence of the population may account for the increase in aortic valve endocarditis reported in many studies. The next most commonly affected valves in descending order of prevalence are the mitral and aortic valves together, the tricuspid valve, mixed right- and left-sided infection, and the pulmonic valve.

Microbiology

About 90% of community-acquired, native valve infective endocarditis is due to staphylococci, streptococci, or enterococci, each of which is a normal inhabitant of the skin, oropharynx, and urogenital tract with frequent access to the blood stream. These organisms express specific receptors for attachment and adherence to damaged valve surfaces. Streptococcal species (Chapter 298) are the most common cause in community-dwelling patients with no history of injection drug use or health care contact. In patients with either of these epidemiologic risk factors, *S. aureus* (Chapter 298) is the predominant cause of infective endocarditis. Because of the emergence of health care contact as the predominant risk factor for blood stream infections, *S. aureus* is now the most common cause of infective endocarditis in many regions of the world.

Viridans streptococci (Chapter 298) are the most common streptococci implicated in native valve infective endocarditis. This group of organisms, which normally inhabit the oropharynx, includes species such as *Streptococcus sanguis, Streptococcus mutans,* and *Streptococcus mitis*. Group B streptococci, β-hemolytic organisms that are also normal oropharyngeal and urogenital flora, most frequently cause infective endocarditis in patients with cirrhosis or diabetes mellitus and in injection drug users. By contrast, group A streptococci, although also β-hemolytic, rarely cause infective endocarditis. *Streptococcus bovis*, a group D streptococcus, is now a leading cause of infective endocarditis in some parts of the world; for example, its incidence in France has increased significantly in recent years. Its presence should prompt endoscopic evaluation for adenocarcinoma of the colon or other malignant lesions of the gastrointestinal tract.

Pneumococcal endocarditis is decreasing in incidence but is quite fulminant when present. It may occur as part of Austrian's (or Osler's) triad of endocarditis, meningitis, and pneumonia and is associated with high morbidity and mortality.

S. aureus (Chapter 296) is the pathogen of primary concern among injection drug users or patients with health care contact. The clinical course of *S. aureus* endocarditis is typically acute, with a rapid progression over the course of several days. Because approximately 12% of nonselected patients with *S. aureus* bacteremia have infective endocarditis, the possibility of cardiac involvement should always be considered in any patient with *S. aureus* bacteremia; those with persistent bacteremia or fever, community acquisition, or cutaneous findings are at particular risk for infective endocarditis and other complications. Coagulase-negative staphylococci are an unusual cause of native valve disease but are an important pathogen in prosthetic valve endocarditis; presentation is usually subacute.

Enterococcal bacteremia is far more common, particularly in hospitalized patients, than enterococcal endocarditis; however, enterococci are responsible for a significant number of cases of both community-acquired and nosocomial endocarditis. In most cases, the source of the bacteria is thought to be the genitourinary tract, and the presentation is usually subacute. Enterococcal endocarditis, as opposed to enterococcal bacteremia, is suggested by community acquisition of infection, the absence of a clear source of infection, preexistent valvular heart disease, and the absence of polymicrobial bacteremia. As in most enterococcal infections, the overwhelming majority of cases (>90%) are due to *Enterococcus faecalis*.

The HACEK group of gram-negative organisms (*Haemophilus* spp, *Actinobacillus actinomycetemcomitans, Cardiobacterium hominis, Eikenella corrodens,* and *Kingella* spp) accounts for about 5% of cases of endocarditis. Because these fastidious organisms usually grow in blood cultures within 7 days using current methods, prolonged incubation is no longer required to isolate HACEK strains. Many other gram-negative bacilli have been reported to cause infective endocarditis but are even more unusual. Traditionally, injection drug use has been regarded as the primary risk factor for enteric gram-negative bacterial endocarditis. However, recent experience from large multinational studies shows that health care contact, not injection drug use, is the most common risk factor for enteric gram-negative endocarditis.

Fungal endocarditis is difficult to diagnose and treat; it is most commonly found in patients with a history of injection drug use, recent cardiac surgery, or prolonged use of indwelling vascular catheters, especially those used for total parenteral nutrition. The most common fungi found in infective endocarditis are *Aspergillus* and *Candida* species. *Aspergillus* (Chapter 347) rarely grows in blood cultures and must usually be cultured from a pathologic specimen (either an embolic site or vegetation); by contrast, *Candida* (Chapter 346) frequently grows out of blood cultures. Mortality is very high, and valve replacement surgery is usually necessary.

Special Situations: Health Care–Associated Infective Endocarditis and Prosthetic Valves

Health care–associated infective endocarditis is defined as endocarditis occurring in the presence of extensive health care contact. Traditionally, this definition was synonymous with nosocomial in-hospital acquisition; however, the increased complexity of outpatient therapy and the increase in the number of patients in long-term care facilities have resulted in a growing number of nonhospitalized patients with health care–associated bacteremia and infective endocarditis. Such patients have many of the same risk factors (e.g., long-term intravascular catheters, extensive instrumentation) and are infected with the same array of pathogens (e.g., high rates of methicillin-resistant *S. aureus* [MRSA]) as patients with nosocomial infection. Health care–associated infective endocarditis now constitutes about one quarter of all cases and is most frequently associated with indwelling vascular catheters; as a result, the most common organisms implicated in nosocomial infective endocarditis are *S. aureus* and coagulase-negative staphylococci.

Prosthetic valve endocarditis can be classified into one of three groups based on the time between valve surgery and disease onset: early (<2 months after surgery), intermediate (2 to 12 months), and late (>12 months) (Table 76-2). Staphylococci, particularly *S. aureus*, predominate during the early period, when most episodes of infective endocarditis are thought to be related to perioperative infection. The intermediate period has a fairly similar microbiologic spectrum, with unusual gram-negative organisms and diphtheroids decreasing and streptococci increasing. In the late period, 1 year or more after surgery, the spectrum of organisms becomes more akin to that of community-acquired native valve disease, in which *S. aureus* and streptococci predominate. Of note, approximately 50% of prosthetic valve recipients with *S. aureus* bacteremia develop infective endocarditis.

TABLE 76-2 CAUSES OF PROSTHETIC VALVE ENDOCARDITIS*

EARLY (<2 MO POSTOPERATIVELY)	LATE (>12 MO POSTOPERATIVELY)
Staphylococcus aureus	Coagulase-negative staphylococci
Coagulase-negative staphylococci	*Staphylococcus aureus*
Gram-negative bacilli	Coagulase-negative staphylococci
Enterococci	Enterococci
Fungi	
Diphtheroids	

*Listed in order of relative frequency.
Adapted from Wang A, Athan E, Pappas PA, et al. Contemporary clinical profile and outcome of prosthetic valve endocarditis. *JAMA*. 2007; 297:1354-1361.

PATHOBIOLOGY

Experimental models of infective endocarditis have demonstrated that the disease follows a predictable sequence: endocardial damage, aggregation of platelets and fibrin to create a sterile vegetation, transient bacteremia resulting in seeding of the vegetation, microbial proliferation on and invasion of the endocardial surface, and metastatic infection to visceral organs and brain.

Most cases of infective endocarditis begin with a damaged endocardial surface. Damage to the endocardium may be caused by a number of factors, ranging from rheumatic disease to senile degeneration and calcification; indeed, any excessive turbulence or high-pressure gradient can cause injury to the nearby endocardium. Next, fibrin-platelet aggregates develop at the site of damage to form sterile vegetations, also termed *nonbacterial thrombotic endocarditis*. Nonbacterial thrombotic endocarditis may occur spontaneously in patients with systemic illnesses (e.g., the marantic endocarditis of malignancy [Chapter 60] or other wasting diseases, or Libman-Sacks endocarditis in systemic lupus erythematosus [Chapter 274]). When transient bacteremia occurs—for example, as a result of distant infection or gingival disease—the previously sterile vegetation may be seeded. Some bacterial species, such as staphylococci and streptococci, are more avidly adherent than others to vegetations and therefore more frequently cause endocarditis. The bacteria then proliferate within the vegetation and may ultimately achieve an organism load of 10^9 to 10^{11} colony-forming units per gram of tissue. The surfaces of cardiac valves and vegetations are avascular, making antibiotic therapy and healing difficult.

CLINICAL MANIFESTATIONS

History

The initial presentation of infective endocarditis varies enormously from patient to patient, so it is sometimes difficult to make the diagnosis. Some cases develop acutely, with symptoms progressing rapidly over several days. Other cases develop insidiously and present with nonspecific symptoms that

TABLE 76-3 PHYSICAL EXAMINATION AND LABORATORY FINDINGS IN INFECTIVE ENDOCARDITIS

FINDING	% OF CASES
Fever	96
Worsening of old murmur	20
New murmur	48
Vascular embolic event	17
Splenomegaly	11
Splinter hemorrhages	8
Osler's nodes	3
Janeway's lesions	5
Roth's spots	2
Elevated ESR	61
Hematuria	26
Positive rheumatoid factor	5
Abnormal CXR (effusion, infiltrate, septic emboli)	67-85 (right-sided infective endocarditis)

CXR = chest x-ray; ESR = erythrocyte sedimentation rate.
Adapted from Murdoch DR, Corey GR, Hoen B, et al. Clinical presentation, etiology, and outcome of infective endocarditis in the 21st century: International Collaboration on Endocarditis—Prospective Cohort Study. *Arch Intern Med.* 2009;169:463-473.

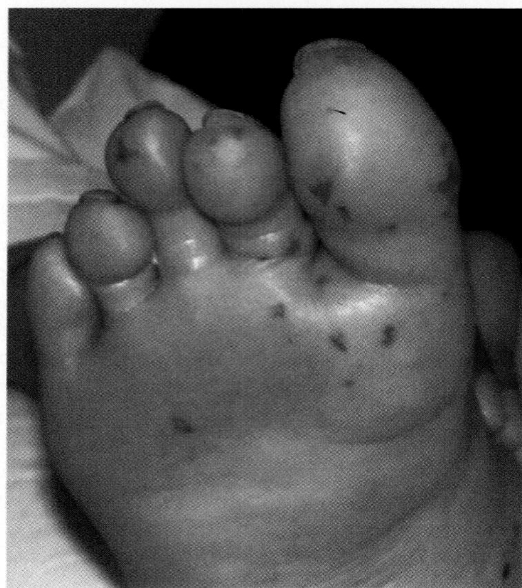

FIGURE 76-1. Petechiae in infective endocarditis.

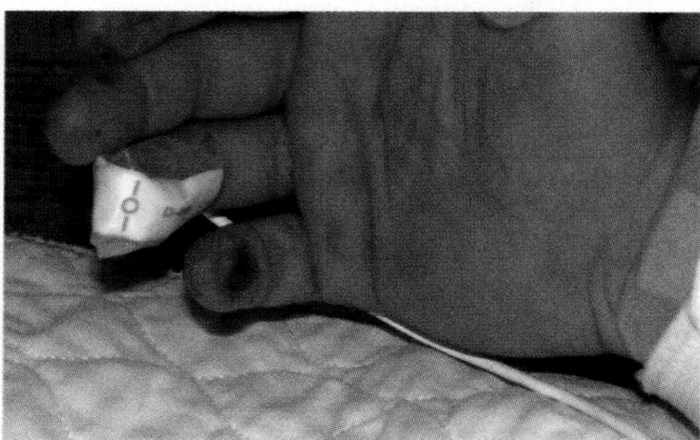

FIGURE 76-2. Osler's node in infective endocarditis.

have been progressing for weeks or months. In patients suspected of having infective endocarditis, the initial history should include a complete review of systems, a travel history, and a thorough discussion of health-related behaviors such as illicit drug use and sexual activity. Most patients complain of fever and nonspecific constitutional symptoms such as fatigue, malaise, or weight loss. Nearly 50% of patients complain of musculoskeletal symptoms ranging from frank arthritis to diffuse myalgias; 5 to 10% of patients have low back pain as their chief complaint, even in the absence of osteomyelitis or epidural abscess. Many intravenous drug users with endocarditis complain of pleuritic chest pain, because tricuspid valve endocarditis mimics pneumonia. Health care–associated infective endocarditis is more likely to be clinically occult and requires a high index of suspicion.

Physical Examination

A thorough physical examination should be performed, including a search for the peripheral stigmata of infective endocarditis (Table 76-3). Fever is present in nearly 50% of patients in most studies; however, elderly patients and those with renal failure or heart failure may be less likely to mount a febrile response. A widened pulse pressure should alert the clinician to the possibility of acute aortic insufficiency (Chapter 75). The skin and nails should be carefully examined for embolic phenomena such as petechiae, Osler's nodes, Janeway's lesions, and splinter hemorrhages; these findings are uncommon in infective endocarditis in the current era but are extremely helpful diagnostic clues when present. Petechiae are most often found on the conjunctiva, palate, and extremities; like the other peripheral stigmata of infective endocarditis, they are a nonspecific but suggestive finding (Fig. 76-1). Osler's nodes are small, painful nodules found most often on the palmar surfaces of the fingers and toes; they frequently wax and wane (Fig. 76-2). Classically considered to be an immunologic phenomenon, Osler's nodes may have an immune complex–mediated component but are most likely initiated by microemboli. Janeway's lesions (Fig. 50-11 in Chapter 50) are hemorrhagic, nonpainful macules also found primarily on the palms and soles; they are embolic in origin and are less frequently noted than the other cutaneous stigmata. Splinter hemorrhages (see Fig. 50-11 in Chapter 50) are nonblanching, linear, brownish red lesions in the nail beds perpendicular to the direction of nail growth; they are nonspecific and may also be found in a significant percentage of hospitalized patients without infective endocarditis.

Funduscopic examination should be performed to look for Roth's spots (see Fig. 431-28 in Chapter 431), chorioretinitis, or endophthalmitis; the latter two are present in a substantial proportion of cases of fungal endocarditis. A careful cardiac examination should be performed to detect any systolic or diastolic murmurs or evidence of heart failure, which is an ominous sign. Of note, patients with health care–associated infective endocarditis are less likely than others to have a pathologic murmur on initial presentation.

The abdomen should be examined for evidence of splenomegaly (Chapter 171), a finding that is more common in patients with a subacute form of infective endocarditis. Finally, a thorough neurologic examination should be performed, both to assess for any focal neurologic deficits and to serve as a baseline during the patient's hospital stay. The neurologic examination may demonstrate evidence of major vessel embolism, cranial nerve palsies, visual field defects, or generalized toxic-metabolic encephalopathy with altered mental status.

Laboratory Findings

Initial laboratory tests should include a complete blood count with differential, serum electrolytes, measurement of renal function, urinalysis, chest radiograph, and electrocardiogram (ECG). All patients should receive at least three sets of blood cultures as well, and many require an echocardiogram (see later). Most patients with subacute infective endocarditis have anemia of chronic disease. The white blood cell count may or may not be elevated; it is more frequently elevated in cases of acute infective endocarditis, particularly if *S. aureus* or a fungus is the causative organism. Microscopic hematuria is noted in many cases, as is proteinuria. The chest radiograph is abnormal—demonstrating consolidation, atelectasis, pleural effusion, or clear septic emboli—in the overwhelming majority of patients with right-sided endocarditis; in others, it may provide evidence of heart failure. The ECG should be carefully examined for evidence of atrioventricular conduction blocks, especially a prolonged PR interval (see Figs. 64-7 through 64-11 in Chapter 64), suggestive of an aortic ring abscess or frank myocardial infarction (see Figs. 73-1 and 73-2 in Chapter 73). Other ancillary tests might include an erythrocyte sedimentation rate, which is elevated in nearly all cases of infective endocarditis, with a mean value of 57 mm/hour. Rheumatoid factor is positive in about half of cases, particularly in subacute endocarditis.

Complications

The complications of infective endocarditis can be divided into four groups for ease of classification: direct valvular damage and consequences of local invasion, embolic complications, metastatic infections from bacteremia, and immunologic phenomena. Local damage to the endocardium or myocardium is a dreaded complication that can be difficult to diagnose and treat. Infection may directly erode through the involved cardiac valve or adjacent myocardial wall, resulting in hemodynamically significant valvular perforations or cardiac fistulas. Such local complications typically present clinically with the acute onset of heart failure and carry a poor prognosis, even with prompt cardiac surgery. Valve ring abscesses also require surgical intervention and are more frequent in patients with prosthetic valves. Although a conduction defect on ECG may suggest the diagnosis, transesophageal echocardiography (TEE) is the diagnostic technique of choice for paravalvular abscess, valve perforation, or intracardiac fistula. Frank myocardial abscess has been found in up to 20% of cases on autopsy; *Aspergillus* endocarditis invades the myocardium in more than 50% of cases. Pericarditis is rare and is associated with myocardial abscess in most cases. Myocardial infarction, thought to be due to embolism of vegetative material in the coronary arteries, has been found in 40 to 60% of cases on autopsy, although most cases are clinically silent and lack characteristic ECG changes. However, up to 16% of elderly patients may present with clinical evidence of acute myocardial infarction, with potentially disastrous complications if the myocardial infarction is thought to be the primary event and the patient is given thrombolytic therapy. Heart failure is the leading cause of death in infective endocarditis, usually related to direct valvular damage.

Embolic events are less common now than in the preantibiotic era; nevertheless, about 35% of patients have at least one clinically evident embolic event. In fungal endocarditis, the majority of patients have at least one embolic event, frequently with a large embolus. The presence of large (>10 mm), mobile vegetations on the echocardiogram, particularly when the anterior mitral valve leaflet is involved, predicts a high risk of embolic complications. Most of the classic peripheral stigmata of infective endocarditis are probably embolic in nature; in addition, patients may have frank infarction of cutaneous tissue from emboli. In addition to the skin, emboli most commonly lodge in the lungs (in right-sided endocarditis), kidneys, spleen, large blood vessels, or central nervous system (CNS). Vegetations of right-sided endocarditis usually embolize to the lungs, resulting in an abnormality on the chest radiograph.

Renal abscesses are rare in infective endocarditis, but renal infarction is seen in more than 50% of cases at autopsy. Similarly, splenic infarction occurs in up to 44% of autopsy-confirmed cases; although frequently silent, such emboli may cause left upper quadrant pain radiating to the left shoulder, sometimes as the presenting symptom of infective endocarditis. Splenic infarction progressing to abscess may be a cause of persistent fever in patients with infective endocarditis; patients with infective endocarditis and unexplained persistent fever should undergo abdominal computed tomography to exclude this complication. Vascular aneurysms, which frequently occur at bifurcation points, may be clinically silent until they rupture (which may be months to years after apparently successful antibiotic treatment of infective endocarditis) and have been found in 10 to 15% of cases at autopsy. The presence of large emboli occluding major vessels can suggest the presence of fungal infective endocarditis. Peripheral mycotic aneurysms require surgical resection; intracerebral aneurysms should be resected if they bleed or if they are causing a mass effect.

Finally, many patients have evidence of cerebrovascular emboli, which have a predilection for the middle cerebral artery distribution and may be devastating. Most emboli to the CNS occur early in the course of the disease and are evident at the time of presentation or shortly thereafter. Cerebrovascular accidents related to these emboli are prone to catastrophic hemorrhagic transformation. The possibility of right-sided infective endocarditis leading to a paradoxical CNS embolism through a patent foramen ovale (Chapter 69) should not be neglected. Of note, the majority of patients with fungal endocarditis have a CNS embolic event.

Some complications of infective endocarditis are a result of bacteremic seeding causing metastatic infection at a distant site. Patients may present with osteomyelitis, septic arthritis, or epidural abscess. Purulent meningitis (Chapter 420) is a rare complication except in pneumococcal endocarditis, although many patients with *S. aureus* infective endocarditis who undergo lumbar puncture have a pleocytosis. Importantly, the finding of one metastatic complication of infective endocarditis does not exclude the possibility of additional sites of hematogenous infection, particularly in *S. aureus* endocarditis. Thus, the need for additional diagnostic evaluations should be guided by the patient's clinical course. Intracranial abscesses are uncommon in bacterial endocarditis but frequent in *Aspergillus* endocarditis; such a finding in the setting of culture-negative endocarditis should prompt the consideration of *Aspergillus* as an etiologic agent.

Multiple immunologic phenomena may occur, many of which are directly related to the circulating immune complexes characteristic of the disease. Renal biopsies performed in the setting of active infective endocarditis show some abnormality in nearly all cases. Infective endocarditis classically causes a hypocomplementemic glomerulonephritis. Histopathologically, the glomerular changes may be focal, diffuse, or membranoproliferative, or they may be akin to the immune complex disease found in systemic lupus erythematosus. In addition, many of the musculoskeletal conditions associated with infective endocarditis, including monoarticular and oligoarticular arthritides, are probably immune mediated.

DIAGNOSIS

The "gold standard" for the diagnosis of infective endocarditis is culture of a pathologic organism from a valve or other endocardial surface. However, unless the patient undergoes valve replacement or postmortem examination, the diagnosis is made clinically. As a result, various clinical criteria have been proposed over the years, the most widely accepted of which are the modified Duke criteria (Table 76-4), which have an estimated 76 to 100% sensitivity and 88 to 100% specificity, with a negative predictive value of at least 92%.

TABLE 76-4 MODIFIED DUKE CRITERIA FOR THE DIAGNOSIS OF INFECTIVE ENDOCARDITIS

MAJOR CRITERIA

1. Blood culture positive
   a. Typical organism (α-hemolytic streptococcus, *Streptococcus bovis*, HACEK organisms, or community-acquired *Staphylococcus aureus* or enterococcus without a primary focus) from 2 separate blood cultures
   or
   b. Persistent bacteremia with any organism (2 positive cultures >12 hr apart or 3 positive cultures or a majority of ≥4 cultures positive >1 hr apart)
   or
   c. Bacteremia with *S. aureus*, regardless of whether the bacteremia was nosocomially acquired or whether a removable focus of infection is found
2. Evidence of endocardial involvement
   a. Echocardiographic findings: mobile mass attached to valve or valve apparatus, abscess, or new partial dehiscence of prosthetic valve
   b. New valvular regurgitation
3. Serology: single positive blood culture for *Coxiella burnetii* or antiphase 1 IgG antibody titer >1 : 800

MINOR CRITERIA

1. Predisposing condition: intravenous drug use or predisposing cardiac condition
2. Fever ≥38° C
3. Vascular phenomena: arterial embolism, septic pulmonary emboli, mycotic aneurysm, intracranial hemorrhage, conjunctival hemorrhages, Janeway's lesions
4. Immunologic phenomena: glomerulonephritis, Osler's nodes, Roth's spots, rheumatoid factor
5. Echocardiogram findings consistent with endocarditis but not meeting major criteria
6. Microbiologic evidence: positive blood cultures not meeting major criteria or serologic evidence of active infection consistent with endocarditis

DEFINITIVE INFECTIVE ENDOCARDITIS

1. Pathologically proven infective endocarditis

or

2. Clinical criteria meeting
   a. Two major criteria *or*
   b. One major and one minor criteria *or*
   c. Three minor criteria

POSSIBLE INFECTIVE ENDOCARDITIS

Findings that fall short of definitive infective endocarditis but do not reject it

REJECTED INFECTIVE ENDOCARDITIS

1. Firm alternative diagnosis *or*
2. Resolution of infective endocarditis syndrome with antibiotic therapy for ≤4 days
   or
3. No pathologic evidence of infective endocarditis at surgery or autopsy with antibiotic therapy for ≤4 days

HACEK = *Haemophilus* spp, *Actinobacillus actinomycetemcomitans, Cardiobacterium hominis, Eikenella corrodens*, and *Kingella* spp; IgG = immunoglobulin G.
Adapted from Li JS, Sexton DJ, Mick N, et al. Proposed modifications to the Duke criteria for the diagnosis of infective endocarditis. *Clin Infect Dis.* 2000;30:633-638.

TABLE 76-5 ORGANISMS CAUSING "CULTURE-NEGATIVE" ENDOCARDITIS*

ORGANISM	EPIDEMIOLOGY	DIAGNOSTIC TESTS
HACEK spp	Mostly oral flora, so often preceded by dental work or history of periodontal disease	Prolonged incubation of standard blood cultures; may need to be subcultured onto blood or chocolate agar
Nutritionally variant streptococci	Slow and indolent course	Supplemented culture media or growth as satellite colonies around *Staphylococcus aureus* streak
Coxiella burnetii (Q fever)	Worldwide; exposure to raw milk, farm environment, or rural areas	Serologic tests (high titers of antibody to both phase 1 and phase 2 antigens); also PCR on blood or valve tissue
Brucella spp	Ingestion of contaminated milk or milk products; close contact with infected livestock	Bulky vegetations usually seen on echocardiography; blood cultures positive in 80% of cases with incubation time of 4-6 wk; lysis-centrifugation technique may expedite growth; serologic tests are available
Bartonella spp	*B. henselae:* transmitted by cat scratch or bite or by cat fleas *B. quintana:* transmitted by human body louse; predisposing factors include homelessness and alcohol abuse	Bulky vegetations usually seen on echocardiography; serologic testing (may cross-react with *Chlamydia* spp); PCR of valve or emboli is best test; lysis-centrifugation technique may be useful
Chlamydia psittaci	Exposure to birds; lawn mowing	Serologic tests available, but must exclude *Bartonella* because of cross-reactivity; monoclonal antibody direct stains on tissue may be useful; PCR now available
Tropheryma whippelii (Whipple's disease)	Systemic symptoms include arthralgias, diarrhea, abdominal pain, lymphadenopathy, weight loss, CNS involvement; however, endocarditis may be present without systemic symptoms	Histologic examination of valve with PAS stain; valve cultures may be done using fibroblast cell lines; PCR on vegetation material
Legionella spp	Contaminated water distribution systems; often nosocomial outbreaks; usually prosthetic valves	Lysis-centrifugation technique; also periodic subcultures onto buffered charcoal yeast extract medium; serologic tests and PCR available
Aspergillus and other noncandidal fungi	Prosthetic valve	Lysis-centrifugation technique; also culture and direct examination of any emboli

*Listed in approximate order of relative frequency.
CNS = central nervous system; HACEK = *Haemophilus* spp, *Actinobacillus actinomycetemcomitans, Cardiobacterium hominis, Eikenella corrodens,* and *Kingella* spp; PAS = periodic acid–Schiff; PCR = polymerase chain reaction.

The Duke criteria rely heavily on the appropriate use of blood cultures and echocardiographic data. At least three sets of blood cultures, with each set consisting of one aerobic and one anaerobic bottle, should be obtained from separate sites, with careful attention to aseptic technique. Ideally, these sets should be collected at least 1 hour apart to document continuous bacteremia; however, when patients are critically ill, this approach may not be feasible.

In most cases of endocarditis, in the absence of prior antibiotic therapy, every blood culture is positive because the bacteremia of endocarditis is continuous. Blood cultures are truly negative in less than 5% of cases of endocarditis; however, prior antibiotic administration may decrease the yield of blood cultures by up to 35%. Accordingly, most "culture-negative" cases of endocarditis occur in patients who have recently received antimicrobial agents. These cases are probably caused by the same organisms responsible for most native valve endocarditis; viridans streptococci and the HACEK organisms are the most likely suspects because they are much more fastidious than staphylococci and enterococci and are therefore more likely to be affected by previous antibiotic administration. Ultimately, however, when blood cultures are negative and endocarditis is suspected, especially when a history of recent antimicrobials is lacking, consideration should be given to fastidious organisms, fungi, and noncultivatable organisms (Table 76-5). This possibility should receive particular attention when the patient's history suggests exposure to farm animals or unpasteurized milk *(Coxiella burnetii, Brucella)*, cats *(Bartonella henselae)*, or body lice *(Bartonella quintana)* or contact with birds or frequent lawn mowing *(Chlamydia psittaci)*. It is important to notify the microbiology laboratory that endocarditis is suspected because special culture techniques can increase the yield for the HACEK species, nutritionally variant streptococci (*Abiotrophia* and *Granulicatella* spp), *Brucella, Legionella,* and some fungi. The traditional practice of "holding" blood cultures for 2 to 4 weeks to investigate culture-negative endocarditis is no longer required routinely. Specific serologic tests can be used to diagnose endocarditis related to *C. burnetii* (the agent of Q fever), *Brucella* species, *Bartonella*, and *C. psittaci*. *Tropheryma whippelii*, the etiologic agent in Whipple's disease, and multiple other organisms may be diagnosed by polymerase chain reaction. If the search for a causative organism is fruitless, noninfectious causes such as marantic or Libman-Sacks endocarditis and atrial myxoma (Chapter 60) should be considered.

Both transthoracic echocardiography (TTE) and TEE (Chapter 55) are highly specific tests (≈98%) when used as part of the diagnostic evaluation of suspected endocarditis. By contrast, TEE has a sensitivity of 90 to 95% in this setting, which is significantly better than TTE's usual sensitivity of 48 to 63%. Significant controversy still exists over whether the diagnostic evaluation of suspected infective endocarditis should begin with TTE or TEE. In most cases in which endocarditis is a serious diagnostic consideration, the evaluation should begin with TEE because negative TTE is not sensitive enough to exclude endocarditis (Fig. 76-3). If TEE is unavailable, technically impossible, or considered too invasive by the patient, it is reasonable to begin with TTE.

Some special situations may also dictate whether to begin with TTE or TEE. TEE is the only relatively noninvasive means of detecting perivalvular extension of infection; the esophageal probe's proximity to the aortic root and basal septal wall of the myocardium allows better visualization of these structures, which are most frequently involved in local spread of infection. For this reason, any patient with a new conduction system abnormality or persistent fever—clinical predictors of perivalvular extension—should be evaluated with TEE. Likewise, TEE's heightened sensitivity is especially important in the evaluation of suspected prosthetic valve endocarditis; TEE provides superior definition of prosthetic valve vegetations and valve ring abscesses. Finally, the high sensitivity of TEE in detecting valvular vegetations on native valves may be used in combination with clinical parameters (e.g., prompt resolution of bacteremia and defervescence) to support the clinical decision to abbreviate therapy in patients with vascular catheter–associated *S. aureus* bacteremia.

The combination of negative TTE and negative TEE has a negative predictive value of 95%. Nevertheless, when clinical suspicion of endocarditis is high and the initial TEE is negative, repeat TEE in 7 to 10 days may reveal the diagnosis.

TREATMENT Rx

Definitive antibiotic treatment of infective endocarditis (Table 76-6) is guided by antimicrobial susceptibility testing of the responsible pathogen isolated from clinical cultures. Although it is often advisable to begin empirical treatment before definitive culture results are available, not all patients admitted to rule out endocarditis need to be treated empirically. Patients who are clinically stable, with a subacute presentation of disease and without evidence of heart failure or other end-organ complications, can be closely observed without antibiotics so that serial blood cultures can be obtained. Likewise, stable patients who were started on empirical antibiotics before

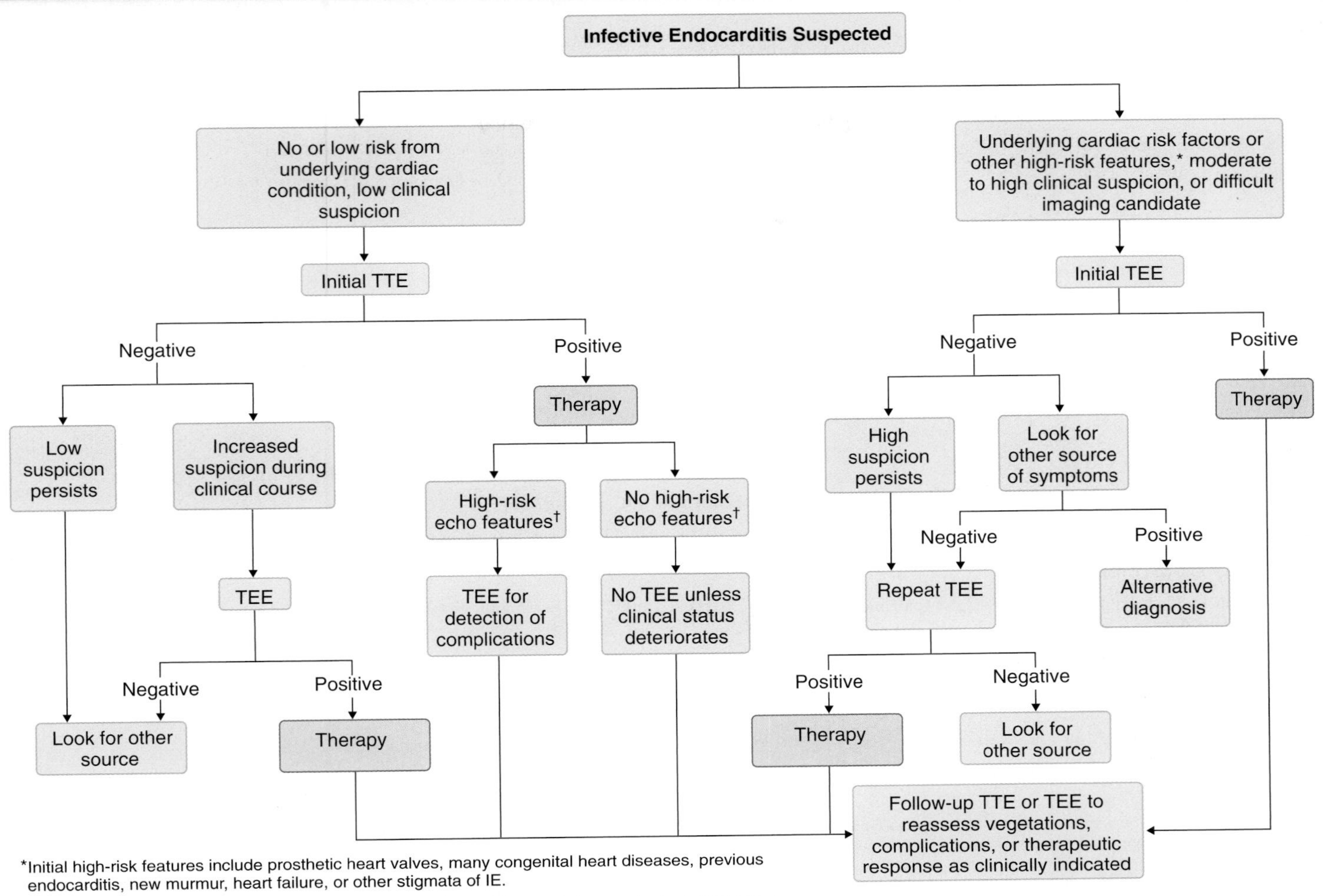

FIGURE 76-3. **Algorithm for the diagnostic use of echocardiography in suspected cases of infective endocarditis (IE).** TEE = transesophageal echocardiography; TTE = transthoracic echocardiography. (Adapted from Bayer AS, Bolger AF, Taubert KA, et al. Diagnosis and management of infective endocarditis and its complications. *Circulation.* 1998;98:2936-2948.)

hospitalization and before blood was drawn for cultures can discontinue the antibiotics so that blood cultures can be obtained, preferably as long as possible after stopping the antibiotics. By contrast, acutely ill patients, those with evidence of complications of endocarditis, and patients who are at high risk for endocarditis should be treated empirically with antibiotics pending culture results. In most cases of infective endocarditis, it is advisable to seek consultation from an infectious diseases specialist to assist in designing an appropriate antibiotic regimen.

Either of two regimens provides appropriate empirical coverage for patients with suspected native valve endocarditis: nafcillin (or oxacillin)-penicillin-gentamicin or vancomycin-gentamicin (Table 76-7). Nafcillin-penicillin-gentamicin is suitable in most cases of suspected native valve endocarditis, providing optimal coverage for streptococci, staphylococci, enterococci, and HACEK organisms. If MRSA is an important consideration, as it is for injection drug users and those with health care contact, empirical therapy should consist of vancomycin and gentamicin. This regimen is also acceptable for patients with a severe penicillin allergy. Patients with prosthetic valves should be empirically treated with vancomycin, gentamicin, and rifampin for adequate coverage of *S. aureus* (including MRSA), coagulase-negative staphylococci, and gram-negative organisms.

Treatment of Specific Organisms

When the organism is definitively identified, antibiotic treatment must be narrowed accordingly. Standardized regimens have been developed and validated for the most common organisms, and these protocols should be followed assiduously (see Table 76-6). More controversy exists over the treatment of unusual organisms, and consultation with infectious disease specialists is advisable in such circumstances. Of note, these regimens recommend low-dose gentamicin, which reduces the risk of toxicity while providing adequate levels for synergism. In cases in which the risk of aminoglycoside toxicity is significantly increased (e.g., elderly people, patients with preexisting renal disease or hearing impairment, diabetics), exposure to gentamicin should be minimized or avoided entirely. In fact, for the organisms listed in Table 76-6, gentamicin is critical for cure only in cases of enterococcal endocarditis. As a result, current American Heart Association guidelines classify even low-dose, short-course gentamicin therapy as "optional" for the treatment of native valve *S. aureus* endocarditis. Since the publication of these guidelines, a post hoc analysis of the data from a large randomized trial showed that a decrease in creatinine clearance occurred in 22% of patients receiving initial low-dose gentamicin, compared with 8% of patients not receiving it. Based on these results and on the minimal data supporting its benefit, initial low-dose gentamicin probably should not be used for *S. aureus* bacteremia in patients without prosthetic valves and should not be used for native valve endocarditis except when enterococcal or gram-negative infection is suspected.

In uncomplicated viridans streptococcal endocarditis, outpatient therapy with once-daily ceftriaxone is as effective as more complex regimens, provided the patient has been observed in the hospital for the development of complications.[1] The decision to administer antimicrobial therapy in the outpatient setting must, of course, take into account the patient's social situation, likelihood of compliance, and other risks involved with either an indwelling intravenous line or recurrent peripheral intravenous placement.

Standard therapy for infective endocarditis caused by fully susceptible enterococci includes penicillin or ampicillin plus either streptomycin or gentamicin. Although gentamicin is preferred over streptomycin, the choice of a specific aminoglycoside should be based on in vitro susceptibility testing, and the duration of aminoglycoside therapy can be as short as 2 to 3 weeks in some clinical settings. Although the optimal therapy for infective endocarditis due to ampicillin-sensitive aminoglycoside-resistant enterococci is undefined, in vitro and experimental data suggest the potential efficacy of a combination of ceftriaxone plus ampicillin for such infections.

Optimal therapy for enterococci that are "resistant" (e.g., to aminoglycosides and/or vancomycin) is not well defined. Endocarditis caused by vancomycin-resistant strains of enterococci may be treatable with daptomycin, quinupristin-dalfopristin (7.5 mg/kg intravenously every 8 hours), or linezolid (600 mg

TABLE 76-6 DEFINITIVE THERAPY OF BACTERIAL ENDOCARDITIS

ORGANISM/REGIMEN*	COMMENTS
PCN-SUSCEPTIBLE VIRIDANS STREPTOCOCCI (MIC ≤0.1 μg/mL) AND *STREPTOCOCCUS BOVIS*	
1. PCN 2-3 million units IV q4h × 4 wk	1. Also effective for other PCN-susceptible nonviridans streptococci
2. Ceftriaxone 2 g IV qd × 4 wk	2. Uncomplicated infection with viridans streptococci in a candidate for outpatient therapy; also for those with PCN allergy
3. PCN 2-3 million units IV q4h × 2 wk plus gentamicin 1 mg/kg IV q8h × 2 wk	3. Uncomplicated infection with none of the following features: renal insufficiency, eighth cranial nerve deficit, prosthetic valve infection, CNS complications, severe heart failure, age >65 yr; also not acceptable for nutritionally variant streptococci
4. PCN 2-4 million units IV q4h × 4 wk plus gentamicin 1 mg/kg IV q8h × 2 wk	4. Nutritionally variant strain; for prosthetic valve, give 6 wk of PCN
5. Vancomycin 15-20 mg/kg IV q8-12h × 4 wk	5. For PCN allergy; goal trough level of 15-20 mg/L
RELATIVELY PCN-RESISTANT VIRIDANS STREPTOCOCCI (MIC 0.12-<0.5 μg/mL)	
1. PCN 4 million units IV q4h × 4 wk plus gentamicin 1 mg/kg IV q8h × 2 wk	—
2. Vancomycin 15-20 mg/kg IV q8-12h × 4 wk	2. For PCN allergy or to avoid gentamicin; goal trough level of 15-20 mg/L
ENTEROCOCCI† AND PCN-RESISTANT VIRIDANS STREPTOCOCCI (PENICILLIN MIC >0.5 μg/mL)	
1. PCN‡ 18-30 million units IV per day in divided doses × 4-6 wk or ampicillin 12 g/24 hr IV in 6 equally divided doses plus gentamicin 1 mg/kg IV q8h × 4-6 wk	1. Increase duration of both drugs to 6 wk for prosthetic valve infection or symptoms >3 mo in enterococcal infection
2. Vancomycin 15-20 mg/kg IV q8-12h × 6 wk plus gentamicin 1 mg/kg q8h × 6 wk§	2. For PCN allergy; PCN desensitization is also an option; high risk of nephrotoxicity with this regimen
STAPHYLOCOCCUS AUREUS	
1. Nafcillin 2 g IV q4h × 4-6 wk with optional addition of gentamicin 1 mg/kg IV q8h × 3-5 days	1. Methicillin-susceptible strain; omit gentamicin if significant renal insufficiency
2. Vancomycin 15-20 mg/kg IV q8-12h × 6 wk	2. PCN allergy (immediate hypersensitivity or anaphylaxis) or MRSA
3. Nafcillin 2 g IV q4h × 2 wk plus gentamicin 1 mg/kg IV q8h × 2 wk	3. Methicillin-susceptible strain; 2-wk regimen only for use in IV drug abusers with only tricuspid valve infection, no renal insufficiency, and no extrapulmonary infection
4. Nafcillin 2 g IV q4h × >6 wk plus gentamicin 1 mg/kg IV q8h × 2 wk plus rifampin 300 mg PO/IV q8h × ≥6 wk	4. Prosthetic valve infection with methicillin-susceptible strain; use vancomycin instead of nafcillin for MRSA
5. Cefazolin 2 g IV q8h × 4-6 wk with optional addition of gentamicin 1 mg/kg IV q8h × 3-5 days	5. PCN allergy other than immediate hypersensitivity
6. Daptomycin 6 mg/kg IV qd × 14-42 days	Daptomycin is FDA-approved for treatment of right-sided *S. aureus* infective endocarditis; for adults, some experts recommend 8-10 mg/kg IV
COAGULASE-NEGATIVE STAPHYLOCOCCI, PROSTHETIC VALVE INFECTION	
Vancomycin 15-20 mg/kg IV q8-12h × >6 wk plus gentamicin 1 mg/kg IV q8h × 2 wk plus rifampin 300 mg PO/IV q8h × >6 wk	Can substitute nafcillin in above doses for vancomycin if isolate is methicillin sensitive
HACEK STRAINS	
1. Ceftriaxone 2 g IV qd × 4 wk; 6 wk for prosthetic valves	—
2. Ampicillin-sulbactam 3 g IV q6h × 4 wk; 6 wk for prosthetic valves	2. HACEK strains increasingly may produce β-lactamase
NON-HACEK GRAM-NEGATIVE BACILLI	
Enterobacteriaceae	
Extended-spectrum PCN or cephalosporin plus aminoglycosides for susceptible strains	Treat for a minimum of 6-8 wk; some species exhibit inducible resistance to third-generation cephalosporins; valve surgery is required for most patients with left-sided endocarditis caused by gram-negative bacilli; consultation with a specialist in infectious diseases is recommended
Pseudomonas aeruginosa	
High-dose tobramycin (8 mg/kg/day IV or IM in once-daily doses) with maintenance of peak and trough concentrations of 15 to 20 μg/mL and ≤2 μg/mL, respectively, in combination with an extended-spectrum penicillin (e.g., ticarcillin, piperacillin, azlocillin); ceftazidime, cefepime, or imipenem in full doses; or imipenem	Treat for a minimum of 6-8 wk; early valve surgery usually required for left-sided *Pseudomonas* endocarditis; consultation with a specialist in infectious diseases is recommended
Fungi	
Treatment with a parenteral antifungal agent (usually an amphotericin B–containing product) and valve replacement	Long-term/lifelong suppressive therapy with oral antifungal agents often required; consultation with a specialist in infectious diseases is recommended

*Dosages are for patients with normal renal function; for those with renal insufficiency, adjustments must be made for all drugs except nafcillin, rifampin, and ceftriaxone. Gentamicin doses should be adjusted to achieve a peak serum concentration of approximately 3 μg/mL 30 min after dosing and a trough gentamicin level of <1 μg/mL.
†Enterococci must be tested for antimicrobial susceptibility. These recommendations are for enterococci sensitive to PCN, gentamicin, and vancomycin.
‡Ampicillin 12 g/day can be used instead of PCN.
§The need to add an aminoglycoside has not been demonstrated for PCN-resistant streptococci.
HACEK = *Haemophilus* spp, *Actinobacillus actinomycetemcomitans, Cardiobacterium hominis, Eikenella corrodens,* and *Kingella* spp; MIC = minimum inhibitory concentration; MRSA = methicillin-resistant *Staphylococcus aureus*; PCN = penicillin.
Adapted from Baddour LM, Wilson WR, Bayer AS, et al. Infective endocarditis: diagnosis, antimicrobial therapy, and management of complications. *Circulation.* 2005;111:e394-e433.

TABLE 76-7 EMPIRICAL TREATMENT OF ENDOCARDITIS

CHARACTERISTICS OF PATIENTS	TREATMENT REGIMEN*
Native valve, community-acquired infection, MRSA unlikely	Nafcillin 2 g IV q4h plus penicillin 4 million units IV q4h plus gentamicin 1 mg/kg IV q8h
Any of the following: health care–associated infection or other reason to suspect MRSA; severe penicillin allergy	Vancomycin 15-20 mg/kg IV q8-12h† plus gentamicin 1 mg/kg IV q8h
Prosthetic valve	Vancomycin 15-20 mg/kg IV q8-12h† plus gentamicin 1 mg/kg IV q8h plus rifampin 300 mg PO/IV q8h

*Dosages are for patients with normal renal function; for those with renal insufficiency, adjustments must be made for all drugs except nafcillin.
†Goal is trough level of 15-20 mg/L.
MRSA = methicillin-resistant *Staphylococcus aureus*.

orally or intravenously twice daily); however, clinical experience with these agents is limited. In this situation, relapse or failure rates are likely to be high, and many cases require surgical intervention (discussed later).

Data suggest that patients with MRSA endocarditis treated with vancomycin have higher rates of bacteriologic failure than those treated with nafcillin. Therefore, every attempt should be made to treat MRSA endocarditis with an antistaphylococcal β-lactam. In a recent randomized trial, daptomycin 6 mg/kg/day for 10 to 42 days, depending on the severity of infection, was as effective as either semisynthetic antistaphylococcal penicillin or vancomycin for the treatment of *S. aureus* bacteremia and right-sided infective endocarditis,[2] and it is approved by the Food and Drug Administration for these indications.

Fungal endocarditis is usually a consequence of extensive health care contact. Traditionally, fungal endocarditis was regarded as an indication for valvular surgery, and amphotericin B (Chapter 339) was considered the treatment of choice. However, the high mortality associated with fungal endocarditis and the availability of new classes of antifungals suggest that these principles should be re-evaluated. The management of fungal endocarditis should always involve the collaboration of an experienced infectious diseases specialist.

Zoonotic endocarditis is usually culture-negative and most commonly caused by *Bartonella* species (Chapter 323), *C. burnetii* (Chapter 335), or *Brucella* species (Chapter 318). The treatments of choice for these fastidious pathogens are based on limited data, but documented *Bartonella* endocarditis is treated with doxycycline for 6 weeks and gentamicin for 2 weeks.

In cases of presumed culture-negative endocarditis in which unusual organisms (see Table 76-5) and other infections have been reasonably excluded, an empirical course of treatment may be undertaken. In this situation, most authorities recommend a 4- to 6-week regimen of ceftriaxone alone, vancomycin-ceftriaxone, or vancomycin-gentamicin (if the clinical setting suggests enterococci).

Continuing Care of the Patient with Endocarditis

In addition to antibiotics, appropriate inpatient care includes careful surveillance for the development of complications. Repeat echocardiography, as clinically indicated in the acute setting and at the end of antibiotic therapy, and serial ECGs should be obtained to look for the development of conduction system disease that might herald perivalvular extension, especially in patients with prosthetic valves and persistent fever. Widening pulse pressure should alert the clinician to the possible development of acute aortic insufficiency (Chapter 75). Similarly, a careful cardiac examination should be performed on a daily basis to assess for new regurgitant murmurs. Any new neurologic findings should prompt a search for evidence of CNS complications such as embolic events, cerebral hemorrhage, mycotic aneurysm, and brain abscess. Renal function should be closely monitored so that antibiotic doses can be adjusted, if necessary. If gentamicin is used for more than a few days, the patient should be alerted to watch for the signs and symptoms of vestibular or otic toxicity. Audiometric testing at baseline and periodically thereafter should be considered in patients at high risk for aminoglycoside-induced ototoxicity, including the elderly, patients with preexisting renal dysfunction or hearing damage, and patients receiving prolonged courses of gentamicin. Serum gentamicin trough concentrations should also be assayed at regular intervals (e.g., twice weekly, and more often if renal function is changing) and should be less than 1 μg/mL; higher concentrations should lead to lower or less frequent dosing or both. Follow-up blood cultures may be indicated toward the end of the first week of therapy in patients whose infective endocarditis is caused by organisms that commonly fail first-line treatment, such as *S. aureus* and enterococci. Positive cultures in this setting might suggest the need to change therapy or intervene surgically, whereas negative cultures are reassuring.

Patients with infective endocarditis may continue to be febrile for some time after the institution of appropriate antibiotic treatment. About 50% of patients defervesce within 3 days of starting antibiotics, 75% by 1 week, and 90% by 2 weeks. Patients whose endocarditis is caused by *S. aureus*, gram-negative organisms, or fungi tend to defervesce more slowly than patients infected with other organisms. Prolonged fever (>1 week after the institution of appropriate antibiotics) should prompt repeat blood cultures. If such cultures are negative, several possibilities should be considered: myocardial abscess, extracardiac infection (e.g., mycotic aneurysm, psoas or splenic abscess, vertebral osteomyelitis, septic arthritis), immune complex–mediated tissue damage, or a complication of hospitalization and therapy (e.g., drug fever, nosocomial superinfection, pulmonary embolism). Appropriate studies might include TEE, computed tomography of the abdomen, bone scan, and urinalysis with microscopy (to elicit evidence of interstitial nephritis). Intravenous line sites should be carefully examined for evidence of infection, and indwelling central lines should be changed.

Anticoagulation in individuals with infective endocarditis is controversial. Although new anticoagulation in the setting of native valve endocarditis does not appear to provide a benefit, continuing ongoing anticoagulation may be advisable. Some authorities recommend continuing anticoagulation in patients with mechanical prosthetic valve endocarditis. However, discontinuation of all anticoagulation for at least the first 2 weeks of antibiotic therapy is generally advised in patients with *S. aureus* prosthetic valve endocarditis who have experienced a recent CNS embolic event; this allows the thrombus to organize and potentially prevents the acute hemorrhagic transformation of embolic lesions. Reintroduction of anticoagulation in these patients must be cautious, and the international normalized ratio must be monitored carefully. The best option for patients with other indications for anticoagulation, such as deep venous thrombosis, major vessel embolization, or atrial fibrillation, is less clear and should be decided in a multidisciplinary fashion that balances the risks and benefits for each individual patient. Aspirin does not prevent embolic events and tends to increase the incidence of bleeding.[3]

Surgery

Some patients require surgical treatment, either to cure infective endocarditis or to prevent death from it (Table 76-8). Most patients with evidence of direct extension of infection to myocardial structures, prosthetic valve dysfunction, or heart failure from endocarditis-induced valvular damage should undergo surgery. In addition, many cases of endocarditis caused by fungi or by gram-negative or resistant organisms (e.g., vancomycin- or gentamicin-resistant enterococci) require surgical management. Progression of disease or persistence of fever and bacteremia for more than 7 to 10 days in the presence of appropriate antibiotic therapy may indicate the need for surgery; however, a thorough search must first be conducted to exclude other foci of infection. Surgical management should also be considered for patients with recurrent (two or more) embolic events or those with large vegetations (>10 mm) on echocardiography and one embolic event, although the data in these situations are less convincing. The presence of *S. aureus* endocarditis involving the anterior mitral valve leaflet and large vegetations (>10 mm) may be a special circumstance calling for early surgical intervention to reduce the high risk of CNS emboli, especially when mitral valve repair, rather than valve replacement, can be accomplished.

Delaying surgery in patients with deteriorating cardiac function in an attempt to "sterilize" the affected valve is ill advised because the risk of progressive heart failure or further complications usually outweighs the relatively small risk of recurrent infective endocarditis after prosthetic valve implantation. Relative contraindications to valve replacement include recent CNS emboli or bleed (because of the risk of bleeding in the perioperative period, when anticoagulation is required), multiple prior valve replacements (because of the difficulty of sewing a new valve into tissue already weakened from previous surgeries), and ongoing injection drug use. On occasion, patients have both a compelling indication for valve replacement (e.g., acute heart failure) and a recent CNS embolic event. The risk of hemorrhagic transformation of such lesions during cardiac bypass–associated anticoagulation is controversial. However, it appears that the greatest risk of such transformation events is in larger (>2 cm) emboli, especially those that have exhibited a hemorrhagic component. In these latter scenarios, it is prudent to try to delay surgery for at least 2 to 4 weeks to allow organization and resolution of such emboli. It appears that valve replacement can be performed safely without such delays in patients with smaller, nonhemorrhagic CNS emboli.

After definitive surgical treatment, most patients should receive further antibiotic therapy unless a full course of antibiotics was administered before surgery and there is no evidence of ongoing infection. If the patient received antibiotics for less than 1 week before surgery or the culture from the operative site is positive, the patient should receive the equivalent of a full initial course of antibiotics appropriate for the organism. If the patient received antibiotics for 2 weeks or more and the culture from the operative site is negative, the patient should receive whatever remains of the originally planned course of appropriate antibiotic therapy.

TABLE 76-8 INDICATIONS FOR SURGERY IN ENDOCARDITIS

INDICATION	CLASS*
NATIVE VALVE ENDOCARDITIS	
Acute aortic insufficiency or mitral regurgitation with heart failure	I
Acute aortic insufficiency with tachycardia and early closure of the mitral valve on echocardiogram	I
Fungal endocarditis	I
Evidence of annular or aortic abscess, sinus or aortic true or false aneurysm, valvular dehiscence, rupture, perforation, or fistula	I
Evidence of valve dysfunction and persistent infection after a prolonged period (7-10 days) of appropriate therapy, provided there are no noncardiac causes for infection	I
Recurrent emboli after appropriate antibiotic therapy	I
Infection with gram-negative organisms or organisms with a poor response to antibiotics in patients with evidence of valve dysfunction	I
Anterior mitral leaflet vegetation (especially with size >10 mm) or persistent vegetation after systemic embolization	IIa
Increase in vegetation size despite appropriate antimicrobial therapy	IIb
Early infections of the mitral valve that can probably be repaired	III
Persistent fever and leukocytosis with negative blood cultures	III
PROSTHETIC VALVE ENDOCARDITIS	
Early prosthetic valve endocarditis (<2 mo after surgery)	I
Heart failure with prosthetic valve dysfunction	I
Nonstreptococcal endocarditis	I
Evidence of perivalvular leak, annular or aortic abscess, sinus or aortic true or false aneurysm, fistula formation, or new-onset conduction disturbances	I
Persistent bacteremia after 7-10 days of appropriate antibiotic therapy, with no noncardiac causes for bacteremia	IIa
Recurrent peripheral embolus despite therapy	IIa
Vegetation of any size seen on or near the prosthesis	IIb

*Class I = conditions for which there is evidence and/or general agreement that a given procedure or treatment is useful and effective; class II = conditions for which there is conflicting evidence and/or a divergence of opinion about the usefulness or efficacy of a procedure or treatment; class IIa = weight of evidence or opinion is in favor of usefulness or efficacy; class IIb = usefulness or efficacy is less well established by evidence or opinion; class III = conditions for which there is evidence and/or general agreement that the procedure or treatment is not useful and in some cases may be harmful.
Adapted with permission from Bonow RO, Carabello B, de Leon AC, et al. Guidelines for the management of patients with valvular heart disease. *Circulation.* 1998;98:1949-1984.

TABLE 76-9 HIGH-RISK CARDIAC CONDITIONS FOR WHICH ENDOCARDITIS PROPHYLAXIS WITH DENTAL PROCEDURES IS REASONABLE

Prosthetic cardiac valve or prosthetic material used for cardiac valve repair
Previous endocarditis
Complex congenital heart disease involving unrepaired cyanotic congenital heart disease (including palliative shunts and conduits), completely repaired congenital heart disease with prosthetic material within 6 mo of the procedure, or repaired congenital heart disease with residual defects at the site or adjacent to the site of prosthetic material
Cardiac transplantation recipients who develop cardiac valvulopathy

Adapted from Wilson W, Taubert KA, Gewitz M, et al. Prevention of infective endocarditis guidelines from the American Heart Association: a guideline from the American Heart Association Rheumatic Fever, Endocarditis, and Kawasaki Disease Committee, Council on Cardiovascular Disease in the Young, and the Council on Clinical Cardiology, Council on Cardiovascular Surgery and Anesthesia, and the Quality of Care and Outcomes Research Interdisciplinary Working Group. *Circulation.* 2007;116:1736-1754.

TABLE 76-10 RECOMMENDATIONS FOR ENDOCARDITIS PROPHYLAXIS

PROPHYLAXIS IS REASONABLE*

Dental: All dental procedures involving manipulation of gingival tissue or the periapical region of teeth or perforation of the oral mucosa
Respiratory: Procedures involving incision or biopsy of the respiratory mucosa, such as tonsillectomy and adenoidectomy
Other: Infected skin, skin structures, or musculoskeletal tissue

PROPHYLAXIS IS NOT RECOMMENDED

Dental: Routine anesthetic injections through noninfected tissue, dental radiographs, placement of removable prosthodontic or orthodontic appliances, adjustment of orthodontic appliances, placement of orthodontic brackets, shedding of deciduous teeth, bleeding from trauma to the lips or oral mucosa
Respiratory: Procedures not involving incision or biopsy of the respiratory mucosa, including bronchoscopy (unless the procedure involves incision of the respiratory tract mucosa)
Genitourinary: Antibiotic prophylaxis solely to prevent infective endocarditis is not recommended
Gastrointestinal: Antibiotic prophylaxis solely to prevent infective endocarditis is not recommended

*Only in patients with underlying cardiac conditions associated with the highest risk for adverse outcome from endocarditis (listed in Table 76-9).
Adapted from Wilson W, Taubert KA, Gewitz M, et al. Prevention of infective endocarditis guidelines from the American Heart Association: a guideline from the American Heart Association Rheumatic Fever, Endocarditis, and Kawasaki Disease Committee, Council on Cardiovascular Disease in the Young, and the Council on Clinical Cardiology, Council on Cardiovascular Surgery and Anesthesia, and the Quality of Care and Outcomes Research Interdisciplinary Working Group. *Circulation.* 2007;116:1736-1754.

PREVENTION

Although the administration of prophylactic antibiotics to patients with known risk factors for infective endocarditis before undergoing procedures known to cause bacteremia is widespread, the efficacy of this practice has not been established. In 2007 the American Heart Association substantially reduced the situations in which prophylactic antibiotics were recommended. These revised recommendations were based on the following points: (1) endocarditis is much more likely to result from frequent exposure to random bacteremias associated with daily activities than from bacteremia caused by a dental, gastrointestinal tract, or genitourinary tract procedure; (2) prophylaxis may prevent an exceedingly small number of infective endocarditis cases, if any, in individuals who undergo dental, gastrointestinal tract, or genitourinary tract procedures; (3) the risk of antibiotic-associated adverse events often exceeds the benefit, if any, from prophylactic antibiotic therapy; and (4) maintenance of optimal oral health may reduce the incidence of bacteremia from daily activities and is more important than prophylactic antibiotics for a dental procedure to reduce the risk of infective endocarditis.

Prophylaxis is now judged to be reasonable for patients with the highest risk of adverse outcomes from endocarditis (Table 76-9) who must undergo dental procedures that involve manipulation of gingival tissue or the periapical region of teeth or perforation of the oral mucosa; an invasive procedure of the respiratory tract that involves incision or biopsy of the respiratory mucosa, such as tonsillectomy and adenoidectomy; or invasive procedures involving infected skin, skin structures, or musculoskeletal tissue (Table 76-10). The new recommendations focus on single-dose oral regimens in most clinical scenarios.

The antibiotics chosen for pre-procedure prophylaxis should be active against the organisms most likely to be released into the blood stream by the procedure (Table 76-11). Antibiotics that cover primarily oral flora are recommended. For patients with the conditions listed in Table 76-9 who undergo a procedure for infected skin, skin structure, or musculoskeletal tissue, it may be reasonable that the therapeutic regimen administered to treat the infection contain an agent active against staphylococci and β-hemolytic streptococci.

PROGNOSIS

Untreated, infective endocarditis is uniformly fatal. Aggressive medical and surgical management, however, has dramatically improved the outcome. Mortality overall from both native and prosthetic valve endocarditis remains fairly high, ranging from 17 to 36%. Certain subgroups carry a lower risk of death (endocarditis related to viridans streptococci), whereas *S. aureus*, fungal, and zoonotic endocarditis have higher mortalities. Heart failure and CNS events are the most frequent causes of death.

Endocarditis recurs in 12 to 16% of patients and is more common in injection drug users, elderly people, and patients with prosthetic valves. The rate

TABLE 76-11 SUGGESTED ANTIBIOTICS FOR ENDOCARDITIS PROPHYLAXIS FOR DENTAL OR RESPIRATORY TRACT PROCEDURES* IN PATIENTS WITH HIGH-RISK CARDIAC CONDITIONS†

PATIENT CHARACTERISTICS	REGIMEN‡
Able to take oral medications	Amoxicillin 2 g PO
Unable to take oral medications	Ampicillin 2 g IV or IM; or cefazolin or ceftriaxone 1 g IM or IV
Allergic to penicillin or ampicillin and able to take oral medications	Cephalexin 2 g PO (or other first- or second-generation oral cephalosporin in equivalent adult doses); clindamycin 600 mg PO; azithromycin 500 mg PO; or clarithromycin 500 mg PO Cephalosporins should not be used in an individual with a history of anaphylaxis, angioedema, or urticaria with penicillin or ampicillin
Allergic to penicillin or ampicillin and unable to take oral medications	Cefazolin or ceftriaxone 1 g IM or IV; or clindamycin 600 mg IM or IV

*For the applicable procedures, see Table 76-10.
†For the applicable conditions, see Table 76-9.
‡All regimens consist of a single dose 30-60 min before the procedure.
Adapted from Wilson W, Taubert KA, Gewitz M, et al. Prevention of infective endocarditis guidelines from the American Heart Association: a guideline from the American Heart Association Rheumatic Fever, Endocarditis, and Kawasaki Disease Committee, Council on Cardiovascular Disease in the Young, and the Council on Clinical Cardiology, Council on Cardiovascular Surgery and Anesthesia, and the Quality of Care and Outcomes Research Interdisciplinary Working Group. *Circulation.* 2007;116:1736-1754.

of relapse also varies depending on the causative organism. Easily treated infections, such as those with α-hemolytic streptococci, have a low rate of relapse (5%), whereas more difficult to eradicate organisms may have significantly higher rates.

FUTURE DIRECTIONS

As cardiac imaging technology continues to improve, the duration of treatment of endocarditis may be dictated in part by the characteristics of visualized vegetations. In addition, now that large vegetations have been demonstrated to cause more embolic events, interventions to remove vegetations (e.g., valve repair, vegectomy) or to introduce agents that prevent the formation or promote the dissolution of vegetations may be feasible. Finally, novel therapeutic approaches (e.g., antibacterial antibodies and cell wall–specific enzymes) that act as adjuncts to antibiotics in facilitating bacteriologic clearance are currently in development.

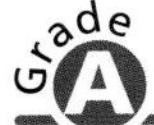

1. Sexton DJ, Tenenbaum MJ, Wilson WR, et al. Ceftriaxone once daily for four weeks compared with ceftriaxone plus gentamicin once daily for two weeks for treatment of endocarditis due to penicillin-susceptible streptococci. Endocarditis Treatment Consortium Group. *Clin Infect Dis.* 1998;27:1470-1474.
2. Fowler VG Jr, Boucher HW, Corey GR, et al. Daptomycin versus standard therapy for *Staphylococcus aureus* bacteremia and endocarditis. *N Engl J Med.* 2006;355:653-665.
3. Chan KL, Dumesnil JG, Cujec B, et al. A randomized trial of aspirin on the risk of embolic events in patients with infective endocarditis. *J Am Coll Cardiol.* 2003;42:775-780.

SUGGESTED READINGS

Prendergast BD, Tornos P. Surgery for infective endocarditis: who and when? *Circulation.* 2010;121:1141-1152. *Review.*

Snygg-Martin U, Rasmussen RV, Hassager C, et al. Warfarin therapy and incidence of cerebrovascular complications in left-sided native valve endocarditis. *Eur J Clin Microbiol Infect Dis.* 2011;30:151-157. *Data suggesting that patients with native valve endocarditis who are already taking and continue warfarin anticoagulation have fewer cerebrovascular complications than patients who are not.*

Tissari P, Zumla A, Tarkka E, et al. Accurate and rapid identification of bacterial species from positive blood cultures with DNA-based microarray platform: an observational study. *Lancet.* 2010;375:224-230. *The DNA-based microarray platform is more sensitive and faster than the culture-based method.*

77

PERICARDIAL DISEASES

WILLIAM C. LITTLE AND JAE K. OH

The pericardium, which is a relatively avascular fibrous sac that surrounds the heart, has two layers: the visceral and parietal pericardium. The potential space between the two layers normally contains only 10 to 50 mL of fluid, which is an ultrafiltrate of plasma. The pericardium is well innervated, so pericardial inflammation may produce severe pain and trigger vagally mediated reflexes.

As a result of its relatively inelastic physical properties, the pericardium limits acute cardiac dilation and enhances mechanical interactions of the cardiac chambers. In response to long-standing stress, the pericardium dilates to allow a slowly accumulating pericardial effusion to become quite large without compressing the cardiac chambers and to allow left ventricular remodeling to occur without pericardial constriction. Conversely, a scarred or thickened pericardium can limit the filling of the heart, resulting in pericardial constriction. Despite the important functions of the normal pericardium, congenital absence or surgical resection of the pericardium does not appear to have any major untoward effects.

ACUTE PERICARDITIS

EPIDEMIOLOGY AND PATHOBIOLOGY

Acute inflammation of the pericardium, with or without an associated pericardial effusion, can occur as an isolated clinical problem or as a manifestation of systemic disease. Although about 85% of isolated cases of acute pericarditis are idiopathic or viral, the list of other potential causes is quite extensive (Table 77-1). Patients with fever greater than 38° C or a subacute course or who fail to respond promptly to therapy are most likely to have pericarditis caused by a systemic autoimmune disease, malignancy, or viral or bacterial infection.

Pericarditis can occur after an acute myocardial infarction (MI). It occurs 1 to 3 days after a transmural MI, presumably owing to the interaction between the healing necrotic epicardium and the overlying pericardium. Dressler's syndrome, which is another form of pericarditis associated with MI, typically occurs weeks to months after MI. It is similar to the pericarditis that can occur days to months following traumatic pericardial injury, surgical manipulation of the pericardium, or pulmonary infarction. This syndrome is presumed to be mediated by an autoimmune mechanism and is associated with signs of systemic inflammation, including fever and polyserositis.

CLINICAL MANIFESTATIONS

Most patients with acute pericarditis experience sharp retrosternal chest pain (see Table 50-2 in Chapter 50), which can be quite severe and debilitating. In some cases, however, pericarditis is asymptomatic, such as when it accompanies rheumatoid arthritis. Pericardial pain is usually worse with inspiration and when supine, and it is generally relieved by sitting and leaning forward. Typically, pericardial pain is referred to the scapular ridge, presumably owing to irritation of the phrenic nerves, which pass adjacent to the pericardium. The chest pain of acute pericarditis must be differentiated from pulmonary embolism and myocardial ischemia or infarction (Table 77-2).

The pericardial friction rub is the classic finding in patients with acute pericarditis. A friction rub is a high-pitched, scratchy sound that can have one, two, or three components occurring when the cardiac volumes are most rapidly changing: during ventricular ejection, during rapid ventricular filling in early diastole, and during atrial systole. A pericardial rub, which is differentiated from a murmur by its scratchy quality, is sometimes localized to a small area on the chest wall and may come and go spontaneously or with changes in position. To hear a rub, it may be necessary to auscultate the heart with the patient in multiple positions, especially using the diaphragm with the patient learning forward and not breathing. The pericardial friction rub must be differentiated from a pleural rub, which is absent during suspended respiration, whereas the pericardial rub is unaffected.

DIAGNOSIS

Early in the course of acute pericarditis, the electrocardiogram (ECG) typically displays diffuse ST elevation in association with PR depression (Fig. 77-1). The ST elevation is usually present in all leads except for aVR, but the

TABLE 77-1 CAUSES OF PERICARDITIS: INFECTIOUS AND NONINFECTIOUS

INFECTIOUS PERICARDITIS (⅔ OF CASES)

Viral (most common): echovirus and coxsackievirus (usual), influenza, EBV, CMV, adenovirus, varicella, rubella, mumps, HBV, HCV, HIV, parvovirus B19, human herpesvirus 6 (increasing reports)
Bacterial: tuberculosis (4-5%)* and *Coxiella burnetii* (most common); other bacterial causes (rare) include pneumococcosis, meningococcosis, gonococcosis, *Haemophilus*, staphylococci, chlamydia, *Mycoplasma, Legionella, Leptospira, Listeria*
Fungal (rare): histoplasmosis more likely in immunocompetent patients; aspergillosis, blastomycosis, candidiasis more likely in immunosuppressed patients
Parasitic (very rare): *Echinococcus, Toxoplasma*

NONINFECTIOUS PERICARDITIS (⅓ OF CASES)

Autoimmune pericarditis (<10%)*
- Pericardial injury syndromes: post–myocardial infarction syndrome, post-pericardiotomy syndrome, post-traumatic pericarditis, including iatrogenic pericarditis (e.g., after percutaneous coronary interventions, pacemaker insertion, ablation)
- Pericarditis in systemic autoimmune and autoinflammatory diseases: more common in systemic lupus erythematosus, Sjögren's syndrome, rheumatoid arthritis, systemic sclerosis, systemic vasculitides, Behçet's syndrome, sarcoidosis, familial Mediterranean fever
- Autoreactive pericarditis*

Neoplastic pericarditis (5-7%)*
- Primary tumors (rare): pericardial mesothelioma
- Secondary metastatic tumors (common): lung and breast cancer, lymphoma

Metabolic pericarditis: uremia, myxedema (common); others rare
Traumatic pericarditis (rare)
- Direct injury: penetrating thoracic injury, esophageal perforation, iatrogenic
- Indirect injury: nonpenetrating thoracic injury, radiation injury

Drug-related pericarditis (rare): procainamide, hydralazine, isoniazid, and phenytoin (lupus-like syndrome), penicillins (hypersensitivity pericarditis with eosinophilia), doxorubicin, and daunorubicin (often associated with cardiomyopathy; may cause pericardiopathy)

*Percentages refer to unselected cases.
The diagnosis of autoreactive pericarditis is established using the following criteria: (1) increased number of lymphocytes and mononuclear cells >5000/mm^3 (autoreactive lymphocytic) or the presence of antibodies against heart muscle tissue (antisarcolemmal) in the pericardial fluid (autoreactive antibody mediated); (2) signs of myocarditis on epicardial or endomyocardial biopsies by ≥14 cells/mm^2; and (3) exclusion of infections, neoplasia, and systemic and metabolic disorders.
CMV = cytomegalovirus; EBV = Epstein-Barr virus; HBV = hepatitis B virus; HCV = hepatitis C virus; HIV = human immunodeficiency virus.
From Imazio M, Spodick DH, Brucato A, et al. Controversial issues in the management of pericardial diseases. *Circulation.* 2010;121:916-928.

TABLE 77-2 DIFFERENTIATION OF PERICARDITIS FROM MYOCARDIAL ISCHEMIA OR INFARCTION AND PULMONARY EMBOLISM

FINDINGS	MYOCARDIAL ISCHEMIA OR INFARCTION	PERICARDITIS	PULMONARY EMBOLISM
CHEST PAIN			
Character	Pressure-like heavy, squeezing	Sharp, stabbing, occasionally dull	Sharp, stabbing
Change with respiration	No	Worsened with inspiration	In phase with respiration (absent when the patient is apneic)
Change with position	No	Worse when supine; improved when sitting up or leaning forward	No
Duration	Minutes (ischemia); hours (infarction)	Hours to days	Hours to days
Response to nitroglycerin	Improved	No change	No change
PHYSICAL EXAMINATION			
Friction rub	Absent (unless pericarditis is present)	Present in most patients	Pleural friction rub may occur
ELECTROCARDIOGRAM			
ST segment elevation	Localized convex	Widespread concave	Limited to leads III, aVF, and V_1
PR segment depression	Rare	Frequent	None

Modified from Little WC, Freeman GL. Pericardial disease. *Circulation.* 2006;113:1622-1632.

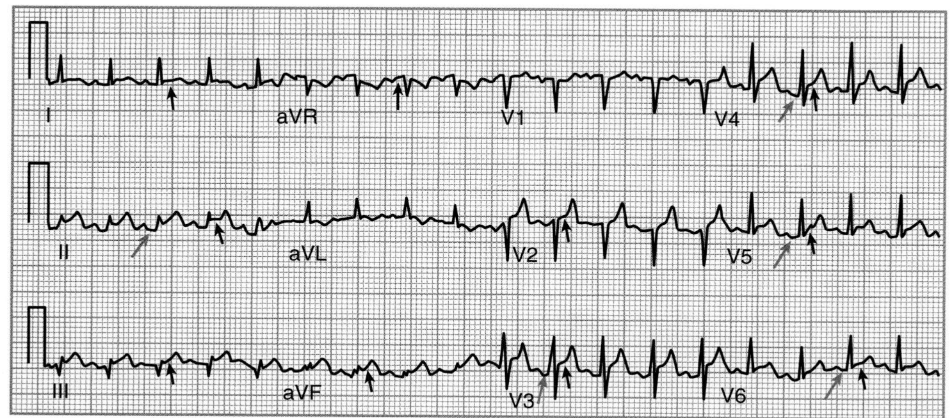

FIGURE 77-1. **Electrocardiogram demonstrating typical features of acute pericarditis on presentation.** There is diffuse ST elevation and PR depression except in aVR, where there is ST depression and PR elevation.

changes may be more localized in post-MI pericarditis. Classically, the ECG changes of acute pericarditis evolve over several days; resolution of the ST elevation is followed by widespread T wave inversion that subsequently normalizes. Uremic pericarditis frequently occurs without the typical electrocardiographic abnormalities.

Patients with acute pericarditis usually have evidence of systemic inflammation, including leukocytosis, an elevated erythrocyte sedimentation rate, and increased C-reactive protein level. A low-grade fever is common, but a temperature greater than 38° C is unusual and suggests the possibility of bacterial pericarditis.

About 85% of cases of acute pericarditis are idiopathic or viral. Viral causes include echoviruses and group B coxsackieviruses, but obtaining specific viral titers does not alter patient management. About 6% of cases are neoplastic in origin, about 4% are caused by tuberculosis, about 3% are caused by other bacterial or fungal infections, and about 2% are caused by collagen vascular disease. A targeted evaluation (Table 77-3) can help identify the various causes (Table 77-4).

Troponin levels typically are minimally elevated in acute pericarditis owing to some involvement of the epicardium by the inflammatory process. An elevated troponin level in acute pericarditis usually returns to normal within 1 to 2 weeks and is not associated with a worse prognosis. Although the elevated troponin level may lead to the misdiagnosis of an ST elevation MI (Chapter 73), most patients with elevated troponin levels and acute pericarditis have normal coronary angiograms. An echocardiogram (Chapter 55) can help avoid a misdiagnosis of MI.

Echocardiography may demonstrate a small pericardial effusion in the presence of acute pericarditis, but a normal echocardiogram does not exclude the diagnosis of acute pericarditis. An echocardiogram is critical, however, in excluding the diagnosis of cardiac tamponade (see later). When the diagnosis of acute pericarditis is unclear, cardiac magnetic resonance imaging (MRI) can demonstrate pericardial inflammation as delayed enhancement of the pericardium (Fig. 77-2). Diagnostic pericardiocentesis is indicated in suspected purulent tuberculosis or malignant pericarditis or if the patient has cardiac tamponade.

TABLE 77-3 SELECTED DIAGNOSTIC TESTS IN ACUTE PERICARDITIS

IN ALL PATIENTS
Tuberculin skin test (plus control skin test to exclude anergy)
BUN and creatinine to exclude uremia
Erythrocyte sedimentation rate
Electrocardiogram
Chest radiograph
Echocardiogram
IN SELECTED PATIENTS
Cardiac magnetic resonance imaging
ANA and rheumatoid factor to exclude systemic lupus erythematosus or rheumatoid arthritis in patients with acute arthritis or pleural effusion
TSH and T_4 to exclude hypothyroidism in patients with clinical findings suggestive of hypothyroidism and in asymptomatic patients with unexplained pericardial effusion
HIV test to exclude AIDS in patients with risk factors for HIV disease or a compatible clinical syndrome
Blood cultures in febrile patients to exclude infective endocarditis and bacteremia
Fungal serologic tests in patients from endemic areas or in immunocompromised patients
ASO titer in children or teenagers with suspected rheumatic fever
Heterophil antibody test to exclude mononucleosis in young or middle-aged patients with a compatible clinical syndrome or acute fever, weakness, and lymphadenopathy

AIDS = acquired immunodeficiency virus; ANA = antinuclear antibody; ASO = antistreptolysin O; BUN = blood urea nitrogen; HIV = human immunodeficiency virus; T_4 = thyroxine; TSH = thyroid-stimulating hormone.
Modified from Nishimura RA, Kidd KR. Recognition and management of patients with pericardial disease. In: Braunwald E, Goldman L, eds. *Primary Cardiology*, 2nd ed. Philadelphia: WB Saunders; 2003:625.

TABLE 77-4 PRESENTATION AND TREATMENT OF THE MOST COMMON CAUSES OF PERICARDITIS

TYPE	PATHOGENESIS OR ETIOLOGY	DIAGNOSIS	TREATMENT	COMPLICATIONS	COMMENTS
Viral	Coxsackievirus B Echovirus type 8 Epstein-Barr virus	Leukocytosis Elevated erythrocyte sedimentation rate Mild cardiac biomarker elevation	Symptomatic relief, NSAIDs	Tamponade Relapsing pericarditis	Peaks in spring and fall
Tuberculous	*Mycobacterium tuberculosis*	Isolation of organism from biopsy fluid Granulomas not specific	Triple-drug antituberculosis regimen Pericardial drainage followed by early (4-6 wk) pericardiectomy if signs of tamponade or constriction develop	Tamponade Constrictive pericarditis	1-8% of patients with tuberculosis pneumonia; rule out HIV infection
Bacterial	Group A streptococcus *Staphylococcus aureus* *Streptococcus pneumoniae*	Leukocytosis with marked left shift Purulent pericardial fluid	Pericardial drainage by catheter or surgery Systemic antibiotics Pericardiectomy if constrictive physiology develops	Tamponade in one third of patients	Very high mortality rate if not recognized early
Post–myocardial infarction	12 hr–10 days after infarction	Fever Pericardial friction rub Echo: effusion	Aspirin Prednisone	Tamponade rare	More frequent in large Q wave infarctions Anterior > inferior
Uremic	Untreated renal failure: 50% Chronic dialysis: 20%	Pericardial rub: 90%	Intensive dialysis Indomethacin: probably ineffective Catheter drainage Surgical drainage	Tamponade Hemodynamic instability on dialysis	Avoid NSAIDs About 50% respond to intensive dialysis
Neoplastic	In order of frequency: lung cancer, breast cancer, leukemia and lymphoma, others	Chest pain, dyspnea Echo: effusion CT, MRI: tumor metastases to pericardium Cytologic examination of fluid positive in 85%	Catheter drainage Subxiphoid pericardiectomy Chemotherapy directed at underlying malignant neoplasm	Tamponade Constriction	

CT = computed tomography; HIV = human immunodeficiency virus; MRI = magnetic resonance imaging; NSAIDs = nonsteroidal anti-inflammatory drugs.
Modified from Malik F, Foster E. Pericardial disease. In: Wachter RM, Goldman L, Hollander H, eds. *Hospital Medicine*, 2nd ed. Philadelphia: Lippincott Williams & Wilkins; 2005:449.

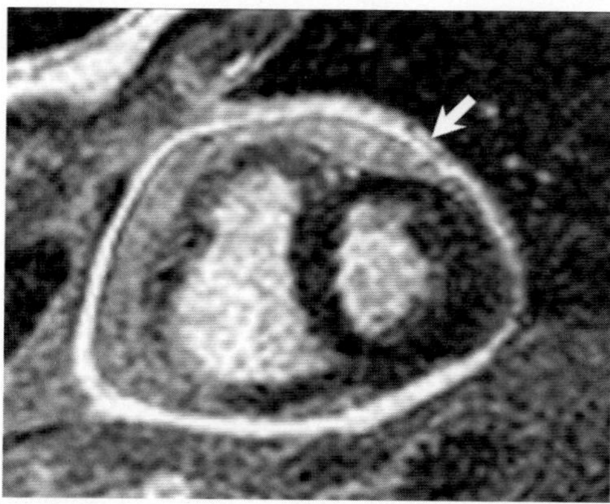

FIGURE 77-2. Cardiac magnetic resonance image of a patient with acute pericarditis shows late gadolinium hyperenhancement of the pericardium and epicardium.

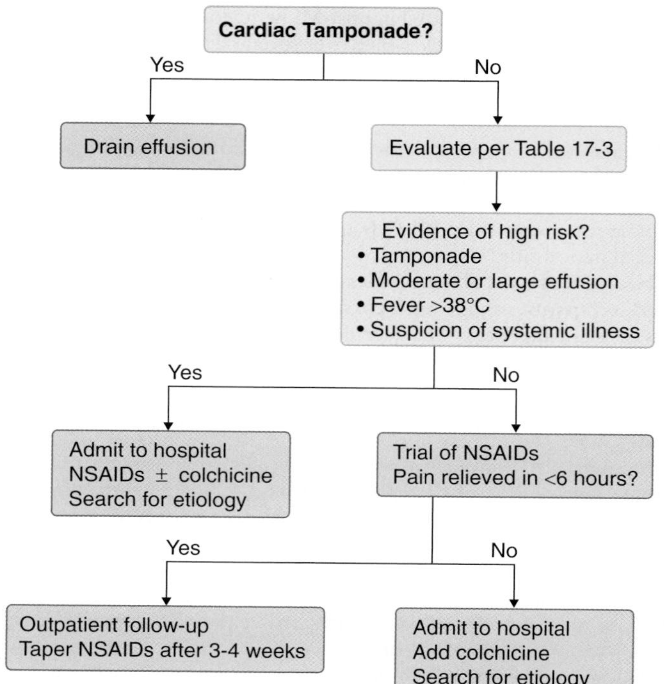

FIGURE 77-3. **Initial management of patients with pericarditis.** NSAIDs = nonsteroidal anti-inflammatory drugs.

TREATMENT Rx

Acutely ill patients with fever should be hospitalized, as should patients with suspected acute MI (Chapter 73), large effusions, evidence of impending hemodynamic compromise, or a cause other than viral or idiopathic pericarditis, because of the risk of a rapidly accumulating effusion with potential tamponade. Patients without effusions can usually be followed as outpatients (Fig. 77-3).

If acute pericarditis is a manifestation of an underlying disease, it often responds to treatment of the primary condition. Most cases of acute idiopathic or viral pericarditis are self-limited and respond to treatment with aspirin (650 mg every 6 hours) or another nonsteroidal anti-inflammatory drug (NSAID) such as ibuprofen (300 to 800 mg every 6 to 8 hours). The dose of NSAID should be tapered once symptoms or the pericardial effusion have resolved, but the medication should be taken for at least 3 to 4 weeks to minimize the risk of recurrent pericarditis.

If the pericardial pain and inflammation do not respond to NSAIDs or if the acute pericarditis recurs, colchicine (0.6 mg once or twice daily) for 3 months is effective in relieving pain and preventing recurrent pericarditis.[1] Alternatively, colchicine can be started in all patients to increase the likelihood of a favorable response to treatment. A major side effect is diarrhea. Colchicine should be avoided in patients with abnormal renal or hepatic function and in those being treated with macrolide antibiotics, which alter its metabolism.

Although acute pericarditis usually responds dramatically to systemic corticosteroids, observational studies strongly suggest that the use of steroids increases the probability of relapse in patients treated with colchicine. Accordingly, systemic steroids should be considered only in patients with recurrent pericarditis unresponsive to NSAIDs and colchicine or when needed to treat an underlying inflammatory disease. If steroids are used, low-dose prednisone (0.2 to 0.5 mg/kg) appears to be as effective as higher doses and is less likely to be associated with recurrence. Steroids should be continued for at least 1 month prior to slow tapering.

A proton pump inhibitor, such as omeprazole (20 mg/day), should be considered to improve the gastric tolerability of NSAIDs. Warfarin and heparin should be avoided to minimize the risk of hemopericardium, but anticoagulation may be required if the patient is in atrial fibrillation or has a prosthetic heart valve. It is prudent to avoid exercise until after the chest pain completely resolves. If pericarditis reoccurs, the patient can be reloaded with colchicine and intravenous ketorolac (20 mg) and then continued on an oral NSAID and colchicine for at least 3 months. Every effort should be made to avoid the use of steroids, reserving low-dose steroids for patients who cannot tolerate aspirin and other NSAIDs or whose recurrence is not responsive to colchicine and intravenous NSAIDs. Pericardiocentesis is not recommended unless purulent or tuberculous pericarditis is clinically suspected or the patient fails to respond to 2 to 3 weeks of NSAID therapy.

PROGNOSIS

The course of viral and idiopathic pericarditis is usually self-limited, and most patients recover completely. About 25% of patients, however, have recurrent pericarditis weeks to months later, probably due to an immune response, and some patients may have multiple debilitating episodes. Recurrent pericarditis is more common in patients treated with steroids for the acute episode, especially during a rapid steroid taper. In these patients, prolonged high-dose NSAID treatment (e.g., ibuprofen 300 to 600 mg three times a day) plus colchicine (0.6 mg twice daily, declining to once daily after 3 to 6 months) is recommended.[2] In patients who cannot tolerate colchicine or who have recurrent episodes despite high-dose NSAID treatment (e.g., indomethacin 50 mg three times a day or ibuprofen 800 mg four times a day), oral steroids (e.g., prednisone 0.2 to 0.5 mg/kg/day for 2 to 4 weeks, then slowly tapered over several months) are generally recommended, with pericardiectomy reserved for refractory cases. Patients who have recurrent pericarditis are at increased risk for progression to constrictive pericarditis (see later).

TABLE 77-5 CAUSES OF MODERATE TO LARGE ASYMPTOMATIC PERICARDIAL EFFUSIONS

CAUSE	% OF CASES
Idiopathic/viral	37
Neoplastic	19
Iatrogenic/trauma	13
Tuberculous or purulent	6
Acute myocardial infarction	6
Collagen vascular disease	4
Heart failure	4
Uremia	4
Radiation induced	2
Aortic dissection	2
Hypothyroidism	1
Other	2

Modified from Nishimura RA, Kidd KR. Recognition and management of patients with pericardial disease. In: Braunwald E, Goldman L, eds. *Primary Cardiology*, 2nd ed. Philadelphia: WB Saunders; 2003:625.

CARDIAC EFFUSION AND TAMPONADE

EPIDEMIOLOGY

A pericardial effusion can be caused by any disease that causes acute pericarditis (see Table 77-1), but a majority of cases are caused by conditions other than viral or idiopathic pericarditis (Table 77-5). For example, tamponade occurs in about 10 to 15% of patients with idiopathic pericarditis, but it develops in more than 50% of patients with malignant, tuberculous, or purulent pericarditis. Tuberculosis and neoplastic disease are typically associated

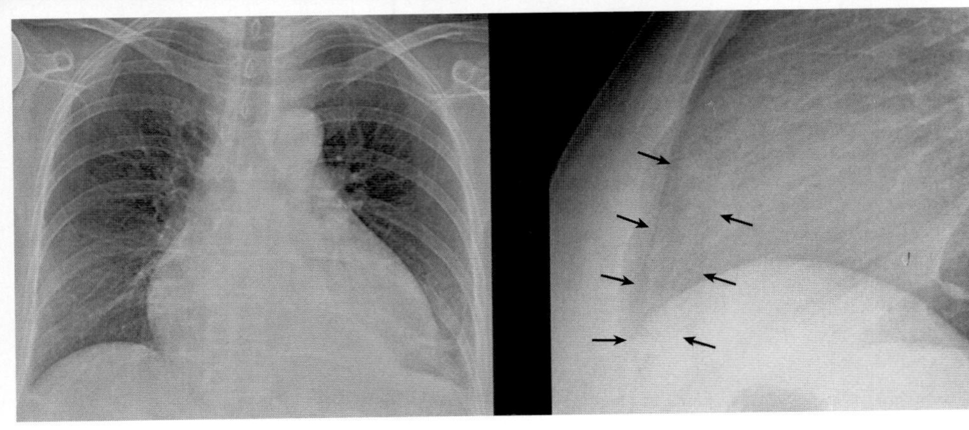

FIGURE 77-4. **Chest radiographs in a patient with a large pericardial effusion.** The cardiac silhouette on the posteroanterior view *(left)* is enlarged with a "water bag" configuration. The lateral view *(right)* shows a separation between the pericardial and epicardial fat stripes *(arrows)*.

with serosanguineous effusions, but such effusions can also be seen with typical viral or idiopathic pericarditis; with uremia, and after mediastinal irradiation. Hemopericardium is seen most commonly with trauma, myocardial rupture after MI, catheter-induced myocardial or epicardial coronary artery rupture, aortic dissection with rupture into the pericardial space, or primary hemorrhage in patients receiving anticoagulant therapy, often after cardiac valve surgery. Chylopericardium is rare and results from leakage or injury to the thoracic duct.

PATHOBIOLOGY

Under normal conditions, the space between the parietal and visceral pericardium can accommodate only a small amount of fluid before the development of tamponade physiology. The clinical consequences of a pericardial effusion depend on the rate of increase. A rapidly accumulating effusion, as in hemopericardium caused by trauma or aortic dissection, may result in tamponade physiology with just 100 to 200 mL of fluid. It is not surprising, therefore, that cardiac perforation quickly results in tamponade. By comparison, a more slowly developing effusion, as is typical with uremia and hypothyroidism, may allow the gradual stretching of the pericardium, with asymptomatic or minimally symptomatic effusions of 1500 mL or more.

Tamponade physiology occurs when fluid accumulation in the intrapericardial space is sufficient to compress the heart, resulting in impaired cardiac filling. The increased pericardial pressure in cardiac tamponade accentuates the interdependence among the cardiac chambers as the total cardiac volume is limited by the pericardial effusion. With normal inspiration, right ventricular filling is enhanced, the intraventricular septum is displaced toward the left ventricle, and left ventricular filling and the resulting stroke volume are reduced. Because of its lower pressures, the right ventricle is most vulnerable to compression by a pericardial effusion, and abnormal right heart filling is the earliest sign of a hemodynamically significant pericardial effusion. In tamponade, left heart filling occurs preferentially during expiration, when there is less filling of the right heart. The small normal respiratory increase in right ventricular volume, with a concomitant decrease in left ventricular stroke volume and systolic arterial pressure, is markedly accentuated in cardiac tamponade and results in the clinical finding of "paradoxical pulse." A small (<10 mm Hg) pulsus paradoxus, which is a decline in systemic blood pressure during inspiration, is normal and is related to the ventricles being confined within the pericardium and sharing a common septum. In cardiac tamponade, this phenomenon is exaggerated, and systemic blood pressure falls by more than 10 mm Hg during inspiration. A pulsus paradoxus also may be present with hypovolemic shock, chronic obstructive pulmonary disease, and bronchospasm.

CLINICAL MANIFESTATIONS

A slowly accumulating, isolated pericardial effusion is often completely asymptomatic. The physical examination may be normal, but the heart sounds may be muffled. The diagnosis is usually suggested by a chest radiograph that shows cardiomegaly with a globular heart (Fig. 77-4; see also Fig. 53-12 in Chapter 53) or by an echocardiogram, computed tomography (CT) scan, or MRI performed for another indication. Patients with hypothyroidism, uremia, or collagen vascular disease may have asymptomatic effusions discovered during comprehensive evaluations.

Patients with impending or early tamponade are usually anxious and tachycardic, and they may complain of dyspnea, orthopnea, and chest pain. The

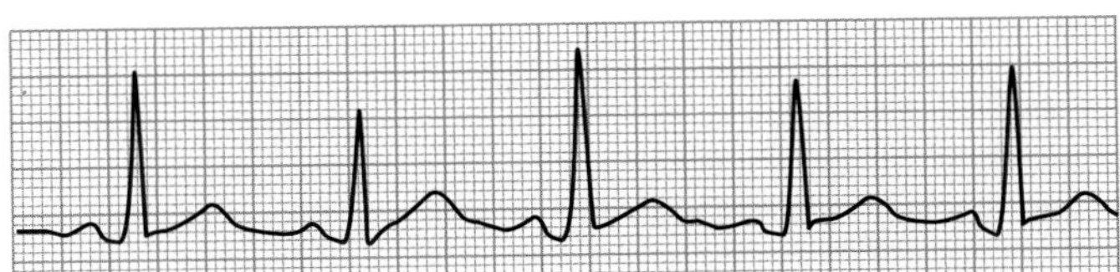

FIGURE 77-5. **Electrical alternans.** Lead V_5 rhythm strip from a patient with a large pericardial effusion and tamponade physiology. Note the relatively low voltage and electrical alternans.

increased venous pressure is usually apparent as jugular venous distention. The x descent (during ventricular systole) is typically the dominant jugular venous wave, with little or no y descent (during early diastole) (Chapter 50). The heart sounds are classically soft or muffled, especially if there is a large pericardial effusion. In rapidly developing cardiac tamponade, especially hemorrhagic cardiac tamponade, the jugular veins may not be distended because the time course has been insufficient for a compensatory increase in venous pressure. Such "low-pressure" tamponade may also occur with uremic pericarditis in volume-depleted patients. The patient may have signs of right heart failure, with peripheral edema, right upper quadrant pain caused by hepatic congestion, or abnormal liver enzymes and serum bilirubin level.

The hallmark of cardiac tamponade is a paradoxical pulse, which is defined as more than a 10 mm Hg drop in systolic arterial pressure during inspiration. When severe, the paradoxical pulse may be apparent as the absence of a palpable brachial or radial pulse during inspiration. A paradoxical pulse can also occur when there are wide swings in intrathoracic pressure, pulmonary embolism (Chapter 98), or hypovolemic shock (Chapter 106). A paradoxical pulse may be difficult to recognize in the presence of severe shock.

DIAGNOSIS

Cardiac tamponade, which is a treatable cause of shock (Chapter 107), can be rapidly fatal if unrecognized. As such, cardiac tamponade should be considered in the differential diagnosis of any patient with shock or pulseless electrical activity.

Cardiac tamponade is usually suspected based on jugular venous distention, sinus tachycardia with hypotension, narrow pulse pressure, elevated (>10 mm Hg) pulsus paradoxus, and distant heart sounds. Pulsus paradoxus may be obvious by palpation; it is more accurately measured with a sphygmomanometer during slow inspiration.

The ECG often shows low voltage and sometimes electrical alternans (Fig. 77-5) when the heart swings within a large pericardial effusion. The chest radiograph shows a globular, enlarged cardiac shadow (see Fig. 53-12 in Chapter 53 and Fig. 77-4) without pulmonary venous congestion.

Echocardiography, which is the key diagnostic test for cardiac tamponade, must be performed without delay in any patient suspected of having this condition. Echocardiography visualizes pericardial effusions as an echo-free space around the heart (Fig. 77-6), demonstrates the presence and size of the pericardial effusion, and reflects its hemodynamic consequences. The inferior vena cava is almost always enlarged, right atrial and right ventricular collapse indicates cardiac compression, and enhanced respiratory variation of ventricular filling is a manifestation of increased ventricular interdependence. Right ventricular collapse is more specific for tamponade than is right atrial

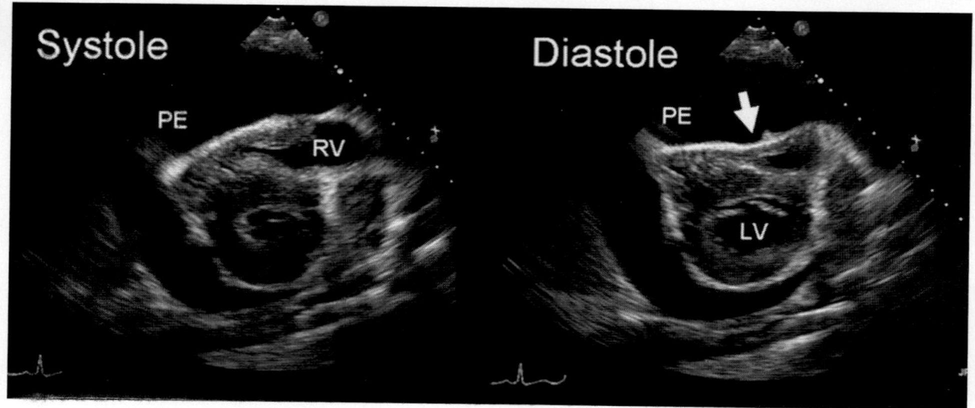

FIGURE 77-6. Two-dimensional echocardiogram from a patient with cardiac tamponade. A large pericardial effusion (PE) is apparent as an echo-free space surrounding the left ventricle (LV) and right ventricle (RV). In diastole, there is collapse of the right ventricle *(arrow)*.

collapse, but the right-sided chambers may not collapse when tamponade occurs in patients with pulmonary hypertension. Cardiac tamponade can result from a loculated pericardial effusion after cardiac surgery or trauma. A loculated effusion may not be apparent on transthoracic echocardiography, but transesophageal echocardiography and thoracic CT or MRI can delineate loculated pericardial effusions.

On Doppler study, mitral inflow velocity (especially early diastolic velocity) normally increases with expiration and decreases with inspiration; the opposite respiratory variation is seen in tricuspid inflow velocity. Doppler findings for tamponade, which are more sensitive than two-dimensional echocardiography, include augmented respiratory variation of mitral and tricuspid inflow velocities as a function of ventricular interdependence. These changes may be seen even before frank hemodynamic compromise due to pericardial effusion. Although Doppler echocardiography provides important information, it must be emphasized that cardiac tamponade is ultimately a clinical diagnosis.

The routine evaluation should include an assessment of renal function, a thyroid-stimulating hormone level, a complete blood count with differential, a platelet count, coagulation parameters, and a tuberculin skin test. Common medications that can cause a pericardial effusion include cromolyn, isoniazid, and phenytoin; hydralazine, procainamide, and reserpine are others. Blood cultures are indicated if an infectious cause is suspected. Complement levels, antinuclear antibodies, and the sedimentation rate can suggest systemic lupus erythematosus (Chapter 274), which rarely presents initially as an isolated pericardial effusion.

- Moderate-large pericardial effusion
  - Cardiac tamponade or suspicion of infection?
    - Yes → Drain effusion
    - No → Large effusion (>20 mm)?
      - No → Treat pericarditis
      - Yes → Present for <1 month or suspicion of malignancy?
        - No → Treat pericarditis
        - Yes → Drain effusion

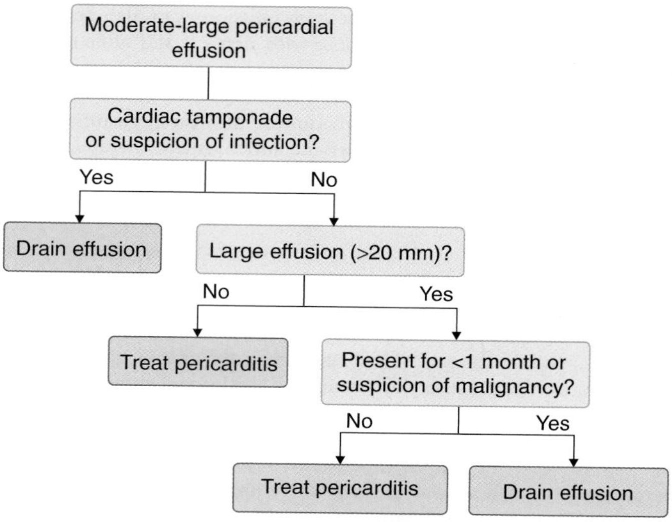

FIGURE 77-7. Algorithm for managing patients with moderate to large pericardial effusions. (Modified from Little WC, Freeman GL. Pericardial disease. *Circulation.* 2006;113:1622-1632.)

TREATMENT Rx

Pericardial Effusion without Tamponade

Acute pericarditis is often accompanied by a small pericardial effusion that does not produce tamponade. If there is no hemodynamic compromise and the diagnosis can be established by other means, pericardiocentesis is not necessary (Fig. 77-7). Even small pericardial effusions may be related to underlying systemic illnesses such as systemic lupus erythematosus (Chapter 274), cardiac amyloid (Chapter 194), scleroderma (Chapter 275), hypothyroidism (Chapter 233), or AIDS, so it is important to consider and treat associated illnesses. Chylous pericardial effusion, which is usually related to obstruction of the thoracic duct, may require a surgical procedure for relief.

For suspected pericardial effusion, transthoracic echocardiography is the initial test of choice, although loculated effusions may be identified better by CT or MRI. If a small (0.5 to 1 cm) echolucent or "organized" pericardial effusion is observed, a follow-up echocardiogram in 1 to 2 weeks, or sooner if the patient deteriorates, is recommended. If the effusion is getting smaller, subsequent echocardiograms are not necessary unless the patient's clinical condition changes.

For moderate (1 to 2 cm) or large (>2 cm) effusions in patients who are hemodynamically stable and in whom tamponade is not suspected, a follow-up echocardiogram should be performed in 7 days and then every month until the effusion is minimal. If bacterial or malignant pericarditis is suspected, diagnostic pericardiocentesis should be performed immediately, even in the absence of clinical instability or suggestion of tamponade; tuberculous pericarditis is diagnosed best by pericardial biopsy. Anticoagulation with heparin or warfarin should be discontinued unless the patient has a mechanical heart valve or atrial fibrillation.

In hypothyroidism (Chapter 233), the effusion and the coexistent cardiomyopathy respond to hormone replacement, sometimes over several months. Uremic pericardial effusions often respond to initiation of dialysis or more intensive dialysis (Chapter 132).

Cardiac Tamponade

The treatment of cardiac tamponade is urgent drainage of the pericardial effusion, especially when there is hemodynamic compromise. Fluid resuscitation may be of transient benefit if the patient is volume depleted (hypovolemic cardiac tamponade), but inotropic agents are usually ineffective because there is already intense endogenous adrenergic stimulation. The initiation of mechanical ventilation in a patient with tamponade may produce a sudden drop in blood pressure because the positive intrathoracic pressure further impairs cardiac filling.

Echocardiographic-guided percutaneous pericardiocentesis, which can be performed at the bedside by experienced operators (Fig. 77-8), is indicated if a patient is in dire circumstances and at least 1 cm of fluid is seen anterior to the mid-right ventricular free wall throughout diastole. The ideal entry site (usually the apex) is defined using echocardiography as the minimal distance from skin to pericardial fluid without intervening structures. The pericardial space is entered with a needle and then drained through a catheter. As much fluid as possible should be removed. The pericardial fluid should be sent for pH, glucose, lactate dehydrogenase, protein, cell count, and cytology as well as staining and culture for bacteria, fungi, and tuberculosis. Continued drainage of the pericardial fluid through an indwelling catheter minimizes the risk of recurrent effusion. For hemodynamically significant effusions of less than 1 cm, organized or multiloculated effusions, and focal effusions, a limited thoracotomy-mediastinoscopy and creation of a pericardial window are advised.

Surgical drainage may be the preferred treatment if pericardial tissue is required for diagnosis or in the case of recurrent effusions or bacterial pericarditis. Malignant pericardial effusions frequently reoccur and, like other recurrent pericardial effusions, may necessitate the surgical creation of a pericardial window that allows the effusion to drain into the pleural space, preventing

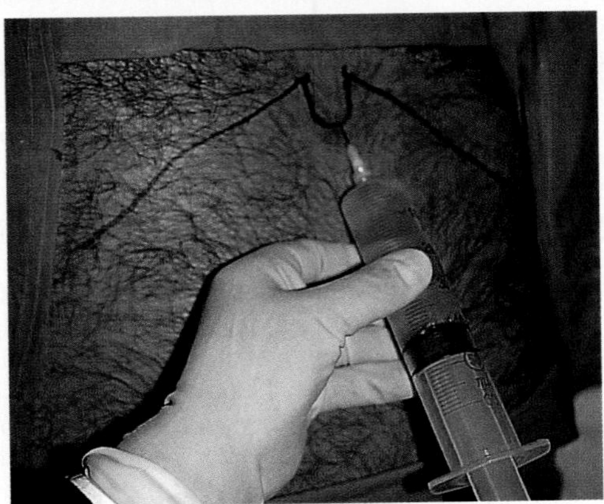

FIGURE 77-8. Aspiration of pericardial fluid is indicated in cardiac tamponade or to obtain fluid for diagnostic purposes. A wide-bore needle is inserted in the epigastrium below the xiphoid process and advanced in the direction of the medial third of the right clavicle. An alternative site is over the left ventricular apex. The procedure should be performed under echocardiographic guidance, but it may need to be performed emergently for life-saving purposes in other settings. Complications of the procedure include puncture of the heart, arrhythmias, vasovagal attack, and pneumothorax. (From Forbes CD, Jackson WF. *Color Atlas and Text of Clinical Medicine,* 3rd ed. London: Mosby; 2003.)

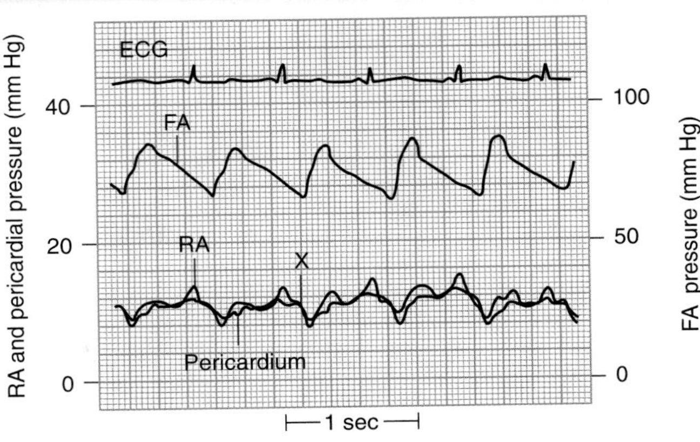

FIGURE 77-9. Right atrial (RA) pressure recording from a patient with constrictive pericarditis. Note the elevation in pressure and the prominent y descent, corresponding to rapid, early diastolic right atrial emptying. ECG = electrocardiogram; FA = femoral artery. (From Lorell BH. Profiles in constriction, restriction and tamponade. In: Baim DS, Grossman W, eds. *Cardiac Catheterization, Angiography, and Intervention,* 6th ed. Philadelphia: Williams & Wilkins; 2000: 832.)

reoccurrence of cardiac tamponade. An attractive alternative in these patients, especially if their overall prognosis is poor from the malignancy, is the percutaneous creation of a pericardial window by balloon dilation. Hemorrhagic effusions related to cardiac trauma or aortic dissection are best managed by emergency surgery.

PROGNOSIS

A pericardial effusion may recur or persist. Symptoms are usually weight loss, fatigue, dyspnea on exertion, and whatever symptoms are associated with the specific cause. Treatment of chronic or recurrent idiopathic effusions is similar to the treatment of recurrent pericarditis. If medical therapy is unsuccessful, creation of a pericardial window is indicated.

A large idiopathic, asymptomatic effusion that persists for 6 months or longer can unpredictably result in tamponade in as many as 30% of patients over long-term follow-up; diagnostic pericardiocentesis occasionally detects a neoplastic or tuberculous cause. Pericardiocentesis with prolonged drainage resolves many chronic large pericardial effusions, but pericardiectomy is often required. Long-term prognosis depends on the cause of the effusion. With pericardial tamponade, the in-hospital mortality rate is less than 10%, but the subsequent mortality rate is about 75% with a malignant effusion, compared with only 3 to 5% subsequent annual mortality for other causes.

PERICARDIAL CONSTRICTION

EPIDEMIOLOGY AND PATHOBIOLOGY

Pericardial constriction, which is usually the result of long-standing pericardial inflammation, occurs when a scarred, thickened, and/or calcified pericardium impairs cardiac filling, thereby limiting the total cardiac volume. The most frequent causes in the developed world are previous cardiac surgery, chronic idiopathic or viral pericarditis, and mediastinal radiation. Constriction may follow cardiac surgery by several weeks to months and may occur decades after chest wall irradiation. In developing countries, tuberculous pericarditis is a more common cause of constrictive pericarditis. Other less common causes include malignant disease, especially lung cancer, breast cancer, or lymphoma; histoplasmosis; rheumatoid arthritis; and uremia. However, a specific cause may not be identified in many patients.

With chronic constriction, the pericardium may thicken from its normal 3 mm or less to 6 mm or more, calcify, and adhere to the epicardium. In subacute constriction, the pericardium may be only minimally thickened and less calcified. Fibrous scarring and adhesions of both pericardial layers obliterate the pericardial cavity. The ventricles are unable to fill because of physical constraints imposed by a thickened, rigid, and sometimes calcified pericardium. The pathophysiologic hallmark of pericardial constriction is the exaggerated interventricular dependence and differential ventricular filling with respiration.

Although both cardiac tamponade and pericardial constriction impair diastolic ventricular filling and elevate venous pressure, the impairment in ventricular filling with constriction is minimal in early diastole until cardiac volume reaches the anatomic limit set by the noncompliant pericardium, at which time diastolic pressure rises abruptly and remains elevated until the onset of systole. This prominent y descent with an elevated plateau of ventricular pressure, which has been termed the "square root" sign (Fig. 77-9), differentiates constriction from tamponade, in which the y descent is absent. Stroke volume and cardiac output are reduced because of impaired filling, but the intrinsic systolic function of the ventricles can be normal.

CLINICAL MANIFESTATIONS

Patients with pericardial constriction typically present with manifestations of elevated systemic venous pressures and low cardiac output. Because there is equalization of all cardiac pressures (including right and left atrial pressures), systemic congestion is much more marked than pulmonary congestion. Typically, patients develop marked jugular venous distention, hepatic congestion, ascites, and peripheral edema, but their lungs remain clear. The limited cardiac output typically presents as exercise intolerance and may progress to cardiac cachexia with muscle wasting. In long-standing pericardial constriction, pleural effusions, ascites, and hepatic dysfunction may be prominent clinical features. Patients with pericardial constriction are much more likely to have left-sided or bilateral pleural effusions than right-sided effusions. Because of the prominent clinical symptoms of ascites and liver enzyme abnormalities, patients may be evaluated for hepatic disease before constrictive pericarditis is recognized.

The jugular veins are distended with prominent x and y descents. The normal inspiratory drop in jugular venous distention may be replaced by a rise in venous pressure (Kussmaul's sign). The classic auscultatory finding of pericardial constriction is a pericardial knock (Chapter 50), which is a high-pitched sound early in diastole when there is the sudden cessation of rapid ventricular diastolic filling, coinciding with the nadir of the y descent.

DIAGNOSIS

Pericardial constriction should be considered in any patient with unexplained systemic venous congestion. Pericardial calcification, seen best on the lateral plain chest radiograph, is a classic finding but is present in only 25% of patients with constrictive pericarditis, mostly in those with long-standing constriction. Similarly, most patients with pericardial constriction have a thickened pericardium (>2 mm) that can be imaged by echocardiography, CT, and MRI (Fig. 77-10). It is important to recognize, however, that pericardial constriction can be present without pericardial calcification and, in about 20% of patients, without any obvious pericardial thickening.

Transesophageal Doppler echocardiography may demonstrate pericardial thickening and calcification, but increased pericardial thickness can be missed on a transthoracic echocardiogram. Echocardiography also differentiates pericardial constriction from right heart failure caused by tricuspid valve disease and/or associated pulmonary hypertension.

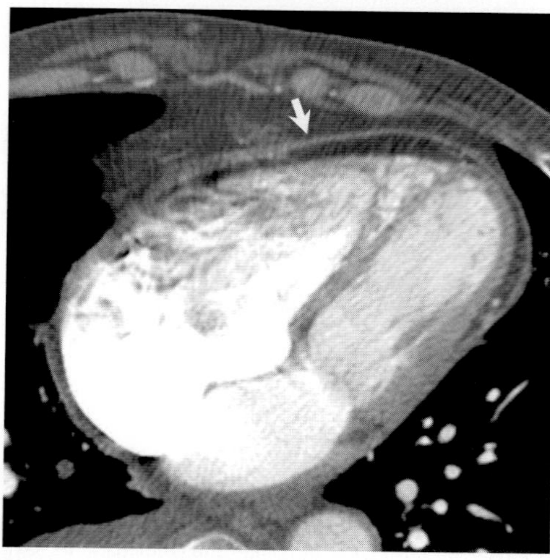

FIGURE 77-10. Computed tomography in a patient with constrictive pericarditis shows a thickened pericardium *(arrow)*.

TABLE 77-6 DIFFERENTIATION OF PERICARDIAL CONSTRICTION FROM RESTRICTIVE CARDIOMYOPATHY

FINDINGS	PERICARDIAL CONSTRICTION	RESTRICTIVE CARDIOMYOPATHY
PHYSICAL EXAMINATION		
Pulmonary congestion	Usually absent	Usually present
Early diastolic sound	Pericardial knock	S_3 (low pitched)
ECHO/DOPPLER		
Respiratory variation in E wave	>25%	<20%
Mitral septal annular early diastolic velocity	>7 cm/sec	<7 cm/sec
CT/MRI		
Pericardial thickness	>2 mm (but <2 mm in 20%)	<2 mm
BIOMARKER		
B-type natriuretic peptide	<200 pg/mL	>600 pg/mL
HEMODYNAMICS		
PA systolic pressure	<60 mm Hg	>60 mm Hg
PCW-LV diastolic pressure	Respiratory variation with reduction in inspiration	No variation
Respiratory variation in RV/LV peak systolic pressure	Discordant	Concordant

CT = computed tomography; LV = left ventricular; MRI = magnetic resonance imaging; PA = pulmonary artery; PCW = pulmonary capillary wedge; RV = right ventricular.
Modified from Little WC, Freeman GL. Pericardial disease. *Circulation.* 2006;113:1622-1632.

Differential Diagnosis

The most difficult differentiation is between pericardial constriction and restrictive cardiomyopathy (Chapter 60), the clinical manifestations of which may be very similar to those of pericardial constriction (Table 77-6). Doppler echocardiography is the most useful method to distinguish constriction from restriction. Patients with pericardial constriction usually have pronounced respiratory variation (>25%) of mitral inflow, whereas patients with restrictive cardiomyopathies do not. In some patients with pericardial constriction and markedly elevated venous pressures, the respiratory variation may be present only after head-up tilt. The Doppler measurement of early diastolic septal mitral annular velocity is almost always reduced in patients with myocardial restriction, whereas it remains normal or increased in patients with pericardial constriction. A prominent diastolic reversal of hepatic vein flow velocity during expiration is characteristic of constriction, whereas the reversal flow velocity occurs during inspiration in patients with right heart failure from other causes. Patients with pericardial constriction usually have only minimally elevated (<200 pg/mL) B-type natriuretic peptide (BNP), but BNP levels are typically markedly increased (>600 pg/mL) in patients with restrictive cardiomyopathy.

Confirmation of the diagnosis of constriction may require cardiac catheterization in patients whose noninvasive evaluation is not clear-cut. Traditional invasive hemodynamic findings of equalized end-diastolic pressures in the right and left ventricles and the "dip and plateau" pattern of left ventricular diastolic pressure do not reliably differentiate constriction from restrictive cardiomyopathy. More specific invasive hemodynamic features of constriction and restriction are based on the respiratory variation in ventricular filling; the simultaneous measurement of left and right ventricular pressures demonstrates discordant changes in their systolic pressures with respiration in constrictive pericarditis. By comparison, the direction of these pressures is concordant (both left and right sides increase with expiration and decrease with inspiration) in restrictive cardiomyopathy.

All patients with documented but otherwise unexplained pericardial constriction should be evaluated for potential tuberculosis.

TREATMENT AND PROGNOSIS Rx

In some patients with pericardial constriction of less than 3 months' duration, the symptoms and constriction may resolve over several weeks with medical therapy consisting of NSAIDs (e.g., ibuprofen 300 to 800 mg every 6 to 8 hours), colchicine (0.6 mg once or twice daily), and the cautious use of diuretics. For more chronic pericardial constriction or cases that do not respond to medical therapy, the definitive treatment is surgical pericardial decortication, with a wide resection of both the visceral and parietal pericardium. This operation is a major undertaking with substantial risk (>6% mortality even in the most experienced centers). In many patients, surgery does not immediately restore normal cardiac function; it may take weeks after removal of the constricting pericardium to return to normal. Empirical treatment of tuberculosis (Chapter 332) may be required in patients with constriction and a high suspicion of tuberculosis, even without a definitive diagnosis.

Effusive-Constrictive Pericarditis

In some patients (<10%) who present with cardiac tamponade, the elevated right atrial pressure and jugular venous distention do not resolve after removal of the pericardial fluid. In these patients, pericardiocentesis converts the hemodynamics from those typical of tamponade to those of constriction. Thus, the restriction of cardiac filling is due not only to pericardial effusion but also to pericardial constriction, predominantly involving the visceral pericardium. Effusive-constrictive pericarditis most likely represents an intermediate transition from acute pericarditis with pericardial effusion to pericardial constriction. Frequently, the symptoms resolve after several weeks of treatment with an NSAID (e.g., ibuprofen 300 to 800 mg every 6 to 8 hours).

SPECIFIC FORMS OF PERICARDIAL DISEASE

Postcardiotomy Syndrome

Postcardiotomy syndrome is acute pericarditis occurring weeks to months after open heart surgery. Patients have typical symptoms of acute pericarditis, which is associated with antimyocardial antibodies. A similar clinical picture is seen with the postperfusion syndrome caused by cytomegalovirus infection (Chapter 384) in patients who were previously uninfected but were exposed to cytomegalovirus-positive blood during cardiopulmonary bypass or transfusions. Atypical lymphocytes and elevated liver enzymes are often seen. Treatment of postcardiotomy syndrome is similar to the treatment of acute pericarditis.

Some patients who have undergone cardiac surgery develop late pericardial constriction without preceding acute pericarditis owing to bleeding in and around the open pericardium, followed by inflammation, scarring, and fibrosis. If active inflammation is present, a trial of anti-inflammatory agents may be instituted; however, surgical removal of the blood clot, usually accompanied by more extensive pericardiectomy, is typically required.

Post–Myocardial Infarction Pericarditis

Acute pericarditis can develop several days after an acute MI (Chapter 73), usually because of transmural extension of the infarction to the pericardial surface. This syndrome is uncommon in the reperfusion era. Anticoagulation should be temporarily withheld to avoid a bloody effusion that might progress to cardiac tamponade.

A late autoimmune pericarditis, termed *Dressler's syndrome*, can develop weeks to months after MI. Diagnosis and treatment are as for acute pericarditis.

Uremic Pericarditis

Pericardial effusions develop in patients with severe renal failure, especially those on dialysis (Chapter 133). Aggressive dialysis may decrease the pericardial effusion, but sometimes the effusion persists and requires drainage or even pericardiectomy.

Infectious Pericarditis

BACTERIAL PERICARDITIS

Purulent bacterial pericarditis may result from direct extension of bacterial pneumonia, direct extension of pleural empyema, or, rarely, peritonitis or a subphrenic abscess. Most patients are acutely ill with systemic sepsis and develop acute tamponade. The most common organisms are streptococci, pneumococci, and staphylococci. Urgent pericardiocentesis, which is required for both diagnosis and therapy, shows leukocytosis and frank pus, and the fluid glucose level is markedly depressed. Persistent or recurrent drainage with an indwelling catheter or repeated taps combined with antimicrobial therapy lead to a high survival rate, but late constrictive pericarditis requiring pericardiectomy develops in 30 to 40% of patients.

TUBERCULOUS PERICARDITIS

Tuberculous pericarditis is common in developing countries but accounts for less than 5% of cases of acute pericarditis in developed countries, usually in patients who are immunosuppressed. Symptoms are often nonspecific, and acute painful pericarditis is rare. Most patients have an effusive-constrictive physiology or pericardial constriction. The chest radiograph suggests active pulmonary tuberculosis is about 30% of cases, and a pleural effusion is present in 40 to 60% of cases. The echocardiogram typically shows fibrinous strands in the pericardial effusion, with multiple echo densities adherent to the pericardial surface. Pericardiocentesis is mandatory if tuberculous pericarditis is suspected. About 75% of patients have a positive culture, and a pericardial fluid adenosine deaminase level of 40 U/L or greater is seen in 75% of patients. Polymerase chain reaction testing and pericardial biopsy are recommended when tuberculous pericarditis is strongly suspected but not otherwise confirmed.

Aggressive antituberculosis therapy (Chapter 332) yields a cure rate of about 85 to 90%. Empirical treatment may be required in patients with a consistent clinical picture but without a confirmed diagnosis.

Even with prompt treatment, 30 to 60% of patients develop constrictive pericarditis, for which surgical pericardiectomy is the treatment of choice. In cases of suspected tuberculous constriction, antituberculosis therapy (Chapter 332) should be administered before and after pericardial surgery.

FUNGAL PERICARDITIS

The most common fungal pericarditis is histoplasmosis, which usually resolves in several weeks and can be treated successfully with NSAIDs. Specific antifungal therapy (Chapter 340) is recommended only in patients with disseminated histoplasmosis.

Malignant Pericarditis

About 6% of cases of acute pericarditis that initially have no obvious cause and about 20% of cases of moderate to large pericardial effusions are related to malignant diseases; in patients with cardiac tamponade, the percentage is even higher. About 80% of malignant pericarditis is linked to breast cancer (Chapter 204), lymphoma (Chapters 191 and 192), and leukemia (Chapters 189 and 190). Melanoma (Chapter 210) is an uncommon cause of malignant pericarditis, but a large proportion of patients with melanoma have pericardial involvement.

Most patients have direct tumor extension from an adjacent malignant lesion or a tumor from hematogenous or lymphatic spread. Pericardial effusions also may be caused by pericardial irritation or compromised lymphatic drainage in patients with mediastinal lymphoma.

Pericardiocentesis is key to diagnosis and management. Fluid cytology is positive in about 85% of patients. Complete drainage with an indwelling catheter for 2 or 3 days is the treatment of choice; if the effusion does not resolve, pericardiectomy is recommended. The prognosis depends on the treatment of the underlying malignancy, but the 1-year mortality rate is 80% or higher.

Post-Radiation Pericarditis

Post-radiation pericarditis develops in about 2% of patients after mantle radiation for Hodgkin's disease (Chapter 192) and in 0.4 to 5% of patients after irradiation for breast cancer. Pericardial injury occasionally manifests during treatment, but it more commonly appears months or even a decade later. The initial pericarditis and effusion may resolve spontaneously, but constrictive pericarditis, adjacent myocarditis, and even coronary artery damage can develop. Pericardiocentesis is critical to distinguish post-radiation pericarditis from malignant pericardial disease. Pericardiectomy is recommended for recurrent pericarditis and for large recurrent pericardial effusions.

Autoimmune Pericarditis

Up to 50% of patients with systemic lupus erythematosus (Chapter 274) have pericarditis, usually during an acute flare. Patients usually present with acute pericarditis or an asymptomatic effusion; cardiac tamponade is uncommon, and constrictive pericarditis is rare. If purulent pericarditis is not suspected, pericardiocentesis is not usually required. The underlying disease should be treated aggressively.

Acute pericarditis or asymptomatic pericardial effusions can develop in patients with advanced rheumatoid arthritis (Chapter 272), scleroderma (Chapter 275), or mixed connective tissue disease (Chapter 275). The process is usually self-limited or responds to aggressive treatment of the underlying disease, although cardiac tamponade can develop.

Myopericarditis

Concomitant myopericarditis (Chapter 60) may develop in patients with pericarditis, probably owing to direct extension of the inflammatory process. It is often manifested by ECG conduction delays, ventricular arrhythmias, and elevated troponin levels. No specific treatment is available.

Acute ventricular dilation and sudden or progressive heart failure develop in some patients after pericardiectomy for constrictive pericarditis or even after drainage of a large pericardial effusion. The syndrome may be underlying myocarditis.

Congenital Abnormalities

Congenital total absence of the pericardium is asymptomatic and clinically unimportant. However, partial or localized absence of the pericardium around the left atrium can cause focal herniation and lead to strangulation. CT or MRI can establish the diagnosis. Patients may present with atypical chest pain or sudden death. Surgical repair is often recommended for a partial pericardial defect.

Benign Cysts

Benign pericardial cysts are rare and are usually asymptomatic, but they can be associated with chest pain. They are typically seen as rounded or lobulated structures adjacent to the heart on the chest radiograph or adjacent to the right atrium on transthoracic echocardiography (Chapter 55). Thoracic CT and MRI are useful for the diagnosis. Cysts rarely rupture and do not require treatment unless they become symptomatic with chest pain. In this situation, the cyst can be removed surgically or drained percutaneously or with a thoracoscope.

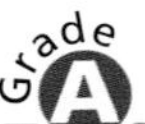

1. Imazio M, Bobbio M, Cecchi E, et al. Colchicine in addition to conventional therapy for acute pericarditis: results of the colchicine for acute pericarditis (COPE) trial. *Circulation.* 2005;112:2012-2016.
2. Imazio M, Bobbio M, Cecchi E, et al. Colchicine as first-choice therapy for recurrent pericarditis. Results of the CORE (Colchicine for Recurrent Pericarditis) trial. *Arch Intern Med.* 2005;165:1987-1991.

SUGGESTED READINGS

Imazio M, Spodick DH, Brucato A, et al. Controversial issues in the management of pericardial diseases. *Circulation.* 2010;121:916-928. *Review of causes and treatments.*

Khandaker MH, Espinosa RE, Nishimura RA, et al. Pericardial disease: diagnosis and management. *Mayo Clin Proc.* 2010;85:572-593. *Review.*

Mitiku TY, Heidenreich PA. A small pericardial effusion is a marker of increased mortality. *Am Heart J.* 2011;161:152-157. *After adjustment for other characteristics, even a small pericardial effusion is associated with about a 17% higher mortality.*

78

DISEASES OF THE AORTA

ERIC M. ISSELBACHER

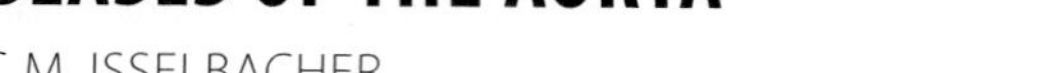

The aorta is composed of three tissue layers. The intima is a thin inner layer lined with endothelial cells. The middle layer, or media, is the thickest layer of the aortic wall and is composed of sheets of elastic tissue that give the aorta tremendous tensile strength. The outermost layer, or adventitia, is composed mostly of collagen and carries the vasa vasorum, which nourish the aortic wall.

The ascending aorta is about 3 cm wide and 5 cm long and is located in the anterior mediastinum. Its most proximal portion (just above the aortic valve) is called the *aortic root* and is composed of the three sinuses of Valsalva. In the superior mediastinum, the ascending aorta meets the aortic arch and gives rise to the brachiocephalic arteries. The descending thoracic aorta courses posteriorly and is about 2.5 cm in diameter and 20 cm long. After crossing the diaphragm, it becomes the abdominal aorta, which is normally 2 cm wide and about 15 cm long; it then bifurcates into the two common iliac arteries.

AORTIC ANEURYSMS

DEFINITION

An aortic aneurysm is pathologic dilation of the aorta. Aneurysms are described in terms of their location, size, shape, and cause. The shape of an aneurysm is *fusiform* when there is symmetrical dilation of the aorta and *saccular* when the dilation involves mainly one wall. In addition, there may be a *false aneurysm* or *pseudoaneurysm* when the aorta is enlarged as a consequence of dilation of only the outer layers of the vessel wall, such as occurs with a contained rupture of the aortic wall.

EPIDEMIOLOGY

Aneurysms can involve any part of the aorta, but abdominal aortic aneurysms are much more common than thoracic aneurysms. Abdominal aortic aneurysms are 5 to 10 times more frequent in men than in women and have a prevalence of at least 3% in persons older than 50 years. Among thoracic aortic aneurysms, those of the ascending aorta are most common, followed by aneurysms involving the descending aorta; aneurysms of the aortic arch are uncommon. If a descending thoracic aortic aneurysm extends distally and involves the abdominal aorta, a thoracoabdominal aortic aneurysm is created.

Smoking is the strongest risk factor associated with the development of abdominal aortic aneurysms, followed by age, hypertension, and hyperlipidemia. In addition, there appears to be a genetic predisposition to their development because up to 28% of first-degree relatives of patients with abdominal aortic aneurysms may be similarly affected.

PATHOBIOLOGY

Atherosclerosis has long been considered the common underlying cause of abdominal aortic aneurysms. Indeed, the infrarenal aorta tends to be most severely affected by the atherosclerotic process and is accordingly a common site for aortic aneurysm formation. However, although aortic atherosclerosis clearly contributes to the process, the pathogenesis of abdominal aortic aneurysms is multifactorial, with genetic, environmental, hemodynamic, and immunologic factors all contributing to the development and progressive growth of aneurysms.

The strength of the aortic wall lies in its extracellular matrix, the most important components of which are elastin and collagen. Consequently, degradation of these structural proteins weakens the aortic wall, allowing aneurysms to develop. There is histologic evidence of inflammatory infiltrates—in particular, macrophages and T lymphocytes—within the media and adventitia of aneurysms, and this inflammation may lead to degradation of the extracellular matrix. Furthermore, matrix metalloproteinases—enzymes produced by smooth muscle and inflammatory cells that can degrade elastin and collagen—are significantly elevated in the walls of abdominal aortic aneurysms and probably contribute to their formation. As the wall begins to dilate, tension on the wall increases according to Laplace's law (tension is proportional to the product of pressure and the radius), thereby promoting further expansion of the aneurysm.

Atherosclerosis is also a common cause of aneurysms of the descending thoracic aorta. However, the most important cause of aneurysms of the ascending thoracic aorta is a process known as *cystic medial degeneration*, which histologically appears as smooth muscle cell necrosis and degeneration of elastic layers within the media. Cystic medial degeneration is found in almost all patients with Marfan syndrome (Chapter 268), who are at very high risk for thoracic aortic aneurysms. Among patients without overt evidence of connective tissue disease, a bicuspid aortic valve and familial thoracic aortic aneurysm syndrome are important congenital causes (Chapter 69). A long-standing history of hypertension is a common risk factor in older patients. Syphilis (Chapter 327), once a common cause of thoracic aortic aneurysms, is now rarely a factor. Other uncommon causes of thoracic aortic aneurysms include infectious aortitis (Chapter 76), great vessel arteritis, aortic trauma (Chapter 112), and aortic dissection (see later). Many thoracic aortic aneurysms are idiopathic.

CLINICAL MANIFESTATIONS

The large majority of abdominal and thoracic aortic aneurysms are asymptomatic and are discovered incidentally on routine physical examination or imaging study. When patients with abdominal aortic aneurysms experience symptoms, pain in the hypogastrium or lower part of the back is the most frequent complaint. The pain tends to have a steady, gnawing quality that may last hours or days. Expansion or impending rupture of an aneurysm may be heralded by new or worsening pain, often of sudden onset. With rupture, the pain is frequently associated with hypotension and a pulsatile abdominal mass.

Patients with thoracic aortic aneurysms may have chest pain or, less often, back pain. Vascular complications include aortic insufficiency (sometimes with secondary heart failure), hemoptysis, and arterial thromboembolism. An enlarging aneurysm may produce local mass effects as a result of compression of adjacent mediastinal structures, with symptoms including coughing, wheezing, dyspnea, hoarseness, recurrent pneumonia, or dysphagia.

DIAGNOSIS

Abdominal aortic aneurysms may be palpable on physical examination, although obesity can obscure even large aneurysms. Typically, abdominal aortic aneurysms are hard to size accurately by physical examination alone because adjacent structures frequently make an aneurysm feel larger than it really is. Thoracic aortic aneurysms usually cannot be palpated at all.

Definitive diagnosis of an aortic aneurysm is made by radiographic examination. Abdominal aortic aneurysms can be detected and sized by either abdominal ultrasonography or computed tomography (CT). Ultrasound is extremely sensitive and is the most practical screening method for aortic aneurysms. Screening is recommended in men aged 65 years or older and women aged 65 years or older who have smoked or have a family history. Such ultrasound screening programs are cost-effective and have been shown to reduce mortality in men aged 65 to 79.[1] CT is even more accurate (Fig. 78-1)

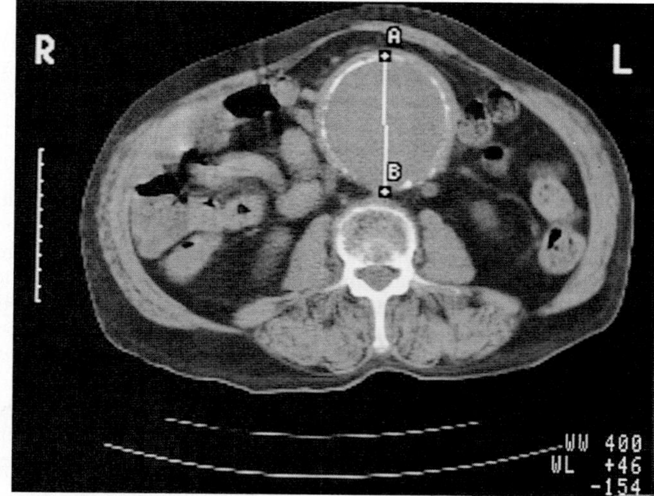

FIGURE 78-1. Abdominal aortic aneurysm on computed tomography. This sensitive imaging method allows precise measurement of size (point A to point B) and demonstrates the thickened wall of the aneurysm. (From Forbes CD, Jackson WF. *Color Atlas and Text of Clinical Medicine,* 3rd ed. London: Mosby; 2003.)

and can size an aneurysm to within a diameter of 2 mm. Although CT is less practical than ultrasound as a screening tool, it is the preferred modality for monitoring serial changes in size over time after the diagnosis has been made.

Thoracic aortic aneurysms are frequently recognized on chest radiographs; they often produce widening of the mediastinal silhouette, enlargement of the aortic knob, or displacement of the trachea from midline. CT is an excellent modality for detecting and sizing thoracic aneurysms and is particularly useful for monitoring size over time. Transthoracic echocardiography, which generally visualizes the aortic root and ascending aorta well, is useful for screening patients with Marfan syndrome, who are at particular risk for aneurysms involving this portion of the aorta.

TREATMENT

Rx

The goal of therapy for patients with aortic aneurysms is to reduce the risk for expansion and rupture of the aneurysm. Although blood pressure control is generally recommended, β-blockers do not reduce the rate of growth of abdominal aortic aneurysms. Nonrandomized data suggest a potential benefit from statins, angiotensin-converting enzyme inhibitors, and even macrolide antibiotics, which may act as matrix metalloproteinase inhibitors. However, no specific medical therapy can be recommended at the current time. Aneurysms should be monitored closely with serial imaging studies (e.g., CT) to detect any progressive enlargement over time, which may indicate the need for surgical repair.

Aortic aneurysms that produce symptoms secondary to expansion, vascular complications, or compression of adjacent structures should be repaired. Substantial evidence confirms a strong correlation between a surgeon's and hospital's aneurysm surgery volume and the outcome of abdominal aortic aneurysm repair.

Size is the major indicator for repair of asymptomatic aortic aneurysms. Abdominal aortic aneurysms larger than 5.5 cm should be repaired,[2,3] as should aneurysms larger than 5 cm in good operative candidates. Abdominal aneurysms of 3.5 to 4.4 cm should be monitored every 12 months, and those 4.5 to 5.4 cm should be monitored every 6 months. Descending thoracic aortic aneurysms larger than 6 cm should undergo surgical repair. Aneurysms of the ascending thoracic aorta should be repaired at 5.5 cm or larger, except that patients with Marfan syndrome or a bicuspid aortic valve should undergo repair when the aneurysm is 5 cm or larger because of the high risk of rupture in these patients.

Open surgical repair consists of insertion of a synthetic prosthetic tube graft. When aneurysms involve branch vessels, such as the renal or mesenteric arteries, the vessels must be reimplanted into the graft. Similarly, when a dilated aortic root must be replaced in the repair of an ascending thoracic aortic aneurysm, the coronary arteries must be reimplanted. An alternative approach for repair of abdominal aortic aneurysms (and some descending thoracic aneurysms) is the percutaneous placement of an expandable endovascular stent graft inside the aneurysm. This endovascular technique is associated with a better short-term outcome,[4,5] but there is no survival advantage after 2 years when compared with open repair.[4-6] In patients who are not candidates for open repair because of comorbid diseases or high surgical risk (Chapter 439), endovascular repair reduces aneurysm-related mortality substantially but does not reduce all-cause mortality compared with conservative medical management.[7]

PROGNOSIS

The chief concern in managing an aortic aneurysm is its tendency to rupture. Most aneurysms expand over time, and the risk for rupture increases with size.

Abdominal aortic aneurysms less than 4.0 cm have only a 0.3% annual risk for rupture, whereas aneurysms 4.0 to 4.9 cm have a 1.5% annual risk for rupture, and aneurysms 5.0 to 5.9 cm have a 6.5% annual risk for rupture. The overall mortality in patients with abdominal aortic aneurysm rupture is 80%, including 50% mortality even among those who reach the hospital.

Thoracic aneurysms smaller than 5 cm typically expand slowly and rarely rupture, but the rate of growth and risk of rupture increase significantly when thoracic aneurysms are 6 cm or larger. Similar to abdominal aneurysms, rupture of thoracic aneurysms has a high early mortality of 76% at 24 hours.

INTRAMURAL AORTIC HEMATOMA AND AORTIC DISSECTION

DEFINITION

An intramural aortic hematoma occurs when bleeding from the vasa vasorum or a tiny intimal tear causes a hematoma within the aortic media. Aortic dissection occurs when the media of the blood vessel is cleaved longitudinally to form a false lumen that communicates with the true lumen.

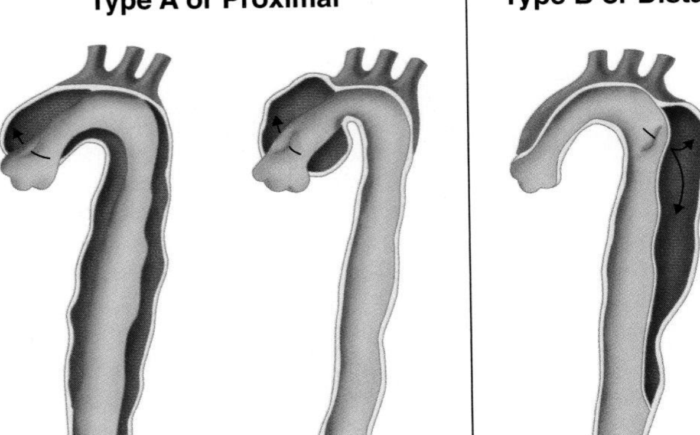

FIGURE 78-2. **Classification systems for aortic dissection.** (From Isselbacher EM. Diseases of the aorta. In: Braunwald E, Zipes DP, Libby P, Bonow RO, eds. *Braunwald's Heart Disease: A Textbook of Cardiovascular Medicine*, 7th ed. Philadelphia: Saunders; 2004:1416.)

The location of an intramural aortic hematoma or dissection may be described according to one of several classification systems (Fig. 78-2). Two thirds of aortic dissections are type A (proximal), and the other third are type B (distal). All the classification schemes serve the same purpose, which is to distinguish dissections that involve the ascending aorta from those that do not. Involvement of the ascending aorta carries a high risk for early rupture and death from cardiac tamponade, so the prognosis and management differ according to the extent of aortic involvement. Hematomas and dissections are also classified according to their duration: less than 2 weeks is considered acute, whereas 2 weeks or more is considered chronic.

The peak incidence of aortic dissection in patients without Marfan syndrome occurs in individuals in their 60s and 70s, and men are affected twice as often as women. A history of hypertension is present in most cases, whereas a bicuspid aortic valve or known preexisting thoracic aortic aneurysm is less common. Rarely, aortic dissection occurs in a young woman during the peripartum period. Iatrogenic trauma from intra-aortic catheterization procedures or cardiac surgery may also cause aortic dissection.

PATHOBIOLOGY

Disease of the aortic media, with degeneration of the medial collagen and elastin, is the most common predisposing factor for aortic dissection. Patients with Marfan syndrome have classic cystic medial degeneration and are at particularly high risk for aortic dissection at a relatively young age. Aortic dissection classically begins either with a tear in the aortic intima, thereby exposing the diseased medial layer to the systemic pressure of intraluminal blood, or with an intramural hematoma and subsequent rupture of the overlying intima. This hematoma may propagate longitudinally along a variable length of the aorta. If the intimal layer remains intact, the hematoma does not communicate with the aortic lumen; however, if open communication occurs, the result is no different than for a dissection that began with an intimal tear. The media cleaves into two layers longitudinally, producing a blood-filled false lumen within the aortic wall. This false lumen propagates distally (or sometimes retrogradely) a variable distance along the aorta from the site of the intimal tear.

CLINICAL MANIFESTATIONS

Pain, which is typically severe and occurs in 96% of cases of both aortic intramural hematoma and dissection, is the most common initial symptom. The pain may be retrosternal, in the neck or throat, interscapular, in the lower part of the back, abdominal, or in the lower extremities, depending on the location of the aortic hematoma or dissection. The pain may migrate as the dissection propagates distally. Thoracic pain is often of sudden onset and most severe at the start. It is sometimes described as "tearing," "sharp," or "stabbing." Although an isolated hematoma rarely causes symptoms other

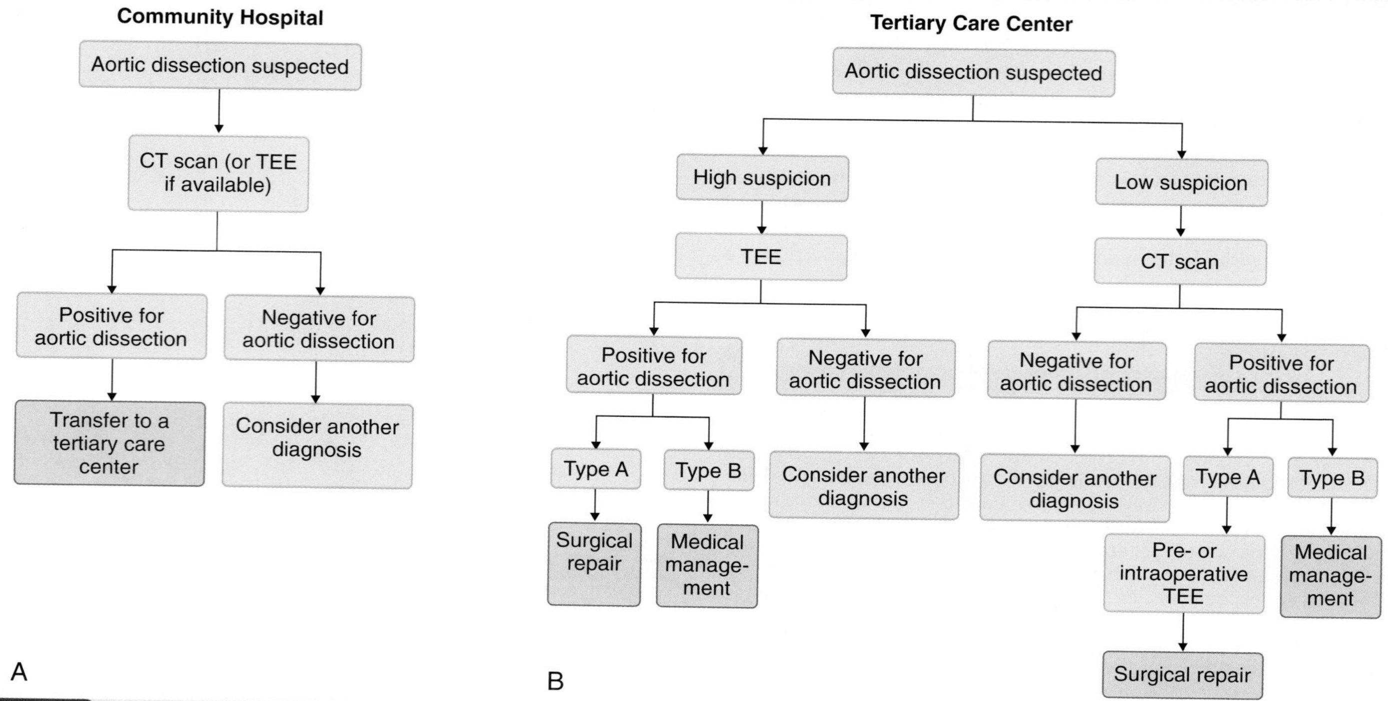

FIGURE 78-3. **Algorithms for the evaluation of suspected acute aortic dissection. A,** This approach is used in many community hospitals where cardiac surgery is not performed. **B,** This approach is used in many tertiary care centers where transesophageal echocardiography (TEE) and cardiac surgery are available. CT = computed tomography.

than pain, a dissection, regardless of how it starts, may also result in acute aortic insufficiency (Chapter 75), right coronary artery occlusion, hemopericardium (Chapter 77), syncope (Chapters 50 and 62), cerebrovascular accident (Chapter 414), mesenteric ischemia (Chapter 145), or ischemic peripheral neuropathy (Chapter 428).

Hypertension is a common finding on physical examination and is present in 70% of patients with distal aortic dissection. Hypotension may also occur, particularly in patients with proximal dissections, and is usually due to rupture into the pericardium or severe aortic insufficiency. Pseudohypotension occurs when a falsely low measure of upper extremity blood pressure is obtained because of involvement of the subclavian artery by the dissection. Similarly, pulse deficits are a common finding on physical examination, particularly in patients with proximal aortic dissections with involvement of the subclavian, carotid, or femoral arteries. Aortic insufficiency occurs in more than a third of patients with a proximal dissection; paradoxically, however, when acute aortic insufficiency is severe, the murmur may not be appreciable, so finding a widened pulse pressure and heart failure should raise suspicion of its presence.

Vascular complications from aortic dissection include compromise of a coronary artery, with subsequent myocardial ischemia or infarction. Involvement of the brachiocephalic arteries may produce a stroke or coma, whereas compromise of the spinal arteries may produce paraplegia. When a dissection extends into the abdominal aorta, flow to one or both renal arteries may be compromised and produce acute renal failure, which may exacerbate the hypertension. Mesenteric ischemia or frank infarction may manifest as abdominal pain. Finally, the dissection may extend distally to the aortic bifurcation and compromise or occlude one of the common iliac arteries and thereby produce a femoral pulse deficit and ischemia of the lower extremities.

An abnormality on a chest radiograph often raises the first suspicion of aortic dissection. The findings on chest radiography are nonspecific, however, and rarely diagnostic. An enlarged mediastinal silhouette is the most common finding, but it may be present in as few as 65% of patients in whom dissection is ultimately diagnosed. A left pleural effusion is commonly seen in patients with involvement of the descending thoracic aorta; when small, this typically represents an exudate from the inflamed aortic wall. A normal chest radiograph does not exclude the diagnosis of aortic dissection. Electrocardiographic findings in aortic dissection are nonspecific.

DIAGNOSIS

When there is clinical suspicion of aortic dissection, it is essential to confirm or exclude the diagnosis promptly with an imaging study (Fig. 78-3). Several

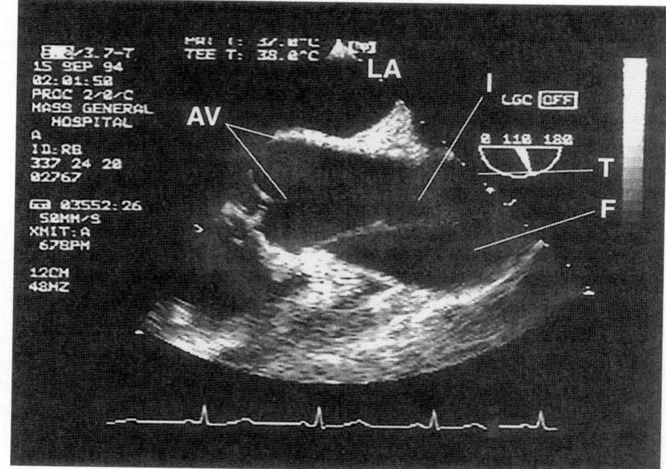

FIGURE 78-4. **Transesophageal echocardiogram of the ascending aorta in the long axis in a patient with type A aortic dissection.** The aortic valve (AV) is on the left, and the ascending aorta extends to the right. Within the aorta is an intimal flap (I) that originates at the level of the sinotubular junction. The true (T) and the false (F) lumens are separated by the intimal flap. LA = left atrium. (From Isselbacher EM. Diseases of the aorta. In: Braunwald E, Zipes DP, Libby P, Bonow RO, eds. *Braunwald's Heart Disease: A Textbook of Cardiovascular Medicine*, 7th ed. Philadelphia: Saunders; 2004:1423.)

imaging modalities can be used to diagnose the presence of aortic dissection accurately, including aortography, CT (Chapter 56), magnetic resonance imaging (Chapter 56), and transesophageal echocardiography (TEE; Chapter 55). Each institution must determine which of these modalities is most appropriate as an initial diagnostic approach, based on their availability and the skill and experience of the clinicians who perform and interpret the studies.

Nevertheless, when suspicion of aortic dissection is high, TEE (Fig. 78-4) is the most rapid means of providing sufficient detail to proceed directly to the operating room. When clinical suspicion is low (i.e., when the goal is to rule out aortic dissection), contrast-enhanced CT (Fig. 78-5) is preferred because it is entirely noninvasive. If TEE is not readily available, contrast-enhanced CT is the imaging modality of choice in both high-probability and low-probability patients.

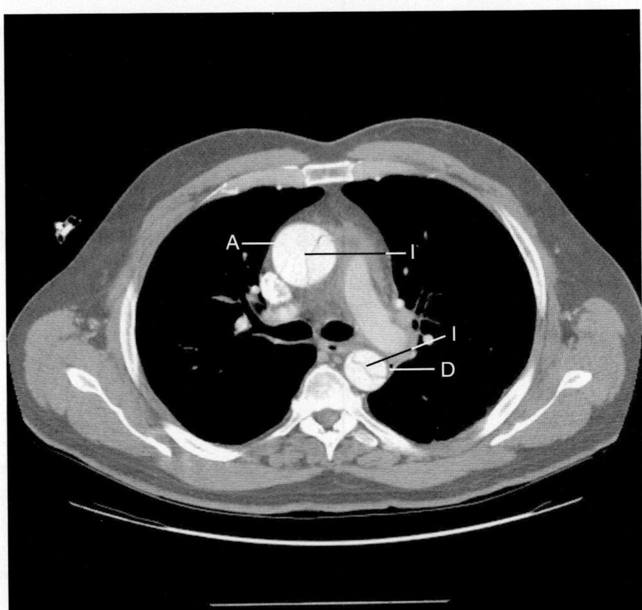

FIGURE 78-5. Aortic dissection. Contrast-enhanced computed tomography scan of the chest at the level of the pulmonary artery shows an intimal flap (I) separating the two lumens of the ascending (A) and descending (D) thoracic aorta in a type A aortic dissection.

On cross-sectional imaging, an isolated intramural hematoma appears as a crescentic thickening around the aortic wall rather than true and false lumens separated by an intimal flap (Fig. 78-6). The presence of an intramural hematoma may be missed on aortography.

TREATMENT Rx

The goal of initial medical therapy for acute aortic intramural hematoma or dissection is to halt further progression and reduce the risk for rupture. Acute management of an isolated hematoma should be the same as for dissection because of the risk that the hematoma will propagate.

Whenever there is suspicion of aortic intramural hematoma or dissection, therapy should be instituted immediately while imaging studies are ordered, rather than waiting until the diagnosis is confirmed. The initial goal is to reduce the force of ventricular contraction and reduce systolic blood pressure to 100 to 120 mm Hg or to the lowest level that maintains cerebral, cardiac, and renal perfusion. Intravenous labetalol (20 mg administered over a 2-minute period, followed by additional doses of 20 to 80 mg every 10 to 15 minutes, up to a maximum total dose of 300 mg, and then a continuous infusion at 2 to 8 mg/minute), which acts as an α-blocker and a β-blocker, may be particularly useful in aortic dissection for controlling hypertension and contractile force. After labetalol or a pure β-blocker (e.g., intravenous propranolol at 1-mg boluses every 3 to 5 minutes to start, followed by a continuous infusion at rates up to 20 mg/hour) has been administered, intravenous nitroprusside (0.5 to 8 μg/kg/minute) should be added to titrate blood pressure minute by minute as needed. If β-blockers are contraindicated, calcium-channel blockers (e.g., intravenous diltiazem with an initial bolus of 20 mg over a 2-minute period, followed by a continuous infusion of 5 to 15 mg/hour) may be useful.

When patients have significant hypotension, pseudohypotension should be carefully excluded first. True hypotension may be due to hemopericardium and cardiac tamponade as a result of rupture of the dissection into the pericardium. These patients should be treated with volume expansion and taken to surgery as quickly as possible because early mortality is extremely high. Pericardiocentesis should be performed only as a last resort because it may precipitate hemodynamic collapse and death.

After initial medical therapy has been instituted and the diagnosis of aortic dissection confirmed, definitive therapy must be determined. Whenever an acute dissection involves the ascending aorta, surgical repair is indicated to minimize the risk of life-threatening complications such as rupture, cardiac tamponade, severe aortic insufficiency, or stroke. Patients with acute dissections confined to the descending aorta are at much lower risk for these complications and tend to fare as well with medical therapy as they do with endovascular repair[8] or surgical repair. When a type B dissection is associated with a serious complication, however, such as end-organ ischemia, intervention is indicated with either endovascular techniques or open surgery. Patients

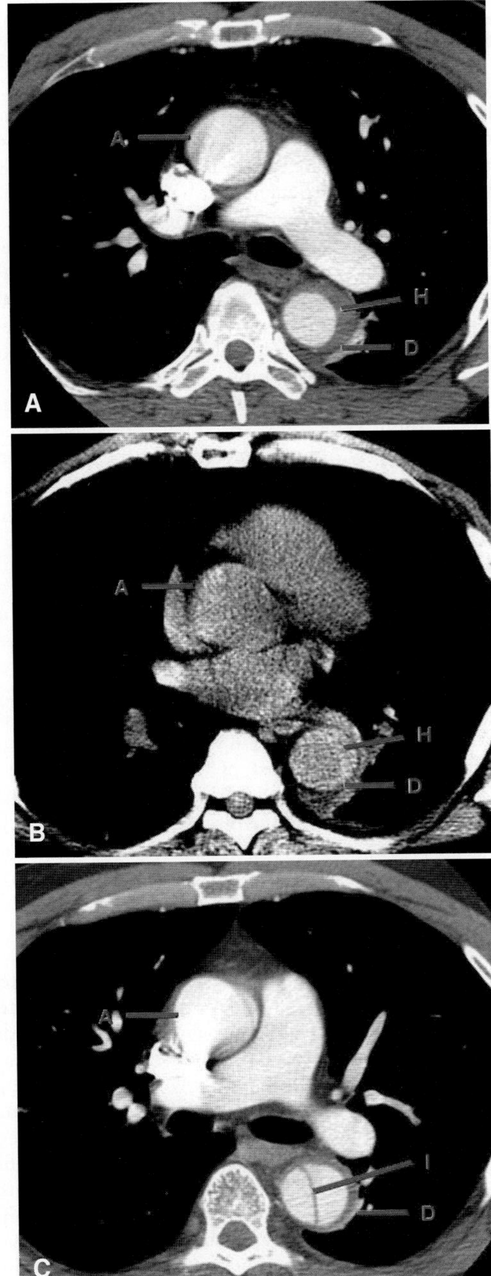

FIGURE 78-6. Intramural aortic hematoma. A, Contrast-enhanced computed tomography scan of the chest at the level of the pulmonary artery demonstrates an intramural hematoma (H) of the descending thoracic aorta (D). The hematoma appears as a crescentic thickening of the aortic wall that does not enhance from the contrast within the aortic lumen. The ascending thoracic aorta (A) is unaffected. **B,** Corresponding image from a non-contrast-enhanced computed tomography scan in which the intramural hematoma appears as a bright crescentic thickening of the aortic wall because the density of the hematoma is greater than that of the blood within the aortic lumen. **C,** Corresponding image from a contrast-enhanced computed tomography scan performed 1 week later for surveillance, in which the intramural hematoma has evolved into a classic aortic dissection with an intimal flap (I) and contrast evident within a patent false lumen.

with chronic type A dissections can often be managed medically because they have already survived the early period of high mortality associated with acute proximal dissections.

For an isolated intramural hematoma, the likelihood of progressive dissection or other complications is lower than in patients who initially have a frank dissection, especially those with smaller hematomas and normal aortic dimensions. Although the 25 to 50% risk of progression may warrant early surgery, serial imaging, with surgery reserved for progressive disease, is reasonable in patients at increased risk with surgery. For distal intramural hematomas, management is generally the same as for distal dissection.

PROGNOSIS

Acutely, the mortality rate from untreated aortic dissection is about 1% per hour. Patients with acute aortic dissection who survive the initial hospitalization generally do well thereafter, whether treated medically or surgically. Late complications such as aortic insufficiency, recurrent dissection, aneurysm formation, and aneurysm rupture can occur, however. Medications to control hypertension and reduce ventricular contractility can dramatically reduce the incidence of late complications and should be continued indefinitely. β-Blockers (e.g., metoprolol 25 to 200 mg twice daily or atenolol 25 to 200 mg/day) are the drugs of choice in this setting, but typically a second (e.g., lisinopril 5 to 40 mg/day) or third (amlodipine 2.5 to 10 mg/day or hydrochlorothiazide 12.5 to 50 mg/day) agent needs to be added to achieve the goal of systolic blood pressure less than 120 mm Hg (Chapter 67).

Patients are at highest risk for complications during the first 2 years after an intramural hematoma or aortic dissection. Progressive aortic expansion typically occurs without symptoms, so patients must be observed closely with serial aortic imaging at 6-month intervals for the first 2 years and annually thereafter, provided the anatomy is stable.

TAKAYASU'S ARTERITIS

DEFINITION

Takayasu's arteritis, which is a chronic inflammatory disease of unknown cause, involves the aorta and its branches. The mean age at onset is 29 years, with women affected eight times as often as men. It occurs more often in Asia and Africa than in Europe or North America. An early stage characterized by active inflammation involving the aorta and its branches progresses at a variable rate to a later sclerotic stage with intimal hyperplasia, medial degeneration, and obliterative changes. Most of the resulting arterial lesions are stenotic, but aneurysms may also occur. The aortic arch and brachiocephalic vessels are affected most often, and the disease tends to be most pronounced at branch points in the aorta. The abdominal aorta is also commonly involved, and the pulmonary artery is sometimes involved. The disease may be diffuse or patchy, with affected areas separated by lengths of normal aorta.

CLINICAL MANIFESTATIONS

Most patients initially have symptoms of a systemic inflammatory process, such as fever, night sweats, arthralgia, and weight loss. There is often a delay of months to years, however, between the onset of symptoms and diagnosis. At the time of diagnosis, 90% of patients have entered the sclerotic phase and have symptoms of vascular insufficiency, typically with pain in the upper (or, less often, lower) extremities. There are often absent pulses and diminished blood pressure in the upper extremities, and the condition has earned the name *pulseless disease.* There may be bruits over affected arteries. Significant hypertension (secondary to renal artery involvement) occurs in more than half the patients, but its presence may be difficult to recognize because of the diminished pulses. Aortic insufficiency may result from proximal aortic involvement. Heart failure may result from either hypertension or aortic insufficiency. Involvement of the ostia of the coronary arteries may cause angina or myocardial infarction. Carotid artery involvement may cause cerebral ischemia or stroke. Abdominal angina may result from mesenteric artery compromise.

The overall 15-year survival rate in patients diagnosed with Takayasu's arteritis is 83%, with most deaths being caused by stroke, myocardial infarction, or heart failure. The survival rate in patients with major complications of the disease is 66%; the survival rate in patients without a major complication is 96%.

DIAGNOSIS

Laboratory abnormalities during the acute phase include an elevated erythrocyte sedimentation rate, elevated C-reactive protein level, mild leukocytosis, anemia, and elevated immunoglobulin levels. The diagnosis is best made by aortography, CT angiography, or magnetic resonance angiography, which reveal stenosis of the aorta and stenosis or occlusion of its branch vessels, often with post-stenotic dilation or associated aneurysms.

TREATMENT Rx

Corticosteroids (e.g., prednisone 60 to 100 mg/day, often for months and tapered after symptoms or evidence of inflammation subside) are the primary therapy for the acute inflammatory stage and may be effective in improving constitutional symptoms, lowering the erythrocyte sedimentation rate, and slowing disease progression. Cyclophosphamide (2 mg/kg/day) or methotrexate (15 to 25 mg/week) may be used when corticosteroid therapy alone is ineffective. It is unknown whether medical therapy reduces the risk for major complications or prolongs life.

Percutaneous balloon angioplasty can effectively dilate short stenotic lesions of the aorta and its branch arteries, although restenosis is common. Surgery may be necessary to bypass or reconstruct key segments, such as the coronary, carotid, or renal arteries, or to treat aortic insufficiency. Ideally, surgery should not be performed during the inflammatory phase.

GIANT CELL ARTERITIS

Giant cell arteritis (Chapter 279) is more common than Takayasu's arteritis. Its cause is also unclear, but it tends to occur in an older population with a mean age of 67 years. It typically affects medium-sized arteries, but in 15% of cases it involves the aorta and branches of the aortic arch. Narrowing of the aorta is rare, but weakening of the ascending aortic wall may lead to localized thoracic aortic aneurysms and secondary aortic insufficiency. Narrowing of the branches of the aortic arch produces symptoms similar to those seen in Takayasu's arteritis. Because the temporal artery is commonly involved, the diagnosis is usually made by temporal artery biopsy. Management involves high-dose corticosteroid therapy (e.g., prednisone 60 to 100 mg/day, often for months and tapered after symptoms or evidence of inflammation subside), to which the disease is usually responsive.

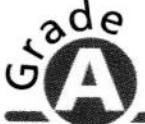

1. Thompson SG, Ashton HA, Gao L, et al. Screening men for abdominal aortic aneurysm: 10 year mortality and cost effectiveness results from the randomised Multicentre Aneurysm Screening Study. *BMJ.* 2009;338:b2307-b2312.
2. United Kingdom Small Aneurysm Trial Participants. Long-term outcomes of immediate repair compared with surveillance of small abdominal aortic aneurysms. *N Engl J Med.* 2002;346:1445-1452.
3. Ashton HA, Buxton MJ, Day NE, et al. The Multicentre Aneurysm Screening Study (MASS) into the effect of abdominal aortic aneurysm screening on mortality in men: a randomised controlled trial. *Lancet.* 2002;360:1531-1539.
4. Lederle FA, Freischlag JA, Kyriakides TC, et al. Outcomes following endovascular vs open repair of abdominal aortic aneurysm: a randomized trial. *JAMA.* 2009;302:1535-1542.
5. United Kingdom EVAR Trial Investigators. Endovascular versus open repair of abdominal aortic aneurysm. *N Engl J Med.* 2010;362:1863-1871.
6. De Bruin JL, Bass AF, Buth J, et al. Long-term outcome of open or endovascular repair of abdominal aortic aneurysm. *N Engl J Med.* 2010;362:1881-1889.
7. United Kingdom EVAR Trial Investigators. Endovascular repair of aortic aneurysm in patients physically ineligible for open repair. *N Engl J Med.* 2010;362:1872-1878.
8. Nienaber CA, Rousseau H, Eggebrecht H, et al. Randomized comparison of strategies for type B aortic dissection: the INvestigation of STEnt Grafts in Aortic Dissection (INSTEAD) trial. *Circulation.* 2009;120:2519-2528.

SUGGESTED READINGS

Braverman AC. Acute aortic dissection: clinician update. *Circulation.* 2010;122:184-188. *Review.*

Hiratzka LF, Bakris GL, Beckman JA, et al. 2010 ACCF/AHA/AATS/ACR/ASA/SCA/SCAI/SIR/STS/SVM Guidelines for the diagnosis and management of patients with thoracic aortic disease: a report of the American College of Cardiology Foundation/American Heart Association Task Force on Practice Guidelines, American Association for Thoracic Surgery, American College of Radiology, American Stroke Association, Society of Cardiovascular Anesthesiologists, Society for Cardiovascular Angiography and Interventions, Society of Interventional Radiology, Society of Thoracic Surgeons, and Society for Vascular Medicine. *Circulation.* 2010;121:e266-e369. *Consensus guidelines.*

Moll FL, Powell JT, Fraedrich G, et al. Management of abdominal aortic aneurysms: clinical practice guidelines of the European Society for Vascular Surgery. *Eur J Vasc Endovasc Surg.* 2011;41:S1-S58. *Consensus guidelines.*

79 ATHEROSCLEROTIC PERIPHERAL ARTERIAL DISEASE

CHRISTOPHER J. WHITE

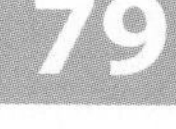

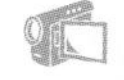

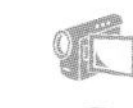

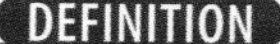

DEFINITION

Lower extremity atherosclerotic peripheral arterial disease is one subset of a larger group of peripheral vascular diseases that includes all noncoronary vascular disorders that may affect the arterial, venous (Chapter 81), or lymphatic circulation. Atherosclerotic arterial diseases are characterized by arterial narrowing or occlusion caused by the accumulation of atherosclerotic

How to Perform and Calculate the ABI

Partners Program ABI Interpretation
Above 0.90—Normal
0.71–0.90—Mild Obstruction
0.41–0.70—Moderate Obstruction
0.00–0.40—Severe Obstruction

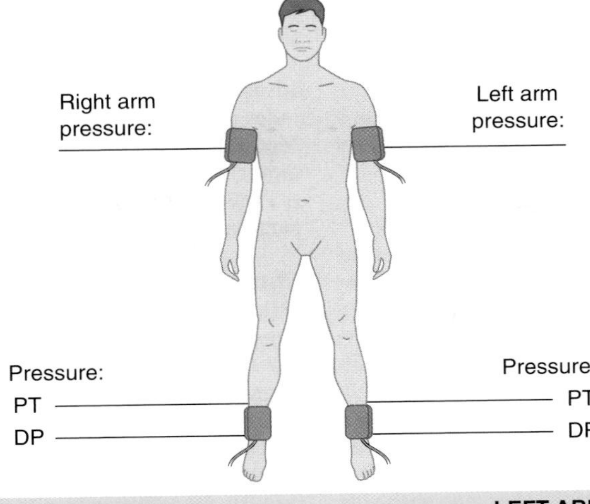

RIGHT ABI

Higher right ankle pressure / Higher arm pressure = mm Hg / mm Hg = ______

LEFT ABI

Higher left ankle pressure / Higher arm pressure = mm Hg / mm Hg = ______

EXAMPLE

Higher ankle pressure / Higher arm pressure = 92 mm Hg / 164 mm Hg = 0.56 See ABI Chart

FIGURE 79-1. Performing pressure measurements and calculating the ankle-brachial index (ABI). To calculate the ABI, systolic pressures are determined in both arms and both ankles with the use of a handheld Doppler instrument. The highest readings for the dorsalis pedis (DP) and posterior tibial (PT) arteries are used to calculate the index.

plaque elements in the vessel wall (Chapter 70). Atherosclerotic vascular disease can also lead to aneurysm formation, which is the pathologic enlargement of arterial segments, and may result in rupture, dissection, or thromboembolism (Chapter 78).

EPIDEMIOLOGY

The prevalence of lower extremity peripheral arterial disease in the United States, Europe, and Asia continues to increase as the population ages and is exposed to atherosclerotic risk factors (Chapter 51). The presence of peripheral arterial disease is defined as an ankle-brachial index (ABI)—the ratio of the systolic blood pressure in the ankle divided by the systolic blood pressure in the arm (Fig. 79-1)—less than 0.90. Among individuals aged 40 years and older, the prevalence is 4.3% (95% confidence interval [CI] 3.1 to 5.5%), but the prevalence in diabetic individuals ranges from 20 to 30%.

Risk factors for atherosclerosis (Chapter 51) increase the likelihood of developing lower extremity peripheral arterial disease. More than 95% of individuals with peripheral arterial disease have at least one traditional cardiovascular risk factor, and most have multiple risk factors. More than one third of patients with peripheral arterial disease have significant coronary disease, and up to one quarter have carotid artery disease. As a result, the risk of heart attack, stroke, and death are increased several-fold in patients with peripheral arterial disease.

Among conventional atherosclerotic risk factors, cigarette smoking is two to three times more likely to cause lower extremity peripheral arterial disease than to cause coronary artery disease. Hypertension is also associated with lower extremity peripheral arterial disease. The development of peripheral arterial disease is more likely in patients with lipid abnormalities (elevated total and low-density lipoprotein cholesterol, decreased high-density lipoprotein cholesterol, and hypertriglyceridemia), and the risk increases by 5 to 10% for each 10 mg/dL rise in total cholesterol. Increased homocysteine levels are associated with a two- to three-fold increased risk for developing atherosclerotic peripheral arterial disease. Diabetes mellitus increases the risk of lower extremity peripheral arterial disease by two- to four-fold, and the risk of developing lower extremity peripheral arterial disease is proportional to the severity and duration of diabetes. Tight control of diabetes is important, and the risk of developing peripheral arterial disease increases by 28% for every 1% increase in glycosylated hemoglobin (Chapters 236 and 237). Diabetic patients with lower extremity peripheral arterial disease are 7- to 15-fold more likely to undergo a major amputation than nondiabetics with lower extremity peripheral arterial disease.

Peripheral arterial disease disproportionately affects older individuals (Fig. 79-2), non-Hispanic blacks, current smokers, diabetics, and those with abnormal renal function. The overall prevalence of peripheral arterial disease

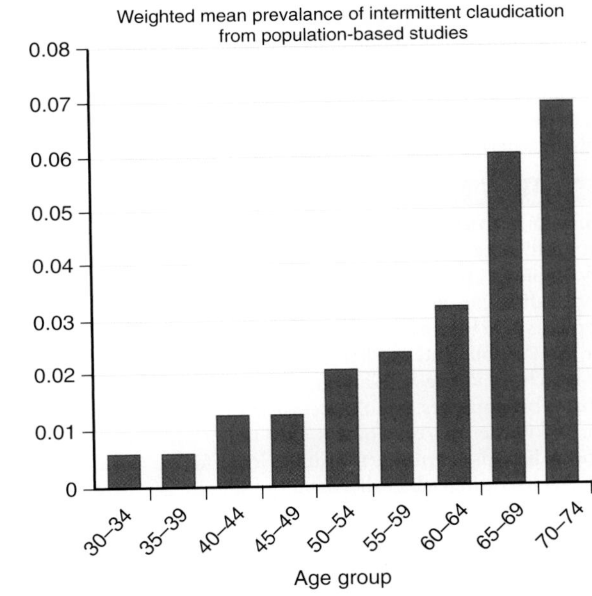

FIGURE 79-2. Weighted mean prevalence of intermittent claudication. (Modified from Dormandy JA, Rutherford RB. Management of peripheral arterial disease. TransAtlantic Inter-Society Consensus (TASC) Working Group. *J Vasc Surg.* 2000;31:S1-S296.)

in the United States among persons aged 70 years and older is 14.5% (95% CI 10.8 to 18.2%), which corresponds to approximately 4 million individuals.

PATHOBIOLOGY

Acute Limb Ischemia

Acute limb ischemia occurs when blood flow to an extremity is abruptly halted or markedly diminished, resulting in hypoperfusion that threatens the viability of the limb. Acute limb ischemia is most commonly caused by either thrombosis or embolism. Thrombosis of a lower extremity arterial bypass graft is the most common clinical scenario. Most emboli originate from the heart as a mural thrombus from a recent myocardial infarction (Chapter 73) or from the atrial appendage in a patient with atrial fibrillation (Chapter 64). A less common cause of lower extremity emboli is an atherosclerotic or aneurysmal abdominal aorta (Chapter 78) that serves as the source of cholesterol emboli (Chapter 80).

Arterial in situ thrombosis as a result of plaque rupture usually represents the final stage of a chronically diseased artery, most commonly the femoral or popliteal artery. Conditions such as severe dehydration or low-output heart failure promote thrombosis at the site of stenosis. If native artery thrombosis occurs in the absence of a preexisting stenosis, a thorough search for a hypercoagulable state should be undertaken. Acutely thrombosed femoral or popliteal aneurysms may present as acute limb ischemia.

Chronic Limb Ischemia

Chronic, stable lower extremity peripheral arterial disease, manifested by the symptoms of intermittent claudication, may be due to atherosclerosis, thromboembolism, inflammatory disease, trauma, aneurysmal disease, adventitial cysts, entrapment syndromes, or congenital abnormalities. Aneurysms may be associated with atherosclerosis, or they may be due to underlying hereditary (familial) or acquired (e.g., due to smoking or trauma) causes.

Patients with critical limb ischemia have inadequate blood flow to sustain viability in the distal tissue bed. Critical limb ischemia is most often caused by atherosclerosis, but it can also be caused by atheroembolic or thromboembolic disease, vasculitis, in situ thrombosis related to hypercoagulable states, thromboangiitis obliterans, cystic adventitial disease, popliteal entrapment, or trauma. Patients presenting with critical limb ischemia typically have multisegment disease along the length of the limb.

Inflammation plays a fundamental role in the development and progression of atherosclerosis (Chapter 70). Elevated levels of C-reactive protein (CRP) are strongly associated with the development of peripheral arterial disease. Markers of inflammation such as interleukin-6, tumor necrosis factor-α, CRP, and platelet activation are increased compared with normal subjects.

No specific genetic markers have been confirmed for peripheral arterial disease, although one study identified a linkage on chromosome 1p. The proportion of low ABIs attributable to heritability is estimated at 20%. Concordance rates among twins are about 33% for monozygotic pairs and about 31% for dizygotic pairs, suggesting a limited role for heritability. Taken together, these data studies suggest a modest but significant heritability factor for peripheral arterial disease.

CLINICAL MANIFESTATIONS

Acute Limb Ischemia

A patient with acute limb ischemia classically presents with a cool, painful extremity. Typically, the major muscle groups below the level of obstruction are symptomatic. The absence of a pulse may help localize the site of occlusion, but pulses may be normal in cases of microemboli or cholesterol emboli (Chapter 80). Venous and capillary filling is an indicator of the severity of acute limb ischemia. The leg should be carefully examined for color and temperature abnormalities. Pallor is seen early on, but with time, cyanosis is common. Poikilothermia, or coolness, is an important finding, particularly if the opposite limb is warm. A transition level for color and temperature changes, which is often clinically obvious, should be correlated with the pulses and denoted as a baseline reference at the initial examination for comparison with subsequent examinations.

Sensory changes include numbness and paresthesias. Paralysis indicates advanced, limb-threatening ischemia. The extent of any motor deficit is a good index of the degree of tissue anoxia and correlates well with the prognosis. Motor deficits progress from distal to more proximal muscle groups, so early motor weakness is seen in the intrinsic foot muscles. Complete motor paralysis is a late symptom that suggests impending irreversible injury. In due course, paralysis progresses to rigor when irreversible ischemia has developed.

Chronic Stable Lower Limb Ischemia

Patients with chronic peripheral arterial disease may be clinically stable and report no symptoms, atypical symptoms, or symptoms of exertional discomfort (claudication). If they are clinically unstable with pain at rest or with ulceration or spreading gangrene, they have critical limb ischemia that threatens the limb (Table 79-1). The majority of patients with chronic peripheral arterial disease are asymptomatic and are identified by abnormal pulse examinations, investigation of vascular bruits, or routine measurement of the ABI (see Fig. 79-1). Patients with typical symptoms of intermittent claudication are only the tip of the iceberg, representing no more than 20% of patients with objective evidence of peripheral arterial disease.

Claudication is defined as exertional discomfort, relieved with rest, in specific muscle groups at risk for ischemia during exercise. Symptoms usually begin one segment below the level of the arterial narrowing. For example, vascular blockages (occlusions or stenoses) of the iliac vessels typically cause hip, thigh, and calf pain, whereas femoral and popliteal artery obstructions typically cause symptoms in the calf and foot muscles. Claudication, which is a specific vascular syndrome, must be distinguished from other conditions that cause exertional leg pain, which have been termed *pseudoclaudication* (Table 79-2).

TABLE 79-1 FONTAINE'S AND RUTHERFORD'S CLINICAL CLASSIFICATIONS OF CHRONIC LOWER LIMB ISCHEMIA

Fontaine		Rutherford		
STAGE	CLINICAL	GRADE	CATEGORY	CLINICAL
I	Asymptomatic	0	0	Asymptomatic
IIa	Mild claudication	I	1	Mild claudication
IIb	Moderate to severe claudication	I I	2 3	Moderate claudication Severe claudication
III	Rest pain	II	4	Rest pain
IV	Ulceration or gangrene	III IV	5 6	Minor tissue loss Ulceration or gangrene

Adapted from Norgren L, Hiatt WR, Dormandy JA, et al. Inter-society consensus for the management of peripheral arterial disease (TASC II). *Eur J Vasc Endovasc Surg.* 2007;33:S1-S75.

TABLE 79-2 DIFFERENTIATION OF TRUE CLAUDICATION FROM PSEUDOCLAUDICATION

	INTERMITTENT CLAUDICATION	SPINAL STENOSIS	ARTHRITIS	VENOUS CONGESTION	COMPARTMENT SYNDROME
Character of discomfort	Cramping, tightness, or tiredness	Same as claudication or tingling, weakness, clumsiness	Aching	Tightness, bursting pain	Tightness, bursting pain
Location of discomfort	Buttock, hip, thigh, calf, foot	Buttock, hip, thigh	Hip, knee	Groin, thigh	Calf
Exercise-induced discomfort	Yes	Variable	Variable	After walking	Excessive exercise
Walking distance to discomfort	Reproducible	Variable	Variable	Variable	Excessive exercise
Occurs with standing	No	Yes	Yes, but positional	Yes, but positional	Yes, but positional
Relief of discomfort	Rapid relief with rest	Relief with sitting or changing position	Slow relief with avoidance of weight bearing	Slow relief with leg elevation	Slow relief with leg elevation
Other	Associated with atherosclerosis and decreased pulses	History of lower back problems	Discomfort at joint	History of deep vein thrombosis, signs of venous congestion	Typical in athletes

From White C. Intermittent claudication. *N Engl J Med.* 2007;356:1241-1250.

TABLE 79-3 CLINICAL CATEGORIES OF ACUTE LIMB ISCHEMIA

CATEGORY	DESCRIPTION	SENSORY LOSS	MUSCLE WEAKNESS	DOPPLER ARTERIAL	DOPPLER VENOUS
I. Viable	Not immediately threatened	None	None	Audible	Audible
IIa. Threatened marginally	Salvageable if promptly treated	Minimal or none	None	Inaudible	Audible
IIb. Threatened immediately	Salvageable if immediately treated	More than toes, associated with rest pain	Mild to moderate	Inaudible	Audible
III. Irreversible	Major tissue loss inevitable	Profound, anesthetic	Profound, paralysis, rigor	Inaudible	Inaudible

Adapted from Rutherford RB, Baker JD, Ernst C, et al. Recommended standards for reports dealing with lower extremity ischemia: revised version. *J Vasc Surg.* 1997;26:517-538.

Symptoms in individual patients are remarkably variable despite similar degrees of vascular stenosis, in part owing to collateral vessel formation. A patient with superficial femoral artery occlusion but robust collateral formation via the deep femoral artery and geniculate collaterals, which supply blood to the infrapopliteal vessels, may have minimal or no symptoms. Another patient with similar anatomy but poor collaterals may have severe symptoms.

Chronic Critical Lower Limb Ischemia

Critical limb ischemia develops in about 10% of all patients with peripheral arterial disease; it presents as resting limb pain or impending limb or tissue loss, as manifested clinically by nonhealing lower extremity ulcers or the presence of gangrene. These patients' limbs are in jeopardy, and even the most minor trauma from a poorly fitting shoe or a carelessly clipped toenail may cause a nonhealing wound or infection necessitating amputation. Critical limb ischemia can be exacerbated by conditions that reduce blood flow to the microvascular bed, such as diabetes, severe low cardiac output states, and, rarely, vasospastic diseases.

DIAGNOSIS

Acute Limb Ischemia

In patients with acute limb ischemia, the history and physical examination are important steps not only in assessing the cause and severity of ischemia but also in determining the diagnostic and therapeutic path. Upon completion of the history and physical examination, the physician should be able to answer the following questions about the severity of acute limb ischemia: Is the limb viable? Is its viability immediately threatened? Are there already irreversible changes that may preclude salvage of the limb? Three findings that help differentiate "threatened" from "viable" extremities are the presence of persistent pain, sensory loss, and muscle weakness (Table 79-3).

Chronic Limb Ischemia

The clinical severity of acute and chronic limb ischemia can be semiquantitatively assessed using either the Fontaine or the Rutherford classification (see Table 79-1). The clinician must distinguish intermittent claudication from nonvascular causes that may mimic claudication (i.e., pseudoclaudication), such as neurogenic pain from spinal stenosis or nerve root compression (Chapter 407), musculoskeletal or arthritic pain, or discomfort from venous congestion or a compartment syndrome (see Table 79-2). A typical history of claudication has a low sensitivity but a high specificity for peripheral arterial disease.

Patients presenting with peripheral arterial disease should be assessed for atherosclerotic risk factors (Table 79-4) and undergo a complete vascular physical examination, including measurement of the ABI (see Fig. 79-1). In healthy adults without arterial occlusive disease, ankle systolic pressure is typically 10 to 15 mm Hg greater than arm (brachial) systolic pressure, owing to the effect of pulse wave reflection. A truly normal ABI is greater than 1.10, although peripheral arterial disease is generally defined as a resting ABI of 0.90 or less.

Imaging

Duplex imaging combines ultrasound imaging and Doppler blood velocity measurements to localize vascular obstructions and estimate lesion severity. The sensitivity and specificity of duplex ultrasound for the diagnosis of a 50% or greater stenosis in the lower extremity are 90% or higher. Duplex ultrasound has proved useful for the surveillance of post-surgical vein graft patency in the lower extremities, although the specific utility of ultrasound surveillance after synthetic bypass grafting or after endovascular therapy has not been demonstrated.

TABLE 79-4 INITIAL LABORATORY EVALUATION OF A PATIENT WITH PERIPHERAL ARTERIAL DISEASE

Serum electrolytes, including fasting serum glucose
Renal function (serum creatinine, blood urea nitrogen, estimated glomerular filtration rate)
Complete blood count
Fasting lipid profile
High-sensitivity C-reactive protein
Ankle-brachial index

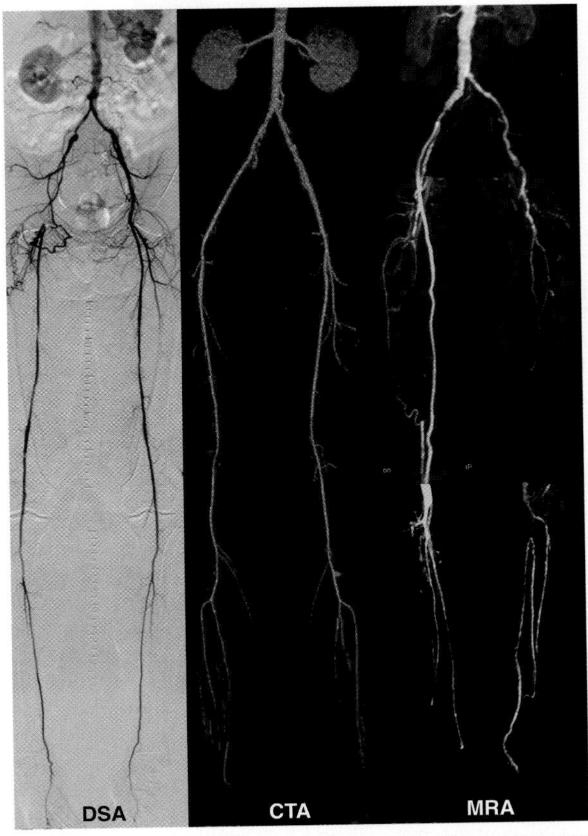

FIGURE 79-3. **Aortography with distal run-off in three different patients by three different methods: digital subtraction angiography (DSA), computed tomography angiography (CTA), and magnetic resonance angiography (MRA).** (From White C. Intermittent claudication. *N Engl J Med.* 2007;356:1241-1250.)

Computed tomography angiography (CTA) and magnetic resonance angiography (MRA) obtain cross-sectional images that can be reconstructed into a three-dimensional angiogram (Fig. 79-3). CTA requires iodinated intravenous contrast material and ionizing radiation, whereas MRA uses gadolinium contrast and does not expose the patient to ionizing radiation. The major toxicity of gadolinium is an uncommon but potentially lethal systemic disorder called nephrogenic systemic fibrosis or nephrogenic sclerosing dermopathy (Chapter 275); chronic kidney disease with a glomerular filtration rate of 60 mL/minute or less is the major risk factor for the development of nephrogenic sclerosing dermopathy.

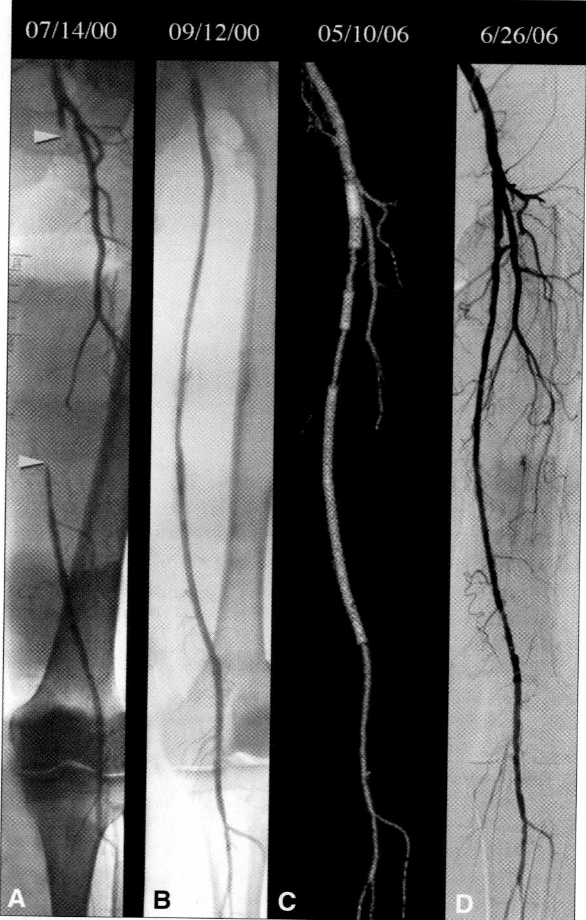

FIGURE 79-4. **A,** Baseline angiogram of left leg showing occlusion *(arrowheads)* of the femoral-popliteal segment. **B,** Post-treatment angiogram after balloon angioplasty and stent placement. **C,** More than 5 years later, the patient returns with claudication and a reduced ankle-brachial index. Follow-up computed tomography angiogram shows narrowing of the superficial femoral artery between the two stents. **D,** Final angiogram following balloon angioplasty and stent placement in the femoral narrowings.

An advantage of CTA over MRA is its ability to visualize metallic stents and stent-grafts (Fig. 79-4). CTA requires only about one fourth the radiation required for invasive digital angiography, and it can be performed more quickly and with less pretreatment planning than MRA. Vascular calcification may be a source of artifact with CTA but is inconsequential with MRA. MRA tends to overestimate lesions at the ostia of arteries owing to turbulent flow, and MRA cannot be performed in patients with ferromagnetic metallic implants. In a randomized trial comparing MRA with CTA for initial imaging in peripheral arterial disease, there was no difference between the two techniques in terms of ease, clinical utility, or patient outcome, but CTA reduced total diagnostic costs.[1]

Invasive digital angiography remains the "gold standard" for the diagnosis and evaluation of peripheral arterial disease (see Fig. 79-3), despite the need for iodinated contrast material and the exposure to ionizing radiation. Another limitation is the two-dimensional nature of the images, given the vascular system's tortuous, three-dimensional structure and detailed morphology, which may be obscured by the overlap of side branches. Invasive angiographic procedures (Chapter 57) are associated with a relatively small but nontrivial rate of complications, including severe contrast allergy in 0.1%, access-related bleeding complications, contrast-induced nephropathy, and, very rarely, infection.

TREATMENT

The treatment of patients with atherosclerotic lower extremity peripheral arterial disease is directed at salvaging the limb, improving walking distance, and reducing the patient's risk for life-threatening cardiovascular complications of atherosclerosis. The decision to perform a percutaneous or surgical revascularization procedure for the relief of claudication is based on a risk-benefit assessment that weighs the patient's disability and discomfort against the estimated short- and long- term success and risks of the procedure. Because very few patients with claudication are in danger of losing their limbs, the primary goal of revascularization is long-lasting relief of symptoms, not limb salvage.

Revascularization strategies now emphasize percutaneous endovascular treatments rather than traditional open surgical approaches because of their lower morbidity (see Fig. 79-4). Stenting has made catheter-based procedures safer, more durable, and more predictably successful.

Acute Limb Ischemia

Patients with irreversible limb ischemia should not undergo angiography and should be scheduled for amputation (Fig. 79-5). All other patients with acute limb ischemia should undergo emergent angiography. Before angiography, anticoagulation to prevent thrombus propagation and/or embolization (e.g., unfractionated heparin 5000 IU bolus, then 1000 IU/hour infusion) and analgesia (e.g., morphine 2 mg intravenously, as needed) should be initiated, and any underlying medical comorbidities (e.g., heart failure) should be managed aggressively to stabilize the patient. The method used for direct revascularization must be tailored to the patient and to the physician's skills (operative or endovascular).

The options for prompt revascularization consist of endovascular therapies with intra-arterial thrombolysis (e.g., recombinant tissue plasminogen activator 0.5 mg/hour intra-arterially) or thrombectomy, or surgical thrombectomy with or without arterial bypass. In general, endovascular therapy is recommended for patients with an onset of acute symptoms less than 14 days earlier, and surgical revascularization is recommended for patients with a duration of symptoms greater than 14 days. These treatments are often complementary, each with its own advantages and limitations. The less invasive endovascular therapy allows simultaneous angiography to guide reperfusion therapy, but it may be difficult to pass the guidewire across a total occlusion. Surgery offers definitive restoration of blood flow with thrombectomy or bypass surgery, but it carries higher short-term risks. When choosing a treatment, consideration should be given to the location of the occlusion, the type of occlusion (thrombus or embolus), the duration of ischemia, patient-related risks, the type of conduit to be recanalized (artery or graft), and therapy-related risks and outcomes. For example, an in situ thrombus is more amenable to thrombolysis than is an embolus, which may require thrombectomy.

Chronic Stable Lower Limb Ischemia

The treatment of patients with claudication is directed at both improving the walking distance and, perhaps more importantly, reducing the patient's risk for life-threatening cardiovascular complications of atherosclerosis. Risk factor modification (Chapter 51), antiplatelet therapy (Chapter 37), and an exercise prescription are the basic elements of treating peripheral arterial disease.

Exercise Therapy

Improvement in walking distance can often be achieved with pharmacologic management, discontinuation of tobacco use, and a regular, supervised exercise program. Patients should be reassured that exercising, even though it may precipitate their claudication symptoms, is not harmful and is the preferred initial treatment.[2] A meta-analysis of eight randomized trials demonstrated that a supervised, as opposed to unsupervised, exercise program improved symptoms of claudication.[3] Supervised exercise commonly involves walking on a treadmill, with the initial workload set to elicit symptoms within 3 to 5 minutes of walking. The patient is permitted to rest until the symptoms resolve but then resumes exercising. Maximal benefits are associated with programs that require the patient to continue walking until the pain is near maximal and with sessions that last more than 30 minutes, occur three or more times per week, and continue for more than 6 months. It typically takes 1 to 2 months for the patient to begin to notice benefits, which gradually increase over several months.

Pharmacology

Currently, two medications are approved in the United States for the symptomatic treatment of intermittent claudication: pentoxifylline and cilostazol. In randomized clinical trials, pentoxifylline has not consistently improved treadmill walking distance, so it cannot be recommended. Cilostazol (50 to 100 mg twice daily), a phosphodiesterase inhibitor, improves maximal walking distance by 40 to 50% compared with placebo.[4] Cilostazol is contraindicated in patients with heart failure. Oral vasodilating prostaglandins, vitamin E, and chelation therapy with EDTA have not been effective in improving either symptoms or walking distance.

Risk Factor Treatment

Antiplatelet therapy with aspirin (usually 81 mg/day) has an established role in the secondary prevention of cardiovascular events in patients at high risk, based on clinical evidence of either coronary artery disease or stroke (Chapter 414). However, the role of aspirin in other populations, such as those with peripheral arterial disease but no clinical evidence of coronary artery disease or stroke, has not been established. The thienopyridines, such as

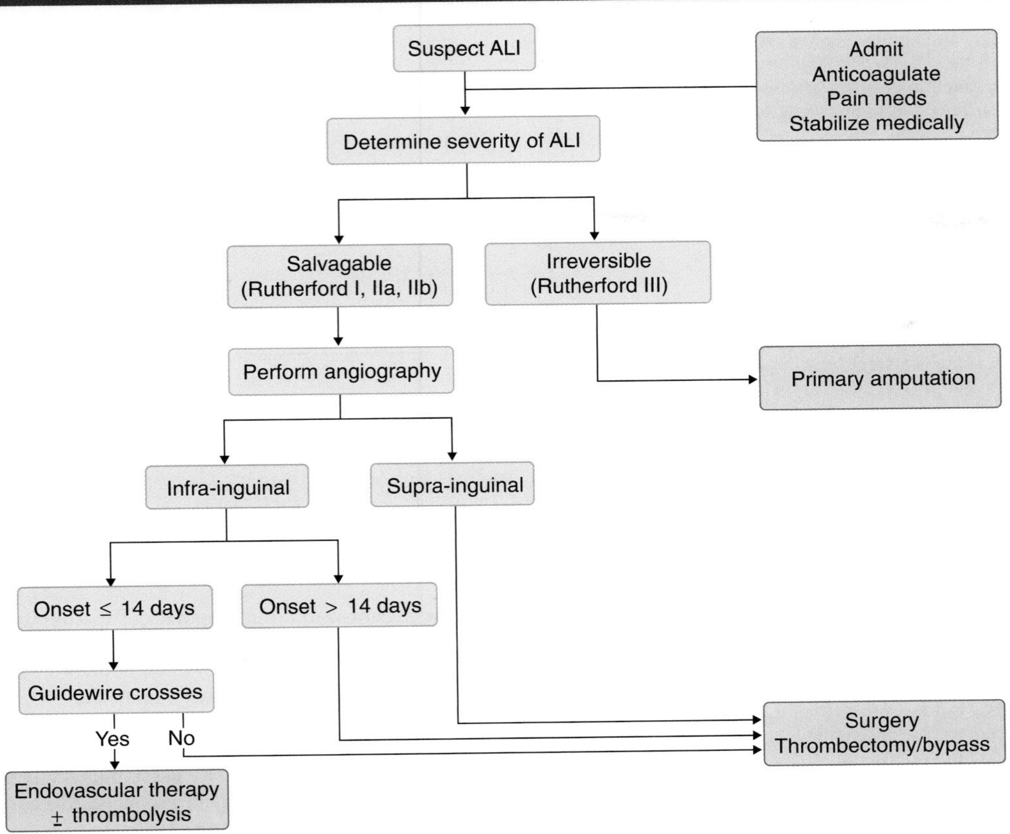

FIGURE 79-5. Treatment algorithm for acute limb ischemia (ALI). (Modified from Gray BH, Conte MS, Dake MD, et al. Atherosclerotic Peripheral Vascular Disease Symposium II: lower-extremity revascularization: state of the art. *Circulation.* 2008;118:2864-2872.)

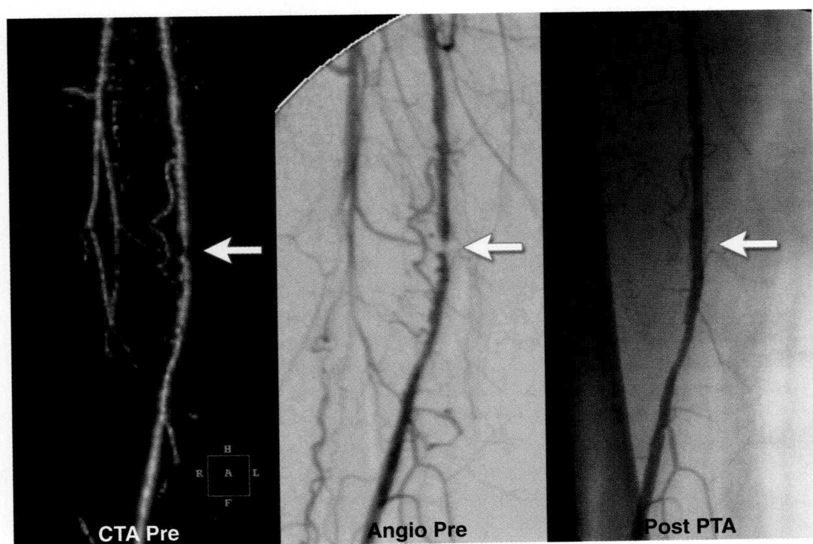

FIGURE 79-6. Discrete stenosis *(arrows)* of the left superficial femoral artery seen on computed tomography angiography (CTA; left), digital subtraction angiography (middle), and digital angiography after percutaneous transluminal angioplasty (PTA; right). (From White C. Intermittent claudication. *N Engl J Med.* 2007;356:1241-1250.)

clopidogrel (usually 75 mg/day), are indicated only if aspirin is not tolerated, based on clopidogrel's efficacy compared with aspirin among patients with peripheral arterial disease.[5]

Patients with known peripheral arterial disease should be encouraged to modify or eliminate atherosclerotic risk factors such as diabetes (Chapter 237), tobacco use (Chapter 31), hyperlipidemia (Chapter 213), and hypertension (Chapter 67) and to exercise regularly (Chapter 15). Medical therapy, dietary modification, and exercise should all be tailored to meet current guidelines for controlling hyperlipidemia (Chapter 213) and hypertension (Chapter 67).

For patients with severe peripheral arterial disease and elevated CRP levels, statin therapy substantially improves overall survival.[6] This finding in patients with peripheral arterial disease is consistent with findings in other studies of patients with a history of vascular disease, with or without peripheral arterial disease, and with either elevated low-density lipoprotein cholesterol levels or elevated CRP levels. Blood pressure control is very important, especially in patients with coexisting diabetes.[7] β-Blockers are effective antihypertensive therapy and are not contraindicated in peripheral arterial disease. Angiotensin-converting enzyme inhibitors reduce the risk of cardiovascular death in patients with peripheral arterial disease.[8]

Revascularization

Patients selected for revascularization to relieve symptoms of intermittent claudication should have significant lifestyle limitations or be unable to work and should have failed to respond to pharmacologic and exercise therapy. They should also have a favorable risk-benefit ratio and favorable vascular anatomy for the planned revascularization procedure.

Superficial femoral artery stenosis or occlusion is the most common lesion associated with claudication (Fig. 79-6). Revascularization with surgery or percutaneous transluminal angioplasty is indicated for the relief of vocational or lifestyle-limiting claudication in patients who have failed exercise and pharmacologic therapy. Angioplasty with stenting is preferred when possible in patients younger than 50 years, as they have a higher risk of surgical graft failure than do older patients.

Clinical trials comparing medical therapy and percutaneous transluminal angioplasty with and without stenting for patients with claudication and for those with femoral-popliteal arterial disease demonstrate substantially better early relief of symptoms and long-term vessel patency with angioplasty. A meta-analysis comparing exercise therapy with balloon angioplasty in claudicants found no difference in quality-of-life measures at 3 and 6 months, but the ABI and functional capacity improved more with angioplasty than with exercise therapy.[9]

Some randomized trials comparing surgery with percutaneous transluminal angioplasty show similar rates of mortality, amputation, and patency at 4 years in patients with lower extremity ischemia. Percutaneous transluminal angioplasty is preferred in amenable lesions because of its lower periprocedural mortality and morbidity. Percutaneous transluminal angioplasty is more cost-effective than surgery if the expected 5-year patency rate of the treated vessel is 30% or greater. Outcomes following femoral-popliteal percutaneous transluminal angioplasty have improved over time, with current patency rates of 87, 69, and 55% at 1, 3, and 5 years, respectively.

Clinical success for patients with claudication caused by femoral lesions depends on obtaining a durable, long-lasting result. Although one option is angioplasty followed by provisional "bailout" stenting if the angioplasty itself is not successful, primary stenting with nitinol self-expanding stents is superior to provisional stent replacement for longer femoral lesions (7 to 10 cm) in terms of restenosis, improvement in ABI, and longer walking distance.[10] At 2 years follow-up, the benefit of primary stenting remained statistically significant, but the restenosis rate for femoral stents is about 50%. In more discrete femoral lesions (mean, 4.5 cm), a strategy of balloon angioplasty first, with stenting only for bailout, is as good as routine stenting.[11,12] The difference in outcomes for short versus long lesions is because stenting is equally good for long and short lesions, but longer lesions are more prone to restenosis after balloon angioplasty; as a result, stents improve outcomes in longer lesions. For shorter superficial femoral artery lesions, a strategy of percutaneous transluminal angioplasty with bailout stenting is preferable.

Adjunctive angioplasty devices such as atherectomy, cryotherapy, and the cutting balloon have not been meaningfully tested in any population, and there are few data to support their use versus less expensive, more conventional therapies. In randomized trials, laser angioplasty is not superior to conventional percutaneous transluminal angioplasty and/or stent placement in the superficial femoral artery. Given the substantial additional expense associated with these devices, more evidence of their efficacy is needed before widespread adoption can be justified.

Attempts to use drug-eluting stents in the femoral artery to reduce recurrence rates have failed. However, two randomized controlled trials using paclitaxel-coated balloons in femoral lesions showed lower restenosis rates compared with control balloons. Despite the small number of patients tested, these two trials provide reason for optimism.

Chronic Critical Lower Limb Ischemia

Patients with critical limb ischemia who have extensive necrosis or infectious gangrene or who are nonambulatory may best be served by primary amputation. For other patients with critical limb ischemia, the optimal treatment is prompt revascularization. The therapeutic goal is to reestablish pulsatile, straight-line flow to the distal extremity. Establishment of uninterrupted flow to at least one infrapopliteal vessel (i.e., the anterior or posterior tibial or peroneal arteries) is a prerequisite for wound healing. When treating patients with potential tissue or limb loss, transient restoration of flow to the extremity may effectively heal an ulcer. The healed ulcer usually does not recur, even if restenosis occurs after several months, if there is no recurrent injury.

In patients with critical limb ischemia caused by infrainguinal disease, percutaneous transluminal angioplasty and surgery are comparable as first-line therapies, but angioplasty is less costly and is associated with a lower morbidity.[13] Percutaneous transluminal angioplasty should be tried first if a patient is a candidate for either procedure, particularly if the patient's life expectancy is less than 2 years. Primary stenting with a drug-eluting stent may be preferable to regular angioplasty[14] compared with percutaneous transluminal angioplasty with "provisional" bailout stenting in patients with occlusions and critical limb ischemia.

PROGNOSIS

Peripheral arterial disease is a major cause of acute and chronic illness associated with impaired functional capacity, reduced quality of life, limb loss, and increased risk of death (Fig. 79-7). Approximately two thirds of patients with peripheral arterial disease have at least one severely diseased coronary artery, and up to one quarter of patients have significant carotid artery stenosis. Consequently, patients with peripheral arterial disease face an increased risk of cardiovascular ischemic events such as myocardial infarction, ischemic stroke, and death. It is estimated that coronary and cerebrovascular adverse events occur two- to four-fold more commonly than do limb adverse events in patients with peripheral arterial disease.

The annual mortality for patients with peripheral arterial disease is about 5%, but it is higher for patients with severe disease. For example, the estimated 1-year mortality rate for patients with critical limb ischemia is 25%, but this can climb to 45% for patients requiring amputation; in contrast, annual mortality for patients with intermittent claudication is only 1 to 2%. For patients presenting with acute limb ischemia, the 30-day amputation rate is as high as 40%, and mortality rates up to 30% have been reported.

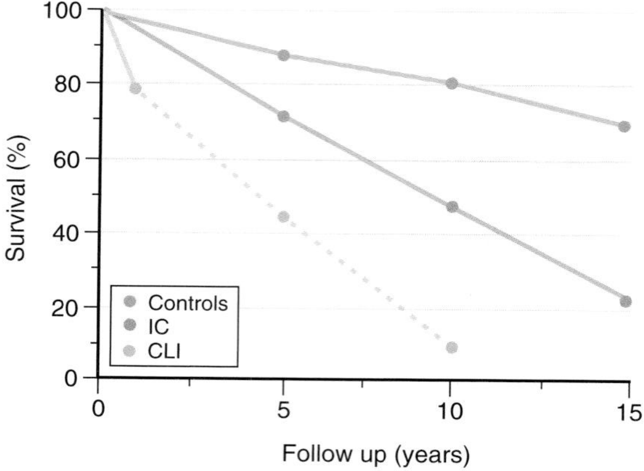

FIGURE 79-7. Survival curve of patients with intermittent claudication (IC) versus critical limb ischemia (CLI). (Modified from Norgren L, Hiatt WR, Dormandy JA, et al. Inter-society consensus for the management of peripheral arterial disease (TASC II). *Eur J Vasc Endovasc Surg.* 2007;33:S1-S75.)

Patients with lower extremity claudication should be reassured that the risk of limb loss is low and that claudication usually does not worsen or improve at a rapid rate. Moreover, a history of claudication, by itself, only slightly increases the risk of amputation after 10 years. However, a reduced ABI and diabetes mellitus are associated with the development of ischemic rest pain and ischemic ulceration, which may lead to limb loss. Among patients with peripheral arterial disease, those who have diabetes are 15 times more likely to have an amputation than are patients without diabetes, whose annual amputation rate is about 0.6%.

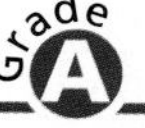

1. Ouwendijk R, de Vries M, Pattynama PM, et al. Imaging peripheral arterial disease: a randomized controlled trial comparing contrast-enhanced MR angiography and multi-detector row CT angiography. *Radiology.* 2005;236:1094-1103.
2. Mazari FA, Gulati S, Rahman MN, et al. Early outcomes from a randomized, controlled trial of supervised exercise, angioplasty, and combined therapy in intermittent claudication. *Ann Vasc Surg.* 2010;24:69-79.
3. McDermott MM, Ades P, Guralnik JM, et al. Treadmill exercise and resistance training in patients with peripheral arterial disease with and without intermittent claudication: a randomized controlled trial. *JAMA.* 2009;301:165-174.
4. Dawson DL, Cutler BS, Hiatt WR, et al. A comparison of cilostazol and pentoxifylline for treating intermittent claudication. *Am J Med.* 2000;109:523-530.
5. A randomised, blinded, trial of clopidogrel versus aspirin in patients at risk of ischaemic events (CAPRIE). CAPRIE Steering Committee. *Lancet.* 1996;348:1329-1339.
6. Schillinger M, Exner M, Mlekusch W, et al. Statin therapy improves cardiovascular outcome of patients with peripheral artery disease. *Eur Heart J.* 2004;25:742-748.
7. Mehler PS, Coll JR, Estacio R, et al. Intensive blood pressure control reduces the risk of cardiovascular events in patients with peripheral arterial disease and type 2 diabetes. *Circulation.* 2003;107:753-756.
8. Yusuf S, Sleight P, Pogue J, et al. Effects of an angiotensin-converting-enzyme inhibitor, ramipril, on cardiovascular events in high-risk patients. The Heart Outcomes Prevention Evaluation Study Investigators. *N Engl J Med.* 2000;342:145-153.
9. Whyman MR, Fowkes FG, Kerracher EM, et al. Is intermittent claudication improved by percutaneous transluminal angioplasty? A randomized controlled trial. *J Vasc Surg.* 1997;26:551-557.
10. Schillinger M, Sabeti S, Loewe C, et al. Balloon angioplasty versus implantation of nitinol stents in the superficial femoral artery. *N Engl J Med.* 2006;354:1879-1888.
11. Kasapis C, Henke PK, Chetcuti SJ, et al. Routine stent implantation vs. percutaneous transluminal angioplasty in femoropopliteal artery disease: a meta-analysis of randomized controlled trials. *Eur Heart J.* 2009;30:44-55.
12. Laird JR, Katzen BT, Scheinert D, et al. Nitinol stent implantation versus balloon angioplasty for lesions in the superficial femoral artery and proximal popliteal artery twelve-month results from the RESILIENT Randomized Trial. *Circulation.* 2010;3:267-276.
13. Conte MS. Bypass versus angioplasty in severe ischaemia of the leg (BASIL) and the (hoped for) dawn of evidence-based treatment for advanced limb ischemia. *J Vasc Surg.* 2010;51:69S-75S.
14. Feiring AJ, Krahn M, Nelson L, et al. Preventing leg amputations in critical limb ischemia with below-the-knee drug-eluting stents: the PaRADISE (PReventinig Amputations using Drug eluting StEnts) trial. *J Am Coll Cardiol.* 2010;55:1580-1589.

SUGGESTED READING

Hamburg NM, Balady GJ. Exercise rehabilitation in peripheral artery disease: functional impact and mechanisms of benefits. *Circulation.* 2011;123:87-97. *Review.*

80

OTHER PERIPHERAL ARTERIAL DISEASES

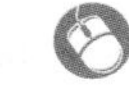

JEFFREY W. OLIN

LIVEDO RETICULARIS

Livedo reticularis is characterized by a reticular, fishnet, or lacy pattern on the skin of the lower extremities and other parts of the body. This pattern is red or blue and is caused by deoxygenated blood in the surrounding horizontally arranged venous plexus.

Primary or benign livedo reticularis occurs most commonly in young women between the ages of 20 and 40 years. Ulceration generally does not occur with this form of the disease, which may result from vasomotor instability or increased sensitivity (e.g., to cold, stress, tobacco) of the dermal blood vessels. It is intensified by cold exposure and is relieved by rewarming, and it may occur in association with Raynaud's phenomenon. The benign variety of livedo reticularis often needs no treatment other than measures to keep the body as warm as possible.

Secondary livedo reticularis occurs in association with atheromatous embolization (Fig. 80-1), polyarteritis nodosa (Chapter 278), systemic lupus erythematosus (Chapter 274), leukocytoclastic vasculitis (Chapter 278), cryoglobulinemia (Chapter 193), other connective tissue diseases, therapy with amantadine, and various neoplastic, neurologic, or endocrine diseases and in patients receiving large doses of vasopressors such as epinephrine, norepinephrine, and dopamine. Livedo reticularis is also one of the many skin manifestations of the antiphospholipid antibody syndrome (Chapter 179). In patients with secondary livedo reticularis, therapy should be directed at the underlying cause.

Livedoid Vasculopathy

In livedoid vasculopathy or livedoid vasculitis, extensive livedo reticularis surrounds a painful, ischemic-appearing ulceration located on the anterior or posterior portion of the lower leg (Fig. 80-2). Pathologically, thrombosis of the microvasculature occurs, with little or no active inflammatory component. Small doses of tissue plasminogen activator (10 mg intravenously daily for 14 days) may be effective in treating the ulcerations. Atrophie blanche (Fig. 80-3) is a variant of livedoid vasculopathy. These ulcerations generally occur around the ankle or foot. They have a white or yellowish base with poor granulation tissue and are exquisitely painful and difficult to heal.

ATHEROMATOUS EMBOLIZATION

DEFINITION

Atheromatous embolization (cholesterol embolization) refers to the embolization of cholesterol crystals or platelet fibrin aggregates to the extremities or to one or more organs. Atheromatous emboli usually originate from ulcerated or stenotic atherosclerotic plaques or from aneurysms that are primarily in the thoracic or abdominal aorta, iliac artery, or carotid artery.

EPIDEMIOLOGY AND PATHOBIOLOGY

Atheromatous embolization of the kidneys (Chapter 127) is a common histologic finding and may occur in 15 to 30% of patients with severe aortic atherosclerosis or aneurysm of the abdominal aorta. Increasing aortic plaque thickness, protruding aortic atheroma, and mobile aortic atheroma are associated with a high likelihood of atheromatous embolization. Atheromatous embolization may be spontaneous, but it occurs most often after percutaneous coronary, peripheral, or cerebrovascular intervention. Pathologically, biconvex cholesterol crystals lodge in the arterioles and lead to a foreign body reaction in which polymorphonuclear leukocytes, macrophages, and multinucleated giant cells appear several days to several weeks after the inciting event.

CLINICAL MANIFESTATIONS

The most common clinical manifestations are skin changes. These changes occur in more than one third of patients and are generally found in the lower extremities, but they may also be seen in the trunk, over the buttocks, and rarely in the upper extremities. These manifestations include livedo reticularis (embolization to the dermal blood vessels), purple or blue toes (see Fig. 80-1), splinter hemorrhages, gangrenous digits or ulcerations, and nodules in the presence of palpable foot pulses. The pain associated with ischemic lesions is disproportionate to the amount of tissue involvement.

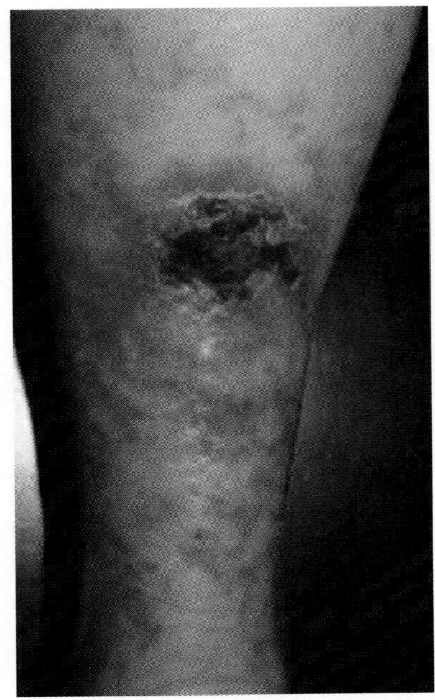

FIGURE 80-2. Livedoid vasculitis. Ischemic ulceration is evident on the posterior portion of the calf, surrounded by a livedoid pattern on the skin.

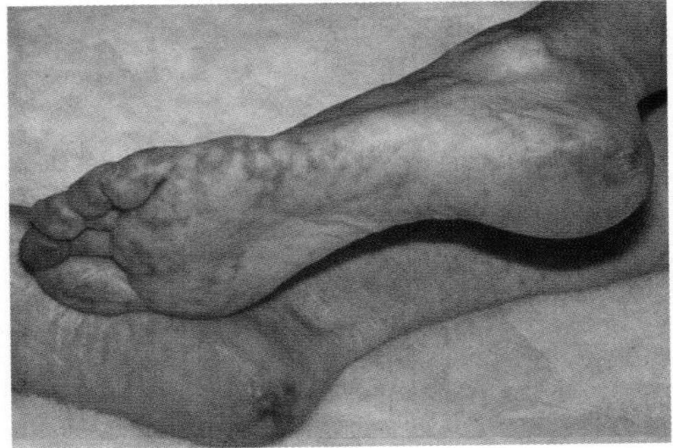

FIGURE 80-1. Typical livedo reticularis on the lateral portion of the left foot and both heels. The second and fourth toes are cyanotic. These findings are typical of atheromatous embolization, and the fact that both feet are involved indicates a source above the aortic bifurcation. (From Bartholomew JR, Olin JW. Atheromatous embolization. In: Young JR, Olin JW, Bartholomew JR, eds. *Peripheral Vascular Diseases,* 2nd ed. St. Louis: Mosby; 1996.)

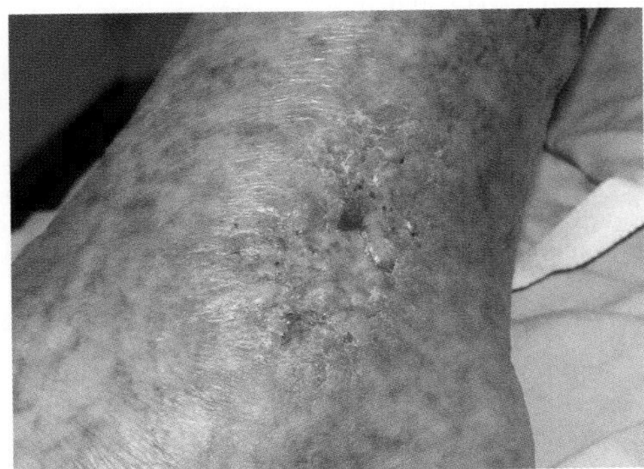

FIGURE 80-3. Atrophie blanche. Typical appearance of atrophie blanche. Note the pearly white plaque surrounded by prominent venules and a shallow ulceration. These lesions are quite painful and notoriously difficult to heal.

Atheroembolic renal disease is a small vessel occlusive disease leading to uncontrolled hypertension and advanced or end-stage renal disease. Atheromatous embolization may also involve the gastrointestinal tract and may produce ischemic bowel, with generalized abdominal pain, nausea, vomiting, melena, or hematochezia. Cholesterol emboli to the gallbladder may produce acute gangrenous cholecystitis, whereas emboli to the pancreas can cause acute pancreatitis.

Cardiac manifestations of atheroemboli include angina pectoris (Chapter 71) and myocardial infarction (Chapter 73). Patients may develop amaurosis fugax or blindness caused by retinal artery occlusion. A Hollenhorst plaque (yellow, highly refractile atheromatous material) may be present at the bifurcation of retinal blood vessels. Stroke, headache, confusion, organic brain syndrome, dizziness, and spinal cord infarction can occur. Constitutional signs and symptoms such as fever, weight loss, anorexia, fatigue, myalgia, headache, nausea, vomiting, or diarrhea may suggest necrotizing vasculitis, infection, or malignant disease.

DIAGNOSIS

Atheromatous embolization is frequently overlooked or misdiagnosed. No single laboratory test is diagnostic. Nonspecific findings such as elevation in the erythrocyte sedimentation rate, leukocytosis, or anemia may be present. Increased levels of serum amylase, hepatic transaminases, blood urea nitrogen, or serum creatinine may be noted if the pancreas, liver, or kidney is involved. The urine sediment may be abnormal but is nonspecific. Eosinophilia and eosinophiluria may be present early in the course, and hypocomplementemia has been reported in a small number of series. Biopsy is the most specific way to make the diagnosis, but it is often not required because the clinical findings are so highly suggestive of atheromatous embolization.

A markedly irregular and shaggy aorta may be observed on various imaging techniques. Transesophageal echocardiography may detect mobile, protruding atheroma, which are associated with a very high risk for future embolization.

Atheromatous embolization may mimic vasculitis, such as polyarteritis nodosa or leukocytoclastic vasculitis, or it may suggest an underlying malignant disease, nonbacterial thrombotic endocarditis, subacute bacterial endocarditis, multiple myeloma, antiphospholipid antibody syndrome, or atrial myxoma. A cardiac source of emboli should always be excluded.

TREATMENT Rx

The treatment of atheromatous embolization has three goals: (1) removal of the source of atheromatous material (by surgical exclusion and bypass, percutaneous transluminal angioplasty, stent implantation, or stent grafting), (2) symptomatic care of the end organs in which the emboli are located, and (3) optimal treatment of cardiovascular risk factors (Chapter 51) to prevent myocardial infarction, stroke, and cardiovascular death.

Pain control and local care of ischemic ulcers are critical to the management of patients with atheromatous embolization. Intravenous prostaglandin analogues (iloprost 0.5 to 2.0 ng/kg/minute continuously for 10 to 14 days, followed by 8-hour infusions three times a week for an additional 2 to 3 weeks) may be useful in the healing of ischemic ulcerations and in controlling pain secondary to atheromatous embolization. Patients should be given antiplatelet therapy with aspirin (81 mg/day) and clopidogrel (75 mg/day). Use of anticoagulants such as heparin or warfarin should be avoided unless a compelling reason exists to use this class of drugs. If a vasospastic component is present, a dihydropyridine calcium-channel blocker (amlodipine 2.5 to 10 mg/day or nifedipine extended release 30 to 120 mg/day) may be effective in relieving some of the symptoms. Chemical or surgical sympathectomy or spinal cord stimulators have been helpful for ulcer healing and pain relief in some patients.

Covered stents or stent grafts, which can be inserted in the thoracic or abdominal aorta for aneurysms or occlusive disease, are now the treatment of choice to prevent future embolic events when such approaches are technically feasible. In other cases, surgical bypass therapy is an alternative, although patients who are poor surgical risks may require ligation of the common femoral arteries followed by extra-anatomic bypass, such as axillobifemoral bypass.

PROGNOSIS

Patients with atheromatous embolization generally have advanced atherosclerosis and a poor prognosis. Patients should receive appropriate risk factor modification (Chapter 71) to slow the progression of atherosclerosis and to improve overall cardiac and cerebrovascular morbidity and mortality. Statins may reduce the risk of embolic events.

THROMBOANGIITIS OBLITERANS (BUERGER'S DISEASE)

DEFINITION

Thromboangiitis obliterans (Buerger's disease) is a nonatherosclerotic, segmental inflammatory disease that most commonly affects the small and medium-sized arteries and veins in the upper and lower extremities. The origin of Buerger's disease is unknown, but there is an extremely strong association with tobacco use, and progression of the disease is closely linked to continued tobacco use.

EPIDEMIOLOGY

Buerger's disease has a worldwide distribution, but it is more prevalent in the Middle East, Near East, and Far East than in North America and western Europe. The prevalence of Buerger's disease is decreasing as the consumption of tobacco products declines.

PATHOBIOLOGY

Patients with Buerger's disease may be hypercoagulable, and some patients have anti–endothelial cell antibodies, anticollagen antibodies, circulating immune complexes, and/or impaired endothelial-dependent vasorelaxation. Patients with thromboangiitis obliterans also have an increase in cellular sensitivity to type I and III collagen (normal constituents of human arteries).

In the acute phase of thromboangiitis obliterans, a highly inflammatory thrombus may affect both the arteries and the veins. The lesion is characterized by acute inflammation involving all layers of the vessel wall in association with occlusive inflammatory cellular thrombosis. Around the periphery of the thrombus, one may see polymorphonuclear leukocytes with karyorrhexis, the so-called microabscess that may contain one or more multinucleated giant cells. The acute phase lesion is followed by an intermediate phase characterized by progressive organization of the acute occlusive thrombus in the arteries and veins; a prominent, inflammatory cellular infiltrate may persist within the thrombus. The chronic phase or end-stage lesion is characterized by complete organization of the occlusive thrombus, with extensive recanalization, prominent vascularization of the media and adventitia, and perivascular fibrosis.

CLINICAL MANIFESTATIONS

Classically, Buerger's disease occurs in young male smokers, with the onset of symptoms before age 40 to 45 years; however, 20 to 30% of patients with Buerger's disease may be women. Buerger's disease usually begins with ischemia of the toes, feet, fingers, and hands (Fig. 80-4). As the disease progresses, it may involve more proximal arteries, but involvement of large arteries is unusual.

Patients may present with claudication of the feet, the legs, and occasionally the arms and hands. Foot or arch claudication may be the presenting manifestation and is often mistaken for an orthopedic problem. Seventy-five to 80% of patients present with ischemic rest pain and/or ulcerations. Two or more limbs are always involved, and angiographic abnormalities are consistently found in limbs that are not yet clinically involved. Superficial thrombophlebitis and Raynaud's phenomenon each occur in approximately 40% of patients.

A positive Allen test indicates the distal nature of thromboangiitis obliterans and its involvement of the lower and upper extremities, helping to differentiate it from atherosclerosis. In this test, the physician simultaneously occludes both the radial and the ulnar arteries. When pressure is released from either artery, one should note prompt filling from that artery, with the return of color to the hand. A positive test result occurs when color does not return to the blanched hand.

DIAGNOSIS

No specific laboratory tests aid in the diagnosis of Buerger's disease, but tests should exclude vasculitis, connective tissue diseases, hypercoagulable states, and a proximal source of emboli. On arteriography, the proximal arteries are normal, and the disease is most often infrapopliteal in the lower extremities and distal to the brachial artery in the upper extremities. Multiple vascular occlusions with collateralization around the obstruction (corkscrew collaterals) may occur, similar to what may be seen in other small vessel occlusive diseases such as the CREST syndrome (calcinosis cutis, Raynaud's phenomenon, esophageal motility disorder, sclerodactyly, and telangiectasias) or

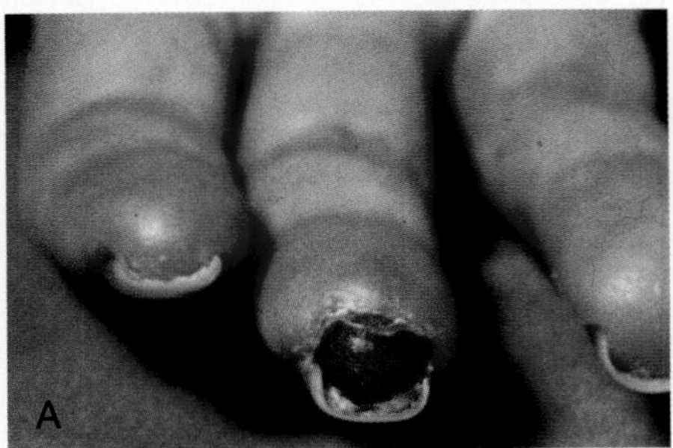

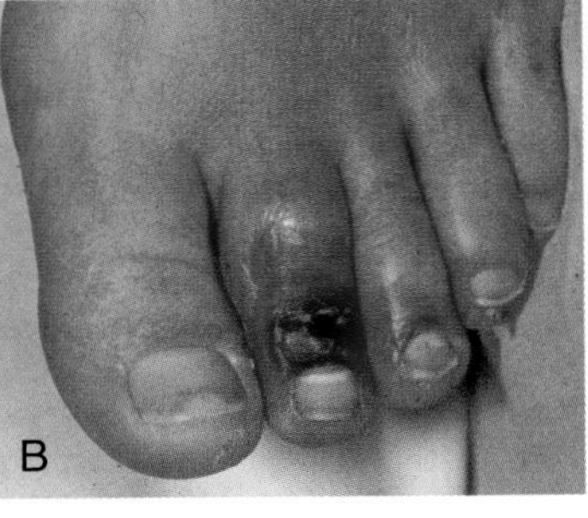

FIGURE 80-4. Buerger's disease. Ischemic finger of a young male patient **(A)** and ischemic toe of a 28-year-old woman **(B)** with Buerger's disease.

scleroderma (Chapter 275). However, the arteriographic appearance of Buerger's disease may also be similar to that of systemic lupus erythematosus (Chapter 274), rheumatoid vasculitis (Chapter 272), mixed connective tissue diseases (Chapter 275), and antiphospholipid antibody syndrome (Chapter 179), although the diagnosis of these other diseases can usually be established or excluded by other tests. Because cocaine and cannabis use (Chapter 33) may produce a clinical and angiographic picture identical to that of thromboangiitis obliterans, a toxicology screen may be indicated if the diagnosis in not clear-cut. Patients with Takayasu's arteritis (Chapter 78) or giant cell arteritis (Chapter 279) present with proximal vascular involvement and can readily be distinguished from patients with Buerger's disease.

TREATMENT Rx

The cornerstone of therapy for thromboangiitis obliterans is the complete discontinuation of cigarette smoking and tobacco use in any form. Patients who stop using tobacco almost always avoid amputation, whereas 40% or more of patients who continue to use tobacco progress to one or more amputations.

In a randomized trial, intravenous iloprost was superior to aspirin at 28 days in relieving rest pain and in healing ischemic ulcerations. At 6 months, 88% of patients receiving iloprost (0.5 to 2.0 ng/kg/minute, maintaining hemodynamic stability for 6 hours daily for up to 28 days) responded to therapy, compared with 21% in the aspirin-treated group; only 6% underwent amputation in the iloprost-treated group, compared with 18% in the aspirin-treated group.[1] Other treatments such as calcium-channel blockers (amlodipine, 2.5 to 10 mg/day or nifedipine extended release 30 to 120 mg/day), antibiotics, and anticoagulants, as well as sympathectomy, are palliative.

Surgical bypass is not a viable option in most patients because they may not have a distal target vessel with which to bypass. Sympathectomy and implantable spinal cord stimulators may help some patients, but iloprost is more effective than lumbar sympathectomy.[2] Stem cell and gene therapy have helped in healing ischemic ulcers and preventing amputation in patients with Buerger's disease. The use of intermittent pneumatic compression (arterial pump device) enhances blood flow to the foot and is useful in relieving rest pain and healing ulcers in patients with small vessel occlusive disease.

VASCULAR DISEASES ASSOCIATED WITH CHANGES IN TEMPERATURE

Raynaud's Phenomenon

DEFINITION

Raynaud's phenomenon is the abrupt onset of a triphasic color (white, blue, and red) response: well-demarcated pallor of the digits progresses to cyanosis with pain and often numbness, followed by reactive hyperemia on rewarming. This vasospastic phenomenon is often precipitated by cold exposure or stress. *Primary Raynaud's phenomenon* denotes patients who have no underlying cause, whereas *secondary Raynaud's phenomenon* is associated with or caused by some other systemic illness or disease process (Fig. 80-5).

EPIDEMIOLOGY

Raynaud's phenomenon is common in patients with connective tissue diseases. Approximately 90% of patients with scleroderma (Chapter 275) experience Raynaud's phenomenon, and it may be a presenting manifestation in many of them. Raynaud's phenomenon is also a component of the CREST syndrome. These patients have small vessel occlusive disease that may lead to digital pitting or ulceration and eventual amputation.

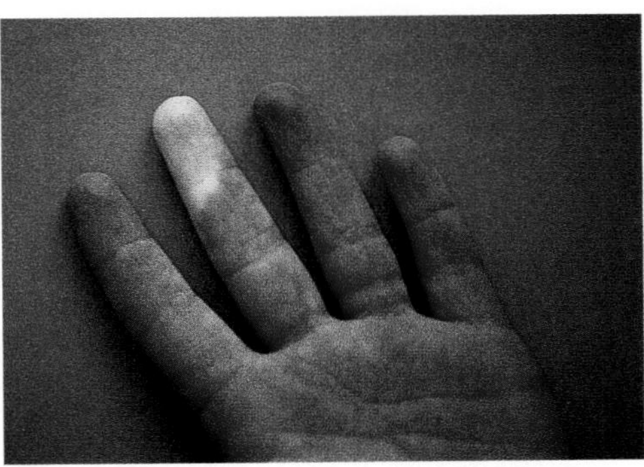

FIGURE 80-5. Raynaud's phenomenon in the acute phase, with severe blanching of the tip of one finger. (From Forbes CD, Jackson WF. *Color Atlas and Text of Clinical Medicine,* 3rd ed. London: Mosby; 2003.)

The β-adrenergic receptor antagonists are most commonly associated with Raynaud's phenomenon because they block the vasodilatory β-receptors and thus leave the vasoconstrictive α-receptors unopposed. Ergotamine preparations, polyvinyl chloride, and several cancer chemotherapeutic agents can also cause Raynaud's phenomenon.

Raynaud's phenomenon occurs frequently in individuals who use vibratory tools such as pneumatic hammers, chain saws, sanders, and grinders. This has been termed the *hand-arm vibration syndrome,* and the prevalence of Raynaud's phenomenon may exceed 90% at 10 years in individuals with heavy exposure. Continued use of vibratory tools can lead to chronic occlusive small vessel disease. The syndrome has also been described in typists, pianists, meat cutters, and sewing machine operators.

Trauma to the distal ulnar artery (several centimeters distal to the wrist) may occur with pounding the palm of the hand, karate, or other activities that traumatize the hypothenar eminence and lead to an aneurysm or pseudoaneurysm of the distal ulnar artery (hypothenar hammer syndrome). Thrombus within the aneurysm may then embolize to the fingers, or the distal ulnar artery may thrombose.

PATHOBIOLOGY

The initial manifestation of Raynaud's phenomenon occurs when the digits turn white as a result of the intense vasoconstriction or spasm of the digital arteries. At this point, blood flow ceases totally, and the digits are often numb and painful. As the arterial vasoconstriction abates, subsequent postcapillary venule constriction causes the blood in the capillaries and veins to become deoxygenated, producing the cyanotic appearance. When rewarming occurs, blood flow is markedly increased due to marked vasodilation, producing reactive hyperemia to the digits (red color).

The pathophysiologic factors operative in Raynaud's phenomenon include vascular, neural, and intravascular abnormalities. Vascular factors include small vessel occlusive disease, such as is seen in scleroderma, and functional abnormalities, such as impaired endothelium-dependent (nitric oxide–mediated) and endothelium-independent vasodilation, reduced production of vasodilators, and increased vasoconstriction. Neural abnormalities include impaired sympathetic nervous system activity that disturbs the balance between vasoconstriction and vasodilation. Intravascular factors such as platelet activation, impaired fibrinolysis, white blood cell activation, reduced red blood cell deformability, and oxidative stress may play important roles in some patients.

TABLE 80-1 DIFFERENTIATING PRIMARY FROM SECONDARY RAYNAUD'S PHENOMENON

CHARACTERISTICS	PRIMARY	SECONDARY
Associated diseases	No	Yes
Age at onset	Younger (<30 yr)	Older (>30 yr)
Nail-fold capillaries	Normal	Large, tortuous with "dropout"
Autoantibodies	Negative or low titers	Frequent
Endothelial cell activation	Yes	Yes
Endothelial damage	No	Frequent
Structural occlusion	No	Yes
Digital gangrene	Rare; only superficial	Common
α_2-Adrenergic activity	High	High
Calcitonin gene-related peptide	Low	Low

From Block JA, Sequeira W. Raynaud's phenomenon. *Lancet.* 2001;357:2042-2048.

CLINICAL MANIFESTATIONS

The signs of Raynaud's phenomenon may include pallor (see Fig. 80-5), cyanosis, and rubor. The triphasic color response occurs in 4 to 65% of patients. Exposure to the cold is the typical precipitating factor, but emotional lability may also cause or exacerbate attacks in some patients. Vasospastic attacks usually occur only in the fingers, but vasospasm can occur in the toes, nose, ears, lips, and other body parts.

In primary Raynaud's phenomenon, the physical examination is normal between attacks. However, in secondary Raynaud's phenomenon, pits or ulcerations on the fingertips may be present in patients with scleroderma, CREST syndrome, or thromboangiitis obliterans. An abnormal Allen test on physical examination indicates fixed arterial obstruction.

DIAGNOSIS

The diagnosis of Raynaud's phenomenon is not difficult when it is based on the patient's description of the attacks. Patients with persistent cyanosis or persistent hyperemia generally have some condition other than Raynaud's phenomenon. In primary Raynaud's phenomenon, vasospastic attacks are precipitated by exposure to the cold or emotional stimuli; there is bilateral involvement of the extremities without gangrene; and, after a careful search, no evidence indicates an underlying systemic disease that could be responsible for the vasospastic attacks (Table 80-1).

To evaluate systemic illnesses, a serologic evaluation should include a complete blood cell count, multiphasic serologic analysis, urinalysis, erythrocyte sedimentation rate, C-reactive protein, antinuclear antibody, extractable nuclear antigen (anti-Smith and ribonuclear protein), anti-DNA, cryoglobulins, complement, anticentromere antibodies, and SCL70 scleroderma antibodies. In addition, nail-fold capillaroscopy can be performed to help confirm a diagnosis of CREST syndrome or scleroderma in patients whose symptoms are not clear. Abnormal nail-fold capillaroscopy indicates that the patient does not have primary Raynaud's phenomenon.

The noninvasive vascular laboratory (pulse volume recordings) is useful in identifying the degree of digital arterial occlusive disease (fixed ischemia) and in predicting whether ischemic ulcerations on the digits will heal. Arteriography is not routinely performed.

TREATMENT Rx

In patients with mild vasospastic attacks, reassurance about the benign nature of the disease and instructions on how to prevent attacks are often all that is needed. Patients should limit their exposure to the cold and should dress warmly and protect not only the extremities but also the entire body. Mittens are better than gloves for keeping the hands warm. Patients need to be especially careful when they handle cold objects. Hand- and foot-warming devices (battery operated or chemical) may be helpful. Smoking should be avoided because nicotine causes intense vasoconstriction. β-Blocking agents may exaggerate the symptoms of Raynaud's phenomenon. Conditioning techniques and biofeedback are sometimes helpful in controlling vasospastic episodes.

The dihydropyridine calcium-channel blockers are the most effective pharmacotherapeutic agents for Raynaud's phenomenon.[3] Patients who have infrequent attacks may benefit from a short-acting calcium-channel blocker such as nifedipine 10 to 20 mg, given 30 minutes to 1 hour before cold exposure. When vasospasm occurs more frequently, the extended-release preparations of nifedipine (30 to 120 mg/day) or amlodipine (2.5 to 10 mg/day) should be used. α_1-Adrenergic receptor antagonists such as prazosin (1 to 10 mg twice daily) or terazosin (2 to 20 mg/day) are also highly effective in decreasing the severity, frequency, and duration of vasospastic attacks. Nitroglycerin or its analogues can be used topically (0.1 to 0.8 mg/hour),[4] whereas prostacyclin can be given intravenously (0.5 ng/kg/minute for 6 hours/day for 21 days).[5] Dual endothelin receptor blockade (e.g., bosentan 62.5 to 125 mg twice daily) has been beneficial in randomized trials.[6] Angiotensin-converting enzyme inhibitors, angiotensin receptor blockers, phosphodiesterase-5 inhibitors, niacin, and papaverine are not of proven benefit. Several reports have suggested a beneficial effect from selective serotonin reuptake inhibitors such as fluoxetine (20 to 40 mg/day). Small case series suggest that cilostazol (100 mg twice daily, 30 minutes before breakfast and 30 minutes before dinner) may improve ulcer healing in patients with secondary Raynaud's phenomenon. L-Arginine (2 to 8 g/day) and sildenafil (50 mg twice daily) have been used with variable success.

Although sympathectomy may be beneficial in the short term, with about a 50% improvement rate, the vasospastic attacks may recur in 6 months to 2 years. Some patients with severe disease have had success with digital sympathectomy.

PROGNOSIS

The prognosis in patients with primary Raynaud's phenomenon is excellent. No mortality is associated with this condition. In a long-term study involving 307 patients with primary Raynaud's phenomenon, 38% had stable disease, 36% were improved, 16% were worsened, and the syndrome disappeared in 10%. The prognosis associated with secondary Raynaud's phenomenon depends on the underlying condition that caused it.

Pernio (Chilblains)

DEFINITION AND EPIDEMIOLOGY

Pernio is a Latin word that means "frostbite"; its synonym *chilblains* is an Anglo-Saxon term that means "cold sore." It is a localized inflammatory lesion of the skin caused by an abnormal response to the cold. Whereas in Raynaud's phenomenon there is acute and readily reversible vasospasm, in pernio the vasospasm is more prolonged. Pernio is frequently encountered in the temperate, humid climates of northwestern Europe and in the northern United States.

PATHOBIOLOGY

Pernio develops in susceptible individuals who are exposed to nonfreezing cold. The pathologic changes include edema of the papillodermis, vasculitis characterized by perivascular infiltration (with lymphocytes) of the arterioles and venules of the dermis, thickening and edema of the blood vessel walls, fat necrosis, and a chronic inflammatory reaction with giant cell formation.

CLINICAL MANIFESTATIONS AND DIAGNOSIS

Pernio most commonly occurs in young women between the ages of 15 and 30 years, but it may occur in older individuals or in children. Acute pernio may develop 12 to 24 hours after exposure to the cold. Single or multiple erythematous, purplish, edematous lesions appear, accompanied by intense itching or burning. These lesions may have a yellowish or brownish discoloration and may be associated with some flaking. They tend to affect the toes and dorsum of the proximal phalanges. The lesions of acute pernio are usually self-limited, although they may lead to recurrent disease. The arterial circulation is normal on physical examination and in the noninvasive vascular laboratory. Chronic pernio occurs when repeated exposure to the cold results in the persistence of lesions, with subsequent scarring and atrophy. Characteristically, the lesions begin in the fall or winter and disappear in the spring or early summer. In advanced cases, the seasonal variation may disappear, and chronic occlusive vascular disease may develop.

In the typical form, the patient develops violet or yellow-brown blisters and shallow toe ulcers that burn and itch (Fig. 80-6). The differential diagnosis of pernio includes recurrent, erythematous, nodular, and ulcerative lesions such as erythema induratum, nodular vasculitis, erythema nodosum, and cold panniculitis. The skin lesions of pernio may resemble those of atheromatous embolization (see earlier).

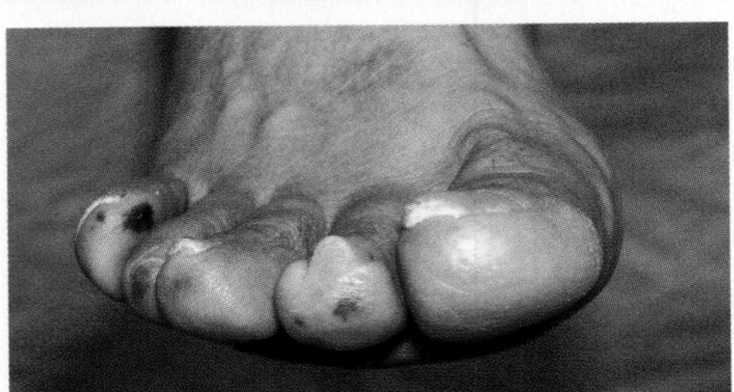

FIGURE 80-6. Pernio on the toes of the right foot. The lesions on the second, third, and fourth toes are the typical red, brown, and yellow scaling lesions. The lesion on the fifth toe can be confused with atheromatous embolization.

PREVENTION AND TREATMENT Rx

Prevention is the best form of therapy. Cold exposure should be minimized as much as possible. In randomized trials, nifedipine (20 to 60 mg/day)[7] and pentoxifylline (400 mg three times daily)[8] reduce pain and facilitate the healing process. The severe itching may be treated with local application of an antipruritic agent.

Acrocyanosis

Acrocyanosis, which is a persistent blue or cyanotic discoloration of the digits, occurs most commonly in the hands and may worsen with exposure to cold and improve with rewarming. The primary form is a benign cosmetic condition, but it may also be seen in patients with connective tissue diseases, thromboangiitis obliterans, and diseases associated with central cyanosis. The exact pathophysiologic abnormality is not clear, but it may be vasospasm in the cutaneous arteries and arterioles, with compensatory dilation and oxygen desaturation in the postcapillary venules.

Ulceration or tissue loss is unusual, and the overall prognosis is excellent. Patients should be advised to keep their entire body and extremities warm. Drugs such as α-adrenergic blocking agents (prazosin 1 to 10 mg twice daily or terazosin, 2 to 20 mg/day) or calcium-channel blockers (amlodipine 2.5 to 10 mg/day or nifedipine extended release 30 to 120 mg/day) may be helpful.

Frostbite

EPIDEMIOLOGY AND PATHOBIOLOGY

Frostbite is the freezing of tissues resulting from exposure to cold. It may occur in above-freezing temperatures under circumstances such as wetness, strong wind, or high altitude.

A person's response to cold is aimed at conserving the core (internal body) temperature as well as the viability of the extremities. Heat loss is reduced by peripheral vasoconstriction caused by sympathetic stimulation and catecholamine release. Maintenance or augmentation of body heat is accomplished by muscular activity such as shivering. However, the heat production from shivering cannot be sustained for more than a few hours because of the depletion of glycogen, which is the source of heat during shivering. The extremities are also protected by the "hunting reaction," which consists of irregular, 5- to 10-minute cycles of alternating vasoconstriction and vasodilation that protect the extremities against excessive sustained vasoconstriction with minimal loss of internal body temperature. However, when the body is exposed to cold of a magnitude or a duration that threatens the internal body temperature, this mechanism fails. Because the disruption of core temperature is more deleterious to the body than is peripheral vasoconstriction, conservation of core temperature takes precedence over rewarming of the extremities, and the hunting response is replaced by continuous and more intense vasoconstriction that promotes frostbite by means of ice crystal formation, cellular dehydration, and thrombosis of the microvasculature.

CLINICAL MANIFESTATIONS AND DIAGNOSIS

Soon after exposure to the cold, pain develops and gradually progresses to numbness; the frozen part turns white because of intense vasoconstriction (Fig. 80-7). With rewarming or thawing, the circulation is restored, and the affected parts become hyperemic. Edema may first occur within hours of thawing and persist for days or weeks. Blisters appear within the first 24 hours and are reabsorbed within 1 to 2 weeks, after which a black eschar may persist. Overactivity of the sympathetic nervous system is manifested by hyperhidrosis or a burning sensation.

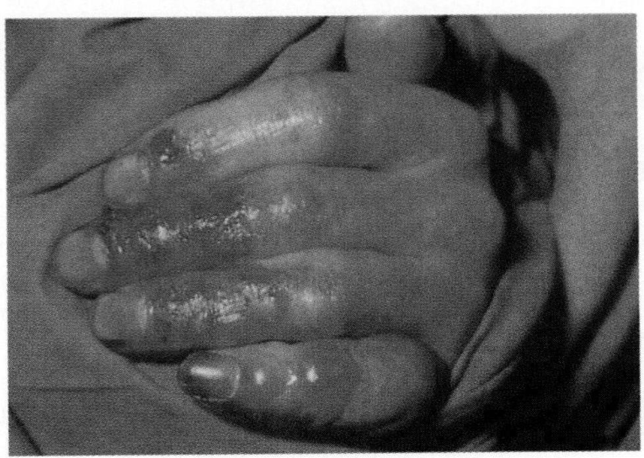

FIGURE 80-7. Frostbite of the hand in a mountaineer. On rewarming, the hand became painful, red, and edematous, with signs of probable gangrene in the fifth finger. (From Forbes CD, Jackson WF. *Color Atlas and Text of Clinical Medicine,* 3rd ed. London: Mosby; 2003.)

Seventy percent of frostbite victims develop chronic sequelae, including cold sensitivity, pain, and sensory disturbances, often resembling complex regional pain syndrome (Chapter 428). Frostbite arthritis may occur in particularly severe cases.

It is important to establish the depth of the frostbite and determine whether the tissue is viable. This may not be obvious on initial clinical examination; it is usually determined weeks or months after the cold injury, when the demarcation zone appears and the dead tissue is sloughed.

TREATMENT 

In mild cases of frostbite, the only treatment necessary may be daily whirlpool baths and bedrest. However, treatment of deep frostbite should be considered a medical emergency because the early institution of therapy may reduce the amount of tissue loss. Thawing, the mainstay of therapy, should not be implemented if the patient may be exposed to cold again, because refreezing of thawed tissue promotes further tissue damage. Walking on a frozen limb produces substantially less damage than walking on a thawed limb.

After the patient's transfer to a medical facility, frozen tissue should be rapidly rewarmed in a water bath of 40 to 42° C (104 to 108° F) for 15 to 30 minutes until complete thawing has occurred. After thawing, reappearance of normal color signifies the reestablishment of blood flow. Thawing is often a painful process and may require the administration of narcotics.

After thawing, the extremity should be cleansed twice daily in a whirlpool bath with an aseptic solution at 35 to 37° C (95 to 99° F). Care should be taken to prevent and treat secondary infections. Tetanus prophylaxis should be administered. A frostbite protocol consisting of débridement of clear blisters with a topical application of aloe vera, oral ibuprofen, and daily hydrotherapy is highly effective. An important principle is to avoid early débridement or amputation, which is indicated only when infected gangrene or generalized sepsis occurs.

ERYTHROMELALGIA

DEFINITION AND EPIDEMIOLOGY

Erythromelalgia literally means "red, painful extremities." It may be classified as primary (or idiopathic) or secondary. The primary form may be nonfamilial or familial. Secondary erythromelalgia is associated with other diseases, the most common being myeloproliferative disorders such as polycythemia vera and essential thrombocythemia. Other diseases associated with secondary erythromelalgia include hypertension, diabetes, rheumatoid arthritis, gout, spinal cord disease, multiple sclerosis, systemic lupus erythematosus, cutaneous vasculitis, and viral infection; it also may result from therapy with various drugs (e.g., nifedipine, nicardipine, verapamil, bromocriptine, pergolide).

PATHOBIOLOGY

Families with autosomal dominant erythromelalgia have demonstrated mutations in the sodium channel $Na_v1.7$, which is selectively expressed within the nociceptive dorsal root ganglion and sympathetic ganglion neurons. The histologic features vary from normal findings to arterial occlusion with thrombus formation.

CLINICAL MANIFESTATIONS AND DIAGNOSIS

Erythromelalgia is characterized by the clinical triad of erythema, burning pain, and increased temperature, usually of the extremities. The feet, especially the soles, are more commonly involved than the hands. The peripheral pulses are generally normal in the primary type and variable in secondary erythromelalgia. The symptoms may occur in "attacks" that last for minutes to hours or occasionally days and are precipitated by a warm environment. Exercise and dependency tend to exacerbate symptoms. Patients seek relief by exposing the affected extremity to a cooler environment, such as placing it in cold water, walking on a cold floor barefoot, or running an air conditioner even in the winter. This response often leads to a cold-induced vascular injury superimposed on the erythromelalgia. Erythromelalgia may precede the clinical appearance of a myeloproliferative disorder by several years, so patients older than 30 years should be monitored periodically with blood cell counts.

TREATMENT Rx

The treatment of erythromelalgia is often difficult and frustrating. Symptoms can be so debilitating that they lead to suicide. In secondary erythromelalgia, treatment of the underlying disease (phlebotomy in patients with polycythemia vera, and normalization of the platelet count in patients with thrombocythemia) may relieve the symptoms. Aspirin (81 to 325 mg/day) is the most effective treatment available, particularly for patients with erythromelalgia secondary to myeloproliferative disorders. Other therapies with variable success in case reports include methysergide, ephedrine, nonsteroidal anti-inflammatory drugs, phenoxybenzamine, nitroglycerin, sodium nitroprusside, corticosteroids, and surgical sympathectomy. Lidocaine transdermal patches (Lidoderm) on the feet and thalamic stimulation have also been used anecdotally.

POPLITEAL ARTERY ENTRAPMENT SYNDROME

In popliteal artery entrapment syndrome, the popliteal artery is compressed by a congenital anatomic abnormality or an abnormal muscle or fibrous band. In the most common abnormality, the medial head of the gastrocnemius muscle compresses the popliteal artery and causes its medial deviation.

The clinical presentation consists of a healthy, "athletic-type" patient complaining of typical claudication symptoms in the absence of premature atherosclerosis. Disappearance of the pulse with passive dorsiflexion of the foot or active plantar flexion against resistance may suggest the diagnosis. Duplex ultrasound may help, and computed tomography or magnetic resonance imaging can confirm the diagnosis. On arteriography, the characteristic finding is medial deviation of the popliteal artery with post-stenotic dilation. Other diseases that can cause mid-popliteal occlusion include cystic adventitial disease, thrombosed popliteal artery aneurysm, and atherosclerosis of the superficial femoral and popliteal arteries. The primary treatment of popliteal artery entrapment syndrome is surgical resection of the abnormal muscle or fibrous band.

CYSTIC ADVENTITIAL DISEASE

In cystic adventitial disease, gelatinous fluid accumulates in an arterial wall cyst, and the cyst encroaches on the vessel lumen, with resulting stenosis or occlusion. The cyst arises in the outer portion of the media or subadventitial layer, most commonly in the popliteal artery. Cystic adventitial disease is an isolated lesion not associated with a systemic process, and the precise pathophysiologic mechanism is unknown.

The disease predominates in men, with an approximate male-female ratio of 5 : 1, and the mean age at diagnosis is about 45 years. Claudication is the most frequent symptom. The pulses may disappear on flexion of the knee (Ishikawa's sign). However, if the artery is occluded, no pulses are palpable.

Pulse volume recordings may show the characteristic decrease in blood pressure and the change in waveform configuration in the affected limb. A perivascular cystic structure may be visualized on duplex ultrasound, computed tomography, or magnetic resonance imaging. Computed tomography–guided needle aspiration can partially but usually not completely remove the highly viscous and gelatinous fluid. Surgical resection is indicated when claudication interferes with a patient's lifestyle or ischemic rest pain is present.

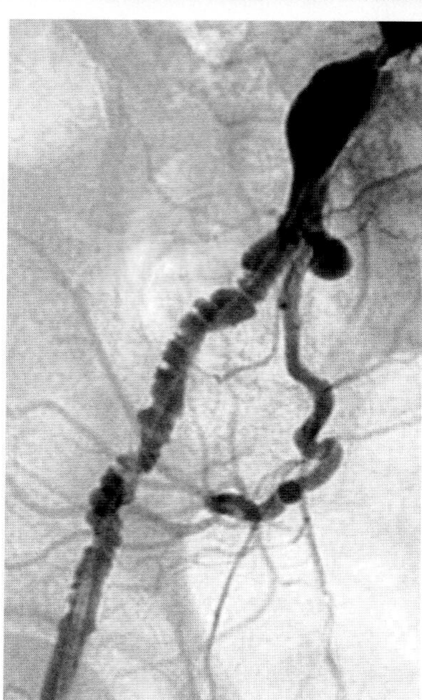

FIGURE 80-8. Fibromuscular dysplasia. Note the "string of beads" or "accordion" appearance in the external iliac artery. This radiographic appearance is diagnostic of fibromuscular dysplasia of the medial type. Also note the aneurysm proximal to the area of dysplasia.

FIBROMUSCULAR DYSPLASIA OF THE EXTREMITIES

Although fibromuscular dysplasia (in particular, medial fibroplasia) is most common in the renal and carotid arteries (Chapters 67 and 127), it may also occur in peripheral arteries of the extremity (iliac, superficial femoral, popliteal, tibial, subclavian, axillary, radial, and ulnar). These lesions may be asymptomatic, or they may produce a difference in blood pressure between the two limbs, with paresthesias, claudication, or critical limb ischemia.

The typical arteriographic appearance of a "string of beads" is virtually pathognomonic of medial fibroplasia (Fig. 80-8). Long, smooth areas of narrowing are characteristic of intimal fibroplasia, but they may also be seen in Takayasu's arteritis (Chapter 78) and giant cell arteritis (Chapters 78 and 279).

Therapy should be reserved for patients with lifestyle-interfering claudication or critical limb ischemia. Under most circumstances, percutaneous balloon dilation is the treatment of choice.

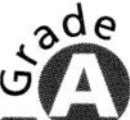

1. Fiessinger JN, Schafer M. Trial of iloprost versus aspirin treatment for critical limb ischaemia of thromboangiitis obliterans: The TAO Study. *Lancet.* 1990;335:555-557.
2. Bozkurt AK, Köksal C, Demirbas MY, et al. A randomized trial of intravenous iloprost (a stable prostacyclin analogue) versus lumbar sympathectomy in the management of Buerger's disease. *Int Angiol.* 2006:25:162-168.
3. Thompson AE, Shea B, Welch V, et al. Calcium-channel blockers for Raynaud's phenomenon in systemic sclerosis. *Arthritis Rheum.* 2001;44:1841-1847.
4. Chung L, Shapiro L, Fiorentino D, et al. MQX-503, a novel formulation of nitroglycerin, improved the severity of Raynaud's phenomenon: a randomized, controlled trial. *Arthritis Rheum.* 2009; 60:870-877.
5. Kawald A, Burmester GR, Huscher D, et al. Low versus high-dose iloprost therapy over 21 days in patients with secondary Raynaud's phenomenon and systemic sclerosis: a randomized, open, single-center study. *J Rheumatol.* 2008;35:1830-1837.
6. Nguyen VA, Eisendle K, Gruber I, et al. Effect of the dual endothelin receptor antagonist bosentan on Raynaud's phenomenon secondary to systemic sclerosis: a double-blind prospective, randomized, placebo-controlled pilot study. *Rheumatology (Oxford).* 2010;49:583-587.
7. Rustin MH, Newton JA, Smith NP, et al. The treatment of chilblains with nifedipine: the results of a pilot study, a double-blind placebo-controlled randomized study and a long-term open trial. *Br J Dermatol.* 1989;120:267-275.
8. Noaimi AA, Fadheel BM. Treatment of perniosis with oral pentoxifylline in comparison with oral prednisone plus topical clobetasol ointment in Iraqi patients. *Saudi Med J.* 2008;29:1762-1764.

SUGGESTED READINGS

Heidrich H. Functional vascular diseases: Raynaud's syndrome, acrocyanosis and erythromelalgia. *Vasa.* 2010;39:33-41. *Review.*

Olin JW, Sealove BA. Diagnosis, management, and future developments of fibromuscular dysplasia. *J Vasc Surg*. 2011;53:826-836. *Comprehensive review of the clinical manifestations and treatment.*
Piazza G, Creager MA. Thromboangiitis obliterans. *Circulation*. 2010;121:1858-1861. *Clinical review.*
Prakash S, Weisman MH. Idiopathic chilblains. *Am J Med*. 2009;122:1152-1155. *Clinical review.*

81

PERIPHERAL VENOUS DISEASE

JEFFREY GINSBERG

DEEP VEIN THROMBOSIS

DEFINITION

Deep vein thrombosis (DVT), which is the most important disease affecting the peripheral veins, has an estimated annual incidence of 0.1% in whites. Most pulmonary emboli (Chapter 98) arise from DVT of the legs. In fact, DVT and pulmonary embolism are usually considered different clinical manifestations of one disease, venous thromboembolism (VTE), because up to 50% of patients who present with proximal (popliteal vein or more proximal) DVT have abnormal lung scans suggestive of clinically silent pulmonary emboli, whereas up to 90% of patients with proven pulmonary emboli have DVT, even though only 15% of them have leg symptoms. For the most part, the cornerstones of management of DVT and pulmonary embolism are the same: immediate and long-term anticoagulation.

Superficial thrombophlebitis consists of thrombosis and inflammation of one or more superficial veins. Provided the associated thrombus has not extended into the deep veins, affected patients have a negligible risk for development of pulmonary emboli and can often be effectively managed conservatively with ice, elevation, and anti-inflammatory medication.

EPIDEMIOLOGY

In nonpregnant patients, DVT usually originates in one of the distal or calf veins, where it has little or no potential to cause clinically important pulmonary emboli. The true incidence of calf vein thrombosis is not known because many affected patients remain asymptomatic while the thrombus forms and spontaneously resolves. On the basis of results of studies of *symptomatic* patients with suspected DVT, about 10 to 25% actually have a diagnosable DVT, of whom about 15% have isolated calf DVT. Approximately one fourth of these thrombi that are initially isolated to a calf vein subsequently extend into the proximal veins, usually within 1 week of presentation, where they *then* have the potential to cause pulmonary emboli.

In pregnancy, most (~90%) thrombi occur in the deep veins of the left leg and frequently involve the ileofemoral veins but not the calf or popliteal veins. These findings suggest an anatomic predisposition to left leg ileofemoral DVT, which may be a result of compression of the left iliac vein by the fetus, an exaggeration of the "obstruction" that occurs where the right iliac artery crosses the left iliac vein, and an increase in venous webs at the left iliac vein (May-Thurner syndrome). These observations strongly suggest that most if not all of the increase in VTE during pregnancy is attributable to the increase in left iliac DVT.

From a clinical perspective, risk factors can be subdivided by duration, that is, transient and finite duration (e.g., fractured fibula treated with plaster immobilization) compared with permanent or long-term duration (e.g., congenital antithrombin deficiency, metastatic cancer), and according to the magnitude of the risk, that is, major (hip or knee replacement surgery) or minor (long-distance air travel, use of oral contraceptives). Classification of patients according to the presence or absence and type of risk factor is predictive of the risk of recurrence after a prolonged (≥3 months) course of anticoagulant therapy and provides key information that helps determine the optimal duration of anticoagulant therapy. Patients in whom DVT develops in association with a major risk factor that has resolved have a much lower risk of recurrence after a 3-month course of anticoagulants than do patients whose DVT was associated with a transient minor risk factor that has resolved or patients whose DVT was apparently idiopathic or associated with an ongoing risk factor.

PATHOBIOLOGY

Virchow's triad of hypercoagulability, venous stasis, and injury to the vessel wall provides a model for understanding many of the risk factors that lead to the formation of thrombosis. For example, in patients who have total hip or knee replacement surgery, there is venous endothelial injury caused by surgery, venous stasis due to perioperative immobilization, and hypercoagulability as a result of postoperative fibrinolytic shutdown. In other patients, an identifiable "thrombophilia" or "tendency to clot," such as congenital antithrombin (formerly antithrombin III) deficiency or the presence of factor V Leiden (Chapter 179), combined with use of oral contraceptives results in DVT in women of childbearing age. However, a relatively high proportion of patients have unexplained DVT without "clinical" risk factors that cause endothelial damage or venous stasis or identifiable thrombophilias that cause hypercoagulability. Undoubtedly, some of these patients have yet to be determined thrombophilias, but the DVT currently is labeled idiopathic.

CLINICAL MANIFESTATIONS

The clinical features of lower extremity DVT include leg pain, tenderness, swelling (Fig. 81-1), palpable cord, discoloration, venous distention, prominence of the superficial veins, and cyanosis. In most patients in whom DVT is clinically suspected, the symptoms and signs are nonspecific, and DVT is confirmed in less than 50% of cases. Conversely, patients with relatively minor symptoms and signs may have extensive DVT.

In some patients, DVT may be asymptomatic, but the patient will present with pulmonary embolism. Conversely, pulmonary embolism occurs in 50% of patients with objectively documented proximal leg vein thrombosis, but many of the emboli are asymptomatic. Usually, only part of the thrombus embolizes, so 50 to 70% of patients with angiographically documented pulmonary emboli have detectable DVT of the legs at the time of initial evaluation.

DIAGNOSIS

By itself, clinical diagnosis of DVT is inaccurate because no individual symptom or sign is sufficiently sensitive or specific for the diagnosis to be made or excluded. Clinical assessment can categorize patients according to their pretest probability of DVT with reasonable accuracy. By combining a validated prediction rule (Table 81-1) to assess this pretest probability with the results of noninvasive tests, diagnostic accuracy can be improved, thereby often limiting or eliminating the need for further investigation (Fig. 81-2).

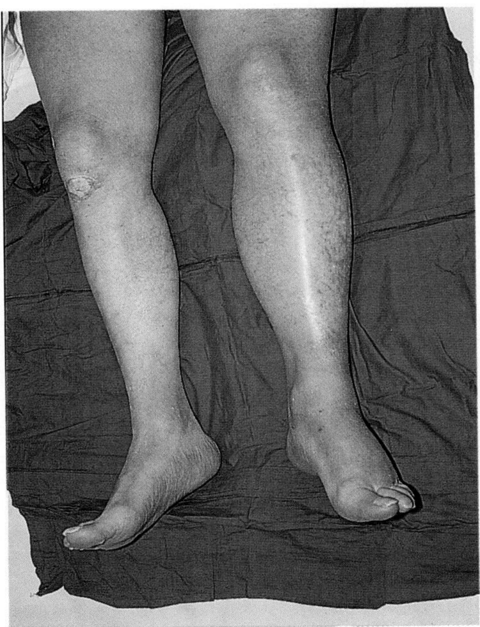

FIGURE 81-1. Deep vein thrombosis (DVT) presenting as an acutely swollen left leg. Note the dilation of the superficial veins. The leg was hot to the touch, and palpation along the line of the left popliteal and femoral veins caused pain. Less than 50% of DVTs present in this way, and other conditions may mimic DVT, so further investigation is always indicated. Note the coincidental psoriatic lesion below the patient's right knee. (From Forbes CD, Jackson WF. *Color Atlas and Text of Clinical Medicine*, 3rd ed. London: Mosby; 2003.)

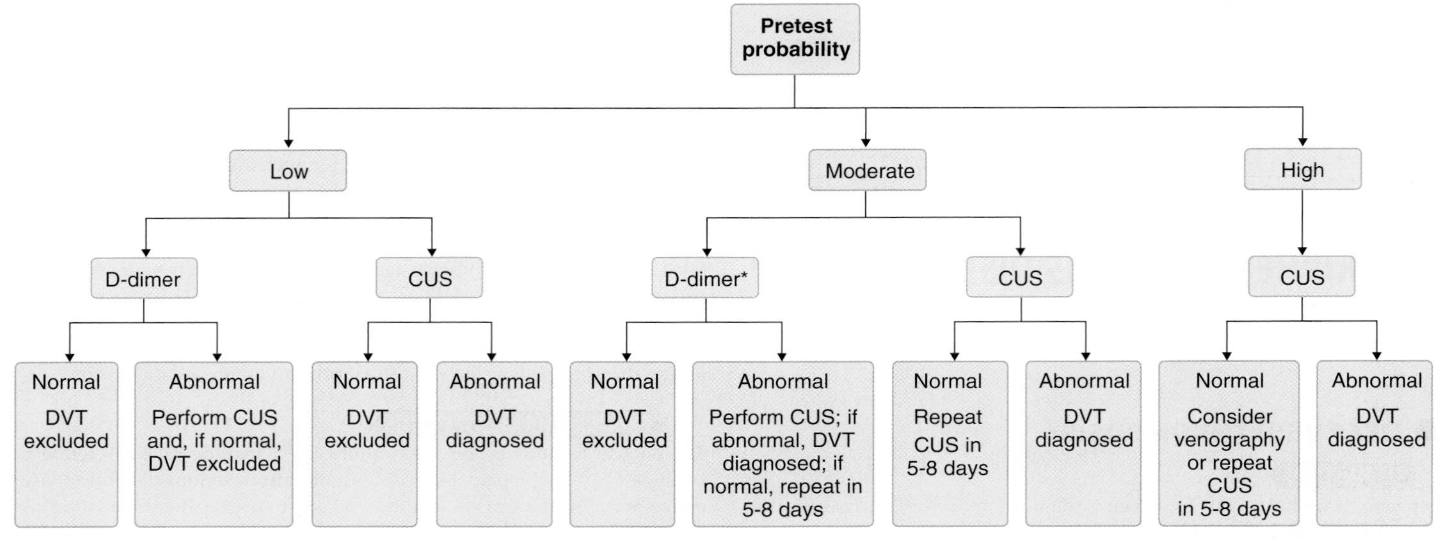

FIGURE 81-2. Diagnostic algorithm for suspected deep vein thrombosis. This algorithm uses evaluation of pretest probability based on a clinical prediction rule (see Table 81-1) and D-dimer testing to complement compression ultrasonography (CUS). The *asterisk* indicates use of a highly sensitive (>95%) D-dimer.

TABLE 81-1 PREDICTION RULE FOR DEEP VEIN THROMBOSIS

CLINICAL CHARACTERISTIC	SCORE*
Active cancer (treatment ongoing within previous 6 mo or palliative)	1
Paralysis, paresis, or recent plaster immobilization of the lower extremities	1
Recent bed rest of >3 days or major surgery within 3 mo requiring anesthesia	1
Localized tenderness of the deep veins of the leg	1
Entire leg swollen	1
Calf swelling of >3 cm larger than asymptomatic side measured 10 cm below tibial tuberosity	1
Pitting edema confined to the symptomatic leg	1
Collateral superficial veins (not varicosed)	1
Previously documented deep vein thrombosis	1
Alternative diagnosis as likely as or more likely than deep vein thrombosis	−2

*A score of 0 or less indicates low probability, 1 or 2 indicates moderate probability, and 3 or more indicates high probability.
Modified from Wells PS, Anderson DR, Bormanis J, et al. Value of assessment of pretest probability of deep-vein thrombosis in clinical management. *Lancet.* 1997;350:1795-1798.

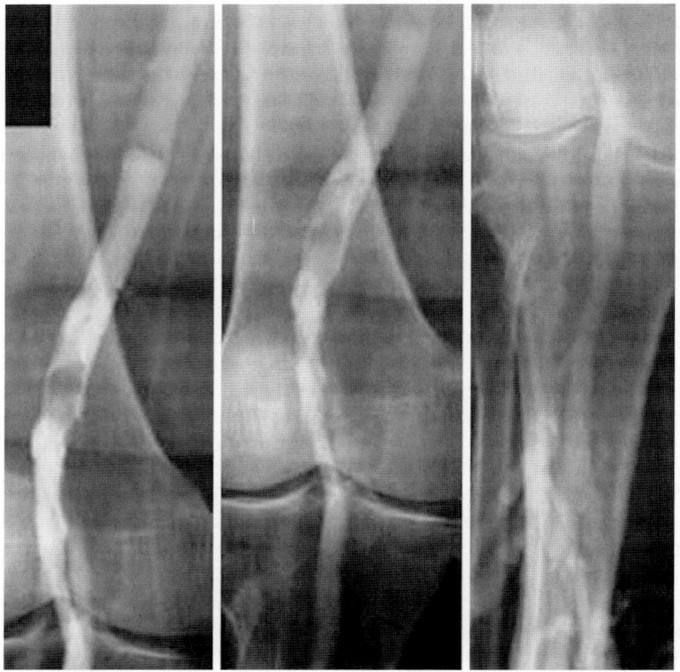

FIGURE 81-3. Abnormal venogram demonstrates a persistent (two or more different views) intraluminal filling defect in the popliteal vein.

Imaging

Contrast Venography

Ascending contrast venography remains the "gold standard" for diagnosis, but because of its expense, discomfort to the patient, and potential for adverse experiences, venography is currently indicated in symptomatic patients only when diagnostic uncertainty persists after noninvasive testing or if noninvasive testing is unavailable. A constant intraluminal filling defect is diagnostic of acute thrombosis (Fig. 81-3), and DVT can essentially be excluded in patients who have a normal, adequately performed venogram. Minor side effects of local pain, nausea, and vomiting are not uncommon, whereas more serious adverse reactions, such as bronchospasm, are rare; however, venography itself can also induce DVT.

Compression Ultrasonography

Compression venous ultrasonography is currently the most widely used noninvasive test for suspected DVT because of its accuracy in detection of thrombus involving the popliteal or more proximal veins; absence of compressibility (Fig. 81-4) of the proximal leg veins on ultrasonography has a sensitivity of 97% and a specificity of 96% for symptomatic patients with suspected DVT. Thus, the finding of a noncompressible venous segment, particularly in the popliteal or common femoral vein, has a high positive predictive value for DVT in symptomatic patients and is an indication for treatment. Of patients with symptoms suggestive of DVT but with normal findings on initial ultrasound examination of the proximal veins, about 15% will have undetected isolated calf DVT; progression into the proximal veins occurs in a minority of patients, usually within a week of presentation. Isolated calf DVT that does not extend into the proximal veins is rarely if ever associated with clinically important pulmonary embolus. The sensitivity of ultrasonography for calf DVT is well below 90%, with a wide range of accuracies reported for different populations of patients.

Imaging of the calf veins is time-consuming and potentially inaccurate. Rather, two-point (common femoral and popliteal) or three-point (two-point plus the calf "trifurcation") ultrasonography should be performed and, if the results are normal, repeated in 1 week after the initial examination. This approach will identify the 20 to 25% of patients who have had proximal

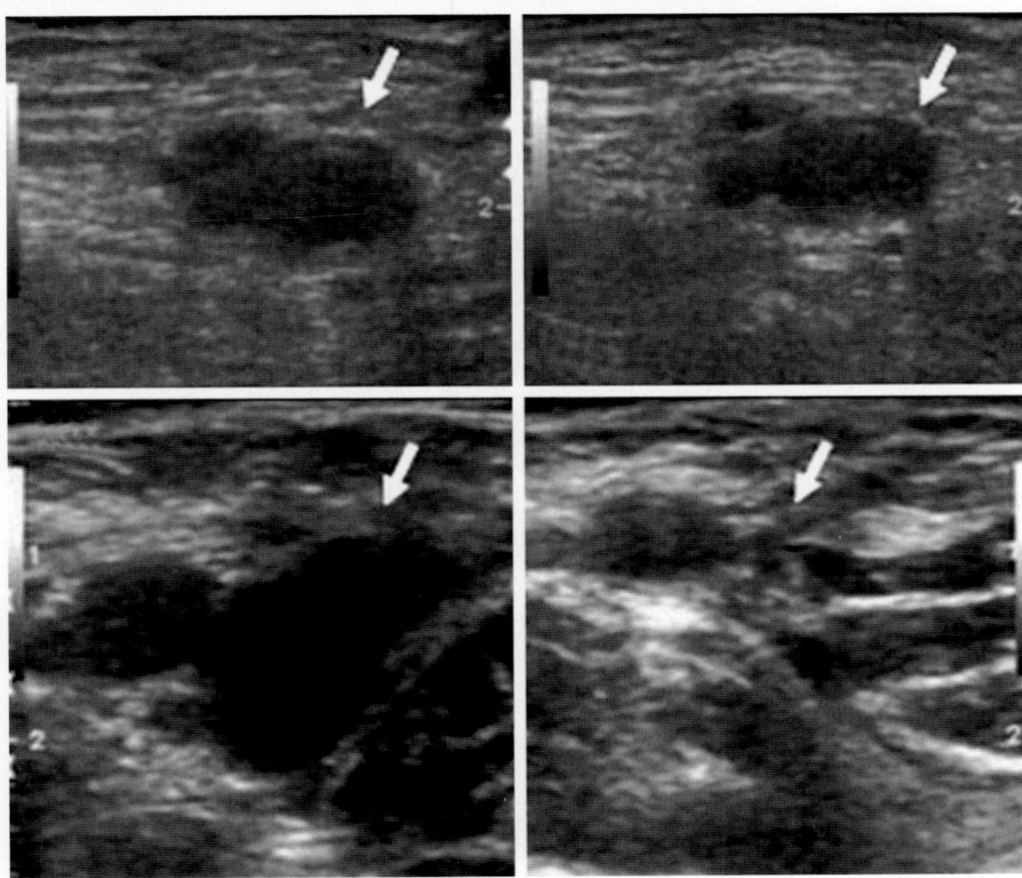

FIGURE 81-4. Compression venous ultrasonography demonstrates thrombosis of the popliteal vein. The sonograms in the *top row* demonstrate examination without *(left side)* and with *(right side)* gentle probe compression of the skin overlying the popliteal vein. The lack of compressibility is diagnostic of deep vein thrombosis. The *bottom row* shows analogous views of the femoral vein, which shows partial compressibility.

extension of distal clot in the calf veins. If the repeated ultrasound examination 1 week later also is normal, further investigation and therapy can be safely withheld. In centers with highly skilled operators, however, one normal ultrasound of the proximal and calf veins at presentation may be sufficiently accurate to exclude clinically important DVT and eliminate the need for follow-up testing, especially in patients with either a normal D-dimer test result or a low clinical pretest probability (see later).

Magnetic Resonance Venography

Magnetic resonance venography (MRV), which uses the difference in magnetic resonance signals between flowing blood and stationary clot, has a high sensitivity and specificity for proximal DVT. Recent interest has focused on magnetic resonance for direct imaging of the thrombus because a thrombus produces a positive image without the use of contrast material owing to its methemoglobin content. Although MRV is undoubtedly accurate in diagnosing and excluding DVT, it is expensive and not readily available in most centers outside of the United States.

Laboratory Findings

D-Dimer

D-dimer is a plasma protein specifically produced after lysis of cross-linked fibrin by plasmin. Levels are almost invariably elevated in the presence of acute VTE, so measurement of D-dimer levels is a sensitive test for recent DVT and pulmonary emboli. Unfortunately, numerous nonthrombotic conditions, including sepsis, pregnancy, surgery, and cardiac or renal failure, can also cause elevated levels. As a result of this nonspecificity, the role of D-dimer assays is limited to helping exclude VTE when levels are not raised.

Laboratory tests for D-dimer use enzyme-linked immunosorbent assay (ELISA) or agglutination techniques, both involving specific monoclonal antibodies. Sensitivity and cut points vary among assays, so results cannot be generalized. Highly sensitive tests, consisting of new rapid ELISA or immunoturbidimetric assays, have sensitivities of 95 to 100% for acute VTE but in general have low specificities (20 to 50%). Moderately sensitive tests, of which the SimpliRED red cell agglutination assay is the main example, have a reported sensitivity of approximately 90% but a higher specificity (~75%) for acute VTE. Serial two-point ultrasonography plus D-dimer is as good as whole-leg color-coded Doppler ultrasonography for diagnosing suspected symptomatic DVT. Highly sensitive D-dimer assays can be employed as "stand-alone tests" for exclusion of DVT, but clinicians must be aware of the accuracy of the assay in their institution before using the D-dimer assay to make management decisions. A point-of-care D-dimer test can help exclude DVT, which is rare in patients with less than four points using the following scale: male sex, use of hormonal contraceptives, active cancer in prior 6 months, surgery in prior month, absence of leg trauma, distention of collateral veins (1 point each); greater than 3-cm difference in calf circumference (2 points), and abnormal D-dimer assay (6 points).

D-dimer measured after a 3-month (or longer) initial treatment with warfarin also appears to be predictive of recurrent or persistent DVT. In addition, an elevated D-dimer level 1 month after stopping warfarin predicts a clinically and statistically significant higher recurrence rate than is seen in patients in whom the D-dimer levels were normal or low.

Algorithms for Diagnosis of Deep Venous Thrombosis

A number of diagnostic algorithms have been tested in prospective management trials (see Fig. 81-2).

Clinical Assessment and Venous Ultrasonography

It is safe to perform only a single ultrasound examination in patients with a low pretest probability by a validated clinical prediction rule (Table 81-2). Other patients require serial ultrasonographic testing if only clinical assessment and ultrasonography are used. Venography should be considered in patients with a high pretest probability and normal compression ultrasonography because the probability of DVT is still approximately 20% in such patients.

Clinical Assessment, D-Dimer Testing, and Venous Ultrasonography

Diagnostic imaging and treatment can be safely withheld in patients who have (1) a low pretest probability based on a validated clinical prediction rule and a negative value on a moderately sensitive D-dimer assay or (2) a low or intermediate pretest probability and a negative value on a highly sensitive D-dimer assay. Patients with a high pretest probability require ultrasonography regardless of the D-dimer result. A normal D-dimer result with use of either a moderately or highly sensitive assay can safely obviate the need for

TABLE 81-2 ALTERNATIVE DIAGNOSES IN 87 CONSECUTIVE PATIENTS WITH CLINICALLY SUSPECTED VENOUS THROMBOSIS AND NORMAL VENOGRAMS*

DIAGNOSIS	PATIENTS (%)
Muscle strain	24
Direct twisting injury to the leg	10
Leg swelling in paralyzed limb	9
Lymphangitis, lymphatic obstruction	7
Venous reflux	7
Muscle tear	6
Baker's cyst	5
Cellulitis	3
Internal abnormality of the knee	2
Unknown	26

*The diagnosis was made once venous thrombosis was excluded by venography.

repeated imaging in patients with normal findings on the initial ultrasound examination.

Differential Diagnosis

A number of conditions can mimic DVT (see Table 81-2), but DVT often can be excluded only by accurate diagnostic testing. In some patients, however, the cause of pain, tenderness, and swelling remains uncertain.

Suspected Recurrent Deep Venous Thrombosis

Approximately 10% of patients with unprovoked VTE will experience recurrent thromboembolism in the first year after ceasing anticoagulant therapy. In addition, many patients will have positional leg swelling and pain early during treatment as a result of venous outflow obstruction or later (≥6 months after diagnosis) because of the post-thrombotic syndrome when venous valvular incompetence is manifested. These and other nonthrombotic disorders can produce symptoms that are similar to acute recurrent DVT, so accurate diagnostic testing to confirm recurrence is mandatory. However, residual venous abnormalities are common after an initial event; persistent abnormalities are seen on compression ultrasonography in approximately 80% of patients at 3 months and 50% of patients at 1 year after a documented proximal DVT. Therefore, comparison with previous ultrasound images is required in patients with suspected recurrence. Although an increase in diameter of 4 mm or more in the compressed vein strongly suggests recurrent DVT, a new noncompressible proximal venous segment is the most reliable criterion for the diagnosis of recurrence. When compression ultrasonography is inconclusive, venography should be considered; a new intraluminal filling defect is diagnostic of acute DVT, and the absence of a filling defect excludes the diagnosis. Nonfilling of venous segments may mask recurrent DVT and is considered a nondiagnostic finding. A normal D-dimer test result is useful in excluding recurrent DVT.

Pregnancy

Symptoms of leg pain or swelling, shortness of breath, and atypical chest pain are common during pregnancy, so objective testing is needed to diagnose VTE. As in nonpregnant patients, compression ultrasonography is the initial test of choice. A normal D-dimer test is also reassuring in excluding DVT. Because isolated iliac and iliofemoral DVT is more common in pregnancy and has the potential to be missed by ultrasonography, venography should be considered when clinical suspicion is high even if the findings of the initial ultrasound examination are normal. MRV, which is sensitive for pelvic DVT, may be useful in this circumstance.

TABLE 81-3 GUIDELINES FOR ANTICOAGULATION WITH LOW-MOLECULAR-WEIGHT HEPARIN AND FONDAPARINUX

INDICATIONS	GUIDELINES
VTE suspected	Obtain baseline aPTT, PT, CBC Check for contraindication to heparin therapy Order imaging study; consider giving IV unfractionated heparin (5000 IU) or LMWH
VTE confirmed	Give LMWH (dalteparin,* enoxaparin,† nadroparin,‡ tinzaparin,§ fondaparinux‖) Start warfarin therapy on day 1 at 5 mg and adjust the subsequent daily dose according to INR Check platelet count between days 3 and 5 Stop LMWH therapy after at least 4 or 5 days of combined therapy when the INR is >2 Anticoagulate with warfarin for at least 3 months at an INR of 2.5, range of 2-3

*Dalteparin sodium, 200 anti-Xa IU/kg/day subcutaneously. A single dose should not exceed 18,000 IU (approved in Canada).
†Enoxaparin sodium, 1 mg/kg q12h subcutaneously, or enoxaparin sodium, 1.5 mg/kg/day subcutaneously. A single daily dose should not exceed 180 mg (approved in both the United States and Canada).
‡Nadroparin calcium, 86 anti-Xa IU/kg two times a day subcutaneously for 10 days (approved in Canada), or nadroparin calcium, 171 anti-Xa IU/kg subcutaneously daily. A single dose should not exceed 17,100 anti-Xa IU.
§Tinzaparin sodium, 175 anti-Xa IU kg/day subcutaneously daily (approved in Canada and the United States).
‖Fondaparinux subcutaneously according to weight: <50 kg, 5 mg once daily; 50-100 kg, 7.5 mg; and >100 kg, 10 mg.
aPTT = activated partial thromboplastin time; CBC = complete blood count; INR = international normalized ratio; LMWH = low-molecular-weight heparin; PT = prothrombin time; VTE = venous thromboembolism.
Modified from Hyers TM, Agnelli G, Hull RD, et al. Antithrombotic therapy for venous thromboembolic disease. *Chest*. 2001;119:176S-193S.

TREATMENT Rx

Anticoagulant therapy, which is the treatment of choice in most patients with VTE, reduces the extension and recurrence of symptomatic proximal and calf DVT and reduces mortality in patients with pulmonary emboli (Fig. 81-5). Coumarin derivatives (e.g., warfarin) are usually the drugs of choice for long-term anticoagulant therapy, but such drugs have a delayed onset of anticoagulant effect (Chapter 37). Therefore, initial short-term therapy with a rapid-acting heparin or heparin derivative for approximately 1 week is necessary to provide an immediate antithrombotic effect and to reduce the risk of thrombus growth or embolization in patients with acute DVT. Initial outpatient therapy with a low-molecular-weight heparin (LMWH) or fondaparinux is preferred to inpatient treatment with intravenous unfractionated heparin whenever feasible in patients with DVT. Rarely, medical therapy is unsuccessful or cannot be tolerated; such patients may require procedural therapy.

Initial Treatment

LMWH preparations, which are produced by either enzymatic or chemical depolymerization of unfractionated heparin, have lower mean molecular weights ranging from 4000 to 6000. The reduced molecular size provides a sufficient pentasaccharide moiety to antithrombin to inhibit factor Xa but reduces the ability of LMWH to inhibit thrombin in comparison with unfractionated heparin. Therefore, LMWH has an increased ratio of anti–factor Xa to anti–factor IIa (thrombin) inhibitory activity. The reduced size of LMWH also decreases charge-related nonspecific protein binding, thereby resulting in improved subcutaneous bioavailability, more predictable anticoagulant response, and predominantly dose-independent renal clearance. These qualities have made outpatient management of DVT with unmonitored, weight-based subcutaneous LMWH feasible and preferable.

LMWH products differ in their method of production, molecular weight, and anticoagulant effect. Few trials have directly compared different LMWH preparations for treatment of acute VTE, and definitive conclusions with regard to comparative efficacy and safety cannot be made. Dosage regimens differ for the various LMWH formulations (Table 81-3), but once-daily administration of LMWH is thought to be as safe and effective as twice-daily administration.

Because the antithrombotic response to weight-based dosing of LMWH is predictable, laboratory monitoring during LMWH treatment is usually unnecessary. There are, however, three populations of patients in whom anti–factor Xa monitoring should be considered: (1) patients with renal insufficiency (calculated creatinine clearance of less than 30 mL/minute); (2) obese patients, in whom the volume of distribution of LMWH might be different, so weight-adjusted dosing might not be appropriate; and (3) pregnant women, in whom it is unclear whether the dose should be adjusted according to the woman's weight change. Levels are usually determined on blood samples drawn 4 hours after subcutaneous injection; therapeutic ranges of 0.6 to 1.0 U/mL for twice-daily administration and 1.0 to 2.0 U/mL for once-daily treatment have been proposed.

Meta-analyses have documented that unmonitored, fixed-dose subcutaneous injection of LMWH is as effective and safe as adjusted-dose intravenous administration of unfractionated heparin for the treatment of acute DVT, with a trend toward a significant difference in mortality benefit favoring

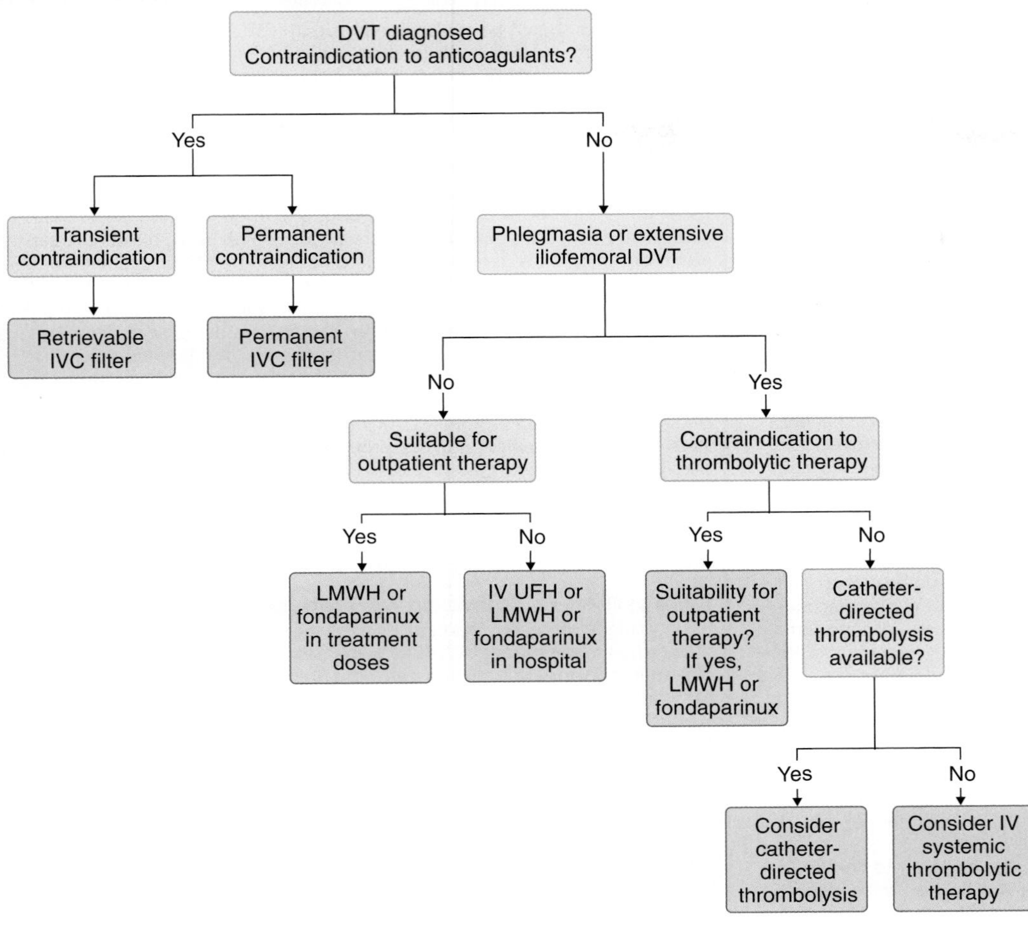

FIGURE 81-5. **Guidelines for treatment of deep vein thrombosis (DVT).** IVC = inferior vena cava; IV = intravenous; LMWH = low-molecular-weight heparin; UFH = unfractionated heparin.

LMWH, probably because of improved survival in patients with malignant disease.[2] However, patients with extensive iliofemoral DVT have often been excluded from trials of LMWH, and extended-duration (i.e., more than 5 days) intravenous unfractionated heparin therapy is often administered to such patients. Outpatient therapy with LMWH is as good as inpatient treatment, thereby making LMWH more cost-effective than intravenous unfractionated heparin in most health care settings.

Fondaparinux

Fondaparinux is a synthetic analogue of the critical pentasaccharide sequence required for binding of heparin molecules to antithrombin (Chapter 37). Chemically engineered, it has minor modifications from the natural pentasaccharide moiety, thereby improving stability and resulting in enhanced binding to antithrombin. Given subcutaneously, fondaparinux demonstrates 100% bioavailability, with peak plasma concentrations occurring 1.7 hours after dosing. Once-daily subcutaneous administration of fondaparinux (5.0 mg daily if weight is less than 50 kg; 7.5 mg daily if weight is 50 to 100 kg; 10 mg daily if weight is more than 100 kg) is an effective and safe alternative to LMWH for the initial 5 to 10 days of treatment of DVT.[3] Clearance is predominantly renal, with approximately 70% of the initial dose recovered in the urine in an unchanged form. Patients with reduced creatinine clearance, such as elderly patients, have higher peak drug levels and longer drug half-life, so their dose may need to be adjusted downward.

Unfractionated Heparin

Unfractionated heparin is a sulfated glycosaminoglycan that exerts its anticoagulant effect predominantly by binding to antithrombin and inducing a conformational change that accelerates the rate at which antithrombin inhibits coagulation enzymes (Chapter 37). It consists of a heterogeneous group of molecules ranging in molecular weight from 3000 to 30,000, and only one third of unfractionated heparin molecules contain the unique pentasaccharide sequence required for binding to antithrombin. This molecular heterogeneity, along with variable charge-related nonspecific binding of unfractionated heparin to other plasma proteins such as von Willebrand factor and platelet factor 4, contributes to the large variability in the anticoagulant response in individual patients.

Unfractionated heparin is usually administered by continuous intravenous infusion, a route that has been shown to be effective in reducing recurrence and extension of thrombus. The use of validated nomograms (Table 81-4), with either fixed initial dosing or dosing according to a patient's weight, results in more rapid achievement of therapeutic activated partial thromboplastin time (aPTT) levels and improves outcome, although adjustment according to the sensitivity of local aPTT methods is required. The initial aPTT level should be measured 6 hours after therapy is commenced. Up to 25% of patients with acute VTE have resistance to heparin, defined as a requirement for greater than expected doses of unfractionated heparin to achieve a "therapeutic" aPTT. If it is available, anti–factor Xa monitoring is recommended in patients with heparin resistance. Larger doses (front-loaded and weight-adjusted follow-up doses) of subcutaneous, 12-hourly unfractionated heparin are as safe and efficacious as LMWH without requiring monitoring of the aPTT. However, this regimen has not been widely embraced by clinicians because of a bias toward monitoring unfractionated heparin with frequent aPTT adjustments.

TABLE 81-4 WEIGHT-BASED NOMOGRAM FOR INITIAL INTRAVENOUS HEPARIN THERAPY

aPTT	DOSE (IU/kg)
Initial dose	80 bolus, then 18/h
<35 sec (<1.2×)*	80 bolus, then 4/h
35-45 sec (1.2-1.5×)	40 bolus, then 2/h
46-70 sec (1.5-2.3×)	No change
71-90 sec (2.3-3×)	Decrease infusion rate by 2/h
>90 sec (>3×)	Hold infusion 1 h, then decrease infusion rate by 3/h

*Figures in parentheses show comparison with control.
aPTT = activated partial thromboplastin time. In general, with contemporary aPTT reagents, the target therapeutic range is more than 1.2 to 2.3 times control.
Modified from Raschke RA, Reilly BM, Guidry JR, et al. The weight-based heparin dosing nomogram compared with a "standard care" nomogram: a randomized controlled trial. *Ann Intern Med.* 1993;119:874-881.

Transition to Oral Treatment

Coumarin Derivatives (Warfarin)

Warfarin is a vitamin K antagonist that inhibits the production of clotting factors II (prothrombin), VII, IX, and X as well as the naturally occurring anticoagulants protein C and protein S. In patients with DVT, the drug should be started within 24 to 48 hours of initiation of heparin with a goal of achieving international normalized ratio (INR) results between 2.0 and 3.0 (Chapter 37). A higher target INR of 3.0 to 4.0 is associated with more bleeding but no better efficacy, even in patients with the antiphospholipid antibody syndrome (Chapter 179),4 and lower intensity warfarin therapy (target INR, 1.5 to 1.9) is significantly less effective at preventing recurrent VTE despite similar rates of major bleeding.5

The dose is empirical, but a starting dose of 5 to 10 mg is suitable for most patients. Warfarin doses are adjusted according to the prothrombin time, expressed as the INR, performed daily or every other day until the results are in the therapeutic range for at least 24 hours. After initial dosing, warfarin can be monitored two or three times per week for 1 to 2 weeks and then less frequently, depending on the stability of INR results, up to intervals as long as 4 to 6 weeks. If dose adjustment is needed, such as when medications that can interact with warfarin are introduced, the cycle of more frequent monitoring is repeated until a stable dose response is again achieved.

It is now clear that pharmacogenetics have a large impact on the relatively wide range of warfarin dose requirements among different populations as well as the variability of warfarin requirements over time in any individual patient. Polymorphisms in the gene encoding cytochrome P-450 2C9 enzyme, the enzyme that primarily clears the S-enantiomer of warfarin, contribute to variable responses to warfarin; some genetic variants result in an increased sensitivity to warfarin and a lower required dose of warfarin. Vitamin K epoxide reductase (VKORC1) recycles vitamin K epoxide to the reduced form of vitamin K and is the target of warfarin. Its common genetic variants result in altered sensitivity to warfarin, and *VKORC1* polymorphisms are associated with a need for lower doses of warfarin during long-term therapy. Routine pharmacogenetic testing may ultimately be recommended in candidates for long-term (>3 months) warfarin therapy to identify individuals who are likely to require higher or lower warfarin doses.

Side Effects of Anticoagulants

Bleeding is the most common side effect of anticoagulant therapy. Major bleeding (e.g., intracranial [Chapter 415], gastrointestinal [Chapter 137], or retroperitoneal) leading to hospitalization or transfusion or death occurs in approximately 2% of patients treated with intravenous unfractionated heparin for acute VTE. Factors such as recent surgery, trauma, and concurrent aspirin or thrombolytic therapy increase the risk of bleeding.

The risk of major bleeding with warfarin in doses adjusted to achieve a target INR of 2.0 to 3.0 ranges from 1 to 3% per year and appears to be highest soon after treatment is started or if anticoagulation is difficult to control. The risk of major bleeding increases according to individual characteristics, such as older age, the presence of comorbid conditions (e.g., diabetes, hypertension, renal insufficiency, previous gastrointestinal bleeding, or cancer), and the use of concomitant drugs, in particular antiplatelet therapy.

Heparin-induced thrombocytopenia, which is a relatively common nonhemorrhagic complication of therapy with unfractionated heparin and a very uncommon complication of LMWH, is manifested typically with thrombocytopenia and new thrombosis (Chapter 37). Monitoring of the platelet count is recommended every other day until day 14 in patients receiving therapeutic unfractionated heparin but is not routinely recommended with LMWH or fondaparinux because of the extremely low risk with these newer medications.

Long-Term Treatment

The preferred long-term treatment of DVT for most patients is warfarin or another coumarin derivative (e.g., acenocoumarol), continued until the benefits of treatment for reducing recurrent VTE no longer outweigh its risks of major bleeding. The decision to prolong or to stop anticoagulation should be individualized, and a patient's preferences should be considered.

Patients with symptomatic proximal DVT or pulmonary emboli should be treated for at least 3 months, even if the VTE was associated with a transient risk factor,6 but the optimal duration of treatment for patients whose VTE is not associated with a transient risk factor is controversial. Three months of treatment is associated with a 10 to 27% risk of a recurrence during the 12 months after anticoagulant therapy is stopped, whereas 6 months of anticoagulant therapy reduces the risk of recurrence in the first year after stopping to about 10%. In patients whose VTE developed in association with minor risk factors (e.g., air travel, pregnancy, within 6 weeks of estrogen therapy, after leg injury or immobilization), the risk of recurrence is probably lower than 10%. Continuation of treatment beyond 6 months reduces the risk of recurrent VTE during the course of therapy, but the benefit is lost after warfarin is discontinued.

The most convincing association of thrombophilia with the risk of recurrent VTE is the antiphospholipid antibody (lupus anticoagulant or anticardiolipin antibody; Chapter 179), which is associated with a two-fold increase in the risk of recurrence. Homozygous factor V Leiden, elevated levels of homocysteine, and deficiencies of antithrombin, protein C, and protein S also have been associated with an increased risk of recurrence in some reports, but other data suggest that testing for heritable thrombophilia does not predict recurrent VTE in the first 2 years after anticoagulant therapy is stopped. In the absence of randomized trials to assess different durations of anticoagulation in patients with VTE and thrombophilia, routine testing for thrombophilias need not be performed but should be considered in young (<50 years) patients, patients with venous thrombosis in unusual sites, and patients with a strong family history of VTE (i.e., one or more first-degree relatives with a history of VTE).

The decision to extend anticoagulant therapy beyond 3 months must balance the risk of recurrent VTE with the risk of bleeding. The annual risk of major bleeding when warfarin is adjusted to achieve a target INR of 2.0 to 3.0 is 1 to 3%, with a case-fatality rate of 10% when major bleeding occurs in patients who received treatment for more than 3 months. By comparison, the case-fatality rate for recurrent VTE is about 5%. In patients whose VTE was associated with a transient risk factor or who are at high risk of bleeding, treatment for 3 months is generally adequate because the risk of fatal recurrent VTE is lower than the risk of fatal bleeding if warfarin treatment is prolonged. Among patients without a reversible or transient cause, however, prolonged warfarin therapy for more than 6 months can be considered because the risk of fatal hemorrhage is counterbalanced by the risk of fatal recurrence. The argument to prolong therapy is stronger in patients with high-risk thrombophilia (e.g., homozygous factor V Leiden; antiphospholipid antibody; deficiency of antithrombin, protein C, or protein S; or combined heterozygous state for factor V Leiden and the prothrombin gene mutation). Indefinite therapy (preferably with LMWH) should be considered in patients with cancer-related VTE (Chapter 187) if the risk of bleeding is not high because the risk of recurrent VTE is more than 10% in the first year after anticoagulation is stopped. In motivated and capable patients, self-management of warfarin therapy is better than management by a physician or nurse.7

Alternatives to Coumarin Derivatives

For patients in whom warfarin is impractical or contraindicated and for those who have recurrent VTE while being treated with appropriate doses of oral anticoagulants, therapeutic doses of LMWH are as effective as warfarin. For patients with cancer-related VTE (DVT, pulmonary embolus, or both), weight-based LMWH that is decreased to 75% of the initial dose after 1 month of treatment reduces the risk of recurrent VTE compared with warfarin, with similar bleeding rates.8

Therapeutic strategies to manage patients in whom symptomatic VTE recurs while they are receiving conventional-intensity warfarin include unfractionated heparin, LMWH, higher-intensity warfarin (e.g., INR range of 3.0 to 4.0), and insertion of a vena caval filter. However, the optimal management of such patients is unknown because no randomized studies have been performed.

Thrombolytic Therapy

Although thrombolytic therapy results in increased rates of early patency of leg veins after DVT, it has not been conclusively shown to decrease the subsequent rate of post-thrombotic syndrome or pulmonary emboli. Except for patients who have life-threatening limb ischemia due to massive thrombosis, thrombolysis is not recommended in patients with DVT. An ongoing trial of catheter-directed thrombolysis versus "standard therapy" should provide the definitive evidence about the relative efficacy of catheter-directed thrombolysis for the prevention of post-thrombotic syndrome.

Vena Caval Filters

In a randomized trial of 400 patients with DVT, the incidence of pulmonary emboli at day 12 was lower in patients who received an inferior vena caval filter plus therapeutic anticoagulation than in those who received anticoagulation alone. However, filters did not reduce early or late mortality and are not recommended in patients who can receive therapeutic anticoagulation because this benefit did not persist at 2 years and was offset by an almost doubling of the risk of recurrent DVT. Inferior vena caval filters should be used in patients who have contraindications to anticoagulant therapy or develop major bleeding while receiving it as well as in patients who develop recurrent VTE while receiving appropriate anticoagulation. Retrievable or removable inferior vena caval filters can be retrieved and removed within 14 days to several weeks after insertion or can be left in permanently. These filters are ideal for a patient who has a reversible cause of or the potential for major bleeding (e.g., DVT after craniotomy, DVT late in pregnancy).

Oral Direct Thrombin and Factor Xa Inhibitors

Ximelagatran is an oral direct thrombin inhibitor that does not require anticoagulant monitoring. When it is used for the acute and long-term treatment of patients with acute VTE, ximelagatran is as effective and safe as unfractionated heparin or LMWH followed by warfarin in preventing recurrent VTE. However, elevation in liver enzymes, especially the alanine aminotransferases, has been reported in 5 to 10% of patients with long-term use. Although the clinical implications of these elevated levels, which may decrease to normal with continued treatment, are unclear, the drug has been removed from the market by the manufacturers.

Rivaroxaban, an oral factor Xa inhibitor, is effective at 15 mg twice daily for 3 weeks then 20 mg daily for up to 12 months, but it also is associated with elevated aminotransferase levels. These and other thrombin inhibitors are under development for acute and chronic treatment of VTE. Although none has yet been approved for use in North America for the treatment of DVT and pulmonary embolism, some have already been approved for other indications.

PREVENTION

In one large randomized trial, rosuvastatin reduced the rate of DVT by 55%.[9] It is unknown at present whether this benefit can be achieved with other statins. Despite the plethora of large randomized trials demonstrating the efficacy and safety of mechanical and pharmacologic measures in reducing the risk of VTE in a wide range of hospitalized populations of patients, prophylaxis remains grossly underused. Factors that increase the risk of DVT include surgery (particularly major hip and knee surgery, as well as neurosurgery; Chapters 439 and 441), major trauma (Chapter 112), prolonged bed rest or immobilization, previous episodes of VTE, presence of malignant disease, paralysis, morbid obesity, and increasing age.

Comprehensive consensus guidelines have been developed for the prevention of VTE in different populations of patients (see Table 37-2 in Chapter 37). In general, mechanical prophylaxis (antiembolic stockings and intermittent pneumatic compression) should be used as an adjunct to pharmacologic prophylaxis or in patients with a high risk of bleeding. For general medical patients admitted to the hospital with a major illness and in whom mobility is likely to be reduced for 72 hours or longer, low-dose unfractionated heparin or LMWH (see Table 37-2 in Chapter 37) should be considered. In patients who undergo major hip or knee surgery, warfarin (to an INR of 2.0 to 3.0), subcutaneous LMWH, subcutaneous fondaparinux (2.5 mg once daily), or oral rivaroxaban (10 mg once daily) should be used for at least 7 to 14 days postoperatively. In patients with continued immobility, prophylaxis should be considered until the patient regains preoperative mobility.

Management of Deep Vein Thrombosis in Pregnancy

The management of pregnant women with DVT (Chapter 247) is problematic because all coumarin derivatives cross the placenta and have the potential to cause warfarin embryopathy, consisting of nasal hypoplasia and epiphyseal stippling, if the newborn is exposed to warfarin between 6 and 12 weeks of gestation. Consequently, parenteral unfractionated heparin and LMWH, which do not cross the placenta and are safe for the fetus, are the agents of choice. The easiest approach is to initiate therapy with weight-adjusted "treatment" doses of LMWH (see Table 81-3), continued for the duration of the pregnancy. Although it is not proved, it is likely that the dose of LMWH can be safely decreased to approximately 80% of the therapeutic dose after 3 months of therapy. As pregnancy progresses, women normally gain weight and generally require higher doses of LMWH to achieve an anti–factor Xa level similar to that achieved at the time of diagnosis. The adequacy of the dose can be assessed by measuring a 4-hour postinjection anti–factor Xa level and targeting the dose to achieve a level of 0.5 to 1.0 U/mL for twice-daily LMWH and 0.8 to 1.5 U/mL for once-daily LMWH. Alternatively, the dose of LMWH can simply be adjusted periodically on the basis of the woman's weight.

Unfractionated heparin is less attractive than LMWH because it is associated with a greater reduction of bone density and a higher risk of heparin-induced thrombocytopenia. Unfractionated heparin can be initiated either by continuous intravenous infusion in doses adjusted to maintain an aPTT in the therapeutic range, followed by 12-hourly subcutaneous injections, or simply with 12-hourly subcutaneous injections throughout the course of pregnancy. The dose should be adjusted to target a mid-interval (6-hour postinjection) aPTT in the therapeutic range.

Pregnant women with a DVT should probably be treated for the duration of pregnancy and for at least 6 weeks postpartum. If the DVT occurred early in pregnancy, elective induction of delivery at about 37 weeks with discontinuation of the heparin 24 hours earlier is recommended. If the DVT occurs in the latter part of the third trimester, intravenous heparin should be administered by continuous infusion until approximately 6 hours before the expected time of delivery. Intravenous unfractionated heparin or subcutaneous LMWH should be started postpartum as soon as hemostasis has been achieved. Maternal warfarin therapy is safe for the breast-fed infant because warfarin and its metabolites are not secreted into breast milk in doses sufficient to cause an anticoagulant effect. Consequently, warfarin (with bridging LMWH or unfractionated heparin until the INR is 2.0 or higher) can be used after delivery.

Venous Thrombosis of the Upper Extremities

DVT of the upper extremities (including the arm and the axillary, subclavian, and internal jugular veins as well as the superior vena cava) is much less common than DVT of the legs, but it is not rare. Factors associated with upper extremity DVT include central venous catheters, acquired or hereditary thrombophilias, and anatomic (cervical rib) and physiologic (muscular individuals) impingement of the vein. The incidence of clinically important post-thrombotic syndrome is not high if patients are treated with anticoagulants alone.

Contrast venography is the gold standard for the diagnosis of upper extremity DVT, but venous ultrasonography is accurate and less invasive. Because it is not feasible to test for compression of the subclavian vein, a diagnosis of subclavian DVT by ultrasonography is based on flow abnormalities or direct visualization of thrombus by B-mode ultrasonography. Upper extremity DVT can cause pulmonary emboli, although the exact frequency is not known.

Considerable controversy exists about the management of patients in whom DVT develops in association with a central venous catheter. If the line is not necessary or is nonfunctional, some recommend simply removing the line without subsequent anticoagulant therapy, whereas others treat with full-dose anticoagulants (a heparin-related compound, followed by 1 to 3 months of warfarin). If the line is functional and must stay in place (e.g., no alternative venous access), full-dose anticoagulants should be given. Otherwise, anticoagulant therapy should be given in all patients with upper extremity DVT, with medications, doses, regimens, and durations identical to those for treatment of DVT of the leg.

SUPERFICIAL THROMBOPHLEBITIS

Superficial thrombophlebitis usually presents with pain, swelling, redness, and tenderness of superficial veins. Varicose veins (Fig. 81-6) can be red, warm, and clustered in a circumscribed area. When superficial thrombophlebitis occurs in the short or long saphenous veins, there is usually redness, tenderness, and often linear induration that follow the course of the involved vein (medial calf or thigh). Superficial thrombophlebitis can also occur at the insertion site of an intravenous catheter. Invariably, superficial thrombophlebitis is associated with thrombosis of the corresponding vein, and particularly when the long saphenous vein is involved, venous ultrasonography should be performed to exclude extension into the deep veins, which occurs in up to 19% of patients.

Nonsteroidal anti-inflammatory drugs and either moderate or full doses of LMWH are each about 70% better than placebo for treating superficial thrombophlebitis.[10] LMWH relieves symptoms more quickly and prevents growth of thrombus more effectively than do nonsteroidal anti-inflammatory drugs. Fondaparinux, 2.5 mg daily for 45 days, reduces the risk of DVT or pulmonary embolism from about 1.3% to 0.2% without adverse effects.[11] Thus, it is reasonable to use moderate doses of LMWH or fondaparinux for the initial treatment of acute, symptomatic superficial thrombophlebitis, particularly for patients with severe symptoms, proximal

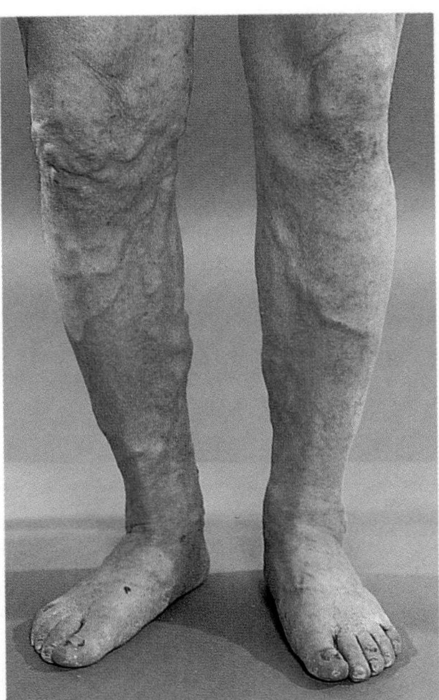

FIGURE 81-6. **Varicose veins are a risk factor for deep vein thrombosis and may result from it.** (From Forbes CD, Jackson WF. *Color Atlas and Text of Clinical Medicine*, 3rd ed. London: Mosby; 2003.)

saphenous vein thrombosis, recurrent disease, or evidence of thrombophilia. Alternatively, and particularly for intravenous catheter-induced superficial thrombophlebitis, a nonsteroidal anti-inflammatory drug can be tried.

POST-THROMBOTIC SYNDROME

The initial pain and swelling in many patients with DVT are due to the venous obstruction or the inflammatory process mediated by the acute thrombus. Once anticoagulant therapy is initiated, the acute obstruction usually resolves during a period of several months as recanalization occurs and collateral venous channels develop, thereby leading to initial improvement in pain and swelling. However, in the long term, probably because of venous valvular incompetence produced when the thrombosed venous segments recanalize and sometimes because of residual chronic obstruction, venous hypertension and sometimes pain and swelling can recur.

This post-thrombotic syndrome develops in up to 50% of patients with proximal DVT, usually within the first 1 to 2 years after DVT. The syndrome is often a chronic, progressive disease with pain, swelling, and occasionally ulceration of the leg in patients with previous DVT.

PREVENTION AND TREATMENT

The use of below-knee graduated compression stockings for 2 years after acute DVT reduces the risk of the post-thrombotic syndrome by about 50%.[12] Some experts recommend routine stocking therapy in all patients with DVT. Others recommend waiting until the acute inflammatory process and acute outflow obstruction have subsided (usually up to 6 months) and then prescribing stockings if the patient's symptoms persist at that time. The use of graduated compression stockings does not significantly reduce DVT after stroke, however, and results in adverse skin events.[13]

However, stockings are hot in the summer, relatively expensive, difficult for many patients to put on in the morning, and cosmetically unappealing to many patients. In addition, simple lifestyle alteration (such as frequent leg elevation, avoidance of prolonged standing or sitting, and occasional use of analgesics) suffices in relieving symptoms in many patients. If symptoms are severe, it is usually because of extensive thrombus causing massive edema. In such patients, a lightweight stocking (such as support hose) can be helpful until the edema improves. If symptoms persist or worsen despite these measures, or if ulceration seems imminent (as evidenced by severe skin changes), a full-strength stocking (30 to 40 mm Hg of pressure at the ankle) can be prescribed. However, if symptoms subside and the patient remains asymptomatic or has only trivial persistent signs or symptoms with little or no effect on quality of life, stockings can be avoided, and the patient can be observed for clinically important signs and symptoms of the post-thrombotic syndrome.

VENOUS ULCERS

Venous ulcers, which are the most severe complication of post-thrombotic syndrome, typically occur in the perimalleolar area of the leg. The best management is prevention by application of graduated compression stockings either at the time of diagnosis of DVT or, at the latest, when skin changes develop in association with leg swelling. When an ulcer occurs, treatment with an emollient and regular wrapping should be commenced. Once the ulcer heals, the patient should be prescribed graduated compression stockings and watched for recurrent ulceration. Surgical closure or removal of the incompetent saphenous veins plus dressing management in patients with chronic venous ulceration does not reduce healing time of the acute ulcer compared with dressing management alone but significantly reduces the rate of recurrent ulceration for at least the next 4 years.[14]

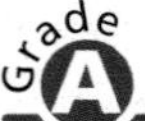

1. Bernardi E, Camporese G, Büller HR, et al. Serial 2-point ultrasonography plus D-dimer vs whole-leg color-coded Doppler ultrasonography for diagnosing suspected symptomatic deep vein thrombosis: a randomized controlled trial. *JAMA.* 2008;300:1653-1659.
2. Hull RD, Pineo GF, Brant RF, et al. Long-term low-molecular-weight heparin versus usual care in proximal-vein thrombosis patients with cancer. *Am J Med.* 2006;119:1062-1072.
3. Buller HR, Davidson BL, Decousus H, et al. Fondaparinux or enoxaparin for the initial treatment of symptomatic deep venous thrombosis: a randomized trial. *Ann Intern Med.* 2004;140:867-873.
4. Crowther MA, Ginsberg JS, Julian J, et al. A comparison of two intensities of warfarin for the prevention of recurrent thrombosis in patients with the antiphospholipid antibody syndrome. *N Engl J Med.* 2003;349:1133-1138.
5. Kearon C, Ginsberg JS, Kovacs MJ, et al. Comparison of low-intensity warfarin therapy with conventional-intensity warfarin therapy for long-term prevention of recurrent venous thromboembolism. *N Engl J Med.* 2003;349:631-639.
6. Kearon C, Ginsberg JS, Anderson DR, et al. Comparison of 1 month of anticoagulation with 3 months of anticoagulation for a first episode of venous thromboembolism provoked by a transient risk factor. *J Thromb Haemost.* 2003;2:743-749.
7. Bloomfield HE, Krause A, Greer N, et al. Meta-analysis: effect of patient self-testing and self-management of long-term anticoagulation on major clinical outcomes. *Ann Intern Med.* 2011;154:472-482.
8. Lee AY, Levine MN, Baker RI, et al. Randomized comparison of low-molecular-weight heparin versus oral anticoagulant therapy for the prevention of recurrent venous thromboembolism in patients with cancer. *N Engl J Med.* 2003;349:109-111.
9. Glynn RJ, Danielson E, Fonseca FA, et al. A randomized trial of rosuvastatin in the prevention of venous thromboembolism. *N Engl J Med.* 2009; 360:1851-1861.
10. Di Nisio N, Wichers IM, Middeldorp S. Treatment for superficial thrombophlebitis of the leg (Review). *Cochrane Database Syst Rev.* 2007;2:CD004982.
11. Decousus H, Prandoni P, Mismetti P, et al, for the CALISTO Study Group. Fondaparinux in the treatment of lower-limb superficial-vein thrombosis. *N Engl J Med.* 2010;363:1222-1232.
12. Prandoni P, Lensing AW, Prins MH, et al. Below-knee elastic compression stockings to prevent the post-thrombotic syndrome: a randomized, controlled trial. *Ann Intern Med.* 2004;141:249-256.
13. Dennis M, Sandercock PA, Reid J, et al, for the CLOTS Trials Collaboration. Effectiveness of thigh-length graduated compression stockings to reduce the risk of deep vein thrombosis after stroke (CLOTS trial 1): a multicentre, randomised controlled trial. *Lancet.* 2009;373:1958-1965.
14. Gohel MS, Barwell JR, Taylor M, et al. Long term results of compression therapy alone versus compression plus surgery in chronic venous ulceration (ESCHAR): randomised controlled trial. *BMJ.* 2007;335:55-56.

SUGGESTED READINGS

Decousus H, Quéré I, Presles E, et al. Superficial venous thrombosis and venous thromboembolism: a large, prospective epidemiologic study. *Ann Intern Med.* 2010;152:218-224. *About 25% of patients who have superficial venous thrombosis have concurrent deep venous thrombosis at the time of presentation, and about 3% of the others will subsequently develop deep venous thrombosis or pulmonary embolism in the next 3 months.*

Goldhaber SZ, Piazza G. Optimal duration of anticoagulation after venous thromboembolism. *Circulation.* 2011;123:664-667. *Review.*

Kucher N. Clinical practice. Deep-vein thrombosis of the upper extremities. *N Engl J Med.* 2011;364:861-869. *Case-based review.*

Watson HG, Baglin TP. Guidelines on travel-related venous thrombosis. *Br J Haematol.* 2011;152:31-34. *Review.*

82

CARDIAC TRANSPLANTATION

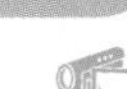

MARIELL JESSUP

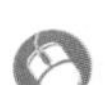

Cardiac transplantation is the treatment of choice for suitable patients with refractory heart failure (Chapters 59, 60, and 107). The number of heart transplantation procedures worldwide reached a peak of about 4500 in 1994 but has subsequently declined because the rate of identification of potential donors has not kept pace with the increased number of patients on waiting lists, where the annual mortality is 10 to 20% (Fig. 82-1). Because newer therapeutic options have usually failed and they now lack other alternatives, patients referred for heart transplantation are becoming progressively older and more ill, with increasing medical comorbidities, which have significantly increased the risk of cardiac transplantation. In many institutions, at least one third of patients are sustained on a ventricular assist device while awaiting transplantation. At the same time, the selection criteria for donors have been broadened to increase the number of organs available. As a result, sicker recipients are now receiving less ideal organs than in the past.

POPULATION OF PATIENTS

Evaluation of the Potential Recipient

The purposes of heart transplantation are to prolong life and to improve quality of life, so the referring physician must understand the potential benefits of transplantation as well as comorbidities that may portend an unsatisfactory outcome. Suitable patients for consideration have cardiogenic shock requiring mechanical support or high-dose inotropic or pressor drugs (Chapter 107); stage D heart failure symptoms despite maximal therapy (Chapter 59); recurrent life-threatening arrhythmias despite maximal interventions, including implanted defibrillators (Chapters 63 and 65); or, rarely, refractory angina without the potential for revascularization (Chapter 71) (Table 82-1). The most potent predictor of outcome in ambulatory patients with heart failure is a symptom-limited metabolic stress test to calculate peak oxygen consumption; a peak of less than 12 mL/kg/minute indicates a lower survival with medical therapy than after transplantation.

An extensive medical and psychosocial evaluation must be performed to exclude contraindications to transplantation. In the setting of fixed

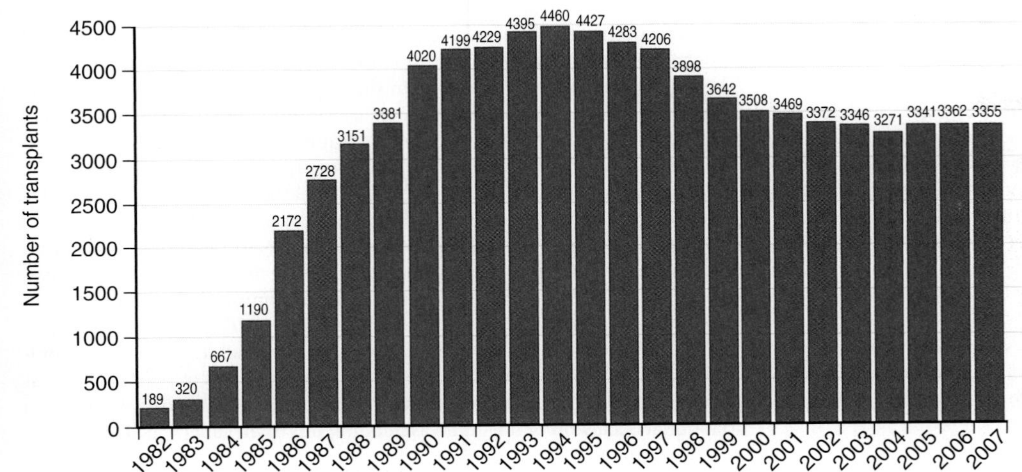

FIGURE 82-1. The number of heart transplantation procedures by year. (Data from the Registry of the International Society for Heart and Lung Transplantation. Reproduced with permission.)

TABLE 82-1 EVALUATION OF THE POTENTIAL HEART TRANSPLANT RECIPIENT

INDICATIONS FOR HEART TRANSPLANTATION

Cardiogenic shock requiring mechanical support or high-dose inotropic drugs
Stage D heart failure symptoms despite maximal therapy
Recurrent life-threatening arrhythmias despite maximal interventions and implanted defibrillator
Refractory angina without potential for revascularization

CONTRAINDICATIONS TO HEART TRANSPLANTATION

	ALTERNATIVE TREATMENT	OPTIONS
Age > 70 yr	Consider permanent mechanical support	End-of-life considerations or investigational therapy
Active or recent malignant disease	End-of-life considerations or investigational therapy	
Diabetes with severe end-organ damage	Consider permanent mechanical support	End-of-life considerations or investigational therapy
FEV/FVC < 40%	Consider heart-lung transplantation	End-of-life considerations or investigational therapy
BMI < 20 or BMI > 35	Nutritional modification; BMI > 35, consider permanent mechanical support or weight loss	
Irreversible pulmonary hypertension (≥4 Wood units)	Consider heart-lung transplantation	End-of-life considerations or investigational therapy
Other comorbidities: cirrhosis, vascular disease, addictions, hepatitis C, human immunodeficiency virus infection, social or psychiatric disorders	Individual transplantation team decisions	

BMI = body mass index; FEV = forced expiratory volume; FVC = forced vital capacity.

pulmonary hypertension, such patients are occasionally considered for combined heart-lung transplantation.

An immunologic evaluation includes determination of ABO blood type, antibody screen, panel-reactive antibody level, and human leukocyte antigen (HLA) typing. Using virtual crossmatch methods, flow cytometry–based single-antigen bead assays can identify prospective donors with undesirable antigens without the need for a prospective crossmatch, thereby allowing for matches outside the recipient's geographic area.

Management of the Patient Waiting for Cardiac Transplantation

A patient's priority status according to the United Network for Organ Sharing is based on the recipient's acuity status, blood type, body size, and duration of time at a particular status level. Patients who can be managed successfully outside the hospital are the lowest priority. Intermediate priority is given to patients who require hospitalization and some continuous inotropic support. The highest priority, status 1A, is given to patients requiring high-dose inotropic support or mechanical support, such as intra-aortic balloon counterpulsation or ventricular assist device. Hearts are offered geographically, by the location of the donor, and limited by an ischemic time of approximately 4 hours. Patients who are waiting for transplantation are regularly reevaluated for a change in status or the development or worsening of a comorbidity that would preclude transplantation.

THE CARDIAC TRANSPLANTATION PROCEDURE

The Cardiac Donor

Relevant history for the assessment of cardiac donors includes the presence or absence of thoracic trauma, hemodynamic stability, pressor and inotropic requirements, duration of cardiac arrest, need for cardiopulmonary resuscitation, and assessment of hypotensive episodes. In many potential donors, brain death causes hemodynamic deterioration that requires inotropic support and substantial fluid administration. Donors up to the age of 50 to 55 years are considered safe by most centers. The final decision to accept a heart for transplantation is made at the time of harvest, after direct examination for myocardial infarction, trauma, and coronary calcification.

Currently, the acceptable cold ischemia time between explant and implant is approximately 4 hours. One of the main reasons for early graft failure after transplantation is inadequate myocardial protection during prolonged ischemic periods.

Surgical Considerations

The biatrial anastomosis technique consists of four suture lines: left atrium, pulmonary artery, aorta, and right atrium. The bicaval anastomosis technique, introduced to minimize distortion of the heart and to preserve atrial conduction, has five anastomoses: left atrium, pulmonary artery, aorta, inferior vena cava, and superior vena cava. To date, there has been no prospective trial to establish the superiority of either technique. Failure to wean a heart transplant recipient from cardiopulmonary bypass is most commonly the result of right-sided heart failure, which is evidenced by low cardiac output in the face of a rising central venous pressure. Native heart pacemakers and cardiac defibrillators are usually surgically removed at the end of the operation after the chest has been closed.

POSTOPERATIVE MANAGEMENT

Early Postoperative Management

Cardiovascular Issues

Management of the heart transplant recipient early after surgery does not differ substantially from management after other cardiac procedures

(Chapter 74). Cardiac transplant patients typically need chronotropic and inotropic support for a few days in the intensive care unit.

Because the donor heart is denervated, bradycardia is a frequent problem. It is usually treated with titrated isoproterenol to maintain a heart rate above 90 beats per minute for the first several days after transplantation. Temporary pacing leads are necessary for all patients, and as many as 10 to 15% of patients require a permanent pacemaker after transplant surgery.

Inhaled nitric oxide, in a usual dose of 20 to 60 parts per million, is a potent vasodilator that has a selective effect on the pulmonary vasculature, reduces pulmonary vascular resistance, and improves right ventricular function in patients with pulmonary hypertension. Intravenous epoprostenol, an alternative, is typically used at 5 to 50 ng/kg/minute.

Immunosuppression

Most immunosuppressive regimens begin with the simultaneous use of three classes of drugs: glucocorticoids, calcineurin inhibitors, and antiproliferative agents. In addition, patients may receive a variety of drugs during induction therapy (Chapter 48).

Perioperative Induction Therapy

The goal of perioperative induction therapy is to inhibit only those T cells that respond to donor antigen, thus achieving immunologic unresponsiveness to the transplant in the face of a fully functioning immune system, called donor-specific tolerance. Agents include the polyclonal anti-thymocyte antibodies, the interleukin-2 receptor antagonists daclizumab and basiliximab, and, less often, the anti-CD3 antibody OKT3.

Acute and Maintenance Immunosuppression

Patients initially receive high doses of intravenous corticosteroids (e.g., 500 mg of intravenous [IV] methylprednisolone at the end of cardiopulmonary bypass, followed by 150 mg IV every 8 hours for three additional doses), then oral steroids that are gradually tapered during the next 6 months in an attempt to minimize side effects (Chapter 34). Corticosteroids also are usually the drug of first choice to treat acute rejection.

The calcineurin inhibitors tacrolimus and cyclosporine act specifically on the immune system and do not affect other rapidly proliferating cells. In a meta-analysis, tacrolimus was as good as cyclosporine in terms of survival and significantly reduced episodes of acute rejection.[1] Important and often limiting side effects include nephrotoxicity, which occurs in up to 40 to 70% of patients, and hypertension. Target therapeutic levels 2 hours after a dose improve outcome.

Mycophenolate mofetil has replaced azathioprine as the first-line antiproliferative drug, with several randomized trials demonstrating superiority to azathioprine.[2] Mycophenolate mofetil may cause leukopenia, debilitating diarrhea, and nausea.

Sirolimus (often called rapamycin) and everolimus are complementary to calcineurin inhibitors, and both drugs have been used as alternatives to standard maintenance immunosuppression and as rescue drugs for rejection. In one randomized trial using cyclosporine and steroids, addition of sirolimus halved the number of patients with acute rejection and reduced the development of vasculopathy in the donor heart compared with addition of azathioprine.[3]

Other Potential Management Issues

The transplant recipient is often debilitated or malnourished. Depression (Chapter 404) is common, and many patients exhibit a marked emotional lability that is aggravated by high-dose steroids. Successful heart transplantation teams must include dedicated physical therapists, nutritionists, and social workers or psychologists, in addition to the nurses and physicians, so that all these needs may be addressed.

Long-Term Care of the Cardiac Transplant Recipient

Rejection

Rejection is categorized histologically and immunologically into three major types: hyperacute, acute (cellular or humoral), and chronic. Hyperacute rejection, which results when an abrupt loss of allograft function occurs within minutes to hours after circulation is established in the allograft, is rare in modern-day transplantation. The phenomenon is mediated by preexisting antibodies to allogeneic antigens on the vascular endothelial cells of the donor organ. These antibodies fix complement, which promotes intravascular thrombosis, leading to rapid occlusion of graft vasculature and swift rejection.

Acute cellular rejection, which is a predominantly lymphocytic mononuclear inflammatory response directed against the cardiac allograft, commonly occurs from the first week to several years after transplantation. The key event in both the initiation and the coordination of the rejection is T-cell activation. The risk of acute cellular rejection in the first 6 months is 40 to 70%. Acute cellular rejection after 6 months occurs most often in patients who have had substantial rejection early after transplantation, recent reduction in immunosuppression, intercurrent infection, or noncompliance with medication.

Acute humoral rejection occurs days to weeks after transplantation and is initiated by alloantibodies directed against donor HLA or endothelial cell antigens rather than by T cells. Patients at greatest risk for humoral rejection are women and patients with a high panel-reactive antibody screen or a positive crossmatch. It is estimated that significant humoral rejection occurs in about 7% of patients, but the rate may be as high as 20%.

Chronic rejection, or late graft failure, is an irreversible gradual deterioration of graft function occurring in many allografts months to years after transplantation. It is characterized by intimal thickening and fibrosis, which lead to luminal occlusion of the graft vasculature; it is often called cardiac allograft vasculopathy.

DIAGNOSIS

Allograft rejection is most frequent within the first month after cardiac transplantation and declines progressively thereafter. Clinical symptoms of rejection are often vague and relatively late in terms of immune injury to myocytes. Endomyocardial biopsy has been the "gold standard" for the diagnosis of rejection. Biopsies are performed by a transjugular approach weekly for 3 or 4 weeks, then every other week for several months; monthly biopsies continue for 6 to 12 months in many transplant programs. Biopsy grading of cellular rejection is based on the severity of lymphocyte infiltration and myocyte necrosis (Table 82-2). In one randomized trial, gene expression profiling of peripheral blood reduced the number of biopsies and provided equivalent outcomes over a mean follow-up of 19 months among patients who were stable 6 months to 5 years after transplantation.[4]

Humoral rejection is usually suspected clinically when there is evidence of suboptimal graft function but the endomyocardial biopsy specimen shows either no evidence of cellular rejection or only mild rejection. The pathologic markers of humoral rejection identifiable in endomyocardial biopsy tissue include deposits of immunoglobulin M, immunoglobulin G, or complement in the microvasculature or myocytes. In particular, C4d, which is a degradation product of the classic complement pathway and which binds to the endothelial and collagen basement membrane, is increasingly used as a marker of antibody-mediated rejection. Evidence for antibodies in the circulation with specificity for non-HLA antigens on the graft also supports the diagnosis of humoral rejection.

PROGNOSIS

Acute rejection causes approximately 12% of deaths in the first year after transplantation, but cardiac allograft vasculopathy represents a substantial portion of annual mortality beyond 3 years. Moreover, efforts to avert rejection with potent immunosuppressive therapy are responsible for other common complications after cardiac transplantation.

Infection

Infections cause approximately 20% of deaths within the first year after transplant surgery and continue to be a common cause of morbidity and mortality throughout the recipient's life. Infections of any type during the first month after transplantation also increase the risk of a subsequent fatal cytomegalovirus (CMV) infection (Chapter 384).

TABLE 82-2 STANDARDIZED CARDIAC BIOPSY GRADING: ACUTE CELLULAR REJECTION* 2004

Grade	Description
Grade 0 R	No rejection
Grade 1 R, mild	Interstitial and/or perivascular infiltrate with up to one focus of myocyte damage
Grade 2 R, moderate	Two or more foci of infiltrate with associated myocyte damage
Grade 3 R, severe	Diffuse infiltrate with multifocal myocyte damage, ± edema, ± hemorrhage, ± vasculitis

*International Society for Heart and Lung Transplantation.

Prophylaxis against CMV infection, *Pneumocystis jiroveci* pneumonia, herpes simplex virus infection, and oral candidiasis is now routine during the first 6 to 12 months after transplantation. As a result, the most common infections seen in the first month after surgery are nosocomial bacterial and fungal infections related to mechanical ventilation, catheters, the surgical site, and residual infections from prior implantation of ventricular assist devices.

The prophylactic use of trimethoprim-sulfamethoxazole, typically for the first year after transplantation, has virtually eliminated *P. jiroveci* pneumonia (Chapter 349) and also prevents nocardial infections and toxoplasmosis. The combination drug is generally reinstituted during subsequent episodes of increased risk, such as enhanced immunosuppression. Aspergillosis and candidiasis (Chapters 346 and 347) are the most common fungal infections after heart transplantation; oral nystatin solution or clotrimazole troches are routinely used in the first 6 to 12 months. Viral infections, especially CMV infection (Chapter 384), can increase immunosuppression, resulting in additional opportunistic infections. Prophylactic intravenous ganciclovir or oral valganciclovir is generally given for variable amounts of time in the CMV-seronegative recipient of a CMV-positive donor.

Health Maintenance

After 5 years, 95% of recipients have hypertension, 81% have hyperlipidemia, and 32% have diabetes. In addition, 25% to 50% have cardiac allograft vasculopathy, and up to 33% have renal insufficiency. Lifelong immunosuppression makes all recipients more susceptible to a number of malignant neoplasms, so careful follow-up is mandatory.

In many centers, recipients are given daily aspirin to reduce vascular disease, but no randomized trial has evaluated the benefits of antiplatelet therapy in heart transplant patients. Likewise, most recipients are given vitamins, stool softeners, iron supplements, and proton pump inhibitors early after surgery on an empirical basis.

Surveillance

New Health Problems

Because osteoporosis (Chapter 251) is a major problem, in part related to use of corticosteroids, prophylaxis with calcium and vitamin D is usually initiated. Depression occurs in up to 25% of recipients. A number of antidepressants may be used, but the potential for adverse drug interactions must be considered. The management of gout is difficult because colchicine may increase the risk of myoneuropathy, nonsteroidal anti-inflammatory drugs often worsen renal insufficiency and hyperkalemia, and allopurinol used with azathioprine can cause life-threatening neutropenia. Minimizing diuretic use and judicious use of colchicine with allopurinol will usually alleviate most patients' symptoms.

Risk factors for malignant disease (Chapter 183) include impaired immunoregulation, a synergistic effect with other carcinogens such as nicotine or ultraviolet light exposure, and oncogenic causes such as Epstein-Barr virus and papillomavirus. The cumulative amount of immunosuppression is positively correlated with risk for malignant change. Lymphoproliferative diseases, skin and lip cancers, and Kaposi's sarcoma are particularly common. Malignant neoplasms account for 24% of deaths after 5 years.

TRANSPLANT VASCULOPATHY

EPIDEMIOLOGY AND PATHOBIOLOGY

Transplant vasculopathy remains the most daunting long-term complication of heart transplantation, with an annual incidence rate of 5 to 10%. After the first postoperative year, cardiac allograft vasculopathy becomes increasingly important as a cause of death. The risk of transplant vasculopathy increases as the number of HLA mismatches and the number and duration of rejection episodes increase. CMV infection and ischemia-reperfusion injury also increase the risk, as do classic risk factors for atherosclerotic disease (Chapter 51), such as smoking, obesity, diabetes, dyslipidemia, and hypertension. Transplant vasculopathy can develop as early as 3 months after transplantation and is detected angiographically in 20% of grafts at 1 year and in 40 to 50% at 5 years.

CLINICAL MANIFESTATIONS

In contrast to eccentric lesions seen in atheromatous disease, cardiac allograft vasculopathy produces concentric narrowing from neointimal proliferation of vascular smooth muscle cells and affects the entire length of the coronary tree, from the epicardial to the intramyocardial segments, leading to rapid tapering, pruning, and obliteration of third-order branch vessels. Most patients will not experience anginal symptoms because of denervation of coronary arteries, so the first clinical manifestation may be myocardial infarction, heart failure, ventricular arrhythmia, or sudden death. As a result, most transplantation centers screen patients annually for possible transplant vasculopathy.

DIAGNOSIS

Intravascular ultrasonography, which is currently the most sensitive imaging technique to study early transplant vasculopathy, provides quantitative data on intimal thickness, luminal cross-sectional area, and external elastic membrane cross-sectional area. An increase in intimal thickness of at least 0.5 mm in the first year after transplantation is a reliable indicator of both cardiac allograft vasculopathy and 5-year mortality. However, increased invasiveness and cost of intravascular ultrasonography preclude its widespread application. Dobutamine stress echocardiography (Chapter 55) has a high sensitivity (83 to 95%) and specificity (between 53 and 91%) compared with angiography. Most transplantation centers do one of the screening tests on an annual basis to assess the risk of new cardiac allograft vasculopathy.

TREATMENT

Rx

The only definitive treatment of transplant vasculopathy is repeated transplantation. The statins pravastatin and simvastatin repress the induction of class II major histocompatibility complex antigen expression by interferon-γ and thereby inhibit T-cell proliferation and have a direct influence on the expression of genes for growth factors that are essential for the proliferation of smooth muscle cells. Randomized controlled trials have shown that either drug significantly reduces rates of severe rejections and transplant vasculopathy while also significantly reducing cholesterol levels and improving survival (see later).5 It is not clear whether all statin drugs have the same benefit in this population. Sirolimus and everolimus are also being evaluated to prevent the development or progression of cardiac allograft vasculopathy, but their role has not yet been determined.

Diabetes

Diabetes (Chapter 237) occurs in 32% of transplant recipients, and patients who develop new-onset diabetes mellitus after transplantation are at increased risk for morbidity and mortality. Although impaired B-cell function appears to be the primary mechanism of calcineurin inhibitor-induced new-onset diabetes, impaired peripheral glucose use also appears to contribute to insulin resistance and abnormal glucose metabolism. Risk factors include obesity, increased age, family history of diabetes, abnormal glucose tolerance, and African American or Hispanic descent. Management is generally similar to that of the nontransplant patient.

Hypertension and Renal Insufficiency

The 5-year incidence of hypertension (Chapter 67) in the population of cardiac transplant recipients is 95%. Excess risk of hypertension is attributable primarily to the use of calcineurin inhibitors because of both direct effects and the associated renal insufficiency. Treatment often requires a combination of agents and is generally as in the nontransplant patient.

The risk of chronic renal failure is about 16% at 10 years, largely related to direct calcineurin inhibitor–mediated renal arteriolar vasoconstriction, increased levels of endothelin-1, decreased nitric oxide production, and alterations in the kidney's ability to adjust to changes in serum tonicity. Once early renal insufficiency occurs, no single treatment has yet been shown to be effective.

Hyperlipidemia

Hyperlipidemia (Chapter 213) occurs in more than 80% of cardiac transplant recipients and is associated with the development of cardiac allograft vasculopathy, cerebrovascular disease, and peripheral vascular disease. Characteristically, total cholesterol, low-density lipoprotein cholesterol, apolipoprotein B, and triglyceride levels increase by 3 months after transplantation and then generally fall somewhat after the first year. Corticosteroids, cyclosporine, sirolimus, and mycophenolate mofetil all have unfavorable effects on lipid levels, whereas tacrolimus probably causes less hyperlipidemia.

In heart transplant recipients, pravastatin and simvastatin have been associated with better outcomes, but there are no long-term data in this population demonstrating that lowering of low-density lipoprotein cholesterol levels to less than 100 mg/dL (compared with 100 to 130 mg/dL) with more potent

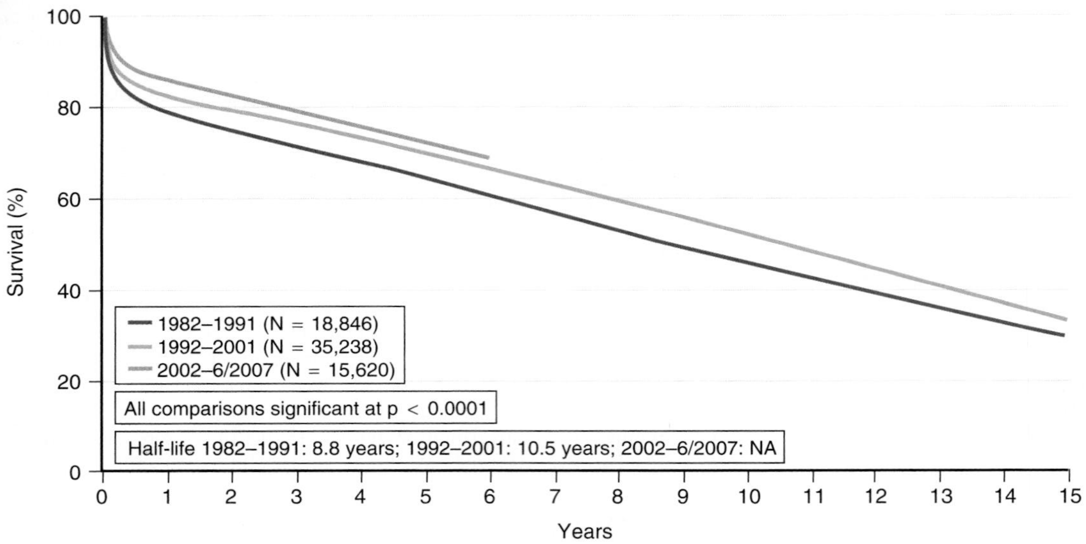

FIGURE 82-2. The Kaplan-Meier survival by era for heart transplantations performed between January 1982 and June 2007. The graph shows a significant improvement in survival over time. (Data from the Registry of the International Society for Heart and Lung Transplantation. Reproduced with permission.)

or higher-dose statin therapy improves outcomes. Different statins are metabolized differently, so caution must be exercised in the prescription of statins beyond the doses used in the randomized trials: simvastatin, 20 to 40 mg daily, and pravastatin, 10 to 20 mg daily.

OUTCOME OF TRANSPLANTATION

During the first year after transplantation, early causes of death are graft failure, infection, and rejection, with an overall survival of 87.7% at 1 year and 79.1% at 3 years (Fig. 82-2). The percentage of patients dying of early graft failure, malignant disease, and infection has remained relatively stable during the past decade. After 5 years, cardiac allograft vasculopathy and late graft failure (33% together), malignant disease (23%), and non-CMV infection (11%) are the most prominent causes of death. With advances in immunosuppression, the average half-life of the cardiac allograft increased approximately 15 months (8.8 years to 10.5 years) from 1986-1990 to 1992-2001.

Hemodynamic and Functional Outcomes

The transplanted heart markedly improves cardiac hemodynamics, but there may be a slightly diminished maximal cardiac output during exercise secondary to denervation, limited atrial function, decreased myocardial compliance from rejection or ischemic injury, and donor-recipient size mismatch. Immediately after surgery, a restrictive hemodynamic pattern is frequently observed, but it gradually improves during a few days to weeks. Some 10 to 15% of recipients develop a chronic restrictive cardiomyopathy (Chapter 60) that may produce fatigue and breathlessness during exercise. Because parasympathetic innervation, which normally lowers the heart rate, is absent, the typical resting heart rate of a recipient is 90 to 115 beats per minute.

At 1 year, 90% of surviving patients report no functional limitations, and approximately 35% return to work. Adapting to life after transplantation depends on many factors, including the patient's condition and duration of illness before transplantation and the patient's personality, intelligence, social support, and financial well-being.

Other Key Long-Term Issues for the Nontransplantation Physician

Drug Interactions

The physician outside the transplanting hospital may be reluctant to interact at all with the heart transplant recipient, a fear that complicates the comprehensive care of these patients. Often a phone call placed to the transplantation center to clarify any proposed medications or new symptoms will obviate the need for the recipient to travel to the transplanting hospital. The most common errors made by nontransplantation physicians are the addition of new drugs that result in adverse drug interactions; examples include acyclovir, allopurinol, amlodipine, antacids, antidepressants, cimetidine, clarithromycin, clotrimazole, colchicine, diltiazem, erythromycin, felodipine, ganciclovir, grapefruit juice, iron, ketoconazole, phenobarbital, phenytoin, primidone, rifampin, statin drugs, St. John's wort, trimethoprim-sulfamethoxazole, valganciclovir, and verapamil. In addition, the index of suspicion must be higher in evaluating the possibility of infection in a transplant recipient (Chapter 289).

FUTURE DIRECTIONS IN CARDIAC TRANSPLANTATION

It is not surprising that uniform agreement has not been achieved among transplantation centers regarding the precise indications for and timing of listing for cardiac transplantation. The basic tenet of organ allocation embraces two axioms that are at times contradictory: equity, or equal access of all patients to donor organs, with priority given to patients closest to death; and utility, an allocation policy for organs that maximizes survival of the patient and graft. As newer therapies, such as cell transplantation and better permanent mechanical devices, become available, the role of heart transplantation will need to be redefined.

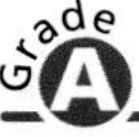

1. Ye F, Ying-Bin X, Yu-Guo W, et al. Tacrolimus versus cyclosporine microemulsion for heart transplant recipients: a meta-analysis. *J Heart Lung Transplant.* 2009;28:58-66.
2. Eisen HJ, Kobashigawa J, Keogh A, et al. Three-year results of a randomized, double-blind, controlled trial of mycophenolate mofetil versus azathioprine in cardiac transplant recipients. *J Heart Lung Transplant.* 2005;24:517-525.
3. Keogh A, Richardson M, Ruygrok P, et al. Sirolimus in de novo heart transplant recipients reduces acute rejection and prevents coronary artery disease at 2 years: a randomized clinical trial. *Circulation.* 2004;110:2694-2700.
4. Pham MX, Teuteberg JJ, Kfoury AG, et al. Gene-expression profiling for rejection surveillance after cardiac transplantation. *N Engl J Med.* 2010;362:890-900.
5. Kobashigawa JA, Moriguchi JD, Laks H, et al. Ten-year follow-up of a randomized trial of pravastatin in heart transplant patients. *J Heart Lung Transplant.* 2005;24:1736-1740.

SUGGESTED READINGS

Mancini D, Lietz K. Selection of cardiac transplantation candidates in 2010. *Circulation.* 2010;122:173-183. *Review.*

Singh TP, Almond C, Givertz MM, et al. Improved survival in heart transplant recipients in the United States: racial differences in era effect. *Circ Heart Fail.* 2011;4:153-160. *Early survival has improved across all ethnic groups, but long-term survival has improved in white but not black or Hispanic recipients.*

Zimmer RJ, Lee MS. Transplant coronary artery disease. *JACC Cardiovasc Interv.* 2010;3:367-377. *Review of pathogenesis and treatment.*

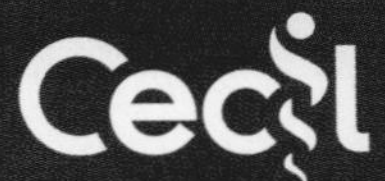

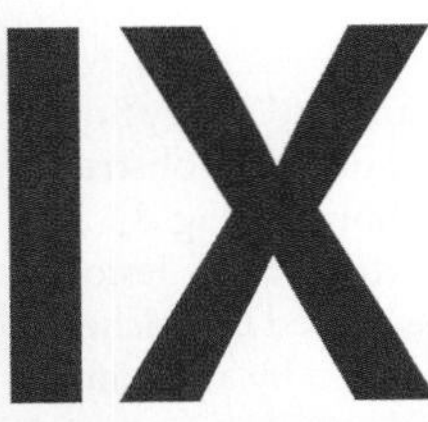

IX RESPIRATORY DISEASES

83

APPROACH TO THE PATIENT WITH RESPIRATORY DISEASE

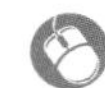

MONICA KRAFT

Respiratory symptoms, which are among the most common reasons why patients seek medical care, are responsible for about 20% of office visits to a primary care physician. Key common respiratory complaints include cough, wheezing, dyspnea, and hemoptysis.

APPROACH TO THE PATIENT WITH COUGH

Cough is the single most common respiratory complaint for which patients seek care. Referrals of patients with persistently troublesome chronic cough of unknown etiology account for 10 to 38% of outpatient visits to respiratory specialists.

For acute cough, defined as coughing that has been present for less than 8 weeks, a careful medical history and physical examination will usually reveal the diagnosis (Table 83-1). Although most acute coughs are of minor consequence, cough can occasionally be a sign of a potentially life-threatening illness, such as pulmonary embolism (Chapter 98), pneumonia (Chapter 97), or heart failure (Chapter 58).

Up to 98% of all cases of chronic cough, defined as a cough that persists for more than 8 weeks, in immunocompetent adults are caused by eight common conditions: postnasal drip syndrome from a variety of rhinosinus conditions (Chapter 259), asthma (Chapter 87), gastroesophageal reflux disease (GERD) (Chapter 140), chronic bronchitis (Chapter 88), eosinophilic bronchitis, bronchiectasis (Chapter 90), use of angiotensin-converting enzyme (ACE) inhibitors, and postinfectious cough. Postinfectious cough is usually nonproductive and lasts for 3 to 8 weeks following an upper respiratory infection; patients have a normal chest radiograph. Uncommon causes of chronic cough include bronchogenic carcinoma (Chapter 197), chronic interstitial pneumonia (Chapter 92), sarcoidosis (Chapter 95), left ventricular failure (Chapter 58), and aspiration (Chapter 94).

DIAGNOSIS

In chronic cough (Fig. 83-1), the character and timing are not of diagnostic help. A chest radiograph should be obtained in all patients, but other tests should not be ordered in current smokers or patients taking ACE inhibitors until the response to smoking cessation or discontinuation of the drug for at least 4 weeks can be assessed. Sinus radiographs, barium esophagography, methacholine challenge, esophageal pH, and bronchoscopy can be ordered as part of the initial evaluation, depending on the history and physical examination (Table 83-2; see Fig. 83-1). If a test points toward a possible diagnosis, a trial of treatment for that condition is needed to confirm the diagnosis.

TREATMENT Rx

The specific cause of cough can be diagnosed and treated successfully 84 to 98% of the time, so nonspecific therapy aimed to suppress the cough per se is rarely indicated. There is no strong evidence that nonspecific therapies such as antitussives, mucolytics, decongestants, or antihistamine-decongestant combinations are efficacious for acute cough in the setting of an upper respiratory tract infection.[1] For nonspecific persistent cough, effective treatment of chronic gastroesophageal reflux disease with a proton pump inhibitor (Chapter 140) provides no more than modest benefit, with about one in five patients improving.[2]

APPROACH TO THE PATIENT WITH WHEEZING

Wheeze is a continuous musical sound that lasts longer than 80 to 100 msec, likely generated by flow though critically narrowed collapsible bronchi. Although expiratory wheezing is a common physical finding in asthma (Chapter 87), the many causes of wheezing (Table 83-3) (e.g., chronic obstructive pulmonary disease [COPD; Chapter 88], pulmonary edema [Chapter 58], bronchiolitis [Chapter 92], bronchiectasis [Chapter 90], and less common entities such as carcinoid [Chapter 240] and parasitic infections) often can be distinguished based on the history, physical examination, and pulmonary function testing (Chapter 85).

DIAGNOSIS

On pulmonary function testing, the shape of inspiratory and expiratory flow-volume loops provides key information about the presence of airway obstruction and whether the obstruction is extrathoracic or intrathoracic (Fig. 83-2). An important cause of extrathoracic obstruction is vocal cord lesions (Chapter 196). Variable intrathoracic obstruction can be caused by tracheomalacia, whereas fixed upper airway obstruction can be caused by a proximal tracheal tumor.

TREATMENT 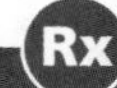

Treatment of the specific cause will usually lead to complete or at least partial resolution of wheezing. However, treatment of associated asymptomatic or minimally symptomatic gastroesophageal reflux disease is not beneficial.[3]

APPROACH TO THE PATIENT WITH DYSPNEA

Dyspnea is the sensation of difficult, labored, or unpleasant breathing. The word *unpleasant* is very important to this definition because the labored or difficult breathing encountered by healthy individuals while exercising does not qualify as dyspnea because it is at the level expected for the degree of exertion. The sensation of dyspnea is often poorly or vaguely described by the patient. The physiology of dyspnea remains unclear, but multiple neural pathways can be involved in processes that lead to dyspnea.

In acute dyspnea, or shortness of breath of sudden onset, the history, physical examination, and laboratory testing must first focus on potential life-threatening conditions, including pulmonary embolism (Chapter 98), pulmonary edema (Chapters 58 and 59), acute airway obstruction from anaphylaxis or foreign bodies, pneumothorax (Chapter 99), or pneumonia (Chapter 97). For chronic dyspnea, specific conditions to consider include COPD (Chapter 88), asthma (Chapter 87), interstitial lung disease (Chapter 92), heart failure (Chapter 58), cardiomyopathy (Chapter 60), GERD (Chapter 140), other respiratory diseases, or hyperventilation syndrome.

DIAGNOSIS

A chest radiograph, electrocardiogram, pulmonary function testing, and an exercise test with electrocardiographic (ECG) monitoring and pulse oximetry at rest and during exercise are key tests to assess patients with unexplained dyspnea (Fig. 83-3). For acute dyspnea, B-type natriuretic peptide testing can be extremely helpful in distinguishing heart failure from other causes.[4] The utility of more detailed pulmonary testing with maximal inspiratory and expiratory pressures, flow-volume loops, with or without methacholine challenge, computed tomographic screening of the chest, and echocardiography depends on history and physical examination and the results of these tests. When GERD is a suspected cause of dyspnea, a modified barium esophagogram or 24-hour esophageal pH monitoring, or both, should be considered (Chapter 140). Other more invasive tests such as cardiac catheterization or lung biopsy may be indicated when the results of less invasive tests have not been conclusive.

TREATMENT Rx

Whenever possible, the final determination of the cause of dyspnea is made by observing which specific therapy eliminates it. Because dyspnea may be simultaneously due to more than one condition, it may be necessary to treat more than one condition.

APPROACH TO THE PATIENT WITH HEMOPTYSIS

Hemoptysis is the expectoration of blood from the lung parenchyma or airways. Hemoptysis may be scant, with just the appearance of streaks of bright red blood in the sputum, or massive, with the expectoration of a large volume of blood. Massive hemoptysis, which is defined as the expectoration of at least 600 mL of blood in 24 to 48 hours, may occur in 3 to 10% of patients with hemoptysis. Dark red clots may also be expectorated when the blood has been present in the lungs for days.

Pseudohemoptysis, which is the expectoration of blood from a source other than the lower respiratory tract, may cause diagnostic confusion when patients cannot clearly describe the source of their bleeding. Pseudohemoptysis can occur when blood from the oral cavity, nares, pharynx, or tongue clings to the back of the throat and initiates the cough reflex, or when patients who have hematemesis aspirate into the lower respiratory tract. When the oropharynx is colonized with *Serratia marcescens*, a red-pigment-producing aerobic gram-negative rod, the sputum can also be red and be confused with hemoptysis.

Hemoptysis can be caused by a wide variety of disorders. Virtually all causes of hemoptysis (Table 83-4) may result in massive hemoptysis, but massive hemoptysis is most frequently caused by infection (e.g., tuberculosis [Chapter 332], bronchiectasis and lung abscess [Chapter 90], and cancer [Chapter 197]). Infections with aspergilloma (Chapter 347) and in patients with cystic fibrosis (Chapter 89) also are associated with massive hemoptysis. Iatrogenic causes of massive hemoptysis include rupture of a pulmonary

TABLE 83-1 SPECTRUM OF CAUSES AND FREQUENCIES OF COUGH IN IMMUNOCOMPETENT ADULTS

COMMON	LESS COMMON
ACUTE COUGH	
Common cold	Asthma
Acute bacterial sinusitis	Pneumonia
Pertussis	Heart failure
Exacerbations of COPD	Aspiration syndromes
Allergic rhinitis	Pulmonary embolism
Environmental irritant rhinitis	Exacerbation of bronchiectasis
CHRONIC COUGH	
Rhinosinus conditions	Bronchogenic carcinoma
Asthma	Chronic interstitial pneumonia
Gastroesophageal reflux	Sarcoidosis
Chronic bronchitis	Left heart failure
Eosinophilic bronchitis	
Bronchiectasis	
ACE inhibitors	
Postinfection	

ACE = angiotensin converting enzyme; COPD = chronic obstructive pulmonary disease.

TABLE 83-2 TESTING CHARACTERISTICS OF DIAGNOSTIC PROTOCOL FOR EVALUATION OF CHRONIC COUGH

TESTS	DIAGNOSIS	POSITIVE PREDICTIVE VALUE, %	NEGATIVE PREDICTIVE VALUE, %
Sinus radiograph	Sinusitis	57-81	95-100
Methacholine inhalation challenge	Asthma	60-82	100
Modified barium esophagography	GERD, esophageal stricture	38-63	63-93
Esophageal pH*	GERD	89-100	<100
Bronchoscopy	Endobronchial mass/ lesion	50-89	100

*24-Hour esophageal pH monitoring.
GERD = gastroesophageal reflux disease.

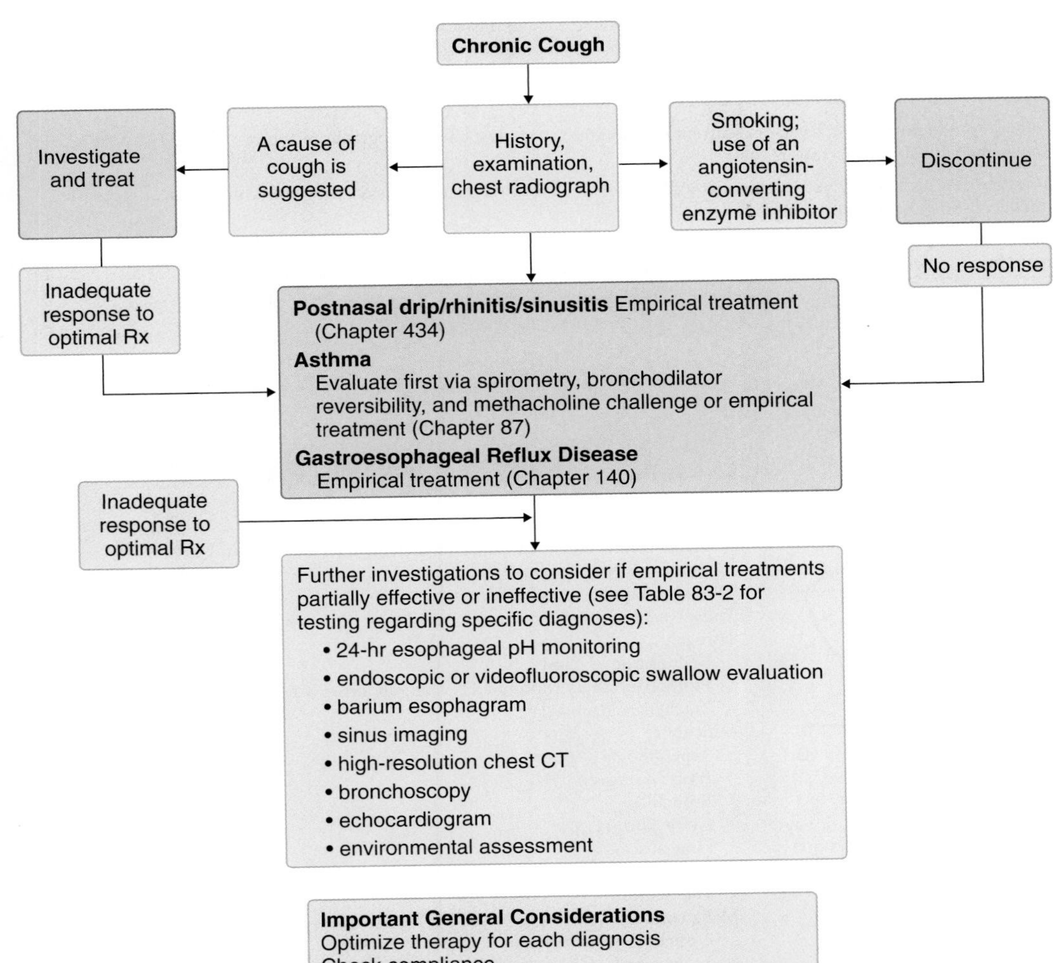

FIGURE 83-1. **Algorithm for the management of chronic cough lasting >8 weeks.** CT = computed tomography; Rx = prescription.

TABLE 83-3 DIAGNOSIS OF SELECTED WHEEZING ILLNESSES OTHER THAN ASTHMA

	DISTINGUISHING FEATURES
UPPER AIRWAY DISEASES	
Postnasal drip syndrome	History of postnasal drip, throat clearing, nasal discharge; physical exam shows oropharyngeal secretions or cobblestone appearance to mucosa.
Epiglottis	History of sore throat out of proportion to pharyngitis. Evidence of supraglottitis on endoscopy or lateral neck radiographs.
Vocal cord dysfunction syndrome	Lack of symptomatic response to bronchodilators, presence of stridor plus wheeze in absence of increased $P(A\text{-}a)O_2$; extrathoracic variable obstruction on flow-volume loops; paradoxical inspiratory and/or early expiratory adduction of vocal cords on laryngoscopy during wheezing. This syndrome can masquerade as asthma, be provoked by exercise, and often coexists with asthma.
Retropharyngeal abscess	History of stiff neck, sore throat, fever, trauma to posterior pharynx; swelling noted by lateral neck or CT radiographs.
Laryngotracheal injury due to tracheal cannulation	History of cannulation of trachea by endotracheal or tracheostomy tube; evidence of intrathoracic or extrathoracic variable obstruction on flow-volume loops, neck and chest radiographs, laryngoscopy, or bronchoscopy.
Neoplasms	Bronchogenic carcinoma, adenoma, or carcinoid tumor is suspected when there is hemoptysis, unilateral wheeze, or evidence of lobar collapse on chest radiograph or combinations of these; diagnosis is confirmed by bronchoscopy.
Anaphylaxis	Abrupt onset of wheezing with urticaria, angioedema, nausea, diarrhea, and hypotension, especially following insect bite, in association with other signs of anaphylaxis such as hypotension or hives, or administration of drug or IV contrast, or family history.
LOWER AIRWAY DISEASES	
COPD	History of dyspnea on exertion and productive cough in cigarette smoker. Because productive cough is nonspecific, it should only be ascribed to COPD when other cough-phlegm syndromes have been excluded, forced expiratory time to empty more than 80% of vital capacity >4 sec, and there is decreased breath sound intensity, unforced wheezing during auscultation, and irreversible, expiratory airflow obstruction on spirometry.
Pulmonary edema	History and physical exam consistent with passive congestion of the lungs, ARDS, impaired lung lymphatics; abnormal chest radiograph, echocardiogram, radionuclide ventriculography, cardiac catheterization, or combinations of these.
Aspiration	History of risk for pharyngeal dysfunction or gastroesophageal reflux disease; abnormal modified barium swallow and/or 24-hr esophageal pH monitoring.
Pulmonary embolism	History of risk for thromboembolic disease, positive confirmatory tests.
Bronchiolitis	History of respiratory infection, connective tissue disease, transplantation, ulcerative colitis, development of chronic airway obstruction over months to a few years rather than over many years in a nonsmoker; mixed obstructive and restrictive pattern on PFTs and hyperinflation; may be accompanied by fine nodular infiltrates on chest radiograph.
Cystic fibrosis	Combination of productive cough, digital clubbing, bronchiectasis, progressive COPD with *Pseudomonas* species colonization and infection, obstructive azoospermia, family history, pancreatic insufficiency, and two sweat chloride determinations of >60 mEq/L; some patients are not diagnosed until adulthood, in one instance as late as age 69 yr; when sweat test is occasionally normal, definitive diagnosis may require nasal transepithelial voltage measurements and genotyping.
Carcinoid syndrome	History of episodes of flushing and watery diarrhea; elevated 5-hydroxyindoleactic acid level in 24-hr urine specimen.
Bronchiectasis	History of episodes of productive cough, fever, or recurrent pneumonias; suggestive chest radiographs or typical chest CT findings; ABPA should be considered when bronchiectasis is central.
Lymphangitic carcinomatosis	History of dyspnea or prior malignancy; reticulonodular infiltrates with or without pleural effusions; suggestive high-resolution chest CT scan; confirmed by bronchoscopy with biopsies.
Parasitic infections	Consider in a nonasthmatic patient who has traveled to an endemic area and complains of fatigue, weight loss, fever; peripheral blood eosinophilia; infiltrates on chest radiograph; stools for ova and parasites for nonfilarial causes; blood serologic studies for filarial causes.

ABPA = allergic bronchopulmonary aspergillosis; ARDS = acute respiratory distress syndrome; COPD = chronic obstructive pulmonary disease; CT = computed tomography; IV = intravenous; $P(A\text{-}a)O_2$ = alveolar-arterial oxygen tension gradient; PFTs = pulmonary function tests.

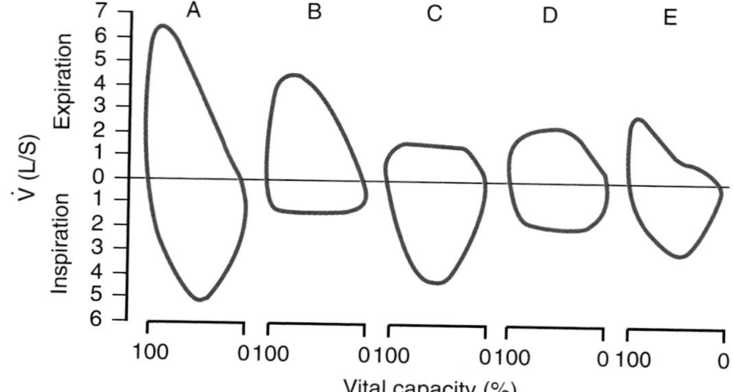

FIGURE 83-2. Schematic flow-volume loop configurations in a spectrum of airway lesions. *A* is normal; *B* is variable extrathoracic upper airway obstruction; *C* is variable intrathoracic upper airway lesion; *D* is fixed upper airway obstruction; and *E* is small airway obstruction. L/S = liters per second; $\dot{V}$ = ventilation.

TABLE 83-4 COMMON CAUSES OF MASSIVE HEMOPTYSIS

- Cardiovascular
  - Arterial bronchial fistula
  - Heart failure, especially from mitral stenosis
  - Pulmonary arteriovenous fistula
- Diffuse intrapulmonary hemorrhage
- Diffuse parenchymal disease
- Iatrogenic
  - Malposition of chest tube
  - Pulmonary artery rupture following pulmonary arterial catheterization
  - Tracheoarterial fistula
- Infections
  - Aspergilloma
  - Bronchiectasis
  - Bronchitis
  - Cystic fibrosis
  - Lung abscess
  - Sporotrichosis
  - Tuberculosis
- Malignancies
  - Bronchogenic carcinoma
  - Leukemia
  - Metastatic cancer
- Trauma

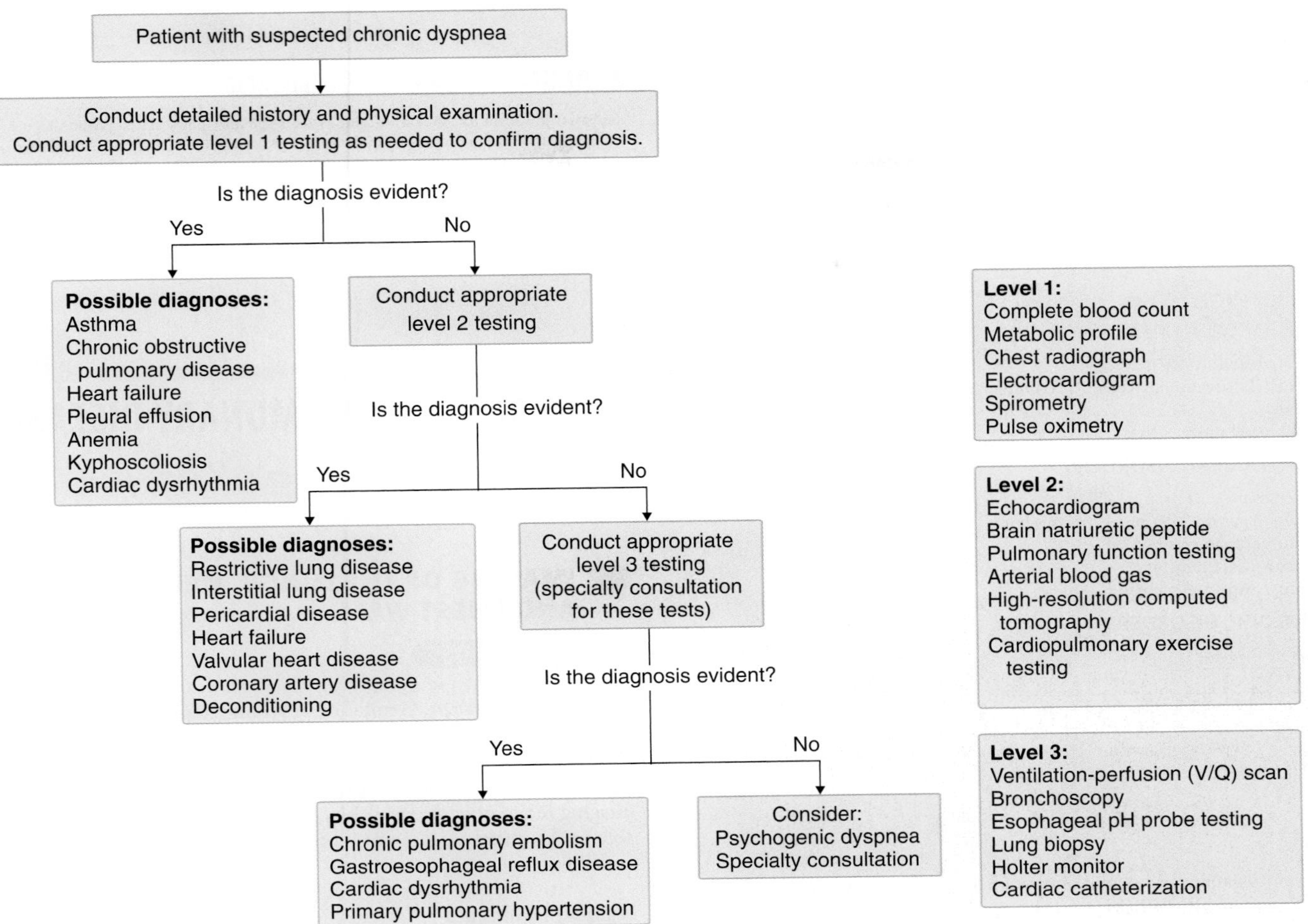

FIGURE 83-3. **Algorithm outlining the approach to chronic dyspnea.** (Modified from Karnani NG, Reisfield GM, Wilson GR. Evaluation of chronic dyspnea. *Am Fam Phys.* 2005;71:1529-1537.)

artery after less than 0.2% of cases of balloon-guided flotation catheterization and tracheal artery fistula as a complication of tracheostomy.

In nonmassive hemoptysis, the etiology is bronchitis in more than one third of cases (Chapter 88), bronchogenic carcinoma (Chapter 197) in one fifth of cases, tuberculosis (Chapter 332) in 7%, pneumonia (Chapter 97) in 5%, and bronchiectasis in 1% (Chapter 90). Using a systematic diagnostic approach (see later), the cause of hemoptysis can be found in 68 to 98% of cases. The remaining 2 to 32% have idiopathic or central hemoptysis, which occurs most commonly in men between the ages of 30 and 50 years. Prolonged follow-up of idiopathic hemoptysis almost always fails to reveal the source of bleeding, even though 10% continue to have occasional episodes of hemoptysis.

DIAGNOSIS

The diagnostic evaluation for hemoptysis begins with a detailed medical history and a complete physical examination. Information on the amount of bleeding should be obtained, as well as details about the frequency, timing, and duration of hemoptysis. For example, repeated episodes of hemoptysis occurring over a period of months to years suggest a bronchial adenoma or bronchiectasis as the cause, whereas small amounts of hemoptysis occurring every day for weeks are more likely to be caused by bronchogenic carcinoma. A travel history can suggest coccidioidomycosis (Chapter 341) and histoplasmosis (Chapter 340) in the United States, paragonimiasis and ascariasis (Chapter 366) in the Far East, and schistosomiasis (Chapter 363) in South America. Orthopnea and paroxysmal nocturnal dyspnea suggest heart failure (Chapter 58), especially from mitral stenosis (Chapter 75). In patients who have occupational exposure to trimellitic anhydride, which occurs when heated metal surfaces are sprayed with a corrosion-resistant epoxy resin, hemoptysis can be part of the postexposure syndrome. In a patient with the triad of upper airway disease, lower airway disease, and renal disease, Wegener's granulomatosis (Chapter 278) should be suspected. Pulmonary hemorrhage may also be a presenting manifestation of systemic lupus erythematosus (Chapter 274). Goodpasture's syndrome, which typically occurs in young men, is also associated with renal disease (Chapter 123). Diffuse alveolar hemorrhage occurs in 20% of cases during autologous bone marrow transplantation (Chapter 181) and should be suspected in patients who have undergone recent bone marrow transplantation (Chapter 181) when they present with cough, dyspnea, hypoxemia, and diffuse pulmonary infiltrates.

On physical examination, inspection of the skin and mucous membranes may show telangiectasias suggesting heredity hemorrhagic telangiectasia (Chapter 176) or ecchymoses and petechiae, suggesting a hematologic abnormality (Chapter 175). Pulsations transmitted to a tracheostomy cannula should heighten suspicion of a tracheal artery fistula. Inspection of the thorax should show evidence of recent or old chest trauma, and unilateral wheeze or rales may herald localized disease such as a bronchial adenoma or carcinoma. Although pulmonary embolism (Chapter 98) cannot be definitively diagnosed on physical examination, tachypnea, phlebitis, and pleural friction rub suggest this disorder. If rales are heard on the chest examination, heart failure as well as other diseases causing diffuse pulmonary hemorrhage (see earlier) or idiopathic pulmonary hemosiderosis (Chapter 92) should be considered. Careful cardiovascular examination may help diagnose mitral stenosis (Chapter 75), pulmonary artery fistulas, or pulmonary hypertension (Chapter 68).

Routine laboratory studies should include a complete blood count, urinalysis, and coagulation studies. The complete blood count may suggest an infection, hematologic disorder, or chronic blood loss. Urinalysis may reveal hematuria and suggest the presence of a systemic disease (e.g., Wegener's granulomatosis, Goodpasture's syndrome, systemic lupus erythematosus) associated with renal disease. Coagulation studies may uncover a hematologic disorder that is primarily responsible for hemoptysis or that contributes to excessive bleeding from another disease. The ECG may help suggest the presence of a cardiovascular disorder. Although as many as 30% of patients

TABLE 83-5 EXAMPLES OF SPECIAL EVALUATIONS FOR HEMOPTYSIS ACCORDING TO CATEGORY OF DISEASE*

TRACHEOBRONCHIAL DISORDERS
Expectorated sputum for TB, parasites, fungi, and cytology Bronchoscopy (if not done) Bronchography High-resolution chest CT scan
LOCALIZED PARENCHYMAL DISEASES
Expectorated sputum for TB, parasites, fungi, and cytology Chest CT scan Lung biopsy with special stains
DIFFUSE PARENCHYMAL DISEASES
Expectorated sputum for cytology Blood for BUN, creatinine, ANA, RF, complement, cryoglobulins, ANCA, anti-GBM antibody Lung or kidney biopsy with special stains
CARDIOVASCULAR DISORDERS
Echocardiogram Arterial blood gas on 21% and 100% oxygen Ventilation-perfusion scans Pulmonary arteriogram Aortogram, contrast-enhanced CT scan
HEMATOLOGIC DISORDERS
Coagulation studies Bone marrow

*This table is not meant to be all inclusive.
ANA = antinuclear antibody; ANCA = antineutrophil cytoplasmic antibody; BUN = blood urea nitrogen; CT = computed tomography; GBM = glomerular basement membrane; RF = rheumatoid factor; TB = tuberculosis.

with hemoptysis have a normal chest radiograph, routine chest radiographs may be diagnostically valuable.

Bronchoscopy can localize the bleeding site in up to 93% of patients by fiberoptic bronchoscopy and in up to 86% with rigid bronchoscopy. It may establish sites of bleeding different from those suggested by the chest radiograph. The best results are obtained when bronchoscopy is performed during or within 24 hours of active bleeding, and rates of diagnosis fall to about 50% by 48 hours after bleeding. When there is no active bleeding, bronchoscopy with bronchoalveolar lavage can be helpful in patients thought to have diffuse intrapulmonary hemorrhage. Typical findings include bright red or blood-tinged lavage fluid from multiple lobes in both lungs or a substantial number of hemosiderin-laden macrophages (i.e., at least 20% of the total number of alveolar macrophages).

Depending on the results of the initial evaluation and the likely categories of hemoptysis, additional diagnostic tests can be helpful (Table 83-5). Bronchoscopy may not be needed in patients who have stable chronic bronchitis (Chapter 88) with one episode of blood streaking or who have acute tracheobronchitis (Chapter 88). Bronchoscopy may also not be needed with obvious cardiovascular causes of hemoptysis, such as heart failure and pulmonary embolism.

TREATMENT Rx

Treatment is targeted toward the cause of hemoptysis. Bronchoscopic approaches (Chapter 101) are increasingly used for endobronchial lesions.

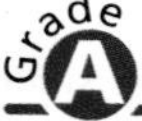

1. Smith SM. Over-the-counter medications for acute cough in children and adults in ambulatory settings. *Cochrane Database Syst Rev.* 2008;1:CD001831.
2. Chang AB, Lasserson TJ, Kiljander TO, et al. Systematic review and meta-analysis of randomised controlled trials of gastro-oesophageal reflux interventions for chronic cough associated with gastro-oesophageal reflux. *BMJ.* 2006;332:11-17.
3. Mastronarde JG, Anthonisen NR, Castro M, et al, for the American Lung Association Asthma Clinical Research Centers. Efficacy of esomeprazole for treatment of poorly controlled asthma. *N Engl J Med.* 2009;360:1487-1499.
4. Lam LL, Cameron PA, Schneider HG, et al. Meta-analysis: effect of B-type natriuretic peptide testing on clinical outcomes in patients with acute dyspnea in the emergency setting. *Ann Intern Med.* 2010;153:728-735.

SUGGESTED READINGS

Benbassat J, Baumal RV. Should teaching of the respiratory physical examination be restricted only to signs with proven reliability and validity? *J Gen Intern Med.* 2010;25:865-872. *Review of value of the full range of respiratory physical findings.*
Burki NK, Lee LY. Mechanisms of dyspnea. *Chest.* 2010;138:1196-1201. *Review.*
Pavord ID, Chung KF. Management of chronic cough. *Lancet.* 2008;371:1375-1384. *Useful review.*
Sakr L, Dutau H. Massive hemoptysis: an update on the role of bronchoscopy in diagnosis and management. *Respiration.* 2010;80:38-58. *Review.*

84 IMAGING IN PULMONARY DISEASE

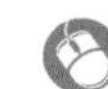

PAUL STARK

IMAGING OF THE LUNGS, MEDIASTINUM, AND CHEST WALL

EPIDEMIOLOGY

Worldwide, chest radiography is the most commonly performed imaging procedure; more than 75 million chest radiographs are performed every year in the United States alone. Chest radiographs provide useful information about the patient's anatomy and disease at a minimal monetary cost and with radiation exposure that most experts agree is negligible. Although many novel imaging techniques are available, the plain chest radiograph remains invaluable in the initial assessment of disorders of the lung, pleura, mediastinum, and chest wall.

Imaging Techniques

Chest radiographs, although classically obtained with cassettes and x-ray film, are now commonly acquired by digital imaging with electronic display at workstations and distribution of data through networks. Regardless of the image processing approach used, the standard chest radiograph is performed at 2 m from the x-ray tube focal spot to the image detector, in frontal and lateral projections. If possible, the radiographs should be obtained with the patient inhaling to total lung capacity. These images provide views of the lungs, mediastinum, and chest wall simultaneously.

Portable Radiography

Although bedside or portable radiography accounts for a large number of chest radiographs, the images obtained are generally of lower technical quality, cost more, and are more difficult to interpret. Lung volumes are low, thereby leading to crowding of vascular structures, and the low kilovoltage technique required for the mobile equipment yields radiographs with overexposed lungs and an underpenetrated mediastinum. The anteroposterior projection and the slightly lordotic angulation of the x-ray beam combine to distort the basal lung structures and magnify the cardiac silhouette. Recumbent studies also make recognition of pleural effusions or pneumothoraces more difficult.

Computed Tomography

Computed tomography (CT) has multiple advantages over conventional radiography. It displays cross-sectional anatomy free of superimposition, with a ten-fold higher contrast resolution. Multislice CT scanners acquire a continuous, volumetric, isotropic data set with possibilities for high-quality two-dimensional or three-dimensional reformatting (volume rendering) in any plane. High-resolution CT of the lung parenchyma is an important application; narrow collimation of the beam combined with an edge-enhancing high spatial frequency algorithm results in exquisite detail of normal and abnormal lungs, and correlation with pathologic anatomy is high.

Magnetic Resonance Imaging

Magnetic resonance imaging (MRI) depends on the magnetic properties of hydrogen atoms. Magnetic coils and radio frequency coils lead to induction,

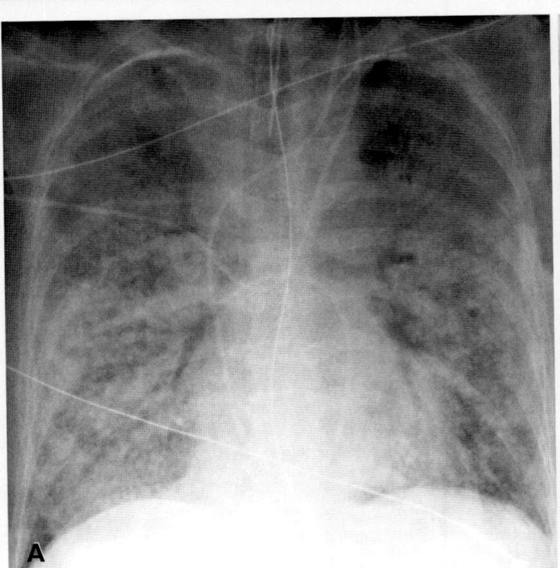

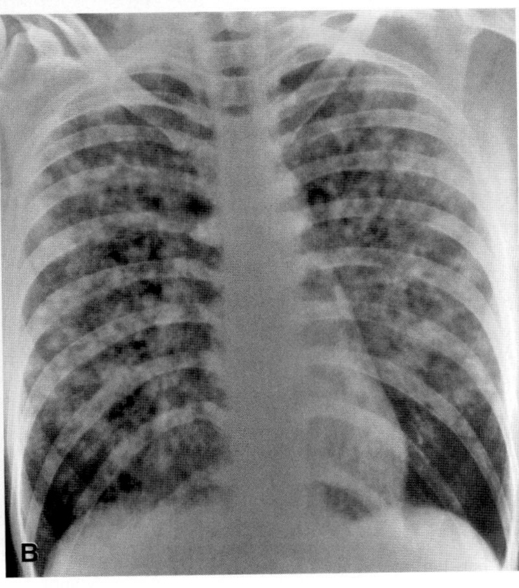

FIGURE 84-1. **A, Patient with diffuse alveolar damage.** Chest radiograph shows diffuse homogeneous opacification of both lungs with clearly visible air bronchograms. **B,** Patient with acute varicella pneumonia. Chest radiograph demonstrates multiple "acinar" nodules with tendency for confluence, yielding multifocal patchy parenchymal opacification.

excitation, and eventual readout of magnetized protons. The molecular environment of hydrogen atoms will affect the rate at which they release energy; this energy yields a spatial distribution of signals that is converted into an image by computer algorithms, similar to CT. Because of its soft tissue specificity, MRI has applications in the assessment of chest wall invasion, mediastinal infiltration, and diaphragmatic involvement by lung cancer or malignant mesothelioma.

Positron Emission Tomography

Fluorodeoxyglucose positron emission tomography (FDG-PET) uses labeled fluorodeoxyglucose to image the glycolytic pathway of tumor cells or other metabolically active tissues with affinity for glucose. This technique has proved helpful in studying intrathoracic tumors and has facilitated the work-up of solitary pulmonary nodules. Integrated PET-CT scans have improved the diagnosis and staging of intrathoracic tumors. 1

Ultrasonography

Outside the heart, ultrasonography plays only a limited role in thoracic imaging. Its primary use is to localize pleural effusions and to guide their drainage.

Evaluation of Chest Images

Images of the chest are best evaluated by examining regions of the lung for specific findings and relating these findings to known diagnostic groups. A number of critical radiographic features should be considered, with an appreciation for the known causes of these changes.

Diffuse Lung Disease

Diffuse lung disease is an overall term for a number of related abnormal parenchymal radiographic patterns. Although radiologists have attempted to separate alveolar from interstitial lung disease radiographically, this distinction is no longer recommended because the correlation between the radiographic localization to a compartment and the actual histopathologic findings is relatively poor. For example, nodular patterns can be produced by either interstitial or alveolar disease. Conversely, so-called alveolar disease processes can induce an interstitial reaction. Ground-glass opacities can be induced by either alveolar or interstitial disease. Air bronchograms, the presumed paradigm of air space disease, can be identified in a small percentage of patients with predominantly interstitial lung disease, such as sarcoidosis, pulmonary lymphoma, and pulmonary calcinosis.

Because of such limitations, a graphically descriptive approach that combines analysis of predominant opacities, assessment of lung expansion, and distribution and profusion of disease yields a differential diagnosis. The term *infiltrate* should be avoided; instead, pulmonary opacities are classified as large (i.e., >1 cm in largest dimension) or small (i.e., <1 cm in diameter).

TABLE 84-1 CLASSIFICATION OF LARGE PULMONARY OPACITIES

Diffuse homogeneous
Multifocal patchy
Lobar without atelectasis
Lobar with atelectasis
Perihilar
Peripheral

Large Opacities

Large opacities (Table 84-1) are characterized according to their distribution. Diffuse homogeneous opacities are typical for diffuse alveolar damage (Fig. 84-1A), increased permeability (noncardiogenic) pulmonary edema, diffuse viral pneumonia, or *Pneumocystis jirovecii* pneumonia. Multifocal patchy opacities (see Fig. 84-1B) are found in multifocal bronchopneumonia, recurrent aspiration, or vasculitis. Lobar opacities without atelectasis are typically seen in lobar pneumonia. Lobar opacities with atelectasis often result from obstruction of a lobar bronchus by foreign bodies, tumors, or mucous plugs. Perihilar opacities are seen in hydrostatic pulmonary edema due to left-sided heart failure (Fig. 84-2), renal failure, volume overload, or pulmonary hemorrhage.

Small Opacities

In contrast to the large pulmonary opacities, a number of radiographic patterns characterize small pulmonary opacities in diffuse lung disease. It is helpful to differentiate small nodular, linear, reticular, or combined patterns (Table 84-2). Micronodular opacities, which include nodules 1 mm and smaller in diameter, can result from talc granulomatosis in intravenous drug abusers (Chapter 33), alveolar microlithiasis, rare cases of silicosis, talcosis, coal workers' pneumoconiosis (Chapter 93), and beryllium-induced lung diseases (Chapter 93) as well as from occasional cases of sarcoidosis (Chapter 95) or hemosiderosis. The nodular pattern includes nodules up to 1 cm in diameter. Frequent causes include infections or inflammatory granulomas such as miliary tuberculosis (Chapter 332), sarcoidosis (Chapter 95), fungal diseases, extrinsic allergic alveolitis, and Langerhans cell histiocytosis (Chapter 92).

Linear Patterns

Linear patterns, also called Kerley's lines, are mostly a reflection of thickened interlobular septa. Kerley's A lines, which radiate 2 to 4 cm from the hilum toward the pulmonary periphery and particularly toward the upper lobes (Fig. 84-3), reflect thickening of the axial interstitial compartment and can be a feature of left ventricular failure or allergic reactions. Kerley's B lines,

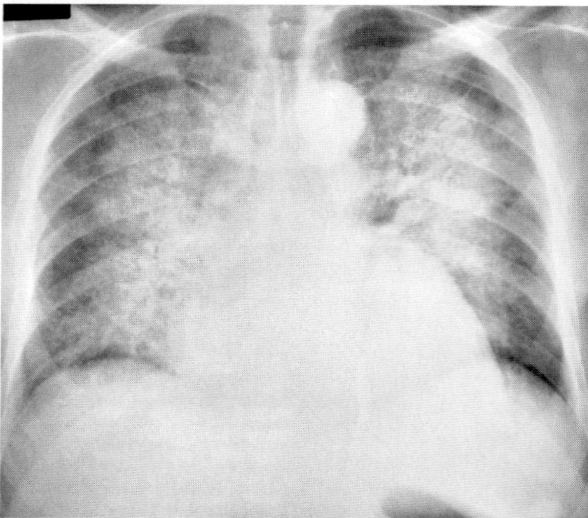

FIGURE 84-2. Patient with hydrostatic pulmonary edema due to left-sided heart failure. Chest frontal radiograph demonstrates classic "batwing" distribution of pulmonary edema.

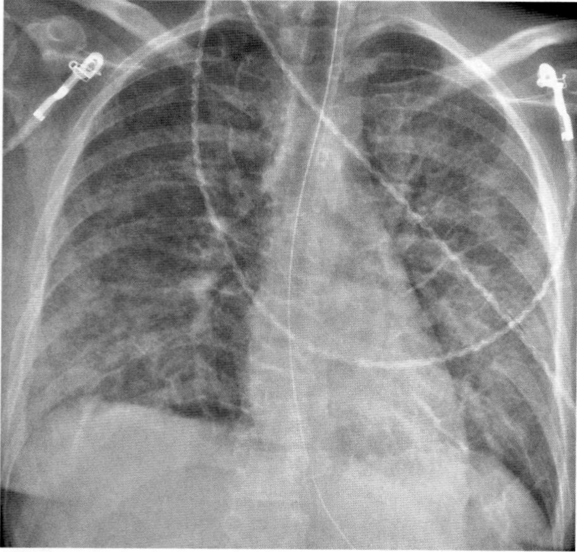

FIGURE 84-3. Patient with known transfusion reaction. Chest radiograph displays ground-glass opacification of both lungs and bilateral Kerley's A lines, presenting as long linear structures extending from the hilar regions into the pulmonary periphery.

TABLE 84-2 PATTERNS OF SMALL PULMONARY OPACITIES

Micronodular
Acinar
Linear
Reticular
Bronchial
Arterial
Destructive

which reflect thickening of the subpleural interstitial compartment, typically are about 1 cm in length and 1 mm in thickness and usually found in the periphery of the lower lobes, abutting the pleura. The B lines are characteristic of subacute and chronic left ventricular failure (Chapter 58), mitral valve disease (Chapter 75), lymphangitic carcinomatosis, viral pneumonia, and pulmonary fibrosis (Chapter 92). Kerley's C lines, which are rarely diagnosed by radiologists, result from thickening of the lung parenchymal interstitium and form a reticular pattern on chest radiographs.

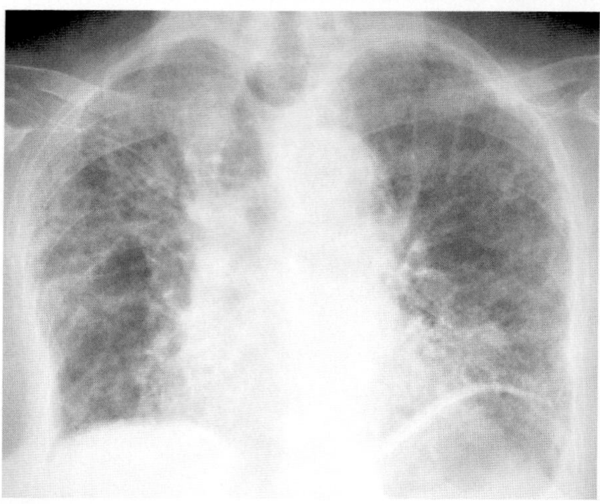

FIGURE 84-4. Diffuse reticular lung disease. Chest radiograph in a 94-year-old patient with diffuse reticular opacities due to idiopathic pulmonary fibrosis with honeycombing and traction bronchiectases. The lung volumes are typically reduced by a decreased pulmonary compliance.

Reticular Patterns

Reticular patterns are small polygonal, irregular, or curvilinear opacities on chest radiographs (Fig. 84-4). The differential diagnosis varies according to the timeline of the pathologic change. Acute onset of a reticular pattern can occur in interstitial edema (e.g., due to left-sided heart failure), atypical pneumonitides (e.g., viral or mycoplasmal pneumonia), early exudative changes in a connective tissue disorder (e.g., systemic lupus erythematosus; Chapter 274), and acute allergic reactions (e.g., transfusion reactions [Chapter 180] or reactions to *Hymenoptera* stings). The common chronic processes resulting in a reticular pattern are idiopathic interstitial pneumonias (Chapter 92), connective tissue diseases (particularly scleroderma and rheumatoid lung), asbestosis (Chapter 93), radiation fibrosis (Chapter 92), end-stage hypersensitivity pneumonia (Chapters 92 and 93), drug reactions, lymphangitic spread of cancer, end-stage granulomatous infection, lymphoma in its bronchovascular form, Kaposi's sarcoma in its bronchovascular manifestation, and sarcoidosis.

Honeycombing

Honeycombing, which is an indication of end-stage interstitial lung disease (Chapter 92), reflects a restructuring of pulmonary anatomy accompanied by bronchiolectasis. Honeycombs form a multilayer of small subpleural spaces between 3 and 10 mm in diameter. They can be distinguished from paraseptal emphysema by their thicker wall and multiple layers.

Alveolar Pattern

An alveolar (Chapter 91) or air space pattern is characterized by acinar nodules, 0.6 to 1 cm in diameter. These nodules encompass more than the acinus, in the strict anatomic sense, with surrounding peribronchiolar lung tissue. Other patterns include ground-glass opacities (a reflection of incomplete alveolar filling), coalescent large opacities, consolidation involving whole lobes or segments, opacification in a bronchocentric distribution, air bronchograms, and air alveolograms. These radiographic features are helpful in placing a disease into a particular radiologic category, but the radiographic pattern called *alveolar* does not simply correspond to exclusive histologic alveolar filling because the interstitial compartment is involved as well in most cases. A more accurate description is parenchymal rather than alveolar opacification or consolidation.

Bronchial Patterns

Bronchial patterns, as best depicted by diffuse bronchiectasis (Chapter 90), are seen on conventional radiographs as linear, tubular, or cystic lucencies and opacities that follow the expected path of bronchi, so-called tramlines because they resemble tram tracks. Mucoid impaction, as seen in patients with asthma, allergic bronchopulmonary aspergillosis, or plastic bronchitis, leads to opacities described as toothpaste, cluster of grapes, or finger-in-glove. The "dirty lung" pattern seen in smokers with chronic bronchitis (Chapter 88) results from bronchial wall thickening, peribronchial fibrosis, respiratory bronchiolitis, and pulmonary arterial hypertension.

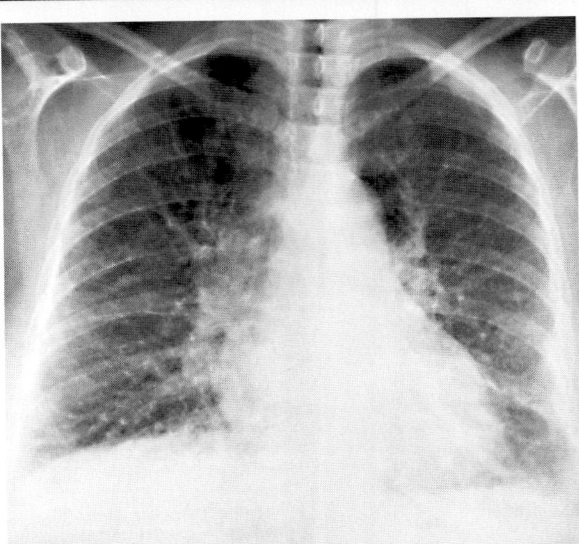

FIGURE 84-5. Patient with left ventricular failure. Chest frontal radiograph shows cephalization of pulmonary blood flow.

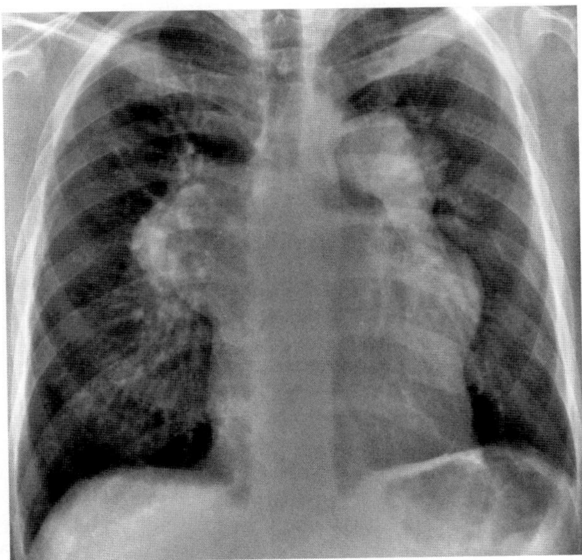

FIGURE 84-6. Patient with primary pulmonary arterial hypertension. Chest frontal radiograph shows centralization of flow with pulmonary artery aneurysms and peripheral pulmonary oligemia.

Vascular Patterns

Arterial patterns reflect changes in pulmonary perfusion. The term *caudalization* reflects the normal blood flow distribution pattern in an upright person in which the basilar pulmonary vessels are two to three times wider than the upper lobe vasculature. *Cephalization,* in which the ratios of diameters of vessels are reversed, is frequently seen in recumbent persons, in whom it may be considered normal; however, when it is present in individuals imaged in the upright position, it indicates left ventricular failure, mitral valve disease, or basilar emphysema (Fig. 84-5). Equalization, or balanced flow with well-demonstrated vessels to upper and lower lung zones, is found in hyperkinetic circulation due to anemia, obesity, pregnancy, Graves' disease, or left-to-right shunts. Equalization or balanced flow with oligemia can be seen in hypovolemia, diffuse emphysema, or right-to-left shunts. Centralization reflects dilation of central pulmonary vessels, with accompanying normal or diminished peripheral circulation. Typically, it is seen in pulmonary arterial hypertension (Fig. 84-6). Lateralization of flow, favoring one lung over the other, also called *asymmetrical perfusion,* is visible with unilateral emphysema, unilateral bronchiolitis obliterans (Swyer-James-McLeod syndrome), or unilateral obstruction of the pulmonary artery. Locally enlarged vessels occur in patchy emphysema, multiple pulmonary emboli, arteriovenous malformations, and

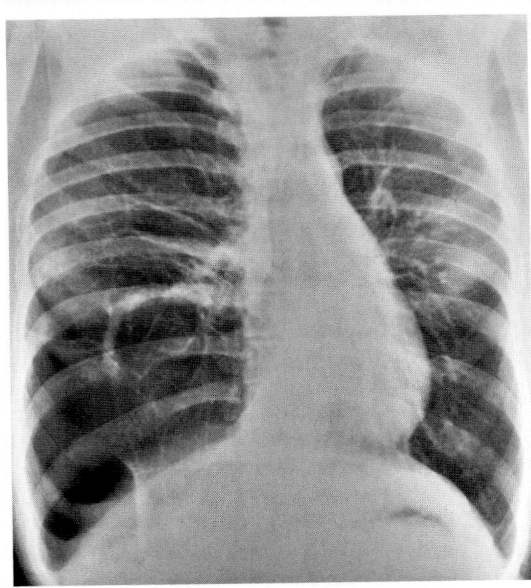

FIGURE 84-7. Patient with severe emphysema. Chest radiograph shows hyperexpansion of both lungs with bullous changes at the right lung base and leftward mediastinal shift.

TABLE 84-3 CONDITIONS ASSOCIATED WITH VARIOUS LUNG VOLUMES IN PATIENTS WITH AN UNDERLYING DIFFUSE LUNG DISEASE PATTERN

LARGE LUNG VOLUMES
Emphysema Chronic asthma Diffuse bronchiolitis obliterans Highly trained athletes Lymphangioleiomyomatosis
SMALL LUNG VOLUMES
End-stage lung fibrosis Bilateral diaphragmatic paralysis Massive ascites
NORMAL LUNG VOLUMES
Sarcoidosis Langerhans cell histiocytosis Neurofibromatosis Emphysema with pulmonary fibrosis

nonuniform bronchiolitis obliterans. This pattern produces a mosaic perfusion on high-resolution CT scanning.

Lung Volume

Conventional radiographs and CT scans are taken during a breath hold at full inspiration. Low lung volumes are inferred by the high position of the diaphragm and the crowding of basal vascular structures (Table 84-3). Lung volumes larger than expected are commonly found in patients with diffuse emphysema (Fig. 84-7) (Chapter 88), chronic asthma (Chapter 87), or diffuse bronchiolitis and in highly trained athletes. With a few rare exceptions, chronic diffuse infiltrative lung diseases (Chapter 92) lead to loss of volume.

Anatomic Distribution

The anatomic distribution of disease can significantly facilitate the approach to diagnosis (Table 84-4 and Fig. 84-8). Upper-zone lung disease predominates in tuberculosis, fungal disease, sarcoidosis, pneumoconiosis (except asbestosis), Langerhans cell histiocytosis, ankylosing spondylitis, cystic fibrosis, cystic *P. jirovecii* pneumonia, radiation pneumonitis, and end-stage hypersensitivity pneumonia. Basal lung disease is preferentially found in bronchiectases, aspiration, desquamative interstitial pneumonia, nonspecific interstitial pneumonia, usual interstitial pneumonia, drug reactions, asbestosis, scleroderma, and rheumatoid arthritis. However, any diffuse lung

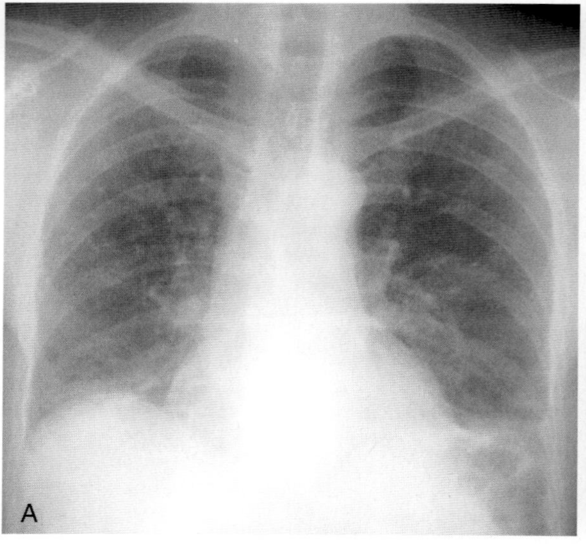

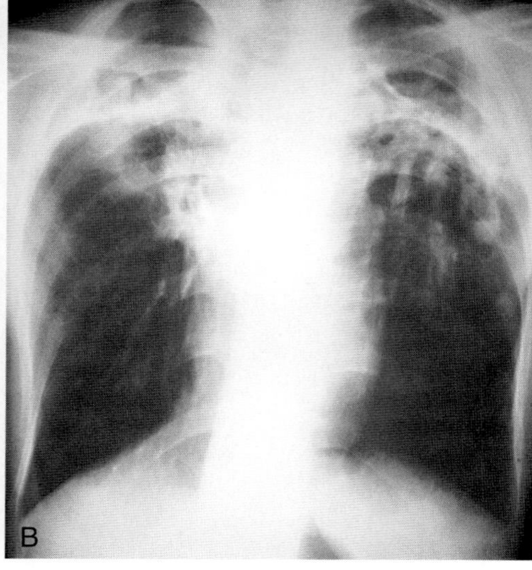

FIGURE 84-8. **A, Basilar pulmonary disease.** Chest radiograph in a 48-year-old patient with known scleroderma. Bibasilar fine reticular opacities and parenchymal bands are visible in both lower lobes. **B,** Apical lung disease. Chest radiograph in a 42-year-old patient with ankylosing spondylitis. Severe architectural distortion with cicatrizing atelectasis of both upper lobes, retraction of both pulmonary arteries cephalad, and bilateral bulla formation containing fungus balls are evident.

TABLE 84-4 CONDITIONS ASSOCIATED WITH DISEASE DISTRIBUTION PATTERNS

UPPER ZONE LUNG DISEASE
Tuberculosis
Fungal disease
Sarcoidosis
Pneumoconioses
Langerhans cell histiocytosis
Cystic fibrosis
End-stage hypersensitivity pneumonitis
Ankylosing spondylitis
Radiation pneumonitis
BASILAR LUNG DISEASE
Bronchiectasis
Aspiration
Drug reactions
Interstitial pulmonary fibrosis, nonspecific interstitial pneumonitis, desquamative interstitial pneumonitis, cryptogenic organizing pneumonia, bronchiolitis obliterans with organizing pneumonia
Asbestosis
Scleroderma

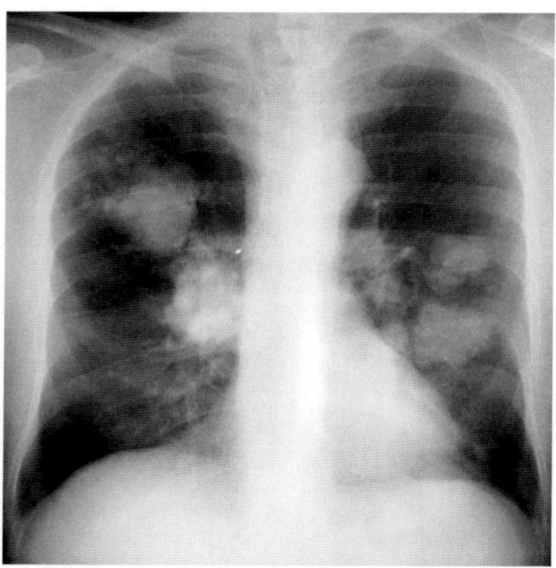

FIGURE 84-9. **Multifocal pulmonary opacities.** Chest radiograph in a 70-year-old patient with known carcinoma of the thyroid gland widening the superior mediastinum and displacing the cervical trachea to the right. Bilateral large and small pulmonary nodules and masses due to metastatic tumor are present.

process will eventually progress to involve both lungs irrespective of zonal boundaries.

Lymph Nodes

Enlarged lymph nodes that are visible on chest CT scans and, when larger, on chest radiographs can provide diagnostic information (Table 84-5). The following entities can be associated with diffuse lung disease and concurrent enlarged lymph nodes: sarcoidosis (Chapter 95); lymphoma; fungal disease; tuberculosis (Chapter 332); pneumoconioses (Chapter 93), particularly silicosis and beryllium-associated lung disease; lung cancer; and metastatic malignant disease other than lung cancer.

TABLE 84-5 CONDITIONS ASSOCIATED WITH HILAR AND MEDIASTINAL LYMPH NODE ENLARGEMENT

Sarcoidosis
Lymphoma
Fungal disease
Tuberculosis
Metastatic cancer
Silicosis, coal worker's pneumoconiosis, beryllium lung

Pulmonary Nodules

Solitary pulmonary nodules are covered in Chapter 197. Most patients with multiple pulmonary nodules larger than 1 cm in diameter have metastatic disease from primary cancers either within or outside the lung (Fig. 84-9). These lesions have a predilection for subpleural lung regions, including the interlobar fissures. In patients with human immunodeficiency virus infection, Kaposi's sarcoma and lymphoma can induce the formation of such nodules. Infectious processes that present with multiple nodules include multiple abscesses from recurrent aspiration (Chapter 94) or septic emboli (Chapter 76); tuberculous and nontuberculous mycobacterial granulomas (Chapters 332 and 333); fungal processes, including histoplasmosis (Chapter 340), coccidioidomycosis (Chapter 341), and cryptococcosis (Chapter 344); and infection with flukes, such as *Paragonimus westermani* (Chapter 364). Noninfectious inflammatory conditions that can present with multiple pulmonary nodules include Wegener's granulomatosis (Chapter 278), rheumatoid nodules (Chapter 272), sarcoidosis (Chapter 95), and amyloidosis (Chapter 194).

Pleural Disease

Pleural diseases are covered in Chapter 99. Abnormalities of the pleural space easily can be displayed by conventional radiographic methods supplemented by CT scanning. The volume of pleural effusions can be reliably estimated on standard posteroanterior films: 75 mL obscures the posterior costophrenic sulcus, 150 mL obscures the lateral costophrenic sulcus, 200 mL produces a

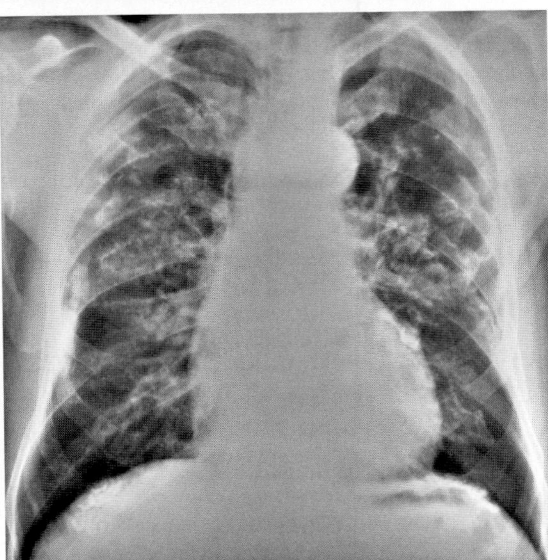

FIGURE 84-10. **Patient with known prior occupational asbestos exposure.** Chest radiograph shows extensive bilateral calcified plaques seen en face, in profile, and along the diaphragmatic contour.

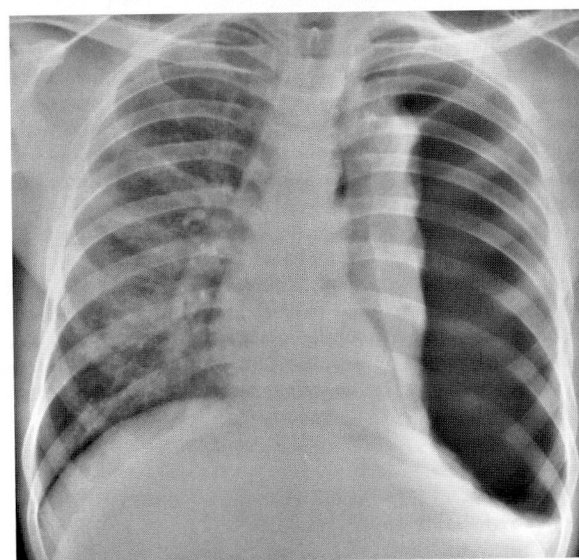

FIGURE 84-11. **Patient with spontaneous tension hydropneumothorax.** Chest radiograph shows complete atelectasis of the left lung with a large pneumothorax and a left basilar gas-liquid level. The patient had primary tuberculosis.

rind of 1 cm in thickness on decubitus films, 500 mL obscures the diaphragm and is visible on supine radiographs, and 1000-mL effusions reach the level of the fourth anterior rib on upright chest radiographs. An effusion of 200 mL or more can be sampled by thoracentesis. The smallest amount visible on decubitus radiographs is 10 mL. With care, as little as 175 mL of effusion can be detected on supine images. Free layering effusions produce a veil of opacity or filter effect superimposed on the aerated lung; pulmonary vessels are clearly visible through the added opacity generated by the effusion, and air bronchograms are absent.

Subpulmonic Effusions

Subpulmonic effusions elevate the lung base, mimicking a high-riding hemidiaphragm. The highest curvature point of the pseudodiaphragm is shifted laterally. Large effusions can lead to diaphragmatic inversion. Separation of the lung base from the gas-containing stomach is indicative of a subpulmonic effusion, particularly when the stomach gas bubble is displaced inferomedially. Loculated pleural effusions suggest the presence of pleural adhesions. Such encapsulated collections have obtuse angles of interface with the chest wall and have a sharply defined border with the adjacent lung.

Pleural Plaques

Pleural plaques result from parietal pleural accumulation of hyalinized collagen fibers (Fig. 84-10); their presence suggests asbestos exposure (Chapter 93). Plaques preferentially involve the parietal pleura adjacent to ribs six through nine and the diaphragm. They are less pronounced in the intercostal spaces and spare the costophrenic sulci as well as the apices. Calcifications are visible on chest radiographs in 20% and on CT scans in 50% of individuals with plaques. Imaged in profile, pleural plaques produce focal areas of apparent pleural thickening. Over the diaphragm, they appear as curvilinear calcifications or scalloping. Pleural plaques viewed en face can simulate lung disease. Their appearance has been likened to holly leaves, sunburst patterns, "geographic" patterns, or stippled or irregular structures. Rare visceral pleural plaques that occur in interlobar fissures can mimic pulmonary nodules.

Diffuse Pleural Thickening

Diffuse pleural thickening is a response observed after exposure to any of a number of stimuli including infection, inflammation, trauma, tumor, thromboembolism, radiation, and asbestos. Severe involvement results in formation of a generalized pleural peel with smooth margins, usually less than 2 cm in thickness. Radiologically diffuse pleural thickening is characterized by a smooth, noninterrupted pleural opacity involving at least one fourth of the chest wall circumference, obliterating the costophrenic sulci and encompassing also the apices. The CT criteria for diffuse pleural thickening include a thickness of at least 3 mm.

Malignant Disease

Malignant tumors of the pleura are more common than benign ones, and metastatic disease is more frequent than primary pleural mesothelioma. Primary tumors originate from pleural membranes. Pleural invasion by lung cancer, subpleural plaques in lymphoma, hematogenous dissemination to the pleura, and direct pleural seeding are other mechanisms of pleural involvement by tumor. Benign pleural tumors include lipomas, fibrous tumors, and neurogenic tumors. Lipomas are most common; their diagnosis is facilitated by CT scanning. Fibrous tumors of the pleura originate from pluripotent mesenchymal cells found in the visceral pleura or, less commonly, in the parietal pleura. They can induce paraneoplastic syndromes such as hypertrophic osteoarthropathy (Chapter 187) or hypoglycemia and only rarely invade or metastasize. In nearly half of these patients, the tumor can be on a pedicle and be mobile as a patient changes position.

Pneumothorax

Pneumothorax means gas in the pleural space (Chapter 99). The most important radiologic feature of a pneumothorax is a visceral pleural line or edge that is convex or straight toward the chest wall and produces a lucent separation of the visceral and parietal pleura (Fig. 84-11). In most cases, no pulmonary vascular structures are visible beyond the visceral pleura. On upright chest radiographs, gas is primarily found in the apicolateral pleural space. Expiratory chest radiographs are not necessary for the detection of small pneumothoraces because all pneumothoraces are visible on inspiratory films. On supine chest radiographs, pleural gas accumulates in a subpulmonic location; it outlines the costophrenic sulcus, forming the deep sulcus sign. A tension pneumothorax leads to a marked shift of the mediastinum to the contralateral side and to flattening or inversion of the ipsilateral hemidiaphragm.

Imaging of the Mediastinum

The mediastinum encompasses midline thoracic structures that are delineated by mediastinal pleura, the diaphragm, the sternum, the spine, and the thoracic inlet. The mediastinum is commonly divided into an anterior compartment, a visceral middle compartment, and a paraspinal, posterior mediastinal compartment (Table 84-6). Each compartment contains specific pathologic entities.

Imaging Techniques

On well-penetrated chest radiographs, the anterior junction line, the posterior-superior junction line, the azygoesophageal stripe, the pleuroesophageal stripe, the paratracheal stripe, and the para-aortic and the paraspinal stripes or lines should be assessed (Fig. 84-12). Mediastinal masses need to be detected and localized first. Their obtuse angles of interface with the mediastinal pleura, as well as extension into both hemithoraces, indicate the mediastinal origin of such lesions.

CT facilitates localization of a mass to a specific mediastinal compartment. When it is known whether the mass is predominantly fat, cystic, soft tissue, or calcified, the differential diagnosis can be limited. MRI of the mediastinum has a role in diagnosis of vertebral disease or neurogenic tumors with extension into the spinal canal. It is as good as CT in diagnosis of aortic aneurysms and dissections (Chapter 78).

Mediastinal Compartments

The anterior mediastinum is actually a potential space that may contain the fatty replaced thymus and small normal lymph nodes. Space-occupying lesions in this compartment typically include thymomas, lymphomas, teratomas and other germ cell tumors, substernal thyroid goiters, lipomas, and other connective tissue tumors as well as hemangiomas or lymphangiomas (Fig. 84-13A).

TABLE 84-6 CLASSIFICATION OF MEDIASTINAL COMPARTMENTS

ANTERIOR MEDIASTINUM
Retrosternal
MIDDLE MEDIASTINUM—VISCERAL COMPARTMENT
Subcarinal space Paratracheal region Retrotracheal space Aortic-pulmonic window Retrocardiac space
POSTERIOR MEDIASTINUM
Paraspinal region

The middle mediastinum is subdivided into the subcarinal space, paratracheal region, retrotracheal region, aortic-pulmonic window region, and retrocardiac space. Characteristic lesions are enlarged lymph nodes and bronchopulmonary foregut malformations (see Fig. 84-13B).

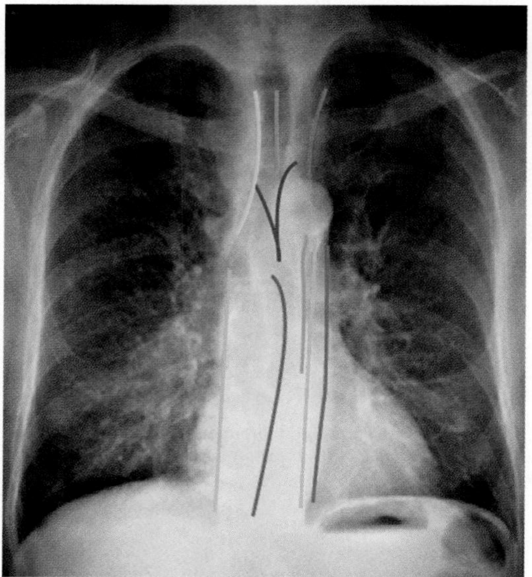

FIGURE 84-12. Chest radiograph with superimposed mediastinal stripes. *Yellow:* right paratracheal stripe. *Light blue:* right and left paraspinal stripes. *Red:* azygoesophageal stripe. *Brown:* pleuroesophageal stripe. *Purple:* anterior junction line complex. *Pink:* left subclavian artery border. *Light green:* posterior-superior junction line. *Dark green:* para-aortic line.

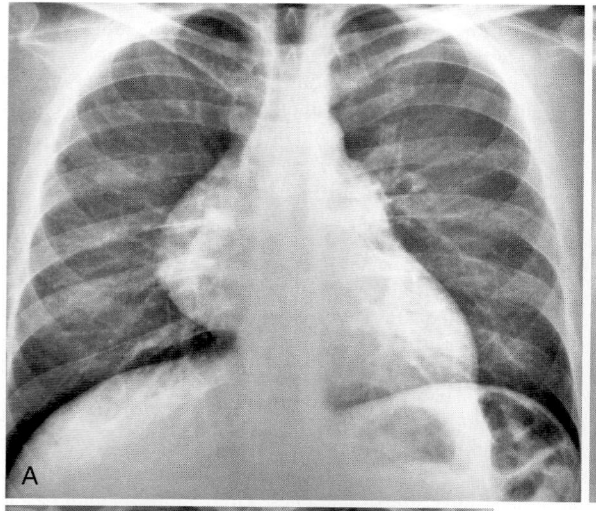

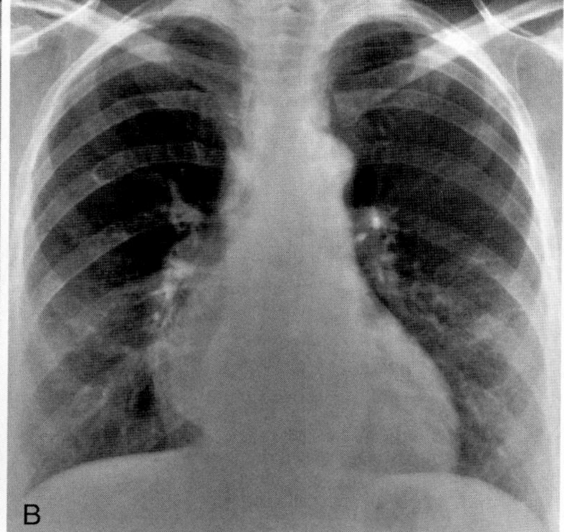

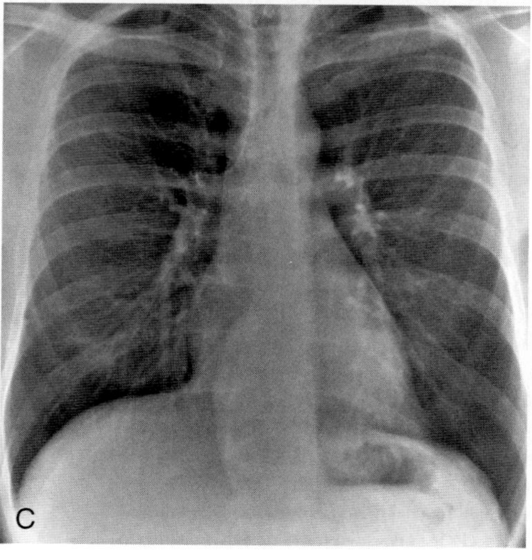

FIGURE 84-13. A, Patient with anterior mediastinal teratoma. Chest radiograph shows a mediastinal contour abnormality due to projection of the mass into the right hemithorax. Note the obtuse angle of interface formed by the pleura covering the mass with the mediastinum. **B,** Patient with Castleman's giant lymph node hyperplasia. Chest frontal radiograph shows large subcarinal middle mediastinal mass that projects lateral to the right atrium. **C,** Patient with paraspinal ganglioneuroma. Chest radiograph shows right lower paraspinal contour abnormality widening the right paraspinal region and encompassing the height of three thoracic vertebrae.

In the retrotracheal region, aberrant right subclavian arteries, posterior descending goiters, esophageal tumors, diverticula, or thoracic duct cysts can be found. In the aortic-pulmonic window, ductus diverticula, bronchopulmonary foregut malformations, or aortic or pulmonic artery aneurysms can form compartment-specific space-occupying lesions.

The paraspinal region is considered radiologically to belong to the posterior mediastinum. Important masses in that space include neurogenic tumors that originate from the sympathetic chain or from segmental nerve roots (see Fig. 84-13C). Extramedullary hematopoiesis in patients with severe anemia can result in paravertebral masses formed by hypertrophied bone marrow that extrudes from ribs or vertebral bodies. Enlarged lymph nodes due to lymphoma or metastatic disease are occasionally seen in a paraspinal location. Vertebral disease, including bacterial or tuberculous spondylitis, tumors, and post-traumatic hematomas, can widen the paraspinal region and produce contour abnormalities.

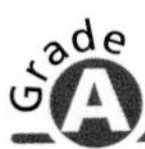

1. Fischer B, Lassen U, Mortensen J, et al. Preoperative staging of lung cancer with combined PET-CT. *N Engl J Med*. 2009;361:32-39.

SUGGESTED READINGS

Oba Y, Zaza T. Abandoning daily routine chest radiography in the intensive care unit: meta-analysis. *Radiology*. 2010;255:386-395. *Chest radiography can be ordered selectively without increasing adverse outcomes.*

Petinaux B, Bhat R, Boniface K, et al. Accuracy of radiographic readings in the emergency department. *Am J Emerg Med*. 2011;29:18-25. *Approximately 3% of radiographs are incorrectly read by the emergency physician, with air-space disease and pulmonary nodules most commonly misread on chest radiographs.*

85

RESPIRATORY STRUCTURE AND FUNCTION: MECHANISMS AND TESTING

HERBERT Y. REYNOLDS

The lungs are designed for oxygen uptake and carbon dioxide elimination through the process of ventilation and molecular diffusion. To maintain health, purified air must be presented to the alveolar epithelial surface to aerate pulmonary capillary blood. Ambient air, which contains environmental debris, microbes, and possibly solubilized toxins and is admixed at times with aspirated oropharyngeal secretions, must be cleansed. Inspired ambient air encounters a system of host defenses that usually removes these contaminants mechanically (by sneezing, rhinorrhea, coughing, and mucociliary clearance), through innate (natural) immunity mechanisms, or immunologically through adaptive (acquired) immunity. This nonventilatory function can be missing (primary host defects) or compromised by systemic illness or the side effects of other medical therapy. Because ventilation and nonventilatory function are so intertwined, both are described together; methods for assessment of clinical function then follow.

RESPIRATORY STRUCTURE AND FUNCTION

Respiratory Tract Structure

Although the respiratory tract is a continuum of branching tubes leading to the air exchange-alveolar surface, it functionally has four distinct anatomic segments: naso-oropharynx or upper airways, conducting airways (larynx, trachea, and bronchi that branch to terminal bronchioles), respiratory bronchioles, and alveolar ducts and alveoli. Vascular and neural structures are integral to each segment; lymphatic channels begin at the level of respiratory bronchioles and flow upward or cephalad into the hilar nodes. But much still remains unknown about various cell lineages contributing to development of the lung, the phenotype and function of perhaps half of the approximately 40 resident cells that compose the human respiratory tract, and the roles of neuroendocrine cells and various progenitor cells that can replenish structural cells after injury.

The airways and their accompanying blood supply develop from an evagination of the foregut and primitive esophagus. The conducting airways form a continuum of approximately 14 generations of branches, which are extended by another 10 or so branches within the acinar airways, finally ending as alveolar sacs. This anatomic structure has been described as a tree with irregular, dichotomously branching tubes. Later developments in the fetus initiate progressive thinning of the mucosal epithelial layer in distal bronchi and then the respiratory bronchioles to a single cell surface, which defines the beginning of the gas exchange unit within the acinar-alveolar structures. Mechanisms to cleanse inspired air are dispersed along the entire tract.

The *naso-oropharynx* includes the upper airways and associated sinuses (Chapter 434). It begins at the nares and lips and extends back through a richly vascular, undulant mucosal covering of the nasal passage, through the glottis, into the extrathoracic trachea. Nasal hairs and turbinates filter out large particles (>10 μm diameter) as inspired air passes over the nasal surface in a turbulent flow pattern. In this process, air is humidified and warmed as it passes through the nose and over the soft palate; it typically is fully conditioned before it reaches the posterior pharynx. Because sinus and posterior nasal secretions can collect in the posterior pharynx, deglutition and respiration are coordinated exquisitely by the epiglottis and laryngeal musculature to direct fluids and food into the esophagus and air into the subglottic trachea. Control is not perfect, however, and microaspiration can occur in normal persons during sleep. Esophageal reflux can cause cough in normal individuals and asthma symptoms in patients with more hyperreactive airways (Chapters 87 and 140). Mucociliary clearance declines with age, explaining in part the more frequent occurrence of respiratory infections in elderly patients.

The *conducting airways* begin with the trachea, a flexible tube held open by cartilaginous, horseshoe-shaped rings with a posterior muscular face that abuts the esophagus. The trachea is about 10 cm in length and contains about 15 rings. At the carina, it divides into two major bronchi, and thereafter multiple smaller bronchial branches diverge through many generations of smaller divisions. In aggregate, however, the branching creates a much greater overall cross-sectional area that not only reduces resistance to airflow but also decelerates the velocity of air molecules as they prepare to enter the acinar ducts and alveolar sacs. Airflow beyond the conducting airways is largely laminar; the slower movement further cleanses the air by allowing the settling out of any 0.5- to 3-μm particulates that still are present and would be impacted at branching points. This action seems especially important in the respiratory bronchioles, which serve as the transition segment between the conducting airways and alveoli, where several adaptations facilitate further removal of particulates or antigens. Throughout the conducting airways (E-Fig. 85-1), the mucosal surface provides a barrier function because of the tight apical junctions between epithelial cells. About half of the epithelial cells are ciliated; a fluid film and mucus cover the beating cilia, creating the mucociliary apparatus. The thickness of the mucosal surface attenuates as the pseudostratified cell layer flattens to become a single cell layer in the terminal bronchioles. Here the less protected surface may become more vulnerable to injury from inhaled toxins and microbes and more susceptible to ravages of chronic inflammation (bronchiolitis).

The airway layer of pseudostratified epithelial cells creates a physical barrier by forming tight apical junctions that control permeability and promote pericellular ion and fluid flux. About half of the epithelial cells have cilia to propel a covering layer of fluid and admixed mucus that can collect airway debris and eliminate it by a process known as *mucociliary clearance*. These epithelial cells have dynamic turnover of several days, with continuous self-renewal from progenitor stem cells, but the normal replication rate may vary at different locations along the airways. If airway injury has destroyed epithelial cells and denuded the surface, regeneration begins quickly from reservoirs of self-renewing stem cells found in niches in the ducts of submucosal glands in the trachea or bronchi and within the surface epithelium of more distal airways.

The *respiratory bronchioles*, which are positioned between the distal conducting airways and the alveolized air exchange surface, functionally separate the upper and lower respiratory tracts. This segment is a bottleneck for airflow and a last surface to capture small particulates and microbial or antigenic debris before the alveolar space; immune responses can be initiated here. The respiratory bronchioles can be the site of airway obstruction, caused by inflammation; a common form is termed *bronchiolitis obliterans* (Chapter 92) and is associated with several lung diseases, such as chronic graft rejection after lung transplantation (Chapter 101) and lung involvement by collagen vascular diseases (Chapter 92). In this transition region of the airway, several changes occur: the single-layer cuboidal epithelial surface further differentiates into alveolar type I cells that cover the alveolar lining surface;

mucus-secreting cells disappear, although goblet cells can develop in cigarette smokers; and another secretory cell type emerges, the Clara cells. Pulmonary brush cells with a tuft of squat microvilli are dense in this area and may be involved with chemosensing or trapping of inhaled particles and pollutants as well as with regulation of fluid and solute absorption. Also, many dendritic macrophage-like cells, which may constitute 1% of the cells, are present to capture antigens. Surface host defenses change from mucociliary clearance to macrophage phagocytes, inflammatory cells (neutrophils or eosinophils), and opsonins. Lymphatic channels form to collect the lymphatic fluid squeezed up from the interalveolar interstitial spaces into lymphatic capillaries that course along pulmonary capillaries and venules in the alveolar walls. The bronchial arterial circulation supplies the conducting airways, whereas the pulmonary arterial to pulmonary capillary circulation encompasses the alveoli and is the locus for diffusion of oxygen into the blood and carbon dioxide from the blood.

The *air exchange* compartment, or the alveolar space, is composed of about 480 million alveoli supported by a fibrous scaffolding and intertwined with a meshwork of pulmonary artery capillaries that permit air-blood contact. Oxygen uptake and carbon dioxide elimination occur across a thin tissue layer of type I epithelial cells and capillary endothelium that in aggregate creates a large surface area of approximately 130 square feet. To increase the likelihood that respiratory function will support a healthy human lifespan despite pollutants, infections, or systemic diseases that affect the lungs, an intricate system of host defenses has evolved. The system specialized for the alveoli is different from the system described in the proximal airways. Although an alveolus is reasonably protected from airborne debris by aerodynamic filtration that occurs in the upper respiratory tract, small particles (<0.5 μm) can remain suspended in air or toxic gases can gain access to the alveoli directly.

Cellular Host Defenses

Respiratory host defenses balance two mechanisms that eliminate or detoxify microbes and other antigenic materials that enter the airways (E-Fig. 85-2). First is an innate or quick response reaction that produces inflammation as an end point (bronchitis or pneumonitis) with subsequent apoptosis of neutrophils and suppression of inflammation to limit the reaction. Second is a more deliberate approach that stimulates lymphocytic pathways, creating a versatile and adaptive response involving specific T-cell activity or production of immunoglobulins (antibodies).

Microbes can be contained in aspirated fluid or carried intravascularly to the parenchyma (septicemia). A microbe entering an alveolus may encounter an antigen-presenting cell or several opsonins in the epithelial lining fluid, including immunoglobulin (Ig) G antibodies (IgG1 and IgG3 subtypes) and nonimmune substances (type II cell-secreted surfactant proteins A and D, fibrinogen, and complement fragments [C3b]) that can promote receptor-mediated uptake or phagocytosis by macrophages. Alveolar T lymphocytes can stimulate the macrophage with cytokines, such as interleukin (IL)-1 and interferon-γ, that enhance its bactericidal activity or, if microbes are too numerous or too virulent, can create an inflammatory response quickly. Chemokines, derived from macrophages or epithelial cells, including IL-8, leukotriene B_4, and tumor necrosis factor, can attract neutrophils and other inflammatory products from adjacent capillaries into the alveolus. If inflammation, or pneumonitis, is successful in eradicating infection, neutrophils undergo apoptosis, the inflammation resolves, and normal lung tissue function is restored. If the inflammatory process is prolonged, a smoldering, chronic inflammatory response can persist and lead to tissue injury that causes fibrosis and scarring, or depending on the antigen-particle or microbe involved, a granulomatous reaction may develop from IL-2 stimulating T_H1 lymphocytes. If this wound-type healing occurs after substantial injury, respiratory function can be lost permanently.

Epithelial cells have about the same repertoire of proinflammatory chemokines as alveolar macrophages, including IL-8, leukotriene B_4, transforming growth factor-β, monocyte chemotactic protein 1, and RANTES. They also can inhibit or downregulate inflammation. This dual capability to help initiate inflammation and then suppress it makes the epithelium crucial for the pathogenesis of diseases such as asthma (Chapter 87), bronchitis, emphysema (Chapter 88), and pulmonary fibrosis (Chapter 92). Chronic inflammatory changes can cause bronchiectasis (Chapter 90) or cell atypia that leads to endobronchial cancer (Chapter 197).

Dendritic cells or surface macrophages process antigens, using Toll-like receptors such as TLR2 and TLR4, and present them to major histocompatibility complex–compatible but naive $CD4^+$ lymphocytes, a process facilitated with the stimulatory cytokine IL-12. IL-2 produced by $CD4^+$ T cells subsequently can direct Th1 lymphocytes to develop and proliferate. Th1 cells can produce IL-1 and interferon-γ, which can stimulate macrophages for heightened activity (phagocytic uptake) in the inflammatory pathway. Also, IL-2 can induce clonal expansion of $CD4^+$ lymphocytes that contributes to creating granulomas for containment of certain microbes, such as mycobacteria, or particles (silica or beryllium).

ASSESSMENT OF PULMONARY VENTILATORY FUNCTION

Pulmonary physiologic function can be measured by examining the relationships between expired airflow and volume or time or by using tests that measure exercise capacity or the distance that can be walked in a prespecified amount of time (typically 6 minutes). These functional tests provide measures of physiologic function and may be used to reproduce clinical symptoms, such as breathlessness or dyspnea, and to correlate these symptoms with the degree of physical limitation. These tests are used to measure baseline status, to monitor treatment, and to estimate prognosis.

Pulmonary Function Tests

Lung function tests (Table 85-1) measure a person's ventilatory capacity in comparison with that of normal subjects. By adjusting for sex, height, ethnicity, and age, the values for a given individual can be compared with those from otherwise normal individuals. Basic tests for preliminary assessment and for monitoring disease progression include spirometry, which is a record of exhaled volume versus time during a forced exhalation (with or without determination of the response to an inhaled bronchodilator for possible reversible airflow); diffusion capacity, which measures the transfer of carbon monoxide to indicate how well inspired gases cross the alveolar-interstitial-capillary endothelial interface into blood; and noninvasive pulse oximetry, for oxygen saturation measured at rest or during ambulation. Pulmonary function tests (PFTs) performed after graduated exercise on a treadmill or a timed walking test on a level surface provides a more dynamic assessment of pulmonary function and correlates well with prognosis in patients with chronic pulmonary conditions such as lung fibrosis and chronic obstructive disease. More specialized tests include body plethysmography to determine total lung volumes and airway resistance as well as maximal cardiopulmonary exercise testing to assess cardiac function and oxygen uptake and consumption. The clinical utility of these tests can be appreciated by understanding how they can be applied to representative types of patients (Table 85-2).

Spirometry

A tracing of the relationship between maximal expiratory airflow and time, termed a *spirogram,* is the most common measure of ventilatory lung

TABLE 85-1 PULMONARY FUNCTION TESTS

LUNG VOLUME	
TLC	Total lung capacity (volume of gas in lungs at the end of maximal inspiration)
FRC	Functional residual capacity (volume of gas in the lungs when elastic inward pull is balanced by outward pull of the chest wall and diaphragm)
ERV	Expiratory reserve volume (volume of gas expired from FRC to maximal expiration)
RV	Residual volume (FRC − ERV, volume of gas left in lungs after maximal exhalation)
EXPIRATORY FLOW	
FEV_1	Forced expiratory volume (in 1 second)
FVC	Forced vital capacity
FEV_1%	FEV_1/FVC ratio (expressed as percentage)
DIFFUSING CAPACITY	
DLCO	Diffusing capacity for carbon monoxide
ARTERIAL BLOOD GASES	
PaO_2	Arterial oxygen pressure
$PaCO_2$	Arterial carbon dioxide pressure
pH	

TABLE 85-2 CLINICAL EXAMPLES OF TESTING IN REPRESENTATIVE TYPES OF PATIENTS WITH COMMON PULMONARY COMPLAINTS

CLINICAL PRESENTATION	PHYSICAL FINDINGS AND CHEST RADIOGRAPH	PULMONARY FUNCTION TESTS	RESULTS OF VENTILATORY FUNCTION (% PREDICTED)	CHARACTERISTIC ABNORMALITIES	DIAGNOSIS	MONITORING OR PREDICTIVE USE OF TESTS
Young adult with episodic attacks of cough, wheezing, and anxiety	Rapid respiratory rate Wheezing and prolonged expiration Thorax hyperresonant Radiograph normal or hyperinflated	Spirometry (but cough and dyspnea may preclude complete results) Oximetry Arterial blood gas analysis (only if the episode is prolonged or severe)	PEFR > 60% FEV_1, 45-75% MMEFR, 30-50% ABG (while breathing ambient air): Pa_{O_2}, 70 mm Hg, Pa_{CO_2}, 30 mm Hg	Decreased PEFR, FEV_1, MMEFR to grade as mild, moderate, or severe attack Hypoxemia, hypocapnia, and pH changes on blood gas analysis during an attack	Asthma exacerbation of moderate intensity	Spirometry after bronchodilator treatment or challenge testing Daily peak flow measurements (keep diary of results) FEV_1 may return to normal range after episode or therapy
Middle aged, male, former smoker	Abdominal obesity (large waist circumference) BP, 140/85 mm Hg BMI, 32 kg/m^2 Hyperglycemia Dyslipidemia	Spirometry	FEV_1, 80% FVC, 84% FEV_1/FVC, 82%	FEV_1 and FVC decreased; restrictive function	Metabolic syndrome with lung restriction from abdominal obesity	Regular spirometry not indicated
Middle aged, moderate smoker (20 cigarettes per day), mild dyspnea, occasional cough and sputum	Examination findings and radiograph are likely to be normal	Baseline spirometry and oximetry Optional baseline cardiorespiratory exercise test	FEV_1 > 80% FEV_1/FVC, 70% DLCO, 80%	Slight decrease in FEV_1 and perhaps FVC	Normal smoker with occasional episodes of acute bronchitis Mild COPD	Spirometry with health maintenance visit/yearly Daily peak flow monitoring Reduce or stop smoking
Older middle aged, moderate smoker for 30-40 yr, dyspnea (with moderate exertion), morning cough and phlegm, mild weight loss	Respiratory rate is likely to be increased at rest Thorax hyperinflated Breath sounds decreased Scattered wheezes and crackles Nail-bed cyanosis Radiograph normal or hyperinflated; no mass lesions evident	Spirometry and oximetry or arterial blood gas analysis Timed walk test Cardiopulmonary exercise testing (especially if heart failure is evident)	FEV_1 > 30% but <50% FEV_1/FVC < 70% DLCO, 30% TLC and RV ~100% Timed walk test shows less than predicted for age and sex	Decreased FEV_1 (usually about 40% predicted), FVC, and FEV_1/FVC (<0.70); increased residual volume and total lung capacity DLCO decreased Hypoxemia CO_2 retention perhaps	COPD of moderate severity	Spirometry yearly and after exacerbations on return to baseline Daily peak flow monitoring Blood gas analysis yearly (if FEV_1 < 40% predicted) Echocardiogram with signs of CHF Chest radiograph yearly Reduce or stop smoking Observe nutritional status and weight
Elderly patient, prior smoker, with insidious onset of dyspnea (occurs only with exertion for past 2 years) and mild nonproductive cough, without prior, relevant occupational exposures	Gaunt Respiratory and heart rates increased Coarse crackles heard at lung bases Mild clubbing Radiograph with diffuse infiltrates, decreased lung volume, and cystic areas at bases	Spirometry DLCO Timed walking, with oximetry and arterial blood gas analysis Cardiopulmonary exercise test advised Baseline ABGs	TLC, 65% FVC, 65% DLCO, 45% Pa_{O_2}, 70% (RA) Timed walk test shows values about 50% of predicted	Reduced lung volumes (vital capacity, total lung capacity) FEV_1/FVC ratio increased DLCO reduced Hypoxemia, but normal CO_2 Exercise tolerance limited	Pulmonary fibrosis	Spirometry at each visit every 6-12 mo Oximetry Timed velocity walk (with oxygen if O_2 < 88% at rest) Echocardiogram with signs of CHF
Patient above, seemingly stable for past 1 yr, and on no therapy, developed worsening dyspnea over 3 wk	As above Afebrile Radiograph with more diffuse ground-glass opacities No clear etiology	Spirometry DLCO ABG	FVC, 52% DLCO, 30% Tests difficult to obtain because of respiratory distress	As above, but tests may be difficult to obtain Will find more restriction and worsened gas exchange	Acute exacerbation Pulmonary fibrosis	Occurs in 10% of patients per year with 70% mortality Resume tests above, pending recovery
Middle-aged female with scleroderma and diffuse skin thickening disease for 3 yr; now exertional dyspnea Nonsmoker Taking prednisone 10 mg/day dose	Thickened skin, has Raynaud's, dry cough No overt cardiac failure HRCT with ground-glass opacities No pulmonary artery enlargement	Spirometry DLCO ABG	TLC, 70% predicted FVC, 68% FEV_1/FVC, 83% FRC, 74% RV, 70% DLCO, 47% (RA)	Ventilatory restriction with FVC between 45% and 80% DLCO, 40-50%	Scleroderma-related interstitial lung fibrosis, possible mild pulmonary hypertension	Spirometry and DLCO with health maintenance exams FVC decline of about 10%/year expected

ABG = arterial blood gases; CHF = congestive heart failure; COPD = chronic obstructive pulmonary disease; DLCO = diffusing capacity of lung for carbon monoxide; FEV_1 = forced expiratory volume in 1 second; FVC = forced vital capacity; FRC= functional reserve capacity; MMEFR = maximum mid-expiratory flow rate; PEFR = peak expiratory flow rate, RV = residual volume; TLC = total lung capacity.

TABLE 85-3 BRONCHOALVEOLAR LAVAGE CELL AND FLUID FINDINGS

STATUS OR ILLNESS	CELL PROFILE	NONCELLULAR COMPONENTS	OTHER ILLNESSES IN THE DIFFERENTIAL DIAGNOSIS WITH OVERLAPPING FINDINGS
Normal nonsmokers Mean, 1.3×10^5 cells/mL of recovered BAL fluid (range, 0.6-2.1)	Differential cell count (mean %): AM, 85%; lymphocytes, 7-12%; PMN, 1-2%; eosinophils-basophils, <1%; ciliated cells, 1-5%, 1% dendritic cells Lymphocyte subsets: CD4 helper, 50%; CD8 suppressor or cytotoxic, 30%; CD4/CD8 ratio, 1.5; B lymphocytes (plasma cells), 5%	95% as IgA (40% as IgA2), 90% IgA in dimeric form with secretory component, almost no IgM, IgG (IgG1-3/albumin ratios similar to serum), increased IgG4 Low concentrations of cytokines (IL-6, IL-8) Adhesion molecules detectable Histamine detectable Surfactant present	
Healthy moderate smokers Mean, 3.6×10^5 cells/mL of recovered BAL fluid (range, 2.2-4.8)	Three-fold increase of total cells, 95% AM, 3- to 5-fold increased AM, PMNs approximately 3% Lymphocytes 3% in differential cell count	Increased IgG as IgG/albumin ratio with serum, increased IgG3 and IgG4, decreased FSC, less surfactant recovered (lipid component profile same as that of nonsmoker) Decreased A_1AT elastase inhibitory activity Increased ACE (in AM) may be found	
INTERSTITIAL LUNG DISEASES			
Sarcoidosis	Lymphocytes, >30% total cells, increased CD4 cells, increased CD4/CD8 ratio AM-lymphocytes (T cells) form spontaneous rosettes PMNs > 3% may indicate deterioration and need for therapy Considerable increase in T lymphocytes as CD4 or T_H1 cells and a raised CD4/CD8 ratio is a common finding A raised neutrophil count may correlate with more severe disease on chest radiograph	Increased IL-2, IL-6, IL-8, IL-10, IL-12, MCP-1, TNF-α, interferon-γ ACE level can be increased Increased adhesion molecule ICAM-1 Increased fibronectin PPARγ deficient in AM MMP-12 and ADAMDECI gene and protein expression increased	Extrathoracic granulomatous diseases (e.g., Crohn's disease), primary biliary cirrhosis, extrinsic allergic alveolitis, idiopathic pulmonary fibrosis, collagen vascular disease
Extrinsic allergic alveolitis (hypersensitivity pneumonitis) Acute and chronic forms	Increased lymphocytes to >40-60% of total cells, often increased CD8 with slight reversal of CD4/CD8 ratio Foamy cytoplasm of AM Increased plasma cells, sometimes increased mast cells or basophils Striking increase of T lymphocytes with most as CD8 cells is usual	Increased IgM and IgG; IgG fraction may have specific precipitating antibody activity against etiologic antigens (thermophilic microbes) Increased IL-4, IL-10, interferon-γ, MIF, MCP	Drug-induced hypersensitivity Fibrotic form of NSIP
Idiopathic pulmonary fibrosis	Increased PMN; approximately 5-15% of cells Increased eosinophils, approximately 3-6% Increased lymphocytes, 15% in some cases A raised percentage of neutrophils and eosinophils is characteristic An increase of lymphocytes and neutrophils could indicate an NSIP pattern in lung biopsy	Increased IgG, increased monomeric IgA Increased IL-4, IL-6, IL-8, IL-13, TGF-β, MIF, galactin-1, CC Chemokines (CCL 2, CCL 17, CCL 22) Increased collagenase and histamine levels Increased fibronectin, decreased interferon-γ, metalloproteinases MMP7, MMP1, and their genes overexpressed	Usually diagnosis of exclusion (occupational, environmental) Increased lymphocytes may indicate EAA (HP) or NSIP
Bronchiolitis obliterans after lung transplantation	Increased PMNs that persist, CD4 T_H17 cells Persistence of neutrophils >3% in serial BAL cell count samples is a clue	Increased IL-1β, IL-6, IL-8, TNF-α, IL-17, fibronectin, collagenase	Autoimmune response to type V collagen in donor lung
Scleroderma (systemic sclerosis)	Increased PMNs to approximately 3-10% of cells Increased eosinophils to approximately 3% of cells Lymphocytes about 10%, but CD8 cells may be increased Myofibroblasts can be recovered BAL cell eosinophilia > 4% may indicate more severe lung fibrosis	Increased IL-4, IL-8, IL-10, IL-12, MCP-1, PDGF, TGF-β, CTGT, and thrombin activity Interferon-γ increased in 15%	
Langerhans cell histiocytosis	Cell profile similar to that of smokers: increased $CD1^+$ cells (>5% AM) Cytoplasmic X body or Birbeck granule on EM		Most patients are smokers
Alveolar lipoproteinosis (pulmonary alveolar proteinosis)	Foamy cytoplasm of AM	Milky, turbid fluid with altered phospholipid proportions; increased surfactant protein A	Extrinsic allergic alveolitis, lipoid pneumonia, drug-induced hypersensitivity (e.g., amiodarone), silicosis
Eosinophilic pneumonia	Increased percentage of eosinophils to 40% of cells	Increased IL-5, IL-18, and VEGF	Churg-Strauss, allergic bronchopulmonary aspergillosis, drug-induced hypersensitivity
Alveolar hemorrhage (Goodpasture's, Wegener's)	Hemosiderin-laden AM		
Inhalation exposure (asbestosis, fiber, silica)	Asbestos bodies or fiber in AM Modest increase in PMNs		Subclinical exposure must be considered in asymptomatic subjects

A_1AT = α_1-antitrypsin protease; ACE = angiotensin-converting enzyme; AM = alveolar macrophages; BAL = bronchoalveolar lavage; CD4 = helper T-lymphocyte subset; CD8 = suppressor T lymphocyte; CTGT = connective tissue growth factor; EM = electron microscopy; FSC = free secretory component; ICAM-1 = intercellular adhesion molecule 1; Ig = immunoglobulin; IL = interleukin; MCP = monocyte chemotactic protein; MIF = macrophage migration inhibition factor; MMP-12 and ADAMDECI = matrix metalloproteinases; NSIP = nonspecific interstitial pneumonia; PDGF = platelet-derived growth factor; PMN = polymorphonuclear neutrophil; PPARγ = peroxisome proliferator-activated receptor γ; TGF-β = transforming growth factor-β; TNF-α = tumor necrosis factor-α; VEGF = vascular endothelial growth factor.

function. It is used to make a preliminary diagnostic assessment or to monitor patients as lung or cardiac disease evolves and responds to treatment. Spirometry is recorded by having a seated subject breathe calmly several times at tidal volume, draw a maximal inhalation, perform a forced exhalation that is continued for at least 6 seconds with sustained vigorous effort (forced vital capacity [FVC]), and finally make a vigorous full inspiration (inspiratory vital capacity). These maneuvers are represented as a volume-time loop or as a flow-volume loop (plotting flow against FVC and inspiratory vital capacity). Flow-volume loops are scrutinized for special patterns that can indicate various clinical or anatomic conditions (E-Fig. 85-3). Considerable physical effort and attentiveness are required for adequate spirometry. Patients, especially during hospitalization, after medical procedures, or if they are deconditioned, often cannot give maximal effort or cooperate or coordinate well, and their test results will not be optimum. PFTs in a patient who is still under treatment for an exacerbation of chronic obstructive pulmonary disease (COPD) or asthma but who is not yet back to pre-illness status will show results that reflect their current status but not their baseline status. Recent treatment with a bronchodilator often improves PFT results and does not reflect intrinsic pulmonary function; about 8 to 12 hours should elapse from the last treatment to provide the most useful data. Reproducibility of several test attempts (at least three) is important and is a criterion for valid interpretation of test results. Other medical problems that can confuse spirometric testing include pulmonary congestion, coughing, thyroid dysfunction, neurologic illness, poor nutrition, and corticosteroid-associated muscle weakness. Serial testing is required to assess improvement, a return to baseline, or the need for intensified treatment in an outpatient.

Among the most common measures made from a spirometric tracing are FVC (liters), forced expiratory volume in the first second of exhalation (FEV_1, liters), ratio of FEV_1 to FVC (percentage), and forced expiratory flow in the middle of expiration ($FEF_{25-75\%}$, liters/second). Residual volume (liters) cannot be determined by spirometry and often is measured by helium dilution or plethysmographic methods. Residual volume is necessary to compute total lung capacity (liters), which is a measure of the air capacity of the maximally inflated lung. FEV_1, although recorded as a volume, is equated with a measure of airflow and is effort dependent.

FEV_1 values, when expressed as a percentage of predicted values, correlate with the amount of physical activity a patient can sustain. Peak flow can be measured from a spirographic tracing or using a portable device made for the outpatient monitoring of lung function; these devices are commonly prescribed for patients with asthma, COPD, or interstitial lung diseases. Encouraging a patient to keep a daily log of peak flow rates to share with the physician or medical staff can improve compliance with therapy and monitor improvement or the lack of it.

Although a healthy young person can produce a peak flow of 500 to 600 L/minute, many people with COPD are unable to achieve a peak flow greater than 200 to 350 L/minute and experience significant exertional dyspnea when peak flow decreases to less than 200 L/minute. Patients whose peak flow is about 150 L/minute are usually sedentary.

Analysis of measured values for FEV_1 and FVC (and their ratio) and total lung capacity allows the physician to make ventilatory diagnosis of the presence of obstructive or restrictive physiology (E-Fig. 85-4). A reduced FEV_1 and low FEV_1/FVC ratio combined with a large total lung capacity indicate obstructive disease of large airways and bronchi, a pattern typically observed in patients with COPD and asthma. FVC is preserved, but the time of exhalation is prolonged. After the administration of bronchodilators, the FEV_1 and FVC may increase by 10 to 15%, especially in asthma, indicating reversibility of airway obstruction. A lesser degree of improvement often is found, however, in patients who are already using inhaled bronchodilators regularly. A decrease in the $FEF_{25-75\%}$ with relatively preserved values of FEV_1 and FVC typically is found in patients with obstruction of small airways. If a person's postbronchodilator FEV_1 is less than 80% of the predicted value and FEV_1/FVC is less than 70%, airflow limitation is not fully reversible—the defining characteristic of COPD (Chapter 88). In patients with restrictive lung disease, the FEV_1 and FVC are reduced, as is total lung capacity, but the FEV_1/FVC ratio is usually normal or increased. Causes of restrictive interstitial lung disease include fibrosis of the lung parenchyma due to many toxic and inhalation exposures and toxic drug reactions (Chapter 94) and idiopathic interstitial lung diseases (Chapter 92). Restrictive physiology with a normal or low FEV_1 may reflect the chest wall habitus, chest wall muscle weakness or deformity, and pleural thickening (Chapter 99).

Diffusion Capacity

Diffusion capacity assesses how well a tracer gas in inspired air can cross from the air into the blood. The test measures the absorption of a low concentration of carbon monoxide in inhaled air by hemoglobin in red blood cells that circulate through pulmonary capillaries. Results must be corrected for reduced lung volumes, anemia, increased carbon monoxide levels in cigarette smokers, and high altitude. The diffusion capacity provides a general assessment of the air-blood interface; reduced values are obtained when interstitial fibrosis is extensive or when the capillary surface is compromised by vascular obstruction or nonperfusion (e.g., pulmonary embolism; Chapter 98) or is destroyed as in emphysema (Chapter 88).

Site-Specific Sampling, Including Bronchoalveolar Lavage

An assessment of airway inflammation can be made by measuring the fraction of nitric oxide in exhaled air or the pH of exhaled air condensates. It is also possible to measure endogenously produced biomarkers of oxidative stress in condensates (i.e., reactive oxygen and nitrogen species or aldehydes of lipid peroxides damaged in cell membranes). Mediators of inflammation can be measured in induced sputum (e.g., IL-8, leukotriene B_4, myeloperoxidase, IL-6, and elastase products). For example, as COPD worsens, induced sputum specimens or exhaled breath condensates provide evidence of neutrophilic inflammation with higher concentrations of exhaled nitric oxide, tumor necrosis factor-α, IL-6, transforming growth factor-β, IL-8, and growth-related oncogene-α as well as more leukotriene B_4.

Site-specific sampling to detach cells by washing or abrading the mucosal surface, coupled with endobronchial or transbronchial biopsy, can provide contiguous samples containing viable cells, noncellular secretions, and adjacent tissue. Multiple sites can be sampled; mucosal cell function can be compared between the nose and lower airways to assess allergic diseases. Bronchoalveolar lavage retrieves cells and secretions from the distal airways and the alveolar space surface. In combination with a thorough clinical evaluation and lung imaging studies, distinctive cellular patterns sometimes can obviate the need for lung biopsy (Table 85-3). Lung biopsy tissue can be microdissected with laser capture of specific cell types, and cells recovered in bronchoalveolar lavage fluid can be prepared for microarray analysis; gene chips created specifically for gene expression patterns may prove helpful for determining genetic susceptibility, aiding diagnosis, predicting response to certain therapeutic agents, and monitoring clinical activity.

Visit expertconsult.com for e-expanded chapter

SUGGESTED READINGS

Burney PG, Hooper R. Forced vital capacity, airway obstruction and survival in a general population sample from the USA. *Thorax*. 2011;66:49-54. *Forced vital capacity, but not airway obstruction, predicts survival in asymptomatic adults without chronic respiratory diagnoses or symptoms.*

Konishi K, Gibson KF, Lindell KO, et al. Gene expression profiles of acute exacerbations of idiopathic pulmonary fibrosis. *Am J Respir Crit Care Med*. 2009;180:167-175. *Potential for using genomic patterns as early indications of serious impending disease.*

Reynolds HY. Present status of bronchoalveolar lavage in interstitial lung disease. *Curr Opin Pulm Med*. 2009;15:479-485. *An overview of research and clinical uses.*

Woodruff PG, Modrek B, Choy DF, et al. T-helper type 2 driven inflammation defines major subphenotypes of asthma. *Am J Respir Crit Care Med*. 2009;180:388-395. *How gene expression can identify molecular mechanisms that identify clinical types of eosinophilic driven T_H2 innate immunity diseases.*

DISORDERS OF VENTILATORY CONTROL

ATUL MALHOTRA

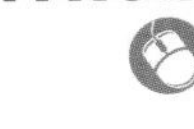

DEFINITIONS AND PATHOGENESIS

Ventilatory Control

Ventilation is controlled by complex interactions between central chemoreceptors, which predominantly are responsive to carbon dioxide (CO_2) tensions in arterial blood, and peripheral chemoreceptors, which predominantly are responsive to CO_2 and oxygen (O_2) tensions (Table 86-1). Disorders of ventilatory control are caused by derangements in these control mechanisms.

TABLE 86-1 CLASSIFICATION OF CENTRAL SLEEP APNEA

CENTRAL SLEEP APNEA SYNDROME	MECHANISM	THERAPY
Sleep transition apneas	CO_2 fluctuations during transitions from sleep to wake to sleep	Reassurance, occasionally hypnotics or oxygen
Chronic narcotic therapy	Lack of central drive	Reduce narcotic dose Consider positive-pressure device
Cheyne-Stokes breathing	High loop gain from robust chemosensitivity and ventilatory drive	Optimize medical therapy for heart failure, consider PAP devices
Idiopathic central apnea	Unknown	Supportive, bilevel PAP; consider ventilatory stimulants
Treatment of emergent central apnea or "complex apnea"	Lowering upper airway resistance at CPAP initiation improves efficiency of CO_2 excretion	Reassurance, generally resolves spontaneously
Sleep hypoventilation syndromes	Fall in drive with loss of wakefulness stimulus, loss of accessory muscle activity during REM sleep	Noninvasive ventilation

CPAP = continuous positive airway pressure; PAP = positive airway pressure; REM = rapid eye movement.

TABLE 86-2 CLASSIFICATION OF HYPERCAPNIC DISEASES

HYPERCAPNIC DISEASE	MECHANISM	DIAGNOSIS	TREATMENT
Narcotic overdose	Reduced central drive	History, narcotized pupils, toxicology	Supportive care, naloxone
Acute severe asthma	Severe airflow obstruction, high dead space	Typical history, wheezing on exam, low FEV_1/FVC	Bronchodilators, anti-inflammatories, mechanical ventilation (usually invasive)
Acute exacerbation of COPD	Airflow obstruction, high dead space	History, cigarette smoking, low FEV_1/FVC, infectious etiology	Bronchodilators, anti-inflammatories, noninvasive ventilation
Obesity-hypoventilation syndrome	Low respiratory system compliance, high upper airway resistance, low central drive	High BMI, lack of other diagnoses; blunted CO_2 response	Weight loss, nocturnal bilevel positive airway pressure
Central congenital hypoventilation syndrome	*PHOX2B* mutation, lack of central drive	Genetic testing	Supportive care, mechanical ventilation (usually noninvasive)
Neuromuscular disease (e.g., myasthenia gravis, ALS, polymyositis, GBS/AIDP)	Lack of respiratory muscle force	Immediate orthopnea, low VC, low MIPs/MEPs	Underlying cause; nocturnal noninvasive ventilation; supportive care
Severe parenchymal lung disease, e.g., COPD	Lack of alveolar surface area; high pulmonary dead space and work of breathing	Typical history, smoking, low FEV_1 and FEV_1/FVC	Bronchodilator, anti-inflammatory therapy, possible nocturnal noninvasive ventilation, smoking cessation
Kyphoscoliosis	Low respiratory system compliance	Physical examination	Supportive care, noninvasive ventilation

AIDP = acute inflammatory demyelinating polyneuropathy; ALS = amyotrophic lateral sclerosis; BMI = body mass index; COPD = chronic obstructive pulmonary disease; FEV_1 = forced expiratory volume in 1 second; FVC = forced vital capacity.

HYPOVENTILATION SYNDROMES

Hypoventilation syndromes are defined by a lack of adequate alveolar ventilation to maintain an arterial CO_2 tension of 40 mm Hg. The two most common clinical settings that result in hypoventilation are severe chronic obstructive pulmonary disease (COPD; Chapter 88) and morbid obesity (Chapters 100 and 227); less common etiologies include chronic opiate therapy, neuromuscular weakness (Chapters 429 and 430), and severe kyphoscoliosis (Chapter 99). The epidemiology of these hypoventilation syndromes is poorly studied, but about 15% of patients with severe COPD or morbid obesity have an elevated $Paco_2$. Regardless of the cause, patients with hypoventilation frequently have further worsening of their ventilation at the onset of sleep, owing to loss of the wakefulness stimulus, which is the normal drive to breathe while awake, and some degree of upper airway collapse after the onset of sleep (Chapter 100).

Patients with central sleep apnea (Chapter 100), which is a group of conditions in which cessation of airflow occurs because of a lack of respiratory effort, are classified into those with inadequate ventilatory drive and those with excessive drive. The paradox of how excessive drive leads to central apnea is explained by the concept of loop gain. A system with a high loop gain is prone to instability that leads to periods of excessive breathing followed by periods of apnea (Table 86-2). The prototype of a condition with high loop gain is periodic breathing or Cheyne-Stokes breathing (Fig. 86-1).

Cheyne-Stokes Breathing

Cheyne-Stokes breathing is a waxing and waning pattern of breathing that often includes periods of central apnea. It is seen most commonly during sleep in patients with heart failure.

EPIDEMIOLOGY

Cheyne-Stokes breathing is a form of ventilatory instability that occurs in 30 to 40% of patients with left ventricular systolic dysfunction and heart failure. Male sex, advanced age, low baseline $Paco_2$, and atrial fibrillation are risk factors for Cheyne-Stokes breathing among patients with heart failure. Controversy remains regarding whether this breathing pattern itself is deleterious or whether it is simply a marker of the underlying severity of cardiac disease. Cheyne-Stokes breathing represents about 5 to 10% of all cases of sleep apnea (Chapter 100) and is uncommon among patients who do not have heart failure.

PATHOBIOLOGY

Individuals with Cheyne-Stokes breathing have robust chemosensitivity as evidenced by marked increases in ventilation with small changes in $Paco_2$. The drive to breathe may be further increased by neural reflexes that are triggered by extravascular lung fluid and an elevated left atrial pressure. Intermittent hypoxemia and catecholamine surges, which are frequent in these patients, contribute to oxidative stress and neuroendocrine activation, both of which are thought to contribute to worsening of the underlying heart failure.

CLINICAL MANIFESTATIONS AND DIAGNOSIS

Patients with Cheyne-Stokes breathing can sometimes be diagnosed at the bedside by careful observation of their breathing pattern. During sleep or exercise, breathing becomes more dependent on metabolic stimuli. Patients may complain of fatigue or sleepiness because arousals from sleep tend to occur during the hyperpneic phase. Paroxysmal nocturnal dyspnea, a classic symptom of heart failure (Chapter 58), most commonly reflects underlying Cheyne-Stokes breathing. Patients often are diagnosed in the sleep laboratory while undergoing investigation for possible obstructive sleep apnea.

The diagnosis of Cheyne-Stokes breathing, if not readily apparent, can be made during overnight polysomnography, when the typical oscillatory pattern of tidal volume is seen in the absence of ventilatory efforts during the apneic periods. When evaluating such recordings, it is important to note that

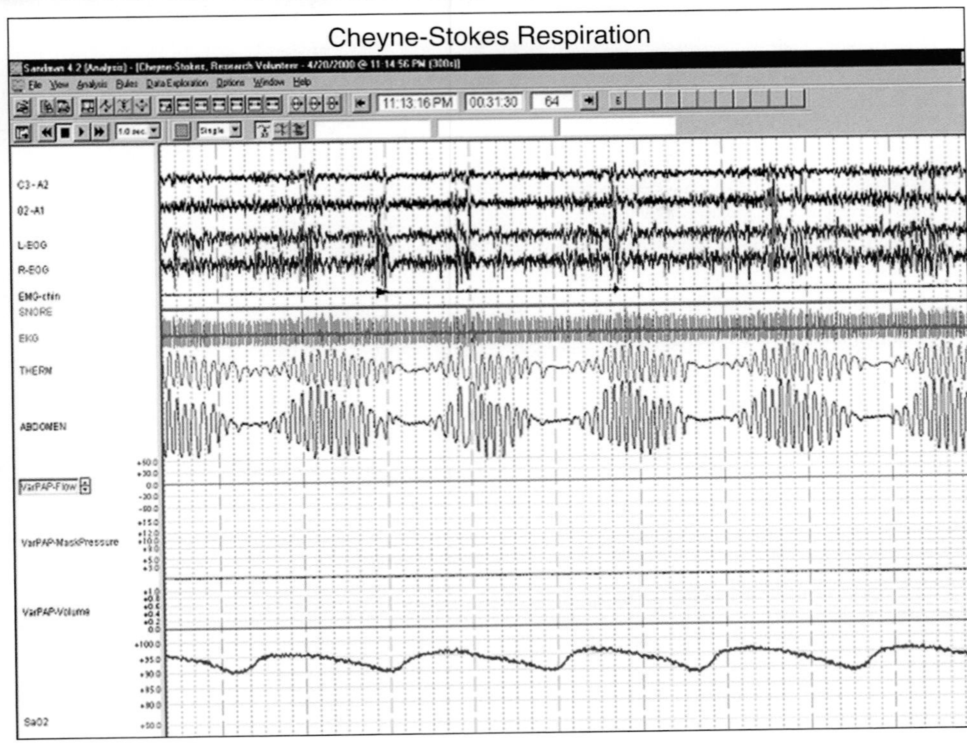

FIGURE 86-1. Cheyne-Stokes breathing with crescendo-decrescendo pattern of breathing. The thermistor detects air temperature changes at the mouth and nose. Note absences in airflow without respiratory effort seen in the abdominal belts. This breathing pattern leads to intermittent desaturations, arousals from sleep, and bursts of tachycardia. The loop gain concept can be understood by considering the thermostat analogy in which a control system is working to regulate a stable room temperature (e.g., 20° C). By analogy, the respiratory control system is working primarily to maintain a stable Pa_{CO_2} of 40 mm Hg and stable pH. Situations in which marked fluctuations in room temperature might occur would include one in which the thermostat is excessively sensitive (i.e., furnace turns on if room temperature falls to 19.999° C); if the furnace is too powerful, a marked overshoot in room temperature will be followed by a prolonged period when the furnace does not run. In the analogy to Cheyne-Stokes breathing, CO_2 is equated to room temperature and would be predicted to be unstable if chemoresponsiveness (i.e., the thermostat) were excessively robust (i.e., a marked increase in ventilation for small change in CO_2), if the efficiency of CO_2 excretion were high (i.e., marked fall in Pa_{CO_2} with increased ventilation), or if the end-expiratory lung volume were small. Situations that increase the propensity for CO_2 fluctuations lead to elevated loop gain and thus increase the risk for Cheyne-Stokes breathing.

Cheyne-Stokes breathing usually resolves during rapid eye movement (REM) sleep, that arousals on the electroencephalogram typically occur during the hyperpneic phase, and that Cheyne-Stokes breathing generally does not resolve immediately when nasal continuous positive airway pressure (CPAP) is applied.

TREATMENT

Medical management of Cheyne-Stokes breathing most often is treatment of the underlying heart failure (Chapter 59). Many patients with clinically significant Cheyne-Stokes breathing are taking inadequate doses of angiotensin-converting enzyme inhibitors, β-adrenergic blockers, or diuretics. After optimization of medical management, the Cheyne-Stokes breathing pattern frequently resolves. By comparison, CPAP is no better than standard medical therapy. 1

Central Congenital Hypoventilation Syndrome

DEFINITION AND EPIDEMIOLOGY

Central congenital hypoventilation syndrome is a rare congenital condition, previously referred to as Ondine's curse, characterized by a diminished ventilatory response to CO_2. The central congenital hypoventilation syndrome was traditionally diagnosed in neonates, but it is increasingly noted in adults.

PATHOBIOLOGY

The syndrome is now defined by a mutation in the *PHOX2B* gene, located on chromosome 4p12. Because most parents of affected children with the central congenital hypoventilation syndrome do not carry a *PHOX2B* mutation, the mutations are de novo. About 90% of patients are heterozygous for a polyalanine repeat expansion mutation, in which the affected allele has 24 to 33 alanines rather than the normal 20 alanines. The remaining 10% of central congenital hypoventilation syndrome patients have missense, nonsense, or frameshift mutations in the *PHOX2B* gene.

The *PHOX2B* gene is a paired-like homeobox that encodes a highly conserved transcription factor key to autonomic development in mice. Mice that are genetically modified for *PHOX2B* have irregular breathing, do not respond to hypercapnia, and die soon after birth from central apnea. These mice have neuronal loss in the retrotrapezoid nucleus and parafacial region of the brain stem, thereby suggesting the importance of this medullary region in normal breathing. Abnormalities in *PHOX2B* genes have also been associated with Hirschsprung's disease (Chapter 138), neural crest tumors, cardiac asystole (Chapter 63), and other abnormalities of the autonomic nervous system (Chapter 427).

CLINICAL MANIFESTATIONS AND DIAGNOSIS

Neonates can present with cyanosis at birth, recurrent central apneas, or both. Adults can present with idiopathic central sleep apnea, unexplained hypercapnia, or autonomic abnormalities (Chapter 427). Confirmation of the diagnosis requires the demonstration of an abnormality in the *PHOX2B* gene.

TREATMENT

There are currently no specific therapies for central congenital hypoventilation syndrome beyond supportive care. Genetic counseling is required for afflicted individuals and their families given the autosomal dominant pattern of inheritance. Patients must be cautioned against the use of sedatives, which could precipitate respiratory failure. Mechanical ventilation during sleep either invasively (through tracheostomy) or noninvasively (through bilevel positive airway pressure support [Chapter 100]) is required in most patients. Some patients remain fully ventilator dependent. Alternative treatments, such as ventilatory stimulants and diaphragmatic pacing, are generally ineffective.

Acquired Hypoventilation Syndromes

DEFINITION AND EPIDEMIOLOGY

Patients with hypoventilation syndromes cannot maintain adequate minute ventilation to keep their Pa_{CO_2} at 40 mm Hg. Patients can be classified into those who lack central ventilatory drive and those who have a pulmonary mechanical or neuromuscular abnormality that prevents adequate gas exchange. The case frequency is unknown, but hypercapnic respiratory failure is one of the more common admission diagnoses in intensive care units.

PATHOBIOLOGY

Patients with conditions characterized by the lack of central drive have reasonably normal lungs and respiratory muscle function but lack adequate response to CO_2 and hypoxia. In contrast, most patients with mechanical or neuromuscular abnormalities have a larger work of breathing compared with normal individuals; the most common underlying conditions are severe

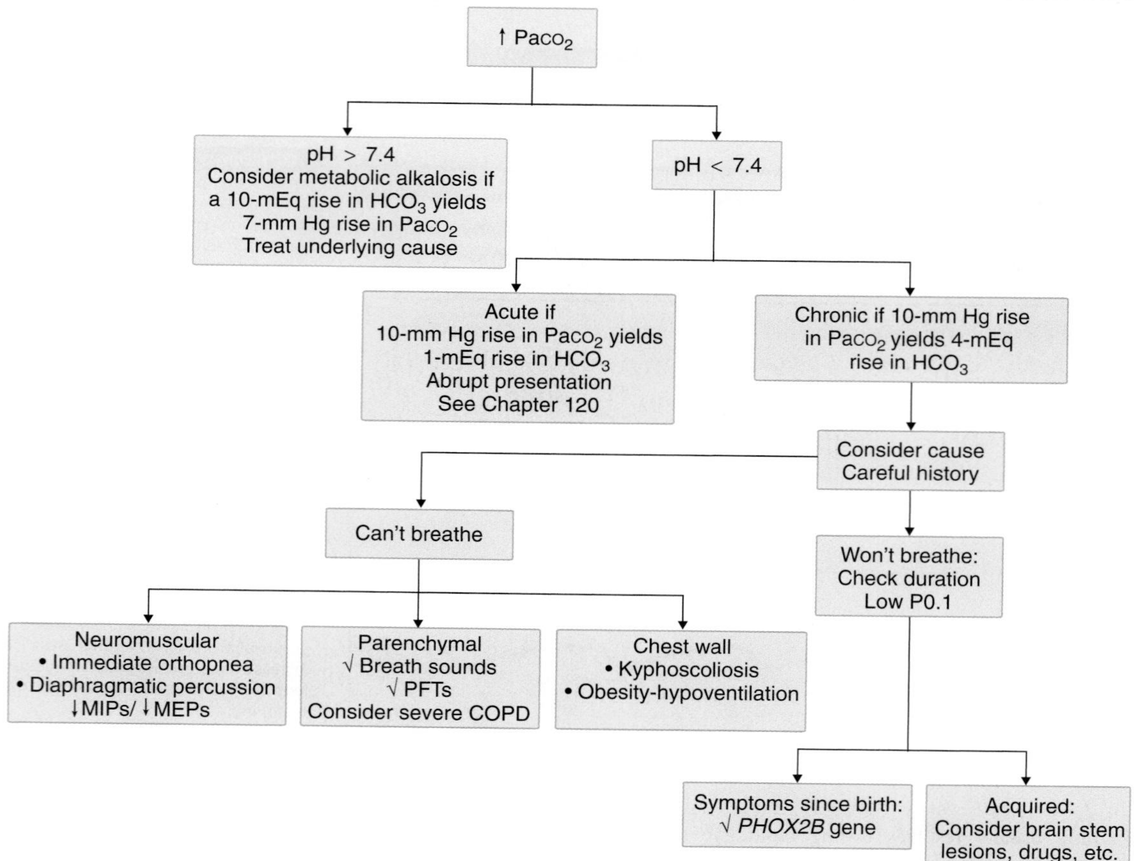

FIGURE 86-2. A flow chart of a systematic approach to hypercapnia and various causes of hypoventilation. The change in pH can help determine the cause and chronicity. A careful history and physical examination, coupled with pulmonary function testing, can help classify patients into those who "can't breathe" owing to neuromuscular or mechanical abnormalities of the respiratory system as compared with those who "won't breathe" owing to central nervous system pathology. COPD = chronic obstructive pulmonary disease; MEP = maximal expiratory pressure; MIP = maximal inspiratory pressure; P0.1 = the negative mouth pressure generated during the first 100 msec of an occluded inspiration; PFT = pulmonary function test.

COPD (Chapter 88) or morbid obesity (Chapter 227) with the obesity-hypoventilation syndrome. Such individuals have diminished but not absent chemoresponsiveness. Another cause of inadequate gas exchange is neuromuscular disease; common causes include disorders of neuromuscular transmission (Chapter 430), severe muscle weakness (Chapter 429), the residua from poliovirus infection (Chapter 423), Guillain-Barré syndrome (Chapter 428), or acute poisoning (Chapter 110).

CLINICAL MANIFESTATIONS AND DIAGNOSIS

Patients with hypoventilation have a myriad of presentations ranging from asymptomatic abnormalities in laboratory testing (e.g., elevated Pa_{CO_2}, unexplained low Sa_{O_2}, or an elevated serum bicarbonate level) to respiratory failure in the intensive care unit (e.g., respiratory infection with laboratory evidence of chronic abnormalities, such as acute-on-chronic respiratory acidosis). Patients who acutely overdose on sedative-hypnotic or narcotic agents may present with acute respiratory acidosis and loss of consciousness. Other patients may present with central sleep apnea-hypopnea or otherwise unexplained oxygen desaturation at night.

Once suspected, the diagnosis of hypoventilation is confirmed by the finding of Pa_{CO_2} higher than 42 mm Hg on analysis of an arterial blood sample. If the increase in Pa_{CO_2} is of short duration so that renal compensation has not yet occurred (Chapter 120), the serum bicarbonate level is increased by 1 mEq/liter for every 10-mm Hg rise in Pa_{CO_2}. By comparison, if the respiratory acidosis is of sufficient duration for renal compensation to occur, the serum bicarbonate level will be increased by 4 mEq for every 10-mm Hg rise in Pa_{CO_2} (Fig. 86-2).

Once an elevated Pa_{CO_2} is established, it is appropriate to distinguish patients who "can't breathe" from those who "won't breathe." "Can't breathe" implies that a respiratory mechanical problem or neuromuscular weakness is causing the elevation in Pa_{CO_2}. Abnormalities in pulmonary function testing (e.g., a markedly diminished vital capacity) are consistent with a pulmonary parenchymal or chest wall disorder.

Patients who "won't breathe" have central nervous system abnormalities that affect central drive or chemosensitivity, or both.

TREATMENT AND PROGNOSIS

Rx

The treatment of hypoventilation should focus on the underlying cause. Acute poisonings can be managed supportively or, in some cases, with specific antidotes (Chapter 110). Chronic conditions can be treated by addressing the underlying cause, such as weight loss in obesity hypoventilation syndrome or cholinesterase inhibitors in myasthenia gravis (Chapter 430). For parenchymal lung disease, treatment is directed at the underlying cause (Chapters 88 and 92).

Sedative medications should be used cautiously because they can occasionally precipitate acute respiratory failure. Although profound hypoxemia can clearly be deleterious, oxygen occasionally can precipitate severe acute respiratory acidosis, particularly in patients with acute exacerbations of COPD (Chapter 88). As a result, hypoventilating patients with COPD require the careful administration of supplemental oxygen, which should be titrated to an arterial oxygen saturation of 90% or an arterial oxygen tension of 60 mm Hg.

Severe hypoventilation requires mechanical ventilation (Chapter 105), such as noninvasive ventilation for an acute exacerbation of COPD.[2] For other presentations in which the Pa_{CO_2} is believed to be acutely elevated, endotracheal intubation and mechanical ventilation are frequently used, especially in patients with impaired consciousness. For chronic hypoventilation in hypercapnic COPD, noninvasive bilevel positive airway pressure through a face mask during sleep can maintain alveolar ventilation and improve outcome.[3] However, the considerable difficulty of adhering to nocturnal bilevel therapy in COPD emphasizes the need for discussions with patients and families regarding its risks and benefits. Other chronic hypoventilation syndromes are also commonly treated with bilevel positive airway pressure, although data are less compelling. In some chronic conditions, such as motor neuron disease (Chapter 418), tracheostomy should be discussed, although the impact of such interventions on quality of life should be carefully considered. Regardless of the underlying cause, an elevation in the Pa_{CO_2} level is considered a poor prognostic sign. End-of-life discussions are also important in such cases because the prognosis of chronic respiratory failure patients is generally poor.

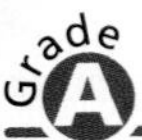

1. Bradley TD, Logan AG, Kimoff RJ, et al. Continuous positive airway pressure for central sleep apnea and heart failure. *N Engl J Med.* 2005;353:2025-2033.
2. Lightowler JV, Wedzicha JA, Elliott MW, et al. Non-invasive positive pressure ventilation to treat respiratory failure resulting from exacerbations of chronic obstructive pulmonary disease: Cochrane systematic review and meta-analysis. *BMJ.* 2003;326:185.
3. McEvoy RD, Pierce RJ, Hillman D, et al. Nocturnal non-invasive nasal ventilation in stable hypercapnic COPD: a randomised controlled trial. *Thorax.* 2009;64:561-566.

SUGGESTED READINGS

Brown LK. Hypoventilation syndromes. *Clin Chest Med.* 2010;31:249-270. *Review of mechanisms and syndromes.*

Pack AI. Central sleep apnea. *Handb Clin Neurol.* 2011;98:411-419. *Review.*

Weese-Mayer DE, Berry-Kravis EM, Ceccherini I, et al. An official ATS clinical policy statement. Congenital central hypoventilation syndrome: genetic basis, diagnosis, and management. *Am J Respir Crit Care Med.* 2010;181:626-644. *Review of the condition, which is defined by the presence of a* PHOX2B *mutation.*

87

ASTHMA

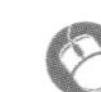

JEFFREY M. DRAZEN

DEFINITION

Asthma is a clinical syndrome of unknown etiology characterized by three distinct components: (1) recurrent episodes of airway obstruction that resolve spontaneously or as a result of treatment; (2) exaggerated bronchoconstrictor responses to stimuli that have little or no effect in nonasthmatic subjects, a phenomenon known as *airway hyperresponsiveness*; and (3) inflammation of the airways as defined by a variety of criteria. Although airway obstruction is largely reversible, it is currently thought that changes in the asthmatic airway may be irreversible in some settings.

EPIDEMIOLOGY

Asthma is an extremely common disorder affecting boys more commonly than girls and, after puberty, women slightly more commonly than men; approximately 8% of the adult population of the United States has signs and symptoms consistent with a diagnosis of asthma. Although most cases begin before the age of 25 years, new-onset asthma may develop at any time throughout life.

The worldwide prevalence of asthma has increased more than 45% since the late 1970s. The greatest increases in asthma prevalence have occurred in countries that have recently adopted an "industrialized" lifestyle. Data from many sources now show that children raised in a farming environment have a much lower risk of asthma than their peers raised in an urban environment; the specific exposures responsible for this decreased disease burden are not known.

Asthma is among the most common reasons to seek medical treatment. In the United States, it is responsible for about 15 million annual outpatient visits to physicians and for nearly 2 million annual inpatient hospital days of treatment. The yearly direct and indirect costs of asthma care are more than $25 billion; more than half of these costs are attributable to direct expenditures on medical care encounters or asthma medications.

PATHOBIOLOGY

Genetics

In twin studies, asthma has about 60% heritability, indicating that both genetic and environmental factors are important in its etiology. A locus on chromosome 17q21, at or near the locus for *ORMDL3*, a member of a gene family that encodes endoplasmic reticulum transmembrane proteins, has been associated with childhood-onset asthma. Although the exact functional variant in this region has not been identified, the isolation of a locus for childhood-onset asthma supports the clinical observation that adult- and childhood-onset asthma appear to be distinct disorders. Genetic variants that influence the response to treatment also have been identified and widely replicated.

Pathology

The pathology of mild asthma, as delineated by bronchoscopic and biopsy studies, is characterized by edema and hyperemia of the mucosa and by infiltration of the mucosa with mast cells, eosinophils, and lymphocytes bearing the T_H2 phenotype. Small placebo-controlled trials with daclizumab, an antibody against CD25, in patients with asthma of moderate severity provides solid evidence for the pathobiologic role of lymphocyte activation in asthma. Chemokines such as eotaxin, RANTES, macrophage inflammatory protein 1α, and interleukin-8 (IL-8), produced by epithelial and inflammatory cells, and the loss of the T-cell signaling molecule T-bet serve to amplify and to perpetuate the inflammatory events within the airway. The role of IL-4 and IL-13 as critical signaling molecules has been confirmed through small randomized controlled trials with pitakinra, an agent that inhibits binding of these cytokines to their receptors. As a result of these inflammatory stimuli coupled with the mechanical deformation of the epithelium from airway smooth muscle constriction, the airway wall is thickened by the deposition of type III and type V collagen below the true basement membrane. In addition, in severe chronic asthma, there is hypertrophy and hyperplasia of airway glands and of both surface and glandular secretory cells as well as hyperplasia of airway smooth muscle. Morphometric studies of airways from asthmatic subjects have demonstrated airway wall thickening of sufficient magnitude to increase airflow resistance and enhance airway responsiveness. During a severe asthmatic event, the airway wall is thickened markedly; in addition, patchy airway occlusion occurs by a mixture of hyperviscous mucus and clusters of shed airway epithelial cells.

The episodic airway narrowing that constitutes an asthma attack results from obstruction of the airway lumen to airflow. Although it is now well established that asthma is associated with infiltration of the airway by inflammatory cells, the links between these cells and the pathobiologic processes that account for asthmatic airway obstruction have not been clearly delineated. Three possible but not mutually exclusive links have been postulated: (1) the constriction of airway smooth muscle, (2) the thickening of airway epithelium, and (3) the presence of liquids within the confines of the airway lumen. Among these mechanisms, the constriction of airway smooth muscle due to the local release of bioactive mediators or neurotransmitters is the most widely accepted explanation for the acute reversible airway obstruction in asthma attacks. Several bronchoactive mediators are thought to be the agents that initiate the airway obstruction characteristic of asthma.

Mediators of the Acute Asthmatic Response

Acetylcholine

Acetylcholine released from intrapulmonary motor nerves causes constriction of airway smooth muscle through direct stimulation of muscarinic receptors of the M_3 subtype. The potential role for acetylcholine in the bronchoconstriction of asthma primarily derives from the observation that tiotropium bromide can be used as an effective asthma treatment.

Histamine

Histamine, or β-imidazolylethylamine, was identified as a potent endogenous bronchoactive agent 100 years ago. Mast cells, which are prominent in airway tissues obtained from patients with asthma, constitute the major pulmonary source of histamine. Clinical trials with novel potent antihistamines indicate a minor role for histamine as a mediator of airway obstruction in asthma.

Leukotrienes and Lipoxins

The cysteinyl leukotrienes, namely, LTC_4, LTD_4, and LTE_4, as well as the dihydroxy leukotriene LTB_4, are derived by the lipoxygenation of arachidonic acid released from target cell membrane phospholipids during cellular activation. 5-Lipoxygenase, the 5-lipoxygenase-activating protein, and LTC_4 synthase make up the cellular protein and enzyme content needed to produce the cysteinyl leukotrienes. The production of LTB_4 requires 5-lipoxygenase, the 5-lipoxygenase-activating protein, and LTA_4 epoxide hydrolase. Mast cells, eosinophils, and alveolar macrophages have the enzymatic capability to produce cysteinyl leukotrienes from their membrane phospholipids, whereas polymorphonuclear leukocytes produce exclusively LTB_4, which is predominantly a chemoattractant molecule; LTC_4 and LTD_4 are among the most potent contractile agonists ever identified for human airway smooth muscle. Clinical trials with leukotriene receptor antagonists or synthesis inhibitors have shown significant clinical efficacy in the treatment of chronic persistent asthma, leading to the conclusion that the leukotrienes are important but not exclusive mediators of the asthmatic response. Lipoxins, which are double lipoxygenase products of arachidonic acid metabolism, have been shown to be endogenous downregulators of the inflammatory response. The amounts of lipoxins are decreased in the airways of patients with severe asthma.

Nitric Oxide

Nitric oxide (NO•) is produced enzymatically by airway epithelial cells and by inflammatory cells found in the asthmatic lung. Free NO• has a half-life on the order of seconds in the airway and is stabilized by conjugation to thiols to form RS-NO. Both NO• and RS-NO have bronchodilator actions and may play a homeostatic role in the airway. Paradoxically, high levels of NO•, when it is coavailable with superoxide anion, may form toxic oxidation products, such as peroxynitrite ($OONO^-$), which could damage the airway. Patients with asthma have higher than normal levels of NO• in their expired air, and these levels decrease consistently after treatment with corticosteroids.

Physiological Changes in Asthma

An increased resistance to airflow is the consequence of the airway obstruction induced by smooth muscle constriction, thickening of the airway epithelium, or free liquid within the airway lumen. Resistance to airflow is manifested by increased airway resistance and decreased flow rates throughout the vital capacity. At the onset of an asthma attack, obstruction occurs at all airway levels; as the attack resolves, these changes are reversed—first in the large airways (i.e., mainstem, lobar, segmental, and subsegmental bronchi) and then in the more peripheral airways. This anatomic sequence of onset and reversal is reflected in the physiological changes observed during resolution of an asthmatic episode (Fig. 87-1). Specifically, as an asthma attack resolves, flow rates first normalize at a high point in the vital capacity and only later at a low point in the vital capacity. Because asthma is an airway disease, not an air space disease, no primary changes occur in the static pressure-volume curve of the lungs. However, during an acute attack of asthma, airway narrowing may be so severe as to result in airway closure, with individual lung units closing at a volume that is near their maximal volume. This closure results in a change of the pressure-volume curve such that for a given contained gas volume within the thorax, elastic recoil is decreased, which in turn further depresses expiratory flow rates.

Additional factors influence the mechanical behavior of the lungs during an acute attack of asthma. During inspiration in an asthma attack, the pleural pressure becomes more negative than the 4- to 6-cm H_2O subatmospheric pressure usually required for tidal airflow. The expiratory phase of respiration also becomes active as the patient tries to force air from the lungs. As a consequence, peak pleural pressures during expiration, which normally are, at most, only a few centimeters of water above atmospheric pressure, may be as high as 20 to 30 cm H_2O above atmospheric pressure. The low pleural pressures during inspiration tend to dilate airways, whereas the high pleural pressures during expiration tend to narrow airways. During an asthma attack, the wide pressure swings, coupled with alterations in the mechanical properties of the airway wall, lead to a much higher resistance to expiratory airflow than to inspiratory airflow.

The respiratory rate is usually rapid during an acute asthmatic attack. This tachypnea is driven not by abnormalities in arterial blood gas composition but rather by stimulation of intrapulmonary receptors with subsequent effects on central respiratory centers. One consequence of the combination of airway narrowing and rapid airflow rates is a heightened mechanical load on the ventilatory pump. During a severe attack, the load can increase the work of breathing by a factor of 10 or more and can predispose to fatigue of the ventilatory muscles. The patchy nature of asthmatic airway narrowing results in a maldistribution of ventilation (V) relative to pulmonary perfusion (Q). A shift occurs from the normal preponderance of V/Q units, with a ratio of near unity, to a distribution with a large number of alveolar-capillary units, with a V/Q ratio of less than unity. The net effect is to induce arterial hypoxemia. In addition, the hyperpnea of asthma is reflected as hyperventilation with a low arterial Pco_2.

CLINICAL MANIFESTATIONS

History

During an acute asthma attack, patients seek medical attention for shortness of breath accompanied by cough, wheezing, and anxiety. The degree of breathlessness experienced by the patient is not closely related to the degree of airflow obstruction but is often influenced by the acuteness of the attack. Dyspnea may occur only with exercise (exercise-induced asthma), after aspirin ingestion (aspirin-exacerbated respiratory disease), after exposure to a specific known allergen (extrinsic asthma), or for no identifiable reason (intrinsic asthma). Variants of asthma exist in which cough, hoarseness, or inability to sleep through the night is the only symptom. Identification of a provoking stimulus through careful questioning helps establish the diagnosis of asthma and may be therapeutically useful if the stimulus can be avoided. Most patients with asthma complain of shortness of breath when they are exposed to rapid changes in the temperature and humidity of inspired air. For example, during the winter months in less temperate climates, patients commonly become short of breath on leaving a heated house; in warm humid climates, patients may complain of shortness of breath on entering a cold dry room, such as an air-conditioned theater.

An important factor to consider in taking a history from a patient with asthma is the potential for occupational exposures in asthma (Chapter 93). Asthma that is brought on by occupational exposures is termed *occupational asthma*; preexisting asthma that is exacerbated by workplace exposures is termed *workplace-exacerbated asthma*. In reactive airway dysfunction syndrome (RADS), a single large exposure leads to a persistent asthma-like phenotype in a previously normal individual.

Physical Examination

Vital Signs

Common features noted during an acute attack of asthma include a rapid respiratory rate (often 25 to 40 breaths per minute), tachycardia, and pulsus paradoxus (an exaggerated inspiratory decrease in the systolic pressure). The magnitude of the pulsus is related to the severity of the attack; a value greater than 15 mm Hg indicates an attack of moderate severity. Pulse oximetry, with the patient respiring ambient air, commonly reveals an oxygen saturation near 90%.

Thoracic Examination

Inspection may reveal that patients experiencing acute attacks of asthma are using their accessory muscles of ventilation; if so, the skin over the thorax may be retracted into the intercostal spaces during inspiration. The chest is usually hyperinflated, and the expiratory phase is prolonged relative to the inspiratory phase. Percussion of the thorax demonstrates hyperresonance, with loss of the normal variation in dullness due to diaphragmatic movement; tactile fremitus is diminished. Auscultation reveals wheezing, which is the cardinal physical finding in asthma but does not establish the diagnosis (Chapter 83). Wheezing, commonly louder during expiration but heard

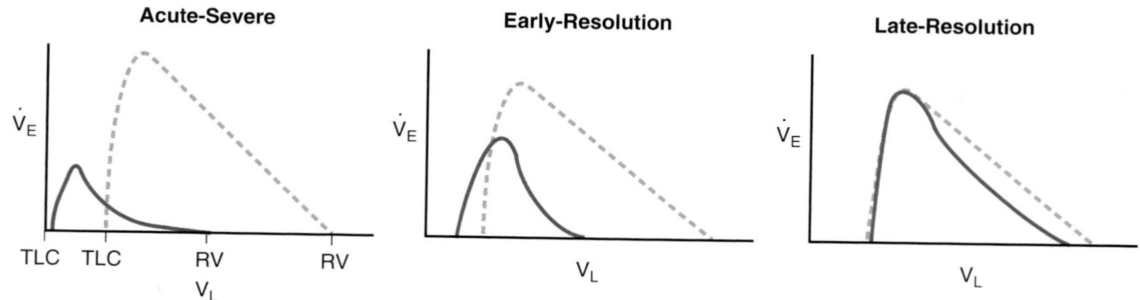

FIGURE 87-1. Schematic flow-volume curves in various stages of asthma. In each figure, the *dashed line* depicts the normal flow-volume curve. Predicted and observed total lung capacity (TLC) and residual volume (RV) are shown at the extremes of each curve. $\dot{V}_E$ = expiratory flow rate; V_L = lung volume.

TABLE 87-1 RELATIVE SEVERITY OF AN ASTHMATIC ATTACK AS INDICATED BY PEFR, FEV_1, AND MMEFR

TEST	PREDICTED VALUE (%)	SEVERITY OF ASTHMA
PEFR	>80	
FEV_1	>80	No spirometric abnormalities
MMEFR	>80	
PEFR	>80	
FEV_1	>70	Mild asthma
MMEFR	55-75	
PEFR	>60	
FEV_1	45-70	Moderate asthma
MMEFR	30-50	
PEFR	<50	
FEV_1	<50	Severe asthma
MMEFR	10-30	

FEV_1 = forced expiratory volume in the first second; MMEFR = maximal mid-expiratory flow rate; PEFR = peak expiratory flow rate.

during inspiration as well, is characterized as polyphonic in that more than one pitch may be heard simultaneously. A recording of wheezing from a patient with asthma can be heard at *www.expertconsult.com*. Accompanying adventitious sounds may include rhonchi, which are suggestive of free secretions in the airway lumen, or rales, which should raise the suspicion of an alternative diagnosis and are indicative of localized infection or heart failure. The loss of intensity or the absence of breath sounds in a patient with asthma is an indication of severe airflow obstruction.

DIAGNOSIS

Laboratory Findings

Pulmonary Function Findings

A decrease in airflow rates throughout the vital capacity is the cardinal pulmonary function abnormality during an asthmatic episode. The peak expiratory flow rate (PEFR), the forced expiratory volume in the first second (FEV_1), and the maximal mid-expiratory flow rate (MMEFR) are all decreased in asthma (Chapter 85). In severe asthma, dyspnea may be so severe as to prevent the patient from performing a complete spirogram. In this case, if 2 seconds of forced expiration can be recorded, useful values for PEFR and FEV_1 can be obtained. Gradation of attack severity (Table 87-1) *must* be assessed by objective measures of airflow; no other methods yield accurate and reproducible results. As the attack resolves, the PEFR and the FEV_1 increase toward normal together while the MMEFR remains substantially depressed; as the attack resolves further, the FEV_1 and the PEFR may normalize while the MMEFR remains depressed (see Fig. 87-1). Even when the attack has resolved clinically, residual depression of the MMEFR is not uncommon; this depression may resolve during a prolonged course of treatment. If the patient is able to cooperate such that more complete measurements of lung function can be made, lung volume measurements made during an attack demonstrate an increase in both total lung capacity and residual volume; the changes in total lung capacity and residual volume resolve with treatment. Because of the extra cooperation needed for this testing, it is not advised during an acute asthmatic event; such testing is, however, indicated between episodes of asthma.

Exhaled NO•

The fraction of NO• in the exhaled air (FE_{NO}) is elevated in patients with asthma. Although the exact concentration considered "elevated" will vary with the details of the technique, a concentration of 15 parts per billion is a convenient and reliable level that can be used to distinguish normal subjects from patients with untreated asthma. However, the measurement of exhaled nitric oxide has not been shown to be of value in the day-to-day management of asthma. 1-3

Arterial Blood Gases

Blood gas analysis need not be undertaken in individuals with mild asthma. If the asthma is of sufficient severity to merit prolonged observation, however, blood gas analysis is indicated; in such cases, hypoxemia and hypocapnia are the rule. With the subject breathing ambient air, the PaO_2 is usually between 55 and 70 mm Hg and the $PaCO_2$ between 25 and 35 mm Hg. At the onset of the attack, an appropriate pure respiratory alkalemia is usually evident; with attacks of prolonged duration, the pH returns toward normal as a result of a compensatory metabolic acidemia. A normal $PaCO_2$ in a patient with moderate to severe airflow obstruction is reason for concern because it may indicate that the mechanical load on the respiratory system is greater than can be sustained by the ventilatory muscles and that respiratory failure is imminent. When the $PaCO_2$ increases in such settings, the pH decreases quickly because the bicarbonate stores have become depleted as a result of renal compensation for the prolonged preceding respiratory alkalemia. Because this chain of events can take place rapidly, close observation is indicated for asthmatic patients with "normal" $PaCO_2$ levels and moderate to severe airflow obstruction.

Other Blood Findings

Asthmatic subjects are frequently atopic; thus, blood eosinophilia is common but not universal. In addition, elevated serum levels of immunoglobulin E (IgE) are often documented; epidemiologic studies indicate that asthma is unusual in subjects with low IgE levels. If indicated by the patient's history, specific radioallergosorbent tests, which measure IgE directed against specific offending antigens, can be conducted. In rare instances during severe asthma attacks, serum concentrations of aminotransferases, lactate dehydrogenase, muscle creatine kinase, ornithine transcarbamylase, and antidiuretic hormone may be elevated.

Radiographic Findings

The chest radiograph of a subject with asthma is often normal. Severe asthma is associated with hyperinflation, as indicated by depression of the diaphragm and abnormally lucent lung fields. Complications of severe asthma, including pneumomediastinum or pneumothorax, may be detected radiographically. In mild to moderate asthma without adventitious sounds other than wheezing, a chest radiograph need not be obtained; if the asthma is of sufficient severity to merit hospital admission, a chest radiograph is advised.

Electrocardiographic Findings

The electrocardiogram, except for sinus tachycardia, is usually normal in acute asthma. However, right axis deviation, right bundle branch block, "P pulmonale," or even ST-T wave abnormalities may arise during severe asthma and resolve as the attack resolves.

Sputum Findings

The sputum of the asthmatic patient may be either clear or opaque with a green or yellow tinge. The presence of color does not invariably indicate infection, and examination of a Gram-stained and Wright-stained sputum smear is indicated. The sputum often contains eosinophils, Charcot-Leyden crystals (crystallized eosinophil lysophospholipase), Curschmann's spirals (bronchiolar casts composed of mucus and cells), or Creola bodies (clusters of airway epithelial cells with identifiable cilia that, in fresh samples, can often be seen to beat), which can affect color without the presence of infection.

DIAGNOSIS

Differential Diagnosis

Asthma is easy to recognize in a young patient without comorbid medical conditions who has exacerbating and remitting airway obstruction accompanied by blood eosinophilia. A rapid response to bronchodilator treatment is usually all that is needed to establish the diagnosis. However, in the patient with cryptic episodic shortness of breath, an elevated FE_{NO} can help establish a diagnosis of asthma. However, in the absence of an elevated FE_{NO}, other causes of wheezing (see Table 83-3 in Chapter 83) should be investigated.

PREVENTION AND TREATMENT Rx

There is currently no way to prevent a patient from developing an asthmatic diathesis. For example, trials of allergen avoidance in childhood have not been successful. If a patient has such a diathesis with an allergic component, avoidance of allergens can reduce the frequency of asthma attacks. For example, removal of indoor mold can improve symptoms by 25% and reduce medication use by 50%.

The treatment of asthma is directed at the airway obstruction and the propensity for the airways to narrow too much and too easily in response to inhaled bronchoconstrictors. It is not acceptable practice to manage patients with asthma without objective measures of lung function. The best measure is FEV_1, but measures of PEFR can be substituted. Inexpensive and easy-to-use peak flowmeters make the measurement feasible in virtually all cases.

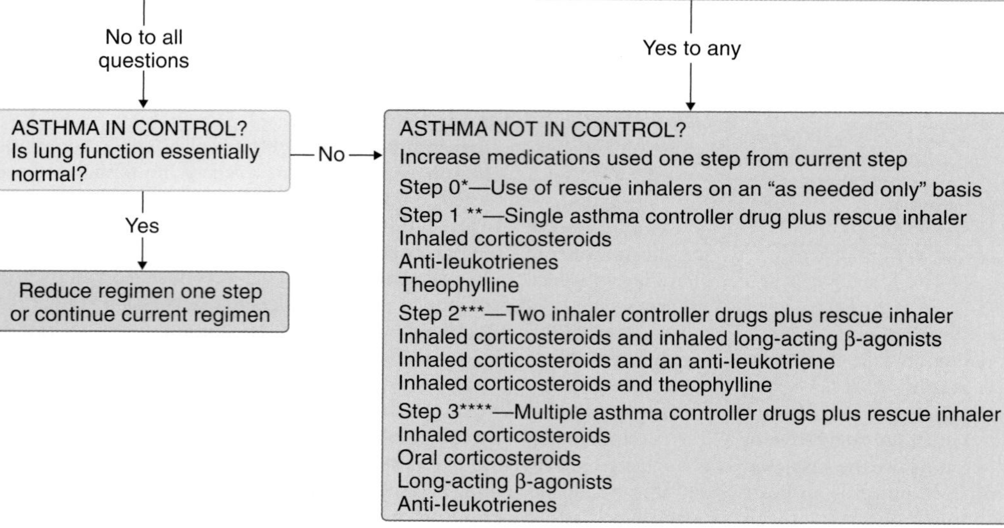

Have your activities of daily life been limited or interrupted because of asthma?
Has asthma caused you to awake from sleep more than one night in two weeks?
Have you had to use your rescue inhaler more than two or three times a day because of asthma symptoms?
Have you had to seek emergent medical care for your asthma since your last visit?
Is the fraction of nitric oxide in the exhaled air greater than 15 parts per billion? (In centers where this test is available)
No to all questions
Yes to any
ASTHMA IN CONTROL? Is lung function essentially normal?
No
Yes
Reduce regimen one step or continue current regimen
ASTHMA NOT IN CONTROL?
Increase medications used one step from current step
Step 0*—Use of rescue inhalers on an "as needed only" basis
Step 1 **—Single asthma controller drug plus rescue inhaler
Inhaled corticosteroids
Anti-leukotrienes
Theophylline
Step 2***—Two inhaler controller drugs plus rescue inhaler
Inhaled corticosteroids and inhaled long-acting β-agonists
Inhaled corticosteroids and an anti-leukotriene
Inhaled corticosteroids and theophylline
Step 3****—Multiple asthma controller drugs plus rescue inhaler
Inhaled corticosteroids
Oral corticosteroids
Long-acting β-agonists
Anti-leukotrienes

FIGURE 87-2. Approach to chronic control of asthma as well as to treatment of acute asthma symptoms. *Inhaled albuterol or, in patients predisposed to adverse effects from this treatment, inhaled ipratropium bromide. **The choice between these two agents as first-line therapy is up to the patient and provider. Inhaled corticosteroids are more potent for improving lung function but have adverse effects when used at high doses for extended periods. Efforts should be made to use the lowest doses possible. Although antileukotrienes are less effective, some patients prefer oral to inhaled treatment and wish to avoid the potential side effects of inhaled steroids. If a response to one treatment is not achieved, it makes sense to try the other. ***The best documented combination is a long-acting β-agonist plus an inhaled steroid, but the dose of inhaled steroids should be at least the median dose (see Table 87-2) before long-acting β-agonists are added. ****The use of multiple medications indicates asthma of substantial severity. Unless success is easily achieved, consultation with an asthma specialist may be appropriate.

Treatment of asthma has two components. The first is the use of acute reliever (rescue) agents (i.e., bronchodilators) for acute asthmatic airway obstruction. The second is the use of controller treatments, which modify the asthmatic airway environment so that acute airway narrowing, requiring rescue treatments, occurs much less frequently.

In a given individual, the intensity of asthma treatment is adjusted, for the most part, to achieve five goals:

1. Allow the patient to pursue the activities of his or her daily life without excessive interference from asthma
2. Allow the patient to sleep without awakening because of asthmatic symptoms
3. Minimize the use of rescue bronchodilator treatment
4. Prevent the need for unscheduled medical care
5. Maintain lung function reasonably near normal

A patient who meets these standards is said to be "in control," whereas a patient whose disease activities prevent these goals from being met is said to be "out of control." Treatment is titrated to achieve reasonable control in each patient. The recommendations given herein for chronic control of asthma are based on the Global Initiative for Asthma, 2009 revision (Fig. 87-2), but are not taken verbatim from them. Based on a directed history and physical examination, the patient's current degree of control can be determined, and then recommendations for future treatment can be made.

Rescue Treatments

All patients with asthma should be prescribed a rescue inhaler to use if they develop acute asthmatic airway obstruction.

β-Adrenergic Agents

Short-acting β-adrenergic agents given by inhalation are the mainstay of bronchodilator treatment of asthma. Constricted airway smooth muscle relaxes in response to stimulation of β_2-adrenergic receptors. β-Adrenergic agonists with varying degrees of β_2-selectivity are available for use in inhaled (by nebulizer or metered-dose inhaler; Fig. 87-3), oral, or parenteral preparations. Most patients with mild intermittent asthma should be treated with a short-acting β_2-selective inhaler (such as albuterol) on an as-needed basis. Regardless of the specific type of medication used, rescue treatment should consist of two "puffs" from the inhaler, with the first and second puffs separated by a 3- to 5-minute interval, which is thought to allow enough time for the first puff to dilate narrowed airways, thus giving the agent better access to affected areas of the lung. Patients should be instructed to exhale to a comfortable volume, to breathe in very slowly (such as they would when sipping hot soup), and to actuate the inhaler as they inspire. Inspiration to near total lung capacity is followed by holding the breath for 5 seconds to allow the deposition of smaller aerosol particles in more peripheral airways. This treatment can be repeated every 4 to 6 hours; patients should be instructed to "advance" their asthma treatment as noted in Figure 87-2 if they need to use more than 12 puffs of a β-agonist in a 72-hour period.

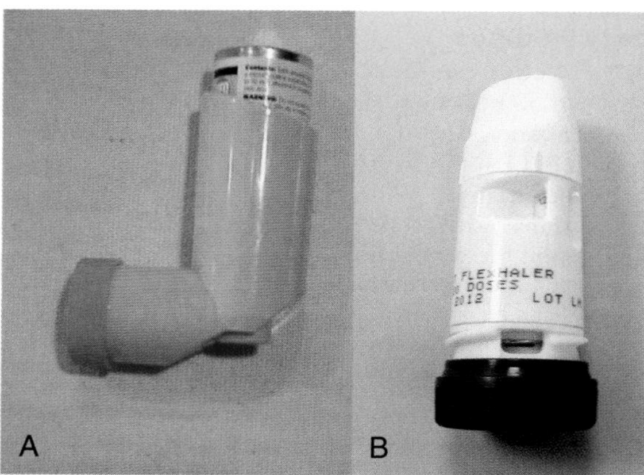

FIGURE 87-3. Commonly used inhalers. A, A pressurized metered-dose inhaler for a branded form of albuterol. Such inhalers propel the medication by means of a pressurized gas; many inhalers use propellants that do not harm the ozone layer. **B,** One of many types of dry powder inhalers; the one shown is a Flexhaler and dispenses budesonide. When this type of inhaler is activated, the active agent is released as a dry powder into a chamber. The patient creates the energy for airflow by means of an inspiratory effort that is directed through the device and that entrains medication into the inhaled airway.

Patients should receive specific instructions for correct inhaler use. Aerosol "spacers" are available from many manufacturers for patients who have difficulty coordinating their inspiratory effort and inhaler actuation. There is definitive evidence from prospective, randomized, placebo-controlled trials that the regularly scheduled use of prophylactic inhaled β-agonists has no deleterious effects in most patients with asthma.

In 2008, albuterol inhalers containing chlorofluorocarbon propellants were withdrawn from the market and replaced by inhalers powered by hydrofluoroalkanes. These inhalers have a lower velocity aerosol plume, so patients will notice a subjective difference in how the aerosol feels as it is dissipated into the mouth; nevertheless, clinical trials document that most hydrofluoroalkane inhalers will have nearly identical therapeutic effects.

Anticholinergics

Atropinic agents inhibit the effects of acetylcholine released from the intrapulmonary motor nerves that run in the vagus and innervate airway smooth muscle. Ipratropium bromide, the atropinic agent used therapeutically in asthma, is available in a metered-dose inhaler; the recommended dose is two puffs from a metered-dose inhaler every 4 to 6 hours. In adults with uncontrolled asthma, inhaled tiotropium (18 μg every morning) added to an

TABLE 87-2 ESTIMATED EQUIPOTENT DAILY DOSE FOR INHALED GLUCOCORTICOSTEROIDS FOR ADULTS

DRUG	LOW DAILY DOSE (μg)	MEDIAN DAILY DOSE (μg)	HIGH DAILY DOSE (μg)
Beclomethasone dipropionate	200-500	500-1000	>1000-2000
Budesonide*	200-400	400-800	>800-1600
Ciclesonide*	80-160	160-320	>320-1280
Flunisolide	500-1000	1000-2000	>2000
Fluticasone	100-250	250-500	>500-1000
Mometasone furoate*	200-400	400-800	>800-1200
Triamcinolone acetonide	400-1000	1000-2000	>2000

*Once-a-day dosing is acceptable.
Note: Some doses may be outside package labeling. Metered-dose inhaler doses are expressed as the amount of drug leaving the valve, not all of which is available to the patient. Dry powder inhaler doses are expressed as the amount of drug in the inhaler after activation.
Modified from 2010 Global Initiative for Asthma guidelines (*www.ginasthma.com*).

inhaled glucocorticoid is more effective than a double dose of glucocorticoids and similar in effect to salmeterol.[4]

Controller Treatments

Inhaled Corticosteroids

Inhaled corticosteroids (see Fig. 87-3), which have less systemic impact for a given level of therapeutic effect than systemic steroids, are effective controller treatments for improving lung function and preventing asthmatic exacerbations in patients with persistent asthma.[5] Accumulating data[6,7] indicate that treatment of patients whose disease can be categorized as "mild persistent asthma" can be limited to periods when the patients have increased asthma symptoms rather than requiring an inhaled corticosteroid on a regularly scheduled basis. However, inhaled corticosteroids do not change the natural history of asthma. A wide variety of inhaled corticosteroid products are on the market (Table 87-2). All available products are effective treatments of persistent asthma but differ in terms of cost, the magnitude of adrenal suppression, and the potential for systemic effects, including growth retardation in children, loss of bone mineralization, cataracts, and glaucoma. Overall, no convincing data are available to suggest that there is reason to prefer one corticosteroid over the others. Adverse effects common to all inhaled corticosteroids are oral thrush and hoarseness (attributed to myopathy of the laryngeal muscles); the risk and severity can be reduced by aerosol spacers and good oropharyngeal hygiene (i.e., rinsing out the mouth by gargling after dosing).

Antileukotrienes

Agents with the capacity to inhibit the synthesis of the leukotrienes (zileuton—controlled release [Zyflo-CR], 1200 mg twice daily) or the action of leukotrienes at the $CysLT_1$ receptor (montelukast [Singulair], 10 mg once a day; pranlukast [Onon, Ultair], 225 mg twice a day, not available in the United States; and zafirlukast [Accolate], 20 mg twice a day) are effective oral controller medications for patients with mild or moderate persistent asthma. In patients treatment with zileuton, function should be monitored for the first 3 to 6 months of treatment; if levels rise to more than three times the upper limit of normal, the drug should be stopped. Theophylline metabolism is slowed by zileuton, so monitoring of levels is indicated if both are prescribed. These treatments can be used on their own for mild persistent asthma or in combination with inhaled steroids for more severe asthma.

Long-Acting β-Agonists

In contrast to medium-acting β-agonists, long-acting β-agonists currently available in the United States (salmeterol [Serevent, 42 μg per puff; the same dose is labeled 50 μg per puff outside of the United States; one or two puffs should be delivered every 12 hours] and formoterol [Foradil, 12 μg through a proprietary dry powder inhaler every 12 hours]) have a duration of action of nearly 12 hours; they are considered a controller rather than a bronchodilator agent. Randomized controlled trials demonstrate that long-acting β-agonists should not be used as a sole controller agent. Other trials have shown that there are excess asthma deaths (about one for every 650 patient years of treatment) when long-acting β-agonists are used.[8] Therefore, long-acting β-agonists should be used only when they are given in concert with inhaled corticosteroids. Combination products with both inhaled steroids and long-acting β-agonists in the same aerosol device are available. These products prevent patients with asthma from using inhaled long-acting β-agonists without inhaled corticosteroids. When prescribing a combination inhaler, the physician should determine the inhaled dose of corticosteroids (fluticasone, budesonide, or beclomethasone) that the patient requires and then choose a combination product that will deliver a dose of long-acting β-agonist with the inhaled corticosteroid when given as two puffs twice per day. The dose of long-acting β-agonist varies with brand and type of inhaler used.

Theophylline

Theophylline and its more water-soluble congener aminophylline are moderately potent bronchodilators that are useful in both inpatient and outpatient management of asthma. The mechanism by which theophylline exerts its effects has not been established with certainty but is probably related to the inhibition of certain forms of phosphodiesterase. Theophylline is not widely used because of its toxicity and the wide variations in the rate of its metabolism, both in a single individual over time and among individuals in a population. Because blood levels need to be monitored for optimal dosing, most physicians have reserved theophylline for third- or fourth-line therapy. For most preparations, the starting dose should be about 300 mg/day; the frequency will depend on the preparation used.

Acceptable plasma levels for therapeutic effects are between 10 and 20 μg/mL; higher levels are associated with gastrointestinal, cardiac, and central nervous system toxicity, including anxiety, headache, nausea, vomiting, diarrhea, cardiac arrhythmias, and seizures. These last catastrophic complications may occur without antecedent mild side effects when plasma levels exceed 20 μg/mL. Because of these potentially life-threatening complications of treatment, plasma levels need to be measured with great frequency in hospitalized patients receiving intravenous aminophylline and less frequently in stable outpatients receiving one of the long-acting theophylline preparations. Most asthma care providers use dosing amounts and intervals to achieve steady-state theophylline levels of 10 to 14 μg/mL, thereby avoiding the toxicity associated with decrements in metabolism. Treatment with theophylline is recommended only for patients who have moderate or severe persistent asthma and who are receiving controller medications, such as inhaled steroids or antileukotrienes, but whose asthma is not adequately controlled.

Systemic Corticosteroids

Systemic corticosteroids are effective for the treatment of moderate to severe persistent asthma as well as for occasional severe exacerbations of asthma in a patient with otherwise mild asthma, but the mechanism of their therapeutic effect has not been established. No consensus has been reached on the specific type, dose, or duration of corticosteroid to be used in the treatment of asthma. In nonhospitalized patients with asthma refractory to standard therapy, a steroid "pulse" with initial doses of prednisone on the order of 40 to 60 mg/day, tapered to zero during 7 to 14 days, is recommended. For patients who cannot stop taking steroids without having recurrent uncontrolled bronchospasm despite the addition of multiple other controller treatments, alternate-day administration of oral steroids is preferable to daily treatment. For patients whose asthma requires in-hospital treatment but is not considered life-threatening, an initial intravenous bolus of 2 mg/kg of hydrocortisone, followed by continuous infusion of 0.5 mg/kg/hour, has been shown to be beneficial within 12 hours. In attacks of asthma that are considered life-threatening, the use of intravenous methylprednisolone (125 mg every 6 hours) has been advocated. In each case, as the patient improves, oral steroids are substituted for intravenous steroids, and the oral dose is tapered during 1 to 3 weeks; addition of inhaled steroids to the regimen is strongly recommended when oral steroids are started.

Monoclonal Antibody Treatment

Omalizumab

Subcutaneous administration of omalizumab, a humanized murine monoclonal antibody that binds circulating IgE, is associated with decreased serum free (not total) IgE levels. In patients who have moderate to severe allergic asthma with elevated levels of serum IgE and who are receiving inhaled corticosteroids, omalizumab treatment improves asthma control even as doses of inhaled steroids are decreased. Dosing is guided by weight and by pretreatment IgE levels: a monthly subcutaneous dose of 0.016 mg × body weight (kg) × IgE level (IU/mL). For example, in a patient weighing 70 kg with a pretreatment total IgE level of 300 IU/mL, 336 mg of omalizumab would be administered monthly by subcutaneous injection. Dosing calculators can be found online (e.g., *http://www.xolairhcp.com/xolairhcp/determining-the-dose.html*). Anti-IgE antibodies can reduce exacerbations and improve quality of life in patients with severe allergic asthma, but their place in treatment schema has not been established. Because of the potential for anaphylaxis, all patients need to be monitored after injection; the duration of the monitoring period is not specified by the U.S. Food and Drug Administration (FDA), but most physicians monitor for 30 to 60 minutes.

Mepolizumab

Mepolizumab is a monoclonal antibody directed against IL-5. Although it is not approved for clinical use, in small randomized trials it reduced asthma exacerbations among relatively rare patients with moderately severe asthma who still had sputum eosinophilia despite treatment with oral and inhaled corticosteroids. Among patients with more conventional asthma, however, mepolizumab treatment did not have a salutary effect.

Other Controller Drugs

Cromolyn sodium (one or two puffs from a metered-dose inhaler three or four times a day) and nedocromil sodium (two puffs from a metered-dose inhaler three or four times a day) are nonsteroid inhaled treatments that have proved beneficial in the management of mild to moderate persistent asthma. They appear to be most useful in pediatric populations or when an identifiable stimulus (such as exercise or allergen exposure) elicits an asthmatic response.

The use of systemic gold (as in rheumatoid arthritis), methotrexate, or cyclosporine has been suggested as adjunctive treatment of patients with severe chronic asthma who cannot otherwise discontinue high-dose corticosteroid treatment. However, these agents are experimental, and their routine use is not advocated. Despite initial encouraging trials, agents that inhibit the action of tumor necrosis factor-α do not benefit patients with asthma and should not be used.

Based on the concern that asthma could be caused by silent gastroesophageal reflux disease, treatment with a proton pump inhibitor has been advocated in patients with mild to moderate asthma even if in the absence of gastrointestinal symptoms. Adequately powered clinical studies suggest that this approach provides no benefit for asthma control. 9

Vaccination for Seasonal Influenza and Pneumococcal Disease

Vaccination of patients for seasonal influenza is safe and not associated with enhanced asthma exacerbations. Vaccination against seasonal influenza and pneumococcal disease is recommended in patients with asthma.

Radio Frequency Ablation of Airway Smooth Muscle

A proprietary system to ablate airway smooth muscle by delivering radio frequency energy through a bronchoscopically placed probe has reduced asthma exacerbations in sham controlled trials among patients whose asthma remained out of control despite the use of multiple controller medications. A device for such treatment was recently approved by the FDA.

Control-Driven Asthma Therapy

Because all asthma treatment is symptomatic (i.e., no current treatment changes the disease history), the approach to the management of asthma is to titrate treatment to achieve an adequate level of control. If a patient's asthma is well controlled, treatment can be continued or "stepped down" (see Fig. 87-2). 10 If a patient's asthma is poorly controlled, treatment intensity should be stepped up. At the mild end of the spectrum, a patient who has rare limitations in activities of daily life, has nearly normal lung function, and sleeps without interruption from asthma can be prescribed nothing more than inhaled rescue treatment on an as-needed basis. In general, if a patient can control his or her asthma with the use of a single metered-dose inhaler of rescue treatment dispensed every 7 to 8 weeks or less frequently, there is no need for background controller treatment. If a patient has a requirement for more rescue treatment, has symptoms that interfere with sleeping through the night, or has moderately deranged lung function, controller therapy should be added.

Single-agent controller therapy should consist of an inhaled corticosteroid or an antileukotriene. If control is not achieved with one of these agents, the patient can be switched to the other or have a second agent added. The best studied two-agent combination is inhaled corticosteroids and a long-acting inhaled β_2-adrenergic agonist, available in a single inhaler under the trade names of Symbicort and Advair in the United States. These combinations provide excellent disease control and often allow a reduction in the dose of inhaled corticosteroids. Data indicate that another combination, an antileukotriene and inhaled steroid, is more effective than either treatment alone, but this regimen does not have as substantial an evidence base as the combination of inhaled corticosteroids and a long-acting β-agonist.

Specific Treatment Scenarios

Concurrent Pulmonary Infection

In some patients, acute exacerbations of asthma may be due to concurrent infection, which requires targeted therapy (Chapters 88, 90, and 97).

Aspirin-Exacerbated Respiratory Disease (Previously Termed Aspirin-Induced Asthma)

Approximately 5% of patients with moderate to severe persistent asthma develop asthma when they ingest agents that inhibit cyclooxygenase, such as aspirin and other nonsteroidal anti-inflammatory drugs (Chapter 36). Inhibitors of cyclooxygenase 2 are less likely to cause these reactions, but aspirin-type reactions have been reported in sensitive patients treated with selective cyclooxygenase 2 inhibitors. Although the physiologic manifestations of laboratory-based aspirin challenge can be blocked by leukotriene pathway inhibitors, these agents do not prevent clinical aspirin-exacerbated respiratory disease. Thus, patients with this form of asthma must avoid aspirin and other nonsteroidal anti-inflammatory drugs.

Asthma in the Emergency Department

When a patient with asthma presents for acute emergency care, objective measures of the severity of the attack, including quantification of pulsus paradoxus and measurement of airflow rates (PEFR or FEV_1), should be evaluated in addition to the usual vital signs. If the attack has been prolonged and failed to respond to treatment with bronchodilators (e.g., albuterol by metered-dose inhaler, two puffs every 2 to 3 hours) and high-dose inhaled steroids (e.g., more than 2000 μg per day of beclomethasone or half that amount of fluticasone) before arrival at the emergency department, intravenous steroids (40 to 60 mg of methylprednisolone or its equivalent) should be administered. If the patient has not been receiving treatment with a leukotriene receptor antagonist, such agents should be administered (10 mg of montelukast or 20 mg of zafirlukast) as soon as possible. 11 Treatment with inhaled β-agonists (either nebulized albuterol, 0.5 mL of a 0.5% solution—repeated at 20- to 30-minute intervals, or albuterol by metered-dose inhaler, two puffs every 30 minutes) should be used until the PEFR or FEV_1 increases to greater than 40% of the predicted values. If this point is not reached within 2 hours, admission to the hospital for further treatment is strongly advocated.

When patients have PEFR and FEV_1 values that are greater than 60% of their predicted value on arrival in the emergency department, treatment with inhaled β_2-agonists alone, albuterol (0.5 mL of an albuterol 0.083% solution) or equivalent, is likely to result in an objective improvement in airflow rates. If significant improvement takes place in the emergency department, such patients can usually be treated as outpatients with inhaled β_2-agonists and a controller agent (see Fig. 87-2). A good strategy is to add inhaled corticosteroids if the patient has not been receiving this treatment or has been using a single controller therapy.

For patients whose PEFR and FEV_1 values are between 40% and 60% of the values predicted at the time of initial evaluation in the emergency care setting, a plan of treatment varying in intensity between these two plans is indicated. Failure to respond to treatment by objective criteria (PEFR or FEV_1) within 2 hours of arrival at the emergency department is an indication for the use of systemic corticosteroids.

Status Asthmaticus

The asthmatic subject whose PEFR or FEV_1 does not increase to greater than 40% of the predicted value with treatment, whose $PaCO_2$ increases without improvement of indices of airflow obstruction, or who develops major complications such as pneumothorax or pneumomediastinum should be admitted to the hospital for close monitoring. Frequent treatments with inhaled β-agonists (0.5 mL of an albuterol 0.083% solution every 2 hours), intravenous aminophylline (at doses to yield maximal acceptable plasma levels, that is, 15 to 20 μg/mL; 500- to 1000-mg loading dose given during an hour followed by an infusion of 30 to 60 mg/hour), and high-dose intravenous steroids (methylprednisolone, 40 to 60 mg every 4 to 6 hours) are indicated. Oxygen should be administered by face mask or nasal cannula in amounts sufficient to achieve SaO_2 values between 92 and 94%; a higher FIO_2 promotes absorption atelectasis and provides no therapeutic benefit. If objective evidence of an infection is present, appropriate treatment should be given for that infection. If no improvement is seen with treatment and if respiratory failure appears imminent, bronchodilator treatment should be intensified to the maximum tolerated by the patient as indicated by the maximum tolerated heart rate, usually 130 to 140 beats per minute. If indicated, intubation of the trachea and mechanical ventilation can be instituted; in this case, the goal should be to provide a level of ventilation just adequate to sustain life but *not sufficient to normalize arterial blood gases*. For example, a $PaCO_2$ of 60 to 70 mm Hg, or even higher, is acceptable for a patient in status asthmaticus.

Asthma in Pregnancy

Asthma may be exacerbated, remain unchanged, or remit during pregnancy (Chapter 247). There need not be substantial departures from the ordinary management of asthma during pregnancy. However, no unnecessary medications should be administered; systemic steroids should be used sparingly to avert fetal complications, and certain drugs should be avoided, including tetracycline (as a treatment of intercurrent infection), ipratropium bromide (which may cause fetal tachycardia), terbutaline (which is contraindicated during active labor because of its tocolytic effects), and iodine containing mucolytics (such as saturated solution of potassium iodide). Moreover, use of prostaglandin $F_2\alpha$ as an abortifacient should be avoided in asthmatic patients.

PROGNOSIS

Asthma is a chronic relapsing disorder. Most patients have recurrent attacks without a major loss in lung function for many years. A minority of patients experience a significant irreversible loss in lung function over and above the normal pulmonary senescence. Methods to distinguish these various clinical phenotypes have not been developed.

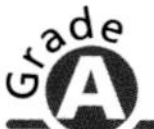

1. Shaw DE, Berry MA, Thomas M, et al. The use of exhaled nitric oxide to guide asthma management: a randomized controlled trial. *Am J Respir Crit Care Med.* 2007;176:231-237.
2. de Jongste JC, Carraro S, Hop WC, et al, for the CHARISM Study Group. Daily telemonitoring of exhaled nitric oxide and symptoms in the treatment of childhood asthma. *Am J Respir Crit Care Med.* 2009;179:93-97.

3. Szefler SJ, Mitchell H, Sorkness CA, et al. Management of asthma based on exhaled nitric oxide in addition to guideline-based treatment for inner-city adolescents and young adults: a randomised controlled trial. *Lancet*. 2008;372:1065-1072.
4. Peters SP, Kunselman SJ, Icitovic N, et al. Tiotropium bromide step-up therapy for adults with uncontrolled asthma. *N Engl J Med*. 2010;363:1715-1726.
5. Busse WW, Pedersen S, Pauwels RA, et al, for the START Investigators Group. The Inhaled Steroid Treatment As Regular Therapy in Early Asthma (START) study 5-year follow-up: effectiveness of early intervention with budesonide in mild persistent asthma. *J Allergy Clin Immunol*. 2008;121:1167-1174.
6. Boushey HA, Sorkness CA, King TS, et al, for the National Heart, Lung, and Blood Institute's Asthma Clinical Research Network. Daily versus as-needed corticosteroids for mild persistent asthma. *N Engl J Med*. 2005;352:1519-1528.
7. Papi A, Canonica GW, Maestrelli P, et al, for the BEST Study Group. Rescue use of beclomethasone and albuterol in a single inhaler for mild asthma. *N Engl J Med*. 2007;356:2040-2052.
8. Nelson HS, Weiss ST, Bleecker ER, et al, for the SMART Study Group. The Salmeterol Multicenter Asthma Research Trial: a comparison of usual pharmacotherapy for asthma or usual pharmacotherapy plus salmeterol. *Chest*. 2006;129:15-26.
9. Mastronarde JG, Anthonisen NR, Castro M, et al, for the American Lung Association Asthma Clinical Research Centers. Efficacy of esomeprazole for treatment of poorly controlled asthma. *N Engl J Med*. 2009;360:1487-1499.
10. Peters SP, Anthonisen N, Castro M, et al, for the American Lung Association Asthma Clinical Research Centers. Randomized comparison of strategies for reducing treatment in mild persistent asthma. *N Engl J Med*. 2007;356:2027-2039.
11. Silverman RA, Nowak RM, Korenblat PE, et al. Zafirlukast treatment for acute asthma-evaluation in a randomized, double-blind, multicenter trial. *Chest*. 2004;126:1480-1489.

SUGGESTED READINGS

Gibson PG, McDonald VM, Marks GB. Asthma in older adults. *Lancet*. 2010;376:803-813. *Review.*
Lazarus SC. Emergency treatment of asthma. *N Engl J Med*. 2010;363:755-764. *Review.*
Morjaria JB, Proiti M, Polosa R. Stratified medicine in selecting biologics for the treatment of severe asthma. *Curr Opin Allergy Clin Immunol*. 2011;11:58-63. *An approach to the use of newer biologic agents.*

88 CHRONIC OBSTRUCTIVE PULMONARY DISEASE

DENNIS E. NIEWOEHNER

DEFINITIONS

Chronic obstructive pulmonary disease (COPD) is now the preferred term for a condition that is characterized by progressive, largely irreversible airflow obstruction, usually with clinical onset in middle-aged or elderly persons with a history of cigarette smoking, and which cannot be attributed to another specific disease, such as bronchiectasis (Chapter 90) or asthma (Chapter 87). Commonly used terms for this condition in the past included *chronic bronchitis* and *emphysema*. That terminology is outdated because nearly all patients with a clinical diagnosis of COPD have both air space destruction (i.e., emphysema) and pathologic changes of the conducting airways consistent with chronic bronchitis.

Emphysema is defined pathologically by abnormal enlargement of the air spaces owing to destruction and deformation of alveolar walls. The severity of emphysema may vary widely in COPD patients with similar degrees of airflow obstruction. Chronic bronchitis is defined clinically as persistent cough and sputum production and pathologically as abnormal enlargement of the mucous glands within the central cartilaginous airways. Chronic bronchitis was once thought to be a key element in the pathogenesis of chronic airflow obstruction, but it is now known that increased airflow resistance in COPD can be attributed principally to a variety of pathologic changes within the distal airways of the lung ("small airways disease").

EPIDEMIOLOGY

COPD represents a growing global public health problem, although estimates vary widely according to the definition used. Cigarette smoking (Chapter 31) is the principal risk factor for COPD, so prevalence tends to reflect societal smoking habits with a lag phase of 20 to 30 years. Cigarette consumption has leveled off or decreased in large segments of North America and Europe, but the prevalence of COPD may continue to increase as these populations age. A greater future burden of COPD may be anticipated in Asia and other regions of the world because of rapidly increasing cigarette consumption.

More than 10% of the population older than 45 years in the United States has airflow obstruction of at least moderate severity as judged by spirometric criteria. COPD is the fourth leading cause of death in the United States, with mortality in women now exceeding that in men. COPD is projected to become the third leading cause of death worldwide by 2020. In 2007, medical costs and lost productivity attributable to COPD exceeded $40 billion in the United States. Direct medical costs rise precipitously as COPD becomes more severe, with hospitalization for exacerbations accounting for more than one half of the total.

Cigarette Smoking

Cigarette smoking is the principal cause of COPD, but the relationship between smoking and COPD is complex and incompletely understood. Airflow obstruction is the sentinel physiologic disturbance in COPD, and the forced expiratory volume in the first second (FEV_1) is the single best indicator of severity. Cigarette smoking causes declines in lung function that exceed those expected from aging alone, and the magnitude of loss is dependent on both the intensity and duration of exposure to cigarette smoke. Thus, the cumulative effects of smoking largely account for the increasing prevalence of COPD with advancing age.

Individual losses of lung function vary widely, even after adjustment for smoking intensity. After age 30 years, everyone loses lung function on a yearly basis, but smoking further impacts the rate of lung function loss. The mean annual reduction in the FEV_1 (Chapter 85) in normal nonsmoking white men is about 25 mL per year, but the loss increases to an average of about 40 mL per year among smokers (Fig. 88-1). A small minority of smokers, "susceptible smokers," suffer annual FEV_1 losses of 100 mL or more and may develop clinically significant airflow obstruction in the fourth and fifth decades of life. Factors that distinguish the susceptible smoker from the average smoker remain largely unknown.

Adverse effects of cigarette smoke on lung function may extend as far back as fetal development. Maternal smoking during pregnancy, secondhand cigarette smoke exposure during early childhood, and active smoking during adolescence impair lung growth. As a consequence, the lower lung function in early adulthood constitutes a significant risk factor for COPD later in life.

Other Environmental Exposures

Workers exposed to dust in certain workplace environments, such as mines, cotton mills, and grain-handling facilities, commonly develop respiratory symptoms and may suffer permanent loss of lung function (Chapter 93). In some regions of the world, repeated exposures to biomass combustion in confined living quarters causes airflow obstruction. Current urban air pollution in economically advanced countries appears to have little effect on the prevalence of airflow obstruction, but this factor may be more important in heavily polluted urban centers in industrializing countries.

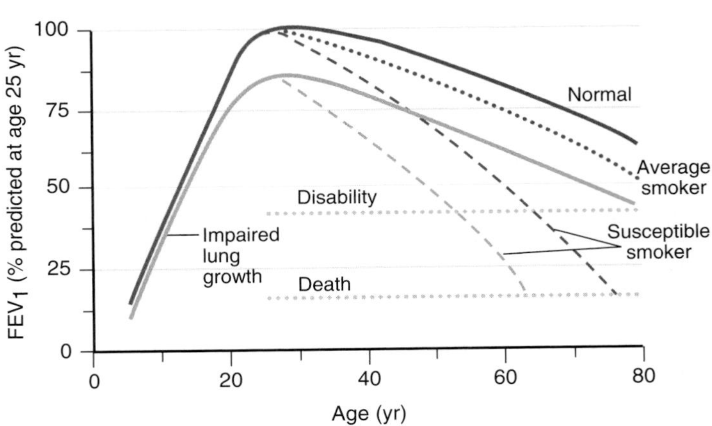

FIGURE 88-1. Lung growth occurs during childhood and adolescence with the forced expiratory volume in one second (FEV_1) reaching a maximum at about 25 years of age. Thereafter, the FEV_1 steadily declines owing to normal aging effects. Lung function declines more rapidly in smokers, but the average effect is so small that clinically significant airflow obstruction would never develop. However, a proportion of "susceptible smokers" lose lung function much faster than the average, so they develop disabling chronic obstructive pulmonary disorder (COPD). If lung growth is impaired, lung function reserve is less as a young adult, and a susceptible smoker will develop disabling COPD at an earlier age.

Respiratory Infections

Recurrent respiratory infections were once thought to be a major factor in the development of airflow obstruction, but longitudinal cohort studies have yielded inconclusive findings. An effect, if present, appears weak relative to cigarette smoking. Whether childhood respiratory infections leave residual effects on adult lung function is similarly unclear.

Airway Responsiveness

Acute bronchoconstriction after inhalation of dilute concentrations of methacholine or histamine, termed *bronchial hyperresponsiveness* (Chapter 87), is a defining feature of asthma but is also present in many COPD patients. Bronchial hyperresponsiveness independently predicts accelerated loss of lung function in persons with mild to moderate COPD, especially among persons who continue to smoke.

Genetic Factors

A severe deficiency of α_1-antitrypsin, which is the only proven genetic risk factor for COPD, is found in about 1-2% of patients with an established diagnosis of COPD. Alpha-1-antitrypsin, which is a serine protease inhibitor that is secreted into the circulation from the liver, is thought to protect lung tissue against digestion by neutrophil elastase and related serine proteinases that have been implicated in the pathogenesis of human emphysema. The most common allele at the α_1-antitrypsin genetic locus is M, and MM homozygotes have what are considered normal levels of α_1-antitrypsin (100 to 300 mg/dL). Numerous variant alleles have been identified, but severe deficiency is most commonly found in persons who are homozygous for the Z allele, in whom serum levels are generally less than 20 to 30% of the lower range of normal. Affected persons are very susceptible to cigarette smoke–induced damage and may develop severe COPD at a relatively early age. The risk for clinically important emphysema appears to be much less if patients with the risk alleles do not smoke. Emphysema associated with severe α_1-antitrypsin deficiency is characteristically of the panacinar type with a predominant basal distribution.

About 2 to 3% of northern European populations possess the MZ heterozygote serum and have α_1-antitrypsin levels about half of normal. Whether these individuals are at greater risk for developing COPD remains unclear. Familial aggregations of COPD not attributed to α_1-antitrypsin deficiency states suggest additional genetic risks. Women with severe COPD appear to have relatively more airway disease and less emphysema compared with men with similar airflow obstruction.

PATHOBIOLOGY

Pathology

Emphysema

Emphysema is characterized by abnormal enlargement of the air spaces distal to the terminal bronchiole, with destruction of the alveolar walls but without obvious fibrosis. The terminal bronchiole, which is the most distal nonalveolated airway within the bronchial tree, supplies ventilation to a lung unit that is termed the *acinus*. Distal to the terminal bronchiole are two or three generations of partially alveolated respiratory bronchioles, and then the alveolar zone, where most gas exchange occurs. Air spaces may enlarge throughout the alveolated zone owing to destruction or rearrangement of their walls.

Human emphysema consists of two major subtypes. Centriacinar emphysema localizes to the respiratory bronchioles just distal to the terminal bronchiole, whereas the remainder of the acinus is largely spared. Individual lesions, which may be up to 10 mm in diameter, tend to be more prominent in the upper lobe. Severe centriacinar emphysema is almost always related to cigarette smoking, but mild centriacinar emphysema can occur from other environmental exposures. Focal areas of inflammation, fibrosis, and carbonaceous pigment are commonly present in adjacent alveolar and bronchiolar walls.

In panacinar emphysema, alveolar ducts are diffusely enlarged; adjacent alveoli may become effaced to the extent that individual units can no longer be identified. With progression of the disease, individual lesions can coalesce to form large bullae. Panacinar emphysema, which is typical of severe α_1-antitrypsin deficiency, also commonly occurs in patients in whom the major risk factor for COPD is cigarette smoking. Most patients with severe COPD appear to have mixed elements of centriacinar and panacinar emphysema, and individual subtypes cannot be reliably distinguished in advanced disease.

Chronic Bronchitis and Bronchiolitis

Mucous glands, located between the epithelial basement membrane and the cartilage plates within the central bronchial tree, and goblet cells in the airway epithelium secrete mucus into the bronchial lumen to aid in host defenses. Enlargement of the bronchial mucous glands and expansion of the epithelial goblet cell population, which occur commonly in COPD, are correlated with clinical symptoms of cough and excess sputum production but not with airflow obstruction. A low-grade inflammatory response, consisting of neutrophils, macrophages, and $CD8^+$ T lymphocytes, may also be seen in the cartilaginous airways of COPD patients.

The principal sites of increased airflow resistance in COPD are the small distal airways that have an internal diameter near the lung's functional residual capacity of less than 2 mm. The earliest pathologic changes identified in young cigarette smokers consist of focal collections of brown-pigmented macrophages in the respiratory bronchiole and a sparse infiltrate of neutrophils and lymphocytes in the walls of the terminal bronchiole. In older patients with established COPD, the inflammatory response is more intense, but still with a similar mix of neutrophils, macrophages, and lymphocytes. Other pathologic changes in the distal airways include fibrosis, goblet cell and squamous cell metaplasia of the lining epithelium, smooth muscle enlargement within the airway walls, and scattered regions of mucous plugging. Compared with normal subjects, distal airways in patients with COPD have thicker airway walls and smaller lumens.

Pulmonary Vasculature

Hypoxemia causes vasoconstriction in small pulmonary arteries and a consequent increase in pulmonary vascular resistance. Vascular remodeling in response to chronic hypoxemia results in irreversible pulmonary hypertension (Chapter 68). Medial smooth muscle enlargement and intimal fibrosis in small pulmonary arteries are the most important vascular changes. Additionally, a substantial portion of the capillary bed may be destroyed by severe emphysema.

Pathogenesis

Emphysema appears to be caused by an elastase-antielastase imbalance in the lung, due either to elastase excess or to antielastase deficiency. Human lungs contain a rich network of elastin-containing fibers and other matrix proteins that confer structural integrity and elasticity to alveolar walls. Intratracheal instillation of proteinases, particularly those capable of hydrolyzing native elastin, induce lesions with morphologic and functional features of human emphysema in experimental animals. Chronic inflammation induced from cigarette smoke increases the burden of inflammatory cell-derived proteinases within lung parenchyma. Severe deficiencies of α_1-antitrypsin, a potent inhibitor of neutrophil elastase and other serine proteinases, is associated with development of severe panacinar emphysema in humans. In addition to neutrophil elastase, other neutrophil-derived serine proteinases, such as proteinase 3 and cathepsin G, and matrix metalloproteinases degrade elastin and other matrix components, including collagen, proteoglycans, and fibronectin. A macrophage-derived metalloproteinase, MMP-12, is essential to the development of cigarette smoke–induced emphysema in an animal model, and genetic studies show a linkage with the region of the genome containing DNA encoding MMP-12.

Relatively less is understood about the pathogenesis of distal airways disease. Particulate matter and toxic gases from inhaled cigarette smoke initiate an inflammatory response composed primarily of macrophages and neutrophils. This early inflammatory response may be mediated by the innate defense system as a response to cell injury. In more advanced disease, inflammation persists even after the patient has stopped smoking. At this stage, humoral and cellular components of the adaptive immune system may predominate, possibly in response to infection or specific antigens from other sources. Infiltration of airway walls with $CD4^+$, $CD8^+$, and B lymphocytes is a prominent feature of more advanced COPD. Repair from either type of immune response might cause airway remodeling by stimulating connective tissue matrix synthesis and smooth muscle formation and by increasing the proportion of mucus-secreting goblet cells within the epithelial layer.

Pathophysiology

Lung and Heart Mechanics

Elastic recoil refers to the lung's intrinsic tendency to deflate following inflation. A dense labyrinth of elastic fibers and other matrix elements within the lung parenchyma, along with surface tension at the alveolar air-liquid interface, confers this important mechanical property. Elastic recoil maintains the patency of small airways through radial alveolar attachments, similar to the way a tent is held up by its guy ropes, and provides a portion of the driving pressure during expiration. Age-related loss of lung elasticity largely explains the normal decline in FEV_1 with advancing age. In emphysema, loss of lung elastic recoil results from damage to elastic fibers and loss of alveolar surface area.

An increase in bronchial airflow resistance is another sentinel feature of lung mechanics in COPD. The increased resistance in COPD is due primarily to changes in the small airways of less than 2 mm diameter. Compared with normal lungs, peripheral airflow resistance of COPD is larger by an order of magnitude or more. In contrast, airflow resistance in the central airways of lungs from COPD patients differs little from that of normal lungs. One of the key physiologic aspects of COPD is limitation of this expiratory airflow (Fig. 88-2) owing to loss of lung elastic recoil and increased viscous resistance to airflow in the small airways (Chapter 85). The severity of emphysema and airflow obstruction is directly related to impaired left ventricular filling, reduced stroke volume, and lower cardiac output without reducing the ejection fraction.

Gas Exchange

Mild hypoxemia may be detected in the early stages of COPD, and hypoxemia often becomes more prominent as airflow obstruction worsens. Hypercapnia usually appears only with severe COPD but is sometimes absent even in late-stage disease. Ventilation-perfusion mismatching, owing to changes in both the airways and pulmonary vessels, is largely responsible for hypoxemia, with uneven ventilation being the primary event. Gas exchange is most efficient when the ratio of ventilation to perfusion is uniform in all lung regions. In COPD, there is "wasted ventilation" because some lung regions have inadequate pulmonary blood flow for the ventilation. The calculated A-a gradient for oxygen is larger than anticipated for the patient's age (Chapter 103). Thus, in most cases of COPD, modest increases in the fraction of inspired oxygen result in a resolution of clinical hypoxemia.

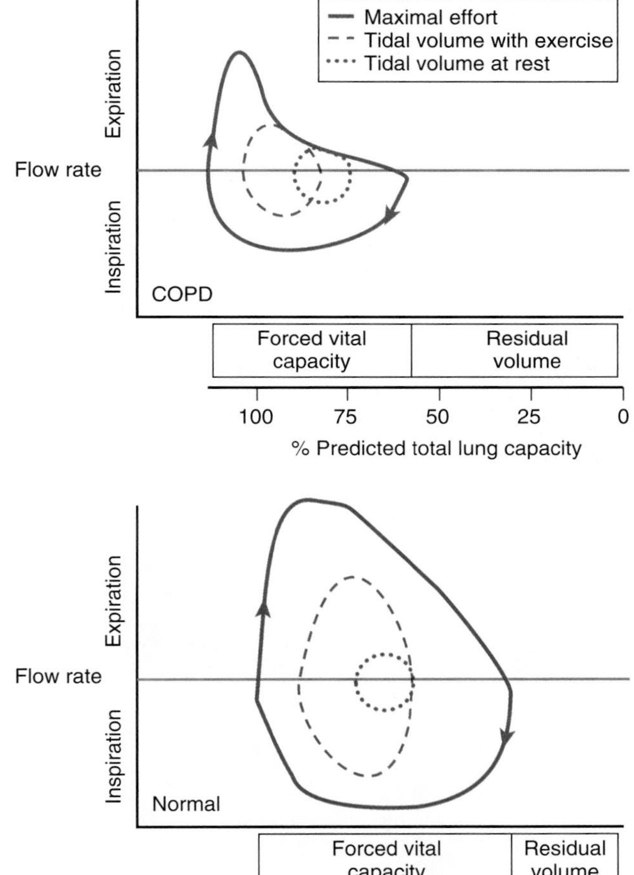

FIGURE 88-2. Inspiratory and expiratory flow-volume loops at rest, with exercise, and with maximal effort in a normal subject are compared with those in a patient with chronic obstructive pulmonary disorder (COPD). The normal subject can easily increase both tidal volume and breathing frequency to match the metabolic requirements of vigorous exercise. In contrast, the COPD patient exhibits maximal expiratory flow limitation even at rest and must breathe at larger lung volumes to optimize expiratory airflow. Lung hyperinflation requires greater respiratory work because the lung and chest wall become stiffer at larger volumes. This effect is accentuated during exercise, which causes end-expiratory lung volume to increase further. This phenomenon is described as *dynamic hyperinflation* and is an important mechanism in limiting exercise and causing dyspnea.

CLINICAL MANIFESTATIONS

History and Physical Examination

COPD should be suspected in all adults who complain of chronic respiratory symptoms, particularly dyspnea (Chapter 83) that limits activities of daily living. Clinical features that increase the likelihood of COPD include older age, current or past cigarette use, insidious onset of dyspnea with slow progression, history of acute bronchitis for which medical care is sought, and symptoms of chronic cough, sputum production, or wheezing. Symptoms of cough and sputum may antedate dyspnea by many years. Some patients date the onset of dyspnea to a respiratory infection, but careful questioning usually elicits some history of impaired exercise tolerance before that event. Absence of cigarette smoking does not preclude a diagnosis of COPD because a few persons develop severe irreversible airflow obstruction without smoking history and even without known genetic predispositions. Some nonsmokers may relate a history of occupational dust or noxious gas exposure (Chapter 94), but sometimes no putative cause can be discerned.

The physical examination is usually normal in patients with mild to moderate disease, and characteristic physical signs may be absent even in severe disease. Physical examination findings commonly present in severe COPD include the appearance of a barrel-shaped chest, low diaphragm detected by percussion, prolonged expiratory phase, and use of accessory muscles of respiration. Heart sounds are usually distant, and auscultation of the chest may reveal diminished breath sounds or a variety of rhonchi, wheezes, and rattles. Auscultatory wheezes may be prominent, particularly during exacerbations, but this physical sign does not reliably differentiate COPD from asthma. With severe hypoxemia, cyanosis may be clinically evident. Clubbing is not associated with COPD, and its presence should suggest another diagnosis. Pedal edema, distended jugular veins, and hepatic congestion are signs of pulmonary hypertension and cor pulmonale (Chapter 68). Patients with advanced COPD may be cachectic, with loss of muscle mass and subcutaneous fat.

Clinical Phenotypes

One of the more enduring efforts to categorize COPD into subtypes is the description of the patients as either "pink puffers" or "blue bloaters." The pink puffer is described as a cachectic individual with unrelenting dyspnea, clinical and radiographic signs of severe lung hyperinflation, and normal or near-normal arterial blood gases at rest. Salient features of the blue bloater are a stout body habitus, chronic cough and sputum, less troubling dyspnea, and severe hypoxemia and hypercapnia resulting in polycythemia and signs of cor pulmonale. In the original description of these phenotypes, the pink puffer phenotype was equated with severe emphysema, whereas the blue bloater was thought to have predominant chronic bronchitis.

Selected COPD patients do fit one or the other of these clinical subtypes, but most cannot be simply categorized. Limited information from clinical and pathologic correlative studies fails to show a consistent association of either clinical subtype with distinguishing pathologic features in lung parenchyma or airways. The blue bloater phenotype may now be less common, possibly because hypoxemia is recognized and treated earlier or because some COPD patients once described as blue bloaters may have had coexisting obstructive sleep apnea (Chapter 100).

COPD patients with similar degrees of airflow obstruction vary greatly with respect to severity of dyspnea, impairment of exercise tolerance, frequency of exacerbations, body habitus, and severity of arterial blood gas disturbances. There is limited understanding about the mechanisms underlying these clinical characteristics.

DIAGNOSIS

Pulmonary Function Tests

Airflow obstruction can be determined only by spirometry. If the ratio of FEV_1 to FVC is less than 0.70 (Chapter 85) after administration of an inhaled bronchodilator, an obstructive defect is present (Table 88-1). A large improvement of perhaps 30 to 40% in FEV_1 after treatment with an inhaled bronchodilator may help identify a patient with predominant asthma, but the test otherwise has little clinical utility and cannot reliably identify patients who will benefit from any particular form of therapy.

Lung volume measurements may help distinguish obstructive and restrictive lung diseases in selected patients, but they are unnecessary in most COPD patients. The diffusing capacity for carbon monoxide (DLCO; Chapter 85) measures the uptake of carbon monoxide between inspired air and the blood stream. Decreases in the DLCO reflect the loss of alveolar surface area that is available for gas transfer and roughly correspond to the severity of emphysema. However, the test provides information of no practical value in the customary management of COPD.

After the diagnosis is established, follow-up spirometry may help determine whether worsening breathlessness is due to COPD, as indicated by a decrease in FEV_1, or to another cause, such as heart failure (Chapter 58). However, repeated spirometry should not be used as a guide to drug therapy because the background variability of the measurement is large relative to treatment effects.

Oximetry

Hypoxemia and hypercapnia become increasingly common as COPD worsens. Because treatment with supplemental oxygen improves mortality, patients with severe COPD should be tested for hypoxemia at regular intervals. Hypoxemia can be detected and quantified by oximetry or arterial blood gases. Oximetry is generally preferred because it is simpler, cheaper, and causes no discomfort. The added information from a set of arterial blood gases (Chapter 103) is most helpful in COPD patients with severe exacerbations.

TABLE 88-1 STAGE AND SEVERITY OF COPD ACCORDING TO POSTBRONCHODILATOR SPIROMETRY

STAGE AND SEVERITY	DEFINITION
I: Mild	$FEV_1/FVC < 0.70$, $FEV_1 \geq 80\%$ of predicted
II: Moderate	$FEV_1/FVC < 0.70$, $50\% \leq FEV_1 < 80\%$ of predicted
III: Severe	$FEV_1/FVC < 0.70$, $30\% \leq FEV_1 < 50\%$ of predicted
IV: Very severe	$FEV_1/FVC < 0.70$, $FEV_1 < 30\%$ of predicted or $FEV_1 < 50\%$ of predicted plus chronic respiratory failure

Data from the Global Initiative for Chronic Obstructive Lung Disease. http://www.goldcopd.com.

Radiographic Studies

Common signs of severe COPD on a chest radiograph include hyperinflated lungs, flattened diaphragms, and increased retrosternal clear space (Fig. 88-3). The walls of large emphysematous bullae may be visualized as thin curvilinear lines, and severe emphysema may appear as regions of relative hyperlucency. Chest radiographs are usually normal in mild to moderate COPD and sometimes in severe COPD. Hence, a chest radiograph is not an adequate diagnostic test for COPD, and it is used mostly to exclude other pulmonary diseases. Chest computed tomography (CT), which is a superior imaging modality to assess the magnitude and distribution of emphysema (Fig. 88-4), is not helpful in the usual management of COPD.

Other Studies

Measurement of the serum level of α_1-antitrypsin deficiency may be considered, particularly if the patient has a strong family history of COPD or if the onset of airflow obstruction occurs at an early age. If the α_1-antitrypsin level is less than 20 to 30% of normal, further testing with specialized phenotyping and genotyping studies is required to confirm the diagnosis.

Differential Diagnosis

COPD is most commonly confused with asthma (Chapter 87), particularly in older patients. Clinical features that favor asthma over COPD include onset of disease at an early age, presence of atopy, lack of a smoking history, substantial variability of symptoms over time, and largely reversible airflow obstruction. However, new onset of asthma may occur in elderly people, some asthmatics smoke, an atopic history is not a requisite for developing asthma, and airflow obstruction may become fixed in patients with severe, long-standing asthma. Because treatment is much the same, distinguishing asthma from COPD may not be so important.

Bronchiectasis (Chapter 90) is characterized by chronic inflammation and abnormal dilation of airways associated with chronic cough and expectoration of purulent sputum. It can be distinguished from COPD with a predominant bronchitis component by chest CT imaging.

Bronchiolitis obliterans is characterized by cicatricial narrowing of the distal airways with severe irreversible airflow obstruction. The condition may occur in association with collagen vascular diseases (Chapters 272 and 274) and is commonly seen after lung transplantation (Chapter 101). A similar

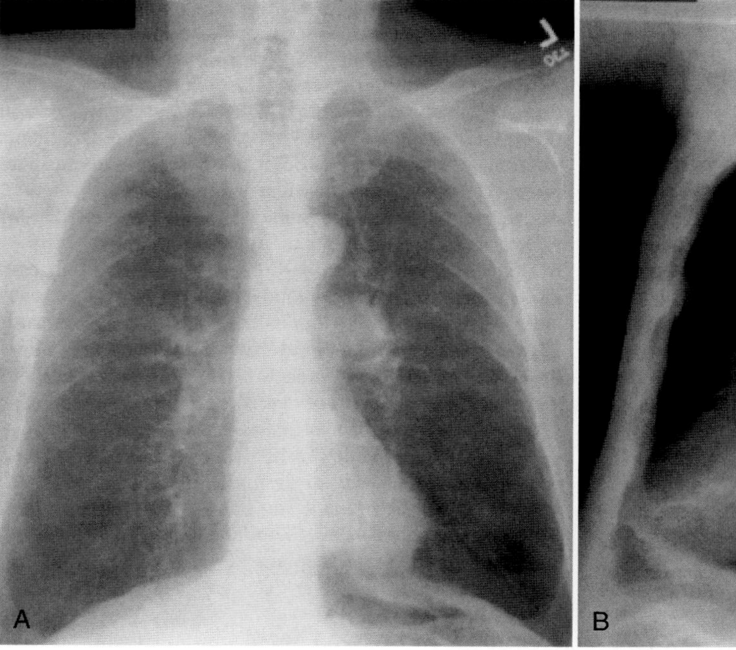

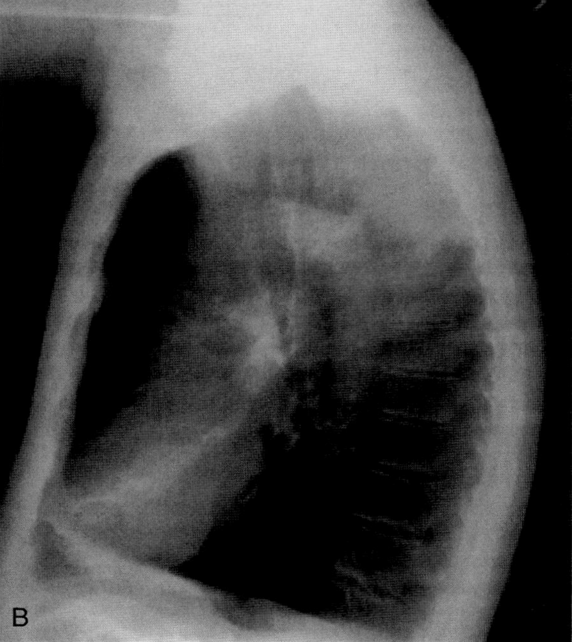

FIGURE 88-3. Posteroanterior (A) and lateral (B) radiographs of the thorax in a patient with emphysema. The most obvious abnormalities are those associated with increased lung volume. The lungs appear dark because of their increased air relative to tissue. The diaphragms are caudal to their normal position and appear flatter than normal. The heart is oriented more vertically than normal because of caudal displacement of the diaphragm, and the transverse diameter of the rib cage is increased; as a result, the width of the heart relative to the rib cage on the posteroanterior view is decreased. The space between the sternum and heart and great vessels is increased on the lateral view.

disorder has been described with certain industrial inhalants, such as diacetyl, a butter-like flavoring manufactured for use with microwavable popcorn (Chapter 93). In nonsmokers, the diagnosis of bronchiolitis obliterans can be reliably inferred from history, the presence of irreversible airflow obstruction, and the absence of emphysema or other explanatory conditions on chest CT images. Attribution of cause in smokers is more difficult because the airway pathology with diacetyl exposure is similar to that found with cigarette smoke.

TREATMENT Rx

Stable Disease

Smoking Cessation

Smoking cessation (Chapter 31) reduces symptoms of cough and sputum production in many patients with COPD, but it improves lung function to only a small extent (Fig. 88-5). Most important, after smoking cessation, the rate of decline of FEV_1 in patients with mild to moderate disease reverts back to that seen in lifelong nonsmokers, thereby making it unlikely that these former smokers will ever develop severe COPD. Smoking cessation in patients with mild to moderate COPD also improves long-term mortality by reducing both respiratory and cardiovascular deaths.[1] It is not known whether smoking cessation slows the decline in lung function or improves mortality in patients with severe COPD.

Limited information indicates that counseling and pharmacotherapy achieve the same low success rates in COPD patients as in the general population. COPD patients tend to quit smoking as the disease progresses, possibly because they have greater awareness of their disease or because cigarette smoke makes their respiratory symptoms worse. Information regarding abnormal spirometry does not motivate patients to quit smoking.

Bronchodilators

Both β_2-adrenergic agonists and anticholinergics are widely used to treat COPD (Table 88-2). Short-acting β_2-adrenergic agonists, such as albuterol and the short-acting anticholinergic ipratropium bromide, can be administered either by oral inhaler devices or by nebulization, with little objective superiority of one delivery device over the other if a spacer is used with oral inhaler devices. Longer-acting bronchodilators have largely replaced shorter-acting drugs, but a short-acting bronchodilator, such as albuterol, is still recommended for "rescue" or "as-needed" use in patients who experience bothersome dyspnea.

The inhaled long-acting bronchodilators widely used for COPD include the β_2-adrenergic agonists salmeterol and formoterol, both administered by one inhalation twice daily, and the anticholinergic tiotropium, administered by one inhalation once or twice daily. Compared with placebo, they consistently provide clinically meaningful improvement in respiratory health status in only about 10 to 15% of patients.[2] Tiotropium (18 µg once daily) appears to be superior to salmeterol (50 µg twice daily) for reducing exacerbations.[3]

Compared with placebo, both classes of long-acting bronchodilators reduce exacerbation rates by about 15 to 20% in relative terms. Because the average patient with severe COPD has about one serious exacerbation per year, the number of patients that need to be treated to prevent one exacerbation is about six.

Adverse symptomatic events of both classes of long-acting bronchodilators in COPD patients are generally minor. Despite concerns about their long-term safety, the largest and longest trials to date have shown no serious safety issues when long-acting β_2-adrenergic agonists or long-acting anticholinergics are used to treat COPD.

Theophylline is a poor bronchodilator that largely has been replaced with inhaled drugs, but its effect is additive when given along with inhaled bronchodilators. Theophylline may also reduce exacerbations. To be used effectively and safely, it should be started with an oral daily dose of between 150 and 300 mg and titrated to achieve serum levels of 8 to 12 µg/mL. Higher levels are poorly tolerated, especially in older patients. Theophylline interacts with numerous other drugs (e.g., allopurinol, diazepam, cimetidine, ciprofloxacin), and conditions such as heart failure and liver disease may reduce its elimination rates. Patients' drug levels must be monitored on a regular basis, and even a patient on a stable dose can develop toxic levels. Oral roflumilast, a phosphodiesterase-4 inhibitor at 500 µg once daily, can increase FEV_1 by 50 mL and reduce moderate to severe exacerbations of COPD, even in patients already treated with tiotropium.[4]

Corticosteroids

Inhaled corticosteroids produce marginal improvements in lung function and respiratory health status in COPD patients, and they reduce COPD exacerbation rates by about 15 to 20% in relative terms.[5] Inhaled corticosteroids combined with an inhaled long-acting β_2-agonist provide added benefit over that seen with either monotherapy. However, multiple large trials found little effect of inhaled corticosteroids on FEV_1 loss over periods of several years.

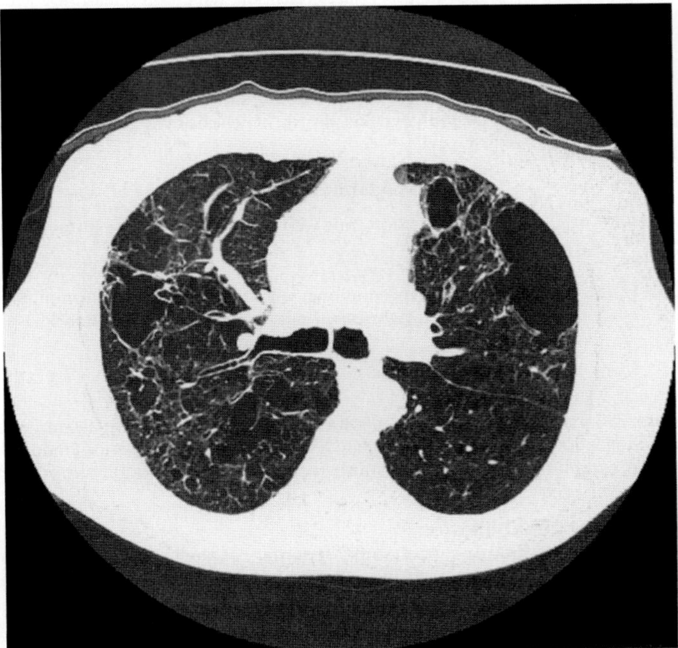

FIGURE 88-4. High-resolution axial computed tomography scan of a 1-mm section of the thorax of a patient with emphysema at the level of the tracheal carina. The right lung is on the *left*. Multiple large bullae—black holes—are evident. Many smaller areas of similar tissue destruction are also present in both lungs. The right upper lobe bronchus is seen entering the lung; its walls are thickened, suggesting chronic inflammation. (Courtesy of Dr. Bruce Maycher.)

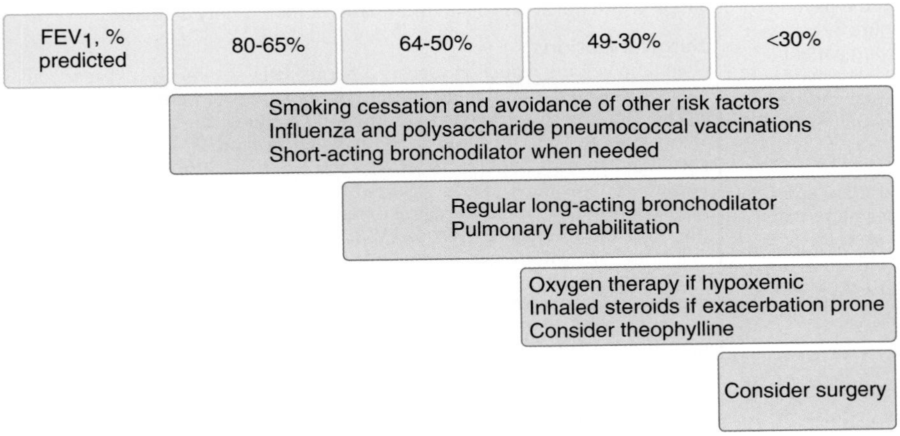

FEV_1, % predicted	80-65%	64-50%	49-30%	<30%

Smoking cessation and avoidance of other risk factors
Influenza and polysaccharide pneumococcal vaccinations
Short-acting bronchodilator when needed

Regular long-acting bronchodilator
Pulmonary rehabilitation

Oxygen therapy if hypoxemic
Inhaled steroids if exacerbation prone
Consider theophylline

Consider surgery

FIGURE 88-5. The flow diagram illustrates step management of stable COPD; more therapies are added as the disease becomes more severe. The percent predicted FEV_1 provides only a rough guide to the severity of the disease so other factors, such as exercise limitations and the frequency of exacerbations, should also be considered in the global assessment.

TABLE 88-2 COMMONLY USED MEDICATIONS FOR STABLE COPD

	MODE OF DELIVERY	DOSE AND FREQUENCY	POSSIBLE ADVERSE REACTIONS
SHORT-ACTING INHALED BRONCHODILATORS			
Albuterol (β_2-adrenergic agonist)	Inhaler	100 μg per inhalation; 1-2 inhalations every 4-6 hours, as needed	Palpitations, tachycardia, tremor, hypersensitivity reaction
	Nebulizer	2.5 mg; every 4-6 hours, as needed	
Ipratropium (anticholinergic)	Inhaler	17 μg per inhalation; 2 inhalations 4 times daily, up to 12 inhalations a day	Dry mouth, cough, blurred vision, hypersensitivity reaction
	Nebulizer	0.5 mg; every 6-8 hours	
Albuterol, ipratropium	Inhaler device	90 μg/18 μg per inhalation; 2 inhalations 4 times daily, up to 12 inhalations per day	All those occurring with either albuterol or ipratropium
	Nebulizer	2.5 mg/0.5 mg; 4 times daily, up to 2 additional doses daily	
LONG-ACTING INHALED BRONCHODILATORS			
Formoterol (β_2-adrenergic agonist)	Inhaler	12 μg; 1 inhalation twice daily	Dizziness, tremor, throat irritation, hypersensitivity reaction
	Nebulizer	20 μg; twice daily	
Salmeterol (β_2-adrenergic agonist)	Inhaler	50 μg; 1 inhalation twice daily	Headache, tremor, throat irritation, hypersensitivity reaction
Tiotropium (anticholinergic)	Inhaler	18 μg; one inhalation each morning	Dry mouth, urinary retention, symptoms of narrow-angle glaucoma, hypersensitivity reaction
INHALED CORTICOSTEROIDS			
Fluticasone powder	Inhaler	250 μg; 1-2 inhalations twice daily	Sore throat, dysphonia, headache, hypersensitivity reaction
Budesonide	Inhaler	160 μg; 1-2 inhalations twice daily	Nasopharyngitis, thrush, hypersensitivity reactions
COMBINATION β-ADRENERGIC AGONIST BRONCHODILATOR AND INHALED CORTICOSTEROID			
Fluticasone/salmeterol	Inhaler	250 μg/50 μg; 1 inhalation twice daily	All those occurring with either fluticasone or salmeterol
Budesonide/formoterol	Inhaler	160 μg/4.5 μg; 2 inhalations twice daily	All those occurring with either budesonide or formoterol
METHYLXANTHINES			
Theophylline (24-hour sustained release)	Pill	200-800 mg, once daily; start with daily dose of 150-300 mg and titrate to blood level of 8-12 μg/mL	Nausea and vomiting, seizures, tremor, insomnia, multifocal atrial tachyarrhythmia, hypersensitivity reaction

The most common adverse effects of inhaled corticosteroids are dysphonia and upper airway thrush. Observational studies suggest that inhaled corticosteroids may cause osteoporosis (Chapter 251) and cataracts (Chapter 431).

A few COPD patients are prescribed systemic corticosteroids on a regular basis, usually in doses of 10 to 15 mg per day of prednisone or its equivalent. These patients are sometimes considered "prednisone dependent" because it is frequently difficult to wean them completely off drug. There are no proven benefits of chronic, low-dose prednisone in COPD, and adverse effects involving bone, eyes, and other organs are well documented (Chapter 34). Consequently, efforts should be made to reduce or discontinue chronic systemic corticosteroids while optimizing other treatment.

Oxygen

Chronic hypoxemia in patients with COPD can induce irreversible pulmonary hypertension and cor pulmonale (Chapter 68). Long-term oxygen therapy extends life in patients who are persistently hypoxemic.[6] The principal qualifying criteria are an arterial PaO_2 of less than 56 mm Hg or an arterial oxygen saturation of less than 89%, both while breathing ambient air at rest in a stable clinical state. Patients should also be considered for home oxygen if their PaO_2 is less than 60 mm Hg in the presence of right heart failure or polycythemia. Treatment should consist of home oxygen to be used for at least 18 hours daily, to include sleep time. To determine an appropriate prescription, the oxygen flow rate should be adjusted in 1-L/minute increments at 15-minute intervals until the resting oxygen saturation remains above 90%. In qualifying patients, long-term oxygen may also decrease polycythemia and pulmonary hypertension and improve neuropsychiatric function. Oxygen does not improve mortality in patients with similarly severe airflow obstruction but milder hypoxemia.

Many patients with severe COPD may be normoxemic at rest while breathing ambient air but exhibit oxygen desaturation with exercise. Physicians commonly prescribe ambulatory oxygen in this setting, with the expectation that it will improve exercise tolerance and increase daily activity. Ambulatory oxygen modestly improves exercise endurance for such patients in a laboratory setting, but efforts to show benefit during activities of daily living have been mostly unsuccessful. It is also unclear whether COPD patients with isolated nocturnal hypoxemia benefit from oxygen therapy.

Immunizations

An annual influenza vaccination (Chapter 17) is recommended for all patients with COPD, although few trials have targeted this patient population. Observational studies suggest that influenza vaccination substantially reduces hospitalization and mortality rates in COPD patients. Polysaccharide pneumococcal vaccination (Chapter 17) is also recommended, although supporting evidence is weak.

Pulmonary Rehabilitation

COPD patients become increasingly sedentary as their disease progresses. Lack of physical activity causes muscular and cardiovascular deconditioning, which further complicates the ability to perform routine tasks. The principal goal of pulmonary rehabilitation is to reverse this process with a program of exercise endurance training. Educational and behavior modification elements are usually included in an effort to improve coping skills and psychological functioning. Most programs are hospital based and consist of 3- to 4-hour sessions, three times a week, over a 6- to 12-week period. Patients who become breathless with minimal activity or who have exercise limiting comorbidities are not suitable candidates.

Numerous randomized, controlled trials have shown that pulmonary rehabilitation confers substantial improvements in respiratory health status and in walking distance and possibly in reduction of health care use.[7] Unfortunately, the benefits of pulmonary rehabilitation erode rapidly in the absence of a continuation plan after completion of the initial program. Pulmonary rehabilitation is also not accessible to most patients for a variety of reasons.

Surgical Options

In lung volume reduction surgery (Chapter 101), severely emphysematous tissue is resected from the upper lobes of both lungs to permit less diseased portions of unresected lung to expand and function more normally. Patients who are severely disabled from COPD and who have no other major comorbid conditions may be candidates for this procedure if CT imaging shows that severe emphysema is mostly localized to the upper lobes. Compared with controls receiving no surgical treatment, lung volume reduction surgery improves lung function, exercise capacity, and respiratory health status in COPD patients with severe emphysema.[8] There is no mortality benefit from this procedure, with a possible exception in the subset of patients with both predominant upper lobe emphysema and low exercise capacity.

Lung transplantation is an option for patients who are severely incapacitated from COPD and have no major comorbid conditions (Chapter 101). Median survival after lung transplantation is only about 5 years, primarily because of the development of bronchiolitis obliterans, a form of chronic graft rejection causing severe airflow obstruction in the peripheral airways. It is unclear whether lung transplantation extends survival in patients with COPD, but patients who are fortunate enough to avoid complications are able to resume normal daily activities.

Exacerbations

Exacerbations represent an important element in the natural history of COPD. An exacerbation is defined as some combination of dyspnea, cough, and productive sputum, each of which has worsened from the stable state or has newly appeared. Exacerbations may also be associated with symptoms of rhinorrhea, sore throat, fever, and chest congestion. A symptom-based clinical event, as described previously, coupled with administration of an antibiotic or a systemic corticosteroid or admission to a hospital, is a definition that has been widely used in clinical trials.

Patients with severe COPD experience an average of about one such exacerbation per year along with additional milder exacerbations that meet the symptomatic definition but do not require a medical intervention. Exacerbations are acute in onset, but recovery may require several weeks. Severe exacerbations have a major adverse impact on health status and may cause permanent loss of lung function. Hospitalization for exacerbations consumes more than half of total medical costs for COPD. For poorly understood reasons, some patients suffer frequent exacerbations, whereas others have very few, despite similar degrees of airflow obstruction. Independent risk factors include low lung function, older age, history of frequent exacerbations and hospitalizations, presence of productive cough, and presence of cardiovascular comorbidities.

Respiratory infections are thought to cause most exacerbations, although many of these implicated microorganisms may be recovered from sputum during periods of stable disease. Bacteria commonly implicated include *Haemophilus influenzae* (Chapter 308), *Streptococcus pneumoniae* (Chapter 297), and *Moraxella catarrhalis* (Chapter 308). *Pseudomonas aeruginosa* (Chapter 314) and enteric gram-negative bacilli (Chapters 312 and 313) are less common but are seen in patients with very severe COPD who were recently hospitalized or intubated. Putative viral pathogens include rhinoviruses (Chapter 369), influenza (Chapter 372), parainfluenza (Chapter 371), and respiratory syncytial virus (Chapter 370). Periods of increased airborne pollution with diesel particulates, sulfur dioxide, ozone, and nitrogen dioxide are associated with more COPD hospitalizations, but no cause can be assigned to many exacerbations.

Evaluation and management of a patient with a suspected exacerbation varies according to severity. Mild exacerbations encountered in an office setting can be diagnosed and treated on the basis of a brief history and physical examination. Patients seen in emergency department or hospital settings generally are sicker and require a more extensive evaluation (Table 88-3). A chest radiograph should be obtained to look for signs of pneumonia (Chapter 97), pneumothorax (Chapter 99), and heart failure (Chapter 58). If pulmonary embolism (Chapter 98) is suspected, spiral CT of the chest is the test of choice. Arterial blood gases should be measured if there is any suspicion of hypercarbia because this information influences subsequent therapy. Sputum cultures need not be done routinely because they are unproven guides to antibiotic therapy. During seasonal outbreaks of influenza (Chapter 372), type A and B viruses can be identified with rapid commercially available assays. However, the sensitivity of these assays is only about 50 to 70%, so they should not be relied on to withhold antiviral therapy if there is a strong clinical suspicion of influenza.

Cardiac disease is a common comorbidity in COPD patients, and distinguishing a COPD exacerbation from left ventricular failure (Chapter 58) by history and physical examination alone is often problematic. Dyspnea (Chapter 83) is common to both conditions. Peripheral edema (Chapter 50) and elevated jugular venous pressure may occur with either left ventricular failure or with cor pulmonale secondary to COPD. Echocardiography (Chapter 55) and serum brain natriuretic peptide (BNP) levels (Chapter 58) are very useful in this clinical setting, although echocardiography is more difficult to perform in patients with severe COPD. BNP levels may be modestly elevated in both stable and exacerbated COPD in the absence of left ventricular dysfunction. A normal BNP level excludes a diagnosis of left heart failure with a high level of confidence, but an elevated level does not confirm its presence unless markedly elevated.

Decisions about the need for hospitalization rely mostly on clinical judgment because there are no well-validated guidelines. Clinical assessment should consider intensity of dyspnea, use of accessory muscles of respiration, arterial blood gas disturbances, hemodynamic stability, and mental alertness.

TABLE 88-3 GUIDELINE RECOMMENDATIONS FOR HOSPITAL MANAGEMENT OF COPD EXACERBATIONS

	GLOBAL INITIATIVE FOR CHRONIC OBSTRUCTIVE LUNG DISEASE*	AMERICAN THORACIC SOCIETY/ EUROPEAN RESPIRATORY SOCIETY†	NATIONAL INSTITUTE FOR CLINICAL EXCELLENCE‡
Date of statement	2010	2004	2010
Diagnostic testing	Chest radiograph, oximetry, ABGs, and ECG. Other testing as warranted by clinical indication.	Chest radiograph, oxygen saturation, ABGs, ECG, sputum Gram stain and culture.	Chest radiograph, ABG, ECG, complete blood count, sputum smear and culture, blood cultures if febrile.
Bronchodilator therapy	Inhaled short-acting β_2-agonist is recommended. Consider ipratropium if inadequate clinical response. Consider theophylline or aminophylline as second-line intravenous therapy.	Inhaled short-acting β_2-agonist and/or ipratropium with spacer or nebulizer, as needed.	Administer inhaled drugs by nebulizer or hand-held inhaler. Specific agents and dosing regimens not specified. Consider theophylline if inadequate response to inhaled bronchodilators.
Antibiotics	Recommended if (1) increases in dyspnea, sputum volume, and sputum purulence all are present; (2) increase in sputum purulence along with increase in either dyspnea or sputum volume; or (3) need for assisted ventilation. See original document for complex treatment algorithm.	Base choice on local bacterial resistance patterns. Consider amoxicillin/clavulanate or respiratory fluoroquinolones. If *Pseudomonas* species and/or other Enterobacteriaceae are suspected, consider combination therapy.	Administer only if history of purulent sputum. Initiate with an aminopenicillin, a macrolide, or a tetracycline, taking into account local bacterial resistance patterns. Adjust therapy according to sputum and blood cultures.
Systemic corticosteroids	Daily prednisolone 30-40 mg (or its equivalent) orally for 7-10 days.	Daily prednisone 30-40 mg orally for 10-14 days. Equivalent dose intravenously if unable to tolerate oral intake. Consider inhaled corticosteroids.	Daily prednisolone 30 mg (or its equivalent) orally for 7-14 days.
Supplemental oxygen	Maintain oxygen saturation >90%. Monitor ABGs for hypercapnia and acidosis.	Maintain oxygen saturation >90%. Monitor ABGs for hypercapnia and acidosis.	Maintain oxygen saturation within the individualized target range. Monitor ABGs.
Assisted ventilation	Indications for NPPV include severe dyspnea, acidosis (pH $\leq$ 7.35) and/or hypercapnia (P_{CO_2} > 45 mm Hg), and respiratory rate >25 breaths/min. Contraindications to NPPV include respiratory arrest, hemodynamic instability, impaired mental status, copious bronchial secretions, and extreme obesity. Intubate if contraindication to NPPV or failure of NPPV (worsening ABGs or clinical status). Consider likelihood of recovery and patient's wishes and expectations before intubation.	Consider with pH < 7.35 and P_{CO_2} > 45-60 mm Hg and respiratory rate > 24 breaths/min. Institute NPPV in a controlled environment, unless there are contraindications (e.g., respiratory arrest, hemodynamic instability, impaired mental status, copious bronchial secretions, and extreme obesity). Intubate if contraindication to NPPV or failure of NPPV (worsening ABGs or clinical status).	NPPV treatment of choice for persistent hypercapnic respiratory failure. Consider functional status, body mass index, home oxygen, comorbidities, prior ICU admissions, age, and FEV_1 when assessing suitability for intubation and ventilation.

*Data from http://www.goldcopd.com.
†Data from MacNee W. Standards for the diagnosis and treatment of patients with COPD: a summary of the ATS/ERS position paper. *Eur Respir J.* 2004;23:932-946.
‡Data from http://www.nice.org.uk.
ABGs, arterial blood gases; ECG, electrocardiogram; ICU, intensive care unit; NPPV, noninvasive positive pressure ventilation.

Guideline recommendations (see Table 88-3) for treatment of patients hospitalized for COPD exacerbations emphasize that antibiotics hasten recovery.[9] Antibiotics are most effective when cough and purulent sputum are present, but there are no well-validated methods for determining which patients should be treated. If patients are sufficiently ill to seek medical attention for an exacerbation, most should probably receive an antibiotic.

Most randomized placebo-controlled trials evaluated first-generation antibiotics, such as amoxicillin, trimethoprim-sulfamethoxazole, and tetracyclines, and it is unclear whether newer classes of antibiotics, such as macrolides and fluoroquinolones, are more effective. Choice of an antibiotic should be made with considerations to cost, safety, and local patterns of antibiotic resistance among the bacterial species commonly isolated from sputa during exacerbations. Doxycycline, 100 mg twice daily for 7 to 10 days, or trimethoprim/sulfamethoxazole, 160–800 mg twice daily for 7 to 10 days, would be reasonable choices for initial therapy in many locales.

Systemic corticosteroids improve lung function, shorten the recovery period, and prevent relapse when given to patients who are hospitalized or present to an emergency department with a COPD exacerbation.[10] Severely symptomatic patients seen in other clinical settings are also likely to benefit. Prednisone, 40 mg once daily for 10 to 14 days, is appropriate for most patients. Longer courses of systemic corticosteroid therapy are strongly discouraged because they are no more effective and they increase the likelihood of adverse effects. Parenteral corticosteroids should be given if gastrointestinal absorption is thought to be impaired. The major adverse effect of systemic corticosteroids is transient hyperglycemia, which may require treatment, particularly in patients with known diabetes mellitus (Chapter 237).

Patients should be encouraged to increase their use of short-acting bronchodilators during outpatient treatment of an exacerbation. For hospitalized patients, a short-acting bronchodilator should be administered on a regular schedule, every 4 to 6 hours and more frequently as needed. Anticholinergic and β_2-agonist agents are similarly effective, and a few small trials found no significant additive effect during exacerbations. Some patients express a preference for a nebulizer delivery system, although equivalent objective results can be achieved when inhalers are used with a spacer.

Sufficient oxygen should be provided to maintain arterial oxygen saturations just above 90%, usually with oxygen flow rates of 2 to 3 L/minute delivered through a nasal cannula. Even at low flow rates, oxygen therapy can be expected to increase $Pa{CO_2}$ by an average of about 5 to 10 mm Hg in patients with chronic hypercapnia. It is prudent to use the lowest flow of oxygen that achieves the desired result. If oxygen is prescribed for hypoxemia during an exacerbation, it is important to retest the patient several weeks later after recovery to determine when long-term oxygen is needed.

The introduction of noninvasive positive-pressure ventilation (NIPPV) has significantly improved the care of patients with severe COPD exacerbations who have respiratory failure. With NIPPV, the patient wears a tightly fitting nasal or full facial mask that is attached to a positive-pressure ventilator, avoiding the need for an endotracheal tube or a tracheostomy (Chapter 105). Compared with usual care, treatment with NIPPV is associated with fewer intubations, a shorter hospital stay, and improved all-cause mortality.

PROGNOSIS

Severe COPD is associated with excess mortality, and lung function, usually expressed as the percent of predicted FEV_1, is the single strongest predictor of death. Only about one half of patients with an FEV_1 that is about 40% of predicted will survive 5 years. Additional risk factors include the severity of dyspnea, weight loss, limited walking distance, hospitalization for exacerbation, hypoxemia, hypercapnia, and impaired quality of life. The only interventions shown to reduce mortality are smoking cessation in patients with mild to moderate COPD and home oxygen therapy for the subset of patients with chronic hypoxemia.

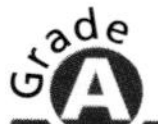

1. Anthonisen NR, Skeans MA, Wise RA, et al. The effects of a smoking cessation intervention on 14.5-year mortality: a randomized clinical trial. *Ann Intern Med.* 2006;142:233-239.
2. Tashkin DP, Celli B, Senn S, et al. A 4-year trial of tiotropium in chronic obstructive pulmonary disease. *N Engl J Med.* 2008;359:1543-1554.
3. Vogelmeier C, Hederer B, Glaab T, et al. Tiotropium versus salmeterol for the prevention of exacerbations of COPD. *N Engl J Med.* 2011;364:1093-1103.
4. Calverley PM, Rabe KR, Goehring UM, et al. Roflumilast in symptomatic chronic obstructive pulmonary disease: two randomized clinical trials. *Lancet.* 2009;374:685-694.
5. Drummond MB, Dasenbrook EC, Pitz MW, et al. Inhaled corticosteroids in patients with stable chronic obstructive pulmonary disease: a systematic review and meta-analysis. *JAMA.* 2008;300:2407-2416.
6. Cranston JM, Crockett A, Moss J, et al. Domiciliary oxygen for chronic obstructive pulmonary disease. *Cochrane Database Syst Rev.* 2005;4:CD001744.
7. Lacasse Y, Goldstein R, Lasserson TJ, et al. Pulmonary rehabilitation for chronic obstructive pulmonary disease. *Cochrane Database Syst Rev.* 2006;4:CD003793.
8. National Emphysema Treatment Trial Research Group. A randomized trial comparing lung volume reduction surgery with medical therapy for severe emphysema. *N Engl J Med.* 2003;348:2059-2073.
9. Ram FSF, Rodriguez-Roisin R, Granados-Navarrete A, et al. Antibiotics for exacerbations of chronic obstructive pulmonary disease. *Cochrane Database Syst Rev.* 2006;2:CD004403.
10. Walters JA, Gibson PG, Wood-Baker R, et al. Systematic corticosteroids for acute exacerbations of chronic obstructive pulmonary disease. *Cochrane Database Syst Rev.* 2009;1:CD001288.

SUGGESTED READINGS

Hurst JR, Vestbo J, Anzueto A, et al. Susceptibility to exacerbation in chronic obstructive pulmonary disease. *N Engl J Med.* 2010;363:1128-1138. *Exacerbations become more frequent as COPD progresses.*

Moullec G, Laurin C, Lavoie KL, et al. Effects of pulmonary rehabilitation on quality of life in chronic obstructive pulmonary disease patients. *Curr Opin Pulm Med.* 2011;17:62-71. *Rehabilitation provides modest benefits.*

Niewoehner DE. Clinical practice: outpatient management of severe COPD. *N Engl J Med.* 2010;362:1407-1416. *Case-based review.*

Salvi SS, Barnes PJ. Chronic obstructive pulmonary disease in non-smokers. *Lancet.* 2009;374:733-743. *Review emphasizing indoor and outdoor air pollution and occupational exposures.*

CYSTIC FIBROSIS

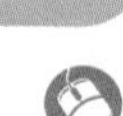

FRANK J. ACCURSO

DEFINITION

Cystic fibrosis is an autosomal recessive disease largely caused by mutations in the gene that encodes the cystic fibrosis transmembrane conductance regulator (CFTR) protein. Cystic fibrosis affects the lungs, pancreas, intestines, liver, sweat glands, sinuses, and vas deferens, and it results in substantial morbidity and premature mortality, with progressive lung disease as the cause of death in 90% of patients.

EPIDEMIOLOGY

The incidence of cystic fibrosis in the United States, Europe, and Australia is 1 in 3000 to 5000 births. Cystic fibrosis is most common in the non-Hispanic white population but also occurs in significant numbers in Hispanics (1 in 7000), African Americans (1 in 12,000), and some Native American populations. It also occurs rarely in individuals of Asian origin.

Approximately 30,000 persons in the United States have cystic fibrosis, so the prevalence is approximately 1 in 10,000. Worldwide, an estimated 100,000 individuals are affected. Exacerbations, particularly those requiring hospitalization, are associated with enormous social and monetary costs.

PATHOBIOLOGY

Lung and Sinus

The pathobiology of cystic fibrosis is based on the ion transport functions of the CFTR, which is a membrane glycoprotein that functions as a chloride channel but is also involved in the regulation of transepithelial sodium and bicarbonate transport. In the airway, CFTR dysfunction reduces chloride secretion from the epithelial lining cell into the airway lumen. In addition, sodium absorption from the lumen into the cell is markedly increased. The net effect is a thinning of the airway surface's liquid lining layer, thereby crucially impairing mucociliary clearance. The subsequent chronic infection leads to an intense neutrophil-dominated inflammatory response. Neutrophil products, including proteolytic enzymes and oxidants, are thought to mediate the subsequent pathologic changes in the airway, including bronchiectasis, bronchiolectasis, bronchial stenosis, and fibrosis. Mucous plugging of airways, likely from chronic infection and inflammation, is another prominent feature of airway disease. Because CFTR is expressed in relatively high concentration in the ductal portions of submucosal glands, speculation exists that mucus is abnormal in cystic fibrosis, but no abnormality has been identified.

The origin of sinus disease is believed to be similar to that in the lung. Impaired mucociliary clearance leads to chronic infection and inflammation. Nasal and sinus polyps are common, but their cause is poorly understood.

Pancreas

Pathologic studies of the pancreas in infants demonstrate ductal obstruction and dilation as well as acinar dilation. The CFTR is expressed in ductal tissue, suggesting that impairment of chloride and bicarbonate secretion into the lumen of the ducts leads to the viscous secretions that obstruct the ducts and cause acinar dilation. The exposure of pancreatic tissue to proteolytic enzymes of acinar origin leads to a cystic and fibrotic pancreas in the first few years of life. Unlike the lung, injury to the exocrine pancreas does not involve infection. Almost complete exocrine pancreatic insufficiency is seen in 85% of patients and is related to genotype.

Intestine and Liver

CFTR is expressed throughout the intestine. In approximately 15% of cases, cystic fibrosis is accompanied by meconium ileus as a manifestation of severe intestinal obstruction at birth. The incidence of jejunal and ileal stenoses and atresias is greatly increased compared with normal individuals. It is unclear how these severe abnormalities arise, but mucous obstruction in intestinal crypts is frequently seen at birth and suggests that abnormalities in CFTR lead to viscous meconium that interferes with normal intestinal development.

In the liver, bile duct obstruction is the first pathologic change noted. Focal areas of sclerosis ensue, probably owing to obstructed bile ducts. Infection is not involved in hepatic injury.

Sweat Gland

In the sweat gland, CFTR dysfunction leads to a failure of chloride absorption from the lumen into the sweat ductal lining cell. In contrast, the abnormality in the lung involves chloride secretion. The failure to absorb chloride and, by electroneutrality, sodium results in marked elevations in the chloride and sodium content of sweat. This abnormality is not accompanied by tissue destruction. The histology of the sweat gland is normal.

Male Reproductive Tract

The vas deferens appears to be the organ that is most sensitive to CFTR dysfunction. It often becomes obstructed in the fetus or in infancy. Resorption of the vas deferens occurs very early in life, and the vas is ultimately not identifiable in most males.

Other Organ Involvement

The primary abnormalities in cystic fibrosis result in secondary involvement of a number of other systems. Diabetes (Chapters 236 and 237), which is increasingly common in adolescents and adults, is thought to result when extensive scarring of the exocrine pancreas extends to the islets of Langerhans. Osteopenia and osteoporosis (Chapter 251), which are common in adults, result from a combination of malnutrition and chronic infection. Delayed puberty (Chapters 242 and 243) is also common. Patients can experience recurrent vasculitis and/or arthralgias that are believed to be caused by the host response to chronic infection. Exocrine pancreatic insufficiency leads to impaired growth and to a multitude of potential nutritional complications, including deficiencies in fat-soluble vitamins and trace elements (Chapter 225).

Genetics

The gene that encodes the CFTR spans more than 250,000 base pairs on the long arm of chromosome 7. The CFTR (ABCC7), which is a protein of 1480 amino acids, belongs to the ATP-binding cassette transporter family. More than 1500 mutations of five different classes have been described (Table 89-1). In the United States, only five mutations are present in more than 1% of cases. The F508δ mutation is by far the most common and is present in approximately 90% of patients in the United States. The next most common mutation, G542X, is present in only 4 to 5% of patients.

In class 1 mutations, protein is not produced because of nonsense mutations. Class II mutations lead to defective protein processing; in the case of 508δF, protein trafficking to the cell membrane is disrupted because the protein is recognized as being defective by cellular quality-control mechanisms, which direct it to the proteasome for degradation. In class III mutations, a protein is produced and processed correctly, but the channel remains closed in response to physiologic stimuli. Class IV mutations are present in the membrane and result in a channel that opens only partially in response to stimuli. In class V mutations, normal CFTR is produced, but in reduced amounts because of defective splicing.

Different mutations lead to differing levels of CFTR dysfunction. Severe mutations may reduce CFTR activity to 1 to 3% of normal, whereas mild mutations may be associated with CFTR activity that is 10 to 20% of normal. An important clinical correlation of CFTR activity is in the exocrine pancreas: patients with severe mutations almost always have pancreatic insufficiency, whereas some patients with milder mutations may retain pancreatic sufficiency. Patients with mild mutations tend, on average, to have less severe lung disease as well.

The clinical course of cystic fibrosis is variable, however, even after controlling for the type of mutation in CFTR, suggesting additional heritable and environmental influences. The genes that code for transforming growth factor-β, mannose-binding lectin, and interferon-related developmental regulator 1 have been identified as modifier genes. Each appears to modify the host response to infection and/or the development of fibrosis, rather than modifying the ion transport function of CFTR.

CLINICAL MANIFESTATIONS

Without specific supportive care, most patients succumb in infancy or early childhood because of malnutrition or lung disease. With the use of pancreatic enzyme replacement therapy, better pulmonary care, and the establishment of specialized centers of expertise, most patients live into the third or fourth decade of life.

TABLE 89-1 CLASSES OF CFTR MUTATIONS

CLASS	MECHANISM	GENETIC AND MOLECULAR ABNORMALITIES	REPRESENTATIVE GENOTYPE
I	Defective protein production	Unstable mRNA Truncated protein Premature stop mutations Frameshift Splicing variants	W1282X Del394TT 1717-1G to A
II	Defective protein processing	Trafficking abnormality Protein degraded in proteasome Deletion	F508del
III	Defective regulation	Protein at membrane Failure of gating Amino acid substitution	G551D
IV	Defective conductance	Protein at membrane Decreased gating Amino acid substitution	R117H
V	Decreased active CFTR	CFTR has normal activity at membrane but is decreased in amount Splice variant Substitution	3849+10kb C to T A455E

LUNG DISEASE

Cough, often persistent after viral infections, is the most prominent early feature of the disease. Viral infection may require more frequent hospitalization in children with cystic fibrosis than in normal children.

Although the lung disease begins in infancy, pulmonary function is often preserved until adolescence, when a steep decline frequently begins; at this time, pulmonary exacerbations become common. Most patients with cystic fibrosis have a daily productive cough by late adolescence or young adulthood.

Cystic fibrosis causes obstructive lung disease, initially with decreased flows at low lung volumes. Forced expiratory volume in 1 second (FEV_1) (Chapter 85) is the best correlate of outcome and starts to differ markedly from normal during adolescence. The rate of decline in FEV_1 often predicts the clinical course.

Early in the disease, the chest radiograph demonstrates hyperinflation and peribronchial thickening. Computed tomography can demonstrate bronchiectasis (Chapter 90) early in the course of the disease.

Airway infection, which is the key clinical manifestation, can be detected by sputum culture or bronchoalveolar lavage. *Pseudomonas aeruginosa* (Chapter 314) is the primary pathogen, although its prevalence is decreasing in the United States, likely owing to improved treatment. *Staphylococcus aureus* (Chapter 296), which is another prominent pathogen, can be methicillin resistant and exist in a small-colony variant form that makes antibiotic treatment difficult.

Most infections remain endobronchial and rarely cause invasive disease, although *Burkholderia* infection can result in sepsis that leads to death. *Burkholderia* infection can also lead to an accelerated decline in lung function and result in death over months to years. Nontuberculous mycobacterial infection can cause granulomatous disease in the airway. *Aspergillus* (Chapter 347) and other fungal species, which are often identified in sputum samples, can cause allergic bronchopulmonary mycoses, but whether they contribute to endobronchitis apart from allergy is unknown.

The polymicrobial nature of airway disease is increasingly appreciated. *Stenotrophomonas maltophilia, Achromobacter xylosoxidans,* and *Inquilinus limosus* are frequently identified serially in airway cultures. Anaerobic infection may also be important.

Individuals with cystic fibrosis are subject to acute exacerbations characterized by cough, dyspnea, decreased exercise tolerance, fatigue, increased sputum production, and change in sputum color that may last days to weeks. Frequently crackles are increased on physical examination, and both the resting oxygen saturation and lung function may decline. Increasing evidence suggests that the permanent loss of lung function is accelerated during periods of exacerbation.

Pulmonary complications can also include pneumothorax (Chapter 99), hemoptysis (Chapter 83), and pulmonary hypertension (Chapter 68). Some patients with more advanced disease exhibit acute ventilatory failure with infection.

GASTROINTESTINAL DISEASE

Exocrine pancreatic insufficiency, which is apparent in the first year of life in most patients, results in impaired growth and lifelong difficulty in maintaining normal weight. Patients at all ages may exhibit signs of malabsorption, including bulky, foul-smelling stools and flatulence. Fat-soluble vitamin and trace element deficiencies are not uncommon and are difficult to diagnose without regular laboratory monitoring.

About 15% of patients retain exocrine pancreatic sufficiency, most of whom have mild mutations associated with 10 to 20% of CFTR function. About one sixth of these patients are subject to recurrent episodes of pancreatitis (Chapter 146) that can lead to pancreatic pseudocysts or ultimately result in exocrine pancreatic insufficiency.

Intestinal obstruction can occur at any age. Frequently the blockage is at the ileocecal valve, but generalized chronic constipation (Chapter 138) is even more common. Intussusception of the appendix can also occur. Inflammatory bowel disease (Chapter 143) and gastrointestinal malignancies (Chapters 198 and 199) appear to be more common than in the general population. Chronic abdominal pain can occur at any time of life, and its cause is often difficult to identify.

Most patients who develop liver disease do so in childhood or adolescence. Liver abnormalities are often first appreciated when a physical examination reveals splenomegaly or a palpable, firm liver. Occasionally, hematemesis leads to the identification of esophageal or gastric varices that are indicative of portal hypertension. Splenic sequestration can lead to neutropenia or thrombocytopenia. Decreased hepatic production of clotting factors can also contribute to bleeding. Occasionally, jaundice is a presenting sign of hepatobiliary disease. Except for γ-glutamyl transpeptidase (GGT) levels, liver enzymes are frequently normal, even in patients with advanced disease. Gallstones (Chapter 158) are common and may or may not lead to symptoms. The hepatopulmonary syndrome (Chapter 157) can occur.

OTHER ORGAN INVOLVEMENT

Although most patients have radiographic evidence of sinus disease, acute or chronic sinusitis occurs in only a minority of individuals. Sinusitis can be accompanied by debilitating headache and anosmia. Nasal or sinus polyposis can lead to obstructed breathing during sleep.

Hypoelectrolytemia can occur at any age. Symptoms range from nausea, vomiting, and decreased appetite to seizures and circulatory collapse with fatal consequences. Sweat electrolyte loss is often an underappreciated problem in cystic fibrosis.

Almost all males are sterile because of the changes in the vas deferens. Spermatogenesis is normal, however.

Cystic fibrosis–related diabetes (Chapter 236) increases in frequency with age. By 30 years of age, approximately one third of patients have diabetes. Although patients rarely develop ketoacidosis, the microvascular and macrovascular complications of diabetes can occur. In addition, patients with diabetes appear to have an accelerated decline in lung function. Osteoporosis (Chapter 251), osteopenia, and increased fractures also increase in frequency with age. Vasculitis accompanied by rash or arthralgia can occur at any time of life. Chronic pain and depression are other important complications that increase with age.

DIAGNOSIS

Newborn Screening and Diagnosis

In the United States, all 50 states require newborn screening to allow early diagnosis and immediate treatment. All newborn screening programs currently measure immunoreactive trypsinogen, a marker of pancreatic injury, from a dried blood spot taken during the first few days of life as the first step in the screening process. This biochemical screen identifies a large number of infants, only a fraction of whom have cystic fibrosis. Most programs perform genetic mutation analysis as the next step. Sweat testing is required to establish the diagnosis if suspected patients carry only one identifiable mutation, but most programs perform confirmatory sweat testing even if two mutations are present.

Sweat testing measures the chloride concentration in sweat that is stimulated by pilocarpine iontophoresis. The result is considered abnormal in adults and children when the concentration of chloride in the sweat is greater than 60 mmol/L; in infants, a concentration greater than 40 mmol/L is considered diagnostic. A family history of cystic fibrosis also provides supportive evidence. In parts of the world where genetic testing is not readily available, the appearance in infancy or childhood of intestinal obstruction or recurrent pulmonary problems should prompt sweat testing.

Diagnosis in Adulthood

Five percent of patients are diagnosed after 18 years of age, mostly on the basis of recurrent pancreatitis, nasal polyposis, chronic sinusitis, bronchiectasis, male infertility, allergic bronchopulmonary mycoses, and nontuberculous mycobacterial infection (Table 89-2). If the predominant symptoms are respiratory, the differential diagnosis includes primary ciliary dyskinesia, immune deficiency, or postinfectious bronchiectasis (Chapter 90). If the predominant symptom is recurrent pancreatitis (Chapter 146), the differential diagnosis includes hereditary pancreatitis with abnormalities in the *SPINK* gene. Transepithelial potential differences are altered in cystic fibrosis because of abnormal transport of sodium and chloride. The measurement of nasal potential difference, therefore, can sometimes be used as a diagnostic tool, particularly in adults.

It is increasingly recognized that some patients appear to have cystic fibrosis on clinical grounds but do not meet the criteria for diagnosis, usually because their sweat test is in the normal range or two genetic mutations cannot be identified. These patients are sometimes diagnosed as having atypical cystic fibrosis, nonclassical cystic fibrosis, or variant cystic fibrosis. Full analysis of the CFTR coding and flanking regions may be helpful in making the diagnosis. Such patients should be followed at a cystic fibrosis center so that their lung disease can be treated and they can be monitored for other complications of cystic fibrosis.

TABLE 89-2 APPROACH TO DIAGNOSIS OF CYSTIC FIBROSIS IN ADULT PATIENTS

CONDITIONS SUGGESTING THE DIAGNOSIS OF CYSTIC FIBROSIS IN ADULTS
Recurrent pancreatitis
Male infertility
Chronic sinusitis
Nasal polyposis
Nontuberculous mycobacterial infection
Allergic bronchopulmonary mycosis
Bronchiectasis
RECOMMENDED DIAGNOSTIC STUDIES
Sweat electrolyte determination
Extended CFTR mutation analysis
Nasal potential difference
High-resolution CT scan to identify bronchiectasis
CT scan of sinuses for polyposis
Sputum induction or bronchoalveolar lavage to identify bacterial and fungal pathogens

CFTR = cystic fibrosis transmembrane conductance regulator; CT = computed tomography.

TREATMENT

Rx

The general consensus is that treatment is best conducted at specialized centers that use a team approach. Much of their success is based on the education of patients and families with regard to the range of symptoms and complications, as well as the close monitoring of pulmonary function and rapid intervention for any detected abnormalities.

Pulmonary Infections

Pulmonary infections can be treated with oral, inhaled, or systemic antibiotics. Increase in cough or other respiratory symptoms should be addressed with the introduction of antibiotics or a change in antibiotics within a few days. Nebulized antibiotics (4 weeks of either aztreonam 75 mg two or three times a day[1] or tobramycin 300 mg twice daily[2]), alone or in combination with oral antibiotics, improve lung function and decrease exacerbations in patients with chronic *Pseudomonas* infection.[3] Chronic oral macrolide treatment (e.g., azithromycin 5 to 15 mg/kg/day, 500 mg three times per week, or 1250 mg once per week[4,5]) can reduce exacerbations for up to 6 months. It is not yet clear whether the chronic use of antibiotics in this setting leads to the development of more resistant organisms.

More severe changes in symptoms or an acute fall in lung function requires intravenous antibiotics aimed at the cultured pathogen (Chapter 97). Nontuberculous mycobacterial infections are treated for 6 months or longer using multiple antibiotic agents (Chapter 333). Allergic bronchopulmonary mycoses are treated with corticosteroids and antifungal agents (Chapter 339).

Agents to alter the viscosity of respiratory secretions include inhaled hypertonic (7%) saline, which can increase pulmonary function and reduce exacerbations.[6] Daily use of inhaled rhDNase (2.5 mg) is associated with improvement in lung function and fewer exacerbations.[7] Conversely, nebulized thiol derivatives do not appear to be beneficial.[8]

Many patients have hyper-reactive airways and may benefit from inhaled bronchodilators (Chapter 87). Inhaled corticosteroids are controversial and do not have proven benefit.[9] Oral corticosteroid "bursts" (e.g., 5 days of prednisone, 1 mg/kg twice a day in children and 30 mg/kg twice a day in adults) are often useful, but chronic administration of oral corticosteroids can result in severe complications, including diabetes and stunted growth. Most patients perform physical means of airway secretion clearance one or more times a day.

Even passive smoke exposure is deleterious. Oxygen therapy is often required to maintain saturation and prevent the development of pulmonary hypertension. Noninvasive ventilation is used mainly in patients with more advanced disease. Pneumothorax almost always requires pleurodesis. Persistent or recurrent hemoptysis is treated with bronchial artery embolization. Occasionally, lobectomy is required. Patients in acute ventilatory failure should receive mechanical ventilation unless they have decided against such treatment. The possible need for ventilation should be addressed in patients with advanced disease before the need arises.

Lung transplantation (Chapter 101) is an option for many adult patients. Individuals with cystic fibrosis have survival rates after transplantation comparable to or better than those of other patients.

Gastrointestinal Diseases

Pancreatic enzyme replacement (Chapter 146) is the mainstay of treatment for exocrine pancreatic insufficiency. Because gastric acid decreases enzyme activity, H_2-blockers (e.g., ranitidine 150 mg twice daily in children weighing >30 kg and in adults) or proton pump inhibitors (e.g., lansoprazole 30 mg orally once daily in children weighing >30 kg and in adults) are often used. Children and adolescents frequently use multiple nutritional supplements every day to maintain weight. Fat-soluble vitamin replacement therapy is necessary in most patients. Between 10 and 20% of patients may require gastrostomy feeding to aid growth or maintain weight.

To prevent intestinal obstruction, dietary fiber should be increased, and polyethylene glycol at varying doses (e.g., 17 mg orally with 8 ounces of water one to three times per day) is frequently used on a daily basis. Acute obstructions can be treated with more intensive use of polyethylene glycol or Gastrografin enema. Occasionally, refractory constipation (Chapter 138) requires surgical approaches that can result in loss of intestine.

Other Organ Systems

A combination of nasal rinses and topically applied corticosteroids and antibiotics is used to treat sinus disease (Chapter 434). Surgery is often required, however, especially for polyps.

Many pediatric patients receive daily salt supplementation. Adults should be counseled on the symptoms of salt depletion and encouraged to increase the amount of salt in their diet if there are no medical contraindications to doing so.

Regular screening for the onset of impaired glucose homeostasis or frank diabetes is required in all patients older than 10 years. Diabetes is treated with insulin (Chapter 236) because the safety and efficacy of oral antihyperglycemic agents have not been demonstrated in cystic fibrosis. Bone health is addressed through vitamin D supplementation, calcium supplementation, and oral bisphosphonate therapy (Chapter 251). Delayed puberty and short stature require consultation with endocrinologists and sometimes hormonal administration. Most clinics believe that both aerobic exercise and strength training can have beneficial effects, although the implementation of exercise programs has been difficult in clinical practice. Males with cystic fibrosis can father children through the use of epididymal aspiration to retrieve sperm, followed by in vitro fertilization.

General Care

Given all the pulmonary, nutritional, and other therapies prescribed for individuals with cystic fibrosis, their care amounts to several hours a day. This burden has a major influence on the quality of life in patients and their families and may contribute to the increasing incidence of depression observed in this population.

End-of-life care encompasses many complex issues. Patients are often depressed and experience chronic pain. They are asked to perform increasingly intense therapeutic regimens. They may have changed locations to await transplantation. Family, medical, and professional relationships are disrupted. Excellent communication with caregivers about advance directives and other planning is necessary.

PREVENTION

Prenatal carrier screening, which is offered in many countries, can decrease the incidence of cystic fibrosis by approximately 25%. Newborn screening programs may also help decrease the incidence by influencing the future reproductive decisions of parents of an affected child.

PROGNOSIS

Prognosis is now greatly improved compared with the natural history of the disease. The median expected survival in the United States is 37 years, but the peak age at death is 26 years, demonstrating that some patients are particularly vulnerable to devastating lung disease. Late adolescence and early adulthood are high-risk times for pulmonary insufficiency. Patients who survive to their 30s and beyond are often more stable, with a very slow decline in lung function.

This variability in prognosis is related to patients' ability to sustain lung function, recognizing that those with severe mutations succumb in adolescence or young adulthood, whereas patients with "milder" mutations often live longer.

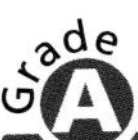

1. McCoy KS, Quittner Al, Oermann CM, et al. Inhaled aztreonam lysine for chronic airway *Pseudomonas aeruginosa* in cystic fibrosis. *Am J Respir Crit Care Med.* 2008;178:921-928.
2. Ramsey BW, Pepe MS, Quan JM, et al. Intermittent administration of inhaled tobramycin in patients with cystic fibrosis. *N Engl J Med.* 1999;340:23-30.
3. Langton Hewer SC, Smyth AR. Antibiotic strategies for eradicating *Pseudomonas aeruginosa* in people with cystic fibrosis. *Cochrane Database Syst Rev.* 2009;7:CD004197.
4. Kabra SK, Pawaiya R, Lodha R, et al. Long-term daily high and low doses of azithromycin in children with cystic fibrosis: a randomized controlled trial. *J Cyst Fibros.* 2010;9:17-23.
5. Steinkamp G, Schmitt-Grohe S, Doring G, et al. Once-weekly azithromycin in cystic fibrosis with chronic *Pseudomonas aeruginosa* infection. *Respir Med.* 2008;102:1643-1653.

6. Elkins MR, Robinson M, Rose BR, et al. A controlled trial of long-term inhaled hypertonic saline in patients with cystic fibrosis. *N Engl J Med.* 2006;354:229-240.
7. Fuchs HJ, Borowitz DS, Christiansen DH, et al. Effect of aerosolized recombinant human DNase on exacerbations of respiratory symptoms and on pulmonary function in patients with cystic fibrosis. *N Engl J Med.* 1994;331:637-642.
8. Nash EF, Stephenson A, Ratjen F, et al. Nebulized and oral thiol derivatives for pulmonary disease in cystic fibrosis. *Cochrane Database Syst Rev.* 2009;21:CD007168.
9. Balfour-Lynn IM, Welch K. Inhaled corticosteroids for cystic fibrosis. *Cochrane Database Syst Rev.* 2009;21:CD001915.

SUGGESTED READINGS

Accurso FJ, Rowe SM, Clancy JP, et al. Effect of VX-770 in persons with cystic fibrosis and the G551D-CFTR mutation. *N Engl J Med.* 2010;363:1991-2003. *In a safety/efficacy trial of adults with cystic fibrosis, VX-770 at various doses improved CFTR function and also improved forced expiratory volume in one second by about 9%.*

Sears EH, Gartman EJ, Casserly BP. Treatment options for cystic fibrosis: state of the art and future perspectives. *Rev Recent Clin Trials.* 2011. [Epub ahead of print.] *Review.*

Simmonds NJ, Macneill SJ, Cullinan P, et al. Cystic fibrosis and survival to 40 years: a case-control study. *Eur Respir J.* 2010;36:1277-1283. *Survival is better in patients with a higher body mass index and forced vital capacity and no history of pneumothorax or* Pseudomonas *infection.*

90 BRONCHIECTASIS, ATELECTASIS, CYSTS, AND LOCALIZED LUNG DISORDERS

ANNE E. O'DONNELL

BRONCHIECTASIS

DEFINITION

Bronchiectasis is an abnormal permanent dilatation of the bronchi and bronchioles caused by repeated cycles of airway infection and inflammation. The distal airways become thickened; the mucosal surfaces develop edema, inflammation, and suppuration; ultimately, there is neovascularization of the adjacent bronchial arterioles. Bronchiectasis, which can be focal or diffuse, is triggered by a variety of genetic, anatomic, and systemic processes. Abnormalities of cilia, mucus clearance, mucus rheology, airway drainage, and host defenses can result in bronchiectasis. Regardless of the cause, patients with bronchiectasis develop chronic infections, which may lead to progressive lung destruction.

EPIDEMIOLOGY

Based on insurance claims reviews, it is estimated that there are at least 110,000 persons in the United States receiving treatment for bronchiectasis that is not related to cystic fibrosis (Chapter 89). The prevalence in the United States has been reported as 4.2 per 100,000 persons age 18 to 34 years and 272 per 100,000 among those older than 75 years. In the older age category, women are disproportionally represented. In Hong Kong, bronchiectasis results in a hospital admission rate of 14.4 per 100,000 persons. Other epidemiologic surveys suggest that there is increased risk for the development of bronchiectasis in individuals with reduced access to health care and higher rates of pulmonary infection in childhood.

PATHOBIOLOGY

In up to one third of cases, the cause of bronchiectasis is not identified. Other cases are related to pulmonary infections, genetic causes, anatomic abnormalities, and immune and autoimmune diseases.

Pulmonary Infections

Approximately one third of patients with bronchiectasis have an infectious trigger, usually years before the onset of the disease. Childhood viral infections, such as pertussis (Chapter 321) and bacterial infection, can cause permanent damage to the airways, leading to bronchiectasis years after the initial infection. Mycobacterial tuberculosis with its resultant granulomatous inflammation of the airway, lung parenchyma, and lymph nodes can cause subsequent bronchiectasis (Chapter 332), and *Mycobacterium avium-intracellulare* (MAI) infections have been recognized as an increasing cause and complication of bronchiectasis, particularly in white women older than 55 years (Chapter 333). MAI-related bronchiectasis typically involves the right middle lobe and lingula and can be associated with the "tree-in-bud" pattern of bronchiolar infection as well.

Genetics

Cystic fibrosis (Chapter 89) is characterized by bilateral diffuse bronchiectasis. Although many cystic fibrosis patients are diagnosed in childhood with multisystem disease, older patients may present with only pulmonary or pulmonary and sinus manifestations.

In primary ciliary dyskinesia, abnormalities in the dynein arms prevent normal ciliary beating. Patients with primary ciliary dyskinesia generally have significant sinopulmonary disease and infertility, and approximately half of these patients have Kartagener's syndrome with situs inversus (Chapter 69). Patients with α_1-antitrypsin deficiency also may develop bronchiectasis.

Anatomic Causes

Patients with chronic abnormalities of their swallowing mechanism or with esophageal dysfunction may develop focal or diffuse bronchiectasis with lower lobe predominance (Chapter 140). Direct lung injury due to acid or particulate matter aspiration or recurrent pneumonia may lead to bronchiectasis.

Chronic obstructive pulmonary disease is sometimes complicated by bronchiectasis (Chapter 88). Patients with chronic lower airway bacterial colonization and increased airway inflammation may develop areas of bronchiectasis. Rarely, patients with asthma (Chapter 87) have been found to have bronchiectasis. Allergic bronchopulmonary aspergillosis (Chapter 347) can cause a distinct "finger-in-glove" central bronchiectasis owing to chronic inflammation and mucous plugging. Airway abnormalities such as endobronchial tumors (Chapter 197), extrinsic compression by lymph nodes (right middle lobe syndrome), and foreign bodies are also rare causes of focal bronchiectasis. Tracheobronchomegaly (Mounier-Kuhn syndrome) is associated with distal bronchiectasis.

Immune and Autoimmune Diseases

Primary hypogammaglobulinemia (Chapter 258) leads to recurrent pulmonary infections that may result in bronchiectasis. Patients with immunoglobulin G subclass deficiencies may develop bronchiectasis if the deficiency leads to reduction in antibody production. Defects of neutrophil adhesion and chemotaxis (Chapter 172) have been found to cause bronchiectasis. Patients with human immunodeficiency virus infection (Chapter 394) have a higher prevalence of bronchiectasis than individuals with a normally functioning immune system.

Bronchiectasis is an increasingly recognized complication of collagen vascular diseases, particularly rheumatoid arthritis (Chapter 272) and Sjögren's syndrome (Chapter 276). The airway injury is likely due to chronic inflammation or esophageal dysfunction. Inflammatory bowel disease (Chapter 143) also causes bronchiectasis by undetermined mechanisms.

CLINICAL MANIFESTATIONS

Patients present with chronic cough and usually have mucopurulent or purulent sputum production. Occasionally, a dry nonproductive cough is the primary manifestation. Other symptoms include dyspnea, intermittent hemoptysis, and pleuritic chest pain. Weight loss, malaise, and fatigue sometimes develop. When patients have infectious exacerbations, they may develop fever as well as an increase in their baseline symptoms. Physical findings in patients with bronchiectasis are nonspecific: an abnormal chest examination with wheezing or crackles, or both. Clubbing of the digits is rare.

The clinical course of patients with bronchiectasis is variable. Some patients have few to no symptoms, others have daily cough with sputum production, and some patients have occasional to frequent exacerbations. A slow decline in pulmonary function is seen with bronchiectasis; decline is more rapid in patients infected with *Pseudomonas aeruginosa* (Chapter 314) and in patients who have more frequent exacerbations.

DIAGNOSIS

Imaging Studies

Although the diagnosis may be suspected by plain chest radiography, high-resolution computed tomography (HRCT) is the current "gold standard" for confirming bronchiectasis. The characteristic computed tomography (CT) findings are lack of bronchial tapering, bronchi visible in the peripheral 1 cm of the lungs, and an internal bronchial diameter greater than the diameter of the accompanying bronchial artery. Other associated HRCT findings are

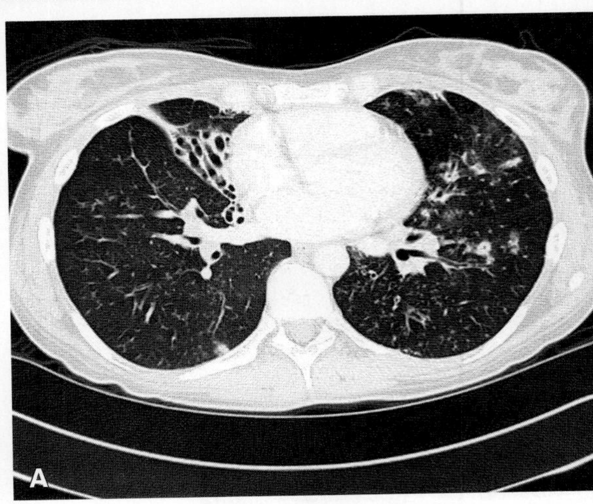

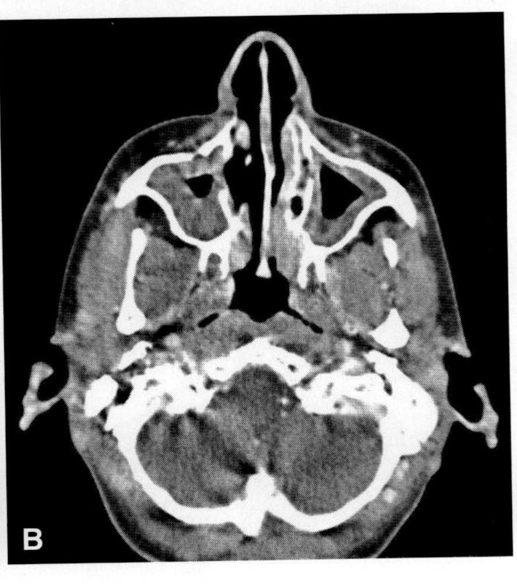

FIGURE 90-1. A and B, High-resolution computed tomographic images of bilateral bronchiectasis in a patient with primary ciliary dyskinesia.

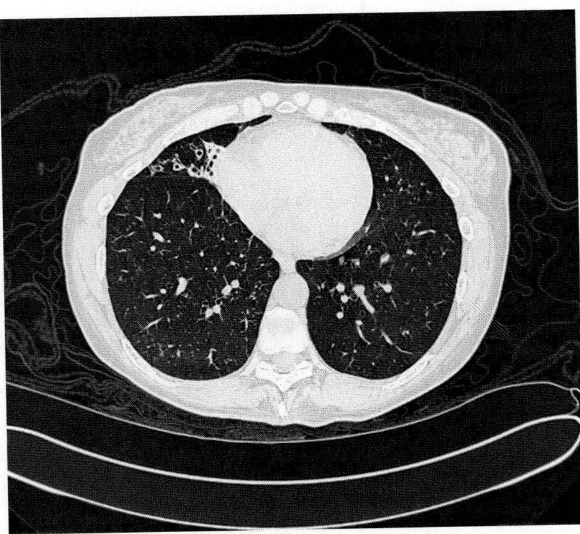

FIGURE 90-2. High-resolution computed tomographic image of nodular bronchiectasis due to nontuberculous mycobacterium infection.

cysts off the end of a bronchus, tree-in-bud irregular branching lines indicating mucus impaction, and occasionally associated consolidation (Fig. 90-1). The location of the bronchiectatic airways may suggest the cause: upper lobe predominance is seen in cystic fibrosis; lower lobe predominance in aspiration syndromes. Right middle lobe and lingula involvement suggests the presence of nontuberculous mycobacterial infection (Fig. 90-2), whereas central bronchiectasis is seen with allergic bronchopulmonary aspergillosis (Fig. 90-3).

Pulmonary function testing, which should be performed on all patients with suspected bronchiectasis, usually shows airflow obstruction as measured by the ratio between the forced expiratory volume in 1 second (FEV_1) and forced vital capacity (FVC) (Chapter 85). The severity of the airflow obstruction and the rate of decline correlate with radiographic extent of disease and frequency of exacerbation. Bronchoscopy will detect airway abnormalities including tumors, structural deformities, and foreign bodies and hence should be considered in the evaluation of localized bronchiectasis.

Cultures of sputum and of bronchoalveolar lavage when expectorated sputum is not available have an important role in assessing the infectious complications of bronchiectasis. The presence of *P. aeruginosa* portends a worse prognosis and more frequent exacerbations. Patients with no identifiable pathogens have the mildest disease. The presence of *Staphylococcus aureus* in the airway may suggest cystic fibrosis as the cause of the bronchiectasis. Nontuberculous mycobacteria are found with increasing frequency in the airways of patients with bronchiectasis, usually as a complication of preexisting bronchiectasis but occasionally as its primary cause. The laboratory evaluation of patients with bronchiectasis should be individualized. All patients should have sputum cultures for bacterial and mycobacterial testing. Other tests that should be considered include measurement of serum immunoglobulin levels and screening for genetic diseases, particularly in patients with diffuse bronchiectasis. Cystic fibrosis (Chapter 89) is diagnosed by elevated sweat chloride levels and by genetic testing. Primary ciliary dyskinesia is confirmed by electron microscopic evaluation of airway mucosal cilia. α_1-Antitrypsin deficiency is diagnosed by measuring levels and performing phenotyping (Chapter 88). Screening for rheumatoid arthritis (Chapter 272) or Sjögren's syndrome (Chapter 276) also may be reasonable in patients with diffuse bronchiectasis.

TREATMENT

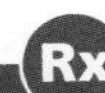

The goals of treatment are to reduce the numbers of exacerbations and potentially to improve quality of life, reduce symptoms, and alter the natural history of the disease (Table 90-1). Currently, maintenance treatment is considered for patients with more advanced disease or more frequent exacerbations. Exacerbations are treated based on clinical acuity. Because patients are heterogeneous and therapeutic trials are few, therapy is commonly individualized in patients with bronchiectasis.

Preventing Exacerbations

The 23-valent pneumococcal vaccination is recommended for patients with bronchiectasis. Routine seasonal influenza vaccination is also standard. At present, no vaccines are available for prevention of the other infectious complications of bronchiectasis.

Treatment of the Underlying Etiology

For treatable conditions, such as immunoglobulin deficiency, replacement therapy (Chapter 258) should be considered even though there are few data on whether that alters the natural history of the lung disease. Patients with allergic bronchopulmonary aspergillosis (Chapter 347) should be treated with steroids to mitigate the inflammatory process that leads to the bronchiectasis.

Antimicrobial Therapy

Nebulized gentamicin (80 mg twice daily) for 12 months can provide sustained bacteriologic and clinical benefit.[1] Clinical trials have demonstrated microbiologic benefits with inhaled tobramycin, 300 mg twice per day as a 4-week trial for one cycle and a 2-week-on/2-week-off trial for three cycles,[2] but clinical benefit was not firmly established, and some patients experienced unacceptable respiratory side effects. Antimicrobial resistance is also a concern. In a retrospective study, radiographic stability was achieved in a limited number of patients who received cycles of alternating antibiotics, including a quinolone, over 6 to 84 months. At present, there is no firm evidence to support the use of routine maintenance antibiotics, although such therapy may be considered in patients with frequent exacerbations and progressive lung destruction. When mycobacterial species are cultured from patients with bronchiectasis, decisions regarding whether to treat and which antimicrobial agents to use are based on published guidelines (Chapters 332 and 333).

Reduction of Airway Inflammation

In two randomized trials of patients treated for 3 and 12 months, inhaled fluticasone, 500 μg twice daily, improved clinical status compared with placebo.[3,4] Small pilot trials of twice- or thrice-weekly oral erythromycin

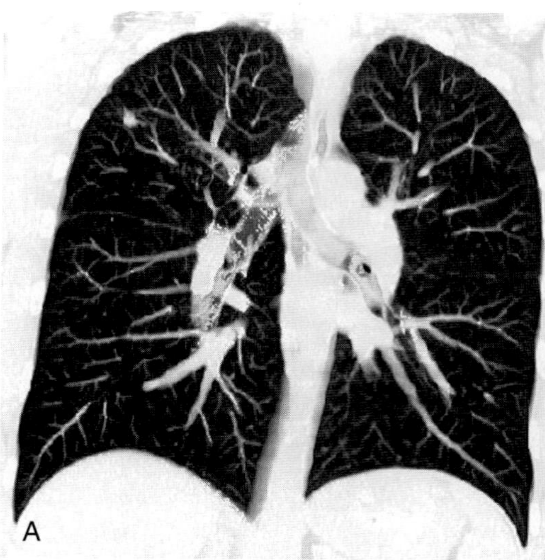

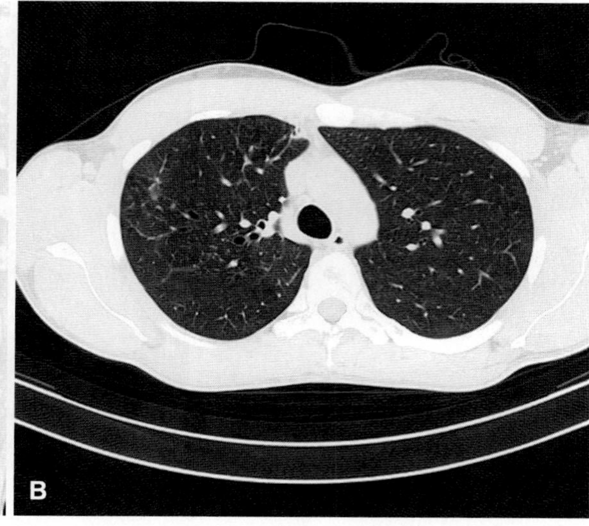

FIGURE 90-3. A and B, High-resolution computed tomographic images of finger-in-glove central bronchiectasis due to allergic bronchopulmonary aspergillosis.

TABLE 90-1 POTENTIAL THERAPIES FOR BRONCHIECTASIS

Treat underlying condition, if possible
Antimicrobial therapy
Pathogen specific
Anti-inflammatory therapy
Inhaled steroids
Macrolides
Mobilization of secretions
Pharmacologic
Mechanical
Surgery
Localized or refractory disease
Transplantation
End-stage disease

Reprinted with permission from O'Donnell A. *Chest.* 2008;134:815-823.

(500 mg twice daily for 8 weeks) and azithromycin (500 mg twice weekly for 6 months) suggest that macrolide therapy can be beneficial in bronchiectasis, but these agents should not be used alone in the presence of infection because they may result in resistant nontuberculous mycobacterial organisms. Oral steroids, although sometimes used in bronchiectasis, have never been tested in a clinical trial setting.

Other Medical Treatments

Chest physiotherapy and the use of devices to aid mucociliary clearance appear to be beneficial in non–cystic fibrosis bronchiectasis. In a randomized trial, twice daily use of an oscillatory positive expiratory pressure device (Acapella) improved sputum volume and quality of life end points compared with no routine physiotherapy.[5] Other techniques that may also have a role for airway clearance include traditional chest physical therapy with postural drainage and the use of chest wall oscillator vests. At least one clinical trial[6] has demonstrated improvement in overall clinical status for bronchiectasis patients enrolled in a pulmonary rehabilitation program.

Inhaled therapy with nebulized hypertonic saline (7%) may enhance airway clearance and decrease exacerbations, but long-term clinical trials have not been performed in patients with non–cystic fibrosis bronchiectasis. Preliminary data suggest that inhalation of mannitol may enhance secretion clearance by improving sputum physical properties. Although recombinant human DNase is efficacious in cystic fibrosis bronchiectasis, a large clinical trial showed it had deleterious effects in patients with non–cystic fibrosis bronchiectasis when given as maintenance therapy, so it should not be used.

No randomized trials support the use of routine β-agonist or anticholinergic bronchodilators in bronchiectasis. However, a subset of patients with airway reactivity likely benefit from use of these agents (Chapter 87).

Surgery and Transplantation

Resectional surgery may have a role for patients who have focal disease or for patients who have hemoptysis that cannot be controlled by embolization of the bleeding vessels (Chapter 101). Surgical resection can also benefit some patients who have diffuse bronchiectasis unresponsive to conventional therapy and some patients infected with nontuberculous mycobacteria.

Double-lung transplantation (Chapter 101) has been successfully performed in patients with end-stage lung disease due to non–cystic fibrosis bronchiectasis, and the clinical outcomes parallel those seen with transplantation for other end-stage lung diseases.

Treatment of Acute Exacerbations of Bronchiectasis

When the bronchiectasis patient experiences an acute exacerbation, antimicrobial treatments should be targeted to the known infecting organisms. Mild to moderate exacerbations can be treated with oral antibiotics, targeted to the results of the sputum culture, for 2 to 3 weeks. More severe exacerbations or exacerbations due to resistant organisms generally require intravenous antibiotics administered in hospital or at home. No benefit has yet been demonstrated by adding an inhaled antibiotic to systemic therapy for an acute exacerbation. Patients experiencing an acute exacerbation likely benefit from airway clearance modalities and the other nonantibiotic therapies discussed previously.

PROGNOSIS

Non–cystic fibrosis bronchiectasis is a heterogeneous disease with a widely variable prognosis. Patients with more severe obstructive and restrictive findings on pulmonary function tests, poor gas transfer, and chronic pseudomonal infection have the worst prognosis. Radiographic extent of disease, hypoxemia, hypercapnia, and evidence of right heart failure are also predictors of outcome. Bronchiectasis patients who are admitted to an intensive care unit for respiratory failure have been reported to have a 60% 4-year survival rate.

ATELECTASIS

DEFINITION

Atelectasis, or collapse, is due to hypoventilation of lung units. Atelectasis may involve an entire lung or a lobe, segment, or subsegment. Atelectasis can be caused by intrinsic obstruction of an airway or external compression from lymph nodes, parenchymal masses, or other entities. When lung units are atelectatic, ventilation-perfusion mismatch leads to hypoxemia. Infection may result from sustained atelectasis.

EPIDEMIOLOGY AND PATHOBIOLOGY

The lung bases and posterior segments are vulnerable to dependent atelectasis, which is caused by inadequate ventilation, particularly in the immobilized or postoperative patient. Patchy atelectasis is caused by alveolar filling processes, such as hemorrhage and edema (Chapter 91). Passive, relaxation, or compression atelectasis occurs when the lung recoils to a smaller volume because of fluid or air in the adjacent pleural space.

Obstructive or resorptive atelectasis is due to bronchial block to the entry of air, with resultant retractile consolidation. Intrinsic airway obstruction may be caused by mucous plugs, foreign bodies, or tumors in the airway. Extrinsic airway obstruction results from compression of the airway owing to peribronchial lymph node enlargement or other masses impinging on the airway.

Rounded atelectasis is caused by pleural thickening that invaginates and traps adjacent lung. Any chronic pleural disease can cause rounded atelectasis, particularly asbestos-related pleural disease.

CLINICAL MANIFESTATIONS AND DIAGNOSIS

Atelectasis is typically asymptomatic and diagnosed on chest imaging, but it may cause dyspnea and tachypnea and result in hypoxemia. In postoperative patients, atelectasis may be a cause of low-grade fever. Plain chest radiography shows loss of lung volume and the displacement of the lobar fissure, mediastinum, or diaphragm toward the involved lung unit (Figs. 90-4 and 90-5). Platelike or discoid atelectasis manifests as horizontal or curvilinear lines on plain chest radiography. Rounded atelectasis is an ovoid masslike density abutting the pleura. The type and cause of atelectasis can sometimes be elucidated by CT or ultrasonography. Bronchoscopy is required to confirm intrinsic versus extrinsic compression in obstructive-resorptive atelectasis and to determine the exact pathology of the obstruction. An oxygen saturation concentration can help assess the severity of the atelectasis and overall lung dysfunction.

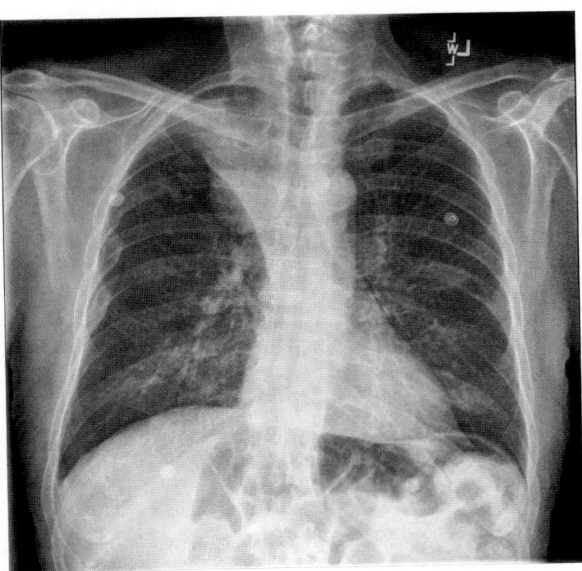

FIGURE 90-4. Plain chest radiograph demonstrating right upper lobe atelectasis (due to endobronchial tumor).

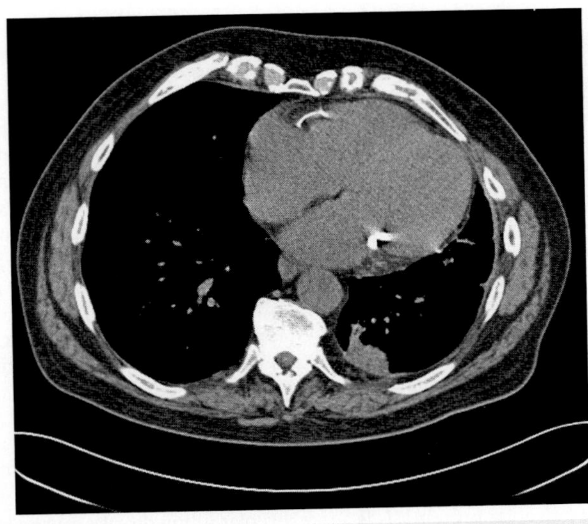

FIGURE 90-5. Computed tomographic image of rounded atelectasis.

PREVENTION AND TREATMENT Rx

Incentive spirometry is commonly prescribed to prevent or treat atelectasis in patients with limited mobility due to recent surgery, neuromuscular weakness, or any prolonged immobilization, but there are no randomized controlled trials that prove its effectiveness. Preoperative inspiratory muscle training reduces atelectasis in patients undergoing upper abdominal surgery,[7] and prophylactic use of noninvasive ventilation may reduce pulmonary dysfunction after lung resection surgery.[8] Other modalities such as positive expiratory pressure devices and high-frequency chest wall oscillation airway clearance are of uncertain benefit.

Patchy atelectasis is treated by addressing the underlying disease process in the lung parenchyma. Compression atelectasis is treated by alleviating the pleural space process.

Obstructive or resorptive atelectasis often requires bronchoscopy for diagnosis and treatment. In patients with obstruction owing to retained secretions, multiple bronchoscopies are sometimes required, but the mucus often rapidly reaccumulates and will resolve only when the patient's overall status improves.

Rounded atelectasis does not require treatment. CT is helpful in distinguishing rounded atelectasis from parenchymal tumor.

CONGENITAL CYSTIC DISEASES OF THE THORAX

Thoracic cysts, which are exceedingly rare, develop because of abnormal development or branching of the foregut. Cysts may develop in the mediastinum at an early stage of gestation or in the lung parenchyma at a later stage. Abnormalities include bronchogenic cysts (mediastinal and parenchymal), congenital pulmonary airway malformation, and pulmonary sequestrations. The cysts are lined with airway and alveolar epithelium but do not communicate in a normal fashion with the airways or lung tissue.

Most patients with thoracic cysts present in childhood, but the cysts can remain asymptomatic and unnoticed until adulthood. In the absence of symptoms, these cystic lesions sometimes present as an incidental finding on chest imaging performed for another indication. Congenital cystic diseases can cause recurrent pneumonia, hemoptysis, or compression of normal structures.

CT scanning with CT angiography can usually detect congenital cystic lesions of the thorax, but pulmonary or bronchial angiography is sometimes necessary to define the blood flow to the lesion.

Bronchogenic cysts are usually found in the right paratracheal or subcarinal areas of the mediastinum but are occasionally seen in the lung parenchyma. These cysts are often asymptomatic, but they can cause wheezing, dyspnea, and cough when they compress adjacent structures. Secondary infection may develop in the cysts, and there are a few case reports of malignant transformation. Complete surgical resection is generally recommended, but partial excision with de-epithelization of the cysts has also been performed. Observation is also an option when the cysts are asymptomatic.

Congenital pulmonary airway malformation, previously called *congenital cystic adenomatoid malformation of the lung*, is an exceedingly rare abnormality with reported incidence of 1 in every 25,000 to 35,000 pregnancies. The abnormality is caused by arrested development of the bronchial tree. Most patients are diagnosed prenatally by ultrasound, but a few adults have first presented with complications, including pneumothorax and air embolism. Treatment is anatomic surgical resection.

Pulmonary sequestrations are areas of nonfunctioning pulmonary parenchyma with no communication to the tracheobronchial tree and abnormal arterial supply and venous drainage (Fig. 90-6). Intralobar sequestration, which accounts for about 75% of cases, does not have visceral pleura and is generally found in a lower lobe, left more frequently than right. Extralobar sequestrations have their own visceral pleura, are separate from the normal lobes, and may even be found below the diaphragms. Sequestrations usually have a feeding vessel that arises from the aorta. Patients with sequestrations may be asymptomatic but sometimes develop recurrent infections and or hemoptysis. Surgical excision with special care for the management of the feeding vessel is curative. Embolization of the feeding vessel is sometimes a successful treatment option.

Hyperlucent lungs are diagnosed by a paucity of vascular and interstitial markings noted on chest imaging. Lung parenchymal air collections can be caused by congenital parenchymal cysts, congenital lobar emphysema (almost exclusively diagnosed in infancy), giant bullous emphysema (vanishing lung syndrome), or Swyer-James syndrome. Lung parenchymal cysts may be a bullous alveolar type or may contain bronchial wall elements such as

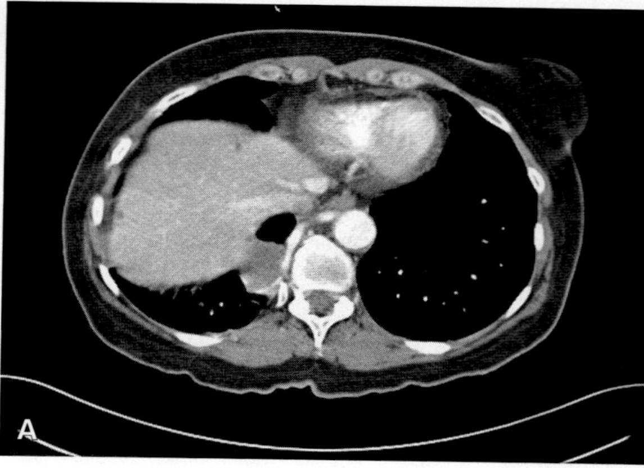

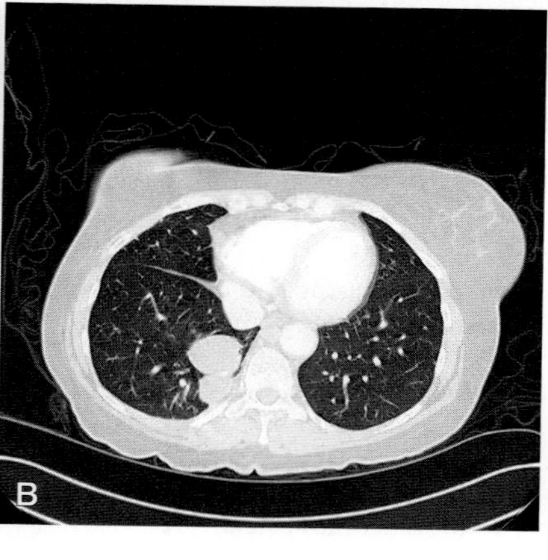

FIGURE 90-6. **Pulmonary sequestration. A,** Computed tomographic image of pulmonary sequestration in right lower lobe. **B,** Feeding vessel visible arising from the aorta.

cartilage, smooth muscle, and glands. They may become infected and may rupture to cause pneumothorax. Surgical resection is generally recommended unless the lesions are small. Congenital lobar emphysema, otherwise known as *congenital large hyperlucent lobe*, may cause severe respiratory distress in infants owing to compression of surrounding lung tissue. Giant bullous emphysema is a rare condition that usually affects the upper lobes of young male smokers. Compression of normal lung parenchyma from these overdistended lobes may require surgical resection.

Swyer-James-Macleod syndrome, which is characterized by unilateral lucency of an entire lung, is caused by childhood bronchiolitis obliterans owing to viral or bacterial infection or toxic inhalation. CT shows air trapping and hyperlucency of the affected lung, with a normal contralateral lung. No therapy is required.

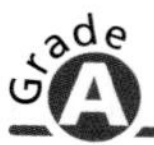

1. Murray MP, Govan JR, Doherty CJ, et al. A randomized controlled trial of nebulised gentamicin in non-cystic fibrosis bronchiectasis. *Am J Respir Crit Care Med.* 2011;183:491-499.
2. Scheinburg P, Shore E. A pilot study of the safety and efficacy of tobramycin solution for inhalation in patients with severe bronchiectasis. *Chest.* 2005;127:1420-1426.
3. Martinez-Garcia MA, Perpina-Tordera M, Roman-Sanchez P, et al. Inhaled steroids improved quality of life in patients with steady state bronchiectasis. *Respir Med.* 2006;100:1623-1632.
4. Tsang KW, Tan KC, Lam WK, et al. Inhaled fluticasone in bronchiectasis: a 12 month study. *Thorax.* 2005;60:239-243.
5. Murray MP, Pentland JL, Hill AT. A randomized crossover trial of chest physiotherapy in non-cystic fibrosis bronchiectasis. *Eur Respir J.* 2009;34:1086-1092.
6. Newall C, Stockley RA, Hill SL. Exercise training and inspiratory muscle training in patients with bronchiectasis. *Thorax.* 2005;60:943-948.
7. Guimaraes MM, El Dib R, Smith AF, et al. Incentive spirometry for prevention of postoperative pulmonary complications in abdominal surgery. *Cochrane Database Syst Rev.* 2009;3:CD0006058.
8. Perrin C, Jullien V, Venissac N, et al. Prophylactic use of noninvasive ventilation in patients undergoing lung resectional surgery. *Respir Med.* 2007;101:1572-1578.

SUGGESTED READINGS

Gursoy S, Ozturk AA, Ucvet A, et al. Surgical management of bronchiectasis: the indications and outcomes. *Surg Today.* 2010;40:26-30. *Review of surgery for bronchiectasis.*

King PT. The pathophysiology of bronchiectasis. *Int J COPD.* 2009;4:411-419. *Overview of pathobiology.*

Lai PS, Cohen DW, DeCamp MM, et al. A 40 year old woman with an asymptomatic cystic lesion in her right lung. *Chest.* 2009;136:622-627. *Review of congenital pulmonary airway abnormality.*

Pasteur MC, Bilton D, Hill AT. British Thoracic Society guideline for non-CF bronchiectasis. *Thorax.* 2010;65(Suppl 1):i1-i58. *Consensus guidelines.*

91 ALVEOLAR FILLING DISORDERS

STEPHANIE M. LEVINE

DEFINITION

Alveolar filling disorders (Table 91-1) are characterized by chest radiographic findings of alveolar involvement ranging from a ground-glass appearance to consolidation; the pathologic process shows primary involvement of the alveolar air spaces distal to the terminal bronchioles. For example, in pulmonary alveolar proteinosis, the alveoli are filled by proteinaceous fluid; in bronchioloalveolar cell cancer, the alveolar walls are lined by adenocarcinoma cells. In acute interstitial pneumonia, exudative organizing fibroproliferative infiltrates fill the alveolar space; in the alveolar hemorrhage disorders, blood fills the alveolar space. Alveolar spaces filled with acute inflammatory cells, as in bacterial pneumonia (Chapter 97), or water, as in cardiogenic or hydrostatic pulmonary edema (Chapter 58), or high-protein fluid, as in noncardiogenic or increased permeability pulmonary edema (Chapter 104), are also part of the radiographic differential diagnosis of alveolar filling disorders and must be excluded.

TABLE 91-1 ALVEOLAR FILLING DISORDERS

DISEASES	PATHOPHYSIOLOGY	RADIOGRAPHIC FINDINGS
Pulmonary alveolar proteinosis	Impaired processing of surfactant by alveolar macrophages due to defects in GM-CSF signaling	Bilateral alveolar infiltrates with "crazy paving" and diffuse areas of ground-glass attenuation on CT scan
Acute interstitial pneumonia	Diffuse alveolar damage with temporal uniformity	Diffuse alveolar filling process similar to the acute respiratory distress syndrome
Diffuse alveolar hemorrhage	Bleeding from the pulmonary microcirculation, usually from the capillaries	Acute development of bilateral alveolar infiltrates
Bronchioloalveolar cell carcinoma	Cancer cells growing along the alveolar septa	Pneumonic infiltrate or nodules (either solitary or multiple)

CT = computed tomographic; GM-CSF = granulocyte-macrophage colony-stimulating factor.

A general approach to these suspected alveolar filling diseases (Fig. 91-1) can be stratified by time since the onset of symptoms. The typical patient may present with the onset of cough (usually dry) and dyspnea of variable duration, depending on the disease process. Hemoptysis is a frequent presenting symptom in the alveolar hemorrhagic disorders. With the exception of acute interstitial pneumonia, acute infectious symptoms such as fever, leukocytosis, and productive cough are usually absent. If the initial chest radiograph or chest computed tomographic (CT) scan is consistent with a possible alveolar filling process (Chapter 84), and acute pneumonia and pulmonary edema are excluded, bronchoscopy with bronchoalveolar lavage (Chapter 85) and transbronchial biopsy should be performed, particularly if pulmonary alveolar proteinosis, bronchioloalveolar cell cancer (Chapter 197), or alveolar hemorrhage is suspected. When these tests are nondiagnostic and in most cases of suspected acute interstitial pneumonia, a surgical lung biopsy obtained by thoracoscopy or an open surgical procedure is indicated.

PULMONARY ALVEOLAR PROTEINOSIS

EPIDEMIOLOGY

Pulmonary alveolar proteinosis is a rare alveolar filling disease caused by the accumulation of phospholipoproteinaceous material in the alveoli. The

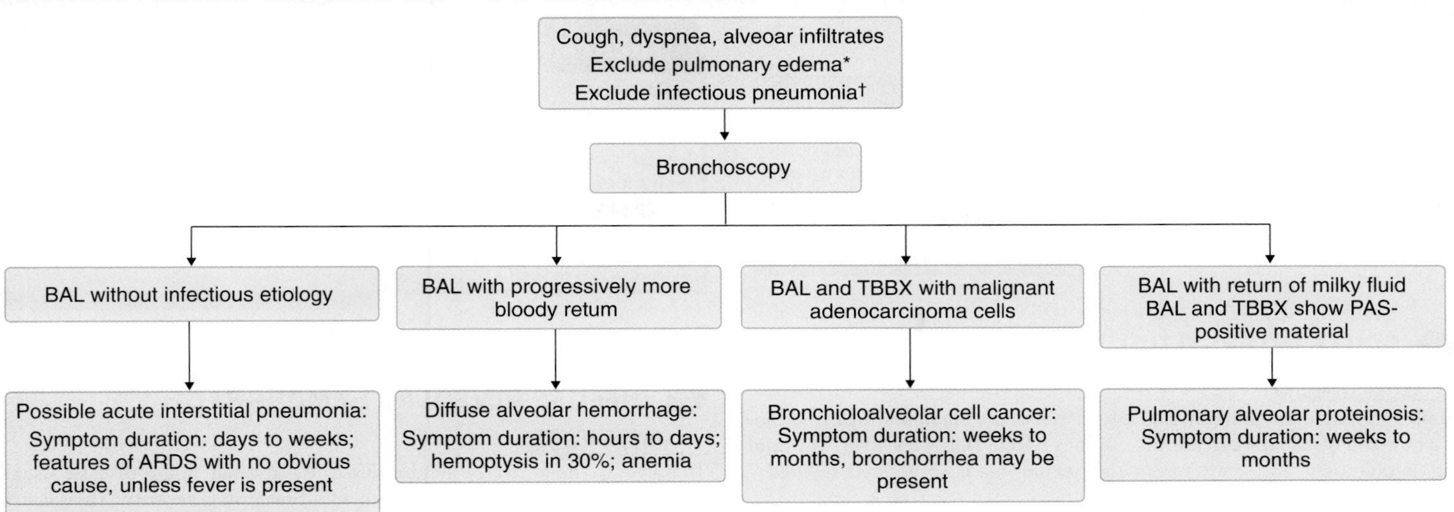

FIGURE 91-1. **A general approach to the alveolar filling disorders.** *See Chapter 58. †See Chapter 97. ARDS = acute respiratory distress syndrome; BAL = bronchoalveolar lavage; PAS = periodic acid–Schiff; TBBX = transbronchial biopsy.

incidence is estimated to be 3.7 cases per million people. Pulmonary alveolar proteinosis in adults is an acquired primary disorder in more than 90% of cases, but similar histopathologic features may be found with identifiable causes, such as acute silicosis (silicoproteinosis; Chapter 93), aluminum dust exposure (Chapter 93), immunodeficiency disorders (e.g., immunoglobulin G monoclonal gammopathy and severe combined immunodeficiency syndrome), hematologic malignant neoplasms (particularly myeloid leukemias; Chapters 189 and 190), and certain infections (e.g., *Pneumocystis* pneumonia). Pulmonary alveolar proteinosis has also been described after bone marrow transplantation (Chapter 181).

PATHOBIOLOGY

The pathogenesis of pulmonary alveolar proteinosis is related to impaired processing of surfactant by alveolar macrophages due to defects in granulocyte-macrophage colony-stimulating factor (GM-CSF) signaling. This impairment may be due to autoantibodies against GM-CSF or GM-CSF receptor gene mutations, but it is not thought to be due to a problem with GM-CSF production. An autosomal recessive congenital form of pulmonary alveolar proteinosis, caused by a mutation in the genes encoding surfactant protein B or C, results in abnormal surfactant function and severe respiratory distress in homozygous infants. The result of this impairment is accumulation of surfactant-rich material and progressive dysfunction in phagocytosis due to excessive production or diminished clearance of surfactant by alveolar macrophages.

Histologic examination in pulmonary alveolar proteinosis reveals alveoli filled with lipoproteinaceous material that stains pink (positive reaction) with periodic acid–Schiff stain. Classically, there is no destruction of alveolar architecture. Electron microscopy reveals lamellar (phospholipid-containing) myelin bodies.

CLINICAL MANIFESTATIONS

Pulmonary alveolar proteinosis presents in patients in the third to fourth decade with a 2:1 male predominance. Most patients (72%) are smokers. Patients present with the insidious onset of dyspnea and cough, which may be dry or occasionally productive of grayish material. The duration of symptoms before diagnosis is typically 6 weeks to 6 to 8 months. Low-grade fevers, malaise, and weight loss may also be present. Hemoptysis is unusual. On physical examination, rales are present in 50% of cases. Clubbing is an unusual finding until later stages of disease.

DIAGNOSIS

Mildly elevated leukocyte counts and mildly to moderately elevated lactate dehydrogenase levels may be found in more than 80% of patients; lactate dehydrogenase levels may correlate with the severity of disease. The chest radiograph (Fig. 91-2) and chest CT scans demonstrate a diffuse symmetrical alveolar filling process with predominance in the lower two thirds of the lung fields; the radiographic appearance may mimic pulmonary edema. The

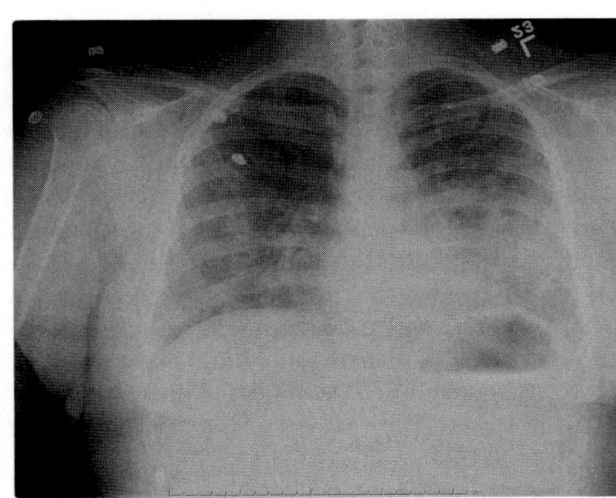

FIGURE 91-2. **A chest radiograph showing bilateral alveolar infiltrates in a patient with pulmonary alveolar proteinosis.**

characteristic CT pattern is often described as "crazy paving," which is due to scattered or diffuse areas of ground-glass attenuation with thickening of intralobular structures and interlobular septa in polygonal shapes (Fig. 91-3). This radiographic pattern is not specific for this disorder and can be seen with acute respiratory distress syndrome (ARDS; Chapter 104), *Pneumocystis jirovecii* pneumonia (Chapter 349), bronchioloalveolar cell carcinoma (Chapter 197), lipoid pneumonia (Chapter 94), sarcoidosis (Chapter 95), organizing pneumonia (Chapter 92), drug reactions, and pulmonary hemorrhage as well as with cardiogenic pulmonary edema (Chapter 59) and acute interstitial pneumonias. Pulmonary function tests often but not always show a restrictive pattern, with a reduced diffusing capacity. Arterial blood gas analyses reveal hypoxemia.

Bronchoscopy should be the initial procedure when pulmonary alveolar proteinosis is suspected. The diagnosis of pulmonary alveolar proteinosis can be established in most cases by the recovery of milky white to sandy-colored or light brown fluid on bronchoalveolar lavage. When it is subjected to microscopic analysis, the bronchoalveolar lavage fluid has a positive reaction on periodic acid–Schiff staining. Transbronchial biopsy or thoracoscopic biopsy can confirm the diagnosis by providing tissue that has similar staining characteristics.

TREATMENT Rx

About 8 to 30% of cases of pulmonary alveolar proteinosis resolve spontaneously, and smoking cessation may contribute to spontaneous resolution. A second group of patients will progress to respiratory failure. The remainder will have stable disease. Superinfection with *Nocardia* species, atypical mycobacteria, and other opportunistic organisms can occur in more than 15% of patients as a result of macrocyte phagocytic dysfunction.

Therapy begins with multistage or sequential whole lung lavage performed under general anesthesia with a double-lumen endotracheal tube. This procedure may have to be repeated at variable intervals. A small open-label trial using GM-CSF resulted in improved quality of life, oxygenation, pulmonary function, and exercise capacity in 48% of patients studied. Lung transplantation can be performed, but recurrent pulmonary alveolar proteinosis has been reported.

Survival rates at 5 years approach 75%.

ACUTE INTERSTITIAL PNEUMONIA

DEFINITION

Acute interstitial pneumonia, also referred to as the *Hamman-Rich syndrome*, is a rare and often fatal disease that mimics ARDS (Chapter 104). The etiology is unknown, and acute interstitial pneumonia is sometimes defined as the development of ARDS in the absence of known triggers. A similar acute presentation may be seen in patients with idiopathic pulmonary fibrosis (Chapter 92), but most investigators believe that acute interstitial pneumonia is a separate disease process.

PATHOBIOLOGY

The pathogenesis of acute interstitial pneumonia is damage to the epithelium of the alveolar membranes by a neutrophil-mediated mechanism; the result is pouring of exudate into the air space in the initial exudative phase of disease. Histologic examination reveals diffuse alveolar damage with intra-alveolar hyaline membrane formation, interstitial and intra-alveolar edema, acute inflammation, and epithelial cell necrosis with a nonspecific distribution and temporal uniformity. This process progresses to the organizing phase, characterized by alveolar septal thickening, type II pneumocyte hyperplasia, and fibroblast proliferation along the interstitium and alveolar spaces. In situ thrombi of small pulmonary arteries may be present. Finally comes a fibrotic phase with alveolar septal thickening from organizing fibrosis. One of the key pathologic findings in acute interstitial pneumonia is the temporal uniformity of the diffuse alveolar damage and of organizing and proliferating connective tissue. This uniformity supports a single acute injury at a particular point in time. Long-standing fibrosis is not a typical pathologic finding in acute interstitial pneumonia.

CLINICAL MANIFESTATIONS

Acute interstitial pneumonia manifests with equal frequency in men and women, typically in previously healthy individuals in the 50- to 55-year age range. It develops acutely to subacutely during a few days to a few weeks. The mean duration of symptoms is 15 days. Dry cough, shortness of breath, malaise, and fever (in 50% of patients) are typical clinical findings. A virus-like prodrome period has been described. Pulmonary rales are heard on physical examination, and hypoxemia is characteristic. Acute interstitial pneumonia often progresses to hypoxemic ventilatory failure, and intensive care unit admission with mechanical ventilation is usually required. Early mortality is high. Radiographic features of acute interstitial pneumonia are diffuse alveolar infiltrates and air space consolidation similar to the appearance of ARDS; CT scans reveal bilateral air space consolidation with areas of ground-glass opacities with little honeycombing. Septal thickening and a subpleural distribution of the opacities may also be present.

DIAGNOSIS

The diagnosis of acute interstitial pneumonia is made in the appropriate clinical setting in a patient who has a clinical presentation compatible with ARDS but without a clear etiology. The differential diagnosis histologically and clinically includes other causes of ARDS (Chapter 104), such as severe infection, trauma, and sepsis, and other causes of acute lung injury (Chapter 94), such as drug toxicity, inhalation injury, and collagen vascular diseases. The presentation is clinically and radiographically similar to that of diffuse alveolar hemorrhage, acute hypersensitivity pneumonitis, acute exacerbation of pulmonary fibrosis, acute eosinophilic pneumonia, and cryptogenic organizing pneumonia. Bronchoscopy with bronchoalveolar lavage is often performed to exclude alveolar hemorrhage, eosinophilic pneumonias, and infectious causes of lung injury. In a small number of cases, transbronchial biopsy may yield the diagnosis, but definitive diagnosis in most cases of acute interstitial pneumonia requires a surgical lung biopsy.

TREATMENT Rx

Treatment includes supportive intensive care unit management. In small case series, corticosteroids at doses of 1 g of methylprednisolone intravenously per day for three consecutive days followed by prednisone or equivalent at 1 mg/kg/day with a taper during several weeks to months, with or without cyclophosphamide, may be of benefit, but mortality remains higher than 60% during the subsequent 6 months. Patients also can have recurrences in months to years. Some cases of acute interstitial pneumonia may resolve without sequelae, but in some series, more than 50% of survivors may be left with residual fibrosis.

DIFFUSE ALVEOLAR HEMORRHAGE

DEFINITION

The alveolar hemorrhage syndromes cause alveolar filling disease, usually with an acute onset and often with life-threatening severity. They can be associated with vasculitides, such as microscopic polyangiitis (Chapter 278) and c-ANCA-associated (Wegener's) vasculitis (Chapter 278); immunologic diseases, such as Goodpasture's syndrome (anti–glomerular basement membrane antibody disease; Chapter 123); collagen vascular diseases, such as systemic lupus erythematosus (Chapter 274); cocaine inhalation (Chapter 33); drugs (including penicillamine, mitomycin C, trimellitic anhydride, all-*trans* retinoic acid, propylthiouracil, and isocyanates); bone marrow transplantation (Chapter 181); coagulopathy (Chapter 177); and mitral stenosis (Chapter 75). A small percentage of idiopathic and recurrent cases are termed *idiopathic pulmonary hemosiderosis*. In Goodpasture's syndrome, there is a strong association with tobacco use and a male predominance, with young men most frequently affected. A viral syndrome and exposure to hydrocarbons may simulate Goodpasture's disease. Idiopathic pulmonary hemosiderosis most often occurs in children and young adults.

PATHOBIOLOGY

Alveolar hemorrhage is caused by bleeding from the pulmonary microcirculation, including the capillaries, arterioles, and venules. It may be associated with injury or neutrophilic inflammation of the capillaries or a capillaritis, usually when it is associated with collagen vascular or vasculitic processes. In Goodpasture's syndrome, for example, the circulating anti–glomerular basement membrane antibodies are directed against the α_3 chain of type IV collagen in the glomerular basement membrane, where they cause glomerulonephritis; these core antibodies can cross-react with the alveolar capillary basement membranes, resulting in alveolar hemorrhage. Alternatively, alveolar hemorrhage may be associated with relatively bland pathologic changes with red blood cells in the alveolar spaces. Idiopathic pulmonary hemosiderosis is an example of bland hemorrhage.

CLINICAL MANIFESTATIONS

Patients present acutely (usually in hours to a week) with dyspnea, shortness of breath, hemoptysis (which may not be present in all patients), and cough. Some patients also have low-grade fever. Lung examination reveals rales.

Laboratory examination may reveal anemia. In Goodpasture's syndrome and the ANCA-associated vasculitides, hematuria and renal insufficiency due to glomerulonephritis are typically present.

Radiographic features include the acute development of bilateral alveolar filling disease similar to pulmonary edema but without cardiomegaly or pleural effusions. Rapid remission and recurrences are seen with repeated episodes of bleeding, which also may result in chronic interstitial changes on the chest radiograph. Pulmonary function testing may reveal an increase in the diffusion capacity for carbon monoxide because of the presence of hemoglobin in the alveolar spaces.

DIAGNOSIS

The diagnosis of alveolar hemorrhage is usually made in the appropriate clinical setting by the triad of diffuse alveolar infiltrates (see Fig. 91-3), hemoptysis (in two thirds of patients), and anemia. Bronchoalveolar lavage typically demonstrates the return of progressively more bloody aliquots of fluid, and cytologic analysis reveals that more than 20% of the macrophages are hemosiderin laden. Goodpasture's syndrome is diagnosed by circulating anti–glomerular basement membrane antibodies, which are present in more than 90% of patients, or by the demonstration of linear deposition

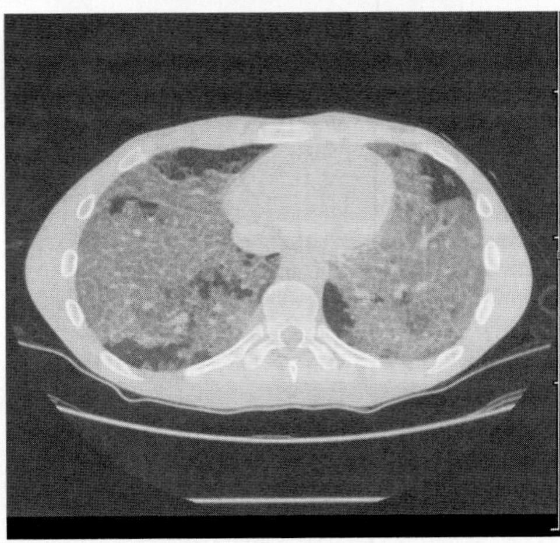

FIGURE 91-3. A chest computed tomographic scan showing the "crazy paving" pattern characteristic of pulmonary alveolar proteinosis.

of immunoglobulin G antibodies along the alveolar or renal capillary basement membrane tissue when it is viewed by direct immunofluorescence. c-ANCA-associated vasculitis causes a focal, segmental, necrotizing glomerulonephritis and is associated with the presence of proteinase 3 antineutrophilic cytoplasmic antibodies in 90% of active cases (Chapter 278). Necrotizing granulomatous inflammation is often found in the upper airway in addition to the lungs and kidneys. A perinuclear myeloperoxidase antineutrophilic antibody is often present in association with microscopic polyarteritis (Chapter 278). Patients with systemic lupus erythematosus usually have antinuclear antibodies (Chapter 274). Idiopathic pulmonary hemosiderosis is a diagnosis of exclusion after other causes of diffuse alveolar hemorrhage have been eliminated.

TREATMENT Rx

Treatment of alveolar hemorrhage varies according to its underlying cause. Massive hemoptysis from any cause of alveolar hemorrhage should be managed as needed. In the case of drug- or toxin-related alveolar hemorrhage, the offending agent should be withdrawn, and supportive care is indicated. In Goodpasture's syndrome, the ANCA-associated vasculitides, and other vasculitides (Chapter 278), treatment typically includes immunosuppressant agents such as corticosteroids (methylprednisolone, 500 to 2000 mg/day in divided doses for 3 to 5 days followed by a prednisone taper beginning at 1 mg/kg/day during the next 6 to 9 months) and cyclophosphamide (2 mg/kg/day orally or 0.75 g/m^2 intravenously for one dose). In Goodpasture's syndrome, plasmapheresis is also a mainstay of therapy to remove the offending circulating antibody. Plasmapheresis (3 to 14 exchanges) may also be used in some cases of alveolar hemorrhage from ANCA-associated vasculitis and systemic lupus erythematosus.

PROGNOSIS

Recurrent alveolar hemorrhage from any cause, such as idiopathic pulmonary hemosiderosis, can be associated with the development of pulmonary fibrosis. Alveolar hemorrhage related to collagen vascular disease, vasculitides, and idiopathic pulmonary hemosiderosis can have mortality rates ranging from 25 to 50%. With Goodpasture's syndrome, renal failure is common, and the degree of renal impairment may correlate with outcome.

BRONCHIOLOALVEOLAR CELL CARCINOMA

DEFINITION

Bronchioloalveolar cell carcinoma, which is a subtype of bronchogenic adenocarcinoma, is characterized by well-differentiated, malignant cells lining the alveolar cell wall (Chapter 197). Of bronchogenic carcinomas, bronchioloalveolar cell carcinoma is the least strongly associated with tobacco use, and patients are more likely to be nonsmokers. Unlike other non–small cell lung cancers, the female-to-male ratio approaches 1:1, and younger patients may be affected. Using the strict pathologic definition described later, the

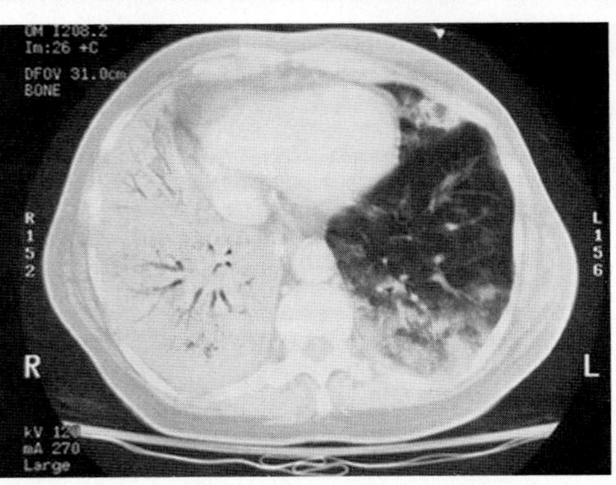

FIGURE 91-4. A chest computed tomographic scan in a patient with bronchioloalveolar cell cancer revealing the pneumonic form of the disease.

prevalence of bronchioloalveolar carcinoma among the non–small cell carcinomas is less than 5%.

PATHOBIOLOGY

Bronchioloalveolar cell carcinoma usually arises in the periphery of the lung and is characterized by pure lepidic growth, which means contiguous growth along the intact alveolar septa, without stromal, pleural, vascular, or lymphatic invasion and without a known primary adenocarcinoma elsewhere. Bronchioloalveolar cell carcinoma can be categorized into mucinous and nonmucinous forms histologically; the mucinous type is thought to derive from respiratory goblet cells, and the nonmucinous type from type II pneumocytes or Clara cells.

CLINICAL MANIFESTATIONS

Patients present with the gradual onset of shortness of breath and cough. The duration of symptoms is usually several months. Constitutional symptoms such as malaise and weight loss may be present. An unusual but unique clinical finding is bronchorrhea, with patients reporting the production of copious amounts of clear sputum daily. This finding is more common in the pneumonic form of disease. Nodal involvement and extrathoracic metastases are less frequent than in other forms of non–small cell lung cancer.

DIAGNOSIS

Radiographic patterns vary and can include localized disease with peripheral solitary or multiple nodules or masses in 60% of cases or a persistent pneumonic pattern in 40% of cases (Fig. 91-4). The radiographic findings are often thought to be consistent with pneumonia, and a typical clinical presentation is that of a nonresolving peripheral density on chest radiograph. In addition, computed tomography may show areas of ground-glass attenuation. Positron emission tomography may be normal because of the low glucose uptake of this lesion. The diagnosis of bronchioloalveolar cell carcinoma is most often made by bronchoscopy with transbronchial biopsy.

TREATMENT Rx

For staging and treatment, bronchioloalveolar cell carcinoma is approached like other types of non–small cell lung cancers (Chapter 197), although bronchioloalveolar carcinoma may respond to epidermal growth factor receptor (EGFR) agents. Bilateral lung transplantation has been performed, but recurrence in the transplanted lungs has been reported.

PROGNOSIS

Prognosis correlates with disease stage and probably with the histologic and radiographic patterns. Patients with a single focus of disease (i.e., a solitary nodule) who undergo surgical resection have a prognosis better than that of patients with nonbronchioloalveolar adenocarcinomas of like stage. Multinodular, pneumonic, and diffuse forms of disease have a worse prognosis, as does the mucinous histologic subtype.

SUGGESTED READINGS

Das M, Salzman GA. Pulmonary alveolar proteinosis: an overview for internists and hospital physicians. *Hosp Pract (Minneap)*. 2010;38:43-49. *Overview.*

Lara AR, Schwarz MI. Diffuse alveolar hemorrhage. *Chest*. 2010;137:1164-1171. *Review.*

Luisetti M, Kadija Z, Mariani F, et al. Therapy options in pulmonary alveolar proteinosis. *Ther Adv Respir Dis*. 2010;4:239-248. *Emphasizes utility of whole lung lavage and of approaches to supplement GM-CSF or reduce autoantibodies against it.*

Perlman CE, Lederer DJ, Bhattacharya J. Micromechanics of alveolar edema. *Am J Respir Cell Mol Biol*. 2011;44:34-39. *Overview of the causes and implications.*

Suzuki T, Maranda B, Sakagami T, et al. Hereditary pulmonary alveolar proteinosis caused by recessive CSF2RB mutations. *Eur Respir J*. 2011:37:201-204. *Gene that can be responsible for adult onset hereditary disease.*

92

INTERSTITIAL LUNG DISEASE

GANESH RAGHU

DEFINITION

In an apparently immunocompetent host, interstitial lung disease (ILD) is a clinical term for a heterogenous group of lower respiratory tract disorders with many potential causes. However, clinical and physiologic features common to all ILDs include exertional dyspnea, a restrictive pattern on pulmonary function testing (Chapter 85), coexistent airflow obstruction, decreased diffusing capacity (DLCO), increased alveolar-arterial oxygen difference (PAO_2-PaO_2) (Chapter 103) at rest or during exertion, and absence of pulmonary infection or neoplasm. ILDs comprise several acute and chronic lung disorders with variable degrees of pulmonary fibrosis (Table 92-1). The term *interstitial* is a misnomer because the pathologic processes are not restricted to the interstitium, which is the microscopic space bounded by the basement membranes of epithelial and endothelial cells. Rather, all of the several cellular and soluble constituents that make up the gas exchange units (alveolar wall, capillaries, alveolar space, and acini) and the bronchiolar lumen, terminal bronchioles, and pulmonary parenchyma beyond the gas exchange units (as well as the pleura, lymphatics, and sometimes the lymph nodes) are involved in the pathogenesis and manifestations of ILD.

EPIDEMIOLOGY

Among persons 18 years or older, the prevalence of all ILDs in the United States is about 81 per 100,000 men and 67 per 100,000 women. The overall incidence is also higher in men (31.5 per 100,000 per year) than in women (26.1 per 100,000 per year). Moreover, the prevalence of undiagnosed or early ILD is estimated to be 10 times that of clinically recognized disease; as physicians' awareness of these entities increases, it is expected that the frequency of the diagnosis of ILD will rise. Among the ILDs, the most common is idiopathic pulmonary fibrosis, which represents at least 30% of incident cases; in the United States, its annual incidence is estimated to be 6.8 to 16.3 per 100,000, with a prevalence of 14.0 to 42.7 per 100,000.

TABLE 92-1 CLINICAL CLASSIFICATION OF INTERSTITIAL LUNG DISEASE

IDIOPATHIC INTERSTITIAL PNEUMONIAS
Idiopathic pulmonary fibrosis
Nonspecific pulmonary fibrosis
Respiratory bronchiolitis–associated interstitial lung disease
Desquamative interstitial pneumonia
Acute interstitial pneumonia
Cryptogenic organizing pneumonia
Lymphoid interstitial pneumonia
INTERSTITIAL LUNG DISEASE ASSOCIATED WITH COLLAGEN VASCULAR DISEASE
Progressive systemic sclerosis
Rheumatoid arthritis
Systemic lupus erythematosus
Dermatomyositis and polymyositis
Sjögren's syndrome
Mixed connective tissue disease
Ankylosing spondylitis
HYPERSENSITIVITY PNEUMONITIS
Occupational and environmental factors (e.g., farmer's lung; bird fancier's lung)
Iatrogenic
DRUG-INDUCED AND IATROGENIC INTERSTITIAL LUNG DISEASE
See Table 92-2
ALVEOLAR FILLING DISORDERS (CHAPTER 91)
Goodpasture's syndrome
Pulmonary alveolar proteinosis
Pulmonary hemosiderosis
Alveolar hemorrhage syndromes
Chronic eosinophilic pneumonia
INTERSTITIAL LUNG DISEASE ASSOCIATED WITH PULMONARY VASCULITIS
Pulmonary capillaritis
Wegener's granulomatosis
Churg-Strauss syndrome
OTHER SPECIFIC FORMS OF INTERSTITIAL LUNG DISEASE
Sarcoidosis
Langerhans cell histiocytosis (histiocytosis X)
Lymphangioleiomyomatosis
INHERITED FORMS OF INTERSTITIAL LUNG DISEASE
Familial idiopathic pulmonary fibrosis
Familial pulmonary fibrosis or interstitial pneumonia
Tuberous sclerosis
Neurofibromatosis
Gaucher's disease
Niemann-Pick disease
Hermansky-Pudlak syndrome

PATHOBIOLOGY

ILDs are thought to result from an unknown tissue injury and attempted repair in the lung of a genetically predisposed person. Genetic variants within the *hTERT* or *hTR* components of the telomerase gene and surfactant protein gene have been associated in a subset of familial pulmonary fibrosis and in some sporadic cases. An *MUC5B* promotor polymorphism is associated with familial interstitial pneumonia and idiopathic pulmonary fibrosis.

In *idiopathic pulmonary fibrosis,* varying degrees of acute, subacute, and chronic fibroproliferation are present in the lungs at the time of diagnosis. Ultimately, progressive fibrosis results in honeycombing, an end-stage finding that is often associated with increased pulmonary vascular resistance and secondary pulmonary hypertension. As a reflection of these dynamic processes, histopathologic examination of lung tissue often reveals highly heterogeneous findings; for example, a single biopsy specimen may show normal alveoli adjacent to abnormal areas of inflammation and fibrosis, with or without granulomas, vasculitis, or secondary vascular changes within the pulmonary parenchyma.

CLINICAL MANIFESTATIONS

ILDs are typically characterized by progressive dyspnea. Nonproductive cough and fatigue are also common complaints. Pleuritic chest pain may occur with certain collagen vascular or drug-induced ILDs, whereas acute pleuritic chest pain with dyspnea may represent a spontaneous pneumothorax (Chapter 99) in association with lymphangioleiomyomatosis, tuberous sclerosis (Chapter 426), neurofibromatosis, or Langerhans cell histiocytosis. Hemoptysis suggests a diffuse alveolar hemorrhagic syndrome, systemic lupus erythematosus (Chapter 274), lymphangioleiomyomatosis, Wegener's granulomatosis (Chapter 283), or Goodpasture's syndrome (Chapter 123); it is rare in other ILDs. In patients with existing ILD, new hemoptysis should prompt consideration of a superimposed malignancy, pulmonary embolus, or infection such as aspergillosis.

In some patients, the first and the only clue to the presence of an ILD may be the finding of coarse rales (crackles) on auscultation of the lungs. These coarse crackles must be distinguished from the finer rales typical of heart failure (Chapter 58) or noncardiogenic pulmonary edema (Chapter 104). Unlike patients with obstructive lung disease, wheezes are not common. A history of wheezing suggests the coexistence of occult hyperactive airways and airflow obstruction and raises the possibility of allergic bronchopulmonary aspergillosis (Chapter 347), Churg-Strauss syndrome (Chapter 278), chronic eosinophilic pneumonia (see later), or parasitic infection (Chapter 352). In some patients, the initial presentation may be with peripheral cyanosis, clubbing, or the signs and symptoms of an underlying systemic disease (see later).

DIAGNOSIS

The first key in patients with an ILD is to establish the syndromic diagnosis and then pursue the differential diagnosis of its specific cause (Fig. 92-1). However, a conclusive cause often may not be identified despite an exhaustive medical history and invasive diagnostic interventions, including sufficiently large and multiple lung biopsy specimens. Thus, the cause of several of the ILDs, even when diagnosed as specific entities, remains unknown.

History

The patient's age, sex, and cigarette smoking history may provide useful clues to the diagnosis. Idiopathic pulmonary fibrosis is an adult disorder that usually occurs in patients older than 50 years. Pulmonary sarcoidosis (Chapter 95), in contrast, is more common in young adults and middle-aged persons. Pulmonary Langerhans cell histiocytosis (previously known as pulmonary histiocytosis X or eosinophilic granuloma) characteristically occurs in young cigarette-smoking men, whereas lymphangioleiomyomatosis occurs exclusively in women of childbearing age. Respiratory bronchiolitis-associated interstitial lung disease is seen almost exclusively in cigarette smokers but occurs in both men and women of all ages.

The medical history also should focus on environmental factors, especially changes in environmental exposure (domestic, recreational, hot tub, whirlpool baths, indoor swimming pool, ventilation system at home, automobiles, and workplace), occupational exposure, medications, and drug use (Chapters 93 and 94). A family medical history should address possible familial ILD. Environmental risk factors that may suggest the diagnosis of hypersensitivity pneumonitis include farming or exposure to avian antigens ("bird fancier's lung" or "pigeon breeder's lung"), visible molds, water leaks, or humidifiers in the domestic environment (hypersensitivity to thermophilic actinomycetes). Other at-risk occupations include mining (pneumoconioses), machine tool grinding, sandblasting and working with granite (silicosis), welding and working in a shipyard (asbestosis), and working in the aerospace or electronic industries (berylliosis) (Chapters 93 and 94). Because of the long interval between the exposure and the onset of symptoms in many occupations associated with ILD, it is important to take a lifelong occupational history (Chapter 18) as well as to establish the interval between exposure and the onset of symptoms. Because the list of medications known to cause ILD is long and continues to grow (Table 92-2), a careful history regarding recent use of prescription and over-the-counter products is essential. Risk factors for immunosuppression, including infection with human immunodeficiency virus, raise the possibility of opportunistic lung infections (Chapter 398), neoplasm (Chapter 197), and transplant-related pulmonary complications.

Particular attention should be paid to the onset and duration of symptoms, the rate of disease progression, and association with hemoptysis, fever, or extrathoracic symptoms. Symptoms that persist 4 weeks or less and the presence of fever suggest cryptogenic organizing pneumonia, drug-induced pulmonary injury, or acute hypersensitivity pneumonitis, whereas idiopathic pulmonary fibrosis, ILD associated with connective tissue diseases, and Langerhans cell histiocytosis tend to have a more subacute onset. Extrapulmonary symptoms suggests that the ILD may be associated with systemic disorders (e.g., sarcoidosis; Chapter 95), and symptoms such as dysphagia, dry eyes or mouth, skin rashes, or arthritis may suggest a collagen vascular disorder (Chapters 274 and 278). Proximal muscle aches or weakness suggests the possibility of polymyositis or dermatomyositis (Chapter 277), and recurrent sinusitis suggests Wegener's granulomatosis (Chapter 278). Extrathoracic manifestations present in tuberous sclerosis (Chapter 426) include hematuria, epilepsy, and mental retardation.

Physical Examination

Physical examination of the respiratory system is rarely helpful in the diagnostic evaluation of ILD because findings such rhonchi and rales on auscultation and digital clubbing are nonspecific. Findings on cardiac examination, such as an accentuated P_2, a right ventricular heave, or tricuspid insufficiency, are suggestive of pulmonary hypertension (Chapter 68) and cor pulmonale in patients with advanced lung disease. However, extrathoracic findings such as skin abnormalities, peripheral lymphadenopathy, and hepatosplenomegaly may be more specifically associated with underlying sarcoidosis (Chapter 95); muscle tenderness and proximal muscle weakness may point to coexisting polymyositis (Chapter 277); and signs of arthritis may indicate collagen vascular disease (Chapters 272, 274, and 278) or sarcoidosis (Chapter 95).

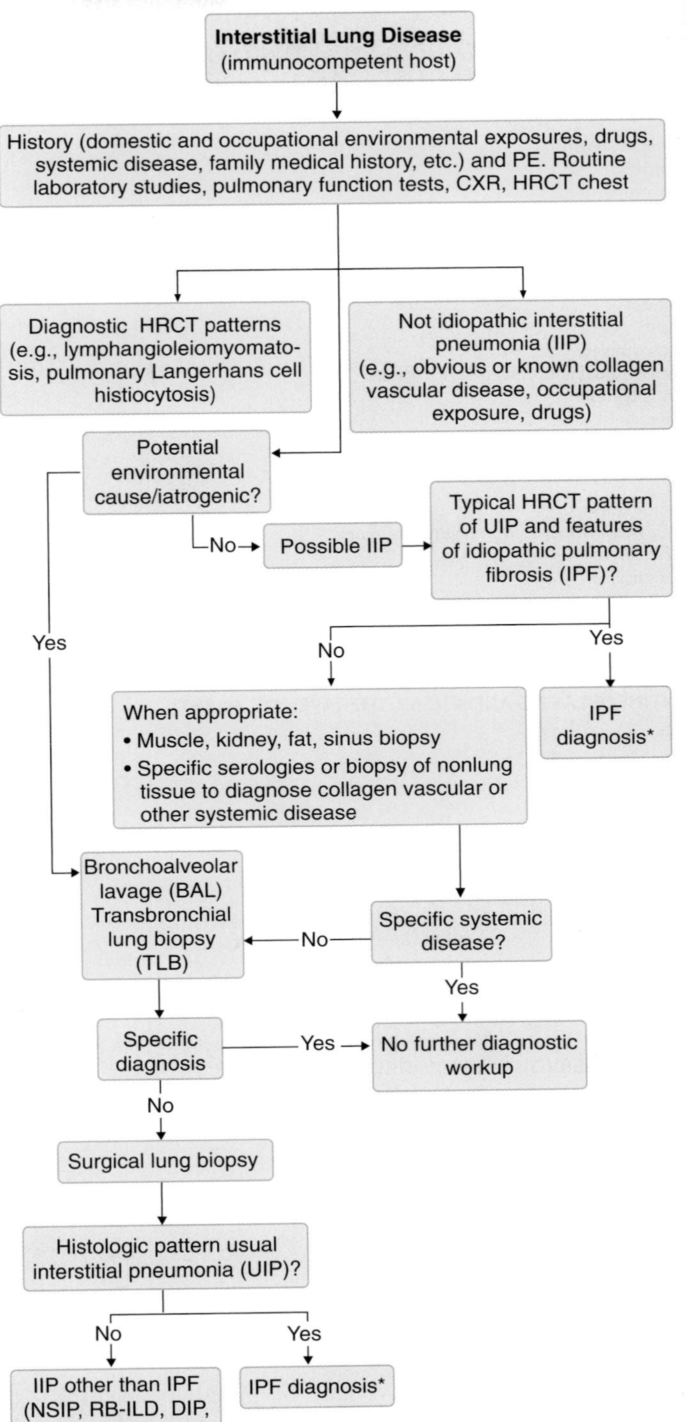

FIGURE 92-1. **An approach to interstitial lung disease.** DAD = diffuse alveolar damage; DIP = desquamative interstitial pneumonia; HRCT = high-resolution computed tomography; LIP = lymphoid interstitial pneumonia; NSIP = nonspecific interstitial pneumonia; OP = organizing pneumonia; PE = physical examination; RB-ILD = respiratory bronchiolitis–associated interstitial lung disease; UIP = usual interstitial pneumonia. *Adapted from American Thoracic Society/European Respiratory Society: International multidisciplinary consensus classification of idiopathic interstitial pneumonias. *Am J Respir Crit Care Med.* 2002;165:277-304 and Raghu G, Collard HR, Egan JJ, et al. An official ATS/ERS/JRS/ALAT statement: idiopathic pulmonary fibrosis: evidence-based guidelines for diagnosis and management. *Am J Respir Crit Care Med.* 2011;183:788-824.

Characteristic rashes occur in several collagen vascular diseases, disseminated Langerhans cell histiocytosis, tuberous sclerosis, and neurofibromatosis. Ophthalmologic findings (Chapter 431) such as iridocyclitis, uveitis, or conjunctivitis may be a clue to the diagnosis of sarcoidosis or a collagen vascular disease, whereas central nervous system abnormalities may be present in sarcoidosis, systemic lupus erythematosus, Langerhans cell histiocytosis, or tuberous sclerosis.

TABLE 92-2 DRUG-INDUCED AND IATROGENIC INTERSTITIAL LUNG DISEASE*

ANTIMICROBIAL AGENTS
Cephalosporins
Isoniazid
Nitrofurantoin
Penicillins
Sulfonamides
ANTI-INFLAMMATORY AGENTS
Aspirin
Gold
Methotrexate
Nonsteroidal anti-inflammatory agents
Penicillamine
Phenylbutazone
Zafirlukast
CARDIOVASCULAR DRUGS
Amiodarone
Angiotensin-converting enzyme inhibitors
β-Blockers
Hydralazine
Hydrochlorothiazide
Procainamide
Protamine sulfate
Tocainide
ANTINEOPLASTIC AND CHEMOTHERAPEUTIC AGENTS
Bleomycin
Busulfan
Chlorambucil
Cyclophosphamide
Erlotinib
Gefitinib
Gemcitabine
Imatinib
Melphalan
Mercaptopurine
Methotrexate
Mitomycin
Nitrosoureas
Procarbazine
CENTRAL NERVOUS SYSTEM DRUGS
Carbamazepine
Chlorpromazine
Imipramine
Phenytoin
ORAL HYPOGLYCEMIC AGENTS
Chlorpropamide
Tolazamide
Tolbutamide
ILLICIT DRUGS
Cocaine
Heroin
Methadone
Propoxyphene
OTHER AGENTS
Antithymocyte globulin
All-*trans*-retinoic acid
Colony-stimulating factors
Interferon-α and -β
Irradiation
Mycophenolate mofetil
Tumor necrosis factor-α modulating agents
High fraction of inspired oxygen (FIO_2) with mechanical ventilation

*This list contains examples only and is not meant to be exhaustive.

Laboratory Testing

Routine laboratory testing should include a complete blood count, leukocyte differential, erythrocyte sedimentation rate, chemistry panel (calcium, liver enzymes, electrolytes, creatinine), and urinalysis. Although these data rarely yield a specific diagnosis, they may provide helpful clues. When appropriate, patients should be screened for systemic lupus erythematosus (e.g., antinuclear antibodies), rheumatoid arthritis (rheumatoid factor, anticitrullinated peptide antibody), scleroderma (ScL 70), dermatomyositis or polymyositis (creatine kinase, aldolase, and anti-Jo-1 antibody), Wegener's granulomatosis (antineutrophil cytoplasmic antibodies), and Goodpasture's syndrome (anti–basement membrane antibodies).

Mild hypoxemia is typically present on arterial blood gas analysis because of abnormal ventilation-perfusion ratios, especially in moderate to severe cases of ILD. However, carbon dioxide retention is rare and suggests possible coexisting emphysema (Chapter 88) or a hypoventilatory disorder (Chapter 86).

Noninvasive Evaluation

Chest Radiograph

The distribution and appearance of radiographic abnormalities (Chapter 84) may prove useful in differentiating the clinicopathologic syndromes in patients with ILD (Table 92-3). Comparison of previous chest radiographs with the current one is important in establishing the rate of progression of the patient's disease. A diffuse ground-glass pattern is often observed early in the course of ILD, followed by progression to reticular (linear) infiltrates with nodules (reticulonodular infiltrates) or, in the case of alveolar filling disorders, ill-defined nodules (acinar rosettes) with air bronchograms. Most ILDs cause infiltrates in the lower lung zones, but upper lobe predominance is typically present in sarcoidosis, berylliosis, Langerhans cell histiocytosis, silicosis, chronic hypersensitivity pneumonitis, cystic fibrosis, and ankylosing spondylitis, whereas the middle and lower lung zones show the most prominent abnormalities in lymphangitic carcinomatosis, idiopathic pulmonary fibrosis, subacute eosinophilic pneumonia, asbestosis, and pulmonary fibrosis caused by rheumatoid arthritis or progressive systemic sclerosis. Hilar adenopathy and mediastinal adenopathy are not common in ILDs; their presence should suggest sarcoidosis, berylliosis, silicosis, lymphocytic interstitial pneumonia, amyloidosis, or Gaucher's disease. A pattern of peripherally located pulmonary infiltrates in the upper and middle lung zones with relatively clear perihilar and central zones is a clue to chronic eosinophilic pneumonia. Recurrent infiltrates raise the possibility of cryptogenic organizing pneumonia, chronic eosinophilic pneumonia, or drug- or radiation-induced pneumonitis, whereas fleeting or migratory infiltrates may occur in Churg-Strauss syndrome (allergic angiitis), allergic bronchopulmonary aspergillosis, tropical eosinophilic pneumonia, or Löffler's syndrome. Localized pleural plaques may indicate asbestosis, whereas diffuse pleural thickening can result from asbestosis, rheumatoid arthritis, progressive systemic sclerosis, radiation pneumonitis, nitrofurantoin, or malignancy. In the absence of left ventricular failure, the presence of a pleural effusion (Chapter 99) raises the possibility of rheumatoid arthritis, systemic lupus erythematosus, acute hypersensitivity pneumonitis, sarcoidosis, asbestosis, amyloidosis, lymphangioleiomyomatosis, or lymphangitic carcinomatosis. Reduction of lung volumes is typical in most ILDs; the presence of preserved lung volumes or hyperinflation should raise suspicion for chronic hypersensitivity pneumonitis, Langerhans cell histiocytosis, lymphangioleiomyomatosis, neurofibromatosis, sarcoidosis, or tuberous sclerosis. However, plain chest radiographs may be normal in about 10% of patients with ILD.

High-Resolution Computed Tomography

Because of its increased sensitivity and ability to distinguish ground-glass changes, which are generally considered to be reversible areas of lung disease, from irreversible fibrotic and honeycomb changes, high-resolution computed tomography (HRCT) is essential in both the diagnosis and staging of ILD. Although microscopic ILD cannot be excluded by a normal HRCT, HRCT allows recognition of abnormalities not apparent in plain chest radiographs and may lead to an earlier diagnosis, help narrow the differential diagnosis patterns (Table 92-4), aid in selecting the site or sites for bronchoalveolar lavage and lung biopsy, and assist in choosing among therapeutic options and in estimating the response to treatment. The presence of patchy subpleural reticular and basilar septal fibrosis, traction bronchiectasis, and honeycombing increases the level of diagnostic confidence for the pattern of usual interstitial pattern, which is characteristic of idiopathic pulmonary fibrosis. The finding of bilateral cysts, including their size, configuration, distribution, and appearance, helps differentiate among lymphangioleiomyomatosis, tuberous sclerosis, and pulmonary Langerhans cell histiocytosis. HRCT can detect ILD despite normal chest radiographs in patients with asbestosis, silicosis, sarcoidosis, and scleroderma. Patients with respiratory bronchiolitis-associated interstitial lung disease typically have patchy ground-glass

TABLE 92-3 CHARACTERISTIC CHEST RADIOGRAPHIC PATTERNS IN PATIENTS WITH INTERSTITIAL LUNG DISEASE

PATTERN	SUGGESTED DIAGNOSES*
Decreased lung volumes	Idiopathic pulmonary fibrosis, nonspecific interstitial pneumonia, desquamative interstitial pneumonia, collagen vascular disease, chronic eosinophilic pneumonia, asbestosis, chronic hypersensitivity pneumonitis, or drug-induced interstitial lung disease (ILD)
Increased or preserved lung volumes	Idiopathic pulmonary fibrosis with emphysema, respiratory bronchiolitis-associated ILD, cryptogenic organizing pneumonia, hypersensitivity pneumonitis, lymphangioleiomyomatosis, Langerhans cell histiocytosis, sarcoidosis, neurofibromatosis, tuberous sclerosis
Micronodules	Infection, hypersensitivity pneumonitis, sarcoidosis, respiratory bronchiolitis-associated ILD
Septal thickening	Malignancy, infection, chronic congestive heart failure, pulmonary veno-occlusive disease
Honeycombing	Idiopathic pulmonary fibrosis, fibrotic nonspecific interstitial pneumonia, collagen vascular disease, asbestosis, chronic hypersensitivity pneumonitis, sarcoidosis
Recurrent infiltrates	Cryptogenic organizing pneumonia, chronic eosinophilic pneumonia, drug- or radiation-induced ILD
Migratory or fleeting infiltrates	Cryptogenic organizing pneumonia, hypersensitivity pneumonitis, Churg-Strauss syndrome, Löffler's syndrome, allergic bronchopulmonary aspergillosis
Pleural disease	Collagen vascular disease, asbestosis, malignancy, radiation-induced ILD, amyloidosis, sarcoidosis, lymphangioleiomyomatosis, nitrofurantoin-induced ILD
Pneumothorax	Langerhans cell histiocytosis, lymphangioleiomyomatosis, tuberous sclerosis, neurofibromatosis
Mediastinal and/or hilar adenopathy	Lymphocytic interstitial pneumonia, collagen vascular disease, silicosis, chronic berylliosis, malignancy, infection, sarcoidosis, amyloidosis, Gaucher's disease
Normal (rare)	Cellular nonspecific interstitial pneumonia, respiratory bronchiolitis–associated interstitial lung disease, collagen vascular disease, hypersensitivity pneumonitis, sarcoidosis
LOCATION OF RADIOGRAPHIC ABNORMALITY	**SUGGESTED DIAGNOSES***
Mid to upper lung zone	Hypersensitivity pneumonitis, chronic berylliosis, ankylosing spondylitis, silicosis, Langerhans cell histiocytosis, sarcoidosis, cystic fibrosis
Lower lung zone	Idiopathic pulmonary fibrosis, nonspecific interstitial pneumonia (fibrotic), collagen vascular disease, asbestosis, chronic hypersensitivity pneumonitis
Peripheral	Idiopathic pulmonary fibrosis, nonspecific interstitial pneumonia (fibrotic), cryptogenic organizing pneumonia, chronic eosinophilic pneumonia

*This list is not intended to be comprehensive.
Adapted from Raghu G, Brown K. Clinical issues: patient evaluation. In: Baughman RP, du Bois RM, eds. *Diffuse Lung Disease: A Practical Approach*. New York: Oxford University Press; 2004.

attenuation on HRCT in concert with bilateral interstitial prominence, fine nodular radiographic infiltrates, and normal lung volumes. Images obtained in the supine and prone positions and on deep inspiration and exhalation sometimes help to differentiate fibrosis from atelectasis.

Pulmonary Function Tests

The most characteristic physiologic abnormalities in patients with ILD, regardless of etiology, are a restrictive lung defect and decreased DLCO

TABLE 92-4 RADIOGRAPHIC FEATURES OF IDIOPATHIC INTERSTITIAL PNEUMONIAS

CLINICAL DIAGNOSIS	USUAL RADIOGRAPHIC FEATURES	TYPICAL FINDINGS ON HRCT
Idiopathic pulmonary fibrosis	Basal-predominant reticulation abnormality with volume loss	Peripheral, basal, subpleural reticulation with honeycombing, traction bronchiectasis, and focal ground-glass attenuation
Nonspecific interstitial pneumonia	Ground-glass and reticular opacification	Peripheral, basal, subpleural, symmetrical ground-glass attenuation with irregular lines and consolidation
Cryptogenic organizing pneumonia	Patchy bilateral consolidation	Subpleural or peribronchial patchy consolidation and/or nodules
Acute interstitial pneumonia	Diffuse ground-glass density/consolidation	Diffuse consolidation and ground-glass opacification, often with lobular sparing and late traction bronchiectasis
Desquamative interstitial pneumonia	Ground-glass opacity	Peripheral, lower lung zone ground-glass attenuation with reticulation and/or small cysts
Respiratory bronchiolitis-associated interstitial lung disease	Bronchial wall thickening, ground-glass opacification	Diffuse bronchial wall thickening with poorly defined centrilobular nodules and patchy ground-glass opacification
Lymphocytic interstitial pneumonia	Reticular opacities and nodules	Diffuse centrilobular nodules, ground-glass attenuation, septal and bronchovascular wall thickening, and thin-walled cysts

HRCT = high-resolution computed tomography.
Adapted from American Thoracic Society/European Respiratory Society. International multidisciplinary consensus classification of the idiopathic interstitial pneumonias. *Am J Respir Crit Care Med*. 2002;165:277-304.

(Chapter 85). Forced expiratory volume in 1 second (FEV_1) and forced vital capacity (FVC) are decreased proportionally such that the ratio of the two remains normal or may even be increased. Both total lung capacity and lung volumes measured by body plethysmography are reduced. Pulmonary function tests (PFTs) may be useful in monitoring the progression of disease and prognosis; significant changes in FVC, DLCO (corrected to hemoglobin), and physiologic measurements (FVC, DLCO) at 1 year portend a worse survival in patients with idiopathic pulmonary fibrosis.

Certain PFT findings may also aid in the differential diagnosis. A mixed obstructive-restrictive pattern occurs in patients with Churg-Strauss syndrome, allergic bronchopulmonary aspergillosis, endobronchial sarcoidosis, hypersensitivity pneumonitis, cryptogenic organizing pneumonia, tropical pulmonary interstitial eosinophilia, coexisting chronic obstructive pulmonary disease or asthma, or secondary bronchiectasis. Diseases associated with respiratory muscle weakness, such as polymyositis, progressive systemic sclerosis, and systemic lupus erythematosus, may exhibit a decrease in maximal voluntary ventilation and increased residual volume out of proportion to the decrease in FEV_1.

Exercise Testing

The magnitude of the increase in PAO_2-PaO_2 on exercise correlates well with the severity of disease and the degree of pulmonary fibrosis in patients with idiopathic pulmonary fibrosis. Other exercise-induced physiologic abnormalities in ILD include a decrease in work rate and maximal oxygen consumption, abnormally high minute ventilation at submaximal work rates, decreased peak minute ventilation, and failure of tidal volumes to increase at submaximal levels of work while the respiratory rate increases disproportionately. The 6-minute walk test, performed on a flat surface, can provide quantitative data on exercise capacity and oxygen desaturation with exercise.

Invasive Evaluation

A collegial interaction and multidisciplinary discussions among the pulmonary clinician, chest radiologist, thoracic surgeon, and pathologist can help determine the best diagnostic approach for an individual patient (see Fig. 92-1).

Findings on bronchoalveolar lavage (BAL) can be diagnostic in some patients with ILD and can narrow the differential diagnosis in others (see Table 85-3 in Chapter 85). For example, a lymphocyte-predominant cellular pattern raises the possibility of sarcoidosis or hypersensitivity pneumonitis in the appropriate clinical setting. Eosinophils are seen in pulmonary Langerhans cell granulomatosis, an asbestos body count greater than 1 fiber per milliliter of BAL fluid is seen in asbestosis, and specially staining surfactant material is seen in pulmonary alveolar proteinosis. A transbronchial lung biopsy may reveal noncaseating granulomas in sarcoidosis, "loose" noncaseating granulomas in hypersensitivity pneumonitis, giant cell granulomas in hard metal pneumoconiosis, or smooth muscle proliferation in lymphangioleiomyomatosis. However, failure to establish a diagnosis on BAL and transbronchial lung biopsy does not exclude these entities.

Video-assisted thoracoscopic biopsy (Chapter 101) or open lung biopsy may be required to obtain an adequate sample for histologic evaluation of a patient with unexplained signs and symptoms when other studies have failed to establish a diagnosis, but most patients with idiopathic pulmonary fibrosis do not need to have a biopsy to confirm the diagnosis. The mortality rate for the procedure is generally less than 1%, and the morbidity is less than 3%.

TABLE 92-5 INTERSTITIAL LUNG DISEASE: CLINICAL RESPONSE TO SYSTEMIC CORTICOSTEROIDS ALONE*

GENERALLY RESPONSIVE	UNRESPONSIVE†
Sarcoidosis	Idiopathic interstitial pneumonia
Acute hypersensitivity pneumonitis	Idiopathic pulmonary fibrosis (usual interstitial pneumonia)
Drug induced	Desquamative interstitial pneumonia (subset)
Environmental causes (some)	Chronic secondary and advanced pulmonary fibrosis
Idiopathic interstitial pneumonia	Chronic hypersensitivity pneumonitis (subset)
Cryptogenic organizing pneumonia	Chronic radiation fibrosis
Nonspecific interstitial pneumonia (cellular)	Cryptogenic organizing pneumonia (subset)
Respiratory bronchiolitis-associated ILD	Acute interstitial pneumonia (?)
Lymphocytic interstitial pneumonia	Chronic pulmonary hemorrhage syndromes
Desquamative interstitial pneumonia (subset)	Pulmonary veno-occlusive disease
Acute interstitial pneumonia (?)	Environmental (e.g., asbestosis, pneumoconiosis)
Acute pulmonary capillaritis	End-stage ILDs, pulmonary fibrosis coexisting or associated with pulmonary hypertension
Eosinophilic pneumonia (acute and chronic)	Pulmonary Langerhans cell granulomatosis
Acute radiation pneumonitis‡	Lymphangioleiomyomatosis
Organizing pneumonia associated with collagen vascular diseases	ILD in inherited disorders (?)

*The dosage plus duration of corticosteroids used is variable and based on anecdotal experience, individual expert opinion, clinical judgment, and response as judged by objective measurements (clinical, radiologic, and/or physiologic). Oral prednisone/prednisolone is the most common corticosteroid used. Most patients who respond during the first few weeks of 20 to 60 mg of prednisone per day require maintenance low-dose oral prednisone at 5 to 10 mg/day beyond 6 months. Some patients who require maintenance of oral prednisone doses higher than 20 mg/day beyond 4 to 6 months may tolerate lower doses of prednisone if other immune-modulating agents (e.g., azathioprine, mycophenolate) are used in combination. There is no evidence to recommend a specific regimen. Patients should be monitored carefully and regularly for known side effects of corticosteroid use (e.g., osteoporosis, glucose intolerance), and preventive and therapeutic measures must be undertaken appropriately.

†Some patients unresponsive to oral corticosteroids alone may respond to combined treatment with corticosteroids and other immune-modulating drugs (e.g., azathioprine, mycophenolate).

‡Although most patients respond to modest doses of oral prednisone (initially, 40 to 60 mg/day), it is important to taper the prednisone very slowly to reach a maintenance dose of 5 to 10 mg/day beyond 6 months; rapid taper of oral prednisone has been associated with "rebound"—an exaggerated lung injury beyond the irradiated segment of the lung and in the contralateral lung.

ILD = interstitial lung disease.

TREATMENT (Rx)

When the cause of the ILD is clearly known (e.g., acute or subacute hypersensitivity pneumonitis, occupational ILD, iatrogenic), further avoidance of the inciting agent or agents is essential (Chapter 93). Although systemic corticosteroids are generally indicated and are associated with a favorable response in some ILDs, the dosage and duration are unclear and essentially based on anecdotal experience (Table 92-5).

Supportive oxygen supplementation is dictated by clinical needs. For selected patients with end-stage ILDs, such as those associated with significant pulmonary fibrosis and pulmonary hypertension, lung transplantation (Chapter 101) may be a feasible and viable option. Treatments for pulmonary hypertension (Chapter 68) are generally recommended, although their utility for ILD patients is unproved.

SPECIFIC TYPES OF INTERSTITIAL LUNG DISEASE

Idiopathic Interstitial Pneumonias

Idiopathic interstitial pneumonias, which are a subset of acute or chronic ILDs of unknown etiology, are characterized by the presence of varying degrees of interstitial and alveolar inflammation and fibrosis. Distinct clinicopathologic forms of idiopathic interstitial pneumonia include idiopathic pulmonary fibrosis, nonspecific interstitial pneumonia, respiratory bronchiolitis-associated ILD, desquamative interstitial pneumonia, acute interstitial pneumonia, cryptogenic organizing pneumonia, and lymphocytic interstitial pneumonia.

Although clinical severity may vary, the idiopathic interstitial pneumonias tend to manifest as an insidious onset of exertional dyspnea and a nonproductive cough. Chest pain and systemic symptoms such as weight loss and fatigue may be present. Bibasilar end-inspiratory crackles are often heard on auscultation. Clubbing, although not specific, is found in 25 to 50% of patients with idiopathic pulmonary fibrosis. Findings on the chest radiograph are most often nonspecific, and the presence of normal lung markings on the chest radiograph does not exclude ILD. On HRCT, many pathologic entities have characteristic image patterns that have greatly aided diagnosis (see Table 92-4).

IDIOPATHIC PULMONARY FIBROSIS

EPIDEMIOLOGY AND CLINICAL MANIFESTATIONS

Idiopathic pulmonary fibrosis accounts for 50 to 60% of all idiopathic interstitial pneumonias. Idiopathic pulmonary fibrosis occurs in adult men and women with a mean age at onset of 62 years. It is a distinct entity limited to the lungs in adults, usually older than 50 years, and generally occurs in men with a history of cigarette smoking. Typical manifestations include a gradual onset and progression of exertional dyspnea, restrictive abnormalities on PFTs (Chapter 85), and a distinct pattern of bilateral pulmonary fibrosis on HRCT. Most often patients have otherwise been in good health and have no known collagen vascular disease or exposure to drugs or environmental factors known to cause pulmonary fibrosis, although patients with significant cigarette smoking history may have coexisting emphysema.

The natural course of idiopathic pulmonary fibrosis in most patients is a slow and steady decline with a median survival of 3 to 5 years after the diagnosis. A small subset of patients decline at a rapid rate over several months. Another subset of patients remain stable over several years before declining. About 5 to 10% of patients experience acute exacerbation that requires hospitalization and intensive care. There are no known risk factors or biomarkers that accurately identify which patients will have various clinical courses.

DIAGNOSIS

Chest radiographs typically show basal-predominant reticular abnormalities with low lung volumes. The diagnostic features on HRCT are peripheral, predominantly basilar patchy intralobular reticulation, often with subpleural honeycomb cysts, traction bronchiectasis, and traction bronchiolectasis as the disease becomes more advanced (Fig. 92-2A). Reticulation may progress to honeycombing, although neither alveolar consolidation nor parenchymal nodules are present. When compared with the other idiopathic interstitial pneumonias, the HRCT appearance of idiopathic pulmonary fibrosis is distinguished by a greater extent of fibrotic abnormality, by its hallmark honeycombing, and by a notable absence of extensive ground-glass opacification, micronodules, cysts, consolidation, and extensive mediastinal adenopathy, all of which are typical of *usual interstitial pneumonia.*

PFTs usually show a progressive restrictive pattern. However, patients with milder disease may have normal lung volumes and a small decrease in DLCO; rarely, PFTs may be normal.

The cellular pattern in BAL fluid, which is nonspecific, is marked by an excess of neutrophils in proportion to the extent of reticular change on HRCT; the percentage of eosinophils may be mildly increased. The histopathologic pattern of usual interstitial pneumonia consists of patchy interstitial changes alternating with zones of honeycombing, fibrosis, minimal inflammatory cells, collagen deposition, and normal lung (see Fig. 92-2B). Subepithelial fibroblastic foci, small aggregates of myofibroblasts, and fibroblasts within myxoid matrix are invariably present and represent areas of active fibrosis. The presence of temporal heterogeneity, or areas at different stages of fibrosis transitioning with normal areas and honeycomb cysts, along with fibrotic foci within the lung, is an essential feature of usual interstitial pneumonia that distinguishes it from other processes such as nonspecific interstitial pneumonia. Interstitial cellular inflammation is minimal in usual interstitial pneumonia. Although usual interstitial pneumonia characterizes the microscopic abnormality in idiopathic pulmonary fibrosis, the same histologic and radiologic pattern can also be seen in patients with rheumatologic lung diseases and asbestosis (Chapter 93).

In the appropriate clinical setting (and after exclusion of other known clinical conditions associated with ILD) (see later), a definitive diagnosis of idiopathic pulmonary fibrosis is based on the presence of a pattern of usual interstitial pneumonia on HRCT and/or surgical lung biopsy (Table 92-6).

TABLE 92-6 DIAGNOSIS OF IDIOPATHIC PULMONARY FIBROSIS: CRITERIA

The diagnosis of idiopathic pulmonary fibrosis requires the presence of usual interstitial pneumonia (UIP) in the absence of other causes of interstitial lung disease (e.g., domestic, occupational, and environmental exposures, connective tissue disease, and drug toxicity) AND

a. The presence of a UIP pattern on HRCT of the chest in the absence of a lung biopsy or
b. Specific combinations* of patterns on HRCT of the chest (UIP, possible UIP, inconsistent with UIP) and histopathologic features (UIP, probable UIP, possible UIP, not UIP) on surgical lung biopsy

HRCT FEATURES OF UIP	HISTOPATHOLOGIC FEATURES OF UIP
• Subpleural, basal predominance • Reticular abnormality • Honeycombing with or without traction bronchiectasis • Absence of peribronchovascular predominance, extensive ground-glass abnormality, diffuse micronodules, discrete cysts, diffuse mosaic attenuation, or consolidation	• Evidence of marked fibrosis/ architectural distortion, +/− honeycombing in a predominantly subpleural/ paraseptal distribution • Presence of patchy involvement of lung parenchyma by fibrosis • Presence of fibroblast foci • Absence of features against a diagnosis of UIP suggesting an alternate diagnosis*

*From Raghu G, Collard HR, Egan JJ, et al. An official ATS/ERS/JRS/ALAT statement: idiopathic pulmonary fibrosis: evidence-based guidelines for diagnosis and management. *Am J Respir Crit Care Med.* 2011;183:788-824.
HRCT = high-resolution computed tomography.

TREATMENT Rx

Because no treatment to date has been proved to improve survival or other clinically relevant outcomes, all treatments for idiopathic pulmonary fibrosis should be considered experimental. Physicians are urged to enroll their patients with idiopathic pulmonary fibrosis into one of the many ongoing clinical trials. The physician must spend adequate time to tailor treatment to individual patients' preferences and values.

A recent clinical trial demonstrated better preservation of PFT results after 1 year of treatment with combined oral prednisone (initiated at 0.5 mg/kg ideal body weight per day during the first month and tapered to a maintenance dose of 0.1 to 0.2 mg/kg of ideal body weight per day, or about 10 mg/day, over the subsequent 3 to 4 months), azathioprine (maintenance dose of 2 mg/kg of ideal body weight per day, or 100 to 150 mg/day), and *N*-acetylcysteine (600 mg three times daily) than with prednisone and azathioprine.[1] However, no randomized trials have compared the results of a triple-drug regimen with no treatment at all.

Pirfenidone (1800 mg daily for 1 year), a novel antifibrotic agent, reduced the loss of lung function and improved progression-free survival in one randomized trial in Japan, where it is approved for the treatment of idiopathic pulmonary fibrosis.[2] Interferon-γ1b,[3] cyclophosphamide, colchicine, D-penicillamine, and oral corticosteroids as monotherapy or in combination with immunosuppressive agents are not beneficial.

Despite the absence of data, patients who require hospitalization and intensive care for an acute exacerbation with loss of respiratory function in the absence of infection or other complications are usually treated with empirical intravenous corticosteroids (e.g., methylprednisolone 1.0 g intravenously as a pulse dose once a day for 3 days and followed by hydrocortisone, 125 mg every 6 hours for another 3 to 5 days), with further dosing dependent on the clinical response. Ancillary treatment measures, including supplemental oxygen (based on clinical and physiologic needs), prompt detection and treatment of respiratory tract infections and pulmonary embolism (Chapter 98), pulmonary rehabilitation, and immunization for influenza, herpes zoster, and pneumococcus, are all appropriate. Pulmonary hypertension, if present, may be treated (Chapter 68). Lung transplantation (Chapter 101) is indicated in selected patients, but about two thirds of patients with idiopathic pulmonary fibrosis are older than 60 to 65 years, which is a relative contraindication to lung transplantation. Gastroesophageal reflux, which is more common in patients with idiopathic pulmonary fibrosis, should receive appropriate treatment (Chapter 140). It is important to initiate discussion of palliative care measures before patients reach the terminal stages of the disease.

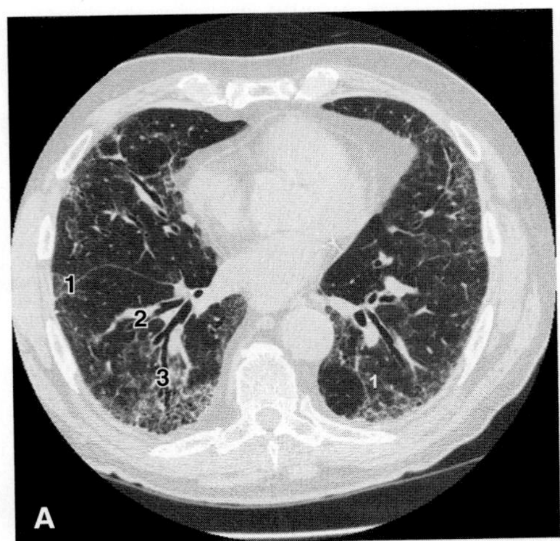

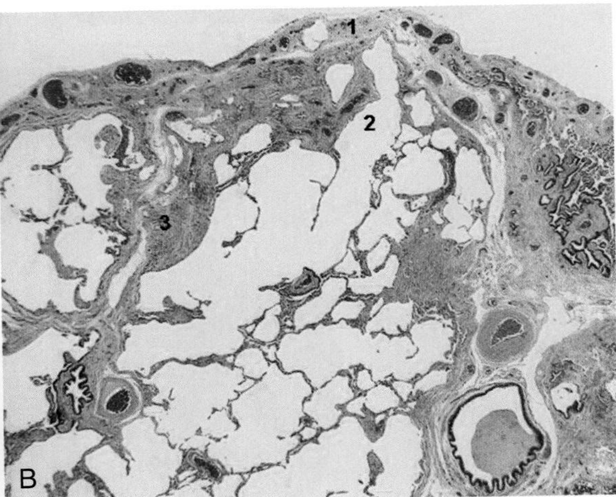

FIGURE 92-2. Diagnosis of idiopathic pulmonary fibrosis. A, The usual interstitial pneumonia pattern of idiopathic pulmonary fibrosis in the lower lobes on high-resolution computed tomography consists of (1) subpleural fibrotic changes with (2) traction bronchiectasis and (3) honeycomb cysts in the lower lobes. **B,** Usual interstitial pneumonia pattern of idiopathic pulmonary fibrosis. Note the presence of (1) subpleural fibrosis with (2) traction emphysema, (3) fibroblastic foci, and temporal heterogeneity of microscopic abnormalities at low magnification. (Courtesy of Dr. Kevin Leslie.)

PROGNOSIS

The usual clinical course is progressive impairment of lung function and gas exchange with a fatal outcome, unless the patient undergoes lung transplantation. Median survival is 3 to 5 years after diagnosis. Patients who survive longer generally have less fibrosis on HRCT, less functional impairment, no evidence of pulmonary hypertension, and no significant oxygen desaturation during a modified version of the 6-minute walk test. Patients with coexisting emphysema, pulmonary hypertension, or episodes of acute exacerbation have even shorter survival times.

NONSPECIFIC INTERSTITIAL PNEUMONIA

Nonspecific interstitial pneumonia is an ILD that is often associated with collagen vascular diseases or hypersensitivity pneumonitis; it may also occur as an idiopathic entity. Two subgroups have been described: cellular and fibrotic. Because the average age at onset is about 10 years earlier in nonspecific interstitial pneumonia than in idiopathic pulmonary fibrosis, and because the clinical features of idiopathic fibrotic nonspecific interstitial pneumonia are very similar to early cases of idiopathic pulmonary fibrosis, questions persist as to whether idiopathic fibrotic nonspecific interstitial pneumonia is a separate clinical entity or represents an early form of idiopathic pulmonary fibrosis.

DIAGNOSIS

Chest radiographs show bilateral patchy pulmonary infiltrates with a lower lung zone predominance in all forms of nonspecific interstitial pneumonia. HRCT reveals a predominant ground-glass pattern of attenuation, usually bilateral and often associated with subpleural reticulation and loss of volume in the lower lobe. In cellular nonspecific interstitial pneumonia, HRCT shows ground-glass opacification, consolidation or both, whereas the biopsy shows mild to moderate lymphoplasmacytic interstitial chronic inflammation. The major differential diagnosis to consider as an alternative to cellular nonspecific interstitial pneumonia is acute or subacute hypersensitivity pneumonitis, so a thorough history regarding environmental exposures is crucial. In contrast, fibrotic nonspecific interstitial pneumonia has a bilateral lower lobe distribution with architectural derangement on HRCT; histopathologically, it has uniformly dense interstitial fibrosis and may sometimes be difficult to distinguish from idiopathic pulmonary fibrosis and usual interstitial pneumonia in the early clinical stages. In these circumstances, the diagnosis of fibrotic nonspecific interstitial pneumonia can be ascertained only by the histologic features in a surgical lung biopsy specimen.

TREATMENT AND PROGNOSIS Rx

Patients with cellular nonspecific interstitial pneumonia usually respond to treatment with corticosteroids (see Table 92-5), and their prognosis is generally better than that of patients with idiopathic pulmonary fibrosis. Given its similarities with idiopathic pulmonary fibrosis, treatment approaches to fibrotic nonspecific interstitial pneumonia have been extrapolated from studies in idiopathic pulmonary fibrosis. However, no clinical trials document this approach.

RESPIRATORY BRONCHIOLITIS–ASSOCIATED INTERSTITIAL LUNG DISEASE

This ILD is almost invariably associated with chronic and current cigarette smoking, and it usually manifests clinically during the fourth or fifth decade of life. However, it may also be detected incidentally on radiographs in relatively younger and asymptomatic persons with a previous history of cigarette smoking or in people passively exposed to chronic cigarette smoke.

DIAGNOSIS

PFTs show varying degrees of airway obstruction, mildly decreased or preserved total lung capacity, and decreased DLCO. The chest radiograph typically reveals bronchial wall thickening and areas of ground-glass attenuation. HRCT reveals centrilobular nodules with an upper lobe predominance, patchy ground-glass attenuation, and peribronchial alveolar septal thickening (Fig. 92-3A). Areas of hypoattenuation (mosaic attenuation) represent air trapping as a result of small airways disease. The characteristic finding on BAL is numerous brown-pigmented alveolar macrophages, often with a modest increase in neutrophils. The hallmark histopathologic feature on biopsy is the accumulation of pigmented alveolar macrophages with glassy eosinophilic cytoplasm and granular pigmentation within respiratory bronchioles, typically with a chronic inflammatory cell infiltrate in the bronchioles and surrounding alveolar walls (see Fig. 92-3B). Fibroblastic foci and honeycomb change are not present, but centrilobular emphysema is frequent.

TREATMENT AND PROGNOSIS Rx

Progression to honeycomb lung and end-stage fibrosis seldom occurs, and the prognosis is good with cessation of smoking. Discontinuation of cigarette smoking is essential, and patients may benefit from low-dose corticosteroids (e.g., prednisone, 10 to 20 mg/day) for a few months.

DESQUAMATIVE INTERSTITIAL PNEUMONIA

Desquamative interstitial pneumonia is a rare entity (<3% of all ILDs) that may represent a more extensive form of respiratory bronchiolitis-associated ILD. Although most affected individuals are cigarette smokers, the histologic pattern of desquamative interstitial pneumonia may also occur in pneumoconiosis, rheumatologic disease, and drug-associated ILD. Patients are often initially seen with advanced disease and striking hypoxemia.

DIAGNOSIS

PFTs reveal a restrictive lung defect and decreased DLCO with or without coexisting airway obstruction. The chest radiograph shows patchy basal consolidation with a lower lobe and peripheral predominance. HRCT shows bilateral symmetrical ground-glass opacities with a predominantly basal and peripheral distribution as well as diffuse alveolar septal thickening (Fig. 92-4A). Irregular linear opacities, typically associated with traction bronchiectasis, may be noted. The finding of small discrete cysts, believed to represent trapped air in dilated bronchioles, within areas of ground-glass

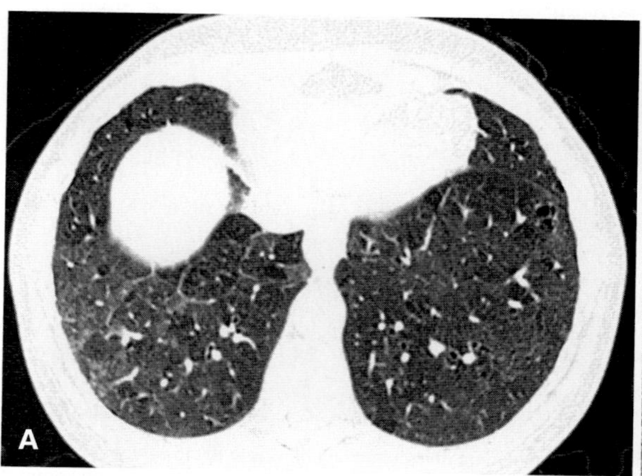

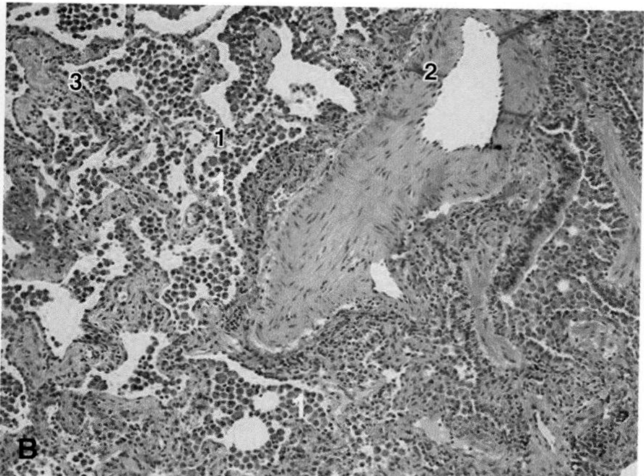

FIGURE 92-3. Respiratory bronchiolitis–associated interstitial lung disease. A, Ground-glass attenuation with a mosaic pattern on high-resolution computed tomography. **B,** Note the dense aggregates of (1) pigmented macrophages present in the air spaces around the terminal airways with (2) variable bronchiolar metaplasia and (3) interstitial fibrosis.

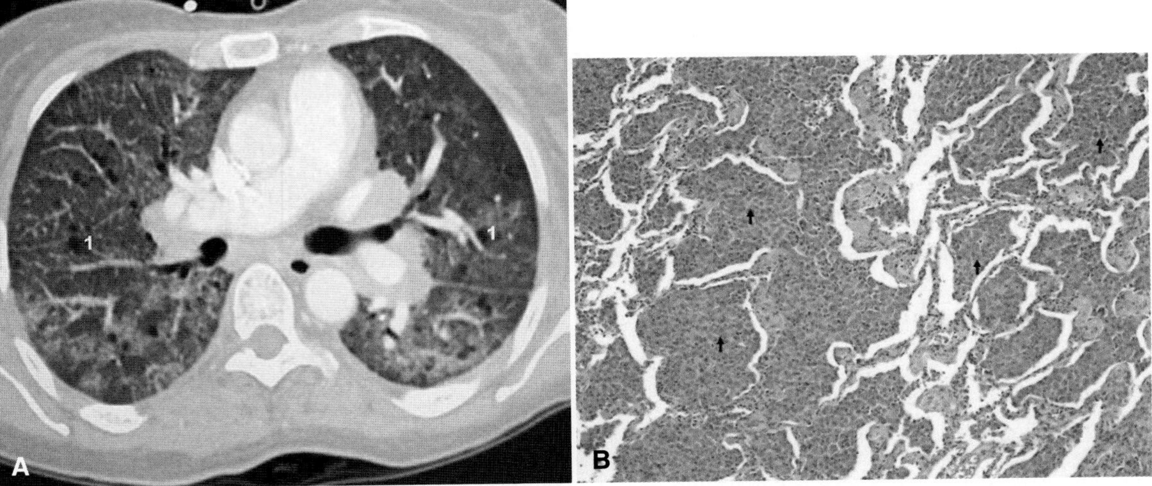

FIGURE 92-4. **Desquamative interstitial pneumonia. A,** Ground-glass attenuation with (1) cystic spaces on high-resolution computed tomography. **B,** Note that the alveolar spaces are densely filled with macrophages *(arrowheads)*.

changes and intervening normal lung parenchyma is highly suggestive of desquamative interstitial pneumonia. Fluid recovered from BAL quite often shows increased numbers of pigmented alveolar macrophages, frequently with increased neutrophils. Histopathologic findings on biopsy include diffuse alveolar septal thickening, hyperplasia of type II pneumocytes, and intense accumulation of intra-alveolar granular pigmented macrophages in a uniform manner (see Fig. 92-4B); fibrosis is minimal.

TREATMENT AND PROGNOSIS (Rx)

Therapeutic outcomes are generally good, particularly with cessation of smoking and administration of oral corticosteroid therapy (see Table 92-5); the estimated overall survival rate is 70% at 10 years. However, a subset of patients may progress despite cessation of cigarette smoking, and a trial of corticosteroid therapy and lung transplantation is an appropriate consideration for selected patients.

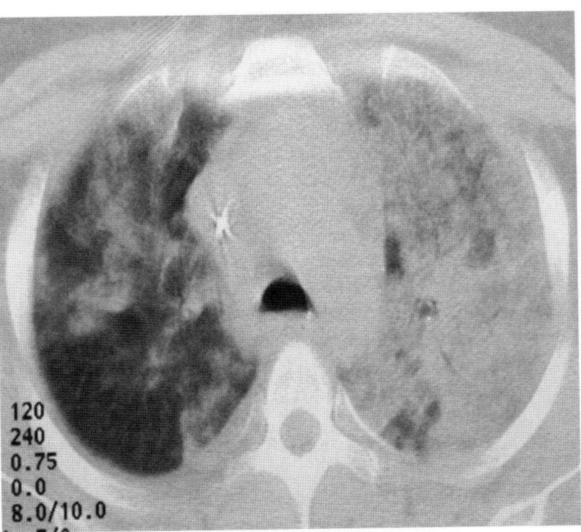

FIGURE 92-5. **Acute interstitial pneumonia with diffuse alveolar damage histologically.** Note the dense air space consolidation.

ACUTE INTERSTITIAL PNEUMONIA

Acute interstitial pneumonia is seen in otherwise healthy persons immediately after an apparent viral upper respiratory infection (Fig. 92-5). The syndrome, historically known as Hamman-Rich syndrome (Chapter 91), mimics the acute respiratory distress syndrome.

TREATMENT AND PROGNOSIS (Rx)

Most patients recover rapidly and completely when treated with oral corticosteroids (see Table 92-5) for 6 months but may relapse after discontinuation and require oral corticosteroids indefinitely, often with adjunct immunosuppressive agents such as azathioprine. A small subset of patients in whom pulmonary fibrosis develops despite corticosteroids and azathioprine behave similarly to patients with idiopathic pulmonary fibrosis. Spontaneous remissions are known to occur.

CRYPTOGENIC ORGANIZING PNEUMONIA

Cryptogenic organizing pneumonia, previously referred to as bronchiolitis obliterans organizing pneumonia of unknown cause (BOOP), is an idiopathic pneumonia that most commonly manifests as a flulike illness with a nonproductive cough, followed by exertional dyspnea.

DIAGNOSIS

PFTs show a restrictive defect, but 20% of patients, most of whom are current or past smokers, also have an obstructive defect. Chest radiography reveals patchy unilateral or bilateral alveolar opacities that may be peripheral or migratory; small nodular opacities are seen in 10 to 50% of cases. In about 90% of patients, HRCT shows areas of air space consolidation with lower lung zone predominance, frequently in a subpleural or peribronchial distribution; other features include small nodules along bronchovascular bundles and ground-glass attenuation. BAL is nonspecific; increased lymphocytes, neutrophils, and eosinophils may be seen. On biopsy, key histologic features are excessive proliferation of granulation tissue within the small airways and alveolar ducts as well as chronic inflammation in the surrounding alveoli.

LYMPHOID AND LYMPHOCYTIC INTERSTITIAL PNEUMONIA

This condition is more common in women, especially in the fifth decade of life, but it may occur at any age. Concurrent collagen vascular disease or an autoimmune disorder (especially Sjögren's syndrome) should be sought because idiopathic lymphocytic interstitial pneumonia is very rare. Symptoms are nonspecific and include a gradual onset of cough and exertional dyspnea.

DIAGNOSIS

Chest radiographs show a reticular or reticulonodular pattern predominantly involving the lower lung zones. HRCT reveals bilateral ground-glass attenuation, small or large nodules, and scattered cysts; perivascular honeycombing and reticular abnormalities may also be seen. Increased numbers of lymphocytes are found on BAL, and biopsy reveals a dense interstitial lymphocytic infiltrate.

TREATMENT AND PROGNOSIS

Some patients respond to or stabilize with oral corticosteroids (see Table 92-5). The prognosis is variable, with more than one third of patients progressing to diffuse pulmonary fibrosis.

Interstitial Lung Disease Associated with Collagen Vascular Disease

Many of the collagen vascular diseases, including progressive systemic sclerosis (Chapter 275), rheumatoid arthritis (Chapter 272), systemic lupus erythematosus (Chapter 274), dermatomyositis and polymyositis (Chapter 277), Sjögren's syndrome (Chapter 276), and mixed connective tissue disorder (Chapter 275), may have ILD as one of their manifestations. In fact, up to 20% of patients with collagen vascular disease may initially be thought to have an ILD alone. Therefore, these diagnoses must be considered in patients with ILD, even in the absence of extrathoracic findings. Conversely, because pulmonary involvement is a major cause of death in patients with collagen vascular disease, the presence of ILD should be carefully sought in affected patients. All forms of idiopathic interstitial pneumonia can occur in patients with collagen vascular disease. The natural history of ILD complicating collagen vascular diseases is variable, especially because coexisting pulmonary vascular disease or nonparenchymal pulmonary involvement may be present.

PROGRESSIVE SYSTEMIC SCLEROSIS

Of the collagen vascular diseases, progressive systemic sclerosis is most frequently associated with ILD. Pulmonary symptoms may antedate cutaneous or digital manifestations of the disease by several years. Most patients affected have nonspecific interstitial pneumonia, with a minority having a usual interstitial pneumonia pattern, and DLCO levels correlate with mortality. Pulmonary hypertension, which can occur in the absence of pulmonary fibrosis, may result in cor pulmonale. The chronic pulmonary fibrosis also increases the risk for bronchogenic carcinoma, usually either bronchoalveolar cell carcinoma or adenocarcinoma. In a controlled trial, treatment with cyclophosphamide (50 to 100 mg/day orally) for 1 year stabilized the PFT findings and improved health-related quality of life in patients with scleroderma-related interstitial lung disease.[4]

RHEUMATOID ARTHRITIS

Although rheumatoid arthritis is more common in women (2:1 to 4:1 ratio), ILD associated with rheumatoid arthritis is more common in men (3:1 ratio). Most cases occur at 50 to 60 years of age, and pulmonary symptoms follow the onset of arthritis in about 75% of cases. Lung involvement in rheumatoid arthritis may take many forms, but bronchiectasis, bronchiolitis, idiopathic interstitial pneumonias, and pleural effusions or pleural thickening are some of the most common. Early in the course, the histologic changes are similar to those of idiopathic interstitial pneumonias, including pulmonary fibrosis, but are distinguished by a prominent lymphocytic infiltrate that may contain germinal follicles adjacent to vessels and airways. As the disease progresses, the infiltration becomes less pronounced and is replaced by fibrous tissue, honeycomb changes, or both. Other pulmonary manifestations include pulmonary nodules, vasculitis, pulmonary hypertension, and Caplan's syndrome (progressive upper lobe nodular pulmonary fibrosis in a coal miner with rheumatoid arthritis) but are relatively rare. Treatment is directed at the underlying rheumatoid arthritis (Chapter 272).

SYSTEMIC LUPUS ERYTHEMATOSUS

Pulmonary abnormalities complicating systemic lupus erythematosus (Chapter 274) may vary greatly. Pleural disease or pleural effusions (or both) are commonly present in lung disease that complicates systemic lupus erythematosus. Acute lupus pneumonitis may mimic acute interstitial pneumonia, with widespread ground-glass attenuation admixed with consolidation, or it may manifest as diffuse alveolar hemorrhage. Chronic ILD may also occur. Infection must always be considered in acutely ill patients who have received steroids or other immunosuppressive therapy. Rarely, the restrictive lung defect, which may be predominantly a result of diaphragmatic weakness, leads to a chest radiographic pattern of small-appearing lungs that may look progressively smaller over time. This so-called shrinking lung is generally resistant to corticosteroids or other immunosuppressive agents used to treat systemic lupus erythematosus. Otherwise, treatment of the ILD is similar to treatment of the underlying systemic lupus erythematosus.

DERMATOMYOSITIS AND POLYMYOSITIS

In contrast to progressive systemic sclerosis, the pattern of lung involvement in dermatomyositis and polymyositis is more heterogeneous. Usual interstitial pneumonia, nonspecific interstitial pneumonia, and organizing pneumonia have all been reported. Most patients have anti-Jo-1 antibody, and the disease is typically progressive over time. An acute interstitial pneumonia–like syndrome occurs in a subset of patients and is associated with high mortality rate despite aggressive immunosuppressive agents and high-dose corticosteroids. ILD may precede the muscular manifestations by months to years or be superimposed on established muscle disease. The severity of the muscular disease does not correlate with that of the ILD. Treatment is directed at the underlying disease (Chapter 277).

SJÖGREN'S SYNDROME

ILD is seen in patients with Sjögren's syndrome, particularly those with the primary form of the disease. Lymphocytic interstitial pneumonia is the most frequent subtype, but cryptogenic organizing pneumonia may also be present. Respiratory infections and bronchiectasis are common in advanced stages, perhaps because of inspissated mucus. Response to corticosteroid or immunosuppressive therapy is usually good (Chapter 275).

MIXED CONNECTIVE TISSUE DISEASE

This overlap syndrome (Chapter 275) combines features of progressive systemic sclerosis, systemic lupus erythematosus, rheumatoid arthritis, and polymyositis or dermatomyositis. Pulmonary disease is common, but it is most often subclinical and identified only radiographically. Treatment includes corticosteroids and other immune-modulating agents for the underlying disease.

ANKYLOSING SPONDYLITIS

The most common pulmonary manifestation of ankylosing spondylitis (Chapter 273) is upper lobe, bilateral reticulonodular infiltrates with cyst formation as a result of parenchymal destruction. There is no known effective therapy for this apical fibrobullous disease.

Hypersensitivity Pneumonitis

EPIDEMIOLOGY AND PATHOBIOLOGY

Hypersensitivity pneumonitis, also known as extrinsic allergic alveolitis, is a syndrome caused by repeated inhalation of specific antigens from occupational or environmental exposure (Chapters 93 and 94) in sensitized individuals. Within a short period after inhalation of an inciting agent, patients develop a nonspecific diffuse pneumonitis with inflammatory cell infiltration of the bronchioles, alveoli, and interstitium. In the subacute and chronic stages, loosely formed, noncaseating, epithelioid cell granulomas may be dispersed in the interstitium. Hypersensitivity pneumonitis can occur with exposure to a wide range of inhaled antigens (Chapters 93 and 94). Some of the more common exposures are farmer's lung, bird fancier's lung, parakeet keeper's lung, and pigeon breeder's lung. Hobbies (woodworker's lung) and recreational activities (sauna taker's lung) may be implicated as well as occupations (Chapter 93).

CLINICAL MANIFESTATIONS

The clinical features and severity of symptoms vary according to the frequency and intensity of exposure. A history of exposure to potential agents or changes in the domestic and other environments (or both) is essential to diagnosis and treatment (Chapters 18 and 93). The interval between exposure to the antigen and the clinical manifestations of lung disease is unknown, although symptoms can occur as soon as 4 to 12 hours after exposure. In such cases, fever and chills are common symptoms, are often temporally related to the workplace or to hobbies, and may actually disappear on vacations or during absence from the site of exposure, only to recur when exposure is resumed. In more chronic and low-level exposures, however, the onset is insidious.

DIAGNOSIS

Findings on chest radiography are diverse, with focal patchy consolidation or a diffuse ground-glass appearance in acute hypersensitivity pneumonitis, micronodular and reticular shadowing in subacute forms, and diffuse, predominantly upper lung zone reticulation with honeycombing in the chronic form. Chest radiographs may be normal in up to 30% of patients with significant physiologic abnormalities.

On HRCT, small centrilobular ill-defined nodules of ground-glass densities are seen, along with evidence of mosaic attenuation (trapped air) as a result of concomitant bronchiolitis. Chronically, findings of lung fibrosis may be indistinguishable from the patterns seen in usual interstitial pneumonia and idiopathic pulmonary fibrosis.

BAL may be quite helpful by showing the most marked increase in lymphocytes of any of the ILDs as well as increased numbers of plasma cells. The characteristic histologic triad in hypersensitivity pneumonitis is cellular nonspecific interstitial pneumonia, cellular bronchiolitis, and granulomatous inflammation; however, this triad is seen in no more than 75% of affected patients. Differentiation from cellular nonspecific interstitial pneumonia may be challenging.

Precipitating serum antibodies for potential causes of hypersensitivity pneumonitis confirm exposure but not cause and effect, and the absence of antibodies does not exclude hypersensitivity pneumonitis. In some cases, a thorough investigation of the patient's home and workplace by an industrial hygienist may reveal molds, spores, thermoactinomycetes species, and other precipitating causes.

TREATMENT AND PROGNOSIS

Further avoidance of exposure to the antigen or antigens and treatment with corticosteroids (see Table 92-5) are important if improvement is to be obtained. Continued exposure to the unidentifiable antigens or prolonged exposure to antigens, or both, can lead to chronic hypersensitivity pneumonitis and irreversible fibrosis that may not respond to any treatment regimen. In the fibrotic stages, the prognosis may be similar to that for idiopathic pulmonary fibrosis.

Occupational Interstitial Lung Diseases

ILDs associated with specific occupations generally involve the inhalation and deposition of dust in the lungs, followed by a tissue reaction that ultimately results in fibrosis. Examples include silicosis (inhalation of silica in crystalline form or silicon dioxide as quartz, cristobalite, or tridymite; at-risk occupations include sandblasting and working with granite), coal workers' pneumoconiosis (inhalation of coal dust), asbestosis (deposition of fibers during mining, milling, or other handling of asbestos; welding and working in a shipyard are two at-risk occupations), berylliosis (seen in aerospace workers and in electronic industries), and hard metal disease (Chapter 93). Radiographic features vary depending on the inciting inhalant. Cessation of the exposure is important, but the fibrosis is generally irreversible.

Drug-Induced Interstitial Lung Disease

More than 300 drugs, biomolecules, or homeopathic remedies (see Table 92-2) can cause acute, subacute, or chronic ILD, and the list continues to increase as new medications are introduced. The clinical and radiographic manifestations are quite varied. Examples of known syndromes include chronic nitrofurantoin-induced ILD that mimics idiopathic pulmonary fibrosis (and is fatal in approximately 8% of cases), granulomatous pneumonitis secondary to methotrexate (<5%), sarcoid-like granulomatous ILD induced by interferon-α and tumor necrosis factor modulating agents, nonspecific bilateral alveolar and interstitial inflammatory and fibrotic abnormalities caused by bleomycin and other chemotherapeutic agents, and alveolar and interstitial abnormalities and nodular densities in acute and chronic amiodarone pulmonary toxicity. Most drug-induced ILD is reversible if recognized early and if use of the responsible drug is discontinued. In addition to discontinuing the implicated drug, treatment with corticosteroids (see Table 92-5) is indicated in patients with moderate to severe functional impairment.

Alveolar Filling Disorders

In alveolar filling disorders (Chapter 91), air spaces distal to the terminal bronchioles are filled with blood, lipid, protein, water, or inflammatory cells. The radiographic appearance is that of an alveolar infiltrate with small nodular densities and ill-defined margins; hence, the radiographic picture is similar to an ILD, and virtually all the alveolar filling disorders may result in ILD, including Goodpasture's syndrome, pulmonary alveolar proteinosis (primary and secondary), alveolar hemorrhage syndromes (Chapter 91), acute interstitial pneumonia, and bronchoalveolar cell carcinoma (Chapter 197).

IDIOPATHIC PULMONARY HEMOSIDEROSIS

This rare disorder of children and young adults is characterized by intermittent, diffuse alveolar hemorrhage without evidence of vasculitis, inflammation, granulomas, or necrosis. The etiology is poorly understood. Anemia and hepatosplenomegaly may be present. Hemosiderin-laden macrophages in BAL fluid and lung tissue are part of the diagnostic picture. The chest radiograph reveals diffuse, bilateral alveolar infiltrates. A chronic interstitial infiltrate may develop after repeated episodes, infrequently with hilar and mediastinal adenopathy. Systemic corticosteroids (see Table 92-5) may be beneficial in treating acute disease.

CHRONIC EOSINOPHILIC PNEUMONIA

The clinical manifestation of chronic eosinophilic pneumonia varies over a wide spectrum, from asymptomatic to respiratory failure. The disease often occurs in women in the second to fourth decades of life; such women often manifest constitutional symptoms of fevers, sweats, weight loss, fatigue, dyspnea, and cough. Peripheral blood eosinophilia (Chapter 173), usually at levels of 10 to 40%, is common but may be absent in up to one third of affected patients at initial evaluation. On chest radiography and HRCT, the cardinal feature is peripheral multifocal consolidation, predominantly in the upper and mid lung zones. These dense peripheral infiltrates, which have sometimes been called the "photographic negative of pulmonary edema," often resolve dramatically after treatment with corticosteroids. Ground-glass attenuation commonly accompanies the consolidation. BAL fluid may show greater than 40% eosinophils during exacerbations. Treatment with corticosteroids (see Table 92-5) results in rapid response, frequently within hours; in fact, such a dramatic resolution of symptoms with radiographic clearance of infiltrates shortly after initiation of corticosteroid therapy is considered "diagnostic." However, the rate of relapse is high, so most patients require prolonged treatment with low-dose corticosteroids (prednisone, 5 to 10 mg/day) to stay in remission.

Interstitial Lung Disease Associated with Pulmonary Vasculitides

Wegener's Granulomatosis

Wegener's granulomatosis (Chapter 278) is the most common form of vasculitis that involves the lung. The systemic necrotizing granulomatous inflammation and small-vessel vasculitis are often manifested first in the upper respiratory tract as chronic rhinitis or sinusitis (or both), epistaxis, oropharyngeal ulcerations, gingival hyperplasia with clefting, or serous otitis media. Destruction of the nasal cartilage may lead to septal perforation or a saddle nose deformity. Ulcerative lesions of the tracheobronchial tree, cavitating nodules within the lung parenchyma, and diffuse alveolar hemorrhage caused by pulmonary capillaritis are lower respiratory tract manifestations. Focal segmental necrotizing glomerulonephritis is the most common extrathoracic manifestation, although pulmonary involvement may occur without renal disease. Chest radiography usually reveals multiple nodular or cavitating infiltrates, but single nodules may be found as well. The diagnosis is most commonly made serologically, with demonstration of antineutrophil cytoplasmic antibodies, although a negative test does not exclude the disease. Treatment is usually with cyclophosphamide (50 to 100 mg/day or 2 mg/kg of ideal body weight per day, but not more than 150 mg/day) in conjunction with oral corticosteroids (prednisone, 10 to 40 mg/day). Initial remission occurs in more than 90% of patients, but most patients require treatment for several years. Relapses may occur in up to 30% of patients, especially when treatment is tapered; such patients may need treatment indefinitely. Rituximab is an alternative if cyclophosphamide is unsuccessful or not tolerated (Chapter 278). Prophylaxis for *Pneumocystis carinii* infection is indicated in patients receiving chronic treatment.

CHURG-STRAUSS SYNDROME (ALLERGIC ANGIITIS)

This systemic necrotizing vasculitis (Chapter 291) affects both the upper and lower respiratory tracts and is almost invariably preceded by allergic disorders such as asthma, allergic rhinitis, sinusitis, or a drug reaction. Peripheral and lung eosinophilia, bronchospasm, increased immunoglobulin E levels, and rashes are common manifestations. The pulmonary radiographic findings are bilateral patchy, fleeting infiltrates, diffuse nodular infiltrates, or diffuse reticulonodular disease. Histopathologic examination of lung tissue is generally diagnostic with features of granulomatous angiitis or vasculitis. Although treatment with corticosteroids is indicated, the dosage and duration are unclear (see Table 92-5).

IDIOPATHIC PULMONARY CAPILLARITIS

Idiopathic pulmonary capillaritis may involve the pulmonary vasculature within the alveolar walls and be manifested as ILD. Patients may also have subclinical alveolar hemorrhage, often associated with the presence of perinuclear antineutrophilic cytoplasmic antibodies. Corticosteroids are the mainstay of treatment, but the doses and duration of treatment are unclear. Frequently, patients need adjunctive treatment with cyclophosphamide or rituximab, similar to patients with vasculitis and Wegener's granulomatosis (Chapter 278).

Other Forms of Interstitial Lung Disease

Sarcoidosis

See Chapter 95.

PULMONARY LANGERHANS CELL HISTIOCYTOSIS

This condition, previously known as pulmonary histiocytosis X or eosinophilic granuloma of the lung, is an idiopathic, granulomatous ILD that typically occurs in the second or third decade of life; there is a male preponderance. The currently accepted term is *Langerhans cell histiocytosis*. Pulmonary Langerhans cell histiocytosis is rare, with an estimated incidence of two to five cases per million population. The large majority (~90%) of affected individuals are smokers, and current evidence suggests that the disorder results from an abnormal immune response to a component or derivative of cigarette smoke.

CLINICAL MANIFESTATIONS

The clinical findings are variable and range from an abnormal chest radiograph in an asymptomatic patient to progressive dyspnea with a nonproductive cough. Systemic symptoms of malaise, fever, and weight loss may be present. Hemoptysis is rare. Spontaneous pneumothorax, which occurs in approximately 25% of patients and is due to rupture of subpleural cysts, may be an initial finding. Langerhans cell histiocytosis may be confined to the lung or may be a component of a multisystem disease that includes painful cystic bone lesions and diabetes insipidus (Chapter 232).

DIAGNOSIS

The chest radiograph shows diffuse symmetrical reticulonodular opacities superimposed on multiple small cysts in the upper and mid lung zones. HRCT reveals subpleural nodules, scattered ground-glass densities, and irregular cysts of varying number, size, and configuration in both lungs, with sparing of the lung bases; in the appropriate clinical setting, this pattern may be pathognomonic. As the disease progresses, the increase in fibrosis and cysts may lead to honeycombing of the lung. PFTs are characterized by a mixed restrictive and obstructive pattern, including a reduction in diffusing capacity. Vital capacity is disproportionately reduced compared with total lung capacity because of air trapping within the cysts; the result is an increased residual volume. BAL reveals Langerhans cells (atypical histiocytes) that have the characteristic "x body" (i.e., Birbeck granule) on electron microscopy; immunostaining shows CD1 antigen on the cell surface and S-100 protein in the cytoplasm. However, the absence of these findings does not exclude the diagnosis. The diagnosis is usually made by transbronchial biopsy or open lung biopsy, which reveals interstitial and peribronchiolar collections of histiocytes, eosinophils, and lymphocytes; peribronchiolar nodules; and cysts with areas of central stellate fibrosis.

TREATMENT AND PROGNOSIS Rx

Although definitive regression after discontinuation of smoking has not been proved, small series report improvement, so patients should be encouraged to discontinue smoking. The prognosis in pulmonary Langerhans cell histiocytosis is usually favorable, with approximately 75% of patients improving or stabilizing, especially with cessation of smoking; some patients, however, may progress to end-stage lung disease. In patients with progressive disease, corticosteroids (see Table 92-5) with or without vincristine, cyclosporine, cyclophosphamide, and azathioprine have been used with some anecdotal reports of success. Lung transplantation has been performed, but recurrent disease has been reported in the allograft.

LYMPHANGIOLEIOMYOMATOSIS

This rare interstitial lung disease is limited to women, primarily of childbearing age. Proliferation of abnormal smooth muscle around bronchioles leads to bilateral small cysts, which give an appearance of ILD on chest radiographs, and progressive impairment of lung function. Hemoptysis, pneumothorax (from rupture of subpleural cysts), and chylothorax (from lymphatic obstruction) may be initial symptoms that distinguish this disorder from other diffuse lung diseases. Although lymphangioleiomyomatosis is usually limited to the lungs, an association with angiomyolipomas of the mediastinal and retroperitoneal lymph nodes and kidney has been described, so the disease may mimic the manifestations of tuberous sclerosis (Chapter 426). Coarse reticulonodular infiltrates, often with cysts or bullae, are typically seen on chest radiographs. In contrast to most other ILDs, increased lung volumes may be present and should prompt consideration of this diagnosis in a nonsmoking woman of reproductive age. HRCT shows characteristic diffuse thin-walled cysts, generally less than 2 cm in diameter. BAL may show occult alveolar hemorrhage. Lung biopsy reveals abnormal smooth muscle cells lining the airways, lymphatics, and blood vessels, with concurrent airflow obstruction and replacement of the lung parenchyma with cysts.

TREATMENT AND PROGNOSIS Rx

In a randomized trial, sirolimus, an inhibitor of rapamycin signaling, initially at 2 mg per day and titrated to maintain trough levels between 5 and 15 ng/mL, was safe and stabilized lung function. Treatment with progesterone or tamoxifen has been tried, but no randomized trials support the use of interventions to alter the estrogen-progesterone balance. Although lung transplantation is indicated as the patient reaches severe functional impairment, the disease may recur in the transplanted lung. Most patients currently die of respiratory failure about 10 years after the onset of symptoms.

Inherited Disorders

Several rare genetic disorders are associated with ILD and pulmonary fibrosis. Inheritance is autosomal dominant with variable penetrance for most cases of familial idiopathic pulmonary fibrosis and idiopathic interstitial pneumonia and for tuberous sclerosis (Chapter 426), neurofibromatosis (Chapter 426), and familial hypocalciuric hypercalcemia (Chapter 253). Inheritance is autosomal recessive for Gaucher's disease (Chapter 215), Niemann-Pick disease (Chapter 215), and Hermansky-Pudlak syndrome (Chapter 215). The congenital form of the alveolar filling disorder pulmonary alveolar proteinosis also is inherited in an autosomal recessive manner.

Tuberous sclerosis (Chapter 426), an autosomal dominant disease of variable penetrance, is characterized pathologically by the presence of hamartomas in multiple organs. The most well-known clinical manifestations include epilepsy, mental retardation, adenoma sebaceum, and renal angiomyolipomas. ILD occurs in only 1% of patients with tuberous sclerosis, usually in women older than 30 years with little or no mental retardation. The pulmonary involvement, which is indistinguishable from lymphangioleiomyomatosis both radiographically and histopathologically, may be manifested as exertional dyspnea, recurrent pneumothorax, and hemoptysis. HRCT reveals thin-walled cysts and a diffuse reticulonodular infiltrate. Recurrent parenchymal hemorrhage may lead to hemosiderin deposition and interstitial pulmonary fibrosis. There is no cure, and treatment is supportive.

Neurofibromatosis (Chapter 426) may affect all age groups and both sexes. Type 1 (von Recklinghausen's disease) is characterized by cafe au lait spots, neurofibromas, optic glioma, and bony lesions; the more rare type 2 is associated with bilateral acoustic neuromas. Diffuse ILD is manifested as bilateral lower lobe fibrosis as well as bullae or cystic changes. Interstitial fibrosis and alveolitis with thickening of the alveolar septa, accompanied by a cellular infiltrate, are seen on lung biopsy. Management is as for idiopathic pulmonary fibrosis.

Gaucher's disease (Chapter 215), a lysosomal glycolipid storage disorder, has a predilection for the Ashkenazi Jewish population. Pulmonary manifestations, which occur most frequently in type 2 disease, may be a result of interstitial infiltration by Gaucher cells with fibrosis, alveolar consolidation, and filling of alveolar spaces; capillary plugging by Gaucher cells may cause secondary pulmonary hypertension. Treatment is as for the systemic disease, and the general approaches for idiopathic interstitial pneumonias and pulmonary arterial hypertension may be followed for these patients.

Niemann-Pick disease (Chapter 215) is a rare lipid storage disease that may cause infiltration of the characteristic "foam cell" throughout the pulmonary lymphatics, the pulmonary arteries, and the pulmonary alveoli. Patients with type B may survive into adulthood. Treatment is as for the systemic disease.

Hermansky-Pudlak syndrome (Chapter 215) is characterized by oculocutaneous albinism, a bleeding diathesis, and ceroid inclusions in macrophages. Most patients are of Puerto Rican ancestry, and women are affected more frequently than men. Pulmonary fibrosis, with onset in the third or fourth decade, is slowly progressive. Treatment principles and interventions are largely supportive and extrapolated from other related conditions, especially idiopathic pulmonary fibrosis.

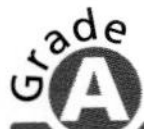

1. Demedts M, Behr J, Buhl R, et al. High dose acetyl cysteine in idiopathic pulmonary fibrosis. *N Engl J Med.* 2005;353:2229-2242.
2. Taniguichi H, Ebina M, Kondoh Y, et al. Pirfenidone in idiopathic pulmonary fibrosis. *Eur Respir J.* 2010;35:821-829.
3. King TE Jr, Albera C, Bradford WZ, et al. Effect of interferon gamma-1b on survival in patients with idiopathic pulmonary fibrosis (INSPIRE): a multicentre, randomised, placebo-controlled trial. *Lancet.* 2009;374:222-228.
4. Tashkin DP, Elashoff R, Clements PJ, et al. Cyclophosphamide versus placebo in scleroderma lung disease. *N Engl J Med.* 2006;354:2655-2666.
5. McCormack FX, Inoue Y, Moss J, et al. Efficacy and safety of sirolimus in lymphangioleiomyomatosis. *N Engl J Med.* 2011;364:1595-1606.

SUGGESTED READINGS

Chan AL, Rafil R, Louie S, et al. Therapeutic update in idiopathic pulmonary fibrosis. *Clin Rev Allergy Immunol.* 2011. [Epub ahead of print.] *Review.*

Fernández Pérez ER, Daniels CE, Schroeder DR, et al. Incidence, prevalence, and clinical course of idiopathic pulmonary fibrosis: a population-based study. *Chest.* 2010;137;129-137. *Median survival was about 4 years.*

Raghu G, Collard HR, Egan JJ, et al. An official ATS/ERS/JRS/ALAT statement: idiopathic pulmonary fibrosis: evidence-based guidelines for diagnosis and management. *Am J Respir Crit Care Med.* 2011; 183:788-824. *Consensus guidelines.*

93 OCCUPATIONAL LUNG DISEASE

SUSAN M. TARLO

Occupational lung diseases include a wide spectrum of respiratory disorders with symptoms, signs, and diagnostic test results that often present with features similar to nonoccupational diseases (Table 93-1). For example, adult-onset asthma (Chapter 87) may be occupational asthma, presumed sarcoidosis (Chapter 95) may actually be chronic beryllium disease, apparent idiopathic pulmonary fibrosis may be asbestosis, or a suspected viral pneumonia (Chapter 97) may be hypersensitivity pneumonitis from an occupational cause such as contaminated metal-working fluid.

When evaluating any respiratory disease, the clinician should consider the possibility of an occupational cause or contribution (see E-Fig. 18-1 in Chapter 18; see Table 93-1). The onset of disease after an occupational exposure may occur with a short latency period, as for an acute toxic inhalation injury, or over a period of months to years, as for occupational asthma or hypersensitivity pneumonitis. Latency can be 20 years or more in chronic beryllium disease or lung cancer from chromium, asbestos, or other carcinogens. The most relevant job and occupational exposure history will therefore depend in part on the type of lung disease: for acute syndromes, the recent job exposure is most relevant; for asthma or hypersensitivity pneumonitis, the exposures at the onset of symptoms and ongoing exposures are most relevant; but for chronic diseases or diseases that may result from a long latency exposure, a full working history is essential. Consideration also should be given to potentially relevant exposures that may be related to a patient's hobbies or avocations (e.g., woodworking, model building, or insect collecting).

The clinical relevance of a correct occupational attribution is most apparent for diseases with a close temporal relationship between exposure and the onset of symptoms because intervention to reduce or remove exposure may reverse the disease or prevent progression. In addition, interventions in the workplace may reduce or prevent disease in other workers. However, even for diseases with a potential long latency, such as chronic beryllium disease, identification of disease in one worker should be regarded as a sentinel event that can lead to investigation of the workplace exposures and introduction of preventive measures. With the assistance of their physicians, workers with occupational lung diseases also often can qualify for workers' compensation.

EPIDEMIOLOGY

No reliable figures exist for the total incidence or prevalence of occupational lung diseases, and regional variation in occupations and exposures is substantial. Work-related asthma has become the most common chronic occupational lung disease in developed countries, where occupational asthma (asthma caused by work) accounts for about 15% of all adult-onset asthma, and work-exacerbated asthma occurs in 25 to 52% of asthmatic workers. The occupational contribution of workplace dusts, fumes, and gases to chronic obstructive pulmonary disease (COPD) is estimated at 15%.

In contrast, pneumoconiosis from silica or coal dust, although still important in developing countries, is declining in incidence in developed countries (E-Fig. 93-1) as a result of occupational hygiene measures. For example, approximately 100,000 Americans received benefits from the Federal Black Lung Program in 2005, compared with about 500,000 in 1980, and the percentage of coal miners with pneumoconiosis has fallen from 11% in the mid-1970s down to 3%. However, newer exposures that lead to silicosis include the textile industry's use of jet silica blasting of denim jeans, reported from Turkey. Newly recognized asbestos-related diseases continue to occur, owing to the long latency period between exposure and clinical disease, despite the declining exposure to asbestos in developed countries. Although annual deaths from asbestosis have now reached a plateau in North America and will likely decline, new cases of mesothelioma, which has a latency of up to 35 years or more, are not estimated to plateau until 2020.

Chronic beryllium disease declined in frequency and severity after the elimination of beryllium from fluorescent lightbulbs in the 1950s, but then increased because of the increasing use of beryllium in nuclear facilities, aerospace, electronics, dental ceramics, metal alloys, recycling of metals, and products such as golf clubs and bicycles. The beryllium lymphocyte proliferation test can identify beryllium sensitization, which can be found in up to 10% of exposed workers and facilitates earlier diagnosis of chronic beryllium disease.

SPECIFIC OCCUPATIONAL LUNG DISORDERS

Occupational lung diseases are often misdiagnosed as other common nonoccupational diseases, but a careful history and appropriate investigations can lead to a correct diagnosis. For many occupational lung diseases, the diagnosis can significantly improve prognosis and lead to measures to prevent illness in other workers.

Work-Related Asthma

Work-related asthma includes both occupational asthma that is caused by work and asthma that is not caused by work but is exacerbated by work exposures.

SENSITIZER-INDUCED OCCUPATIONAL ASTHMA

EPIDEMIOLOGY

Occupational asthma is most commonly associated with a specific immune response to a high- or low-molecular-weight sensitizer (Table 93-2). Sensitizer-induced occupational asthma usually affects no more than 5 to 10% of workers exposed to the sensitizing agent, but exposure to complex platinum salts or detergent enzymes may result in symptoms in about 50% of highly exposed workers. In most studies, higher levels of exposure are associated with higher rates of sensitization in the exposed populations, but there is no clear threshold exposure below which all workers are protected from the risk of sensitization.

PATHOBIOLOGY

Genetic factors increase the risk of sensitization, but the risks appear to be polygenic and may differ for different allergens and sensitizers. Underlying atopy, as exemplified by a history of allergy or positive skin tests to common environmental allergens (Chapter 257), carries an increased risk of

TABLE 93-1 EXAMPLES OF OCCUPATIONAL RESPIRATORY DISEASES THAT COULD BE MISDIAGNOSED AS COMMON NONOCCUPATIONAL RESPIRATORY DISEASE

DISEASE THAT IS MIMICKED	POSSIBLE OCCUPATIONAL DISEASE	EXAMPLES OF SUGGESTIVE FEATURES LEADING TO A CORRECT DIAGNOSIS
Asthma	Occupational asthma from a work sensitizer	Asthma symptoms begin and are worse during a working period, with some improvement on days or weeks off work. Exposure to a high- or low-molecular-weight workplace sensitizer
	Occupational asthma—irritant-induced, including reactive airways dysfunction syndrome	Asthma begins within days after a high-level (accidental) workplace exposure
	Work-exacerbated asthma	Asthma usually began before starting the job or exposure, but severity is worse on days of work, or work exposures to expected asthma triggers or common allergens at work
COPD	Occupational COPD	Prolonged exposure at work to dusts, fumes, or gases
Pneumonia	Acute hypersensitivity pneumonitis	Symptoms typically resolve within days and recur on re-exposure to the same work trigger (e.g., metal-working fluid, moldy hay, humidifiers)
Acute viral respiratory illness or pneumonia	Humidifier fever, organic dust toxic syndrome, metal fume fever, polymer fume fever, cotton dust fever	Exposure triggers the episodes
Sarcoidosis	Chronic beryllium disease	History of exposure to beryllium dust or fumes up to 30 years or more before onset of disease
	Silicosis	History of exposure; typical radiographic findings of rounded opacities with upper lobe predominance and progressive massive fibrosis, biopsy
Idiopathic pulmonary fibrosis	Asbestosis	History of moderate or high previous asbestos exposure and appropriate latency period, often with other markers of asbestos exposure, such as radiographic evidence of pleural plaques
	Chronic hypersensitivity pneumonitis	± Work exposure to a known trigger, ± improvement during periods away from exposure
	Flock-worker's lung	Lymphocytic bronchiolitis and interstitial lung disease from nylon/synthetic textile microfibers
Idiopathic pulmonary fibrosis or hypersensitivity pneumonitis	Hard metal disease	History of exposure to hard metal (tungsten, cobalt), and histologic findings of giant cell pneumonitis on lung biopsy
Chest infections	Occupational causes of chest infections, e.g., SARS or TB in health care workers, histoplasmosis in construction workers, anthrax in wool workers or farmers	History of occupation and exposures
Pleural effusion	Asbestos-related benign pleural effusion	Previous asbestos exposure with appropriate latency; pleural plaques commonly present
Incidental pulmonary nodule	Rounded atelectasis from asbestos	Previous asbestos exposure with appropriate latency; pleural plaques commonly present
Multiple nodules	Silicosis or pneumoconiosis	History of exposure, distribution of nodules, presence of progressive massive fibrosis
Lung cancer	Occupational lung cancer	History of exposure to carcinogens at work, with an appropriate latency period (e.g., asbestos, radon, chromium)
Bronchiolitis obliterans	Popcorn lung	History of working with microwave popcorn or flavorings

COPD = chronic obstructive pulmonary disease; SARS = severe acute respiratory syndrome; TB = tuberculosis.

sensitization to the high-molecular-weight allergens, and smoking (Chapter 31) has been reported as a risk factor for sensitization to complex platinum salts. Currently, no host factors are sufficiently specific to justify exclusion of workers from settings with exposure to potential sensitizers.

Occupational asthma from a high-molecular-weight allergen is associated with specific immunoglobulin E (IgE) antibody production. Low-molecular-weight sensitizers may act as haptens or may induce neoantigens by reacting with proteins in vivo, but specific IgE antibodies have been demonstrated with only a few low-molecular-weight sensitizers, such as complex platinum salts and acid anhydrides used in epoxy compounds.

CLINICAL MANIFESTATIONS

Sensitizer-induced occupational asthma has a latency period ranging from weeks to several years before it develops, but most patients develop symptoms within the first few years of exposure. Once a patient has become sensitized and has developed asthma, even very small subsequent exposures can trigger asthma, sometimes including exposures that may be below the limit of measurable detection. Pulmonary function and histologic changes are similar to those in nonoccupational asthma (Chapter 87). Sensitizer-induced occupational asthma from a high-molecular-weight agent sensitizer typically causes a prompt asthmatic response within minutes after exposure with or without a late asthmatic response starting 4 to 6 hours after exposure. By comparison, responses to low-molecular-weight sensitizers typically start 4 to 6 hours after exposure.

DIAGNOSIS

The diagnosis of sensitizer-induced occupation asthma is clinically suspected by history and should be considered in all cases of new-onset asthma in patients who work. Supportive features include symptomatic improvement when away from work, such as weekends off work or holidays, but not necessarily in the evenings after a work shift, when symptoms from a late asthmatic response may occur. In patients who are exposed to high-molecular-weight sensitizers, allergic rhinitis or conjunctivitis associated with work frequently appears before the development of asthma. A detailed occupational history (Chapter 18) or review of material safety data sheets or occupational hygiene reports may reveal a known occupational sensitizer. However, more than 300 occupational respiratory sensitizers are currently known, and new agents or exposures are reported each year; as a result, the absence of a recognized sensitizer does not exclude occupational asthma.

Although the history can be very helpful, the evaluation should always include objective pulmonary function testing (Chapter 85) to confirm asthma, either when the patient has symptoms or within 24 hours of the typical suspected work exposure (Fig. 93-1). Allergy skin-prick tests, blood samples, or both should be obtained to test for specific IgE antibodies to any relevant sensitizer if feasible. Serial monitoring of peak expiratory flow rates, symptom diaries, or use of rescue inhalers can provide supportive information. The results of a methacholine challenge test (Chapter 87) toward the

TABLE 93-2 COMMON CAUSES OF SENSITIZER-INDUCED OCCUPATIONAL ASTHMA

OCCUPATION	ALLERGEN BY SETTING
Bakers	Wheat, rye, fungal amylase in flour
Laboratory workers	Animal allergens, e.g., proteins in rat urine, mouse or rabbit dander
Detergent-making, medical instrument cleaning, pharmaceuticals or laboratory workers	Enzymes: e.g., *Bacillus subtilis*, pancreatic enzymes
Farmers	Grains, plant, and animal allergens; mites
Greenhouse workers and florists	Pollen, fungi, mites
Food workers	Airborne food allergens, e.g., powdered milk or eggs and vegetables
Some office workers	Fungal allergens in moldy or "sick" buildings
Health care workers	Latex allergens from gloves, glutaraldehyde, orthophthaldehyde, aerosolized medications
Factory or other industrial workers	Chemicals in spray paints, glues, polyurethane, coatings and spray insulation, adhesives
Electronic workers	Soldering flux with colophony

end of a typical work week can help when compared with results after 10 days or more without exposure. A comparison of eosinophil counts in induced sputum at work and after a period away from exposure, showing higher levels when exposed, provides supportive diagnostic information. If the diagnosis is still in doubt, a carefully controlled specific inhalation challenge with the suspected workplace sensitizer can be performed. Each investigation can be falsely positive or negative, so a combination of investigations is advised while the patient continues to work until the diagnosis is confirmed. Given the specialized nature of many of these studies, consultation with a specialist is recommended. The main differential diagnosis for patients with confirmed asthma is the coincidental onset of asthma with subsequent work-exacerbated asthma. Other conditions, such as vocal cord dysfunction, may explain symptoms or may coexist with asthma and confound the diagnosis.

TREATMENT AND PREVENTION Rx

The optimal management of patients with sensitizer-induced occupational asthma includes complete removal from further exposure to the sensitizer and cross-reacting agents combined with the usual pharmacologic approach to the treatment of asthma (Chapter 87) and advocacy for appropriate workers' compensation. Consideration of the other exposed workers typically includes communication with the workplace or public health officials, in the hope that measures may be instituted to protect other workers from similar exposures and symptoms. Recommendations for primary prevention have been to reduce exposures to occupational sensitizers as far as possible, removing unnecessary sensitizing agents (e.g., removing high-powdered and high-protein latex gloves) and limiting exposures to sensitizers with occupational hygiene measures. Ongoing medical surveillance measures in the workplace may also be of value.

PROGNOSIS

Outcome is best if an early diagnosis results in removal from further exposure while asthma is relatively mild. Improvement may continue to occur up to 10 years after removal from exposure, but asthma does not completely resolve in most patients. For patients with occupational asthma from natural rubber latex, use of powder-free, low-protein latex gloves by coworkers and direct avoidance of natural rubber products by the sensitized worker results in improvement that is similar to the improvement in patients who are completely removed from work.

Work-Exacerbated Asthma

EPIDEMIOLOGY AND CLINICAL MANIFESTATIONS

Work-exacerbated asthma is defined as asthma that is not caused by work but is aggravated or exacerbated by work conditions. Asthma may have been present before starting employment or may begin coincidentally during employment, but it is not caused by work. Work exposures that commonly exacerbate asthma include extreme temperature or humidity, exertion, dusts, fumes, and gases. Patients may be exposed at work to common environmental allergens (e.g., fungal allergens in an office setting or dust mites or animals in domestic settings) that exacerbate asthma in patients who are sensitized to these allergens. Symptoms of work-exacerbated asthma may occur transiently with an unusual work exposure (e.g., during renovation in a work building) or may occur on a daily basis (e.g., daily exposure to fumes while performing physical exertion in an industrial setting).

DIAGNOSIS AND TREATMENT Rx

Transient work-exacerbated asthma is commonly diagnosed on the basis of the history of work exposures and the associated increase in asthmatic symptoms, medication requirements, or unscheduled physician visits. The recommended evaluation of patients with daily or frequent work exacerbations of asthma is similar to that for patients with suspected occupational asthma. Work-related changes in serial peak flow recordings mimic those seen in occupational asthma, but sputum eosinophil counts typically show less of a work-related increase than is observed with occupational asthma. If the workplace exposure includes a potential work sensitizer, immunologic testing or a controlled challenge exposure may confirm whether respiratory sensitization has occurred.

Management includes the same pharmacologic measures as for non-work-related exacerbations, including the optimization of pharmacologic asthma management (Chapter 87) and, when needed, adjusting the work exposures to avoid ongoing exacerbations. Occupational hygiene measures can reduce exposures, but some patients require a change in job description or work area. Workers' compensation may be available for some patients who miss work owing to work-exacerbation of asthma.

IRRITANT EXPOSURE AND REACTIVE AIRWAYS DYSFUNCTION SYNDROME

A high level of usually accidental exposure to an irritant agent can cause asthma. Although the clinical manifestations can be dramatic, irritant-induced occupational asthma represents a relatively small proportion of all occupational asthma. The most definitive criteria for this condition are those applied to the term *reactive airways dysfunction syndrome*: the onset of asthma symptoms within 24 hours of the exposure, generally severe enough to lead to an unscheduled physician visit; exposure to a single high-level irritant; asthma symptoms that persist for at least 3 months; pulmonary function testing that confirms asthma with a significant beneficial response to bronchodilators or a bronchoconstrictor response to a methacholine challenge; and the lack of preexisting lung disease or other conditions to explain the symptoms. When these criteria are not completely met (e.g., symptoms start later than 24 hours after exposure or resolve within weeks after exposure), the term *irritant-induced asthma* is commonly applied, recognizing that this diagnosis is less certain than reactive airways dysfunction syndrome.

Irritant-induced asthma and reactive airways dysfunction syndrome may clear after weeks or months. Management is the same as for other causes of asthma (Chapter 87), although these patients are often less responsive to the usual pharmacologic treatment.

Occupational hygiene measures at the workplace should be improved to prevent similar future exposures. Affected patients may need a modified work environment to prevent subsequent exacerbations of asthma.

OCCUPATIONAL CHRONIC OBSTRUCTIVE PULMONARY DISEASE

Chronic exposure to dusts, fumes, and gases can cause occupationally induced COPD, with pathophysiologic changes essentially identical to those seen in COPD that is related to smoking (Chapter 88). Symptoms of chronic bronchitis, including chronic cough and sputum production, may occur with or without changes on pulmonary function testing. Causes include mineral dusts such as silica and organic dust exposures such as those of farmers and woodworkers; particulate matter in diesel exhaust fumes; and nitrogen oxides, ozone, and ultrafine particles in welding fumes.

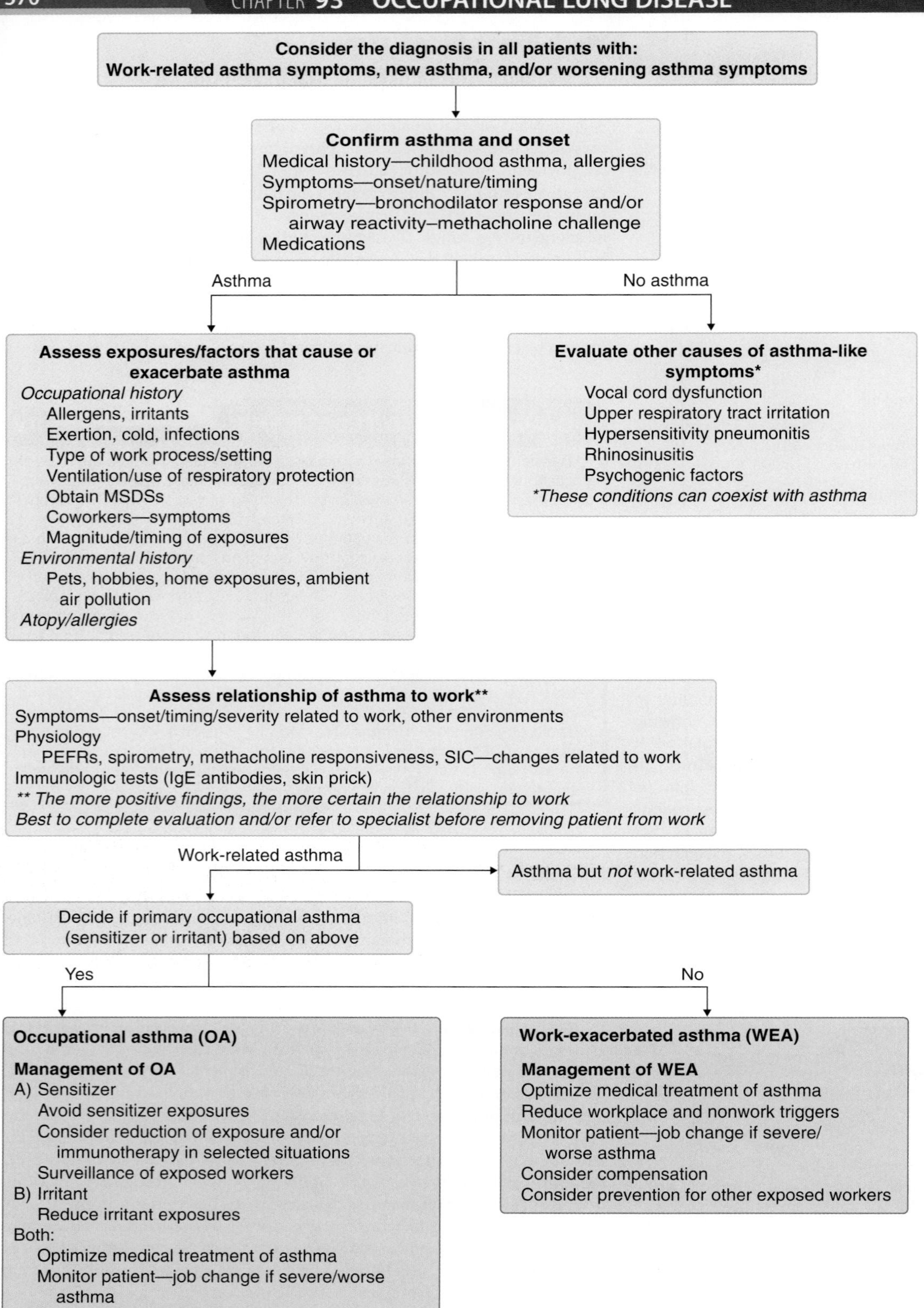

FIGURE 93-1. Clinical evaluation and management of work-related asthma. IgE = immunoglobulin E; MSDS = Material Safety Data Sheets; PEFR = peak expiratory flow rates; SIC = specific inhalation challenge. (From American College of Chest Physicians. Consensus statement: diagnosis and management of work-related asthma. *Chest.* 2008;134:1S-41S.)

No specific diagnostic tests distinguish an occupational from a nonoccupational cause of COPD. The history of exposure, with objective documentation, is helpful. Confirmation of the absence of a smoking history can assist in determining probability of an occupational cause, but a positive smoking history does not exclude an occupational contribution.

Management is the same as for patients with nonoccupational COPD (Chapter 88). In addition, however, further exposure to dusts, fumes, and gases that are likely to worsen disease should be minimized.

HYPERSENSITIVITY PNEUMONITIS

Many exposures that lead to hypersensitivity pneumonitis (Chapter 92) occur in the workplace, and several bear the name of the occupation or job associated with them: farmer's lung; maple bark stripper's lung; cheese washer's lung; thatcher's lung; mushroom worker's lung, and metal-working fluid hypersensitivity pneumonitis (Table 93-3). Occupational causes also include exposure to contaminated humidifiers (with protozoa or fungi) in factories

TABLE 93-3 EXAMPLES OF OCCUPATIONAL CAUSES OF HYPERSENSITIVITY PNEUMONITIS

OCCUPATION	CAUSE
Farmer	Thermophilic actinomycetes in moldy hay
Metal worker	Contamination of metal-working fluids with microorganisms such as *Mycobacteria immunogens* or fungi
Worker exposed to humidifiers	Contamination with microorganisms such as protozoa or fungi
Sugarcane worker	Moldy sugarcane (bagassosis)
Maple bark stripper	Fungi
Chicken or turkey worker	Avian proteins
Pharmaceutical worker	Penicillin
Food handler	Soybeans
Office worker	Microorganisms contaminating air conditioners or humidifiers
Swimming pool attendant	Fungal contamination in sprays around pool area
Animal worker	Rat proteins
Mushroom worker	Fungi
Wheat farmer or handler	Weevil-infested flour
Greenhouse worker	Fungi
Workers spraying urethane paint or adhesives/sealants (or less often, other workers using diisocyanate)	Methylene diphenyl diisocyanate, hexamethylene diisocyanate, toluene diisocyanates
Chemical worker using plastics, resins, paints	Trimellitic anhydride

or office buildings (humidifier lung), as well as lifeguards exposed to sprays of water from pool fountains contaminated with microorganisms. Metal workers or machinists can develop hypersensitivity pneumonitis from recirculated coolants that can become contaminated with gram-negative bacteria or atypical mycobacteria, which then are aerosolized in the coolant mist and inhaled.

PATHOBIOLOGY

Most antigenic exposures that lead to hypersensitivity pneumonitis are organic, especially thermophilic actinomycetes (Chapter 337), fungi, atypical mycobacteria (Chapter 333), and protozoa. Other common antigens include avian and rat proteins. Less commonly, hypersensitivity pneumonitis can be induced by low-molecular-weight chemical antigens, such as penicillin or methylene diphenyl diisocyanate (MDI), which is used as a sealant or binder. Small particles, commonly 3 to 5 μm in mass median aerodynamic diameter, reach the small airways and alveoli, where the immune response leads to hypersensitivity pneumonitis. This immune response is associated with specific IgG antibodies and T lymphocytes, and it recurs with repeated exposures.

CLINICAL MANIFESTATIONS AND DIAGNOSIS

The acute form of disease manifests as cough, dyspnea, chills, and malaise, typically 4 to 8 hours after exposure and clearing by 12 to 24 hours. On examination, patients typically are febrile and tachypneic, with reduced chest expansion and basal crackles. Neutrophilia is common, and the chest radiograph shows acute infiltrates. Pulmonary function testing may show a restrictive pattern, with a reduced diffusing capacity, and arterial blood gases may show hypoxemia owing to ventilation-perfusion mismatch.

Chronic hypersensitivity pneumonitis may follow repeat acute episodes or start de novo. It causes a chronic dry cough, progressive dyspnea, and often significant weight loss. The physical examination typically reveals reduced chest expansion and basal crackles. Results on pulmonary function testing and radiographic findings may be similar to nonspecific idiopathic pulmonary fibrosis (Chapter 92), and ground-glass opacities are often seen on a computed tomography (CT) scan of the chest. Bronchoalveolar fluid typically shows an increase in the lymphocyte count, and there may be a predominance of CD8 T lymphocytes (Chapter 85).

The specific occupational cause for hypersensitivity pneumonitis may be suspected from a temporal relationship to work exposures. The differential diagnosis in the chronic form includes idiopathic pulmonary fibrosis, although clubbing is less common in hypersensitivity pneumonitis. Radiographic and pulmonary function test findings may also mimic idiopathic pulmonary fibrosis, but a distinguishing finding is often a bronchoalveolar lavage that shows lymphocytes as high as 60 to 80% of the cells, usually with a predominance of $CD8^+$ T lymphocytes, but sometimes with $CD4^+$ cells in chronic forms of disease.

Laboratory investigations include determining the presence of serum IgG antibodies to the suspected antigen. However, IgG antibodies may also be present in exposed individuals who do not have disease and are therefore not specific to the diagnosis. Conversely, failure to demonstrate specific antibodies is not uncommon in hypersensitivity pneumonitis because the limited number of antigens used for testing may not include the relevant occupational antigen. Specific challenge with the suspected antigen in a laboratory setting is occasionally needed if the diagnosis is in doubt.

Some patients can safely undergo "work challenge" that monitors changes in symptoms, fever, blood neutrophil count, radiographic findings, and pulmonary function with and without exposure to the suspected agent. Lung biopsy, if performed, may show granulomas and foreign body giant cells. If other findings are supportive of hypersensitivity pneumonitis, however, open biopsy and challenges usually are not needed.

TREATMENT AND PROGNOSIS Rx

Treatment principles are the same as for nonoccupational hypersensitivity pneumonitis (Chapter 94). Removal from exposure to the causative agent is the primary treatment measure. As with occupational asthma from a sensitizer, the removal must be complete and often requires a change in work if the causative agent cannot be removed. Reduction of exposure by use of respiratory protective devices is generally not practical and not effective, with the exception of air-supplied helmet respirators for occasional short-term exposures. Patients with acute hypersensitivity pneumonitis may not require any medications in addition to removal from antigen exposure, but if acute episodes are severe, they may need supportive measures, including corticosteroids (e.g., 20 to 60 mg of prednisone orally per day), supplemental oxygen, and intensive care (Chapter 94). Chronic hypersensitivity pneumonitis may require additional oral corticosteroid treatment (e.g., 5 to 10 mg of prednisone orally per day) as for nonoccupational chronic hypersensitivity pneumonitis, and severe end-stage fibrosis may lead to need for lung transplantation. Prognosis is better with early diagnosis and complete removal from exposure to the causative agent. Preventive measures include occupational hygiene measures to avoid contamination of aerosolized fluid or dusts with bio-organisms and use of appropriate respiratory protective devices.

CHRONIC BERYLLIUM DISEASE

EPIDEMIOLOGY AND PATHOBIOLOGY

Acute toxic pneumonitis was described in workers who had high exposure to beryllium in the manufacture of fluorescent lightbulbs in the 1940s, and a hypersensitivity response causing chronic beryllium disease was described in the 1950s. Acute toxic effects are now rare, but chronic beryllium disease remains a problem because of the expanded use of beryllium (Table 93-4) and better recognition of sensitization by development of an immunologic blood test.

Chronic beryllium disease is a hypersensitivity disease with a strong genetic association with HLA-DPB1 gene variants that code for Glu69 and that have been identified in 83 to 97% of patients with disease. However, this gene variant occurs in 30 to 48% of the general population and, as a result, is not useful as a screening test.

CLINICAL MANIFESTATIONS

The pulmonary clinical features of chronic beryllium disease are similar to those of sarcoidosis (Chapter 95), ranging from asymptomatic histologic or radiographic findings, to potential progression, to severe granulomatous restrictive lung disease. Onset can occur up to 20 years or more after exposure to beryllium, even if the patient no longer is exposed. The clinical history in all patients with apparent sarcoidosis must include inquiry about possible beryllium exposure, even many years ago.

DIAGNOSIS AND TREATMENT Rx

The chest radiograph shows changes that appear identical to sarcoidosis with enlarged hilar or mediastinal lymph nodes or multiple lung nodules, or both (Fig. 93-2). Sensitization to beryllium can be detected by a beryllium lymphocyte proliferation test that demonstrates the presence of sensitized lymphocytes in blood or bronchoalveolar lavage fluid. This test also can detect sensitization to beryllium among asymptomatic exposed workers, who can then be evaluated to assess possible chronic beryllium disease and provided with advice for reducing or eliminating further work exposures.

After disease develops, removal from exposure is advised, but the disease may still worsen. Progressive deterioration in lung function is treated similarly to sarcoidosis (Chapter 95), with oral corticosteroids and supportive measures.

ASBESTOS-RELATED DISEASES

Although the use of asbestos has declined, and better protective equipment has been mandated, asbestos-related disease has continued to occur owing to the long latency between exposure and disease. Chrysotile asbestos has less effect on the lungs than other forms of asbestos, that is, amphiboles. Effects of exposure include benign and malignant disease.

Benign asbestos disease is often asymptomatic and identified on chest imaging. Pleural thickening and pleural plaques, commonly with calcification, can occur 20 to 30 years after first exposure and may initially appear on the chest radiograph as calcified linear opacities over the hemidiaphragms and cardiac border (see Fig. 84-10 in Chapter 84). If extensive, it may be difficult to exclude intrapulmonary opacities except by CT scan. Pleural plaques are a marker of asbestos exposure but do not occur in all workers with significant asbestos exposure. They generally do not cause significant changes in lung function, except diffuse pleural thickening may result in exertional dyspnea and extrapulmonary restrictive lung disease. Pleural thickening may cause rounded atelectasis (Chapter 90) when encasement of a portion of the peripheral lung tissue by thickened pleura causes an apparent lung nodule, typically with a "comet sign" showing the thickened pleura. Benign pleural effusion can develop, typically about 10 to 15 years after asbestos exposure. It requires further investigation because the differential diagnosis includes malignant pleural effusion (Chapter 99).

Asbestosis is the term for interstitial lung disease caused by asbestos. The clinical presentation is usually with dry cough and dyspnea on exertion. Physical examination usually reveals digital clubbing and basal crackles on lung auscultation. Chest imaging shows basal interstitial lung disease, with or without additional pleural changes as described earlier. Pulmonary function testing shows restrictive lung disease (Chapter 85), and histologic findings are the same as in usual interstitial pneumonia (Chapter 92). Findings supporting the diagnosis of asbestosis rather than usual interstitial pneumonia include a significant duration and level of exposure to asbestos, an appropriate latency of usually 20 to 40 years after first exposure, and the finding of ferruginous asbestos bodies in sputum or lung tissue (Fig. 93-3). Unfortunately, pharmacologic treatment is not effective, and the lung disease may progress to end-stage fibrosis. Management is supportive, including supplemental oxygen and consideration for lung transplantation (Chapter 101). As with the other diseases of long latency, preventing exposure is paramount.

Mesothelioma (Chapter 197), a malignant tumor of the pleura, peritoneum, or both, is the one complication of asbestos exposure that can occur after even relatively minor exposure, such as second-hand exposure from dust on clothing in the families of those working with exposure. It typically occurs 30 to 40 years after exposure to asbestos and may present incidentally on chest imaging or with chest pain or weight loss. Radiographs show pleural thickening, and a pleural effusion may be present. Mesothelioma often is difficult to distinguish from benign pleural thickening without a biopsy. No treatment has proved effective (Chapter 197), so routine screening to detect mesothelioma in exposed persons is not currently recommended. The risk of lung cancer (Chapter 197) increases after significant exposure to asbestos, with a usual latency period of 20 to 30 years. Smoking and asbestos exposure have multiplicative effects on the risk of lung cancer.

TABLE 93-4 POTENTIAL EXPOSURES TO BERYLLIUM

OCCUPATIONAL EXPOSURES
Metal and alloy production (alloys of aluminum, copper, and nickel; recently includes golf clubs and metal pen clips)
Ceramic manufacturing
Metal casting, including dental technicians (crowns, bridges)
Electronics, including computer components, transistors, microwave and x-ray windows, heat sinks, telecommunications
Aerospace and atomic engineering (rocket fuels, heat shields, nose cones, and metal parts)
Aircraft manufacture and repair
Nuclear reactors, nuclear weapons and defense industry
Coating of cathode ray tubes for radar and similar installations
Laboratories
Extraction from ore
Metal reclamation and recycling
NONOCCUPATIONAL EXPOSURES
Family members exposed to dust from workers' clothing
Breakage of old fluorescent lamps (made before 1950 in North America)
Downwind exposure from industrial accidents (e.g., from a nuclear processing plant in Kazakhstan, in the former Soviet Union in 1990)

From Tarlo SM, Rhee K, Powell E, et al. Marked tachypnoea in siblings with chronic beryllium disease due to copper-beryllium alloy. *Chest*. 2001;119:647-650.

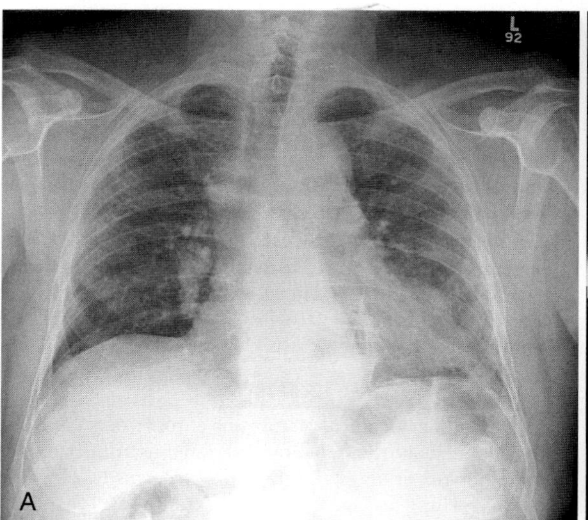

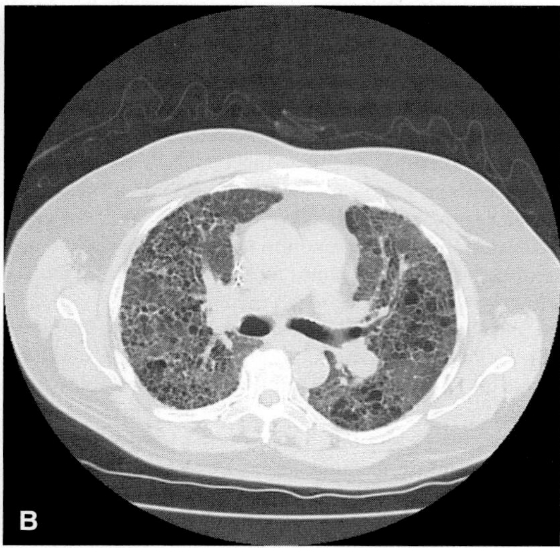

FIGURE 93-2. Posteroanterior chest radiograph (A) and high-resolution computed tomography scan (B) from patients with chronic beryllium disease. The chest radiograph demonstrates hilar adenopathy and infiltrates, and the scan shows air space destruction and infiltrates.

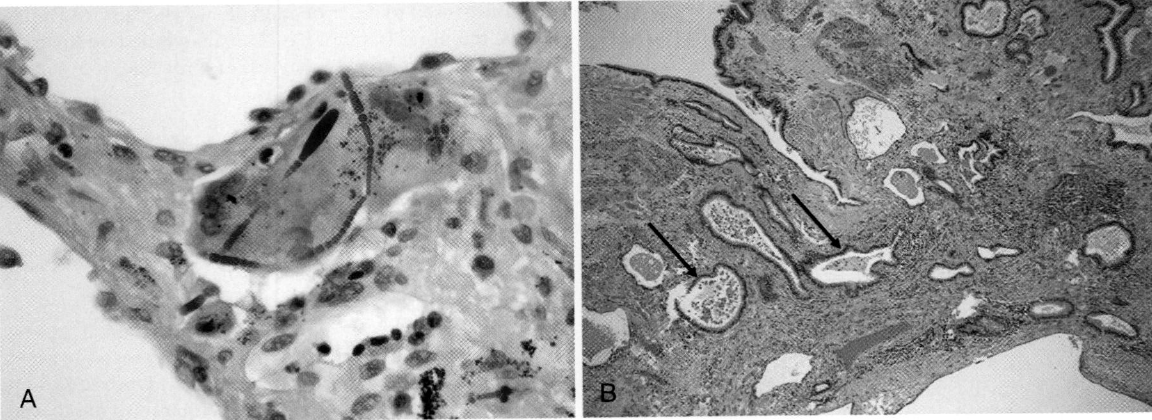

FIGURE 93-3. **Histology from a lung biopsy showing asbestos bodies.** Ferruginous bodies consisting of asbestos fibers coated by iron-protein-mucopolysaccharide material with typical golden-brown, beaded appearance. The two longest asbestos bodies at the centre of the figure are present within a multinucleated giant cell. (Hematoxylin and eosin stain, × 400). (Courtesy of Dr. David Hwang, Toronto General Hospital.)

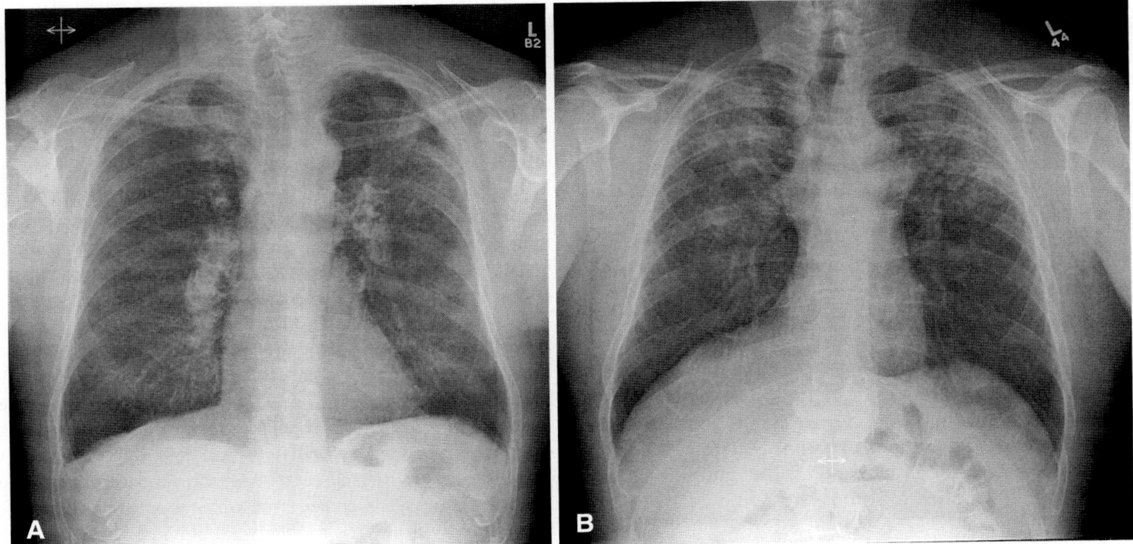

FIGURE 93-4. **Posteroanterior chest radiographs from two patients with silicosis. A**, Small nodules and eggshell calcification of hilar lymph nodes. **B**, Progressive massive fibrosis of the upper lung zones with compensatory emphysema.

SILICOSIS AND OTHER PNEUMOCONIOSES

The incidences of silicosis and other inorganic dust diseases of the lungs (Table 93-5) have declined substantially in recent decades owing to better worksite protection in mines, sandblasting, and other settings. There is an association between silicosis and the development of collagen-vascular disease, especially rheumatoid arthritis. Patients with pneumoconiosis and rheumatoid arthritis may be at higher risk of developing rheumatoid nodules in the lung, so-called Caplan's syndrome, and mycobacterial infections.

Patients may initially be identified incidentally during a medical surveillance program or by a chest radiograph that shows multiple small lung nodules, often with enlarged mediastinal lymph nodes that can mimic sarcoidosis (Fig. 93-4). Nodules can coalesce and lead to progressive massive fibrosis, especially in the upper lungs, with compensatory emphysema in the lower lung fields. On chest imaging, mediastinal lymph nodes may have a characteristic "eggshell" calcification in silicosis. Treatment is supportive. Patients with exposure to silica or coal dust may develop COPD from the dust exposure. Patients who develop end-stage lung disease may be considered for lung transplantation.

TABLE 93-5 JOBS THAT CAN LEAD TO SILICOSIS

Mining: surface or underground mining (tunneling)
Milling: ground silica for abrasives and filler
Quarrying
Sandblasting: e.g., of buildings, preparing steel for painting
Pottery; ceramic or clay work
Grinding, polishing using silica wheels
Stone work
Foundry work: grinding, molding, chipping
Refractory brick work
Glass making: to polish and as an abrasive
Boiler work: cleaning boilers
Manufacture of abrasives

ACUTE FEBRILE SYNDROMES

A variety of occupational exposures can cause acute febrile respiratory syndromes that may mimic acute viral respiratory illnesses (Table 93-6). The mechanism of these syndromes is incompletely understood, but they are associated with systemic neutrophilia and cytokine activation, often with increased interleukin-6 (IL-6) and IL-8.

CLINICAL MANIFESTATIONS AND DIAGNOSIS

Typically, chills, fever, malaise, dry cough, and chest tightness start about 6 to 8 hours after onset of an exposure at work and generally resolve by the next day. Occasionally, shortness of breath and other respiratory symptoms are

TABLE 93-6 OCCUPATIONAL CAUSES OF AN ACUTE FEBRILE SYNDROME

SYNDROME	CAUSE
Polymer fume fever or Teflon fever	Polytetrafluoroethylene and other fluorocarbon polymer fumes
Metal fume fever	Zinc fumes from welding of galvanized steel, less commonly other metal fumes
Cotton mill fever	Dust and endotoxins from bacterial contamination of unprocessed cotton, flax, and hemp
Humidifier fever	Microorganisms found in reservoirs, e.g., humidifiers, air conditioners, aquariums
Organic dust toxic syndrome	Grain dust, moldy wood chips

severe enough for patients to seek emergency medical attention. Infiltrates on the chest radiograph can occur with neutrophilia and hypoxemia that can mimic acute pneumonia or acute hypersensitivity pneumonitis. Symptoms and signs generally resolve in 24 to 48 hours without antibiotics and recur with further exposures, although the clinical manifestations generally become milder with repeated daily exposures (e.g., Monday morning fever in cotton mill workers). Workers are often familiar with the syndrome because it commonly affects up to 30% of exposed workers. If the diagnosis is not provided by the patient, however, careful elicitation of potential work exposures is needed.

TREATMENT Rx

Treatment is supportive. If the causative exposure can be removed (e.g., cleaning a contaminated humidifier), symptoms can be prevented. If the cause cannot be removed and symptoms are severe, the patient may need reduction or change of the work exposure.

OCCUPATIONAL LUNG CANCER

A significant duration and level of exposure to a recognized carcinogen such as asbestos, hexavalent chromium (as in chromate production and the pigment industry), soluble radon compounds or radon gas, polycyclic aromatic hydrocarbons, chloromethyl ethers, arsenic, or silica can increase the risk of lung cancer (Chapter 197). Such a history should be elicited in all patients. The International Agency for Research on Cancer provides a listing of occupational lung carcinogens and the likelihood of their association with cancer (*http://monographs.iarc.fr/ENG/Monographs/PDFs/index.php*).

SUGGESTED READINGS

CDC NIOSH Work-Related Lung Disease (WoRLD) Surveillance System. http://www2.cdc.gov/drds/WorldReportData. Accessed Oct. 27, 2010. *Information on the prevalence of occupational lung diseases in the United States.*

Peden DB, Bush RK. Advances in environmental and occupational respiratory diseases in 2009. *J Allergy Clin Immunol.* 2010;125:559-562. *Review.*

Sawyer RT, Maier LA. Chronic beryllium disease: an updated model interaction between innate and acquired immunity. *Biometals.* 2011;24:1-17. *Review of how beryllium drives chronic inflammation and granuloma formation.*

94 PHYSICAL AND CHEMICAL INJURIES OF THE LUNG

DAVID C. CHRISTIANI

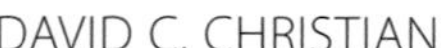

SUBMERSION INCIDENTS: DROWNING

DEFINITION

Drowning is defined as "the process of experiencing respiratory impairment from submersion/immersion in liquid." The term *near-drowning* was previously used to describe individuals who survived a submersion incident, at least temporarily, but it has been abandoned on the basis of recommendations of the First World Congress of Drowning in Amsterdam in 2002.

EPIDEMIOLOGY

The estimated annual number of deaths worldwide due to drowning is 500,000. About 4200 persons are treated per year for nonfatal drowning in U.S. emergency departments, and about another 3400 suffer fatal drowning. Alcohol use, age younger than 4 years, and male gender are associated with increased rates of both nonfatal and fatal drowning.

PATHOBIOLOGY

The initial response to submersion/immersion is apnea, followed almost invariably by aspiration. Laryngospasm may result in aspiration of a variable quantity of liquid medium into the lungs. Hypoxemia, hypercapnia, and acidemia develop acutely. Aspiration of either fresh or salt water results in occlusion of the airway, reduced surfactant activity, direct alveolar injury, and bronchospasm. Acute lung injury or the acute respiratory distress syndrome (ARDS), associated with noncardiogenic pulmonary edema and severe hypoxemia, may develop hours or days after the incident. Mortality is primarily due to cardiovascular effects as a result of severe early or late hypoxia. The most serious secondary consequence of hypoxia is anoxic brain injury. Acute renal failure may also occur. Alcohol consumption also increases the risk for hypothermia. Changes to serum electrolytes with drowning in either fresh water or salt water are not clinically significant.

CLINICAL MANIFESTATIONS

The initial presentation of a drowning victim varies widely. Hypothermia, which is common in drowning victims, may be associated with bradycardia or cardiac arrest due to asystole or ventricular fibrillation. Tachypnea, tachycardia, and low-grade fever are typical in nonhypothermic patients. Cyanosis may be present, and a coughing patient may produce pink frothy sputum. Neurologic evaluation may reveal agitation with or without intoxication or coma. The patient should be examined carefully for signs of associated trauma.

Expected laboratory findings include mild electrolyte abnormalities independent of whether submersion occurs in salt water or fresh water, moderate leukocytosis, slight decrease in hematocrit in the first 24 hours or slight increase in free hemoglobin with a stable hematocrit in fresh water submersion due to hemolysis, severe hypoxemia, and metabolic acidosis. Evidence of disseminated intravascular coagulation may occur. Initial electrocardiographic changes include sinus tachycardia and nonspecific ST segment and T wave changes, which revert to normal within hours. Life-threatening ventricular arrhythmias, complete heart block, or evidence of myocardial infarction can occur early or late in the course. Chest radiographs may initially be normal, despite severe respiratory impairment. Bilateral patchy alveolar infiltrates indicating progression to acute lung injury or ARDS may develop.

DIAGNOSIS

The diagnosis of drowning is made on clinical history of submersion in liquid medium with resulting respiratory impairment. Patients with unusual presenting circumstances should be carefully examined for evidence of trauma or assault.

PREVENTION

Drowning incidents are largely preventable, particularly in children. Pool fencing is a proven, effective strategy to prevent drowning. The primary cause of drowning of infants and toddlers is lack of adult supervision, and supervision of all young children near any form of water is strongly recommended. The role of alcohol in teenage and adult drowning incidents is substantial, and all individuals participating in water-based activities should restrict alcohol intake. The use of personal flotation devices is recommended for children and adults.

TREATMENT Rx

Once the victim has been recovered from submersion, treatment should focus on basic life support algorithms, including notification of emergency response personnel and establishment of an adequate airway and cardiopulmonary resuscitation, if necessary (Chapter 63). If the victim is apneic, rescue breathing should occur immediately, even before removal from the water. Cervical spine stabilization is needed if there is a history of diving, use of a water slide, signs of injury, or signs of alcohol intoxication. Spinal cord injury

(Chapter 406) is otherwise unlikely, and cervical spine stabilization techniques and equipment may impede timely and effective treatment. Attempts to remove water from the airway are unnecessary. Cardiac arrhythmias should be treated with Advanced Cardiac Life Support (ACLS) protocols, including the use of automated external defibrillators when appropriate (Chapter 63). Most drowning victims who receive cardiopulmonary resuscitation or rescue breathing will vomit; if vomiting occurs, the head should be turned to the side and the vomitus removed with a finger. When vomiting occurs in patients who may have spinal cord injury, log rolling techniques are recommended for turning the patient to the side.

All victims of a submersion incident should be transported to a hospital for further evaluation, treatment of potential respiratory failure (Chapter 104), and monitoring for up to 24 hours. Bronchoscopy may be required to evaluate localized wheezing or persistent atelectasis. Prophylactic antibiotics are not useful, but evidence of pneumonia (Chapter 97) should be treated with appropriate antibiotics. Because unusual microorganisms may be isolated from the lower airways, efforts should be made to identify specific microbial flora pertinent to the locus of the drowning incident.

Treatment of neurologic injury is focused on supportive care while the extent of cerebral edema is minimized. To decrease cerebral edema and intracranial pressure, intravenous 23% hypertonic saline (30 mL initially then 75 to 100 mL/hour; goal serum sodium level of 155 mM/L) through a central line may be preferred to mannitol (1 g/kg bolus of 20% solution initially, with repeated doses of 0.25 to 0.5 g/kg every 6 to 8 hours). Hyperventilation to a $PaCO_2$ of 34 to 36 mm Hg may be helpful. Intracranial pressure may increase in response to shivering or purposeless movements, which should be reduced. Induced therapeutic hypothermia improves neurologic outcome after cardiac arrest (Chapter 109), and current recommendations for drowning victims who remain comatose after rescue are to avoid rewarming to core or tympanic temperatures above 34° C and to maintain temperature of 32° to 34° C for 24 to 48 hours. Hyperthermia should be avoided at all times.

PROGNOSIS

The mortality rate for drowning victims who present alive to an emergency department is about 25%. Long-term neurologic deficits persist in approximately 6% of nonfatal drowning victims. Although prolonged duration of submersion is associated with a worse prognosis, young children who are hypothermic when they are rescued after submersion times of up to 60 minutes have recovered without neurologic damage. Other factors associated with poor prognosis include hypotension, persistent apnea, coma, more than a 10-minute delay in receiving basic life support, and duration of resuscitation of more than 25 minutes.

DISEASES OF HIGH ALTITUDE

DEFINITION

Neurologic and pulmonary disturbances, primarily due to direct tissue effects of hypoxia, occur in individuals who either ascend to or reside at altitudes of 7000 feet (2133 meters) or more (Table 94-1).

EPIDEMIOLOGY

Acute mountain sickness is the most common high-altitude syndrome. It occurs in approximately 20% of individuals who ascend to altitudes of 7000 to 9000 feet, 40% at 10,000 to 14,000 feet, and more than 50% above 14,000 feet. The incidence of chronic mountain sickness, also known as Monge's disease, is thought to be between 5 and 18%. More severe neurologic disturbances due to high-altitude cerebral edema are rare, occurring in approximately 1 to 2% of individuals who ascend to altitudes above 15,000 feet. High-altitude pulmonary edema occurs in approximately 2 to 6% of otherwise healthy individuals who ascend to altitudes of 8000 to 15,000 feet. However, the incidence in individuals with a prior history of high-altitude pulmonary edema may be as high as 60%, or higher during rapid ascents. The occurrence of high-altitude retinal hemorrhage is approximately 33% among individuals who ascend to very high altitudes (up to 19,000 feet) and is thought to be common at lower altitudes as well. High-altitude retinal hemorrhage is not associated with high-altitude cerebral edema or long-term visual consequences.

TABLE 94-1 HIGH-ALTITUDE SYNDROMES

SYNDROME	CLINICAL DESCRIPTION
Acute mountain sickness	Recent ascent to altitudes above 7000 feet; headache, anorexia, and malaise; common
Chronic mountain sickness	Dwelling above 10,000 feet; headache, fatigue, dyspnea, and digestive disturbances; incidence: 5-18%
High-altitude cerebral edema	Above 15,000 feet; confusion, ataxia, hallucinations, coma, or death; rare
High-altitude pulmonary edema	Above 9500 feet; dyspnea, cough, and tachycardia; incidence: 2-6%
High-altitude retinal hemorrhage	Above 15,000 feet; asymptomatic or reversible vision changes; common

PATHOBIOLOGY

Clinically significant hypoxemia is the underlying factor in all high-altitude diseases. The decrease in barometric pressure during an ascent to altitude causes a decrease in the alveolar pressure of oxygen (PAO_2). For example, PAO_2 drops from 105 mm Hg at sea level to 60 mm Hg at 10,000 feet and to 40 mm Hg at 18,000 feet. Below 60 mm Hg, oxygen dissociates from hemoglobin more readily (see Fig. 161-2 in Chapter 161), thereby decreasing oxygen saturation and oxygen delivery to tissues. The effect is even more noticeable in individuals with impaired diffusion capacity, for example, emphysema, interstitial lung diseases, or heart failure. Furthermore, increased ventilatory drive induces an acute respiratory alkalosis. In the brain, hypoxia causes cerebral vasodilation, whereas hypobaria causes cerebral vasoconstriction. In severe hypoxia, vasodilation is the likely cause of cerebral edema in susceptible individuals. The response to hypoxia in the lungs is primarily increased pulmonary arterial pressures due to hypoxic pulmonary vasoconstriction, which results in reversible injury to pulmonary capillaries, increased capillary permeability, and eventually pulmonary edema. Reduced oxygen consumption also occurs, perhaps from impaired mitochondrial function in the presence of hypoxia. Periodic breathing during sleep is also noted but has minimal if any clinical significance.

CLINICAL MANIFESTATIONS

Symptoms of acute mountain sickness begin 2 to 3 hours after ascent and include breathlessness, lightheadedness, fatigue, nausea, anorexia, headache, and insomnia. Most symptoms resolve within 2 to 3 days, although insomnia may persist. Chronic symptoms of headache, fatigue, sleep disturbances, dyspnea, and digestive complaints are seen with chronic mountain sickness in individuals residing at higher elevations. Chronic mountain sickness may be associated with polycythemia (hemoglobin concentrations above 21 g/dL). Severe neurologic symptoms with high-altitude cerebral edema include ataxia and confusion that may progress to coma or death. Symptoms of high-altitude pulmonary edema that usually begin 2 to 4 days after ascent to higher altitudes include dyspnea, cough, and tachycardia. Funduscopic changes of flame-shaped hemorrhages are seen with high-altitude retinal hemorrhage.

DIAGNOSIS

Diagnosis of most high-altitude disease is made on the basis of clinical manifestations at high altitude. Diagnosis of chronic mountain sickness, and a milder form often called subacute mountain sickness, is more challenging because it may mimic other cardiopulmonary, neurologic, or psychiatric disease. Individuals with chronic mountain sickness typically have higher hemoglobin concentrations, higher serum erythropoietin levels, higher nocturnal heart rates, lower nocturnal oxygen saturation, and higher systolic and diastolic arterial pressure than normal individuals living at similar altitude.

PREVENTION

Prevention of high-altitude disease can be achieved by avoidance in high-risk individuals, such as young children and persons with a history of high-altitude disease. Gradual ascent and acclimatization are crucial to prevention of high-altitude illness, particularly at extreme altitudes. At altitudes up to 10,000 feet, 2 to 3 days or more may be needed for adjustment to the effects of hypoxia. For mountaineers, current recommendations are to ascend no more than approximately 984 feet (300 m) per day at altitudes higher than 9843 feet (3000 m).

When rapid ascent is unavoidable, such as flights to high-altitude locales, the carbonic anhydrase inhibitor acetazolamide (250 mg orally once or twice daily) provides effective prophylaxis of acute mountain sickness, and 125 mg at night may improve sleep.[1] Dexamethasone (given in doses of 4 mg twice daily)[2] and prednisolone (20 mg daily) have been shown to decrease the severity of acute mountain sickness. The long-acting β-adrenergic agonist salmeterol (125 μg inhaled twice daily) also reduces the risk for high-altitude pulmonary edema.[3] Sumatriptan, 50 mg, after ascent is useful for reducing symptoms.[4] The calcium-channel blocker nifedipine (20 mg of slow-release formulation) is useful for preventing recurrent high-altitude pulmonary edema in individuals with previous episodes.

TREATMENT

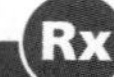

For acute, life-threatening symptoms such as high-altitude pulmonary edema and high-altitude cerebral edema, the best treatment is immediate descent, if possible, combined with supplemental oxygen therapy and, if needed, use of a portable hyperbaric chamber. For individuals who develop less severe symptoms, sildenafil (50 mg) can increase exercise capacity at altitude by 10 to 35%.[5] Increasing inspired oxygen concentrations in high-altitude working facilities also improves productivity and quality of sleep. Sustained-release theophylline (375 mg twice daily) significantly reduces the symptoms of acute mountain sickness compared with placebo.[6] Acetazolamide (250 mg or 500 mg once daily) is also useful in treating symptoms of chronic mountain sickness.[7] Milder forms of acute mountain sickness, such as headache, can be treated with typical doses of nonsteroidal anti-inflammatory medications, including aspirin and acetaminophen.

PROGNOSIS

Symptoms of high-altitude disease respond rapidly to immediate descent. However, high-altitude cerebral edema and high-altitude pulmonary edema can be fatal, particularly at extreme altitudes and weather when descent may be impossible.

DECOMPRESSION ILLNESS: DECOMPRESSION SICKNESS, BAROTRAUMA, AND ARTERIAL GAS EMBOLISM

DEFINITION

Exposures to changes in ambient pressure cause a spectrum of illness, either (1) by increasing or decreasing the volume of gas in air-filled body cavities, or (2) by causing the release of inert gas bubbles from solution in tissues or blood vessels. Symptoms associated with decreasing ambient pressure, which occur most commonly with ascent from depth during recreational or occupational diving, are known as decompression illness. The most common form of decompression illness is decompression sickness, which is classified as either type I (mild symptoms, such as general fatigue or joint pain) or type II (more severe neurologic or cardiopulmonary disturbances). Life-threatening forms of decompression illness include pulmonary barotrauma and arterial gas embolism syndromes. During the descent of a dive, increasing ambient pressure may cause mild symptoms of facial or sinus pain, often called "the squeezes."

EPIDEMIOLOGY

In addition to the approximately 9 million recreational divers in the United States, aviators, astronauts, and compressed air workers are also exposed to changes in ambient pressure that may cause decompression illness. Among recreational divers, the annual incidence rate for either type I or type II decompression sickness is estimated at 1 case per 5000 to 10,000 dives. Approximately 1000 episodes of decompression illness severe enough to warrant recompression therapy occur each year, up to 10% of which are fatal. Well-recognized risk factors for decompression illness include long duration of dives, deep dives, repetitive dives, heavy exertion at depth, cold water, and rapid ascent. Additional risk occurs in individuals who experience further decreases in ambient pressure after the dive, such as on commercial or private aircraft or driving over mountainous areas.

PATHOBIOLOGY

The principles of Boyle's law and Henry's law describe the properties of gases during changes in ambient pressure. Boyle's law states that the volume of a gas varies inversely to changes in pressure, $P_1V_1 = P_2V_2$. During the descent of a dive, pain due to the "squeezes" is caused by increasing ambient pressures that are not equalized by an increase in gas volume. The resulting negative pressure causes a vacuum effect in the mask associated with engorgement of the blood vessels in adjacent tissues, such as periorbital and ocular vessels, and may result in swelling, pain, and subconjunctival hemorrhages. Facial sinuses, the middle ear, and the external auditory canal may also be affected.

Barotrauma in sinus, otic, or pulmonary tissues may be due to changes in ambient pressures and the resulting increase or decrease in the volume of gas. During descent, the decreasing volume of gas causes vascular engorgement in the sinuses and otic compartments and may result in rupture of the tympanic or inner ear membranes. During ascent, breath-holding, particularly with compressed air devices (SCUBA diving), and the presence of obstructive lung disease with delayed exhalation times and air trapping impair equilibration and increase the risk for pulmonary barotrauma. If the expanding volume of gas causes a pressure gradient between the alveoli and pulmonary interstitium that exceeds the compliance of the lung, alveolar disruption will lead to pulmonary interstitial emphysema. Further extension of gas along pulmonary tissues may cause additional barotrauma, leading to pneumothorax, mediastinal emphysema, pneumopericardium, and soft tissue emphysema.

Arterial gas embolism, which is a serious consequence of pulmonary barotrauma, results in the development of free gas in the pulmonary arterial circulation. The resulting bubbles may then enter the systemic circulation by overwhelming the filtering mechanism of the pulmonary capillaries or through a right-to-left intracardiac shunt (Chapter 69), such as a patent foramen ovale. Bubbles may then migrate to the brain, spinal cord, heart, lung, or kidney and lead to tissue ischemia or infarct.

Henry's law states that the solubility of a gas in liquid is proportional to the partial pressure of that gas above the liquid. An increase in partial pressure of gases during descent will therefore cause the amount of gas dissolved in the pulmonary capillaries to increase. Dissolved oxygen is used during normal body metabolism; however, inert nitrogen, which is abundant in inspired air, becomes dissolved in the blood and tissues, particularly in fat, where it is five-fold more soluble than in water. During ascent, decreasing ambient pressure causes tissues to become supersaturated with nitrogen, and nitrogen is subsequently released into blood vessels and tissues as gas bubbles. Decompression-induced gas bubbles cause decompression illness by either mechanical compression of tissues or embolization through blood vessels to end organs. Bubbles that obstruct capillaries or venules damage the endothelium and cause tissue ischemia, which leads to activation of inflammatory mediators or tissue reperfusion injury. Although not well understood, toxic effects due to increased partial pressure of gases also are likely to contribute to symptoms of decompression illness, possibly by denaturing of proteins and release of fatty acids from cell membranes.

CLINICAL MANIFESTATIONS AND DIAGNOSIS

Symptoms of decompression illness can occur within minutes and up to 24 hours or more after exposure to changes in ambient pressure associated with dives of 20 feet in depth or more. The severity of symptoms depends on the rate and the magnitude of the change of ambient pressure and can vary among individuals. Diagnosis is based on clinical manifestations, which can be classified according to whether they are caused by formation of inert nitrogen gas bubbles or the localized toxic effects of gas (associated with decompression sickness), barotrauma associated with descent (sinus or otic barotrauma), barotrauma associated with ascent (pulmonary barotrauma), or more severe arterial gas embolism syndromes.

Symptoms vary according to location of bubble formation. For example, type I decompression sickness, also known as the bends or caisson disease, is typically associated with pain in the joints, from mild to severe, and numbness of the extremities. Rashes and lymphedema may also occur. Symptoms of type II decompression sickness may be systemic (fatigue, hypovolemic shock), cardiopulmonary (cough, substernal chest pain, tachypnea, asphyxia), otic (vertigo, hearing loss), or neurologic (ataxia, aphasia, speech disturbances, incontinence, confusion, personality changes, depression, paralysis, and loss of consciousness).

Otic barotrauma, which typically occurs during descent, can affect the external, middle, or inner ear (Chapter 434). External ear symptoms, such as a sensation of ear fullness or otalgia, are caused by a blockage of the canal, for example, with the use of ear plugs or presence of cerumen. Middle ear symptoms of otalgia, vertigo, tinnitus, transient conductive hearing loss, and facial nerve palsy occur when inadequate equalization of pressures results from blocked eustachian tubes, typically in association with allergic rhinitis or upper respiratory infections. Inner ear barotrauma, which is a more serious form of otic barotrauma, is associated with elevated intracranial pressure and rupture of the inner ear membrane. Inner ear barotrauma causes symptoms of sensorineural deafness, tinnitus, vertigo, nausea, and vomiting. Sinus barotrauma typically occurs during descent, is associated with facial pain and epistaxis, and occurs more frequently in individuals with mucosal inflammation from allergies or infection.

Pulmonary barotrauma, which is the second leading cause of death among divers, should be suspected in postdive individuals, particularly at-risk individuals, with symptoms of sudden pleuritic pain, dyspnea, or coughing. Physical examination findings include tachypnea, subcutaneous emphysema, and dullness to percussion or decreased breath sounds over a pneumothorax. Development of tension pneumothorax (Chapter 99) or severe pneumomediastinum may lead to decreased venous return of systemic blood and reduced cardiac preload, a situation that is characterized by hypotension and may lead to refractory shock or cardiac arrest. Chest and neck radiographs are recommended for diagnosis, particularly because pneumothoraces must be treated with chest tube thoracostomy before recompression therapy.

Because arterial gas embolism syndromes are caused by pulmonary barotrauma, careful neurologic assessment is critical. The neurologic findings are similar to those of an acute stroke (Chapter 414), with manifestations of focal or unilateral motor deficits, visual disturbances, sensory deficits, speech difficulties, and cognitive disturbances, including loss of consciousness. Symptoms typically occur within 10 minutes after ascent. Delayed neurologic symptoms are more likely to be due to type II decompression sickness.

PREVENTION

Education is the most effective method of preventing decompression illness. Before participation in diving-related activities, all individuals should undergo a thorough and intensive training program. Instruction of proper pressure equalization techniques is critical in the prevention of decompression illness. Persons with asthma who wish to dive should be assessed by a physician (preferably knowledgeable in the field of diving medicine), have no wheezing on physical examination, and have normal spirometry before and after exercise. The presence of structural lung disease (e.g., lung cysts or bullae) is associated with a significant increase in the risk for pneumothorax and is a contraindication to diving. Presence of a known right-to-left intracardiac shunt, such as a patent foramen ovale, is not an absolute contraindication to diving, although conservative diving is recommended, and patients should be cautioned that they are at increased risk for decompression illness.

TREATMENT Rx

Symptoms of decompression illness at altitude should be treated with supplemental oxygen and return to the lowest attainable altitude. Serious decompression illness associated with diving requires immediate medical evaluation by emergency personnel, including basic and advanced life support (Chapter 63) when hemodynamic instability is present. Pneumothorax (Chapter 99) should be treated immediately with needle decompression or chest tube thoracostomy. Symptoms that persist for more than 2 hours or increase in intensity require recompression therapy, preferably with 100% oxygen or transfer to a facility with a hyperbaric chamber, where standard protocols should be followed. Tenoxicam (20 mg daily) decreases the number of recompression treatments needed in divers with decompression illness.[8]

PROGNOSIS

Survival of patients with decompression illness depends on prompt medical evaluation and treatment. Immediate hyperbaric oxygen therapy per standard protocols is associated with resolution of symptoms in 95% of cases. However, symptoms of decompression illness, even neurologic deficits, may respond to recompression therapy after delays of 24 hours or more.

SMOKE INHALATION

Smoke Inhalation and Thermal Injury

DEFINITION

Pulmonary complications, largely caused by smoke inhalation, occur in a large proportion of burn victims (Chapter 112) and account for a substantial number of deaths in these patients. Even patients who do not sustain surface burns in a fire can inhale sufficient smoke to result in injury to the lungs or airways.

EPIDEMIOLOGY

Modern building codes and the widespread presence of firefighting personnel in communities have decreased the importance of fire as a cause of death in the United States. However, fire continues to cause several thousand deaths annually. Also, larger-scale fires with mass casualties and wildfires that affect large geographic areas still occur occasionally.

PATHOGENESIS

Smoke loses heat rapidly as it traverses the upper airway, so direct thermal injury is often limited to the mucosa of the supraglottic airway. A notable exception is steam inhalation, which can produce thermal injury throughout the airways. Smoke inhalation injury affects the entire respiratory tract. The pathogenesis of smoke inhalation is complicated by the wide variety of pulmonary irritants in smoke, many of which are directly toxic to respiratory epithelial or alveolar cells: aldehydes such as acrolein, acetaldehyde, and formaldehyde; acids such as hydrochloric, hydrofluoric, and hydrocyanic acid; and ammonia, nitrogen oxides, and phosgene.

Irritants can rapidly induce intense neutrophilic inflammation, which evolves during 12 to 24 hours after injury and is characterized by mucosal edema and ulceration, abnormally increased permeability of pulmonary capillaries with resultant capillary leak, and epithelial, alveolar, and immune cellular dysfunction. Bronchospasm or bronchorrhea may occur, and the processes may result in ARDS. In addition, because oxygen is consumed in fires, breathing of hypoxic air for prolonged periods may potentiate other injuries or cause clinically significant hypoxia in its own right.

CLINICAL MANIFESTATIONS

Thermal injury to upper airway mucosa can cause airway compromise, particularly due to laryngeal edema, sometimes rapidly and sometimes after 12 to 24 hours. Burns to the face, mouth, and neck can externally damage and distort structures of the upper airway and cause airway compromise, both subacutely and late in the course. Inhalation injury manifests primarily with bronchospasm and bronchorrhea, which cause cough, dyspnea, or wheezing and may progress rapidly to respiratory failure. Accumulation of secretions, failure of mucociliary clearance and immune mechanisms, and epithelial necrosis predispose to pulmonary infection, particularly 3 to 5 days after injury. Late pulmonary complications can also be caused indirectly by eschar formation and restriction of thoracic motion.

DIAGNOSIS

Patients with apparent or suspected burn injuries (Chapter 112) should be assessed emergently for airway patency. Head or neck burns, respiratory distress, stridor, or visibly erythematous or edematous oral mucosa should prompt immediate laryngoscopic evaluation of the oropharynx and supraglottic airway. Hypoxemia may develop and may be severe enough to meet criteria for ARDS. Chest radiography should be performed serially to detect the evolution of lung injury or superinfection.

TREATMENT

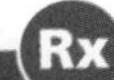

If airway patency is threatened, endotracheal intubation should be performed immediately. Delay can result in increased edema and greater technical difficulty of intubation. Patients who cannot be intubated should have emergent tracheostomy performed surgically. Because of the risk for ARDS, mechanical ventilation with a goal tidal volume of 3 to 6 mL/kg of ideal body weight should be considered. All patients should receive supplemental oxygen with the goal of providing a high fractional concentration of inspired oxygen (F_{IO_2}) to reverse the effects of hypoxia and carbon monoxide inhalation (see later).

Pulmonary toilet is essential to clear secretions in the face of bronchorrhea and epithelial sloughing. Because of the risk for superinfection, surveillance for infection should be vigilant, including diagnostic bronchoscopy if ventilator-associated pneumonia is suspected.

PROGNOSIS

Patients who survive burns and recover generally do not have long-term pulmonary sequelae. Tracheostomies placed at the time of injury can usually be removed later, unless airway structures are damaged or distorted. Impaired pulmonary function is uncommon but may be manifested as airway hyperresponsiveness that has been termed *reactive airway dysfunction syndrome.*

Carbon Monoxide Poisoning

DEFINITION AND EPIDEMIOLOGY

Carbon monoxide is a colorless, odorless gas produced by the combustion of carbon-based fuels. Because of the ubiquity of these substances, carbon monoxide inhalation is often coincident with smoke inhalation in fires or may occur accidentally in association with malfunctioning equipment or improper venting of emissions from heaters, stoves, combustion motors, or other similar devices. In addition, intentional inhalation of carbon monoxide is a method commonly used in suicide attempts (404). Carbon monoxide inhalation is the leading cause of death from poisoning (Chapter 110) worldwide.

PATHOBIOLOGY

Carbon monoxide readily diffuses across the alveolar-capillary interface and binds to hemoglobin with extremely high affinity. When the resulting carboxyhemoglobin molecule undergoes an allosteric change at oxygen-binding sites, the ability of bound oxygen to dissociate and to be delivered to peripheral tissues is greatly reduced. This tissue hypoxia can cause severe functional impairment and ischemic injury of oxygen-sensitive tissues, particularly in the brain and heart.

CLINICAL MANIFESTATIONS

Mild carbon monoxide intoxication may go unrecognized because the symptoms are nonspecific and may include headache, nausea, malaise, fatigue, and dizziness. With more severe intoxications, neuropsychiatric symptoms may range from minor disturbances in attention and cognition to agitation, confusion, hallucination, or, in the worst intoxications, seizures or frank coma. Physical findings, which are generally nonspecific, can include tachycardia or hyperthermia. The classic cherry-red skin thought to be associated with carbon monoxide intoxication is rarely seen. Other manifestations of severe intoxications may include lactic acidosis, cardiac dysfunction with arrhythmia or ischemia, pulmonary edema, and rhabdomyolysis.

DIAGNOSIS

A high index of suspicion is required for diagnosis because clinical findings are nonspecific. All patients known to have been involved in fires, suicide attempts, or other scenarios compatible with exposures should have arterial carboxyhemoglobin levels checked by co-oximetry. Although levels do not correlate well with clinical findings or risk for complications, symptoms generally occur at carboxyhemoglobin concentrations of 10% or higher.

TREATMENT Rx

All patients should be treated with 100% supplemental oxygen, which competes with carbon monoxide for hemoglobin-binding sites and gradually eliminates it from the blood. If patients require mechanical ventilation because of depressed neurologic status or respiratory problems, 100% oxygen should be administered by endotracheal tube. Treatment with hyperbaric oxygen at a pressure of 2.5 to 3.0 atm can increase the dissolved oxygen content of blood by more than ten-fold, and at least one treatment of approximately 2 hours should be considered in severe cases to reverse the effects of acute intoxication; three hyperbaric oxygen treatments within 24 hours of diagnosis reduce neurocognitive sequelae. A small, but intriguing, randomized trial of seven healthy volunteers examined normocapnic hyperpnea and CO elimination and showed that persons randomized to normocapnic hyperpnea (compared with those getting 100% O_2 at normal minute ventilation) had a significantly faster half-time of decrease in carboxyhemoglobin.

PROGNOSIS

The mortality rate is highly variable according to the severity of intoxication but can approach 30% in severe cases. Approximately two thirds of patients who survive acute intoxication will recover without sequelae. Many of the remainder will suffer from long-term neuropsychiatric symptoms including cognitive dysfunction, abnormal mood or affect, memory disturbances, and other motor or sensory abnormalities, which can often occur within the first month but may be delayed for up to 6 to 9 months.

Cyanide and Other Gases

PATHOBIOLOGY

In addition to carbon monoxide and pulmonary irritants, cyanide gas may be formed when a number of commonly found substances, particularly plastics and textiles, are combusted. This gas is highly toxic and can rapidly cause morbidity and death by binding to cytochrome enzymes and inhibiting cellular respiration.

Other inhaled gases that can injure the lungs in occupational settings include ammonia, chlorine, nitrogen dioxide, organic dust, paraquat, phosgene (which has also been used as a chemical weapon), sulfur dioxide, and toxic metal fumes such as cadmium and mercury.

CLINICAL MANIFESTATIONS AND DIAGNOSIS

Cyanide intoxication typically includes shock, lactic acidosis, and coma; it can rapidly lead to death before results of laboratory studies are available. In the setting of possible exposure, an elevated venous oxygen saturation indicates that cyanide is preventing cells from extracting oxygen from arterial blood.

Other inhaled gases that can produce potent irritant responses include ammonia, chlorine, and nitrogen dioxide ("silo-filler's lung"). Phosgene is notable for its propensity to cause delayed symptoms, up to 24 hours after exposure. Other inhalants may produce an acute chemical pneumonitis with respiratory distress (Chapter 93). A diverse group of inhaled toxins can cause syndromes of inhalational fever, including heavy metal fumes, polymer fumes, and organic dust aerosols that contain thermophilic bacteria, gram-negative bacteria and their associated endotoxins, and fungal elements. These inhalations are characterized by fever and malaise with mild respiratory symptoms and are also notable for tachyphylaxis with repeated exposure (and thus referred to as Monday morning fever in some professions).

TREATMENT Rx

Cyanide intoxication is treated by use of a Taylor Cyanide Antidote Package (Taylor Pharmaceuticals) that contains amyl nitrite gas ampules (one 0.3-mL ampule each minute until sodium nitrite infusion begins) for inhalation. This treatment is followed by intravenous administration of sodium nitrite (300 mg), which acts by converting hemoglobin to methemoglobin. Finally, patients are treated with intravenous sodium thiosulfate (12.5 g), which converts cyanide to less harmful thiocyanate ions. If carboxyhemoglobinemia is present, sodium thiosulfate should be used alone because of the additive toxicity of this condition with methemoglobinemia.

Hydroxocobalamin, which directly binds cyanide, can be used in conjunction with sodium thiosulfate. It is thought to be safer than the amyl nitrate gas ampules because it does not cause methemoglobinemia and is better suited to prehospital care.

The mainstay for treatment of other irritating inhalations is to remove the patient immediately from the toxic environment and to provide supportive care for respiratory injury. Depending on the intensity and duration of exposure, most patients will recover completely without sequelae.

OXYGEN TOXICITY

DEFINITION

Hypoxic respiratory failure often requires treatment with supplemental oxygen to maintain tissue oxygenation. In some settings, such as ARDS, patients may require high FIO_2 for prolonged periods to combat severe hypoxia. However, it has long been recognized that oxygen may be toxic to the lungs when it is present in concentrations higher than those found in ambient air.

PATHOBIOLOGY

When the concentration of oxygen in the airways is high, formation of reactive oxygen species and free radicals is increased. Under normal circumstances, innate antioxidant mechanisms in airway epithelia and alveoli are sufficient to abrogate the effect of these molecules. However, under conditions of critical illness, prolonged exposure to increased concentrations of these toxins may overwhelm these defenses. Superoxide, hydrogen peroxide, and hydroxyl radicals may directly oxidize cellular components. Cellular damage potentiates inflammation and may be synergistic with inflammatory processes already under way in the diseased lung; the result can be alveolar edema, formation of hyaline membranes, hypoxemia, and progression to fibrosis and obliteration of alveolar and capillary structures. In addition, washout of nitrogen from air spaces can result in absorptive atelectasis if oxygen is removed by the circulation faster than it can be replenished by ventilation (especially in the setting of ventilation-perfusion mismatch). Hyperoxia can also worsen hypercapnia through multiple mechanisms, as occurs in patients with chronic obstructive pulmonary disease who suffer from carbon dioxide retention.

CLINICAL MANIFESTATIONS AND DIAGNOSIS

Although the exact levels of hyperoxia that cause lung injury are unclear, it appears to occur with exposure to FIO_2 of 50 to 60% after exposures as short as 6 hours in duration. Because of the high flow of supplemental oxygen required to deliver this F_{IO_2}, oxygen toxicity is observed primarily in mechanically ventilated patients being treated for hypoxic respiratory failure. This level of exposure can cause a clinically detectable tracheobronchitis, demonstrable by symptoms of cough and dyspnea, as well as airway erythema that is visible macroscopically on bronchoscopy. This syndrome may impair mucociliary clearance and result in impaction of secretions, especially in conjunction with absorptive atelectasis.

Patients who may be susceptible to oxygen toxicity generally already have a significant degree of parenchymal injury from other processes. Thus, although some patients may appear to display a syndrome of worsening air space disease, atelectasis, consolidation, hypoxia, and diffuse alveolar damage, it is not clear when these changes are related to oxygen therapy or merely occur as part of the acute lung injury from other causes.

TREATMENT Rx

Because the threshold level for oxygen toxicity is unknown, a general guideline for treatment of hypoxemic respiratory failure (Chapter 104) is that patients be ventilated with the lowest possible F_{IO_2} that is required to restore an acceptable oxygen saturation. An Sa_{O_2} of 90%, corresponding to Pa_{O_2} of 55 to 60 mm Hg, is generally considered the minimum acceptable level. Unfortunately, under conditions of severe hypoxia, as in ARDS, patients often require an F_{IO_2} approaching 100% to achieve this oxygen level. Maneuvers to improve oxygenation without increasing F_{IO_2} include red blood cell transfusions to improve the delivery of oxygen; alternative ventilatory strategies, such as high-frequency oscillatory ventilation, airway pressure-release ventilation, inverse-ratio ventilation, and prone positioning; and alveolar recruitment maneuvers using positive end-expiratory pressure or transiently increased inflation pressures (Chapter 105).

PROGNOSIS

Patients who sustain oxygen toxicity in the setting of prior bleomycin exposure may be left with residual pulmonary fibrosis. In other patients, the incremental impact of oxygen toxicity on prognosis is unknown.

LUNG INJURY

Radiation Lung Injury

DEFINITION

Accidental or occupational radiation exposures (Chapter 19) are generally characterized by systemic toxicity that outweighs any injury to the lungs. As such, radiation lung injury refers to a pneumonitis that can progress to pulmonary fibrosis and that results from therapeutic use of ionizing radiation, usually in the treatment of malignant neoplasms.

EPIDEMIOLOGY

As many as 50% of patients receiving thoracic radiation will display radiographic abnormalities after treatment; duration and dose of therapy affect the odds for development of lung injury. However, most of these patients will never have clinically significant radiation lung injury. For unclear reasons, the incidence of lung injury appears to vary by the type of underlying malignant disease and modality of treatment. The highest frequency appears to be found in patients with lung cancer (10 to 15%).

PATHOBIOLOGY AND CLINICAL MANIFESTATIONS

The pathogenesis of radiation lung injury is often divided into three or four phases on the basis of time course. Typically, the early phase occurs immediately after exposure and is characterized by injury to alveolar cells, resulting in mild alveolitis, recruitment of inflammatory cells, capillary leak, and pulmonary edema. These changes are usually asymptomatic; patients do not usually come to clinical attention, although the chest radiograph will be abnormal if it is performed. In most patients, these changes resolve without progression within 1 to 3 months.

A minority of patients will progress to the next phase, in which alveolar cells desquamate and the air spaces fill with protein-rich fluid. In this phase, referred to as radiation pneumonitis, patients complain of cough, dyspnea, and occasionally fever or pleuritic chest pain. Severe cases may present with hypoxemic respiratory failure. This phase generally resolves within 3 to 6 months after exposure and is followed by an organizing phase, in which alveolar edema resolves and the damaged alveoli heal. Clinically, patients generally show improvement in symptoms during this period. However, this phase is also characterized by fibroblast proliferation and deposition of collagen in the lung. In a minority of patients, this process will proceed unchecked and result in clinically significant fibrosis, with progressive loss of alveolar-capillary surface and development of restrictive lung disease.

DIAGNOSIS

Clinical history and radiographic evaluation are often sufficient for diagnosis of radiation lung injury because patients typically present with respiratory symptoms and opacities on chest radiography after undergoing radiation therapy. Radiography may show air space disease with alveolar filling or consolidation during the pneumonitis phase, which may progress to an interstitial pattern and eventual honeycombing with parenchymal distortion in the chronic phase. Because radiation characteristically causes injury only within directly affected lung tissue, radiography may show opacities that are well delineated and form straight lines that cross anatomically distinct regions of lung. This finding is rarely if ever seen in other conditions.

The differential diagnosis may include pneumonia, recurrence, and metastatic malignant disease. On occasion, invasive evaluation with bronchoalveolar lavage or even biopsy is required to exclude these possibilities if the clinical history and imaging do not provide a diagnosis.

TREATMENT AND PREVENTION Rx

Corticosteroids such as prednisone, 1 mg/kg body weight/day followed by a slow taper over several weeks or months, are the mainstay of therapy. Patients often show a dramatic response to treatment, and symptoms may recur after treatment is discontinued. Other immunosuppressive agents have been used successfully in case reports of patients who failed to respond to corticosteroids. Prophylactic amifostine, a cytoprotective agent (340 mg/m^2 given 15 minutes before irradiation), significantly reduces the risk for radiation pneumonitis in patients who receive radiation treatment for lung cancer. 

PROGNOSIS

Within 2 years after initial exposure, progression will usually slow, and symptoms and lung function will stabilize and improve. After this time, further improvement or worsening is uncommon. In severe cases that become chronic, patients may develop features of advanced interstitial lung disease, including pulmonary hypertension and hypoxic respiratory failure.

Aspiration Injury

DEFINITION

Aspiration, which is defined as the inhalation of any nongaseous foreign substance into the lungs, generally refers specifically to the inhalation of gastric contents or secretions from the oropharynx. Aspiration is a common occurrence, and in most cases it resolves spontaneously without clinical manifestations. Clinically significant aspiration can range from acute pneumonitis and respiratory failure caused by a single massive aspiration to chronic symptoms of respiratory disease caused by recurrent small-scale aspiration. These syndromes may overlap with pneumonia that occurs when the lungs are exposed to bacteria from the gastrointestinal tract (Chapter 97).

PATHOBIOLOGY

The common element of clinically significant aspiration is impairment of normal airway protective mechanisms. Under normal circumstances, the airway is protected by the normal swallowing mechanism, the cough reflex, and the anatomy of the supraglottic airway. However, even healthy individuals experience microaspiration despite having functional protective mechanisms. These secretions are handled by normal pulmonary clearance mechanisms.

Any disturbance of these protective mechanisms can result in aspiration injury to the lungs. An altered level of consciousness can impair normal swallowing and suppress the cough reflex. Even in patients who are alert, neurologic injury can result in dysphagia and concomitant aspiration, as in patients who have bulbar neurologic deficits in association with ischemic stroke. Patients with altered airway or oropharyngeal anatomy, such as patients who have received surgical or radiation therapy for head and neck malignant neoplasms, may also be highly susceptible to aspiration of oral secretions.

The nature of the aspirated material is also important in determining whether an injury occurs. Materials with a pH lower than 2.5, such as acidic gastric contents, are much more likely to cause a significant chemical pneumonitis.

Particulate matter also increases the likelihood for development of clinically significant inflammation. A large-volume aspiration with distribution throughout the lungs is more likely to produce an acute, severe pneumonitis.

Once material has been aspirated into the lungs, the injury that occurs is similar to a chemical burn. Acid rapidly injures airway epithelial and alveolar cells; within hours, cells become dysfunctional and capillary leak occurs, resulting in profound noncardiogenic pulmonary edema. In severe cases, diffuse alveolar damage may result.

CLINICAL MANIFESTATIONS

The classic eponym applied to aspiration pneumonia is Mendelsohn's syndrome, which refers to a single, large-volume aspiration of gastric contents followed by rapidly progressive hypoxemic respiratory failure that develops within hours. Patients may suffer from cough, dyspnea, fever, and respiratory distress. Physical examination may reveal diffuse crackles, wheezing, cyanosis, and hypotension. Chest radiography may show a pattern of alveolar filling with diffuse bilateral involvement or involvement of dependent regions, particularly the right lower lobe. In many patients, this period of acute deterioration is followed by stabilization and resolution within 2 or 3 days. In other patients, deterioration may continue, and patients may meet clinical criteria for ARDS. If the volume of aspirated material is large enough, the initial aspiration may be sufficient to cause tracheal obstruction and asphyxiation.

In patients who initially improve, a small percentage will show further deterioration after 2 or 3 days. This deterioration should prompt an investigation for bacterial superinfection.

DIAGNOSIS

The clinical history and presentation are generally sufficient for diagnosis of aspiration pneumonitis. Bacterial pneumonia and other causes of ARDS also should be considered, as should cardiogenic pulmonary edema. Airway erythema and edema on bronchoscopy can be suggestive of aspiration. Bronchoalveolar lavage may help evaluate for the presence of bacterial infection.

PREVENTION

Prevention should focus on identification of patients who are at risk for aspiration and then use of strategies to minimize the risk. Patients with swallowing dysfunction or airway abnormalities can work with speech pathologists to learn effective strategies for swallowing. Patients who are unsuccessful or not suitable for this approach may benefit from tracheostomy or enteral tube feedings, which do not prevent microaspiration but can prevent large-volume aspiration. In hospitalized patients, particularly patients with an altered mental status due to illness or sedation, simple strategies such as avoidance of oral feeding and semirecumbent positioning can effectively reduce the risk for aspiration. Use of histamine-2 blockers or proton pump inhibitors (Chapter 141) can alter gastric pH to reduce the risk for injury from acidic secretions.

TREATMENT Rx

Because of the acuity and severity of aspiration pneumonitis, immediate attention should be paid to maintaining a patent airway. The oropharynx and trachea should be suctioned to clear any potentially obstructing material, and endotracheal intubation should be performed if necessary (Chapter 105). Bronchoscopy is often performed to clear residual particulate or solid matter, but it cannot remove acidic secretions, which damage airways and parenchyma quickly and then are rendered neutral. Oxygen supplementation should be provided as needed for hypoxia. Corticosteroids have not been shown to be beneficial. Antibiotics should be reserved for patients who appear to have developed bacterial superinfection (Chapter 97).

PROGNOSIS

For patients with severe respiratory failure or ARDS, mortality can be high. In others, improvement should be expected within days. If the underlying factor that led to aspiration is irreversible, patients have an increased likelihood of recurrent episodes.

Lipoid Pneumonia

DEFINITION

Lipoid pneumonia is a chronic inflammatory reaction of the lungs to the presence of lipid substances. Exogenous lipoid pneumonia results from the aspiration of vegetable, animal, or (most commonly) mineral oils.

PATHOBIOLOGY

The most frequently implicated agent is mineral oil used as a laxative and to reduce dysphagia, either in clear liquid form or as petroleum jelly. Mineral oil is bland and, when introduced into the pharynx, can enter the bronchial tree without eliciting the cough reflex. It also mechanically impedes the ciliary action of the airway epithelium. The risk for mineral oil aspiration is increased in debilitated or senile patients, in those with neurologic disease that interferes with deglutition, and in patients with esophageal disease. Mineral oil taken as nose drops to relieve nasal dryness can also cause lipoid pneumonia. Inhalation of mineral oil mist by airplane and automobile mechanics has also been implicated as a cause.

Mineral oils, which cannot be hydrolyzed in the body, provoke a chronic inflammatory reaction that may not become clinically overt until years later. In the alveolar spaces, macrophages accumulate and phagocytose the emulsified oil. Some macrophages disintegrate, releasing their lysosomal enzymes and oil. The alveolar septa become thickened and edematous, containing lymphocytes and lipid-laden macrophages. Oil droplets are seen in the pulmonary lymphatics and hilar nodes. Later, fibrosis develops, and the normal lung architecture is effaced. A single pathologic specimen may include both the early inflammatory and the later fibrotic picture, in keeping with repetitive aspirations during many months or years. Nodular lesions may grossly resemble tumor and be called paraffinomas.

CLINICAL MANIFESTATIONS

Most patients are asymptomatic and come to the physician's attention because of an abnormal chest radiograph. When patients are symptomatic, cough and exertional dyspnea are the most frequent complaints. Chest pain (sometimes pleuritic), hemoptysis, fever (usually low grade), chills, night sweats, and weight loss may occur. Findings on physical examination may be completely normal, but fever, tachypnea, dullness on percussion of the chest, bronchial or bronchovesicular breath sounds, rales, and rhonchi may be found. Clubbing and cor pulmonale are rare.

DIAGNOSIS

In mild lipoid pneumonia, arterial blood gas values may be normal with the patient at rest but may show hypoxemia after exercise. In more severe disease, resting hypoxemia, hypocapnia, and mild respiratory alkalosis develop. Pulmonary function testing reveals a restrictive ventilatory defect; lung compliance is decreased. The only specific laboratory finding is the presence in sputum of macrophages with clusters of vacuoles that are 5 to 50 μm in diameter and that stain deep orange with Sudan IV; extracellular droplets may stain similarly.

On radiographic examination, the earliest abnormalities are air space infiltrates, most often in the dependent portions of the lung. The infiltrates may be unilateral or bilateral, localized or diffuse. Air bronchograms may be seen. Hilar adenopathy and pleural reaction are rare. As fibrosis develops, volume loss occurs, and linear and nodular infiltrates appear. A solid lesion that closely resembles bronchogenic carcinoma may develop. High-resolution computed tomography usually shows consolidated areas of low attenuation and "crazy paving" (Fig. 94-1).

The differential diagnosis is extensive, particularly in the late phase, when multiple other causes of pulmonary fibrosis must be considered. The key to the correct diagnosis before biopsy is the history of chronic oral or intranasal use of an oil- or a lipid-based product or an occupational exposure to oil mists. The presence of lipid-laden macrophages in sputum or bronchoalveolar lavage fluid also can be used to confirm the diagnosis, particularly in conjunction with typical findings on high-resolution computed tomography.

TREATMENT AND PREVENTION Rx

Once the diagnosis has been made and the aspiration stopped, the subsequent course is variable. Because the only way the lung can dispose of mineral oil is by expectoration, the patient should be instructed in coughing exercises to be performed many times each day for months. Expectorants have not been shown to help. In some uncontrolled case reports, systemic corticosteroids at varying doses and durations have been associated with a successful outcome, but they cannot be routinely recommended for treatment.

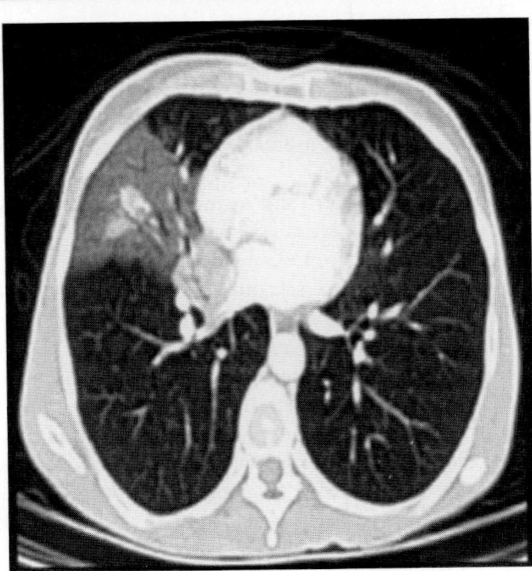

FIGURE 94-1. Lipoid pneumonia on a computed tomographic scan.

Transfusion-Related Acute Lung Injury

DEFINITION

The syndrome of transfusion-related acute lung injury (TRALI; Chapter 180) involves the rapid onset of respiratory distress within minutes to hours after the transfusion of blood products (fresh-frozen plasma, platelets, and red blood cells). The initial clinical picture is indistinguishable from acute lung injury or ARDS due to other causes, such as sepsis, multiple trauma, and lung injury. TRALI may similarly be confused with pulmonary edema due to volume overload (Chapter 58).

EPIDEMIOLOGY

The true incidence of TRALI is unknown; incidence rates are underestimated because of the difficulty in distinguishing TRALI from other causes of acute respiratory failure and the labor-intensive and costly diagnostic evaluation required. Reported incidences range from 1 in 1000 to 1 in 100,000 units of blood products transfused. The risk for TRALI varies according to the type of blood product transfused, with pooled products associated with a higher incidence. Only 8 to 21 TRALI-related deaths are reported to the U.S. Food and Drug Administration annually, and even liberal estimates accounting for under-reporting suggest the number may be only as high as 300 per year of an estimated 25 million transfusions in the United States.

PATHOBIOLOGY

The physiologic manifestations of TRALI are caused by alveolar filling with fluid and protein. This alveolar process is the result of increased microvascular permeability due to pulmonary endothelial damage mediated by either leukocyte antibodies or the priming and activation of neutrophils in the pulmonary circulation by bioactive substances.

TRALI most commonly occurs when human leukocyte antigen (HLA) type I or II or neutrophil-specific antigen antibodies from the donor attach to the recipient's leukocytes, leading to the release of injurious oxidative and nonoxidative products. Development of HLA antibodies occurs commonly in women during pregnancy, and increasing parity in female blood donors is associated with an increased risk for TRALI.

Episodes of TRALI occurring in patients without HLA or neutrophil-specific antigen antibodies in either the donor or recipient are thought to be caused by a two-hit process of neutrophil priming and activation. Neutrophils are primed and sequestered in the lung by conditions that often occur in patients requiring blood products, such as multiple trauma, surgery, or sepsis. Primed neutrophils are then activated by bioactive lipids and cytokines stored in the blood products, thereby leading to lung injury and alveolar damage. Levels of these bioactive lipids or cytokines may increase after prolonged storage of blood products.

CLINICAL MANIFESTATIONS

Although most cases of TRALI present within 1 to 2 hours after the transfusion of blood products, tachypnea, hypoxemia, cyanosis, dyspnea, and fever can develop during the transfusion or up to 6 hours later. Hypertension or hypotension commonly occurs, depending on the severity of the reaction. Copious amounts of pink, frothy edema fluid may be present. Lung auscultation generally reveals bilateral crackles and decreased breath sounds in dependent lung zones.

DIAGNOSIS

Bilateral patchy infiltrates consistent with alveolar edema are found on plain chest radiographs, typically without effusions. Arterial blood gas analysis demonstrates reduced PO_2, and further laboratory testing may reveal thrombocytopenia or a transient leukopenia. Diagnosis of TRALI requires the presence of the following: acute onset of hypoxemia with PaO_2/FIO_2 of 300 or less, or room air oxygen saturation less than 90% during or within 6 hours after a transfusion; bilateral infiltrates on the chest radiograph; no evidence of left atrial hypertension; no preexisting acute lung injury before transfusion; and no temporal relationship to an alternative risk factor for acute lung injury.

The diagnosis of "possible TRALI" is made in patients who have a concurrent diagnosis of another risk factor for acute lung injury, including (1) direct lung injury due to aspiration, pneumonia, toxic inhalation, lung contusion, or nonfatal drowning; and (2) indirect lung injury due to severe sepsis, shock, multiple trauma, burn injury, acute pancreatitis, cardiopulmonary bypass, or drug overdose. Absolute confirmation of the diagnosis requires testing for HLA and neutrophil-specific antigen antibodies, usually performed first in female donors, then in male donors, and finally in the recipient.

TREATMENT

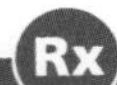

Most cases are self-limited and resolve within hours to days with supplemental oxygen and supportive care. Volume resuscitation, with or without vasopressors, is required for hypotension. Mechanical ventilation should be managed as for any other case of acute lung injury, with the implementation of a low tidal volume ventilation strategy to prevent further ventilator-induced lung injury. Diuresis should be attempted cautiously and may even be detrimental because intravascular filling pressures are often low.

PROGNOSIS

The mortality rate of TRALI is approximately 5%. If an implicated donor can be identified, the recipient should not receive any further transfusions from that donor, but patients are not at increased risk for further episodes of TRALI from nonimplicated donor transfusions.

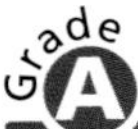

1. van Patot MC, Leadbetter G 3rd, Keyes LE, et al. Prophylactic low-dose acetazolamide reduces the incidence and severity of acute mountain sickness. *High Alt Med Biol.* 2008;9:289-293.
2. Fischler M, Maggiorini M, Dorschner L, et al. Dexamethasone but not tadalafil improves exercise capacity in adults prone to high-altitude pulmonary edema. *Am J Respir Crit Care Med.* 2009;180:346-352.
3. Sartori C, Allemann Y, Duplain H, et al. Salmeterol for the prevention of high-altitude pulmonary edema. *N Engl J Med.* 2002;346:1631-1636.
4. Jafarian S, Gorouhi F, Salimi S, et al. Sumatriptan for prevention of acute mountain sickness: randomized clinical trial. *Ann Neurol.* 2007;62:273-277.
5. Ghofrani HA, Reichenberger F, Kohstall MG, et al. Sildenafil increased exercise capacity during hypoxia at low altitudes and at Mount Everest base camp: a randomized, double-blind, placebo-controlled crossover trial. *Ann Intern Med.* 2004;141:169-177.
6. Küpper TE, Strohl KP, Hoefer M, et al. Low-dose theophylline reduces symptoms of acute mountain sickness. *J Travel Med.* 2008;15:307-314.
7. Richalet JP, Rivera-Ch M, Maignan M, et al. Acetazolamide for Monge's disease: efficiency and tolerance of 6-month treatment. *Am J Respir Crit Care Med.* 2008;177:1370-1376.
8. Bennett MH, Lehm JP, Mitchell SJ, et al. Recompression and adjunctive therapy for decompression illness: a systematic review of randomized controlled trials. *Anesth Analg.* 2010;111:757-762.
9. Sasse AD, Clark LG, Sasse EC, et al. Amifostine reduces side effects and improves complete response rate during radiotherapy: results of a meta-analysis. *Int J Radiat Oncol Biol Phys.* 2006;64:784-791.

SUGGESTED READINGS

Divers Alert Network. Available at *http://www.diversalertnetwork.org/index.asp. This website includes a link to a 24-hour hotline for diving emergencies.*

Nasrullah M, Muazzam S. Drowning mortality in the United States, 1999-2006. *J Community Health.* 2011;36:69-75. *About 3500 Americans drown annually, with males and minorities most at risk.*

Sololovic M, Pastores SM. Transfusion therapy and acute lung injury. *Expert Rev Respir Med.* 2010;4:387-393. *Review.*

95

SARCOIDOSIS

MICHAEL IANNUZZI

DEFINITION

Sarcoidosis, a systemic granulomatous disease of unknown cause, is characterized by a variable clinical presentation and course. More than 90% of patients exhibit thoracic involvement with mediastinal and hilar lymph node enlargement or parenchymal lung disease, but any organ may be involved. The presentation and course vary from asymptomatic disease with spontaneous resolution to organ system failure and even death.

EPIDEMIOLOGY

Sarcoidosis occurs worldwide, affects people of all racial and ethnic groups, and may present at any age. Sarcoidosis usually develops before the age of 50 years with the incidence peaking at 20 to 39 years. The incidence of sarcoidosis fluctuates throughout the world, most likely because of differences in the presentation of the disease and the surveillance methods used. The annual incidence of sarcoidosis is highest in northern European countries, where it is 5 to 40 cases per 100,000 people. The incidence in Japan is about 1 to 2 cases per 100,000 people. In the United States, the adjusted annual incidence among black Americans is about 3.5 times higher than among white Americans (35.5 cases per 100,000 compared with 10.9 per 100,000). Regardless of ethnic or racial group, sarcoidosis affects women more often. The reportedly low incidence in certain regions such as Africa, China, India, and Russia may be due to decreased access to health care, minimal surveillance, and misdiagnosis of sarcoidosis as tuberculosis or leprosy.

Black women in the United States have the highest lifetime risk of developing sarcoidosis (2.7%). In both black men and women, sarcoidosis occurs later in life, peaks in the fourth decade, and is more likely to be chronic and fatal. Socioeconomic status does not affect the incidence of sarcoidosis, but low income and other financial barriers to care are associated with more severe sarcoidosis, even after adjustment for age, sex, and race or ethnic group.

Sarcoidosis clusters in families and monozygotic twins are more often concordant for disease than are dizygotic twins. Familial sarcoidosis occurs in 10% of cases from the Netherlands, 7.5% from Germany, 6% from the United Kingdom, 4.7% from Finland, and 0.8% from Spain. In the United States, sarcoidosis patients are five times as likely to have siblings or parents with sarcoidosis as control subjects. However, less than 1% of the first-degree relatives of patients with sarcoidosis are affected, so screening for disease in asymptomatic relatives is ineffective.

PATHOBIOLOGY

The development and accumulation of granulomas represent the basic pathologic abnormality in sarcoidosis. Sarcoidal granulomas are tightly organized collections of macrophages and macrophage-derived epithelioid cells encircled by lymphocytes. Fused epithelioid cells, which become multinucleated giant cells, are often found scattered throughout the granuloma. This appearance suggests that the granuloma is meant to contain an inciting agent, but no such agent has been identified.

Granuloma formation begins with HLA-mediated processing of antigens by macrophages. T-cell activation follows, with oligoclonal expansion of $CD4^+$ (helper-inducer) lymphocytes. These $CD4^+$ cells, primarily of the T_H1 phenotype, produce interleukin-2 (IL-2) and interferon-γ (IFN-γ). A complex interplay of cytokines, along with macrophage-derived tumor necrosis factor-α, organizes the inflammatory cells into granulomas. In some cases, fibroblasts and collagen encase the granulomas with subsequent fibrosis. Fibrosis has been associated with a shift in the involved lymphocytes from the T_H1 (IL-2 and IFN-γ) to the T_H2 phenotype (IL-4, -10, and -13). This fibrotic process irreversibly alters organ architecture and function. Increased 1-α hydroxylase activity in macrophages within granulomas and the alveoli converts 25-hydroxyvitamin D to the biologically active form 1,25-dihydroxyvitamin D (calcitriol), thereby resulting in increased intestinal absorption of calcium.

In sarcoidosis, an immune paradox exists: patients often develop anergy as indicated by a suppressed response to tuberculin, despite active granulomatous inflammation. This anergy results in part from an expansion of $CD25^{bright}$ regulatory T cells, which are a subgroup of $CD4^+$ T lymphocytes and which can abolish production of IL-2 and inhibit T-cell proliferation. Although sarcoidosis is predominantly a T-cell-driven disease, the presence of polyclonal hyperglobulinemia indicates that B lymphocytes may also play a role.

Multiple inciting agents rather than a single pathogen are likely to cause sarcoidosis. Airborne antigens are suspected because the lungs, followed by the eyes and skin, are the most commonly involved organs. A microbial origin of the antigens is favored because sarcoidosis occurs sporadically in clusters and is worldwide. Furthermore, sarcoidosis may recur in transplanted organs and can develop in recipients of tissues from donors with sarcoidosis.

Several environmental exposures are modestly associated with the risk for sarcoidosis, each with odds ratios of about 1.5: mold or mildew, musty odors at work, agricultural employment, and pesticide-using industries. Highly sensitive methods for detecting microbial DNA and proteins, such as polymerase chain reaction and mass spectrometry, have yielded potential etiologic agents. One promising candidate of microbial origin is the mycobacterial KatG protein.

Major histocompatibility complex (MHC) genes and non-MHC genes located on the short arm of chromosome 6p have been implicated as genetic risk factors for sarcoidosis. HLA-DQB1*0201 and HLA-DRB1*0301 alleles are strongly associated with acute disease and good prognosis. The HLA-DRB1*1501/DQB1*0602 haplotype predicts a chronic course and severe pulmonary sarcoidosis. Genome-wide scans have identified the gene candidates *BTNL2* (butyrophilin-like 2 gene) and *ANXA11* (annexin A11).

CLINICAL MANIFESTATIONS

Patients may present with any organ involved, with or without concomitant intrathoracic involvement. The severity of symptoms and organ dysfunction also varies, and as many as 30 to 50% of patients have no symptoms at the time of diagnosis. Clinical manifestations also vary by ethnicity, race, and sex as well as by the particular organ system predominantly affected.

Sarcoidosis often first comes to attention during routine screening when enlarged mediastinal and hilar lymph nodes are detected on a chest radiograph (Fig. 95-1). Symptomatic individuals commonly experience fatigue, night sweats, and weight loss. Fatigue often remains a prominent problem and can lead to impaired quality of life.

Symptomatic sarcoidosis may present insidiously or as an acute illness. Löfgren's syndrome, an acute form of the disease, consists of erythema nodosum (see Fig. 448-23 in Chapter 448), arthritis, and bilateral hilar adenopathy. Fever and uveitis may also accompany Löfgren's syndrome. Erythema nodosum occurs predominantly in women, whereas arthritis predominates in men.

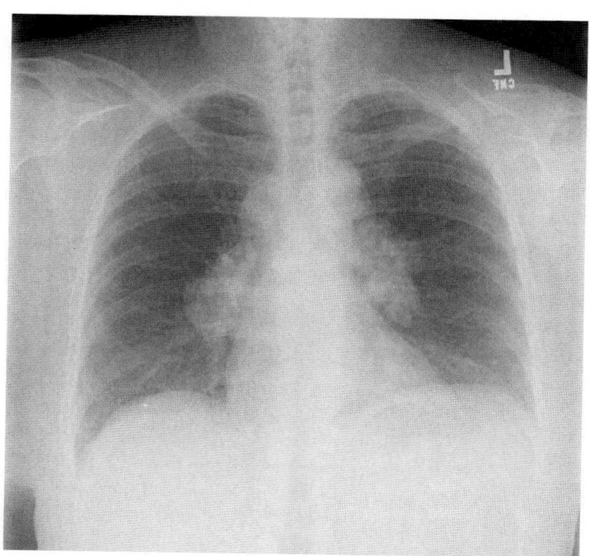

FIGURE 95-1. Chest radiograph demonstrating a stage I disease with enlarged mediastinal and hilar lymph nodes.

Respiratory System Disease

More than 90% of patients have respiratory tract involvement, sometimes with symptoms and sometimes with asymptomatic radiographic abnormalities. The most common respiratory symptoms are dry cough and dyspnea. Chest pain, when present, is vague and nonspecific.

Upper respiratory tract involvement occurs in from 2 to 6% of patients, with most having nasal mucosal involvement. Severe upper respiratory tract disease may lead to anosmia, erosion of septal cartilage, and nasal deformity. Supraglottic and glottic involvement can lead to stridor, dysphonia, cough, and dysphagia.

Examination of the chest often reveals few or no findings. Localized wheezing suggests endobronchial granulomatous disease, whereas diffuse wheezing suggests hyperreactive airways disease. Crackles may be heard when bronchiectasis and fibrosis are present. Hemoptysis may occur with bronchiectasis or cavitary disease.

The most common radiographic finding is intrathoracic lymph node enlargement with or without parenchymal lung involvement. Mediastinal lymphadenopathy without hilar adenopathy is extremely rare. Hilar lymph node enlargement is usually symmetrical, and less than 3% of patients have unilateral enlargement. Concurrent enlargement of right paratracheal and aortic-pulmonary window lymph nodes is common.

The chest radiograph is traditionally categorized into five stages (Table 95-1), but these stages do not necessarily denote the severity or chronologic progression of disease, particularly when extrathoracic involvement is present. Furthermore, 50 to 94% of patients will have hilar or mediastinal lymphadenopathy on computed tomographic (CT) scans irrespective of their stage on a plain chest radiograph.

Chest CT may demonstrate nodules, ground-glass opacities, bronchiectasis, cysts, and thickening of the pleural surface (Fig. 95-2). CT scanning, however, generally adds little to diagnosis and management, particularly for those with a stage I chest radiograph. CT scanning can be justified when atypical clinical and chest radiographic findings are present, a normal chest radiograph is found during the evaluation of suspected extrathoracic disease, or complications are suspected.

Endobronchial sarcoidosis may lead to bronchial stenosis and recurrent obstructive pneumonias. Pleural effusions on plain radiography are uncommon (1 to 3% of patients). Pulmonary hypertension (Chapter 68) may complicate sarcoidosis, particularly when pulmonary fibrosis is present.

TABLE 95-1 CHEST RADIOGRAPHIC STAGING

Stage 0: Normal
Stage 1: Bilateral hilar adenopathy, often with right paratracheal adenopathy
Stage 2: Bilateral hilar adenopathy and parenchymal infiltration
Stage 3: Parenchymal infiltration without lymphadenopathy
Stage 4: Advanced parenchymal disease demonstrating fibrosis and may include honeycombing, cysts, bullae, and traction bronchiectasis

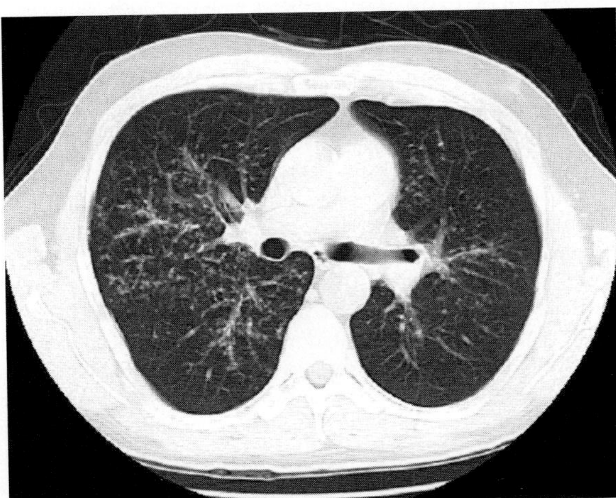

FIGURE 95-2. High-resolution chest computed tomography scan demonstrating numerous small nodules in a predominantly bronchovascular distribution.

Skin Disease

Skin involvement occurs in 25 to 35% of patients, but lesions are commonly misdiagnosed because they can present as macules, papules, plaques, subcutaneous lesions, areas of increased or decreased pigmentation, and ulcerations. Lesions are commonly found on the upper back, the nape of the neck, and extremities (Fig. 95-3) and have a predilection for scars and tattoos. The most common skin manifestation is a maculopapular eruption, consisting of firm, flesh-colored to violaceous lesions that have a predilection for the eyelids and perioral area. Scalp involvement with alopecia may occur. Skin lesions in black American patients frequently leave scars and pale or depigmented areas.

Erythema nodosum occurs in about 10% of patients and commonly occurs as part of Löfgren's syndrome. It presents as raised, red, hot, tender subcutaneous nodular lesions, most commonly on the shins, but sometimes also on the arms and buttocks (see Fig. 448-3 in Chapter 448). Lesions persist for 1 to 3 weeks and may recur. The lesions of erythema nodosum typically show nonspecific septal panniculitis without sarcoidal granulomas, so biopsy is not usually helpful. Erythema nodosum portends a good prognosis, with up to 85% of patients resolving their sarcoidosis within 2 years.

Lupus pernio (Fig. 95-4) consists of chronic, lumpy, violaceous, indurated plaques and nodules distributed around the nose, cheeks, lips, and ears; it is specific to sarcoidosis. Patients with lupus pernio more commonly have a chronic course, fibrotic lung disease, and upper respiratory tract involvement.

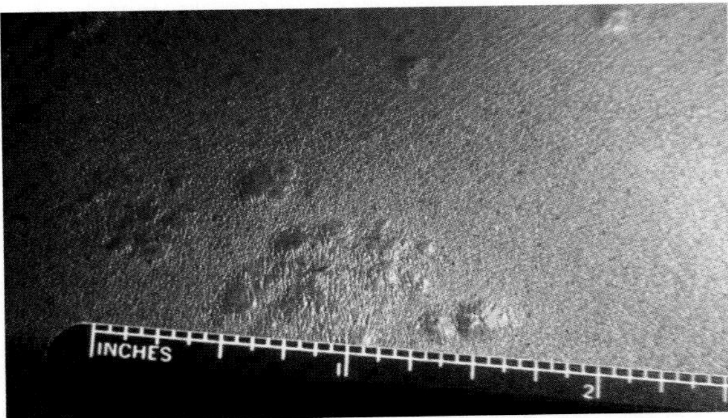

FIGURE 95-3. **Skin lesions of sarcoidosis.** Sarcoidal lesions may occur at any site. This patient's papules have a waxy appearance and are located on the upper part of the back.

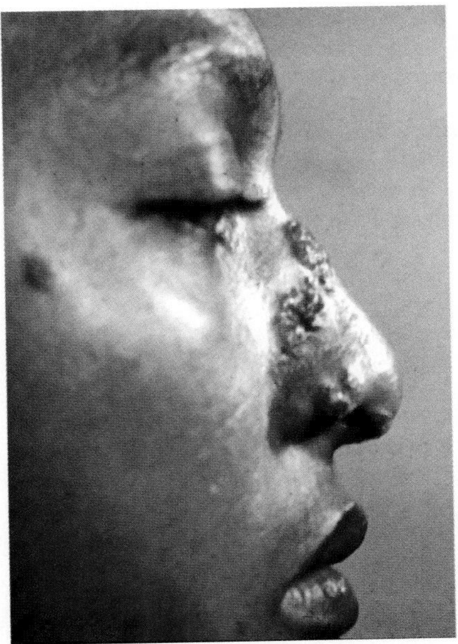

FIGURE 95-4. Lupus pernio is the term used to describe infiltrative skin lesions affecting the nose, cheeks, and ears in chronic sarcoidosis.

Eye Disease

More than 25% of patients have ocular involvement (Chapter 431), and any part of the eye and adnexa may be involved. Lacrimal gland enlargement and conjunctival involvement are common. Conjunctival involvement consists of pale yellow nodules, which demonstrate granulomas on biopsy. Corneal involvement is rare. Acute anterior uveitis presents with pain, photophobia, lacrimation, and redness. Chronic anterior uveitis, which is more common than acute uveitis, may have minimal symptoms. Posterior uveitis, which occurs in about 30% of patients with ocular sarcoidosis, is frequently accompanied by central nervous system involvement. Choroidal lesions may occur anywhere in the fundus and may be multifocal. In 10 to 15% of patients with uveitis, both the anterior and posterior segments are affected.

Uveitis can herald the nonocular signs of sarcoidosis and may precede the diagnosis of sarcoidosis by decades. Chronic anterior uveitis may lead to cataracts and glaucoma. Heerfordt's syndrome consists of anterior uveitis accompanied by parotid gland enlargement and fever.

Cardiac Disease

Cardiac granulomas are found in about 25% of sarcoidosis patients who are examined at autopsy, but cardiac sarcoidosis is suspected in only about 5% of patients. In cardiac sarcoidosis (Chapter 60), granulomas most often infiltrate the left ventricular free wall. Next most frequently, sarcoidal granulomas infiltrate the intraventricular septum, where they often involve the conduction system. Cardiac manifestations include atrioventricular block, ventricular arrhythmias, left ventricular dysfunction, and sudden death.

Neurologic Disease

Nervous system granulomas are found in up to 25% of sarcoidosis patients who undergo autopsy, but only 10% of patients present with neurologic symptoms (Table 95-2). In patients with neurologic involvement, the neurologic signs or symptoms precede the diagnosis of sarcoidosis in up to 75% of patients and may be the only manifestation of sarcoidosis.

Neurosarcoidosis has a predilection for the base of the brain, hypothalamus, and pituitary gland. Myelopathy may occur anywhere in the spinal cord and carries a poor prognosis. Peripheral neuropathy (Chapter 428) may manifest as mononeuropathy or polyneuropathy.

Liver and Spleen

Liver involvement is twice as common in black Americans as in white Americans. Symptoms due to liver disease are infrequent, but abdominal pain and pruritus are the most common symptoms. Fever, weight loss, and jaundice are present in less than 5% of those with liver involvement. About 20% of patients will have hepatomegaly on physical examination, and 35% will have an elevated serum aminotransferase or alkaline phosphatase level. Sarcoidosis can rarely (<1%) cause progressive liver disease that leads to portal hypertension with variceal bleeding; the hepatopulmonary syndrome, with refractory hypoxemia, cirrhosis, and liver failure, may also occur.

Splenomegaly is found on physical examination in 5 to 15% of patients with sarcoidosis. Massive splenomegaly is rare.

Bone and Joint

Most patients complain of arthralgias, but only about 35% develop arthritis. Acute sarcoid arthritis (Chapter 283) consists of large joint periarthritis, particularly involving the ankles and knees, and commonly occurs with Löfgren's syndrome. These patients often report difficulty walking related to joint pain. Acute sarcoid arthritis usually persists for up to 3 months but is self-limited. Chronic sarcoid arthritis with direct granulomatous synovial infiltration is rare. Osseous sarcoidosis usually does not produce symptoms.

TABLE 95-2 NEUROSARCOIDOSIS

Cranial neuropathies
- VII—Facial nerve palsy (unilateral, bilateral)
- II—Optic nerve (unilateral and bilateral)
- VIII—Hearing loss
- Other cranial neuropathies

Myelopathy (sensory and motor)
Seizure
Basilar meningitis
Central diabetes insipidus
Panhypopituitarism
Intraparenchymal mass
Hydrocephalus
Peripheral neuropathy

Calcium Metabolism

Aberrant calcium and vitamin D metabolism occurs in up to 50% of patients and may result in renal stones (Chapter 128), nephrocalcinosis with renal insufficiency, and hypercalciuria (urine calcium > 300 mg/24 hours) with or without hypercalcemia (Chapter 253). In chronic sarcoidosis, 10 to 14% of patients have at least one symptomatic renal stone.

Renal Involvement

Renal involvement, other than as a result of dysregulated calcium metabolism, occurs in less than 1% of patients. Renal disease may include granulomatous interstitial nephritis, glomerular disease, renal tubular dysfunction, renal vascular disease, and obstructive uropathy. Granulomatous interstitial nephritis is more common in white men.

DIAGNOSIS

The diagnosis of sarcoidosis should be based on compatible clinical and radiographic findings supported by histologic evidence of noncaseating granulomas in one or more organs in the absence of any foreign particles or organisms. An occupational history consistent with beryllium exposure (Chapter 93), such as employment in the aerospace, automotive, ceramic, or computer industries, requires further investigation because chronic beryllium disease cannot be clinically or histologically distinguished from sarcoidosis.

A diagnosis of sarcoidosis is reasonably certain even without histologic confirmation in patients who present with Löfgren's syndrome. In all other cases, a biopsy specimen from an involved organ should be obtained. The organ for which biopsy is safest, such as the skin, peripheral lymph nodes, lacrimal glands, or conjunctiva, should be sampled.

If diagnosis requires intrathoracic sampling, transbronchial biopsy by means of bronchoscopy has a diagnostic yield of at least 85%. Even when pulmonary parenchymal involvement is not visible on plain chest radiography, transbronchial lung biopsy has an excellent diagnostic yield when multiple lung segments are sampled. Bronchoalveolar lavage sampling demonstrates lymphocytosis with normal or low granulocyte counts in more than 85% of patients (Chapter 85). The CD4/CD8 ratio is increased in bronchoalveolar lavage in about 50% of patients with sarcoidosis, but bronchoalveolar lavage findings are nonspecific and should not be used to diagnose sarcoidosis. Bronchoalveolar lavage findings also cannot predict prognosis or responsiveness to corticosteroid therapy.

Fine-needle aspiration of enlarged intrathoracic lymph nodes guided by endobronchial ultrasound has an 80% diagnostic yield and is significantly more likely to make the diagnosis than in unguided transbronchial biopsy.[1] Endobronchial ultrasound allows visualization of mediastinal structures, including the subcarinal region, paraesophageal space, and aortopulmonary window. Bronchoscopy and endobronchial ultrasound-guided fine-needle aspiration generally make the need for more invasive approaches, such as mediastinoscopy or video-assisted thoracoscopic surgical biopsies, unnecessary.

Sarcoidal granulomas produce angiotensin-converting enzyme (ACE). Although serum ACE levels are elevated in 60% of patients with sarcoidosis, the value of a serum ACE level in diagnosing sarcoidosis remains limited because positive and negative predictive values are only about 84% and 74%, respectively.

Patients should routinely undergo pulmonary function testing, which often does not correlate with the chest radiographic stage. For example, pulmonary function tests may be abnormal even in patients with a normal chest radiograph. Diffusion capacity for carbon monoxide (DLCO) is usually the first abnormality detected and the last to normalize on remission. A DLCO of less than 50% of predicted is associated with exercise-induced oxygen desaturation and should prompt formal oxygen saturation testing with exercise.

About two thirds of patients have airflow limitation at presentation. Spirometry usually indicates restrictive ventilatory dysfunction with a reduced forced vital capacity (FVC) and reduced forced expiratory volume in 1 second (FEV_1). At least 50% of patients have concurrent obstructive airways disease. Airway hyperreactivity, as measured by increased responsiveness to methacholine, occurs in up to 83% of patients. In patients with abnormal spirometric findings at diagnosis, spirometry returns to normal in 80%.

Alterations in cardiopulmonary exercise testing have been reported in nearly 50% of patients with sarcoidosis. Abnormalities, including a ventilatory limitation with exercise and a widened alveolar-arterial O_2 gradient, may be present. FVC is the single best test for following respiratory involvement and correlates well with FEV_1, total lung capacity, and DLCO.

Because ocular involvement is common and vision loss may occur, complete ocular evaluation with slit lamp and funduscopic examinations should be routinely performed during the initial evaluation and then annually in patients with active systemic disease.

An electrocardiogram (ECG) should be performed at the initial encounter. Screening for cardiac symptoms (palpitations, dizziness, and syncope) should be performed during the initial evaluation and routinely during follow-up visits if the disease is active. Any cardiac symptoms or abnormalities on the ECG should prompt further cardiac event monitoring (Chapter 62) and testing by echocardiography (Chapter 55). Endomyocardial biopsy has less than 20% diagnostic yield because cardiac involvement is patchy and is usually most dense in the left ventricle and basal ventricular septum where endomyocardial biopsies are avoided. If cardiac involvement is suspected, positron emission tomography (PET) or cardiac magnetic resonance imaging (MRI) with contrast should be performed. For significant symptoms, such as arrhythmias, decreased ventricular function, or septal involvement detected on MRI or PET, electrophysiologic studies should be considered and the need for an automatic implantable cardioverter-defibrillator (AICD) should be evaluated (Chapters 65 and 66).

The criteria for the diagnosis of neurosarcoidosis in the absence of histologic confirmation are not established. Compatible MRI findings, a characteristic presentation, and exclusion of other neurologic diseases are required. Histologic confirmation of disease elsewhere supports the diagnosis of neurosarcoidosis. Cerebrospinal fluid (CSF) analysis typically demonstrates nonspecific lymphocytic inflammation (Chapter 420). The CSF glucose can be as low as 14 mg/dL, with a white blood cell count as high as 350 cells/µL and a protein concentration as high as 670 mg/dL. CSF ACE levels are neither sensitive nor specific. CSF oligoclonal immunoglobulin bands are elevated in one third of patients, thereby making it difficult to differentiate sarcoidosis from multiple sclerosis (Chapter 419).

Up to 65% of patients will have granulomas on liver biopsy, but hepatic granulomas (Chapter 154) occur commonly with other disorders such as infection and drug-induced hepatitis. As a result, the diagnosis of sarcoidosis should not be based solely on detection of hepatic granulomas.

On plain radiographic images, most skeletal lesions of sarcoidosis are seen in the small bones of the hands and feet. MRI and PET scanning show much greater involvement of the axial skeleton and long bones, and osseous sarcoidosis may appear similar to metastatic disease on a PET scan.

Sarcoidosis Complicating Type 1 Interferon Therapy

Type 1 interferons, IFN-α and IFN-β, used to treat viral hepatitis (Chapter 151), multiple sclerosis (Chapter 419), and autoimmune and malignant disease may increase the T_H1 cytokines, IFN-γ, and IL-2 and rarely (<1 to 5%) result in sarcoidosis. Most reported cases of interferon-induced sarcoidosis occur within 6 months of therapy and manifest primarily with lung and skin involvement.

TABLE 95-3 TREATMENT

ORGAN	CLINICAL FINDINGS	TREATMENT
Respiratory	Dyspnea, persistent cough, FVC < 70%	Prednisone, 20-40 mg/day
	Mild cough, wheezing	Inhaled corticosteroid
Skin	Lupus pernio	Prednisone, 20-40 mg/day Hydroxychloroquine, 400 mg/day Methotrexate, 10-15 mg/wk Infliximab, 3-5 mg/kg every 2-4 weeks
	Maculopapular eruptions	Topical corticosteroid Hydroxychloroquine, 400 mg/day Prednisone, 20-40 mg/day
	Erythema nodosum	NSAID*
Eyes	Anterior uveitis	Topical corticosteroid
	Posterior uveitis	Prednisone, 20-40 mg/day
Cardiac	Complete heart block, ventricular arrhythmias	AICD, prednisone, 20-40 mg/day
	Decreased LVEF (<35%)	AICD, prednisone, 20-40 mg/day
Central nervous system	Cranial nerve palsies	Prednisone, 20-40 mg/day
	Myelopathy	Prednisone, 40-60 mg/day, and azathioprine, 150 mg/day (or mycophenolate mofetil, or cyclophosphamide)
	Intracerebral involvement	Prednisone, 40-60 mg/day, and azathioprine, 150 mg/day (or mycophenolate mofetil, or cyclophosphamide)
Liver	Cholestatic hepatitis	Prednisone, 20-40 mg/day
Bone and joint	Arthralgias	NSAID
	Granulomatous arthritis	Prednisone, 20-40 mg/day Methotrexate, 10-15 mg/wk
	Bone destruction/pain	Prednisone, 20-40 mg/day Methotrexate, 10-15 mg/wk
Hypercalciuria and hypercalcemia	Kidney stones	Prednisone, 20-40 mg/day Hydroxychloroquine, 400 mg/day

*For example, ibuprofen, 200-800 mg three times a day.
AICD = automatic implantable cardioverter-defibrillator; FVC = forced vital capacity; LVEF = left ventricular ejection fraction; NSAID = nonsteroidal anti-inflammatory drug.

PREVENTION AND TREATMENT Rx

Because the inciting agent has not yet been identified nor genetic risk factors firmly established, no means exist to prevent sarcoidosis. Most patients with sarcoidosis are not disabled by their illness, so the decision to recommend treatment should weigh the risks of using corticosteroids (Chapter 34), which are the most common treatment, against potential benefits (Table 95-3). Hypercalcemia, cardiac disease, and neurologic disease are indications for treatment, and immediate treatment is appropriate whenever organ function is threatened or when symptoms are severe. Detection of granulomatous inflammation on physical examination, biopsy, or imaging or the presence of an elevated serum ACE level is not a mandate to provide treatment.

Oral prednisone at a dose of 20 to 40 mg per day for 3 months is usually the initial recommended therapy. Response to treatment is indicated by improvement in symptoms or objective measures, such as decreased size and number of skin lesions, increased FVC, or a reduction of detectable cardiac or brain lesions. For pulmonary involvement, steroids improve symptoms, pulmonary function test results, and chest radiographic findings. [2] If a response is noted at 3 months, the prednisone dose should be tapered to 10 to 15 mg per day for an additional 6 to 9 months and then tapered off. Because recurrence may occur, patients should be followed closely for 1 to 2 years after discontinuing treatment. The indications for restarting treatment are the same as those used to begin treatment. Lack of response after a 3-month trial suggests nonadherence to therapy, an inadequate dose of prednisone, or irreversible fibrotic disease. Inhaled corticosteroids should be used only in patients with bronchial hyperreactivity or persistent cough.

Cytotoxic and immunosuppressive drugs have been used to treat patients who do not respond to corticosteroid therapy or who cannot tolerate it (see Table 95-3), but data on their benefit are inconclusive, [3] and no large randomized trials confirm an optimal agent. Generally, 3 to 6 months of cytotoxic and immunosuppressive treatment is required to determine whether a response has occurred. For patients who respond, the duration of treatment should be 9 to 12 months. In patients who are steroid dependent but have ongoing extrapulmonary disease, the addition of infliximab, 3 to 5 mg/kg for 24 weeks, can be efficacious. [4]

Moderate doses of corticosteroids (15 to 20 mg prednisone) reduce the elevated serum and urinary calcium within a few days of starting treatment. Failure of serum calcium to normalize within 2 weeks should alert the clinician to an alternative diagnosis such as hyperparathyroidism or malignancy (Chapter 253). With treatment, most patients with granulomatous interstitial nephritis regain renal function but are often left with chronic kidney disease of varying severity.

Less than 1% of heart and liver and about 3% of lung transplantations are performed in patients with sarcoidosis. The 1- and 5-year graft survival rates for lung, liver, and heart transplantations in patients with sarcoidosis compare favorably with the results obtained for patients with other disorders.

PROGNOSIS

Patients with Löfgren's syndrome have a good prognosis characterized by spontaneous resolution with few consequences. Overall, spontaneous remission with few or no consequences occurs in more than 50% of patients within 3 years of diagnosis and in two thirds of patients within a decade. After one or more years of remission without treatment, recurrence occurs in fewer than 5% of patients. Up to one third of patients have unrelenting disease that leads to significant organ impairment, but less than 5% of patients die from sarcoidosis. Black Americans tend to have a worse prognosis with more chronic disease and more extrathoracic involvement of the eyes, liver, bone marrow, extrathoracic lymph nodes, and skin. Patients with neurologic and cardiac involvement have a poorer prognosis.

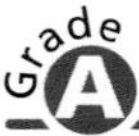

1. Tremblay A, Stather DR, Maceachern P, et al. A randomized controlled trial of standard vs endobronchial ultrasonography-guided transbronchial needle aspiration in patients with suspected sarcoidosis. *Chest.* 2009;136:340-346.
2. Paramothayan NS, Lasserson TJ, Jones PW. Corticosteroids for pulmonary sarcoidosis. *Cochrane Database Syst Rev.* 2000;18:CD001114.
3. Paramothayan S, Lasserson TJ, Walters EH. Immunosuppressive and cytotoxic therapy for pulmonary sarcoidosis. *Cochrane Database Syst Rev.* 2006;3:CD003536.
4. Judson MA, Baughman RP, Costabel U, et al. Efficacy of infliximab in extrapulmonary sarcoidosis: results from a randomized trial. *Eur Respir J.* 2008;31:1189-1196.

SUGGESTED READINGS

Dubrey SW, Falk RH. Diagnosis and management of cardiac sarcoidosis. *Prog Cardiovasc Dis.* 2010;52:336-346. *Review of clinical manifestations, diagnosis, and treatment.*

Iannuzzi MC, Fontana JR. Sarcoidosis: clinical presentation, immunopathogenesis, and therapeutics. *JAMA.* 2011;305:391-399. *Review.*

Jones N, Mochizuki M. Sarcoidosis: epidemiology and clinical features. *Ocul Immunol Inflamm.* 2010;18:72-79. *Review with emphasis on eye involvement.*

Kollert F, Geck B, Suchy R, et al. The impact of gas exchange measurement during exercise in pulmonary sarcoidosis. *Respir Med.* 2011;105:122-129. *Impaired gas exchange during exercise reflects disease activity and a prolonged need for immunosuppressive treatment.*

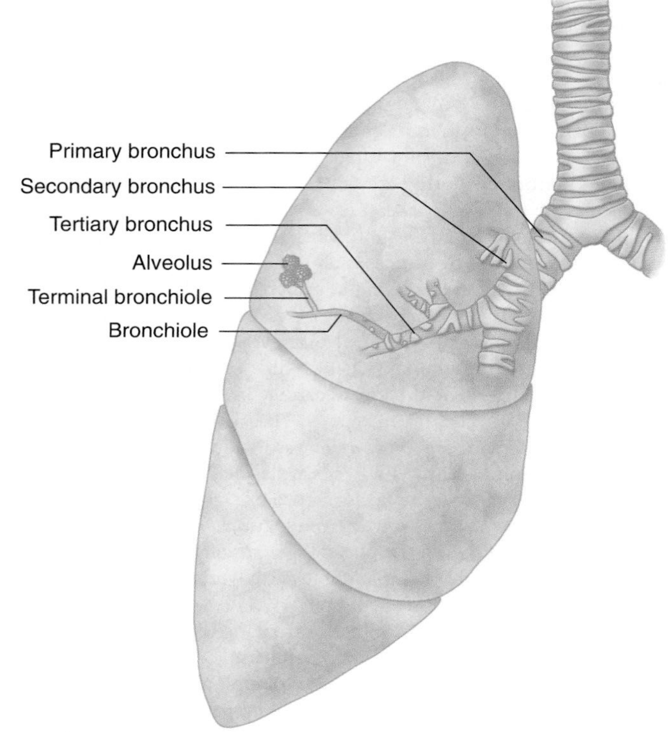

FIGURE 96-1. Many infecting agents that cause bronchitis and tracheitis can infect both large and small airways of the lung and occasionally the alveoli. Not surprisingly, a wide spectrum of signs and symptoms are associated with bronchitis, including cough, wheezing, and shortness of breath.

96 ACUTE BRONCHITIS AND TRACHEITIS

RICHARD P. WENZEL

DEFINITION

The term *acute bronchitis and tracheitis* defines a self-limited (1 to 3 weeks) inflammation of the large airways of the lung that extends to the tertiary bronchi (Fig. 96-1). In patients with a primary symptom of cough (Chapter 83), the diagnosis is made if there is no clinical or radiologic evidence of pneumonia. At the bedside, the absence of criteria for systemic inflammatory response syndrome (SIRS) (Chapter 108) suggests bronchitis and tracheitis and makes a diagnosis of pneumonia (Chapter 97) unlikely. The SIRS criteria are met if the patient has more than two of the following: temperature lower than 36° C or higher than 38° C, pulse greater than 90 beats/minute, respiratory rate higher than 20 breaths/minute, or white blood cell count less than 4000 cells/mm^3 or higher than 12,000 cells/mm^3 or with greater than 10% bands.

The definition of acute bronchitis and tracheitis also seeks to differentiate the illness from acute inflammation of the small airways (bronchiolitis), even though the accompanying symptoms with the former may include sputum production, wheezing, and shortness of breath. Among patients with primarily small airways disease, some might be expected to have prominently decreased breath sounds in the areas involved. Acute bronchitis and tracheitis is also different from bronchiectasis (Chapter 90), which is associated with permanent dilation of bronchi and a chronic cough. Furthermore, a diagnosis of chronic bronchitis (Chapter 88) is reserved for patients who have prolonged cough and sputum production: at least 3 months of the year for 2 consecutive years.

EPIDEMIOLOGY

Occurring at a rate of 44 per 1000 adults per year, acute bronchitis and tracheitis affects approximately 5% of adults annually. A higher incidence is observed in the winter and fall than in the summer and spring. In the United States, acute bronchitis and tracheitis is the ninth most common illness in outpatients as reported by physicians.

The disorder is thought to be viral in origin almost all the time. However, viruses have been isolated in only 8 to 37% of patients. Thus, the true causes of the illness are unknown in most cases. Nevertheless, at least 70% of patients with acute bronchitis and tracheitis in the United States receive antibacterial antibiotics after visiting a physician. Importantly, although the same bacteria that are commonly implicated in community-acquired pneumonia are also isolated from the sputum in half the patients, their role in the pathobiology of acute bronchitis and tracheitis or its attendant symptoms is unclear, and bronchial biopsies have not shown bacterial invasion.

PATHOBIOLOGY

Infections of the epithelium of the bronchi and trachea are thought to incite an inflammatory response. Pathologically, there is an accompanying microscopic thickening of bronchial and tracheal mucosa corresponding to the inflamed areas. Such pathologic findings are also consistent with the occasional case report of upper airway inflammation confined to the bronchi and trachea detected by ^{18}F-labeled fluorodeoxyglucose positron emission tomography (FDG-PET).

In human experimental rhinovirus infections (Chapter 369), virus was detected in all subjects in induced sputum samples and also in approximately one third of bronchial biopsy specimens, almost one fourth of bronchoalveolar lavage samples, and more than one third of biopsy and brushing samples. Such data indicating viral infection of the lower airways may help explain the relationship observed between rhinovirus infection and exacerbations of asthma (Chapter 87). Furthermore, pathologic islands of inflammation have been found in the trachea with rhinovirus infection, thus supporting the idea of a patchy distribution. The viruses implicated in acute bronchitis and tracheitis include influenza A and B (Chapter 372), parainfluenza (Chapter 371), respiratory syncytial virus (Chapter 370), coronavirus (Chapter 374), adenovirus (Chapter 373), and rhinoviruses (Chapter 369), usually in this order from the most to the least common. However, a recent French study of influenza-vaccinated adults found a viral cause in 37% of 164 cases of acute bronchitis, 21% of which were rhinovirus. Thus, at least three variables can influence the yield of specific pathogens: the presence of epidemics, the season of the year, and the population's influenza vaccination status. More recently, human metapneumovirus (Chapter 369) has been identified as an etiologic agent.

Up to 10% of cases of acute bronchitis and tracheitis may be due to "atypical" bacteria: *Bordetella pertussis* (Chapter 321), *Chlamydophila (Chlamydia) pneumoniae* (Chapter 325), and *Mycoplasma pneumoniae* (Chapter 326). Severe bronchiolitis has also been reported with *M. pneumoniae,* even though this pathogen is usually associated with either pneumonia or acute bronchitis and tracheitis in adults. In children, bronchiolitis has been associated with respiratory syncytial virus, influenza virus, parainfluenza virus, and metapneumovirus (Chapter 369). Thus, there are probably wide variations in the anatomic distribution of all pathogens causing acute bronchitis and tracheitis, extending from the nasal mucosa to the bronchiolar epithelium.

CLINICAL MANIFESTATIONS

The cardinal clinical symptom is cough (Chapter 83) of recent onset. Because most upper respiratory infections resolve within 1 week, a more extended period of cough is useful for considering the diagnosis of acute bronchitis. Patients usually seek care from their physician after 4 to 7 days of coughing that is not resolving. With acute bronchitis, there is often a continued cough and sometimes a worsened cough that lasts an initial 1 to 3 weeks. Associated symptoms vary and include sputum production, fever, malaise, wheezing, and dyspnea. Adults with pertussis may exhibit paroxysms of coughing, whooping, or vomiting, although less commonly than seen in children with this infection.

DIAGNOSIS

Acutely ill patients may not be able to distinguish their early symptoms from those accompanying very mild upper respiratory infections. However, with acute bronchitis and tracheitis, a protracted phase of coughing persists beyond 1 to 5 days, during which time pulmonary function tests may become abnormal. A substantial proportion of patients will have significant declines in forced expiratory volume in the first second (FEV_1) (Chapter 85).

Rapid diagnostic tests exist for most viruses linked to acute bronchitis and tracheitis. However, their value lies in identifying a virus for which there is therapy or avoiding antibacterial antibiotics if any virus is identified. Not all rapid tests are widely available, and they are expensive and rarely cost-effective in an outpatient setting.

When "atypical" bacteria are identified by culture or serology, patients tend to be seen later in the course of their illness than patients with viral causes and more often have wheezing. In some studies, 12 to 32% of patients with coughing that persists for longer than 1 week had pertussis. In other studies, however, pertussis has been confirmed in only 1% of such patients.

Polymerase chain reaction (PCR) testing of nasopharyngeal swabs or aspirates is the easiest and most sensitive way to diagnose infections by *B. pertussis, M. pneumoniae,* and *C. pneumoniae;* most experts recommend calcium alginate swabs for pertussis because cotton inhibits growth. Dacron swabs with aluminum handles are preferred for specimens used to diagnose *Chlamydophila* because cotton, calcium alginate, and the wooden shaft can all inhibit growth of the organism. Cultures for *M. pneumoniae* are slow and insensitive. In general, testing for atypical organisms should not be done because of the cost of PCR and both the insensitivity and slowness of cultures. However, if the clinician suspects an outbreak in the community or the likelihood of pertussis, rapid testing with PCR may be quite beneficial.

TREATMENT

Rx

In a meta-analysis of nine randomized trials of antibacterial antibiotics for acute bronchitis, patients receiving antibiotics were significantly less likely to have a cough, but their 0.58 fewer days with cough, 0.52 fewer days of productive cough, and 0.58 fewer days of feeling ill were not statistically significant.[1] A large clinical trial in a population with a high prevalence of human immunodeficiency virus infection found that amoxicillin for 7 days was no better than placebo.[2]

These results are not surprising because, at most, about 50% of cases are probably caused by bacterial pathogens. Nevertheless, antibiotics are used in 50 to 85% of cases worldwide.

Antibiotics may be used in patients with known atypical pathogens, but even then their effect on outcomes is not clear except to limit the spread of pertussis, especially during a defined outbreak. In adults suspected of having pertussis, erythromycin, 500 mg four times a day for 14 days, is thought to be most effective. However, many patients cannot tolerate erythromycin, and either doxycycline, 100 mg every 12 hours, or a newer macrolide such as azithromycin, 500 mg on day 1 and 250 mg/day thereafter, is effective. The latter two drugs are also active against *C. pneumoniae* and *M. pneumoniae,* although the optimal duration of therapy for acute bronchitis is unknown. A useful range is 5 to 14 days.

During influenza season, anti-influenza agents may be useful in decreasing symptoms by approximately 1 day and may lead to a 0.5-day earlier return to normal activity in patients with influenza. The first-generation drugs amantadine and rimantadine are ineffective against H3N2 influenza A viruses and are not recommended. Second-generation drugs such as zanamivir (two inhalations of 5 mg each, twice a day) or oseltamivir (75 mg twice a day) can be given for 5 days. Up to 20% of patients given oseltamivir will have nausea or vomiting.

Antihistamines and over-the-counter antitussives and expectorants have no apparent value. Subsets of patients with bronchial hyperresponsiveness may benefit from β-agonists, but no data support the use of inhaled steroids. Mucolytic agents may be of small benefit.[3]

In experimental rhinovirus colds, nonsteroidal drugs, alone or in combination with antihistamines, reduce the severity of symptoms, including cough. However, the widespread use of either type of drug alone or as a combination in naturally occurring, community-acquired bronchitis and tracheitis has not been evaluated. In patients with acute bronchitis, a meta-analysis of four placebo-controlled clinical trials suggested that *Pelargonium sidoides* (a herbaceous perennial widely used in Europe) reduced bronchitis symptom scores by day 7.[4]

PROGNOSIS

Coughing usually lasts 10 to 14 days, during which time the illness causes significant transient decrements in vitality and social functioning. Limited data on short- and long-term outcomes show that up to 20% of patients have persistent or recurrent symptoms for a month. Antibiotics may reduce symptoms by a fraction of a day, but side effects, the emergence of antibiotic resistance, and cost must be weighed against their modest benefits. The mean duration of an office visit for adults in the United States with upper respiratory tract infections is 14.2 minutes when patients are prescribed antibiotics versus 15.2 minutes without prescription of antibiotics, but antibiotic use is not an independent predictor of visit length. Future widespread use of rapid diagnostic tests for specific bacterial and viral pathogens will be useful in targeting effective therapies.

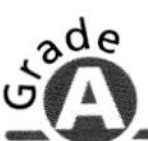

1. Smucny J, Fahey T, Becker L, et al. Antibiotics for acute bronchitis. In: The Cochrane Collaboration. New York: J Wiley & Sons; 2005:1-26. Available at *http://www.cochrane.org/reviews/en/ab000245.html.*
2. Nduba VN, Mwachari CW, Margaret AS, et al. Placebo found equivalent to amoxicillin for treatment of acute bronchitis in Nairobi, Kenya: a triple-blind randomized, equivalence trial. *Thorax.* 2008;63:999-1105.
3. Poole P, Black PN. Mucolytic agents for chronic bronchitis or chronic obstructive pulmonary disease. *Cochrane Database Syst Rev.* 2010;2:CD001287.
4. Agbabiaka TB, Guo R, Edzard E. *Pelargonium sidoides* for acute bronchitis: a systematic review and meta-analysis. *Phytomedicine.* 2008;15:378-385.

SUGGESTED READINGS

Fahy JV, Dickey BF. Airway mucus function and dysfunction. *N Engl J Med.* 2010;363:2233-2247. *Review.*

Sethi S. Antibiotics in acute exacerbations of chronic bronchitis. *Expert Rev Anti Infect Ther.* 2010;8:405-417. *Review of guidelines.*

97

OVERVIEW OF PNEUMONIA

ANDREW H. LIMPER

It is a useful distinction to separate pneumonias, which are infections of the lung parenchyma and thus distinct from infections limited to the trachea or large bronchi (Chapter 96), into those acquired in the community (community-acquired pneumonia) and those arising in institutional settings, with the second group being composed of hospital-acquired pneumonia, ventilator-associated pneumonia, and health care–associated pneumonia. These two major pneumonia categories are considered separately in this chapter. Additional consideration should be given to pneumonia caused by recurrent aspiration of oropharyngeal contents.

The term *pneumonia* itself, however, includes other causes of inflammation of the lower respiratory air spaces, particularly the alveoli, such as acute or chronic eosinophilic pneumonia, cryptogenic organizing pneumonia, and usual interstitial pneumonia, all of which are presented in more detail elsewhere (Chapter 92).

COMMUNITY-ACQUIRED PNEUMONIA

DEFINITION

Community-acquired pneumonia includes cases of infectious pneumonia in patients living independently in the community. Patients who have been hospitalized for other reasons for less than 48 hours before the development of respiratory symptoms are also considered to have community-acquired pneumonia because it is likely that the inoculation had occurred before admission. However, patients who have previously been hospitalized for at least 2 days within the 90 days before infection; patients from nursing homes who received intravenous antibiotic therapy, chemotherapy, or wound care within the past 30 days; and patients from hemodialysis centers are considered to have health care–associated pneumonia and are therefore excluded from the case definition of community-acquired pneumonia. Patients contracting pneumonia more than 48 hours after the institution of endotracheal intubation and mechanical ventilation are also excluded inasmuch as they are considered to have ventilator-associated pneumonia. These distinctions are important because they help define the most likely infectious agents and hence strongly influence appropriate choices for the initial antibiotic therapy.

EPIDEMIOLOGY

More than 10 million cases of infectious pneumonia occur annually in the United States and result in more than 1 million hospitalizations. Pneumonia is a leading cause of death worldwide, the sixth leading cause of death in the United States, and the most common lethal infectious disease. The mortality rate associated with community-acquired pneumonia ranges from less than 5% in mildly ill outpatients to somewhat greater than 12% overall in patients who are admitted to a hospital. Mortality is even greater in patients who have severe invasive disease, which is often associated with bacteremia, and in elderly nursing home patients. Mortality from pneumonia can exceed 40% in patients who require management in the intensive care unit (ICU). It costs approximately $7000 to manage an uncomplicated case of pneumonia in the hospital, or about 20-fold more than treating it in the outpatient setting.

PATHOBIOLOGY

Aspiration of Oropharyngeal Contents

The most common mechanism by which the lung is inoculated with pathogenic organisms is through microaspiration of oropharyngeal contents, a process that occurs in otherwise healthy individuals during sleep (Chapter 94). Colonization of the oral pharynx with pathogenic organisms, such as *Streptococcus pneumoniae* (Chapter 297), can thereby lead to delivery of sufficient quantities of organisms to infect the lung. In contrast, gross aspiration normally occurs only in individuals with altered sensorium, depressed consciousness, abnormalities in protective cough or gag reflexes, or substantial gastroesophageal reflux. Gross aspiration, which can also deliver large numbers of anaerobic bacteria to the lower respiratory tract, is a major contributing factor to anaerobic lung infection and abscess formation (Chapter 90).

Inhalation of Aerosolized Droplets

The second most frequent mechanism of lung infection is the inhalation of small, suspended aerosolized droplets ranging in size from 0.5 to 1 μm that may contain microorganisms. In view of the limited number of organisms delivered in such a manner, only relatively aggressive pathogenic organisms such as *Mycobacterium tuberculosis* (Chapter 332), *Legionella pneumophila* (Chapter 322), *Yersinia pestis* (plague; Chapter 320), *Bacillus anthracis* (anthrax; Chapter 302), and some viral infections can be transmitted in this manner.

Blood Stream Infection

Less commonly, the lung may become infected as a consequence of a blood stream infection. Blood-borne pneumonia is seen especially in staphylococcal sepsis (Chapter 296) or right-sided endocarditis (Chapter 76), both of which are more common in intravenous drug users (Chapter 33), and in gram-negative bacteremias, particularly in an immunocompromised host. The lung may also rarely be inoculated directly by penetrating chest trauma or by local spread from a nearby infected organ (bacterial or amoebic liver abscess or paragonimiasis; Chapters 360 and 364) or a contiguous soft tissue infection.

Fortunately, the lung is well equipped to defend against inoculation with most microbes. When large droplets of infected material reach the airways, they are removed by the mucociliary escalator, which sweeps entrapped contents up to the oropharynx, where they are swallowed or expectorated. Smaller particles, in the range of 0.5 to 2.0 μm, are deposited in the alveoli, where alveolar macrophages phagocytize and destroy most pathogens. These macrophages are further activated to release potent cytokines and chemokines, including tumor necrosis factor-α, interleukin-8, and leukotriene B_4, which help recruit neutrophils from the blood stream into the alveolar spaces, where they participate in the uptake and degradation of microorganisms. For many microorganisms such as *S. pneumoniae* (Chapter 297), clearance of infection is greatly facilitated by the development of specific immunoglobulin G that binds the surface of the organisms or their polysaccharide capsule. These specific antibodies, which act as immune opsonins, greatly augment the ability of neutrophils and macrophages to phagocytize and destroy the bacteria. In addition, pattern recognition receptors and other nonimmune opsonins, including surfactant proteins A and D, fibronectin, and vitronectin, also bind to specific epitopes on the surface of organisms that reach the lower respiratory tract and assist in their recognition and elimination. Only when organisms overwhelm or evade these multiple host defense systems does inoculation of the lung result in clinically significant pneumonia.

CLINICAL MANIFESTATIONS

The possibility of pneumonia should be considered in any patient who has new respiratory symptoms, including cough, sputum, or dyspnea, particularly when these symptoms are accompanied by fever or abnormalities on physical examination of the chest, such as rhonchi and rales. The initial manifestation is frequently more subtle in patients who are elderly or have an altered immunologic status; in such patients, nonspecific symptoms, including loss of appetite, confusion, dehydration, worsening of symptoms or signs of other chronic illnesses, or failure to thrive, may be the initial manifestation of pneumonia. Pneumonia is also increasingly prevalent in patients with specific comorbid conditions, including smoking, chronic obstructive pulmonary disease (COPD; Chapter 88), diabetes mellitus, malignancy, heart failure, neurologic diseases, narcotic and alcohol use, and chronic liver disease.

The initial symptoms and signs are often variable from patient to patient and cannot be reliably used to establish a specific (microbiologic) diagnosis. The classic physical findings in lobar pneumonia include evidence of consolidation with altered transmission of breath sounds, egophony, crackles, and changes in tactile fremitus. However, in many patients, the physical findings are subtler and may be limited to scattered rhonchi. A thorough physical examination, posteroanterior and lateral chest radiographs, and a blood leukocyte count with a differential cell count should be performed when pneumonia is suspected. An assessment of gas exchange (oximetry or arterial blood gas determination) should be obtained for all patients who are admitted to the hospital. The clinician needs to be mindful of competing diagnoses that can mimic the findings of pneumonia, such as pulmonary embolism (Chapter 98), bronchogenic and bronchoalveolar carcinoma (Chapter 197), drug-induced lung diseases (Chapter 94), and idiopathic interstitial lung diseases (Chapter 92).

DIAGNOSIS

Even with intensive laboratory investigation, the specific microbiologic cause can be established with certainty only in approximately 50% of patients with pneumonia. The probable predominant organism varies with the host's epidemiologic factors, the severity of illness, and which laboratory approach is used to establish the diagnosis.

Bacterial Pneumonia

S. pneumoniae (Chapter 297) is the organism most frequently detected by culture of sputum or blood. In contrast, *Mycoplasma pneumoniae* (Chapter 325) is frequently detected with serologic tests. Additional bacterial agents include *Haemophilus influenzae* (Chapter 308), *Staphylococcus aureus* (Chapter 296), enteric gram-negative bacilli (Chapters 290 and 314), and *L. pneumophila* (Chapter 322). *Chlamydia* and respiratory viruses have also been implicated in up to 10% of cases. The so-called atypical pathogens,

TABLE 97-1 HOST FACTORS ASSOCIATED WITH SPECIFIC PATHOGENIC CAUSES OF PNEUMONIA

UNDERLYING CONDITION	ASSOCIATED MICROORGANISM
Active smoking/chronic obstructive lung disease	*Streptococcus pneumoniae, Haemophilus influenzae, Legionella pneumophila, Moraxella catarrhalis, Pseudomonas aeruginosa, Chlamydophila pneumonia*
Nursing home residents	*S. pneumoniae*, gram-negative bacilli, *H. influenzae, Staphylococcus aureus, Chlamydophila pneumonia*, anaerobes, *Mycobacterium tuberculosis*
Alcoholism	*S. pneumoniae* (including drug-resistant strains), gram-negative bacilli, anaerobes, *Mycobacterium tuberculosis, Klebsiella pneumoniae, Acinetobacter* species
Gross aspiration/poor dentition	Anaerobes, gram-negative enteric pathogens
Travel to southwestern United States	*Coccidioides immitis*
Exposure to bats	*Histoplasma capsulatum*
Exposure to birds	*Cryptococcus neoformans, Chlamydia psittaci, H. capsulatum*
Exposure to rabbits	*Francisella tularensis*
Exposure to farm animals	*Coxiella burnetii* (Q fever)
Viral influenza	Influenza, *S. aureus, S. pneumoniae, H. influenzae*
Bronchiectasis, cystic fibrosis	*Pseudomonas aeruginosa, Burkholderia cepacia, S. aureus, Aspergillus* species, *Mycobacterium avium* complex
Lung abscess	CA-MRSA, oral anaerobes, endemic fungal pneumonia, *M. tuberculosis*, atypical mycobacteria
Intravenous drug use	*S. aureus*, anaerobes, *M. tuberculosis, S. pneumoniae*
Endobronchial obstruction	Anaerobes
Recent antibiotic therapy	Drug-resistant *S. pneumoniae, P. aeruginosa*
HIV (early)	*S. pneumoniae, H. influenza, M. tuberculosis*
HIV (late)	The pathogens listed for early HIV infection, plus *Pneumocystis jirovecii, Cryptococcus, Histoplasma, Aspergillus*, atypical mycobacteria (especially *M. kansasii* and *M. avium* complex), *P. aeruginosa, H. influenza*
In the context of bioterrorism	*Bacillus anthracis* (anthrax), *Yersinia pestis* (plague), *Francisella tularensis* (tularemia)

CA-MRSA = community-acquired methicillin-resistant *Staphylococcus aureus*; HIV = human immunodeficiency virus.
Adapted from Infectious Diseases Society of America/American Thoracic Society. Consensus guidelines on the management of community acquired pneumonia in adults. *Clin Infect Dis.* 2007;44:S27-S72.

including *M. pneumoniae, Chlamydia pneumoniae,* and *Legionella* species, are increasingly being recognized as important and prevalent causes of pneumonia. Mixed infections, particularly those related to coinfection with these "atypical" pathogens in addition to the usual bacterial pathogens, have been reported in up to one third of patients with lower respiratory tract infection.

Specific host factors also influence the relative risk for infection with specific microorganisms (Table 97-1). For instance, smokers and those with COPD are at increased risk for invasive *S. pneumoniae,* as well as *H. influenzae, Moraxella catarrhalis* (Chapter 308), and *Legionella* species. Alcoholism is associated with increased risk for drug-resistant *S. pneumoniae,* anaerobic lung infection, and tuberculosis.

The clinician also should solicit information about household and workplace exposure, such as to other ill persons. The clinician should ask about recent travel to specific geographic regions, such as the central United States, where histoplasmosis is endemic (Chapter 340), the Southwest, where coccidioidomycosis is found (Chapter 341), and selected northern and central regions of the United States, where blastomycosis is found (Chapter 342). Recent travel to regions with epidemic viral respiratory infections, including seasonal influenza, avian influenza, H1N1 (swine) influenza, and severe acute respiratory syndrome (SARS), or travel to Asia, Africa, and central and eastern Europe, which are highly endemic for tuberculosis, should be considered (Chapter 332). In addition, environmental exposure, such as to birds (psittacosis), bird droppings (histoplasmosis), bats (histoplasmosis), rabbits (tularemia, Chapter 319), and farm animals (Q fever, Chapter 335), is additional data that should be obtained during the history.

Viral Pneumonia

Although most attention traditionally focuses on bacterial causes of severe community-acquired pneumonia, viruses can also cause serious lower respiratory tract infections. The predominant respiratory viruses that can cause severe pneumonia include various influenza viruses and respiratory syncytial virus (RSV) (Chapter 370). Both influenza virus and RSV can be detected in respiratory secretions, which should be obtained in suspected cases. It is estimated that influenza infections are responsible for in excess of 36,000 respiratory- and circulatory-related deaths annually in the United States, predominantly in elderly patients and those with underlying cardiopulmonary or metabolic disease. Influenza-associated pneumonia should be considered in the differential diagnosis of respiratory infections in high-risk patients with underlying disease and in residents of nursing homes or other chronic care facilities during the season of October through May, especially in patients who have not received appropriate vaccination.

It is also increasingly being appreciated that RSV and parainfluenza (Chapter 371) viruses, although formerly considered mainly infections of pediatric populations, can lead to serious lower respiratory tract infections in adults during the winter season. Host immunity to RSV infection in childhood is incomplete, and recurrent infections can occur in both immune-competent and immune-impaired adults, particularly in elderly patients. It is estimated that RSV is associated with more than 11,000 deaths each year in the United States, with most deaths occurring in elderly people and in patients with chronic cardiopulmonary disease.

Emerging influenza infections must also be considered. Although typical seasonal influenza tends to occur in North America during the months of October to May, novel influenza viruses do not always follow that epidemiology. In particular in the spring and summer of 2009, a novel H1N1 (swine) influenza virus occurred in epidemic proportions in Mexico and rapidly spread over the world. In contrast to many other influenza outbreaks, the virus continued to circulate over the summer months in both the northern and southern hemispheres. H1N1 generally produced a typical syndrome with fever, headaches, cough, malaise, and myalgias. Most cases were mild or self-limited. However, excess hospitalization and mortality from H1N1 infection has been observed in infants, children, and adults younger than 24 years. Pregnant women and children, in particular those who are immunosuppressed, are at particular risk.

Avian influenza A (H5N1; Chapter 372) generally infects wild birds, which carry the H5N1 virus in their intestines, but usually are not made very sick by the virus. However, avian influenza can be highly contagious and fatal among domesticated birds, including chickens, turkeys, and ducks. Transmission to humans has been relatively uncommon, despite the lack of immunity against the virus, but human outbreaks have occurred from contact with infected birds (e.g., domesticated chicken and turkeys) or with secretions or excretions from infected birds.

SARS emerged as an additional form of life-threatening atypical pneumonia that was first detected in the Guangdong Province of China in late 2002, with major outbreaks in Hong Kong, Guangdong, Singapore, and Toronto and Vancouver, Canada. The disease is caused by a novel coronavirus (Chapter 374) with an incubation period of 2 to 10 days. The initial source of the infection remains uncertain, although palm civet cats and Chinese ferret badgers harbor a coronavirus with greater than 99% similarity to human SARS isolates. Worldwide, however, the illness is largely a nosocomial disease, with health care workers representing a significant fraction of the infected individuals. SARS is characterized by an insidious onset of fever, chills, headache, cough, malaise, and dyspnea, with radiologic evidence of pneumonia. Although upper respiratory symptoms are uncommon, voluminous watery diarrhea without mucus or blood develops in up to 70% of patients. SARS is believed to be principally transmitted by respiratory droplets. Current treatment is supportive, with no antiviral agent yet having been proved to be efficacious. SARS pneumonia tends to resolve slowly and spontaneously, usually by the third week of illness. However, the estimated case-fatality rate remains approximately 10%. SARS is highly contagious, and lethal transmission to health care workers has been documented. Isolation procedures and equipment appropriate for SARS include standard, contact, and airborne isolation precautions such as scrupulous hand hygiene, gowning, disposable gloves, the use of N95 respirators, and eye protection. Suspected cases of SARS require notification of local public health departments and the Centers for Disease Control and Prevention.

Agents of Bioterrorism

Physicians should also be vigilant for clues of pneumonia related to agents of bioterrorism (Chapter 20). These clues can include outbreaks of severe illness and pneumonia in multiple, otherwise healthy individuals or the isolation of unusual organisms in patients with pneumonic illness. The microorganisms most likely to be associated with severe pneumonia during bioterrorism-related inhalation exposure include *B. anthracis* (Chapter 302), *Francisella tularensis* (Chapter 319), and *Y. pestis* (Chapter 320). Inhalational anthrax always indicates a bioterrorism threat, whereas pneumonic plague or tularemia may or may not be associated with bioterrorism.

Radiography

Clinical suspicion of pneumonia should prompt standard posteroanterior and lateral chest radiography. Although the pattern of infiltration can rarely establish a specific microbiologic etiology, chest films are most useful for providing essential information on the distribution and extent of involvement, as well as potential pneumonic complications. Many bacterial pneumonias result in localized alveolar infiltrates and consolidation. Even though pneumococcal pneumonia is classically described as having a lobar distribution, the pattern can be multilobar (Fig. 97-1) or bilateral. The "bulging" fissure sign, which represents lobar filling and consolidation, has traditionally been attributed to *Klebsiella pneumoniae,* but this finding is not specific and can be observed with *S. pneumoniae* and other bacteria and even with bronchoalveolar carcinoma. Diffuse interstitial and alveolar infiltrates should suggest viral infections (cytomegalovirus, influenza virus, or RSV), *L. pneumophila,* or enteric gram-negative pneumonia, particularly in neutropenic patients. These diffuse pulmonary infiltrations can be indistinguishable from other causes of acute respiratory distress syndrome. Diffuse alveolar and interstitial infiltration can also be observed in patients with *Pneumocystis jirovecii* pneumonia (Chapter 349) related to immune suppression, such as in those with acquired immunodeficiency syndrome. Cavitary lesions often indicate a necrotizing infection related to *S. aureus, M. tuberculosis* (Fig. 97-2), and certain endemic fungi such as *Coccidioides immitis, Aspergillus* species infection in an immunocompromised patient (Chapter 347), or anaerobic lung infection with abscess formation. Mediastinal adenopathy and widening have been observed in inhalational anthrax infections.

The chest radiograph provides further important information about potential infectious complications of pneumonia. Pleural effusions (Chapter 99), which occur in a variety of respiratory infections, are best documented with lateral decubitus views or with computed tomography (CT) imaging of the thorax. The discovery of any pleural effusion greater than 10 mm in thickness on a lateral decubitus film or any loculated effusion should prompt thoracentesis to aid in the identification of a complicated parapneumonic effusion or empyema, which may require definitive drainage (Chapter 99). Enlargement of mediastinal and hilar lymph nodes, which is rare in acute bacterial infection, suggests fungal or mycobacterial infection or an underlying lung cancer. Loss of volume of a lung segment or lobe should raise suspicion of postobstructive pneumonia distal to an endobronchial lesion caused by a neoplasm, occult foreign body, or broncholithiasis.

Laboratory Findings

Sputum Gram Stain and Culture

Considerable controversy exists over the appropriate microbiologic evaluation of patients with suspected pneumonia. Despite intensive microbiologic evaluation, a specific organism may not be discovered in half the patients with pneumonia. Furthermore, most patients with pneumonia satisfactorily respond to simple, relatively nontoxic antibiotic regimens based on the most likely organisms causing infection. Thus, the necessity to document the precise cause of the process remains uncertain.

Debate continues over the need to perform a sputum examination with Gram staining in every patient with community-acquired pneumonia. An American Thoracic Society consensus panel has recommended that a sputum Gram stain and culture be obtained primarily if an organism that is resistant to the usual empirical treatment regimens is suspected. To be useful, sputum should contain fewer than 10 squamous cells and more than 25 leukocytes per low-power field; a well-performed Gram stain may reveal a single, predominant organism such as encapsulated gram-positive cocci (pneumococci) or small pleomorphic gram-negative coccobacilli *(Haemophilus).* However, current data have not clearly correlated Gram stain findings with the results of culture of alveolar materials in large numbers of patients with community-acquired pneumonia. Nevertheless, sputum examination can strongly support the diagnosis of certain specific infections, including *M. tuberculosis* (acid-fast stain), endemic fungi (KOH preparations), *P. jirovecii* (methenamine silver or fluorescent antibody stain), or *Legionella* species (direct fluorescent antibody staining). In most cases of community-acquired pneumonia, the general intent of sputum Gram stain examination, if it is performed, should be to detect additional or unusual pathogens and hence to expand rather than narrow the initial antibiotic therapy. All too often, an adequate sputum specimen cannot be obtained, and the Gram stain interpretation may be equivocal. Therefore, the initial therapeutic plan must be based on the most likely pathogens responsible for the pneumonia.

If unusual or drug-resistant pathogens are suspected, sputum specimens should be sent for culture before antibiotic therapy is initiated. When the culture results are available, they should be compared with the predominant organisms observed on Gram stain. Unfortunately, the sensitivity and specificity of sputum culture are not optimal, each being roughly 50%. Antibiotic susceptibility information on an isolated pathogenic organism can, however, be useful both for epidemiologic surveillance and for management of patients who do not respond to initial empirical therapy.

Other Bacterial Cultures

Cultures of normally sterile body fluids such as blood, pleural fluid, or occasionally cerebrospinal fluid (CSF) are highly specific when positive.

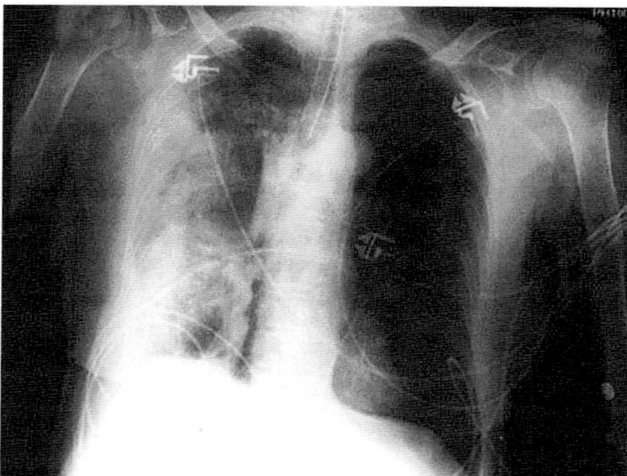

FIGURE 97-1. Radiologic diagnosis of pneumonia. A standard posteroanterior radiograph in a 70-year-old woman demonstrates chronic obstructive pulmonary disease complicated by right multilobar *Streptococcus pneumoniae* pneumonia and empyema.

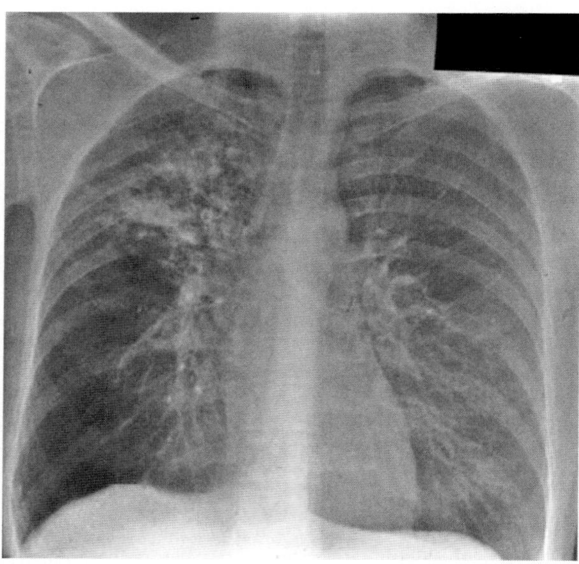

FIGURE 97-2. Cavitary lesions. A posteroanterior radiograph in a 54-year-old man with cough and fever shows a right upper lobe cavitary process caused by *Mycobacterium tuberculosis* infection.

Approximately one fourth of patients with bacterial pneumonia have demonstrable bacteremia. Blood should be drawn for culture before administration of antibiotics in patients with serious illness attributable to pneumonia, and diagnostic thoracentesis should be performed if an effusion is large enough to be aspirated safely. CSF examination is generally reserved for patients with additional signs and symptoms of meningeal irritation (Chapter 420) or abnormalities on neurologic examination.

Testing for Suspected Bioterrorism

Recommended testing for suspected anthrax includes blood culture and chest CT scanning. For the diagnosis of pneumonic plague, blood culture as well as sputum Gram stain and culture are advised. For tularemic pneumonia, cultures should be obtained from blood, sputum, and the pharynx. Culture of these extremely virulent organisms should be undertaken in a level 3 (BL3) biocontainment laboratory.

Immunologic Studies

Immunologic techniques such as immunofluorescence, enzyme-linked immunosorbent assay, antigen detection, polymerase chain reaction, and DNA hybridization may be considered when specific organisms are strongly suspected on clinical grounds, but these tests are not routinely indicated in most cases of community-acquired pneumonia. For example, *Legionella* urinary antigen screening and acute and convalescent serologic evaluation may be helpful when *L. pneumophila* pneumonia is suspected (Chapter 322). *Legionella* urinary antigen testing may underdiagnose infections caused by organisms other than *Legionella* serogroup 1. Furthermore, the judicious use of fungal serology can detect endemic mycoses, particularly histoplasmosis and coccidioidomycosis (Chapters 340, 341, and 342). Histoplasmosis can also be confirmed by urinary antigen testing with high sensitivity. The measurement of *Aspergillus galactomannan* antigen in serum can be a useful adjunct in the diagnosis of invasive *Aspergillus* pneumonia in various immunocompromised patients. Bronchoscopy with lavage for immunostaining may, in selected circumstances, provide enhanced sensitivity, such as in the diagnosis of *P. jirovecii* pneumonia (Chapter 349).

Viral Studies

Rapid antigen detection tests are now available, with tests that distinguish between influenza A and B being preferred. These tests are currently recommended for epidemiologic purposes in the community and also help direct individual therapy. RSV antigen detection tests are likewise available, but they are relatively less sensitive when applied to sputum in adult patients. A variety of other assays, including polymerase chain reaction (PCR) and specialized antigen testing, are available in reference laboratories for detection of diagnosis of novel H1N1 (swine) influenza, H5N1 (avian) influenza, and the SARS coronavirus.

Bronchoscopy

Invasive sampling of respiratory secretions is not usually necessary in patients with community-acquired pneumonia. Flexible fiberoptic bronchoscopy with a protected catheter brush and bronchoalveolar lavage (BAL) sampling has largely supplanted transtracheal and transthoracic needle aspiration. Bronchoscopy is indicated in selected clinical situations in which a delay in accurate diagnosis may have serious consequences, such as in immunocompromised hosts or patients whose condition has worsened despite initial antimicrobial therapy. Other indications for bronchoscopy in the setting of apparent community-acquired pneumonia include either lung abscess detected on a chest radiograph (Chapter 84) or evidence of volume loss and distal consolidation suggesting endobronchial obstruction.

PREVENTION

In light of the significant morbidity and potential mortality of pneumonia, appropriate measures should be instituted to reduce the possibility of lung infection. Important but often neglected interventions include smoking cessation (Chapter 31) and avoidance of illicit drugs (Chapter 33) or excess alcohol (Chapter 32), which may impair consciousness. Optimizing the patient's nutritional status is also important in that markedly underweight or obese patients are at increased risk. Finally, the appropriate and consistent use of vaccines can strongly reduce the risk for pneumonia in appropriate patient populations (Chapter 17). The current pneumococcal vaccine contains 23 purified capsular polysaccharides from the serotypes of *S. pneumoniae* that are responsible for more than 85% of invasive pneumococcal infections. Overall, this vaccine is approximately 50 to 80% effective in preventing death from invasive infection. Accordingly, current recommendations are that it should be administered to all patients older than 65 years and to patients younger than 65 years who have chronic pulmonary disease, heart disease, diabetes mellitus, alcoholism, chronic liver disease, CSF leaks, or asplenia and to patients who live in certain settings, including Alaskan natives, high-risk Native American populations, and patients in long-term care facilities. Current pneumococcal vaccines have little toxicity, limited mainly to local site irritation. Individuals generally receive one dose of vaccine, but a single revaccination 5 years later should be considered in those who received their vaccination before 65 years of age or who are at increased risk for severe pneumonia. Pneumococcal vaccine can safely be administered at the time of hospitalization for community-acquired pneumonia.

Vaccination (Chapter 17) should also be considered for viral influenza (Chapter 372). Although usually manifested as an upper respiratory tract infection, influenza can itself cause pneumonia in both immunocompetent and immunosuppressed individuals. More commonly, influenza may precipitate a subsequent bacterial infection, often with *S. aureus, H. influenzae,* and *S. pneumoniae*. Influenza vaccines are developed annually against the current influenza strains, so annual revaccination is necessary (Chapter 17). Influenza vaccines are estimated to be roughly 80% effective in preventing mortality related to influenza. The vaccine should be considered in all patients older than 50 years; residents of nursing homes and chronic care facilities; persons with chronic pulmonary, cardiac, or other diseases requiring ongoing medical care; pregnant women in the second or third trimester during influenza season; and all health care workers with direct patient contact. A weakened virus vaccine, which is administered through a nasal application, does not cause influenza and is approved for healthy people 2 years to 49 years of age who are not pregnant. An inactivated vaccine containing killed virus, administered by injection, is approved for people 6 months of age and older, including healthy people, people with chronic medical conditions, and pregnant women. Both have demonstrated efficacy in preventing influenza and its related complications, including pneumonia.

Contraindications to influenza vaccine include allergy to raw eggs or thimerosal. Side effects are generally self-limited and include injection site soreness, myalgias, mild fever, and malaise. Seasonal influenza vaccination does not lead to exacerbations of asthma. The vaccine should be administered in the fall of the year, but it can also be administered during local epidemics.

TREATMENT Rx

Oversight agencies are increasingly focused on objective measures of optimal care for community-acquired pneumonia, particularly in the hospital setting. Although recommendations are evolving and sometimes vary, current recommendations are that hospitalized patients with community-acquired pneumonia should undergo assessment of oxygenation, initiation of antibiotic therapy in the emergency department, drawing of blood for culture before antimicrobial initiation, smoking cessation intervention, and review and update of immunization status. Most experts also advise chest radiography at the time of admission. The use of biomarkers for bacterial infection, such as levels of procalcitonin, may prove to be helpful when determining which patients can avoid immediate antibiotics or discontinue initial empirical antibiotics because of a low likelihood of bacterial infection. [1]

Initial Empirical Therapy

Because the microbiologic etiology of community-acquired pneumonia is determined in only approximately 50% of cases and the diagnosis may take a day or two, the clinician must institute appropriate empirical therapy based on the most likely agents contributing to the lung infection (Table 97-2). When possible, empirical therapy should be initiated as soon as possible after the diagnosis is established—immediately in the outpatient setting and in the emergency department if the patient is hospitalized. Empirical antimicrobial therapy is based on the severity of illness (inpatient or outpatient setting) and should broadly cover the most likely organisms. The most common bacterial pathogens are *S. pneumoniae* (Chapter 297) and *H. influenzae* (Chapter 308); however, the so-called atypical pathogens, including *M. pneumoniae, C. pneumoniae,* and *Legionella* species (Chapters 325, 326, and 322, respectively), can be the primary or coinfecting agents in up to 40% of community-acquired pneumonia and must be covered in empirical antibiotic regimens. Therapy can be narrowed later after any relevant culture information is obtained.

Guidelines for Hospital and Intensive Care Unit Admission and Treatment

Under current guidelines, patients are stratified with respect to where treatment is initiated (outpatient, inpatient, or ICU setting), the presence of underlying cardiopulmonary disease, and other modifying factors, such as whether

TABLE 97-2 MOST COMMON MICROBIOLOGIC CAUSES OF COMMUNITY-ACQUIRED PNEUMONIA IN APPROXIMATE ORDER OF FREQUENCY

OUTPATIENTS	HOSPITALIZED PATIENTS	SEVERE PNEUMONIA/ICU
Streptococcus pneumoniae	*S. pneumoniae*	*S. pneumoniae*
Mycoplasma pneumoniae	*M. pneumoniae*	*Staphylococcus aureus*
Haemophilus influenzae	*C. pneumoniae*	*Legionella* species
Chlamydophila pneumoniae	*H. influenzae*	Gram-negative bacilli
Respiratory viruses	*Legionella* species Aspiration Respiratory viruses	*H. influenzae*

Adapted from Infectious Diseases Society of America/American Thoracic Society. Consensus guidelines on the management of community acquired pneumonia in adults. *Clin Infect Dis.* 2007;44:S27-S72.

TABLE 97-3 TRIAGE GUIDELINES FOR COMMUNITY-ACQUIRED PNEUMONIA

DECISION TO ADMIT TO THE HOSPITAL

Follow CURB-65 Guidelines and admit patients who have two or more of the following:
Confusion
Uremia (with blood urea nitrogen ≥20 mg/dL)
Respiratory rate >30 breaths/min
Blood pressure ≤90 mm Hg systolic or <60 mm Hg diastolic
Age ≥65 yr

INDICATIONS FOR ICU ADMISSION (1 MAJOR AND ≥3 MINOR)

Major Criteria

Hypotension requiring vasopressors
Respiratory compromise requiring mechanical ventilation

Minor Criteria

Respiratory rate >30 breaths/min
PaO_2/FIO_2 ratio ≤250
Multilobar infiltrate
Confusion/disorientation
Uremia (blood urea nitrogen ≥20 mg/dL)
Leukopenia (white blood cell count ≤4000 cells/mm^3)
Thrombocytopenia (platelets ≤100,000 cells/mm^3)
Hypothermia (≤36° C)
Hypotension requiring aggressive fluid resuscitation

the patient is likely to be infected with drug-resistant *S. pneumoniae*, gram-negative enteric bacilli, or *Pseudomonas aeruginosa*. Following these guidelines reduces the number of hospital admissions without adversely affecting outcomes.

The decision to admit a patient to the hospital must be made on clinical grounds. Patients can be effectively and safely managed as outpatients if they are mildly ill, are younger than 65 years, and do not have coexisting cardiopulmonary disease, malignancy, immune compromise, or renal, liver, or other significant systemic diseases (Table 97-3).

In general, outpatients who are mildly ill and do not have any underlying cardiopulmonary disease or other modifying factors are usually infected with *S. pneumoniae, M. pneumoniae, C. pneumoniae, H. influenzae,* respiratory viruses, or *Legionella* species. These uncomplicated outpatient cases can be managed with an oral advanced-generation macrolide, such as azithromycin or clarithromycin, both of which are better tolerated and provide better coverage of *Haemophilus* species than erythromycin. 2 Alternatively, doxycycline may be used in patients who are intolerant of macrolides, although this option is less optimal because of increasing levels of tetracycline resistance in *S. pneumoniae* isolates. Outpatients who have underlying comorbidities (e.g., chronic heart, lung, liver, or renal disease, diabetes mellitus, alcoholism, asplenia, immunosuppressive conditions or drugs, use of antibiotics within the past 3 months, or exposure to a child in a daycare center) are at higher risk of having drug-resistant *S. pneumoniae*. If their pneumonia is not sufficiently severe to warrant admission, and any comorbid illnesses are stable and compensated, patients can be treated either with respiratory fluoroquinolones (e.g., moxifloxacin, gemifloxacin, or levofloxacin) or with a β-lactam plus a macrolide (e.g., high-dose amoxicillin or amoxicillin-clavulanate is preferred; alternatives

TABLE 97-4 EMPIRICAL TREATMENT GUIDELINES FOR COMMUNITY-ACQUIRED PNEUMONIA

OUTPATIENT MANAGEMENT

1. Previously healthy patients without comorbidities and no use of antimicrobials within the prior 3 months
   A macrolide (preferred) (e.g., clarithromycin, extended release, 1000 mg orally each day for at least 5 days, or azithromycin, 500 mg orally on day 1, followed by 250 mg orally each day on days 2-5)
   Doxycycline, 100 mg orally twice daily for at least 5 days
2. Presence of comorbidities such as chronic cardiopulmonary, liver, or renal disease; diabetes mellitus; alcoholism; malignancies; asplenia; immunosuppressive conditions or drugs; or use of antimicrobials in the prior 3 months (if so, select an alternative agent from a different class)
   A respiratory fluoroquinolone (oral moxifloxacin, 400 mg/day, or gemifloxacin, 320 mg/day, or levofloxacin, 750 mg daily for at least 5 days), *or*
   A β-lactam (e.g., ceftriaxone, 1-2 g IM each day for at least 5 days) *plus* a macrolide (e.g., azithromycin, 500 mg orally on day 1, followed by 250 mg orally each day on days 2-5)
3. In regions with a high rate (>25%) of infection with high-level (MIC ≥16 mg/mL) macrolide-resistant *Streptococcus pneumoniae*, consider an alternative agent as noted under (2) for patients without comorbidities.

INPATIENTS, NON-ICU MANAGEMENT

1. A respiratory fluoroquinolone (moxifloxacin, 400 mg/day, or gemifloxacin, 320 mg/day, or levofloxacin, 750 mg IV for 2 days followed by oral for at least 5 days total), *or*
2. A β-lactam (e.g., ceftriaxone 1-2 g IV daily for at least 1-2 days, followed by 1-2 g IM daily for at least 5 days total), *plus*
   A macrolide (azithromycin, 500 mg IV each day for at least 2 days, followed by 500 mg orally each day for a total of at least 5 days)

INPATIENTS—ICU MANAGEMENT

1. A β-lactam (cefotaxime, 1-2 g IV every 6-8 hr, or ceftriaxone, 1-2 g IV each day, or ampicillin-sulbactam, 1.5-3 g IV every 6 hours, up to maximum of 4 g of sulbactam/day, for 7-14 days, *plus*
   Either azithromycin, 500 mg IV each day for at least 2 days, followed by 500 mg orally each day for a total of at least 5 days, or a respiratory fluoroquinolone (e.g., moxifloxacin, 400 mg/day, or gemifloxacin, 320 mg/day, or levofloxacin, 750 mg IV daily for 7-14 days)
2. For penicillin-allergic individuals, a respiratory fluoroquinolone (e.g., moxifloxacin, 400 mg/day, or gemifloxacin, 320 mg/day, or levofloxacin, 750 mg IV daily for 7-14 days) and aztreonam, 2 g IV every 6-8 hr for 7-14 days, are recommended.

SPECIAL CONCERNS

If *Pseudomonas* species infection is a concern:

1. An antipneumococcal, antipseudomonal β-lactam (piperacillin-tazobactam, 3.375 g IV every 6 hr, or cefepime, 1-2 g every 12 hr, or imipenem, 500 mg every 6 hr or 1 g every 8 hr, or meropenem, 1 g IV every 8 hr), *plus* either ciprofloxacin, 400 mg IV every 8 hr, or levofloxacin, 500-750 mg IV every day, for 7-14 days, *or*
2. The above β-lactam plus an aminoglycoside (e.g., gentamicin, 7 mg/kg/day in three divided doses, with monitoring to maintain trough levels lower than 1 μg/mL, or tobramycin, 7 mg/kg/day in three divided doses, with monitoring to maintain trough levels lower than 1 μg/mL) and azithromycin (500 mg IV each day for at least 2 days, followed by 500 mg orally each day) for 7-14 days, *or*
3. The above β-lactam plus an aminoglycoside (as described above) and an antipneumococcal fluoroquinolone (ciprofloxacin, 400 mg IV every 8 hr, or levofloxacin, 500-750 mg IV every day) for 7-14 days

For penicillin-allergic patients, use aztreonam, 2 g IV every 6-8 hr for 7-14 days, instead of the β-lactam.

If community-acquired methicillin-resistant *Staphylococcus aureus* is a consideration, add vancomycin, 15 mg/kg every 12 hr with monitoring to maintain trough at 15-20 μg/mL, or linezolid, 600 mg every 12 hr, for 7-14 days.

Adapted from Infectious Diseases Society of America/American Thoracic Society. Consensus guidelines on the management of community acquired pneumonia in adults. *Clin Infect Dis.* 2007;44:S27-S72.

include ceftriaxone, cefpodoxime, and cefuroxime; doxycycline is an alternative to the macrolide) (Table 97-4). In regions that have a high incidence of macrolide-resistant (>25%) *S. pneumoniae,* the alternative agents should be used. When pneumonia is treated on an outpatient basis, patients require careful monitoring to be certain that they respond over the first 72 hours of therapy. The clinician must maintain vigilance about the need to hospitalize patients who deteriorate or fail to respond to the initial empirical therapy.

Patients who have more severe respiratory illnesses, significant unstable or uncompensated comorbid illnesses, or a poor initial response to otherwise appropriate outpatient therapy generally should be admitted to the hospital promptly. Patients who require hospitalization but not intensive care should be treated initially with either an intravenous respiratory fluoroquinolone, such as levofloxacin or moxifloxacin,[3] or with the combination of an intravenous β-lactam plus a macrolide.

Patients who have respiratory insufficiency, septicemia, shock, or significant multiorgan dysfunction, with or without the need for mechanical ventilatory support, require management in an ICU and evaluation to exclude infection with *P. aeruginosa* (Chapter 314). ICU admission should also be considered for patients who exhibit three or more of the minor criteria for severe community-acquired pneumonia (see Table 97-3).

Among patients with severe community-acquired pneumonia, those at increased risk for *P. aeruginosa* infection include patients with structural lung disease (particularly bronchiectasis), greater than 10 mg/day of previous corticosteroid therapy, neutropenia, malnutrition, or previous broad-spectrum antibiotics for more than 7 days in the past month. ICU patients who are *not* considered at risk for *P. aeruginosa* infection can be treated initially with a β-lactam (cefotaxime, ceftriaxone, or ampicillin-sulbactam) plus either azithromycin or a respiratory fluoroquinolone (moxifloxacin or levofloxacin) (see Table 97-4). In penicillin-allergic patients, a respiratory fluoroquinolone and aztreonam is a reasonable regimen. Fluoroquinolone monotherapy is not considered appropriate in the setting of severe community-acquired pneumonia. In the ICU population considered to be at risk for *P. aeruginosa* infection, combination antipseudomonal therapy should be used, including an antipneumococcal, antipseudomonal β-lactam (piperacillin-tazobactam, cefepime, imipenem, or meropenem) plus either ciprofloxacin or levofloxacin or a β-lactam plus an aminoglycoside and azithromycin. If community-acquired methicillin-resistant *S. aureus* (MRSA) infection is a consideration, vancomycin or linezolid should be added to the regimen.

Suspected or Proven Viral Infection

Therapies for suspected and proven viral infection are relatively limited when compared with those for bacterial infections. Early treatment of influenza A or B within the first 48 hours of symptoms with oseltamivir (75 mg orally taken twice daily for 5 days), or zanamivir (two inhalations of 5 mg per inhalation every 12 hours for 5 days) is effective in reducing symptoms and the duration of illness (Chapter 368). Both agents have been used for novel H1N1 swine influenza, and oseltamivir may also have activity against H5N1 bird flu. Empirical antibiotic treatment of possible bacterial superinfection in addition to influenza should include agents effective against *S. pneumoniae* (Chapter 297), *S. aureus* (Chapter 296), and *H. influenzae* (Chapter 308). In these considerations, amoxicillin-clavulanate, cefpodoxime, cefprozil, cefuroxime, or a respiratory fluoroquinolone would be appropriate. Pneumonias caused by varicella-zoster and herpes simplex virus should be treated with parenteral acyclovir (10 mg/kg intravenously every 8 hours for 7 days) (Chapters 382 and 383). No antiviral agents have established efficacy against RSV in adults, parainfluenza virus, adenovirus, metapneumovirus, the SARS coronavirus, or hantavirus. Treatment is largely supportive, with oxygen and ventilator therapy as necessary.

Duration of Therapy

Most patients respond to empirical antibiotic regimens over the first 3 days of therapy. In general, it is not advisable to alter the antibiotic program in the first 72 hours unless the patient is deteriorating or culture results indicate alternative therapy. Patients initially begun on parenteral therapy may be switched to an oral regimen when they are afebrile (temperature less than 38° C [100° F] on two occasions 8 hours apart) and demonstrate improvement in cough, dyspnea, and leukocytosis.

Patients with community-acquired pneumonia should be treated for at least 5 days,[4] should be afebrile for at least 48 to 72 hours, and should not show signs of clinical instability before discontinuation of antibiotic therapy. Accordingly, the total duration of antimicrobials should be individualized to the patient's clinical response. Initial multiagent regimens of a β-lactam with the addition of macrolides for the coverage of *Legionella* and *Mycoplasma* can frequently be de-escalated after several days to the β-lactams alone if *Legionella* urinary antigen and *Mycoplasma* serology prove negative. The clinical caveat remains, however, that macrolides may still be required in clinical situations in which a strong clinical suspicion for *Legionella* persists because urinary antigen testing does not detect organisms other than *Legionella* serogroup 1. Furthermore, in situations in which a causative organism is isolated from a normally sterile site, such as blood or pleural fluid, antibiotic therapy should be simplified and directed by susceptibility testing. Finally, when alternative clinical diagnoses other than pneumonia are proved to be the cause of the respiratory symptoms and all cultures remain negative over the first 72 hours, antibiotic therapy may be safely discontinued.

Treatment Failure

Treatment failures occur in approximately 10% of patients with community-acquired pneumonia, and complications occur in roughly 25% of patients. Adherence to treatment guidelines, such as those described earlier, increases the likelihood of a good outcome.

For patients who do not respond to initial empirical coverage, an aggressive search should be undertaken to detect unusual pathogens, alternative diagnoses such as pulmonary embolism (Chapter 98), or complications of pneumonia such as a complicated pleural effusion (Chapter 99), empyema, or lung abscess (Chapter 90). Additional diagnostic testing may include a chest CT scan, sampling of pleural fluid, and bronchoscopy with collection of respiratory secretions, brushings, and BAL fluid for microbiologic analysis.

Follow-Up after Treatment

Even when the patient appears to respond to the initial antibiotic regimen, the chest radiograph signs resolve more slowly (over a period of 6 to 8 weeks) than other clinical signs and symptoms. The physician must document that abnormalities on the chest radiograph have resolved completely or, in some cases, have led to the formation of a fibrotic scar. Usual practice includes performing repeat radiography 6 to 8 weeks after completion of the antibiotic regimen. Persistence of abnormalities on the chest radiograph or the development of recurrent pneumonia in a similar distribution should prompt a careful search for an underlying endobronchial obstruction such as an occult neoplasm (Chapter 197), foreign body, bronchostenosis, or broncholithiasis. Follow-up CT scanning is usually the prelude to formal pulmonary consultation for consideration of bronchoscopy and other further diagnostic tests.

ASPIRATION PNEUMONIA

EPIDEMIOLOGY AND PATHOBIOLOGY

Although microaspiration is the mechanism underlying most cases of pneumonia, the clinician is occasionally confronted with recurrent bacterial pneumonia in a patient experiencing repeated gross aspiration of oropharyngeal contents. Most of these patients have difficulty swallowing related to either underlying neuromuscular disorders or altered sensorium as a result of medications, drugs or alcohol, or underlying neurologic diseases. Common clinical scenarios associated with recurrent aspiration pneumonia include tracheobronchial fistulas secondary to esophageal or tracheal malignancies, esophageal obstruction related to esophageal cancer and its treatment (Chapter 198), and a wide variety of neurologic disorders, including amyotrophic lateral sclerosis (Chapter 418), multiple sclerosis (Chapter 419), stroke (Chapter 414), and other myopathic processes. Other patients with severe esophageal reflux (Chapter 140) may also experience significant aspiration during sleep despite apparently normal deglutition mechanisms and protective reflexes during wakefulness. Patients with neuromuscular disorders tend to have greater difficulty swallowing thin or liquid materials, whereas patients with obstruction from either malignancy or benign strictures tend to have the greatest difficulty swallowing solid food.

CLINICAL MANIFESTATIONS

Aspiration pneumonias tend to have a less acute manifestation than the usual bacterial pneumonias, with the onset of fever, dyspnea, purulent sputum, malaise, and other systemic symptoms, including loss of appetite, evolving over a number of days. Physical examination of the chest generally reveals only coarse rhonchi in the lower lobes or dependent lung regions.

DIAGNOSIS

The diagnosis of aspiration pneumonia relies foremost on maintaining a high clinical index of suspicion. Recovery of tracheal secretions containing food particles or lipid-laden macrophages strongly supports the diagnosis. In patients receiving tube feedings, the respiratory secretions should be tested for glucose because these secretions normally contain low levels of glucose. Alternatively, methylene blue or similar tracer dyes can be added to tube feeding materials to confirm the presence of aspiration. Additional diagnostic modalities include the use of cineradiographic swallowing studies with thin liquid water-soluble contrast agents to confirm the aspiration event. Radionuclide imaging studies may also document aspiration in adults whose neurologic status precludes them from cooperating fully with the cineradiographic studies. Overnight esophageal pH monitoring may be undertaken in individuals who are suspected of having recurrent esophageal reflux and aspiration events at night. However, except in the most severe cases, it remains difficult to predict which patients with gastroesophageal reflux will actually experience aspiration pneumonia.

Chest radiographs should be reviewed in light of the patient's probable position during aspiration. The lower lobes, particularly the superior segments of the right lower lobe, and the posterior segments of the upper lobes are frequently involved. However, unilateral aspiration or aspiration into virtually any pulmonary segment has been reported, depending on the patient's position during the aspiration event. The radiographic appearance usually reflects a parenchymal bronchopneumonia process. Pleural involvement is uncommon initially, unless aggressive anaerobic infection is present. Nonresolving or inadequately treated aspiration pneumonia can result in lung abscess and empyema formation.

Bronchoscopy, although not routinely necessary, can confirm the presence of aspiration by recovering food particles or lipid-laden macrophages derived from fats present in the aspirated food. Bronchoscopy with BAL can be useful in providing quantitative counts of aerobic bacteria, and protected specimen brush sampling can document anaerobic organisms, although negative cultures do not exclude the presence of anaerobes.

Microbiology

Oropharyngeal secretions contain massive numbers of microorganisms, with counts of aerobic bacteria ranging between 10^6 and 10^8 and anaerobic organisms being as high as 10^9 per milliliter of saliva. Accordingly, aspiration pneumonia should be viewed as a polymicrobial infection, with the clinical manifestations being driven by the predominant and most aggressive organisms in the mixture. Oropharyngeal colonization is strongly influenced by the clinical setting in which the patient was dwelling at the time of aspiration (outpatient versus hospital or institutional). In otherwise healthy outpatients, aggressive organisms such as *S. pneumoniae, S. aureus,* and *H. influenzae* may also be present. In contrast, the oropharyngeal secretions of hospitalized patients and residents of long-term care facilities include aerobic gram-negative bacteria and *P. aeruginosa.* Anaerobic organisms, which are a major consideration in both settings, include anaerobic and microaerophilic streptococci, *Bacteroides* species, *Fusobacterium nucleatum,* and *Prevotella* species. Cultures of sputum and tracheal secretions probably document such mixed flora.

TREATMENT

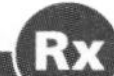

Empirical antibiotic therapy should be initiated rapidly once the diagnosis of aspiration pneumonia is made; the regimen can be modified later after culture information from sputum, tracheal secretions, or bronchoscopic sampling is available. Otherwise healthy individuals with isolated aspiration pneumonia related to trauma, seizures, or oversedation may be treated initially with either oral amoxicillin-clavulanate (amoxicillin, 875 mg, and clavulanate acid, 125 mg, orally every 12 hours for at least 5 days), intravenous clindamycin (600 mg intravenously [IV] every 8 hours for at least 5 days), or intravenous piperacillin-tazobactam (3.375 g IV every 6 hours for at least 5 days), depending on the severity of illness. In uncomplicated mild to moderate aspiration pneumonia in elderly patients, intravenous clindamycin is as effective, less expensive, and associated with a lower rate of post-treatment occurrence of MRSA. 5 For patients with underlying chronic diseases, intravenous piperacillin-tazobactam (3.375 g IV every 6 hours for 7 to 14 days) or intravenous fluoroquinolones that cover anaerobes, such as moxifloxacin (400 mg IV each day for 7 to 14 days), can be considered. In seriously ill individuals, particularly patients requiring intubation and mechanical ventilation, as well as patients experiencing aspiration in the hospital or long-term care setting, coverage must be extended to aerobic gram-negative bacteria and *Pseudomonas* species; treatment considerations would include extended-spectrum β-lactam/β-lactamase inhibitor combinations such as piperacillin-tazobactam (3.375 g IV every 6 hours for 7 to 14 days) or ticarcillin-clavulanate (3 g of ticarcillin, and 0.1 g of clavulanic acid IV every 4 to 6 hours for 7 to 14 days), or carbapenems such as imipenem (500 mg IV every 6 to 8 hours for 7 to 14 days). Intravenous clindamycin (600 mg IV every 8 hours) can also be added in these settings, or alternatively, intravenous clindamycin can be given in combination with ciprofloxacin (400 mg IV every 8 hours for 7 to 14 days) or aztreonam (2 g IV every 6 to 8 hours for 7 to 14 days). In patients with concern about organisms with high levels of antibiotic resistance, such as *P. aeruginosa,* an antipseudomonal β-lactam such as ceftazidime (2 g IV every 8 hours for 7 to 14 days) or cefepime (1 to 2 g every 12 hours for 7 to 14 days) can be combined with an antipseudomonal fluoroquinolone such as ciprofloxacin or an aminoglycoside (e.g., gentamicin 7 mg/kg/day in three divided doses IV for 7 to 14 days, measuring drug levels and adjusting doses to achieve a trough level of <1 μg/mL). Again, addition of extended anaerobic coverage with clindamycin should be considered. Finally, if the patient is known or suspected to harbor MRSA, intravenous vancomycin (15 mg/kg every 12 hours IV and measuring drug level and adjusting doses to achieve trough levels of 15 to 20 μg/mL) or linezolid (600 mg IV every 12 hours) for 10 to 14 days should be added to the regimen.

Surgical Therapy

Adequate nutrition is a concern in patients with multiple episodes of aspiration pneumonia and underlying neurologic disease or malignancy. Endoscopic or surgical placement of a gastrostomy or jejunostomy feeding tube can be considered to aid in providing nutrition, fluids, and medications in the palliation of such patients. Of greater challenge are patients who continue to have pneumonia related to aspiration of saliva, sometimes around cuffed endotracheal and tracheostomy tubes. If aggressive therapy is considered appropriate, ligation of the submaxillary and parotid salivary ducts can decrease the production of saliva.

HOSPITAL-ACQUIRED PNEUMONIA, VENTILATOR-ASSOCIATED PNEUMONIA, AND HEALTH CARE–ASSOCIATED PNEUMONIA

EPIDEMIOLOGY

Hospital-acquired pneumonia, ventilator-associated pneumonia, and health care–associated pneumonia represent the second most common nosocomial infections in the United States. Hospital-acquired pneumonia on average increases the length of hospital stay from 7 to 9 days, at an additional cost of more than $40,000 per patient; it is responsible for one fourth of all ICU infections and half of all antibiotic use. Early-onset hospital-acquired pneumonia and ventilator-associated pneumonia, defined as infections occurring within the first 4 hospital days, tend to be caused by antibiotic-susceptible bacteria, whereas late-onset infections are more frequently caused by multidrug-resistant (MDR) organisms (Table 97-5), which are associated with greater morbidity and mortality. The overall mortality attributed to hospital-acquired pneumonia may be as high as 30 to 50%.

PATHOBIOLOGY

Gram-negative bacterial pneumonias are fairly uncommon in previously healthy outpatients, except in patients with impaired immunity or underlying structural lung disease such as chronic obstructive pulmonary disease. However, aerobic gram-negative bacilli, including *P. aeruginosa, Escherichia coli, K. pneumoniae,* and *Acinetobacter* species, play major roles in patients with hospital-acquired pneumonia, ventilator-associated pneumonia, and health care–associated pneumonia. Many cases are polymicrobial, and gram-positive agents such as *S. aureus,* particularly MRSA strains, are also increasingly common. The frequency of MDR bacteria varies by the patient population, hospital, ICU, and local use of antimicrobial agents, so routine surveillance and monitoring of local pathogens and drug susceptibilities are key to adjusting antibiotic use appropriately.

P. aeruginosa, Acinetobacter species, *Stenotrophomonas maltophilia,* and *Burkholderia cepacia* complex are of particular concern because these organisms rapidly become resistant to multiple classes of antibiotics. MDR organisms are most commonly found in patients with severe underlying chronic disease, in patients with health care–associated pneumonia, and in those with late-onset hospital-acquired pneumonia and ventilator-associated pneumonia. Although considerable emphasis is placed on gram-negative bacteria in the hospital setting, more traditional bacterial pathogens such as *S. pneumoniae* and *H. influenzae* must also be considered as potential causes.

TABLE 97-5 HOST RISK FACTORS ASSOCIATED WITH DEVELOPMENT OF MULTIDRUG-RESISTANT INFECTION DURING HAP, VAP, AND HCAP

Antibiotic therapy in the past 90 days
High incidence of antibiotic resistance in the community or in the specific hospital unit
Current hospitalization for 5 or more days
Immunosuppressive disease or therapy
Presence of risk factors for HCAP
Hospitalization for 2 or more days in the past 90 days
Resident in a nursing home or extended care facility
Home infusion therapy (including antibiotics)
Chronic dialysis within the past 30 days
Home wound care
Family member with an MDR pathogen

HAP = hospital-associated pneumonia; HCAP = health care-associated pneumonia; MDR = multidrug resistant; VAP = ventilator-associated pneumonia.
Adapted from American Thoracic Society and Infectious Diseases Society of America. Guidelines for management of adults with hospital-acquired, ventilator-associated, and health care-associated pneumonia. *Am J Respir Crit Care Med.* 2005;171:388-416.

L. pneumophila also occasionally occurs as a nosocomial infection, particularly where there is contaminated water or during construction.

CLINICAL MANIFESTATIONS

Hospital-acquired pneumonia, ventilator-associated pneumonia, and health care–associated pneumonia are often first suspected with the demonstration of new or worsening radiographic infiltrates along with other clinical signs of infection, including fever, leukocytosis, and purulent sputum. Oxygenation may have also worsened. In general, two of the three major clinical features (fever, leukocytosis, purulent sputum) should be present. In patients with acute respiratory distress syndrome, however, a single clinical factor alone should prompt additional investigation and microbiologic culture.

DIAGNOSIS

All patients with suspected hospital-acquired pneumonia, ventilator-associated pneumonia, and health care–associated pneumonia should receive a comprehensive history and physical examination to define the severity of disease and potential sources of infection. Chest radiography is essential to determine the extent of pneumonia, particularly whether it is focal or multilobar. Some patients without new or evolving radiographic infiltrates but with other signs of infection may have purulent tracheobronchitis (Chapter 96), which may require antibiotic therapy if clinical signs of infection are present. Arterial blood gases, complete blood count, electrolytes, and liver and renal function should also be evaluated. Blood should be obtained for culture, although it is positive in only a minority of patients, before instituting new antibiotics whenever possible.

Lower respiratory tract secretions should be obtained for culture from all patients by endotracheal aspiration, BAL, or protected specimen brush whenever possible before changes in antibiotic therapy; a reliable Gram stain can help direct initial empirical therapy. A sterile culture of lower respiratory tract secretions in the absence of a new antibiotic in the past 72 hours essentially excludes most bacterial pneumonias with a 94% negative predictive value, although *Legionella* and viral infection are still possible in this situation. The quantitative diagnostic threshold for significant bacterial infection, in the absence of recent (<72 hours) changes in antibiotic regimens, is as follows: greater than 10^6 colony-forming units (cfu)/mL for tracheal aspirates, greater than 10^4 or 10^5 cfu/mL for quantitative BAL fluid, and greater than 10^3 cfu/mL for protected specimen brushings. The use of bronchoscopically obtained specimens and quantitative bacterial culture in directing therapy reduces the 14-day mortality in suspected ventilator-associated pneumonia.

TREATMENT Rx

Initial Empirical Therapy

If the patient is unstable or has evidence of sepsis, or if there is a high suspicion for hospital-acquired pneumonia, ventilator-associated pneumonia, or health care–associated pneumonia, prompt antibiotic therapy is required regardless of whether bacteria are found on the initial microscopic examination of lower respiratory tract samples because delays in antimicrobial therapy increase mortality. The choice of initial empirical therapy is based on several factors, including whether the pneumonia is early onset, whether there are risk factors for MDR bacterial infections (Table 97-6), and local surveillance data on bacterial prevalence and susceptibilities.

Suspected or Early-Onset Disease

For patients with suspected hospital-acquired or ventilator-associated pneumonia, with early-onset disease, and with no identifiable risk factors for MDR organisms, initial empirical therapy can include either ceftriaxone, an intravenous fluoroquinolone (levofloxacin, moxifloxacin, or ciprofloxacin), ampicillin/sulbactam, or ertapenem. These options will cover *S. pneumoniae,*

TABLE 97-6 EMPIRICAL ANTIBIOTIC TREATMENT OF HOSPITAL-ACQUIRED PNEUMONIA, VENTILATOR-ASSOCIATED PNEUMONIA, AND HEALTH CARE–ASSOCIATED PNEUMONIA

GROUP A: PATIENTS WITH EITHER HAP OR VAP, WITHOUT RISK FACTORS FOR MDR PATHOGENS, AND WITH EARLY-ONSET PNEUMONIA	
POTENTIAL PATHOGENS	**RECOMMENDED THERAPY**
Streptococcus pneumoniae *Haemophilus influenzae* Methicillin-sensitive *Staphylococcus aureus* Antibiotic-sensitive enteric gram-negative bacilli *Escherichia coli* *Klebsiella pneumoniae* *Enterobacter* species *Proteus* species *Serratia marcescens*	Ceftriaxone, 1-2 g IV/IM every 12-24 hr, maximum of 4 g/day, with duration dependent on clinical response and individualized, as discussed in text *or* Levofloxacin, 500-750 mg IV every day, with duration dependent on clinical response and individualized; or ciprofloxacin, 400 mg IV every 8 hr, with duration dependent on clinical response and individualized; or moxifloxacin, 400 mg IV or orally every 24 hr, with duration dependent on clinical response and individualized *or* Ampicillin-sulbactam, 1.5-3 g (1-2 g ampicillin and 0.5-1 g sulbactam) IV/IM every 6 hr, maximum of 4 g sulbactam/day, depending on type and severity of infection, with duration dependent on clinical response and individualized *or* Ertapenem, 1 g IV/IM once a day, with duration dependent on clinical response and individualized
GROUP B: PATIENTS WITH HAP, VAP, OR HCAP AND WITH LATE-ONSET PNEUMONIA OR WITH RISK FACTORS FOR MDR PATHOGENS	
ORGANISMS	**THERAPY**
Streptococcus pneumoniae *Haemophilus influenzae* Methicillin-sensitive *S. aureus* Antibiotic-sensitive enteric gram-negative bacilli *E. coli* *K. pneumoniae* *Enterobacter* species *Proteus* species *S. marcescens* MDR pathogens *Pseudomonas aeruginosa* *K. pneumoniae* (extended spectrum β-lactamase producing) *Acinetobacter* species Methicillin-resistant *S. aureus* *Legionella pneumophila*	Antipseudomonal cephalosporin (ceftazidime, 2 g IV every 8 hr, or cefepime, 1-2 g every 8-12 hr, with duration dependent on clinical response and individualized) *or* Antipseudomonal carbapenems (meropenem, 1 g every 8 hr, or imipenem, 500 mg every 6 hr or 1 g every 8 hr, with duration dependent on clinical response and individualized) *or* β-Lactam/β-lactamase inhibitor (piperacillin-tazobactam, 4.5 g IV every 6 hr, with duration dependent on clinical response and individualized) *plus* Antipseudomonal fluoroquinolone (levofloxacin, 750 mg IV every day, or ciprofloxacin, 400 mg IV q8h, with duration dependent on clinical response and individualized) *or* Aminoglycoside (amikacin, 15-20 mg/kg/day, divided every 8-12 hours, with monitoring to maintain trough lower than 4-5 μg/mL; or gentamicin, 7 mg/kg/day as a single daily dose, with monitoring to maintain trough levels lower than 1 μg/mL; or tobramycin, 4-7 mg/kg/day as a single daily dose, with monitoring to maintain trough levels lower than 1 μg/mL and duration dependent on clinical response and individualized) *plus* Vancomycin (15 mg/kg IV every 12 hr, with monitoring to maintain trough at 10-15 μg/mL and duration dependent on clinical response and individualized) or linezolid (600 mg IV every 12 hr, with duration dependent on clinical response and individualized)

HAP = hospital-associated pneumonia; HCAP = health care–associated pneumonia; MDR = multidrug resistant; VAP = ventilator-associated pneumonia.
Adapted from American Thoracic Society. Guidelines for management of adults with hospital-acquired ventilator associated, and healthcare-associated pneumonia. *Am J Respir Crit Care Med.* 2005:171:388-416.

H. influenzae, MRSA, and most antibiotic-sensitive gram-negative bacilli, including *E. coli*, *K. pneumoniae*, *Proteus* species, *Enterobacter* species, and *Serratia marcescens*.

Late-Onset Disease

In contrast, with late-onset hospital-acquired pneumonia, ventilator-associated pneumonia, or health care–associated pneumonia, or when risk factors for MDR infection have been identified, multiagent regimens should be used initially. Options include an antipseudomonal cephalosporin such as ceftazidime or cefepime, an antipseudomonal carbapenem (meropenem or imipenem), or a β-lactam/β-lactamase inhibitor agent such as piperacillin-tazobactam; in addition, either an antipseudomonal fluoroquinolone (ciprofloxacin or levofloxacin) or an aminoglycoside such as amikacin, gentamicin, or tobramycin should be used. In combination, these agents should empirically address most MDR pathogens, including *P. aeruginosa*, *Acinetobacter* species, and *K. pneumoniae* strains with extended-spectrum β-lactamase production. Most *L. pneumophila* isolates will also be covered, but if *Legionella* is strongly suspected, a macrolide such as azithromycin should be included. Finally, either vancomycin or linezolid should be added for coverage of MRSA if risk factors are present or the risk for MRSA is high locally.

Duration of Treatment

The initiation of empirical antibiotic therapy mandates careful daily reassessment. If the patient improves over the first 48 to 72 hours, strong consideration should be given to de-escalating antibiotic therapy based on culture results. If lower respiratory cultures remain negative but the patient has not improved, an extrapulmonary site of infection should be considered. Additional radiographic imaging and cultures from the lung, pleura, and other sites may be helpful. The total duration of therapy, therefore, must be individualized. In general, aminoglycoside use should be limited to 5 to 7 days. Overall antibiotic therapy can be as short as 7 days if the patient has improved, but patients with sluggish improvement may require 14 to 21 days of therapy.

PREVENTION

Sources of pathogens for hospital-acquired pneumonia include the environment, health care devices, and transfer of microbes by patients, staff, and visitors. Thus, scrupulous hand hygiene is essential for reducing these infections. Colonization plus aspiration of oropharyngeal pathogens or leakage of secretions around endotracheal tubes is the usual route of inoculation. The stomach and sinuses may be additional sites harboring pathogens. Infected biofilms on endotracheal tubes may also serve as an important reservoir for these infections. In this light, aggressive measures should be enforced to reduce the risk for hospital-acquired pneumonia and ventilator-associated pneumonia. Prevention centers first on staff education and compliance with alcohol-based hand disinfection, which must be used before and after each patient interaction. In addition, patients with documented MDR organisms should be isolated to reduce the risk for patient cross-contamination. Microbiologic surveillance within the hospital environment is also necessary to identify MDR organisms and determine antibiotic use and susceptibility patterns. Within the ICU, intubation and reintubation rates should be monitored and reduced as feasible, the duration of mechanical ventilation should be minimized to reduce the risk for ventilator-associated pneumonia, and methods known to reduce infection rates should be followed (Chapter 105). Ventilator-associated pneumonia can be reduced by elevation of the head of the patient's bed, daily "sedation vacations," daily assessment of the patient's readiness for extubation, peptic ulcer disease prophylaxis, and deep vein thrombosis prophylaxis. In addition, continuous aspiration of subglottic secretions is a safe procedure that also reduces the use of antimicrobial agents and the incidence of ventilator-associated pneumonia in patients who are at risk.[6]

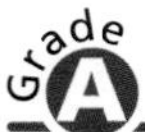

1. Schuetz P, Albrich W, Christ-Crain M, et al. Procalcitonin for guidance of antibiotic therapy. *Expert Rev Anti Infect Ther*. 2010;8:575-587.
2. Paris R, Confalonieri M, Dal Negro R, et al. Efficacy and safety of azithromycin 1 g once daily for 3 days in the treatment of community-acquired pneumonia: an open-label randomized comparison with amoxicillin-clavulanate 875/125 mg twice daily for 7 days. *J Chemother*. 2008;20:77-86.
3. Vardakas KZ, Siempos II, Grammatikos A, et al. Respiratory fluoroquinolones for the treatment of community-acquired pneumonia: a meta-analysis of randomized controlled trials. *CMAJ Can Med Assoc J*. 2008;179:1269-1277.
4. Shorr AF, Zadeikis N, Xiang JX, et al. A multicenter, randomized, double-blind, retrospective comparison of 5- and 10-day regimens of levofloxacin in a subgroup of patients aged > or = 65 years with community-acquired pneumonia. *Clin Ther*. 2005;27:1251-1259.
5. Kadowaki M, Demura Y, Mizuno S, et al. Reappraisal of clindamycin IV monotherapy for treatment of mild-to-moderate aspiration pneumonia in elderly patients. *Chest*. 2005;127:1276-1282.
6. Bouza E, Perez MJ, Munoz P, et al. Continuous aspiration of subglottic secretions in the prevention of ventilator-associated pneumonia in the postoperative period of major heart surgery. *Chest*. 2008;134:938-946.

SUGGESTED READINGS

Fung HB, Monteagudo-Chu MO. Community-acquired pneumonia in the elderly. *Am J Geriatr Pharmacother*. 2010;8:47-61. *Review*.

McCabe C, Kirchner C, Zhang H, et al. Guideline-concordant therapy and reduced mortality and length of stay in adults with community-acquired pneumonia: playing by the rules. *Arch Intern Med*. 2009;169:1525-1531. *Compliance with the current IDSA and ATS community-acquired pneumonia guidelines improves mortality and length of hospitalization.*

Mortensen EM, Copeland LA, Pugh MJ, et al. Diagnosis of pulmonary malignancy after hospitalization for pneumonia. *Am J Med*. 2010;123:66-71. *About 9% of patients hospitalized with pneumonia were diagnosed with a pulmonary malignancy within the next year.*

Ruuskanen O, Lahti E, Jennings LC, et al. Viral pneumonia. *Lancet*. 2011;377:1264-1275. *Review*.

98

PULMONARY EMBOLISM

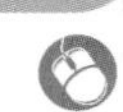

JEFFREY I. WEITZ

DEFINITIONS

Pulmonary embolism (PE) refers to an obstruction of a pulmonary artery by material that has traveled to the lungs from elsewhere in the body through the blood stream. Thrombus from the deep veins of the legs or arms represents the most common type of material to embolize to the lungs—a process known as venous thromboembolism (VTE). In addition to thrombotic pulmonary emboli, nonthrombotic material also can embolize to the lungs. Such material includes fat, air, amniotic fluid, tumor cells, talc in intravenous drug users, and various medical devices. Regardless of the type of embolic material, blockage of blood flow through the lungs and the resultant increased pressure in the right ventricle are responsible for the symptoms and signs of PE.

THROMBOTIC PULMONARY EMBOLISM

EPIDEMIOLOGY

VTE, which includes deep vein thrombosis (DVT; Chapter 81) and PE, represents the third most common cause of cardiovascular death after myocardial infarction and strokes. A first episode of VTE occurs in about 1 person per 1000 each year in the United States. The incidence rises exponentially with age, with 5 cases per 1000 persons per year by the age of 80 years. Although men and women are affected equally, the incidence is higher in whites and African Americans than in Hispanic persons and Asian-Pacific Islanders.

Approximately one third of patients with symptomatic VTE present with PE, whereas the remainder present with DVT alone. Up to half of the patients with a first episode of VTE have no identifiable risk factors and are described as having unprovoked or idiopathic VTE. The remainder develop VTE secondary to well-recognized, transient risk factors, such as surgery or immobilization. PE accounts for an estimated 15% of deaths in hospitalized patients, with at least 100,000 deaths from PE each year in the United States.

PATHOBIOLOGY

PE and DVT are part of the spectrum of VTE and share the same genetic and acquired risk factors, which determine the intrinsic risk of VTE for each individual (Fig. 98-1). Genetic risk factors include abnormalities associated with hypercoagulability of the blood (Chapter 174), the most common of which are factor V Leiden and the prothrombin 20210 gene mutation. Acquired risk factors include advanced age, history of previous VTE, obesity, and active cancer, all of which limit mobility and may be associated with hypercoagulability. Superimposed on this background risk, VTE often occurs in the presence of a triggering factor, which increases the risk above the critical threshold. The triggering factors, including surgery and pregnancy or estrogen therapy, lead to vascular damage, stasis, and hypercoagulability, which are the components of Virchow's triad.

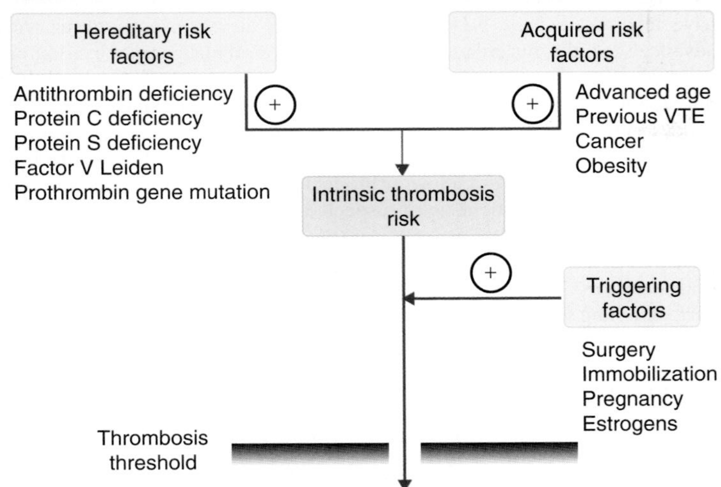

FIGURE 98-1. Thrombosis threshold. Hereditary and acquired risk factors combine to create an intrinsic risk of thrombosis for each individual. This risk is increased by extrinsic triggering factors. If the intrinsic and extrinsic forces exceed a critical threshold where thrombin generation overwhelms protective mechanisms, thrombosis occurs. VTE = venous thromboembolism.

In at least 90% of patients, PE originates from DVT in the lower limbs, and up to 70% of patients with proven PE still have demonstrable DVT on presentation. Thrombi usually start in the calf veins. About 20% of these calf vein thrombi then extend into the popliteal and more proximal veins of the leg, from which they are more likely to embolize. Although often asymptomatic, PE can be detected in about 50% of patients with proximal DVT (Chapter 81). Upper extremity DVT involving the axillary or subclavian veins also can give rise to PE, but only 10 to 15% of such patients develop PE. Upper extremity DVT most often occurs in patients with cancer (Chapter 187), particularly those with indwelling central venous catheters. Unprovoked upper extremity DVT, usually involving the dominant arm, can occur with strenuous effort—the so-called Paget-Schroetter syndrome.

PE often involves both lungs, with the lower lobes affected more frequently than the upper. Larger emboli tend to lodge in the main pulmonary artery or its branches, whereas smaller emboli occlude in more peripheral arteries. Peripheral PE can lead to pulmonary infarction, which is characterized by intra-alveolar hemorrhage and necrosis that may be pleura based. Because the circulation to the lungs arises from bronchial as well as pulmonary arteries, pulmonary infarction occurs in only about 10% of patients without underlying cardiopulmonary disease. In contrast, pulmonary infarction occurs in up to 30% of patients who have compromised oxygenation of the affected areas of lung because of preexisting disorders such as airways disease or increased pulmonary venous pressure because of left ventricular dysfunction.

The clinical impact of PE depends on the extent of reduction in pulmonary blood flow, the time frame over which vascular obstruction occurs, and the absence or presence of underlying cardiopulmonary disease. With acute PE, most patients develop tachypnea and some degree of hypoxemia. Stimulation of irritant receptors in the lungs likely accounts for the increase in respiratory rate. Obstruction of pulmonary arteries contributes to the hypoxemia and the increase in alveolar-arterial oxygen tension gradient, which reflects inefficient oxygen transfer across the lungs. These abnormalities result mainly from the increase in alveolar dead space that occurs because ventilation to alveoli exceeds blood flow in the adjacent capillaries in parts of the lung affected by PE. Other contributing factors to the hypoxemia include ventilation-perfusion mismatch because of relative overperfusion of normal areas of the lung, and shunting of blood through nonventilated atelectatic or collapsed areas of lung that retain at least some perfusion.

Pulmonary vascular resistance increases with PE because of vascular occlusion by thrombi. In addition, humoral mediators, such as serotonin and thromboxane, are released from activated platelets and may trigger vasoconstriction in unaffected areas of lung. Consequently, the increase in pulmonary vascular resistance may be disproportionate to the extent of pulmonary vascular occlusion. With obstruction of less than 50% of the pulmonary vascular bed, the mean pulmonary artery pressure rarely exceeds 25 mm Hg. Under these circumstances, the right ventricle maintains its output, so cardiac output and systemic blood pressure remain normal.

With acute occlusion of more than 50% of the pulmonary circulation, the pulmonary artery systolic pressure increases, thereby increasing right ventricular afterload. The pulmonary artery systolic pressure rarely exceeds 55 mm Hg with sudden occlusion because of insufficient time for right ventricular hypertrophy to occur. If the thin-walled right ventricle fails to maintain output in the face of the increased pulmonary artery pressure, it dilates, and right heart failure ensues. Right ventricular end-diastolic and right atrial pressures increase as the right ventricle fails. Dilation of the right ventricle may result in tricuspid regurgitation, which can compromise left ventricular filling and lead to reduced cardiac output and subsequent hypotension. Rightward bulging of the interventricular septum may also contribute to left ventricular diastolic dysfunction. The decrease in aortic pressure, together with the increase in right ventricular pressure, can produce right ventricular ischemia because of decreased perfusion of the right coronary artery despite increased demand by the dilated right ventricle. If this process occurs over a rapid time frame, syncope or sudden death, often associated with electromechanical dissociation, may be the first manifestation of severe PE.

With multiple pulmonary emboli over an extended period of time, the right ventricle has an opportunity to adapt to the increased pulmonary vascular resistance. The subsequent increase in right ventricular systolic pressure results in less right heart failure than occurs with acute large PE. Patients with multiple smaller PEs over an extended period of time often have increasing dyspnea with progressively decreasing exercise tolerance. With maintained cardiac output, hypotension does not develop. Additional emboli, however, may convert the clinical picture to one of severe acute PE.

Patients who have underlying cardiopulmonary disease or who are elderly, frail, and debilitated will be more sensitive to the effects of PE than patients who were previously healthy. Consequently, even a small PE may be fatal in patients with limited reserve.

CLINICAL MANIFESTATIONS

Patients with PE most often present with a history of dyspnea, which may be sudden in onset and tends to progress in severity over time. Dyspnea may be associated with pleuritic chest pain, cough, and hemoptysis, particularly in patients with pulmonary infarction. Although the symptoms and signs of PE can be nonspecific, the diagnosis should be suspected in patients with risk factors for VTE, such as prolonged immobility, recent surgery, or active malignancy. Patients with associated DVT (Chapter 81) may present with recent onset of leg pain or with swelling and tenderness along the course of the deep veins. The superficial veins of the leg may be dilated, and the affected leg may be warm to touch, with skin that is red or dusky blue in color.

Most patients with PE have tachypnea and tachycardia associated with hypoxemia, but these findings also can occur with disorders such as heart failure, pneumonia, or chronic obstructive pulmonary disease. Other nonspecific symptoms include palpitations, anxiety, and lightheadedness.

Patients with acute severe PE often complain of dyspnea at rest or with minimal exertion, and they may present with syncope (Chapters 50 and 62) because of hypoxemia and low cardiac output. The combination of hypotension, hypoxemia, and increased cardiac work load may trigger angina (Chapter 72) or overt myocardial infarction (Chapter 73).

Central and peripheral cyanosis can occur, and a gallop rhythm may develop as a consequence of heart failure. The jugular veins may be distended if right heart failure develops. The second heart sound can be widely split, with a loud pulmonic component because of delayed emptying of the right ventricle. A right ventricular heave may be present with massive PE and acute pulmonary hypertension.

DIAGNOSIS

Most patients with PE will have one or more of the following clinical features: dyspnea, often of sudden onset; tachypnea, with a respiratory rate of more than 20 breaths per minute; and chest discomfort, which is usually substernal and often pleuritic in nature. When patients present with these features, the differential diagnosis includes pulmonary disorders, such as pneumonia (Chapter 97), an exacerbation of chronic obstructive lung disease (Chapter 88), or asthma (Chapter 87); pleurisy secondary to connective tissue disease (Chapter 99); cardiac disorders, such as heart failure (Chapter 58), acute coronary syndrome (Chapter 72), or pericarditis (Chapter 77); and musculoskeletal disorders, such as rib fracture.

Because the clinical features are nonspecific, the diagnosis of PE requires objective testing. Patients who require such testing can be identified by their pretest likelihood of PE using validated clinical prediction rules (Table 98-1) that include components of the clinical assessment, presence of risk factors for VTE, and absence of an alternative diagnosis to explain the symptoms and signs. Some clinical prediction rules also include the results of simple tests, such as the electrocardiogram (ECG) and the chest radiograph.

Based on the results of such an assessment, the pretest likelihood of PE can be designated as low, moderate, or high, and this likelihood then guides the subsequent selection of blood tests, such as the D-dimer assay, and noninvasive or invasive tests for diagnosis of PE or DVT (Fig. 98-2) (Chapter 81). Tests for diagnosis of DVT are relevant because a diagnosis of DVT in patients with suspected PE provides sufficient grounds for initiation of treatment, and the treatment of DVT and PE is usually the same. Noninvasive tests include computed tomography (CT) pulmonary angiography or ventilation-perfusion lung scanning for diagnosis of PE and venous compression ultrasound for diagnosis of DVT. These tests have largely replaced pulmonary angiography to diagnose PE and venography to diagnose DVT.

Diagnostic Tests

D-Dimer

A plasmin-derived degradation product of cross-linked fibrin, D-dimer can be measured in whole blood or plasma to provide an indirect index of ongoing activation of the coagulation system. An elevated D-dimer level has an 85% to 98% sensitivity for the diagnosis of PE, but all available D-dimer assays have low specificities. False-positive D-dimer elevations can occur with advanced age, chronic inflammatory conditions, and malignancy. In addition, hospitalized patients are more likely to have an elevated D-dimer level than outpatients. Because of this lack of specificity, the value of the D-dimer assay resides with its high negative predictive value and the ability of a normal D-dimer to reduce the probability of PE sufficiently to avoid further diagnostic testing in patients with a low or moderate pretest likelihood,[1] who represent up to 30% of patients with suspected VTE.

Computed Tomography Pulmonary Angiography

Multidetector CT pulmonary angiography has largely replaced ventilation-perfusion lung scanning for PE diagnosis because of its wide availability and the rapidity of its results. In contrast to lung scanning, CT pulmonary angiography not only permits direct visualization of thrombi in the pulmonary arteries of patients with PE (Fig. 98-3) but also provides an alternative diagnosis in many of those who prove not to have PE. With the evolution from single-detector to multidetector CT scanners, the sensitivity and specificity of CT pulmonary angiography are sufficient for its use as a stand-alone test: a CT pulmonary angiogram showing thrombus in pulmonary arteries up to

TABLE 98-1 WELLS' CLINICAL PREDICTION RULE FOR LIKELIHOOD OF PULMONARY EMBOLISM

VARIABLE	POINTS
PREDISPOSING FACTORS	
Previous VTE	1.5
Recent surgery or immobilization	1.5
Cancer	1
SYMPTOMS	
Hemoptysis	1
SIGNS	
Heart rate over 100 beats/min	1.5
Clinical signs of DVT	3
CLINICAL JUDGMENT	
Alternative diagnosis less likely than PE	3
CLINICAL PROBABILITY	**TOTAL POINTS**
Low	<2
Moderate	2-6
High	>6

DVT = deep vein thrombosis; PE = pulmonary embolism; VTE = venous thromboembolism.
Adapted from Wells PS, Ginsberg JS, Anderson DR, et al. Use of a clinical model for safe management of patients with suspected pulmonary embolism. *Ann Intern Med*. 1998;129:997-1005.

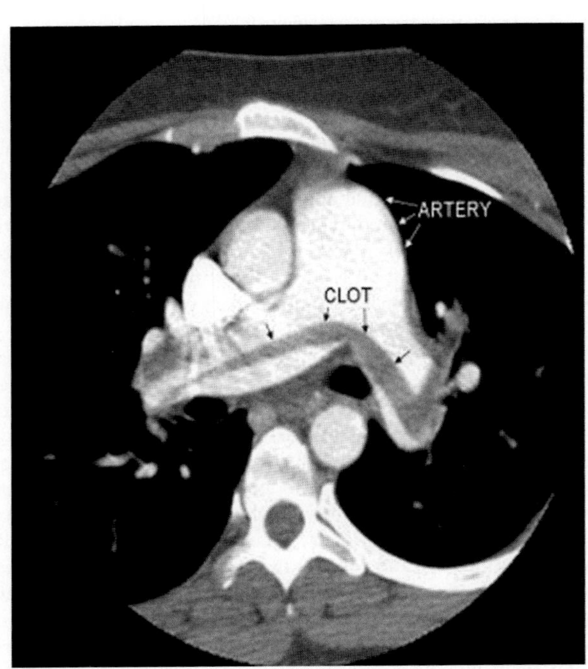

FIGURE 98-3. Computed tomographic pulmonary arteriogram demonstrating a pulmonary embolus.

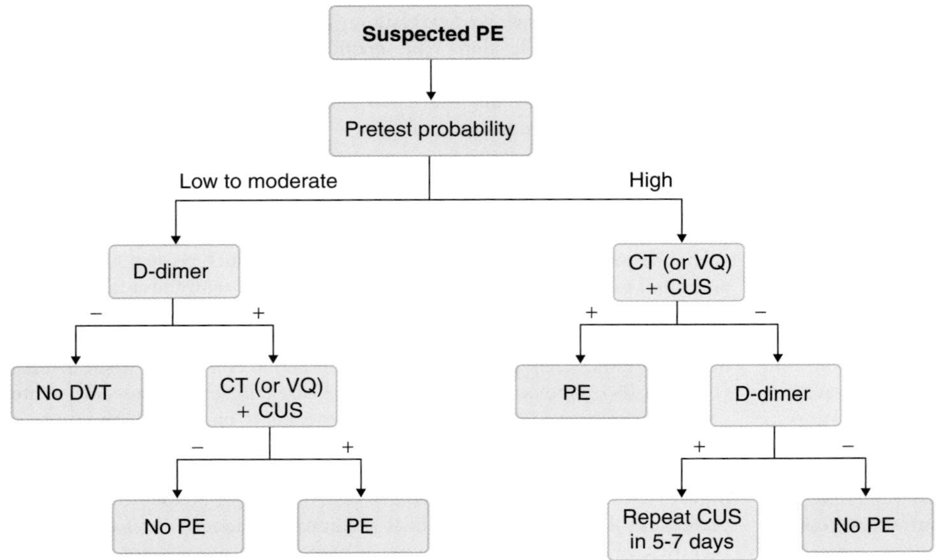

FIGURE 98-2. Clinical management of patients with suspected pulmonary embolism (PE). CT = computed tomography; CUS = venous compression ultrasound; DVT = deep vein thrombosis; VQ = ventilation-perfusion lung scan.

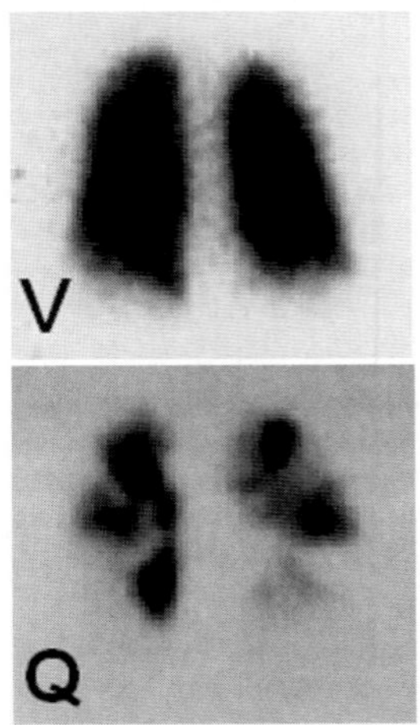

FIGURE 98-4. Ventilation-perfusion lung scan demonstrating pulmonary emboli.

the segmental level provides evidence of PE, whereas a negative CT pulmonary angiogram excludes PE with subsequent clinical outcomes at least as good as with lung scanning.[2] Compared with lung scanning, CT pulmonary angiography detects more isolated subsegmental thrombi in about 1 to 5% of patients, but the importance of such thrombi is unclear because patients with isolated subsegmental defects have uneventful outcomes despite withholding treatment. A negative D-dimer or a normal venous compression ultrasound examination may help to exclude the possibility of VTE in this setting.

Ventilation-Perfusion Lung Scanning

In this two-part test; the ventilation phase involves inhalation of an aerosol form of xenon or technetium to assess air delivery to the various parts of the lung, whereas the perfusion phase involves the intravenous injection of technetium-labeled macroaggregates of albumin, which enables assessment of blood flow within the lungs once the aggregates lodge in the pulmonary microcirculation. Images for both parts of the test are acquired using a gamma counter. Areas of lung affected by PE do not light up on the perfusion scan because the macroaggregates of albumin fail to reach sites where the pulmonary arteries are occluded (Fig. 98-4). In contrast, areas with abnormal perfusion ventilate normally yielding a ventilation-perfusion mismatch.

A normal lung scan effectively excludes the diagnosis of PE, but only 25% of patients with suspected PE have a normal scan. One or more segmental or larger perfusion defects that ventilate normally characterize a high probability lung scan, which establishes the diagnosis of PE, but even use of single-photon emission CT technology identifies only about 10% of patients with suspected PE as having a high probability lung scan. The remaining 65% of lung scans exhibit smaller areas of mismatch or matched defects and fall within the non-high-probability category. Because up to 40% of patients with non-high-probability scans have PE, such patients require additional investigations to exclude the diagnosis.

Although CT pulmonary angiography has largely replaced lung scanning, the lung scan remains the diagnostic test of choice for patients with renal impairment or a history of allergy to angiographic contrast media. For diagnosis of PE in pregnancy, lung scanning produces less maternal and fetal radiation exposure and is preferred over CT pulmonary angiography.

Magnetic Resonance Imaging

In contrast to CT pulmonary angiography, gadolinium-enhanced magnetic resonance imaging (MRI) does not subject patients to ionizing radiation, and gadolinium can safely be given to patients with a history of allergy to contrast dye. Although originally promoted as the test of choice to diagnose PE in patients with renal impairment, the emergence of nephrogenic systemic fibrosis (Chapter 275) as a complication of gadolinium administration in patients with renal impairment has tempered enthusiasm for the test. The accuracy of MRI for the detection of PE appears to be similar to that of CT pulmonary angiography, but magnetic resonance (MR) pulmonary angiography is more technically demanding. The combination of MR pulmonary angiography with MR venography has a higher sensitivity than MR pulmonary angiography alone for the diagnosis of PE. With these limitations, MRI should be used to diagnose PE only in centers with experience with the test and in patients for whom standard tests are contraindicated.

Pulmonary Angiography

Pulmonary angiography requires direct contrast injection into the pulmonary arteries, followed by imaging using digital subtraction technology to provide high-quality images. Presence of a thrombus, which appears as a filling defect or as a sudden cutoff of blood flow in a pulmonary arterial branch, establishes the diagnosis of PE. Although direct angiography allows visualization of small thrombi in subsegmental pulmonary arteries, high interobserver variability in the interpretation of isolated findings at this level limits the specificity of this finding. As an invasive test, the mortality rate associated with pulmonary angiography is 0.2%, with deaths usually occurring in patients with hemodynamic compromise or respiratory failure. Because of its associated risks and because CT pulmonary angiography offers similar or better information, direct pulmonary angiography is now rarely performed, except in the patient who may undergo pulmonary embolectomy.

Diagnostic Strategies

The diagnosis of DVT (Chapter 81) is usually based on venous compression ultrasound, which has a sensitivity and specificity of about 95% for the diagnosis of proximal DVT. In patients with suspected PE, the venous compression ultrasound examination can be limited to the proximal veins, which are the sources of most PE.

CT venography can be combined with CT pulmonary angiography as a simple test to diagnose DVT because both tests require only one injection of contrast dye. Compared with CT pulmonary angiography alone, the combination of CT pulmonary angiography and CT venography increases the sensitivity from 83 to 90%, but the specificity remains unchanged, thereby resulting in only a modest increase in negative predictive value. CT venography adds significant radiation exposure and only marginally increases the overall detection rate, so venous compression ultrasound is preferred because it provides the same information without exposing patients to ionizing radiation. Standard venography is not recommended in patients with suspected PE.

In summary, patients with a low to moderate pretest likelihood should undergo D-dimer testing (see Fig. 98-2). A negative D-dimer test excludes the diagnosis of PE in these patients, whereas a positive test should prompt multidetector CT pulmonary angiography. Patients with a high pretest likelihood of PE should be sent directly for multidetector CT pulmonary angiography. A positive CT pulmonary angiogram establishes the diagnosis of PE, whereas a negative test excludes it.

The role of venous compression ultrasound remains controversial. Because of the suboptimal sensitivity of single-detector CT pulmonary angiography for the diagnosis of PE, bilateral venous compression ultrasound should also be performed if multidetector technology is not available. Although a negative multidetector CT pulmonary angiogram safely excludes PE, at least in patients with low to moderate pretest likelihood, bilateral venous compression ultrasound can still be helpful. For example, the finding of proximal DVT obviates the need for further testing, a result that can be particularly helpful in patients who are poor candidates for CT pulmonary angiography, such as those with renal impairment or a history of allergy to contrast dye. Patients with a non-high-probability lung scan or with equivocal CT pulmonary angiographic findings should undergo serial venous compression ultrasound examination to exclude the possibility of calf DVT, which then extends into the proximal veins.

Other Tests

Blood markers of right ventricular dysfunction, which is seen in more severe pulmonary emboli, include brain natriuretic peptide (BNP) or its precursor, N-terminal proBNP, which are released in response to myocardial stretching. Although elevated levels of these markers in patients with PE are associated with a worse prognosis, their positive predictive value is low.

Elevated levels of troponin I or T and fatty acid–binding protein provide evidence of myocardial injury in PE patients with right ventricular infarction. In PE patients without hemodynamic compromise, elevated levels of these markers are associated with increased mortality.

The ECG may show new changes suggestive of right ventricular strain, such as T wave inversion in leads V_1 to V_4; the classic S1, Q3, T3 pattern (Fig. 98-5); and complete or incomplete right bundle branch block. However, these ECG changes have limited sensitivity and are seen predominantly in patients with more severe pulmonary emboli.

Echocardiography findings suggestive of right ventricular dysfunction include right ventricular dilation or hypokinesis, increased right ventricular diameter relative to that of the left ventricle, and increased velocity of the jet of tricuspid regurgitation. Echocardiography can also detect a right-to-left shunt through a patent foramen ovale and may provide evidence of right ventricular thrombus, both of which are associated with increased mortality in patients with PE. With no universal criteria for the diagnosis of right ventricular dysfunction, however, the utility of routine echocardiography remains uncertain. In general, routine echocardiography is recommended only in patients with severe hypoxia or other evidence to suggest hemodynamic compromise.

Other routinely ordered tests should include a complete blood count, platelet count, and international normalized ratio (INR) to help guide anticoagulation. A creatinine level and blood urea nitrogen level provide useful baseline information, as do serum electrolytes and liver enzymes.

TREATMENT Rx

Although anticoagulant therapy remains the mainstay of treatment of PE, patients with severe PE may require reperfusion therapy to increase blood flow quickly to the pulmonary arteries and to reduce pulmonary artery pressure. 3 Therefore, rapid risk stratification is crucial to help guide treatment. PE patients who have contraindications to anticoagulant therapy may require insertion of a filter.

Severe Pulmonary Embolism

High-risk patients can be identified at the bedside (Table 98-2) based on the presence or absence of hemodynamic compromise, right ventricular dysfunction, and elevated biomarkers. Patients with severe PE usually die because they develop acute right ventricular failure, which causes low systemic output. Patients with severe PE require hemodynamic and respiratory support and may require reperfusion therapy. Patients with right ventricular failure often require modest fluid expansion and may need inotropic agents, such as dobutamine (starting at a dose of 0.5 to 1.0 μg/kg/minute and then titrated according to the blood pressure), dopamine (starting at a dose of 5 μg/kg/minute and then increased gradually in 5- to 10-μg/kg/minute increments, according to the blood pressure, up to 20 to 50 μg/kg/minute) or norepinephrine (starting at a dose of 2 to 4 μg/minute and then titrated according to the blood pressure) for severe hypotension or shock. Emerging data raise the possibility that endothelin antagonists and phosphodiesterase-5 inhibitors may attenuate the pulmonary hypertension in patients with severe PE, but these drugs are not currently approved for use in PE.

Patients with PE frequently have hypoxemia and hypocapnia. Hypoxemia can usually be reversed with nasal oxygen. Measures to reduce fever and agitation with acetaminophen and mild sedation may help minimize oxygen consumption. In patients who have severe PE and who require mechanical ventilation, low tidal volumes should be used, and positive end-expiratory pressure should be applied with caution because it can reduce venous return and worsen right ventricular failure (Chapter 105).

Reperfusion Therapy

Patients with severe PE associated with hypotension or shock may benefit from pharmacologic, mechanical, or surgical reperfusion therapy. Pharmacologic reperfusion therapy involves the systemic administration of a fibrinolytic agent (Table 98-3), preferably within 48 hours of the onset of symptoms, but later treatment may still be of benefit. Up to 13% of patients who receive fibrinolytic therapy experience a major bleed, and the rate of intracranial or fatal bleeding can reach 1.8%. Consequently, fibrinolytic therapy currently is justified only in patients who have severe PE and no contraindications (Table 98-4). It remains unclear whether the benefits of fibrinolytic therapy outweigh the risks in patients at intermediate risk.

Mechanical reperfusion includes percutaneous catheter embolectomy with thrombus fragmentation, an approach that avoids the need for fibrinolytic drugs altogether, or catheter-directed fibrinolytic therapy, which requires lower doses of fibrinolytic agents than used for systemic administration. In some centers, surgical pulmonary embolectomy may be an option for patients who have severe PE and who are at high risk for bleeding with systemic fibrinolytic therapy or who have failed such treatment. Mechanical techniques require skilled operators but provide useful alternatives to systemic fibrinolytic therapy for patients who have severe PE and who are at high risk for bleeding.

Anticoagulation Therapy

Anticoagulation therapy is the cornerstone of PE treatment and should be initiated immediately with parenteral anticoagulants, such as heparin, low-molecular-weight heparin (LMWH), or fondaparinux, even while patients with suspected PE are awaiting the results of confirmatory tests. Patients with severe PE should be treated with heparin because neither LMWH nor fondaparinux has been extensively evaluated in this setting. Heparin should be used in patients with severe renal impairment (creatinine clearance < 30 mL/minute) because LMWH and fondaparinux are cleared by the kidneys. If LMWH or fondaparinux is used in patients with moderate renal impairment (creatinine clearance of 30 to 50 mL/min), anti–factor Xa levels should be measured at trough to ensure there is no accumulation.

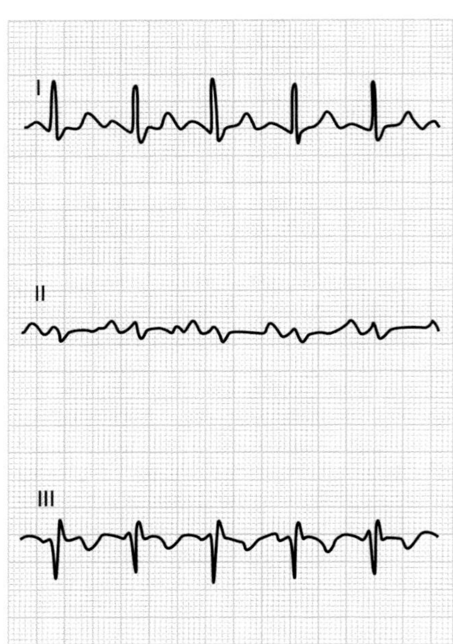

FIGURE 98-5. Classic electrocardiogram of pulmonary embolus. Note the "S1, Q3, T3" pattern.

TABLE 98-3 APPROVED REGIMENS FOR FIBRINOLYTIC THERAPY FOR TREATMENT OF SEVERE PULMONARY EMBOLISM

AGENTS	RECOMMENDED REGIMENS
Streptokinase	250,000 IU as a loading dose over 30 min, followed by 100,000 IU/hr over 12 to 24 hr
Tissue plasminogen activator	100 mg over 2 hr, or 0.6 mg/kg over 10 to 15 min (maximal dose of 50 mg)

TABLE 98-2 RISK STRATIFICATION OF PATIENTS WITH PULMONARY EMBOLISM AND TREATMENTS IN ADDITION TO ANTICOAGULATION

CLASSIFICATION	HEMODYNAMIC COMPROMISE	RIGHT VENTRICULAR DYSFUNCTION	INCREASED TROPONIN AND/OR BNP LEVELS*	TREATMENT
Severe	Yes	Yes	Yes	Fibrinolytic therapy
Moderate	No	Yes	Yes	May consider fibrinolytic therapy if very symptomatic
Mild	No	No	No	Consider outpatient treatment

*Blood markers include troponin, brain natriuretic peptide (BNP), and N-terminal proBNP.

TABLE 98-4 CONTRAINDICATIONS TO FIBRINOLYTIC THERAPY

ABSOLUTE CONTRAINDICATIONS
Any hemorrhagic stroke or stroke of unknown origin
Central nervous system damage or neoplasm
Major trauma, surgery, or head injury in past 3 weeks
Gastrointestinal bleeding in past month
Significant ongoing bleeding
RELATIVE CONTRAINDICATIONS
Ischemic stroke or transient ischemic attack in past 6 months
Treatment with a vitamin K antagonist
Pregnancy or within 1 week of delivery
Noncompressible puncture site
Traumatic resuscitation
Advanced liver disease
Infective endocarditis
Active peptic ulcer disease

TABLE 98-5 LOW-MOLECULAR-WEIGHT HEPARIN AND FONDAPARINUX REGIMENS FOR TREATMENT OF PULMONARY EMBOLISM

AGENT	DOSE	INTERVAL
Enoxaparin	1 mg/kg 1.5 mg/kg	Twice daily Once daily
Dalteparin	100 U/kg 200 U/kg	Twice daily Once daily
Tinzaparin	175 U/kg	Once daily
Fondaparinux	5 mg (weight < 50 kg) 7.5 mg (weight 50-100 kg) 10 mg (weight > 100 kg)	Once daily Once daily Once daily

Heparin should be administered by continuous intravenous infusion and dosed using weight-based nomograms (see Table 81-4 in Chapter 81). Typically, an 80 U/kg bolus is followed by an infusion at the rate of 18 U/kg per hour, and subsequent doses are adjusted based on the results of the activated partial thromboplastin time (aPTT). Rapid achievement and maintenance of a therapeutic aPTT are important to reduce the risk of recurrent PE. In addition to monitoring the aPTT, the platelet count should be measured frequently because of the risk of heparin-induced thrombocytopenia (Chapter 37).

LMWH or fondaparinux can be used for intermediate- or low-risk PE patients (see Table 98-2) using the regimens illustrated in Table 98-5.[4,5] Unlike heparin, these agents do not require coagulation monitoring. In addition, the risk of heparin-induced thrombocytopenia is lower with LMWH than with heparin, and the risk is minimal with fondaparinux. Outpatient management of PE is safe for low-risk PE patients. In PE patients at intermediate risk (see Table 98-2), outpatient management can be considered, but brief admission to hospital may be a safer approach.

After initial treatment with a parenteral anticoagulant, most patients with PE receive extended therapy with a vitamin K antagonist, such as warfarin (Chapter 81), to prevent recurrent DVT and PE. In PE patients at low or intermediate risk (see Table 98-2), warfarin can be started on the same day that parenteral anticoagulant therapy is initiated. Parenteral anticoagulant therapy should be continued for at least 5 days and should only be stopped when the INR has been within the therapeutic range of 2 to 3, which is needed for long-term therapy, for 2 consecutive days. Initiation of warfarin therapy should be delayed in patients with severe PE; such patients should receive heparin until they have stabilized.

An emerging option is unmonitored, fixed-dose dabigatran etexilate (150 mg twice daily) for patients with VTE, including PE. The rates of recurrent VTE and bleeding are similar with dabigatran and warfarin, but dabigatran is superior to warfarin for preventing stroke in patients with atrial fibrillation.[6] This agent and oral factor Xa inhibitors (e.g., rivaroxaban, apixaban, and edoxaban) have the potential to replace warfarin, thereby simplifying long-term anticoagulant treatment.

Patients who develop PE as a complication of a reversible risk factor, such as surgery, trauma, or medical illness, have a low risk of recurrence when anticoagulant therapy is stopped. Consequently, a 3-month course of warfarin therapy represents adequate treatment in such patients provided that their risk factors have resolved. Women who develop PE with estrogen therapy also can be treated for 3 months, provided that hormonal treatment is withdrawn. In contrast, patients with unprovoked PE have a higher rate of recurrent VTE when anticoagulant therapy stops and require longer treatment; some experts recommend indefinite anticoagulant therapy provided that the risk of bleeding remains low. One month after stopping anticoagulant therapy, an elevated D-dimer level or residual venous compression ultrasound abnormalities identify patients at higher risk for recurrence who require indefinite anticoagulation therapy.[7,8] After a minimum 3-month course of usual-intensity warfarin (target INR between 2 and 3), a lower-intensity regimen (target INR between 1.5 and 2.0) may simplify management by decreasing the frequency of INR monitoring and reducing the risk of bleeding,[9] but the risk of recurrent VTE is slightly higher with this lower-intensity warfarin regimen.[10]

Caval Filters

Filters, which are inserted percutaneously, are usually placed below the level of the renal veins but can be placed higher for thrombus in the inferior vena cava. Both permanent and retrievable filters reduce the risk of recurrent PE but have not been shown to prolong survival, in part because permanent filters can be associated with long-term complications, including inferior vena cava occlusion because of thrombus, recurrent DVT, and post-thrombotic syndrome.[11] Retrievable filters, designed to be removed within 2 to 4 weeks of implantation, can circumvent these long-term complications, but device migration or thrombosis occurs in up to 10% of patients with temporary filters because most are not removed. Because of these potential problems, caval filters should be restricted to patients who have high risk for recurrent PE and an absolute contraindication for anticoagulation, such as patients who develop a PE after major surgery, patients who experience major bleeding with anticoagulant therapy, and pregnant women who have a PE shortly before delivery. Retrievable filters should be used in these cases, and the devices should be removed as soon as anticoagulant therapy can safely be administered. Permanent filters are suitable for patients who have ongoing contraindications to anticoagulation.

Specific Patient Subgroups

Patients with PE in the setting of active cancer, women who suffer a PE during pregnancy, and patients with chronic thromboembolic pulmonary hypertension (Chapter 68) require special treatment.

Cancer

Active cancer and its treatment with chemotherapy, radiation therapy, and growth factors or other biological agents increase the risk of VTE (Chapter 187). Patients with advanced cancer often have limited mobility, which adds to their risk of VTE. In addition, indwelling central venous access catheters can trigger upper extremity DVT, which can lead to PE. Therefore, the index of suspicion should be high in cancer patients who present with symptoms and signs suggestive of PE or DVT, or both. With advances in diagnostic imaging, incidental PE may be discovered on CT scans performed for staging purposes or for monitoring response to treatment. Although 20% of patients with VTE have an underlying malignancy, patients with PE should not undergo routine extensive screening for cancer.

Like patients without cancer, initial treatment of PE in cancer patients involves administration of a rapidly acting parenteral anticoagulant. For extended treatment, however, LMWH reduces the risk of recurrent VTE to a greater extent than warfarin. In addition, in the face of poor nutritional intake, severe nausea and vomiting, transient thrombocytopenia, or invasive procedures, LMWH is easier to manage than warfarin.

Cancer patients who develop PE after curative surgery or with adjuvant chemotherapy for limited-stage disease should be treated for at least 3 months or until they have completed their chemotherapy. Those with PE on the background of advanced cancer have a risk of recurrence of at least 20% in the first year after stopping anticoagulant therapy, so they require lifelong treatment.

Pregnancy

Treatment of PE in pregnancy (Chapter 247) centers mainly on heparin or LMWH because, unlike warfarin, these agents do not cross the placenta. Although both agents can be given subcutaneously, weight-adjusted LMWH has advantages over heparin because it can be given once daily without routine monitoring and because the risks of heparin-induced thrombocytopenia and osteoporosis are lower with LMWH than with heparin. Anti–factor Xa monitoring of LMWH should be considered in women at extremes of body weight and in those with renal impairment. Fondaparinux should be considered for pregnant women who have a history of heparin-induced thrombocytopenia or who develop injection-site reactions to heparin or LMWH.

Heparin or LMWH should be continued throughout pregnancy. Warfarin must be avoided because it crosses the placenta and can cause bone and central nervous system abnormalities, fetal hemorrhage, or placental abruption. During labor and delivery, epidural analgesia should be avoided unless prophylactic LMWH has been stopped at least 12 hours before insertion of the epidural catheter and therapeutic LMWH has been stopped at least 24 hours before. Treatment can be resumed within 6 hours of catheter withdrawal. After delivery, anticoagulation therapy should be continued for at least 3 months; warfarin can be used because it does not appear in breast milk.

Fibrinolytic agents have been used successfully for treatment of severe PE in pregnancy but can cause bleeding, usually from the genital tract. If PE develops late in pregnancy, a retrievable filter may prevent recurrence during delivery when anticoagulant therapy must be withheld.

Chronic Thromboembolic Pulmonary Hypertension

A complication of PE, chronic thromboembolic pulmonary hypertension develops in 0.5 to 5% of patients over the course of months or years when emboli in major pulmonary arteries are replaced by fibrous tissue that becomes incorporated into the vessel wall, thereby narrowing or obstructing it. Chronic obstruction of the pulmonary vascular bed increases pulmonary arterial resistance and can lead to right heart failure. Although patients initially may be asymptomatic, they experience increasing dyspnea on exertion and hypoxemia as the disease progresses. Chronic thromboembolic pulmonary hypertension should be suspected in patients with pulmonary hypertension (Chapter 68), and the diagnosis can be established with a combination of echocardiography and lung scanning or CT pulmonary angiography.

Medical therapy focuses on treatment of right heart failure and the use of prostacyclin, endothelin receptor antagonists, or phosphodiesterase-5 inhibitors, or a combination of these, to lower pulmonary artery pressure (see Table 68-2 and Fig. 68-7 in Chapter 68). These agents may be of limited utility, however, because of the fibrotic nature of the obstructing material. Definitive treatment involves surgical thromboendarterectomy to remove the occluding material from the pulmonary arteries. This procedure is associated with a perioperative mortality rate that can be as high as 4%, depending on the severity of the disease, and a 3-year survival rate of about 80%.

PREVENTION

At least half of the outpatients with newly diagnosed VTE have a history of recent hospitalization, and most failed to receive thromboprophylaxis during their hospital stay; as a result, PE is the most common preventable cause of death in hospitalized patients in the United States. Guidelines for primary prophylaxis are available and should be followed (see Tables 37-2 and 37-3 in Chapter 37).

PROGNOSIS

With the diagnosis established and adequate anticoagulant therapy initiated, most patients with PE survive. Case-fatality rates 1 month after diagnosis of DVT or PE are 6% and 12%, respectively. Patients with severe PE who present with shock have the highest mortality rate, and many die within an hour of presentation. Although the case-fatality rate in patients with PE is twice that in those with DVT, many of the deaths are the result of comorbid conditions rather than the PE itself. Factors associated with early mortality after VTE include presentation as PE, advanced age, cancer, and underlying cardiovascular disease. The most serious long-term complication of PE is chronic thromboembolic pulmonary hypertension (Chapter 68), a rare condition associated with significant morbidity and mortality.

Despite anticoagulant therapy, recurrent VTE occurs in about 6% of patients during the first 6 months. While on anticoagulation treatment, patients with unprovoked VTE and those with secondary VTE have similar risks of recurrence. In contrast, when anticoagulant therapy is stopped, patients with unprovoked VTE have a risk of recurrence of 10% at 1 year and 30% at 5 years, whereas those with secondary VTE have recurrence rates of 3% at 1 year and 10% at 5 years. Recurrent events often mirror the index events; after an initial PE, about 60% of recurrences are PE. Because of the high risk of recurrence in patients with unprovoked VTE, many experts recommend indefinite anticoagulant therapy for such patients. In contrast, because of the lower risk of recurrence, anticoagulation therapy can be stopped after 3 months in patients with secondary VTE whose risk factors have resolved.

NONTHROMBOTIC PULMONARY EMBOLISM

DEFINITION

Nonthrombotic material that can embolize to the lungs includes fat, air, amniotic fluid, tumor cells, talc in intravenous drug abusers, and medical devices.

Fat Embolism Syndrome

EPIDEMIOLOGY

Fat embolism syndrome usually occurs in the setting of trauma, particularly after fracture of long bones or the pelvis. The risk increases with the number of fractured bones, and the syndrome occurs more often with closed fractures than with open ones. Fat embolism also can complicate orthopedic surgery or trauma to tissues rich in fat, such as may occur with liposuction.

PATHOBIOLOGY

Characterized by a combination of respiratory, neurologic, hematologic, and cutaneous manifestations, fat embolism syndrome reflects a combination of vascular obstruction by fat globules, as well as the deleterious effects of free fatty acids released from these fat globules by the action of lipoprotein lipases. These free fatty acids increase vascular permeability, induce a capillary leak syndrome, and can trigger platelet aggregation.

CLINICAL MANIFESTATIONS

Symptoms typically develop 24 to 72 hours after trauma or surgery. Patients often complain of vague chest pain and shortness of breath. Tachypnea and fever associated with disproportionate tachycardia are common. The syndrome can rapidly progress to severe hypoxemia that requires mechanical ventilation. Neurologic manifestations, which often start after the respiratory distress, include drowsiness, confusion, decreased level of consciousness, and seizures. Patients may have petechiae, particularly involving the conjunctiva, oral mucosa, and upper half of the body.

DIAGNOSIS

Fat embolism syndrome should be suspected when respiratory distress occurs a day or more after major trauma or orthopedic surgery, particularly when there are associated neurologic defects and petechiae. The chest radiograph may reveal diffuse alveolar infiltrates. Although fat droplets may be found in bronchoalveolar lavage fluid, this finding lacks specificity for the fat embolism syndrome.

PREVENTION, TREATMENT, AND PROGNOSIS (Rx)

Early stabilization of long bone fractures reduces the risk of fat embolization. Supportive treatment should be provided, including oxygen and mechanical ventilation. The utility of corticosteroids remains controversial.

Although mortality rates as high as 10% have been reported, the prognosis is generally good.

Venous Air Embolism

EPIDEMIOLOGY

Venous air embolism, which involves entrapment of environmental air or exogenous gas in the venous system, requires direct communication between the air and a vein, as well as a pressure gradient that favors entry of the air into the vein. Air can be introduced through indwelling central venous catheters as a consequence of invasive surgical or medical procedures or after barotrauma.

PATHOBIOLOGY

Large venous air emboli obstruct the right ventricular pulmonary outflow tract, whereas mixtures of air bubbles and fibrin thrombi can obstruct pulmonary arterioles. In either case, right ventricular failure can result. With a patent foramen ovale (Chapter 69), venous air emboli can enter the coronary, cerebral, or systemic circulation.

CLINICAL MANIFESTATIONS

Symptoms and signs depend on the volume of air and the rapidity of its entry into the circulation. Large, rapid boluses of air are tolerated less well than slow entry of smaller amounts. Small air emboli may be asymptomatic. With larger emboli, patients often complain of dyspnea and retrosternal chest discomfort, and they may feel lightheaded. Physical findings include tachypnea, tachycardia, and evidence of respiratory distress. Patients may have signs of right heart failure. A continuous, drumlike, mill-wheel murmur, which reflects air in the right ventricle, may be heard.

DIAGNOSIS

Patients may present with ECG evidence of right ventricular dysfunction associated with elevated levels of troponin, indicative of myocardial injury. Echocardiography or chest CT may reveal air in the right ventricle. Patients may have hypoxemia and hypercapnia, and the platelet count may be low.

PREVENTION AND TREATMENT

All catheters should be removed using techniques that minimize air embolism, air should be removed from syringes before injection, and care should be taken during surgery to ensure that air bubbles do not form in blood vessels. To avoid air embolism associated with barotrauma, divers require training in how to dive and surface safely (Chapter 94).

The source of any air embolism should be identified so that further embolism can be prevented. Left lateral decubitus positioning may benefit patients who have a large air bubble trapped in the right ventricular outflow tract; such positioning places the outflow tract below the right ventricular cavity, thereby allowing the air bubble to migrate into a nonobstructing position. Aspiration of the right ventricle through a central venous catheter may also be of benefit. Patients should receive high-flow supplemental oxygen, and hyperbaric oxygenation should be considered for patients with cardiac or neurologic dysfunction.

PROGNOSIS

The outcome depends on the extent of air embolism. With good supportive care, the mortality rate can be less than 10%, even in patients with major air emboli. However, residual neurologic defects often persist.

Amniotic Fluid Embolism

EPIDEMIOLOGY AND PATHOBIOLOGY

Amniotic fluid embolism is a rare but catastrophic complication of pregnancy, occurring in about 1 in 8000 to 1 in 80,000 pregnancies. The syndrome develops when amniotic fluid and fetal cells enter the maternal blood stream through small tears in the uterine veins during labor. Emboli to the heart and lungs cause cardiac dysfunction and respiratory distress. In addition, amniotic fluid and other debris activate the coagulation system, and the resultant thrombin then triggers fibrin formation and platelet activation to induce disseminated intravascular coagulation.

CLINICAL MANIFESTATIONS AND DIAGNOSIS

The syndrome often starts with the abrupt onset of dyspnea, cyanosis, and hypotension that can rapidly progress to cardiovascular collapse and death. Patients who survive this stage often develop manifestations of disseminated intravascular coagulation (Chapter 178) characterized by diffuse bleeding, petechiae, and ecchymoses.

The diagnosis should be suspected in women late in pregnancy, often in labor, who present with sudden onset of respiratory distress followed by cyanosis, hypotension, and shock. These findings are often associated with confusion or reduced level of consciousness, seizures, and evidence of a consumptive coagulopathy.

TREATMENT

Supportive measures include oxygen, mechanical ventilation, and hemodynamic support. Fresh-frozen plasma, cryoprecipitate, and platelets transfusion can be given to replace consumed clotting factors and platelets. Heparin, often in low therapeutic doses, may be useful in some cases. If amniotic fluid embolism occurs before or during delivery, the fetus often has a poor outcome. As soon as the mother stabilizes, therefore, every attempt should be made to deliver the fetus.

PROGNOSIS

Although rare, amniotic fluid embolism remains the leading cause of maternal death during labor and the first few hours after delivery. Despite advances in critical care management, maternal and fetal mortality rates continue to be about 60% and 20%, respectively, with up to half of the survivors, both mother and baby, suffering from permanent hypoxia-induced neurologic dysfunction.

Other Embolic Material

Many substances, such as talc, starch, and cellulose are used as fillers in the manufacture of drugs. Some of these drugs are ground up by drug users (Chapter 33), mixed in liquids, and then injected intravenously. The filler particles can then be trapped in the pulmonary vasculature, where they can induce granuloma formation.

Tumor emboli (Chapter 179) in the lung can mimic pneumonia, tuberculosis, or interstitial lung disease on the chest radiograph. Cancers of the prostate and breast are the most common sources of such emboli, followed by hepatoma and cancers of the stomach and pancreas. Although found in up to 26% of autopsies in patients with advanced cancer, tumor emboli are infrequently identified before death.

Various types of intravascular devices can embolize to the lungs, including vena cava filters, broken catheter tips, guidewires, stent fragments, and coils used for embolization. Many of these devices lodge in the right atrium, right ventricle, or pulmonary arteries. Intravascular retrieval can recover most of these devices; open surgery may be required for the remainder.

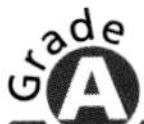

1. Kearon C, Ginsberg JS, Douketis J, et al, for the Canadian Pulmonary Embolism Diagnosis Study (CANPEDS) Group. An evaluation of D-dimer in the diagnosis of pulmonary embolism: a randomized trial. *Ann Intern Med.* 2006;144:812-821.
2. Anderson DR, Kahn SR, Rodger MA, et al. Computed tomographic pulmonary angiography vs ventilation-perfusion lung scanning in patients with suspected pulmonary embolism: a randomized controlled trial. *JAMA.* 2007;298:2743-2753.
3. Wan S, Quinlan DJ, Agnelli G, et al. Thrombolysis compared with heparin for the initial treatment of pulmonary embolism: a meta-analysis of the randomized controlled trials. *Circulation.* 2004;110:744-749.
4. Quinlan DJ, McQuillan A, Eikelboom JW. Low-molecular-weight heparin compared with intravenous unfractionated heparin for treatment of pulmonary embolism: a meta-analysis of randomized, controlled trials. *Ann Intern Med.* 2004;140:175-183.
5. Büller HR, Davidson BL, Decousus H, et al, for the Matisse Investigators. Subcutaneous fondaparinux versus intravenous unfractionated heparin in the initial treatment of pulmonary embolism *N Engl J Med.* 2003;349:1695-1702.
6. Schulman S, Kearon C, Kakkar AK, et al, for the RE-COVER Study Group. Dabigatran versus warfarin in the treatment of acute venous thromboembolism. *N Engl J Med.* 2009;361:2342-2352.
7. Palareti G, Cosmi B, Legnani C, et al, for the PROLONG Investigators. D-dimer testing to determine the duration of anticoagulation therapy. *N Engl J Med.* 2006;355:1780-1789.
8. Prandoni P, Prins MH, Lensing AW, et al, for the AESOPUS Investigators. Residual thrombosis on ultrasonography to guide the duration of anticoagulation in patients with deep venous thrombosis: a randomized trial. *Ann Intern Med.* 2009;150:577-585.
9. Ridker PM, Goldhaber SZ, Danielson E, et al, for the PREVENT Investigators. Long-term, low-intensity warfarin therapy for the prevention of recurrent venous thromboembolism. *N Engl J Med.* 2003;348:1425-1434.
10. Kearon C, Ginsberg JS, Kovacs MJ, et al, for the Extended Low-Intensity Anticoagulation for Thrombo-Embolism Investigators. Comparison of low-intensity warfarin therapy with conventional-intensity warfarin therapy for long-term prevention of recurrent venous thromboembolism. *N Engl J Med.* 2003;349:631-639.
11. The PREPIC Study Group. Eight year follow-up of patients with permanent vena cava filters in the prevention of pulmonary embolism. *Circulation.* 2005;112:416-422.

SUGGESTED READINGS

Agnelli G, Becattini C. Acute pulmonary embolism. *N Engl J Med.* 2010;363:266-274. *Review.*

Bourjeily G, Paidas M, Khalil H, et al. Pulmonary embolism in pregnancy. *Lancet.* 2010;375:500-512. *Review.*

Ceylan N, Tasbakan S, Bayraktaroglu S, et al. Predictors of clinical outcome in acute pulmonary embolism: correlation of CT pulmonary angiography with clinical, echocardiography and laboratory findings. *Acad Radiol.* 2011;18:47-53. *Neither CT pulmonary angiographic findings nor echocardiography predicts in-hospital mortality.*

Jakobsson C, Jimenez D, Gomez V, et al. Validation of a clinical algorithm to identify low-risk patients with pulmonary embolism. *J Thromb Haemost.* 2010;8:1242-1247. *Validates an easy-to-use risk scoring system to identify low-risk patients whose pulmonary emboli might be treated on an outpatient basis.*

Piazza G, Goldhaber SZ. Management of submassive pulmonary embolism. *Circulation.* 2010;122:1124-1129. *Review.*

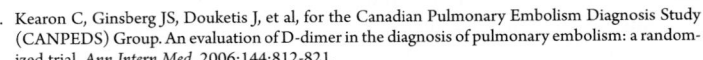

99 DISEASES OF THE DIAPHRAGM, CHEST WALL, PLEURA, AND MEDIASTINUM

F. DENNIS MCCOOL

DIAPHRAGM

The diaphragm is a dome-shaped structure that separates the thorax from the abdomen. It consists of a central tendon and a peripheral muscular component that inserts into the rib cage laterally along the inner surface of the lower six ribs, the costal cartilages anteromedially, and the upper three lumbar vertebral bodies posteriorly. The diaphragm is innervated by the phrenic nerve, which originates from cervical nerve roots 3 through 5.

DIAPHRAGMATIC WEAKNESS AND PARALYSIS

EPIDEMIOLOGY AND PATHOBIOLOGY

When the diaphragm is activated, it contracts and descends caudally. The downward descent of the diaphragm expands the lower rib cage and lowers pleural pressure, thereby resulting in lung inflation. It is the major muscle of inspiration, and its action accounts for approximately 70% of the inspired tidal volume in the normal individual. Diaphragm function can be impaired by disorders that affect the brain (Chapter 411), spinal cord (Chapter 407), phrenic nerve (Chapter 428), neuromuscular junction (Chapter 430), and muscle itself (Chapter 429). The incidence and prevalence of diaphragm paralysis and weakness are unknown.

CLINICAL MANIFESTATIONS

Diaphragmatic weakness or paralysis can involve either one or both hemidiaphragms. With unilateral diaphragmatic paralysis, patients are generally asymptomatic at rest but may have dyspnea with exertion or when supine. If they are asymptomatic, the abnormality may be discovered as an incidental finding of an elevated hemidiaphragm on chest radiography.

Bilateral diaphragmatic paralysis is not as common as unilateral paralysis. Generally, the disability with bilateral paralysis is more dramatic than with unilateral paralysis. Orthopnea is an especially prominent symptom, and patients are often unable to sleep in the supine position. These individuals also experience significant dyspnea with exertion and are at an increased risk to hypoventilate during sleep, especially during rapid eye movement (REM) sleep. Consequently, initial symptoms of individuals with bilateral or unilateral diaphragm weakness or paralysis may be related to nocturnal hypoventilation and include frequent nocturnal awakenings, nocturia, vivid nightmares, night sweats, daytime hypersomnolence, depression, and morning headaches.

The physical examination is remarkable for use of accessory muscles of inspiration and paradoxical inward motion of the abdominal wall during inspiration, which is especially noticeable when these individuals are asked to lie flat. Percussion during inspiration and expiration can detect the absence of diaphragmatic movement.

DIAGNOSIS

Disorders that can cause unilateral diaphragmatic weakness or paralysis (Table 99-1) include traumatic phrenic nerve injury, herpes zoster (Chapter 383), cervical spinal disease (Chapter 407), compressive tumors, and phrenic nerve injury related to cardiac or thoracic surgery. Diagnosis is often suggested by elevation of a hemidiaphragm on a chest radiograph. The diagnosis can be confirmed by performing a "sniff test" using fluoroscopy, in which paradoxical (cephalad) movement of the hemidiaphragm occurs during a sniff maneuver.

The presence of bilateral diaphragmatic paralysis can be much more difficult to ascertain than unilateral paralysis. Chest radiography, which typically shows elevation of both hemidiaphragms, may be interpreted as a "poor inspiratory effort" or "low lung volumes."

Tests that can support or refute the diagnosis include pulmonary function testing (Chapter 85), which typically shows a moderate to severe reduction of vital capacity (VC) and total lung capacity (TLC) (30 to 60% predicted). The restriction becomes more severe (10 to 30% further decrease for unilateral and 30 to 50% further decrease for bilateral paralysis) when the individual assumes the supine position. Maximal static inspiratory pressure measured at the airway opening (PI_{max}) is reduced to 20 to 30% of predicted in individuals with bilateral diaphragmatic paralysis. The diagnosis can be confirmed if measurements of transdiaphragmatic pressure (the pressure difference between the thoracic and abdominal cavity) do not change with inspiration. Diaphragm electromyography and phrenic nerve conduction studies may be useful to distinguish neuropathy or myopathy. Unlike unilateral diaphragmatic paralysis, a sniff test is not helpful in individuals with bilateral diaphragmatic paralysis because it can yield both false-negative and false-positive results. Using two-dimensional ultrasound, the normal thickening of the diaphragm during inspiration will not be observed. If the diagnosis of bilateral diaphragmatic paralysis is confirmed, an evaluation for nocturnal hypoventilation (Chapter 86) should be undertaken.

TABLE 99-1 CAUSES OF DIAPHRAGMATIC WEAKNESS AND PARALYSIS

TRAUMA
Cardiac surgery with cold cardioplegia
Blunt trauma
Spinal cord injury
Cervical manipulation
Scalene and brachial nerve block
TUMOR COMPRESSION
Lung cancer
Metastatic mediastinal tumor
METABOLIC
Diabetes
Vitamin deficiency (B_6, B_{12}, folate)
Hypothyroidism
Acid maltase deficiency
INFLAMMATORY NEURITIS
Neuralgic amyotrophy (Parsonage-Turner)
Mononeuritis multiplex
Vasculitis
Paraneoplastic
MUSCULAR DYSTROPHIES
Limb-girdle
Duchenne's and Becker's
MISCELLANEOUS
Amyloidosis
Malnutrition
Radiation injury
Cervical spondylosis
Poliomyelitis
Amyotrophic lateral sclerosis
IDIOPATHIC

TREATMENT AND PROGNOSIS (Rx)

Bilateral diaphragmatic paralysis may not be reversible unless the underlying cause is treatable. For example, myopathies (Chapter 429) related to metabolic disturbances may be improved by correcting electrolyte imbalances or replacing thyroid hormone. Toxic or metabolic disturbances related to diabetes, alcohol, or viral infections may resolve with treatment of the underlying disease. Idiopathic diaphragmatic paralysis or paralysis due to neuralgic amyotrophy (brachial plexus neuritis) may spontaneously improve or resolve completely in approximately 60% of individuals, but recovery can take 18 months to 3 years. Phrenic nerve damage related to cardiac surgery usually resolves spontaneously. For a high spinal cord injury, in which the phrenic nerve roots remain intact (injury above C-3), phrenic nerve pacing can provide ventilation.

As in sleep-disordered breathing (Chapter 100), noninvasive positive-pressure ventilation (NPPV) is the preferred method of treatment for patients with diaphragmatic paralysis because it can improve both symptoms and physiologic derangements.

Nocturnal positive-pressure ventilation is associated with a number of benefits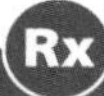 in patients with neuromuscular disease (Table 99-2). The improvement in ventilation may be related to resting the diaphragm during periods of mechanical ventilation; this reduced work appears to reverse chronic respiratory muscle fatigue and improve daytime function. Other benefits may be related to changes in the control of breathing by reversing the brain's adaptation to high levels of CO_2 by "resetting" the central controller toward normal. When patients with unilateral paralysis have severe symptoms, surgical plication of the paralyzed hemidiaphragm may improve vital capacity.

MISCELLANEOUS DIAPHRAGMATIC DISORDERS

Diaphragmatic eventration results from localized atrophy of the diaphragm muscle or from part of the diaphragm being replaced with fibroelastic tissue. Eventration most often results in an elevation of the right anteromedial portion of the diaphragm. Metastatic tumors to the diaphragm usually are related to direct extension of lung cancer. Primary tumors of the diaphragm are very rare. Lipomas are the most common benign tumor, and fibrosarcomas are the most common malignant neoplasm.

CHEST WALL

The chest wall is a key component of the "inspiratory pump" and allows for maintenance of normal alveolar ventilation. It consists of the bony structures

TABLE 99-2 THERAPEUTIC BENEFITS OF NONINVASIVE MECHANICAL VENTILATION IN PATIENTS WITH CHEST WALL AND NEUROMUSCULAR DISORDERS*

GAS EXCHANGE INDICES	
Pa_{O_2}	Increase
Pa_{CO_2}	Decrease
Bicarbonate	Decrease
RESPIRATORY MECHANICS	
MIP, MEP	No change or slight increase
HEMODYNAMIC PARAMETERS	
PAP	Decrease
VENTILATORY CONTROL	
Hypercapnic ventilatory response	Increase
SLEEP	
Epworth sleepiness score	Decrease
OTHER PARAMETERS	
Quality of life	Improvement
Survival	Increase

*Efficacy data derived from mostly nonrandomized, noncontrolled studies.
MEP = maximal expiratory pressure; MIP = maximal inspiratory pressure; PAP = pulmonary artery pressure.

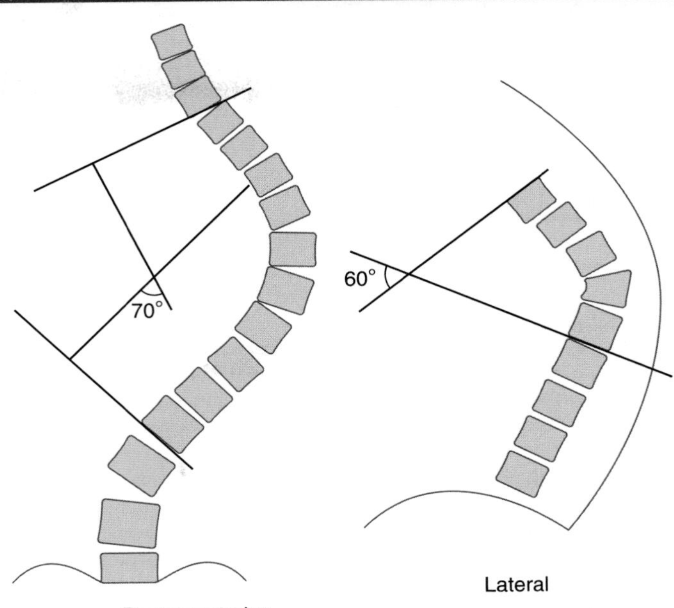

FIGURE 99-1. Schematic drawings of the spine illustrating the lines constructed to measure the Cobb angle of scoliosis and kyphosis. The angle can be calculated either from the intersection of the lines parallel to the vertebrae (as shown for kyphosis, on the *right*) or from the intersection of lines perpendicular to these lines (as shown for scoliosis, on the *left*).

of the rib cage, the articulations between the ribs and the vertebrae, the diaphragm, intercostal muscles, and the abdomen. Disorders that affect any of the components of the chest wall can result in impaired breathing.

KYPHOSCOLIOSIS

EPIDEMIOLOGY AND PATHOBIOLOGY

Kyphoscoliosis, which is a common spinal disorder, affects approximately 1 in 1000 individuals, and about 1 in 10,000 affected individuals has a severe spinal deformity. Deformities include excessive spinal curvature in the coronal (scoliosis) and sagittal (kyphosis) planes as well as rotation of the spinal axis. Kyphoscoliosis can be idiopathic or can be secondary (paralytic) and associated with neuromuscular diseases, such as muscular dystrophy and polio (Chapters 423 and 429).

Idiopathic kyphoscoliosis, in which there may be a familial predominance, usually manifests in late childhood or early adolescence and involves females more than males with a ratio of 4:1. Although a defect in the chromatin-remodeling gene family (*CHD7*) has been associated with idiopathic kyphoscoliosis, other genes have also been identified.

Kyphoscoliosis produces one of the most severe restrictive impairments of all the chest wall diseases. Total lung capacity and vital capacity may be reduced to as low as 30% of predicted values. This restrictive pathology becomes most severe as the degree of spinal angulation increases. The patient's age, degree of spinal rotation, presence of respiratory muscle weakness, and involvement of the thoracic vertebrae are all factors that promote the restrictive process. Respiratory failure is a common cause of morbidity and mortality in patients with kyphoscoliosis.

CLINICAL MANIFESTATIONS

Individuals with mild to moderate kyphoscoliosis may have complaints of back pain and have psychosocial problems as a result of their deformity. Adolescents with mild idiopathic kyphoscoliosis usually have normal exercise capacity, whereas those with moderate idiopathic kyphoscoliosis have reduced exercise capacity with additional exercise limitation due to deconditioning. With severe deformities, patients may experience dyspnea with minimal exertion or at rest.

Severe kyphoscoliosis can be readily diagnosed on physical examination. Typical findings are the dorsal hump, which is due to the angulated ribs and shoulder asymmetry, as well as the hip tilt that is related to the spinal rotation. In younger individuals with milder spinal deformities, the initial changes may be subtle. The Adams forward bend test, in which the examiner observes for thoracic or lumbar region asymmetry while the patient bends forward at the waist until the spine becomes parallel to the floor, can help detect minor deformities. With severe kyphoscoliosis, signs of right heart failure (Chapter 58) may be present such as cyanosis, distended neck veins, peripheral edema, and hepatomegaly.

Individuals with kyphoscoliosis are particularly prone to hypoventilation during sleep, especially REM sleep. Because sleep-related abnormalities and their effects on cardiorespiratory function are potentially treatable, individuals with kyphoscoliosis should be evaluated for nocturnal hypoventilation well in advance of the development of daytime hypercapnia.

DIAGNOSIS

Although spinal deformity is often readily apparent on physical examination, the degree of spinal deformity should be assessed by calculation of the angle of spinal curvature (the Cobb angle) from radiographs. This angle is formed by the intersection of lines parallel to the top and bottom vertebrae of the scoliotic or kyphotic curves (Fig. 99-1). Angles more than 100 degrees are usually associated with respiratory symptoms, and angles more than 120 degrees with respiratory failure. Factors associated with progression of the spinal deformity include inspiratory muscle weakness, a large spinal curvature at the time of presentation, skeletal immaturity, and a thoracic location of the curve apex. Individuals with inspiratory muscle weakness and kyphoscoliosis are more prone to develop respiratory failure than those with normal inspiratory muscle strength.

TREATMENT

Rx

Patients should be encouraged to remain physically active to minimize peripheral muscle deconditioning. In addition, general supportive measures including immunizations against influenza and pneumococci (Chapter 17), smoking cessation (Chapter 31), maintenance of a normal body weight (Chapter 227), and treatment of respiratory infections in a timely fashion should be instituted. Patients with severe kyphoscoliosis and Cobb angles of more than 100 degrees should be monitored closely for respiratory complications. Respiratory failure may be precipitated by respiratory infections or by medications that produce central nervous system depression.

Nocturnal hypoventilation typically precedes findings of daytime hypercapnia and hypoxemia and should be treated with NPPV. Indications for instituting NPPV include symptoms of nocturnal hypoventilation or signs of cor pulmonale (Chapter 68) with either an elevated daytime Pa_{CO_2} or nocturnal oxygen saturation of less than 89% for 5 consecutive minutes. Supplemental oxygen will be needed if hypoxemia persists despite correction of hypoventilation. NPPV can reduce the number and duration of hospitalizations and improve gas exchange, daytime blood gases, quality of life, and survival (see Table 99-2).

Surgical and nonsurgical (back-brace) treatments have been used in skeletally immature patients with idiopathic kyphoscoliosis in an effort to correct or prevent progression of the spinal deformity. Braces have been used for growing children with Cobb angles between 25 and 40 degrees, whereas surgery has been used for adolescents with a Cobb angle of more than 45 degrees. The overall role of surgical management in restoring function to that of nonscoliotic individuals and minimizing the possibility of respiratory failure is not clear.

PROGNOSIS

Idiopathic kyphoscoliosis has a better prognosis than kyphoscoliosis secondary to neuromuscular diseases. In general, individuals with mild idiopathic kyphoscoliosis have an overall benign course. Patients with moderate or severe deformities are at higher risk of developing respiratory complications.

In secondary kyphoscoliosis, factors such as an early age of onset, rapid curve progression during growth, progression of scoliosis after skeletal maturity, large curves at the time of presentation, and a thoracic rather than a thoracolumbar or lumbar location of the curve apex are risk factors for respiratory complications. Respiratory failure may occur in individuals with mild or moderate kyphoscoliosis owing to concurrent respiratory muscle dysfunction. Muscle strength should be evaluated in individuals with respiratory failure and Cobb angles of less than 100 degrees. When cor pulmonale develops (Chapter 68), the prognosis is poor, and death may occur within 1 year without therapy.

PECTUS EXCAVATUM

EPIDEMIOLOGY AND PATHOBIOLOGY

Pectus excavatum, a chest wall deformity that occurs in approximately 0.5 to 2% of the population, is characterized by excessive depression of the sternum and its adjacent costal cartilages. The ratio of affected males to females is 4:1, and a family history is common. Pectus excavatum produces minimal functional impairment of the respiratory system. Occasionally, a restrictive defect will be present with mild reductions in VC and TLC. Individuals with the most severe pectus deformities may exhibit a mild reduction in maximal exercise capacity.

CLINICAL MANIFESTATIONS

Cosmetic concerns are the usual reason for seeking medical attention. Dyspnea with activity or exercise may be present but is usually out of proportion to any measurable abnormality in cardiopulmonary function. On physical examination, sternal depression is readily apparent, and there is normal excursion of the rib cage during inspiration. A mild degree of scoliosis may be present in 40 to 60% of individuals.

DIAGNOSIS

Chest computed tomography (CT) is the best means of assessing the sternal deformity. The anteroposterior diameter of the rib cage and the transverse diameter of the rib cage are measured at the level of the deepest sternal depression. Normally, the transverse-to-anteroposterior diameter ratio is 2.5. A ratio of greater than 3.5 signifies a significant pectus deformity.

TREATMENT AND PROGNOSIS Rx

Surgical correction of the deformity is considered for patients with a CT ratio of more than 3.5 in conjunction with symptoms of dyspnea or laboratory evidence of cardiac or pulmonary restriction. However, there is no convincing evidence that correction of the deformity improves either cardiopulmonary function or exercise capacity. Invasive surgical approaches include resecting costal cartilage and repositioning the sternum. Sternal necrosis and infection may complicate invasive surgical procedures, and sternal osteotomy should be avoided in early childhood because it may be complicated by arrested growth of the rib cage. Minimally invasive approaches insert curved metal rods into the sternum through small incisions on each side of the rib cage; over time, the rod is rotated to force the sternum outward. After approximately 2 years, the rods are removed. The prognosis is excellent in individuals who have only mild deformity and patients who have undergone minimally invasive surgical correction of more severe deformities.

FLAIL CHEST

EPIDEMIOLOGY AND PATHOBIOLOGY

Flail chest occurs following trauma in which there have been either double fractures of three or more contiguous ribs or combined sternal and rib fractures. The result is an unstable segment of the chest wall, which moves paradoxically inward with inspiration and outward with expiration. In adults, flail chest is most commonly a consequence of blunt chest wall trauma owing to automobile accidents or falls (Chapter 112).

With a flail chest, inspiratory capacity is limited, and VC may be reduced by 50% or more. Reductions in lung compliance, owing to concomitant pulmonary contusion or microatelectasis, will worsen the restrictive dysfunction and impair gas exchange. The most common location for a flail segment is the lateral chest wall, and this location is generally associated with more clinical derangement. By contrast, a posterior flail segment has less impact on the respiratory system because of splinting provided by the paraspinal muscles.

Hypoventilation and flail-induced changes in respiratory muscle function are key factors to the development of respiratory failure in individuals with flail chest (E-Fig. 99-1). Excessive shortening of the inspiratory muscles related to the flail segment increase the work of breathing. The increased work, in concert with reduced oxygen supplies due to pulmonary contusion or hypoventilation, predisposes these individuals to developing respiratory muscle fatigue. Pain associated with the rib fractures and the disordered motion of the flail segment during expiration impair cough.

DIAGNOSIS

Bedside inspection and gentle palpation of the rib cage and abdomen can reveal the characteristic paradoxical movement of the flail segment during spontaneous breathing. Chest radiographs will confirm the presence of multiple rib fractures, but a three-dimensional reconstruction of a thoracic CT can provide better visualization of thoracic injuries, including lung contusion. The diagnosis may be less apparent in a sedated mechanically ventilated patient, in whom paradoxical motion of a segment of the rib cage may not occur because the positive alveolar and pleural pressures act as a "pneumatic splint" and allow for uniform inflation of the chest wall. However, after withdrawal of sedation, spontaneous breathing should reveal the flail segment.

TREATMENT Rx

Nonsurgical management of flail chest consists of adequate analgesia, clearance of bronchial secretions, and mechanical ventilatory assistance if needed. Pain relief (Chapter 29) can be accomplished by oral medications, patient-controlled analgesic pumps, intercostal nerve blocks, or epidural anesthesia. These interventions often produce a successful outcome with avoidance of respiratory failure and mechanical ventilation, and as the rib cage heals, function is restored. If respiratory failure ensues, not only will mechanical ventilation enhance gas exchange, but also the positive pleural pressure provided by the ventilator during inspiration will stabilize the flail segment. Ventilation delivered by a nasal or face mask to patients who are spontaneously breathing improves gas exchange and may allow for early mobilization and access to physical therapy.

Surgical techniques, none of which is supported by randomized clinical trial evidence, include open thoracotomy with stabilization of the fractured ribs. The indications for operative fixation are not fully defined, but patients who are unable to wean from mechanical ventilation owing to chest wall instability or patients who are undergoing thoracotomy for concomitant injuries may be candidates for surgical fixation.

PROGNOSIS

The overall mortality from chest wall trauma is high, ranging from 7 to 14%. If concomitant lung contusion is present, the mortality rate increases further and may be as high as 70%. The associated high mortality rate is also partly due to the coexistence of other injuries, such as fractures of the long bones, head trauma, or rupture of major vascular structures (Chapter 112). Older age is another poor prognostic factor.

In patients with flail chest without lung contusion, the restrictive impairment can resolve, and the VC can return to baseline values within 6 months after the acute injury. By contrast, individuals with flail chest and concomitant lung contusion often have persistent impairment of pulmonary function, which may persist for up to 4 years after injury. Operative fixation of the chest wall may reduce long-term respiratory dysfunction in these individuals.

ANKYLOSING SPONDYLITIS

EPIDEMIOLOGY AND PATHOBIOLOGY

Ankylosing spondylitis (Chapter 273) is an inflammatory disease that involves the ligamentous structures of the spine, sacroiliac, and large peripheral joints. It affects men more than women, with the most common age of onset between 15 and 25 years. There is a genetic predisposition, with the HLA-B27 antigen present in 95% of whites with ankylosing spondylitis. Chronic inflammation of the spine and peripheral joints may cause fibrosis and ossification of structures adjacent to the spine. Fusion of the costovertebral and sternoclavicular joints produces relative fixation of the rib cage in an inspiratory position, with limited motion of the rib cage during inspiration and a mild restrictive respiratory impairment. The degree of restriction is proportional to disease activity and duration as well as to the degree of spinal and rib cage immobility. Concomitant kyphosis, which may occur in advanced disease or be secondary to osteoporosis, will further impair respiratory function. Because the rib cage is less distensible, the diaphragm shortens to a greater degree for a given tidal volume, thereby increasing the work performed by the diaphragm. Intercostal muscle atrophy secondary to decreased rib cage mobility may cause inspiratory muscle weakness.

About 1 to 4% of patients with ankylosing spondylitis develop fibrobullous upper lobe disease. The cause of this apical disease is unknown, but its presence may impair gas exchange. Occasionally, individuals with ankylosing spondylitis develop nonapical interstitial lung disease (Chapter 92).

CLINICAL MANIFESTATIONS AND DIAGNOSIS

Ankylosing spondylitis is diagnosed when there is a history of low back pain and stiffness for more than 3 months, limited chest wall expansion, limited lumbar spine motion in the sagittal and frontal planes, and radiographic evidence of sacroiliitis. Radiographic findings include calcifications and ossifications of the vertebrae and paravertebral tissues.

Low back pain and spinal stiffness are the most common presenting symptoms. Dyspnea may be present as the disease progresses and chest wall expansion becomes more restricted. Physical examination may reveal loss of lateral flexion of the lumbar spine, tenderness over the sacroiliac joints, and kyphosis.

TREATMENT AND PROGNOSIS (Rx)

Exercise and physiotherapy programs can enhance cardiorespiratory fitness and spinal mobility. Ankylosing spondylitis is treated with nonsteroidal anti-inflammatory agents and biological agents, such as tumor necrosis factor antagonists that relieve symptoms, reduce spinal inflammation, and improve quality of life. These agents also are associated with improvements in rib cage expansion. Corticosteroids do not prevent the progression of fibrobullous disease, which can be complicated by major hemoptysis. Thoracic surgery may be indicated for hemoptysis, but surgical intervention carries major risk, with 50 to 60% of patients developing bronchopleural fistulas. Ankylosing spondylitis rarely leads to disability unless individuals develop fibrobullous disease.

OBESITY

PATHOBIOLOGY

The degree of obesity (Chapter 227) can be assessed by measuring the body mass index (BMI), which is the ratio of body weight (BW) in kilograms to the square of the height (Ht) in meters (BW/Ht^2). Individuals with a BMI between 18.5 and 24.9 kg/m^2 are normal, whereas those with a BMI greater than 40 kg/m^2 are considered morbidly obese.

Obesity can be accompanied by changes in pulmonary function or alterations in respiratory control. Obesity characteristically reduces end-expiratory lung volume or functional reserve capacity (FRC) and expiratory reserve volume (ERV). TLC and VC may be normal or only mildly reduced except in the most severe cases. Obesity can be accompanied by alterations in respiratory control resulting in elevated levels of $Paco_2$ (Chapter 86).

Dyspnea and exercise intolerance, which are the most frequent respiratory complaints of obese individuals, may be related to disordered chest wall mechanics, restrictive pulmonary dysfunction, altered respiratory control, or the presence of inflammatory mediators, such as those linking obesity to airway hyper-responsiveness. Weight loss (Chapter 227) is the optimal therapy, and it improves lung volumes, respiratory muscle performance, gas exchange, dyspnea, and sleep apnea. In individuals with obesity-hypoventilation syndrome (Chapter 100), nocturnal positive-pressure ventilation can reverse gas exchange abnormalities.

PLEURA

The pleura, which is a thin membrane that covers the inner surfaces of the thoracic cavity, consists of a layer of mesothelial cells supported by a network of connective and fibroelastic tissue. The visceral pleura lines the lung, whereas the parietal pleura lines the rib cage, diaphragm, and mediastinal structures. The closed space between the visceral and parietal pleura is referred to as the pleural space. The vascular supply of the parietal pleural surface is from the systemic circulation, and it contains sensory nerves and lymphatics. By contrast, the visceral pleura is supplied with blood vessels from the pulmonary circulation and has no sensory nerves.

PLEURAL EFFUSION

EPIDEMIOLOGY AND PATHOBIOLOGY

The overall frequency of pleural effusion on a chest radiograph ranges from 0.3 to 1% but varies widely depending on the underlying disease. Pleural effusions occur most frequently in patients with pneumonia (Chapter 97) or heart failure (Chapter 58).

Normally, a small amount of fluid in the pleural space forms a thin layer between the visceral and parietal pleural surfaces and acts as a lubricant to minimize friction between the chest wall and lung as they move against each other during inspiration and expiration. There is continual movement of fluid into and out of the pleural space. This flux of fluid depends on the oncotic and hydrostatic pressures within the parietal and visceral pleura as well as the pressure within the pleural space itself. Hydrostatic pressure in the parietal pleura is similar to systemic circulation (30 cm H_2O), whereas that of the visceral pleura is similar to the pulmonary circulation (10 cm H_2O). Accordingly, most fluid in the pleural space is filtered from the higher-pressure vascular structures in the parietal pleura. Because the pressure within the pleural space itself is more subatmospheric at the apex than at the base, most of the fluid filters in from the less dependent upper lung zones. Fluid is drained out primarily through lymphatics in the parietal pleura. The fluid enters through lymphatic stomas on the surface of the parietal pleura, which are located beneath the mesothelial monolayer. The normal turnover of fluid within the pleural space is 10 to 20 mL/day, with only 0.2 to 1 mL remaining in the pleural space.

Under abnormal circumstances, fluid can accumulate within the pleural space. An increase in hydrostatic pressure, a decrease in oncotic pressure, decreased pressure in the pleural space, increased pleural membrane permeability, or obstruction of pleural lymphatics will promote pleural fluid accumulation (Table 99-3).

An increase in hydrostatic pressure or decrease in oncotic pressure will result in a low-protein collection of pleural fluid characterized as *transudates* (Table 99-4). For example, heart failure (Chapter 58) can produce transudates by increasing hydrostatic pressure in the pulmonary venous system, atelectasis (Chapter 90) can promote transudates by making pleural pressure more subatmospheric, and occasionally, oncotic pressure may be sufficiently reduced to cause transudates (e.g., with hypoalbuminemia). Changes in pleural membrane permeability can produce high-protein effusions, which are characterized as *exudates* and can be seen in inflammatory states such as pneumonia, tuberculosis, or rheumatoid arthritis. Tumors can disrupt the

TABLE 99-3 MECHANISMS PROMOTING PLEURAL FLUID ACCUMULATION

MICROVASCULAR CIRCULATION
Increased hydrostatic pressure (heart failure) Decreased oncotic pressure (severe hypoalbuminemia) Increased permeability (pneumonia)
PLEURAL SPACE
Decreased pressure (lung collapse)
LYMPHATICS
Impaired lymphatic drainage (malignant effusion)
DIAPHRAGM
Movement of fluid from the peritoneal space (hepatic hydrothorax)

TABLE 99-4 CONDITIONS THAT CAUSE PLEURAL EFFUSION

TRANSUDATES

Heart failure
Nephrotic syndrome
Hepatic hydrothorax
Superior vena cava syndrome
Peritoneal dialysis
Atelectasis
Urinothorax

EXUDATES

Parapneumonic effusions
- Simple
- Complicated
- Empyema

Other infections
- Tuberculosis
- Fungal
- Parasites
- Nocardia

Esophageal rupture
Malignancy
- Carcinoma
- Lymphoma
- Mesothelioma
- Metastatic disease

INFLAMMATORY DISORDERS

Connective tissue disease
- Rheumatoid arthritis
- Systemic lupus erythematosus
- Churg-Strauss syndrome
- Wegener's granulomatosis
- Familial Mediterranean fever

Abdominal disease
- Subdiaphragmatic abscess (hepatic, splenic)
- Pancreatitis, pancreatic pseudocyst
- Postoperative

Iatrogenic
- Drug induced
- Misplacement of enteral feeding tube
- Esophageal endoscopic interventions

Miscellaneous
- Asbestos exposure
- Atelectasis
- Cholesterol effusion
- Chylothorax
- Dressler's syndrome
- Meigs' syndrome
- Pulmonary embolus
- Radiation
- Sarcoidosis
- Trapped lung
- Uremia
- Yellow nail syndrome

integrity of the mesothelial layer or the integrity of the capillary epithelium, thereby resulting in exudative effusions, or they may block lymphatic drainage either through interference with stomal openings into the pleural space or obstruction of lymphatic channels.

CLINICAL MANIFESTATIONS

Patients with pleural effusions may be asymptomatic or may experience dyspnea. When the parietal pleura is actively inflamed, pain can be present, and it is generally unilateral, sharp, and worsens with inspiration. At times, effusions may be sufficiently large to contribute to respiratory failure. Physical findings include dullness to percussion in the area of the effusion, along with diminished breath sounds and absent tactile fremitus.

DIAGNOSIS

Chest radiography is often the first imaging method used to detect an effusion (Fig. 99-2). The volume of fluid in the pleural space needs to exceed 250 mL to be visualized on the chest radiograph. When an effusion is present, there is blunting of the costophrenic angle on the posteroanterior chest radiograph (Fig. 99-3), and a meniscus can be seen posteriorly on the lateral chest radiograph (see Fig. 99-2B). Fluid may also collect in either the minor or major fissures. Occasionally, pleural fluid collections in the major or minor fissures may appear as a pulmonary mass and are referred to as *pseudotumors*. A lateral decubitus chest radiograph can be obtained to determine whether fluid is free flowing or loculated. Chest CT provides much better characterization of pleural and parenchymal abnormalities by better defining loculated effusions, distinguishing between atelectasis and effusion, and distinguishing loculated effusion from lung abscess (Fig. 99-4).

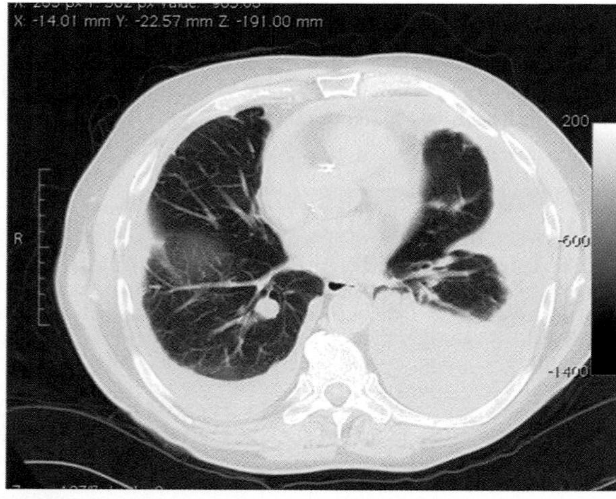

FIGURE 99-3. Chest computed tomography showing pleural effusion in the same patient as in Fig. 99-2.

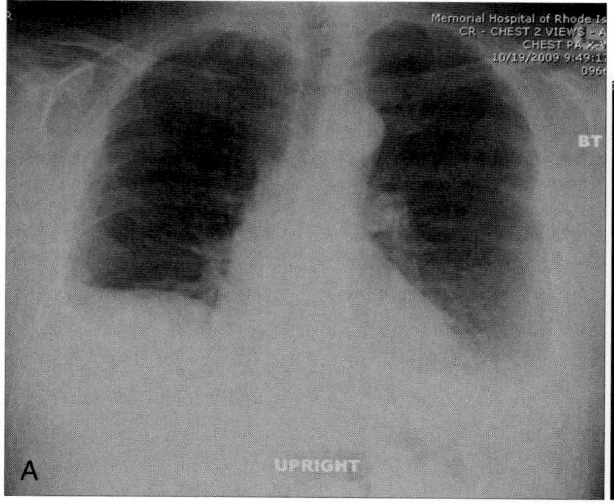

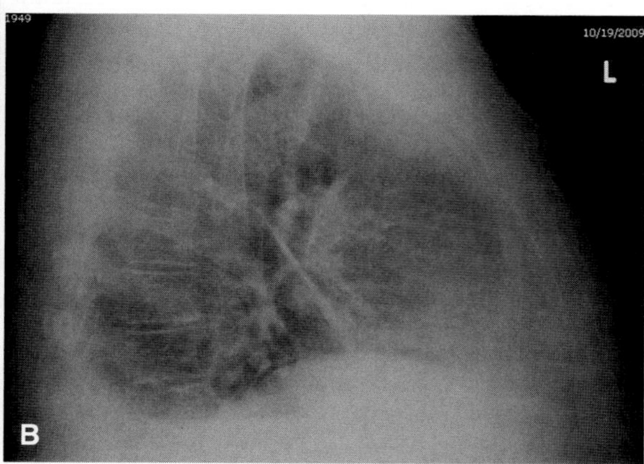

FIGURE 99-2. Patient with bilateral pleural effusions as seen on the posteroanterior radiograph of the chest (A) and lateral radiograph of the chest (B).

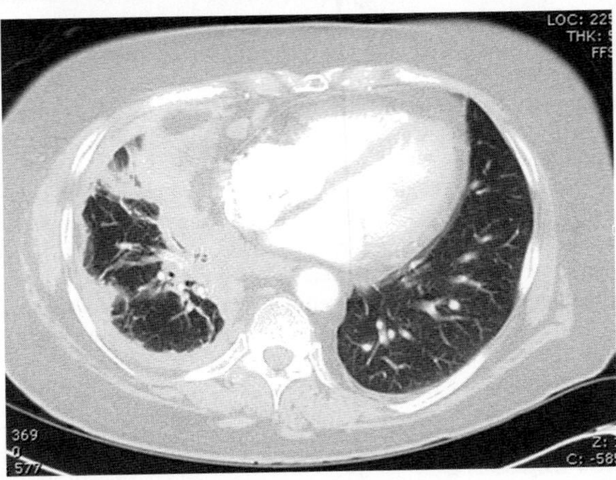

FIGURE 99-4. Computed tomographic angiogram of the chest in a patient with mesothelioma. There is diffuse thickening of the pleura and pericardium on the right with a rindlike appearance.

TABLE 99-6 CORRELATION OF THE CHARACTERISTICS OF PLEURAL EXUDATES WITH SPECIFIC DISEASE

TEST	DISEASE
pH < 7.2	Empyema, malignancy, esophageal rupture; rheumatoid, lupus, and tuberculous pleuritis
Glucose (<60 mg/dL)	Infection, rheumatoid pleurisy, tuberculous and lupus effusions, esophageal rupture
Amylase (>200 μg/dL)	Pancreatic disease, esophageal rupture, malignancy, ruptured ectopic pregnancy
RF, ANA, LE cells	Collagen vascular disease
↓ Complement	SLE, RA
RBCs (>5000/μL)	Trauma, malignancy, pulmonary embolus
Chylous effusion (triglycerides > 110 mg/dL)	Tuberculosis, disruption of thoracic duct (trauma, malignancy)
Cytology or biopsy (+)	Malignancy
ADA (>50 μg/L)	Tuberculosis

ADA = adenosine deaminase; ANA = antinuclear antibody; RA = rheumatoid arthritis; RBC = red blood cell; RF, rheumatoid factor; SLE = systemic lupus erythematosus.

TABLE 99-5 PLEURAL FLUID CHARACTERISTICS OF EXUDATES

LIGHT'S CRITERIA	
Protein	>0.5 pleural fluid/serum value
LDH	>0.6 pleural fluid/serum value
LDH	>2/3 upper limit of normal serum value
TWO-TEST RULE	
LDH	>0.45 upper limit of normal serum value
Cholesterol	>45 mg/dL
THREE-STEP CRITERIA	
LDH	>0.45 upper limit of normal serum value
Cholesterol	>45 mg/dL
Protein	>2.9 g/dL

LDH = lactate dehydrogenase.

A sample of fluid from the pleural space by thoracentesis is the key to determining the etiology of a pleural effusion. The tests needed to make a diagnosis require a relatively small amount of fluid (30 to 50 mL). Larger volumes of fluid can be removed (1 to 1.5 L) in an attempt to alleviate symptoms. Removing volumes greater than 1.5 L may result in re-expansion pulmonary edema. Most thoracenteses can be performed at the bedside, using ultrasound guidance to enhance the procedure's safety. In instances when the effusion is small or fluid is loculated, a CT scan can help direct the thoracentesis catheter into fluid that would otherwise be difficult to drain. Relative contraindications to a diagnostic thoracentesis include a bleeding diathesis, a very small volume of pleural fluid, and a low benefit-to-risk ratio.

Once fluid is obtained, a definitive diagnosis may be achieved, and the fluid can be classified as either a transudate or exudate (Table 99-5). To differentiate an exudate from a transudate, the pleural fluid needs to be analyzed for protein and lactate dehydrogenase (LDH). Simultaneous serum values of protein and LDH also need to be obtained. A pleural fluid exudate is characterized by a pleural fluid–to–serum protein ratio greater than 0.5, a pleural fluid–to–serum LDH ratio greater than 0.6, and a pleural fluid LDH greater than two thirds the normal serum value for LDH. An exudate can also be defined if the pleural fluid cholesterol is higher than 45 mg/dL, protein higher than 2.9 g/dL, or LDH higher than 0.45 upper limit of normal serum value.

Transudates

Effusions that accumulate owing to changes in osmotic and hydrostatic forces usually form transudates. Transudative effusions are most commonly due to heart failure, in which the effusions are often bilateral or, if unilateral, preferentially involve the right hemithorax. Transudates may also be seen in cirrhosis (Chapter 156), nephrotic syndrome (Chapter 123), myxedema (Chapter 233), pulmonary embolism (Chapter 98), superior vena caval obstruction, and peritoneal dialysis (Chapter 133). With cirrhosis, ascites may cross from the peritoneum into the pleural space through small defects in the diaphragm (hepatic hydrothorax) (see Table 99-4). Unusual causes of transudates include peritoneal dialysis and atelectasis. Although malignancy typically causes an exudate, it can occasionally produce a transudate. Urinothorax, which is a rare cause of transudate, results from obstruction of the urinary system.

Exudates

An effusion is characterized as an exudate if it meets one of the following criteria: pleural fluid–to–serum protein ratio higher than 0.5, pleural fluid–to–serum LDH ratio higher than 0.6, or a pleural fluid LDH concentration higher than two thirds the normal serum value. Cholesterol levels also may be increased in exudates (>45 mg/dL). The pleural fluid analysis helps distinguish among the causes of pleural exudates (Table 99-6).

Parapneumonic Effusions

Parapneumonic effusions, which are the most common type of exudative pleural effusion, occur in up to 40% of patients with pneumonia. They typically occur in patients with bacterial pneumonia (Chapter 97) and can be classified as uncomplicated or complicated. With uncomplicated parapneumonic effusion, the pH is generally greater than 7.3, the glucose content more than 60 mg/dL, and the pleural fluid LDH less than 1000 IU/L. Uncomplicated parapneumonic effusions are usually free flowing, do not require drainage, and will respond to the same antibiotic therapy as the pneumonia itself. However, uncomplicated parapneumonic effusions can, at times, transition to complicated effusions. Complicated effusions are characterized by a pH of less than 7.2 and often have a low glucose content. These effusions generally will not respond to antibiotic therapy alone but require drainage to prevent formation of an empyema or a thick pleural peal.

Empyema

An empyema is present when frank pus is aspirated from the pleural space or when the Gram stain of the fluid is positive for bacteria. Pneumonia due to *Streptococcus pneumoniae* (Chapter 297) or *Staphylococcus aureus* (Chapter 296) infection can cause empyema. Individuals who aspirate are at high risk for empyema caused by anaerobic organisms, and patients with tuberculosis (Chapter 332) can develop a tuberculous empyema. Methicillin-resistant staphylococci, *Klebsiella* species pneumonia, and *Pseudomonas* species infections may cause an empyema that is difficult to treat. Uncommon infectious causes of effusions include *Actinomyces* species (Chapter 337), *Nocardia* species (Chapter 338), amebiasis (Chapter 360), *Echinococcus* species (Chapter 362), and paragonimiasis (Chapter 364).

Individuals with empyema often complain of pleuritic chest pain and have refractory fevers several days or more into the course of their pneumonia, but immunocompromised patients may develop empyema sooner and more rapidly. When an empyema is present, it requires prompt chest tube drainage. If chest tube drainage is unsuccessful in resolving the empyema, video-assisted thoracic surgery (Chapter 101) is preferred, with intrapleural streptokinase reserved for patients who are poor candidates for video-assisted thoracic surgery or are in situations in which it is not available. 3

Tuberculous Effusions

Tuberculosis (Chapter 332) can cause pleural effusion in up to 30% of patients who reside in endemic locations for tuberculosis. The pleural effusion typically is not due to direct mycobacterial infection itself, but rather to increased vascular permeability of the pleural membrane because of a hypersensitivity reaction to mycobacterial proteins. The pleural fluid is generally lymphocyte predominant and culture negative for acid-fast bacilli. Adenosine deaminase levels higher than 50 U/L may be helpful in identifying tuberculous pleural effusions. A tuberculous empyema, which is distinct from a tuberculous effusion, is characterized by direct extension of the infection from thoracic lymph nodes or hematogenous spread of tuberculosis into the pleural space.

Malignancy

Malignant effusions are the second most common cause of exudative pleural effusions. Rarely, a malignant effusion may be transudative. Lung cancer (Chapter 197) is the most frequent cause of malignant pleural effusion, and other malignancies that can involve the pleural space include breast cancer (Chapter 204), ovarian cancer (Chapter 205), gastric cancer (Chapter 198), and lymphoma (Chapters 191 and 192). When malignancy involves the pleural space, the prognosis is poor. However, the finding of a pleural effusion in an individual with underlying malignancy does not necessarily imply that there is a metastatic malignant process involving the pleural space. Benign effusions in patients with underlying malignancy may be due to atelectasis, postobstructive pneumonia, hypoalbuminemia, pulmonary emboli (Chapter 98), lymphatic obstruction, and complications from radiation (Chapter 19) or chemotherapy. For this reason, it is important to obtain a sample of pleural fluid in these individuals. The diagnosis of malignant pleural effusion is established by demonstrating malignant cells in the pleural fluid. Approximately 60% of malignant pleural effusions can be diagnosed with one thoracentesis, and the yield increases to 80% with repeat thoracenteses. If needed, a biopsy of the pleura may be useful in identifying the malignancy. Pleural biopsies are optimally obtained either by medical or surgical thoracoscopy (Chapter 101) rather than in a blind fashion (e.g., using a Cope or Abrams needle).

Systemic Inflammatory Disorders

Effusions may be seen in as many as 15% of patients with rheumatoid arthritis (Chapter 272), with a male preponderance to the development of effusions. Effusions typically appear within 5 years after the onset of disease but occasionally occur before the onset of joint disease. Rheumatoid factor in the pleural fluid is often greater than 1:320, and pleural fluid glucose is low (<60 mg/dL, or the pleural fluid–to–serum glucose ratio is <0.5). Other causes of low pleural fluid glucose include complicated parapneumonic effusions or empyema, malignant effusions, tuberculous pleurisy, lupus pleuritis, and esophageal rupture. Pleural effusions can be seen in 15 to 50% of patients with systemic lupus erythematosus (SLE). Lupus erythematosus cells and low levels of complement (C3 and C4) can be seen in effusions due to SLE. Wegener's granulomatosis, Sjögren's syndrome, and sarcoidosis are less common causes of pleural effusions.

Pancreatitis

Patients with pancreatitis or pancreatic pseudocysts (Chapter 146) may develop exudative pleural effusions that often involve the left hemithorax. A pleural fluid amylase concentration that is greater than the upper limits of normal for serum amylase is consistent with acute or chronic pancreatitis as a cause of the effusion. Amylase also may be seen in the pleural fluid with an esophageal rupture or malignancy. Pancreatic disease is associated with pancreatic isoenzyme amylase, whereas malignancy and esophageal rupture are characterized by a predominance of salivary amylase isoenzymes.

Chylothorax

A chylothorax has a milky-white appearance and is characterized by high levels of triglycerides (>110 mg/dL) and chylomicrons. A chylothorax is caused by leakage of lymph from the thoracic duct into the pleural space, most commonly related to mediastinal malignancy but also occurring after trauma to the thoracic duct. Major complications from a chylothorax are malnutrition and immunologic compromise when fat, protein, and lymphocytes are depleted by repeated thoracentesis or chest tube drainage. Chylous effusions must be distinguished from pseudochylous effusions, which have a white appearance but are devoid of chylomicrons, and are indicative of a chronic long-standing effusion.

Hemothorax

Blood in the thorax is easily recognized during a thoracentesis. A hemothorax has a pleural fluid hematocrit that is at least half that of the circulating hematocrit. By contrast, a bloody pleural effusion will appear red but have a lower hematocrit. A bloody effusion often suggests a malignant process. Other causes include trauma, pulmonary infarction (Chapter 98), tuberculosis (Chapter 332), collagen vascular disease (Chapters 272 and 274), and hematologic disorders. Generally, blood removed from the pleural space does not clot, whereas blood due to the trauma of the thoracentesis itself will clot when collected. Because blood in the pleural space does not clot, it can be removed by lymphatics if the volume is small. Larger hemothoraces may require chest tube drainage.

Asbestos Exposure

Pleural effusion may occur following exposure to asbestos. The effusion is often small, unilateral, and serosanguineous, with fewer than 6000 cells/mL. The effusion tends to resolve within a year, resulting in pleural plaques that may calcify over time. Malignant mesothelioma should be excluded in these individuals.

Other Causes of Pleural Exudates

Meigs' syndrome is the triad of ovarian tumor (Chapter 205), ascites, and pleural effusion. The effusion, which is usually large and on the right side, is formed when fluid moves from the abdomen to the pleural space through diaphragmatic defects. Meigs' syndrome usually occurs in postmenopausal women and resolves following removal of the tumor.

Dressler's syndrome may occur from 3 to 30 days following open heart surgery or myocardial infarction. The patient usually experiences pleuritic pain and has a small to moderate left-sided effusion. Treatment is as for the accompanying pericardial effusion (Chapter 77).

Uremia (Chapter 132), which can cause a polyserositis with effusion, must be distinguished from the transudate that commonly is seen in the nephrotic syndrome (Chapter 123). Subdiaphragmatic processes, such as hepatic or splenic abscesses (Chapter 154), may cause effusions. Trapped lung occurs when a lobe or segment is unable to re-expand owing to a restrictive visceral pleural peel or an endobronchial mass. Increased negative intrapleural pressures associated with trapped lung promote the formation of an effusion. A number of drugs, including amiodarone, bleomycin, dantrolene, hydralazine, isoniazid, methotrexate, methysergide, mitomycin, procainamide, and procarbazine, can cause pleural effusions. Treatment consists of discontinuing the offending agent, although treatment with oral corticosteroids may be needed (Chapter 262).

TREATMENT AND PROGNOSIS Rx

Empyemas and complicated parapneumonic effusions require drainage by tube thoracostomy in concert with appropriate antibiotic therapy. Treatment options for malignant pleural effusion include observation, chemical pleurodesis with talc or tetracycline derivatives, ambulatory drainage catheter, and treatment of underlying malignancy. A complete response occurs in perhaps 50% of patients. A low pleural fluid pH (<7.2) tends to impart a poor response to chemical pleurodesis. Malignant effusions with a tendency to respond to generalized chemotherapy include those related to breast cancer (Chapter 204) and small cell carcinoma of the lung (Chapter 197). Malignant effusions related to lymphomas and obstruction of lymphatic drainage of the pleural space may also respond to treatment of the underlying disease. Treatment of inflammatory effusions centers on the use of anti-inflammatory agents and corticosteroids (Chapters 272 and 274). Treatment of chylous effusions may involve chest tube drainage, although fat malnutrition may ensue. Attempts to decrease chyle formation can be accomplished by intravenous hyperalimentation, decreased oral fat intake, and the intake of medium- and light-chain fatty acids, which are absorbed directly into the portal circulation. Ligation of the thoracic duct should be considered for traumatic chylous effusions.

MESOTHELIOMA

EPIDEMIOLOGY AND PATHOBIOLOGY

Malignant mesotheliomas are neoplasms arising from the serosal membrane of body cavities. Eighty percent of mesotheliomas originate in the pleural space, and most others arise from the peritoneum. Individuals are usually older than 55 years and often have a history of asbestos exposure in the distant past (frequently, 30 to 40 years ago). Smoking is not a risk factor for developing mesothelioma, but smoking in concert with asbestos exposure increases the risk of lung cancer. Approximately 3000 cases of mesothelioma occur in the United States each year. The annual incidence is decreasing in the United States owing to better control of occupational exposure, but it may still be increasing in other countries where there are fewer regulations.

CLINICAL MANIFESTATIONS AND DIAGNOSIS

Patients with mesothelioma often complain of dyspnea, weight loss, and pain. Malignant mesothelioma may present as an extremely large mass or pleural effusion occupying the entire hemithorax at times. Chest CT may demonstrate either localized or circumferential pleural thickening associated with various amounts of calcified pleural plaque (see Fig. 99-4). Thoracoscopy is the most efficient means of obtaining the diagnosis. Elevated levels of hyaluronic acid in the pleural fluid, as well as special stains and electron microscopy of biopsy tissue, may help to make the difficult distinction between metastatic adenocarcinoma and mesothelioma.

A fraction of mesotheliomas are benign. Benign mesotheliomas are usually large and often pedunculated at the time of diagnosis.

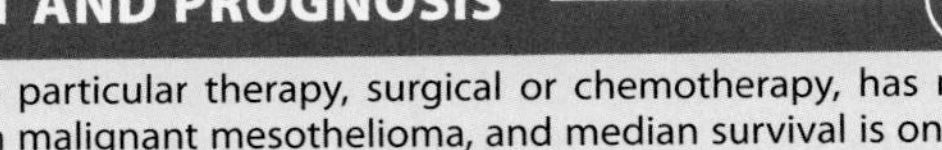

TREATMENT AND PROGNOSIS Rx

Unfortunately, no particular therapy, surgical or chemotherapy, has met with great success in malignant mesothelioma, and median survival is only 8 to 12 months after diagnosis. Pleurodesis with talc or pleurectomy is usually performed for palliation and control of symptoms related to any pleural effusion. In highly selected patients with localized disease and no comorbid illnesses, surgical resection or radical extrapleural pneumonectomy may be attempted. Radiation therapy can provide symptom palliation and has been used following attempts at curative surgery. Treatment of benign mesothelioma involves surgical resection.

PNEUMOTHORAX

Pneumothorax refers to the accumulation of air in the pleural space. Normally, the pressure within the pleural space is slightly subatmospheric. However, when more than a very small amount of air accumulates within the pleural space, pressure within it becomes positive, and there is compression of underlying lung.

EPIDEMIOLOGY AND PATHOBIOLOGY

Pneumothorax is often associated with blunt or penetrating trauma. With penetrating trauma, air may leak into the pleural space through the injured chest wall or into the pleural space from the injured lung. Patients with underlying lung disease undergoing mechanical ventilation may acutely develop a pneumothorax when high local pressures disrupt lung tissue, thereby leading to a leak (Chapter 105).

Pneumothorax also may occur spontaneously or be secondary to underlying lung disease. Typically, spontaneous pneumothorax occurs in tall, young, thin men, presumably as a result of rupture of preexisting apical blebs. Diseases that are associated with pneumothorax include emphysema (Chapter 88), cystic fibrosis (Chapter 89), granulomatous inflammation, necrotizing pneumonia, pulmonary fibrosis (Chapter 92), eosinophilic granulomatous disease, sarcoidosis (Chapter 95), and endometriosis (Chapter 244).

CLINICAL MANIFESTATIONS AND DIAGNOSIS

Symptoms typically include acute shortness of breath and sharp chest pain. Physical examination is characterized by tachycardia, decreased breath sounds, decreased tactile fremitus, a pleural friction rub, subcutaneous emphysema, hyper-resonance to percussion, and a tracheal shift toward the uninvolved hemithorax.

Air within the pleural space will separate the visceral from parietal pleura and appears as an area of lucency on the chest radiograph (Fig. 99-5). With a small pneumothorax, the lucency is best appreciated at the lung apex when the patient is upright (see Fig. 84-11 in Chapter 84). An end-expiratory radiograph is particularly helpful in diagnosing a small pneumothorax. During expiration, the density of the lung will increase because of a reduction in volume, thereby highlighting the difference between lung parenchymal and pleural gas. When a portable chest radiograph is obtained with the patient in the supine position, such as a patient in an intensive care unit, the lucent area may be most noticeable over the lower rib cage (superior sulcus sign).

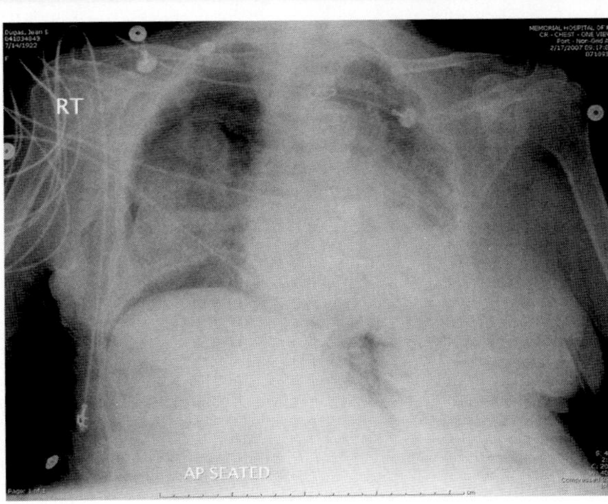

FIGURE 99-5. A portable anteroposterior chest radiograph demonstrating a right-sided pneumothorax. Note that the right lung has collapsed to less than half the size of the right hemithorax. In addition, there is a pneumoperitoneum best seen as a collection of air under the right hemidiaphragm.

A tension pneumothorax is defined as a pneumothorax associated with a mediastinal shift and hemodynamic compromise, usually because high intrathoracic pressures compress the vena cava and atrium. This physiology implies an ongoing leak of air into the pleural space.

TREATMENT AND PROGNOSIS

If the pneumothorax is small and the patient is not in distress, tube thoracostomy is not needed, and observation alone may be sufficient. If a pneumothorax occupies more than 50% of the hemithorax, the patient develops symptoms, or a tension pneumothorax develops, tube thoracostomy and suction followed by water-seal drainage are indicated. If there is a continuing leak despite tube thoracostomy, a bronchopleural fistula may be suspected. In this instance, chemical pleurodesis or surgical correction, usually by video-assisted thoracoscopic surgery, may be necessary (Chapter 101).

MEDIASTINUM

The mediastinum, which is the central part of the thoracic cavity, lies between the right and left lung. It contains the heart and aorta, esophagus, trachea, lymph nodes, thymus, and great vessels. It is bordered by the two pleural cavities laterally, the diaphragm inferiorly, and the thoracic inlet superiorly.

MEDIASTINAL MASSES

PATHOBIOLOGY

For clinical purposes, the mediastinum has been divided into three compartments: anterior, middle, and posterior (E-Fig. 99-2). The anterior compartment contains the thymus, substernal extensions of the thyroid, blood vessels, pericardium, and lymph nodes. The middle compartment contains the heart, great vessels, trachea, main bronchi, lymph nodes, and the phrenic and vagal nerves. The posterior compartment contains the vertebrae, descending aorta, esophagus, thoracic duct, azygous and hemizygous veins, lower portion of the vagus, sympathetic chain, and lymph nodes.

CLINICAL MANIFESTATIONS

Mediastinal masses usually are not accompanied by symptoms, and most masses are incidentally found on either a chest radiograph or a chest CT scan. If present, however, symptoms include chest pain, cough, hoarseness, stridor, dysphasia, and dyspnea. One third of patients with a mediastinal thymoma have symptoms or weakness owing to myasthenia gravis (Chapter 430), and individuals with mediastinal lymphoma (Chapters 191 and 192) may have systemic symptoms such as fever, night sweats, and weight loss. Occasionally, a mass may produce superior vena cava obstruction with resultant facial edema and dilated neck and chest veins (Fig. 99-6).

DIAGNOSIS

Once a mass is identified by chest radiography or chest CT, further evaluation is mandatory. If a benign process is suspected, a follow-up CT may be

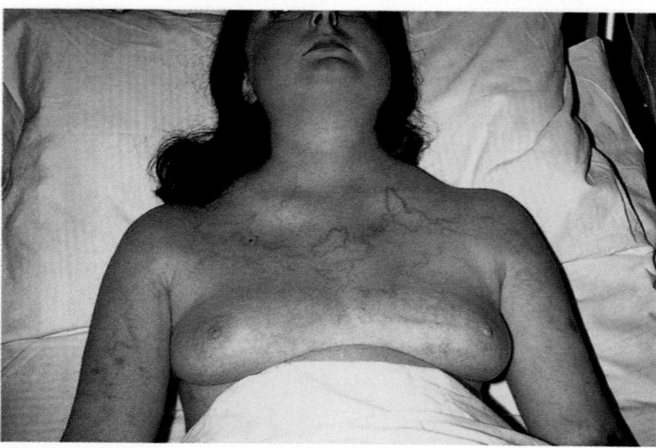

FIGURE 99-6. Superior vena cava obstruction in bronchial carcinoma. Note the swelling of the face and neck and the development of collateral circulation in the veins of the chest wall.

TABLE 99-7 CAUSES OF MEDIASTINAL MASSES

ANTERIOR	MIDDLE	POSTERIOR
Teratoma	Pericardial cyst	Neurogenic tumor
Thymoma	Lymph node hyperplasia	Esophageal tumor
Thyroid tumor	Bronchogenic tumor	Bronchogenic tumor
Goiter	Bronchogenic cyst	Bronchogenic cyst
Aneurysm	Aneurysm	Aneurysm
Lymphoma	Lymphoma	Lymphoma
Parathyroid tumor		Meningocele
Lipoma		Enteric cyst
Morgagni's diaphragm hernia		Esophageal diverticula
		Bochdalek's diaphragm hernia

indicated. If a malignant process is suspected, radiologic evaluation may include angiography, positron emission tomography, or magnetic resonance imaging. Biopsies can be obtained either with mediastinoscopy, mediastinotomy, or ultrasound-guided transbronchial needle aspiration biopsy. Direct sampling by transthoracic CT-guided needle aspiration may be useful in evaluating anterior or posterior mediastinal masses. The evaluation and differential diagnosis of mediastinal masses are guided by the compartment in which they arise (Table 99-7). The *anterior mediastinal compartment* includes lesions such as thymomas, germ cell tumors (teratomas), lymphomas, and intrathoracic thyroid tissue. Thymomas make up about 20% of mediastinal neoplasms in adults, in whom they are the most common anterior mediastinal primary neoplasm. Patients with systemic lymphoma often have involvement of the mediastinum, but only 5 to 10% of patients with lymphoma present with primary mediastinal lesions. Teratomas, which account for 10% of mediastinal tumors, may contain squamous cells, hair follicles, sweat glands, cartilage, and linear calcifications; about one third are malignant. Intrathoracic goiters (Chapter 233) (Fig. 99-7) may compress the trachea and cause stridor, cough, dyspnea, and, occasionally, superior vena cava obstruction. Anterior masses in the right cardiophrenic angle, which are rare and may be associated with pericardial defects or obesity, may be due to herniation of liver or intestinal contents through the foramina of Morgagni.

In the posterior mediastinum, neurogenic tumors are the most common lesions. Many of these tumors are benign and originate in the nerve sheath or sympathetic ganglion cells (ganglioneuroma). Posterior mediastinal masses also include cysts, meningocele, lymphoma (Chapter 191 and 192), aortic aneurysm (Chapter 78), and esophageal disorders (Chapter 140) such as diverticula and neoplasm. Herniation of abdominal contents into the thorax can result in posterior mediastinal masses. Herniation of abdominal contents through the foramina of Bochdalek results in a mass in the posterolateral area of the diaphragm, usually on the left side; it is the most common congenital hernia and may contain spleen or kidney. Herniation of the stomach through the esophageal hiatus (Chapter 140), which is the most common type of diaphragmatic herniation, produces a mass posterior to the heart, often with an air-fluid level.

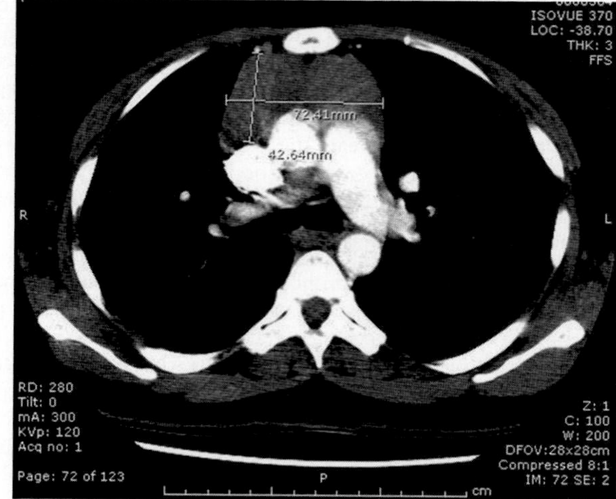

FIGURE 99-7. Chest computed tomography of a patient with an anterior mediastinal mass that proved to be a substernal goiter.

Benign cysts can occur in the anterior, middle, or posterior compartments. Pericardial cysts, which are often located in the cardiophrenic angle, contain clear liquid. Bronchogenic cysts occur in the middle or posterior compartments and are filled with liquid and lined with respiratory epithelium; they often develop around the paratracheal area or carina and do not communicate with the tracheal bronchial tree.

TREATMENT

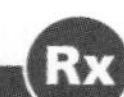

The treatment of a mediastinal mass depends on the underlying pathology. Some lesions, such as thymomas, teratomas, cysts, neurogenic tumors, and hernias, require surgical resection. Others, such as lymphoma, are treated with radiation or chemotherapy. Some can be monitored over time.

MEDIASTINITIS

Acute mediastinitis is most commonly caused by bacterial infection. Mediastinal infections may be iatrogenic after sternotomy or invasive procedures involving the esophagus or tracheobronchial tree. Rupture of the esophagus or trachea from trauma or tissue necrosis can cause mediastinitis. Treatment of acute mediastinitis requires antibiotics, pleural drainage, and evacuation of necrotic tissue. Chronic mediastinitis (fibrosing mediastinitis) is a progressive illness that may be idiopathic or can be caused by granulomatous infection, neoplasm, radiotherapy, or drugs (such as methysergide). Patients with chronic mediastinitis remain asymptomatic until vascular or neurologic structures are affected, and the diagnosis and treatment often require surgical exploration.

PNEUMOMEDIASTINUM

Pneumomediastinum occurs when air infiltrates the mediastinal structures after a rupture of the esophagus, trachea, or lung dissects into the mediastinum. Loss of esophageal or tracheal integrity often results from trauma, whereas leaks from alveoli may result from trauma, occur spontaneously, or be a complication of mechanical ventilation. The diagnosis can be made by seeing thin columns of hyperlucency between mediastinal structures on chest radiography or CT scan. Pneumomediastinum may present as a sore throat, neck pain, or shortness of breath. Often, the mediastinal air dissects into the subcutaneous tissues of the neck and chest wall, where it results in subcutaneous emphysema. A characteristic crepitus is palpable when subcutaneous emphysema is present. Spontaneous pneumomediastinum generally resolves without treatment. When more severe collections of subcutaneous air occur, surgical decompression is often warranted.

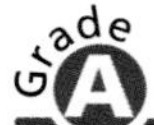

1. Consensus Conference. Clinical indications for noninvasive positive pressure ventilation in chronic respiratory failure due to restrictive lung disease, COPD, and nocturnal hypoventilation—a consensus conference report. *Chest.* 1999;116:521-534.

2. van der Heijde D, Kivitz A, Schiff MH, et al. Efficacy and safety of adalimumab in patients with ankylosing spondylitis: results of a multicenter, randomized, double-blind, placebo-controlled trial. *Arthritis Rheum*. 2006;54:2136-2146.
3. Maskell N, Davies C, Nunn A, et al. U.K. controlled trial of intrapleural streptokinase for pleural infection. *N Engl J Med*. 2005;351:865-874.
4. Muers MF, Stephens RJ, Fisher P, et al. Symptom control with or without chemotherapy in the treatment of patients with malignant pleural mesothelioma (MS01): a multicentre randomized trial. *Lancet*. 2008:371:1685-1694.

SUGGESTED READINGS

Mishra EK, Davies RJ. Advances in the investigation and treatment of pleural effusions. *Expert Rev Respir Med*. 2010;4:123-133. *Review.*
Uzbeck MH, Almeida FA, Sarkiss MG, et al. Management of malignant pleural effusions. *Adv Ther*. 2010;27:334-347. *Review of pharmaceutical and nonpharmaceutical approaches.*
Volpicelli G. Sonographic diagnosis of pneumothorax. *Intensive Care Med*. 2011;37:224-232. *Ultrasound can accurately diagnose or exclude pneumothorax at the bedside in most patients.*

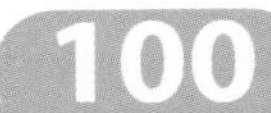

OBSTRUCTIVE SLEEP APNEA

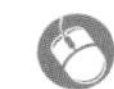

ROBERT C. BASNER

DEFINITION

Obstructive sleep apnea (OSA) is a chronic condition of cyclic obstruction of the upper airway during sleep, combined with associated symptoms or signs of disturbed sleep (Chapter 412), the most common being excessive daytime sleepiness and loud snoring. A frequency of at least five obstructive events per hour of sleep is a minimal criterion for diagnosing OSA in adults, although a higher frequency of obstructive events is more consistently correlated with an increased risk of cardiovascular and neurocognitive disorders.

EPIDEMIOLOGY

OSA is underrecognized by clinicians and underreported by patients. It is estimated that most adults with moderate to severe OSA remain undiagnosed. In adults, OSA is characteristically found in overweight persons, although other anatomic (primarily upper airway and craniofacial) and ventilatory abnormalities may also predispose to development of the syndrome. The presence of at least five obstructive events per hour of sleep has been found in 9 to 28% of persons without specific risk factors for, or symptoms of, OSA. Its overall prevalence appears to be much greater in men than in women, but postmenopausal and obese women are at increased risk. Populations with a particularly high prevalence of OSA include those older than 60 years; patients with systemic hypertension, particularly those with poorly controlled hypertension (Chapter 67); patients who have had strokes (Chapter 414); patients with heart failure (Chapter 58); and patients with medically refractory epilepsy (Chapter 410). African Americans, particularly those younger than 25 and older than 65 years; adult Hispanics; and Asians have a higher incidence and/or greater severity of OSA than whites. There is a strong familial disposition to OSA, such that the presence of OSA in a given patient more than doubles the chance of family members having the disorder when compared with controls. Mean annual medical costs for patients with untreated OSA are almost double those of otherwise normal people, and the costs increase in proportion to the severity of the OSA.

PATHOBIOLOGY

Genetics

Most identified candidate genes linked to OSA share linkages to body mass index (BMI). Similarly, most polymorphic DNA sequences related to expression of OSA appear to be linked to characteristics that predispose to the disorder, including obesity, serotonin transport, and craniofacial structure, or to correlates of the disorder, such as elevated blood pressure. Thus, no specific genes or genetic loci for OSA have been identified to date.

Pathogenesis

OSA involves complete or partial closure of the collapsible segments of the pharynx, including the velopharynx, oropharynx, and hypopharynx. *Obstructive apnea* is defined by absent airflow for at least 10 seconds associated with continued ventilatory effort. Partial obstruction is referred to as *hypopnea* and is recognized functionally by a discrete decrease in rather than cessation of airflow for at least 10 seconds, associated with either a pathologic decrease in the oxygen saturation of hemoglobin (Sao_2) or an abrupt arousal from sleep, typically with progressive ventilatory effort and/or crescendo snoring. Respiratory effort–related arousal occurs when such limitations of airflow and decrease in Sao_2 are not severe enough to cause hypopnea but the progressive ventilatory effort is nevertheless associated with abrupt arousal from sleep.

Both excess weight and increasing weight are closely linked to the development of OSA and the worsening of existing OSA in adults. Conversely, weight loss, both surgical and nonsurgical, has been associated with improvement in OSA (see Treatment). Anatomic and physiologic explanations of how excess weight contributes to OSA include restriction of chest wall movement, with resultant mechanical and reflex upper airway narrowing; increased compliance and narrowing of the upper airway; ventilatory instability; and impaired ability to compensate for increased upper airway resistance at sleep onset.

The final common pathway in each obstructive event is attainment of a critical pharyngeal closing pressure. Once collapsed, the pharynx is more difficult to expand during the next inspiratory effort, resulting in the characteristic generation of progressively more forceful inspiratory efforts against the obstructed upper airway and increasingly negative intrathoracic pressure excursions. The subsequent arousal is usually associated with reopening of the airway. After several hyperpneic breaths, re-transition into sleep generally occurs. The cycling of blood gases and the recurrent awake-to-asleep transitions interfere with the respiratory controllers' need to find a set point during sleep. Hypopnea or outright apnea followed by hyperpnea is the hallmark of OSA.

The pathogenic importance of respiratory periodicity in OSA varies by sleep stage (Chapter 412). The transition into "light" stages of sleep, termed *stages N1* and *N2 non–rapid eye movement* (NREM) *sleep*, is characterized by a tendency for arousal and sleep-wake cycling. These stages are most likely to demonstrate the periodic obstructive events characteristic of OSA. In contrast, "deep" NREM sleep, termed *stage N3* or *slow-wave sleep*, is characteristically a time of relatively regular central nervous system output, with a decreased tendency for arousal, a regularization of breathing, and a relative paucity of obstructive events, even with generally increased upper airway resistance when compared with N1 and N2 sleep. During rapid eye movement (REM) sleep, descending neural inhibition of accessory respiratory muscles may lead to severe alveolar hypoventilation. Severe hypoxemia, caused by a combination of obstructive events and ventilation-perfusion mismatch, is characteristic of REM sleep in patients with OSA.

Pathophysiology

With each obstructive event, the combination of progressive asphyxia, increasingly negative intrathoracic pressure, and sudden autonomic and behavioral arousal leads to acute cardiac and cerebrovascular perturbations, including increased afterload of both the left and right ventricles, decreased left ventricular compliance, increased pulmonary artery pressure, decreased coronary artery blood flow, and increased myocardial oxygen demand (Chapter 52). The abrupt arousal at the termination of the majority of obstructive events is associated with sympathetic discharge, leading to peripheral vasoconstriction and an abrupt increase in the heart rate and in systolic and diastolic blood pressure, even as cardiac output continues to fall when ventilation resumes with the airway reopened. Accordingly, systemic blood pressure characteristically fluctuates; it is relatively low during apnea and acutely elevated at termination of the obstructive event (Chapter 67). Electrocardiographic abnormalities include sinus bradycardia during obstructive events and acceleration at arousal; in REM sleep, which is a time of increased vagal tone, sinoatrial and atrioventricular block may be seen. Ventricular and supraventricular ectopy and atrial fibrillation occur with OSA. At the termination of obstructive apnea, cerebral blood flow and oxygenation are decreased. The recurrent abrupt, transient arousal from sleep at the termination of each obstructive event is associated with fragmented sleep and a decreased ability to consolidate restorative sleep.

CLINICAL MANIFESTATIONS

Symptoms and Signs

The cardinal manifestations of OSA include loud, chronic snoring; excessive daytime somnolence; and apneas witnessed by third parties. Snoring in OSA reflects vibratory noise from partially occluded pharyngeal soft tissue, usually

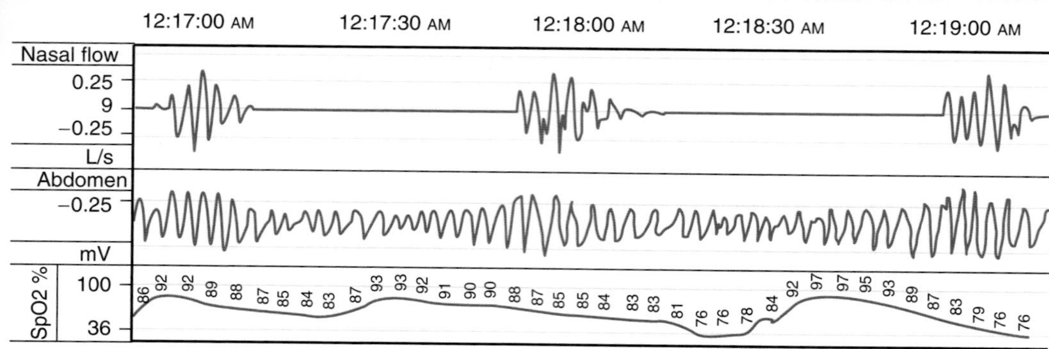

FIGURE 100-1. Polysomnographic tracing of a patient with obstructive sleep apnea during 2 minutes of non–rapid eye movement sleep. Displayed are airflow in the upper airway ("nasal flow"), recorded with a nasal pressure transducer; respiratory effort ("abdomen"), recorded by inductance plethysmography; and oxygen saturation of hemoglobin (Spo_2), recorded with pulse oximetry.

with the mouth open, and it typically occurs in a crescendo pattern, with a burst of louder noise at resolution of the event. Loud snoring without OSA may progress to OSA, particularly if the patient gains weight.

In the hospital setting, OSA may be detected because of apnea or refractory decreases in Sao_2 during surgical or endoscopic procedures that require sedation or anesthesia. In other cases, the diagnosis may be suspected when hospital staff note nocturnal heart block or dysrhythmias during sleep.

Excessive Daytime Somnolence

Patients with excessive daytime somnolence (Chapter 412) fall asleep unexpectedly; this is typically microsleep rather than sustained sleep episodes. Excessive daytime somnolence may be quantified by laboratory tests that monitor the propensity to fall asleep during the day or by questionnaires or subjective scales that assess sleepiness or decrements in quality of life. Resolution of OSA does not necessarily resolve excessive daytime somnolence, suggesting the possibility of sustained neurologic perturbation from chronic intermittent hypoxemia. However, many patients with significant OSA do not complain of excessive daytime somnolence, nor are patients typically aware of their degree of sleep fragmentation. Mood disorders, including depression and irritability, as well as perturbations in visual memory and working memory appear to be related to the severity of sleep fragmentation and hypoxemia.

Obstructed Breathing

The bed partners of OSA patients often describe breathing cessation rather than obstructed breathing; close questioning usually elicits the obstructive nature of the breathing. Patients may be aware of their own snoring or complain of choking or dyspnea, particularly in relation to an inability to sleep supine. Morning dry mouth is a common symptom, as is morning headache.

Insomnia and Parasomnia

Insomnia, which is the subjective complaint of difficulty falling asleep or staying asleep (Chapter 412), is associated with the consistent sleep interruption characteristic of OSA. Transient arousals during N3 sleep may result in confusional parasomnias, such as sleep walking and sleep talking. Arousals and increased work of breathing may result in restless sleep and night sweats. Nocturia, possibly mediated via atrial natriuretic receptors, may resolve with treatment of OSA.

Upper Airway Abnormalities

Nasal congestion, rhinitis, chronic sinusitis, and nasopharyngeal anatomic abnormalities are often associated with OSA, as are craniofacial abnormalities such as micrognathia and retrognathia. Large tonsils, redundant soft palate tissue, and a large tongue may all be associated with a "crowded" oropharynx, but the precise role of these upper airway abnormalities in the pathogenesis of adult OSA is unclear.

DIAGNOSIS

The spectrum of sleep-related breathing disorders other than OSA includes hypoventilation and gas exchange disorders that may worsen with sleep, including nocturnal asthma (Chapter 87), chronic obstructive pulmonary disease (Chapter 88), neuromuscular and chest wall disorders (Chapter 99), and obesity-hypoventilation syndrome (Chapter 227), as well as other disorders in which central apnea (Chapter 412) is prominent, such as idiopathic central apnea, Cheyne-Stokes breathing, and central alveolar hypoventilation (Chapter 86). Patients with OSA alone characteristically do not hypoventilate while awake, unlike patients with other disorders of hypoventilation. Disorders associated with hypersomnia, such as narcolepsy, insufficient sleep, poor sleep hygiene, periodic limb movement disorder, and circadian rhythm disorders such as shift work sleep disorder, must also be considered in patients with suspected OSA (Chapter 412).

Polysomnography

The definitive diagnostic study is polysomnography (Fig. 100-1), which generally involves all-night monitoring in a sleep laboratory via electroencephalography, electro-oculography (primarily to determine rapid eye movements characteristic of REM sleep), electrocardiography, leg and chin electromyography, and measures of respiratory effort, airflow, Sao_2, and alveolar or arterial carbon dioxide (usually end-tidal or transcutaneous CO_2). Audiovisual recordings can identify crescendo snoring and thoracoabdominal paradoxical breathing efforts to help differentiate obstructive from nonobstructive hypopnea.

The severity of OSA is usually described by the apnea-hypopnea index (AHI), which is the number of obstructive apneas plus hypopneas per hour of sleep (Fig. 100-2). The term *respiratory disturbance index* includes obstructive apneas and hypopneas, as well as obstructive events that do not meet the threshold for hypopnea but nevertheless result in a discrete arousal that appears to be associated with abnormal indices of oxygen desaturation. Oxygen desaturation more directly reflects the chronic intermittent hypoxia that has been increasingly linked to adverse cardiovascular effects and outcomes.

It is possible to diagnose OSA by means of unattended home studies that include cardiorespiratory monitoring and/or use of an autotitrating positive airway pressure (PAP) machine, which continuously self-adjusts the level of positive pressure delivered to the airway on a breath-to-breath basis in response to upper airway impedance changes. Such autotitration allows the immediate diagnosis and treatment of a patient suspected of having severe OSA.

TREATMENT

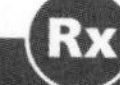

The goal of treatment is to decrease sleep fragmentation and repetitive asphyxia, the resultant cardiovascular and cerebrovascular stress, and the increased work of breathing associated with OSA.

Mechanical Therapy

Positive Airway Pressure

PAP, which is the current first-line therapy for OSA, consistently lowers the AHI, decreases oxygen desaturation, decreases diurnal and nocturnal blood pressure, and improves sleep efficiency, daytime sleepiness, and quality of life at a reasonable cost compared with oral appliances or no treatment,[1] especially in patients with an AHI greater than 30/hour. For patients with less severe OSA, continuous positive airway pressure (CPAP) is generally recommended in those with prominent oxygen desaturation, daytime sleepiness, or concurrent respiratory, cardiovascular, or cerebrovascular disease. CPAP improves cognitive function, improves left ventricular function in patients with heart failure and decreases the risk of motor vehicle accidents.

The major equipment required to administer PAP includes an interface with appropriate headgear, anchoring straps, and hosing and a compact airflow generator (Fig. 100-3). With CPAP, the fixed level of positive pressure delivered to the upper airway acts as a physiologic splint throughout the respiratory cycle, allowing the patient to achieve normal ventilation as well as more continuous and deeper sleep. CPAP does not supply ventilation above this

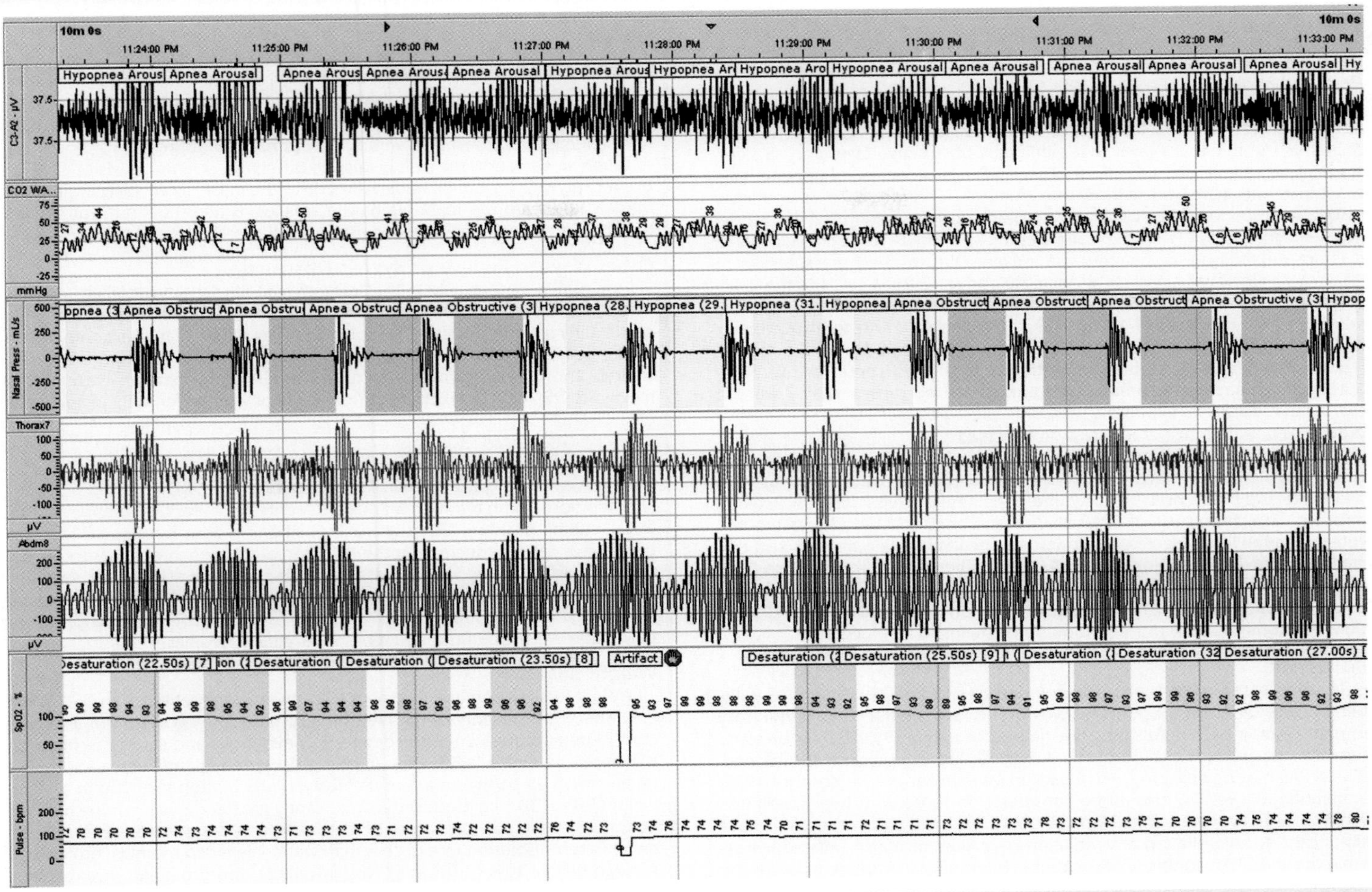

FIGURE 100-2. Continuous 10-minute polysomnographic tracing in a patient with severe obstructive sleep apnea. The 14 repetitive obstructive apneas constitute an apnea-hypopnea index of 84/hour. Each obstructive event is associated with a cyclic waxing-waning respiratory effort (seen in the thoracic and abdominal effort tracings), absent airflow (in the nasal pressure transducer), electroencephalographic arousal (C3-A2, top tracing), oxygen desaturation, and increased end-tidal P_{CO_2}.

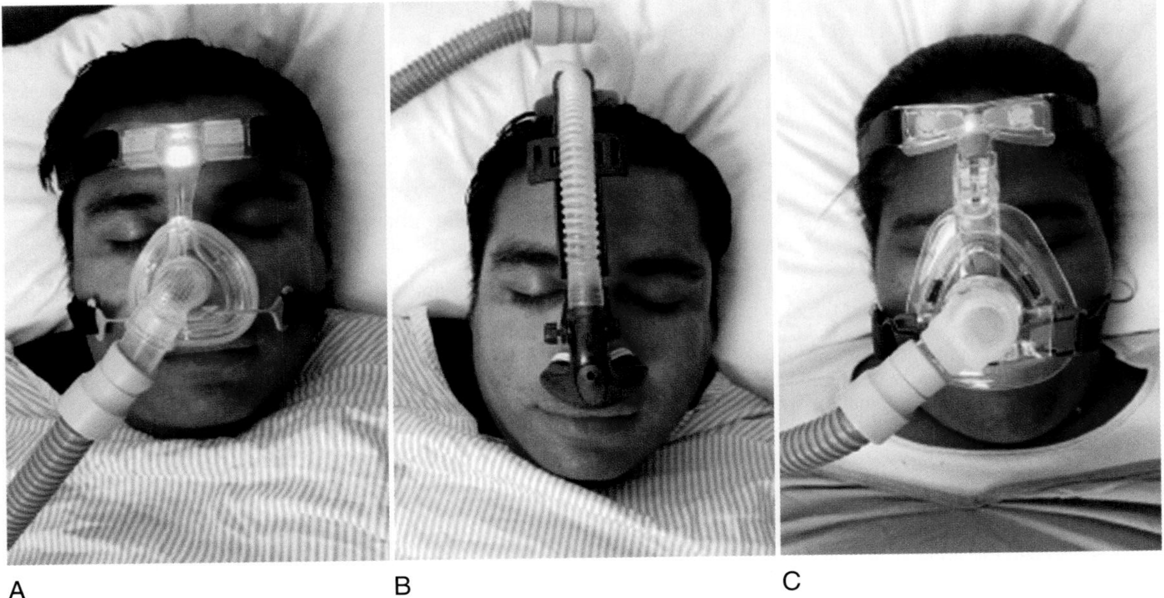

FIGURE 100-3. Positive airway pressure–patient interfaces. A, Subject wearing a nasal mask and headgear with positive airway pressure being delivered. Positive pressure is delivered only to the nasal airway; opening of the mouth may cause air to leak and decrease the efficacy of the positive-pressure regimen. **B,** Subject wearing nasal pillows. Positive pressure is delivered directly into the nares rather than covering the nose or mouth; only minimal headgear is necessary to anchor the interface in place. **C,** Subject wearing a full face mask. Positive pressure is delivered to both the nose and the mouth based on the subject's own breath-to-breath partitioning of nasal and oral airflow.

splinting; the positive end-expiratory pressure may, however, result in improved oxygenation.

Prescribing PAP

PAP is typically prescribed after therapeutic titration in the sleep laboratory, beginning with CPAP of 2 to 4 cm H_2O and increasing by 1- to 2-cm H_2O increments to the minimum level that eliminates obstructive events in all sleep stages. Such a level should reduce other evidence of increased upper airway resistance and increased work of breathing (e.g., snoring, use of accessory inspiratory muscles, thoracoabdominal paradoxical respiration), while improving sleep. Although CPAP is typically prescribed in the 8- to 12-cm H_2O range, it is not uncommon for patients with severe OSA to need pressures up to 20 cm H_2O. However, as pressures increase above 12 to 14 cm H_2O, the likelihood of air leak and discomfort rises. When laboratory titration is not available, starting CPAP at a level of 10 cm H_2O is reasonable. Short-term outcomes, including AHI, symptomatic sleepiness, and quality of life, are similar, regardless of whether CPAP is guided by titration at a sleep center or use of an autotitrating machine at home to determine a fixed pressure.[2,3] Adding a feature that decreases expiratory pressure ("pressure relief") does not improve outcomes or adherence or reduce side effects.[4]

The first night of CPAP is generally associated with a "rebound" of slow-wave NREM sleep and REM sleep, along with amelioration of acute fluctuations in heart rate and blood pressure. Daytime sleepiness and vigilance consistently improve with chronic use of CPAP; diurnal and nocturnal blood pressure and catecholamine levels decrease, and left ventricular ejection fraction and diastolic function improve. However, OSA returns when CPAP is removed, so CPAP must be used nightly throughout sleep. The term *complex sleep apnea* refers to the commonly noted emergence of central apneas during initial CPAP titration; the significance of this phenomenon remains to be elucidated.

Bilevel PAP

In some cases, a more ventilatory mode of pressure delivery—generally, bilevel PAP, wherein inspiratory pressure is set higher than expiratory pressure—may be helpful after the degree of expiratory positive pressure necessary to prevent closure of the airway during expiration is established. Bilevel PAP may be delivered with a backup rate, similar to assist/control mode ventilation. Bilevel PAP should be considered in those with hypoventilation syndromes that overlap OSA, such as obese patients who continue to have significant hypoventilation or ventilation-perfusion mismatch–related hypoxemia despite CPAP. For most OSA patients beginning treatment, however, no high-quality data show improved outcomes or cost-effectiveness of bilevel PAP compared with CPAP, even when bilevel PAP is used as secondary therapy when CPAP is unsuccessful; numerous randomized controlled trials have demonstrated similar adherence with CPAP and bilevel PAP.[5]

Autotitrating PAP

Both CPAP and bilevel PAP can be delivered so that the pressure automatically adjusts to the patient's breathing, based on either breath-to-breath detection of changes in airway resistance or the pattern of breathing. However, autotitrating PAP does not improve adherence or outcomes compared with fixed-pressure CPAP.[5]

PAP-Patient Interface

The choice of interface is important for achieving optimal efficacy and adherence. Aside from many different shapes, sizes, and consistencies of nasal masks (Fig. 100-3A), flexible nasal "pillows" or "prongs" (Fig. 100-3B) can fit directly into the nares, avoiding the discomfort of a mask over the nose and pain and pressure at the bridge of the nose and over the upper teeth. Although nasal PAP is most commonly used, nasal delivery is often ineffective because of nasal congestion, nasopharyngeal anatomic abnormalities, or inability to keep the mouth closed, allowing air to leak from the mouth so that ineffective pressure is delivered to the collapsible airway. Soft "hybrid" interfaces, which have a mouthpiece and nasal prongs to permit both mouth and nose breathing, are often used in such settings. Full face masks (Fig. 100-3C) may also improve CPAP efficacy in such situations, but gastrointestinal bloating secondary to air swallowing is a common side effect, and the risks of vomiting and aspiration are a concern. Regardless of the interface used, the patient must be vigilant to maintain the interface throughout sleep, particularly after changes in position. Cold or heated humidification may be added directly to the circuit to improve comfort and adherence, but contamination of the humidifier with pathogenic organisms must be avoided.

Adherence and Outcome

Adherence to PAP is generally similar to that for treatments of other chronic medical disorders, although most studies suggest that CPAP is not used optimally for maximizing restorative sleep. Adherence may be improved by systematic cognitive behavioral and educational strategies, as well as strategies that address the specific issues of individual patients.[6] Treatment with PAP should be objectively monitored by tracking the amount of time that physiologically successful PAP levels are delivered.

Oxygen

Although supplemental oxygen alone during sleep may ameliorate hypoxemia and improve sleep quality in OSA, such treatment alone may lengthen apneas, cause paradoxical worsening of Sao_2, and fail to improve sleep fragmentation. Therefore, oxygen alone should not be used as first-line treatment for suspected or proven OSA without nocturnal monitoring.

When sleep Sao_2 remains low despite otherwise optimal levels of CPAP or bilevel PAP, oxygen can be added directly to the mask, to an adapter near the mask, or beneath the mask via nasal cannulae. Higher flow rates of oxygen may be necessary as PAP levels increase, particularly if bilevel PAP is used.

Other Ways to Relieve or Bypass Obstruction

Oral appliances, usually in the form of mandibular advancement devices fitted by an expert, improve symptoms in patients with mild to moderate OSA, particularly with predominantly supine OSA. However, such devices are generally less effective than CPAP in improving AHI and oxygen desaturation during sleep,[7] and they are currently recommended only for patients with mild or moderate OSA who do not benefit from CPAP or who prefer such an appliance over CPAP.

General Measures

Sleep Positioning and Nasal Treatments

Sleep positioning may benefit many patients who have OSA predominantly in the supine position, although such positioning does not appear to be as effective as CPAP in decreasing the AHI.[8] Treatment of chronic nasal congestion and inflammation with nasal steroids, saline washes, and systemic antihistamine-decongestant regimens may ameliorate OSA in many cases. Otolaryngologic consultation can be useful to identify treatable nasopharyngeal disorders, including the rare nasopharyngeal neoplasm.

Weight Loss

Weight loss is a primary treatment in an overweight patient with OSA. It not only affects the severity of the breathing disorder during sleep but also may contribute to regression of the deleterious metabolic and cardiovascular perturbations associated with OSA. In obese diabetic patients with a mean BMI greater than 35 kg/m^2, an intensive lifestyle intervention resulting in a mean weight loss of 10.8 kg produced a significantly greater decrease in the number of apneic-hypopneic events per hour, less oxygen desaturation during sleep, and a better resolution rate of OSA than was achieved in a control group with a mean weight loss of 0.6 kg.[9] Non–morbidly obese patients who achieve nonsurgical weight loss also have significantly greater improvements in OSA than do controls without such weight loss. In severely obese patients with marked OSA, weight loss achieved with bariatric surgery significantly ameliorates but usually does not resolve OSA.[10]

Treatment of Other Underlying Conditions

It is important to treat underlying conditions such as diabetes (Chapter 237) and heart failure (Chapter 59) in patients with OSA, but such treatment does not substitute for treating the OSA itself. For example, in patients with OSA and heart failure, cardiac atrial overdrive pacing provides small improvements in the AHI and sleep-related oxygen desaturation, but it is not as effective as CPAP.

Surgery

Tracheostomy

Tracheostomy, which bypasses the site of upper airway obstruction, decreases morbidity and mortality and improves blood gas abnormalities in OSA. However, tracheostomy makes speech difficult and is reserved for only the most severe cases and for patients with concomitant hypoventilation syndromes that do not respond to noninvasive forms of PAP.

Uvulopalatopharyngoplasty

Procedures to reduce uvular or palatal tissue, which were once widely recommended, have not shown a consistent benefit in high-quality studies.[11] As a result, surgical uvulopalatopharyngoplasty, radio frequency volumetric tissue reduction of the palate or tongue (or both), and laser-assisted uvuloplasty are not recommended as first-line therapy to treat symptomatic OSA patients.

Medical Therapy

At this time, there is no acceptably efficacious pharmacologic therapy for OSA. Respiratory stimulants, including medroxyprogesterone and acetazolamide, have not proved effective in patients with normal $Paco_2$ levels. Selective serotonin re-uptake inhibitors, including fluoxetine and paroxetine, have been associated with a decreased apnea index during NREM but not REM sleep in a small number of patients. Tricyclic antidepressants have shown some utility in predominantly REM sleep–associated OSA by decreasing REM volume, although side effects have hindered the use of such agents. Hormone replacement therapy may ameliorate the breathing disorder in postmenopausal women.

PROGNOSIS

Population studies show an increased risk of all-cause and cerebrovascular and coronary mortality in patients with untreated severe OSA and in patients with AHIs of 30 or more per hour, independent of other major risk factors. When patients with severe OSA are prescribed CPAP, 5-year survival rates are significantly higher in those with good CPAP adherence (>6 hours/day) than in those with poor adherence. Like other patients with sleep disorders (Chapter 412), patients with OSA are at greater risk for morbidity and mortality from motor vehicle accidents compared with drivers without OSA.

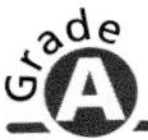

1. Giles T, Lasserson TJ, Smith BH, et al. Continuous positive airways pressure for obstructive sleep apnoea in adults. *Cochrane Database Syst Rev.* 2006.1.CD001106.
2. Mulgrew AT, Fox N, Ayas NT, et al. Diagnosis and initial management of obstructive sleep apnea without polysomnography: a randomized validation study. *Ann Intern Med.* 2007;146:157-166.
3. Berry RB, Hill G, Thompson L, et al. Portable monitoring and autotitration versus polysomnography for the diagnosis and treatment of sleep apnea. *Sleep.* 2008;31:1423-1431.
4. Nilius G, Happel A, Domanski U, et al. Pressure-relief continuous positive airway pressure vs constant continuous positive airway pressure: a comparison of efficacy and compliance. *Chest.* 2006;130:1018-1024.
5. Smith I, Lasserson TJ. Pressure modification for improving usage of continuous positive airway pressure machines in adults with obstructive sleep apnoea. *Cochrane Database Syst Rev.* 2009.4.CD003531.
6. Smith I, Nadig V, Lasserson TJ. Educational, supportive and behavioural interventions to improve usage of continuous positive airway pressure machines for adults with obstructive sleep apnoea. *Cochrane Database Syst Rev.* 2009.4.CD007736.
7. Lim J, Lasserson TJ, Fleetham J, et al. Oral appliances for obstructive sleep apnoea. *Cochrane Database Syst Rev.* 2006.1.CD004435.
8. Skinner MA, Kingshott RN, Filsell S. Efficacy of the "tennis ball technique" versus nCPAP in the management of position-dependent obstructive sleep apnoea syndrome. *Respirology.* 2008;5:708-715.
9. Foster GD, Borradaile KE, Sanders MH, et al. A randomized study on the effect of weight loss on obstructive sleep apnea among obese patients with type 2 diabetes. The Sleep Ahead Study. *Arch Intern Med.* 2009;169:1619-1626.
10. Greenburg DL, Lettieri CJ, Eliasson AH. Effects of surgical weight loss on measures of obstructive sleep apnea: a meta-analysis. *Am J Med.* 2009;122:535-542.
11. Aurora RN, Casey KR, Kristo D, et al. Practice parameters for the surgical modifications of the upper airway for obstructive sleep apnea in adults. *Sleep.* 2010;33:1408-1413.

SUGGESTED READINGS

Kasai T, Bradley TD. Obstructive sleep apnea and heart failure: pathophysiologic and therapeutic implications. *J Am Coll Cardiol.* 2011;57:119-127. *Review.*

Pack AI, Pien GW. Update on sleep and its disorders. *Annu Rev Med.* 2011;62:447-460. *Review focusing on obstructive sleep apnea.*

101 INTERVENTIONAL AND SURGICAL APPROACHES TO LUNG DISEASE

ARMIN ERNST AND MALCOLM M. DECAMP

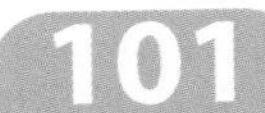
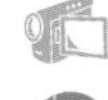
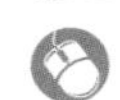

Currently available interventional and surgical procedures can provide diagnostic and staging information and sometimes definitively treat or effectively palliate patients with benign, infectious, and malignant lung diseases.

BRONCHOSCOPY

Bronchoscopy affords a direct view of the major airways and access to lung parenchyma for blind biopsy. Endobronchial therapy has conventionally been used for the management of central airway obstruction, but newer technologic developments permit minimally invasive diagnosis and staging of lung cancer with endobronchial ultrasound (US) and endoscopic approaches to diseases such as emphysema.

Bronchoscopy for Central Airway Obstruction

Airway disorders that cause central airway obstruction of the trachea, mainstem bronchi, and bronchus intermedius are a common indication for therapeutic bronchoscopy. The airway obstruction may be caused by malignant

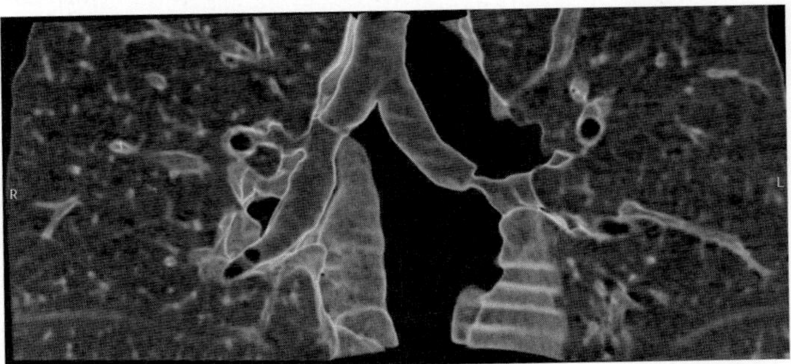

FIGURE 101-1. Three-dimensional reconstruction of a computed tomographic scan in a 20-year-old woman status after bilateral lung transplantation. The image clearly shows the high-grade stenosis at the level of the left mainstem anastomosis. The right-sided airways are normal.

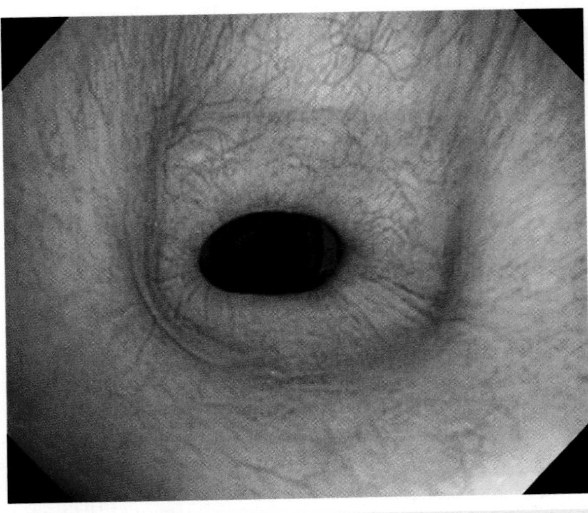

FIGURE 101-2. Bronchoscopic view of the proximal trachea in a 54-year-old man with shortness of breath and stridor. Significant circumferential narrowing is noted in the subglottic space, consistent with gastric reflux–induced subglottic stenosis.

conditions (e.g., bronchogenic carcinoma or metastatic malignancy to the bronchi) and benign disorders (e.g., sarcoidosis, amyloidosis, goiters). The reduction in the airway lumen may remain asymptomatic until a critical airway diameter (5 to 8 mm) is reached or a new event (infection, bleeding, or mucous plugging) exacerbates the underlying narrowing.

CLINICAL MANIFESTATIONS AND DIAGNOSIS

A high index of suspicion is mandatory because patients with central airway obstruction often do not have specific symptoms. Stridor is usually a sign of impending respiratory failure that requires urgent intervention.

Hemoptysis may be prominent in patients with malignancies. Some patients may present with a postobstructive pneumonia that responds poorly to antibiotic treatment or recurs. Most patients, however, present with nonspecific symptoms, including dyspnea and cough.

Patients who have risk factors for chronic airway obstruction and present with symptoms consistent with obstruction unresponsive to conventional therapy should undergo airway imaging by computed tomography (CT) scanning (Fig. 101-1) and flexible bronchoscopy (Fig. 101-2). Because loss of airway patency can be lethal, evaluation of these patients must be performed by individuals experienced in the management of critical airway disorders.

TREATMENT

Removal of obstructing tissue is a key objective in the relief of airway obstruction. Mechanical débridement, which is accomplished by "coring-out" the tissue with the barrel of the rigid bronchoscope, is the safest approach to patients with chronic airway obstruction. Although laser and electrocautery can be used to vaporize tumor tissue, the preferred technique is to use electrocautery or argon plasma coagulation before mechanical débridement, in a fashion known as *heat-assisted mechanical debulking.*

Airway stenting is the primary treatment for airway obstruction caused by extrinsic compression, as may be seen by patients with large malignant mediastinal masses. However, airway stenting is associated with long-term complications, including stent and airway fractures, secondary airway occlusion, infection, and migration, so it should be considered primarily as a palliative procedure for malignant diseases.

For malignant disease, local débridement may temporize the clinical situation while extirpative options are considered. If the lesion or patient is deemed inoperable, such procedures, with or without stenting, are usually a complement to definitive radiation therapy. Patients with endoscopically relieved malignant airway obstruction usually experience a significant improvement in their of quality of life and are more likely to succumb to distant disease than to a local recurrence.

Endobronchial Ultrasound

Bronchoscopy is a standard component of the evaluation and staging of patients with thoracic tumors. Endobronchial US incorporated into the tip of special endoscopes provides ultrasonographic visualization of peri-airway abnormalities and allows transbronchial needle biopsies to be targeted at abnormal areas instead of being taken blindly. Endobronchial ultrasound with biopsy of enlarged nodes has largely obviated the need for mediastinoscopy for the biopsy of mediastinal lymph nodes for staging or diagnosis of cancer and can be useful for the diagnosis of sarcoidosis (Chapter 95). For example, adding endobronchial ultrasound to surgical staging improves the sensitivity for finding nodal metastases and can reduce the unnecessary thoracotomy rate from 18 to 7%.[1]

Surgical Approaches

Open Approaches

Thoracotomy has been the standard approach to evaluate the contents of the pleural space, lung parenchyma, pulmonary hilum, and ipsilateral mediastinum and diaphragm. Selective lung ventilation, achieved by use of a double-lumen endotracheal tube or mainstem bronchial blocker, allows one lung to be collapsed and visualized. Given the precision and accuracy of contemporary preprocedure CT and magnetic resonance imaging (MRI), many procedures can be performed using smaller targeted incisions, with a muscle-sparing technique that allows specific access to regional pathology. Many lung processes can also be approached through a median sternotomy, which affords access to both lungs, although access to the left lower lobe through this approach can be challenging.

Video-Assisted Thoracoscopic Surgery

Thoracoscopy, or video-assisted thoracoscopic surgery (VATS), requires two or three incisions, termed *ports,* to place instruments in any intercostal space. A common configuration is to place one port for the video thoracoscope and two ports for endoscopic instrumentation. With the VATS approach, recovery is shorter than following an open thoracotomy because little if any muscle is divided and no mechanical rib spreading retractors are used.

The size of the surgical incisions depends on the goals of the procedure and the anatomic findings at the time of exploration. Unexpected pleural symphysis or incomplete lobar fissures may require extension of the incision to facilitate visualization. In patients undergoing anatomic resection, such as segmentectomy or lobectomy, at least one of the port incisions is extended to 4 to 8 cm in length to permit extraction of the resected lung from the hemithorax.

SURGERY FOR BENIGN LUNG DISEASE

A variety of benign lung diseases present as focal parenchymal lesions that require a tissue biopsy for diagnosis. Thoracoscopy has essentially replaced a limited thoracotomy and wedge resection for this purpose. VATS provides a more complete view of the ipsilateral hemithorax, including the visceral, parietal, and mediastinal pleura. In addition, subpleural nodules that are too small to be visualized by preoperative radiography can be identified so that representative biopsy samples can be obtained.

Spontaneous Pneumothorax

Although most spontaneous pneumothoraces (Chapter 99) are uncomplicated, up to 20% of patients with pneumothoraces experience complications such as tension pneumothorax, persistent air leak despite tube drainage, or recurrent pneumothoraces either ipsilaterally or contralaterally. Patients in whom a second pneumothorax develops have a 70 to 80% chance of a third recurrence within 2 years. The current surgical approach to the treatment of recurrent pneumothoraces is VATS resection of the subpleural blebs responsible for the pneumothorax, usually combined with mechanical abrasion of the parietal pleura or chemical pleurodesis with insufflated talc to cause an inflammatory reaction that will allow the lung to adhere to the chest wall.

Giant Bullae

Most patients with chronic obstructive pulmonary disease (COPD) have diffuse parenchymal disease, but a small number of patients with COPD have dominant or giant bullae that may occupy 50% or more of the volume of the hemithorax and that compress relatively preserved lung parenchyma. The indications for bullectomy include progressive symptoms with demonstrated disability, obstructive spirometry (Chapter 85), and a single or dominant bullous lesion with radiographic demonstration of compression of the surrounding preserved lung parenchyma. Either excision or plication can remove the bullous lesion.

Malignant Lung Disease

Solitary Pulmonary Nodules

Most small pulmonary nodules (see Fig. 197-5 in Chapter 197) present in the periphery of the lung beyond the reach of diagnostic bronchoscopy. For such lesions, VATS excisional biopsy of a small pulmonary nodule leads to a definitive diagnosis in almost all cases and is generally preferred over transthoracic needle biopsy. Furthermore, thoracoscopy can allow concurrent nodal staging should a primary malignancy (Chapter 197) be confirmed. In the absence of regional adenopathy, patients with primary malignant lesions can undergo definitive resection at the same time.

Primary Lung Cancer

In patients with node-negative primary lung cancer and adequate pulmonary reserve, lobectomy or pneumonectomy is indicated to obtain optimal survival and to decrease the risk of local recurrence. Lobectomy can be achieved by thoracotomy or VATS with similar outcomes. Although VATS wedge resection of primary lung cancer has not been specifically studied in randomized trials, available evidence suggests that an open wedge resection may not be as good as lobectomy for staging or for tumor-free prognosis.

Metastatic Cancer

The lung is a frequent site of metastatic recurrence. Common histologies include colorectal cancer (Chapter 199), renal cell carcinoma (Chapter 203), sarcoma (Chapter 209), melanoma (Chapter 210), breast cancer (Chapter 204), and head and neck cancer (Chapter 196). VATS is often the diagnostic procedure of choice to detect and locate nodules too small for reliable percutaneous biopsy.

The role of pulmonary metastectomy as therapy for advanced disease remains controversial. Five-year survival rates of 20 to 30% have been reported for selected patients, especially if the disease-free interval from original diagnosis to lung metastasis is greater than 3 years. These cases often require resection of bilateral lung nodules, which in turn mandate either a median sternotomy, clamshell incision, or staged, bilateral VATS.

SURGERY FOR ADVANCED LUNG DISEASES: LUNG VOLUME REDUCTION SURGERY

Emphysema (Chapter 88) is the most common chronic progressive disabling lung disease treated by pulmonologists and thoracic surgeons. In eligible patients (Table 101-1), lung volume reduction surgery confers durable symptomatic, physiologic, and survival benefits compared with medical therapy (Fig. 101-3) for patients who have severe emphysema but who do not have a forced expiratory volume in 1 second (FEV_1) measure of less than 20% of predicted with either a homogeneous distribution of emphysema on CT or a diffusing capacity of less than 20% of predicted.[2] However, subgroup analyses suggest that the benefit is mainly in patients with upper lobe predominant disease.

For eligible patients, most programs require a 6- to 10-week preoperative pulmonary rehabilitation followed by a cardiopulmonary exercise test to assess the risks and benefits of surgery. Patients with upper lobe predominant emphysema and a low preoperative exercise capacity have a nearly 50% lower risk of death after lung volume reduction surgery compared with continued

TABLE 101-1 INCLUSION AND EXCLUSION CRITERIA FOR LUNG VOLUME REDUCTION SURGERY

INCLUSION CRITERIA
Radiographic evidence of emphysema, especially involving upper lobes
Hyperinflation evidenced by TLC > 100% predicted and RV > 150% predicted
FEV_1 > 20 and < 45% predicted (after bronchodilator)
DLCO > 20% predicted
Severe dyspnea
Restricted activities of daily living
Decreased quality of life
Abstinence from tobacco
EXCLUSION CRITERIA
Active smoking
Bronchiectasis
Pulmonary nodule requiring evaluation
Excessive daily sputum production
Previous thoracotomy
Obvious pleural disease
Active or inducible coronary ischemia
Pulmonary hypertension
Depressed LVEF (<45%)
Obesity (BMI > 32)
Unable or unwilling to participate in pulmonary rehabilitation
Systemic steroids, ≥20 mg prednisone/day

BMI = body mass index; DLCO = diffusion capacity for carbon monoxide; FEV_1 = first second forced expiratory volume; LVEF = left ventricular ejection fraction; RV = residual capacity; TLC = total lung capacity.

Adapted from DeCamp MM Jr, McKenna RJ Jr, Deschamps CC, et al. Lung volume reduction surgery: technique, operative mortality and morbidity. *Proc Am Thorac Soc.* 2008;5:442-446; and DeCamp MM Jr, Lipson D, Krasna M, et al. The evaluation and preparation of the patient for lung volume reduction surgery. *Proc Am Thorac Soc.* 2008;5:427-431.

TABLE 101-2 DECISION GUIDE FOR SELECTION OF LUNG VOLUME REDUCTION SURGERY VERSUS TRANSPLANTATION FOR SEVERE CHRONIC OBSTRUCTIVE PULMONARY DISEASE

FACTORS FAVORING LVRS	FACTORS FAVORING TRANSPLANTATION
Age > 65 yr	FEV_1 ≤ 20% predicted
Upper lobe predominant disease	DLCO ≤ 20% predicted
Chronic medical conditions	Homogeneous or lower lobe distribution of disease
Hepatitis B and/or C	TLC < 100% predicted
HIV infection	RV < 150% predicted
Renal insufficiency	$Paco_2$ > 60 mm Hg
Cirrhosis	Pao_2 < 45 mm Hg
Neuropathy	6 MWD < 140 m or
Poorly controlled diabetes	< 3 min unloaded pedaling cycle ergometer
Osteoporosis	Pulmonary hypertension
Severe GERD	Bronchiectasis
Poor esophageal motility	Recurrent pulmonary infections
Malignancy	
Unable to maintain long-term follow-up	
Psychiatric issues limiting compliance	
Insufficient social support	

6 MWD = six-minute walk distance; DLCO = diffusion capacity of carbon monoxide; FEV_1 = first second forced expired volume; GERD = gastroesophageal reflux disease; HIV = human immunodeficiency virus; LVRS = lung volume reduction surgery; RV = residual volume; TLC = total lung capacity.

Adapted from Patel N, DeCamp M, Criner GJ. Lung transplantation and lung volume reduction surgery versus transplantation in chronic obstructive pulmonary disease. *Proc Am Thorac Soc.* 2008;5:447-453.

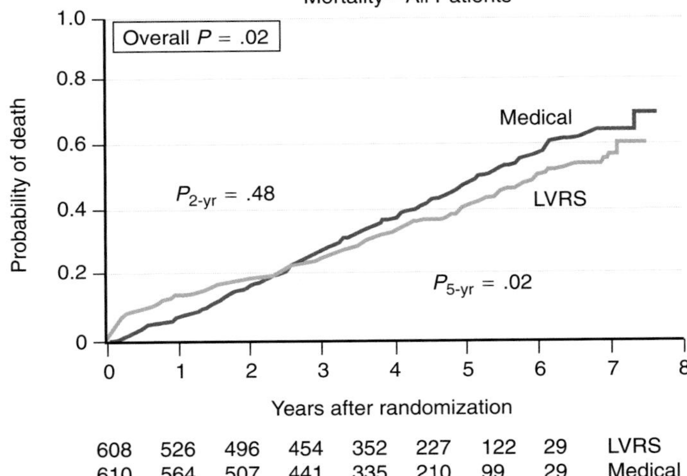

FIGURE 101-3. Long-term mortality of all patients treated with lung volume reduction surgery (LVRS) versus maximal medical therapy in the National Emphysema Treatment Trial. Note the statistically significant (P = .02) reduction in relative risk of death (RR = 0.85) for the surgical cohort. (Adapted from Naunheim KS, Wood DE, Mohsenifar Z, et al, for the National Emphysema Treatment Trial Research Group. Long-term follow-up of patients receiving lung-volume-reduction surgery versus medical therapy for severe emphysema in the National Emphysema Treatment Trial. *Ann Thorac Surg.* 2006;82:431-443.)

medical therapy. High-risk patients with severe airflow obstruction (FEV_1 < 20%) should be assessed for lung transplantation evaluation unless their disease is localized to the upper lobes and their gas exchange as defined by diffusing capacity is preserved (Table 101-2).

In experienced centers, bilateral stapled resection approaches yield nearly twice the physiologic benefit of unilateral lung volume reduction surgery without adversely affecting operative morbidity or mortality. Bilateral lung volume reduction surgery using the VATS approach reduces hospital length of stay and increases the likelihood of living independently 60 days after surgery. 3

ENDOSCOPIC MANAGEMENT OF EMPHYSEMA

Endoscopic approaches to lung volume reduction include airway valves, blockers, stents, sealants, and implants. Unlike lung volume reduction surgery, which causes peridiaphragmatic pleural scarring and can restrict diaphragmatic movement when lower lobe emphysema is treated, endobronchial lung volume reduction does not cause such scarring and may result in better post-operative functional outcomes. Endobronchial lung volume reduction may permit stepwise and gradual therapy that may facilitate weaning of COPD patients from ventilators. Furthermore, some endobronchial lung volume reduction modalities, such as endobronchial valves, are reversible and can be removed if they are not beneficial or if complications arise.

Endobronchial valves are designed to exclude the most affected emphysematous regions from ventilation and reduce dynamic air trapping. If segmental or lobar atelectasis can be induced, a physiologic effect similar to lung volume reduction surgery can be obtained. In a randomized trial, bronchoscopic implantation of endobronchial valves to allow air to escape from but not enter emphysematous lung areas resulted in a 7% relative improvement in FEV_1 but at the expense of more hemoptysis, pneumonia, and exacerbations of COPD. 4 Endobronchial valve therapy for emphysema is safer than lung volume reduction surgery, with a reported mortality rate of approximately 1% and with most patients being discharged within 2 to 4 days. Postobstructive pneumonia has not been a commonly reported complication.

The bronchoscopic creation of extra-anatomic bronchial fenestrations allows trapped air to escape by bypassing obstructed airways, thereby partially deflating emphysematous lung segments through enhanced collateral ventilation.

Biological sealants induce localized irreversible atelectasis by sealing off highly damaged areas of lung. Unlike endobronchial valves or bypass, sealants work at the alveolar level, where air space inflammation and remodeling leads to scarring and contraction of lung parenchyma. Within 6 to 8 weeks, a mature scar and functional lung volume reduction reduce dead space and residual volume to a degree similar to what can be achieved with lung volume reduction surgery.

LUNG TRANSPLANTATION

About 150 worldwide lung transplant centers perform more than 2700 transplantations per year. Lung transplantation is now an accepted therapy for all forms of advanced lung disease.

TABLE 101-3 INDICATIONS AND CONTRAINDICATIONS FOR LUNG TRANSPLANTATION

SINGLE-LUNG TRANSPLANT	PATIENTS (%)	DOUBLE-LUNG TRANSPLANT	PATIENTS (%)
INDICATIONS			
COPD	49	CF, bronchiectasis	31
Pulmonary fibrosis, sarcoid	31	Emphysema	26
α_1-Antitrypsin deficiency	6	α_1-Antitrypsin deficiency	8
PPH, Eisenmenger's	1.2	PPH, Eisenmenger's	6
CF, bronchiectasis	2.4	Pulmonary fibrosis, sarcoid	17
Retransplantation	3	Retransplantation	2
Other*	7	Other*	10

ABSOLUTE CONTRAINDICATIONS

Untreatable advanced extrapulmonary organ dysfunction (e.g., heart, liver, kidney)
- CAD not amenable to PCI or bypass
- Poor LV function (could consider heart-lung transplantation)

Malignancy within 2 years (excludes cutaneous squamous or basal cell carcinoma)
- 5-year disease-free interval preferred

Noncurable extrapulmonary infection
- Infection with human immunodeficiency virus
- Hepatitis B antigen positivity
- Hepatitis C with histologic evidence of active liver disease

Active substance abuse (including cigarettes)
Severe musculoskeletal disease affecting the thorax
Documented noncompliance
Untreatable psychiatric condition which impairs compliance
Absence of consistent and reliable social support

RELATIVE CONTRAINDICATIONS

Physiologic age > 65 years
Poor nutritional status (<70% ideal body weight)
Severe obesity (BMI > 30 kg/m)
Symptomatic osteoporosis
Colonization with highly virulent and/or highly resistant fungi, mycobacteria, or bacteria
Requirement for invasive ventilation and/or circulatory support
Uncontrolled chronic medical conditions (e.g., diabetes, hypertension, GERD)
Severely limited functional status with poor rehabilitation potential
Psychosocial problems likely to affect the outcome adversely
High-dose (>20 mg of prednisone daily) corticosteroid use

*Other includes lymphangioleiomatosis, non-retransplantation-related obliterative bronchiolitis, and miscellaneous indications.
BMI = body mass index; CAD = coronary artery disease; CF = cystic fibrosis; COPD = chronic obstructive pulmonary disease; GERD = gastroesophageal reflux disease; LV = left ventricle; PCI = percutaneous coronary intervention; PPH = primary pulmonary hypertension.
Adapted from Registry of the International Society for Heart and Lung Transplantation. Twenty-second official adult lung and heart-lung transplant report—2009. *J Heart Lung Transplant.* 2009;28:989-1049; and Orens JB, Estenne M, Arcasoy S, et al. International guidelines for the selection of lung transplant candidates: 2006 update. A consensus report from the Pulmonary Scientific Council of the International Society for Heart and Lung Transplantation. *J Heart Lung Transplant.* 2006;25:745-755.

The most common indications for transplantation (Table 101-3) are diseases or conditions that share the following features: they produce extreme disability in affected patients, they are unresponsive to medical therapy, and they are responsible for limited life expectancy in affected patients. With the exception of a small number of cases of sarcoidosis and lymphangioleiomyomatosis, the original lung disease does not usually recur after lung transplantation.

Types of Procedures

Currently, four types of lung transplantation procedures are performed. *Single-lung transplantation,* which is typically performed through a posterolateral thoracotomy incision, requires three anastomoses: the mainstem bronchus, pulmonary artery, and pulmonary veins and left atrium. The contralateral lung is not removed, so single-lung transplantation is not performed in patients with bilaterally infected lungs (e.g., patients with cystic fibrosis or bronchiectasis) (see Table 101-3).

Bilateral lung transplantation is performed in a sequential fashion that is functionally equivalent to two single-lung transplantations completed during a single operation, most commonly through a transverse sternotomy ("clamshell") incision. It requires six anastomoses: both mainstem bronchi, both pulmonary arteries, and both sets of pulmonary veins. It is the procedure of choice for patients with bilaterally infected lungs and is also performed in certain patients with emphysema, primary pulmonary hypertension, and other diseases (see Table 101-3). Bilateral transplantations are preferred for nearly all indications because a double-lung recipient can expect a half-life of 6.6 years compared with 4.6 years for a single-lung recipient.

Heart-lung transplantation is now performed in only about 75 cases per year. It is an en bloc procedure with right atrial, aortic, and distal tracheal anastomoses. It is performed in patients with advanced lung disease and coexistent irreparable cardiac disease, usually associated with fixed pulmonary hypertension, and Eisenmenger's syndrome (Chapter 69).

Living donor lobar transplantation involves the removal of a lower lobe from each of two living donors. One is implanted into each hemithorax of the recipient in a manner similar to bilateral lung transplantation.

Evaluation of Potential Transplant Recipients

The ideal candidate for lung transplantation has lung disease unresponsive to medical therapy but is in otherwise good health. Patients who experience critical illness as a result of lung disease often have poor nutritional status, coexistent major organ dysfunction, refractory infection, or other contraindications to transplantation. The specific evidence-based recommendations for referral for transplant evaluation vary with the underlying disease.

In the United States, the lung allocation system is based on expected disease-specific and patient-specific survival during the waiting period and following engraftment, thereby reflecting net transplant benefit. Early evaluations of the system, which was introduced in 2005, indicate shorter waiting times, an increase in the total number of transplantations performed, a decreased waitlist mortality, and an unchanged overall survival after transplantation.

Post-transplantation Issues

Most of the medical issues that patients and physicians face after lung transplantation are the consequence of the transplantation and post-transplantation medication rather than the underlying disease for which the transplantation was performed. Examples include immunosuppression, infections and their prophylaxis, acute allograft rejection, chronic allograft rejection, and nonpulmonary complications of transplantation.

Immunosuppression

The standard chemotherapeutic regimen for immunosuppression after lung transplantation consists of a calcineurin inhibitor such as cyclosporine or tacrolimus, azathioprine or mycophenolate mofetil, and corticosteroids. Some centers add an antilymphocyte antibody preparation in the first days after transplantation, although this addition has not been demonstrated to improve outcome.

Infections and Prophylaxis after Lung Transplantation

Lung transplant recipients are at high risk for bacterial, viral, fungal, and protozoal infections; infections are the leading causes of death during the early post-transplantation period. In the first 3 months after transplantation, bacterial infections are responsible for most deaths. In approximately one third of patients, pneumonia is diagnosed in the first weeks after transplantation, with gram-negative organisms as the cause in 75% of cases. Colonization and recurrent infections, usually with *Pseudomonas* species, often develop in patients with chronic rejection.

Among potential viral pathogens, *cytomegalovirus* (CMV; Chapter 384) is the most important in lung transplant recipients. Seronegative patients who receive an allograft from a seropositive donor are at particularly high risk for the development of a clinically significant CMV infection. Seronegative patients who have a seronegative donor are at low risk for infection if they are treated with seronegative blood products. Epstein-Barr virus (EBV) has been associated with the development of post-transplantation lymphoproliferative disorder.

Aspergillus species are the most common cause of invasive fungal infection (Chapter 347). Colonized patients and those deemed at risk may receive prophylactic inhaled amphotericin B.

Because of the nature of the immunosuppressive chemotherapeutic regimen used, patients are at high risk for infection by the protozoan *Pneumocystis jirovecii* (Chapter 349). The use of trimethoprim-sulfamethoxazole prophylaxis (typically 1 double-strength tablet three times weekly indefinitely) has virtually eliminated *Pneumocystis* pneumonia.

Acute Rejection

Histologically, the initial manifestation of acute rejection is a lymphocyte-predominant inflammatory response, usually centered around blood vessels, airways, or both. By convention, acute rejection is graded histologically from 0 (normal) to 4 (severe), with subclasses defined by the presence or absence of airway inflammation.

The risk for acute allograft rejection is highest in the early months after transplantation and declines with time. Multiple episodes of acute rejection are the major risk factor for the subsequent development of chronic rejection.

Clinically, patients may have fever, cough, and exertional dyspnea. Evaluation may demonstrate rales or rhonchi on chest examination, a decline in pulmonary function by spirometry, leukocytosis, opacities on chest radiography, and exertional desaturation. The clinical manifestation is often indistinguishable from infectious pneumonia, and the clinical impression is accurate in only 50% of cases.

Treatment of acute rejection most often consists of high-dose corticosteroids (typically, 1 g/day of methylprednisolone administered intravenously for 3 days).

Chronic Rejection

PATHOBIOLOGY

The bronchiolitis obliterans syndrome is thought to be a manifestation of chronic rejection. Risk factors for development of the syndrome include the number of acute rejection episodes and, in some series, previous symptomatic CMV infection. Pathologically, "early" lesions demonstrate inflammation and disruption of the epithelium of small airways, followed by growth of granulation tissue into the airway lumen and subsequent complete or partial obstruction. The granulation tissue then organizes in a stereotypical pattern with resultant fibrosis that obliterates the lumen of the airway.

CLINICAL MANIFESTATIONS

Clinically, bronchiolitis obliterans is accompanied by nonspecific symptoms. Progressive exertional breathlessness typically develops, and pulmonary function testing usually demonstrates evidence of progressive airflow obstruction (Chapter 85). Bronchiolitis obliterans is classified according to the FEV_1: 0 (no significant abnormality) if FEV_1 is greater than 80% of baseline; 1 (mild) if FEV_1 is 65 to 80% of baseline; 2 (moderate) if FEV_1 is 50 to 65% of baseline; and 3 (severe) if FEV_1 is 50% or less of baseline. In early stages, chest radiography is notable only for hyperinflation, but it may show bronchiectasis as the syndrome progresses. Later stages of bronchiolitis obliterans may include a syndrome of bronchiectasis with chronic productive cough and airway colonization with *Pseudomonas* species.

DIAGNOSIS

The diagnosis of bronchiolitis obliterans is made on both clinical and pathologic grounds. Transbronchial biopsy has a low yield for demonstrating histologic evidence of bronchiolitis obliterans, but when such evidence is seen, it is diagnostic. In patients with a compatible clinical syndrome, exclusion of anastomotic stenosis and occult pulmonary infection is sufficient to establish the diagnosis.

TREATMENT Rx

A variety of therapies have been tried, including pulse corticosteroids, antilymphocyte antibodies, total lymphoid irradiation, photopheresis, and nebulized cyclosporine, but none has been clearly established as effective. Most patients with bronchiolitis obliterans experience a progressive decline in pulmonary function despite immunosuppression.

PROGNOSIS

Bronchiolitis obliterans is the leading cause of late mortality after lung transplantation. Half of lung transplant recipients surviving to 5 years will have either biopsy-proven bronchiolitis obliterans or the clinical diagnosis of bronchiolitis obliterans syndrome.

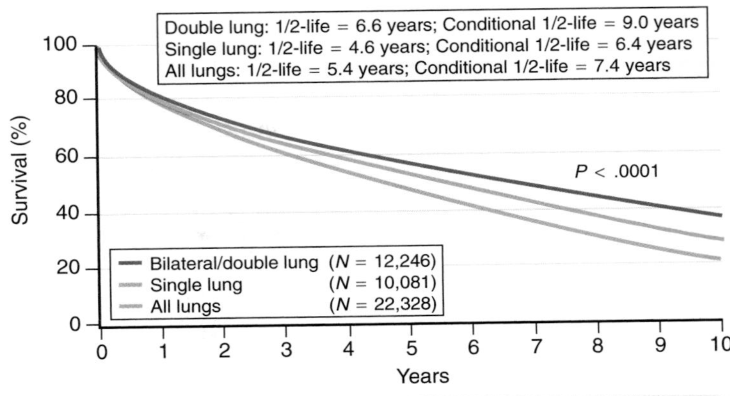

FIGURE 101-4. Kaplan-Meier survival estimates for all lung transplantations reported to the International Registry for Heart and Lung Transplantation from 1994 to 2007. Note the highly statistically significant survival advantage conferred by double lung grafts. (Adapted from Registry of the International Society for Heart and Lung Transplantation. Twenty-second official adult lung and heart-lung transplant report—2009. *J Heart Lung Transplant.* 2009;28:989-1049.)

Nonpulmonary Medical Complications of Lung Transplantation

Most of the nonpulmonary medical complications that arise in patients after lung transplantation are the result of immunosuppressive therapy. One or more of these complications develop in virtually all lung transplant recipients.

Osteoporosis (Chapter 251) is common because of the long-term use of corticosteroids and cyclosporine. Bone density should be monitored periodically, and pharmacologic therapy should be instituted if excessive bone loss is identified.

Chronic renal insufficiency (Chapter 132) is common and is the result of therapy with the calcineurin inhibitors cyclosporine or tacrolimus, both of which affect afferent vascular tone in the kidneys and result in an average 50% drop in the glomerular filtration rate in the first 12 months after lung transplantation. Systemic arterial hypertension is also common and is caused by corticosteroids and cyclosporine. Calcium-channel blockers, which are often used to treat hypertension, raise serum cyclosporine levels; appropriate monitoring and dose adjustment are needed when starting such therapy. Both corticosteroids and tacrolimus contribute to the development of diabetes mellitus and hyperlipidemia.

Solid organ transplantation is associated with an increased incidence of malignancy, thought to be due to pharmacologic immunosuppression and alteration in immune surveillance. Patients are at increased risk for lymphoproliferative malignancies and other types of cancers. Post-transplantation lymphoproliferative disorders occur in about 4% of patients after organ transplantation; most are associated with EBV. These syndromes can be polyclonal or monoclonal. Reduction in immunosuppression is sometimes therapeutic in those with polyclonal disease. The prognosis in patients with monoclonal disease is poor, with little response to modification of immunosuppression or antineoplastic chemotherapy. Patients are also at increased risk for skin, cervical, anogenital, and hepatobiliary malignancy after solid organ transplantation.

Outcomes after Lung Transplantation

Currently, the annual mortality following lung transplantation is 8 to 10% per year, largely owing to bronchiolitis obliterans syndrome. The median survival after lung transplantation is about 5.4 years (Fig. 101-4).

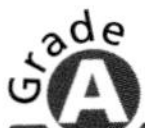

1. Annema JT, van Meerbeeck JP, Rintoul RC, et al. Mediastinoscopy vs endosonography for mediastinal nodal staging of lung cancer: a randomized trial. *JAMA.* 2010;304:2245-2252.
2. Naunheim KS, Wood DE, Mohsenifar Z, et al, for the National Emphysema Treatment Trial Research Group. Long-term follow-up of patients receiving lung-volume-reduction surgery versus medical therapy for severe emphysema in the National Emphysema Treatment Trial. *Ann Thorac Surg.* 2006;82:431-443.

3. National Emphysema Treatment Trial Research Group. Safety and efficacy of median sternotomy versus video-assisted thoracic surgery for lung volume reduction surgery. *J Thorac Cardiovasc Surg.* 2004;127:1350-1360.
4. Sciurba FC, Ernst A, Herth FJF, et al: A randomized study of endobronchial valves for advanced emphysema. *N Engl J Med.* 2010;363:1233-1244.

SUGGESTED READINGS

Ernst A, Anantham D. Endoscopic management of emphysema. *Clin Chest Med.* 2010;31:117-126. *Review.*

Floreth T, Bhorade SM. Current trends in immunosuppression for lung transplantation. *Semin Respir Crit Care Med.* 2010;31:172-178. *Review.*

Kreisel D, Krupnick AS, Puri V, et al. Short- and long-term outcomes of 1000 adult lung transplant recipients at a single center. *J Thorac Cardiovasc Surg.* 2011;141:215-222. *Five-year survival is improving but is limited by the development of bronchiolitis obliterans.*

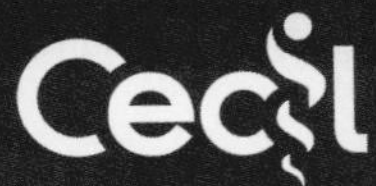

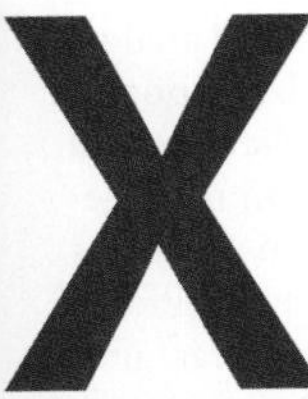

X CRITICAL CARE MEDICINE

102

APPROACH TO THE PATIENT IN A CRITICAL CARE SETTING

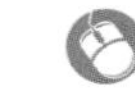

DEBORAH J. COOK

THE INTENSIVIST-LED MULTIDISCIPLINARY TEAM

Patients with critical illness in the intensive care unit (ICU) usually require advanced life support such as mechanical ventilation, inotropic agents, or dialysis. Morbidity associated with critical illness includes complications of both acute and chronic diseases, nosocomial and iatrogenic consequences, and impaired quality of life among survivors. Critically ill patients are at a higher risk of death than any other hospital population. Accordingly, the goals of critical care are to reduce morbidity and mortality, maintain organ function, and restore health. Unlike many other specialties, critical care medicine is not limited to a particular population, disease, diagnosis, or organ system.

Staffing of ICUs with critical care physicians, often referred to as *intensivists*, who provide mandatory consultations or principal ongoing care is associated with a significantly reduced ICU and hospital mortality and reduced ICU and hospital lengths of stay. These findings emphasize the value of the on-site availability of trained physicians who are dedicated to appropriate triaging, prevention, diagnosis, monitoring, treatment, and palliation of critically ill patients.

In addition, daily rounds by an ICU physician who leads a multidisciplinary team appear to improve outcomes. Emerging evidence suggests that leadership, communication, and organizational culture can streamline the process of critical care. These favorable findings may be due to the intensivist-coordinated teamwork of physicians, nurses, respiratory therapists, dieticians, and pastoral care workers to meet the needs of patients and families.

FLUID RESUSCITATION

Intravenous fluids to maintain or restore intravascular volume are an important component of ICU therapy. Both crystalloid and colloid solutions are in widespread use. Crystalloids are readily available and inexpensive, whereas colloids generally require less volume to achieve a specific physiologic goal. Albumin is a naturally occurring protein colloid that increases intravascular oncotic pressure, but its use also carries a small risk of transmitting infection.

In a large randomized trial of fluid replacement with either normal saline or 4% albumin, mortality was the same (21%) in both groups, and there were no differences in organ failure, duration of mechanical ventilation, renal replacement therapy, or length of ICU or hospital stay[1]; however, crystalloid resulted in lower mortality for the pre-specified subgroup of patients with traumatic brain injury. Based on these data, either crystalloid- or albumin-based fluid resuscitation is recommended for most critically ill patients, but crystalloids are recommended for head-injured patients.

Intravenous hydroxyethyl starch, which, like albumin, draws extravascular fluid into the intravascular space, appears to be associated with an increased risk of adverse outcomes, especially the need for renal replacement therapy in the setting of severe sepsis and septic shock.[2] Although starch has not been shown to increase overall mortality, it should be avoided in patients with severe sepsis and septic shock pending ongoing randomized trials.

SEDATION, ANALGESIA, AND SPONTANEOUS BREATHING TRIALS

Endotracheal intubation, central venous catheterization, postoperative pain management, and other ICU procedures require that most patients receive sedation, analgesia, or both. Continuous infusion of sedatives and analgesics is preferable to intermittent boluses, because infusions ensure ongoing tolerance to mechanical ventilation and provide consistent relief of pain and anxiety.

Daily interruption of the infusion of sedatives and analgesics, using protocols that provide an opportunity for the patient to be observed in a less sedated state, is associated with a shorter duration of mechanical ventilation and ICU length of stay.[3] A standardized approach to sedation and analgesia, combining a drug titration protocol with a sedation scale, can favorably impact ICU outcomes and resource consumption.

Discontinuation of ventilatory support is affected by sedation and analgesic infusions, and vice versa. A daily sedation vacation followed by a spontaneous breathing test increases the days of breathing without assistance and shortens ICU stay and hospital stay compared with usual sedation management plus a daily spontaneous breathing test.[4] Although sedation vacations may theoretically increase the risk of self-extubation, the number of patients requiring reintubation does not appear to be increased. In the year after enrollment, patients who were treated with a "wake up and breathe" protocol, which linked daily sedation vacation periods with daily spontaneous breathing trials, had a 32% better survival rate. Based on these data, a nurse-implemented sedation and analgesic management scale with daily drug interruption and daily spontaneous breathing trials are recommended for mechanically ventilated critically ill patients.

LONG-TERM OUTCOMES FOR SURVIVORS

For survivors of critical illness, triggers for ICU discharge are restoration of hemodynamic stability, ability to protect the airway, and spontaneous breathing. However, biomarkers of inflammation, residual organ dysfunction, and functional disabilities persist in most ICU survivors. Treatments administered in the ICU also have serious sequelae. For example, neuromuscular blockers and corticosteroids may contribute to critical illness polyneuropathy. These problems have particularly serious adverse consequences for elderly critically ill patients who are deconditioned before hospitalization.

In addition, anxiety, post-traumatic stress, and major mood disorders are common among patients and their caregivers during recovery. Therefore, although ICU discharge and hospital discharge are milestones in a patient's trajectory, sequelae of critical illness have rarely resolved completely when patients are on the regular hospital floor or at home. Accordingly, multidimensional rehabilitation may optimize the long-term outcomes of survivors of critical illness and their families.

Sedative-induced immobility is now understood to be a preventable contributor to ICU-acquired weakness and functional impairment in the recovery phase of critical illness. This concept has prompted multifaceted interventions to improve long-term outcomes. In a randomized trial of previously independent patients who received mechanical ventilation for 72 hours or less, the addition of graduated, individualized, early physical therapy and occupational therapy during daily sedation vacation periods improved functional capacity at hospital discharge, reduced the duration of delirium, and reduced the number of ventilator days during the 28-day follow-up.[5] Discontinuation of therapy as a result of patient instability, usually patient-ventilator asynchrony, occurred in only 4% of all sessions. This trial highlights how the recovery of critically ill patients can be improved by coordinated multidisciplinary care, including the interruption of sedation, physical therapy, and occupational therapy in the early days of critical illness.

APPLYING EVIDENCE TO PREVENT COMPLICATIONS OF CRITICAL ILLNESS

Considerable evidence of effective preventive and therapeutic ICU interventions has emerged in randomized trials over the past decade. However, barriers to applying this evidence in fast-paced ICUs can lead to a lack of responsibility and decisional authority and to errors of omission.

Analysis of most clinical practices has shown that passive dissemination of information, whether written or verbal, is generally ineffective in modifying physicians' behavior. More effective strategies to encourage the implementation of evidence-based recommendations are interactive education, audit and feedback, reminders (written or computerized), involvement of local opinion leaders, and multifaceted approaches. In the high-acuity ICU setting, pre-printed physician orders may help guide (but never dictate) management (Table 102-1). Highlights of evidence-based management include low tidal volume ventilation, high positive end-expiratory pressure,[6] inotrope or vasopressor infusion, low-dose corticosteroids, early enteral small bowel nutrition, head of bed elevation, oral antisepsis, stress ulcer prophylaxis, thromboprophylaxis, and insulin therapy aimed at avoiding marked hyperglycemia but not achieving normoglycemia (Chapters 104 and 105).[7,8] Another useful management strategy is oral decontamination with nonabsorbable antiseptic agents such as chlorhexidine, which decreases the risk of pneumonia. This antiseptic approach is favored over using antibiotics

TABLE 102-1 ICU ADMISSION ORDERS: EXAMPLE FOR A PATIENT WITH UROSEPSIS AND ARDS

MANAGEMENT STRATEGY	ORDERS	REEVALUATE
ACUTE PHASE		
Mechanical ventilation	Target TV 5-7 mL/kg of ideal body weight, PC 16 cm, rate 12, F_{IO_2} 0.7, PEEP 18 cm, plateau pressure <30 cm	PRN
Maintenance fluid	Ringer's lactate 75 mL/hr IV	PRN
Norepinephrine	Titrate to mean arterial pressure >65 mm Hg	PRN
Corticosteroids	Hydrocortisone 50 mg IV q6h while vasopressor dependent	Daily
Sedation	Midazolam 2-8 mg/hr IV, bolus 2-4 mg PRN	PRN
Analgesia	Morphine 1-4 mg IV PRN	PRN
Antibiotics	Ampicillin 2 g IV q6h	Daily
Head of bed	45-degree elevation from horizontal	PRN
Oral antisepsis	Chlorhexidine 15 mL q6h	Daily
Small bowel enteral nutrition	10 mL/hr of a commercial balanced feed containing about 1 kcal/mL; increase by 10 mL q6h to 70 mL/hr	Daily
Stress ulcer prophylaxis	Ranitidine 50 mg IV q8h	Daily
Thromboprophylaxis	Unfractionated heparin 5000 U SC q12h	Daily
Intensive insulin therapy if glucose >180 mg/dL	50 U insulin in 50 mL NS; start at 0.5 U/hr, repeat glucose q1h for 4 hr, and reassess; target 110-150 mg/dL	Daily
Glucometer calibration	Calibrate glucose from glucometer and central laboratory every morning	Daily
Tests	Glucose q4h when stable, ABG with each ventilator change, other tests as per ICU team	PRN
Monitoring	Arterial catheter for systolic blood pressure, central venous catheter for central venous pressure and mixed venous oxygen saturation, ECG, oximetry, ABGs, sedation scale, Foley catheter, others as per ICU monitoring protocols	PRN
RECOVERY PHASE		
Sedation vacation	Daily interruption of sedation from 0700 h until 0900 h; restart at half prior infusion at 0900 h as tolerated	Daily
Spontaneous breathing trials	Spontaneous breathing trial when weaning readiness criteria met	Daily
Early mobility	Physiotherapy and occupational therapy when able	Daily

ABG = arterial blood gas; ARDS = acute respiratory distress syndrome; ECG = electrocardiogram; F_{IO_2} = fraction of inspired oxygen; ICU = intensive care unit; IV = intravenous; NS = normal saline; PC = pressure control; PEEP = positive end-expiratory pressure; PRN = as needed; SC = subcutaneous; TV = tidal volume.

for conventional selective digestive tract decontamination, given concerns about global microbial antibiotic resistance.[9] In mechanically ventilated adults, chest radiographs on demand provide equivalent clinical outcomes as do routine radiographs, despite about one-third fewer radiographs.[10] Later during the recovery phase of critical illness, evidence-based management includes daily interruption of sedation infusions, daily spontaneous breathing trials, and early mobilization.

For example, in a statewide study, the creation and coaching of local safety teams to lead multidisciplinary education, central venous catheter carts stocked with necessary equipment, a five-step procedural checklist to decrease blood stream infections (handwashing, full barrier precautions for catheter insertion, chlorhexidine skin cleansing, avoidance of the femoral site, and removal of unnecessary catheters), and periodic site-specific feedback on infection rates decreased catheter-related blood stream infections from 7.7 per 1000 catheter-days at baseline to 1.4 at 18 months' follow-up.[11]

PREDICTIONS, PREFERENCES, AND END-OF-LIFE CARE

As the population ages and new technologies are developed, the use of basic and advanced life support will increase. Since demand for ICU beds is outstripping supply, the selection of patients to receive critical care is challenging. Three common but not mutually exclusive approaches to rationing ICU beds are admitting the sickest patients; admitting on a first-come, first-served basis; and triaging on the grounds of likely relative benefit. When ICU beds are rationed, patients who are refused ICU admission owing to a perceived minimal potential to benefit have a three-fold higher hospital mortality than those admitted. However, when ICU beds are reduced because of bed closures, admitted patients are sicker, are less frequently admitted for monitoring, and have shorter stays without adverse effects.

Once in the ICU, the prognosis of many critically ill patients improves. For others, treatment responsiveness is delayed or not realized, organ dysfunction evolves but does not resolve, and complications arise. Despite best efforts of the multidisciplinary ICU team, critical illness proves fatal to between 5 and 40% of adults. When a therapeutic trial of critical care is started, and particularly when it is failing, it is crucial to discuss prognosis openly with families. Families bring key information about the patients' prior function and preferences. In the shared decision-making model that dominates today, these exchanges often result in plans to withhold or withdraw basic or advanced life support.

Mechanical ventilation is the most frequent life support administered to, and withdrawn from, critically ill patients. Ventilator withdrawal very often precedes death in the ICU. Patients undergoing ventilator withdrawal or who die while mechanically ventilated have a shorter ICU stay than patients successfully weaned from the ventilator. Such withdrawal may be guided by the severity of the illness and other physiologic characteristics, but it is more heavily influenced by the contemporary life support model that is attentive to a patient's values and the physician's predictions about future quality of life. This complexity underscores the need for ICU teams to be expert communicators, sensitive in eliciting patients' preferences, timely in relieving suffering, and compassionate in providing dignity to the dying while administering culturally competent, family-centered end-of-life care.

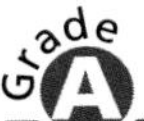

1. The SAFE Study Investigators. A comparison of albumin and saline for fluid resuscitation in the intensive care unit. *N Engl J Med.* 2004;350:2247-2256.
2. Zarychanski R, Turgeon AF, Fergusson DA, et al. Renal outcomes following hydroxyethyl starch resuscitation in critically ill patients: a meta-analysis of randomized trials. *Open Med.* 2009;3:196-209.
3. Kress JP, Pohlman AS, O'Connor MF, et al. Daily interruption of sedative infusions in critically ill patients undergoing mechanical ventilation. *N Engl J Med.* 2000;342:1471-1477.
4. Girard T, Kress JP, Fuchs BD, et al. Efficacy and safety of a paired sedation and ventilator weaning protocol for mechanically ventilated patients in intensive care (Awakening and Breathing Controlled trial): a randomised controlled trial. *Lancet.* 2008;371:126-134.
5. Schweickert WD, Pohlman MC, Pohlman AS, et al. Early physical and occupational therapy in mechanically ventilated, critically ill patients: a randomised controlled trial. *Lancet.* 2009;373:1874-1882.
6. Briel M, Meade M, Zhou Q, et al. Higher versus lower positive end-expiratory pressure in patients with acute lung injury and acute respiratory distress syndrome: systematic review and individual patient data meta-analysis. *JAMA.* 2010;303:865-873.
7. The NICE-SUGAR Study Investigators. Intensive versus conventional glucose control in critically ill patients. *N Engl J Med.* 2009;360:1283-1297.
8. Soylemez Wiener R, Wiener DC, Larson RJ. Benefits and risks of tight glucose control in critically ill adults: a meta-analysis. *JAMA.* 2008;300:933-944.
9. Chaney E, Ruest A, Meade MO, et al. Oral decontamination for prevention of pneumonia in mechanically ventilated adults: systematic review and meta-analysis. *BMJ.* 2007;334:889.

10. Hejblum G, Chalumeau-Lemoine L, Ioos V, et al. Comparison of routine and on-demand prescription of chest radiographs in mechanically ventilated adults: a multicentre, cluster-randomized, two-period crossover study. *Lancet*. 2009;374:1687-1693.
11. Pronovost P, Needham D, Berenholtz S, et al. An intervention to decrease catheter-related bloodstream infections in the ICU. *N Engl J Med*. 2006;355:2725-2732.

SUGGESTED READINGS

Magder S. Hemodynamic monitoring in the mechanically ventilated patient. *Curr Opin Crit Care*. 2011;17:36-42. *Review*.

Pronovost PJ, Goeschel CA, Colantuoni E, et al. Sustaining reductions in catheter related bloodstream infections in Michigan intensive care units: observational study. *BMJ*. 2010;340:c309. *Multi-modality intervention to reduce bloodstream infections showed continued benefit 18 months after the intervention ended.*

Scales DC, Dainty K, Hales B, et al. A multifaceted intervention for quality improvement in a network of intensive care units. *JAMA*. 2011;305:363-372. *In community ICUs, a multifaceted quality improvement intervention improved adoption of beneficial care practices.*

Wunsch H, Guerra C, Barnato AE, et al. Three-year outcomes for Medicare beneficiaries who survive intensive care. *JAMA*. 2010;303:849-856. *Survivors of the ICU had a higher mortality rate than controls, especially if they required mechanical ventilation.*

103 RESPIRATORY MONITORING IN CRITICAL CARE

JAMES K. STOLLER AND NICHOLAS S. HILL

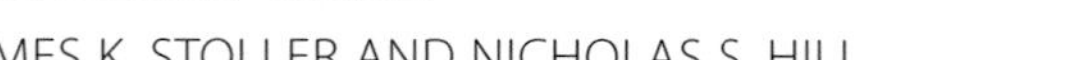

Monitoring the respiratory system involves a broad array of assessment techniques, ranging from low-technology approaches like a careful physical examination to using very sophisticated technologies to monitor oxygenation and ventilation.

PHYSICAL EXAMINATION

The physical examination can provide important information regarding the patient's ventilation and oxygenation. Ventilation can be assessed by recording the respiratory rate (normally 12 to 20 breaths/minute in adults) as well as by closely inspecting the pattern of chest wall movement during inspiration and by noting the use of accessory inspiratory muscles (e.g., the scalene, trapezius, and sternocleidomastoid muscles). Hypopnea (shallow or slow breathing) or a slowed respiratory rate (bradypnea) can indicate decreased ventilation. Shallow breathing may relate to muscle weakness (Chapter 429) or increased lung stiffness, which is commonly accompanied by a compensatory increase in the ratio of the respiratory rate to maintain ventilation. Bradypnea may relate to a suppressed respiratory drive (e.g., excessive use of narcotics, slowing the respiratory rate). Conversely, sustained tachypnea (e.g., >35 breaths/minute in an adult) can indicate ongoing increased work of breathing, impending respiratory failure, and the need for mechanical assistance, such as noninvasive ventilation or intubation and mechanical ventilation, depending on the etiology of the respiratory failure.

Contraction of the sternocleidomastoid muscles or scalene muscles, often with a seated, bent posture, is called the *tripod sign* (E-Fig. 103-1). This response indicates inadequate diaphragmatic function, most commonly in the setting of emphysema with associated diaphragmatic flattening, which causes a mechanical disadvantage of diaphragmatic contraction. In this circumstance, patients may demonstrate Hoover's sign, which is inspiratory retraction of the rib cage at the level of the zone of apposition, where the diaphragm inserts on the chest wall.

The physical examination of the nail beds and lips may also reveal cyanosis, which suggests hypoxemia. Cyanosis occurs when saturation falls, but it requires the presence of 5 g of desaturated hemoglobin. As such, polycythemic patients may show cyanosis with relatively high oxyhemoglobin saturation values, whereas patients with profound anemia may not demonstrate cyanosis even in the face of low values of oxyhemoglobin saturation.

SYSTEMIC ARTERIAL BLOOD GAS ANALYSIS

Sampling arterial blood, either through a percutaneous arterial puncture or by withdrawing blood from an indwelling arterial catheter, provides important information about the patient's oxygenation and ventilation status as well as the acuity of and compensation for derangements. The partial pressure of carbon dioxide ($Paco_2$) reflects ventilation, the elimination of carbon dioxide. In many but not all cases, $Paco_2$ is close to the mixed alveolar Pco_2.

The $Paco_2$ in the arterial blood is closely related to the ratio of metabolic CO_2 production to alveolar ventilation:

$$Paco_2 = (K)(CO_2 \text{ production rate})/(\text{alveolar ventilation}[V_A]) \quad (1)$$

The partial pressure of oxygen (Pao_2) reflects the level of oxygenation, with normal levels of oxygenation defined by the alveolar-arterial oxygen gradient, $P(A\text{-}a)O_2$, which is calculated as:

$$P(A\text{-}a)O_2 = Fio_2(P_B - P_{H_2O \text{ at standard pressure and body temperature}}) - (Pao_2 + Paco_2/\text{respiratory quotient}) \quad (2)$$

where the respiratory quotient equals the number of moles of CO_2 produced for each mole of oxygen consumed (generally ~0.8 under normal metabolic conditions at rest, but variable with dietary intake and metabolic rate). The normal value of the alveolar-arterial oxygen gradient varies with age and position and can be approximated by the simple equation:

$$P(A\text{-}a)O_2 = (\text{age}/4) + 4 \quad (3)$$

Normal age-related values of Pao_2 in the sitting position can be determined by the equation:

$$Pao_2 \text{ sitting} = 104.2 - (0.27 \times \text{age in years}) \quad (4)$$

Normal values of Pao_2 are generally in the range of 70 to 95 mm Hg, depending on the patient's age.

The $Paco_2$ helps assess the adequacy of the patient's ventilation. At sea level, normal values of $Paco_2$ range from 35 to 45 mm Hg. Values of $Paco_2$ below 35 mm Hg indicate hyperventilation, either as a primary respiratory event (e.g., with anxiety) or in response to another insult (e.g., hypoxemia, sepsis, liver disease). Similarly, values of $Paco_2$ exceeding 45 mm Hg indicate hypoventilation, hypercapnia, and respiratory acidosis, which may result either from suppression of the ventilatory drive (Chapter 86) (e.g., excess narcotics; Chapter 33) or from respiratory insufficiency (e.g., respiratory muscle weakness; Chapter 429).

Assessment of the patient's bicarbonate level (HCO_3^-) helps define the chronicity of changes in the patient's Pco_2, where the value of bicarbonate is defined by the Henderson-Hasselbalch equation:

$$pH = 6.1 + \log_{10}[HCO_3^-]/0.003\,Paco_2 \quad (5)$$

Acute increases in $Paco_2$ drive the normal kidney to retain bicarbonate (Chapter 120), whereas acute decreases in $Paco_2$, as in hyperventilation from anxiety or liver disease, would be expected to cause the normal kidney to waste bicarbonate in order to preserve the body's pH (normally 7.35 to 7.45).

The clinician can also assess whether the patient's ventilatory response to metabolic acidosis is appropriate or inadequate by using the Winter equation, which predicts the expected $Paco_2$ in the face of a decreased bicarbonate from a metabolic acidosis (Equation 6). Specifically, a measured $Paco_2$ above the expected value indicates an inadequate ventilatory response, whereas a value of $Paco_2$ that falls within the expected range indicates an expected, appropriate ventilatory response to the metabolic derangement (i.e., the acidosis).

$$Paco_2 = (1.5[HCO_3^-] + 8) \pm 2 \quad (6)$$

When the patient is hypercapnic and hypoxemic, a useful step is to calculate the ambient air $P(A\text{-}a)O_2$ and to determine whether it is normal or increased for the patient's age. Of the six mechanisms of hypoxemia, only two (hypoventilation and breathing decreased ambient oxygen, as at altitude or from a hypoxic gas mixture) are associated with a preserved $P(A\text{-}a)O_2$ (Table 103-1). Under clinical circumstances at sea level, hypoxemia in the face of a normal $P(A\text{-}a)O_2$ indicates that the patient's hypoxemia is caused by hypoventilation and should prompt the clinician to consider the various etiologies of suppressed respiratory drive (Chapter 86) or respiratory insufficiency that interferes with a normal ventilatory response (e.g., respiratory muscle weakness; Chapter 429).

PULSE OXIMETRY

Pulse oximetry is a noninvasive method to assess arterial blood oxygenation. The percentage of hemoglobin that is oxygenated is measured by passing light of two different wavelengths (660 nm [for deoxyhemoglobin] and 940 nm [for oxyhemoglobin]) through a blood-carrying tissue (e.g., finger, earlobe, forehead), identifying the pulsatile component (which contains arterial blood and background tissue elements), and subtracting the nonpulsatile component to isolate the arterial component. The device can estimate the percent of oxygenated hemoglobin over the range of 100% to about 75%. Most clinicians regard the output of pulse oximeters to be inaccurate for percent saturation values of less than 70%, although the probability of a low saturation should not be discounted (Fig. 103-1). Pulse oximetry measurements may help identify significant drops in Pao_2 below 60 to 65 mm Hg but are relatively insensitive to changes in Pao_2 from 90 to 65 mm Hg.

CARBON DIOXIDE MONITORING: CAPNOMETRY AND TRANSCUTANEOUS CARBON DIOXIDE MEASUREMENT

The fraction of CO_2 in exhaled air can be measured in real time by infrared capnometry. Partial pressures can then be calculated based on knowledge of atmospheric pressure. The expiratory capnogram (see Fig. 103-1) represents a continuous plot of exhaled Pco_2 versus time or exhaled volume and reflects the sequential appearance of gas from various compartments (e.g., the endotracheal tube, central airways, and finally the alveoli, where the Pco_2 is in equilibrium with end-capillary blood). The shape of the capnogram provides clues to the presence of chronic obstructive pulmonary disease, in that emptying of areas of lung with increased dead space (see later) can cause the capnogram to have a rising contour (see Fig. 103-1A), whereas the attainment of a so-called alveolar plateau on the normal capnogram (see Fig. 103-1B) indicates that alveolar gas is composed of a mix with a relatively small contribution from areas of increased dead space. The value of $P_{E}co_2$ measured at the end of expiration on the capnometer (i.e., the highest value recorded) represents the end-tidal $P_{ET}co_2$. Notably, the value of $P_{ET}co_2$ is always below the $Paco_2$ because there is a normal component of dead space ventilation (VD/VT) related to the anatomic dead space of the conducting airways (i.e., the trachea and airways to the level of gas-exchanging alveolar ducts and alveoli). The numerical difference between the $Paco_2$ and the mixed exhaled CO_2 tension ($P_{E}co_2$, defined as the partial pressure of carbon dioxide that would be measured in a balloon in which the entire exhaled volume is gathered) is related to the magnitude of dead space ventilation (i.e., areas of the lung that are ventilated without accompanying blood flow, normally ~0.3 to 0.4) as defined by the Bohr equation:

$$V_D/V_T = (Paco_2 - P_{E}co_2)/Paco_2 \qquad (7)$$

The difference between $Paco_2$ and $P_{E}co_2$ may be as low as several millimeters of mercury, but changing conditions of ventilation-perfusion matching (e.g., with pulmonary embolism [Chapter 98], atelectasis [Chapter 90]) may change the gradient over time. Measurement of the $P_{ET}co_2$ can be clinically useful to assess trends, to help detect esophageal intubation, to detect disconnection from the ventilator, and to detect perfusion during cardiopulmonary resuscitation, but it is not a reliable surrogate for $Paco_2$. Furthermore, measurement of the dead space fraction has prognostic value in patients with early acute respiratory distress syndrome (Chapter 104), in whom rising dead space is linearly related to increased mortality risk.

Measurement of transcutaneous Pco_2 using heated probes applied to the skin represents an alternative noninvasive method for estimating $Paco_2$. This approach is less widely used clinically, at least in adults, because of technical requirements, such as site rotation for the probes and repetitive calibration, and its generally lower accuracy in estimating $Paco_2$.

TABLE 103-1 PHYSIOLOGIC MECHANISMS OF HYPOXEMIA AND ACCOMPANYING VALUES OF THE ALVEOLAR-ARTERIAL OXYGEN GRADIENT BREATHING ROOM AIR

MECHANISM/ PHYSIOLOGIC PROCESS	EXAMPLE	ALVEOLAR-ARTERIAL OXYGEN GRADIENT ON ROOM AIR
Ventilation-perfusion mismatch	Pneumonia	Increased
Diffusion impairment	Interstitial lung disease	Increased
Anatomic right-to-left shunt	Pulmonary arteriovenous malformation	Increased
Hypoventilation	Neuromuscular weakness	Normal
Breathing decreased ambient oxygen (from either hypobaric conditions [e.g., altitude] or breathing a gas mixture with decreased inspired oxygen fraction)	Altitude exposure	Normal
Diffusion-perfusion impairment	Hepatopulmonary syndrome	Increased

ARTERIAL OXYGEN CONTENT AND SYSTEMIC OXYGEN DELIVERY

Arterial (Cao_2) and venous oxygen content (Cvo_2) are used to calculate cardiac output using the Fick equation (Equation 8), which is an alternative to determining cardiac output by the thermodilution method using a flow-directed pulmonary artery (Swan-Ganz) catheter (Chapter 57). The Fick equation is:

$$\text{Oxygen consumption (mL } O_2\text{/min)} = \text{cardiac output} \times (Cao_2 - Cvo_2) \qquad (8)$$

where oxygen content has the units of mL O_2/100 mL of blood and is calculated as:

$$\text{Oxygen content} = 1.34(\text{hemoglobin})(\%\ \text{saturation}) + 0.0031(Pao_2) \qquad (9)$$

Under normal conditions (with, for example, an arterial percent saturation of 95% and a hemoglobin of 15 g/100 mL and an oxygen consumption of 250 mL/minute), arterial oxygen content is about 20 mL/100 mL and, because mixed venous oxygen saturation is about 75%, central venous oxygen content is about 15 mL/100 mL, making the normal arteriovenous oxygen content difference with a normal cardiac output about 5 mL/100 mL.

Systemic oxygen transport defines the amount of oxygen delivered to the tissues and multiplies the arterial oxygen content by the cardiac output:

$$\text{Systemic oxygen transport (mL/min)} = \text{cardiac output} \times Cao_2 \qquad (10)$$

where the normal value is about 1000 mL/minute.

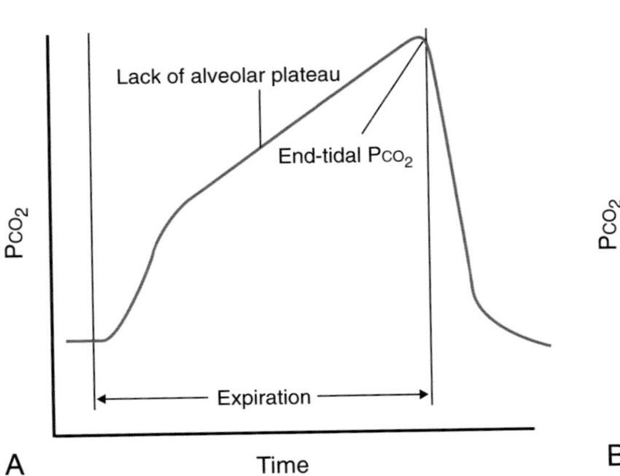

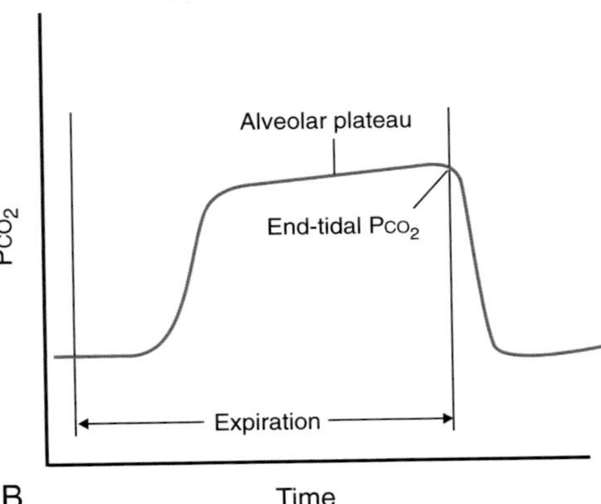

FIGURE 103-1. **Abnormal and normal end-tidal capnograms. A,** Illustration of a capnogram from a patient with chronic obstructive pulmonary disease in which the end-tidal Pco_2 rises throughout expiration as CO_2 excretion varies from different parts of the lung. **B,** Illustration of a normal capnogram in which the end-tidal Pco_2 reaches a plateau with more uniform CO_2 excretion. The end-tidal Pco_2 ($P_{ET}CO_2$) is the highest point of the alveolar plateau.

MEASURING VENTILATION: MINUTE VENTILATION AND ALVEOLAR VENTILATION

Minute ventilation (VE), which is the amount of gas exhaled from the airway per minute, is the product of the respiratory rate times the exhaled tidal volume, measured at body temperature and standardized to barometric pressure at sea level, saturated with water vapor (BTPS). The BTPS is a standard condition under which many measurements for most pulmonary function equipment and mechanical ventilators are made. These devices use an airflow meter to measure exhaled airflow and integrate the signal to derive tidal volume. An alternative way to measure tidal volume in an intensive care setting is respiratory impedance plethysmography, which uses calibrated magnetic coils in belts strapped around the chest and abdomen to monitor respiratory frequency and changes in thoracic volume.

Alveolar ventilation is the rate of gas delivery in liters per minute to gas-exchanging areas of the lung (i.e., the alveoli and alveolar ducts). The portion of minute ventilation that fails to undergo gas exchange is dead space ventilation (VD) and is determined by Equation 7 above. Minute, alveolar (VA), and dead space ventilation are related as follows:

$$V_E = V_A + V_D \quad (11)$$

It follows that conditions such as acute lung injury or acute respiratory distress syndrome (ARDS; Chapter 104) that are associated with very high dead space ratios require high VE to achieve a sufficient VA. Conversely, conditions that cause neuromuscular weakness (Chapter 429) are associated with small tidal volumes and have a high VD/VT ratio because the anatomic dead space is fixed and constitutes a higher fraction of the diminished tidal volume.

MEASURING CARBON DIOXIDE PRODUCTION

Measurement of CO_2 production is sometimes referred to as *indirect calorimetry* because it provides an index of metabolic rate and permits estimation of caloric requirements. Metabolic "carts" that simultaneously measure not only CO_2 production but also O_2 consumption and respiratory quotient are commonly used clinically to estimate metabolic needs in order to prescribe nutritional repletion (Chapter 223). The normal baseline CO_2 production is in the range of 200 mL/minute but is subject to wide variation because of hypermetabolic states commonly encountered in critically ill patients, such as sepsis or the systemic inflammatory response syndrome. A high CO_2 production might be used as an indication to increase caloric delivery.

The respiratory quotient also gives insight into the composition of feedings because carbohydrates yield a respiratory quotient of 1, whereas fatty acids yield a ratio of 0.8 and amino acids a ratio of 0.7. Thus, balanced nutrition should yield a respiratory quotient of approximately 0.85. A respiratory quotient of 1 in combination with a high CO_2 production suggests that the dietary proportion of carbohydrates is excessive.

MEASURING RESPIRATORY COMPLIANCE

Respiratory compliance is the change in respiratory system volume induced by a change in applied pressure (i.e., inspiratory pressure) and is the inverse of elastance. Compliance diminishes in conditions like lung injury and ARDS (Chapter 104) or pulmonary fibrosis (Chapter 92), in which diffuse inflammation and scarring alter lung structure and contribute to increased lung "stiffness." Static respiratory compliance is measured in patients receiving volume-limited mechanical ventilation by imposing a brief inspiratory hold at end inspiration. Assuming the patient has no spontaneous breathing effort, the airway pressure measured when airflow ceases is referred to as the plateau pressure ($P_{plateau}$). The difference between this pressure and the positive end-expiratory pressure (PEEP) is taken as the driving pressure required to deliver the tidal volume (Fig. 103-2). Static respiratory system compliance (CRS) is then calculated as:

$$C_{RS} = \Delta V(\text{exhaled tidal volume})/\Delta P(P_{plateau} - \text{PEEP}) \quad (12)$$

This compliance not only reflects the status of the lung but also includes contributions of the chest wall and abdomen. Thus, patients with chest wall deformities or morbid obesity have lower values of respiratory compliance even in the absence of lung abnormalities (Chapter 99). The normal respiratory compliance is in the range of 50 to 70 mL/cm H_2O, and patients with ARDS usually have values of CRS of less than 30 cm H_2O. If respiratory compliance is below 20 to 25 cm H_2O, weaning from mechanical ventilation (Chapter 105) is unlikely because of the high work of breathing requirements (see later).

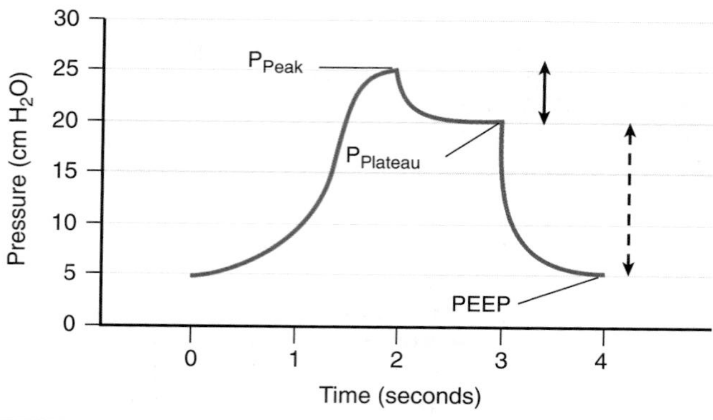

FIGURE 103-2. Illustration of inspiratory hold maneuver to determine plateau pressure ($P_{plateau}$). Airway pressure during volume-targeted mechanical ventilation rises as the tidal volume is delivered and reaches a peak. An inspiratory hold is initiated at peak pressure that prevents exhalation, so pressure falls to a "plateau" of about 20 cm H_2O. The drop in pressure reflects the pressure needed to overcome airway resistance. After slightly more than 1 second, the inspiratory hold is released, and airway pressure falls to positive end-expiratory pressure (PEEP). The difference between ($P_{plateau}$) and PEEP is used to calculate static compliance by dividing the difference into the tidal volume.

MEASURING RESPIRATORY DRIVE

The respiratory center, located in the pons and medulla, regulates respiratory drive. Hypercapnia is a strong stimulus to ventilation (Chapter 86). This response may be blunted by chronic CO_2 retention or by drugs like narcotics. Hypoxemia is a weaker ventilatory stimulus that is potentiated by hypercapnia and blunted by hypocapnia.

Thus, respiratory drive can be assessed as the response to CO_2 in the blood in the hypercapnic ventilatory response. In one technique to measure respiratory drive, the patient rebreathes his or her exhaled air while minute ventilation and $P_{ET}CO_2$ are monitored; a graph relating $P_{ET}CO_2$ with minute ventilation is used to measure respiratory drive. However, this technique is impractical in an intensive care unit (ICU) setting. Another technique is to measure the negative swing in airway pressure during the first 100 msec of inspiration (P_{100}). This technique avoids the problem of diminished ventilatory response due to airway obstruction, but it is still subject to blunting by some drugs and still underestimates drive in patients with respiratory muscle weakness, a very common problem in the ICU. In patients who are failing to wean from mechanical ventilation, a practical way to assess the integrity of respiratory drive is to determine whether the respiratory rate increases, usually into the 30s or 40s, as $Pa{CO_2}$ rises after the patient is removed from ventilatory support.

MEASURING RESPIRATORY MUSCLE STRENGTH

Respiratory muscle weakness has long been recognized as a contributor to respiratory failure and failure to wean from mechanical ventilation in the ICU (Chapter 105). This recognition has intensified in recent years with the increased awareness of ICU-acquired weakness following critical illness. However, measurement of respiratory muscle strength remains challenging because of the need to differentiate between actual weakness and reduced muscle performance owing to inability to cooperate or to exert a full inspiratory effort.

The most commonly used measures of respiratory muscle strength are the maximal inspiratory and expiratory pressures (PI_{max} or MIP and PE_{max} or MEP). These values are obtained by measuring the pressure change with a manometer when the patient inhales with maximal force from residual volume and exhales with maximal force from total lung capacity. Normal MIP is usually more negative than −75 cm H_2O, and normal MEP is usually more positive than 125 cm H_2O. When the value for MIP is less negative than −20 or −30 cm H_2O, weaning may be difficult, and values less positive than 60 cm H_2O suggest cough insufficiency. However, these values have poor predictive value in mechanically ventilated patients because many of these patients are unable to cooperate. This problem may be addressed by attaching a one-way valve to the end of endotracheal tube that permits exhalation but not inhalation and then measuring the inspiratory pressure efforts for 20 to 25 seconds.

MEASURING WORK OF BREATHING

Work of breathing is the product of pressure and volume for each breath (Fig. 103-3). The components include work needed to overcome elastic recoil of

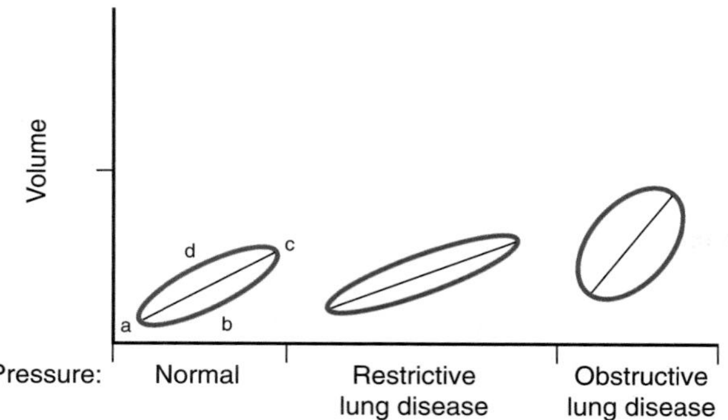

FIGURE 103-3. Pressure-volume curves illustrating components of work in a normal subject and in patients with restrictive or obstructive disease. The line between **a** and **c** represents elastic work as the lung expands, but this work is a net zero because static forces return the lung to its neutral position. The restrictive curve is flatter than normal because the lung is stiffer and volume changes less for a given unit change in pressure. The obstructive curve has a greater slope because (e.g., in emphysema) the lung is more compliant and starts inhalation from a higher volume. The **abc** curve represents resistive work during inspiration, and **cda** represents resistive work during exhalation. Resistive work during exhalation is greater in patients with obstructive lung disease.

the lung and to displace the chest wall and abdomen as well as work needed to overcome airway resistance and lung viscosity and work needed to overcome inertia. With restrictive lung diseases, the inspiratory work of breathing is increased because of the decreased lung elasticity. With obstructive diseases, the work of breathing is increased because of increased airway resistance.

In clinical settings, a more practical way to assess the inspiratory work of breathing is to calculate the pressure-time product (PTP) in cm H_2O-seconds. The PTP can be calculated using the decrease in airway pressure during inspiration, esophageal pressure (measured using an esophageal balloon manometer), or transdiaphragmatic pressure (measured using esophageal and gastric balloon manometers)—as an index of diaphragmatic work. The work can be calculated as work of breathing per breath or as work of breathing per minute by multiplying the work per breath by the respiratory frequency. Commercially available devices using esophageal manometry automatically calculate the inspiratory work of breathing, which may be of some value in assessing the likelihood of weaning from mechanical ventilation. If the drop in inspiratory pressure necessary to achieve an adequate tidal volume is too large, the calculated work of breathing will be high, and the likelihood of successful weaning will be reduced.

SUGGESTED READINGS

De Wit M, Miller K, Green D, et al. Ineffective triggering predicts increased duration of mechanical ventilation. *Crit Care Med.* 2009;37:2740-2745. *Graphic waveforms from the mechanical ventilator are correlated with the duration of mechanical ventilation.*

Gattinoni L, Carlesso E, Cressoni M. Assessing gas exchange in acute lung injury/acute respiratory distress syndrome: diagnostic techniques and prognostic relevance. *Curr Opin Crit Care.* 2011;17:18-23. *Dead space and CO_2 retention are most closely associated with outcome.*

See KC, Phua J, Mukhopadhyay A. Monitoring of extubated patients: are routine arterial blood gas measurements useful and how long should patients be monitored in the intensive care unit? *Anaesth Intens Care.* 2010;38:96-101. *Data suggesting that blood gases at 1 and 3 hours are not useful predictors of successful extubation.*

104

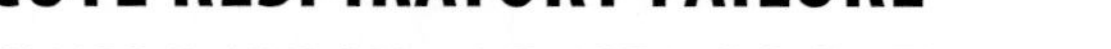

ACUTE RESPIRATORY FAILURE

LEONARD D. HUDSON AND ARTHUR S. SLUTSKY

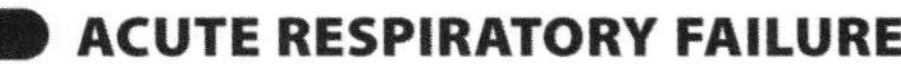

ACUTE RESPIRATORY FAILURE

DEFINITION

Acute respiratory failure occurs when dysfunction of the respiratory system results in abnormal gas exchange that is potentially life-threatening. Each element of this definition is important to understand. The term *acute* implies a relatively sudden onset (from hours to days) and a substantial change from the patient's baseline condition. Dysfunction of the respiratory system indicates that the abnormal gas exchange may be caused by abnormalities in any element of the respiratory system (e.g., a central nervous system abnormality affecting the regulation of breathing or a musculoskeletal thoracic abnormality affecting ventilation; Chapter 83), in addition to abnormalities of the lung itself. The term *respiration* refers, in a broad sense, to the delivery of oxygen (O_2) to metabolically active tissues for energy usage and the removal of carbon dioxide (CO_2) from these tissues (Table 104-1). Respiratory failure is a failure of the process of delivering O_2 to the tissues and/or removing CO_2 from the tissues. Abnormalities in the periphery (e.g., cyanide poisoning, pathologic distribution of organ blood flow in sepsis) can also lead to tissue

TABLE 104-1 ABBREVIATIONS COMMONLY USED IN ACUTE RESPIRATORY FUNCTION

ABG	Arterial blood gas or arterial blood gas analysis
ALI	Acute lung injury
ARDS	Acute respiratory distress syndrome
ARF	Acute respiratory failure
cm H_2O	Centimeters of water
$Ca{O_2}$	Content of oxygen in arterial blood
$Cc{O_2}$	Content of oxygen in end-capillary blood
CO_2	Carbon dioxide
COPD	Chronic obstructive pulmonary disease
CPAP	Continuous positive airway pressure (used when positive pressure during exhalation is applied with spontaneous ventilation)
$Cv{O_2}$	Content of oxygen in mixed venous blood
$FI{O_2}$	Fraction of inspired oxygen
g/dL	Grams per deciliter
HbO_2	Saturation of hemoglobin by oxygen
L/min	Liters per minute
mL/kg	Milliliters per kilogram
mL/min	Milliliters per minute
mm Hg	Millimeters of mercury
NIPPV	Noninvasive positive-pressure ventilation
O_2	Oxygen
$P(A\text{-}a)O_2$	Difference of partial pressure of oxygen between mean alveolar gas and arterial blood (alveolar-to-arterial oxygen difference)
$PA{CO_2}$	Partial pressure of carbon dioxide in alveolar gas
$Pa{CO_2}$	Partial pressure of carbon dioxide in arterial blood
$PA{O_2}$	Partial pressure of oxygen in alveolar gas
$Pa{O_2}$	Partial pressure of oxygen in arterial blood
$Pa{O_2}/FI{O_2}$	Ratio of partial pressure of oxygen in arterial blood to fraction of inspired oxygen
PBW	Predicted body weight
$Pc{CO_2}$	Partial pressure of carbon dioxide in end-capillary blood
$Pc{O_2}$	Partial pressure of oxygen in end-capillary blood
PEEP	Positive end-expiratory pressure (used when positive pressure during exhalation is applied with mechanical ventilation)
P/F	$Pa{O_2}/FI{O_2}$ ratio
$PI{O_2}$	Partial pressure of oxygen in inspired gas
PO_2	Partial pressure of oxygen
$Pv{CO_2}$	Partial pressure of carbon dioxide in mixed venous blood
$Pv{O_2}$	Partial pressure of oxygen in mixed venous blood
Q	Blood flow or perfusion
RR	Respiratory rate
$Sa{O_2}$	Percentage of saturation of hemoglobin by oxygen in arterial blood
$\dot{V}$	Ventilation
$\dot{V}/\dot{Q}$	Ventilation-to-perfusion ratio
V_T	Tidal volume

TABLE 104-2 SYSTEMS TO CLASSIFY ACUTE RESPIRATORY FAILURE

HYPOXIC VERSUS HYPERCAPNIC-HYPOXIC ARF	ARF WITH AND WITHOUT CHRONIC LUNG DISEASE
Causes of Hypoxic ARF	**With Chronic Lung Disease**
Acute lung injury/ARDS Pneumonia Pulmonary thromboembolism Acute lobar atelectasis Cardiogenic pulmonary edema Lung contusion Acute collagen vascular disease (Goodpasture's syndrome, systemic lupus erythematosus)	COPD Asthma Parenchymal lung diseases Restrictive lung/chest wall diseases **Without Chronic Lung Disease**[‡] Acute lung injury/ARDS Pneumonia Pulmonary thromboembolism
Causes of Hypercapnic-Hypoxic ARF	**ARF BY ORGAN SYSTEM INVOLVED**
Pulmonary disease COPD Asthma: advanced, acute, severe asthma Drugs causing respiratory depression Neuromuscular Guillain-Barré syndrome Acute myasthenia gravis Spinal cord tumors Metabolic derangements causing weakness (including hypophosphatemia, hypomagnesemia) Musculoskeletal Kyphoscoliosis Ankylosing spondylitis Obesity hypoventilation syndrome (often with additional acute, superimposed abnormality as cause of ARF)	**Respiratory (Lungs and Thorax)** Airway/airflow obstruction COPD Asthma Pulmonary parenchyma Pneumonia Acute lung injury/ARDS Acute flare of chronic collagen vascular disease (e.g., Goodpasture's syndrome, systemic lupus erythematosus) **Central Nervous System** Respiratory depression Increased sedatives, tranquilizers with respiratory effect; opiates; alcohol Brain stem and spinal cord involvement Tumors, trauma, vascular accidents
ETIOLOGIC MECHANISMS OF HYPOXEMIA	
Normal $P(A\text{-}a)O_2$*	**Neuromuscular**
$\downarrow PIO_2$ High altitude; inadvertent administration of low FIO_2 gas mixture Hypoventilation See causes of hypercapnic-hypoxic ARF above	Guillain-Barré syndrome Myasthenia gravis **Cardiovascular** Cardiogenic pulmonary edema Pulmonary thromboembolism
Increased $P(A\text{-}a)O_2$*	**Renal/Endocrine**
Ventilation-perfusion ($\dot{V}/\dot{Q}$) mismatch Airway disease Vascular disease, including pulmonary thromboembolism Shunt Acute lung injury/ARDS Pneumonia Parenchymal lung disease Cardiogenic pulmonary edema Pulmonary infarction Diffusion limitation[†]	Volume overload Metabolic abnormalities

*Calculated using the alveolar-air equation; see text for description.
[†]See text for discussion.
[‡]These can also be superimposed on chronic disease.
ARDS = acute respiratory distress syndrome; ARF = acute respiratory failure; COPD = chronic obstructive pulmonary disease; FIO_2 = fraction of inspired oxygen; $P(A\text{-}a)O_2$ = alveolar-to-arterial oxygen difference; PIO_2 = partial pressure of inspired oxygen; $\dot{V}/\dot{Q}$ = ventilation-to-perfusion ratio.

hypoxia; although these conditions represent forms of respiratory failure in the broadest terms, this chapter focuses on respiratory failure resulting from dysfunction of the lungs, chest wall, and control of respiration.

PATHOBIOLOGY

Abnormal gas exchange is the physiologic hallmark of acute respiratory failure, which can be classified in several ways (Table 104-2). Although gas exchange can be abnormal for either oxygenation or CO_2 removal, significant hypoxemia is nearly always present when patients with acute respiratory failure breathe ambient air. If CO_2 is retained at a potentially life-threatening level, this is usually accompanied by significant hypoxemia (see later). The *life-threatening* aspect of the condition places the degree of abnormal gas exchange in a clinical context and calls for urgent treatment.

The diagnosis of acute respiratory failure requires a significant change in blood gases from baseline. Many patients with chronic respiratory problems can function with blood gas tensions that would be alarming in a physiologically normal individual. Over time, these patients with so-called chronic respiratory failure or chronic respiratory insufficiency develop mechanisms to compensate for inadequate gas exchange. Conversely, this chronic condition makes patients vulnerable to insults that could be easily tolerated by a previously healthy individual.

In acute respiratory failure, the O_2 content in the blood (available for tissue use) is reduced to a level at which the possibility of end-organ dysfunction increases markedly. The value of the partial pressure of O_2 in the arterial blood (PaO_2) that demarcates this vulnerable zone is the point of the oxyhemoglobin dissociation relationship at which any further decrease in the PaO_2 results in sharp decreases in the amount of hemoglobin saturated with O_2 (SaO_2) and in the arterial blood O_2 content (CaO_2). Although arbitrary, acute respiratory failure is often defined in practice as occurring when the PaO_2 is less than 55 mm Hg (Fig. 104-1). In general, the locus on the curve that indicates the partial pressure at which O_2 is being unloaded to the tissues is the most important determinant of how much O_2 is available for the cells and their mitochondria. Usually, the ability to unload O_2 at the tissue level more than compensates for small decreases in the amount of O_2 picked up in the lungs when the oxyhemoglobin dissociation curve is shifted rightward. With a leftward shift in the curve, O_2 is bound more tightly to hemoglobin, so less O_2 is available for tissue delivery.

These clinical considerations imply that any definition of acute respiratory failure based on an absolute level of PaO_2 is arbitrary. A healthy, young, conditioned individual climbing at high altitude may have a PaO_2 of less than 50 mm Hg because of the reduction in inspired O_2 pressure. This individual is not in acute respiratory failure, even though the PaO_2 may be in the low 40s. A patient who has chronic obstructive pulmonary disease (COPD) and whose usual range of PaO_2 is 50 to 55 mm Hg would not be considered to be in acute respiratory failure if the PaO_2 was 50 mm Hg. However, if a patient's usual PaO_2 was 60 to 70 mm Hg, a PaO_2 of 50 mm Hg would be associated

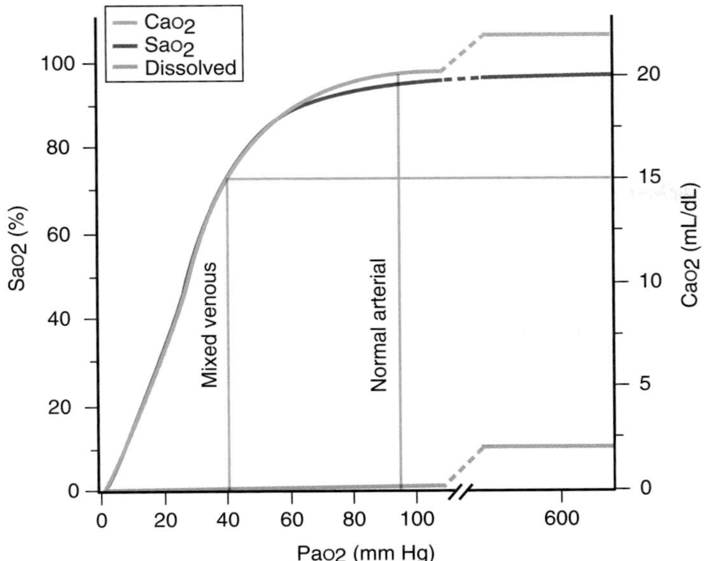

FIGURE 104-1. **Oxyhemoglobin association-dissociation curve.** The axis for oxygen saturation in the arterial blood (SaO_2) is on the left, and the axis for arterial content of oxygen (CaO_2) is on the right. CaO_2 is the sum of the oxygen dissolved in plasma (denoted as "Dissolved" in the figure) plus the oxygen bound to hemoglobin. At a normal hemoglobin, most of the oxygen is carried in combination with hemoglobin, with only a relatively small amount of oxygen dissolved in plasma. When the value of the arterial partial pressure of oxygen (PaO_2) is on the "flat" portion of the curve (PaO_2 ≥60 to 65 mm Hg, normal partial pressure of carbon dioxide [PCO_2], and normal pH), raising the PaO_2 further has relatively little effect on total oxygen content. Increases in temperature, PCO_2, hydrogen ion concentration, or 2,3-diphosphoglycerate cause a rightward shift in the oxyhemoglobin association-dissociation curve.

with a substantial risk for a further life-threatening reduction in oxygenation; this patient should be considered to have acute respiratory failure.

Traditionally, the level of arterial CO_2 partial pressure ($PaCO_2$) that defines acute respiratory failure has been 50 mm Hg or greater, if accompanied by arterial acidosis with a pH of 7.30 or less. The $PaCO_2$ is linked to pH because it is generally thought that acidosis leads to tissue dysfunction and symptoms. Patients with severe COPD may have chronic CO_2 retention, but renal compensation for the respiratory acidosis protects them against abnormalities related to the elevation in CO_2. A further acute rise in $PaCO_2$ can precipitate symptoms and other organ dysfunction; however, even severe respiratory acidosis (pH 7.1) seems to be better tolerated than metabolic acidosis of the same pH in most previously healthy individuals if arterial and tissue oxygenation is adequate.

Pathophysiology

Five mechanisms can lead to a reduction in PaO_2: (1) decreased inspired partial pressure of O_2 (PIO_2) (e.g., at high altitude or when breathing a reduced percentage O_2 mixture); (2) hypoventilation; (3) ventilation-perfusion ($\dot{V}/\dot{Q}$) mismatch; (4) shunting of blood from the pulmonary to systemic circulation, bypassing the alveoli anatomically or functionally; and (5) abnormal diffusion of O_2 from the alveoli into the capillary blood. In essence, a shunt is an extreme $\dot{V}/\dot{Q}$ mismatch in which blood perfuses alveoli with *no* ventilation; it is differentiated clinically from other $\dot{V}/\dot{Q}$ mismatching by the response to breathing supplemental O_2 (see later).

For clinical purposes, diffusion abnormalities are not an important cause of hypoxemia at sea level because there is sufficient time for adequate diffusion of O_2 during the transit of a red blood cell through the pulmonary capillary bed, even in the presence of severe lung disease. Even when diffusion abnormalities are present and contribute to hypoxemia, $\dot{V}/\dot{Q}$ mismatch and shunting nearly always coexist and are quantitatively more important causes of hypoxemia. Except at high altitude or when a subject is breathing a gas mixture low in O_2, hypoventilation, $\dot{V}/\dot{Q}$ mismatch, and shunting are the dominant causes of acute respiratory failure.

If only hypoventilation is present, the resulting hypoxemia is associated with a normal difference between the calculated alveolar and the measured arterial oxygenation levels ($P(A\text{-}a)O_2$). In this setting, an elevated $PaCO_2$ suggests disease processes that affect nonpulmonary respiratory function (e.g., central respiratory depression resulting from drug overdose, neuromuscular diseases such as Guillain-Barré syndrome, or chest wall disease such as flail chest; Chapter 86). In contrast, $\dot{V}/\dot{Q}$ mismatch and shunting are associated with an elevated $P(A\text{-}a)O_2$, which may or may not coexist with hypoventilation. The normal value for $P(A\text{-}a)O_2$ varies as a function of the fraction of inspired O_2 (FIO_2), increasing as FIO_2 increases.

When $\dot{V}/\dot{Q}$ mismatch or shunting is the cause of hypoxemia, some alveolar regions have increased $PACO_2$ and reduced PAO_2; the blood in the vessels perfusing these alveoli reflects these abnormal gas tensions. The increased $PACO_2$ usually can be reversed by increasing overall ventilation, but hyperventilation does not correct the decreased PaO_2.

$\dot{V}/\dot{Q}$ mismatch is distinguished from shunting by assessing the PaO_2 response to enhanced O_2 administration. Hypoxemia caused by $\dot{V}/\dot{Q}$ mismatch can be corrected to a nearly complete O_2 saturation of the hemoglobin in most patients by a relatively small increase in FIO_2, such as from 0.24 to 0.28 by face mask or 1 to 2 L/minute O_2 by nasal prongs, in patients with acute exacerbations of COPD. If the airways to poorly ventilated alveoli remain open and the enriched O_2 mixture is administered for an adequate length of time (ranging from a few minutes to 20 minutes, depending on the degree of $\dot{V}/\dot{Q}$ inequality), the increased PIO_2 is reflected by an increased PAO_2 and an increased PaO_2. When a shunt is present (no ventilation but continued perfusion), a relatively small increase in the FIO_2 has little or no effect on the PaO_2, and even large increases in FIO_2 up to 1.0 result in only modest increases in PaO_2 (Fig. 104-2).

CLINICAL MANIFESTATIONS

The hallmark of acute respiratory failure is the inability to maintain adequate oxygenation or the inability to maintain an appropriate $PaCO_2$. Patients are typically dyspneic and tachypneic, unless progressive respiratory failure causes fatigue—sometimes leading to respiratory arrest—or a drug overdose or neuromuscular condition prevents an appropriate respiratory response to hypoxia and/or the hypercapnic acidosis. Neurologic function may deteriorate, and myocardial ischemia or even infarction may be precipitated by the hypoxemia. In addition, each cause has its own specific manifestations (see later).

DIAGNOSIS

As part of the diagnosis of acute respiratory failure, the physician has three objectives: (1) confirm the clinical suspicion that acute respiratory failure is present, (2) classify the type of acute respiratory failure (e.g., hypoxemia caused by hypoventilation vs. hypoxemia caused by $\dot{V}/\dot{Q}$ mismatch or shunting), and (3) determine the specific cause (e.g., acute lung injury secondary to sepsis or decompensated COPD because of acute bronchitis). Defining the type of acute respiratory failure and determining the specific cause are prerequisites to optimal management.

The initial approach to diagnosis consists of considering information from four sources: (1) clinical history and physical examination; (2) physiologic abnormalities, particularly arterial blood gas derangements, which help establish the pathophysiologic mechanisms of hypoxemia; (3) chest radiographic findings; and (4) other tests aimed at elucidating specific causes. In many cases, the clinical picture from the history is so clear that the presumptive type of acute respiratory failure (and sometimes the cause) is obvious, so treatment can be started while confirmatory laboratory studies are ordered. In other cases, a clinician may be asked to see a patient because of an abnormal chest radiograph or abnormal arterial blood gases ordered by someone else and may elicit the pertinent history based on these clues. When the degree of hypoxemia is life-threatening, therapeutic decisions must be made quickly, even if data are limited. The clinician must obtain updated information continually and should view most therapeutic decisions as therapeutic trials, with careful monitoring to assess desired benefits and possible detrimental effects.

Clinical Evaluation

The presentation often reflects one of three clinical scenarios: (1) the effects of hypoxemia and/or respiratory acidosis, (2) the effects of primary (e.g., pneumonia) or secondary (e.g., heart failure) diseases involving the lungs, and (3) the nonpulmonary effects of the underlying disease process. The clinical effects of hypoxemia and/or respiratory acidosis manifest mainly in the central nervous system (e.g., irritability, agitation, changes in personality, depressed level of consciousness, coma) and the cardiovascular system (e.g., arrhythmias, hypotension, hypertension) (Table 104-3). In patients with underlying COPD (Chapter 88) with a gradual onset of acute respiratory failure, central nervous system abnormalities may be the major presenting

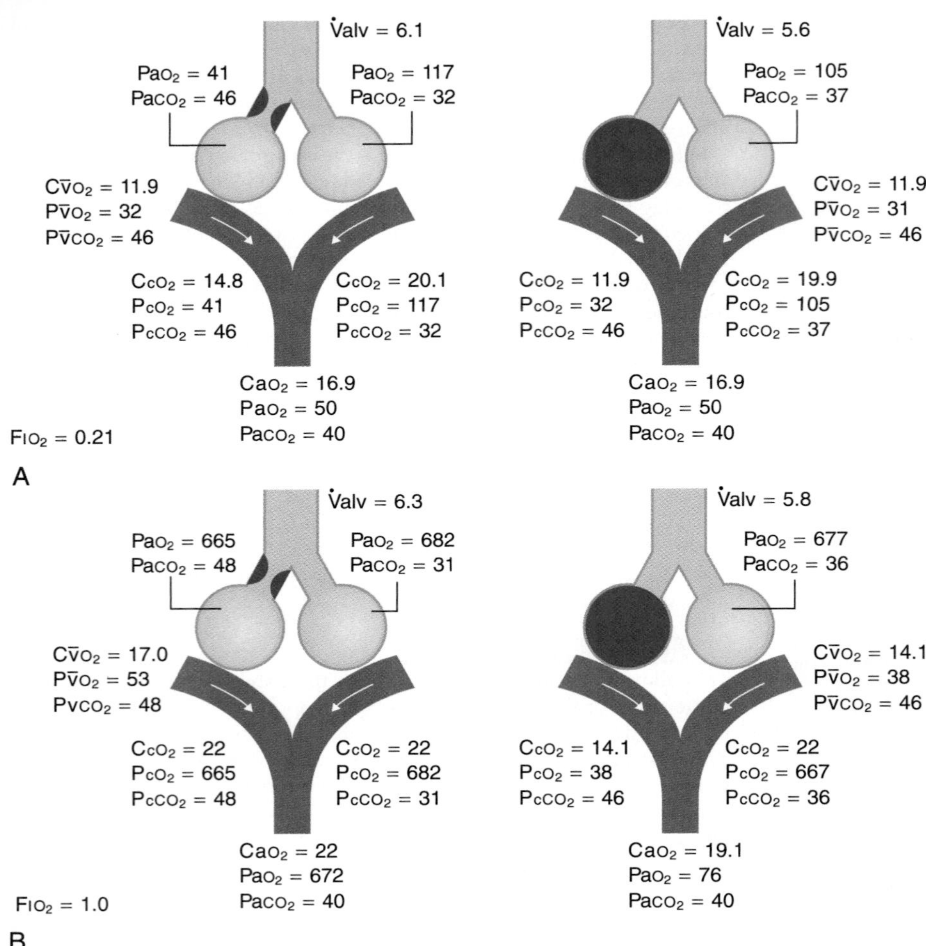

FIGURE 104-2. **Arterial oxygenation.** Comparison of the effect on arterial oxygenation of increasing the fraction of inspired oxygen (F_{IO_2}) from breathing ambient air (F_{IO_2} = 0.21) **(A)** and breathing 100% oxygen (F_{IO_2} = 1.0) **(B)** with a low ventilation-to-perfusion ratio ($\dot{V}/\dot{Q}$) (left) and a shunt (right), using a two-compartment lung model. Shunting and decreased $\dot{V}/\dot{Q}$ can lead to identical arterial blood gases (partial pressure of oxygen in arterial blood [Pa_{O_2}] = 50 mm Hg; partial pressure of carbon dioxide in arterial blood [Pa_{CO_2}] = 40 mm Hg). The response to supplemental oxygen administration is markedly different. Hypoxemia is only partially corrected by breathing 100% oxygen when a shunt is present because arterial oxygenation represents an average of the end-capillary oxygen content (Cc_{O_2}) from various parts of the lung, not an average of the partial pressures of oxygen (partial pressure of carbon dioxide in the end-capillary blood [Pc_{CO_2}]). When the Cc_{O_2} values are mixed, the Pa_{O_2} is determined from the resultant content of oxygen in the arterial blood (Ca_{O_2}) by the oxyhemoglobin association-dissociation relationship (see Fig. 104-1). With low $\dot{V}/\dot{Q}$ (as is often the case in patients with chronic obstructive pulmonary disease), an increase in F_{IO_2} increases the alveolar partial pressure of oxygen (P_{O_2}) of the low $\dot{V}/\dot{Q}$ unit and leads to a marked increase in arterial P_{O_2}. The values in this figure were generated from modeling to result in the same Pa_{CO_2} (40 mm Hg) for all four situations shown; this is the reason for slight changes in alveolar ventilation ($\dot{V}/\dot{Q}$ alv) for some of the conditions. Several assumptions are made: (1) no diffusion limitation is present; (2) oxygen consumption = 300 mL/minute, and CO_2 production = 240 mL/minute; (3) cardiac output = 6.0 L/minute; (4) the low $\dot{V}/\dot{Q}$ regions in the left panels represent 60% of the cardiac output perfusing alveoli with a $\dot{V}/\dot{Q}$ 25% of normal; and (5) the shunts in the right panels represent a 37% shunt (i.e., 37% of the cardiac output is perfusing alveoli with no ventilation).

TABLE 104-3 CLINICAL MANIFESTATIONS OF HYPOXEMIA AND HYPERCAPNIA

HYPOXEMIA	HYPERCAPNIA
Tachycardia	Somnolence
Tachypnea	Lethargy
Anxiety	Restlessness
Diaphoresis	Tremor
Altered mental status	Slurred speech
Confusion	Headache
Cyanosis	Asterixis
Hypertension	Papilledema
Hypotension	Coma
Bradycardia	Diaphoresis
Seizures	
Coma	
Lactic acidosis*	

*Usually requires additional reduction in oxygen delivery because of inadequate cardiac output, severe anemia, or redistribution of blood flow.

findings. Cyanosis, which requires at least 5 g/dL of unsaturated hemoglobin to be detectable, may not be seen before serious tissue hypoxia develops, especially in patients with underlying anemia.

Pulmonary symptoms and signs often reflect the respiratory disease causing the acute respiratory failure. Examples include cough and sputum with pneumonia (Chapter 97) or chest pain from pulmonary thromboembolism with infarction (Chapter 98). Dyspnea and respiratory distress are nonspecific reflections of the respiratory system's difficulty in meeting the increased demands from pulmonary and nonpulmonary diseases.

Physical findings may be associated with a particular pathologic lung process, such as pneumonia, causing bronchial breathing and crackles on auscultation, or the crackles (rales) of cardiogenic pulmonary edema (Chapter 58). Abnormal findings may be minimal or absent in patients with acute lung injury or pulmonary thromboembolism.

In some patients, the clinical picture is dominated by the underlying disease process, particularly with diseases that cause acute lung injury, such as sepsis (Chapter 108), severe pneumonia (Chapter 97), aspiration of gastric contents (Chapter 94), and trauma. In these conditions the physical examination is often nonspecific, with no obvious clues except, for example, fever with sepsis or pneumonia and hypotension with septic shock.

Assessment of Physiologic Abnormalities

The clinical suspicion of acute respiratory failure must be addressed by arterial blood gas analysis to answer several questions.

1. *Is hypoxemia present?* The answer is based largely on the value of the Pa_{O_2} or Sa_{O_2}, and the degree of the hypoxemia not only confirms the diagnosis of acute respiratory failure but also helps define its severity.
2. *Is hypoventilation present?* If the Pa_{CO_2} is elevated, alveolar hypoventilation is present.
3. *Does the degree of hypoventilation explain the hypoxemia?* If the $P(A\text{-}a)_{O_2}$ is normal, hypoventilation explains the presence and degree of hypoxemia. In this case, the most likely causes of acute respiratory failure are central nervous system abnormalities and a chest wall abnormality. If the $P(A\text{-}a)_{O_2}$ is increased but hypoventilation does not explain the hypoxemia, another condition must be present; common diagnoses include COPD, severe asthma, and early-stage acute respiratory distress syndrome (ARDS).
4. If hypoxemia exists without hypoventilation, an elevated $P(A\text{-}a)_{O_2}$ should be confirmed, and the response to breathing an enhanced O_2 mixture would answer this question: *Is the increase in $P(A\text{-}a)_{O_2}$ the result of a $\dot{V}/\dot{Q}$ abnormality or of shunting?* If hypoxemia is primarily the result of a $\dot{V}/\dot{Q}$ abnormality, the likely cause is an airway disease, either COPD or acute severe asthma, or a vascular disease, such as pulmonary

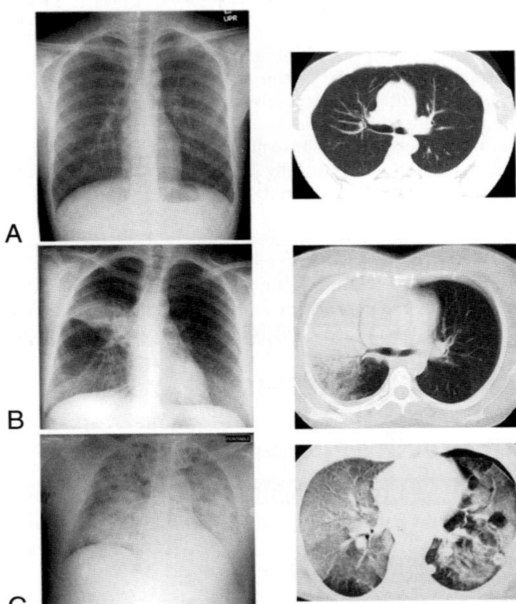

FIGURE 104-3. **Chest radiographs (left) and computed tomography (CT) scans (right) of the three most common findings in diseases causing acute respiratory failure. A,** Relatively clear chest, consistent with an acute exacerbation of airway disease (e.g., asthma, chronic obstructive pulmonary disease) or a central nervous system or neuromuscular disease as the cause of acute respiratory failure. **B,** Localized alveolar filling opacity, most commonly seen with acute pneumonia. **C,** Diffuse bilateral alveolar filling opacities consistent with acute lung injury and acute respiratory distress syndrome. The CT scan in C shows a small left pneumothorax and cavities or cysts that are not apparent on the anteroposterior chest radiograph.

thromboembolism. If shunting is the major explanation for the hypoxemia, processes that fill the air spaces (e.g., cardiogenic pulmonary edema, noncardiogenic pulmonary edema in acute lung injury or ARDS, or purulent pulmonary secretions in acute pneumonia) or, less commonly, an intracardiac or anatomic intrapulmonary shunt is the likely cause. Conditions that fill air spaces should be confirmed by an abnormal chest radiograph; if the radiograph is normal, an intracardiac shunt should be considered and confirmed by echocardiography.

Chest Radiography

The chest radiograph in acute respiratory failure is likely to show one of three patterns (Fig. 104-3): (1) normal (or relatively normal), (2) localized alveolar filling opacities, or (3) diffuse alveolar filling opacities. Diffuse interstitial opacities are also possible, but diseases that cause this pattern usually have a more gradual onset and are associated with chronic respiratory failure. If the chest radiograph is normal (i.e., it is clear or relatively clear), airway diseases, such as COPD and asthma, or pulmonary vascular diseases, such as thromboembolism, are more likely. If a localized alveolar filling abnormality is present, pneumonia is the major consideration, but pulmonary embolism and infarction should also be considered. When diffuse (bilateral) alveolar filling abnormalities are present, cardiogenic pulmonary edema, acute lung injury (e.g., as seen in sepsis, trauma, or aspiration of gastric contents), and diffuse pneumonia are the major considerations. The combination of the chest radiograph and the arterial blood gas interpretation can be helpful. The finding of a significant shunt may suggest acute lung injury in a patient in whom this diagnosis was not clinically obvious; the chest radiograph should help to confirm that possibility.

Other Evaluations

All patients with acute respiratory failure should have a complete blood count, including a platelet count; routine blood chemistry tests; prothrombin time; and urinalysis to screen for possible underlying causes and comorbid conditions. Other blood tests should be guided by the clinical picture. Examples include a serum amylase level if pancreatitis is a possible cause of ARDS and thyroid indices if severe hypothyroidism is a possible cause of hypoventilation. Blood cultures are recommended whenever sepsis is suspected.

Any abnormal fluid collections, especially pleural effusion (Chapter 99), should be aspirated for diagnostic purposes. Sputum Gram stain and culture are indicated when pneumonia is suspected.

Other specific tests should be directed by the history, physical examinations, arterial blood gas levels, and chest radiograph. An abdominal computed tomography (CT) scan may be indicated to search for the source of infection in a patient with sepsis and acute lung injury. A chest CT scan may help define pulmonary disease if the chest radiograph is not definitive. A CT arteriogram of the pulmonary circulation may diagnose pulmonary thromboembolism (Chapter 98). A head CT scan may be indicated if a stroke involving the respiratory center is suspected. Routine blood chemistry studies can detect diabetic ketoacidosis or renal failure as contributing causes.

TREATMENT Rx

General Measures

The management of acute respiratory failure depends on its cause, its clinical manifestations, and the patient's underlying status. Certain goals apply to all patients: (1) improvement of the hypoxemia to eliminate or markedly reduce the acute threat to life, (2) improvement of the acidosis if it is considered life-threatening, (3) maintenance of cardiac output or improvement if cardiac output is compromised, (4) treatment of the underlying disease process, and (5) avoidance of predictable complications.

The precise methods for improving hypoxemia depend on the cause of the acute respiratory failure. An increase in the inspired O_2 concentration is a cornerstone of treatment for nearly all patients, however.

The level of acidosis that requires treatment other than for the underlying disease process is not clear. Although normalization of the arterial pH was suggested in the past, respiratory acidosis is apparently well tolerated in many patients with severe ARDS, so a patient with a pH of 7.15 or greater may not require bicarbonate therapy. If the acidemia coexists with clinical complications, such as cardiac arrhythmias or a decreased level of consciousness, that have no other obvious cause, treatments to increase pH should be considered. The therapeutic goal is alleviation or reduction of the accompanying complications by improving the level of acidosis; it usually is not necessary to normalize the pH (Chapter 120).

The maintenance of cardiac output is crucial for O_2 delivery in acute respiratory failure, especially because mechanical ventilation and positive end-expiratory pressure (PEEP) may compromise cardiac output. Placement of a pulmonary artery catheter allows measurement of cardiac output and filling pressures, but patients who have these catheters do no better than similar patients managed without them.[1]

Many therapeutic interventions that improve short-term physiologic variables may worsen long-term, clinically important outcomes. Transfusing all patients to maintain a hemoglobin greater than 10 g/dL increases mortality in critically ill patients who have not had an acute myocardial infarction and do not have unstable angina, even though the O_2 carrying capacity of the blood is acutely increased. Use of a relatively large tidal volume (e.g., 12 mL/kg predicted body weight, which is equivalent to approximately 10 to 10.5 mL/kg measured body weight in patients who are somewhat overweight) increases mortality in patients with ARDS when compared with a lower tidal volume (6 mg/kg predicted body weight), even though it raises PaO_2 more in the short term than does a lower tidal volume. Conservative use of fluids improves lung function and shortens the duration of mechanical ventilation and intensive care.[2]

Improvements in oxygenation, acid-base status, and cardiac output are of no more than temporary benefit unless the underlying disease processes are diagnosed and treated properly. In patients with acute lung injury, sepsis may worsen injury to the lung and other organs despite optimal supportive care. Similarly, if the precipitating cause of acute respiratory failure in a patient with COPD is not identified and treated, supportive care is likely to be futile. Complications may arise from the physiologic effects of the gas exchange abnormality, from the disease processes causing the acute respiratory failure, from being critically ill and its associated incursions on homeostasis (e.g., sleep deprivation), or from iatrogenic complications of therapy.

Mechanical Therapy to Improve Oxygenation

A PaO_2 greater than 60 mm Hg is usually adequate to produce an SaO_2 in the low to middle 90s. The PaO_2 can be increased by the administration of supplemental O_2, by pharmacologic manipulations, by continuous positive airway pressure (CPAP), by mechanical ventilation with or without maneuvers such as PEEP, and by the prone position. PEEP, pharmacologic manipulations, and positioning are used primarily in patients with acute lung injury (see later).

The initial choice of the concentration and amount of supplemental O_2 is based on the severity of the hypoxemia, the clinical diagnosis, the likely mechanism causing the hypoxemia, and the O_2 delivery systems available. For the tracheal FIO_2 to be the same as the delivered FIO_2, the O_2 delivery system must deliver a flow that matches the patient's peak inspiratory flow rate with gas of a known FIO_2. High-flow O_2 blenders can achieve this goal by delivering gas at 80 L/minute or greater to a nonintubated patient. These systems require a large flow of O_2 (from a wall unit or tank), however, and are not universally available. Other systems for nonintubated patients (including nasal prongs, simple face masks, and non-rebreather and partial rebreather masks) use a simple regulator that mixes room air with O_2 at 12 L/minute from a wall unit or tank, with resulting flows that are frequently unable to match the patient's peak inspiratory flow rate. The patient entrains more air from the environment, and the resulting tracheal F_{IO_2} or partial pressure of oxygen in inspired gas (P_{IO_2}) is unknown. The amount of air entrained depends on the patient's inspiratory pattern and minute ventilation. Although the resulting F_{IO_2} is unknown, these systems are satisfactory if the delivery is constant and if they result in adequate arterial O_2 saturation, as monitored by arterial blood gases or oximetry. Nasal prongs can deliver a tracheal F_{IO_2} of approximately 0.50, and non-rebreather masks can deliver 50 to 100% O_2; in both cases, this depends on the inspiratory pattern and flow rate. If only hypoventilation or $\dot{V}/\dot{Q}$ mismatch is present, only a small increment in F_{IO_2} (e.g., an F_{IO_2} of 0.24 or 0.28 delivered by a Venturi principle face mask or by mechanical ventilation; or 1 to 2 L/minute O_2 delivered by nasal prongs) is likely to be required. By comparison, if marked shunting or many lung units with low but not zero $\dot{V}/\dot{Q}$ are the cause of hypoxemia, a considerably higher F_{IO_2} (e.g., >0.7) may be required, and even this high F_{IO_2} may not reverse the hypoxemia. A common practice when a significant shunt is suspected is to give an F_{IO_2} of 1.0, then adjust the F_{IO_2} downward as guided by the resulting Pa_{O_2} or Sa_{O_2}.

The O_2 concentration that is toxic to the lungs in critically ill patients is not known, but prior injury may provide tolerance to O_2 toxicity, whereas other conditioning agents, such as bleomycin, may enhance oxidative injury. An F_{IO_2} of 0.7 or higher is generally considered injurious to the normal human lung. Because it is unknown what lower concentration is safe, however, patients should be given the lowest F_{IO_2} that provides an adequate Sa_{O_2} (≥90%). If an F_{IO_2} equal to or greater than 0.5 to 0.7 is required for adequate oxygenation, other measures, especially PEEP or CPAP, should be considered. Even a lower F_{IO_2} of about 0.5 may be associated with impaired ciliary action in the airways and impaired bacterial killing by alveolar macrophages, but the clinical importance of these effects is not known.

A low concentration of supplemental O_2 can be administered by nasal prongs or nasal cannula, which most patients find comfortable and allows them to cough, speak, eat, and drink while receiving O_2. When the nasal passages are open, the P_{IO_2} does not depend too much on whether the patient breathes through the nose or the mouth because O_2 is entrained from the posterior nasal pharynx during a breath taken through the mouth. The level of O_2 can be adjusted by the flow rate to the nasal prongs. In patients with COPD, flows as low as 0.5 to 2 L/minute are usually adequate unless an intrapulmonary shunt is contributing to the hypoxemia, as usually occurs in acute pneumonia. At flows greater than approximately 6 L/minute, only a small further augmentation in the P_{IO_2} can be achieved. Because gas flow through the nose has a drying and irritating effect, a face mask should be considered at high flow rates. O_2 face masks using the Venturi principle allow the regulation of F_{IO_2} and can be particularly useful when COPD is suspected, and it is important to avoid the CO_2 retention that can be associated with the unregulated administration of O_2. A higher F_{IO_2} of 0.5 to nearly 1.0 can be administered through a non-rebreathing face mask with an O_2 reservoir. If an F_{IO_2} equal to or greater than 0.70 is required for more than several hours, particularly in an unstable patient, endotracheal intubation should be considered so O_2 can be administered by a closed system with reliable maintenance of the patient's Sa_{O_2}. Indications for placing an artificial airway in a patient with acute respiratory failure include airway protection against massive aspiration of gastric contents, delivery of an increased F_{IO_2}, facilitation of prolonged mechanical ventilation, and to aid in the control of respiratory secretions (Chapter 105).

Ventilatory maneuvers that may increase arterial oxygenation include mechanical ventilation itself and the administration of PEEP or CPAP, all of which allow ventilation of areas of the lung that were previously poorly ventilated or unventilated. Although large tidal volumes with mechanical ventilation may open areas of atelectasis and may improve oxygenation initially, these higher tidal volumes can cause lung injury, particularly if the lung is already injured (Chapter 105).

CPAP refers to the maintenance of positive pressure during the respiratory cycle while breathing spontaneously. PEEP refers to the maintenance of positive pressure throughout the expiratory cycle when it is applied together with mechanical ventilation (Chapter 105). CPAP and PEEP can result in recruitment of microatelectatic regions of the lung that are perfused but were not previously ventilated, thus contributing substantially to hypoxemia. CPAP and PEEP have the theoretical advantage of keeping some of these regions open during exhalation, thus preventing cyclic closure and reopening of lung units, which can result in alveolar wall stress and injury.

Supportive Measures

Every patient with acute respiratory failure is at risk for deep vein thrombosis, pulmonary thromboembolism, and gastric stress ulceration. Prophylactic anticoagulation is recommended in patients who are not at high risk for bleeding complications; sequential leg compression therapy may be preferred for high-risk patients (Chapter 81).

The best means of preventing stress ulceration is not known, but current evidence indicates that the use of an H_2-blocker is superior to the gastric administration of sucralfate, based on a large randomized, controlled trial that found a higher incidence of significant bleeding in patients receiving sucralfate than in those receiving ranitidine. Evidence also indicates that proton pump inhibitors may be useful in the acute care setting. There is little firm evidence to guide nutritional management in patients with acute respiratory failure (Chapters 221 and 224).

Current evidence supports maintaining the head of the bed at a 45-degree angle to reduce aspiration in critically ill patients. Attempts should be made to ensure a normal day-night sleep pattern, including minimizing activity and reducing direct lighting at night. The patient should change position frequently, including sitting in a chair and walking short distances if possible, even while receiving mechanical ventilatory support. Mobilization can enhance the removal of secretions, help maintain musculoskeletal function, reduce the risk of deep vein thrombosis, and provide psychological benefits.

SPECIFIC ACUTE RESPIRATORY FAILURE SYNDROMES

Chronic Obstructive Pulmonary Disease

EPIDEMIOLOGY AND PATHOBIOLOGY

The epidemiology and pathobiology of COPD are discussed in Chapter 88.

CLINICAL MANIFESTATIONS

When COPD causes acute respiratory failure, patients commonly have a history of increasing dyspnea and sputum production. Acute respiratory failure may manifest in more cryptic ways, however, such as changes in mental status, arrhythmias, or other cardiovascular abnormalities. Acute respiratory failure must be considered whenever patients with COPD have significant nonspecific clinical changes.

DIAGNOSIS

The diagnosis can be confirmed or excluded by arterial blood gas analysis. The pH is helpful in assessing whether the hypoventilation is partly or exclusively acute: The pH drops by approximately 0.08 for each 10 mm Hg rise in the Pa_{CO_2} in acute respiratory acidosis without renal compensation. By comparison, in chronic respiratory acidosis with normal renal compensation, the pH drops only about 0.03 for each 10 mm Hg rise in the Pa_{CO_2}.

TREATMENT Rx

General Care

As soon as acute respiratory failure is confirmed in a patient with COPD, attention must focus on detecting any precipitating events (Table 104-4), including decreased ventilatory drive, commonly because of oversedation; decreased muscle strength or function, often related to electrolyte abnormalities, including hypophosphatemia and hypomagnesemia; decreased chest wall elasticity, possibly related to rib fracture, pleural effusion, ileus, or ascites; atelectasis, pneumonia, or pulmonary edema; increased airway resistance, caused by bronchospasm or increased secretions; or increased metabolic O_2 requirements, such as with systemic infection. Many of these abnormalities can impair the cough mechanism, diminish the clearance of airway secretions, and precipitate acute respiratory failure.

Infection

The most common specific precipitating event is airway infection, especially acute bronchitis. The role played by viral agents, *Mycoplasma pneumoniae,* chronic contaminants of the lower airway such as *Haemophilus influenzae* and *Streptococcus pneumoniae,* and other acute pathogens is difficult to determine on a clinical or even microbiologic basis. Acute exacerbations of COPD commonly result from new infections rather than re-emergence of an infection from preexisting colonization. Antibiotics modestly shorten the duration of the exacerbation, with no significant increase in toxicity, compared with placebo; the impact of antibiotics on the subsequent emergence of resistant organisms is not known. It is standard practice to use antibiotics to treat a patient with COPD who has an exacerbation severe enough to cause acute respiratory failure and who has evidence consistent with acute tracheobronchitis (Chapters 88 and 96). Pneumonia may account for 20% of cases of acute respiratory failure in patients with COPD. Compared with the physiologically normal population, patients with COPD who have community-acquired pneumonia are more likely to have gram-negative enteric bacteria or *Legionella* infections and are more likely to have antibiotic-resistant organisms.

Other Precipitating Causes

Other common precipitating causes of acute respiratory failure include heart failure and worsening of the underlying COPD, often related to noncompliance with medications. Less common and often difficult to diagnose in this setting is pulmonary thromboembolism.

TABLE 104-4 KEY PRINCIPLES IN THE MANAGEMENT OF CHRONIC OBSTRUCTIVE PULMONARY DISEASE PATIENTS WITH ACUTE RESPIRATORY FAILURE

1. Monitor and treat life-threatening hypoxemia (these measures should be performed virtually simultaneously).
   a. Assess the patient clinically, and measure oxygenation by arterial blood gases and/or oximetry.
      (1) If the patient is hypoxemic, initiate supplemental oxygen therapy with nasal prongs (low flows [0.5-2. L/min] are usually sufficient) or by Venturi face mask (24 or 28% oxygen delivered).
      (2) If the patient needs ventilatory support, consider noninvasive ventilation.
      (3) Determine whether the patient needs to be intubated; this is almost always a clinical decision. Immediate action is required if the patient is comatose or severely obtunded.
   b. A reasonable goal in most patients is Pao_2 of 55-60 mm Hg or Sao_2 of 88-90%.
   c. After changes in Fio_2, check blood gases and check regularly for signs of carbon dioxide retention.
2. Start to correct life-threatening acidosis.
   a. The most effective approach is to correct the underlying cause of ARF (e.g., bronchospasm, infection, heart failure).
   b. Consider ventilatory support, based largely on clinical considerations.
   c. With severe acidosis, the use of bicarbonate can be considered, but it is often ineffective, and there is little evidence of a clinical benefit.
3. If ventilatory support is required, consider noninvasive mechanical ventilation.
   a. The patient must have intact upper airway reflexes and be alert, cooperative, and hemodynamically stable.
   b. Careful monitoring is required; if the patient does not tolerate the mask, becomes hemodynamically unstable, or has a deteriorating mental status, consider intubation.
4. Treat airway obstruction and the underlying disease process that triggered the episode of ARF.
   a. Treat airway obstruction with pharmacologic agents: systemic corticosteroids and bronchodilators (ipratropium and/or β-adrenergic agents).
   b. Improve secretion clearance: encourage the patient to cough, administer chest physical therapy if cough is impaired and a trial appears effective.
   c. Treat the underlying disease process (e.g., antibiotics, diuretics).
5. Prevent complications of the disease process and minimize iatrogenic complications.
   a. Pulmonary thromboembolism prophylaxis: use subcutaneous heparin if no contraindications exist.
   b. Gastrointestinal complications: administer prophylaxis for gastrointestinal bleeding.
   c. Hemodynamics: if the patient is ventilated, monitor and minimize auto-PEEP.
      (1) Treat the underlying obstruction.
      (2) Minimize minute ventilation; use controlled hypoventilation.
      (3) Use small tidal volumes; increase the inspiratory flow rate to decrease the inspiratory time and lengthen the expiratory time.
   d. Cardiac arrhythmias: maintain oxygenation and normalize electrolytes.

ARF = acute respiratory failure; Fio_2 = fraction of inspired oxygen; Pao_2 = partial pressure of oxygen in arterial blood; PEEP = positive end-expiratory pressure; Sao_2 = oxygen saturation.

TABLE 104-5 DISORDERS ASSOCIATED WITH ACUTE LUNG INJURY AND ACUTE RESPIRATORY DISTRESS SYNDROME

COMMON

Sepsis (gram-positive or gram-negative bacterial, viral, fungal, or parasitic infection)
Diffuse pneumonia (bacterial, viral, or fungal)
Aspiration of gastric contents
Trauma (usually severe)

LESS COMMON

Near-drowning (fresh or salt water)
Drug overdose
  Acetylsalicylic acid
  Heroin and other narcotic drugs
Massive blood transfusion (likely a marker of severe trauma, but also seen with severe gastrointestinal bleeding, especially in patients with severe liver disease)
Leukoagglutination reactions
Inhalation of smoke or corrosive gases (usually requires high concentrations)
Pancreatitis
Fat embolism

UNCOMMON

Miliary tuberculosis
Paraquat poisoning
Central nervous system injury or anoxia (neurogenic pulmonary edema)
Cardiopulmonary bypass

Site of Care

Many patients with COPD and acute respiratory failure can be managed on a general medical hospital floor rather than in an intensive care unit if the precipitating cause of acute respiratory failure has been diagnosed and is potentially responsive to appropriate therapy, if any blood gas abnormalities respond to O_2 therapy and are not life-threatening, if the patient can cooperate with the treatment, and if appropriate nursing and respiratory care can be provided (Chapter 88). An unstable patient who requires closer observation and monitoring should be admitted to an intensive care unit.

Mechanical Therapy

The decision to use mechanical ventilation in patients with COPD and acute respiratory failure must be made on clinical grounds and is not dictated by any particular arterial blood gas values. In general, if the patient is alert and is able to cooperate with treatment, mechanical ventilation is unlikely to be necessary. If ventilatory support is required (Chapter 105), the decision is whether to use noninvasive positive-pressure ventilation therapy (without endotracheal intubation) or endotracheal intubation with positive-pressure ventilation. Many studies have demonstrated that noninvasive positive-pressure ventilation is preferred for patients with COPD and can decrease mortality if applied in appropriate patients with no factors that are likely to lead to complications.[3]

PROGNOSIS

Acute respiratory failure in patients with severe COPD is associated with an in-hospital mortality of 6 to 20%. The severity of the underlying disease and the severity of the acute precipitating illness are important determinants of hospital survival. Hospital mortality is higher if the respiratory failure is associated with a pH less than 7.25. The pH, the $Paco_2$, and other clinical characteristics are not very reliable in predicting a particular patient's chances of survival.

Acute Lung Injury/Acute Respiratory Distress Syndrome

DEFINITION

ARDS was first described in 1967 as the abrupt onset of diffuse lung injury characterized by severe hypoxemia (shunting) and generalized pulmonary infiltrates on the chest radiograph in the absence of overt cardiac failure. In the early 1990s the term *acute lung injury* was officially introduced to include traditional ARDS and less severe forms of lung injury. Both acute lung injury and ARDS, by definition, require bilateral pulmonary infiltrates compatible with pulmonary edema in the absence of clinical heart failure (usually determined by the lack of elevated left atrial pressures). The two are differentiated by the degree of abnormal oxygenation: Patients are defined as having acute lung injury if the Pao_2 divided by the Fio_2 (Pao_2/Fio_2, also called the P/F ratio) is less than or equal to 300. When the Pao_2/Fio_2 is less than or equal to 200, the patient meets the criteria for ARDS.

EPIDEMIOLOGY

Acute lung injury and ARDS are major public health problems and major causes of death. The annual incidence of acute lung injury is about 80 cases per 100,000 adult population. Case-fatality rates are 30 to 50% and are highly dependent on disease severity and the underlying predisposing condition.

ETIOLOGY

Acute lung injury is a clinical syndrome triggered by some other cause (Table 104-5). This underlying precipitating factor may affect and injure the lungs directly, such as in diffuse pneumonia or aspiration of gastric contents, or it may affect the lungs indirectly, such as in severe sepsis (Chapter 108) or severe nonthoracic trauma (Chapter 112). Severe sepsis is the most common precipitating cause of acute lung injury worldwide. The organisms vary widely, ranging from gram-negative and gram-positive bacteria and viruses (e.g., H1N1 influenza in 2009) to leptospiral infections or malaria. It may be difficult to determine whether pneumonia is diffuse, with endobronchial spread involving most of the lungs, or whether localized pneumonia has precipitated a sepsis syndrome, with secondary injury to other parts of the lung.

PATHOBIOLOGY

Pathology

Despite the variety of underlying disease processes leading to acute lung injury, the response to these insults in the lung is monotonously characteristic, with similar clinical findings, physiologic changes, and morphologic abnormalities. The pathologic abnormalities in acute lung injury and ARDS are nonspecific and are described as *diffuse alveolar damage* by pathologists. The initial process is inflammatory, with neutrophils usually predominating in the alveolar fluid. Hyaline membranes develop, similar to those seen in premature infants with infant respiratory distress syndrome, presumably related to the presence of large-molecular-weight proteins that have leaked into the alveolar space. Alveolar flooding leads to impairment of surfactant, which is abnormal in quantity and quality. The result is microatelectasis, which may be associated with impaired immune function. Cytokines and other inflammatory mediators are usually markedly elevated, although with different patterns over time in the bronchoalveolar lavage fluid and the systemic blood. Lung repair is also disturbed; early evidence of pro-fibrotic processes includes the appearance of breakdown products of pro-collagen in the bronchoalveolar lavage fluid, followed by scarring. The pulmonary fibrosis observed on lung biopsy or at autopsy is identical to that seen in patients with idiopathic pulmonary fibrosis (Chapter 92). Because lung function improves over time in survivors of ARDS, however, it has been assumed that this scarring is often reversible.

Pathophysiology

The physiologic abnormalities are dominated by severe hypoxemia with shunting, decreased lung compliance, decreased functional residual capacity, and increased work of breathing. Initially, the $Paco_2$ is low or normal, usually associated with increased alveolar ventilation. The initial abnormalities in oxygenation are thought to be related to alveolar flooding and collapse. As the disease progresses, especially in patients who require ventilatory support, fibroproliferation develops; the lungs (including alveoli, blood vessels, and small airways) remodel and scar, with a loss of microvasculature. These changes may lead to pulmonary hypertension and increased dead space; marked elevations in minute ventilation are required to achieve a normal $Paco_2$, even as oxygenation abnormalities are improving.

CLINICAL MANIFESTATIONS

In most cases of acute lung injury, the onset either coincides with or occurs within 72 hours of the onset of the underlying disease process; the mean time from onset of the underlying cause to onset of acute lung injury is 12 to 24 hours. The presenting picture is dominated by respiratory distress and the accompanying laboratory findings of severe hypoxemia and generalized infiltrates or opacities on the chest radiograph. Alternatively, it may be dominated by manifestations of the underlying disease process, such as severe sepsis with hypotension and other manifestations of systemic infection.

DIAGNOSIS

The key to diagnosis is to distinguish ARDS from cardiogenic pulmonary edema (Table 104-6). No specific biochemical test exists to define ARDS. Certain blood or bronchoalveolar lavage (Chapter 85) abnormalities are frequent but are not sufficiently specific to be useful clinically.

TABLE 104-6 FEATURES ASSOCIATED WITH NONCARDIOGENIC AND CARDIOGENIC PULMONARY EDEMA*

NONCARDIOGENIC EDEMA (ARDS)	CARDIOGENIC EDEMA/VOLUME OVERLOAD
PRIOR HISTORY	
Younger	Older
No history of heart disease	Prior history of heart disease
Appropriate fluid balance (difficult to assess after resuscitation from shock or trauma)	Hypertension, chest pain, new-onset palpitations; positive fluid balance
PHYSICAL EXAMINATION	
Flat neck veins	Elevated neck veins
Hyperdynamic pulses	Left ventricular enlargement, lift, heave, dyskinesis
Physiologic gallop	S_3 and S_4; murmurs
Absence of edema	Edema: flank, presacral, legs
ELECTROCARDIOGRAM	
Sinus tachycardia, nonspecific ST-T wave changes	Evidence of prior or ongoing ischemia, supraventricular tachycardia, left ventricular hypertrophy
CHEST RADIOGRAPH	
Normal heart size	Cardiomegaly
Peripheral distribution of infiltrates	Central or basilar infiltrates; peribronchial and vascular congestion
Air bronchograms common (80%)	Septal lines (Kerley's lines), air bronchograms (25%), pleural effusion
HEMODYNAMIC MEASUREMENTS	
Pulmonary artery wedge pressure <15 mm Hg, cardiac index >3.5 L/min/m^2	Pulmonary capillary wedge pressure >18 mm Hg, cardiac index <3.5 L/min/m^2 with ischemia, may be >3.5 L/min/m^2 with volume overload

*These features are neither highly sensitive nor specific. Although the findings are more commonly associated with the type of pulmonary edema as listed, they do not have high positive or negative predictive value.
ARDS = acute respiratory distress syndrome.

TREATMENT Rx

Treatment for acute lung injury and ARDS consists predominantly of respiratory support and treatment of the underlying disease (Fig. 104-4). Although sepsis is a common predisposing condition for the development of acute lung injury, a small study examining the usefulness of activated protein C in patients with acute lung injury did not demonstrate any beneficial effects in terms of ventilator-free days or mortality.

Mechanical Therapy

Current recommendations for mechanical ventilation via endotracheal intubation (Table 104-7) emphasize lower tidal volumes based on the patient's predicted body weight (Chapter 105).[4] PEEP is a mainstay in the ventilatory strategy for acute lung injury; although the method for determining the optimal level of PEEP has not been established, higher PEEP levels appear to benefit patients with ARDS.[4,5] PEEP may allow a lower Fio_2 to provide adequate oxygenation, thus avoiding O_2 toxicity. It also may prevent the cyclic collapse and reopening of lung units, a process that is thought to be a major cause of ventilator-induced lung injury, even when adequate oxygenation can be obtained at relatively low levels of Fio_2. The early use of cisatracurium besylate (15 mg rapid infusion followed by 37.5 mg/hr for 48 hours), a neuromuscular blocker, can reduce ARDS mortality rates by about 25%.[6] In patients with severe ARDS who do not respond to standard therapy but otherwise have a reasonable life expectancy, extracorporeal membrane oxygenation can improve the 6-month survival from 47 to 63% at an acceptable cost of about $35,000 per quality-adjusted year of life saved.[7]

Acute Respiratory Failure without Lung Disease

Acute respiratory failure without pulmonary abnormalities (see Table 104-2) is seen in patients with depressed ventilatory drive secondary to central nervous system dysfunction and in patients with severe neuromuscular disease. The prototypical patient with suppressed ventilatory drive has taken an overdose of a sedative or tranquilizing medication (Chapter 110). The prototypical patient with neuromuscular disease has Guillain-Barré syndrome (Chapter 428). The treatment for both types of patients is supportive. In the case of a patient with a sedative overdose, the threshold for intubation with mechanical ventilatory support should be low because this temporary condition is quickly reversible when the responsible drug is eliminated. Such a patient may require intubation for airway protection against aspiration of gastric contents.

Patients with Guillain-Barré syndrome or other forms of progressive neuromuscular disease should be monitored with serial measurements of vital capacity. In general, when the vital capacity decreases to less than 10 to 15 mL/kg body weight, intubation and mechanical ventilatory support should be considered without regard to the patient's $Paco_2$.

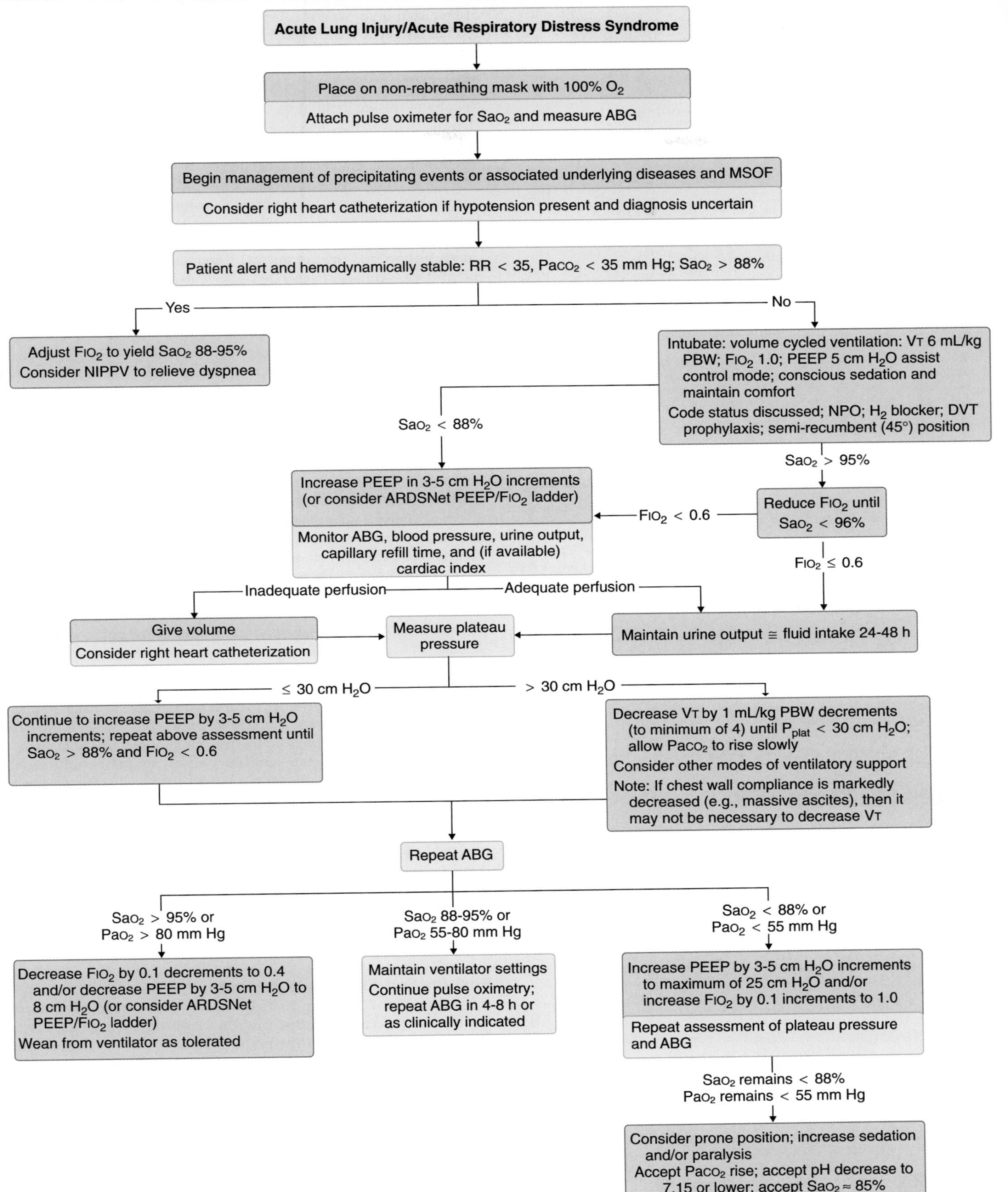

FIGURE 104-4. Algorithm for the initial management of acute respiratory distress syndrome. ABG = arterial blood gas analysis; CO_2 = carbon dioxide; DVT = deep vein thrombosis; F_{IO_2} = inspired oxygen concentration; MSOF = multisystem organ failure; NIPPV = noninvasive intermittent positive-pressure ventilation; O_2 = oxygen; Pa_{CO_2} = arterial partial pressure of carbon dioxide; Pa_{O_2} = arterial partial pressure of oxygen; PBW = predicted body weight; PEEP = positive end-expiratory pressure; P_{plat} = plateau pressure; RR = respiratory rate; Sa_{O_2} = arterial oxygen saturation; V_T = tidal volume.

TABLE 104-7 ARDSNet VENTILATORY MANAGEMENT PROTOCOL FOR TIDAL VOLUME AND PLATEAU PRESSURE

Calculate PBW:
Male PBW: 50 + 2.3 (height in inches − 60) or 50 + 0.91 (height in centimeters − 152.4)
Female PBW: 45.5 + 2.3 (height in inches − 60) or 45.5 + 0.91 (height in centimeters − 152.4)
Select assist control mode
Set initial VT at 8 mL/kg PBW
Reduce VT by 1 mL/kg at intervals < 2 hr until VT = 6 mL/kg PBW
Set initial RR to approximate baseline minute ventilation (maximum RR = 35/min)
Set inspiratory flow rate higher than patient's demand (usually > 80 L/min)
Adjust VT and RR further to achieve P_{plat} and pH goals
If P_{plat} > 30 cm H_2O: decrease VT by 1 mL/kg PBW (minimum = 4 mL/kg PBW)
If pH ≤ 7.30, increase RR (maximum = 35)
If pH < 7.15, increase RR to 35; consider sodium bicarbonate administration or increase VT

PBW = predicted body weight; P_{plat} = plateau pressure (airway pressure at the end of delivery of a tidal volume breath during a condition of no airflow); RR = respiratory rate; VT = tidal volume. See the ARDSNet website *(http://www.ardsnet.org)* for further details about the protocol, including the approach for setting positive end-expiratory pressure and fraction of inspired oxygen.

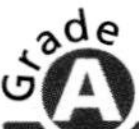

1. Wheeler AP, Bernard GR, Thompson BT, et al. National Heart, Lung, and Blood Institute Acute Respiratory Distress Syndrome (ARDS) Clinical Trials Network: pulmonary-artery versus central venous catheter to guide treatment of acute lung injury. *N Engl J Med.* 2006;354:2213-2224.
2. The National Heart, Lung, and Blood Institute Acute Respiratory Distress Syndrome (ARDS) Clinical Trials Network. Comparison of two fluid-management strategies in acute lung injury. *N Engl J Med.* 2006;354:2564-2575.
3. Ram FS, Lightowler JV, Wedzicha JA. Non-invasive positive pressure ventilation for treatment of respiratory failure due to exacerbations of chronic obstructive pulmonary disease. *Cochrane Database Syst Rev.* 2004.3.CD004104.
4. Putensen C, Theuerkauf N, Zinserling J, et al. Meta-analysis: ventilation strategies and outcomes of the acute respiratory distress syndrome and acute lung injury. *Ann Intern Med.* 2009;151:566-576.
5. Briel M, Meade M, Mercat A, et al. Higher vs lower positive end-expiratory pressure in patients with acute lung injury and acute respiratory distress syndrome: systematic review and meta-analysis. *JAMA.* 2010;303:865-873.
6. Papazian L, Forel JM, Gacouin A, et al. Neuromuscular blockers in early acute respiratory distress syndrome. *N Engl J Med.* 2010;363:1107-1116.
7. Peek GJ, Mugford M, Tiruvoipati R, et al. Efficacy and economic assessment of conventional ventilatory support versus extracorporeal membrane oxygenation for severe adult respiratory failure (CESAR): a multicentre randomized controlled trial. *Lancet.* 2009;374:1351-1363.

SUGGESTED READINGS

Del Sorbo L, Slutsky AS. Acute respiratory distress syndrome and multiple organ failure. *Curr Opin Crit Care.* 2011;17:1-6. *Review.*

Esan A, Hess DR, Raoof S, et al. Severe hypoxemic respiratory failure: part 1—ventilatory strategies. *Chest.* 2010;137:1203-1216. *Review.*

Raoof S, Goulet K, Esan A, et al. Severe hypoxemic respiratory failure: part 2—nonventilatory strategies. *Chest.* 2010;137:1437-1448. *Review.*

105

MECHANICAL VENTILATION

ARTHUR S. SLUTSKY AND LEONARD D. HUDSON

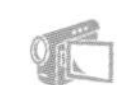

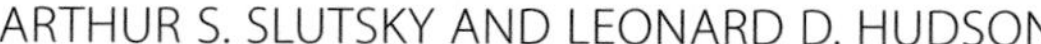

DEFINITION

Mechanical ventilation, a life-sustaining therapy for patients with respiratory failure (Chapter 104), is provided partially or fully by external sources through a variety of mechanical strategies termed *modes of ventilation.* In addition to providing ventilation, the treating physician can also alter the inspired oxygen tension, the pressure at the airway opening at the end of a breath, and other facets of the volume or pressure time pattern imposed on the patient. Current approaches focus on ventilatory strategies that minimize iatrogenic injury through the use of tidal volumes on the order of 6 mL/kg of predicted body weight or end-inspiratory airway pressures of 25-30 cm H_2O or less, even if the arterial blood gases achieved are not in the "normal range."

TYPES OF MECHANICAL VENTILATORS

Negative-Pressure Ventilators

Delivery of gas to the lungs requires a hydrostatic pressure gradient between the airway opening and the airways and alveoli. During spontaneous breathing, this pressure gradient is generated by development of a negative pleural pressure as a result of contraction of the respiratory muscles. Some ventilators operate by generating negative pressure around the chest wall (e.g., cuirass) or the entire body below the neck (e.g., iron lung). Such ventilators have two major advantages: there is no need to intubate the patient to apply mechanical ventilation, and the detrimental hemodynamic consequences are minimized if the ventilators generate negative pressure solely around the chest wall. However, these ventilators have several difficulties. First, the device around the chest wall or the patient's body used to apply the negative pressure must have an adequate seal so that the negative pressure is not dissipated to the room—a task that is not always easy to accomplish in a manner that is comfortable for the patient. Second, the nursing care of patients in such ventilators can be difficult, especially with iron lungs, which enclose the entire patient from the neck down. Although this type of ventilator was widely used during the polio epidemic of the mid-1950s, its only current use is for patients who have relatively normal lungs but who require long-term ventilation for neuromuscular problems.

Positive-Pressure Ventilators

The most widely used mechanical ventilation approach is to deliver gas to the lung using positive-pressure ventilation (PPV) applied through an endotracheal tube, a tracheostomy, or a tight-fitting mask. The approach using a mask is considered noninvasive ventilation (NIV) and is considered separately.

The most basic mode of PPV is *controlled ventilation,* in which a preset tidal volume at a predetermined rate is delivered to the patient regardless of the patient's requirements or efforts. This form of ventilation is usually used in patients who cannot initiate spontaneous breaths (e.g., heavily sedated or paralyzed patients) or in those who need full ventilatory support because of extremely severe pulmonary or cardiovascular disease (e.g., severe shock). This mode is not routinely used in patients who are able to make spontaneous ventilatory efforts because it can lead to asynchrony between the patient's efforts and the breaths generated by the ventilator. *Assisted ventilation* is the term used when spontaneous ventilatory efforts are present; the onset of a breath is triggered by the patient's respiratory efforts, rather than being based strictly on the time between breaths.

Mechanical ventilation can be applied using either volume-controlled or pressure-controlled modes. In volume-controlled ventilation, the desired tidal volume and respiratory rate are set by the user, and the airway pressure is the dependent variable that changes with the mechanical properties of the patient's respiratory system and with the flow settings on the ventilator. In pressure-controlled ventilation, the pressure imposed at the airway opening and the respiratory rate are set by the user, and the tidal volume becomes the dependent variable.

Positive End-Expiratory Pressure

A key characteristic that can be used with any of the modes of ventilation is the level of the end-expiratory pressure. Positive end-expiratory pressure (PEEP) is used in patients with diffuse pulmonary diseases (e.g., pulmonary edema, acute respiratory distress syndrome [ARDS]) to recruit collapsed alveolar regions and to maintain them in a recruited state, to reopen collapsed airways, to redistribute fluid in the lung, to increase functional residual capacity, and to redistribute ventilation to dependent regions. All these changes can improve the ratio of ventilation to perfusion as well as oxygenation, thereby allowing the fractional inspiratory concentration of oxygen (FIO_2) to be reduced. PEEP does not usually improve alveolar ventilation and, in fact, may increase dead space by overdistending alveoli, with a concomitant decrease in alveolar capillary blood flow in certain regions of the lung. PEEP can also be administered to spontaneously breathing subjects by using a technique termed *continuous positive airway pressure.* Continuous positive airway pressure and PEEP can be used in patients with exacerbations of chronic obstructive pulmonary disease (COPD) to overcome auto-PEEP (see later) and to minimize the work of breathing, provided the magnitude of the PEEP is low enough that it does not cause additional hyperinflation.

Volume-Controlled Ventilation

The term *volume-controlled ventilation* (or *volume-limited ventilation*) refers to mechanical ventilation in which the tidal volume is preset. The major advantage is that the delivered tidal volume is maintained even if lung mechanics change, thereby ensuring a more constant partial pressure of arterial carbon dioxide ($PaCO_2$). The potential disadvantage is that if lung mechanics deteriorate, higher pressures may be required to achieve the tidal volume goal, and regions of overinflation with lung injury may result. Although controlled ventilation as described earlier can be either volume limited (preset tidal volume) or pressure limited (preset peak airway pressure), clinicians usually use the term *controlled mechanical ventilation* to refer to volume-limited ventilation with a set rate. In volume-controlled ventilation, an upper limit to applied airway pressure is commonly included for safety reasons.

The most common form of volume-controlled ventilation is one in which the patient assists the ventilator, thus triggering at least some of the breaths. The term *assisted mechanical ventilation* can refer either to volume-limited ventilation or to pressure-limited ventilation when the patient triggers some or all of the breaths, but the ventilator will always deliver a minimum number of breaths if apnea occurs. This mode is also referred to as *assist/control* (A/C).

Intermittent Mandatory Ventilation

The term *intermittent mandatory ventilation* (IMV) refers to a mode in which the patient is allowed to breathe spontaneously through an endotracheal tube or tracheostomy but also receives some preset (and thus mandatory) volume-limited breaths from the ventilator. In current ventilators, the mandatory breaths are triggered by the patient and thus are synchronized (synchronized IMV); however, if the patient ceases spontaneous ventilatory efforts, breaths at the rate set on the ventilator will still be delivered. Synchronized IMV is a form of partial ventilatory support because some breaths are spontaneous, rather than full ventilatory support, in which all breaths are delivered by the ventilator. This mode allows the patient to do a variable amount of the respiratory work but with the security of a set minimal backup rate should spontaneous ventilatory efforts stop.

Pressure-Control Ventilation

Pressure-control ventilation is a type of ventilation in which the ventilator delivers pressure-limited breaths to the patient; delivered volume becomes a dependent variable. The initiation of each breath may be triggered by the patient (assisted breaths) or may be initiated by the ventilator (controlled breaths). The delivered tidal volume depends on the preset pressure, the ventilatory rate, the inspiratory-to-expiratory ratio, and the patient's respiratory mechanics (resistance, compliance, and auto-PEEP). At a fixed preset pressure and inspiratory-to-expiratory ratio, tidal volume decreases as respiratory frequency increases. In patients with COPD, the tidal volume at low frequencies is relatively high but decreases substantially as the respiratory rate is increased, whereas in patients with stiff respiratory systems (e.g., ARDS), the tidal volume does not change much with respiratory frequency because the lung fills with gas quickly.

Pressure-Support Ventilation

Pressure-support ventilation is a pressure-limited, patient-triggered ventilatory mode. Once the patient triggers the ventilator, by creating either a small negative pressure or a low inspiratory flow at the airway, the ventilator switches to inspiratory mode and provides the airflow needed to maintain a preset level of pressure. In contrast to pressure-control ventilation, inspiration terminates when the inspiratory airflow decreases to a threshold level (the specific algorithm varies from ventilator to ventilator). This mode provides flexibility for the patient with respect to tidal volume, inspiratory flow, and ratio of time allowed for inspiration as compared with expiration. Tidal volume depends on patient-related factors (effort), respiratory system mechanics, and the level of pressure set for support. Pressure-support ventilation is a form of partial ventilatory support in which the size of each breath is determined partially by the patient's muscular effort and partially by the ventilator. This mode can compensate for the added work of breathing imposed by the resistance of the endotracheal tube compared with the natural airway. Pressure-support ventilation has largely been used to wean patients from ventilatory support because it provides a simple way to reduce the magnitude of mechanical support while the patient assumes a larger fraction of the ventilatory work than with most other modes of assisted ventilation.

High-Frequency Ventilation

The term *high-frequency ventilation* refers to certain ventilatory modes that have the common feature of providing ventilation using frequencies that are substantially greater than those used during normal breathing. Several different approaches are used for the delivery of high-frequency ventilation: high-frequency PPV, high-frequency jet ventilation, and high-frequency oscillatory ventilation. During high-frequency ventilation, tidal volumes may be less than the dead space, so adequate gas transport takes place by various convective and diffusive mechanisms. Interest in using these modes of ventilation has waxed and waned over the past 2 decades. In recent years, interest in high-frequency ventilation has had a resurgence, based on the concept that it may be the ideal way to minimize ventilator-induced lung injury because the small tidal volumes make it easier to avoid both overdistention of lung units and injury that occurs during ventilation at low lung volumes. Animal data in support of this approach are very strong in models of acute lung injury. Recent data in infants with respiratory distress syndrome and in adults with ARDS suggest that high-frequency ventilation may be as effective as conventional mechanical ventilatory assistance.

Proportional Assist Ventilation and Neurally Adjusted Ventilatory Assist

One of the difficulties when providing assisted ventilation to patients is ensuring that there is adequate synchrony between the patient's respiratory drive and the delivery of each breath from the ventilator. This issue is particularly problematic for patients with severe obstructive airways disease, especially if they have significant auto-PEEP. Two newer modes of ventilation, proportional assist ventilation (PAV) and neurally adjusted ventilatory assist (NAVA), have been developed and implemented on some ventilators in part to address this concern. Both these modes deliver ventilation in proportion to the instantaneous effort of the patient, but the underlying principles are different. Although both of these modes improve patient-ventilator synchrony, data are insufficient to know whether either will improve clinically important outcomes.

PAV is based on the mathematical relationships between airway pressure and airflow; these state that the pressure applied by the respiratory muscles is used to overcome the elastic forces (i.e., compliance) and the resistive forces of the respiratory system. With PAV, the pressure that is applied during inspiration varies based on the patient's inspiratory effort and respiratory system mechanics. This form of ventilation is not in widespread use currently, in part because of its complexity and the need to estimate the patient's compliance and resistance on a regular basis. This latter issue has been addressed in new versions of the technique in which intermittent measurements of compliance and resistance are automatically measured repeatedly.

By contrast, NAVA makes use of the electrical activity of the diaphragm (Edi) as measured by an array of electrodes attached to a nasogastric tube inserted into the esophagus. Pressure is then delivered by the ventilator in direct proportion to the (virtually) instantaneous Edi. Because the initiation and delivery of the breath by the ventilator is not dependent on measurement of pressures in the lung, patient-ventilator synchrony is improved in patients with auto-PEEP. The mode is relatively easy to use; the only parameter to set is the proportionality factor linking the Edi and the pressure delivered by the ventilator.

Noninvasive Positive-Pressure Ventilation

Since the mid-1990s, interest in providing PPV through a mask rather than through an endotracheal tube has increased. This method has been termed *noninvasive* because the patient is not intubated. This approach, although conceptually simple, requires appropriate implementation and monitoring for its successful application. Of particular importance are the selection of patients and the appropriate training of hospital personnel. Patients must be alert, cooperative, and hemodynamically stable. Patients must also have intact upper airway reflexes, so they do not aspirate upper airway materials into the lung, and they must not have any facial trauma that would preclude the use of a mask. Once patients are started on NIV, they should be carefully monitored, and NIV should be discontinued if the patient does not tolerate the mask, if it becomes clear from clinical examination that the patient may aspirate, if cardiovascular instability exists, or if the patient's mental status is deteriorating. NIV can also be delivered through a "helmet" that avoids some of the problems associated with the use of face masks.

NIV has certain potential advantages compared with invasive ventilation. It is relatively easy to apply and can be used for short intervals because it can be started and stopped very easily. The major advantages are that it avoids the complications associated with intubation, it is usually more comfortable for the patient, and it reduces the need for sedation. Patients receiving NIV are able to communicate verbally with medical staff and family members, are likely able to sleep better, and are able to eat if they are sufficiently stable to remove the mask for short periods of time.

However, NIV has several disadvantages. Implementation of NIV takes more time from caregivers at the bedside initially, and the time course of correction of blood gases is slower than usually occurs in patients who are intubated and ventilated. Gastric distention is an unusual occurrence; medical staff should be aware of this complication and should watch for signs of abdominal distention. Data strongly support the use of NIV for patients with COPD (see later), and it is preferred in cardiogenic pulmonary edema,[1] but whether it provides better outcomes in other forms of respiratory failure is uncertain.

COMPLICATIONS

Intubation

Endotracheal intubation can be used to secure a patient's airway, to act as a conduit to deliver gas from the ventilator to the patient, to prevent aspiration, and to help with pulmonary toilet when secretions are increased. However, intubation can be associated with certain complications, including upper airway trauma, disruption of normal host defense mechanisms, and the risk of aspiration during insertion of the endotracheal tube. Pressure from the cuff of the tube that provides a pneumatic seal between the tube and trachea can lead to regions of tracheal ischemia and may eventually cause tracheal stenosis as a result of injury repair processes. The endotracheal tube causes an increase in airway resistance because its diameter is smaller than the airway into which it is inserted. The magnitude of the increase depends on the length, diameter, and shape of the tube as well as the buildup of secretions and mucus that narrow the tube's diameter. Furthermore, the upper airway is normally a very effective means of heating and humidifying inspiratory gases. This natural system is bypassed by an endotracheal tube; inadequately humidified inspiratory gases can reduce mucociliary clearance and can lead to inspissation of tracheal secretions.

Cough is impaired in patients in whom an endotracheal tube has been placed. Normally, cough involves an increase in airway pressure as respiratory muscles are contracted against a closed glottis. When the glottis opens, expiratory flow sharply increases, resulting in dynamic compression of major airways. The presence of an endotracheal tube limits the buildup of airway pressure and alters the dynamics of expiratory flow, thereby greatly impairing the efficacy of the patient's cough.

A cuffed endotracheal tube helps to prevent gross aspiration, but pharyngeal secretions that pool at the top of the cuff often seep into the lungs and increase the probability of developing nosocomial pneumonia (Chapter 97). Endotracheal tubes also make swallowing and communication difficult. Silver-coated tubes reduce the risk of ventilator-associated pneumonia but are considerably more expensive than conventional endotracheal tubes and are unlikely to be used routinely for initial intubation. Endotracheal tubes with a port that allows suctioning of secretions above the cuff may also reduce the incidence of ventilator-associated pneumonia, although results of studies have been mixed.

Hemodynamic Compromise

The major mechanical determinants of cardiovascular hemodynamics during mechanical ventilation are intrathoracic pressure, changes in lung volume, and the patient's circulatory volume status. An increase in lung volume can cause a beneficial decrease in pulmonary vascular resistance, if lung units that had been closed are opened as a result of mechanical ventilation, or it can lead to a detrimental increase in pulmonary vascular resistance related to overdistention of the lung with concomitant compression and lengthening of alveolar vessels.

PPV can have a major impact on cardiovascular hemodynamics through its effect on pleural pressure, an effect that is directly related to changes in lung volume and not necessarily directly reflected in measurements of airway pressure; the relation between alveolar pressure and lung volume depends on respiratory system mechanics. For example, in a patient with stiff lungs (e.g., ARDS), a given increase in plateau pressure (Pplat) will lead to much less of an increase in lung volume than in a patient with COPD, so the increase in pleural pressure will be much less in the patient with ARDS. As a result, patients with ARDS tolerate relatively high PEEP levels, whereas similarly high levels in patients with normal lungs (e.g., in a drug overdose) or in patients with COPD would markedly reduce cardiac output. At very high lung volumes, a direct effect of the pressure of the lung on the heart can increase pericardial pressure and can thereby decrease cardiac filling.

Auto-PEEP and Dynamic Hyperinflation

A key factor that affects cardiovascular hemodynamics and other physiologic variables during mechanical ventilation is the development of *auto-PEEP*, defined as the difference between alveolar pressure and airway pressure at the end of expiration. Auto-PEEP leads to dynamic hyperinflation, which is an increase in the end-expiratory lung volume higher than the value that would be obtained if there were complete exhalation to the static functional residual capacity. This phenomenon occurs whenever time is insufficient for a complete exhalation to occur; the respiratory system is thus prevented from reaching its static end-expiratory volume. The major determinants of auto-PEEP and hence dynamic hyperinflation are increased expiratory airway resistance, high minute ventilation, increased respiratory system compliance, and decreased expiratory time.

Auto-PEEP is more likely to occur in patients with airway obstruction. Avoidance of high levels of auto-PEEP using approaches such as controlled hypoventilation is a fundamental principle when ventilating patients with airways obstruction.

Auto-PEEP may not be detected by routine measurements of pressure at the airway opening because the major pressure drop occurs across the airways. Moreover, measurements of auto-PEEP are difficult to make in spontaneously breathing patients. When patients are not making spontaneous breathing efforts, auto-PEEP can be assessed as the difference in pressure between the set PEEP and the pressure obtained when the airway opening is occluded at the end of expiration (Fig. 105-1). It can also be assessed using the change in Pplat after a prolonged pause during volume cycle ventilation. If it is considered safe for the patient, a rapid estimate of the effect of auto-PEEP on cardiovascular hemodynamics can be obtained by transiently disconnecting the ventilator and allowing the auto-PEEP to approach zero during a long expiration. If the auto-PEEP is less than 5 cm H_2O, it is unlikely to cause clinically important changes in the measured intravascular pressures.

If auto-PEEP is not considered in the interpretation of respiratory mechanics, measurements of respiratory system compliance will be falsely low.

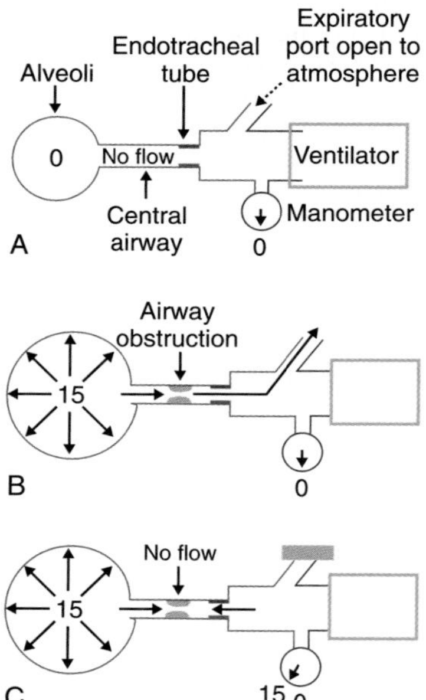

FIGURE 105-1. The relationships among alveolar, central airway, and ventilator circuit pressure at the end of exhalation under the following conditions: A, Normal conditions (no auto–positive end-expiratory pressure [auto-PEEP]). **B,** Severe dynamic airway obstruction with the expiratory port open. **C,** Severe dynamic airway obstruction with the expiratory port occluded at the end of exhalation. The auto-PEEP level is identified by creating an end-expiratory hold, thereby allowing the alveolar, central airway, and ventilator circuit pressures to equilibrate because there is no flow in the circuit. During equilibration, the level of auto-PEEP can be read on the manometer in the ventilator circuit (Adapted from Pepe PE, Marini JJ. Occult positive end-expiratory pressure in mechanically ventilated patients with airflow obstruction: the auto-PEEP effect. *Am Rev Respir Dis.* 1982;126:166-170.)

Dynamic hyperinflation can be measured as the volume of gas that is released when the expiratory time of a given breath is lengthened by 20 to 30 seconds. These techniques are based on the assumptions that no respiratory efforts are made and that the alveoli communicate with the airway opening, thereby allowing equilibration of pressures or exhalation of trapped gas. However, this assumption is not necessarily correct in patients with very severe airways obstruction (e.g., status asthmaticus).

Auto-PEEP should be suspected whenever flow at the end of expiration is detectable or when a patient fails to trigger the ventilator consistently with inspiratory efforts. This failure to trigger the ventilator occurs because the patient must generate sufficient pressure to overcome the level of auto-PEEP before a negative deflection of pressure or generation of inspiratory flow (either of which may be used by the ventilator to detect the onset of inspiration) is sensed at the airway opening.

Auto-PEEP and dynamic hyperinflation have numerous detrimental consequences. In a patient who is not breathing spontaneously, the dynamic hyperinflation increases pleural pressure and right atrial pressure, thereby leading to a decrease in the driving pressure for venous return, with a concomitant decrease in cardiac output. This effect can be magnified in the patient with airway obstruction immediately after intubation and initiation of mechanical ventilation because compensatory mechanisms to enhance venous return are impaired by pharmacologic agents that are often used to prepare the patient for endotracheal tube insertion and that also reduce venous and arterial tone. In such patients, auto-PEEP can also lead to gross misinterpretation of vascular pressures. For example, the absolute value of capillary wedge pressure will be directly affected by the increase in intrathoracic pressure during auto-PEEP. The clinician may interpret this high (absolute) capillary wedge pressure as indicating adequate ventricular filling, when, in fact, transmural capillary wedge pressure is low because intrathoracic pressure is also high. This misinterpretation, coupled with the decreased cardiac output related to the high intrathoracic pressure, may suggest the diagnosis of cardiogenic shock, rather than the correct diagnosis of auto-PEEP.

Treatment of the detrimental hemodynamic consequences of auto-PEEP include decreasing the level of auto-PEEP by increasing the expiratory time, decreasing airway resistance (e.g., bronchodilators, when appropriate), or decreasing minute ventilation. The last approach is usually the most effective ventilatory maneuver but results in an increase in the Pa_{CO_2}. Cardiovascular hemodynamics can also usually be restored by infusion of fluids.

In a spontaneously breathing patient, dynamic hyperinflation can markedly increase the oxygen cost of breathing for two reasons. First, because the respiratory system is stiffer at higher lung volumes, more energy is required to complete each ventilatory cycle. Second, to initiate flow into the lung, the patient must generate a pressure in the alveolar zone that is lower than atmospheric pressure. However, if dynamic hyperinflation is present, the patient first has to generate an inspiratory effort sufficient to overcome the (positive) end-expiratory alveolar pressure before he or she begins to lower alveolar pressure to less than atmospheric pressure to initiate airflow. The increase in lung volume associated with dynamic hyperinflation also has an impact on the effectiveness of the ventilatory muscles: at high lung volumes, the diaphragm is relatively flat, so it is at a mechanical disadvantage in producing changes in pleural pressure. Mechanical ventilation for just 18 to 69 hours causes extensive atrophy of diaphragmatic muscle fibers.

Ventilator-Induced Lung Injury

Mechanical ventilation itself can lead to numerous types of lung injuries (Fig. 105-2). The term *barotrauma* refers to large pulmonary air leaks, such as pneumothorax and pneumomediastinum. However, a much more subtle injury, *diffuse alveolar damage* presenting as pulmonary edema, also occurs. For both types of injuries, the critical factor is the degree of overdistention of the lung, best assessed by the transpulmonary pressure (Ptp, the airway opening minus pleural pressure). The esophageal pressure, measured using an esophageal balloon, estimates pleural pressure (Ppl), although this measurement has not been routinely performed in clinical practice.

The usual pressures measured during mechanical ventilation are airway pressures referenced to atmospheric pressure. The peak inspiratory pressure (PIP) is easy to measure, but its interpretation is not always simple. PIP represents the sum of the pressure required to inflate the lungs plus the pressure needed to overcome the resistance to flow. Thus, a high PIP does not necessarily indicate an increased propensity to the development of ventilator-induced lung injury. For example, if inspiratory flow is constant and a smaller endotracheal tube is used, PIP will increase even though the danger of pulmonary overdistention is no greater than would be present with

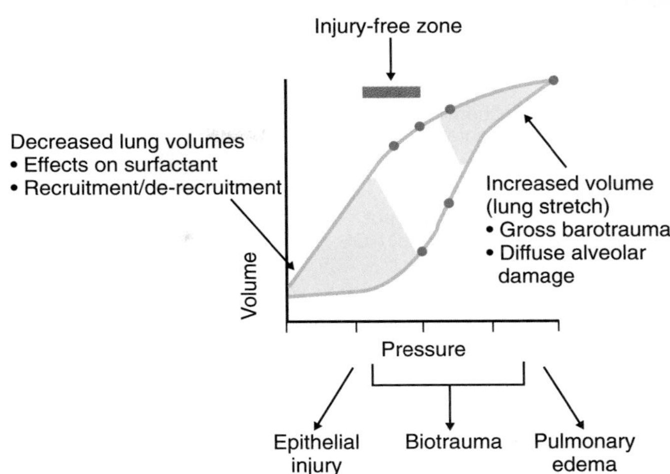

FIGURE 105-2. Schematic representation of the pressure-volume curve of a lung with diffuse alveolar edema. Mechanical ventilation can induce or worsen lung injury by numerous mechanisms when ventilation occurs at high lung volumes or when ventilation occurs at low lung volumes. Lung-protective strategies during ventilation of patients with acute respiratory distress syndrome should try to keep the ventilatory pattern in the *injury-free zone.* Data in patients confirm the benefit of ensuring that overdistention does not occur.

ventilation using a larger-bore tube. The Pplat, which is the airway pressure at the end of an end-inspiratory pause (>0.5 second), is the pressure that can be most easily measured at the bedside and that bears some relationship, depending on Ppl, to the development of overdistention; however, there is no single value of Pplat that is "dangerous" from a lung injury perspective because Ppl can vary so much. However, based on the ARDS Clinical Network (ARDSNet) study, a reasonable maximal value of Pplat in patients with acute lung injury is 30 cm H_2O. Certain caveats should be noted in interpreting Pplat and PIP, related to associated changes in Ppl. If the patient is breathing spontaneously, Ppl will be negative, and overdistention may occur even with a Pplat lower than 30 cm H_2O. Conversely, in a patient who is either paralyzed or not making ventilatory efforts and who has a very stiff chest wall (e.g., due to ascites, obesity, pregnancy), as airway pressure increases, most of the pressure drop will be dissipated across the chest wall, thus leading to values of Ppl that are positive. In this setting, a high Pplat may not be indicative of a high Ptp and hence may not indicate increased lung distention. Thus, the physician caring for a patient receiving mechanical ventilatory support must analyze the measured airway pressures within their clinical context. Measurement of Ppl, as noted earlier, may help resolve these difficulties.

During mechanical ventilation, some areas of the lung may undergo cyclic recruitment and derecruitment. This process, which is of particular importance in patients who have acute lung injury or ARDS, has been termed *atelectrauma* and can cause significant lung injury. The precise mechanisms of injury are not entirely clear but are thought to result from shear stress owing to opening and closing of lung units, regional hypoxia in atelectatic lung units, and effects on surfactant. Prevention of this type of injury provides part of the rationale for the use of PEEP to maintain recruitment of lung units during tidal ventilation.

Finally, evidence suggests that mechanical ventilation strategies that promote overdistention and atelectrauma can lead to an inflammatory response in the lung, a mechanism of injury termed *biotrauma,* through the release of certain pro-inflammatory cytokines and chemokines. To the extent that these mediators can translocate from the lung into the systemic circulation, they could potentially lead to dysfunction of other organs (Fig. 105-3). This concept suggests that optimal ventilatory strategies are important not only for maintenance of lung function but also for preventing the development of multiple-organ dysfunction (Chapter 104) that commonly occurs in this setting. This hypothesis may explain the decreased mortality recently observed with a strategy designed to avoid overdistention in a large randomized trial of mechanical ventilation in patients with ARDS.

SPECIFIC COMMON TREATMENT SCENARIOS

Initiation of Mechanical Ventilation

The initiation of mechanical ventilation involves several steps in clinical decision making (Table 105-1). Despite the utility of such guidelines, each

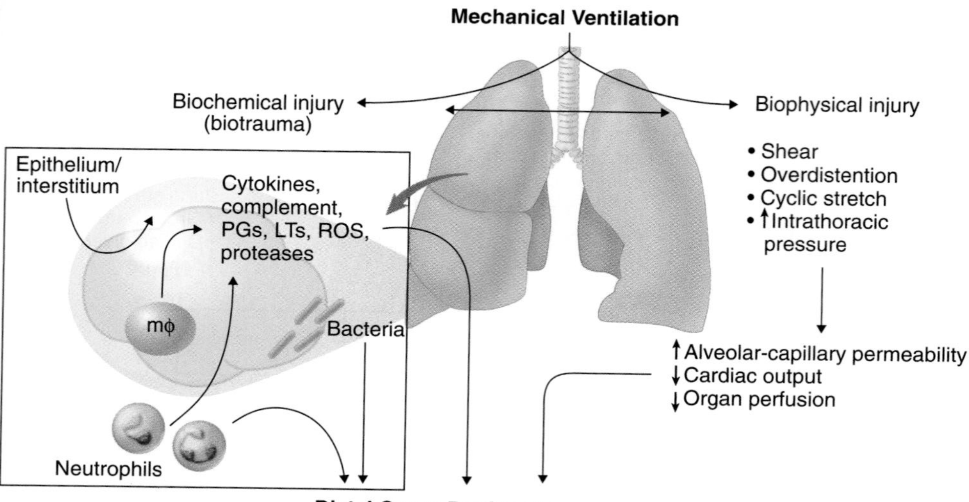

FIGURE 105-3. Mechanisms by which mechanical ventilation may lead to distal organ dysfunction. LTs = leukotrienes; mø = macrophages; PGs = prostaglandins; ROS = reactive oxygen species. (Adapted from Slutsky AS, Tremblay LN. Multiple system organ failure: is mechanical ventilation a contributing factor? *Am J Respir Crit Care Med.* 1998;157:1721-1725.)

TABLE 105-1 STEPS AND GUIDELINES FOR INITIATING MECHANICAL VENTILATION*

1. Ventilatory mode
   Unintubated patients:
   - NIV for patients with COPD and acute hypercapnic respiratory failure if alert, cooperative, and hemodynamically stable
   - NIV not routinely recommended for acute hypoxemic respiratory failure

   Intubated patients:
   - Assist/control with volume-limited ventilation as initial mode
   - Consider specific indications for PCV or HFOV (see text) in acute lung injury
   - SIMV: consider if some respiratory effort, dyssynchrony
   - PSV: consider if patient's effort good, ventilatory needs moderate to low, and patient more comfortable during PSV trial
2. Oxygenation
   - If infiltrates on chest radiograph, then
     FIO_2: begin with 0.8-1.0, reduce according to SpO_2
     PEEP: begin with 5 cm H_2O, increase according to PaO_2 or SpO_2, FIO_2 requirements, and hemodynamic effects; consider PEEP/FIO_2 "ladder" (see Fig. 105-4); goal of SpO_2 >90%, $FIO_2 \leq 0.6$
   - No infiltrates on chest radiograph (COPD, asthma, PTE),
     FIO_2: start at 0.4 and adjust according to SpO_2 (consider starting higher if pulmonary embolism is strongly suspected)
3. Ventilation
   - Tidal volume: begin with 8 mL/kg PBW (see Fig. 105-4 for formulas); decrease to 6 mL/kg PBW over a few hours if acute lung injury present (see Fig. 105-4)
   - Rate: begin with 10-20 breaths/min (10-15 if not acidotic; 15-20 if acidotic); adjust for pH; goal pH > 7.3 with maximal rate of 35; may accept lower goal if minute ventilation high
4. Secondary modifications
   - Triggering: in spontaneous modes, adjustment of sensitivity levels to minimize effort
   - Inspiratory flow rate of 40-80 L/min; higher if tachypneic with respiratory distress or if auto-PEEP present, lower if high pressure in ventilator circuit leads to a high-pressure alarm
   - Assessment of auto-PEEP, especially in patients with increased airways obstruction (e.g., asthma, COPD)
   - I/E ratio: 1:2, either set or as function of flow rate; higher (1:3 or more) if auto-PEEP present
   - Flow pattern: decelerating ramp reduces peak pressure
5. Monitoring
   - Clinical: blood pressure, ECG, observation of ventilatory pattern including assessment of dyssynchrony, effort or work by the patient; assessment of airflow throughout expiratory cycle
   - Ventilator: tidal volume, minute ventilation, airway pressures (including auto-PEEP), total compliance
   - Arterial blood gases, pulse oximetry

*Decisions within this algorithm will be influenced by the specific conditions of the individual patient.
COPD = chronic obstructive pulmonary disease; ECG = electrocardiogram; FIO_2 = fraction of inspired oxygen; HFOV = high-frequency oscillatory ventilation; I/E ratio = inspiratory-to-expiratory ratio; NIV = noninvasive ventilation; PaO_2 = partial pressure of oxygen in arterial blood; PBW = predicted body weight; PCV = pressure control ventilation; PEEP = positive end-expiratory pressure; PSV = pressure support ventilation; PTE = pulmonary thromboembolism; SIMV = synchronized intermittent mandatory ventilation; SpO_2 = arterial oxygen saturation by pulse oximetry.

patient must be evaluated for specific factors that could modify the recommendation or mandate an alternative.

Acute Respiratory Distress Syndrome

Patients with ARDS (Chapter 104) have noncardiogenic pulmonary edema, with a reduced functional residual capacity and a mortality rate of 30 to 60%. Although therapy may be available for the underlying disease process that led to the development of ARDS (e.g., antibiotics for a predisposing pneumonia), no effective therapy is directly aimed at the diffuse alveolar damage. These patients require mechanical ventilation as supportive therapy to improve oxygenation and to decrease the oxygen cost of breathing until their lungs recover from the primary insult that led to the alveolar damage.

The lungs in a patient with ARDS are stiff and are characterized on computed tomographic scans by patchy, heterogeneous infiltrates that consist of airless atelectatic or consolidated regions. Many patients have a dependent region that is consolidated, atelectatic, or fluid filled; a nondependent region that looks relatively normal; and a middle region that has some areas that look like the dependent regions but can be recruited to resemble the nondependent regions if high enough tidal volumes or increased levels of airway pressure are used transiently; these latter approaches are called *recruitment maneuvers.*

The challenge in ventilating patients with ARDS is to provide adequate gas exchange while at the same time not causing further lung injury (see earlier), an approach termed *lung protective ventilation strategy*. Arterial oxygen saturation can often be increased by high tidal volumes but at the expense of regional overdistention of those lung units that were not affected by the disease process itself, thereby improving oxygen saturation initially but, over time, worsening lung injury and clinical outcome.

The injury caused by mechanical ventilation can be reduced by using ventilatory strategies that avoid or minimize regional lung overdistention: limiting inspiratory pressure to some "safe" level or using smaller tidal volumes to limit end-inspiratory stretch, or both. However, in some patients, this lower "dose" of ventilation results in higher levels of $PaCO_2$ (so-called permissive hypercapnia) and a lower pH. Higher tidal volumes (12 mL/kg predicted body weight) yielded more normal blood gases, but lower tidal volumes (6 mL/kg predicted body weight) decreased mortality by 22% (from an absolute value of 40 to 31%) in a large clinical trial (Fig. 105-4).

Data also suggest that limiting tidal volume in ventilated patients who are intubated for reasons other than acute lung injury prevents injury later in the course of their intensive care unit stay. A lung protective strategy with limitation of tidal volume should be considered in ventilated patients who are at high risk of developing acute lung injury or ARDS.

Positive End-Expiratory Pressure

PEEP has been used traditionally to improve oxygenation while at the same time allowing reduction in FIO_2 to relatively nontoxic levels. Within the context of the current paradigm of trying to minimize iatrogenic complications of mechanical ventilation, PEEP is viewed as a therapy that potentially can abrogate or minimize the injury caused by ventilation at low lung volumes, by recruiting lung units and keeping them open. No definitive answer exists regarding how PEEP levels should be set in patients with ARDS; outcomes

Ventilatory Strategy for Patients with ARDS*

Goal 1: Low Vt/Pplat

Initiation:

Calculate PBW
—Male:
50 + 2. 3 (height [inches] − 60)
—Female:
45.5 + 2.3 (height [inches] − 60)

Initiate volume assist control
—start with 8 mL/kg, and ↓ to 6 mL/kg over a few hours

↓

Keep Pplat (based on 0.5-sec pause) <35 cm H_2O

If Pplat > 30 cm H_2O, ↓ Vt by 1 mL/kg to 5 or 4 mL/kg

If Pplat < 25 AND Vt < 6 mL/kg, ↑Vt by 1 mL/kg until Pplat > 25 cm H_2O OR Vt = 6 mL/kg

If patient severely distressed and/or breath stacking, consider ↑Vt to 7 or 8 mL/kg, as long as Pplat ≤ 30 cm H_2O†

Goal 2: Adequate Oxygenation

Specific goal:

$Pa{O_2}$ 55-80 mm Hg
or
$Sp{O_2}$ 88-95%

Use only $FI{O_2}$/PEEP combinations shown below to achieve this target

- if oxygenation is low, choose $FI{O_2}$/PEEP combination (from $FI{O_2}$/PEEP table) to the right
- if oxygenation is high, choose $FI{O_2}$/PEEP combination to the left

Goal 3: Arterial pH

Goal:

pH: 7.30–7.45

Acidosis algorithm

If pH 7.15–7.30

- ↑ set rate until pH > 7.30 or $Pa{CO_2}$ < 25 mm Hg (max RR = 35)
- if RR = 35 & pH < 7.30 $NaHCO_3$ may be given

If pH < 7.15

- ↑ set RR to 35
- if set RR = 35 & pH < 7.15, Vt may be ↑ in 1 mL/kg steps until pH > 7.15

(Pplat target may be exceeded)

Alkalosis algorithm

If pH > 7.45

- ↓ set RR until patient RR > set RR

(minimum set RR = 6/min)

$FI{O_2}$/PEEP Table

$FI{O_2}$	0.3	0.4	0.4	0.5	0.5	0.6	0.7	0.7	0.7	0.8	0.9	0.9	0.9	1.0
PEEP	5	5	8	8	10	10	10	12	14	14	14	16	18	20–24

*Based on ARDS Network Algorithm

† If compliance of the chest wall is markedly decreased (e.g., massive ascites), it may not be reasonable or necessary (if the patient is very hypoxemic) to allow a Pplat >30 cm H_2O.

FIGURE 105-4. **Ventilatory strategy for patients with the acute respiratory distress syndrome (ARDS).** Several caveats should be considered when using the low tidal volume strategy: (1) tidal volume (Vt) is based on predicted body weight (PBW),[1] not actual body weight; PBW tends to be about 20% lower than actual body weight; (2) the protocol mandates decreases in the Vt lower than 6 mL/kg of PBW if the plateau pressure (Pplat) is greater than 30 cm H_2O and allows for small increases in Vt if the patient is severely distressed and/or if there is breath stacking, as long as Pplat remains at 30 cm H_2O or lower; (3) because arterial carbon dioxide (CO_2) levels will rise, pH will fall; acidosis is treated with increasingly aggressive strategies dependent on the arterial pH; (4) the protocol has no specific provisions for the patient with a stiff chest wall, which in this context refers to the rib cage and abdomen; in such patients, it seems reasonable to allow Pplat to increase to more than 30 cm H_2O, even though it is not mandated by the protocol; in such cases, the limit on Pplat may be modified based on analysis of abdominal pressure, which can be estimated by measuring bladder pressure. RR = respiratory rate; $Sp{O_2}$ = oxygen saturation based on pulse oximeter.

appear to be similar with the routine use of higher (≈13 cm H_2O) and lower (≈8 cm H_2O) levels of PEEP. The critical issues are how to assess the level of PEEP in an individual patient and how to determine whether the procedures to recruit the lung units and keep them open are less harmful than allowing the lung units to remain de-recruited. One experimental option is chest computed tomography to assess whether areas of the lung are recruited, but this technique is not practical for routine assessment. A second approach is to measure the mechanical properties of the respiratory system by generating a pressure-volume curve (see Fig. 105-2). Investigators have suggested that the optimal strategy is to set PEEP just higher than the lower inflection point, which is thought to represent the opening pressure of the lung, and to adjust tidal volume so that Pplat is just lower than the upper inflection point, at which compliance decreases. Although lung continues to be recruited well above the lower inflection point, and the upper inflection point may not indicate overdistention, two clinical studies that based their lung protection strategies on the pressure-volume curve demonstrated reductions in mortality; however, both studies also included other features to reduce lung injury, so use of the pressure-volume curve to set PEEP levels and tidal volume (or pressure limits) cannot be recommended at this time. In the trial that demonstrated the benefit of lower tidal volumes, PEEP levels were individualized based on a PEEP/$FI{O_2}$ table (see Fig. 105-4); a subsequent trial using PEEP about 5 cm H_2O higher found no additional benefit. Higher PEEP (to achieve a plateau pressure of 28 to 30 cm of H_2O) can reduce the duration of ventilation and organ failure but not mortality compared with moderate PEEP (5 to 9 cm H_2O).[2] Multifaceted ventilation therapy protocols using low tidal volumes, recruitment maneuvers, and high PEEP can improve oxygenation but not reduce barotrauma or mortality compared with conventional therapy.[3] PEEP guided by esophageal pressure measured by an intraesophageal balloon may result in significantly higher PO_2 levels and better respiratory compliance than treatment guided by a standard protocol.[4] Pooled results of all trials suggest higher PEEP improves survival only in patients with ARDS.[5]

Obstructive Airways Diseases

The major pathophysiologic abnormality in patients with obstructive airways diseases is an increase in airway resistance leading to expiratory airflow limitation; patients may also have a concomitant increase in minute ventilation. These factors may lead to dynamic hyperinflation, which is associated with numerous complications, including respiratory muscle compromise, an increased oxygen cost of breathing, and hemodynamic compromise. Thus, the main goals in the ventilatory support of patients with obstructive airway diseases (COPD, asthma) are to minimize auto-PEEP, to rest the respiratory muscles, to maintain adequate gas exchange, and to decrease the oxygen cost of breathing while simultaneously minimizing the iatrogenic complications of mechanical ventilation and allowing time for the successful diagnosis and treatment of the primary cause of the exacerbation and the resulting increase in airway obstruction (Chapters 87 and 88).

Noninvasive Ventilation

For patients with acute respiratory failure resulting from an exacerbation of COPD, the preferred approach is NIV if the patient is hemodynamically stable, alert, and cooperative and does not need to be intubated to protect the airway. It is important to choose a comfortable mask and to reassure the patient because some patients find the mask difficult to tolerate. This strategy may be applied using several ventilation modes, including pressure support or bilevel positive airway pressure. The ventilation settings are adjusted to improve gas exchange and to ensure the patient's comfort. Despite this approach, some patients with COPD require intubation and ventilation because of cardiac or respiratory arrest, agitation, increased sputum, or other concomitant severe disorders.

Intubation and Ventilation

The key goal after intubation is to minimize the detrimental effects of dynamic hyperinflation. The most effective way to minimize dynamic hyperinflation is to decrease the minute ventilation, even if this means an increase in $Pa{CO_2}$, a strategy known as *permissive hypercapnia* or *controlled hypoventilation*. Judicious use of sedation may decrease carbon dioxide production and improve patient-ventilator synchrony, although the avoidance of sedation can reduce the duration of ventilation and hospitalization.[6] In a randomized study, no difference was found between dexmedetomidine and midazolam in time at targeted sedation level, but dexmedetomidine resulted in less time on mechanical ventilation, less delirium, and less hypertension and with less tachycardia but more bradycardia.[7] Care must be taken in the use of paralytic agents, especially when patients with asthma are also receiving corticosteroids. However, early neuromuscular blockade using cisatracurium besylate (15 mg rapid infusion followed by 37.5 mg/hr for 48 hours) can reduce mortality by 25% in patients with ARDS.[8]

Increasing expiratory time by using a higher peak inspiratory flow may be somewhat helpful, but it is not nearly as effective as decreasing minute ventilation. What level of $Paco_2$ (and pH) should be tolerated is not known with certainty, but maintaining pH higher than approximately 7.15 is a reasonable target, although much lower values have been reported in clinical studies.

In patients with COPD who are spontaneously breathing, the addition of external (set) PEEP at a level that is just less than what is necessary to overcome the auto-PEEP fully may not increase Pplat and may decrease the inspiratory effort that the patient needs to generate to initiate inspiratory airflow. This strategy does not appear to be as effective in patients with status asthmaticus, in whom it may cause an increase in Pplat. Measurements of auto-PEEP by airway occlusion may be inaccurate in some patients with status asthmaticus, likely because of gas trapping at the end of expiration with closed-off lung regions that do not communicate with the central airways.

ADJUNCTS

Tracheal gas insufflation involves washing out the carbon dioxide–rich gas in the anatomic dead space with fresh gas through a special catheter or endotracheal tube, thereby allowing a reduction in tidal volume while maintaining the same $Paco_2$. A clinically significant outcome benefit has not yet been demonstrated with tracheal gas insufflation.

The prone position compared with the supine position in patients with acute lung injury results in improved oxygenation in approximately 70% of patients and has a rationale (through more even distribution of pleural pressure) for preventing ventilator-induced lung injury and decreasing Fio_2. Trials in adults, however, have not demonstrated an outcome benefit, including a trial of prone positioning for 16 hours per day with all patients ventilated with the so-called lung-protective ventilation strategy used in the ARDSNet trial. Based on current studies, the prone position cannot be recommended for routine use but should be considered in patients with severe gas exchange abnormalities (e.g., $P/F \leq 100$) who require high PEEP and high Fio_2.

Inhaled nitric oxide is a potent vasodilator and bronchodilator that can enhance arterial oxygenation. It has not been shown to improve outcome in clinical trials, however, so its routine use cannot be recommended.

DISCONTINUATION OF MECHANICAL VENTILATION

To minimize the iatrogenic consequences of intubation and mechanical ventilation, discontinuation of ventilatory support and extubation should occur as expeditiously as possible. However, if discontinuation is attempted too early, patients may deteriorate and require urgent reintubation.

From the moment that mechanical ventilation is instituted, it is important for the clinician to start planning for eventual discontinuation of ventilatory support. A key aspect of this approach is serial evaluation, with aggressive treatment of the factors contributing to the patient's ventilatory dependence, including respiratory systems factors (e.g., respiratory muscles), cardiovascular factors (e.g., myocardial ischemia), neurologic factors (e.g., respiratory muscle weakness), and metabolic factors (e.g., increased oxygen consumption).

Two major types of weaning strategies have been used historically: (1) a ventilatory mode thought to hasten the weaning process and (2) daily monitoring of the patient for criteria to suggest the likelihood of successful weaning and a trial of spontaneous breathing for those deemed likely to succeed. Studies of ventilatory modes of weaning have included trials in which patients are allowed to breathe spontaneously from a fresh gas supply delivered to the endotracheal tube (a so-called T-tube), trials of IMV, and studies of pressure-support ventilation. With all approaches, the level of support is gradually decreased until extubation is tolerated by the patient. These methods have been compared in randomized controlled trials, with mixed results, although weaning with IMV appeared less favorable in most trials. Likewise, using ventilatory criteria to predict weaning success has been disappointing, mainly because some patients who fail to meet the criteria will be successfully weaned if they are given the opportunity to breathe spontaneously. The

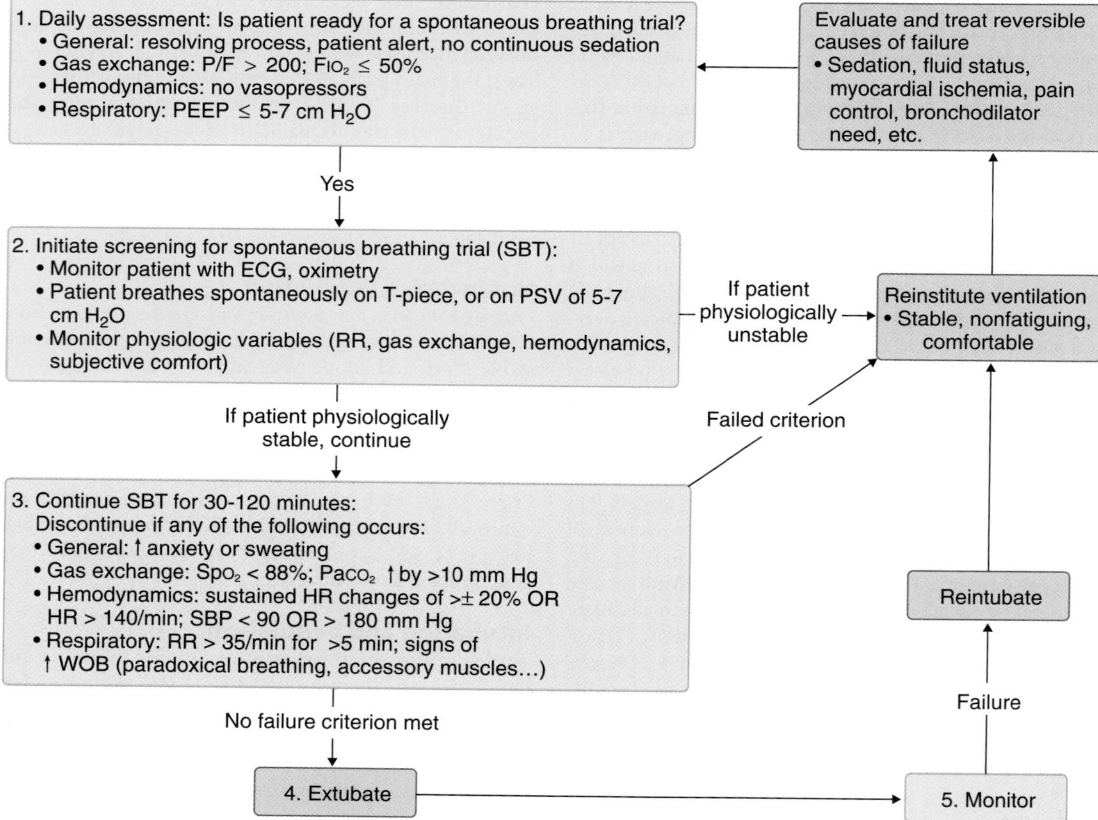

FIGURE 105-5. **Algorithm for assessing whether a patient is ready to be liberated from mechanical ventilation and extubated.** ECG = electrocardiogram; HR = heart rate; P/F = Pao_2/Fio_2 ratio; PSV = pressure support ventilation; RR = respiratory rate; SBP = systolic blood pressure; Spo_2 = oxygen saturation based on pulse oximeter; WOB = work of breathing.

criterion with the greatest predictive accuracy is the so-called rapid shallow breathing index, in which the respiratory rate is divided by tidal volume (in liters), with a value less than 105 suggesting the ability to wean; however false-negative and false-positive test results occur.

More recently, the approach to weaning has been based on the concept that a patient is ready to be removed from ventilatory support when the underlying disease process that led to the intubation has resolved or improved substantially. Rather than applying rigorous ventilatory criteria, the only requirements are that the patient be clinically stable (i.e., has shown improvement in the underlying process), be hemodynamically stable, and have oxygen requirements that can be met by face mask once the patient is extubated. If the patient meets these general criteria, a spontaneous breathing trial is recommended (Fig. 105-5); if the patient passes the trial, the patient can be extubated. A corollary is that a gradual weaning is not necessary; instead, patients should be assessed on a daily basis regarding their suitability to be removed from ventilatory support, and, if they are not ready, a comfortable, nonfatiguing form of mechanical ventilation should be used between the assessments. Assisted modes of ventilation are preferred between the spontaneous breathing trials.

An important recommendation in relation to weaning or discontinuing mechanical ventilation relates to evidence that intensive care units should develop weaning or discontinuation protocols that are designed to be implemented by health care professionals other than physicians. Three large randomized trials demonstrated that protocols implemented by health care professionals other than physicians improved care and were associated with substantial savings in costs compared with standard management approaches, even though the specifics of the protocols were different. More recently, a strategy that paired spontaneous awakening, based on the interruption of sedatives, with spontaneous breathing trials improved extubation rates, reduced intensive care length of stay, and decreased mortality by 32%.[9]

A major issue to assess before extubation is the patency of the patient's airway and whether the patient will be able to clear secretions after extubation. Assessment of the likely patency of the upper airway can be achieved using the *cuff-leak volume,* which is the difference between the inspiratory and expiratory tidal volume when the cuff of the endotracheal tube is deflated. If this volume is greater than 110 mL, it is usually an indication that major upper airway obstruction will not occur after extubation. Although this test is not required before extubation, a low *cuff-leak volume* warrants added precautions, such as the availability of equipment and personnel for managing a difficult intubation, when extubating the patient. In patients who have been ventilated for more than 36 hours, methylprednisolone (20 mg intravenously) started 12 hours before a planned extubation and repeated every 4 hours until tube removal substantially reduces postextubation laryngeal edema and reduces the need for reintubation by 50%.[10]

Despite the use of all these techniques, approximately 5 to 25% of patients will have to be reintubated and have mechanical ventilation reinstituted. Once a patient is reintubated, it is again necessary to reevaluate the respiratory and nonrespiratory reasons for the failure.

The choice of the specific weaning protocol should be left to the individual institution and should be individualized to the specific group of patients considered. In instituting such protocols, several key issues should be recognized. First, protocols are guides that should not replace clinical judgment. If a clinician does not follow some aspect of the protocol, there should be a mechanism in place for keeping track of what recommendations were not accepted, with an explanation of the rationale; these data should be collated and used to reassess the protocol. Second, protocols should be viewed as dynamic structures that are open to change and should be reevaluated on a regular basis. Third, implementation of a protocol requires adequate resources, and an institution must make a commitment not only to develop protocols but also to implement and assess them.

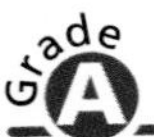

1. Gray A, Goodacre S, Newby DE, et al. Noninvasive ventilation in acute cardiogenic pulmonary edema. *N Engl J Med.* 2008;359:142-151.
2. Mercat A, Richard JC, Vielle B, et al. Positive end-expiratory pressure setting in adults with acute lung injury and acute respiratory distress syndrome: a randomized controlled trial. *JAMA.* 2008;299:646-655.
3. Meade MO, Cook DJ, Guyatt GH, et al. Ventilation strategy using low tidal volumes, recruitment maneuvers, and high positive end-expiratory pressure for acute lung injury and acute respiratory distress syndrome: a randomized controlled trial. *JAMA.* 2008;299:637-645.
4. Talmor D, Sarge T, Malhotra A, et al. Mechanical ventilation guided by esophageal pressure in acute lung injury. *N Engl J Med.* 2008;359:2095-2104.
5. Briel M, Meade M, Mercat A, et al. Higher vs lower positive end-expiratory pressure in patients with acute lung injury and acute respiratory distress syndrome: systematic review and meta-analysis. *JAMA.* 2010;303:865-873.
6. Strom T, Martinussen T, Toft P. A protocol of no sedation for critically ill patients receiving mechanical ventilation: a randomized trial. *Lancet.* 2010;375:475-480.
7. Riker RR, Shehabi Y, Bokesch PM, et al. Dexmedetomidine vs midazolam for sedation of critically ill patients: a randomized trial. *JAMA.* 2009;301:489-499.
8. Papazian L, Forel JM, Gacouin A, et al. Neuromuscular blockers in early acute respiratory distress syndrome. *N Engl J Med.* 2010;363:1107-1116.
9. Girard TD, Kress JP, Fuchs BD, et al. Efficacy and safety of a paired sedation and ventilator weaning protocol for mechanically ventilated patients in intensive care (Awakening and Breathing Controlled trial): a randomised controlled trial. *Lancet.* 2008;371:126-134.
10. Francois B, Bellisant E, Gissot V, et al. 12-h Pretreatment with methylprednisolone versus placebo for prevention of postextubation laryngeal oedema: a randomised double-blind trial. *Lancet.* 2007;369:1083-1089.

SUGGESTED READINGS

Bouferrache K, Viellard-Baron A. Acute respiratory distress syndrome, mechanical ventilation, and right ventricular function. *Curr Opin Crit Care.* 2011;17:30-35. *The up to 25% incidence of acute cor pulmonale may be prevented by keeping the plateau pressure below 27-28 cm H_2O, controlling hypercapnia, avoiding intrinsic PEEP, and keeping the applied PEEP low.*

Burns KE, Adhikari NK, Keenan SP, et al. Use of non-invasive ventilation to wean critically ill adults off invasive ventilation: meta-analysis and systematic review. *BMJ.* 2009;338:b1574. *Review of data to support this approach.*

Magder S. Hemodynamic monitoring in the mechanically ventilated patient. *Curr Opin Crit Care.* 2011;17:36-42. *A practical approach.*

Phoenix SI, Paravastu S, Columb M, et al. Does a higher positive end expiratory pressure decrease mortality in acute respiratory distress syndrome? A systematic review and meta-analysis. *Anesthesiology.* 2009;110:1098-1105. *Evidence favors the use of high PEEP when ventilating patients with severe ARDS syndrome.*

106 APPROACH TO THE PATIENT WITH SHOCK

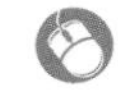

EMANUEL P. RIVERS

DEFINITION

The key feature of shock is tissue hypoperfusion, not a specific level of systemic arterial blood pressure. The clinical picture may be cryptic or obvious.

EPIDEMIOLOGY

More than 1 million patients present in shock or develop shock in U.S. hospitals each year, at an annual cost of more than $100 billion. Shock can be categorized as hypovolemic, cardiogenic (Chapter 107), extracardiac/obstructive, distributive, or dissociative.

PATHOBIOLOGY

The delivery and utilization of oxygen are essential for cellular viability, and the failure to deliver or utilize oxygen is central to the concept of shock and its pathogenesis (Fig. 106-1). Systemic oxygen delivery—that is, the amount of oxygen delivered to tissues by the arterial blood—depends on the concentration of hemoglobin in the blood, the fractional saturation of the hemoglobin with oxygen ($Sa{O_2}$), the amount of oxygen dissolved in the blood ($Pa{O_2}$), and cardiac output. Cardiac output is a product of stroke volume and heart rate. Stroke volume is determined by ventricular preload and afterload, as well as contractility of the right or left heart. Systemic vascular resistance (SVR), the force resisting cardiac contraction, can be calculated using equation 1:

$$SVR = (MAP - CVP) * 80 / CO \quad (1)$$

$$MAP = \text{Diastolic blood pressure} + (\text{Systolic} - \text{Diastolic blood pressure})/3 \quad (2)$$

MAP denotes the mean systemic arterial blood pressure, CVP denotes central venous pressure, and CO denotes cardiac output. SVR is determined primarily by the degree of vasomotor tone in the precapillary smooth muscle sphincters.

The systemic circulation is normally autoregulated, so that when systemic arterial pressure increases, vessel diameter decreases to maintain flow at a steady level. The clinical significance of these relationships is apparent when

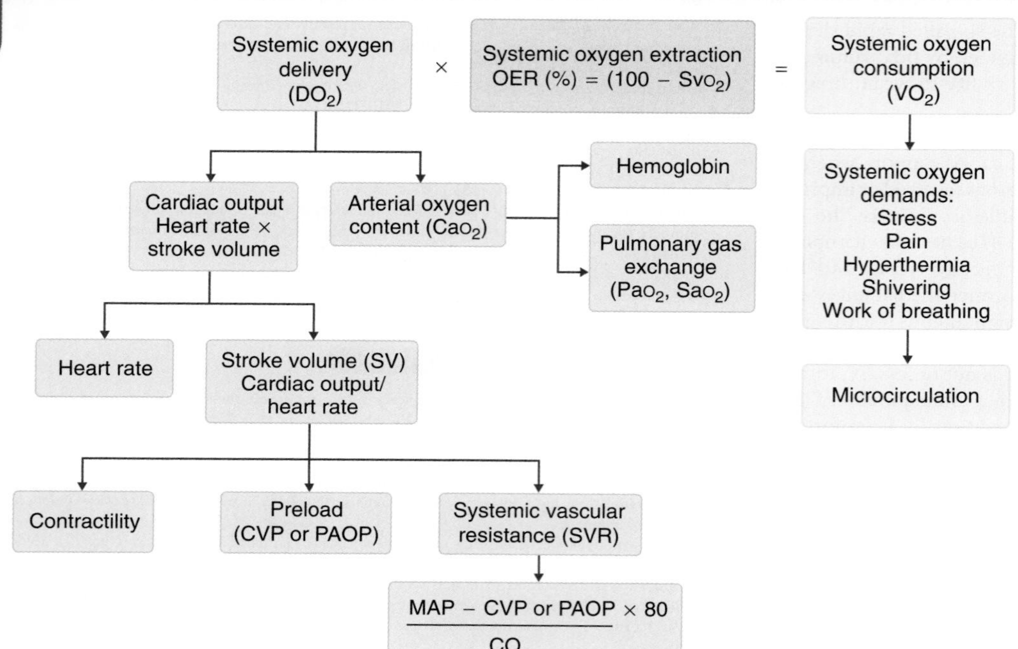

FIGURE 106-1. The hemodynamic, oxygen transport, and oxygen utilization components of shock management. Systemic oxygen delivery is impacted by cardiac output (CO) and arterial oxygen content. The cardiac, pulmonary, and blood determinants of systemic oxygen delivery are shown. CVP = central venous pressure; MAP = mean arterial pressure; PAOP = pulmonary artery occlusion pressure.

a patient presents with a decrease in cardiac output, but a compensatory increase in systemic vascular resistance maintains a near-normal mean arterial blood pressure. Despite the near-normal blood pressure, however, the patient is in "cryptic shock" because of tissue hypoperfusion. Compensatory mechanisms are organ specific. Blood flow to organs such as the heart and brain is carefully regulated and maintained over a wide range of blood pressures. In other organs, however, such as the intestine or liver, autoregulation is not as tightly maintained.

Systemic oxygen consumption, which is the amount of oxygen consumed by the body per minute, is calculated as the systemic oxygen delivery multiplied by the systemic oxygen extraction ratio. Oxygen demand is the amount of oxygen required by the tissues to avoid anaerobic metabolism. Normally, systemic oxygen delivery is sufficient so that systemic oxygen consumption is not altered by or dependent on changes in delivery. However, if systemic oxygen delivery drops below a critical value, a compensatory increase in the oxygen extraction ratio maintains systemic oxygen consumption at adequate levels to meet systemic oxygen demands. When this compensatory response in the oxygen extraction ratio is inadequate to meet systemic oxygen demands, a switch occurs from aerobic metabolism to the less efficient anaerobic metabolism. The result is depletion of adenosine triphosphate (ATP) and intracellular energy reserves. Intracellular acidosis occurs, and anaerobic glycolysis leads to the production of lactate. Below this critical value of systemic oxygen delivery, systemic oxygen consumption is dependent on systemic oxygen delivery, a relationship termed *physiologic oxygen supply dependency.*

A pathologic oxygen delivery dependency exists in patients with sepsis, trauma, and acute respiratory distress syndrome (ARDS) and after resuscitation from prolonged cardiac arrest. These patients have systemic oxygen delivery in the normal or elevated range but an impairment of oxygen utilization. This condition of cytopathic tissue hypoxia is a result of maldistribution of blood flow or a defect in the utilization of substrate at the microcirculatory or subcellular level. This pathologic supply dependency is accompanied by very high mixed venous oxygen saturation levels or venous hyperoxia, as well as by elevated lactate levels. This process is believed to be an important mechanism of cellular damage in various forms of shock.

Compensatory Responses

Minor decreases in arterial blood pressure and systemic oxygen delivery activate the baroreceptor reflex via stretch receptors or sensing mechanisms located in the carotid sinus, splanchnic vasculature, aortic arch, right atrium, and juxtaglomerular apparatus of the kidney, as well as chemoreceptors sensitive to concentrations of carbon dioxide or oxygen located in the central nervous system, mostly in the medulla. These compensatory responses mediated by activation of the sympathetic nervous system include (1) release of cortisol, aldosterone, and epinephrine; (2) activation of the renin-angiotensin system; (3) release of arginine vasopressin (AVP) from the posterior pituitary; (4) augmentation of myocardial contractility and heart rate; (5) constriction of arterial and venous capacitance vessels, particularly in the splanchnic bed, thereby augmenting venous return; (6) redistribution of blood flow away from skeletal muscle beds and the splanchnic viscera; and (7) creation of a local tissue environment to enhance the unloading of oxygen to tissues and improve its extraction because of acidosis, pyrexia, and increased red blood cell 2,3-diphosphoglycerate.

Noncompensatory Responses

Noncompensatory responses develop when physiologic adjustments are exaggerated or lead to pathologic results. Vasodilatory shock results from many sources, including unregulated nitric oxide synthesis, inadequate ATP synthesis in vascular smooth muscle cells, activation of the enzyme poly (ADP ribosyl) polymerase (PARP)-1, lipid mediators, and opening of ATP-sensitive potassium channels in vascular smooth muscle cells. This multifaceted insult leads to interstitial fluid and cellular edema, which impairs oxygen diffusion from capillary to cell, causing a failure of energy-dependent ion transport, the production of lactate, and the inability to maintain normal transmembrane gradients of potassium, chloride, and calcium. Cells lose their ability to utilize available oxygen as a result of mitochondrial dysfunction, abnormal carbohydrate metabolism, and failure of many energy-dependent enzyme reactions.

Acidosis commonly accompanies shock. When a molecule of ATP is hydrolyzed to adenosine diphosphate (ADP) and inorganic phosphate, the reaction also generates a proton. The net yield of protons is positive when ATP is hydrolyzed in the cell and then regenerated only by the anaerobic breakdown of glucose. Thus, during anaerobic glycolysis, the use of ATP to power cellular processes, coupled with the anaerobic production of ATP by substrate-level phosphorylation reactions, results in the development of acidosis.

Cells in organs such as the kidneys, liver, and brain can convert lactate into glucose via gluconeogenesis or oxidize lactate to pyruvate and then, ultimately, to carbon dioxide and water.

Lactate levels are a reflection of tissue hypoxia, clearance, and alternative sources of production. When the splanchnic circulation is compromised in shock, hepatic lactate clearance is impaired, contributing to the buildup of lactate levels in the circulation. In sepsis, however, the rate of glycolysis increases even in the absence of tissue hypoxia. This phenomenon, which has been termed *accelerated aerobic glycolysis,* may reflect a change in the ratio of the active to the inactive form of pyruvate dehydrogenase, which is the rate-limiting step for the entry of substrate into the mitochondrial tricarboxylic acid cycle.

When systemic oxygen delivery continues to fail to meet systemic oxygen demands, the oxygen debt accumulates. Three stages of shock can ensue. The first stage, which is called early, reversible, or compensated shock, is characterized by compensatory responses to minimize tissue injury. This stage of shock can be self-limited, with full recovery and minimal residual morbidity, if the cause is recognized and treated early. If substantial oxygen debt persists without timely repayment or resolution, inflammation and cellular and microvascular injury define the second stage of shock, which is associated with a prolonged recovery and is typically complicated by organ failure, including acute lung injury and acute tubular necrosis. The third stage is late, irreversible, or decompensated shock. In this situation, the oxygen debt is large, and repayment is slow to nonexistent. When shock reaches this point, cellular and tissue injury is extensive and largely irreversible. Progression to multisystem organ failure and/or death is inevitable, regardless of therapy.

CLINICAL MANIFESTATIONS

The five general types of shock are cardiogenic, distributive, hypovolemic, obstructive, and dissociative. The distinction among these five shock syndromes can be made by combining the history, clinical picture, and hemodynamic measurements. Cardiogenic shock (Chapter 107) and shock syndromes related to sepsis (Chapter 108) are covered in detail elsewhere.

The clinical manifestation of shock is variable and depends on the initiating cause and the response of multiple organs. Shock typically presents as absolute or relative systemic arterial hypotension and evidence of end-organ dysfunction (Table 106-1). The extremities are cool and pale if shock is associated with peripheral vasoconstriction, which is typical of hypovolemic, cardiogenic, and obstructive shock, but they are typically warm and pink with the peripheral vasodilation of distributive shock and dissociative shock (cyanide poisoning).

The most frequent neurologic finding in shock is alteration in the level of consciousness, ranging from confusion to coma. Many of the clinically apparent manifestations of cardiac involvement in shock result from sympathoadrenal stimulation, with tachycardia being the most sensitive indicator that shock is present. Acute lung injury causes impaired gas exchange; the work of breathing is increased, and respiratory muscle fatigue and ventilatory failure require mechanical ventilation. Hypovolemia with or without acute tubular necrosis results in oliguria, although polyuria may be seen in early shock.

Typical clinical manifestations of gut involvement during shock include abdominal pain, ileus, erosive gastritis, pancreatitis, acalculous cholecystitis, and submucosal hemorrhage. If the integrity of the gut barrier is compromised, bacteria and their toxins are translocated into the blood stream. The most common manifestation of liver involvement in shock is a mild increase in serum levels of aminotransferases and lactate dehydrogenase. With severe hypoperfusion, shock liver may manifest with massive aminotransferase elevations and extensive hepatocellular damage.

Thrombocytopenia may result from dilution during volume repletion or from immunologic platelet destruction, which is especially common during septic shock. Activation of the coagulation cascade can lead to disseminated intravascular coagulation (Chapter 178), which results in thrombocytopenia, decreased fibrinogen, elevated fibrin split products, and microangiopathic hemolytic anemia.

Hypovolemic Shock

Hemorrhagic shock, be it from internal or external bleeding, is the most common cause of hypovolemic shock (Table 106-2). Nonhemorrhagic hypovolemic shock can be caused by severe dehydration owing to massive urinary or gastrointestinal fluid losses. Such losses are common in conditions such as diabetic ketoacidosis (Chapters 236) or diarrhea from some infectious diseases, such as cholera (Chapter 310). Massive insensible losses of water or perspiration can precipitate shock in patients with major burn injuries (Chapter 112) or heatstroke (Chapter 109). Sequestration of fluid in the extravascular compartment, commonly referred to as "third spacing," can cause shock in patients as a result of surgery, bowel obstruction, hepatic failure (Chapter 157), systemic inflammation, acute pancreatitis (Chapter 146), or thermal injuries (Chapter 112). Regardless of whether hypovolemic shock is due to hemorrhage or fluid losses, the rate of loss is a critical component of the presentation. If volume is lost at a slow rate, compensatory mechanisms are usually effective, and any given amount of volume depletion is often better tolerated than if the same volume were lost acutely. In addition, underlying diseases, especially those that limit cardiac reserve, can substantially influence the clinical severity of a hypovolemic insult.

TABLE 106-1 PHYSICAL EXAMINATION AND SELECTED LABORATORY SIGNS IN SHOCK

Central nervous system	Acute delirium, restlessness, disorientation, confusion, and coma, which may be secondary to decreased cerebral perfusion pressure (mean arterial pressure minus intracranial pressure). Patients with chronic hypertension or increased intracranial pressure may be symptomatic at normal blood pressures. Cheyne-Stokes respirations may be seen with severe decompensated heart failure. Blindness can be a presenting complaint or complication.
Temperature	Hyperthermia results in excess tissue respiration and greater systemic oxygen delivery requirements. Hypothermia can occur when decreased systemic oxygen delivery or impaired cellular respiration decreases heat generation.
Skin	Cool distal extremities (combined low serum bicarbonate and high arterial lactate levels) aid in identifying patients with hypoperfusion. Pallor, cyanosis, sweating, and decreased capillary refill and pale, dusky, or clammy extremities indicate systemic hypoperfusion. Dry mucous membranes and decreased skin turgor indicate low vascular volume. Low toe temperature correlates with the severity of shock.
General cardiovascular	Neck vein distention (e.g., heart failure, pulmonary embolus, pericardial tamponade) or flattening (e.g., hypovolemia), tachycardia, and arrhythmias. Decreased coronary perfusion pressures can lead to ischemia, decreased ventricular compliance, and increased left ventricular diastolic pressure. A "mill wheel" heart murmur may be heard with an air embolus.
Heart rate	Usually elevated. However, paradoxical bradycardia can be seen in patients with preexisting cardiac disease and severe hemorrhage. Heart rate variability is associated with poor outcomes.
Systolic blood pressure	May actually increase slightly when cardiac contractility increases in early shock and then fall as shock advances. A single episode of undifferentiated hypotension with a systolic blood pressure <80 mm Hg carries an in-hospital mortality of 18%.
Diastolic blood pressure	Correlates with arteriolar vasoconstriction and may rise early in shock and then fall when cardiovascular compensation fails.
Pulse pressure	Defined as systolic minus diastolic pressure and related to stroke volume and the rigidity of the aorta. Increases early in shock and decreases before systolic pressure decreases.
Pulsus paradoxus	An exaggerated change in systolic blood pressure with respiration (systolic blood pressure declines >10 mm Hg with inspiration) seen in asthma, cardiac tamponade, and air embolus.
Mean arterial blood pressure	Diastolic blood pressure + [pulse pressure/3]
Shock index	Heart rate/systolic blood pressure. Normal = 0.5 to 0.7. A persistent elevation of the shock index (>1.0) indicates impaired left ventricular function (as a result of blood loss and/or cardiac depression) and is associated with increased mortality.
Respiratory	Tachypnea, increased minute ventilation, increased dead space, bronchospasm, hypocapnia with progression to respiratory failure, acute lung injury, and adult respiratory distress syndrome.
Abdomen	Low-flow states may result in abdominal pain, ileus, gastrointestinal bleeding, pancreatitis, acalculous cholecystitis, mesenteric ischemia, and shock liver.
Renal	Because the kidney receives 20% of cardiac output, low cardiac output reduces the glomerular filtration rate and redistributes renal blood flow from the renal cortex toward the renal medulla, leading to oliguria. Paradoxical polyuria in sepsis may be confused with adequate hydration.
Metabolic	Respiratory alkalosis is the first acid-base abnormality, but metabolic acidosis occurs as shock progresses. Hyperglycemia, hypoglycemia, and hyperkalemia may develop.

TABLE 106-2 CLASSIFICATION OF HEMORRHAGIC SHOCK*

	CLASS I	CLASS II	CLASS III	CLASS IV
Blood loss (mL)	Up to 750	750-1500	1500-2000	>2000
% Volume	Up to 15	15-30	30-40	>40
Pulse rate (per min)	<100	>100	>120	>140
Blood pressure	Normal	Normal	Decreased	Decreased
Pulse pressure	Normal or increased	Decreased	Decreased	Decreased
Respiratory rate (per min)	14-20	20-30	30-40	>35
Urine output (mL/hr)	>30	20-30	5-15	Negligible
Mental status	Slightly anxious	Mildly anxious	Anxious, confused	Confused, lethargic
Fluid replacement	Crystalloid	Crystalloid	Crystalloid and blood	Crystalloid and blood

*Estimates based on a 70-kg patient.
From Committee on Trauma of the American College of Surgeons. *Advanced Trauma Life Support for Doctors*. Chicago: American College of Surgeons; 1997:108.

Distributive Shock

The most important and prevalent cause of distributive shock is septic shock (Chapter 108), but anaphylaxis (Chapter 261), drug overdose (Chapter 33), neurogenic insults, and addisonian crisis (Chapter 234) can also produce vasodilatory shock. Sepsis can be a combination of hypovolemia, vasodilation, myocardial suppression, and impaired tissue oxygen use (dissociative shock). In approximately 10 to 15% of septic shock patients, myocardial dysfunction results in a low-cardiac-output form of shock. Early interventions (Chapter 108) can improve outcomes substantially.

Cardiogenic Shock

Cardiogenic shock (Chapter 107) is defined by a decrease in systemic oxygen delivery caused by an acute or chronic deterioration of cardiac function owing to myocardial, valvular, structural, toxic, or infectious causes. The clinical picture of cardiogenic shock is variable, depending on which structural component of the ventricle is impaired.

Extracardiac Obstructive Shock

This form of shock results from acute obstruction to flow in the circulation. Examples include impaired diastolic filling of the right ventricle (e.g., superior vena cava syndrome; Chapter 187), obstruction of right ventricular output (e.g., massive pulmonary embolism; Chapter 98), or an air embolus from cardiopulmonary bypass or central line placement (Chapter 98). Systemic arterial hypertension (Chapter 67) severe enough to impair left ventricular function or acute pericardial tamponade or constrictive pericarditis (Chapter 77) can also produce an obstructive shock pattern.

Dissociative Shock

Dissociative shock results from microvascular abnormalities, with maldistribution or shunting of blood flow, or cytopathic tissue hypoxia. Dissociative shock includes disorders that inhibit oxygen utilization, such as cyanide poisoning, sodium nitroprusside use, and sepsis.

Mixed Shock States

Shock may arise from multiple causes. For example, a patient with pneumonia and a history of ischemic cardiomyopathy may present in a hypodynamic rather than a hyperdynamic state when combined with sepsis. Thus, a mixture of hypovolemic, distributive, and cardiogenic shock can be seen in the same patient.

DIAGNOSIS

A key element in the approach to shock is a problem-directed history and physical examination. Some patients present with few symptoms other than generalized weakness, lethargy, or altered mental status. A discussion with the patient and family members should specifically address symptoms that suggest volume depletion, including bleeding, vomiting, diarrhea, excessive urination, insensible losses due to fever, or orthostatic lightheadedness. The history should also inquire about prior or current evidence of cardiovascular disease, especially episodes of chest pain (Chapter 50) or symptoms of heart failure (Chapter 58). Prior neurologic diseases can render patients more susceptible to complications from hypovolemia. Medication use, both prescribed and nonprescribed, must be ascertained. Some medications cause volume depletion (e.g., diuretics), whereas others depress myocardial contractility (e.g., β-blockers, calcium-channel blockers). The possibility of an anaphylactic reaction to a new medication or cardiovascular depression owing to drug toxicity should be considered. A recent or remote history of steroid use may suggest adrenal insufficiency (Chapter 34).

Findings on the physical examination can provide critical information to aid in the diagnosis (see Table 106-1). Traditionally, shock is defined by a systolic blood pressure less than 90 mm Hg or 40 mm Hg less than the baseline systolic blood pressure if the patient has a history of hypertension.

Acidosis

A common theme in shock is that tissue hypoxia leads to acidosis (Chapter 120), which develops as a consequence of anaerobic metabolism and generally parallels the severity of shock. Laboratory manifestations may include a base deficit, low arterial and venous pH levels, and an elevated serum lactate level. Base deficit is the absolute decrease in the serum concentration of bicarbonate (normal minus the patient's bicarbonate). A mild base deficit is −2 to −5, moderate is −6 to −14, and severe is −15 mM/L or greater. When patients are resuscitated using large volumes of normal saline, the large fluid load can cause a dilutional acidosis, and the large chloride load can induce metabolic acidosis even in the absence of tissue hypoxia and anaerobic metabolism. Base deficit can also be caused by cocaine, alcohol, and diabetic ketoacidosis. Despite its limitations, base deficit provides the clinician with a quick indicator to assess the severity of tissue hyperfusion and the adequacy of resuscitation in relieving anaerobic metabolism and oxygen debt.

The low pH of metabolic acidosis can result from different acids. Acidosis caused by lactate and unidentified anions produces an ion gap. The blood lactate concentration rises with increased anaerobic metabolism, as is seen in shock but also in diabetic ketoacidosis (Chapter 236) , total parenteral nutrition (Chapter 224), seizures (Chapter 410), thiamine deficiency (Chapter 225), treatment of HIV infection with protease inhibitors (Chapter 396), and administration of metformin, salicylate, isoniazid, propofol, and cyanide (Chapter 110). A lactate concentration greater than 4 mmol/L is unusual in normal and non–critically ill hospitalized patients and warrants concern. A lactate concentration greater than 4 mmol/L is associated with an in-hospital mortality exceeding 25%, regardless of the cause, and failure to decrease lactate levels over the first 6 hours of shock is associated with an increased inflammatory response, the development of organ failure, and mortality.

Urine Output

The kidneys normally receive 20% of the systemic oxygen delivery, and because of this large amount of blood flow per gram of tissue, they are highly sensitive to changes in renal blood flow. Urine output is a valuable indicator of renal perfusion and vital organ blood flow. Although a significant drop in urine output indicates reduced renal blood flow, an adequate urine output does not always indicate successful resuscitation. Other factors that may affect urine output include the use of mannitol or diuretics. Preexisting conditions, such as renal failure, may also limit the ability of this measure to reflect the adequacy of resuscitation.

TREATMENT

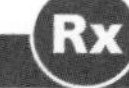

The goal of initial management is to restore global and microvascular perfusion to levels that sustain aerobic cellular respiration. Multiple randomized trials have shown significant and consistent reductions in mortality when shock is reversed aggressively before organ failure develops. Once this initial management is accomplished, the definitive diagnosis leads to more specific therapy based on the cause of shock.

Markers of shock serve not only as diagnostic tools for risk stratification but also as targets or end points for the early restoration of adequate tissue perfusion. Clinical monitoring of tissue oxygenation and organ function commonly involves measuring traditional end points of resuscitation, such as heart rate, blood pressure, mentation, urine output, and skin perfusion. Many clinicians continue to use these parameters as indicators that systemic oxygenation imbalances have been corrected. However, there is increasing evidence that clinical parameters may be poor indicators of the ongoing tissue hypoxia that is associated with increased mortality.

Initial Management

The initial management of shock requires immediate diagnostic and therapeutic interventions, including attention to airway, breathing, circulation, and definitive diagnosis and treatment (Chapter 63). The first step to optimize systemic oxygen delivery is to provide supplemental oxygen to increase arterial oxygen content. If any doubt exists about the patency of the airway or the adequacy of ventilation, endotracheal intubation should be performed and mechanical ventilation initiated (Chapter 105). Mechanical ventilation helps provide adequate oxygenation and carbon dioxide elimination and decreases oxygen utilization by the respiratory muscles, which may be responsible for up to 40% of systemic oxygen consumption and lactate production.

Although endotracheal intubation and mechanical ventilation may be critical for patients in shock, the sudden increase in airway pressure can lead to a series of deleterious hemodynamic complications, especially in patients who are hypovolemic or vasodilated or have compromised cardiac function. In such patients, the resulting decreased venous return, increased pulmonary vascular resistance, and decreased ventricular compliance may lead to hypotension and cardiovascular collapse. Furthermore, when sedatives, anxiolytics, or induction agents are used during and after intubation, the decrease in catecholamine levels, peripheral vascular resistance, and cortisol levels may result in hypotension. If possible, preparations should be made to monitor physiologic variables, ensure adequate fluid administration, and provide rapid access to vasopressors should systemic arterial pressure fall to dangerously low levels.

Upon initial presentation, it is good practice to place one or two large-bore (≥16 gauge) peripheral intravenous catheters and to administer a crystalloid solution (normal saline or Ringer's lactate solution). If MAP is less than 60 to 65 mm Hg, systolic blood pressure is less than 90 mm Hg, or evidence of tissue hypoperfusion is present, an intravenous fluid challenge (20 to 40 mL/kg crystalloid or colloid) should be given rapidly. A bolus of 500 mL every 30 minutes titrated to MAP or measurement of preload is recommended. In an 80-kg person, the average intravascular volume is 5 L. In shock states, such as septic shock, in which intravascular hypovolemia is a predominant feature, 5 to 6 L of fluid over the first 6 hours is considered an average volume resuscitation. If hemorrhage is the likely cause of shock, blood should be used to replace volume. Fluids should not be withheld, even in patients with end-stage renal disease.

Central venous access and arterial blood pressure monitoring should be established to monitor hemodynamics and venous and arterial blood gases, respectively. Electrocardiographic monitoring and continuous measurement of oxygen saturation by pulse oximetry are useful adjuncts. Because the Trendelenburg position may impair gas exchange and promote aspiration, an alternative is to raise the patient's legs above the level of the heart with the patient in the supine position.

If the patient remains hypotensive, vasopressors such as norepinephrine, dopamine, or Neo-Synephrine (Table 106-3) should be administered to restore adequate systemic arterial pressure while the diagnostic evaluation is ongoing. Treatment with vasopressors should not be postponed while trying to achieve euvolemia by using fluid boluses, because patients with cerebrovascular and coronary artery disease may be intolerant of the hypotensive interval. However, vasopressors may also mask hypovolemia when they increase blood pressure. If the volume status remains undefined or the hemodynamic condition requires repeated fluid challenges or vasopressor treatment, a central venous catheter should be placed to determine central venous oxygen saturation, ventricular filling pressures, and intravascular volume status while echocardiography is performed. Based on these data, patients can usually be classified and managed according to their hemodynamic and oxygen transport patterns (Figs. 106-2 and 106-3).

Fluid Replacement

Rapid and appropriate restoration of vascular volume decreases the need for vasopressor therapy, adrenal replacement therapy, and invasive monitoring; in addition, it modulates the inflammation that arises when a patient progresses to severe shock. The goal of fluid resuscitation is not merely to achieve a predetermined volume but rather to titrate fluid to optimize systemic oxygen delivery and meet tissue oxygen demands.

To assess the adequacy of cardiac preload during the resuscitation of a patient with shock, a central venous catheter is as good as a pulmonary artery catheter.[1] However, the CVP does not correlate well with left ventricular end-diastolic volume: although a low CVP indicates hypovolemia, a "normal" CVP does not exclude inadequate preload as a cause of shock. A fluid challenge in a volume-responsive patient increases cardiac output by about 20% for each 2 cm H_2O change in CVP; by comparison, cardiac output does not change if the CVP is raised in a patient with adequate left ventricular volume.

When intrathoracic pressure increases during the application of positive airway pressure in a mechanically ventilated patient, venous return decreases and, as a consequence, left ventricular stroke volume also decreases. The variation in pulse pressure or stroke volume during a positive-pressure breath can also predict the responsiveness of cardiac output to changes in preload. Pulse pressure variation is defined by equation 3:

$$100 \times (PPmax - PPmin)/[(PPmax + PPmin)/2] \qquad (3)$$

PPmax and PPmin are the maximal and minimal pulse pressures, respectively, in a respiratory cycle. Pulse pressure variation values of 13 to 15% suggest that hypovolemia is present and that the cardiac index will increase by at least 15% after the rapid infusion of 500 mL of crystalloid. Pulse pressure variation is generally the best predictor of volume status and response to fluids, although atrial arrhythmias can interfere with the usefulness of this technique.

Types of Fluids

The two most commonly used crystalloid solutions are 0.9% sodium chloride solution (normal saline) and Ringer's lactate solution. Although these two solutions have been regarded as essentially interchangeable, accumulating data suggest that large volumes of normal saline, but not Ringer's lactate solution, promote the development of hyperchloremic metabolic acidosis and coagulopathy (Table 106-4).

Colloids are higher-molecular-weight solutions that increase plasma oncotic pressure; they are classified as natural (albumin) or artificial (starches, hetastarch, pentastarch, dextrans, and gelatins). Colloids are dissolved in either normal saline or a balanced salt solution. There are no clinically significant differences among the various colloid solutions when they are used for shock resuscitation. When compared with saline-based solutions, hetastarch dissolved in a calcium-containing, low-chloride, balanced salt solution may be

TABLE 106-3 VASOPRESSOR AGENTS

		Peripheral Vasculature		*Cardiac Effects*			
AGENT	**DOSE RANGE**	**VASOCONSTRICTION**	**VASODILATION**	**HEART RATE**	**CONTRACTILITY**	**DYSRHYTHMIAS**	**TYPICAL USE**
Dopamine	1-4 μg/kg/min	0	1+	1+	1+	1+	"Renal dose" does not improve renal function; may be used with bradycardia and hypotension
	5-10 μg/kg/min	1-2+	1+	2+	2+	2+	
	11-20 μg/kg/min	2-3+	1+	2+	2+	3+	Vasopressor range
Vasopressin	0.04-0.1 units/min	3-4+	0	0	0	1+	Septic shock, post–cardiopulmonary bypass shock state, no outcome benefit in sepsis
Phenylephrine	20-200 μg/min	4+	0	0	0	1+	Vasodilatory shock, best for supraventricular tachycardia
Norepinephrine	1-20 μg/min	4+	0	2+	2+	2+	First-line vasopressor for septic shock, vasodilatory shock
Epinephrine	1-20 μg/min	4+	0	4+	4+	4+	Refractory shock, shock with bradycardia, anaphylactic shock
Dobutamine	1-20 μg/kg/min	1+	2+	1-2+	3+	3+	Cardiogenic shock, septic shock
Milrinone	37.5-75 μg/kg bolus followed by 0.375-0.75 μg/min	0	2+	1+	3+	2+	Cardiogenic shock, right heart failure, dilates pulmonary artery; caution in renal failure

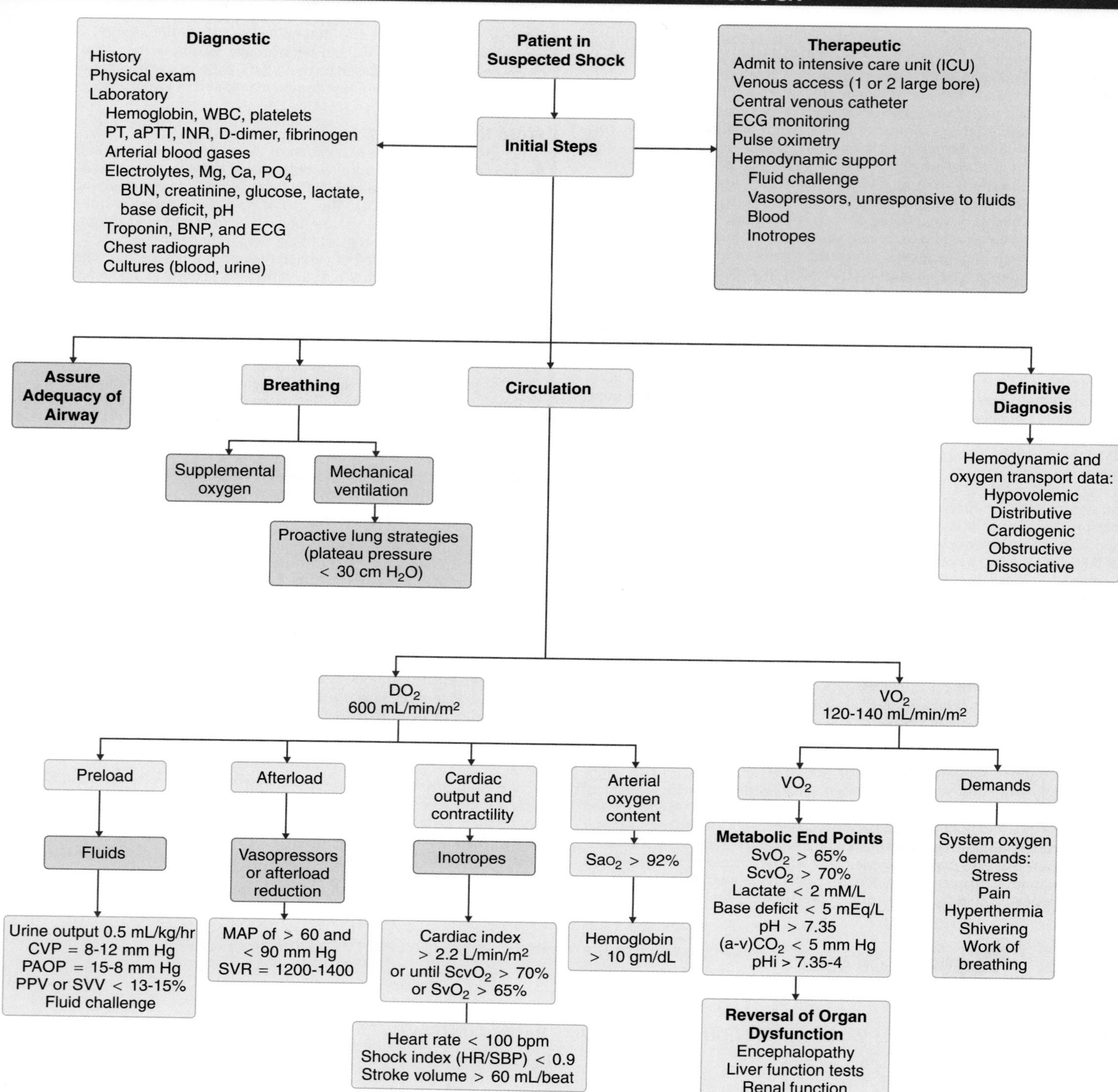

FIGURE 106-2. General hemodynamic management. aPTT = activated partial thromboplastin time; BNP = brain natriuretic peptide; bpm = beats per minute; CVP = central venous pressure; DO_2 = (systemic) oxygen delivery; ECG = electrocardiogram; HR = heart rate; INR = international normalized ratio; MAP = mean arterial pressure; PAOP = pulmonary artery occlusion pressure; pHi = intestinal mucosal pH; PPV = pulse pressure variation; PT = prothrombin time; SBP = systolic blood pressure; SVR = systemic vascular resistance; SVV = stroke volume variation; VO_2 = (systemic) oxygen eonsumption; WBC = white blood cell.

associated with less acidosis and less use of blood products, but its use in severe sepsis and septic shock has been associated with increased renal failure and mortality.[2]

Colloids stay in the intravascular space significantly longer than crystalloids do, with an intravascular half-life of 16 hours for albumin versus 30 to 60 minutes for normal saline and lactated Ringer's. When titrated to the same volume status, colloids and crystalloids restore tissue perfusion to the same magnitude, but a two to four times greater volume of crystalloids is required to achieve the same end point. Various types of fluids have potential advantages and disadvantages, but the outcomes of patients with hypovolemic shock are equivalent for crystalloids and albumin (see Table 106-4).[3]

Fluid Management Strategies

Initial aggressive fluid resuscitation usually occurs within 6 hours of presentation, but different strategies are needed for the longer-term management of fluid status, especially in patients with acute lung injury. For example, conservative volume therapy (euvolemia) beginning an average of 47 hours after admission to the intensive care unit (ICU) and 24 hours after the establishment of acute lung injury results in significantly better lung and central nervous system function and a decreased need for sedation, mechanical ventilation, and ICU care.[4] However, patients who receive conservative volume replacement transiently may need more vasopressor support.

Optimal Hemoglobin

In hemorrhagic shock, the rapid administration of packed red blood cells and, if indicated, platelets and thawed fresh-frozen plasma can be lifesaving. Whenever possible, fully cross-matched packed red blood cells are preferable, but type-specific blood can often be given safely when immediate therapy is warranted (Chapter 180). In dire emergencies, type O Rh-negative blood can be administered to women of childbearing potential, and type O

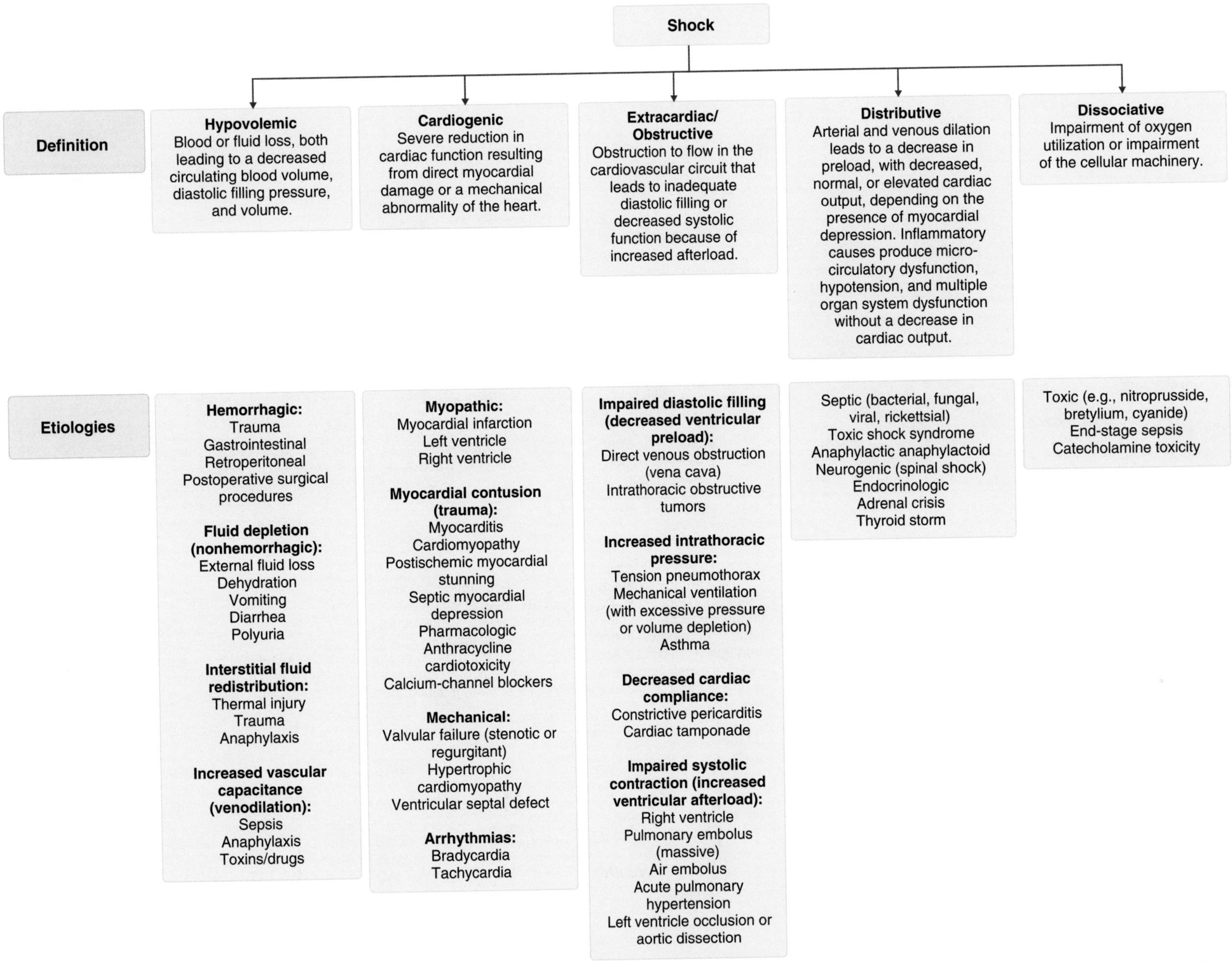

Shock

	Hypovolemic	Cardiogenic	Extracardiac/Obstructive	Distributive	Dissociative
Definition	Blood or fluid loss, both leading to a decreased circulating blood volume, diastolic filling pressure, and volume.	Severe reduction in cardiac function resulting from direct myocardial damage or a mechanical abnormality of the heart.	Obstruction to flow in the cardiovascular circuit that leads to inadequate diastolic filling or decreased systolic function because of increased afterload.	Arterial and venous dilation leads to a decrease in preload, with decreased, normal, or elevated cardiac output, depending on the presence of myocardial depression. Inflammatory causes produce micro-circulatory dysfunction, hypotension, and multiple organ system dysfunction without a decrease in cardiac output.	Impairment of oxygen utilization or impairment of the cellular machinery.
Etiologies	**Hemorrhagic:** Trauma Gastrointestinal Retroperitoneal Postoperative surgical procedures **Fluid depletion (nonhemorrhagic):** External fluid loss Dehydration Vomiting Diarrhea Polyuria **Interstitial fluid redistribution:** Thermal injury Trauma Anaphylaxis **Increased vascular capacitance (venodilation):** Sepsis Anaphylaxis Toxins/drugs	**Myopathic:** Myocardial infarction Left ventricle Right ventricle **Myocardial contusion (trauma):** Myocarditis Cardiomyopathy Postischemic myocardial stunning Septic myocardial depression Pharmacologic Anthracycline cardiotoxicity Calcium-channel blockers **Mechanical:** Valvular failure (stenotic or regurgitant) Hypertrophic cardiomyopathy Ventricular septal defect **Arrhythmias:** Bradycardia Tachycardia	**Impaired diastolic filling (decreased ventricular preload):** Direct venous obstruction (vena cava) Intrathoracic obstructive tumors **Increased intrathoracic pressure:** Tension pneumothorax Mechanical ventilation (with excessive pressure or volume depletion) Asthma **Decreased cardiac compliance:** Constrictive pericarditis Cardiac tamponade **Impaired systolic contraction (increased ventricular afterload):** Right ventricle Pulmonary embolus (massive) Air embolus Acute pulmonary hypertension Left ventricle occlusion or aortic dissection	Septic (bacterial, fungal, viral, rickettsial) Toxic shock syndrome Anaphylactic anaphylactoid Neurogenic (spinal shock) Endocrinologic Adrenal crisis Thyroid storm	Toxic (e.g., nitroprusside, bretylium, cyanide) End-stage sepsis Catecholamine toxicity

FIGURE 106-3. Definitions, etiologies, and therapies of various shock states. CI = cardiac index; CO = cardiac output; CT = computed tomography; CVP = central venous pressure; DO_2 = systemic oxygen delivery; ECG = electrocardiogram; IABP = intra-aortic balloon pumping; LV = left ventricular; MAP = mean arterial pressure; MRI = magnetic resonance imaging; PA = pulmonary artery; PAOP = pulmonary artery occlusion pressure; RA = right atrial; RV = right ventricular; SVR = systemic vascular resistance; US = ultrasonography; VSD = ventricular septal defect.

Continued

Hemodynamic Characterization	CVP/RA ↓ PAOP ↓ $CO/CI/DO_2$ ↓ SVR ↑ $SvO_2/ScvO_2$ ↓ Comments: Preexisting heart disease may alter the filling pressures	CVP/RA ↑ PAOP ↓ early ↑ later $CO/CI/DO_2$ ↓↓ SVR ↑ $SvO_2/ScvO_2$ ↓ Comments: If there is a VSD, there may be $ScvO_2/SvO_2$ or a step up from the right atrium to right ventricle to the pulmonary artery. Large V wave is seen on PA catheter with mitral regurgitation.	CVP/RA ↑↑ PAOP ↓ $CO/CI/DO_2$ ↕ SVR ↑ $SvO_2/ScvO_2$ ↓ Comments: Equalization of intracardiac diastolic pressure is consistent with pericardial tamponade. A rapid x and blunted y descent on CVP wave form indicates the inability of the heart to fill.	CVP/RA ↓ early normal later PAOP ↓ early normal later $CO/CI/DO_2$ ↓ early ↑ later SVR ↑ early ↓ later $SvO_2/ScvO_2$ ↓ early ↑ later Comments: In the early stage, filling pressures are low, leading to low to normal cardiac output and variable $ScvO_2/SvO_2$. If myocardial depression accompanies, then a similar profile of cardiogenic shock is seen. After resuscitation a hyperdynamic circulation is seen.	CVP/RA ↓ early normal to ↑ later PAOP ↓ early normal to ↑ later $CO/CI/DO_2$ ↓ early ↑ later SVR ↑ early ↓ later $SvO_2/ScvO_2$ ↑ early ↑↑ later Comments: Filling pressures can be variable, depending on stage of the disease. Cardiac output is generally increased. SVR is decreased and $ScvO_2/SvO_2$ and lactate are increased.
Therapy	Rapid replacement of blood, colloid or crystalloid Identify source of blood/fluid loss Replace deficient coagulation factors Consider factor VIIa Endoscopy/colonoscopy Angiography CT/MRI/US or other	LV infarction: intra-aortic balloon pump (IABP) coronary angiography Recanalization: thrombolytic therapy, angioplasty, coronary bypass surgery RV infarction: fluids and inotropes with PA catheter Mechanical abnormality: echocardiography, cardiac catheterization Corrective surgery: mechanical assist devices, transplantation	Pericardial tamponade: pericardiocentesis, surgical drainage (if needed) Pneumothorax: chest tube Pulmonary embolism: heparin ventilation-perfusion lung scan pulmonary angiography consider thrombolytic therapy, embolectomy Severe hypertension: afterload reduction	Identify site of infection Antimicrobial agents Early goal-directed therapy fluids vasopressors inotropic agents Goals: $ScO_2 > 70\%$ CVP > 8 mm Hg MAP > 65 mm Hg Improving organ function Decreasing lactate levels Consider activated protein C Requiring vasopressors, consider corticosteroids	Toxin antidote or remove agent, hyperbaric oxygen therapy Recombinant activated protein C Nitroglycerin (speculative) Prostacyclin (speculative)

FIGURE 106-3, cont'd.

TABLE 106-4 FLUID THERAPY

Normal saline	Normal saline is a slightly hyperosmolar solution containing 154 mEq/L of both sodium and chloride. Owing to the relatively high chloride concentration and low pH, normal saline carries a risk of inducing hyperchloremic metabolic acidosis when given in large amounts.
Lactated Ringer's solution (LR)	Lactate is metabolized to carbon dioxide (CO_2) and water by the liver, leading to the release of CO_2 in the lungs and excretion of water by the kidneys. LR is preferred over normal saline and buffers acidemia. Because LR contains a very small amount of potassium, there is a small risk of inducing hyperkalemia in patients with renal insufficiency or renal failure. LR may be incompletely metabolized in severe hepatic failure.
Albumin	Albumin is a protein derived from human plasma and is available in varying concentrations from 4 to 25%. A study comparing fluid resuscitation with albumin versus saline found similar 28-day mortalities and secondary outcomes in each arm.[3] However, a post-hoc subset analysis of patients with sepsis and acute lung injury resuscitated with albumin showed a trend toward a decrease in mortality. There was a significant increase in mortality in trauma patients, particularly those with head injury.
Hydroxyethyl starch (HES)	HES, which is a synthetic colloid derived from hydrolyzed amylopectin, causes renal impairment at recommended doses and impaired long-term survival at high doses. HES can also cause coagulopathy and bleeding complications from reduced factor VIII and von Willebrand factor levels, as well as impaired platelet function. HES increases the risk of acute renal failure and reduces the probability of survival in patients with sepsis.
Dextrans	Dextrans are artificial colloids synthesized by *Leuconostoc mesenteroides* bacteria grown in sucrose media. Dextrans are used more frequently to lower blood viscosity than for rapid plasma expansion. They can cause renal dysfunction as well as anaphylactoid reactions.
Gelatins	Gelatins are produced from bovine collagen. Because they have a small molecular weight, they are not very effective at expanding plasma volume, but they cost less than other options. They have been reported to cause renal impairment as well as allergic reactions ranging from pruritus to anaphylaxis. Gelatins are not currently available in North America.

Rh-negative or Rh-positive blood can be given to men or postmenopausal women.

The appropriate hemoglobin level in shock remains controversial, but a value of 10 mg/dL is often recommended as long as the patient has increased lactate levels, decreased venous oxygen saturation, or evidence of systemic hypoperfusion. A more conservative transfusion strategy (hemoglobin value of 7 to 10 mg/dL) is appropriate when the patient is in the more convalescent phase of critical illness.

Vasopressor Therapy

To optimize end-organ perfusion, the second phase of intervention after adequate fluid therapy is to maintain perfusion pressure. A specific MAP goal has not been established for all shock states, but a MAP of at least 60 to 65 mm Hg is a reasonable target.

The most common vasopressors are agonists at various adrenergic receptors. Receptors include peripheral α-adrenergic receptors that lead to vasoconstriction, cardiac β_1 receptors with both chronotropic and inotropic effects, β_2 receptors located in the circulation and airways that mediate vasodilation and bronchodilation, and dopaminergic receptors located throughout the cardiovascular, mesenteric, and renal circulations. Based on these mechanisms, therapy can be tailored to a specific circumstance. For example, a patient with severe tachycardia would be best served by an agent with more α-selective activity and less β activity to avoid tachycardia and increased myocardial oxygen consumption (see Table 106-3).

Norepinephrine, which is a vasoconstrictor and an inotrope, provides better splanchnic oxygen utilization compared with dopamine. It is generally considered the first-line vasopressor for treating persistent hypotension in septic patients despite adequate resuscitation,[5] and it may be superior to dopamine in treating cardiogenic shock. For example, a randomized trial comparing dopamine with norepinephrine in patients with shock showed no significant difference in mortality for hypovolemic and septic shock but a significant benefit of norepinephrine in cardiogenic shock.[5] In addition, there was a significant two-fold increase in arrhythmic events with dopamine compared with norepinephrine (24.1 vs. 12.4%).

Dopamine's effects result from transduction at dopaminergic receptors in the renal, mesenteric, coronary, and systemic circulations. The positive chronotropic and inotropic effects of dopamine can lead to tachycardia and tachyarrhythmias; this effect frequently limits its dosing because the increased myocardial oxygen requirements promote the development of myocardial ischemia, especially in the presence of coronary artery disease.

Phenylephrine is a synthetic catecholamine that is a selective α-adrenergic agonist and is ideal in patients with tachycardia. However, the resulting increase in myocardial oxygen consumption, decrease in splanchnic blood flow, and decrease in cardiac output can be detrimental for patients with septic shock.

Epinephrine, which is a potent α-, β_1-, and β_2-adrenergic agonist, increases peripheral arteriolar tone as well as cardiac contractility. It is the first-line agent for the treatment of anaphylactic shock and is used to support myocardial contractility following cardiac surgery. Epinephrine increases the white blood cell count and the blood lactate concentration because of accelerated aerobic glycogenolysis and/or maldistribution of blood flow.

Vasopressin deficiency accompanies vasodilatory shock. Vasopressin is not a potent vasopressor in normal subjects, but very low doses (0.04 unit/minute) markedly increase arterial blood pressure in septic patients with intractable hypotension. In addition, vasopressin enhances the pressor response to catecholamines.

Adrenal Dysfunction

Beyond their metabolic functions, glucocorticoids are required to maintain responsiveness to vasopressors, intravascular volume, vascular permeability, and myocardial contractility. If the hypothalamic-pituitary-adrenocortical axis is depressed in shock, clinical findings can include unexplained fever, hypoglycemia, metabolic acidosis, hypotension refractory to fluid resuscitation, and eosinophilia. Cortisol levels and the results of cosyntropin stimulation testing may not be clinically helpful. If adrenal insufficiency is strongly suspected, or if patients have refractory hypotension despite vasopressors and hemodynamic optimization, stress doses of intravenous hydrocortisone (e.g., 50 mg every 6 hours) are recommended.[6]

PROGNOSIS

Clinical characteristics associated with a poor outcome include the severity of shock; its temporal duration, underlying cause, and reversibility; and preexisting vital organ dysfunction. Direct noninvasive measurement of maximal oxygen uptake predicts outcome in patients who have cardiogenic shock. Persistently elevated lactate levels are prognostic in trauma, septic shock, and after cardiac arrest, and an anion gap acidosis is associated with significantly higher hospital mortality than is hyperchloremic acidosis. Regional measurements of pH are highly predictive of outcome; for example, if the gastric mucosal pH remains below 7.3 for 24 hours, the hospital mortality rate is about 50%. The severity of the base deficit correlates with the development of multisystem organ failure in trauma. The mortality for an undiagnosed patient who is sent to a general medical floor and develops shock is three times higher than for a patient who is admitted directly to the ICU.

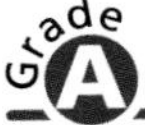

1. The National Heart, Lung, and Blood Institute Acute Respiratory Distress Syndrome (ARDS) Clinical Trials Network. Pulmonary-artery versus central venous catheter to guide treatment of acute lung injury. *N Engl J Med*. 2006;354:2213-2224.
2. Brunkhorst FM, Engel C, Bloos F, et al. Intensive insulin therapy and pentastarch resuscitation in severe sepsis. *N Engl J Med*. 2008;358:125-139.
3. Finfer S, Bellomo R, Boyce N, et al. A comparison of albumin and saline for fluid resuscitation in the intensive care unit. *N Engl J Med*. 2004;350:2247-2256.
4. The National Heart, Lung, and Blood Institute Acute Respiratory Distress Syndrome (ARDS) Clinical Trials Network. Comparison of two fluid-management strategies in acute lung injury. *N Engl J Med*. 2006;354:2564-2575.
5. De Backer D, Biston P, Devriendt J, et al. Comparison of dopamine and norepinephrine in the treatment of shock. *N Engl J Med*. 2010;362:779-789.
6. Sprung CL, Annane D, Keh D, et al. Hydrocortisone therapy for patients with septic shock. *N Engl J Med*. 2008;358:111-124.

SUGGESTED READINGS

Barbee RW, Reynolds PS, Ward KR. Assessing shock resuscitation strategies by oxygen debt repayment. *Shock*. 2010;33:113-122. *Incorporates the concept of the oxygen supply and delivery relationship with that of oxygen debt and shows the relevance to shock and resuscitation.*

Greer R. The temporal evolution of acute respiratory distress syndrome following shock. *Eur J Anaesthesiol*. 2010;27:3:226-232. *Comprehensive overview.*

Groeneveld AB, Navickis RJ, Wilkes MM. Update on the comparative safety of colloids: a systematic review of clinical studies. *Ann Surg*. 2011;253:470-483. *Among colloids, albumin is safer than hydroxyethyl starch solutions.*

Strehlow MC. Early identification of shock in critically ill patients. *Emerg Med Clin North Am.* 2010; 28:57-66. *Reviews the physiologic definition, the importance of early intervention, and the clinical and diagnostic signs clinicians can use to identify patients in shock.*

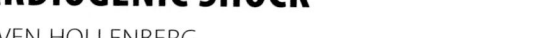

107

CARDIOGENIC SHOCK

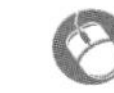

STEVEN HOLLENBERG

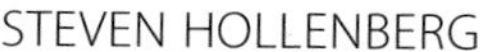

DEFINITION

Cardiogenic shock is the syndrome that ensues when the heart is unable to deliver enough blood to maintain adequate tissue perfusion. The hemodynamic picture includes sustained systemic hypotension, pulmonary capillary wedge pressure (PCWP) greater than 18 mm Hg, and cardiac index less than 2.2 L/minute/m^2 (Table 107-1). Although systolic blood pressure less than 90 mm Hg is a commonly accepted threshold for shock, a decrease of 30 mm Hg from baseline can also be used. The diagnosis of cardiogenic shock is often made on clinical grounds—hypotension combined with signs of poor tissue perfusion, including oliguria, clouded sensorium, and cool extremities, all in the setting of myocardial dysfunction. To make the diagnosis, it is important to document myocardial dysfunction and to exclude or correct factors such as hypovolemia, hypoxemia, and acidosis.

EPIDEMIOLOGY

The predominant cause of cardiogenic shock (Fig. 107-1) is left ventricular failure secondary to acute myocardial infarction (MI)—an extensive first acute MI, cumulative loss of myocardial function in a patient with previous MI or cardiomyopathy, or a mechanical complication of MI (Chapter 73). However, any cause of severe left ventricular (LV) or right ventricular (RV) dysfunction can lead to cardiogenic shock, including end-stage cardiomyopathy (Chapter 60), prolonged cardiopulmonary bypass, valvular disease (Chapter 75), myocardial contusion (Chapter 112), sepsis with unusually profound myocardial depression (Chapter 108), and fulminant myocarditis (Chapter 60) (Table 107-2). Stress-induced (takotsubo) cardiomyopathy (Chapter 60), a syndrome of acute apical LV dysfunction that occurs after emotional distress, may also present with cardiogenic shock. Acute valvular regurgitation, most often caused by endocarditis (Chapter 76) or chordal rupture (Chapter 75), can lead to shock, as can physiologic stress in the setting of severe valvular stenosis. Cardiac tamponade (Chapter 77) and massive pulmonary embolism (Chapter 98) with acute RV failure can cause shock without pulmonary edema.

The incidence and mortality associated with cardiogenic shock appear to be declining. In the past 30 years the incidence has fallen from about 8% to 6% of MIs, largely because of the benefit of early perfusion strategies (Chapter 73). In parallel, mortality from cardiogenic shock has decreased from 70 to 80% to 50% or less, suggesting that increasingly effective early treatment and more widespread adoption of early revascularization have improved the outcomes of patients in whom shock has already developed.

TABLE 107-1 DIAGNOSIS OF CARDIOGENIC SHOCK

CLINICAL SIGNS
Hypotension
Oliguria
Clouded sensorium
Cool and mottled extremities
HEMODYNAMIC CRITERIA
Systolic blood pressure < 90 mm Hg or > 30 mm Hg decrease from baseline for > 30 min
Cardiac index < 2.2 L/min/m^2
Pulmonary capillary wedge pressure > 18 mm Hg
OTHER
Documented myocardial dysfunction
Exclusion of hypovolemia, hypoxia, and acidosis

Risk factors for the development of cardiogenic shock in MI parallel those for LV dysfunction and the severity of coronary artery disease. Patient characteristics include older age, anterior MI, diabetes, hypertension, multivessel coronary artery disease (CAD), previous MI, and peripheral vascular and cerebrovascular disease. Clinical risk factors include decreased ejection fractions, larger infarctions, and lack of compensatory hyperkinesis in myocardial territories remote from the infarction. Clinical harbingers of impending shock include the degree of hypotension and tachycardia at hospital presentation. The factors that predict mortality reflect the severity of the acute insult as well as comorbid conditions.

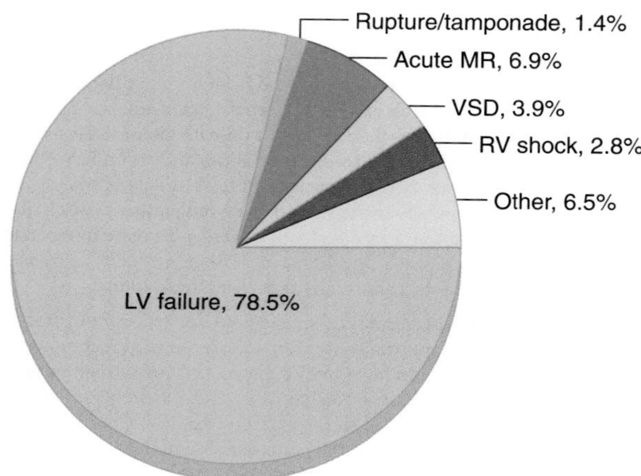

FIGURE 107-1. Causes of cardiogenic shock in patients with myocardial infarction in the SHOCK trial registry. LV = left ventricular; MR = mitral regurgitation; RV = right ventricular; VSD = ventricular septal defect. (Adapted from Hochman JS, Boland J, Sleeper LA, et al. Current spectrum of cardiogenic shock and effect of early revascularization on mortality. Report of an international registry. SHOCK registry investigators. *Circulation.* 1995;91:873-881).

TABLE 107-2 CAUSES OF CARDIOGENIC SHOCK

ACUTE MYOCARDIAL INFARCTION
Pump failure
Large infarction
Smaller infarction with preexisting left ventricular dysfunction
Infarct extension
Reinfarction
Infarct expansion
Mechanical complications
Acute mitral regurgitation due to papillary muscle rupture
Ventricular septal defect
Free wall rupture
Pericardial tamponade
Right ventricular infarction
CARDIOMYOPATHY
Myocarditis
Peripartum cardiomyopathy
End-stage low-output heart failure
Hypertrophic cardiomyopathy with outflow tract obstruction
Stress cardiomyopathy
VALVULAR HEART DISEASE
Acute mitral regurgitation (chordal rupture)
Acute aortic regurgitation
Aortic or mitral stenosis with tachyarrhythmia or other comorbid condition causing decompensation
Prosthetic valve dysfunction
TACHYARRHYTHMIA
OTHER CONDITIONS
Prolonged cardiopulmonary bypass
Septic shock with severe myocardial depression
Penetrating or blunt cardiac trauma
Orthotopic transplant rejection
Massive pulmonary embolism
Pericardial tamponade

Coronary angiography most often demonstrates multivessel CAD. About 30% of patients have a left main coronary artery occlusion, about 60% have three-vessel coronary disease, and only about 20% have single-vessel disease. Multivessel CAD helps explain the failure to develop compensatory hyperkinesis in remote myocardial segments, because of either previous infarction or high-grade coronary stenoses.

Only one fourth of patients who develop cardiogenic shock are in shock when they initially present to the hospital; in the others, shock usually evolves over several hours, suggesting that early treatment may prevent shock. Comparison of the clinical characteristics of patients with early and late shock shows similar demographic, historical, clinical, and hemodynamic characteristics, but shock tends to develop earlier in patients with single-vessel CAD than in those with triple-vessel disease. This finding suggests that early shock in the setting of acute MI may be more amenable to revascularization of the culprit vessel via thrombolysis or angioplasty (Chapter 73), whereas shock developing later may require more complete revascularization with multivessel percutaneous coronary intervention (PCI) or coronary artery bypass graft (CABG) surgery (Chapter 74).

TABLE 107-3 CLINICAL SIGNS OF VOLUME STATUS AND PERFUSION

SIGNS AND SYMPTOMS OF CONGESTION
Orthopnea, paroxysmal nocturnal dyspnea
Jugular venous distention
Abdominojugular reflux
Rales
Hepatomegaly
Edema
Right upper quadrant tenderness
POSSIBLE EVIDENCE OF LOW PERFUSION
Narrow pulse pressure
Obtundation
Cool extremities
Cachexia, muscle loss
Decreased exercise tolerance
Renal/hepatic dysfunction
Hypotension with angiotensin-converting enzyme inhibition

PATHOBIOLOGY

Cardiogenic shock is characterized by a downward cascade in which myocardial dysfunction reduces stroke volume, cardiac output, and blood pressure; these changes compromise myocardial perfusion, exacerbate ischemia, and further depress myocardial function, cardiac output, and systemic perfusion. Concomitant diastolic dysfunction increases left atrial pressure, which leads to pulmonary congestion and hypoxemia and exacerbates myocardial ischemia and impairs ventricular performance.

Compensatory mechanisms include sympathetic stimulation, which increases heart rate and contractility, and renal fluid retention, which increases preload. Increases in heart rate and contractility increase myocardial oxygen demand and exacerbate ischemia. Another compensatory mechanism, vasoconstriction to maintain blood pressure, increases myocardial afterload, further impairing cardiac performance and increasing myocardial oxygen demand. In the face of inadequate perfusion, this increased demand can worsen ischemia and perpetuate a vicious circle that, if unbroken, may culminate in death. Interrupting this circle of myocardial dysfunction and ischemia is the basis for therapeutic regimens for cardiogenic shock.

In cardiogenic shock, LV dysfunction is not always severe. In one large study, the mean LV ejection fraction was 30%, indicating that mechanisms other than primary pump failure were operative. Furthermore, systemic vascular resistance is not always elevated, suggesting that compensatory vasoconstriction is not universal. Inflammatory responses may contribute to the vasodilation and myocardial dysfunction in cardiogenic shock.

Patients in cardiogenic shock may have areas of nonfunctional but viable myocardium owing to stunning or hibernation. Myocardial stunning represents postischemic dysfunction that persists despite restoration of normal blood flow. Hibernating myocardial segments have persistently impaired function at rest owing to severely reduced coronary blood flow; function in these segments might be normalized by improving blood flow. Although hibernation is conceptually different from stunning, the two conditions may not differ much clinically. Repetitive episodes of myocardial stunning can occur in areas of viable myocardium subtended by a critical coronary stenosis. Such episodes can recapitulate the hibernation phenotype, blurring the distinction between myocardial stunning and hibernation. Regardless of the degree of overlap, the therapeutic implications make distinguishing the two conditions vital in patients with cardiogenic shock. The contractile function of hibernating myocardium improves with revascularization, whereas stunned myocardium retains inotropic reserve and can respond to inotropic stimulation. In addition, the severity of the antecedent ischemic insult determines the intensity of stunning, providing a rationale for reestablishing the patency of occluded coronary arteries in patients with cardiogenic shock. Finally, the notion that some myocardial tissue may recover function emphasizes the importance of measures to support the patient hemodynamically and minimize myocardial necrosis in patients with shock.

CLINICAL MANIFESTATIONS

The physical examination should be geared toward evaluating congestion and systemic perfusion to characterize the patient's hemodynamic profile (Table 107-3). An assessment of whether the patient is "wet" or "dry" and "cold" or "warm" is integral to management. Signs of congestion (Chapter 58) include jugular venous distention (see Fig. 50-3 in Chapter 50) and pulmonary rales and may include peripheral edema and ascites. Whether the patient is "cold" or "warm" is an indication of systemic perfusion.

The majority of the cardiogenic shock patients present "wet" and "cold." Patients with shock are usually ashen or cyanotic, and they have cool skin and mottled extremities. Cerebral hypoperfusion may cloud the sensorium. Pulses, which are rapid and faint, may be irregular in the presence of arrhythmias. Jugular venous distention and pulmonary rales are usually present, although their absence does not exclude the diagnosis. A precordial heave resulting from LV dyskinesis may be palpable. The heart sounds may be distant, and third and/or fourth heart sounds are usually present. A systolic murmur of mitral regurgitation or a ventricular septal defect may be heard, but either complication can occur without an audible murmur (Chapter 73).

DIAGNOSIS

After recognizing the clinical manifestations of apparent cardiogenic shock, the clinician must confirm its presence and assess its cause while simultaneously initiating supportive therapy before there is irreversible damage to vital organs. The clinician must balance overzealous pursuit of an etiologic diagnosis before achieving stabilization with overzealous empirical treatment without establishing the underlying pathophysiology.

An electrocardiogram (ECG) should be performed immediately. In cardiogenic shock caused by acute MI, the ECG most commonly shows ST elevation, but ST depression or nonspecific changes are found in 25% of cases. If RV infarction is suspected, ST elevation in modified right-sided leads may be diagnostic (Chapter 73). The ECG may also provide information on previous MIs and rhythm abnormalities. A relatively normal ECG or one showing only diffuse, nonspecific changes in a patient with clinical cardiogenic shock should suggest myocarditis (Chapter 60), especially if the patient has arrhythmias. In end-stage heart failure, the ECG may show Q waves and/or bundle branch block, indicative of extensive disease.

Other initial diagnostic tests include a chest radiograph, complete blood count, and measurement of arterial blood gases, electrolytes, and cardiac biomarkers. A high-quality chest film can assess signs of pulmonary edema and is helpful when signs suggest an alternative diagnosis, such as a widened mediastinum indicative of aortic dissection (Chapter 78).

Echocardiography

Echocardiography should be performed as early as possible, preferably with color flow Doppler, to provide an expeditious assessment of cardiac chamber size, LV and RV function, valvular structure and motion, atrial size, and the pericardium (Chapter 55). Echocardiography can also assess or diagnose overall and regional systolic function, diastolic function, papillary muscle rupture, acute ventricular septal defect, free wall rupture, degree of mitral regurgitation, presence of RV infarction, cardiac tamponade, and valvular stenosis.

Right Heart Catheterization

If the history, physical examination, chest radiograph, and echocardiogram demonstrate systemic hypoperfusion, low cardiac output, and elevation of venous pressures, right heart catheterization may not be necessary for diagnosis. However, therapy with vasopressors and inotropic agents is best optimized using hemodynamic measurements. Right heart catheterization can exclude other causes of shock such as volume depletion and sepsis, and it helps diagnose mechanical complications. A step-up in oxygen saturation between the right atrium and pulmonary artery can indicate a ventricular septal defect (Chapter 69), and large "V" waves in the PCWP waveform can reflect acute severe mitral regurgitation. RV infarction should be suspected when the PCWP is normal but right-sided filling pressures are notably elevated.

Right heart catheterization is most useful, however, to optimize therapy in unstable patients. In such patients, clinical estimates of filling pressures can be unreliable, and changes in myocardial performance or therapeutic interventions can change cardiac output and filling pressures precipitously. Although patients with a low cardiac index ($<$2.2 L/minute/m^2) and a PCWP greater than 18 mm Hg meet the definition of cardiogenic shock, optimal filling pressures may be even higher in individual patients with LV diastolic dysfunction.

TREATMENT Rx

Initial Management

Initial stabilization of the patient with suspected cardiogenic shock consists of venous access, supplemental oxygen, and continuous ECG monitoring (Fig. 107-2). Many patients require endotracheal intubation and mechanical ventilation (Chapter 105), if only to reduce the work of breathing and facilitate sedation and stabilization before cardiac catheterization. Electrolyte abnormalities should be corrected. Morphine (1 to 2 mg every 5 minutes) relieves pain and anxiety, reduces excessive sympathetic activity, and decreases oxygen demand, preload, and afterload. Atrial bradyarrhythmias or tachyarrhythmias (Chapter 64) or ventricular tachyarrhythmias can reduce cardiac output and should be corrected promptly with antiarrhythmic drugs (see Table 64-7 in Chapter 64), cardioversion, or pacing (Chapter 66).

If the cause is likely an acute MI, aspirin and heparin should be given immediately (Chapter 73). Some therapies routinely used in acute MI (e.g., nitrates, β-blockers, angiotensin-converting enzyme inhibitors) have the potential to exacerbate hypotension in cardiogenic shock and should be avoided in patients with a tenuous hemodynamic status until they stabilize.

An initial assessment of fluid status and systemic perfusion should be performed. Patients are commonly diaphoretic, and relative hypovolemia may be present. Ischemia produces diastolic dysfunction, so high filling pressures may be necessary to maintain stroke volume in some patients. Some patients may benefit from judicious fluid replacement with predetermined rapid infusions of 100 to 200 mL of normal saline titrated to clinical end points. Patients who do not respond rapidly to initial treatment should be considered for invasive hemodynamic monitoring to identify the filling pressure at which cardiac output is maximized. Maintenance of adequate preload is particularly important in patients with RV infarction.

Following initial stabilization and restoration of adequate blood pressure, tissue perfusion should be assessed. If tissue perfusion is adequate but significant pulmonary congestion remains, low-dose diuretics may be used, taking care not to remove too much fluid. If tissue perfusion remains inadequate, inotropic support or an intra-aortic balloon pump (IABP) should be initiated.

Vasopressors and Inotropes

Maintenance of adequate blood pressure is essential to break the vicious circle of progressive hypotension and further myocardial ischemia. When arterial pressure remains inadequate, therapy with vasopressor agents, titrated not only to blood pressure but also to clinical indices of perfusion and mixed venous oxygen saturation, may be required. Norepinephrine and dopamine are considered first-line drugs for hypotension in this situation. Dopamine acts as both an inotrope (particularly at 3 to 10 μg/kg/minute) and a vasopressor (10 to 20 μg/kg/minute). Norepinephrine (0.02 to 1.0 μg/kg/minute) acts primarily as a vasoconstrictor, has a mild inotropic effect, and increases

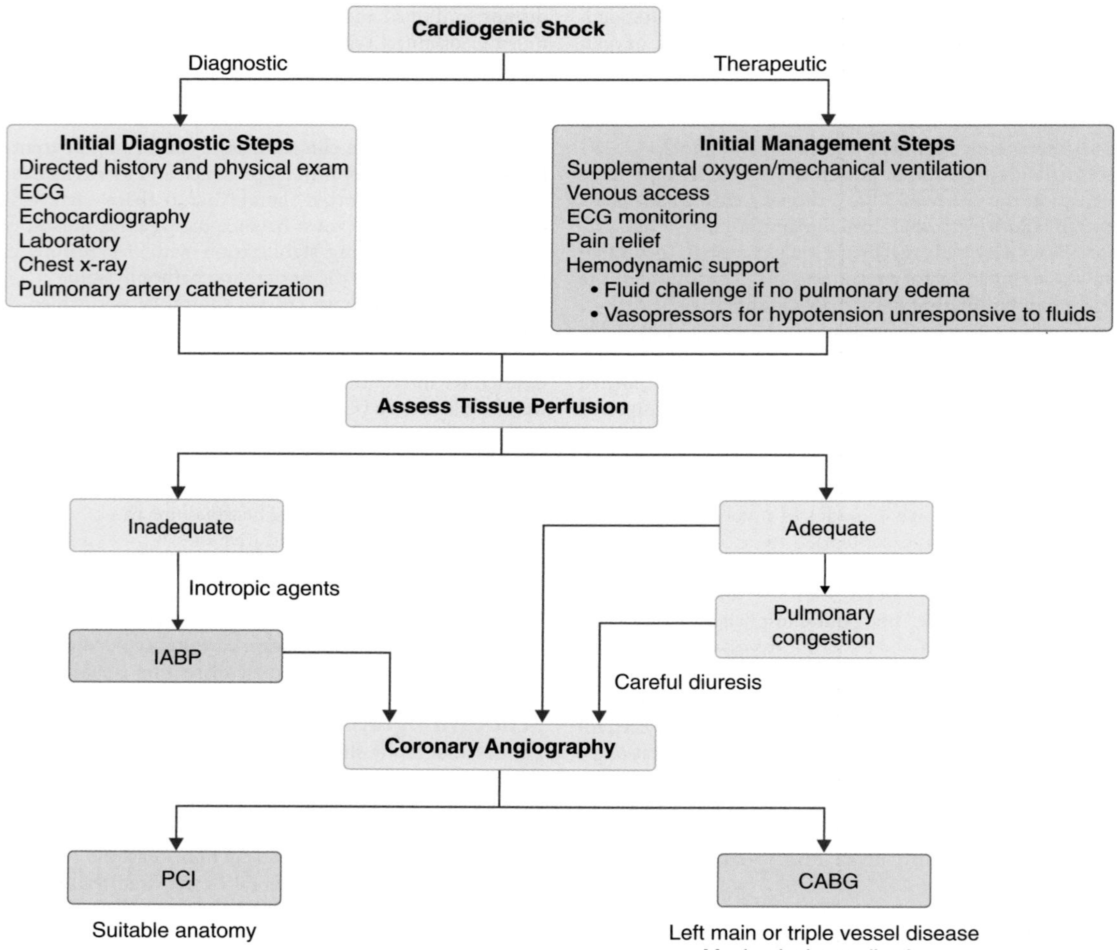

FIGURE 107-2. Approach to the diagnosis and treatment of cardiogenic shock caused by myocardial infarction. Right ventricular infarction and mechanical complications are discussed in the text. CABG = coronary artery bypass graft; ECG = electrocardiogram; IABP = intra-aortic balloon pump; PCI = percutaneous coronary intervention. Adapted from Hochman JS, Boland J, Sleeper LA, et al. Current spectrum of cardiogenic shock and effect of early revascularization on mortality: results of an International Registry. SHOCK Registry Investigators. *Circulation.* 1995;91:873-881.

coronary flow. In a randomized trial of patients with shock, there was no significant difference overall in 28-day mortality between those receiving dopamine and those receiving norepinephrine, but norepinephrine reduced mortality in a prespecified subgroup of patients with cardiogenic shock.[1] Vasopressor infusions need to be titrated carefully in patients with cardiogenic shock to maximize coronary perfusion pressure with the least possible increase in myocardial oxygen demand. Invasive hemodynamic monitoring with an arterial line and right heart catheterization are advisable during the initial titration of vasoactive agents.

If tissue perfusion remains inadequate despite norepinephrine, inotropic therapy should be initiated. Dobutamine (2.5 to 20 μg/kg/minute), a selective β_1-adrenergic receptor agonist, can improve myocardial contractility and increase cardiac output, and it is the initial agent of choice in patients with a low-output syndrome and systolic blood pressures greater than 90 mm Hg. Dobutamine may exacerbate hypotension in some patients owing to its vasodilatory effects, and it can precipitate tachyarrhythmias. Milrinone (0.125 to 0.75 μg/kg/minute), a phosphodiesterase inhibitor, has fewer chronotropic and arrhythmogenic effects than catecholamines, but it has a long half-life and can cause hypotension; in patients whose clinical status is tenuous, it is usually reserved for situations in which other agents have proved ineffective. Levosimendan (0.05 to 0.2 μg/kg/minute) is a calcium sensitizer that has both inotropic and vasodilatory properties and does not increase myocardial oxygen consumption. Levosimendan is more effective than dobutamine in treating low-output heart failure,[2] but it may cause hypotension, and it must be used with caution in patients with cardiogenic shock. Attempts to inhibit nitric oxide synthase have not been beneficial.

Intra-aortic Balloon Counterpulsation

An IABP reduces systolic afterload and augments diastolic perfusion pressure. In contrast to the effects of inotropic or vasopressor agents, these benefits occur without an increase in oxygen demand. IABPs do not, however, produce a significant improvement in blood flow distal to a critical coronary stenosis; thus, they act as a bridge, helping patients through a critical period of shock, but they are not definitive therapy.

An IABP should be used for MI patients when cardiogenic shock is not quickly reversed with pharmacologic therapy. Although it has not been shown to improve mortality when used alone, use of an IABP in cardiogenic shock complicating acute MI improves survival at 30 days and 1 year,[3] suggesting its efficacy as a stabilizing measure before angiography and prompt revascularization in appropriately selected patients.

Reperfusion

Supportive therapy may improve blood pressure and cardiac output in cardiogenic shock, but it does not interrupt the vicious circle of myocardial dysfunction and ischemia. Rapid restoration of myocardial blood flow is the cornerstone of therapy for patients with cardiogenic shock due to MI (Chapter 73). Fibrinolytic therapy (see Table 73-5 in Chapter 73) restores patency of the infarcted artery and decreases the likelihood of progression to cardiogenic shock. After cardiogenic shock has already developed, however, fibrinolytic therapy is less effective at achieving and maintaining reperfusion, likely due to a combination of hemodynamic, mechanical, and metabolic factors that prevent the achievement and maintenance of patency in the infarct-related artery.

Prompt revascularization is the only intervention that consistently reduces mortality rates in patients with cardiogenic shock. In a randomized trial of patients with LV failure complicating ST elevation MI, cardiac catheterization with PCI or CABG within 48 hours of presentation reduced all-cause mortality marginally at 30 days (47% in the revascularization group vs. 56% in the medical therapy group; $P = 11$) and significantly at 6 months, 1 year,[4] and 6 years[5] compared with optimal medical management, including IABP, in 86% of patients. Subgroup analyses also revealed benefits in patients younger than 75 years, those with prior MI, and those randomized less than 6 hours from the onset of infarction. Another trial with a similar design was terminated early owing to difficulties in patient recruitment, but it also showed a trend toward reduced 30-day and 1-year mortality. Together, these trials suggest that for each 100 patients treated, 9 lives will be saved at 30 days and 13.2 lives will be saved at 1 year.

On the basis of these results, emergent coronary revascularization, most often with PCI and stents, is the standard of care for cardiogenic shock due to pump failure in acute MI. Outcomes are best when PCI is performed within 6 hours after the onset of symptoms, but survival benefits are still demonstrable up to 48 hours after the onset of MI and 18 hours after the onset of shock. Elderly patients who are suitable for aggressive therapy also appear to benefit.

CABG surgery is more likely to provide complete revascularization and achieves long-term survival rates comparable to PCI, often despite worse coronary anatomy and a higher prevalence of diabetes. In practice, however, emergency CABG is performed less than 10% of the time.

When cardiogenic shock results from mechanical complications of MI (Chapter 73), surgery is recommended when feasible. For acute mitral regurgitation owing to papillary muscle rupture, supportive therapy with an IABP and vasoactive agents is a temporizing measure; definitive therapy requires expeditious surgical valve repair or replacement (Chapter 75). Although mortality is 20 to 40%, survival and ventricular function are improved compared with medical therapy.

Timely surgery is also critical in patients whose cardiogenic shock is caused by ventricular septal or free wall rupture. Because perforations are exposed to shear forces, the rupture site can expand abruptly. Repair can be technically difficult owing to the need to suture in areas of necrosis. Surgical mortality is 20 to 50% and is especially high for serpiginous inferoposterior ruptures, which are typically less well circumscribed than anteroapical ruptures. RV function is an important determinant of outcome in this setting. Timing of surgery has been controversial, but guidelines now recommend that operative repair be undertaken early, within 48 hours of the rupture. Placement of a septal occluding device may be helpful in selected patients.

Circulatory Support

Mechanical support with a left ventricular assist device (LVAD; Chapter 73) can interrupt the downward spiral of myocardial dysfunction, hypoperfusion, and ischemia in cardiogenic shock, allowing time for stunned or hibernating myocardium to recover. In cardiogenic shock after acute MI, percutaneous LVADs can be placed in the catheterization laboratory. These devices provide short-term support and are usually intended as a bridge to recovery or, occasionally, as a bridge to transplantation. Extracorporeal support has been used in selected patients.

Management of Special Conditions

At the end stage of a dilated or restrictive cardiomyopathy (Chapter 60), low cardiac output can result in cardiogenic shock. A search for reversible precipitating causes should be undertaken. Some patients will respond to inotropic therapy and will have a brief period of relative improvement. Appropriate candidates should be referred for evaluation for possible cardiac transplantation (Chapter 82). In selected patients, a surgically placed LVAD, such as a continuous-flow device, can provide 45% two-year survival free of device surgery or disabling stroke.[6] LVADs can be used either as a bridge to transplantation or as destination therapy. A discussion about end-of-life care is also warranted.

Acute myocarditis (Chapter 60) can have a fulminant course leading to shock in 10 to 15% of cases. Patients with acute myocarditis are typically younger than those with cardiogenic shock due to MI, and they present more commonly with dyspnea rather than chest pain. Echocardiography usually shows global LV dysfunction. Supportive therapy is indicated; some patients may require circulatory support and even consideration of cardiac transplantation. Immunosuppressive therapy does not improve outcome in this setting.

Patients with hypertrophic cardiomyopathy (Chapter 60) may present with severe outflow tract obstruction and shock. Recognition of this condition is important, because diuretic and inotropic therapy may worsen the obstruction. Careful volume resuscitation and use of a pure α-agonist, such as phenylephrine (0.1 to 0.3 mg/kg/minute), can increase afterload and cavity size. β-Blockers (esmolol 0.05 to 0.2 mg/kg/minute; metoprolol 2.5 to 5 mg IV every 2 to 5 minutes, up to 15 mg) and/or calcium blockers with negative inotropic properties (e.g., diltiazem 5 mg IV every 2 minutes, up to 20 mg) can also be helpful.

Some patients with stress (takotsubo) cardiomyopathy (Chapter 60) may have LV dysfunction severe enough to produce shock. Because the presentation is similar to that of acute MI, with chest pain and ECG changes, the diagnosis is usually made in the catheterization laboratory, when significant coronary obstruction is excluded and the characteristic apical hypokinesis or dyskinesis is documented. Treatment is supportive and may include an IABP. Most patients have recovery of LV function within days to weeks, and the long-term prognosis is excellent.

Acute valvular regurgitation (Chapter 75) presents with pulmonary edema and decreased forward cardiac output. The regurgitant murmur may be soft or inaudible, and the diagnosis is best made by echocardiography. Acute ischemic mitral regurgitation is usually associated with rupture of the posterior papillary muscle, which has a single blood supply. Other causes include spontaneous chordal rupture, infective endocarditis (Chapter 76), rheumatic fever (Chapter 298), and trauma (Chapter 112). Immediate management includes afterload reduction (Chapter 59) and an IABP as temporizing measures. Inotropic or vasopressor therapy may also be needed to support cardiac output and blood pressure. Definitive therapy, however, consists of surgical valve repair or replacement (Chapter 75).

Acute aortic regurgitation most commonly results from infective endocarditis (Chapter 76) with leaflet destruction, but it may also be due to traumatic injury (Chapter 112) or acute aortic dissection (Chapter 78). The pulse pressure is usually narrow, indicating decreased forward stroke volume, and the bounding pulsations seen with chronic aortic regurgitation are usually absent. Temporizing measures include afterload reduction, with vasopressor and inotropic support as needed. IABP is contraindicated, and excessive slowing of the heart rate may worsen hemodynamics by prolonging diastole. Definitive therapy is surgical.

PROGNOSIS

Cardiogenic shock is still the most common cause of death in acute MI. Survival rates are improving, however, coincident with the increasing use of reperfusion therapy in appropriately selected patients. Hemodynamics predict short-term but not long-term mortality. Among patients undergoing revascularization, age, time to revascularization, and restoration of coronary blood flow independently predict survival, but the benefits of revascularization are seen at every level of risk, with an average 1-year survival of 50 to 55%. Encouragingly, the survival benefit of early revascularization is maintained at 6-year follow-up, with 5-year survival approaching 45%. The quality of life in survivors is usually excellent, with 83% either asymptomatic or having only mildly symptomatic heart failure. For patients with end-stage nonischemic myocardial disease, the prognosis is very poor in the absence of heart transplantation.

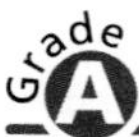

1. De Backer D, Biston P, Devriendt J, et al. Comparison of dopamine and norepinephrine in the treatment of shock. *N Engl J Med.* 2010;362:779-789.
2. Follath F, Cleland JGF, Just H, et al. Efficacy and safety of intravenous levosimendan compared with dobutamine in severe low-output heart failure (the LIDO study): a randomised double-blind trial. *Lancet.* 2002;360:196-202.
3. Stone GW, Marsalese D, Brodie BR, et al. A prospective, randomized evaluation of prophylactic intra-aortic balloon counterpulsation in high-risk patients with acute myocardial infarction treated with primary angioplasty: Second Primary Angioplasty in Myocardial Infarction (PAMI-II) Trial Investigators. *J Am Coll Cardiol.* 1997;29:1459-1467.
4. Hochman JS, Sleeper LA, White HD, et al. One-year survival following early revascularization for cardiogenic shock. *JAMA.* 2001;285:190-192.
5. Hochman JS, Sleeper LA, Webb JG, et al. Early revascularization and long-term survival in cardiogenic shock complicating acute myocardial infarction. *JAMA.* 2006;295:2511-2515.
6. Slaughter MS, Rogers JG, Milano CA, et al. Advanced heart failure treated with continuous-flow left ventricular assist device. *N Engl J Med.* 2009;361:2241-2251.

SUGGESTED READINGS

Goldstein D, Neragi-Miandoab S. Mechanical bridge to decision: what are the options for the management of acute refractory cardiogenic shock? *Curr Heart Fail Rep.* 2011;8:51-58. *Review.*

Sarswat N, Hollenberg SM. Cardiogenic shock. *Hosp Pract (Minneap).* 2010;38:74-83. *Review.*

108

SHOCK SYNDROMES RELATED TO SEPSIS

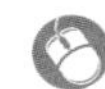

JAMES A. RUSSELL

DEFINITION

Sepsis is defined by presence of at least two of the four signs of the systemic inflammatory response syndrome (SIRS): (1) fever (>38°C) or hypothermia (<36°C); (2) tachycardia (>90 beats/minute); (3) tachypnea (>20 breaths/minute), hypocapnia (partial pressure of carbon dioxide <32 mm Hg), or the need for mechanical ventilatory assistance; and (4) leukocytosis (>12,000 cells/mm^3), leukopenia (<4000 cells/mm^3), or a left shift (>0% immature band cells) in the circulating white cell differential and suspected or proven infection. *Bacteremia* is defined as the growth of bacteria in blood cultures, but infection does not have to be proved to diagnose sepsis at the onset. *Severe sepsis* is sepsis in addition to dysfunction of one or more organ systems (e.g., hypoxemia, oliguria, lactic acidosis, thrombocytopenia, decreased Glasgow Coma Scale score). *Septic shock* is defined as severe sepsis in addition to hypotension (systolic blood pressure <90 mm Hg or a >40 mm Hg decrease from baseline) despite adequate fluid resuscitation.

EPIDEMIOLOGY

Approximately 750,000 cases of severe sepsis or septic shock occur every year in the United States. Sepsis causes as many deaths as acute myocardial infarction, and septic shock and its complications are the most common causes of death in noncoronary intensive care units (ICUs). The medical care costs associated with sepsis are approximately $16.7 billion a year in the United States alone. The frequency of septic shock is increasing as physicians perform more aggressive surgery, as more resistant organisms are present in the environment, and as the prevalence of immune compromise resulting from disease and immunosuppressive drugs increases. Recent studies suggest that African Americans have a higher incidence of severe sepsis than whites (6.0 vs. 3.6 per 1000 population) and a higher mortality in ICUs (32.1 vs. 29.3%; $P < .0001$), even after adjusting for poverty levels. The mechanisms of this apparent difference in risk for and mortality from sepsis are not known.

Gram-positive or gram-negative bacteria, fungi, and, very rarely, protozoa or rickettsiae can cause septic shock. Increasingly common causes of septic shock are gram-positive bacteria, especially methicillin-resistant *Staphylococcus aureus*, vancomycin-resistant enterococci, penicillin-resistant *Streptococcus pneumoniae*, and resistant gram-negative bacilli.

The common infections causing septic shock are pneumonia, peritonitis, pyelonephritis, abscess (especially intra-abdominal), primary bacteremia, cholangitis, cellulitis, necrotizing fasciitis, and meningitis. Nosocomial pneumonia is the most common cause of death from nosocomial infection.

PATHOBIOLOGY

At onset, septic shock activates inflammation, leading to enhanced coagulation, activated platelets, increased neutrophils and mononuclear cells, and diminished fibrinolysis (Table 108-1). After several days, a compensatory anti-inflammatory response with immunosuppression may contribute to death. Several pathways amplify one another: inflammation triggers coagulation, and coagulation triggers inflammation, resulting in a positive feedback loop that is pro-inflammatory and pro-coagulant. Tissue hypoxia in septic shock also amplifies inflammation and coagulation. Many mediators that are critical for the homeostatic control of infection may be injurious to the host (e.g., tumor necrosis factor-α [TNF-α]), so therapies that fully neutralize such mediators are largely ineffective.

Widespread endothelial injury is an important feature of septic shock; an injured endothelium is more permeable, so the flux of protein-rich edema fluid into tissues such as the lung increases. Injured endothelial cells release nitric oxide, a potent vasodilator that is a key mediator of septic shock. Septic shock also injures epithelial cells of the lung and intestine. Intestinal epithelial injury increases intestinal permeability; this leads to epithelial translocation of intestinal bacteria and endotoxin, which further augments the inflammatory phenotype of septic shock.

Early Infection, the Innate Immune Response, Inflammation, and the Endothelium

Host defense is organized into innate and adaptive immune responses. The innate immune system responds by using pattern recognition receptors (e.g., Toll-like receptors [TLRs]) to pathogen-associated molecular patterns, which are extremely well-conserved molecules of microorganisms. Surface molecules of gram-positive and gram-negative bacteria (peptidoglycan and lipopolysaccharide, respectively) bind to TLR-2 and TLR-4, respectively (Fig. 108-1). TLR-2 and TLR-4 binding initiates an intracellular signaling cascade that culminates in nuclear transport of the transcription factor nuclear factor kappa B (NFκB), which triggers transcription of cytokines such as TNF-α and interleukin (IL)-6. Cytokines upregulate adhesion molecules of neutrophils and endothelial cells, and neutrophil activation leads to bacterial killing. However, cytokines also directly injure host endothelial cells, as do activated neutrophils, monocytes, and platelets. Inhibition of early cytokine mediators of sepsis, such as TNF-α and IL-1β, has not proved successful, likely because TNF-α and IL-1β peak and then decline quickly, before these antagonist therapies can be applied clinically.

After the early cytokine inflammatory response, immune cells, including macrophages and neutrophils, release later mediators, such as high-mobility group box-1 (HMGB-1). HMGB-1 activates neutrophils, monocytes, and endothelium. Unlike TNF-α antagonists, inhibitors of HMGB-1 decrease mortality even when they are given 24 hours after the induction of experimental peritonitis.

Adaptive Immunity Adds Specificity and Amplifies the Immune Response

Microorganisms stimulate specific humoral and cell-mediated adaptive immune responses that amplify innate immunity. B cells release immunoglobulins that bind to microorganisms and thereby facilitate delivery of microorganisms to natural killer cells and neutrophils. In sepsis, type 1 helper T (T_H1) cells generally secrete pro-inflammatory cytokines (TNF-α, IL-1β),

TABLE 108-1 PATHWAYS; MEDIATORS; AND POSITIVE, NEGATIVE, AND POTENTIALLY ATTRACTIVE TRIALS IN SEPTIC SHOCK

PATHWAYS	MEDIATORS	POSITIVE RCTs*	NEGATIVE RCTs	EXAMPLES OF POTENTIAL THERAPIES
Organism features	Superantigens: TSST-1 Streptococcal exotoxins (pyrogenic exotoxin A) Lipopolysaccharide (endotoxin)		Anti-lipopolysaccharide	Anti-TSST1 Polymyxin B hemoperfusion[†] Anti-exotoxins
Innate immunity	TLR-2, TLR-4 Monocytes, macrophages Neutrophils			TLR agonists; TLR antagonists GM-CSF, interferon-γ G-CSF[‡]
Adaptive immunity	B cells, plasma cells, immunoglobulin T cells: CD4, T_H1, T_H2			Immunoglobulin G
Pro-inflammatory pathway	TNF-α		Anti–TNF-α	
	IL-1β		IL-1 receptor antagonist	
	IL-6			IL-6 antagonist
	Prostaglandins, leukotrienes		Ibuprofen, high-dose corticosteroids	
	Bradykinin		Bradykinin antagonist	
	Platelet-activating factor		Platelet-activating factor acetylhydrolase	
	Proteases (e.g., elastase)		Elastase inhibitor[§]	
	Oxidants			Antioxidants (e.g., *N*-acetylcysteine)
	Nitric oxide		Nitric oxide synthase inhibitor	
Pro-coagulant pathway	↓ Protein C	Activated protein C[14]		
	↓ Protein S			Protein S
	↓ Antithrombin		Antithrombin	
	↓ Tissue factor pathway inhibitor		Tissue factor pathway inhibitor	
	↑ Tissue factor			Tissue factor antagonist
	↑ Plasminogen activator inhibitor (PAI-1)			Tissue plasminogen activator
			Heparin[‖]	
Anti-inflammatory pathway	IL-10		IL-10[¶]	
	TNF-α receptors		TNF-α receptors	
Tissue hypoxia	HIF-1α, VEGF	Early goal-directed therapy[3]	Supernormal oxygen delivery Epinephrine, norepinephrine, dobutamine[††]	Erythropoietin[**]
Immunosuppression/ apoptosis	Lymphocyte apoptosis			Anti-caspases
	Intestinal epithelial cell apoptosis			Anti-caspases
Endocrine dysfunction	Adrenal insufficiency		Corticosteroids[‡‡]	Corticosteroids[§§]
	Vasopressin deficiency			Vasopressin[‖‖]
	Hyperglycemia			Intensive insulin[¶¶]
Renal dysfunction	Metabolites with renal clearance		Intensive renal support[***]	

*Positive RCTs are pivotal randomized controlled trials powered for mortality as the primary end point.
[†]In a small RCT, polymyxin B hemoperfusion decreased mortality compared with usual care.
[‡]G-CSF is effective in septic patients with profound neutropenia.
[§]Elastase inhibitor was ineffective in a phase II trial in acute lung injury.
[‖]Unfractionated heparin did not decrease mortality in acute sepsis.
[¶]IL-10 was ineffective in a phase II trial in acute lung injury.
[**]Erythropoietin does not decrease red blood cell transfusions in the critically ill and may increase the risk of thrombotic events.
[††]In an RCT of norepinephrine plus dobutamine versus epinephrine alone, there was no difference in mortality.
[‡‡]In a randomized placebo-controlled trial, corticosteroids did not change mortality in septic shock, regardless of whether there was an abnormal corticotropin stimulation test.
[§§]Corticosteroids, which have no effect on overall 28-day mortality, decreased mortality in a subgroup of nonresponders to corticotropin in one study[12] but not another.[2]
[‖‖]In an RCT, vasopressin compared with norepinephrine did not change overall mortality, but it was associated with decreased mortality in patients who had less severe septic shock (norepinephrine infusion 5-15 μg/min).
[¶¶]Intensive insulin (compared with conventional insulin) did not change mortality in one RCT and increased mortality in another.
[***]In an RCT, intensive renal support (six times/wk) compared with conventional renal support (three times/wk) did not change mortality in critically ill patients with acute kidney injury (many of whom had sepsis).
↑ = increased; ↓ = decreased; G-CSF = granulocyte colony-stimulating factor; GM-CSF = granulocyte-macrophage colony-stimulating factor; HIF-1α: hypoxia-inducing factor-1α; IL = interleukin; RCT = randomized controlled trial; T_H1 and T_H2 = type 1 and 2 helper T cell, respectively; TNF-α = tumor necrosis factor-α; TLR = Toll-like receptor; TSST-1 = toxic shock syndrome toxin-1; VEGF = vascular endothelial growth factor.

and type 2 helper T (T_H2) cells secrete anti-inflammatory cytokines (IL-4, IL-10).

Coagulation Response to Infection

Septic shock activates the coagulation system (Fig. 108-2) and ultimately converts fibrinogen to fibrin, which is bound to platelets to form microvascular thrombi. Microvascular thrombi further amplify endothelial injury by the release of mediators and by tissue hypoxia because of obstruction to blood flow.

Normally, natural anticoagulants (protein C, protein S, antithrombin, and tissue factor pathway inhibitor) dampen coagulation, enhance fibrinolysis, and remove microthrombi. Thrombin-α binds to thrombomodulin, which activates protein C when protein C is bound to the endothelial protein C receptor (EPCR). Activated protein C dampens the pro-coagulant phenotype because it inactivates factors Va and VIIIa and inhibits the synthesis of plasminogen activator inhibitor-1 (PAI-1). Activated protein C also decreases apoptosis, leukocyte activation and adhesion, and the production of cytokines.

Septic shock decreases the levels of the natural anticoagulants protein C, protein S, antithrombin, and tissue factor pathway inhibitor. Furthermore, lipopolysaccharide and TNF-α decrease thrombomodulin and EPCR, thereby limiting the activation of protein C. Lipopolysaccharide and TNF-α also increase levels of PAI-1, inhibiting fibrinolysis.

Tissue Hypoxia in Septic Shock

Tissue hypoxia independently activates inflammation (by activation of NFκB and cytokines, synthesis of nitric oxide, and activation of HMGB-1), induces coagulation (through tissue factor and PAI-1), and activates neutrophils,

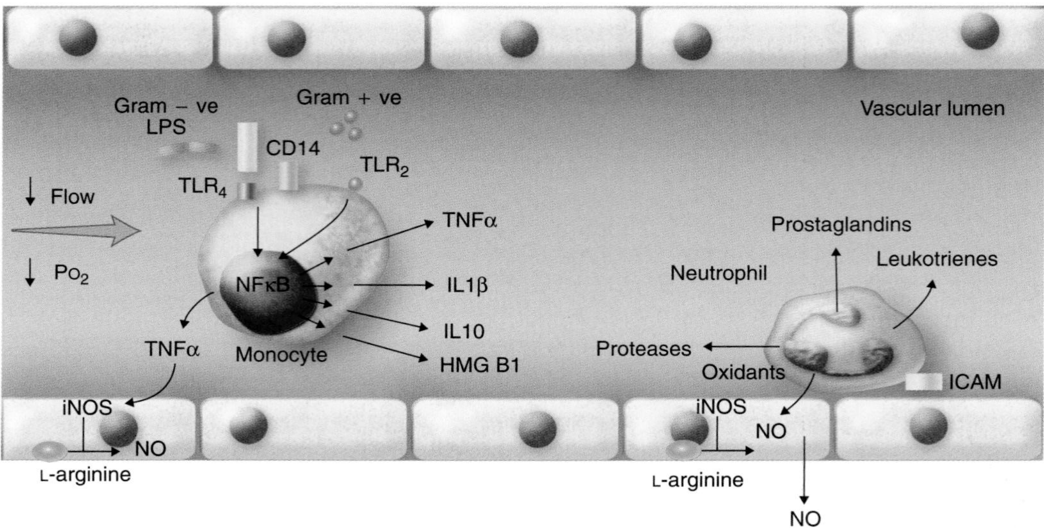

FIGURE 108-1. **Inflammatory responses to sepsis.** Gram-positive and gram-negative bacteria, viruses, and fungi have unique cell wall molecules called pathogen-associated molecular patterns that bind to pattern recognition receptors (called Toll-like receptors [TLRs]) on the surface of immune cells. The lipopolysaccharide (LPS) of gram-negative bacilli binds to LPS-binding protein–CD14 complex. The peptidoglycan of gram-positive bacteria and the LPS of gram-negative bacteria bind to TLR-2 and TLR-4, respectively. TLR-2 and TLR-4 binding activates intracellular signal transduction pathways that lead to the activation of the cytosolic transcription factor nuclear factor kappa B (NFκB). Activated NFκB moves from the cytoplasm to the nucleus, binds to transcription start sites, and increases the transcription of cytokines such as tumor necrosis factor-α (TNF-α), interleukin-1β (IL-1β), and interleukin-10 (IL-10). TNF-α and IL-1β are pro-inflammatory cytokines that activate the adaptive immune response but also cause both direct and indirect host injury. IL-10 is an anti-inflammatory cytokine that inactivates macrophages and has other anti-inflammatory effects. Sepsis increases the activity of inducible nitric oxide synthase (iNOS), which increases the synthesis of nitric oxide (NO), a potent vasodilator. Cytokines activate endothelial cells by upregulating adhesion receptors such as intercellular adhesion molecule (ICAM), and they injure endothelial cells by the activation and binding of neutrophils, monocytes, macrophages, and platelets to endothelial cells. These effector cells release mediators such as proteases, oxidants, prostaglandins, and ICAM leukotrienes. Cytokines also activate the coagulation cascade.

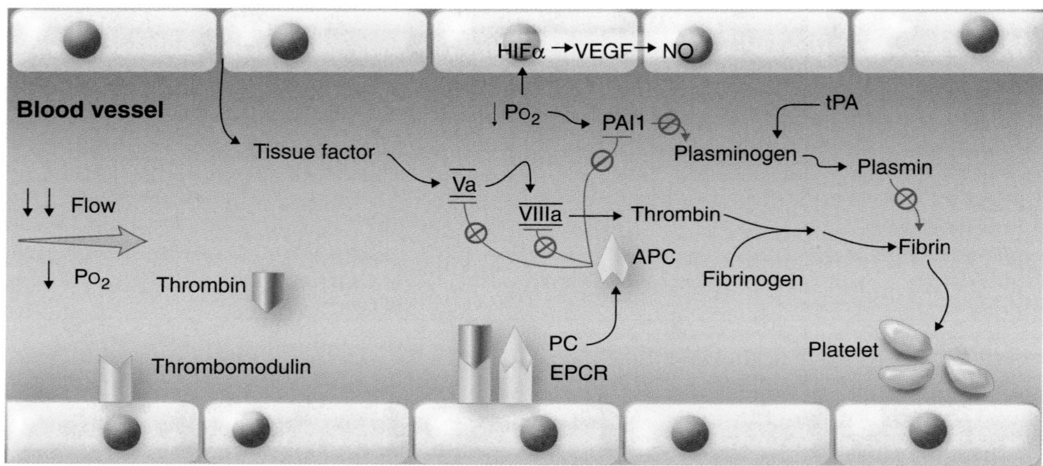

FIGURE 108-2. **Pro-coagulant response in sepsis.** Sepsis initiates coagulation by activating the endothelium to increase tissue factor. Activation of factors Va and VIIIa leads to the formation of thrombin-α, which converts fibrinogen to fibrin. Fibrin binds to platelets that adhere to endothelial cells, forming microvascular thrombi. Microvascular thrombi amplify injury by the release of mediators and by microvascular obstruction, which causes distal ischemia and tissue hypoxia. Normally, natural anticoagulants—protein C (PC), protein S (PS), antithrombin, and tissue factor pathway inhibitor (TFPI)—dampen coagulation, enhance fibrinolysis, and remove microthrombi. Thrombin-α binds to thrombomodulin on endothelial cells and thus activates the binding of PC to endothelial PC receptor (EPCR). PC forms a complex with its cofactor PS. PC binding to EPCR increases the activation of PC to activated PC (APC). APC proteolytically inactivates factors Va and VIIIa and decreases the synthesis of plasminogen activator inhibitor-1 (PAI-1). Sepsis decreases levels of PC, PS, antithrombin, and TFPI. Lipopolysaccharide and tumor necrosis factor-α (TNF-α) decrease thrombomodulin and EPCR, thus decreasing the activation of PC. Lipopolysaccharide and TNF-α also inhibit PAI-1, so fibrinolysis is inhibited. HIFα = hypoxia-inducing factor-α; NO = nitric oxide; tPA = tissue plasminogen activator; VEGF = vascular endothelial growth factor.

monocytes, and platelets. Hypoxia induces hypoxia-inducing factor-1α (HIF-1α), which upregulates erythropoietin, and vascular endothelial growth factor (VEGF). Erythropoietin is protective to brain and other tissues. VEGF inhibits fibrinolysis and increases inducible nitric oxide synthase, which augments nitric oxide–induced vasodilation. Nitric oxide has a further injurious effect: excessive nitric oxide inhibits the beneficial actions of HIF-1α (e.g., upregulating synthesis of erythropoietin) during hypoxia.

Late Septic Shock, Immunosuppression, and Apoptosis of Immune and Epithelial Cells

After about 1 week of septic shock, death can result from immunosuppression, which is suggested by anergy, lymphopenia, hypothermia, and nosocomial infection. Multiple organ dysfunction may be an anti-inflammatory phenotype because of the apoptosis of immune, epithelial, and endothelial cells. Activated $CD4^+$ T cells evolve into either a T_H1 pro-inflammatory (TNF-α, IL-1β) or a T_H2 anti-inflammatory (IL-4, IL-10) phenotype. Sepsis leads to migration from a T_H1 to a T_H2 phenotype; for example, persistent elevation of IL-10 is associated with an increased risk of death. Immunosuppression also develops because of apoptosis of lymphocytes. Pro-inflammatory cytokines, activated B and T cells, and glucocorticoids induce lymphocyte apoptosis, whereas TNF-α and endotoxin induce apoptosis of lung and intestinal epithelial cells. The fact that glucocorticoids also stimulate apoptosis could be the biologic explanation for the observation that patients with septic shock who are treated with hydrocortisone have more superinfections than do patients treated with placebo.[1]

Death from infectious disease appears to be highly heritable. Sepsis is a prime example of a polygenic disease related to the interaction of multiple

TABLE 108-2 HEMODYNAMIC VARIABLES, ABBREVIATIONS, AND NORMAL VALUES

Arterial pressure: systolic pressure (SAP) (>100 mm Hg), diastolic pressure, pulse pressure, mean arterial pressure (MAP) (>65 mm Hg)
Central venous pressure (CVP): normal 6-12 mm Hg
Pulmonary artery pressure (PAP): normal 25/15 mm Hg
Pulmonary vascular resistance (PVR): normal 150-250 dynes/sec/cm

$$\left(\equiv \frac{\text{PAP} - \text{PAOP}}{\text{CO}} \times 80\right)$$

Pulmonary artery occlusion pressure (PAOP) or pulmonary artery wedge pressure (PAWP): normal 8-15 mm Hg
Systemic vascular resistance (SVR): normal 900-1400 dynes/sec/cm

$$\left(\equiv \frac{\text{MAP} - \text{CVP}}{\text{CO}} \times 80\right)$$

Cardiac output (CO): normal 5 L/min
Left ventricular stroke work index (LVSWI): normal (60-100 grams × meters/beats) = (SV × [MAP − PAWP] × 0.0136)
Oxygen delivery (Do_2): normal 1 L/min (= CO × [Hg × 1.38 × Sao_2] + [0.003 × Po_2])
Oxygen consumption (Vo_2): normal 250 mL/min (= CO × Hg × 1.38 × [Sao_2 − Svo_2] + [0.003 × (Pao_2 − Pvo_2)])
Oxygen extraction ratio: normal 0.23-0.32 (= Vo_2/Do_2)
Hemodynamic variables are often normalized to account for different body mass by dividing by body surface area (BSA):
Pulmonary vascular resistance index (PVRI): normal (= PVR/BSA)
Systemic vascular resistance index (SVRI): normal (= SVR/BSA)
Cardiac index (CI): normal 2.5-4.2 L/min/m^2 (= CO/BSA)
Left ventricular stroke work index (LVSWI): normal (= LVSW/BSA)
Oxygen delivery index (Do_2I): normal 460-650 mL/min/m^2 (= Do_2/BSA)
Oxygen consumption index (Vo_2I): normal 95-170 mL/min/m^2 (= Vo_2/BSA)

genes and an environmental insult (infection). Single nucleotide polymorphisms of cytokines (TNF-α, IL-6, IL-10), coagulation factors (protein C, fibrinogen-β), the catecholamine pathway (β-adrenergic receptor), and innate immunity genes (CD14, TLR-1, TLR-2) have been variably associated with an increased risk of death from sepsis.

Cardiovascular Dysfunction

Inadequate tissue perfusion and tissue hypoxia are the cardinal features of all types of shock. Early in septic shock, most patients have sinus tachycardia and, by definition, decreased blood pressure (<90 mm Hg systolic, a decrease of ≥40 mm Hg from baseline systolic pressure, or mean arterial pressure <65 mm Hg; Table 108-2). Septic shock is the classic form of distributive shock (Chapter 106), characterized by increased pulse pressure (bounding pulses), decreased systemic vascular resistance (warm, flushed skin), and functional hypovolemia (low jugular venous pressure). Distributive shock means that the distribution of systemic blood flow is abnormal, such that areas of both low flow (and low venous oxygen saturation) and high flow (and increased venous oxygen saturation) are present. Nevertheless, about one third of patients with septic shock initially present with findings more typical of hypovolemic shock (low central venous pressure and low central venous oxygen saturation), because the clinical features depend on the stage and severity of septic shock as well as on the degree of fluid resuscitation that has occurred. After fluid resuscitation, patients typically develop the characteristic clinical and hemodynamic features of classic distributive shock.

Ventricular preload is commonly decreased in early septic shock, for several reasons. First, patients may be volume depleted because of decreased fluid intake and because of increased fluid losses as a result of fever, vomiting, and diarrhea if gastrointestinal disease is present. Second, fluid loss from the intravascular to the interstitial space (capillary leak) is caused by mediators that induce widespread endothelial injury, which increases capillary permeability. Increased capillary permeability leads to loss of protein-rich edema fluid into the interstitial space. In the lung, increased permeability is a key component of acute lung injury. A third reason that ventricular preload is decreased in septic shock is venodilation induced by mediators such as nitric oxide. Venodilation increases venous capacitance, leading to relative volume depletion, which compounds the absolute volume depletion. Ventricular afterload is decreased because of excessive release of potent vasodilators such as nitric oxide, prostaglandin I_2, adenosine diphosphate, and other vasodilators.

In addition to abnormal vasodilation, patients have concurrent microvascular vasoconstriction. Microvascular vasoconstriction may not be apparent clinically or hemodynamically, but it can lead to tissue hypoxia, detected by increased arterial lactate concentrations. Microvascular vasoconstriction is caused by increased norepinephrine, thromboxanes, and other local vasoconstrictors. Microvascular vasoconstriction causes focal hypoxia, which is exacerbated by microvascular obstruction by platelets and leukocytes.

The abnormal mismatch of oxygen delivery to oxygen demand can disturb the global relationship of oxygen delivery to oxygen consumption. Normally, oxygen consumption is independent of oxygen delivery over a wide range. When oxygen delivery decreases to less than the critical oxygen delivery level, oxygen consumption decreases and leads to a state in which oxygen consumption depends on oxygen delivery. At levels lower than the critical oxygen delivery level, arterial lactate increases as a result of tissue hypoxia. The clinical implication is that oxygen delivery should be increased (e.g., by increasing cardiac output by volume resuscitation, infusion of dobutamine, or transfusion of erythrocytes) to more than the critical level.

Cardiovascular function is further compromised in septic shock because of decreased ventricular contractility. Decreased ventricular contractility may be difficult to detect clinically and may be diagnosed only by hemodynamic or echocardiographic assessment. Numerous circulating mediators of sepsis, including endotoxin, cytokines (e.g., IL-6, TNF-α), and nitric oxide (locally released into the coronary circulation), decrease contractility. Endotoxin signals via TLRs to upregulate the expression of proteins such as S110A8 and S100A9 to cause a receptor for advanced glycation end products (RAGE)–dependent decrease in calcium flux, which decreases the ejection fraction. Coronary ischemia resulting from microvascular obstruction by leukocytes and oxygen free radicals, which are released by neutrophils adherent to the coronary capillary endothelium, is another mechanism of decreased contractility.

Early in septic shock, patients who survive have increased left ventricular end-diastolic volume, which likely allows them to maintain cardiac output despite decreased contractility. In contrast, nonsurvivors do not have increased left ventricular end-diastolic volume, so their cardiac output is compromised. In some patients with septic shock, concurrent acute lung injury and secondary pulmonary hypertension increase right ventricular afterload, with a secondary shift of the interventricular septum from right to left. This septal shift decreases left ventricular end-diastolic volume and can also limit cardiac output.

CLINICAL MANIFESTATIONS

Cardiovascular dysfunction in septic shock is characterized by decreased preload (because of decreased intake, fluid losses, third spacing resulting from increased permeability, and venodilation), decreased afterload, and often decreased ventricular contractility. Decreased ventricular volume is detected clinically by low jugular venous pressure and hemodynamically by decreased central venous pressure. Left ventricular resistance, or afterload, is also commonly decreased and is detected clinically by warm, flushed skin and hemodynamically by decreased systemic vascular resistance.

DIAGNOSIS

Even as the diagnostic evaluation is beginning, the initial assessment of a critically ill patient must focus immediately on the airway (need for intubation), breathing (respiratory rate, respiratory distress, pulse oximetry), circulation (heart rate, blood pressure, jugular venous pressure, skin perfusion), and rapid initiation of resuscitation (Fig. 108-3). Vital signs and the leukocyte count quickly establish whether the patient has SIRS (two of the four criteria). Arterial blood gases and lactate levels are useful complementary tests. A secondary survey is designed to determine the likely source of infection and the status of organ function. Pneumonia (Chapter 97) is suggested by cough, sputum, and respiratory distress; empyema (Chapter 99) is suggested by pleuritic chest pain. Signs of peritonitis, an abdominal mass, and right upper quadrant tenderness suggest abdominal sepsis. Pyelonephritis (Chapter 292) is likely in patients with dysuria and costovertebral angle tenderness. Integumentary assessment for erythema (cellulitis), line site erythema (line sepsis), tenderness (necrotizing fasciitis), crepitus (anaerobic myonecrosis), and petechiae and purpura (meningococcemia) can be illuminating. Headache, stiff neck, and signs of meningismus raise the suspicion of meningitis (Chapter 420). Focal neurologic signs suggest brain abscess (Chapter 421).

Laboratory investigations that are helpful to identify the source of infection include appropriate cultures and Gram stains (blood, sputum, urine, fluids, and cerebrospinal fluid). Blood cultures are positive in 40 to 60% of patients who have septic shock. The chest radiograph aids in the diagnosis of

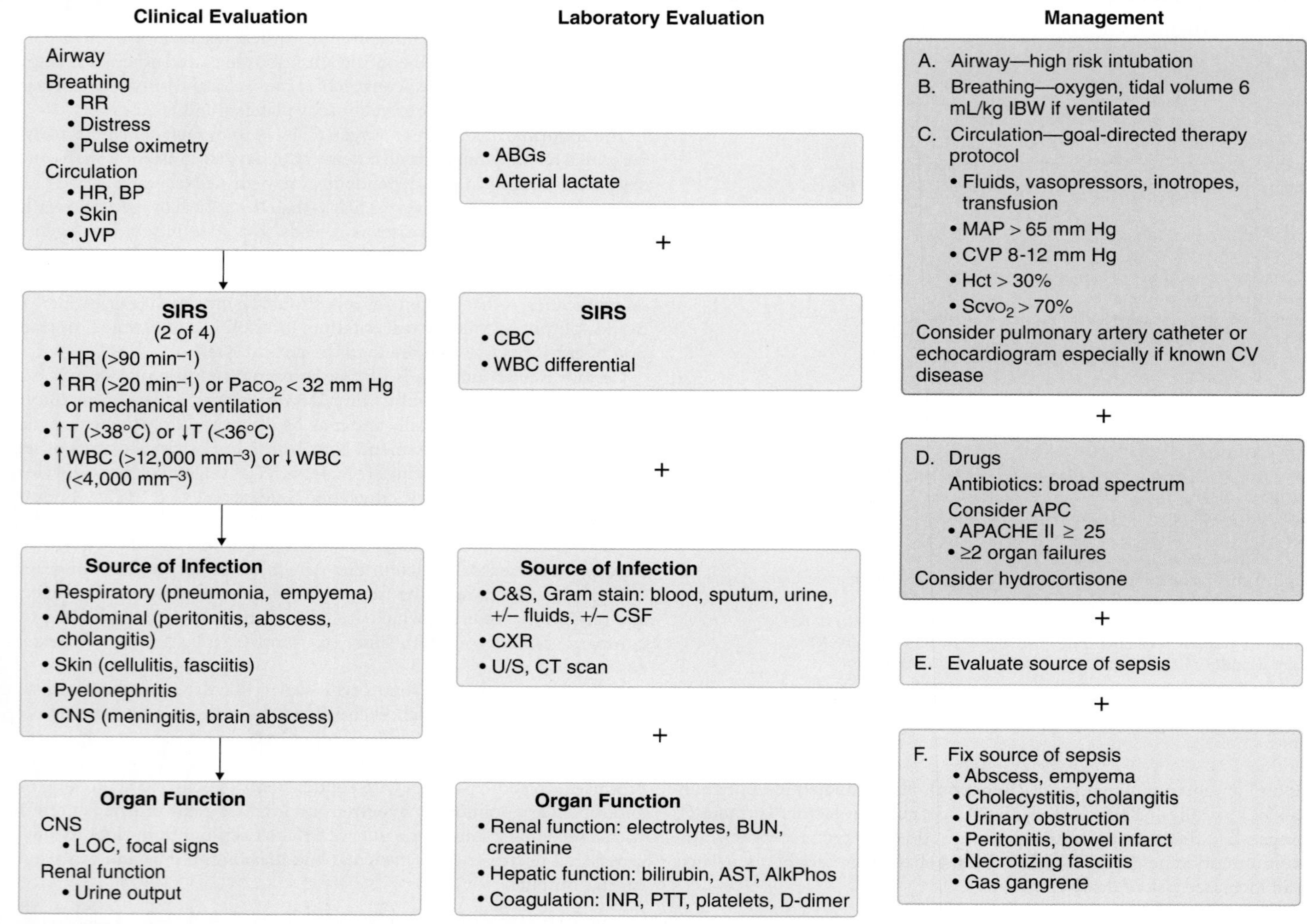

Clinical Evaluation
Laboratory Evaluation
Management
Airway
Breathing
• RR
• Distress
• Pulse oximetry
Circulation
• HR, BP
• Skin
• JVP
• ABGs
• Arterial lactate
+
A. Airway—high risk intubation
B. Breathing—oxygen, tidal volume 6 mL/kg IBW if ventilated
C. Circulation—goal-directed therapy protocol
• Fluids, vasopressors, inotropes, transfusion
• MAP > 65 mm Hg
• CVP 8-12 mm Hg
• Hct > 30%
• $Scvo_2$ > 70%
Consider pulmonary artery catheter or echocardiogram especially if known CV disease
SIRS
(2 of 4)
• ↑HR (>90 min^{-1})
• ↑RR (>20 min^{-1}) or $Paco_2$ < 32 mm Hg or mechanical ventilation
• ↑T (>38°C) or ↓T (<36°C)
• ↑WBC (>12,000 mm^{-3}) or ↓WBC (<4,000 mm^{-3})
SIRS
• CBC
• WBC differential
+
D. Drugs
Antibiotics: broad spectrum
Consider APC
• APACHE II ≥ 25
• ≥2 organ failures
Consider hydrocortisone
Source of Infection
• Respiratory (pneumonia, empyema)
• Abdominal (peritonitis, abscess, cholangitis)
• Skin (cellulitis, fasciitis)
• Pyelonephritis
• CNS (meningitis, brain abscess)
Source of Infection
• C&S, Gram stain: blood, sputum, urine, +/– fluids, +/– CSF
• CXR
• U/S, CT scan
+
E. Evaluate source of sepsis
+
F. Fix source of sepsis
• Abscess, empyema
• Cholecystitis, cholangitis
• Urinary obstruction
• Peritonitis, bowel infarct
• Necrotizing fasciitis
• Gas gangrene
Organ Function
CNS
• LOC, focal signs
Renal function
• Urine output
Organ Function
• Renal function: electrolytes, BUN, creatinine
• Hepatic function: bilirubin, AST, AlkPhos
• Coagulation: INR, PTT, platelets, D-dimer

FIGURE 108-3. Algorithm for the clinical and laboratory evaluation and management of septic shock. ABGs = arterial blood gases; AlkPhos = alkaline phosphatase; APACHE II = Acute Physiology and Chronic Health Evaluation II; APC = activated protein C; AST = aspartate aminotransferase; BP = blood pressure; BUN = blood urea nitrogen; C&S = culture and sensitivity; CBC = complete blood count; CNS = central nervous system; CSF = cerebrospinal fluid; CT = computed tomography; CV = cardiovascular; CVP = central venous pressure; CXR = chest radiograph; Hct = hematocrit; HR = heart rate; IBW = ideal body weight; INR = international normalized ratio; JVP = jugular venous pressure; LOC = level of consciousness; MAP = mean arterial pressure; $Paco_2$ = partial pressure of carbon dioxide; PTT = partial thromboplastin time; RR = respiratory rate; $Scvo_2$ = central venous oxygen saturation; SIRS = systemic inflammatory response syndrome; T = temperature; U/S = ultrasound; WBC = white blood cell count.

pneumonia, empyema, and acute lung injury. Abdominal ultrasound and computed tomography are indicated if abdominal sepsis is suspected.

Hemodynamic assessment of the patient includes insertion of a central venous or pulmonary artery catheter. In early septic shock, central venous pressure is usually low and increases in response to volume resuscitation. Central venous oxygen saturation, cardiac output, and ventricular filling pressures may be determined continuously. Pulmonary artery pressure is usually normal but may be increased because septic shock can cause pulmonary hypertension. Pulmonary artery occlusion (or wedge) pressure is usually low before resuscitation, but it may be normal or increased if the patient has underlying preexisting heart disease (e.g., heart failure or coronary artery disease with prior myocardial infarction) or if left ventricular contractility is decreased by sepsis. Cardiac output may be low or normal before fluid resuscitation and typically increases to higher than normal after fluid resuscitation. If fluid resuscitation increases central venous pressure and pulmonary artery occlusion pressure but cardiac output does not increase, left ventricular dysfunction is presumably present.

Echocardiographic features of decreased ventricular contractility include decreased right and left ventricular ejection fractions and increased end-diastolic and end-systolic volumes. Early in septic shock, the left ventricular ejection fraction is decreased, and it remains low in nonsurvivors. In survivors, the left ventricular ejection fraction usually returns to normal over 5 to 10 days.

Renal, hepatic, and coagulation function tests are helpful to evaluate organ function. After determining the source of sepsis, it is crucial to address that source by draining abscesses and empyemas; radiologically or surgically correcting urinary tract obstruction; and surgically managing peritonitis, bowel infarction, cholecystitis, cholangitis, necrotizing fasciitis, and gas gangrene.

Differential Diagnosis

The major differential diagnoses of classic septic shock are other nonseptic causes of SIRS, such as acute pancreatitis (Chapter 146), acute respiratory distress syndrome (Chapter 104), aspiration pneumonitis (Chapter 94), multiple trauma (Chapter 112), and recent major surgery without infection (Chapter 441). Other causes of distributive shock are anaphylactic shock (suggested by angioedema and hives; Chapter 448), spinal shock (recent trauma and paraplegia; Chapter 406), acute adrenal insufficiency ("tanned skin," hyperkalemia, metabolic alkalosis; Chapter 234), and acute or acute-on-chronic hepatic failure (jaundice, ascites, encephalopathy; Chapter 157).

The differential diagnosis of septic shock must include the other causes of shock: hypovolemic, cardiogenic, and obstructive shock (Chapters 106 and 107). Patients with hypovolemic shock (from internal or external fluid losses, hemorrhage) present with a suggestive history and signs of hypovolemia (low jugular venous pressure) and skin hypoperfusion (cool, clammy, cyanotic extremities). Cardiogenic shock (resulting from myocardial infarction or acute-on-chronic congestive heart failure or occurring after cardiovascular surgery) is suggested by the history, signs of increased filling pressure (increased jugular venous pressure, crackles, S_3, pulmonary edema, cardiomegaly), and skin hypoperfusion (Chapter 107). Some patients who have acute myocardial infarction and cardiogenic shock have features of SIRS

TABLE 108-3 RELEVANT RANDOMIZED CONTROLLED TRIALS IN SEVERE SEPSIS, SEPTIC SHOCK, AND ACUTE LUNG INJURY

PATIENT GROUP	INTERVENTION	CONTROL	INTERVENTION MORTALITY (%)*	CONTROL MORTALITY (%)*	NNT
ALI/ARDS† [2]	Low tidal volume (6 mL/kg)	High tidal volume (12 mL/kg)	31	40	11
Sepsis and septic shock [3]	Early goal-directed therapy	Usual therapy	33	49	6
Severe sepsis and septic shock [14]	Activated protein C	Placebo	25	31	16
Severe sepsis and septic shock at increased risk of death‡ [14]	Activated protein C	Placebo	31	44	7.7
Septic shock [12]	Hydrocortisone and fludrocortisone	Placebo	53§	63§	10

*28-day mortality.
†Many also had sepsis.
‡As defined by Acute Physiology and Chronic Health Evaluation (APACHE) II quartiles 3 and 4, APACHE II ≥ 25.
§Nonresponders to a 250-μg corticotropin stimulation test.
ALI/ARDS = acute lung injury/acute respiratory distress syndrome; NNT = number needed to treat to save one life.

without infection. Obstructive shock (from pulmonary thromboembolism, cardiac tamponade, pneumothorax) manifests similarly to cardiogenic shock.

PREVENTION

Measures to prevent sepsis include handwashing, elevation of the head of the bed, scrupulous sterile techniques for the insertion of catheters, and possibly the use of antibiotic-impregnated catheters. New catheter insertion sites for catheter changes, isolation of patients who have resistant organisms, and isolation of significantly immunocompromised patients may also prevent infection.

Preventing the progression from sepsis to septic shock requires early diagnosis and aggressive resuscitation. Early goal-directed therapy, lung-protective ventilation, antibiotics, and consideration of activated protein C are critical therapies in early septic shock (Table 108-3).

TREATMENT Rx

Respiratory Therapy

All patients in septic shock require oxygen initially, and many require mechanical ventilation. Mechanical ventilation is required in most patients who have septic shock because acute lung injury is the most common complication. Lung-protective ventilation (mechanical ventilation that minimizes lung injury by using a relatively low tidal volume, such as <6 mL/kg of predicted body weight) decreases mortality from acute lung injury and acute respiratory distress syndrome (Chapter 105). [2]

Patients who require ventilation need adequate but not excessive sedation, which can worsen hemodynamic instability, prolong ventilation, and increase the risk of developing nosocomial pneumonia. Sedation should be titrated using objective assessment. Daily interruption of sedation decreases the duration of mechanical ventilation and intensive care. Neuromuscular blocking agents should be avoided because of the risk of prolonged neuromuscular dysfunction.

Circulatory Therapy

Early goal-directed therapy is the cornerstone of emergency management, and this approach decreases hospital, 28-day, and 60-day mortality rates dramatically (see Table 108-3). [3] In general, the goal of resuscitation is to increase tissue oxygen delivery by increasing profoundly low blood pressure, increasing inadequate blood flow, increasing low arterial oxygen saturation, and increasing mixed venous oxygen saturation. Although oxygen delivery is higher in survivors than in nonsurvivors, it is not clear that a specific oxygen delivery target is more beneficial than clinical end points. Several trials have shown that supernormal global oxygen delivery does not decrease mortality rates in sepsis and septic shock. Goal-directed therapy requires continuous monitoring of central venous oxygen saturation, with resuscitation directed to increase and then maintain central venous oxygen saturation greater than 70%.

In patients who have acute lung injury, no difference in outcomes is seen with management using a pulmonary artery catheter versus a central venous catheter; this finding suggests that there is no advantage to using a pulmonary catheter to guide the hemodynamic management of acute lung injury. [4] Patients whose acute lung injury is managed after 24 to 48 hours with a conservative fluid strategy (compared with a liberal fluid strategy) have significantly improved lung function and shorter duration of ventilation and ICU stay. [5]

Fluids should be used to maintain central venous pressure at 8 to 12 mm Hg; at present, no convincing data indicate that albumin is better than normal saline solution. [6] In patients with severe sepsis, modified Ringer's lactate is preferred over 10% hetastarch (a colloid) because of lower rates of both acute kidney injury and the need for renal replacement therapy. [7] If central venous oxygen saturation is less than 70%, packed red cell transfusions should be used to maintain a hematocrit greater than 30%.

Vasopressors (e.g., norepinephrine 1 to 50 μg/minute; epinephrine 1 to 30 μg/minute) should be added if the mean arterial pressure is less than 65 mm Hg. Dobutamine (2.5 to 20 μg/kg/minute) is required if central venous pressure, mean arterial pressure, and hematocrit are optimized but the central venous oxygen saturation remains less than 70%. In a randomized trial of patients with septic shock, the combination of norepinephrine plus dobutamine resulted in a similar mortality as epinephrine alone, with no differences in organ dysfunction, time to resolution of shock, or adverse events. [8] In another randomized trial, norepinephrine was slightly but not significantly better than dopamine for reducing mortality when used as the first-line vasopressor for patients with septic shock [9]; however, norepinephrine was associated with a lower rate of arrhythmias, especially atrial fibrillation. These accumulated data suggest that norepinephrine may be preferable to dopamine as the first vasopressor in septic shock.

Clinicians can use epinephrine alone, norepinephrine alone, or norepinephrine plus dobutamine in patients with low cardiac output.

As a strategic approach to persistent hypotension despite adequate fluid resuscitation, a vasopressor such as norepinephrine (1 to 50 μg/minute) can be added first. If the cardiac index is low or if the mixed venous oxygen saturation is low (<70%) despite an adequate central venous pressure, an inotropic agent such as dobutamine should be added, initially at approximately 2 to 5 μg/kg/minute and increasing until the mixed venous oxygen saturation is adequate. In some patients in septic shock, the cardiac index is inadequate, as reflected by a low mixed venous oxygen saturation despite a high central venous pressure (>12 mm Hg) and/or pulmonary artery wedge pressure (>18 mm Hg), because of underlying cardiovascular dysfunction or because of acute left ventricular dysfunction resulting from sepsis. In such patients, earlier use of an inotropic agent such as dobutamine should be considered to increase left ventricular contractility. The overall goal is to achieve an adequate mean arterial pressure (>65 mm Hg), central venous pressure, and mixed venous oxygen saturation while other indices of adequate perfusion are monitored, such as hourly urine output (>0.5 mL/kg/hour), arterial lactate levels (<2 mmol/L), mental status, and skin perfusion. To assess the adequacy of early resuscitation of severe sepsis and septic shock and to guide ongoing therapy, a central venous oxygen saturation goal greater than 70% or a lactate clearance of at least 10% is an equally good measure. [10]

Transfusion of Erythrocytes and Erythropoietin

Anemia is common in septic shock, but the optimal hemoglobin level for resuscitation is controversial. Goal-directed therapy aims for a hematocrit of 30%, whereas a randomized trial of transfusion in critically ill patients found that a hemoglobin range of 7 to 9 g/dL was equivalent to or better than a higher hemoglobin (10 to 12 g/dL), except possibly in patients with acute myocardial infarction or unstable angina. A reasonable approach is to use a hematocrit level of 30% as the threshold for erythrocyte transfusion for the first 6 hours and then to lower the threshold to a hemoglobin of 7 to 9 g/dL for the rest of the hospital course, except in patients with underlying cardiac disease. Recombinant erythropoietin decreases the need for transfusion in critically ill patients, but it does not decrease mortality.

Drugs

Antibiotics

The infected site and infecting organisms of septic shock are often not known initially. After appropriate cultures are obtained, intravenous broad-spectrum antibiotics should be administered on an emergency basis (within 1 hour) while considering host factors such as immune and allergic status (Chapters 288 and 289; see Fig. 108-3). Outcomes in patients with septic shock are worse if the organisms causing the sepsis are not sensitive to the initial antibiotic regimen.

Emergency, empirical antibiotic therapy (Table 108-4) should be guided by the greater frequency of gram-positive bacteria, the possibility of resistant organisms, and local bacteriologic features. If a causative organism is identified (<20% of septic patients have negative cultures), the antibiotic regimen should be narrowed to decrease the emergence of resistant organisms. Empirical fluconazole treatment does not result in better outcomes in critically ill, non-neutropenic patients at risk for invasive candidiasis.[11] The duration of antibiotics should be guided by the cause of septic shock, but patients generally require 10 to 14 days of therapy.

Corticosteroids

High-dose corticosteroids do not improve outcomes in the full spectrum of patients with sepsis or acute respiratory distress syndrome, but the evidence supporting the use of low-dose corticosteroids in septic shock is controversial. In one trial, corticosteroids (hydrocortisone 50 mg intravenously every 6 hours, plus fludrocortisone 50-µg tablet/day per nasogastric tube or orally for 7 days) increased survival in septic patients whose serum cortisol response after stimulation with an intravenous infusion of 250 µg corticotropin was 9 µg/dL or less.[12] In a subsequent randomized trial of hydrocortisone (50 mg every 6 hours intravenously for 5 days) versus placebo, however, mortality was not improved, regardless of the patient's response to corticotropin stimulation.[2] Adding fludrocortisone to hydrocortisone does not appear to be better than hydrocortisone alone, and aggressive insulin therapy to address the hyperglycemia that often accompanies corticosteroid treatment is no better than usual glucose control.[13] Hydrocortisone treatment is often associated with a shorter duration of septic shock but can increase the risk of superinfections. Current sepsis guidelines suggest that corticosteroids should be considered only in patients who are poorly responsive to vasopressors.

Corticosteroids administered before antibiotics also decrease the neurologic sequelae of bacterial, especially pneumococcal, meningitis (Chapter 420). Enthusiasm for corticosteroid therapy must be tempered by the risk of complications such as superinfection, neuromyopathy, hyperglycemia, immune suppression, and impaired wound healing.

Recombinant Human Activated Protein C

Activated protein C infusion (24 µg/kg/hour for 96 hours) decreases mortality, improves organ dysfunction, and decreases biomarkers of inflammation and coagulation in severe sepsis and septic shock.[14] Activated protein C is approved for patients who have severe sepsis and a high risk of death, as defined by an Acute Physiology and Chronic Health Evaluation (APACHE) II score of 25 or higher and/or two or more dysfunctional organs (see Fig. 108-3). By comparison, activated protein C is not beneficial in low-risk patients.[15] Activated protein C has not been tested in patients with major trauma, recent surgery (within 12 hours), active hemorrhage, coagulopathy, thrombocytopenia, or recent stroke because of the increased risk of hemorrhage. Even in patients without these risk factors, treatment increases the risk of serious hemorrhage nearly two-fold, and about 0.5% of treated patients develop intracranial hemorrhage. Activated protein C should not be used in surgical patients who have severe sepsis with single-organ dysfunction. If patients are receiving subcutaneous low-dose heparin prophylaxis and activated protein C is to be used, discontinuation of heparin should be weighed carefully: although its discontinuation while using activated protein C reduces bleeding, discontinuation also increases the risk of stroke[16] and may increase the risk of death. The use of activated protein C in septic shock is being reevaluated in

TABLE 108-4 POTENTIAL ANTIBIOTIC REGIMENS FOR PATIENTS WITH SEPTIC SHOCK*

SOURCE OF SEPSIS	INITIAL ANTIBIOTIC REGIMEN	ALTERNATIVE ANTIBIOTIC REGIMEN
Community-acquired pneumonia	Third-generation cephalosporin: cefotaxime 2 g IV q6h; ceftriaxone 2 g IV q12h; ceftizoxime 2 g IV q8h PLUS Fluoroquinolone (e.g., ciprofloxacin 400 mg IV q12h, levofloxacin 750 mg IV q24h, moxifloxacin 400 mg IV q24h) OR Macrolide (azithromycin 500 mg IV q24h)	Piperacillin-tazobactam 3.375 g IV q6h PLUS Fluoroquinolone OR Macrolide
Hospital-acquired pneumonia	Imipenem 0.5 g IV q6h OR Meropenem 1 g IV q8h	Fluoroquinolone (ciprofloxacin 400 mg IV q12h) PLUS Vancomycin 1.5 g IV q12h OR Piperacillin-tazobactam 3.375 g IV q6h PLUS Tobramycin 1.5 mg/kg q8h PLUS Vancomycin
Abdominal (mixed aerobic/anaerobic)	Piperacillin-tazobactam 3.375 g IV q6h OR Imipenem 0.5 g IV q6h (or meropenem 1 g IV q8h)	Ampicillin 2 g IV q4h PLUS Metronidazole 500 mg IV q8h PLUS Fluoroquinolone (ciprofloxacin 400 mg IV q12h)
Urinary tract	Fluoroquinolone (ciprofloxacin 400 mg IV q12h)	Ampicillin 2 g IV q4h PLUS Gentamicin 1.5 mg/kg IV q8h OR Third-generation cephalosporin (cefotaxime 2 g IV q6h, ceftriaxone 2 g IV q12h, OR ceftizoxime 2 g IV q8h)
Necrotizing fasciitis	Imipenem 0.5 g IV q6h	Penicillin G (if confirmed group A streptococci)
Primary bacteremia (normal host)	Piperacillin-tazobactam 3.375 g IV q6h PLUS Vancomycin 1.5 g IV q12h	Imipenem 0.5 g IV q6h PLUS Vancomycin 1.5 g IV q12h
Primary bacteremia (intravenous drug user)	Vancomycin 1.5 g IV q12h PLUS Fluoroquinolone (ciprofloxacin 400 mg IV q12h)	Piperacillin-tazobactam 3.375 g IV q6h PLUS Vancomycin 1.5 g IV q12h
Febrile neutropenia	Cefepime 2 g IV q8h PLUS Vancomycin 1.5 g IV q12h	Piperacillin-tazobactam 3.375 g IV q6h PLUS Gentamicin 1.5 mg/kg q8h OR Imipenem 0.5 g IV q6h PLUS Gentamicin 1.5 mg/kg q8h
Bacterial meningitis	Ceftriaxone 2 g IV q12h PLUS Ampicillin 3 g IV q6h PLUS Vancomycin 1.5 g IV q12h PLUS Dexamethasone 0.15 mg/kg IV q6h for 2-4 days	Gram-positive cocci: Vancomycin PLUS Ceftriaxone 2 g IV q12h Gram-negative diplococci: Cefotaxime 2 g IV q4-6h Gram-positive bacilli: Ampicillin 3 g IV q6h PLUS Gentamicin Gram-negative bacilli: Ceftazidime 2 g IV q8h PLUS Gentamicin 1.5 mg/kg IV q8h All above PLUS Dexamethasone
Cellulitis	Ciprofloxacin 400 mg IV q12h PLUS Clindamycin 900 mg IV q8h	Imipenem 0.5 g IV q6h

*Most antibiotic doses must be adjusted if there is hepatic or renal dysfunction. Some antibiotics require adjustment based on levels (e.g., gentamicin). When selecting a drug, carefully consider the patient's history of antibiotic (especially penicillin) allergy.

a large, multicenter, randomized controlled trial; until that study is completed, activated protein C is still recommended for patients who meet the criteria and have no contraindications to its use.

Controversial Therapies in Septic Shock

Vasopressin Deficiency and Use of Vasopressin

Vasopressin deficiency and downregulation of vasopressin receptors are common findings in septic shock. Vasopressin selectively dilates renal afferent but not efferent glomerular arterioles, and it also dilates pulmonary, cerebral, and coronary arterioles. Low-dose vasopressin infusion (0.03 to 0.04 U/minute) increases blood pressure, urine output, and creatinine clearance while dramatically decreasing the dosage of norepinephrine required to maintain blood pressure in patients with septic shock. In a randomized trial, low-dose vasopressin added to norepinephrine was not significantly better than as-needed norepinephrine alone,[17] although added vasopressin may be useful in patients with less severe shock. Complications of vasopressin include gastrointestinal ischemia, decreased cardiac output, skin or digital necrosis, and cardiac arrest (especially at doses >0.04 U/minute).

Hyperglycemia and Intensive Insulin Therapy

Hyperglycemia and insulin resistance are common in septic shock. Hyperglycemia is a pro-coagulant and pro-apoptotic stimulus; it impairs neutrophil function, increases the risk of infection, impairs wound healing, and is associated with increased mortality. However, the risks of unrecognized hypoglycemia and cerebral injury may be increased in septic shock because of unstable endocrine function and the use of sedation. In addition, brain ischemia and hypoxia increase sensitivity to even transient hypoglycemia. At present, the appropriate glucose range and insulin doses are controversial. Intensive insulin therapy to control hyperglycemia is not beneficial in patients in medical ICUs because of significantly higher rates of hypoglycemia[7,18] and perhaps increased mortality.[18] Therefore, intensive insulin therapy cannot be recommended for patients with septic shock.

Renal Dysfunction and Dialysis

Acute renal failure is an important complication of septic shock because of its associated morbidity, mortality, and resource use (Fig. 108-4). Continuous renal replacement therapy induces less hemodynamic instability compared with intermittent hemodialysis, but no conclusive evidence indicates that continuous renal replacement therapy or more intensive dialysis changes the mortality of acute renal failure. In critically ill patients who have acute kidney injury, hemodialysis six times per week is no better than conventional hemodialysis, and intensive renal replacement therapy is no better than standard therapy overall or in patients who have sepsis.[19]

Low-dose dopamine (2 to 4 μg/kg/minute) does not decrease the need for renal support, does not improve outcomes, and is not recommended. Lactic acidosis is a common complication of septic shock, but administration of sodium bicarbonate in the setting of lactic acidosis does not improve hemodynamics or the response to vasopressors.

A small randomized controlled trial evaluated the use of polymyxin B hemoperfusion in patients with abdominal sepsis to reduce blood endotoxin levels. Polymyxin B hemoperfusion increased blood pressure, decreased vasopressor requirements, improved organ dysfunction, and reduced mortality by one third.[20] However, this intervention requires further evaluation before it can be recommended.

Other Therapies

Deep vein thrombosis prophylaxis using low-dose heparin, which can be administered in combination with activated protein C, is recommended for patients who do not have active bleeding, coagulopathy, or a contraindication to heparin (see Fig. 108-4). Stress ulcer prophylaxis using H_2-receptor antagonists decreases the risk of gastrointestinal hemorrhage. Proton pump inhibitors may also be effective, but they have not been fully evaluated in septic shock.

Enteral nutrition is generally safer and more effective than total parenteral nutrition, but total parenteral nutrition is sometimes required in patients with abdominal sepsis, surgery, or trauma. The use of sedation, neuromuscular blocking agents, and corticosteroids should be minimized because they can exacerbate septic encephalopathy and the polyneuropathy or myopathy of sepsis. Neutropenic patients may benefit from granulocyte colony-stimulating factor (Chapter 170). The risk of nosocomial infection is decreased by narrow-spectrum antibiotics, early weaning from ventilation, and periodic removal and replacement of catheters (Chapter 290).

B. Breathing—Oxygen, with a tidal volume 6 mL/kg IBW if ventilated. Wean according to ARDSNet protocol (Chapters 105 and 106)

C. Circulation
- Fluids, vasopressors, inotropes, transfusion; goals include:
  - MAP > 65 mm Hg
  - CVP 8-12 mm Hg
  - Hg 70-90 g/L
  - $ScvO_2$ > 70%

Consider pulmonary artery catheter or echocardiogram especially if known cardiovascular disease; goals include:
- Wedge pressure 8-15 mm Hg
  - Cardiac index: normal or increased

D. Drugs:
- Antibiotics: Narrow spectrum to cause of infection
- APC (if indicated): 24 μg/kg/hour infusion for 96 hours
- Hydrocortisone (if evidence of relative adrenal insufficiency [see text]): hydrocortisone 50 mg intravenously every 6 hours and fludrocortisone 50-μg tab orally or per NG tube daily for 7 days

Other Organ Support
- Renal function: Continuous renal replacement
- DVT prophylaxis: Low-dose heparin 5000 IU subcutaneously every 12 hours
- Stress ulcer prophylaxis: H_2-receptor antagonist (e.g., ranitidine 50 mg intravenously every 8 hours)
- Nutrition: Enteral preferred
- Sedation: Intermittent with daily awakening

FIGURE 108-4. Ongoing critical care support and management in septic shock. APC = activated protein C; CVP = central venous pressure; DVT = deep vein thrombosis; Hg = hemoglobin; IBW = ideal body weight; MAP = mean arterial pressure; NG = nasogastric; $ScvO_2$ = central venous oxygen saturation.

PROGNOSIS

The 28-day mortality of septic shock is 40 to 70%. Early deaths (in the first 72 hours) are usually the result of refractory, progressive shock despite escalating life support. Later deaths from septic shock (after day 3) are usually secondary to multiple organ dysfunction. The number of dysfunctional organs and the progression or lack of improvement of organ dysfunction are indicators of increased risk of death. Other factors that portend a poor prognosis are increased age, underlying medical conditions, high APACHE II score, increased arterial lactate concentrations, and lack of response to vasopressors. Furthermore, recent evidence indicates that a delay in achieving the goals of early goal-directed therapy is associated with increased mortality. Survivors of sepsis who also had acute lung injury (Chapter 104) can have weakness, fatigue, and dyspnea on exertion after hospital discharge owing to pulmonary dysfunction, neuromuscular dysfunction, or other persistent organ dysfunction.

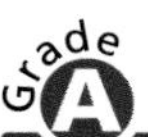

1. Sprung CL, Annane D, Keh D, et al. Hydrocortisone therapy for patients with septic shock. *N Engl J Med.* 2008;358:111-124.
2. Acute Respiratory Distress Syndrome Network. Ventilation with lower tidal volumes as compared with traditional tidal volumes for acute lung injury and the acute respiratory distress syndrome. *N Engl J Med.* 2000;342:1301-1308.
3. Rivers E, Nguyen B, Havstad S, et al. Early goal-directed therapy in the treatment of severe sepsis and septic shock. *N Engl J Med.* 2001;345:1368-1377.
4. Wheeler AP, Bernard GR, Thompson BT, et al. National Heart, Lung, and Blood Institute Acute Respiratory Distress Syndrome (ARDS) Clinical Trials Network: pulmonary-artery versus central venous catheter to guide treatment of acute lung injury. *N Engl J Med.* 2006;354:2213-2224.
5. Wiedemann HP, Wheeler AP, Bernard GR, et al. Comparison of two fluid management strategies in acute lung injury. *N Engl J Med.* 2006;354:2564-2575.
6. SAFE. A comparison of albumin and saline for fluid resuscitation in the intensive care unit. *N Engl J Med.* 2004;350:2247-2256.
7. Brunkhorst FM, Engel C, Bloos F, et al. Intensive insulin therapy and pentastarch resuscitation in severe sepsis. *N Engl J Med.* 2008;358:125-139.
8. Annane D, Vignon P, Renault A, et al. Norepinephrine plus dobutamine versus epinephrine alone for management of septic shock: a randomized trial. *Lancet.* 2007;370:676-684.
9. De Backer D, Biston P, Devriendt J, et al. Comparison of dopamine and norepinephrine in the treatment of septic shock. *N Engl J Med.* 2010;362:779-789.
10. Jones AE, Shapiro NI, Trzeziak S, et al. Lactate clearance vs. central venous oxygen saturation as goals of early sepsis therapy: A randomized clinical trial. *JAMA.* 2010;303:739-746.
11. Schuster MG, Edwards JE Jr, Sobel JD, et al. Empirical fluconazole versus placebo for intensive care unit patients: a randomized trial. *Ann Intern Med.* 2008;149:83-90.
12. Annane D, Sebille V, Charpentier C, et al. Effect of treatment with low doses of hydrocortisone and fludrocortisone on mortality in patients with septic shock. *JAMA.* 2002;288:862-871.

13. The COIITS Study Investigators. Corticosteroid treatment and intensive insulin therapy for septic shock in adults: a randomized controlled trial. *JAMA.* 2010;303:341-348.
14. Bernard GR, Vincent JL, Laterre PF, et al. Efficacy and safety of recombinant human activated protein C for severe sepsis. *N Engl J Med.* 2001;344:699-709.
15. Abraham E, Laterre PF, Garg R, et al. Drotrecogin alfa (activated) for adults with severe sepsis and a low risk of death. *N Engl J Med.* 2005;353:1332-1341.
16. Levy M, Levy M, Williams M, et al. Prophylactic heparin in patients with severe sepsis treated with drotrecogin alfa (activated). *Am J Resp Crit Care Med.* 2007;176:483-490.
17. Russell JA, Walley KR, Singer J, et al. Vasopressin versus norepinephrine infusion in patients with septic shock. *N Engl J Med.* 2008;358:877-887.
18. NICE SUGAR. Intensive versus conventional glucose control in critically ill patients. *N Engl J Med.* 2009;360:1283-1297.
19. VA/NIH Network. Intensity of renal support in critically ill patients with acute kidney injury. *N Engl J Med.* 2008;359:7-20.
20. Cruz DN, Antonelli M, Fumagalli R, et al. Early use of polymyxin B hemoperfusion in abdominal septic shock. *JAMA.* 2009;301:2445-2452.

SUGGESTED READINGS

Angus DC. Management of sepsis: a 47-year-old woman with an indwelling intravenous catheter and sepsis. *JAMA.* 2011;305:1469-1477. *Case-based review.*

Funk DJ, Kumar A. Antimicrobial therapy for life-threatening infections: speed is life. *Crit Care Med.* 2011;27:53-76. *Emphasizes that early recognition of life-threatening infection and rapid initiation of appropriate antimicrobial therapy is the critical element in reducing mortality.*

Levy MM, Dellinger RP, Townsend SR, et al. The Surviving Sepsis campaign: results of an international guidelines-based performance improvement program targeting severe sepsis. *Crit Care Med.* 2010;38:367-374. *Suggests that the use of guidelines improves quality of care and may decrease mortality of severe sepsis and septic shock.*

Winters BD, Eberlein M, Leung J, et al. Long-term mortality and quality of life in sepsis: a systematic review. *Crit Care Med.* 2010;38:1276-1283. *Survivors have increased mortality and impaired quality of life for at least 2 years.*

109

DISORDERS DUE TO HEAT AND COLD

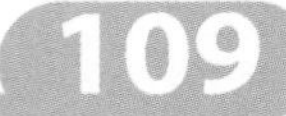

WILLIAM WINKENWERDER JR. AND MICHAEL N. SAWKA

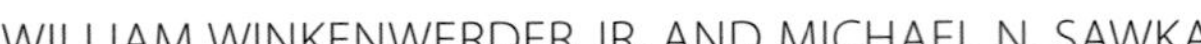

TEMPERATURE REGULATION

Body temperature is regulated through two parallel processes that modify body heat balance: behavioral (clothing, shelter, physical activity) and physiologic (skin blood flow, sweating, shivering). Both peripheral (skin) and central (core) thermal receptors provide afferent input to a central nervous system integrator (hypothalamic thermoregulatory center), and any deviation between the controlled variable (body temperature) and a reference variable ("set point" temperature) results in a heat loss or conservation response (Fig. 109-1).

Humans normally regulate body (core) temperature at about 37° C (98.6° F), and fluctuations within the narrow range of 35 to 41° C (95 to 105.8° F) can be tolerated by healthy acclimatized persons; core temperatures outside this range can induce morbidity and mortality. There is no single core temperature because it varies at different deep body sites and during rest and physical exercise. Arterial blood temperature provides the best invasive measurement of core temperature. The most accurate noninvasive index of core temperature is esophageal temperature, followed in order of preference by rectal, gastrointestinal tract (telemetry pill), and oral temperature. Ear (tympanic and auditory meatus) or scanned temporal artery temperature should not be relied on for clinical judgment.

HEAT ILLNESS

DEFINITIONS

Minor heat-related illnesses include miliaria rubra, heat syncope, and heat cramps. Serious heat illness represents a continuum from heat exhaustion to heat injury and heatstroke.

EPIDEMIOLOGY

Body temperature can increase from exposure to environmental heat (impeded heat dissipation), physical exercise (increased heat production), and fever (elevated set point). Febrile persons have accentuated elevations in core temperature when exposed to high ambient temperature, physical exercise, or both. Serious heat illness is associated with a variety of individual factors, health conditions, drugs, and environmental factors (Table 109-1). Anticholinergic and sympathomimetic poisoning (Chapter 110) can induce hyperthermia. Malignant hyperthermia (Chapter 440) is caused by rapid and massive skeletal muscle contraction from exposure to anesthesia. Neuroleptic malignant syndrome (Chapter 442) is hyperthermia caused by skeletal muscle rigidity from treatment with neuroleptic medications (e.g., antipsychotics, antidepressants, antiemetics).

Heat illness can also occur in low-risk individuals who have taken appropriate precautions relative to situations they have been exposed to in the past. Historically, such unexpected cases were attributed to dehydration (which impairs thermoregulation and increases hyperthermia and cardiovascular strain), but it is now suspected that a previous heat exposure or event (e.g., sickness or injury) might make these individuals more susceptible to serious heat illness. One theory is that previous heat injury or illness primes the acute phase response and augments the hyperthermia of exercise, inducing unexpected serious heat illness. Another theory is that previous infection produces pro-inflammatory cytokines that deactivate the cells' ability to protect against heat shock.

PATHOBIOLOGY

Environmental and exercise heat stress challenges the cardiovascular system to provide high blood flow to the skin, where blood pools in warm, compliant vessels such as those found in the extremities. When blood flow is diverted to the skin, reduced perfusion of the intestines and other viscera can result in ischemia, endotoxemia, and oxidative stress. In addition, excessively high

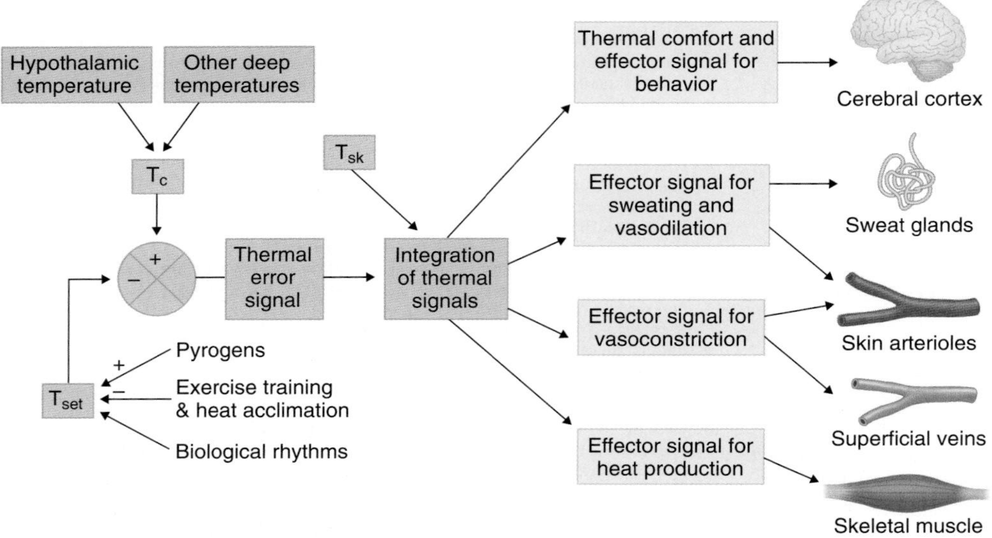

FIGURE 109-1. **Control of human thermoregulation.** (From Sawka MN, Young AJ. Physiological systems and their responses to conditions of heat and cold. In: Tipton CM, Sawka MN, Tate CA, Terjung RL, eds. *ACSM's Advanced Exercise Physiology.* Baltimore: Lippincott Williams & Wilkins; 2005:535-563.)

TABLE 109-1 FACTORS PREDISPOSING TO SERIOUS HEAT ILLNESS

INDIVIDUAL FACTORS
Lack of acclimatization
Low physical fitness
Excessive body weight
Dehydration
Advanced age
Young age
HEALTH CONDITIONS
Inflammation and fever
Viral infection
Cardiovascular disease
Diabetes mellitus
Gastroenteritis
Rash, sunburn, and previous burns to large areas of skin
Seizures
Thyroid storm
Neuroleptic malignant syndrome
Malignant hyperthermia
Sickle cell trait
Cystic fibrosis
Spinal cord injury
DRUGS
Anticholinergic properties (atropine)
Antiepileptic (topiramate)
Antihistamines
Glutethimide (Doriden)
Phenothiazines
Tricyclic antidepressants
Amphetamines, cocaine, "Ecstasy"
Ergogenic stimulants (e.g., ephedrine, ephedra)
Lithium
Diuretics
β-Blockers
Ethanol
ENVIRONMENTAL FACTORS
High temperature
High humidity
Little air motion
Lack of shade
Heat wave
Physical exercise
Heavy clothing
Air pollution (nitrogen dioxide)

TABLE 109-2 COMPARISON OF CLASSIC AND EXERTIONAL HEATSTROKE

PATIENT CHARACTERISTICS	CLASSIC	EXERTIONAL
Age	Young children or elderly	15-55 yr
Health	Chronic illness	Usually healthy
Fever	Unusual	Common
Prevailing weather	Frequent in heat waves	Variable
Activity	Sedentary	Strenuous exercise
Drug use	Diuretics, antidepressants, anticholinergics, phenothiazines	Ergogenic stimulants or cocaine
Sweating	Often absent	Common
Acid-base disturbances	Respiratory alkalosis	Lactic acidosis
Acute renal failure	Uncommon	Common (≈15%)
Rhabdomyolysis	Uncommon	Common (≈25%)
CK	Mildly elevated	Markedly elevated (500-1000 U/L)
ALT, AST	Mildly elevated	Markedly elevated
Hyperkalemia	Uncommon	Common
Hypocalcemia	Uncommon	Common
DIC	Mild	Marked
Hypoglycemia	Uncommon	Common

ALT = alanine aminotransferase; AST = aspartate aminotransferase; CK = creatine kinase; DIC = disseminated intravascular coagulation.

tissue temperatures (heat shock: >41° C [105.8° F]) can produce direct tissue injury; the magnitude and duration of the heat shock influence whether cells respond by adaptation (acquired thermal tolerance), injury, or death (apoptotic or necrotic). Heat shock, ischemia, and systemic inflammatory responses can result in cellular dysfunction, disseminated intravascular coagulation, and multiorgan dysfunction syndrome. In addition, reduced cerebral blood flow, combined with abnormal local metabolism and coagulopathy, can lead to dysfunction of the central nervous system.

CLINICAL MANIFESTATIONS AND DIAGNOSIS

Mild heat illness is common and can be recognized by its clinical features. Miliaria rubra (heat rash) results from the occlusion of eccrine sweat gland ducts and can be complicated by secondary staphylococcal infection. Heat syncope (fainting) is caused by temporary circulatory insufficiency as a result of blood pooling in the peripheral veins, especially the cutaneous and lower extremity veins. Heat cramps (skeletal muscles cramps) occur during and after intense exercise and are believed to result from excessive loss of sodium in sweat.

Serious heat illness is often not apparent at the initial evaluation. Patients who exhibit symptoms (e.g., dizziness, unsteady gait, ataxia, headache, confusion, weakness, fatigue, nausea, vomiting, diarrhea) should have an immediate assessment of their mental status, core (rectal) temperature, and other vital signs. Heatstroke should be the working diagnosis in anyone who is a heat casualty and has an altered mental status.

Heat exhaustion is a mild to moderate illness characterized by an inability to sustain cardiac output with moderate (>38.5° C [101° F]) to high (>40° C [104° F]) body temperatures. It is frequently accompanied by sweaty hot skin, dehydration, and collapse. Heat injury is a moderate to severe illness characterized by organ (e.g., liver, renal) and tissue (e.g., gut, muscle) injury with high body temperatures, usually but not always greater than 40° C (104° F).

Heatstroke is a severe illness characterized by mental status changes with high body temperatures, usually but not always greater than 40° C (104° F). However, patients with a core temperature higher than 40° C do not universally have a heat injury or heatstroke, and the entire clinical picture, including mental status and laboratory results, must be considered. Heatstroke is often categorized as classic or exertional, with the former observed primarily in otherwise sick and compromised individuals and the latter observed primarily in apparently healthy and physically fit individuals (Table 109-2). Heatstroke victims have profound neuropsychiatric impairments that develop early and universally. In addition, heatstroke can be complicated by liver damage, rhabdomyolysis, disseminated intravascular coagulation, water and electrolyte imbalance, and renal failure.

PREVENTION, TREATMENT, AND PROGNOSIS (Rx)

Heat illness can be prevented by heat acclimatization and acquired thermal tolerance, maintenance of adequate hydration, and avoidance of overwhelming heat exposure. Adequate fluid intake is critical, and oral rehydration solutions may be preferable to other forms of hydration.[1]

Management of serious heat illness includes cooling, rehydration, and monitoring (Table 109-3). Body cooling should be initiated immediately and continued until the core temperature falls below 38.8° C (102° F). Body cooling lowers tissue temperatures and reduces cardiovascular stress by causing vasoconstriction in the skin. Immersion or soaking the skin in cool or iced water with skin massage is the most effective method, but other effective methods include soaking the skin followed by accelerated evaporation with fans or the use of ice sheets or ice packs. Cooling can induce shivering, which is usually not sufficient to increase body temperature, so shivering need not be treated.

Fluid and electrolyte deficits should be corrected; restoration of plasma volume with isotonic fluids sufficient to sustain adequate perfusion, as judged by urine output, is a priority. Rapid overcorrection of serum electrolytes (e.g., sodium) should be avoided. If rhabdomyolysis (Chapter 115) and myoglobinuria are present, maintaining urine flow helps minimize renal injury. Patients should be monitored for cardiac arrhythmia and acute respiratory failure. Medications to be avoided include antipyretics and sedatives with hepatic toxicities. Lorazepam (1 to 2 mg administered intravenously over a

TABLE 109-3 MANAGEMENT OF HEAT ILLNESS

HEAT EXHAUSTION

Rest and shade
Loosen and remove clothing
Supine position and elevate legs
Actively cool skin
Fluids by mouth
Monitor core temperature
Monitor mental status

HYPERTHERMIA

Protect the airway
Insert at least two large-bore intravenous lines
Monitor core temperature; options include pulmonary artery, rectal probe, esophageal probe
Actively cool the skin until core temperature reaches 39° C (102.2° F)
Ice baths or cool water (≈22° C [71.6° F]) immersion
Wetting with water (avoid alcohol rubs)
Continuous fanning
Exposure to cool environment
Axillary or perineal ice packs and ice sheets
Infusion of room-temperature saline
Gastric or colonic iced saline lavage
Peritoneal lavage with cool saline
Monitor electrocardiogram for arrhythmia
Obtain serial diagnostic studies*

*Electrocardiogram, chest radiograph, complete blood count with differential, platelet count, urinalysis, aminotransferases, alkaline phosphatase, bilirubin, creatine kinase, blood urea nitrogen, creatinine, phosphate, calcium, glucose, electrolytes, uric acid, prothrombin time and partial thromboplastin time, fibrin split products, fibrinogen, arterial blood gases, toxicology screen.

2- to 5-minute period, repeated if necessary) is a safe sedative because of its low hepatotoxicity and rapid metabolism.

A single episode of heat exhaustion does not imply a predisposition to heat illness, and most patients recover within several hours after cooling and rehydration. In contrast, heat injury and heatstroke patients should not be re-exposed to heat until recovery is complete, and about 10% of heatstroke patients remain intolerant of heat. The long-term consequences of heatstroke likely include sustained organ damage, which presumably explains why patients have a higher long-term mortality from cardiovascular, liver, and digestive diseases.

COLD INJURY

DEFINITIONS

Cold injuries are classified as hypothermia and peripheral cold injuries. Hypothermia is whole body cooling, whereas peripheral cold injuries are localized to the extremities and exposed skin. Peripheral cold injuries can be divided into nonfreezing (chilblain, trench foot) and freezing (frostbite). Both hypothermia and peripheral cold injuries often occur simultaneously.

EPIDEMIOLOGY

A variety of individual factors, health conditions, medications, and environmental factors are associated with a predisposition to cold injury (Table 109-4). In trauma patients (Chapter 112), hypothermia is associated with increased morbidity and mortality.

PATHOBIOLOGY

Cold exposure elicits peripheral vasoconstriction to reduce heat transfer between the body's core and shell (skin, subcutaneous fat). If sufficiently cold, the underlying tissues (e.g., muscle) constrict to thicken the isolative shell while reducing the body's core area. This vasoconstrictor response defends core temperature, but at the expense of declining peripheral tissue temperatures, which contribute to peripheral cold injuries. Hypothermia depresses enzymatic activity, interferes with physiologic functions (e.g., clotting, respiration, cardiac conduction and rhythm), impairs the expression of cytokines, and can induce cellular injury and death.

CLINICAL MANIFESTATIONS AND DIAGNOSIS

Hypothermia is a core temperature below 35° C (95° F), and clinical manifestations are related to the core temperature achieved (Table 109-5). The classic J wave on the electrocardiogram (Fig. 109-2) appears at a core temperature below about 33.8° C (93° F).

Chilblain (Chapter 80) appears as localized inflammatory lesions of the skin most often involving the dorsal surface of fingers, but the ears, face, and exposed shins are other common areas. Trench foot is caused by prolonged

TABLE 109-4 FACTORS PREDISPOSING TO COLD INJURY

INDIVIDUAL FACTORS

Inadequate clothing and shelter
Lean and low body fat
Low physical fitness
Advanced age
Young age
Black race (men and women)

HEALTH CONDITIONS

Burns
Diabetes mellitus
Hypoglycemia
Neurologic lesions
Dementia
Hypoadrenalism, hypopituitarism, hypothyroidism
Prior frostbite or trench foot
Raynaud's phenomenon
Sickle cell trait
Trauma
Spinal cord injury

DRUGS

Alcohol
Anesthetics
Antidepressants
Antithyroid agents
Sedatives and narcotics

ENVIRONMENTAL FACTORS

Cold temperatures
High air motion
Rain and immersion
Skin contact with metal and fuels
Repeated cold exposure
Physical fatigue
Immobility
High-altitude and low-oxygen-tension environments

TABLE 109-5 HYPOTHERMIA: STAGES AND ASSOCIATED CLINICAL MANIFESTATIONS

STAGE	Core Temperature ° F	Core Temperature ° C	CLINICAL MANIFESTATIONS
Normothermia	98.6	37.0	
Mild hypothermia	95.0	35.0	Cold diuresis, maximal shivering
	93.0	33.8	Ataxia, poor judgment, J wave
	91.0	32.7	Amnesia, blood pressure difficult to measure
Moderate hypothermia	89.0	31.6	Stupor, pupils dilated
	87.0	30.5	Shivering ceases
	85.0	30.0	Cardiac arrhythmias, insulin inactive
	82.0	27.8	Unconsciousness, ventricular fibrillation likely
	80.0	26.6	No muscle reflexes
Profound hypothermia	78.0	25.5	Acid-base disturbances, no response to pain
	75.0	23.8	Pulmonary edema, hypotension
	73.0	22.7	No corneal reflexes
	66.0	18.8	Heart standstill
	62.0	16.6	Isoelectric electrocardiogram
	57.6	14.2	Lowest infant survival from accidental hypothermia
	48.2	9.0	Lowest adult survival from accidental hypothermia

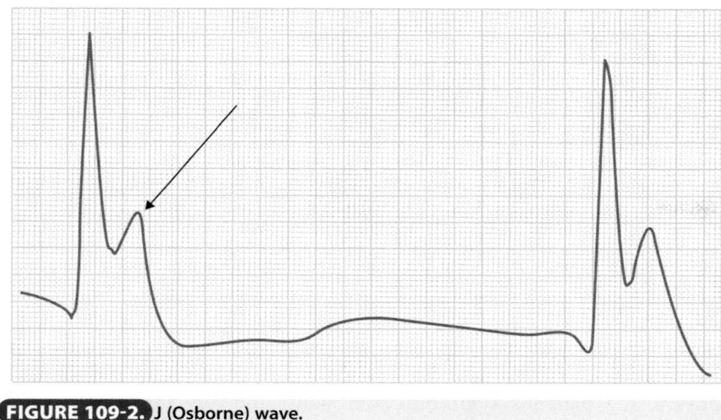

FIGURE 109-2. J (Osborne) wave.

TABLE 109-6 TREATMENT OF HYPOTHERMIA

STAGE	MANAGEMENT	BODY REWARMING
Mild hypothermia	Monitor vital signs Warm intravenous saline Oxygen Monitor electrocardiogram for arrhythmia	Insulate Shivering Warm bath Active warming blanket
Moderate hypothermia	Diagnostic studies* Intensive care Anticipate infection and multiorgan dysfunction	Prevent extra heat loss by supplementing with airway rewarming Colonic irrigation Peritoneal dialysis
Profound hypothermia	Diagnostic studies*	Central rewarming

*See Table 109-3. Also lactate dehydrogenase, serum lactate, cortisol, thyroid-stimulating hormone, T_3, and T_4.

cold, wet exposure (e.g., wet socks or gloves), which can cause skin breakdown and nerve damage. Trench foot is often accompanied by infection and increased sensitivity to pain. Frostbite is the freezing of tissues and can be categorized as first degree (superficial, "frostnip"), second degree (full skin), third degree (subcutaneous tissue), and fourth degree (extensive tissue and bone). It may take many days to weeks to determine the severity of frostbite. Frostbite requires early surgical consultation once the diagnosis is made.

PREVENTION, TREATMENT, AND PROGNOSIS (Rx)

Humans demonstrate minimal cold acclimatization, so prevention depends primarily on avoiding cold exposure and having adequate protection and caloric intake to support metabolism. Management of hypothermia depends on the core temperature (Table 109-6). Patients' wet clothing should be removed, and they should be provided with dry insulation. Shivering is an effective physiologic rewarming mechanism and should not be pharmacologically suppressed. Moderately and profoundly hypothermic patients require active rewarming. Rewarming at a rate of 0.5 to 1.0° C (0.9 to 1.8° F) per hour is acceptable in most cases, except that aggressive rewarming is warranted in patients with significant trauma (because coagulation is hindered by hypothermia) or cardiac arrest.

Patients should be warmed gently because ventricular fibrillation is easily precipitated. When ventricular fibrillation is present, repeated electrical shocks should not be attempted until the patient has been rewarmed to a core temperature higher than 30° C (86° F); instead, cardiopulmonary resuscitation should be maintained during this period. Arrhythmias can be treated with lidocaine, propranolol, or bretylium (Chapter 63). Body cooling induces cold diuresis, so plasma volume needs to be reestablished to support adequate perfusion: patients should receive an intravenous infusion of 250 to 1000 mL of heated (40 to 42° C [104 to 108° F]) 5% dextrose in normal saline. Lactated Ringer's solution should be avoided because the liver cannot metabolize lactate efficiently during hypothermia. Patients should be monitored for disturbances in potassium and glucose. If hypoglycemia, alcohol, or opiate intoxication is contributing to hypothermia, intravenous glucose (10 to 25 g), thiamine (100 mg), or naloxone (1 to 2 mg), respectively, may be indicated.

Frostbitten tissues should be protected from friction or trauma and gently rewarmed in a water bath (38 to 43° C [100 to 108° F]). Frostbitten tissues should not be thawed until there is confidence in the ability to maintain warmth, because refreezing causes more injury. Patients should receive ibuprofen, antibiotics if infection is suspected, and possibly an analgesic.

Hypothermic Syndromes

Exercise-induced bronchospasm (Chapter 87) can be triggered by exercise in cold air, particularly in patients with asthma. Livedo reticularis (Fig. 80-2 in Chapter 80) is patchy mottling of the limbs with cold exposure. Cryoglobulinemia (Chapter 193) occurs when immunoglobulins (IgM, IgG) reversibly precipitate after being cooled and contribute to impaired capillary blood flow in hypothermic tissues. Cold urticaria (Chapters 260 and 448) is the development of localized and general erythema and wheals in skin exposed to cold. Paroxysmal hypothermia is periodic lowering of the thermoregulatory set point and is often associated with hypothalamic abnormalities. Raynaud's phenomenon (Fig. 80-5 in Chapter 80) is intense vasoconstriction with sensitivity to pain in limbs exposed to cold.

Trauma Hypothermia

In trauma patients (Chapter 112), unintended hypothermia (<34° C [93° F]) is associated with increased morbidity and mortality due to impaired coagulation, peripheral vasoconstriction, respiratory depression, and increased risk for cardiac arrhythmias. Shivering aggravates perfusion problems by requiring blood flow to support increased metabolism in contracting muscles. Trauma patients become hypothermic because of heat loss from exposed cavities, environmental exposure, infusion of cool fluids, and ischemia, which depletes cell energy stores. Body temperature should be measured, and appropriate actions should be taken to restore normothermia during the early treatment of trauma patients.

THERAPEUTIC HYPOTHERMIA AND HYPERTHERMIA

Therapeutic Hypothermia

Therapeutic hypothermia provides benefits by suppressing metabolism, free radical production, lipid peroxidation, inflammatory products, excitatory amino acid release, and calcium release. Induction of mild hypothermia (32 to 34° C [89 to 93° F]) for 12 to 24 hours provides long-term benefits to patients after a cardiac arrest (Chapter 63).[2] It is being tested for spinal cord injury but has not consistently shown a benefit in neonates with traumatic brain injury or hypoxic-ischemic encephalopathy.[3,4] Mild hypothermia may be beneficial for patients suffering from hemorrhagic shock, brain injury, or stroke.

Therapeutic hypothermia should be initiated as soon as possible by either skin cooling (e.g., cooling packs to the axilla, groin, head, and neck while simultaneously treating the patient with a cooling blanket, water mattress, or fan), endovascular cooling, or both. Endovascular cooling can be achieved either by the infusion of cool fluids (e.g., 30 mL/kg crystalloids at 4° C [40° F]) or by indwelling heat transfer devices. Cooling by peritoneal and pleural lavage is not generally used. Endovascular cooling provides a more rapid and better-controlled cooling than skin cooling. Thermoregulatory responses (shivering and peripheral vasoconstriction) will resist induced hypothermia and elevate blood pressure and should therefore be pharmacologically blunted. Low-dose meperidine (e.g., 12.5 mg intravenously) can blunt shivering without excessive toxicity.

Hyperthermia Treatment

Hyperthermia treatment (whole body or regional) is an experimental technique used as an adjunct to chemotherapy or radiation therapy in advanced cancer patients. Hyperthermia (40 to 43° C [104 to 109° F]) alone can damage or kill cancer cells, but more importantly, hyperthermia might potentiate the effectiveness of chemotherapy and radiation by softening the tumor tissue, thus reducing its interstitial pressure.

Whole body hyperthermia is usually induced by externally applied radiant heat, microwaves, or extracorporeal circulation. Target temperatures are usually achieved over 1 to 2 hours and then maintained for approximately 1 hour, followed by a 1-hour cooling phase. Patients are usually sedated while core and skin temperatures are monitored. In regional hyperthermia, the part of the body where the tumor is located is heated while being perfused or bathed by a warmed solution containing anticancer drugs.

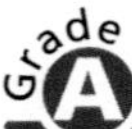

1. Ishikawa T, Tamura H, Ishiguro H, et al. Effect of oral rehydration solution on fatigue during outdoor work in a hot environment: a randomized crossover study. *J Occup Health*. 2010;52:209-215.
2. Janata A, Holzer M. Hypothermia after cardiac arrest. *Prog Cardiovasc Dis*. 2009;52:168-179.
3. Azzopardi DV, Strohm B, Edwards AD, et al. Moderate hypothermia to treat perinatal asphyxia encephalopathy. *N Engl J Med*. 2009;361:1349-1358.
4. Hutchison JS, Ward RE, Lacroix J, et al. Hypothermia therapy after traumatic brain injury in children. *N Engl J Med*. 2008;358:2447-2456.

SUGGESTED READINGS

Holzer M. Targeted temperature management for comatose survivors of cardiac arrest. *N Engl J Med*. 2010;363:1256-1264. *Review.*

Metzger KB, Ito K, Matte TD. Summer heat and mortality in New York City: how hot is too hot? *Environ Health Perspect*. 2010;118:80-86. *Risk rises abruptly at a heat index between 95 and 100° F.*

Nelson NG, Collins CL, Comstock RD, et al. Exertional heat-related injuries treated in emergency departments in the U.S. 1997-2006. *Am J Prev Med*. 2011;40:54-60. *Review of about 55,000 cases.*

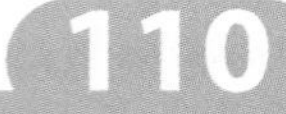

110 ACUTE POISONING

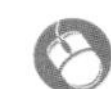

MARSHA D. FORD

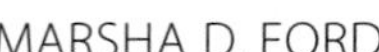

EPIDEMIOLOGY

Each year, more than 4 million poisoning cases, suspected or verified, and 300,000 related hospital admissions occur in the United States. Poisoning-related deaths total more than 30,000 per year and are increasing. Unintentional poisonings are now the second leading cause of injury-related death in the United States, and they exceed motor vehicle accidents as the leading cause of injury-related death in adults 34 to 56 years of age. Ninety-two percent of these deaths involve drugs, predominantly prescription opioid analgesics. The incidence of recurrent, purposeful self-poisoning is 12 to 18%, with most events occurring within 3 months of the original attempt. These facts emphasize the need for regulatory measures to improve the safety of opioid analgesic drugs, including appropriate prescribing, and aggressive treatment of poisoned patients, including early psychiatric intervention for suicidal behavior, to reduce fatalities and repeat attempts (Chapter 404).

DIAGNOSIS

Diagnosis and management of poisoned patients require knowledge and skill in five areas to identify and treat the factors that contribute to the risk for death or long-term disability: (1) history taking; (2) physical examination, with recognition of specific toxic syndromes, or *toxidromes;* (3) appropriate use of diagnostic tests; (4) treatment, including initial stabilization and critical care, decontamination, and administration of antidotes for specific poisonings; and (5) use of methods to enhance the elimination of specific toxicants.

History

Details elicited about toxic exposures should include the involved drugs and other toxicants, their estimated or known amounts, the time and routes of exposure, the patient's symptoms and signs, and any treatment already administered. Intoxication may result from acute, chronic, or acute-on-chronic exposure. A *toxicant* is defined as a chemical capable of harming a biologic organism; this definition encompasses toxins, which are derived from living organisms, as well as drugs and industrial and other chemicals. Determination of chronicity is important because signs and symptoms of chronic intoxication (Chapter 21) can differ from those of acute and acute-on-chronic intoxication. For example, a history of acute collapse narrows the toxicant possibilities to a few gases, chemicals, and drugs. A listing of available medications (e.g., medications of the patient, spouse, relatives, or friends); use of nonprescription medications, herbal or dietary supplements, or ethnic remedies; and occupational and avocational activities should be obtained. Occupational and avocational histories should include present and all past jobs and hobbies, with a focus on chemicals, metals, and gases. Known medical conditions may suggest classes of medications available to the patient. The patient's history, which may be incomplete if the patient is confused or suicidal, should be correlated with the clinical manifestations and course. Further history from relatives and friends and findings from the scene as reported by the transporting emergency medical services personnel may be relevant.

Physical Examination

The physical examination should focus on vital signs; the eye, ear, nose, and throat examination; and the neurologic, cardiopulmonary, gastrointestinal, and dermatologic systems. Findings can suggest certain toxidromes, which are clusters of signs and symptoms typical of poisoning with adrenergic, anticholinergic, cholinomimetic, opioid, and sedative-hypnotic agents (Table 110-1). Patients may have some or all of these signs and symptoms; an incomplete clinical picture does not exclude a particular toxidrome, but it can still assist the clinician in identifying the correct category of toxicant involved.

TABLE 110-1 TOXIDROMES AND ASSOCIATED DRUGS AND TOXICANTS

	Syndrome Features		
TOXIDROME	**VITAL SIGNS**	**END ORGAN**	**COMMON DRUGS/TOXICANTS**
Adrenergic	Hypertension, hyperthermia, tachycardia, tachypnea	Agitation, arrhythmias, diaphoresis, mydriasis, seizures	Amphetamines, caffeine, cathinone derivatives, cocaine, ephedrine, pseudoephedrine, *Ephedra* sp, phenylpropanolamine,* theophylline
Anticholinergic	Hyperthermia, tachycardia	Agitation, delirium, decreased or absent bowel sounds, dry flushed skin and mucous membranes, mydriasis or blurred vision, seizures, urinary retention	First-generation H_1-receptor antagonists (e.g., classic antihistamines), belladonna alkaloids (e.g., scopolamine, hyoscyamine) from plants (e.g., *Datura* sp—deadly nightshade, henbane), benztropine, cyclic antidepressants, dicyclomine, muscle relaxants (e.g., orphenadrine, cyclobenzaprine), trihexyphenidyl
Cholinomimetic	Tachycardia or bradycardia†	Agitation, delirium, coma; bronchorrhea, bronchospasm; diaphoresis; fasciculations; lacrimation; miosis; urination; diarrhea, vomiting; seizures	Carbamates, cholinesterase inhibitors (e.g., physostigmine, neostigmine, edrophonium), *Inocybe* or *Clitocybe* mushroom sp, nerve gases (e.g., soman, sarin), organophosphorus compounds
Opiate, opioid	Bradycardia, bradypnea or apnea, hypotension (rare), hypothermia	CNS depression; hypotonia; miosis; mydriasis (dextromethorphan, meperidine, pentazocine)	Codeine, fentanyl, designer fentanyls, heroin, opioids (e.g., hydrocodone, oxycodone, meperidine, morphine), propoxyphene, central α_2-agonists (e.g., clonidine, imidazolines)
Sedative-hypnotic	Bradypnea or apnea, hypotension, hypothermia	Ataxia, CNS depression, hyporeflexia, slurred speech, stupor, or coma	Barbiturates, benzodiazepines, bromides, chloral hydrate, ethanol, ethchlorvynol, etomidate, glutethimide, meprobamate, methaqualone, methyprylon, propofol, zolpidem

*Reflex bradycardia can occur as a result of a pure α-adrenergic agonist effect.
†Tachycardia can occur early as a result of a preganglionic nicotinic effect; as toxicity progresses, postganglionic muscarinic effects predominate, and bradycardia develops.
CNS = central nervous system.

Vital Signs

Tachycardia can occur with numerous toxicants and with anxiety and other nontoxicologic conditions and is not a helpful finding. The limited differential diagnosis for toxicant-induced *bradycardia* includes baclofen, β-adrenergic receptor antagonists, L-type calcium-channel antagonists (diltiazem or verapamil), cardiac glycosides, α-adrenergic receptor agonists (e.g., phenylpropanolamine, whose effects are mediated by baroreceptor reflexes), γ-hydroxybutyric acid, opioids, some sedative-hypnotics, central α_2-agonists, organophosphorus compounds, carbamates, cyanide, muscarine-containing mushrooms (*Clitocybe, Inocybe* sp), plant- and animal-derived toxins (aconitine, andromedotoxin, ciguatoxin, veratridine), therapeutic cholinesterase inhibitors (e.g., physostigmine), cyclic antidepressants (bradycardia is a preterminal sign), and some antiarrhythmic drugs (e.g., procainamide, flecainide, other class IA and IC drugs such as amiodarone, sotalol).

Many toxicants cause *hypotension* (Chapter 7). The primary mechanisms are decreased peripheral vascular resistance, decreased myocardial contractility, hypovolemia secondary to vomiting or loss of intravascular volume, and, occasionally, arrhythmias. Common causes of *hypertension* (Chapter 67) include amphetamines, cocaine, ephedrine and similar agents, ergots, phencyclidine, nicotine, phenylpropanolamine, thyroid hormones, chronic yohimbine use, and chronic lead toxicity. Blood pressure can rise early in poisoning with cyclic antidepressants, central α_2-adrenergic agonists, and monoamine oxidase inhibitors.

Hyperthermia (Chapter 109) occurs with toxicants that cause agitation or excessive motor activity (e.g., cocaine, phencyclidine, monoamine oxidase inhibitors, strychnine), uncouple oxidative phosphorylation (e.g., salicylates, 2,4-dinitrophenol), increase the metabolic rate (thyroid hormones), impair sweating (e.g., first-generation antihistamines, anticholinergics, cocaine, phenothiazines, zonisamide), cause vasoconstriction (e.g., amphetamines, ephedrine), or impair vasodilation and alter perception of heat (cocaine). Other toxicant-induced states associated with hyperthermia include malignant hyperthermia, neuroleptic malignant syndrome, serotonin syndrome, metal fume fever, and hydrocarbon aspiration. Toxicant-induced *hypothermia* is typically due to sedative-hypnotics, opioids, barbiturates, ethanol, phenothiazines, or hypoglycemic agents such as insulin, sulfonylureas, meglitinides, or unripe akee fruit. Oxygen saturation (Figure 161-2 in Chapter 161) as measured by *pulse oximetry*, decreases with true hypoxemia (Figure 104-1 in Chapter 104) or methemoglobinemia (Chapter 161) but remains normal or may be increased in carbon monoxide poisoning (Chapter 94).

Eyes, Ears, Nose, and Throat

Toxicant-induced bilateral miosis (Fig. 110-1) has a limited differential diagnosis that includes central α_2-agonists such as clonidine, guanfacine, and the imidazolines; olanzapine; opioids; organophosphorus compounds or carbamates; therapeutic cholinesterase inhibitors (e.g., physostigmine); topical miotic ophthalmic drugs (e.g., pilocarpine, carbachol); and, variably, phencyclidine, phenothiazines, ethanol, and some sedative-hypnotics (Chapter 432). Pontine hemorrhage is the major nontoxicologic diagnosis to consider in a comatose patient with miotic pupils (Chapter 415). Mydriasis is a nonspecific finding. A unilateral dilated pupil may be due to topical ocular application of sympathomimetics (e.g., phenylephrine), antihistamines, or anticholinergic agents (e.g., inhaled anticholinergics such as ipratropium or tiotropium, dust or sap from *Datura* sp) and can be caused by a postauricular scopolamine patch. Failure of topical 4% pilocarpine ophthalmic drops to constrict the pupil supports the diagnosis of pupillary dilation from a topical mydriatic agent. Visual disturbances, including partial or total blindness as a result of systemic toxicity, have been reported with anticholinergic agents, carbon monoxide, digitalis, ethambutol, methanol, methyl bromide, quinine, and agents that are associated with pseudotumor cerebri, including antimicrobials (e.g., ampicillin, metronidazole, nalidixic acid, nitrofurantoin, sulfa drugs, tetracycline), glucocorticosteroids, lead, lithium, oral contraceptives, phenothiazines, phenytoin, and vitamin A. Nonarteritic anterior ischemic optic neuropathy has developed after the use of sildenafil and other related drugs (Chapter 242); the causal relationship is unknown.

Acute hearing loss (Chapter 436) can occur as a toxic effect of aminoglycosides, bromates, chloroquine, cisplatin, carboplatin, high-dose loop diuretics, nitrogen mustard, quinine, salicylates, vinblastine, and vincristine. Nasal septal erosions and perforations may be due to chronic exposure to intranasal cocaine (Chapter 33) or inhalation of fumes from chromium and nickel (Chapters 93 and 94).

Neurologic Signs

Many toxicants affect the central nervous system (CNS) and can produce agitated delirium, depression, or seizures (Table 110-2). Distinguishing features of various toxicants may assist in making the correct diagnosis. Patients withdrawing from opioids are alert and oriented, whereas patients withdrawing from alcohol, barbiturates, benzodiazepines, and other sedative-hypnotics can be disoriented. Initial CNS depression can also develop with large ingestions of acetaminophen or ibuprofen. Isoniazid and theophylline are noted for producing seizures refractory to the usual doses of benzodiazepines and barbiturates. Pyridoxine treats isoniazid-induced seizures by increasing CNS γ-aminobutyric acid; phenytoin is relatively ineffective for theophylline-induced seizures. Plant or mushroom ingestion can also produce CNS depression (e.g., *Rhododendron* sp, *Solanum* [bittersweet], *Taxus* [yew], *Sophora* [mescal bean]), CNS stimulation (e.g., *Catha edulis* [khat], *Strychnos nux vomica* [contains strychnine], *Cicuta* sp [water hemlock], *Ephedra* [Mormon tea]), atropine-like effects (e.g., *Atropa belladonna* [deadly

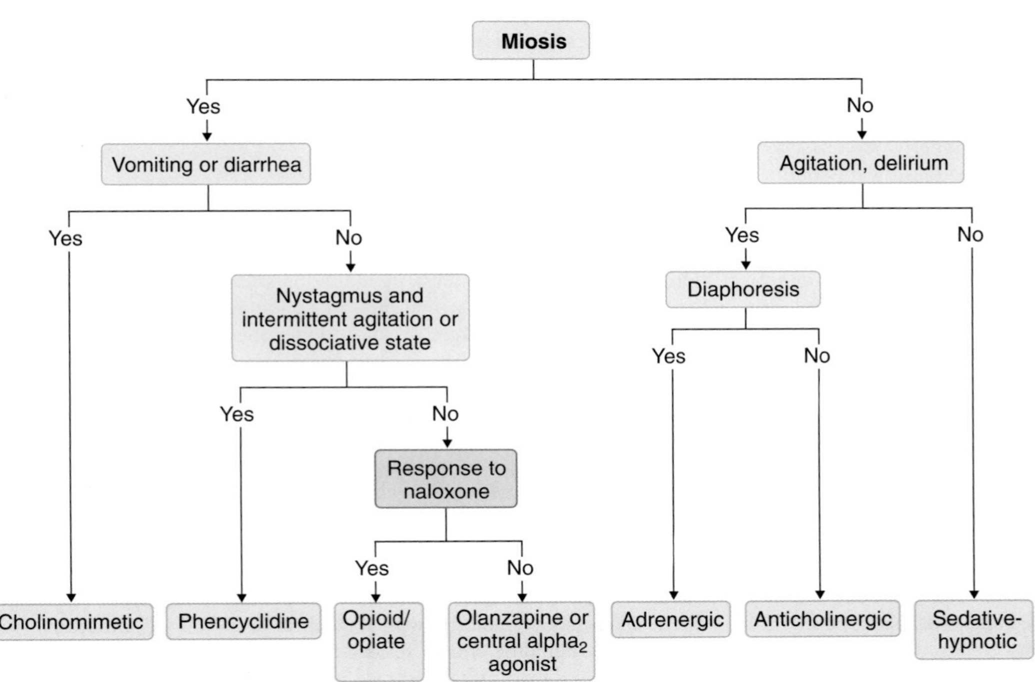

FIGURE 110-1. Diagnostic algorithm using the size of the pupils.

TABLE 110-2 CENTRAL NERVOUS SYSTEM EFFECTS OF TOXICANTS

	CNS Effects		
TOXICANT CATEGORIES/AGENTS	**AGITATED DELIRIUM**	**DECREASED LEVEL OF CONSCIOUSNESS**	**SEIZURES**
CATEGORIES			
Adrenergic agonists	•		•
Anticholinergic agents	•	•	•
Anticonvulsants		•	• (paradoxical with some agents)
Antipsychotic drugs	•	•	•
β-Adrenergic receptor antagonists		•	•
Hallucinogenic agents	•		•
Monoamine oxidase inhibitors	•	•	•
Opioids	• (propoxyphene, normeperidine, tramadol)	•	• (propoxyphene, normeperidine, tramadol)
Sedative-hypnotics		•	• (rare)
Serotonin agonists	•	•	•
AGENTS			
Amphetamines, cocaine	•	•	•
Antidepressants	•	•	• (can be delayed with bupropion)
Antihistamines (first generation, e.g., diphenhydramine)	•	•	•
Barbiturates		•	
Benzodiazepines		•	
Cytochrome oxidase inhibitors (e.g., carbon monoxide, cyanide, hydrogen sulfide, azides)		•	•
Ephedra alkaloids and similar agents			•
Ethylene glycol, methanol	•	•	•
γ-Hydroxybutyrate and precursors	•	•	• (rare)
Lithium	•	•	•
Organophosphorus compounds, carbamates (e.g., diazinon, malathion, fenthion, carbaryl)		•	•
Salicylates	•	•	•
SSRIs/SRIs	•	•	• (uncommon)
Withdrawal from alcohol, barbiturates, benzodiazepines, other sedative-hypnotics	•	•	•
Withdrawal from opioids			• (reported only in neonates)

CNS = central nervous system; SRIs = serotonin re-uptake inhibitors; SSRIs = selective serotonin re-uptake inhibitors.

nightshade], *Datura* sp [jimsonweed]), and cholinomimetic effects (e.g., *Nicotiana* genus [tobacco], *Conium maculatum* [poison hemlock], *Inocybe* and *Clitocybe* mushrooms). Seizures can also occur with many of these plants and with mushrooms that contain gyromitrins (e.g., *Gyromitra* sp) and muscimol (e.g., *Amanita muscaria, Amanita pantherina*).

Distal axonopathy, a primary degeneration of peripheral nervous system axons with secondary degeneration of the myelin sheath, is the predominant type of toxicant-induced peripheral neuropathy. Common causative agents include acrylamide monomer, allyl chloride, arsenic (inorganic), capsaicin, carbon disulfide, chloramphenicol, cisplatin, colchicine, cyanate, dapsone, dideoxycytidine (ddC), dideoxyinosine (ddI), disulfiram, ethambutol, ethanol, ethylene oxide, gold salts, hexachlorophene, *n*-hexane, hydralazine, interferon, isoniazid, lead, linezolid, mercury, methyl bromide, methyl *n*-butyl ketone, metronidazole, nitrofurantoin, nitrous oxide, some organophosphorus compounds, phenol, platinum, podophyllotoxin, polychlorinated biphenyls, pyridoxine, tacrolimus, taxoids, thalidomide, thallium, vidarabine, vinca alkaloids, and vinyl chloride. Amiodarone, arsenic, and trichloroethylene can produce a demyelinating neuropathy, whereas pyridoxine can produce a sensory neuronopathy.

Neuronal transmission can be altered by aminoglycosides; the venom of *Latrodectus* species (widow spiders), scorpions (only the bark scorpion, *Centruroides exilicauda*, in the United States), and crotaline (e.g., rattlesnakes) and elapid snakes; brevetoxin (shellfish) and ciguatoxin (various fish); neuromuscular blocking drugs; nicotine and related alkaloids; paralytic shellfish toxins; saxitoxin (shellfish); organophosphorus compounds and carbamates; tetrodotoxin (puffer fish [fugu], blue-ringed octopus, salamanders, newts, and others); and veratridine (e.g., false hellebore). Cranial nerves can be affected by carbon disulfide, ciguatoxin, domoic acid (shellfish), elapid venom, ethylene glycol metabolites, paralytic shellfish toxins, bark scorpion, saxitoxin, tetrodotoxin, thallium, and trichloroethylene. Mononeuropathies and vasculitic neuropathies are unlikely to be induced by toxicants (Chapters 113 and 114).

Cardiopulmonary Effects

The examination should focus on blood pressure, heart rate, electrocardiographic abnormalities (e.g., rhythm, conduction, depolarization, repolarization), and pulmonary findings, including pulse oximetry. Drugs and other toxicants that can cause arrhythmias or conduction abnormalities include β-adrenergic receptor antagonists, butyrophenones (e.g., droperidol), L-type calcium-channel antagonists, cardiac glycosides (e.g., digoxin; bufadienolides, found in toxic toad venom and incorporated into some illicit aphrodisiacs; cardenolides, found in plants such as oleander and lily of the valley), chloral hydrate, chloroquine, cocaine, cyclic antidepressants, ethanol, halogenated hydrocarbons (e.g., halothane, trichloroethylene), magnesium, potassium, propoxyphene, thioridazine or mesoridazine, and antiarrhythmics and other agents that affect the myocardial voltage-gated sodium channels (e.g., bupivacaine, chloroquine, cocaine, cyclic antidepressants, flecainide, mexiletine, quinidine, procainamide, propafenone) and potassium channels (e.g., astemizole, cisapride, citalopram, erythromycin [especially when taken concomitantly with cytochrome P-450 A inhibitors; see Chapter 28], quinidine, sotalol, terfenadine). Bedside echocardiography may reveal depressed myocardial contractility as a result of agents that block the myocardial voltage-gated sodium channel, β-adrenergic receptor antagonists, calcium-channel antagonists, cyclic antidepressants, magnesium, arsenic, ciguatoxin, cyanide, ethanol, iron, scorpion venom, and tetrodotoxin.

Toxicants can produce myriad pulmonary effects, including airway irritation; parenchymal, pleural, and vascular diseases; and barotrauma. Immediate life-threatening toxic effects include acute lung injury and pulmonary edema, acute respiratory distress syndrome (ARDS; Chapter 104), and rapidly developing pulmonary fibrosis or bronchiolitis obliterans. Typical syndromes and etiologic agents include pulmonary edema (β-adrenergic receptor antagonists, calcium-channel antagonists, antiarrhythmics, daunorubicin, doxorubicin), acute lung injury or ARDS (amphetamines, cadmium, chlorine, cocaine, ethchlorvynol, methotrexate, opioids, heroin, paraquat, salicylates; inhalation of smoke, zinc chloride, methyl bromide, methyl chloride), and rapidly developing pulmonary fibrosis or bronchiolitis obliterans (nitrogen dioxide, paraquat).

Gastrointestinal Effects

Symptoms of nausea, vomiting, diarrhea, and abdominal pain are nonspecific and must be interpreted in the context of other findings. Agents that produce severe or life-threatening toxicity with early gastrointestinal findings include acid or large alkali ingestions; cardiac glycosides, colchicines, and other microtubular toxicants; iron; metals such as arsenic, acute high-level lead, mercury salts, or thallium; mushrooms containing amanitine (*Amanita phalloides, Amanita virosa, Amanita verna, Lepiota chlorophyllum*), gyromitrins (*Gyromitra esculenta*), orellanines (*Cortinarius orellanus*), or allenic norleucine (*Amanita smithiana*); nicotine; organophosphorus compounds; and theophylline. Severe abdominal pain and rigidity can occur with envenomation by *Latrodectus* species (widow spiders). Right upper quadrant tenderness develops with toxic hepatitis. Hepatotoxicity can occur as an adverse effect of the therapeutic use of many drugs; in the United States, acetaminophen and ethanol are the most common causes of toxicant-induced hepatotoxicity (Chapter 152). Other notable hepatotoxicants include aflatoxins (in food contaminated with *Aspergillus flavus*), arsenicals, carbon tetrachloride, copper sulfate, cyclopeptide mushrooms (e.g., *Amanita phalloides*), *Ephedra* species (e.g., ma huang), iron, methamphetamine, pennyroyal oil, pyrrolizidine alkaloids (various plant species used in herbal teas), and vitamin A in chronic excessive doses.

Dermatologic Signs

The skin, hair, nails, and mucous membranes should be examined for evidence of intravenous drug use; the presence or absence of skin and mucous membrane moisture; abnormal skin coloration, including erythema and cyanosis; alopecia; and nail abnormalities. Bullous skin lesions have been reported with chronic barbiturate use, glutethimide, carbon monoxide, meprobamate, methadone, and valproic acid. Cyanosis may reflect hypoxemia or methemoglobinemia. Commonly used agents that can cause methemoglobinemia include aniline dyes, benzocaine and other amide anesthetics, dapsone, naphthalene, nitrates, nitrites, phenazopyridine, rifampin, and sulfonamides. Skin erythema or flushing occurs with anticholinergic agents, boric acid ingestion, monosodium glutamate, niacin, scombroid toxicity as a result of the ingestion of inadequately refrigerated fish with a high histidine content (e.g., tuna, mahi-mahi, amberjack), vancomycin, and interactions between ethanol and numerous agents that produce disulfiram or disulfiram-like reactions (e.g., carbon disulfide, some cephalosporins, *Coprinus atramentarius* mushroom, disulfiram, griseofulvin, metronidazole, thiuram herbicides, trichloroethylene).

Specific Toxicants

Some common toxicants can be suspected from their characteristic manifestations (Table 110-3). These suspicions should guide specific diagnostic and therapeutic strategies that complement general decontamination and supportive treatments.

Diagnostic Tests

Drug testing should be guided by the history and physical examination, with emphasis on tests that can influence management. Rapid qualitative urine drug screening tests are readily available in most hospitals, but their clinical value is limited by the number of drugs that can be tested and the reliability of the tests themselves. A positive test result may be unrelated to the patient's condition because drug analytes may be detectable within hours to more than 30 days after drug use, depending on the drug, dose, and frequency of use. False-positive and false-negative results occur (Table 110-4), and the screening result must be verified with a second method, such as gas chromatography–mass spectrometry. The type of drug use in a population should be considered when determining the drugs to be screened to decrease the incidence of false-positive results. A test with 99% specificity for a drug with a prevalence of 0.1% in a population would produce 10 false-positive results for every true-positive result. Clinically irrelevant true-positive findings also occur, such as when poppy seeds produce a positive opiate test. Failure to consider these limitations of drug screens can result in misdiagnosis.

For a limited number of drugs and toxicants, levels in blood or urine are useful for diagnosis, therapy, or monitoring (Table 110-5). Threshold levels of certain toxicants indicate the need for specific therapies: acetaminophen (*N*-acetylcysteine), ethylene glycol (fomepizole and hemodialysis), iron (deferoxamine), methanol (fomepizole and hemodialysis), methemoglobin (methylene blue), salicylates (urine alkalinization and hemodialysis), and theophylline (hemoperfusion or hemodialysis). In chronic poisoning with some drugs, such as salicylates or theophylline, these therapies may be indicated at lower drug levels. In general, any end-organ toxicity that is evident or anticipated (based on the toxicant, amount ingested, and time required to produce toxic effects) is more important than a specific level in determining the need for treatment.

Occult acetaminophen ingestion with toxic serum levels occurs in 0.3 to 1.9% of intentional ingestions. Given that these patients may be asymptomatic until hepatotoxicity develops and that administration of an antidote can prevent this hepatotoxicity, the current recommendation is to test for acetaminophen in all patients with intentional ingestions.

Other Blood Tests

Anion gap metabolic acidosis resulting from primary lactic acidosis can be caused by cyanide, hydrogen sulfide, iron, isoniazid, metformin, nucleoside reverse transcriptase inhibitors, phenformin, sodium azide, and, rarely, acetaminophen with high serum levels. Anion gap metabolic acidosis not related to lactic acidosis occurs with diethylene glycol, ethylene glycol, nonsteroidal anti-inflammatory drugs (NSAIDs), methanol, salicylates, theophylline, and toluene. In poisonings resulting from ibuprofen, methanol, propylene glycol, and salicylates, lactic acid can also be produced, but the level is insufficient to account for the anion gap. Anion gap metabolic acidosis can also develop in patients with ongoing agitation, hyperthermia, and muscle rigidity, such as in neuroleptic malignant syndrome (Chapter 442), or in some cases of rhabdomyolysis (Chapter 115) secondary to toxicants such as doxylamine, phencyclidine, strychnine, cocaine, and amphetamines. Elevated serum creatinine and blood urea nitrogen levels indicative of declining renal function may be seen with numerous toxicants. Direct toxicity occurs with acetaminophen, aminoglycosides, cadmium, Chinese weight-loss botanicals (containing *Stephania tetrandra* or *Magnolia officinalis*), chromium, *Crotalus durissus* venom, diethylene glycol, diquat, ethylene glycol, fluorinated anesthetics, gold, heroin, lithium (diabetes insipidus), mercury salts, mushrooms (*Amanita smithiana* and *Cortinarius* sp), paraquat, radiocontrast agents, solvents (e.g., carbon tetrachloride, trichloroethylene, tetrachloroethylene, toluene), and sulfonamides. Agents that decrease glomerular perfusion by reducing renal blood flow include amphotericin, angiotensin-converting enzyme inhibitors, angiotensin receptor blockers, cocaine, cyclosporine, mannitol (excessive chronic doses), methotrexate, and NSAIDs.

Imaging

A computed tomographic scan of the head can detect life-threatening cerebral edema secondary to toxicant-induced hepatic failure, ethylene glycol, and methanol. It also detects intracranial bleeding caused by anticoagulant drugs and rodenticides, scorpion venom, and sympathomimetics (e.g., amphetamines, cocaine, phenylpropanolamine). An abdominal radiograph can reveal radiopaque ferrous sulfate tablets or metals such as arsenic, lead, mercury, and thallium.

Diagnostic Syndromes

Given the myriad combinations of signs, symptoms, and laboratory findings, making the correct diagnosis in a noncommunicative patient can be daunting. A thorough history from bystanders, friends, and prehospital medical personnel may yield crucial information. Additionally, the diagnostic possibilities can be narrowed by noting a finding to limit that list. For example, consider a patient with sudden loss of consciousness, anion gap metabolic acidosis, and bradycardia without hypoxemia. Among the possible causes of anion gap metabolic acidosis (see earlier) and sudden loss of consciousness

TABLE 110-3 PATHOPHYSIOLOGY, CLINICAL EFFECTS, AND MANAGEMENT OF SPECIFIC DRUGS AND TOXICANTS

DRUG OR TOXICANT	PATHOPHYSIOLOGY	CLINICAL EFFECTS	LABORATORY	SPECIFIC THERAPY
Acetaminophen	NAPQI (toxic metabolite) binds hepatic and renal tubular cells; acetaminophen itself induces transient decrease in functional factor VII	Initial: nausea, vomiting, coma, lactic acidosis in severe cases Days 1-3: elevated INR, aminotransferase, and bilirubin levels; RUQ tenderness; increased creatinine level in severe cases Days 4-14: gradual recovery or continued increase in INR and creatinine, lactic acidosis, coma, cerebral edema, death	Potentially toxic level ≥ 150 μg/mL 4 hr after ingestion* INR may be transiently elevated in first 24 hr because of decrease in functional factor VII; further increases indicate hepatic necrosis; elevated aminotransferase and bilirubin levels not predictive of hepatic failure Creatinine elevated in severe cases	NAC (see dosing guidelines in Table 110-6); NAC can increase INR but not aPTT†
Amphetamines	Increased release of presynaptic norepinephrine and dopamine Increased serotonin release (especially MDMA, PMA, DOB, other synthetic amphetamines)	Mild: euphoria, decreased appetite, repetitive behavior Moderate: vomiting, agitation, hypertension, tachycardia, mydriasis, bruxism, diaphoresis Severe: hypertension or hypotension, arrhythmias, hyperthermia, seizures, coma, hepatotoxicity, rhabdomyolysis, DIC, hyponatremia (SIADH), renal failure, cerebral infarction or hemorrhage	Not helpful; many false-positives and false-negatives on screening tests (see Table 110-4)	IV crystalloids External cooling Benzodiazepines or barbiturates to control agitation or seizures Benzodiazepines or nitroprusside for hypertension See SSRIs/SRIs for features and treatment of serotonin syndrome
β-Adrenergic receptor antagonists	Blocks catecholamines from β-adrenergic receptors α- and β-adrenergic receptor antagonism: carvedilol, labetalol Delayed rectifier potassium-channel blockade: sotalol	Bradyarrhythmias, decreased myocardial contractility, hypotension, respiratory depression, decreased consciousness with seizures or coma (lipophilic agents, e.g., propranolol), prolonged QT interval (sotalol)	ECG No specific tests	IV glucagon, 3.5-5 mg over 2-min period; if no increase in BP or HR, can repeat up to 10 mg; if effective, immediately start continuous infusion at 2-10 mg/hr; if still unstable, options include (1) regular insulin, 1 U/kg by IV bolus, followed by 1 U/kg/hr, plus dextrose to maintain euglycemia; (2) norepinephrine or dobutamine infusion titrated to desirable BP and HR; (3) IV milrinone, 50 μg/kg over 10-min period, then 0.375-0.75 μg/kg/min based on hemodynamic status‡ Electrical pacing and IABP in refractory cases
L-type calcium-channel antagonists	Blocks L-type voltage-sensitive calcium channels, thereby decreasing calcium entry into myocardial and vascular smooth muscle cells Decreases pancreatic insulin release and increases insulin resistance	Bradyarrhythmias (verapamil, diltiazem), hypotension, hyperglycemia	ECG No specific tests	IV 10% calcium chloride, 10-20 mg/kg (0.1-0.2 mL/kg); can repeat once; if BP improves, continuous infusion at 0.2-0.5 mL/kg/hr (20-50 mg/kg/hr) Ionized Ca^{2+} levels should not exceed 2× normal (severe cases will be refractory to calcium therapy) Glucagon, high-dose insulin and dextrose, catecholamines, and milrinone (as for β-adrenergic antagonists)
Cardiac glycosides, including digoxin, bufadienolides (toxic toad venom), or cardenolides (e.g., oleander, lily of the valley, dogbane)	Inhibits Na^+,K^+-ATPase Decreased CNS sympathetic output Decreased baroreceptor sensitivity Increased vagal acetylcholine discharge	Bradyarrhythmias, including second- and third-degree AV block and asystole Ventricular ectopy, tachycardia, fibrillation Junctional tachycardia, paroxysmal atrial tachycardia with block Weakness, visual disturbances, nausea, vomiting	Serum digoxin level Serum potassium (hyperkalemia occurs in acute poisoning; hypokalemia may be present in chronic poisoning), magnesium, and creatinine levels	Correct hypokalemia and hypomagnesemia; do not give calcium Digoxin-specific antibody fragments (Fab) indicated if patient has hemodynamically significant arrhythmias, serum potassium ≥5 mg/L, Mobitz II or third-degree AV block, ingestion of bufadienolide- or cardenolide-containing agents, or renal insufficiency Empirical dose Chronic: 2-5 vials Acute: 10-20 vials Calculated dose Chronic: number of vials = 2 × serum digoxin level (ng/mL) × 5.6 × weight (kg)/1000 Acute: number of vials = 2 × oral digoxin dose (mg) × 0.8
Cyclic antidepressants	Myocardial sodium- and potassium-channel blockade Blockade of α-adrenergic and cholinergic muscarinic receptors Inhibition of norepinephrine re-uptake	Decreased level of consciousness (can develop rapidly), myoclonus, seizures, coma Anticholinergic toxidrome (see Table 110-1) Sinus tachycardia, ventricular conduction delays, ventricular arrhythmias, asystole Hypotension	Serum levels not helpful in management	Intermittent IV boluses of $NaHCO_3$ (1 mEq/kg) to maintain arterial pH at 7.5 because acidemia can worsen cardiovascular complications Intubation and neuroparalytic drugs may be useful to ameliorate acidemia from muscular hyperactivity while seizures are being treated Contraindicated drugs: types IA and IC antiarrhythmic agents, physostigmine, flumazenil

TABLE 110-3 PATHOPHYSIOLOGY, CLINICAL EFFECTS, AND MANAGEMENT OF SPECIFIC DRUGS AND TOXICANTS—cont'd

DRUG OR TOXICANT	PATHOPHYSIOLOGY	CLINICAL EFFECTS	LABORATORY	SPECIFIC THERAPY
Ethylene glycol, methanol (e.g., antifreeze, window cleaners, camping stove fuels)	Ethylene glycol: toxic metabolites produce cytotoxicity in CNS, kidneys, lungs, heart, liver, muscles; metabolic acidosis is due to glycolate accumulation; oxalate complexes with calcium, so hypocalcemia can develop Methanol: metabolized to formic acid, which is responsible for metabolic acidosis and inhibition of cytochrome aa_3; target organs include retina, optic nerve, CNS	Ethylene glycol: CNS depression, cerebral edema, seizures, anion gap metabolic acidosis, renal failure with acute tubular necrosis, pulmonary edema, myositis Methanol: nausea, vomiting; cerebral edema, hemorrhage, infarcts; necrosis of thalamus and putamen; anion gap metabolic acidosis; visual disturbances, papilledema, hyperemic optic disc, nonreactive pupils	Serum ethylene glycol and methanol levels; levels may be low or undetectable if significant metabolism has occurred Ethylene glycol: serum calcium, creatinine, BUN levels; examine urine for calcium oxalate crystals; false hyperlactatemia occurs with certain analyzers using L-lactate oxidase, which cross-reacts with glycolic and glyoxylic acids	For both: fomepizole (which inhibits alcohol dehydrogenase and blocks formation of toxic metabolites), 15 mg/kg IV loading dose, then 10 mg/kg IV for 4 doses during the next 48 hr, then 15 mg/kg for subsequent doses; interval dosing is q12h (q4h during hemodialysis, with dosing interval adjustments at start and finish); continue until ethylene glycol or methanol is no longer detectable Use of ethanol is no longer recommended Hemodialysis: initiate if level is ≥50 mg/dL or metabolic acidosis with end-organ toxicity; continue until acidosis resolves and serum level of ethylene glycol or methanol is undetectable Monitor for cerebral edema with possible herniation Ethylene glycol: IV calcium for symptomatic hypocalcemia Methanol: folinic acid, 50 mg IV q4h until methanol not detectable and acidosis cleared
γ-Hydroxybutyrate (GHB) and its precursors (γ-butyrolactone and 1,4-butanediol [1,4-BD])	Agonist effect on CNS GHB receptors; indirect action with opioid receptors (may increase proenkephalins); metabolized to GABA, interacts with $GABA_B$ receptors; decreases dopamine release	CNS: rapid loss of consciousness, with recovery typical within 2-4 hr; myoclonus (possible seizures) Respiratory depression; bradycardia; nausea, vomiting	No specific tests	Supportive care, including respiratory support as needed Withdrawal resembles sedative-hypnotic withdrawal and can be treated with benzodiazepines or pentobarbital
Lithium	Decreases brain inositol; alters CNS serotonin, dopamine, and norepinephrine; inhibits adenylate cyclases, including those that mediate vasopressin-induced renal concentration and thyroid function	Chronic toxicity usually more severe than acute toxicity: tremor, hyperreflexia, drowsiness, incoordination, clonus, confusion, ataxia; in severe cases, seizures, coma, death; recovery may take weeks, and CNS deficits may persist Sinus node dysfunction, QT prolongation, T wave abnormalities, U waves Nephrogenic diabetes insipidus, hypothyroidism, hyperthyroidism, hypercalcemia, pseudotumor cerebri Acute toxicity: nausea, vomiting, diarrhea, and milder neurologic findings	Peak serum levels: Normal dose 2-3 hr; up to 5 hr for sustained-release lithium Acute overdose Peak may be delayed ≥4-12 hr	Replenish intravascular volume, maintain urinary output at 1-2 mL/kg/hr Consider GI decontamination with oral polyethylene glycol electrolyte solution within 1-2 hr after acute overdose of sustained-release drug Hemodialysis[§] in patients with altered mental status, ataxia, seizures, or coma or in patients with mild symptoms in the setting of acute overdose or renal insufficiency Ineffective or contraindicated therapies include oral activated charcoal, diuretics, and aminophylline
Opioids (e.g., heroin, morphine, oxycodone, fentanyl)	Agonist effect at CNS μ, κ, and δ opioid receptors; result is cell hyperpolarization and decreased neurotransmitter release	CNS depression, respiratory depression, miosis (see Table 110-1) Dextromethorphan increases CNS serotonin and inhibits NMDA receptors, which causes hallucinations Propoxyphene and its metabolite norpropoxyphene block sodium channels and can cause seizures and wide-complex arrhythmias similar to cyclic antidepressants; $NaHCO_3$ treats arrhythmias Seizure risk with tramadol, meperidine, propoxyphene Rapid, powerful heroin-like effect when sustained-release oxycodone is crushed before ingestion, snorting, or smoking QTc prolongation and torsades de pointes with methadone	Rapid urine drug screens detect morphine and codeine but may not detect semisynthetic and synthetic opioids; some interferents/irrelevants (see Table 110-4)	IV naloxone, 0.4-2 mg; can repeat up to 10 mg if no response Continuous infusion for recurrent symptoms or sustained-release opioid ingestion; give 50% of dose that produces desired effect 15 min after initial effect is obtained, then infuse two thirds of this dose every hr; infusion rate can be increased or decreased to maintain normal respiration and avoid withdrawal symptoms Contraindicated therapies: nalmefene and naltrexone should not be used for acute opioid reversal

TABLE 110-3 PATHOPHYSIOLOGY, CLINICAL EFFECTS, AND MANAGEMENT OF SPECIFIC DRUGS AND TOXICANTS—cont'd

DRUG OR TOXICANT	PATHOPHYSIOLOGY	CLINICAL EFFECTS	LABORATORY	SPECIFIC THERAPY
Organophosphorus compounds and carbamates (e.g., diazinon, mevinphos, fenthion, aldicarb)	Inhibits acetylcholinesterase, resulting in excessive acetylcholine stimulation of nicotinic and muscarinic receptors in autonomic and somatic motor nervous systems and CNS	Nicotinic-mediated effects: tachycardia, mydriasis, hypertension, delirium, coma, seizures, muscle weakness, fasciculations Muscarinic-mediated effects: salivation, lacrimation, urination, vomiting, defecation, miosis, bronchorrhea, bronchospasm, bradycardia	Serum (butyrylcholinesterase) or RBC (acetylcholinesterase) activity <50% of normal (see Table 110-6) Clinical recovery occurs before serum cholinesterase levels normalize	Atropine, 1-2 mg by initial IV bolus; double the dose every 5 min (2 mg, 4 mg, 8 mg, 16 mg, etc) until drying of bronchial secretions, adequate oxygenation, pulse >80 bpm, systolic blood pressure >80 mm Hg achieved; continuous infusion at 10- 20% of total stabilizing dose per hr; stop infusion if patient develops any signs or symptoms of anticholinergic toxidrome (see Table 110-1); restart infusion at lower rate when signs or symptoms abate Pralidoxime[‖] chloride 30 mg/kg (maximum 2 g) IV bolus over 30 min, then 8-10 mg/kg/hr (maximum 650 mg/hr) continuous infusion; administer as soon as possible after poisoning; continue 12-24 hr after atropine no longer required and symptoms resolve[2]
Salicylates	Inhibits cyclooxygenase; decreases formation of prostaglandins and thromboxane A_2; stimulates CNS medullary respiratory receptor and chemoreceptor trigger zone; impairs platelet function; disrupts carbohydrate metabolism; uncouples oxidative phosphorylation; increases vascular permeability	Acute toxicity Mild: nausea, vomiting, diaphoresis, tinnitus, decreased hearing, hyperpnea, tachypnea Moderate–severe: confusion, delirium, coma, seizures, hyperthermia, ALI; death can occur within hours of overdose Chronic toxicity: same as acute, but may not have diaphoresis or vomiting Consider diagnosis in patients with new-onset confusion, anion gap metabolic acidosis, or ALI	Serum salicylate level: toxic ≥30 mg/dL; level ≥100 mg/dL indicates life-threatening toxicity with possible sudden, rapid clinical deterioration; in chronic toxicity, levels may be minimally elevated (>30 mg/dL), and clinical evaluation is more reliable for gauging degree of toxicity Arterial blood gases: respiratory alkalosis with metabolic acidosis Anion gap metabolic acidosis Prolonged PT and PTT, ketonuria, ketonemia	Multidose activated charcoal q2-3h in acute overdose with progressive symptoms or rising salicylate level
SSRIs/SRIs	Inhibits re-uptake of serotonin SRIs have additional effects (e.g., duloxetine inhibits norepinephrine re-uptake, nefazodone inhibits serotonergic 5-HT2 receptors, trazodone inhibits peripheral α-adrenergic receptors, venlafaxine inhibits norepinephrine and dopamine re-uptake)	Vomiting, blurred vision, CNS depression, tachycardia Seizures and coma rare Torsades de pointes reported with citalopram Serotonin syndrome: clonus, agitation, tremor, diaphoresis, hyperreflexia; hyperthermia and hypertonicity in severe cases	No specific tests If serotonin syndrome suspected: electrolytes, BUN, glucose, liver enzymes, coagulation panel, blood gases, chest radiograph	Respiratory support as needed Benzodiazepines for agitation or seizures Serotonin syndrome: consider cyproheptadine, 12 mg PO initial dose, then 2 mg PO q2h (to a maximum of 32 mg/day) until symptoms resolve Critical care therapies for hyperthermia, rhabdomyolysis, DIC, ARDS, renal and hepatic dysfunction, torsades de pointes

*A nomogram to evaluate the potential toxicity of levels drawn more than 4 hours after ingestion is provided in Rumack BH, Matthew H. Acetaminophen poisoning and toxicity. *Pediatrics.* 1975;55:871-876. The nomogram is valid only for levels drawn after a single acute ingestion.

†NAC can be discontinued in patients with uncomplicated disease after a loading dose plus six maintenance doses if hepatic aminotransferase levels are normal and acetaminophen is not detected; otherwise, the full regimen should be administered.

‡Adjust infusion for reduced renal function.

§Continue hemodialysis until the serum lithium level is less than 1 mEq/L. Recheck the level 8 hours after dialysis, and restart hemodialysis if the level is higher than 1 mEq/L. Repeat this cycle until the serum lithium level remains lower than 1 mEq/L.

‖A double-blind, randomized, placebo-controlled trial of pralidoxime in acute organophosphorus poisoning found no significant difference in mortality rates or need for intubation.[2]

ALI = acute lung injury; aPTT = activated partial thromboplastin time; ARDS = acute respiratory distress syndrome; AV = atrioventricular; BP = blood pressure; bpm = beats per minute; BUN = blood urea nitrogen; CNS = central nervous system; DIC = disseminated intravascular coagulation; DOB = 4-bromo-2,5-dimethoxyamphetamine; ECG = electrocardiogram; GABA = γ-aminobutyric acid; GI = gastrointestinal; HR = heart rate; IABP = intra-aortic balloon counterpulsation; INR = international normalized ratio; IV = intravenous; MDMA = 3,4-methylenedioxymethamphetamine; Na^+,K^+-ATPase = sodium, potassium adenosine triphosphatase; NAC = *N*-acetylcysteine; NAPQI = *N*-acetyl-p-benzoquinone imine; NMDA = *N*-methyl-D-aspartate; PMA = paramethoxyamphetamine; PT = prothrombin time; PTT = partial thromboplastin time; RBC = red blood cell; RUQ = right upper quadrant (abdomen); SIADH = syndrome of inappropriate antidiuretic secretion; SRI = serotonin re-uptake inhibitor; SSRI = selective serotonin re-uptake inhibitor.

are hydrogen sulfide, cyanide, and severe poisoning with sodium azide; however, sinus bradycardia in the absence of acute ischemic injury is typical only of cyanide poisoning.

TREATMENT Rx

Initial Stabilization

Intubation and Respiratory Support

Appropriate airway management should be instituted to correct hypoxemia and respiratory acidosis and to protect against pulmonary aspiration (Fig. 110-2); intubation should be considered if the patient has depressed consciousness and a decreased gag reflex. Rapid-sequence intubation facilitates airway management. Anatomic difficulties should be anticipated in patients with caustic ingestions (hypopharyngeal burns that may perforate); angioedema caused by angiotensin-converting enzyme inhibitor therapy or envenomation by some rattlesnakes, such as the canebrake (*Crotalus horridus atricaudatus*) and eastern diamondback (*Crotalus adamanteus*) (Chapter 113); and swelling secondary to direct tissue injury (e.g., huffing Freon, snakebite on the tongue) or secondary to anaphylactoid and anaphylactic reactions. Endotracheal intubation via flexible fiberoptic nasopharyngoscopy may be indicated in these cases. Hypoxemia can occur with toxicants that produce CNS depression, such as antidepressants, barbiturates, sedative-hypnotics, and central α_2-adrenergic receptor agonists (clonidine), or agents causing peripheral neuromuscular impairment, such as nicotine, organophosphorus

TABLE 110-4 QUALITATIVE URINE DRUG SCREENS: CAUSES OF ERRONEOUS RESULTS*

DRUG/TOXICANT	INTERFERENTS/IRRELEVANTS[†]	COMMENTS
Amphetamines	Amantadine, bupropion, chlorpromazine, ephedrine, pseudoephedrine, desoxyephedrine, *Ephedra* sp, mexiletine, phenylephrine, phenylpropanolamine, selegiline, trazodone	Vicks nasal inhaler (desoxyephedrine) and selegiline also cause positive GC-MS findings; chiral confirmation is required; newer immunoassays have eliminated false-positive results from desoxyephedrine Interferents in older assays include labetalol and ranitidine
Benzodiazepines	Oxaprozin, sertraline	Poor detection of parent drugs with absent or low concentration of oxazepam metabolite (e.g., alprazolam, lorazepam, triazolam)
Cocaine	Coca leaf teas	Urine is most reliable for detecting true positives
Opiates, opioids	Dextromethorphan, poppy seeds, quinine, quinolones, rifampin	Does not detect semisynthetic or designer opioids (e.g., fentanyls, meperidine, methadone, propoxyphene)
Phencyclidine	Dextromethorphan, diphenhydramine, doxylamine, ibuprofen, ketamine, meperidine, mesoridazine, thioridazine, tramadol, venlafaxine	
Tetrahydrocannabinol	Dronabinol, efavirenz, proton pump inhibitors	Positive result is seldom clinically relevant; synthetic cannabinomimetics are not detected
Tricyclic antidepressants	Carbamazepine, cyclobenzaprine, cyproheptadine, diphenhydramine, phenothiazines, quetiapine	

*Advances in drug screening and variability in immunoassay results should be considered by the clinician when interpreting qualitative drug screening results. Consultation with the testing laboratory is advised. Positive screening results are considered presumptive and should be verified by GC-MS.
[†]Irrelevants are agents causing true-positive but clinically irrelevant results on laboratory screening tests; they vary, depending on the screening method.
GC-MS = gas chromatography–mass spectrometry.

TABLE 110-5 CLINICALLY IMPORTANT QUANTITATIVE DRUG LEVELS

	Levels	
DRUG OR TOXICANT	**THERAPEUTIC**	**TOXIC**
SOURCE: BLOOD OR SERUM		
Acetaminophen*	10-30 μg/mL	≥150 g/mL 4 hr after ingestion[†]
Carbamazepine	4-12 μg/mL	>15 g/mL
Carboxyhemoglobin	Nonsmoker: 0.5-1.5% Smoker: 4-9%	>20%[‡]
Cholinesterase[§]		
Serum (butyrylcholinesterase)	3100-6500 U/L	<50% of normal value
Red blood cell (acetylcholinesterase)	26.7-49.2 U/g of hemoglobin	<50% of normal value
Digoxin (≥12 hr after dose for long-term therapy)	0.8-2.0 ng/mL[‖]	>2.0 ng/mL
Ethanol	None measured	>80-100 mg/dL
Ethylene glycol	None measured	>25 mg/dL
Iron	50-175 μg/dL	>350 g/dL
Lead	<10 μg/dL	>25 g/dL
Lithium	0.6-1.2 mEq/L	>1.2 mEq/L[¶]
Methanol	None measured	>20 mg/dL
Methemoglobin	1-2%	>15%
Phenobarbital	15-40 μg/mL	>40 g/mL
Phenytoin	10-20 μg/mL	>20 g/mL
Salicylates	≤30 mg/dL	>30 mg/dL
Theophylline	8-20 μg/mL	>20 g/mL
Valproic acid	50-100 μg/mL	>100 g/mL
SOURCE: URINE		
Arsenic	None measured	>100 g/24-hr urine[¶]
Mercury	None measured	>20 g/L[¶]
Thallium	None measured	>200 g/L[¶]

*False-positive levels of 16-28 μg/mL have been reported in patients with bilirubin levels greater than 17 mg/dL.
[†]Levels drawn more than 4 hours after ingestion should be plotted on the nomogram provided by Rumack and Matthew (Rumack BH, Matthew H. Acetaminophen poisoning and toxicity. *Pediatrics.* 1975;55:871-876) to assess the potential for toxicity.
[‡]Lower levels may be toxic in pregnant patients and in those with prolonged exposure to carbon monoxide.
[§]Consult a reference laboratory for normal values; results are assay dependent.
[‖]Some patients may require levels above the therapeutic range to control symptoms.
[¶]Lower values may indicate toxicity if appropriate clinical findings are present.

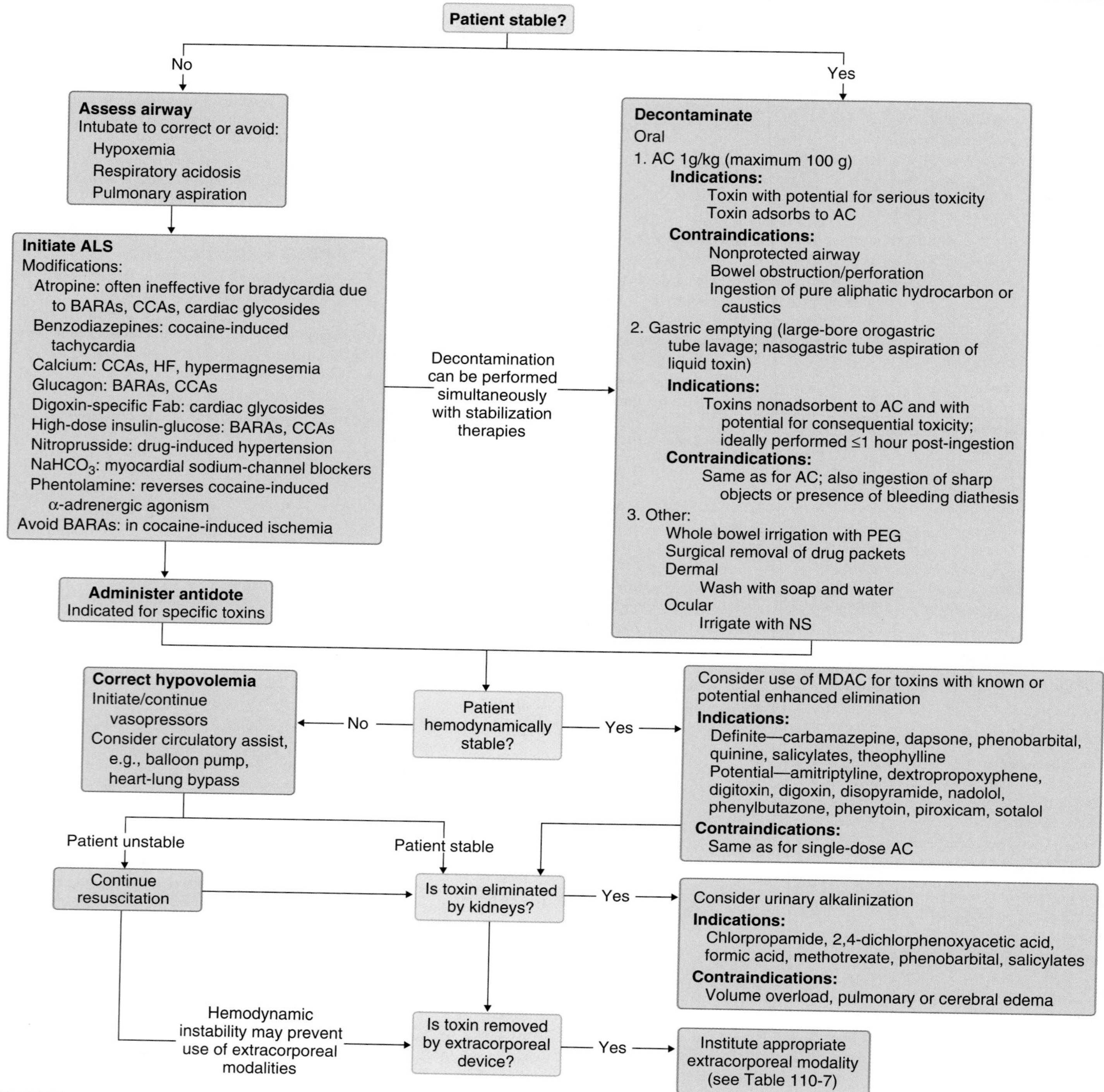

FIGURE 110-2. Algorithm for the management of acute poisoning. AC = activated charcoal; ALS = advanced life support; BARAs = β-adrenergic receptor antagonists; CCAs = L-type calcium-channel antagonists; HF = hydrofluoric acid; MDAC = multidose activated charcoal; NS = 0.9% saline solution; PEG = nonabsorbable polyethylene glycol solution.

compounds, strychnine, tetrodotoxin (puffer fish, blue-ringed octopus), botulinum, or envenomation from elapids (coral snake), Mojave rattlesnakes, or certain coelenterates (box jellyfish, Portuguese man-of-war) (Chapters 113 and 114).

Respiratory acidosis can rapidly worsen the toxicities of cyclic antidepressants and salicylates; sedation of these patients should be accompanied by immediate airway support. Intoxicated patients may have an increased risk for pulmonary aspiration because of concomitant CNS depression, attenuated airway reflexes, full stomachs, and delayed gastric emptying.

Succinylcholine can cause prolonged paralysis in patients with organophosphorus poisoning and can exacerbate hyperkalemia from cardiac glycosides, hydrofluoric acid, or rhabdomyolysis (Chapter 115). Rhabdomyolysis has been reported with adrenergic agents, doxylamine, phencyclidine, heroin, *Tricholoma equestre* mushrooms, and envenomation by crotaline snakes, scorpions, or widow spiders (*Lactrodectus* sp); short-acting nondepolarizing agents, such as vecuronium and rocuronium, are preferable in these cases.

Advanced Life Support

Standard emergency cardiovascular care algorithms (Chapter 63) must be modified for effects caused by specific poisons. Atropine often does not reverse bradycardia secondary to β-adrenergic receptor antagonists, L-type calcium-channel antagonists, or cardiac glycosides. In these cases, more specific therapy with intravenous calcium (calcium-channel antagonists), high doses of glucagon (β-adrenergic receptor antagonists, calcium-channel antagonists), or digoxin-specific Fab antibody (cardiac glycosides) is indicated. High-dose insulin-glucose therapy can successfully reverse myocardial depression and conduction abnormalities in humans poisoned with β-adrenergic receptor antagonists and calcium-channel antagonists. Intravenous sodium bicarbonate may reverse cardiac conduction delays caused by antiarrhythmic drugs with sodium-channel blockade recovery rates of greater than 1 second (Vaughn-Williams classification IA and IC), cocaine, cyclic antidepressants, diphenhydramine, propoxyphene, and quinine. β-Adrenergic receptor antagonists are contraindicated in patients with cocaine-induced myocardial syndromes, but phentolamine can reverse the agonistic effects of cocaine on α-adrenergic receptors. Benzodiazepines can reverse significant sinus tachycardia from sympathomimetic agents. Calcium may also be life-saving in systemic hydrofluoric acid poisoning and severe hypermagnesemia, and it is indicated for symptomatic hypocalcemia caused by ethylene glycol toxicity. Drug-induced hypertension may be transitory; nitroprusside should be used if treatment is clinically indicated. In patients with toxicant-induced circulatory collapse refractory to maximal therapy, including vasopressors, circulatory assist devices may support the patient until sufficient toxicant is eliminated (Chapter 107).

Decontamination

Activated Charcoal

Single-dose activated charcoal without prior gastric emptying has been the preferred method of treatment for the ingestion of substances that have the potential to cause moderate to life-threatening toxicity and are known to adsorb to activated charcoal. The absence of clinical signs and symptoms does not preclude administering activated charcoal, because drug absorption and toxicity can be delayed. Activated charcoal can also be administered when the ingested toxicant cannot be identified but significant toxicity is a concern. Activated charcoal consists of pyrolysis products that have been specially cleaned to produce an internal pore structure to which substances can reversibly adsorb, thus preventing their absorption by the gastrointestinal tract. Activated charcoal can be administered with antiemetic drugs or given through a nasogastric tube, when necessary. The oral dose is approximately 1 g/kg body weight, with a maximum single dose of 100 g. Efficacy in preventing toxicant absorption declines with time, so activated charcoal should be given as soon as possible after ingestion. A large randomized trial in Sri Lankan hospitals showed no benefit of activated charcoal in reducing mortality,[1] but 87% of the study patients had ingested a pesticide or yellow oleander (which contains a cardiac glycoside); the applicability of this study's findings to populations in which other toxicants are more commonly ingested is unknown. Activated charcoal should not be used in patients with CNS depression until the airway is secure to minimize aspiration; the patient's head should also be elevated unless contraindicated. Activated charcoal is contraindicated in patients with a perforated bowel, functional or mechanical bowel obstruction, ingestion of a pure aliphatic hydrocarbon such as gasoline or kerosene (no benefit and increased risk for aspiration), and ingestion of caustic acid and alkali (no benefit and obscures endoscopy). Certain agents, such as lithium, iron, metals, and ethanol, do not adsorb significantly to activated charcoal, but its use is not precluded if the patient has ingested other toxicants that do adsorb to activated charcoal. Pulmonary aspiration and bowel obstruction from inspissated activated charcoal are the most common complications; both occur more frequently when multidose activated charcoal is administered, but they can be avoided by withholding treatment in patients who have suboptimal bowel function or decreased fecal elimination.

Gastric Emptying

Two methods of gastric emptying, syrup of ipecac and orogastric lavage via a large-bore tube, are no longer routinely used. Both are relatively ineffective therapies that potentially increase the risk for aspiration. No well-designed study has documented any benefit of gastric emptying, either by lavage or by syrup of ipecac, when compared with the use of activated charcoal alone. Gastric emptying via lavage or, rarely, by syrup of ipecac may be of benefit and should be performed in patients who have ingested toxicants that do not adsorb to activated charcoal and are known to produce significant morbidity, or for which aggressive decontamination may offer the best chance for survival (e.g., colchicine, sodium azide, sodium fluoroacetate). Removal of a liquid toxicant, such as ethylene glycol, may be accomplished by aspiration of gastric contents via a nasogastric tube. Contraindications to gastric emptying include those for activated charcoal, a bleeding diathesis, and the ingestion of sharp objects. Placement of an endotracheal tube before gastric lavage may be necessary to protect the airway in patients who have a decreased level of consciousness and impaired gag reflex; major complications of gastric emptying include pulmonary aspiration, esophageal tears and perforations, and laryngospasm (with lavage).

Whole Bowel Irrigation

Whole bowel irrigation with a nonabsorbable polyethylene glycol solution has been recommended for iron and sustained-release medications, for agents not adsorbed to activated charcoal, and for body packers (smugglers who swallow packets of illicit drugs). The most common complication is vomiting, and whole bowel irrigation is contraindicated in patients with bowel perforation, obstruction, hemorrhage, or hemodynamic or respiratory instability. The initial recommended dose is 500 mL/hour given orally or via nasogastric tube, with titration to 2000 mL/hour as tolerated; treatment continues until the rectal effluent clears. Rarely, surgery may be necessary to remove packets in smugglers who have symptoms of drug toxicity; endoscopic removal of these packets should never be attempted because of the risk of packet rupture.

Antidotes

Few toxicants have specific therapies (Table 110-6). Although antidotes may be essential in treating patients exposed to certain toxicants, their use does not preclude the need for ongoing supportive care and, in some cases, extracorporeal elimination.

Enhanced Elimination

Three methods are used to accelerate the elimination of toxicants or drugs from the body: (1) multiple doses of oral activated charcoal, (2) urinary alkalinization, and (3) extracorporeal removal. A fourth method using the oral ion exchange resins sodium polystyrene sulfonate and cholestyramine has experimentally enhanced the elimination of lithium, digoxin, digitoxin, and organochlorines but has limited clinical usefulness.

Multiple Doses of Oral Activated Charcoal

The rationale for administering multiple doses of oral activated charcoal includes the adsorption of any toxic agent remaining in the gastrointestinal tract (e.g., sustained-release drugs, drugs that retard their absorption); interference with the enterohepatic and enteroenteric recirculation of toxicants; and enhancement of the elimination of drugs with a long half-life, a volume of distribution less than 1 L/kg body weight, and low protein binding. The existing evidence shows enhanced elimination of carbamazepine, dapsone, phenobarbital, quinine, salicylates, and theophylline, but multiple doses of activated charcoal may also be effective for amitriptyline,

Text continues on p. 684

TABLE 110-6 ANTIDOTES AND INDICATIONS FOR USE

ANTIDOTE	INDICATION FOR USE	DOSE*	TREATMENT END POINT	COMMENTS
Antivenom (Fab)[†]	Crotalines	4-6 vials; repeat for persistent or worsening clinical condition; repeat doses of 2 vials at 6, 12, and 18 hr after initial antivenom dose(s) are recommended	Halt in progression of circumferential and proximal swelling Resolving systemic effects	Better safety profile than equine-derived antivenom Repetitive dosing indicated for recurrent soft tissue swelling
Antivenom, *Latrodectus* (equine)[†]	Black widow spider (*Latrodectus* sp)	1 vial diluted in 100 mL NS, infused over 1 hr; can repeat	Resolution of symptoms, vital signs normal	Dilution and slow infusion rate are **critical** to avoid anaphylactoid reaction Indications include severe pain unresponsive to opioids and severe hypertension Serum sickness can occur IV calcium is ineffective
Atropine	Carbamates Nerve agents Organophosphorus compounds	2 mg IV; double the dose every 5 min to achieve atropinization and hemodynamic stability; then start continuous infusion of 10-20% of total stabilizing dose per hr	Cessation of excessive oral and pulmonary secretions, >80 bpm, systolic blood pressure >80 mm Hg	Doubling of the dose every 5 min (e.g., 2 mg, 4 mg, 8 mg, 16 mg) estimated to achieve atropinization within 30 min Stop infusion if patient develops any signs or symptoms of anticholinergic toxidrome (see Table 110-1); restart infusion at lower rate when signs or symptoms abate

TABLE 110-6 ANTIDOTES AND INDICATIONS FOR USE—cont'd

ANTIDOTE	INDICATION FOR USE	DOSE*	TREATMENT END POINT	COMMENTS
Calcium[†]	Calcium-channel antagonists	Calcium chloride 10%, 20-50 mg (0.2-0.5 mL)/kg/hr	Reversal of hypotension; may not reverse bradycardia	*All indications:* Monitor ionized calcium levels IV extravasation causes tissue necrosis, especially with calcium chloride Can administer at faster than stated rates for immediate life-threatening conditions Taper infusions and monitor for relapse of toxicity when discontinuing therapy Calcium chloride contains three times more elemental calcium than calcium gluconate does Calcium-channel antagonists: may be ineffective in severe toxicity
	Hydrofluoric acid	Systemic toxicity: calcium gluconate 10%, 1-3 g (10-30 mL) per dose IV over 10-min period; repeat as needed every 5-10 min	Reversal of life-threatening manifestations of hypocalcemia and hyperkalemia	Can dilute and give intra-arterially or IV with a Bier block for extremity exposures and burns
	Hyperkalemia (except cardiac glycosides)	Calcium gluconate 10%, 1 g (10 mL) per dose IV over 10-min period; repeat as needed every 5-10 min	Reversal of myocardial depression and conduction delays	May precipitate ventricular arrhythmias
	Hypermagnesemia	Calcium gluconate 10%, 1-2 g (10-20 mL) per dose IV over 10-min period; repeat as needed every 5-10 min	Reversal of respiratory depression, hypotension, and cardiac conduction blocks	Simultaneous therapies to increase magnesium elimination should be instituted
	Hypocalcemia (e.g., ethylene glycol)	Calcium gluconate 10%, 0.5-1.0 g (5-10 mL) per dose over 10-min period; repeat as needed every 10 min	Reversal of tetany	Correct symptomatic hypocalcemia; avoid excessive administration that may increase production of calcium oxalate crystals in ethylene glycol poisoning
L-Carnitine	Valproate-induced hyperammonemia or hepatotoxicity	100 mg/kg (maximum 6 g) IV over 30 min, then 15 mg/kg IV over 30-min period q4h (max 6 g/day)	Treat until clinical improvement occurs	Levocarnitine is active form Adjust dose for end-stage renal disease
Cyanide antidote kit Amyl nitrite Sodium nitrite Sodium thiosulfate	Cyanide	Amyl nitrite: 0.3-mL pearls, crush and inhale over 30-sec period Sodium nitrite 3%: 10 mL IV over 10-min period Sodium thiosulfate 25%: 50 mL (12.5 g) IV over 10-min period	Resolution of lactic acidosis and moderate to severe clinical signs and symptoms: seizures, coma, dyspnea, apnea, hypotension, bradycardia	Coordinate amyl nitrite with continued oxygenation and give only until sodium nitrite infusion is begun; nitrites may produce hypotension and excess methemoglobinemia Sodium nitrite dose must be adjusted if patient has hemoglobin <12 g/dL Sodium thiosulfate dosing can be repeated
Deferoxamine	Iron	15 mL/kg/hr IV (max 8 g/day) Mild to moderate: administer for 6-12 hr Severe toxicity: administer 24 hr	Resolution of clinical signs and symptoms Do not use urine color, which is an unreliable marker for iron clearance	Indications: symptomatic patients with lethargy, severe abdominal pain, hypovolemia, acidosis, shock; any symptomatic patient with peak serum iron level >350 g/dL Prolonged therapy can cause pulmonary toxicity
Digoxin-specific antibody fragments (Fab)	Digoxin Digitalis Other cardiac glycosides (e.g., bufodienalides [Bufo toads], oleander)	Unknown digoxin dose or serum level or for plant or toad source: acute toxicity—10-20 vials; chronic toxicity—3-6 vials Digoxin dose known: number of vials = (mg ingested × 0.8) ÷ 0.5 Digoxin serum level known: number of vials = [serum level (ng/mL) × weight (kg)] ÷ 100	Resolution of hyperkalemia, symptomatic bradydysrhythmias, ventricular arrhythmias, Mobitz II or third-degree heart block	Each vial binds 0.5 mg of digoxin or digitoxin Monitor ECG and potassium levels Digoxin serum levels unreliable after antidote administered unless test is specific for free serum digoxin

TABLE 110-6 ANTIDOTES AND INDICATIONS FOR USE—cont'd

ANTIDOTE	INDICATION FOR USE	DOSE*	TREATMENT END POINT	COMMENTS
Dimercaprol (BAL)	Arsenic Lead Mercury, elemental and inorganic salts	Arsenic: 3-5 mg/kg IM q4h Lead: 75 mg/m^2 (4 mg/kg) IM q4h for 5 days Inorganic mercury: 5 mg/kg IM, then 2.5 mg/kg IM q12h for 10 days or until patient clinically improved	Arsenic: 24-hr urinary arsenic <50 μg/L Lead: encephalopathy resolved, blood lead level <100 μg/dL, and succimer therapy can be started Mercury, elemental and inorganic: 24-hr urinary mercury <20 μg/L	Maximum adult dose is 3 g/day BAL started 4 hr before initiation of concomitant $CaNa_2EDTA$ for lead encephalopathy Dosing not well established for arsenic and elemental or inorganic mercury toxicity; not used for organic mercury poisoning Adverse effects: painful injections, fever, diaphoresis, agitation, headache, salivation, nausea and vomiting, hemolysis in G6PD-deficient patients, chelation of essential metals Check essential metal levels if chelation is prolonged Succimer is replacing BAL for many indications except lead encephalopathy Treatment end points for arsenic and mercury include improving clinical condition
Edetate calcium disodium ($CaNa_2EDTA$)	Lead	1500 mg/m^2/24 hr (max 3 g) by continuous infusion	Treat for 5 days, followed by 2-day hiatus; repeat until encephalopathy resolved, lead level <100 μg/dL, and succimer therapy can be started	Use in patients with lead encephalopathy or lead level >100 g/dL Administer BAL 4 hr before initiating $CaNa_2EDTA$ Hydrate patient and establish good urinary output before starting therapy Avoid thrombophlebitis by diluting in NS or D_5W to a concentration ≤0.5% Substitution of Na_2EDTA can cause fatal hypocalcemia
Flumazenil	Benzodiazepines Venlafaxine	0.1 mg/min IV to a total dose of 1 mg	Reversal of respiratory depression	Limit use to reversal of inadequate respiration in benzodiazepine-toxic patients Increases intracranial pressure and risk for seizures in presence of underlying seizure disorder or ingestion of seizure-producing toxicants Monitor for resedation up to 2 hr after last dose
Folinate (tetrahydrofolic acid [leucovorin])	Methanol Methotrexate	Methanol: 50 mg IV q4h Methotrexate: 100 mg/m^2 IV q3-6h	Methanol: methanol undetectable, metabolic acidosis cleared Methotrexate: serum level $<1 \times 10^{-8}$ mol/L	Essential therapy for both toxicants Methotrexate: large ingestions may require increased dose Glucarpidase administered 2-4 hr before or after folinate
Fomepizole	Ethylene glycol Methanol	Dose 1: 15 mg/kg IV Doses over next 48 hr: 10 mg/kg IV All subsequent doses: 15 mg/kg IV Administer q12h, except when HD performed: HD initiation: ½ next dose if >6 hr since last dose HD ongoing: q4h End of HD (based on time of last dose): <1 hr, no dose; 1-3 hr, ½ next dose; >3 hr, next dose	For both: serum level <20 mg/dL and metabolic acidosis resolved	Start immediately if toxic alcohol suspected, without waiting for confirmatory levels Dose amount is not affected by interval timing of doses
Glucagon	β-Adrenergic receptor antagonists Calcium-channel antagonists	Bolus of 3.5-5 mg IV; can repeat to achieve clinical effect, then infusion of 2-10 mg/hr	Reversal of hypotension and bradycardia; taper infusion	Can precipitate vomiting; be prepared to protect airway Mild hyperglycemia occurs Maximum dosing amounts unknown; bolus doses up to 30 mg reported Duration of effect is 15 min; thus infusion must be started immediately
Hydroxocobalamin	Cyanide	Initial: 5 g IV over 15-min period Second dose: 5 g IV over 15 min-2 hr; maximum total dose is 10 g Follow each hydroxocobalamin dose with sodium thiosulfate 25%: 50 mL (12.5 g) IV over 10-min period	Resolution of lactic acidosis and moderate to severe clinical signs and symptoms: seizures, coma, dyspnea, apnea, hypotension, bradycardia	Can be administered IV push if patient is in cardiac arrest Do not give hydroxocobalamin and sodium thiosulfate through the same IV line Adverse effects: red discoloration of plasma, urine, mucous membranes, skin; transient hypertension Interference with laboratory colorometric assays: Levels increased: bilirubin; creatinine; glucose; hemoglobin; magnesium; co-oximetry total Hb, COHb%, MetHb% Levels decreased: AST, ALT, creatinine, co-oximetry O_2Hb%

TABLE 110-6 ANTIDOTES AND INDICATIONS FOR USE—cont'd

ANTIDOTE	INDICATION FOR USE	DOSE*	TREATMENT END POINT	COMMENTS
Hyperbaric oxygen (HBO)	Carbon monoxide Experimental: carbon tetrachloride, cyanide, hydrogen sulfide	3.0 atm pressure for 60 min (25 min O_2, 5 min air, 25 min O_2, 5 min air), then 2.0 atm for 65 min (30 min O_2, 5 min air, 30 min O_2), then "surface" to 1.0 atm	One treatment Second treatment rarely administered (controversial)	Carbon monoxide: treatment protocols may vary HBO indicated for loss of consciousness; seizures; cerebellar dysfunction; impaired cognition; headache, nausea/vomiting persisting after 4 hr O_2 therapy regardless of carboxyhemoglobin level Experimental indications: treatment protocols not established
Insulin-glucose	Calcium-channel antagonists β-Adrenergic receptor antagonists	Regular insulin, 1 U/kg bolus, followed by 0.5-1 U/kg/hr Titrate 50% dextrose IV to avoid hypoglycemia	Reversal of myocardial depression	Beneficial in case series and reports Initiate if glucagon and vasopressor or inotropic drugs fail to reverse myocardial depression; more effective if used before onset of cardiogenic shock Monitor glucose and potassium; hypoglycemia can occur during and after therapy Hyperglycemia results from toxicant-induced insulin resistance, and initial dextrose requirements may be less than anticipated. Recovery may be heralded by normalization of glucose levels, with increased dextrose required to avoid hypoglycemia
Intralipid	Cardiac toxicity from local anesthetics (e.g., bupivacaine, ropivacaine) Experimental: verapamil, diltiazem, tricyclic antidepressants, bupropion, propranolol	Use 20% formulation Initial bolus: 1.5 mL/kg IV over 1 min, followed immediately by infusion of 0.25 mL/kg/min for 30-60 min Can repeat bolus for asystole	Return of hemodynamic stability	Use based on animal experiments and human case reports; numerous dosing regimens have been used Use if advanced life support measures fail; continue CPR as needed during drug administration
Methylene blue	Methemoglobin-producing agents	1-2 mg/kg body weight (0.1-0.2 mL/kg) of 1% methylene blue is administered over 5-min period; repeat dose for persistent or recurrent symptoms or signs	Resolution of dyspnea and altered mental status	Use if patient is symptomatic (i.e., dyspneic, altered mental status) Maximum dose should not exceed 7 mg/kg (0.7 mL/kg) Contraindicated in G6PD-deficient patients; may cause hemolysis Some toxicants (e.g., dapsone) may require prolonged therapy
N-acetylcysteine (NAC)	Acetaminophen Experimental: carbon tetrachloride, chloroform, pennyroyal oil	Oral: Load—140 mg/kg Maintenance (starting 4 hr after load)—70 mg/kg q4h IV: Load—150 mg/kg over 1-hr period Maintenance infusion—12.5 mg/kg over 4-hr period, then 6.25 mg/kg per hour as continuous infusion	Administer 24 hr of NAC and repeat AST and APAP levels: if AST normal and APAP not detected, stop NAC; if AST normal and APAP detected, continue NAC for 12 hr, then reassess AST and APAP levels; if AST elevated, continue NAC for total of 72 hr of therapy After 72 hr of therapy, if INR <2.0, stop NAC After patient has received 72 hr of therapy, if INR ≥2.0 or severe hepatotoxicity present, continue NAC until INR <2.0	Most effective if initiated within 8 hr after ingestion; may be started any time after ingestion and is beneficial in severe hepatotoxic states Use IV in patients unable to tolerate PO or with severe hepatotoxicity; the dose and timing differ from the oral regimen Dosage and administration of FDA-approved IV formulation assumes early treatment of acute overdose without hepatotoxicity; longer duration of treatment required in patients with hepatotoxicity Treatment end points simplified for ease of use INR result not valid indicator if FFP recently administered
Naloxone	Opioids	Bolus: 0.4-2 mg via IV, sublingual injection, or endotracheal instillation; 0.4-0.8 mg SC Continuous infusion: establish bolus dose required to reverse respiratory depression Begin infusing two thirds of reversal dose every hour, and titrate to maintain adequate respirations Rebolus with half of reversal dose 15 min after reversing respiratory depression	Initial: reversal of respiratory depression with resolution of hypoxia and hypercapnia Final: resolution of CNS and respiratory depression	Preventilate patients with respiratory depression by bag-valve mask or intubation before administration Use smaller doses in opioid-dependent patients; some opioids (e.g., propoxyphene, pentazocine, fentanyls) may require larger doses of naloxone; use continuous infusion for recurrent symptoms and prolonged action of some formulations (e.g., sustained-release morphine, methadone) Resedation can occur Do not use nalmefene or naltrexone to reverse acute toxicity
Octreotide	Sulfonylureas	50 mg SC q6h	Resolution of hypoglycemia and dextrose not required	Maintain dextrose infusion as needed

TABLE 110-6 ANTIDOTES AND INDICATIONS FOR USE—cont'd

ANTIDOTE	INDICATION FOR USE	DOSE*	TREATMENT END POINT	COMMENTS
Physostigmine	Anticholinergic agents (e.g., diphenhydramine, jimsonweed [*Datura* sp], scopolamine)	1-2 mg IV over 5-min period; can repeat once after 10-15 min if no effect	Reversal of anticholinergic effects	Duration of effect is 60-90 min Benzodiazepine used for subsequent treatment of agitation and seizures; additional physostigmine used rarely (e.g., refractory seizures or agitation) Adverse effects include seizures, excessive oral secretions, bradyarrhythmias; contraindicated in cyclic antidepressant toxicity
Pralidoxime chloride	Organophosphorus compounds Nerve agents—sarin, VX	30 mg/kg IV bolus (max 2 g) over 30 min, followed by continuous infusion of 8-10 mg/kg/hr (max 650 mg/hr)	Resolution of signs and symptoms, atropine no longer required	Can give initial dose over 2-min period for life-threatening clinical effects Administer early when diagnosis known or strongly suspected Efficacy variable, depending on the organophosphate Fat-soluble organophosphates may require prolonged treatment
Pyridoxine	Ethylene glycol (theoretical efficacy) Isoniazid Monomethylhydrazine mushrooms	100 mg IV 5 g IV, repeat for refractory seizures	One dose Resolution of seizures	Efficacy theoretical Pyridoxine may stop seizures, but patient can remain comatose (isoniazid, mushrooms); use benzodiazepines and phenobarbital concomitantly to manage seizures Excessive dosing can cause neuropathy
Sodium bicarbonate ($NaHCO_3$)	Reversal of myocardial sodium-channel blockers (e.g., cyclic antidepressants, cocaine, propoxyphene, sodium-channel-blocking antiarrhythmics with $\tau_{recovery}$ >1 sec, piperidine phenothiazines (thioridazine, mesoridazine)	1-2 mEq $NaHCO_3$/kg via intermittent bolus; repeat as needed	Narrowing of prolonged QRS, resolution of ventricular arrhythmias, reversal of hypotension	Monitor blood pH (optimal pH approximately 7.50); avoid pH > 7.55
	Altered tissue distribution or enhanced elimination of salicylates; may be used in chlorophenoxy herbicides, chlorpropamide, formic acid, methotrexate, phenobarbital	1-2 mEq $NaHCO_3$/kg, followed by 3 ampules (150 mL) $NaHCO_3$ (44 mEq per 50 mL) in 850 mL of D_5W, infused at 2-3 times normal maintenance fluid rate	Serum salicylate <30 mg/dL and patient clinically stable	Monitor urinary pH hourly; adjust infusion to maintain urine pH of 7.5-8.0 (avoid blood pH >7.55) Monitor ABGs Maintain normokalemia
Succimer (DMSA)	Arsenic Lead Mercury, all forms	10 mg/kg/dose q8h for 5 days, followed by q12h for 14 days Drug holiday for 2 wk; repeat if treatment end point not reached	Arsenic: 24-hr urinary arsenic <50 µg/L Lead: resolution of encephalopathy, gastrointestinal symptoms, neuropathy, nephropathy, arthralgias, myalgias, and blood lead level <70 µg/dL Mercury, elemental and inorganic: 24-hr urinary mercury <20 µg/L Mercury, organic: end point not well established	Oral chelator; adverse effects include rash, transient AST and alkaline phosphatase elevations, and gastrointestinal distress; minimal chelation of essential metals occurs Dosing for arsenic and mercury not well established Therapeutic end point for organic mercury not established; neurotoxicity not responsive to chelation therapy; suggest chelation until blood mercury level within normal value range for reference laboratory
Vitamin K	Anticoagulants (e.g., warfarin, long-acting anticoagulant rodenticides [LAARs])	Subcutaneous: AquaMEPHYTON (K_1), 10-25 mg, repeat every 6-12 hr until oral vitamin K_1 started Oral: 25-50 mg q6h; larger doses may be required	INR is normal 48-72 hr after stopping vitamin K_1 therapy Can also monitor factor VII activity	Anaphylactoid reaction can occur with IV administration Severe bleeding may also require FFP or factor concentrates Base decision to treat on finding of elevated INR; do not administer prophylactic vitamin K_1 Oral therapy has been required for months with LAAR poisoning because of lipophilicity of toxicant, with slow body clearance

*Dose concentrations and infusion times are not given. Drug dosages may require adjustment in patients with renal or hepatic failure.
†Administer antivenom in a monitored setting; antivenom must be reconstituted and then diluted; initially infuse at a rate of 2 to 5 mL/hr, and double the infusion rate every 5 minutes as tolerated to administer antivenom over a 1-hour period.
‡Ten percent calcium chloride solution = 100 mg/mL (27.2 mg/mL elemental calcium); 10% calcium gluconate solution = 100 mg/mL (9 mg/mL elemental calcium).
ABG = arterial blood gas; ALT = alanine aminotransferase; APAP = acetyl-para-aminophenol (acetaminophen); AST = aspartate aminotransferase; BAL = British antilewisite; bpm, beats per minute; CNS = central nervous system; COHb% = percent carboxyhemoglobin; CPR, cardiopulmonary resuscitation; D_5W = 5% dextrose in water; DMSA = 2,3-dimercaptosuccinic acid; ECG = electrocardiogram; FDA = Food and Drug Administration; FFP = fresh-frozen plasma; G6PD = glucose-6-phosphate dehydrogenase; Hb = hemoglobin; HD = hemodialysis; IM = intramuscular; INR = international normalized ratio; IV = intravenous; MetHb% = percent methemoglobinemia; NS = normal saline; PO = per os (by mouth); SC = subcutaneous; ; $\tau_{recovery}$ = drug blockade recovery rate.

TABLE 110-7 COMMON TOXICANTS REMOVED BY HEMODIALYSIS

TOXICANT	INDICATIONS	COMMENTS
Ethylene glycol	Serum level ≥50 mL/dL, or lower levels with concomitant metabolic acidosis and evidence of end-organ toxicity	May not be required in a patient with normal creatinine clearance and acid-base status who is receiving fomepizole
Lithium*	Clinical indications	Clinical indication is CNS toxicity (e.g., decreased mental status, ataxia, coma, seizures) Use dialysate containing bicarbonate to decrease Na^+/K^+ antiporter intracellular sequestration of lithium
Methanol	Serum level ≥50 mL/dL, or lower levels with concomitant metabolic acidosis and evidence of end-organ toxicity	Usually required because of slow elimination half-life in presence of fomepizole (mean, 52 hr; range, 22-87 hr), even in patients with no metabolic acidosis or evidence of end-organ toxicity
Phenobarbital	Clinical indications	Rarely necessary except when a patient is hemodynamically unstable despite aggressive support
Salicylates	Acute toxicity: serum level ≥100 mL/dL or <100 mg/dL in the presence of a clinical indication Chronic toxicity: any clinical indication	Serum protein binding decreases with increasing toxic levels, increasing the amount of free salicylate available for HD removal; clinical indications are one or more of the following: altered mental status, seizures, pulmonary edema, intractable acidosis, renal failure
Theophylline	Acute toxicity: serum level ≥90 μg/mL or <90 μg/mL plus any clinical indication Chronic toxicity: serum level ≥40 μg/dL and not declining despite MDAC; any clinical indication	Clinical indications for HD: seizures, hypotension, ventricular arrhythmias
Valproic acid	Severe intoxication with serum concentration >850 mg/L	Clinical indications include hepatic dysfunction; coma, especially with hyperammonemia; deteriorating clinical status despite aggressive support

*Hemodiafiltration removes lithium; the clinical benefit of this technique is unknown.
CNS = central nervous system; HD = hemodialysis; MDAC = multidose activated charcoal.

dextropropoxyphene, digitoxin, digoxin, disopyramide, nadolol, phenylbutazone, phenytoin, piroxicam, and sotalol. Whether enhanced elimination translates into decreased morbidity and mortality has not been examined in controlled clinical trials. The usual recommendations are an average dose of 12.5 g of activated charcoal (after the initial dose) administered every 1, 2, or 4 to 6 hours after the previous dose. The contraindications to single-dose activated charcoal also apply to multidose activated charcoal. Reported complications include pulmonary aspiration, bowel obstruction, and fluid and electrolyte imbalance from multiple doses of a simultaneously administered cathartic.

Urinary Alkalinization

Alkalinization of the urine, which increases the renal elimination of weak acids, is used primarily to enhance the elimination of salicylates, but the elimination of chlorpropamide, 2,4-dichlorophenoxyacetic acid, formic acid, methotrexate, and phenobarbital may be increased with this method. Urinary alkalinization is accomplished by an intravenous bolus of 1 to 2 mEq of sodium bicarbonate per kilogram body weight, followed by three ampules (150 mL) of sodium bicarbonate (44 mEq/50 mL) in 850 mL of 5% dextrose in water infused at two to three times the normal maintenance fluid rate. Urinary pH should be checked hourly, and the infusion should be adjusted to maintain a urine pH of 7.5 to 8.0. Potassium should be administered simultaneously to avoid hypokalemia, which would result in urinary acidification because the distal tubule excretes hydrogen ion in exchange for potassium (Chapter 112). Serum pH should be monitored to avoid excessive alkalemia. Contraindications to this therapy include volume overload and cerebral or pulmonary edema. Urinary acidification is no longer recommended to enhance the elimination of weak bases, such as amphetamines, because of the danger of precipitating tubular myoglobin in patients with rhabdomyolysis.

Extracorporeal Removal

Extracorporeal techniques enhance the elimination of a few drugs and toxicants that exhibit single-compartment kinetics, a volume of distribution less than 1 L/kg, and endogenous clearance of less than 4 mL/minute/kg (Table 110-7). For hemodialysis, the toxicant must be water soluble, have a molecular weight less than 500 D, and exhibit low protein binding. For hemoperfusion, the toxicant must adsorb to activated charcoal. For continuous renal replacement therapy, the toxicant must have a molecular weight less than the permeability limit of the filter membrane. Rarely, extracorporeal removal has been used for aminoglycosides, atenolol, bromide, carbamazepine, diethylene glycol, isopropanol, magnesium, metformin, methotrexate, *N*-acetylprocainamide, phenobarbital, procainamide, sotalol, and trichloroethanol (chloral hydrate).

PROGNOSIS

Almost all patients who reach the hospital alive survive with appropriate care. Inpatient mortality rates are 0.2 to 0.5%.

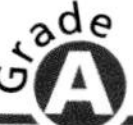

1. Eddleston M, Juszczak E, Buckley NA, et al. Multiple-dose activated charcoal in acute self-poisoning: a randomised controlled trial. *Lancet*. 2008;371:579-587.
2. Eddleston M, Eyer P, Worek F, et al. Pralidoxime in acute organophosphorus insecticide poisoning—a randomized controlled trial. *PLOS Med*. 2009;6:e1000104.

SUGGESTED READINGS

Brent J. Fomepizole for ethylene glycol and methanol poisoning. *N Engl J Med*. 2009;360:2216-2223. *Review*.

Eddleston M, Buckley NA, Eyer P, et al. Management of acute organophosphorus pesticide poisoning. *Lancet*. 2008;371:597-607. *Clinical review*.

Hill GE, Ogunnaike B, Nasir D. Patients presenting with acute toxin ingestion. *Anesthesiol Clin*. 2010;28:117-137. *Review*.

Miech R, Koester S, Dorsey-Holliman B. Increasing U.S. mortality due to accidental poisoning: the role of the baby boom cohort. *Addiction*. 2011;106:806-815. *Emphasizes the need to bolster overdose prevention programs and policies*.

Yarema MC, Johnson DW, Berlin RJ, et al. Comparison of the 20-hour intravenous and 72-hour oral acetylcysteine protocols for the treatment of acute acetaminophen poisoning. *Ann Emerg Med*. 2009;54:606-614. *In this retrospective study, the relative risk of hepatotoxicity was lower in the 20-hour group when acetylcysteine was started within 12 hours of ingestion*.

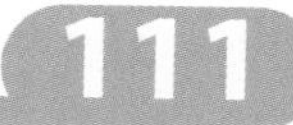

ELECTRIC INJURY

BASIL A. PRUITT JR.

ELECTRIC CURRENT INJURY

DEFINITION

The tissue damage caused by electric current ranges from a transient increase in cell membrane permeability to immediate coagulation necrosis of large volumes of tissue. The clinical consequences include disturbances in the physiologic electrical conduction systems, which may cause cardiopulmonary arrest; tetanic muscle contractions, with resulting compression fractures of vertebrae; and delayed tissue damage, such as cataract formation.

EPIDEMIOLOGY

As the use of electricity has increased worldwide, the number of electric injuries has increased. The precise incidence of electric injury is unknown, but the National Centers for Health and Centers for Disease Control and Prevention have estimated that each year in the United States there are 52,000 trauma admissions for electric injuries. During a recent 86-month period, 5.3% of patients admitted to the U.S. Army Burn Center had an electric injury; at other burn centers, the percentage of admissions related to electric injury ranges from 0.04 to 6.7% in developed countries and as high as 32 to 42% in developing countries.

PATHOBIOLOGY

Environmental conditions, duration of contact, pathway of the current, type of current (and, if alternating current, its frequency), and voltage all influence the effects of electricity on tissue. Voltage greater than 40 is potentially dangerous, and the likelihood of sudden death and remote tissue injury increases as voltage increases to 1000. Voltages greater than 1000 are considered to be high tension and are associated with immediate severe tissue damage. Alternating current is more dangerous than direct current because of its likelihood to produce cardiac arrest or cessation of respiration and its tetanic effect, which may prevent the patient from breaking contact with the source of electricity. As the frequency of alternating current increases to greater than 60 cycles per second, tissue injury decreases. The path of the current through the body between the points of contact is important in determining tissue damage; a course through the heart or the respiratory center of the brain is especially dangerous. Ventricular fibrillation can be produced by current flow of only 100 mA from a hand to the feet. Rapid separation from the source of electricity is crucial, because tissue damage increases in proportion to the duration of contact. Resistance to current flow at the point of contact is influenced by environmental conditions; dry and thickened palmar or plantar skin is more resistant to the passage of current than is skin moistened by perspiration or other liquid.

Heat is the principal mediator of tissue damage in electric injury, the severity of which is related to voltage and duration of contact. Tissue-specific differences in resistance to the flow of current (neural tissue least; blood vessels, muscle, and skin intermediate; bone greatest) may explain differences in tissue injury caused by low-voltage current. Because all body tissues and fluids are conductive, the soft tissues between bone and skin can be viewed as a volume conductor. Heat is produced in tissues as a function of voltage drop and current flow per unit of cross-sectional area (i.e., density of the current). The inverse relationship between the density of the current and the tissue's cross-sectional area accounts for the frequency of severe injury to the digits and extremities and the rarity of major injury to the trunk in patients with high-tension electric injury (Fig. 111-1). Contact with less than 1000 V causes injuries that are self-limited because at the contact points, where the density of the current is greatest, the skin is severely injured and chars, which results in a rapid increase in resistance and reduction in the passage of current. When the source is greater than 1000 V, arcing is so intense that tissue destruction is increased markedly as relatively constant levels of current are maintained. Arcing, which may occur across the flexor surfaces of joints, can char the skin in these areas and ignite the patient's clothing. After cessation of the flow of current, the heated tissue acts like a volume radiator and cools unevenly, with the superficial portions cooling more rapidly than the deeper portions; deeper tissues are therefore more prone to severe injury.

Tissue damage can also be caused by low-voltage direct current (e.g., contact with automobile battery terminals or with defective or inappropriately used medical equipment, such as electrosurgical devices, external pacing devices, or defibrillators). Direct-current injuries are reportedly common during laparoscopy with high-voltage coagulation.

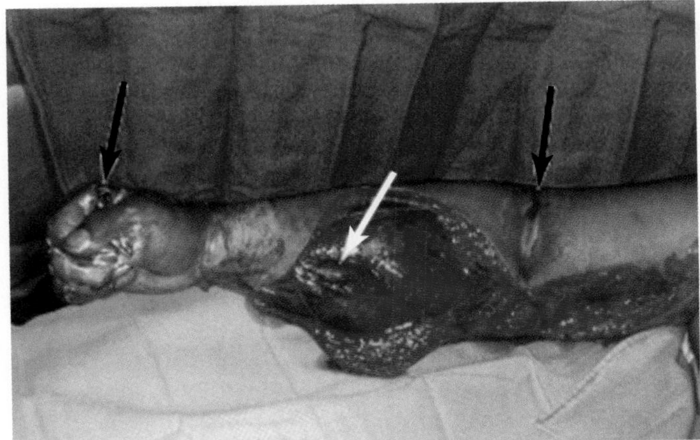

FIGURE 111-1. Charring at the contact site in the first web space and at the site of arcing in the antecubital space *(black arrows)* of a victim of electric injury. The fixed flexion deformity of the thumb and other digits is characteristic of severe high-voltage injury to the hand and forearm. The severity of the injury is indicated by the marked edema of the forearm muscles, bulging above the cut edges of the fasciotomy incision, and by the patchy dark discoloration of the muscles of the arm and the forearm, particularly the deeper muscle exposed in the central portion of the forearm incision *(white arrow)*.

CLINICAL MANIFESTATIONS AND DIAGNOSIS

Cardiopulmonary arrest can be caused by low-voltage electric injury but is more common with high-voltage electric injury. Extensive tissue necrosis may also liberate enough potassium to cause cardiac dysfunction. Because cardiac arrhythmias may recur after resuscitation or develop 24 to 48 hours after injury, all patients who have sustained high-voltage electric injury should undergo continuous electrocardiogram (ECG) monitoring for at least 48 hours after the last ECG-documented arrhythmia. Early imaging of the heart with technetium-99m tetrofosmin has been proposed as a means of detecting myocardial perfusion defects requiring cardiac monitoring and predicting the possibility of long-term cardiac effects. Renal failure may occur in patients with high-voltage electric injury if inapparent deep tissue injury with accompanying occult edema results in an underestimation of fluid requirements, inadequate resuscitation, and oliguria. Additionally, the destruction of muscle and red blood cells liberates hemochromes, which may precipitate in the renal tubules unless adequate urinary output is maintained (Chapter 122).

Muscle Damage

High-voltage electric injury commonly causes edema beneath the investing fascia of the involved muscle compartments, thereby compromising nutrient blood flow to muscles within the compartments and to distal unburned tissue. Clinical indications for the surgical release of intracompartmental pressure by fasciotomy and surgical exploration of a limb include impaired capillary refilling of distal unburned skin or nails, cyanosis of distal unburned skin, stony hardness of a muscle compartment on palpation, and diminished or absent pulsatile flow in the distal arteries as assessed by Doppler ultrasound. Tissue pressures 30 mm Hg or higher above atmospheric pressure, as measured by a catheter placed in the compartment, indicate the need for immediate decompression. If clinical signs are consistent with deep tissue injury but large-vessel pulses are intact, arteriography can determine the need for operative intervention, including amputation of the affected limb. "Pruning" of the arterial tree, with a decrease in the density of nutrient branches in the muscles of an involved limb, identifies the level of amputation required to remove muscle that has been irreversibly damaged. Muscle blood flow of 1 mL/minute/100 g of tissue, as determined by xenon-133 "washout," has been proposed as the minimum level required for ultimate tissue viability. In patients with high-voltage electric injury, myoglobinemia and elevation of serum creatine phosphokinase reflect significant muscle damage, and myoglobinuria is a strong predictor of the need for fasciotomy in the first 24 hours after injury.

Neurologic Examination

On admission and at scheduled intervals thereafter, a detailed neurologic examination must be performed on all patients with high-voltage electric injury; all nerve deficits should be documented fully. Central nervous system or peripheral nerve dysfunction may be apparent immediately after electric injury or may appear later. Recovery of function after direct electrical nerve damage is rare. Conversely, the spontaneous resolution of immediate and early functional deficits of nerves not injured directly (motor nerves are more sensitive to nondestructive injury than are sensory nerves) is common. A polyneuritic syndrome of relatively late onset can cause deficits in the function of peripheral nerves far removed from the points of contact. Direct nerve damage of the spinal cord causes immediate deficits, which are more likely to be transient than are deficits with a later onset. Delayed-onset spinal cord deficits can manifest as quadriplegia, hemiplegia, localized nerve deficits with signs of ascending paralysis, transverse myelitis, and even an amyotrophic lateral sclerosis–like syndrome. The cause of delayed paresthesias and nerve dysfunction after electric injury is unknown, but an increase in permeability of the cell membrane and an associated loss of cell contents induced by exposure to a millivoltage electric field (electroporation) have been implicated. Children have greater improvement in neurologic function than adults do, owing to their greater neurologic plasticity. Children with electric injuries that cause full-thickness destruction of the calvaria may have direct brain injury, with affective and/or cognitive difficulties that can persist for a year or longer.

Remote Organ Injury

Direct liver injury, focal pancreatic and gallbladder necrosis, and intestinal perforation have been reported after electric injury, but all are uncommon. Delayed hemorrhage from moderate to large blood vessels has been ascribed to an arteritis caused by the electric injury, but this hemorrhage seems to be related to inadequate débridement of injured tissue or to vascular wall necrosis as a consequence of exposure after débridement.

Compression fractures of vertebral bodies may be produced by tetanic contractions of the paraspinous muscles. Fractures of the skull and the long bones of both the upper and lower extremities may be caused by falls after the electric shock.

TREATMENT Rx

Cardiopulmonary arrest must be treated by immediate institution of cardiopulmonary resuscitation (Chapter 63). In patients with high urinary hemochrome concentrations, a urinary output of 75 to 100 mL/hour should be maintained (Chapter 115). If the hemochromes do not clear promptly or the patient remains oliguric despite the administration of resuscitation fluids at more than twice the required rate, as estimated based on the extent of the burn and the patient's weight (Chapter 112), 25 g of mannitol should be given as an intravenous bolus, and 12.5 g of mannitol should be added to each liter of intravenous fluid until the pigment has cleared from the urine. Hyperkalemia is treated as in any other patient (Chapter 119).

If the electric injury is limited to the skin and subcutaneous tissue, an antibacterial cream such as Sulfamylon should be applied twice daily to the burned tissue until débridement is performed. The antimicrobial (mafenide acetate) in Sulfamylon readily diffuses into the nonviable tissue to limit microbial proliferation. As soon as resuscitation has restored hemodynamic stability, severely damaged limbs or other areas of tissue necrosis should be surgically explored. The viability of vital structures and the extent of deep tissue damage are assessed to determine the need for amputation. If amputation is not required, all necrotic tissue is débrided to eliminate the source of hyperkalemia and reduce the risk for infection. It is imperative to examine the periosseous muscles, which may be necrotic because of delayed heat dissipation but overlain by more superficial viable muscles. After débridement or amputation, the operative wound is dressed but not surgically closed, and the patient is scheduled for re-exploration of the wound 24 to 72 hours later. At that time, residual necrotic tissue is débrided, and the wound is closed by skin grafts, tissue transfer, or biologic dressings, depending on the condition, extent, and site of the wound. An exception to early excision of questionably viable tissue is the conservative removal of only obviously necrotic tissue from low-voltage oral commissure wounds that result from a child's biting or sucking on exposed wires or house current outlets (Fig. 111-2).

PROGNOSIS

Cardiopulmonary and fluid resuscitation combined with monitoring of limb tissue pressure and wound care have maximized tissue salvage, reduced renal failure, and increased the survival of patients with electric injuries. Overall, current treatment is associated with a 96% survival rate.

Among the patients with serious high-voltage electric injuries hospitalized at the U.S. Army Burn Center over the past decade or so, about 8% died and another 22% had permanent neurologic deficits at discharge. High-voltage electric injury has been associated with the subsequent formation of cataracts, most frequently when the contact site was on the head or neck. Cataracts may form rapidly, but they more commonly develop 3 years or more after the injury. Rarely, exfoliative debris may be evident in the anterior chamber of the eye immediately after injury. Cholelithiasis and gastrointestinal dysfunction have been reported after high-voltage injury, but they appear to be rare.

Most patients with low-voltage injuries, many caused by electric flash burns, develop long-term sequelae. The neurologic symptoms (memory loss, numbness, headache, chronic pain, weakness), psychological symptoms (depression, insomnia, post-traumatic stress syndrome, nightmares, anxiety), and musculoskeletal symptoms (pain, reduced range of motion, contracture) often have a delayed onset (1.6 to 29.5 months), persist on average for 300 days after injury, and limit return to work in more than 40% of patients.

LIGHTNING INJURY

An estimated 300 to 350 persons are struck by lightning each year, and about 30% of them die. The duration of a lightning bolt is $\frac{1}{100}$ to $\frac{1}{1000}$ of a second, but it may have a voltage of approximately 1 billion V and induce currents ranging from 12,000 to 200,000 A. The temperature in a lightning bolt, which may be 30,000 K, dissipates in a few microseconds.

CLINICAL MANIFESTATIONS

Cardiopulmonary arrest, which can be secondary to either asystole or ventricular fibrillation, is common in patients struck by lightning. Cardiopulmonary resuscitation (Chapter 63) must be instituted immediately; recovery has been reported in some patients who were apparently without life signs for 15 minutes or longer. Although signs of acute myocardial damage may become evident later, persistent or recurrent ECG abnormalities are uncommon. Coma is common immediately after injury and typically resolves in a few hours. Abdominal signs of peritonitis with free air in the peritoneal cavity should alert one to the possibility of intestinal perforation, which must be treated by prompt primary closure. Keraunoparalysis (lightning paralysis), which is characterized by paresthesias and paralysis, usually involves the lower limbs, often develops over a period of several days after lightning injury, is typically associated with vasomotor disorders, and is usually transient. Myoglobinuria is uncommon; when present, it is treated as described earlier for other electric injuries. Tympanic membrane rupture and hearing loss may

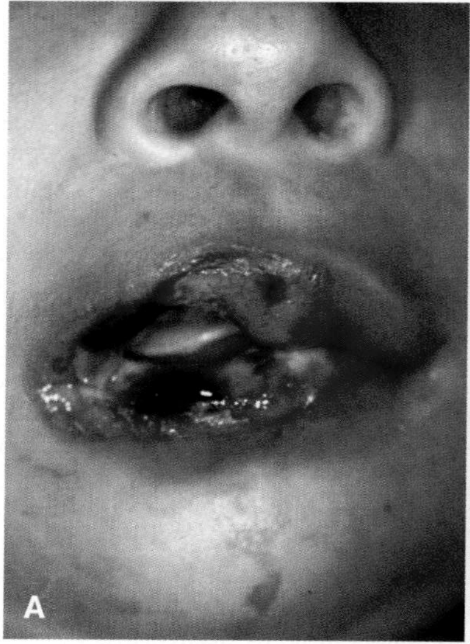

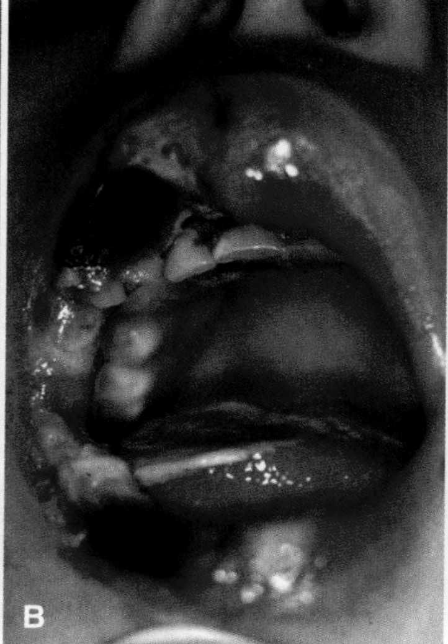

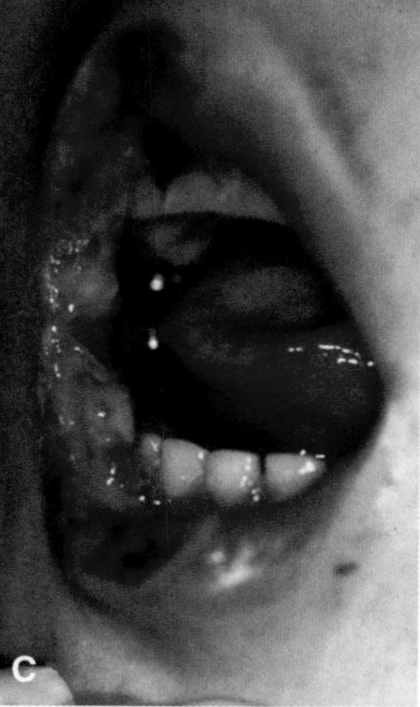

FIGURE 111-2. **A,** This child sustained a potentially disfiguring injury by biting on wires carrying house current. **B,** Note the extent of the injury, with black areas of necrotic tissue on each lip and the white plaque of nonviable tissue on the upper surface of the tongue. **C,** Spontaneous separation and removal of only unequivocally dead tissue minimizes disfigurement and reduces the magnitude of surgical reconstruction required to restore lip function.

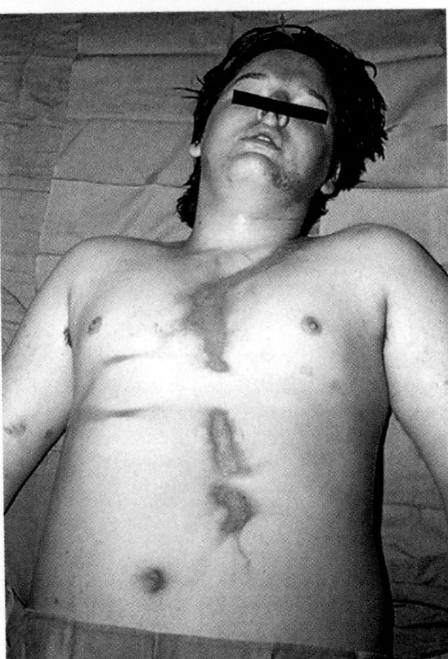

FIGURE 111-3. The arborescent current markings on the face, neck, and anterior trunk of this young patient, which are characteristic of lightning injury, healed without the need for grafting. Note the focal lesions on the right arm, indicating the spread of the current that produced the marks on the right anterolateral aspect of the chest wall.

also be caused by lightning injury. Cutaneous burns of the trunk and proximal areas of the limbs caused by lightning injury, called *Lichtenberg figures*, typically have a "splashed on" arborescent and spidery appearance and are generally superficial (Fig. 111-3). Small, circular, full-thickness burns of the tips of the toes are also common and have been termed the *tiptoe sign*. Mottling of the skin and other signs of vasoconstriction previously considered specific to lightning injury generally resolve with adequate resuscitation.

TREATMENT AND PROGNOSIS

Rx

Current treatment, which emphasizes immediate cardiopulmonary resuscitation, has decreased mortality significantly, and two thirds of lightning-injured patients now survive. Persistent nerve deficits and long-term problems are relatively uncommon in survivors. However, Guillain-Barré syndrome, with neurologic deficits persisting beyond hospital discharge, has been reported.

SUGGESTED READINGS

Li AL, Gomez M, Fish JS. Effectiveness of pain management following electrical injury. *J Burn Care Res.* 2010;31:73-82. *Review emphasizing the chronic need for pain medications in many patients.*

Ritenour AE, Morton MJ, McManus JG, et al. Lightning injury: a review. *Burns.* 2008;34:585-594. *Describes the epidemiology, treatment, and sequelae.*

Vierhapper MF, Lumenta DB, Beck H, et al. Electrical injury: a long-term analysis with review of regional differences. *Ann Plast Surg.* 2011;66:43-46. *Review of 56 hospitalized cases, with mean burn surface area of 26% and a 4% mortality rate.*

112

MEDICAL ASPECTS OF TRAUMA AND BURN CARE

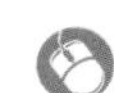

ROBERT H. DEMLING AND JONATHAN D. GATES

MEDICAL ASPECTS OF TRAUMA

EPIDEMIOLOGY

Trauma is the third leading cause of death in people of all ages in the United States, surpassed only by cancer and atherosclerosis. Trauma is the leading cause of death in children, adolescents, and young adults aged 1 to 44 years.

More than 140,000 deaths and twice as many permanent disabilities occur annually in the United States from injuries. Fatal injuries have a trimodal distribution. Half of all fatalities occur within minutes of the injury as a result of massive hemorrhage from the heart, lacerations of large blood vessels, or catastrophic neurologic injury. In such cases, there is insufficient time for medical intervention to alter the outcome; the only method to reduce this category of trauma-related morbidity and mortality is through prevention and education programs. Of the fatalities, 30% occur within a few hours after injury from airway obstruction, shock, or neurologic dysfunction. This interval represents an opportunity during which appropriate and timely medical or surgical intervention is most likely to influence outcome. Fatalities within this second peak occur as a result of epidural and subdural hematomas, chest injuries, liver lacerations, splenic rupture, pelvic fractures, or the accumulation of multiple injuries resulting in significant blood loss. The third peak of trauma fatalities is due to multisystem organ dysfunction or overwhelming infection weeks later. This delayed systemic response is related to the degree of the initial insult, the individual response to the injury, and the cumulative effect of any additional complications that arise after injury.

Motor vehicle crashes, firearms, and falls are major contributors to injury in the United States. In 2008, an estimated 2.35 million people were injured in motor vehicle traffic crashes, which resulted in approximately 38,000 fatalities. About 50% of all traffic deaths in 15- to 34-year-olds are alcohol related (Chapter 32). About 35,000 gun-related deaths, unintentional and intentional, occur annually. Of all injury deaths, 8% are related to falls, and fall from a height is responsible for one third of all injury-related hospitalizations.

PATHOBIOLOGY

Mechanism of Injury

Trauma produces a structural or physiologic alteration as a result of an external force, whether it is mechanical, chemical, electrical, or thermal energy. The force that initiated the motion of an object must be absorbed or dissipated in an effort to decelerate that object. When an automobile traveling at a given speed strikes an immobile object, a tremendous amount of energy in the moving vehicle is transmitted to the immobile object and the structure of the vehicle, deforming both until the automobile stops. These same forces are imparted to the occupants of the vehicle with potentially dire consequences. In a head-on impact, the driver continues to move forward until impeded by objects inside the automobile or until the energy is dissipated by the restraint of a seat belt or air bag. Deceleration forces are imparted to individual organs. These same physical principles apply to injury after a fall from a height. Compression, shear, and overpressure from these and other forces injure internal organs.

Penetrating injuries, which are described as either low velocity or high velocity, result from the kinetic energy of the missile. In the case of a bullet discharged from a gun, the tissue immediately contacted by the bullet is crushed to create a permanent cavity. Transfer of energy farther away from the bullet path creates a temporary cavity beyond the boundary of the permanent tract, the so-called blast effect. A simple stab wound from a knife or sharp object is considered a low-velocity injury in which the wound is confined to the tract itself. Virtually no temporary cavity is created, but the consequences may be just as devastating as a high-velocity injury if a vital structure is affected.

Pathophysiology of Injury

Shock (Chapter 106) results in inadequate organ perfusion and subsequent failure to deliver sufficient oxygen to maintain aerobic metabolism. Poor peripheral perfusion results in cellular hypoxia and slowing of oxidative phosphorylation, with the accumulation of H^+ ion in the extracellular fluid, resulting in metabolic acidosis. The initial step in managing shock associated with trauma is to recognize inadequate organ perfusion. The second step is to identify and treat the probable cause. The four general categories of shock in trauma are hemorrhagic, compressive, neurogenic, and cardiogenic; however, most shock is hypovolemic in nature. Adrenal insufficiency (Chapter 234), anaphylaxis (Chapter 261), and septic shock (Chapter 108) are less common but may occur during the recovery period. The goal of treatment is restoration of cellular and organ perfusion with adequately oxygenated blood volume.

Hemorrhagic Shock

Hemorrhagic shock results from a decline in cardiac filling pressure as blood is lost (Chapter 106). Cardiac output is preserved through compensatory mechanisms when the loss of blood is about 10% of blood volume. Endogenous neurogenic and endocrine responses result in peripheral vasoconstriction and shunting of blood from the nonessential areas of skin, muscle, and abdominal viscera to maintain perfusion to the heart and brain. Cardiac output decreases with a blood volume loss of 20 to 40%, with a resultant decrease in systolic blood pressure. Additional compensatory mechanisms to maintain perfusion pressure in the face of a sudden decrease in intravascular volume result in a shift of proteins and fluids from the extracellular space to the intravascular compartment. The relative decrease in volume and increase in osmolarity of the extracellular space stimulate movement of fluid out of the cells to replace it.

It is imperative to identify a patient in shock or compensated shock. A normal systemic arterial blood pressure or absence of tachycardia may lead an inexperienced physician to believe that the patient is hemodynamically stable when in fact the patient may be in the precarious situation of partially compensated shock. A high index of suspicion and early aggressive diagnostic evaluation and treatment minimize the possibility that occult blood loss may be missed and lead to appropriate volume resuscitation and possible surgical correction.

Compressive Shock

Compressive shock arises when external compression of the lungs or heart from air, fluid, or blood either compromises diastolic filling of the right ventricle or prevents adequate ventilation and oxygenation. The two most notable forms of compressive shock are tension pneumothorax (Chapter 99) and pericardial tamponade (Chapter 77).

In tension pneumothorax, air within the pleural space impedes expansion of the ipsilateral lung and shifts the mediastinum. Compression of the inferior and superior vena cava leads to inadequate filling of the right atrium and ventricle, which decreases cardiac output. Identification of the injury is paramount; typical findings include absence of breath sounds in the ipsilateral chest, jugular venous distention, and tracheal deviation to the opposite side. Appropriate intervention involves release of air under tension in the pneumothorax by means of needle or tube thoracentesis.

Cardiac tamponade occurs because of extrinsic compression of the chambers of the heart from blood within the pericardial space, which is normally a potential space filled with less than 50 mL of pericardial fluid (Chapter 77). An external chest wound that penetrates the pericardium and the heart may create a rent in the pericardium too small to vent the accumulated blood; as a result, blood collects in the noncompliant pericardial sac, and pressure is directed inward toward the hollow chambers of the heart. The external compression inhibits diastolic filling of the chambers and reduces stroke volume. Pericardial tamponade should be suspected in patients who have wounds in the vicinity of the precordium and epigastrium, hypotension, tachycardia, jugular venous distention, and muffled heart sounds. Treatment is immediate evacuation of the pericardial space by needle pericardiocentesis, followed by sternotomy or left thoracotomy.

Neurogenic Shock

Complete injury to the cervical or upper thoracic spinal cord may result in sympathetic denervation manifested as loss of vasomotor tone in the periphery. Neurogenic shock should be considered in any trauma patient who is hypotensive but not actively bleeding. Only about 20% of patients with a complete high spinal cord injury have neurogenic shock, however, and patients with incomplete motor or sensory deficits (or both) rarely have hypotension directly caused by neurologic injury.

Cardiogenic Shock

Cardiogenic shock (Chapter 107) implies inadequate peripheral perfusion as a result of pump failure. It may be caused by arrhythmias, valvular dysfunction, or failing myocardial contraction. The latter may be seen with cardiac contusion or ischemic dysfunction of a previously damaged myocardium with marginal reserve.

DIAGNOSIS AND TREATMENT Rx

An organized approach to a trauma patient is mandatory to avoid confusion or missing life-threatening injury. A randomized trial found no benefit in advanced prehospital life support, whereby paramedics in the field perform endotracheal intubation and administer intravenous therapy, compared with basic prehospital life support and rapid transfer to a trauma center.[1] The American College of Surgeons Advanced Trauma Life Support (ATLS) guidelines divide management into the primary survey for rapid diagnosis and treatment of life-threatening injuries and the secondary survey for a more complete, in-depth evaluation of the whole patient for definitive therapy.

The initial management of a trauma patient requires immediate intravenous access for volume resuscitation. The type and rapidity of solution delivered are determined by the patient's hemodynamic stability, as reflected by the degree of intravascular depletion or blood loss. Four classes of hemorrhage are widely accepted (Table 112-1). Intravenous access also allows the administration of analgesics, sedatives, and antibiotics. The rapidity of volume resuscitation with isotonic crystalloid and blood products is determined by the initial degree or class of shock. The guidelines are based on the "three-to-one" rule, which derives from the empirical observation that most patients in hemorrhagic shock require 300 mL of electrolyte solution for each 100 mL of blood loss because crystalloid equilibrates in the entire extracellular space.

More recently, the experience of the U.S. military had led to the concept of damage control resuscitation, which focuses on the strategy of transfusing blood products (red cells, plasma, and platelets) early and often in the exsanguinating patient while limiting the use of crystalloids to avoid hemodilution of coagulation products. Despite the absence of randomized trials, a 1:1 ratio of plasma and platelets to packed red blood cells appears to result in higher survival among patients with exsanguinating injury. Use of leukoreduced blood provides no advantage over standard blood products.[2] Tranexamic acid (loading dose 1 g over 10 minutes then infusion of 1 g over 8 hours), which inhibits thrombolysis, beginning within 8 hours of injury reduces mortality by 9% in trauma patients who require blood transfusions.[3]

Primary Survey

The primary survey (airway, breathing, circulation) is the same whether the mechanism of injury was blunt, penetrating, or thermal. Evaluation of the airway is paramount. Supplemental oxygen is given to all trauma patients to maximize delivery of oxygen to the periphery. If the patient is hemodynamically unstable or is unable to maintain a patent airway because of mental status changes or airway debris, endotracheal intubation should be performed. There is little role for the use of oral airways or nasal trumpets in a trauma patient. Care must be taken to avoid movement of the cervical spine during intubation so that exacerbation of an undiagnosed cervical spine fracture or ligamentous disruption is avoided. Inability to perform endotracheal intubation in a trauma patient should lead to rapid surgical control of the airway by cricothyroidotomy. Tracheostomy is a poor second choice because

TABLE 112-1 CATEGORIZATION AND INITIAL TREATMENT OF HEMORRHAGIC SHOCK*

	CLASS I	CLASS II	CLASS III	CLASS IV
Blood loss (mL)	≤750	750-1500	1500-2000	≥2000
Blood loss (% of blood volume)	≤15	15-30	30-40	≥40
Pulse rate	<100	>100	>120	≥140
Blood pressure	Normal	Normal	Decreased	Decreased
Capillary refill test	Normal	Positive	Positive	Positive
Respiratory rate	14-20	20-30	30-40	>35
Urine output (mL/hr)	≥30	20-30	5-15	Negligible
Mental status	Slightly anxious	Mildly anxious	Anxious and confused	Confused and lethargic
Fluid replacement (3:1 rule)	Crystalloid	Crystalloid	Crystalloid + blood	Crystalloid + blood

*Based on a 70-kg adult.

it is more time-consuming and potentially bloody, especially if the landmarks are obscured by trauma.

The primary survey should observe the symmetry of chest wall movement, determine whether breath sounds are equal bilaterally and adequate, and assess the chest wall for crepitus, instability, or tenderness. If a tension pneumothorax or massive hemothorax is suspected (and the findings are not caused by intubation of the right mainstem bronchus), a large-bore chest tube is placed in the ipsilateral anterolateral fifth intercostal space. Chest tube insertion is diagnostic and therapeutic. Return of greater than 1500 mL of blood suggests a significant injury within the ipsilateral hemothorax; this magnitude of initial output or ongoing hourly blood loss of 200 to 250 mL through the chest tube may warrant urgent thoracic surgical exploration.

Adequacy of the circulation is determined clinically by noting the presence of carotid, radial, and femoral pulses. Brisk capillary refill, as elicited by transient compression of the nail bed, and a warm, well-perfused patient suggest good peripheral perfusion. A patient in extremis may have a barely palpable carotid pulse, mental status changes, and mottled, cold, clammy skin. During this evaluation, simultaneous insertion of short, large-caliber intravenous catheters into the antecubital veins is recommended for the initial administration of lactated Ringer's solution.

The primary survey should include an evaluation of neurologic function. The Glasgow Coma Scale (Chapter 406) grades the patient's eye movement, best motor response, and best verbal response on a scale from 1 to 5, with a total score of 15 indicating the best function. For patients with brain trauma (Chapter 406), resuscitation with a saline solution provides better outcomes than using albumin.[4]

The patient should be assessed for all evidence of traumatic injury. This assessment should include an examination of the back with the patient log-rolled under cervical spine precautions.

Secondary Survey

The secondary survey is the head-to-toe physical examination of the patient to evaluate the airway, reassess the adequacy of breathing and circulation, and look for any injuries or underlying conditions that were not immediately apparent during the primary survey. At this stage, pertinent radiographs, blood tests, and other tests (e.g., an electrocardiogram) are obtained, and a Foley catheter can be inserted if needed.

Head and Neck

Evaluation of neurologic function should determine whether there is evidence of closed head injury (Chapter 406). Physical examination should assess for skull and facial fractures and eye and ear injuries. The physician should have a low threshold for performing computed tomography (CT) of the head, which is preferred over magnetic resonance imaging in this situation.

The management of neck injuries that penetrate the platysma is dependent on the anatomic level of injury. The neck is divided into threes zones. Zone I injury, including the thoracic inlet up to the level of the cricothyroid membrane, is treated as an upper thoracic injury. In a stable patient, injuries in zone I require an arteriogram or CT angiography to define the injury and plan the surgical approach; hemodynamically unstable patients should undergo immediate surgical exploration.

Zone III injury, from the angle of the mandible to the base of the skull, is treated as a head injury. Most patients with injuries in this region are hemodynamically stable. Arteriography, bronchoscopy, esophagoscopy, and sometimes direct laryngoscopy should be performed to evaluate the type and extent of injury.

Zone II injuries, which are in the most exposed area of the neck between the other two zones, must be evaluated locally to determine whether the platysma muscle has been penetrated. Both selective operative management and mandatory exploration of penetrating injuries to zone II of the neck appear to be equally justified and safe. Selective operative management of a patient with penetrating wounds deep to the platysma requires nonoperative evaluation with arteriography and diagnostic upper endoscopy and bronchoscopy, with operative intervention reserved for situations in which the evaluation reveals pathology. Spiral CT with intravenous contrast material can define arterial injuries and has replaced angiography except where CT cannot define the arterial anatomy. Hemodynamically unstable patients should be resuscitated and explored surgically without further testing.

Chest

Life-threatening injuries of the chest include tension pneumothorax, massive hemothorax, cardiac tamponade (see earlier), flail chest, open pneumothorax, and disruption of the thoracic aorta. Flail chest implies an unstable segment of the chest wall as a result of multiple rib fractures. The negative pleural pressure required for inspiration pulls the unstable segment of the chest wall inward while the remainder of the chest moves in the opposite direction. An open pneumothorax implies air entering the pleural space through an external chest wound. The wound should be covered with a partially occlusive dressing, and a chest tube should be inserted to prevent the accumulation of air and the development of tension pneumothorax. Large open chest wounds require endotracheal intubation, operative débridement, chest tube drainage, chest wall stabilization, and closure. Although not usually considered life-threatening, there are a myriad of chest injuries, including simple pneumothorax, pulmonary contusions (Fig. 112-1), rib fractures, and minor to moderate hemothorax, that may play a major role in the duration of lung dysfunction or the need for ventilatory support, or both.

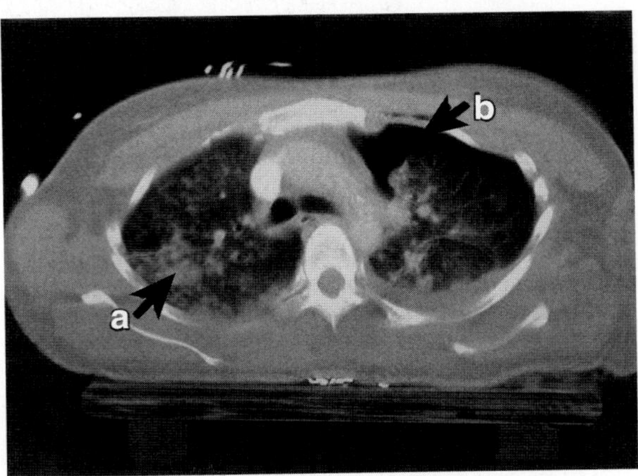

FIGURE 112-1. Chest evaluation. A chest computed tomographic scan shows bilateral pulmonary contusions *(arrow a)* and effusions with a small pneumothorax on the left *(arrow b)*.

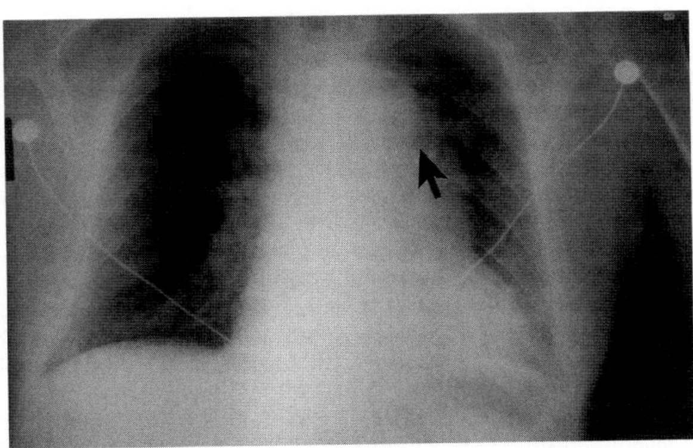

FIGURE 112-2. Widened superior mediastinum on an upright chest radiograph. Note the loss of normal contour of the aortic knob *(arrow)*.

All trauma patients should have a supine chest radiograph taken to examine the lung fields, the mediastinal contour, and the chest wall. Thoracic aortic injury, which is a feared complication of severe acceleration-deceleration injury, results in the immediate death of 90% of persons with this injury. Survivors who reach medical care often have a contained mediastinal hematoma that appears as a widened superior mediastinum or loss of the aortic contour on the chest radiograph, or both (Fig. 112-2). These patients have historically been evaluated by arteriography (Fig. 112-3), but now chest CT is used to screen for this injury. A contained mediastinal hematoma is an unstable condition that demands timely evaluation and possible endovascular or open operative intervention.

Myocardial Injury

Myocardial contusion results from transmission of force to the myocardium in the form of compression, blast, or sudden deceleration. The true incidence is difficult to define given the absence of consensus on a reliable test to identify myocardial contusion. A high degree of suspicion is needed because there are no specific clinical signs of myocardial injury. Sternal fracture, anterior rib fractures, and aortic injuries are all examples of trauma that may suggest underlying cardiac contusion. Life-threatening myocardial contusion (5%) is manifested within the first 6 to 12 hours after injury as malignant arrhythmias or, if enough of the left ventricle is damaged, cardiogenic shock. Myocardial rupture is uncommon and typically involves the right ventricle because of the thin muscular wall and close proximity to the sternum. More commonly, arrhythmias or conduction disturbances may occur with elevation of cardiac biomarkers. Electrocardiographic findings include ST-T wave anomalies, supraventricular and ventricular arrhythmias, and atrioventricular nodal dysfunction. The echocardiogram may show left ventricular wall motion abnormalities, valvar dysfunction, or pericardial effusion. There is no evidence to support prophylactic treatment of arrhythmias, and emergency surgery for other injuries does not appear to carry a risk for increased morbidity or mortality in the presence of minor abnormalities.

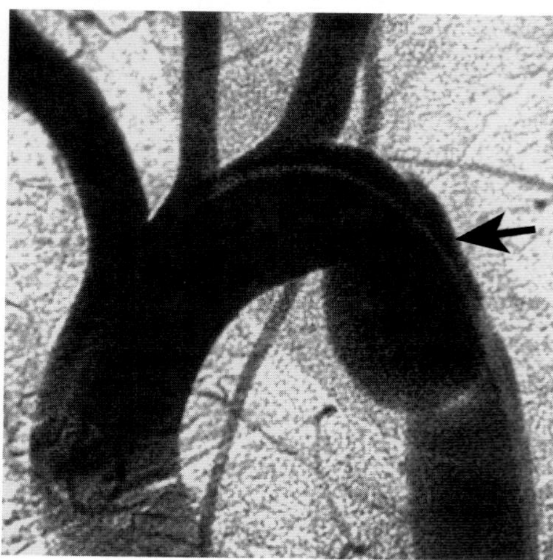

FIGURE 112-3. Arteriography of the chest. An arteriogram shows thoracic aortic disruption *(arrow)* beyond the left subclavian artery in the patient depicted in Fig. 112-2.

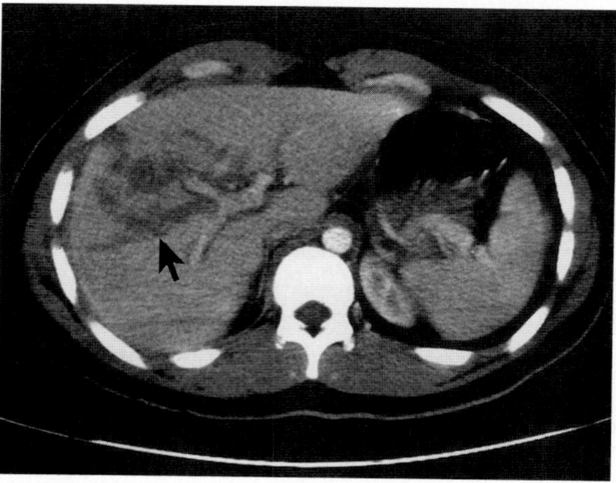

FIGURE 112-4. Abdominal injury. An abdominal computed tomographic scan shows an injury to the right lobe of the liver *(arrow)*.

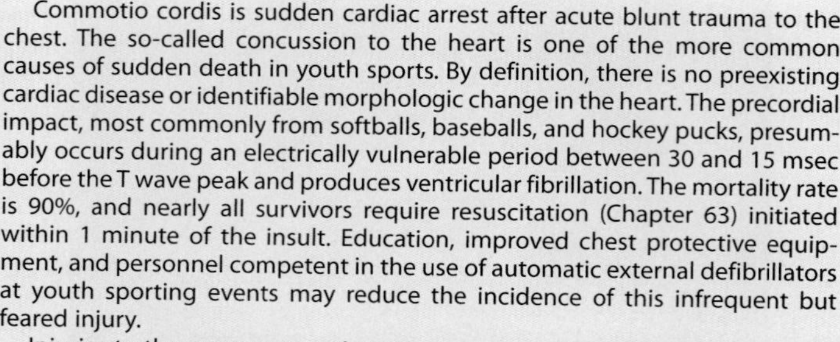

Commotio cordis is sudden cardiac arrest after acute blunt trauma to the chest. The so-called concussion to the heart is one of the more common causes of sudden death in youth sports. By definition, there is no preexisting cardiac disease or identifiable morphologic change in the heart. The precordial impact, most commonly from softballs, baseballs, and hockey pucks, presumably occurs during an electrically vulnerable period between 30 and 15 msec before the T wave peak and produces ventricular fibrillation. The mortality rate is 90%, and nearly all survivors require resuscitation (Chapter 63) initiated within 1 minute of the insult. Education, improved chest protective equipment, and personnel competent in the use of automatic external defibrillators at youth sporting events may reduce the incidence of this infrequent but feared injury.

Injuries to the coronary arteries are uncommon. Potential vascular injuries include laceration, intimal disruption with dissection, and vasospasm. The sequelae and treatment are similar to those for myocardial ischemia from atherosclerotic occlusion (Chapter 73).

Back

Palpation of the thoracic and lumbar spine combined with a thorough history is sufficient to exclude a thoracolumbar spine fracture in an alert patient. Ongoing back discomfort or a mechanism suggestive of the possibility of injury should lead to radiographic examination of the spine.

Abdomen

The abdominal contents may be injured by blunt or penetrating mechanisms. The ability to identify intra-abdominal injury is limited on physical examination. If the patient is hemodynamically stable, has a normal abdominal examination, and has sustained no other injuries that warrant operative repair, serial abdominal examination, a complete blood count, and amylase and lipase levels suffice. If there is any question about the normality of the abdominal examination or the ability to monitor the patient reliably, further evaluation is warranted.

Abdominal CT has proved a reliable determinant of intra-abdominal injury in a stable patient (Fig. 112-4). It identifies both intraperitoneal and retroperitoneal injury (Fig. 112-5). CT evaluation can identify sources of blood loss and help decide whether the problem requires operative exploration.

The most frequently injured intra-abdominal organ is the spleen. Left-sided rib fractures, left upper quadrant pain or tenderness, and pain referred to the left shoulder secondary to diaphragmatic irritation are suggestive of splenic injury. CT allows definition of the grade of splenic injury and detection of free intraperitoneal blood. Hemodynamic instability, ongoing blood loss, and CT findings of a high-grade injury to the spleen are all indications for splenectomy or, preferably, splenorrhaphy for salvage of the damaged spleen with preservation of splenic function.

Blunt injury to the liver is often associated with right-sided rib fractures and right upper quadrant tenderness with or without peritonitis. An abdominal CT scan with intravenous contrast material allows classification of the liver injury according to the location, depth, and extent of the hematoma or laceration. Currently, most (85%) blunt liver injuries are managed successfully nonoperatively if other intra-abdominal injuries do not require surgery.

Focused abdominal sonography in trauma (FAST) has a sensitivity of 95% for detecting free blood in the abdomen (Fig. 112-6). FAST sequentially surveys for the presence or absence of blood in the pericardial sac and dependent abdominal regions, including the right upper quadrant, left upper quadrant, and pelvis. Evaluation of the pericardial sac also allows the operator to identify tamponade physiology (Chapter 77). FAST is limited in its ability to identify the

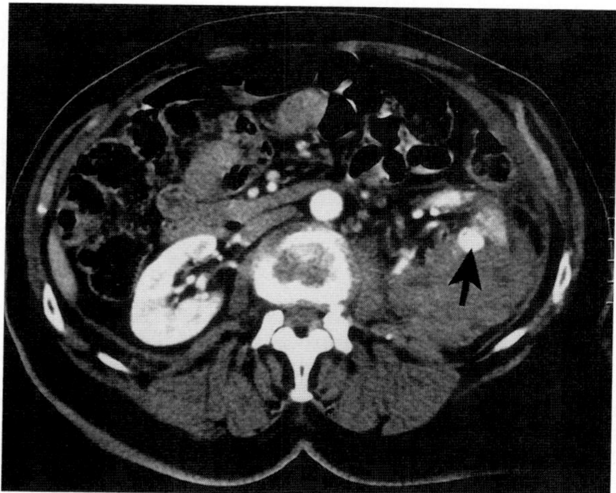

FIGURE 112-5. Intraperitoneal and retroperitoneal injury. An abdominal computed tomographic scan shows blood in the retroperitoneum surrounding a shattered left kidney, with pooling of contrast *(arrow)* in the kidney parenchyma. These findings are consistent with a pseudoaneurysm of a branch of the left renal artery.

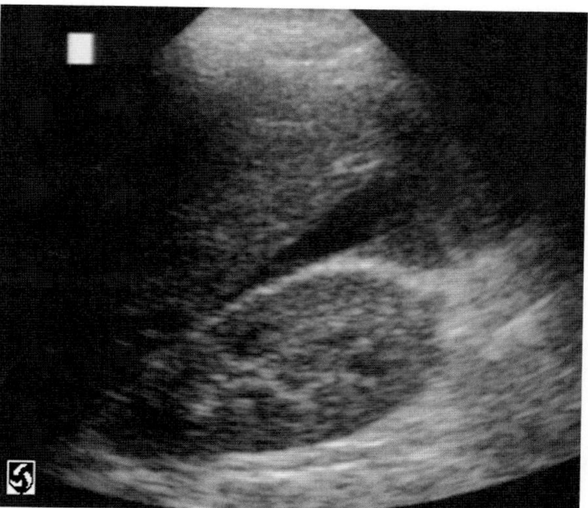

FIGURE 112-6. Positive focal abdominal sonography in trauma (FAST) study. There is a collection of fluid that shows up as a black strip between the liver and kidney. The white appearance is fat around the kidney. These findings are consistent with a fluid collection in Morrison's pouch.

source of bleeding and the retroperitoneal structures. It is effective in a pregnant trauma patient and allows evaluation of the fetus.

An alternative to FAST is diagnostic peritoneal aspiration or lavage. In this approach, a small midline infraumbilical incision is made in the peritoneum to allow sampling of fluid in the peritoneal cavity. If blood is found, laparotomy is necessary to identify and correct the source.

Wounds that penetrate the anterior abdominal region are further divided into low-velocity stab wounds and gunshot wounds, each of which has a different management algorithm. Because mandatory laparotomy for stab wounds results in a high number of negative explorations, many institutions have adopted a selective approach. An unstable victim of an abdominal stab wound should be explored immediately in the operating room. In contrast, a stable patient can undergo local exploration of the wound to determine the depth of penetration. If the wound is superficial, it is irrigated and the patient is observed; if the wound extends beneath the fascia, the patient should undergo exploratory laparotomy to exclude intra-abdominal injury. All gunshot wounds to the anterior abdominal region, except injuries with tangential trajectories, are now routinely explored, but this approach may change in the future.

In an unstable patient or a patient with clinical signs of peritonitis, penetrating wounds to the flanks and posterior abdominal region require exploratory laparotomy. In a stable patient without peritoneal signs, a CT scan with oral, intravenous, and occasionally rectal contrast material may help identify injury to retroperitoneal structures, the ascending and descending colon, the duodenum, the pancreas, and the kidneys.

Pelvis, Perineum, and Buttocks

Clinical evaluation of the pelvis is accomplished through compression of the lateral and anterior aspect of the pelvis to elicit tenderness or bony instability. Rectal examination is essential to exclude bony fragments or blood. Bladder catheterization can identify hematuria and monitor urinary output as a reflection of intravascular volume. Scrotal hematoma, meatal blood, or a high-riding boggy prostate indicates potential urethral injury and requires a urethrogram before insertion of a Foley catheter. All patients with major trauma require an anteroposterior plain film of the pelvis to exclude pelvic or hip fractures. A wound in the perineum in the presence of a pelvic fracture represents an open fracture until proven otherwise.

Penetrating wounds of the buttocks should not be overlooked or underestimated. The likelihood of concomitant peritoneal penetration is 25%, with a mortality rate of 5%. Structures at risk include the retroperitoneal rectum, bladder, ureters, and major arterial and venous structures within the pelvis.

Extremities

Palpation of the long bones is performed to determine whether there is any tenderness or deformity. Range of motion should be assessed in all joints of the upper and lower extremities. Areas of concern on examination should be evaluated radiographically. If there is any suspicion of vascular injury, angiographic examination should be performed.

The compartments of the lower part of the leg are most prone to intracompartmental swelling from direct trauma, long bone fracture, or arterial injury with ischemia or bleeding. Palpation of rigid compartments suggests elevated compartment pressures, which may be measured directly; if pressures are elevated, four-compartment fasciotomies should be performed.

Penetrating wounds to an extremity require operative exploration if they are associated with an enlarging hematoma, active arterial bleeding, or absent arterial pulses. Penetrating wounds resulting in diminished or fluctuating pulses require arteriography to document arterial injury. Otherwise, extremity wounds in proximity to major arterial structures do not require an arteriogram, but the vascular territory should be observed for 24 hours.

MEDICAL ASPECTS OF BURNS

EPIDEMIOLOGY

The National Fire Prevention and Control Administration estimates that 2.6 million fires are reported annually in the United States. About 500,000 burn injuries occur per year and result in about 4000 deaths. About 75% of these deaths occur at the scene of the incident or during initial transport. The most common age groups involved are toddlers (2 to 4 years), for whom scalding is the most common cause, and young adults (17 to 25 years), usually male, for whom the most common cause is a flammable liquid. Structural fires account for less than 5% of hospital admissions but are responsible for more than 45% of burn-related deaths.

Burns can be categorized as scalds, contact burns, and flame burns. Scald burns are the predominant injury in children, whereas contact and flame burns are most common in adults. The major cause of the injury to the skin is exposure to high temperature, which destroys surface tissue. Flames result in temperatures of several thousand degrees Fahrenheit, especially in a closed space. Because water can conduct heat 1000 times better than air, a much lower temperature (about 48 to 55° C, or 120 to 130° F) is required to produce a deep burn from hot liquid.

Chemical and electrical burns (Chapter 111), although often severe, account for less than 5% of burn admissions. The mechanism of a chemical burn is protein coagulation of skin caused by the acid or alkali. The injury progresses until the chemical is removed by aggressive water lavage. An electrical burn produces tissue coagulation along the course of passage of the current. This deeper injury is hidden from view and must be anticipated to make an early diagnosis and initiate effective treatment.

PATHOBIOLOGY

The skin is the largest organ of the body and ranges from 0.25 m^2 in a newborn to more than 2 m^2 in an adult (Chapter 443). The outermost layer of the epidermis is composed of dead, cornified cells that act as a tough protective barrier against the environment. The second, thicker layer, the corneum (0.06 to 0.12 mm), is composed chiefly of fibrous connective tissue. The dermis contains the blood vessels and nerves to the skin and the epithelial appendages of specialized function. The nerve endings that mediate pain are found in the dermis. Partial-thickness injuries are extremely painful because the nerve endings are exposed. Full-thickness burns are usually anesthetic because of destruction of the nerves.

The skin is also the barrier that prevents loss of body heat and fluids by evaporation. Sweat glands help maintain body temperature by controlling the amount of heat lost by evaporation. Increased loss of water and heat through burned skin is a major problem early after a burn. In addition, the skin is the primary protective barrier against invasive infection. The skin also detects the sensations of touch, pressure, pain, cold, and heat; loss of this function leads to long-term impairment.

TREATMENT

Rx

A burned patient undergoes many dramatic physiologic and metabolic changes over the course of the injury. The burn injury is divided into four phases, each of which has many different physiologic and metabolic characteristics: (1) resuscitation phase (0 to 36 hours), (2) postresuscitation phase (2 to 6 days), (3) inflammation and infection phase (7 days to wound closure), and (4) rehabilitation and wound-remodeling phase (admission to 1 year afterward).

Resuscitation Phase (0 to 36 hours)

Life-threatening airway and breathing problems are of major immediate concern, with the effects of smoke inhalation injury being the most concerning problem (Chapter 94). The initial phase is also characterized by hypovolemia as plasma volume is lost into the burned tissue. The burn itself is of less immediate concern except for initial assessment regarding its severity and depth and the selected need for escharotomy. Wound management becomes a higher priority in later phases. The adequacy of initial treatment of pulmonary and circulatory abnormalities sets the stage for subsequent management.

Smoke Inhalation Injury

The first priority in managing a burn victim is recognition and treatment of smoke exposure. Inhalation injury can be divided into three components based on the onset of symptoms and pathophysiology (Table 112-2).

Carbon Monoxide Toxicity

Carbon monoxide and sometimes cyanide toxicity is evident immediately, with peak symptoms occurring at the scene of the inhalation (Chapter 94). Carbon monoxide rapidly displaces oxygen from hemoglobin and produces carboxyhemoglobin, which impairs oxygen delivery to tissues. The peak level

TABLE 112-2 SMOKE INHALATION COMPLEX

CARBON MONOXIDE (CYANIDE) TOXICITY
Onset of peak symptoms is immediate Symptoms are systemic
SUPRAGLOTTIC INJURY
Onset of peak symptoms is delayed (hours) Problem is upper airway edema
INFRAGLOTTIC INJURY
Onset of peak symptoms is delayed (days) Problem is lower airway mucosal injury

of carboxyhemoglobin also occurs at the scene of the burn; its half-life is about 20 minutes. Treatment is 100% oxygen. Symptoms, which range from confusion to coma, resolve with oxygen therapy unless the patient also suffered severe anoxic injury. The use of hyperbaric oxygen remains controversial in this situation.

Cyanide, which is present in smoke, is absorbed rapidly through the lung and causes systemic toxicity. Cyanide levels are difficult to obtain, but an unexplained base deficit can be assumed to be due to cyanide mitochondrial toxicity; treatment consists of oxygen along with sodium thiosulfate and hydroxocobalamin.

Supraglottic Injury

Smoke injures the mucosa above the glottis because of the combination of superheated air and the toxins in smoke. Mucosal edema, which usually develops over a period of several hours, impedes and potentially obstructs the upper airway. Early endotracheal intubation is indicated if significant edema is evident on direct laryngoscopy, especially if the edema is increasing on subsequent examinations. Upper airway edema generally resolves in 3 to 4 days.

Infraglottic Injury

Toxins in the inhaled air or coating the inhaled soot particles damage the tracheobronchial mucosa, but heat does not usually reach this level. The extent of damage depends on the toxicity of the chemicals and the duration of exposure. Symptoms vary from transient bronchospasm to sloughing of the airway mucosa, which results in plugging and infection. Bronchoscopic evidence of erythema and edema indicates that an injury has occurred but does not predict the degree of injury or time course to recovery.

Endotracheal intubation and positive-pressure ventilation are indicated if symptoms increase, especially if there is an early and progressive impairment in gas exchange. Aggressive pulmonary toilet is necessary to avoid respiratory failure. The time course to resolution may be days or weeks.

Burn Shock and Resuscitation

Adequate volume resuscitation is crucial to survival of the victim of a major body burn. Hypovolemia can also rapidly lead to conversion of viable burned tissue to a nonviable, full-thickness burn, thus further increasing mortality. With modern treatment in burn centers, the failure rate of initial volume restoration is less than 5%, even for large burns involving greater than 85% of the total body skin surface.

Two processes lead to postburn hypovolemia: an increase in microvascular permeability in the burn wound and an increase in the osmolarity of surface burn tissue. A large intravascular-to-extravascular plasma shift occurs. The phase of rapid loss of intravascular fluid persists for about 24 to 36 hours.

Isotonic crystalloid, preferably lactated Ringer's solution, is used in the first 24 hours. Normal saline in large amounts predictably leads to hyperchloremic metabolic acidosis. A volume of 4 mL/kg is given for each percent of body surface burned, with 50% given in the first 8 hours and 50% in the subsequent 16 hours. Isotonic crystalloid is used for the first 24 hours in view of the change in skin capillary permeability for protein. Albumin can be added to the resuscitation fluid to maintain a serum albumin level greater than 2.5 g/dL. After the acute injury, the major fluid loss is water from the injured skin surface, which is no longer able to act as a barrier to the evaporation of water.

Burn Wound

The initial management of a burn wound is based on knowledge of the anatomy of the skin and the functional losses with injury. The major objectives are to decrease the potential for further local damage and the systemic abnormalities that can be produced by loss of the barrier function. Early treatment focuses on neutralizing the source of burn injury, avoiding excess heat loss, determining the extent of the injury, cleaning and débriding the wound, controlling infection with topical antibiotics, and maintaining tissue perfusion.

Assessment of Burn Depth and Size

Burns are categorized as partial thickness or full thickness. A partial-thickness burn is defined by destruction of the epidermis and a portion of the dermis; a superficial partial-thickness burn is confined to the upper third of the dermis, a mid partial-thickness burn involves the middle third, and a deep partial-thickness burn leaves only a portion of the dermis viable. For management purposes, a deep partial-thickness burn is managed similarly to a full-thickness burn: wound excision and skin grafting are required. The approach to superficial partial-thickness burns is to provide for optimal healing, which is initiated by the remaining viable epidermal cells in the hair follicles. Burn size in older children and adults is determined by the percentage of total skin surface area that is involved by the burn (Fig. 112-7).

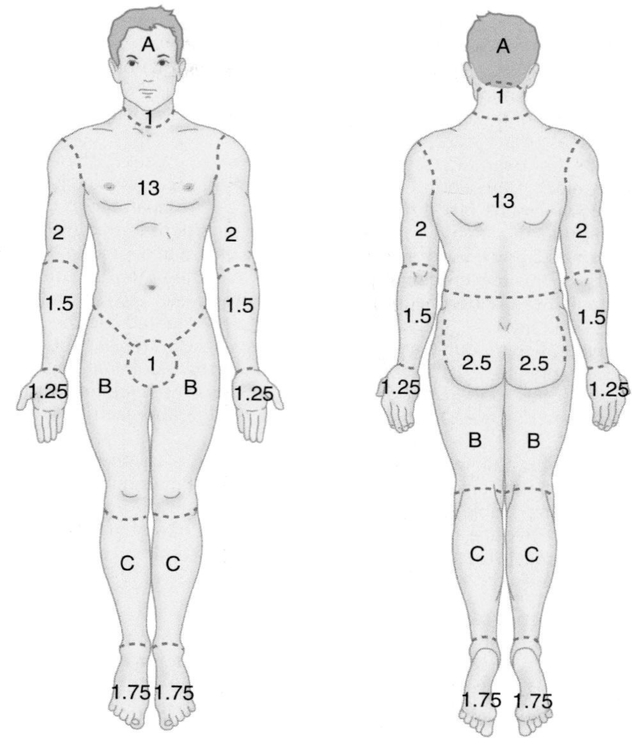

Relative percentages of areas affected by growth			
	Age		
Area	10	15	Adult
A = half of head	5.5	4.5	3.5
B = half of one thigh	4.25	4.5	4.75
C = half of one leg	3	3.25	3.5

FIGURE 112-7. Assessment tool for assessing burn size as a percentage of total body surface area.

Postresuscitation Phase (2 to 6 days)

The early postresuscitation phase is a period of transition from the shock phase to the hypermetabolic phase. In general, cardiopulmonary stability is optimal during this period because wound inflammation and infection have not yet developed. Early wound excision and grafting are initiated during this period. Operative risks, especially blood loss and septicemia, are substantially less than later, when inflammation and infection are common.

Pulmonary Support

Continued upper airway maintenance with an endotracheal tube may be required. Placement of the patient with the head elevated 30 to 45 degrees allows faster resolution of edema. Deciding when to extubate is difficult, and the degree of lower airway injury dictates the timing. Laryngoscopy to determine the presence of cord edema is helpful. Extubation should not be performed unless reintubation is feasible. Lower airway injury is managed by aggressive pulmonary toilet for increased sputum production and microbial overgrowth. Progressive tracheobronchitis and bronchopneumonia are common. The predicted extravascular-to-intravascular fluid shift results in an increased risk for pulmonary edema. Increased levels of antidiuretic stress hormones can prevent appropriate diuresis.

Hemodynamic Stability

The postresuscitation period is characterized by major fluid shifts mainly from the extravascular to the intravascular fluid space. Edema in burned tissue is maximum between 24 and 30 hours after injury in patients with well-controlled fluid resuscitation. The red blood cell mass continues to decrease. Electrolyte and acid-base changes are prominent.

Evaporation from the surface of the burn is a major source of water loss that persists until the wound is closed. The loss is measured in terms of water vapor pressure at the surface. In normal skin, vapor pressure is 2 to 3 mm Hg, whereas the pressure is about 32 mm Hg in a full-thickness burn in which the eschar is soft and hydrated. The rate of loss is increased with increasing surface blood flow. A reasonable estimate of the average loss per hour can be obtained from the following formula: evaporative water loss (mL/hr) = (25 + % total body surface burn) × body surface area (m^2).

Burn Wound

The wound undergoes dramatic changes during the next several days as inflammation develops. Of particular importance is the potential for change in the zone of injured, but still viable, tissue. Changes in local wound microcirculatory blood flow as a result of vasoactive inflammatory agents or local infection can convert this zone of ischemia to a zone of necrosis.

TABLE 112-3 MOST COMMON ORGANISMS IN BURN INFECTIONS

	STAPHYLOCOCCUS AUREUS	PSEUDOMONAS AERUGINOSA	CANDIDA ALBICANS
Wound appearance	Loss of wound granulation	Surface necrosis, patchy black	Minimal exudates
Course	Slow onset, 2-5 days	Rapid onset, 12-36 hr	Slow onset, days
Central nervous system	Disorientation	Modest changes	Often no change
Temperature	Marked increase	High or low	Modest changes
White blood cells	Marked increase	High or low	Modest changes
Hypotension	Modest	Often severe	Minimal change
Mortality	5%	20-30%	30-50%

Hypermetabolic-Sepsis Phase (7 Days to Recovery)

The generalized inflammation of the final phase alters organ function and magnifies any preexisting organ dysfunction. The burn wound is now colonized with bacteria, so wound sepsis is of prominent concern. Infection, whether in the lung or burn wound, becomes increasingly difficult to diagnose because of the continued presence of a non-infection-induced hyperdynamic state. Multisystem organ failure, if it is to occur, is seen during this period.

Burn Wound Infection

Burn wounds are never sterile, even with the administration of topical agents or systemic antibiotics. The presence of bacteria just on the wound surface is termed *colonization*. Colonization may be with a single type of organism or with multiple types. Infection of the wound (Table 112-3) indicates invasion of the underlying viable tissue; this process is diagnosed by eschar biopsy and quantitative culture showing greater than 10^5 organisms per gram of tissue. With progression, viable tissue and its blood vessels are invaded, and septicemia develops. Wound infections require systemic antibiotics. Because all patients have a hyperdynamic state with an elevated temperature and leukocytosis, it is difficult to make a diagnosis of infection based on systemic symptoms. Optimally, most of the eschar should be removed in the first week to avoid burn wound sepsis. *Staphylococcus aureus* is the most common organism isolated from the burn, especially during the first week.

Hypermetabolic State

Beginning at day 5 or 6, there is a gradual increase in the metabolic rate from a normal of 35 to 40 cal/m²/hr (25 cal/kg/day) to levels twice this value at about 10 days. The increase in metabolic rate after burns is far in excess of that seen after any other severe injury, including sepsis. The magnitude of the increase is related to the size of the burn. The hypermetabolic state is characterized by increased oxygen consumption, increased heat production, increased body temperature, and increased protein catabolism. Body temperature increases from normal to 38 to 38.5° C (100 to 101° F) because of resetting of the hypothalamic temperature center as a result of the altered hormonal environment (Chapter 288).

Marked and sustained increases in circulatory catecholamines lead to hypermetabolism, and treatment with β-blockers (e.g., propranolol titrated to reduce the resting heart rate by 20%)[5] may reduce muscle catabolism. Sustained increases in glucagon and glucocorticoids result in excessive gluconeogenesis and an insulin-resistant state. Increased glucocorticoids also lead to a severe catabolic state, especially because anabolic hormones (growth hormone and testosterone) are decreased after a burn injury.

Nutritional Support

Optimal nutritional support is essential and can decrease net catabolism by about 50%. Currently, there is no recognized ideal nutritional program because of evolving changes with new research findings on postburn nutrient processing. Decreasing stress by wound closure and control of pain, heat loss, and hypovolemia further controls the hypermetabolism. Caloric requirements can be measured with indirect calorimetric techniques. Because more than 95% of the energy generated requires oxygen, there is a direct relationship between oxygen consumption and the metabolic rate. Caloric needs can be estimated by the formula whereby energy requirements = basal metabolic rate × 1.25 × stress factor; the stress factor is 1.2 for a 10% burn, 1.5 for a 20% burn, 1.7 for a 30% burn, 1.8 for a 40% burn, and 2.0 for a 50% or greater burn. If the activity level is increased markedly or additional stress (e.g., severe pain) is present, the metabolic rate can be increased further.

Nutrients Required

Carbohydrate is the preferred fuel for most tissues, but there is a limit to the amount that is used, especially in a hypermetabolic or septic patient (Chapters 221, 223, and 224). Current recommendations are that carbohydrate infusions not exceed 5 to 7 mg/kg per minute, or approximately 1800 to 2200 carbohydrate calories per day. Excess carbohydrate results in the formation of fat, which requires energy rather than produces energy. Approximately 50% of the estimated calorie requirements is usually given as glucose to spare nitrogen. Fat is used as a calorie source, but fat should account for no more than 30% of the total calories. Protein represents 20 to 25% of infused calories. A standard estimate of 1.5 to 2 g of protein per kilogram of body weight can be used for all major burns. Necessary vitamins and trace elements should be provided in the form of high-potency multivitamin-mineral pills or liquid.

Route of Administration of Nutrition

Nutritional support is best managed during this period by the enteral route, generally through a combination of balanced tube feeding and voluntary intake (Chapter 223). Parenteral hyperalimentation (Chapter 224) through a central vein is occasionally required if for some reason the gastrointestinal tract is not functioning adequately, as sometimes occurs in a patient on a ventilator or a patient with sepsis.

Use of Anabolic Agents

An increase in anabolic activity can decrease the catabolic response to burns, thereby preserving lean body mass, which improves all aspects of wound healing. Glutamine, a conditionally essential amino acid, is invariably deficient several days after a burn because of increased utilization and decreased intake. Glutamine supplementation in major burns, at a dose of 0.4 g/kg body weight, improves wound healing and decreases infections and mortality.[6] Endogenous levels of anabolic human growth hormone and testosterone are decreased after burn surgery, and insulin resistance often develops. These intrinsic changes are all detrimental to wound healing. Supplemental human growth hormone significantly decreases the rate of muscle loss and increases wound healing.[7] Similarly, insulin infusion with glucose in burn patients increases lean mass loss and improves outcome.

The only anabolic steroid approved by the U.S. Food and Drug Administration to treat weight loss and catabolism is oxandrolone, which is given orally (10 mg twice a day), is excreted by the kidney, and has no effects on metabolism other than protein synthesis. Oxandrolone acts on androgenic receptors in lean mass, especially on skin fibroblasts. A number of studies have demonstrated its ability to preserve lean mass after burn injury and thereby improve local healing.[8] In addition, several recent studies have demonstrated direct wound-healing properties.

Rehabilitation after burns is critical to recovery. An augmented exercise program can effectively treat deconditioning and improve subsequent aerobic capacity.[9]

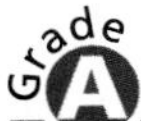

1. Stiell IG, Nesbitt LP, Pickett W, et al. The OPALS Major Trauma Study: impact of life-support on survival and morbidity. *CMAJ*. 2008;178:1141-1152.
2. Watkins TR, Rubenfeld GD, Martin TR, et al. Effects of leukoreduced blood on acute lung injury after trauma: a randomized controlled trial. *Crit Care Med*. 2008;36:1493-1499.
3. Shakur H, Roberts R, Bautista R, et al, for the CRASH-2 Trial Collaborators. Effects of tranexamic acid on death, vascular occlusive events, and blood transfusion in trauma patients with significant haemorrhage (CRASH-2): a randomised, placebo-controlled trial. *Lancet*. 2010; 376:23-32.
4. SAFE Study Investigators, Australian and New Zealand Intensive Care Society Clinical Trials Group, Australian Red Cross Blood Service, et al. Saline or albumin for fluid resuscitation in patients with traumatic brain injury. *N Engl J Med*. 2007;357:874-884.
5. Herndon DN, Hart DW, Wolf SE, et al. Reversal of catabolism by beta-blockade after severe burns. *N Engl J Med*. 2001;345:1223-1229.
6. Garrel D, Patenaude J, Nedelec B, et al. Decreased mortality and infectious morbidity in adult burn patients given enteral glutamine: a prospective controlled randomized clinical trial. *Crit Care Med*. 2003;10:2444-2449.
7. Ramirez R, Wolf S, Herndon D. Growth hormone treatment in pediatric patients: a safe therapeutic approach. *Ann Surg*. 1998;4:439-448.
8. Demling R, Orgil D. The anticatabolic and wound-healing effects of the testosterone analog oxandrolone after severe burn injury. *J Crit Care*. 2000;15:12-17.
9. de Lateur BJ, Magyar-Russell G, Bresnick MG, et al. Augmented exercise in the treatment of deconditioning from major brain injury. *Arch Phys Med Rehabil*. 2007;88:S18-S23.

SUGGESTED READINGS

Milia DJ, Brasel K. Current use of CT in the evaluation and management of injured patients. *Surg Clin North Am.* 2011;91:233-248. *Review.*

Moore CL, Copel JA. Point-of-care ultrasonography. *N Engl J Med.* 2011;364:749-757. *Review emphasizing its utility in the emergency department and in seriously ill patients.*

Rafla K, Tredget EE. Infection control in the burn unit. *Burns.* 2011;37:5-15. *Review of epidemiology, diagnosis, management, and prevention.*

Roppolo LP, Wigginton JG, Pepe PE. Intravenous fluid resuscitation for the trauma patient. *Curr Opin Crit Care.* 2010;16:283-288. *Review including evidence for plasma and factor VIIa.*

Wolf SJ, Bebarta VS, Bonnett CJ, et al. Blast injuries. *Lancet.* 2009;374:405-415. *Review.*

113 VENOMOUS SNAKE BITES

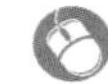

STEVEN A. SEIFERT, JAMES O. ARMITAGE, AND G. RALPH COREY

About 500 of the approximately 2900 species of snakes are venomous, and more than 200 species have caused fatal envenomation in humans. It has been estimated that, worldwide, there are up to 5 million snake bites annually, causing up to 125,000 deaths.

EPIDEMIOLOGY

The incidence of venomous snake bites varies enormously throughout the world. Snake-free areas consist primarily of islands, and Europe continues to be the continent with the lowest incidence of venomous snake bites. In the United States, it is estimated that up to 8000 venomous bites by native species occur each year, mostly by pit vipers (rattlesnakes, copperheads, cottonmouths), with fewer than 100 bites by coral snakes, the only native elapid. Fortunately, the number of fatalities, primarily caused by rattlesnakes, is less than 10 per year. Children and possibly pregnant women are at highest risk for complications. In addition, there are approximately 50 venomous snake bites a year in the United States by non-native (exotic) species; most of these snakes are in private collections, but also in zoos and academic institutions. In the past 10 years, human envenomation by more than 90 different non-native species has occurred. The majority of bites are by viperids, with about 40% by elapids, mostly cobras. The case-fatality rate of exotic envenomation is an order of magnitude higher than that of native species, because of both the number of highly venomous animals that are kept and the logistical issues of management. Most bites occur on extremities when snakes are threatened by being trod on, by someone reaching without looking, or by intentional handling of venomous snakes. Because the crotaline antivenom in the United States is effective against all U.S. crotaline species (and because coral snakes are easily identifiable), there is no need to capture or kill the offending snake for purposes of genus or species identification; such actions only increase the risk of a second envenomation or additional victims. Prevention of snake bite is better than therapy.

Venomous snakes belong to one of five families: Viperidae, with its two subfamilies—Viperinae, or Old World vipers, and Crotalinae, or pit vipers (e.g., rattlesnakes, copperheads, cottonmouths [water moccasins]); Elapidae (e.g., cobras, mambas, kraits, coral snakes); Hydrophiidae (e.g., sea snakes); Atractaspididae (e.g., asps); and Colubridae (e.g., garter snakes, corn snakes, boomslangs). Although all five families contain venomous species, the two responsible for more than 90% of venomous bites are Viperidae and Elapidae. In North America, pit vipers, named for the heat-sensitive organ between the eye and nostril used for hunting warm-blooded prey, are responsible for the majority of venomous snake bites. Fatalities are rare because of a well-developed health care system and the ready availability of antivenom.

In Europe, the only snake of importance is the adder, a viperid snake. Bites are uncommon and rarely fatal. Australia is home to numerous very dangerous Elapidae, including the taipan, death adder, tiger snake, and eastern brown snake. As a result, there are many serious bites each year, despite the low-density population. Fatalities are infrequent, however.

In Central and South America, pit vipers are the primary subfamily responsible for human envenomation; rattlesnakes (Crotalinae, *Sistrurus*) and the *Bothrops* species (*Bothrops jararaca,* fer-de-lance) are responsible for the high morbidity and mortality. The largest venomous snake in the Americas is the bushmaster (*Lachesis muta muta*).

Africa is home to a large number of venomous species. Elapids (cobras and mambas) and the Old World vipers (e.g., saw-scaled viper, puff adder) are among the most prevalent and dangerous of all the world's snakes.

Asia produces the largest number of fatalities from snake envenomation. In India and its eastern neighbors, elapids and viperids are prominent. Cobras, kraits, pit vipers, saw-scaled vipers, and Russell's viper inflict most of the injuries. Although antivenoms are available for most African and Asian snakes of clinical importance, mortality remains high because the health care system is less well developed in these regions.

PATHOBIOLOGY

Snake venoms are complex poisons and often consist of dozens of components that immobilize and digest prey. The effects of venom may be neurotoxic, cardiotoxic, hemotoxic, or myotoxic. Particular species generally produce a characteristic envenomation profile, but the presence or absence of particular components may be variable even within a single species.

Local swelling and bruising after a bite are caused by increased vascular permeability as a result of endothelial cell damage and are mediated by hydrolases, proteases, phospholipase A_2, polypeptide toxins, metalloproteinases, and the release of endogenous autacoids such as bradykinin and histamine. Snakes from the Viperidae and Elapidae families are primarily responsible for these effects.

Hemostatic abnormalities are frequent and varied. Pro-coagulants activate factors V, IX, and X, protein C (Russell's viper), and prothrombin (vipers) and cleave fibrinopeptide A from fibrinogen. Fibrinolytic activators result in a disseminated intravascular coagulation (DIC)–like picture, although there are key differences from true DIC, including the absence of thrombin formation and the failure of heparin therapy in snake evenomation. Snake venom hemorrhagins damage endothelium and increase the potential for serious bleeding, especially after viper bites. Intravascular hemolysis, which can occur after bites by *Bothrops* (e.g., fer-de-lance) and other species, results in severe anemia and acute renal failure.

Paralysis is the primary function of many types of venom of the Elapidae and Hydrophiidae families and of some Viperidae snakes. Presynaptic neurotoxins (e.g., β-bungarotoxins, crotoxin, taipoxin) prevent acetylcholine release, and postsynaptic toxins (e.g., α-bungarotoxins, cobrotoxin) bind to acetylcholine receptors on the motor end plate.

Rhabdomyolysis (Chapter 115) occurs most commonly from the presynaptic neurotoxins of sea snakes, but myotoxins have also been found in Australasian elapids, Russell's viper, and selected rattlesnakes. Acute renal failure, hyperkalemia, and death often result. Other mechanisms of renal failure after envenomation include a direct renal toxin, hemoglobinuria after massive intravascular hemolysis, hypotension, and DIC-like defects.

Toxins that do not immobilize prey through neurotoxins may immobilize by causing hypotension. Some snakes (primarily vipers) produce an acute hypotensive syndrome within minutes after envenomation through the release of vasodilating autacoids. *Bothrops* species inhibit the breakdown of bradykinin and angiotensinogen (angiotensin-converting enzyme inhibitors). Vasodilation, diffuse vascular permeability, myocardial depression, and atrioventricular block all play roles in the hypotension caused by crotalines and elapids. Individuals who handle snakes or who have been bitten previously may develop an immunoglobulin (Ig) E–mediated anaphylactic reaction. A non-IgE-mediated anaphylactoid response may be seen with the rapid introduction of foreign proteins into circulation; nonspecific effects, such as vagal reactions and hypovolemia secondary to massive tissue fluid accumulation as a result of local venom injury, may also produce hypotension.

CLINICAL MANIFESTATIONS

Pit Viper Envenomation

Swelling and pain are the first and most important findings of early pit viper envenomation. These symptoms often occur within minutes and are followed by progressive proximal swelling and ecchymosis in the bitten extremity, although onset of the latter may be delayed for hours. Local swelling, usually extracompartmental, may be massive, and elevated tissue or compartmental pressures may occur from tension created by the skin's limited elasticity. Necrosis may develop as a consequence of direct venom-related tissue injury or possibly as a result of pressure-mediated vascular compromise. Necrosis typically occurs over a period of several days, with the potential for permanent tissue loss. Progression of local injury usually ceases within 24 to 36 hours. Secondary infection of snake bites is rare, but the presence of necrosis increases its likelihood. The development of systemic symptoms such as nausea, diaphoresis, paresthesias, metallic taste, and dizziness may indicate more severe envenomation. Hypotension and bleeding manifestations (e.g., distant petechiae; hematuria; gingival, gastrointestinal, central nervous system bleeding) may also occur early and pose the greatest risk for death. During the first 24 hours, the white blood cell count is often increased. Various coagulation abnormalities, alone or in combination, may be seen, including thrombocytopenia; elevated D-dimer or fibrin-fibrinogen degradation products, with or without hypofibrinogenemia; and prolongation of the international normalized ratio or activated partial thromboplastin time. Hematologic effects are more common with rattlesnake bites but can occur with copperhead or cottonmouth envenomation as well. Spontaneous bleeding is more likely with combined and severe coagulation system abnormalities. In patients with persistent hypotension, the presence of coma, acidosis, and oliguric renal failure presages death.

Progression of local injury may recur in the first 24 hours, particularly in patients treated with a Fab antivenom. This occurs as protective levels of circulating antivenom decline rapidly secondary to their larger volume of distribution compared with IgG or $F(ab')_2$ antivenoms and the renal clearance of unbound antivenom. This recurrence is not associated with a recurrence of detectable blood venom antigens and appears to be the result of a lack of adequate amounts of neutralizing antivenom at the leading margin of envenomated tissue. Coagulation system disorders may persist despite antivenom and may also recur. Recurrence of coagulation defects typically occurs several days after treatment with a Fab antivenom and is associated with the loss of protective circulating antivenom secondary to renal clearance, thereby allowing unneutralized venom still entering the circulation to exert its toxic effects. This recurrence is associated with detectable blood venom antigens. The specific hematologic abnormalities (e.g., thrombocytopenia) seen early in the course tend to recur, with similar degrees of severity ("like predicts like in kind and degree"). The ultimate severity of envenomations treated within 1 to 2 hours may have been masked, and such patients are also at risk of severe recurrence, despite apparently mild early effects. Recurrent coagulation abnormalities may persist or continue to recur following additional treatment, for up to 3 weeks.

Coral Snake Envenomation

Unlike the pit vipers, local symptoms after coral snake bites are often confined to paresthesias around the bite and mild swelling in a minority of patients. Systemic symptoms are often delayed for 1 to 6 hours. Because of species differences, coral snake bites in Florida (*Micrurus fulvius*) tend to be more severe than those in Texas (*Micrurus tener*). In the bordering states (Louisiana, Alabama), which may have either species, the risk of toxicity may be difficult to determine. Coral snake bites in Arizona and New Mexico (*Micruroides euryxanthus*) do not produce significant clinical effects. With severe envenomation, perioral paresthesias, nausea, vomiting, hypersalivation, and euphoria give way to cranial nerve paralysis (e.g., ptosis, diplopia, dysphagia) and respiratory failure. Respiratory failure may develop within minutes of the onset of neurologic signs.

TREATMENT Rx

Expert assistance in managing a snake bite of any kind can be obtained by contacting the regional poison center at 1-800-222-1222.

Snake bite is primarily a medical rather than a surgical condition. On a patient's arrival at an emergency care facility, primary attention should be given to assessing and establishing the airway, breathing, and circulation. Management might include antivenom administration, management of type I hypersensitivity reactions to snake venom or antivenom (e.g., epinephrine, H_1- and H_2-blockers), intravenous fluids, tetanus toxoid, airway protection, mechanical ventilation, pressors, pain medications, radiographs of the wound to rule out retained foreign bodies (fangs or teeth), and, later, physical therapy. Late surgical débridement of necrotic tissue, if any, may be required. Surgical treatment of elevated tissue or compartment pressures is very rarely indicated. Because of the inability of prophylactic antibiotics to prevent infection[1] and the potential of an adverse drug reaction occurring simultaneously with venom toxicity, antibiotics should be reserved for documented infection, a clinical appearance that cannot be easily distinguished from infection, or frank tissue necrosis.

A wide variety of ineffective and potentially harmful therapies for snake bite have been and, in some cases, continue to be popular (Table 113-1). Use of these methods in true envenomations may contribute to venom injury and could result in tragedy if they delay or supplant effective therapy.

TABLE 113-1 INEFFECTIVE OR POTENTIALLY HARMFUL REMEDIES FOR SNAKE BITE

LOCAL WOUND MEASURES
Aloe vera leaves
Cold
Electricity
Heat
Incision
Kerosene
Pineapple concentrate
Suction
Tourniquets (arterial or venous)
SYSTEMIC OR LOCAL MEASURES
Castor oil
Chinese herbs
Colloidal silver
Drinking water
Echinacea
Ethanol
Euphorbia
Grape juice
Impatiens
Lantana
Turmeric
Vitamin C

Pit Viper Envenomation

Prehospital

Appropriate care consists of immobilization of a bitten extremity, consideration of the need to slow systemic absorption by dependent positioning or lymphatic obstruction, and, most important, rapid transit to a hospital emergency department. Any treatment that increases or prolongs the local concentration of venom may result in greater local injury and should be used only when life-threatening systemic effects (e.g., profound hypotension, anaphylaxis, severe bleeding) are occurring. The application of a lymphatic constriction band (15 to 25 mm Hg) or a pressure immobilization bandage requires training and proper equipment and is rarely required. Popular prehospital treatments such as arterial or venous tourniquets, incision, suction, heat, cold, and electric shock are not helpful, can delay definitive treatment, and can cause additional trauma.

Hospital

The chance of a North American crotaline bite resulting in envenomation is around 80%. The onset of symptoms of pit viper envenomation is usually rapid and obvious but may be delayed for many hours. Potentially "dry" bites should be observed for at least 10 to 12 hours.

The ultimate severity of envenomation becomes apparent only over time, and "mild" envenomation may progress to "severe," depending on the venom load, venom components, and host factors. Definitive therapy for systemic symptoms of snake bite, including hypotension and coagulation abnormalities, is antivenom, which should be used for any significant or progressive envenomation. The starting dose is based on the severity of symptoms or signs and the rapidity of progression. Administration of blood product components is usually futile in the absence of adequate venom neutralization. With neutralization, the body replenishes platelets, fibrinogen, and clotting factors on its own. Blood products should be reserved for life-threatening bleeding and should be given in conjunction with additional antivenom.

The crotaline snake antivenom available in the United States, CroFab, consists of Fab antibodies to specific crotaline venoms that were raised in sheep. It is indicated and efficacious for all North American crotaline snakes.[2] Because antivenom contains foreign proteins, type I (immediate) hypersensitivity reactions are possible, including anaphylaxis. With Fab antivenom, predominantly mild type I hypersensitivity reactions have been reported to date in less than 7% of patients. Cutaneous sensitivity testing before administration is not recommended and does not adequately predict the likelihood of a type I reaction in other settings. Type I hypersensitivity reactions are managed by stopping or slowing the rate of infusion and by administering H_1-blockers (e.g., diphenhydramine 50 mg IV), H_2-blockers (e.g., ranitidine 50 mg IV or cimetidine 300 mg IV), and epinephrine (0.3 mg SC as a 1:1000 dilution) as needed. It is usually possible to restart the infusion at a slower rate after treatment and to give the complete dose, although a risk-benefit reassessment should be made regarding the ongoing need for antivenom. Means of treating anaphylaxis should always be immediately available.

The initial dose of Fab antivenom is 4 to 6 vials, regardless of the patient's weight, because the objective is to neutralize a specific quantity of injected venom. Children may, in fact, require higher doses because of higher serum venom levels (a larger venom dose relative to weight) and particular

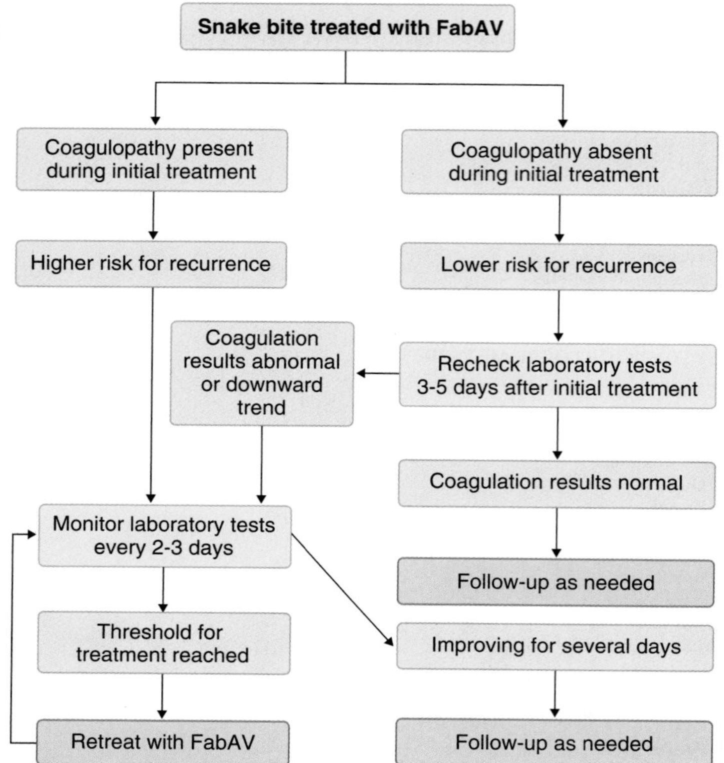

FIGURE 113-1. Monitoring for coagulopathy in patients treated with Crotalidae polyvalent immune Fab (ovine) (FabAV).

vulnerabilities, such as smaller airway size and the increased proportion of vascular volume lost into tissues. Additional antivenom doses may be administered as needed to obtain initial control of the signs and symptoms of envenomation. Initial control includes reversal of systemic symptoms, cessation of progression of proximal swelling or a reduction in circumferential swelling and tissue pressures, and cessation of worsening or evidence of improvement in coagulation components. Repeated dosing of Fab antivenom after initial control (2 vials every 6 hours for three doses) is recommended to prevent the recurrence of local effects (Fig. 113-1). Additional doses (2 vials) may be required for breakthrough local recurrences.

Management of elevated tissue or compartmental pressures (Chapter 115) is controversial. Dermotomy may be considered in areas without true compartments (e.g., fingers) if the degree of swelling compromises circulation; however, additional antivenom and elevation may reduce the swelling, making this procedure unnecessary. In practice, dermotomy is very rarely required. If there is concern about significantly elevated tissue or compartmental pressures, they should be measured directly. In general, additional antivenom and elevation are recommended for increased pressure (>30 mm Hg). Elevation is controversial because it decreases local tissue perfusion in the typical compartment syndrome. After snake bites, however, elevated compartmental pressures may be entirely secondary to subcutaneous edema and may respond to elevation with a proximal redistribution of tissue fluid and a reduction in tissue pressures. Conversely, in true compartment syndrome, owing to either direct intracompartmental injection of venom or lymphatic drainage of venom into the compartment, elevation may be harmful. Nevertheless, judicious elevation seems reasonable to see whether a reduction in pressures can avoid fasciotomy, which does not appear to be beneficial in compartment syndrome caused by venom injection.

Patients with early, severe coagulopathic abnormalities are at risk for recurrence of severe abnormalities of the same kind; about 70% of those with early coagulation defects return with late recurrences. Optimal management of severe recurrence is undetermined, but patients with severe abnormalities in multiple coagulation systems (e.g., platelets and fibrinogen) or with comorbid conditions (e.g., advanced age, hypertension, bleeding diathesis, risk-taking behavior) are at increased risk for significant bleeding and are candidates for repeat dosing of Fab antivenom (Table 113-2). Two vials should be given intravenously, and the patient should be monitored and possibly treated daily until a clear improving trend is observed (see Fig. 113-1).

Postacute Phase

In an effort to improve functional outcome, physical therapy should begin as soon as the acute phase of local injury has subsided, usually in 36 to 48 hours. Type III hypersensitivity reactions ("serum sickness," occurring 5 to 21

TABLE 113-2 RECOMMENDATIONS FOR RETREATMENT WITH ANTIVENOM FOR PERSISTENT OR RECURRENT HEMATOLOGIC ABNORMALITIES

Active, significant bleeding (in conjunction with blood products as needed)
Fibrinogen < 50 μg/mL
Platelet count < 25,000/mm^3
INR > 3.0 sec or aPTT > 50 sec
Multicomponent effects with lesser abnormalities
Worsening trend in a patient at risk for severe recurrence
High-risk behaviors for trauma in a patient with lesser abnormalities
Comorbid conditions that increase bleeding risk

aPTT = adjusted partial thromboplastin time; INR = international normalized ratio.

days after treatment) are usually mild with Fab antivenom but occur in up to 5% of cases. For management of mild type III hypersensitivity reactions, treatment is with nonsteroidal anti-inflammatory drugs (e.g., ibuprofen 200 to 800 mg orally four times a day as needed for arthralgia, myalgia, and fever) and antihistamines (e.g., diphenhydramine 25 to 50 mg orally four times a day as needed for urticaria). For more severe reactions, corticosteroids (e.g., prednisone 20 to 40 mg/day orally, with a taper over 2 weeks if treatment is needed for more than 5 days) are recommended. Type III reactions are self-limited and typically have a duration of 2 to 10 days, rarely lasting more than 3 to 4 weeks.

Coral Snake Envenomation

Prehospital

Appropriate care consists of immobilization of a bitten extremity and efforts to slow systemic absorption with the use of a pressure immobilization bandage. Proper application of this bandage requires training, and it is frequently misapplied by untrained providers; therefore, a lymphatic constriction band (blood pressure cuff inflated to 15 to 25 mm Hg) may be safer but possibly less effective. Most important is rapid transit to a hospital emergency department. Because local effects are minimal and neurologic toxicity may progress rapidly, there is little risk in the use of a properly applied pressure immobilization bandage or lymphatic constriction band. Popular prehospital treatments such as tourniquets, incision, suction, heat, cold, and electric shock are not helpful, can delay definitive treatment, and can cause additional trauma.

Hospital

The chance of a bite from an eastern coral snake resulting in envenomation is around 75%. The onset of neurologic symptoms may be quickly evident, but it may also be delayed for many hours. Because of minimal local effects and potentially delayed neurotoxicity, envenomation and the seriousness of such bites can easily be underestimated. The snake bite severity score is not valid for these snake bites. Potentially "dry" bites should be closely observed for at least 24 hours.

In the United States, the Food and Drug Administration–approved monovalent, equine IgG antivenom (manufactured by Wyeth) should be given at the first signs of envenomation by bites of the eastern coral snake (*Micrurus fulvius*) or the Texas coral snake (*Micrurus tener*). However, Wyeth ceased production in 2006, and supplies are limited and dwindling in endemic areas. It is estimated that replacement supplies will no longer be available in 2010 or 2011, after which remaining antivenom stocks, currently distributed primarily to hospitals in endemic areas, will gradually be consumed.

Skin testing is suggested by the manufacturer, although such testing is not adequately predictive of the risk for type I (immediate) hypersensitivity reactions, and an expert consensus panel has concluded that skin testing should not be performed. Regardless, testing should not delay administration in the event of life-threatening effects. When available, the initial dose is 3 to 6 vials, repeated as needed until progression of signs and symptoms ceases. Rarely are more than 10 vials required. Type III hypersensitivity reactions ("serum sickness") may occur; management is as described earlier.

If fresh Wyeth antivenom is not available, some advocate using expired Wyeth antivenom, despite medicolegal concerns. Neostigmine (infants, 0.025 to 0.1 mg/kg/dose; children, 0.025 to 0.08 mg/kg/dose; adults, 0.5 to 2.5 mg/dose, total dose not to exceed 5 mg) is efficacious against the neurotoxicity of other elapids, including several South American species of coral snake; doses can be repeated as needed to maintain reversal of blockade. Neostigmine may be considered a temporizing measure, adjunctive therapy, or monotherapy; however, there are no published reports on its use in U.S. coral snake envenomations. If neostigmine is used, atropine (0.4 mg per 1 mg of neostigmine) should be given several minutes before the neostigmine to counter unwanted cholinergic effects. Foreign antivenoms, which may have efficacy against U.S. coral snakes, can be located and obtained through the Antivenom Index, which can be accessed via the regional poison center (1-800-222-1222). If respiratory compromise results in intubation, days to weeks of respiratory support may be required.

Bites by Non-native Species

Management of bites by non-native species is challenging because of both their unfamiliarity and potential delays in obtaining appropriate antivenom, which is usually kept by zoos that have specimens of the biting species. Poison centers have access to information about zoo supplies of antivenom through an online listing, the Antivenom Index. Assistance in locating and obtaining species-specific antivenom and clinical case management can be obtained through the regional poison center (1-800-222-1222).

PROGNOSIS

In general, the prognosis is good if timely access to antivenom is possible. For coral snake bites, the mortality rate before the introduction of antivenom in 1967 was between 10 and 15%. Age and underlying disease can increase morbidity, particularly if hemorrhage and hypotension develop.

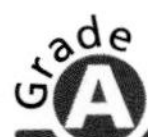

1. Kularatne SA, Kumarasiri PV, Pushpakumara SK, et al. Routine antibiotic therapy in the management of the local inflammatory swelling in venomous snakebites: results of a placebo-controlled study. *Ceylon Med J.* 2005;50:151-155.
2. Dart RC, Seifert SA, Boyer LV, et al. A randomized multicenter trial of crotalinae polyvalent immune Fab (ovine) antivenom for the treatment for crotaline snakebite in the United States. *Arch Intern Med.* 2001;161:2030-2036.

SUGGESTED READINGS

Kasturiratne A, Wickremasinghe AR, de Silva N, et al. The global burden of snakebite: a literature analysis and modelling based on regional estimates of envenoming and deaths. http://www.plosmedicine .org/article/info:doi/10.1371/journal.pmed.0050218. *Review of the worldwide morbidity and mortality burden of snake bite.*

Warrell D. Snake bite. *Lancet.* 2010;375:77-88. *Review of management.*

Weinstein SA, Dart RC, Staples A, et al. Envenomations: an overview of clinical toxinology for the primary care physician. *Am Fam Phys.* 2009;80:793-802. *Management of envenomation.*

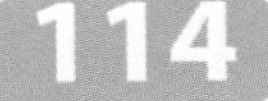

114 VENOMS AND POISONS FROM MARINE ORGANISMS

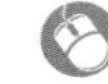

JAY W. FOX

The term *envenomation* implies penetration of a target by an organism for delivery of venom containing one or more toxins. In contrast, poisons are toxins acquired from the environment by mechanisms such as absorption, inhalation, and ingestion. In the marine environment, both forms of intoxication cause effects ranging from mild irritation and discomfort to death (Table 114-1). Severe outbreaks of poisoning can result from the ingestion of marine organisms that contain toxins, and such outbreaks have become more frequent as microorganisms in coastal waters increase, owing to a combination of global sea warming, eutrophication, aquaculture, and discharge of organisms from ship ballasts. Encroachment on the marine environment for recreation, living space, and food sources increases the frequency of adverse encounters with venomous and poisonous marine organisms.

VENOMOUS MARINE ORGANISMS

Venomous marine organisms deliver their venom by bites and stings. Envenomation involves penetration of the skin and may be complicated by secondary bacterial infections, especially after deep puncture wounds and bites.

Chordata

Sea Snakes

Sea snakes, which are members of the family *Hydrophiidae*, are generally found in tropical and subtropical waters, especially the coastal waters of Thailand, Indonesia, the Persian Gulf, Australia, and India. One species, the yellow-bellied sea snake (*Pelaramis platurus*), is found in the Pacific coastal waters of Central America. Sea snakes, which are very capable swimmers and are relatively immobile on land, inject their venom with two small maxillary fangs (2 to 4 mm long) that contain ducts connected to venom glands located posterior and ventral to the maxillary bone. The relatively short length of the fangs prevents effective envenomation through most protective clothing such as dive suits. If the subject reacts to envenomation by forceful retraction, the fangs are often dislodged from the maxillary bone of the snake and may remain in the site—a condition that imposes an additional risk for infection.

Because of the nature of the venom and the size of the fangs, the sea snake bite itself is not generally painful. One or two small prick marks are present at the envenomation site, occasionally with additional marks from the other teeth in the snake's mouth. The primary toxin in sea snake venom is a postsynaptic peptide neurotoxin that functions by blocking the acetylcholine receptor at neuromuscular junctions (Fig. 114-1). Ptosis, dysphagia, and nonrigid paralysis, which are the most common symptoms of sea snake envenomation, typically appear within 30 minutes to 2 hours after the bite. In severe cases, respiratory failure may develop, and respiratory support may be necessary. Antivenom is available.

Weeverfish, Lionfish, Scorpionfish, and Stonefish

Weeverfish belong to the *Trachinidae* family, whereas scorpionfish, stonefish, and lionfish all belong to the family *Scorpaenidae*. Members of the *Scorpaenidae* family are found mostly in tropical and subtropical waters, but weeverfish are in European and African waters. All of these fish sting by using dorsal spines. The anal spines of *Scorpaenidae* fish and the opercular spines of *Trachinidae* fish can also deliver venom. The spines are encased in an integumentary sheath that is torn when the spine punctures the victim's skin. Venom glands are located at the base of the spine.

Few details are known regarding the biochemistry and pharmacology of the toxins in weeverfish venom. The sting of the weeverfish is extremely painful and may produce systemic effects such as aphonia, fever, chills, dyspnea, cyanosis, nausea, syncope, hypotension, and arrhythmias. The wound is edematous, erythematous, and ecchymotic. Bacterial infection is typical, and gangrene has developed in severe cases of infection. The venom may be somewhat heat labile, and soaking in tolerably hot water may reduce pain and attenuate the effects of the venom. Death from an untreated weeverfish sting is rare.

Scorpaenidae envenomation symptoms are generally less severe for lionfish (*Pterois*), more severe for scorpionfish (*Scorpaena*), and most severe for stonefish (*Synanceia*). Lionfish (turkey fish, dragon fish, butterfly cod), which are found worldwide, have long thin spines. Scorpionfish have shorter, thicker spines and are primarily found in tropical and subtropical waters and the Mediterranean. The local consequences of edema and erythema from stings of these fish are very similar to those of the weeverfish. Immersion in hot water is generally effective to alleviate pain associated with envenomation.

The stonefish (*Synanceja*) group has short strong spines and is found throughout the Indo-Pacific area, China, Australia, and the Indian Ocean. Their toxins are high-molecular-weight, multimeric, heat-labile proteins. Symptoms of envenomation are similar to those from the stings of members of the other groups. A lethal toxin, stonustoxin, from the venom of *Synanceja horrida* causes muscle relaxation by producing nitric oxide and also causes hemolysis, platelet aggregation, and inhibition of neuromuscular function. Trachynilysin, a pore-forming neurotoxin from *Synanceja trachynis,* causes massive presynaptic release of acetylcholine. Soaking of the wound site in hot water (45° C) is recommended. In cases of severe blistering, the blisters should be excised to flush residual active venom from the blister fluid to ameliorate dermal necrosis. As with all fish stings, care should be taken to ensure that no broken portions of the spines remain in the wound; vigilance against bacterial infections is imperative. Antivenom should be used only if it is clear that envenomation has occurred.

Stingrays

Stingrays (family Dasyatidae) are found in most seas but are predominant in the Indo-Pacific area. Some members of the family are also found in fresh water. Venom containing serotonin is delivered by stings from spines (one or more) on the tail of the stingray. Stingray spines are retroserrated on the margins and are covered by an integumentary sheath. Venomous glandular tissue is located at the base of the spines. On puncture of the skin, the sheath is torn by the serrated spine, and venom flows along the two ventrolateral grooves of the spine into the surrounding tissue. The spines are often deeply embedded in the tissue and difficult to extract because of the retroserration. Care must be taken to remove all spine and sheath fragments. Depending on the location of the spine and the depth of penetration, specialized care may

TABLE 114-1 SIGNIFICANT VENOMOUS AND POISONOUS MARINE ORGANISMS

ORGANISM	MECHANISM OF INTOXICATION (EVENOMING/POISONING)	PRIMARY TOXINS	ANTIVENOM AVAILABLE (SOURCE)
Sea snakes (Hydrophiidae)	Bite	Postsynaptic neurotoxins	Yes (CSL, Ltd.)
Blue-ringed octopus (Octopodidae)	Bite	Tetrodotoxin (neurotoxin)	No
Cone shell (Conidae)	Sting	Presynaptic and postsynaptic neurotoxins	No
Box jellyfish *(Chironex fleckeri, Chiropsalmus quadrigatus)*	Sting	Hemolysins, proteinases, cardiotoxin, necrotoxins	Yes (CSL, Ltd.)
Portuguese man-of-war *(Physalia physalis)*	Sting	Hemolysins, proteinases, cardiotoxin, necrotoxins	No
Sea nettles *(Chrysaora quinquecirrha, Cyanea capillata)*	Sting	Hemolysins, proteinases, cardiotoxin, necrotoxins	No; generally no need
Sea anemone *(Anemonia sulcata)*	Sting	Neurotoxins	No; generally no need
Scorpionfish (Scorpaenidae)	Sting puncture	Hemolysins, necrotoxins?	Yes (CSL, Ltd.)
Lionfish (Scorpaenidae)	Sting puncture	Hemolysins, necrotoxins?	No
Stonefish (Scorpaenidae)	Sting puncture	Hemolysins, necrotoxins?	Yes (CSL, Ltd)
Weeverfish (Trachinidae)	Sting puncture	Hemolysins, necrotoxins?	No
Stingrays (Rajiformes)	Sting puncture	Uncertain	No
Dinoflagellates	Ingestion (found in seafood)	Ciguatera poisoning	No
Gambierdiscus toxicus	Ingestion (found in fish)	Ciguatoxins, maitotoxin (neurotoxins)	No
Ptychodiscus brevis	Ingestion (found in shellfish)	Neurotoxic shellfish poisoning, neurotoxins	No
Gonyaulax species	Ingestion (found in shellfish)	Paralytic shellfish poisoning	No
Pyrodinium species	Ingestion (found in shellfish)	Saxitoxin, neosaxitoxin, and gonyautoxin	No
Jania species	Ingestion (found in shellfish)	Okadaic acid (phosphatase inhibitors)	No
Pufferfish (Tetraodontiformes)	Ingestion	Tetrodotoxin (neurotoxin)	No
Porcupinefish (Tetraodontiformes)	Ingestion	Tetrodotoxin (neurotoxin)	No
Sunfish (*Mola* species)	Ingestion	Tetrodotoxin (neurotoxin)	No

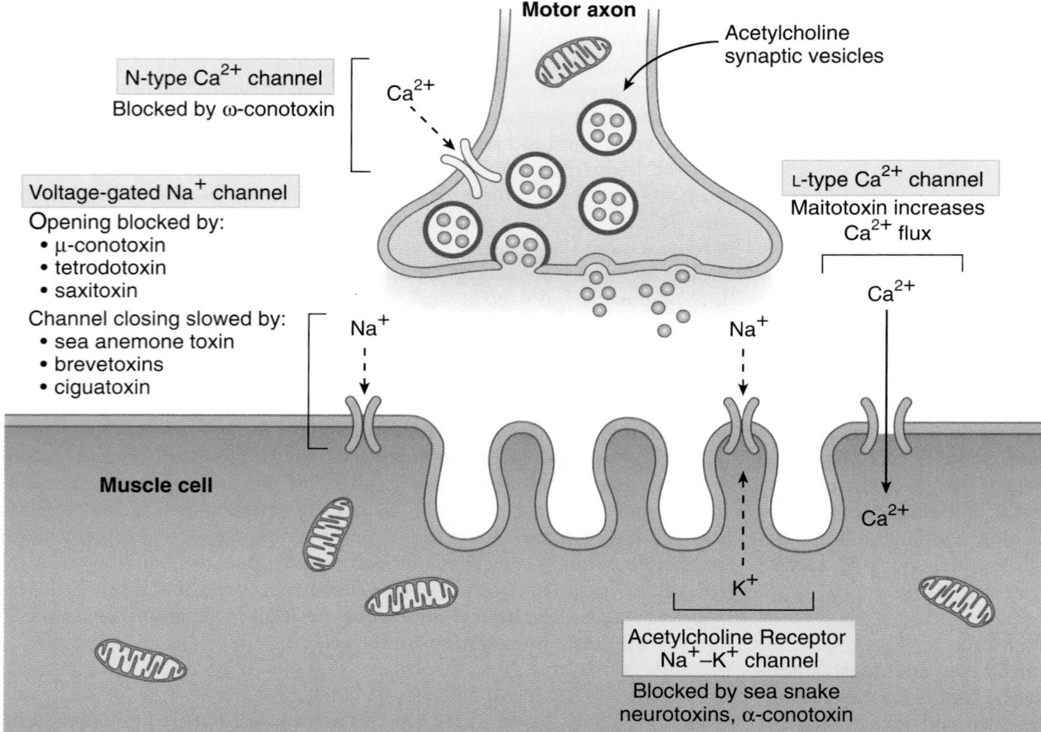

FIGURE 114-1. Schematic representation of a motor axon synapse and the sites of action of various marine neurotoxins.

be necessary to extract the spine and cleanse the wound. A sting produces severe pain and edema, which in extreme cases is accompanied by hemorrhage, syncope, vomiting, hypotension, and cardiac arrhythmias. In rare cases, death can occur, especially if the pericardial, peritoneal, or pleural cavities are penetrated. Soaking the wound in hot water inactivates some of the heat-labile toxins in the venom.

Mollusca

Cone Snails

Cone snail (Conidae) venom is injected into victims through a hollow, harpoon-like tooth. The venom, which is primarily neurotoxic, causes paresthesias, hypotension, and respiratory impairment or failure. Fourteen superfamilies of conopeptide toxins have been identified in cone snail venom:

A, I, M, O, P, S, T, I2, J, L, O2, O3, V, and Y. All of the conopeptides are short polypeptides that demonstrate a variety of neurotoxic actions by targeting specific subtypes of ion channels, neurotransmitter receptors, or transporters (see Fig. 114-1). The bite is very painful and may be followed by systemic symptoms such as dysphagia, aphonia, pruritus, blurred vision, syncope, muscular paralysis, and respiratory and cardiac failure. Treatment is supportive; in cases of severe envenomation, preparation for cardiovascular and respiratory support should be made. Rare cases of coagulopathy have been reported, and fatal envenomation has occurred.

Octopuses

The two species of blue-ringed octopuses (*Hapalochlaena maculosa* and *Hapalochlaena lunulata*), found in Australian waters, inject their venom by a relatively painless bite that produces two small puncture wounds. Hemorrhage at the site may occur. The major toxic component in the venom is tetrodotoxin, a neurotoxin that blocks action potentials of voltage-activated sodium channels and causes perioral and intraoral paresthesias, dysphagia, nausea, ataxia, aphonia, flaccid muscular paralysis, and respiratory distress or failure. Fatal envenomation has occurred, and urgent respiratory support may be required in severe cases.

Cnidaria

Jellyfish and Anemones

Jellyfish and anemones belong to the Cnidaria phylum, so named because of their venomous organelles called *cnidae*. The cnidae found in jellyfish and anemones (called *nematocysts* and *spirocysts*, respectively) are located on exposed tentacles. On tactile stimulation, the tentacles send forth a tethered projectile to deliver venom through the dermis. As the victim's surrounding musculature contracts, the venom is disseminated. Hemolysins, DNAase, and histamine releasers have been identified in some venoms. A number of peptide toxins of sea anemones mostly function by binding to sodium channel receptor site 3 to delay the inactivation phase of the channel. Other peptide toxins from anemones target the Kv3 potassium channel.

Stings by jellyfish and anemones typically produce immediate pain at the site of envenomation, followed by erythematous and urticarial lesions. Anaphylaxis is not common unless the patient has previously been sensitized. Depending on the severity of the sting, wheals and whiplike patterns may appear at the sites of envenomation within a few minutes or be delayed by several hours, followed in some cases by dermal necrosis. Eruptions sometimes recur days after the envenomation. Systemic reactions may include muscle spasms and cramps, vomiting, nausea, diarrhea, diaphoresis, and, in rare cases, cardiorespiratory failure.

Unfired nematocysts on tentacles adhering to the skin may be neutralized by vinegar or baking soda, depending on the species of jellyfish. Vinegar appears to be most useful for Australian blue bottle *(Physalia utriculus)* stings, whereas baking soda appears more efficacious for sea nettle *(Chrysaora quinquecirrha)* stings.

The box jellyfish *(Chironex fleckeri)* found in Australian waters is perhaps the most venomous jellyfish; it produces very severe stings that may cause death from hypotension, muscular and respiratory paralysis, and ultimately, cardiac arrest. Treatment of box jellyfish stings may require respiratory support and administration of antivenom.

The Portuguese man of war (*Physalia physalis*) is not a true jellyfish, and its venom differs from true jellyfish. It stings through nematocysts that cause intense pain and, occasionally, an allergic reaction. Flushing with salt water (sea water) followed by application of heat may ease the pain.

Sponges

Some sponges colonized by coelenterates produce toxins that can cause a pruritic, allergic dermatitis or an irritant dermatitis. These toxins are delivered by the sharp spicules, which penetrate the dermis. The toxins can cause the typical sponge diver's disease, which is characterized by local burning and itching and may be accompanied by soft tissue edema and purulent vesiculation. Serious illness is rare.

Corals

Fire coral *(Millepora alcicornis)* is found in shallow tropical waters. Stings are a common consequence of brushing or rubbing against the coral. Envenomation produces a burning or stinging sensation, followed by severe pruritus. Edematous wheals may develop but generally dissipate over the course of several days. The site of envenomation should be soaked in vinegar (5% acetic acid) or 70% isopropanol to relieve pain.

Annelida

Bristle worms

Bristle worms are segmented invertebrates found in tropical Pacific waters and the Gulf of Mexico. The bristles can penetrate the skin and produce severely painful envenomation, with pruritus and burning that may persist for several days. Local paresthesia is typical and may linger for weeks. Treatment is symptomatic, with consideration of possible tetanus infection (Chapter 304). Little is known regarding the chemistry of bristle worm venom.

Echinodermata

Sea Urchins

Of the echinoderms, sea urchins and sea stars are responsible for most stings in humans. The venom is delivered by the long spines and pedicellaria protruding from the sea urchin body. The spines are covered at the tips with a venom sac that is broken when it penetrates the skin. The pedicellaria, present on some species of sea urchins, are pincer-like appendages carrying venom glands. The toxins of sea urchin venom are not well characterized. Stings can produce pain, hemorrhage, aphonia, paresthesias, paralysis, hypotension, nausea, syncope, and respiratory distress. Immersion in hot water helps inactivate heat-labile toxins in the venom. Attached pedicellaria and embedded spines must be removed to prevent additional envenomation and infection.

POISONOUS MARINE ORGANISMS

Unlike envenomation, marine poisoning nearly always results from consumption of fish or shellfish that have accumulated various toxins from dinoflagellates. Most marine poisonings cause neurologic and gastrointestinal effects associated with the specific toxins found in the food source. Diagnosis is clinical, based on the type of fish ingested and the clinical symptoms presented. Neurotoxic marine poisoning is generally caused by one of six different toxins.

Neurotoxic Marine Toxins

Ciguatoxins

Ciguatoxins are occasionally found in reef fish of the Caribbean and Pacific. These toxins are cyclic polyethers that act as excitatory agents by binding to sodium channels. Maitotoxin, from the same dinoflagellate, is a water-soluble polyether that acts by enhancing calcium entry through L-type calcium channels. Symptoms of ciguatera poisoning generally appear within 2 to 12 hours after the ingestion of contaminated fish. Gastrointestinal symptoms, including diarrhea, abdominal pain, nausea, and vomiting, appear first, followed by neurologic and cardiovascular symptoms. Neurologic symptoms include aphonia, dental dysesthesias, fatigue, tremor, ataxia, pruritus, extremity and perioral dysesthesia, vertigo, headache, myalgia, arthralgia, temperature reversal, and hyporeflexia. Cardiovascular symptoms, such as bradycardia and hypotension, are less common. Treatment of ciguatera poisoning is supportive, with symptom-based therapy as indicated. Death from ciguatera poisoning is rare.

Tetrodotoxin

Pufferfish (i.e., blowfish, balloonfish, and toadfish), porcupinefish, and sunfish (*Mola* species) have a very potent toxin, tetrodotoxin, in their livers, gonads, intestines, and skin. The flesh of the fish (fugu) is a delicacy in Japan, where it is prepared by specially trained chefs to avoid serving significant amounts of toxins. Tetrodotoxin is a heterocyclic compound that binds at voltage-sensitive sodium channels to block sodium-channel conduction, thereby preventing nerve and muscle action potentials and resulting in paralysis. Symptoms occur rapidly (several minutes to several hours), beginning with circumoral paresthesias and progressing to descending widespread paresthesias. After the initial paresthesias, additional symptoms soon follow, including ataxia, weakness, aphonia, diaphoresis, excess salivation, dyspnea, dysphagia, weakness, and respiratory distress or failure. Gastrointestinal symptoms include nausea, vomiting, and diarrhea. Coagulopathies also may develop. Respiratory intervention is crucial because of the potential for complete flaccid paralysis. Without respiratory assistance, death is not unusual with severe intoxication.

Palytoxin

Palytoxin is an extremely potent toxin produced in sea anemones (*Palythoa* species) and accumulated in sharks, crabs, and marine turtles. The toxin functions by targeting sodium-potassium ion pumps, thereby disrupting ion gradients. Symptoms include tachycardia, hemolysis, and angina-like chest pain. Treatment is generally symptomatic and supportive.

Saxitoxin and Gonyautoxin

Paralytic shellfish poisoning is typically associated with the ingestion of mussels, clams, and oysters. The two toxins associated with this poisoning, saxitoxin and gonyautoxin, are produced by marine microalgae dinoflagellates that are associated with harmful algal blooms, such as "red tides," and are then accumulated in bivalve shellfish to give rise to "paralytic" shellfish poisoning. The primary paralytic shellfish poisoning toxins are heterocyclic compounds that block nerve and muscle action potentials by binding to sodium channels at the same site as tetrodotoxin, thereby resulting in paralysis.

Paralytic shellfish poisoning, which is significantly more severe than neurotoxic shellfish poisoning, predominantly involves neurologic symptoms with less pronounced nausea, vomiting, or diarrhea. Symptoms appear soon after the consumption of contaminated shellfish (minutes to hours), beginning with circumoral and extremity paresthesias. Additional neurologic symptoms such as ataxia, arthralgia, dysphagia, dysmetria, diaphoresis, and tachycardia soon follow the initial paresthesias. Respiratory depression or failure can result in death, usually within 12 hours of the onset of symptoms. As with other shellfish poisoning, therapy is supportive, with close attention to potential respiratory distress or failure.

Brevetoxins

Neurotoxic shellfish poisoning is caused by eating shellfish that contain brevetoxins, which are produced by the annual blooms of the red tides that are associated with the dinoflagellate *Karenia brevis.* Brevetoxins are cyclic polyethers that function similarly to ciguatoxins. Gastrointestinal and neurologic symptoms of intoxication appear within 3 hours after toxic shellfish is eaten and are similar to those of ciguatera poisoning. Treatment is supportive. No deaths have been reported after neurotoxic shellfish poisoning.

Domoic Acid

Domoic acid is a neurotoxin produced by the algae *Nitzschia* during harmful algae blooms and causes amnesic shellfish poisoning following ingestion of contaminated shellfish. The toxin disrupts neuron function by altering calcium influx into cells. Symptoms include headaches, dizziness, loss of short-term memory, confusion, seizures, and coma. After about 24 hours, gastrointestinal symptoms may include diarrhea, vomiting, and abdominal cramping. Death is rare.

Non-neurotoxic Poisoning

Histamine

Scrombroid fishes, such as mackerel, bonito, and tuna, can contain an inordinate amount of histamines in their tissues as a result of bacterial destruction of fish proteins associated with spoilage. Ingestion of spoiled fish with high histamine concentrations can result in pseudoallergic symptoms such as diarrhea, flushing, headache, rash, and vomiting. A metallic taste in the mouth may be reported by some patients. Treatment usually is not necessary for scombrotoxic fish poisoning, and the symptoms usually resolve in several hours. For more severe cases, antihistamines or epinephrine have been reported to be effective.

SUGGESTED READINGS

James KJ, Carey B, O'Halloran J, et al. Shellfish toxicity: human health implications of marine algal toxins. *Epidemiol Infect.* 2010;138:927-940. *Review.*

Shiomi K. Novel peptide toxins recently isolated from sea anemones. *Toxicon.* 2009;54:1112-1118. *A review of peptide toxins found in sea anemones and their structures.*

Stewart I, Lewis RJ, Eaglesham GK, et al. Emerging tropical diseases in Australia. Part 2. Ciguatera fish poisoning. *Ann Trop Med Parasitol.* 2010;104:557-571. *Review.*

115

RHABDOMYOLYSIS

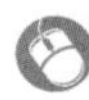

FRANCIS G. O'CONNOR AND PATRICIA A. DEUSTER

DEFINITION

Rhabdomyolysis, an acute, potentially fatal clinical syndrome, reflects the dissolution and disintegration of striated muscle, with the release of muscle cell contents into the systemic circulation. Myoglobinemia and myoglobinuria are common. Skeletal muscle destruction can cause systemic effects mediated by substances released from affected muscle cells (e.g., myoglobin, calcium, potassium). Prerenal azotemia, complicated by the toxicity of free myoglobin on the renal tubules, may lead to acute renal failure, which exacerbates other metabolic abnormalities. At the extreme, arrhythmias, caused by the release of intracellular potassium and organic acids, coupled with hypocalcemia may be fatal.

EPIDEMIOLOGY

Approximately 26,000 hospitalized cases of rhabdomyolysis are reported each year in the United States. Rhabdomyolysis, which precipitates acute kidney injury in 13 to 67% of affected individuals, accounts for 5 to 10% of all cases of acute renal failure in the United States.

ETIOLOGY

Rhabdomyolysis is a complex and multifactorial clinical disorder, with multiple potential inherited and acquired causes (Table 115-1). In urban adults, alcohol (and other drug) abuse, muscle compression, and status epilepticus are common causes of rhabdomyolysis. In pediatric patients, the most common cause is trauma, followed by nonketotic hyperosmolar coma, viral myositis, dystonia, and malignant hyperthermia. However, exercise-induced rhabdomyolysis from repetitive exercise is also a concern in children. Importantly, children and adolescents with recurrent rhabdomyolysis are increasingly being recognized as possibly having inherited metabolic disorders.

Drugs and Intoxications

Among intoxications, which are a common cause of rhabdomyolysis, the most frequent illegal drug-associated causes are cocaine and heroin (Chapter 33), with nearly 20% of cocaine overdoses complicated by rhabdomyolysis. Other substances that can induce rhabdomyolysis include ethanol (Chapter 32), amphetamines, phenylalkylamine derivatives, caffeine, and statins. Statins (Chapter 213) may result in myalgias in up to 10% of patients receiving treatment, but reported rates of statin-induced rhabdomyolysis are only 0.1 to 0.2 cases per 1000 person years.

Exertional Rhabdomyolysis

Rhabdomyolysis can also be a consequence of excessive exertion, prolonged heat exposure (Chapter 109), coexisting sickle cell trait (Chapter 166), and the use of dietary supplements (e.g., ephedra). In one series, 35 of 225,000 emergency department visits to an urban tertiary care center were for exertional rhabdomyolysis. The average creatine kinase (CK) level was 40,000 U/L, but no patient developed acute renal failure. In another series, 57% of participants in an ultramarathon had evidence of myoglobinemia, but none progressed to acute renal failure. Rhabdomyolysis has also been diagnosed in other sports settings (e.g., baseball, football, track, wrestling), but none with a higher frequency than that seen with endurance events.

In the military, acute exertional rhabdomyolysis occurs in 2 to 40% of individuals undergoing basic training, usually within the first 6 days. Resolution of myoglobinuria typically occurs within 2 to 3 days, with clinical improvement within 1 week. Consistent risk factors are low levels of physical fitness and early introduction of repetitive exercises (e.g., squats, push-ups, sit-ups). Although most cases are self-limited, with no long-term evidence of renal or muscle injury, patients who demonstrate systemic signs, generalized clinical findings, or acute renal failure often have an underlying metabolic myopathy. Importantly, 25% of all cases of heatstroke in the military between 1980 and 2000 were associated with rhabdomyolysis; acute renal failure developed in 33%. A retrospective review of deaths in a military basic trainee

TABLE 115-1 INHERITED AND ACQUIRED CAUSES OF RHABDOMYOLYSIS

INHERITED	ACQUIRED
Glycolytic/glycogenolytic, e.g., McArdle's disease (myophosphorylase deficiency)	Exertion, e.g., exercise, status epilepticus, delirium, electrical shock, status asthmaticus, cardiopulmonary resuscitation (see also Table 115-2)
Fatty acid oxidation, e.g., carnitine palmitoyltransferase II deficiency	Crush, e.g., external weight, prolonged immobility, bariatric surgery
Krebs cycle, e.g., aconitase deficiency	Ischemia, e.g., arterial occlusion, compartment syndrome, sickle cell disease, disseminated intravascular coagulation
Pentose phosphate pathway, e.g., glucose-6-phosphate dehydrogenase deficiency	Extremes of body temperature, e.g., fever, exertional heatstroke, burns, malignant hyperthermia, hypothermia, lightning
Purine nucleotide cycle, e.g., myoadenylate deaminase deficiency	Metabolic, e.g., hypokalemia, hypernatremia or hyponatremia, hypophosphatemia, pancreatitis, diabetic ketoacidosis, renal tubular acidosis, hyperthyroidism or hypothyroidism, nonketotic hyperosmolar states
Mitochondrial respiratory chain, e.g., succinate dehydrogenase deficiency	Drugs or toxins, e.g., anticholinergics, amphetamines, antihistamines, arsenic, ethanol, opiates, statins, cocaine, succinylcholine, halothane, corticosteroids, cyclosporine, itraconazole, phenothiazines
Malignant hyperthermia susceptibility, e.g., familial malignant hyperthermia (*RyR1*) mutations, myotonic dystrophy, Duchenne's and Becker's dystrophies	Infections, e.g., Epstein-Barr virus, human immunodeficiency virus, herpes simplex, influenza A and B, *Borrelia burgdorferi*, tetanus
Other, e.g., familial recurrent myoglobinuria	Inflammatory and autoimmune disorders, e.g., polymyositis, dermatomyositis

Adapted and reproduced with permission from Warren JD, Blumbergs PC, Thompson PD. Rhabdomyolysis: a review. *Muscle Nerve.* 2002;25:332-347.

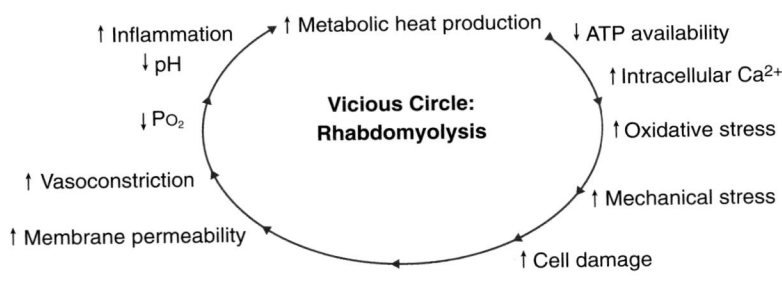

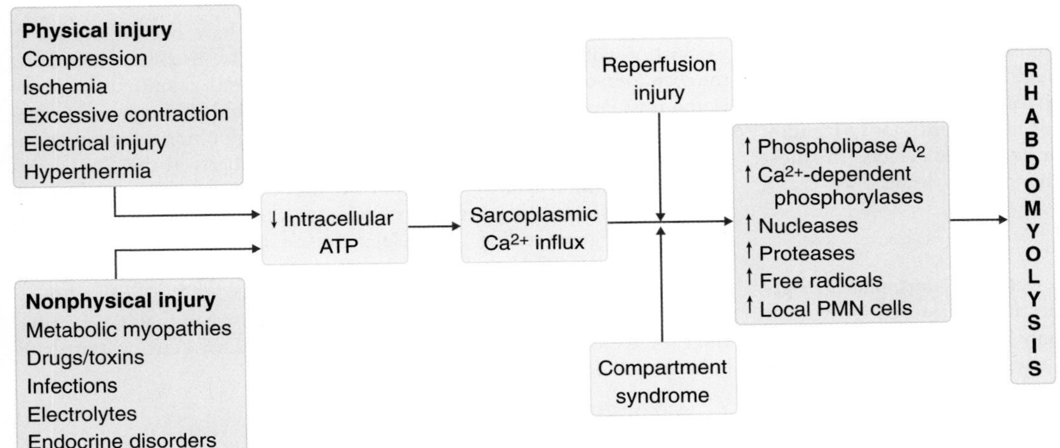

FIGURE 115-1. **A,** Pathogenesis of rhabdomyolysis. **B,** Vicious circle of rhabdomyolysis. ATP = adenosine triphosphate; PMN = polymorphonuclear.

population found an increased risk for nontraumatic exertional sudden death in African Americans with sickle cell trait.

The extreme exertion characteristics of military service carry over to the population of correctional inmates and civil servants. Reports indicate that unsupervised repetitive exercise in prison populations has led to exertional rhabdomyolysis. Among New York City firefighters, 32 of 16,506 candidates (0.2%) were hospitalized for rhabdomyolysis after a physical fitness test, with 4 requiring hemodialysis. In a group of 50 prospective police officers from Massachusetts, 13 trainees were hospitalized with rhabdomyolysis and CK levels greater than 32,000 U/L; 6 required dialysis, and 1 died 44 days later as a result of complications of heatstroke, rhabdomyolysis, and renal and hepatic failure.

PATHOBIOLOGY

Pathophysiology

The final common pathway for all cases of rhabdomyolysis is destruction of muscle cells as a result of direct or indirect injury, with displacement of their intracellular contents into extracellular fluid, the circulation, or both (Fig. 115-1). Cell function is critically dependent on the relationship between intracellular calcium (Ca^{2+}) and sodium (Na^+) concentrations. Sarcolemmal Na^+, K^+-ATPase regulates extracellular Ca^{2+} concentrations by exchanging Na^+ for Ca^{2+} across the sarcolemma. A low intracellular Na^+ concentration creates a gradient that actively results in efflux of Ca^{2+} as it is exchanged for Na^+ ions. This process maintains intracellular Ca^{2+} levels at several orders of magnitude lower than extracellular Ca^{2+}.

When the cell is subjected to mechanical stress, stretch-activated channels in the sarcolemma can open and cause an influx of Na^+ and Ca^{2+}. With excessive intracellular Ca^{2+}, several pathologic processes begin. Excessive intracellular Ca^{2+} results in persistent contraction of myofibers, depletion of adenosine triphosphate (ATP), production of free radicals, activation of vasoactive molecules, release of proteases, and, ultimately, cell death. Cell death is followed by an invasion of neutrophils, which amplify the damage by further release of proteases and increased production of free radicals. Rather than simple necrosis, a self-sustaining, inflammatory myolytic reaction develops.

Rhabdomyolysis can be further complicated by reperfusion injury and compartment syndrome. In reperfusion injury, ischemia for a prolonged period is followed by restoration of vascular flow. The increase in blood flow results in the delivery of activated neutrophils in combination with an abundance of oxygen, which contributes to the development of highly reactive free radicals. Because most muscle groups are contained within rigid fascial compartments, rhabdomyolysis can quickly precipitate a secondary acute compartment syndrome. The swelling associated with traumatized tissue can also lead to increased intracompartmental pressure, which can provoke additional damage by compromising both venous and arterial blood flow. Thus, compartment syndrome can also lead to rhabdomyolysis.

Inherited and Acquired Rhabdomyolysis

Rhabdomyolysis can be classified into two major categories: inherited and acquired (see Table 115-1). Metabolic myopathies, though not the most common cause, should be carefully considered in patients who have recurrent episodes triggered by low levels of stress or exertion. A number of pathways that lead to the formation of ATP can be disrupted by genetic defects (e.g., inherited disorders of glycogenolysis, glycolysis, and lipid and purine metabolism). In one series of 77 patients who underwent biopsy for idiopathic myoglobinuria, 47% were found to have enzymatic defects. The most common disorders were deficiencies of carnitine palmitoyltransferase II and myophosphorylase.

Inherited Rhabdomyolysis

Malignant hyperthermia is a potentially fatal, heterogeneous, pharmacogenetic disorder triggered by volatile anesthetics in predisposed individuals (Chapter 440). The disorder is most commonly inherited in an autosomal dominant pattern. Evidence from molecular studies indicates that 25% of patients who are susceptible to malignant hyperthermia have mutations in the ryanodine receptor (*RyR1*) gene, which is responsible for coding proteins for one of the primary Ca^{2+} release channels involved in triggering muscle contraction. When a susceptible patient is exposed to a triggering agent, excessive release of Ca^{2+} into the myoplasm leads to a hypermetabolic state manifested by hypercapnia, tachycardia, and metabolic acidosis. Whether the genetic predisposition to malignant hyperthermia is related to exertional rhabdomyolysis and exercise-induced heat injury has not been proved.

Acquired Rhabdomyolysis

DRUGS AND TOXINS. Drugs and toxins, also common causes of rhabdomyolysis, operate through a number of mechanisms, including direct membrane toxicity (e.g., herbicides), indirect metabolic derangements (e.g., anticholinergics), ischemia (e.g., cocaine), and agitation (e.g., hemlock). The most commonly cited drugs precipitating rhabdomyolysis are alcohol, statins, cocaine, amphetamines, and phenothiazines. Alcohol can induce rhabdomyolysis through a combination of mechanisms, including immobilization, direct myotoxicity, and electrolyte abnormalities. Statins, which inhibit 3-hydroxy-3-methylglutaryl-coenzyme A (HMG-CoA) reductase, can be directly myotoxic and appear to trigger sustained increases in intracellular Ca^{2+}. Although the precise mechanisms underlying statin-induced myopathy are currently incompletely understood, it can be aggravated by the concomitant administration of cytochrome P-450 3A4 inhibitors (e.g., itraconazole, erythromycin, cyclosporine, danazol) and fibrates, as well as by physical exercise, excessive alcohol intake, and preexisting comorbid medical conditions. Amphetamines and phenothiazines may lead to a clinical picture of rhabdomyolysis through the serotonin syndrome (Chapter 442) and the neuroleptic malignant syndrome (Chapter 427), respectively.

INFECTIONS. Both viral and bacterial infections can trigger rhabdomyolysis. Either cellular invasion or generation of various toxins may precipitate infection-induced rhabdomyolysis by the virus or bacterium. Influenza A and B (Chapter 372) are the most common viral causes, followed by human immunodeficiency virus (Chapter 394), coxsackievirus (Chapter 387), and Epstein-Barr virus (Chapter 385). The most common bacterial organisms that induce rhabdomyolysis are *Legionella* species (Chapter 322), followed by *Francisella tularensis* (Chapter 319) and *Streptococcus pneumoniae* (Chapter 297). Acute renal failure develops in approximately 57% (33 to 100%) of bacterial cases and 34% (0 to 100%) of viral cases of rhabdomyolysis.

TRAUMA. Trauma is traditionally thought of as the principal cause of rhabdomyolysis. Wars, natural disasters, and traffic and occupational accidents are frequent causes of trauma-induced "crush injury syndrome" (Chapter 112). Other less common causes of trauma- or compression-induced rhabdomyolysis include struggling against restraints, direct blows, child abuse, torture, prolonged immobilization (e.g., anesthesia, coma, drug- or alcohol-induced stupor), and bariatric and other forms of surgery. The primary mechanism of crush syndrome and compression-induced rhabdomyolysis is reperfusion of damaged tissue after a period of ischemia.

Exertional rhabdomyolysis can result from excessive exercise in fit and unfit individuals, particularly eccentrically based activities (lengthening contractions, such as lowering a weight), but it can also be triggered by exertion in combination with thermal stress, sickle cell trait, altitude, or the use of medications (e.g., anticholinergics) or ergogenic substances (e.g., caffeine, ephedra). Exertional rhabdomyolysis may also reveal or provide evidence of an underlying inherited disorder in certain individuals. The spectrum of exertional rhabdomyolysis is broad and can range from a subclinical event to catastrophic collapse and death. The underlying mechanisms may be either mechanical or metabolic in nature, but exertional rhabdomyolysis is associated with elevated myoplasmic Ca^{2+} concentrations.

A number of genetic mutations (Table 115-2) have been identified in association with metabolic myopathies, with exercise usually precipitating the rhabdomyolysis. Multiple mutations in the carnitine palmitoyltransferase II and myophosphorylase genes have been found, and although each mutation has been associated with exercise-induced myoglobinuria, the mutations alone may not explain the clinical episodes. Mutations in the *RyR1* gene, which are common in malignant hyperthermia (Chapter 440), have also been noted in persons with exertional rhabdomyolysis. Two single-point mutations in the gene coding for skeletal muscle myosin light chain kinase (*C37885A* and *C49T*) have been associated with an exaggerated CK response to an exercise challenge, but the role of these mutations in exertional rhabdomyolysis is not known. Yet to be identified are genes that can be used clinically to predict susceptibility to infection-, toxin-, exertion-, or drug-induced rhabdomyolysis.

CLINICAL MANIFESTATIONS

The classic manifestation of rhabdomyolysis includes acute myalgia and pigmenturia as a result of myoglobinuria in association with elevated serum muscle enzymes (CK in particular). Many clinical features are nonspecific, however, and the course and initial signs, symptoms, and laboratory abnormalities are clearly dependent on the underlying cause and severity of the event.

TABLE 115-2 GENETIC MUTATIONS ASSOCIATED WITH EXERTIONAL RHABDOMYOLYSIS

GENE	
Ryanodine receptor 1	*RyR1*
Myoadenylate deaminase	*AMPDA1*
Carnitine palmitoyltransferase II	*CPT2*
Myophosphorylase	*PYGM*
Phosphofructokinase	*PFKM*
Phosphorylase *b* kinase	*PHKA1*
Very long chain acyl coenzyme-A dehydrogenase	*ACAD9*
Phosphoglycerate mutase	*PGAMM*
Phosphoglycerate kinase	*PGK1*
Lactate dehydrogenase	*LDHA*
Cytochrome *c* oxidase	*COX I, II,* and *III*
Cytochrome *b* (complex III)	*CYTB*
Mitochondrial tRNA	*Mt-tRNA*
β-Sarcoglycan	*SGCB*

Rhabdomyolysis can be accompanied by both local and systemic features. Local features, generally noted in the area of the traumatized muscle groups, can occur within hours of the trauma and include muscle pain, tenderness, and swelling. Systemic features include tea-colored urine, chills, fever, and malaise. In extreme cases, patients complain of nausea and vomiting and demonstrate confusion, agitation, or delirium. Whenever systemic features such as chills, fever, malaise, or generalized muscular involvement are observed, an underlying metabolic myopathy should be considered.

Clinical findings may also include compartment syndrome, which can occur in muscle groups encased by fascia, especially the lower leg, forearm, and thigh muscle groups. Sensory abnormalities caused by nerve compression are an early manifestation of compartment syndrome; the loss of a pulse as a result of vascular compromise is a later finding. If compartment syndrome is not addressed within 6 to 8 hours, irreversible ischemic muscle and nerve damage may occur.

Laboratory findings are related to the degree of muscle involvement. Early findings include elevated blood levels of CK, myoglobin, potassium, urea, and phosphorus. CK levels typically peak 2 to 5 days after the initial insult; levels higher than 16,000 U/L are more likely to be associated with renal failure than are lower levels. Hypocalcemia, caused by the influx and deposition of Ca^{2+} in damaged muscle tissue, may accompany rhabdomyolysis. Moreover, an anion gap metabolic acidosis may develop because of the release of organic acids from damaged muscle. With resolution of rhabdomyolysis, sequestered Ca^{2+} may be released back into the circulation and cause hypercalcemia.

DIAGNOSIS

Creatine Kinase Levels

A diagnosis of rhabdomyolysis is made when there is clinical evidence of myonecrosis and release into the systemic circulation of muscle cell contents, including myoglobin, creatinine, CK, organic acids, potassium, aldolase, lactate dehydrogenase, and hydroxybutyrate dehydrogenase. The skeletal muscle subtype CK-MM is abundantly present in skeletal muscle and released as a result of muscle destruction. Serum levels exceeding 100,000 U/L are not uncommon with rhabdomyolysis. Because CK remains in the circulation longer than myoglobin does and can be detected clinically both easily and efficiently, it is the most frequently used marker to diagnose rhabdomyolysis. No universally accepted clinical or laboratory definition of rhabdomyolysis currently exists, but CK elevations ranging from more than 5 times to more than 50 times the upper limits of normal, as well as varying requirements for serum creatinine elevation, have been proposed. Importantly, gender, ethnicity, and baseline physical activity levels all affect individual baseline CK levels. African American males and young athletic men have the highest baseline CK levels, and non–African American women have the lowest. Thus, gender, ethnicity, and prior activity must be considered when using CK for the diagnosis of rhabdomyolysis. In general, CK levels in excess of 5 times normal, with the appropriate clinical presentation, are accepted as evidence of muscle breakdown, which may be consistent with a diagnosis of rhabdomyolysis.

Myoglobin Testing

Because myoglobinuria does not occur in the absence of rhabdomyolysis, myoglobin should be the best marker and the diagnostic cornerstone. However, testing for serum or urine myoglobin is problematic and is not always consistent. Myoglobin is normally bound to plasma globulins; therefore, only a small fraction reaches the glomeruli. In the presence of severe muscle damage, blood levels of myoglobin overwhelm the binding capacity of the circulating proteins, so free myoglobin reaches the glomeruli and eventually the renal tubules. Elevations in serum myoglobin occur before the rise in serum CK, but the elimination kinetics of serum myoglobin is more rapid than that of CK, which makes the often evanescent rise in serum myoglobin a less reliable marker of muscle injury. Furthermore, the liver can quickly metabolize myoglobin. Diagnostic tests for urine myoglobin are often not readily available; in addition, it may take more than 24 hours to obtain results, and urine myoglobin is not an accurate predictor of acute kidney injury. Nevertheless, urine screening for rhabdomyolysis may be performed by dipstick if the urine sediment is also examined. The orthotoluidine portion of the dipstick turns blue in the presence of hemoglobin or myoglobin, so if the urine sediment does not contain erythrocytes, one can assume, in the appropriate clinical setting, that a positive dipstick reading reflects the presence of myoglobin. Other associated laboratory findings in acute rhabdomyolysis can include hypocalcemia or hypercalcemia, hyperphosphatemia, metabolic (lactic) acidosis, thrombocytopenia, and disseminated intravascular coagulation.

Differential Diagnosis

The clinical findings of acutely swollen muscles or muscle weakness (or both) with reddish brown urine are not always the result of rhabdomyolysis, and the examining clinician must be careful to scrutinize all information. The differential diagnosis includes disorders that may indirectly affect myocytes, such as Guillain-Barré syndrome and periodic paralysis. Guillain-Barré syndrome (Chapter 428) is distinguished from rhabdomyolysis in that it is characterized as a fulminant polyneuropathy, usually after an antecedent viral infection. Periodic paralysis (Chapter 429) is frequently associated with transient electrolyte disturbances and is distinguished from rhabdomyolysis in that most cases follow periods of rest or sleep.

Myoglobinuria causes the urine to be reddish brown, but tea-colored (or cola-colored) urine does not necessarily indicate the presence of myoglobin. Other conditions associated with discoloration of urine include hemoglobinuria from hemolysis, intrinsic renal disease, porphyria, acute glomerulonephritis, "athletic pseudonephritis," or external factors such as ingestion of beets and various drugs (e.g., phenytoin, rifampin, vitamin B_{12}).

The diagnosis of rhabdomyolysis is complete when the clinician determines the cause. This step, though frequently established during the history and physical examination, may require further diagnostic assessment after initiating clinical treatment during the acute phase. Clinical issues that are both controversial and poorly defined include which patients warrant further testing and what tests to perform. Individuals with recurrent rhabdomyolysis, a positive family history of rhabdomyolysis or malignant hyperthermia, low exercise tolerance, no apparent cause, or a fulminant or explosive form of rhabdomyolysis appear to warrant further testing.

Testing may include a nonischemic forearm test, which involves isometric exercise at 70% of maximal voluntary contraction for 30 seconds under nonischemic conditions; electromyography; blood tests for muscle enzymes (e.g., mitochondrial myopathies [Chapter 429], fatty acid transport defects [Chapter 429], glycogen storage diseases [Chapter 214], diseases associated with myoglobinuria); muscle biopsy to investigate specific metabolic myopathies and other enzyme or genetic defects; or any combination of such testing. The forearm exercise test may help identify metabolic and genetic causes of rhabdomyolysis. Patients who have had an episode of malignant hyperthermia or exertional heat illness may be candidates for a caffeine halothane contracture test, which evaluates the force produced in small muscle biopsy samples after exposure to caffeine and separate exposure to halothane in the laboratory. Isolated, perfused muscle fibers must show an increase in tension of at least 0.2 g when exposed to 2 mM of caffeine or at least 0.7 g of tension after exposure to 3% halothane. Additionally, genetic investigation for mutations of the *RyR1* receptor gene may be warranted.

PREVENTION

Approaches for preventing rhabdomyolysis induced by infections, medications, toxins, heat stress, or exercise may emerge in the future, but no definitive guidelines can be presented at this time. To prevent further muscle injury, blood flow to ischemic areas must be promptly restored to minimize ischemia-reperfusion damage. Administration of free radical scavengers to prevent rhabdomyolysis may prove useful in the future.

TREATMENT Rx

Treatment of rhabdomyolysis begins with a careful history and physical examination to identify and manage any underlying illness; it then focuses on preserving renal function. All patients require aggressive early management because it is difficult to stratify risk initially (Table 115-3). Careful observation plus treatment of potential early and late complications is critical. Accordingly, vital signs, urine output, serial electrolyte levels, and CK levels should be obtained as soon as possible. Intensive care monitoring may be required, depending on the clinical situation.

Hydration

Hydration is the cornerstone of preserving renal function in patients with rhabdomyolysis. Providing fluids addresses the early threats to survival: hypovolemic shock and hyperkalemia. Currently, there is no way to accurately predict or stratify overall risk or risk of acute renal failure among patients with rhabdomyolysis, but CK levels greater than 15,000 U/L are thought to portend an increased risk. Patients with mild symptoms and serum CK levels less than 3000 U/L are considered to be at low risk and may be treated as outpatients with hydration, limited physical activity, and careful follow-up. Victims of collapse, trauma, or exertional heat injury, or patients who demonstrate moderate early symptoms with more than mild elevations in CK or abnormal

TABLE 115-3 STEPS IN THE PREVENTION AND TREATMENT OF RHABDOMYOLYSIS-INDUCED ACUTE KIDNEY INJURY

Check for extracellular volume status, central venous pressure, and urine output.*
Measure serum creatine kinase levels. Measurement of other muscle enzymes (myoglobin, aldolase, lactate dehydrogenase, alanine aminotransferase, aspartate aminotransferase) adds little information relevant to diagnosis or management.
Measure levels of plasma and urine creatinine, potassium, and sodium; blood urea nitrogen; total and ionized calcium, magnesium, and phosphorus; and uric acid and albumin. Evaluate acid-base status, blood cell count, and coagulation.
Perform a urine dipstick test, and examine the urine sediment.
Initiate volume repletion with normal saline promptly at a rate of approximately 400 mL/hr (200-1000 mL/hr, depending on the setting and severity), and monitor the clinical course or central venous pressure.
Target urine output of approximately 3 mL/kg body weight/hr (200 mL/hr).
Check serum potassium levels frequently.
Correct hypocalcemia only if symptomatic (e.g., tetany, seizures) or if severe hyperkalemia occurs.
Investigate the cause of rhabdomyolysis.
Check urine pH: if it is <6.5, alternate each liter of normal saline with 1 L 5% dextrose or 0.45% saline plus 100 mmol bicarbonate. Avoid potassium- and lactate-containing solutions.
Consider treatment with mannitol (up to 200 g/day; cumulative dose up to 800 g). Check for plasma osmolality and plasma osmolal gap. Discontinue if diuresis (>20 mL/hr) is not established.
Maintain volume repletion until myoglobinuria is cleared (as evidenced by clear urine or urine dipstick test that is negative for blood).
Consider renal replacement therapy if there is resistant hyperkalemia (>6.5 mmol/L) that is symptomatic (as assessed by electrocardiography), rapidly rising serum potassium levels, oliguria (<0.5 mL of urine/kg/hr for 12 hr), anuria, volume overload, or resistant metabolic acidosis (pH < 7.1).

*In the case of the crush syndrome (e.g., earthquake, building collapse), institute aggressive volume repletion promptly before evacuating the patient.
From Bosch X, Poch E, Grau JM. Rhabdomyolysis and acute kidney injury. *N Engl J Med.* 2009;361:62-72.

metabolic panels, should be treated with intravenous hydration in an inpatient setting. Hydration is accomplished by aggressive intravenous fluid therapy with isotonic fluids at a rate that results in a urine output of 200 mL/hour until CK levels begin to decrease. When fluid resuscitation fails to correct intractable hyperkalemia and acidosis, renal replacement therapy should be considered (Chapter 122).

Specific Therapeutic Measures

Several retrospective clinical studies and case reports, as well as animal models, promote the addition of bicarbonate and mannitol, but no prospective clinical trials have been conducted to support or refute their benefit in patients with rhabdomyolysis. Alkalinization of the urine decreases cast formation, minimizes the toxic effects of myoglobin on the renal tubules, inhibits lipid peroxidation, and decreases the risk for hyperkalemia. However, this approach can cause Ca^{2+} to precipitate and be deposited in the soft tissues, as well as contributing to a hyperosmolar state. Mannitol serves as an osmotic diuretic, volume expander, and free radical scavenger; it should be used very carefully in patients with marginal cardiac function, and only after adequate renal function is established.

Despite the absence of definitive evidence in humans, both mannitol and a forced alkaline diuresis are recommended for rhabdomyolysis caused by crush syndrome when CK levels are greater than 20,000 U/L. The treatment goals are to (1) achieve a urine output of 200 mL/hour, (2) maintain urine pH between 6 and 7, (3) keep serum pH below 7.50, and (4) achieve hemodynamic stability and prevent volume overload. Fluid resuscitation begins with a bolus of 1 L of 5% dextrose plus 0.22% NaCl and 100 mEq $NaHCO_3$ over a 30-minute period, followed by an infusion at 2 to 5 mL/kg/hour. A 20% mannitol infusion at a dose of 0.5 g/kg is given over a 15-minute period, followed by an infusion at 0.1 g/kg/hour. Adjustments are made to maintain urine output above 200 mL/hour. Urinary and serum pH levels should be monitored, with acetazolamide added if the serum pH exceeds 7.45 or urinary pH remains below 6.0. However, the use of mannitol and forced alkaline diuresis in patients with crush syndrome, as well as other clinical manifestations of rhabdomyolysis, has not been tested in randomized trials.

Management of Metabolic Abnormalities

Deposition of Ca^{2+}, which occurs early in rhabdomyolysis, is directly related to the degree of muscle destruction and administration of Ca^{2+}. Reversal of hypocalcemia may in fact worsen ectopic calcification and exacerbate hypercalcemia during the resolution phase. Accordingly, hypocalcemia should be treated only when clinical symptoms, signs of tetany, or severe hyperkalemia develops.

Management of Compartment Syndrome

Compartment syndrome (Chapter 112) is a well-described late complication as well as a potential cause of rhabdomyolysis. Compartment syndrome can occur as a direct consequence of muscle injury with increased vascular permeability, aggressive fluid resuscitation, or restoration of reperfusion. When a compartment syndrome is suspected, such as when the muscles are tense and swollen or there is evidence of neurovascular compromise, compartment pressures should be measured; in the proper clinical setting, pressures in excess of 30 mm Hg should prompt consideration of fasciotomy. However, late fasciotomy (>12 hours after the onset of symptoms) may be counterproductive by converting a closed injury to an open wound, with an increased risk of uncontrollable infection. Accordingly, late fasciotomy is relatively contraindicated.

Management of Crush Injury

Management of crush injury victims (Chapter 112) is unique, in that many individuals have the opportunity to receive treatment before extrication and reperfusion. Current recommendations for on-site management of trauma victims before extrication include aggressive hydration with intravenous normal saline. In the event of massive damage, amputation of the extremity may be required to protect the patient's overall health. A Mangled Extremity Severity Score (MESS) may be used to identify nonsalvageable extremities prospectively. The MESS is a grading system based on four groups of clinical criteria, including the degree of skeletal and soft tissue injury, rating of blood pressure (shock) and pulse (ischemia), and age. Scores from each group are added to obtain a total score that ranges from 0 to 14; higher scores indicate more severe involvement, and a score of 7 or greater has a positive predictive value of nearly 100% for amputation. It is hoped that ongoing clinical trials in this population will elucidate the roles of *N*-acetylcysteine, continuous renal replacement therapy, and deferoxamine in reducing the direct toxic effects of myoglobin on the kidneys.

Malignant Hyperthermia

One cause of rhabdomyolysis that requires rapid and aggressive management is malignant hyperthermia (Chapter 440). Episodes of malignant hyperthermia occur most commonly in the operating room and are recognized by the anesthesiologist. The typical clinical features represent an uncontrolled, exaggerated, hypermetabolic state; an increase in end-tidal carbon dioxide during ventilation is the most sensitive sign. With the clinical recognition of impending malignant hyperthermia, anesthetics should be discontinued, and the patient should be treated with dantrolene sodium. The usual initial dose is 2.5 to 4 mg/kg, followed by about 1 mg/kg every 4 hours for up to 48 hours to avoid recrudescence.

PROGNOSIS

The most serious consequence of rhabdomyolysis is acute renal failure, which occurs in up to 67% of all cases, regardless of cause. Although acute renal failure may be relatively benign, the mortality rate from myoglobinuric renal failure reportedly ranges from 3 to 80%. Various clinical factors are used to predict the risk for acute renal failure, including serum CK, creatinine, potassium, and Ca^{2+}, as well as the urine myoglobin level, but no single parameter has been established. However, mortality appears to be significantly higher in patients with CK values in excess of 75,000 U/L and in those with hyperkalemia or hypocalcemia. For compartment syndrome, a poor prognosis is associated with an ischemic period lasting longer than 6 hours.

The prognosis of patients with rhabdomyolysis improves markedly when treatment is started soon after the diagnosis is made. With mild episodes, the prognosis is customarily excellent, and the patient can typically resume usual activities within several weeks after CK levels have normalized. However, some patients do not return to normal and continue to experience extreme fatigue and muscle pain on exertion. These patients require additional testing (nonischemic forearm test, electromyography, muscle disease enzyme panel, muscle biopsy) to determine whether an underlying metabolic myopathy exists. The results of these tests will help determine future recommendations, but the patient's tolerance of and response to light and more strenuous exercise are important factors.

For patients with statin-induced myopathy, deciding when to discontinue statin therapy remains controversial. However, most authorities agree that suspension should occur with either intolerable muscle symptoms or evidence of rhabdomyolysis.

FUTURE DIRECTIONS

Although a number of genetic mutations have already been defined, the prevalence of such mutations is unknown. Moreover, a genetic linkage in individuals susceptible to exertional or drug-induced rhabdomyolysis (or both) has not been thoroughly investigated. It is likely that the greatest progress will come from prospective trials that evaluate both diagnostic and treatment modalities for myoglobinuric renal failure.

SUGGESTED READINGS

Bosch X, Poch E, Grau JM. Rhabdomyolysis and acute kidney injury. *N Engl J Med*. 2009;361:62-72. *A comprehensive review.*

Cervellin G, Comelli I, Lippi G. Rhabdomyolysis: historical background, clinical, diagnostic and therapeutic features. *Clin Chem Lab Med*. 2010;48:749-756. *Review.*

Graziani G, Calvetta A, Cucchiari D, et al. Life-threatening hypercalcemia in patients with rhabdomyolysis-induced oliguric acute renal failure. *J Nephrol*. 2011;24:128-131. *Review of this unusual but serious complication.*

Joy TR, Hegele RA. Narrative review: statin-related myopathy. *Ann Intern Med*. 2009;150:858-868. *Rhabdomyolysis remains rare.*

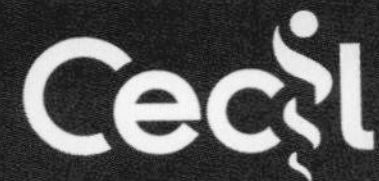

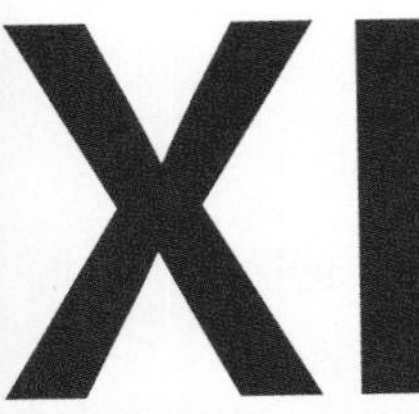

XI RENAL AND GENITOURINARY DISEASES

116

APPROACH TO THE PATIENT WITH RENAL DISEASE

DONALD W. LANDRY AND HASAN BAZARI

DIAGNOSIS

The prominent functions of the kidney include the excretion of nitrogenous waste; the regulation of the excretion of sodium, potassium, and acid; and the synthesis of a variety of hormones, including 1,25-dihydroxyvitamin D, erythropoietin, and renin. A patient can have an isolated failure in a particular function, such as in acid excretion (Chapter 120), in which case the "approach to the patient" is distinct for the isolated defect. First and foremost, however, the kidney is a filtration organ, and acute kidney injury (Chapter 122) and chronic kidney disease (Chapter 132) refer specifically to defects in the filtration function of the kidney. In the context of impaired filtration, many of the individual functions may fail.

The approximately 2 million renal glomeruli normally filter about 180 L/day. The renal glomerulus is not simply a filter, but rather a size- and charge-dependent ultrafilter that excludes not only cells but also proteins larger than 60 kD from the ultrafiltrate. Smaller proteins are variably filtered at the glomerulus and endocytosed in the proximal tubule, so that the protein concentration of the urine is normally quite low. Kidney disease reflects a failure in the quantity or quality of the glomerular ultrafiltrate.

The normal glomerular filtration rate (GFR) may decline in hours or a few days in acute kidney injury or over months and years in chronic kidney disease. An acute decline in glomerular filtration is the necessary and sufficient condition for the diagnosis of acute kidney injury, but abnormal urinary findings can assist with elucidating of the etiology of the injury. Proteinuria, ranging from microscopic to the nephrotic range (Chapter 123), and urinary findings, from a few cells per microscopic high-power field to gross hematuria or pyuria, may be the only evidence of the earliest stages of chronic kidney disease. As chronic kidney disease advances, the decline in the GFR progresses until dialysis or transplantation (Chapter 133) is required to forestall or treat the syndrome of uremia.

Serum creatinine is, to a first approximation, neither secreted nor reabsorbed, so the amount appearing in the urine per unit time is a measure of the amount that was filtered at the glomerulus during that period. As a result, the rate of creatinine clearance is, at first approximation, equivalent to the GFR. A decrement in the GFR diminishes creatinine clearance but has no immediate effect on creatinine production by muscle; as a result, the serum creatinine concentration rises. The change in serum creatinine over time indicates the tempo of the renal disease and can distinguish acute injury from chronic kidney disease. Advanced chronic kidney disease (Chapter 132) is commonly associated with anemia, renal osteodystrophy, and a small kidney size on ultrasonography, although kidney size may be normal or increased with amyloidosis or diabetes mellitus. Hyperphosphatemia, which develops within 1 or 2 weeks after acute kidney injury, is less useful as a discriminator of acute versus chronic renal injury.

The serum creatinine level is elevated in both acute and chronic kidney disease, but an actively rising serum creatinine level confirms an acute or acute-on-chronic insult to kidney function. As a blood filtration organ, the kidney is susceptible to an acute compromise of renal arterial perfusion (Chapter 127), such as prerenal kidney injury, or blockage in urine outflow, such as urinary obstruction owing to benign prostatic hypertrophy (Chapter 131). The intrarenal causes of acute kidney injury (Chapter 122) include acute tubular necrosis, acute interstitial nephritis, acute glomerulonephritis, and acute vasculitis and vascular disease. Dysmorphic red blood cells in the urine or clumps of cells in the form of the renal tubules, so-called tubular casts, suggest the site of the lesion and narrow the range of potential etiologies.

Most of the diagnoses of renal disease can be made with a careful history and physical examination supplemented by review of basic laboratory tests, especially the urinary sediment. The specificity of the diagnosis can be improved by the use of serologic analysis, imaging, and, occasionally, invasive procedures such as angiography and renal biopsy.

History

The history reviews potential factors that contribute to the development of renal disease and identifies the systemic features of diseases that may affect the kidney. These factors include the following:

- Medication use
- Family history of renal disease
- The time of onset of symptoms of renal dysfunction
- Changes in bladder function, including nocturia, polyuria, and hesitancy
- Fatigue and weakness
- Dyspnea on exertion, a manifestation of fluid overload or acidosis
- Systemic features of vasculitis

A systemic vasculitis may present in a variety of ways, with skin manifestations including petechial rash, purpura, digital gangrene, and splinter hemorrhages. Otitis, sinusitis, epistaxis, hemoptysis, and nasal septal ulcers are common manifestations of Wegener's granulomatosis (Chapter 278). Pulmonary hemorrhage can be a catastrophic manifestation of Goodpasture's syndrome (Chapter 123) or anti–glomerular basement membrane (anti-GBM) disease. Abdominal distention may be seen in nephrotic syndrome with ascites, as well as in autosomal polycystic kidney disease (Chapter 129). Abdominal pain and tenderness and gastrointestinal hemorrhage may be observed in Henoch-Schönlein purpura and classic polyarteritis nodosa (Chapter 278). Lower extremity edema is common in cirrhosis (Chapter 156), heart failure (Chapter 58), and nephrotic syndrome (Chapter 123). Neurologic symptoms may be a manifestation of vasculitis, such as microscopic polyangiitis (Chapter 278) and cryoglobulinemia (Chapter 193).

Physical Examination

The vital signs are crucial. A patient with a "normal blood pressure" may be relatively hypotensive in the setting of renovascular disease. Orthostatic hypotension may explain the acute decompensation of kidney function in a patient with chronic kidney disease (Chapter 132). Pulsus paradoxus may reflect cardiac tamponade (Chapter 77).

The eyes may exhibit conjunctivitis, episcleritis, or uveitis. In the abdomen, ascites may be seen in cirrhosis, nephrosis, and heart failure. Hepatomegaly is seen in passive congestion and amyloidosis (Chapter 194). Splenomegaly may be seen in amyloidosis, endocarditis (Chapter 76), and lymphoma (Chapters 191 and 192). Kidney and liver enlargement may be seen in autosomal dominant polycystic kidney disease. Lower extremity edema can be seen in cirrhosis, nephrotic syndrome, and heart failure. Splinter hemorrhages, as well as Osler nodes and Janeway lesions, may represent bacterial endocarditis. Rashes can be seen in many of the vasculitides.

Cardiovascular Signs

Assessment of the jugular venous pressure (Chapter 50) can play a crucial role in the bedside evaluation of volume status. The presence of a pericardial friction rub can be observed in the serositis associated with systemic lupus erythematosus (SLE; Chapter 274) or the pericarditis associated with uremia (Chapter 132). Infiltrative diseases, such as amyloidosis and sarcoidosis (Chapter 95), can lead to restrictive cardiomyopathy with associated heart failure. The presence of a fourth heart sound (S_4) may be a sign of cardiac hypertrophy, and S_3 may be a sign of heart failure. Vascular bruits reflect generalized atherosclerosis, and the presence of an abdominal bruit may be an important clue to the presence of renovascular disease (Chapter 127).

Neurologic Signs

Peripheral neuropathy may be seen in vasculitis with involvement of the nerves as mononeuritis multiplex. Frank cerebrovascular accidents may be seen in SLE and in the antiphospholipid antibody syndrome (Chapter 179).

The signs and symptoms of chronic renal failure are shown in Figure 116-1.

Laboratory Findings

Measurement of Renal Function

Renal function is routinely assessed in clinical practice by the measurement of serum creatinine. Creatine is released as a waste product from myocytes and converted to creatinine in the liver. The normal range of serum creatinine is 0.6 to 1.5 mg/dL, and the value for a given patient is relatively fixed in the absence of a change in renal function. About 90% of the daily production of creatinine is excreted through glomerular filtration and the remainder by tubular secretion. Mild elevations of the plasma creatinine concentration can

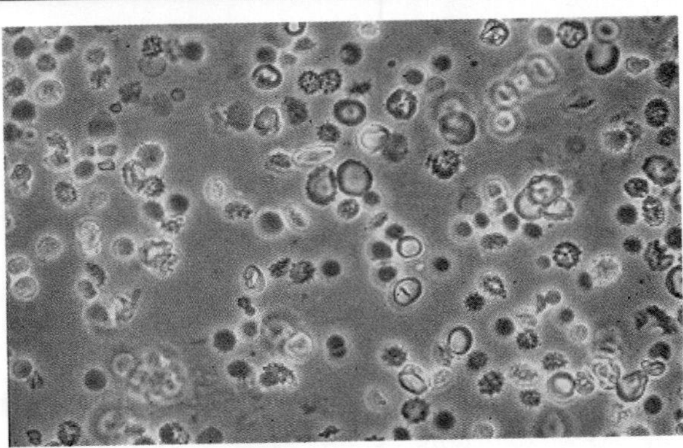

FIGURE 116-2. Dysmorphic erythrocytes. These dysmorphic erythrocytes vary in size, shape, and hemoglobin content and reflect glomerular bleeding. (From Johnson RJ, Feehally J. *Comprehensive Clinical Nephrology*. London: Mosby; 2000.)

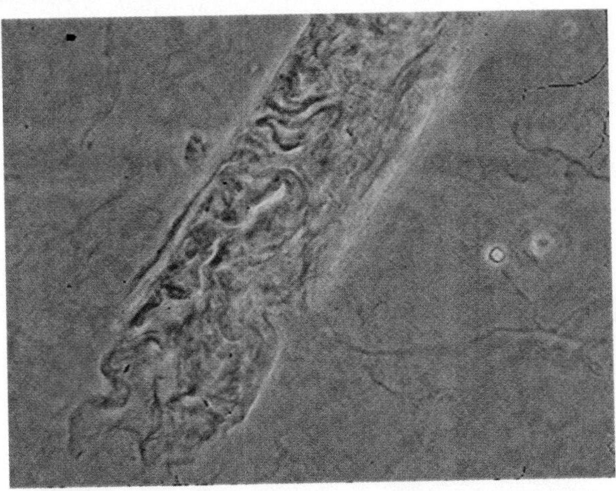

FIGURE 116-4. Hyaline cast of the type seen in small numbers in normal urine. (From Johnson RJ, Feehally J. *Comprehensive Clinical Nephrology*. London: Mosby; 2000.)

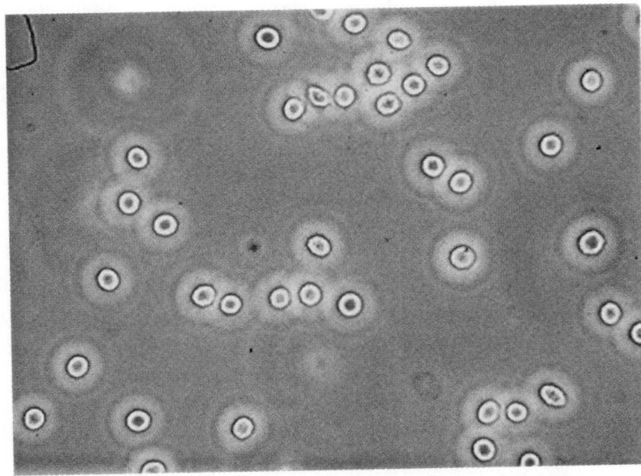

FIGURE 116-3. Isomorphic erythrocytes. These erythrocytes are similar in size, shape, and hemoglobin content. Isomorphic cells reflect nonglomerular bleeding from lesions such as calculi or papillomas or hemorrhage from cysts in polycystic renal disease. (From Johnson RJ, Feehally J. *Comprehensive Clinical Nephrology*. London: Mosby; 2000.)

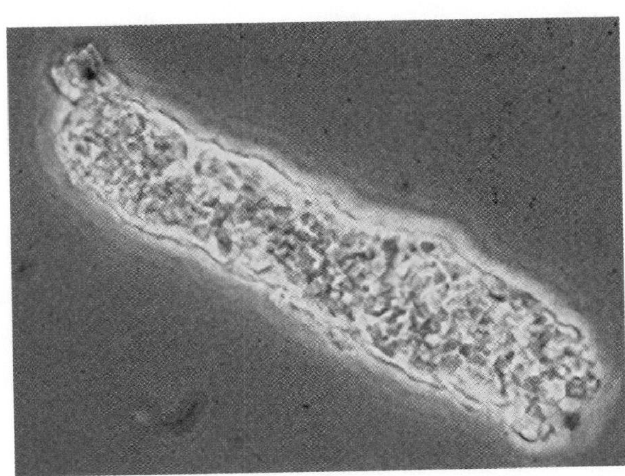

FIGURE 116-5. Number and type of granules and their density in the cast vary in different casts. The presence of erythrocytes in this cast may mean that the granules are derived partly from disrupted erythrocytes. (From Johnson RJ, Feehally J. *Comprehensive Clinical Nephrology*. London: Mosby; 2000.)

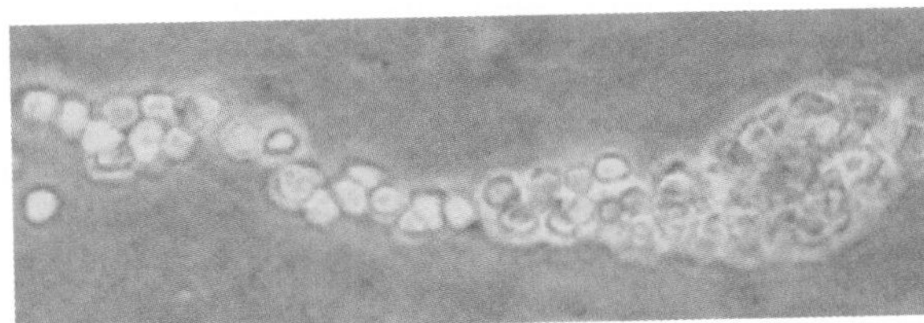

FIGURE 116-6. A cast composed entirely of erythrocytes reflects heavy hematuria and active glomerular disease. Crescentic nephritis is likely to be present if erythrocyte cast density is greater than 100/mL. (From Johnson RJ, Feehally J. *Comprehensive Clinical Nephrology*. London: Mosby; 2000.)

a majority of dysmorphic RBCs in a urine sediment points to a glomerular origin of the hematuria. The presence of RBC casts is often conclusive evidence for the presence of glomerulonephritis.

WBCs are seen most commonly in urinary tract infections, but they also can be seen in acute interstitial nephritis, with *Legionella* (Chapter 322) and *Leptospira* (Chapter 331) species infections, chronic infections such as tuberculosis (Chapter 332), allergic interstitial nephritis (Chapter 124), atheroembolic diseases (Chapter 127), and granulomatous diseases such as sarcoidosis (Chapter 95) and tubulointerstitial nephritis uveitis syndrome. Mononuclear cells often appear with transplant rejection. Tubular cells, which are seen in many conditions involving tubulointerstitial diseases, also are seen in ischemic and nephrotoxic injury, such as with myeloma kidney (Chapter 193) or cast nephropathy. Eosinophils require special stains, with the Giemsa stain being much less sensitive than the Hansel stain (Chapter 124). Urine eosinophils classically are seen in allergic interstitial nephritis (Chapter 124), but they also are seen in atheroembolic disease (Chapter 127), prostatitis (Chapter 131), and vasculitis.

Other Elements

Bacteria may be seen in the urine sediment. A spun urine sediment may show rods or cocci in chains, but bacteria are identified best by Gram staining of the urine sediment. Budding yeast forms, which are highly refractile, trichomonads, and spermatozoa also may be seen in the urinary sediment.

Casts

Casts, which are formed in tubules, are characterized by the arrangement of the cells in a clearly formed matrix composed of Tamm-Horsfall protein. Because casts are formed in the renal parenchyma, they may give a clue to the origin of accompanying cellular elements.

Hyaline casts are composed of Tamm-Horsfall proteins that are formed normally and are seen in increased numbers after exercise (Fig. 116-4). *Granular casts* are degenerated tubular cell casts that are seen in the setting of tubular injury (Fig. 116-5). *Pigmented granular casts* are seen in rhabdomyolysis (Chapter 115) with myoglobinuria or, rarely, hemoglobinuria. *RBC casts* (Fig. 116-6) are rarely seen in allergic interstitial nephritis and diabetic nephropathy, but they are frequently seen in acute glomerulonephritis (Chapter 123). The presence of RBC casts in a patient with microscopic hematuria can narrow the focus of the evaluation to a glomerular lesion. *WBC casts* are seen commonly in pyelonephritis (Chapter 292) and in acute and chronic nonbacterial infections. They also are seen in other conditions in which WBCs are associated with parenchymal renal processes, such as allergic interstitial nephritis (Chapter 124), atheroembolic diseases (Chapter

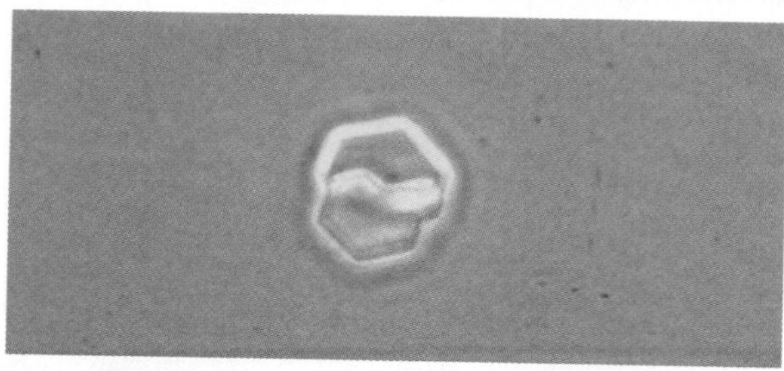

FIGURE 116-7. **Typical hexagonal cystine crystal.** A single crystal provides a definitive diagnosis of cystinuria. (From Johnson RJ, Feehally J. *Comprehensive Clinical Nephrology*. London: Mosby; 2000.)

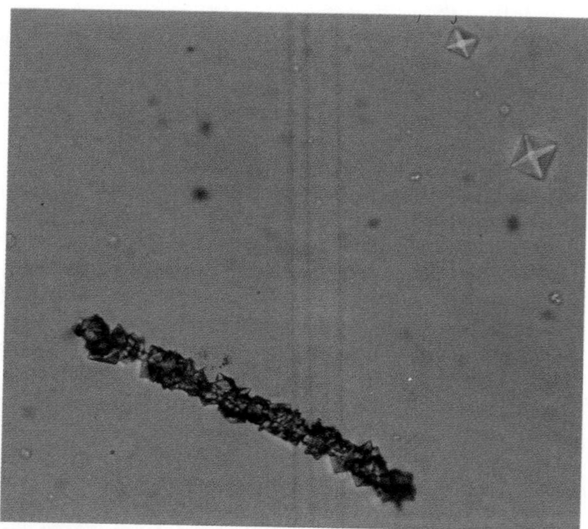

FIGURE 116-8. **Oxalate crystals.** A pseudocast of calcium oxalate crystals accompanied by crystals of calcium oxalate dehydrate. (From Johnson RJ, Feehally J. *Comprehensive Clinical Nephrology*. London: Mosby; 2000.)

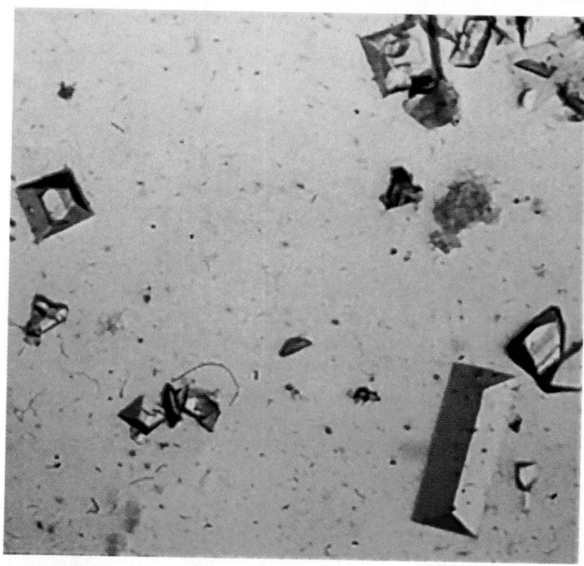

FIGURE 116-9. **Coffin-lid crystals of magnesium ammonium phosphate (struvite).** (From Johnson RJ, Feehally J. *Comprehensive Clinical Nephrology*. London: Mosby; 2000.)

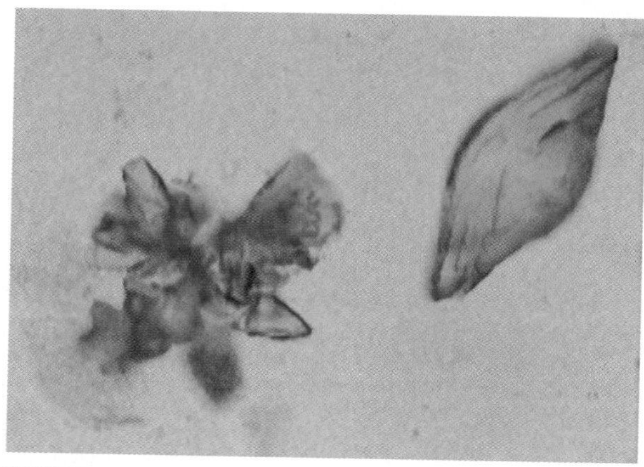

FIGURE 116-10. **Urate crystals.** Complex crystals suggestive of acute urate nephropathy or urate nephrolithiasis. (From Johnson RJ, Feehally J. *Comprehensive Clinical Nephrology*. London: Mosby; 2000.)

127), and granulomatous diseases such as sarcoidosis (Chapter 95). Rarely, WBC casts can be a dominant feature of many diseases that traditionally are thought of as glomerular diseases, such as SLE (Chapter 274) and Wegener's granulomatosis (Chapter 278). *Tubular cell casts* are seen with any acute tubular injury and are the dominant cellular casts in ischemic acute tubular necrosis (Chapter 122). They also can be seen with nephrotoxic injury, such as with aminoglycosides and cisplatin. Some casts may contain both leukocytes and tubular cells or be difficult to distinguish.

Crystals

Crystals can be a normal finding in the urine or serve as clues to pathophysiologic processes. Certain crystals, such as the hexagonal crystals seen with cystinuria (Chapter 130), are always abnormal (Fig. 116-7). Others, such as the octahedral calcium oxalate crystals (Fig. 116-8), may be a normal finding or may be evidence for ethylene glycol intoxication (Chapter 110). Triple phosphate crystals, which are composed of ammonium magnesium phosphate and are coffin shaped (Fig. 116-9), are seen in urinary tract infections with urea-splitting organisms (Chapter 292). Uric acid crystals, sodium urate crystals (Fig. 116-10), and calcium phosphate amorphous crystals are common and do not have pathologic significance.

Serologies for the Evaluation of Renal Disease

The evaluation of renal dysfunction has to follow a stepwise progression from noninvasive serologic evaluation to a definitive or confirmatory diagnostic evaluation, such as a renal biopsy. Sometimes an expeditious diagnosis is needed, and a biopsy may be done relatively early in the evaluation. Serologic diagnostic markers for certain diseases, such as Wegener's granulomatosis (Chapter 278), can sometimes avoid the need for a diagnostic renal biopsy in patients with renal insufficiency.

Antinuclear Antibody

An antinuclear antibody (ANA) can be useful to evaluate glomerular disease, especially the nephrotic syndrome. A high ANA titer (e.g., 1:320), especially if it is accompanied by a more specific finding such as anti-double-stranded DNA (anti-dsDNA) antibody or anti-Smith antibody, can be highly specific for the diagnosis of SLE renal disease (Chapter 274), which usually requires a renal biopsy. Lower titers (e.g., 1:80 or 1:40) are nonspecific.

Rheumatoid Factor

A rheumatoid factor titer will usually be elevated in patients with rheumatoid arthritis, but vasculitis is a relatively late and rare event. Rheumatoid factor can be detected in cryoglobulinemia (Chapter 193); immunoglobulin M (IgM), which is present in type II and type III cryoglobulinemia, has rheumatoid factor activity. Rheumatoid factor also can be seen as a nonspecific finding in bacterial endocarditis (Chapter 76) and systemic vasculitis (Chapter 278).

Complement

The levels of complement components C3 and C4 and the 50% hemolyzing dose of complement (CH_{50}) usually are measured in the evaluation of suspected rapidly progressive glomerulonephritis (Chapter 123). Complement levels are usually low in active SLE (Chapter 274), poststreptococcal glomerulonephritis (Chapter 123), endocarditis (Chapter 76), membranoproliferative glomerulonephritis, cryoglobulinemia (Chapter 193), shunt nephritis, and glomerulonephritis associated with visceral abscesses. A particularly depressed C4 compared with C3 should raise the suspicion of cryoglobulinemia.

Serum and Urine Immunoelectrophoresis and Bence Jones Protein

Elevated polyclonal IgA levels are seen in about 50% of cases of IgA nephropathy (Chapter 123) and Henoch-Schönlein purpura (Chapter 123). Polyclonal elevation of IgG may occur in a variety of systemic diseases and is a nonspecific finding. The presence of a monoclonal protein in the serum should raise the suspicion for a monoclonal gammopathy–associated disease (Chapter 193). The differential diagnosis includes monoclonal gammopathy of uncertain significance, myeloma kidney, lymphomas (Chapter 191), amyloidosis (Chapter 194), light chain deposition disease, heavy chain deposition disease, immunotactoid glomerulonephritis, and cryoglobulinemia. The concentration of the monoclonal protein is higher when the diagnosis of multiple myeloma is made, but even small quantities of Bence Jones proteins in the serum can have clinical significance. Because a substantial fraction of multiple myelomas can have no heavy chain excretion and small quantities of light chains may be hard to detect by serum immunoelectrophoresis, a urine immunoelectrophoresis always should be obtained concomitantly to ensure a complete evaluation. A new, more sensitive assay for serum free light chains and an assessment of the ratio of kappa to lambda lights chains increase the sensitivity for detecting monoclonal gammopathies.

A urine test for Bence Jones protein complements the serum immunoelectrophoresis. Patients may have Bence Jones proteinuria even in the absence of an M component in the serum immunoelectrophoresis. Bence Jones proteinuria may be present in myeloma kidney, amyloidosis, light chain deposition disease, lymphoma, or, occasionally, monoclonal gammopathy of uncertain significance. However, many patients with systemic amyloidosis have a normal serum immunoelectrophoresis and no Bence Jones proteinuria (Chapter 193).

Antineutrophil Cytoplasmic Antibody

The antineutrophil cytoplasmic antibody (ANCA) assay has allowed for earlier and more definitive recognition of one of the most common causes of rapidly progressive glomerulonephritis. The ANCA test, when confirmed by enzyme-linked immunosorbent assay (ELISA), is highly sensitive and specific for a group of vasculitides (Chapter 278). The antibodies are present in the serum of the affected patient and cause two different patterns of staining: perinuclear staining (p-ANCA) and cytoplasmic staining (c-ANCA). Both antigens actually have a cytoplasmic distribution, and the former pattern is an artifact of the fixation method. The antigen for p-ANCA is myeloperoxidase, and the antigen for c-ANCA is proteinase-3. p-ANCA is associated with microscopic polyangiitis, idiopathic crescentic glomerulonephritis, or Churg-Strauss syndrome (Chapter 278). The c-ANCA serology result often correlates with the classic disease of Wegener's granulomatosis (Chapter 278). Immunofluorescence is highly sensitive but is not specific, unless used with ELISA and Western blotting. In the appropriate clinical setting, it can avoid the need for renal biopsy. Anti-GBM antibody staining also may occur in the presence of a positive ANCA, the significance of which is unclear. It is speculated that exposure of the Goodpasture antigen, as a result of the glomerular injury, leads to anti-GBM antibody formation as a secondary process.

Anti–Glomerular Basement Membrane Antibody

Anti-GBM antibodies are autoantibodies to the Goodpasture antigen, which resides in a domain of the α chain of type 4 collagen. An early and accurate diagnosis of Goodpasture's syndrome can be made by immunofluorescence and confirmed by Western blot analysis.

Cryoglobulins

Cryoglobulins (Chapter 193) are thermolabile immunoglobulins of single monoclonal type (type I cryoglobulinemia); in type II and type III cryoglobulinemia, the mixture of immunoglobulins includes one with rheumatoid factor activity against IgG. Type I and type II cryoglobulins are more likely to be associated with clinical disease, especially at higher titers. In type II cryoglobulinemia, the monoclonal component has rheumatoid factor activity and is often an IgM κ M component. Type III cryoglobulinemia is often of less clinical significance. Type I cryoglobulinemia is seen with Waldenström's macroglobulinemia and multiple myeloma (Chapter 193); type II, with hepatitis C infection (Chapters 150 and 151), Sjögren's syndrome (Chapter 276), lymphomas (Chapters 191 and 192), and SLE (Chapter 274); and type III, with hepatitis C (Chapters 150 and 151), chronic infections, and inflammatory conditions. When cryoglobulinemia is associated with hepatitis C, the hepatitis C virus (HCV) RNA is concentrated in the cryoprecipitate; the diagnosis can be made by an RNA assay of the cryoprecipitate at 37° C.

Other Serologies

Membranous nephropathy is associated with chronic hepatitis B infection with hepatitis B surface antigenemia (Chapter 151). Classic polyarteritis nodosa (Chapter 278) occasionally is seen with chronic hepatitis B infection, often with surface antigenemia and hepatitis B e-antigenemia.

Hepatitis C serology is associated with a variety of renal entities, including cryoglobulinemia, membranoproliferative glomerulonephritis, and membranous nephropathy. The evaluation may include the antibody test and an assay for HCV RNA. Occasionally, the HCV RNA analysis may have to be conducted on the cryoprecipitate at 37° C.

Human immunodeficiency virus (HIV)-associated nephropathy (Chapter 123) is associated with nephrotic syndrome and acute kidney injury. In the appropriate clinical setting, HIV serology and viral titers are appropriate tests for both clinical syndromes.

Streptococcal infection can be confirmed as the cause of postinfectious glomerulonephritis (Chapter 123) with an anti-DNase or antistreptolysin assay. Acute and convalescent serology assays are used to confirm recent infection.

Erythrocyte Sedimentation Rate

The erythrocyte sedimentation rate (ESR) is a relatively nonspecific test in the evaluation of renal disease. However, a high ESR often points to systemic vasculitis (Chapter 278), multiple myeloma (Chapter 193), or malignancy as the underlying cause. However, the ESR often is elevated in the nephrotic syndrome (Chapter 123), including diabetic nephropathy (Chapter 126).

Noninvasive Imaging

A variety of renal imaging techniques can assist in the evaluation of diseases of the kidney. Of note is that plain films and intravenous pyelography largely have been replaced by renal ultrasonography and computed tomography (CT) for the evaluation of renal size and the detection of stones and masses.

Renal Ultrasonography

Ultrasonography, which is the most commonly used renal imaging study (Fig. 116-11), provides reliable information regarding obstruction, renal size, the presence of masses, and renal echotexture. The study has only 90% sensitivity for the detection of hydronephrosis, however, and is not sufficient to exclude obstruction with certainty. Additionally, its inability to detect stones in the ureters and bladder limits its utility in the evaluation for kidney stones. Doppler imaging permits evaluation of the renal vessels and resistive index.

Computed Tomography

A stone protocol CT scan of the kidneys, ureter, and bladder has become the study of choice for the detection of kidney stones (Chapter 128) because of its ability to detect stones of all kinds, including uric acid stones and nonobstructing stones in the ureters (Fig. 116-12). Masses in the kidney can be evaluated using either contrast CT or a renal ultrasound. CT angiography with iodinated contrast material can assess possible renal artery stenosis

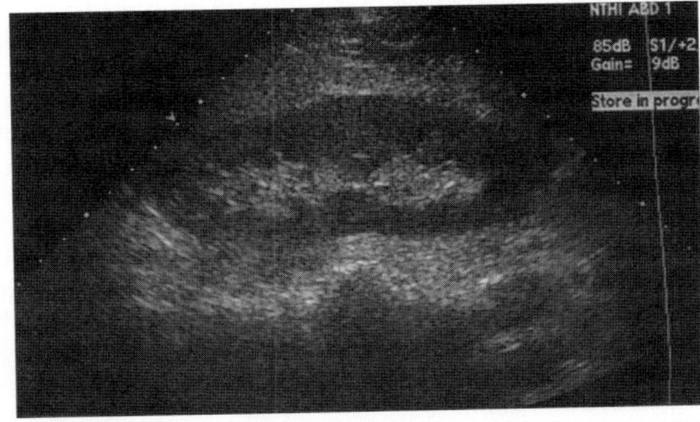

FIGURE 116-11. Normal sagittal renal ultrasound. The cortex is hypoechoic compared with the echogenic fat containing the renal sinus. (From Johnson RJ, Feehally J. *Comprehensive Clinical Nephrology*. London: Mosby; 2000.)

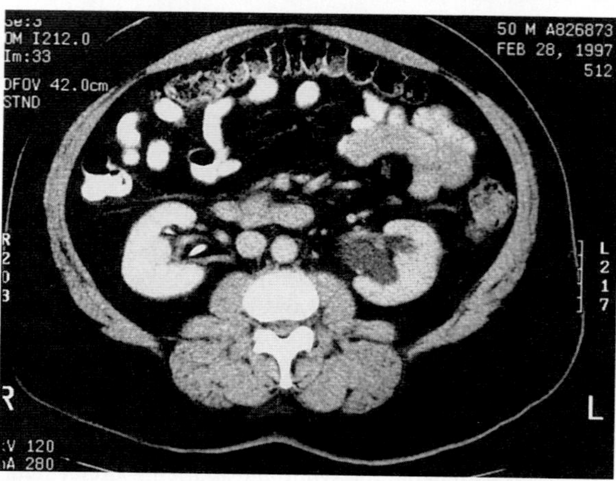

FIGURE 116-12. Delayed excretion in the left kidney secondary to a distal calculus. Contrast-enhanced computed tomography scan shows dilated left renal pelvis. (From Johnson RJ, Feehally J. *Comprehensive Clinical Nephrology*. London: Mosby; 2000.)

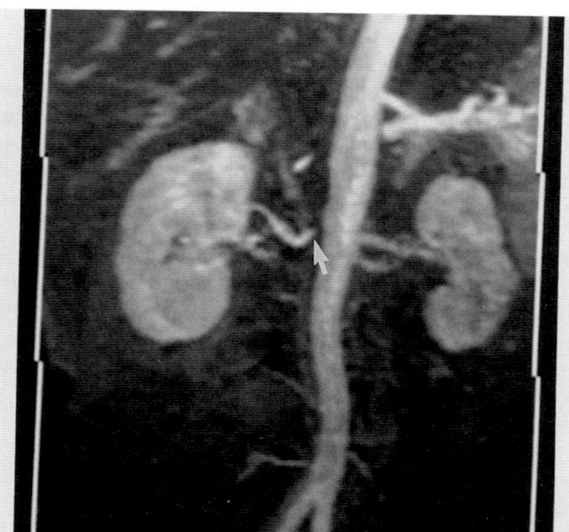

FIGURE 116-13. Magnetic resonance angiography. Coronal three-dimensional image shows right renal artery stenosis *(arrow)*. (From Johnson RJ, Feehally J. *Comprehensive Clinical Nephrology*. London: Mosby; 2000.)

(Chapter 127) with an accuracy comparable to magnetic resonance (MR) angiography.

Magnetic Resonance Imaging with Magnetic Resonance Angiography

Magnetic resonance imaging (MRI) with MR angiography (Fig. 116-13) is highly sensitive for detecting atherosclerotic renovascular disease (Chapter 127), but it tends to overestimate the degree of stenosis. Its accuracy in detecting fibromuscular dysplasia, however, is less well validated. MRI also can be used to evaluate renal masses. MRI does not require iodinated contrast material, but gadolinium-based contrast agents for vascular studies are associated with the syndrome of nephrogenic systemic fibrosis in patients with renal failure (Chapter 275).

Renography

The uptake by the kidneys of ^{99m}Tc-DTPA, as a marker of GFR, and mercaptoacetyl triglycine, as a marker of renal blood flow, can help evaluate patients with suspected renovascular disease. However, neither is commonly used now that CT angiography and MR angiography are widely available.

Invasive Evaluation

Renal Angiography

Renal arteriography, which is the gold standard in the evaluation of renal artery stenosis (Chapter 127), also is used for the evaluation of arteriovenous malformations, polyarteritis nodosa, and other vascular lesions of the kidneys. This invasive study uses iodinated contrast material and incurs a small risk for atheroembolic disease (Chapter 127). Therapeutic angioplasty and stenting can be done at the time of the angiogram.

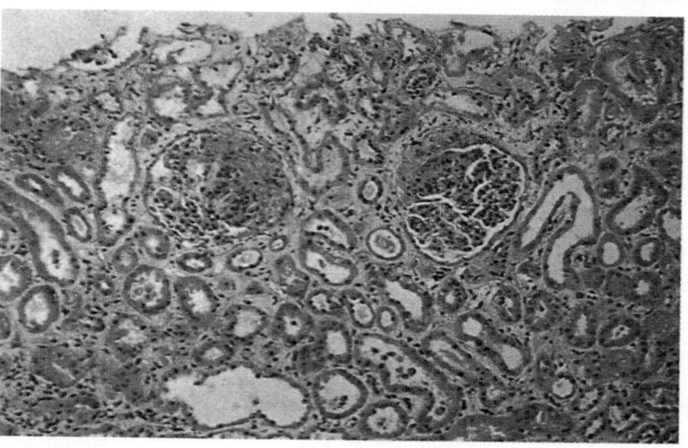

FIGURE 116-14. Systemic lupus erythematosus. This renal biopsy specimen shows proliferative change and crescent formation in both glomeruli (hematoxylin and eosin stain; magnification, 116×). (From Johnson RJ, Feehally J. *Comprehensive Clinical Nephrology*. London: Mosby; 2000.)

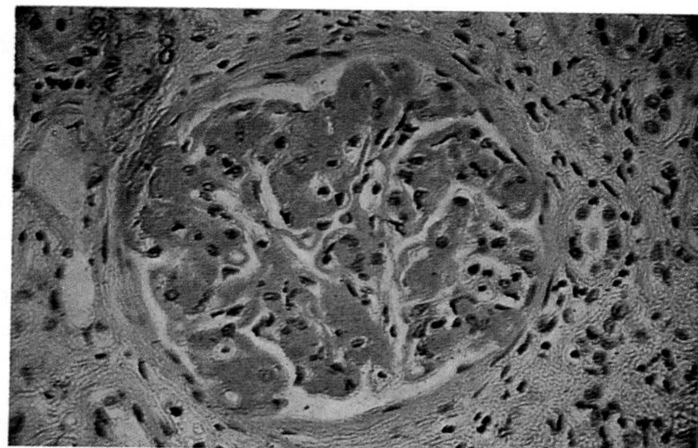

FIGURE 116-15. Renal amyloidosis. The glomerulus shows amyloid deposition, stained by Congo red, in the glomerular capillaries (magnification, 330×). (From Johnson RJ, Feehally J. *Comprehensive Clinical Nephrology*. London: Mosby; 2000.)

Renal Biopsy

Renal biopsy usually is performed percutaneously with real-time ultrasound or CT guidance. The risk for bleeding that requires a transfusion is 1 to 2% in patients without coagulopathy. The transjugular approach can be used in patients in whom the risks for bleeding are high. Current indications for renal biopsy include the following:

1. Rapidly progressive glomerulonephritis. Biopsy is generally indicated for ANCA-related vasculitis unless the case is classic, such as red blood cell casts and renal dysfunction. For patients with cryoglobulinemia and SLE, biopsy is recommended to stratify patients before therapy.
2. SLE with renal involvement to categorize the degree of nephropathy, which cannot be assessed based on clinical criteria (Fig. 116-14). A repeat biopsy is indicated if a change in immunosuppressive therapy is planned and the clinical picture is at all ambiguous (e.g., serum creatinine, urine sediment, and proteinuria are in good control but anti-DNA antibody titers remain high).
3. Nephrotic syndrome without an obvious cause. In childhood nephrotic syndrome, empirical steroid therapy is used routinely because of the high prevalence of steroid-responsive minimal change disease. In adults, the approach generally is to use the biopsy to guide appropriate therapy (Fig. 116-15).
4. Unexplained renal failure of any cause, especially if immunosuppressive therapy is contemplated. Patients with hospital-acquired renal failure rarely require renal biopsy.
5. Unexplained proteinuria below the nephrotic range to exclude nephrosis in evolution. Biopsy is recommended if proteinuria exceeds 1 g per 24 hours or occurs in the setting of a reduced GFR.

6. Renal transplantation with acute and chronic renal failure, in which the biopsy information can be crucial in guiding diagnosis and treatment.

MAJOR RENAL SYNDROMES

Renal disease can be divided logically into major overlapping categories, which are used to characterize the most common renal syndromes.

Acute Kidney Injury

Acute kidney injury (Chapter 122) is a syndrome in which glomerular filtration declines over a period of hours to days. The patient with acute renal failure is approached best by evaluation for prerenal, renal, and postrenal causes. Most cases of acute renal failure in the hospital have hemodynamic or toxic etiologies. The careful and systematic evaluation of the patient should start with a thorough history and physical examination, which should be followed by selected laboratory tests and often an imaging test, such as renal ultrasonography.

Nephritic Syndrome

The acute nephritic syndrome is an uncommon but dramatic presentation of an acute glomerulonephritis (Chapter 123). The hallmark of the acute nephritic syndrome is the presence of dysmorphic RBCs and RBC casts, but their absence does not exclude the syndrome. The acute nephritic syndrome can be caused by any of the rapidly progressive glomerulonephropathies, all of which warrant urgent and usually inpatient evaluation.

Nephrotic Syndrome

The nephrotic syndrome (Chapter 123) is characterized by the presence of proteinuria of greater than 3.5 g/day/1.73 m^2, with accompanying edema, hypertension, and hyperlipidemia. Other consequences include a predisposition to infection and hypercoagulability. In general, the diseases associated with nephrotic syndrome do not cause acute kidney injury, although acute kidney injury may be seen with minimal change disease, HIV-associated nephropathy, and bilateral renal vein thrombosis (Chapter 127). The causes of primary idiopathic nephrotic syndrome, in decreasing order of prevalence, are focal and segmental glomerulosclerosis, membranous nephropathy, minimal change disease, and membranoproliferative glomerulonephritis. Secondary causes of the nephrotic syndrome include diabetic nephropathy (Chapter 126), amyloidosis (Chapter 194), and SLE (Chapter 274) with membranous nephropathy.

Tubulointerstitial Diseases

Tubulointerstitial diseases (Chapter 124) vary in presentation from acute kidney injury to chronic kidney dysfunction that manifests as asymptotic mild renal insufficiency (Table 116-2). The urine sediment often contains small-to-moderate amounts of proteinuria, usually less than 1 g/day, as well as WBCs, RBCs, tubular cells, and WBC casts. RBC casts are rare in acute interstitial nephritis and are more characteristic of glomerular disease.

Vascular Diseases of the Kidney

Vascular diseases of the kidney can be divided into large-vessel obstruction and medium- to small-vessel diseases (Chapter 127). Renovascular disease is a common cause of hypertension, heart failure, and renal insufficiency. About 90% of renal artery stenosis is atherosclerotic in origin, with most of the remaining caused by fibromuscular dysplasia, which is more common in women 20 to 50 years of age. Medium-sized arterial vessel diseases include polyarteritis nodosa, which is seen in patients with hepatitis B, HIV infection, or, rarely, hepatitis C. Symptoms include abdominal pain, hypertension, and mild renal insufficiency, often with a benign sediment; diagnostic findings include microaneurysms at the bifurcation of medium-sized arteries. Other diseases involving small vessels include atheroembolic disease (Chapter 127), which is seen either spontaneously or after arteriography or surgery; this syndrome typically affects the kidneys, gastrointestinal tract, and lower extremities, but it can also involve the central nervous system when the aortic arch is affected.

The thrombotic microangiopathies include hemolytic-uremic syndrome and thrombotic thrombocytopenic purpura (Chapter 174). Thrombocytopenic purpura is associated with an acquired inhibitor to, or the congenital inherited absence of, a protease that cleaves large-molecular-weight von Willebrand multimers. Hemolytic-uremic syndrome is caused by endothelial injury induced by Shiga toxin from *Escherichia coli* O157:H7 infection. The antiphospholipid antibody syndrome (Chapter 179) can cause large vessel thrombosis and stenosis as well as a thrombotic microangiopathy with proteinuria, hypertension, and renal insufficiency. Scleroderma renal crisis, which is a manifestation of systemic sclerosis (Chapter 275), often leads to an inexorable progression to end-stage renal insufficiency if it is untreated.

TABLE 116-2 MAJOR CAUSES OF TUBULOINTERSTITIAL DISEASE

Ischemic and toxic acute tubular necrosis
Allergic interstitial nephritis
Interstitial nephritis secondary to immune complex–related collagen vascular disease, such as Sjögren's disease or systemic lupus erythematosus
Granulomatous diseases: sarcoidosis, tubulointerstitial nephritis with uveitis
Pigment-related tubular injury: myoglobulinuria, hemoglobinuria
Hypercalcemia with nephrocalcinosis
Tubular obstruction: drugs such as indinavir, uric acid in tumor lysis syndrome
Myeloma kidney or cast nephropathy
Infection-related interstitial nephritis: *Legionella, Leptospira* species
Infiltrative diseases, such as lymphoma

Papillary Necrosis

Acute necrosis of the renal papilla is associated with sickle cell anemia (Chapter 166), analgesic nephropathy (Chapter 124), diabetic nephropathy (Chapter 126), and obstructive pyelonephritis (Chapter 125). In sickle cell disease (Chapter 166), the hypoxic and hypertonic milieu of the inner medulla promotes sickling, and chronic sickling at the vasa recta results in medullary ischemia. Massive and prolonged consumption of analgesics, particularly the combination of aspirin, caffeine, and acetaminophen, is associated with chronic interstitial nephritis and a predisposition to papillary necrosis (Chapter 124); medullary ischemia is thought to be caused by inhibition of synthesis of vasodilatory prostaglandins by aspirin, and direct toxicity is attributed to metabolites of phenacetin. Similarly, medullary perfusion is thought to be compromised in diabetic nephropathy (Chapter 126) and obstructive pyelonephritis (Chapter 125).

The clinical manifestations of papillary necrosis can include flank pain and hematuria. If the papilla is sloughed, obstruction may occur at the renal pelvis or ureter of the affected kidney, with referred pain migrating from the flank to the groin. A sloughed papilla may precipitate frank renal failure if the function of the contralateral kidney is impaired or if obstruction occurs at the level of the bladder or urethra (Chapter 125).

Classically, papillary necrosis is diagnosed on an excretory pyelogram as a calyceal defect after sloughing of a papilla, but CT with contrast is as good for advanced lesions. If the necrotic papilla is retained, however, the defect will be more subtle. Transitional cell carcinoma (Chapter 203) can occur in the setting of papillary necrosis or can mimic its appearance. Obstruction, if present, must be relieved, but treatment otherwise is limited to pain control and hydration.

Chronic Kidney Disease

Chronic kidney disease, which is defined as either kidney damage or a GFR of less than 60 mL/min/1.73 m^2 for longer than 3 months, includes five stages (Table 116-3). Kidney damage is defined as pathologic abnormalities or markers of kidney damage, including abnormalities in the composition of blood or urine or abnormalities on imaging tests. The excretion of 30 to 300 mg of albumin in a 24-hour period defines microalbuminuria. An estimated 12% of the adult U.S. population has abnormal albumin excretion in the urine, and the frequency increases with age. Kidney failure is defined as either a GFR of less than 15 mL/min/1.73 m^2 that is accompanied by signs and symptoms of uremia or a need for initiation of kidney replacement therapy for treatment of complications of decreased GFR. End-stage renal disease includes all cases requiring treatment by dialysis or transplantation regardless of the level of GFR.

Patients with chronic kidney disease warrant referral to a nephrologist. Care of these patients should focus on efforts to slow disease progression, optimize medical management, and make a seamless transition to renal replacement therapy (Chapter 132). The care should include optimal blood pressure control, use of angiotensin-converting enzyme inhibitors and angiotensin receptor blockers if indicated, dietary counseling, careful management of calcium and phosphorus levels, control of the parathyroid hormone level, and management of anemia with the use of erythropoietin and iron supplements. Early referral for placement of access for dialysis and initiation of

TABLE 116-3 STAGES OF CHRONIC KIDNEY DISEASE*

STAGE	DESCRIPTION	GFR (mL/min/1.73 m²)
1	Kidney damage with normal or ↑GFR	≥90
2	Kidney damage with mild or ↓GFR	60-89
3	Moderate ↓GFR	30-59
4	Severe ↓GFR	15-29
5	Kidney failure	<15 (or dialysis)

*Chronic kidney disease is defined as either kidney damage or GFR <60 mL/min/1.73 m² for ≥3 months. Kidney damage is defined as pathologic abnormalities or presence of markers of damage, including abnormalities in blood or urine tests or image studies.
GFR = glomerular filtration rate.
From http://www.kidney.org/kidneydisease/ckd/knowGFR.cfm. Accessed Jan. 31, 2010.

transplant evaluation (Chapter 133) are important components of the care of patients with chronic kidney disease.

SUGGESTED READINGS

Abboud H, Henrich WL. Stage IV chronic kidney disease. *N Engl J Med.* 2010;362:56-65. *Treatment guidelines to slow the progression of advanced kidney disease and prepare for renal replacement therapy.*

James MT, Hemmelgarn BR, Tonelli M. Early recognition and prevention of chronic kidney disease. *Lancet.* 2010;375:1296-1309. *Review.*

Kidney Foundation Disease Outcomes Quality Initiative (DOQI) Guidelines. http://www.kidney.org/professionals/KDOQI/index.cfm. Accessed Dec. 13, 2010. *A periodically updated source of consensus guidelines for the management of chronic kidney disease.*

Poff JA, Hecht EM, Ramchandani P. Renal imaging in patients with renal impairment. *Curr Urol Rep.* 2011;12:24-33. *Suggestions for choosing studies to minimize the adverse effects of contrast media.*

Tonelli M, Muntner P, Lloyd A, et al. Using proteinuria and estimated glomerular filtration rate to classify risk in patients with chronic kidney disease: a cohort study. *Ann Intern Med.* 2011;154:12-21. *The combination of proteinuria and estimated GFR is effective for risk stratification.*

117

STRUCTURE AND FUNCTION OF THE KIDNEYS

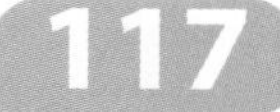

QAIS AL-AWQATI AND JONATHAN BARASCH

The kidney regulates the ionic composition and volume of body fluids, the excretion of nitrogenous waste, the elimination of exogenous molecules (e.g., many drugs), the synthesis of a variety of hormones (e.g., erythropoietin), and the metabolism of low-molecular-weight proteins (e.g., insulin). Befitting such an array of responsibilities, the kidney receives 25% of the cardiac output. The gross anatomy of the kidney is notable for a weight of approximately 150 g and a characteristic bean shape with approximate dimensions of 11 × 6 × 2.5 cm. On bisection, a simple gross structure is evident with an outer cortex and a more central medulla that narrows to multiple papillae at the apices of so-called pyramids (Fig. 117-1).

Understanding the kidney, however, requires an appreciation of the intricate microstructure that underlies its complex functions. The kidney is a composite organ comprising approximately 1 million essentially identical functional units termed *nephrons*. All the functions of the kidney are performed by each individual nephron, and at a first approximation, all nephrons are independent of each other because they have their own innervation and blood supply. The nephron is made up of two functional subunits, the glomerulus and the following tubules and ducts (Fig. 117-2). The glomerulus begins with the branching of the afferent arteriole, an end artery of the corresponding renal artery, to a tuft of capillaries. The glomerular capillaries invaginate an epithelium with the visceral epithelial cells adjacent to the capillary and the parietal epithelial cells outside this tuft. The space between the epithelial layers is the urinary space. The fenestrated glomerular capillary endothelium, the intervening basement membrane, and the foot processes of the visceral epithelium, so-called podocytes, make up the glomerular filtration barrier. The balance of hydrostatic and oncotic pressures drives the extrusion of a protein-free filtrate through this barrier into the urinary space. The urinary space then leads to a series of tubules and ducts: the proximal tubule, the thin limb of the loop of Henle, the thick limb of the loop of Henle,

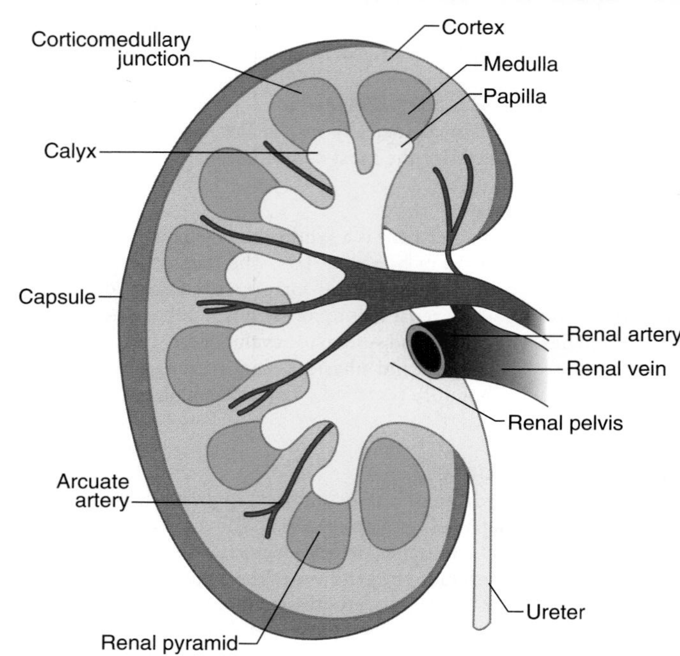

FIGURE 117-1. Sagittal section of the human kidney depicting gross anatomy and organization.

the distal convoluted tubule, the cortical collecting duct, and the medullary collecting duct. The papillary collecting duct empties through the renal papilla into the renal pelvis and then to the ureter. The glomerular capillary bed coalesces to form the efferent arteriole, a vessel that is exquisitely sensitive to angiotensin II, and then to the peri (proximal) tubular capillaries. This system allows efferent arteriole constriction to regulate proximal tubule reabsorption, as described later.

The nephron regulates homeostasis by three actions. First, in the glomerulus, nephrons produce as much as 120 mL/minute of an ultrafiltrate of blood. Second, in different segments of the nephron, the composition of the filtrate is altered by the transfer of nearly 99% of its components (e.g., glucose, NaCl, water) from the lumen to the blood. Third, additional electrolytes (e.g., NH_4^+, K^+, HCO_3^-) are secreted from the blood into the lumen.

To perform these functions, each nephron segment, with the exception of the collecting ducts, is composed of a single epithelial cell type whose luminal or apical surface (facing the urine) and basolateral surface (facing the blood) differentially express various proteins and lipids. For example, the apical membrane often has microvilli or cilia, whereas the basolateral membrane does not. Apical polarized endocytosis and exocytosis are often important in the regulation of the number of transport proteins on the apical surface. In addition, epithelia are connected to one another by tight junctions, which confer a characteristic ionic permeability on the epithelial sheet. Transepithelial transport occurs largely through the cell, but transport through the tight junction (the *paracellular pathway*) can also be important in different segments of the tubule. For instance, Na transport begins with entry at the luminal surface down an electrochemical gradient, whereas its exit at the basolateral surface is uphill and requires adenosine triphosphate (ATP) hydrolysis. The Na^+, K^+-ATPase is located at the basolateral surface of all epithelia, and all "active" energy-consuming transport is coupled directly or indirectly to it with the exception of H^+ transport. Each segment has a distinct composition of channels, carriers, and ATPases, and each segment is regulated by different chemical and physical sensors, so the "final urine" contains the components that must be discarded to maintain constancy of body composition.

THE KIDNEY REGULATES EXTRACELLULAR FLUID VOLUME BY REGULATING ITS SODIUM CONTENT

Filtration of 180 L/day containing 24,000 mEq of Na^+ is followed by the reabsorption of more than 99% of the filtered Na^+. Na^+ reabsorption accounts for more than 90% of oxygen consumed by the kidney. Na^+ reabsorption is regulated by volume receptors, which are located in the carotid artery and

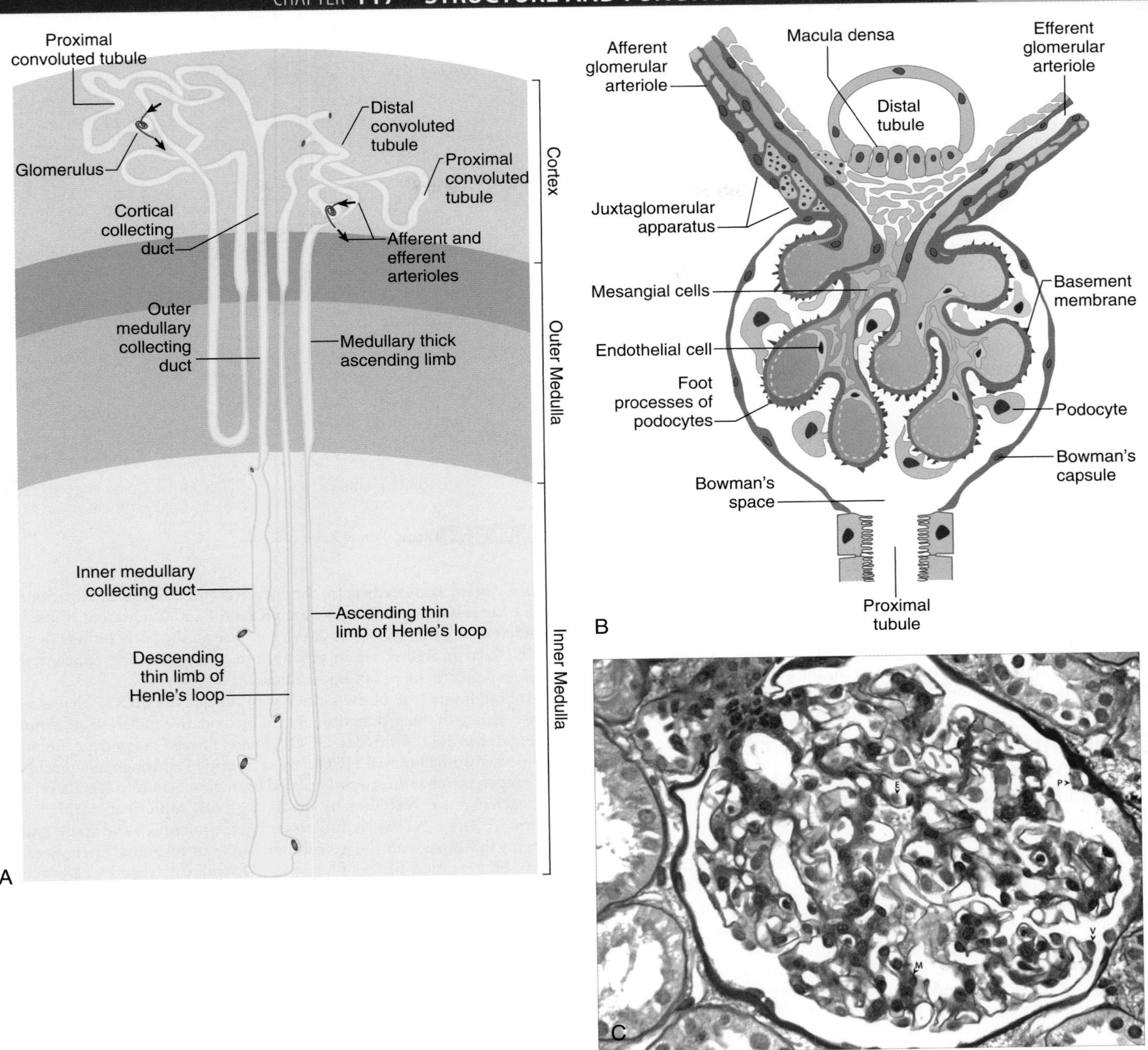

FIGURE 117-2. Structure of the nephron. A, Components of the cortical and juxtaglomerular nephrons. **B,** Anatomy of the glomerulus. **C,** Light micrograph of a human glomerulus. E = endothelial cell; M = mesangial cell; P = parietal epithelial cell; V = visceral epithelial cell. (**C,** Courtesy of Dr. Glen Markowitz.)

increase β-sympathetic output, which in turn release renin, an aspartate protease from the granular cells of the juxtaglomerular apparatus. The renin-releasing cells are close to the afferent arterioles, where renin cleaves angiotensinogen to angiotensin I, which is then converted locally to angiotensin II. Angiotensin II binds to angiotensin receptors and constricts the efferent arteriole, thereby affecting glomerular hemodynamics. The increased hydrostatic pressure within the glomerular capillaries drives the formation of an ultrafiltrate of plasma. As filtration progresses, a protein-rich, oncotically active solution in the capillary opposes the glomerular capillary hydrostatic pressure until a pressure equilibrium is achieved before the efferent arteriole is reached. Consequently, angiotensin II may not change glomerular filtration rate (GFR) markedly, but it can increase proximal reabsorption by reducing the hydrostatic pressure and increasing the oncotic pressure in the peritubular capillaries that surround the proximal tubule in a plexus, thereby favoring reabsorption of water and solutes such as urea.

The glomerular filtrate next enters the tubular portion of the nephron, where Na^+ traverses the cell by entering the apical membrane either through a cotransporter or countertransporter or through an Na^+ channel, depending on the specific mechanisms of different segments. In the apical membrane of the proximal tubule, an Na^+/H^+ (NHE_3) exchanger, an Na-coupled glucose carrier, and an Na^+-coupled amino acid and phosphate cotransporter are present. Subsequently, Na^+ is actively transported by the basolateral Na^+, K^+-ATPase into the paracellular space, thereby resulting in local hypertonicity, which causes osmosis through low-resistance tight junctions of the initial segments of the proximal tubule (Fig. 117-3).

In the thick ascending limb of Henle, Na^+ is absorbed by an NaK-2Cl cotransporter. The driving force for this neutral carrier allows Na^+ and Cl^- to enter the cell, but K^+ is then recycled across the apical membrane, thereby resulting in depolarization of the transepithelial membrane potential. In the distal convoluted tubule, Na^+ is absorbed by a thiazide-sensitive cotransporter, which conducts Na^+ and Cl^- in a strict 1:1 stoichiometry. Na^+ exits as usual by the Na^+, K^+-ATPase, but there is also a basolateral Na/Ca exchanger. In this short segment, the macula densa helps control the GFR by regulating renin release through secretion of adenosine and prostaglandins.

In the principal cells of the collecting duct, aldosterone, derived from the zona glomerulosa of the adrenal cortex, increases reabsorption of the final 50 to 100 mEq/day of Na^+ remaining in the lumen by increasing the number of open Na^+ channels (ENac), by activating expression of α-subunits, and by

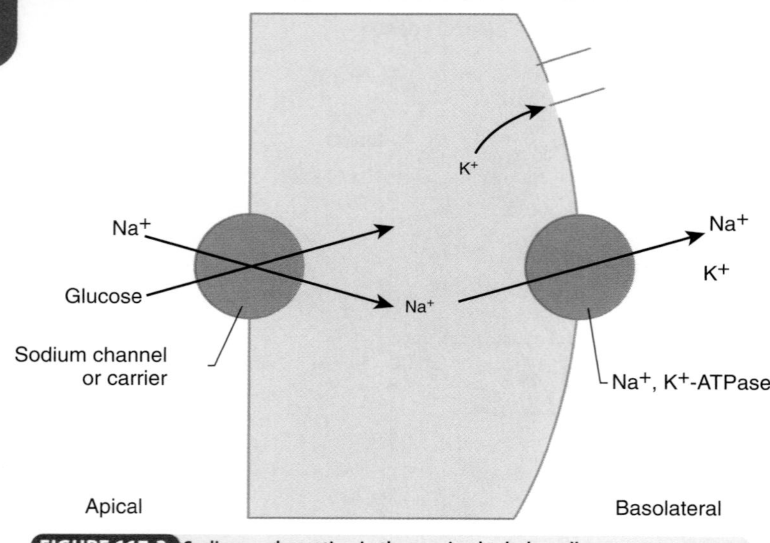

FIGURE 117-3. Sodium reabsorption in the proximal tubular cell.

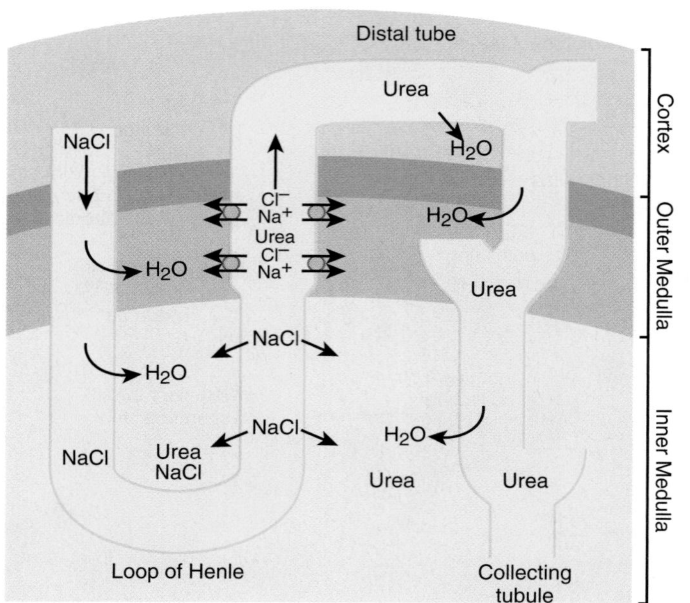

FIGURE 117-4. Regulation of water content.

increasing the activity of the basolateral Na^+, K^+-ATPase. Aldosterone is the final critical regulator of Na^+ balance.

A number of the steps that regulate Na^+ reabsorption can be counteracted by atrial natriuretic peptide (ANP), which is released from the atria in response to volume overload. ANP increases filtration in the glomerulus by dilating the afferent arteriole, thereby increasing glomerular capillary pressure and lowering the oncotic pressure. Additionally, ANP increases Na^+ excretion by inhibiting the release of renin, the production of aldosterone, and the tubular reabsorption of Na^+ in the terminal collecting duct.

THE KIDNEY REGULATES BODY FLUID OSMOLARITY BY REGULATING ITS WATER CONTENT

Water moves freely among all cells and compartments of the body, and its concentration, or osmolarity, is strictly regulated to prevent cells from swelling or contracting. The kidney regulates water content by varying the osmolarity of urine. It can dilute the urine by absorbing Na^+ without water in the thick ascending limb, the distal tubule, and the collecting duct. Conversely, the absorbed NaCl and urea provide a hyperosmotic region in the medulla, where the limited blood flow maintains an osmotic gradient. To concentrate the urine, water is removed from the filtrate by this osmotic gradient as it passes through the cortical and medullary collecting tubules.

Antidiuretic hormone (ADH), also called *vasopressin*, is a critical component of water reclamation. The neurohypophysis releases ADH as a result of activation of Trvp1 channels, which are responsive to cell shrinkage caused by changes in osmolarity of as little as 1%. In the kidney, ADH binds to the V2R receptor Trvp1 on collecting tubules and increases water permeability by reversibly inserting a water channel, called *aquaporin-2*, in the apical membrane by the fusion of vesicles. During states of water deprivation, the dilute urine generated by the thick ascending limb enters vasopressin-sensitive segments in the cortical collecting tubule, where the bulk of the water is absorbed into the cortex to increase the osmolarity of the urinary filtrate to 300 mOsm, which is the osmolarity of plasma. Subsequently, the urine becomes concentrated when it equilibrates with the osmolarity of the medulla as the urine courses down the medullary collecting duct (Fig. 117-4).

THE KIDNEY REGULATES PLASMA pH BY REGULATING HCO_3 CONTENT

The concentration of free H^+ in the intracellular and extracellular fluids is maintained at about 40 nM (pH 7.4) by the daily excretion of acid or base in amounts equal to what is generated by dietary intake and by cellular activity. The complete oxidation of carbohydrates and fats generates approximately 15 to 20 mol/day of the volatile acid CO_2, and nonvolatile acids generated by the metabolism of protein-rich diets account for 60 to 80 mEq/day. HCO_3^- is the most important buffer not only because it is consumed by metabolic acid, thereby producing CO_2 that can be exhaled, but also because it can be regenerated by the kidney. The overall relationship of this buffer system is described by the Henderson-Hasselbalch equation: $pH = pKa + \log [HCO_3^-]/\alpha\, P_{CO_2}$, where pKa is 6.1 and α represents the solubility coefficient of P_{CO_2} (which is 0.03). Because all the body buffers (e.g., bone, intracellular proteins) are in equilibrium, changes in the concentration of HCO_3^- regulate the pH of body fluids.

Although one task of the kidney is to replace the HCO_3^- that is lost as a consequence of the production of acid by oxidative metabolism, it must first reabsorb the 5000 mEq/day HCO_3^- that is filtered every day. The proximal tubule reabsorbs luminal HCO_3^- by secreting H^+ through an apical Na^+/H^+ exchanger, which is directly stimulated by angiotensin II to secrete H^+ in strict 1:1 exchange for Na^+, thereby mediating both sodium absorption and H^+ secretion. An H^+-ATPase is also present in the microvilli and apical endocytic vesicles that fuse with the apical membrane in response to elevated blood P_{CO_2}. H^+ secretion titrates filtered HCO_3 and, catalyzed by carbonic anhydrase, converts it to CO_2 and water, thereby allowing CO_2 reabsorption. H^+ secretion leads to an excess of OH^- in the cell, where it combines with this CO_2 to produce cellular HCO_3^-, which then exits across the basolateral membrane through an Na-HCO_3^- cotransporter (Fig. 117-5).

Given that the proximal tubule regulates bicarbonate reabsorption, the collecting duct must produce "new" HCO_3 to replace what is lost during titration by nonvolatile acids. The cortical and medullary collecting tubules contain intercalated cells that mediate H^+-HCO_3 transport; α- and β-cell types are present in the cortex, whereas only α cells are present in the medulla. H^+ secretion is mediated by the α-intercalated cell, where the H^+-ATPase is delivered to the apical membrane by fusion of apical vesicles as stimulated by ambient P_{CO_2} (Fig. 117-6).

In a reaction catalyzed by carbonic anhydrase II, the excess OH^- is carboxylated by CO_2 to form HCO_3^-. HCO_3^- is subsequently transported across the basolateral surface in exchange for Cl^- by an alternately spliced form of the red cell anion exchanger (band 3). In contrast, β cells secrete HCO_3^- by an apical Cl/HCO_3 exchanger (pendrin) and a basolateral H^+-ATPase. An H^+, K^+-ATPase in the collecting tubule also may play a role in K absorption and perhaps in H^+ secretion.

The collecting tubule is a "tight epithelium" that can maintain electrical and concentration gradients. Secretion of H^+ reduces the pH of the filtrate; the maximal gradient is 3 pH units or 180 mV, but both the size of the pH gradient and its transepithelial membrane potential can be modified to regulate H^+ secretion. For example, Na^+ absorption by the principal cell hyperpolarizes the membrane and can drive H^+ transport. Aldosterone can stimulate not only Na^+ absorption but also independently H^+ secretion—hence, it is the major hormone that stimulates acid secretion in the collecting tubule. Finally, chronic metabolic acidosis converts the β-intercalated cells into α-intercalated cells, thereby increasing the number of acid-secreting cells and reducing the amount of HCO_3^- secretion in this segment.

The secreted H^+ titrates urinary NH_3, and HPO_4^{2-}. NH_3, which is synthesized by the conversion of glutamine to α-ketoglutarate, is secreted into the proximal lumen. In the loop of Henle and distal segments, the protonated ammonium ion is transferred into the interstitium, from where it reenters the nephron as ammonia gas. Once in the lumen, ammonia gas becomes reprotonated to ammonium, thus trapping a proton. The amount of NH_3 generated from glutamine increases up to four- to five-fold in the setting of metabolic acidosis. Net acid secretion is consequently urinary NH_4^+ plus titratable weak acids (such as HPO_4^{2-}) minus urinary HCO_3^-. Each of these components is regulated by the kidney.

THE KIDNEY REGULATES PLASMA POTASSIUM BY EXCRETION AND THE CONTROL OF EXTRACELLULAR PH

Because the membrane potential of most cells is governed by the ratio of intracellular to extracellular K, the plasma K concentration must be heavily regulated. Most dietary K^+ is pumped into the cell by the Na/K-ATPase, but about 90% of ingested K^+ eventually must be excreted into the urine. K^+ is filtered but is then reabsorbed by the proximal tubule and loop of Henle. K^+ is then secreted by the distal convoluted tubule and the principal cells through apical potassium inwardly rectifying (ROMK) and potassium large conductance calcium-activated (BK) channels. K^+ is secreted in response to a gradient, with cell K^+ greater than lumen K^+, which drives K^+ into the lumen. Secretion is enhanced by the increased entry of K^+ into the principal cell as a result of high extracellular concentration, by metabolic alkalosis, and by aldosterone. Aldosterone increases the synthesis of Na^+, K^+-ATPase and increases the probability that the ROMK channels will be open. Aldosterone also enhances Na^+ reabsorption by ENaC and thereby hyperpolarizing the transepithelial membrane potential, which increases the driving force for K secretion. High urinary flow rates deliver a large volume of fluid that is essentially K^+ free, thereby providing a concentration gradient. However, the flow rate also activates mechanosensory flagella that lead to an increase in cell calcium, which in turn activates BK channels. K^+ reabsorption is not regulated to the same extent as Na^+ retention, and profound K^+ depletion may be required for K^+ excretion by the kidneys to be eliminated completely.

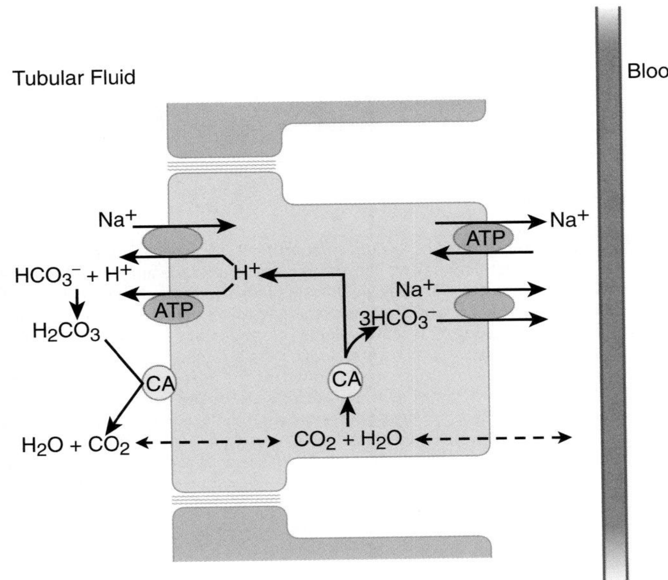

FIGURE 117-5. **Ion transport in the proximal tubule.** ATP = adenosine triphosphate; CA = carbonic anhydrase.

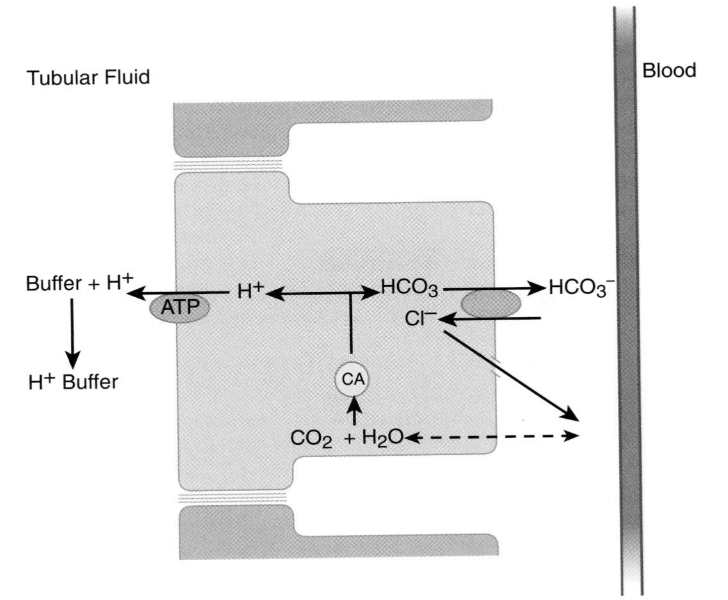

FIGURE 117-6. **Mechanism of acid secretion in the collecting duct.** ATP = adenosine triphosphate; CA = carbonic anhydrase.

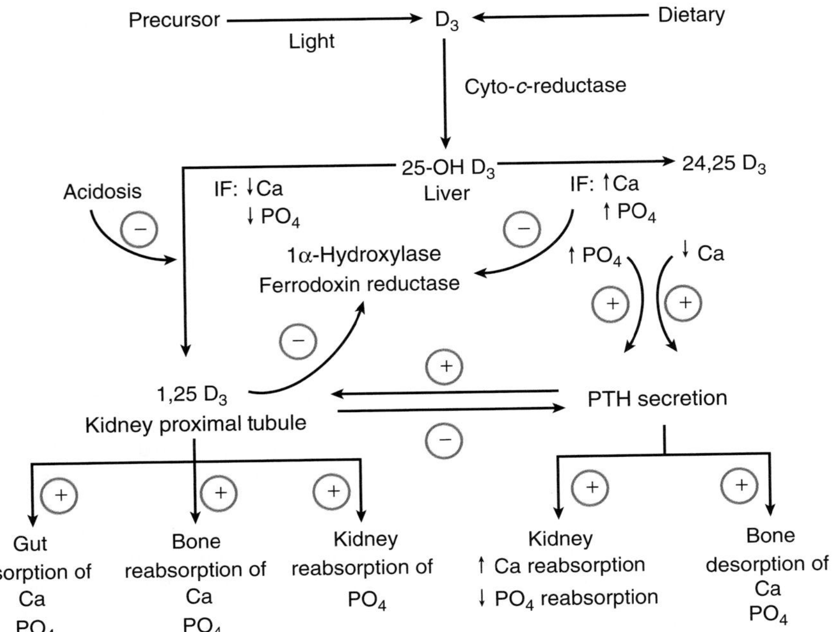

FIGURE 117-7. **Calcium and phosphate metabolism.** PTH = parathyroid hormone.

THE KIDNEY REGULATES PLASMA PO_4 AND CA^{2+} BY EXCRETION AND BY SYNTHESIZING VITAMIN D_3

The level of PO_4 also critically regulates serum Ca^{2+} because their plasma concentrations are close to their saturation, at which point crystallization occurs. Thus, any significant increase in PO_4 results in precipitation of $CaPO_4$.

The level of PO_4 is regulated by glomerular filtration. Initially, about 85% is reabsorbed by the proximal tubule NaPi-2a/c cotransporter. Parathyroid hormone and the heteromeric receptor FGFR/Klotho, which binds FGF23, inhibit the expression of NaPi and hence increase excretion of PO_4. Conversely, the proximal tubule generates vitamin D_3 [1,25-$(OH)_2$ cholecalciferol] by capturing 25-OH cholecalciferol, bound to its filtrable transport protein with brush boarder megalin (Fig. 117-7), after which 1α-hydroxylation is stimulated by low Ca^{2+} and PO_4. 1,25-vitamin D_3 inhibits parathyroid hormone and stimulates PO_4 reabsorption in gut and kidney, thereby counteracting parathyroid hormone and FGF23-Klotho. Nonetheless, Klotho signaling blocks 1,25-vitamin D_3 synthesis, thereby suggesting that it dominates the control of PO_4.

The level of serum calcium is also regulated by the kidney. Approximately 60% of serum Ca^{2+} is filtered, after which it follows Na^+ reabsorption in the proximal tubule and in the loops of Henle, where Ca^{2+} absorption is driven by the positive membrane potential generated by the Na-K-2Cl/K recycling transporter. In contrast, Ca^{2+} and Na^+ are regulated independently in the distal convoluted tubule by parathyroid hormone and Klotho, which increase reabsorption. Phosphate and calcium metabolism are regulated by Na^+ reclamation, parathyroid hormone, 1,25-$(OH)_2$ cholecalciferol, and Klotho in different segments of the nephron.

SUGGESTED READINGS

Hamm LL, Feng Z, Hering-Smith KS. Regulation of sodium transport by ENaC in the kidney. *Curr Opin Nephrol Hypertens.* 2010;19:98-105. *A review of the role of the amiloride-sensitive epithelial sodium channel in regulating sodium transport and balance.*

Riccardi D, Brown EM. Physiology and pathophysiology of the calcium-sensing receptor. *Am J Physiol Renal Physiol.* 2010;298:F485-F499. *Overview of the role of the extracellular calcium-sensing receptor in calcium regulation, kidney physiology, and pathophysiology.*

Toda N, Okamura T. Modulation of renal blood flow and vascular tone by neuronal nitric oxide synthase–derived nitric oxide. *J Vasc Res.* 2011;48:1-10. *Overview of the control of renal blood flow.*

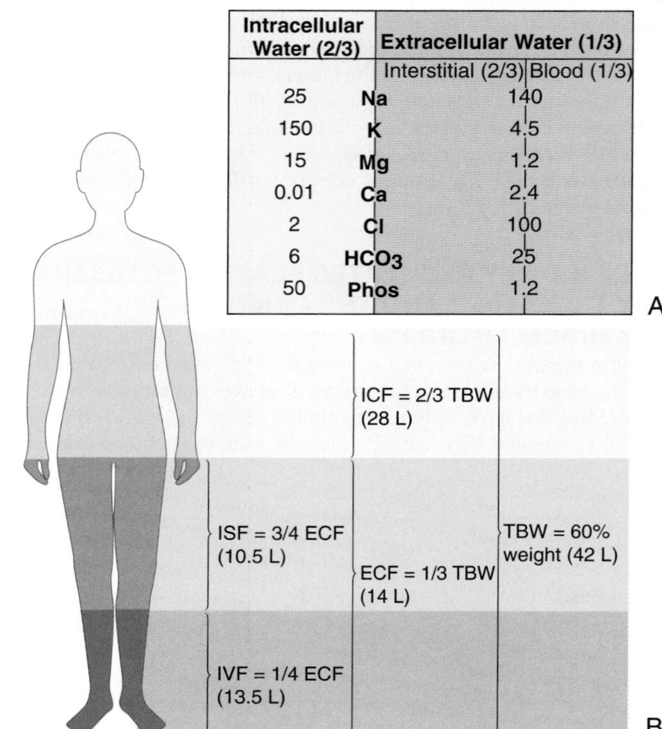

FIGURE 118-1. Composition of body fluid compartments. A, Schematic representation of body fluid compartments in humans. The *shaded areas* depict the approximate size of each compartment as a function of body weight. The figures indicate the relative sizes of the various fluid compartments and the approximate absolute volumes of the compartments (in liters) in a 70-kg adult. **B,** Relative volumes of various body fluid compartments. In a normally built individual, the total body water content is roughly 60% of body weight. Because adipose tissue has a low concentration of water, the relative water-to-total body weight ratio is lower in obese individuals. Intracellular electrolyte concentrations are in millimoles per liter and are typical values obtained from muscle. ECF = extracellular fluid; ICF = intracellular fluid; ISF = interstitial fluid; IVF = intravascular fluid; TBW = total body water. (**A,** From Verbalis JG. Body water osmolality. In: Wilkinson B, Jamison R, eds. *Textbook of Nephrology*. London: Chapman & Hall; 1997:89-94. Reproduced with permission of Hodder Arnold.)

118

DISORDERS OF SODIUM AND WATER HOMEOSTASIS

KARL SKORECKI AND DENNIS AUSIELLO

SODIUM AND WATER HOMEOSTASIS

EPIDEMIOLOGY

Disturbances in sodium and water balance or distribution, with attendant perturbations in the volume or solute composition of body fluid compartments, are among the most frequently encountered abnormalities in clinical medicine. The principal clinical manifestations of these disturbances are *hypovolemia, hypervolemia, dysnatremia (hyponatremia* or *hypernatremia),* and *polyuria*. Disturbances in body tonicity, reflected by hyponatremia or hypernatremia, are estimated to affect up to 15 to 20% of hospitalized patients, with severe disturbances (>10% deviation from normal values) affecting 1 to 2% of patients. Prevalence rates for these abnormalities in ambulatory populations are lower, and elderly individuals and patients treated with multiple medications are the most susceptible.

PATHOBIOLOGY

Approximately 60% of body mass is composed of solute-containing fluid solutions that are divided into extracellular fluid (ECF) and intracellular fluid (ICF) compartments. Water flows freely across cell membranes through specific water channels (aquaporin family of transmembrane proteins) according to the dictates of osmotic forces, thereby maintaining near equality of the solute-to-water ratio (osmolality) in the ICF and ECF. However, the composition of the major solutes differs between the ECF and ICF (Fig. 118-1). Sodium and potassium are the major cations in the ECF and ICF, respectively. Chloride and bicarbonate are the major accompanying anions in the ECF, and negative charges on organic molecules maintain electroneutrality with potassium in the ICF. The difference in cationic solute composition between these two compartments is maintained by a pump-leak mechanism involving the activity of Na^+, K^+-adenosine triphosphate (ATPase) operating in concert with cell membrane sodium and potassium conductance pathways. The free movement of water ensures that the sodium concentration in ECF is nearly equivalent to the potassium concentration in ICF. *Osmolality* refers to the concentration of all solutes, whereas *tonicity* refers to the concentration of solutes that are "effective" in eliciting a water shift between body fluid compartments. Addition or removal of solutes causes a sustained shift of water to restore the near equality of concentrations, and they are thus considered effective solutes that contribute to body fluid tonicity. The restriction of sodium to the ECF compartment by virtue of the pump-leak mechanism, together with maintenance of osmotic equilibrium between the ECF and ICF, ensures that ECF volume is determined principally by the total body fluid sodium content and governs the partitioning of fluid between the ECF and ICF compartments. In contrast, solutes that permeate across most cell membranes, such as urea, do not elicit a sustained shift in water and therefore do not contribute to the steady-state partitioning of fluid volumes across body compartments. However, urea and glucose do contribute to the laboratory measurement of fluid osmolality. The addition or removal of water without solutes results in a proportionate reduction or increase, respectively, in both osmolality and tonicity of all body fluid compartments.

The mechanisms that govern body fluid homeostasis preserve near constancy of the volumes of the ECF and ICF compartments despite variations in dietary intake and extrarenal losses of sodium and water and adjust this balance in response to variations in the capacity of these compartments. Thus, the overriding principle of body fluid and solute homeostasis is mass balance of total body intake and output of water as well as balance of osmotically active particles. Even the slightest perturbations in these parameters activate neural and hormonal mediators for restoration of balance. This restoration of balance is achieved through adjustments in the urinary excretion of sodium and water in response to perceived changes in ECF or ICF volume. Constancy of ECF volume, together with control of vascular capacitance, ensures a high degree of circulatory stability.

Sodium Balance

Sodium balance refers to the difference between intake and excretion. In the nonclinical setting, sodium intake is controlled by dietary habits. In the clinical setting, prescribed adjustments in sodium intake or the administration of sodium-containing medications or solutions cause variation to overall sodium intake. Although nonrenal loss is under some regulatory influence (e.g., aldosterone-mediated regulation of sodium concentration in stool and sweat), the fine adjustment of sodium balance in response to changes in intake is mediated by regulation of urinary sodium excretion. In the steady state, urinary excretion of sodium is closely matched to dietary salt intake. This balance depends on a series of afferent mechanisms that sense the volume of the ECF compartment relative to its capacitance and trigger effector mechanisms that modify the rate of renal sodium excretion to maintain ECF volume homeostasis. Normal functioning of these mechanisms in turn is impacted by the partitioning of the ECF into two subcompartments: intravascular and extravascular (interstitial) (see Fig. 118-1). The composition and concentration of small, noncolloid electrolyte solutes in these two ECF subcompartments are nearly equivalent, but there is a higher concentration of colloid osmotic particles, mostly molecules of albumin and globulin proteins, in the intravascular compartment. Opposing transcapillary hydraulic and colloid osmotic (oncotic) pressure gradients (Starling forces) favor the net transudation of fluid from the intravascular to the interstitial compartment. At the same time, lymphatic fluid movement from interstitial sites back to the circulation through the thoracic duct ensures that the intravascular subcompartment is replenished and maintains a nearly constant proportion of approximately 25% of the overall ECF, which corresponds to 3.5 L of plasma. The remaining approximately 75% of ECF volume (equivalent to 10.5 L in a normal 70-kg male) is contained in the interstitial spaces. Because intravascular volume is one of the key determinants of circulatory integrity, preservation of the constancy of ECF volume, and appropriate partitioning of the ECF volume between the intravascular and interstitial subcompartments are critical for hemodynamic stability.

Effective Arterial Blood Volume

The circulatory network is composed of central and peripheral venous compartments as well as renal and extrarenal arterial compartments. Each compartment reflects a unique characteristic of overall circulatory function (e.g., cardiac filling, tissue perfusion, renal perfusion, and transudation of fluid into the interstitial space) (Table 118-1).

The concept of effective arterial blood volume (EABV) is crucial to understanding the afferent mechanisms that govern the regulation of sodium homeostasis. Unlike ICF, ECF, and intravascular volume, EABV is not measurable as an anatomically defined space but rather is best understood in functional terms as an integration of hemodynamic parameters that emanate from specific sites in the arterial circuit that monitor tissue perfusion and trigger appropriate changes in urinary sodium excretion. These sites include the carotid baroreceptor and intrarenal mechanisms located at the glomerular afferent arterioles, the juxtaglomerular apparatus, and peritubular capillaries. EABV often, but not always, varies directly with actual ECF volume.

TABLE 118-1 MECHANISMS FOR SENSING REGIONAL CHANGES IN BODY FLUID VOLUME

Cardiopulmonary volume sensors
Atria (neural and humoral pathways)
Ventricular and pulmonary sensing sites
Arterial volume sensors
Carotid and aortic arch baroreceptors
Renal volume sensors
Central nervous system sensors
Hepatic and gastrointestinal tract sensors

Low-pressure sensors (e.g., cardiac atrial transmural stretch and tension receptors) respond to the state of cardiac filling and tend to protect against overfilling of the ECF compartment, but they also have a role in renal sodium retention in states of perceived underfilling. Taken together, the integrated ECF volume-sensing signals elicit an appropriate renal response for modulating sodium excretion in an effort to maintain a constant ECF volume.

The filtered load of sodium vastly exceeds net intake, so tubular reabsorption usually serves as the principal modulator of urinary sodium excretion, the preservation of sodium balance, and the maintenance of a constant ECF volume. Specific luminal membrane sodium transporters or channels at each tubular segment mediate movement of sodium from the luminal fluid into the cell in a carefully regulated manner, followed by extrusion of sodium across the basolateral surface through Na^+, K^+-ATPase and other sodium transporters. Among many others, these regulated luminal transporters include the Na/H exchanger (proximal tubule), the Na-K-2Cl (NKCC2) cotransport pathway (loop of Henle), the NaCl cotransporter (NCCT) along the distal convoluted tubule, and the apical sodium channel (ENaC) along the connecting and cortical collecting tubule. At some nephron sites, sodium reabsorption is isotonic (e.g., proximal tubule), whereas at other sites, sodium reabsorption exceeds water resorption, so tubular fluid has a sodium concentration less than that of plasma (e.g., thick ascending limb of the loop of Henle). Sodium reabsorptive transport pathways are subject to a series of regulatory influences that sense EABV, including the renin-angiotensin-aldosterone pathway, natriuretic peptides, endothelium-derived endothelins and nitric oxide, the eicosanoid-prostaglandin system, guanylin peptides of gut origin, and urotensins. This redundancy of multiple hormonal mediators, which act together with the sympathetic nervous system, renal neural stimulation, and intrarenal physical factors (e.g., peritubular capillary Starling forces, tubule lumen sodium chloride delivery, and tubuloglomerular feedback), underscores the evolutionary importance of regulating urinary sodium excretion to maintain volume homeostasis.

Water Balance

Water balance refers to the difference between intake (oral, enteral, or parenteral) and excretion (insensible, gastrointestinal, perspiratory, and renal). Maintaining equivalency of intake and excretion of water ensures constancy of body fluid tonicity (osmoregulation). Osmoregulation ensures that the content of effective solutes in each body fluid compartment determines the volume of that compartment. Positive water balance or negative water balance and the corresponding changes in tonicity and cell volume are sensed by osmoreceptor and thirst center cells in the hypothalamus. The osmoreceptors are situated in the supraoptic and paraventricular nuclei of the hypothalamus; the thirst center is situated in the organum vasculosum of the anterior hypothalamus. Just a 2% change in effective osmolality or tonicity elicits a change in release of the hormone arginine vasopressin (AVP) from the posterior pituitary gland and the perception of thirst. Endothelin-1 also is released from the posterior pituitary in response to water deprivation and increases plasma AVP levels. Stimulation of thirst depends on centrally produced angiotensin II. A reduction of more than approximately 8% of ECF volume serves as an overriding afferent signal (carried by the ninth and tenth cranial nerves) for the nonosmotically driven release of AVP and also stimulates thirst by means of angiotensin II, even when body tonicity is not elevated (Fig. 118-2A).

The urinary excretion of water depends on the delivery of isotonic sodium-containing filtrate to the thick ascending limb of the loop of Henle, reabsorption of sodium and accompanying electrolytes in the thick ascending limb of the loop of Henle and the distal tubule, and the AVP-regulated reabsorption of the appropriate volumes of solute-free water through aquaporin-2 water channels in the cells of the collecting tubule. The hydro-osmotic movement of water from the collecting tubule lumen to the hyperosmotic milieu of the renal medulla minimizes urinary excretion of the hypotonic fluid generated in the thick ascending limb of the loop of Henle and the distal tubule, thereby promoting positive water balance. In the *absence* of AVP, this hypotonic fluid is excreted, and negative water balance ensues. Typical levels of urine osmolality that can be achieved in the human kidney by fluctuations in AVP action range between 50 and 1200 mOsm/kg, but this range narrows at the extremes of age or in the presence of intrinsic renal disease. Laboratory measurement of urine osmolality reflects overall renal concentrating ability, including the hydro-osmotic action of AVP. However, not all solutes that contribute to the laboratory measurement of urine osmolality correspond to effective solutes in terms of body fluid tonicity. Thus, excretion of urine with high concentrations of urea and low concentrations of sodium, potassium, and chloride

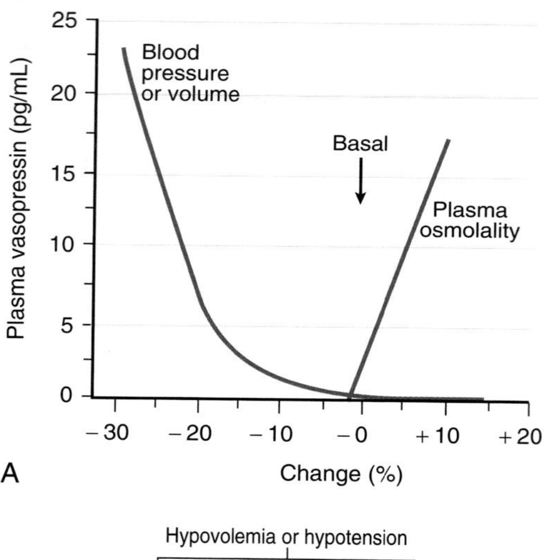

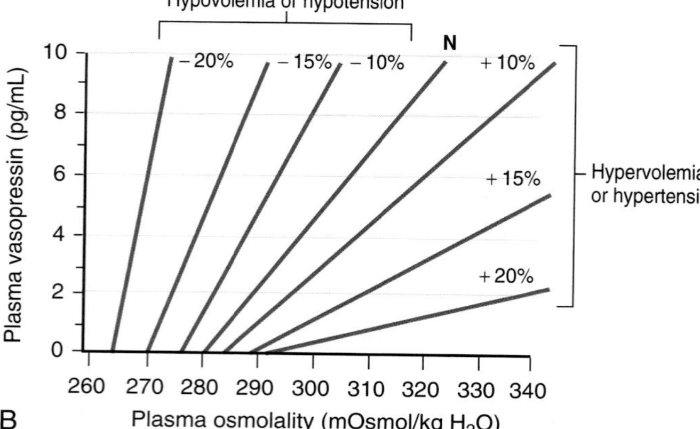

FIGURE 118-2. **Relationship between arginine vasopressin (AVP) and osmolality.** **A**, Comparative sensitivity of AVP secretion in response to increases in plasma osmolality versus decreases in blood volume or blood pressure in human subjects. The *arrow* indicates the low plasma AVP concentrations found at basal plasma osmolality. Note that AVP secretion is much more sensitive to small changes in blood osmolality than to changes in volume or pressure. **B**, The relationship between the osmolality of plasma and the concentration of AVP in plasma is modulated by blood volume and pressure. The line labeled N shows plasma AVP concentrations across a range of plasma osmolality in an adult with normal intravascular volume (euvolemic) and normal blood pressure (normotensive). The lines to the left of N show the relationship between plasma AVP concentration and plasma osmolality in adults whose low intravascular volume (hypovolemia) or blood pressure (hypotension) is 10%, 15%, and 20% below normal. Lines to the right of N are for volumes and blood pressure 10%, 15%, and 20% above normal. Note that hemodynamic influences do not disrupt the osmoregulation of AVP but rather raise or lower the set point and possibly also the sensitivity of AVP secretion in proportion to the magnitude of the change in blood volume or pressure.

indicates a strong renal concentrating capacity but contributes less to positive water balance than does excretion of urine with the same measured osmolality and higher concentrations of these electrolytes.

PATHOPHYSIOLOGY

Disturbances in sodium balance primarily affect ECF volume, and disturbances in water balance primarily affect body fluid tonicity. A cumulative negative balance of sodium (sodium deficit) in the absence of a change in tonicity results in ECF volume contraction (hypovolemia), whereas a cumulative positive balance of sodium (sodium surfeit) results in ECF volume expansion (hypervolemia). In contrast, a cumulative positive body water balance (water surfeit) results in volume expansion of all the body fluid compartments, whereas negative water balance (water deficit) results in volume contraction of all the body fluid compartments. However, because ICF volume is double that of ECF at baseline, the more prominent expansion or contraction in absolute volume terms involves the ICF compartment. Furthermore, maintenance of a surfeit or deficit of water relative to solutes results in a uniform decrease or increase in body fluid tonicity in all fluid compartments. Because the solute composition of the plasma component of the ECF compartment is sampled, a disturbance in tonicity is most commonly detected as an abnormality in plasma sodium concentration (hyponatremia for water surfeit and hypernatremia for water deficit). Frequently, disturbances in water and sodium balance occur together, and all combinations of surfeit or deficit can occur (Table 118-2). The clinical approach to a patient with a sodium or water balance disturbance (or both) can be facilitated by careful consideration of which states apply.

TABLE 118-2 PATHOGENIC PROCESSES LEADING TO DISORDERS OF BODY SODIUM AND FLUID HOMEOSTASIS

CLINICAL STATE	EXTRACELLULAR FLUID VOLUME	BODY FLUID TONICITY	PATHOGENIC PROCESS
Normal	↔	↔	
Hypervolemic normonatremia	↑	↔	Isotonic net gain of sodium and water
Hypervolemic hyponatremia	↑	↓	Hypotonic net gain of sodium and water
Hypervolemic hypernatremia	↑	↑	Hypertonic net gain of sodium and water
Normovolemic hyponatremia	↔	↓	Net water gain ± sodium loss
Normovolemic hypernatremia	↔	↑	Net water loss ± sodium gain
Hypovolemic hypernatremia	↓	↑	Net loss of water in excess of sodium
Hypovolemic normonatremia	↓	↔	Isotonic net loss of sodium and water
Hypovolemic hyponatremia	↓	↓	Net loss of sodium in excess of water

↔ = Unchanged.

SODIUM BALANCE DISORDERS

Hypovolemia

DEFINITION

Hypovolemia is a reduction in the volume of the ECF compartment in relation to its capacitance. In states of absolute hypovolemia, a deficit in sodium reflects past or ongoing negative sodium balance. The volume of the ECF intravascular and extravascular (interstitial) subcompartments may vary in the same or opposite directions. ICF volume is reflected by the measurement of plasma osmolality and sodium concentration and may be concomitantly disturbed (see Table 118-2).

EPIDEMIOLOGY

Causes of absolute and relative hypovolemia (Table 118-3) can be categorized into extrarenal and renal causes. Bleeding is the most frequent and direct cause of a reduction in the absolute volume of the intravascular subcompartment of the ECF (Chapters 106 and 137). Other causes of absolute hypovolemia include fluid loss from the kidney or from the gastrointestinal, integumentary, or respiratory systems. Infectious diarrhea remains a leading cause of death from hypovolemia in many areas of the world. Burns allow the loss of large volumes of plasma and interstitial fluid and can rapidly lead to profound hypovolemia similar to what is seen with bleeding (Chapter 112). Enhanced evaporative water loss from the respiratory tract can occur with exercise, in response to heat stress (Chapter 109), in febrile states, and in patients undergoing mechanical ventilation with inadequate humidification.

ECF also can be sequestered into compartments within the body without an evident history of loss. Such pathologic conditions are often referred to as third space loss and include gastrointestinal obstruction, sequestration of fluids in subcutaneous tissue after trauma or burns (Chapter 112), and sequestration in the retroperitoneal or peritoneal space in patients with pancreatitis (Chapter 146) or peritonitis (Chapter 144), respectively. The accumulation of ascites may also compromise intravascular volume.

In any form of kidney disease in which tubular reabsorption of the filtered sodium load does not match the sum of this filtered load plus dietary intake, a renal sodium-wasting state may ensue. Most of the widely used diuretic medications inhibit specific pathways for sodium reabsorption at various sites along the nephron and should more properly be referred to as natriuretic medications. Loop diuretics (furosemide, bumetanide, torsemide, and ethacrynic acid) are the most potent diuretics, and their potential to induce renal

TABLE 118-3 CAUSES OF ABSOLUTE AND RELATIVE HYPOVOLEMIA

EXTRARENAL
Absolute
Bleeding
Gastrointestinal fluid loss (diarrhea, vomiting, ileostomy or colostomy secretions)
Fluid loss from skin (burns, sweat)
Respiratory fluid loss
Relative
Third space loss
Sepsis
Edema states (heart failure, cirrhosis)
RENAL
Absolute
Diuretics
Inherited sodium-wasting tubulopathies
Tubulointerstitial diseases
Partial obstruction or postobstruction etiology
Endocrine disorders (e.g., hypoaldosteronism, adrenal insufficiencies)
Relative
Nephrotic syndrome

sodium loss is augmented when they are combined with other classes of diuretic agents (thiazides, carbonic anhydrase inhibitors, aldosterone antagonists, and distal epithelial sodium-channel blockers).

Natriuretic medications often are used to treat hypervolemic states, but their overuse or inappropriate use can result in hypovolemia. Tubular sodium reabsorption also may be disrupted by inherited or acquired renal tubulopathies, such as various forms of proximal tubulopathy and different forms of Bartter's and Gitelman's syndromes (Chapter 130).

Impairment of renal tubule sodium reabsorption may also occur with nonoliguric acute kidney injury and the recovery phase after oliguric acute kidney injury or after release of urinary obstruction (Chapters 122 and 125). Interstitial renal disease (Chapter 124) may result in fluid and electrolyte abnormalities, which can include renal sodium wasting. Nonelectrolyte urinary solutes such as glucose (in severe hyperglycemia) and mannitol cause polyuria and hypovolemia. Mineralocorticoid deficiency and resistance, including adrenal insufficiency (Chapter 234), should always be considered in a patient with evidence of urinary sodium loss in the face of hypovolemia. In cerebral salt wasting (also referred to as renal salt wasting), tubular sodium reabsorption is impaired in the setting of acute head injury (Chapter 406) or intracranial hemorrhage.

In *relative hypovolemia*, ECF volume is not reduced in absolute terms, but the capacitance of the ECF or intravascular compartment is expanded, thereby leading to clinical manifestations that mimic those of absolute hypovolemia. Relative hypovolemic states can be classified into two categories: states of vasodilation and states of generalized edema. Vasodilation occurs in response to endogenous endothelial substances (e.g., nitric oxide) and to exogenous agents that induce vasodilation (e.g., vasodilator drugs). Peripheral vasodilation occurs in sepsis (Chapter 108) and in normal pregnancy. Relative hypovolemia also occurs in patients with a positive sodium and water balance and generalized edema but a reduced intravascular volume. Examples include heart failure (Chapters 58 and 59), decompensated cirrhosis with ascites (Chapter 156), and the nephrotic syndrome (Chapter 123).

PATHOBIOLOGY

Extrarenal Causes of Absolute Hypovolemia

The immediate effect of bleeding is a proportionate net loss in plasma and erythrocytes and hence an isotonic reduction in ECF volume. Compensatory hemodynamic responses include tachycardia and vasoconstriction, followed by a shift of fluid from the interstitial to the intravascular compartment because of altered transcapillary Starling hydraulic forces. Additional neural and hormonal responses result in renal sodium and water retention, with the aim of restoring intravascular volume and stabilizing the circulation.

Besides dietary intake, approximately 7 L of isotonic fluid enters the gastrointestinal tract on a daily basis, the bulk of which is reabsorbed to minimize fecal fluid loss. Because these fluids contain varying concentrations of sodium and accompanying anions, enhanced secretion or impaired reabsorption causes absolute ECF volume depletion. The composition of the fluid and electrolyte loss differs according to the cause and source of gastrointestinal fluid loss (Chapters 134 and 142).

Given its large surface area, it is not surprising that fluid losses from the integumentary system can be an important cause of hypovolemia. In the absence of medical intervention, hemoconcentration and hypoalbuminemia ensue; however, because of the isotonic composition of the lost fluid, no changes in plasma osmolality or sodium concentration are expected. Exertion in hot environments increases thermoregulatory fluid losses from the skin in the form of sweat. Fluid loss through perspiration can reach 1 L/hour or more, depending on exertion and environment. The sodium concentration in sweat varies among individuals (range of approximately 20 to 50 mmol/L). Thus, although the fluid loss is hypotonic, a significant sodium deficit and ECF volume contraction can ensue. The extent of hypovolemia and the resulting body fluid composition (plasma osmolality and sodium concentration) will depend on fluid replacement, which is determined primarily by thirst and availability.

All extrarenal causes of hypovolemia are expected to invoke a renal response, whose hallmark is sodium and fluid conservation. Obviously, this expected response is absent when the kidney itself is responsible for sodium loss, whether owing to the effect of pharmacologic or hormonal influences or to intrinsic renal disease.

Renal Causes of Hypovolemia

When the glomerular filtration rate (GFR) and plasma sodium concentration are normal, approximately 24,000 mmol of sodium are filtered per day. Even when the GFR is markedly impaired, the quantities of sodium filtered far exceed normal dietary intake. Thus, the small quantities of sodium excreted in urine relative to the filtered load depend on the integrity of tubular sodium reabsorptive mechanisms to match urinary sodium excretion to dietary intake through volume sensing and effector mechanisms. Impairment in the integrity of one or more of these sodium reabsorptive mechanisms can result in a profound sodium deficit and absolute volume depletion.

An underappreciated but frequent clinical setting for renal sodium loss occurs after the iatrogenic administration of high volumes of volume-expanding, salt-containing solutions to hospitalized patients. Such patients are usually in the postoperative or post-trauma setting and are frequently administered many liters of saline or other sodium-containing maintenance intravenous fluids for several consecutive days, during which tubule reabsorption of sodium is downregulated. There may be a lag in the restoration of full tubule reabsorptive capacity, when intravenous fluids are discontinued, and high volumes of urine rich in sodium continue to be excreted. During this lag phase, the patient may become mildly, but transiently, hypovolemic. This scenario can be avoided by a graduated reduction in administered sodium-containing fluids, at a pace that allows sodium reabsorptive tubular pathways to be upregulated and restored to their normal reabsorptive levels.

Diabetes insipidus represents a spectrum of conditions resulting from deficiency or tubular resistance to the action of AVP. However, because it is the tubular reabsorption of water and not solutes that is impaired, the impact on ECF volume is generally a minor consideration in comparison to the impact on ICF and body fluid tonicity.

CLINICAL MANIFESTATIONS

The clinical manifestations of hypovolemia depend on the magnitude and rate of volume loss, the solute composition of the net fluid loss (taking into account ingested or administered fluids), and vascular and renal responses. A detailed history is often helpful in assessing bleeding, vomiting, diarrhea, polyuria, medications, and diaphoresis.

However, the absence of symptoms does not exclude mild to moderate hypovolemia, especially if the volume loss has occurred gradually. Intravascular volume contraction of less than 5% does not usually elicit symptoms and readily escapes detection by physical examination. With greater degrees of absolute hypovolemia (corresponding to intravascular volume contraction in the 5 to 15% range), symptoms and signs begin to appear. Patients may exhibit nonspecific symptoms related to end-organ hypoperfusion, including weakness, muscle cramps, and postural lightheadedness. Thirst may be an early manifestation but more likely reflects a concomitant hypertonic state.

A number of clinical scenarios illustrate the relationship of clinical manifestations to causes of hypovolemia. For example, a patient with an acute *gastrointestinal hemorrhage* (Chapter 137) of 0.5 L of whole blood can experience tachycardia, postural hypotension, peripheral vasoconstriction with cool extremities, lightheadedness, and oliguria, with high urine osmolality and low urine sodium concentration. Hemoglobin and albumin will probably remain constant initially, and then a drop in hemoglobin will ensue after movement of ECF from the interstitial to the intravascular compartment. The plasma solute composition (sodium and potassium concentration, acid-base parameters) is not likely to change initially. The plasma concentration of urea may rise somewhat as a result of increased proximal tubular reabsorption of urea, increased proximal reabsorption of salt and water, and the increased nitrogen load from the destruction of erythrocytes in the gastrointestinal tract. Jugular venous pressure is expected to fall, and central venous pressure (CVP) will generally be less than 5 cm H_2O in the absence of confounding factors. Urine output is expected be low, with a high specific gravity and osmolality and a low urine sodium concentration.

In another scenario, a patient inappropriately receiving potent *loop diuretics* over a period of many days for localized peripheral edema may suffer a cumulative net ECF loss of 3 L, or about 20%; approximately one third of this lost volume will have originated from the intravascular compartment, with the remainder coming from the interstitial compartment. This degree of intravascular loss usually induces weakness, tachycardia, low jugular venous pressure, and hypotension. However, because the deficit may have accumulated over time, a degree of adaptation would attenuate the severity of these clinical manifestations and lead the clinician to underestimate the extent of hypovolemia. The plasma sodium concentration may remain unaltered because disruption of the urine-concentrating mechanism by loop diuretics attenuates the tendency to water retention, and an intact thirst mechanism prevents hypertonicity. Because loop diuretics enhance urinary potassium and ammonium excretion, hypokalemic metabolic alkalosis is expected. The ongoing effect of the loop diuretic would mitigate oliguria and lead to inappropriately high concentrations of solutes including sodium and potassium in urine. After cessation of the loop diuretic, the appropriate renal response of oliguria, high urine osmolality, and sodium concentration would be expected.

A third scenario is a patient with relative hypovolemia owing to the vasodilation that typically accompanies *bacteremic sepsis* (Chapter 108). No source of fluid loss would be identified in the history, but the patient would usually manifest symptoms of weakness and even prostration, accompanied tachycardia and hypotension. The extremities may be warm, but reduced tissue perfusion may reduce the level of consciousness and cause oliguria, elevated plasma urea and creatinine levels, and lactic acidosis.

DIAGNOSIS

The most readily appreciated physical findings related to contraction of the intravascular compartment include tachycardia, orthostatic hypotension, and reduced jugular venous pressure. Although low CVP often reliably reflects intravascular volume contraction, an elevated CVP does not necessarily exclude hypovolemia because of the possible confounding influence of cardiac or lung disease. Severe degrees of hypovolemia (corresponding to intravascular volume contraction exceeding 10 to 20%) cause hypotension (even in the supine position), peripheral cyanosis, cold extremities, and reduced levels of consciousness (extending even to coma) as a result of end-organ and cerebral hypoperfusion. Hemodynamic collapse (hypovolemic shock; Chapter 106) also can occur with more rapid volume loss, comorbid conditions, and greater degrees of hypovolemia. When the source of volume loss is purely extrarenal, oliguria is expected. Physical findings such as reduced skin or eyeball turgor and dry mucous membranes are not reliable indicators of hypovolemia.

Laboratory Findings

Laboratory measurements are an adjunct to clinical assessment but do not replace symptoms and physical examination findings as a primary diagnostic tool. Decreases in *hemoglobin* indicate past or ongoing bleeding, but a normal or stable hemoglobin does not exclude acute bleeding. Hemoconcentration is often observed when hypovolemia is not the consequence of bleeding, but comorbid disease processes that produce anemia may mitigate this rise.

The *albumin* concentration may rise with gastrointestinal, urinary, or skin losses of albumin-free fluids. Conversely, fluid losses that are accompanied by albumin loss (e.g., proteinuria, protein-losing enteropathy) may mitigate this rise or even result in hypoalbuminemia. Similarly, burns and hepatic disease are often accompanied by hypoalbuminemia as a result of the loss or third spacing of protein-rich fluid.

Serum levels of *sodium* and *other electrolytes* also can vary widely. Even subtle and subclinical degrees of hypovolemia trigger urinary water retention and result in a hypotonic hyponatremic plasma composition if the patient is exposed to solutions that are more hypotonic than that of the fluid lost. In contrast, loss of hypotonic fluids with inadequate water ingestion or replacement results in a hypertonic plasma composition and hypernatremia.

Acid-base (Chapter 120) and *potassium* (Chapter 119) changes point to specific causes. For example, hypokalemia with metabolic alkalosis frequently accompanies vomiting and some causes of diarrhea (e.g., a villous adenoma). More often, diarrheal fluid loss is associated with a non–anion gap metabolic acidosis. Loop and thiazide diuretic-induced hypovolemia is often associated with hypokalemic metabolic alkalosis, as are the inherited tubulopathies (Bartter's and Gitelman's syndromes) (Chapter 130), which disrupt sodium reabsorptive mechanisms at the loop of Henle and distal convoluted tubule, respectively. Severe hypovolemia with circulatory compromise and tissue hypoperfusion is often accompanied by lactic acidosis.

Increases in *plasma urea* and *creatinine* concentrations are frequently observed in hypovolemic states and reflect reduced renal plasma flow. If acute tubule injury does not supervene, the rise in plasma urea concentration is often disproportionate to the rise in plasma creatinine concentration (see Prerenal Azotemia in Chapter 122). The rise in plasma urea and creatinine concentrations is particularly common when hypovolemia is a consequence of urinary fluid losses. In such conditions, the patient is not oliguric, even though renal plasma flow and GFR are compromised. Other forms of urinary sodium loss, such as occur with adrenal insufficiency or aldosterone unresponsiveness, are accompanied by a tendency toward hyperkalemia and mild metabolic acidosis.

Urinary biochemical parameters may also help in the clinical assessment of hypovolemic states. When fluid loss is extrarenal, the expected renal response of water and sodium conservation results in oliguria with an elevated urine specific gravity (>1.020) and osmolality (>400 mOsm/kg) and a sodium concentration less than 20 mmol/L because of enhanced renal tubule reabsorptive activity. More complex indices of the appropriate renal response to hypovolemia include fractional excretion of sodium less than 1% and fractional excretion of urea less than 30 to 35%. Intrinsic renal injury confounds the diagnostic value of these urinary indices.

Differential Diagnosis

Relative hypovolemia secondary to arterial vasodilation mimics some of the clinical manifestations of absolute hypovolemia. With vasodilation, as seen for example in sepsis (Chapter 108), tachycardia and hypotension are common, but the extremities may be warm. However, tissues are actually underperfused, as reflected by reduced renal and cerebral function and lactic acidosis.

TREATMENT

Rx

Absolute Hypovolemia

The major goal in treatment of hypovolemia is to restore hemodynamic integrity and tissue perfusion. The treatment approach includes treatment of the underlying disease state when possible, replacement of the volume deficit, and fluid administration to maintain ECF volume in the event of continuing losses. Beyond the specific treatments, the mainstay of therapy involves fluid administration. The important issues are the volume, rate of administration, and composition of the replacement and maintenance fluids. These decisions may vary during different stages of treatment and should be adjusted according to the patient's response as determined by closely monitored clinical parameters.

The choice of oral or intravenous replacement fluids (or both) for hypovolemic states is dictated principally by the disturbances in other electrolyte and acid-base parameters. The rate of replacement is a function of the urgency of the threat to circulatory integrity and consideration of complications related to overzealous or too rapid correction.

Fluid therapy for hypovolemic states sometimes begins with a diagnostic fluid challenge. In situations in which clinical parameters do not permit a firm diagnosis of hypovolemia, the response to a fluid challenge can be informative and serve as the initial treatment step. For example, a patient with known long-standing compensated heart failure who is being maintained on a therapeutic regimen that includes diuretics may have tachycardia, a reduction in blood pressure from baseline values, poor cognition, and renal dysfunction. Such a clinical scenario could have a number of different explanations, including superimposed volume depletion with inadequate left ventricular filling volume. CVP, whether measured directly or assessed by jugular venous pressure, may be misleading in the face of right ventricular dysfunction, but direct measurement of pulmonary capillary wedge pressure does not significantly improve clinical outcomes.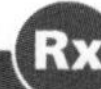 In such a case, a carefully monitored diagnostic fluid challenge can minimize the risk for fluid overload. Such monitoring should include clinical assessment of parameters indicating pulmonary venous hypertension (pulmonary congestion or edema by physical examination or chest radiograph). Reversal of the disturbed clinical parameters would support the diagnosis of volume depletion.

Another example is a patient with hyponatremia in the setting of suspected volume depletion. Often the degree of volume depletion is too subtle to be detected by clinical examination, and a therapeutic challenge with fluid of the appropriate composition can be informative.

The initial volume and rate of therapeutic replacement fluid should be determined by ongoing monitoring of clinical parameters rather than a priori estimates of volume deficit. In some settings, the clinical state will dictate rapid fluid replacement, as in a patient with unambiguous hypovolemic shock and life-threatening circulatory collapse. In such cases, fluids can be administered at the most rapid rate possible, limited only by intravenous access, until blood pressure and tissue perfusion are restored. However, in most cases, much slower rates are indicated, especially in elderly patients, patients whose medical background is unclear, or those with known comorbid conditions. It is important to note that replacement fluids of different compositions have quite disparate volumes of distribution in the body fluid compartments and therefore differ in their efficiency of restoring ECF volume. *Crystalloid solutions* with sodium as the principal cation are the mainstay in fluid replacement therapy for hypovolemic states and are indicated primarily for hypovolemic states that are caused by renal, gastrointestinal, or sweat-based sodium losses. These solutions also are useful initial agents and adjuncts to therapy for the hypovolemia of hemorrhage and burns. *Isotonic saline* is confined to the ECF compartment (except in cases of severe dysnatremia). Thus, retention of 1 L of infused isotonic saline increases plasma volume by about 300 mL, with the remaining portion distributed in the interstitial subcompartment of the ECF. In contrast, a solution of *5% dextrose in water (D_5W)* is equivalent to administering solute-free water and distributes uniformly throughout all body fluid compartments (one third of the retained volume of infusate remains in the ECF compartment and only approximately 10 to 15% in the intravascular compartment). Infusing a given volume of *half isotonic saline (0.45% sodium chloride plus 5% glucose)* can be considered equivalent to infusing half that volume as solute-free water (distributed throughout body fluid compartments) and the other half as isotonic saline (confined to the ECF compartment). The retained solute-free volume reduces body tonicity and the plasma sodium concentration, potential benefit in the follow-up treatment of patients whose hypovolemia is accompanied by hypertonicity and hypernatremia, but a detriment for patients with normotonic or hypotonic hypovolemia.

When hypovolemia is accompanied by hypobicarbonatemia (metabolic acidosis), it may be appropriate to design a solution in which a portion of the sodium is accompanied by bicarbonate (Chapter 120). For example, it is possible to add a given quantity of hypertonic sodium bicarbonate to a solution of half isotonic saline (in which chloride is the anion accompanying sodium) to obtain an isotonic replacement fluid appropriate for the given acid-base status of the patient. Similarly, in patients with concomitant potassium depletion (Chapter 119), especially when accompanied by metabolic alkalosis, addition of potassium chloride to the replacement solution may be indicated. A number of crystalloid solutions with predetermined concentrations of potassium, lactate (converted to bicarbonate by the liver), and other electrolytes are commercially available, but it is more appropriate to begin with a sodium chloride–containing solution at a concentration appropriate to body tonicity, then to add other solutes as indicated or at a separate intravenous administration site. This approach provides maximal flexibility in tailoring individualized fluid replacement therapy to patient needs.

Colloid-containing solutions include albumin or high-molecular-weight carbohydrate molecules (e.g., hydroxyethyl starch or dextran) at concentrations that exert a colloid osmotic pressure equal to or greater than that of plasma. Banked human plasma is also considered a colloid solution. Because large molecules such as albumin and high-molecular-weight carbohydrates do not readily cross the transcapillary barrier, they are thought to expand the intravascular compartment more rapidly and efficiently than crystalloid solutions. However, a randomized trial showed no benefit of colloids compared with crystalloids for fluid resuscitation.[2] Nevertheless, albumin-containing solutions may be useful in hypovolemia associated with burns (Chapter 112), when cutaneous protein losses are appreciable. Furthermore, because of the capacity for rapid intravascular volume expansion with just a small volume of replacement fluid, colloid-containing solutions are frequently used when rapid intravascular expansion is desired, such as at trauma sites outside of the hospital setting. Some large-molecular-weight carbohydrates are nephrotoxic and should be used with caution in patients with renal impairment. In patients with multiorgan system failure and capillary leakage, albumin is both rapidly catabolized and redistributed into the interstitial compartment, so it can aggravate interstitial edema without providing an intravascular volume repletion benefit. It is for these reasons that crystalloid-containing solutions remain the mainstay of volume replacement therapy.

Blood products can be used for volume replacement in hypovolemic states, and a unit of packed red blood cells remains entirely in the vascular compartment. However, erythrocytes are actually considered part of the intracellular compartment and do not contribute to organ plasma flow. The role of packed red cells in the treatment of hemorrhage is to restore the principal function of the erythrocyte in oxygen carriage and delivery, not as a means of ECF volume replacement.

In addition to replacement fluids, maintenance fluids must be provided to counteract ongoing losses. Such ongoing losses may be a continuation of the underlying disease state (e.g., continued vomiting, diarrhea, polyuric states, or severe burns). The volume, rate of administration, and composition of these replacement fluids are best determined by actual measurements of the corresponding ongoing fluid losses, with appropriate adjustments for the patient's clinical assessment parameters.

Relative Hypovolemia

The treatment approach to relative hypovolemia is more complex than for absolute hypovolemia. When relative hypovolemia is the result of peripheral vasodilation, therapy should be directed toward reversal of the underlying cause and restoration of normal vascular reactivity. Bridging to maintain circulatory integrity until the underlying cause is successfully reversed can be achieved by infusion of an *isotonic crystalloid solution* such as normal saline. In such situations, selection of volumes and rates must be done with extreme caution because there is no absolute deficit and the administered volume will have to be excreted or removed once systemic vascular resistance and vascular capacitance are restored to normal. Furthermore, it is more difficult to estimate an increase in vascular capacitance than it is to estimate an absolute volume deficit. Occasionally, it is appropriate to consider the use of vasoconstrictor agents. When relative hypovolemia occurs in the setting of an edema state, therapy must take into account the fact that the patient actually has a total body sodium surfeit with excess ECF volume, but a maldistribution of that volume away from the EABV. When crystalloid solutions are provided to such patients, a variable, but usually substantial, proportion of administered fluid is distributed into the interstitial compartment and consequently does not contribute to restoration of EABV. This vicious cycle emphasizes the importance of treatment directed at the underlying disease state.

Hypervolemia

DEFINITION

Hypervolemia refers to expansion of ECF volume, which varies, even in normal individuals, with dietary sodium intake. Thus, an individual in steady state with low daily dietary sodium intake (e.g., 20 mmol/day, corresponding to approximately 1.2 g of table salt per day) will have correspondingly low urinary sodium excretion, equivalent to dietary intake minus extrarenal losses. A shift to much higher sodium intake (e.g., 200 mmol/day, corresponding to approximately 12 g of table salt per day) will bring the individual to a new steady state characterized by a correspondingly higher urinary sodium excretion rate. This shift is accompanied by an increase in ECF volume, which triggers the sensor and effector mechanisms for increased urinary sodium excretion (described earlier). In most individuals, this increase in ECF volume is not clinically detectable and does not have pathologic consequences. In some individuals, however, this upward shift in ECF volume increases systemic arterial blood pressure. When the sodium surfeit expands the ECF volume beyond the range necessary for the adjustment needed to restore sodium balance, a state of pathologic hypervolemia ensues.

EPIDEMIOLOGY

Primary and secondary renal sodium retention (Table 118-4) can lead to hypervolemia. Patients with oliguric renal failure of any cause (Chapters 122 and 132) have a limited ability to excrete both sodium and water. Urinary sodium retention can be one of the cardinal manifestations of primary glomerular diseases (Chapter 123), even when the GFR is well preserved. States of *mineralocorticoid excess* (Chapter 234) or enhanced activity are associated with a phase of sodium retention; however, because of the phenomenon of "mineralocorticoid escape," the clinical manifestation is generally that of hypertension rather than hypervolemia. Both heart failure (Chapter 58) and cirrhosis (Chapter 156) are associated with renal sodium retention.

PATHOBIOLOGY

Two pathophysiologic mechanisms can lead to sodium retention with ECF volume expansion. The first involves renal sodium retention that is primary and unrelated to the activation of afferent sensor mechanisms. This category includes primary renal diseases and endocrine disorders characterized by excess mineralocorticoid action. In the second category, EABV is reduced, and afferent sensory mechanisms activate effector responses that drive renal sodium retention. In these conditions, ECF volume is expanded; intravascular volume may be expanded, normal, or contracted; but the volume homeostatic mechanisms of the body mimic those of hypovolemia because of the perception of reduced EABV. The degree of solute-free water retention that

TABLE 118-4 PRIMARY AND SECONDARY RENAL SODIUM-RETAINING STATES

Oliguric renal failure
Chronic kidney disease
Glomerular disease, including nephrotic syndrome
Severe bilateral renovascular obstruction
Mineralocorticoid excess
Inherited sodium-retaining tubulopathies
Cardiac failure
Cirrhosis
Idiopathic edema

accompanies the sodium surfeit has a relatively small influence on the extent of hypervolemia but influences the accompanying tonicity state and determines whether the hypervolemia is hypotonic or isotonic.

When the ECF volume is expanded, the relative distribution between the intravascular and extravascular (interstitial) compartments depends on a number of factors. When cardiac and hepatic functions are normal and peripheral transcapillary Starling forces are intact, the excess ECF volume is evenly distributed between the intravascular and interstitial fluid compartments. In such cases, edema does not occur until there is a substantial surfeit of sodium, and hypertension is expected. In contrast, concomitant disruption of transcapillary Starling forces in a given microcirculatory bed would favor the accumulation of retained fluid at one or more such interstitial locations (e.g., dependent edema progressing to anasarca, ascites, pleural effusion, pulmonary congestion).

Primary Renal Sodium Retention

Patients who retain ingested or administered sodium and water loads expand their ECF volume. In patients with chronic kidney disease, the filtered load of sodium remains well above dietary intake until very late stages of severely reduced GFR: even when the GFR is decreased by as much as 90%, the daily filtered load of approximately 2400 mmol still greatly exceeds dietary intake. Nevertheless, the relationship between tubular reabsorption and filtered load may be disrupted in kidney disease.

Monogenic disorders that cause or mimic enhanced mineralocorticoid activity or are associated with enhanced activity of the distal nephron sodium reabsorptive pathways include Liddle's syndrome and pseudohypoaldosteronism type II (Chapters 67, 119, and 130). In these conditions and in other causes of mineralocorticoid excess, the only clue to mild hypervolemia may be hypertension, which can be severe. Mineralocorticoid excess, glucocorticoid remediable hypertension, apparent mineralocorticoid excess, and Liddle's syndrome are associated with hypokalemia, whereas pseudohypoaldosteronism type II or Gordon's syndrome are often accompanied by hyperkalemia.

Secondary Renal Sodium Retention

With both low-output and high-output heart failure, and both systolic and diastolic dysfunction, sodium retention is typical (Chapter 58). Low cardiac output, diversion of cardiac output away from arterial intravascular volume-sensing sites, or a high cardiac output that still is not sufficient to meet tissue demands appears to be a necessary and sufficient condition for initiating renal sodium retention. In the case of cirrhosis with ascites (Chapter 156), hepatic intrasinusoidal hypertension is a sufficient and necessary condition for initiating renal sodium retention. These pathophysiologic disturbances in cardiac or hepatic function disrupt afferent signals that govern normal sodium homeostasis and trigger effector mechanisms that lead to enhanced tubular reabsorption of sodium at multiple nephron sites. At the very earliest stages of disease, sodium retention occurs independently of any measurable or detectable reduction in the volume of the intravascular compartments or any of its measurable subcompartments. At more advanced stages of disease, reduced intravascular volume serves as the overriding stimulus for renal sodium retention and thereby leads to a decompensated state of intractable ECF volume accumulation. The more advanced stages, which often are accompanied by a disproportionate degree of positive water balance and consequent hyponatremia, herald imminent compromise of the GFR. Among the many neuronal and humoral abnormalities that characterize the sodium retention associated with heart failure and cirrhosis are endothelial dysfunction, enhanced sympathetic nerve activity, activation of the renin-angiotensin-aldosterone axis, and resistance to natriuretic peptides. In cirrhosis with ascites (Chapter 156), portosystemic shunting together with translocation of intravascular volume to the splanchnic and venous circulation further compromise EABV. In addition, synthetic dysfunction with resulting hypoalbuminemia favors transudation of fluid into the interstitial compartment. At the level of intrahepatic hemodynamics, intrasinusoidal hypertension results in enhanced hepatic lymph formation. When the rate of enhanced hepatic lymph formation exceeds the capacity for return to the intravascular compartment through the thoracic duct, hepatic lymph accumulates in the form of ascites, and the intravascular compartment is further compromised.

CLINICAL MANIFESTATIONS

In addition to the clinical manifestations of the underlying disease, the clinical manifestations of *hypervolemia* depend on the amount and relative distribution of accumulated fluid in the various ECF subcompartments, including the venous and arterial components of the intravascular compartment (jugular venous distention and hypertension), the interstitial spaces of the extremities, subcutaneous tissues of the lower back and the periorbital region (peripheral pitting edema, whose predominant location depends on the patient's position), the peritoneal and pleural spaces (ascites and pleural effusion, respectively), and the alveolar space (pulmonary edema). When cardiac and hepatic function is normal and the transcapillary Starling forces are not disrupted, the excess volume is distributed proportionately throughout the ECF compartment. *Hypertension* may be an early manifestation depending on cardiac function and the state of systemic vascular resistance. Jugular venous distention (see Fig. 50-3 in Chapter 50) and peripheral edema (see Fig. 50-7 in Chapter 50) may be present. Clinically detectable pitting peripheral edema usually signifies the accumulation of at least 3 L of excess interstitial volume. Because intravascular plasma volume is itself only 3 L, any state of generalized peripheral edema must signify ECF volume expansion and therefore past or ongoing renal sodium retention, or both.

When cardiac function is impaired because of myocardial disease, valvular disease, or pericardial disease, pulmonary and systemic venous hypertension predominates, and systemic arterial pressure may be low as a result of disproportionate accumulation of intravascular volume in the venous as opposed to the arterial circulation (Chapter 58). The presence of transudative ascites (see Fig. 148-5 in Chapter 148) signifies the substantial accumulation of excess ECF volume in the peritoneal cavity, most commonly secondary to disruption of intrahepatic hemodynamics in the setting of liver disease. Pleural effusions can also be a manifestation of hypervolemia, particularly in the setting of heart failure or advanced cirrhosis with ascites.

DIAGNOSIS

Hypervolemia usually is easily detected by findings of generalized edema, ascites, elevated jugular venous pressure, inspiratory pulmonary crackles, or evidence of the presence of pleural effusion. The prevailing systemic arterial blood pressure often provides a clue about whether the hypervolemic state is secondary to reduced EABV or instead due to primary renal sodium retention. The history and physical examination are often sufficient to yield the diagnosis of an underlying secondary cause of sodium retention, such as heart failure or cirrhosis. Adjunctive laboratory tests providing evidence of cardiac dysfunction or liver disease may be helpful. The presence of glomerular-range proteinuria with hypoalbuminemia indicates a glomerular cause of the sodium retention and hypervolemia. Elevated creatinine points to renal failure, which can be intrinsic or may occur in association with advanced stages of some of the aforementioned conditions, such as heart failure or hepatic cirrhosis (hepatorenal failure). Hypoalbuminemia is characteristic of both cirrhosis and nephrotic syndrome.

A low urine sodium concentration and low fractional excretion of sodium confirm renal sodium retention secondary to a perceived decrease in EABV in the edema states, even in the face of overall hypervolemia. More recently, elevated concentrations of brain natriuretic peptide have been used to support the diagnosis of hypervolemia, particularly in the setting of cardiac failure and renal disease.

TREATMENT

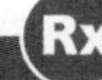

Recognition and treatment of the underlying disease is the most important step in ameliorating renal sodium retention. Optimization of hemodynamic parameters in heart failure (Chapter 59), improvement of liver function (Chapter 157), or remission of nephrotic syndrome (Chapter 123) improves or reverses sodium retention. Therapeutic intervention to reduce ECF volume without addressing the underlying disease is often met by complications, especially when ECF volume expansion is associated with decreased intravascular volume or EABV. Nevertheless, three treatment modalities are available to reduce ECF volume directly by inducing negative sodium balance: dietary sodium restriction, diuretics, and extracorporeal fluid removal by ultrafiltration. The modality and the desired rate of sodium removal vary with the clinical setting and depend on the relative distribution of the sodium surfeit and excess volume in the body fluid compartments. Therefore, before initiating any treatment, the clinician should identify the specific disturbances that are harmful to the patient in clinical parameters and monitor the improvement in these parameters during the course of treatment. Harmful manifestations of hypervolemia include hypertension, pulmonary congestion and edema or pleural effusions with compromised respiratory function, hepatic congestion and ascites, and degrees of peripheral edema that compromise skin integrity and predispose the patient to cellulitis. Once ECF volume reduction has removed these threats to the patient's well-being, rates of sodium removal should be slowed significantly. Thus, a patient with mild peripheral edema, small pleural effusions, minimal ascites, jugular venous distention, and normal blood pressure might be managed with sodium restriction and limited use of natriuretic medications to induce a gradual negative sodium balance over a period of many days to weeks. In contrast, a patient with limb- or life-threatening anasarca, pulmonary congestion, or hypervolemia-induced hypertension might require the continuous intravenous infusion of natriuretics or in some cases extracorporeal ultrafiltration therapy.

Sodium Restriction

Other modalities are futile if not accompanied by restriction of sodium intake because renal sodium avidity results in the reaccumulation of ECF fluid as soon as the influence of diuretics has ceased. Dietary sodium restriction in the range of 20 to 40 mmol/day is often recommended and requires abstention from added salt as well as from foods rich in sodium. Sodium substitutes can be useful, although caution needs to be exercised in patients with a tendency to hyperkalemia because some salt substitutes contain potassium. Caloric intake and nutritional parameters should be monitored to ensure that an overly draconian diet does not induce protein-energy malnutrition. In hospitalized patients, it is particularly important to ensure that the sodium content of administered intravenous fluids and sodium-containing medications is monitored and reduced to the minimum possible. The practice of infusing sodium-containing solutions on the one hand and simultaneously treating with diuretics has no sound physiologic or therapeutic basis. Furthermore, water restriction is not appropriate in hypervolemic edema states unless severe (plasma sodium concentration <135 mmol/L) or symptomatic hyponatremia supervenes.

Diuretics

Diuretics and other natriuretic medications (Table 118-5) enhance the urinary excretion of sodium-containing fluid by inhibiting tubule reabsorption at specific nephron sites (Fig. 118-3).

Proximal Tubule Natriuretics

The cardinal example of a proximal tubule natriuretic is acetazolamide, a carbonic anhydrase inhibitor that blocks proximal reabsorption of sodium bicarbonate. Consequently, prolonged use of acetazolamide may lead to hyperchloremic acidosis, in contrast to all other natriuretics, which act at loci before the late distal nephron. Metolazone, a congener of the thiazide class of natriuretics, blocks sodium chloride absorption in the proximal tubule as well as the early distal tubule. Because the major locus for phosphate absorption is in the proximal nephron, the phosphaturia accompanying metolazone administration considerably exceeds that observed with other thiazide-class diuretics. Proximal tubule natriuretics rarely are used as primary therapy but are used as supplements to loop natriuretics when loop natriuretics alone are ineffective.

Loop Natriuretics

Loop natriuretics, such as furosemide, bumetanide, torsemide, and ethacrynic acid, induce natriuresis by inhibiting the coupled entry of Na^+, Cl^-, and K^+ across apical plasma membranes in the thick ascending limb of the loop of Henle, which is responsible for the reabsorption of approximately 25% of filtered sodium. Loop diuretics, which are the most potent diuretics, continue to be effective even in patients with relatively compromised kidney function.

Distal Tubule Natriuretics

Distal tubule natriuretics, such as hydrochlorothiazide, chlorthalidone, and metolazone, interfere primarily with sodium chloride absorption in the earliest segments of the distal convoluted tubule, where they block the sodium chloride cotransport mechanism across apical plasma membranes. Distal tubule natriuretics generally are used in the same conditions as loop natriuretics, but not in chronic kidney disease and in disorders of calcium metabolism. Whereas loop natriuretics are calciuretic and are valuable for managing acute hypercalcemia (Chapter 253), thiazide natriuretics promote hypocalciuria and calcium retention and are useful in managing hypercalciuric states. With the exception of acetazolamide, which impairs bicarbonate absorption, tubule natriuretics can cause hypokalemia and metabolic alkalosis.

Collecting Duct Natriuretics

Spironolactone and eplerenone compete with aldosterone and inhibit sodium absorption in the collecting duct, while concomitantly suppressing potassium and proton secretion. Triamterene and amiloride directly block sodium uptake by collecting duct cells and concomitantly suppress potassium and proton secretion. These agents are used in combination with thiazide and loop natriuretics to offset hypokalemia. However, hyperkalemia and hyperchloremic metabolic acidosis may complicate the injudicious use of any of these agents. Spironolactone and eplerenone are useful in managing disorders characterized by secondary hyperaldosteronism, such as cirrhosis with ascites, in promoting natriuresis in hypokalemic patients, and in competitively blocking nonepithelial mineralocorticoid receptors in patients with left ventricular dysfunction (Chapter 59).

Nesiritide is the recombinant version of a naturally occurring brain natriuretic peptide with unique vasodilator and natriuretic actions. Nesiritide may compromise renal function, especially when high levels are achieved after an initial bolus, so its usefulness appears to be quite limited and to require frequent monitoring of urine output, plasma urea, and creatinine concentrations.

Patients with severe degrees of renal sodium avidity can be resistant to conventionally recommended doses of individual classes of diuretic agents. In such patients, combinations of diuretic agents acting at different sites along the nephron may overcome this resistance and induce a natriuretic response.

TABLE 118-5 DIURETICS AND OTHER NATRIURETIC MEDICATIONS

DIURETICS IN COMMON USE	DAILY DOSE RANGE	ADVERSE REACTIONS	COMMENTS
Thiazides (oral)		Rash, neutropenia, thrombocytopenia, hyperglycemia, hyperuricemia	Usually not effective below GFR of 30-40 mL/mm (metolazone 20-30 mL/mm)
Hydrochlorothiazide	25-100 mg		
Metolazone	2.5-5 mg		
Chlorthalidone	20-50 mg		
Loop diuretics (oral or intravenous)			Rapid onset, short duration: split doses in normal renal function, give intravenously in acute situations or if reduced GI absorption; can use up to 500 mg furosemide (or equivalent) in severe renal insufficiency
Furosemide	20-320 mg	Ototoxicity at high doses	
Bumetanide	1-8 mg		
Torsemide	20-200 mg		
Potassium sparing		Hyperkalemia	Not very potent
Spironolactone	25-400 mg		
Triamterene	25-100 mg		
Amiloride	5-20 mg		
Eplerenone	25-50 mg		

GI = gastrointestinal; GFR = glomerular filtration rate.

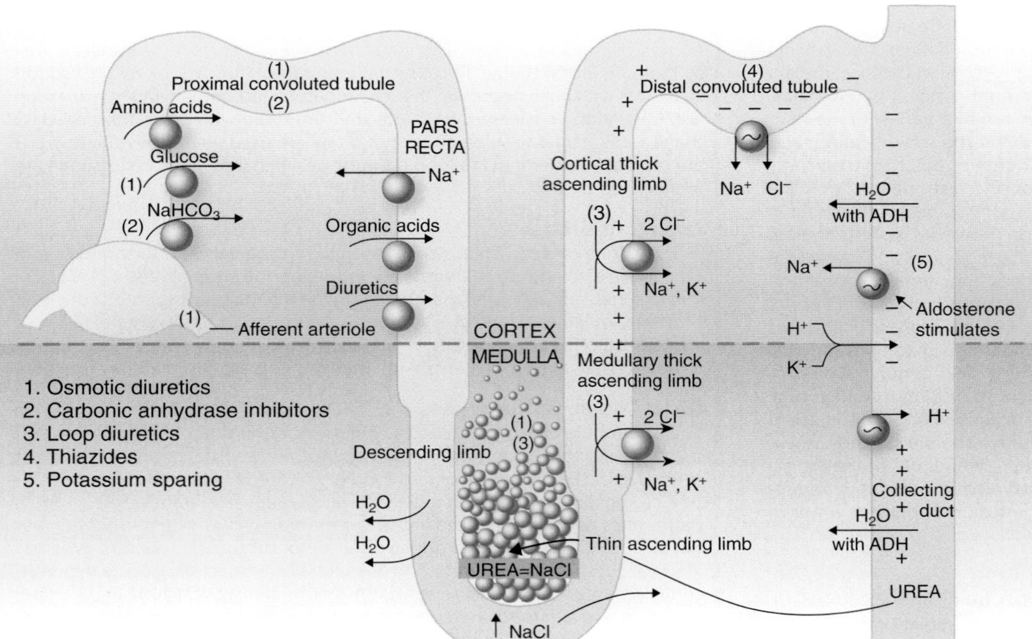

FIGURE 118-3. Major transport processes along the nephron segment and primary sites of action of diuretics. The numbers next to the diuretics in the insert refer to the site of action along the nephron. ADH = antidiuretic hormone. (From Kokko JP. Diuretics. In: Alexander RW, Schlant RC, Fuster V, eds. *The Heart*, 9th ed. New York: McGraw-Hill; 1998.)

The continuous intravenous infusion of furosemide, sometimes in conjunction with intermittent bolus infusions of albumin, also can overcome natriuretic resistance in some hospitalized patients. Monitoring of plasma sodium, potassium, magnesium, calcium, and phosphate concentrations is mandatory in patients treated with high or frequent doses or continuous infusions of natriuretic agents. Besides body tonicity and electrolyte disturbances, other potential adverse consequences include a reduction in GFR. Drug-specific idiosyncratic adverse responses such as allergic cutaneous reactions, interstitial nephritis, pancreatitis, and blood dyscrasias are much less common.

Extracorporeal Ultrafiltration

In a small subset of patients, either superimposed renal impairment or extreme resistance to natriuretic action requires the direct removal of excess ECF volume by hemofiltration or peritoneal dialysis (Chapter 133). Chronic ambulatory peritoneal dialysis has been used for the symptomatic relief of pulmonary congestion and anasarca in some patients with chronic heart failure who are unresponsive to other therapeutic modalities and are not candidates for cardiac transplantation.

WATER BALANCE DISORDERS

Water balance disorders generally come to medical attention because of one or more of three clinical manifestations: hyponatremia, hypernatremia, or polyuria.

Hyponatremia

DEFINITION

Hyponatremia, which is defined as a plasma sodium concentration less than 136 mmol/L, is the most frequently encountered electrolyte abnormality in hospitalized patients.

EPIDEMIOLOGY AND PATHOBIOLOGY

Hyponatremia does not necessarily signify a hypotonic state. *Hypertonic hyponatremia* occurs when there is an accumulation in the ECF compartment of non-sodium-containing effective solutes such as very high concentrations of glucose in diabetic patients or exogenously administered mannitol or glycerol. These hypertonic hyponatremic states are characterized by a shift of water from the ICF to the ECF compartments, with ICF shrinkage rather than swelling. The accumulation of a solute such as urea, which contributes to the measured plasma osmolality but is not an osmotically effective solute in terms of transcellular water shift, should not be included in the category of hypertonic hyponatremic states. *Isotonic hyponatremia* signifies the laboratory finding of hyponatremia in patients with no disturbances in body fluid tonicity and almost always reflects the interference of marked hyperlipidemia or marked hyperglobulinemia with certain laboratory techniques for the measurement of the plasma sodium concentration; these situations are termed *pseudohyponatremia* and should not prompt diagnostic or therapeutic measures to alter water balance or body tonicity.

True *hypotonic hyponatremia* always reflects an important underlying disorder that leads to abnormal body water balance, and the hypotonic state indicates either past or ongoing expansion of ICF volume. Even in chronic hypotonic hyponatremic states, in which cell volume has been restored to normal by osmotic adaptive mechanisms, the compensation occurs at the price of loss of intracellular solutes and compromised cell function.

Heart failure (Chapter 59) and cirrhosis with ascites (Chapter 156) are examples of hypervolemic hyponatremia. In these conditions, reduced EABV stimulates the release of AVP and also may limit the delivery of glomerular ultrafiltrate to the diluting segments of the nephron.

Most fluid lost from the body is hypotonic compared with plasma, so sweat, most gastrointestinal losses, and even many cases of urinary fluid loss do not cause hyponatremia. However, if the replacement fluid that is ingested or administered is more hypotonic than the lost fluid (e.g., ingestion of water or intravenous administration of D_5W), the net result is to decrease body tonicity. Another important consideration is the potassium concentration in the lost fluid. For example, diarrheal fluid and natriuretic-medication-induced polyuric urine are often rich in potassium as well as sodium; even if the concentration of sodium alone is less than that in the ECF, combined loss of sodium plus potassium can cause hypotonicity.

CLINICAL MANIFESTATIONS

The finding of hyponatremia is often incidental on routine laboratory testing, on laboratory testing of patients with nonspecific complaints, or as part of the investigation of other clinical syndromes. The symptoms of hypotonic hyponatremia depend on its duration. In the first hours to days, the major clinical manifestations are neurologic and are due to acute brain swelling or cerebral edema. Symptoms include headache, lethargy, seizures, and a progressively decreased level of consciousness that can progress to coma and death. The severity of these neurologic manifestations depends more on the rate of the hypotonic decline in plasma sodium concentration than on the absolute concentration. In addition, women between menarche and menopause are particularly susceptible to the life-threatening neurologic manifestations of acute hyponatremia, even of relatively mild degree. If a patient survives the acute hyponatremia, osmotic adaptation tends to mitigate the symptoms of cerebral edema.

DIAGNOSIS

After immediate assessment of the clinical urgency of the situation, the first step in the diagnostic approach to a patient with the laboratory finding of hyponatremia is to confirm the presence of true hypotonic hyponatremia. A repeat set of plasma determinations, including electrolytes, osmolality, urea, and glucose, allows comparison of the measured with the calculated plasma osmolality according to the following equation:

$$\text{Plasma osmolality (mOsm/kg)} = 2\text{Na}^+ \text{(mmol/L)} + (\text{blood urea nitrogen [mg/dL]}/2.8) + (\text{glucose [mg/dL]}/18)$$

A careful history, including a search of the medical record for previous measured concentrations of plasma sodium, is critical. The history, together with the physical examination, usually provides important clues to underlying disorders, disease states, or medication exposures that can inform the diagnosis. A history of weight gain or loss also can be helpful in the assessment of recent fluid mass balance. The physical examination should focus on attempts to establish the state of ECF volume. The presence of generalized edema with jugular venous distention and ascites, especially in the setting of heart or liver disease, points quite clearly to hypervolemic hyponatremia. Orthostatic hypotension and tachycardia, particularly in the setting of a history of natriuretic medication use or gastrointestinal fluid losses, suggests hypovolemia, but the absence of these findings does not exclude hypovolemia.

Laboratory tests should include a repeat set of plasma electrolyte concentrations, including potassium and chloride levels, which together with determination of acid-base parameters (pH, $P\text{CO}_2$, and bicarbonate) can point to processes not always elicited in the history, such as vomiting, diarrhea, or natriuretic medication exposure. Other laboratory tests should include liver function tests and measurement of plasma urea, creatinine, uric acid, thyroid-stimulating hormone, cortisol concentrations, and, if indicated, an adrenocorticotropic hormone stimulation test. High levels of both urea and creatinine point to intrinsic renal disease, whereas a disproportionate elevation of urea over creatinine might support hypovolemia with a tendency to prerenal azotemia (Chapter 122). In contrast, very low levels of urea and uric acid are typical of both the syndrome of inappropriate antidiuretic hormone secretion (SIADH) and the cerebral salt-wasting syndrome.

Marked elevation in the plasma glucose concentration increases both measured and calculated plasma osmolality and indicates a state of hypertonic hyponatremia that should be approached as a state of body fluid hypertonicity with cell shrinkage (see later) rather than hypotonicity. The plasma sodium concentration declines by approximately 1.6 mmol/L for each 100-mg/dL (5.5-mmol/L) increase in plasma glucose concentration. However, the value of approximately 1.6 is quite variable and is greater in states of progressively severe hyperglycemia. In contrast to hyperglycemia, an elevated urea concentration should not be considered as contributing to plasma or ECF tonicity, even though urea does contribute to the laboratory measurement of plasma osmolality. Thus, a hyponatremic patient with a normal or elevated laboratory measurement of plasma osmolality, which can be fully attributed to an increased urea concentration, should be considered as having hypotonic hyponatremia. A discrepancy in which measured plasma osmolality exceeds calculated plasma osmolality and cannot be attributed to either glucose or urea indicates the presence of an unidentified small solute (osmolar gap), including alcohols (e.g., ethanol, methanol, ethylene glycol, and isopropyl alcohol), and the organic anions of weak acids, which raise the plasma anion gap. Because these small solutes are not effective solutes in terms of water movement, the water balance and tonicity status of the patient is determined by the plasma sodium concentration. Just as for urea, a patient with hyponatremia and normal or elevated measured plasma osmolality as a result of one of these small solutes should be approached as having a true hypotonic hyponatremia, notwithstanding the normal or elevated plasma osmolality measurement. However, the finding of such an osmolar gap should prompt a thorough investigation for poisoning, intoxication, or an organic acidosis (Chapter 120).

Once a state of true hypotonic hyponatremia has been established, determination of the cause and further diagnostic approach follows a classification into one of three categories based on assessment of the volume status of the patient (Fig. 118-4). Abnormal liver function test results can provide adjunctive support for hepatic disease and a hypervolemic hyponatremic state. The diagnosis of heart failure should be made clinically, but it can be assisted by a brain natriuretic peptide level, chest radiograph, or echocardiograph (Chapter 58). A radiograph or chest computed tomography (CT) scan may help identify intrathoracic lesions that are associated with SIADH.

Approximately 85% of hyponatremic inpatients have true hypotonic hyponatremia; among these patients, about 25% are hypovolemic, about 25% have an edema state, about one third are normovolemic, and most of the remainder have renal failure.

In the absence of a clinically obvious edema state, a low urine sodium concentration (<20 mmol/L) or a low fractional excretion of sodium (<1%) supports the diagnosis of hypovolemic hyponatremia secondary to extrarenal losses or past renal losses that have since abated. If hypovolemia is due to ongoing renal losses, the urine sodium concentration may remain high in the face of hypovolemia, but a low fractional excretion of urea (<35%) may still be evident. High urinary concentrations of potassium point to persistent vomiting or the ongoing effect of potassium-depleting natriuretic drugs. In

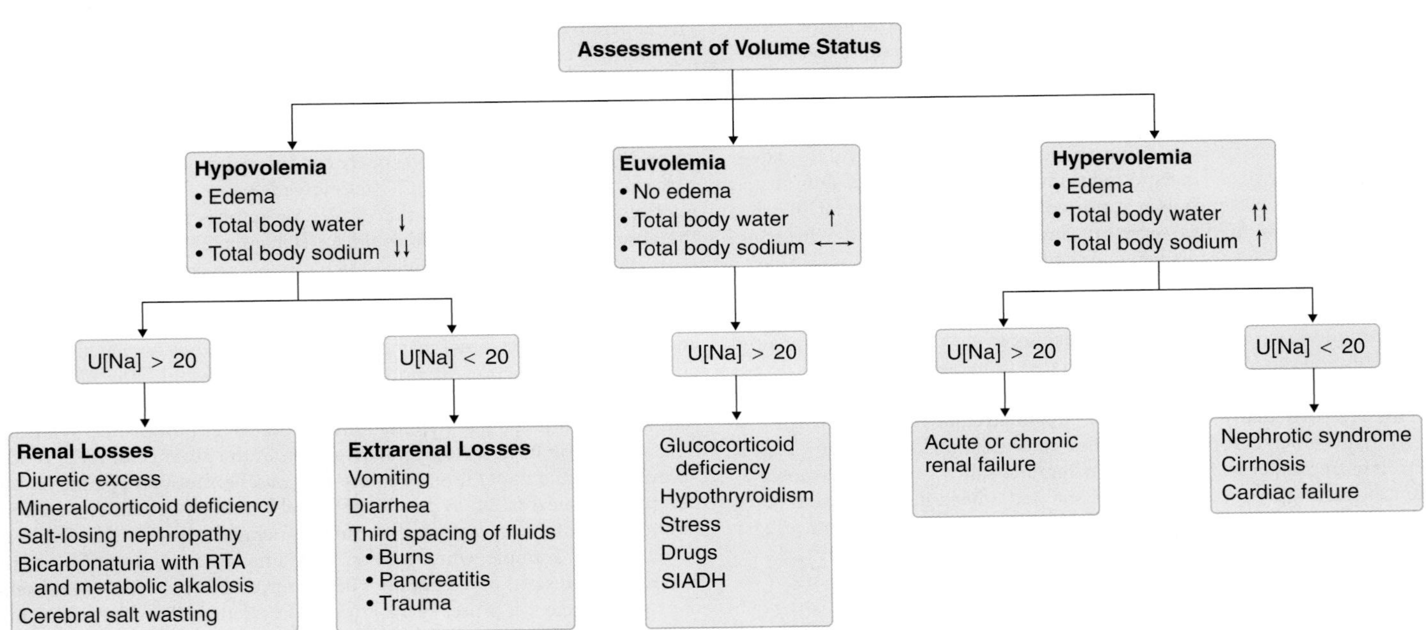

FIGURE 118-4. Diagnostic approach to hyponatremia. RTA = renal tubular acidosis; SIADH = syndrome of inappropriate antidiuretic hormone secretion. (Modified from Halterman R, Berl T. Therapy of dysnatremic disorders. In: Brady H, Wilcox C, eds. *Therapy in Nephrology and Hypertension*. Philadelphia: Saunders; 1999:256.)

SIADH, the urine sodium concentration often reflects sodium intake, as well as mild volume expansion, and is therefore most often greater than 40 mmol/L and frequently higher than 100 mmol/L. The combination of hypotonic hyponatremia in a patient without evidence of either hypovolemia or hypervolemia, together with low plasma urea and uric acid concentrations without hypothyroidism or adrenal insufficiency, strongly suggests SIADH. If there is any doubt about the presence of hypovolemia, a carefully monitored volume challenge can be of diagnostic as well as therapeutic benefit (see later). Lack of sustained improvement after an adequate salt-containing volume challenge lends further support to the diagnosis of SIADH. Once the diagnosis of SIADH has been established in this manner, the cause should be sought, including a thorough review of medication exposure, review of the history for symptoms and signs of malignancy, and magnetic resonance imaging (MRI) or CT of the brain and chest (see Table 118-5).

Hypervolemic Hyponatremia

A patient with hypervolemic hyponatremia suffers from a surfeit of both sodium and water, but the surfeit of water is disproportionate to that of sodium. As for any hypervolemia, the clinical approach is to establish that the patient is hypervolemic and to determine the cause of the sodium surfeit. The most frequently diagnosed causes are heart failure, decompensated cirrhosis with ascites, and renal failure. The occurrence of hyponatremia in any of these conditions often signifies either advanced disease or overzealous sodium deprivation and natriuretic medications. Patients who have heart failure or cirrhosis with ascites experience avid renal sodium retention with urine sodium concentrations less than 20 mmol/L and fractional sodium excretion less than 1% in the face of clear-cut clinical evidence of ECF volume expansion, usually with generalized edema. However, these urine parameters can be masked by the ongoing influence of medications. The edema state of the nephrotic syndrome is less commonly associated with hyponatremia, unless the patient has been exposed to severe salt restriction and natriuretic therapy. Water retention with hyponatremia is a feature of renal failure only in its more advanced stages (stages IV and V chronic kidney disease; Chapter 132).

TABLE 118-6 CAUSES OF THE SYNDROME OF INAPPROPRIATE ANTIDIURETIC HORMONE SECRETION

MALIGNANT NEOPLASIA
Carcinoma: bronchogenic, pancreatic, duodenal, ureteral, prostatic, bladder
Lymphoma and leukemia
Thymoma and mesothelioma
CENTRAL NERVOUS SYSTEM DISORDERS
Trauma
Infection
Tumors
Porphyria
PULMONARY DISORDERS
Tuberculosis
Pneumonia
Fungal infections
Lung abscesses
Mechanical positive-pressure ventilation
DRUG INDUCED
Carbamazepine
Desmopressin
Oxytocin
Vincristine
Chlorpropamide
Nicotine
Cyclophosphamide
Morphine
Amitriptyline
Selective serotonin reuptake inhibitors

Normovolemic and Hypovolemic Hyponatremia

It is often difficult to distinguish normovolemic from hypovolemic hyponatremia because mild hypovolemia can easily escape clinical detection. The initial history and physical examination should try to establish or exclude a cause of hypovolemia. In extrarenal hypovolemia, a low urine sodium concentration and low fractional excretion of sodium are characteristic. When the hypovolemia is due to urinary loss, the urine sodium concentration is usually elevated rather than decreased.

Hypovolemic hyponatremia always signifies past or ongoing sodium loss (often with potassium), accompanied by a degree of net water loss that does not match the electrolyte loss and hence leaves the patient hypotonic. The high levels of AVP that are associated with hypovolemic hyponatremia are usually an appropriate response to the physiologic stimulus of hypovolemia. The most common extrarenal causes of hypovolemia leading to hyponatremia are gastrointestinal fluid losses and excessive sweating. In gastrointestinal fluid losses, any concomitant nausea and vomiting may be independent triggers for the central release of AVP. Clues to vomiting include the characteristic plasma and urine biochemical parameters of metabolic alkalosis (Chapter 120), often with higher than expected urinary concentrations of sodium and bicarbonate. Hyponatremia is a more common complication of diarrhea when the diarrheal fluid is secretory and rich in electrolytes. Sweating-induced hyponatremia occurs when individuals ingest high volumes of hypotonic fluid, often pure water, while losing sodium in sweat.

The renal causes of hyponatremic hypovolemia (see Fig. 118-4) include thiazide-induced hyponatremia, which occurs when patients with impaired urinary diluting capacity excrete concentrated urine because thiazides do not affect the ability of the renal medulla to concentrate urine. Thiazide-treated patients are particularly susceptible to hyponatremia when they ingest or receive hypotonic solutions that exceed their maximal capacity to excrete electrolyte-free water in their urine. In cerebral salt wasting (also known as renal salt wasting), patients who have suffered a head injury or intracranial hemorrhage experience a state of negative sodium balance because urinary fluid loss stimulates the release of AVP, coupled with the ingestion or administration of hypotonic fluids. In these patients, urine sodium concentrations can be impressively high, and the syndrome can be difficult to distinguish from hyponatremia caused by the syndrome of inappropriate secretion of AVP (see later). Persistent uricosuria, even after correction of the hyponatremia, remains an unexplained distinguishing feature of this syndrome.

In normovolemic hypotonic hyponatremia, there is neither an osmolar nor a volume stimulus to the release of AVP. Thus, concentrated urine, usually containing high concentrations of sodium (often >40 mmol/L as a result of dietary intake plus the effects of mild ECF volume expansion), indicates either inappropriate secretion or an augmented renal response to AVP. Conditions that can result in inappropriate AVP secretion or responsiveness include tumors, central nervous system lesions or disorders, intrathoracic or chest wall disease, and numerous drugs and medications (Table 118-6). All syndromes in which AVP levels or the kidney's responsiveness are inappropriately high and not attributable to osmolar or volume stimuli are known collectively as SIADH (Chapter 232). Patterns of abnormal AVP secretion (Fig. 118-5) include erratic release of AVP from the neurohypophysis without any apparent coordination with incoming volume or osmotic stimuli (type A pattern), a constant low-level leak of AVP from the neurohypophysis (type B pattern), a reduced threshold for osmotic release of AVP at a lower than normal plasma osmolality (type C pattern), or an abnormal renal response to circulating AVP in patients whose neurohypophysial regulation is intact (type D pattern). However, no consistent correlation between these various patterns and an underlying cause has emerged. A specific monogenic disorder involves a mutation in which the V_2 AVP receptor is constitutively active in the absence of ligand. Hypothyroidism (Chapter 233) and adrenal glucocorticoid insufficiency (Chapter 234) can be associated with hypotonic hyponatremia without clinically evident hypovolemia and with a clinical and biochemical profile that mimics SIADH; abnormal regulation of the aquaporin-2 water channel may be involved. Pregnancy, which also is associated with a reduction in both the osmotic threshold for AVP release and thirst, results in mild hyponatremia (Chapter 247). Another unusual setting for normovolemic hyponatremia is the "beer potomania" syndrome. Because the minimal urine osmolarity, even in the absence of AVP, is 30 to 50 mOsm/L, the upper limit of solute-free water excretion depends on total obligate solute excretion. A paucity of available urinary solutes sets an upper limit on the total water intake that can be tolerated without inducing hyponatremia. For example, when patients consume large volumes of beer (rich in carbohydrates and water, but poor in sodium and electrolytes), the absence of protein intake limits urea production and excretion, thereby limiting non-electrolyte urinary solutes and hence urinary water excretion. Together with the large volumes of beer ingested, the result is the unusual combination of a normovolemic hypotonic hyponatremic state with low urine osmolality.

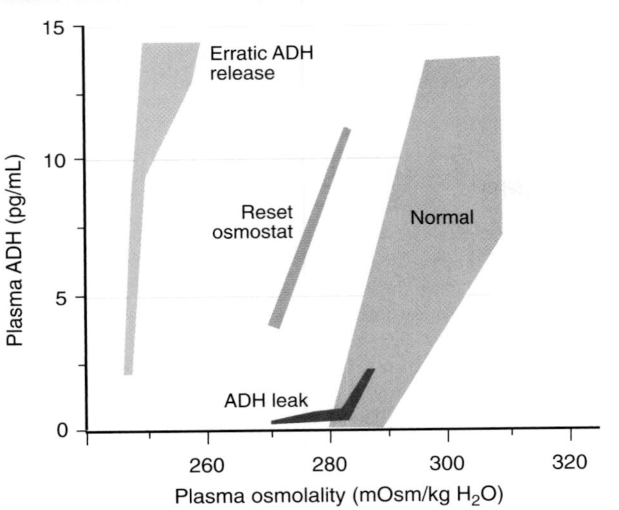

FIGURE 118-5. Patterns of serum antidiuretic hormone (ADH) abnormalities in the syndrome of inappropriate ADH secretion (SIADH). The *shaded areas* indicate the normal relationship between increases in effective extracellular osmolality and ADH levels; the normal osmotic threshold is lower than the normal serum osmolality. The *three shaded areas* indicate ADH patterns in SIADH. (Adapted from Zerbe R, Strope L, Robertson G. Vasopressin function in the syndrome of inappropriate diuresis. *Annu Rev Med.* 1980;31:315-327.)

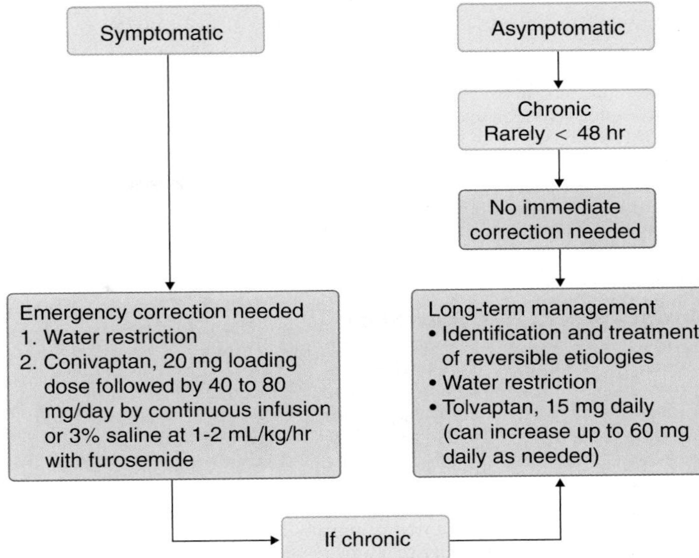

FIGURE 118-6. Treatment of severe normovolemic hyponatremia. (From Thurman J, Halterman R, Berl T. Therapy of dysnatremic disorders. In: Brady H, Wilcox C, eds. *Therapy in Nephrology and Hypertension*, 2nd ed. Philadelphia: Saunders; 2003.)

TREATMENT

Rx

Treatment of hyponatremia varies depending on the category and underlying diagnosis (Fig. 118-6). The overall treatment approach can be divided into the immediate approach to newly appreciated hypotonic hyponatremia and the long-term management of chronic persistent hyponatremia.

The first principle is the importance of identifying and treating any underlying disorder. Thus, in a patient with hypervolemic hyponatremia associated with heart failure, measures to optimize cardiac function are the most appropriate and effective means of restoring normal sodium concentration. Indeed, restoration of normal sodium concentration provides one of the most reassuring indices for successful management of this underlying disorder.

Another principle common to all causes of hypotonic hyponatremia, irrespective of the underlying cause, is that the sodium concentration and the rate of correction should be guided by the patient's age, gender, neurologic status, and any information about recent past plasma sodium concentrations or osmolality values. Delayed correction of hyponatremia can perpetuate cerebral edema and result in irreversible neurologic damage and death, especially in women of reproductive age and in patients whose hyponatremia developed at a rapid pace that outstripped the rate of osmotic adaptation by brain cells. In contrast, too rapid correction or correction to a sodium concentration that is above the level needed to safeguard the patient from the neurologic sequelae of cerebral edema can result in the *osmotic demyelination syndrome.* This devastating and often irreversible syndrome is characterized by fluctuating levels of consciousness, pseudobulbar palsy, ataxia, dysarthria, difficulty swallowing, and characteristic MRI abnormalities in the region of the brain stem. Osmotic demyelination syndrome can be fatal, and recovery in nonfatal cases is either slow or incomplete, often with irreversible residual neurologic sequelae.

Hypotonic Hyponatremia

Current guidelines suggest that if the hyponatremia is known to be acute (<24 to 48 hours) and is accompanied by severe neurologic symptoms such as seizures or decreased level of consciousness, correction should be rapid and should reach a target sodium concentration based on amelioration of neurologic symptoms. However, even under these circumstances, the desired rise in sodium concentration should not exceed 2 mmol/L/hour, and the total increase in sodium concentration during the first 12 to 24 hours of treatment should not exceed 12 mmol/L. The only exceptions to these guidelines would be an unusual patient who has suffered documented severe acute water intoxication, such as occurs during the inadvertent instillation of a glycine-containing irrigation solution during prostate surgery or the administration of hypotonic solutions to a patient who is anuric.

Chronic Hyponatremia

If the rate of decline in plasma sodium concentration has been slow, brain cells have the opportunity to undergo osmotic adaptation by extruding or eliminating intracellular solutes. It is this subgroup of patients who are most susceptible to osmotic demyelination after too rapid or overzealous correction of hyponatremia. Patients in whom there is no previous record of sodium concentration or osmolality should be considered in the same category and treated accordingly. In such cases, the targeted rate of increase in sodium concentration should not exceed 0.5 mmol/L/hour, and the total rise in sodium concentration should not exceed 8 mmol/L in the first 24 hours, even (and especially) if the initial sodium concentration is extremely low (<110 mmol/L), provided that the hyponatremia is not accompanied by severe neurologic symptoms. Patients with severe degrees of chronic hyponatremia in the setting of malnutrition, alcoholism, or chronic illness are particularly susceptible to osmotic demyelination. Frequent monitoring of the plasma sodium concentration and osmolality is crucial, and osmotic demyelination can be prevented by slowing the rate of correction, or even returning to a lower plasma sodium concentration by the judicious readministration of hypotonic solutions or administration of vasopressin analogues (see later).

Having established a target goal and rate of correction, the specific approach varies with the underlying diagnosis. Mild degrees of hyponatremia can be tolerated over long periods, and only symptomatic hyponatremia or sodium concentrations below 125 to 130 mmol/L require specific additional treatment. In hypervolemic hyponatremia, there is a surfeit of both sodium and water, but in tonicity terms, the excess water is disproportionate to the excess sodium. Thus, the goal of treatment is to remove both sodium and water, but to replace proportionately less water than sodium. Water restriction is helpful but is often inadequate or impractical because patients are thirsty, and their adequate nutrition requires caloric intake that is accompanied by obligate water ingestion and metabolic water production. The AVP V_2-receptor antagonist tolvaptan (starting at 15 mg once daily, with a maximal dose of 60 mg once daily) 3 ameliorates hyponatremia and improves symptoms and outcomes in patients with hypervolemic hyponatremic syndromes, including decompensated heart failure and hepatic cirrhosis. It is useful in normovolemic hyponatremic states, such as SIADH (see later), but should be assiduously avoided in hypovolemic hyponatremic states. Two related oral drugs, lixivaptan and conivaptan, have not been proved to be as effective in reducing symptoms of heart failure.

Hypovolemic Hypotonic Hyponatremia

A frequent diagnostic dilemma is the distinction between hypovolemic and normovolemic hypotonic hyponatremia. When hypovolemia is clearly evident (appropriate clinical history, orthostatic hypotension, low urine sodium concentration in the setting of extrarenal fluid losses, elevated plasma urea and uric acid concentrations), administration of volume repletion in the form of isotonic saline is the treatment of choice. The salutary effect of saline derives mostly from the effect of volume repletion to remove the hypovolemic stimulus to release of AVP, thereby inducing a water diuresis, with a minor contribution of the osmolar effect of the infused solute. However, great caution should be exercised in the administration of isotonic saline to these patients because sometimes the administration of small volumes of isotonic saline can induce a brisk and rapid decrease in urine osmolality and an accompanying water diuresis, with an overly rapid correction of hyponatremia. Accordingly, whenever isotonic saline or other forms of volume repletion therapy are administered to patients with known or suspected hypovolemic hyponatremia, careful hour-by-hour monitoring of urine output, urine osmolality, the plasma concentration of sodium, and plasma osmolality are required. A rapid drop in urine osmolality accompanied by water diuresis should prompt cessation of volume repletion and, in some cases, administration of hypotonic solutions or even analogues of AVP itself (see later) to halt or reverse the rapid rise in sodium concentration to within the recommended guidelines so as to prevent osmotic demyelination. When hypovolemia is not clearly evident but cannot be excluded, a brisk drop in urine osmolality in response to a saline challenge confirms the suspicion of hypovolemia and simultaneously initiates therapy. In contrast, failure to induce such a response lends support to the diagnosis of normovolemic hyponatremia.

Normovolemic Hyponatremia

In patients with normovolemic hyponatremia, the appropriate therapeutic approach is to address the underlying disease. Hypothyroidism (Chapter 233) and adrenal insufficiency (Chapter 234) should be corrected with appropriate hormonal replacement therapy. Medication-induced SIADH mandates identification and cessation of the offending medication when possible. If the underlying disease cannot be identified or reversed, treatment is aimed at removing the water surfeit. The therapeutic outcome depends on the minimal urine osmolality that can be achieved, which in turn depends on the severity of SIADH. In many cases, when urine osmolality cannot be suppressed below certain high levels, the severity of water restriction required would not be consistent with the need for caloric intake nor compatible with reasonable expectations for patient adherence. Therefore, maneuvers to generate a gradual net negative water balance are required. In such cases, titrated dose oral tolvaptan (beginning at 15 mg once daily and increasing to a maximum of 60 mg once daily) and reliance on an intact thirst mechanism are crucial to avoid polyuria or hypernatremia. In rare cases with an urgent need to correct the hyponatremia because of a neurologic emergency or definitive documentation that the sodium concentration has decreased acutely over a 24- to 72-hour period, intravenous conivaptan (20 mg loading dose followed by 40 to 80 mg/day by continuous infusion)[4] can be used cautiously to avoid overly rapid correction of hyponatremia. When in doubt about volume status, however, these agents are better avoided until the possibility of hypovolemic hyponatremia has been addressed. Hemodialysis, which can rapidly raise the plasma sodium concentration, should be reserved for the most extreme cases of acute-life threatening hyponatremia for which no other solution is available (Chapter 133).

Hypernatremia

DEFINITION

Hypernatremia, defined as a plasma sodium concentration greater than 144 mmol/L, always reflects a state of hypertonicity, with an increase in the ratio of the concentration of osmotically active solutes to water throughout all body fluid compartments because sodium is an osmotically effective ECF solute.

EPIDEMIOLOGY AND PATHOBIOLOGY

Hypernatremic patients have undergone a process whereby water has moved from the ICF to the ECF compartment, accompanied by a reduction in ICF volume and cell shrinkage. Cell shrinkage in the brain is associated with intracerebral hemorrhage, which often punctates but sometimes disrupts blood vessels, particularly at the brain surface and arachnoid interface. In an effort to restore their cell volume, brain cells undergo osmotic adaptation by accumulating sodium and other electrolytes and then subsequently producing nonelectrolyte small solutes (osmolytes) such as inositol, taurine, glutamine, and glutamate, among others. This process partially reverses cell shrinkage, but at the price of an altered intercellular solute composition with consequent perturbations in neuronal function.

Hypernatremia is the most frequent but not the only hypertonicity state in clinical medicine. Glucose, mannitol, and glycerol can produce hypertonicity states that may not be accompanied by hypernatremia and, in fact, are frequently accompanied by hyponatremia (see earlier). In hypertonicity states, the measured plasma osmolality is always high, but the converse is not necessarily true because a number of solutes that contribute to the measured plasma osmolality are not osmotically effective in terms of movement of water from the ICF to the ECF compartment. Thus, patients with high concentrations of urea or small alcohols (e.g., methanol, ethylene glycol, ethanol) often have elevated plasma osmolality but should not be considered to have a hypertonicity state.

TABLE 118-7 CAUSES OF HYPERNATREMIA CLASSIFIED BY TOTAL BODY SODIUM CONTENT

Hypervolemia	Hypertonic saline excess Hypertonic sodium bicarbonate solutions
Hypertonicity with near normovolemia	Diabetes insipidus Febrile fluid loss
Hypovolemia	Gastrointestinal loss (diarrhea, vomiting) Skin fluid loss (burn, sweat) Loop diuretics Osmotic diuresis Impaired thirst perception

Although hypernatremia can be diagnosed as an incidental laboratory abnormality, it most commonly occurs in the setting of a severe underlying disease with other accompanying disturbances in body fluid homeostasis (Table 118-7).

In *hypervolemic hypernatremia*, a disproportionate excess of sodium as opposed to water expands ECF volume, but ICF volume is decreased because cells shrink. Hypervolemic hypernatremia usually occurs in the hospital setting because inadvertent or overzealous administration of hypertonic saline, the administration of hypertonic sodium bicarbonate solutions during cardiopulmonary resuscitation, or dialysis against a hypertonic dialysate can lead to hypervolemic hypernatremia in the clinical setting.

In *normovolemic hypernatremia*, a pure water deficit with no disturbance in body sodium content does not generally result in a clinically perceptible decrease in ECF volume because the predominant (approximately two thirds) origin of the water deficit is in the ICF rather than the ECF compartment. Thus, for example, a 3-L pure net water deficit will reduce ECF volume by only 1 L, approximately 300 mL of which emanates from plasma water. Yet a 3-L or greater deficit certainly increases body fluid tonicity and the measured plasma sodium concentration. Therefore, such pure net water deficits with no change in body sodium content often are considered to be approximately normovolemic. Clinical conditions that fit this category require a source of fluid loss that has a relatively low content of osmotically effective solutes (principally sodium and potassium and their accompanying anions), such as the various forms of diabetes insipidus or use of vaptan drugs without adequate monitoring. In these conditions, profuse volumes of low osmolality urine are excreted. However, hypernatremia is actually uncommon as long as thirst perception and availability of water remain intact. The principal clinical manifestation is polyuria and polydipsia (see later). Insensible evaporative losses from the skin and respiratory tract also are a source of hypotonic fluid loss. Increased fluid loss can occur in febrile patients (skin and respiratory tract), patients on mechanical ventilation (respiratory tract), and patients with profuse sweating. The sweat sodium concentration decreases with increasing volumes of perspiration. These conditions will lead to hypernatremia with body fluid hypertonicity only if the thirst mechanism or access to water is impaired.

Hypovolemic hypernatremia is by far the most common hypertonicity state. Patients with hypovolemic hypernatremia have lost both sodium and water, but the net loss of water is disproportionately greater than the net loss of sodium. The actual plasma sodium concentration resulting from loss of hypotonic fluid depends not only on the sodium concentration of the fluid lost but also on the concentration of other osmotically active solutes, such as potassium, and on the solute composition of concomitantly ingested or administered fluids. The extrarenal and renal causes of such fluid losses are similar to those of hypovolemia. Among gastrointestinal causes of hypovolemic hypernatremia, diarrhea is more common than vomiting, and osmotic diarrheas result in disproportionately greater loss of water than electrolytes, with a greater propensity to hypernatremia than for secretory diarrheas. Among the renal sources of sodium and water loss, the two most common causes are loop natriuretic medications and osmotic diuresis. Loop natriuretic agents interfere with the countercurrent mechanism and generate large volumes of urine with an iso-osmolar composition. Because some of the solutes are nonelectrolyte (urea), the impact on body tonicity may be to increase tonicity, unless there is concomitant intake or administration of hypotonic fluids. In contrast, thiazides do not interfere with the countercurrent mechanism and therefore rarely promote hypernatremia. The presence of nonelectrolyte solutes in urine causes an osmotic diuresis. Such solutes can be of either endogenous origin (e.g., urea or glucose) or exogenous origin (e.g., mannitol or glycerol). The presence of these solutes in tubular fluid impairs both sodium and water reabsorption, but the excretion of urine that is relatively rich in nonelectrolyte solutes tends to promote body fluid hypertonicity, unless sufficient hypotonic fluids are ingested or administered concomitantly.

Failure to replace hypotonic fluid losses generally reflects either impairment in thirst, disability, or infirmity that prevents the patient from responding to thirst, or failure of the clinician to recognize the need for hypotonic fluid replacement. Rarely, impaired thirst in patients who are awake and alert can be caused by damage to the hypothalamic osmoreceptors that control thirst perception and response, a condition known as *primary hypodipsia*. Usually this condition tends to be associated with an abnormality in the osmotic regulation of AVP secretion. However, cases have been described in which the osmotic regulation of AVP secretion has been dissociated from the osmotic regulation of thirst. Such patients suffer hypernatremia only when extrarenal fluid losses exceed their habitual water intake, as might occur in settings of thermal stress or exercise.

CLINICAL MANIFESTATIONS

The clinical features of patients with hypernatremia can be divided into those associated with the underlying disease state, those associated with a concomitant disturbance in ECF volume, and those associated with an increase in body fluid tonicity. The main clinically relevant consequence of increased body fluid tonicity is decreased brain cell volume, with the attendant risk for intracerebral hemorrhage. Thus, the major symptoms are neurologic and include confusion, seizures, focal neurologic deficits, and a progressively decreasing level of consciousness that can progress to coma. In the absence of an underlying neurologic problem or disturbance in the thirst mechanism, the patient would be expected to complain of thirst unless the neurologic injury has disturbed consciousness.

In patients with hypernatremia of sufficient duration to enable brain cells to undergo osmotic adaptation, the risk for intracerebral hemorrhage from cell shrinkage is decreased, but a hypertonic intracellular environment with the accumulation of new intracellular solutes can perturb normal cellular function.

DIAGNOSIS

The diagnosis of hypernatremia is made by laboratory testing of the sodium concentration, which always should be repeated to confirm its accuracy, corroborated by measurement of plasma osmolality, which is expected to be elevated in all cases. The underlying cause of the hypernatremia is usually evident from the history and physical examination. The history should include a review of recent and current medication use and questions regarding exercise, heat exposure, sweating, vomiting, diarrhea, urine output, recent fluid intake, and the presence of thirst. Physical examination should include an assessment of ECF volume and a complete neurologic evaluation. Urine volume should be monitored, urine osmolality should be measured in several spot urine samples, and 24-hour urine osmolar excretion should be measured if polyuria is present. In the less common situation of hypervolemic hypernatremia, there is often an antecedent history of the administration of sodium-containing solutions, and the findings on physical examination are consistent with ECF volume expansion. In the absence of underlying intrinsic renal disease or diuretic action, urine osmolality should be high because of the hypertonic stimulus to AVP release, which overrides the attenuating effect of hypervolemia. In such patients, the urine sodium concentration should be elevated in response to hypervolemia.

In the more common condition of hypovolemic hypernatremia with extrarenal fluid loss, urine output should be reduced to less than 500 mL/day, and urine osmolality should be the maximum expected for age (urine osmolality >1000 mOsm/kg in young adulthood and decreasing to >600 mOsm/kg by the seventh decade of life and beyond). Polyuria with a submaximal urine osmolality in the presence of hypernatremia suggests impaired urine-concentrating ability, such as occurs with preexisting or underlying intrinsic renal disease or exposure to diuretic agents. A spot urine osmolality measurement less than 100 to 200 mOsm/kg or polyuria (>3 L/day), together with 24-hour urine solute excretion less than 600 mOsm/day in the face of hypernatremia, suggests diabetes insipidus. In contrast, daily solute excretion exceeding 800 to 1000 mOsm/day suggests an osmotic diuresis, which can be confirmed by measuring glucose and urea in urine.

TREATMENT

Rx

The main components of treatment are to treat the underlying disorder, correct the abnormality in ECF volume, replace the water deficit, and provide maintenance fluids to match continuing ongoing fluid losses if they persist.

The therapeutic approach to serious symptomatic hypovolemic hypernatremia is challenging and often controversial. It is best to divide the therapeutic approach into two separate phases: rapid correction of the depleted ECF volume, followed by gradual replacement of the water deficit, including provision for ongoing fluid losses. When ECF volume contraction is severe, as evidenced by tissue hypoperfusion and shock, administered fluid should have a sodium concentration as close as possible to that of the patient and should distribute to the ECF or even the intravascular compartment. Isotonic saline is generally the fluid of choice, and the volume and rate of administration should be guided by clinical parameters related to reversal of hypovolemia. After the patient's tissue perfusion has been restored, further fluid replacement should be aimed at correcting the estimated water deficit. This estimate begins with a simple calculation of the percent deficit based on the measured sodium concentration:

$$\text{Total body water deficit} = 0.6 \times \text{premorbid weight} \times (1 - [140/\text{Na}^+])$$

Total body water is used because the sodium concentration reflects tonicity in all body fluid compartments, including the ICF. Unlike the isotonic fluid replacement for ECF volume, the water replacement should be administered gradually over a period of hours to days, unless there is clear documentation that the hypernatremia has itself evolved over minutes to hours. The necessity for gradual replacement is dictated by the process of osmotic adaptation described previously, and ideally, the rate of water replacement should match the rate at which brain intracellular solutes can be adaptively extruded or removed. More rapid rates of administration could result in brain cell swelling with attendant dangerous neurologic consequences. It is recommended that the estimated volume of the water deficit be replaced at a rate that will lead to an approximately 0.5 to 1.0 mmol/L reduction in measured plasma sodium concentration per hour. In addition to the estimated water deficit, the estimated ongoing water loss during replacement should include at least 1 L per 24 hours of insensible fluid losses (greater volumes in patients who are febrile or mechanically ventilated), supplemented with any ongoing water losses (renal or gastrointestinal) resulting from continuation of the underlying disease process. Because of the need to distribute replacement of the initial water deficit, which can amount to several liters over a number of days during which ongoing water losses continue, it is not unusual for patients to require large volumes of water, sometimes reaching 5 to 10 L, over the duration of the correction period. This water deficit, together with ongoing losses, can be replaced by the dietary ingestion of tap water if the patient's condition is suitable or by an enteral feeding tube. If a gastrointestinal or other disease process precludes these preferred routes, a hypotonic intravenous solution such as D_5W or half-normal saline can be used. When D_5W is used, the glucose is either stored as glycogen or fat or metabolized into carbon dioxide and water, thus effectively providing the patient with solute-free water replacement. In the case of half-normal saline, for any given liter administered, only half can be considered as replacement of the water deficit, and the sodium content will either replace any remaining sodium deficit that has not been fully corrected in the first phase of treatment or be excreted if there is no impairment in urinary sodium excretion. In elderly patients with known or possible underlying cardiac, hepatic, or renal disease, caution should be exercised in the provision of excessive volumes of salt-containing solutions. In any case, the sodium concentration should be monitored at regular intervals of no less than every 4 hours to avoid too slow or too rapid correction, and ECF volume parameters should be monitored to avoid hypervolemic complications.

Special considerations apply for hypertonic states in the setting of uncontrolled diabetes with hyperglycemia (Chapters 236 and 237). The unusual cases of patients with hypervolemic hypernatremia in the hospital setting also need special attention and sometimes require continuous infusions of loop diuretics together with the administration of hypotonic solutions or, in some cases, extracorporeal means to remove both the sodium and water excess in a controlled and safe manner under careful monitoring, often in the intensive care unit.

The route of administration should change in accordance with the patient's response. Although an initial parenteral or nasogastric enteral route might be appropriate when the patient's neurologic status is compromised, subsequent therapy can consist of simple dietary intake of water. Once a patient is awake and alert and if thirst mechanisms are intact, the patient will generally correct the hypertonic state by spontaneous oral fluid intake.

Polyuria

Polyuria (Table 118-8), which is defined as a urine output greater than 3 L/day, should be distinguished from urinary frequency, which can occur with frequent voiding of small volumes totaling less than this amount per day. Polyuria occurs when urine-concentrating mechanisms are not being used at any time during the day (water diuresis) or urine solute excretion is excessive (solute diuresis).

SOLUTE DIURESIS

Solute diuresis is defined as the excretion of greater than 800 to 1000 mOsm of urinary solute per day. The composition of these excess solutes can be electrolyte or nonelectrolyte. Electrolyte solute diuresis usually occurs in response to the iatrogenic administration of high volumes of electrolyte-containing solutions, which are disposed by the kidney through normal physiologic mechanisms. Nonelectrolyte solute diuresis is equivalent to osmotic diuresis in which the presence of a nonreabsorbable nonelectrolyte solute in the tubule fluid prevents reabsorption of sodium and other electrolytes as well as water. The result is the excretion of large volumes of urine with a urine osmolality close to that of plasma osmolality.

WATER DIURESIS

When polyuria is associated with 24-hour urine solute excretion greater than 600 mOsm/day, a defect in urine concentrating ability is generally suggested. In some cases, this defect occurs in association with a more general state of intrinsic renal injury and can be part of the spectrum of interstitial injury in chronic renal disease. More specific defects in urine-concentrating ability fall into the category of the diabetes insipidus disorders (Chapter 232).

TABLE 118-8 REASONS FOR POLYURIA

WATER DIURESIS
Diabetes insipidus
Central (neurogenic)
Inherited
Acquired (e.g., tumors, trauma, hypoxia)
Nephrogenic
Hypercalcemia
Amyloidosis
Drugs (e.g., lithium, foscarnet, cidofovir, vaptans)
Sjögren's syndrome
Sickle cell disease
Inherited
Polydipsia
Primary (e.g., hypothalamic)
Psychogenic
SOLUTE DIURESIS
Sodium
Excess sodium intake (oral, enteral, parenteral)
Renal sodium wasting (e.g., inherited tubulopathies, interstitial nephritis, natriuretic drugs)
Anion-based (usually sodium is the associated cation)
Chloride excretion (e.g., Bartter's syndrome, loop diuretic)
Bicarbonate excretion (e.g., exogenous bicarbonate, carbonic anhydrase inhibition)
Glucose/ketoacids
Diabetic ketoacidosis
Hyperglycemic-hyperosmolar syndrome
Renal glycosuria
Sugar alcohols
External loading (e.g., mannitol, glycerol)
Urea
Exogenous loading (e.g., urea, protein, amino acids)
Diuretic phase of acute kidney injury
Post-obstructive diuresis
Hypercatabolic states
Hemoglobin/myoglobin driven (post-rhabdomyolysis or reabsorption of a hematoma)
Other
Radiocontrast agents

TREATMENT 

Once a patient with polyuria has been classified as having abnormally increased excretion of solute (solute diuresis) or water (water diuresis) (see Table 118-8), the clinical manifestations and treatment will be those of the underlying disease, and the consequences of changes in ECF volume and tonicity are the same as discussed earlier. Depending on the nature of fluid intake and medication used at the onset of polyuria, a significant percentage of polyuric patients will have alterations in serum sodium and ECF volume and will need attention to the underlying disease, as well as correction of fluid and electrolyte abnormalities. Thus, for example, although antihyperglycemic treatment effectively corrects the solute diuresis and polyuric state of uncontrolled diabetes mellitus, initial correction of the concomitant electrolyte and ECF volume disorders takes precedence (Chapters 236 and 237).

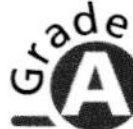

1. Wheeler AP, Bernard GR, Thompson BT, et al. for the National Heart, Lung, and Blood Institute Acute Respiratory Distress Syndrome (ARDS) Clinical Trials Network. Pulmonary-artery versus central venous catheter to guide treatment of acute lung injury. *N Engl J Med.* 2006;354:2213-2224.
2. The Saline versus Albumin Fluid Evaluation (SAFE) study investigators. A comparison of albumin and saline for fluid resuscitation in the intensive care unit. *N Engl J Med.* 2004;350:2247-2256.
3. Schrier RW, Gross P, Gheorghiade M, et al. Tolvaptan, a selective oral vasopressin V2-receptor antagonist, for hyponatremia. *N Engl J Med.* 2006;355:2099-2012.
4. Zeltser D, Rosansky S, van Rensburg H, et al. Assessment of the efficacy and safety of intravenous conivaptan in euvolemic and hypervolemic hyponatremia. *Am J Nephrol.* 2007;27:447-457.

SUGGESTED READINGS

Elhassan EA, Schrier RW. Hyponatremia: diagnosis, complications, and management including V2 receptor antagonists. *Curr Opin Nephrol Hypertens.* 2011;20:161-168. *Review.*

King JD, Rosner MH. Osmotic demyelination syndrome. *Am J Med Sci.* 2010;339:561-567. *Review of clinical manifestations and of potential role of corticosteroids and the reintroduction of hyponatremia in preventing the syndrome.*

Neville KA, Sandeman DJ, Rubinstein A, et al. Prevention of hyponatremia during maintenance intravenous fluid administration: a prospective randomized study of fluid type versus fluid rate. *J Pediatr.* 2010;156:313-319. *The risk of hyponatremia was decreased by isotonic saline solution but not fluid restriction.*

Sterns RH, Hix JK, Silver S. Treatment of hyponatremia. *Am J Kidney Dis.* 2010;56:774-779. *Review including newer vasopressin antagonists.*

119 POTASSIUM DISORDERS

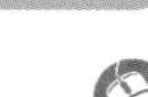

JULIAN L. SEIFTER

DEFINITION

Potassium is ubiquitous in both plant and animal sources of nutrition, so it is difficult to avoid eating potassium in a normal diet. Plant cells have cytosolic potassium concentrations of approximately 80 mmol/L, whereas animal cells may have as much as 140 mmol/L.

EPIDEMIOLOGY

Maintenance of a normal and narrow range of serum potassium, usually on the order of 3.5 to 5.0 mmol/L, is vital for health. The actual concentration may vary during the day, according to a circadian rhythm of decreased excretion in the morning and dietary intake. Insulin-deficient diabetic patients have a greater tendency to develop hyperkalemia, especially if other factors, such as a high-potassium diet, renal disease, or treatment with medications that interfere with renal excretion also are at work. Athletes may have chronically mild decreases in serum potassium. β-blockers may be associated with increased potassium during exercise, particularly in patients with renal failure.

PATHOBIOLOGY

Potassium Balance

Within the human body, potassium is not equally distributed in the total body water. Approximately two thirds of body water is intracellular, and within that compartment, potassium is the major cation. Most cells express sodium-potassium adenosine triphosphatase (Na^+, K^+-ATPase) on the cell plasma membranes and by this enzyme utilize metabolic energy in the form of adenosine triphosphate (ATP) to establish gradients of potassium and sodium. As a result, the potassium concentration of the cell may reach 140 mmol/L, compared with the extracellular potassium concentration of approximately 4 mmol/L. These established ion gradients, and the associated electrical gradients that follow, provide the essential mechanisms for electrical activity in excitable cells such as muscle and neural tissue, cellular nutrient uptake, and transcellular solute transport in polarized epithelial cells in the kidney and intestine.

If there is a ratio of 35:1 intracellular-to-extracellular potassium and a 2:1 ratio of intracellular-to-extracellular water, it is apparent that more than 98% of potassium resides within cells. The total amount of potassium is usually on the order of 50 mmol/kg of body weight, so a 70-kg individual has a store of about 3500 mmol of potassium. In the entire extracellular fluid, which is approximately 20% of body weight, or 14 L in a 70-kg person, the total potassium content is 50 to 60 mmol.

From these calculations, several important issues of potassium homeostasis emerge. First, total body potassium balance may be poorly reflected by the extracellular or serum potassium concentration. This fact dissociates hypokalemia from potassium depletion or hyperkalemia from potassium excess. Changes in the distribution between the cells and extracellular fluid can occur rapidly, within minutes, in contrast to the matching of dietary intake of potassium to potassium elimination from the body, which occurs within hours. It is also apparent that potassium ingestion at the time of a meal may be equal to a large fraction of the total extracellular potassium. An average daily consumption may be on the order of 50 to 100 mmol. Because this potassium cannot be eliminated instantaneously, there is the potential danger of rapid rises in extracellular potassium concentration after meals. Protection against this eventuality comes from the ability of potassium to distribute from the extracellular to intracellular spaces. The intracellular space, given its large volume and potassium content, can accommodate, or buffer, an extra load of potassium without significant changes in concentration. Distribution of potassium from extracellular to intracellular spaces is known as *internal balance*, and the matching of intake to losses from the body is known as *external balance*.

Importance of Potassium

Potassium is essential for a number of critical body functions, including enzymatic reactions that regulate protein synthesis, glycogen synthesis, cell growth, and cell division. The ability of cells to take up or extrude potassium contributes to the regulation of cell volume during periods of osmotic stress. In excitable cells, such as cardiac myocytes, the relationship of intracellular to extracellular potassium concentrations is critical in establishing the resting membrane potential, which normally may approach the Nernst equilibrium potential for potassium. Because larger percentage changes can occur in the extracellular potassium concentration compared with the intracellular concentration, changes in extracellular potassium have the greatest impact on the electrical potential difference across cell membranes. The serum potassium itself has effects on conductance of potassium through specific K^+ channels.

Potassium is also an important local mediator of vascular tone in muscle beds. During exercise, local extracellular potassium concentrations may rise to as high as 10 mmol/L, thereby causing local vasodilation to allow more blood supply to the exercising muscle. Very little of that potassium remains within the total extracellular fluid, so severe hyperkalemia does not usually occur with exercise. The trained athlete develops an adaptive increase in Na^+, K^+-ATPase to allow for efficient reuptake of potassium into muscle cells. The importance of adequate potassium stores to muscle function is well known to experienced marathoners, and overexertion of muscles in a state of potassium depletion can lead to rhabdomyolysis.

Renal Potassium Handling

In the kidney, potassium excretion begins with filtration. Because the extracellular potassium concentration is approximately 4 mmol/L, and that of sodium is 140 mmol/L, far less potassium is filtered than sodium (about 3%). The renal proximal tubule reabsorbs potassium in the process of reabsorbing sodium and water. In the thick ascending limb of the loop of Henle, potassium is reabsorbed both by the apical sodium-potassium-2-chloride cotransporter (NKCC) and, like calcium and magnesium, by paracellular reabsorption of the cation. The latter mechanism is a consequence of the luminal electropositivity created by recycling of potassium through K^+ channels from the cell to the lumen. Luminal ammonium (NH_4^+) can substitute for potassium on the NKCC cotransporter; the resulting increase in medullary interstitial fluid NH_4^+ concentrations enhances medullary collecting duct net acid excretion. In hyperkalemic states, less NH_4^+ appears in the urine because the high concentration of luminal potassium competes with NH_4^+ for reabsorption in the thick limb. As a consequence, a renal mechanism exists for metabolic acidosis to develop in hyperkalemic states, and this in part accounts for the success in treating acidosis by lowering the elevated serum potassium level.

In hypokalemia, whether through proximal tubule intracellular acidosis or other mechanisms, glutaminase enzymes are increased, and more ammonia is produced. This ammonia leads to greater medullary interstitial fluid concentrations and therefore to enhanced net acid elimination. Ammonium production in hypokalemia could be considered an adaptation to allow for potassium to be reabsorbed as NH_4^+ accompanies excreted anions into the urine. The increase in ammonia production can have a deleterious effect in that it may contribute to the chronic tubulointerstitial nephritis of chronic hypokalemia.

By the time the tubular fluid reaches the distal tubule and collecting duct, more than 90% of potassium has been reabsorbed. In potassium depletion, an increase in the apical membrane hydrogen-potassium H^+, K^+-ATPase of the collecting duct intercalated cell allows near-complete removal of potassium from the urine. However, potassium reabsorption is seldom as complete as that of sodium. It is unusual to see potassium concentrations in the urine lower than 5 to 10 mmol/L.

When dietary potassium is abundant, the reabsorption of 90% of filtered potassium by the proximal and distal nephron is followed by net potassium secretion. The urinary potassium most closely reflects potassium secreted by the distal nephron. The major regulatory site for potassium secretion resides in the principal cells of the cortical collecting duct. Three major mechanisms control overall potassium secretion (Fig. 119-1), which may vary depending on the need by as much as 400%: (1) development of a lumen-negative transepithelial potential difference that provides the driving force for potassium secretion into the lumen, (2) adequacy of a variety of apical membrane secretory potassium channels, and (3) flow-dependent movement of fluid through the lumen.

Mechanism of Potassium Secretion

First, sodium must be delivered in ample amounts (depending on the flow rate and sodium concentration of the tubular fluid) to result in sodium reabsorption through the apical epithelial sodium channel (ENaC) in the principal cell. In severely prerenal states of avid sodium reabsorption, sodium delivery may become rate limiting for potassium secretion. Low urinary sodium concentrations limit K^+ secretion in the hepatorenal syndrome or severe heart failure. Assuming that sodium delivery is not limiting, reabsorption of the sodium cation creates a lumen-negative transepithelial potential difference. The reabsorption of sodium in turn is dependent on the low intracellular sodium concentrations resulting from the energy-requiring Na^+, K^+-ATPase on the basolateral membrane. Although K^+ secretion is increased by Na^+ reabsorption, most of the potassium that enters the principal cell from the extracellular fluid through the Na^+, K^+-ATPase is recycled back to the extracellular fluid by basolateral potassium transport mechanisms.

Extracellular potassium is also a regulator of potassium secretion in the kidney. As plasma potassium increases, Na^+, K^+-ATPase increases, bringing more potassium into the cells for transepithelial secretion.

Another determinant of the transepithelial potential difference is the effect of anions in the collecting duct lumen. Non-reabsorbable anions maximize lumen negativity. To the extent that anions such as chloride are reabsorbed, the effect on luminal negativity will be reduced as sodium is reabsorbed. As a consequence, there will be less driving force for potassium (and hydrogen) secretion.

Aldosterone affects the transepithelial potential difference in several ways. The intracellular mineralocorticoid receptor functions to increase the density of ENaC and of basolateral Na^+, K^+-ATPase enzymes. Cortisol, which is normally present in higher concentrations than aldosterone, has equal affinity for the aldosterone receptor and therefore could lead to enhanced potassium secretion. However, the enzyme 11β-hydroxysteroid dehydrogenase type 2 is present in the collecting duct cells and converts cortisol to inactive cortisone.

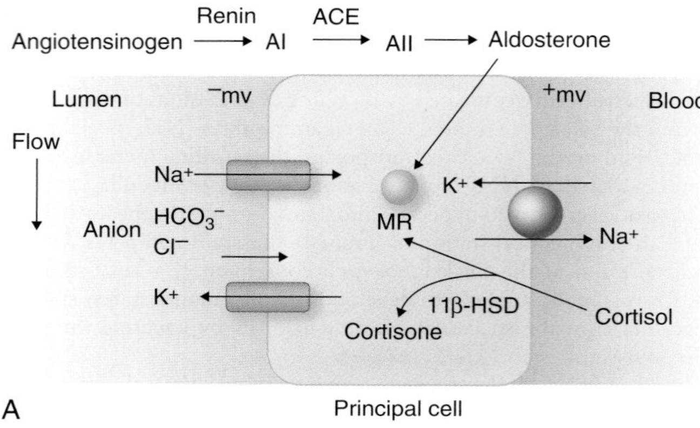

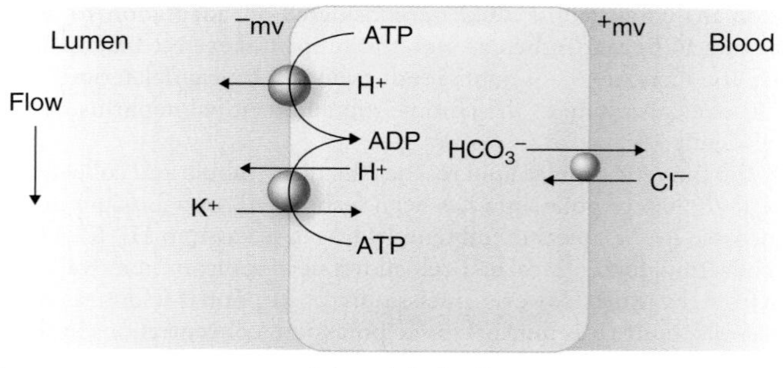

FIGURE 119-1. **Two cell types in the cortical collecting duct. A,** The principal cells mediate sodium (Na^+) reabsorption energized by the basolateral Na^+, K^+ pump. Entry from the lumen is through the epithelial Na^+ channel (ENaC), which renders the lumen negatively charged (⁻mv). This transepithelial voltage stimulates secretion of potassium (K^+) through K^+ channels. Reabsorbable anions such as chloride (Cl^-) lessen the luminal negativity and decrease K^+ secretion. Bicarbonate (HCO_3^-) has an effect to increase K^+ secretion. High flow rates increase net K^+ secretion by preventing development of high lumen K^+ concentrations. The effects of the renin-angiotensin-aldosterone axis are shown: increased mineralocorticoid receptor (MR) activation increases ENaC, the Na^+, K^+ pump, and K^+ channels, thereby increasing Na^+ reabsorption and K^+ secretion. Cortisol would also increase MR activity, but it is inactivated by the enzyme, 11β-hydroxysteroid dehydrogenase (11β-HSD). AI = angiotensin I; AII = angiotensin II; ACE = angiotensin-converting enzyme; mv = millivolts. **B,** Intercalated cells are carbonic anhydrase–rich cells that secrete acid and reabsorb HCO_3^-. The H^+-ATPase secretes H^+ in a way favored by the negatively charged lumen in conjunction with the aldosterone-stimulated effect on Na^+ reabsorption in neighboring principal cells. The K^+, H^+-ATPase is an electroneutral pump. The K^+/H^+ exchanger, reabsorbing K^+, is important in states of K^+ depletion when urinary K^+ is decreased. ADP = adenosine diphosphate; ATP = adenosine triphosphate.

Role of Potassium Secretory Channels

The second mechanism for collecting duct potassium secretion is adequate function of several types of potassium secretory channels on the luminal membrane of the principal cell. Among many factors regulating these channels, antidiuretic hormone (ADH) and intracellular pH are likely of most significance. The increase in K^+ channel activity in response to ADH, combined with an ADH effect to increase ENaC, allows for the highest possible potassium concentration in the urine under circumstances of low flow that accompanies increased water reabsorption. Cellular acidification, as occurs in metabolic acidosis, inhibits potassium secretion through an effect on potassium secretory channels, thereby contributing to potassium retention in metabolic acidosis.

Flow Rate Dependence of Potassium Secretion

The third mechanism for regulating K^+ secretion in the collecting duct is the flow rate of urine. Increasing flow allows for greater sodium delivery and, hence, greater sodium reabsorption through ENaC; it also maintains optimal K^+ gradients for further secretion into the lumen. Conversely, in conditions of water diuresis, the decreased ADH diminishes the net amount of potassium secreted. Yet, because the urine cannot fully be free of potassium, polyuria over a prolonged period is likely to lead to significant potassium losses.

Because potassium excretion is highly dependent on flow rate, conditions in which high urine flow rates are accompanied by high aldosterone levels may result in substantial potassium losses. Such is the case with diuretic use (e.g., acetazolamide, thiazide, and loop diuretics). Increased urinary flow rates contribute to the hypokalemia in osmotic diuresis, Fanconi's syndrome, and metabolic alkalosis from vomiting. Conversely, low urinary flow rates make potassium excretion difficult and may contribute to hyperkalemic states. The increase in aldosterone and ADH that accompanies prerenal states may offset the K^+ retention that would otherwise accompany oliguria.

Excretion Mechanisms and Normal Function

Taken together, three feedback loops are relevant to normal function. First, drinking excessive water does not acutely lead to large losses of potassium because there is a simultaneous decrease in ADH. Second, expansion of the extracellular fluid with isotonic sodium chloride does not necessarily result in potassium depletion because the renin-angiotensin-aldosterone axis is suppressed. Third, in metabolic acidosis, intracellular acidification limits potassium secretion, favoring more acid secretion to compensate for the acidosis.

Diuretics such as furosemide and thiazides are well known and common causes of hypokalemia. The potassium-losing effects of thiazides are greater than those of loop diuretics.

Proximal tubule disorders associated with Fanconi's syndrome increase the delivery of solute, with an osmotic diuresis and bicarbonaturia that increase potassium secretion The volume depletion increases renin and aldosterone. Increased bicarbonate delivery from the proximal tubule overwhelms the capacity to reabsorb bicarbonate by the collecting duct. Bicarbonate acts as a non-reabsorbable anion that stimulates potassium secretion. For example, marked potassium wasting associated with vomiting is caused by renal losses when the urine is alkaline, not by lost potassium from the gastrointestinal tract.

The feedback mechanism coupling aldosterone with serum potassium is important in regulating the degree of potassium losses in the urine. For example, hyperaldosteronism results in K^+ loss, and then the resulting hypokalemia reduces aldosterone production and subsequent K^+ losses. Hyperkalemia has the opposite effect: it is an important stimulus of aldosterone synthesis and release. Thus, with volume expansion and low angiotensin II, the rise in K^+ stimulates aldosterone release from the zona glomerulosa of the adrenal cortex, thereby allowing for K^+ to be secreted into the urine.

Potassium Depletion and Excess

Potassium has critical effects on excitable tissues, especially cardiac and skeletal muscle. Low serum potassium not only hyperpolarizes most cells, thereby leading to an increase in the resting potential, but also alters potassium channels required for repolarization. Thus, hypokalemia decreases or slows potassium conductance.

Because of an increased potassium conductance, hyperkalemia antagonizes the normal slow depolarization of pacemaker tissue that is usually associated with a decrease in potassium conductance. Certain muscle-depolarizing anesthetic agents, such as succinylcholine, may potentiate effects of hyperkalemia, as may gentamicin, particularly in patients with renal failure.

Potassium is as important a body fluid osmole as sodium, and losses of potassium obligate sodium to replace it in the intracellular space, thereby resulting in hyponatremia. Hypokalemia contributes to the hyponatremia associated with thiazide diuretics. Isoosmotic losses of combined potassium and sodium salts in watery diarrhea may result in isotonic extracellular volume depletion. Similarly, if potassium chloride is added to isotonic saline, a hypertonic solution results, and potassium may enter cells as sodium exits, thereby contributing to hypernatremia.

Internal Potassium Balance

Because of the delay in hours before renal excretion matches dietary intake and because potassium first enters the extracellular fluid from the gastrointestinal tract, it is critical that the process of cellular buffering be effective (Table 119-1). Essentially, increases in postprandial blood potassium are minimized before potassium is eliminated from the body. A major factor in this regulation after meals is the feedback loop involving insulin and potassium. An increase in serum potassium stimulates insulin release from the β cells of the pancreatic islets. Insulin increases potassium uptake into cells, primarily muscle, independent of its effect on glucose uptake. Potassium uptake is chiefly the result of increased Na^+, K^+-ATPase trafficking to the plasma membranes in these cells.

Another important mechanism of regulating the distribution of potassium between extracellular and cellular spaces involves the sympathoadrenal system. β-Adrenergic activation, particularly through the β_2-receptor,

TABLE 119-1 FACTORS REGULATING INTERNAL POTASSIUM BALANCE

Insulin
β-Adrenergic activity
Acid-base balance
Magnesium
Osmolality
Thyroid hormone
Potassium

increases potassium uptake into muscle and fat cells. As with insulin, potassium uptake is the consequence of increased Na^+, K^+-ATPase activity associated with increased intracellular cyclic adenosine monophosphate (AMP). The adrenergic effect is important in regulating the serum potassium concentration during exercise and is independent of the additional effect that catecholamines may have on blood sugar with the expected increases in insulin. In the trained athlete, a chronic increase in Na^+, K^+-ATPase on cell membranes may cause a transient lowering of the serum potassium concentration after exertion. Conversely, a severe stress may contribute to hypokalemia, through both direct β_2 effects and insulin action secondary to the blood sugar rise.

Phenylephrine, an α-adrenergic agonist, increases serum potassium. Importantly, epinephrine, which also has α-adrenergic effects, is associated with a transient increase in potassium release from the liver before a more prolonged period of decreased serum potassium mediated by the β_2-receptor.

Metabolic acidosis raises the potassium level more than does respiratory acidosis; both metabolic alkalosis and respiratory alkalosis lower the potassium level. Anion gap acidosis does not raise the potassium level, probably because of the movement of the organic anion (e.g., lactate) from cells into the extracellular space with an accompanying proton, whereas the ingestion of chloride salts has the most profound effect on the potassium level because chloride is restricted to the extracellular space and protons enter cells in exchange for the exit of the potassium cation. The ingestion of excessive chloride salts of arginine and lysine is associated with hyperkalemic acidosis. ε-Aminocaproic acid has also been associated with hyperkalemia and is hypothesized to exchange for cellular potassium, much like the other cationic amino acids.

Just as multiple simultaneous acid-base disturbances lead to a single blood pH level, many processes that affect potassium can be simultaneously present. Metabolic acidosis may be associated with diarrheal or urinary losses of potassium, so that the potassium concentration is low, not high. Metabolic acidosis in diabetes can also be associated with insulin deficiency and renal failure, in which case the serum potassium level might be elevated despite osmotically driven urinary losses of potassium and total body potassium depletion.

Other hormonal effects on potassium include thyroid and growth hormone, but patients with disorders of these hormones do not usually have significant changes in their blood potassium levels. Some patients with hyperthyroidism may have mild hypokalemia, perhaps related to increased sympathetic activity. Growth states are associated with a greater need for potassium; for example, in normal pregnancy, the maternal potassium concentration may fall as the developing fetus grows.

Hypomagnesemia frequently accompanies hypokalemia. Both magnesium and potassium are found predominantly in cells, but Na^+, K^+-ATPase requires magnesium for function. If magnesium is deficient, potassium distributes more to the extracellular fluid, thereby masking the degree of potassium deficiency. Moreover, magnesium deficiency leads to renal potassium wasting, so potassium depletion is hard to correct until magnesium is repleted.

External Potassium Balance and Associated Disorders

Normally, no more than 10 to 20% of total potassium excretion is accomplished by the gastrointestinal tract, but colonic excretion is increased in renal failure, primarily through potassium-induced increases in epithelial Na^+, K^+-ATPase activity and aldosterone. In renal failure, the normal mechanisms to distribute potassium acquire increased importance.

Some conditions that cause the greatest losses of gastrointestinal potassium include secretory diarrheas of the colon, the result of infection or laxative abuse. Disorders of the small intestine, which may lead to large quantities of liquid stool with a low potassium concentration, engender favorable gradients for marked potassium secretion by the colon. A syndrome of watery diarrhea and hypokalemia is associated with neuroendocrine tumors (Chapter 211) that secrete vasoactive intestinal peptide. Rectosigmoid secretion of potassium may result in particularly high potassium losses, and potassium deficiency is seen in patients who have ureterosigmoidostomies. Potassium can be lost from a variety of other sources, including excess sweat or salivation, vomiting, and diarrhea.

Potassium can be depleted by vomiting or diarrhea. Urinary losses may exceed intake in renal tubular disorders, when excessive quantities of osmotic or anionic products are excreted in the urine, or in patients who take diuretics.

It is unusual for hyperkalemia to be caused by excessive potassium intake unless the patient has renal dysfunction. However, patients who have brisk hemolysis, internal hemorrhage, or rhabdomyolysis, particularly if the hemoglobinuria or myoglobinuria also results in acute kidney injury, can quickly develop life-threatening hyperkalemia owing to rapid release of cellular potassium stores.

CLINICAL MANIFESTATIONS

Hypokalemia

Clinical manifestations of potassium depletion include hypertension, decreased growth, and muscle symptoms such as weakness, cramps, fasciculations, and even paralysis. In severe cases, the diaphragm may be paralyzed, leading to respiratory failure. Cardiac arrhythmias are a critical component of low potassium states and are usually seen when the serum potassium falls below 3 mmol/L or when ischemia, hypercalcemia, or drugs such as digoxin are simultaneously present. A patient who has a chronically low potassium level (e.g., from diuretic use) may be particularly vulnerable to supraventricular and ventricular tachyarrhythmias during periods of stress, such as head trauma, or during the acute coronary syndrome, to which cardiac ischemia also contributes. The prolonged cardiac repolarization phase of hypokalemia accounts for the characteristic electrocardiographic findings of broad, flattened T waves. U waves are also indicative of this delay in repolarization (Fig. 119-2). In the intestine, hypokalemia may result in paralytic ileus, which may interfere with oral replacement. Hypokalemia may result in acute skeletal muscle weakness and even paralysis.

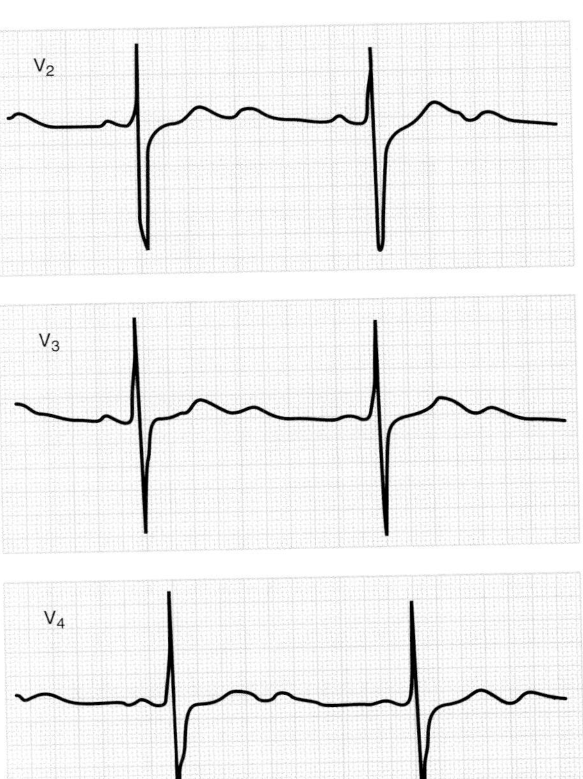

FIGURE 119-2. **The electrocardiographic manifestations of hypokalemia.** The serum potassium concentration was 2.2 mEq/L. The ST segment is prolonged, primarily because of a U wave following the T wave, and the T wave is flattened.

In addition to these systemic effects of potassium imbalance, the kidney is particularly sensitive to depletion of potassium. Structural changes in the glomeruli and tubules lead to a decreased glomerular filtration rate (GFR), increased proximal tubule ammoniagenesis, increased sodium bicarbonate reabsorption, and net acid excretion. A condition of nephrogenic diabetes insipidus results when potassium depletion decreases expression of vasopressin-dependent water channels (aquaporin-2) in the collecting duct luminal plasma membranes. Hypokalemia diminishes insulin secretion and may be associated with glucose intolerance.

Hyperkalemia

In hyperkalemia, the depolarizing effect on the resting membrane potential and increased potassium channel conductance lead to the classic electrocardiographic changes of hyperacute peaked T waves associated with rapid repolarization (Fig. 119-3). Hyperkalemia commonly results in sinus bradycardia. Heart block, loss of P waves on the electrocardiogram, and prolonged QRS intervals are all seen in cases of severe hyperkalemia, usually in excess of 6 mmol/L. The electrocardiogram, however, is not a sensitive indicator of severe hyperkalemia, and cardiac arrest may occur without warning. Like hypokalemia, severe hyperkalemia can cause skeletal muscle paralysis; unlike hypokalemic paralysis, it is often ascending in nature.

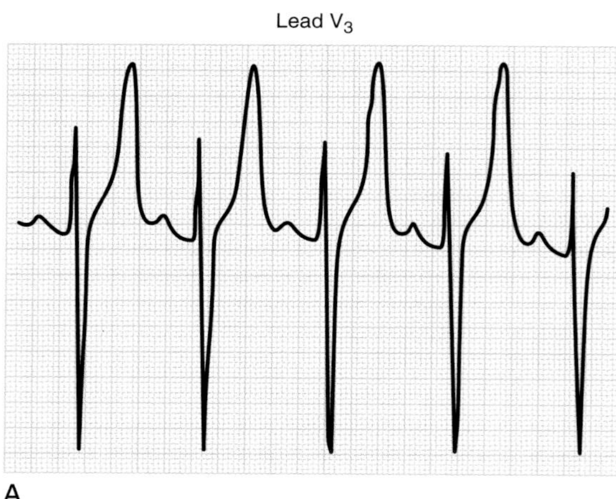

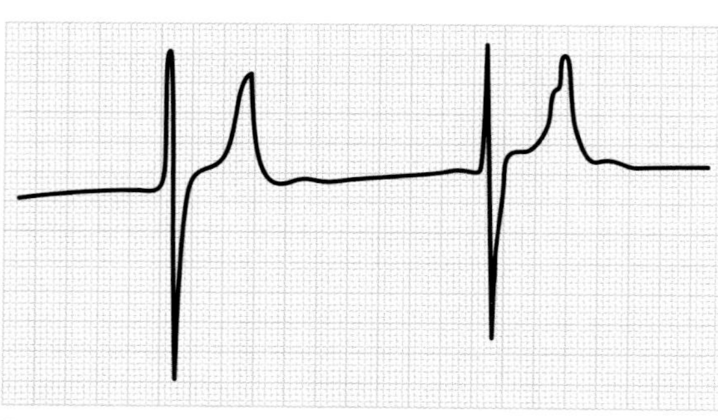

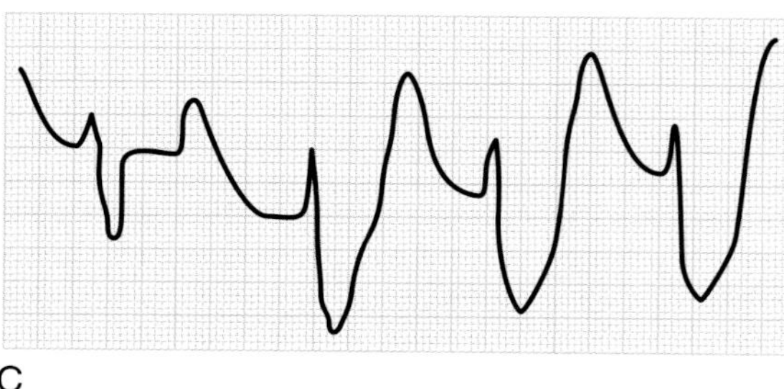

FIGURE 119-3. The effects of progressive hyperkalemia on the electrocardiogram. All of the illustrations are from lead V_3. **A,** Serum potassium concentration ($[K^+]$) = 6.8 mEq/L; note the peaked T waves together with normal sinus rhythm. **B,** Serum $[K^+]$ = 8.9 mEq/L; note the peaked T waves and absent P waves. **C,** Serum $[K^+]$ = >8.9 mEq/L; note the classic sine wave with absent P waves, marked prolongation of the QRS complex, and peaked T waves.

DIAGNOSIS

The first clue to a disorder in potassium balance usually is an abnormal serum potassium concentration obtained as part of a laboratory evaluation, not because an abnormal potassium level itself is suspected. When the potassium is elevated above normal, it is imperative to exclude common artifacts, known as pseudohyperkalemia. Hemolysis in the test tube is a common artifact; in cases of cold-induced hemolysis (Chapter 164), it is important to collect the blood and allow it to clot in a warm environment. Some patients have pseudohyperkalemia resulting from high platelet counts, usually in excess of 1 million/μL, or myelogenous leukemia (Chapters 189 and 190); in such cases, plasma potassium levels should be within the normal range. Sometimes the serum potassium level may be elevated because of local ischemia related to application of the tourniquet and clenching of the fist.

A detailed medical history should focus on medications, family history, and sources of potassium excess or loss. The physical examination should pay particular attention to blood pressure, extracellular volume status, heart rate and rhythm, and muscle strength and reflexes.

Laboratory testing should include a complete blood count as well as serum levels of sodium, chloride, bicarbonate, creatinine, and blood urea nitrogen. In more serious cases, arterial blood gases and levels of creatine kinase and magnesium should be obtained. A 12-lead electrocardiogram also should be obtained.

A low urinary potassium level is expected in hypokalemia. In a hypokalemic patient, a urinary potassium concentration greater than 30 mEq/L suggests renal potassium wasting, whereas extrarenal losses are usually reflected by concentrations lower than 20 mEq/L. In a state of potassium excess, urinary potassium excretion should exceed about 35 mEq/L, unless urinary underexcretion was the cause of the hyperkalemia. A high aldosterone level causes a high urinary potassium-to-sodium ratio, whereas hypoaldosteronism may cause the opposite. Another way to determine the appropriateness of urinary potassium content is to calculate the transtubular potassium gradient (TTKG) as follows:

$$\text{TTKG} = (\text{urinary potassium concentration} \div \text{plasma potassium concentration}) / (\text{urine osmolality} \div \text{plasma osmolality})$$

Correct use of the TTKG requires the urine Na^+ to be greater than 25 mEq/L and the urine osmolality as high as or higher than the serum osmolality.

In a hyperkalemic patient, a TTKG of more than 7 to 8 would be expected. Lower values suggest renal underexcretion as the cause of the hyperkalemia. In a hypokalemic patient, a healthy kidney should conserve potassium, so the TTKG should be less than 2 to 3; if it is more than 3, urinary potassium wasting would be suspected as the cause of the hypokalemia.

Hypokalemic Disorders

The most common cause of hypokalemia (Table 119-2) in medical practice is the use of thiazide diuretics or loop diuretics. Patients may have low, normal, or high blood pressures depending on their volume status and whether the diuretics were prescribed for hypertension or heart failure. The most common acute causes of hypokalemia are diarrhea or vomiting.

Hypokalemic Hypertensive Syndromes

If the renal collecting duct cells develop a transepithelial electrical gradient that is more lumen negative than is needed to maintain potassium balance, urinary potassium wasting, inappropriate to the blood potassium level, occurs. Because a parallel increase in H^+ secretion will occur, it is common to see an accompanying metabolic alkalosis. If the abnormality is related to a primary increase in sodium reabsorption, hypertension or extracellular volume expansion also will develop.

Evaluation of plasma renin and aldosterone levels can help distinguish among specific diagnoses (see Table 119-2). Primary hyperaldosteronism is associated with low renin levels owing to volume expansion. If corrected for serum potassium, an aldosterone-to-renin ratio of 30:1 suggests a primary adrenal cortical tumor (aldosteronoma) or hyperplasia (Chapter 234). The tubular delivery of large amounts of sodium chloride in a setting of volume expansion and nonsuppressible aldosterone results in hypokalemia, which improves after sodium restriction and worsens with the administration of intravenous saline. In congenital adrenal hyperplasia (Chapter 234), such as 11β-hydroxylase deficiency, hypokalemic alkalosis is associated with excessive androgen production. In patients with renin-secreting tumors or unilateral renal artery stenosis, high renin levels stimulate angiotensin and then

TABLE 119-2 CAUSES OF HYPOKALEMIA AND INCREASED POTASSIUM EXCRETION

CAUSES OF INCREASED K^+ EXCRETION AND HYPOKALEMIA	RENIN	ALDOSTERONE	EXTRACELLULAR VOLUME OR BLOOD PRESSURE	ACID-BASE STATUS
Increased ENaC: Liddle's syndrome	Low	Low	High	Alkalosis
Decreased β-OH steroid dehydrogenase: apparent mineralocorticoid excess, licorice	Low	Low	High	Alkalosis
Adrenal tumor or hyperplasia	Low	High	High	Alkalosis
Ectopic ACTH; Cushing's syndrome	Low	Low	High	Alkalosis
Congenital adrenal hyperplasia	Low	High	High	Alkalosis
Unilateral renal artery stenosis	High	High	High	Alkalosis
Renin-secreting tumor	High	High	High	Alkalosis
Diuretics:				
Acetazolamide	High	High	Variable	Acidosis
Furosemide, thiazides	High	High	Low	Alkalosis
Bartter's syndrome	High	High	Low	Alkalosis
Gitelman's syndrome	High	High	Low	Alkalosis
Fanconi's syndrome	High	High	Low	Acidosis
Distal RTA	High	High	Low	Acidosis

ACTA = adrenocorticotropic hormone; β-OH = β-hydroxy; ENaC = epithelial Na^+ channel; RTA = renal tubular acidosis.

aldosterone secretion, with a resulting increase in sodium reabsorption, hypertension, and hypokalemic metabolic alkalosis.

In some patients with overproduction of adrenocorticotropic hormone (ACTH), as in ectopic production from lung and other malignancies (Chapter 187), cortisol may overwhelm the aldosterone receptor and result in hypertensive hypokalemic alkalosis. The patient may not show signs of Cushing's syndrome, unless the syndrome is prolonged. In glucocorticoid-remediable aldosteronism, which is a familial disorder in which episodes of hypokalemia and hypertension develop, a chimeric gene duplication couples the ACTH-responsive 11β-hydroxylase promoter to the coding region of aldosterone synthase.

Glycyrrhizic acid, which is found in licorice or anisette, inhibits the renal enzyme 11β-hydroxysteroid dehydrogenase and thereby causes hypokalemia, metabolic alkalosis, and hypertension. A rare genetic disorder known as apparent mineralocorticoid excess syndrome produces the same effect owing to deficiency of 11β-hydroxysteroid dehydrogenase. The syndrome produces a high ratio of cortisol to cortisone; as a result, renin and aldosterone are suppressed by the volume expansion.

Activating mutations of ENaC cause increased Na^+ reabsorption (Liddle's syndrome; Chapter 130). The syndrome can be distinguished from primary or secondary hyperaldosteronism by a decrease in renin and aldosterone levels.

Hypokalemic Hypotensive Syndromes

In contrast to the hypokalemic hypertensive syndromes, in which an increased sodium reabsorption is a primary event, many hypokalemic alkaloses are associated with extracellular volume depletion. With a physiologic response to volume depletion, the K^+ losses may be a result of appropriate Na^+ reabsorption; signs of hypotension or extracellular volume depletion will be observed. Secretory diarrheas, whether associated with hypochloremic alkalosis or hyperchloremic acidosis, lead to extracellular volume depletion and secondary increases in renin and aldosterone; the result is both gastrointestinal and urinary K^+ losses.

Diuretic use, Bartter's syndrome (Chapter 130), and Gitelman's syndrome (Chapter 130) are renal tubular causes of extracellular volume depletion, hypotension, and hypokalemic alkalosis; sodium and chloride are lost in the urine, and secondary rises in renin and aldosterone occur. Increased urinary flow rates are important contributors to the increased potassium losses in each of these examples. Bartter's syndrome affects the function of the thick ascending limb through mutations in NKCC or in K^+ or Cl^- channels, whereas Gitelman's syndrome is characterized by inactivating mutations or dysregulation of the sodium-chloride cotransporter (NCC) in the distal tubule. The hypokalemia in Gitelman's syndrome may be caused by secondary hyperaldosteronism, bicarbonaturia, and, hypomagnesemia.

Classic type 1 distal renal tubular acidosis (Chapter 130) is often associated with hypokalemia, which may improve with correction of the acidemia. In contrast, proximal renal tubular acidosis, when corrected with bicarbonate, often results in worsening of the hypokalemia owing to greater bicarbonate wasting associated with increases in the filtered bicarbonate load.

Acetazolamide, when given to an alkalotic patient, is a particularly potent kaliuretic agent. Volume depletion and hyperaldosteronism contribute to the potassium losses, as does the bicarbonate wasting, which appears to have a direct effect on potassium secretion. Whenever the urine is alkaline, potassium will usually be present in significant amounts.

Tubular toxins that may be associated with severe potassium losses include aminoglycosides, cisplatinum, and ifosfamide. Amphotericin B results in significant potassium wasting accompanied by renal tubular acidosis. In many of these conditions, simultaneous use of amiloride may diminish potassium losses by as much as 50%.

Patients who present with unexplained hypokalemia and alkalosis with volume depletion should have urinary electrolytes measured to determine whether the urine chloride is low, as with vomiting or laxative abuse. If the urine contains chloride, a diuretic screen should be considered; Gitelman's syndrome and Bartter's syndrome are other possibilities.

Hyperkalemic Disorders

In clinical practice, acute hyperkalemia is seen most commonly with renal failure (Chapter 133), with acidosis (Chapter 120), and with acute muscle damage from rhabdomyolysis (Chapter 115) (Table 119-3). Chronic hyperkalemia is most commonly seen with medications that reduce potassium secretion and with renal tubular disorders.

Hyperkalemic Hypotensive or Normotensive Syndromes

Type IV renal tubular acidoses (Chapter 130) that are associated with an inability to acidify the urine are caused by diseases that disrupt distal nephron function, including systemic lupus erythematosus (Chapter 274), urinary tract obstruction (Chapter 125), amyloidosis (Chapter 194), the nephropathy associated with kidney and bone marrow transplantation (Chapters 133 and 181), and sickle cell nephropathy (Chapter 127). Males who present with hyperkalemia and renal insufficiency of unknown cause should be evaluated for possible prostatic obstruction (Chapter 131). Each of these conditions may also be associated with failure to concentrate the urine (nephrogenic diabetes insipidus) or with a hyperchloremic metabolic acidosis caused by abnormalities in acid secretion.

Primary selective hypoaldosteronism or complete adrenal cortical deficiency (Chapter 234) is associated with elevated renin and low aldosterone. Secondary hypoaldosteronism may be seen in hyporenin states caused by β-blockers, renin antagonists, or nonsteroidal anti-inflammatory drugs (NSAIDs). Angiotensin-converting enzyme inhibitors and angiotensin receptor blockers increase renin and decrease aldosterone. Heparin, including low-molecular-weight and fractionated forms (Chapter 37), can lead to hyperkalemia even in small subcutaneous doses.

Disorders that affect the transepithelial potential difference and can result in hyperkalemia, acidosis, and extracellular volume depletion include

TABLE 119-3 CAUSES OF HYPERKALEMIA AND DECREASED POTASSIUM EXCRETION

CAUSE OF DECREASED K^+ EXCRETION AND HYPERKALEMIA	RENIN	ALDOSTERONE	EXTRACELLULAR VOLUME OR BLOOD PRESSURE	ACID-BASE STATUS
Decreased ENaC: Drugs: amiloride, triamterene, trimethoprim, lithium Pseudohypoaldosteronism type 1 autosomal recessive ENaC mutation	High	High	Low or normal	Normal or acidosis
Pseudohypoaldosteronism type 1 autosomal dominant MR mutation	High	High	Low	Acidosis
MR blockade: spironolactone, eplerenone, progesterone	High	High	Low	Acidosis
Hypoaldosteronism: Adrenal insufficiency	High	Low	Low	Acidosis
Hyporenin-hypoaldosteronism: NSAIDs, β-blockers, autonomic neuropathy	Low	Low	Low	Acidosis
Pseudohypoaldosteronism type 2	Low	Low	High	Acidosis

ENaC = epithelial Na^+ channel; MR = mineralocorticoid receptor; NSAIDs = nonsteroidal anti-inflammatory drugs.

inactivating mutations of ENaC (autosomal recessive pseudohypoaldosteronism type 1), which may be accompanied by high renin and aldosterone levels. The ENaC may also be inhibited by the potassium-sparing diuretics (i.e., amiloride and triamterene) and certain medications secreted by the proximal tubule organic cation transporters, such as trimethoprim and pentamidine, as well as by lithium. Inhibition of the aldosterone receptor may be the result of antagonists such as spironolactone and eplerenone.

Hyperkalemic Hypertensive Syndromes

NSAIDs can cause hyperkalemia, particularly in patients with renal disease, by decreasing sodium delivery, increasing water reabsorption, and decreasing renin and aldosterone. Hypertension with the NSAIDs is most likely caused by renal salt and water retention.

Cyclosporine or tacrolimus may produce a hyperkalemic acidosis. The mechanism may involve inhibition of cyclooxygenase 2 (COX2) and therefore hyporenin-hypoaldosteronism. There may also be a decrease in apical potassium secretion in the collecting duct. Gordon's syndrome is a genetic disorder (pseudohypoaldosteronism type 2) associated with hyperkalemia, volume expansion, and metabolic acidosis; it is highly responsive to thiazide diuretics.

TREATMENT Rx

It may be difficult to determine the exact state of total body potassium stores from the serum potassium level because as much as 100 to 300 mmol of potassium may be lost from the body with a fall in serum potassium of only 1 mmol/L.

Hypokalemia

The goal of acute therapy for hypokalemia is to prevent or manage potentially life-threatening arrhythmias or paralysis. Patients at greatest risk are elderly patients, patients with known liver disease or cardiac disturbances, and patients who have had an abrupt fall in serum K^+ to less than 2.5 mEq/L. Potassium must traverse the extracellular space before repleting intracellular stores, so it is dangerously easy to replete potassium too quickly. Oral potassium should be given, if possible. If the K^+ is greater than 3 mEq/L, increasing dietary K^+ can be considered, along with removing the underlying cause of hypokalemia. Usual oral replacement is with KCl at a dose of 40 to 100 mmol per day. The Cl salt has the advantage of treating concomitant metabolic alkalosis, but other available forms include K citrate (in the acidotic patient) and K phosphate (in patients with a phosphate deficit). Giving potassium with a nonreabsorbable anion, such as gluconate, may not replace the potassium deficit adequately. Intravenous potassium is reserved for patients who are unable to take enteral potassium and patients with symptomatic hypokalemia, paralysis, or cardiac arrhythmias. It is usually given as a solution of 20 to 40 mmol of K^+ in 1 L of solution at a rate that does not exceed 10 to 20 mmol/hour. In some cases of severe hypokalemia (<2.5 mEq/L) and in symptomatic patients, higher concentrations (up to 40 mmol in 100 mL) have been used. If the potassium level is less than 3 mmol/L or if more than 10 mmol/hour is to be delivered, it may be best to treat the patient in a monitored setting to observe for cardiac complications. A central venous catheter may be required for these higher concentrations. In these unusual circumstances, it is best to consult with a renal specialist and the pharmacy.

In patients who have prerenal azotemia associated with hyperglycemia or severe metabolic alkalosis, volume expansion with sodium chloride solutions alone can result in life-threatening potassium losses, despite improvement in the extracellular volume. Potassium must be given in anticipation of such events.

In a hypokalemic patient, care must be exercised when glucose-containing solutions are given because the resulting increase in insulin may further decrease the blood potassium level. Attention to the urine output and ongoing losses is crucial. If ongoing losses of potassium are severe, it may be necessary to provide a potassium-sparing diuretic (e.g., amiloride, 5 to 10 mg orally) and to treat the cause of the ongoing losses (e.g., diarrhea). Magnesium should be measured and replaced, if necessary, in any hypokalemic patient.

In the outpatient setting, hypokalemia is a common side effect of diuretic therapy. The serum potassium level should be maintained within the normal range (>3.5 mEq/L), especially in high-risk patients. Addition of 40 to 100 mmol of K^+ per day as the chloride salt is the usual treatment, depending on the patient's response.

Hyperkalemia

If hyperkalemia is severe, the goal is to achieve a rapid reduction in potassium concentration. If hyperkalemia is associated with cardiac arrhythmias, however, the cardiac effects of the hyperkalemia require interim treatment in a monitored setting, before the serum potassium can be expected to decline, even with aggressive therapy. Calcium gluconate, 10 mL of a 10% solution (8.9 mg calcium) over 10 to 20 minutes, is often indicated to stabilize electrical effects on cardiac excitation. Calcium chloride (3 to 4 mL of a 10% solution) is used as another alternative, but it should be administered through a central access line because extravasation of the chloride salt may result in tissue necrosis.

However, calcium does not lower the potassium concentration. Nebulized or inhaled β-agonists and intravenous insulin and glucose, either alone or the two in combination, are the best treatments. [1] To lower the potassium within 15 minutes, 10 units of regular insulin should be given, with glucose given as a 10% solution over 1 hour for a total of 30 to 50 g in the normoglycemic patient. The blood glucose level should be monitored. Albuterol by nebulizer (10 to 20 mg in 4 mL saline over 10 minutes) can redistribute potassium acutely but should not be the sole treatment because some patients are not responsive. In some cases, intravenous β-adrenergic agonists (e.g., albuterol, 0.5 mg in 100 mL of 5% dextrose over 15 minutes) have been used to lower the serum potassium level by about 1 mmol/L within minutes to hours. Sodium bicarbonate, as an isotonic mixture calculated to correct acid-base status, should be reserved for acidemic patients who otherwise require alkalinization, while being careful to avoid hypocalcemia; complications of sodium bicarbonate infusions include hypernatremia, volume expansion, and decreased ionized calcium, potentially resulting in tetany. Diabetic patients may be potassium depleted even though they present with hyperkalemia; as they are volume repleted, they typically require potassium replacement (Chapter 236).

Over the longer term, potassium loss can be sustained by using cation exchange resins such as sodium polystyrene sulfonate, given orally or as an enema (Chapter 133). A dose of 30 to 50 g can reduce potassium levels over several hours. This resin will also provide a sodium load and bind calcium, thereby resulting in volume expansion and hypocalcemia. These resins may interfere with the absorption of lithium and thyroxine. A serious complication of sodium polystyrene sulfonate resins when used in combination with sorbitol is colonic ulceration and necrosis. These resins also should not be given in combination with aluminum-based antacids because the resulting concretions can obstruct the gastrointestinal tract. If the patient is volume expanded, furosemide (40 to 100 mg), chlorothiazide (500 mg) or, if the patient is also alkalotic, acetazolamide (250 to 500 mg) may enhance renal potassium clearance. If the patient is volume depleted, isotonic saline expansion may improve urine output and, with it, potassium excretion.

Specific Clinical Syndromes

Hypokalemia

Patients with pernicious anemia who receive vitamin B_{12} to stimulate erythropoiesis may deplete extracellular potassium and suffer from hypokalemia as a cost of producing new red blood cells. Leukemias with rapid growth rates (Chapter 189) also may cause a drop in the serum potassium level, and some forms of myelogenous leukemia are associated with a high level of lysozyme, which leads to urinary potassium loss as well (Chapter 190).

Familial hypokalemic periodic paralysis is caused by a variety of mutations in a cellular calcium channel, with resulting reduced activity of an ATP-regulated K^+ channel that extrudes potassium from skeletal muscle cells. Without the ability to recycle potassium to the extracellular space, the hypokalemic effect of the Na^+, K^+-ATPase is unopposed. The presentation is usually in the teenage years or early adulthood. In some cases, a progressive proximal myopathy may develop. A form is seen in Asian patients with hyperthyroidism; it manifests as episodic paralysis brought out by high-carbohydrate meals (insulin secretion). Another aggravating factor is rest after exercise, a time when blood potassium falls owing to reuptake of potassium by the ATPase pumps. The condition is treated by a high potassium diet as well as with β_2-blockers (e.g., propranolol, 20 to 40 mg twice daily) and carbonic anhydrase inhibitors (e.g., acetazolamide, 125 to 500 mg), which in part work by creating a hyperchloremic acidosis that offsets the urinary potassium wasting they cause.

Hyperkalemia

The abnormal distribution of potassium between cells and the extracellular space results in the hyperkalemia that is associated with acidosis, insulin-deficient states, and β_2-adrenergic blockade. Although it is not always possible, it is best to know the levels of serum glucose and potassium in an unconscious diabetic patient before infusing concentrated glucose solutions, because of the risk for aggravating an already elevated potassium concentration.

Familial hyperkalemic periodic paralysis is a myopathy caused by a genetic defect in voltage-gated Na^+ channels in skeletal muscle. Exercise or dietary increases in plasma potassium result in mild depolarization of skeletal muscle that then unmasks the sodium channel defect, rendering the cells unexcitable. Treatment is frequent meals and acetazolamide (125 to 500 mg).

Potassium competes with digoxin-binding sites on the Na^+, K^+-ATPase, so that, if hypokalemia coexists, digoxin will have an intensified effect and may lead to drug toxicity. In extreme cases of digitalis overdose, severe hyperkalemia develops owing to generalized blockade of Na^+, K^+-ATPase.

PROGNOSIS

The prognosis of patients with hypokalemia and hyperkalemia depends on the severity and underlying illness. Most hypokalemic cases are mild (K^+, 3 to 3.5 mEq/L). However, mortality of hospitalized patients with hypokalemia is increased ten-fold. Hyperkalemia is reported in 1 to 10% of hospitalized patients, of whom 10% have severe hyperkalemia (K^+, >6.0 mEq/L). Hyperkalemia is associated with increased mortality (14 to 41%), and it accounts for 2 to 5% of deaths in patients with end-stage renal disease.

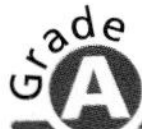

1. Mahoney BA, Smith WA, Lo DS, et al. Emergency interventions for hyperkalemia. *Cochrane Database Syst Rev*. 2005;2:CD003235.

SUGGESTED READINGS

Einhorn LM, Zhan M, Hsu VD, et al. The frequency of hyperkalemia and its significance in chronic kidney disease. *Arch Intern Med*. 2009;169:1156-1162. *Emphasizes the association of hyperkalemia with adverse outcomes.*

Khanna A, White WB. The management of hyperkalemia in patients with cardiovascular disease. *Am J Med*. 2009;122:215-221. *Review.*

Lippi G, Favaloro EJ, Montagnana M, et al. Prevalence of hypokalaemia: the experience of a large academic hospital. *Intern Med J*. 2010;40:315-316. *Review.*

Sterns RH, Rojas M, Bernstein P, et al. Ion-exchange resins for the treatment of hyperkalemia: are they safe and effective? *J Am Soc Nephrol*. 2010;21:733-735. *Review of usefulness and potential complications when used with sorbitol or aluminum-based antacids.*

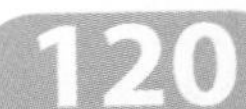

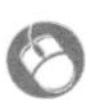

ACID-BASE DISORDERS

JULIAN L. SEIFTER

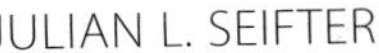

DEFINITION

The pH is defined as the negative log of the hydrogen ion concentration. At a pH of 7.40, the hydrogen ion concentration is 40 nanoequivalents (nEq) per liter, a very small concentration in comparison to serum sodium at 140 mEq/L. The hydrogen ion concentration of body fluids is in equilibrium with each of multiple buffers, such as proteins, phosphate, and hemoglobin (the isohydric principle), but acid-base equilibria in the body are often analyzed by using the CO_2/HCO_3^- system and the relationship of the proton concentration (thus pH) to the ratio of HCO_3^- to CO_2. The Henderson-Hasselbalch equation is a logarithmic expression of the relationship.

$$CO_2 + H_2O \rightarrow H_2CO_3 \rightarrow H^+ + HCO_3^-$$

$$pH = pK + \log[HCO_3]/0.03(PCO_2)$$

In this equation, pK, or the dissociation constant, is 6.1; 0.03 (mM/mm Hg) is the solubility factor for CO_2 in solution. The product of $0.03 \times PCO_2$ represents dissolved CO_2; the "total CO_2" in plasma is the sum of HCO_3^-, normally about 25 mM, and $0.03 \times PCO_2$, normally about 1.2 mM. It is important to note that pH is a function of the *ratio* of HCO_3^- to PCO_2. The HCO_3^- concentration in the numerator is regulated by the kidney, and PCO_2 is regulated by the lung, the major organ systems involved in acid-base balance.

EPIDEMIOLOGY

If the production of acid exceeds elimination, a state of acidosis exists, whereas if elimination exceeds production, alkalosis will develop. In metabolic acidosis, production could exceed excretion through a marked excess in the production rate, as might be seen with diabetic ketoacidosis (Chapter 236) or lactic acidosis, or it could develop even with a normal rate of metabolic acid production if the kidney were unable to eliminate acid normally, as in kidney failure (Chapters 122 and 132).

In most humans, particularly those who eat animal protein or an acid-ash diet, the requirement for net acid excretion dominates. However, vegetarians can have an overall alkaline-ash diet, for which net alkali must be excreted to match intake.

Hypochloremic alkalosis might be anticipated in a patient with a history of vomiting or the use of thiazide or loop diuretics. Metabolic acidosis might be anticipated in hypotensive shock, sepsis, diarrhea, and renal failure. Chronic lung disease can be associated with respiratory acidosis, whereas fever, infection, stroke, or acute pulmonary disease may be a cause of acute respiratory alkalosis.

PATHOBIOLOGY

Normal Acid-Base Physiology

Many of the body's metabolic and physiologic functions are pH dependent or pH sensitive. The range of normal arterial pH is 7.38 to 7.42. Intracellular pH is lower than extracellular pH because cells are electronegative with respect to extracellular fluid and metabolically produced acids are constantly being transported to extracellular fluid for eventual elimination from the body. Net acid production must equal net acid excretion. When the diet calls for excretion of acids, urine pH will fall to a value as low as 5.0, and the urine will become nominally free of bicarbonate. When there is an alkaline load, the kidney will reject the excess filtered HCO_3^-, and urine pH may approach a maximal value of 8.0 to 8.5.

In severe disease states, arterial pH may fall as low as 6.8 and rise as high as 7.8. Strenuous exercise with the metabolic production of lactate may transiently but severely lower pH, even in normal healthy individuals.

Production of Acids and the Elimination of CO_2 by the Lung

Volatile acid is the term used for the carbon dioxide produced by metabolic processes in all tissues, an amount that approximates 20,000 mmol/day. This CO_2 is carried from tissues to the lung, where it is eliminated by alveolar ventilation. Steady-state PCO_2 is normally 38 to 42 mm Hg.

Nonvolatile acid is a term used to describe acids other than carbonic acid that are formed primarily from protein metabolism. The usual amount of formation is approximately 1 to 2 mEq of H^+ per kilogram of body weight per day. Most diets that contain animal protein have a net positive quantity of nonvolatile acids, primarily from the sulfur-containing amino acids cysteine and methionine; phosphates from phosphoproteins, phospholipids, and phosphonucleotides; nonmetabolizable organic acids, such as uric acid, and inorganic sources; and HCl derived from chloride salts of lysine, arginine, and histidine. The addition of protons to body fluids by these acid end products consumes bicarbonate, which then must be replenished by the kidney as it eliminates the proton. The kidney must excrete any nonvolatile acid or alkali load to maintain a steady-state serum HCO_3^- concentration in the 22- to 28-mM range.

Oxidation of carbohydrates and fats results in the production of water and CO_2, but not nonvolatile acids. To maintain a steady state, any acid or base produced per day must be equivalent to what is excreted. If CO_2 production exceeds CO_2 excretion by the lungs, respiratory acidosis characterized by a high P_{CO_2} will develop. If the rate of CO_2 excretion exceeds production, respiratory alkalosis develops. By the equation,

$$\text{alveolar ventilation} \sim CO_2 \text{ elimination} \div P_{CO_2}$$

the inverse relationship of alveolar ventilation to P_{CO_2} is obvious. At steady state, CO_2 production by tissues must equal CO_2 elimination by the lungs for a constant P_{CO_2} to be maintained. The changes in P_{CO_2} are almost always caused by changes in alveolar ventilation rather than production of CO_2. Thus, respiratory acidosis is nearly always a consequence of decreased pulmonary ventilation because of lung or central nervous system (CNS) disease and not a consequence of increased production of CO_2. Similarly, respiratory alkalosis develops because of hyperventilation rather than decreased CO_2 production. In either case, when the elimination rate of CO_2 (alveolar ventilation × P_{CO_2}) again equals CO_2 production, a new steady state will prevail, with no net retention or loss of carbonic acid.

Bicarbonate and the Kidney in Acid-Base Balance

The first role of the kidney in acid-base balance is to reabsorb all filtered HCO_3^- (Fig. 120-1). At a normal glomerular filtration rate (i.e., ~180 L/day in an adult) and serum HCO_3^- concentration of 25 mEq/L, about 4500 mEq of HCO_3^- is filtered in 1 day. Loss of even a small fraction of that amount would result in metabolic acidosis if not replaced by intake.

The Proximal Tubule

About 80 to 90% of HCO_3^- reabsorption is accomplished in the proximal tubule by a proton secretory process. The brush border membranes facing the lumen of the proximal tubule cell contain transporters known as Na/H exchangers (NHE3 is the abundant isoform). Through the normal function of basolateral membrane Na^+,K^+-adenosine triphosphatase (ATPase), cell Na^+ is kept at low concentration so that filtered Na^+ in the lumen will be favored to enter the cell in exchange for H^+ secreted into the lumen. This H^+ rapidly combines with filtered HCO_3^- to form H_2CO_3, which then dehydrates in the lumen to form CO_2 and H_2O. This last process is greatly facilitated by luminal carbonic anhydrase (CA_{IV}). The CO_2 diffuses into the proximal cell, where it reforms HCO_3^-, a reaction catalyzed by intracellular carbonic anhydrase (CA_{II}). The HCO_3^- is then transported back to the blood by a sodium bicarbonate cotransporter (NBC), which couples 1Na and $3HCO_3^-$, thereby completing net Na^+ and HCO_3^- reabsorption. The entire process requires a mitochondrial source of adenosine triphosphate (ATP) for the Na/K pump, intact NHE3 and NBC, and two isoforms of carbonic anhydrase. Additionally, there must be favorable ion gradients for luminal Na^+ entry, H^+ secretion, and basolateral HCO_3^- transport. A disturbance in any of these factors may disrupt proximal HCO_3^- reabsorption enough to cause loss of HCO_3^- in urine. Another 10 to 15% of HCO_3^- is reabsorbed in the thick ascending limb of Henle through a similar mechanism so that only small amounts of the filtered HCO_3^- are normally delivered to more distal nephron segments.

The Cortical Collecting Duct

The cortical connecting tubule and collecting duct reabsorb less than 10% of the filtered HCO_3^-. In principal cells, Na^+ is reabsorbed from lumen to cell by the epithelial Na^+ channel (ENaC), driven by the inwardly directed Na^+ gradient and favorable electrical potential. With the reabsorption of Na^+, the lumen becomes electronegative, thus favoring the secretion of both K^+, through K^+ channels, and H^+, through vacuolar H^+-ATPases on the luminal

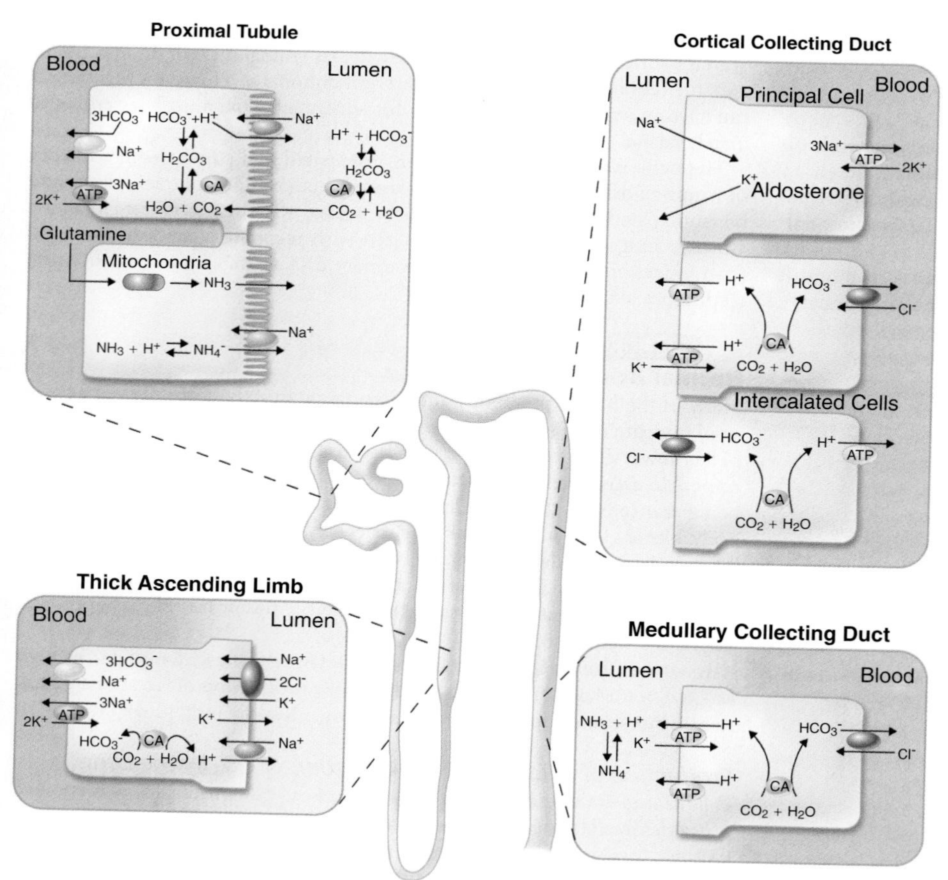

FIGURE 120-1. **Renal acidification mechanisms.** ATP = adenosine triphosphate; CA = carbonic anhydrase.

surface of neighboring α-intercalated cells, which are acid-secreting cells. The secreted H^+ will combine with the remaining HCO_3^- in the lumen to generate CO_2, with subsequent reabsorptive diffusion of CO_2, re-formation of cellular HCO_3^- with the help of cellular carbonic anhydrase (CA_{II}), and then exchange of HCO_3^- from cell to blood for entry of Cl^- through Cl/HCO_3 exchangers. It is at this distal site that tubular fluid pH starts to fall to levels below pH 6.0.

Some collecting duct cells have reverse polarity and secrete HCO_3^- into the lumen in exchange for Cl^- entry into the cell. In these cells, the H^+-ATPase faces the blood side of the cell (β-intercalated cells). An elevated extracellular HCO_3^- concentration, as seen with an alkaline-ash diet or alkalosis, will increase HCO_3^- secretion by these cells.

The Medullary Collecting Duct

The medullary collecting duct continues to secrete protons into the luminal fluid, where the pH reaches its lowest values of close to 5.0. The mechanism is based on continued function of H^+-ATPases with an additional role of an ATP-dependent K/H exchanger, a member of the family of K^+, H^+-ATPases found in the stomach and colon.

Once the filtered HCO_3^- is fully reabsorbed, the kidney is still required to eliminate an additional net amount of acid equivalent to that produced in metabolism. Most of this net acid excretion is in the form of ammonium (NH_4^+), which is derived from the renal synthesis of ammonia from glutamine in the proximal tubule and the titration of filtered phosphate to acid phosphate (titratable acidity).

$$NH_3 + H^+ \rightarrow NH_4^+ \text{ pK 9.1, and}$$

$$HPO_4^{2-} + H^+ \rightarrow H_2PO_4^- \text{ pK 6.8}$$

Urinary Buffers

As the collecting duct cells continue to secrete H^+ into urine with a diminishing luminal HCO_3^- concentration and decreasing pH, H^+ is captured by the urinary buffers. The resulting alkalinization of the cells after H^+ leaves results in the formation of HCO_3^- ready for transport into blood. This process generates "new" HCO_3^- that is not a result of the reabsorption of filtered HCO_3^-. The amount of new HCO_3^- matches the amount of net acid eliminated and is also equal to each of the following: the amount of acid produced, the amount of body buffer consumed by that acid, and the amount of fixed acid anions, such as sulfate, phosphate, and Cl^-, that accompanied the H^+. The result is maintenance of normal acid-base equilibrium.

The ability of the kidney to lower urinary pH to values as low as 5.0 enables the buffers to capture a proton. Net acid excretion in urine is accomplished not simply by a decrease in urine pH but mostly by titration of these important urinary buffers. For example, a typical daily urine volume of 1 liter at pH 5.0 contains only 10^{-5} molar hydrogen ion, or 0.01 mmol, a trivial amount compared with the amount of produced acid (~1 mmol/kg/day). In chronic kidney disease, it is the failure to produce enough ammonium that leads to a poorly buffered, though acid, urine and an inability to excrete enough net acid to stay in normal balance.

Regulation of Urinary Acid Secretion

Renal mechanisms of urinary acidification are adaptable. Transport processes such as H^+-ATPases, Na/H exchange, and Cl/HCO_3 exchange can increase or decrease their capacity to handle acid-base equivalents, depending on the challenge presented. Renal ammoniagenic mechanisms are also critically regulated to serve the acid-base needs of the individual. Metabolic acidosis and respiratory acidosis increase the capacity to reabsorb HCO_3^-, including increased expression of the transporters involved in acidifying the urine. At the same time, increased glutamine uptake into proximal cells and ammonia production enables increased acid excretion and the generation of new HCO_3^- in the distal nephron. Metabolic alkalosis and respiratory alkalosis have the opposite effects.

Carbonic anhydrase is important in acid-secreting epithelia as well as in other cells, such as red blood cells, in which rapid interconversion of large quantities of CO_2 to HCO_3^- is required. In the proximal tubule, carbonic anhydrase exists not only within cells but also on the luminal brush border membrane, where it accelerates the dehydration of carbonic acid to CO_2, thereby allowing the large amount of HCO_3^- reabsorption in that segment. The distal nephron, which has a smaller requirement for bicarbonate reabsorption, lacks luminal carbonic anhydrase. However, intracellular carbonic anhydrase is present in all cells that transport CO_2 and HCO_3^-.

In acid-secreting cells, bicarbonate exits back to blood across the basolateral membrane as protons exit across the apical membrane. These processes are reversed in bicarbonate-secreting cells. In addition, the mechanisms of proton secretion and bicarbonate reabsorption may vary in different cell types.

Ammoniagenesis, which is a key element in urinary acid excretion, provides the major acceptor for protons. Ammonia is produced predominantly in the proximal tubule cell by mitochondrial glutaminase enzymes. Production is increased by increasing the metabolic acid load in the body, respiratory acidosis, and hypokalemia. NH_4^+ can preserve potassium in the hypokalemic state by serving as a counter-ion for anion excretion. Similarly, in response to metabolic acidosis, the kidney would ideally excrete chloride with ammonium and preserve Na^+ and K^+.

Ammonia can be secreted by nonionic diffusion into the proximal fluid, where it will pick up a proton and form ammonium (NH_4^+), or it could form ammonium within the proximal tubule cell and be secreted by Na/NH_4 exchange, a mode of operation of the Na/H exchanger. Ammonium may be reabsorbed by the thick ascending limb of Henle on the Na/K/2Cl transporter, where it can substitute for K^+. By countercurrent multiplication, NH_4^+ concentrates in the medullary interstitial fluid rather than remaining in the ascending limb fluid as it reaches the highly perfused renal cortex, where it could otherwise dissipate into renal venous blood. The countercurrent mechanism also allows for ammonia to diffuse into the lumen of the medullary collecting duct, where it will be trapped as ammonium in the acid tubular fluid. Collecting duct cells also secrete NH_3 by way of glycoproteins that are in the family of the Rh factor, red blood cell ammonia transporters.

Regulation is accomplished at a number of levels. Hormones such as angiotensin II and catecholamines stimulate Na^+ reabsorption in the proximal tubule by increasing Na/H exchange. Aldosterone increases H^+-ATPase in the distal collecting duct cell and stimulates Na^+ reabsorption, thereby increasing proton secretion. Low extracellular fluid volume increases proximal HCO_3^- reabsorption, as does hypokalemia and high P_{CO_2}. Hyperkalemia (Chapter 119) may limit urinary acidification by several mechanisms, including decreased ammonia synthesis, decreased NH_3 entering the countercurrent multiplier in the loop of Henle, and decreased H^+ secretion by ATPases in the collecting duct as the need to secrete K^+ predominates.

CLINICAL MANIFESTATIONS AND DIAGNOSIS

An acid-base disturbance never should be considered an isolated problem but always should alert the clinician to the possible presence of an important underlying condition. Anion gap acidoses usually represent important underlying metabolic conditions, ranging from sepsis (Chapter 108) to uremia (Chapter 132) to diabetic ketoacidosis (Chapter 236) to serious poisonings (Chapter 110). Specific renal abnormalities as well as diarrhea (Chapter 142) can cause hyperchloremic acidosis (Table 120-1). Metabolic alkaloses are commonly caused by renal abnormalities or the loss of acid from the stomach owing to vomiting or nasogastric suction (Table 120-2). Respiratory acidosis and alkalosis are related to ventilation, which is increased by conditions such as sepsis (Chapter 108) and anxiety and decreased in many pulmonary conditions (Chapter 86).

Assessment of clinical acid-base disturbances usually begins with measurement of arterial blood gases (Fig. 120-2 and Table 120-3). In some situations, venous blood can be used as an alternative, accounting for the fact that the normal venous pH is approximately 0.05 pH units more acid than arterial pH, and P_{CO_2} is 5 to 6 mm Hg higher than that of arterial blood. Venous bicarbonate concentrations are normally greater than arterial concentrations.

If arterial pH is below 7.35, acidemia is said to exist. If pH is greater than 7.45, alkalemia exists. However, several processes may simultaneously drive the pH upward or downward; these individual processes are known as *acidoses* or *alkaloses*. Because multiple processes may coexist, an abnormal pH is not always noted in acid-base disturbances. Because pH is related to the ratio of HCO_3^- to P_{CO_2}, the finding of an abnormal bicarbonate level alone also cannot define acidemia or alkalemia.

It is customary to define acid-base balance in terms of the hydrogen ion concentration, bicarbonate, and P_{CO_2}, where

$$CO_2 + H_2O \longleftrightarrow H_2CO_3 \longleftrightarrow H^+ + HCO_3^-$$

The addition of CO_2, as in respiratory acidosis, will increase the hydrogen and bicarbonate concentrations. Removal of CO_2, as in respiratory alkalosis, will decrease CO_2, protons, and bicarbonate. The addition of protons with an anion other than HCO_3^-, as in metabolic acidosis, will lead to increased

TABLE 120-1 CAUSES OF HYPERCHLOREMIC ACIDOSIS

TYPE	CAUSE
Renal with hypokalemia	Proximal RTA, type 2 Distal RTA, type 1 Some anion gap acidoses with high anion clearance
Renal with hyperkalemia	Type 4 RTA; hyporenin-hypoaldosteronism
Nonrenal with hypokalemia	Diarrhea Urinary diversions: ureteroileostomy, ureterosigmoidostomy
Nonrenal with hyperkalemia	NaCl, KCl, NH_4Cl, $CaCl_2$, Arg-HCl, Lys-HCl

RTA = renal tubular acidosis.

TABLE 120-2 CAUSES OF METABOLIC ALKALOSIS

TYPE	CAUSES
Renal, hypochloremic alkalosis: Cl responsive with urine Cl > 20	Loop and distal tubule diuretics Bartter's syndrome Gitelman's syndrome Posthypercapnic status
Nonrenal, hypochloremic alkalosis: Cl responsive with urine Cl < 20	Vomiting, nasogastric suction Chloridorrhea Villous adenoma
Renal, alkalosis with extracellular expansion: Cl unresponsive with urine Cl > 20	Hyperaldosteronism, primary and secondary Liddle's syndrome
Nonrenal alkalosis, Cl unresponsive	$NaHCO_3$, acetate, citrate, lactate
Other causes of metabolic alkalosis	Excessive non-reabsorbable anion excretion Hypoproteinemia

TABLE 120-3 LABORATORY STEPS IN IDENTIFYING ACID-BASE DISORDERS

EVALUATE pH	ACIDEMIC	ALKALEMIC
Elevated P_{CO_2}	Respiratory acidosis	Metabolic alkalosis
Elevated HCO_3	Respiratory acidosis	Metabolic alkalosis
Decreased P_{CO_2}	Metabolic acidosis	Respiratory alkalosis
Decreased HCO_3	Metabolic acidosis	Respiratory alkalosis
EVALUATE FOR EXPECTED COMPENSATION		
Meets expectation: simple disorder with compensation or could be offsetting metabolic alkalosis and acidosis *Does not meet expectation:* complex disorder, but pH indicates whether acidosis or alkalosis is dominant *If a metabolic disorder is dominant,* a P_{CO_2} greater than predicted indicates an additional respiratory acidosis. A P_{CO_2} less than predicted indicates an additional respiratory alkalosis. *If a respiratory disorder is dominant,* an HCO_3 concentration greater than predicted indicates additional metabolic alkalosis. An HCO_3 concentration less than predicted indicates an additional metabolic acidosis.		
ASSESS ANION GAP		
Elevated: metabolic acidosis is present whether acidemic or alkalemic. If alkalemic, an additional metabolic or respiratory alkalosis is present. *If the gap is greater than the fall in HCO_3,* consider an additional metabolic alkalosis or respiratory acidosis. *If the gap is less than the fall in HCO_3,* consider an additional nongap acidosis or respiratory alkalosis.		

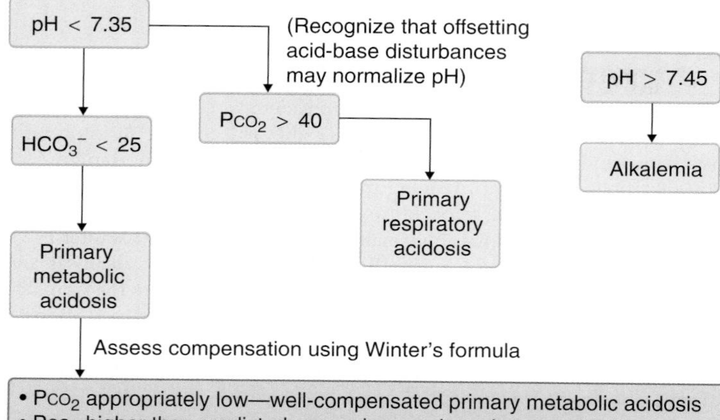

FIGURE 120-2. Evaluation of acidemia.

concentrations of protons and a decreased bicarbonate concentration. This increase in CO_2 can be rapidly removed by the lungs because it constitutes a small additional amount of CO_2 over the usually produced quantities. Removal of HCO_3^- with a cation such as Na^+, also a cause of metabolic acidosis, will increase the proton concentration and lower the HCO_3^- concentration. Metabolic alkalosis might be caused by the addition of $NaHCO_3$ with a resulting decrease in the proton concentration or by removal of H^+ with chloride, thereby leading to a decreased proton concentration and increased HCO_3^-.

Compensatory Changes

Few patients have an isolated acid-base disturbance. In nearly all cases, a respiratory or renal compensation (or both) occurs in response to counteract a primary acid-base disturbance.

With normal organ function, the lungs may maintain a normal pH and P_{CO_2} during changes in volatile acid production. The kidneys will also help maintain normal acid-base balance during changes in fixed acid production. Only excesses beyond the capacity to eliminate an acid or alkali load will lead to clinical disturbances. It follows that patients with renal or lung disease may do less well in response to metabolic and respiratory disorders.

When an acid-base disturbance develops, the initial response to modulate its severity depends on the titration of various body buffer pairs. For example, phosphate, hemoglobin, and albumin change their protonated and unprotonated concentrations. The body will then further attempt to correct the extracellular pH toward normal but usually not to normal. For metabolic disturbances caused by increased or decreased nonvolatile acid, the response is respiratory; for primary respiratory acidosis and alkalosis, the compensation is renal (Table 120-4). The direction of change in HCO_3^- and P_{CO_2} is the same when the primary disturbance is compensated; the ratio of HCO_3^- to P_{CO_2} and thus pH becomes more normal. These compensations tend to take time, so acid-base disturbances, particularly the respiratory conditions, are classified as acute (lasting less than 24 to 48 hours) or chronic.

Peripheral blood does not demonstrate complete compensation for most acid-base disturbances, with the occasional exception of chronic respiratory alkalosis. Yet the CNS closely regulates its pH, with nearly full correction within 1 to 2 days. Before this compensation occurs, acute alkalemia may be associated with cerebral vasoconstriction and ischemia, whereas acidemia may result in vasodilation and cerebral edema. Rapid changes in P_{CO_2} affect the CNS chemosensors more quickly than do changes in HCO_3^- because of the more rapid movement of nonionic CO_2 across the blood-brain barrier. Increases in CNS CO_2 lead to acidification of the medullary center interstitial fluid and an increased ventilatory drive. Decreases in CNS CO_2 lead to hypoventilation.

In metabolic acidosis, peripheral chemosensors in the carotid body stimulate the CNS to increase ventilation to reduce P_{CO_2}. The fall in peripheral P_{CO_2} will lead to dissolved CO_2 leaving the CNS ahead of HCO_3^-; the alkalinization of the medullary center interstitial fluid will then slow the hyperventilatory response until a new steady state of hypocapnia is achieved.

TABLE 120-4 EXPECTED DEGREES OF COMPENSATION IN ACID-BASE DISORDERS

DISORDER	EXPECTED COMPENSATION
Metabolic acidosis	Steady state in 12-36 hr Expected Pco_2 = 1.5 (measured HCO_3) + 8 ± 2
Metabolic alkalosis	Less predictable Expected Pco_2 increases 0.5 mm Hg per 1-mEq/L increase in HCO_3
Respiratory acidosis	
Acute	Expected 1-mEq/L increase in HCO_3 per 10-mm Hg rise in Pco_2
Chronic, 24-36 hr	Expected 3- to 5-mEq/L increase in HCO_3 per 10-mm Hg rise in Pco_2
Respiratory alkalosis	
Acute	Expected 1- to 2-mEq/L fall in HCO_3 per 10-mm Hg fall in Pco_2
Chronic, after 24-36 hr	Expected 5-mEq/L fall in HCO_3 per 10-mm Hg fall in Pco_2

Patients may sense dyspnea or air hunger acutely with rapid and shallow respirations. In severe cases of metabolic acidemia, the respirations are deep and gasping, typical of Kussmaul breathing.

When the bicarbonate concentration increases as a result of metabolic alkalosis, a hypoventilatory response, signaled from the peripheral chemosensors, raises Pco_2. As Pco_2 rises, the dissolved CO_2 will enter the cerebrospinal fluid (CSF) and will acidify the medullary respiratory center. The stimulus to breathe will, in part, antagonize the peripheral signal until a steady state of hypoventilation is reached.

The acute stimulus of hypercapnia to increase net renal acid excretion disappears in chronic respiratory acidosis when, at the elevated Pco_2, carbonic acid production and elimination are again equal. However, the hypochloremia, brought about by the compensatory early excretion of NH_4Cl, and elevated serum HCO_3^-, maintained by the high Pco_2, persist.

In respiratory alkalosis, the primary event is a fall in Pco_2 because of increased alveolar ventilation. Upon transition from acute to chronic respiratory alkalosis, the compensatory mechanisms that initially helped maintain a more normal systemic pH are no longer required as CO_2 production and elimination become equal. Thus, the initial compensatory decrease in renal acid excretion brought about by increased loss of filtered $NaHCO_3$ ceases, but low serum HCO_3^- and high serum Cl^- concentrations are still maintained.

In identifying whether an acid-base disturbance is simple (a single disturbance with its compensation) or complex (multiple processes simultaneously present), it is useful to compare the expected compensation with the observed parameters of the blood gases (see Table 120-3). For example, if Pco_2 is lower than would be predicted in a patient with a simple, compensated metabolic acidosis, an additional respiratory alkalosis must be driving the Pco_2 down. If Pco_2 is higher than what would be predicted for a low bicarbonate level in a patient with metabolic acidosis, a coexistent respiratory acidosis is present.

METABOLIC ACIDOSIS

EPIDEMIOLOGY AND PATHOBIOLOGY

In metabolic acidosis, the primary change is a fall in serum bicarbonate. The compensatory response is to increase ventilation to reduce Pco_2. Worsening acidosis elicits increasing alveolar ventilation.

Primary metabolic acidosis results from an imbalance between net acid production and net acid excretion (NAE) in the form of urinary ammonium and acid phosphate. Consider the following relationship, where U_x represents the urinary concentration and $\dot{V}$ the urinary flow rate:

$$NAE = (U_{NH_4^+}\,\dot{V}) + (U_{phos}\,\dot{V}) - (U_{bicarb}\,\dot{V})$$

In a normal steady-state condition, the rate of excretion of net acid must be equal to the rate of production. The normal production rate depends on diet. If net acid production is normal, metabolic acidosis could occur because of a failure to reabsorb bicarbonate or a failure to elaborate enough urinary buffers, as is the case in renal failure and renal tubular acidosis. An inequality also could develop if net acid production were excessive or if large extrarenal bicarbonate losses were unable to be matched by maximal adaptive increases in net acid excretion. Endogenous sources of acid include ketoacidosis and lactic acidosis, whereas exogenous sources are metabolic products of ingested ethylene glycol or methanol. On occasion, strong inorganic acids may be ingested. When net acid is retained in body fluids, the serum bicarbonate concentration falls. However, maintenance of a constant serum HCO_3^- concentration does not guarantee that there is a new steady state in which net acid production is equal to net acid excretion because body buffers such as carbonate salts of bone may become depleted by relentless acid retention, as in renal failure and distal renal tubular acidosis.

The causes of metabolic acidosis are usually categorized according to the presence of either a normal or an elevated serum anion gap. The serum anion gap is the net charge difference when the sum of chloride and bicarbonate is subtracted from the serum sodium concentration.

$$\text{Anion gap} = Na^+ - (Cl^- + HCO_3^-)$$

The normal anion gap is due to the unmeasured anionic charge associated predominantly with albumin. When acidemia is present, albumin is in a more protonated form, which lowers the normal gap. In alkalemia, the effect of pH is to increase the gap attributed to albumin. Each 1 g/dL of albumin contributes approximately 2.8 mEq/L to the normal anion gap. The anion gap may be low with hypoalbuminemia or with an increase in unmeasured cations, such as immunoglobulin G myeloma paraproteins, calcium, lithium, or magnesium. When the anion gap is increased above the normal value of approximately 10 to 12 mEq/L by a nonchloride acid anion, an anion gap metabolic acidosis exists. The accompanying proton is responsible for lowering the serum bicarbonate concentration. The degree of increase in the anion gap, sometimes referred to as the *gap delta*, may be estimated by the difference between the observed anion gap and a normal value of 10 to 12 mEq/L. A similar calculation for a change in serum HCO_3^- can be made by subtracting the observed HCO_3^- from the normal value of about 25 mEq/L. Comparison of the two values (the *delta-delta*) may help identify more complicated acid-base disorders. If the increase in the anion gap is larger than the decrease in serum HCO_3^-, a process is raising the HCO_3^- level. The patient may have a coexisting metabolic alkalosis or be compensating for chronic respiratory acidosis. If the decreases in serum HCO_3^- are larger than the increases in the anion gap, a sign that another process is lowering the HCO_3^- level, the patient may have an additional hyperchloremic acidosis or respiratory alkalosis.

CLINICAL MANIFESTATIONS

The effects of metabolic acidosis depend on its rapidity of onset and severity. Patients often complain of fatigue and dyspnea, particularly on exertion. Nausea and vomiting are common. On examination, deep respirations, often labored with the use of accessory muscles, may be detected acutely, but hyperventilation may be less notable with long-standing metabolic acidemia. Metabolic acidemia also may be associated with vasodilation, tachycardia, and hypotension (Chapter 106). The negative inotropic effect of acidemia on the heart can exacerbate septic shock (Chapter 108). The stress of either an underlying illness or an increase in adrenergic and corticosteroid activity associated with acidemia may elevate the peripheral white blood cell count and cause hyperglycemia. Other laboratory findings include variable degrees of hyperkalemia, hyperphosphatemia, and hyperuricemia, as well as hypocalcemia as a result of decreased renal synthesis of 1,25-dihydroxyvitamin D.

Anion Gap Metabolic Acidoses

A variety of abnormalities can cause anion gap acidosis (Table 120-5). Other organic anions that may be detectable by special screening include hereditary disorders of methylmalonic aciduria or 5-oxoprolinuria. In patients who ingest acetaminophen and deplete intracellular glutathione, acquired 5-oxoprolinuria anion gap acidosis may occur.

UREMIC ACIDOSIS

The metabolic acidosis of advanced chronic kidney disease (Chapter 132) may be due to tubular leakage of HCO_3^-, but it is often present when inadequate ammonia production is unable to facilitate excretion of the normal metabolic acid load. Many patients with renal failure can acidify their urine, but the lack of buffering capacity diminishes net acid excretion. Many organic and inorganic anions, such as phosphate and sulfates, are retained at glomerular filtration rates of less than 25 mL/minute and constitute an increased anion gap in association with the metabolic acidosis. The magnitude of the gap is usually less than 20 mEq/L.

The systemic acid-base disturbance in renal diseases that particularly target the renal tubules is attributable to the kidney's inability to secrete hydrogen

TABLE 120-5 CAUSES OF INCREASED ANION AND OSMOLAL GAPS

ANION GAP METABOLIC ACIDOSIS	OSMOLAL GAP
Uremia	No
Lactic acidosis	Variable/no
D-Lactic acidosis	No
Diabetic ketoacidosis	No
Starvation ketoacidosis	No
Alcoholic ketoacidosis	If ethanol is present
Ethylene glycol	Yes
Methanol	Yes
Salicylates	No
5-Oxoprolinuria (acetaminophen)	No

and to reabsorb and generate HCO_3^-. It is particularly pronounced in oliguric acute renal failure and is exacerbated by hypercatabolic states such as infection. A significant metabolic acidosis in a patient with chronic kidney disease of unknown cause should raise the possibility of urinary tract obstruction (Chapter 125) or chronic tubulointerstitial diseases (Chapter 124), including amyloidosis (Chapter 194), myeloma (Chapter 193), autoimmune disorders and analgesic nephropathy (Chapter 124).

The presentation and approach to uremia are discussed in Chapters 132 and 133. It is important to treat the metabolic acidosis of chronic kidney disease. Maintaining the serum HCO_3^- concentration above 20 to 22 mEq/L, by administering $NaHCO_3$ at a rate of 1 mEq HCO_3^-/kg/day, will slow the progression of chronic kidney disease, delay end-stage renal failure, and improve nutritional state.[1]

OVERPRODUCTION OF ENDOGENOUS ACIDS

Lactic Acidosis

EPIDEMIOLOGY AND PATHOBIOLOGY

Lactic acidosis is caused by an imbalance in the rates of lactate production and its clearance, primarily in the liver. Lactic acidosis, which increases the anion gap, is most often due to impaired lactate clearance owing to circulatory failure, hypoxia, and mitochondrial dysfunction that increase anaerobic glycolysis and the rate of conversion of pyruvate to lactate. Other causes are thiamine deficiency (Chapter 221), hypophosphatemia (Chapter 121), isoniazid toxicity (Chapter 110), and hypoglycemic states (Chapter 238). Metformin may cause lactic acidosis, particularly in elderly patients with cardiac, hepatic, or renal dysfunction. Nucleoside antivirals (Chapter 396), including zidovudine, may cause lactic acidosis and abnormal liver function as a result of toxic mitochondrial effects. Abnormal mitochondrial function is also a feature of aspirin overdose (Chapter 36) or toxicity with hypoglycin from ingestion of the unripe akee fruit (Jamaican vomiting sickness).

Lactic acidosis can also be caused by the overproduction of lactate, which may occur with severe exertion and malignancies, particularly with a large tumor burden from lymphoma or widely metastatic cancer. Malignant cells can upregulate glycolytic activity, which may increase their uptake of glucose and decrease their dependence on mitochondrion-derived energy.

Lactate, the final product in the anaerobic pathway of glucose metabolism, is produced from pyruvate by the following reaction catalyzed by lactate dehydrogenase:

$$\text{NADH} + \text{pyruvate} + \text{H}^+ \rightarrow \text{lactate} + \text{NAD}$$

CLINICAL MANIFESTATIONS

Symptoms and signs are related to the underlying cause as well as to the metabolic acidosis itself (see earlier). Sepsis (Chapter 108) is associated with an elevated lactate level because of poor clearance and impaired gluconeogenesis. Lactic acidosis can also result from seizure activity (Chapter 410) when lactate is released from muscle cells that have sustained a period of anaerobic metabolism.

A high reduced nicotinamide adenine dinucleotide (NADH)/NAD ratio will favor lactate formation. Conversion of ethanol to acetaldehyde and conversion of β-hydroxybutyrate to acetoacetate uses NAD and produces NADH. Alcohol metabolism may be associated with excessive β-hydroxybutyrate and lactic acidosis.

DIAGNOSIS

In any patient with an anion gap acidosis, the serum lactate level should be directly measured. Glucose, creatinine, and blood urea nitrogen levels also should be obtained. In cases in which a toxic ingestion is suspected (see Table 120-5), a screen for such toxins in the serum should be performed.

TREATMENT Rx

Treatment of lactic acidosis is aimed at correcting the underlying cause. Tissue perfusion and ventilation should be restored if possible. Sodium bicarbonate therapy should be considered when the arterial pH is below 7.0 or when acidemia has resulted in decreased cardiac inotropy or systemic vasodilation and shock. It is preferable to give $NaHCO_3$ as an isotonic mixture in 5% dextrose and water, rather than as a hypertonic bolus, because the latter carries the risk of pulmonary edema and hypernatremia. The quantity of administered sodium bicarbonate to raise arterial pH to 7.2 should be estimated by multiplying the desired minus observed bicarbonate concentration by the estimated total body water. Full correction should be avoided. Bicarbonate treatment of less severe lactic acidosis is controversial. In a randomized trial of patients with lactic acidosis (pH 6.9 to 7.2 and an average 7.8-mM lactate level) in an intensive care unit, sodium bicarbonate infused at a rate of 2 mEq/kg per 15 minutes did not improve hemodynamics, despite improvement in pH, but adversely lowered ionized serum calcium compared with saline.[2]

In patients with a metabolic acidosis after seizures (Chapter 410), the lactate is quickly metabolized to HCO_3^- by the liver and kidneys, and the acidosis often resolves within 60 minutes. The administration of HCO_3^- is usually unnecessary and may precipitate an overshoot metabolic alkalosis as the lactate is metabolized, which lowers the seizure threshold.

In patients with intestinal bacterial overgrowth (Chapter 142), a syndrome of disorientation, ataxia, and anion gap metabolic acidosis may develop after a carbohydrate meal because of bacterial production of D-lactate. This isomer of the mammalian L-lactate can be measured only by a specific D-lactate assay. The condition is treated with oral antibiotics and appropriate diet.

PROGNOSIS

Lactic acidosis when severe is associated with a high early mortality. When the pH is less than 7.2, only 17% of patients who are admitted to an intensive care unit are ultimately discharged from the hospital.

Diabetic Ketoacidosis

EPIDEMIOLOGY AND PATHOBIOLOGY

Diabetic ketoacidosis is defined as hyperglycemia with metabolic acidosis resulting from generation of the acid anions β-hydroxybutyrate and acetoacetate in response to insulin deficiency and elevated counter-regulatory hormones such as glucagon. It is most commonly seen in cases of type 1 diabetes mellitus (Chapter 236) but can occasionally be seen in type 2 diabetes mellitus (Chapter 237).

The lack of insulin increases lipolysis in adipose tissue; free fatty acids are transported to the liver, where hepatic mitochondria produce ketone bodies, including acetoacetate, from acetyl coenzyme A. In the presence of high NADH/NAD ratio, the more reduced form of β-hydroxybutyrate is produced.

CLINICAL MANIFESTATIONS

Symptoms include nausea, vomiting, anorexia, polydipsia, and polyuria. Patients often exhibit Kussmaul respirations and volume depletion. Neurologic symptoms include fatigue and lethargy with depression of the sensorium. CSF exhibits a change in acid-base status with treatment of diabetic ketoacidosis. Even without bicarbonate administration, CSF pH falls as a result of the ventilatory response to the correction of acidosis and the sudden rise in P_{CO_2}. However, no correlation between decreased CSF pH and depression of sensorium has been established. Ketoacidosis is also seen in cases of starvation, in which it is generally mild and not associated with hyperglycemia.

Ketoacids in the urine may be accompanied by cations, including sodium and potassium, thereby contributing to volume depletion, potassium depletion, relative chloride retention, and a mixed anion gap and hyperchloremic acidosis. The "delta HCO_3^-" will exceed the "delta anion gap," especially if the glomerular filtration rate and the filtered load of ketoacids are high. The serum anion gap in general will be greatest when renal failure is present because the additional anions cannot be cleared from extracellular fluid.

DIAGNOSIS

The urinary dipstick nitroprusside test for ketones may underestimate the degree of ketosis because it does not detect β-hydroxybutyrate; in fact, the ketone test may become more positive as treatment helps metabolize β-hydroxybutyrate to acetoacetate. This problem should be addressed by direct measurement of serum β-hydroxybutyrate. Diabetic patients also are more prone to lactic acidosis because an increase in NADH favors the formation of lactate from pyruvate, and pyruvate dehydrogenase is inhibited in the absence of insulin.

TREATMENT

Rx

Treatment of diabetic ketoacidosis (Chapter 236) consists of volume repletion, insulin administration with dextrose if necessary to avoid hypoglycemia, and potassium replacement (Chapter 119). Bicarbonate administration should be considered only if ketoacidosis is accompanied by shock or if arterial pH is less than 7.0 or 7.1, and bolus infusion should be avoided. The administration of bicarbonate occasionally results in cerebral edema significant enough to lead to loss of consciousness and even death.

PROGNOSIS

Most patients with diabetic ketoacidosis recover. In the less than 0.5% of patients who present with coma from cerebral edema, the mortality rate ranges from 20% to as high as 90%. The cerebral edema may be exacerbated by bicarbonate administration, which is discouraged in this situation.

Salicylate Intoxication

EPIDEMIOLOGY AND PATHOBIOLOGY

Salicylate intoxication can be caused by accidental overdose, therapeutic overdose, or a suicide attempt (Chapters 36 and 110). Salicylate functions as an uncoupler of oxidative phosphorylation and consequently results in increased oxygen consumption and CO_2 production. However, the increase in alveolar ventilation resulting from stimulation of central chemoreceptors overcomes this increase in CO_2.

CLINICAL MANIFESTATIONS AND DIAGNOSIS

The most common clinical manifestation is a combined anion gap metabolic acidosis and respiratory alkalosis, although the condition also can be manifested as either one or the other only. Children are often seen with metabolic acidosis, whereas adults often have predominant respiratory alkalosis. Hypoglycemia, ketoacidosis, and lactic acidosis may result. Other manifestations of intoxication include hemorrhage, fever, nausea and vomiting, hyperventilation, diaphoresis, tinnitus, and occasionally polyuria followed by oliguria. Severe cases may lead to seizures, respiratory depression, and coma. Noncardiogenic pulmonary edema is sometimes seen in adults.

Respiratory alkalosis is the result of a direct stimulatory effect of salicylate on the medullary respiratory control center. Salicylate intoxication also increases the metabolic rate. Diagnosis is suspected by the clinical presentation and confirmed by the salicylate level (Chapters 36 and 110).

Treatment of salicylate intoxication (Chapter 110) is aimed at correcting the metabolic acidosis and removing salicylate. Bicarbonate as a sodium salt should be administered according to an estimated calculation of the deficit if metabolic acidosis predominates. Salicylates are removed by alkaline diuresis because the less reabsorbable salicylate anion will predominate when the urine pH increases. Urinary alkalinization with acetazolamide is not advised because carbonic anhydrase inhibition may impair CO_2 transport from tissue to blood and potentially worsen acidosis in the respiratory center. In severe intoxication (salicylate concentrations greater than 35 mg/dL) or when renal failure is present, dialysis may be required.

PROGNOSIS

The prognosis of salicylate toxicity is better with early diagnosis and prompt management, in which case most patients do well. Patients who ingest oil of wintergreen (methylsalicylate) may have more severe deterioration because of the highly lipid soluble form of the drug.

Alcoholic Ketoacidosis

EPIDEMIOLOGY AND PATHOBIOLOGY

Alcoholic ketoacidosis occurs in a patient who has been drinking very heavily without eating. The pathophysiology is based on the overproduction of β-hydroxybutyrate and, to a lesser extent, acetoacetate because of an increased production of free fatty acids. Alcohol inhibits the conversion of lactate to glucose in the liver. The oxidation of ethanol increases the ratio of NADH to NAD^+ and favors the production of β-hydroxybutyrate. Damage to mitochondria by alcohol can further elevate the ratio of β-hydroxybutyrate to acetoacetate by preventing reoxidation of NADH to NAD. The oxidative metabolism of ethanol favors the reaction of dehydrogenase enzymes to form β-hydroxybutyrate and lactate (opposing glucose production).

CLINICAL MANIFESTATIONS

Alcoholic ketoacidosis usually follows binge drinking and may be associated with withdrawal symptoms (Chapters 32 and 425) and the associated hyperadrenergic state. Alcoholic ketoacidosis is associated with abdominal pain, vomiting, starvation, and volume depletion. In contrast to diabetic ketoacidosis, coma is rare. Blood glucose levels are generally low or normal, and the insulin level is frequently low, with elevated glucagon and cortisol levels. Some patients have hyperglycemia because of the increased catecholamine response.

DIAGNOSIS

Patients typically have a high osmolal gap initially (defined as the difference between the measured and the calculated serum osmolality).

$$\text{Calculated osmolality} = 2(\text{Na}^+) + (\text{Glucose [mg/dL]} \div 18) + (\text{Blood urea nitrogen [mg/dL]} \div 2.8)$$

Blood alcohol levels may be absent or elevated on initial evaluation. A clue to the diagnosis of toxic alcohol ingestion is the simultaneous presence of an anion gap metabolic acidosis and an osmolal gap. This osmolal gap, if secondary to ethanol, should be equal to the ethanol concentration in milligrams per deciliter divided by 4.6. If this calculation does not yield the expected gap based on the ethanol concentration, ingestion of another alcohol such as methanol, isopropanol, or ethylene glycol should be suspected (see Table 120-2).

The serum osmolality should be measured by a freezing point depression technique and compared with the calculated osmolality. If possible, ethanol, ethylene glycol, propylene glycol, and methanol levels should be measured directly; each is associated with a metabolic acidosis. In contrast, isopropanol metabolizes to acetone and causes ketosis without acidosis.

TREATMENT

Treatment of alcoholic metabolic acidosis consists of volume repletion with normal saline in dextrose; the administration of thiamine (50 to 100 mg intravenously) and enough glucose to treat hypoglycemia; and the correction of any hypophosphatemia (Chapter 121), hypokalemia (Chapter 119), and hypomagnesemia (Chapter 121) that may be present. The acid-base disturbance usually resolves after several hours. Both hypophosphatemia and thiamine deficiency, which may not be apparent until 12 to 24 hours after the initiation of treatment in an undernourished patient, are exacerbated by glucose administration.

PROGNOSIS

The prognosis of alcoholic ketoacidosis is usually favorable. The long-term outlook is more closely tied to other complications of continued alcohol abuse.

Ethylene Glycol

Ethylene glycol (Chapter 110) is commonly found in antifreeze and is used as an industrial solvent. It has a sweet taste, and patients occasionally ingest it as a substitute for ethanol. Although ethylene glycol itself is not particularly damaging, its highly toxic metabolites include glyoxylate, glycolate, oxalic acid, and ketoaldehydes. Glycolic acid appears to be primarily responsible for the metabolic acidosis observed in this condition.

Intoxication is characterized by profound CNS symptoms, including seizures and coma, severe metabolic acidosis, and cardiac, pulmonary, and renal failure. Patients are often dehydrated because of osmotic diuresis from the renal excretion of the alcohol.

An increased anion gap is attributable to ethylene glycol metabolites. A high osmolal gap will also be present because of the uncharged alcohol. However, an osmolal gap may not be present if all of the alcohol has been converted to the toxic anionic forms. Calcium oxalate crystals in the urine may cause intratubular obstruction and acute renal failure. Treatment is aimed at rehydration with saline and correction of acidosis with $NaHCO_3$ based on an estimate of the bicarbonate deficit. When an osmolal gap exists, competitive inhibition of alcohol dehydrogenase should be initiated with fomepizole at a loading dose of 15 to 20 mg/kg intravenously in 100 mL normal saline over 30 minutes to 1 hour, followed by a maintenance dose of 10 mg/kg every 12 hours (Chapter 110). If ethanol is used, a solution of 10% ethanol in 5% dextrose can be given as a loading dose of 0.6 g/kg intravenously followed by a maintenance dose of 150 mg/kg per hour in alcoholic patients, or 65 mg/kg per hour in nonalcoholic patients. The ethanol level should be maintained at a 100 to 200 mg/dL. The goal of therapy is early recognition to prevent metabolism of the uncharged glycol to acidic products. Hemodialysis is required in severe cases. If the diagnosis is made promptly and appropriate therapy is instituted, outcomes are favorable. Renal failure may be reversible.

Methanol

Methanol, wood alcohol, is a component of shellac and windshield wiper fluid and is highly toxic to the CNS after metabolism to formaldehyde and formic acid. Optic papillitis may cause blindness. Treatment consists of competitive inhibitors for alcohol dehydrogenase, including ethanol or fomepizole, in similar amounts as for ethylene glycol poisoning, to reduce the formation of acid anions and the anion gap while maintaining a higher level of methanol in the blood (Chapter 110). Hemodialysis may be necessary to increase elimination.

Early diagnosis and treatment are associated with a favorable outcome, but visual loss may be permanent. Late presentation is associated with a poor prognosis, particularly if the amount consumed exceeds 30 mL. As with ethylene glycol, the simultaneous presence of ethanol on presentation may help slow the metabolism of methanol and improve outcome.

Isopropyl Alcohol

Toxic ingestion of isopropyl alcohol, as in rubbing alcohol, does not cause an increased anion gap or ketoacidosis because the metabolite is acetone, but tests for ketones are positive and a high osmolal gap will be present.

Propylene Glycol

Occasionally, patients in the intensive care unit setting are given high doses of intravenous benzodiazepines, such as lorazepam or diazepam, that contain propylene glycol as a diluents. Other intravenous medications that also contain this diluent include phenobarbital, phenytoin, nitroglycerine, and esmolol. Propylene glycol has also been used as a less toxic substitute for methanol in windshield wiper fluid. A high osmolal gap may develop because of the propylene glycol and lead to a clinical picture of sedation, failure to wean from the respirator, and an increased lactate level. Propylene glycol metabolites include lactate and pyruvate. Treatment, which consists of early recognition and withdrawal of the offending agent, usually results in a favorable prognosis.

Hyperchloremic (Normal Anion Gap) Acidosis

Hyperchloremic metabolic acidoses (see Table 120-1) can be caused by renal or nonrenal mechanisms and can be associated with an elevated, normal, or low serum potassium level.

Hyperchloremic Metabolic Acidosis of Nonrenal Origin Associated with Normal or Increased Potassium

Hyperchloremic metabolic acidoses with a normal or elevated potassium concentration can develop as a result of the addition of chloride salts such as NaCl, KCl, $CaCl_2$, NH_4Cl, arginine and lysine hydrochlorides, or HCl itself. If the quantity of Cl^- introduced exceeds the ability of the kidney to eliminate Cl^- salts in urine, hyperchloremia will develop. Electroneutrality is maintained by a decrease in the serum HCO_3^- concentration, and a hyperchloremic acidosis ensues. Renal production of NH_3 increases in an attempt to improve HCl excretion. Hyperkalemia can occur because the acidemia favors the exit of K^+ from cells. Hyperkalemia also inhibits K^+ secretion in the renal collecting duct.

Hyperchloremic Metabolic Acidosis of Nonrenal Origin Associated with Hypokalemia

Hypokalemic, hyperchloremic acidosis may result from loss of a body fluid that is low in Cl^- relative to Na^+ and K^+ when compared with the ratio of Cl^- to Na^+ in extracellular fluid. For example, stool losses of Na^+, K^+, and HCO_3^- in small bowel diarrhea or organic acid anions of bacterial origin in colonic diarrhea lead to hyperchloremic acidosis (Chapter 142). Pancreatic secretions (Chapter 201) or heavy losses from ileostomy sites may lead to loss of bicarbonate-containing fluids. Secretagogues such as vasoactive intestinal peptide (VIP), which is associated with neoplasms of the pancreas or sympathetic chain (Chapter 201), cause large losses of HCO_3^- in stool, with a resulting hypokalemic, hyperchloremic metabolic acidosis. Concomitant gastric achlorhydria is part of the syndrome known as *watery diarrhea, hypokalemic, hypochlorhydric acidosis*. Urinary diversions, such as ureterosigmoidostomies and ileal loops, may increase chloride absorption in exchange for bicarbonate in the intestinal segment and lead to hyperchloremic acidosis.

RENAL TUBULAR ACIDOSIS TYPES 1 AND 2

Proximal Renal Tubular Acidosis

Renal tubular acidosis causes the cations Na^+ and K^+ to be lost in the urine with HCO_3^- rather than Cl^-, thereby leading to hyperchloremia. Proximal renal tubular acidosis (type 2) is characterized by a decreased threshold for bicarbonate reabsorption. HCO_3^- wasting and concomitant urinary losses of potassium occur until a lower level of serum bicarbonate reduces the filtered HCO_3^- to a level that the renal tubule can completely reabsorb.

Isolated proximal renal tubular acidosis may result from mutations of specific transporters of the proximal tubule, such as the $NaHCO_3$ cotransporter, or from hereditary deficiency of carbonic anhydrase. More commonly, proximal renal tubular acidosis is associated with generalized proximal tubule dysfunction. Causes (Table 120-6) include genetic diseases such as glucose-6-phosphatase deficiency (Chapter 164), cystinosis (Chapter 130), hereditary fructose intolerance (Chapter 212), and Wilson's disease (Chapter 218). Multiple myeloma (Chapter 193) and Sjögren's syndrome (Chapter 276) should be considered in an adult patient. Primary hyperparathyroidism (Chapter 253) results in proximal renal tubular acidosis and hypophosphatemia secondary to inhibition of Na/H exchange and sodium phosphate cotransport in the proximal tubule. Drug toxicity with aminoglycosides, tenofovir, cisplatin, and ifosfamide may cause proximal tubule dysfunction. The syndrome also may be seen after kidney transplantation (Chapter 133).

Distal Renal Tubular Acidosis

In distal renal tubular acidosis (type 1), failure to produce ammonia leads to an inability to excrete net acid, thereby leading to continuous retention of acid in the body. The degree of acidemia is often severe, with pH reaching values as low as 7.2, whereas urine pH usually exceeds 5.3.

Kindreds have been described in which mutations in genes for the distal vacuolar H^+-ATPase cause an autosomal recessive distal renal tubular acidosis with deafness. Mutations resulting in defective Cl/HCO_3 exchange protein (AE1) have been linked to an autosomal dominant form of distal renal tubular acidosis.

Distal renal tubular acidosis (see Table 120-6) is also associated with autoimmune disorders, including systemic lupus erythematosus (Chapter 274) and Sjögren's syndrome (Chapter 276), and genetic diseases, including sickle cell anemia (Chapter 166), Wilson's disease (Chapter 218), Fabry's disease (Chapter 215), cystic kidney diseases (Chapter 129), and hereditary elliptocytosis (Chapter 164). Hypercalciuria and hyperoxaluria may cause distal renal tubular acidosis; nephrocalcinosis may be present. Amyloidosis (Chapter 194) may be manifested as severe acidemia and other tubular dysfunction, including nephrogenic diabetes insipidus. Tubulointerstitial disease of the kidney (Chapter 124), including reflux nephropathy and urinary obstruction, may result in renal tubular acidosis with hypokalemia or hyperkalemia. Drugs such as amphotericin B can cause hypokalemic distal renal tubular acidosis.

HYPERCHLOREMIC METABOLIC ACIDOSIS OF RENAL ORIGIN ASSOCIATED WITH HYPERKALEMIA

Hyperkalemic, hyperchloremic acidosis (type 4) suggests dysfunction of the cortical collecting duct, where acidification of urine and disorders in potassium secretion may occur. Some patients with high blood potassium and hyperchloremic acidosis can lower urinary pH below 5.3, whereas others appear to have defects in both potassium balance and urinary acidification. Hyperkalemia itself may worsen metabolic acidosis by decreasing NH_3 accumulation by countercurrent multiplication in the medullary interstitium.

TABLE 120-6 CAUSES OF RENAL TUBULAR ACIDOSIS*

HYPOKALEMIC DISTAL (TYPE 1) RTA
Hereditary tubule disorders
Vacuolar H^+/ATPase β-subunit gene mutations
Carbonic anhydrase type II deficiency
Cl/HCO_3 exchanger (AE-1) mutations
Genetic causes
Sickle cell
Fabry's disease
Wilson's disease
Elliptocytosis
Paroxysmal nocturnal hemoglobinuria
Medullary cystic kidneys
Autoimmune disorders
Systemic lupus erythematosus
Sjögren's syndrome
Multiple myeloma and amyloidosis
Drugs: amphotericin, cisplatinum, aminoglycosides
Nephrocalcinosis and hypercalcemic disorders
Tubulointerstitial diseases
Acute tubulointerstitial nephritis
Reflux nephropathy
Analgesic nephropathy
PROXIMAL (TYPE 2) RTA
Hereditary tubule disorders
Na HCO_3 cotransport (NBC) mutations
Carbonic anhydrase deficiency
Generalized proximal tubular dysfunction
Hereditary Fanconi's syndrome
Genetic diseases: cystinosis, glycogen storage disease (glucose-6-phosphatase deficiency), Wilson's disease
Hormonal: hyperparathyroidism, vitamin D deficiency
Multiple myeloma, lysozymuria
Sjögren's syndrome
Renal transplantation
Heavy metals: cobalt, mercury, lead
Drugs: ifosfamide, outdated tetracycline, tenofovir, tacrolimus, aminoglycosides
HYPERKALEMIC (TYPE 4) RTA
Renal diseases-aldosterone resistance
Diabetes mellitus
Amyloidosis
Systemic lupus erythematosus
Urinary tract obstruction
Hyporeninism
Autonomic neuropathy (diabetic)
Sickle cell anemia
Primary hypoaldosteronism
Adrenal insufficiency: Addison's disease,
Tubular mutations: pseudohypoaldosteronism
Drugs: K-sparing diuretics, amiloride, triamterene, spironolactone, nonsteroidal anti-inflammatory drugs, lithium, trimethoprim, cyclosporine, tacrolimus, renin inhibitors, angiotensin-converting enzyme inhibitors, angiotensin II receptor antagonists

*Type 3 renal tubular acidosis (RTA) is not listed separately because it is an overlap of proximal and distal dysfunction.

Causes include hyporenin-hypoaldosteronism, as seen in diabetic renal disease (Chapter 126); other tubulointerstitial diseases (Chapter 124), usually with some renal impairment; sickle cell anemia (Chapter 166); or the use of drugs such as β-blockers and nonsteroidal anti-inflammatory drugs. Low renin and aldosterone levels can also be found in cases of volume expansion with hypertension. Cyclosporine and tacrolimus may lead to decreased electrical driving forces for K^+ and H^+ secretion. Hyperkalemic acidosis with elevated renin and low aldosterone is found in adrenal insufficiency (Chapter 234), isolated hypoaldosteronism (Chapter 234), and the use of angiotensin-converting enzyme inhibitors, renin inhibitors, and angiotensin II receptor blockers. High renin and aldosterone levels are anticipated when the renal collecting duct cell is insensitive to aldosterone, as in urinary tract obstruction, sickle cell anemia, amyloidosis, and systemic lupus erythematosus. Inhibition of aldosterone action with spironolactone or eplerenone may cause hyperkalemic acidosis, as does ENaC inhibition by amiloride and triamterene.

Pseudohypoaldosteronism type 1 is due to autosomal recessive, inactivating mutations of the Na^+ channel ENaC, whereas autosomal dominant pseudohypoaldosteronism type 1 is due to mutations of the mineralocorticoid receptor. Both cause hypovolemia, metabolic acidosis, and hyperkalemia with secondary increases in renin and aldosterone. In Gordon's syndrome (pseudohypoaldosteronism type 2), increases in Na^+ and Cl^- reabsorption through increased activity of the distal thiazide-sensitive NaCl transporter lead to hypertension, hyperkalemic acidosis, volume expansion, and consequently, low renin and aldosterone. Type 3 renal tubular acidosis is the syndrome of combined proximal and distal renal tubular acidosis.

CLINICAL MANIFESTATIONS AND DIAGNOSIS

The urinary anion gap helps distinguish renal tubular acidosis from extrarenal bicarbonate loss (e.g., from diarrhea). Because the normal renal response to metabolic acidosis is an increase in ammoniagenesis, the urine should contain large amounts of NH_4Cl while the kidney retains sodium and potassium; the urinary anion gap, which is $(Na^+ + K^+) - Cl^-$, should be strongly negative because of the unmeasured NH_4^+.

In renal diseases such as distal renal tubular acidosis, however, the urinary anion gap will be zero or positive because of either the failure of ammoniagenesis or the excretion of sodium plus potassium with bicarbonate. With type 2 (proximal) renal tubular acidosis, patients often have Fanconi's syndrome with glycosuria, phosphaturia, aminoaciduria, and uricosuria. In proximal renal tubular acidosis, the steady-state urine pH is usually less than 5.3, the acidosis is not severe (i.e., HCO_3^- usually not less than 16), and acid excretion may balance acid production at this new steady state.

In contrast to proximal renal tubular acidosis, distal renal tubular acidosis (type I) is generally a more severe metabolic disorder that may be accompanied by hypercalciuria, nephrocalcinosis, calcium phosphate kidney stones (Chapter 128), and bone disease that includes rickets in children and osteomalacia in adults. Although rarely necessary to perform, the NH_4Cl loading test can confirm the diagnosis of distal renal tubular acidosis. In this test, the plasma bicarbonate is lowered by an acid challenge. If urine pH remains above 5.3, a distal abnormality is suspected. Proximal and distal renal tubular acidoses usually can be distinguished by a careful clinical evaluation (Fig. 120-3). Helpful findings include the presence of a urine pH greater than 5.3 in distal but not proximal renal tubular acidosis during acidemia; a fractional excretion of bicarbonate as high as 10 to 15% in proximal renal tubular acidosis; and the lowering of serum potassium upon correction of proximal but not distal tubular acidosis.

In patients with an elevated serum anion gap, unmeasured anions such as ketoacids and lactate, rather than NH_4^+, are present in urine, so a positive urinary anion gap does not indicate renal tubular acidosis. On occasion, however, the prompt renal excretion of organic anions with sodium and potassium may minimize the increase in the serum anion gap. In the metabolic acidosis of glue sniffers, hippurate, which is a product of toluene, is rapidly excreted, thus giving the appearance of a nongap metabolic acidosis with a positive urinary anion gap.

TREATMENT Rx

If possible, treatment of metabolic acidosis should focus on correcting the underlying cause and permitting the body's homeostatic mechanisms to correct the acid-base disturbance. Patients whose pH is less than 7.2 are typically treated with infusions of sodium bicarbonate, guided by the estimated base deficit in milliequivalents, calculated using the serum HCO_3^- concentration in milliequivalents per liter:

$$\text{Amount of } HCO_3^- = (25 - [HCO_3^-]) \times \text{wt (kg)}/2$$

In general, the correction of metabolic acidemia should be based on a calculated amount, with not more than 50% of the estimate given before recalculation. Moreover, this equation is used for deficit correction only; the ongoing losses of 1 to 2 mEq/kg per day, equivalent to the daily acid load, should be replaced in distal renal tubular acidosis with $NaHCO_3$, $KHCO_3$, or citrate salts in divided doses. Hypokalemia may accompany distal renal tubular acidosis and may improve with treatment.

Proximal renal tubular acidosis in children may affect growth and require large quantities of bicarbonate in excess of 1 to 2 mEq/kg per day to correct the acidosis because ingested alkali is promptly excreted in alkaline urine. In adults, treatment is often deferred because the steady state acidosis allows for a normal acid excretion rate. Hypokalemia may worsen with bicarbonate treatment of proximal tubular acidosis.

In type 4 renal tubular acidosis, treatment of hyperkalemia with a low potassium diet, thiazide, or loop diuretics or sodium polystyrene sulfonate often improves urinary acidification without the use of bicarbonate salts.

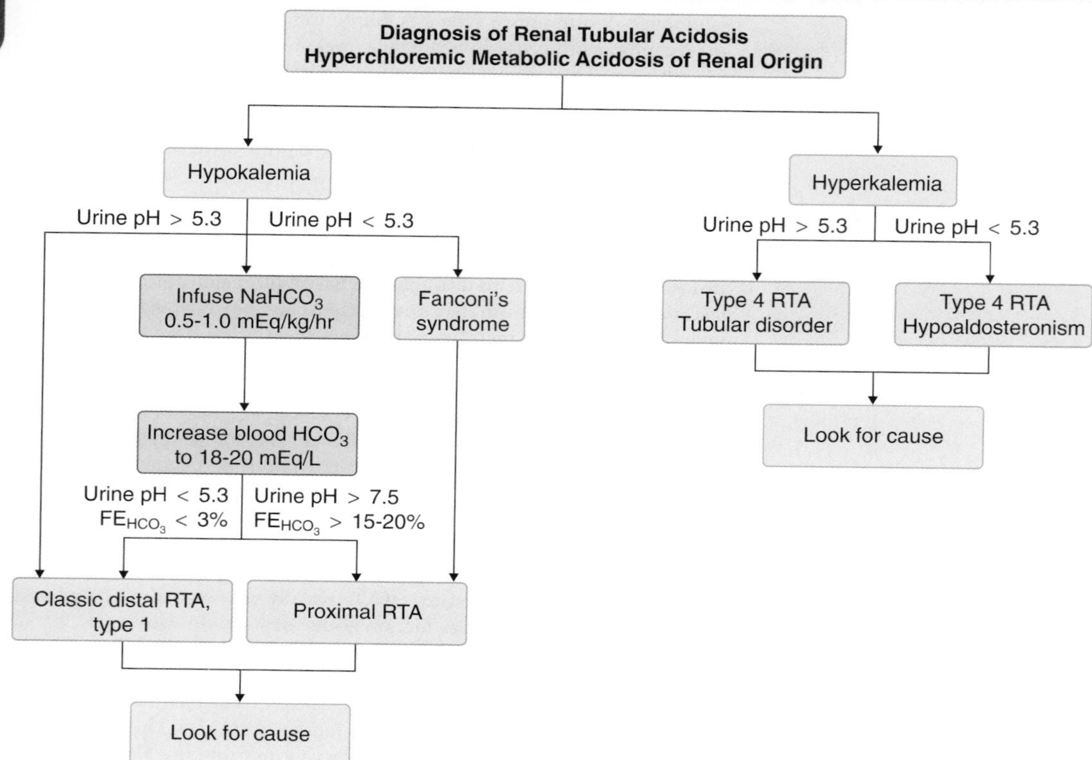

FIGURE 120-3. Diagnosis of renal tubular acidosis (RTA). FE = fractional excretion; $NaHCO_3$ = sodium bicarbonate.

PROGNOSIS

The prognosis of renal tubular acidosis generally depends on the presence of an underlying systemic disease, such as myeloma (Chapter 193). In children, disorders such as medullary cystic kidney disease (Chapter 129) or cystinosis (Chapter 130) usually result in renal failure by the teenage years. These patients are candidates for renal replacement therapy, including transplantation. Chronic metabolic acidosis in children, if not well treated, is associated with rickets (Chapter 252) and short stature.

METABOLIC ALKALOSIS

EPIDEMIOLOGY AND PATHOBIOLOGY

In metabolic alkalosis, the primary event is elevation of the plasma bicarbonate concentration. In response to increased systemic pH, alveolar ventilation is decreased to increase P_{CO_2} and thereby decrease pH. However, respiratory compensation is generally less effective in cases of metabolic alkalosis than in cases of metabolic acidosis. Contributing factors may include the fact that hypoventilation also decreases P_{O_2}, which is a potent stimulus for the peripheral chemoreceptors to increase alveolar ventilation when P_{O_2} falls below about 60 mm Hg. A second mechanism that may blunt respiratory compensation is intracellular acidosis in the brain in the setting of hypokalemia. In acute metabolic alkalosis, an initial paradoxical acidotic shift in CSF pH secondary to a sudden increase in P_{CO_2}, similar to the alkaline shift in CSF pH in acute metabolic acidosis, may activate central chemoreceptors and increase ventilatory drive despite peripheral stimulation to decrease alveolar ventilation. In chronic metabolic alkalosis, CSF pH may return to normal, so respiratory drive is controlled entirely by the peripheral chemoreceptors. The result is that the ventilatory response to metabolic alkalosis is highly varied: many patients with metabolic alkalosis maintain nearly normal P_{CO_2} levels, and the level rarely rises above 60 mm Hg.

Metabolic alkalosis requires a generation phase, in which new HCO_3^- is added to the extracellular fluid, and a maintenance phase, in which the new elevated serum HCO_3^- concentration is sustained. Without the latter phase, a kidney with normal filtration and tubular function has a high capacity to excrete HCO_3^-, thereby preventing alkalosis. Maintenance of a high HCO_3^- concentration usually occurs because of volume depletion, a reduced glomerular filtration rate, hypokalemia, or low chloride levels.

Metabolic Alkalosis of Renal Origin Associated with Volume Depletion

Metabolic alkalosis of renal origin may be the result of excessive urinary chloride excretion, most commonly related to diuretics that inhibit reabsorption of Cl^-. The Cl^- loss results in hypochloremia, with a compensatory increase in plasma HCO_3^- to maintain electroneutrality. Extracellular volume depletion stimulates the renin-angiotensin-aldosterone pathway, and high aldosterone levels superimposed on increased distal urinary flow rates results in increased K^+ excretion and hypokalemia. The volume depletion and hypokalemia enhance proximal HCO_3^- reabsorption, thereby maintaining the alkalosis, and the prerenal fall in the glomerular flow rate limits HCO_3^- filtration.

Important but rare genetic syndromes characterized by urinary chloride wasting include Bartter's syndrome and Gitelman's syndrome. Bartter's syndrome is an autosomal recessive salt-losing state associated with extracellular volume depletion and excessive urinary chloride loss that results in hypokalemia and hypochloremic metabolic alkalosis. Secondary increases of plasma renin and aldosterone occur, as does renal juxtaglomerular cell hyperplasia. The syndrome resembles the effects of furosemide on the thick ascending limb of Henle; gene mutations in the Na-K-2Cl cotransporter, K^+ channel, and Cl^- channels have been described. Because calcium reabsorption occurs in the thick ascending limb of Henle, Bartter's syndrome, like furosemide, causes hypercalciuria as well as polyuria.

Gitelman's syndrome is an autosomal recessive cause of extracellular volume depletion, urinary chloride wasting, and hypokalemic metabolic alkalosis. It is due to inactivating mutations in the *SLC12A3* gene encoding the thiazide-sensitive NaCl cotransporter of the renal distal tubule. Urinary concentrating ability is preserved, and patients are hypocalciuric because decreased NaCl reabsorption in the distal tubule is associated with a decrease in calcium excretion. Hypomagnesemia may also be severe.

Metabolic Alkalosis of Nonrenal Origin with Extracellular Volume Depletion

Metabolic alkalosis may develop as a result of gastrointestinal Cl^- loss from vomiting, nasogastric suctioning, or secretory diarrhea. In such cases, extracellular volume is usually contracted, hypochloremia develops, and the urinary chloride level is usually less than 20 mEq/L.

In Zollinger-Ellison syndrome (Chapter 201), excessive gastrin-induced gastric acid secretion may result in an acidic stool with high chloride content. Diarrhea does not cause metabolic alkalosis unless the stool electrolytes $[(Na^+ + K^+) - Cl^-]$ are less than plasma HCO_3^-.

Infectious gastroenteritis, congenital chloridorrhea, and villous adenomas also cause chloride losses in stool. Congenital chloridorrhea is an autosomal recessive disorder of defective colonic, apical Cl/HCO_3 exchange associated with the downregulated adenoma *(DRA)* gene.

With vomiting, the initiating event is loss of HCl. This secretion of HCl into the stomach lumen by the parietal cell is coupled to the absorption of HCO_3^- in exchange for chloride at the basolateral membrane. When gastric acid is normally secreted, a mild increase in serum HCO_3^- spills into urine and causes an "alkaline tide." With vomiting, however, the net loss of HCl generates the alkalosis. Initially, this increased HCO_3^- is filtered by the glomeruli and excreted in urine accompanied by Na^+ and K^+; volume depletion begins to develop. As vomiting continues, extracellular volume depletion worsens, glomerular filtration falls, HCO_3^- filtration is limited, volume depletion increases the renin-angiotensin II–aldosterone system, proximal fluid and HCO_3^- reabsorption increase, distal Na^+ reabsorption increases under the influence of aldosterone, and greater H^+ secretion enhances HCO_3^- reabsorption. These effects reduce renal Na^+ loss but at the expense of maintaining the metabolic alkalosis. Significant K^+ losses, which occur as a result of the bicarbonaturia and hyperaldosteronism, lead to hypokalemia, which is actually due to renal, not gastrointestinal, losses as a consequence of attempts to maintain extracellular volume. The hypokalemia further increases proximal $NaHCO_3$ reabsorption, distal H^+ secretion, and K^+ reabsorption, all at the expense of further reabsorption of HCO_3^-. At the new steady state after vomiting or nasogastric suctioning ceases, the paradoxical aciduria of metabolic alkalosis develops as HCO_3^- reabsorption is complete, and the urine contains low levels of Na^+, K^+, and Cl^-. The patient may be hypovolemic, hypokalemic, and alkalemic, but because Na^+, K^+, and acid-base balance are intrinsically linked, life-threatening volume depletion, K^+ depletion, and alkalemia are usually avoided.

Most nonrenal metabolic alkaloses with volume depletion are due to gastrointestinal losses. However, some patients with cystic fibrosis (Chapter 89) may develop hypochloremic alkalosis as a consequence of excessive sweat chloride content related to the *CFTR* gene mutation.

Metabolic Alkalosis of Renal Origin with Volume Expansion and Hypertension

The renal conditions that cause metabolic alkalosis and volume expansion are due to a proportionately greater increase in Na^+ reabsorption above what is required to maintain a steady state of Na^+ balance, rather than primary loss of the Cl^- anion. As Na^+ is reabsorbed, electroneutrality is maintained by an increase in plasma HCO_3^-. The plasma Na^+ concentration may be increased, and Cl^- balance is normal; Cl^- appears in urine, and hypochloremia is not present. In the kidney, the loss of net acid as NH_4Cl in excess of the acid produced generates a metabolic alkalosis, in which the new bicarbonate generated is due to proton secretion by the distal nephron through H^+-ATPases. The H^+ then combines with NH_3 to form NH_4^+ in urine.

Na^+ is reabsorbed independently of Cl^- in the cortical collecting duct through the aldosterone-sensitive cells containing the ENaC. When Na^+ is reabsorbed by the principal cells of the cortical collecting duct, the tubule lumen becomes electronegative and stimulates both K^+ and H^+ secretion by the electrogenic H^+-ATPases. To the extent that HCO_3^- remains in the lumen, the secreted protons complete HCO_3^- reabsorption. Additional secreted protons combine with NH_3 and phosphates and lead to net acid excretion. Any increase in the distal H^+ secretory mechanism will produce more urinary net acid; more "new" HCO_3^- will be generated and returned to the now expanded extracellular fluid, and metabolic alkalosis will develop. The increased plasma HCO_3^- will be filtered, but in the absence of a stimulus to increase proximal HCO_3^- reabsorption, the HCO_3^- will flow distally to be reabsorbed by the increased H^+ secretion of the collecting duct. At first, the alkalosis is mild, but increased cortical collecting duct Na^+ reabsorption will also lead to increased K^+ secretion and hypokalemia. Hypokalemia increases the capacity for proximal HCO_3^- reabsorption, thereby opposing the effect of volume expansion, so that distal delivery of HCO_3^- decreases. The higher than normal distal H^+ secretion titrates urinary buffers so further "new" HCO_3^- is formed and the alkalosis worsens. Metabolic alkaloses in the hypermineralocorticoid syndromes are sustained by hypokalemia.

Metabolic Alkalosis of Nonrenal Origin Associated with Normal or Expanded Volume

If an alkalotic patient is not hypochloremic, electroneutrality must be maintained either by depletion of an alternative anion or by an excessive concentration of a cation. An example of a metabolic alkalosis associated with depletion of a nonchloride anion is hypoproteinemic alkalosis, with hypoalbuminemia and a small anion gap. Chloride balance is normal and chloride appears in urine.

Alkalosis also may result from the addition of alkali salts of organic anions. The normal response to the ingestion of $NaHCO_3$ is rapid urinary alkalinization because of an unaltered threshold for HCO_3^- reabsorption. However, a marked excess of HCO_3^-, as may be administered in an attempt to alkalinize a patient's urine, expands volume and causes an alkalemia, especially in the presence of volume depletion or low glomerular filtration. Milk-alkali syndrome, usually seen when patients in renal failure ingest milk or calcium antacids, is associated with hypercalcemia, alkalemia, and normal Cl^-.

Other situations in which intake of alkali salts results in metabolic alkalosis include infusion of large quantities of sodium salts of metabolizable organic compounds such as acetate, citrate, lactate, or bicarbonate; hyperalimentation with acetate salts; chronic peritoneal dialysis with acetate or lactate dialysate; or excessive transfusions or plasmapheresis, in which large quantities of citrate, used as an anticoagulant, are delivered.

CLINICAL MANIFESTATIONS

Mild metabolic alkalosis up to a pH of 7.50 *is* usually asymptomatic. When the pH exceeds 7.55, however, the alkalosis itself and the compensatory hypoventilation are frequently associated with metabolic encephalopathy. Symptoms include confusion, obtundation, delirium, and coma. The seizure threshold is lowered; tetany, paresthesias, muscular cramping, and other symptoms of low calcium are seen. In patients with hypocalcemia, these signs may be seen at pH values above 7.45. Other findings include cardiac tachyarrhythmias and hypotension. Lactate production increases as a result of the increased anaerobic glycolysis.

DIAGNOSIS

In diagnosing the cause of metabolic alkalosis, it is important to distinguish whether the condition is chloride responsive or chloride unresponsive. Metabolic alkalosis is generally divided into two categories based on its responsiveness to chloride (see Table 120-2). Chloride-responsive metabolic alkalosis is associated with extracellular fluid and chloride depletion and is seen in cases of gastric fluid loss and diuretic use. A diagnostic clue comes from the serum electrolytes. HCO_3^- is increased with a corresponding fall in serum chloride (hypochloremic alkalosis). Chloride-unresponsive metabolic alkalosis is seen in patients with extracellular fluid expansion in conditions such as primary aldosteronism and hypokalemia. Entry of hydrogen ions into cells can also lead to metabolic alkalosis in patients with hypokalemia.

Vomiting, nasogastric suction, and diarrhea are usually obvious sources of metabolic alkalosis. However, the Zollinger-Ellison syndrome (Chapter 201), villous adenomas (Chapter 199), and VIPomas (Chapter 201) may be more difficult to diagnose unless the index of suspicion is high.

Patients who present with hypokalemic metabolic alkalosis with normal or low blood pressure and have urinary chloride concentrations above 25 mEq/L may be taking diuretics such as furosemide or thiazides surreptitiously; a diuretic screen can document the presence of the drug. If the screen is negative, Bartter's or Gitelman's syndrome (Chapter 130) should be considered. Bartter's syndrome is less common, usually more severe, and presents in young patients. The presence of hypercalciuria favors Bartter's syndrome, whereas hypocalciuria suggests Gitelman's syndrome.

Specific causes of renal alkalosis with volume expansion and hypertension can be classified according to levels of renin and aldosterone. Primary increases in renin with secondary increases in aldosterone can be seen in patients with unilateral renal artery stenosis (Chapter 127), renin-secreting tumors of the kidney (Chapter 67), and malignant hypertension (Chapter 67). Low renin and elevated aldosterone levels are characteristic of primary hyperaldosteronism from adrenal adenoma or hyperplasia (Chapter 235). A high cortisol level with volume expansion is seen in hypercortisolism (Chapter 234) and adrenocorticotropic hormone-secreting tumors (Chapter 186). Inhibition of the intracellular enzyme 11β-hydroxysteroid dehydrogenase, which normally inactivates cortisol to form cortisone in the cortical collecting duct, will also result in low renin levels, low aldosterone levels, and hypokalemic alkalosis. Both genetic mutations (the apparent mineralocorticoid excess syndrome) and an excess consumption of glycyrrhizic acid found in licorice or anisette are causes of this enzyme block. Another cause of hypertension with hypokalemic alkalosis but with low renin and aldosterone levels is Liddle's syndrome (Chapter 130), in which an activating mutation in the cortical collecting duct Na^+ channel (ENaC) leads to increased Na^+ reabsorption.

Metabolic alkalosis may also develop without volume expansion when a non-reabsorbable anion is presented to the cortical collecting duct lumen. Nitrates, sulfates, and certain antibiotics such as nafcillin, carbenicillin, and ticarcillin may obligate K^+ and H^+ secretion as Na^+ is reabsorbed. Topical administration of silver nitrate to burn victims may result in alkalosis.

TREATMENT Rx

In chloride-responsive patients (see Table 120-2), treatment is directed at increasing urinary excretion of bicarbonate. In patients with mild to moderate alkalosis, liberalizing salt intake and administering potassium chloride is effective in increasing renal HCO_3^- excretion. The K deficit is likely to be at least 100 mEq for every 1 mEq/L decrease in serum potassium. Unless KCl is also replenished, the improvement in filtration and proximal reabsorption will result in severe K^+ wasting as bicarbonaturia develops and aldosterone's effects remain. In addition, complete resolution of alkalosis will not occur until K^+ is normalized. In a patient with renal failure and vomiting, the elevation in HCO_3^- may be more severe because of poor HCO_3^- filtration. In cases of volume expansion and alkalosis, acetazolamide may be administered carefully while monitoring its potential for losing K^+. If this agent fails to work, dilute solutions of HCl (0, 1N HCl) may be cautiously administered. The amount of H^+, in milliequivalents, to be given may be calculated as the product of the desired change in serum HCO_3^- concentration (mEq/L) times the estimated total body water (L). It is likely that the this calculation will overestimate the amount of acid needed for correction, so no more than one third of the amount should be given before recalculating to avoid metabolic acidosis. Full correction of HCO_3^- should not be the goal. In the absence of renal failure, intravenous acetazolamide (250 to 500 mg every 8 hours) may be effective but may greatly increase K^+ losses.

Chloride-unresponsive patients (see Table 120-2) include those with mineralocorticoid excess. In these patients, the metabolic alkalosis can be lessened by potassium replacement or by blocking Na^+ reabsorption with aldosterone antagonists such as spironolactone, starting with 25 mg orally, or amiloride, beginning with 5 mg orally. Indomethacin effectively treats Bartter's syndrome (Chapter 130) by interfering with prostaglandin E_2 to allow greater Na-Cl reabsorption in the thick ascending limb. Gitelman's and Bartter's syndromes are best treated with combinations of KCl, a potassium-sparing diuretic, and magnesium if needed.

RESPIRATORY ACIDOSIS

Respiratory acidosis is characterized by a primary elevation in P_{CO_2} as reflected by reduced arterial pH with variable elevation in the HCO_3^- concentration. It is most frequently caused by a decrease in alveolar ventilation owing to pulmonary disease (Chapter 104), respiratory muscle fatigue (Chapter 99), or abnormalities in ventilatory control (Chapter 86).

CLINICAL MANIFESTATIONS

Clinical findings in respiratory acidosis are related to the degree and duration of the respiratory acidosis and whether hypoxemia is present. A precipitous rise in P_{CO_2} can lead to confusion, anxiety, psychosis, asterixis, seizures, and myoclonic jerks, with progressive depression of the sensorium and coma at an arterial P_{CO_2} greater than 60 mm Hg (CO_2 narcosis). Hypercapnia, which increases cerebral blood flow and volume, can lead to symptoms and signs of elevated intracranial pressure, including headaches and papilledema. Other findings in acute respiratory acidosis include signs of catecholamine release, such as skin flushing, diaphoresis, and increased cardiac contractility and output. Symptoms of chronic hypercapnia include fatigue, lethargy, and confusion, in addition to the findings seen in acute hypercapnia.

The slow time course of many of these diseases allows the kidney to compensate adequately as the disease progresses by increasing its excretion of hydrogen ion as ammonium and generating and reabsorbing bicarbonate to restore systemic pH toward normal values. This compensatory process is not maximal until 3 to 5 days after the onset of respiratory acidosis.

DIAGNOSIS

Disorders that cause a respiratory acidosis include central effects of drugs, stroke, and infection; airway obstruction; primary parenchymal processes such as chronic obstructive pulmonary disease (Chapter 88) and acute respiratory distress syndrome (Chapter 104); disorders of ventilation (Chapter 105); and neuromuscular diseases such as myasthenia gravis (Chapter 430) and muscular dystrophies (Chapter 429). Permissive hypercapnia has been used clinically in patients with acute respiratory distress syndrome to limit pulmonary damage secondary to mechanical ventilation (Chapter 105).

It can be difficult to distinguish the signs of hypercapnia from those of hypoxemia because the two often appear together. If correction of the hypoxemia does not improve the clinical picture, however, it can be surmised that hypercapnia is responsible.

TREATMENT Rx

Treatment of both chronic and acute respiratory acidosis is aimed primarily at correcting the underlying cause and ensuring adequate ventilation. In acute respiratory acidosis, measures to relieve severe hypoxemia and acidemia should be instituted immediately, including intubation and assisted mechanical ventilation (Chapter 105) if necessary.

In patients with chronic respiratory acidosis, however, ventilation may be driven by hypoxemia; oxygen must be carefully titrated because correction of the hypoxemia can worsen the hypercapnia. In patients with compensated chronic respiratory acidosis, rapid and complete correction of hypercapnia can also result in posthypercapnic metabolic alkalosis. Patients recovering from an acute-on-chronic respiratory acidosis should be monitored carefully to correct hypokalemia, hypochloremia, and hypovolemia so that adequate renal excretion of bicarbonate can occur.

Bicarbonate therapy is not indicated for respiratory acidosis unless the pH falls below 7.0 and the patient is about to be intubated. There is a role for bicarbonate therapy in patients with renal failure (Chapter 132), in whom adequate compensatory acid excretion cannot take place.

RESPIRATORY ALKALOSIS

EPIDEMIOLOGY AND PATHOBIOLOGY

In respiratory alkalosis, a primary decrease in P_{CO_2} is reflected by increases in arterial pH and variable decreases in plasma bicarbonate concentration. The most common cause is alveolar hyperventilation, not underproduction of CO_2.

Acute hypocapnia results in an initial increase in the pH of both the CSF and the brain's intracellular environment. However, this increase is quickly offset by a decrease in bicarbonate levels. In acute respiratory alkalosis, one of the primary mechanisms of this fall in bicarbonate appears to be the generation of lactate as a result of vasoconstriction, hypoxia, and increased hemoglobin affinity for oxygen. The combination of increased oxygen demand and decreased oxygen delivery may contribute to adverse clinical outcomes in hypocapnic alkalosis.

Cerebral blood flow is significantly decreased by hypocapnia, which is a potent vasoconstrictor. As in respiratory acidosis, the CNS is immediately affected by decreases in systemic P_{CO_2} because of the blood-brain barrier's permeability to CO_2. In addition, as in respiratory acidosis, CSF and intracellular pH show an initial short-lived response that parallels the systemic increase in pH.

Renal compensation for sustained hypocapnia is complete in 36 to 72 hours. The mechanism rests primarily in the kidney's net reduction of hydrogen ion excretion, which it accomplishes largely by decreasing ammonium and titratable acid excretion. The threshold for bicarbonate excretion is also lowered, and bicarbonaturia develops. As a result, systemic bicarbonate levels decrease, and arterial pH returns toward normal values.

CLINICAL MANIFESTATIONS

The clinical manifestations of respiratory alkalosis depend on the degree and duration of the condition but are primarily those of the underlying disorder. Chronic hypocapnia does not appear to be associated with any significant clinical symptoms.

Symptoms of acute hypocapnia are largely attributable to the alkalemia and include dizziness, perioral or extremity paresthesias, confusion, asterixis, hypotension, seizures, and coma. Most symptoms, which are manifested only when the P_{CO_2} falls below 25 or 30 mm Hg, can be related to decreased cerebral blood flow or reduced free calcium because alkalosis increases calcium's protein-bound fraction. Shortness of breath and chest wall pain, which frequently may be seen when patients hyperventilate because of pain or anxiety, do not appear to be related to hypocapnia.

Adaptation to High Altitude

Acute exposure to high altitude (Chapter 94) results in hypoxia-induced hyperventilation. Compensation requires at least several days and is characterized by a gradual further increase in hyperventilation, a steadily decreasing P_{CO_2}, and an increasing P_{O_2}. The effect of the hypoxic stimulus to ventilate is initially modulated by the effects of alkalosis, both peripherally and centrally. However, as HCO_3^- in CSF falls, inhibition of the central stimulus to ventilate decreases. Once a steady state is achieved, the drive to ventilate is determined by the effects of hypoxemia and alkalemia on the peripheral chemoreceptors.

DIAGNOSIS

Alveolar hyperventilation leading to respiratory alkalosis is seen with hypoxemia from pulmonary disease (Chapter 83), heart failure (Chapter 58), high altitudes (Chapter 94), or anemia. Mechanical ventilation (Chapter 105) is also a common cause of respiratory alkalosis.

Another common cause of respiratory alkalosis is primary stimulation of the central chemoreceptor, as seen in sepsis (Chapter 108), hepatic cirrhosis (Chapter 156), salicylate intoxication (Chapters 36 and 110), correction of metabolic acidosis, hyperthermia (Chapter 109), and pregnancy, as well as cortical hyperventilation from anxiety and pain. In these situations, central signals override peripheral chemoreceptors until the primary stimulus is removed.

Primary neurologic diseases that can stimulate alveolar hyperventilation include acute stroke, infection, trauma, and tumors. Two patterns of respiration are seen: central hyperventilation and Cheyne-Stokes respiration (Chapter 86). Central hyperventilation, which is associated with lesions at the pontine-midbrain level, is regular, but with an increased rate and tidal volume. Cheyne-Stokes breathing, which is characterized by periods of hyperventilation alternating with apnea, is seen in patients with bilateral cortical and upper pontine lesions and in patients with heart failure.

TREATMENT

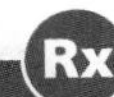

Treatment of respiratory alkalosis must address the underlying cause of the disturbance. Hyperventilation syndrome is a diagnosis of exclusion, but patients who exhibit symptoms, such as tetany and syncope, and who do not have more serious causes of hyperventilation can be treated with a rebreathing mask. Hypophosphatemia can be seen in these patients, but it usually improves with treatment of the alkalosis. Patients with respiratory alkalosis associated with mountain sickness can be pretreated with acetazolamide to induce a metabolic acidosis, thereby preventing extreme elevations in pH (Chapter 94).

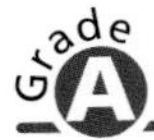

1. de Brito-Ashurst I, Varagunam M, Raftery MJ, et al. Bicarbonate supplementation slows progression of CKD and improves nutritional status. *J Am Soc Nephrol.* 2009;20:1869-1870.
2. Cooper DJ, Walley KR, Wiggs BR, et al. Bicarbonate does not improve hemodynamics in critically ill patients who have lactic acidosis: a prospective, controlled clinical study. *Ann Intern Med.* 1990;112:492-498.

SUGGESTED READINGS

Karet FE. Disorders of water and acid-base homeostasis. *Nephron Physiol.* 2011;118:28-34. *Review.*

Yaqoob MM. Acidosis and progression of chronic kidney disease. *Curr Opin Nephrol Hypertens.* 2010;19:489-492. *Review of data supporting the concept that correction of acidosis by sodium bicarbonate in patients with advanced CKD attenuates the decline of renal function.*

Yunos NM, Bellomo R, Story D, et al. Bench-to-bedside review: chloride in critical illness. *Crit Care.* 2010;14:226. *Review.*

121 DISORDERS OF MAGNESIUM AND PHOSPHORUS

ALAN S. L. YU

MAGNESIUM METABOLISM

Magnesium is an important mineral component of the bony skeleton, a cofactor for many metabolic enzymes, and a regulator of ion channels and transporters in excitable tissues.

Normal Magnesium Metabolism

The majority of total body magnesium is intracellular or in bone, with only 1% in extracellular fluid. The normal serum magnesium concentration is 1.8 to 2.3 mg/dL (1.5 to 1.9 mEq/L). The average daily intake of magnesium is 300 mg, the main sources of which are green vegetables, nuts, whole grain cereals, milk, and seafood. Magnesium is absorbed mainly in the jejunum and ileum. In the kidney, 70 to 80% of serum magnesium is filtered at the glomerulus, with the majority being reabsorbed along the length of the tubule, particularly in the thick ascending limb of Henle. In states of magnesium deficiency or excess, renal tubule reabsorption is tightly regulated so that magnesium excretion is adjusted accordingly.

Magnesium Deficiency

PATHOBIOLOGY

Magnesium deficiency is usually detected when hypomagnesemia becomes evident. However, because magnesium is stored primarily intracellularly, substantial depletion of total body magnesium can occur before serum magnesium levels drop appreciably.

Magnesium deficiency may be due to nutritional deficiency, intestinal malabsorption, redistribution into bone, or losses via cutaneous, lower gastrointestinal, or renal routes (Table 121-1). The recommended daily allowance of magnesium is 420 mg for males and 320 mg for females. Approximately 25% of alcoholics are chronically hypomagnesemic because of a combination of poor nutritional intake and increased renal loss. Magnesium deficiency can rarely occur in protein-calorie malnutrition and may be associated with acute hypomagnesemia during refeeding because of rapid cellular magnesium

TABLE 121-1 CAUSES OF MAGNESIUM DEFICIENCY

Nutritional deficiency
Alcoholism*
Malnutrition
Refeeding syndrome
Intestinal malabsorption*
Proton pump inhibitors
Lower gastrointestinal losses
Colonic diarrhea*
Intestinal fistula
Laxative abuse
Cutaneous losses
Burns*
Exercise-induced sweating
Redistribution into bone
Hungry bone syndrome
Renal losses
Polyuria (including diabetes mellitus)*
Volume expansion
Hyperaldosteronism
Bartter's and Gitelman's syndromes
Hypercalcemia
Loop and thiazide diuretics*
Nephrotoxins (cisplatin, amphotericin, aminoglycosides, pentamidine, cyclosporine)*
Epidermal growth factor monoclonal antibodies (cetuximab, panitumumab)*

*Common causes.

uptake. Fat malabsorption in conditions such as celiac disease, Crohn's disease, and small intestinal resection causes magnesium deficiency because free fatty acids accumulate in the intestinal lumen, where they combine with magnesium to form insoluble soaps. Proton pump inhibitors can also cause hypomagnesemia, which is thought to be due to inhibition of intestinal absorption. Lower gastrointestinal secretions are rich in magnesium, so diarrhea of colonic origin is a common cause of hypomagnesemia. Sweat contains significant amounts of magnesium, and transient hypomagnesemia can occur after prolonged, intense exercise such as marathon runs. Magnesium is also lost from burned skin surfaces, and 40% of patients with severe burns (Chapter 112) are hypomagnesemic.

In patients with severe hyperparathyroidism (Chapter 253) and high bone turnover, continued sequestration of minerals within bone may continue for several days after parathyroidectomy and cause transient hypocalcemia, hypomagnesemia, and hypophosphatemia. Renal magnesium losses can occur in any polyuric state, including the recovery phase of acute tubular necrosis or urinary tract obstruction. Hypomagnesemia is common in diabetes mellitus (Chapters 236 and 237), where it is thought to be due to a combination of poor intestinal absorption owing to autonomic neuropathy, osmotic diuresis, and decreased renal tubule reabsorption. Failure of sodium reabsorption in the thick ascending limb of Henle as a result of the use of loop diuretics and in the distal convoluted tubule as a result of thiazide diuretics inhibits tubular magnesium reabsorption and leads to urinary magnesium wasting. Drugs that are tubular toxins are also common causes of renal magnesium wasting. Such drugs include cisplatin, amphotericin B, and aminoglycosides, which are commonly associated with hypokalemia and rarely with renal tubule acidosis, as well as calcineurin inhibitors such as cyclosporine and tacrolimus, which also cause hyperkalemia. Antibodies to the epidermal growth factor receptor, such as cetuximab and panitumumab, which are used to treat metastatic colorectal cancer, downregulate a distal tubule magnesium channel and are an increasing cause of isolated severe hypomagnesemia.

Inherited hypomagnesemia is usually caused by renal magnesium loss and can be subdivided into three main types, depending on the coexistence of other electrolyte disturbances: Bartter's and Gitelman's syndromes, which are associated with renal salt wasting and hypokalemic metabolic alkalosis; familial hypomagnesemia with hypercalciuria and nephrocalcinosis; and isolated hypomagnesemia, which is usually associated with hypocalcemia.

CLINICAL MANIFESTATIONS

Mild to moderate hypomagnesemia or magnesium deficiency is frequently asymptomatic. Manifestations of increased neuronal excitability are the most common symptoms, including paresthesias, tetany, and seizures. These may be associated with Chvostek's sign (twitching of the cheek muscles in response to tapping the facial nerve in front of the ear) or Trousseau's sign (carpal spasm induced by compressing the upper arm with a tourniquet or blood pressure cuff). Cardiac disturbances may also occur and range in severity from mild electrocardiographic abnormalities (nonspecific T wave changes, U waves, prolonged QT interval, and repolarization alternans) to ventricular tachycardia, torsades de pointes, and ventricular fibrillation (Chapter 65).

Coexistent hypokalemia is very common, for two reasons: many of the causes of hypomagnesemia are also causes of potassium loss, and hypomagnesemia itself causes renal potassium wasting. Severe hypomagnesemia also impairs parathyroid hormone secretion and induces tissue resistance to its actions, thereby leading to hypocalcemia.

DIAGNOSIS

The cause of the magnesium deficiency is often obvious from the history. In difficult diagnostic cases, 24-hour urinary magnesium excretion should be measured. With extrarenal magnesium loss (usually malabsorption or laxative abuse), urinary magnesium excretion is appropriately suppressed (<25 mg/day). Higher urinary magnesium levels indicate renal magnesium wasting, often secondary to surreptitious diuretic use or one of the familial magnesium-wasting disorders.

TREATMENT Rx

It is unclear whether mild, asymptomatic hypomagnesemia needs to be treated. Magnesium repletion is recommended in hypomagnesemic patients if they are symptomatic, have underlying cardiac or seizure disorders, exhibit concurrent severe hypocalcemia or hypokalemia, or have severe hypomagnesemia (<1.4 mg/dL). In mild cases or in the outpatient setting, oral magnesium salts such as magnesium oxide (250 to 500 mg four times daily) can be used for repletion, but these substances frequently cause diarrhea, particularly at high doses. In the inpatient setting, intravenous magnesium sulfate (1 to 2 g every 6 hours) can be used for repletion. Because the redistribution of magnesium from extracellular to intracellular compartments is relatively slow, the serum magnesium concentration may normalize before total body magnesium stores are replete. It is therefore prudent to continue intravenous magnesium for an additional 1 to 2 days after restoration of normomagnesemia. In patients with normal renal function, any excess magnesium is simply excreted renally. Adverse effects from intravenous magnesium administration are primarily due to transient hypermagnesemia and include flushing, hypotension, and flaccid paralysis. Amiloride (10 to 20 mg orally once daily) abrogates renal magnesium wasting in some patients with this problem, but the mechanism is unknown.

PROGNOSIS

In patients with a self-limited cause of magnesium deficiency, repletion is easily accomplished. However, in patients with persistent magnesium wasting, such as in Gitelman's syndrome (Chapter 119), it can be difficult to keep up with the ongoing losses with oral therapy. Fortunately, these individuals tend to adapt to their chronic hypomagnesemia and tolerate it fairly well.

Hypermagnesemia

Transient hypermagnesemia can occur in patients given large doses of intravenous magnesium, for example, in the setting of preeclampsia. It has also been reported in individuals taking large doses of magnesium-containing antacids or cathartics, particularly in settings in which intestinal absorption is enhanced, such as inflammatory bowel disease and intestinal obstruction. However, the kidney has a very large capacity to excrete excess magnesium. Thus, persistent hypermagnesemia is seen almost exclusively in patients who have chronic renal insufficiency (Chapter 132) who are also taking excessive amounts of magnesium in the form of antacids, cathartics, or enemas.

CLINICAL MANIFESTATIONS

Magnesium toxicity is a serious and potentially fatal condition. Mild hypermagnesemia (serum magnesium level >4 to 6 mg/dL) causes hypotension, nausea, vomiting, facial flushing, urinary retention, and ileus. Above serum levels of 8 to 12 mg/dL, flaccid skeletal muscle paralysis and hyporeflexia may ensue, along with bradyarrhythmias, respiratory depression, coma, and cardiac arrest. A low or even negative serum anion gap is sometimes seen.

TREATMENT Rx

Mild hypermagnesemia in a patient with good renal function usually requires no treatment because renal clearance is rapid and the normal serum half-life of magnesium is about 1 day. In the event of serious toxicity, the effects of magnesium can be temporarily antagonized by the administration of intravenous calcium salts (5 to 10 mL of 10% calcium chloride). Renal magnesium excretion can be enhanced by administering furosemide (20 to 40 mg every 4 hours) together with a saline infusion (0.9% NaCl at 150 mL/hour, titrated to replace urinary losses). In patients with advanced renal insufficiency, the most effective method of magnesium removal is hemodialysis.

PROGNOSIS

Severe hypermagnesemia is potentially fatal. Lesser degrees of hypermagnesemia usually respond well to treatment.

PHOSPHORUS METABOLISM

Phosphorus has many critical roles. It is a major component of bone mineral, of phospholipids in cell membranes, and of nucleic acids. It forms high-energy phosphate bonds in compounds such as adenosine triphosphate (ATP), is post-translationally bound to proteins as an intracellular signal, and acts as a major pH buffer in serum and urine.

Normal Phosphorus Metabolism

Of the total body phosphorus content, 85% is in bone, 14% is in intracellular compartments, and only 1% is in extracellular fluid. The normal concentration of phosphorus in plasma is 3 to 4.5 mg/dL (1 to 1.5 mM). Daily intake of phosphorus is 800 to 1500 mg. Phosphorus is present in many foods, including dairy products, meats, and grains, and it is absorbed in the small intestine. The kidneys excrete excess phosphorus, which is the principal mechanism by which the body regulates extracellular phosphate balance. Ninety percent of serum phosphate is filtered at the glomerulus, of which 80 to 97% is reabsorbed along the nephron, primarily in the proximal tubule. Parathyroid hormone increases renal phosphate excretion by inhibiting the sodium-phosphate cotransporter in the proximal tubule, whereas vitamin D enhances intestinal phosphate absorption.

Hypophosphatemia

PATHOBIOLOGY

Hypophosphatemia may be caused by decreased intake, impaired intestinal absorption, redistribution into cells or bone, and renal losses (Table 121-2). Phosphate is frequently depleted in alcoholism (Chapter 32) because of the intake of a carbohydrate-rich, phosphate-poor diet, as well as renal phosphate wasting. Divalent cation-containing antacids bind phosphate in the intestinal lumen to form insoluble salts, thereby preventing their absorption. Vitamin D deficiency also leads to decreased intestinal phosphate absorption and hence to hypophosphatemia. Respiratory but not metabolic alkalosis (Chapter 120) may cause transient hypophosphatemia. In this disorder, intracellular pH is increased, thereby stimulating glycolysis, which depletes the intracellular inorganic phosphate pool and leads to a shift of phosphate into cells.

Insulin is also a strong stimulus for shifting phosphate into cells. Patients with diabetic ketoacidosis (Chapter 120) are often hyperphosphatemic because of a shift of phosphate out of cells under insulinopenic conditions, but their total body phosphate is actually depleted as a result of urinary losses. Subsequent treatment with insulin may uncover severe hypophosphatemia. Similarly, in malnourished patients (Chapter 222), whose total body phosphate stores may be depleted, overzealous intravenous refeeding with carbohydrate-rich fluids may stimulate insulin release and cause acute hypophosphatemia. The tyrosine kinase inhibitors imatinib and sorafenib, which are used in the treatment of various cancers (Chapter 190), can cause profound hypophosphatemia, which appears to be due to inhibition of bone resorption.

Renal phosphate wasting is usually due to impaired proximal tubule phosphate reabsorption. In primary hyperparathyroidism (Chapter 253), hypercalcemia is typically associated with hypophosphatemia. Fanconi's syndrome is a generalized proximal tubule disorder characterized by hypophosphatemia in association with glycosuria, aminoaciduria, hypokalemia, and type II renal tubular acidosis; it can be caused by a variety of inherited metabolic disorders, multiple myeloma (Chapter 193), heavy metal intoxication (Chapter 21), and drugs such as ifosfamide, cidofovir, and tenofovir. Phosphaturia can also occur with diuretics, particularly carbonic anhydrase inhibitors, and with antimicrobial agents such as pentamidine and foscarnet.

Oncogenic osteomalacia is a paraneoplastic syndrome (Chapter 187) associated primarily with mesenchymal tumors that secrete a variety of phosphaturic factors collectively known as phosphatonins. A similar phenotype is found in X-linked and autosomal dominant hypophosphatemic rickets; these inherited disorders are characterized by an increase in a circulating phosphatonin called fibroblast growth factor-23. Phosphatonins inhibit both renal tubular phosphate reabsorption and 1α-hydroxylation of 25-hydroxycholecalciferol, thereby leading to hypophosphatemia, rickets or osteomalacia (Chapter 252), and inappropriately low serum levels of 1,25-dihydroxycholecalciferol.

TABLE 121-2 CAUSES OF HYPOPHOSPHATEMIA

Nutritional deficiency
Alcoholism*
Impaired intestinal absorption
Antacids
Vitamin D deficiency*
Redistribution into cells
Respiratory alkalosis*
Insulin*
Refeeding syndrome
Burns*
Redistribution into bone
Hungry bone syndrome
Tyrosine kinase inhibitors (imatinib, sorafenib)
Renal losses
Hyperparathyroidism*
Renal tubulopathy
Fanconi's syndrome
Drugs (pentamidine, foscarnet, acetazolamide)
Phosphatonin excess syndrome
Oncogenic osteomalacia
Familial hypophosphatemic rickets

*Common causes.

CLINICAL MANIFESTATIONS

Clinical complications, which are usually observed only with severe hypophosphatemia (<1 mg/dL), are thought to be due to the disruption of cell membrane composition, depletion of ATP (which particularly affects high energy-consuming tissues such as skeletal and cardiac muscle), and depletion of 2,3-diphosphoglycerate in erythrocytes, with impaired tissue oxygen delivery. Manifestations of severe hypophosphatemia include encephalopathy, dilated cardiomyopathy, generalized muscle weakness that can lead to respiratory failure, rhabdomyolysis, and hemolysis. Hypophosphatemia also impairs renal ammoniagenesis and reduces the availability of urinary buffer, thereby impairing renal acid excretion and causing metabolic acidosis. Chronic hypophosphatemia leads to resorption of bone and osteomalacia.

DIAGNOSIS

The cause of hypophosphatemia is often evident from the history and physical examination. If not, measurement of either 24-hour urinary phosphate excretion or fractional excretion of phosphate (F_EPO_4) in a spot urine sample is often helpful.

$$F_EPO_4 = \frac{\text{Urine phosphate} \times \text{Serum creatinine}}{\text{Serum phosphate} \times \text{Urine creatinine}}$$

In the setting of hypophosphatemia, the normal response of the kidney is to reduce urinary phosphate excretion to less than 100 mg/day or to reduce F_EPO_4 to less than 5%. Higher values suggest one of the causes of renal phosphate wasting.

TREATMENT Rx

Patients with asymptomatic mild to moderate hypophosphatemia, normal total body phosphorus stores, and minimal ongoing phosphorus losses (e.g., a patient with hypophosphatemia as a result of acute respiratory alkalosis) do not require treatment. Phosphate should be repleted in patients who are symptomatic, are suspected of having severely depleted intracellular phosphorus stores (malnourished or alcoholic patients), have ongoing gastrointestinal or renal losses, or have severe hypophosphatemia (<1 mg/dL). Oral repletion can be accomplished with sodium or potassium phosphate salts (1 to 2 g/day) or with skimmed milk. Intravenous phosphorus repletion at a dose of 0.16 to 0.64 mmol/kg over 4 to 8 hours is recommended for severe hypophosphatemia but is contraindicated in patients with renal insufficiency or hypercalemia. Complications of phosphate therapy include hypocalcemia, metastatic calcification, hypotension, acute renal failure, and arrhythmias, as well as concomitant hypernatremia or hyperkalemia, depending on which salt is administered.

PROGNOSIS

Most patients with hypophosphatemia respond well to treatment.

Hyperphosphatemia

PATHOBIOLOGY

Pseudohyperphosphatemia may occur in blood specimens that are hemolyzed or hyperglobulinemic, such as in multiple myeloma (Chapter 193). True hyperphosphatemia is caused by excessive phosphate intake, increased intestinal absorption, redistribution from intracellular stores, or impaired renal excretion (Table 121-3). Overzealous phosphate repletion can obviously cause hyperphosphatemia. The phosphorus in some laxatives and enemas may be absorbed and cause hyperphosphatemia. Intoxication with vitamin D or its analogues increases intestinal absorption of both calcium and phosphorus. Conditions associated with massive cell lysis, such as rhabdomyolysis (Chapter 115) and tumor lysis syndrome (Chapter 182), cause the release of intracellular phosphate into the extracellular fluid. Patients with diabetic ketoacidosis (Chapters 236 and 237) are often hyperphosphatemic at initial evaluation because of the redistribution of phosphate out of cells in the insulin-deficient state. Decreased phosphate excretion is most commonly

TABLE 121-3 CAUSES OF HYPERPHOSPHATEMIA

Phosphate intake
- Phosphate repletion
- Phosphate-containing laxatives and enemas*

Increased intestinal absorption
- Vitamin D toxicity

Redistribution from intracellular stores
- Rhabdomyolysis
- Tumor lysis syndrome
- Diabetic ketoacidosis

Decreased renal excretion
- Renal failure*
- Hypoparathyroidism

*Common causes.

TABLE 121-4 MEDICATIONS FOR HYPERPHOSPHATEMIA

MEDICATION	USUAL DOSE WITH EACH MEAL	COMMENTS
CALCIUM SALTS		
Calcium acetate	1334 mg	Calcium level will increase about 0.5 mg/dL
Calcium carbonate	500-1000 mg	Calcium level will increase about 0.5 mg/dL
MAGNESIUM SALTS		
Magnesium hydroxide	311-622 mg	Can cause diarrhea or hypermagnesemia
Magnesium carbonate	63-126 mg	Can cause diarrhea or hypermagnesemia
ALUMINUM SALTS		
Aluminum hydroxide	300-600 mg	Encephalopathy and osteomalacia with prolonged use
OTHERS		
Sevelamer hydrochloride	800-1600 mg	Gastrointestinal side effects
Sevelamer carbonate	800-1600 mg	Gastrointestinal side effects
Lanthanum carbonate	250-500 mg	Monitor serum bicarbonate and chloride levels as well as folic acid and vitamin D, E, and K levels

due to acute or chronic renal failure (Chapter 132). With a normal diet, serum phosphate levels can be maintained within the normal range until the glomerular filtration rate falls below 25 mL/minute. However, even mild degrees of renal insufficiency may predispose to hyperphosphatemia if there is a concurrent excessive intake of phosphate-containing compounds such as laxatives. Finally, because parathyroid hormone stimulates proximal tubule phosphate excretion, primary hypoparathyroidism (Chapter 253) is often associated with mild hyperphosphatemia together with hypocalcemia.

CLINICAL MANIFESTATIONS

Acute hyperphosphatemia increases the risk of precipitation of calcium phosphate and subsequent metastatic calcification in soft tissues, including the kidney, where it can cause acute renal failure. The resultant hypocalcemia (Chapter 253) can cause tetany, hypotension, seizures, and cardiac arrhythmias. In the chronic hyperphosphatemia of chronic renal insufficiency, patients with a serum phosphate concentration greater than 6.5 mg/dL have higher mortality. Hyperphosphatemia in this setting is a risk factor for coronary and other vascular calcification, which is associated with increased mortality.

TREATMENT Rx

Acute hyperphosphatemia in an asymptomatic patient with normal renal function often resolves spontaneously as excess phosphate is excreted. In symptomatic patients and those with impaired renal function, phosphate should be removed by extracorporeal therapy. Because of the slow rate of phosphate mobilization from intracellular stores, continuous venovenous hemodiafiltration is considerably more effective than intermittent hemodialysis. Chronic hyperphosphatemia (Chapter 132) can be managed by minimizing dietary phosphorus intake and administering oral phosphate binders such as calcium salts (e.g., calcium acetate 1334 mg with each meal), lanthanum carbonate (500 mg with each meal), or sevelamer (800 to 1600 mg with each meal) (Table 121-4). Aluminum hydroxide (300 to 600 mg with meals) is also a very effective phosphate binder, but prolonged use leads to aluminum accumulation and results in encephalopathy and osteomalacia. Cinacalcet (30 to 180 mg/day), a calcimimetic used in patients with chronic renal insufficiency to treat secondary hyperparathyroidism, also reduces the serum phosphate concentration and calcium-phosphate product.

PROGNOSIS

Severe acute hyperphosphatemia can be life-threatening owing to metastatic calcification and multiorgan failure, but it generally responds well to prompt therapy. Chronic hyperphosphatemia in patients with chronic kidney failure (Chapter 132) is often fairly resistant to treatment, particularly in poorly compliant individuals, and is associated with increased long-term mortality.

SUGGESTED READINGS

Geerse DA, Bindels AJ, Kuiper MA, et al. Treatment of hypophosphatemia in the intensive care unit: a review. *Crit Care*. 2010;14:147. *Review.*

Musso CG. Magnesium metabolism in health and disease. *Int Urol Nephrol*. 2009;41:357-362. *Review.*

Tonelli M, Pannu N, Manns B. Oral phosphate binders in patients with kidney failure. *N Engl J Med*. 2010;362:1312-1324. *Review suggesting that calcium carbonate, calcium acetate, magnesium hydroxide, and magnesium carbonate are as good as sevelamer or lanthanum and much less expensive.*

Zeki S, Culkin A, Gabe SM, et al. Refeeding hypophosphataemia is more common in enteral than parenteral feeding in adult in patients. *Clin Nutr*. 2011. [Epub ahead of print.] *Refeeding hypophosphatemia may occur in up to one third of patients.*

122 ACUTE KIDNEY INJURY

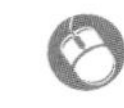

BRUCE A. MOLITORIS

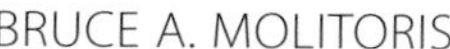

DEFINITION

Acute kidney injury (AKI) describes the clinical syndrome formerly called acute renal failure (ARF). This nomenclature defines AKI as a functional or structural abnormality of the kidney that manifests within 48 hours, as determined by blood, urine or tissue tests or by imaging studies. Diagnostically, the reduction in kidney function in AKI is associated with either an absolute increase in serum creatinine of 0.3 mg/dL or a percentage increase in serum creatinine of 50%. In addition, a reduction in urine output with oliguria (<0.5 mL/kg/hour) for more than 6 hours also fulfills the diagnostic criteria for AKI.

EPIDEMIOLOGY

Most episodes of AKI occur in the hospital, with an incidence ranging from 5 to 7% among all hospitalized patients and 15 to 40% among patients in intensive care units (ICUs). By contrast, the incidence of community-acquired AKI is no more than 1%.

Both conceptually and diagnostically, the various causes of AKI are divided broadly into three anatomic categories: prerenal, intrarenal or intrinsic, and postrenal (Fig. 122-1). Each of the categories represents a unique pathophysiologic process with distinctive diagnostic parameters and prognosis.

Prerenal Azotemia

Prerenal azotemia, which is the most common cause of AKI, accounts for approximately 60 to 70% of community-acquired and 40% of hospital-acquired cases. Decreased renal perfusion is seen in disease states that reduce intravascular volume, such as sepsis (Chapter 108), heart failure (Chapter 58), or liver failure (Chapter 157). Additionally, medications that reduce glomerular capillary perfusion, such as angiotensin-converting enzyme (ACE) inhibitors, angiotensin-receptor blockers (ARBs), and nonsteroidal anti-inflammatory drugs (NSAIDs), can also cause prerenal AKI.

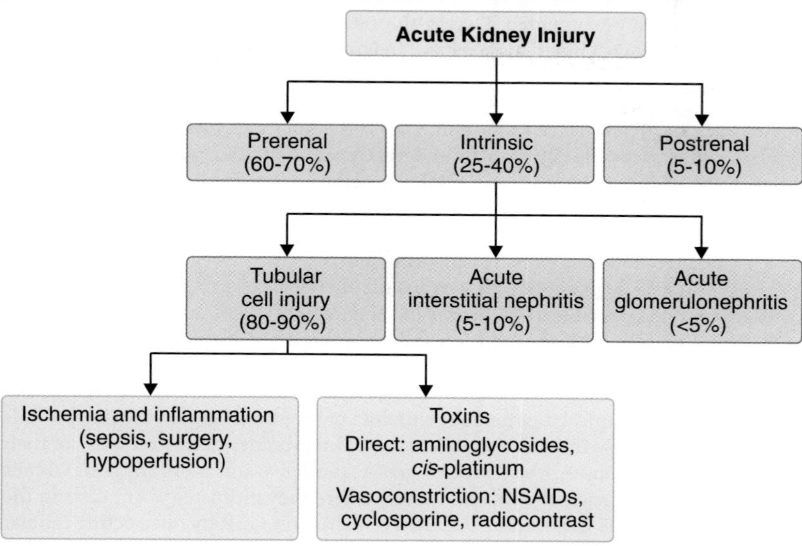

FIGURE 122-1. **Main categories of acute kidney injury.** NSAIDs = nonsteroidal anti-inflammatory drugs.

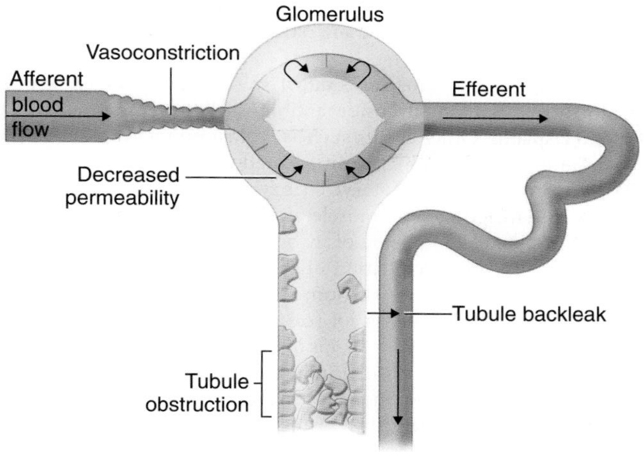

FIGURE 122-2. **Mechanisms of prerenal and intrinsic acute renal injury.** See text for descriptions.

TABLE 122-1 COMMON RENAL TUBULAR TOXINS

Aminoglycosides
Radiocontrast agents
Acyclovir
Cisplatin
Sulfonamides
Methotrexate
Cyclosporine
Tacrolimus
Amphotericin B
Foscarnet
Pentamidine
Ethylene glycol
Toluene
Cocaine
HMG-CoA reductase inhibitors

HMG-CoA = 3-hydroxy-3-methylglutaryl coenzyme A.

TABLE 122-2 MEDICATIONS ASSOCIATED WITH ACUTE INTERSTITIAL NEPHRITIS

β-LACTAM ANTIBIOTICS
Penicillin
Cephalosporins
Ampicillin
Methicillin
Nafcillin
DIURETICS
Furosemide
Hydrochlorothiazide
Triamterene
OTHER ANTIBIOTICS
Sulfonamides
Vancomycin
Rifampin
Acyclovir
Indinavir
NSAIDS
Ibuprofen
Naproxen
Indomethacin

NSAIDs = nonsteroidal anti-inflammatory drugs.

Intrinsic Acute Kidney Injury

Intrarenal AKI is often the result of untreated or untreatable prerenal azotemia that leads to ischemic AKI. The diverse causes of intrinsic AKI can involve any portion of the renal vasculature, nephron, or interstitium (Fig. 122-2). Ischemic and septic injury are major causes. Renal toxins also can damage tubules both directly and indirectly (Table 122-1). Fortunately, AKI does not develop in every patient exposed to these agents, but elderly patients with diabetes mellitus, hypotensive patients, and patients with a reduced effective arterial volume (heart failure, burns, cirrhosis, hypoalbuminemia) are the most susceptible to toxic renal injury. In fact, the incidence of aminoglycoside antibiotic nephrotoxicity increases from 3 to 5% to 30 to 50% in these high-risk patients.

AKI secondary to injury to the renal interstitium is termed *acute interstitial nephritis*. Commonly implicated medications for interstitial nephritis include penicillins, cephalosporins, sulfonamides, and NSAIDs (Table 122-2) (Chapter 124). Bacterial and viral infections can be the causative agents. Interstitial nephritis is also associated with a kidney-confined or systemic autoimmune process, such as systemic lupus erythematosus (Chapter 274), Sjögren's syndrome (Chapter 276), cryoglobulinemia (Chapter 193), and primary biliary cirrhosis (Chapter 156).

Postrenal Acute Kidney Injury

Postrenal AKI can occur in the setting of bilateral urinary outflow obstruction or in a patient with a solitary kidney when a single urinary outflow tract is obstructed (Chapter 125). Most commonly, this type of outflow obstruction is observed in patients with prostatic hypertrophy (Chapter 131), prostatic or cervical cancer (Chapter 205), or retroperitoneal disorders. A functional obstruction can be observed in patients with a neurogenic bladder. In addition, intraluminal obstruction can be seen in patients with bilateral renal calculi (Chapter 128), papillary necrosis, blood clots, and bladder carcinoma, whereas extraluminal obstruction can develop in connection with retroperitoneal fibrosis, colon cancer, and lymphomas. Finally, intratubular crystallization of compounds such as uric acid, calcium oxalate, acyclovir, sulfonamide, and methotrexate, as well as myeloma light chains, can result in tubular obstruction.

PATHOBIOLOGY

The etiology of AKI is diverse, and it can arise from a number of physiologic insults that injure the kidney and reduce the glomerular filtration rate (GFR). Decreased kidney perfusion and a reduced GFR can occur with or without cellular injury; toxic, ischemic, or obstructive injury to the renal tubule; inflammation and edema of the tubulointerstitium; and a primary glomerular disease process.

Prerenal Acute Kidney Injury

The precipitating event for prerenal AKI is renal hypoperfusion (see Fig. 122-2), which can be caused by a reduction in the volume of extracellular fluid or disease states associated with normal or even increased extracellular fluid volumes but decrements in effective arterial volume, such as in sepsis, heart failure, and advanced cirrhosis. Prerenal azotemia is also divided functionally into volume responsive and nonresponsive azotemia, based on the etiology. For example, in severe heart failure (Chapter 58), additional intravascular volume may not improve kidney perfusion, whereas afterload reduction may. Early in the course of prerenal AKI, the renal parenchyma remains intact and functional. During this initial phase, the GFR remains largely intact because renal hypoperfusion initiates a neurohormonal cascade that results in afferent arteriolar dilation and efferent arteriolar constriction. Because prerenal azotemia is often easily reversible and mortality rates are low, early diagnosis and correction of the underlying pathophysiology are of critical importance. However, without early medical corrective intervention, prerenal azotemia progresses, ischemia worsens, and the resulting injury to tubular epithelial cells further decreases the GFR. This progression from prerenal azotemia to ischemic AKI is a continuum that depends on the severity and duration of the physiologic insult.

Intrarenal Acute Kidney Injury

Intrinsic AKI is classified according to the primary histologic site of injury: tubules, interstitium, vasculature, or glomerulus. Renal tubular epithelial cell injury, commonly termed *acute tubular necrosis* (ATN), occurs more commonly in the setting of ischemia, although the renal tubules can also be damaged by specific renal toxins. Ischemia can arise from a number of different clinical scenarios, but the common underlying pathogenesis is reduced renal blood flow (Table 122-3) with progression from prerenal azotemia to ischemic AKI in four distinct clinical and cellular phases: initiation, extension, maintenance, and recovery. Each of these phases encompasses distinct cellular events and declines in GFR as the kidneys respond to the insult and attempt to maintain and reestablish function (Fig. 122-3). The initiation phase, which marks the transition from prerenal to tubular cell injury and dysfunction, is characterized by severe cellular depletion of adenosine triphosphate. Renal tubular epithelial cell injury is a prominent feature during this phase; however, endothelial and vascular smooth muscle cell injury has also been documented. During the extension phase, microvascular congestion with continued hypoxia and inflammation are most pronounced in the corticomedullary junction of the kidney, where reperfusion is limited owing to endothelial dysfunction at the capillary and postcapillary venule levels, with white blood cell adhesion. The GFR is at its ebb during the maintenance phase, but cells continue to undergo repair, migration, and proliferation, as the kidney attempts to reestablish cellular and tubular integrity. Finally, during the recovery phase, the GFR begins to improve as cellular differentiation continues and normal cellular and organ function returns. This last phase is often heralded by increasing urine output.

The S3 segment of the proximal tubule is located in the outer stripe of the medullary region of the nephron. This region is particularly susceptible to continued reduced perfusion following injury, and ongoing or worsening hypoxia results in continued cellular injury. Proximal tubular cell injury during the initiation phase of renal ischemia is first manifested as bleb formation in the apical membranes, with loss of the brush border. Proximal tubule cells also lose the polarity of the surface membrane and the integrity of their tight junctions. As the injury progresses, both live and necrotic proximal cells detach and enter the tubular lumen, where they ultimately form casts in the distal tubule. Casts contribute to a reduction in GFR by obstructing tubular urine flow, thereby preventing further filtration into that nephron. In addition, loss of the epithelial cell barrier and cell tight junctions allows backleak of the glomerular filtrate into the interstitium, thus further compromising GFR (see Fig. 122-2).

Common agents that can cause direct tubular cell toxicity (see Table 122-1) include the aminoglycoside antibiotics, intravenous radiocontrast agents, and cisplatin. Other agents such as radiocontrast dyes, NSAIDs, and cyclosporine induce vasoconstriction and reduce renal perfusion. Cocaine and the 3-hydroxy-3-methylglutaryl coenzyme A (HMG-CoA) reductase inhibitors can damage skeletal muscle and cause *rhabdomyolysis* (Chapter 115), which results in the release of myoglobin that is toxic to the tubular epithelium. Finally, the precipitation of some compounds or their metabolites can cause intratubular obstruction; agents in this category include acyclovir, sulfonamides, ethylene glycol (calcium oxalate metabolite; Chapter 110), methotrexate, and the light chains of multiple myeloma (Chapter 193).

In AKI caused by the interstitial injury, a mixed inflammatory infiltrate composed of T lymphocytes, monocytes, and macrophages, is seen. These inflammatory lesions can be diffuse or patchy in distribution. Granulomas can also occasionally be observed, especially in drug hypersensitivity reactions. Acute interstitial nephritis that persists and becomes chronic is characterized by interstitial fibrosis and tubular atrophy, although foci of inflammatory cells can persist. This process can lead to chronic and even end-stage kidney disease requiring chronic dialysis.

Vascular causes of intrinsic AKI can include microvascular and macrovascular processes. Classic microvascular disorders, which include thrombotic thrombocytopenic purpura (Chapter 175), sepsis (Chapter 108), hemolytic-uremic syndrome (Chapter 127), and the HELLP syndrome (*h*emolysis, *e*levated *l*iver enzymes, and *l*ow *p*latelet count; Chapter 153), cause AKI as a

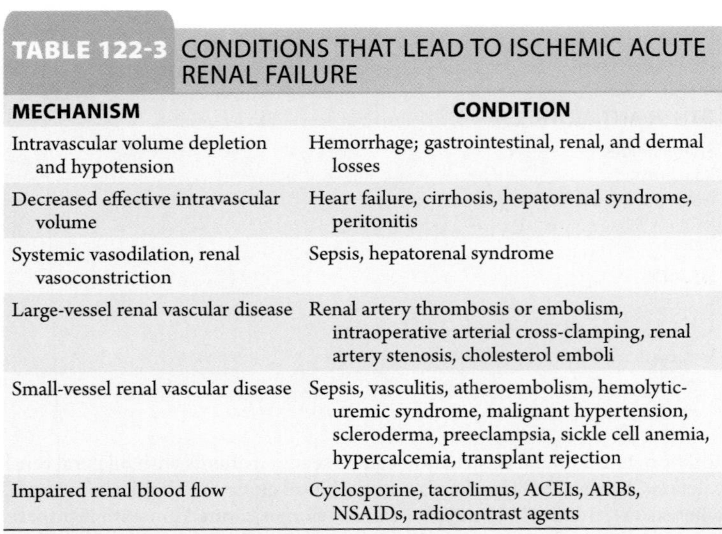

TABLE 122-3 CONDITIONS THAT LEAD TO ISCHEMIC ACUTE RENAL FAILURE

MECHANISM	CONDITION
Intravascular volume depletion and hypotension	Hemorrhage; gastrointestinal, renal, and dermal losses
Decreased effective intravascular volume	Heart failure, cirrhosis, hepatorenal syndrome, peritonitis
Systemic vasodilation, renal vasoconstriction	Sepsis, hepatorenal syndrome
Large-vessel renal vascular disease	Renal artery thrombosis or embolism, intraoperative arterial cross-clamping, renal artery stenosis, cholesterol emboli
Small-vessel renal vascular disease	Sepsis, vasculitis, atheroembolism, hemolytic-uremic syndrome, malignant hypertension, scleroderma, preeclampsia, sickle cell anemia, hypercalcemia, transplant rejection
Impaired renal blood flow	Cyclosporine, tacrolimus, ACEIs, ARBs, NSAIDs, radiocontrast agents

ACEIs = angiotensin-converting enzyme inhibitors; ARBs = angiotensin-receptor blockers; NSAIDs = nonsteroidal anti-inflammatory drugs.

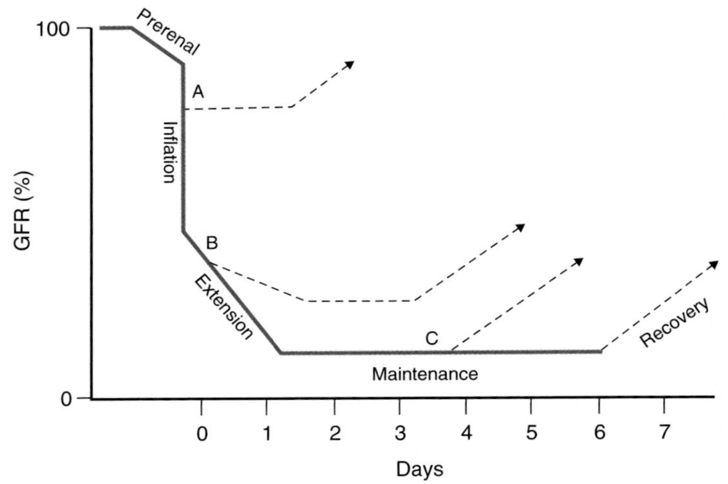

FIGURE 122-3. **Phases of acute kidney injury.** GFR = glomerular filtration rate. (From Sutton TA, Fisher CJ, Molitoris BA. Microvascular endothelial injury and dysfunction during ischemic acute renal failure. *Kidney Int.* 2002;62:1539-1549.)

result of glomerular capillary thrombosis and microvascular occlusion. Macrovascular disease such as atherosclerosis can cause AKI secondary to atheroembolization (Chapter 126), especially during or after an invasive or interventional vascular procedure in a patient with preexisting atherosclerotic disease.

A less common cause of AKI is glomerulonephritis (Chapter 123), which can be seen in systemic lupus nephritis (Chapter 274), Wegener's granulomatosis (Chapter 278), polyarteritis nodosa (Chapter 278), Goodpasture's syndrome (Chapter 123), Henoch-Schönlein purpura (Chapter 278), and hemolytic-uremic syndrome (Chapter 176). AKI in this setting is termed *rapidly progressive glomerulonephritis* and results from direct inflammatory glomerular or vascular injury.

Postrenal Acute Kidney Injury

Postrenal AKI is caused by obstruction to luminal flow of the glomerular filtrate. This obstruction results in a relatively complex pathophysiology that begins with transmission of backpressure to Bowman's space of the glomerulus. Intuitively, this backpressure would be expected to reduce the GFR. However, by dilation of the glomerular afferent arteriole, the GFR remains largely preserved. Unfortunately, such compensation is only transient, and the GFR will begin to attenuate if the obstruction is not rapidly relieved. With continued obstruction for more than 12 to 24 hours, renal blood flow and intratubular pressure decline, and large unperfused and underperfused areas of the renal cortex result in a reduction in GFR.

CLINICAL MANIFESTATIONS

AKI, even when advanced, frequently is first diagnosed by abnormalities observed in a patient's laboratory studies and not by any specific symptom or sign. The clinical manifestations associated with AKI are frequently protean, occur late in the course, and are often not apparent until the renal dysfunction has become severe. The clinical findings of AKI also depend on the stage at which it is diagnosed. Patients with AKI may report symptoms such as anorexia, fatigue, nausea and vomiting, and pruritus, as well as a decline in urine output or dark-colored urine. Furthermore, if the patient has become volume overloaded, shortness of breath and dyspnea on exertion may be noted.

A thorough physical examination with special emphasis on determination of volume status and effective arterial volume is essential. If volume overload is present, jugular venous distention, pulmonary crackles, and peripheral edema may be found (Chapter 58). Findings such as asterixis, myoclonus, or a pericardial rub may be seen in severe AKI.

DIAGNOSIS

A systematic approach that considers each of the three major categories in the pathogenesis of AKI will ensure that an accurate diagnosis and an appropriate therapeutic plan will be achieved. An appropriate diagnostic strategy is to exclude prerenal and postrenal causes first and then, if needed, begin an evaluation for possible intrinsic causes.

Laboratory analysis of blood and urine samples of patients with AKI reveals the level of dysfunction, will frequently suggest a cause, and may also direct the rapidity with which a specific therapy needs to be instituted. All patients with clinical findings of AKI should be evaluated with serum measurements of electrolytes, creatinine, calcium, and phosphorus; a blood urea nitrogen level; and complete blood count with differential. In addition, urine studies, including sodium, potassium, chloride, and creatinine (Cr) determinations for calculation of the fractional excretion of sodium (FE_{Na}), are important. The formula for calculating FE_{Na} is as follows:

$$FE_{Na} = \frac{\text{Urine Na} \times \text{Plasma Cr}}{\text{Plasma Na} \times \text{Urine Cr}} \times 100$$

The numerical value of FE_{Na} can be helpful in determining the potential cause of the AKI (Table 122-4). In some cases, it is better to use FE_{Cl} because urinary sodium can be elevated during systemic alkalosis when a high urinary bicarbonate level obligates the loss of sodium. Urine dipstick and microscopy (Table 122-5) should be performed on a fresh urine sample because important cellular elements that could indicate potential causes degrade rapidly with time. Finally, renal ultrasound to determine the presence or absence of outlet obstruction should also be included in the initial evaluation. Measurement of serum levels of structural biomarkers, such as kidney injury molecule 1 (KIM-1) and neutrophil gelatinase-associated lipocalin (NGAL), may aid in the diagnosis of AKI, although the data are not yet conclusive.

TABLE 122-4 FE_{Na} VALUES FOR THE VARIOUS CAUSES OF ACUTE KIDNEY INJURY

ETIOLOGY OF ACUTE KIDNEY INJURY	FE_{Na}	BUN-TO-SERUM CREATININE RATIO
Prerenal	<1%	>20
Intrarenal		<10-15
Tubular necrosis	≥1%	
Interstitial nephritis	≥1%	
Glomerulonephritis (early)	<1%	
Vascular disorders (early)	<1%	
Postrenal	≥1%	>20

TABLE 122-5 COMMON URINALYSIS FINDINGS IN ACUTE KIDNEY INJURY

CAUSE OF ACUTE KIDNEY INJURY	URINALYSIS
Prerenal	Normal or hyaline casts
Intrarenal	
Tubular cell injury	Muddy-brown, granular, epithelial casts
Interstitial nephritis	Pyuria, hematuria, mild proteinuria, granular and epithelial casts, eosinophils
Glomerulonephritis	Hematuria, marked proteinuria, red blood cell casts, granular casts
Vascular disorders	Normal or hematuria, mild proteinuria
Postrenal	Normal or hematuria, granular casts, pyuria

PRERENAL AZOTEMIA

Prerenal azotemia, which is the most common cause of renal dysfunction, can often be determined by the patient's history. Common historical features in patients with prerenal azotemia include vomiting, diarrhea, and poor oral intake. Heart failure can suggest a possible prerenal cause of reduced renal perfusion from overdiuresis or as exacerbation of the heart failure itself. Other medications that can attenuate renal perfusion, such as NSAIDs, ACE inhibitors, and ARBs, can cause prerenal azotemia. Common physical examination findings include tachycardia, systemic or orthostatic hypotension (or both), and dry mucous membranes.

Laboratory studies in patients with prerenal azotemia demonstrate elevated serum creatinine and blood urea nitrogen (BUN) levels. FE_{Na} is typically less than 1%. However, in a patient taking diuretics such as furosemide, FE_{Na} may be greater than 1% even though the patient has prerenal azotemia because of diuretic-induced natriuresis. For these clinical situations, the fractional excretion of urea can be used and is calculated in similar fashion:

$$FE_{urea} = \frac{\text{Urine urea} \times \text{Plasma Cr}}{\text{Plasma urea} \times \text{Urine Cr}} \times 100$$

FE_{urea} less than 35% suggests prerenal AKI. Other causes of an FE_{Na} greater than 1% include the presence of a non-reabsorbable solute such as bicarbonate, glucose, or mannitol. Chronic kidney disease, ATN, and late obstructive nephropathy are also associated with FE_{Na} greater than 1%. Therefore, in these disease states, FE_{Na} cannot provide reliable diagnostic information regarding AKI unless the FE_{Na} is less than 1%. Moreover, FE_{urea} has not been validated for these clinical entities.

Another laboratory parameter to assist in diagnosing prerenal AKI is the ratio of BUN to serum creatinine. Commonly, a patient with prerenal azotemia will have a BUN-to-serum creatinine ratio of greater than 20 : 1.

INTRARENAL ACUTE KIDNEY INJURY

A history of hypotension or exposure to a nephrotoxin or medication is a common finding in patients with intrarenal AKI. The nephrotoxin can be a specific tubular toxin that causes ATN or a medication that causes an allergic reaction as in acute interstitial nephritis (see Tables 122-1 and 122-2). Physical examination may reveal signs and symptoms of fluid overload. Rash may accompany acute interstitial nephritis. Cholesterol embolism in patients with severe atherosclerotic disease (Chapter 127) may manifest classically as cyanotic digits and AKI; this finding is frequently seen after invasive vascular surgery or an interventional study.

Laboratory studies will demonstrate elevated serum creatinine and BUN levels in intrarenal AKI. ATN and acute interstitial nephritis are frequently associated with FE_{Na} greater than 1, whereas FE_{Na} is typically less than 1 in glomerulonephritis and vascular disorders. Peripheral eosinophilia and urinary eosinophils may be present in acute interstitial nephritis, although the latter are neither sensitive nor specific for this type of AKI. Urinary eosinophils are also associated with cholesterol microembolic disease (Chapter 127). Intrarenal AKI has specific urinalysis findings that can be helpful in making diagnostic and therapeutic decisions (see Table 122-5).

POSTRENAL ACUTE KIDNEY INJURY

A history of prostatic hypertrophy (Chapter 131), prostate cancer (Chapter 207), lymphoma (Chapter 191), cervical cancer (Chapter 205), or retroperitoneal disease can often be found in patients with postrenal AKI. Postrenal AKI should always be in the differential diagnosis of patients with severe oliguria (urine output < 450 mL/day) or anuria (urine output < 100 mL/day). However, many patients with postrenal AKI are neither oliguric nor anuric. Beyond an elevation in a patient's serum creatinine and BUN levels, laboratory studies generally yield benign results. Bladder catheterization can be both diagnostic and therapeutic in postrenal AKI. However, renal ultrasound is the diagnostic test of choice, although it may be falsely negative early in postrenal AKI.

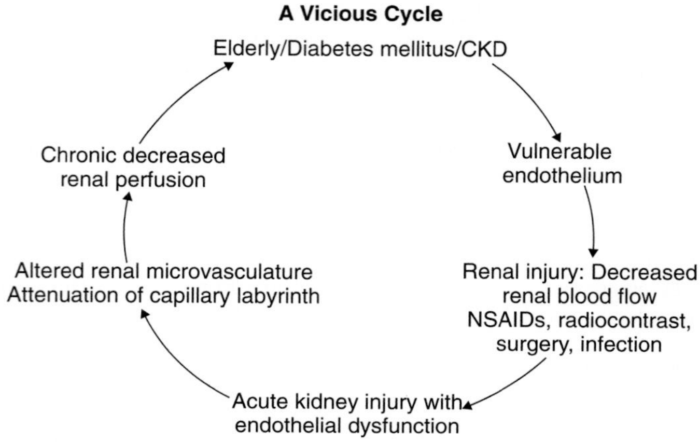

FIGURE 122-4. A vicious cycle exists between acute kidney injury (AKI) and chronic kidney disease (CKD), with CKD increasing the risk of developing AKI, and AKI accelerating progression of CKD.

TREATMENT Rx

The cornerstones of therapy for AKI are rapid recognition and correction of reversible causes, avoidance of any further renal injury, and correction and maintenance of a normal electrolyte and fluid volume milieu. Preventive therapy or medical interventions performed during the initiation and extension phases of AKI provide the greatest chance for minimizing the extent of injury (see Fig. 122-3, lines A and B) and hastening renal recovery (see Fig. 122-3, line B); interventions provided during the maintenance phase of AKI have not proved beneficial (see Fig. 122-3, line C). If prerenal AKI is not addressed early in a patient's course or if the patient is seen late in the course, ATN may occur and markedly increase morbidity and mortality.

Prerenal azotemia in its early stages often can be rapidly corrected by aggressive normalization of effective arterial volume, although more care must be taken during volume resuscitation in patients with a history of heart failure. Key approaches include administering volume (e.g., normal saline) to achieve euvolemia, improving cardiac output by afterload reduction (Chapter 59), or normalizing systemic vascular resistance.

Postrenal AKI secondary to prostatic hypertrophy can frequently be corrected by placement of a bladder catheter. However, outlet obstruction from a neoplastic process will usually require urologic consultation for consideration of ureteral stenting or placement of a percutaneous nephrostomy tube.

Intrarenal AKI can be the most complex and difficult to treat. AKI caused by glomerulonephritis (Chapter 123) or vasculitis (Chapters 274 and 278) will frequently require immunosuppressive therapy. For suspected acute interstitial nephritis, the offending medication must be determined and discontinued; a 2-week tapering course of glucocorticoids, beginning with 1 mg/kg of prednisone for 3 days, is commonly recommended despite the absence of definitive data.

General supportive measures include avoiding any further nephrotoxins and paying careful attention to the patient's fluid balance by monitoring weight and daily input and output. In addition, serum electrolytes, creatinine, and BUN should be monitored at least daily, more frequently if the patient's renal function appears to be tenuous. Patients with AKI should also receive a low sodium, potassium, and protein diet, which can be liberalized as the patient's renal function improves. A phosphate binder (e.g., calcium acetate [1334 mg], lanthanum carbonate [500 mg], sevelamer [300 to 1000 mg], or aluminum hydroxide [300 to 600 mg] with each meal; see Table 121-4) is also usually helpful in controlling the serum phosphate level by minimizing the absorption of dietary phosphate.

Early nephrology consultation will ensure that the patient receives optimal care. Some patients will warrant urgent hemodialysis because of marked metabolic acidosis unresponsive to sodium bicarbonate infusions; electrolyte abnormalities, such as hyperkalemia that is unresponsive to medical management; pulmonary edema not responding to diuretic therapy; and uremic symptoms of encephalopathy, seizures, and pericarditis. In the absence of acute indications, however, when to initiate dialysis in AKI remains unresolved.

For AKI, intensive dialytic renal support therapy is no better than standard dialytic therapy,[1] and intermittent hemodialysis and continuous renal replacement therapy lead to similar clinical outcomes in acute renal failure.[2] Neither furosemide[3] nor low-dose dopamine[4] improve outcome, even though low-dose dopamine may temporarily improve metrics of renal physiology.

PREVENTION

Given the marked increase in morbidity and mortality associated with AKI, especially for critically ill patients, potential measures to prevent AKI are essential. The first step in prevention, however, is being aware of patients who are at highest risk for AKI because of known kidney disease or comorbid medical conditions, such as diabetes, hypertension, nephrotic syndrome, heart failure, and peripheral vascular disease.

Of all the risk factors for acquiring AKI, the presence of preexisting chronic kidney disease is the most predictive. Recent data document a vicious cycle involving AKI and CKD (Fig. 122-4). Appropriate hospital surveillance measures include avoiding nephrotoxic medications (e.g., NSAIDs and aminoglycosides); minimizing diagnostic procedures that require radiocontrast material, especially in the prerenal patient; and careful monitoring of urinary output with daily determination of serum electrolytes and creatinine levels after any procedures known to induce AKI. Additionally, educating the patient regarding common nonprescription nephrotoxins such as NSAIDs can reduce the risk for AKI in outpatients.

Before a potentially nephrotoxic exposure, early consultation with a nephrologist is warranted for this high-risk group to advise whether a specific medication or intervention may reduce the risk of AKI or whether an alternative medication or procedure, such as magnetic resonance imaging instead of computed tomography with intravenous radiocontrast agents, may be preferred. All potential nephrotoxins, such as NSAIDs, should be discontinued before a potentially nephrotoxic procedure and avoided after it. The patient's volume and hemodynamic status must be maximized.

In high-risk patients, a renal protective intervention is often instituted before exposure to the agent. Interventions that may be useful for preventing AKI associated with intravenous radiocontrast agents include sodium bicarbonate[5] (e.g., 15 mEq/L infused at 3 mL/kg/hour for 1 hour before the procedure and at 1 mL/kg/hour for 6 hours after it) and N-acetylcysteine[6] (usually 600 mg orally or intravenously 4 hours before the procedure), although the data for each individually or even the two together remain controversial.[7]

PROGNOSIS

Typically, AKI secondary to prerenal causes, if diagnosed and treated early, has the best prognosis for renal recovery. Patients with prerenal AKI commonly return to their baseline level of renal function and have a mortality rate of less than 10%. Similarly, patients with postrenal AKI also have a good prognosis for renal recovery if the outlet obstruction is promptly diagnosed and definitively treated.

In contrast, patients with intrarenal AKI have a less predictable renal outcome, and mortality in this group varies between 30 and 80%, depending on the severity of injury. Higher mortality rates occur in older patients with hospital-acquired AKI admitted to ICUs. Furthermore, mortality in patients with AKI is incremental, and seemingly modest increases in serum creatinine can result in marked increases in the mortality rate. Even a rise in serum creatinine of only 0.3 mg/dL results in a significantly increased risk of mortality.

The clinical course after recovery from ATN is subsequent tubular regeneration with recovery of renal function. However, this outcome is less ensured in patients with preexisting kidney disease. In addition, given the frequent systemic nature of their illness, patients with ATN, glomerulonephritis, and vasculitic causes of AKI may not fully recover to their baseline renal function. Patients who have a severe episode of AKI requiring hemodialysis may not recover their renal function and may need hemodialysis indefinitely (Chapter 133), especially if they have a preexisting history of chronic kidney disease. AKI hastens progression of chronic kidney disease to end-stage kidney disease and is often the major factor that causes such progression.

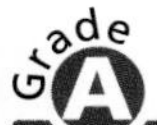

1. Palevsky PM, Zhang JH, et al. VA/NIH Acute Renal Failure Trial Network. Intensity of renal support in critically ill patients with acute kidney injury. *N Engl J Med.* 2008;359:7-20.
2. Pannu N, Klarenbach S, Wiebe N, et al. Renal replacement therapy in patients with acute renal failure: a systematic review. *JAMA.* 2008;299:793-805.
3. Ho KM, Sheridan DJ. Meta-analysis of furosemide to prevent or treat acute renal failure. *BMJ.* 2006;333:420.
4. Friedrich JO, Adhikary N, Herridge MS, et al. Meta-analysis: low-dose dopamine increases urine output but does not prevent renal dysfunction or death. *Ann Intern Med.* 2005;142:510-524.
5. Zoungas S, Ninomiya T, Huyley R, et al. Systematic review: sodium bicarbonate treatment regimens for the prevention of contrast-induced nephropathy. *Ann Intern Med.* 2009;151:631-638.
6. Trivedi H, Daram S, Szabo A, et al. High-dose N-acetylcysteine for the prevention of contrast-induced nephropathy. *Am J Med.* 2009;122:874.
7. Brown JR, Block CA, Malenka DJ, et al. Sodium bicarbonate plus N-acetylcysteine prophylaxis: a meta-analysis. *JACC Cardiovasc Interv.* 2009;2:1116-1124.

SUGGESTED READINGS

Anderson S, Eldadah B, Halter JB, et al. Acute kidney injury in older adults. *J Am Soc Nephrol.* 2011;22:28-38. *Review.*

Brochard L, Abroug F, Brenner M, et al. An Official ATS/ERS/ESICM/SCCM/SRLF Statement: prevention and management of acute renal failure in the ICU patient. An international consensus conference in intensive care medicine. *Am J Respir Crit Care Med.* 2010;181:1128-1155. *Review.*

Devarajan P. Biomarkers for the early detection of acute kidney injury. *Curr Opin Pediatr.* 2011;23:194-200. *Overview including the potential usefulness of neutrophil gelatinase-associated lipocalin (NGAL).*

Solomon P, Dauerman HL. Contrast-induced acute kidney injury. *Circulation.* 2010;122:2451-2455. *Review recommending hydration with normal saline or sodium bicarbonate.*

123

GLOMERULAR DISORDERS AND NEPHROTIC SYNDROMES

GERALD B. APPEL AND JAI RADHAKRISHNAN

GLOMERULAR DISORDERS

DEFINITION

Each *glomerulus,* the basic filtering unit of the kidney, consists of a tuft of anastomosing capillaries formed by the branching of the afferent arteriole. Approximately 1 million glomeruli comprise about 5% of the kidney weight and provide almost 2 m^2 of glomerular capillary filtering surface. The glomerular basement membrane provides both a size- and charge-selective barrier to the passage of circulating macromolecules. Renal pathology involving all glomeruli is called *diffuse* or *generalized;* if only some glomeruli are involved, the process is called *focal.* When dealing with the individual glomerulus, a process is *global* if the whole glomerular tuft is involved and *segmental* if only part of the glomerulus is involved. The modifying terms *proliferative, sclerosing,* and *necrotizing* are often used (e.g., focal and segmental glomerulosclerosis; diffuse global proliferative lupus nephritis). Extracapillary proliferation or crescent formation is caused by the accumulations of macrophages, fibroblasts, proliferating epithelial cells, and fibrin within Bowman's space. In general, crescent formation in any form of glomerular damage conveys a serious prognosis. Scarring of the tissue between the tubules and glomeruli, interstitial fibrosis, is also a poor prognostic sign in every glomerular disease.

EPIDEMIOLOGY

At present, about 17% of the U.S. population has proteinuria or renal dysfunction, and many, if not most, cases are caused by glomerular diseases. More than 500,000 Americans are in end-stage renal disease (ESRD) programs, and chronic kidney disease costs about $60 billion per year and accounts for about 28% of all Medicare spending, largely as a result of renal involvement by glomerular diseases. Diabetic renal damage alone affects many millions of persons and is the major cause of ESRD in the United States (Chapter 126). Worldwide, glomerular diseases associated with infectious agents such as malaria (Chapter 353) and schistosomiasis (Chapter 363) are still major health problems. The emergence of glomerular diseases linked to human immunodeficiency virus (HIV) and the hepatitis B and C viruses (Chapter 151) has focused new attention on the patterns and mechanisms of glomerular injury. Manifestations of glomerular injury range from asymptomatic microhematuria and albuminuria to rapidly progressive oliguric renal failure. Some patients develop massive fluid retention and edema at onset of their glomerular disease, whereas others present with only the slow insidious signs and symptoms of chronic renal failure (Chapter 132).

PATHOBIOLOGY

Common mechanisms such as breaks in the glomerular capillary wall and loss of the selective barrier to particles based on size and charge underlie the proteinuria and hematuria that are characteristic of glomerular diseases. Nevertheless, the nature of the initiating processes varies among different glomerular diseases. In some glomerular disorders, such as diabetes and amyloidosis, structural and biochemical alterations are present in the glomerular capillary wall. In others, immune-mediated renal injury is caused by deposition of circulating immune complexes, the localized effects of anti–glomerular basement membrane (anti-GBM) antibodies, or other mechanisms.

CLINICAL MANIFESTATIONS

Findings indicative of a glomerular origin of renal disease include erythrocyte casts and dysmorphic red blood cells (RBCs) in the urinary sediment as well as large amounts of albuminuria. Persistent urinary excretion of more than 500 to 1000 erythrocytes per milliliter (or greater than two RBCs per high-power field on microscopy) is abnormal. Dysmorphic RBCs, which are deformed as a result of their passage through the glomerular capillary wall and tubules, and red blood cell casts, which are formed when these erythrocytes become enmeshed in a proteinaceous matrix in the lumen of the tubules, are also indicative of glomerular disease.

In a normal person, the urinary excretion of albumin is less than 30 mg/day, and the total urinary excretion of protein is less than 150 mg/day. Although increases in urinary protein excretion may come from the filtration of abnormal circulating proteins (e.g., light chains in multiple myeloma) or from the deficient proximal tubular reabsorption of normal, filtered low-molecular-weight proteins (e.g., β_2-microglobulin), the most common cause of proteinuria, and specifically albuminuria, is glomerular injury. Proteinuria associated with glomerular disease may range from several hundred milligrams to more than 30 g daily. In some diseases, such as minimal change nephrotic syndrome, albumin is the predominant protein in the urine. In others, such as focal sclerosing glomerulonephritis and diabetes, the proteinuria, although still largely composed of albumin, is nonselective and contains many higher-molecular-weight proteins.

DIAGNOSIS

Some patients have asymptomatic microhematuria or proteinuria discovered by routine evaluations. Microscopic hematuria associated with deformed RBCs or RBC casts is likely to be glomerular in origin. Subnephrotic levels of proteinuria may arise from orthostatic proteinuria, hypertension, tubular disease, or glomerular damage.

In patients with asymptomatic urinary abnormalities of glomerular origin, the underlying glomerular lesion may represent the early phase of one of the progressive glomerular diseases or may be due to a benign, nonprogressive glomerular lesion. In general, if patients have less than 1 g of proteinuria daily or glomerular microhematuria but a normal glomerular filtration rate (GFR) and no evidence of systemic disease based on a careful history, physical examination, and serologic tests, it is not necessary to proceed to a renal biopsy to establish a diagnosis, because most of these patients need no immunosuppressive therapy. The patient can be followed closely, and biopsy need be performed only in patients with progressively increasing proteinuria or evidence of a decreasing GFR.

TABLE 123-1 TYPICAL FINDINGS OF NEPHROTIC SYNDROME VERSUS NEPHRITIS

NEPHROTIC SYNDROME	NEPHRITIS
RENAL INSUFFICIENCY	
Uncommon	Common at presentation
PROTEINURIA	
Typically high (>3 g/day)	Variable
URINE RBCs	
Few	Prominent
URINE RBC CASTS	
Unlikely	Likely

RBCs = red blood cells.

TABLE 123-2 CAUSES OF IDIOPATHIC NEPHROTIC SYNDROME IN ADULTS

	INCIDENCE (%)
Minimal change disease	5-10
Focal segmental glomerulosclerosis	20-25
Membranous nephropathy	25-30
Membranoproliferative glomerulonephritis	5
Other proliferative and sclerosing glomerulonephritides	15-30

TABLE 123-3 NEPHROTIC SYNDROME ASSOCIATED WITH SPECIFIC CAUSES ("SECONDARY" NEPHROTIC SYNDROME)

SYSTEMIC DISEASES

Diabetes mellitus
Systemic lupus erythematosus and other collagen diseases
Amyloidosis (amyloid AL- or AA-associated)
Vasculitic-immunologic disease (mixed cryoglobulinemia, Wegener's granulomatosis, rapidly progressive glomerulonephritis, polyarteritis, Henoch-Schönlein purpura, sarcoidosis, Goodpasture's syndrome)

INFECTIONS

Bacterial (post-streptococcal, congenital and secondary syphilis, subacute bacterial endocarditis, cerebral ventriculoatrial shunt nephritis)
Viral (hepatitis B, hepatitis C, HIV infection, infectious mononucleosis, cytomegalovirus infection)
Parasitic (malaria, toxoplasmosis, schistosomiasis, filariasis)

MEDICATION RELATED

Gold, mercury, and the heavy metals
Penicillamine
Nonsteroidal anti-inflammatory drugs including COX2 inhibitors
Lithium
Paramethadione, trimethadione
Captopril
"Street" heroin
Others: probenecid, chlorpropamide, rifampin, tolbutamide, phenindione, pamidronate

ALLERGENS, VENOMS, AND IMMUNIZATIONS

NEOPLASMS

Hodgkin's lymphoma and leukemias/lymphomas (with minimal change lesion)
Solid tumors (with membranous nephropathy)

HEREDITARY AND METABOLIC DISEASE

Alport's syndrome
Fabry's disease
Sickle cell disease
Congenital (Finnish type) nephrotic syndrome
Familial nephrotic syndrome
Nail-patella syndrome
Partial lipodystrophy

OTHER

Pregnancy related (includes preeclampsia)
Transplant rejection
Serum sickness
Accelerated hypertensive nephrosclerosis
Unilateral renal artery stenosis
Massive obesity–sleep apnea
Reflux nephropathy

THE NEPHROTIC SYNDROME

DEFINITION

The nephrotic syndrome (Table 123-1) is defined by albuminuria in amounts of more than 3 to 3.5 g/day accompanied by hypoalbuminemia, edema, and hyperlipidemia. In practice, many clinicians refer to "nephrotic range" proteinuria regardless of whether their patients have the other manifestations of the full syndrome, which is a consequence of the proteinuria.

EPIDEMIOLOGY

Many cases of the nephrotic syndrome are idiopathic (Table 123-2), but others are caused by known underlying conditions (Table 123-3). Although minimal change disease is the most common cause of nephrotic syndrome in children, idiopathic membranous nephropathy and focal segmental glomerular sclerosis are the most common causes in adults. In England, men account for about 58% of hospitalizations for nephrotic syndrome, and the mean hospital length of stay for nephrotic syndrome is about 6 days.

PATHOBIOLOGY

Hypoalbuminemia is largely a consequence of urinary protein loss. It also can be due to the catabolism of filtered albumin by the proximal tubule, the redistribution of albumin within the body, and the reduced hepatic synthesis of albumin. As a result, the relationship among urinary protein loss, the level of the serum albumin, and other secondary consequences of heavy albuminuria is inexact.

The salt and volume retention in the nephrotic syndrome may occur through at least two different major mechanisms. The classic teaching is that hypoalbuminemia reduces the oncotic pressure of plasma, the resulting intravascular volume depletion leads to activation of the renin-angiotensin-aldosterone axis, and this activation increases the retention of renal sodium and fluid. However, primary salt retention in the distal nephron also may occur independently of the renin-angiotensin-aldosterone axis.

CLINICAL MANIFESTATIONS

Patients may present with weight gain, peripheral edema, and periorbital edema. Hypertension is common. The urinalysis shows more than 3+ of proteinuria and varying degrees of hematuria, depending on the cause. A 24-hour urine usually shows 3 to 5 mg/kg/day of proteinuria.

Nephrotic patients often have a hypercoagulable state and are predisposed to deep vein thrombosis (Chapter 81), pulmonary emboli (Chapter 98), and renal vein thrombosis (Chapter 127). Patients with the nephrotic syndrome have increased risk of atherosclerotic complications. Most nephrotic patients have elevated levels of total and low-density lipoprotein (LDL) cholesterol with low or normal high-density lipoprotein (HDL) cholesterol. Lipoprotein(a) levels are elevated as well and return to normal with remission of the nephrotic syndrome.

DIAGNOSIS

Initial evaluation of the nephrotic patient includes laboratory tests to define whether the patient has primary idiopathic nephrotic syndrome (see Table 123-2) or a secondary cause related to a systemic disease, toxin, or medication (see Table 123-3). Common screening tests include the fasting blood sugar and glycosylated hemoglobin tests for diabetes, an antinuclear antibody test for collagen vascular disease, and a serum complement level, which screens for many immune complex–mediated diseases (Table 123-4). In selected patients, cryoglobulins, hepatitis B and C serologies, HIV testing, antineutrophil cytoplasmic antibodies (ANCAs), anti-GBM antibodies, serum protein electrophoresis, and other tests may be useful.

After exclusion of secondary causes, a renal biopsy is often required in the adult nephrotic patient. Biopsy results in patients with heavy proteinuria and the nephrotic syndrome are likely to provide a specific diagnosis, determine prognosis, and guide therapy.

TABLE 123-4 SERUM COMPLEMENT LEVELS IN GLOMERULAR DISEASES

DISEASES WITH A REDUCED COMPLEMENT LEVEL
Post-streptococcal glomerulonephritis
Subacute bacterial endocarditis, visceral abscess, shunt nephritis
Systemic lupus erythematosus
Cryoglobulinemia
Idiopathic membranoproliferative glomerulonephritis
DISEASES ASSOCIATED WITH A NORMAL SERUM COMPLEMENT
Minimal change nephrotic syndrome
Focal segmental glomerulosclerosis
Membranous nephropathy
Immunoglobulin A nephropathy
Henoch-Schönlein purpura
Anti–glomerular basement disease
Pauci-immune rapidly progressive glomerulonephritis
Polyarteritis nodosa
Wegener's granulomatosis

TREATMENT Rx

Treatment varies by the specific cause. Elevated lipid levels should be treated (Chapter 213). Anticoagulation is not recommended routinely but is needed if any thrombotic complications occur. Edema is treated with diuretics, and the combination of furosemide plus albumin is more effective than furosemide alone for patients with refractory edema.[1]

Idiopathic Nephrotic Syndrome

MINIMAL CHANGE DISEASE

Minimal change disease, which is the most common pattern of nephrotic syndrome in children, accounts for only about 5 to 10% of cases of idiopathic nephrotic syndrome in adults. A similar histologic pattern may be seen as an adverse reaction to certain medications (nonsteroidal anti-inflammatory drugs [NSAIDs], lithium) or in association with certain tumors (e.g., Hodgkin's disease).

CLINICAL MANIFESTATIONS

Patients typically present with weight gain and periorbital and peripheral edema related to the proteinuria, which is usually well into the nephrotic range. Additional findings in adults are hypertension and microscopic hematuria, each in about 30% of patients. However, active urinary sediment with RBC casts is not found. Many adult patients have mild to moderate azotemia, which may be related to hypoalbuminemia and intravascular volume depletion. Complement levels and serologic test results are normal.

DIAGNOSIS

In true minimal change disease, histopathology typically reveals no glomerular abnormalities on light microscopy (Fig. 123-1). The tubules may show lipid droplet accumulation from absorbed lipoproteins (hence the older term *lipoid nephrosis*). Immunofluorescence staining and electron microscopy (Fig. 123-2) show no immune-type deposits. By electron microscopy, the GBM is normal, and effacement or "fusion" of the visceral epithelial foot processes is noted along virtually the entire distribution of every capillary loop.

TREATMENT Rx

The course of minimal change nephrotic syndrome is often one of remissions, relapses, and responses to additional treatment. When treated with corticosteroids for 8 weeks, 85 to 95% of children experience a remission of proteinuria. In adults, the response rate is somewhat lower, with 75 to 85% of patients responding to regimens of daily (1 mg/kg, maximum 80 mg) or alternate-day (2 mg/kg, maximum 120 mg) prednisone therapy, tapered after 2 months of treatment for a total of 5 to 6 months of therapy. The time to clinical response is slower in adults, and they are not considered steroid resistant until they have failed to respond to 16 weeks of treatment. Tapering of the steroid dose after remission should be gradual over 1 to 2 months. Approximately 40% of adults relapse by 1 year and 50% by 5 years. Most clinicians treat the first relapse similarly to the initial episode. Patients who relapse a

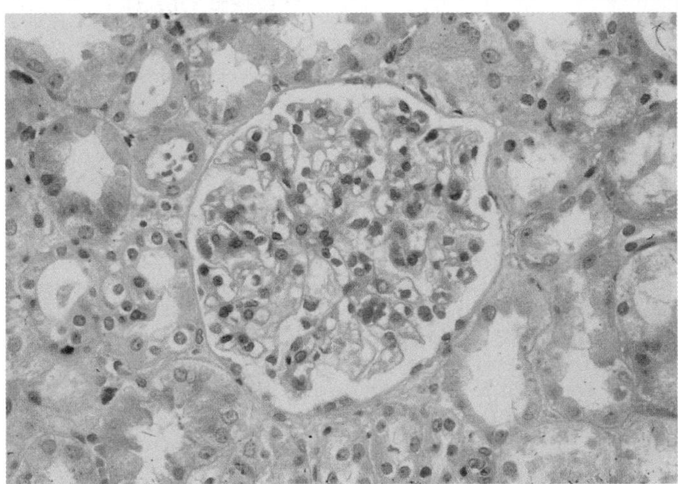

FIGURE 123-1. Unremarkable light microscopic appearance of minimal change disease glomerulopathy. Glomerular basement membranes are thin, and there is no glomerular hypercellularity.

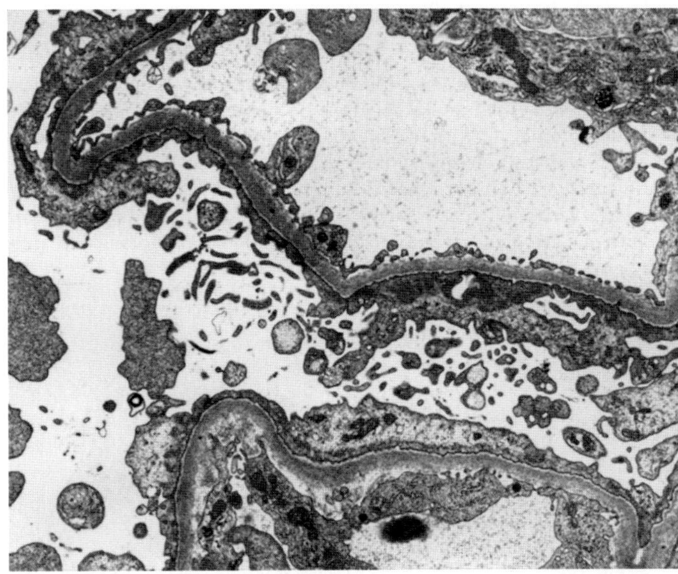

FIGURE 123-2. Minimal change disease. Electron micrograph shows widespread effacement of foot processes with microvillous transformation of the visceral epithelium. No electron-dense deposits are present (uranyl acetate, lead citrate stain; ×6000).

third time or who become corticosteroid dependent (unable to decrease the prednisone dose without proteinuria recurring) may be treated with a 2- to 3-month course of the alkylating agent cyclophosphamide at a dose of up to 2 mg/kg/day. Up to 50% of patients will have a remission of at least 5 years, but the response rate is lower in corticosteroid-dependent patients. Other alternative treatments for patients who frequently relapse or are steroid resistant include low-dose cyclosporine (3 to 5 mg/kg/day in divided doses for 4 months), tacrolimus (0.05 to 0.1 mg/kg/day in divided doses), and mycophenolate mofetil (750 to 1000 mg twice daily). All provide approximately equivalent remission and relapse rates, but cyclosporine and tacrolimus increase the risk of nephrotoxicity, so their blood levels must be carefully monitored.

PROGNOSIS

The prognosis of minimal change disease is excellent in terms of kidney function, and most patients who have a decline in kidney function have focal segmental glomerulosclerosis on a subsequent kidney biopsy. However, more than 50% of patients have relapses, and 10 to 20% may become steroid dependent.

FOCAL SEGMENTAL GLOMERULOSCLEROSIS

About 20 to 25% of adults with idiopathic nephrotic syndrome are found on biopsy to have focal segmental glomerulosclerosis (FSGS). The incidence of FSGS is increasing in all races, but it is especially common in African Americans. FSGS may be either idiopathic or secondary to a number of different causes (e.g., heroin abuse, HIV infection, sickle cell disease, obesity, reflux of urine from the bladder to the kidneys, and lesions associated with single or remnant kidneys). FSGS can occur in multiple family members owing to genetic defects in components of the visceral epithelial cell: an autosomal recessive pattern caused by mutations in the structural protein podocin; and autosomal dominant forms, caused by mutations in the structural protein α-actinin 4, the TRPC6 glomerular slit diaphragm-associated channel, or INF2, which encodes a formin (actin-regulating protein). The predisposition of African Americans to FSGS is related to alleles in the genes for myosin heavy chain 9 (MYH9) and apolipoprotein L1.

CLINICAL MANIFESTATIONS

Patients with idiopathic FSGS typically present with either asymptomatic proteinuria or edema. Although criteria for the nephrotic syndrome are met in two thirds of patients at presentation, proteinuria may vary from less than 1 to more than 30 g/day. Hypertension is found in 30 to 50% of patients, and microscopic hematuria occurs in about one half of all patients. The GFR is decreased at presentation in 20 to 30% of patients. Complement levels and other serologic test results are normal.

DIAGNOSIS

By light microscopy, only some glomeruli initially have areas of segmental scarring (Fig. 123-3). As renal function declines, repeat biopsy specimens show more glomeruli with segmental sclerosing lesions and increased numbers of globally sclerotic glomeruli. By immunofluorescence staining, immunoglobulin M (IgM) and C3 commonly are trapped in the areas of glomerular sclerosis. Electron microscopy shows no deposits and only visceral epithelial cell foot process effacement. The histopathologic variants of FSGS are associated with epidemiologic, clinical, and prognostic differences. For example, the "tip lesion" variant has a relatively benign course, whereas the collapsing variant progresses more rapidly to renal failure.

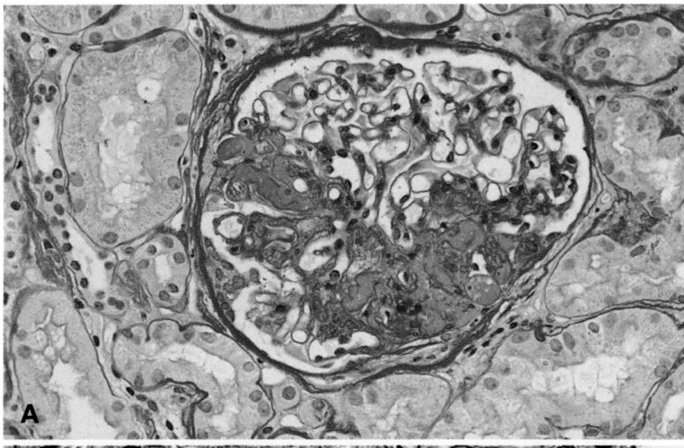

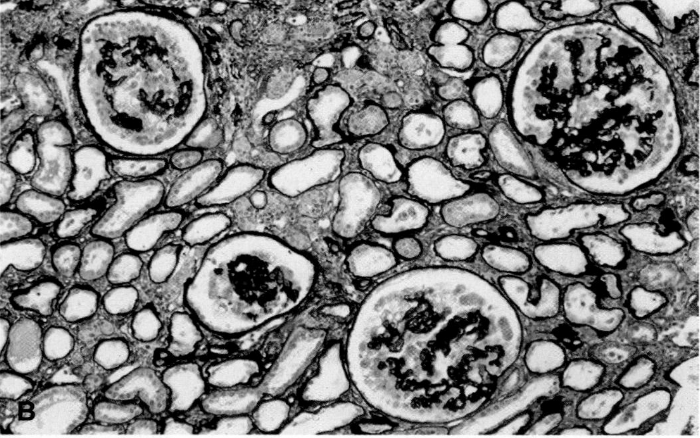

FIGURE 123-3. **Focal segmental glomerulosclerosis. A,** Light micrograph of classic focal segmental glomerulosclerosis. **B,** Silver stain of collapsing focal segmental glomerulosclerosis showing collapse of the glomerular tufts.

TREATMENT Rx

For primary (idiopathic) FSGS, corticosteroids are used as initial therapy (e.g., prednisone, 1 mg/kg/day, maximum 80 mg, or 2 mg/kg every other day, maximum 120 mg, as tolerated) for a minimum of 3 to 4 months and slowly tapered over the next 3 to 6 months if remission is achieved. A complete or partial remission may be seen in up to 40 to 60% of patients, with preservation of long-term renal function. In patients who relapse after initial therapy, oral cyclophosphamide (2 to 2.5 mg/kg/day for 12 weeks) or cyclosporine (4 mg/kg/day in divided doses) is used for 12 to 24 months, with slow tapering thereafter. With cyclosporine, careful monitoring of renal function and cyclosporine levels are necessary to avoid nephrotoxicity. In patients who are steroid resistant after 4 months of high-dose prednisone, the dose of prednisone should be tapered and patients should be treated with cyclosporine (3.5 mg/kg/day in divided doses adjusted to serum levels 125 to 225 μg/L) plus prednisone (0.15 mg/kg/day in divided doses, maximum 15 mg/day) for 6 months.[2]

PROGNOSIS

The course of untreated FSGS is usually one of progressive proteinuria and declining GFR. Only a minority of patients experiences a spontaneous remission of proteinuria, and most untreated patients eventually develop ESRD within 5 to 20 years from presentation. Patients with a sustained remission of their nephrotic syndrome are unlikely to progress to ESRD, whereas those with unremitting nephrotic syndrome are likely to progress.

In general, patients with genetic forms of the disease are steroid resistant, have a progressive course, and do not experience recurrences of the FSGS when they receive a renal transplant. Overall, however, focal sclerosis recurs in the transplanted kidney in up to 30% of cases, often in association with elevated levels of a circulating permeability factor. Younger patients, those with a rapid course to renal failure, and those with a prior recurrence are more likely to have recurrence in the allograft.

MEMBRANOUS NEPHROPATHY

Membranous nephropathy is the most common pattern of idiopathic nephrotic syndrome in white patients. It may also be associated with infections (syphilis [Chapter 327] and hepatitis B and C [Chapter 151]), systemic lupus erythematosus (SLE; Chapter 274), medications (gold salts, NSAIDs), and certain tumors (solid tumors and lymphomas). In many cases of what was previously classified as idiopathic membranous nephropathy, the antigen is the M-type phospholipase A_2 receptor in the podocyte.

CLINICAL MANIFESTATIONS

Membranous nephropathy typically presents as proteinuria and edema. Hypertension and microhematuria are not infrequent findings, but renal function and GFR are usually normal at presentation. Despite the finding of complement in the glomerular immune deposits, serum complement levels are normal. Membranous nephropathy is the most common pattern of the nephrotic syndrome to be associated with a hypercoagulable state and renal vein thrombosis (Chapter 127). The presence of sudden flank pain, deterioration of renal function, or symptoms of pulmonary disease in a patient with membranous nephropathy should prompt an investigation for renal vein thrombosis and pulmonary emboli.

DIAGNOSIS

On light microscopy, the glomerular capillary loops often appear rigid or thickened (Fig. 123-4), but there is no cellular proliferation. Immunofluorescence staining and electron microscopy show subepithelial immune dense deposits all along the glomerular capillary loops (Fig. 123-5). The presence of circulating antibodies to the M-type phospholipase A_2 receptor are 75% sensitive and 100% specific for idiopathic membranous nephropathy.

TREATMENT

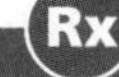

Studies using corticosteroids to treat membranous nephropathy have given conflicting results, and proof of their benefit is lacking. By comparison, corticosteroid therapy (methylprednisolone, 1 g intravenously daily for 3 days, then oral prednisone, 0.5 mg/kg/day for 27 days, in months 1, 3, and 5) and oral cytotoxic therapy (chlorambucil, 0.2 mg/kg/day, or cyclophosphamide,

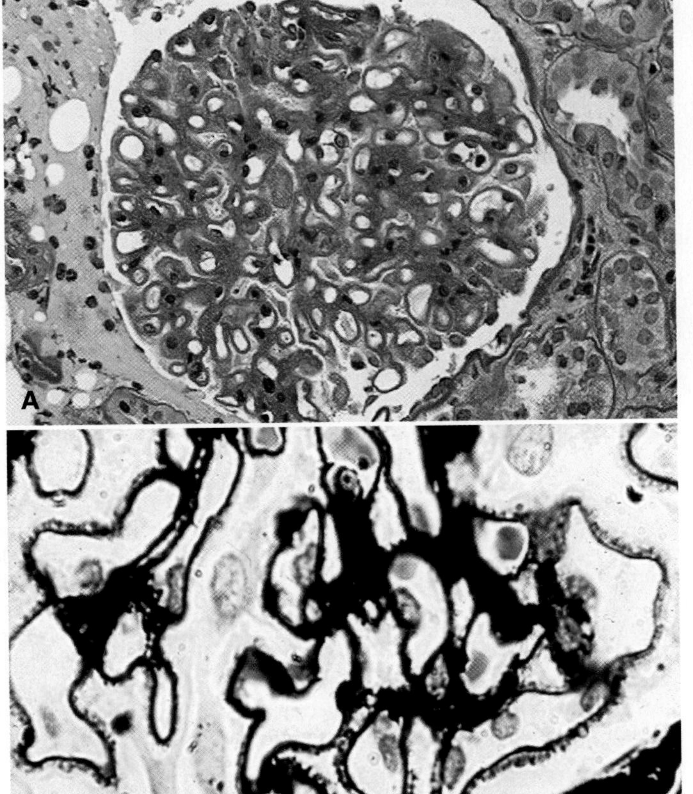

FIGURE 123-4. **Membranous nephropathy. A,** Light micrograph of membranous nephropathy demonstrating thickening of the glomerular capillary wall but no hypercellularity. **B,** Silver stain of idiopathic membranous nephropathy showing spike formation along the outer aspect of the glomerular basement membrane corresponding to projections of the basement membrane between the epimembranous deposits.

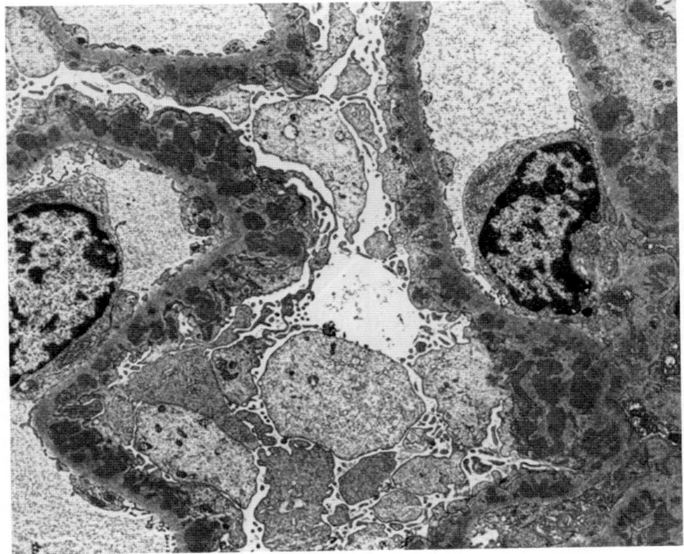

FIGURE 123-5. **Membranous glomerulopathy.** On ultrastructural examination, there are numerous, closely apposed epimembranous electron-dense deposits separated by basement membrane spikes (uranyl acetate, lead citrate stain; ×2500).

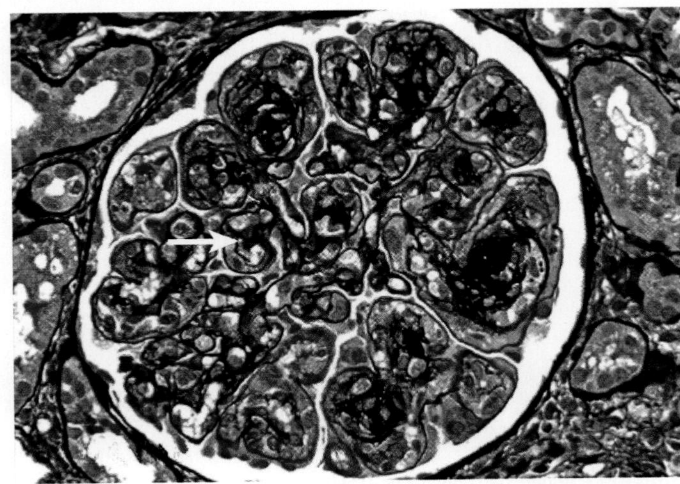

FIGURE 123-6. **Membranoproliferative glomerulonephritis with lobulation of the glomerular tuft and splitting of the basement membrane as seen by silver stain.**

2.5 mg/kg/day, for 30 days in months 2, 4, and 6) given in alternating months over 6 months results in more total remissions and better preservation of renal function compared with symptomatic therapy. [3] The combination of cyclosporine (3.5 mg/kg/day adjusted to serum levels of 125 to 225 µg/L) plus prednisone (0.15 mg/kg/day up to a maximum of 15 mg/day) for 6 months also is more likely to induce remission of the nephrotic syndrome compared with placebo or prednisone alone. [4] Other agents used successfully in uncontrolled or small controlled trials in membranous nephropathy include mycophenolate mofetil, adrenocorticotropic hormone, and the monoclonal anti-CD20 antibody, rituximab.

PROGNOSIS

In most large series, renal survival is more than 75% at 10 years, with a spontaneous remission rate of 20 to 30%. In general, older patients, males, and those with heavy persistent proteinuria are most likely to progress to renal failure and hence to benefit from therapy.

Membranoproliferative Glomerulonephritis

Idiopathic type I membranoproliferative or mesangiocapillary glomerulonephritis (MPGN) is an uncommon primary glomerular disease that represents only a small percentage of renal biopsy results. However, by light microscopy, similar patterns of glomerular damage commonly have been seen in association with hepatitis C (Chapter 151), SLE (Chapter 274), monoclonal gammopathies, and thrombotic microangiopathy associated with antiphospholipid antibodies (Chapter 179). All these stimuli have been proposed to incite the glomerular mesangial cells to grow out along the capillary wall and split the glomerular basement membrane.

Type II MPGN, or dense deposit disease, is an even less common disease that is associated with uncontrolled systemic activation of the alternative complement pathway. The cause may be C3 nephritic factor, which is an autoantibody directed against the C3 convertase of the alternate complement pathway, deficiencies of factor H or I or other inhibitors of the alternate complement cascade. Dense deposit disease may be associated with partial lipodystrophy. Because the histology of dense deposit disease may show patterns other than what are typical in MPGN (e.g., mesangial proliferation, sclerosis, crescents) and its pathogenesis is unique, many investigators feel it should be categorized independently of the other forms of MPGN.

CLINICAL MANIFESTATIONS AND DIAGNOSIS

Most patients with idiopathic MPGN are children or young adults who present with proteinuria or the nephrotic syndrome. A low serum complement level is found intermittently in type I MPGN, whereas the C3 level is usually reduced in dense deposit disease. The diagnosis of type II MPGN requires a renal biopsy that shows complement C3 in a characteristic ribbon-like pattern around the capillary loop by light microscopy (Fig. 123-6).

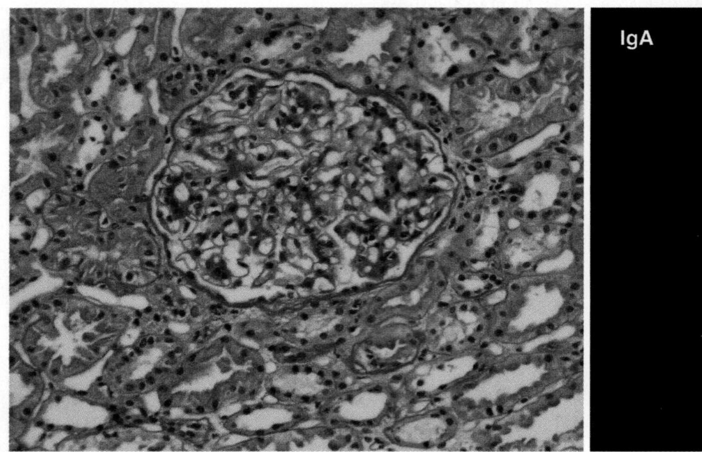

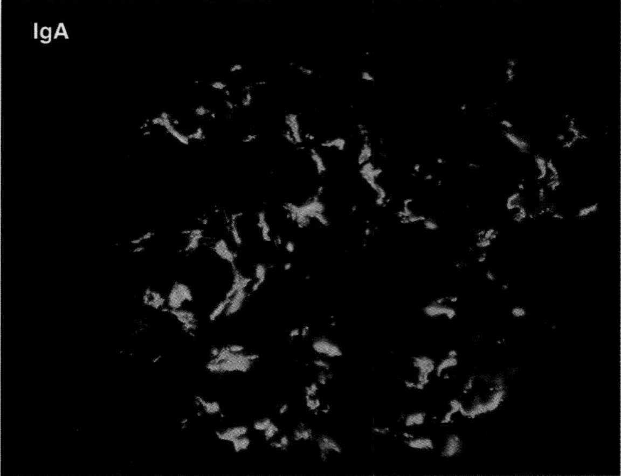

FIGURE 123-7. Immunoglobulin A (IgA) nephropathy with mesangial cell proliferation by light microscopy and IgA deposition on immunofluorescence.

TREATMENT AND PROGNOSIS (Rx)

Attempts to treat idiopathic type I MPGN have included corticosteroids, other immunosuppressive medications, anticoagulants, and antiplatelet agents. No therapy has been proved effective in a randomized trial in adults, but corticosteroids have had some success in children at a dose of 40 mg/m^2 every other day for a mean period of 41 months. Most studies have found a similar course and prognosis for the various patterns of MPGN, with half of the patients progressing to ESRD within 10 years of diagnosis.

ACUTE GLOMERULONEPHRITIS AND THE NEPHRITIC SYNDROME

EPIDEMIOLOGY AND PATHOBIOLOGY

Known inciting causes of acute glomerulonephritis include infectious agents, such as type 12 and type 49 "nephritogenic" strains of group A streptococci and endocarditis caused by *Staphylococcus aureus* and *Streptococcus viridans*. Acute glomerulonephritis can also be caused by the deposition of immune complexes in autoimmune diseases such as SLE (Chapter 274), and the damaging effect of circulating antibodies directed against the GBM, as in Goodpasture's syndrome.

Invading neutrophils and monocytes, as well as resident glomerular cells, can damage the glomerulus through a number of mediators, including oxidants, chemoattractant agents, proteases, cytokines, and growth factors. Some factors, such as transforming growth factor-β, have been related to eventual glomerulosclerosis and chronic glomerular damage.

CLINICAL MANIFESTATIONS AND DIAGNOSIS

Patients with acute glomerulonephritis often present with a nephritic picture characterized by a decreased GFR, azotemia, oliguria, hypertension, and an active urinary sediment (see Table 123-1). Hypertension is common and is caused by intravascular volume expansion, although renin levels may not be appropriately suppressed for the degree of volume expansion. Patients may note dark, smoky, or cola-colored urine in association with an active urinary sediment, which is composed of erythrocytes, leukocytes, and a variety of casts, including RBC casts. Although many patients with acute glomerulonephritis have proteinuria, sometimes even in the nephrotic range, most patients have lesser degrees of albumin leakage into the urine, especially when the GFR is markedly reduced. Regardless of the inciting cause, acute glomerulonephritis is characterized on light microscopy by hypercellularity of the glomerulus, which may be composed of infiltrating inflammatory cells, proliferation of resident glomerular cells, or both.

Immunoglobulin A Nephropathy

EPIDEMIOLOGY AND PATHOBIOLOGY

IgA nephropathy, which is now recognized as the most frequent form of idiopathic glomerulonephritis worldwide, represents 15 to 40% of primary glomerulonephritides in parts of Europe and Asia. In geographic areas where renal biopsies are commonly performed for milder urinary findings, a higher incidence of IgA has been noted. In the United States, some centers report this diagnosis in up to 20% of all primary glomerulopathies. Affected males outnumber females, and the peak occurrence is in the second to third decades of life.

In IgA nephropathy, the predominant antibody is composed of polymeric IgA1, but the antigen—whether infectious, dietary, or other—to which it is directed is unknown in most cases. The pathogenesis may involve abnormal O-linked galactosylation of the IgA molecule at the hinge region, with resultant abnormal binding of IgA complexes to the glomerular mesangial cells.

CLINICAL MANIFESTATIONS AND DIAGNOSIS

IgA nephropathy often presents either as asymptomatic microscopic hematuria with or without proteinuria (the most common presentation in adults) or as episodic gross hematuria following an upper respiratory tract infection or exercise (the most common presentation in children and young adults). Hypertension is present in 20 to 50% of all patients. Increased serum IgA levels, noted in one third to one half of cases, do not correlate with the course of the disease. Serum complement levels are normal. The diagnosis of IgA nephropathy is established by finding glomerular IgA deposits as either the dominant or the codominant immunoglobulin on immunofluorescence microscopy (Fig. 123-7). Deposits of C3 and IgG also are often found. The light microscopy picture varies from the most common picture of mild mesangial proliferation to severe crescentic glomerulonephritis. By electron microscopy, immune-type dense deposits are typically found in the mesangial and paramesangial areas.

TREATMENT (Rx)

Because the pathogenesis of IgA nephropathy is thought to involve abnormal antigenic stimulation of mucosal IgA production and subsequent immune complex deposition in the glomeruli, treatment has been directed at these sites. Efforts to treat the disease by preventing antigenic stimulation, including broad-spectrum antibiotics (e.g., doxycycline), tonsillectomy, and dietary manipulations (e.g., gluten elimination), generally have been controversial or unsuccessful. Most physicians choose to treat only patients at high risk for progression to renal failure. Trials using fish oils to decrease proteinuria and slow progressive disease have given conflicting results. Controlled studies suggest that glucocorticoids (e.g., pulse methylprednisolone, 1 g daily for three doses in months 0, 2, and 4, followed by prednisone, 0.5 mg/kg every other day for 6 months) may decrease proteinuria and progressive renal failure in some patients.[5] The benefit of immunosuppressive agents (e.g., cyclophosphamide, azathioprine, mycophenolate mofetil) is far from clear. For the few patients with crescentic IgA nephropathy, cytotoxic agents have been used. Angiotensin-converting enzyme (ACE) inhibitors and angiotensin receptor blockers (ARBs) have reduced proteinuria and the progression of renal disease in small randomized studies and appear to have incremental benefit when added to glucocorticoid therapy.

PROGNOSIS

The course is variable, with some patients showing no decline in GFR over decades and others developing the nephrotic syndrome, hypertension, and renal failure. Factors predictive of a poor outcome in IgA nephropathy include older age at onset, absence of gross hematuria, hypertension, persistent proteinuria greater than 1 g/day, male gender, an elevated serum creatinine level, and the histologic features of severe proliferation and sclerosis or tubulointerstitial damage and crescent formation. Renal survival rates are estimated at 75 to 85% at 10 years and 70 to 75% at 20 years. A significant percentage of transplant recipients have a morphologic recurrence in the allograft, but graft loss owing to the disease is uncommon.

Henoch-Schönlein Purpura

Henoch-Schönlein purpura (HSP; Chapter 278) is characterized by a small-vessel vasculitis with arthralgias, skin purpura, and abdominal symptoms as well as a proliferative acute glomerulonephritis. HSP is predominantly a disease of childhood, although cases occur in adults. Despite the finding of circulating IgA-containing immune complexes, no infectious agent or allergen has been defined as causative, and serum complement levels are normal.

CLINICAL MANIFESTATIONS AND DIAGNOSIS

The clinical manifestations of HSP (Chapter 278) include dermatologic, gastrointestinal, rheumatologic, and renal findings. Skin involvement typically starts with a macular rash that coalesces into purpuric lesions (see Fig. 278-2 in Chapter 278) on the ankles, legs, and occasionally arms and buttocks. Gastrointestinal symptoms include cramps, diarrhea, nausea, and vomiting, with melena and bloody diarrhea in the most severely involved cases. Although arthralgias of the knees, wrists, and ankles are common, true arthritis is uncommon. Symptoms of different organ system involvement may occur concurrently or separately, and recurrent episodes during the first year are not uncommon. The renal histopathology of HSP is similar to that of IgA nephropathy. In the skin, there is a small-vessel leukocytoclastic angiitis with immune deposition of IgA.

TREATMENT AND PROGNOSIS Rx

Like IgA nephropathy, HSP has no proven therapy. Episodes of rash, arthralgias, and abdominal symptoms usually resolve spontaneously. Some patients with severe abdominal findings have been treated with short courses of high doses of corticosteroids. Patients with severe glomerular involvement may benefit by modalities used to treat patients with severe IgA nephropathy. Although most patients with HSP recover fully, patients with a more severe nephritic or nephrotic presentation and more severe glomerular damage on renal biopsy have an unfavorable long-term prognosis.

Post-streptococcal Glomerulonephritis

Acute post-streptococcal glomerulonephritis may occur in either an epidemic form or as sporadic cases after infection with nephritogenic strains of group A β-hemolytic streptococci (Chapter 298). Post-streptococcal glomerulonephritis is largely a disease of childhood, but severe disease in adults has been well documented. The disease is most common after episodes of pharyngitis, but it can follow streptococcal infections at any site, and subclinical cases greatly outnumber clinical cases. Post-streptococcal glomerulonephritis is an acute immune complex disease characterized by the formation of antibodies against streptococci with the localization of immune complexes with complement in the kidney.

CLINICAL MANIFESTATIONS AND DIAGNOSIS

Most cases are diagnosed by detecting hematuria, proteinuria, hypertension, and the nephritic syndrome (see Table 123-1) 10 days to several weeks after a streptococcal infection. Throat cultures and skin cultures of suspected sites of streptococcal involvement often may not be positive for group A β-hemolytic streptococci. A variety of antibodies (e.g., antistreptolysin O [ASLO], antihyaluronidase [AHT]) and a streptozyme panel of antibodies against streptococcal antigens (which includes ASLO, AHT, antistreptokinase, and anti-DNase) often show high titers, but a change in titer over time is more indicative of a recent streptococcal infection. More than 95% of patients with post-streptococcal glomerulonephritis secondary to pharyngitis and 85% of patients with streptococcal skin infections have positive antibody titers. The serum total hemolytic complement levels and C3 levels are decreased in more than 90% of patients during the episode of acute glomerulonephritis.

In a patient with a classic acute nephritic episode after a documented streptococcal infection, a change in streptococcal antibody titer, and a depressed serum complement level, a renal biopsy adds little to the diagnosis. In other cases, a biopsy may be necessary to confirm or refute the diagnosis. On light microscopy (Fig. 123-8), glomeruli are markedly enlarged and often fill Bowman's space. Glomeruli exhibit hypercellularity owing to an infiltration of monocytes and polymorphonuclear cells and a proliferation of the glomerular cellular elements. The capillary lumens often are compressed by the glomerular hypercellularity. Some cases demonstrate extracapillary proliferation with crescent formation. On immunofluorescence microscopy, there is coarse granular deposition of IgG, IgM, and complement, especially C3, along the capillary wall. Electron microscopy shows large dome-shaped, electron-dense subepithelial deposits resembling the humps of a camel at isolated intervals along the GBM.

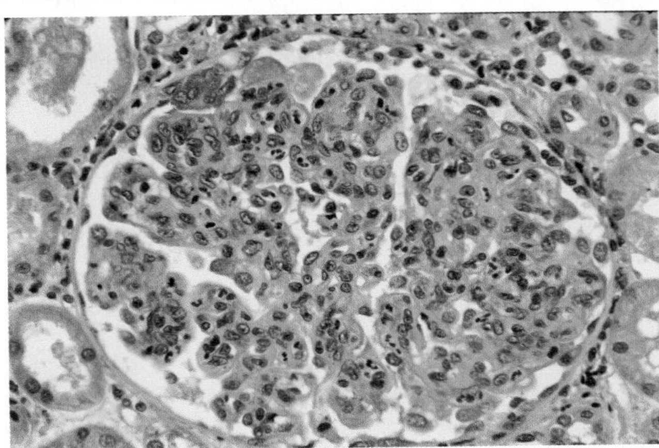

FIGURE 123-8. Post-streptococcal glomerulonephritis with hypercellular glomerulus filling Bowman's space and infiltrated by polymorphonuclear and other cells.

TREATMENT AND PROGNOSIS Rx

Therapy is symptomatic and directed at controlling the hypertension and fluid retention with antihypertensive agents (see Tables 67-5 and 67-7 in Chapter 67) and diuretics. In most patients, post-streptococcal glomerulonephritis is a self-limited disease, with recovery of renal function and disappearance of hypertension in several weeks. However, the presence of underlying renal disease, especially diabetic nephropathy, is associated with a worse prognosis. Proteinuria and hematuria may resolve more slowly over months.

Glomerulonephritis with Endocarditis and Visceral Abscesses

Various glomerular lesions are found in patients with acute and chronic bacterial endocarditis (Chapter 76). Although embolic phenomena can lead to glomerular ischemia and infarcts, a common finding is an immune complex glomerulonephritis. With *S. viridans* endocarditis, both focal and diffuse proliferative glomerulonephritides are common. With the increased incidence of *S. aureus* endocarditis, 40 to 80% of patients with endocarditis have clinical evidence of an immune complex proliferative glomerulonephritis. Glomerulonephritis is now more common with acute than subacute bacterial endocarditis, and the duration of illness is not an important determinant of the renal disease.

Patients often have hematuria and RBC casts in their urinary sediment, proteinuria ranging from less than 1 g/day to nephrotic levels, and progressive renal failure. Serum total complement and C3 levels are usually reduced. Renal insufficiency may be mild and reversible with appropriate antibiotic therapy, or it may be progressive and lead to dialysis and irreversible renal failure.

A proliferative immune complex glomerulonephritis can occur in patients with deep visceral bacterial abscesses and infections, such as empyema of the lung (Chapter 99) and osteomyelitis (Chapter 296). Immune complex forms of acute glomerulonephritis also have been noted in patients with bacterial pneumonias, including *Mycoplasma* (Chapter 325), and patients with chronically infected cerebral ventriculoatrial shunts for hydrocephalus. Many patients have nephrotic-range proteinuria and only mild renal dysfunction. With appropriate antibiotic therapy, most patients' glomerular lesions heal, and renal function recovers.

TABLE 123-5 CLASSIFICATION OF RAPIDLY PROGRESSIVE ("CRESCENTIC") GLOMERULONEPHRITIS

PRIMARY
Type I: Anti–glomerular basement membrane antibody disease, Goodpasture's syndrome (with pulmonary disease)
Type II: Immune complex mediated
Type III: Pauci-immune (usually antineutrophil cytoplasmic antibody-positive)
SECONDARY
Membranoproliferative glomerulonephritis
Immunoglobulin A nephropathy, Henoch-Schönlein purpura
Post-streptococcal glomerulonephritis
Systemic lupus erythematosus
Polyarteritis nodosa, hypersensitivity angiitis

TABLE 123-6 COMMON RENAL DISEASES WITH ASSOCIATED PULMONARY DISEASES

DISEASE	MARKER
Goodpasture's syndrome	+Anti–glomerular basement membrane antibodies
Wegener's granulomatosis, polyarteritis	+Antineutrophil cytoplasmic antibodies
Systemic lupus erythematosus	+Anti-DNA antibodies, low complement
Nephrotic syndrome, renal vein thrombosis, pulmonary embolus	+Lung scan or +CT angiography
Pneumonia with immune complex glomerulonephritis	Low complement, circulating immune complexes
Uremic lung	Elevated creatinine level

CT = computed tomography.

Rapidly Progressive Glomerulonephritis

Rapidly progressive glomerulonephritis (RPGN) represents a variety of glomerular diseases that are notable for progression to renal failure in a matter of weeks to months (Table 123-5). Patients with primary RPGN can be divided into three patterns as defined by immunologic pathogenesis: type I, with anti-GBM disease (e.g., Goodpasture's syndrome); type II, with immune complex deposition (e.g., SLE, Henoch-Schönlein purpura, post-streptococcal); and type III, without immune deposits or anti-GBM antibodies (so-called pauci-immune, usually ANCA-positive RPGN). The renal biopsy in all RPGN shows extensive extracapillary proliferation, that is, crescent formation.

ANTI–GLOMERULAR BASEMENT MEMBRANE DISEASE

The disease has two peaks of occurrence: in the third decade of life in men and in women after 60 years of age. Anti-GBM disease (Table 123-6) is caused by circulating antibodies that are directed against the noncollagenous domain of the α_3 chain of type IV collagen and that damage the GBM. The result is an inflammatory response, breaks in the GBM, and the formation of a proliferative and often crescentic glomerulonephritis. If the anti-GBM antibodies cross-react with and damage the basement membrane of pulmonary capillaries, the patient develops pulmonary hemorrhage and hemoptysis, an association called *Goodpasture's syndrome.*

CLINICAL MANIFESTATIONS AND DIAGNOSIS

Patients present with a nephritic picture (see Table 123-1). Renal function may deteriorate from normal to dialysis-requiring levels in a matter of days to weeks. Patients with pulmonary involvement may have life-threatening hemoptysis with dyspnea and with diffuse alveolar infiltrates on chest radiograph.

The pathology of anti-GBM disease shows a proliferative glomerulonephritis, often with severe crescentic proliferation in Bowman's space. There is linear deposition of immunoglobulin (usually IgG) along the GBM by immunofluorescence (Fig. 123-9), but electron microscopy does not show any electron-dense deposits.

Although the treatment of this rare disease has not been studied in large controlled trials, intensive immunosuppressive therapy with cyclophosphamide (e.g., 2 mg/kg/day as tolerated) and corticosteroids (e.g., pulse methylprednisolone, 15 to 30 mg/kg to a maximum of dose of 1000 mg intravenously daily for three doses, followed by oral prednisone, 1 mg/kg per day to a maximum of 60 to 80 mg/day and slowly tapered after achieving clinical remission) to reduce the production of anti-GBM antibodies, combined with daily plasmapheresis to remove circulating anti-GBM antibodies, has been successful in many patients. Rapid treatment is recommended to prevent irreversible renal damage and is necessary in patients with pulmonary hemorrhage. The optimal duration of therapy is uncertain, but daily plasmapheresis should be performed, preferably until anti-GBM antibody is undetectable, and corticosteroids and cyclophosphamide should be continued until clinical remission is achieved, typically between 3 and 6 months. Patients who already require dialysis at the time of treatment generally do not regain renal function despite aggressive therapy.

IMMUNE COMPLEX RAPIDLY PROGRESSIVE GLOMERULONEPHRITIS

Type II RPGN, which is associated with immune complex–mediated damage to the glomeruli, may occur with idiopathic glomerulopathies, such as IgA nephropathy and MPGN, or with postinfectious glomerulonephritis and SLE. The therapy for IgA nephropathy and MPGN was discussed earlier.

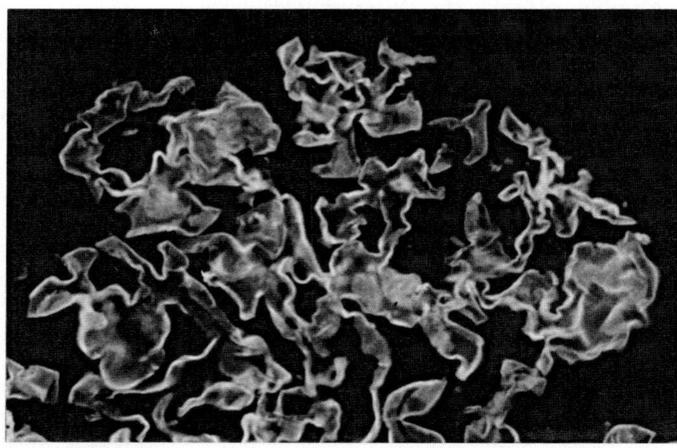

FIGURE 123-9. Anti–glomerular basement membrane (GBM) glomerulonephritis. An immunofluorescence micrograph of a portion of a glomerulus with anti-GBM glomerulonephritis shows linear staining of GBM for immunoglobulin G (IgG) (fluorescein isothiocyanate anti-IgG stain, ×600). (From Falk RJ, Jennette JC, Nachman PH. Primary glomerular disease. In: Brenner BM, ed. Brenner and Rector's The Kidney. 7th ed. Philadelphia: Elsevier; 2004.)

Many cases of crescentic postinfectious glomerulonephritis resolve with successful treatment of the underlying infection. For the treatment of severe SLE, see later.

PAUCI-IMMUNE AND VASCULITIS-ASSOCIATED RAPIDLY PROGRESSIVE GLOMERULONEPHRITIS

Pauci-immune type III RPGN includes patients with and without evidence of systemic vasculitis. Most patients have circulating ANCAs that are directed against components of neutrophil primary granules.

CLINICAL MANIFESTATIONS AND DIAGNOSIS

Patients often present with progressive renal failure and a nephritic picture (see Table 123-1). Patients who are perinuclear ANCA positive (antibodies usually directed against granulocyte myeloperoxidase) more often have a clinical picture akin to that of microscopic polyangiitis (Chapter 278) with arthritis, leukocytoclastic angiitis, and constitutional and systemic signs. Patients who are cytoplasmic ANCA positive (antibodies usually directed against a granulocyte serine proteinase, anti-PR3) more often have Wegener's granulomatosis (Chapter 278) associated with their glomerulonephritis. However, there is considerable overlap among these groups, and some patients have both ANCA and anti-GBM antibodies (Fig. 123-10). Although there is no direct correlation between ANCA titers and disease activity, patients with high titers (especially high anti-PR3 titers) and those with a four-fold increase in titers are more likely to have flares of their disease.

TREATMENT AND PROGNOSIS Rx

For induction therapy, combination therapy with corticosteroids (e.g., pulse methylprednisolone, 10-15 mg/kg/day up to a maximum of 500-1000 mg intravenously daily, for 3 days, followed by oral prednisolone, 1 mg/kg/day)

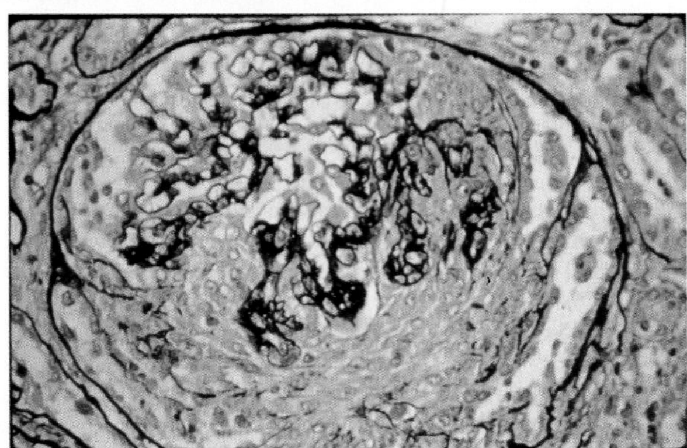

FIGURE 123-10. Crescentic glomerulonephritis typical of both anti–glomerular basement membrane disease and antineutrophil cytoplasmic antibody–positive pauci-immune glomerulonephritis.

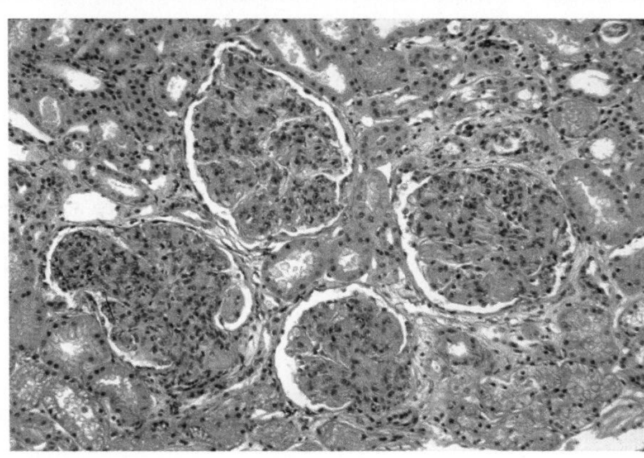

FIGURE 123-11. Diffuse proliferative lupus nephritis with involvement of all glomeruli.

and cyclophosphamide (e.g., 15 mg/kg intravenously every 2 to 3 weeks or 1.5 to 2 mg/kg/day orally), with or without plasmapheresis, has markedly improved renal and patient survival rates in patients with Wegener's granulomatosis (Chapter 278) and microscopic polyangiitis (Chapter 278). Methotrexate (20 to 25 mg per week orally for 12 months) is as effective as cyclophosphamide in achieving remission but leads to a higher relapse rate, so it should be limited to non-organ- or non-life-threatening disease, in which it is a less toxic alternative to cyclophosphamide. In severe renal vasculitis, renal survival, but not patient survival, is improved with the addition of plasmapheresis.6 Rituximab (375 mg/m^2 weekly for 4 weeks) is as effective as cyclophosphamide at 6-month follow-up.7 Maintenance regimens using azathioprine (1.5 mg/kg/day) or methotrexate (20 to 25 mg/week) should be administered for 12 to 18 months after achieving remission.8 Corticosteroids should be slowly tapered off, as determined by the presence of clinical symptoms. Ongoing trials include the comparison of mycophenolate mofetil to azathioprine for maintenance therapy of ANCA-positive vasculitis.

As in all forms of RPGN, renal function may deteriorate rapidly. In pauci-immune RPGN, high-risk patients include older patients, patients with severe pulmonary involvement, and patients with severe renal failure. Analyses have found no difference in prognosis in patients with or without documented true arterial vasculitis or with crescentic or focal segmental necrotizing glomerulonephritis.

GLOMERULAR DISEASES ASSOCIATED WITH GENETIC DEFECTS

Some patients, often with a history of similar findings in siblings and other relatives, have a hereditary nephritis.

Alport syndrome is a hereditary form of glomerulonephritis that often presents with asymptomatic urinary findings. In approximately 85% of cases, it is an X-linked condition with hematuria and proteinuria, often in association with high-pitched hearing loss and abnormalities of the lens of the eye (lenticonus). The defect in most of these cases is localized to a mutation in the α_5 chain of type IV collagen (COL4A5). Other families have different patterns of inheritance, more often with mutations in the α_3 and α_4 chains of type IV collagen (COL4A3, COL4A4). Although the light microscopy findings vary from mild mesangial proliferative to advanced sclerosing lesions depending on the stage of biopsy, electron microscopy typically shows areas of GBM thinning and areas of basement membrane splitting with lamellations. Some patients with mutations in the collagen IV gene have microhematuria and proteinuria with areas of extreme basement membrane thinning on electron microscopy. In males, Alport's syndrome often leads to progressive glomerulosclerosis and ESRD.

Fabry's disease (Chapter 215), which is caused by an X-linked recessive genetic defect of α-galactosidase, leads to the deposition of ceramide trihexose in the kidneys and other organs. It may cause progressive proteinuria and renal insufficiency in males and in some female carriers. It also is associated with telangiectasias of the skin, typically in the bathing suit area; acroparesthesias; cardiac abnormalities; and eye changes.

Nail-patella syndrome, associated with skeletal and nail deformities, is a rare cause of the nephrotic syndrome in children. It is due to an autosomal dominant mutation in the LMX1B transcription factor that regulates collagen, nephrin, and podocin gene expression.

TABLE 123-7 CLASSIFICATION OF LUPUS NEPHRITIS

CLASS	CLINICAL FEATURES
I. Minimal mesangial LN	No renal findings
II. Mesangial proliferative LN	Mild clinical renal disease; minimally active urinary sediment; mild to moderate proteinuria (never nephrotic) but may have active serology
III. Focal proliferative LN < 50% glomeruli involved A. Active A/C. Active and chronic C. Chronic	More active sediment changes; often active serology; increased proteinuria (about 25% nephrotic); hypertension may be present; some evolve into class IV pattern; active lesions require treatment, chronic do not
IV. Diffuse proliferative LN (>50% glomeruli involved); all may be with segmental or global involvement (S or G) A. Active A/C. Active and chronic C. Chronic	Most severe renal involvement with active sediment, hypertension, heavy proteinuria (frequent nephrotic syndrome), often reduced glomerular filtration rate; serology very active. Active lesions require treatment
V. Membranous LN glomerulonephritis	Significant proteinuria (often nephrotic) with less active lupus serology
VI. Advanced sclerosing LN	More than 90% glomerulosclerosis; no treatment prevents renal failure

LN = lupus nephritis.

Systemic Lupus Erythematosus

Renal involvement may greatly influence the course and therapy of SLE (Chapter 274). Although the incidence of clinical renal disease in SLE varies from 15% to 75%, histologic evidence of renal involvement is found in most biopsy specimens.

The International Society of Nephrology classification of lupus nephritis uses light microscopy, immunofluorescence, and electron microscopy to classify each biopsy in order to separate milder mesangial lesions and bland membranous lupus nephritis from true proliferative lupus nephritis (Table 123-7). In general, class I and II patients have mild lesions that require no therapy directed at the kidney. All patients with class IV lesions on biopsy deserve some form of vigorous therapy for their lupus nephritis. Many class III patients, especially those with active necrotizing lesions and large amounts of subendothelial deposits (Fig. 123-11), also benefit from therapy. For class V patients, the optimal therapy is less clear, and recommendations vary from vigorous treatment of all patients with membranous lupus nephritis to reserving such therapy for those with serologic activity or more severe nephrotic syndrome. Vigorous therapy of lupus nephritis now emphasizes monthly high-dose intravenous cyclophosphamide therapy (0.5 to 1 g/m^2) for 6 months combined with intravenous methylprednisolone (1000 mg/m^2) as the best regimen for preventing flares of disease or progression to renal failure. Daily oral mycophenolate mofetil (target dose, 1500 mg twice daily) appears to be equally effective in inducing remissions of severe lupus nephritis.9 Maintenance therapy with mycophenolate mofetil (500 to 1000 mg twice daily) or azathioprine (1 to 3 mg/kg/day) is more effective and less toxic than continued intravenous cyclophosphamide therapy after the 6-month induction period. Rituximab, an anti-CD20 monoclonal antibody, has not proved beneficial when added to full doses of other immunosuppressive agents in controlled trials of patients with SLE renal disease. Other agents under investigation include blockers of T- and B-cell costimulatory molecules, and anti-B LyS therapy.

Many patients with lupus nephritis (40 to 50%) produce autoantibodies against certain phospholipids, including anticardiolipin antibodies. If these patients experience clotting in the glomeruli and arterioles, they require anticoagulation or antiplatelet agents, or both, as well as immunosuppressive medications.

Diabetes Mellitus

Diabetic nephropathy, which is the most common form of glomerular damage seen in developed countries, is discussed in detail in Chapter 126.

Amyloidosis

Renal amyloid deposits, whether due to AL or to AA amyloid, are predominantly found within the glomeruli, where they often appear as amorphous eosinophilic extracellular nodules (Chapter 194) that stain positively with Congo red and display apple-green birefringence under polarized light. By electron microscopy, amyloid appears as nonbranching rigid fibrils 8 to 10 nm in diameter.

Although almost 80% of patients with AL amyloid have renal disease, amyloidosis is a disease with multisystem involvement. Renal manifestations include albuminuria and renal insufficiency. Approximately 25% of patients with AL amyloid present with the nephrotic syndrome, which eventually is diagnosed in up to one half of patients. Patients may present with symptoms referable to cardiac involvement (Chapter 60) or neuropathy (Chapter 428), as well as with renal symptoms. Diagnosis may be made from organ biopsy other than the kidney (e.g., gingival biopsy, rectal biopsy, or fat pad biopsy). Treatment strategies for renal AL amyloidosis are similar to those for multiple myeloma and other plasma cell dyscrasias (Chapter 193).

AA amyloid is usually associated with chronic inflammatory conditions such as rheumatoid arthritis (Chapter 272), familial Mediterranean fever (Chapter 269), inflammatory bowel disease (Chapter 143), osteomyelitis (Chapter 296), and other chronic infections. Treatment is directed at the underlying inflammatory process. Specific therapy against the primary inflammatory disease (e.g., anti–tumor necrosis factor therapy in rheumatoid arthritis and colchicine in familial Mediterranean fever) can prevent fibrillogenesis in AA amyloid patients. Eprodisate, a compound that inhibits polymerization and deposition of amyloid fibrils (800 to 2400 mg/day based on renal function), can slow the progression of renal disease in patients with AA amyloidosis. [10]

Light Chain Deposition Disease

Light chain deposition disease, like AL amyloidosis, is a systemic disease caused by the overproduction and extracellular deposition of a monoclonal immunoglobulin light chain (Chapter 193). However, the deposits do not form β-pleated sheets, do not stain with Congo red, and are granular rather than fibrillar. Most patients with light chain deposition disease have a lymphoplasmacytic B-cell disease similar to multiple myeloma (Chapter 193).

Albuminuria is common, and the nephrotic syndrome is found in one half of patients at presentation, often accompanied by hypertension and renal insufficiency. On light microscopy, most glomeruli contain eosinophilic mesangial glomerular nodules. Some biopsies show associated light chain cast nephropathy with eosinophilic laminated casts obstructing the tubules, as seen in myeloma. By immunofluorescence, a single class of immunoglobulin light chain (κ in 80% of cases) stains in a diffuse linear pattern along the GBM, in the nodules, and along the tubular basement membranes. The treatment for most patients with light chain deposition disease is chemotherapy similar to that for myeloma (Chapter 193).

Fibrillary Glomerulopathy-Immunotactoid Glomerulopathy

Some patients with renal disease have glomerular lesions with deposits of nonamyloid fibrillar proteins ranging in size from 12 to more than 50 nm. Patients with these lesions have been divided into two groups: those with fibrillary glomerulonephritis with fibrils of 20 nm in diameter, and those with immunotactoid glomerulonephritis, a much rarer disease often associated with lymphoproliferative disorders, in which the fibrils are much larger (30 to 50 nm). Proteinuria is found in almost all patients, and hematuria, the nephrotic syndrome, and renal insufficiency eventually develop in most. There is no proven therapy for fibrillary glomerulopathy at this time.

Human Immunodeficiency Virus–Associated Nephropathy

Infection with human immunodeficiency virus (HIV) (Chapter 394) is associated with a number of patterns of renal disease, including acute renal failure and a unique form of glomerulopathy now called HIV-associated nephropathy. HIV-associated nephropathy is characterized by heavy proteinuria and rapid progression to renal failure. On light microscopy, findings on renal biopsy include diffuse global collapse of the glomerular tufts, severe tubulointerstitial changes with interstitial inflammation, edema, microcystic dilation of tubules, and severe tubular degenerative changes. On electron microscopy, tubuloreticular inclusions can be seen in the glomerular endothelium. The use of ACE inhibitors, in doses needed to achieve a target systolic blood pressure of 120 mm Hg or lower as tolerated (see Table 67-5 in Chapter 67), and highly active antiretroviral therapy (HAART) may slow the progression to renal failure and decrease proteinuria. Corticosteroids (e.g., prednisone, 1 mg/kg for 1 month followed by a taper over several months) may be beneficial in selected patients with HIV-associated nephropathy.

Mixed Cryoglobulinemia

Cryoglobulinemia (Chapter 193) is caused by the production of circulating immunoglobulins that precipitate on cooling and resolubilize on warming. Cryoglobulinemia may be found in association with many types of diseases, including infections, collagen-vascular disease, and lymphoproliferative diseases such as multiple myeloma and Waldenström's macroglobulinemia. Many patients with what was originally described as glomerulonephritis due to essential mixed cryoglobulinemia have been found to have hepatitis C–associated renal disease. Some patients develop an acute nephritic picture with acute renal insufficiency. Most patients have proteinuria, and about 20% present with the nephrotic syndrome. Most patients with renal disease have a slow, indolent course characterized by proteinuria, hypertension, hematuria, and renal insufficiency. Hypocomplementemia, especially of the early components C1q to C4, is a characteristic finding in cryoglobulinemic glomerulonephritis whether hepatitis C–related or idiopathic. Treatment of hepatitis C–associated cryoglobulinemia includes antiviral therapy (Chapter 151). When significant renal disease is present, various combinations of corticosteroids with or without rituximab or cyclophosphamide or plasmapheresis can be tried.

Thrombotic Microangiopathies

A number of systemic diseases, including hemolytic-uremic syndrome (Chapters 127 and 175), thrombotic thrombocytopenic purpura (TTP; Chapter 175), and the antiphospholipid syndrome (Chapter 179), as well as microangiopathy associated with drugs such as mitomycin and cyclosporine, are characterized by microthromboses of the glomerular capillaries and small arterioles. The renal findings may be dominant or only part of a more generalized picture of microangiopathy.

Renal manifestations of the thrombotic microangiopathies may include gross or microscopic hematuria, proteinuria that is typically less than 2 g/day but may reach nephrotic levels, and renal insufficiency. Patients may have oliguric or nonoliguric acute renal failure. The histologic findings in all of the microangiopathies resemble each other and include glomerular capillary thromboses, areas of ischemic damage, and intimal proliferation with luminal narrowing by thrombi of arterioles and small arteries. In all thrombotic microangiopathies, treatment includes correcting hypovolemia, controlling hypertension, and the use of dialytic support for those with severe renal failure. In TTP associated with an acquired or hereditary deficiency of the von Willebrand's convertase ADAMTS-13 and in some other cases, plasmapheresis with fresh-frozen plasma is beneficial (Chapter 175). In the antiphospholipid syndrome, anticoagulation with heparin and then warfarin is useful (Chapter 37).

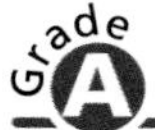

1. Dharmaraj R, Hari P, Bagga A. Randomized cross-over trial comparing albumin and frusemide infusions in nephritic syndrome. *Pediatr Nephrol.* 2009;24:775-782.
2. Cattran DC, Appel GB, Hebert LA, et al. A randomized trial of cyclosporine in patients with steroid-resistant focal segmental glomerulosclerosis. North America Nephrotic Syndrome Study Group. *Kidney Int.* 1999;56:2220-2226.

3. Ponticelli C, Altieri P, Scolari F, et al. A randomized study comparing methylprednisolone plus chlorambucil versus methylprednisolone plus cyclophosphamide in idiopathic membranous nephropathy. *J Am Soc Nephrol.* 1998;9:444-450.
4. Cattran DC, Appel GB, Hebert LA, et al. Cyclosporine in patients with steroid-resistant membranous nephropathy: a randomized trial. *Kidney Int.* 2001;59:1484-1490.
5. Samuels JA, Strippoli GF, Craig JC, et al. Immunosuppressive treatments for immunoglobulin A nephropathy: a meta-analysis of randomized controlled trials. *Nephrology (Carlton).* 2004;9:177-185.
6. Jayne DR, Gaskin G, Rasmussen N, et al. Randomized trial of plasma exchange or high dosage methyl-prednisolone as adjunctive therapy for severe renal vasculitis. *J Am Soc Nephrol.* 2007;18:2180-2188.
7. Stone JH, Merkel PA, Spiera R, et al, for the RAVE-ITN Research Group. Rituximab versus cyclophosphamide for ANCA-associated vasculitis. *N Engl J Med.* 2010;363:221-232.
8. Jayne D, Rasmussen N, Andrassy K, et al, for the European Vasculitis Study Group. A randomized trial of maintenance therapy for vasculitis associated with ANCA. *N Engl J Med.* 2003;349:36-44.
9. Kamanamool N, McEvoy M, Attia J, et al. Efficacy and adverse events of mycophenolate mofetil versus cyclophosphamide for induction therapy of lupus nephritis: systematic review and meta-analysis. *Medicine (Baltimore).* 2010;89:227-235.
10. Dember LM, Hawkins PN, Hazenberg BP, et al. Eprodisate for the treatment of renal disease in AA amyloidosis. *N Engl J Med.* 2007;356:2349-2360.

SUGGESTED READINGS

Ayodele OE, Okpechi IG, Swanepoel CR. Predictors of poor renal outcome in patients with biopsy-proven lupus nephritis. *Nephrology (Carlton).* 2010;15;482-490. *Baseline serum creatinine, no-remission following therapy, and higher blood pressure predict poor renal outcome.*

Beck LH Jr, Salant DJ. Membranous nephropathy: recent travels and new roads ahead. *Kidney Int.* 2010;77:765-770. *Circulating antibodies to the M-type phospholipase A2 receptor are 75% sensitive and 100% specific for idiopathic membranous nephropathy.*

Eison TM, Ault BH, Jones DP, et al. Post-streptococcal acute glomerulonephritis in children: clinical features and pathogenesis. *Pediatr Nephrol.* 2011;26;165-180. *Review.*

Kaufman L, Collins SE, Klotman PE. The pathogenesis of HIV-associated nephropathy. *Adv Chronic Kidney Dis.* 2010;17:36-43. *Review.*

Peto P, Salama AD. Update on antiglomerular basement membrane disease. *Curr Opin Rheumatol.* 2011;23:32-37. *Review.*

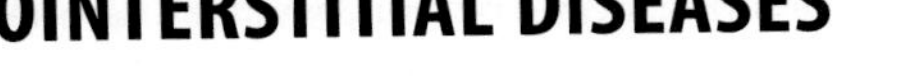

124 TUBULOINTERSTITIAL DISEASES

ERIC G. NEILSON

TUBULOINTERSTITIAL NEPHRITIS

DEFINITION

Interstitial nephritis can be primary and begin in the tubulointerstitium or appear as a secondary event and spread from blood vessels, including the glomerular capillaries. Although injury to the tubulointerstitial compartment can be the result of autoimmunity, a toxic insult, an infection, or exposure to a drug, the inflammatory process always has an immunologic component that leads to the release of tissue cytokines, which eventually convert tubular epithelia into fibroblasts to produce fibrosis.

Tubulointerstitial nephritis can be arbitrarily divided into acute and chronic types. The acute form of interstitial nephritis often begins abruptly. When inciting events subside, so does the nephritis, and the glomerular filtration rate tends to normalize, with little residual damage except in patients with preexisting disease. Chronic interstitial nephritis is persistent and over time reduces the number of functioning nephrons by encasing and dismantling them, with irreversible fibrosis. So-called toxic nephropathy is similar to this form of nephritis. Sometimes acute and chronic injury are difficult to distinguish because global destruction of the tubulointerstitium can occur within a matter of weeks.

EPIDEMIOLOGY

Acute interstitial nephritis appears unexpectedly in otherwise healthy individuals from a variety of causes. About 1% of patients with hematuria and proteinuria have acute interstitial nephritis, and it is seen in 1 to 15% of autopsy series.

The development of acute interstitial nephritis is largely due to the use of pharmaceuticals. Other important causes include infection and idiopathic autoimmune diseases (Table 124-1). Penicillin moieties (less so nafcillin and piperacillin), cephalosporins, sulfa-like drugs, and nonsteroidal anti-inflammatory drugs (NSAIDs) top the list. NSAIDs cause both acute interstitial nephritis and chronic analgesic nephropathy. Diphtheria in children (Chapter 300), legionellosis (Chapter 322), leptospirosis (Chapter 331), histoplasmosis (Chapter 340), tuberculosis (Chapter 332), and DNA viruses such as cytomegalovirus (Chapter 384) and Epstein-Barr virus (Chapter 385) are well-recognized agents of acute interstitial nephritis. Anti–tubular basement membrane disease is a rare cause of autoimmune interstitial nephritis. Although sarcoidosis or the tubulointerstitial nephritis and uveitis (TINU) syndrome can manifest as acute interstitial nephritis on biopsy, they often quickly evolve into chronic disease.

TABLE 124-1 CAUSES OF ACUTE INTERSTITIAL NEPHRITIS

DRUGS
Antibiotics
Penicillins
Rifampin, ethambutol
Sulfa
Vancomycin
Ciprofloxacin
Cephalosporins
Erythromycin
Trimethoprim-sulfamethoxazole
Acyclovir
Nonsteroidal anti-inflammatory drugs
Selective and nonselective cyclooxygenase-2 inhibitors
Diuretics
Thiazides
Furosemide
Triamterene
Miscellaneous
Captopril
Ranitidine
Omeprazole
Phenobarbital
Phenytoin
Sodium valproate
Carbamazepine
Allopurinol
Interferon
Interleukin-2
All-*trans*-retinoic acid
INFECTIONS
Bacteria
Legionella
Brucella
Diphtheria
Streptococcus
Staphylococcus
Yersinia
Salmonella
Escherichia coli
Campylobacter
Viruses
Epstein-Barr virus
Cytomegalovirus
Hantaan virus
Human immunodeficiency virus (HIV)
Herpes simplex virus
Hepatitis B virus
Other
Mycoplasma
Rickettsia
Leptospira
Mycobacterium tuberculosis
Schistosoma mekongi
Toxoplasma
Chlamydia
AUTOIMMUNE DISEASES
Anti–tubular basement membrane disease
Tubulointerstitial nephritis and uveitis (TINU) syndrome
Kawasaki disease

All forms of injury to the kidney, regardless of origin, progress to end-stage renal disease through a terminal phase of chronic interstitial nephritis. In addition to glomerulonephritides (Chapter 123), cystic diseases (Chapter 129), and diabetes (Chapters 236 and 237), a wide variety of renal conditions start slowly in the tubulointerstitium and often go unrecognized until late in the course, when biopsy shows chronic interstitial nephritis.

TABLE 124-2 CAUSES OF CHRONIC INTERSTITIAL NEPHRITIS

HEREDITARY DISEASES
Mitochondrial mutations
METABOLIC DISTURBANCES
Hypercalcemia, nephrocalcinosis
Hyperoxaluria
Hypokalemia
Hyperuricemia
Cystinosis
Methylmalonicacidemia
DRUGS AND TOXINS
Analgesics
Cadmium
Lead
Health food botanicals, herbs
Lithium
Cyclosporine, tacrolimus
Cisplatin, methotrexate
Nitrosoureas
AUTOIMMUNE DISEASES
Renal allograft rejection
Wegener's granulomatosis
Sjögren's syndrome
Systemic lupus erythematosus, vasculitis
Progressive glomerular disease
Sarcoidosis
HEMATOLOGIC DISTURBANCES
Multiple myeloma, light chains
Lymphoma
Sickle cell disease
INFECTIONS
Complicated pyelonephritis
Human immunodeficiency virus (HIV)
Epstein-Barr virus
Malacoplakia
Xanthogranulomatous pyelonephritis
OBSTRUCTIVE NEPHROPATHY
Tumors
Stones
Outlet obstruction
Vesicoureteral reflux
MISCELLANEOUS
Age-related vascular disease
Hypertension
Ischemia
Balkan (endemic) nephropathy
Radiation nephritis

Primary chronic interstitial nephritis can be caused by a variety of toxic, metabolic, hematologic, obstructive, and infectious processes. Ingestion of six or more tablets per day of acetaminophen, aspirin, or NSAIDs, alone or together, for at least 3 years puts patients at risk for analgesic nephropathy. A careful history of drug or toxin exposure, previous renal images, and a family history often point to a probable diagnosis (Table 124-2).

PATHOBIOLOGY

Pathophysiology

Regardless of the origin of renal inflammation, the kidneys do not fail until interstitial nephritis, fibrosis, and tubular atrophy develop. Interstitial nephritis is the pathologic equivalent of clinical progression because it is the final common pathway to permanent tissue damage. The degree of reduction in the glomerular filtration rate correlates with the degree of interstitial injury. Urinary flow is impeded by tubular obstruction. Increased vascular resistance causes progressive tubular injury and fibrosis. A net reduction in the cross-sectional area of peritubular vessels increases postglomerular resistance to the extent that the compensatory increase in glomerular hydrostatic pressure cannot fully restore filtration to normal levels. Tubuloglomerular feedback assumes increasing importance in the transition from acute to chronic glomerulonephritis when autoregulation of renal blood flow is disrupted by tubulointerstitial fibrosis. Loss of autoregulation by tubuloglomerular feedback results from the absence or insensitivity of the afferent arteriole. Perhaps more significant is the effect of interstitial pressure on the sensitivity of the feedback mechanism. Tubular atrophy may disrupt the normal renal osmotic gradient by decreasing sodium chloride transport along the proximal tubule or thick ascending loop of Henle. The result is poor abstraction of water from the filtrate, with hyposthenuria and polyuria. Such an increase in solute and water within the tubular fluid results in adaptive downregulation of the glomerular filtration process.

The antigen targets for the immune system in interstitial nephritis are poorly understood. Drugs act as haptens, mimic endogenous structures in the interstitium, alter regulation of the immune system, or function in some combination of the foregoing. Bacteria, fungi, and viruses can infect the kidney and cause mononuclear cell infiltration or activate Toll-like receptors on tubular epithelia, which subsequently educate the adaptive immune response to events in the interstitium. Autoimmune diseases such as anti–tubular basement membrane disease or spontaneous interstitial nephritis remain confined to the kidney, whereas systemic diseases spread to the kidney where they cause persistent, chronic interstitial nephritis.

Although the adaptive immune response is similar to that of other tissues, T-cell activation figures prominently in interstitial nephritis. Antibodies (anti–tubular basement membrane disease) and immune complex deposition along the tubular basement membrane (systemic lupus erythematosus) are rarely seen. Antigens presented by class II major histocompatibility complex molecules on macrophages, dendritic cells, and adjacent tubular epithelia, in conjunction with associative recognition molecules, engage the CD4/CD8 T-cell repertoires. The resultant cytokine and protease activity injures tubular nephrons and basement membranes and causes fibroblasts to form locally by epithelial-mesenchymal transition. Transforming growth factor-β (TGF-β), fibroblast growth factor 2, and platelet-derived growth factor are particularly active in this transition. If the nephritis persists, fibrogenesis dismantles nephrons and causes tubular atrophy; in late stages, the inflammatory reaction outgrows its survival factors, and lymphocytes and fibroblasts disappear by apoptosis and leave an acellular fibrotic scar.

Viruses, including Epstein-Barr virus, have long been suspected of contributing to idiopathic, chronic interstitial nephritis. Malacoplakia and xanthogranulomatous pyelonephritis are probably not defects in nephrogenesis but rather are destructive responses to bacterial inflammation in the interstitium. Focal abnormalities in kidney structure can be a nidus for infections associated with perinephric, psoas, or peritoneal abscesses. Children with vesicoureteral reflux can have chronic or repeating episodes of pyelonephritis, but whether the reflux or the infection is more important to progression to renal failure is unclear. There is also no agreement on whether recurrent pyelonephritis by itself produces chronic interstitial nephritis in adults.

Pathology

Both kidneys are typically involved, except in cases of unilateral infection, obstruction, or trauma. The inflammatory reaction in acute interstitial nephritis consists mainly of T lymphocytes and monocytes, but neutrophils, plasma cells, and eosinophils can be present. The T cells are of a mixed phenotype with a distinct preference for $CD4^+$ lymphocytes. The infiltrative process is associated with interstitial edema, which displaces tubules away from one another and causes the kidneys to swell. The tubular basement membrane may be disrupted in more severe cases, but immune deposits are rarely found by immunofluorescence.

In chronic interstitial nephritis, the kidney assumes an irregular or contracted appearance. The tubular epithelia sit on thickened or disrupted tubular basement membranes and are often effaced against dilated lumens, and the tubules eventually dismantle and atrophy. *Chronic* is a relative term, because fibrotic changes can be seen within 7 to 10 days of continuing inflammation. Normal glomeruli in primary interstitial nephritis are eventually surrounded by periglomerular fibrosis and subsequently undergo segmental or global sclerosis. Chronic vascular thickening and glomerular changes are present in advanced stages of disease, so pathologic determination of the primary cause may be difficult in some biopsy samples. Progressive glomerular sclerosis also occurs with aging and must be factored in when interpreting the biopsy findings.

A third pathologic category, granuloma formation, can be seen in either acute or chronic interstitial nephritis. In acute granulomatous interstitial nephritis, granulomas are sparse and non-necrotic, and giant cells are rare. The granulomas in chronic interstitial nephritis contain an abundance of giant cells, and those caused by tuberculosis may become necrotic. Drugs are a common cause of this lesion in the acute setting, and most of the drugs associated with acute interstitial nephritis have been reported to cause granuloma formation. In the absence of drug exposure, sarcoidosis (Chapter 95), Wegener's granulomatosis (Chapter 278), histoplasmosis (Chapter 340), or tuberculosis (Chapter 332) should be considered, depending on the context, when numerous granulomas are present. The renal granulomas seen in Wegener's granulomatosis are almost always accompanied by glomerular and vascular pathology.

ACUTE INTERSTITIAL NEPHRITIS

CLINICAL MANIFESTATIONS

Most patients present with an asymptomatic rise in the serum creatinine level or an abnormal urinalysis, and it is important to consider acute interstitial nephritis in any patient with an unexplained precipitous diminution in renal function. Because injury is often asymptomatic, patients may already have substantial renal failure on initial presentation. Patients may also present with nonspecific symptoms such as lethargy or weakness, and many patients have fever and oliguria owing to severe acute kidney injury (Chapter 122).

Several features can distinguish acute interstitial nephritis from acute tubular necrosis (Chapter 122) or glomerulonephritis (Chapter 123) (Table 124-3). Fever and occasional flank pain over the kidneys occur in infection or with drug-induced acute interstitial nephritis. Lumbar pain, sometimes unilateral, is due to distention of the renal capsule. Allergic reactions are associated with maculopapular rash, fever, and eosinophilia, but the entire triad is seen in less than 33% of patients, and such signs are uncommon when NSAIDs cause acute interstitial nephritis.

The course of renal failure in acute interstitial nephritis takes several days to weeks and follows the kinetics of the primary immune response. However, renal failure can be precipitous, especially in patients re-exposed to a previous agent. Rarely, the course can be protracted, with the glomerular filtration rate declining over a period of months if the diagnosis is not recognized. This protracted course is more common with diuretic-induced interstitial nephritis. The onset of drug-induced nephritis ranges from days to weeks after the initiation of therapy, and a previous allergic history is rare. The classic setting for a drug reaction is a febrile patient with an infectious process and who defervesces while taking antibiotics but then develops recurrent fever several days later.

DIAGNOSIS

Urinalysis is particularly helpful. Mild to moderate proteinuria and hematuria are seen in most cases, and gross hematuria is observed occasionally. The sediment typically shows red and white blood cells, and white blood cell casts are commonly seen. Conversely, red blood cell casts suggest a glomerular diagnosis. The finding of eosinophils in the urine supports the diagnosis of allergic interstitial nephritis, but the absence of eosinophiluria does not exclude the diagnosis of acute interstitial nephritis.

An elevated serum creatinine level is usually the first abnormal laboratory result in renal injury. The normal serum creatinine of 0.6 to 1.3 mg/dL varies with muscle mass, age, and gender. Early recognition of acute interstitial nephritis requires a high degree of clinical suspicion because the serum creatinine level may be only mildly elevated even after the kidneys lose half their function.

The magnitude of proteinuria in acute interstitial nephritis is nearly always less than 3 g/24 hours and is typically less than 1 g/24 hours. Nephrotic-range proteinuria is not seen unless there is a coexisting glomerular lesion, such as a concurrent minimal-change lesion, or after exposure to NSAIDs. Many patients with acute interstitial nephritis also have a fractional excretion of sodium (FE_{Na}) greater than 1, but occasionally they are oliguric.

Imaging is of little diagnostic value. The kidney in acute interstitial nephritis is usually normal or slightly increased in size on echographic or tomographic images. Increased cortical echogenicity may correlate with diffuse interstitial infiltrates on renal biopsy. Gallium scanning is not particularly useful because a variety of other renal processes can cause gallium uptake, including minimal change glomerulonephritis, cortical necrosis, and acute tubular necrosis; in addition, acute interstitial nephritis can be found on biopsy in those with a normal scan.

Differential Diagnosis

It is sometimes difficult to distinguish among nonoliguric acute tubular necrosis, acute interstitial nephritis, and glomerulonephritis without a biopsy. Selective tubular defects and tubular syndromes such as proximal acquired Fanconi's syndrome (bicarbonaturia with a plasma carbon dioxide [CO_2] content <20 mEq/L, aminoaciduria, phosphate wasting, uricosuria, and glycosuria) or distal renal tubular acidosis type 1 (urine pH >5.6, plasma CO_2 content <20 mEq/L, with low or high potassium) can be seen in subacute or chronic interstitial nephritis but argue against acute interstitial nephritis.

Biopsy

Ultimately, the diagnosis can be established with certainty only by renal biopsy, which confirms and assesses the extent of acute interstitial inflammation. A biopsy should be performed in patients with acute renal failure who have suggestive signs or symptoms of an interstitial process and in whom prerenal azotemia and obvious acute tubular necrosis cannot be excluded on clinical grounds (Table 124-4). In primary acute interstitial nephritis, the biopsy demonstrates inflammatory cells that typically spare the glomeruli until late in the course (Fig. 124-1A). Lesions that reduce renal function are usually diffuse, but drug-induced interstitial injury is often patchy, beginning deep in the cortex before spreading.

TREATMENT Rx

Biopsy is important to confirm acute interstitial nephritis, because chronic interstitial fibrosis rarely responds to aggressive treatment. The principal intervention for acute interstitial nephritis is to remove the inciting drug or treat the infection. Switching to different derivatives of a suspected drug is unwise. Concomitantly, or if the serum creatinine concentration does not fall after a few days, steroids (prednisone 0.75 to 1.0 mg/kg orally) can be given daily for approximately 1 week. If no further improvement occurs, oral cyclophosphamide (1 to 2 mg/kg/day) can be added for several more weeks. In patients who respond, cyclophosphamide can be steroid sparing, particularly in those with persistent sarcoidosis. It is important not to continue high-dose immunosuppression without some evidence of benefit because immunosuppressive drugs in patients with azotemia can lead to serious infection and even death. It is better to reserve these drugs for use with kidney transplantation if the primary disease does not respond.

PROGNOSIS

The prognosis for acute interstitial nephritis is good if it is recognized early. Early removal of offending agents or prompt treatment with antibiotics or immunosuppressive drugs can be renoprotective.

CHRONIC INTERSTITIAL NEPHRITIS

CLINICAL MANIFESTATIONS

Patients with primary chronic interstitial nephritis typically have elevated levels of serum creatinine and signs and symptoms of renal failure, including

TABLE 124-3 TYPICAL CLINICAL MANIFESTATION OF ACUTE INTERSTITIAL NEPHRITIS

History of drug hypersensitivity or recent infection and taking antibiotics
Sudden onset of fever lasting several days to weeks
Variable degrees of hypertension
Rise in creatinine with FE_{Na} >1.0; no expected acute tubular necrosis or glomerulonephritis
Kidney size normal or increased
Hematuria with mild proteinuria (<1.0 g)
Presence of WBC casts and WBCs on urinalysis; rarely eosinophils

FE_{Na} = fractional excretion of sodium; WBC = white blood cell.

TABLE 124-4 WHEN TO CONSIDER A RENAL BIOPSY TO DIAGNOSE NEPHRITIS

The setting, history, or clinical findings do not support a diagnosis of acute tubular necrosis or volume depletion
The clinical setting warrants a tissue diagnosis to determine the type of lesion, the extent of involvement, or the degree of fibrosis
The patient is stable enough to undergo biopsy and receive immunosuppressive drugs
The physician believes that the choice of therapy or the length of treatment is partially determined by the type of tissue injury

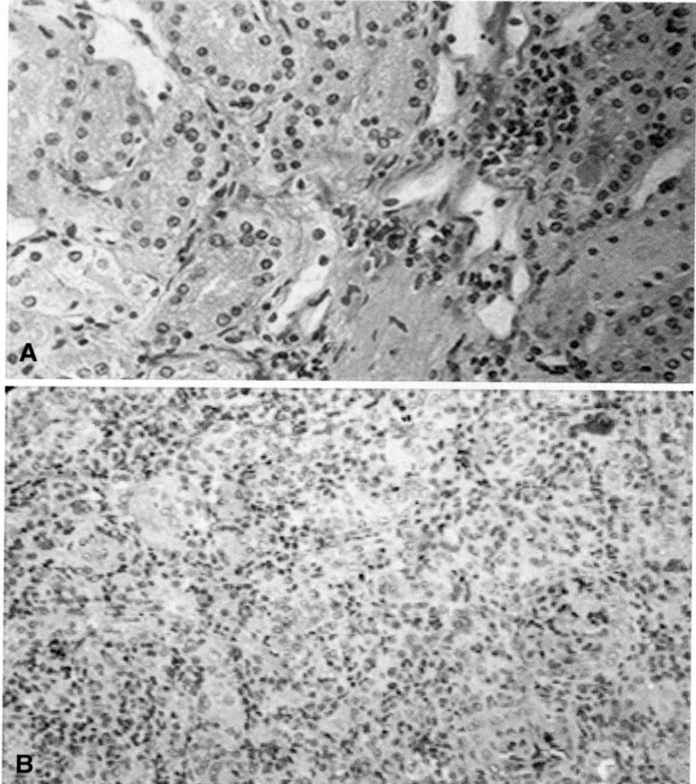

FIGURE 124-1. **Tubulointerstitial nephritis on biopsy. A,** Acute interstitial nephritis can be most aggressive when the interstitium is crowded with mononuclear cells and giant cells that destroy nearly all tubular nephrons (hematoxylin-eosin). **B,** Chronic interstitial nephritis is a slower process, with substantial collagen deposition (blue color; trichrome), tubular dropout, and fibroblasts in the interstitial spaces widened by fibrosis.

hematuria, hyposthenuria, nocturia, fatigue, and nausea. Urinalysis shows a fixed specific gravity of about 1.010, occasional glycosuria, and non-nephrotic–range proteinuria (often <1 g/L), with red and white blood cells and granular casts. Pyuria and positive urine cultures for bacteria are seen occasionally, and varying degrees of metabolic acidosis and hyperphosphatemia may be present. Before the glomerular filtration rate falls below 25 to 30 mL/minute, tubular acidosis is common. Anemia is often out of proportion to the degree of renal failure, and many patients have hypertension but only minimal edema until advanced stages of renal failure. Acquired Fanconi's syndrome can be seen in patients with a serum creatinine level less than 2.5 mg/dL in the setting of drug exposure, myeloma, human immunodeficiency virus (HIV) infection, lead exposure, and herbal nephropathy.

DIAGNOSIS

A careful dietary history is critical. As for any patient with evidence of renal failure, the evaluation includes laboratory tests to determine possible causes and severity. These tests include measures of renal function(serum creatinine level and blood urea nitrogen level), as well as levels of serum electrolytes, calcium, phosphate, uric acid, and albumin. Urinalysis shows a fixed specific gravity of about 1.010, occasional glycosuria, proteinuria (often <1 g/L), and red cells, white cells, and granular casts. Depending on the clinical situation, the search for specific causes may include serum and urine protein electrophoresis, blood cultures, and serologic tests for autoimmune diseases (e.g., cryoglobulin level, antinuclear antibodies [see Table 265-1 in Chapter 265], anti–neutrophil cytoplasmic antibody, and anti–glomerular basement membrane antibody levels).

Classic images of analgesic nephropathy on tomography are quite specific (Fig. 124-2) and show a decrease in overall kidney size, with atrophic scars and an irregular cortical contour, sometimes accompanied by papillary necrosis.

On biopsy (see Table 124-4), chronic interstitial nephritis is manifest by a cellular infiltrate that is eventually replaced by tubulointerstitial fibrosis (Fig. 124-1B). Infiltrates of lymphocytes and rare neutrophils are scattered and less abundant than in acute interstitial nephritis.

Specific Causes

Analgesics

Aspirin, acetaminophen, and NSAIDs alone or together are a source of toxic metabolites and can induce medullary ischemia and papillary necrosis, sometimes with papillary calcification. The likelihood of analgesic nephropathy from taking acetaminophen alone is much less than with the others. Uroepithelial malignancies also occur with increased frequency in this group of patients.

Aristolochic Acid Nephropathy

Aristolochic acid has been implicated as a cause of Balkan nephropathy and so-called Chinese herbal nephropathy. A growing number of people are taking vitamins and herbal preparations purchased from health food stores (Chapter 38). Some of these remedies contain botanicals that produce chronic interstitial nephritis. Patients who are dieting often use these remedies and are first seen when they already have late-stage disease, which increases the risk for uroepithelial malignancies.

Vascular Disease

Chronic renal ischemia from vascular injury can lead to interstitial nephritis, nephrosclerosis, and fibrosis. This is the classic renal lesion of untreated essential hypertension (Chapter 67). Similar injury is seen with aging, diabetes (Chapter 126), sickle cell disease (Chapter 166), and radiation nephritis (Chapter 19). This tubulointerstitial injury from the vascular diseases just mentioned is quite different from the aggressive necrosis seen with acute vasculitis. In patients taking calcineurin inhibitors such as cyclosporine or tacrolimus, renal ischemia from vasoconstriction can cause interstitial fibrosis that is sometimes difficult to distinguish from chronic allograft rejection.

Obstruction

Significant urinary obstruction (Chapter 125) owing to occlusion of both ureters by bladder tumors, cervical carcinoma, ureteral valve disease, or bladder outlet obstruction is an important cause of chronic interstitial nephritis. Complete or partial urinary tract obstruction is accompanied by a decline in glomerular filtration and classic tubular abnormalities, including diminished reabsorption of solutes, impaired excretion of H^+ and K^+, and a vasopressin-resistant concentrating defect in the medulla. Obstruction is associated with a fall in the glomerular filtration rate because of reduced plasma flow and hydraulic pressure associated with the release of angiotensin II, leukotrienes, and nitric oxide, a process leading to mononuclear cell infiltration. Growth factors such as TGF-β, released by infiltrating cells, may contribute to the interstitial and glomerular fibrosis. Obstruction is more common in men than in women and is part of the routine assessment of renal failure by renal ultrasound (Chapters 122 and 125). Almost all obstructed kidneys eventually become infected if the obstruction is not relieved.

Hypercalcemia

Hypercalcemia can decrease glomerular filtration through renal vasoconstriction, a decrease in the glomerular ultrafiltration coefficient, and volume depletion as a result of a vasopressin-resistant concentrating defect associated with nephrocalcinosis and calcium deposition around the basement membranes of the distal tubules and collecting ducts. Such deposition secondarily leads to mononuclear cell infiltration and tubular death. Nephrocalcinosis also occurs in normocalcemic disorders of augmented calcium absorption through the gut (sarcoidosis [Chapter 95], vitamin D intoxication [Chapter 253]), skeletal breakdown (neoplasms or multiple myeloma [Chapter 193]), or classic distal renal tubular acidosis.

Myeloma

The chronic renal failure of multiple myeloma (Chapter 193) is caused by several mechanisms, including cast nephropathy ("myeloma kidney"), coexistent volume depletion, hypercalcemia (Chapter 253), nephrocalcinosis (Chapter 253), and uric acid nephropathy. Proteinaceous casts form in dilated, atrophic distal nephron segments that are surrounded by multinucleated giant cells in interstitial infiltrates. The casts typically contain both Tamm-Horsfall protein and a pathologic light chain. Interstitial plasma cells and mononuclear infiltrates, calcifications in the interstitium, and amyloid deposits in the vessels and glomeruli are often present. Light chains are nephrotoxic by direct injury to tubular cells or through intrarenal obstruction from cast formation. In the setting of excess light chain production, the proximal tubule reabsorptive capacity is overwhelmed, leading to their urinary excretion as Bence Jones

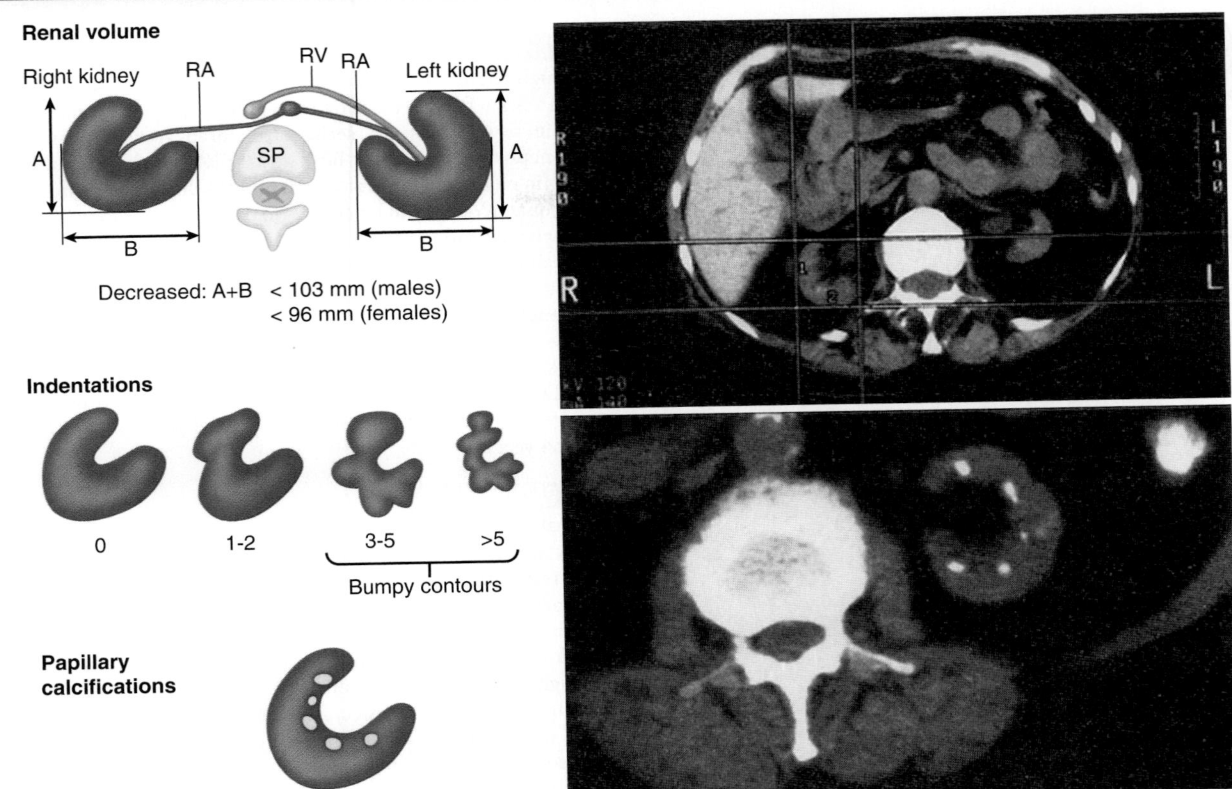

FIGURE 124-2. **Renal changes in analgesic nephropathy seen by tomographic imaging.** Structural changes, including reduced volume, nodularity, and calcifications, are seen on computed tomography. RA = right artery; RV = right vein; SP = spinal vertebra. (From Elseviers MM, De Schepper A, Corthouts R, et al. High diagnostic performance of CT scan for analgesic nephropathy in patients with incipient to severe renal failure. *Kidney Int.* 1995;48:1316.)

proteins. An elevated intratubular pressure partly accounts for the decline in glomerular filtration in experimental cast nephropathy.

Lead Toxicity

Epidemiologic analyses support the association between excess lead burden (Chapter 21) and chronic renal failure. Blood lead levels reflect only recent, not chronic, exposure and can be normal in patients with a significant lead burden. Lead preferentially deposits in the proximal tubule, and nuclear inclusions within proximal tubular cells are characteristic of lead nephropathy.

Ingestion of moonshine liquor, with its high lead content, can be an important historical clue to the diagnosis. In adults, lead nephropathy produces chronic interstitial nephritis, fibrosis, and nephrosclerosis. Proximal tubular dysfunction may produce isolated tubule defects or a full Fanconi's syndrome. Patients often have recurrent gout, and hyperuricemia and hypertension may be present. Some laboratories can measure δ-aminolevulinic acid dehydratase, which is inhibited by lead. Although chelation studies may document lead burden, this test is difficult to perform in patients with renal failure. X-ray fluorescent measurements of in vivo skeletal lead stores correlate well with ethylenediaminetetraacetic acid (EDTA) chelation tests and have the advantage of being rapid and noninvasive.

Cadmium Toxicity

Cadmium nephropathy (Chapter 21) is seen in regions with contamination from smelters that result in prolonged low-level exposure. Cadmium is bound to metallothionein, and proximal tubular cells take up these complexes. The liver and kidney are the two major organs in which cadmium accumulates. Its half-life in the body is longer than 10 years. Like blood levels of lead, blood levels of cadmium fall after acute exposure because of extensive tissue deposition. Once a threshold of renal deposition is exceeded, excess cadmium is excreted in urine. Cadmium intoxication produces irreversible proximal tubular dysfunction, hypercalciuria, nephrolithiasis, and metabolic bone disease with pain (called "ouch-ouch" disease in Japan).

Hyperuricemia

Hyperuricemia, especially in acutely treated myeloproliferative disease, can cause acute renal failure. Many patients with chronic renal failure have serum uric acid levels higher than 10 mg/dL, attributable to diminished glomerular filtration and the effects of diuretics. However, most studies have not demonstrated an independent association of hyperuricemia with chronic interstitial disease that could not otherwise be attributed to hypertension, vascular disease, calculi, or aging.

TREATMENT Rx

Chronic interstitial nephritis tends to progress slowly. Inciting factors such as obstruction, infection, drugs, or toxins should be removed whenever possible. Angiotensin-converting enzyme inhibitors or angiotensin II receptor blockers (see Table 67-5 in Chapter 67) are used early to slow disease progression, with a systolic blood pressure goal of 130 mm Hg or less (Chapters 67 and 132), except when hyperkalemia limits their use. Early treatment of acidosis with oral sodium bicarbonate, starting at 600 mg three times daily.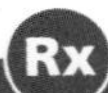 Anemia with erythropoietin (e.g., darbepoetin alfa 0.45 μg/kg weekly to keep the hemoglobin concentration between 10 and 12 g/L), hyperphosphatemia with oral phosphate binders (see Table 121-4 in Chapter 121), and hyperparathyroidism with calcitriol (starting at 0.25 μg/day) can improve performance status and protect against bone loss (Chapters 132 and 133). There is no clear role for immunosuppressive drugs in the treatment of chronic interstitial nephritis, except perhaps in early sarcoidosis (Chapter 95).

For certain specific causes of chronic interstitial nephritis, specific therapeutic approaches are warranted. For analgesic nephropathy, stopping analgesic use can help reduce progression. For hypercalcemia (Chapter 253), therapy is directed toward the primary disease: reduction of the serum calcium concentration, when appropriate, and correction of acid-base disturbances.

Appropriate therapy for presumed cast nephropathy in multiple myeloma includes chemotherapy to ameliorate excess light chain production (Chapter 193); treatment of hypercalcemia (Chapter 253); alkalinization of the urine with the addition of bicarbonate to hypotonic fluids; and avoidance of radiocontrast agents, which may enhance the nephrotoxicity of light chains. Loop diuretics should be used with caution, particularly in the setting of volume depletion.

EDTA is advocated as chelation therapy for lead toxicity (Chapter 21). The goal of chelation is to normalize the EDTA mobilization test. In occasional patients, this may arrest or reverse the progression of the renal failure.

PROGNOSIS

The prognosis for chronic interstitial nephritis is highly variable and depends on the underlying condition and on comorbid conditions, including cardiovascular disease and diabetes mellitus, which become increasingly common in these patients over time.

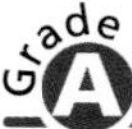

1. de Brito-Ashurst I, Varagunam M, Raftery MJ, et al. Bicarbonate supplementation slows progression of CKD and improves nutritional status. *J Am Soc Nephrol.* 2009;20:2075-2084.

SUGGESTED READINGS

Perazella MA, Markowitz GS. Drug-induced acute interstitial nephritis. *Nat Rev Nephrol.* 2010;6:462-470. *Review, including the potential role for corticosteroids.*

Praga M, González E. Acute interstitial nephritis. *Kidney Int.* 2010;77:956-961. *Review suggesting a role for early corticosteroid therapy.*

Tanaka T, Nangaku M. Pathogenesis of tubular interstitial nephritis. *Contrib Nephrol.* 2011;169:297-310. *Review.*

125

OBSTRUCTIVE UROPATHY

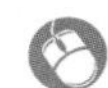

MARK L. ZEIDEL

DEFINITION

Each day in the average adult, 1.5 to 2 L of urine flows from the kidneys to the end of the urethra, a process that requires proper functioning of each renal pelvis, the ureters, bladder, and urethra. *Obstructive uropathy* occurs when a defect (structural or functional) in the urinary tract blocks or reduces urine flow. When obstructive uropathy impairs renal function, *obstructive nephropathy* ensues. Increased hydrostatic pressure from obstruction downstream may cause dilation of upstream elements of the urinary tract, or *hydronephrosis*. Because recovery of renal function is inversely related to the duration and severity of the obstruction, prompt recognition and treatment of obstructive uropathy can preserve renal function in this condition.

EPIDEMIOLOGY

Although there are few studies of unselected populations, autopsy series reveal a 3.1% frequency of hydronephrosis in all subjects (2.9% in females, 3.3% in males). Autopsy series of children younger than 16 years reveal hydronephrosis in 2.2% of boys and 1.5% of girls; 80% of hydronephrosis occurs in children younger than 12 months. In adults, hydronephrosis occurs with equal frequency in both sexes in those younger than 20 years, but owing to pregnancy and uterine cancer, it is more common in women than in men between the ages of 20 and 60 years. In those older than 60 years, obstructive uropathy is more common in men because of prostate disease. The annual frequency of hospitalization for obstructive uropathy in the United States is 166 per 100,000. Each year, about 2000 patients with a presumed diagnosis of obstructive nephropathy begin treatment for end-stage renal disease (ESRD), representing 2% of ESRD patients. Among these patients, 4% are younger than 20 years, 44% are aged 20 to 64 years, and the balance are older than 64 years.

PATHOBIOLOGY

Normal urine flow from the renal papilla requires the orderly contraction of the renal pelvis, which "milks" the urine into the proximal end of the ureter. The ureter drives the urine to the bladder by rhythmic peristalsis coupled with periodic opening of the ureterovesical junction. As the bladder fills, stretch is detected in the wall and possibly the urothelium, thereby activating relaxation reflexes that suppress contraction of the bladder wall musculature and tighten the urethral sphincter to allow the bladder to expand without large increases in intravesicular pressure (Fig. 125-1; Chapter 25). When filling reaches a critical level, the voiding reflex is initiated. Suppression of detrusor muscle contraction ends, and stimulation begins, while the urethral sphincter is relaxed, leading to the buildup of pressure needed for voiding. Obstructive uropathy may occur as a result of functional or mechanical defects. Functional failures include an inability to open the ureteropelvic or ureterovesical junction, failure to open the urethrovesical junction, or failure of bladder reflexes. Partial or complete mechanical blockade of the urinary tract at any level can lead to obstruction.

Obstruction can occur at any point along the urinary tract from the renal pelvis and proximal urethra to the end of the urethra (phimosis). Because diagnosis and treatment depend heavily on the location of the obstruction, disorders are classified by anatomic location and whether the obstruction is due to factors within the urinary tract (intrinsic obstruction) or factors outside the tract (extrinsic obstruction) (Table 125-1). Intrinsic obstruction

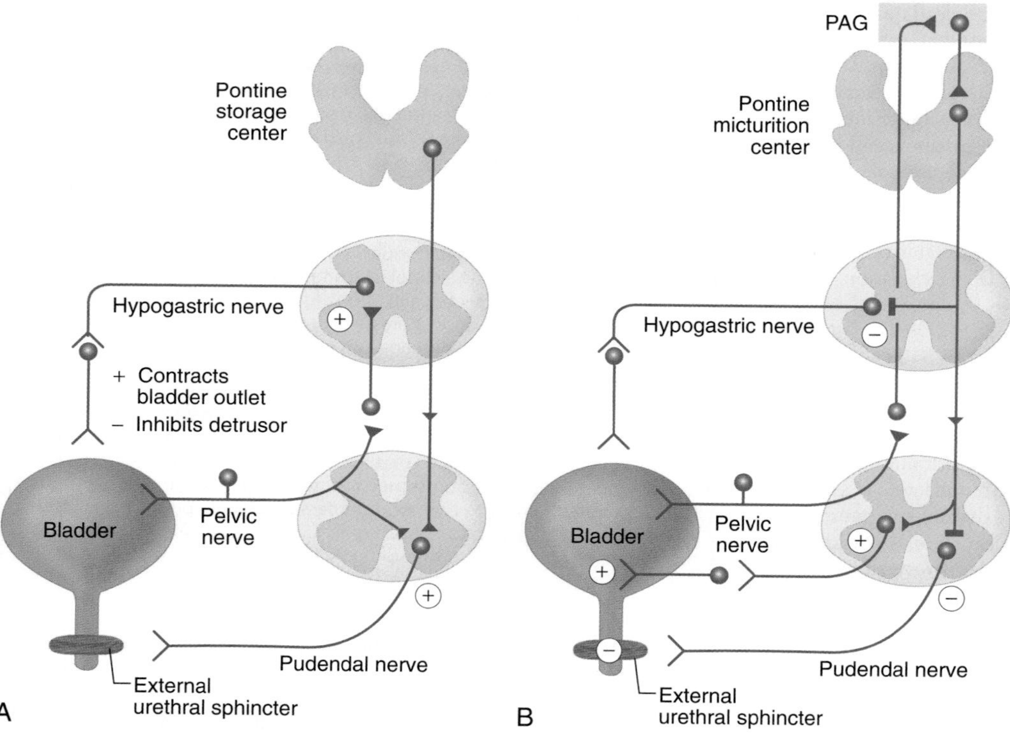

FIGURE 125-1. Neural circuits controlling continence and micturition. A, Reflexes mediating urine storage and continence. As the bladder fills, distention stimulates low-level firing of vesical afferents (pelvic nerve), which in turn stimulate sympathetic outflow to the bladder outlet (hypogastric nerve to contract the internal sphincter and inhibit detrusor activity) and pudendal outflow to the external urethral sphincter. These responses occur by spinal reflex pathways that promote continence. The pontine storage center in the rostral pons augments pudendal nerve firing to enhance external urethral sphincter activity. **B,** Voiding reflexes. As the bladder becomes fuller, afferents fire more intensely and activate spinobulbospinal reflex pathways passing through the pontine micturition center. These reflexes stimulate parasympathetic outflow to the bladder and urethral smooth muscle (hypogastric nerve) and inhibit sympathetic and pudendal outflow to the urethral outlet. Ascending afferent input from the spinal cord may pass through the periaqueductal gray (PAG) matter before reaching the cortex, leading to the sensation of urgency. (Modified from DeGroat WC. Integrative control of the lower urinary tract: a preclinical perspective. *Br J Pharmacol.* 2006;147[Suppl 2]:S25-S40.)

TABLE 125-1 CAUSES OF URINARY TRACT OBSTRUCTION

INTRARENAL
Uric acid nephropathy
Sulfonamide precipitates
Acyclovir, indinavir precipitates
Multiple myeloma
URETERAL
Intrinsic
Intraluminal
Nephrolithiasis
Papillary necrosis
Blood clots
Fungus balls
Intramural
Ureteropelvic junction dysfunction
Ureterovesical junction dysfunction
Ureteral valve, polyp, or tumor
Ureteral stricture
Schistosomiasis
Tuberculosis
Scarring from instrumentation
Drugs (e.g., nonsteroidal anti-inflammatory agents)
Extrinsic
Vascular system
Aneurysm: abdominal aorta or iliac vessels
Aberrant vessels: ureteropelvic junction
Venous: retrocaval ureter
Gastrointestinal tract
Crohn's disease
Diverticulitis
Appendiceal abscess
Colon cancer
Pancreatic tumor, abscess, or cyst
Reproductive system
Uterus: pregnancy, prolapse, tumor, endometriosis
Ovary: abscess, tumor, ovarian remnants
Gartner's duct cyst, tubo-ovarian abscess
Retroperitoneal disease
Retroperitoneal fibrosis: radiation, drugs, idiopathic
Inflammatory: tuberculosis, sarcoidosis
Hematoma
Primary tumor (e.g., lymphoma, sarcoma)
Metastatic tumor (e.g., cervix, ovarian, bladder, colon)
Lymphocele
Pelvic lipomatosis
BLADDER
Neurogenic bladder
Diabetes mellitus
Spinal cord defect
Trauma
Multiple sclerosis
Stroke
Parkinson's disease
Spinal anesthesia
Anticholinergics
Bladder neck dysfunction
Bladder calculus
Bladder cancer
URETHRA
Urethral stricture
Prostate hypertrophy or cancer
Obstruction from instrumentation

may be due to intraluminal or intramural causes. Intraluminal causes include stones or sludging of material, such as sloughed papillae or clots in papillary necrosis. Intramural causes may be anatomic (e.g., tumors or strictures) or functional (e.g., uncoordinated ureteral peristalsis or failure to open the ureteropelvic or ureterovesical junction). Extrinsic causes of obstruction are grouped according to the organ system causing the obstruction.

PATHOLOGY AND PATHOPHYSIOLOGY

Acute obstruction of urine flow out of the nephron reversibly alters renal blood flow, glomerular filtration, and tubular function. Acute unilateral obstruction may cause minimal clinical disturbance because, in the absence of other disease, the contralateral kidney compensates for the loss of function in the affected kidney. Obstructive uropathy is most often partial and of prolonged duration; this chronic obstruction leads to fibrosis and permanent damage.

In acute complete obstruction, glomerular filtration ceases and tubular transport is markedly reduced. Immediately after the onset of complete ureteral obstruction, blockage of urine flow markedly increases tubular intraluminal pressure, which is transmitted back to the glomerulus. Initial dilation of the afferent arteriole maintains glomerular filtration. However, local production of the potent vasoconstrictors angiotensin II and thromboxane A_2 soon decreases the renal blood flow, glomerular filtration pressure, and glomerular filtration rate. Angiotensin and thromboxane also contract glomerular mesangial cells, reducing the glomerular capillary bed surface area available for filtration. At the same time, prostaglandin E_2 and I_2 levels rise and attenuate the level of vasoconstriction.

Obstruction also disrupts the ability of renal tubules (including the proximal tubule, the medullary thick ascending limb of Henle, and the cortical and medullary collecting ducts) to absorb sodium, secrete potassium and acid, and concentrate and dilute the urine. Reduced tubular transport results from the local release of mediators, such as prostaglandin E_2, that inhibit transport, the local accumulation of macrophages, and the release of inflammatory mediators, as well as mechanisms intrinsic to tubular epithelial cells. When urine flow is halted or markedly slowed, reduced delivery of solutes to tubular cells slows the rate of apical sodium entry, resulting in reduced synthesis and deployment to the plasma membrane of crucial transporter proteins, such as Na^+, K^+-ATPase, and apical sodium entry pathways, such as the epithelial sodium channel and Na/K/Cl cotransporter. As obstruction becomes more prolonged, renal fibrosis and permanent damage ensue. In addition to attenuation of salt reabsorption, reduced solute reabsorption in the thick ascending limb leads to loss of high solute concentrations in the medullary interstitium. Obstruction also markedly reduces the synthesis and membrane trafficking of aquaporins, especially aquaporin 2. The combined impact of the absence of medullary solute accumulation and reduced aquaporin activity leads to an inability to concentrate and dilute the urine.

With bilateral complete obstruction, the loss of function of both kidneys leads to the accumulation of salt, water, and uremic toxins; acidosis; and hyperkalemia. Accumulation of salt and water leads to elevated levels of salt-wasting hormones, such as atrial natriuretic peptide, kinins, and prostaglandins, and reduced levels of salt-retaining hormones, such as angiotensin II, catecholamines, and aldosterone. These hormonal changes act synergistically with the postobstructive state of the kidneys to enhance glomerular filtration and reduce tubular salt reabsorption.

Obstructive nephropathy markedly attenuates the ability of distal nephron segments to secrete potassium and acid, leading to hyperkalemia and a non–anion gap metabolic acidosis. With acidemia, failure to acidify the urine may be revealed by a high urine pH (>5.5) and a positive urine anion gap (urine sodium and potassium higher than urine chloride), which indicates distal nephron failure to excrete ammonium in urine. In elderly patients, especially those with azotemia, chronic partial obstruction is associated with hyporeninemic hypoaldosteronism. In this condition, hyperkalemia and non–anion gap metabolic acidosis result from a combination of inadequate aldosterone production for the level of potassium and blood pH and an inadequate tubular response to aldosterone secondary to tubular dysfunction.

Chronic partial urethral obstruction, such as that caused by prostatic hypertrophy in men, can lead to dilation and remodeling of the bladder. Under normal circumstances, as the bladder fills, stretch receptors in the bladder wall and possibly in the epithelium sense the filling. Signaling via afferents to brain stem centers transmits efferent impulses to inhibit bladder wall contraction, permitting the bladder to fill with a modest increase in hydrostatic pressure (see Fig. 125-1). These bladder-filling reflexes also tighten the internal urethral sphincter and allow the maintenance of continence without the need for voluntary contraction of the external sphincter. However, bladder filling to volumes of 200 to 300 mL in women and 300 to 400 mL in men activates additional stretch receptors, stimulating brain stem micturition centers (see Fig. 125-1). Efferents from these centers augment reflex contraction of the bladder detrusor musculature, relax the internal sphincter, and alert the cortex of the need to void. As the bladder fills further, the micturition reflex becomes stronger, the urge to void becomes uncomfortable and urgent, and the bladder begins to contract against the voluntary, external sphincter, rendering it difficult to maintain continence.

With chronic urethral obstruction, micturition requires higher contractile pressure, resulting in detrusor muscle hypertrophy. The bladder empties less completely, and residual volumes increase. Initially, retained urine owing to incomplete emptying diminishes the volume capacity of the bladder between micturitions, thereby resulting in frequency and nocturia. Over time, with bladder remodeling and changes in autonomic reflexes, the transition from bladder accommodation to the micturition reflex may be delayed and occur at increasingly higher bladder-filling volumes. When the micturition reflex is suddenly activated in patients whose bladders are dilated, urgency, dribbling, and frank incontinence ensue. Some of these same features occur in women with pelvic floor disturbances that impede normal bladder function. Bladder wall remodeling and elevated pressures on voiding may increase back pressure up the ureters and result in the physiologic changes of chronic obstruction, including diminished ability to acidify and concentrate the urine, as well as reduced glomerular filtration.

The renal response to the release of obstruction depends on several factors, including whether the obstruction is unilateral or bilateral and the extent and duration of the obstruction. Release of acute unilateral obstruction leads to gradual reversal of renal vasoconstriction and rapid recovery of the glomerular filtration rate. Because tubular transport mechanisms may still be inhibited, postobstructive salt wasting, inability to secrete potassium and acid, and inability to concentrate and dilute the urine persist and lead to the production of a high quantity of isosthenuric urine (urine with a tonicity similar to that of plasma) from the affected kidney. However, the normal contralateral kidney compensates for these abnormalities in tubular transport. Release of an acute bilateral obstruction can lead to high volumes of urine output and striking salt wasting.

CLINICAL MANIFESTATIONS

The clinical appearance of obstructive uropathy depends on the extent (partial or complete), duration (acute or chronic), and location of the obstruction, as well as on whether one or both kidneys are affected (Table 125-2). Patients may be asymptomatic even with severe obstruction, especially when the obstruction has developed gradually.

Symptoms

In patients with acute obstruction, bladder distention caused by the inability to relax the urethral sphincter (e.g., postoperatively) gives rise to sharp pain. By contrast, significant bladder stretching may occur without pain in the setting of gradual urethral obstruction from prostatic enlargement.

Renal colic from the abrupt distention of the ureter is a common manifestation of the passage of a renal calculus (Chapter 128), with or without acute ureteral obstruction. Renal colic is a severe, stabbing pain localized to the flank (when the stone is in the upper third of the ureter) or radiating to the groin or pelvic structures (when the stone is located in the lower two thirds of the ureter).

Patients with chronic partial obstruction may have no symptoms or may have intermittent pain. Chronic partial ureteral obstruction may cause intermittent flank pain. Abdominal pain that radiates to the flank during voiding may indicate vesicoureteral reflux. Increasing the urine volume with the administration of fluid loads or diuretics may elicit pain in patients with partial obstruction by stretching the ureteral wall.

Symptoms such as reduced force and caliber of the urine stream, urinary frequency, hesitancy, incontinence, nocturia, postvoid dribbling, and urgency often arise with urethral obstruction. A neurogenic bladder may alter micturition and result in frequency, urgency, and incontinence. Incontinence may occur because an inadequate sensation of bladder fullness or an inability to void properly leads to overfilling of the bladder and reflex emptying (overflow incontinence).

In patients with complete bilateral ureteral obstruction, complete obstruction of a solitary functioning kidney, or complete obstruction to urine flow beyond the bladder, anuric acute renal failure occurs. Patients with partial obstruction may have normal urine volumes or polyuria. In some cases, partial obstruction prevents urinary concentration, leading to polyuria, increased thirst, and sometimes hypernatremia. Although unusual, a history of oligoanuria alternating with polyuria or the sudden onset of anuria strongly suggests obstructive uropathy.

Bilateral complete obstruction or complete obstruction of a single functioning kidney may cause signs, symptoms, and laboratory evidence of acute renal failure (Chapter 122), with volume overload, hypertension, and metabolic disturbances. By contrast, unilateral obstruction with a functioning contralateral kidney usually does not lead to manifestations of renal failure because the functioning kidney may compensate in large part for the failure of filtration and tubular transport in the obstructed kidney. If the obstruction affects both kidneys, patients may have symptoms of impaired renal function, including nocturia and polyuria from failure to concentrate the urine and increased levels of potassium, phosphate, creatinine, and blood urea nitrogen (Chapter 122).

TABLE 125-2 CLINICAL MANIFESTATIONS AND LABORATORY FINDINGS IN URINARY TRACT OBSTRUCTION

No symptoms (chronic hydronephrosis)
Intermittent pain (chronic hydronephrosis)
Elevated levels of blood urea nitrogen and serum creatinine with no other symptoms (chronic hydronephrosis)
Renal colic (usually caused by ureteral stones or papillary necrosis)
Changes in urinary output
- Anuria or oliguria (acute renal failure)
- Polyuria (incomplete or partial obstruction)
- Fluctuating urinary output

Hematuria
Palpable masses
- Flank (hydronephrotic kidney, usually in infants)
- Suprapubic (distended bladder)

Hypertension
- Volume dependent (usually caused by chronic bilateral obstruction)
- Renin dependent (usually caused by acute unilateral obstruction)

Repeated urinary tract infections or infection refractory to treatment
Hyperkalemic, hyperchloremic acidosis (usually caused by defective tubular secretion of hydrogen and potassium)
Hypernatremia (seen in infants with partial obstruction and polyuria)
Polycythemia (increased renal production of erythropoietin)
Lower urinary tract symptoms: hesitancy, urgency, incontinence, postvoid dribbling, decreased force and caliber of the urinary stream, nocturia

Physical Examination

In patients with acute ureteral obstruction, the physical examination may be normal or it may reveal flank tenderness. Flank tenderness can denote obstruction or pyelonephritis. Renal colic may cause abdominal distention and evidence of reduced peristalsis with diminished bowel sounds. Kidneys enlarged by chronic hydronephrosis may be palpable on the abdominal examination or may cause costovertebral angle tenderness and flank rigidity. In patients with acute obstruction below the bladder, acute bladder distention may be detectable as a suprapubic mass, and the bladder may be tender. In the setting of bladder distention, the rectal examination in men may reveal prostatic enlargement, whereas the pelvic examination in women may reveal pelvic masses. Obstructive uropathy may cause hypertension owing to salt and water retention. Examination of the sensory and reflex pathways of the sacral nerves may reveal neurologic causes of urinary retention.

Hematuria

Laboratory Findings

Patients with obstruction may exhibit gross hematuria, especially in the setting of ureteral stones, which may cause bleeding by abrading the ureteral epithelium (urothelium) as they pass. Microscopic examination of the urine reveals round, regular red cells; this is different from hematuria from glomerular disease, in which red cells (because they cross the glomerulus and remain for prolonged periods in the tubules) appear dysmorphic. Gross hematuria from any cause may lead to clots, which themselves can cause obstruction.

A urinary tract infection in a younger man or repeated urinary tract infections without apparent cause suggest a structural lesion in the urinary tract and are often associated with partial or complete obstruction. Infection occurs more commonly in patients with obstruction involving the bladder or urethra, likely due to disruption of normal defenses against bacterial access and adherence to the bladder urothelium. The finding of unusual organisms (e.g., *Pseudomonas* or *Proteus* species) in noninstrumented patients suggests the disruption of normal defense mechanisms and possible obstruction.

Depending on the extent and duration of obstruction, obstructive uropathy impairs renal function. Hyperkalemia and a nonanion acidosis, owing to distal renal tubular acidosis (Chapter 130), commonly develop. Chronic and

TABLE 125-3 DIAGNOSTIC TESTS FOR OBSTRUCTIVE UROPATHY

UPPER URINARY TRACT OBSTRUCTION
Sonography (ultrasound)
Plain films of the abdomen (KUB)
Excretory or intravenous pyelography
Retrograde pyelography
Isotopic renography
Computed tomography*
Magnetic resonance imaging*
Pressure flow studies (Whitaker test)
LOWER URINARY TRACT OBSTRUCTION
Tests marked with an asterisk above
Cystoscopy
Voiding cystourethrography
Retrograde urethrography
Urodynamic tests
Cystometrography
Electromyography
Urethral pressure profile

KUB = kidneys, ureter, bladder.
From Klahr S. Obstructive uropathy. In: Jacobson HR, Striker GE, Klahr S, eds. *The Principles and Practice of Nephrology*. Toronto: BC Decker; 1991:432-441.

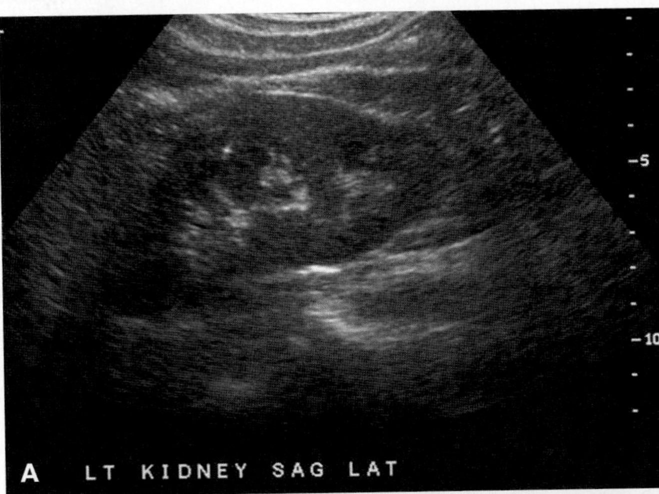

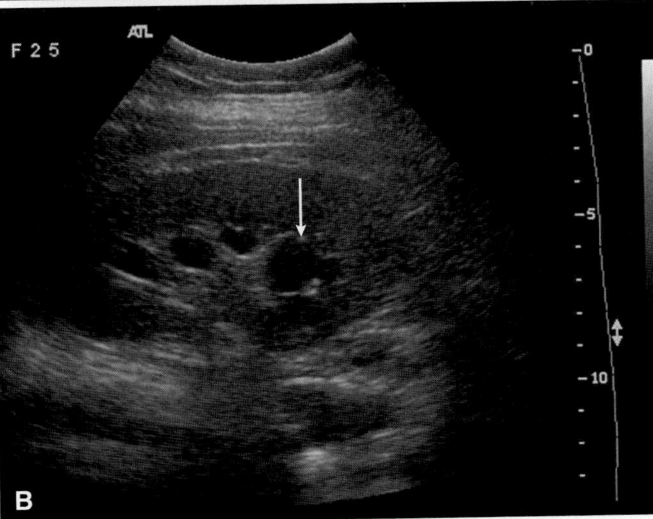

FIGURE 125-2. **A,** Renal ultrasound of a normal kidney. The outline of the kidney is clearly seen, and the calyces (darker areas) are small and somewhat indistinct. **B,** Renal ultrasound of an obstructed kidney. The arrow points directly at a dilated renal calyx. Other dilated calyces are seen as large, round, dark areas adjacent to the calyx pointed out by the arrow. For orientation, the tail end of the arrow overlies the margin of the renal cortex. (Courtesy Jonathan Kruskal, MD.)

more complete obstruction causes permanent renal damage and can lead to ESRD. Any patient with no previous history of kidney disease who has significant renal impairment should be evaluated for obstructive uropathy, especially if the urinary sediment is bland (Chapter 122). In addition, obstruction should be considered as a potential cause of accelerating deterioration of renal function in patients with underlying disease. In some obstructed kidneys, vasoconstriction may reduce cortical blood flow and oxygen tension, leading to increased erythropoietin production and polycythemia, which reverses with relief of the obstruction.

DIAGNOSIS

Because obstructive uropathy may be asymptomatic or may manifest in many different ways, the diagnosis may not be apparent. However, early diagnosis (Table 125-3) and prompt treatment reduce the extent of long-term renal damage.

Age, gender, and concomitant conditions often help identify the cause of obstruction. In children, congenital sources of obstruction at the ureteropelvic or ureterovesical junction are a major cause of ESRD. In adult women, complications of pregnancy or reproductive malignancies such as cervical or uterine cancer may cause obstruction due to compression of the ureters or ureterovesical junction. In older men, prostatic hypertrophy or cancer often causes urethral obstruction.

In outpatients, a history of renal colic, flank pain, or hematuria may suggest stone disease leading to ureteral obstruction. Changes in the volume or frequency of urination, including anuria, polyuria, or swings from oligoanuria to polyuria, may suggest obstruction. Bladder dysfunction is suggested by symptoms of frequency, urgency, and nocturia. In addition, a history of conditions that predispose to obstructive uropathy, such as sickle cell disease, chronic ingestion of high levels of pain relievers (papillary necrosis), previous stone disease, or abdominal cancer (which may lead to ureteral obstruction), should raise the suspicion of obstruction. Finally, the presence of a single functioning kidney should raise the possibility that unilateral obstruction may be causing azotemia. In the inpatient setting, monitoring the pattern of urine output may reveal oligoanuria or polyuria.

Laboratory Studies

Initial laboratory evaluation includes a careful urinalysis and standard chemistry panel. The urine may reveal hematuria in the case of stones, bacteriuria, numerous granulocytes in the setting of obstruction and infection, or a urine pH greater than 7.5 in the case of chronic infection with urea-splitting organisms. Serum chemistries may reveal hyperkalemia, non–anion gap acidosis, and, more rarely, hypernatremia. Corresponding urine chemistry evaluation may reveal a pH higher than 5.5, lack of a negative anion gap (see earlier), and isosthenuria. The urine sediment may also reveal evidence of crystals (uric acid or calcium oxalate), suggestive of stone disease. In addition, laboratory measurements should include blood urea nitrogen and creatinine to assess the adequacy of glomerular filtration.

Diagnostic Testing

When obstructive uropathy is suspected, ultrasonography is the best screening modality because it is highly sensitive, safe, and inexpensive and does not expose the patient to contrast material or ionizing radiation. Because of its safety and low cost, ultrasonography is often used in patients with acute renal failure to rule out obstruction. Ultrasound may reveal dilation of the calyces, renal pelvis, and, on occasion, proximal ureter (Fig. 125-2). It is also the preferred test to diagnose a renal calculus (Chapter 128; see Fig. 125-2). False-positive findings (dilation in the absence of obstruction) occur in patients with congenital anomalies, during diuresis, and in many patients with ileal conduits. False-negative findings may occur because the pelvis and calyces fail to dilate despite obstruction, as may occur with retroperitoneal fibrosis or volume depletion. Because of the possibility of false-negative ultrasound results, computed tomography (CT) is warranted when the clinical setting strongly suggests obstruction and the ultrasound findings are negative. CT scanning may define the anatomic location of obstruction in patients found to have hydronephrosis on ultrasound, or it may identify obstruction in patients with negative ultrasound studies. In the setting of cancer or other structural lesions obstructing the ureters or invading the bladder, CT may help identify the cause of obstruction.

Diffusion-weighted magnetic resonance imaging (MRI) can noninvasively detect changes in renal perfusion and in tissue density that occur during acute ureteral obstruction, but the role of MRI in patients with suspected obstructive uropathy remains unclear. MRI is limited by the risk of nephrogenic systemic fibrosis in azotemic patients, especially if the glomerular filtration rate is below 30 mL/minute. Definitive diagnosis of the location of obstruction can be obtained by retrograde pyelography, in which contrast material is injected directly into the ureters via catheters inserted into the urethra and bladder, or by antegrade pyelography, in which the contrast material is injected into the renal pelvis via a percutaneous catheter. Retrograde pyelography is performed when obstruction has been diagnosed or is strongly suggested. This procedure precisely localizes the site of obstruction and guides the urologist in the placement of stents to clear the obstruction.

When bladder dysfunction or lesions in the bladder have been identified, retrograde cystograms may define bladder anatomy. In addition, cystometrography with urodynamic testing can define the force of detrusor function, determine whether the detrusor and sphincter act in a coordinated fashion (lack of coordination is referred to as *dyssynergy*), and define the extent to which pressure within the bladder is elevated and is causing obstruction to urine flow (Chapter 25).

Differential Diagnosis

Because obstructive uropathy may have subtle manifestations that mimic many other conditions, the differential diagnosis depends on the initial clinical symptoms and signs. Though suggestive of obstructive uropathy, anuria and acute renal failure (Chapter 133) may result from intrarenal diseases such as glomerulonephritis or acute tubular necrosis. Patients with polyuria, hypernatremia, and dilute urine may have nephrogenic or central diabetes insipidus (Chapters 236 and 237). Obstructive uropathy is a rare cause of nephrogenic diabetes insipidus. Patients with hyperkalemic hyperchloremic metabolic acidosis may have hyporeninemic hypoaldosteronism, which is associated with chronic mild obstruction or other tubular disorders (Chapter 124). Renal colic may resemble abdominal pain secondary to diseases of the gastrointestinal or reproductive tract, such as appendicitis (Chapter 144) or an ovarian cyst (Chapter 243), especially when the colic is associated with nausea, vomiting, and diaphoresis.

TREATMENT

Rx

Once obstructive nephropathy has been identified, therapy focuses on the rapid restoration of normal urine flow, treatment of any accompanying infection, and management of postobstructive complications. The degree to which renal function recovers depends on several factors, including the extent and duration of the obstruction and the extent of previous renal dysfunction.

Acute Obstruction

Complete obstruction causes acute renal failure. Because the extent and rate of recovery of renal function depend on the speed of relief, prompt resolution of obstruction obviates the complications of uremia and the need for acute dialysis in patients with bilateral obstruction or obstruction of a single functioning kidney. In the setting of antecedent renal disease, partial obstruction may lead to permanent renal damage, so prompt relief can salvage significant renal function. In all cases of obstruction, the urine should be examined and cultured to identify and treat infections (Chapter 292). In patients with urinary sepsis and obstruction, the sepsis cannot be treated successfully until the obstruction is relieved; in such patients, it is also crucial to look for perinephric abscesses and drain them if present.

The site of the obstruction and its cause determine the therapeutic approach. Obstruction in the urethra or owing to bladder dysfunction may be relieved by placement of a urethral catheter. If catheters cannot be passed through the urethra, urgent suprapubic cystotomy is needed, followed by a more permanent approach, such as surgical diversion or ileal conduits, to prevent recurrent obstruction. If the obstruction is in the upper urinary tract, retrograde ureteral catheters with stents or nephrostomy tubes may be needed to relieve the obstruction. Retrograde catheters have the advantage that internal stents can be left in place to restore normal voiding, avoiding the need to maintain percutaneous drainage tubes.

Acute Obstruction Caused by Calculi

Calculi (Chapter 128) are the most common cause of ureteral obstruction. The cornerstones of therapy include analgesia, relief of the obstruction, and treatment of concomitant infections (Chapter 292). Stones smaller than 6 mm often pass without procedural intervention, but larger (7 to 15 mm) stones are more likely to cause complete obstruction and are unlikely to pass without intervention. If the stone is above the pelvic brim and is less than 15 mm, extracorporeal shock wave or ultrasonic lithotripsy is 90% effective, with passage of the fragments within 3 months. It is important to increase the volume of urine flow after these approaches to help the patient pass the fragments. For stones located below the pelvic brim or for larger stones, endoureteroscopy with direct removal may be performed via catheters passed through the urethra. In all patients with stone disease, it is crucial to identify the cause and initiate appropriate measures to prevent further stones (Chapter 128). The common practice of routinely placing a ureteral stent after ureteroscopy increases irritative lower urinary symptoms without any demonstrable clinical benefit. [1]

Chronic Partial Obstruction

Although patients with chronic partial obstruction may do well for prolonged periods, the obstructive process should be relieved because it poses a long-term threat to renal function. Prompt relief is mandatory when partial obstruction progresses to frank urinary retention, the obstruction is accompanied by urinary sepsis or repeated urinary tract infections, the obstruction is causing renal damage, or the patient has symptoms such as voiding dysfunction, flank pain, or dysuria. Most often, chronic partial obstruction results from lesions in the lower urinary tract, including urethral blockage from prostate enlargement (Chapter 131). In men, benign prostatic hypertrophy, which may remain stable for long periods, usually responds to medications, but therapeutic decisions, including surgery, depend on symptoms, the presence of infection, and the risk for permanent bladder or renal dysfunction (Chapter 131). The possibility of prostate cancer also must be assessed (Chapter 207).

Chronic obstruction at the bladder neck or urethra can lead to bladder dilation and remodeling, with attendant persistence of dysfunction and symptoms even after relief of the obstruction. On this basis, it may be appropriate to relieve the obstruction before infection, major symptoms, or renal dysfunction occurs. Urethral strictures can be treated by dilation or urethrotomy.

Postobstructive Diuresis

Though usually self-limited, postobstructive diuresis can last several days to a week and may result in clinically important depletion of sodium, potassium, and chloride. Because postobstructive diuresis is prolonged and promoted by excessive fluid replacement, administration of volume is justified only when excessive losses result in clear volume depletion. Proper replacement is guided by measurement of urine chemistries and osmolality. Because the urine is generally isosthenuric, with relatively high sodium levels as a result of residual tubular dysfunction, appropriate replacement fluid is often 0.45% saline given at a rate somewhat slower than that of urine output. By careful monitoring of vital signs, volume status, urine output, and serum and urine chemistry and osmolality, coupled with judicious fluid replacement, the diuresis can be limited and will not cause serious volume or electrolyte abnormalities.

PROGNOSIS

The recovery of renal function depends on the duration and completeness of the obstruction. If the obstruction involves only one kidney and the other kidney has relatively normal function, the preserved kidney will compensate for the loss of function in the obstructed kidney. If obstruction is of relatively short duration and is partial, renal function will likely improve, leaving the patient with no symptoms of renal failure. However, if obstruction is bilateral, complete, or near-complete and persists for a week or more, significant permanent renal damage ensues, particularly if renal function was impaired before the onset of obstruction. Following restoration of urine flow, it may take weeks for renal function to recover, and recovery may be partial or negligible. In these cases, patients may need chronic renal replacement therapy (Chapter 133).

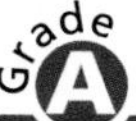

1. Nabi G, Cook J, N'Dow J, et al. Outcomes of stenting after uncomplicated ureteroscopy: systemic review and meta analysis. *BMJ*. 2007;334:572-584.

SUGGESTED READINGS

Chung DE, Sandhu JS. Overactive bladder and outlet obstruction in men. *Curr Urol Rep*. 2011;12:77-85. *Review*.

Rodrigues P, Hering F, Meller A, et al. Outline of 3830 male patients referred to urodynamic evaluation for lower urinary tract symptoms: how common is infravesical outlet obstruction? *Urol Int*. 2009;83:404-409. *Infravesical obstruction explains less than 50% of lower urinary tract symptoms in men.*

Swartz, RD. Idiopathic retroperitoneal fibrosis: a review of the pathogenesis and approaches to treatment. *Am J Kidney Dis*. 2009;54:546-553. *Review*.

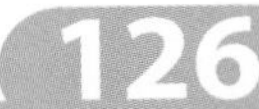

DIABETES AND THE KIDNEY

RAYMOND C. HARRIS

EPIDEMIOLOGY

In the industrialized world, diabetes mellitus is the single leading cause of end-stage renal disease (ESRD). Both the incidence and the prevalence of ESRD secondary to diabetes continue to rise. In the United States, more than 30% of patients undergoing either dialysis or renal transplantation have ESRD as a result of diabetic nephropathy, and 40% of the new (incident) cases of ESRD are attributable to diabetes.

In the United States, Europe, and Japan, more than 90% of patients with diabetes have type 2 (Chapter 237) rather than type 1 (Chapter 236) (insulinopenic) diabetes. Correspondingly, more than 80% of the ESRD secondary to diabetes is also seen in patients with type 2 diabetes. Although it was previously supposed that ESRD was less common in type 2 diabetes than in type 1 diabetes, when cohorts of patients with both types are monitored for an extended period, the incidence of renal disease is equivalent. The demographics of ESRD secondary to type 2 diabetes mirror the prevalence of type 2 diabetes in the U.S. population, with a higher incidence in females and in African Americans, Hispanic Americans, Native Americans, and Asian Americans and a peak incidence in the fifth to seventh decades of life. Given the global epidemic of obesity in developed countries, an increasing incidence of diabetic nephropathy is being widely appreciated.

PATHOBIOLOGY

Hyperglycemia

Increasing evidence implicates the metabolic sequelae of hyperglycemia as the most important causative factor in the development of diabetic nephropathy. Nearly 20 years ago, randomized clinical trials first demonstrated that aggressive control of blood sugar decreases the development of nephropathy, as well as other microvascular complications, in type 1 diabetes. Furthermore, repeat renal biopsies have documented that the renal lesions of diabetic nephropathy may reverse after long-term (10 years) functioning pancreas transplantation. Hyperglycemia leads to increased generation of reactive oxygen species; depletion of the reduced form of nicotinamide dinucleotide (phosphate); activation of the polyol pathway, which can lead to de novo synthesis of diacylglycerol and increased protein kinase C activity; alterations in the hexosamine pathway; and nonenzymatic protein glycation (advanced glycosylation end products), all of which have been implicated in development of diabetic nephropathy as well as other diabetic microvasculopathies.

Hemodynamics

Patients with type 1 and, to a lesser extent, type 2 diabetes exhibit an increased glomerular filtration rate (GFR)—so-called hyperfiltration—that is mediated by proportionately greater relaxation of the afferent arteriole than the efferent arteriole; such hyperfiltration leads to increased glomerular blood flow and elevated glomerular capillary pressure. With poorly controlled diabetes, patients develop glomerular hypertrophy, with an increased glomerular capillary surface area. These intraglomerular hemodynamic and structural alterations may contribute to the beginning or progression (or both) of diabetic renal injury. Because angiotensin-converting enzyme (ACE) inhibitors and decreased dietary protein reduce intraglomerular capillary pressure in experimental animals, the hyperfiltration hypothesis provides one rationale for the success of these interventions in resisting the progression of diabetic nephropathy (see later).

Hormones and Cytokines

Studies in experimental animals have implicated a number of cytokines, hormones, and intracellular signaling pathways in either the development or the progression of diabetic nephropathy, notably transforming growth factor-β (TGF-β), connective tissue growth factor, angiotensin II, vascular endothelial growth factor (VEGF), endothelin, prostaglandins, and nitric oxide. Because these factors have also been implicated in a variety of nondiabetic kidney diseases, it is likely that they are not specific for diabetic nephropathy. However, agents that interrupt angiotensin II production and signaling are very effective in slowing the progression of diabetic nephropathy. Furthermore, agents that interrupt intracellular pathways activated by these factors or by other consequences of hyperglycemia may provide future therapeutic opportunities.

Genetics

At present, it is impossible to predict in which patients diabetic nephropathy will develop. Although poor glycemic and blood pressure control undoubtedly contributes, nephropathy may or may not develop in an individual patient even after many years of hypertension and hyperglycemia. Type 1 diabetics with siblings who have diabetic nephropathy have a greater than 70% lifetime risk of developing diabetic nephropathy. There also appears to be a hereditary predisposition for the development of diabetic nephropathy in patients with type 2 diabetes.

Diabetic nephropathy is likely to be a polygenic disease. Various genetic linkage analyses have provided conflicting results, likely owing to genetic heterogeneity and the relatively small number of cases examined in individual studies. For example, in some (but not all) studies, an ACE insertion (I)/deletion (D) polymorphism has been associated with an increased incidence of the D allele, which predisposes to increased levels of ACE and the development or greater severity of a variety of nondiabetic renal diseases. Similarly, some but not all linkage studies have suggested the involvement of angiotensinogen polymorphisms and angiotensin II type 1 (AT1) receptor polymorphisms in the development of diabetic nephropathy.

Endothelial dysfunction in diabetes is associated with impaired vascular nitric oxide synthesis. Linkage studies have suggested that polymorphisms in endothelial nitric oxide synthase (eNOS) are associated with nephropathy in Pima Indians with type 2 diabetes, and some but not all linkage studies in other populations with diabetic nephropathy have identified eNOS polymorphisms. Polymorphisms in apolipoprotein E have also been linked to a predisposition to develop diabetic nephropathy in some studies. A variety of other genes, including those for the receptor for advanced glycosylation end products (RAGE), the glucose transporter Glut1, plasminogen activator inhibitor 1 (PAI-1), TGF-β, the B2 bradykinin receptor paroxonase, the homocysteine metabolism-related enzyme methylenetetrahydrofolate reductase, atrial natriuretic peptide, RANTES (regulated on activation, T-cell expressed and secreted), superoxide dismutase, lipoprotein lipase, decorin, VEGF, and peroxisome proliferator-activated receptor-γ (PPAR-γ), have also been linked in some but not all studies.

CLINICAL MANIFESTATIONS

Natural History

Although a minority of patients with diabetic nephropathy have type 1 diabetes, the natural history of the disease is best exemplified in this population. This is true because the onset of diabetes is more clearly definable, and initially, patients with type 1 diabetes usually do not have the comorbid conditions often associated with type 2 diabetes, including essential hypertension, atherosclerotic cardiovascular disease, and obesity, which may independently produce chronic renal injury. Furthermore, the relatively advanced age of onset of type 2 diabetes and the increased cardiovascular mortality in this population may preclude the development of all manifestations of diabetic nephropathy. In type 1 diabetes, diabetic nephropathy progresses in four relatively distinct stages (Fig. 126-1).

Stage I

In stage I, which commences soon after the overt manifestations of diabetes, the kidney undergoes hypertrophy of both the glomeruli and the tubules in comparison with age- and weight-matched normal control subjects. Despite up to a 50% increase in renal blood flow and GFR, macroalbuminuria is not yet detectable, but transient microalbuminuria (measurable by radioimmunoassay, enzyme-linked immunosorbent assay, or special dipsticks) is occasionally evident, especially when induced by stress, physical exertion, concurrent illness, or poor glycemic control. Hypertension is usually absent in the early stages of type 1 diabetes but is often present in type 2 diabetes at its initial detection.

Stage II

Approximately 30% of type 1 diabetic patients progress to clinically silent stage II, characterized by fixed microalbuminuria of at least 30 mg/24 hours, after having diabetes for a median of 10 years. Although the GFR remains elevated or is within the normal range, abnormal renal histology manifests as glomerular and tubular basement membrane thickening and expansion of the

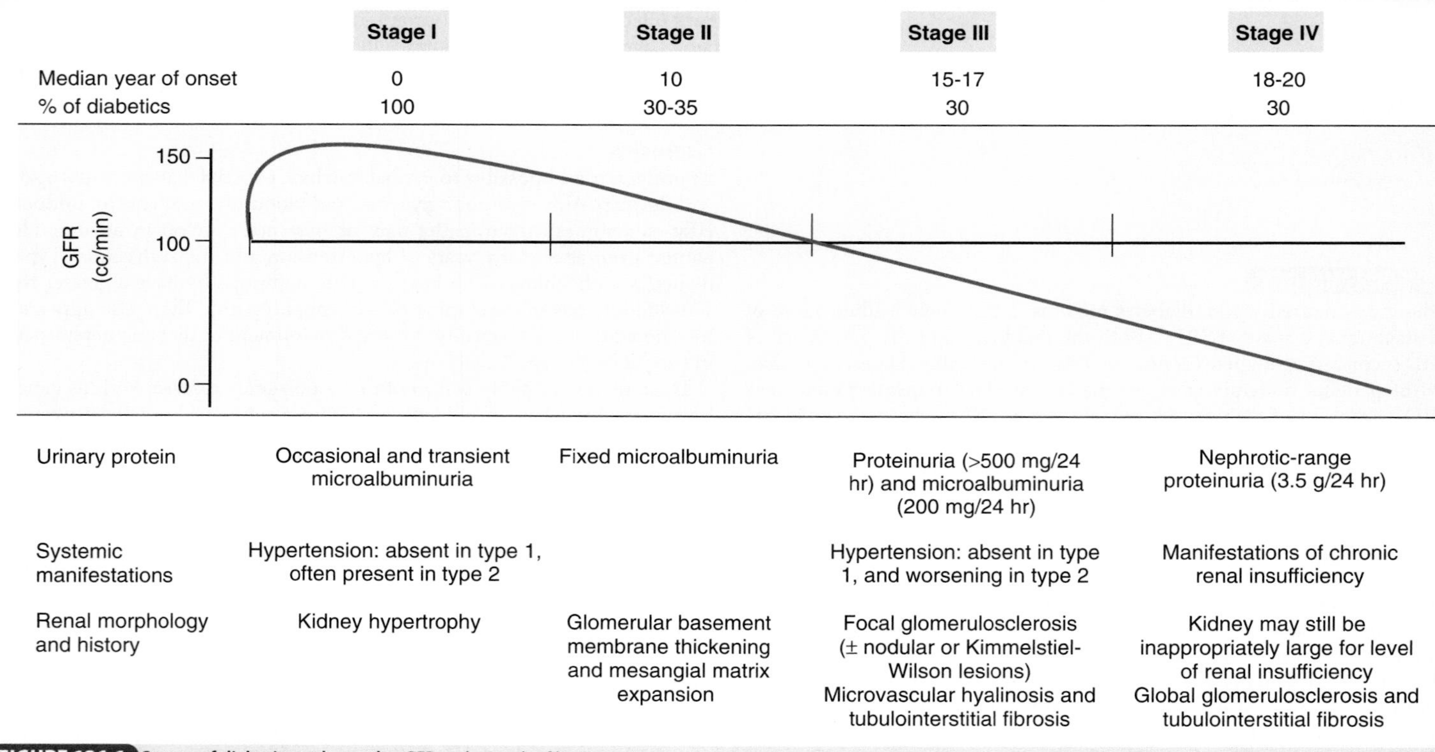

Stage I
Stage II
Stage III
Stage IV
Median year of onset
0
10
15-17
18-20
% of diabetics
100
30-35
30
30
150
100
0
GFR (cc/min)
Urinary protein
Occasional and transient microalbuminuria
Fixed microalbuminuria
Proteinuria (>500 mg/24 hr) and microalbuminuria (200 mg/24 hr)
Nephrotic-range proteinuria (3.5 g/24 hr)
Systemic manifestations
Hypertension: absent in type 1, often present in type 2
Hypertension: absent in type 1, and worsening in type 2
Manifestations of chronic renal insufficiency
Renal morphology and history
Kidney hypertrophy
Glomerular basement membrane thickening and mesangial matrix expansion
Focal glomerulosclerosis (± nodular or Kimmelstiel-Wilson lesions)
Microvascular hyalinosis and tubulointerstitial fibrosis
Kidney may still be inappropriately large for level of renal insufficiency
Global glomerulosclerosis and tubulointerstitial fibrosis

FIGURE 126-1. **Stages of diabetic nephropathy.** GFR = glomerular filtration rate.

mesangial matrix. Microalbuminuria is more likely to develop in patients with other microvascular insults, especially proliferative retinopathy. Microalbuminuria is more likely to be caused by diabetic nephropathy in type 1 than in type 2 diabetes, in which hypertension itself may lead to microalbuminuria.

Stage III

The great majority of patients who initially have fixed microalbuminuria progress within 5 to 7 years to overt nephropathy (stage III), with proteinuria (>500 mg of total protein per 24 hours) and macroalbuminuria (>200 mg/24 hours) detectable on a routine urinary protein dipstick. Blood pressure begins to rise in type 1 patients and becomes more problematic in type 2 patients.

Renal biopsy reveals diffuse or nodular (Kimmelstiel-Wilson) glomerulosclerosis. Although the Kimmelstiel-Wilson lesion is considered pathognomonic of advanced diabetic nephropathy, only about 25% of patients manifest this lesion. A nodular pattern of glomerulopathy mimicking Kimmelstiel-Wilson lesions may also be seen in light chain nephropathy (Chapter 193), amyloidosis (Chapter 194), and membranoproliferative glomerulonephritis type II (Chapter 123). Also pathognomonic of diabetic nephropathy is the finding of both afferent and efferent arteriolar hyalinosis; this differs from the arteriolar lesion of essential hypertension, which is restricted to the afferent arteriole. In overt diabetic nephropathy, progressive tubulointerstitial fibrosis correlates most closely with the decline in renal function. The GFR begins to fall from the normal range, but the serum creatinine level may remain in the normal range.

Stage IV

Stage IV, or advanced diabetic nephropathy, is characterized by a relentless decline in renal function to end-stage disease. Patients manifest nephrotic-range proteinuria (>3.5 g/24 hours) and systemic hypertension but have no evidence of inflammatory glomerular (red blood cell casts) or tubulointerstitial (white blood cells, white blood cell casts) lesions. The kidneys may be inappropriately large for the observed degree of renal insufficiency.

Other Renal Complications

Type IV (hyporeninemic, hypoaldosteronemic) renal tubular acidosis (Chapter 124) with hyperkalemia is commonly encountered in patients with diabetes and mild to moderate renal insufficiency. These patients should be carefully monitored for the development of severe hyperkalemia (Chapter 119) in response to volume depletion or after the initiation of drugs that interfere with the renin-angiotensin system, such as ACE inhibitors, angiotensin receptor blockers (ARBs), β-adrenergic blockers, both nonselective and selective cyclooxygenase 2 nonsteroidal anti-inflammatory agents, and heparin, as well as potassium-sparing diuretics.

Patients with diabetes have an increased incidence of bacterial and fungal infections of the genitourinary tract (Chapter 292), as well as an increased risk for developing intrarenal and perinephric abscesses. Unilateral or bilateral renal artery stenosis (Chapter 127) is more frequent in type 2 diabetes and should be considered if a diabetic patient has intractable hypertension or a rapidly rising serum creatinine level immediately after initiation of therapy with an ACE inhibitor or AT1 receptor blocker. Other causes of acute deterioration in renal function include papillary necrosis with ureteral obstruction owing to sloughing of a papilla, obstructive uropathy (Chapter 125) caused by bladder dysfunction as a result of autonomic neuropathy, and contrast media–induced acute tubular necrosis (Chapter 124). In addition, prerenal azotemia or acute tubular necrosis may develop in diabetic patients as a result of heart failure or volume depletion owing to vomiting induced by gastroparesis (Chapter 236) or diarrhea from autonomic neuropathy.

PREVENTION

Tight glycemic control (Chapter 236) significantly lessens but does not completely eliminate the incidence of diabetic nephropathy.[1] Elevated blood pressure is an important risk factor for the progression of diabetic nephropathy, and blood pressure targets for patients with diabetes are lower (130/80 mm Hg) than those for those without diabetes. However, blood pressure control does not prevent the development of microalbuminuria.[2]

TREATMENT

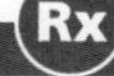

Latent (Stage II) and Overt (Stage III) Diabetic Nephropathy

Tight glycemic control in type 1 diabetes may not prevent progression to macroalbuminuria, but it prevents other microvascular complications such as retinopathy and peripheral neuropathy (Fig. 126-2). It also slows the progression of nephropathy in type 2 as well as type 1 diabetic patients (Chapter 236).[3,4]

Optimal blood pressure control does not retard the progression of renal disease in patients without macroalbuminuria,[5] but it does retard the progression of frank diabetic nephropathy. In addition to lowering systemic blood pressure, both ACE inhibitors and ARBs have the additional benefit of delaying

Stage I	Tight glucose control BP control—consider use of ACEI or ARB
Stage II	Tight glucose control ACEI or ARB BP control Smoking cessation Weight reduction Exercise Annual eye examination
Stage III	ACEI or ARB BP control Restriction of dietary protein (to 0.8g/kg of ideal body weight/day) Antihyperlipidemic medications
Stage IV	Treat manifestations of nephrotic syndrome and chronic renal insufficiency Prepare for renal replacement therapy, including prevention of abnormalities in calcium/phosphorus metabolism and prevention of anemia by early use of erythropoietin

FIGURE 126-2. Treatment of diabetic nephropathy. ACEI = angiotensin-converting enzyme inhibitor; ARB = angiotensin receptor blocker; BP = blood pressure.

the progression of nephropathy in both type 1 and type 2 patients.[6,7] The combination of a direct renin inhibitor and an ARB may further decrease proteinuria in patients with diabetic nephropathy.[8]

When administering ACE inhibitors or ARBs to patients with diabetic nephropathy, serum potassium and creatinine levels should be monitored closely for the first week because of the possibility of associated type IV renal tubular acidosis or renal artery stenosis. If blood pressure control is not achieved with these agents, diuretics and other antihypertensive agents, including cardioselective β-blockers, α-blockers, and nondihydropyridine calcium-channel blockers (CCBs), can be added (Chapter 67). Although dihydropyridine CCBs may increase intraglomerular capillary pressure, control of systemic blood pressure is essential, and both dihydropyridine and nondihydropyridine CCBs can effectively treat hypertension in these patients without accelerating renal injury.

Judicial restriction of dietary protein (to 0.8 g/kg of ideal body weight per day) is recommended. Although further dietary protein restriction may retard the progression of diabetic nephropathy, an individual's nutritional requirements must be considered. Smoking cessation (Chapter 31) and the use of antihyperlipidemic medications in patients with documented lipid abnormalities (Chapter 213) should be encouraged.

The efficacy of treatment can be determined by monitoring albuminuria and/or total proteinuria. For patients with deteriorating renal function, GFR determined by creatinine clearance and plots of the reciprocal of serum creatinine versus time (1/sCr) are effective indicators of whether interventions are slowing the progression of nephropathy.

Renal Replacement Therapy

In general, management of a diabetic patient nearing ESRD is similar to that of a nondiabetic patient. The patient should be under the care of a nephrologist, and planning for dialysis should be initiated. Although dialysis is generally started when the GFR declines to approximately 10 to 15 mL/minute, early initiation of dialysis is sometimes necessary in diabetic patients when either volume-dependent hypertension or hyperkalemia is not manageable by nondialytic therapy or when uremia, combined with gastroparesis, leads to anorexia, malnutrition, or uncontrollable emesis. Ultimately, more than 80% of patients with end-stage diabetic nephropathy require dialysis (Chapter 133), with about six times as many undergoing hemodialysis as peritoneal dialysis. Approximately 25% of the renal transplant recipients (Chapter 133) in the United States are diabetic patients. The vast majority (>90%) are type 1 diabetics, given their younger age and less severe macrovascular comorbidities in comparison with type 2 patients. Pancreas or combined kidney-pancreas transplantation has a significant effect on quality of life among patients with diabetic nephropathy by improving autonomic neuropathy, either retarding or possibly correcting retinopathy, and avoiding the potential complications of insulin administration. However, all transplantation options remain limited by organ availability.

PROGNOSIS

Because of the associated macrovascular complications (cardiovascular, cerebrovascular, peripheral vascular) and the increased risk for infection, the mortality of diabetic patients who receive either type of dialysis is 1.5 to 2.0 times that of nondiabetic patients, with a 5-year survival rate of less than 20%. The survival of diabetic patients is slightly worse with peritoneal dialysis than with hemodialysis, although it is not clear whether this is related to the type of dialysis or reflects the severity of illness among patients treated with peritoneal dialysis.

Long-term survival and quality of life are generally superior in patients undergoing transplantation compared with those receiving only dialysis. However, the other microvascular complications (retinopathy, neuropathy) are not improved by renal transplantation alone.

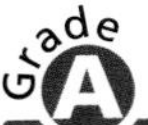

1. The Diabetes Control and Complications Trial Research Group. The effect of intensive treatment of diabetes on the development and progression of long-term complications in insulin-dependent diabetes mellitus. *N Engl J Med.* 1993;329:977-986.
2. Bilous R, Chaturvedi N, Sjølie AK, et al. Effect of candesartan on microalbuminuria and albumin excretion rate in diabetes: three randomized trials. *Ann Intern Med.* 2009;151:11-20.
3. UKPDS Group. Intensive blood-glucose control with sulphonylureas or insulin compared with conventional treatment and risk of complications in patients with type 2 diabetes. *Lancet.* 1998;352:837-852.
4. Writing Team for the Diabetes Control and Complications Trial/Epidemiology of Diabetes Interventions and Complications Research Group. Sustained effect of intensive treatment of type 1 diabetes mellitus on development and progression of diabetic nephropathy: the Epidemiology of Diabetes Interventions and Complications (EDIC) study. *JAMA.* 2003;290:2159-2167.
5. Mann JF, Schmieder RE, Dyal L, et al. Effect of telmisartan on renal outcomes: a randomized trial. *Ann Intern Med.* 2009;151:1-10.
6. Strippoli GF, Bonifati C, Craig M, et al. Angiotensin converting enzyme inhibitors and angiotensin II receptor antagonists for preventing the progression of diabetic kidney disease. *Cochrane Database Syst Rev* 2006.4.CD006257.
7. Brenner BM, Cooper ME, de Zeeuw D, et al. RENAAL Study Investigators: Effects of losartan on renal and cardiovascular outcomes in patients with type 2 diabetes and nephropathy. *N Engl J Med.* 2001;345:861-869.
8. Parving HH, Persson F, Lewis JB, et al. Aliskiren combined with losartan in type 2 diabetes and nephropathy. *N Engl J Med.* 2008;358:2433-2446.

SUGGESTED READINGS

Decleves E, Sharma K. New pharmacological treatments for improving renal outcomes in diabetes. *Nat Rev Nephrol.* 2010;6:371-380. *Review.*

Matheson A, Willcox MD, Flanagan J, et al. Urinary biomarkers involved in type 2 diabetes: a review. *Diabetes Metab Res Rev.* 2010;26:150-171. *Potential of newer, more sensitive biomarkers to monitor the development and progression of diabetic nephropathy.*

Van Buren PN, Toto R. Hypertension in diabetic nephropathy: epidemiology, mechanisms, and management. *Adv Chronic Kidney Dis.* 2011;18:28-41. *Review.*

127

VASCULAR DISORDERS OF THE KIDNEY

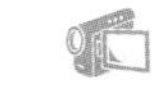

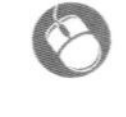

THOMAS D. DUBOSE JR. AND RENATO M. SANTOS

Vascular disorders that significantly alter renal perfusion can impact the glomerular filtration rate (GFR), tubular function, and, ultimately, kidney function. Stenosis, thrombosis, emboli, atherosclerosis, inflammation, or hypertension may involve the renal arteries, arterioles, microvasculature, and renal veins.

ARTERIES

Renal Artery Stenosis

DEFINITION

Renal artery stenosis, which is a narrowing of the renal arteries, leads to hypoperfusion of one or both of the kidneys. The two most common forms of renal artery stenosis are atherosclerotic disease and fibromuscular dysplasia. The two differ in prevalence, pathophysiology, clinical presentation, prognosis, and management.

EPIDEMIOLOGY

Atherosclerotic disease, which is much more common than fibromuscular dysplasia, accounts for 90% of renal artery stenosis. The prevalence of renal artery stenosis in the Medicare population is only 0.5%, but it is 2 to 4% in patients with hypertension (Chapter 67) and about 5.5% in patients with chronic kidney disease. Atherosclerotic disease is also more common in the elderly and in patients with typical cardiovascular risk factors such as coronary artery disease, heart failure, carotid or peripheral vascular disease, and dyslipidemia. In patients with established coronary artery disease or peripheral vascular disease and hypertension, the prevalence of some degree of renal artery stenosis may be as high as 20 to 40%.

Fibromuscular dysplasia is 2 to 10 times more common in women than in men. It is an important cause of treatable hypertension in young patients without cardiovascular risk factors, and it is pathologically and angiographically distinct from atherosclerotic disease. Although the cause is unknown, there appears to be a genetic predisposition to fibromuscular dysplasia. Other possible pathogenetic factors include hormonal influences (most patients are women of childbearing age), mechanical factors, and ischemia of the vessel wall.

PATHOBIOLOGY

The pathobiology of atherosclerotic renal artery stenosis is identical to that of atherosclerotic disease in other arterial beds (Chapter 70). Fibromuscular dysplasia includes four distinct histopathologic types: medial fibroplasia, which is the most common type and accounts for 75 to 80% of cases; perimedial fibroplasia, with irregular thickening of the media; medial hyperplasia, with smooth muscle hyperplasia without fibrosis; and intimal fibroplasia. Unlike atherosclerotic disease, which localizes at the ostial and proximal segments of the renal arteries, fibromuscular dysplasia more commonly involves the middle and distal arterial segments.

Models of renovascular hypertension using renal artery clips in animals have elegantly demonstrated that activation of the renin-angiotensin-aldosterone system by renal hypoperfusion causes an increase in systemic blood pressure. This mechanism is further supported by the ability of angiotensin-converting enzyme (ACE) inhibitors and angiotensin receptor blockers (ARBs) to control the resulting hypertension in animals and in patients with fibromuscular dysplasia. The mechanism for the development of hypertension with renal artery stenosis, however, appears to be more complex. Although atherosclerotic renal activation of the renin-angiotensin-aldosterone system by renal hypoperfusion is essential for initiating the pressor response, it is transient. Over time, the pathobiology transitions to pressor mechanisms independent of angiotensin II, including vasoconstriction owing to oxidative stress, endothelial dysfunction, endothelin release, and sympathetic activation. Confounding risks including smoking, advanced age, dyslipidemia, diabetes, and hypertension itself, which can contribute to vascular injury. The uncertain cause-and-effect relationship of these confounding risks may explain the inconsistent blood pressure response to renal revascularization for atherosclerotic renal artery stenosis compared with fibromuscular dysplasia.

Renal artery stenosis leads to ischemic nephropathy, defined as an impairment of renal function beyond the occlusive disease in the main renal arteries. However, the pathophysiologic basis of renal injury is likely multifactorial. Unlike cardiac or cerebral tissue, perfusion of the kidneys is determined by glomerular ultrafiltration and the autoregulation of the GFR and renal blood flow rather than metabolic needs. Less than 10% of renal blood flow is required to meet the oxygen demands of the kidneys. Therefore, a severe reduction in perfusion to the entire renal parenchyma is necessary to affect kidney function materially. This relationship is supported by the observation that hemodynamically significant lesions of fibromuscular dysplasia are rarely associated with renal dysfunction. Conversely, a decline in kidney function is common in atherosclerotic renal artery stenosis. Atherogenic stimuli such as hypercholesterolemia can magnify oxidative stress and activate pro-inflammatory and pro-fibrogenic pathways. Repetitive bouts of hypoperfusion in atherosclerotic disease may lead to renal tubular injury and, over time, can lead to tubulointerstitial fibrosis. Thus, a combination of repetitive perfusion insults superimposed on atherogenic risk factors contributes to renal dysfunction.

CLINICAL MANIFESTATIONS

The clinical features of renal artery stenosis are related primarily to renovascular hypertension and ischemic nephropathy (Table 127-1). A significant percentage of patients has resistant hypertension that is unresponsive to high doses of multiple antihypertensive agents. Malignant phase hypertension, though rarely seen with contemporary antihypertensive drugs, still occurs.

Hemodynamically significant renal artery stenosis can also lead to end-organ manifestations remote from the kidneys. A common association is "flash" pulmonary edema (Chapter 58) that cannot be explained by other cardiac problems, particularly if left ventricular function is preserved. Severe hypertension can also precipitate the acute coronary syndrome (Chapter 72), stroke (Chapter 414), transient ischemic attack (Chapter 414), intracranial hemorrhage (Chapter 415), encephalopathy, or papilledema.

TABLE 127-1 CLINICAL FEATURES OF RENAL ARTERY STENOSIS

Onset of hypertension before 30 or after 50 years of age
Absence of a family history of hypertension
Short duration or recent worsening of hypertension
Severe hypertension or retinopathy
Resistance to antihypertensive therapy
Signs of other cardiovascular disease
Deterioration of renal function with angiotensin-converting enzyme inhibitor or angiotensin receptor blocker therapy
Abdominal bruit
Unexplained hypokalemia with or without metabolic alkalosis
Unexplained progression of kidney disease or failure
Neurofibromatosis

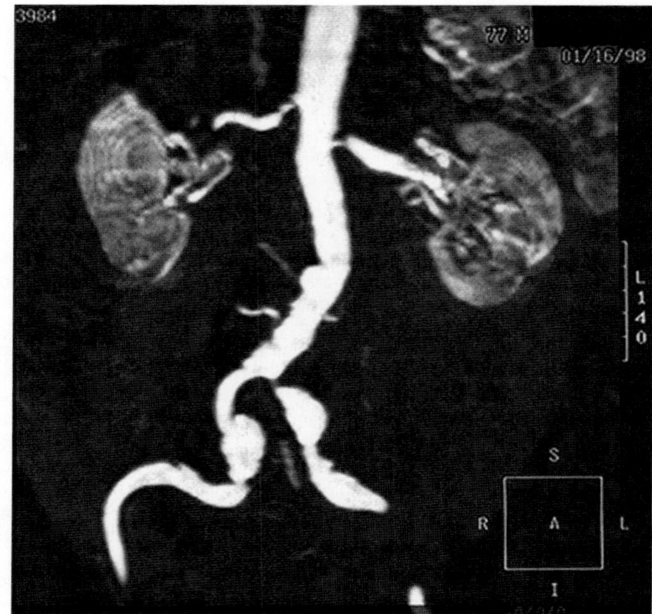

FIGURE 127-1. **Magnetic resonance angiogram of the abdominal aorta showing bilateral renal artery stenosis.** Significant iliac stenosis is also demonstrated.

DIAGNOSIS

There are no universally accepted guidelines for routine screening for renal artery stenosis (see Table 67-4 in Chapter 67), but the decision to perform diagnostic imaging studies depends on the likelihood that revascularization would be beneficial. Incidental renal artery stenosis is a common finding on noninvasive imaging tests obtained for unrelated reasons.

Preferred imaging modalities include renal duplex ultrasonography, computed tomography (CT) angiography, and magnetic resonance angiography (MRA) (Fig. 127-1). Captopril renal scintigraphy is no longer recommended owing to its poor sensitivity and specificity in the presence of renal insufficiency, bilateral disease, or disease in a solitary functioning kidney.

Renal Doppler ultrasonography is an excellent noninvasive screen for either type of renal artery stenosis and is the preferred initial test for fibromuscular dysplasia. However, it is not available in all centers, is highly operator dependent, and is affected by body habitus and bowel gas; therefore, multiple views, such as oblique and flank approaches, may be required to visualize the cortical branches.

In patients with suspected atherosclerotic renal artery stenosis, the choice among ultrasonography, CT angiography, and MRA depends in part on the availability of the technology, the experience of the vascular imaging department, and the preferences and expertise of the institution. CT angiography is rapid and has good spatial resolution but has the distinct disadvantage of requiring a large contrast load. MRA avoids the need for iodinated contrast

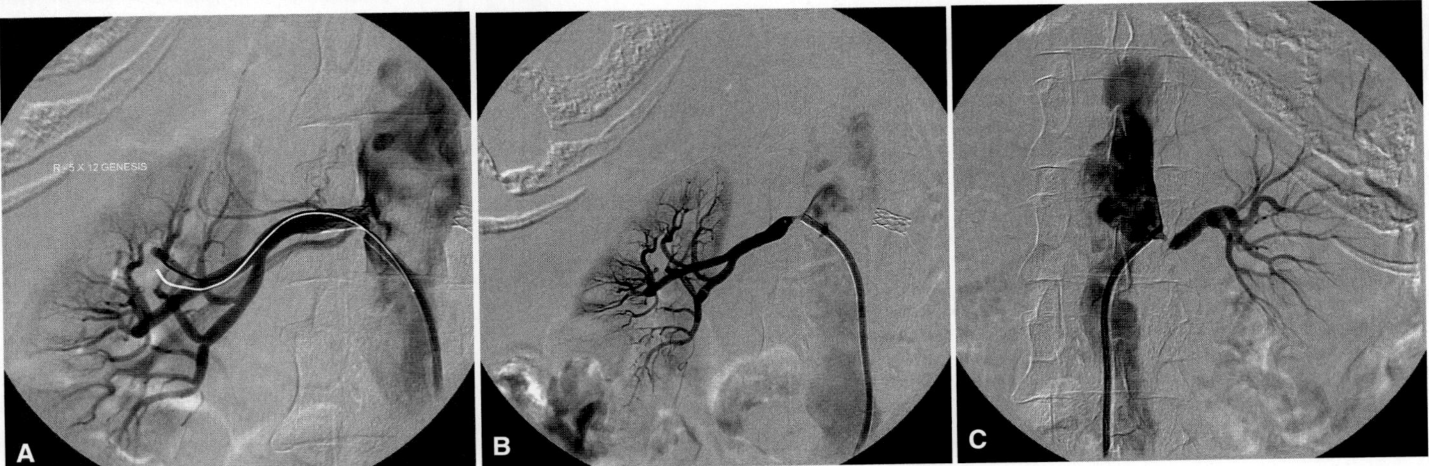

FIGURE 127-2. **Renal angiograms from an elderly patient with heart failure.** Cardiac catheterization revealed normal coronary arteries, but after initiation of therapy with an angiotensin-converting enzyme inhibitor and spironolactone, progressive kidney disease with hyperkalemia and poor blood pressure control ensued. Renal Doppler ultrasonography suggested bilateral renal artery stenosis, as confirmed by angiography (**A** and **B**). The patient underwent successful percutaneous revascularization in stages, leading to a return to normal left ventricular function and improved blood pressure control (**C**).

and can accurately visualize the proximal segment of the renal artery, although motion artifact and spatial resolution limit the ability to image the middle and distal segments. MRA requires gadolinium enhancement, which may precipitate a rare but severe condition called nephrogenic systemic fibrosis (Chapter 275), especially when the linear gadolinium chelate gadodiamide is used in patients with advanced chronic kidney disease or acute kidney injury. Clearly, the risk of nephrogenic systemic fibrosis limits the applicability of enhanced MRA for patients with advanced renal dysfunction. When the diagnosis remains unclear or when renal artery revascularization is being considered, invasive digital subtraction renal angiography (Fig. 127-2), the "gold standard" test, may be required. In addition to providing anatomic information, the translesion gradient can be measured. Although the complication rates are low, the usual risks of catheterization should be considered, including access site trauma, contrast reactions, and contrast nephropathy.

TREATMENT Rx

The goals of therapy are to control blood pressure, stabilize renal function, and reduce cardiovascular complications.

Atherosclerotic renal artery stenosis reflects a high atherosclerotic burden and is a strong predictor of subsequent cardiovascular events and cardiac mortality. Efforts to optimize medical therapy for secondary prevention include aspirin (81 mg/day), statins to treat dyslipidemia (Chapter 213), management of diabetes (Chapter 236), and control of blood pressure (Chapter 67). Medical therapy for blood pressure control should include ACE inhibitors or ARBs because of their proven benefit in renal protection (see Table 67-6 in Chapter 67). The serum creatinine and GFR should be monitored for the first weeks after initiating ACE inhibitor or ARB therapy, particularly in the elderly. An increase in creatinine of 1.0 mg/dL or greater is an indication to discontinue ACE inhibitor or ARB therapy; it suggests bilateral renal artery stenosis, renal artery stenosis in a unilateral functional kidney, or, in a kidney transplant recipient, renal artery stenosis in the allograft. Smoking cessation, weight control, and increased exercise should be universally recommended.

Renal artery revascularization for atherosclerotic renal artery stenosis remains controversial. In a large trial that randomized more than 800 patients with atherosclerotic renal artery stenosis to medical therapy or renal stenting, no difference was found in blood pressure control or recovery of renal function.[1] Similarly, smaller randomized trials of balloon angioplasty or stenting versus medical therapy showed no benefit of revascularization.[2] The potential utility of renal revascularization for atherosclerotic renal artery stenosis remains poorly defined, and the challenge is to identify patients with ischemic nephropathy and viable renal parenchyma who might improve from revascularization—perhaps those with a recent deterioration in blood pressure control, a sudden decline in renal function, a resistive index of less than 0.8, resistant hypertension, or episodes of malignant hypertension.

In patients with fibromuscular dysplasia, medical treatment alone is usually ill-advised because the stenosis can progress to renal artery occlusion despite adequate blood pressure control. Fibromuscular dysplasia responds well to balloon angioplasty; stenting is rarely needed, and restenosis rates are generally low. Close follow-up with serial blood pressure measurements and evaluation of renal function should be performed every 3 to 4 months.

PROGNOSIS

When adjusted for baseline variables, atherosclerotic renal artery stenosis remains an independent predictor of cardiovascular mortality, with a 4-year adjusted mortality rate of 25 to 40%. Factors associated with higher mortality include an elevated baseline creatinine level, more severe renal artery stenosis, worsening renal function, age, diabetes, other cardiovascular disease, and heart failure. Improvement of blood pressure control or renal function after revascularization is associated with improved survival, even though revascularization does not affect overall survival.

For fibromuscular dysplasia, angioplasty cures hypertension in about 45% of patients. Younger age, milder hypertension, and shorter duration of hypertension are associated with successful outcomes. An atrophic kidney (<8 cm), however, is unlikely to recover with revascularization.

Thromboembolic Occlusion of the Renal Arteries

EPIDEMIOLOGY AND PATHOBIOLOGY

Acute occlusion of the renal arteries and segmental branches may arise as a result of intrinsic pathology of the renal arteries, abdominal trauma, or embolization of thrombi arising in the heart or proximal aorta (Table 127-2). Thrombosis can occur as a complication of progressive atherosclerosis, in which case it may be an important cause of progressive renal insufficiency. In other patients, thrombosis may be associated with thrombophilic states (Chapter 179), such as the antiphospholipid antibody syndrome. Thrombosis also may occur as a consequence of inflammatory disorders, including Takayasu's arteritis (Chapter 78), syphilis (Chapter 327), thromboangiitis obliterans (Chapter 80), and systemic vasculitides, especially Wegener's granulomatosis (Chapter 278). In situ thrombosis has been observed in structural lesions of the renal arteries, such as fibromuscular dysplasia or renal artery aneurysms. In patients younger than 60 years, traumatic thrombosis is the most common cause. Blunt trauma and deceleration injuries can cause acute thrombosis as a result of intimal tears, contusion against the vertebral column, or compression from a retroperitoneal hematoma. Iatrogenic causes include diagnostic angiography or arterial intervention in the renal arteries or vessels proximal to the kidneys.

Embolization, which is a more common cause of renal artery occlusion than in situ thrombosis, is generally unilateral but is bilateral in 15 to 30% of cases. Total infarction of the kidney is much less common than segmental infarction or ischemia. Approximately 90% of thromboemboli to the renal arteries originate in the heart. Atrial fibrillation with embolization of atrial thrombus is the most common cause, but left ventricular thrombus, valvular heart disease (Chapter 75), bacterial endocarditis (Chapter 76), nonbacterial (aseptic) endocarditis (Chapter 76), and atrial myxoma (Chapter 60) are other causes. Noncardiac sources include aortic atheroma and mural thrombus, as well as paradoxical emboli through an atrial septal defect or patent foramen ovale (Chapter 69).

TABLE 127-2 CAUSES OF RENAL ARTERY OCCLUSION

THROMBOSIS

Progressive atherosclerosis
Trauma, blunt
Aortic or renal artery aneurysm
Aortic or renal artery dissection
Aortic or renal artery angiography
Superimposed on inflammatory disorders
- Vasculitis
- Thromboangiitis obliterans
- Syphilis

Superimposed on structural lesions
- Fibromuscular dysplasia

THROMBOEMBOLISM

Atrial fibrillation
Mitral stenosis
Mural thrombus
Atrial myxoma
Prosthetic valve
Septic or aseptic valvular vegetations
Paradoxical emboli
Tumor emboli
Fat emboli

ATHEROEMBOLI (CHOLESTEROL EMBOLIZATION)

Elderly patients with advanced atherosclerosis
Abdominal aortic surgery
Trauma, blunt
Angiographic catheters
Angioplasty or stent placement
Excessive anticoagulation

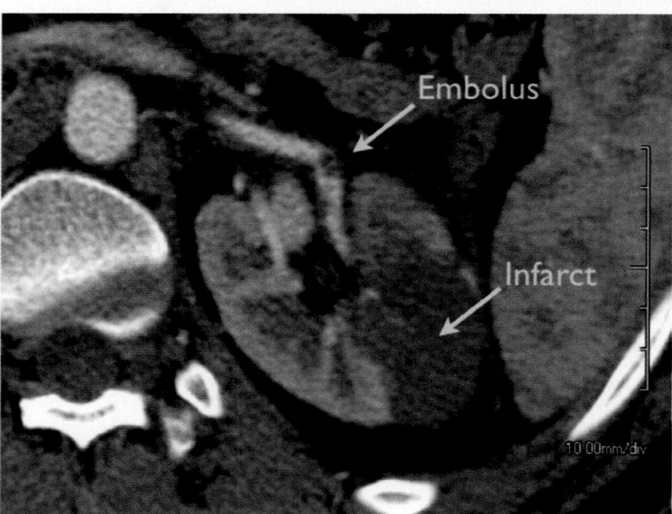

FIGURE 127-3. Computed tomography demonstrating a clot in the main renal artery and segmental renal infarction.

CLINICAL MANIFESTATIONS

The clinical presentation of renal vascular disease can be variable, and the diagnosis is often confused with more common disorders such as renal colic. Occlusion of a primary or secondary branch of the renal artery in a patient with preexisting disease and established collateral circulation, such as in long-standing renal artery stenosis, may produce little or no infarction and minimal symptoms. Acute thrombosis and infarction may cause the sudden onset of flank pain, fever, nausea, vomiting, and, on occasion, hematuria. Pain may be localized to the abdomen, back, or even the chest, but pain is absent in more than 50% of cases. Hypertension, which occurs with infarction as a result of the release of renin from the ischemic renal parenchyma, may be severe.

Anuria suggests bilateral involvement or occlusion of the artery to a solitary kidney. Urinalysis usually, but not always, reveals microscopic hematuria, and mild proteinuria may be seen.

If infarction occurs, leukocytosis usually develops, and serum enzyme levels of aspartate aminotransferase, lactate dehydrogenase, and alkaline phosphatase may be elevated. These laboratory findings are nonspecific, but elevation of the urinary lactate dehydrogenase level is more specific because its concentration should be normal in extrarenal disorders. Blood urea nitrogen and creatinine levels typically increase transiently with unilateral infarction, but more severe and protracted renal dysfunction may follow bilateral renal infarction or infarction of a solitary kidney.

DIAGNOSIS

The diagnosis of renal artery occlusion is most reliably established by CT with and without contrast. CT is accurate, can be performed rapidly, and can identify associated traumatic injury. Findings may include filling defects in the main or segmental renal arteries, as well as the absence of enhancement of renal tissue, indicating a lack of perfusion (Fig. 127-3). The complication of contrast nephropathy is a major concern in patients with a creatinine level of 2.0 mg/dL or greater or an estimated GFR less than 60 mg/dL. Alternatives to contrast administration should be considered in patients with chronic kidney disease, acute renal failure, or diabetes mellitus and in elderly patients. MRA has a high diagnostic accuracy and may be preferable to contrast CT in the elderly or in patients with diabetes mellitus, although it is contraindicated in patients with renal insufficiency. Radioisotope renograms, excretion urograms, and duplex ultrasound scanning are not recommended for the diagnosis of acute occlusions. Invasive angiography carries inherent risks but is occasionally required if the diagnosis remains uncertain or if percutaneous reperfusion is considered.

In patients with suspected embolic renal artery occlusion, echocardiography is indicated to search for a possible intracardiac thrombus. In nontraumatic thrombotic occlusion, evaluation for thrombophilia (Chapter 179), vasculitides (Chapter 278), or progressive atherosclerosis (Chapter 70) should be considered.

TREATMENT Rx

The human kidney can tolerate 60 to 90 minutes of warm ischemia, although the presence of collateral circulation may permit longer ischemic times. As a result, acute renal artery thrombosis requires urgent treatment in an attempt to reopen the artery. Treatment options for nontraumatic renal artery occlusion include systemic anticoagulation with unfractionated heparin (see Table 81-4 in Chapter 81) or low-molecular-weight heparin (see Table 37-3 in Chapter 37 and Table 81-3 in Chapter 81), followed by oral warfarin (Coumadin) to maintain an international normalized ratio of 2.0 to 3.0, or intra-arterial thrombolytic therapy. Surgical revascularization has been associated with higher mortality than medical therapy, without improved renal salvage rates; it is not recommended as primary therapy but can be considered for patients with bilateral renal artery occlusion or occlusion of the renal artery of a solitary kidney. Percutaneous endovascular therapies (e.g., local thrombolysis, thrombectomy, stent placement) have also been successful in acute renal artery occlusion. For iatrogenic occlusion of the renal artery as a result of angiographic manipulations or angioplasty, intra-arterial stent placement may be considered. For traumatic renal artery thrombosis, surgery is the treatment of choice, but it typically can salvage renal function only if accomplished immediately.

Patients with renal artery thrombosis also require close medical care, often with multiple parenteral agents (see Table 67-8 in Chapter 67), to control their hypertension and achieve a blood pressure between 140/90 and 110/70 mm Hg. Adequate hydration is also imperative.

PROGNOSIS

Mortality is high, especially in patients who require hemodialysis, and it correlates with the severity of underlying conditions. For patients undergoing surgical revascularization for complete acute renal artery occlusion, the mortality rate is 11 to 25%. The risk of losing renal function is variable, and rates of 0 to greater than 50% have been reported. Hypertension, which may develop as a late sequela of renal artery occlusion, is preferably treated with ACE inhibitors, ARBs, or nondihydropyridine calcium-channel blockers (see Table 67-5 in Chapter 67).

ARTERIOLES AND MICROVASCULATURE

Atheroembolic Disease of the Renal Arteries

EPIDEMIOLOGY AND PATHOBIOLOGY

Cholesterol crystal embolization is a potential complication of widespread atherosclerosis. The risk factors are similar to those for all atherosclerotic disease (Chapter 51), including smoking, hypertension, hyperlipidemia, diabetes, and age. Atheroembolic disease appears to be more common in whites, but the condition may be underdiagnosed in African Americans owing to the difficulty of assessing livedo reticularis in this population.

The most common triggering events are manipulation of a thrombus or of the abdominal aorta or renal arteries during angiography or transluminal angioplasty. It is therefore not unusual for cholesterol crystal embolization to be mistaken for contrast-induced nephropathy. Atheroemboli can also be associated with anticoagulant or thrombolytic therapy and may be accompanied by the finding of a cyanotic toe on physical examination. Spontaneous atheroembolism after detachment of a mural plaque is uncommon. Cholesterol crystals typically do not occlude arterial flow but induce an inflammatory response and subsequent endothelial proliferation, so the clinical manifestations may occur some time after the initial insult.

CLINICAL MANIFESTATIONS

Although all organ systems can be affected (Chapter 80), the kidneys are most commonly involved, followed by the spleen and gastrointestinal tract. Renal insufficiency, hypertension, or both typically occur. Nonspecific complaints may include fever, myalgias, headaches, and weight loss. Evidence of cholesterol embolization may be present in the retina, muscles, or skin, where livedo reticularis (see Fig. 80-1 in Chapter 80) or blue toes may be seen. Embolization can also result in cerebrovascular events, acute pancreatitis, ischemic bowel, and gangrene of the extremities (Chapter 79).

DIAGNOSIS

Although most atheroembolic events are diagnosed because of an acute clinical change, clinically silent, chronic, low-grade embolization may be overlooked because patients at risk for this complication often have other chronic illnesses associated with renal failure, hypertension, and atherosclerosis. Urinalysis may not be helpful because cholesterol crystals often are not present, although mild proteinuria, eosinophiluria, and increased cellularity are frequently observed. Transient eosinophilia is common, and an elevated erythrocyte sedimentation rate, hypocomplementemia, anemia, and leukocytosis may also be present. As many as 80% of patients may have a serum creatinine level exceeding 2 mg/dL.

Although the demonstration of cholesterol crystals in the renal microvasculature with subsequent vessel occlusion is considered a diagnostic feature, a kidney biopsy generally is not necessary for patients with typical clinical features, including livedo reticularis and violaceous mottling of the toes, eosinophilia, and an elevated erythrocyte sedimentation rate. When uncertainty exists, noninvasive biopsy of the skin of the lower extremity, muscle of the calf or thigh, or gastric mucosa can be diagnostic in up to 80% of patients.

TREATMENT Rx

There is no curative therapy for atheroembolic disease, so supportive care is often all that can be offered. Aggressive control of dyslipidemia with statins (Chapter 213) is recommended and may have the added benefit of stabilizing the endothelial surface. Anticoagulants are of no value and may delay the healing of ulcerating atherosclerotic lesions; if possible, anticoagulant therapy should be discontinued. Adequate hydration is important to sustain renal perfusion. Hypertension should be treated (see Table 67-5 in Chapter 67) with angiotensin II antagonists and vasodilators, and volume should be controlled with diuretics, while being careful not to cause hypotension. Intravascular radiologic procedures and vascular surgery should be avoided if possible.

PROGNOSIS

Recent series suggest up to 80% survival at 1 year. Most patients die of cardiovascular complications. With adequate blood pressure control for several months or years, renal function may recover sufficiently to avoid dialysis. Patients who develop end-stage renal disease have a significantly higher mortality.

Hypertensive Arteriolar Nephrosclerosis

EPIDEMIOLOGY

The risk of nephrosclerosis among hypertensive patients is a function of the severity and duration of hypertension (Chapter 67). Although only a small percentage of patients with hypertensive nephrosclerosis progress to end-stage renal disease, the high prevalence of this condition makes it an important cause. The availability of effective antihypertensive medications has sharply reduced the occurrence of this devastating disorder. However, both benign and malignant hypertensive renal disease and the sequelae of these disorders appear to be more prevalent in African Americans.

PATHOBIOLOGY

The renal vasculature is exquisitely sensitive to damage caused by systemic hypertension when elevated blood pressure is transmitted to the glomerular capillary bed. Unopposed or sustained increases in glomerular capillary hydrostatic pressure eventually result in sclerosis. In benign nephrosclerosis, the kidney is the victim of the adverse effects of chronic hypertension. In malignant or accelerated hypertension, intimal changes in the renal arterial vessels lead to ischemia, increased production of renin, and exacerbation of hypertension, potentially resulting in acute renal failure that, if not treated successfully, will result in end-stage renal disease. Renal vascular lesions similar to those seen in malignant hypertension are also observed in scleroderma (Chapter 275), thrombotic microangiopathy (Chapter 123), and renal transplant rejection (Chapter 133). *MYH9* (myosin, heavy chain 9, nonmuscle) gene polymorphisms are associated with a spectrum of kidney diseases in African Americans with essential hypertension and nephropathy attributed to hypertension, focal segmental glomerulosclerosis, or HIV-associated nephropathy; these data suggest that much of the excess risk of end-stage renal disease in African Americans is linked to genetic susceptibility.

CLINICAL MANIFESTATIONS AND DIAGNOSIS

Typically, patients with benign hypertensive nephrosclerosis have been hypertensive for more than 10 to 15 years. Kidney size is usually reduced, and the urine sediment is unremarkable except for proteinuria, which is generally less than 1.5 g/day. The sudden development of malignant or accelerated hypertension (Chapter 67), either in patients with previously established mild to moderate hypertension or in patients with no previous diagnosis of hypertension, manifests as an abrupt increase in blood pressure (diastolic usually >130 mm Hg). Hypertensive retinopathy (see Fig. 67-1 in Chapter 67) is common, papilledema (see Fig. 431-27) may develop, and renal function may decline rapidly. The kidneys may be enlarged, the urinary sediment may show gross or microscopic hematuria, and proteinuria is often in the nephrotic range. Microangiopathic hemolytic anemia may be present. Abnormalities in the central nervous system are usually evident and include headaches, cerebrovascular accidents, generalized seizures, and coma.

TREATMENT Rx

In benign hypertensive nephrosclerosis, the renal outcome depends on the timely initiation of effective therapy, patient adherence, and careful follow-up. The primary goal is a blood pressure of 130/80 mm Hg or less (Chapter 67). Medications that provide renal protection include ACE inhibitors and ARBs (see Table 67-5 in Chapter 67). Nondihydropyridine calcium-channel blockers do not afford protection from progression of renal insufficiency and should be used only in patients who cannot tolerate ACE inhibitor or ARB therapy. For malignant hypertension, more aggressive therapy is required (see Table 67-8 in Chapter 67).

PROGNOSIS

With the skillful selection of renal-specific antihypertensive agents and control of blood pressure, progression of kidney disease can usually be avoided. Unfortunately, such measures may not be initiated sufficiently early or may not be successful in preventing progression to end-stage renal disease.

SYSTEMIC DISORDERS AFFECTING THE RENAL MICROVASCULATURE

Hemolytic-Uremic Syndrome and Thrombotic Thrombocytopenic Purpura

Renal failure is a common consequence of both hemolytic-uremic syndrome (HUS) and thrombotic thrombocytopenic purpura (TTP) (Chapter 175). These conditions are characterized by platelet and fibrin thrombi within the renal microvasculature, accompanied by thrombocytopenia and microangiopathic hemolytic anemia.

TTP is suggested by the co-occurrence of hemolysis, thrombocytopenia, fever, purpura, and alternating mental status changes. HUS may be associated with acute renal failure, thrombocytopenia, and microangiopathic hemolytic anemia, most commonly in children after an acute diarrheal illness. Either disorder may be observed in the setting of cancer and infection and while administering chemotherapeutic agents. In addition to specific therapies (Chapter 175), acute implementation of renal replacement therapy has significantly improved survival.

Scleroderma

The clinical features and progression of scleroderma are highly variable, but mild proteinuria without loss of renal function or evidence of glomerular disease is the most common sign of renal disease (Chapter 275). Significant renal involvement, which has been reported in 50% of patients with systemic sclerosis of 20 or more years' duration, is the most dreaded complication and has the poorest prognosis. A renal crisis may be associated with the use of corticosteroids and can be precipitated in situations that compromise renal blood flow (e.g., dehydration). An increase in vasomotor tone at the level of the renal vasculature contributes to a reduction in renal blood flow, hypertension, and progressive impairment in renal function. The resulting increase in renin and angiotensin II contributes to the development of worsening hypertension and hypertensive nephrosclerosis. Once azotemia develops, hypertension may become more difficult to manage, and dialysis is required within 1 to 2 years. Conversely, patients may initially come to medical attention with a "renal crisis" manifested by the abrupt onset of malignant hypertension and renal failure, commonly associated with heart failure and microangiopathic hemolytic anemia. This manifestation is seen in approximately 2.8% of all patients with scleroderma but in 14 to 18% of those with diffuse cutaneous disease.

TREATMENT (Rx)

Therapy should be directed primarily toward controlling hypertension, which may require several drugs in combination, such as ACE inhibitors or ARBs, nondihydropyridine calcium-channel blockers, vasodilators (e.g., minoxidil), and other agents (see Table 67-5 in Chapter 67). Renal crisis is an emergency that usually requires intravenous antihypertensive therapy (see Table 67-8 in Chapter 67). Some patients follow a progressive course despite blood pressure control. Patients with an initial serum creatinine level of 3.0 mg/dL or greater have a poorer prognosis. If dialysis is required, aggressive management of hypertension may allow a small but significant percentage of patients to regain sufficient renal function to allow cessation of renal replacement therapy.

Sickle Cell Nephropathy

PATHOBIOLOGY

The hypoxemic and hypertonic environment of the renal medulla (vasa recta) encourages the sickling of red blood cells circulating through this region (Chapter 166). When sickle hemoglobin desaturates, polymerization of hemoglobin can impair or interrupt capillary flow. The major manifestations of sickle cell nephropathy can all be explained by the development of papillary infarction.

CLINICAL MANIFESTATIONS

A defect in urinary concentration results in a tendency toward volume depletion in sickle cell disease and in sickle cell trait. A defect in urinary acidification is common and is manifested as distal renal tubular acidosis with hyperkalemia and hyperchloremic metabolic acidosis (type 4 renal tubular acidosis; Chapter 120). The acidification defect is usually not observed in patients with sickle trait. Microscopic hematuria occurs in most patients with sickle cell anemia. Painless gross hematuria occurs in up to 50% of patients with sickle cell nephropathy and also occurs in patients with hemoglobin SC disease. With recurrent papillary infarction, papillary necrosis can occur and progress. Sickle cell "crisis," dehydration, hypoxemia, and the use of nonsteroidal anti-inflammatory drugs predispose to papillary necrosis. Renal papillary necrosis is often silent, but it may progress to chronic renal insufficiency and predispose the patient to repeated urinary tract infections. Nephrotic syndrome may develop in approximately 4% of patients with sickle glomerulopathy. Findings on renal biopsy usually indicate membranoproliferative glomerulopathy (Chapter 123) with segmental and global sclerosis. As this disorder progresses, glomerulopathy results in sclerosis and progressive loss of glomerular function. In contrast, papillary infarction can result in persistent hematuria.

TREATMENT

Volume depletion should be corrected by the intravenous administration of isotonic or hypotonic saline, as dictated by the serum sodium concentration. Hyperkalemia may require potassium exchange resin (sodium polystyrene [Kayexalate] 50 g in 70% sorbitol) per rectum or orally (15 g in water or 70% sorbitol). When acidosis accompanies the hyperkalemia, alkali may help correct both. Long-term administration of Shohl solution (15 mL two or three times daily) or sodium bicarbonate tablets (two 650-mg [7.6-mEq] tablets orally twice a day) may be necessary, and loop diuretics may be helpful. Potassium-sparing diuretics, nonsteroidal anti-inflammatory drugs, and potassium supplements should be strictly avoided. Rarely, small doses of ε-aminocaproic acid may be necessary for life-threatening hematuria, but this can result in thrombosis or ureteral obstruction.

RENAL VEINS

Renal Vein Thrombosis

EPIDEMIOLOGY

Unilateral or bilateral thrombosis of the major renal veins or their segments is often a subtle disorder that can develop in a variety of conditions (Table 127-3), but especially with nephrotic syndrome (Chapter 123) or renal malignancies (Chapter 203). Cases have also been associated with trauma, oral contraceptive use, hypovolemia, renal transplantation (Chapter 133), and thrombophilic states (Chapter 179). The reported incidence of renal vein thrombosis ranges from 5 to 62% in patients with nephrotic syndrome, including those with membranous nephropathy, membranoproliferative glomerulonephritis, focal glomerular sclerosis, sickle cell nephropathy, amyloidosis, diabetic nephropathy, renal vasculitis, and lupus nephritis. Spontaneous renal vein thrombosis is unusual in patients without underlying risk factors.

PATHOBIOLOGY

The precipitating factors are apparently abnormalities in coagulation or fibrinolysis. Antithrombin III and plasminogen levels may be depressed as a result of urinary excretion of antithrombin III in patients with nephrotic syndrome. Thrombocytosis, increased platelet activation, hyperfibrinogenemia, inhibition of plasminogen activation, and altered circulating levels of proteins S and C in nephrotic syndrome contribute to thromboembolic complications.

Extrinsic compression of the renal veins from retroperitoneal sources such as lymph nodes, fibrosis, abscess, aortic aneurysm, or tumor may cause renal vein thrombosis as a result of sluggish renal venous flow. Acute pancreatitis, trauma, and retroperitoneal surgery also may predispose to renal vein thrombosis. Renal cell carcinoma characteristically invades the renal vein and compromises venous flow, resulting in renal vein thrombosis. Renal vein thrombosis in the setting of severe volume depletion and impaired renal blood flow has been described in young adults.

CLINICAL MANIFESTATIONS

The manifestations of renal vein thrombosis depend on the extent and rapidity of the development of the occlusion. Patients with acute renal vein thrombosis may have nausea, vomiting, flank pain, leukocytosis, hematuria, compromised renal function, and an increase in kidney size. These features may be confused with renal colic or pyelonephritis. Adult patients with nephrotic syndrome and chronic renal vein thrombosis may have more subtle findings, such as a dramatic increase in proteinuria or evidence of tubular dysfunction, including glycosuria, aminoaciduria, phosphaturia, and impaired urinary acidification. Chronic renal vein thrombosis may first present in association with a pulmonary embolus.

TABLE 127-3 CAUSES OF RENAL VEIN THROMBOSIS
Nephrotic syndrome
Renal cell carcinoma with renal vein invasion
Pregnancy or estrogen therapy
Volume depletion (especially in infants)
Extrinsic compression (lymph nodes, tumor, retroperitoneal fibrosis, aortic aneurysm)
Corticosteroids

DIAGNOSIS

For acute renal vein thrombosis, which is typically associated with thrombophilia, contrast-enhanced CT shows an enlarged kidney, stretching of the calyces, and notching of the ureters. A venogram is rarely required but can be considered in cases of acute renal failure in which thrombectomy or thrombolysis is considered. In chronic renal vein thrombosis, an incidentally noted renal vein thrombus may be seen on imaging studies ordered for other reasons. Routine screening for thrombus is not recommended for those with nephrotic syndrome, but contrast-enhanced CT is recommended in patients with suggestive clinical manifestations.

TREATMENT Rx

The most widely accepted form of therapy for both acute and chronic renal vein thrombosis is anticoagulation with low-molecular-weight heparin (see Table 81-3 in Chapter 81) or unfractionated heparin (see Table 81-4 in Chapter 81), which can be converted to oral warfarin after 7 to 10 days and should continue for at least 1 year and to an international normalized ratio of 2.0 to 3.0. In patients with ongoing risk factors, such as persistent nephrotic syndrome, or recurrent thrombosis, anticoagulation should be continued indefinitely. Fibrinolytic therapy may be considered in patients with acute renal vein thrombosis associated with acute renal failure.

PROGNOSIS

The prognosis of renal vein thrombosis depends entirely on the underlying condition causing or associated with it. Renal vein thrombosis associated with membranous glomerulonephritis and nephrotic syndrome (Chapter 123) usually resolves if the underlying condition responds to therapy or spontaneously resolves. In contrast, renal vein thrombosis associated with renal cell carcinoma (Chapter 203) has a very poor prognosis. Renal vein thrombosis associated with trauma or hypovolemia may resolve after appropriate therapy.

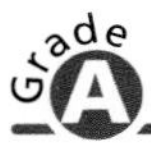

1. Wheatley K, Ives N, Gray R, et al. Revascularization versus medical therapy for renal artery stenosis. *N Engl J Med*. 2009;361:1953-1962.
2. Bax L, Woittiez AJ, Kouwenberg HG, et al. Stent placement in patients with atherosclerotic renal artery stenosis and impaired renal function: a randomized trial. *Ann Intern Med*. 2009;150:840-848.

SUGGESTED READINGS

Colyer WR Jr, Cooper CJ. Management of renal artery stenosis: 2010. *Curr Treat Options Cardiovasc Med*. 2011;13:103-113. *Review.*

Dworkin LD, Cooper CJ. Renal-artery stenosis. *N Engl J Med*. 2009;361:1972-1978. *Review.*

Fries C, Roos M, Gaspert A, et al. Atheroembolic disease—a frequently missed diagnosis: results of a 12-year matched-pair autopsy study. *Medicine (Baltimore)*. 2010;89:126-132. *Review emphasizing an association with intravascular procedures.*

Scolari F, Ravani P. Atheroembolic renal disease. *Lancet*. 2010;375:1650-1660. *Review recommending treatment with a statin and perhaps corticosteroids.*

128

NEPHROLITHIASIS

GARY C. CURHAN

DEFINITION

A kidney stone is a crystalline mass that is formed in the kidney and that is of sufficient size to be clinically detectable, either by symptoms or by imaging. The composition of different types of kidney stones determines the clinical evaluation, treatment, and prognosis. The most common component is calcium oxalate; other types are calcium phosphate, uric acid, struvite, and cystine stones (Fig. 128-1). Infrequently, stones may be composed of medications, including acyclovir, indinavir, and triamterene.

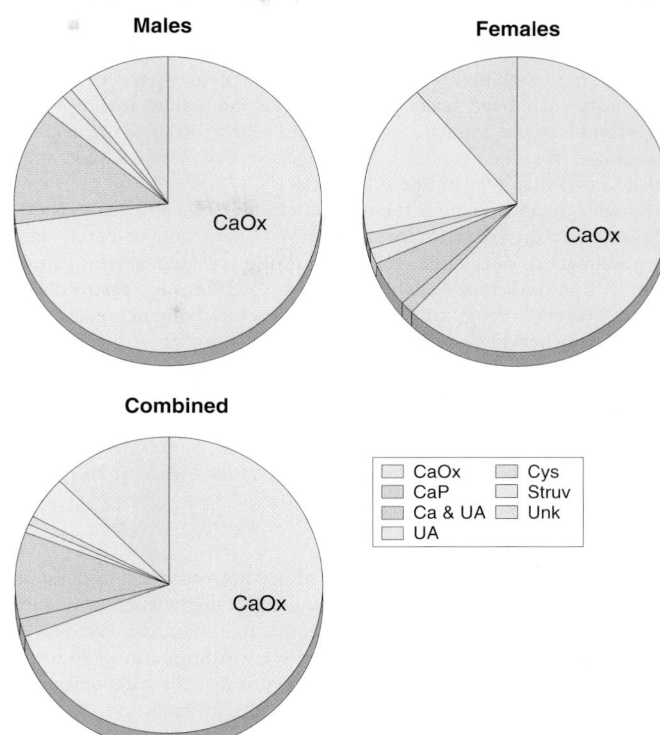

FIGURE 128-1. Types of stones and frequency in adults. Ca & UA = calcium and uric acid; CaOx = calcium oxalate; CaP = calcium phosphate; Cys = cystine; Struv = struvite; UA = uric acid; Unk = unknown. (From Coe F, Parks J, eds. *Nephrolithiasis: Pathogenesis and Treatment*. Chicago: Year Book; 1988. Reprinted in Greenberg A, Cheung AK. *Primer on Kidney Diseases*. Philadelphia: Elsevier; 2005.)

EPIDEMIOLOGY

The prevalence of a history of kidney stone disease increased between the early 1970s and 1990 in both men and women and in whites and blacks. Nephrolithiasis accounts for nearly 2 million physician office visits with estimated annual health care costs of approximately $2 billion. The lifetime risk of stone formation in the United States is approximately 12% in men and 6% in women. The risk in blacks is one fourth that of whites.

Among men who have never had a stone, the incidence is 3 to 4 cases per 1000 men per year between the ages of 30 and 60 years and then slowly declines with age. For women, the incidence is 2 cases per 1000 women per year between the ages of 20 and 30 and then declines to approximately 1 per 1000 women per year for the next four decades.

The risk of recurrent stone formation in untreated patients after the first stone remains uncertain. Earlier studies reported stone recurrence rates ranging from 30 to 50% at 5 years. However, control groups in recent randomized controlled trials of incident calcium oxalate stone formers experienced substantially lower rates of first recurrence (2 to 5 per 100 person years). Unfortunately, no information on sex-specific rates is available from these trials.

Risk Factors

Dietary Factors

Nutrients

Dietary factors that appear to increase the risk for nephrolithiasis include animal protein, oxalate, sodium, sucrose, fructose, and vitamin C. Higher intake of potassium and phytate reduces the risk.

Low dietary calcium intake increases the risk for stone formation. Although the mechanism is uncertain, low calcium intake increases the gastrointestinal absorption and urinary excretion of oxalate. It is also possible that other factors in dairy products, the major source of dietary calcium, may reduce the risk for stone formation. In contrast, calcium supplements appear to increase the risk of incident stone formation. Thus, they should be used with caution in individuals with a history of calcium stone disease.

Higher animal protein intake may raise urinary excretion of calcium and uric acid and decrease urinary excretion of citrate, thereby increasing the risk for stone formation. Higher sodium or sucrose intake increases urinary calcium excretion, and potassium supplementation decreases calcium excretion. In prospective studies, an increased risk for stone formation has been observed in men with higher intakes of animal protein, whereas a decreased risk for stones has been observed with higher potassium intake. Phytate, which is found in cold cereals, dark bread, and beans, can substantially reduce the likelihood of stone formation in younger women. These studies suggest that risk factors may vary by age and gender.

Although calcium oxalate is the most common stone and urine oxalate is clearly an important risk factor for stone formation, the role of dietary oxalate in the pathogenesis of calcium oxalate nephrolithiasis appears to be limited. The proportion of dietary oxalate that is absorbed from the gastrointestinal tract is estimated to range from 10 to 50%. Factors influencing absorption likely include other dietary components (e.g., calcium), genetic factors, and possibly intestinal flora. In addition, the bioavailability of oxalate in food is unknown. Urinary oxalate is also derived from the endogenous metabolism of glycine, glycolate, hydroxyproline, and vitamin C. Individuals who have Crohn's disease (Chapter 143) or who have had gastrointestinal bypass surgery often have very high urinary oxalate values owing to an increased absorption of dietary oxalate.

Fluid Intake

Fluid intake is the primary determinant of urinary volume, and daily urine volume is a crucial factor in stone formation, particularly when urine output is less than 1 L/day. The important protective role of fluid intake has been demonstrated in observational studies and was confirmed in a randomized controlled trial. Because the concentrations, not just the total amounts, of relevant urinary factors are the key determinants of stone formation, fluid intake and subsequent urinary volume are critical.

Systemic Conditions

Systemic conditions that increase the risk for formation of calcium-containing stones include primary hyperparathyroidism (Chapter 253) and renal tubular acidosis (Table 128-1). Primary hyperparathyroidism is found in less than 5% of stone formers. Obesity, gout, and diabetes mellitus are independently associated with stone formation, as are Crohn's disease and surgical treatments for obesity, such as gastric bypass surgery.

PATHOBIOLOGY

Genetics

Individuals with a family history of stone disease have a two-fold higher risk of becoming stone formers. Rare monogenic causes of nephrolithiasis include Dent's disease and cystinuria (Chapter 130). A recent genome-wide association study suggested that a single nucleotide polymorphism in the claudin-14 gene is associated with a higher risk of stone formation. Conversely, studies of specific genes involved in calcium metabolism, such as the calcium-sensing receptor and the vitamin D receptor, have not been conclusive in humans.

Pathogenesis

Supersaturation

Stone formation is the result of a complex physicochemical process that leads to crystallization. Although normal individuals can have crystalluria and not actual stones, the presence of crystalluria substantially increases the likelihood of stone formation. Formation of crystals in urine is largely a function of supersaturation, a concentration above a material's solubility in water.

Evidence suggests that the initial crystal nidus of calcium oxalate stones forms in the *medullary interstitium* and is composed of calcium phosphate. The calcium phosphate crystals then erode through the papilla, forming the classic Randall's plaque, where they act as a nidus for the deposition of calcium oxalate.

TABLE 128-1 SYSTEMIC DISORDERS ASSOCIATED WITH A HIGHER RISK FOR STONE FORMATION

Crohn's disease
Primary hyperparathyroidism
Gout
Diabetes mellitus
Obesity
Gastric bypass procedure
Renal tubular acidosis

Most stones do not contain one single type of crystal but rather are a mixture with one or two types that predominate. Furthermore, kidney stones also contain protein in the stone matrix.

Modifiable factors that influence supersaturation include pH, volume, and inhibitors. Crystallization of uric acid and calcium phosphate is strongly influenced by urinary pH, which has little effect on calcium oxalate. For all types of stones, supersaturation is dependent on urinary volume; increasing daily urine volume (ideally to greater than 2 L) is of practical benefit in reducing the supersaturation and incidence of stones.

The urine of most individuals is supersaturated with respect to calcium oxalate and calcium phosphate. The remarkable ability of urine to inhibit crystallization prevents most of the population from continuously forming stones. The compounds that stabilize and prevent crystallization within the tubules and the urinary tract are incompletely characterized but include citrate and urinary proteins.

Hypercalciuria

The common definition of hypercalciuria is urine calcium excretion greater than 300 mg/day in men, greater than 250 mg/day in women, or greater than 4 mg/kg/day on a 1000-mg/day calcium diet. Although this higher cutoff for men is reasonable from a calcium balance perspective, it is not relevant for stone formation because urine volumes in men and women are similar. Second, a definition based on weight is problematic. For example, if an individual gains 20 kg in weight, the amount of calcium that that person would be "allowed" to excrete would increase by 80 mg, but the risk of forming stones would rise.

Hyperoxaluria

Hyperoxaluria is often defined as urinary oxalate excretion of more than 45 mg/day, but the risk of stone formation begins well below this level. Elevated urinary oxalate excretion may be present in up to 40% of male and 10% of female stone formers, but hyperoxaluria is also frequently found in individuals who do not have a history of stone disease.

Hyperuricosuria

Persons with gout (Chapter 281) have an increased frequency of stone disease, and a double-blind trial about 25 years ago showed that allopurinol successfully decreased recurrence rates of calcium stones in patients with hyperuricosuria, often defined as more than 800 mg/day in men or more than 750 mg/day in women. However, a large study did not find a correlation of 24-hour urine uric acid excretion with an increased risk of calcium oxalate stone formation. Although hyperuricosuria is a risk factor for uric acid stones, its role in calcium oxalate stones is uncertain, and any protective benefit of allopurinol may be through a mechanism other than the lower urine urate.

Hypocitraturia

Citrate inhibits the growth and aggregation of crystals, and individuals with hypocitraturia (<320 mg/day for men and women) are at increased risk for stone formation. It is likely that an increase of urinary citrate above the normal range provides additional protection against stones. Although citrate in normal individuals is influenced by foods that are high in alkali (e.g., fruits, vegetables) or that generate acid (e.g., nondairy animal protein), they do not completely account for the higher renal tubular reabsorption of citrate in patients who have hypocitraturia and idiopathic calcium stones.

Formation of Non-Calcium-Containing Stones

Uric Acid Stones

Although uric acid excretion is important, the major driver of uric acid supersaturation and subsequent uric acid stone formation is low urinary pH. Many patients who form uric acid stones do not have markedly elevated urinary uric acid excretion (defined previously), but they do have persistently acid urine with the urinary pH typically below 5.5 throughout the day. Factors that contribute to lower urinary pH include obesity, type 2 diabetes mellitus, and high nondairy animal protein intake.

Struvite Stones

Struvite stones, also known as infection or triple-phosphate stones, form only when the upper urinary tract is infected with urease-producing bacteria such as *Proteus mirabilis, Klebsiella pneumoniae,* or *Providencia* species. Hydrolysis of urea by urease results in a supraphysiologic urine pH higher than 8.0 and the formation of struvite $[(NH_4)MgPO_4 \cdot 6(H_2O)]$. If the infection is inadequately treated, struvite stones may grow quickly, fill the renal collecting system, and result in a staghorn calculus.

Cystine Stones

Cystine stones form in individuals with an uncommon autosomal recessive disorder of defective proximal renal tubular reabsorption of filtered dibasic amino acids. Cystine is clinically significant because of its poor solubility in urine. Normal cystine excretion is less than 18 mg/day, but heterozygotes with hypercystinuria (Chapter 130) may excrete up to 100 mg/day, and homozygotes may excrete more than 1 g/day. Cystine solubility is about 250 mg/L, so heterozygotes typically do not form cystine stones. Cystine stones are visible on plain radiographs and will often be manifested as staghorn calculi or multiple bilateral stones.

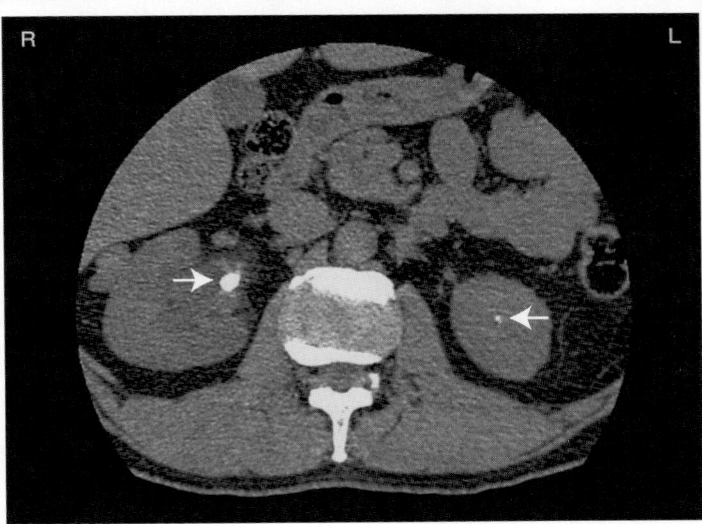

FIGURE 128-2. High-resolution helical computed tomographic (CT) scan of the upper part of the abdomen demonstrating a stone in the right renal pelvis and a smaller stone in the left kidney *(arrowheads)*. There is no hydronephrosis. (From Curhan GC. Clinical crossroads: a 44-year-old woman with kidney stones. *JAMA*. 2005;293:1107-1114.)

CLINICAL MANIFESTATIONS

A kidney stone takes weeks to months (and often much longer) to grow to a clinically detectable size. Although the passage of a stone is a dramatic event, a stone's formation and growth are typically clinically silent. A stone can remain asymptomatic in the kidney for years or even decades. Signs (e.g., hematuria) and symptoms may not become apparent until years after the stone has formed. Thus, it is important to remember that onset of symptoms, typically attributable to a stone moving into the ureter, does not provide insight into when the stone actually formed. The precipitants of movement of a stone are unknown.

Acute Renal Colic

When a stone moves from the renal pelvis into the ureter, the typical symptom is the sudden onset of unilateral flank pain of sufficient severity that the individual eventually seeks medical attention, often at an emergency department. Although the term *colic* is used, the pain does not completely remit but rather waxes and wanes. The pain, which is often accompanied by nausea and occasionally by vomiting, may radiate differently, depending on the location of the stone. If the stone lodges in the upper part of the ureter, pain may radiate anteriorly; if the stone is in the lower part of the ureter, pain can radiate to the ipsilateral testicle in men or the ipsilateral labium in women; and if lodged at the ureterovesical junction, the major symptoms may be urinary frequency and urgency. Occasionally, a patient will have gross hematuria without pain.

DIAGNOSIS

Physical examination alone will rarely make the diagnosis, but it may uncover clues to guide the evaluation. The patient will typically be in obvious pain and unable to find a comfortable position. Ipsilateral costovertebral tenderness is common. If the stone causes urinary obstruction, signs of infection and sepsis may be found. Occasionally, the examination may reveal findings associated with stone formation, such as tophi, but the physical examination rarely is diagnostic for stone disease.

Serum chemistry findings are typically normal, but the white blood cell count may be elevated. Urinalysis will classically reveal red and white blood cells and occasionally crystals. The absence of hematuria does not exclude a stone because no urine will be flowing from a ureter that is completely obstructed by a stone.

The diagnosis often is so clear, based on the history, physical examination, and urinalysis, that urgent radiographic confirmation is not required for acute care to be started. When such stable patients respond to analgesic therapy, imaging studies can be deferred for 2 to 3 weeks and performed only in patients whose stones do not pass or symptoms resolve.[1]

Diagnosis is confirmed by an appropriate imaging study (Fig. 128-2), preferably helical computed tomography (CT) because of its high sensitivity, ability to visualize uric acid stones (traditionally considered "radiolucent"), and ability to avoid radiocontrast. Helical CT detects stones as small as 1 mm, thus identifying small stones that may be missed by intravenous urography. Typically, helical CT will reveal a ureteral stone or evidence of recent passage (e.g., perinephric stranding or hydronephrosis), whereas a plain abdominal radiograph (kidney-ureters-bladder) can miss a stone in the ureter or kidney, even if radiopaque, and provides no information on obstruction. Although abdominal ultrasound has the advantage of avoiding radiation, this technique can image only the kidney and possibly the proximal segment of the ureter, so it misses most ureteral stones.

Differential Diagnosis

Because stone disease is common, a stone in the renal pelvis does not alone confirm the diagnosis in a patient with acute abdominal or flank pain. A stone lodged at the right ureteropelvic junction may mimic acute cholecystitis (Chapter 158), a stone in the distal right ureter may mimic acute appendicitis (Chapter 144), a stone at the ureterovesical junction may mimic acute cystitis (Chapter 292), and a stone in the distal left ureter may mimic diverticulitis (Chapter 144). An obstructing stone with proximal infection may mimic acute pyelonephritis (Chapter 292). Infection in the setting of ureteral obstruction is a medical emergency ("pus under pressure") that requires immediate drainage by placement of either a ureteral stent or a percutaneous nephrostomy tube. Other conditions to consider in the differential diagnosis include muscular or skeletal pain, herpes zoster (Chapter 383), duodenal ulcer (Chapter 141), abdominal aortic aneurysm (Chapter 144), gynecologic causes, ureteral stricture, and ureteral obstruction by materials other than a stone, such as a blood clot or sloughed papilla. Although extraluminal processes, such as extensions of gynecologic malignancies (Chapter 205) or retroperitoneal fibrosis (Chapter 284), can lead to ureteral obstruction, patients with these conditions tend not to have colic because of the usually gradual onset of the obstruction.

Chronic Nephrolithiasis

Among individuals with a documented history of nephrolithiasis, chronic back or flank pain is not infrequently encountered. Clinically, patients with an asymptomatic renal stone often have microscopic hematuria. Because stone disease itself is rarely a cause of chronic pain, the goal should be to determine the source of the pain. The differential diagnosis includes musculoskeletal pain, other intra-abdominal and pelvic conditions, and drug seeking. A thorough urologic evaluation, including appropriate radiologic studies, may curtail the long-term use of narcotics and avert frequent trips to the emergency room.

TREATMENT Rx

Medical Therapy

Renal colic can cause excruciating pain, so pain control is a priority after the definitive diagnosis has been made (Fig. 128-3). Nausea and vomiting often prevent the use of oral medication, so parenteral medication is typically required. Narcotics and parenteral nonsteroidal anti-inflammatory drugs (NSAIDs) have been demonstrated to be equally effective, and NSAIDs are preferred because of fewer side effects.[2] Ketorolac, 30 mg given intravenously (IV), is the usual adult dose. If oral NSAIDs are selected, ibuprofen is the most common choice. Morphine (5 to 10 mg IV) and hydromorphone (1 to 2 mg IV) are the most commonly used parenteral narcotics in adults. Oral oxycodone may be given for pain control after discharge. If antiemetics are required, ondansetron (2 to 4 mg IV) is often used because it is not sedating. However, the risk of parenteral NSAIDs may be increased in the setting of dehydration, decreased renal function, or the use of radiocontrast. Alkalinization of urine may be effective for the acute treatment of ureteral uric acid stones, but these are not nearly as common as calcium stones. Intravenous

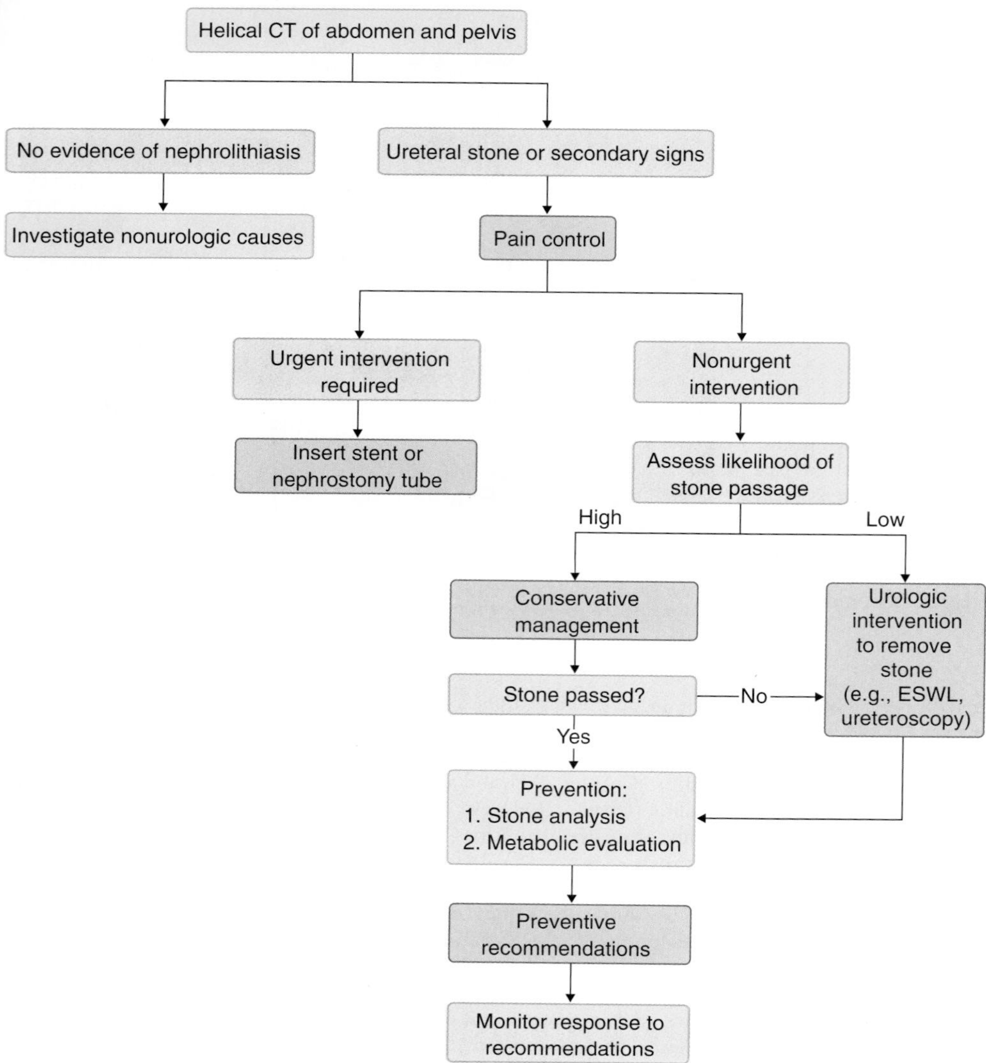

FIGURE 128-3. **Algorithm for evaluation of suspected renal colic.** ESWL = extracorporeal shock wave lithotripsy.

fluids are routinely given in the hope that increased ureteral flow will increase the likelihood that the stone will pass, but hydration status has little, if any, impact on stone passage. [3] Maintenance intravenous fluid replacement, such as half-normal saline with dextrose at 50 to 75 mL/hour, is reasonable for patients who are not able to take fluids orally.

A patient who is able to tolerate oral analgesics does not require admission, but instructions should be given to return if fever or uncontrollable pain develops. A urologist should be involved if infection is suspected, if the patient has persistent or uncontrollable pain, if the stone is not passed within 1 week, if urinary extravasation is detected by imaging, if there is high-grade obstruction with a large stone, or if the patient has a solitary kidney or is pregnant. For distal ureteral stones, meta-analysis suggests that oral calcium-channel blockers (e.g., nifedipine, 30 mg slow-release daily) or α-blockers (e.g., tamsulosin, 0.4 mg daily) administered for up to 28 days can increase the rate of spontaneous stone passage by 65%. [4]

Surgical Therapy

Most urologists usually wait several days before intervening unless there is evidence of urinary tract infection, a low probability of spontaneous stone passage (e.g., stone >6 mm or an anatomic abnormality), or intractable pain. Relief of obstruction is critical. A ureteral stent may be placed cystoscopically, but general anesthesia is typically required. Although the stent can be quite uncomfortable and may cause gross hematuria, it may help with stone passage.

The approach to removing a stone is dictated by its size, location, and composition; urinary tract anatomy; availability of technology; and the experience of the urologist. The least invasive approach is extracorporeal shock wave lithotripsy (ESWL). The ESWL procedure uses shock waves that are generated outside the body and that are focused on the stone using fluoroscopy or ultrasound. The shock waves fragment the stone into smaller pieces that then can be passed more easily. The strength of the shock waves, which is determined by the model of lithotripter machine used, determines the type of anesthesia required. ESWL can be used in the acute setting for upper tract stones, [5] but the success rate depends on the size, location, and composition of the stone. Cystoscopic stone removal, either by basket extraction or by laser fragmentation, is more invasive than ESWL but has a higher success rate, especially for ureteral stones, and is as good as ESWL for removing lower pole renal caliceal stones less than 1 cm in diameter. [6] Percutaneous nephrostolithotomy has the highest likelihood of making a patient stone free but is more invasive than cystoscopic methods. These endoscopic approaches have virtually eliminated the need for open surgical procedures such as ureterolithotomy or pyelolithotomy.

Asymptomatic Stones

With the increasing use of imaging, more incidental stones are being found. The best approach for asymptomatic renal stones is unsettled. Slightly less than 50% of individuals with radiologically documented asymptomatic stones will become symptomatic over a 5-year period. Most urologists would not consider removal of a stone that is 6 mm or smaller. For stones that are 10 mm or larger, many would recommend "prophylactic lithotripsy," but there are no data to support this approach.

Struvite Stones

Struvite stones require urologic intervention to ensure complete removal. The recommended approach is a combination of percutaneous nephrolithotomy and extracorporeal shock wave lithotripsy. Prolonged use of antibiotics alone may slow stone growth but rarely eradicates the infection. Although the medication acetohydroxamic acid inhibits bacterial urease, it is rarely used because of frequent and serious side effects.

PREVENTION

Evaluation after the First Stone

A complete history should include the pace and severity of all prior stone episodes as well as information regarding previous imaging studies (to

TABLE 128-2 LABORATORY EVALUATION

Spot urinalysis	Measure pH and examine the sediment for RBC, WBC, and crystals
24-Hour urine collection	Perform at least two at baseline; measure total volume, calcium, oxalate, citrate, uric acid, sodium, potassium, and creatinine If patient with cystine stones, also measure cystine
Blood	Electrolytes, calcium, phosphorus, BUN, creatinine If urine calcium or serum calcium is high, then measure PTH; if PTH is elevated, measure 25-hydroxyvitamin D to rule out secondary hyperparathyroidism If history of gout or considering use of a thiazide, measure serum uric acid If history of cystine stones, CBC and liver function tests should be performed before starting tiopronin

BUN = blood urea nitrogen; CBC = complete blood count; PTH = parathyroid hormone; RBC = red blood cells; WBC = white blood cells.

TABLE 128-3 DIETARY PRESCRIPTION FOR CALCIUM STONE PREVENTION ACCORDING TO URINARY RISK FACTOR

URINARY ABNORMALITY	DIETARY CHANGES
High calcium	Adequate dietary calcium intake Reduce nondairy animal protein intake (5-7 servings of meat, fish, or poultry/week) Reduce sodium intake to <2.4 g/day Reduce sucrose intake
High uric acid	Reduce purine intake
High oxalate	Avoid high-oxalate foods Avoid vitamin C supplements Adequate dietary calcium intake
Low citrate	Increase fruit and vegetable intake Reduce nondairy animal protein intake
Low volume	Increase total fluid intake to maintain urine volume to >2 L/day

Taylor EN, Curhan GC. Diet and fluid prescription in stone disease. *Kidney Int.* 2006;70:835-839.

distinguish stone passage events from actual new stone formation), surgical interventions, urinary tract infections, bowel disease or surgery, diarrhea or laxative abuse, family history of stone disease, and signs or symptoms suggestive of hyperparathyroidism (Chapter 253). In addition, information should be collected on dietary intake and the use of vitamins (e.g., C and D), minerals, and other supplements, as well as medications (e.g., carbonic anhydrase inhibitors, diuretics). The evaluation should also include appropriate clinical and laboratory evaluation to identify derangements and predict the likelihood of recurrence. Advice should be deferred until after the evaluation is complete; specifically, patients should be encouraged to resume their usual dietary habits while laboratory studies are completed.

Metabolic Evaluation

Every effort should be made to recover a stone that has passed or was removed, and its chemical composition should be analyzed by modern crystallographic methods. Even if the content of the stone is known, the metabolic evaluation for first-time and recurrent stone formers (Table 128-2) should include a serum chemistry profile and two 24-hour urine collections (because of substantial day-to-day variability).

Blood studies should include measurements of creatinine, calcium, phosphorus, albumin, uric acid, potassium, and total CO_2. Measurement of plasma parathyroid hormone level is recommended if serum or urine calcium levels are elevated.

The 24-hour urinary studies should be performed at least 6 weeks after the stone episode to ensure that patients have resumed their usual diet. The 24-hour measurements should include calcium, oxalate, uric acid, citrate, sodium, total volume, and creatinine. The urinary sediment should be examined for crystalluria in a freshly voided sample.

The 24-hour urine composition provides important prognostic information and directs recommendations for stone prevention. Traditionally, patients have been categorized into "normal" and "abnormal" with respect to the amount of lithogenic substances excreted. However, the measured values for the urinary factors are continuous variables, so dichotomization into normal and abnormal is somewhat artificial and potentially misleading. Second, stone formation is a disease of *concentration,* not just absolute amounts. Although a patient may have a normal amount of calcium in the urine over 24 hours, if the volume is low, the concentration of calcium would be abnormally high.

Patients with hypercalciuria can be divided into those with *absorptive* hypercalciuria (increased gastrointestinal calcium absorption), *resorptive* hypercalciuria (increased bone resorption), or *renal* hypercalciuria. However, a substantial proportion of patients do not fit into one category, an individual's classification may change over time, low bone mineral density may not be causally related to stone formation, and this classification approach rarely affects therapy.

All Stones

Dietary Modification

The observed increasing prevalence of nephrolithiasis and the physiologic impact of dietary factors have focused attention on the role of diet in stone formation (Table 128-3). In addition, the strong associations found in prospective studies of diet and initial stone formation (see earlier) suggest that dietary factors play an important role.

Fluid Intake

Stone formation is strongly influenced by urinary concentration, so the risk for stone formation decreases with increasing urine output. A general target is to encourage patients to drink enough fluid to produce more than 2 L of urine each day. The composition of the fluid ingested may be important, and observational studies suggest that higher intakes of coffee, tea, or alcoholic beverages are associated with a decreased risk for stone formation, perhaps because of the known diuretic action of these beverages.

Dietary Measures

Calcium Stones

The most controversial topic in dietary intervention for patients with nephrolithiasis is calcium intake. A low-calcium diet is often inappropriately recommended despite evidence that a low-calcium diet may in fact be *harmful* by increasing oxalate absorption from the intestine and also by leading to negative calcium balance and bone mineral loss. For example, in a randomized trial in men with hypercalciuria and recurrent calcium oxalate stones, a diet containing 1200 mg of calcium with a low intake of sodium and animal protein significantly reduced subsequent stone formation compared with a low-calcium diet (400 mg day). [7] The protective role for adequate dietary calcium intake does not extend to calcium from supplements, which either have no effect or slightly increase the risk of stone formation, and a very high calcium intake (>2 to 3 g/day) should be discouraged. Although the bioavailability of calcium is the same in dairy and calcium supplements, it is possible that dairy products, the major source of dietary calcium, contain some unidentified protective factor.

Other Dietary Factors

Restriction of nondairy animal protein (e.g., meat, chicken, seafood) is a reasonable option and may result in higher excretion of citrate and lower excretion of uric acid and calcium. For patients with high oxalate excretion, restriction of dietary oxalate may be beneficial. Reliable and complete data on the oxalate content of many commonly consumed foods are now available (*https://regepi.bwh.harvard.edu/health/Oxalate/files*). Spinach should be avoided because it is the highest oxalate-containing food. Reducing sodium intake to less than 3 g/day may decrease the obligatory, concurrent urinary excretion of calcium and may be particularly important for patients prescribed a thiazide. Sucrose intake, which may increase urinary calcium excretion, should be minimized. In contrast, potassium-rich foods should be encouraged. Dietary recommendations should be tailored to the patient's urinary chemistry profile, and the impact of the recommendations can be monitored by repeating the urine collections.

Uric Acid Stones

The mainstay of treatment to prevent uric acid stones is increasing urine pH by dietary modification, which should focus on decreasing acid production by reducing the intake of animal flesh and increasing the intake of alkali-rich foods, specifically fruits and vegetables. If dietary modification is unsuccessful, alkalinization with oral bicarbonate, typically requiring 20 to 30 mEq three times per day, or a bicarbonate precursor (e.g., potassium citrate, 20 to 30 mEq three times per day) should be started. The pH goal is 6 to 7 throughout the day and night. Alkali three or four times a day is typically needed to match the endogenous acid production of approximately 1 mEq/kg per 24 hours. However, a urine pH greater than 7 should be avoided to minimize the likelihood of inducing calcium phosphate crystallization. Allopurinol (100 to 300 mg/day) should be prescribed for patients in whom alkalinization fails.

Cystine Stones

The total amount of cystine excreted cannot be easily modified, so treatment is directed at decreasing the urinary cystine concentration below the limit of solubility. Increasing urinary volume is the first approach, but some patients would need more than 4 L of urine per day, which is impractical. Increasing urine pH above 7.5 using oral alkali, such as 20 to 30 mEq of potassium citrate twice daily, will slightly increase cystine solubility, but this pH is often difficult to maintain in the long term. Tiopronin, typically 300 mg orally three times per day, will bind cystine and reduce urine supersaturation. Although side effects are common, tiopronin is first-line therapy in patients with recurrent cystine stone formation because there are no other alternatives.

Medical Prevention

Although nephrolithiasis is a common disease, surprisingly few well-designed prospective double-blind controlled trials have been conducted. Some medications may improve the urinary chemistry profile but not cure the underlying abnormality. Thus, the decision to start medication requires consideration of efficacy, side effects, cost, and adherence of the patient. Certainly, if new stone formation occurs despite dietary recommendations, medication should be prescribed. If urine calcium levels are elevated, a thiazide diuretic is recommended. For patients with hypocitraturia or hyperuricosuria as a sole finding, potassium citrate and allopurinol can be used, respectively. Unfortunately, the optimal duration of treatment is unclear, and long-term adherence remains suboptimal.

Thiazides

Thiazide diuretics, such as hydrochlorothiazide and chlorthalidone, increase calcium reabsorption in the proximal convoluted tubule and distal tubule and effectively lower urinary calcium excretion by 20 to 50%. In some patients, urine calcium levels may rise after a year despite continued therapy. Thiazides can also increase the mineral content of bone. About 30 years ago, two trials showed that thiazides reduced the risk of recurrent calcium oxalate stones in otherwise unclassified patients. The doses required for urinary calcium reduction (25 to 100 mg/day) are higher than those needed for treating hypertension. Side effects are reported in 8 to 35% of patients. Thiazide-induced hypokalemia can be treated with potassium citrate (20 mEq per day) or amiloride (2.5 to 5.0 mg per day). Because of its potential to precipitate in the urine, triamterene should be avoided in these patients. Indapamide (2.5 mg per day), although not strictly a thiazide, will also reduce urine calcium. Monitoring the urine calcium response with subsequent dosage adjustment is recommended.

Allopurinol

Allopurinol (300 mg per day) can reduce urine uric acid excretion by up to 50%, and it was shown 25 years ago to reduce stone recurrence in individuals with hyperuricosuric calcium oxalate stone disease. In patients without hyperuricosuria, allopurinol has no benefit when compared with placebo.

Potassium Citrate

Systemic alkalinization of the urine with bicarbonate (typically 30 mEq twice daily) or citrate (typically 30 mEq twice daily) will lead to an increase in urinary citrate excretion. The most commonly used salt is potassium citrate, which avoids the calciuric effect of a sodium load and restores any potassium deficiency. Citrate supplementation reduces recurrent calcium oxalate stones compared with placebo, but adherence to prescribed dosing is suboptimal.[8]

Magnesium

Oral magnesium from supplements may reduce stone risk by forming soluble complexes with oxalate in the bowel or urine. However, in a 3-year double-blind trial, magnesium was no more effective than placebo. Thus, the role of magnesium supplementation remains uncertain.

Other Genitourinary Stones

Stones can form in other parts of the genitourinary tract, including the bladder and rarely the prostate. In the United States, the most common type of bladder stone is uric acid. Bladder stones are much more common in men because the primary risk factors are urinary stasis owing to bladder outlet obstruction and a persistently low urine pH. As with uric acid stones that form in the kidney, hyperuricosuria is not always present, but the low urine pH dramatically reduces the solubility of uric acid in the urine. Patients with bladder stones often pass stones frequently, sometimes on a daily basis. The stones can range in size from "sand" or "gravel" to several centimeters. Stones of sufficient size are characteristically round because of the rolling that can occur in the bladder. Bladder stones do not cause renal colic but can cause partial or complete acute urinary retention by obstructing the urethra. The rate of stone formation can be dramatically reduced or even halted by improving urine flow by medications or surgery (Chapter 131) or through alkalinization of the urine. Potassium citrate, typically 20 to 30 mEq three times daily, is sufficient to stop stone formation.

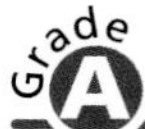

1. Lindqvist K, Hellstrom M, Holmberg G, et al. Immediate versus deferred radiological investigation after acute renal colic: a prospective randomized study. *Scand J Urol Nephrol.* 2006;40:119-124.
2. Holdgate A, Pollock T. Systematic review of the relative efficacy of non-steroidal anti-inflammatory drugs and opioids in the treatment of acute renal colic. *BMJ.* 2004;328:1401.
3. Springhart WP, Marguet CG, Sur RL, et al. Forced versus minimal intravenous hydration in the management of acute renal colic: a randomized trial. *J Endourol.* 2006;20:713-716.
4. Hollingsworth JM, Rogers MAM, Kaufman SR, et al. Medical therapy to facilitate urinary stone passage: a meta-analysis. *Lancet.* 2006;368:1171-1179.
5. Kravchick S, Bunkin I, Stepnov E, et al. Emergency extracorporeal shockwave lithotripsy for acute renal colic caused by upper urinary-tract stones. *J Endourol.* 2005;19:1-4.
6. Pearle MS, Lingeman JE, Leveillee R, et al. Prospective, randomized trial comparing shock wave lithotripsy and ureteroscopy for lower pole caliceal calculi 1 cm or less. *J Urol.* 2005;173:2005-2009.
7. Borghi L, Schianchi T, Meschi T, et al. Comparison of two diets for the prevention of recurrent stones in idiopathic hypercalciuria. *N Engl J Med.* 2002;346:77-84.
8. Ettinger B, Pak CY, Citron JT, et al. Potassium-magnesium citrate is an effective prophylaxis against recurrent calcium oxalate nephrolithiasis. *J Urol.* 1997;158:2069-2073.

SUGGESTED READINGS

Kenny JE, Goldfarb DS. Update on the pathophysiology and management of uric acid renal stones. *Curr Rheumatol Rep.* 2010;12:125-129. *Review.*

Moe OW, Pearle MS, Sakhaee K. Pharmacotherapy of urolithiasis: evidence from clinical trials. *Kidney Int.* 2011;79:385-392. *Comprehensive review.*

Worcester EM, Coe FL. Calcium kidney stones. *N Engl J Med.* 2010;363:954-963. *Clinical review.*

129

CYSTIC KIDNEY DISEASES

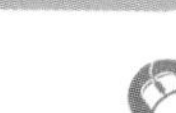

M. AMIN ARNAOUT

DEFINITION AND EPIDEMIOLOGY

The term *cystic kidney diseases* refers to a heterogeneous group of hereditary and acquired disorders characterized by the presence of unilateral or bilateral renal cysts. When acquired singly or in small numbers and in the absence of any other pathology, renal cysts are termed *simple cysts*, which are present in approximately 50% of individuals older than 40 years, are usually not loculated, and tend to bulge out from the renal surface (Fig. 129-1). The *polycystic kidney diseases* (PKDs), by comparison, constitute a clinically important group of genetically mediated disorders characterized by prominent, expanding, bilateral renal cysts. PKDs are classified as dominant, recessive, or X-linked, based on their pattern of inheritance. Autosomal dominant PKD (ADPKD), with a prevalence rate between 1 : 400 and 1 : 1000, is the most common monogenic disease in humans and accounts for about 10% of all end-stage renal disease (ESRD) in the United States. ADPKD develops in an age-dependent manner and affects mainly adults. Autosomal recessive PKD (ARPKD), by contrast, is a relatively rare childhood disorder that appears in 1 in every 6000 to 50,000 live births. Renal cysts are also seen in several other rare hereditary kidney diseases and in several syndromic PKDs (Table 129-1). Collectively, the hereditary PKDs generally affect both genders and all races equally and cost more than $1 billion annually to manage in the

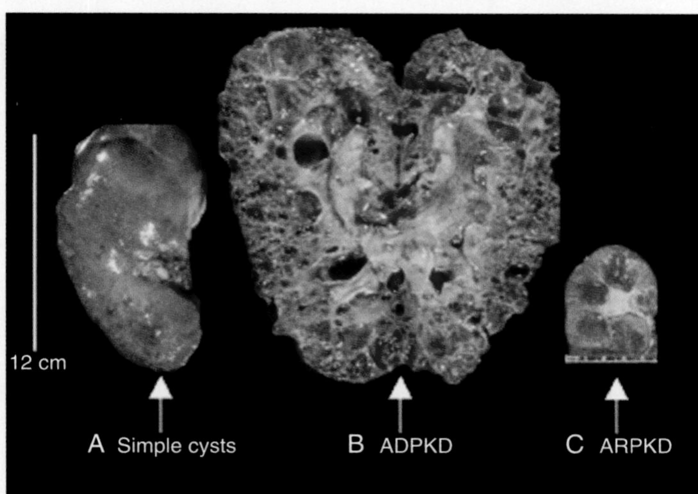

FIGURE 129-1. **Gross pathology of selected cystic kidney diseases. A,** Photograph of a kidney with multiple simple cysts. The cysts bulge out from the surface of a normal-sized kidney. **B,** Sagittal cross section of a kidney from an adult with autosomal dominant polycystic kidney disease (ADPKD). Multiple macroscopic cysts have resulted in an enlarged but still reniform kidney (note the evidence of prior hemorrhage within some of the cysts). **C,** Sagittal cross section of a kidney segment from a neonate with autosomal recessive polycystic kidney disease (ARPKD). The kidney is enlarged, with numerous small cysts. (Courtesy Dr. Robert Colvin, Massachusetts General Hospital.)

United States alone. *Acquired cystic kidney disease* refers to the multiple bilateral renal cysts that develop in patients who already have kidney disease. Cysts occur in 90% of patients who have been receiving renal replacement therapy for 8 years or longer and are associated with increased rates of renal cell carcinoma.

AUTOSOMAL DOMINANT POLYCYSTIC KIDNEY DISEASE

PATHOBIOLOGY

ADPKD is a systemic disorder characterized by cyst formation in multiple organs, including the kidneys, other ductal organs, and the cardiovascular system. Renal cysts originate as outpouchings of tubules and may affect any portion of the nephron, with up to 1% of nephrons involved. The outpouchings expand and eventually separate from the parent tubules, yielding cysts (Fig. 129-2). Expansion of cysts is caused by proliferation of the cyst lining cells, by chloride-driven fluid secretion that outpaces absorption, and by remodeling of the extracellular matrix. The kidneys become massively enlarged.

Genetics

Heterogeneous mutations in two genes, *PKD1* and *PKD2,* cause ADPKD. Mutations in *PKD1* account for approximately 85% of cases of ADPKD. Heterogeneous mutations in *PKD2* contribute an additional 10 to 15% of cases. The onset and severity of the disease are dramatically affected by the developmental stage at which gene inactivation occurs. In a minority of ADPKD cases, no demonstrable *PKD1* or *PKD2* mutations are found, suggesting that a third gene may be involved.

PKD1 is 54 kb long and is located on chromosome 16p13.3, adjacent to the tuberous sclerosis 2 (*TSC2*) gene. *PKD1* has 46 exons, generates a 14-kb transcript, and encodes a 4302- residue protein called polycystin-1, the first described member of an expanding group of polycystins. The 5′ region of human *PKD1* (to exon 33) is replicated on the same chromosome, resulting in approximately six copies of *PKD1*-like pseudogenes, which must be distinguished from the *PKD1* gene in direct mutational analysis. To date, more than 330 truncating mutations have been identified throughout the gene, but especially in the 3′ half. Mutations in the 5′ half of the gene are associated with more severe disease, with only 19% of patients retaining adequate renal function at 60 years of age (vs. 40% of those with 3′ mutations), and they are more likely to be associated with intracerebral aneurysms and aneurysm rupture.

The 68-kb *PKD2* gene is located on chromosome 4q13-23, transcribes 15 exons, and generates a 5-kb transcript, which encodes a protein of 968 residues called polycystin-2. Ninety-five heterogeneous mutations in *PKD2* have been identified to date.

Large intrafamilial variability in the onset and severity of ADPKD may be caused by bilineal inheritance of *PKD1* and *PKD2* mutant alleles or of hypomorphic variants of either gene. Mosaicism in a parent in whom a mutation has arisen de novo could result in one sibling having the disease while another is disease free, despite sharing the identical inherited haplotype at the *PKD* gene. Concomitant mutations affecting other genes can also result in ADPKD in infancy. Because cysts appear from a small number of nephrons, somatic inactivation of the normal allele has been proposed as the main mechanism of disease. *PKD1* or *PKD2* haplo-insufficiency and gene dose effects are associated with a high frequency of genomic instability, which likely increases the incidence of somatic second hits in ADPKD. Genomic instability may also explain the increased rate of apoptosis and the low incidence of renal cell carcinoma in this disease.

PATHOGENESIS

Polycystin-1 comprises a large extracellular modular ectodomain, followed by an 11-pass transmembrane segment and a short cytoplasmic carboxyl terminus (E-Fig. 129-1). The polycystin-1 ectodomain contains multiple functional motifs, suggesting a role in cell-cell and/or cell-matrix adhesion. Polycystin-2 is a six-membrane spanner that acts as a nonselective voltage-dependent, calcium-permeable ion channel with cytoplasmic amino and carboxyl termini. Its six-transmembrane segment bears a topologic and sequence similarity to the carboxyl terminal six-transmembrane segment of polycystin-1. The coiled-coil domains within the carboxyl termini of polycystin-1 and polycystin-2 interact to stabilize the channel activity of polycystin-2 and facilitate its translocation to the plasma membrane. In addition, polycystin-1 interacts with intermediate filaments, E-cadherin, focal adhesion proteins, β-catenin, and tuberin. Polycystin-1 and polycystin-2 also interact with a number of other proteins, and each of these interactions could serve as a modifier of the polycystins' functions.

Polycystin-1 and polycystin-2 are widely expressed in tissues, with some overlap consistent with their direct interaction. Polycystin-1 is found at multiple membrane sites, including adherens junctions, desmosomes and focal adhesions, primary cilia, and intracellular vesicles. Polycystin-2 is found in primary cilia as well as the basolateral membrane, endoplasmic reticulum, centrosome, and mitotic spindles in dividing cells. Both polycystin-1 and polycystin-2 are also found in urinary vesicles. Levels of polycystin-1 expression are highest in fetal tissue and progressively decline thereafter, whereas polycystin-2 levels are maintained throughout development.

Cyst Formation

Both polycystin-1 and polycystin-2 localize to primary cilia, which are found on the apical surface of all renal cells except intercalated cells. The primary cilium consists of an axoneme comprising nine microtubular doublets surrounded by a cell membrane. It is assembled during the interphase from the mother centriole (basal body), which serves as a microtubule-organizing center just beneath the plasma membrane. Transition fibers associated with the basal body regulate protein entry and exit into the cilium. Because cell division requires both centrioles to form the mitotic spindle, the cell is unable to divide until its cilium is resorbed, linking the structural integrity of the cilium to cell cycle regulation. A mechanosensitive cilium is normally deflected by the tubular flow of urine, thereby activating polycystin-1– and polycystin-2–mediated calcium influx, which is amplified by calcium released from internal stores. How this process translates into regulation of tube diameter (cyst formation) is still unclear. It is proposed that calcium influx through normal primary cilia favors the noncanonical Wnt pathway (also known as planar cell polarity) over the mitogenic canonical (β-catenin–dependent) Wnt pathway, thereby maintaining cell polarity and suppressing proliferation. Planar cell polarity couples polarized cell movement and cell division for proper control of tube diameter size during tube elongation. Loss of polycystin-1 or polycystin-2 disrupts this structural link, causing cysts.

Regulation of calcium influx by polycystin-1 and polycystin-2 may not be restricted to the cilium. For example, polycystin signaling also activates the JAK/STAT pathway. Polycystin-1– and polycystin-2–mediated calcium influx suppresses intracellular cyclic adenosine monophosphate (cAMP) signaling by inhibiting adenylyl cyclase and stimulating cAMP phosphodiesterase (E-Fig. 129-2). Loss of the polycystin-1 and polycystin-2 calcium signal may lead to a buildup of cAMP, promoting cell proliferation.

TABLE 129-1 COMPARISON OF CLINICAL FEATURES OF CYSTIC KIDNEY DISEASES

DISEASE	INHERITANCE	FREQUENCY	GENE PRODUCT	AGE OF ONSET	CYST ORIGIN	RENOMEGALY	CAUSE OF ESRD	OTHER MANIFESTATIONS
ADPKD	AD	1:400–1000	Polycystin-1 Polycystin-2	20s and 30s	Anywhere (including Bowman's capsule)	Yes	Yes	Liver cysts Cerebral aneurysms Hypertension Mitral valve prolapse Kidney stones UTIs
ARPKD	AR	1:6000–10,000	Fibrocystin/ polyductin	First year of life	Distal nephron, CD	Yes	Yes	Hepatic fibrosis Pulmonary hypoplasia Hypertension
ACKD	No	90% of ESRD patients at 8 yr	None*	Years after onset of ESRD	Proximal and distal tubules	Rarely	No	None
Simple cysts	No	50% in those older than 40 yr	None*	Adulthood	Anywhere (usually cortical)	No	No	None
Nephronophthisis	AR	1:80,000	Nephrocystins (NPHP1–9)	Childhood or adolescence	Medullary DCT	No	Yes	Retinal degeneration; neurologic, skeletal, hepatic, cardiac malformations
MCKD	AD	Rare	Uromodulin, others	Adulthood	Medullary DCT	No	Yes	Hyperuricemia, gout
MSK	No	1:5000–20,000	None*	30s	Medullary CD	No	No	Kidney stones Hypercalciuria
Tuberous sclerosis	AD	1:10,000	Hamartin (TSC1), tuberin (TSC2)	Childhood	Loop of Henle, DCT	Rarely	Rarely	Renal cell carcinoma Tubers, seizures Angiomyolipoma Hypertension
VHL syndrome	AD	1:40,000	VHL protein	20s	Cortical nephrons	Rarely	Rarely	Retinal angioma, CNS hemangioblastoma, renal cell carcinoma, pheochromocytoma
Oral-facial-digital syndrome-1	XD	1:250,000	OFD1 protein	Childhood or adulthood	Renal glomeruli	Rarely	Yes	Malformation of the face, oral cavity, and digits; liver cysts; mental retardation
Bardet-Biedl syndrome	AR	1:65,000–160,000	BBS 1-14	Adulthood	Renal calyces	Rarely	Yes	Syn- and polydactyly, obesity, retinal dystrophy, male hypogenitalism, hypertension, mental retardation

*No known genetic susceptibility.

ACKD = acquired cystic kidney disease; AD = autosomal dominant; ADPKD = autosomal dominant polycystic kidney disease; AR = autosomal recessive; ARPKD = autosomal recessive polycystic kidney disease; CD = collecting duct; CNS = central nervous system; DCT = distal convoluted tubule; ESRD = end-stage renal disease; MCKD = medullary cystic kidney disease; MSK = medullary sponge kidney; UTI = urinary tract infection; VHL = von Hippel-Lindau; XD = X-linked dominant.

CLINICAL MANIFESTATIONS

ADPKD has a highly variable presentation, even within families. The clinical features of *PKD2*-associated ADPKD are indistinguishable from those of *PKD1*-associated disease. However, *PKD2* disease is milder, with an older average age of onset—74 years versus about 54 years for *PKD1*-associated disease—owing to the development of fewer cysts at an early age rather than to a slower cyst growth rate.

Despite an estimated 100% penetrance by age 90 years, only half the individuals with heterozygous mutations in *PKD1* or *PKD2* are ever diagnosed clinically with ADPKD. Of these patients, the majority present in the third or fourth decade of life with symptoms referable to renal cystic disease. However, ADPKD can develop at any age, including infancy, and it can have a nonrenal presentation. Renomegaly may predominate the clinical picture, with abdominal distention, discomfort, or pain; however, renomegaly can also be discovered incidentally on physical examination or after radiographic studies of the abdomen.

Nocturia, which is one of the earliest signs of abnormal renal function in ADPKD, reflects the early impairment in urinary concentration. The urinary pH is typically low, with hypocitric aciduria. Hematuria is typical, but proteinuria is less prominent than in many other renal diseases. Anemia features less prominently than in other renal diseases, probably because of the relatively well-preserved erythropoietin secretion. Recurrent cyst infection, usually by common urinary tract–infecting organisms, is characterized by flank or abdominal pain, fever, rigors, leukocytosis, and occasionally sepsis. Cyst hemorrhage and sometimes rupture, which can occur spontaneously or after trauma, present as sharp pain and hematuria.

Arterial hypertension is present in approximately 70% of cases before renal dysfunction is detected. Enhanced vascular smooth muscle contractility, reduced endothelial-dependent vasorelaxation, lower constitutive nitric oxide synthase activity, activation of the intrarenal renin-angiotensin system, and increased sympathetic nerve activity are likely causes of the accompanying arterial hypertension. Development of hypertension at a young age is associated with a four-fold increased risk of ESRD and increased cardiovascular morbidity. The risk for preeclampsia is also higher than in the general population.

An estimated 4 to 15% of individuals with ADPKD develop saccular cerebral aneurysms (Chapter 415), a prevalence rate that is 4 to 10 times greater than in the general population. These aneurysms tend to segregate in families, making ADPKD one of a group of diseases characterized by autosomal dominant inheritance of cerebral aneurysms. ADPKD-associated aneurysms tend to rupture at a smaller size and in younger individuals—on average, 10 years younger than among the general population. Although usually clinically silent, intact cerebral aneurysms can present with focal neurologic symptoms and headaches. By contrast, aneurysms that rupture lead to subarachnoid hemorrhage (Chapter 415) and have dramatic presentations that include severe headaches, seizures, altered sensorium, and death. Aortic and coronary

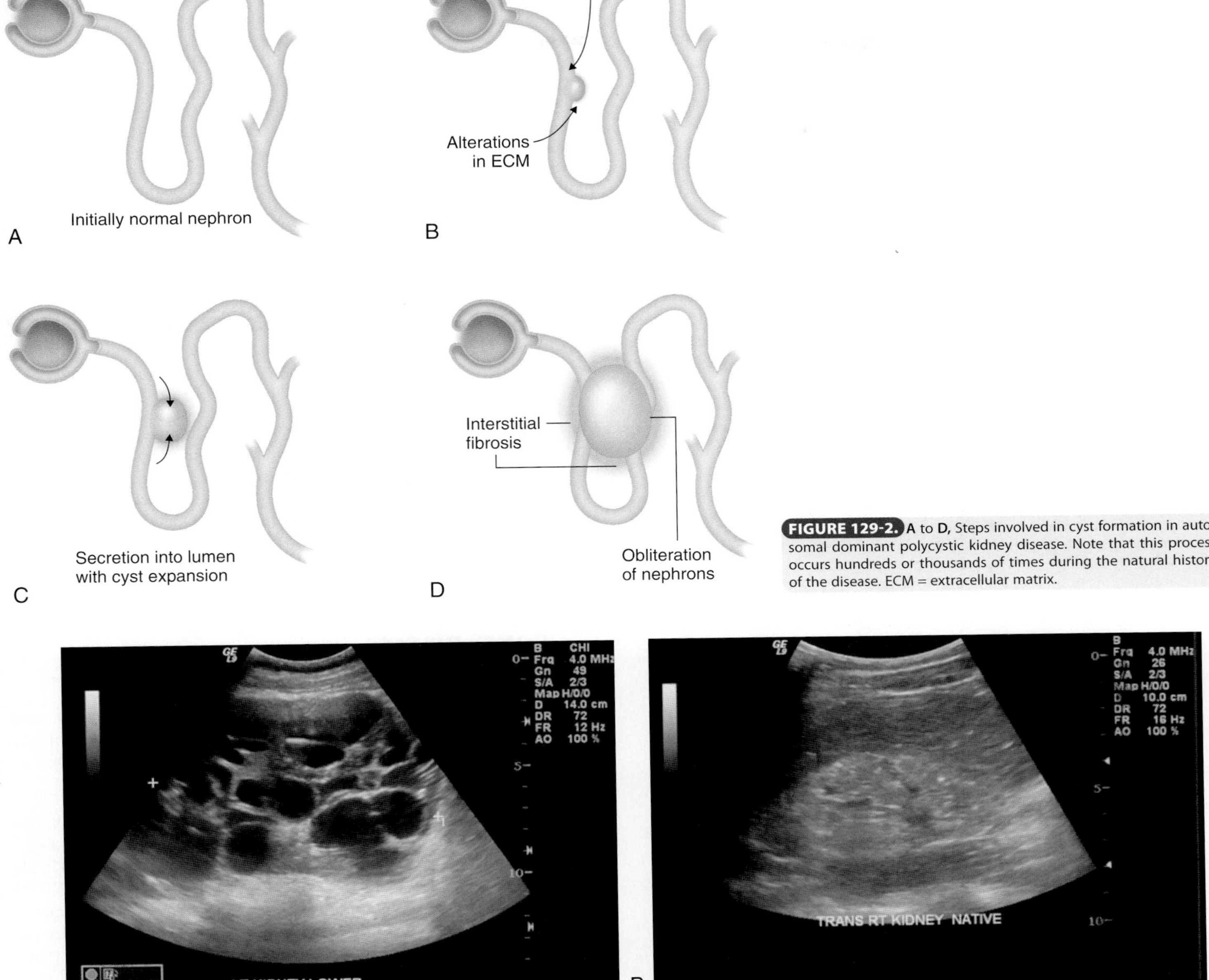

FIGURE 129-2. **A** to **D**, Steps involved in cyst formation in autosomal dominant polycystic kidney disease. Note that this process occurs hundreds or thousands of times during the natural history of the disease. ECM = extracellular matrix.

FIGURE 129-3. **A**, Ultrasound images of a kidney from a patient with autosomal dominant polycystic kidney disease. **B**, Ultrasound images of a kidney from a patient with autosomal recessive polycystic kidney disease. (Courtesy Dr. Javier M. Romero and Jennifer A. McDowell, Massachusetts General Hospital.)

artery aneurysms are also more prevalent in patients with ADPKD, and the frequency of aortic insufficiency is increased.

Although almost never severe enough to cause end-stage liver disease, age-dependent hepatic cysts occur in 30 to 80% of patients with ADPKD and can lead to signs and symptoms of mass effect, infection, hemorrhage, and rupture. Estrogen intake and multiparity in women are risk factors in developing larger and more symptomatic cysts. The cysts that occasionally form in other organs, such as the pancreas, spleen, brain, ovaries, epididymis, and prostate, are usually asymptomatic. Sperm abnormalities and defective motility may occur but rarely cause male infertility. Bronchiectasis (Chapter 90) is three-fold more common, inguinal hernias may be more prevalent, and colonic diverticulosis and diverticulitis are more common in ESRD patients with ADPKD.

DIAGNOSIS

The specific diagnosis of ADPKD requires a consideration of associated extrarenal manifestations, age at presentation, and family history. Because only about 60% of individuals give a family history of PKD, ultrasound screening of asymptomatic parents or grandparents may be required to uncover diagnostically relevant silent PKD. To account for the common age-dependent appearance of simple cysts, ADPKD is diagnosed if at least three renal cysts (distributed in one or both kidneys) are present in individuals 15 to 39 years old, if at least two renal cysts are present in each kidney in individuals aged 40 to 59 years, or if at least four renal cysts are present in each kidney in individuals 60 years and older (Fig. 129-3A). Fewer than two renal cysts in an individual aged 40 years or older from an ADPKD family with an unknown genotype, or the absence of renal cysts in such an individual aged 30 to 39 years, is sufficient to exclude the disease, with negative predictive values of 100 and 99.3%, respectively. A negative ultrasound is less accurate in excluding disease in individuals younger than 30 years, so computed tomography (CT) or magnetic resonance imaging (MRI) is recommended. When a young relative is being considered as a potential kidney donor to a family member with end-stage ADPKD, contrast-enhanced, three-dimensional CT or magnetic resonance angiography (MRA) is required because these tests can detect 3-mm cysts, compared with ultrasound's ability to detect 10-mm cysts.

DNA-based diagnosis of ADPKD by means of direct sequencing is commercially available and detects mutations in more than 90% of affected individuals. Such testing is expensive, however, and the marked allelic heterogeneity of the *PKD1* and *PKD2* mutations, as well as the paucity of phenotype-genotype correlations, contributes to the complexity of DNA-based diagnostics. Testing is recommended when imaging studies are equivocal, in a young transplant donor from an ADPKD family when imaging studies are negative, or to facilitate preimplantation genetic diagnosis.

Monitoring Disease Progression

Despite ongoing renal cyst expansion, the glomerular filtration rate (GFR) and the serum creatinine level are generally maintained within the normal range in ADPKD patients until the fourth to sixth decade of life. As a result, these markers are insensitive for monitoring disease progression, especially in the young. Estimating kidney volume from measurements of kidney length, width, and thickness using MRI, CT, or ultrasonography can reliably monitor disease progression in the early stages of ADPKD, when the GFR is still in the normal range. Although gadolinium-enhanced MRI provides excellent detail of kidney structures, MRI without gadolinium is recommended to monitor kidney volume, especially in ADPKD patients with a reduced GFR, because of concern about nephrogenic systemic fibrosis (Chapter 275) and further impairment of renal function associated with its use. The combined kidney volume in ADPKD patients progressively increases in most cases, but at widely differing rates, ranging from less than 1% to more than 10%. Combined kidney volumes greater than 1500 mL are frequently associated with a decreased GFR and gross hematuria and invariably with arterial hypertension.

PREVENTION AND TREATMENT Rx

Management strategies are aimed at monitoring for complications of ADPKD and treating them, as well as providing counseling. Frequent blood pressure monitoring is recommended because hypertension accelerates the decline in renal function. The goals of blood pressure control are the same as for other patients with renal disease, including the attainment of a symptom-free blood pressure of 125/75 mm Hg or less. Although all available antihypertensive agents have been used with roughly equivalent success, theoretical considerations and preliminary data suggest that angiotensin-converting enzyme (ACE) inhibitors or angiotensin receptor blockers (ARBs) combined with salt restriction may be more efficient in slowing the rate of progression to ESRD (see Tables 67-5 and 67-7 in Chapter 67). If these drugs fail to lower blood pressure sufficiently owing to the associated plasma volume expansion, thiazides or loop diuretics may be added (see Table 67-5 in Chapter 67).

Treatment of urinary tract infection (Chapter 292) and prevention of nephrolithiasis (Chapter 128) are the same as in the general population and include standard antimicrobial therapy and increased fluid intake, respectively. Renal or hepatic cyst infections are optimally treated with lipophilic antibiotics that possess cyst-penetrating capabilities, including ciprofloxacin, trimethoprim, clindamycin, and vancomycin. Blood or urine cultures and sensitivities are used to guide the choice of antibiotic therapy.

Cyst hemorrhage and rupture, with resultant pain and hematuria, are usually managed conservatively with rest and analgesics; nonsteroidal anti-inflammatory drugs (NSAIDs) are avoided, owing to their antiplatelet action and potential renal toxicity. Alternatives include acetaminophen 500 mg up to every 4 hours for mild to moderate pain, nonopiates such as tramadol 50 mg up to every 4 hours for moderate to severe pain, and the addition of an oral or transdermal opioid (see Table 29-4 in Chapter 29) as needed. Patients with enlarged kidneys should be advised to avoid playing contact sports, and those with massively enlarged kidneys should refrain from wearing belts and seatbelts. Some patients with unusually painful cysts respond to cyst fluid aspiration, cyst deroofing, or ethanol-induced sclerosis.

Nephrectomy is rarely indicated before the onset of ESRD. Renal replacement therapies, including renal transplantation (Chapter 133), are at least as effective as in other causes of ESRD.

The massive cystic enlargement of the liver commonly seen by midlife in women with ADPKD makes it prudent to avoid estrogen intake and repeated pregnancies. Partial hepatectomy has been successful in improving the quality of life in patients with massive liver enlargement.

Screening MRA is not routinely recommended for asymptomatic patients without a family history of cerebral aneurysm or subarachnoid hemorrhage, but it is recommended for patients with a positive family history and may be considered in those with high-risk occupations, such as airline pilots, or with incapacitating anxiety. The risk of a patient with a positive family history developing a new aneurysm after an initially negative magnetic resonance angiogram is 2.6% at a mean follow-up of 9.8 years, so rescreening every 5 to 10 years in such cases may be appropriate, especially in patients with early-onset hypertension or a history of heavy smoking. Individuals shown to have cerebral aneurysms should be referred to a neurosurgeon for consideration of clipping (Chapter 415). Annual MRA screening is recommended in all patients with untreated aneurysms to assess for aneurysmal growth.

Patients should be advised that their children have a 50% probability of inheriting a disease-causing germline mutation. DNA-based diagnostics are most useful in identifying the germline mutation prenatally or preimplantation. As DNA-based diagnostics become more widely available and less expensive, and as promising new treatment options are developed, counseling will become an increasingly important component of prevention.

Experimental Therapies

The better understanding of the pathobiology of ADPKD raises the hope of directed therapies to halt or slow the progression of disease. The metabolically stable somatostatin analogue octreotide (at a dose of 40 mg intravenously every 28 days) halted the expansion of renal cysts but did not have a beneficial effect on the GFR in a small trial of ADPKD patients.[1] Neither sirolimus[2] nor everolimus[3] slowed the decline of renal function in ADPKD patients, although everolimus slowed the increase in kidney volume. These data suggest that cyst growth may not be the key determinant of renal function decline. ACE inhibitors and ARBs are currently being tested in large clinical trials, and the vasopressin V2 receptor inhibitor tolvaptan is being evaluated in phase III clinical trials.

PROGNOSIS

The rate of progression of renal disease is highest in men with poorly controlled hypertension, an early age at diagnosis, and mutations in *PKD1*. The presence of one affected family member who developed ESRD by age 60 years is highly predictive of PKD1 disease (positive predictive value, 100%; sensitivity, 75%), whereas the development of ESRD after age 70 years in a family member is highly predictive of PKD2 disease (positive predictive value, 95%; sensitivity, 75%). Approximately 5% of all ADPKD patients with cerebral aneurysms die from aneurysmal rupture.

AUTOSOMAL RECESSIVE POLYCYSTIC KIDNEY DISEASE

DEFINITION AND EPIDEMIOLOGY

ARPKD is a multisystem childhood disorder characterized by severe and early PKD dominated by dilation of the kidney collecting ducts, biliary ductal plate dysgenesis in neonates, and portal tract fibrosis in older children.

PATHOBIOLOGY

ARPKD has been linked to heterogeneous mutations in a single gene, *PKHD1* (polycystic kidney and hepatic disease 1). Located on chromosome 6q21, *PKHD1* has 67 exons and spans a genomic region of approximately 470 kb, the longest open reading frame of which is 12,222 base pairs long. *PKHD1* encodes a unique type I membrane protein, fibrocystin/polyductin, comprising 4074 amino acids, with a large extracellular segment and a short cytoplasmic carboxyl terminus. The precise physiologic function of fibrocystin/polyductin in collecting duct and biliary duct epithelium is not clear, but its domains are known to mediate cell motility and invasion, extracellular protein and carbohydrate binding, and catalysis of polysaccharide hydrolysis. Alternatively-spliced transcripts of *PKHD1* encode a membrane protein with variable extracellular domains, as well as forms lacking the transmembrane segment. Homozygous truncating mutations in *PKHD1* are associated with perinatal renal disease, whereas patients with homozygous missense mutations present later because some functional protein is produced.

PKHD1 messenger RNA is detected mostly in the cortical and medullary collecting ducts and the thick ascending limbs of Henle, but it is also found to a lesser degree in the pancreas, liver, and lungs, which are also affected in ARPKD. In common with many cystogenic proteins, the fibrocystin/polyductin protein is found in basal bodies and primary apical cilia, suggesting that it is important in maintaining the structural integrity of cilia.

Loss of the fibrocystin/polyductin protein downregulates polycystin-2, which is the deficient protein in one form of ADPKD. Fibrocystin/polyductin–polycystin-2 interactions may regulate calcium influx mediated by polycystin-2. These findings suggest that cystogenesis in ADPKD and ARPKD share a common mechanism, with the variability in the ARPKD phenotype traced to the degree of polycystin-2 expression among patients. However, renal cysts can originate from any part of the nephron and are detached from the nephron proper in ADPKD, whereas they originate from and remain attached to the distal nephron in ARPKD, suggesting that additional signaling pathways specific for each disease and gene product likely explain these anatomic differences.

CLINICAL MANIFESTATIONS

Although ARPKD can present as renal cysts discovered radiographically either antenatally or during adulthood, it usually manifests as bilateral abdominal masses and renal insufficiency in infancy. It carries a 30% mortality owing to severe pulmonary hypoplasia; oligohydramnios, presumably linked to in utero renal disease, likely accounts for the pulmonary hypoplasia. Hypertension is almost universal, typically develops before renal impairment is apparent, and probably accelerates the decline in renal function. Findings related to renal tubular dysfunction may be present and include polyuria, enuresis, hyponatremia, and hyperchloremic metabolic acidosis. Cystic complications related to infection and rupture also occur, although hematuria is an infrequent finding. ESRD can take up to 20 years to develop, and in rare instances, it never occurs.

Hepatic fibrosis, secondary to dilation of the intrahepatic and extrahepatic bile ducts, manifests as recurrent ascending cholangitis (Chapter 158) and portal hypertension with splenomegaly and esophageal varices. Pancreatic fibrosis is rarely a clinical concern.

DIAGNOSIS

The demonstration by abdominal ultrasound (Fig. 129-3B) or CT of symmetrically enlarged polycystic kidneys that retain their reniform shape (owing to uniform microcystic dilation of collecting ducts) and hepatic fibrosis is sufficient to diagnose ARPKD. In contrast to ADPKD cysts, ARPKD cysts tend to retain their connections with the originating nephron. Aside from an occasional affected sibling, a family history is often not elicited. Distinguishing ARPKD from ADPKD, especially in patients presenting in childhood or adulthood, may require a liver biopsy to document otherwise undetectable hepatic fibrosis. Gene-based diagnostics in ARPKD are helpful in making a firm diagnosis, especially in patients with late-onset disease, and they are useful in preimplantation and in prenatal diagnosis.

PREVENTION AND TREATMENT

In the absence of specific therapy for ARPKD, management goals focus on early detection and treatment of the complications of hypertension, urinary tract or cyst infection, ESRD, and portal hypertension. Kidney transplantation may be necessary in late childhood in ARPKD patients who present with renal disease perinatally. Treatment of portal hypertension may require liver transplantation or portosystemic shunting (Chapter 157). Treatment of hypertension begins with ACE inhibitors and ARBs (see Tables 67-5 and 67-7 in Chapter 67), which are generally effective. As in all children with ESRD, attention to nutrition and renal osteodystrophy is paramount (Chapter 132). With improving sensitivity of gene-based diagnostics, genetic counseling will play a more active role in prevention.

PROGNOSIS

For patients with ARPKD, the highest mortality rates occur during the first year of life. Approximately 50 to 80% of patients survive to 15 years of age.

NEPHRONOPHTHISIS

DEFINITION AND EPIDEMIOLOGY

The autosomal recessive disorder nephronophthisis is characterized pathologically by renal interstitial fibrosis, tubular atrophy with basement membrane thickening and disruption, and renal cysts and diverticula that are largely restricted to the loops of Henle and distal tubules at the corticomedullary junctions. Nephronophthisis is the most common genetic cause of ESRD in childhood and adolescence, accounting for 5 to 15% of cases. Kidney size is generally normal or reduced, except in the rare infantile form of nephronophthisis that leads to ESRD by 5 years of age.

Patients exhibit extrarenal anomalies, with missense mutations causing a milder phenotype and truncating mutations causing severe disease. The most frequently associated extrarenal abnormalities are retinal degeneration secondary to photoreceptor cell defects (Senior-Loken syndrome), seen in 15% of cases; cerebellar ataxia (Joubert's syndrome and related diseases), observed in 10 to 15% of cases; and hepatic fibrosis (Boichis disease), seen in 5% of cases.

The clinical syndrome of nephronophthisis is caused by recessively acquired homozygotic and compound heterozygotic mutations in nine known genes (*NPHP1* through *NPHP9*), which account for only about 30% of cases, indicating the presence of yet-to-be-discovered genes. Expression of the encoded proteins, called nephrocystins, at extrarenal sites accounts for the associated retinal, neural, liver, and skeletal abnormalities. Each of the nine genes is associated with a somewhat different phenotype, although some share common phenotypes, explained by protein-protein interactions between two or more gene products. Most of the encoded proteins localize to centrosomes or cilia, but some also localize to adherens junctions and/or focal adhesions in epithelia.

CLINICAL MANIFESTATIONS

Presenting symptoms include polyuria, growth failure, and anemia. Polyuria occurs early, owing to reduced urinary concentrating ability and to salt wasting. Decreased growth rate is related to chronic dehydration, and growth failure and anemia occur with the onset of ESRD. Blood pressure is normal and edema is absent before the onset of renal failure. Hematuria and proteinuria are absent or minimal. Patients with mutations in specific nephronophthisis genes may also present with eye defects, oculomotor apraxia, congenital amaurosis, retinitis pigmentosa, neural anomalies, cerebellar ataxia, seizures, liver fibrosis, skeletal defects, scoliosis, cleft palate, and situs inversus.

DIAGNOSIS

Diagnosis relies on clinical suspicion of the disorder in a pediatric or adolescent patient who presents with ESRD and extrarenal manifestations such as abnormal eye movements, blindness, mental retardation, and polydactyly. Abdominal ultrasound, MRI (without gadolinium), electroretinogram, and full neurologic and ophthalmologic evaluations should assess the patient's renal, liver, retinal, and neurologic status. A renal ultrasound showing loss of corticomedullary differentiation, increased parenchymal echogenicity, and occasionally small medullary or corticomedullary cysts in normal-sized or moderately small kidneys is highly suggestive of juvenile nephronophthisis in a child with severe uremia. Genetic testing may be required for a conclusive diagnosis. A renal biopsy showing evidence of chronic tubulointerstitial nephritis may be necessary to confirm the diagnosis if genetic testing is not available.

PREVENTION AND TREATMENT

Rx

Treatment is largely supportive, focusing on the progressive renal failure and the need for dialysis and transplantation. Vasopressin V2 receptor antagonists and rapamycin show promise in animal models, but clinical trials are needed to assess these treatments in patients.

Prenatal genetic testing in families with a genetic diagnosis of nephronophthisis is feasible. DNA-based diagnostics are most useful in identifying the germline mutation prenatally or preimplantation.

MEDULLARY CYSTIC KIDNEY DISEASE

Medullary cystic kidney disease is an autosomal dominant interstitial kidney disease that results in renal failure after the fourth decade of life. It is rarer than autosomal recessive nephronophthisis, with which it shares a number of histologic features, including tubular basement membrane disintegration, tubular cyst formation, and tubulointerstitial inflammation and fibrosis.

At least two genes, *MCKD1* and *MCKD2*, cause medullary cystic kidney disease. *MCKD2* encodes an 85-kD nonciliary protein, uromodulin, which is secreted by the thick ascending limb of the loop of Henle and is the most abundant protein in human urine. The *MCKD1* gene has not yet been identified, but some studies have linked it to chromosome 1q21.

Mutations in *MCKD1* and *MCKD2* result in a similar clinical picture, except for an earlier onset of ESRD and precocious gout with mutations in *MCKD2*. Polyuria and anemia are usually not clinically present in the early stages, and renal failure generally occurs after the fourth decade of life. Hypertension is likely secondary to renal failure.

Corticomedullary cysts, which are present in most adult patients, cannot always be recognized on ultrasonography or CT because they tend to be very small. Except for the treatment of gout (Chapter 281), management is similar to that of patients with nephronophthisis.

MEDULLARY SPONGE KIDNEY

Medullary sponge kidney, which is a rare disorder of unknown pathogenesis, is characterized by congenitally acquired inner medullary and papillary collecting duct dilations, hypercalciuria, and a mild defect in urinary concentration and acidification owing to tubular dysfunction. Patients present with hematuria and recurrent kidney stones, usually by the second or third decade of life. Medullary sponge kidney may also be an incidental finding on an intravenous pyelogram that shows the characteristic pooling of contrast material within the cystic collecting ducts. ESRD is uncommon, and the long-term prognosis is excellent.

OTHER INHERITED CYSTIC SYNDROMES

Bardet-Biedl syndrome is an autosomal recessive disorder characterized by obesity, hypertension, and dystrophy of the hands, eyes, kidneys, and male genitalia. Mutations in 14 different genes encoding proteins that localize to basal bodies have been identified. Calyceal cysts and calyceal clubbing predominate the renal lesion and are best diagnosed by intravenous urography rather than ultrasound. Renal impairment is frequent and is an important cause of death.

Oral-facial-digital syndrome is characterized by malformations of the face, oral cavity, and digits. It is inherited in an X-linked pattern and is caused by defects in the *OFD1* gene, which encodes OFD1 protein expressed in basal bodies but otherwise has an undetermined function. Renal (primarily glomerular) cysts are found in as many as 50% of patients, all of whom are females; males carrying the mutation die in utero. ESRD has been reported in affected females ranging in age from 11 to 72 years.

Autosomal dominant renal cyst formation is also seen in tuberous sclerosis and von Hippel-Lindau syndrome (Chapter 426). In tuberous sclerosis, cyst formation is commonly associated with hypertension; this disorder can resemble ADPKD and is associated with about a 5% incidence of renal cell carcinoma. In von Hippel-Lindau syndrome, cyst formation can also lead to features of ADPKD; more importantly, the syndrome is associated with a 25% incidence of renal cell carcinoma.

ACQUIRED CYSTIC KIDNEY DISEASE

Acquired cystic kidney disease is largely confined to the ESRD population on dialysis (Chapter 133). Cysts arise from proximal and distal tubule dilations in small end-stage kidneys regardless of cause, mode of dialysis, or presence of a functioning kidney transplant. Identifiable risk factors include duration of ESRD, older age, large cysts, male gender, black race, and chronic hypokalemia.

CLINICAL MANIFESTATIONS AND DIAGNOSIS

Acquired cystic kidney disease is usually asymptomatic, but it occasionally leads to enlarged kidneys with associated abdominal discomfort and pain. Cyst hemorrhage, which is more common than cyst infection, presents with flank pain, anemia, or hematuria. The most significant complication of acquired cystic kidney disease is malignant conversion of cysts into renal cell carcinoma (Chapter 203). Carcinomas commonly present as hematuria and are 2 to 200 times more common in patients with acquired cystic kidney disease than in the general dialysis population.

Acquired cystic kidney disease is diagnosed by ultrasound or CT demonstrating multiple and bilateral renal cysts in a patient with preexisting chronic renal failure or ESRD. In contrast to ADPKD and ARPKD, the kidneys are usually not enlarged, and there is no family history of PKD. Renal CT or MRI is preferable to detect cysts in small kidneys and to assess for malignant conversion.

PREVENTION AND TREATMENT Rx

There are no strategies to prevent the appearance or delay the expansion of renal cysts in patients on hemodialysis, but cysts may stabilize or regress following successful renal transplantation. New or frank hematuria raises the concern of renal cell carcinoma (Chapter 203), which should be assessed using ultrasound and contrast-enhanced CT. Any evidence of septa formation, solid material, or contrast enhancement within a cyst is suspicious for renal cell carcinoma and warrants consideration of nephrectomy.

PROGNOSIS

Asymptomatic acquired cystic kidney disease does not affect survival. The incidence of renal cell carcinoma in patients with acquired cystic kidney disease is approximately 0.18% per year. Although metastasis is less common at the time of diagnosis in patients with acquired cystic kidney disease than in other patients with renal cell carcinoma, the 5-year mortality rates are higher, likely related to the almost invariable coexistence of ESRD.

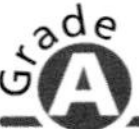

1. Hogan MC, Masyuk TV, Page LJ, et al. Randomized clinical trial of long-acting somatostatin for autosomal dominant polycystic kidney and liver disease. *J Am Soc Nephrol.* 2010;21:1052-1061.
2. Serra AL, Poster D, Kistler AD, et al. Sirolimus and kidney growth in autosomal dominant polycystic kidney disease. *N Engl J Med.* 2010;363:820-829.
3. Walz G, Budde K, Mannaa M, et al. Everolimus in patients with autosomal dominant polycystic kidney disease. *N Engl J Med.* 2010;363:830-840.

SUGGESTED READINGS

Barua M, Pei Y. Diagnosis of autosomal-dominant polycystic kidney disease: an integrated approach. *Semin Nephrol.* 2010;30:356-365. *Review of imaging and molecular-based diagnostic tests.*

Harris PC, Rossetti S. Molecular diagnostics for autosomal dominant polycystic kidney disease. *Nat Rev Nephrol.* 2010;6:197-206. *Review of molecular testing methods to detect mutations in ADPKD.*

Hildebrandt F. Genetic kidney diseases. *Lancet.* 2010;375:1287-1295. *Review.*

Kyongtae T, Bae KT, Grantham JJ. Imaging for the prognosis of autosomal dominant polycystic kidney disease. *Nat Rev Nephrol.* 2010;6:96-106. *Supports imaging as an invaluable tool to monitor the onset and progression of ADPKD.*

Pei Y. Practical genetics for autosomal dominant polycystic kidney disease. *Nephron Clin Pract.* 2011;118:19-30. *Review of clinical predictors of gene types, imaging, and molecular-based diagnostic tests.*

130 HEREDITARY NEPHROPATHIES AND DEVELOPMENTAL ABNORMALITIES OF THE URINARY TRACT

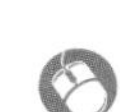

LISA M. GUAY-WOODFORD

HEREDITARY NEPHROPATHIES

The proximal tubule is responsible for reclaiming most of the filtered glucose, amino acids, uric acid, phosphate, bicarbonate, and low-molecular-weight proteins. The loop of Henle and the distal nephron reabsorb approximately 30% of the filtered sodium chloride and 50% of the filtered divalent cations. The collecting duct, under the regulatory control of aldosterone, fine-tunes sodium reabsorption and secretes hydrogen and potassium ions. In the terminal collecting duct, antidiuretic hormone regulates water reabsorption and urinary concentration.

Inherited renal tubular disorders are a group of conditions in which the normal renal tubular reabsorption of ions, organic solutes, and water (Chapter 118) is disrupted. These defects can be categorized by the nephron segment affected (Table 130-1).

Disorders of Proximal Tubule Function

CYSTINURIA

Cystinuria is characterized by defective proximal tubular reabsorption of cystine and dibasic amino acids, resulting in the formation of urinary calculi (Chapter 128). This autosomal recessive trait has an estimated prevalence of 1 in 7000 individuals. Two cystinuria genes have been identified: *SLC7A9*, which encodes the luminal transport channel itself, and *SLC3A1*, which encodes the transporter regulatory subunit. Several large studies indicate that mutations in *SLC3A1* are more common than mutations in *SLC7A9*. Mutations in *SLC3A1* cause cystinuria type A, mutations in *SLC7A9* cause cystinuria type B, and mutations in both genes (compound heterozygotes) cause cystinuria type AB.

Although the severity of the disease is similar in all types of cystinurias, the clinical presentation can be quite variable, and the onset of disease may occur from infancy to the seventh decade of life. Affected children can be identified by elevated urinary cystine levels, but testing must be performed after tubular transport has fully matured (at age 2 years). Cystine stones are radiopaque and often form the nidus for secondary calcium oxalate stones. Symptoms include renal colic, which may be associated with urinary tract obstruction and/or infection. Conservative therapy with high urine volume and urinary alkalinization is sufficient for many patients with cystinuria, but recurrent stone formation may cause renal damage and warrants treatment with thiol agents (e.g., D-penicillamine: pediatric dose, 15 to 20 mg/kg/day; adult dose, 2 g/day in four divided doses) or α-mercaptopropionylglycine

TABLE 130-1 HEREDITARY NEPHROPATHIES BY NEPHRON SEGMENT

DISORDER	INHERITANCE	OMIM*	MAJOR RENAL FEATURES
PROXIMAL TUBULE			
Renal glucosuria	AR	233100	Isolated glucosuria
Proximal renal tubular acidosis	AR	604278	Hyperchloremic, hypokalemic metabolic acidosis
Carbonic anhydrase II deficiency	AR	259730	Mixed proximal and distal renal tubular acidosis
Hartnup disease	AR	234500	Neutral aminoaciduria
Cystinuria	AR	Type A: 220100 Type B: 604144	Urinary calculi
Cystinosis	AR	Infantile: 219800 Late-onset: 219900 Non-nephropathic: 219750	Renal Fanconi's syndrome
Dent disease	X-linked	Dent disease 1: 300009 Dent disease 2: 300555	Nephrocalcinosis, urinary calculi, low-molecular-weight proteinuria
Lowe syndrome	X-linked	309000	Renal Fanconi's syndrome
Hereditary fructose intolerance	AR	229600	Renal Fanconi's syndrome
Tyrosinemia type I	AR	276700	Renal Fanconi's syndrome
Wilson disease	AR	277900	Renal Fanconi's syndrome
LOOP OF HENLE			
Bartter's syndrome	AR AD	Type I: 601678 Type II: 241200 Type III: 607364 Type IV: 602522 Type V: 601199	Hypokalemic, hypochloremic metabolic alkalosis
DISTAL TUBULE			
Gitelman's syndrome	AR	263800	Hypokalemic, hypochloremic metabolic alkalosis
Familial hypomagnesemia with hypercalciuria	AR	248250, 248190	Severe renal magnesium and calcium wasting
Isolated hypomagnesemia	AD	154020	Renal magnesium wasting
COLLECTING DUCT			
Liddle's syndrome	AD	177200	Low-renin hypertension
Glucocorticoid-remediable hyperaldosteronism	AD	103900	Low-renin hypertension
Apparent mineralocorticoid excess	AR	218030	Low-renin hypertension
Pseudohypoaldosteronism type I	AR, AD	AR: 264350 AD: 177735	Hyponatremic, hypokalemic metabolic acidosis
Pseudohypoaldosteronism type II (Gordon's syndrome)	AD	114300	Low-renin hypertension with hyperkalemia
Distal renal tubular acidosis	AR, AD	AR: 602722, 605239 AD: 179800, 611590	Hyperchloremic, hypokalemic metabolic acidosis
Carbonic anhydrase II deficiency	AR	259730	Mixed proximal and distal renal tubular acidosis
Nephrogenic diabetes insipidus	X-linked, AR, AD	X-linked: 304800 AR and AD: 125800	Urinary concentrating defect

*Entries in Online Mendelian Inheritance in Man (OMIM), available at www.ncbi.nlm.nih.gov/omim. Accessed Dec. 15, 2009.
AD = autosomal dominant; AR = autosomal recessive.

(pediatric dose, 10 to15 mg/kg/day; adult dose, 1 to 2 g/day in two divided doses) to form soluble mixed disulfides with cystine and maintain free urine cystine levels below 200 mg/g of creatinine.

CYSTINOSIS

Cystinosis is the most common inherited cause of renal Fanconi's syndrome; it also affects the eyes, muscles, central nervous system, lungs, and various endocrine organs. Cystinosis is an autosomal recessive disorder caused by mutations in the gene *CTNS,* which encodes cystinosin, a lysosomal cystine transporter. Defects in this transporter lead to the accumulation of intralysosomal cystine crystals and widespread cellular destruction.

Three clinical presentations have been described. The most severe is infantile (classic) cystinosis, which manifests in the first year of life with renal tubular acidosis, impaired growth, and evidence of renal Fanconi's syndrome, including aminoaciduria, glucosuria, phosphaturia, and low-molecular-weight proteinuria. Progressive renal failure reaches end-stage renal disease in childhood. A less severe, late-onset (juvenile or intermediate) form causes renal dysfunction in adolescence and involves cystine deposits in the cornea. The mildest form, an ocular, non-nephropathic form, features photophobia but no renal problems.

The mainstay of cystinosis therapy is oral cysteamine (adult dose, 500 mg four times daily), an aminothiol that can lower intracellular cystine content by 90%. In well-treated adolescent and young adult patients, cysteamine delays renal glomerular deterioration, enhances growth, prevents hypothyroidism, and lowers muscle cystine content. Therefore, early diagnosis and prompt, proper treatment are critical for preventing or significantly delaying the complications of cystinosis.

Disorders of Loop of Henle and Distal Tubule Function

THE BARTTER-GITELMAN DISORDERS

The Bartter-Gitelman syndromes are a group of disorders characterized by markedly reduced salt transport in the thick ascending limb of Henle (Bartter's syndrome) or in the distal convoluted tubule (Gitelman's syndrome).

Most patients with Gitelman's syndrome have defects in *SLC12A3,* the gene encoding the sodium-chloride cotransporter NCCT. However, a minority of patients with the Gitelman phenotype have mutations in *CLCNKB.*

Bartter's syndrome can be caused by mutations in one of four genes—*SLC12A2,* encoding the sodium-potassium-chloride cotransporter NKCC2;

TABLE 130-2 FEATURES OF THE INHERITED RENAL TUBULAR ACIDOSES (RTAs)

DISORDER	RENAL TRANSPORT DEFECT	MINIMAL URINE pH DURING ACIDOSIS	ALKALI SUPPLEMENTATION (HCO_3^-)	UAG DURING ACIDOSIS*
Proximal RTA	↓Proximal bicarbonate reabsorption	<5.5	Children: 10-15 mEq/kg/day	0 or +
Carbonic anhydrase II deficiency	↓Proximal bicarbonate reabsorption and ↓distal acidification	Variable	Variable	0 or +
Distal RTA	↓Distal acidification	>5.5	Adults: 1-3 mEq/kg/day Children: 3-6 mEq/kg/day	0 or +

*In RTA, the UAG is usually 0 or positive, whereas in metabolic acidosis associated with diarrheal illness, the UAG is negative.
HCO_3^- = bicarbonate; UAG = urinary anion gap ($[Na^+] + [K^+] - [Cl^-]$).

KCNJ1, encoding the ROMK1 potassium ion channel; *CLCNKB,* encoding the ClC-Kb basolateral chloride ion channel; and *BSND,* encoding barttin, a regulatory subunit required for basolateral chloride channel targeting to the membrane. These mutations cause autosomal recessive Bartter's syndrome types I, II, III, and IV, respectively. Defects in any of these genes disrupt salt transport in the thick ascending limb, causing a furosemide-like effect (E-Fig. 130-1). In addition, severe gain-in-function mutations in *CASR,* the gene encoding the extracellular calcium ion–sensing receptor CaSR, can cause a Bartter-like phenotype (referred to as Bartter's type V) that is distinguished from the others by autosomal dominant transmission and associated hypocalcemic hypercalciuria.

Individuals with Bartter's syndrome exhibit renal salt wasting, lowered blood pressure, polyuria, hypokalemic metabolic alkalosis, and hypercalciuria with a variable risk of nephrocalcinosis. In comparison, individuals with Gitelman's syndrome exhibit milder renal salt wasting, normal blood pressure, hypokalemic metabolic alkalosis, hypomagnesemia, and hypocalciuria. This clinical disorder resembles the effects of long-term thiazide administration. Clinical differences between Bartter's and Gitelman's syndromes relate to the severity of salt wasting, whereas phenotypic differences among Bartter's types I through V correlate with the specific physiologic roles played by the individual transporters or channels in the kidney and other organs.

The mainstay of treatment includes replacing salt and water losses and providing potassium supplementation to maintain serum levels greater than 3 mEq/dL. In patients with perinatal (type I or II) Bartter's syndrome, cyclooxygenase inhibitors (e.g., indomethacin 2-4 mg/kg/day in two to four divided doses) may be beneficial. In patients with Gitelman's syndrome and some patients with Bartter's syndrome type III, oral magnesium supplementation may be required to maintain serum levels above 1.2 mg/dL.

Disorders of Collecting Duct Function

LIDDLE'S SYNDROME (PSEUDOALDOSTERONISM)

Liddle's syndrome, which is an autosomal dominant form of salt-sensitive hypertension (Chapter 67), is caused by mutations in the α, β, or γ subunits of the epithelial sodium channel, which is expressed at the apical surface of collecting duct cells and plays a critical role in maintaining salt balance and blood pressure. Both the β and the γ subunits regulate the channel activity of the α subunit. Mutations in either of these regulatory subunits result in increased epithelial sodium channel activity and Liddle's syndrome.

Severe hypertension typically manifests in childhood, with features of hypokalemic metabolic alkalosis that resemble primary aldosteronism. However, renin and aldosterone secretion is suppressed in this disorder. The clinical abnormalities can be ameliorated by a low-salt diet plus a potassium-sparing diuretic (e.g., amiloride 5 to 10 mg/day), which acts as an antagonist of the epithelial sodium channel.

DISTAL RENAL TUBULAR ACIDOSIS

Distal renal tubular acidosis (dRTA) results from failure of the collecting duct α-intercalated cells to excrete fixed acids (see Fig. 120-1 in Chapter 120). Both autosomal dominant and autosomal recessive forms of dRTA have been described. These heritable disorders include mutations in genes encoding carbonic anhydrase II, the chloride-bicarbonate exchanger AE1, and subunits of the hydrogen–adenosine triphosphatase (H^+-ATPase) proton pump. Mutations in the *SLC4A1* gene encoding AE1 cause autosomal dominant dRTA and are rarely associated with recessive forms of the disease. Mutations in subunits of H^+-ATPase are the primary causes of autosomal recessive dRTA. Vacuolar H^+-ATPases (V-type ATPases) are ubiquitous, multi-subunit protein complexes that mediate the ATP-dependent transport of protons. In the kidney, V-type ATPases are the major proton-secreting pumps in the distal nephron and are involved in net proton secretion (bicarbonate generation) or proton reabsorption (net bicarbonate secretion). Defects in two genes, *ATP6B1* and *ATP6N1B,* cause dRTA with or without associated sensorineural deafness.

Clinical consequences include hypokalemic, hyperchloremic metabolic acidosis; impaired growth; hypercalciuria; hypocitraturia; nephrocalcinosis; nephrolithiasis; rickets in children; and osteomalacia in adults. Classic dRTA can be distinguished from other metabolic acidoses by an inappropriately high urine pH (>5.5), diminished net acid excretion, positive urinary anion gap, and low urinary ammonium concentration (Table 130-2). Treatment with alkali supplementation (1 to 3 mEq/kg/day in adults and 3 to 6 mEq/kg/day in children) is usually effective in correcting the acidosis. In contrast to proximal RTA, urinary potassium wasting can be ameliorated with alkali therapy alone.

DEVELOPMENT OF THE KIDNEY AND URINARY TRACT

The human kidney and urogenital tract develop from three principal embryonic structures: the metanephric mesenchyme, the mesonephric (wolffian) duct, and the cloaca (Fig. 130-1). At 4 to 5 weeks of gestation, the ureteric bud originates as a diverticulum of the mesonephric duct. Reciprocal interactions between the branching ureteric bud and the metanephric mesenchyme induce kidney development, with the metanephros undergoing an epithelial transformation to form the glomeruli and the proximal and distal tubules. The ureteric bud branches give rise to the collecting ducts, the renal pelvis, the ureter, and the bladder trigone. Nephrogenesis is completed by 34 weeks of gestation.

Concurrent with the initial nephrogenic events, the urorectal fold divides the cloaca into the urogenital sinus and the future rectum. The mesonephric duct opening into the bladder becomes the vesicoureteric orifice of the trigone. Between 5 and 6 weeks of gestation, the second genital duct (müllerian duct) appears and runs in parallel with the wolffian duct. In males, the müllerian duct subsequently regresses, the wolffian duct proceeds to form the epididymis, the vas deferens, the seminal vesicle, and the ejaculatory duct. In females, the wolffian duct regresses, and the müllerian ducts fuse to form the ureterovaginal primordium, which merges with the urogenital sinus and eventually gives rise to the uterus, the oviducts, and the proximal vagina. The remnants of the allantois form the urachus, a fibrous cord that connects the bladder to the umbilicus.

Congenital abnormalities of the kidney and urinary tract occur in 1 in 500 newborns and account for approximately 20 to 30% of all anomalies identified in the prenatal period. Some urinary tract anomalies are asymptomatic and inconsequential, but many renal tract malformations are important causes of infant mortality as well as morbidity in older children and adults, including the progression to renal failure.

ABNORMALITIES OF THE URINARY TRACT

Renal Parenchymal Malformations

Congenital defects in renal development may result in the absence of a kidney (agenesis) or abnormalities in kidney size, structure, or position. Irregularities in the renal contour may arise from the persistence of fetal lobulation or

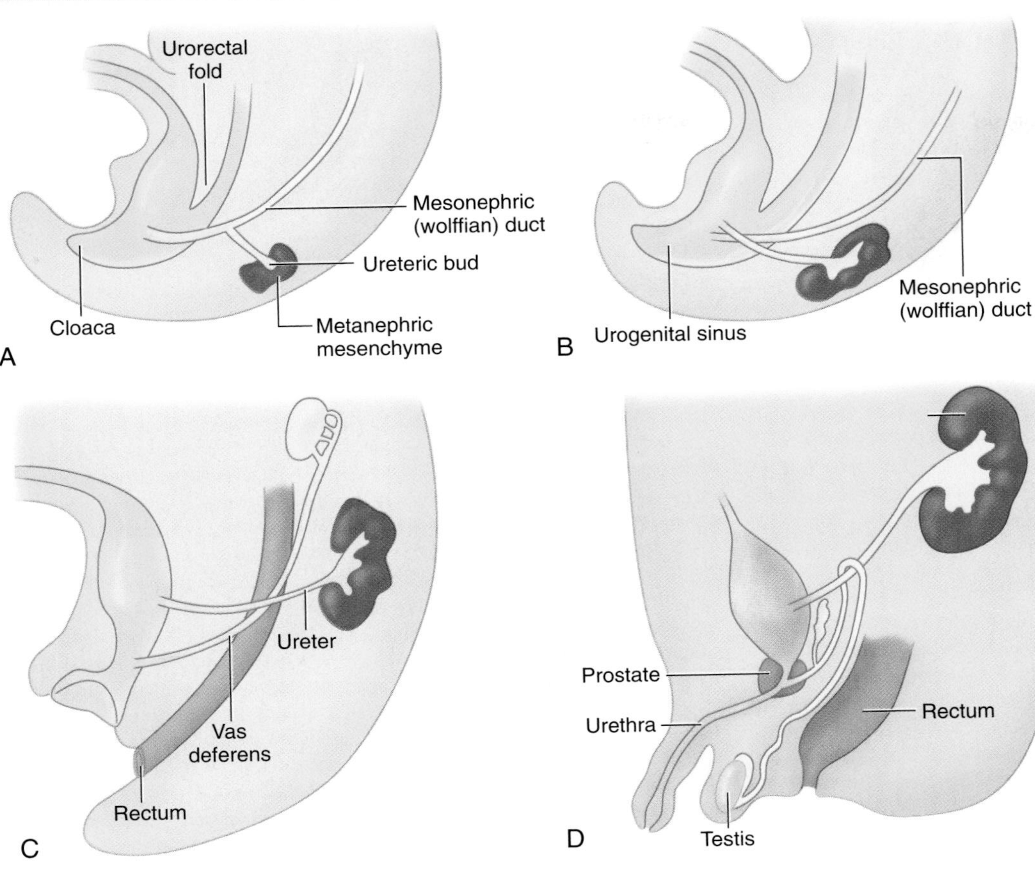

FIGURE 130-1. Key events in the development of the urinary tract. In the 4-week embryo, the ureteric bud emerges from the wolffian duct (**A**). Reciprocal interactions between the branching ureteric bud and the metanephric mesenchyme induce kidney development. Concurrently, the cloaca is divided by the urorectal fold into the urogenital sinus and the future rectum (**B**). In the 8-week male embryo, the wolffian duct begins to give rise to the epididymis, the seminal vesicles, and the caudal part of the vas deferens (**C**). By 9 weeks, axial growth of the fetal spine prompts the developing kidney to ascend from the pelvis to its final lumbar position. The external genitalia develop between 8 and 16 weeks, and testicular descent begins in month 7 of gestation (**D**).

a depression in the midpole of the left kidney caused by the spleen (a "dromedary hump"). Neither irregularity impairs renal function.

RENAL AGENESIS

Renal agenesis reflects a complete failure of nephrogenesis. Unilateral agenesis can occur as an isolated abnormality or as a component of syndromic disorders, such as Turner's syndrome (Chapter 241). As an isolated entity, the complete absence of one kidney occurs in 1 in 5000 individuals. The incidence is higher in males and occurs somewhat more frequently on the left side; in about half the patients, the ipsilateral ureter and hemitrigone are also absent. The remaining kidney is usually enlarged owing to compensatory hypertrophy, but it may be ectopic or malrotated. Vesicoureteral reflux is observed on the contralateral side in about 30% of patients.

Renal agenesis is commonly associated with genital anomalies, suggesting that it represents a developmental field defect. In females, absence of the ipsilateral oviduct and malformation of the uterus and vagina result from maldevelopment of the müllerian duct, whereas in males, wolffian duct–derived structures, such as the vas deferens and the seminal vesicles, are often absent. Other associated anomalies can include cardiovascular malformations, vertebral defects, and imperforate anus.

Bilateral renal agenesis has an estimated incidence of 1 in 10,000 births and is associated with the Potter phenotype, which includes pulmonary hypoplasia, a characteristic facies, and deformities of the spine and limbs. At birth, these neonates have a critical degree of pulmonary hypoplasia that is incompatible with survival. The familial association of unilateral and bilateral renal agenesis, renal dysplasia, and congenital hydronephrosis occurs in hereditary renal adysplasia syndrome (Online Mendelian Inheritance in Man entry 191830), a rare autosomal dominant disorder with variable penetrance.

RENAL HYPOPLASIA

The term *renal hypoplasia* describes small kidneys with normally differentiated nephrons that are reduced in number. *Oligomeganephronia* describes a form of bilateral renal hypoplasia with a marked reduction in nephron number and associated hypertrophy of individual glomeruli and tubules. This abnormality occurs sporadically as an isolated developmental defect that must be differentiated from acquired renal atrophy and the nephronophthisis–medullary cystic disease complex. Renal function declines slowly, with progression to end-stage renal failure in the second to third decade of life.

RENAL DYSPLASIA

Renal dysplasia, which can be associated with various abnormalities of kidney size, results from abnormal metanephric differentiation that causes anomalous and/or incompletely differentiated renal elements. Small dysplastic kidneys are commonly referred to as *aplastic*. Large dysplastic kidneys are often cystic; the most extreme type is referred to as *multicystic dysplastic kidney*.

Unilateral dysplasia may be asymptomatic well into adult life. Small aplastic and large multicystic dysplastic kidneys are nonfunctioning and can be distinguished from renal agenesis by imaging studies. The ipsilateral ureter is typically atretic. Contralateral malformations, including obstruction and vesicoureteral reflux, are common. Unilateral multicystic kidneys involute over time and often disappear. Unilateral aplasia and multicystic dysplasia may be manifestations of the hereditary renal adysplasia syndrome. Bilateral multicystic dysplastic kidneys are incompatible with neonatal survival.

Renal and Ureteral Structural Abnormalities

RENAL MALROTATION AND ECTOPIA

Metanephric kidney development begins caudally. By 9 weeks of gestation, the kidney has ascended to its normal level (L1-L3), and the renal pelvis has rotated 90 degrees toward the midline. Anomalies of ascent and/or failure of rotation are common. Bilateral renal ectopia is often associated with kidney fusion. The most common fusion anomaly is the horseshoe kidney, which occurs in 1 in 500 newborns with a 2 : 1 male predominance. Renal ascent is prevented by the root of the inferior mesenteric artery (Fig. 130-2A). Crossed renal ectopia can occur with or without fusion. Supernumerary (extra) kidneys are typically ectopic and vary in location. Although almost one third of patients with renal ectopia remain asymptomatic, the associated malrotation of the renal pelvis increases the risk of hydronephrosis, infection, and stone formation.

PELVIURETERAL ABNORMALITIES

Obstruction of the ureteropelvic junction impedes the flow of urine from the renal pelvis into the ureter. It is one of the most frequently occurring urinary

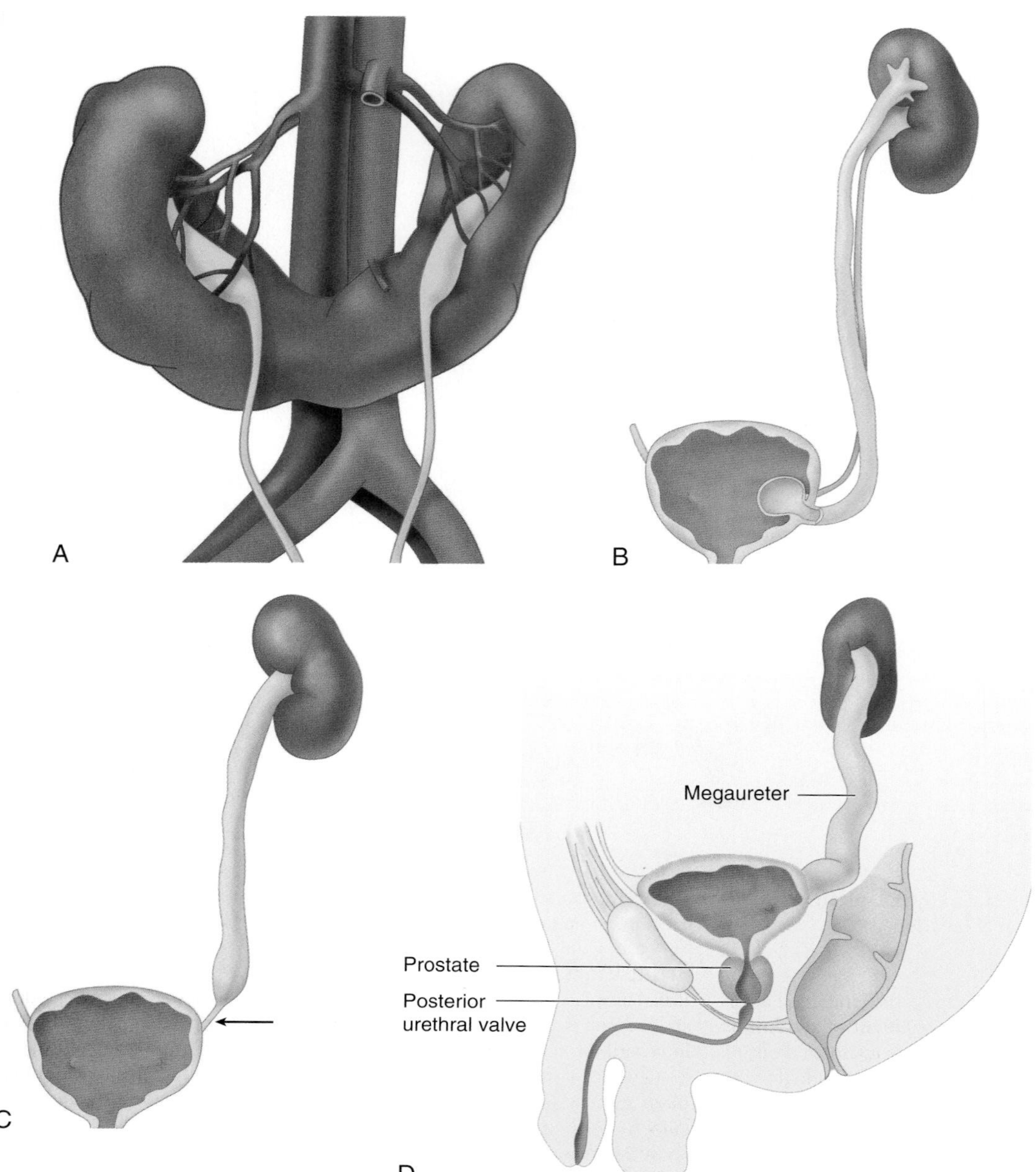

FIGURE 130-2. **Developmental abnormalities of the urinary tract. A,** Horseshoe kidney. **B,** Ectopic ureter associated with a ureterocele. **C,** Megaureter with the aperistaltic segment (arrow). **D,** Bladder outlet obstruction caused by posterior urethral valves.

tract anomalies in children and is the most common cause of collecting system dilation in the fetal kidney. In congenital obstruction of the ureteropelvic junction, urologic anomalies in the contralateral system are common, including renal agenesis, renal dysplasia, multicystic dysplasia, ureteropelvic junction obstruction, and vesicoureteral reflux. Ureteropelvic junction obstruction may occur in adults secondary to external compression, kinking, or stenosis of the proximal ureter. Surgical intervention is indicated if there is associated renal function impairment, pyelonephritis, stones, or pain.

Hydrocalyx or *hydrocalycosis* refers to dilation of a major calyx that occurs in the context of intrinsic obstruction, as in infundibular stenosis, or in the context of extrinsic compression of the pelvis, as caused by a vessel or a parapelvic cyst. In comparison, *megacalycosis* represents a nonobstructive, dysplastic lesion seen primarily in males, in which the calyces are dilated and usually increased in number. Associated renal medullary hypoplasia causes malformation of the renal papillae.

Calyceal diverticula are cystic structures connected by a narrow channel to an adjacent minor calyx. In imaging studies, these diverticula typically fill with contrast material, which distinguishes them from renal parenchymal cysts.

Partial duplication of the renal pelvis and ureter is a common anomaly that occurs more frequently in females, is typically unilateral, and is clinically insignificant.

URETERIC ANOMALIES

Ectopic ureters usually reflect complete ureteric and renal duplication. Approximately 10% are bilateral. The ectopic ureter typically drains the dysplastic upper pole of a duplex kidney and inserts below the normal vesicoureteral junction into the lower trigone or the proximal urethra. Ectopic ureters occur much more frequently in females, and the insertion sites can include the vagina and the vulva, with resulting incontinence. An ectopic ureter is often associated with a ureterocele, a cystic dilation of the terminal ureter (Fig. 130-2B). In children, ureteroceles can be associated with urinary tract infection and obstruction of the bladder neck or even of the contralateral ureter. In adults, the clinical presentation usually involves an associated infection, ureteric stones, or both.

A megaureter, or grossly dilated ureter, has multiple potential causes, including intrinsic ureteric obstruction by a stone, bladder outflow obstruction, vesicoureteral reflux, and external compression of the distal ureter. In contrast, primary megaureter results from a functional obstruction of the distal ureter caused by an aperistaltic segment (Fig. 130-2C).

VESICOURETERAL REFLUX

In the normal urinary tract, urinary reflux from the bladder into the ureters is prevented by a functional valve-like mechanism at the vesicoureteral junction. The competence of this valve is dependent on several critical factors, such as the intramural length of the ureter, the position of the ureteric orifice in the bladder, and the integrity of the bladder wall musculature. Primary vesicoureteral reflux, with an estimated incidence of 1 to 2% in children, results from incompetence of the vesicoureteral junction owing to the shortened length of the ureter's submucosal segment and the lateral, ectopic position of its orifice. Genetic factors appear to contribute to the pathogenesis of primary vesicoureteral reflux, as there is a 30- to 50-fold increased risk in immediate relatives of an index case. As the intramural ureter lengthens with age, primary vesicoureteral reflux tends to remit or disappear. Vesicoureteral reflux can also occur secondary to obstructive maldevelopment of the lower urinary tract, such as in triad syndrome and posterior urethral valves.

In both primary and secondary vesicoureteral reflux, intrarenal reflux can lead to the development of reflux nephropathy, a tubulointerstitial lesion associated with gross scarring at the renal poles. In addition, the development of a glomerular lesion consistent with focal and segmental glomerulosclerosis can cause proteinuria, hypertension, and progressive loss of renal function.

In children younger than 18 years with prior urinary tract infections, daily treatment with trimethoprim (2 mg/kg/day) plus sulfamethoxazole (10 mg/kg/day) reduces recurrent infections by about 40%,[1] but the value of long-term suppression is less clear.[2] Although surgical correction is the current standard of care for severe grades of vesicoureteral reflux, particularly secondary forms associated with maldevelopment of the lower urinary tract, the long-term benefit of either endoscopic or surgical intervention appears to be small and is unlikely to prevent renal damage.[3]

Lower Urinary Tract Abnormalities

TRIAD SYNDROME (PRUNE-BELLY SYNDROME, EAGLE-BARRETT SYNDROME)

Triad syndrome, also referred to as prune-belly syndrome or Eagle-Barrett syndrome, involves a constellation of anomalies including congenital absence or deficiency of the abdominal wall musculature, gross ureteral dilation, bladder wall thickening, prostatic hypoplasia, and bilateral undescended testes (cryptorchidism). The full syndrome is expressed only in males, and surviving individuals are typically infertile. Patients with an incomplete syndrome can have anomalies of the abdominal wall musculature, bladder, and upper urinary tract; 3% of these patients are females. Although the specific molecular events have yet to be defined, defects in mesenchymal development appear to cause poor prostate and bladder differentiation, ureteral smooth muscle aplasia with consequent ureteral aperistalsis, and varying degrees of renal dysplasia. Three fourths of patients with triad syndrome have associated malformations in the cardiopulmonary system, gastrointestinal tract, and skeleton. In the immediate postnatal period, prognosis depends on the severity of extragenitourinary anomalies. Long-term outcome is based on the degree of renal dysplasia and the success of urodynamic management.

BLADDER ABNORMALITIES

Bladder exstrophy results from a midline closure defect involving the lower anterior abdominal wall, the bladder, and the external genitalia. These abnormalities have been attributed to a primary defect in the differentiation of the cloacal membrane, but the precise molecular events are unclear. In severe cases, bladder exstrophy may be associated with imperforate anus and rectal atresia. However, other congenital anomalies are rarely associated. Clinical studies indicate that there is a correlation between the success of bladder reconstruction and long-term preservation of renal function.

In adults, neuropathic or neurogenic bladder (Chapter 25) has numerous etiologic contributors, including central nervous system trauma, stroke, disorders such as Parkinson's disease, spinal trauma, multiple sclerosis, and peripheral nerve damage caused by trauma or surgery. In children, myelomeningocele (spina bifida) is the most common cause of neurogenic bladder dysfunction. Other forms of myelodysplasia, such as spinal dysraphism (spina bifida occulta) and sacral agenesis, are less common causes.

POSTERIOR URETHRAL VALVES

In male infants, posterior urethral valves are the most common cause of bladder outflow obstruction, with resulting bilateral hydronephrosis and megaureters. However, among all infants with hydronephrosis, only 10% have posterior urethral valves. The urethral obstruction results from defective reabsorption of mucosal folds in the posterior urethra, just distal to the verumontanum. As a result, dilation of the proximal urethra, bladder wall hypertrophy and trabeculation, associated vesicoureteral reflux, and varying degrees of renal dysplasia are present (Fig. 130-2D). Surgical management strategies are dictated by the age of the child and the degree of associated renal insufficiency. Survival and long-term renal outcome depend on the severity of the associated renal dysplasia.

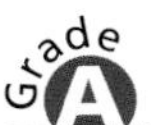

1. Craig JC, Simpson JM, Williams GJ, et al. Antibiotic prophylaxis and recurrent urinary tract infection in children. *N Engl J Med*. 2009;361:1748-1759.
2. Garin EH, Olavarria F, Garcia Nieto V, et al. Clinical significance of primary vesicoureteral reflux and urinary antibiotic prophylaxis after acute pyelonephritis: a multicenter, randomized, controlled study. *Pediatrics*. 2006;117:626-632.
3. Hodson EM, Wheeler DM, Vimalchandra D, et al. Interventions for primary vesicoureteric reflux. *Cochrane Database Syst Rev*. 2007.3.CD001532.

SUGGESTED READINGS

Hildebrandt F. Genetic kidney disease. *Lancet*. 2010;375:1287-1295. *Review*.

Jeck N, Seyberth HW. Loop disorders: insights derived from defined genotypes. *Nephron Physiol*. 2011;118:7-14. *Review*.

Tiselius HG. New horizons in the management of patients with cystinuria. *Curr Opin Urol*. 2010;20:169-173. *Review*.

131

BENIGN PROSTATIC HYPERPLASIA AND PROSTATITIS

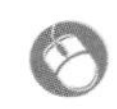

MICHAEL J. BARRY AND MARY MCNAUGHTON COLLINS

The prostate gland, the largest accessory gland in the male reproductive system, surrounds the prostatic urethra below the bladder. Superiorly, its base is contiguous with the bladder neck; inferiorly, its apex adjoins the urogenital diaphragm. The prostatic urethra is angulated at the verumontanum, the union with the two ejaculatory ducts. In younger men, the prostate weighs about 20 g. As men age, the prostate enlarges and develops a characteristic zonal anatomy (Fig. 131-1). Its acini, which communicate with the urethra via prostatic ducts, supply about 20% of semen volume. Prostatic fluid is rich in citrate, zinc, and polyamines, although their roles in reproduction are poorly defined.

BENIGN PROSTATIC HYPERPLASIA

DEFINITION

Benign prostatic hyperplasia (BPH) is defined histologically by hyperplasia of both epithelial and stromal cells, beginning in the periurethral area. With aging, multiple small hyperplastic nodules grow, coalesce, and compress normal tissue outward against the true prostatic capsule, creating a surgical capsule that bounds the expanding adenoma.

EPIDEMIOLOGY

The hyperplastic process often begins in the third decade of life; by age 80 years, 85% of men have BPH. The age-specific prevalence of BPH at autopsy is remarkably similar among men of different ethnicities. Aging and functioning testes are the dominant risk factors. The onset of clinical manifestations of BPH before age 65 in a first-degree relative is also a risk factor. The prevalence of clinical manifestations is uncertain because of a lack of consensus on a working definition. Nevertheless, in the United States, about one third of men aged 40 to 79 years have moderate to severe lower urinary tract symptoms, a majority of which are attributable to BPH.

PATHOBIOLOGY

Testosterone is converted by the 5α-reductase enzyme into dihydrotestosterone, the major intraprostatic androgen. BPH does not develop in men who are castrated before puberty or who have 5α-reductase deficiency. Although the type 2 isoenzyme predominates in the prostate, the type 1 isoenzyme predominates elsewhere. An array of peptide growth factors, along with dihydrotestosterone, mediates stromal-epithelial interactions that alter the balance of cell proliferation and apoptosis and thereby lead to BPH. The mechanisms are poorly understood.

The genetics of BPH are also unclear. An autosomal dominant hereditary form may account for less than 10% of cases.

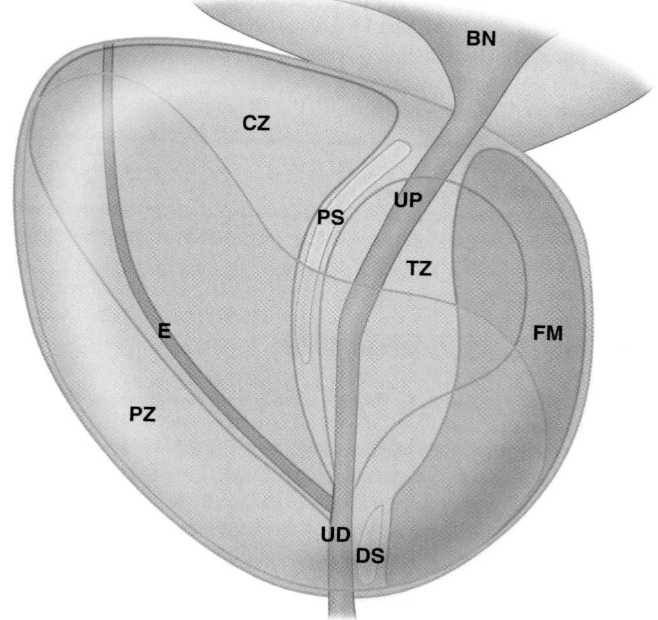

FIGURE 131-1. Anatomy of the prostate. Sagittal diagram of the distal prostatic urethral segment (UD), proximal urethral segment (UP), and ejaculatory ducts (E), showing their relationships to a sagittal section of the anteromedial nonglandular tissues: the bladder neck (BN), anterior fibromuscular stroma (FM), preprostatic sphincter (PS), and distal striated sphincter (DS). These structures are shown in relation to a three-dimensional representation of the glandular prostate: central zone (CZ), peripheral zone (PZ), and transitional zone (TZ). (From McNeal J. Normal histology of the prostate. *Am J Surg Pathol.* 1988;12:619-633.)

CLINICAL MANIFESTATIONS

The morbidity of BPH is conferred through bothersome lower urinary tract symptoms. Traditionally, voiding symptoms such as hesitancy, straining, a sense of incomplete emptying, intermittency, a weak stream, and postvoid dribbling were considered a consequence of mechanical bladder outlet obstruction. Filling symptoms, such as frequency, nocturia, urgency, and urge incontinence (Chapter 25), were thought to be caused by secondary uninhibited detrusor contractions. However, poor correlations among the severity of symptoms, prostatic size, degree of obstruction, and detrusor instability suggest that the pathophysiology is more complex. The key lower urinary tract symptoms of BPH can be quantified by asking the seven symptom questions in the International Prostate Symptom Score (IPSS) (Fig. 131-2).

Bladder outlet obstruction owing to BPH has both static and dynamic components. The static component is due to the enlarged prostate, whereas the dynamic component is due to increased adrenergic tone in the prostate, where α_2-adrenoreceptors predominate.

In the setting of obstruction, increased detrusor pressure can result in detrusor hypertrophy and, eventually, fibrosis. Complications of BPH include acute urinary retention, which may result from prostatic infarction. Postvoid residual urine probably increases the risk of urinary tract infection or stone formation. With long-standing obstruction, hydroureter and hydronephrosis may develop, and renal failure may eventually ensue. Men with BPH may have hematuria because of the complex of veins stretched over the enlarged prostate; however, other causes, especially malignancy (Chapter 203), need to be considered.

DIAGNOSIS

History

Symptoms are commonly attributed to BPH when an older man presents with lower urinary tract symptoms. IPSSs of 0 to 7 represent mild symptoms;

	Not at all	Less than 1 time in 5	Less than half the time	About half the time	More than half the time	Almost always
1. Over the past month or so, how often have you had a sensation of not emptying your bladder completely after you finished urinating?	0 ☐	1 ☐	2 ☐	3 ☐	4 ☐	5 ☐
2. Over the past month or so, how often have you had to urinate again less than two hours after you finished urinating?	0 ☐	1 ☐	2 ☐	3 ☐	4 ☐	5 ☐
3. Over the past month or so, how often have you found you stopped and started again several times when you urinated?	0 ☐	1 ☐	2 ☐	3 ☐	4 ☐	5 ☐
4. Over the past month or so, how often have you found it difficult to postpone urination?	0 ☐	1 ☐	2 ☐	3 ☐	4 ☐	5 ☐
5. Over the past month or so, how often have you had a weak urinary stream?	0 ☐	1 ☐	2 ☐	3 ☐	4 ☐	5 ☐
6. Over the past month or so, how often have you had to push or strain to begin urination?	0 ☐	1 ☐	2 ☐	3 ☐	4 ☐	5 ☐

7. Over the past month, how many times did you most typically get up to urinate from the time you went to bed at night until the time you got up in the morning?

0 ☐ none	1 ☐ 1 time	2 ☐ 2 times	3 ☐ 3 times	4 ☐ 4 times	5 ☐ 5 or more times

Total IPSS Score = sum of questions 1–7 = ________

Quality of life due to urinary symptoms

If you were to spend the rest of your life with your urinary condition just the way it is now, how would you feel about that?

Delighted	Pleased	Mostly satisfied	Mixed—about equally satisfied and dissatisfied	Mostly dissatisfied	Unhappy	Terrible
0 ☐	1 ☐	2 ☐	3 ☐	4 ☐	5 ☐	6 ☐

FIGURE 131-2. International Prostate Symptom Score (IPSS). The seven symptom questions constitute a scale initially developed by the American Urological Association. The eighth question about quality of life is scored separately. (From Barry MJ, Fowler FJ Jr, O'Leary MP, et al. The American Urological Association symptom index for benign prostatic hyperplasia: the Measurement Committee of the American Urological Association. *J Urol.* 1992;148:1549.)

8 to 19, moderate symptoms; and 20 to 35, severe symptoms (see Fig. 131-2). When frequency and nocturia are the dominant symptoms, a voiding diary, in which the patient records the times and amounts of each void over several days, may be helpful. For example, if the diary documents nocturnal polyuria alone, causes other than BPH should be strongly considered. Men with BPH tend to have a balance of voiding and filling symptoms that slowly progress with age. A complete list of medications should be obtained because many drugs, especially over-the-counter antihistamines, sympathomimetics, and anticholinergics, can affect the urinary tract.

Differential Diagnosis

Although lower urinary tract symptoms in older men are often due to BPH, the differential diagnosis includes systemic diseases that cause frequency and nocturia, such as diabetes (Chapter 236 and 237), hypercalcemia (Chapter 253), bladder outlet obstruction due to urethral strictures, and neurologic diseases affecting the bladder (Chapter 25). Rapid onset of symptoms, presentation before age 50, or filling symptoms without voiding symptoms are "red flags" that suggest these alternative causes. Older men can have overactive bladders either primarily or secondary to outlet obstruction. A general medical history and the pattern of symptoms should provide clues to systemic diseases. Men with strictures usually have undergone genitourinary instrumentation or have had sexually transmitted diseases (Chapter 293). Primary bladder problems should be suspected in men with previous stroke (Chapter 414), Parkinson's disease (Chapter 416), or diabetic neuropathy (Chapter 428).

Physical Examination

The physical examination should include a digital rectal examination and a focused neurologic examination to look for evidence of peripheral neuropathy or saddle-area anesthesia (the S2-S4 segments innervate the bladder), which might suggest an underlying neuropathic bladder. The digital rectal examination should assess the size and consistency of the prostate. Classically, BPH causes a symmetrically enlarged, firm prostate, with a consistency similar to that of the tip of the nose. Asymmetry or frank nodules suggest prostate cancer (Chapter 207), but prostate cancer can be present even when the prostate feels normal. Physicians tend to underestimate the prostate's size; if the prostate feels enlarged, it usually is.

Laboratory Findings

Urinalysis should assess possible pyuria or hematuria. Optional studies include measurement of the serum creatinine and prostate-specific antigen (PSA) levels. Peak urinary flow is often measured in urologists' offices, but results are unreliable with low voided volumes (<150 mL). Peak flows less than 10 mL/second are more suggestive of outlet obstruction, whereas peak flows greater than 15 mL/second are less suggestive. Unfortunately, men can have good flows with forceful bladder contractions despite obstruction, and they can have poor flows with weak bladder contractions in the absence of obstruction.

PSA results must be interpreted with caution. Generally, a level greater than 4 ng/mL should trigger an ultrasonography-guided prostate biopsy. About 50% of men with PSA levels greater than 10 ng/mL have prostate cancer at biopsy, about 25% with levels of 4.1 to 10 ng/mL have cancer, and 15% with levels of 4 ng/mL or less have cancer. Most authorities doubt the value of early detection of nonpalpable prostate cancer in men with a life expectancy of less than 10 years or those older than 75 years with average comorbidities. However, for medicolegal reasons, it is wise to discuss the possibility of an underlying prostate cancer with any older man who presents with lower urinary tract symptoms. A PSA level, probably by serving as a proxy for prostate size, can also help stratify the future risk of progression to surgery or acute urinary retention, with higher values predicting greater risk.

The "gold standard" test for the diagnosis of bladder outlet obstruction (Chapter 25) is the documentation of increased bladder pressure relative to urinary flow. Pressure-flow studies should be considered in men who have atypical presentations, diseases that increase their risk of primary bladder problems, or no response to adequate medical therapy.

PREVENTION

There are no documented effective strategies for the prevention of BPH. For the prevention of adverse outcomes from prostate cancer, which may present similarly to BPH, data are still evolving. A PSA level may detect prostate cancer in patients evaluated for suspected BPH, but the PSA level has relatively poor specificity in this situation. Early detection of prostate cancer with routine PSA testing may reduce prostate cancer–specific mortality somewhat, but at the expense, morbidity, and inconvenience of substantial false-positive and overtreatment rates (Chapter 207).[1]

TREATMENT Rx

Men with IPSSs in the mild range are rarely bothered enough by their symptoms to warrant treatment. Similarly, an enlarged prostate alone is not an indication for treatment. The key step in decision making for men with moderate or severe symptoms is to assess the degree to which the patient is bothered. The last IPSS question—"If you were to spend the rest of your life with your urinary condition just the way it is now, how would you feel about that?"—can serve as an entrée to this discussion.

For men whose symptoms cause little inconvenience, "watchful waiting" is appropriate. The patient's situation should be reassessed periodically. Avoidance of offending medications is also wise. Self-managed lifestyle changes, including fluid management (daily intake of 1500 to 2000 mL and fluid restriction before long journeys and within 2 hours of bedtime), avoiding caffeine, and the use of voiding techniques (double voiding, urethral milking, and bladder retraining) can improve symptoms and decrease the need for medical or surgical intervention substantially, at least over the short term.[2]

Medical Therapy

Most men with bothersome symptoms initially choose medical therapy. α_1-Adrenergic blockers and 5α-reductase inhibitors are the prescription options in the United States. When men present with symptomatic BPH, an α-blocker is a reasonable first choice for medical therapy. Finasteride or dutasteride can also be offered to men with palpably enlarged prostates or higher PSA levels for added preventive benefit. Combination α_1-adrenergic blocker and antimuscarinic therapy, though not yet approved by the Food and Drug Administration (FDA), may be effective for men with BPH symptoms related to overactive bladder; however, men need to be monitored closely for acute urinary retention, particularly during the first month of therapy.

α-Blockers (Table 131-1), which attack the dynamic component of BPH, reduce symptoms significantly, independent of prostate size, but they do not significantly reduce the risks of acute retention or progression to surgery over 4 years.[3] In general, doses should be increased toward the maximum until the therapeutic effect is optimal, unless side effects, including orthostatic hypotension, dizziness, and asthenia, are limiting. Tamsulosin, alfuzosin, and silodosin, which appear to be more specific for the α_{1a}-receptor subtype that dominates in the prostate, have little or no effect on blood pressure. However, because α-blocker-related dizziness and asthenia are not mediated primarily through hypotension, it is unclear whether these agents have advantages other than a lower risk of orthostatic hypotension. An intraoperative floppy iris syndrome can complicate cataract surgery in patients taking tamsulosin and other α_1-blockers; preoperative risk assessment (Chapter 439) should consider the use of these medications, but it is unclear whether discontinuation before surgery reduces the occurrence rate.

Finasteride and dutasteride are 5α-reductase inhibitors (see Table 131-1) that block the conversion of testosterone to dihydrotestosterone by the type 2 isoenzyme (finasteride) or both isoenzymes (dutasteride). Prostate size decreases by 15 to 20% over 1 year of treatment with either agent. Compared with placebo, finasteride and dutasteride reduce lower urinary tract symptoms for at least 2 to 4 years.[4] Although relief of symptoms may be more modest than with α-blockers in some men, dutasteride monotherapy produces more symptom relief than tamsulosin alone in men with larger prostate glands.[5] In addition, 5α-reductase inhibitors reduce the rate of progression to surgery or to acute urinary retention in men with larger prostates. The "number needed to treat" for 4 years to prevent an episode of acute retention or surgery is about 30 for men with PSA levels less than 1.4 ng/mL, about 20 for those with PSA levels of 1.4 to 3.2 ng/mL, and about 10 for those with PSA levels greater than 3.2 ng/mL. Given the different mechanisms of α-blockers and 5α-reductase inhibitors, it is not surprising that combination therapy is more effective than monotherapy in preventing progression of symptoms and disease.[5]

The main side effect of finasteride and dutasteride is sexual or ejaculatory dysfunction, which occurs in about 5% of men. Both agents lower PSA levels by about 50% but do not appear to interfere with the detection of prostate cancer if the physician mentally doubles the measured PSA and then interprets this higher value as usual. Finasteride reduces the 7-year cumulative incidence of prostate cancer from 24 to 18% in men who are heavily screened, including routine end-of-study biopsies. However, concerns about the higher risk of high-grade prostate cancer observed in this trial have not been completely allayed.[6]

Some short-term trials have suggested that daily use of a 5-phosphodiesterase inhibitor can reduce lower urinary tract symptoms, but these agents are not FDA approved for this purpose, and their role in the management of lower urinary tract symptoms due to BPH has yet to be defined. Although a variety of plant extracts, such as saw palmetto, have been suggested for the relief of lower urinary tract symptoms, recent results from a high-quality trial were disappointing.[7]

Surgical Therapy

Transurethral prostatectomy (TURP) reduces symptoms significantly more than watchful waiting or any form of medical therapy, without any greater risk of sexual dysfunction or incontinence.[8] Standard TURP, which uses a wire electrode to resect obstructing tissue, generally requires a brief hospital stay and an indwelling catheter for a few days or a week. Newer variations use a rolling electrode or laser energy to vaporize or resect prostate tissue. These procedures appear to result in less short-term bleeding and good short-term symptom improvement, but their long-term effectiveness is undefined.

Minimally invasive transurethral microwave thermotherapy (TUMT) heats and coagulates prostate tissue by using a microwave antenna surrounded by a cooling jacket to protect the urethra. Transurethral needle ablation (TUNA) uses radio frequency needles placed directly into the prostate to generate heat and cause coagulation. The mechanisms by which these treatments work are poorly understood. However, they appear to produce an initial level of symptom relief intermediate between drug therapy and TURP. Their long-term effectiveness remains unclear.

PROGNOSIS

Lower urinary tract symptoms attributable to BPH generally progress slowly over time, but individual experience varies. For example, in one study of men with symptom scores in the moderate range who elected watchful waiting, after 4 years of follow-up, 13% had only mild symptoms, 46% still had moderate symptoms, 17% had severe symptoms, and 24% had opted for surgery. The risk of acute urinary retention for such men is 1 to 2% per year. More serious complications appear to be exceedingly rare.

TABLE 131-1 MEDICATIONS USED IN THE TREATMENT OF MEN WITH LOWER URINARY TRACT SYMPTOMS ATTRIBUTED TO BENIGN PROSTATIC HYPERPLASIA

DRUG	TABLET/CAPSULE SIZE (mg)	RECOMMENDED DOSE STEPS
α-BLOCKERS		
Alfuzosin ER	10	10 mg qd
Doxazosin	1, 2, 4, 8	1, 2, 4, 8 mg qd
Doxazosin XL	4, 8	4, 8 mg qd
Silodosin	4,8	8 mg qd (4 mg qd for moderate renal impairment)
Tamsulosin	0.4	0.4, 0.8 mg qd
Terazosin	1, 2, 5, 10	1, 2, 5, 10 mg qd
5α-REDUCTASE INHIBITORS		
Finasteride	5	5 mg qd
Dutasteride	0.5	0.5 mg qd

PROSTATITIS

DEFINITION

The validity of the traditional etiology-based classification of prostatitis has never been confirmed. The current National Institutes of Health prostatitis classification system incorporates the term *chronic pelvic pain syndrome* to reflect uncertainty about whether chronic nonbacterial prostatitis and prostatodynia are actually related to the prostate (Table 131-2).

EPIDEMIOLOGY

Two million outpatient visits for prostatitis are made annually in the United States. The histologic prevalence ranges widely from 6 to 98%. The prevalence of current prostatitis-like symptoms or a previous physician's diagnosis of prostatitis is about 10%.

PATHOBIOLOGY

Both type I (acute bacterial) and type II (chronic bacterial) prostatitis account for 5 to 10% of cases. Like urinary tract infections, 80% are due to strains of *Escherichia coli*; 10 to 15% are due to *Pseudomonas aeruginosa, Serratia, Klebsiella,* and *Proteus* species; and 5 to 10% are due to enterococci. The remaining cases (>90%) are type III (chronic abacterial/chronic pelvic pain syndrome) prostatitis, for which the pathogenesis remains uncertain. Type III prostatitis is further divided into inflammatory (type IIIA) and noninflammatory (type IIIB) subtypes, based on the presence of leukocytes in expressed prostatic secretions and prostatic urine. Because there appears to be no correlation between the presence of leukocytes and symptoms, the subdivision into types IIIA and IIIB is controversial; many experts believe that both inflammatory and noninflammatory chronic prostatitis/chronic pelvic pain syndrome are the same noninfectious condition, which may or may not be related to the prostate gland.

Theories about the cause of type III prostatitis include infectious agents such as *Mycoplasma hominis, Ureaplasma urealyticum, Trichomonas vaginalis, Chlamydia trachomatis,* viruses, anaerobic bacteria, and coagulase-negative staphylococci; pro-inflammatory cytokines; autoimmune mechanisms; neurogenic processes; increased prostate tissue pressure; chemical irritation; and increased tension in the muscles of the bladder neck and prostatic urethra or from a tension myalgia of the pelvic floor. Psychological factors have also been implicated.

CLINICAL MANIFESTATIONS

Type I prostatitis is characterized by the acute onset of fever, chills, malaise, low back or perineal pain, and urinary symptoms, particularly dysuria, frequency, and urgency. The presentation is generally dramatic, and the patient may appear toxic. Digital rectal examination often reveals a markedly tender gland.

Type II prostatitis generally occurs in older men in association with recurrent urinary tract infections (Chapter 292). The presentation is less dramatic but involves similar lower urinary tract symptoms, pelvic pain, and sexual dysfunction. On digital rectal examination, the prostate may be normal, swollen, firm, or tender.

TABLE 131-2 CLASSIFICATION AND DEFINITION OF PROSTATITIS

Traditional Classification		*National Institute of Diabetes and Digestive and Kidney Diseases Classification*	
CATEGORY	**DEFINITION**	**CATEGORY**	**DEFINITION**
Acute bacterial prostatitis	Recovery of bacteria from prostatic fluid, purulence of fluid, and systemic signs of infectious illness (fever, chills, myalgia)	Type I (acute bacterial prostatitis)	Acute infection of the prostate
Chronic bacterial prostatitis	Recovery of bacteria in significant numbers from prostatic fluid in the absence of concomitant urinary infection or significant systemic signs (as in acute bacterial prostatitis)	Type II (chronic bacterial prostatitis) Type III (chronic abacterial prostatitis/chronic pelvic pain syndrome)	Recurrent infection of the prostate No demonstrable infection
Nonbacterial prostatitis	No recovery of significant numbers of bacteria from prostatic fluid, but the fluid consistently reveals microscopic purulence	Type IIIA (inflammatory chronic pelvic pain syndrome)	Leukocytes in semen, expressed prostatic secretions, or post–prostatic massage urine
Prostatodynia	No recovery of significant bacteria or purulence in the prostatic fluid, but patients have persistent pelvic pain and lower urinary tract symptoms	Type IIIB (noninflammatory chronic pelvic pain syndrome) Type IV (asymptomatic inflammatory prostatitis)	No leukocytes in semen, expressed prostatic secretions, or post–prostatic massage urine No subjective symptoms; detected by prostate biopsy or by the presence of leukocytes in expressed prostatic secretions or semen during evaluation for other disorders

NIH-Chronic Prostatitis Symptom Index (NIH-CPSI)

Pain or Discomfort

1. In the last week, have you experienced any pain or discomfort in the following areas?

	Yes	No
a. Area between rectum and testicles (perineum)	☐1	☐0
b. Testicles	☐1	☐0
c. Tip of the penis (not related to urination)	☐1	☐0
d. Below your waist, in your pubic or bladder area	☐1	☐0

2. In the last week, have you experienced:

	Yes	No
a. Pain or burning during urination?	☐1	☐0
b. Pain or discomfort during or after sexual climax (ejaculation)?	☐1	☐0

3. How often have you had pain or discomfort in any of these areas over the last week?

☐ 0 Never
☐ 1 Rarely
☐ 2 Sometimes
☐ 3 Often
☐ 4 Usually
☐ 5 Always

4. Which number best describes your AVERAGE pain or discomfort on the days that you had it, over the last week?

☐ ☐ ☐ ☐ ☐ ☐ ☐ ☐ ☐ ☐ ☐
0 1 2 3 4 5 6 7 8 9 10
NO PAIN — PAIN AS BAD AS YOU CAN IMAGINE

Urination

5. How often have you had a sensation of not emptying your bladder completely after you finished urinating, over the last week?

☐ 0 Not at all
☐ 1 Less than 1 time in 5
☐ 2 Less than half the time
☐ 3 About half the time
☐ 4 More than half the time
☐ 5 Almost always

6. How often have you had to urinate again less than two hours after you finished urinating, over the last week?

☐ 0 Not at all
☐ 1 Less than 1 time in 5
☐ 2 Less than half the time
☐ 3 About half the time
☐ 4 More than half the time
☐ 5 Almost always

Impact of Symptoms

7. How much have your symptoms kept you from doing the kinds of things you would usually do, over the last week?

☐ 0 None
☐ 1 Only a little
☐ 2 Some
☐ 3 A lot

8. How much did you think about your symptoms, over the last week?

☐ 0 None
☐ 1 Only a little
☐ 2 Some
☐ 3 A lot

Quality of Life

9. If you were to spend the rest of your life with your symptoms just the way they have been during the last week, how would you feel about that?

☐ 0 Delighted
☐ 1 Pleased
☐ 2 Mostly satisfied
☐ 3 Mixed (about equally satisfied and dissatisfied)
☐ 4 Mostly dissatisfied
☐ 5 Unhappy
☐ 6 Terrible

Scoring the NIH-Chronic Prostatitis Symptom Index Domains

Pain: Total of items 1a, 1b, 1c,1d, 2a, 2b, 3, and 4 = ______

Urinary Symptoms: Total of items 5 and 6 = ______

Quality of Life Impact: Total of items 7, 8, and 9 = ______

FIGURE 131-3. National Institutes of Health Chronic Prostatitis Symptom Index.

Type III prostatitis is characterized by pelvic pain, often associated with lower urinary tract symptoms and pain during or after ejaculation. Digital rectal examination findings also vary. Type IV prostatitis is, by definition, asymptomatic.

The hallmark of chronic prostatitis is a complex of symptoms that wax and wane. A brief, self-administered questionnaire (Fig. 131-3) has been developed and validated to quantify symptoms for clinical practice and research protocols.

DIAGNOSIS

Whereas acute prostatitis is relatively straightforward to diagnose, chronic prostatitis is more challenging. The symptom complexes of chronic prostatitis and BPH overlap, and BPH may be misdiagnosed in older men with chronic prostatitis. Although men can and do get both conditions, pain generally distinguishes chronic prostatitis from BPH. A PSA test is not indicated for the evaluation of chronic prostatitis; however, if a PSA test is performed and the level is found to be elevated, this should not be ascribed to chronic prostatitis/chronic pelvic pain syndrome.

Type I prostatitis is diagnosed primarily by clinical findings and a positive urine culture. Prostate massage is not recommended because of concern for precipitating bacteremia.

Type II and type III prostatitis are traditionally diagnosed with the four-glass test. This segmented, quantitative culture technique involves culturing initial-stream urine, midstream urine, expressed prostatic secretions after massage, and post–prostate massage urine. The simplified two-glass test involves culture and microscopic examination of urine obtained before and after prostate massage; it is easier for all concerned, with similar sensitivity and specificity. Type II prostatitis is characterized by the presence of uropathogenic bacteria, whereas type III prostatitis is defined by the absence of uropathogens in the setting of genitourinary pain. Type IV prostatitis is usually diagnosed incidentally by prostate biopsy or by the finding of leukocytes in prostatic secretions collected for infertility evaluations.

Differential Diagnosis

The diagnosis of type III prostatitis is challenging because it is a diagnosis of exclusion; therefore, a careful evaluation is necessary to rule out other causes of pelvic pain that may be associated with lower urinary tract symptoms and sexual dysfunction. The differential diagnosis for type III prostatitis includes BPH and prostate cancer. The patient's sexual history may suggest a sexually transmitted disease (Chapter 293), and a medical history of genitourinary instrumentation or sexually transmitted disease may suggest a urethral stricture. The physical examination may detect a hernia (Chapter 144) or a scrotal mass (Chapter 206). A urinalysis revealing hematuria should prompt evaluation for a kidney stone (Chapter 128) or bladder cancer (Chapter 203). A urine culture is important to exclude urinary tract infection (Chapter 292).

PREVENTION AND TREATMENT

There is no proven preventive strategy for any type of prostatitis.

Type I prostatitis is relatively easy to treat. Antibacterial agents that normally diffuse poorly into prostatic fluid work well, probably because intense inflammation enhances penetration. The choice of antimicrobial is driven by culture results. Parenteral antibiotics (e.g., ciprofloxacin 400 mg IV every 12 hours) are necessary for sicker patients, but oral fluoroquinolones (e.g., ciprofloxacin 500 mg orally every 12 hours or levofloxacin 500 mg orally daily) or trimethoprim-sulfamethoxazole (one double-strength tablet orally every 12 hours) is adequate for outpatients. Treatment for 4 weeks is generally recommended. Modification of the dosing of fluoroquinolones is advised in patients with renal impairment.

Type II prostatitis is more difficult to treat because prostatic fluid becomes alkaline with chronic inflammation, reducing antibiotic penetration. The fluoroquinolones (e.g., ciprofloxacin 500 mg orally every 12 hours or levofloxacin 500 mg orally daily) and trimethoprim-sulfamethoxazole (one double-strength tablet orally every 12 hours) penetrate the prostate, but the penicillins, cephalosporins, aminoglycosides, and nitrofurantoin do not. The duration of treatment is generally 4 weeks.

Type III prostatitis often engenders frustration on the part of the physician and confusion and dissatisfaction on the part of the patient. Because the cause is unknown, affected men receive various empirical therapies. Antibiotics, α-blocker therapy, and pregabalin have not been beneficial.[9,10]

For type IV prostatitis, no treatment is recommended.

PROGNOSIS

The untreated natural history of all types of prostatitis is poorly defined. Most patients with type I prostatitis respond well to antibiotics, but some may progress to chronic prostatitis. Complications of type I prostatitis include prostatic abscess, acute urinary retention, septicemia, and, rarely, vertebral osteomyelitis. Type II prostatitis can cause repeated urinary tract infections. Both type II and type III prostatitis have been associated with decreased fertility, although this relationship is not certain.

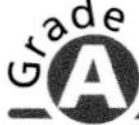

1. Schröder FH, Hugosson J, Roobol MJ, et al. Screening and prostate-cancer mortality in a randomized European study. *N Engl J Med*. 2009;360:1320-1328.
2. Brown CT, Yap T, Cromwell DA, et al. Self management for men with lower urinary tract symptoms: randomised controlled trial. *BMJ*. 2007;334:25-28.
3. Djavan B, Chapple C, Milani S, et al. State of the art on the efficacy and tolerability of alpha-1 adrenoreceptor antagonists in patients with lower urinary tract symptoms suggestive of benign prostatic hyperplasia. *Urology*. 2004;64:1081-1088.
4. McConnell JD, Roehrborn CG, Bautista OM, et al. The long-term effect of doxazosin, finasteride, and combination therapy on the clinical progression of benign prostatic hyperplasia. *N Engl J Med*. 2003;349:2385-2396.
5. Roehrborn CG, Siami P, Barkin J, et al. The influence of baseline parameters on changes in international prostate symptom score with dutasteride, tamsulosin, and combination therapy among men with symptomatic benign prostatic hyperplasia and an enlarged prostate: 2-year data from the CombAT study. *Eur Urol*. 2009;55:461-471.
6. Thompson IM, Goodman PJ, Tangen CM, et al. The influence of finasteride on the development of prostate cancer. *N Engl J Med*. 2003;349:215-224.
7. Bent S, Kane C, Shinohara K, et al. Saw palmetto for benign prostatic hyperplasia. *N Engl J Med*. 2006;354:557-566.
8. Wasson JH, Reda DJ, Bruskewitz RC, et al. A comparison of transurethral surgery with watchful waiting for moderate symptoms of benign prostatic hyperplasia. *N Engl J Med*. 1995;332:75-79.
9. Alexander RB, Propert KJ, Schaeffer AJ, et al. Ciprofloxacin or tamsulosin in men with chronic prostatitis/chronic pelvic pain syndrome: a randomized, double-blind trial. *Ann Intern Med*. 2004;141:581-589.
10. Nickel JC, Krieger JN, McNaughton-Collins M, et al. Alfuzosin and symptoms of chronic prostatitis-chronic pelvic pain syndrome. *N Engl J Med*. 2008;359:2663-2673.

SUGGESTED READINGS

Anothaisintawee T, Attia J, Nickel JC, et al. Management of chronic prostatitis/chronic pelvic pain syndrome: a systematic review and network meta-analysis. *JAMA*. 2011;305:78-86. *Antibiotics and alpha blockers give the best results.*

AUA Practice Guidelines Committee. AUA guideline on management of benign prostatic hyperplasia (2010). http://www.auanet.org/guidelines-and-quality-care/clinical-guidelines.cfm?sub=bph. *Consensus guidelines.*

Lipsky BA, Byren I, Hoey CT. Treatment of bacterial prostatitis. *Clin Infect Dis*. 2010;50:1641-1652. *Review.*

132

CHRONIC KIDNEY DISEASE

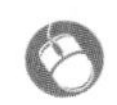

WILLIAM E. MITCH

DEFINITION

Chronic kidney disease (CKD) refers to the many clinical abnormalities that progressively worsen as kidney function declines. CKD results from a large number of systemic diseases that damage the kidney or from disorders that are intrinsic to the kidney (Table 132-1). A glomerular filtration rate (GFR) persistently below 60 mL/minute/1.73 m^2, which is below the level of kidney function expected to occur with aging, defines clinically significant CKD.

In CKD, the damage is rarely repaired, so loss of function persists. This distinguishes CKD from acute kidney damage (Chapter 122), which can be repaired to permit the return of kidney function. The chronic loss of kidney function generates even more kidney damage and more severe clinical abnormalities. As a result, CKD progressively worsens even if the disorder that caused it becomes inactive.

CKD describes a spectrum of clinical dysfunction that ranges from abnormalities detectable only by laboratory testing to uremia. *Uremia*, which literally means "urine in the blood," results from the accumulation of unexcreted waste products and the metabolic abnormalities they induce. When the kidney fails to perform most of its functions, the clinical state is called *end-stage renal disease* (ESRD), and dialysis or transplantation is required to sustain life (Chapter 133). However, the progressive and chronic nature of CKD permits the institution of treatment strategies that can slow the loss of kidney function. In addition, many symptoms of uremia can be ameliorated or eliminated, thereby postponing ESRD.

EPIDEMIOLOGY

The increase in the number of patients with ESRD in the United States and other industrialized countries has features of an epidemic. In the United States, the prevalence of CKD continues to increase (Table 132-2). An estimated 13.1% of the U.S. population, representing about 26 million noninstitutionalized individuals older than 20 years, has stages 1 through 4 CKD, and 65% of these have stage 3 or 4 CKD. The prevalence of albuminuria is nearly 10%, representing approximately 19 million adults. Notably, the prevalence of ESRD (stage 5 CKD) has increased by 82% over the past decade or two, from nearly 800 per million persons in the U.S. population to more than 1400 persons per million.

Two disorders account for more than 70% of all new ESRD patients in the United States: 45% of patients have diabetes mellitus (Chapters 236 and 237), and 27% have hypertension-induced kidney damage (Chapter 67). The increasing prevalence of CKD is due in part to the increasing prevalence of diabetes and obesity, plus the aging of the population and an increase in the proportion of minority populations, who seem to be more susceptible to developing CKD. Other epidemiologic factors that increase the risk of progressive CKD include cardiovascular disease, smoking, albuminuria, hyperlipidemia, and a family history of CKD.

PATHOBIOLOGY

The intact nephron hypothesis helps explain the importance of GFR as a measure of remaining kidney function. The nephron consists of the glomerulus, proximal tubule, loop of Henle, distal tubule, and collecting duct. Individuals are born with 0.75 million to 1.25 million nephrons per kidney. If nephrons are lost, new ones are not regenerated. The intact nephron hypothesis maintains that each nephron functions as an independent unit, so the sum of the function of all remaining nephrons determines the whole kidney's GFR, the most accurate estimate of remaining kidney function.

Physiologic and metabolic functions of the kidney include the regulation of blood pressure, several endocrine functions, and ion concentrations in the extracellular and intracellular fluids, as well as the excretion of waste products (Table 132-3). The breadth of these functions yields several direct and derivative consequences of CKD. For example, a limitation in the ability to excrete acid causes hyperventilation and a decrease in P_{CO_2}. In muscle, acidosis activates the ubiquitin-proteasome enzymatic process to degrade muscle protein, causing loss of muscle mass. In bone, acidosis causes loss of calcium and phosphates; this response, plus the secretion of parathyroid hormone (PTH) and decreased activation of vitamin D, demineralizes bone and makes it susceptible to fracture.

Balance and Steady-State Considerations

Metabolic balance is the state in which the intake or production of a substance equals its elimination. For example, a loss of functioning units (nephrons) impairs the ability to excrete sodium, but remaining nephrons adjust to excrete a greater fraction of the sodium filtered by each glomerulus. Similar phenomena occur in the excretion of other ions and substances, allowing the patient with CKD to avoid their accumulation. The ability to achieve balance has a limit, however; if the intake of sodium or other ions or molecules destined for excretion by the kidney is not regulated, complications of CKD will arise.

A related concept is that of steady state. A patient is in steady state when intake and production equal output and metabolism. A single parameter that integrates input and output may, if stable, be taken as indicative of a steady state. Thus, constant weight indicates that sodium intake is balancing sodium output. A steady state does not, however, indicate a normal state; for example, a patient who is grossly edematous may have a stable weight.

The Tradeoff Hypothesis

Another important principle, the tradeoff hypothesis, refers to the activation of pathophysiologic responses that produce adverse consequences. A classic example in CKD patients involves the responses activated to achieve sodium balance. Kidney damage initially reduces salt excretion, leading to sodium retention, expansion of extracellular fluid, and a rise in blood pressure.

TABLE 132-1 CAUSES OF CHRONIC RENAL FAILURE

Diabetic glomerulosclerosis*
Hypertensive nephrosclerosis
Glomerular disease
- Glomerulonephritis
- Amyloidosis, light chain disease*
- Systemic lupus erythematosus, Wegener's granulomatosis*

Tubulointerstitial disease
- Reflux nephropathy (chronic pyelonephritis)
- Analgesic nephropathy
- Obstructive nephropathy (stones, benign prostatic hypertrophy)
- Myeloma kidney*

Vascular disease
- Scleroderma*
- Vasculitis*
- Renovascular renal failure (ischemic nephropathy)
- Atheroembolic renal disease*

Cystic disease
- Autosomal dominant polycystic kidney disease
- Medullary cystic kidney disease

*Systemic disease involving the kidney.

TABLE 132-3 FUNCTIONS OF THE KIDNEY AND IMPAIRMENT OF KIDNEY FUNCTION IN PATIENTS WITH CHRONIC KIDNEY DISEASE

KIDNEY FUNCTION	CONSEQUENCES OF DYSFUNCTION
Maintain concentration and body content of electrolytes and fluid volume	Hyponatremia, hyperkalemia, low total potassium content, hypocalcemia, hyperphosphatemia, decreased tolerance to electrolyte or mineral loading
Regulate blood pressure	Hypertension, cardiovascular disease
Endocrine mediator	Anemia (low erythropoietin), hypertension (renin system activation), bone disease (secondary hyperparathyroidism), low vitamin D activation, prolonged half-lives of peptide hormones (e.g., insulin)
Waste product excretion	Anorexia, nausea, soft tissue deposition of oxalates and phosphates, neurologic dysfunction, loss of muscle protein

TABLE 132-2 PREVALENCE OF STAGES OF CHRONIC KIDNEY DISEASE AND FREQUENCY OF COMPLICATIONS

STAGE	DESCRIPTION	GFR* (mL/min/1.73 m²)	ADULT PREVALENCE (MILLIONS)†	SYMPTOMS OR SIGNS
1	Chronic kidney damage; normal or increased GFR	>90	3.6	Anemia 4% Hypertension 40% 5-yr mortality 19%
2	Mild GFR loss	60-89	6.5	Anemia 4% Hypertension 40% 5-yr mortality 19%
3	Moderate GFR loss	30-59	15.5	Anemia 7% Hypertension 55% 5-yr mortality 24%
4	Severe GFR loss	15-29	0.7	Hyperphosphatemia 20% Anemia 29% Hypertension 77% 5-yr mortality 46%
5	Kidney failure†	<15 or dialysis	0.5	Hyperphosphatemia 50% Anemia 69% Hypertension >75% 3-yr mortality 14%

*The formula for estimating the glomerular filtration rate (GFR) of adults with chronic kidney disease (CKD) is derived from data obtained during the National Institutes of Health Modification of Diet in Renal Diseases trial: $GFR = 186 \times [\text{serum creatinine}]^{-1.154} \times [\text{age}]^{0.203} \times [0.742 \text{ if patient is female}] \times [1.212 \text{ if patient is black}]$.
†Rate prevalent end-stage renal disease/million; United States Renal Data System Annual Report 2008.
Results based on the CKD Surveillance 2009 Report from the Centers for Disease Control and Prevention (unpublished).

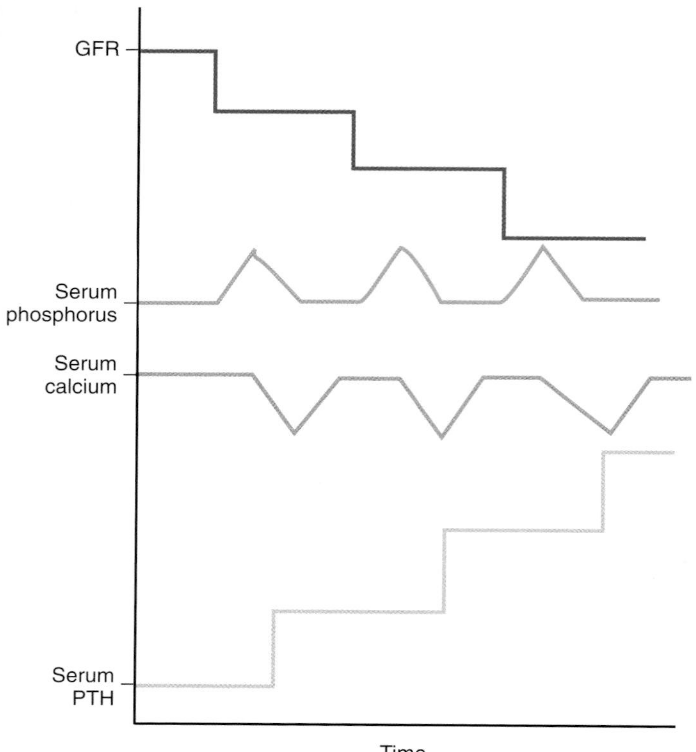

FIGURE 132-1. A decrease in glomerular filtration rate (GFR) is followed by an increase in serum phosphorus and a decrease in serum calcium. An increase in serum parathyroid hormone (PTH) returns phosphorus and calcium to normal levels.

Although a higher blood pressure initially is beneficial because it increases the filtration and excretion of sodium, the tradeoff for maintaining sodium balance is volume-dependent hypertension. Another proposal is that this increased sodium excretion is mediated by an increase in circulating Na^+, K^+-ATPase inhibitors, which increase the sodium concentration in tubular cells, reducing the cells' ability to reabsorb filtered sodium. Thus, the tradeoff for the increased ability to excrete sodium despite a loss of kidney function is that the patient loses the ability to reduce sodium excretion rapidly when salt intake is abruptly reduced. Inappropriately high salt excretion leads to loss of extracellular volume, impaired kidney perfusion, and a decrease in the GFR.

The most extensively studied tradeoff is the adaptation that stimulates secondary hyperparathyroidism (Fig. 132-1). When CKD impairs the kidney's ability to excrete phosphates, they accumulate in extracellular and intracellular fluids and lead to the physicochemical formation of calcium-phosphate complexes that reduce the level of ionized calcium. This process, in turn, stimulates the calcium-sensing receptor to increase the production and release of PTH. PTH release is beneficial because it suppresses the reabsorption of phosphates by the proximal tubule and thereby increases phosphate excretion. As the accumulation of phosphates decreases because of their excretion by the kidney, the ionized calcium rises to suppress PTH production. The tradeoff, however, is that the new steady-state levels of ionized calcium and phosphate can be maintained only as long as the circulating PTH concentration is increased (see Fig. 132-1). This higher level of PTH stimulates osteoclastic activity and leads to renal bone disease (see later).

Hypertension

Hypertension, like anemia, is almost universal in CKD patients and is often the first clinical indication of CKD. The coincidence of CKD and high blood pressure is particularly important because hypertension contributes to the development of cardiovascular disease, which is the leading cause of morbidity and mortality in CKD patients. Hypertension in CKD patients largely reflects an expanded extracellular volume owing to a salt-rich diet plus an impaired capacity to excrete sodium; activation of the renin-angiotensin-aldosterone system also plays a role. The normal response to retained sodium is an increase in extracellular volume, which raises blood pressure and increases sodium excretion, leading to a balance between sodium intake and the excretion of salt. In the renewed steady state, however, salt balance can be maintained only as long as blood pressure is high. Two practical implications arise from these relationships. First, treatment of hypertensive patients with vasodilating drugs alone is frequently unsuccessful; when vasodilator drugs reduce blood pressure, the initial decrease in sodium excretion leads to sodium retention, expansion of extracellular volume, and a rise in blood pressure. Second, hypertension in CKD patients may not respond to diuretic therapy because a salt-rich diet can cancel the benefits of diuretics even in normal adults.

Another mechanism for hypertension in CKD patients is activation of the renin-angiotensin-aldosterone system and the sympathetic nervous system, as evidenced by circulating levels of renin and aldosterone that are too high for individuals who are hypertensive. Inhibitors of the renin-angiotensin-aldosterone system slow the loss of kidney function. Evidence for activation of the sympathetic nervous system includes higher circulating levels of norepinephrine, which not only causes vasoconstriction but also suppresses the production of nitric oxide.

Endocrine Disorders

CKD, even in patients with serum creatinine values as low as 2.5 mg/dL, reduces the ability of insulin to stimulate glucose uptake by muscle and other organs, an abnormality known as *insulin resistance* (Chapter 237). The result is a transient increase in blood glucose that causes a compensatory increase in insulin release to maintain blood glucose levels near normal. In insulin-resistant CKD patients, the failure is due to a post-receptor defect in cell signaling, including an impaired ability to activate phosphatidylinositol 3-kinase and its downstream kinase Akt. The importance of this abnormality is that the reduced function of these enzymes in muscle cells impairs the metabolism of both glucose and protein, causing loss of muscle protein. Insulin resistance in nondiabetic CKD patients is generally associated with blood glucose values within the normal range; blood glucose levels rarely exceed 200 mg/dL.

One possible cause of insulin resistance in CKD is metabolic acidosis (Chapter 120). Acidosis also activates the degradation of muscle protein, impairs the ability of growth hormone to stimulate insulin-like growth factor-I (IGF-I), depresses circulating levels of thyroxine (T_4) and triiodothyronine (T_3), and increases levels of thyroid-stimulating hormone (Chapter 233). Fortunately, most of these adverse metabolic changes can be reversed simply by treating CKD patients with sodium bicarbonate or other alkalizing agents.

Another mechanism that affects endocrine status in CKD patients is the kidney's impaired ability to degrade small proteins, including several hormones. For example, diabetic CKD patients can progressively lose the ability to degrade insulin and may even develop hypoglycemia if they are treated with their usual dose of insulin. Impaired degradation of peptides by the damaged kidney can also affect the interpretation of the circulating PTH concentration because PTH is not fully degraded when the kidney is damaged; the PTH immunoassay may recognize one or more PTH fragments, which may be misinterpreted as representing excessively high levels of PTH.

In patients with stage 4 CKD, normochromic, normocytic anemia (Chapter 161) is almost universal, principally owing to impaired production of erythropoietin by interstitial cells in the kidney. However, anemia may be detected even in patients with stage 2 CKD and serum creatinine values just above the normal range. Other factors contributing to anemia in CKD patients include a shortened half-life of erythrocytes and deficiencies of vitamins and iron.

Renal Bone Disease

Renal bone disease, also called *renal osteodystrophy,* afflicts virtually all CKD patients to different degrees. Bone biopsies of patients with renal bone disease range from features indicative of increased bone turnover (i.e., greater numbers of osteoclasts, osteoblasts, and osteocytes) to abnormalities reflecting low bone turnover (i.e., reduced numbers of osteoclasts and osteoblasts and the accumulation of demineralized matrix). Patients with high bone turnover have high circulating PTH levels, whereas those with low bone turnover exhibit only a mild increase in circulating PTH. A third type of pathology is mixed uremic osteodystrophy, which has features of hyperparathyroidism and defective mineralization, presumably because increased PTH activates osteoclasts to reduce bone mass, while abnormalities in mineralization of bone result in an increase in fibrosis. Specifically, CKD produces hyperphosphatemia (see Fig. 132-1) because the intake of phosphates exceeds their excretion. Hyperphosphatemia stimulates the development of renal bone disease in two ways. First, the physicochemical interaction between phosphates and "free" or ionized calcium lowers the level of ionized calcium and reduces the interaction between calcium and the calcium receptor. Decreased activation of the calcium receptor causes the parathyroid gland to hypertrophy and PTH production to rise; it also stimulates osteoclast activity, resulting in loss of bone mass. Second, hyperphosphatemia acts directly on the parathyroid glands to stimulate PTH production. Other factors that contribute to CKD-induced bone disease include defects in cellular signaling by the calcium receptor and changes in vitamin D metabolism.

A G protein–coupled plasma membrane protein present in chief cells of the parathyroid gland and in certain renal tubular cells responds directly to calcium ions. The interaction of this receptor with calcium or with cinacalcet, which is a small, orally available molecule that activates the calcium receptor, suppresses the expression and release of PTH from parathyroid chief cells. In contrast, hyperphosphatemia and a decreased level of circulating ionized calcium increase the production and release of PTH (see Fig. 132-1). These responses can be negated by cinacalcet because it effectively suppresses the production and release of PTH even when there is hyperphosphatemia and decreased ionized calcium. Consequently, use of this drug requires careful monitoring to avoid hypoparathyroidism and even hypocalcemia.

Another factor that regulates the circulating calcium level and plays a role in the development of renal bone disease is vitamin D. The activation of vitamin D proceeds by repeated hydroxylation of the parent molecule, cholecalciferol (vitamin D_3). The initial hydroxylation occurs in the liver, where 25-hydroxyvitamin D_3 is formed. This form of vitamin D stimulates the absorption of calcium and phosphates from the intestines and is believed to change the function and metabolism of muscle and possibly other organs by mechanisms that are poorly defined. Moreover, recent evidence indicates that CKD patients who have low circulating values of 25-hydroxyvitamin D_3 experience an increase in the risk of all-cause mortality, thereby supporting the conjecture that the function of 25-hydroxyvitamin D_3 extends beyond serving as a precursor for the most active vitamin D, calcitriol.

Calcitriol is produced when a 25-hydroxycholecalciferol 1α-hydroxylase in the proximal tubules of the kidney hydroxylates 25-hydroxyvitamin D_3. The activity of 1α-hydroxylase changes in response to factors that regulate mineral metabolism: for example, its activity is decreased by hyperphosphatemia, and the decrement in calcitriol decreases the intestinal absorption of calcium and phosphates. However, the β-glucuronidase klotho confers the tissue specificity of fibroblast growth factor-23 (FGF-23), a hormone that increases the renal excretion of phosphates. Both klotho and FGF-23 are involved in the regulation of calcitriol production, but exactly how these factors influence the development of renal bone disease has not been defined.

Because the 1α-hydroxylase enzyme is expressed mainly in proximal tubule cells, progressive loss of kidney function causes calcitriol deficiency. This deficiency, in turn, results in impaired absorption of both calcium and phosphates from the intestine; the resulting decrease in calcium should stimulate 1α-hydroxylase activity to produce more calcitriol. If this is not possible because of a decrease in proximal tubular function, serum calcium decreases, thereby increasing PTH production. Depressed calcitriol production also can augment PTH production by reducing the level of vitamin D receptor in the parathyroid gland, promoting the development of hyperparathyroidism even before hypocalcemia has developed.

Soft tissue calcification, which is the deposition of calcium phosphate crystals and inflammation in the vessels and soft tissues, is common when the product of the concentrations of serum calcium and phosphorus exceeds 60 mg^2/dL^2, but it can occur with lower levels. The deposition of crystals seems to be linked most closely to an increase in the local concentration of phosphates, emphasizing why the serum phosphorus level should be kept in the normal range.

Accumulation of Uremic Toxins

In diets containing protein-rich foods, protein is metabolized to amino acids that can be used to build body protein stores (Fig. 132-2). Alternatively, the amino acids are metabolized to form urea or potentially toxic products that are excreted when kidney function is normal. The serum creatinine level is determined by the degree of renal insufficiency and the rate of creatinine production, which is proportionate to lean body mass. As a result, a serum creatinine concentration of 1.4 mg/dL in an adult with a small muscle mass signifies a much greater loss of kidney function than it does in an individual with a large muscle mass. In addition, the amount of creatinine excreted in 24-hour urine collections can vary by up to 25%, making creatinine clearance of limited use in determining the degree of kidney damage in CKD patients.

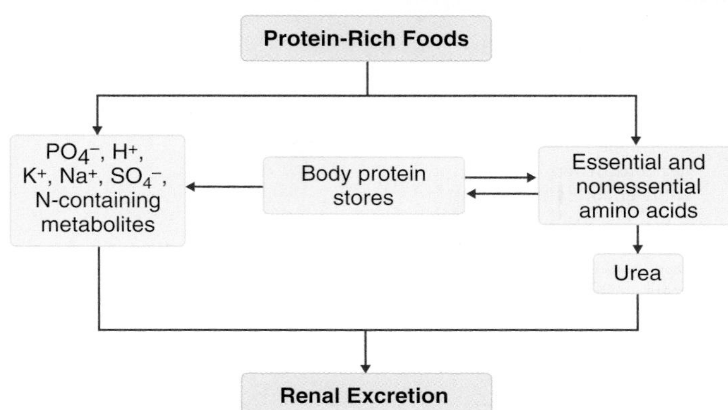

FIGURE 132-2. The breakdown of dietary protein enlarges the pool of essential and nonessential amino acids that can be used to synthesize body protein. Protein breakdown also increases the production of urea and other nitrogenous waste products, and it is accompanied by the increased intake of inorganic ions that must be excreted.

Because creatinine is formed from creatine, which is highly concentrated in muscle, extensive cooking of dietary meat converts creatine to creatinine. Consequently, eating a meal containing a large amount of well-cooked meat raises the amount of creatinine excreted. Even if meat and high-protein foods are eliminated from the diet of CKD patients, at least 4 months are required to reach a new steady state. In terms of extrarenal creatinine clearance, the degradation rate of creatinine, presumably by bacteria in the gut, is so small that it is virtually undetectable in patients with normal kidney function; when serum creatinine rises above 5 mg/dL, however, degradation can contribute to creatinine clearance.

With CKD, the accumulation of peptides (also known as *middle molecules*) is associated with disorders that range from the induction of anorexia to neurologic abnormalities. Another potential toxin is indoxyl sulfate, a product of tryptophan metabolism; it has been linked to progressive kidney damage and the symptoms of uremia. High uric acid levels, which are related to excess protein intake, can cause gout (Chapter 281) and may be linked to the development of hypertension and inflammatory responses in blood vessels. Besides generating potentially toxic metabolites, diets containing protein-rich foods also increase the intake of phosphates, sodium, potassium, acid, and other ions that must be eliminated.

Ideally, circulating levels of uremic toxins should be monitored, but measuring these levels is not practical. The blood urea nitrogen (BUN), however, provides an index of the level of uremic toxins because the production of urea is directly proportional to the metabolism of proteins and hence the production of other unexcreted waste products (see Fig. 132-2). Thus, the load of waste product production can be approximated from the 24-hour excretion of urea nitrogen as long as the patient is in the steady state (i.e., BUN concentration and body water are stable). In general, the ratio of BUN to serum creatinine is 10 : 1 in normal adults or CKD patients. When the BUN concentration is below this ratio, it can be concluded that the patient is eating a protein-restricted diet. If the BUN concentration exceeds 10 times the serum creatinine concentration, three possibilities should be considered. First, the patient may have gastrointestinal bleeding or may be suffering from a severely catabolic condition (e.g., trauma or high-dose glucocorticoid administration). Second, the patient may be eating excessive amounts of protein, yielding more urea than the impaired kidney can excrete. Finally, there may be extracellular volume depletion with active proximal tubular reabsorption of sodium and fluid and concomitant passive reabsorption of urea; the result is a rise in BUN. The corollary is that a decrease in urea production is associated with a decrease in the load of uremic toxins. For this reason, the production of urea should be kept to a minimum that is consistent with maintaining body protein stores. To accomplish this goal, the dietary content of protein should be monitored and manipulated to decrease urea production (see later).

Progression of Chronic Kidney Disease

Persistence of diseases affecting the kidney (e.g., diabetes or inflammatory conditions such as systemic lupus erythematosus) is not the only factor that determines the rapidity of the loss of kidney function. Even when the disease that initially damaged the kidney is no longer active, kidney function continues to decline, probably because systemic hypertension, hemodynamic injury

TABLE 132-4 ANGIOTENSIN II RESPONSES IN CHRONIC KIDNEY DISEASE*

Hemodynamic responses
- Systemic hypertension
  - Vasoconstriction
  - Salt retention (aldosterone)
  - Intraglomerular hypertension
  - Efferent arteriolar vasoconstriction

Nonhemodynamic responses in the kidney
- Macrophage infiltration and inflammation
- Interstitial matrix accumulation
  - Increased transforming growth factor-β
  - Increased plasminogen activator inhibitor type 1
  - Increased aldosterone

*Includes the proposed actions of angiotensin II that can contribute to the development of cardiovascular disease and progressive loss of kidney function.

TABLE 132-5 COMPLICATIONS OF CHRONIC KIDNEY DISEASE

AFFECTED SYSTEM	CAUSE OR MECHANISM	CLINICAL SYNDROME
Systemic symptoms	Anemia, inflammation	Fatigue, lassitude
Skin	Hyperparathyroidism, calcium-phosphate deposition	Rash, pruritus, metastatic calcification
Cardiovascular disease	Hypertension, anemia, homocysteinemia, vascular calcification	Atherosclerosis, heart failure, stroke
Serositis	Unknown	Pericardial or pleural pain and fluid, peritoneal fluid
Gastrointestinal	Unknown	Anorexia, nausea, vomiting, diarrhea, gastrointestinal tract bleeding
Immune system	Leukocyte dysfunction, depressed cellular immunity	Infections
Endocrine	Hypothalamic-pituitary axis dysfunction	Amenorrhea, menorrhagia, impotence, oligospermia, hyperprolactinemia
Neurologic	Unknown	Neuromuscular excitability, cognitive dysfunction progressing to coma, peripheral neuropathy (restless leg syndrome or sensory deficits)

to the kidney, proteinuria, and accumulation of nephrotoxins all contribute to progressive damage.

The belief that hypertension causes progressive loss of kidney function is based on several observations. First, hypertension alone can damage the kidney; malignant hypertension damages the endothelial cells of the afferent arteriole and the glomerulus and may even cause thrombosis in these vessels. Second, chronic hypertension is frequently associated with ischemic injury to glomeruli owing to transmission of the blood pressure into the afferent arteriole and glomerulus, causing glomerulosclerosis. Third, the degree of hypertension is directly correlated with the rate of loss of kidney function. Fourth, effective treatment of hypertension slows the progression of CKD. Although it is sometimes difficult to determine the extent to which hypertension is a cause or an effect of CKD in an individual patient, hypertension is strongly associated with progressive kidney injury and with the development of cardiovascular disorders.

Experimentally, angiotensin II–related, progressive glomerular damage (Table 132-4) arises from preferential constriction of the glomerular efferent arteriole to a greater extent than in the afferent arteriole. The imbalance in arteriolar vasoconstriction increases intracapillary pressure and tends to raise glomerular filtration (the hyperfiltration mechanism), but the tradeoff for any increase in GFR is damage to glomerular capillaries. Because angiotensin II is the mediator of preferential efferent arteriolar constriction, angiotensin-converting enzyme (ACE) inhibitors and angiotensin receptor blockers (ARBs) may prevent both hyperfiltration and damage to the kidney.

The benefits of treatment with ACE inhibitors or ARBs may extend beyond reducing hyperfiltration. Angiotensin II has growth factor properties, and it activates transforming growth factor-β, plasminogen activator inhibitor type 1, and other cytokines, thereby aggravating interstitial damage to the kidney (see Table 132-4). Aldosterone may also contribute to the development of interstitial damage and collagen deposition in the kidney. However, blocking the actions of aldosterone can cause hyperkalemia.

Patients receiving ACE inhibitor or ARB treatment experience a reduction in albuminuria, presumably because of a decrease in the pressure within glomeruli. Experimental evidence suggests that albumin or some component of albumin (e.g., lipids or molecules bound to albumin) may injure kidney cells; therefore, reducing albuminuria may be directly beneficial. Because the degree of albuminuria is related to the rapidity of the loss of kidney function, reducing albuminuria is a treatment goal.

CLINICAL MANIFESTATIONS

Unfortunately, progressive loss of kidney function produces no clinically distinct signs or symptoms. Findings that should raise the possibility of CKD include urinary abnormalities, such as hematuria or repeated urinary infections, or the appearance of hypertension and/or edema. The possibility of CKD should also be considered in patients with chronic hypertension, diabetes, or albuminuria and those with a family member with CKD.

As the GFR declines, clinical abnormalities become more frequent. Even when CKD is advanced (stage 4; see Table 132-2), however, the symptoms are mostly nonspecific. Some patients complain only of exercise intolerance, fatigue, or anorexia. If these symptoms are present, serum creatinine and BUN levels should be measured, and the urine should be examined for albuminuria. As CKD progresses, patients frequently have anemia, metabolic acidosis, hyperkalemia, hyperphosphatemia, hypocalcemia, and hypoalbuminemia, each of which can be associated with specific symptoms (Table 132-5).

Specific syndromes are associated with proteinuria and CKD. For example, severe albumin losses (>3 g/day) plus edema and hypercholesterolemia define the nephrotic syndrome (Chapter 123), which can lead to the loss of the relatively small (59 kD) vitamin D–binding protein plus the attached 25-hydroxyvitamin D_3, thereby aggravating bone disease. Advanced proteinuria can also be associated with losses of clotting factors IX, XI, and XII, causing coagulation defects (Chapter 177). Conversely, urinary losses of antithrombin III can result in thrombosis (Chapter 174), especially when inflammation-induced increases in the levels of acute phase reactant proteins lead to hyperfibrinogenemia.

Bone Disease and Extraosseous Calcification

Some patients with renal bone disease complain of vague, ill-defined pain in the lower back, hips, knees, and other locations. Advanced bone disease can cause such severe pain that it impairs the ability to exercise, aggravating the tendency to lose muscle mass. With advanced renal bone disease, minimal trauma may produce fractures.

Another clinical syndrome related to renal bone disease is the development of vascular calcification, which causes vascular stiffness and increases systolic blood pressure, thereby participating in the development of left ventricular hypertrophy. A more disabling manifestation is the development of calcifications in the tunica media of blood vessels (i.e., Mönckeberg's sclerosis) as well as calcifications that impair the function of multiple organs, including the lungs, myocardium, and skin. Calcification of the skin and cutaneous vessels is seen in the syndrome of calciphylaxis.

DIAGNOSIS

If CKD is suspected, emphasis should be placed on eliciting a history of hypertension, urinary abnormalities, and treatment with drugs that might affect kidney function (Chapter 122). The family history should focus on the presence of family members with kidney diseases, kidney stones, or surgery involving the urinary tract, as well as diabetes and hypertension. The physical examination should include lying and standing blood pressure measurements in both arms and a search for findings associated with CKD, such as skin abnormalities, persistent itching, a palpable polycystic kidney (Chapter 129), evidence of decreased lean body mass, peripheral edema, and neurologic abnormalities.

Staging

The severity of CKD is divided into five stages according to persistent reductions in estimated GFR (see Table 132-2). Two assessments of impaired kidney function are necessary: GFR and degree of albuminuria. Generally, the GFR can be estimated based on the serum creatinine level, age, body weight, gender, and race (see Table 132-2). The serum creatinine concentration is influenced by both kidney function and creatinine production, and the latter is directly proportional to lean body mass plus a small contribution from dietary meat. Notably, the serum creatinine concentration can remain in the nominally normal range until as much as 50% of kidney function is lost. Consequently, an elevated serum creatinine level means that both kidneys are functioning inadequately and that more than 50% of nephrons and nearly 50% of kidney function have been lost. By itself, the serum creatinine level is too variable to be used as a measure of GFR, but repeated values can be used to assess how rapidly changes in GFR are occurring. For example, changes in the reciprocal of the creatinine level (1/serum creatinine) yield a linear relationship with the rate of GFR loss (Fig. 132-3). Deviations from linearity signal a change in the course of CKD.

Other methods of estimating kidney function are not as accurate. For example, the BUN concentration is determined not only by the remaining kidney function but also by the amount of protein in the diet.

A careful microscopic examination of the urine is critical. Erythrocytes and erythrocyte casts in urine sediment are consistent with glomerulonephritis (Chapter 123), fine granular casts plus protein suggest diabetic kidney disease (Chapter 126), leukocytes plus fine and coarse granular casts suggest interstitial nephritis (Chapter 124), and eosinophils in the urine suggest a drug reaction with interstitial damage (Chapter 124).

Microalbuminuria is defined as 30 to 300 mg albumin/24 hours or 30 to 300 mg albumin/g creatinine in an initial morning urine specimen. Albuminuria is defined as excretion rates that are greater than those of microalbuminuria. The measured magnitude of albuminuria in a 24-hour urine collection depends on a full collection. An equally accurate alternative is to measure the ratio of albumin to creatinine concentrations in the first morning urine specimen on 3 separate days.

The urea nitrogen content of the 24-hour urine collection also allows calculation of the amount of dietary protein, which is composed of 16% nitrogen (see Fig. 132-2; Table 132-6). When the amount of urea nitrogen excreted in the steady state (i.e., when weight and BUN are stable) is added to the nonurea nitrogen excreted daily—which can accurately be estimated as 0.031 g nitrogen/kg ideal body weight/day—total daily nitrogen excretion can be calculated. If the total amount of nitrogen excreted exceeds the nitrogen contained in the prescribed diet, possibilities include dietary nonadherence, gastrointestinal bleeding, or a catabolic illness.

Other Laboratory Tests

Blood chemistries that evaluate the consequences of CKD include concentrations of sodium, potassium, chloride, bicarbonate, calcium, and phosphorus, as well as uric acid levels. The blood glucose level and hemoglobin A_{1c} level should be monitored in diabetics, and serum complement levels should be measured in patients with inflammatory diseases of the kidney. The hematocrit and/or hemoglobin level should be assessed and monitored because anemia often appears with even mild renal dysfunction and tends to progress as CKD progresses, owing to reduced erythropoietin production and/or iron deficiency. Iron deficiency can be recognized if the serum iron level is low, the serum ferritin concentration is less than 200 ng/mL, and the transferrin saturation level is less than 20% (Chapter 162). To detect CKD-induced bone disease, levels of PTH, alkaline phosphatase, calcium, and phosphorus should be obtained.

Imaging

The initial evaluation should include an ultrasound examination of the kidney and bladder to ensure that there is no obstruction of urine flow (Chapter 125). Enlarged kidneys suggest that CKD is due to diabetes, HIV-associated nephropathy, or infiltrative diseases (e.g., amyloidosis). Small kidneys, especially with a shrunken kidney cortex, suggest chronic glomerular or interstitial diseases (Chapter 124). If the size of the two kidneys differs substantially, stenosis of the renal artery (Chapter 127) of the smaller kidney should be considered, especially in hypertensive patients.

TABLE 132-6 ESTIMATION OF DIETARY PROTEIN FROM 24-HOUR UREA NITROGEN EXCRETION

ASSUMPTIONS

The patient is in the steady state, and neither the serum urea nitrogen concentration nor body weight is changing; there is no edema.
The patient is in nitrogen balance, so that nitrogen intake equals nitrogen excretion.
Protein is 16% nitrogen.
The nonurea nitrogen excretion (the nitrogen in urinary creatinine, uric acid, and peptides plus feces) is 0.031 g nitrogen/kg/day.

CASE 1

A 50-year-old patient with a stable weight of 70 kg is prescribed a diet containing 0.8 g protein/kg/day. His 24-hr urea nitrogen excretion is 6.8 g nitrogen/day. How much protein is he eating?
His diet should contain 70 kg × 0.8 g protein/kg, or 56 g protein. His intake of nitrogen from this diet is approximately 9 g (56 g protein × 0.16 = 8.96 g nitrogen). His nitrogen excretion is 6.8 g urea nitrogen + 2.17 g nonurea nitrogen/day (70 × 0.031 g nonurea nitrogen/kg/day). The total nitrogen excretion is 8.97 g, so the patient is compliant with the prescribed diet.

CASE 2

A 40-year-old woman weighing 60 kg is confident that she is eating a diet containing 0.6 g protein/kg/day. Her 24-hr urea nitrogen excretion is 10 g nitrogen/kg/day. Does she require additional investigation?
Her diet should contain 60 kg × 0.6 g protein/kg, or 36 g protein. Therefore, her intake of nitrogen is approximately 5.8 g (36 g protein × 0.16 = 5.76 g nitrogen). Her nitrogen excretion is 10 g urea nitrogen + 1.86 g nonurea nitrogen (60 kg × 0.031 g nonurea nitrogen/kg/day). Her total nitrogen excretion is 11.9 g/day, far in excess of the amount of protein she believes she is eating. Consequently, the patient requires investigation for gastrointestinal bleeding.

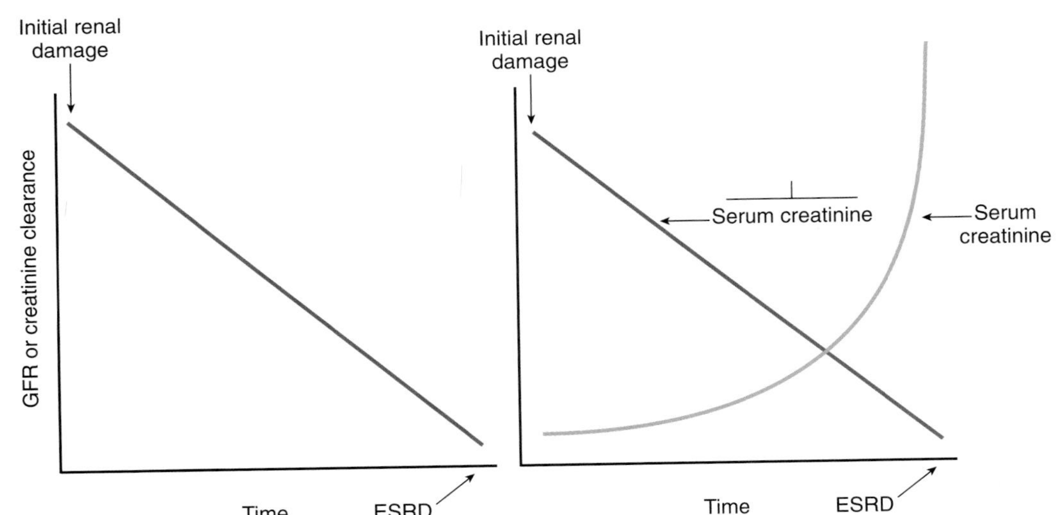

FIGURE 132-3. The course of renal insufficiency from initial renal damage to end-stage renal disease (ESRD; left panel). The course is estimated most easily by the reciprocal of serum creatinine (right panel). (Reprinted, with permission, from *Annual Review of Medicine* 35. ©1984 by Annual Reviews, www.annualreviews.org.)

TREATMENT

Rx

Because the risk of developing cardiovascular disorders is increased in CKD, the first goal of treatment is to reduce blood pressure to reduce mortality.[1] Therapy with an ACE inhibitor or ARB should be started to slow the loss of kidney function.[2-4] The preferred strategy is to begin at the lower recommended doses (see Table 67-5 in Chapter 67) and titrate upward until blood pressure is controlled (usually to a goal of 130/80 mm Hg) and albuminuria is decreased. In patients with type 2 diabetes, a systolic blood pressure goal of 135 to 140 mm Hg is preferable to a goal of less than 120 mm Hg, and a blood pressure of about 140/85 mm Hg is as good as 130/80 mm Hg for reducing the progression of hypertensive renal disease.[5,6] Combining an ACE inhibitor and an ARB provides no additional benefit in terms of protecting the kidney and is associated with more frequent adverse events,[6] so this combination is not recommended. Adverse effects of ACE inhibitors or ARBs include an increase in the serum creatinine level and/or hyperkalemia, especially in patients with bilateral renal artery stenosis. In these cases, the fall in GFR is due to a lowering of intraglomerular blood pressure, which reduces albuminuria and slows the loss of GFR, not to additional kidney damage; therefore, an increase in serum creatinine concentration after starting therapy should not trigger an automatic discontinuation of ACE inhibitor or ARB therapy. However, any unexpected changes in the serum creatinine level should stimulate the consideration of progressive CKD from an increase in blood pressure, infection, drugs that adversely affect kidney function, or exacerbation of the underlying renal disease. If no other reason for a decrease in kidney function is uncovered, the ACE inhibitor or ARB treatment should be continued, but with a 50% reduction in dose.

Hyperkalemia occurs with ACE inhibitors and ARBs because reduced angiotensin II decreases the release of aldosterone. Other causes of an increase in serum potassium should be considered (e.g., treatment with nonsteroidal anti-inflammatory drugs or potassium-sparing diuretics, or an increase in potassium-rich foods) and addressed. If needed, the addition of a loop diuretic (e.g., 40 mg furosemide when the serum creatinine level is <3 mg/dL and higher doses for more advanced CKD) may treat hyperkalemia successfully.

The blood pressure goal of 130/80 mm Hg almost always requires additional therapy, including dietary salt restriction to 2 g sodium/day. This goal is equivalent to 86 mEq sodium/day and is achievable if patients avoid salt-rich foods. For patients who develop problems with inhibitors of the renin-angiotensin system, other vasodilators, such as nondihydropyridine calcium-channel blockers (e.g., diltiazem, verapamil), seem to have fewer side effects than dihydropyridine drugs (e.g., amlodipine). Despite their ability to combat hypertension, vasodilators other than ACE inhibitors and ARBs are not as effective for reducing albuminuria, and they can cause peripheral edema. The loop diuretics are preferred for patients with more advanced CKD because they maintain renal blood flow, have few adverse effects, and, unlike thiazide diuretics, remain effective even at GFRs below 25 mL/minute. As renal insufficiency advances, high daily doses of loop diuretics (e.g., 80 to 160 mg furosemide orally) may be required to reduce extracellular volume. The dose-response relationship of loop diuretics is sigmoidal, so once a dose is identified as being effective in producing loss of edema and body weight, it should not be reduced or given in divided doses.

Stage 1 and Stage 2 Chronic Kidney Disease

In patients with stage 1 or 2 CKD, uremic symptoms are unusual because there is sufficient kidney function to control the levels of potential uremic toxins. Therapy therefore emphasizes reducing blood pressure to 130/80 mm Hg, intensive treatment of the underlying disease (e.g., normalization of blood glucose concentration in diabetic patients), and monitoring changes in albuminuria and loss of GFR (Fig. 132-4).

Dietary salt restriction is routinely recommended, and many patients require a diuretic (see Table 67-5 in Chapter 67) because an ACE inhibitor or ARB rarely controls hypertension unless steps are taken to avoid salt

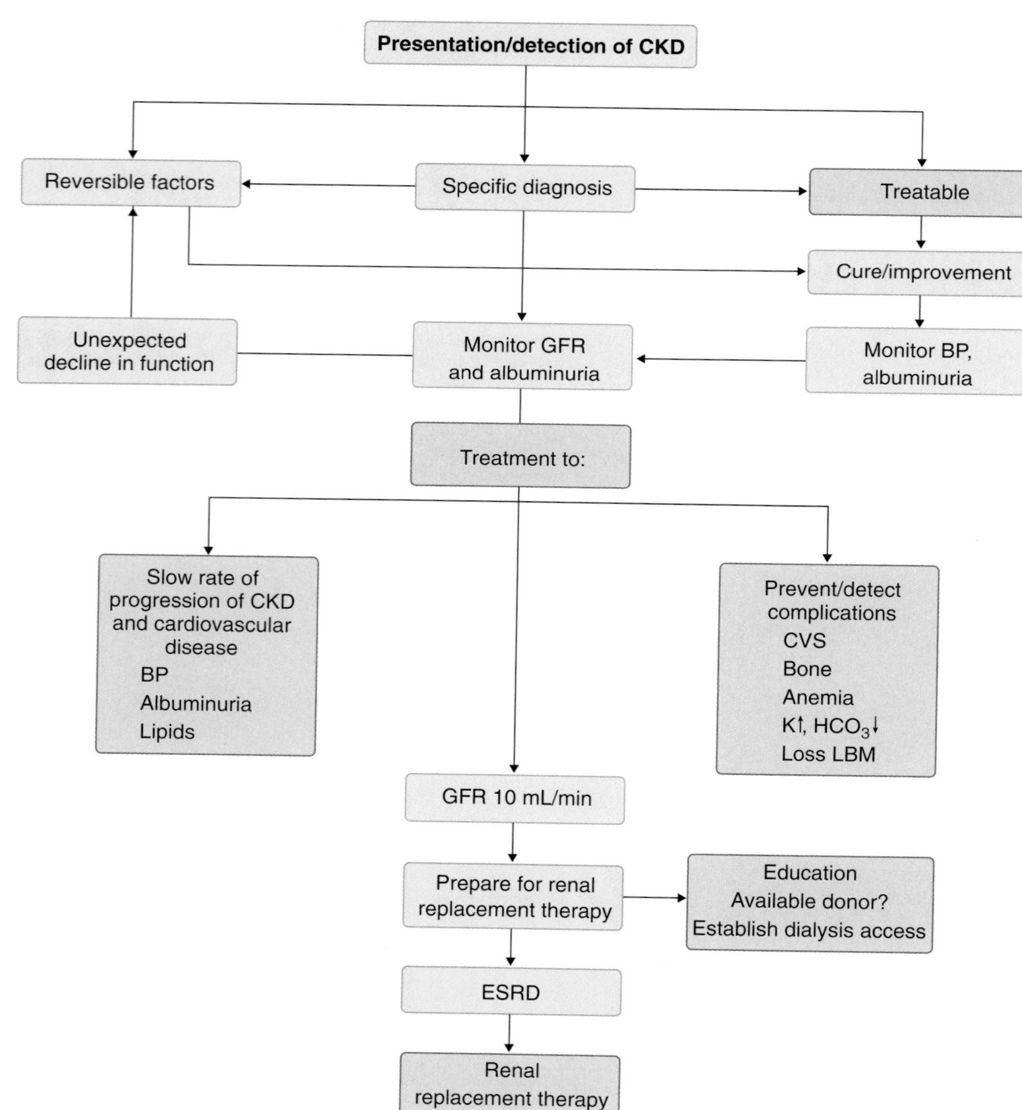

FIGURE 132-4. Management of patients in the various stages of chronic kidney disease (CKD). BP = blood pressure; CVS = cardiovascular system; ESRD = end-stage renal disease; GFR = glomerular filtration rate; LBM = lean body mass.

accumulation. A critical tactic is to monitor body weight; if weight and edema increase, it signifies salt retention. Conversely, a rapid loss of weight and edema would be the first clue that the diuretic dose should be reduced.

Stage 3 and Stage 4 Chronic Kidney Disease

Patients with stage 3 CKD should be referred to a nephrologist to maximize preventive measures and to search for remediable disorders. When stage 4 CKD is reached, a nephrologist should instruct patients about the advantages of therapies such as dialysis or transplantation (Chapter 133).

In stage 3 and stage 4 CKD, the doses of many renally excreted drugs must be adjusted downward to prevent overdosing. Treatable complications of CKD, including hypertension, secondary parathyroidism, acidosis, and uremic symptoms must be addressed. Radiologic tests with nephrotoxic contrast dye should be avoided if possible.

The development of many CKD complications (see Table 132-5) requires modification of the diet. An unrestricted high-protein diet contains an excess of salt, acid precursors, and phosphates and can lead to the development of metabolic acidosis, hyperphosphatemia, edema, hypertension, and uremic symptoms. CKD patients with any of these complications should initiate a diet consisting of 0.8 g protein/kg ideal body weight/day to maintain body protein stores and reduce the likelihood of developing other complications. Calorie intake should be limited to 30 kcal/kg ideal body weight/day for largely sedentary patients, with more for those who still exercise vigorously. If CKD-induced uremic symptoms persist, dietary protein can be restricted to a minimum of 0.6 g protein/kg/day, with a calorie intake of 30 kcal/kg/day. With either diet, successful implementation requires the advice, guidance, and close monitoring of a dietitian to take advantage of the patient's food preferences. Compliance can be monitored by measuring the 24-hour excretion of urea nitrogen (see Table 132-6), and the adequacy of protein stores should be assessed regularly by measuring body weight and serum protein levels. Although low-protein diets may not slow the loss of kidney function, they reduce uremic symptoms and can delay the need for dialysis without compromising the maintenance of protein stores.[7] Most patients on a protein-restricted diet should receive a multivitamin to sustain levels of water-soluble vitamins, but they should take fat-soluble vitamins only for documented deficiencies.

Renal Bone Disease

Treatment of renal bone disease relies on correcting the principal disorder, which is the accumulation of phosphates. This is best detected by measuring the serum phosphorus level after a normal meal. In patients with more advanced CKD (e.g., late stage 3 or stage 4) and an increased PTH level, treatment is directed at reducing the serum phosphorus level to the normal range. Because kidney damage limits the capacity to excrete phosphates, the dietary content of phosphates must be reduced to less than 1000 mg/day. If dietary restriction proves insufficient to control serum phosphorus, "phosphate binders" (see Table 121-4 in Chapter 121) should be added to the treatment regimen to promote the formation of poorly absorbed complexes of phosphates in the gastrointestinal tract. Once complexed, the phosphates are poorly absorbed by the intestine. Aluminum hydroxide binders should be avoided because they are associated with aluminum deposition in bone, where they inhibit normal bone formation and have been associated with neurotoxicity. Other phosphate binders include calcium carbonate (initially one or two 500-mg tablets with each meal), calcium acetate (initially one or two 667-mg tablets with each meal), sevelamer hydrochloride (400- to 800-mg tablets, initially 2 g/day in divided doses), or lanthanum carbonate (750 mg to 1 g/day with meals). Calcium-containing binders must be used cautiously to avoid hypercalcemia and the deposition of calcium phosphate in soft tissues. Conversely, calcium-containing agents are preferred for hyperphosphatemia in association with hyperkalemia (Chapter 119) or neuromuscular irritability, as demonstrated by a positive Trousseau's sign (Chapter 253). The non-calcium-containing phosphate binder sevelamer decreases the progression of aortic and coronary artery calcification when compared with calcium-containing binders. Lanthanum carbonate is a newer binder, and experience with this agent is more limited. For patients with serum phosphorus levels less than 6 mg/dL, calcium-based binders are generally recommended, but the dose should not exceed 2 g calcium/day to reduce the risk of soft tissue calcification. When the serum phosphorus level is higher or higher doses are required, sevelamer is the preferred phosphate binder. If the serum phosphorus level exceeds 7 mg/dL, aluminum-based binders (600 mg of concentrated aluminum hydroxide solution with each meal) can rapidly decrease the serum phosphorus level, but use of this drug should be limited to a week to avoid aluminum toxicity. In all cases, the cornerstone of therapy is to reduce phosphate intake, which generally requires dietary protein restriction because protein-rich foods contain excess phosphates.

Calcitriol, which increases the intestinal absorption of both calcium and phosphates, has the unique ability to suppress the development of hyperparathyroidism. However, calcitriol should not be given to patients who have increased circulating levels of phosphates. Low serum levels of 25-hydroxyvitamin D_3 in CKD patients are associated with increased mortality; patients with low levels of calcitriol and 25-hydroxyvitamin D_3 can be treated with cholecalciferol 1000 units/day. Careful monitoring is needed to avoid hypercalcemia or urinary calcium values above 250 mg/day.

In a patient who develops calciphylaxis, treatment options are few and are directed mainly at reducing serum phosphorus with phosphate binders and aggressively restricting dietary phosphate. If the disorder persists despite correcting the serum phosphorus level, a trial of cinacalcet (initial dose 30 mg, increasing as needed to achieve a reduction in PTH) is warranted. With advanced calciphylaxis, successful treatment requires parathyroidectomy.

Anemia

Because of the decreased absorption of oral iron in patients with advanced CKD, ferumoxytol (two 500-mg IV injections separated by 3 to 8 days) provides a better response than oral iron supplements, with a low risk of side effects.[8] In pre-dialysis patients, treatment with erythropoietin (e.g., weekly injections of darbepoetin alfa 0.45 µg/kg) corrects anemia and improves quality of life.[9] Caution is necessary, however, because fully correcting the hemoglobin concentration has been associated with an increased risk of stroke.[10] Consequently, erythropoietin-stimulating agents should be used to maintain the hemoglobin concentration between 10 and 12 g/dL.

Atherosclerosis

The increased risk of cardiovascular complications is linked, in part, to high circulating levels of homocysteine and low-density-lipoprotein cholesterol (Chapter 51). However, interventions to reduce homocysteine have not decreased the risk of cardiovascular complications in patients with CKD. Statins have not benefited patients on dialysis but appear to benefit patients with stage 2 or early stage 3 CKD,[11] and possibly those with the nephrotic syndrome.

PROGNOSIS

Because the rate of loss of kidney function varies widely, even in patients who have the same type of kidney disease, it is critical to monitor the course of declining kidney function in each CKD patient by plotting the estimated GFR or 1/serum creatinine versus time (see Fig. 132-3). If the serum creatinine level remains unchanged after 4 months, it is likely that the rate of loss of kidney function has been slowed. Monitoring albuminuria provides additional information about the progressive loss of GFR, because the decline in GFR increases with rising degrees of albuminuria; in addition, persistent microalbuminuria, and especially albuminuria, is associated with an increased risk of cardiovascular disease and a more rapid loss of kidney function. Diabetic patients who decrease their albuminuria reduce their risk of major cardiovascular events and slow their rate of loss of kidney function.

Although population data are of limited value for the individual patient with CKD, epidemiologic studies indicate that one third of patients with stage 4 CKD (see Table 132-2) will progress to ESRD within 3 years. Dialysis or transplantation is generally required when the serum creatinine reaches 10 mg/dL; however, patients should be informed about treatment options well before this stage of CKD because the frequency of complications rises sharply when dialysis is initiated on an emergency basis.

Cardiovascular disease is the most common cause of mortality in CKD. It is present in many patients even in the early stages of kidney disease. Other contributors to the high mortality of CKD include diabetes, anemia, increased low-density-lipoprotein cholesterol levels, vascular calcification, and perhaps increased cysteine levels.

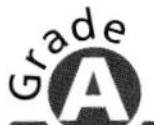

1. Heerspink HJ, Ninomiya T, Zoungas S, et al. Effect of lowering blood pressure on cardiovascular events and mortality in patients on dialysis: a systematic review and meta-analysis of randomised controlled trials. *Lancet*. 2009;373:1009-1015.
2. Jafar TH, Schmid CH, Landa M, et al. Angiotensin-converting enzyme inhibitors and progression of non-diabetic renal disease: a meta-analysis of patient-level data. *Ann Intern Med*. 2001;135:73-87.
3. Hou FF, Zhang X, Zhang GH, et al. Efficacy and safety of benazepril for advanced chronic renal insufficiency. *N Engl J Med*. 2006;354:131-140.
4. Brenner BM, Cooper ME, De Zeeuw D, et al. Effects of losartan on renal and cardiovascular outcomes in patients with type 2 diabetes and nephropathy. *N Engl J Med*. 2001;345:861-869.
5. Cushman WC, Evans GW, Byington RP, et al. Effects of intensive blood-pressure control in type 2 diabetes mellitus. *N Engl J Med*. 2010;362:1575-1585.
6. Appel LJ, Wright JT, Greene T, et al. Intensive blood-pressure control in hypertensive chronic kidney disease. *N Engl J Med*. 2010;363:918-929.
7. Fouque D, Laville M. Low protein diets for chronic renal failure in non-diabetic adults. *Cochrane Database Syst Rev*. 2009;3:CD001892.
8. Lu M, Cohen MH, Rieves D, et al. FDA report: ferumoxytol for intravenous iron therapy in adult patients with chronic kidney disease. *Am J Hematol*. 2010;85:315-319.
9. Cody J, Daly C, Campbell M, et al: Recombinant human erythropoietin for chronic renal failure anaemia in pre-dialysis patients. *Cochrane Database Syst Rev*. 2001;4:CD003266.

10. Palmer SC, Navaneethan SD, Craig JC, et al. Meta-analysis: erythropoiesis-stimulating agents in patients with chronic kidney disease. *Ann Intern Med.* 2010;153:23-33.
11. Tonelli M, Keech A, Shepherd J, et al. Effect of pravastatin in people with diabetes and chronic kidney disease. *J Am Soc Nephrol.* 2005;16:3748-3754.

SUGGESTED READINGS

James MT, Hemmelgarn BR, Tonelli M. Early recognition and prevention of chronic kidney disease. *Lancet.* 2010;375:1296-1309. *Review.*

Tangri N, Stevens LA, Griffith J, et al. A predictive model for progression of chronic kidney disease to kidney failure. *JAMA.* 2011;305:1553-1559. *A predictive model incorporating age, sex, estimated GFR, albuminuria, and serum levels of calcium, phosphate, bicarbonate, and albumin effectively identifies patients who will progress to kidney failure.*

133 TREATMENT OF IRREVERSIBLE RENAL FAILURE

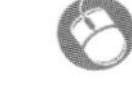

NINA TOLKOFF-RUBIN

Therapeutic options for irreversible end-stage renal disease (ESRD) include hemodialysis, peritoneal dialysis, and renal transplantation. Each of these approaches to renal replacement therapy has its unique risks and benefits. Currently, approximately 350,000 patients are on dialysis in the United States, and the ESRD population is projected to grow by about 7% per year.

The physician and the patient should recognize that these treatment modalities also can be complementary, thereby allowing flexibility of care under different clinical circumstances. The key is early identification of patients with progressive renal failure to enable them to make an educated choice that fits their lifestyle and medical situation. Careful planning can decrease emergency hospitalizations, complications, and costs. Early evaluation also enables identification of potential living donors so that preemptive transplantation can be performed.

INDICATIONS FOR RENAL REPLACEMENT THERAPY

The decision as to when to institute dialysis depends on the patient's signs and symptoms rather than an absolute level of blood urea nitrogen (BUN) or serum creatinine (Table 133-1). The benefits of early initiation of dialysis include the avoidance of malnutrition, fluid overload, and the deleterious effects of prolonged exposure to the accumulation of phosphorus, β_2-microglobulin, and other uremic toxins. However, early initiation of dialysis is no better than standard care.[1]

Hyperkalemia (Chapter 119) unresponsive to diuretics, ion exchange resins, and dietary restriction in the face of electrocardiographic (ECG) changes is an absolute indication for dialysis to avoid life-threatening arrhythmias. Volume overload refractory to intravenous diuretics, increasing lethargy, difficulty concentrating, nausea, and anorexia may be manifestations of the uremic syndrome requiring dialytic therapy. Intervention should occur before the progression of uremic encephalopathy, seizures, and coma or the development of pericarditis or pericardial tamponade (Chapter 77). Emergency hemodialysis is more costly because such patients typically lack vascular access, are sicker, and often require prolonged hospitalization.

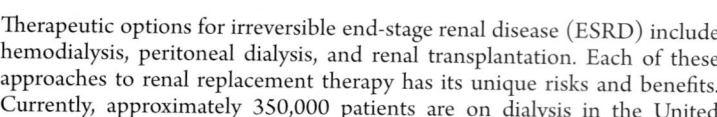

TABLE 133-1 INDICATIONS FOR DIALYSIS IN CHRONIC KIDNEY DISEASE

Uremic encephalopathy or neuropathy
Pericarditis or pleuritis
Bleeding attributable to uremia
Fluid overload refractory to diuretics
Hypertension poorly responsive to medication
Persistent hyperkalemia, metabolic acidosis, hypercalcemia, hypocalcemia, or hyperphosphatemia refractory to medical therapy
Malnutrition or weight loss
Persistent nausea and vomiting

HEMODIALYSIS

Dialysis substitutes two major renal functions: *solute removal* and *fluid removal.* In hemodialysis, solute removal occurs predominantly by diffusive clearance, which is the movement of solutes from the blood compartment to the dialysate compartment across a semipermeable membrane. Several basic principles apply. Clearance is higher for smaller molecules. The greater the concentration gradient between the blood and the dialysis solution, the more rapidly diffusion occurs. The net transfer of solute increases as membrane surface area increases. Membrane permeability is determined by the specific characteristics of the membrane, such as pore size, charge, and quaternary conformation. Higher flow rates allow greater solute removal, especially if the flow of dialysate is countercurrent to blood flow, thereby maximizing the gradient across the membrane.

Solute removal can also occur by the process of convection, the movement of solutes by bulk flow in association with fluid removal (solvent drag). Although the convective mass transfer of solutes may not play a dominant role in conventional hemodialysis, convection does play a significant role in high-flux dialysis and in continuous venovenous hemofiltration (CVVH).

Fluid removal in hemodialysis occurs by the process of ultrafiltration. The ultrafiltration rate is determined by the hydrostatic pressure gradient across the dialysis membrane, called the *transmembrane pressure.* Ultrafiltration increases if positive pressure is applied to the blood compartment or if negative pressure is applied to the dialysate side of the dialysis membrane. During dialysis, the ultrafiltration rate is adjusted to obtain the desired fluid loss.

The hemodialysis machine has three main components: (1) the dialyzer (i.e., the dialysis membrane); (2) a pump that regulates blood flow; and (3) a dialysate solution delivery system. In addition, the machine has many safety devices to monitor arterial and venous pressures, concentration of ions and temperature in the dialysate, and air and blood leaks (Fig. 133-1).

Under most circumstances, solute removal and fluid removal occur simultaneously. However, if vigorous ultrafiltration is attempted during conventional hemodialysis, patients frequently complain of muscle cramping, nausea, and vomiting. Moreover, during aggressive fluid removal systemic vascular resistance may decrease, thereby reducing blood pressure. Separating ultrafiltration from dialysis enables efficient fluid removal with greater hemodynamic stability. Osmotic changes are minimized with isolated ultrafiltration (i.e., fluid removal in the absence of solute removal). As a result, vascular resistance is well maintained, and, consequently, less hypotension occurs despite large fluid shifts.

Performing Hemodialysis

Hemodialyzers

The hollow-fiber dialyzer is composed of thousands of parallel capillary tubes. Blood flows through the capillary tubes, and dialysate flows in a countercurrent direction, bathing the outside of the capillary tubes (see Fig. 133-1). Dialysis membranes made of polycarbonate, polysulfones, polyacrylonitrile, or polymethylmethacrylate are less proinflammatory, provide better filtration rates, and improve survival compared with earlier cellulose-based membranes.

Access

To perform hemodialysis on a repetitive basis, access to the circulation is essential. An arteriovenous fistula involves anastomosis of the radial or brachial artery to the cephalic or basilic veins, with subsequent "arterialization" of the superficial forearm veins to enable blood flow rates up to 400 mL/minute. The most frequent problem is failure of the fistula to mature, particularly in patients with peripheral vascular disease or diabetes. In patients with progressive chronic kidney disease, the nondominant arm should be spared from venipuncture and a fistula should be placed in advance of the need of hemodialysis because the fistula usually takes 6 to 8 weeks to mature. Guidelines recommend elective placement of a fistula when the serum creatinine exceeds 4 mg/dL, the creatinine clearance falls to less than 25 mL/minute, or the initiation of hemodialysis is anticipated within 1 year.

Synthetic arteriovenous grafts, which can be used when a native fistula cannot be placed, have higher rates of thrombosis and infection. A third option is percutaneous dual-lumen catheters, which are placed preferentially in the internal jugular vein with a segment of the line tunneled under the skin.

Anticoagulation

Contact of patient's blood with the dialysis membrane and the tubing leads to activation of the coagulation cascade. Thrombus within the catheter can

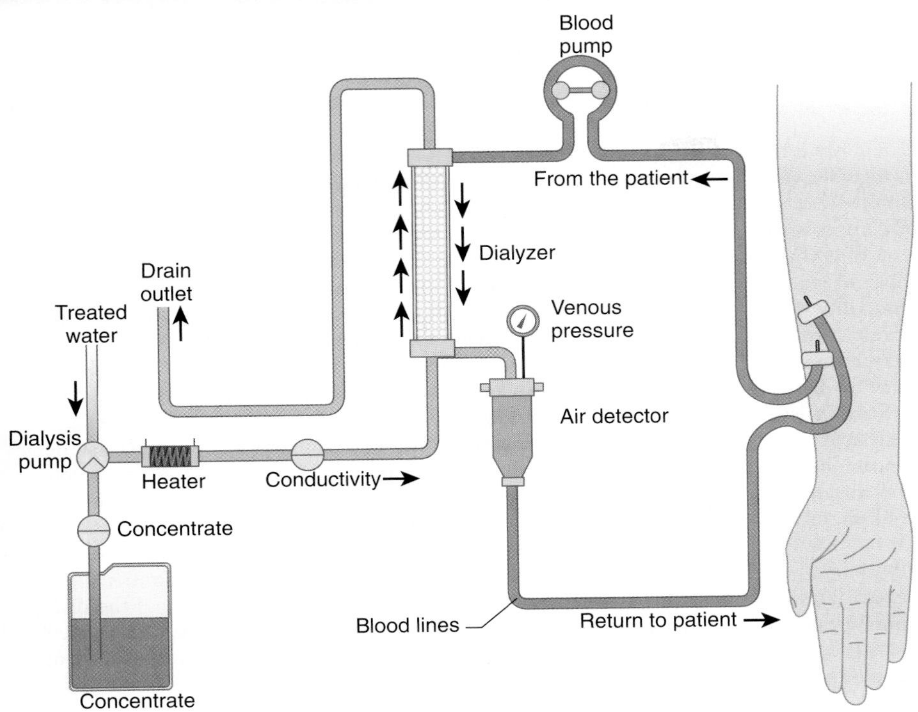

FIGURE 133-1. Hemodialysis. Treated water is mixed with concentrated dialysate. The dialysate solution flows around the fibers of the hollow-fiber dialyzer counter-current to the blood flow through the dialyzer. A computerized ultra-filtration control device regulates fluid removal (Modified from http://www.gml-dialyza.cz/Obrazky/hemodialysis.jpg.)

obstruct blood flow and also serve as a nidus for pathogens. Heparin (dosed at 500 to 1000 units/hour) is usually required to prevent clotting, but it may cause bleeding or heparin-induced thrombocytopenia (Chapter 175).

In patients at high risk for bleeding, hemodialysis can be performed without anticoagulation. Heparin-free dialysis requires a high blood flow rate and frequent flushing of the system with normal saline. Many patients also develop a procoagulant state caused by the development of anticardiolipin (Chapter 177), lupus anticoagulant antibodies, or high homocysteine levels, which may contribute to the tendency for clotting in the dialyzer and vascular access systems.

Dialysate Solution

The dialysate is a balanced solution of sodium, potassium, calcium, magnesium, chloride, and dextrose, with bicarbonate as a buffer. During dialysis, the sodium concentration is usually maintained at 135 to 140 mEq/L. A higher sodium dialysate concentration helps prevent hypotension, muscle cramps, nausea, vomiting, headaches, and seizures during hemodialysis; the sodium concentration can be programmed to return to normal range by the end of hemodialysis. Mannitol can also be used to prevent dialysis disequilibrium syndrome. The potassium concentration in the dialysate can be adjusted from 0 to 4 mEq/L but is generally maintained at 2 mEq/L in chronic outpatient dialysis centers with central delivery systems. The calcium concentration is usually 2.5 mEq/L.

Because patients are exposed to large volumes of water during each hemodialysis treatment, purity of the water is essential. A charcoal filter removes organic toxins such as chloramines, whereas reverse osmosis or de-ionization of the water effectively removes aluminum, fluoride, and copper. Chronic exposure to aluminum can lead to dialysis dementia, bone disease, and erythropoietin-resistant anemia.

Complications

Complications during Hemodialysis

In addition to vascular access problems, the most common complications during hemodialysis are hypotension, muscle cramps, nausea, vomiting, headache, and chest pain. Although excessive fluid removal is the most frequent cause of hypotension, other potential causes if the hypotension persists after fluid replacement include sepsis, myocardial ischemia, pericardial tamponade, arrhythmias, and active bleeding. Antihypertensive agents may need to be withheld before dialysis to avoid hypotension.

Air embolus, which is the most dreaded technical complication of the hemodialysis procedure (Chapter 98), presents with agitation, cough, dyspnea, and chest pain. As soon as the diagnosis is suspected, the patient should be positioned with the left side down in an attempt to trap air in the right ventricle. One hundred percent oxygen should be administered.

Vascular Access Infections

Although tunneled lines provide immediate and convenient access to the circulation, the surrounding skin and the catheter hubs are the primary sources of bacteria. Infectious complications of the vascular access account for nearly 75% of all cases of bacteremia in the ESRD population. If a patient presents with possible catheter-related bacteremia, blood cultures should be obtained both from the catheter and from a peripheral vein.

Because most vascular access infections are caused by staphylococcal organisms (Chapter 296), which carry high rates of mortality, recurrence, and metastatic complications, empirical vancomycin, 1 g every 3 days for at least 2 weeks while monitoring blood levels, is usually used in institutions with an increased incidence of methicillin-resistant staphylococci. However, the indiscriminate and prolonged use of vancomycin should be avoided to prevent the emergence of vancomycin-resistant organisms, especially *Enterococcus* species. If the patient has any evidence of systemic sepsis with hemodynamic instability, the line should be pulled promptly and reinserted only after blood cultures are negative for at least 48 hours and the patient has defervesced. In the interim, dialysis can be performed femorally or through a temporary nontunneled catheter.

In patients with a prompt response to antibiotic therapy, antimicrobial agents should be administered for at least 2 to 3 weeks. A prolonged course of antibiotic therapy (4 to 8 weeks) is recommended if there is persistent bacteremia or fungemia after catheter removal or if there is evidence of endocarditis (Chapter 76), septic arthritis (Chapter 280), osteomyelitis (Chapter 296), epidural abscess (Chapter 421), or other metastatic infection.

Long-Term Complications in Hemodialysis

Anemia

The development of a normochromic normocytic anemia (Chapter 161) parallels the progression of chronic kidney disease, and almost two thirds of patients who start dialysis have hematocrit levels less than 30% and hemoglobin levels less than 10 g/dL. Decreased erythropoietin production is the major cause, but contributing factors include a shortened life span of red blood cells, uremic inhibitors of erythropoiesis, iron deficiency owing to poor iron absorption, gastrointestinal bleeding, loss of blood with frequent blood sampling, and losses during hemodialysis. Folic acid is removed by dialysis, so folate replacement is necessary. Infection, inflammation, malignancy, and high parathyroid hormone levels can also inhibit red blood cell maturation. Aluminum toxicity, either from aluminum contamination of the water supply or through the use of aluminum-containing phosphate binders, has been associated with microcytic anemia in dialysis patients with normal iron stores.

Erythropoietin

The administration of erythropoietin (50 to 100 U/kg intravenously three times weekly depending on the baseline hemoglobin level), together with repletion of iron stores, folic acid supplementation, and treatment of concomitant infection, is effective in correcting the anemia of chronic renal disease. The target hemoglobin level, with or without the use of erythropoietin, should be no higher than 12 g/dL because a number of studies have shown that higher levels are associated with increased mortality rates, particularly due to cardiovascular events and strokes.[2] Failure to provide an adequate supply of iron is the most common cause of erythropoietin treatment failure. The best way to replenish the iron stores in dialysis patients is intravenous iron (Chapter 162). A transferrin saturation level (serum iron ÷ total iron-binding capacity × 100%) of less than 20% and a ferritin level of less than 100 ng/mL are indications for intravenous iron therapy in dialysis patients. Erythropoietin resistance also occurs in the presence of ongoing infection, inflammation, hyperparathyroidism, or aluminum toxicity.

Malnutrition

Hypoalbuminemia is associated with an increased mortality among patients undergoing dialysis. Patients with an albumin level of less than 3.0 g/dL have a 2-year mortality rate of up to 40%, in comparison with the expected mortality rate of 20%. Marked catabolism, anorexia, and severe diet limitations during the predialysis period lead to loss of lean weight. After the initiation of dialysis, patients usually have an improved appetite, and their protein intake should be at least 1.2 g/kg per day for a total caloric intake of 35 cal/kg/day. Water-soluble vitamins, including folic acid, need to be replaced because they are depleted during dialysis.

Chronic Kidney Disease and Cardiovascular Disease

Cardiovascular disease, which is the most important cause of death among patients with chronic kidney disease, accounts for approximately 50% of the deaths among patients on dialysis and among recipients of renal allografts. Two thirds of patients with chronic kidney disease have diabetes mellitus or hypertension, but the rates of cardiovascular disease and mortality are also elevated among patients with primary renal diseases such as glomerulonephritis. Among patients younger than 45 years of age, cardiac mortality is 100 times greater than in the general population.

In patients initiating dialysis, the main cardiac abnormality is left ventricular hypertrophy. A number of studies have shown a direct correlation between an elevated serum phosphorus concentration (>5.5 mg/dL), a calcium-phosphorus product (Ca × P) greater than 56, and mortality in hemodialysis patients. A striking degree of coronary and aortic calcification has been demonstrated in young adults with ESRD using electron-beam tomography (Chapter 56). These findings have led to a decrease in the use of calcium- versus non-calcium-containing phosphate binders, such as sevelamer and lanthanum carbonate.

Decreased synthesis of the active principal form of vitamin D (1,25-$[OH]_2D_3$) contributes to the secondary hyperparathyroidism of dialysis patients, and pulse-dose intravenous activated vitamin D is used to suppress synthesis of parathyroid hormone (PTH) directly and to prevent skeletal complications. However, randomized trials are needed because the aggressive use of vitamin D analogues may also increase vascular calcification or ossification. Recent retrospective studies suggest that therapy with pulse-dose activated vitamin D improves the survival of patients undergoing chronic hemodialysis and that paricalcitol in particular may provide a survival advantage over calcitriol.

Renal Osteodystrophy

Three forms of bone disease are seen in patients with renal failure. *Osteitis fibrosis cystica* is a condition in which there is increased bone turnover owing to secondary hyperparathyroidism. *Osteomalacia* (Chapter 252) is characterized by an increase in unmineralized bone (widened osteoid seam) as well as low bone turnover. *Adynamic bone disease* is a condition in which there is low bone turnover. Although bone biopsy remains the gold standard for determining the form of renal-associated bone disease, the diagnosis is typically made chemically, guided by serum PTH, calcium, phosphorus, and alkaline phosphatase, as well as the clinical scenario.

At present, adynamic bone disease is the principal bone lesion in dialysis patients, mostly as a result of oversuppression of PTH with overzealous use of calcium-containing binders and vitamin D analogues. Fractures and hypercalcemia can occur. Adynamic bone disease, defined by bone biopsy or intact serum PTH less than 100 picograms/mL, is treated by allowing the PTH to rise by avoiding calcium-containing binders and vitamin D analogues and by using non-calcium-containing phosphate binders, such as sevelamer or lanthanum, to control hyperphosphatemia.

Dialysis Dose

The time-averaged concentration of urea and nutritional status, as determined by protein catabolic rate, is an important determinant of morbidity and mortality in hemodialysis. It is better for patients to be dialyzed longer and be well nourished than to have a low BUN value and be dialyzed for shorter periods. The prescription of hemodialysis is tailored to the patient's size and protein intake. The best method for determining the adequacy of hemodialysis is urea kinetic modeling, a dimensionless formula that determines the fractional urea clearance per treatment normalized to the volume of urea distribution. K is the dialyzer clearance, t is the time (duration) of dialysis therapy, and V is the volume of distribution of urea, which is approximately equal to the total body water. When supplied with simple clinical information (predialysis and postdialysis weights, ultrafiltration volume, hematocrit, and predialysis and postdialysis BUN, as well as the dialyzer clearance), computer software programs perform the calculation. Guidelines recommend a single pool Kt/V greater than 1.2 to minimize uremic complications and hospitalizations. Increasing the chronic dose of dialysis beyond a Kt/V of 1.4 does not appear to increase survival,[3] but chronic hemodialysis six times per week generally improves outcomes compared with conventional hemodialysis three times per week.[4] Similarly, nocturnal hemodialysis, performed six or seven nights a week at home for 6 to 8 hours, improves solute clearance, controls serum phosphate, and provides excellent blood pressure control with a reduction in medication requirements.[5] It also can improve kidney-specific measures of quality of life.[6] A family member can help perform the treatment, or the patient can be monitored at a central station through closed-circuit television. This intensive dialysis modality may be a bridge to transplantation or a long-term option when the patient is not a transplantation candidate.

Continuous Renal Replacement Therapy

Critically ill patients with renal failure are frequently hemodynamically unstable, are hypercatabolic (e.g., sepsis, severe burns, brain injury, liver failure, trauma), and require large amounts of fluids (e.g., nutrition, antibiotics). Standard hemodialysis may be complicated by hypotension, in part owing to rapid fluid and solute removal. Slow, low-efficiency hemodialysis performed with low blood flows for 6 to 8 hours daily is one alternative for unstable dialysis patients with renal failure. However, patients with liver failure, traumatic brain injury, or coma do not tolerate the rapid osmolarity changes produced by hemodialysis, which can cause severe brain edema and herniation. In contrast, during CVVH, the rate of fluid removal through venovenous filtration is slower, and solute clearance relies on convection (solvent drag) rather than diffusion, which does not cause such acute changes in osmolarity.

CVVH requires central venous access (double-lumen catheter) and blood flows between 150 and 200 mL/minute. Blood under pressure passes down one side of a highly permeable membrane, thereby allowing both water and solutes up to a molecular weight of about 60 kD to pass across the membrane. In contrast to hemodialysis, urea, creatinine, and phosphate are cleared at similar rates (convective clearance) during hemofiltration. The filtrate is discarded, and the fluid lost is partially replaced with a solution containing the major crystalloid components of the plasma at physiologic levels. However, if further clearance is needed in highly catabolic patients, diffusive dialysis (CVVH) can be added by passing dialysis solution through the dialysate compartment.

Heparin anticoagulation (500 to 1000 U/hour) is usually required to maintain the patency of the CVVH circuit, except in patients who are at high risk for bleeding. An effective method of regional anticoagulation is the use of a calcium-free citrate replacement fluid administered in a separate central line before filtration; citrate chelates calcium in the blood, thereby preventing clotting of the hemofilter. If the patient cannot metabolize citrate, usually because of liver failure, an anion gap metabolic acidosis will develop. The presence of a low ionized calcium and a high total calcium level also is a clue indicating citrate toxicity. Patients who have liver failure and contraindications to heparin often can tolerate CVVH without anticoagulation using bicarbonate-containing replacement solution.

Presently, there is no evidence from randomized trials that demonstrates that CVVH offers a survival advantage compared with intermittent hemodialysis in patients with acute renal failure, despite the advantages of CVVH in enabling the removal of large amounts of fluid with improved hemodynamic stability and excellent metabolic and acid-base control. Increasing the dose of CVVH (ultrafiltration rates of >35 mL/kg/hour versus 25 mL/kg/hour) does not improve survival in critically ill patients with acute renal failure. 7.8

PERITONEAL DIALYSIS

Approximately 10% of patients with ESRD in the United States and more than 50% of those in the United Kingdom, Mexico, Canada, and Australia receive continuous ambulatory peritoneal dialysis (CAPD), which provides survival rates comparable to those of hemodialysis, when adjusted for patient age and comorbid conditions. CAPD obviates the need for vascular access, which is a major challenge in diabetic patients, young children, and patients with severe vascular disease. Moreover, peritoneal dialysis can be performed without anticoagulation, thereby decreasing the possible risk for bleeding. Because peritoneal dialysis is a slow, continuous process, it avoids the marked hemodynamic and osmotic shifts associated with hemodialysis. Patients can be taught to do the procedure at home, thereby giving them a sense of control and independence. Also, peritoneal dialysis enables greater liberalization of diet with respect to salt, potassium, protein, and fluid. Peritoneal dialysis, when feasible, is the treatment modality of choice in children because it avoids frequent needle sticks, and, most importantly, allows children to grow.

Performing Peritoneal Dialysis

Peritoneal dialysis uses the patient's own peritoneal membrane for removal of waste products and fluid (Fig. 133-2). During chronic peritoneal dialysis in an adult, 2 to 3 L of dialysate solution containing electrolytes in physiologic concentrations (to correct acid-base and electrolyte disturbances) and varying concentrations of glucose are infused into the peritoneal cavity through a peritoneal catheter. After a specified dwell time varying between 3 and 6 hours per exchange, the fluid is drained, and the process is repeated. The removal of solute from the body, which depends on a concentration gradient between the blood and peritoneal fluid, occurs by diffusion across the peritoneal membrane. Osmotic ultrafiltration is achieved by the addition of increasing concentrations of glucose to the dialysate solution. The osmotic pressure generated by the glucose draws water from the extracellular fluid and the tissues into the peritoneal fluid. However, the net ultrafiltration rate decreases during the exchange, because of glucose absorption.

In peritoneal dialysis, membrane characteristics vary from one individual to another. The peritoneal equilibration test (PET) is a semiquantitative clinical test commonly used to characterize the transport functions of the peritoneal membrane. The standardized PET procedure consists of a 4-hour dwell using 2 L of 2.5% glucose-containing dialysate solution; equilibration ratios are then determined between plasma and dialysate for creatinine at 0, 2, and 4 hours. The PET also enables measurement of net fluid removal by examining the ratio of dialysate glucose at 4 hours to dialysate glucose at time zero.

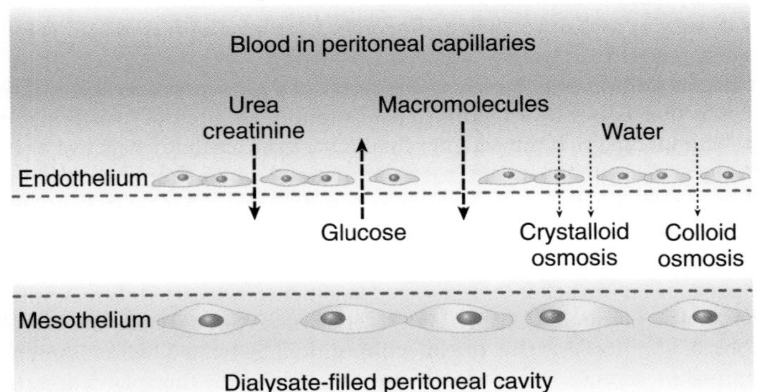

FIGURE 133-2. Solute and water transport in peritoneal dialysis. Various pore systems in the vascular wall. The small interendothelial pores are involved in the transport of low-molecular-weight solutes and in water transport. Large pores allow the passage of macromolecules. Crystalloid osmosis induces water transport partly across the small pores, but also through ultrasmall transcellular water channels. Colloid osmosis induces fluid transport only across the small pore system. The mesothelium is not an osmotic barrier. (From Andreucci VE, Fine LG. *International Yearbook of Nephrology*, 1997. Oxford, UK: Oxford University Press; 1998.)

Patients who have a high dialysate-to-plasma creatinine ratio and achieve rapid equilibration of creatinine and urea across the peritoneal membrane tend to lose their osmotic gradient for fluid removal. Therefore, high or rapid transporters tend to have excellent solute clearance but have difficulty with ultrafiltration. They do well with frequent exchanges and short dwell times that can be achieved with the automated cycler machine, commonly at night while the patient sleeps.

Patients who have low dialysate-to-plasma ratios for creatinine and urea tend to do best with long dwells and high volumes of dialysate to maximize diffusion. These patients usually have excellent ultrafiltration and excellent fluid removal.

Peritoneal Dialysis Dose

Clearance of small solutes is a key predictor of survival in patients undergoing peritoneal dialysis, and residual renal function also plays a critical role. Current guidelines advocate a minimal target Kt/V urea of at least 1.7 per week. Every effort should be made to maintain residual renal function as long as possible by avoiding nephrotoxins such as nonsteroidal anti-inflammatory drugs, iodinated contrast agents, and aminoglycosides. As residual renal function diminishes over time, the peritoneal dialysis prescription needs to be adjusted accordingly.

Complications

Infection

Infection remains the most common problem in patients undergoing CAPD, and it represents the most frequent cause for catheter removal and discontinuation of therapy. Infection can occur at the exit site, with purulent or bloody drainage, erythema, tenderness, or induration; around the subcutaneous tunnel of the catheter, with redness, swelling, or tenderness; or in the peritoneal cavity (peritonitis). The diagnosis of peritonitis should be entertained if a patient presents with abdominal pain and cloudy dialysate; patients frequently have fever, nausea, and vomiting. Abdominal tenderness, often with rebound, is frequently found on physical examination. The major diagnostic criterion is the cell count in the peritoneal fluid. Patients with peritonitis typically show a white blood cell count higher than 100/mm^3 with a predominance of neutrophils. Lymphocytes may predominate with fungal or mycobacterial infections. Prompt recognition and treatment are critical to avoid relapsing or refractory infections that require catheter removal.

For exit site and tunnel infections, *Staphylococcus aureus* is the most common responsible organism. Initial empirical oral or intravenous therapy therefore should cover gram-positive organisms. Oral penicillinase-resistant penicillins (e.g., dicloxacillin, 250 to 500 mg twice daily for 14 days), fluoroquinolones (e.g., ciprofloxacin, 250 to 500 mg twice daily for 14 days), trimethoprim-sulfamethoxazole (e.g., 40/800 mg for 14 days), or cephalosporins (e.g., cephalexin, 500 mg twice daily for 14 days) are recommended. Vancomycin should be avoided as first-line therapy except for methicillin-resistant *S. aureus*. *S. aureus* nasal carriage is a recognized risk factor for exit site and tunnel infections. Mupirocin nasal ointment used twice daily for 5 days every 4 weeks, or mupirocin ointment applied to the exit site, significantly reduces the incidence of *S. aureus* exit site infections.

In patients with peritonitis, *Staphylococcus epidermidis* (Chapter 296) is the most common organism, usually the result of contamination, such as in the introduction of skin bacteria due to breaks in sterile technique. The introduction of disconnect systems has led to a reduction in the overall rate of *S. epidermidis* peritonitis. *Pseudomonas* species infection (Chapter 314) accounts for 5 to 8% of the episodes of CAPD peritonitis; it is often difficult to eradicate because of the development of a biofilm on the catheter, and the catheter often needs to be removed. Fungal infections are extremely difficult to eradicate despite appropriate antifungal therapy because of the development of biofilm, so many institutions remove the peritoneal dialysis catheter as soon as the diagnosis of fungal peritonitis is made.

Another major cause of peritonitis (Chapter 144) is intra-abdominal pathology such as a perforated diverticulum (Chapter 144), ruptured appendix (Chapter 144), ischemic bowel (Chapter 145), incarcerated hernia (Chapter 144), pancreatitis (Chapter 146), or gynecologic conditions (Chapters 205, 243, and 244). The major diagnostic clue is the presence of polymicrobial enteric organisms on culture, particularly the presence of anaerobic organisms in the dialysate. An abdominal computed tomography

(CT) scan may help identify the anatomic site of the lesion. Although free air may be seen in asymptomatic patients undergoing peritoneal dialysis, the presence of free air should raise the possibility of a perforated viscus, which requires emergency surgery.

For the treatment of CAPD-related peritonitis, current guidelines recommend intravenous or intraperitoneal vancomycin (e.g., 1 g every 5 to 7 days, as guided by serum levels, for at least 2 weeks) or a cephalosporin (e.g., cefazolin, 15 mg/kg in one exchange per day) together with intravenous or intraperitoneal administration of a third-generation cephalosporin with antipseudomonal activity (e.g., ceftazidime, 1 to 1.5 g in one exchange per day) or gentamicin (0.6 mg/kg in one exchange per day or 80 mg IV) as initial empirical therapy. Once culture and sensitivities results are available, the antibiotic prescription should be tailored to avoid gentamicin, if possible, to preserve residual renal function. Therapy should be continued for at least 2 weeks.

Other Complications

Mechanical problems of CAPD include catheter malfunction owing to omental wraps and blood or fibrin clots in the catheter lumen, catheter migration, and abdominal hernias caused by increased intra-abdominal pressure with large volumes of dialysate. Metabolic complications include hyperglycemia and hypertriglyceridemia from high glucose loads, weight gain, and protein loss, especially during an episode of peritonitis. Because peritoneal dialysis requires daily multiple exchanges, it is essential to assess for compliance on an ongoing basis and to ensure that the patient has an adequate support system to avoid "burnout."

The high glucose concentration of the standard CAPD dialysate not only contributes to metabolic abnormalities but also inhibits the function of leukocytes and affects the long-term function of the peritoneal membrane. A dialysate that contains 7.5% icodextrin is a safe and effective substitute for hypertonic glucose and is effective in patients with ultrafiltration failure. This alternative may decrease the metabolic consequences of long-term glucose use and help preserve peritoneal membrane function.

PROGNOSIS

Although dialysis acutely prevents death from uremic complications, the mortality rate among patients undergoing chronic dialysis therapy remains high, at about 20% per year in the United States. Age and comorbid conditions such as diabetes, cardiovascular disease, nutritional status, and infection all contribute significantly to the high mortality in this population.

RENAL TRANSPLANTATION

Successful renal transplantation offers patients the best quality of life. They are liberated from potassium and fluid restrictions, are free to travel and work, and achieve correction of metabolic abnormalities and anemia with restoration of normal renal function. Moreover, in comparison with hemodialysis, renal transplantation also improves long-term survival in both diabetic and nondiabetic patients.

Because renal transplantation offers patients the best chance for quality as well as quantity of life, it is essential to evaluate candidates early and, if possible, proceed directly to preemptive transplantation if a living donor can be identified. The ideal form of renal transplantation for patients with type 1 diabetes mellitus (Chapter 236) and nephropathy is from a living related donor, followed by pancreas or islet cell transplantation from a deceased donor. If a living donor is unavailable, simultaneous pancreas and kidney transplantation should be pursued from a deceased donor. Although successful pancreas transplantation does not reverse the established macrovascular and microvascular complications of long-standing diabetes mellitus, it improves blood glucose control and quality of life and may prevent the progression of retinopathy and autonomic neuropathy. Islet cell transplantation after renal transplantation is presently under investigation.

Pretransplantation Evaluation of the Recipient

The potential renal transplant recipient must have irreversible ESRD and no evidence of active infection or malignancy. In addition to a careful history and physical examination, the evaluation must address the likelihood of compliance and exclude unmanageable patients with psychosis, substance abuse, or alcohol abuse.

Systemic Diseases

A careful cardiovascular evaluation is critical, including stress testing with imaging (Chapters 56 and 71) and a coronary angiogram if any evidence of ischemia is demonstrated, particularly in diabetic patients. In view of the increasing recognition of calcific aortic stenosis (Chapter 75) and hypertension in patients with ESRD, an echocardiogram (Chapter 55) should be obtained to assess valve area as well as systolic and diastolic function.

Likewise, a careful evaluation of carotid and peripheral vessels should be undertaken because the new kidney will be anastomosed to the iliac vessels. The new kidney's ureter may be implanted into the recipient's bladder, or the patient's own ureter may be used. Further urologic testing may be needed if a neurogenic bladder is suspected or if there is a history of obstructive uropathy (Chapter 125). Bilateral nephrectomies are required if there is persistent, smoldering infection unresponsive to chronic suppressive antimicrobial therapy or there is severe polycystic kidney disease.

It is recommended that patients with Goodpasture's syndrome (Chapter 123), systemic lupus erythematosus (Chapter 274), or antineutrophil cytoplasmic antibody–positive vasculitis (Chapter 278) become clinically and serologically quiescent before transplantation. A number of primary glomerular diseases (Chapter 123) have been shown to recur in the renal allograft, including focal segmental glomerulosclerosis, membranous glomerulonephritis, membranoproliferative glomerulonephritis, and immunoglobulin A (IgA) nephropathy. Diabetic nephropathy also may recur after transplantation and can be prevented by combined kidney-pancreas transplantation. Combined kidney-liver transplantation can cure oxalosis (Chapter 212).

Infectious Diseases

Serologic determination of human immunodeficiency virus (HIV; Chapter 394) and hepatitis B and C virus infection (Chapter 151) status should be obtained. In this era of highly active antiretroviral therapy, HIV positivity is no longer an absolute contraindication to transplantation. Although patients with hepatitis C do better with renal transplantation than dialysis, with time liver failure is the major cause of morbidity and mortality. It is therefore critical to stage patients with hepatitis C before transplantation, by means of liver biopsy, viral load determination, measurement of the α-fetoprotein level, and a CT scan looking for hepatocellular carcinoma (Chapter 202) and portal hypertension (Chapter 157). The possibility of a combined kidney and liver transplantation needs to be explored. Combined therapy with pegylated interferon and ribavirin may be indicated after transplantation but requires cautious monitoring and usually is not well tolerated. Post-transplantation interferon therapy may trigger allograft rejection, possibly by upregulation of genes for the major histocompatibility complex and various cytokines. Severe hemolytic anemia may occur with ribavirin administration and should be avoided in dialysis patients.

All patients waiting for renal transplantation should be vaccinated against hepatitis B, although the response rate appears to be less than 50%. If a patient is positive for hepatitis B surface antigen, a DNA viral load determination and liver biopsy should be obtained for staging. Lamivudine or entecavir therapy may be initiated either before or after transplantation. Once again, if there is significant cirrhosis (Chapter 156), consideration should be given to combined kidney-liver transplantation.

Patients with a newly positive purified protein derivative (PPD) skin test (Chapter 332) should ideally be treated before transplantation. A patient with positive PPD and negative chest radiograph before transplantation may be closely monitored. If the patient has a positive PPD and a history of previous disease or a positive chest radiograph, treatment with isoniazid is indicated starting 1 to 2 months after transplantation.

Patients also should be evaluated for previous exposure to varicella. If the varicella titer is negative before transplantation, an attempt at vaccination may be undertaken. If the patient remains varicella antibody negative or has not been vaccinated, varicella-zoster immune globulin should be given on exposure to patients with chickenpox or herpes zoster (Chapter 383) because the immunosuppressed host is at risk for fulminant varicella with pulmonary infiltrates, pancreatitis, and liver disease.

Special attention needs to be directed to patients from tropical areas, where *Strongyloides stercoralis* (Chapter 365) is endemic. A *Strongyloides* titer should be obtained; if it is positive, the infection should be treated before immunosuppression because fulminant disease can occur after transplantation. If a patient comes from an area where schistosomiasis (Chapter 363) is endemic, diagnosis and treatment should be initiated before transplantation.

Identifying Donors

Living Donors

The demand for deceased donors far exceeds the supply of organs, and the waiting list for cadaver renal transplants is now 4 to 5 years in all blood groups throughout most of the United States. As a result, living organ donation

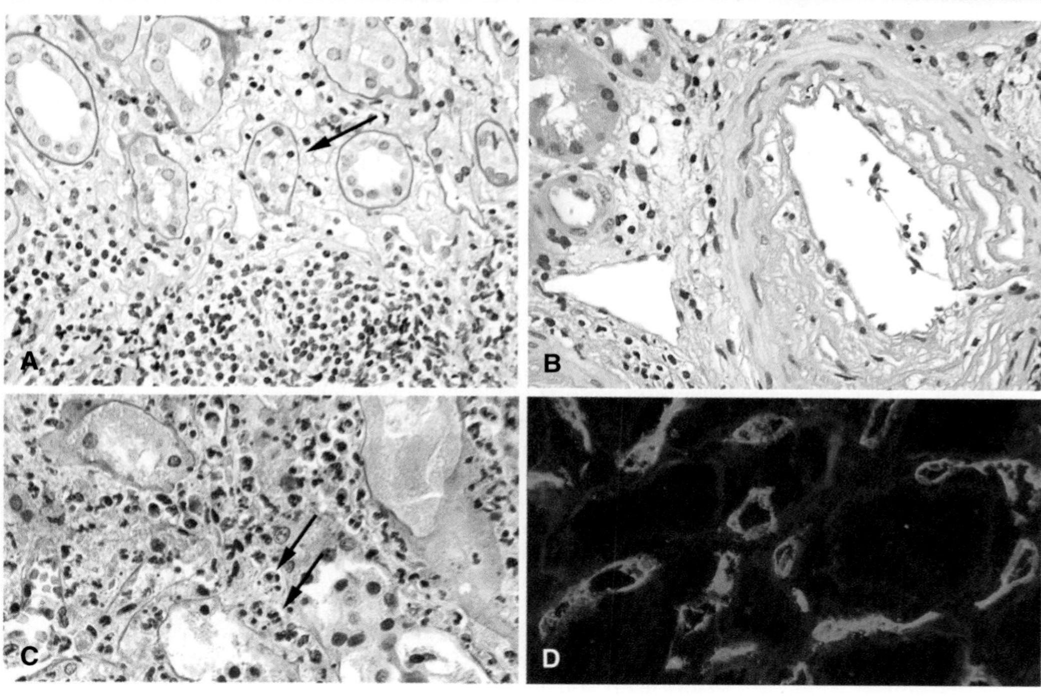

FIGURE 133-3. **Histology of renal allograft with acute cellular rejection (A and B) and acute humoral rejection (C and D). A,** Interstitial mononuclear infiltrate. The *arrow* points to an area with tubulitis. **B,** Arteritis. Note the accumulation of inflammatory cells beneath the intima, which is characteristic of acute cellular rejection type 2 (Banff classification). **C,** Acute humoral rejection. The peritubular space is occupied by an inflammatory infiltrate with the presence of polymorphonuclear neutrophils *(arrows)*. **D,** Positive C4d staining in the peritubular capillaries by immunofluorescence, a hallmark of humoral rejection.

accounts for more than 50% of the transplantations now being performed. Living donation is generally safe, and both the short- and long-term outcomes for the recipient are better with a living donor. Results from a living unrelated donor transplant are equivalent to a one-haplotype parental match, with a 1-year graft survival rate of 92%, thereby suggesting that the quality of the organ is as important as or more important than the closeness of the genetic "match." Donors require a complete medical examination and a psychological evaluation by physicians and psychiatrists independent of the recipient to ascertain their health and the voluntary, altruistic nature of the donor's decision.

For the donor, the immediate risk of surgery is a mortality rate of 0.05%, in addition to the pain, time out of work, and possibility of phlebitis or pulmonary embolus, urinary tract infection, wound infection, or pneumonia. Laparoscopic donor nephrectomy in carefully selected patients allows for a faster recovery and more rapid return to work.

The long-term risks of having one kidney include the slightly increased risk of proteinuria, chance of trauma, and development of cancer in the one remaining kidney. Although isolated cases of chronic renal failure have been reported after donation, for the most part long-term mortality is not affected by kidney donation. Nevertheless, all donors must be carefully monitored long term.

Deceased Donors

The shortage of deceased organs for transplantation has led to the increased use of kidneys from donors older than 55 years of age or with a history of hypertension or cerebrovascular accident. In these situations, a donor kidney biopsy is performed to assess the degree of fibrosis, sclerosis, and vascular disease; if deemed appropriate, these kidneys are then offered with informed consent to older potential recipients or patients with multiple access problems. Although there may be a 10% difference in survival between these kidneys and standard deceased donor kidneys at 3 years, the potential benefit to the recipient is the opportunity to terminate dialysis without waiting on the list for 4 years or longer.

Another alternative is the use of organs from donors who die from traditional cardiac death, known as donation after cardiac death donors. Once the patient's family and the attending physician have decided that life support will be discontinued, the patient is taken to the operating room, the ventilator is discontinued, and cardiac arrest occurs. The patient is pronounced dead only after all signs of respiration have ceased. Patient and graft survival rates are not statistically different from rates with traditional brain death donors.

Tissue Typing

A key element in the evaluation for transplantation is tissue typing. The recipient must receive a transplant from a blood group–compatible donor to avoid hyperacute rejection and immediate irreversible graft loss on the operating table. The donor and recipient need not share the same Rh factor.

HLA typing is performed on all potential recipients and donors. It is critical to determine the recipient's sensitization (i.e., the level of preformed HLA antibodies in the serum of the recipient). These antibodies typically result from previous transplantations, pregnancies, or blood transfusions. The critical test before renal transplantation is the final crossmatch: a complement-dependent cytotoxicity assay performed using the cells of the donor and serum of the recipient. If the crossmatch is positive, the transplantation should not be performed. Another option to increase the availability of organs is the donor exchange program, whereby an incompatible live donor-recipient pair in one institution finds a compatible match at another institution through computerized matching.

Rejection

Allograft rejection is initiated by the recipient's recognition of donor major histocompatibility complex antigens, thereby leading to activation of humoral and cellular immunity (Chapter 48). *Hyperacute humoral rejection*, which is rare, usually causes immediate irreversible necrosis of the allograft on the operating table. Hyperacute rejection is caused by preformed alloantibodies in the recipient directed against donor HLA or ABO antigens, and this form of antibody-mediated rejection can usually be prevented by careful cross-matching techniques.

The clinical manifestations of *acute cellular rejection* (Fig. 133-3), which can occur any time but are generally seen within the first 3 months, may be minimal with the use of newer immunosuppressive agents but may include fever, allograft swelling and tenderness, or oliguria. The BUN and creatinine concentrations are usually elevated. A Doppler ultrasound study should be performed to exclude obstruction or vascular thrombosis (Chapter 127). The diagnosis of acute rejection can be reliably made only with an allograft biopsy (Table 133-2).

Acute humoral rejection (see Fig. 133-3) usually occurs within the first 3 months but can occur at any time, particularly if the patient is noncompliant with medications. It occurs when the recipient develops de novo donor-reactive cytotoxic antibodies after transplantation (i.e., positive crossmatch after but negative before transplantation). These alloantibodies may be reactive with HLA class I or II antigens. Early detection and treatment of acute humoral rejection with plasmapheresis, pooled human immune globulin (e.g., 0.4 to 0.6 g/kg), and rituximab (e.g., 1 g) in addition to tacrolimus (to maintain a level of 8 to 10), mycophenolate mofetil (e.g., 750 to 1000 mg twice daily), and steroids has led to dramatic reversal of the acute allograft dysfunction in approximately 90% of cases. Protocols using plasma exchange, rituximab, and intravenous immune globulin also have been used before transplantation in an attempt to lower the levels of preformed HLA antibody

TABLE 133-2 DIFFERENTIAL DIAGNOSIS OF RENAL ALLOGRAFT DYSFUNCTION

IMMEDIATE/DELAYED GRAFT FUNCTION (1-3 DAYS)
Acute tubular necrosis
Hyperacute humoral rejection
Urinary leak or obstruction
Renal artery or vein thrombosis
Recurrence of disease (e.g., FSGS)
EARLY POST-TRANSPLANTATION PERIOD (FIRST MONTH)
Acute cellular rejection
Acute humoral rejection
Calcineurin inhibitor toxicity
Urinary tract obstruction
Volume depletion
Recurrence of disease
LATE ACUTE DYSFUNCTION
Acute rejection
Cyclosporine or tacrolimus toxicity
Recurrence of primary disease
Tubulointerstitial nephritis, drug-induced
Renal artery stenosis
Infection (bacterial UTI, cytomegalovirus, BK virus)
Hemodynamic (volume; use of ACEI, AIIRB)
CHRONIC DYSFUNCTION
Chronic rejection
Cyclosporine or tacrolimus toxicity
Recurrent renal disease
De novo renal disease
Urinary tract obstruction
Bacterial UTI
Hypertensive nephrosclerosis

ACEI = angiotensin-converting enzyme inhibitor; AIIRB = angiotensin II receptor blocker; FSGS = focal segmental glomerulosclerosis; UTI = urinary tract infection.

in highly sensitized patients. Such protocols often convert a previously positive crossmatch to a negative one, thus enabling transplantation from a living donor.

Another promising approach to the treatment of acute humoral rejection focuses on the depletion of plasma cells with the proteasome inhibitor bortezomib, which is also used in the treatment of multiple myeloma. Long-term studies are needed to determine whether the successful treatment of acute antibody-mediated rejection and chronic humoral rejection will improve long-term graft survival.

Induction Immunosuppression

The goal of immunosuppression therapy (Chapter 48) is to prevent allograft rejection but still allow the immune system to fight infection and malignancy. The multiagent strategy allows for a synergistic effect and reduction of specific drug toxicity (Fig. 133-4). Immunosuppression is initiated at high doses (induction) during the initial period after transplantation, when the risk of rejection is highest, and is reduced over time (maintenance immunosuppression). In recipients with a high risk of rejection (children, retransplant recipients, delayed graft function, multiparous women, and multitransfused patients), induction immunosuppression is often used, consisting of a course of polyclonal antilymphocyte-antithymocyte globulin (ATG) or antilymphocyte globulin; monoclonal anti-CD3 antibodies (OKT3); or anti-interleukin-2 (anti-IL-2) receptor monoclonal antibodies (basiliximab or daclizumab). Appropriate antiviral prophylaxis is essential to reduce the risk of severe cytomegalovirus (CMV) infection and Epstein-Barr virus (EBV)-associated post-transplantation lymphoproliferative disease (PTLD). Likewise, prophylaxis with trimethoprim-sulfamethoxazole has been effective in preventing urinary tract infections as well as *Pneumocystis jirovecii* infection in these highly immunosuppressed patients.

Polyclonal Antibodies

Polyclonal antibodies are raised in various animals (rabbits, goats, horses) using different antigenic preparations (thymocytes, lymphocytes). The polyclonal antilymphocyte antibodies (1.5 mg/kg for three doses) are used for

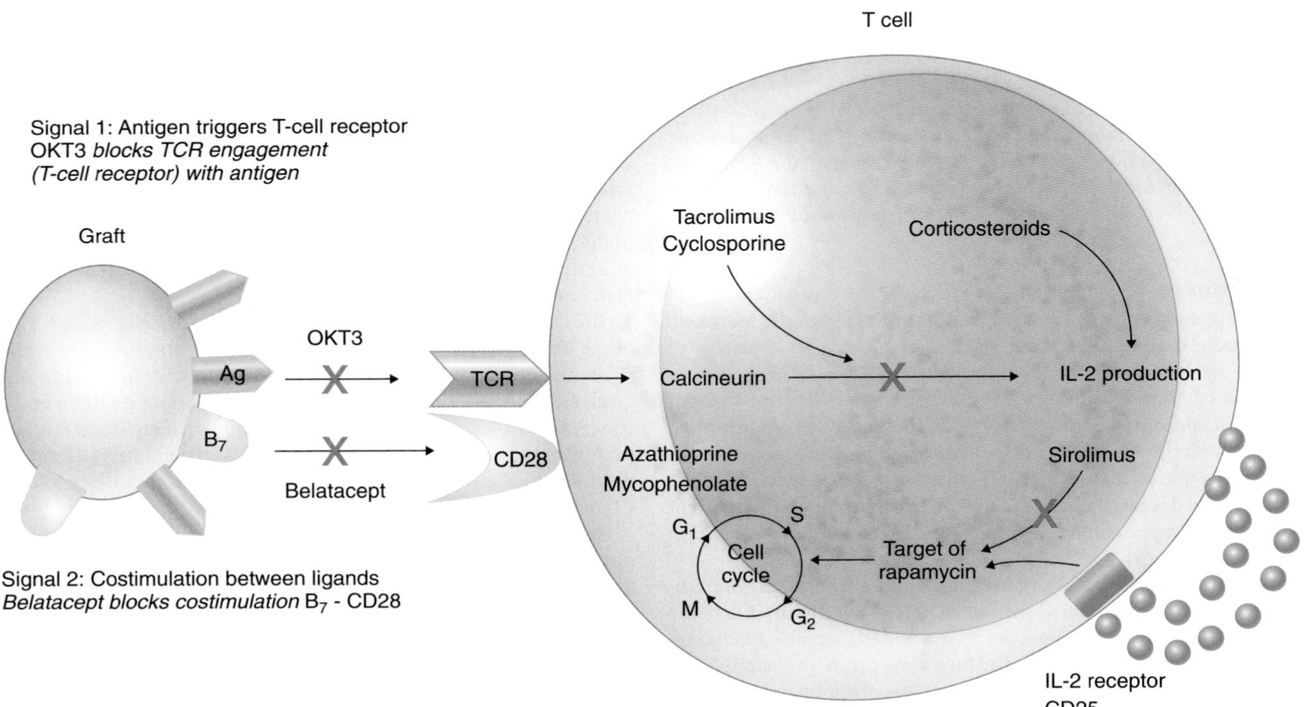

FIGURE 133-4. Targets of immunosuppressive agents. G_1, S, G_2, and M are stages of the cell cycle. Ag = antigen; AZA = azathioprine; B_7 = costimulatory molecule; CsA = cyclosporine; IL = interleukin; MMF = mycophenolate mofetil; SRL = sirolimus; TAC = tacrolimus; TCR = T-cell receptor; TOR = target of rapamycin.

induction therapy in high-risk recipients (i.e., those with high panel-reactive antibodies and those undergoing retransplantation) at the onset of transplantation, for treatment of steroid-resistant acute cellular rejection, and as a calcineurin inhibitor–sparing agent in recipients with delayed graft function. The polyclonal antibodies can cause serum sickness, bone marrow suppression, and hemolysis. The use of these agents also may trigger a potent cytokine response. Most side effects are related either to the degree of purity of the antigenic preparation used to immunize the animals or to the purification of the serum. Serum sickness (Chapter 46) and anaphylactic reactions (Chapter 261) are related to previous exposure to the animal species used to raise the antibody.

OKT3

OKT3, which is a mouse monoclonal antibody directed against the CD3 antigen, is used primarily for treatment of steroid-resistant acute cellular rejection and occasionally as an induction agent. OKT3 can cause myriad side effects, including fever, rigors, nausea, vomiting, diarrhea, severe headache (aseptic meningitis), hypotension, chest pain, dyspnea, wheezing, and, infrequently, pulmonary edema. These symptoms are secondary to massive cytokine release after OKT3 engages the TCR. OKT3 is associated with a higher incidence of severe CMV infections and PTLD, so CMV prophylaxis (Chapter 384) is essential.

Interleukin-2 Receptor Blockers

IL-2 receptor blockers are engineered monoclonal antibodies against the α-chain of the IL-2 receptor. Daclizumab is a humanized molecule consisting of a human IgG1 with antigen-binding regions from a mouse antibody. Basiliximab is a chimeric construct with a murine variable region and human constant regions. Daclizumab and basiliximab are used only as induction agents to prevent rather than treat rejection. They both have a safe side-effect profile, largely because of their human origin.

New Agents

Alemtuzumab is an anti-CD52 monoclonal antibody used as an induction agent at the time of transplantation. Alemtuzumab appears to facilitate minimization of maintenance immunosuppressive protocols (with either sirolimus or low-dose tacrolimus). The dose and frequency of administration remain to be determined.

Maintenance Immunosuppression

Many immunosuppressive agents are available for prevention of rejection in the maintenance phase (Table 133-3). Common regimens consist of low-dose steroids, mycophenolate mofetil, or azathioprine plus a calcineurin inhibitor (either cyclosporine or tacrolimus). Corticosteroids (Chapter 34), which have nonspecific immunosuppressive and anti-inflammatory actions, are used for induction therapy, for maintenance immunosuppression, and in high doses (pulse) for the treatment of acute cellular rejection. Corticosteroids cause many metabolic changes, including diabetes, hypercholesterolemia, osteoporosis, increased risk of cardiovascular events, obesity, and hypertension, and they can cause significant mood swings, irritability, and depression.

The calcineurin inhibitors cyclosporine and tacrolimus inhibit the translocation of nuclear factor of activated T lymphocyte (NFAT) from the cytoplasm to the nucleus. Cyclosporine and tacrolimus levels must be closely monitored to avoid toxicity as well as rejection. The most important nonimmune toxicity of the calcineurin inhibitors is nephrotoxicity, with three distinct patterns. First is an acute hemodynamic effect, which is caused by afferent arteriolar constriction and which may exacerbate ischemic injury and delay graft function, with a reversible decrease in the glomerular filtration rate that improves when the dose of the drug is adjusted. Second is subacute to chronic nephrotoxicity, which may be evidenced by tubular lesions, hyalinosis of small arterioles, or striped fibrosis in the more chronic phase. Third is a thrombotic microangiopathy, which can present a picture similar to the hemolytic-uremic syndrome (Chapter 175) with intimal proliferation, fibrin deposition, and thrombotic occlusion of the arcuate and intralobular arteries. The peripheral smear may show evidence of schistocytes, and thrombocytopenia may or may not be present. Switching from cyclosporine to tacrolimus or vice versa sometimes may be beneficial. Other side effects of the calcineurin inhibitors include neurotoxicity (tremors, mental status changes, irritability, and seizures), hypertension, hyperglycemia, hyperkalemia, hyperuricemia, gout, and an increased incidence of EBV-related B-cell lymphomas (PTLD). Both cyclosporine and tacrolimus are metabolized by the cytochrome P-450 system and excreted by the liver. Therefore, drugs that interact with the P-450 system, such as macrolide antibiotics, diltiazem, imidazole, and triazole antifungals may raise the levels of calcineurin inhibitors. In contrast, agents such as rifampin, phenobarbital, and phenytoin that induce cytochrome P-450 enzymes increase the catabolism of calcineurin inhibitors. Many other significant interactions need to be recognized, including the risk of rhabdomyolysis with statins and interaction with most nephrotoxic agents.

Azathioprine, which was a cornerstone of transplant immunosuppression until the introduction of mycophenolate mofetil, is still useful. Azathioprine inhibits DNA synthesis; its main side effect is bone marrow suppression (see Table 133-3). Azathioprine has also been associated with malignancies, especially skin cancers, and papillomavirus infection. Azathioprine is metabolized by xanthine oxidase, so concomitant administration of allopurinol, a xanthine oxidase inhibitor, should be avoided because significant bone marrow toxicity may occur.

Mycophenolate mofetil, which selectively inhibits lymphocyte proliferation (see Table 133-3), reduces the incidence of acute cellular rejection by 50% and allows for a significant reduction in the use of OKT3/ATG. Gastrointestinal symptoms (e.g., nausea, epigastric discomfort, diarrhea) are the main side effects and usually can be improved by dose reduction. The effect of mycophenolate mofetil on the prevention of chronic rejection is currently under study.

Sirolimus binds to the same immunophilin as tacrolimus but does not affect calcineurin activity (see Table 133-3). Inhibition of mTOR by sirolimus suppresses alloantigen and cytokine-driven T-cell proliferation when it inhibits the cell cycle. Regimens using sirolimus have reduce the incidence of acute cellular rejection. Sirolimus causes hyperlipidemia and also is associated with thrombocytopenia. Sirolimus also interacts with calcineurin inhibitors and may cause an increase in calcineurin inhibitor toxicity.

TABLE 133-3 IMMUNOSUPPRESSIVE AGENTS

AGENT	MECHANISM OF ACTION	SIDE EFFECTS
Corticosteroids	Multiple anti-inflammatory actions, blockade of IL-1, IL-6, TNF-α	Infection, hypertension, glucose resistance, osteoporosis, hyperlipidemia, glaucoma, adrenal suppression
Azathioprine	Blockade of purine synthesis, which affects DNA and RNA synthesis	Bone marrow suppression
Cyclosporine	Binds to cyclophilin, causing calcineurin inhibition, which prevents NFAT activity on IL-2 gene; stimulates production of TGF-β	Hypertension, glucose intolerance, nephrotoxicity, hirsutism, gingival hyperplasia
Tacrolimus	Binds to FKBP-12, causing calcineurin inhibition, which prevents NFAT activity on IL-2 gene	Neurotoxicity, increased incidence of diabetes mellitus (≈20%)
Mycophenolate mofetil	Blocks de novo pathway of purine synthesis by inhibition of IMPDH, selective for lymphocytes	Gastrointestinal symptoms (diarrhea), leukopenia
Sirolimus	Binds to FKBP-12 and mTOR, blocking cell cycle progression	Hyperlipidemia, leukopenia, thrombocytopenia, impaired wound healing

FKBP-12 = FK506-binding protein 12; IL = interleukin; IMPDH = inosine monophosphate dehydrogenase; NFAT = nuclear factor of activated T lymphocyte; TGF-β = transforming growth factor-β; TNF-α = tumor necrosis factor-α; mTOR = mammalian target of rapamycin.

PROGNOSIS

Since 1975, the 1-year deceased donor kidney survival rate has dramatically improved, from approximately 50% to 90% in 2010. The 1-year allograft survival for kidneys from living donors has increased from 88 to 93%. The acute rejection rates are only about 11% with new immunosuppressive regimens, and 1-year allograft survival rates have improved. However, the initial projected long-term improvement in the survival of grafts from living as well as deceased donors has not been realized.

Patients benefit from aggressive control of coronary risk factors because coronary disease is a major cause of death in these patients (Chapters 51 and 73). The ultimate goal of transplantation is tolerance to donor antigens while maintaining the ability to respond to third-party antigens in the absence of ongoing immunosuppression. The induction of mixed hematopoietic chimerism, using nonmyeloablative conditioning, has been successfully accomplished in rodents, miniature swine, and nonhuman primates. These observations now are being extended to patients with multiple myeloma and ESRD.

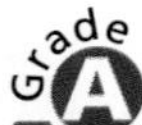

1. Cooper BA, Branley P, Bulfone L, et al. A randomized, controlled trial of early versus late initiation of dialysis. *N Engl J Med.* 2010;363:609-619.
2. Singh AK, Szczech L, Tang KL, et al. Correction of anemia with epoetin alfa in chronic kidney disease. *N Engl J Med.* 2006;355:2085-2098.
3. Eknoyan G, Beck GJ, Cheung AK, et al. Effect of dialysis dose and membrane flux in maintenance hemodialysis. *N Engl J Med.* 2002;347:2010-2019.
4. The FNH Trial Group. In-center hemodialysis six times per week versus three times per week. *N Engl J Med.* 2010;363:2287-2300.
5. Culleton BF, Walsh M, Klarenbach SW, et al. Effect of frequent nocturnal hemodialysis vs conventional hemodialysis on left ventricular mass and quality of life: a randomized controlled trial. *JAMA.* 2007;298:1291-1299.
6. Manns BJ, Walsh MW, Culleton BF, et al. Nocturnal hemodialysis does not improve overall measures of quality of life compared to conventional hemodialysis. *Kidney Int.* 2009;75:542-599.
7. Palevsky PM, Zhang JH, O'Connor TZ, et al. for the VA/NIH Acute Renal Failure Trial Network. Intensity of renal support on critically ill patients with acute kidney injury. *N Engl J Med.* 2008;359:7-20.
8. Renal Replacement Study Investigators. Intensity of continuous renal replacement therapy in critically ill patients. *N Engl J Med.* 2009:361:1627-1638.

SUGGESTED READINGS

Gupta G, Unruh ML, Nolin TD, et al. Primary care of the renal transplant patient. *J Gen Intern Med.* 2010;25:731-740. *Review.*

Himmelfarb J, Ikizler TA. Hemodialysis. *N Engl J Med.* 2010;363:1833-1845. *Review.*

Mehrotra R, Chiu YW, Kalantar-Zadeh K, et al. Similar outcomes with hemodialysis and peritoneal dialysis in patients with end-stage renal disease. *Arch Intern Med.* 2011;171:110-118. *Patients who begin treatment with hemodialysis or peritoneal dialysis now have similar outcomes.*

Nankivell BJ, Alexander SI. Rejection of the kidney allograft. *N Engl J Med.* 2010;363:1451-1462. *Comprehensive review.*

http://www.kidney.org/professionals/kdoqi/guidelines.cfm. Accessed Jan. 2010. *Guidelines for the care of patients with end-stage renal failure—anemia, dialysis adequacy, bone metabolism.*

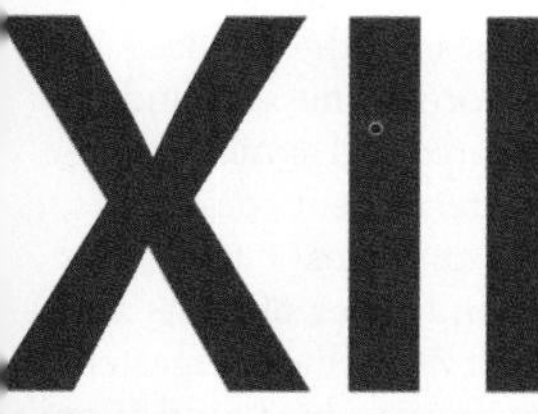

GASTROINTESTINAL DISEASES

134

APPROACH TO THE PATIENT WITH GASTROINTESTINAL DISEASE

KENNETH MCQUAID

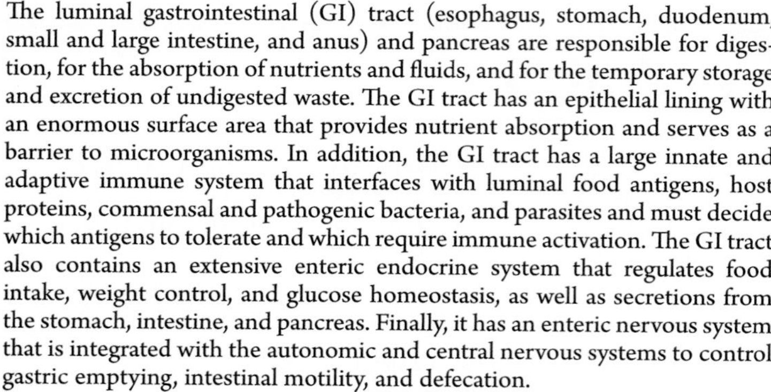

The luminal gastrointestinal (GI) tract (esophagus, stomach, duodenum, small and large intestine, and anus) and pancreas are responsible for digestion, for the absorption of nutrients and fluids, and for the temporary storage and excretion of undigested waste. The GI tract has an epithelial lining with an enormous surface area that provides nutrient absorption and serves as a barrier to microorganisms. In addition, the GI tract has a large innate and adaptive immune system that interfaces with luminal food antigens, host proteins, commensal and pathogenic bacteria, and parasites and must decide which antigens to tolerate and which require immune activation. The GI tract also contains an extensive enteric endocrine system that regulates food intake, weight control, and glucose homeostasis, as well as secretions from the stomach, intestine, and pancreas. Finally, it has an enteric nervous system that is integrated with the autonomic and central nervous systems to control gastric emptying, intestinal motility, and defecation.

Numerous diseases within and outside the GI tract may alter normal function by causing structural damage (erosion, ulceration, perforation, stenosis, or obstruction), bleeding, inflammation, abnormal absorption or secretion of nutrients and electrolytes, or abnormal motility. Despite its anatomic and physiologic complexity, the GI system has only a limited repertoire of symptoms and signs to express conditions that may be either serious or clinically insignificant: abdominal pain, heartburn, regurgitation, dysphagia, odynophagia, dyspepsia, nausea and vomiting, gas and bloating, weight loss, diarrhea, constipation, overt or occult gastrointestinal bleeding, and incontinence.

GENERAL APPROACH TO PATIENTS WITH GASTROINTESTINAL SIGNS AND SYMPTOMS

An appropriate history and physical evaluation usually can narrow the differential diagnosis of GI complaints. A specific diagnosis can almost always be established thereafter by the judicious use of laboratory, endoscopic, or imaging studies (Table 134-1).

Clinical History

The clinician should elicit the nature of the complaint, including its acuity, severity, location, radiation, duration, pattern (steady vs. colicky; abrupt vs. gradual onset), and relationship to food, meals, and bowel movements. Symptoms that arise from the GI tract are almost always improved or worsened by eating or by bowel movements. For symptoms of recent onset, it is important to elicit recent dietary intake, a medication history, potential exposure to enteric infections or sexually transmitted diseases (Chapter 293), and recent travel. It is also useful to establish whether there are signs or symptoms that suggest a systemic illness, including fever, weight loss, arthralgias, fatigue, weakness, or skin rash.

Most nonsurgical GI diseases manifest with mild to moderate symptoms that develop gradually and do not require immediate attention. Acute symptoms that require urgent assessment are severe abdominal pain and overt GI bleeding (Chapter 137) that manifests by hematemesis, melena, or large-volume hematochezia. Severe or dramatic abdominal pain that develops acutely over minutes to hours requires urgent evaluation to determine whether surgical intervention is required. Severe vomiting or diarrhea with signs of dehydration also warrants urgent attention.

Mild to moderate chronic or intermittent symptoms that have been present for a long period can be evaluated in a deliberate fashion. A substantial proportion of chronic GI complaints have no obvious organic or biochemical basis and ultimately are classified as *functional* GI disorders (Chapter 139). Complaints that have been ongoing for years rarely are attributable to readily remedied structural disorders. In patients with chronic GI symptoms, it is important to elicit and address the current reason for seeking evaluation, which may include concern for underlying serious illness (especially cancer), a change in the character or severity of symptoms, life stressors, or depression. Asking the patient what he or she thinks or fears may provide insights into the proportion of the complaint attributable to these amplifying issues, regardless of whether the problem is functional or structural in origin.

A dietary history (Chapter 221) should be obtained. For acute symptoms of nausea, vomiting, diarrhea, or abdominal pain, intake over the previous 24 to 48 hours should be reviewed for clues to a food-borne illness, including possible exposure to a contaminated food or water source and similar symptoms in other people (Chapter 291). For chronic or intermittent complaints, a recall of meals and types of foods eaten over the previous 1 to 2 days provides insight into eating habits and the amounts and types of fruits and vegetables, whole grains, fiber, protein, fat, and dairy products ingested. A relationship between specific foods and symptoms may be found. For example, pain, flatulence, or diarrhea may be caused by dairy products (lactose intolerance), whole grains, legumes or cruciferous vegetables, or fatty meals (malabsorption), and chronic constipation may be due to a low-fiber diet. Recent and long-term changes in body weight should be elicited. Involuntary loss of greater than 5% of body weight over the prior 12 months is worrisome for serious disease and significant malnutrition (Chapter 222).

The number and consistency of bowel movements should be elicited, and any change in bowel habits must be explored. Signs of acute GI bleeding (melena or hematochezia) or inflammatory colitis (blood, mucus, or pus) should be elicited. Improvement in symptoms after passage of flatus or a bowel movement suggests a disorder of the colon or anorectum.

Past Medical History

The past medical history should be reviewed for conditions that may cause acute or chronic GI symptoms, including endocrine disorders such as diabetes (Chapter 237) or thyroid dysfunction (Chapter 233), cardiovascular diseases such as heart failure (Chapter 58) or peripheral vascular disease (Chapter 81), chronic liver disease and portal hypertension (Chapter 156), neurologic conditions such as Parkinson's disease (Chapter 416) or neuromuscular disorders (Chapter 403), and rheumatologic and collagen vascular disorders (Chapter 264). In addition to their impact on GI tract function, the severity of these conditions must be considered when weighing the risks of diagnostic studies, especially endoscopy. Patients with symptomatic or advanced respiratory insufficiency (Chapter 83), sleep apnea (Chapter 100), valvular heart disease (Chapter 75), coronary artery disease (Chapter 50), heart failure (Chapter 58), cirrhosis (Chapter 156), cerebrovascular disease (Chapter 413), neuromuscular disease (Chapter 430), or dementia (Chapter 409) have an increased risk of sedation-related complications during endoscopy.

A list of prescription and nonprescription medications, vitamins, minerals, and other nutritional supplements should be obtained, paying particular attention to any that were recently initiated or changed. Herbal supplements (Chapter 38) are commonly used but are seldom reported without direct questioning. Medications are potential causes of odynophagia, dyspepsia, nausea or vomiting, abdominal pain, diarrhea, and constipation. The use of antiplatelet agents, including aspirin and anticoagulants, should be determined. The risks of stopping versus continuing these medications must be weighed in patients who have acute or chronic GI bleeding or in whom a therapeutic procedure is to be performed.

Social History

The patient's personal relationships, employment history, quality of life, alcohol intake (Chapter 32), and smoking (Chapter 31) history should be determined. It can be very informative to observe both verbal and nonverbal interactions between the patient and a partner or caregiver during an interview. Alcohol may cause heartburn, dyspepsia, nausea, diarrhea, or chronic liver disease. Many patients are reluctant to disclose the full extent of their alcohol intake on direct questioning; therefore, in addition to asking how often they imbibe (days/week and drinks/day), it may be revealing to inquire about their preferred beverage and how it is purchased (location, volume, and frequency). Cigarette smoking is associated with an increased risk of heartburn, peptic ulcer disease, Crohn's disease, and GI malignancies.

Clinicians should inquire about the degree to which GI symptoms are disrupting a patient's life. GI illness may affect dietary and bowel habits, sleep, and sense of vitality. Concerns about dietary intolerances, inability to eat, inability to have comfortable bowel movements, uncontrolled diarrhea or gas, fecal urgency, or fecal incontinence may affect a patient's social life, personal and sexual relationships, employment, and sense of optimism.

The social history should also be reviewed for recent stressors that may precipitate or exacerbate GI symptoms, including marital or interpersonal discord, personal or family illness, bereavement, financial pressures, job loss, or change in employment. To elicit such information, it may be helpful to tell the patient that stress worsens many conditions and to inquire whether they believe stress may be contributing to their problem.

For elderly, disabled, or marginally housed patients, it is important to elicit how they obtain and prepare their meals and how they access toilet facilities. For patients undergoing GI procedures, it is important to determine whether they have mental, physical, or social barriers that would make it difficult to comply with pre-procedure instructions (including bowel preparation) and whether they have an able-bodied adult who can accompany them to the procedure and observe them at home, if necessary, afterward.

Family History

The family history should be reviewed for GI disorders with a heritable component, especially celiac disease (Chapter 142), inflammatory bowel diseases (Chapter 143), and GI, gynecologic, and genitourinary neoplasms.

Physical Examination

Nonabdominal Examination

The nonabdominal examination should assess nutritional status (Chapter 221) and any signs of systemic conditions that may cause GI symptoms or that must be considered when weighing the risks and benefits of further testing, especially endoscopy. Vital signs should be obtained in all patients. Low-grade fever (<100.5° F) is common in inflammatory conditions, including gastroenteritis, inflammatory bowel disease, appendicitis, cholecystitis, and diverticulitis. High fever (>102° F) suggests sepsis, pelvic, or intra-abdominal infections (e.g., cholangitis, pelvic inflammatory disease, pyelonephritis) or peritonitis. Hemodynamic instability (hypotension or tachycardia) suggests intravascular depletion due to poor oral intake, acute GI or intra-abdominal bleeding, severe diarrhea, or peritonitis. A body mass index less than 18 suggests malnourishment.

A general survey should be performed to assess for signs of weight loss (fat and muscle wasting), malnutrition (dry or thin skin, hair loss, edema, anasarca), and vitamin deficiencies (pellagra, scurvy). Skin lesions may provide clues to systemic conditions such as liver disease (jaundice, spider telangiectasias, palmar erythema), inflammatory bowel disease (erythema nodosum, pyoderma gangrenosum), celiac disease (dermatitis herpetiformis), vasculitis, and rare gastrointestinal malignancies, polyposis syndromes, and pancreatic endocrine tumors (Chapters 198, 199, and 201). An oral examination looks for mucocutaneous candidiasis (which may reflect immunosuppression), ulcerations (which may reflect inflammatory bowel disease, vasculitis, viral infection, or vitamin deficiencies), and glossitis or angular cheilitis (which may reflect vitamin deficiencies). With the exception of supraclavicular lymph nodes, peripheral lymph nodes are uninvolved with GI diseases but should be examined when systemic infection or advanced malignancy is suspected (Chapter 171). Examination of the lungs and cardiovascular system should focus on evidence of conditions that might increase the risk of moderate sedation in the event endoscopy is required (respiratory insufficiency, heart failure) and for conditions that increase the risk of intestinal ischemia (atrial fibrillation, valvular heart disease, peripheral vascular disease) (Chapter 145). The extremities should be evaluated for edema and peripheral pulses. Finally, a brief neurologic assessment should be performed to screen for intracranial mass lesions or other neurologic disorders that may present with GI symptoms.

Abdominal Examination

The abdominal examination begins with a visual inspection of the abdomen and inguinal region for scars (due to prior surgeries or trauma), asymmetry (suggesting a mass or organomegaly), distention (due to obesity, ascites, or intestinal ileus or obstruction), prominent periumbilical veins (suggesting portal hypertension), or hernias (umbilical, ventral, inguinal). The examination proceeds with auscultation followed by percussion, and it ends with light and deep palpation.

In patients *without* abdominal pain, auscultation of bowel sounds to assess intestinal motility has limited usefulness and may be omitted. Percussion may be performed before or in conjunction with light and deep palpation. Initial cursory light percussion across the upper, mid-, and lower abdomen is useful to denote areas of dullness and tympany, as well as to elicit unanticipated areas of pain or tenderness before palpation. More extensive percussion provides limited but useful information about the size of the liver and spleen, gastric or intestinal distention, bladder distention, and ascites (Chapters 148 and 156). Gentle, light palpation promotes abdominal relaxation and allows the detection of muscular resistance (guarding), abdominal tenderness, and superficial masses of the abdominal wall or abdomen. Deeper palpation of the abdominal organs (liver, spleen, kidneys, aorta) and abdominal cavity may detect enlargement or abnormal masses. Superficial or deep masses should be assessed for size, location, mobility, content (solid, liquid, or air), and the presence or absence of tenderness. The consistency of a patient's response to palpation with and without distraction is particularly useful in those with suspected chronic functional abdominal discomfort. Superficial masses include hernias, lymph nodes, subcutaneous abscesses, lipomas, and hematomas. Deep abdominal masses may be caused by neoplasms (liver, gallbladder, pancreas, stomach, intestine, kidney), abscesses (appendicitis, diverticulitis, Crohn's disease), or aortic aneurysms.

Examination of the right upper quadrant should assess the liver size, contour, texture, and tenderness. Liver size is crudely estimated by percussion of the upper and lower borders of liver dullness in the midclavicular line. Liver contour and tenderness are best assessed during held inspiration by deep palpation along the costal margin. Examination of the left upper quadrant is useful to detect splenomegaly (Chapter 171), although a normal-sized or even an enlarged spleen often cannot be detected. Percussion in the left upper quadrant near the tenth rib (posterior to the midaxillary line) may detect splenic dullness that is distinct from gastric or colonic tympany. The tip of an enlarged spleen may be palpated during inspiration if the examiner supports the left costal margin with the left hand while palpating below the costal margin with the right hand. Ascites should be suspected in a patient with a protuberant abdomen and bulging flanks. To screen for ascites, percussion of the flanks should be performed to assess the level of dullness. If the level of flank dullness appears to be increased, the most sensitive test for ascites is to check for "shifting" dullness when the patient rolls from the supine to the lateral position.

Digital Rectal and Pelvic Examinations

The digital rectal examination is intrusive and uncomfortable and should be performed only when necessary, such as in patients with perianal or rectal symptoms, incontinence, difficult defecation, suspected inflammatory bowel disease, and acute abdominal pain. The digital examination, with or without fecal occult blood testing, is not a useful screening test for colorectal cancer (Chapter 199). However, in patients with acute or chronic GI bleeding (Chapter 137), it is a rapid means of assessing the stool for color and occult blood. The perianal area should be visually inspected for rashes, soilage (suggesting incontinence or fistula), fistulas, fissures, skin tags, external hemorrhoids, and prolapsed internal hemorrhoids (Chapter 147). After gentle digital insertion, the anal canal should be assessed for resting tone and voluntary squeeze. The distal rectal vault should be swept circumferentially to palpate for mass lesions, tenderness, or fluctuance.

Laboratory Studies

Blood Tests

Blood tests routinely obtained in the evaluation of patients with GI symptoms include a complete blood count, liver tests (Chapter 149), serum chemistries, and, in selected cases, pancreatic enzymes and markers of inflammation. GI causes of anemia include acute or chronic GI blood loss, inflammatory bowel disease, nutrient malabsorption (folate, iron, or vitamin B_{12}), and chronic liver disease. Microcytosis suggests iron deficiency due to chronic GI blood loss or malabsorption. Macrocytosis may be attributable to folate or B_{12} malabsorption, medications (e.g., immunomodulators used for inflammatory bowel disease), or chronic liver disease. An elevated platelet count suggests chronic inflammation (e.g., inflammatory bowel disease) or GI blood loss with compensatory marrow production. A low platelet count may be attributable to portal hypertension with splenic sequestration. Low serum albumin may be caused by chronic GI disorders that result in weight loss, nutrient malabsorption, chronic inflammation, loss of protein across abnormal GI mucosa (i.e., protein-losing enteropathy), or decreased hepatic synthesis (e.g., chronic liver disease). Abnormal liver tests may be due to acute or chronic liver diseases, disorders of the pancreas or biliary tract, and medications (Chapter 149). Serum amylase and lipase are obtained to screen for pancreatitis (Chapter 146) in patients with acute abdominal pain. Increased levels of inflammatory markers, such as an elevated erythrocyte sedimentation rate and C-reactive protein, are nonspecific but useful in the management of patients with inflammatory bowel disease (Chapter 143).

Serum ferritin reflects total body iron and may be decreased in patients with chronic GI blood loss or intestinal malabsorption (e.g., celiac disease).

TABLE 134-1 APPROACH TO COMMON GASTROINTESTINAL SIGNS AND SYMPTOMS

	ABDOMINAL PAIN	GI BLEEDING	DIARRHEA	STEATORRHEA	CONSTIPATION
History (ascertain the following)	Duration: acute vs. chronic Onset: sudden vs. 1-2 hr vs. gradual Character: visceral (vague or dull, steady or cramping, diffuse) or parietal (severe, well localized, worse with movement) Location: upper, middle, or lower; radiation Associated symptoms: vomiting, hematemesis, diarrhea, hematochezia, melena, constipation, obstipation, jaundice Previous episodes Other diseases	Acute vs. chronic (duration); intermittent vs. continuous; quantity; hematemesis, melena, or hematochezia; associated pain and location; symptoms of anemia (e.g., dyspnea, chest pain, lightheadedness); medication use (especially aspirin, NSAIDs, anticoagulants); previous episodes; risk factors for chronic liver disease (alcohol, hepatitis)	Acute (<2 wk) vs. chronic (duration); fever, weight loss, or abdominal pain; stool character: number per 24 hr, watery or bloody, large vs. small volume, change in volume with eating, greasy; dietary history (especially lactose); history of IBD, pancreatic disease, intestinal surgery, DM; recent change in medications or antibiotic use; community outbreak or similar symptoms in family members; potential exposure to contaminated food; elderly immunosuppressed host; risk of HIV or sexually transmitted disease	Duration; weight loss; stool number, consistency (greasy), presence of blood; abdominal pain; flatulence; history of excessive alcohol, chronic liver disease, pancreatitis, intestinal dysmotility, surgery, DM; history of easy bruising, night blindness, bone pain, osteoporosis, dermatitis herpetiformis	Acute vs. chronic (duration); age; number of stools per wk; difficulty with defecation (straining, incomplete evacuation, digital manipulation); bloating or discomfort; blood on stools, weight loss; dietary fiber and fluid intake; chronic illness (DM, neuromuscular, endocrine); abdominal surgeries; medications, impaired mobility
Physical findings (evaluate for the following)	Fever, HR, BP Appearance: calm, restless, motionless Inspect: skin, distention, hernias Bowel sounds: present, absent, roaring Percussion and palpation: organomegaly, mass (abscess), focal tenderness, guarding Peritoneal signs: sharp pain with cough, shaking, percussion, light palpation	HR, BP, orthostatic findings; abdominal pain present or absent; signs of chronic liver disease and portal hypertension (which may indicate varices); jaundice, spider angiomas, hepatosplenomegaly; ascites; examine nasogastric aspirate for blood ("coffee grounds" vs. bright red); examine stool for blood (Hemoccult) and color (melena, maroon, or bright red)	HR, BP, orthostatic findings; fever; wasting; presence of abdominal tenderness or mass; perianal disease; extraintestinal symptoms of IBD (e.g., oral ulcers, arthritis, erythema nodosum)	Wasting, presence or absence of abdominal mass or tenderness; rash (vitamin deficiencies) or excessive bruising (vitamin K deficiency); jaundice or signs of chronic liver disease	Assess mobility and chronic medical conditions; abdominal distention; palpable stool within bowel in left lower quadrant; rectal examination—impacted stool, anal fissure, rectal prolapse, pelvic floor descent with straining, rectocele
Laboratory tests	CBC, BUN, Cr, glucose, amylase, lipase, liver tests (ALT, AST, bilirubin, alkaline phosphatase), albumin, INR, U/A, urine β-HCG	CBC BUN, Cr, liver tests, INR, type and cross	CBC, BUN, Cr, glucose, electrolytes, liver tests, albumin, C-reactive protein Selected cases: consider serum chromogranin A, VIP, calcitonin, gastrin, glucagon, urinary 5-HIAA; stool for culture, ova, parasites; consider fecal weight, fat, electrolytes, laxative screen	CBC, glucose, liver tests, albumin, electrolytes, celiac disease antibodies (anti-tTG or antiendomysial); assessment of vitamin and mineral absorption (A, D) and INR (K is fat soluble), folate, iron, calcium, phosphate, B_{12}; qualitative or quantitative stool for fecal fat; H_2 breath test for bacterial overgrowth	CBC, Chem-7, calcium, magnesium, phosphate, TFTs; selected patients with severe constipation may undergo colonic transit studies and/or anal manometry with balloon expulsion

NAUSEA AND VOMITING	DYSPHAGIA	ODYNOPHAGIA	HEARTBURN AND REGURGITATION	ANOREXIA	WEIGHT LOSS
Nausea with or without emesis; acute vs. chronic (duration); intermittent vs. constant; presence or absence of severe abdominal pain, comorbid illnesses, especially peptic ulcer, endocrine (DM), cardiac, psychiatric; medications; history of excessive alcohol	Oropharyngeal vs. esophageal dysphagia; solids vs. liquids; acute vs. chronic (duration); intermittent vs. progressive; GERD symptoms present or absent; weight loss; history of food impactions, allergies, atopic conditions, skin changes, cold hands (Raynaud's phenomenon)	Duration of pain with swallowing; underlying immunosuppression (e.g., HIV infection, DM); caustic ingestion; use of medications that cause topical injury (especially NSAIDs, KCl, bisphosphonates, iron, antibiotics, zidovudine)	Duration of symptoms; location; relation to meals or specific foods; nocturnal symptoms; dysphagia or chest pain; extraesophageal manifestations: cough, hoarseness, asthma	Acute vs. chronic (duration); association with different foods; psychiatric disease (e.g., depression, dementia); chronic or undiagnosed medical conditions (e.g., DM, thyroid or adrenal disease, COPD, advanced heart failure, renal insufficiency, malignancy, HIV infection); medication use	Acute vs. chronic (duration); age; total amount (>5% is significant); intentional vs. unintentional; appetite increased or decreased; rapid vs. gradual; change in physical activity; documented vs. undocumented; fever or sweats; anorexia, nausea, vomiting; diarrhea, steatorrhea, blood in stool; abdominal pain; history or symptoms of chronic medical, neurologic, or psychiatric illness; medications; alcohol and substance abuse
Acute with severe abdominal pain: evaluate for GI obstruction, pancreatitis, mesenteric ischemia, biliary colic, appendicitis, or other conditions causing peritonitis Acute without abdominal pain: evaluate for pregnancy, medications, food poisoning, infectious gastroenteritis, hepatitis, CNS disease, postoperative ileus Chronic: evaluate for medications, chronic gastric outlet obstruction (due to ulcer disease or malignancy), impaired GI motility (gastroparesis), other chronic medical conditions, intracranial disorders, psychiatric disease (bulimia)	Usually normal; examine oropharynx and neck for lymphadenopathy and masses; evaluate the skin for sclerodermatous changes	Usually normal; evaluate oropharynx for thrush, herpetic lesions, caustic injury; general exam for signs of underlying immunosuppression	Usually normal, unless extraesophageal manifestations are present	Wasting; fever; signs of bulimia (e.g., loss of tooth enamel, knuckle ulcerations and calluses); abdominal masses; enlarged lymph nodes	Wasting; malnutrition; poor dentition or poorly fitting dentures; thyromegaly; COPD or heart failure; abdominal masses; enlarged lymph nodes; pelvic masses in women; diabetic neuropathy; signs of depression, dementia, or bulimia
β-HCG, CBC, serum electrolytes, BUN, Cr, glucose, HbA_{1c}, liver tests, albumin, TFTs, cortisol	CBC; eosinophilia or elevated IgE in some patients with eosinophilic esophagitis	CBC, HIV test, fasting glucose	Usually normal	CBC, Chem-7, liver tests, albumin, HIV test, TFTs	CBC, Chem-7, HbA_{1c}, TFTs, liver tests, C-reactive protein or ESR, calcium, phosphate, albumin, HIV test, morning cortisol

TABLE 134-1 APPROACH TO COMMON GASTROINTESTINAL SIGNS AND SYMPTOMS—cont'd

	ABDOMINAL PAIN	GI BLEEDING	DIARRHEA	STEATORRHEA	CONSTIPATION
Endoscopy	EGD, colonoscopy	EGD, colonoscopy, enteroscopy, wireless capsule study	Colonoscopy (including ileal inspection) with biopsies; EGD with duodenal biopsies; wireless capsule study	EGD with duodenal biopsies	Colonoscopy if recent change in bowel habits
Imaging	CT scan or ultrasound; angiography; small bowel enterography	Tagged RBC scan, angiography	Small bowel enterography: CT, MRI, or barium (Crohn's disease); somatostatin scintigraphy	CT of the abdomen (pancreatic calcifications; biliary dilation)	Usually not necessary; MRI or defecography

ALT = alanine transaminase; AST = aspartate transaminase; BP = blood pressure; BUN = blood urea nitrogen; CBC = complete blood count; CNS = central nervous system; COPD = chronic obstructive pulmonary disease; Cr = creatinine; CT = computed tomography; DM = diabetes mellitus; EGD = esophagogastroduodenoscopy; ESR = erythrocyte sedimentation rate; GERD = gastroesophageal reflux disease; GI = gastrointestinal; HCG = human chorionic gonadotropin; 5-HIAA = 5-hydroxyindoleacetic acid; HIV = human immunodeficiency virus; HR = heart rate; IBD = inflammatory bowel disease; INR = international normalized ratio; MRI = magnetic resonance imaging; NSAIDs = nonsteroidal anti-inflammatory drugs; RBC = red blood cell; TFTs = thyroid function tests; tTG = tissue transglutaminase; U/A = urinalysis; VIP = vasoactive intestinal polypeptide.

Adapted from Proctor DD. Approach to the patient with gastrointestinal disease. In: Goldman L, Ausiello D, eds. *Cecil Textbook of Medicine*, 23rd ed. Philadelphia: Saunders-Elsevier; 2008.

Disorders of malabsorption that result in steatorrhea may lead to deficiencies in the fat-soluble vitamins (A, D, E, K) (Chapter 142). The serum international normalized ratio may be elevated in patients with cholestasis owing to malabsorption of vitamin K or in patients with chronic liver disease due to decreased hepatic synthetic function. Serum B_{12} may be decreased in patients with autoimmune gastritis (pernicious anemia), gastric bypass surgery, or malabsorption due to small bowel bacterial overgrowth or disease of the terminal ileum (e.g., Crohn's).

Specialized laboratory tests that are useful for the diagnosis of specific diseases include antibodies to *Helicobacter pylori* in patients with peptic ulcer disease or dyspepsia, antibodies to tissue transglutaminase in celiac disease, antibodies to microbial antigens or autoimmune markers in inflammatory bowel disease (anti–*Saccharomyces cerevisiae* [ASCA], perinuclear antineutrophil cytoplasmic antibody [pANCA]), and CA-19-9 in pancreaticobiliary malignancy. Owing to their limited sensitivity and specificity, these tests are not useful for screening but may be helpful in circumscribed situations in which the results may shift the diagnostic probability.

Stool Examination

Fecal occult blood testing is useful to evaluate iron deficiency anemia and acute or chronic GI blood loss. In patients with acute diarrhea, assessment of fecal leukocytes or culture of common pathogens is routine, and in selected patients, testing for parasites (*Giardia, Entamoeba histolytica*), *Clostridium difficile, Escherichia coli* O157:H7, or other specific organisms may be warranted. To distinguish among the causes of chronic diarrhea (Chapter 142), stool samples may be sent for assessment of electrolytes, leukocytes, and fecal fat.

Endoscopy and Radiology

Endoscopy (Chapter 136) and radiographic studies (Chapter 135) play a major role in the evaluation and management of many GI disorders. Esophageal manometry and esophageal pH and impedance monitoring can be useful for the evaluation of heartburn, reflux, and other esophageal symptoms (Chapter 140). Anorectal manometry may be useful in some patients with fecal incontinence and defecatory dysfunction (Chapter 147). Breath tests are commonly used to diagnose *H. pylori* infection (Chapter 141), lactose intolerance, and small bowel bacterial overgrowth (Chapter 142).

The diagnosis of a functional GI disorder is made after organic disorders have been excluded by clinical evaluation and limited, directed diagnostic testing. "Overtesting" should be avoided. Thereafter, the emphasis should switch from finding a "cause" of the symptoms to implementing successful coping and adaptive behaviors.

ABDOMINAL PAIN

Abdominal pain, which is a frequent complaint among outpatients in the office setting and emergency department, may be benign and self-limited or the presenting symptom of severe, life-threatening disease. Chronic abdominal pain that has been present for months or years in the absence of other organic illness is almost always functional in origin and does not require urgent evaluation. By contrast, most patients with severe acute abdominal pain require a thorough but emergent evaluation, which may quickly reveal an acute surgical illness.

PATHOBIOLOGY

Stimulation of hollow abdominal viscera is mediated by splanchnic afferent fibers within the muscle wall, visceral peritoneum, and mesentery that are sensitive to distention and contraction. Visceral afferent nerves are loosely organized, innervate several organs, and enter the spinal cord at several levels. Thus, visceral pain is vague or dull in character and diffuse; patients attempting to localize the pain often move their entire hand over the upper, middle, or lower abdomen. Most visceral pain is steady, but cramping, intermittent pain or "colic" results from peristaltic contractions caused by partial or complete obstruction of the small intestine, ureter, or uterine tubes. In contrast to visceral innervation, the parietal peritoneum is innervated unilaterally by a dense network of nerve fibers that follow a spinal T6 to L1 somatic distribution. Pain fibers of the parietal peritoneum are stimulated by stretch or distention of the abdominal cavity or retroperitoneum; direct irritation from infection, pus, or secretions (e.g., caused by a ruptured viscus); or inflammation caused by contact between the parietal peritoneum and an adjacent inflamed organ (e.g., appendicitis). Parietal pain is sharp, well characterized, and localized by the patient to a precise location on the abdomen, often by pointing with one finger.

The gastrointestinal viscera (liver, biliary system, pancreas, and GI tract) arise during embryology from midline structures that have bilateral innervation. Thus, GI visceral pain is typically localized to the abdominal midline.

Acute Abdominal Pain

CLINICAL MANIFESTATIONS

History

The history should determine the time course, character, and location and radiation pattern of the pain (Table 134-2). Severe abdominal pain that begins suddenly over seconds to minutes indicates a catastrophic event such as esophageal rupture, perforated peptic ulcer or viscus, ruptured ectopic pregnancy, ruptured aortic aneurysm, acute mesenteric ischemia, or myocardial infarction. Pain that progresses within 1 to 2 hours is consistent with a rapidly progressive inflammatory disorder (e.g., cholecystitis, appendicitis, pancreatitis), acute obstruction of a viscus (small intestinal obstruction, ureteral colic), or organ ischemia caused by a strangulated blood supply (volvulus, strangulated hernia, ovarian torsion). Pain that is less severe and develops over several hours is more commonly caused by a medical rather than a surgical condition, including upper GI disorders (dyspepsia), intestinal disorders (gastroenteritis, inflammatory bowel disease), liver disorders (hepatitis, abscess), urinary disorders (cystitis, pyelonephritis), or gynecologic infections; however, the slow evolution of surgical disorders such as cholecystitis (Chapter 158), appendicitis or diverticulitis (Chapter 144), and intra-abdominal abscesses must not be overlooked.

The character of the pain provides important information about whether the symptoms are due to visceral stimulation or parietal stimulation

NAUSEA AND VOMITING	DYSPHAGIA	ODYNOPHAGIA	HEARTBURN AND REGURGITATION	ANOREXIA	WEIGHT LOSS
EGD to exclude gastric outlet obstruction	EGD with biopsies and/or dilation, esophageal motility study, 24-hr pH probe	EGD with biopsies	EGD (to detect erosive esophagitis or Barrett's esophagus); 24-hr pH probe	Directed at detecting underlying disease, e.g., if a GI cause is suspected, EGD and/or colonoscopy with biopsies may be helpful	Directed at detecting underlying disease, e.g., if a GI cause is suspected, EGD and/or colonoscopy with biopsies may be helpful
CT of the abdomen; if chronic, also consider head CT, gastric emptying study, small bowel enterography	Esophagogram (barium swallow) will show stricture, Schatzki's ring, mass, etc.	Usually not necessary	Usually not necessary	Directed at detecting underlying disease, e.g., if a GI cause is suspected, abdominal CT may be helpful	Directed at detecting underlying disease, e.g., chest or abdominal CT may be helpful

(peritonitis). Patients with peritonitis may report severe localized pain or irritation with activities or maneuvers that stretch or move the parietal peritoneum, such as walking, moving in bed, and coughing; as a result, they tend to lie quietly to avoid painful stimulation. By contrast, patients with visceral pain may move or walk restlessly or attempt a bowel movement in an effort to relieve their symptoms.

The location of pain in the upper, middle, or lower abdomen is a crude but important indicator of the diagnosis (Fig. 134-1). Visceral pain arising from the foregut (esophagus, stomach, proximal duodenum, bile duct, gallbladder, pancreas) most often manifests in the epigastrium. Pain derived from the midgut (small intestine, appendix, ascending colon, proximal transverse colon) presents in a periumbilical location. Pain derived from the hindgut (distal transverse colon, left colon, rectum) localizes to the lower midline between the umbilicus and symphysis pubis. Paired intra-abdominal organs such as the kidneys, ureters, ovaries, and fallopian tubes have unilateral innervation that localizes pain to the side of the involved organ. As some surgical conditions progress, the character and location of the pain shift from a visceral to a parietal pain pattern. Thus, early cholecystitis (Chapter 158) may present with vague midline epigastric pain that progresses to sharp right upper quadrant pain as localized peritoneal irritation develops. Likewise, appendicitis (Chapter 144) commonly begins with vague, diffuse periumbilical pain that evolves to sharp, well-localized right lower quadrant pain as peritonitis ensues.

Anorexia, vomiting, diarrhea, distention, and constipation are commonly seen with abdominal pain caused by both medical and surgical disorders. Although nonspecific, the *absence* of any of these symptoms is evidence against an emergent surgical or medical disorder because severe illness usually leads to reflex stimulation or inhibition of gastric and intestinal peristalsis. Vomiting is common in medical and surgical disorders involving the upper GI tract, including acute gastroenteritis, pancreatitis, gastric and small intestinal obstruction, and biliary tract disease. Pain that precedes the onset of vomiting is typical of surgical conditions, whereas the reverse is true of medical conditions (e.g., food poisoning, gastroenteritis). Abdominal pain with prominent diarrhea is most commonly caused by a medical condition (e.g., gastroenteritis, inflammatory bowel disease). Although constipation alone is a nonspecific complaint, the absence of stool passage and flatus is consistent with complete bowel obstruction or paralytic ileus.

Jaundice accompanying acute abdominal pain virtually always indicates a hepatobiliary disorder (Chapter 149), including obstruction of the biliary duct (choledocholithiasis, pancreatic carcinoma, cholangiocarcinoma), complications of acute cholecystitis, acute hepatitis (viral, ischemic), or hepatic malignancies. The possibility of cholangitis should be considered and excluded in all patients with acute abdominal pain and jaundice, especially if the patient has fever, chills, hypotension, altered mental status, or leukocytosis. Hematemesis with upper abdominal pain suggests a Mallory-Weiss tear, alcoholic gastritis, or peptic ulcer disease. Hematochezia with abdominal pain is most commonly caused by medical conditions such as infectious gastroenteritis or inflammatory bowel disease, but it also may be caused by ischemic colitis or mesenteric ischemia. Gross hematuria may be due to cystitis (Chapter 292) or a ureteral stone (Chapter 125). Abdominal pain with weight loss may be due to inflammatory bowel disease, chronic mesenteric ischemia, or advanced GI malignancies. In women, a missed menstrual period, adnexal pain, spotting, or cramping may suggest pregnancy, ectopic pregnancy, or spontaneous abortion. Acute pain between cycles may be caused by ovarian follicles or ruptured corpus luteum cysts. Pelvic pain with fever, chills, or cervical discharge suggests pelvic inflammatory disease.

The past medical history and review of systems can provide clues about systemic and extra-abdominal conditions that may present with abdominal pain. Acute coronary syndromes (Chapter 72), heart failure (Chapter 58), pneumonia (Chapter 97), or empyema may cause dyspepsia, epigastric or right or left upper quadrant pain, nausea, and vomiting. Metabolic conditions such as uremia (Chapter 132), diabetes with hyperglycemia or ketoacidosis (Chapter 236), hypercalcemia (Chapter 253), or acute adrenocortical insufficiency (Chapter 234) may cause pain, nausea, vomiting, and diarrhea. Acute intermittent porphyria (Chapter 217) and familial Mediterranean fever (Chapter 283) may cause recurrent episodes of severe pain and peritonitis that may be misdiagnosed, leading to unnecessary surgeries. Other causes of acute abdominal pain include narcotic withdrawal (Chapter 33), insect or reptile bites (Chapter 113), and lead or arsenic poisoning (Chapter 21).

Physical Examination

The physical examination must identify life-threatening illnesses that require urgent surgical evaluation. Nevertheless, the examination must be orderly, careful, and complete. If the examiner immediately palpates the site of maximal pain, the patient is unlikely to relax and cooperate for the remainder of the examination.

First, the patient should be observed and the abdomen inspected. Most patients remain calm, cooperative, and freely capable of moving during the examination. Patients who are writhing or restless may have pain due to visceral distention (e.g., renal colic, intestinal obstruction), whereas patients who lie motionless may have peritonitis. Gentle shaking of the bed or having the patient cough may elicit sharp, well-localized pain in patients with parietal but not visceral pain. Auscultation should be performed before percussion or palpation so that intestinal activity is undisturbed. An abdomen that is quiet except for infrequent squeaks or tinkles suggests peritonitis or ileus. Loud peristaltic rushes that occur in synchrony with abdominal pain suggest small bowel obstruction. Light percussion across the upper, middle, and lower abdomen can determine any site of focal tenderness suggestive of peritonitis. Light palpation should be performed with one or two fingers (not the whole hand), beginning away from where the patient localizes the pain and gradually moving to the site of pain. Thereafter, gentle, deeper palpation of the entire abdomen is performed gradually, including the region of tenderness. An attempt should be made to palpate for an abdominal aortic aneurysm (Chapter 78). Examination also should include the inguinal and femoral canals, umbilicus, and surgical scars for evidence of incarcerating hernias. The presence of focal tenderness indicates parietal peritoneal irritation. Voluntary or involuntary tightening of the muscle wall ("guarding") may occur during

TABLE 134-2 TYPICAL MANIFESTATIONS OF KEY CAUSES OF ACUTE AND CHRONIC ABDOMINAL PAIN

CONDITION	LOCATION	QUALITY	ONSET	AGGRAVATING OR RELIEVING FACTORS	ASSOCIATED SYMPTOMS OR SIGNS	DIAGNOSTIC STUDIES
Peptic ulcer disease (Chapter 141)	Epigastric, occasionally RUQ, rarely LUQ	Dyspepsia: mild to moderate aching discomfort, pain, burning, gnawing, postprandial fullness	Days	Variable relief with antacids; may be relieved by, worsened by, or unrelated to meals	Recurrent; associated factors (e.g., *Helicobacter pylori*, aspirin, NSAIDs)	Anemia, upper endoscopy, *H. pylori* testing
Acute pancreatitis (Chapter 146)	Epigastric, radiates to midback (occasionally RUQ or LUQ)	Diffuse, steady, stabbing, penetrating	1-2 hr	Aggravated by food; better when lying still and with narcotics	Severe nausea and vomiting; reduced or absent bowel sounds; associated factors (e.g., alcohol, gallstones)	Elevated amylase and lipase, CT
Acute cholecystitis (Chapter 158)	Epigastric, then moves to RUQ; may radiate to right scapula	Gradual, steady increase, moderate to severe	Hours	May follow a fatty meal; better with narcotics and surgery	Nausea, some vomiting, fever	Elevated WBC count, US or CT
Acute appendicitis (Chapter 144)	Periumbilical, then moves to RLQ	Vague initially; gradual, steady increase to intense, localized, pain	Hours	Unprovoked; better with narcotics and surgery	Anorexia, nausea, obstipation; occasional vomiting, fever late	Elevated WBC count, US or CT
Diverticulitis (Chapter 144)	LLQ or suprapubic	Moderate to severe, steady or cramping, sharp or aching, localized	Hours to days	Unprovoked; better with narcotics and antibiotics or surgery	Anorexia, nausea, distention, constipation or loose stools; partial relief with passage of flatus or BM; fever late	Elevated WBC count, CT
Ruptured viscus and peritonitis (Chapter 144)	Diffuse	Intense	Minutes to hours	Worse with cough or movement; better when lying still or with narcotics or surgery	Fever, anorexia, nausea, vomiting; lack of bowel sounds; tenderness with percussion, light touch, rebound; guarding and rigidity (late); loath to move	Elevated WBC count, CT
Intestinal ischemia (Chapter 145)	Small intestine—periumbilical; proximal (right) colon—periumbilical or RLQ; distal colon—LLQ	Severe, stabbing pain out of proportion to physical findings	Minutes	Chronic ischemia—occurs after eating; acute ischemia—usually unprovoked; better with narcotics, thrombus dissolution, stenting, surgical resection	Nausea, bloody diarrhea; associated factors (e.g., hypotension, cardiac arrhythmias)	Elevated WBC count, angiography or colonoscopy (colonic ischemia)
Strangulated hernia (Chapter 144)	Localized	Sharp, localized, intense; crampy or steady	Minutes to hours	Previous hernia history; unprovoked; better with narcotics and decompression, including surgery	Anorexia, nausea, vomiting, no stool or flatus passage if obstruction; bowel sounds variable—hyperactive early if obstruction present, but absent bowel sounds late, especially with peritonitis	Elevated WBC count, CT, US
Small or large bowel obstruction (Chapter 144)	Small intestine—periumbilical; proximal (right) colon—periumbilical or right abdomen; distal (left) colon—LLQ	Early—diffuse, colicky, crampy; late—steady and better localized	Hours to days	Aggravated by food; better with narcotics, NGT decompression, and/or surgery	Distention, anorexia, nausea, vomiting; no stool or flatus passage; small intestine—increased hyperperistaltic (rushes) bowel sounds (early) or quiet abdomen (late); large intestine—bowel sounds variable; associated factors (e.g., hernia, previous surgery)	CT

TABLE 134-2 TYPICAL MANIFESTATIONS OF KEY CAUSES OF ACUTE AND CHRONIC ABDOMINAL PAIN—cont'd

CONDITION	LOCATION	QUALITY	ONSET	AGGRAVATING OR RELIEVING FACTORS	ASSOCIATED SYMPTOMS OR SIGNS	DIAGNOSTIC STUDIES
Abdominal abscess (Chapter 144)	Located over the abscess, usually LLQ or RLQ	Insidious, intense, constant	Days	May be aggravated by movement; better with abscess drainage	Fever, anorexia, nausea, abdominal mass	Elevated WBC count, CT
Acute hepatitis (Chapter 150)	RUQ	Dull or intense; localized	Days	Worse with deep inspiration	Jaundice, anorexia, nausea; liver enlarged and tender to palpation; associated factors (e.g., alcohol, infection)	Abnormal liver tests
GERD (Chapter 140)	Substernal or epigastric	Burning, gnawing	Days to years	Provoked by large or fatty meals or recumbency; relief with antacids	Recurrent; may have regurgitation, dysphagia, or extraesophageal manifestations (e.g., asthma, chronic cough, laryngitis)	Upper endoscopy (usually normal), 24-hr pH probe
Nonulcer (functional) dyspepsia (Chapter 139)	Epigastric	Mild to moderate discomfort, pain, burning, gnawing, postprandial fullness	Years	May be worsened by meals; cannot be reliably distinguished from ulcer disease by history alone	Other symptoms of functional disorders (IBS, fibromyalgia, pelvic pain)	Normal EGD
IBS (Chapter 139)	Variable; usually lower abdomen	Vague, crampy, sense of urgency	Years	Pain may be precipitated by dietary factors or stress; associated with change in bowel characteristics (e.g., frequency, form, difficulty with passage); relieved with stool passage	Bloating and abdominal distention	Normal sigmoidoscopy, colonoscopy, and CT, but these are usually not necessary for diagnosis
Chronic pancreatitis (Chapter 146)	Epigastric or periumbilical, radiates to midback	Intense, localized	Days to years	Aggravated by food; better with narcotics	Anorexia, nausea, vomiting; associated factors (e.g., alcohol)	Amylase and lipase may be normal; CT may show calcifications, dilated pancreatic duct, pseudocyst
Inflammatory or infectious enterocolitis (Chapters 142 and 291)	Small intestine—periumbilical; large intestine—right or left side of the abdomen over the colon; rectum—tenesmus	Crampy	Hours to days	Better with stool passage and treatment of underlying cause	Nausea, vomiting, bloody diarrhea; associated factors (e.g., infectious—food transmission, IBD—prolonged duration, family history)	Stool studies for culture, colonoscopy with biopsies
Malignancy (Chapter 199)	Variable, depending on cancer location	Variable; intense and crampy if bowel obstruction; steady and vague if local invasion	Days	Better with narcotics and cancer therapy	Primary vs. metastatic disease	CT and biopsies, PET
Pneumonia/pleurisy (Chapters 97 and 99)	Upper abdomen: epigastric, RUQ, or LUQ	Localized; worse with deep breathing	Hours to days	Painful breathing; better with antibiotics	Cough, fever, dyspnea	CXR
Angina and myocardial infarction (Chapters 71-73)	Retrosternal or epigastric	Pressure, squeezing, heaviness, or intense	Minutes	Worse with exertion; relief with nitroglycerin	Dyspnea, diaphoresis	ECG, cardiac enzymes, stress testing
Genitourinary disorders (Chapters 128 and 293)	Bladder—suprapubic; renal colic—abrupt, excruciating LLQ or RLQ pain radiating to the groin; prostate—dull, suprapubic; kidney—CVA	Constant or colicky; stone passage—restless, cannot find a comfortable position	Minutes to days	Better with antibiotics and pain medications (pyelonephritis or nephrolithiasis)	Hematuria, dysuria, prostate tenderness, fever	Urinalysis, urine culture, CT for stone disease

TABLE 134-2 TYPICAL MANIFESTATIONS OF KEY CAUSES OF ACUTE AND CHRONIC ABDOMINAL PAIN—cont'd

CONDITION	LOCATION	QUALITY	ONSET	AGGRAVATING OR RELIEVING FACTORS	ASSOCIATED SYMPTOMS OR SIGNS	DIAGNOSTIC STUDIES
Ovarian cysts or torsion (Chapters 205 and 243)	LLQ or RLQ	Constant, intense	Minutes	Better with NSAIDs or surgery (torsion)	Nausea, vomiting; may be recurrent	US
Ruptured ectopic pregnancy (Chapter 247)	LLQ or RLQ	Constant, intense, stabbing	Minutes	Better with surgery	Rebound and guarding present, abnormal menses or amenorrhea	Acute anemia, elevated β-HCG, US
Musculoskeletal disorders	Specific muscle groups	Aching	Days	Better with heat or NSAIDs; aggravated by movement	History of muscle injury or exertion	Normal laboratory results
Herpes zoster (Chapter 383)	Dermatomal distribution	Burning, itching, neuropathic, constant	Days	Aggravated by touching the dermatome; better with pain or antiviral medications	Recurrent; rash may or may not be present	Skin culture or biopsy
Metabolic disorders (e.g., DM; Chapter 236)	Epigastric or generalized	Intense, constant	Hours to days	Worse with poor metabolic control (e.g., poor glucose control)	Recurrent; nausea, vomiting, diabetic neuropathy	Specific metabolic parameters abnormal (e.g., elevated glucose in DM)
Abdominal epilepsy (Chapter 410)	Epigastric or umbilical	Constant	Hours to days	Unprovoked; better with antiseizure therapy	Recurrent; may have associated seizure disorder	EEG
Dissecting or leaking abdominal aortic aneurysm (Chapter 78)	Over the aneurysm, radiates to the back or groin	Severe, searing, constant	Minutes to hours to days	History of HTN or CAD	Shock, pulsatile mass; bruit *not* usually present	Acute anemia, CT, angiography

BM = bowel movement; CAD = coronary artery disease; CT = computed tomography; CVA = costovertebral angle; CXR = chest x-ray; DM = diabetes mellitus; ECG = electrocardiogram; EEG = electroencephalogram; EGD = esophagogastroduodenoscopy; GERD = gastroesophageal reflux disease; HCG = human chorionic gonadotropin; HTN = hypertension; IBD = irritable bowel disease; IBS = irritable bowel syndrome; LLQ = left lower quadrant; LUQ = left upper quadrant; NGT = nasogastric tube; NSAIDs = nonsteroidal anti-inflammatory drugs; PET = positron emission tomography; RLQ = right lower quadrant; RUQ = right upper quadrant; US = ultrasonography; WBC = white blood cell.

Adapted from Proctor DD. Approach to the patient with gastrointestinal disease. In: Goldman L, Ausiello D, eds. *Cecil Textbook of Medicine*, 23rd ed. Philadelphia: Saunders-Elsevier; 2008.

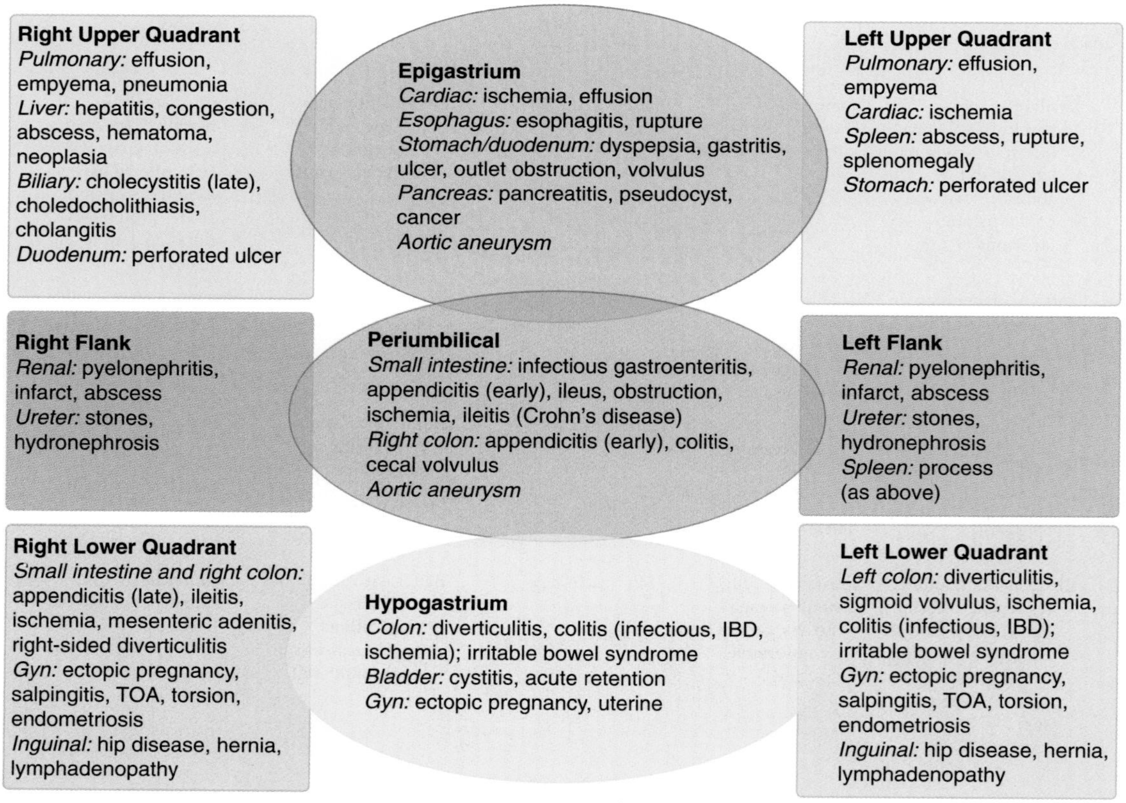

Right Upper Quadrant
Pulmonary: effusion, empyema, pneumonia
Liver: hepatitis, congestion, abscess, hematoma, neoplasia
Biliary: cholecystitis (late), choledocholithiasis, cholangitis
Duodenum: perforated ulcer
Epigastrium
Cardiac: ischemia, effusion
Esophagus: esophagitis, rupture
Stomach/duodenum: dyspepsia, gastritis, ulcer, outlet obstruction, volvulus
Pancreas: pancreatitis, pseudocyst, cancer
Aortic aneurysm
Left Upper Quadrant
Pulmonary: effusion, empyema
Cardiac: ischemia
Spleen: abscess, rupture, splenomegaly
Stomach: perforated ulcer
Right Flank
Renal: pyelonephritis, infarct, abscess
Ureter: stones, hydronephrosis
Periumbilical
Small intestine: infectious gastroenteritis, appendicitis (early), ileus, obstruction, ischemia, ileitis (Crohn's disease)
Right colon: appendicitis (early), colitis, cecal volvulus
Aortic aneurysm
Left Flank
Renal: pyelonephritis, infarct, abscess
Ureter: stones, hydronephrosis
Spleen: process (as above)
Right Lower Quadrant
Small intestine and right colon: appendicitis (late), ileitis, ischemia, mesenteric adenitis, right-sided diverticulitis
Gyn: ectopic pregnancy, salpingitis, TOA, torsion, endometriosis
Inguinal: hip disease, hernia, lymphadenopathy
Hypogastrium
Colon: diverticulitis, colitis (infectious, IBD, ischemia); irritable bowel syndrome
Bladder: cystitis, acute retention
Gyn: ectopic pregnancy, uterine
Left Lower Quadrant
Left colon: diverticulitis, sigmoid volvulus, ischemia, colitis (infectious, IBD); irritable bowel syndrome
Gyn: ectopic pregnancy, salpingitis, TOA, torsion, endometriosis
Inguinal: hip disease, hernia, lymphadenopathy

FIGURE 134-1. **Differential diagnosis of abdominal pain by its initial location.** IBD = inflammatory bowel disease; TOA = tubo-ovarian abscess.

palpation. With gentle, steady compression of the abdomen with one hand, voluntary guarding usually subsides, allowing the examination to proceed. Persistent involuntary guarding indicates peritonitis with reflex muscle wall contraction. Testing for "rebound tenderness" in patients with suspected peritonitis is not recommended because it causes significant pain and is usually not necessary to establish the diagnosis. When the presentation strongly suggests a nonserious GI disorder but the patient has significant tenderness with palpation, it is useful to use the stethoscope ostensibly to listen for bowel sounds but actually to reproduce the pressure of palpation. A significant discrepancy in the tenderness elicited by the stethoscope and by digital palpation may be seen in patients who are anxious, have functional complaints, or are seeking secondary gain. A digital rectal examination should be performed in most patients with acute abdominal pain to evaluate for tenderness or fluctuance that suggests a perirectal abscess and to assess the stool for signs of overt or occult blood. Women with lower abdominal pain should have a pelvic examination by a skilled examiner to evaluate for gynecologic pathology. Some specific and dramatic findings point to particular diagnoses (Table 134-3).

Special Populations

Increased diligence is required in the evaluation of patients in whom abdominal signs and symptoms may be minimal until the disease process is far advanced. Such patients include the elderly (Chapter 24) and patients who have dementia (Chapter 409), psychiatric disturbances (Chapter 404), or spinal cord injuries. An admitting diagnosis of "altered mental status," "failure to thrive," "obstipation," or "fever of unknown origin" may stem from serious intra-abdominal conditions. Disorders that may be overlooked in the elderly include bowel perforation, bowel obstruction, cholecystitis, diverticulitis, volvulus, mesenteric ischemia, and abdominal aortic aneurysm. In patients with chronic liver disease, the presence of ascites may mask the signs and symptoms of serious surgical conditions such as cholecystitis, appendicitis, and diverticulitis. Even in the presence of perforation, signs of peritonitis may be lacking because the ascites fluid separates the visceral peritoneum and parietal peritoneum. Likewise, immunocompromised populations, who are at risk for infectious, drug-related, and iatrogenic complications, may manifest few physical findings or laboratory abnormalities. Owing to the limitations of the clinical evaluation in these vulnerable populations, there should be a low threshold for the use of abdominal imaging.

Abdominal Pain Developing in the Hospital

When pain develops as a new problem in a hospitalized patient, it is usually caused by a limited number of conditions. Postprocedural complications may cause perforation, infection, or bleeding (intraperitoneal, retroperitoneal, or within solid organs). Shunting of splanchnic blood flow in severely ill medical or surgical patients may cause stress gastritis, nonocclusive mesenteric ischemia, or acalculous cholecystitis. Adynamic ileus or acute colonic pseudo-obstruction is common in critically ill or postoperative patients and manifests as diffuse abdominal pain and distention. *Clostridium difficile* (Chapter 304) colitis is a common cause of pain, diarrhea, and distention, especially in patients on antibiotics. Constipation (Chapter 138), which is a common problem in hospitalized patients, may go unnoticed until pain and distention develop. Finally, many medications can cause dyspepsia and abdominal pain.

TABLE 134-3 PHYSICAL SIGNS IN PATIENTS WITH ACUTE ABDOMINAL PAIN

SIGN	DESCRIPTION	DIAGNOSIS
Murphy's sign	Cessation of inspiration during right upper quadrant examination	Acute cholecystitis
McBurney's sign	Tenderness located midway between anterior superior iliac spine and umbilicus	Acute appendicitis
Cullen's sign	Periumbilical bluish discoloration	Retroperitoneal hemorrhage Pancreatic hemorrhage Ruptured abdominal aortic aneurysm
Grey Turner's sign	Bluish discoloration of flanks	Retroperitoneal hemorrhage Pancreatic hemorrhage Ruptured abdominal aortic aneurysm
Kehr's sign	Severe left shoulder pain	Splenic rupture Ectopic pregnancy rupture
Obturator sign	Pain with flexed right hip rotation	Appendicitis
Psoas sign	Pain with straight leg raising against resistance (right side)	Appendicitis

DIAGNOSIS

Patients with acute abdominal pain should have a complete blood count with differential; leukocytosis is present in most acute surgical conditions (Fig. 134-2). A pregnancy test is required in women of childbearing age. Serum electrolytes, glucose, blood urea nitrogen, and creatinine levels assess hydration, acid-base status, and renal function. Liver chemistries and pancreatic enzymes should be obtained in most patients, but especially in those with upper abdominal pain, jaundice, or vomiting. An elevation in aspartate or alanine aminotransferase levels may reflect choledocholithiasis with acute biliary obstruction (Chapter 158), acute gallstone pancreatitis (Chapter 146), or a hepatocellular process (Chapter 150). Painful jaundice with a significant rise in the alkaline phosphatase level usually reflects cholestasis caused by extrahepatic biliary obstruction (Chapter 158). Amylase and lipase levels are elevated in most patients with acute pancreatitis, but minor amylase elevations also occur with a perforated viscus or mesenteric ischemia (Chapter 145). Urinalysis may demonstrate pyuria, hematuria, or bacteriuria owing to ureteral calculi (Chapter 128) or urinary tract infection (Chapter 292).

Imaging

Ultrasound is preferred in suspected pregnancy and to evaluate for other acute gynecologic disorders such as tubo-ovarian abscess, ruptured corpus luteum cyst, or ovarian torsion; it is also preferred for the initial evaluation of suspected acute cholecystitis (Chapter 158) and ureteral stones with hydronephrosis (Chapter 125) and for the bedside evaluation of unstable patients. In most other settings, abdominal computed tomography (CT) with oral and intravenous contrast (when possible) is preferred and can provide a definitive diagnosis in up to 90% of patients with acute severe abdominal pain (Chapter 135). Abdominal CT may be falsely negative early in the course of acute pancreatitis, mesenteric ischemia, cholecystitis, appendicitis, and diverticulitis, especially if performed without contrast.

TREATMENT Rx

Once the diagnosis is clear, treatment of the underlying condition is initiated. In patients with nonspecific acute abdominal pain and no clear diagnosis, early laparoscopy is useful for diagnosis, but outcomes such as complication rates, readmission rates, and length of hospitalization are no better than with a strategy of active observation.[1]

Chronic Abdominal Pain

Chronic or recurrent abdominal pain that has been present for months to years may be caused by structural (organic) disease, but the majority of patients have a functional disorder such as irritable bowel syndrome (Chapter 139). Common organic causes of chronic abdominal pain include medications with GI side effects, peptic ulcer disease (Chapter 141), inflammatory bowel disease (Chapter 143), chronic pancreatitis (Chapter 146), biliary tract disease (Chapter 158), GI cancers (Chapters 198 and 199), and endometriosis (Chapter 244). The clinician should attempt to distinguish patients with symptoms or signs of organic disease, in whom further diagnostic investigation is warranted, from those with probable functional disease (Fig. 134-3). Although functional disorders occur in all age groups, the symptoms usually begin before age 40. "Alarm" features that suggest a structural disorder and are inconsistent with a functional disorder are fever, severe pain, significant weight loss, jaundice, progressive dysphagia, recurrent vomiting, nocturnal pain or diarrhea, and stools that are bloody or positive for fecal occult blood. Laboratory studies should be normal with functional disorders; therefore, an unrevealing evaluation for anemia, leukocytosis, and levels of iron, albumin, C-reactive protein, and vitamins A, D, or B_{12} argues against structural or organic disease.

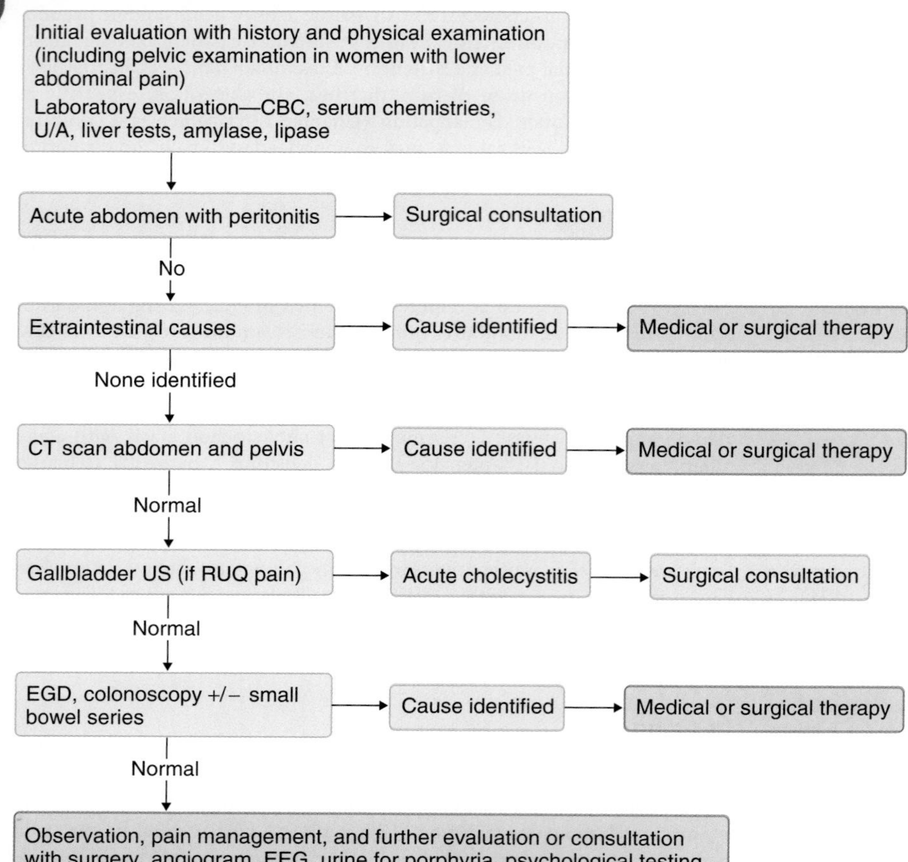

FIGURE 134-2. Approach to the patient with acute abdominal pain. CBC = complete blood count; CT = computed tomography; EEG = electroencephalography; EGD = esophagogastroduodenoscopy; RUQ = right upper quadrant; U/A = urinalysis; US = ultrasonography.

In patients younger than 50 years with a suspected functional disorder and no alarm features (e.g., family history of colon cancer or inflammatory bowel disease or abnormalities on screening blood tests), further testing should be minimized, and the emphasis should be shifted to managing symptoms, coping, and making lifestyle changes (Chapter 139). In patients who may have organic disease, testing often includes a combination of upper GI endoscopy, colonoscopy, and ultrasound or CT imaging.

GAS AND BLOATING

Belching

Belching (eructation), which is the involuntary or voluntary release of gas from the esophagus or stomach, commonly occurs during or after a meal. Virtually all belching is caused by swallowed air, which may be increased by eating quickly, drinking carbonated beverages, chewing gum, and smoking. Gas also may be produced within the stomach by antacids, especially sodium bicarbonate, which rapidly neutralize gastric acid and release carbon dioxide. Belching seldom reflects serious GI dysfunction but may be increased in patients with gastroesophageal reflux (Chapter 140), functional dyspepsia (Chapter 139), or gastroparesis (Chapter 138). Chronic, excessive, repetitive belching is a functional disorder caused by habitual aerophagia (air swallowing) and is treated with behavioral modification.

Flatus

Flatus or "gas" is a normal byproduct of digestion. Otherwise healthy adults pass flatus 10 to 20 times daily and excrete up to 1500 mL. Thus, it is difficult to distinguish patients with abnormal or excessive gas production from those with only a heightened awareness of or sensitivity to normal production. Increased flatulence with diarrhea may be symptomatic of disorders of malabsorption, including celiac disease (Chapter 142), pancreatic insufficiency (Chapter 146), and small intestinal bacterial overgrowth (Chapter 142).

In normal adults, flatus is derived from two sources: swallowed air and colonic bacterial fermentation of carbohydrates that results in the production of carbon dioxide or methane. Carbohydrates that may be incompletely absorbed in the small intestine and pass into the colon include lactose (dairy products), fructose, sorbitol, trehalose (mushrooms), and the α-galactosyl oligosaccharides raffinose, stachyose, and verbascose. The latter are found in increased amounts in cruciferous vegetables (cabbage, broccoli, cauliflower, brussels sprouts, turnips, rutabagas), legumes (beans, soy, lentils, peas), pasta, and whole grains. Fructose is present in fruits, especially apples and pears, and is a major component of corn syrups that are used widely as sweeteners. Sorbitol is a natural sugar in stone fruits (peaches, apricots, plums, prunes) and is a common sweetener in sugar-free candies.

TREATMENT Rx

Patients with long-standing flatulence in the absence of other symptoms or signs of GI disease can be treated conservatively. Avoidance of carbonated beverages, chewing gum, sorbitol- and fructose-containing sweeteners, and gas-producing vegetables improves symptoms in most patients. Lactase deficiency may be confirmed by a lactose breath test. Underlying GI illness is suggested by the recent onset of flatulence with other symptoms of organic disease, including weight loss, abdominal pain, diarrhea, distention, and abnormal laboratory studies (Chapter 142). A positive fecal fat analysis confirms malabsorption and merits further investigation (see Table 142-4 in Chapter 142). Suspected small bowel bacterial overgrowth may be confirmed by carbohydrate breath tests or treated empirically with antibiotics.

Bloating and Distention

Bloating and distention are common complaints among patients with functional GI disorders (Chapter 139). As chronic, isolated symptoms, they are almost never caused by serious structural disease. Functional bloating may be caused by heightened sensitivity to minor increases in intestinal gas or impaired transit of gas, even though the total volume of intestinal gas is within normal limits. The acute onset of distention in conjunction with alarm symptoms such as cramping pain, weight loss, nausea, vomiting, obstipation, or diarrhea warrants further evaluation for disorders that cause intestinal

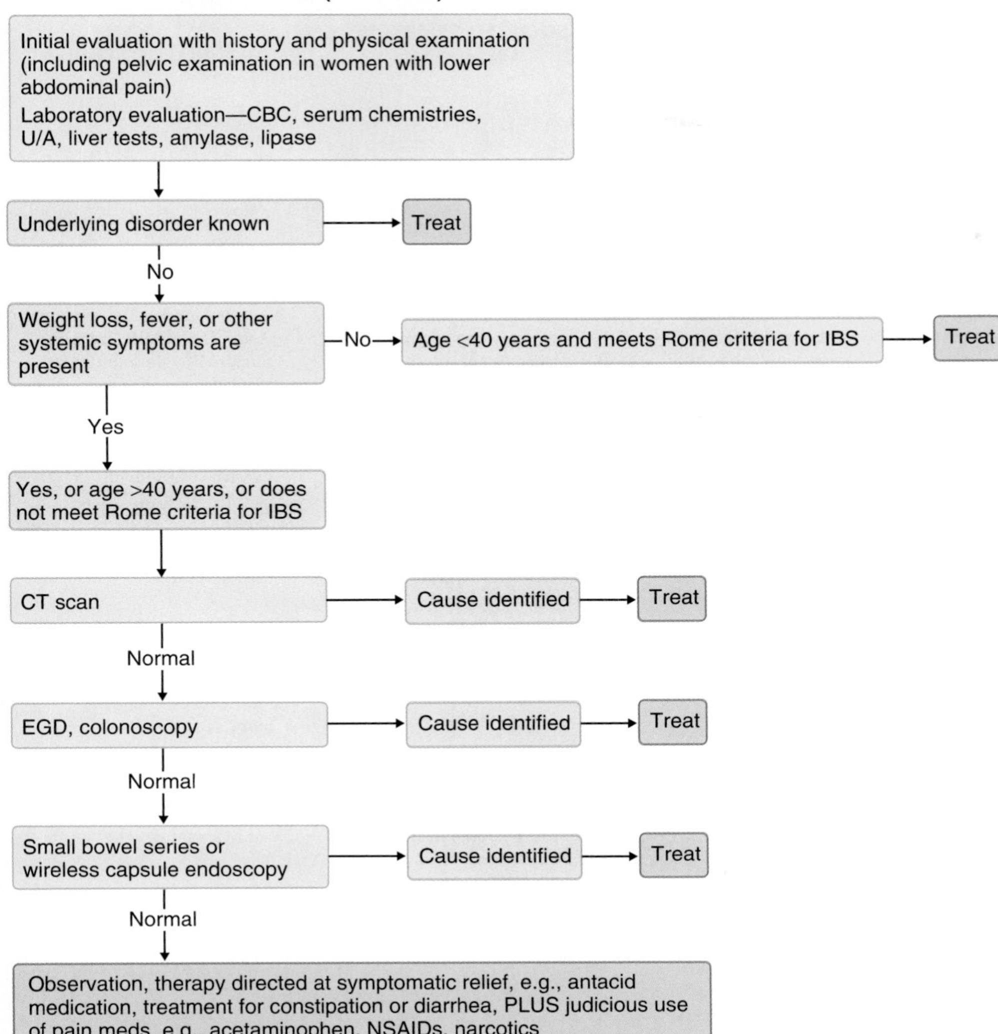

FIGURE 134-3. Approach to the patient with chronic abdominal pain. CBC = complete blood count; CT = computed tomography; EGD = esophagogastroduodenoscopy; ERCP = endoscopic retrograde cholangiopancreatography; IBS = irritable bowel syndrome; NSAIDs = nonsteroidal anti-inflammatory drugs; U/A = urinalysis.

obstruction (Chapter 144) or malabsorption (Chapter 142). Rifaximin (550 mg three times daily for 2 weeks) is effective for functional bloating, pain, and loose or watery stools;[2] but dietary and behavioral changes and reassurance may also be useful.

INVOLUNTARY WEIGHT LOSS

The unintentional loss of more than 5% of baseline weight within a 12-month period is frequently due to a serious underlying medical or psychiatric illness. Weight loss is seldom the sole presenting sign of medical disorders, but it is often revealed during the clinical evaluation of other complaints. Chronic weight loss in the elderly is commonly caused by depression, dementia, difficulty chewing or swallowing, malignancy, medications, alcoholism, or physical and social limitations to procuring, preparing, and eating meals (Table 134-4) (Chapter 23). Gradual, mild weight loss occurs in some elderly patients owing to the loss of lean body mass. In young patients, weight loss is more commonly caused by eating disorders (Chapter 226), endocrine disorders (Chapters 233 and 234), or chronic GI conditions such as inflammatory bowel disease (Chapter 143) or celiac disease (Chapter 142). In chronic medical conditions, involuntary weight loss is usually caused by a combination of decreased appetite (anorexia) and varying degrees of cachexia; examples include advanced malignancy, chronic infections (HIV, tuberculosis), heart failure, chronic kidney or liver disease, end-stage lung disease, and adrenal insufficiency. Weight loss that occurs in the presence of normal or increased appetite suggests increased metabolism and energy expenditure caused by endocrine disorders such as poorly controlled diabetes (Chapter 236) or hyperthyroidism (Chapter 233) or GI disorders that result in food malabsorption (Chapter 142). Chronic GI disorders that cause progressive narrowing or obstruction of the esophagus (cancer, achalasia), stomach (cancer, peptic ulcer disease with gastric outlet obstruction), small intestine (Crohn's disease), or arterial circulation (chronic mesenteric ischemia) may cause weight loss owing to dysphagia, vomiting, or postprandial pain that limits the ability to ingest sufficient calories.

DIAGNOSIS

The cause of weight loss (see Table 134-4) is usually evident from the history, physical examination, and routine laboratory studies, including complete blood count, electrolytes, liver chemistries, thyroid-stimulating hormone, urinalysis, and, when appropriate, HIV serology (Fig. 134-4). A chest radiograph should be obtained in patients who smoke, have any respiratory symptoms, or are older than 40 years. Signs of dehydration or severe malnutrition may require an assessment for nutritional deficiencies (Chapter 221) and nutritional support (Chapters 223 and 224).

The need for further diagnostic testing is determined by other symptoms and signs. Weight loss with increased appetite merits an assessment of thyroid function (Chapter 233), glucose intolerance (Chapter 237), and malabsorption (Chapter 142). Suspected malabsorption may be confirmed by a positive fecal fat analysis. GI symptoms suggesting obstruction or occult GI malignancy can be evaluated with upper GI endoscopy, upper GI radiographic series, colonoscopy, or abdominal CT. Psychiatric evaluation may be

TABLE 134-4 CAUSES OF INVOLUNTARY WEIGHT LOSS

CONDITION	QUALITY	DURATION	AGGRAVATING OR RELIEVING FACTORS	ASSOCIATED SYMPTOMS OR SIGNS	DIAGNOSTIC STUDIES
WEIGHT LOSS SECONDARY TO GASTROINTESTINAL CAUSES					
GI, pancreatic, or hepatobiliary malignancy (Chapters 198-202)	Progressive, fast	Months	Better with cancer therapy (e.g., surgery, XRT, chemotherapy)	Dysphagia (esophageal); anorexia, nausea, vomiting (gastric, small or large bowel obstruction); visible or occult blood in stool; altered bowel habits; jaundice or hepatomegaly (biliary obstruction, hepatic tumor, metastatic disease); iron deficiency anemia	CBC, FOBT, ferritin, CEA, CA19-9, AFP, EGD, colonoscopy, abdominal CT, PET
Malabsorption (Chapter 142) (poor absorption of nutrients due to pancreatic insufficiency, small intestinal mucosal disorders, or bacterial overgrowth)	Progressive, slow	Months to years	Diarrhea or steatorrhea, excessive flatulence; worse with eating and resolves with NPO status	Usually associated with increased appetite; may have anemia (iron, B_{12}, folate), osteoporosis, or osteomalacia (vitamin D, calcium, phosphorus); easy bruising (vitamin K), night blindness (vitamin A)	72-hr stool for fecal fat; vitamins A and D and INR; calcium, ferritin, B_{12}, albumin; celiac disease antibodies (e.g., anti-tTG, antiendomysial antibodies); EGD with small bowel biopsy; breath test for bacterial overgrowth
Inflammatory bowel disease (especially Crohn's disease) (Chapter 143)	Progressive, slow	Months	Eating causes pain, cramps, increased diarrhea and urgency; improved by low-residue diet or NPO status	Bloody stools, abdominal cramps and pain, perianal disease, extraintestinal manifestations (e.g., oral ulcers, uveitis, erythema nodosum, arthralgias)	CBC, albumin, ESR, CRP, colonoscopy with biopsies, CT or MR enterography, wireless capsule study
GI motility disorders (Chapter 138)	Intermittent, slow	Years	Worse with eating	Nausea, vomiting, distention, diarrhea, or constipation may be present	EGD and colonoscopy, gastric emptying study, CT or MR enterography, surgical full-thickness intestinal biopsies
Cirrhosis (Chapter 156)	Muscle wasting with edema, so weight may increase	Months to years	Worse with salt or fluid intake	Ascites, peripheral edema	Liver biopsy
Chronic intestinal ischemia (Chapter 145)	Progressive	Months to years	Worse with eating	Afraid to eat; postprandial abdominal pain, nausea; associated atherosclerotic disease	CT or MR angiography
WEIGHT LOSS SECONDARY TO NONGASTROINTESTINAL CAUSES					
Poor or inadequate caloric intake due to social factors	Intermittent or progressive, acute (hospitalized) or chronic	Days to months to years	Common in elderly, teenagers; exacerbated by poor dentition or poorly fitting dentures	Will eat if food is made available	Review dietary log and how food is obtained and prepared
Medications	Intermittent or progressive	Months	Worse with medication; resolves with discontinuation of offending drug	Anorexia, nausea, vomiting	Review drug profile
Non-GI malignancy	Progressive	Months	Better with cancer therapy (e.g., surgery, XRT, chemotherapy)	Anorexia, nausea, vomiting; pain; metastatic disease	Calcium, cortisol; CT for underlying disease, PET
Endocrine disorders: DM, hyperthyroidism, adrenal insufficiency (Chapters 233-237)	DM—appetite increased or decreased, early satiety; hyperthyroidism—increased appetite	Months to years	Worse with disease chronicity	DM: gastroparesis, neuropathy, retinopathy, nephropathy Adrenal insufficiency: nausea, vomiting, diarrhea, abdominal pain	Serum glucose, TFT, cortisol
Chronic infections, including HIV and TB (Chapters 332 and 397)	Progressive, fast	Months	Better with directed therapy, megestrol acetate (Megace)	Nausea, anorexia, other infections	HIV test, PPD, cultures, biopsies if necessary
Systemic inflammatory disorders	Progressive, moderate	Months to years	Better with directed therapy, megestrol acetate (Megace)	Arthritis, rash, vasculitis	ANA, RF, ESR, CRP
Chronic renal failure (Chapter 132)	Progressive, slow; edema may increase weight	Months to years	Better with dialysis, megestrol acetate (Megace)	Nausea, anorexia, weight gain	BUN, Cr, 24-hr creatinine clearance
Advanced COPD or heart failure (Chapters 58 and 88)	Progressive, slow	Months to years	Better with oxygen and specific treatment	Fatigue, dyspnea, edema, wasting	Pulmonary function testing or two-dimensional echocardiography
Psychiatric illness: depression, manic-depressive illness (Chapter 404)	Progressive, slow	Months to years		Depression common in elderly; flat affect; manic phase associated with hyperactivity and decreased intake	Psychological testing

TABLE 134-4 CAUSES OF INVOLUNTARY WEIGHT LOSS—cont'd

CONDITION	QUALITY	DURATION	AGGRAVATING OR RELIEVING FACTORS	ASSOCIATED SYMPTOMS OR SIGNS	DIAGNOSTIC STUDIES
Psychogenic eating disorders—anorexia nervosa, bulimia (Chapter 226)	Intermittent or progressive	Months to years	Worse with stressors	Refusal to eat, loss of tooth enamel, calluses and healing ulcerations of hand	Psychiatric testing
Substance abuse (alcohol, opiates, CNS stimulants)	Intermittent or progressive	Months	Resolves with discontinuation	Anorexia, nausea, vomiting	Careful interview; patients may deny or minimize

AFP = α-fetoprotein; ANA = antinuclear antibody; BUN = blood urea nitrogen; CBC = complete blood count; CEA = carcinoembryonic antigen; CNS = central nervous system; COPD = chronic obstructive pulmonary disease; Cr = creatinine; CRP = C-reactive protein; CT = computed tomography; DM = diabetes mellitus; EGD = esophagogastroduodenoscopy; ESR = erythrocyte sedimentation rate; GI = gastrointestinal; FOBT = fecal occult blood test; GI = gastrointestinal; HIV = human immunodeficiency virus; INR = international normalized ratio; MR = magnetic resonance; NPO = nothing orally; PET = positron emission tomography; PPD = purified protein derivative; RF = rheumatoid factor; TB = tuberculosis; TFT = thyroid function test; tTG = tissue transglutaminase; XRT = x-ray therapy.
Adapted from Proctor DD. Approach to the patient with gastrointestinal disease. In: Goldman L, Ausiello D, eds. *Cecil Textbook of Medicine*, 23rd ed. Philadelphia: Saunders-Elsevier; 2008.

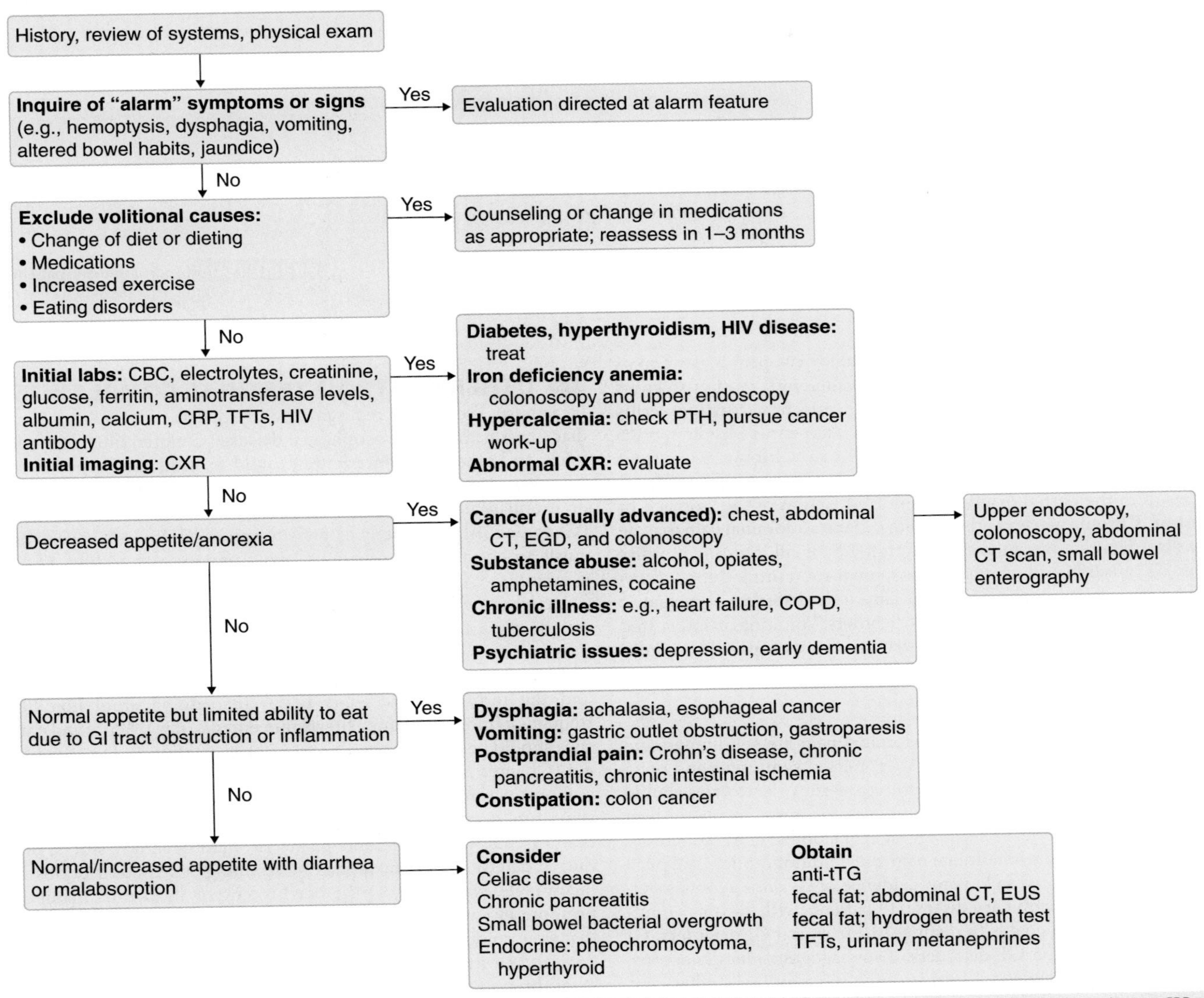

FIGURE 134-4. Approach to the patient with unintentional weight loss greater than 5%. CBC = complete blood count; COPD = chronic obstructive pulmonary disease; CRP = C-reactive protein; CT = computed tomography; CXR = chest radiograph; EGD = esophagogastroduodenoscopy; EUS = endoscopic ultrasound; GI = gastrointestinal; HIV = human immunodeficiency virus; PPD = purified protein derivative; PTH = parathyroid hormone; TFTs = thyroid function tests; tTG = tissue transglutaminase; U/A = urinalysis.

warranted in patients with signs of depression, early dementia, or eating disorders. In up to 25% of patients, no cause of weight loss is found.

NAUSEA AND VOMITING

Nausea is an unpleasant feeling of the impending need to vomit. *Vomiting* is the forceful oral expulsion of gastric contents as a result of retrograde contraction of the duodenum and antrum with compression of the thoracoabdominal musculature. Nausea and vomiting may be caused by a number GI and non-GI disorders, but they are best categorized according to chronicity and the presence of abdominal pain. The acute onset of vomiting *with* severe abdominal pain suggests a serious illness potentially requiring surgical intervention, including GI obstruction (Chapter 144), mesenteric ischemia (Chapter 145), pancreatitis (Chapter 146), biliary colic (Chapter 158), or conditions causing peritonitis (Chapter 144), such as appendicitis

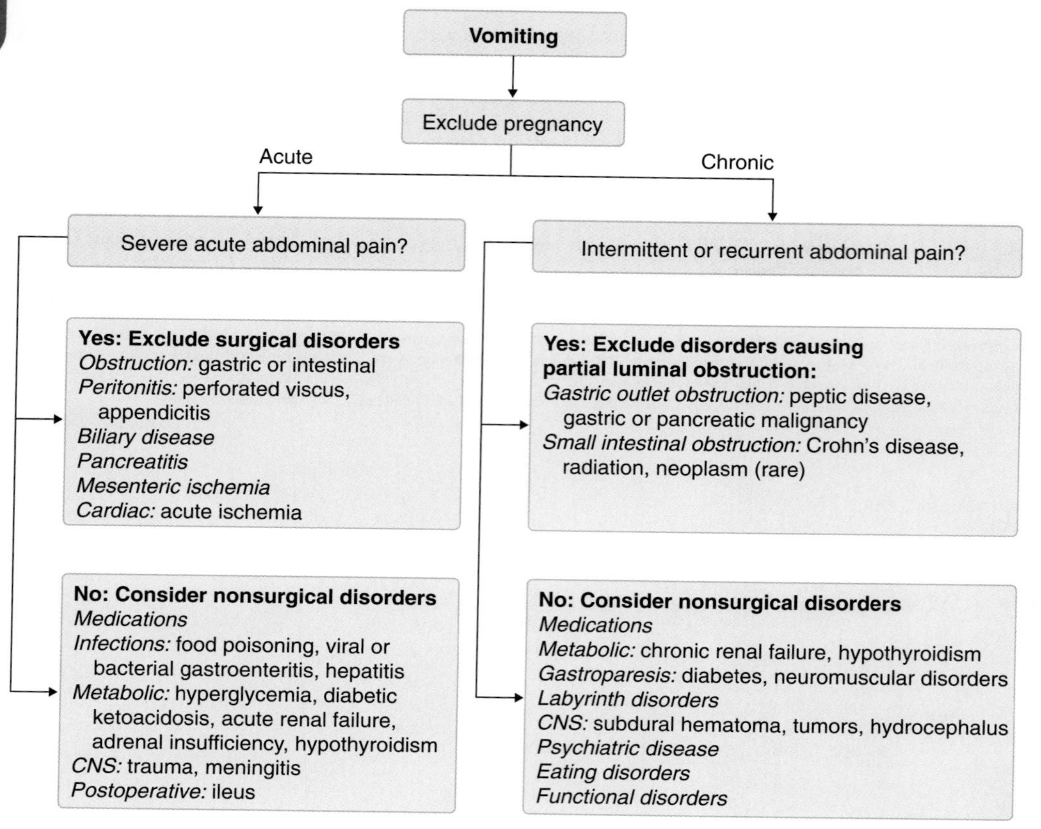

FIGURE 134-5. Approach to the patient with vomiting. CNS = central nervous system.

or a perforated viscus. Acute vomiting *without* abdominal pain is most commonly caused by medications (including chemotherapy), motion sickness (Chapter 436), food poisoning (Chapter 291), infectious gastroenteritis (Chapter 291), hepatitis (Chapters 150 and 151), upper GI bleeding, postoperative ileus, or acute central nervous system disease. Chronic or recurrent nausea and vomiting *with* abdominal pain are commonly caused by GI disorders that result in the partial or intermittent obstruction of the stomach or small intestine. Chronic nausea and vomiting *without* abdominal pain may be caused by disorders that impair gastric emptying or small intestine motility and by non-GI causes including medications, pregnancy, intracerebral disorders, cardiac disease, endocrine disease, labyrinth disorders, psychiatric disease (including bulimia), and functional disorders. Vomiting of undigested food eaten hours earlier suggests gastric obstruction or gastroparesis. Abdominal distention or feculent emesis suggests obstruction of the small intestine.

DIAGNOSIS

Most cases of acute vomiting without abdominal pain are self-limited and require no evaluation (Fig. 134-5). Medication-related symptoms and pregnancy should be excluded. With severe vomiting, serum electrolytes should be obtained. Hyperglycemia may cause acute gastroparesis. Increased liver chemistries or pancreatic enzymes suggest hepatobiliary or pancreatic disease. In patients with acute abdominal pain and vomiting, abdominal plain radiographs or CT is obtained to look for evidence of GI obstruction, a perforated viscus, or pancreaticobiliary disease. In patients with chronic vomiting of uncertain cause, the goal is to distinguish structural GI disorders, GI motility disorders, and non-GI disorders. Esophagogastroduodenoscopy, enterography, abdominal cross-sectional imaging, GI motility studies, and head CT or magnetic resonance imaging may all be indicated.

TREATMENT Rx

The approach to the medical treatment of nausea and vomiting depends on the cause (Table 134-5). Patients who are receiving moderately emetogenic chemotherapy are frequently managed with a 5-HT_3-receptor antagonist and dexamethasone[3]; aprepitant is added for highly emetogenic regimens. For patients with mildly emetogenic regimens or vomiting from other causes, treatment with single or combinations of anti-cholinergic agents, dopamine-receptor antagonists, or 5-HT_3-receptor antagonists usually provides symptomatic relief.[4,5]

OTHER GASTROINTESTINAL COMPLAINTS

Heartburn, esophageal regurgitation, dysphagia, odynophagia, and noncardiac chest pain suggest esophageal disease (Chapter 140). *Dyspepsia,* which refers to bothersome, intermittent, mild to moderate upper abdominal or epigastric symptoms, can be caused by peptic ulcer disease (Chapter 141) or esophageal disease (Chapter 140), or it can be functional in origin (Chapter 139). An orderly diagnostic approach (Fig. 134-6) can help distinguish among the various causes, avoid unnecessary testing, and minimize symptoms.

Diarrhea, which is defined pathophysiologically as an increase in stool weight to greater than 200 g/day, can be caused by malabsorption of osmotically active substances or by increased intestinal secretion of electrolytes and water. In clinical practice, however, stool weight is seldom quantified, and the term *diarrhea* refers to an increase in stool liquidity and/or frequency (more than three bowel movements/day). Acute and chronic diarrhea should be distinguished because the evaluation and treatment are different (Chapter 142).

Constipation (Chapter 138), which is the most common digestive symptom, occurs in 15% of the population. Constipation may refer to fewer than three bowel movements per week; hard or lumpy stools; or difficulty during defecation, characterized by straining, a sensation of obstruction or incomplete evacuation, or the need to engage in manual manipulations to promote evacuation. Constipation may be caused by systemic conditions that slow colonic transit, including neuromuscular disease, endocrine disorders, and electrolyte abnormalities, or by lesions that obstruct the passage of stool through the distal colon or anorectum, such as neoplasms, strictures, prolapse, and agangliosis (Hirschsprung's disease). Most patients, however, do not have an apparent cause and are deemed to have functional constipation.

GI bleeding (Chapter 137) may be acute and clinically apparent (overt) or chronic, slow, and clinically inapparent (occult). The location of acute GI bleeding is described as either upper or lower, according to whether the source is proximal or distal to the ligament of Treitz (distal duodenum). Upper GI bleeding, which is three times more common than lower GI bleeding, is manifested by bloody emesis (hematemesis), coffee ground emesis, and, in most cases, black stools (melena). Common causes of significant bleeding are peptic ulcer disease, esophageal varices, Mallory-Weiss tears, erosive gastritis or esophagitis, and vascular ectasias. Major lower GI bleeding

TABLE 134-5 MEDICAL TREATMENT OF NAUSEA AND VOMITING

DRUG	USUAL INDICATIONS	USUAL DOSE (RANGE)	ROUTE	COMMENTS
ANTICHOLINERGIC-ANTIHISTAMINE AGENTS				Side effects: sedation, dizziness, delirium, blurred vision, glaucoma, bronchospasm, tachycardia, urinary retention Avoid concomitant alcohol or CNS depressants; use with caution in elderly patients
Scopolamine patch	MS	1.5 mg/72 hr	Patch	
Dimenhydrinate	MS	50 mg (50-100 mg) q4-6h	PO, IM, IV	Maximum 400 mg/24 hr
Cyclizine	MS, GIDz	50 mg q8h	PO, IM	Maximum 200 mg/24 hr
Meclizine	MS, V	25-50 mg q24h	PO	
Diphenhydramine	GIDz	25-50 mg q6h 50-100 mg q6h	PO, IV IM	
Promethazine	GIDz, PONV, MS	25 mg (12.5-25 mg) q6-12h 25 mg (12.5-50 mg) q4-6h	PO, PR IV, IM	Phenothiazine derivative, but lacks significant antidopaminergic effects Avoid perivascular extravasation or subcutaneous injection (severe tissue necrosis)
Trimethobenzamide	GIDz, PONV	200 mg q6-8h	IM	
DOPAMINE RECEPTOR ANTAGONISTS				Side effects: neuromuscular (extrapyramidal) symptoms—agitation, restlessness, involuntary movements, dystonia, torticollis, laryngospasm, Parkinson-like features
Prochlorperazine	GIDz, PONV, CTX	5-10 mg q6-8h 25 mg q12h	PO, IV, IM PR	Maximum dose 20-40 mg/24 hr; avoid subcutaneous injection (irritation)
Metoclopramide	GIDz CTX	10 mg (10-20 mg) q6-8h 1-2 mg/kg before and 2 hr after CTX	PO, IV, IM IV	Modest efficacy at these doses High doses infrequently used owing to availability of safer, more effective CTX regimens; use with diphenhydramine to reduce adverse side effects
Droperidol	PONV	2.5 mg (1.25-5 mg) pre-induction and q4-6h as needed	IV, IM	May cause QTc prolongation and torsades de pointes; use is restricted to patients who fail to respond to other agents
CORTICOSTEROIDS				
Dexamethasone	PONV CTX	4-8 mg once pre-induction 8-20 mg on day 1; 8 mg on days 2-4	PO, IV PO, IV	Most beneficial when used with other agents (e.g., 5-HT_3 RA, neurokinin-1 RA)
BENZODIAZEPINES				Used to reduce anxiety and anticipatory vomiting
Lorazepam	CTX	1-2 mg q4-6h	PO, IV	
CANNABINOIDS				May stimulate appetite; adverse side effects (sedation, dizziness, dysphoria, dry mouth) limit use
Dronabinol	GIDz, CTX	5-10 mg q6-8h	PO	
Nabilone	GIDz, CTX	1-2 mg q12h	PO	
5-HT_3 RECEPTOR ANTAGONISTS	PONV, CTX			PONV prevention: give IV immediately before anesthesia induction Prevention of CTX-induced vomiting: give 30 min (IV) to 1 hr (PO) before chemotherapy
Ondansetron	PONV CTX, RadTx	4 mg once 4-8 mg Moderately emetogenic CTX: 8 mg twice daily Highly emetogenic CTX: 24 mg once	IV PO IV or PO IV or PO	
Granisetron	CTX, RadTx	1-2 mg once daily 1 mg once daily	PO IV	
Dolasetron	CTX, PONV	100 mg once daily	PO, IV	
Palonosetron	CTX PONV	0.25 mg 0.5 mg 0.075 mg	IV PO IV	
NEUROKININ-1 RECEPTOR ANTAGONISTS	Highly emetogenic CTX			Used exclusively in combination with a 5-HT_3 RA and/or dexamethasone
Aprepitant		125 mg on day 1 80 mg on days 2-3	PO	
Fosaprepitant		115 mg on day 1	IV	Aprepitant 80 mg PO on days 2-3
ANTIEMETIC REGIMENS FOR CHEMOTHERAPY				
Mildly emetogenic CTX	Option 1 Option 2	Dexamethasone 8 mg Dopamine receptor antagonist	IV or PO	One dose only One dose only

TABLE 134-5 MEDICAL TREATMENT OF NAUSEA AND VOMITING—cont'd

DRUG	USUAL INDICATIONS	USUAL DOSE (RANGE)	ROUTE	COMMENTS
Moderately emetogenic CTX		Day 1: 5-HT_3 RA plus dexamethasone 8 mg	IV or PO	Days 2-3: continue oral 5-HT_3 RA or dexamethasone 8 mg to reduce delayed emesis
Highly emetogenic CTX		Day 1: 5-HT_3 RA plus dexamethasone 12 mg plus neurokinin-1 RA	IV or PO	Give aprepitant 80 mg PO days 2-3 and dexamethasone 8 mg PO days 2-4 to reduce delayed emesis

CNS = central nervous system; CTX = chemotherapy; GIDz = gastrointestinal disorders associated with nausea and vomiting; 5-HT_3 = serotonin 5-hydroxytryptamine$_3$; MS = motion sickness; PONV = postoperative nausea and vomiting; RA = receptor antagonist; RadTx = radiation therapy–induced nausea and vomiting; V = vertigo.

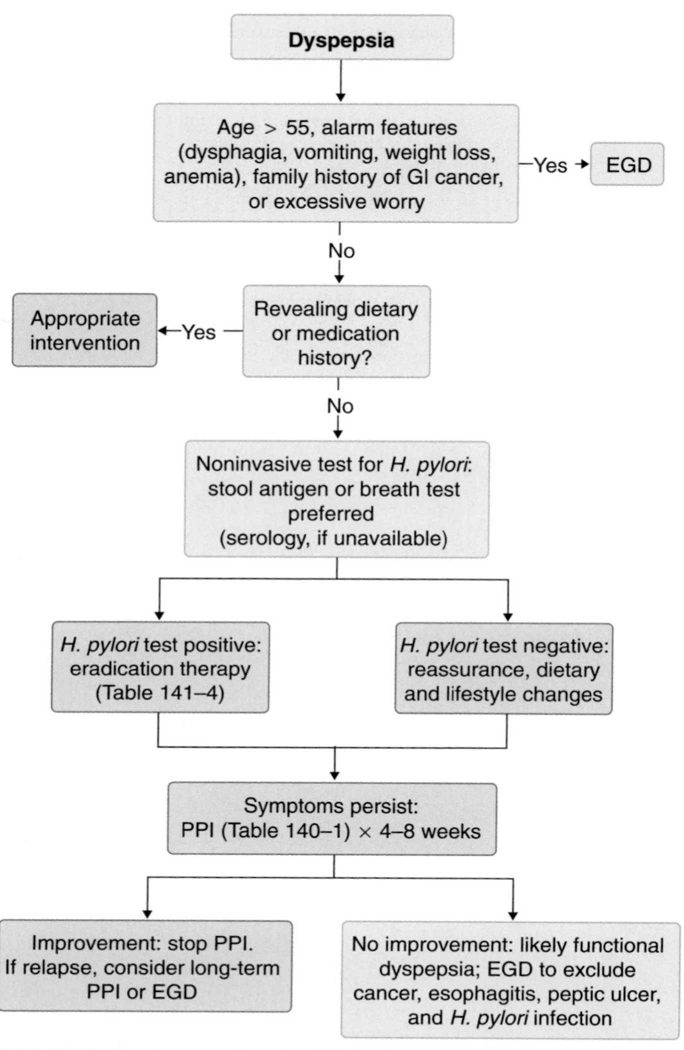

FIGURE 134-6. Approach to the patient with dyspepsia. EGD = esophagogastroduodenoscopy; GI = gastrointestinal; PPI = proton pump inhibitor.

is manifested by large-volume maroon or bright red bloody stools (hematochezia). Although 80 to 90% of patients with hematochezia have a lower source of bleeding, massive upper GI bleeding also may cause hematochezia. Approximately 95% of major lower GI bleeding arises from the colon and 5% from the small intestine. Lower GI bleeding is increased in patients older than 50 years, in whom diverticulosis accounts for 60% of cases; the remainder are due to ischemia, neoplasms, ulcers, vascular ectasias, or hemorrhoids. In patients younger than 50, bleeding is more commonly attributable to inflammatory bowel disease, hemorrhoids, or infectious colitis.

Occult GI bleeding refers to GI blood loss that is small in volume and not apparent to the patient but is detectable by tests for fecal occult blood. Chronic occult bleeding may result in iron deficiency anemia. Both upper endoscopy and colonoscopy should be performed to look for a source of occult bleeding, most commonly gastroesophageal or colonic neoplasia, erosive esophagitis or gastritis, ulcer disease, or vascular ectasia. In patients with recurrent iron deficiency and occult blood loss in whom no source is found on upper and lower endoscopy, video capsule endoscopy or enteroscopy is performed to look for a small bowel source (vascular ectasia, ulcer, or neoplasm).

Fecal incontinence (Chapter 147) is dependent on a number of factors, including a solid or semisolid stool, a compliant and distensible rectal reservoir, the ability to sense rectal fullness, an intact internal anal sphincter (an involuntary muscle innervated by the enteric nervous system), an intact external anal sphincter and puborectalis (voluntary muscles innervated by the pudendal nerve), and the mental and physical ability to reach a toilet facility when needed. Minor incontinence, which occurs in 10% of people older than 70 years, is characterized by the inability to control flatus or by the seepage of fecal matter that results in soiling of the perianal area and undergarments. It tends to be intermittent, occurring after bowel movements; when coughing, lifting, or passing flatus; or when stools are loose. Major incontinence is characterized by the partial or complete inability to reliably control bowel movements, resulting in gross, involuntary loss of feces and the need to wear a diaper. It occurs in less than 1% of the population and is virtually always caused by a central nervous system disorder that results in diminished awareness of bowel needs, neuropathy, or damage to the anal sphincters.

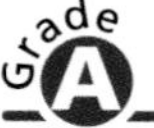

1. Maggio AQ, Reece-Smith AM, Tang TY, et al. Early laparoscopy versus active observation in acute abdominal pain: systematic review and meta-analysis. *Int J Surg.* 2008;6:400-403.
2. Pimentel M, Lembo A, Chey WD, et al. Rifaximin therapy for patients with irritable bowel syndrome without constipation. *N Engl J Med.* 2011;364:22-32.
3. Billio A, Morello E, Clarke MJ. Serotonin receptor antagonists for highly emetogenic chemotherapy in adults. *Cochrane Database Syst Rev.* 2010.1.CD006272.
4. Davis MP, Hallerberg G. Palliative Medicine Study Group of the Multinational Association of Supportive Care in Cancer. A systematic review of the treatment of nausea and vomiting in cancer unrelated to chemotherapy or radiation. *J Pain Symptom Manage.* 2010;39:756-767.
5. Apfel CC, Korttila K, Abdalla M, et al. A factorial trial of six interventions for the prevention of postoperative nausea and vomiting. *N Engl J Med.* 2004;350:2441-2451.

SUGGESTED READINGS

Metalidis C, Knockaert DC, Bobbaers H, et al. Involuntary weight loss. Does a negative baseline evaluation provide reassurance? *Eur J Intern Med.* 2008;19:345-349. *Organic causes were found in 56%, including malignancy in 22%, a psychiatric disorder in 16%, and no cause in 28%.*

Roila F, Herrstedt J, Gralla RJ, et al. Prevention of chemotherapy- and radiotherapy-induced nausea and vomiting: guideline update and results of the Perugia consensus. *Support Care Cancer.* 2011;19:S63-S65. *Consensus guidelines.*

Stoker J, van Randen A, Lameris W. Imaging patients with acute abdominal pain. *Radiology.* 2009;253:31-46. *Abdominal CT scan is recommended, except that ultrasonography is preferred for patients with suspected cholecystitis.*

Strate LL, Naumann CR. The role of colonoscopy and other procedures in the management of lower gastrointestinal bleeding *Clin Gastroenterol Hepatol.* 2010;8:333-343. *Review of lower GI bleeding and the controversies surrounding optimal initial management.*

135

DIAGNOSTIC IMAGING PROCEDURES IN GASTROENTEROLOGY

DAVID H. KIM AND PERRY J. PICKHARDT

A wide range of diagnostic imaging modalities is available for evaluating diseases of the gastrointestinal (GI) tract and the hepatopancreaticobiliary system. Once the workhorse of GI radiology, conventional radiography and fluoroscopy are still relevant but have largely given way to more advanced cross-sectional imaging studies such as ultrasonography, computed tomography (CT), and magnetic resonance imaging (MRI). Many of the visceral vascular evaluations undertaken by conventional angiography have been replaced by these noninvasive modalities as well. These cross-sectional technologies have become the preferred methods of evaluation, allowing more precise and accurate diagnoses. In addition, cross-sectional techniques can be used to guide a wide variety of interventional procedures. With the emergence of molecular imaging, there has been renewed interest in nuclear medicine, most notably positron emission tomography (PET).

CONVENTIONAL RADIOGRAPHY

Conventional radiographs, often referred to as "plain films," remain useful for a limited number of abdominal indications but are generally much less sensitive and specific for pathology compared with techniques such as CT. Advantages of radiography include its wide availability, low cost, and portability, allowing the acquisition of images in acute clinical situations. Supine and upright frontal abdominal radiographs can assess rapidly for bowel obstruction or perforation in the setting of an acute abdomen (Fig. 135-1). Serial abdominal radiographs remain a practical approach for following patients with an abnormal bowel gas pattern suggestive of either evolving small bowel obstruction or adynamic ileus. Conventional radiographs can demonstrate abnormal abdominal calcifications and radiopaque foreign bodies. In each of these cases, however, cross-sectional modalities such as CT have increased sensitivity and provide better delineation of disease processes. CT is often undertaken when the initial plain film evaluation is negative or to provide better information when conventional radiography is positive.

FLUOROSCOPIC PROCEDURES

Standard double-contrast barium examinations that depict the mucosa, particularly of the stomach, duodenum, and colon, have largely been supplanted by endoscopy (Chapter 136) and advanced radiologic techniques. However, a variety of single-column fluoroscopic contrast studies remain quite useful because of their relatively noninvasive nature and their low cost. Real-time fluoroscopic contrast studies can provide a valuable physiologic evaluation, serve as a problem-solving tool when endoscopy is equivocal or contraindicated, and evaluate for suspected leaks, perforations, or fistulas. Depending on the specific indication, either barium or water-soluble iodinated contrast material may be used.

The videofluoroscopic swallowing study and barium esophagram are effective noninvasive means of excluding significant pathology in patients with dysphagia. Endoscopy is generally indicated when an esophageal stricture or mass is encountered on fluoroscopic examination, but it can be avoided in many cases that lack concerning findings. Fluoroscopic contrast evaluation may also avoid the need for endoscopy in symptomatic patients with suspected esophagitis from *Candida* or herpes infection. In the setting of gastroesophageal reflux disease, the barium esophagram is effective for excluding significant complications such as peptic stricture and adenocarcinoma, but it is insensitive to the changes of Barrett's esophagus (Chapter 140).

Although the double-contrast barium upper GI series can identify mucosal abnormalities of the stomach and duodenum, such as erosions, ulcers, polyps, and masses (Fig. 135-2), this function is now largely the domain of esophagogastroduodenoscopy (EGD). Gastroduodenal barium studies still play an important diagnostic role in evaluating for sliding hiatal and/or paraesophageal hernias and in pediatric evaluations for malrotation and hypertrophic pyloric stenosis.

For evaluation of the mesenteric small bowel, capsule endoscopy, CT enterography, and magnetic resonance (MR) enterography have largely replaced barium studies. Although fluoroscopic studies can still provide an anatomic roadmap, assess transit time, and detect fold thickening, the evaluation of unexplained GI bleeding (Chapter 137) or possible Crohn's disease (Chapter 143) is better performed using CT, MRI, or capsule endoscopy.

The single-contrast barium enema remains an important diagnostic tool in such settings as suspected sigmoid volvulus, colonic obstruction, postoperative leak or fistula, and ileocolic intussusception in children (Chapter 144). Many practices continue to perform fluoroscopic defecography to help delineate functional abnormalities in patients with evacuation disorders (Chapter 147), although dynamic MR cine series have replaced defecography at some institutions.

ULTRASONOGRAPHY

The introduction of harmonic and compound imaging, advances in high-resolution transducers, and improvements in color Doppler evaluation have all combined to enhance the diagnostic capabilities of portable ultrasound.

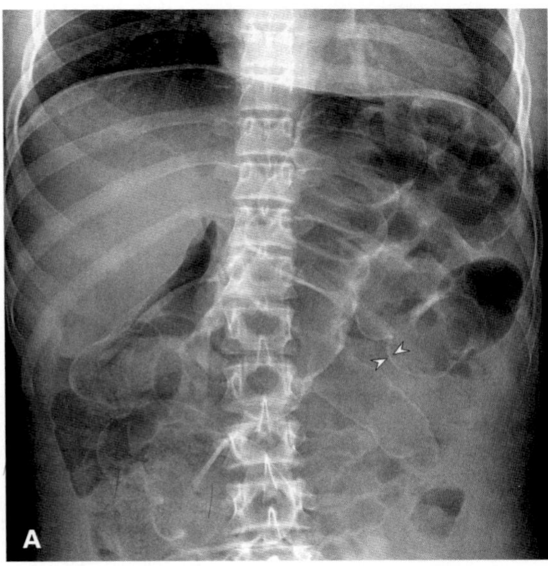

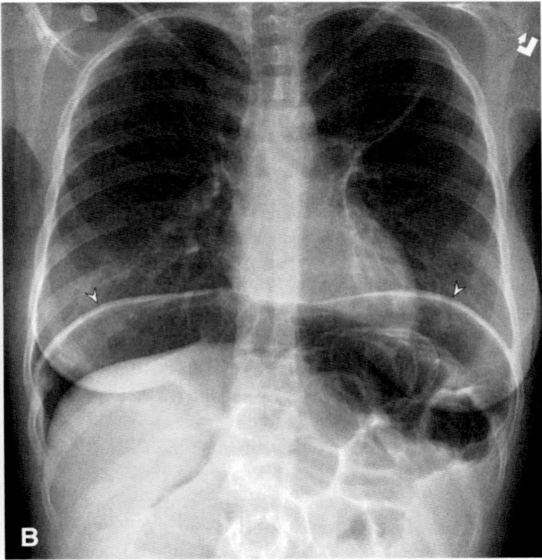

FIGURE 135-1. Pneumoperitoneum from bowel perforation on conventional radiographs. A, Supine abdominal radiograph shows abnormal lucency surrounding multiple bowel loops and the liver. Both sides of the bowel wall *(arrowheads)* are outlined by gas in areas (Rigler's sign), which typically requires a large amount of free peritoneal air to be visible on supine films. **B,** Upright radiograph centered over the diaphragm *(arrowheads)* shows the large amount of free intraperitoneal air (lucent area just inferior to the diaphragm) to better advantage. This view is more sensitive for the detection of pneumoperitoneum.

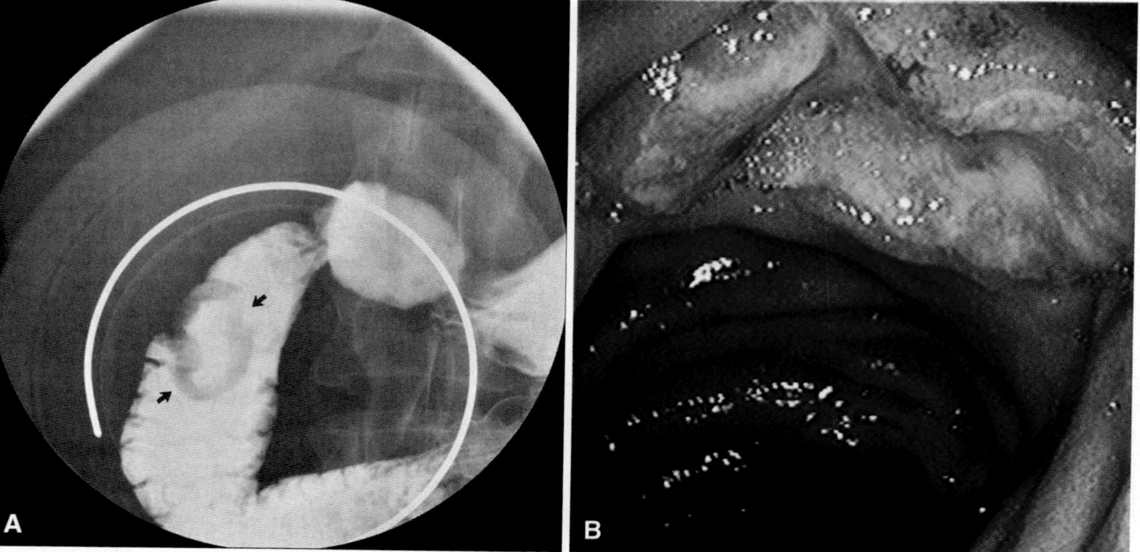

FIGURE 135-2. Metastatic melanoma on barium upper GI study. A, Fluoroscopic spot film image shows a filling defect *(arrows)* within the second portion of the duodenum that has a "bull's-eye" or "target" appearance due to the collection of barium in the center of the lesion. This appearance is characteristic of a submucosal mass with central ulceration and is typical of hematogenous metastatic disease from melanoma. **B,** Digital photograph from EGD confirms the presence of an ulcerated submucosal mass within the duodenum.

In general, ultrasound is useful for imaging solid organs and fluid-filled structures, but it is unable to penetrate gas-filled structures. For example, overlying bowel gas often precludes a complete sonographic evaluation of the pancreas. Ultrasound is a relatively versatile imaging technique, in that it can be performed via many different routes, including transabdominal, endoscopic (as part of EGD), transrectal, intravascular, and endovaginal approaches. In addition, it is excellent for many image-guided interventions because of its real-time evaluation.

With regard to GI pathology, ultrasonography is used most frequently to evaluate the liver and biliary system. Suspected acute cholecystitis (Chapter 158) is a common indication for right upper quadrant sonography; classic findings include cholelithiasis, gallbladder wall thickening, and a sonographic Murphy's sign (reproducible pain when the transducer is pressed over the gallbladder) (Fig. 135-3). The sensitivity for detecting gallstones with ultrasonography exceeds 95%. Acalculous cholelithiasis can be a more challenging diagnosis because the findings overlap with nonspecific gallbladder wall thickening in critically ill patients. Ultrasound is typically the first imaging test obtained in patients with new-onset jaundice or cholestatic laboratory findings because it offers a rapid, noninvasive evaluation of the biliary tree to differentiate obstruction from other causes. If biliary ductal dilation is present, the level and cause of the obstruction can sometimes be demonstrated on ultrasound; common causes include choledocholithiasis and pancreatic head masses. In most cases of biliary obstruction, additional imaging tests will be necessary, consisting of CT, MR cholangiopancreatography (MRCP), endoscopic retrograde cholangiopancreatography (ERCP), or percutaneous transhepatic cholangiography (PTC), depending on the specific circumstances.

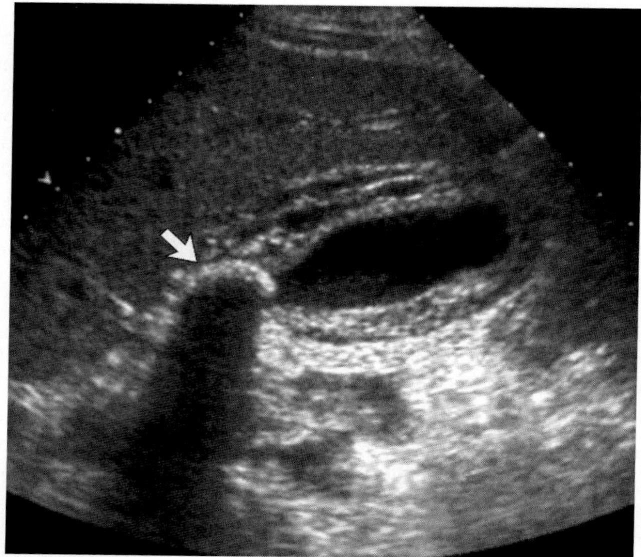

FIGURE 135-3. Acute cholecystitis on ultrasound. Image from right upper quadrant sonography shows diffuse gallbladder wall thickening and a shadowing impacted gallstone *(arrow)*. A sonographic Murphy's sign was present. These findings are diagnostic for acute calculous cholecystitis.

Ultrasonography can be used to detect or further characterize focal liver lesions (Chapter 154), although it is typically less sensitive and specific than CT or MRI. Ultrasound is quite capable of distinguishing cystic from solid lesions. Although not approved for use in the United States, intravenous contrast agents for ultrasound have been studied fairly extensively in other countries and appear to offer similar advantages seen with CT and MRI contrast agents.

In diffuse disease, ultrasound is being used with increased frequency to screen patients with viral hepatitis for cirrhosis and hepatocellular carcinoma (Chapters 156 and 202). Sonographic findings in cirrhosis include a heterogeneously coarsened parenchymal echotexture, nodular surface contour, predominantly right-sided volume loss, and evidence of portal hypertension, including ascites, splenomegaly, and portosystemic collaterals. Focal hepatic lesions in the setting of cirrhosis are concerning for hepatocellular carcinoma, but they may also represent regenerative or dysplastic nodules. In noncirrhotic patients with elevated liver enzymes, ultrasonography can often suggest the diagnosis of hepatic steatosis (fatty liver; Chapter 155) when the parenchyma demonstrates increased echogenicity and decreased penetration of the sound beam. The findings of steatosis can be focal, multifocal, or diffuse; MRI is more specific and can confirm the diagnosis.

Color and power Doppler evaluation allows the noninvasive sonographic assessment of vascular patency. Doppler evaluation of the liver is commonly performed in patients with end-stage liver disease (Chapter 157) to evaluate the portal system and search for portosystemic collaterals. Abnormal portal vein findings include hepatofugal flow and thrombosis (Fig. 135-4). Doppler ultrasound is also used for the evaluation of transjugular intrahepatic portosystemic shunts (TIPS), both before and after stent placement. In orthotopic liver transplant recipients, Doppler evaluation is frequently performed to assess the hepatic vasculature, with particular attention to the hepatic arterial supply.

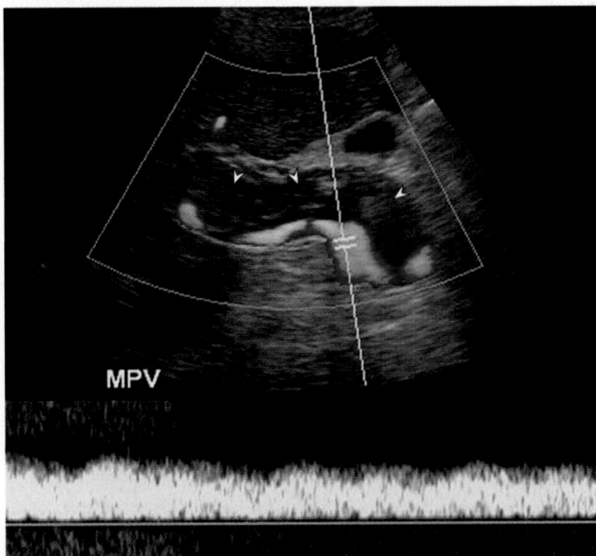

FIGURE 135-4. Portal vein thrombosis on ultrasound. Ultrasound gray-scale image with both power color Doppler and spectral Doppler interrogation shows a tubular hypoechoic structure *(arrowheads)* consistent with nonocclusive thrombus filling the majority of the main portal vein (MPV). Flow patency is seen in the deep peripheral aspect of the vessel.

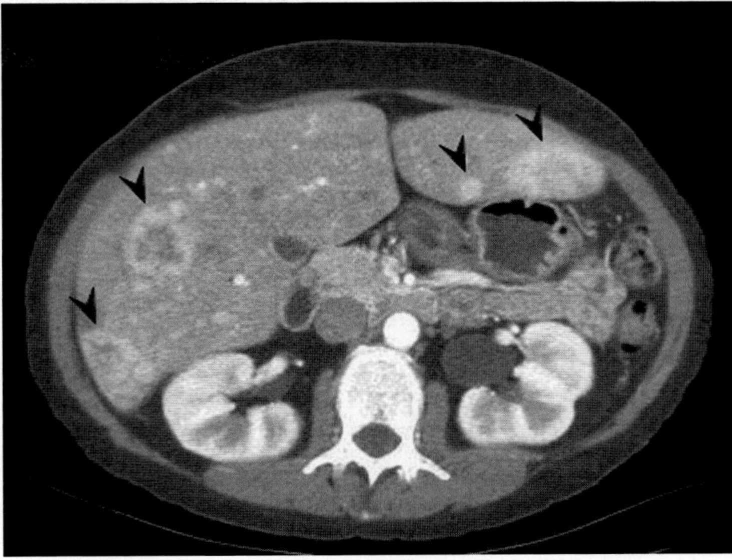

FIGURE 135-5. Multiple hypervascular liver lesions on CT. Dynamic contrast-enhanced CT image obtained during the arterial phase shows multiple hypervascular liver lesions *(arrowheads)*, which proved to be hepatic adenomas in a patient with von Gierke's disease.

COMPUTED TOMOGRAPHY

CT has revolutionized the imaging of abdominal pathology, providing a rapid, reproducible, and comprehensive evaluation. The introduction of single-detector helical or spiral CT, followed by multidetector scanners, has resulted in improved resolution and faster acquisition of true volumetric data. High-resolution scans of the entire abdomen and pelvis can now be easily acquired in a single short breath-hold. With the automated, high-rate injection of intravenous contrast materials and advanced processing, specialized CT examinations are replacing many traditional modalities. A major challenge, however, is to minimize radiation doses as CT use increases. The clinical indications for abdominal CT are very broad. One common use is the diagnostic evaluation of a nontraumatic acute abdomen (Chapter 144). Common inflammatory conditions such as appendicitis and diverticulitis are readily diagnosed by CT. Other common indications include evaluation for intra-abdominal abscess, pancreatitis, and small bowel obstruction. In cases of relatively high-grade bowel obstruction, CT can often localize the transition point, elucidate the underlying cause, and evaluate for vascular compromise. In the setting of an acute abdomen due to blunt trauma (Chapter 112), CT has become invaluable for the prompt detection of significant abdominal injury.

In the nonacute setting, multiphase CT with intravenous contrast can characterize lesions and often results in a noninvasive diagnosis, particularly in combination with the clinical history (Fig. 135-5). Primary abdominal malignancies, such as pancreatic cancer and hepatocellular carcinoma, are often first detected on CT. Abdominal staging for metastatic disease, including hematogenous, lymphatic, peritoneal, and local spread, is commonly performed with CT, as is assessing the response to various therapies.

CT is increasingly being used for primary bowel evaluation, often replacing traditional fluoroscopy because of its increased sensitivity and specificity. CT enterography protocols often combine neutral (i.e., water density) oral contrast with dynamic, high-resolution imaging that provides detailed multiplanar evaluation of the small bowel. Dedicated CT enterography and capsule endoscopy yield a complementary and comprehensive evaluation of the small bowel. CT colonography, also referred to as virtual colonoscopy, combines two- and three-dimensional evaluation of the prepared and distended colon for the detection of colorectal polyps and masses (Fig. 135-6). CT colonography is a promising tool for colorectal evaluation, particularly if it can improve adherence rates associated with screening. Optical colonoscopy is still required for polypectomy.

Visceral CT angiography is largely replacing conventional diagnostic angiography. For example, in many institutions, evaluation of the vascular anatomy before hepatic transplantation (Chapter 157) is now undertaken by CT rather than by catheter angiography (Fig. 135-7).

MAGNETIC RESONANCE IMAGING

The advantages of MRI over CT for abdominal evaluation include superior soft tissue contrast resolution and lack of ionizing radiation. However, for many institutions, MRI remains primarily a problem-solving tool for the abdomen because of several drawbacks, including decreased spatial resolution, longer examination times, increased expense, decreased availability, and inability to scan some patients owing to claustrophobia or implanted devices such as cardiac pacemakers. Imaging artifacts can also make MRI interpretation more difficult and less uniform across different readers.

Contrast-enhanced MRI offers a dynamic evaluation comparable to CT for the solid abdominal organs. In addition, intravenous gadolinium-based agents with hepatocyte-specific uptake increase MRI's diagnostic capabilities in evaluating focal hepatic lesions (Fig. 135-8). The high accuracy of MRI in diagnosing hepatic steatosis (Chapter 155) can sometimes prevent unnecessary biopsy, particularly in cases of nodular focal fatty infiltration that simulates metastatic disease. MRI is also sensitive for detecting iron overload within the liver and other organs related to primary hemochromatosis (Chapter 219) and secondary hemosiderosis (most often due to multiple transfusions). Similar to CT, MRI can provide quality arterial and venous angiographic imaging, such that conventional angiography is generally reserved for therapeutic interventions.

In the past, contrast MRI was considered an alternative to CT in patients with decreased renal function. However, the newly recognized condition of nephrogenic systemic fibrosis (Fig. 135-9) argues against this strategy. Nephrogenic systemic fibrosis, characterized by involvement of the skin, eyes, joints, and internal organs, is associated with intravenous gadolinium administration. Patients with impaired renal function are at risk of developing this rare but often fatal condition related to heavy metal toxicity from free gadolinium that has been dissociated from its chelate. Currently, there is no curative treatment.

Two specialized MR examinations have significantly changed practice patterns in recent years. MRCP, a heavily T2-weighted imaging technique for the noninvasive diagnostic evaluation of the biliary and pancreatic ductal systems, relies not on contrast administration but on the presence of static fluid. MRCP can be a useful screening tool to select appropriate candidates for more invasive therapeutic procedures such as ERCP and PTC. MRCP is useful for diagnosing biliary and pancreatic ductal obstruction, choledocholithiasis, primary sclerosing cholangitis, and cystic conditions such as Caroli's disease (Fig. 135-10). T1-weighted MR cholangiography with intravenous contrast agents that undergo biliary excretion can be useful in evaluating for bile leaks, analogous to hepatobiliary scintigraphy.

MR enterography is increasingly used to monitor patients with Crohn's disease (Chapter 143). Given the lack of ionizing radiation, it is particularly

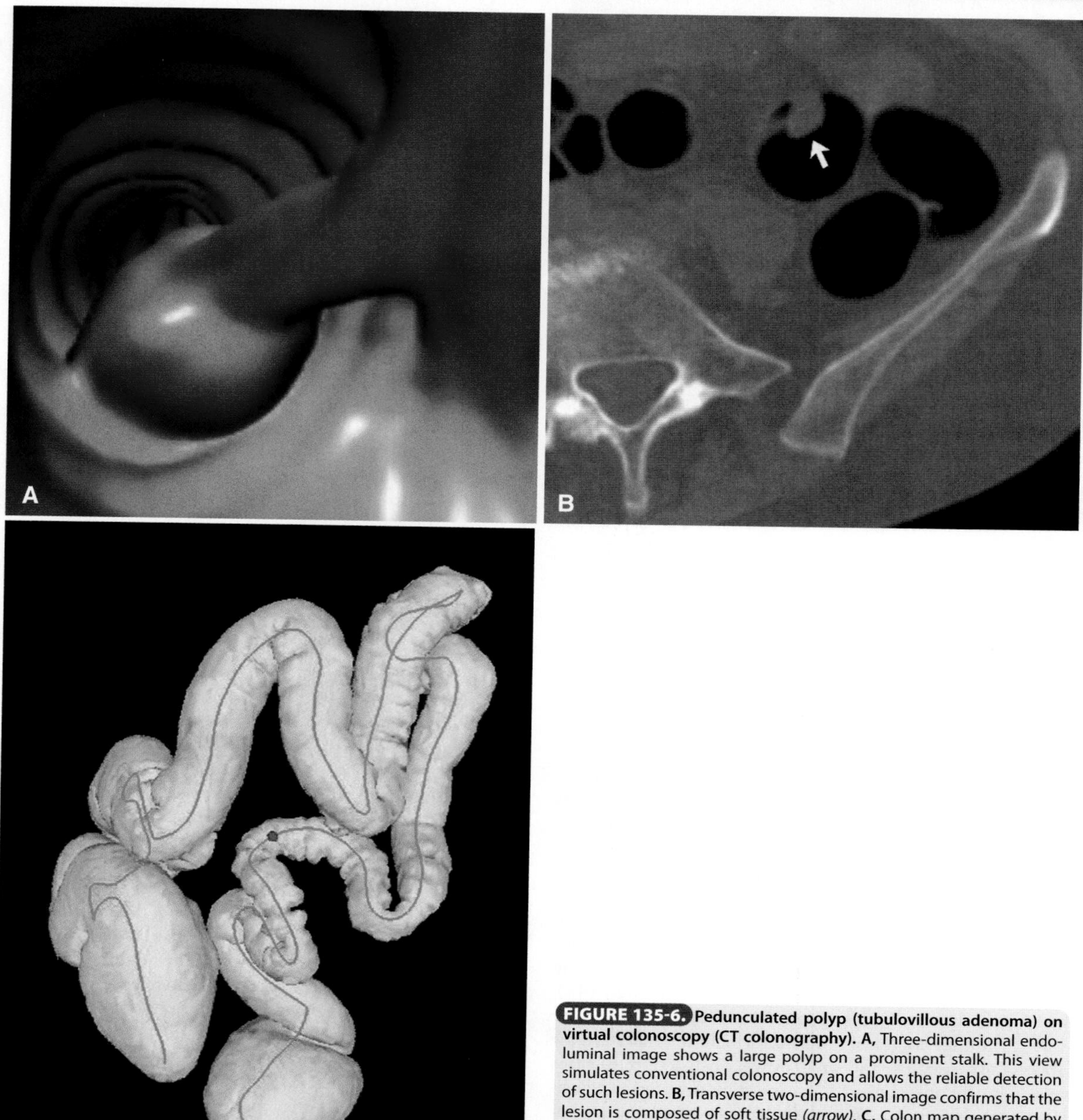

FIGURE 135-6. Pedunculated polyp (tubulovillous adenoma) on virtual colonoscopy (CT colonography). **A,** Three-dimensional endoluminal image shows a large polyp on a prominent stalk. This view simulates conventional colonoscopy and allows the reliable detection of such lesions. **B,** Transverse two-dimensional image confirms that the lesion is composed of soft tissue *(arrow)*. **C,** Colon map generated by the virtual colonoscopy software system allows precise localization of the polyp (red dot in sigmoid colon). The green line represents the centerline for automated navigation.

advantageous in young patients who require multiple examinations over a lifetime. Oral contrast agents such as polyethylene glycol are given to distend the small bowel; spasmolytics are typically administered to decrease bowel peristalsis. Similar to CT, fast breath-held imaging with intravenous contrast administration allows the evaluation of mucosal and wall enhancement or thickening, suggesting active disease. Unlike CT, MRI can assess intrinsic signal characteristics on T2-weighted images to improve specificity and distinguish active inflammation from chronic fibrostenotic disease (Fig. 135-11). Other emerging applications include MR staging for rectal cancer to assess the need for neoadjuvant chemoradiation.

INTERVENTIONAL PROCEDURES

Ultrasound, CT, fluoroscopy, and even MR techniques have been used for guidance when performing a wide variety of abdominal interventional procedures. Percutaneous image-guided biopsy, whether by fine-needle aspiration or core biopsy, is a relatively safe procedure that is commonly performed for tissue diagnosis and has drastically reduced the need for open surgical biopsy. Other common nonvascular procedures that use image guidance include abscess drainage, biliary interventions, gastrostomy, and tumor ablation. In the case of peridiverticular and periappendiceal abscesses, CT-guided drainage can often simplify the ultimate operative approach and turn high-risk emergent surgery into a safer elective procedure. Biliary interventions include transhepatic access of an obstructed system for stenting or external drainage, as well as cholecystostomy tube placement. Percutaneous CT- or ultrasound-guided tumor ablation is a rapidly evolving technique that is particularly useful in poor operative candidates or in conjunction with surgical resection of other lesions. A variety of ablation methods have been employed, including radio frequency, alcohol, microwave, and cryoablation.

Diagnostic conventional angiography has been largely replaced by noninvasive CT and MR techniques, but direct catheter angiography remains an important procedure for directing various therapies. Vascular interventions include angioplasty, stenting, embolization, and thrombolysis. TIPS placement (Chapter 157) is a commonly performed angiographic procedure in patients with portal hypertension complicated by variceal bleeding or intractable ascites. Placement of a TIPS stent creates a low-pressure communication between the portal and hepatic venous systems. Chemoembolization can provide palliation for those with advanced hepatic malignancy, whether primary or metastatic.

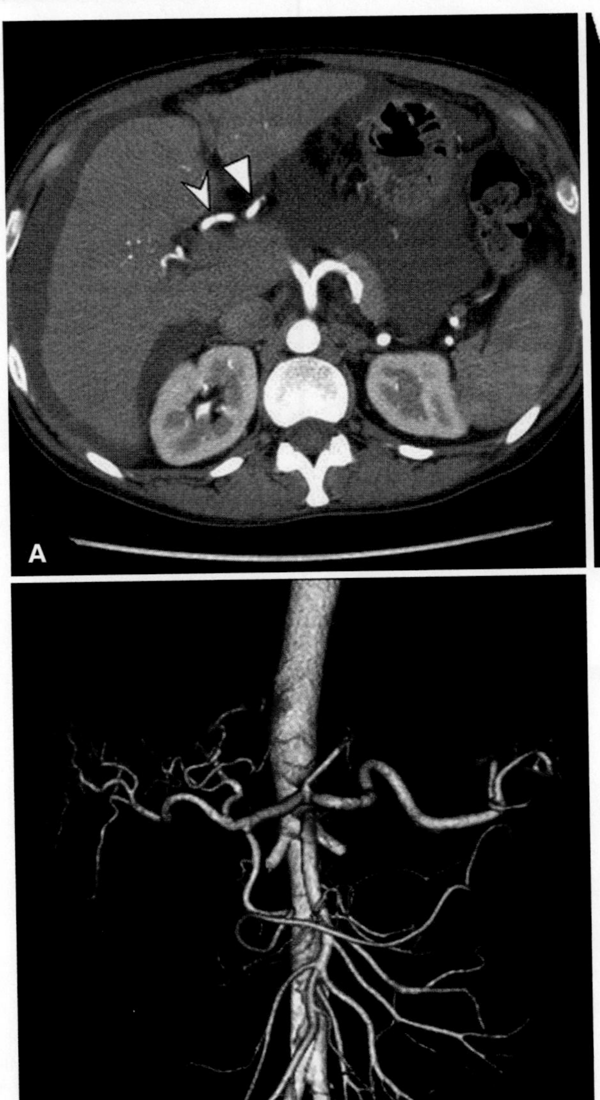

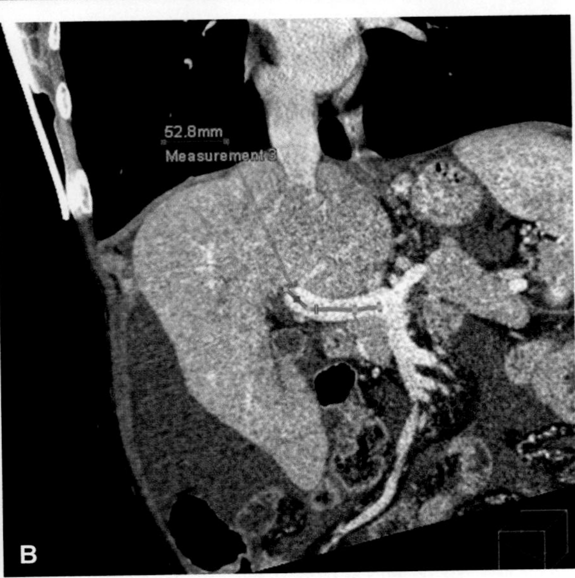

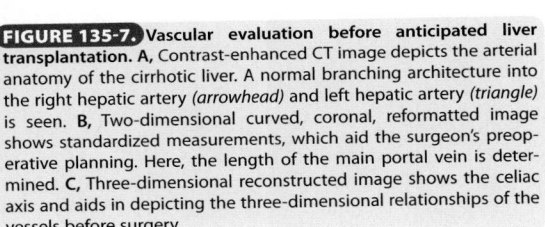

FIGURE 135-7. Vascular evaluation before anticipated liver transplantation. A, Contrast-enhanced CT image depicts the arterial anatomy of the cirrhotic liver. A normal branching architecture into the right hepatic artery *(arrowhead)* and left hepatic artery *(triangle)* is seen. **B,** Two-dimensional curved, coronal, reformatted image shows standardized measurements, which aid the surgeon's preoperative planning. Here, the length of the main portal vein is determined. **C,** Three-dimensional reconstructed image shows the celiac axis and aids in depicting the three-dimensional relationships of the vessels before surgery.

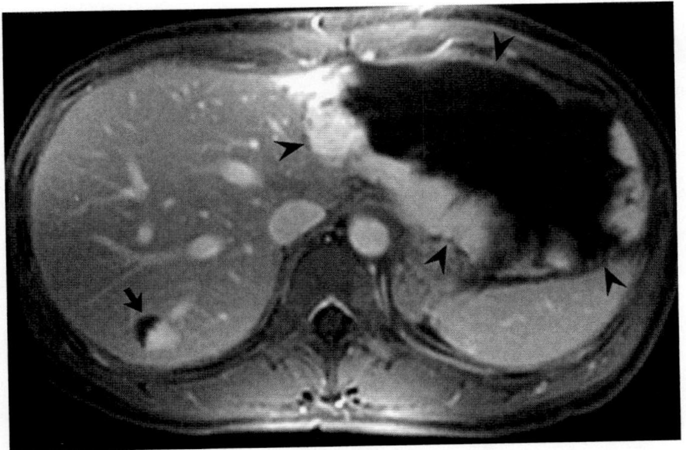

FIGURE 135-8. Hepatic cavernous hemangiomas on MRI. Contrast-enhanced fat-suppressed gradient echo MRI shows the characteristic findings of cavernous hemangiomas, including a giant left hepatic lobe lesion *(arrowheads)* and a smaller right hepatic lobe lesion *(arrow)*. Note the peripheral enhancement of the lesions, which matches the signal intensity of the aortic blood pool. These findings are diagnostic, and tissue biopsy is unnecessary.

NUCLEAR MEDICINE (RADIONUCLIDE SCINTIGRAPHY)

Owing to the emergence of PET-CT for oncologic evaluation, nuclear medicine is more relevant now than ever before in abdominal imaging. PET-CT is a powerful diagnostic tool that combines functional and anatomic imaging. PET is useful for both initial staging and evaluating the response to therapy for a wide range of primary malignant tumors, especially when combined with CT (Fig. 135-12). Currently, clinical PET imaging most often utilizes F^{18}-fluorodeoxyglucose, but other positron-emitting agents may be used for specific purposes.

Several other nuclear medicine studies are used to evaluate GI and hepatobiliary diseases. Injection of red blood cells labeled with technetium-99m provides a useful test for GI bleeding. Advantages of performing this as the initial diagnostic imaging study include its noninvasive nature, high sensitivity for active bleeding, and ability to rescan the patient hours later without the need for repeat injection. Disadvantages include relatively poor anatomic localization and lack of therapeutic ability. The use of tagged red blood cell scintigraphy for the diagnosis of hepatic cavernous hemangioma has decreased significantly owing to advances in CT and MRI. Hepatobiliary scintigraphy remains a useful tool in equivocal cases of cholecystitis, particularly acalculous disease, and it can confirm suspected biliary leaks. Scintigraphic imaging with In^{111}-octreotide is valuable for the diagnosis, staging,

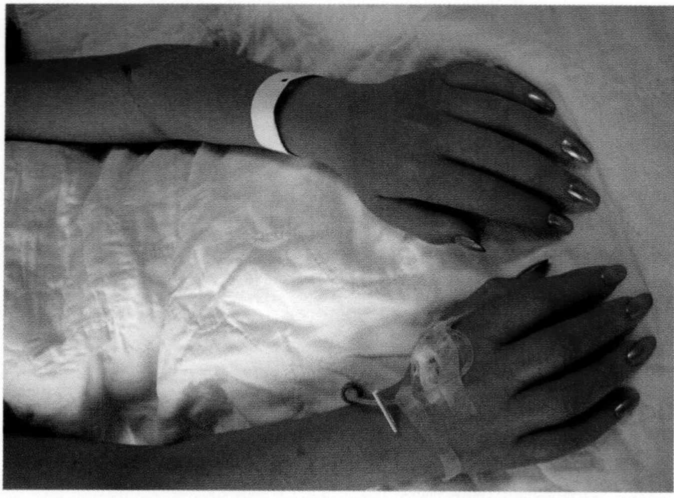

FIGURE 135-9. **Nephrogenic systemic fibrosis (NSF).** Digital photograph of the upper extremities in a patient with NSF shows vague fibrotic plaques that are difficult to visualize but easily palpated. In the skin, NSF presents as bilateral, symmetrical, and variably erythematous fibrotic plaques beginning distally and progressing proximally, often with a reticulated advancing edge. (Courtesy of Dr. Molly A. Hinshaw.)

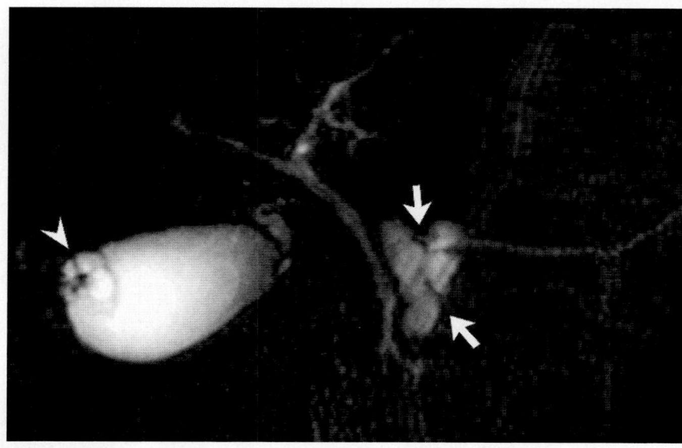

FIGURE 135-10. **Pancreatic intraductal papillary mucinous neoplasm on MRCP.** Heavily T2-weighted MR image shows a lobulated cystic lesion in the pancreatic head region *(arrows)* that represents a side branch intraductal papillary mucinous neoplasm. Note the mild focal irregularity of the gallbladder *(arrowhead)*, consistent with the fundal form of adenomyomatosis. The intra- and extrahepatic biliary ducts are normal.

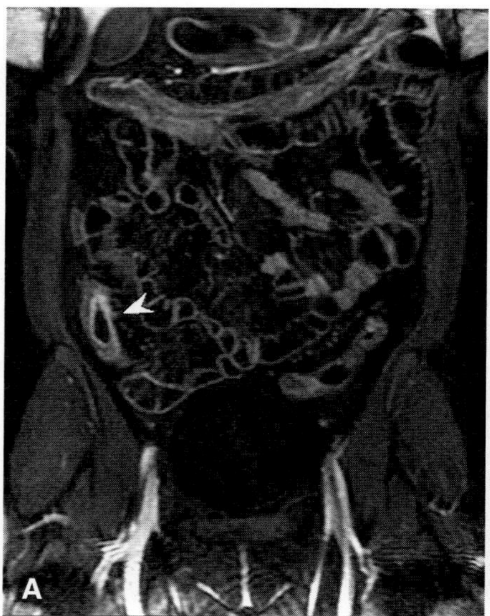

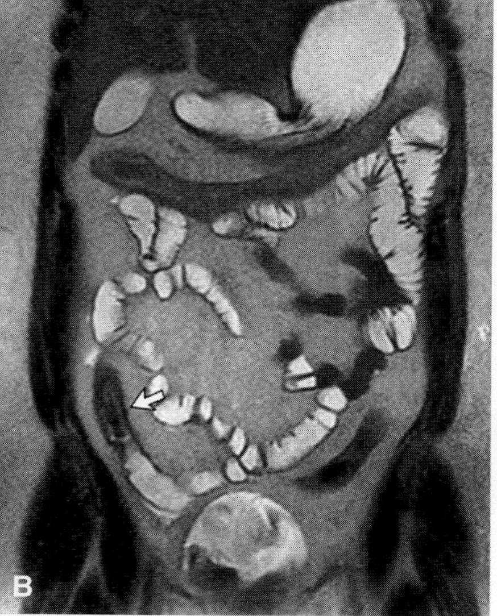

FIGURE 135-11. **Active Crohn's disease on MR enterography.** **A,** Coronal three-dimensional volume-acquired breath-hold, T1-weighted, gradient-echo image with dynamic gadolinium administration and fat saturation shows wall thickening and enhancement *(arrowhead)* of an abnormal segment of terminal ileum. **B,** Coronal two-dimensional single-shot, fast spin-echo, T2-weighted image shows increased signal in this area *(arrow)*, signifying edema and active disease.

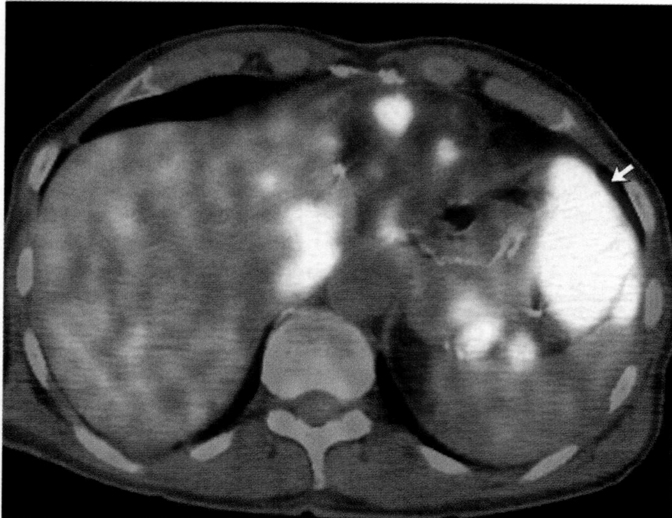

FIGURE 135-12. **Metastatic gastrointestinal stromal tumor (GIST) on fused PET-CT.** Transverse fused PET-CT image shows a dominant hypermetabolic mass *(arrow)* representing a gastric GIST. Multiple smaller peritoneal and hepatic hypermetabolic foci are consistent with metastatic deposits. Note the utility of combining the functional information from PET with the anatomic localization provided by CT.

and follow-up of GI neuroendocrine tumors, such as carcinoid and pancreatic islet cell tumors.

SUGGESTED READINGS

American College of Radiology, Expert Panel on Gastrointestinal Imaging. ACR Appropriateness Criteria. http://www.acr.org/s_acr/sec.asp?CID=1207&DID=15048. *Recommended imaging approaches for various clinical presentations.*

Currie GM, Kiat H, Wheat JM. Scintigraphic evaluation of acute lower gastrointestinal hemorrhage: current status and future directions. *J Clin Gastroenterol.* 2011;45:92-99. *Review.*

Mellinger JD, Bittner JG 4th, Edwards MA, et al. Imaging of gastrointestinal bleeding. *Surg Clin North Am.* 2011;91:93-108. *Review.*

Singh JP, Steward MJ, Booth TC, et al. Evolution of imaging for abdominal perforation. *Ann R Coll Surg Engl.* 2010;92:182-188. *Emphasizes the role of CT.*

136

GASTROINTESTINAL ENDOSCOPY

PANKAJ JAY PASRICHA

IMPORTANCE AND USE OF ENDOSCOPY

Technologic advances in radiologic and endoscopic imaging have transformed medicine in the past few decades. With its remarkable accessibility, the gastrointestinal tract has benefited from the endoscopic approach perhaps more than any other organ system. The major advantages of endoscopy over contrast radiography in evaluating diseases of the alimentary tract include direct visualization, resulting in a more accurate and sensitive evaluation of mucosal lesions; the ability to obtain biopsy specimens from superficial lesions; and the ability to perform therapeutic interventions. These advantages make endoscopy the procedure of choice in most cases in which mucosal lesions or growths are suspected. Conversely, computed tomography (CT) or, occasionally, contrast radiography may be indicated when extrinsic or intrinsic distortions of anatomy are suspected, such as volvulus, intussusceptions, subtle strictures, or complicated postsurgical changes (Chapter 135).

INSTRUMENTS AND PROCEDURES (TABLE 136-1)

Luminal Endoscopy: Conventional and Wireless

The vast majority of endoscopic procedures are intraluminal in nature. The endoscopic shaft not only carries the optical elements for imaging but also contains channels that enable various functions such as air insufflation, water irrigation, suction, and passage of diagnostic and therapeutic devices.

A relatively recent innovation is capsule endoscopy, with a disposable plastic capsule that measures 11 mm by 26 mm and contains a chip camera, batteries, and a radio transmitter that wirelessly sends images to a device that the patient wears as a belt. At the end of the procedure, the information is downloaded to a computer, and the capsule itself passes harmlessly in the stool. Variations of this instrument have been developed for esophageal and colonic imaging, but these are not yet recommended for routine clinical use.

Ancillary Organ Imaging: Endoscopic Retrograde Cholangiography and Pancreatography

Endoscopic retrograde cholangiopancreatography (ERCP) uses a side-viewing endoscope that accesses the second part of the duodenum, where a small catheter is introduced into the bile or pancreatic duct to inject radiographic contrast medium under fluoroscopic monitoring. Successful cannulation and imaging can be achieved in up to 95% of cases. In some instances, a fine-caliber endoscope can also be introduced into the duct of interest (cholangioscopy or pancreaticoscopy) for direct visualization of intraductal disease.

Mural and Transmural Imaging: Endoscopic Ultrasound

An ultrasonic transducer in the tip of a flexible endoscope or a stand-alone ultrasound probe inserted through the channel of a regular endoscope can image lesions within the wall of the gut and beyond. Endoscopic ultrasonography (EUS) can guide fine-needle aspiration more accurately than abdominal ultrasonography or CT.

COMPLICATIONS AND PRE-ENDOSCOPY PREPARATION

Diagnostic endoscopy is usually a remarkably safe and well-tolerated procedure. It can be performed under conscious sedation with a combination of benzodiazepines and narcotics or with propofol, which provides faster and deeper sedation with rapid recovery (Chapter 440). However, potential complications (Table 136-2) must be carefully explained to the patient as part of the informed consent process. In general, routine blood tests, radiographs, or electrocardiograms are not necessary before endoscopy unless a careful history and physical examination suggest possible hematologic, cardiovascular, or pulmonary or airway problems. Women of childbearing age should be questioned about the possibility of pregnancy and tested if there is any doubt.

Diagnostic endoscopies, including those with mucosal biopsies, are considered low risk and do not warrant discontinuation of anticoagulant medication. Similarly, aspirin or other nonsteroidal anti-inflammatory agents can be continued by patients undergoing screening colonoscopy. In high-risk elective procedures, anticoagulants and antiplatelet agents may be discontinued,

TABLE 136-1 ENDOSCOPIC PROCEDURES AND GENERAL APPLICATIONS

ENDOSCOPIC PROCEDURES	THERAPEUTIC APPLICATIONS
LUMINAL ENDOSCOPY	
Common procedures Esophagogastroduodenoscopy Colonoscopy Flexible sigmoidoscopy	Hemostasis Luminal restoration (dilation, ablation, stenting) Lesion removal (e.g., polypectomy, mucosal ablation) Provision of access (percutaneous endoscopic gastrostomy and jejunostomy)
Less common procedures Enteroscopy Capsule endoscopy	Barrier strengthening (antireflux procedures)
PANCREATOBILIARY IMAGING	
Endoscopic retrograde cholangiopancreatography	Lesion (stone) removal Luminal restoration (dilation, stenting) Provision of access (sphincterotomy) Drainage (bile, pancreatic pseudocyst)
TRANSLUMINAL IMAGING	
Endoscopic ultrasonography	Analgesic block Delivery of therapeutic agents (experimental)

TABLE 136-2 COMPLICATIONS OF ENDOSCOPY

ENDOSCOPIC COMPLICATIONS	INCIDENCE (%)	SPECIFIC PROPHYLAXIS
GENERAL COMPLICATIONS		
Complications related primarily to sedation (cardiovascular and respiratory depression, aspiration)	0.6-0.7	Airway protection with massive upper gastrointestinal bleeding Preprocedure medical evaluation, intraprocedure and postprocedure monitoring Anesthesiology consultation for high-risk patients
Perforation	0.14-0.25 (colonoscopy) 0.1-0.3 (upper endoscopy)	None (except careful technique)
Bleeding	0.7-2.5 (polypectomy) 0.3 (upper endoscopy)	Carefully balance risk and benefits Discontinue or reduce anticoagulant use before high-risk procedures
Bacteremia and infectious complications (endocarditis, bacterial ascites)	<0.1	Antibiotics for patients at risk for endocarditis (patients with artificial valves, pulmonary-systemic shunts, previous history of endocarditis), with synthetic vascular grafts, and with bacterial ascites (cirrhotics)
Death	0.2 (colonoscopy) 0.6 (upper endoscopy)	
COMPLICATIONS ASSOCIATED WITH SPECIALIZED PROCEDURES		
Pancreatitis (ERCP)	3-20	Not well established; experimental
Cholangitis (ERCP)	0.1-2	Preprocedure antibiotics
Wound infections (PEG)	3-4	Preprocedure antibiotics

ERCP = endoscopic retrograde cholangiopancreatography; PEG = percutaneous endoscopic gastrostomy.

in consultation with both the prescribing specialist and the gastroenterologist (Chapter 439). For patients with acute bleeding, reversal therapy or platelet replacement may be considered (Chapters 174 through 178).

ERCP is associated with the highest risk of serious complications, and about 1 to 5% of patients develop pancreatitis. Risk factors include young age, female gender, underlying sphincter of Oddi dysfunction, and previous history of pancreatitis. Despite a variety of trials, no pharmacologic prophylaxis has been unequivocally successful. However, most experts place a short-term pancreatic stent in high-risk cases as a reasonable preventive measure.

SPECIFIC INDICATIONS

Most indications for gastrointestinal endoscopy are based on the patient's presenting symptoms (e.g., dysphagia, bleeding, diarrhea). In other instances, endoscopy is required to evaluate specific lesions found by other diagnostic imaging, such as a gastric ulcer or colon polyp discovered by barium radiography. Finally, screening endoscopy is often performed in asymptomatic individuals on the basis of their risk for commonly occurring and preventable conditions, such as colon cancer (see later).

Implicit in the decision to perform endoscopy is the assumption that it will have a bearing on future management strategy. When evaluating gastrointestinal symptoms, several questions need to be addressed by the referring physician and the endoscopist: Which patients need endoscopy? When should the endoscopy be done? What is the endoscopist looking for? What endoscopic therapy, if any, should be planned?

Gastroesophageal Reflux and Heartburn (Chapters 140 and 141)

Gastroesophageal reflux disease (GERD) is an extremely common condition in the general population. The fact that its cardinal symptom, heartburn, is relatively specific for this condition justifies an empirical approach to treatment by a combination of lifestyle modifications and over-the-counter or even prescription drugs. Endoscopy is therefore not necessary to make the diagnosis of GERD. Indeed, normal findings on endoscopy do not rule out the diagnosis because the overall sensitivity of endoscopy in GERD is only about 70%. If necessary, further evaluation with ambulatory esophageal manometry and pH monitoring can establish the diagnosis. However, there are several circumstances in which endoscopy should be considered for patients with reflux, including those with warning symptoms ("red flags") such as dysphagia, odynophagia, regurgitation, weight loss, gastrointestinal bleeding, or frequent vomiting (Fig. 136-1). These symptoms imply either the development of a GERD-related complication (erosive esophagitis, stricture, or adenocarcinoma) or another disorder masquerading as GERD (esophageal cancer or a gastric-duodenal lesion such as cancer or peptic ulcer). Other candidates for endoscopy are those with severe, persistent, or frequently recurrent symptoms that suggest significant esophagitis and hence a risk for complications, such as stricture or Barrett's esophagus, which is intestinal metaplasia of the esophageal epithelium.

If a significant length of Barrett's esophagus (especially >3 cm) is discovered (see Fig. 136-1), most experts recommend some form of periodic surveillance endoscopy because of the increased risk for the development of adenocarcinoma. Control of reflux by either pharmacologic or surgical means does not generally lead to regression of established Barrett's esophagus (Chapter 140). Furthermore, endoscopic techniques to reduce reflux have not resulted in long-term benefits, despite promising initial results.

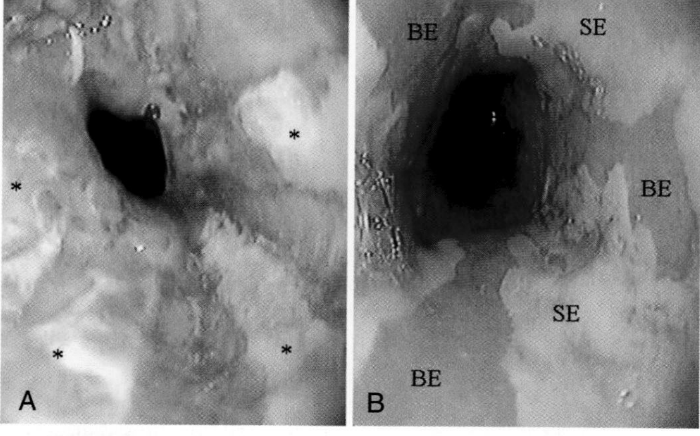

FIGURE 136-1. **Severe reflux esophagitis. A,** Mucosal erythema and linear ulcers with yellow exudates (asterisks). **B,** It is thought that such changes eventually lead to Barrett's esophagus, in which the normal white squamous epithelium *(SE)* is replaced by red columnar epithelium *(BE)*. These examples are from different patients.

For patients in whom high-grade dysplasia associated with Barrett's esophagus poses a serious risk for cancer, endoscopic ablation or resection provides a potentially curative alternative to surgical esophagectomy. Ablation can be achieved by a variety of modalities, including radio frequency, cryotherapy, electrical cautery, argon plasma coagulation, and photodynamic therapy. An alternative to ablation is endoscopic mucosal resection, which is en bloc resection of the mucosa to allow complete pathologic analysis and minimize the risk for regrowth of the abnormal mucosal lining.

Heartburn in immunocompromised patients often indicates an esophageal infection. The most common causes in patients with human immunodeficiency virus (HIV) infection are *Candida albicans,* cytomegalovirus, herpesvirus, and idiopathic esophageal ulcers. Because most patients with acquired immunodeficiency syndrome (AIDS) and esophagitis have candidiasis, an empirical 1- to 2-week course of antifungal therapy may be justified. Patients who do not respond to this approach should almost always have endoscopy and biopsy so that more specific therapy can be instituted.

Dysphagia (Chapter 140)

Dysphagia can often be categorized as oropharyngeal on the basis of the clinical features of nasal regurgitation, laryngeal aspiration, or difficulty moving the bolus out of the mouth. These symptoms are usually associated with a lesion in the central or peripheral nervous system. Although endoscopy is often performed in these patients, videofluoroesophagography (modified barium swallow or cine-esophagogram) is the procedure of choice because it allows a frame-by-frame evaluation of the rapid sequence of events involved in transfer of the bolus from the mouth to the esophagus. Common causes of esophageal dysphagia include malignant as well as benign processes (peptic strictures secondary to reflux, Schatzki's rings) and motility disturbances of the esophageal body or the lower esophageal sphincter. Endoscopic examination is considered mandatory in all patients with esophageal dysphagia. However, contrast esophagography may also be helpful; it can provide guidance in cases in which endoscopy is anticipated to be difficult (e.g., a patient with a complex stricture), suggest a disturbance in motility, and occasionally detect subtle stenoses that are not appreciated on endoscopy (the scope diameter is typically ≤10 mm, whereas some symptomatic strictures can be considerably wider).

Endoscopic treatment options are available for many causes of esophageal dysphagia. Tumors may be dilated mechanically, ablated by thermal means (cautery or laser), or stented with prosthetic devices. Metallic expandable stents have become the palliative procedure of choice for most patients with symptomatic esophageal cancer. Benign lesions of the esophagus, such as strictures or rings, can also be dilated endoscopically, usually with excellent results. Finally, some motility disturbances, such as achalasia, are best approached endoscopically with the use of large balloon dilators for the lower esophageal sphincter or the local injection of botulinum toxin.

Dyspepsia (Chapter 139)

Dyspepsia, which is chronic or recurring pain or discomfort centered in the upper abdomen, is a common condition that can be caused by a variety of disorders, including peptic ulcer, reflux esophagitis, gallstones, gastric dysmotility, and, rarely, gastric or esophageal cancer. However, up to 60% of patients with chronic (>3 months) dyspepsia have a so-called functional disorder in which there is no definite structural or biochemical explanation for the symptoms. Although *Helicobacter pylori* gastritis is found frequently in these patients, there is no evidence of a cause-and-effect relationship between these two findings. If a diagnostic test is to be performed, endoscopy, sometimes with biopsies to detect *H. pylori,* is clearly the procedure of choice (see Fig. 141-2 in Chapter 141); it has an accuracy of about 90%, compared with about 65% for double-contrast radiography. Because dyspepsia is a recurrent condition and patients who do not respond to empirical therapy almost always undergo endoscopy, many gastroenterologists opt for early endoscopy, if only for the reassurance that a normal examination provides.

Upper Gastrointestinal Bleeding (Chapter 137)

Acid peptic disease (including ulcers, erosions, and gastritis), variceal bleeding, and Mallory-Weiss tears account for most cases of upper gastrointestinal bleeding. Other less common but important lesions are angioma, gastric vascular ectasia ("watermelon" stomach), and the rarer Dieulafoy's lesion (a superficial artery that erodes through the gut mucosa). Finally, upper gastrointestinal cancers are occasionally associated with significant bleeding. Endoscopy is mandatory in all patients with upper gastrointestinal bleeding, with the rare exception being a terminally ill patient in whom the outcome is unlikely to be affected. Endoscopy can detect and localize the site of bleeding in 95% of cases and is clearly superior to contrast radiography (with an accuracy of only 75 to 80%). The endoscopic appearance of bleeding lesions can also help predict the risk of rebleeding, thus facilitating the triage and treatment process. Bleeding can be effectively controlled during the initial endoscopic examination itself in the majority of cases. The risk of recurrent bleeding is diminished, resulting in a shorter hospital stay as well as a reduction in the need for surgery.

In general, endoscopy should be performed only after adequate stabilization of hemodynamic and respiratory parameters. The role of gastric lavage before endoscopy is controversial; some endoscopists prefer that it be done, occasionally even with a large-bore tube, whereas others avoid such preparation for fear of producing artifact. The timing of subsequent endoscopy depends on two factors: the severity of the hemorrhage, and the risk status of the patient. Patients with active, persistent, or severe bleeding (>3 units of blood) require urgent endoscopy. In these patients, endoscopy is best performed in the intensive care unit because of the risk for aspiration and the occasional need for emergent intubation to provide respiratory protection and ventilation. Patients with slower or inactive bleeding can be evaluated by endoscopy in a "semielective" manner (usually within 12 to 20 hours), but a case can be made for early endoscopy even in these stable patients (perhaps in the emergency department itself) to allow more confident triage and more efficient resource management.

Most bleeding from upper gastrointestinal lesions can be effectively controlled endoscopically. The endoscopist considers factors such as age (older patients have a higher risk of rebleeding), severity of the initial hemorrhage (which has a direct correlation to the risk of rebleeding), and appearance of the lesion in determining the need for endoscopic therapy. Nonvariceal bleeding vessels can be treated by a variety of means, including injections of various substances (epinephrine, saline, sclerosants), thermal coagulation (laser or electrocautery), and mechanical means (clipping). In the United States, the most popular approach to a bleeding peptic ulcer lesion is a combination of injection with dilute epinephrine and electrocoagulation. Initial hemostasis can be achieved in 90% or more of cases; rebleeding, which may occur in up to 20% of cases, responds about half the time to a second endoscopic procedure. Patients who continue to bleed (typically those with large ulcers in the posterior wall of the duodenal bulb) are usually managed angiographically (with embolization of the bleeding vessel) or surgically.

Variceal bleeding can also be effectively managed endoscopically, with a success rate similar to that for bleeding ulcers (Fig. 136-2) (Chapter 156). Hemostasis is achieved by band ligation (Fig. 136-3), sclerotherapy, or a combination of both. Increasingly, patients who do not respond to endoscopic treatment are considered candidates for a transjugular intrahepatic portosystemic shunt (TIPS); traditional shunt surgery for bleeding varices is rarely performed. Even if initial endoscopic hemostasis is successful, long-term prevention of rebleeding requires a program of ongoing endoscopic sessions until variceal obliteration is complete. Ligation is the preferred approach in this setting because it is associated with fewer side effects. In patients whose large esophageal varices have never bled, β-blockers are considered first-line treatment, but endoscopic band ligation may be useful in selected patients.

Acute Lower Gastrointestinal Bleeding (Chapter 137)

The most common cause of acute lower gastrointestinal bleeding is angiodysplasia, followed by diverticulosis, neoplasm, and colitis. In about 10% of patients presenting with hematochezia, a small bowel lesion may be responsible. In contrast to upper gastrointestinal bleeding, there is no single best test for acute lower gastrointestinal bleeding. In patients younger than 40 years with minor bleeding, findings that are highly suggestive of anorectal origin (e.g., blood on the surface of the stool or on the wipe) may warrant only flexible sigmoidoscopy. Conversely, patients presenting with hemodynamic compromise may need upper endoscopy first to exclude a lesion in the upper gastrointestinal tract (typically postpyloric) that is bleeding so briskly it presents as hematochezia. Colonoscopy was traditionally recommended after bleeding slowed or stopped and the patient had been given an adequate bowel purge. However, a disadvantage of delaying endoscopy is that when a

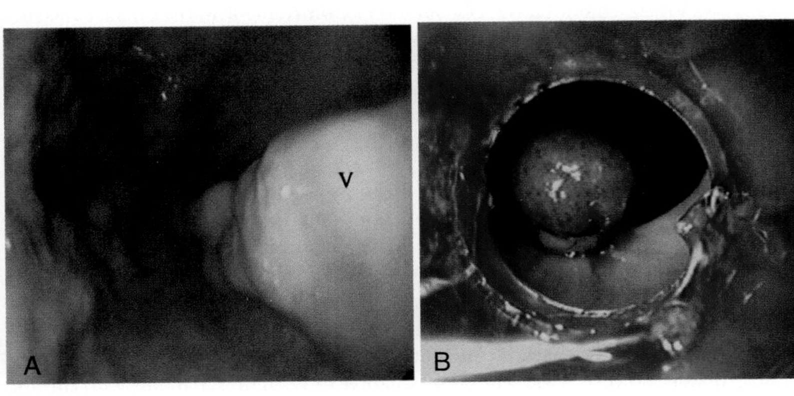

FIGURE 136-2. **Esophageal varices. A,** Endoscopic view of esophageal varices in the wall of the esophagus (V). **B,** Varix that has been endoscopically ligated with a band.

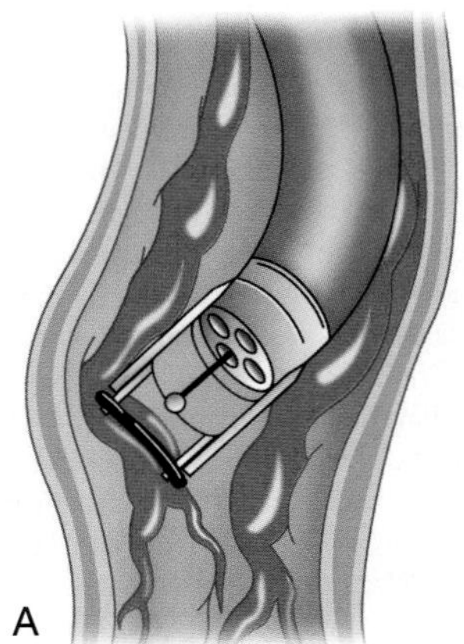

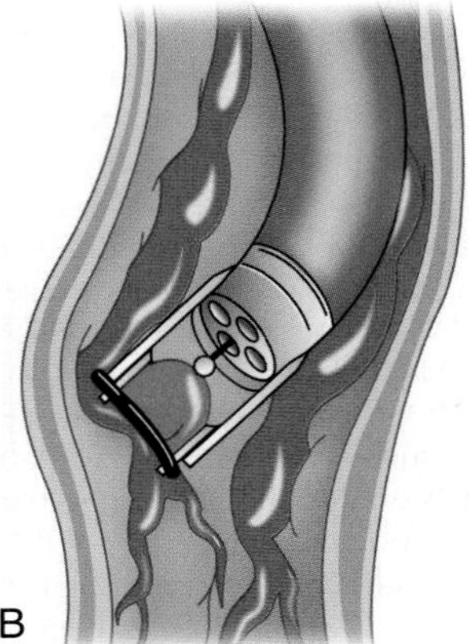

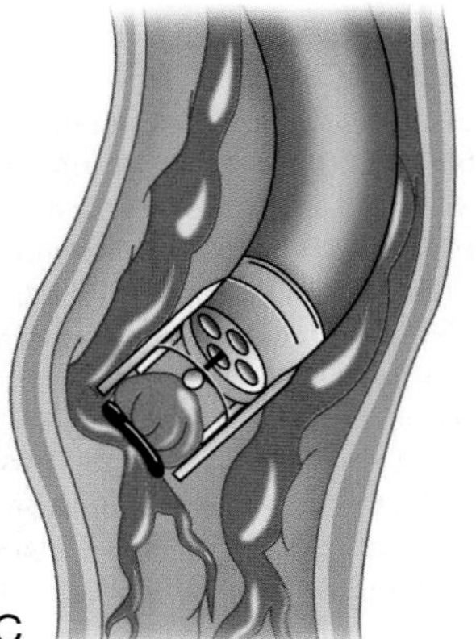

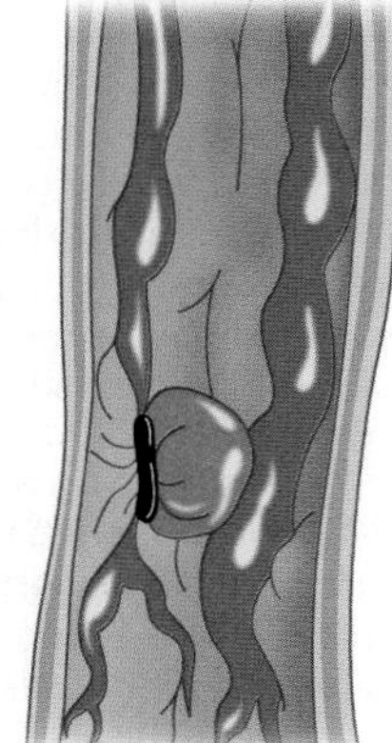

FIGURE 136-3. **Endoscopic variceal ligation technique. A,** The endoscope, with an attached ligating device, is brought into contact with a varix just above the gastroesophageal junction. **B,** Suction is applied, drawing the varix-containing mucosa into the dead space created at the end of the endoscope by the ligating device. **C,** The trip wire is pulled, releasing the band around the aspirated tissue. **D,** Completed ligation.

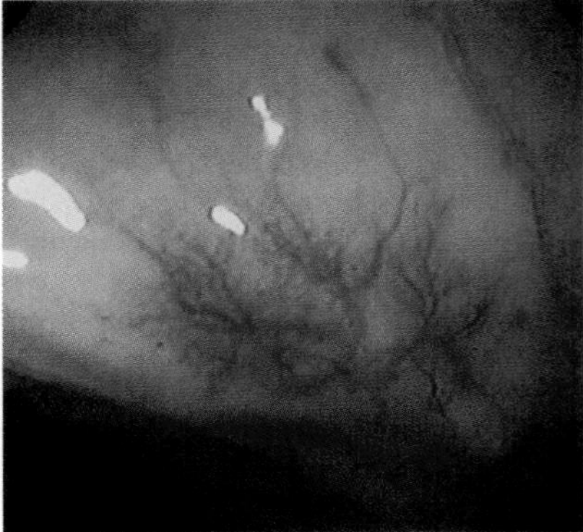

FIGURE 136-4. **Mucosal telangiectasia (arteriovenous malformation) in the colon.** The patient presented with hematochezia. The lesion was subsequently cauterized endoscopically.

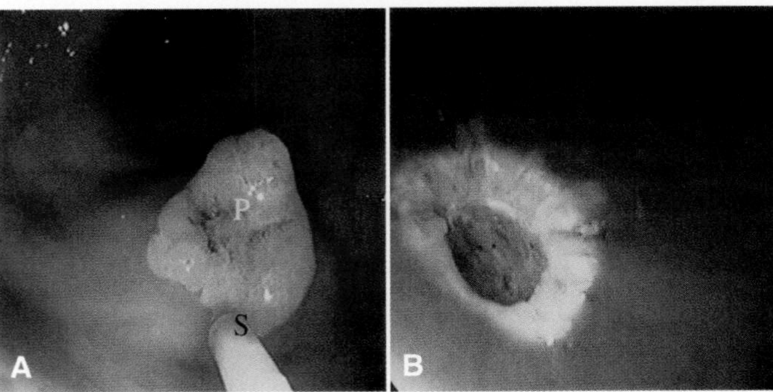

FIGURE 136-5. **Endoscopic polypectomy. A,** A snare *(S)* has been passed through the endoscope and positioned around the polyp *(P)*. **B,** Cautery was applied, and the polyp was guillotined, leaving behind a clean mucosal defect.

pathologic lesion such as an arteriovenous malformation (Fig. 136-4) or diverticulum is found, it may be impossible to implicate it confidently as the site of bleeding (complementary information by radiography or scintigraphy becomes particularly important in this situation). Some experts therefore recommend urgent diagnostic endoscopy with little or no preparation for acute lower gastrointestinal hemorrhages and have reported significant diagnostic as well as therapeutic success rates. However, such recommendations have not been universally accepted and remain logistically difficult to implement in most hospital settings.

It is not uncommon for gastrointestinal bleeding to develop or to be discovered in hospitalized patients who have had a recent myocardial infarction. In many cases, the bleeding is of a microscopic nature, and endoscopic evaluation can be deferred until the patient has fully recovered from the cardiac event. In other cases, however, the bleeding is more significant, and its risks outweigh the potential adverse effects of endoscopic intervention. In patients with recent myocardial infarction, upper endoscopy and colonoscopy are associated with a higher risk of cardiovascular complications, but they are usually transient and minor.

Occult Gastrointestinal Bleeding or Iron Deficiency Anemia (Chapter 137)

Normal fecal blood loss is usually less than 2 to 3 mL/day. Most standard fecal occult blood tests detect only blood loss of 10 mL/day or more. Therefore, even if this test result is negative, patients with iron deficiency anemia and no other obvious source of blood loss should always undergo aggressive gastrointestinal evaluation, which uncovers a gastrointestinal lesion in the majority of cases. Although most lesions that cause overt gastrointestinal bleeding can also cause occult blood loss, occult bleeding should almost never be ascribed to diverticulosis or hemorrhoids. Endoscopy is always preferable to radiographic studies for the evaluation of occult blood loss or iron deficiency anemia because of its ability to detect flat lesions, particularly vascular malformations, which may be found in 6% or more of patients. If the findings on both upper and lower endoscopy are normal, the next test is capsule endoscopy, which may be helpful to detect small bowel lesions such as erosions, tumors, or angiomas. Although it is relatively contraindicated in patients with suspected narrowing or strictures of the small bowel, capsule endoscopy has become the diagnostic procedure of choice in patients with obscure gastrointestinal bleeding (with normal findings on upper and lower endoscopies) and when mucosal lesions of the small bowel are suspected. Findings on capsule endoscopy may prompt the consideration of enteroscopy (using specialized double- or single-balloon endoscopes), which can theoretically access the entire small bowel and permit biopsy and/or therapy of suspected lesions.

Colorectal Neoplasms (Chapter 199)

Colonoscopy is the most accurate test for detecting mass lesions of the large bowel or colon that are suspected on clinical or radiologic grounds. However, endoscopy's greatest impact on colorectal neoplasia may be in the area of screening and prevention. The adenoma to carcinoma sequence of progression in colorectal cancer provides a unique opportunity for prophylaxis. Thus, if screening programs can identify patients with polyps, and if these polyps are removed, cancer can largely be prevented. Various techniques are available for safe and effective polypectomy, depending on the size, presence of a stalk, and location (Fig. 136-5). Colonoscopy is currently recommended for screening patients at average risk—that is, anyone older than 50 years. Adenomatous polyps should be removed, and patients should then enter a surveillance program with follow-up colonoscopies every 3 to 10 years, depending on the nature and number of initial lesions. Patients with no polyps generally do not require follow-up colonoscopies more than every 10 years.

More aggressive screening strategies are required for patients considered at high risk for colorectal cancer, including patients with well-defined hereditary syndromes as well as those with a history of colorectal cancer in a first-degree relative. In addition, patients with ulcerative colitis (Chapter 143) with long-standing (>8 years) disease affecting the entire colon have an increased risk for the development of colon cancer, about 0.5 to 3% after 20 years. Periodic colonoscopic surveillance (every 1 to 2 years with biopsies) is recommended for patients with long-standing disease (8 years with pancolitis, 12 to 15 years with left-sided colitis); the discovery of high-grade dysplasia or cancer is an indication for colectomy.

"Virtual colonoscopy" (Chapter 135), which involves the digital construction of an endoluminal view of the colon on the basis of data from abdominal CT, is fast emerging as a viable alternative to colonoscopy, particularly in patients who have failed previous endoscopic attempts or for whom colonoscopy is a high-risk procedure. Alternative screening techniques, including devices that can be used by nonphysicians, electronically mapped and driven instruments, and even completely self-propelled devices, are currently undergoing clinical trials.

Chronic Diarrhea (Chapter 142)

Endoscopy may be a valuable aid in the evaluation of patients with persistent diarrhea. The timing of the endoscopy in these patients often depends on the clinical features of the illness. Patients with bloody diarrhea should have lower endoscopy as part of an initial evaluation to determine whether inflammatory bowel disease is present (Chapter 143). In most patients with chronic diarrhea, endoscopy is often done when routine testing does not yield a specific diagnosis. Both upper and lower endoscopies may be performed, depending on the clinical presentation. Thus, a patient suspected of having a malabsorptive process may require upper endoscopy with jejunal or duodenal biopsies to look for celiac sprue or rarer lesions such as lymphoma or Whipple's disease; endoscopic biopsy has largely replaced blind intestinal biopsy for these conditions. Conversely, a patient thought to have a secretory cause of diarrhea requires a colonoscopy with biopsies to look for overt inflammatory bowel disease or more subtle variants such as microscopic or lymphocytic colitis, in which case the diagnosis requires careful examination of the biopsy specimens.

The endoscopic approach to diarrhea in immunocompromised patients, such as those with HIV infection, is guided by the degree of immunosuppression and the need to find treatable infections. When the results of routine stool tests are negative, patients with CD4 counts less than 100/mm^3 should undergo endoscopic evaluation to detect pathogens such as cytomegalovirus, *Mycobacterium avium* complex, and microsporidia. Small-volume stools with tenesmus suggest proctocolitis, for which sigmoidoscopy (rather than full colonoscopy) with biopsies is usually adequate. In patients with upper gastrointestinal symptoms (large-volume diarrhea, bloating, and dyspepsia), upper endoscopy with small bowel biopsy may be attempted first.

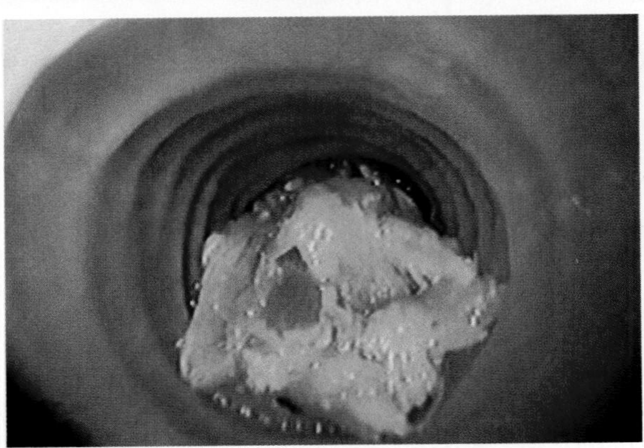

FIGURE 136-6. **Impacted food bolus in a young male patient who was found to have a ringed esophagus on endoscopy.** This presentation is characteristic and may be either congenital or acquired secondary to reflux-induced or eosinophilic esophagitis.

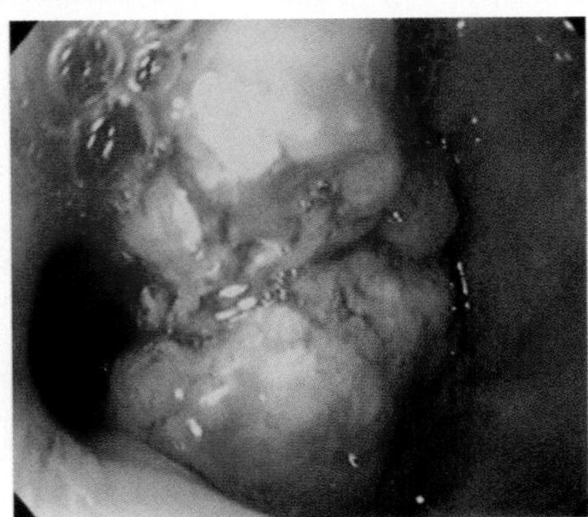

FIGURE 136-7. **Large malignant mass at the gastroesophageal junction, as seen endoscopically.**

Miscellaneous Indications

The upper endoscope has provided a relatively quick and noninvasive means of removing accidentally or deliberately ingested foreign bodies. Timing is critical for removal, however, because objects are usually beyond endoscopic retrieval when they reach the small bowel. Any foreign object that is causing symptoms should be removed, as should all potentially dangerous devices such as batteries and sharp objects. In general, objects larger than 2.5 cm wide or 13 cm long are unlikely to leave the stomach and should be removed. On occasion, patients with food impacted in the esophagus require endoscopic removal (Fig. 136-6). This condition almost always indicates an underlying functional or structural problem (Chapter 140) and should prompt a thorough diagnostic evaluation after the acute problem has been addressed.

Because of the relatively poor correlation between oropharyngeal lesions and more distal visceral injury, upper endoscopy is usually recommended urgently in patients with corrosive ingestion (Chapter 110). Endoscopy allows patients to be divided into high- or low-risk groups with regard to complications, with the institution of appropriate monitoring and therapy. Among the myriad causes of nausea and vomiting, a few, such as mucosal lesions and unsuspected reflux disease, are amenable to endoscopic diagnosis.

Malignant obstruction of the gastrointestinal lumen, including the esophagus (Fig. 136-7), pylorus or duodenum, and colon, can now be safely and effectively palliated endoscopically by expandable metal stents, thereby avoiding surgery. Colonoscopy is also useful in patients with pseudo-obstructive (nonobstructive) colonic dilation or Ogilvie's syndrome (Chapter 138); such patients are at risk for colonic rupture at diameters greater than 9 to 12 cm, and colonoscopic decompression is often required, sometimes on an emergent basis.

A major advance in enteral feeding has been the introduction of percutaneous endoscopic gastrostomy (PEG), a relatively quick, simple, and safe endoscopic procedure that has virtually eliminated the surgical placement of gastric tubes. A variation of PEG is percutaneous endoscopic jejunostomy (PEJ), in which a long tube is passed through the gastric tube, past the pylorus, and into the jejunum. PEJ does not prevent aspiration, but it is effective in patients with a significant impairment of gastric emptying. Retrograde tube migration with PEJ is common, however, and PEJ may require frequent replacement. The most common indication for these procedures is the need for sustained nutrition in patients with neurologic impairment of swallowing or with head and neck cancers. Patients with a short life expectancy are not suitable candidates for PEG and can be managed by nasoenteral tubes. Further, despite its intuitive appeal, there is little or no evidence that PEG feeding alters clinical or nutritional outcomes or significantly improves quality of life.

PANCREATOBILIARY ENDOSCOPY

Suspected Biliary Disease (Chapters 148 and 158)

The diagnostic approach to patients with cholestasis begins with an attempt to differentiate obstructive from hepatocellular causes. The most common causes of obstructive jaundice are common bile duct stones and tumors of the pancreatic and bile ducts. Less invasive conventional imaging with ultrasonography, CT, or magnetic resonance imaging (MRI) demonstrates dilated bile ducts and mass lesions; however, it is not sensitive or specific in the detection or delineation of pathologic change in the distal common bile duct and pancreas, two regions where the majority of obstructing lesions are found. Furthermore, some biliary diseases, such as sclerosing cholangitis, do not result in dilated ducts but have a characteristic appearance on cholangiography. Finally, the ability to use devices such as cytology brushes and biopsy forceps during cholangiography provides an additional aid in the diagnosis of biliary lesions. Both percutaneous and endoscopic cholangiographic techniques are associated with a high rate of success in experienced hands, but the endoscopic approach allows visualization of the ampullary region and the performance of sphincterotomy; it also avoids the small risk of a biliary leak associated with puncture of the liver capsule.

In the past few years, magnetic resonance cholangiopancreatography (MRCP), a digital reconstruction technique based on an abdominal MRI scan, has become a popular imaging modality for the pancreatobiliary system, with excellent sensitivity and specificity. Because of its relative safety, many experts now advocate this procedure for screening patients with a low likelihood of disease. In those with a higher probability, ERCP is still the procedure of choice because of its therapeutic options.

Of the approximately 600,000 patients undergoing cholecystectomy in the United States, 5 to 10% may present with bile duct stones before or after surgery. Endoscopic stone removal is successful in 90% or more of these cases and usually requires a sphincterotomy (Fig. 136-8). The sphincter of Oddi is a band of muscle that encircles the distal common bile duct and pancreatic duct in the region of the ampulla of Vater; cutting of this muscle, or sphincterotomy, is one of the mainstays of endoscopic biliary treatment and is accomplished with a special tool called a papillotome or sphincterotome. This procedure is often sufficient for the treatment of small stones in the bile ducts, but larger stones may require additional procedures such as mechanical, electrohydraulic, or laser lithotripsy, which can be performed endoscopically. In addition, sphincterotomy may be curative for patients with papillary stenosis or muscle spasm (sphincter of Oddi dysfunction). Finally, by enlarging the access to the bile duct, sphincterotomy facilitates the passage of stents and other devices into the bile duct. Sphincterotomy carries an additional small risk of bleeding, but its associated morbidity is about one third that of surgical exploration.

Endoscopic therapy has also revolutionized the palliative approach to malignant biliary obstruction. This technique, which requires the placement of indwelling stents, is superior to both radiologic and surgical techniques. Plastic stents have been the mainstay of treatment, but metal stents last longer and may be preferred in patients with longer life expectancies.

Pancreatic Neoplasms

EUS is probably the single best test for the diagnosis of pancreatic tumors (Chapter 201), particularly the small endocrine varieties, with a sensitivity approaching 95% (Fig. 136-9). It is also the procedure of choice for imaging submucosal and other mural lesions of the gastrointestinal tract (overall accuracy of 65 to 70%) as well as for staging a variety of gastrointestinal tumors (overall accuracy of 90% or more), especially esophageal and pancreatic cancer.

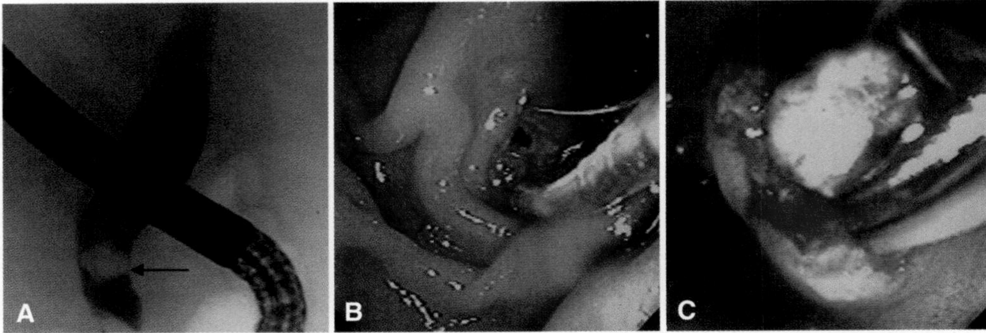

FIGURE 136-8. Biliary sphincterotomy and stone removal from the bile duct. A, Endoscopic retrograde cholangiographic image showing stones (arrow) in the distal common bile duct. **B,** Endoscopic image of a sphincterotome in the bile duct, with the wire cutting the roof of the ampulla (sphincter). **C,** A stone is being removed from the bile duct by an endoscopically passed basket.

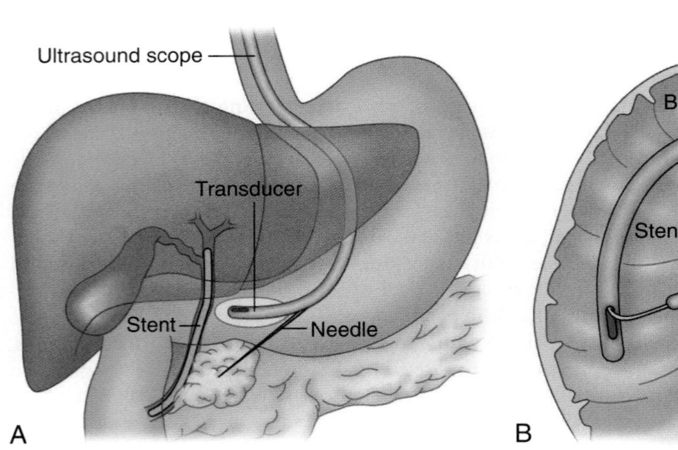

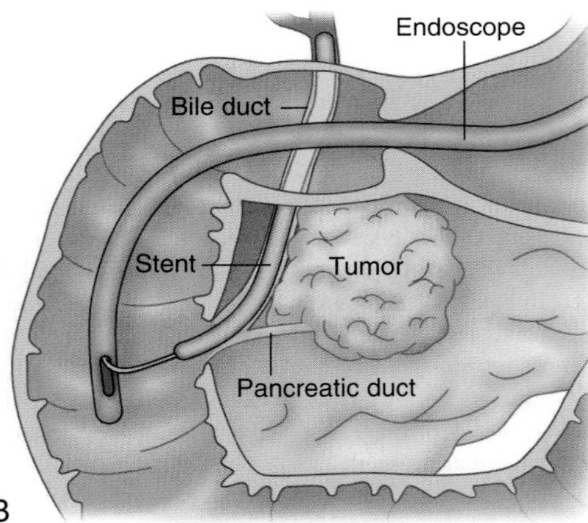

FIGURE 136-9. Diagram of biopsy of a pancreatic mass and stent placement. The biopsy is guided by endoscopic ultrasonography (**A**), and placement of the stent into a malignant bile duct stricture is accomplished with endoscopic retrograde cholangiopancreatography (**B**). (From Brugge WR, Van Dam J. Pancreatic and biliary endoscopy. *N Engl J Med.* 1999;341:1808-1816. Copyright 1999 Massachusetts Medical Society. All rights reserved.)

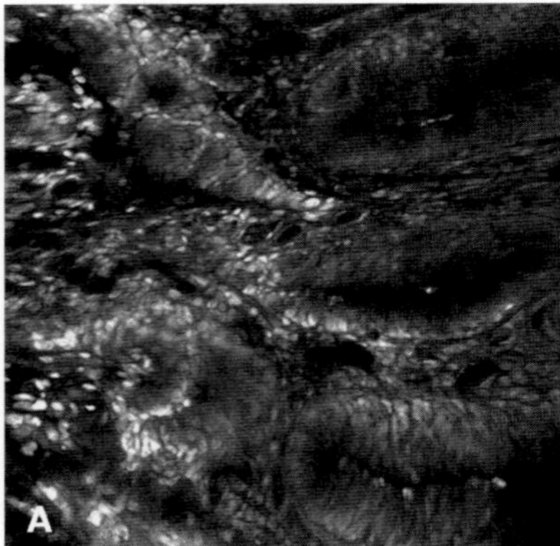

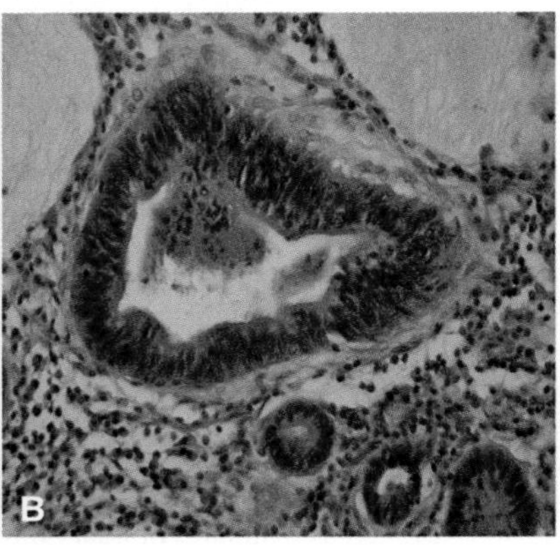

FIGURE 136-10. High-grade intraepithelial neoplasia. A, Confocal microscopy shows high-grade intraepithelial neoplasia of a colorectal polyp during endoscopy. Acriflavine was used as a contrast agent (0.02%), highlighting the cellular and nuclear architecture. **B,** Histologic picture from the same polyp. (Courtesy of Dr. Ralph Kiesselich, University of Mainz.)

EUS-directed celiac plexus neurolysis appears to be effective for the treatment of pain in patients with pancreatic cancer, although it does not work as well in patients with chronic pancreatitis.

Nonmalignant Pancreatic Disease (Chapter 146)

ERCP is indicated for patients with acute or recurrent pancreatitis without any obvious risk factors based on history or routine laboratory evaluation. Imaging of the pancreatic duct may delineate anatomic abnormalities responsible for the pancreatitis, such as congenital variants (pancreas divisum, annular pancreas), intraductal tumors, or possibly sphincter of Oddi dysfunction. In such cases, bile can be collected from the bile duct for microscopic examination for crystals (so-called microlithiasis) that can cause pancreatitis in some patients even in the absence of macroscopic stones. In patients with chronic pancreatitis, which is most often due to excessive alcohol intake, pancreatography can confirm the diagnosis, provide useful information about disease severity, and identify ductal lesions that may be amenable to therapy by either endoscopic or surgical means. In more subtle cases, collection and analysis of pancreatic juice after stimulation with secretin may be useful in establishing exocrine impairment and hence confirming chronic pancreatic injury.

ERCP also has a role in some patients with acute pancreatitis caused by obstructing biliary stones. Patients presenting with severe biliary pancreatitis may benefit from urgent ERCP early in the course of the disease, with the intention being to detect and remove stones from the common bile duct. Similarly, patients with smoldering acute pancreatitis that is not improving satisfactorily with conservative treatment may require ERCP for the identification and treatment of any obstructing lesions in the pancreatic or distal biliary duct.

Therapeutic endoscopy for chronic pancreatic disease is still evolving. Relief of ductal obstruction (e.g., by endoscopic removal of pancreatic stones or dilation of strictures) can provide short- to intermediate-term pain relief in some patients with chronic pancreatitis, although it is probably not as effective as surgery in the long term. Endoscopic pseudocyst drainage by a variety of techniques is now technically feasible, with results that appear to be comparable to those of surgical or radiologic techniques. Patients with ductal disruptions (e.g., pancreatic ascites) can often be treated successfully with endoscopic stent placement. Pancreatic papillotomy may also be useful in some patients with recurrent pancreatitis, such as when pancreas divisum is thought to play a role. Although the ability to approach these difficult clinical entities by less invasive endoscopic techniques represents a major accomplishment, the treatment of pancreatic diseases remains a multidisciplinary effort, with important and in some cases dominant roles played by surgeons and interventional radiologists.

EVOLVING TECHNIQUES AND FUTURE DIRECTIONS

Promising innovations include endoscopic optical coherence tomography, different forms of spectroscopy, and confocal microscopy (Fig. 136-10). These and a variety of other so-called optical biopsy techniques have the ability to provide microscopic images of cells at the surface as well as within deeper layers, thereby providing virtual real-time histology. Further, using targeted probes, it is possible to image function as well as form (E-Fig. 136-1). Innovations in endoscopic therapy include natural orifice transluminal endoscopic surgery (NOTES), by which the endoscopist or surgeon introduces an endoscope through a natural orifice (mouth, vagina, anal canal), traverses the wall of the viscus, and accesses the peritoneal cavity to perform diagnostic and therapeutic procedures.

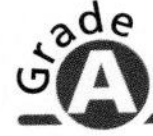

1. Shaheen NJ, Sharma P, Overholt BF, et al. Radiofrequency ablation in Barrett's esophagus with dysplasia. *N Engl J Med.* 2009;360:2277-2288.
2. Cahen DL, Gouma DJ, Nio Y, et al. Endoscopic versus surgical drainage of the pancreatic duct in chronic pancreatitis. *N Engl J Med.* 2007;356:676-684.

SUGGESTED READINGS

ASGE Technology Committee, Kaul V, Adler DG, Conway JD, et al. Interventional EUS. *Gastrointest Endosc.* 2010;72:1-4. *Consensus guidelines.*

The DAVE (Digital Atlas of Video Education) Project. www.daveproject.org. *This website is devoted to videos and other educational material on a variety of endoscopic procedures.*

Laine L, Sahota A, Shah A. Does capsule endoscopy improve outcomes in obscure gastrointestinal bleeding? Randomized trial versus dedicated small bowel radiography. *Gastroenterology.* 2010;138:1655-1688. *Raises questions about whether the improved diagnostic accuracy of capsule endoscopy translates into better outcomes.*

Leighton JA. The role of endoscopic imaging of the small bowel in clinical practice. *Am J Gastroenterol.* 2011;106:27-36. *Review.*

137

GASTROINTESTINAL HEMORRHAGE AND OCCULT GASTROINTESTINAL BLEEDING

DENNIS M. JENSEN

GASTROINTESTINAL HEMORRHAGE

Background

Gastrointestinal (GI) hemorrhage, which is a common clinical problem, has an annual hospitalization rate of 350 per 100,000 population in the United States, thereby resulting in more than 1 million hospitalizations annually. It can manifest clinically as overt bleeding from the upper GI tract (esophagus, stomach, and duodenum) or lower GI tract (colon), or it can emanate from obscure locations, usually in the small intestine. Alternatively, it can present as occult bleeding that is detected by the presence of iron deficiency anemia (Chapter 162) or a positive fecal occult blood test (Chapter 199).

Upper Gastrointestinal Bleeding

CLINICAL MANIFESTATIONS

Upper GI bleeding, which occurs proximal to the ligament of Treitz, accounts for approximately 50% of hospitalizations for GI bleeding. Upper GI bleeding usually presents as either hematemesis (vomiting of blood or coffee-ground material) or melena (black, tarry stool), but about 15 to 20% of patients who present with hematochezia, which is passage of red blood or clots per rectum, have an upper GI source of brisk bleeding. The most common causes are peptic ulcer disease , esophageal or gastric varices (Fig. 137-1), and erosive esophagitis (see Fig. 136-1 in Chapter 136). Variceal bleeding, which occurs in the setting of portal hypertension, is discussed in Chapter 156. Other causes of severe upper GI bleeding include tumors, vascular ectasias, Mallory-Weiss tears (Fig. 137-2), and erosions (Table 137-1). Depending on the severity of bleeding, patients may otherwise be asymptomatic, may present with fatigue or dizziness, or may have hypovolemic shock (Chapter 106).

DIAGNOSIS

Initial assessment includes a medical history, vital signs, and a comprehensive physical examination, including a digital rectal examination. Patients should be asked questions that may help determine the source of the bleeding. For example, peptic ulcer bleeding (Chapter 141) should be suspected in patients taking daily aspirin or nonsteroidal anti-inflammatory drugs (NSAIDs). For patients with known or suspected liver disease, bleeding from varices or gastropathy related to portal hypertension (Chapter 156) should be strongly considered. Heavy alcohol intake or vomiting should suggest a Mallory-Weiss tear (Chapter 140). The presence of a feeding tube or a chronic nasogastric

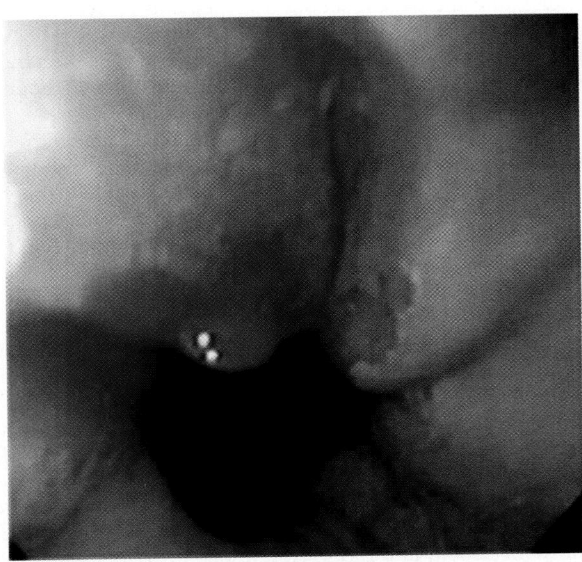

FIGURE 137-1. Bleeding esophageal varix at the gastroesophageal junction. (Courtesy of Pankaj Jay Pasricha, MD.)

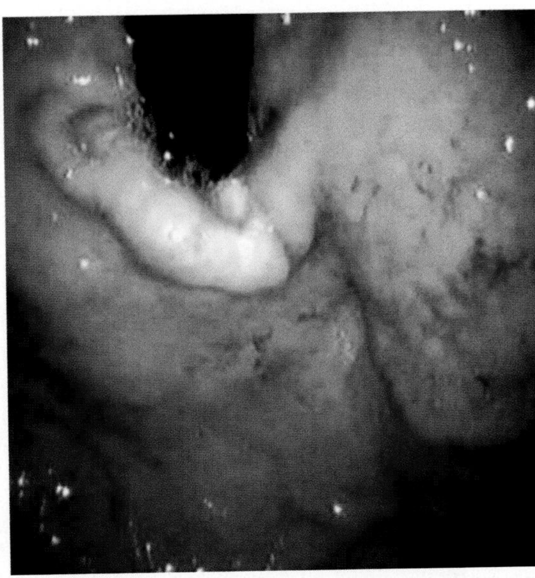

FIGURE 137-2. Retroflexed endoscopic image of a Mallory-Weiss tear at the gastroesophageal junction.

tube or a history of gastroesophageal reflux disease raises the suspicion for erosive esophagitis.

On the vital signs, special attention should be paid to signs of hypovolemia such as hypotension and tachycardia. Evidence of postural tachycardia or hypotension may reveal severe volume depletion that is not appreciated on a supine examination. It is important to examine the skin for petechiae, purpura, spider angiomas, and palmar erythema (see Fig. 148-2 in Chapter 148), and the abdomen for ascites (see Fig. 148-5 in Chapter 148), hepatomegaly, or splenomegaly, which may indicate portal hypertension. Tenderness or a mass may indicate an intra-abdominal tumor.

Placement of a nasogastric or orogastric tube can help localize bleeding to the upper GI tract, determine whether red blood or coffee-ground material is present, and assess how brisk, persistent, and recurrent the bleeding is. However, the sensitivity of nasogastric aspiration for upper GI bleeding is only about 80%, usually because blood in the duodenum is not refluxed into the stomach. Guaiac testing of nasogastric tube aspirates for unseen blood is not useful because the trauma of tube placement often may cause scant bleeding and false-positive results. Patients who have witnessed coffee-ground emesis or fresh bloody emesis do not require a nasogastric tube for diagnostic purposes but may need one to help clear the gastric blood for better endoscopic visualization and to minimize the risk of aspiration.

Blood should be sent for standard hematology, chemistry, liver, and coagulation studies, and the patient should be typed and crossmatched for the potential infusion of packed red blood cells (Chapter 180). The hemoglobin concentration and the hematocrit level may not accurately reflect blood loss because equilibration with extravascular fluid requires 24 to 72 hours. A low platelet count suggests chronic liver disease, dilution, drug reaction, or a hematologic disorder. In upper GI bleeding, the blood urea nitrogen level typically increases to a greater extent than the creatinine level because of increased intestinal absorption of urea after breakdown of blood proteins, but this phenomenon may not be seen in the setting of renal insufficiency or rapid transit of blood. An elevated international normalized ratio (INR) can be seen in chronic liver disease or with the use of warfarin.

Endoscopy

Patients with evidence of active bleeding (red blood by nasogastric lavage or hypotension) should undergo emergency endoscopy as soon as possible after medical resuscitation. Other patients should have endoscopic evaluation within 24 hours of their presentation (Chapter 136). Endoscopy can identify the site of bleeding with a sensitivity of about 92% and a specificity of nearly 100%, and it also can provide therapeutic hemostasis in most patients. An intravenous prokinetic agent (either erythromycin, 250 mg, or metoclopramide, 10 mg) 30 to 60 minutes before endoscopy may help move blood out of the stomach and into the small intestine, thereby improving endoscopic visualization.

In addition to localizing and treating the bleeding source, endoscopic evaluation can provide prognostic information and stratification for the risk of rebleeding, based on the presence or absence of stigmata of recent hemorrhage (Table 137-2). Other poor prognostic factors include older age, bleeding onset in the hospital, medical comorbidities, shock, coagulopathy, fresh blood in the nasogastric lavage, and the need for multiple blood transfusions. Clinical scoring systems, such as the Rockall score (Table 137-3), use clinical information and endoscopic findings to predict clinical outcomes. Similarly a Glasgow-Blatchford bleeding score of zero (urea < 6.5 mmol/L [18.3 g/dL], hemoglobin > 13 g/dL in men or >12 g/dL in women, systolic blood pressure ≥ 110 mm Hg, pulse < 100/minute, and no melena, syncope, heart failure, or liver disease) can identify patients whose upper GI hemorrhage can be treated on an outpatient basis.

Pre-endoscopic proton pump inhibitor therapy has not been shown to alter clinical outcomes, but it may downstage the severity of the lesion and decrease the need for endoscopic intervention. Therefore, in patients with suspected ulcer bleeding, intravenous proton pump inhibitors (e.g., pantoprazole, 80 mg bolus, followed by 8 mg/hour for 72 hours) may be considered while waiting for the endoscopy, but this therapy is no substitute for endoscopy and should not delay it. 1

TREATMENT Rx

Resuscitation efforts should be initiated simultaneously with the initial assessment. Large-bore (14- or 16-gauge) intravenous catheters are recommended for essentially all patients so that normal saline can be infused as fast as necessary to maintain hemodynamic stability (Chapter 106). Blood products should be considered as needed to keep the hemoglobin above 8 g/dL, the platelet count above 50,000/mm^3, and the INR below 2. Endotracheal intubation should be considered in patients with active hematemesis or with altered mental status to prevent aspiration, which can cause considerable morbidity and mortality.

The goal of endoscopic therapy is to stop acute bleeding and reduce the risk of recurrent bleeding. Most endoscopic therapies were designed for peptic ulcer hemorrhage, but they can be used for other causes of nonvariceal upper GI bleeding, in which underlying arteries are the source of bleeding. Available treatments include injection (epinephrine or sclerosant), thermal coagulation (with multipolar, bipolar, or heater probe), and mechanical compression (hemostatic clips). Epinephrine injection therapy is effective, safe, and inexpensive, but it should be combined with either thermal coagulation or hemoclips to achieve hemostasis in more than 95% of patients with active bleeding and to reduce the risk of rebleeding. Endoscopic therapy is reserved for lesions that have high-risk stigmata for rebleeding (e.g., active arterial bleeding, nonbleeding visible vessel, or adherent clot) or moderate-risk stigmata, such as oozing blood without associated clot or a nonbleeding visible vessel; it is not warranted for low-risk stigmata (clean-based ulcer or flat pigmented spot), which have the lowest risk of rebleeding (Fig. 137-3). Repeat or "second-look" endoscopy, usually about 24 hours after the initial endoscopy, may occasionally be useful to confirm adequate hemostasis in high-risk patients but is not generally recommended. Some causes of upper GI bleeding, such as gastric or duodenal erosions and neoplasms, generally are not amenable to endoscopic treatment and require appropriate medical or surgical therapy, or both.

TABLE 137-1 CAUSES OF SEVERE UPPER GASTROINTESTINAL BLEEDING IN A LARGE SERIES

DIAGNOSIS	%
Gastric or duodenal ulcer	38
Gastric or esophageal varices	16
Erosive esophagitis	13
No UGI cause found*	8
UGI tumor	7
UGI angioma†	6
Mallory-Weiss tear	4
Gastric or duodenal erosions	4
Dieulafoy's lesion	2
Other‡	2

*No cause found in esophagus, stomach, or duodenum, but 25% of these patients (2% of all patients) had mouth, nose, or pharyngeal bleeding sites.
†Upper gastrointestinal (UGI) angiomas include single or multiple angiectasias, watermelon stomach, or Osler-Weber-Rendu telangiectasia.
‡Other lesions were surgical anastomoses, Cameron ulcers, aortoenteric fistulas, and hemobilia.

TABLE 137-2 ENDOSCOPIC STIGMATA OF RECENT ULCER HEMORRHAGE AND THEIR ASSOCIATED FREQUENCIES, RISKS OF REBLEEDING, AND REDUCTION IN BLEEDING RISKS AFTER SUCCESSFUL ENDOSCOPIC HEMOSTASIS

ENDOSCOPIC APPEARANCE	FREQUENCY (%)	RISK OF REBLEEDING (%)	REBLEEDING RISK AFTER ENDOSCOPIC HEMOSTASIS (%)*
Active arterial bleeding	12	80-90	15-30
Nonbleeding visible vessel	22	40-50	15-30
Adherent clot	10	30-35	0-5
Oozing without other stigmata	14	10-20	0-5
Flat spot	10	5-10	—†
Clean ulcer base	32	3	—†

*Reduction in the risk of rebleeding is based on the administration of a proton pump inhibitor and successful endoscopic hemostasis.
†Endoscopic hemostasis is not recommended for these stigmata.

TABLE 137-3 COMPLETE ROCKALL SCORING SYSTEM FOR UPPER GASTROINTESTINAL BLEEDING

VARIABLE	0 POINTS	1 POINT	2 POINTS	3 POINTS
Age (yr)	<60	60-79	>80	—
Shock				
Pulse rate (beats/min)	<100	>100	—	—
Systolic blood pressure	>100	>100	<100	—
Comorbidity	None	—	Ischemic heart disease, cardiac failure, other major illness	Renal failure, hepatic failure, metastatic cancer
Endoscopic stigmata of recent hemorrhage	No stigmata or dark spot in ulcer base	—	Blood in upper GI tract, adherent clot, visible vessel, active bleeding	—
Diagnosis	Mallory-Weiss tear or no lesion seen	All other diagnoses	Malignant lesions	—
PRE-ENDOSCOPY SCORE	**MORTALITY (%)**	**POSTENDOSCOPY SCORE**	**REBLEED RATE (%)**	**MORTALITY (%)**
0	0.2	0	4.9	0
1	2.4	1	3.4	0
2	5.6	2	5.3	0.2
3	11	3	11.2	2.9
4	24.6	4	14.1	5.3
5	39.6	5	24.1	10.8
6	48.9	6	32.9	17.3
7	50	7	43.8	27
—	—	8+	41.8	41.1

Rockall TA, Logan RFA, Devlin HB, Northfield TC, for the Steering Committee and Members of the National Audit of Acute Upper Gastrointestinal Haemorrhage. Risk assessment after acute upper gastrointestinal haemorrhage. *Gut.* 1996;38:316-321.

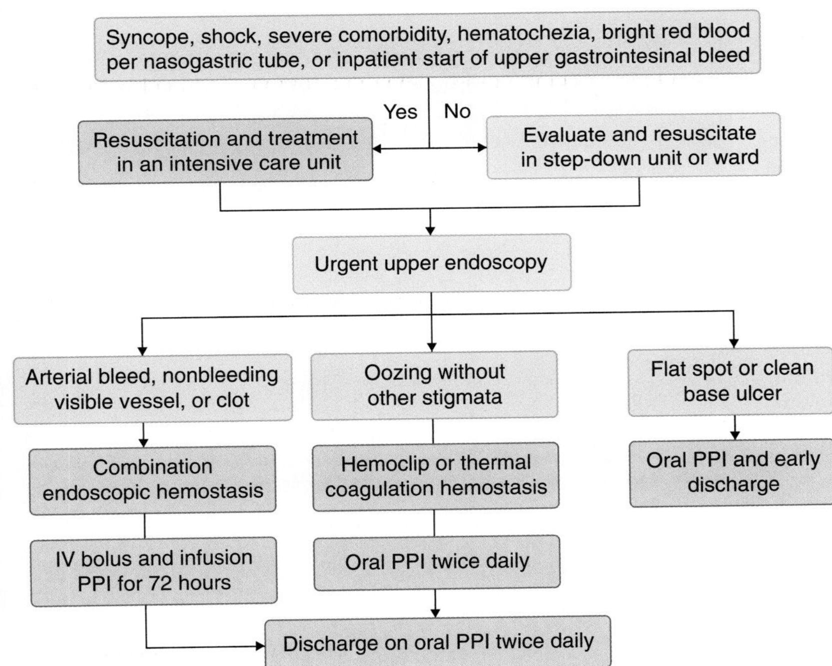

FIGURE 137-3. Management algorithm for nonvariceal upper gastrointestinal hemorrhage. IV = intravenous; PPI = proton pump inhibitor.

Medical Therapy

The most common cause of upper GI bleeding is peptic ulcer disease (Chapter 141), and the most common cause of bleeding peptic ulcers is the use of NSAIDs. Aspirin and other NSAIDs should be discontinued in patients with bleeding peptic ulcers, unless there is a contraindication to doing so (e.g., secondary prophylaxis for stroke). Patients with documented *Helicobacter pylori* infection should be treated with combination antibiotics (see Table 141-4 in Chapter 141) and proton pump inhibitors (see Table 140-1 in Chapter 140). *H. pylori* eradication does not help ulcers heal but reduces the risk of future peptic ulcer disease.

Proton pump inhibitors are the mainstay of medical therapy for hemostasis and healing of peptic lesions. Acid suppression can promote platelet aggregation and clot formation and reduce the risk of rebleeding. High-dose intravenous proton pump inhibitors (e.g., pantoprazole, 80 mg bolus followed by 8 mg/hour for 72 hours) after successful endoscopic hemostasis can reduce rebleeding rates and mortality in patients with high-risk stigmata of recent hemorrhage.[2] Patients with high-risk stigmata should receive proton pump inhibitor infusion for 72 hours before converting to oral proton pump inhibitor therapy. Patients with low-risk or no stigmata can be treated with high-dose oral proton pump inhibitor therapy (see Table 140-1 in Chapter 140) twice daily for 4 to 6 weeks and considered for early discharge. For patients who have upper GI bleeding and who require an NSAID, a proton pump inhibitor combined with a cyclooxygenase-2 inhibitor (e.g., celecoxib; Chapter 36) is preferred to reduce rebleeding. Patients with upper GI bleeding who require secondary cardiovascular prophylaxis should start receiving aspirin plus proton pump inhibitor therapy again as soon as cardiovascular risks outweigh GI risks, usually within 7 days.

Of nonulcer causes of upper GI bleeding, varices (see Fig. 137-1) are the most common cause. Variceal bleeding is treated with a combination of pharmacotherapy (octreotide, somatostatin), endoscopy (band ligation, sclerotherapy), and balloon tamponade (Chapter 156).

A Mallory-Weiss tear (Chapter 140) at the gastroesophageal junction usually stops bleeding spontaneously, but persistent bleeding should be treated similarly to bleeding from peptic ulcers.[3] Bleeding from erosive esophagitis (see Fig. 136-1 in Chapter 136) and gastritis (see Fig. 141-1 in Chapter 141) is generally treated in the same way as ulcer bleeding, although oral liquid sucralfate (1 g twice daily) is another alternative (Chapter 140). Dieulafoy's lesion, which is an aberrant submucosal artery that erodes into the lumen of the stomach, and tumors (Chapter 199) are rare causes of acute upper gastrointestinal bleeding. Vascular lesions commonly present as chronic, low-grade blood loss rather than as acute bleeding. Critically ill patients can bleed from diffuse gastric erosions, which usually do not respond to endoscopy therapy, but may respond to proton pump inhibitors (see Table 140-1 in Chapter 140).

PROGNOSIS

Despite progressive advances in diagnosis, the mortality rate from acute upper intestinal bleeding requiring hospitalization remains about 4% for young patients and has been reported to be as high as 15% for elderly patients.

Lower Gastrointestinal Bleeding

DEFINITION AND EPIDEMIOLOGY

Lower GI hemorrhage generally refers to bleeding from the colon and anorectum. Severe lower GI bleeding occurs with an annual incidence of 20 per 100,000 population, a rate that is much less than upper GI bleeding. Patients are usually older and present with painless hematochezia, typically without orthostasis. If orthostasis is present, a brisk upper GI bleed, which occurs in 15 to 20% of patients with severe hematochezia, should be considered. Among colorectal causes of severe lower GI bleeding, diverticulosis is the most common. Other frequent causes include internal hemorrhoids, neoplasms, and ischemic colitis (Table 137-4).

DIAGNOSIS

Patients with hematochezia should have a careful history, physical examination, and laboratory evaluation as for upper GI bleeding. A history of diverticulosis (see Figs. 144-4 and 144-5 in Chapter 144) should raise the suspicion for a diverticular bleed (Chapter 144). Abdominal cramping followed by bloody diarrhea suggests ischemic colitis (see Fig. 145-2 in Chapter 145). A recent polypectomy makes a postpolypectomy bleed more likely.

After medical resuscitation, most patients need endoscopic evaluation. Flexible sigmoidoscopy or anoscopy, or both, may be performed more rapidly than full colonoscopy in patients who are highly likely to be bleeding from the anorectum or distal colon. Colonoscopy allows for the identification of a luminal source of bleeding as well as for hemostasis of amenable lesions, but urgent colonoscopy may be no better than elective colonoscopy for improving outcomes.[4] To cleanse the colon and see the colonic mucosa adequately, a bowel purge with 6 L or more of a polyethylene glycol solution must be administered.

If colonoscopy does not reveal the source of bleeding, an upper GI endoscopic evaluation should be performed. If both are negative, capsule endoscopy (Chapter 136) can be used to look for a small intestinal source, such as angiectasias. Alternatively, if bleeding persists or is too rapid to perform a colonoscopy, a tagged red blood cell nuclear scan or angiography can localize the bleeding. A red blood cell scan is useful only if bleeding is at a rate of at least 0.1 mL/minute, whereas angiography requires an even faster bleeding rate of at least 0.5 mL/minute. Neither red blood cell scan nor angiogram identifies nonbleeding stigmata, and neither usually yields an etiologic diagnosis.

TREATMENT

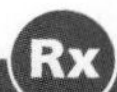

Medical resuscitation is similar as for upper GI bleeding. Colonoscopic treatment (Fig. 137-4) of focal bleeding sources with stigmata of recent hemorrhage relies on the same methods (epinephrine with either thermocoagulation or hemoclips) as for upper GI bleeding. Colonic angiodysplasias (see Fig. 145-5 in Chapter 145) may be a challenge to diagnose, and some patients who are bleeding from them may have their bleeding mistakenly blamed on diverticula. In addition, coagulation of angiectasias and bleeding biopsy sites is feasible during urgent colonoscopy.

Angiographic embolization or the infusion of vasoconstrictors is about 80% successful for treating rapidly bleeding vessels that are diagnosed at angiography, but with a 10% or so risk of causing local ischemia. Surgical management is rarely required for hemostasis of lower GI bleeding because most bleeding is either self-limited or easily managed with medical or endoscopic therapy. The main indications for surgery are malignant lesions (Chapter 199); diffusely bleeding lesions, such as ischemic colitis (Chapter 145) that fail medical therapy; and recurrent diverticular hemorrhage (Chapter 144). If the bleeding source can be localized preoperatively, a segmental colonic resection rather than a subtotal colectomy can be performed.

TABLE 137-4 MOST COMMON COLONIC SOURCES OF SEVERE HEMATOCHEZIA (486 CASES) (EXPRESSED AS PERCENTAGE OF COLONIC SOURCES)*

Source	%
Diverticulosis	32%
Internal hemorrhoids	13%
Ischemic colitis	12%
Rectal ulcers	8%
Colonic angiodysplasia, angiectasia, angiomas, or radiation telangiectasias	7%
Ulcerative colitis, Crohn's colitis, other colitis	6%
Postpolypectomy ulcer	5%
Ulcerated polyps	4%
Colorectal cancer	3%

*Less common causes include surgical anastomotic ulcers or sutures, nonsteroidal anti-inflammatory agent colopathy, metastases, portal hypertensive colopathy, lymphoma, and endometriosis.

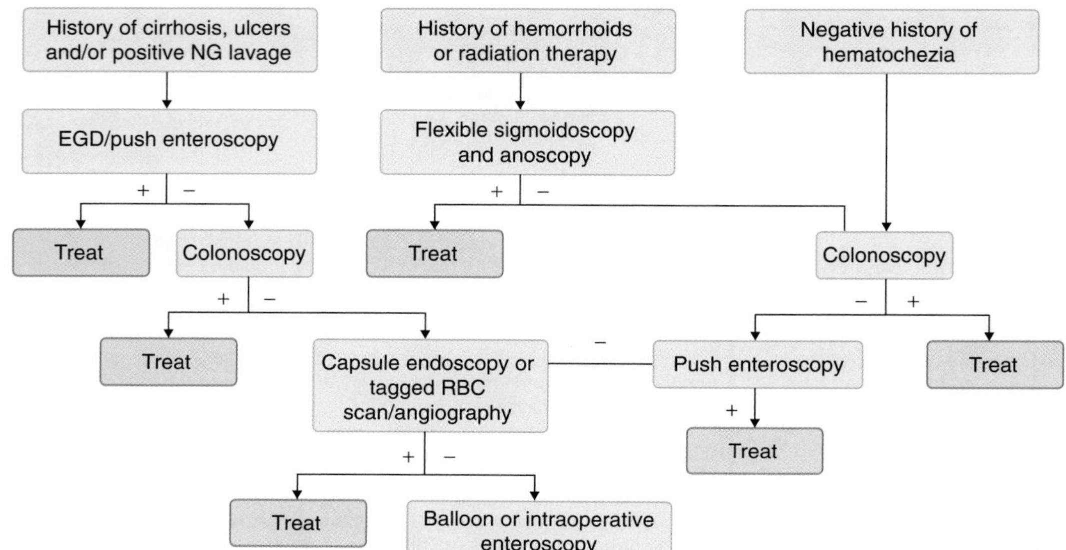

FIGURE 137-4. Management algorithm for severe hematochezia. EGD = esophagogastroduodenoscopy; NG = nasogastric; RBC = red blood cell.

PROGNOSIS

In most patients, the lower GI bleeding stops spontaneously and does not recur. The overall mortality rate from lower GI bleeding is 2 to 4%.

OBSCURE AND OCCULT GASTROINTESTINAL BLEEDING

DEFINITIONS AND EPIDEMIOLOGY

Obscure GI bleeding is persistent or recurrent bleeding, despite a negative initial GI evaluation, including upper endoscopy, colonoscopy, and radiologic evaluation of the small intestine with a small bowel follow-through. Obscure GI bleeding can be classified as either overt bleeding, with melena, maroon stool, or hematochezia, or occult bleeding, with a positive fecal occult blood test, usually in the setting of iron deficiency anemia.

In most large series of hospitalized patients, 5% of overt GI bleeding cases are considered to be obscure, and 75% of these patients have bleeding from the small intestine that is beyond the reach of an upper endoscope or colonoscope. Angiectasias (see Fig. 136-4 in Chapter 136) are the most common source of small intestinal bleeding, followed by ulcers and tumors (Table 137-5). Other causes of obscure GI bleeding include lesions that are within reach of standard endoscopes but that were not recognized as the bleeding site (e.g., a large hiatal hernia with lesions known as Cameron's ulcers on endoscopy, or internal hemorrhoids on colonoscopy) and intermittently bleeding lesions such as a Dieulafoy's lesion (Fig. 137-5), which is an aberrant submucosal vessel without an ulcer.

Iron deficiency (Chapter 162), which has a prevalence of 2 to 5% among adult men and postmenopausal women, can result from overt or occult blood loss (e.g., GI tract lesions, menorrhagia), iron malabsorption (celiac disease, atrophic gastritis), and chronic red blood cell destruction (hemolysis). It should be suspected in patients with low mean corpuscular volume, low ferritin level, or low transferrin saturation.

DIAGNOSIS

The approaches to overt and occult obscure GI bleeding are similar (Fig. 137-6). In cases with recurrent overt bleeding, upper endoscopy and colonoscopy should be repeated, with the type of bleeding dictating which endoscopic procedure to do first; about 30% of cases will be diagnosed by these repeat tests. Colonoscopy with anoscopy should be done first in patients with hematochezia. If there is melena, a push enteroscopy—a long upper-type endoscope that can be passed well beyond the duodenum and into the jejunum—should be

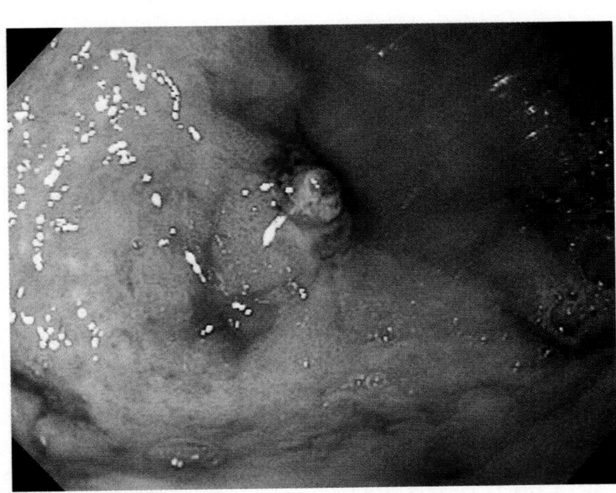

FIGURE 137-5. Dieulafoy's lesion.

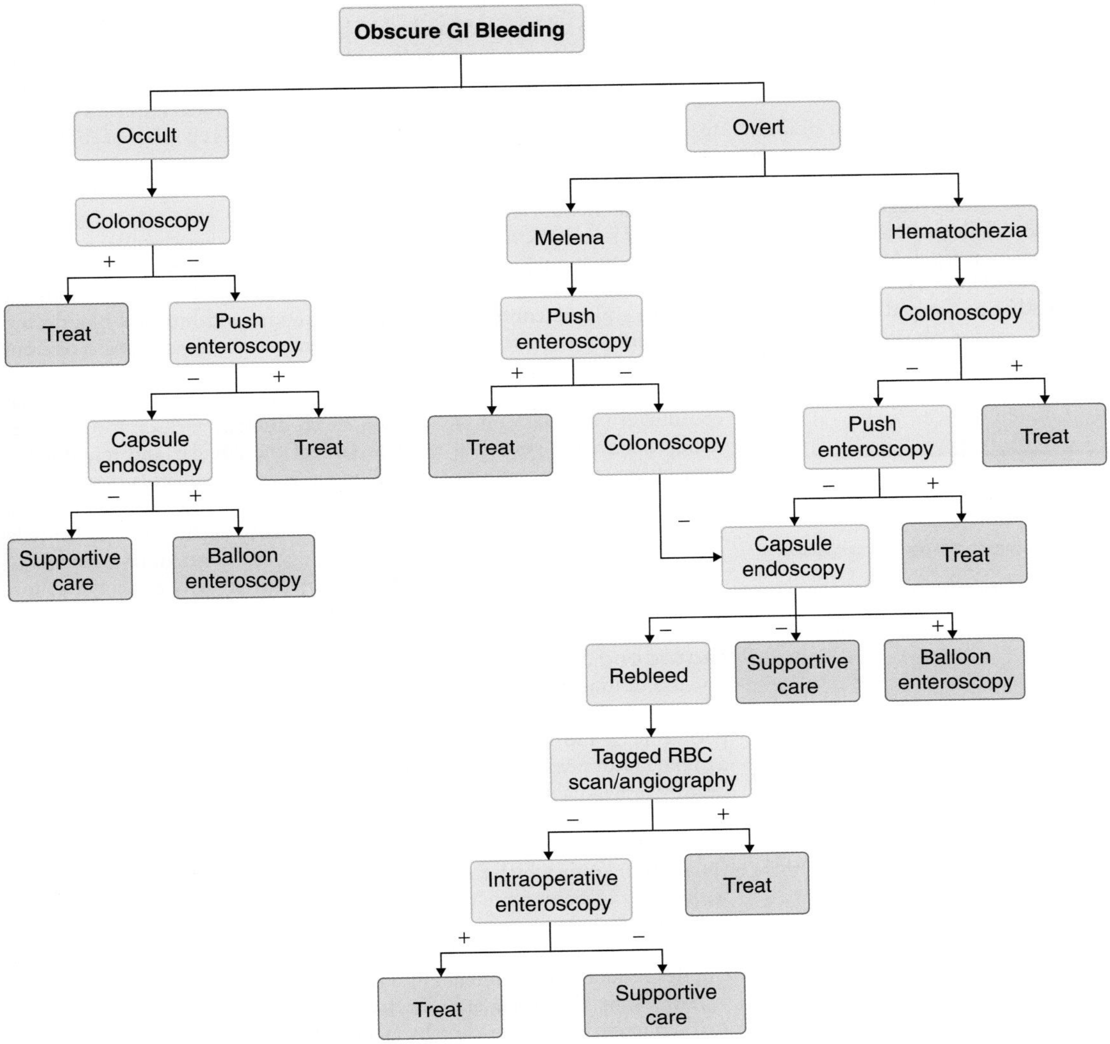

- **Obscure GI Bleeding**
  - Occult
    - Colonoscopy
      - + Treat
      - − Push enteroscopy
        - + Treat
        - − Capsule endoscopy
          - − Supportive care
          - + Balloon enteroscopy
  - Overt
    - Melena
      - Push enteroscopy
        - + Treat
        - − Colonoscopy
          - − Capsule endoscopy
    - Hematochezia
      - Colonoscopy
        - + Treat
        - − Push enteroscopy
          - + Treat
          - − Capsule endoscopy
            - − Rebleed
              - Tagged RBC scan/angiography
                - + Treat
                - − Intraoperative enteroscopy
                  - + Treat
                  - − Supportive care
            - − Supportive care
            - + Balloon enteroscopy

FIGURE 137-6. Management algorithm for obscure gastrointestinal bleeding. GI = gastrointestinal; RBC = red blood cell.

TABLE 137-5 SMALL INTESTINAL LESIONS FOUND DURING DOUBLE-BALLOON ENTEROSCOPY FOR OBSCURE GASTROINTESTINAL BLEEDING IN 488 PATIENTS

LESION	FREQUENCY (RANGE)
None	40% (0-57)
Angiectasias	31% (6-55)
Ulcerations	13% (2-35)
Malignancy	8% (3-26)
Other	6% (2-22)

Rajir GS, Gerson L, Das A, Lewis B. American Gastroenterological Association (AGA) Institute technical review on obscure gastrointestinal bleeding. *Gastroenterology.* 2007;133:1697-1717.

performed. If the first procedure is unremarkable, evaluation should be undertaken from the opposite end. If the second test is negative, capsule endoscopy should be performed. If bleeding from the small intestine is observed on capsule endoscopy, further attempts to diagnose and treat the bleeding should be performed with either balloon enteroscopy, which uses a balloon overtube to slide much farther into the small intestine, or intraoperative enteroscopy. All these long enteroscopes facilitate diagnosis and hemostasis. If the capsule endoscopy is negative, a tagged red blood cell scan or angiography may be used if rebleeding is rapid enough for these tests to be useful.

For occult GI bleeding, colonoscopy should be performed first because fecal occult blood testing was designed to screen for colorectal cancer (Chapter 199). Among patients over age 60 years with positive occult fecal blood tests, about 25 to 35% will have a significant colonic polyp and about 3 to 5% will have a colorectal cancer. Upper endoscopy should follow if the colonoscopy is unremarkable. Afterward, the approach is the same as for overt bleeding; if the capsule endoscopy is negative, however, efforts should be focused toward providing supportive care rather than further invasive evaluation.

Iron Deficiency Anemia

GI evaluation of iron deficiency anemia (Chapter 162) is indicated in all adult men, regardless of age, and all postmenopausal women. Women who have not reached menopause may warrant a GI evaluation after obvious or potential causes of iron deficiency, such as chronic menorrhagia, have been excluded. Colonoscopy should be performed first, followed by upper endoscopy if the colonoscopy was negative. Duodenal biopsies should be taken to look for evidence of celiac disease (Chapter 142). If both endoscopic procedures are unrevealing, capsule endoscopy should be performed. If the capsule study is negative, investigation into non-GI causes for iron deficiency (Chapter 162) may be pursued.

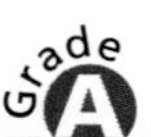

1. Barkun AN, Bardou M, Kuipers EJ, et al. International consensus recommendations on the management of patients with nonvariceal upper gastrointestinal bleeding. *Ann Intern Med.* 2010;152:101-113.
2. Lau JY, Leung WK, Wu JC, et al. Omeprazole before endoscopy in patients with gastrointestinal bleeding. *N Engl J Med.* 2007;356:1631-1640.
3. Sung JJ, Barkun A, Kuipers EJ, et al. Intravenous esomeprazole for prevention of recurrent peptic ulcer bleeding. *Ann Intern Med.* 2009;150:455-464.
4. Laine L, Shah A. Randomized trial of urgent vs. elective colonoscopy in patients hospitalized with lower GI bleeding. *Am J Gastroenterol.* 2010;105:2636-2641.

SUGGESTED READINGS

Halland M, Young M, Fitzgerald MN, et al. Characteristics and outcomes of upper gastrointestinal hemorrhage in a tertiary referral hospital. *Dig Dis Sci.* 2010;55:3430-3435. *The most common nonvariceal causes were ulcers (33%), Mallory-Weiss tear (11%), esophagitis (8%), and malignancy (4%); mortality rate was 4%.*

Kohn A, Ancona C, Belleudi V, et al. The impact of endoscopy and specialist care on 30-day mortality among patients with acute non-variceal upper gastrointestinal hemorrhage: an Italian population-based study. *Dig Liver Dis.* 2010;42:629-634. *Data supporting the benefit of early endoscopy and specialty care.*

Lanas A, Garcia-Rodriguez LA, Polo-Tomás M, et al. The changing face of hospitalisation due to gastrointestinal bleeding and perforation. *Aliment Pharmacol Ther.* 2011;33:585-591. *Hospitalizations due to peptic ulcer bleeding and perforation have decreased significantly, whereas colonic diverticular and angiodysplasia bleeding have increased.*

Riccioni ME, Urgesi R, Spada C, et al. Unexplained iron deficiency anaemia: is it worthwhile to perform capsule endoscopy? *Dig Liv Dis.* 2010;42:560-566. *Lesions were found in about two thirds of patients after negative upper and lower endoscopies.*

138

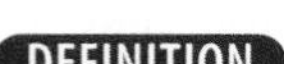

DISORDERS OF GASTROINTESTINAL MOTILITY

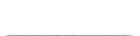

MICHAEL CAMILLERI

DEFINITION

Motility disorders result from impaired control of the neuromuscular apparatus of the gastrointestinal tract. Associated symptoms include recurrent or chronic nausea, vomiting, bloating, abdominal discomfort, and constipation or diarrhea in the absence of intestinal obstruction.

PATHOBIOLOGY

Normal Physiology

Neuroenteric Control

Motor function of the gastrointestinal tract depends on the contraction of smooth muscle cells and their integration and modulation by enteric and extrinsic nerves and by the interstitial cells of Cajal. Extrinsic neural control of gastrointestinal motor function consists of the cranial and sacral parasympathetic outflow (excitatory to nonsphincteric muscle) and the thoracolumbar sympathetic supply (excitatory to sphincters, inhibitory to nonsphincteric muscle). The cranial outflow is predominantly through the vagus nerve, which innervates the gastrointestinal tract from the stomach to the right colon. Parasympathetic innervation of the colon is provided by the vagal fibers coursing along the ileocolonic branches of the superior mesenteric artery and the S2 to S4 parasympathetic supply to the distal colon. Sympathetic fibers to the stomach and small bowel arise from T5 to T10 levels of the intermediolateral column of the spinal cord. Sympathetic innervation of the colon arises from T11 to L3 levels of the spinal cord. The prevertebral ganglia play an important role in the integration of afferent impulses between the gut and the central nervous system and in the reflex control of abdominal viscera.

The enteric nervous system is an independent nervous system comprising approximately 100 million neurons organized into ganglionated plexuses. The larger myenteric or Auerbach's plexus is situated between the longitudinal and circular muscle layers of the muscularis externa; this plexus contains neurons responsible for gastrointestinal motility. The submucosal or Meissner's plexus controls absorption, secretion, and mucosal blood flow. The enteric nervous system also plays an important role in visceral afferent function.

The interstitial cells of Cajal are spontaneously active pacemaker cells that coordinate muscular contraction and sense distortion. They form a nonneural pacemaker system at the interface of the circular and longitudinal muscle layers of the intestine and function as intermediaries between the neurogenic enteric nervous system and the myogenic control system, which regulates the electrical activity generated by gastrointestinal smooth muscle cells. Electrical control activity spreads through the contiguous segments of the gut through neurochemical activation by excitatory (e.g., acetylcholine, substance P) and inhibitory (e.g., nitric oxide, somatostatin) transmitters.

Gastric and Small Bowel Motility

The motor functions of the stomach and small intestine are characterized by distinct manometric patterns of activity in the fasting and postprandial periods (Fig. 138-1). The fasting or interdigestive period is characterized by a cyclic motor phenomenon, the interdigestive migrating motor complex. In healthy individuals, one cycle of this complex is completed every 60 to 90 minutes. The complex has three phases: a period of quiescence (phase I), a period of intermittent pressure activity (phase II), and an activity front (phase III) during which the stomach and small intestine contract at highest frequencies (3 per minute in the stomach, 12 per minute in the duodenum, 8 per minute in the ileum). Another characteristic motor pattern in the distal small intestine is the giant migrating complex, or power contraction, which empties residue from the ileum into the colon in bolus transfers.

With eating, the proximal stomach accommodates food by a vagally mediated reduction in its tone, thereby facilitating the ingestion of food without

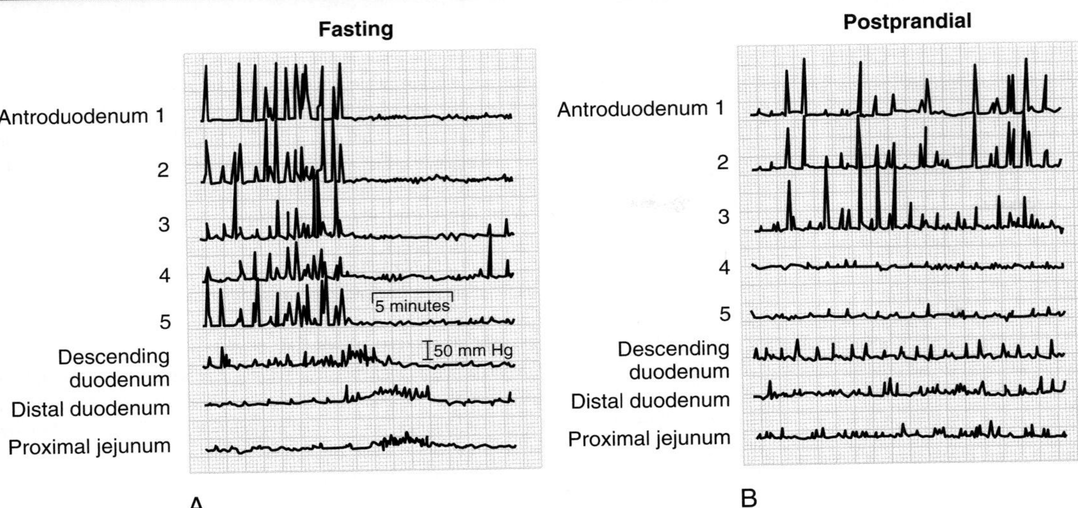

FIGURE 138-1. Fasting and postprandial gastroduodenal manometric recordings in a healthy volunteer. A 535-kcal meal is ingested during the study. Note the cyclic interdigestive migrating motor complex (**A**) and the sustained, high-amplitude but irregular pressure activity after a meal (**B**). (From Coulie B, Camilleri M. Intestinal pseudo-obstruction. *Annu Rev Med*. 1999;50:37-55.)

an increase in pressure. Liquids empty from the stomach in an exponential manner. The half-emptying time for non-nutrient liquids in healthy individuals is usually less than 20 minutes. Solids are retained selectively in the stomach, where they undergo acid and peptic digestion as well as "churning" or trituration by high liquid shearing forces in the antrum. Digestible food particles are emptied after their size is reduced by trituration to less than 2 mm. Gastric emptying of solids is characterized by an initial lag period followed by a linear postlag emptying phase. Secretion of hormones that mediate the motor and digestive process (e.g., gastrin for acid secretion; cholecystokinin for gallbladder contraction and bile and pancreatic secretion; and insulin, glucagon, and incretins such as glucagon-like peptide [GLP] 1 for glucose regulation) is integrated with the arrival of food or chyme at different levels of the gut to ensure optimal digestion.

The small intestine transports solids and liquids at approximately the same rate. As a result of the lag phase for the transport of solids from the stomach, liquids typically arrive in the colon before solids. Chyme moves from ileum to colon intermittently in boluses.

In the postprandial period, the interdigestive migrating motor complex is replaced by an irregular pattern of variable amplitude and frequency. This pattern, which enables mixing, digestion, and absorption, is observed in the gastrointestinal regions in contact with food. The maximum frequency of contractions is lower than during phase III of the interdigestive motor complex, and the duration of this postprandial contractile activity is proportional to the number of calories consumed (about 1 hour for each 200 kcal ingested). Segments of the small intestine that are not in contact with food continue with interdigestive motor patterns.

Vomiting is characterized by a stereotypic sequence of motor events, including contractions of the stomach, abdominal muscles, and diaphragm. This sequence is followed immediately in the proximal small bowel by a propagated, rhythmic contractile response similar to the migrating motor complex.

Colonic Motility

The normal colon displays short-duration (phasic) contractions and a background contractility or tone. Nonpropagated phasic contractions have a role in segmenting the colon into haustra, which compartmentalize the colon and facilitate mixing, retention of residue, and formation of solid stool. High-amplitude propagated contractions, which are characterized by an amplitude greater than 75 mm Hg, propagation over a distance of at least 15 cm, and a propagation velocity of 0.15 to 2.2 cm/second contribute to the mass movements in the colon. In health, these contractions occur on average five or six times per day, most often postprandially and between 6 AM and 2 PM.

Colonic transit is a discontinuous process, slow most of the time and rapid at other times. Residue may be retained for prolonged periods in the right colon, and a mass movement may deliver the contents to the sigmoid colon in seconds. Movement of colonic content is stimulated by feeding (gastrocolonic response). In health, the average mouth-to-cecum transit time is about 6 hours, and transit times through the right colon, left colon, and sigmoid colon are about 12 hours each. As dietary fiber is increased, mean colonic transit time decreases, stool frequency increases, and stool consistency becomes softer. Decreased caloric intake slows colonic transit, whereas a meal (typically >500 kcal) stimulates colonic motor function and propulsion of colonic content. Outlet obstruction in patients with pelvic floor dysfunction or voluntary suppression of defecation often is associated with slow colonic transit and decreased motor response to feeding.

Fluid reabsorption influences gastrointestinal transit. Approximately 9 L of fluid enters the gut from oral intake and endogenous secretions. The small intestine delivers about 1.5 L of fluid to the colon, where most is reabsorbed, leaving a maximum of 200 mL of water excreted in normal stool. Up to 3 L of fluid can be reabsorbed by the colon in a 24-hour period, unless the rate of ileocolonic flow or colonic motility overwhelms the colon's capacity or reabsorptive ability.

Defecation and Continence

Normal defecation requires a series of coordinated actions of the colon, rectum, pelvic floor, and anal sphincter muscles (Fig. 138-2). Filling of the rectum by a volume of 10 mL may be sensed, although the rectum can accommodate 300 mL before a sense of fullness and urge to defecate develop. Distention of the rectum results in the relaxation of the internal anal sphincter (rectoanal inhibitory reflex) and simultaneous contraction of the external anal sphincter to maintain continence. The anal transition zone can sense the difference between solid or liquid stool and gas.

DISEASES OF SLOW TRANSIT THROUGH THE STOMACH AND SMALL BOWEL

PATHOBIOLOGY

Gastrointestinal motility disturbances (Table 138-1) result from disorders of the extrinsic nervous system, enteric nervous system, interstitial cells of Cajal (or intestinal pacemakers), or smooth muscle. Neuropathic patterns are characterized by normal amplitude but incoordinated contractions, whereas myopathies are characterized by low-amplitude contractions (average of less than 40 mm Hg in the antrum and less than 10 mm Hg in the small bowel). Combined disorders occur in systemic sclerosis (Chapter 275), amyloidosis (Chapter 194), and mitochondrial cytopathy (Chapter 429), which initially can manifest with neuropathic patterns and later display myopathic characteristics with disease progression.

Genetic defects that result in congenital dysmotilities include abnormalities of *RET,* the gene that encodes the tyrosine kinase receptor, and abnormalities in the endothelin B system. Neural crest cells migrate from the vagal and sacral crest to the developing gut and, over time, colonize the entire alimentary canal and its appendages. Endothelin B serves to retard maturation of migrating neural crest cells, thus facilitating colonization of the entire gut with nerve cells. Other abnormalities resulting in congenital dysmotility involve other transcription factors, such as Sox10, which enhances maturation of neural precursors, and *KIT,* a marker for the interstitial cells of Cajal. Defects of *RET,* endothelin B, and Sox10 are associated with the phenotypic picture recognized as Hirschsprung's disease, whereas *KIT* defects have been associated with idiopathic hypertrophic pyloric stenosis and congenital megacolon.

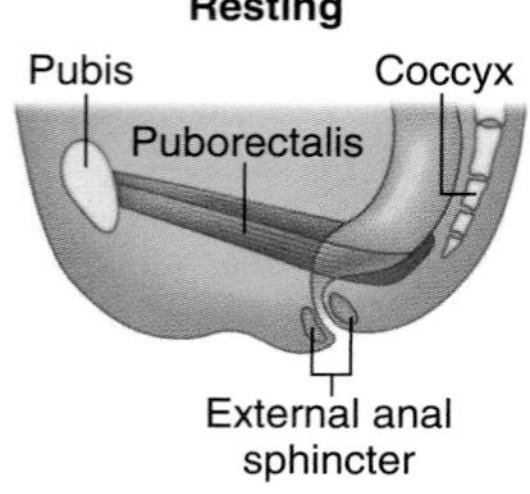

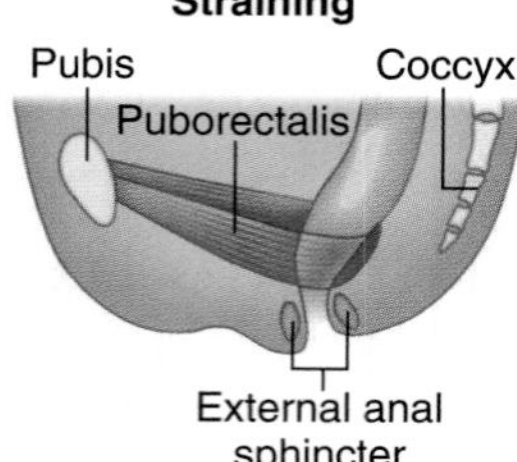

FIGURE 138-2. **Pelvic floor and anorectal functions during continence and defecation.** Sagittal view through the pelvis in the resting (**A**) and straining (**B**) postures. Coordinated functions of pelvic floor (puborectalis) and anal sphincter are essential for continence and defecation.

TABLE 138-1 CLASSIFICATION OF GASTROPARESIS AND PSEUDO-OBSTRUCTION

TYPE	NEUROPATHIC	MYOPATHIC
Infiltrative	Progressive systemic sclerosis Amyloidosis	Progressive systemic sclerosis Amyloidosis Systemic lupus erythematosus Ehlers-Danlos syndrome Dermatomyositis
Familial	Familial visceral neuropathies	Familial visceral myopathies Metabolic myopathies
Idiopathic	Sporadic hollow visceral myopathy	Idiopathic intestinal pseudo-obstruction
Neurologic	Porphyria Heavy metal poisoning Brain stem tumor Parkinson's disease Multiple sclerosis Spinal cord transection	Myotonia Other dystrophies
Infectious	Chagas' disease Cytomegalovirus Norwalk virus Epstein-Barr virus	
Drug induced	Tricyclic antidepressants Narcotic agents Anticholinergic agents Antihypertensives Dopaminergic agents Vincristine Laxatives	
Paraneoplastic	Small cell lung cancer Carcinoid syndrome	
Postsurgical	Postvagotomy with or without pyloroplasty or gastric resection	
Endocrine	Diabetes mellitus Hypothyroidism or hyperthyroidism Hypoparathyroidism	

Extrinsic Neuropathic Disorders

Extrinsic neuropathic processes include vagotomy, trauma, Parkinson's disease (Chapter 416), diabetes (Chapter 236), amyloidosis (Chapter 194), and a paraneoplastic syndrome usually associated with small cell carcinoma of the lung (Chapter 197). Another common "neuropathic" problem in clinical practice results from the effect of medications, such as α_2-adrenergic agonists, GLP-1 analogues, opiates, and anticholinergics, on neural control.

Damage to the autonomic nerves by trauma, infection, neuropathy, and neurodegeneration may lead to motor, secretory, and sensory disturbances, most frequently resulting in constipation. Patients with spinal cord injury (Chapter 406) above the level of the sacral segments have delayed proximal and distal colonic transit attributable to parasympathetic denervation. In these patients, fasting colonic motility and tone are normal, but the response to feeding generally is reduced or absent. Spinal cord lesions involving the sacral segments and damage to the efferent nerves from these segments disrupt the neural integration of rectosigmoid expulsion and anal sphincter control. In patients with these injuries, there is loss of contractile activity in the left colon and decreased rectal tone and sensitivity, which may lead to dilation and fecal impaction. Parkinson's disease (Chapter 416) and multiple sclerosis (Chapter 419) frequently are associated with constipation.

Enteric and Intrinsic Neuropathic Disorders

Disorders of the enteric nervous system are usually the result of a degenerative, immune, or inflammatory process. Virus-induced gastroparesis (e.g., rotavirus, Norwalk virus [Chapter 388], cytomegalovirus [Chapter 384], or Epstein-Barr virus [Chapter 385]) is associated with infiltration of the myenteric plexus with inflammatory cells. In idiopathic chronic intestinal pseudo-obstruction, in which there is no disturbance of the extrinsic neural control, degeneration of the interstitial cells of Cajal, inflammation, or herpesvirus infection may contribute.

Smooth Muscle Disorders

Disturbances of smooth muscle may result in significant disorders of gastric emptying and of transit through the small bowel and colon. These disturbances include, in descending order of prevalence, systemic sclerosis (Chapter 275), amyloidosis (Chapter 194), dermatomyositis (Chapter 277), myotonic dystrophy (Chapter 429), and metabolic muscle disorders (Chapter 429). Motility disturbances may be the result of metabolic disorders, such as hypothyroidism (Chapter 233) and hyperparathyroidism (Chapter 233), but these patients more commonly present with constipation. Scleroderma may result in focal or general dilation, wide-mouthed diverticula in the small bowel and colon, and delayed transit. The amplitude of contractions is reduced, and bacterial overgrowth may result in steatorrhea or pneumatosis intestinalis. Mitochondrial neurogastrointestinal encephalomyopathy, or familial visceral myopathy type II, is an autosomal recessive condition that may present with hepatic failure in neonates, seizures or diarrhea in infants, and hepatic failure or chronic intestinal pseudo-obstruction in adults.

Gastroparesis and Pseudo-obstruction

CLINICAL MANIFESTATIONS

The clinical features of gastroparesis and chronic intestinal pseudo-obstruction are similar and include nausea, vomiting, early satiety, abdominal discomfort, distention, bloating, and anorexia. In severe cases, there may be considerable dilation, as well as weight loss, with depletion of mineral and vitamin stores. Diarrhea and constipation indicate that the motility disorder extends beyond the stomach. Vomiting may be complicated by aspiration pneumonia or Mallory-Weiss esophageal tears, and patients with a generalized motility disorder may have abnormal swallowing or delayed colonic transit.

A careful family and medication history is essential. Review of systems may reveal an underlying collagen vascular disease (e.g., scleroderma) or disturbances of extrinsic autonomic neural control, including orthostatic dizziness, difficulties with erection or ejaculation, recurrent urinary tract infections, dry mouth, dry eyes, dry vagina, difficulties with visual accommodation in bright lights, and absence of sweating.

On physical examination, a succussion splash indicates stasis, typically in the stomach. The hands and mouth may reveal signs of Raynaud's phenomenon (Chapter 275) or scleroderma. Testing of pupillary responses (to light and accommodation), external ocular movements, blood pressure in the lying and standing positions, and general features of a peripheral neuropathy can identify patients with an associated neurologic disturbance (e.g., diabetic neuropathy) or with the oculogastrointestinal dystrophy that typically is found with mitochondrial cytopathies (see under Smooth Muscle Disorders).

The differential diagnosis includes mechanical obstruction, functional gastrointestinal disorders, anorexia nervosa, and the rumination syndrome. The rumination syndrome is a relatively common, underdiagnosed condition that presents with early (0 to 30 minutes) postprandial, effortless regurgitation of undigested food after virtually every meal.

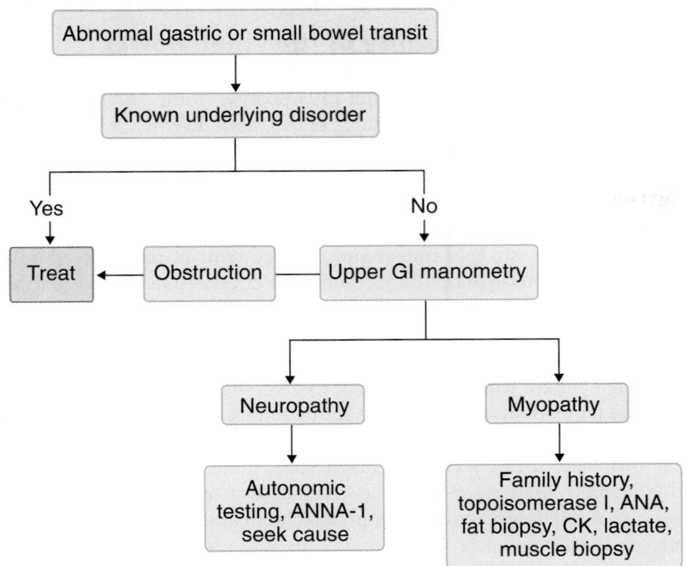

FIGURE 138-3. Flow diagram outlines steps in diagnosis of idiopathic gastroparesis and intestinal pseudo-obstruction. ANA = antinuclear antibody; ANNA-1 = type 1 antineuronal nuclear antibody; CK = creatine kinase; GI = gastrointestinal.

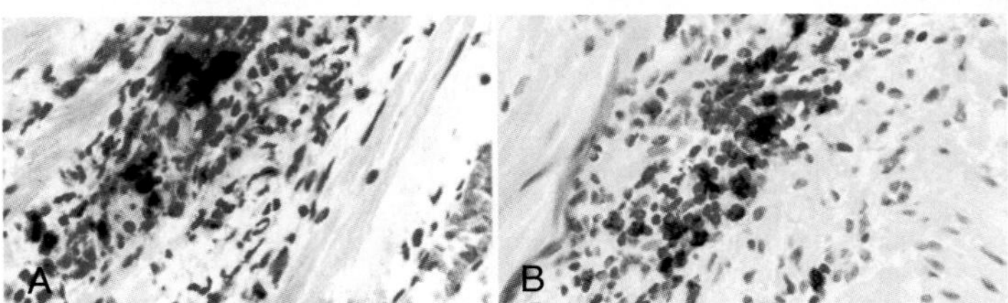

FIGURE 138-4. Micrographs showing both types of T lymphocytes, CD4 (**A**) and CD8 (**B**), detectable within the myenteric plexus of the small intestine (proximal ileum) of a 20-year-old man with chronic intestinal pseudo-obstruction. Note the intense CD4 and CD8 immunoreactivities that represent the predominant component of the immune infiltrate observed in cases of lymphocytic ganglionitis. Alkaline phosphatase anti-alkaline phosphatase immunohistochemical technique (×120) in **A** and **B**. (From De Giorgio R, Camilleri M. Human enteric neuropathies: morphology and molecular pathology. *Neurogastroenterol Motil.* 2004;16:515-531.)

DIAGNOSIS

A motility disorder of the stomach or small bowel should be suspected whenever large volumes are aspirated from the stomach, particularly after an overnight fast, or when undigested solid food or large volumes of liquids are observed during esophagogastroduodenoscopy. The clinician should assess the acuity of the symptoms and the patient's state of hydration and nutrition. The goals of the evaluation are to determine what regions of the digestive tract are malfunctioning and whether the symptoms are due to a neuropathy or a myopathy (Fig. 138-3). Key steps include the following:

1. *Suspect and exclude mechanical obstruction.* In symptomatic patients with pseudo-obstruction, plain radiographs of the abdomen typically show dilated loops of small bowel with associated air-fluid levels. Mechanical obstruction should be excluded by upper gastrointestinal endoscopy and small bowel imaging studies, including a small bowel follow-through or computed tomographic enterography. Barium studies may suggest the presence of a motor disorder, particularly if there is gross dilation, dilution of barium, or retained solid food within the stomach. These studies rarely identify the cause, however, except for systemic sclerosis or mitochondrial cytopathy, which are characterized by megaduodenum, multiple small bowel diverticula, and pneumatosis intestinalis.
2. *Assess gastric and small bowel motility.* After mechanical obstruction and alternative diagnoses such as Crohn's disease (Chapter 143) have been excluded, a transit profile of the stomach or small bowel should be performed. In a gastric emptying study, ingestion of a radiolabeled meal is followed by scanning at 0, 1, 2, 3, 4, and 6 hours. If the cause of the motility disturbance is obvious, such as gastroparesis in a patient with longstanding diabetes mellitus, it is usually unnecessary to pursue further diagnostic testing. If the cause is unclear, gastroduodenal manometry by use of a multilumen tube with sensors in the distal stomach and proximal small intestine can differentiate a neuropathic process (normal-amplitude contractions but abnormal patterns of contractility) from a myopathic process (low-amplitude contractions in the affected segments).
3. *Identify the pathogenesis* (see Table 138-1). In patients with neuropathic causes of uncertain origin, tests should assess autonomic dysfunction (Chapter 427), measure type 1 antineuronal nuclear autoantibodies and other autoantibodies associated with paraneoplastic syndromes, and consider the possibility of a brain stem lesion. In patients with a myopathic disorder of unclear cause, the evaluation should consider amyloidosis (immunoglobulin electrophoresis, fat aspirate, or rectal biopsy; Chapter 194), systemic sclerosis (topoisomerase I; Chapter 275), and thyroid disease (Chapter 233). In appropriate settings, porphyria (Chapter 217) and Chagas' disease (Chapter 355) may need to be excluded. In refractory cases, referral to a specialized center may result in genetic testing or full-thickness biopsy of the small intestine (Fig. 138-4) to identify metabolic muscle disorders and mitochondrial cytopathies.

   Diabetes mellitus (Chapter 236) is associated with gastroparesis, pylorospasm, intestinal pseudo-obstruction, diarrhea, constipation, and fecal incontinence. All of these manifestations may be caused by autonomic dysfunction, although more recent evidence points to acute changes in glycemia and, more important, to changes in the structure and function of the interstitial cells of Cajal and enteric nervous system. The prevalence of constipation is 22% among diabetic patients with neuropathy but only 9.2% in diabetic patients without neuropathy, a rate that is not significantly different from that of healthy controls.
4. *Identify complications of the motility disorder, including bacterial overgrowth, dehydration, and malnutrition.* In patients presenting with diarrhea, it is important to assess nutritional status and to exclude bacterial overgrowth by culture of small bowel aspirates (Chapter 142). Bacterial overgrowth is relatively uncommon in neuropathic disorders but is found more often in myopathic conditions, such as scleroderma, that are associated more often with dilation or low-amplitude contractions. An empirical trial of antibiotics (see later) often is used instead of formal testing.

TREATMENT Rx

Rehydration, electrolyte repletion, and nutritional supplementation are particularly important during acute exacerbations of gastroparesis and chronic intestinal pseudo-obstruction. Initial nutritional measures include low-fiber supplements with the addition of iron, folate, calcium, and vitamins D, K, and B_{12} at the usually recommended daily levels. In patients with more severe symptoms, enteral or parenteral supplementation may be required. If it is anticipated that enteral supplementation may be needed for more than 3 months, a jejunostomy tube is recommended. Gastrostomy tubes should be avoided in patients with gastroparesis except for venting purposes. The rumination syndrome is treated using behavioral approaches such as diaphragmatic breathing in the early postprandial period.

Medical Therapy

Medications increasingly are being used to treat neuromuscular motility disorders, but there is little evidence of effectiveness in myopathic disturbances except for the rare case of dystrophia myotonica affecting the stomach and for small bowel systemic sclerosis. Small randomized trials demonstrate symptomatic benefit of metoclopramide and domperidone over placebo. Metoclopramide is a dopamine antagonist with prokinetic and antiemetic properties. Antiemetic effects are due in part to its anti-5-hydroxytryptamine type 3 (HT_3) antagonist actions. Long-term use of metoclopramide is limited by the side effects of tremor and parkinsonian-like symptoms. It is available in tablet or elixir form or as a parenteral preparation and, typically, is taken orally 30 minutes before meals and at bedtime. Usual doses are 5 to 10 mg four times daily, but patients may experience side effects (changes in affect, anxiety) at relatively low doses (even 30 to 40 mg/day). The U.S. Food and Drug Administration (FDA) recommends its use only in patients who do not respond to other treatments and for periods of less than 3 months.

Domperidone (10-20 mg, three times per day before meals) is another dopamine antagonist that is approved in some countries but not in the United States, where it is available through an application to the FDA and local Institutional Review Board. Its efficacy appears similar to metoclopramide, with a lower incidence of somnolence and much lower incidence of involuntary movements.

Erythromycin, a macrolide antibiotic that stimulates motilin receptors at higher doses (250 to 500 mg) and cholinergic mechanisms at lower doses (40 to 80 mg), results in the dumping of solids from the stomach. It accelerates gastric emptying in gastroparesis, increases the amplitude of antral contractions, and improves antroduodenal coordination. Erythromycin is most effective when it is used intravenously (3 mg/kg every 8 hours by slow infusion) during acute exacerbations of gastroparesis. For oral erythromycin, tolerance and gastrointestinal side effects often prevent use for longer than 1 month, but sometimes liquid erythromycin can be tolerated at 40 to 80 mg three times daily before meals.

Octreotide (50 μg subcutaneously at bedtime), a cyclized analogue of somatostatin, induces small intestinal activity that mimics phase III of the interdigestive migrating motor complex. It retards gastric emptying, decreases postprandial gastric motility, and inhibits small bowel transit. Octreotide appears to be useful in the treatment of dumping syndromes associated with accelerated transit. Octreotide may be used at night to induce migrating motor complex activity and to avoid bacterial overgrowth. If it is required during the daytime, octreotide often is combined with oral prokinetic to "normalize" the gastric emptying rate.

Antiemetics, including diphenhydramine (25 mg orally up to two times per day for up to 3 months), prochlorperazine (orally or by suppository 25 mg up to two times per day), and metoclopramide (5 to 10 mg orally up to three times per day for up to 3 months), can treat nausea and vomiting in patients with gastroparesis and intestinal pseudo-obstruction. The more expensive serotonin 5-HT_3 antagonists (e.g., ondansetron) have not proved to be of greater benefit than these less expensive alternatives in these patients.

Antibiotic therapy is indicated in patients with documented, symptomatic bacterial overgrowth. Although formal clinical trials have not been conducted, it is common practice to use different antibiotics for 7 to 10 days each month, in an attempt to avoid bacterial resistance. Common antibiotics include doxycycline, 100 mg twice daily; metronidazole, 500 mg three times daily; ciprofloxacin, 500 mg twice daily; double-strength trimethoprim-sulfamethoxazole, two tablets twice daily; or rifaximin, 275 mg twice daily. Use of antibiotics in patients with diarrhea and fat malabsorption secondary to bacterial overgrowth results in significant symptomatic relief.

Surgical Therapy

Surgical decompression is rarely necessary in patients with chronic pseudo-obstruction. Venting enterostomy (jejunostomy) is effective, however, in relieving abdominal distention and bloating and in reducing the frequency with which nasogastric intubations and hospitalizations are required for acute exacerbations relative to the period before vent placement. Access to the small intestine by enterostomy also provides nutrients and should be considered in patients with intermittent symptoms. Surgical treatment should be considered whenever the motility disorder is localized to a resectable portion of the gut: completion gastrectomy for patients with post–gastric surgical stasis syndrome, and colectomy with ileorectostomy for intractable constipation associated with chronic colonic pseudo-obstruction.

Gastric electrical stimulation, an approved treatment for humanitarian use, may improve gastric emptying and symptoms in patients with severe gastroparesis, but data on efficacy are inconclusive. Small bowel transplantation currently is limited to patients with intestinal failure who have reversible liver disease induced by total parenteral nutrition or who have life-threatening or recurrent catheter-related sepsis. Isolated transplantation of the small intestine is associated with higher graft and patient survival and fewer complications related to rejection and infection.

DISEASES OF RAPID TRANSIT THROUGH STOMACH AND SMALL BOWEL

Dumping Syndrome and Accelerated Gastric Emptying

Dumping syndrome and accelerated gastric emptying typically follow truncal vagotomy and gastric drainage procedures (Chapter 141) or fundoplication for gastric esophageal reflux disease (Chapter 140). With the widespread use of highly selective vagotomy and the advent of effective antacid secretory therapy, these problems are becoming rare. A high calorie (usually carbohydrate) content of the liquid phase of the meal evokes a rapid insulin response with secondary hypoglycemia. These patients also may have impaired antral contractility and gastric stasis of solids, which paradoxically may result in a clinical picture of gastroparesis (for solids) and dumping (for liquids).

The management of dumping syndrome and accelerated gastric emptying emphasizes dietary maneuvers, such as avoidance of high-nutrient liquid drinks and possibly addition of guar gum or pectin to retard gastric emptying of liquids. Rarely, pharmacologic treatment with octreotide, 25 to 100 μg subcutaneously before meals, is needed to retard intestinal transit and to inhibit the hormonal responses that lead to hypoglycemia.

Rapid Transit Dysmotility of the Small Bowel

Rapid transit of material through the small bowel may occur in the setting of the irritable bowel syndrome (Chapter 139), postvagotomy diarrhea (Chapter 142), short bowel syndrome (Chapter 142), diabetic diarrhea (Chapter 142), and carcinoid diarrhea (Chapter 240). With the exception of irritable bowel syndrome, these conditions may cause severe diarrhea and result in significant losses of fluid and electrolytes. Ileal resection or disease and idiopathic bile acid malabsorption may represent an inability of the distal ileum to reabsorb bile acids because of rapid transit and reduced contact time with the ileal mucosa; this condition may induce colonic secretion and secondary diarrhea. Accelerated transit may be confirmed by scintigraphic studies.

Treatment goals are to restore hydration and nutrition and to slow small bowel transit. Dietary interventions include avoiding hyperosmolar drinks and replacing them with iso-osmolar or hypo-osmolar oral rehydration solutions. The fat content in the diet should be reduced to approximately 50 g/day to avoid delivery of unabsorbed fat to the colon. All electrolyte and nutritional deficiencies of calcium, magnesium, potassium, and water-soluble and fat-soluble vitamins should be corrected. In patients with less than 1 m of residual small bowel, it may be impossible to maintain fluid and electrolyte homeostasis without parenteral support. In patients with a longer residual segment, oral nutrition, pharmacotherapy, and supplements are almost always effective.

The opioid agent loperamide (4 mg 30 minutes before meals and at bedtime for a total dose of 16 mg/day) suppresses the motor response to feeding and improves symptoms but may be ineffective or cause side effects (e.g., hypotension). Bile acid binding (e.g., with cholestyramine (4 g three times daily) or colesevelam (1.875 g twice daily) is indicated for patients with suspected or proven bile acid malabsorption. Verapamil (40 mg twice daily) or clonidine (0.1 mg twice daily), or both, may be used in addition to loperamide. Octreotide (50 μg subcutaneously three times daily before meals) may be used in patients for whom the oral agents are ineffective or poorly tolerated. 5-HT_3 antagonists (e.g., alosetron, 0.5-1 mg orally up to two times per day) may be efficacious in the treatment of carcinoid diarrhea and diarrhea-predominant irritable bowel syndrome, but it should be reserved for patients with severe, unresponsive diarrhea.

COLONIC MOTILITY DISORDERS

Constipation

EPIDEMIOLOGY

Constipation is a common clinical problem, reported by about 20% of the population, and 40% of Americans report needing to strain excessively to pass their bowel movements.

PATHOBIOLOGY

In functional constipation, transit is normal, and there is no evacuation disorder. These patients may have pain in association with constipation, and there is overlap with constipation-predominant irritable bowel syndrome (Chapter 139). In patients with acquired slow-transit constipation, unassociated with colonic dilation, the number of interstitial cells of Cajal in the different layers of the colon is reduced compared with controls.

Idiopathic megarectum and megacolon can be either congenital or acquired; an enteric nervous system defect is suspected. In megacolon, the dilated segment shows normal phasic contractility but decreased colonic tone, with smooth muscle hypertrophy and fibrosis of the muscularis mucosa, circular muscle, and longitudinal muscle layers.

Acquired defects in the enteric nervous system may result in constipation in Chagas' disease (Chapter 355), which is caused by infection with *Trypanosoma cruzi* and results in the destruction of myenteric neurons. Acquired aganglionosis also has been reported with circulating antineuronal antibodies, with or without associated neoplasm.

DIAGNOSIS

It is essential to distinguish an evacuation disorder, also called functional outlet obstruction (Table 138-2), from constipation resulting from slow transit or other causes. In one study in a tertiary center, 50% of 70 patients with severe, unresponsive constipation had impaired evacuation, and the remainder had constipation associated with either normal transit (also called functional constipation) or delayed colonic transit (also called slow-transit constipation). Characterization of constipated patients (Fig. 138-5) relies on the measurement of transit with radiopaque markers or scintigraphy.

TABLE 138-2 CLINICAL CLUES SUGGESTIVE OF AN EVACUATION DISORDER

HISTORY

Prolonged straining to expel stool
Taking up unusual postures on the toilet to facilitate stool expulsion
Support of perineum or digitation of rectum or vagina to facilitate rectal emptying
Inability to expel enema fluid
Constipation after subtotal colectomy for constipation

RECTAL EXAMINATION (WITH PATIENT IN LEFT LATERAL POSITION)

Inspection
Anus "pulled" forward during attempts to simulate strain during defecation
Anal verge descends <1 cm or >4 cm during attempts to simulate strain during defecation
Perineum balloons down during straining, and rectal mucosa prolapses through anus

Palpation
High anal sphincter tone at rest precludes easy entry of examining finger (in absence of painful perianal condition, e.g., anal fissure)
Anal sphincter pressure during voluntary squeeze is minimally higher than tone at rest
Perineum descends <1 cm or >4 cm during attempts to simulate strain during defecation
Puborectalis muscle palpable through posterior rectal wall is tender
Palpable mucosal prolapse during straining
"Defect" in anterior wall of the rectum, suggestive of rectocele

ANORECTAL MANOMETRY AND BALLOON EXPULSION (WITH PATIENT IN LEFT LATERAL POSITION)

Average anal sphincter resting tone >80 cm H_2O or squeeze pressure >240 cm H_2O
Failure of balloon expulsion despite addition of 200 g weight

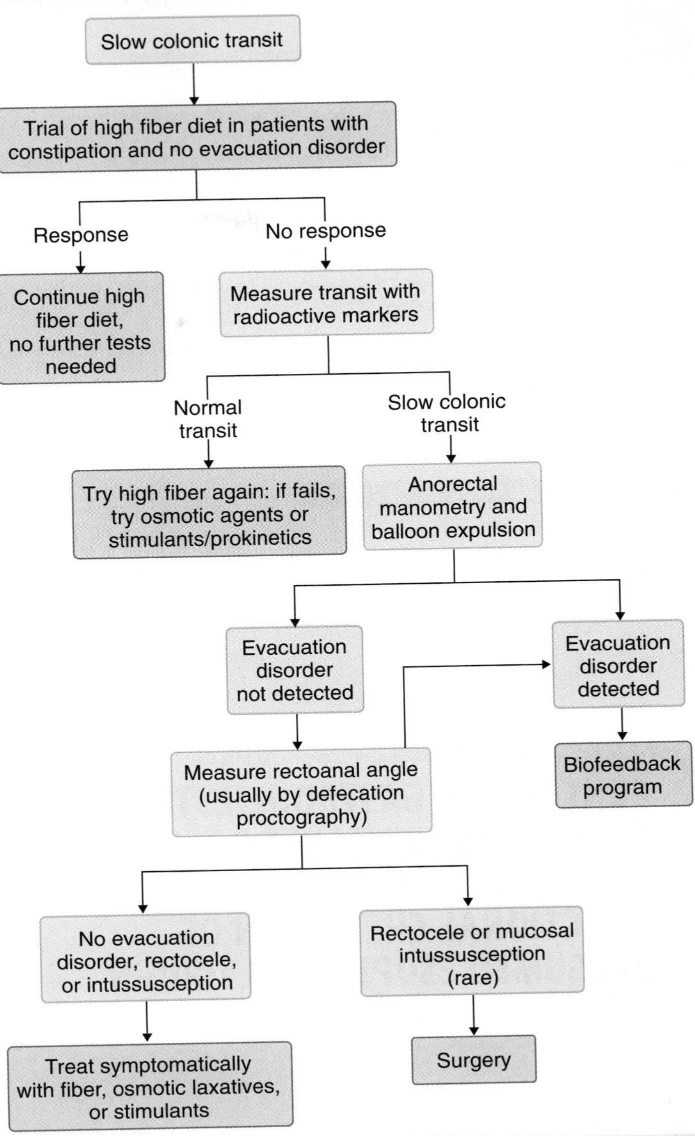

FIGURE 138-5. Flow diagram outlines steps in the management of constipation.

TREATMENT Rx

The average daily fiber intake is around 12 g/day. In patients with normal-transit constipation, 12 to 30 g/day is effective in relief of constipation. In patients with slow-transit constipation, drug-induced constipation, or evacuation disorders, however, supplementation of 30 g of fiber per day does not result in any improvement in constipation. A second step is to add an osmotic laxative, such as a magnesium salt or polyethylene glycol solution, to enhance the retention of fluid within the lumen by osmotic forces, to increase the fluidity, and to ease aboral transport of colonic content. Polyethylene glycol solutions (such as GoLYTELY, NuLYTELY, MiraLAX, OCL solution) are used frequently as a first-line therapy.[1] If these measures do not suffice, a prokinetic or stimulant agent, such as bisacodyl (5 to 10 mg every 1 to 2 days) may be added.

Newer medications that accelerate colonic transit include prucalopride (2 mg daily), which is beneficial in chronic constipation,[2] and lubiprostone (24 μg twice daily), a chloride channel activator that induces fluid secretion. Methylnaltrexone (0.15 mg/kg subcutaneously every other day for 2 weeks) is 33% more effective than placebo in patients with opiate-induced constipation as a complication of advanced illness.[3] Linaclotide, a guanylate cyclase-C receptor activator that results in fluid secretion, improves bowel habits, global symptoms, and quality of life in patients with chronic constipation, but it is not currently approved for use in the U.S.[4]

When these approaches do not work, the patient should be reassessed to exclude an evacuation disorder. For evacuation disorders, a biofeedback treatment program with muscle relaxation of the anal sphincters and pelvic floor results in a 70% or greater cure rate for the constipation. The response to this treatment program is influenced by comorbidity, such as the coexistence of eating disorders or a psychological or psychiatric diagnosis.

Surgical Therapy

In patients whose constipation is not associated with an evacuation disorder and does not respond to aggressive medical therapies (including combinations described earlier), subtotal colectomy with ileorectostomy is effective in relieving constipation. Laparoscopic colectomy with ileorectostomy achieves the same success rate with less morbidity compared with open colectomy with ileorectostomy.

Hirschsprung's Disease

DEFINITION

Hirschsprung's disease occurs in 1 in 5000 live births. It is characterized by a localized segment of narrowing of the distal colon as a result of failure of local development of intrinsic nerves in the myenteric plexus.

PATHOBIOLOGY

A relative deficiency of *KIT*-positive interstitial cells of Cajal has been reported in Hirschsprung's disease and chronic intestinal pseudo-obstruction. Hirschsprung's disease is well characterized histologically by the absence of ganglion cells in the myenteric and submucosal plexus and the presence of hypertrophied nerve trunks in the space normally occupied by the ganglion cells. The lack of nerve growth factor receptors in the muscle layers of the colon involved with Hirschsprung's disease has been shown. The narrowing and failure of relaxation in the aganglionic segment are thought to be due to the lack of neurons containing nitric oxide synthase.

CLINICAL MANIFESTATIONS

Hirschsprung's disease is usually diagnosed at birth because of failure to pass meconium or the presence of megacolon, although it may be identified in childhood as a result of fecal retention, constipation, or abdominal distention. Onset of symptoms or diagnosis after the age of 10 years is rare.

DIAGNOSIS

Diagnosis is based on the typical focal narrowing of the colon, the absence of the rectoanal inhibitory reflex (relaxation of anal sphincter pressure at rest during distention of a balloon in the rectum depends on natural preservation and maturation of intrinsic nerves in the distal bowel), and a deep rectal biopsy specimen showing absence of submucosal neurons with hypertrophied nerve trunks.

TREATMENT

Treatment involves excision of the affected bowel segment or a pull-through procedure by which normal bowel is anastomosed to the cuff of the rectum, just above the anal sphincters.

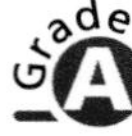

1. Dipalma JA, Cleveland MV, McGowan J, et al. A randomized multicenter, placebo-controlled trial of polyethylene glycol laxative for chronic treatment of chronic constipation. *Am J Gastroenterol.* 2007;102:1436-1441.
2. Camilleri M, Kerstens R, Rykx A, et al. A placebo-controlled trial of prucalopride for severe chronic constipation. *N Engl J Med.* 2008;358:2344-2354.
3. Thomas J, Karver S, Cooney GA, et al. Methylnaltrexone for opioid-induced constipation in advanced illness. *N Engl J Med.* 2008;358:2332-2343.
4. Lembo AJ, Kurtz CB, Macdougall JE, et al. Efficacy of linaclotide for patients with chronic constipation. *Gastroenterology.* 2010;138:886-895.

SUGGESTED READINGS

Camilleri M, Bharucha AE, Farrugia G. Epidemiology, mechanisms, and management of diabetic gastroparesis. *Clin Gastroenterol Hepatol.* 2011;9:5-12. *Review.*

Rao SS, Camilleri M, Hasler WL, et al. Evaluation of gastrointestinal transit in clinical practice: position paper of the American and European Neurogastroenterology and Motility Societies. *Neurogastroenterol Motil.* 2011;23:8-23. *Consensus recommendations.*

139

FUNCTIONAL GASTROINTESTINAL DISORDERS: IRRITABLE BOWEL SYNDROME, DYSPEPSIA, AND FUNCTIONAL CHEST PAIN OF PRESUMED ESOPHAGEAL ORIGIN

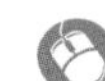

EMERAN A. MAYER

FUNCTIONAL GASTROINTESTINAL DISORDERS

DEFINITIONS

Irritable bowel syndrome (IBS), functional dyspepsia, and functional chest pain of presumed esophageal origin are characterized by chronic, recurrent symptoms of pain and discomfort referred to the lower abdomen, the epigastrium and upper abdomen, and the retrosternum, respectively. They belong to the family of functional gastrointestinal (GI) disorders that comprise a wide spectrum of chronic GI disorders common in both the adult and pediatric populations. In the absence of disease-specific biomarkers, each syndrome is classified by symptoms and the absence of other conditions that can account for the symptoms. Despite the benign prognoses, functional GI diseases can affect health-related quality of life at least as much as organic diseases.

PATHOBIOLOGY

The pathophysiology of functional GI diseases remains incompletely understood, but these diseases are characterized by alterations in bidirectional interactions between the brain and the gut (brain-gut axis; E-Fig. 139-1), with variable contributions of enhanced perception of visceral signals by the central nervous system (visceral hypersensitivity) and altered signaling from the nervous system to the GI tract, through autonomic nervous system activity. Each diagnostic category of functional GI disease is defined by symptomatic criteria that include different subsets of patients who exhibit different patterns of the brain-gut axis dysregulation and that result in varying abnormalities in GI motility, secretion, immune function, or visceral sensitivity. Despite this heterogeneity, however, functional GI diseases all share certain features, including enhanced sensitivity to stress, the frequent coexistence of psychiatric and chronic pain disorders, an enhanced perception of visceral events, and a greater prevalence in women.

Enhanced Perception of Visceral Pain

About 30 to 70% of patients with functional GI diseases have an altered perception of visceral afferent stimuli ("visceral hypersensitivity"), in which normally innocuous stimuli, such as physiologic contractions, distentions, or chemical stimulation of the intestine, stomach, or esophagus, lead to the sensation of pain or discomfort. The stimulus may be spontaneous peristaltic activity or result from distention by luminal contents, such as ingested food, liquids, gas, or feces. Visceral hypersensitivity may be associated with aberrant referral of visceral sensations to a particular body area, and this referral is often atypical in location and larger compared with most individuals.

Altered Stress Responsiveness

Abnormal autonomic and neuroendocrine responses to psychosocial stressors are a key feature of functional GI disease and may play an important role in both its cause and its exacerbation. For example, stressful events are more likely to lead to abdominal pain and a change in stool pattern in patients with IBS compared with healthy controls, and stress has been correlated with bowel symptoms and physician visit. Data also support an association between stress and functional dyspepsia. Patients with functional GI disease report more lifetime stressful events than healthy controls, and this early life stress may interact with a genetic predisposition to determine the vulnerability of an individual to adult stressors and the subsequent development of functional GI diseases.

IRRITABLE BOWEL SYNDROME

DEFINITION

IBS is defined as chronic, recurring abdominal pain or discomfort that is associated with defecation or a change in bowel habits; the diagnosis also requires the absence of detectable organic disease that may explain the symptoms (Table 139-1). Given the high prevalence of IBS in the general population, comorbid organic GI syndromes may coexist with IBS, including ulcerative colitis (Chapter 143), microscopic and collagenous colitis (Chapter 142), and celiac disease (Chapter 142). As a result, some patients may continue to have GI symptoms after their inflammatory bowel disease or other types of colitis have been treated successfully because at least some of their original symptoms were due to comorbid IBS. For example, a small subset of ulcerative colitis patients exhibit IBS-like symptoms and have demonstrable changes in colonic motility when they are in clinical remission.

IBS is further subdivided into IBS with diarrhea, IBS with constipation, or IBS with mixed bowel habits depending on the predominant bowel habit. Another subset is postinfectious IBS, which includes patients who develop persistent IBS symptoms despite the resolution of an episode or episodes of bacterial gastroenteritis. When patients do not fulfill criteria for these subtypes, they are classified as unspecified IBS.

TABLE 139-1 ROME III DIAGNOSTIC CRITERIA FOR IRRITABLE BOWEL SYNDROME

Recurrent abdominal pain or discomfort at least 3 days per month in the last 3 months (but with symptom onset for at least 6 months) associated with 2 or more of the following:
Improvement with defecation
Onset associated with a change in frequency of stool
Onset associated with a change in form (appearance) of stool
Symptoms that cumulatively support the diagnosis of irritable bowel syndrome
Abnormal stool frequency: ≤3 bowel movements per week or >3 bowel movements per day
Abnormal stool form: lumpy/hard stool or loose/watery stool
Defecation straining
Urgency
Feeling of incomplete bowel movement
Passing mucus
Bloating or feeling of abdominal distention
Absence of alarm symptoms
Weight loss
Bloody stool
Anemia
Family history of inflammatory bowel disease
Colon cancer
Celiac disease

EPIDEMIOLOGY

IBS is a common disorder, with a worldwide prevalence that ranges between 10 and 20%. As is the case with many related functional pain disorders, it is more common in women, with a female-to-male ratio of 2 : 1 to 2.5 : 1. It is generally assumed that IBS most commonly presents between the ages of 30 and 50 years, but IBS is also common in the pediatric population, in which such symptoms have traditionally been referred to as recurrent abdominal pain.

The socioeconomic burden of IBS is substantial, with patients taking three times as many days of sick leave compared with individuals without IBS; about 8% of patients retire early because of their symptoms. IBS is estimated to account for about 12% of primary care visits and 19% of GI specialty visits. In the United States, IBS is estimated to account for $1.6 billion in direct costs and $19.2 billion in indirect costs annually.

PATHOBIOLOGY

Although IBS is the most common and best studied functional GI disease, there is no general agreement on its pathophysiology. However, brain-imaging studies in IBS patients strongly suggest enhanced responses to both expected and delivered visceral pain stimuli, including in brain regions concerned with sensory processing, emotional arousal, and cognitive modulation.

Autonomic Nervous System

Converging results from experimental animal and human studies suggest that stress-induced activation of central autonomic circuits plays an important role in the regulation of gut motility, secretion, and immune modulation. Acute stress-induced activation of contractions and secretions of the hindgut is mediated by sacral parasympathetic pathways, and IBS patients have increased activation of these pathways in response to severe laboratory stressors. Tonic upregulation of sympathetic and sacral parasympathetic activity may result in neuroplastic changes in peripheral target mechanisms within the gut, including the enteric nervous system. For example, increased tonic sympathetic influences on the gut may play a role in the development of constipation.

Altered Gastrointestinal Motility and Secretion

GI motility is quantitatively but not qualitatively different in 25 to 75% of IBS patients compared with healthy controls, but these measured differences are not sufficiently reliable to be used as diagnostic markers. Colonic transit is accelerated in IBS with diarrhea, and high-amplitude propagating contractions occur more frequently in such patients than in controls. These high-amplitude propagating contractions correlate with abdominal pain and may be the mechanism underlying urgency, diarrhea, and associated fecal incontinence in this patient subgroup. By contrast, slowed colonic transit is observed in a subgroup of patients with IBS with constipation. Exaggerated or prolonged colonic motility responses to food intake (gastrocolonic response) may be present in approximately 30% of patients who report an exacerbation of abdominal pain after food intake. Secretory abnormalities and alterations in fluid handling by the intestine may also contribute to alterations in bowel habits.

Hypothalamic-Pituitary-Adrenal Axis

Alterations in neuroendocrine responses in IBS patients may be reflected by altered plasma levels of adrenocorticotropic hormone and cortisol. However, the exaggerated cortisol responses in IBS may be more related to a history of adverse early life events rather than to the IBS itself.

Mucosal Immune Activation

In some patients with postinfectious IBS, symptoms persist after the infective gastroenteritis has resolved. Even after resolution of the initial infection, changes in intestinal permeability, as well as small increases in intraepithelial lymphocytes and enterochromaffin cells, can be detected in postinfectious IBS. However, mucosal changes cannot fully account for the pathogenesis because clinical symptoms do not correlate with the observed mucosal inflammatory changes, most patients with bacterial gastroenteritis do not develop IBS symptoms after infection, and the prevalence of IBS is not greater in countries with endemic GI infections. Psychological stress, female gender, a history of other somatic symptoms (somatization), and the duration of the infection all increase the probability of developing postinfectious IBS.

Patients who meet the current diagnostic criteria for IBS but who do not have a prior history of gastroenteritis may have increased inflammatory cells on mucosal biopsy specimens. Fecal calprotectin, which is a surrogate marker of inflammation and which is increased in most patients with proven organic GI disease, has also been detected in a small subset of IBS patients.

Evidence suggests an increased number of mucosal mast cells in the colon and distal small bowel in IBS patients and a closer proximity of these mast cells with enteric nerves. Mast cell degranulation, in response to increased autonomic nervous system activity, and release of histamine, tryptase, and serotonin may increase nerve activity and contribute to symptoms, but a causative role for mast cells remains unproved.

Altered Intestinal Flora

Some data suggest that the intestinal bacterial flora may be altered in patients with IBS and that these alterations may differ among IBS groups according to predominant bowel habits. Small bowel bacterial overgrowth may contribute to IBS symptoms, especially in patients with predominant bloating-type symptoms, in whom treatment with nonabsorbable antibiotics may reduce symptoms. Qualitative changes in colonic flora, such as a decrease in bifidobacteria, have been described in IBS patients.

Genetics

Familial aggregation has been demonstrated in several studies of IBS patients, and the genetic heritability of functional GI diseases has been estimated to be between 22 and 57%. Candidate gene association studies suggest possible association of IBS with polymorphisms in genes related to the serotonin signaling system.

CLINICAL MANIFESTATIONS

Symptoms

The location of abdominal symptoms in IBS is highly variable, but pain is most typically referred to the lower abdomen. Pain and discomfort are frequently aggravated by emotion or stress, poor sleep, and intake of food, but these aggravating factors cannot be elicited in all patients. By definition, abdominal symptoms are relieved by defecation, but this relief may be temporary.

IBS symptoms occur mainly during wakefulness but may also awaken patients from sleep.

If symptoms are unrelated to defecation or food intake and if patients indicate that symptoms are constant and not relievable by any physiologic intervention, other diagnoses should be considered. Weight loss is uncommon in IBS except in patients with depression (Chapter 404) or eating disorders (Chapter 226), and its presence mandates investigation of an underlying organic cause.

IBS symptoms vary widely, from mild to very severe. Most patients seen by primary care physicians have mild symptoms, whereas most patients seen by gastroenterologists have moderate to severe symptoms.

Psychiatric Comorbidity

Psychiatric disorders (Chapter 404), such as anxiety disorders (e.g., generalized anxiety disorder, panic disorder, and posttraumatic stress syndrome), depression, somatization, hypochondriasis, and phobias, are more common in patients with IBS, even mildly symptomatic patients. The prevalence of coexisting psychiatric disorders can be as high as 40% to more than 90% in patients seen in tertiary referral centers but is lower in patients seen in primary care practices. However, stress plays an important role in exacerbating IBS symptoms in patients seen in all settings.

Comorbid Conditions and Extra-intestinal Manifestations

Patients with IBS have a three-fold or higher prevalence of fibromyalgia (Chapter 282) and migraine headaches (Chapter 405) compared with patients without IBS. IBS also frequently coexists with the chronic fatigue syndrome, and 60% or more of patients with chronic fatigue syndrome have IBS symptoms. Interstitial cystitis, chronic prostatitis (Chapter 131), and chronic pelvic pain are also common in IBS patients.

These associations of IBS with comorbid conditions and other symptoms are more common in female patients, but all patients with IBS on average see primary care physicians for non-GI complaints three times more frequently than do healthy subjects. IBS patients also often complain of extra-intestinal symptoms such as dyspareunia, fatigue, loss of energy, impotence, urinary frequency, backache, and dysmenorrhea.

DIAGNOSIS

Clinical Examination

The Rome III criteria (see Table 139-1) can establish the diagnosis of IBS without additional extensive testing. Alarm features raising concern for an

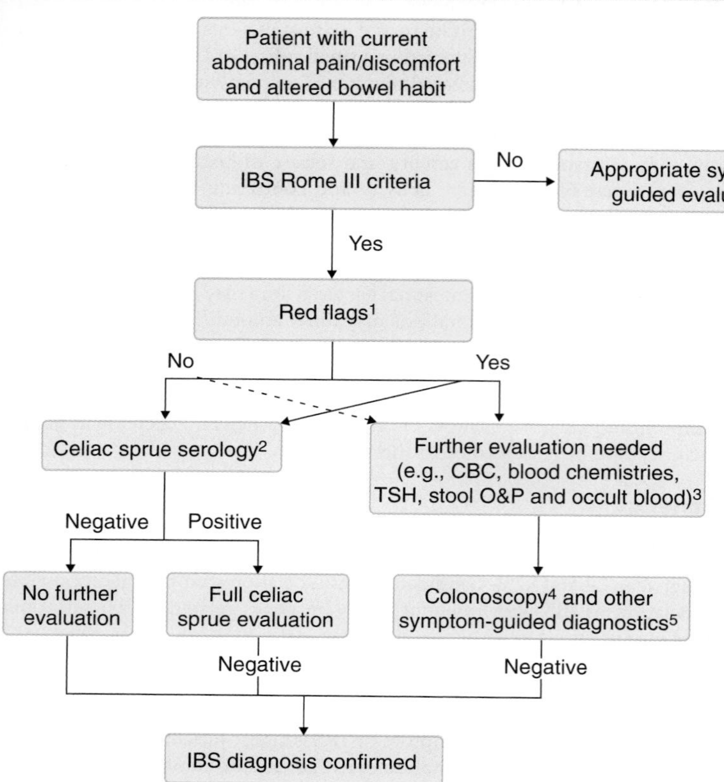

FIGURE 139-1. Diagnostic algorithm for irritable bowel syndrome. (1) Red flags include rectal bleeding, anemia, weight loss, fever, family history of colon cancer, first symptom onset after age 50 years, or major symptom change. (2) Testing for celiac sprue may be useful in patients meeting Rome criteria, in particular in irritable bowel syndrome (IBS) with diarrhea, if there are red flags, and in populations in which the background prevalence of celiac sprue is high. (3) In the absence of red flags, basic complete blood count (CBC), serum biochemistry, stool testing for occult blood and ova and parasites (O&P), and thyroid-stimulating hormone (TSH) levels are only indicated in cases of a supportive clinical history. (4) Colonoscopy is only recommended in the patient with positive red flags. However, according to colon cancer screening guidelines, routine colonoscopy should be performed in irritable bowel syndrome patients at age 50 years or older regardless of irritable bowel syndrome symptoms. (5) If there has been a major qualitative change in the pattern of chronic symptoms, a new comorbid condition producing these symptoms should be suspected and a more comprehensive diagnostic approach is warranted. (From Mayer EA. Clinical perspectives: irritable bowel syndrome. *N Engl J Med.* 2008;358:1692-1699.)

alternative diagnosis include weight loss, bloody stool, anemia, and a family history of inflammatory bowel disease, colon cancer, or celiac disease.

Careful review of medications and dietary supplements may reveal an etiologic agent because many prescribed medications can cause constipation and some diet supplements can lead to the inadvertent ingestion of laxatives. Although specific dietary agents are rarely the cause of IBS symptoms, the presence of lactose malabsorption can be determined by history or by a short trial of a lactose-free diet (Chapter 142). A brief psychosocial assessment is useful in identifying risk factors for chronic pain, such as traumatic early life events or somatization, as well as potential symptom triggers or exacerbating factors, such as anxiety, depression, and life stress.

The physical examination in IBS is usually normal but may reveal abdominal tenderness (most often in the left lower quadrant) or a tender, palpable sigmoid colon. In patients with constipation-predominant IBS and associated defecatory dysfunction, rectal examination may reveal paradoxical contraction of the puborectalis muscle or decreased descent of the pelvic floor when simulating a bowel movement.

Diagnostic Testing

In an otherwise healthy person who is younger than 50 years and who fulfills the ROME III criteria, further diagnostic testing should be minimal and guided by the individual presentation (Fig. 139-1). It remains controversial when to order a complete blood count, sedimentation rate, or thyroid studies, but most agree that it is not cost-effective to obtain these tests in all patients with presumed IBS. Serologic screening for celiac sprue (Chapter 142) should be pursued in patients with diarrhea-predominant or mixed bowel habits and in those with a family history of celiac disease. Colonic biopsies for collagenous or microscopic colitis (Chapter 142) should be considered in the setting of severe persistent diarrhea. The onset of symptoms after age 50 years and the presence of rectal bleeding or unexpected weight loss are indications for colonoscopy to assess for colorectal cancer (Chapter 199). Lower abdominal discomfort occurring with menses or with associated weight loss should trigger gynecologic evaluation. If the duration of diarrhea symptoms is short, it may be useful to assess for giardiasis (Chapter 359) or *Campylobacter* species infection (Chapter 311), but routine stool testing of all patients with diarrhea is not indicated.

Differential Diagnosis

Differential diagnosis for IBS with diarrhea predominance or mixed bowel habit includes inflammatory bowel diseases (e.g., Crohn's disease, ulcerative colitis, collagenous or microscopic colitis) (Chapters 142 and 143), celiac disease (Chapter 142), infection, small bowel bacterial overgrowth (Chapter 142), malabsorptive syndromes (including lactose intolerance) (Chapter 142), bile salt malabsorption (Chapter 142), and pancreatic insufficiency (Chapter 146) or malignancy (including neuroendocrine tumors [Chapter 239] and colorectal adenocarcinoma [Chapter 199]). The differential diagnosis for constipation-predominant IBS includes colonic inertia, pseudo-obstruction, paradoxical pelvic floor contraction, or pelvic outlet obstruction from structural causes such as rectal prolapse, rectocele, or short-segment Hirschsprung's disease (Chapter 138).

TREATMENT Rx

General Principles

Symptomatic treatment attempts to normalize bowel habits and decrease abdominal pain in part by reassurance that the symptoms are real and the prognosis is benign. Dietary intervention can be helpful, and specific medications can be targeted to the management of individual symptoms, such as constipation, diarrhea, and abdominal pain (Table 139-2).

Physician-Patient Relationship and Patient Education

The doctor-patient relationship is of utmost importance in the treatment of IBS and other functional GI diseases. Many patients have been told previously that their symptoms are "all in their head" and have had their concerns dismissed. The physician must listen to and determine the patient's understanding of the illness and related concerns because patients frequently seek validation from the physician that their symptoms are real. Patients with functional GI disease typically visit a physician because of a flare of their usual symptoms, and it is important to identify such triggering factors, in particular various psychosocial stressors or, less commonly, a gastroenteric infection.

A thorough explanation of the symptoms and relationship to functional GI disease should be provided to the patient, including the natural history and benign prognosis of the disorder. Patients who are not properly informed tend to have more health care visits, whereas symptoms generally are reduced when diagnostic and prognostic information is explained. The physician must then set realistic short-term and long-term goals, including methods of adapting to symptoms that are not amenable to treatment. Patients often benefit from being involved in their treatment, and the maintenance of a symptom diary is one such example. Apart from providing the patient with a sense of empowerment, the symptom diary can help identify erroneous beliefs as well as lifestyle or dietary factors that may exacerbate symptoms; lifestyle modifications based on this information may provide symptomatic relief.

TABLE 139-2 MEDICATIONS USED IN THE TREATMENT OF IRRITABLE BOWEL SYNDROME*

SYMPTOMS AND MEDICATION	INITIAL DOSE (mg/day)[†]	TARGET DOSE (mg/day)[†]	COMMON OR SERIOUS SIDE EFFECTS	*Degree of Evidence* OF THE SYMPTOM	*Degree of Evidence* OF IBS	*FDA Approved* FOR THE SYMPTOM	*FDA Approved* FOR IBS
CONSTIPATION							
Laxatives[‡] and Secretory Stimulators							
Polyethylene glycol 3350 (MiraLAX)	17,000	70,000	Diarrhea, bloating, cramping	+++	–		
Lactulose (Kristalose)	10,000-20,000	20,000-40,000	Diarrhea, bloating, cramping	+++	–		
Lubiprostone (Amitiza)		24, twice a day	Nausea, diarrhea, headache, abdominal pain and discomfort	+++	–	Yes[§]	No
Prokinetics							
Tegaserod (Zelnorm)		6, twice a day	Initial diarrhea, abdominal pain, cardiovascular ischemia (rare)	+++	+++	Yes[‖]	Yes[‖]
DIARRHEA							
Loperamide (Imodium)	2	2-8	Constipation	+++	–	Yes	No
Alosetron (Lotronex)			Constipation, ischemic colitis (rare)	–	+++	No	Yes[¶]
BLOATING							
Antibiotics							
Rifaximin		400, three times a day	Abdominal pain, diarrhea, bad taste	–	+	No	No
Probiotics**							
Bifidobacterium infantis 35624		1 capsule per day	None	+	+	No	No
PAIN							
Tricyclic Antidepressants[††]			Dry mouth, dizziness, weight gain				
Amitriptyline (Elavil)	10, at bedtime	10-75, at bedtime		++	+	No	No
Desipramine (Norpramin)	10, at bedtime	10-75, at bedtime		++	+	No	No
Selective Serotonin Reuptake Inhibitors[‡‡]			Sexual dysfunction, headache, nausea, sedation, insomnia, sweating, withdrawal symptoms				
Paroxetine (Paxil CR)		10-60		–	+	No	No
Citalopram (Lexapro)		5-20		+	+	No	No
Fluoxetine (Prozac)		20-40	Somnolence, dizziness, headaches, insomnia	+	–	No	No

*This list is not exhaustive but includes major medications for which there is evidence from well-designed clinical trials of effectiveness for global irritable bowel syndrome (IBS) symptoms or for individual symptoms (e.g., constipation, diarrhea, or abdominal pain and discomfort). In the column about evidence, + denotes some evidence from at least one controlled trial; ++, moderate evidence from several controlled trials or from meta-analysis of such trials; +++, strong evidence from well-designed, controlled clinical trials; and –, no evidence. FDA denotes U.S. Food and Drug Administration.
†Dosages are in milligrams per day unless otherwise noted.
‡A wide range of osmotic and irritant laxatives, including fiber products, are available over the counter.
§Lubiprostone is FDA approved for the treatment of chronic constipation.
‖Zelnorm was suspended by the FDA in March 2005 because of rare cardiovascular side effects but is now available as part of a restricted-access program for women who have constipation-predominant IBS or chronic idiopathic constipation, without known or preexisting heart problems, that is unresponsive to other medications.
¶Lotronex use is restricted for women with severe diarrhea-predominant IBS, unresponsive to other medications, because of side effects.
**Many probiotics are available over the counter and are not listed. Align is a probiotic for which a beneficial effect for IBS symptoms has been shown in a high-quality, randomized, controlled trial.
††A wide range of tricyclic antidepressants with various side effects and side-effect profiles are available. Two commonly prescribed tricyclic antidepressants are listed.
‡‡Many selective serotonin reuptake inhibitors are available. Only those that have been evaluated in IBS trials are listed. Also not listed are serotonin-norepinephrine reuptake inhibitors.

Dietary Modification

Patients with functional GI disease, especially patients with IBS and functional dyspepsia, often complain that certain types of food exacerbate their symptoms. Perceived food sensitivity may be related to a variety of factors, including conditioned fear responses related to anticipatory anxiety, food intake in general, volume of the meal, or sensitivities to certain food items. For example, some IBS patients report an exacerbation of symptoms with high-fat food, gas-producing food, alcohol, and caffeine. It is important to inform the patient that there is no universal diet that is successful for IBS. A therapeutic trial of a lactose-free diet may be beneficial in some patients. Others may benefit from a low-carbohydrate, high-protein diet. It is essential, however, for patients to realize that if the dietary changes are not effective in reducing symptoms, they can resume consumption of the eliminated foods.

Pharmacologic Therapy

Antispasmodics

Antispasmodic medications, which include anticholinergic agents, calcium-channel blockers, and opioid receptor antagonists, may reverse or attenuate tonic contractions of the sigmoid colon or high-amplitude contractions of the colon, thereby relieving contractility. A meta-analysis of several low-quality studies reported a short-term benefit of the smooth muscle relaxants otilonium and hyoscine over placebo, but these agents are not available in the United States.[1] Antispasmodic medications have been combined with anxiolytic agents (e.g., clidinium bromide, 2.5 mg, and chlordiazepoxide, 5 mg, 1 to 2 tablets every 8 to 12 hours), but evidence supporting their benefit is lacking.

Medications for Bowel Habit Abnormalities and Bloating

In IBS patients with constipation, osmotic laxatives, such as polyethylene glycol or lactulose, or secretory stimulators, such as lubiprostone,[2] can be useful. Dietary fiber supplements (see Table 139-2) (e.g., psyllium fiber supplement starting at 3 to 6 g per day and increasing slowly every 1 to 2 weeks up to a total of 15 to 20 g per day in divided doses two or three times per day) may be effective[3] in some patients but often increase symptoms of gas, bloating, and flatulence.

In the IBS patient with diarrhea, loperamide is generally effective in reducing urgency and uncontrollable bowel movements. Several 5-HT$_3$ receptor antagonists and 5-HT$_4$ agonists are effective.[4] For example, alosetron (0.5 to 1 mg orally twice per day) or tegaserod (6 mg orally twice per day)[4] are beneficial, but alosetron should be considered only in patients who have severe bloating and diarrhea and who have failed all other therapies because of its infrequent but potentially serious side effects.

Manipulation of the intestinal flora with antibiotics (rifaximin 550 mg three times daily for 2 weeks),[5] and probiotics[6] may be effective in some patients, particularly patients with abdominal bloating symptoms. Herbal laxatives such as aloe, rhubarb root products, and peppermint oil may be of use in some patients.

Antidepressants and Psychological Therapies

Low doses of tricyclic antidepressants (e.g., nortriptyline or amitriptyline, 10 to 50 mg at bedtime) are frequently used to treat IBS based on data that about one patient in four may benefit.[7] Doses should be started as low as 5 mg once daily and gradually advanced to a maximum of 75 mg once daily. The therapeutic effect should be expected within days to 2 weeks of initiating therapy; if no beneficial effect is observed at 75 mg once daily or if significant side effects are experienced, the drug should be discontinued. Amitriptyline may be most useful in patients with prominent abdominal pain and diarrhea symptoms and in patients with sleep problems.

To maximize compliance and reduce side effects, the patient should be informed about the rationale of the treatment choice (i.e., the goal is the treatment of pain and not psychiatric symptoms) and informed about the much lower risk for side effects at the low dose range compared with full psychiatric doses.

If the treatment goal is aimed at comorbid depression or anxiety disorders, a selective serotonin reuptake inhibitor (SSRI) generally has fewer side effects than tricyclic antidepressants and appears to be beneficial in patients with IBS.[7] In patients with psychiatric comorbidity, a low-dose tricyclic antidepressant and a full therapeutic dose of an SSRI should also be considered, or a nonselective uptake inhibitor such as duloxetine or venlafaxine may be used.

Cognitive-behavioral therapy, which involves relaxation, change in beliefs, and self-management, can reduce gastrointestinal symptoms in at least 50% of patients,[8] although patients with coexisting depression do not respond as well as other patients. Hypnotherapy also has been reported to improve symptoms.

PROGNOSIS

The natural history of IBS is periods of exacerbation followed by periods of remission, but about 50% of IBS patients become asymptomatic. Patients with coexisting psychiatric disorders are less likely to have their IBS symptoms resolve.

FUNCTIONAL DYSPEPSIA

As with other functional GI diseases, the diagnosis of functional dyspepsia is based on specific symptoms (Tables 139-3 and 139-4). Functional dyspepsia is thought to originate from the upper gastrointestinal tract, but no detectable organic disease can explain the symptoms. Symptoms may include epigastric pain, epigastric burning, postprandial fullness, and early satiation. Abdominal bloating and nausea also may be experienced, but they are less specific and are not considered cardinal symptoms of functional dyspepsia. Symptoms overlap with atypical manifestations of gastroesophageal reflux disease (GERD; Chapter 140), and previous studies on functional dyspepsia may have inadvertently included patients with atypical GERD symptoms.

In the current Rome III criteria, symptoms have been divided into meal-related (postprandial distress syndrome) and meal-unrelated (epigastric pain syndrome) symptoms (see Table 139-4). The clinical utility of these subgroups is controversial because there is considerable overlap between them. Moreover, the concept of distinct pathophysiologies correlating with distinct symptom patterns has not been confirmed.

TABLE 139-3 ROME III DIAGNOSTIC CRITERIA FOR FUNCTIONAL DYSPEPSIA*

1. One or more of the following:
   Bothersome postprandial fullness
   Early satiation
   Epigastric pain
   Epigastric burning

and

2. No evidence of structural disease (including at upper endoscopy) that is likely to explain the symptoms

*The criteria must be fulfilled for the last 3 months with symptom onset at least 6 months before diagnosis.

TABLE 139-4 ROME III DIAGNOSTIC CRITERIA FOR SUBGROUPS OF PATIENTS WITH FUNCTIONAL DYSPEPSIA*

POSTPRANDIAL DISTRESS SYNDROME

One or both of the following:
1. Bothersome postprandial fullness, occurring after ordinary sized meals, at least several times per week
2. Early satiation that prevents finishing a regular meal, at least several times per week

Supportive Criteria

1. Upper abdominal bloating or postprandial nausea or excessive belching can be present.
2. Epigastric pain syndrome may coexist.

EPIGASTRIC PAIN SYNDROME

One or more of the following:
1. Pain or burning localized to the epigastrium of at least moderate severity at least once per week
2. Intermittent pain
3. Pain not generalized or localized to other abdominal or chest regions
4. Pain not relieved by defecation or passage of flatus
5. Pain not fulfilling criteria for gallbladder and sphincter of Oddi disorders

Supportive Criteria

1. The pain may be of a burning quality but without a retrosternal component.
2. The pain is commonly induced or relieved by ingestion of a meal but may occur while fasting.
3. Postprandial distress syndrome may coexist.

*The criteria must be fulfilled for the last 3 months with symptom onset at least 6 months before diagnosis.

EPIDEMIOLOGY

Functional dyspepsia is a common disorder, with an estimated prevalence of 15 to 20%. Unlike IBS, there does not appear to be a sex-related difference in prevalence. The socioeconomic burden of functional dyspepsia is substantial; patients with functional dyspepsia take three times as much sick leave as patients with duodenal ulcers. In the United Kingdom, an estimated 2 to 5% of primary care visits and more than 10% of primary care drug expenditures are related to functional dyspepsia. Approximately 1 of 2 individuals with functional dyspepsia seeks health care for symptoms at some time in his or her life. It is therefore not surprising that in the United Kingdom, the annual indirect and direct cost of dyspepsia to society are U.S. $1.46 billion and U.S. $730 million, respectively.

Comorbidity with Irritable Bowel Syndrome

Pain or discomfort in the upper abdomen may at first be assumed to be related to the upper GI tract, but on detailed questioning, the "dyspepsia" may be related to bowel disturbances. One third of patients with functional dyspepsia have concurrent symptoms of IBS, and approximately 40% of IBS patients also report symptoms of functional dyspepsia. Moreover, transitions between the two syndromes in the same patient over time are common. In a 1-year follow-up of patients with IBS or dyspepsia, 22% of IBS patients reported a change in their symptom profile to that of functional dyspepsia, and 16% of patients with functional dyspepsia reported a change to an IBS symptom profile. This transition of patients between different diagnostic categories questions the concept that these symptom-based entities are really distinct pathophysiologic syndromes. Compared with patients with non-life-threatening organic GI disease, patients with functional dyspepsia have higher anxiety but not depression or neuroticism scores.

PATHOBIOLOGY

The pathobiology of functional dyspepsia is not fully understood, and both central and peripheral mechanisms have been proposed. Although enhanced perception of gastric stimuli may be a key central mechanism, the roles of gastric acid, acute and chronic gastric mucosal infections, and gastroduodenal dysmotility remain to be determined. Attempts to classify subtypes of functional dyspepsia based on pathophysiologic abnormalities have been unsuccessful.

As with IBS patients, visceral hypersensitivity is common in functional dyspepsia, and 34 to 65% of patients with functional dyspepsia report pain and discomfort at lower volumes of gastric distention than healthy control subjects or patients with dyspepsia from organic causes. Chemical sensitivity to capsaicin also has been reported. Central pain amplification also is likely to contribute to the observed gastric hypersensitivity. For example, the presence of lipids in the duodenum increases the sensitivity of patients with functional dyspepsia to gastric balloon distention compared with controls. This abnormal modulation of gastric perception thresholds to distention by lipid in a distant site supports the concept of a centrally mediated mechanism. Furthermore, about 50% of patients with functional dyspepsia experience altered viscerosomatic referral patterns in response to gastric balloon distention.

Several large multicenter studies have demonstrated that only 10 to 15% of patients with functional dyspepsia benefit from acid suppression therapy. This finding suggests that such patients are hypersensitive to either intraduodenal or intra-antral acid or that they suffer from atypical manifestations of GERD. Chronic *Helicobacter pylori* infection may be related to dyspeptic symptoms in patients with functional dyspepsia.

Some data suggest the presence of alterations in gastroduodenal motility in patients with functional dyspepsia, but the low concordance between symptoms and altered motility findings argues against such testing except in highly selected patients. For example, about 40% of patients with functional dyspepsia have evidence of impaired gastric accommodation, which may cause rapid transit of food from the proximal stomach, thereby resulting in early antral distention, which in turn results in dyspeptic symptoms. In addition, postprandial antral hypomotility can be demonstrated by manometric studies in about 50% of patients with functional dyspepsia, and this abnormality correlates with delayed gastric emptying, which has been demonstrated in one third of patients with functional dyspepsia. A correlation between delayed gastric emptying and dyspeptic symptoms of postprandial fullness has been reported. About 20% of patients with functional dyspepsia develop their symptoms after an acute episode of presumed viral or bacterial gastroenteritis or *Giardia* species infection.

DIAGNOSIS

Clinical Examination

Dyspepsia can be suspected to be functional based on a clinical history consistent with the ROME III criteria (see Tables 139-3 and 139-4) and the absence of alarm features (see Table 139-1). The presence of anxiety, in particular symptom-related anxiety and comorbid IBS, increases the likelihood of functional dyspepsia.

The physical examination is generally normal, although epigastric tenderness may be present. In contrast to gastroparesis, a succussion splash is typically absent. Although confirmation of the functional dyspepsia diagnosis, as noted in the Rome III criteria, requires a normal upper endoscopic examination, invasive testing in the absence of alarm features should be considered only in a minority of symptomatic patients, such as patients older than 50 years with new-onset or changing symptoms or a poor response to initial therapy (see Fig. 134-6 in Chapter 134). Evaluation for *H. pylori* (Chapter 141) should be performed by stool antigen, urea breath test, or gastric biopsy. If present, the infection should be eradicated, and then symptoms should be reassessed. Young patients who respond well to a trial of proton pump inhibitor therapy or *H. pylori* eradication do not require further investigation unless alarm features are identified. Nonsteroidal anti-inflammatory medications, dietary supplements, and other prescription or over-the-counter medications can trigger dyspeptic symptoms. The patient's medication list should be reviewed, and nonessential treatments should be discontinued. As in the evaluation of IBS, a psychosocial history may reveal underlying stressors that contribute to symptoms.

Differential Diagnosis

Common organic causes of dyspepsia include peptic ulcer disease (Chapter 141) and gastroesophageal reflux disease (Chapter 140). Delayed gastric emptying is present in a small number of patients with functional dyspepsia but is characteristic and more pronounced in patients with diabetic or idiopathic gastroparesis (Chapter 138). Vomiting of undigested food is characteristic of these forms of gastroparesis, but not of dyspepsia. Gastric and esophageal cancers (Chapter 198) may also present with symptoms of dyspepsia but are much less common. Pancreaticobiliary disorders (Chapters 146 and 158) (including sphincter of Oddi dysfunction, chronic pancreatitis, or pancreatic cancer) also occasionally mimic dyspepsia.

TREATMENT Rx

Acid suppression therapy is safe and may have a beneficial effect over placebo in approximately 10% of patients, who presumably have either atypical GERD (Chapter 140) or duodenal hypersensitivity to gastric acid. The choice of acid suppressive agents is open to debate (see Table 140-1 in Chapter 140), and both histamine (H_2)-receptor antagonists (e.g., famotidine, 20 mg twice per day) and proton pump inhibitors (e.g., omeprazole, 20 mg per day) have been reported to be more effective than placebo. A proton pump inhibitor (e.g., omeprazole, 20 mg/day, or lansoprazole, 30 mg/day) is superior to placebo or an H_2 antagonist in functional dyspepsia, especially in patients with epigastric pain. In a randomized study of step-up and step-down treatment with antacids, H_2-receptor antagonists, and proton pump inhibitors in patients with new-onset dyspepsia, the two treatments were equally successful (about 70%), but the step-up approach was more cost-effective.[9]

A subset of patients with functional dyspepsia improve after eradication of *H. pylori* (Chapter 141), and the likelihood of a positive response is comparable to that with acid suppression.[10] This short-duration treatment also can reduce the risk of subsequent peptic ulcer disease, atrophic gastritis, and gastric cancer, and it currently is recommended by consensus guidelines.

The use of prokinetic drugs such as metoclopramide or domperidone, 10 mg three times per day, before meals is of uncertain benefit. Low-dose tricyclic antidepressant therapy has not been as extensively evaluated in functional dyspepsia compared with IBS, but small studies reported a beneficial effect. The benefits of psychological therapy for functional dyspepsia are not well established, but it may be a reasonable option in patients who do not respond to pharmacotherapy.

PROGNOSIS

As with all functional disorders, functional dyspepsia has a benign prognosis, although symptoms can be persistent.

FUNCTIONAL CHEST PAIN OF PRESUMED ESOPHAGEAL ORIGIN

DEFINITION

Functional chest pain of presumed esophageal origin (Table 139-5) is a chronic, unexplained midline chest pain that is thought to be of esophageal origin. To make the diagnosis, cardiac causes, gastroesophageal reflux, and well-defined motility disorders (achalasia, scleroderma) must be excluded.

EPIDEMIOLOGY

Most patients who present to a physician with acute chest pain (see Table 50-2 in Chapter 50) have a noncardiac cause, and many are cases of functional chest pain. Most of these are cases of functional chest pain. Despite its frequency, however, the prevalence of functional chest pain and its natural course are not well understood, likely because most patients undergo a cardiac evaluation but then may have no further evaluation of their symptoms.

Functional chest pain is quite common, with prevalence rates as high as 25%, evenly divided between men and women. Its prevalence appears to decline with advancing age. Risk factors for developing functional chest pain are not well defined but include younger age, adversity in childhood, and a history of other functional gastrointestinal conditions. Once symptoms occur, more than 50% of patients have persisting symptoms for longer than 6 months. Even after the initial diagnosis, however, many patients with chronic pain undergo repeated and unnecessary diagnostic cardiac evaluations. Patients with functional chest pain may have comorbid anxiety or panic attacks, but formal referral for psychological treatment is infrequent. When

TABLE 139-5 ROME III DIAGNOSTIC CRITERIA FOR FUNCTIONAL CHEST PAIN OF PRESUMED ESOPHAGEAL ORIGIN*

Must include all of the following:
- Midline chest pain or discomfort that is not of burning quality
- Absence of evidence that gastroesophageal reflux is the cause of symptoms
- Absence of histopathology-based esophageal motility disorders

*The criteria must be fulfilled for the last 3 months with symptom onset at least 6 months before diagnosis.

compared with patients who have known cardiac chest pain, patients with functional chest pain report greater impairment of health-related quality of life in the domains of mental health and vitality. These findings suggest a link between psychological disturbance and functional chest pain, at least in a subgroup of patients.

PATHOBIOLOGY

Visceral hypersensitivity, altered esophageal motility, and psychological factors have all been implicated in the pathophysiology of functional chest pain. A substantial proportion of patients show enhanced sensitivity to esophageal distention by a balloon. These same patients will often also have increased perceptual responses to intraesophageal acid infusion. The origin of such findings is not clear, although alterations in central processing of pain signals (central pain amplification) has been implicated. In addition, altered esophageal motility can be observed in a subset of patients with functional chest pain, with or without visceral hypersensitivity. Increased contraction of the esophageal muscle has long been considered a source of chest pain, although reproducible studies to prove this hypothesis are lacking.

CLINICAL MANIFESTATIONS

Patients may complain of pain that is typical for myocardial ischemia or of pain with a variety of characteristics that would be considered atypical for ischemia (Chapters 50 and 71). The location of pain is typically substernal, but radiation to the arm and neck can be described. The pain typically is not precipitated by exertion and may persist for hours. Nitroglycerin may sometimes be helpful acutely in patients with coexisting esophageal spasm. Patients may describe the discomfort using a variety of adjectives, and those descriptions may be indistinguishable from angina.

DIAGNOSIS

Patients who present with chest pain suspicious for angina should undergo prompt cardiac evaluation (Chapters 50 and 71). In patients with an initial negative cardiac evaluation, causes of functional chest pain can be categorized based on historical features (Table 139-6), and repeated cardiac evaluation for recurrent pain is of low yield. Patients with prominent chest wall pain and tenderness on palpation or with changes in pain with movement usually have musculoskeletal rather than an esophageal pain.

The remaining patients may have an esophageal source of pain (Chapter 140) and should be divided into patients with and without alarm symptoms, such as weight loss, progressive dysphagia, or anemia. Upper endoscopy is useful in patients with alarm features but is of lower yield in patients without them.

Many patients with functional chest pain will have underlying GERD. Because clinical features, such as association with certain foods or pain location, do differentiate well between acid-induced versus non-acid-related causes, evaluation for atypical GERD is best performed by a proton pump inhibitor trial (e.g., omeprazole, 20 mg daily).[11] Patients who respond to a 1- to 2-week trial of daily proton pump inhibitor likely have acid-related symptoms and should be treated for GERD (Chapter 140). In patients whose response is equivocal, a longer proton pump inhibitor trial of 4 to 8 weeks, endoscopy, or 24-hour pH testing (Chapter 140) can be considered.

For patients who do not respond to a proton pump inhibitor, a disorder of esophageal motility or visceral hypersensitivity may be present. Esophageal motility disorders such as high-amplitude contractions ("nutcracker esophagus") or diffuse esophageal spasm can be identified by esophageal manometry (Chapter 140), but the low concordance between symptoms and manometric findings suggests that such testing should be performed only in highly selected patients based on the advice of a gastroenterologist.

TABLE 139-6 DIFFERENTIAL DIAGNOSIS OF FUNCTIONAL CHEST PAIN

ORGANIC ESOPHAGEAL CAUSES
Gastroesophageal reflux disease
Achalasia
Virus- or pill-induced esophagitis
NONGASTROINTESTINAL CAUSES
Cardiac chest pain
Chest wall pain
Pulmonary disease
Panic attack

TREATMENT

All patients benefit from reassurance regarding the benign course of functional chest pain. Fears of cardiac disease should be addressed explicitly, and the significance of a negative cardiac evaluation must be reinforced. If the functional chest pain is responsive to a proton pump inhibitor trial, patients should be continued on such therapy or treated with alternative acid-suppressing medications. The optimal duration of treatment is unclear, but it is reasonable to attempt withdrawal of medication and observe patients who have remained asymptomatic for several months. Although evidence from well-designed clinical trials is lacking, low-dose tricyclic antidepressants (e.g., desipramine, 10 to 75 mg per day) may be useful, particularly in patients suspected to have visceral hypersensitivity.

Comorbid psychological symptoms should be addressed with either pharmacologic or cognitive behavioral therapy. Even in the absence of a specific psychiatric diagnosis, relaxation therapy or cognitive behavioral therapy may be of benefit for functional chest pain.

PROGNOSIS

Functional chest pain has a benign prognosis, although symptoms may persist and continue to diminish quality of life.

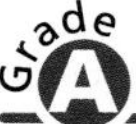

1. Ford AC, Talley NJ, Spiegel BM, et al. Effect of fibre, antispasmodics, and peppermint oil in the treatment of irritable bowel syndrome: systematic review and meta-analysis. *BMJ*. 2008;337:a2313.
2. Drossman DA, Chey WD, Johanson JF, et al. Clinical trial: lubiprostone in patients with constipation-associated irritable bowel syndrome—results of two randomized, placebo-controlled studies. *Aliment Pharmacol Ther*. 2009;29:329-341.
3. Bijkerk CJ, de Wit NJ, Muris JW, et al. Soluble or insoluble fibre in irritable bowel syndrome in primary care? Randomised placebo controlled trial. *BMJ*. 2009;339:b3154.
4. Ford AC, Brandt LJ, Young C, et al. Efficacy of 5-HT3 antagonists and 5-HT4 agonists in irritable bowel syndrome: systematic review and meta-analysis. *Am J Gastroenterol*. 2009;104:1831-1843.
5. Pimentel M, Lembo A, Chey WD, et al. Rifaximin therapy for patients with irritable bowel syndrome without constipation. *N Engl J Med*. 2011;364:22-32.
6. Nikfar S, Rahimi R, Rahimi F, et al. Efficacy of probiotics in irritable bowel syndrome: a meta-analysis of randomized, controlled trials. *Dis Colon Rectum*. 2008;51:1775-1780.
7. Ford AC, Talley NJ, Schoenfeld PS, et al. Efficacy of antidepressants and psychological therapies in irritable bowel syndrome: systematic review and meta-analysis. *Gut*. 2009;58:367-378.
8. Lackner JM, Mesmer C, Morley S, et al. Psychological treatments for irritable bowel syndrome: a systematic review and meta-analysis. *J Consult Clin Psychol*. 2004;72:1100-1113.
9. van Marrewijk CJ, Mujakovic S, Fransen GA, et al. Effect and cost-effectiveness of step-up versus step-down treatment with antacids, H2-receptor antagonists, and proton pump inhibitors in patients with new onset dyspepsia (DIAMOND study): a primary-care-based randomised controlled trial. *Lancet*. 2009; 373:215-225.
10. Moayyedi P, Soo S, Deeks J, et al. Eradication of Helicobacter pylori for non-ulcer dyspepsia. *Cochrane Database Syst Rev* 2006;2:CD002096.
11. Cremonini F, Wise J, Moayyedi P, et al. Diagnostic and therapeutic use of proton pump inhibitors in non-cardiac chest pain: a meta-analysis. *Am J Gastroenterol*. 2005;100:1226-1232.

SUGGESTED READINGS

Chang JY, Talley NJ. Current and emerging therapies in irritable bowel syndrome: from pathophysiology to treatment. *Trends Pharmacol Sci*. 2010;31:326-334. *Review*.

Olafsdottir LB, Gudjonsson H, Jonsdottir HH, et al. Natural history of functional dyspepsia: a 10-year population-based study. *Digestion*. 2010;81:53-61. *Patients are generally stable but continue to have an increased intensity and frequency of gastrointestinal pain*.

Sperber AD, Drossman DA. Review article: the functional abdominal pain syndrome. *Aliment Pharmacol Ther*. 2011;33:514-524. *Comprehensive review*.

140

DISEASES OF THE ESOPHAGUS

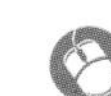

GARY W. FALK AND DAVID A. KATZKA

NORMAL ANATOMY AND PHYSIOLOGY

The esophagus, which averages about 27 cm in length, is a hollow muscular tube consisting of mucosa, submucosa, and muscularis layers and the absence of a serosal layer. The mucosa is a stratified squamous nonkeratinized epithelium that transitions to a columnar epithelium at the gastroesophageal junction. The muscular layer of the esophagus is composed of striated muscle in the upper one third and smooth muscle in the lower two thirds. These muscular components are arranged as an inner circular and an outer longitudinal layer. Located between the circular and longitudinal muscle layers is Auerbach's (myenteric) plexus, whereas Meissner's plexus is located within the submucosa and innervates the muscularis mucosae. The esophagus is bounded by an upper esophageal sphincter proximally and the lower esophageal sphincter distally. The upper esophageal sphincter contains functional contributions from the inferior pharyngeal constrictor proximally and the cricopharyngeus distally. By contrast, the lower esophageal sphincter is anatomically and histologically indistinguishable from the lower esophagus. Blood supply for the cervical portion is derived from branches of the inferior thyroid artery. The intrathoracic segment of the esophagus receives its blood supply from bronchial arteries and direct branches from the aorta, and the short abdominal portion of the esophagus is supplied by the left gastric and the inferior phrenic arteries. Venous drainage follows the arterial supply in the cervical and abdominal portions, whereas the thoracic esophagus drains into the azygous and hemiazygos system. Likewise, the lymphatic drainage of the esophagus is segmental, with the cervical portion draining into deep cervical lymph nodes, the thoracic portion into the superior and posterior mediastinal lymph nodes, and the abdominal portion into the gastric and celiac lymph nodes.

The motor functions of the esophagus are to transport a food bolus from the oropharynx into the stomach and then to keep food from returning to the esophagus after it has entered the stomach. The upper esophageal sphincter and the proximal third of the esophagus compose the first portion of the esophagus. The upper esophageal sphincter, which is approximately 2 to 4 cm in length, is controlled by the recurrent laryngeal nerve inferiorly and a pharyngeal plexus superiorly. The muscle layers close the esophageal lumen and shorten the esophagus to facilitate forward transport through the proximal esophagus. After food traverses the proximal esophagus, it moves into the distal two thirds of the esophagus, where peristalsis is achieved by sequential muscular contraction mediated by an interplay of inhibitory and excitatory neurotransmitters. Peristalsis may be primary, that is, initiated by a swallow, or secondary, that is, stimulated by refluxed gastric contents. Although local mechanisms control most esophageal motor function, vagal input is important in the distal esophagus, where smooth muscle myopathies and autonomic neuropathies can cause dysfunction. The distal esophagus is separated from the stomach by the lower esophageal sphincter, which is 4 to 5 cm in length and is functionally distinct because it maintains a tonic high-pressure zone. This sphincter relaxes nearly completely upon swallowing to allow the passage of food and then regains its tone to provide a barrier against reflux. It also relaxes transiently during normal functions, such as belching and vomiting. The vagus nerve, acetylcholine, and nitric oxide influence tone, but the lower esophageal sphincter tone also is influenced by the crural diaphragm as the esophagus traverses the diaphragmatic hiatus.

Esophageal Functional Testing

Options for esophageal functional testing include barium esophagography, esophageal manometry, and esophageal impedance testing. Barium esophagography (Chapter 135) reveals both anatomic and physiologic information about endoluminal lesions, such as malignancies, ulceration, diverticula, hiatal hernia, and strictures; intramural lesions, such as leiomyomas; and extrinsic lesions, such as occur from vascular (aorta, right atrium, subclavian artery) impingement or solid lesions (pulmonary malignancy, adenopathy) that compress the esophagus. Radiography is also an excellent tool for studying motility patterns, such as peristalsis with either liquid or solid contrast material, while precisely visualizing how the esophagus handles a bolus rather than by implying function from pressure or impedance changes.

Esophageal manometry measures pressure changes generated by esophageal wall contraction using multiple ports that simultaneously measure pressure from the pharynx to the lower esophageal sphincter. Esophageal impedance testing measures conductance between catheter-based electrodes based on the substance that is in contact with each electrode. Air, which is a poor conductor of electric current, will yield high impedance, whereas swallowed or refluxed liquids, which are excellent conductors of electricity, will generate a low impedance signal. From these measurements, the direction and velocity of the transport of air and bolus can help assess peristaltic function and measure reflux of acid and nonacid gastric contents.

Symptoms of Esophageal Disease

The most common symptom of esophageal disease is heartburn, which is defined as a sensation of substernal burning. Chest pain without typical heartburn may occur in a variety of esophageal disorders, including gastroesophageal reflux and motor disorders such as in achalasia. However, esophageal pain and even heartburn can be indistinguishable from cardiac angina (Chapter 50), so care must be taken when a patient at risk for coronary artery disease complains of heartburn for the first time.

Dysphagia, or difficulty swallowing, is another cardinal symptom of esophageal disease. Dysphagia with only solid food tends to occur with structural lesions, which cause esophageal constriction, whereas dysphagia with both liquids and solids occurs more often with motility disorders. Patients with oropharyngeal dysphagia will commonly complain of a feeling of food "sticking" in the throat or the inability to propel the bolus from the mouth to the pharynx; they may also complain of the need for multiple swallowing motions to clear the bolus. Because the cranial nerves that generally control the initial phases of swallowing are responsible for other functions as well, symptoms that may be associated with oropharyngeal dysphagia include drooling, dysarthria (due to tongue dysfunction), nasal regurgitation (due to failure to seal off the nasal passage), or coughing and aspiration (due to failure to elevate and cover the laryngeal vestibule). Dysphagia that results from abnormalities in the body of the esophagus may be referred to the chest or the neck, so the location of pain does not predict the location of the disease. Dysphagia may also lead to a variety of behavioral accommodations, including maneuvers such as slow eating, food aversion, avoidance of hard solid food, and drinking of large amounts of liquids with solid meals.

Regurgitation, which is another typical esophageal symptom, may be described as the feeling of food coming up into the chest or, more dramatically, into the mouth. When regurgitation occurs early in the meal, it suggests a proximal lesion. Regurgitation later in the meal suggests a motility abnormality such as achalasia.

Food impaction is an extreme esophageal symptom. When impaction occurs in the oropharynx, patients may develop a "steakhouse" syndrome, in which an impacted food bolus leads to tracheal impaction or compression. With more distal esophageal lesions, impaction may occur any time during the meal, almost always from a mechanical cause. Patients experience the sudden onset of chest pain and the sensation of food sticking, typically after solids such as meats, raw vegetables, and sometimes sticky rice. With complete impaction, patients who cannot handle secretions because of the obstructing bolus are at risk of aspiration.

GASTROESOPHAGEAL REFLUX DISEASE

DEFINITION

Gastroesophageal reflux disease (GERD) develops when the reflux of stomach contents into the esophagus causes troublesome symptoms or complications.

EPIDEMIOLOGY

It is estimated that GERD, defined as at least weekly heartburn or acid regurgitation, has a prevalence ranging from 10 to 20% in the Western world and less than 5% in Asia. The prevalence also tends to be higher in North America than Europe and higher in northern Europe than in southern Europe. Risk factors for developing GERD include obesity and possibly increasing age. A genetic component may also play a role because GERD is more common in patients with a positive family history and in a monozygotic than in a dizygotic twin.

PATHOBIOLOGY

The esophagus is protected from the harmful effects of refluxed gastric contents by the antireflux barrier at the gastroesophageal junction, by esophageal clearance mechanisms, and by epithelial defensive factors. The antireflux barrier consists of the lower esophageal sphincter, crural diaphragm, phrenoesophageal ligament, and the angle of His, which causes an oblique entrance of the esophagus into the stomach. The attachment of the lower esophageal sphincter to the crural diaphragm results in increased pressure during inspiration and when intra-abdominal pressure increases. Disruption of normal defense mechanisms leads to pathologic amounts of reflux.

Reflux of gastric contents from the stomach into the esophagus occurs in healthy individuals, but refluxed gastric contents are normally cleared in a two-step process: volume clearance by peristaltic function and neutralization of small amounts of residual acid by weakly alkaline swallowed saliva. In normal healthy individuals, physiologic reflux occurs primarily when the lower esophageal sphincter transiently relaxes in the absence of a swallow because of a vagally mediated reflex that is stimulated by gastric distention.

In GERD patients, transient relaxation of the lower esophageal sphincter or a low resting lower esophageal sphincter pressure can result in regurgitation, especially when intra-abdominal pressure is increased.

A hiatal hernia, which results in spatial separation between the augmenting effects of the crural diaphragm and the lower esophageal sphincter, predisposes to reflux events by widening the opening of the gastroesophageal junction and decreasing the pressure of the lower esophageal sphincter. The result is an increased exposure of the esophagus to acid, with increased reflux events during transient physiologic relaxation of the lower esophageal sphincter. Hernias also act as a reservoir for gastric contents when normal esophageal clearance mechanisms result in trapping of fluids in the hernia sac; these contents can reflux into the esophagus when the lower esophageal sphincter relaxes during subsequent swallowing.

Obesity results in an increase in intragastric pressure, which increases the gastroesophageal pressure gradient and the frequency of transient lower esophageal sphincter relaxation, thereby predisposing gastric contents to migrate into the esophagus. In addition, obesity enhances the spatial separation of the crural diaphragm and the lower esophageal sphincter, thereby predisposing obese individuals to a hiatal hernia.

The normal defense mechanisms based on peristalsis and saliva can also be impaired. Peristaltic dysfunction is associated with an increasing severity of esophagitis, and ineffective peristaltic clearance may occur when the amplitude of esophageal contractions is less than 30 mm Hg. Saliva production may be impaired by a variety of mechanisms, such as smoking and Sjögren's syndrome (Chapter 276).

The esophageal mucosa contains several lines of defense. A pre-epithelial barrier is composed of a small unstirred water layer combined with bicarbonate from swallowed saliva and from the secretions of submucosal glands. A second epithelial defense is composed of cell membranes and tight intercellular junctions, cellular and intercellular buffers, and cell membrane ion transporters. The postepithelial line of defense is composed of the blood supply to the esophagus. Acid and acidified pepsin in the refluxate are the key factors that damage the intercellular junctions, increase intracellular permeability, and dilate intercellular spaces. If sufficient quantities of refluxate diffuse into the intercellular spaces, cellular damage may occur. Signs and symptoms of GERD occur when defective epithelium comes into contact with refluxed acid, pepsin, or other noxious gastric contents. In addition to the direct noxious effects of refluxed acid, pepsin, and bile, refluxed gastric juice stimulates esophageal epithelial cells to secrete chemokines that attract inflammatory cells into the esophagus, thereby damaging the esophageal mucosa.

CLINICAL MANIFESTATIONS

The classic symptoms of GERD are heartburn and acid regurgitation; atypical symptoms include chest pain, dysphagia, and odynophagia. Extraesophageal manifestations of reflux disease can include cough (Chapter 83), laryngitis (Chapter 437), asthma (Chapter 87), and dental erosions, but these symptoms can be reliably attributed to reflux only if they are accompanied by classic signs and symptoms of reflux disease. Other proposed associations that are not clearly established include pharyngitis, sinusitis, otitis media, and idiopathic pulmonary fibrosis (Fig. 140-1).

When excessive gastric contents overwhelm the mucosal protective factors in the esophagus, esophagitis may be manifest as erosions or ulceration of the esophagus and may also lead to fibrosis with stricturing, columnar metaplasia (Barrett's esophagus) or esophageal adenocarcinoma (Chapter 198). However, approximately two thirds of individuals with reflux symptoms have no evidence of esophageal damage by endoscopy.

DIAGNOSIS

When GERD presents with typical signs and symptoms, such as heartburn or acid regurgitation, that are responsive to antisecretory therapy, no diagnostic evaluation is warranted. Diagnostic endoscopy is warranted in individuals who fail to respond to therapy or have alarm symptoms or signs such as dysphagia (see Fig. 134-6 in Chapter 134), weight loss, anemia, gastrointestinal bleeding, or persistent heartburn (Fig. 140-2). Endoscopy permits the detection of erosive esophagitis and complications such as a peptic stricture (Fig. 140-3) and Barrett's esophagus (Fig. 140-4); mucosal biopsy, which is crucial in these settings, also excludes conditions that can mimic GERD, such as eosinophilic esophagitis. However, most patients have no mucosal damage seen on endoscopy, regardless of whether they are on or off antisecretory therapy.

Esophageal manometry is useful to exclude achalasia in patients with suggestive symptoms. Esophageal reflux testing by 24-hour transnasal pH monitoring, by 48-hour devices attached to the esophageal lumen, or by 24-hour combined impedance and pH monitoring, may be performed while patients are not on therapy to detect pathologic acid and nonacid reflux as well to correlate reflux events with atypical symptoms, especially in patients with normal endoscopies. Barium radiography has no role in the diagnostic evaluation of patients with reflux disease.

TREATMENT Rx

Although avoidance of foods or beverages that may provoke symptoms, such as alcohol, coffee, spicy foods, and late meals, makes physiologic sense, data from clinical trials to support these maneuvers are lacking. Similarly, elevation of the head of the bed for patients with nocturnal regurgitation or heartburn also is logical. Given the association of obesity and GERD symptoms, weight loss should be part of any treatment program for obese patients.

Inhibition of gastric acid secretion (Table 140-1) is the cornerstone of the acute treatment of GERD, and proton pump inhibitors (PPIs) are superior to histamine (H_2)-receptor antagonists for both the healing of esophagitis and the control of symptoms.[1] However, the healing of esophagitis is more predictable than improvement in heartburn symptoms, even with PPIs.[2] There are no major differences in treatment efficacy among the various PPIs, and once-daily dosing is adequate.

Given the chronicity of reflux symptoms, long-term maintenance therapy with PPIs is typically required, with dosing titrated to the lowest dose necessary to control symptoms. Data to support the use of PPIs in the management of extraesophageal GERD syndromes are weak, although selected patients may benefit. The safety profile of PPIs is excellent, but short-term adverse events such as headaches and diarrhea may occur. Recent epidemiologic studies suggest that long-term PPI use may be associated with an increased risk of *Clostridium difficile* infection, community-acquired pneumonia, hip fracture, and vitamin B_{12} deficiency.

Although PPIs are superior to H_2-receptor antagonists for long-term maintenance therapy as well as for short-term relief, H_2-receptor antagonists are

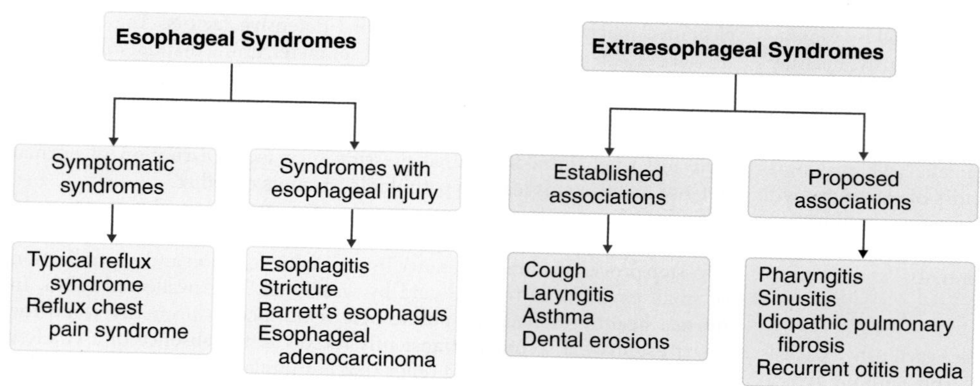

FIGURE 140-1. Montreal classification of gastroesophageal reflux disease (GERD). (From Vakil N, van Zanten S, Kahrilas P, et al. The Montreal definition and classification of gastroesophageal reflux disease: a global evidence-based consensus. *Am J Gastroenterol.* 2006;101:1900-1920.)

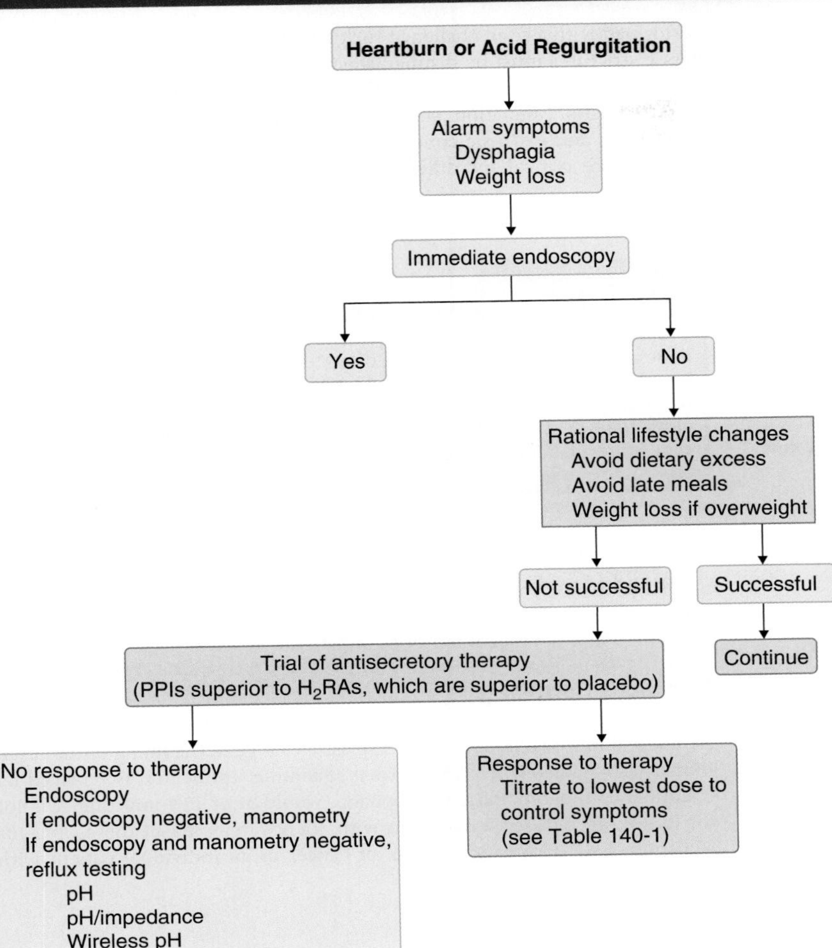

FIGURE 140-2. Algorithm for the management of heartburn or regurgitation symptoms. Surgery is indicated only for patients who are intolerant of antisecretory therapy or who have ongoing symptoms, especially regurgitataion if reflux is well documented. H_2RA = histamine-2 receptor antagonist; PPI = proton pump inhibitor. (Based on Kahrilas PJ, Shaheen NJ, Vaezi MF. American Gastroenterological Association Institute technical review on the management of gastroesophageal reflux disease. *Gastroenterology.* 2008;135:1392-1413.)

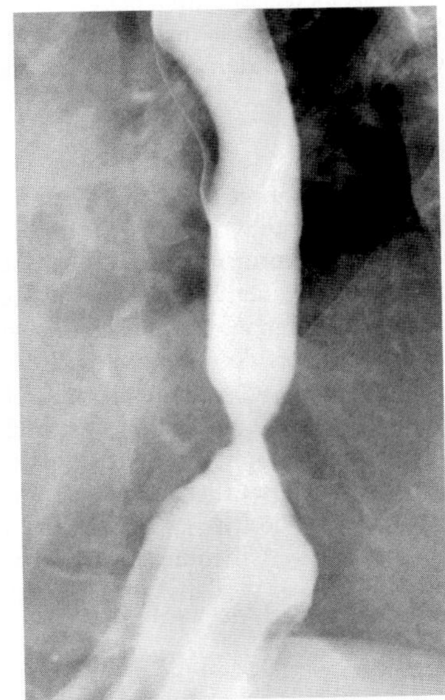

FIGURE 140-3. Barium radiograph of a peptic stricture. (Image courtesy of Marc Levine, MD.)

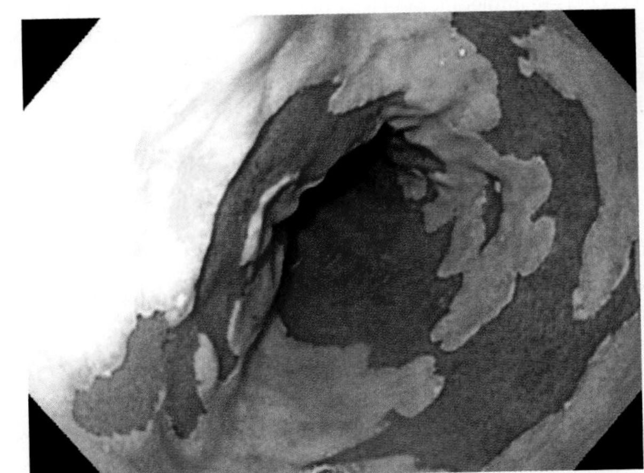

FIGURE 140-4. Endoscopic appearance of Barrett's esophagus. Note the white-appearing normal squamous mucosa displaced above the true end of the esophagus. The intervening mucosa appears salmon-pink.

TABLE 140-1 DRUG THERAPY FOR ESOPHAGEAL DISORDERS

AGENT	DOSE
ANTACIDS: LIQUID (TO BUFFER ACID AND INCREASE LESP)	
For example, Mylanta II/Maalox TC (acid-neutralizing capacity, 25 mEq/5 mL)*	15 mL qid 1 hour after meals and at bedtime or as needed
GAVISCON (TO DECREASE REFLUX VIA A VISCOUS MECHANICAL BARRIER AND BUFFER ACID)	
$Al(OH)_3$, $NaHCO_3$, Mg trisilicate, alginic acid	2-4 tablets qid at bedtime or as needed
H_2-RECEPTOR ANTAGONISTS (TO DECREASE ACID SECRETION)	
Cimetidine	800 mg bid, 400 mg qid, ≈13 mL bid
Ranitidine	150 mg qid or 10 mL qid; maintenance dose, 150 mg bid, 10 mL bid
Famotidine	20-40 mg bid or 2.5-5 mL bid
Nizatidine	150 mg bid
PROTON PUMP INHIBITORS (TO DECREASE ACID SECRETION AND GASTRIC VOLUME)†	
Omeprazole	20 mg/day; maintenance dose, 20 mg/day
Lansoprazole	30 mg/day; maintenance dose, 15 mg/day
Pantoprazole	40 mg/day; maintenance dose, 40 mg/day
Rabeprazole	20 mg/day; maintenance dose, 20 mg/day
Esomeprazole	20-40 mg/day; maintenance dose, 20 mg/day
Dexlansoprazole	30-60 mg/day; maintenance dose, 30 mg/day

*Patients with reflux are not generally hypersecretors of gastric acid, so the therapeutic doses of antacids are based on their capacity to buffer (normal) basal acid secretion rates of approximately 1 to 7 mEq/hr (mean, 2 mEq/hr) and peak meal-stimulated acid secretion rates of about 10 to 60 mEq/hr (mean, 30 mEq/hr).
†High-dose therapy is a twice-daily administration of the usually daily dose.
LESP = lower esophageal sphincter pressure.

superior to placebo, are useful in patients who are intolerant of PPIs, and can be used at bedtime[3] to supplement PPIs in patients who have persistent symptoms. No high-quality data exist to support the common practice of using metoclopramide as either monotherapy or an adjunct to acid suppression therapy[2]; furthermore, its significant adverse effects argue against the use of this drug in any GERD patients.

Antireflux surgery is an option for patients who have documented esophagitis and who are intolerant of PPIs or unresponsive to them. For the healing of esophagitis, laparoscopic fundoplication yields results comparable to continued PPI therapy.[4] However, surgery has a number of serious complications that may affect quality of life, including dysphagia, vagal nerve injury, gas bloat syndrome, and diarrhea. There are inadequate data to support any of the many proposed endoscopic approaches to GERD at present.

PROGNOSIS

Patients with GERD generally do well with conservative antireflux measures and PPI therapy. When surgery is required, the outcome is usually excellent.

Peptic Strictures

Esophageal strictures are a well-recognized complication of GERD, especially in older patients with long-standing reflux symptoms, but population-based studies suggest that the incidence of new and recurrent strictures is declining. Peptic strictures are thought to be a consequence of severe inflammation, which leads to fibrosis, scarring, esophageal shortening, and loss of compliance of the lumen.

CLINICAL MANIFESTATIONS AND DIAGNOSIS

Symptoms are typically dysphagia to solids with or without antecedent symptoms of heartburn or acid regurgitation. Strictures may be diagnosed by barium radiography or with upper endoscopy, but barium esophagrams (see Fig. 140-3) have a higher sensitivity for detecting subtle lesions, especially if performed with a solid challenge such a barium-impregnated pill. However, peptic strictures must be distinguished from a wide variety of other causes of luminal narrowing, including pills, prior nasogastric tube intubation, neoplasia, infection, radiation, surgical anastomosis, systemic diseases, caustic substances, and extrinsic compression. As a result, endoscopic biopsy and cytology are critical for differentiating benign from malignant causes of strictures.

TREATMENT 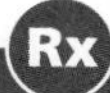

Endoscopic dilation, which remains the cornerstone of therapy, should be done gradually to achieve a luminal diameter that is sufficiently large to relieve symptoms—typically a diameter of 13 mm or greater. After dilation is accomplished, patients should receive chronic PPI therapy (see Table 140-1). For recalcitrant peptic strictures, injection of triamcinolone into the stricture is superior to sham injection in patients who receive balloon dilation and post-procedure PPIs.[5]

PROGNOSIS

Endoscopic dilation will usually alleviate symptoms, but repetitive dilation is required in a significant minority of patients.

Barrett's Esophagus

Barrett's esophagus, which is an acquired condition that results from severe esophageal mucosal injury, is a metaplastic change in the lining of the distal tubular esophagus, where the normal squamous epithelium is replaced by columnar epithelium. Barrett's esophagus would be of little importance if not for its well-recognized association with adenocarcinoma of the esophagus (Chapter 198). However, the risk of cancer in an individual patient with Barrett's esophagus is low.

EPIDEMIOLOGY

It is estimated that Barrett's esophagus is found in approximately 5 to 15% of patients who undergo endoscopy for symptoms of GERD. Population-based studies suggest that the prevalence of Barrett's esophagus is approximately 1.3 to 1.6%, but about 45% of affected patients do not have reflux symptoms. Barrett's esophagus is predominantly a disease of middle-aged white men, but about 25% of patients are women or are less than 50 years of age. The prevalence of Barrett's esophagus increases until a plateau is reached between the seventh and ninth decades. Risk factors include frequent and long-standing reflux episodes, smoking, male gender, older age, and central male pattern obesity.

PATHOBIOLOGY

Barrett's esophagus results from severe esophageal mucosal injury. Patients who develop Barrett's esophagus typically have more esophageal acid exposure, based on 24-hour pH monitoring, and almost always have a hiatal hernia, which is typically longer and associated with larger defects than in patients without Barrett's. However, why some patients with GERD develop Barrett's esophagus whereas others do not remains unclear, as does the cell of origin of columnar metaplasia. Candidates include dedifferentiation of squamous epithelium into columnar epithelium or stimulation of stem cells from either the basal layer of the esophageal epithelium, the esophageal submucosal glands, or the bone marrow. The transcription factor CDX2, which can be induced by both acid and bile salts, appears to play a role in promoting the development of the columnar epithelium. A small subset of patients may have an inherited predisposition, perhaps with an autosomal dominant pattern.

CLINICAL MANIFESTATIONS

The development of reflux symptoms at an earlier age, an increased duration of reflux symptoms, an increased severity of nocturnal reflux symptoms, and prior complications of GERD such as esophagitis, ulceration, stricture, and bleeding may raise the likelihood of Barrett's esophagus. Nevertheless, patients with Barrett's esophagus are difficult to distinguish clinically from patients whose GERD is uncomplicated by a columnar-lined esophagus. Patients with Barrett's esophagus may paradoxically have impaired sensitivity to esophageal acid perfusion compared with patients with uncomplicated GERD.

DIAGNOSIS

Endoscopically, Barrett's esophagus is characterized by displacement of the squamocolumnar junction so that it is now proximal to the gastroesophageal junction, which is defined by the proximal margin of gastric folds (Fig. 140-4). The diagnosis of Barrett's esophagus is established if a biopsy determines that the squamocolumnar junction is displaced proximal to the gastroesophageal junction and if intestinal metaplasia, which is characterized in part by acid mucin-containing goblet cells, is detected.

The precise junction of the stomach and the esophagus may be difficult to determine endoscopically owing to the presence of a hiatal hernia, inflammation, and the dynamic nature of the gastroesophageal junction. If the squamocolumnar junction is above the level of the esophagogastric junction, as defined by the proximal margin of the gastric folds, biopsy specimens should be obtained for confirmation of columnar metaplasia.

Intestinal metaplasia may be seen in the cardia of normal individuals as well as in persons with chronic reflux disease, and the prevalence of intestinal metaplasia at a normal-appearing gastroesophageal junction varies from 5 to 36%. Dysplasia and an increased risk of carcinoma have been reported in patients who have intestinal metaplasia of the gastroesophageal junction or cardia, but the magnitude of that risk appears to be less than that of short-segment Barrett's esophagus.

TREATMENT Rx

Patients who are diagnosed with Barrett's esophagus require surveillance endoscopy at regular intervals (Fig. 140-5). They characteristically worry about cancer risk, which they typically overestimate, face higher life insurance premiums, and may receive conflicting information on how best to treat their condition.

PPIs (see Table 140-1), which are the cornerstone of medical therapy for Barrett's esophagus, consistently relieve symptoms and heal esophagitis. However, PPIs, even at high doses, provide no more than modest regression of Barrett's histology, perhaps because alleviation of reflux symptoms is not necessarily equivalent to normalization of esophageal acid exposure. In fact, abnormal acid exposure persists in approximately 25% of Barrett's esophagus patients despite twice-daily PPIs. The importance of complete control of esophageal acid exposure in patients with Barrett's esophagus remains unknown. Antireflux surgery also effectively alleviates GERD symptoms in these patients, and the indications for surgery are the same as those for patients with GERD without Barrett's esophagus. Surgery should not, however, be viewed as a cancer prevention tool.

Current practice guidelines, based on observational data, recommend endoscopic surveillance of patients with documented Barrett's esophagus in an attempt to detect dysplasia and cancer at an early and potentially curable stage. Before entering into a surveillance program, patients should be advised about risks and benefits, including the limitations of surveillance endoscopy as well as the importance of adhering to appropriate surveillance intervals. Other considerations include age, likelihood of survival over the next 5 years, and ability to tolerate either endoscopic or surgical interventions for early esophageal adenocarcinoma.

Systematic four-quadrant biopsies should be obtained at 2-cm intervals along the entire length of the Barrett's segment after inflammation related to GERD is controlled with antisecretory therapy. Mucosal abnormalities, especially in the setting of high-grade dysplasia, should be resected endoscopically. Surveillance intervals, determined by the presence and grade of dysplasia, are based on a limited understanding of the biology of esophageal adenocarcinoma. Surveillance initially should be annual in patients with metaplasia, but surveillance every 3 years is adequate after two negative examinations. If low-grade dysplasia is found, the diagnosis should be confirmed by an expert gastrointestinal pathologist because of the marked interobserver variability in the interpretation of these biopsies. If confirmed, aggressive PPI therapy (see Table 140-1) is recommended to decrease inflammation and regeneration, which may make pathologic interpretation difficult. A repeat endoscopy

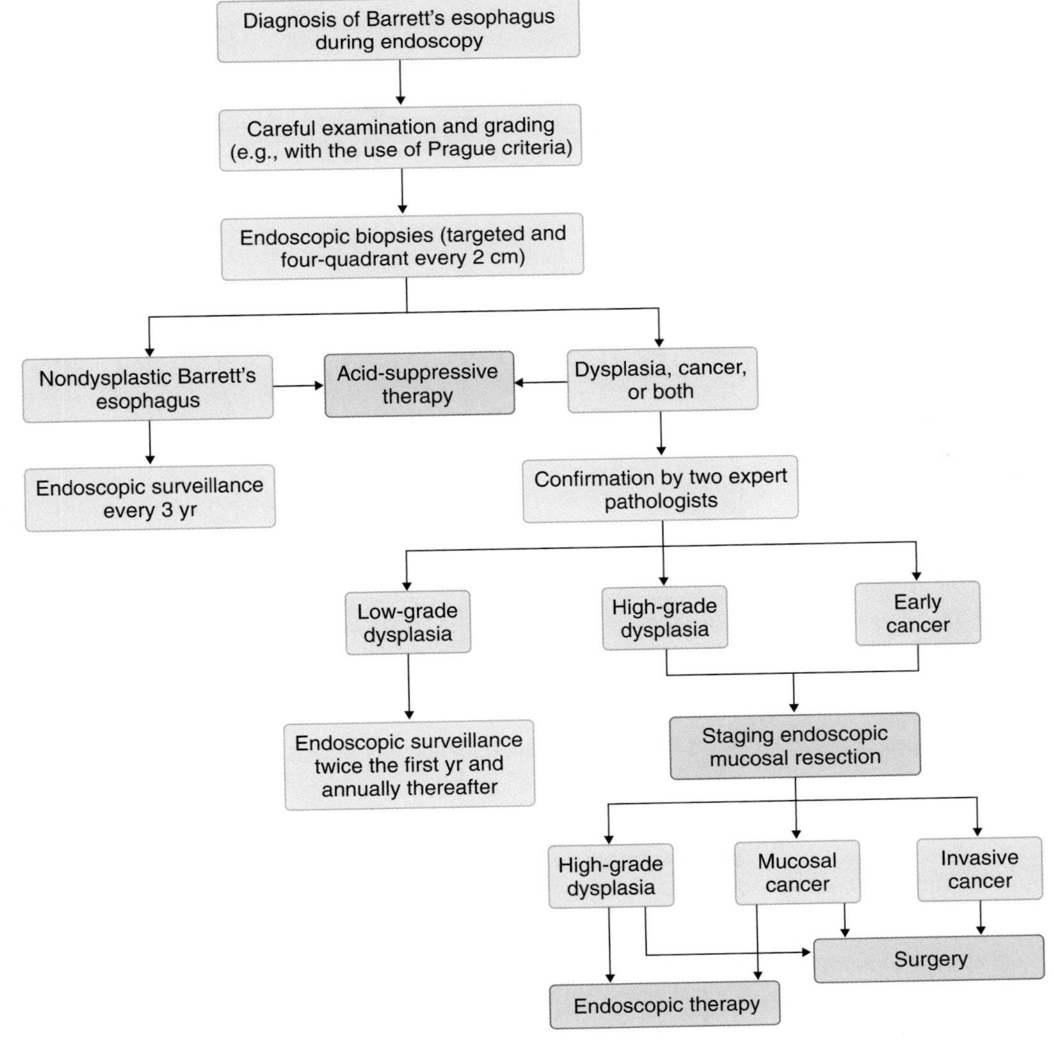

FIGURE 140-5. Proposed treatment algorithm for patients with Barrett's esophagus. (From Sharma P. Barrett's esophagus. *N Engl J Med.* 2009;361:2548-2556, Fig. 3).

should then be performed within 6 months of the initial diagnosis. If low-grade dysplasia is confirmed, annual surveillance is recommended until two consecutive examinations are negative for dysplasia.

If high-grade dysplasia is found, the diagnosis should be confirmed by an experienced gastrointestinal pathologist. Treatment options include continued surveillance, endoscopic therapy by a variety of different methods, or esophagectomy. Factors to consider include the available surgical and endoscopic expertise, age, length of Barrett's epithelium that would require biopsy to eliminate sampling error, compliance with endoscopic surveillance, future need for multiple surveillance endoscopies, and suspicious lesions such as plaque, nodules, and strictures. Currently, endoscopic mucosal resection and radiofrequency ablation 6 are the most promising of the endoscopic methods.

PROGNOSIS

The risk that a patient with Barrett's esophagus will develop esophageal adenocarcinoma is approximately 0.5% to 0.7% annually. These data also emphasize that most patients with Barrett's esophagus will never develop esophageal cancer.

ESOPHAGITIS

Eosinophilic Esophagitis

Eosinophilic esophagitis is probably caused by an aberrant immune or antigenic response to food and aeroallergens that trigger chronic inflammation in the esophageal mucosa. The disease is most common in children and adolescents, but adults are commonly affected as well. Patients often have a personal and family history of other allergic disorders. A genetic predisposition is suggested by the finding of an abnormal eotaxin gene in almost 50% of children with this disorder.

CLINICAL MANIFESTATIONS AND DIAGNOSIS

Children present with dyspeptic symptoms, whereas adults classically present with solid food dysphagia, food impaction, or chest pain. Diagnosis is made by classic findings on endoscopy, such as linear furrowing and multiple rings (Fig. 140-6), accompanied by biopsies demonstrating eosinophilic infiltration (Table 140-2).

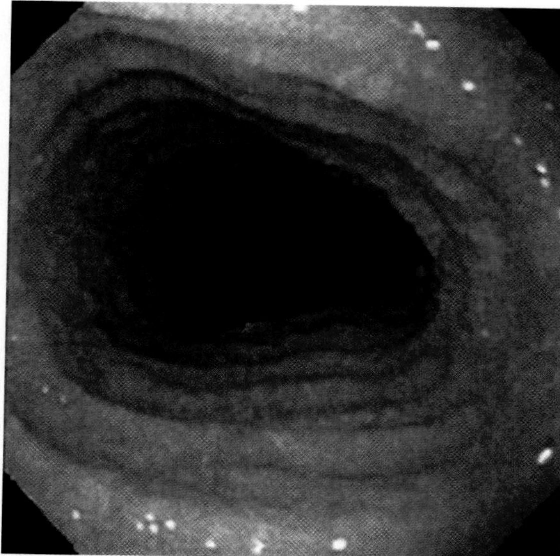

FIGURE 140-6. Endoscopic corrugated (ringed) appearance of esophagus in eosinophilic esophagitis.

TABLE 140-2 GUIDELINES FOR DIAGNOSIS OF EOSINOPHILIC ESOPHAGITIS

Clinical symptoms of esophageal dysfunction
>15 Eosinophils in 1 high-power field
Lack of responsiveness to high-dose proton pump inhibition (see Table 140-1) or normal pH monitoring of the distal esophagus

TREATMENT AND PROGNOSIS Rx

Treatment is a 2-month course of topical steroids, such as swallowed fluticasone (440-880 μg twice daily) or budesonide suspension (1 mg twice daily, for 15 days, followed by 0.25 mg twice daily) 7 or occasionally a 1-month course of systemic steroids (e.g., prednisone, starting at 40 mg and then tapering). Patients also should undergo a formal allergy evaluation (Chapter 257) to determine whether any food trigger can be identified and avoided. Another option is an empirical six-food elimination diet that eliminates cow's milk protein (casein), soy, wheat, egg, peanut/tree nuts, and seafood. Most patients do well after treatment.

Pill-Induced Esophagitis

Pills (Table 140-3) can induce esophageal injury by producing a caustic acid solution (e.g., ascorbic acid and ferrous sulfate), producing a caustic alkaline solution (e.g., alendronate, button batteries), placing a hyperosmolar solution in contact with the esophageal mucosa (e.g., potassium chloride), or causing direct drug toxicity to the esophageal mucosa (e.g., tetracycline). Because prolonged contact is an essential part of the injury, predisposing factors for pill-induced injury include anatomic barriers, such as a stricture, a prominent aortic arch that compresses the esophagus, or improper ingestion of the pill because of inadequate fluid or improper positioning (i.e., lying down directly after taking the pill). The most common medications are tetracycline and its derivatives, but other commonly implicated medications include nonsteroidal anti-inflammatory drugs (NSAIDs), bisphosphonates, ferrous sulfate, quinidine, and potassium chloride.

Patients usually complain of the acute onset of severe odynophagia. Radiographic or endoscopic findings may range from a discrete ulceration to diffuse esophagitis. Treatment is generally supportive with discontinuation of the medication until the injury resolves. Although acid suppression is commonly recommended, there is no proven evidence for its benefit. Patients should be given careful instructions to avoid lying down immediately after ingesting

TABLE 140-3 MEDICATIONS COMMONLY ASSOCIATED WITH ESOPHAGITIS OR ESOPHAGEAL INJURY

ANTIBIOTICS
Tetracycline
Doxycycline
Clindamycin
Penicillin
Rifampin
ANTIVIRAL AGENTS
Zalcitabine
Zidovudine
Nelfinavir
BISPHOSPHONATES
Alendronate
Etidronate
Pamidronate
CHEMOTHERAPEUTIC AGENTS
Dactinomycin
Bleomycin
Cytarabine
Daunorubicin
5-Fluorouracil
Methotrexate
Vincristine
NONSTEROIDAL ANTI-INFLAMMATORY DRUGS
Aspirin
Naproxen
Ibuprofen
OTHER MEDICATIONS
Quinidine
Potassium chloride
Ferrous sulfate
Ascorbic acid
Multivitamins
Theophylline

medication and to drink adequate fluids helps prevent injury. Rarely, pill-induced injury may lead to strictures and even fistulas.

Caustic Injury

Potentially devastating caustic esophageal injuries may be caused by highly alkaline solutions, such as sodium hydroxide, or highly acidic solutions, such as sulfuric acid. The most common products that contain these substances are drain cleaners and industrial strength cleaners, but other corrosive substances include hair relaxers, oven and toilet bowl cleaners, and button batteries. Patients require emergent endoscopy to determine the degree of injury, which helps predict long-term prognosis. No clear evidence supports routine steroids or antibiotics. Many patients will have lifelong disease marked by chronic strictures that require frequent dilation and even esophageal reconstruction. In patients with a severe initial injury, the risk of esophageal cancer is significantly increased.

ESOPHAGEAL MOTOR DISORDERS

Oropharyngeal Dysfunction

The cricopharyngeus and inferior pharyngeal constrictor are composed of striated muscle and innervated by upper motor neurons, the brain stem, and the cerebral cortex. Both primary myopathic and neuropathic disorders can result in dysfunction. The most common neurologic cause of oropharyngeal dysphagia is a cerebrovascular accident (Chapter 414). Other neuropathic disorders that may also affect function include myasthenia gravis (Chapter 430), brain stem tumors (Chapter 195), amyotrophic lateral sclerosis (Chapter 418), Parkinson's disease (Chapter 416), Alzheimer's disease (Chapter 409), postpolio syndrome (Chapter 423), Guillain-Barré syndrome (Chapter 428), and botulism (Chapter 304). Myogenic disorders that cause dysfunction include paraneoplastic antibody-mediated syndromes (Chapter 187), thyroid disease (Chapter 233), primary myopathies (Chapter 429) such as dermatomyositis, and drugs that cause myopathy such as statins and amiodarone.

Patients with oropharyngeal abnormalities experience dysphagia, often accompanied by postprandial coughing, hoarseness, and aspiration pneumonia. Treatment focuses on the underlying myopathic or neurologic cause, but prognosis is often poor owing to limited treatment options.

Achalasia

Achalasia, which is the prototypic esophageal motility disorder, is characterized by a hypertensive lower esophageal sphincter with incomplete relaxation upon swallowing, accompanied by aperistalsis of the esophageal body.

EPIDEMIOLOGY AND PATHOBIOLOGY

Achalasia can occur in patients of almost any age, from infants to nonagenarians, but it most commonly presents between 25 and 60 years of age. The prevalence is 10 per 100,000 in the United States, with all races affected and an equal distribution in men and women. The pathophysiology of achalasia most likely reflects an antibody-mediated autoimmune myenteric plexopathy in the lower esophageal sphincter and a generalized neuropathy in the esophageal body. The triggering event is unclear, but a viral cause is suggested. Injury to the lower esophageal sphincter neurons leads to a relative selective deficiency of nitric oxide. With this loss of the main functional inhibitory neurotransmitter, the sphincter becomes hypertensive and loses its ability to relax. The neurochemical process that leads to aperistalsis is unclear.

CLINICAL MANIFESTATIONS AND DIAGNOSIS

The cardinal symptoms of achalasia are dysphagia to both liquids and solids, regurgitation, and chest pain. Some patients may have more subtle symptoms, including heartburn, presumably caused by esophageal stasis of acidic food content, weight loss, and aspiration pneumonia; in these settings, diagnosis is often delayed.

The diagnosis of achalasia relies on esophageal manometry and barium radiography. The classic radiographic appearance is esophageal dilation, stasis of contrast material, and a "bird's beak" appearance to the lower esophageal sphincter (Fig. 140-7). Manometry demonstrates high residual pressures of the lower esophageal sphincter and either simultaneous contractions or complete absence of peristaltic contractions. Endoscopy is recommended to exclude secondary causes of achalasia, such as cancer of the gastroesophageal junction. Occasional patients present with a massively dilated esophagus and marked persistent food retention. Radiographically, these patients develop a "sigmoid" esophagus with a radiographic picture similar to a sigmoid colon.

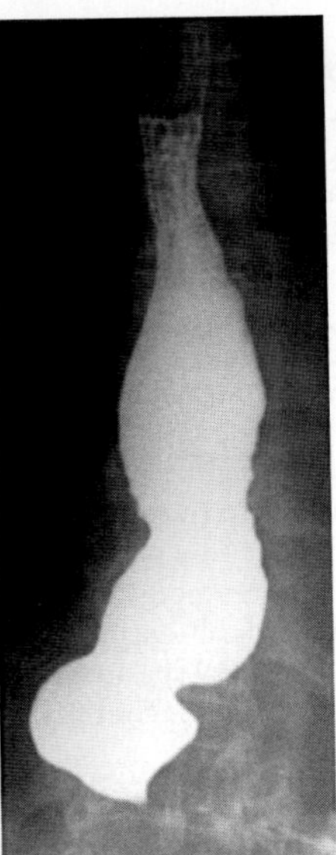

FIGURE 140-7. Esophagogram of a patient with idiopathic achalasia. Note the dilated esophagus with an air-fluid level and distal tapering providing a "bird's beak" deformity in the area of the lower esophageal sphincter. (From Feldman M, Friedman LS, Sleisenger MH, eds. *Sleisenger and Fordtran's Gastrointestinal and Liver Disease: Pathophysiology, Diagnosis, Management*, 7th ed. Philadelphia: Saunders; 2002.)

Achalasia may represent a paraneoplastic presentation of some malignancies, particularly small cell carcinoma of the lung (Chapter 197); in these patients, the tumor produces an antineuronal antibody (anti-Hu) that mediates the autoimmune lower esophageal sphincter plexopathy and produces a syndrome identical to primary achalasia. Some tumors, such as proximal gastric cancer, may also metastasize to or directly extend into the lower esophageal sphincter and produce an achalasia-like picture, possibly owing to extrinsic compression or tumor infiltration.

TREATMENT Rx

Treatment options to decrease the functional obstruction at the level of the lower esophageal sphincter include the intrasphincteric injection of botulinum toxin, pneumatic dilation, and cardiomyotomy. Injection of botulinum toxin during endoscopy reduces symptoms and improves esophageal emptying in up to 90% of patients.[8] Because symptoms typically recur within 1 to 2 years, this treatment is best for patients who are not candidates for more definitive therapies or to confirm the diagnosis of achalasia when clinical, radiographic, and manometric criteria are not conclusive.

In pneumatic dilation, a 30- to 40-mm pneumatic balloon is placed fluoroscopically to straddle the lower esophageal sphincter; the balloon is then inflated to tear the muscle fibers of the lower esophageal sphincter. In general, one dilation will achieve 5 years of symptomatic remission in 40% of patients, and three dilations will succeed in 90% of patients. The downside of this procedure is the risk of perforation, which occurs in up to 5% of patients.

The third approach is a Heller myotomy, which is now typically performed laparoscopically. This long myotomy starts at least 2 cm below the lower esophageal sphincter and extends for about 6 cm upward past the sphincter; a loose fundoplication is performed to prevent gastroesophageal reflux. The 5-year success rate approaches 90%.

In patients with massive dilation, esophageal dysfunction may warrant total esophagectomy because of life-threatening symptoms such as continued weight loss, recurrent aspiration pneumonia, or tracheal compression. In patients with underlying malignancy, treatment of the tumor may be helpful, and botulinum toxin has been tried with anecdotal success.

PROGNOSIS

No treatment approach is curative, and all are palliative. Recurrent symptoms may be related to an incomplete myotomy, herniation or unwrapping of the fundoplication, esophageal strictures, Barrett's esophagus, or just the natural history of the disease. Achalasia patients may also be predisposed to squamous cell carcinoma of the esophagus, and some recommend yearly screening for patients who have a chronically large dilated esophagus.

Diffuse Esophageal Spasm

Diffuse esophageal spasm is found in less than 5% of patients who undergo manometry for symptoms of chest pain, dysphagia, or both. The pathophysiology of diffuse esophageal spasm is not well understood, but a deficiency of nitric oxide in the esophageal body may lead to a loss of control of esophageal peristalsis, high pressures, and rapid velocity contractions.

CLINICAL MANIFESTATIONS AND DIAGNOSIS

Classically, patients have symptoms of intermittent chest pain (Chapter 139), dysphagia, or both. On endoscopic ultrasound, patients may demonstrate thickening of the circular and longitudinal muscle layers. Diffuse esophageal spasm is defined manometrically by simultaneous contractions in at least 20% of all swallows, accompanied by normal peristalsis. Other manometric features include repetitive contractions, high-amplitude contractions with multiple peaks, and variable relaxation of the lower esophageal sphincter. Radiographically, diffuse esophageal spasm is characterized by a "corkscrew" esophagus with multiple simultaneous contractions that obliterate the lumen (Fig. 140-8).

TREATMENT AND PROGNOSIS

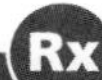

Rx

Treatment of these patients is challenging, and clinical trials have not demonstrated efficacy of any therapy. Empirical therapy may be tried with agents that relax smooth muscle or augment the nitric oxide content, such as hyoscyamine (0.125 mg sublingually), calcium-channel antagonists (nifedipine, 10 mg sublingually), nitroglycerin (0.3 mg sublingually), and sildenafil (50 mg orally). Injection of botulinum toxin into the esophageal body has had equivocal results. Antidepressants, particularly low-dose tricyclics (e.g., imipramine, 10 to 50 mg before bedtime), have had some success. For patients with dysphagia, sphincter options include botulinum toxin injection and pneumatic dilation, but surgery is not indicated unless there is evidence of achalasia. In general, these disorders can be difficult to manage but are not life-threatening.

Other Motility Disorders

Nutcracker esophagus, which is a manometric diagnosis characterized by high-amplitude contractions, likely represents a manometric epiphenomenon of little clinical significance. Antisecretory therapy with PPIs (see Table 140-1) is often warranted.

A hypertensive lower esophageal sphincter is of unknown significance, but isolated incomplete relaxation of the lower esophageal sphincter may represent an achalasia variant and should be treated as such. Patients with manometric findings of low-amplitude contractions, failed contractions, or prolonged nonpropagated contractions have hypotensive peristalsis, which is typically seen in patients with severe underlying GERD.

STRUCTURAL ABNORMALITIES

Cricopharyngeal Bars

A cricopharyngeal bar, which is caused by a prominent impression of the cricopharyngeus, reflects an inability to relax the upper esophageal sphincter maximally during the flow of barium, with a sustained increase in pressure. The decrease in cross-sectional area of the upper esophageal sphincter is likely caused by fibrosis. This condition may be asymptomatic or accompanied by symptoms of oropharyngeal dysphagia to solids. Treatment of symptomatic patients is usually surgical, and the response is generally excellent.

Esophageal Diverticula

Esophageal diverticula are encountered in less than 1% of upper gastrointestinal radiographic studies and account for less than 5% of cases of dysphagia. Esophageal diverticula may occur in one of three locations: above the upper esophageal sphincter, in the mid-esophagus, and just above the lower esophageal sphincter.

Zenker's diverticulum is a pouch that protrudes posteriorly above the upper esophageal sphincter (Fig. 140-9). This protrusion occurs through a triangular region known as Killian's triangle, which is bordered above by fibers of the inferior constrictor muscle and below by the cricopharyngeal muscle. It is thought to be caused by increased hypopharyngeal pressure that results from decreased compliance and impaired opening of the upper esophageal sphincter. Small diverticula may be asymptomatic, but increasing size is associated with such symptoms as globus, dysphagia to solids or liquids, regurgitation of undigested food, halitosis, and aspiration. Although no treatment is needed for asymptomatic patients, open or endoscopic surgery is indicated when symptoms occur. Prognosis after surgery is excellent.

Mid-esophageal diverticula, which are focal outpouchings of the middle of the esophagus, are thought to be related to an underlying abnormality of esophageal motility. Symptoms typically include dysphagia with or without regurgitation, and diagnosis is usually made with barium contrast radiography. Surgical diverticulectomy with myotomy is reserved for patients with symptoms.

Epiphrenic diverticula are herniations of mucosa and submucosa through the muscular layers of the distal 10 cm of the esophagus. They may be caused by functional obstruction, owing to underlying motility abnormalities, such as achalasia or diffuse esophageal spasm, or a mechanical obstruction, owing to a leiomyoma, prior surgery, stenosis, stricture tumor, or web. Epiphrenic diverticula may be asymptomatic or cause dysphagia, regurgitation,

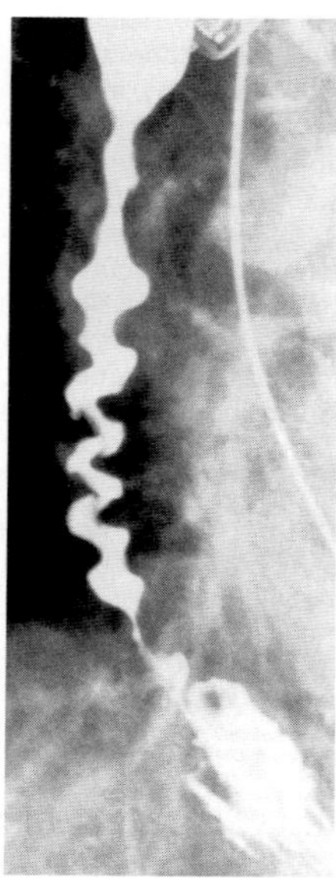

FIGURE 140-8. Barium esophagogram showing a "corkscrew" esophagus in a patient with diffuse esophageal spasm. The patient had dysphagia, chest pain, and normal endoscopic findings. (From Feldman M, ed. *Gastroenterology and Hepatology: The Comprehensive Visual Reference,* New York: Churchill Livingstone; 1997.)

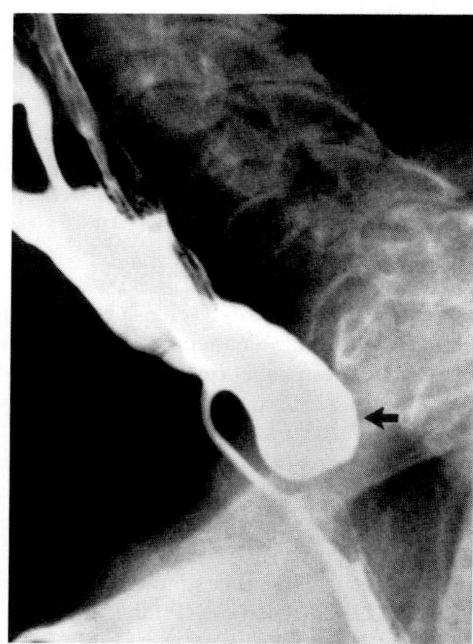

FIGURE 140-9. Barium radiograph of Zenker's diverticulum *(arrow)*. (From Feldman M, ed. *Gastroenterology and Hepatology: The Comprehensive Visual Reference,* New York: Churchill Livingstone; 1997.)

odynophagia, chest pain, heartburn, or aspiration. Diagnosis is typically made by barium radiography (Fig. 140-10), but endoscopy is recommended to exclude a structural cause of obstruction, and esophageal manometry is recommended to evaluate for underlying motility abnormalities. No therapy is warranted in asymptomatic patients, but symptomatic patients generally do well with surgical diverticulectomy, repair of the defect in the esophageal wall, and relief of the underling obstruction, usually with a myotomy and partial fundoplication.

Rings and Webs

Esophageal rings are concentric areas of narrowing, usually in the distal esophagus. *Schatzki's ring* (Fig. 140-11) is a thin, fixed, circumferential membrane-like narrowing at the gastroesophageal junction, typically at the proximal border of a hiatal hernia. The cause may be congenital, secondary to a pleat of redundant mucosa, or related to gastroesophageal reflux. Symptoms typically occur if the ring results in a lumen that is 13 mm or less in diameter. Classic symptoms are intermittent dysphagia to solids or impaction of solid food. Diagnosis is best accomplished with barium radiography, especially for rings larger than 13 mm in diameter, which may be missed at the time of endoscopy. Treatment involves use of large caliber dilators at least 18 mm in diameter, and long-term therapy with PPIs (see Table 140-1) may prevent relapses. Most patients relapse after a single dilation.

Muscular rings, which are located several centimeters above the squamocolumnar junction, are composed of mucosa, submucosa, and muscle. Barium radiography and endoscopy reveal a focal constriction of variable diameter. Optimal therapy is unclear. Dilation leads to only partial or temporary relief. Other treatment modalities include injection of botulinum toxin and anticholinergic agents.

Esophageal webs are thin, eccentric, membranous areas of narrowing that may be found anywhere in the esophagus but most commonly are in the proximal region (Fig. 140-12). The pathogenesis of webs is unknown, but they are associated with a number of systemic diseases, including bullous skin disorders, chronic graft-versus-host disease, and iron deficiency anemia.

Hiatal Hernia

A hiatal hernia involves herniation of elements of the abdominal cavity through the diaphragmatic hiatus. A sliding, or type I hernia, in which the gastroesophageal junction is displaced above the diaphragmatic hiatus, is the most common type. Type I hiatal hernias are typically asymptomatic or present with symptoms of heartburn or acid regurgitation. Treatment is as for GERD (see earlier).

In a type II or true paraesophageal hernia, which is uncommon, the gastroesophageal junction is in its normal location, but the fundus and parts of the greater curvature of the stomach herniate into the mediastinum alongside the esophagus. With type III or mixed paraesophageal hernia, the gastroesophageal junction and a large part of the stomach herniate into the mediastinum. Both types of paraesophageal hernias present with symptoms of postprandial distress, such as epigastric pain, chest pain, substernal fullness, shortness of breath, nausea, or vomiting. Iron deficiency anemia may be seen with large hiatal hernias in which at least one third of the stomach is in the chest; linear gastric erosions at the top of gastric folds at the level of the diaphragm have been implicated as a cause of chronic blood loss. Asymptomatic paraesophageal hernias do not require surgery. Symptomatic paraesophageal hernias warrant surgical therapy because of the risk of strangulation, bleeding, perforation, or obstruction.

THE ESOPHAGUS IN SYSTEMIC DISEASES

Scleroderma

Up to 90% of patients with scleroderma (Chapter 275) have esophageal involvement, thereby making it the most common gastrointestinal abnormality in the disease. The classic manometric and radiologic findings are aperistalsis of the distal two thirds of the esophagus, initially because of neuropathy and later because of the myopathy. The main clinical manifestation is severe gastroesophageal reflux that may cause Barrett's esophagus in up to 20% of patients and often causes esophageal strictures. Delayed gastric emptying

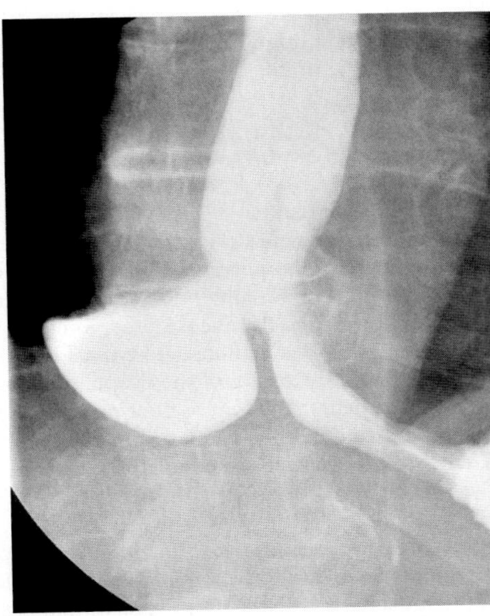

FIGURE 140-10. Barium radiograph of an esophageal epiphrenic diverticulum. (Image courtesy of Marc Levine, MD.)

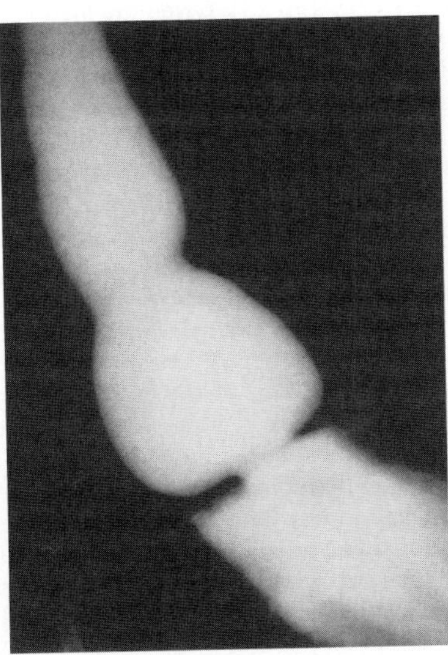

FIGURE 140-11. Barium radiograph of Schatzki's ring. (From Feldman M, ed. *Gastroenterology and Hepatology: The Comprehensive Visual Reference.* New York: Churchill Livingstone; 1997.)

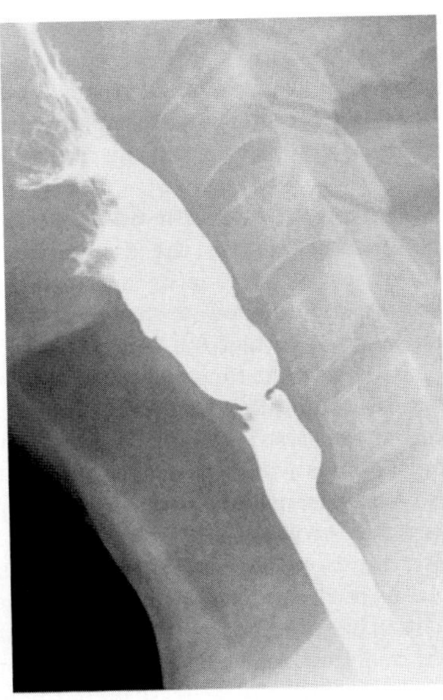

FIGURE 140-12. Barium radiograph of an esophageal web. (Image courtesy of Marc Levine, MD.)

may also occur. Marked esophageal stasis may also lead to candidal esophagitis. The diagnosis is confirmed by a patulous (on radiography) or hypotensive (on manometry) lower esophageal sphincter. PPI therapy (see Table 140-1) is the cornerstone of treatment. Lifestyle changes, including small frequent meals and avoiding nighttime meals, may reduce the gastric symptoms. Antireflux surgery can exacerbate dysphagia by creating a functional high-pressure zone in the distal esophagus and is thus contraindicated. Unfortunately, many patients suffer from chronic GERD and are at risk of developing Barrett's esophagus, recurrent strictures, and adenocarcinoma.

Amyloidosis

Amyloidosis (Chapter 194) may lead to smooth muscle and autonomic nervous system dysfunction that involves the esophagus in a pattern similar to scleroderma. Patients will have both dysphagia and severe reflux because of esophageal aperistalsis and a hypotensive lower esophageal sphincter. Dysphagia may result not only from the motility changes but also from diffuse esophageal rigidity and loss of compliance owing to amyloid infiltration of the esophageal wall. Rarely, an achalasia-like pattern may develop. No treatment improves the esophageal manifestations of amyloidosis, other than treatment for the underlying disease and high-dose PPIs given twice daily.

Other Systemic Diseases

Dermatomyositis (Chapter 277) principally involves the striated muscle of the oropharynx and proximal esophagus, but sometimes the distal esophagus may lose normal peristaltic function. Symptoms can be oropharyngeal or esophageal depending on the site of greatest muscular involvement. Dysphagia may be an early presenting symptom of dermatomyositis, and the esophagus may be involved in 10 to 50% of patients. Treatment is directed at the generalized myositis because there are no specific treatments for the esophagus. Swallowing therapy may sometimes be helpful. Return of swallowing commonly lags behind recovery of other striated muscle symptoms.

Esophageal involvement in *systemic lupus erythematosus* (Chapter 274) is not as prominent as in scleroderma, dermatomyositis, or mixed connective tissue disease. Dysphagia occurs in less than 15% of patients and may be caused by decreased salivation from secondary Sjögren's syndrome or reduced esophageal peristalsis. Other causes of esophageal symptoms in patients with systemic lupus erythematosus include GERD, esophageal ulcers, esophageal infection, and medication-induced esophagitis. *Behçet's disease* (Chapter 278) causes esophageal ulcers in less than 15% of affected patients. Ulcers are typically located in the middle third of the esophagus and are often associated with ulcers in the stomach, ileum, or colon. Rare esophageal lesions include strictures, varices, and fistulas connecting with the trachea. These complications can be severely debilitating.

Esophageal involvement in *Crohn's disease* (Chapter 143) is uncommon but has been described in up to 1 to 2% of patients. Occasionally, isolated esophageal disease may occur. Ulceration is the most common manifestation, but strictures, fissures, esophagobronchial fistulas, mediastinal abscesses, and aphthoid lesions have been described. Patients typically complain of dysphagia and odynophagia. Treatment and prognosis are as for the underlying Crohn's disease.

In the *Ehlers-Danlos syndrome* (Chapter 268), hiatal hernias are common, and structural esophageal defects, such as giant epiphrenic diverticula, megaesophagus, and spontaneous esophageal rupture may also be seen.

Skin Disorders that Involve the Esophagus

Lichen planus (Chapter 446) involves the esophagus. Patients generally present in the fourth to seventh decade of life. Histologically, the lesions in up to 25 to 50% of patients show a characteristic lymphohistiocytic inflammatory infiltrate and apoptotic basal keratinocytes. Lesions classically occur on the buccal mucosa and the tongue, but the disease may also involve other areas of the oral cavity and the esophagus, conjunctiva, nose, larynx, stomach, bladder, and anus. Most patients are asymptomatic or have only minor symptoms, but patients with severe esophageal lichen planus often develop strictures and may present with dysphagia, odynophagia, and weight loss. Strictures are typically proximal but may be variable in length, sometimes involving most of the esophageal body. Rare patients may present with esophageal lichen planus in the absence of extraesophageal disease. Endoscopic findings, which can be subtle and nonspecific, include peeling mucosa, hyperemic focal abnormalities, and submucosal plaque or papules. High-dose systemic steroids, starting with at least 40 mg prednisone and then tapering over 1 to 2 months, are often successful, but relapse is common when steroids are tapered. Dilation and intralesional steroids can alleviate the symptoms associated with strictures, but symptoms frequently recur in less than a year and necessitate repeat dilations. The esophageal lesions of lichen planus may have malignant potential.

Pemphigus vulgaris (Chapter 447) patients who experience acute flares may have upper gastrointestinal symptoms (dysphagia, odynophagia, or retrosternal burning) in 80% of cases and biopsy-proven esophageal pemphigus lesions in nearly 50% of cases. Pemphigus vulgaris may rarely be isolated to the esophagus. Paraneoplastic pemphigus (Chapter 447), most commonly reported with lymphoreticular disease, also may involve the esophagus. Like lesions on the skin, esophageal lesions may be flaccid blisters or erosions, but they may also appear as red longitudinal lines along the entire esophagus. Like cutaneous and oral pemphigus, esophageal pemphigus is generally treated with corticosteroids.

In *mucous membrane pemphigoid* (cicatricial pemphigoid, Chapter 447), the esophagus is the most common site of gastrointestinal involvement, but esophageal disease occurs in less than 15% of patients. The esophageal disease can present as many as 10 years after disease onset and may be the only presentation of the disease. Patients complain of dysphagia and odynophagia. Imaging typically shows erosions, strictures, bullae, or webs. Treatment generally is as for the skin disease.

In *dystrophic epidermolysis bullosa* (Chapter 447), approximately 70 to 95% of patients develop esophageal stenosis or strictures. Strictures are especially common in children with recessive dystrophic epidermolysis bullosa, whereas fewer than 10% of patients with dominant dystrophic epidermolysis bullosa develop strictures by age 50 years.

ESOPHAGEAL INFECTIONS

Herpes Simplex Virus

Herpes simplex virus (HSV; Chapter 382) esophagitis, which is usually caused by HSV-1, is a well-recognized disease in immunocompromised patients but may also occur in immunocompetent hosts. HSV typically presents as severe odynophagia. Endoscopy and radiology characteristically demonstrate multiple ulcers and friable mucosa, predominantly involving the distal esophagus. Mucosal biopsies demonstrate typical intranuclear inclusion bodies. Depending on the severity of the esophageal disease and the underlying health of the patient, treatment options may include intravenous acyclovir, 5 mg/kg every 8 hours for 7 days, or oral acyclovir, 800 mg five times daily for 7 days, combined with symptomatic treatment.

Candidiasis

Esophageal candidiasis is common in patients with HIV infection or with impaired cellular immunity owing to hematologic malignancies, immunosuppressive therapy, or diabetes mellitus. Esophageal candidiasis is also occasionally seen in immunocompetent patients with marked esophageal stasis, such as patients with advanced achalasia or scleroderma. Esophageal candidiasis characteristically presents with symptoms of odynophagia, dysphagia, and chest pain. Endoscopy demonstrates scattered or coalescent yellow-white mucosal plaques (Fig. 140-13). Given the high prevalence of esophageal candidiasis in HIV patients, some recommend treating symptomatic HIV patients empirically and reserving endoscopy for refractory symptoms. Mild oropharyngeal candidiasis may be treated with topical clotrimazole (10 mg troche five times daily for 7 to 14 days) or nystatin (600,000 units four times daily for 7 to 10 days), whereas oral fluconazole (100 mg daily for 7 to 14 days) is needed for moderate to severe oropharyngeal and esophageal candidiasis. Intravenous fluconazole or amphotericin B deoxycholate (Chapter 339) are appropriate options for severe esophageal candidiasis or for patients who cannot tolerate oral therapy.

Cytomegalovirus

Cytomegalovirus (CMV) infection of the esophagus is exclusively found in immunocompromised patients. Patients infected with the HIV virus with low CD4 counts are most commonly affected, but CMV also occurs in transplant recipients on immunosuppressive therapy and in immunosuppressed patients with malignancy. Patients typically have severe odynophagia with evidence of radiographic or endoscopic esophageal ulcers. Treatment is usually with intravenous ganciclovir (5 mg/kg once or twice daily for 10 to 14 days) or foscarnet (90 mg/kg every 8 to 12 hours until healing occurs).

Bacterial Esophagitis

Bacterial infection of the esophagus is uncommon but can occur in immunosuppressed patients, typically those with neutropenia and malignancy.

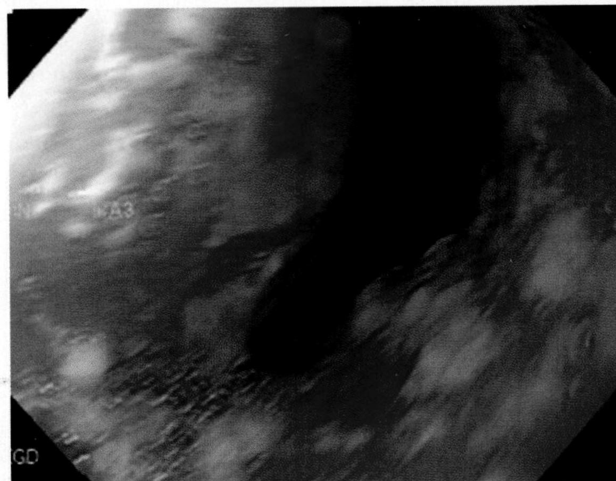

FIGURE 140-13. Candidal esophagitis.

Patients present with chest pain or odynophagia, or both, and endoscopy reveals extensive erosions, usually in the distal esophagus. Biopsy and Gram stain reveal acute and chronic inflammation and bacteria, commonly gram-positive organisms, especially Viridans-group streptococci, *Staphylococcus aureus*, *Staphylococcus epidermidis*, and *Bacillus* species. Treatment is with the appropriate antibiotics administered parenterally.

Human Papillomavirus

Esophageal infections with HPV are typically asymptomatic. HPV lesions are most frequently found in the mid to distal esophagus as erythematous macules, white plaque, nodules, or exuberant frondlike lesions. The diagnosis is made by histologic demonstration of koilocytosis (an atypical nucleus surrounded by a ring), giant cells, or immunohistochemical stains. Treatment is usually not necessary, although large lesions may require endoscopic removal. Other treatments, such as interferon, bleomycin, and etoposide, have yielded varying results. HPV infection is a risk factor for esophageal squamous cell carcinoma, but the value of endoscopic surveillance is not known.

MISCELLANEOUS ESOPHAGEAL CONDITIONS

Esophageal Emergencies

BOERHAAVE'S SYNDROME

Boerhaave's syndrome, or spontaneous rupture of the esophagus, is a transmural full-thickness tear of the esophageal wall. A sudden rise in intraesophageal pressure during forceful vomiting is the cause in most cases. The tear is most commonly in the lower third of the esophagus, 2 to 3 cm proximal to the gastroesophageal junction.

CLINICAL MANIFESTATIONS AND DIAGNOSIS

The classic presentation is vomiting, lower thoracic pain, and subcutaneous emphysema. Other findings may include pleural effusions, especially left sided, tachypnea, abdominal rigidity, fever, and hypotension. Because the condition is rare and classic antecedent vomiting is not always reported, rupture is often recognized only after the development of mediastinitis.

The chest radiograph may demonstrate mediastinal widening, a unilateral pleural effusion, hydropneumothorax, and pneumomediastinum. The esophagram, typically with a water-soluble agent, reveals extravasation, although false-negative results may be encountered. Computed tomography (CT) scanning with an oral contrast agent, which is perhaps the best diagnostic option, typically demonstrates air in the mediastinum.

TREATMENT AND PROGNOSIS (Rx)

Successful therapy depends on early recognition and the underlying condition of the patient. The classic approach is operative repair in conjunction with broad-spectrum antibiotics and nutritional support, especially if the diagnosis is made within the first 24 hours. Aggressive conservative therapy with percutaneous drains, broad-spectrum parenteral antibiotics, and nutrition has also been successful. In selected individuals, endoscopic insertion of self-expanding covered metallic stents is an option. The mortality rate can be as high as 100% without treatment.

MALLORY-WEISS TEAR

A Mallory-Weiss tear (see Fig. 137-2 in Chapter 137) is a mucosal tear, often at the gastroesophageal junction, usually caused by severe vomiting or retching. The syndrome is more common in alcoholic patients. In about 85% of patients, it is associated with acute upper gastrointestinal bleeding, which requires transfusion in about 70% of patients and urgent intervention in about 10% of cases (Chapter 137). Most tears heal spontaneously within about 48 hours.

IATROGENIC PERFORATION

Esophageal perforation may occur as a result of a variety of iatrogenic causes, including endoscopy, dilation, endosonography, or surgery as well as with foreign body ingestion. Typical symptoms include chest pain with or without abdominal pain, subcutaneous emphysema, and fever. Diagnosis may be made immediately at the time of endoscopy or radiography. Chest radiographs may show pneumomediastinum, subcutaneous emphysema, hydrothorax, or hydropneumothorax. A Gastrografin swallow may show a leak, and chest CT may show mediastinal air. Acute perforations are life-threatening emergencies that warrant immediate closure before contamination of the mediastinum. For acute perforation caused by endoscopy, endoscopic clips or stents are an option. Conservative therapy also is an option for well-contained perforations with minimal mediastinal, pleural, or peritoneal contamination and no obvious signs of sepsis. Prognosis is generally good if the perforation is recognized and treated early, preferably within 12 to 24 hours.

FOREIGN BODIES

Impaction of food or foreign bodies is a common gastrointestinal emergency. Meat impaction is most commonly seen in adults, but other foreign objects that also may be ingested accidentally or by design include batteries, coins, or bones. Many patients have an underlying esophageal abnormality, such as a Schatzki's ring, stricture, eosinophilic esophagitis, tumor, or achalasia. The clinical presentation includes dysphagia, odynophagia, foreign body sensation, chest pain, excessive salivation, and difficulty handling secretions. Immediate endoscopic extraction with concomitant airway protection is recommended because prolonged impaction may result in penetration into the esophageal wall followed by perforation and mediastinitis.

ESOPHAGEAL VARICES

Esophageal varices are described in Chapter 137.

ESOPHAGEAL FISTULAS

Tracheoesophageal fistulas may arise from a variety of different causes, including trauma, infectious esophagitis, necrosis after prolonged endotracheal intubation, esophageal cancer, and radiation therapy. Patients are often critically ill and may not tolerate surgery. Metallic stents are a treatment option.

Atrial-esophageal fistulas are a rare complication after radiofrequency ablation (Chapter 66) for atrial fibrillation. The clinical presentation is nonspecific and includes features such as dysphagia, fever, leukocytosis, bacteremia, massive intestinal bleeding, and septic shock. Diagnosis requires a high index of suspicion and is aided by a chest CT scan. Surgery is required; the prognosis is excellent with early recognition and treatment but can be dire if treatment is delayed.

Congenital Abnormalities

ESOPHAGEAL ATRESIA AND TRACHEOESOPHAGEAL FISTULA

Children with congenital esophageal anomalies commonly survive into adulthood after successful surgery. As adults, these patients commonly have gastroesophageal reflux that warrants PPI therapy. Strictures at prior surgical anastomoses are common, and patients may require periodic endoscopic dilation.

HETEROTOPIC GASTRIC MUCOSA (INLET PATCH)

Inlet patches, which are areas of gastric columnar epithelium, are present in up to 4.5% of adults, and are usually found incidentally at the time of routine endoscopy. Typically, a red columnar patch varying in size from a few millimeters to a few centimeters is seen just below the cricopharyngeus. Inlet patches can be associated with hoarseness, sore throat, and globus sensation. Strictures, ulcers, and rare malignant transformation have also been described. Treatment options include PPIs (see Table 140-1) and endoscopic ablation.

OTHER CONGENITAL ESOPHAGEAL DISORDERS

Duplication cysts, which may be located anywhere in the esophagus, may be in continuity with or separate from the esophageal lumen. Symptoms, which may present initially in adulthood, include dysphagia owing to luminal compression, chest pain, and regurgitation. Treatment is surgical.

Dysphagia lusoria is caused by an aberrant right subclavian artery that originates from the right aortic arch and causes partial compression of the esophagus as it crosses over to the left side. Patients may complain of dysphagia. This condition is most commonly detected incidentally during barium radiography, where it is visualized as a crossing diagonal impression at the junction of the proximal and middle thirds of the esophagus. Surgery is rarely indicated because of the complexity of the operation and the difficulty in establishing a clear relationship between the radiographic findings and symptoms.

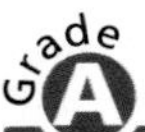

1. Khan M, Santana J, Donnellan C, et al. Medical treatments in the short term management of reflux oesophagitis. *Cochrane Database Syst Rev.* 2007;2:CD003244.
2. van Pinxteren B, Sigterman KE, Bonis P, et al. Short-term treatment with proton pump inhibitors, H2-receptor antagonists and prokinetics for gastro-oesophageal reflux disease-like symptoms and endoscopy negative reflux disease. *Cochrane Database Syst Rev.* 2006;3:CD002095.
3. Wang Y, Pan T, Wang Q, et al. Additional bedtime H2-receptor antagonist for the control of nocturnal gastric acid breakthrough. *Cochrane Database Syst Rev.* 2009;7:CD004275.
4. Lundell L, Miettinen P, Myrvold HE, et al, for the Nordic GEORD Study Group. Seven-year follow-up of a randomized clinical trial comparing proton-pump inhibition with surgical therapy for reflux oesophagitis. *Br J Surg.* 2007;94:198-203.
5. Ramage JI Jr, Rumalla A, Baron TH, et al. A prospective, randomized, double-blind, placebo-controlled trial of endoscopic steroid injection therapy for recalcitrant esophageal peptic strictures. *Am J Gastroenterol.* 2005;100:2419-2425.
6. Shaheen NJ, Sharma P, Overholt BF, et al. Radiofrequency ablation in Barrett's esophagus with dysplasia. *N Engl J Med.* 2009;360:2353-2355.
7. Straumann A, Conus S, Degen L, et al. Budesonide is effective in adolescent and adult patients with active eosinophilic esophagitis. *Gastroenterology.* 2010;139:1526-1537.
8. Leyden JE, Moss AC, MacMathuna P. Endoscopic pneumatic dilation versus botulinum toxin injection in the management of primary achalasia. *Cochrane Database Syst Rev.* 2006;4:CD005046.

SUGGESTED READINGS

Becher A, Dent J. Systematic review: ageing and gastro-oesophageal reflux disease symptoms, oesophageal function and reflux oesophagitis. *Aliment Pharmacol Ther.* 2011;33:442-454. *Review.*

Cook IJ. Oropharyngeal dysphagia. *Gastroenterol Clin N Am.* 2009;38:411-431. *Review.*

Rees JR, Lao-Sirieix P, Wong A, et al. Treatment for Barrett's oesophagus. *Cochrane Database Rev Syst.* 2010;1:CD004060. *Review of evidence for medical and interventional therapies.*

Rothenberg ME. Biology and treatment of eosinophilic esophagitis. *Gastroenterology.* 2009;137:1238-1249. *Review.*

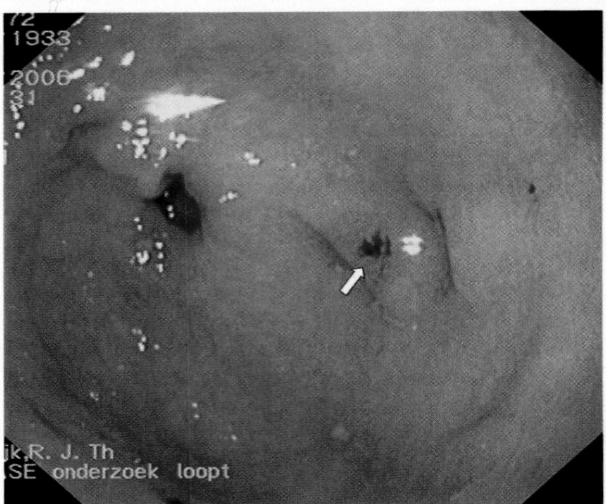

FIGURE 141-1. **Endoscopic view of uncomplicated erosive gastritis.** The erosion appears as a small, superficial mucosal break with a black base *(arrow)*.

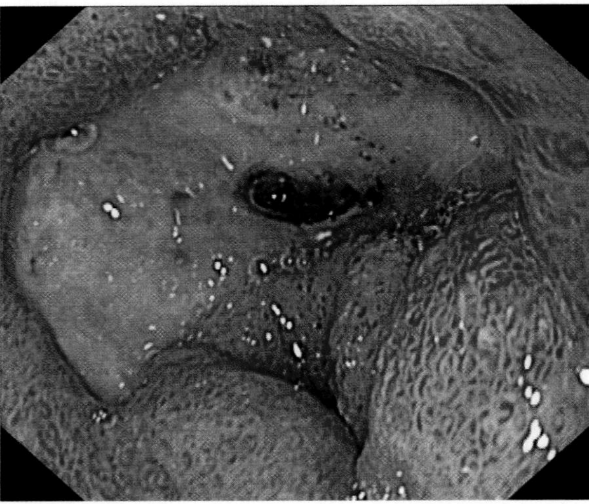

FIGURE 141-2. **Endoscopic view of an ulcer at the anterior wall of the duodenal bulb.** The ulcer has a clean base, with a visible vessel appearing as a dark red protruding spot close to the lower ulcer rim. The surrounding mucosa is inflamed and swollen.

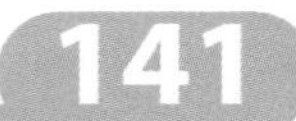

141 ACID PEPTIC DISEASE

ERNST J. KUIPERS AND MARTIN J. BLASER

Acid peptic diseases can involve the esophagus (Chapter 140), the stomach, and the duodenum. Dyspeptic symptoms also can occur in patients who have no endoscopic abnormalities, in whom it is termed *nonulcer dyspepsia* (Chapter 139).

DEFINITIONS

Gastric and duodenal ulcers usually occur in an area of inflamed mucosa. This inflammation, termed *gastritis, duodenitis, or bulbitis,* can sometimes be recognized during endoscopy by signs of edema, reddening, and swelling of the mucosa, but microscopic evaluation of endoscopic biopsy specimens is required for a definitive diagnosis of mucosal inflammation.

Gastritis is categorized by endoscopic and histologic criteria, with granulocytes predominating in active gastritis and mononuclear cells in chronic gastritis. Gastritis is also classified by the segment of involved stomach: antral-predominant gastritis, corpus-predominant gastritis, or pangastritis. Finally, the absence or presence of premalignant stages of damage to the mucosa as a result of long-standing inflammation defines the categories of nonatrophic and atrophic gastritis, respectively. Endoscopic findings are usually nonspecific, unless the gastric mucosa has either a typical miniature cobblestone appearance, termed *nodular gastritis* (a lesion found particularly in children colonized by *Helicobacter pylori*), or grossly enlarged folds without evidence of cancer, termed *hypertrophic gastritis*.

A *peptic ulcer* is a mucosal defect at least 0.5 cm in diameter that penetrates the muscularis mucosae. Smaller mucosal defects are called *erosions* (Fig. 141-1). Gastric ulcers are subdivided into proximal ulcers, located in the body of the stomach, and distal ulcers, located in the antrum and angulus of the stomach. Gastric ulcers are located mainly along the lesser curvature, in particular at the transitional zone of corpus- to antral-type mucosa. This transitional zone is often in the area of the angulus but may shift proximally. Duodenal ulcers usually are located on the anterior or posterior wall of the duodenal bulb (Fig. 141-2), or occasionally at both sites ("kissing" ulcers). Lesions distal to the duodenal bulb are termed *postbulbar ulcers.* Patients who previously underwent a distal gastric resection (Billroth I or II procedure) can develop ulceration at the gastroduodenal anastomosis (anastomotic ulcer). However, ulcers occurring after Billroth II resection are located predominantly in the jejunal mucosa at the junction between the afferent and efferent loops. Other peptic ulcers can occur at sites of metaplastic or heterotopic gastric mucosa, for example, in Meckel's diverticulum, the rectum, or Barrett's esophagus. Patients with a large hiatal hernia can develop gastric ulceration, known as *Cameron's ulcers,* at the level of the herniation. *Dieulafoy's ulcers,* which are small mucosal defects over an intramural arteriole, can lead to severe bleeding. Although these lesions can occur throughout the gastrointestinal tract, two thirds occur in the stomach.

EPIDEMIOLOGY

The worldwide prevalence of gastritis reflects the prevalence of *H. pylori.* Colonization with this bacterium is virtually always associated with chronic active gastritis, which persists as long as an individual remains colonized and only slowly disappears 6 to 24 months after the eradication of *H. pylori.* In developing countries and among first-generation immigrants from these countries, the prevalence of *H. pylori* gastritis is high (often ≥80%) in all age groups, including children. In Western countries, the prevalence of *H. pylori* gastritis increases with age; it is currently less than 20% in young adults but 40 to 60% in elderly persons.

Although peptic ulcer disease is strongly related to *H. pylori* gastritis and duodenitis, the epidemiology of ulcer disease has shown secular variations even when *H. pylori* was ubiquitous. The incidence of peptic ulcer disease rose steeply in Western countries in the late 19th and early 20th centuries and has decreased over the past 30 years, yet peptic ulceration remains a common disorder. The decline in incidence, associated with a decrease in hospital admissions and surgery for ulcer disease, is believed to reflect mainly the decreasing prevalence of gastric colonization with *H. pylori.* The declining incidence of ulcer disease is also the result of the widespread application of eradication therapy, which strongly reduced recurrent ulcers in *H. pylori*–positive patients. Other factors may include the widespread use of acid suppressive medication. Nevertheless, hospital admissions for complications of ulcers and mortality from ulcer disease have remained relatively stable in both the United States and other countries, as the reduction in *H. pylori*–associated ulcers in younger persons has been counterbalanced by an increase in ulcers related to nonsteroidal anti-inflammatory drugs (NSAIDs) in older persons.

In Western countries, duodenal ulcers occur more frequently than gastric ulcers. The predominant age at which duodenal ulcers occur is between 20 and 50 years, whereas gastric ulcers most commonly occur in patients older than 40 years. The incidence of gastroduodenal ulcer disease is approximately 1 to 2 per 1000 inhabitants per year. Two thirds of patients with ulcers are male, and the disease is more common in smokers. The risk of recurrent disease after initial healing is high; more than 50% of patients have a recurrent ulcer within 12 months of healing in the absence of treatment. Maintenance acid suppressive therapy reduces this recurrence rate, but only therapeutic measures that remove the underlying cause of the ulcer can prevent most ulcer recurrences.

PATHOBIOLOGY

Helicobacter pylori

Most peptic ulcers are associated with colonization with *H. pylori* (Fig. 141-3). Initial clinical studies of the association between *H. pylori* and ulcer disease reported that approximately 85% of patients with gastric ulcer disease and 95% of patients with duodenal ulcer disease were colonized by *H. pylori.* Most persons who are *H. pylori* positive do not have any specific complaints, nor do they develop ulcer disease. The estimated risk for the development of ulcer disease during persistent *H. pylori* colonization is 5 to 15%—that is, three- to eight-fold higher than the risk for patients who are *H. pylori* negative. The risk for the development of an ulcer in the presence of *H. pylori* is determined by a combination of host- and bacteria-related factors. Host factors include immune response, smoking, and stress. Bacterial factors that increase the risk of ulcer include a high production of the *VacA* product, which reflects the presence of the s1m1 genotype; a high level of cytokine induction, owing to the presence of genes in the *cag* pathogenicity island; and enhanced adherence, resulting from *babA*.

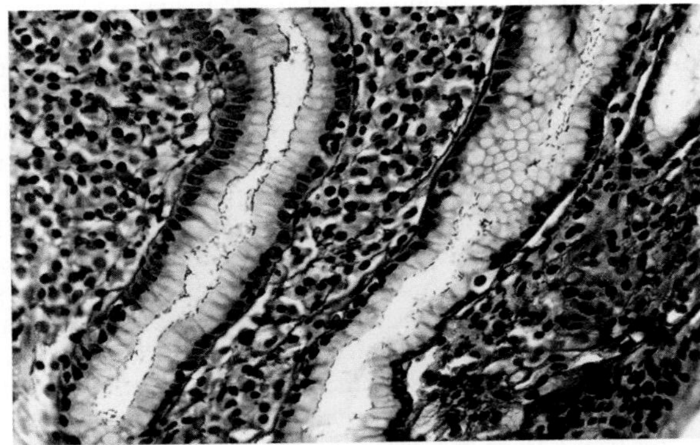

FIGURE 141-3. Gastric mucosa colonized with *Helicobacter pylori* appearing as curved bacilli on the mucosal surface.

Nonsteroidal Anti-inflammatory Drugs and Aspirin

The other common cause of gastroduodenal ulcer disease is the use of NSAIDs. At least 2 to 4% of the population in many countries use acetylsalicylic acid, acetic acid derivatives (diclofenac, indomethacin, sulindac), or propionic acid derivatives (ibuprofen, ketoprofen, naproxen) on a daily basis. Within 14 days after the start of such treatment, about 5% of patients develop mucosal breaks, that is, erosions and ulcers. In patients who continue therapy for 4 weeks or longer, this proportion increases to 10%. The concomitant presence of *H. pylori* infection increases the incidence of NSAID-related ulcers. The risk of developing an ulcer during NSAID use is also higher in patients who are older than 60 years, those with a previous ulcer, patients who use corticosteroids or high-dose NSAIDs, and those with major comorbid diseases. In patients who use anticoagulants, such as warfarin, or who have severe comorbid disease, an NSAID-induced ulcer is more likely to lead to life-threatening gastroduodenal hemorrhage.

On the basis of their activities, NSAIDs are divided into cyclooxygenase 1 (COX1) and COX2 inhibitors (Chapter 36). The COX1 enzyme is involved in the production of prostaglandins, which play a role in normal cell regulation. The COX2 enzyme, which is also involved in the production of prostaglandins, is induced by inflammatory responses. Most NSAIDs have a nonselective COX inhibitory effect; selective COX2 inhibitors are associated with fewer gastroduodenal ulcers, but their use is limited by their adverse coronary effects (Chapter 36). Because of the strong association between NSAIDs and ulcer disease and the risk for recurrence of ulcers with their continued use, patients with ulcers must be thoroughly assessed for the use of NSAIDs.

Helicobacter pylori–Negative, Non-NSAID Ulcer Disease

In most series, *H. pylori* and NSAID use account for 80 to 95% of cases of ulcer disease. The remaining cases are often referred to as *idiopathic* or *H. pylori–negative, non-NSAID* acid peptic disease. The proportion of ulcer disease that is idiopathic is increasing throughout the world as the prevalence of *H. pylori* decreases. Further, it is likely that some ulcers in *H. pylori*–positive patients were not caused by *H. pylori.* Consistent with this notion is the fact that some *H. pylori*–positive patients develop recurrent ulcers after successful bacterial eradication, so presumably their ulcer disease was idiopathic. It is not known whether the increase in idiopathic ulcer disease is simply proportional to the decrease in *H. pylori*–associated ulcers or whether it reflects a true increase in the incidence of idiopathic ulcers.

In patients with idiopathic ulcer disease, specific clues to the underlying cause are often provided by the medical history, including comorbidity and drug use; the endoscopic appearance of the ulcer; and the histologic features of the ulcer's margins and surroundings. In most cases, these initial data can direct further diagnostic studies (Table 141-1).

Malignant Ulcer Disease

Gastroduodenal ulcers can result from underlying malignant disease. In the stomach, these tumors are related to gastric adenocarcinoma and, rarely, to mucosa-associated lymphoid tissue (MALT) lymphomas (Chapter 198). Malignant ulcers in the duodenum may result from primary duodenal carcinomas or from penetrating pancreatic cancers. Duodenal cancers have an association with polyposis syndromes, especially familial adenomatous polyposis and, to a much lesser extent, MUTYH-associated polyposis and Peutz-Jeghers syndrome (Chapter 199). In both the stomach and the duodenum, ulcer disease can also be caused by metastatic tumors, including cancers of the breast, colon, thyroid, or kidney, or by melanoma, disseminated lymphoma, or Kaposi's sarcoma. Malignant ulcers are characteristically irregular in shape with heaped borders, but they may also be flat or depressed lesions. Current high-resolution and magnification endoscopes allow visualization of the altered mucosal structure surrounding an ulcer, including changes in the microvascular pattern. For a definite diagnosis of malignancy, multiple biopsy specimens are needed, usually from the ulcer margins.

Systemic Inflammatory Disorders

A few gastroduodenal ulcers are caused by systemic inflammatory diseases, in particular, Crohn's disease (Chapter 143). Patients with Crohn's disease affecting the proximal gastrointestinal tract often have multiple ulcers

TABLE 141-1 DIFFERENTIAL DIAGNOSIS OF PEPTIC ULCER DISEASE

ORIGIN	CONDITION	FREQUENCY*	DIAGNOSTIC TEST	FINDINGS
Microbes	*Helicobacter pylori*	Very common	*Helicobacter pylori* tests Histology	Bacteria, enzymes, antigens, antibodies Gastritis
	Helicobacter heilmannii	Rare	Histology	Spiral bacteria, gastritis
	Treponema pallidum	Very rare	Serology	Antibodies
	Mycobacterial infection	Very rare	Histology, immune response testing, chest radiograph	Acid-fast bacteria, granuloma, immune response, pulmonary infiltrate
	Cytomegalovirus, herpes simplex virus type 1	Rare	Histology, serology	Virus inclusions, antibodies
Drug use	NSAIDs, aspirin	Very common	History, urine test	NSAID use
	Bisphosphonates	Rare	History	Bisphosphonate use
	Corticosteroids	Rare	History	Corticosteroid use, comorbidity
	Amphetamines, cocaine	Rare	History, drug testing	Drug use
	Anticoagulants, coagulopathy	Rare	Endoscopy	Ulcer after intramural bleed
Malignancy	Gastric cancer	Common	Histology	Malignancy
	Duodenal cancer	Rare	Histology, CT	Malignancy
	Pancreatic cancer	Common	Histology, CT	Malignancy
	Mucosa-associated lymphoid tissue lymphoma	Rare	Histology	Malignancy
	Metastatic cancer	Rare	Histology	Malignancy
Gastritis syndromes	Eosinophilic gastritis	Rare	Histology	Eosinophilic infiltration
	Lymphocytic gastritis	Rare	Histology, celiac disease screening	Lymphocytic infiltration, villous atrophy
Hyperacidic syndromes	Zollinger-Ellison syndrome	Rare	Serum gastrin, secretin test	Extreme hypergastrinemia, positive secretin test
	Antral G-cell hyperfunction	Very rare	Serum gastrin, secretin test	Moderate hypergastrinemia, negative secretin test
	Retained gastric antrum	Very rare	Medical history, gastrin	Billroth II resection, hypergastrinemia
	Systemic mastocytosis	Very rare	Histology of affected sites	Mast cell infiltration
	Chronic myelogenous leukemia	Very rare	Leukemia evaluation	Leukemia
Ischemia	Mesenteric vascular occlusion	Common	Angiography	Vascular disease
	Polycythemia vera	Rare	Blood counts	Polycythemia
Specific ulcer types	Cameron's ulcer	Common	Endoscopy	Ulcer in large hiatal hernia
	Marginal ulcer	Common	Endoscopy	Ulcer at anastomosis
	Dieulafoy's ulcer	Common	Endoscopy	Singular bleeding focus with minimal mucosal disruption
Systemic inflammation	Crohn's disease	Common	Histology, ileocolonoscopy	Inflammation, granulomas
	Vasculitides	Rare	Histology, systemic evaluation	Vasculitis, signs of systemic disease
	Gastric amyloidosis	Very rare	Histology	Amyloid deposition
Other conditions	Stress ulcer	Fairly common in patients in intensive care units	Endoscopy	—
	Radiation therapy, chemotherapy	Rare	Endoscopy, history	—

*Frequency as a cause of gastroduodenal ulcer disease.
CT = computed tomography; NSAID = nonsteroidal anti-inflammatory drug.

characterized by irregular longitudinal shapes. Ulcers in the duodenum occur atop Kerckring's folds. Patients with gastroduodenal ulcers from Crohn's disease do not invariably have evidence of disease elsewhere in the digestive tract, nor do blood tests always suggest an active inflammatory bowel disorder. The demonstration of ulcerative inflammation elsewhere in the digestive tract, in particular in the terminal ileum and colon, strongly supports the diagnosis of Crohn's disease, as do granulomas on a biopsy specimen. However, the absence of granulomas does not exclude Crohn's disease, and these lesions are not specific for Crohn's disease; they are also associated with *H. pylori* gastritis and other conditions, particularly sarcoidosis (Chapter 95). Sarcoidosis can also lead to gastroduodenal ulcer disease.

Other inflammatory disorders that can cause gastritis or gastroduodenal ulcers include various forms of vasculitis affecting the mesenteric system, in particular Behçet's disease (Chapter 278), Henoch-Schönlein purpura (Chapter 278), Takayasu's arteritis (Chapter 278), polyarteritis nodosa (Chapter 278), systemic lupus erythematosus (Chapter 274), Churg-Strauss syndrome (Chapter 278), and Wegener's granulomatosis (Chapter 278). Lymphocytic gastroduodenitis, which is strongly associated with celiac disease (Chapter 142), may lead to duodenal ulceration and subsequent stenotic web formation. Ulcer disease also may occur in patients with polycythemia vera (Chapter 169), possibly in relation to reduced mucosal blood flow. Vasculitis underlying ulcer disease should be considered in patients with chronic or recurrent ulceration in whom other causes have been excluded. Lymphocytic phlebitis, which is a rare vasculitic inflammatory disorder affecting the mesenteric veins, may cause gastric ulcer disease. Systemic amyloidosis (Chapter 194) affecting the stomach wall may lead to gastric ulcer disease. Rare cases of duodenal ulceration have been described in the presence of annular pancreas or congenital bands obstructing the descending duodenum.

Hypergastrinemic Syndromes

Peptic ulcers can result from chronic gastric hyperacidity related to hypergastrinemia. The most important hypergastrinemic disorder is Zollinger-Ellison syndrome (Chapter 201), a condition of marked hyperacidity leading to severe peptic ulcer disease caused by a gastrin-producing endocrine tumor. These patients usually have multiple therapy-resistant bulbar and postbulbar duodenal ulcers. The diagnosis can be confirmed by the presence of a high fasting serum gastrin level (often but not always ≥10-fold increased and >1000 pg/mL). Similar gastrin levels are sometimes seen in patients treated for chronic ulcer disease with high-dose proton pump inhibitors. For clarification, secretin testing can be performed: in patients with Zollinger-Ellison syndrome, the injection of secretin (1 U/kg) increases serum gastrin levels by more than 50%, or 120 pg/mL or greater in those with fasting gastrin levels less than 10-fold above normal. Imaging techniques, such as computed tomography (CT), magnetic resonance imaging, isotope scanning, endoscopic ultrasonography, videocapsule endoscopy, and balloon-assisted enteroscopy, may be used to detect the primary tumor, which is often located in either the pancreas or the proximal small bowel. In some patients, Zollinger-Ellison syndrome occurs as part of multiple endocrine neoplasia (Chapter 239), particularly in association with hyperparathyroidism. Other

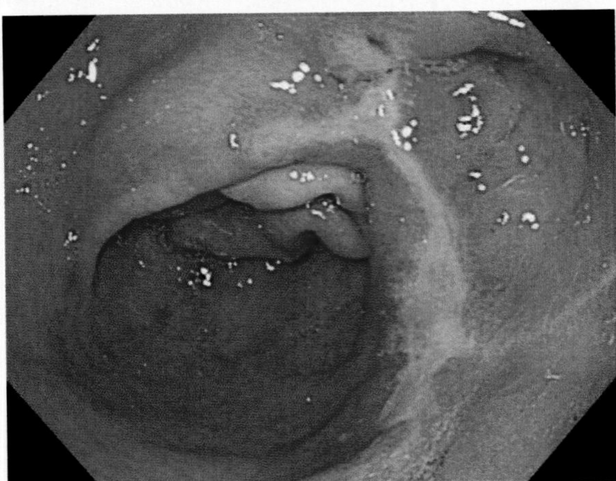

FIGURE 141-4. Endoscopic view of an irregular gastric ulcer at the posterior wall and smaller curvature in a patient with chronic mesenteric ischemia due to subtotal stenosis of the celiac trunk.

hypergastrinemic hyperacidity syndromes are the retained gastric antrum syndrome (see later) and antral G-cell hyperfunction. In the latter, fasting serum gastrin levels are only modestly increased and do not rise after the injection of secretin, but they respond in an exaggerated way to meals, thereby leading to hyperacidity. When the condition occurs in an *H. pylori*–positive patient, bacterial eradication therapy may be curative. However, some patients with G-cell hyperfunction are *H. pylori* negative.

Ischemia

Stenosis or occlusion of the celiac trunk or the superior mesenteric artery (Chapter 145) also can lead to ulceration in the mucosa of the proximal digestive tract (Fig. 141-4). These ulcers typically occur in elderly patients with risk factors for atherosclerosis, but they can also occur in younger subjects with mesenteric obstruction due to other causes. Ischemic ulcers tend to heal slowly and recur. Pallor of the mucosa, consistent with decreased mucosal blood flow, may be noted at endoscopy. Upper mesenteric ischemia is often associated with upper abdominal pain, which can be elicited by a meal or by physical activity. These symptoms may cause patients to decrease their food intake, leading to weight loss before their clinical presentation. The prevalence of upper mesenteric ischemia with secondary ulcer disease is unknown, in part owing to its variable presentation, often with a history of gradual symptoms; the lack of standardized and reliable diagnostic tests; and clinicians' unfamiliarity with the condition. Diagnostic evaluation includes a duplex ultrasound scan for vascular flow and conventional or CT angiography of the affected arteries. Validated functional tests for gastroduodenal mucosal perfusion are not widely available, but a technique for directly measuring mucosal oxygen saturation during endoscopy is investigational.

Stress Ulcers

Patients with severe medical conditions, such as major trauma, sepsis, extensive burns, head injury, or multiorgan failure, can develop stress ulcers in the stomach or duodenum. Major risk factors for stress ulceration in severely ill patients include mechanical ventilation, coagulopathy, and hypotension, but factors such as hepatic and renal failure and the use of ulcerogenic medications may contribute. Stress ulcers occur independently of *H. pylori* colonization. Ulcers associated with head injury are known as Cushing's ulcers, and ulcers associated with extensive burns are known as Curling's ulcers. Stress ulcers were once common in patients in intensive care units, but improvements in overall management, including respiratory and hemodynamic care, acid inhibition, and emphasis on adequate feeding, have reduced the incidence of these ulcers, which currently affect 1 to 2% of these patients. Stress ulcers may be asymptomatic, but they can also cause complications, especially bleeding.

Other Factors

Cameron's Ulcer

Patients with large hiatal hernias (Chapter 140) may present with proximal gastric ulcers, termed *Cameron's ulcers,* at the level of the hiatus, where the stomach is compressed. These ulcers are usually asymptomatic but may cause occult or overt bleeding. During upper gastrointestinal endoscopy, patients with large hiatal hernias and iron deficiency anemia should be carefully examined in normal and retroverted positions for the presence of Cameron's ulcers.

Anastomotic or Marginal Ulceration

Patients who have undergone partial gastrectomy sometimes develop recurrent ulcers, often located at the anastomosis or within the jejunum immediately opposite the anastomosis. Ischemia and chronic inflammation resulting from *H. pylori* and biliary reflux may cause such ulcers, as may underlying cancer. If biopsy excludes cancer, treatment includes acid suppression and *H. pylori* eradication, if needed. Ulcer disease can be caused by the retained gastric antrum syndrome after partial gastrectomy when the antrum is not completely excised from the detached duodenum. Because it then lacks exposure to acid and is thus not physiologically downregulated, it continues to secrete gastrin despite normal or even high acid levels. Marginal ulcers can also occur after bariatric Roux-en-Y gastric bypass surgery.

Other Microbes

Colonization with *Helicobacter heilmannii* (formerly known as *Gastrospirillum hominis*), which is probably a zoonotic organism, is associated with mild gastritis and sometimes with transient ulcer disease. Ulcer disease also may be infectious, resulting from secondary syphilis (Chapter 327), mycobacterial infection (Chapter 332), infection with herpes simplex virus type 1 (Chapter 382), or cytomegalovirus infection (Chapter 384).

Alcohol

Short-term heavy alcohol use or long-term moderate to heavy alcohol use can lead to signs of acute and chronic gastritis. No evidence indicates that this gastritis is associated with a significant risk for peptic ulceration, although alcohol use increases the risk of bleeding in patients with peptic ulcer disease.

Hyperhistaminic Syndromes

Similar to the hypergastrinemic syndromes, persistent elevation of histamine can lead to hyperacidity as a result of the chronic stimulation of parietal cells. Elevated histamine levels are observed in two rare syndromes. *Systemic mastocytosis* (Chapter 263) is characterized by a proliferation of mast cells in the bone marrow, skin, liver, spleen, and gastrointestinal tract, often associated with both spontaneous and trigger-induced (e.g., alcohol) release of histamine and other vasoactive substances. Patients with systemic mastocytosis often have gastrointestinal symptoms, including pain, diarrhea, and blood loss. Ulceration results from chronic gastric acid hypersecretion. Clues to the diagnosis include symptoms of pruritus, urticaria, or rash. The bone marrow and affected organ mast cell infiltrates carry a specific *C-kit* mutation and express CD2 and CD25. Histamine hypersecretion leading to peptic ulcer disease can also occur in *chronic myelogenous leukemia* (Chapter 190) with basophilia.

Other Drugs

Treatment with oral bisphosphonates, widely used for osteoporosis (Chapter 251), is complicated by gastric erosions and ulceration in an estimated 3 to 10% of treated patients. The risk for ulcer disease may be synergistically increased by NSAID use but is probably independent of *H. pylori* colonization. Although corticosteroid treatment can be complicated by peptic ulcer disease, the relative risk is only slightly increased, except in patients with serious comorbid diseases, using long-term or high-dose therapy, or with prior ulcers. Other patients who use corticosteroids are not at serious risk for ulcer disease and therefore do not require measures to prevent ulcers.

Persons who use amphetamines and crack cocaine (Chapter 33) frequently develop ulcer disease, often with perforation, possibly as a result of vascular insufficiency. Chemotherapy, particularly when given selectively as a high-dose intra-arterial infusion in the celiac system, can be complicated by ulcer disease. Patients on anticoagulant therapy and those with other coagulopathies may rarely develop intramural hematoma of the gastrointestinal tract. Depending on the location, these hematomas may cause obstruction, but they can also leave large ulcers when they rupture into the lumen. Radiation therapy of the upper abdomen is sometimes complicated by chronic ischemic ulceration, especially in long-term follow-up.

CLINICAL MANIFESTATIONS

The clinical manifestations of acid peptic disease (Table 141-2) do not always predict the various morphologic presentations found at endoscopy. Indeed,

TABLE 141-2 KEY SYMPTOMS AND SIGNS OF PEPTIC ULCER

UNCOMPLICATED ULCER
No symptoms ("silent ulcer" in up to 40% of cases)
Epigastric pain
Pain may radiate to the back, thorax, other parts of abdomen (cephalad most likely, caudad least likely)
Pain may be nocturnal (most specific), "painful hunger" relieved by food, or continuous (least specific)
Nausea
Vomiting
Heartburn (mimics or associated with gastroesophageal reflex)
COMPLICATED ULCER
Acute perforation
Severe abdominal pain
Shock
Abdominal board-like rigidity (and rebound and other signs of peritoneal irritation)
Free intraperitoneal air
Hemorrhage
Hematemesis and/or melena
Hemodynamic changes, anemia
Previous history of ulcer symptoms (80%)
Gastric outlet obstruction
Satiation, inability to ingest food, eructation
Nausea, vomiting (and related disturbances)
Weight loss

TABLE 141-3 DIAGNOSTIC PATHS AND TOOLS IN ULCER DISEASE

PATH 1: MORPHOLOGIC DIAGNOSIS
Gastroduodenoscopy
Barium contrast (inferior alternative)
Endoscopic ultrasound (selected cases only)
Computed tomography (useful in selected cases)
PATH 2: ETIOLOGIC DIAGNOSIS
***Helicobacter pylori* Testing**
Histologic examination of gastric mucosa
Stool antigen test
Carbon-13 urea breath test
Serum antibodies
Ulcer Associated with Nonsteroidal Anti-inflammatory Drug Use
History of drug ingestion
Decreased platelet adherence
Molecular identification (complex, expensive)
Acid Hypersecretory Syndromes
Serum gastrin elevation
Gastrin provocative tests (intravenous secretin, meal)
Gastric analysis

a silent ulcer may be recognized only when it presents abruptly with a complication, most commonly hemorrhage or perforation, or it may be discovered incidentally when a diagnostic test is performed for other reasons. Nevertheless, the typical presentation of acid peptic disease is recurrent episodes of pain. The pain is almost invariably located in the epigastrium and may radiate to the back or, less commonly, to the thorax or other regions of the abdomen (see Table 141-2). Some patients describe the pain as burning or piercing, whereas others describe it as an uncomfortable feeling of emptiness of the stomach, referred to as *painful hunger.* Indeed, the pain may improve with the ingestion of food, only to return in the postprandial period. The timing of the pain in relation to meals and the soothing effects of food are nonspecific, however, and may also occur in patients with functional dyspepsia without ulcer. Nocturnal epigastric pain that awakens a patient several hours after a late meal is more likely to represent ulcer pain.

Besides the pain during symptomatic episodes, patients may complain of retrosternal burning (heartburn) or acidic regurgitation into the throat, symptoms that reflect associated gastroesophageal reflux (Chapter 140), which is aggravated by hyperacidity or delayed gastric emptying. Nausea and vomiting may also occur but are nonspecific. The presence of significant diarrhea should raise the possibility of Zollinger-Ellison syndrome (Chapter 201), but diarrhea also may result from the heavy use of magnesium-containing antacids. In untreated patients, symptoms tend to be intermittent, with flares of daily pain lasting 2 to 8 weeks, separated by prolonged asymptomatic intervals. During periods of remission, patients may feel well and may be able to eat even heavy or spicy meals without apparent discomfort.

Physical Examination

The physical examination is usually unrevealing. If significant bleeding has occurred (Chapter 137), the patient may present with pallor and may be hypovolemic (Chapter 106). It is always useful to inquire about the characteristics of the stool, because ulcer-related bleeding may manifest not only obviously in the form of hematemesis but also insidiously as melena (black feces). In the case of massive ulcer bleeding with the rapid bowel passage of blood, patients may also present with red rectal blood loss. When a patient has acute perforation, severe epigastric and abdominal pain develops, and the patient appears distressed. Characteristically, intense contracture of the abdominal muscles is apparent on palpation, together with rebound tenderness and other signs of peritoneal irritation. With large amounts of intra-abdominal air, percussion may reveal hypertympany over the liver.

DIAGNOSIS

In a patient who presents with symptoms consistent with ulcer disease, the diagnostic evaluation should proceed along two different but complementary paths: confirmation of the anatomic abnormality and investigation of its cause (Table 141-3). In most patients, it is advisable to follow both diagnostic paths simultaneously, but sometimes it is reasonable to skip the anatomic verification as a cost-saving strategy and proceed to management based on the probable cause.

Anatomic Diagnosis

Endoscopy (Chapter 136) is the primary investigative tool in patients suspected of having acid peptic disease. This technique can detect erosive gastritis (see Fig. 141-1) or an ulcer in the gastric wall or duodenal bulb (see Fig. 141-2). Because of the high prevalence and the often spontaneous improvement of dyspeptic symptoms, endoscopy usually should not be performed immediately; rather its use should be restricted to patients with persistent or recurrent symptoms. However, immediate endoscopy is indicated in patients with alarm symptoms such as weight loss, dysphagia, anorexia, considerable vomiting, anemia, or signs of overt bleeding.

Endoscopy is both highly sensitive and highly specific for the detection of ulcer disease. The most common locations for a peptic ulcer are the stomach and duodenal bulb, but peptic ulcers sometimes occur in the esophagus, the small bowel, and a Meckel's diverticulum lined with heterotopic gastric mucosa. Endoscopic ultrasound may detect an unsuspected submucosal component or enlarged lymph nodes, such as may occur in gastric neoplasia, especially lymphoma and linitis plastica (Chapter 198). Ulcers in the dorsal wall of the duodenal bulb, especially at the transition from the bulb to the postbulbar descending portion of the duodenum, are most difficult to visualize, and they sometimes require a side-viewing endoscope, particularly when endoscopic treatment is needed. Other regions where gastroduodenal ulcers can be easily missed are the cardia and the gastric angulus. Dieulafoy's lesions may be difficult to diagnose because of their small mucosal defects and intermittent bleeding. Some patients require more than one endoscopy, preferably during acute bleeding, to localize the lesion. Endoscopy is also useful for ascertaining the presence of concomitant disorders, including esophagitis and duodenitis, or complications, such as bleeding or a visible vessel (see Fig. 141-2); obtaining biopsy specimens, such as for histologic examination and to assess for *H. pylori* (see Fig. 141-3); and performing therapeutic interventions.

In rare cases, such as stenosis that blocks the advancing endoscope, conventional barium contrast radiographs (Chapter 135) are indicated. Additional investigations by endosonography or CT are needed when an underlying malignant disease is suspected. The endoscopist should obtain biopsy samples from all gastric ulcers, especially those with a suspicious appearance, to exclude potential malignant disease. Because duodenal ulcers are less likely to be malignant, biopsies are usually not required unless malignancy is specifically suspected.

Etiologic Diagnosis

Diagnosis also must focus on establishing the cause of the ulcer. The first step is to determine whether *H. pylori* or NSAID use is present, because these are the major risk factors for peptic ulcers and can be contributing factors in ulcers with other precipitating causes.

Testing for Helicobacter pylori

In populations with a high prevalence of *H. pylori,* nearly all patients with peptic ulcer disease are positive for *H. pylori,* so diagnostic testing has little value except when antimicrobial susceptibility testing is needed. The prevalence of *H. pylori* remains high in immigrants from developing countries, where most people become *H. pylori* positive in youth. In Western countries, approximately 50% of individuals who are older than 65 years are colonized with *H. pylori,* but the prevalence is less than 20% in those younger than 30 years. In these younger persons, the proportion of patients with ulcers who are *H. pylori* negative is higher than in older patients, making diagnostic testing for *H. pylori,* followed by targeted therapy in those who are positive for the bacterium, more attractive than empirical therapy.

The presence of *H. pylori* can be ascertained by four possible approaches. *Histologic examination* of gastric mucosal biopsies, which is the standard procedure when diagnostic endoscopy is initially performed, is quite sensitive and specific for *H. pylori.* However, the accuracy of this technique may be affected by sampling error, improper orientation of the specimen, and recent therapy with proton pump inhibitors or antibiotics.

A second option is *serology,* which is a relatively simple, inexpensive test that has reduced predictive value in areas where the prevalence of *H. pylori* is low. Serology is not helpful to verify whether *H. pylori* has been eradicated with antibiotics because it may take many months or even years for *H. pylori* antibodies to fall to undetectable levels. None of the diagnostic tests that do not involve endoscopy can determine whether an ulcer is present.

A third option is a *stool antigen test,* which is more accurate than serology. Finally, the *carbon-13 or carbon -14 urea breath test,* which relies on the detection of *H. pylori* urease activity, is a noninvasive and relatively simple test, but it is more expensive than stool or blood testing. Although the test becomes negative as soon as *H. pylori* is eradicated, a minimum interval of 4 to 6 weeks after antibiotic treatment is recommended to reduce false-negative results.

Nonsteroidal Anti-inflammatory Drugs

NSAIDs are usually established as the putative cause of an ulcer based on information obtained from the patient. Assessment of NSAID use in an individual patient presenting with ulcer disease can be difficult, both because NSAID use is common and often intermittent and because many different NSAIDs are widely available over the counter in most countries. NSAID use is usually evaluated by detailed medical history, focusing not only on current and recent drug use but also on symptoms of pain, including musculoskeletal complaints. Further information from family members, family practitioners, and pharmacists is sometimes helpful. If surreptitious use of NSAIDs is suspected, direct serum and urine testing for aspirin and NSAID derivatives is feasible, or aspirin use can be assessed indirectly by a platelet adherence assay; however, these tests are not commonly used in clinical practice.

Hypersecretory Syndromes

Hypersecretory syndromes not related to *H. pylori* or NSAIDs are rare causes of ulcer disease and are diagnosed by special tests (see Table 141-3). Zollinger-Ellison syndrome should be strongly considered in patients with multiple ulcers, particularly in atypical locations such as distal to the duodenal bulb, and when diarrhea is present, because these finding are uncommon in *H. pylori*–related peptic ulcer disease. Hypergastrinemic syndromes (e.g., Zollinger-Ellison syndrome, antral G-cell hyperplasia) are best diagnosed by a determination of serum gastrin levels, both basal and after stimulation with intravenous secretin (gastrinoma detection) or a test meal (antral G-cell hyperplasia detection). When detected early, gastrinomas may be resectable (Chapter 201).

Gastric analysis, which is performed by placing a nasogastric tube to aspirate gastric juice and to quantify gastric acid output (both basal and after stimulation with subcutaneous pentagastrin), is indicated in only two rare circumstances: patients with elevated serum gastrin levels suggestive of Zollinger-Ellison syndrome or antral G-cell hyperplasia, but with equivocal responses to standard gastric provocative tests, and patients with indirect signs of gastric hypersecretion (e.g., enlarged folds and abundant clear fluid at endoscopy), normal gastrin levels, and negative provocative gastrin tests but who may still be hypersecretors, such as patients with recurrent ulcer disease despite a prior vagotomy with or without antrectomy. A basal acid output greater than 15 mEq/hour or greater than 5 mEq/hour in a postoperative patient is considered a positive test result.

The diagnosis of Zollinger-Ellison syndrome is best confirmed by gastric analysis showing a basal acid output greater than 15 mEq/hour in conjunction with a fasting serum gastrin level exceeding 1000 pg/mL in the presence of gastric pH less than 2. To skip the cumbersome gastric analysis, a gastric pH determination showing a fasting pH of 2 or less is adequate. For serum gastrin levels in the range 100 to 1000 pg/mL and intragastric pH greater than 2, an increase in the serum gastrin to more than 200 pg/mL after a secretin stimulation test is suggestive of the diagnosis. An elevated serum gastrin level alone is not sufficient to diagnose Zollinger-Ellison syndrome, because serum gastrin levels tend to increase over time with atrophic gastritis and are also increased in patients receiving proton pump inhibitor therapy.

Other Causes

In patients in whom a gastroduodenal ulcer cannot be ascribed to colonization with *H. pylori,* use of NSAIDs, or a hypersecretory syndrome, the establishment of a definite etiologic diagnosis may require a more thorough evaluation, starting with a medical history that focuses on the use of other ulcerogenic agents and the presence of symptoms that could suggest an underlying systemic disease. The next step is to evaluate biopsy samples from ulcer borders and from the antrum, corpus, and duodenum. The ulcer specimens may reveal overt or suspicious signs of malignancy, in particular adenocarcinoma (Chapter 198) or lymphoma. In these cases, further diagnostic evaluation should include staging of the malignancy. Alternatively, the biopsies may provide evidence of other infectious conditions, specific types of gastritis, celiac disease, ischemia, amyloidosis, or a systemic inflammatory condition. These data can be combined with clues provided by the endoscopic evaluation, including the character and location of the ulcer, signs of ischemia, and signs of inflammation at other locations. Further evaluation should focus on the presence of systemic disorders and may include a chest radiograph, angiography, ileocolonoscopy, and abdominal CT.

Differential Diagnosis

The differential diagnosis of ulcer-like symptoms includes many disorders of the upper abdominal organs, including malignant diseases of the stomach (Chapter 198), duodenum (Chapter 199), pancreas (Chapter 200), or bile ducts (Chapter 202). The differential diagnosis of upper abdominal symptoms also includes liver and gallstone disease (Chapter 158), pancreatitis (Chapter 146), and motility disorders (Chapter 138). In many patients with upper abdominal dyspeptic complaints, no underlying cause can be identified. In this "nonulcer" or functional dyspepsia group, complaints characteristic of gastroesophageal reflux, ulcer symptoms, or dysmotility symptoms may be prominent. A few of these patients (generally 5%) benefit from eradication of *H. pylori,* with a slow decrease of dyspeptic complaints over 12 to 24 months, but functional dyspepsia is not a proven or widely accepted indication for treatment of *H. pylori.* If such treatment is considered, both the patient and the physician should be prepared for persistent symptoms despite eradication of *H. pylori.*

Diagnostic Scenarios: Acute or Initial Clinical Presentation

Younger (≤45 years old) patients without alarm symptoms or signs such as anemia, rapid weight loss, or other evidence of serious disease do not necessarily require endoscopy, and evidence indicates that malignant gastric disease is unlikely. When a generalist physician is treating a patient who lives in an area of the world with a relatively high prevalence of *H. pylori* infection (>10% of the population is positive), a test-and-treat approach can begin with an *H. pylori* stool antigen determination, urea breath test, or *H. pylori* serologic examination. If the test is positive, the patient can be treated with the appropriate *H. pylori* eradication drugs (see later) and observed for 4 to 6 weeks. If the patient is also taking an NSAID, either orally or parenterally, the same approach is appropriate, but the NSAID should be discontinued. If the *H. pylori* test is negative in a person taking NSAIDs, these drugs should be discontinued, and the patient should be treated with a proton pump inhibitor for 4 to 6 weeks. In patients who are not taking NSAIDs or who do not improve after these drugs are discontinued, endoscopy is indicated to determine whether an ulcer is present.

Conversely, gastroenterologists more commonly proceed directly to endoscopy. If no abnormalities are apparent or the endoscopic study shows only "gastritis" without an overt ulcer, a biopsy should be obtained to ascertain by histologic examination or urease testing whether *H. pylori* is present. If *H. pylori* is found by endoscopic biopsy, eradication treatment may be given; however, the effect of *H. pylori* eradication on relief of functional dyspeptic symptoms is only about 5% greater than with placebo.[1]

If endoscopic examination shows an ulcer, its location determines the subsequent approach. An ulcer in the duodenal bulb has only a remote chance of representing a malignant lesion and need not routinely be examined by biopsy. By contrast, biopsy is mandatory for a gastric ulcerative lesion identified at endoscopy, because malignant gastric disease may present with similar clinical manifestations and may resemble benign ulcer disease morphologically; even if histologic assessment does not identify a malignant process, repeat endoscopy is recommended about 1 month after therapy to verify complete healing and for biopsy of the scar.

TREATMENT Rx

Helicobacter pylori Infection

H. pylori–associated ulcers often heal spontaneously, but acid suppressive therapy accelerates healing and ameliorates symptoms. Four weeks of acid suppressive therapy heals 70 to 80% of ulcers, and this number increases to more than 90% after 8 weeks of therapy. If *H. pylori* infection persists, however, ulcers recur in 50 to 90% of patients within 12 to 24 months; this rate can be reduced to 20 to 30% with maintenance acid suppression and to less than 5% with *H. pylori* eradication.[2] Eradication treatment is therefore mandatory (Table 141-4). Treatment for 10 to 14 days has about a 5 to 10% advantage over 7- to 10-day therapy,[3] and quadruple drug therapy is probably better than triple therapy.[4] Nevertheless, 7-day treatment may be acceptable in regions where local studies have shown that a particular treatment is very effective, and it is probably the most economical option in countries with low health care budgets. For patients in whom such therapy fails, a 4- to 10-day course of quadruple therapy is advised. This second-line regimen eradicates *H. pylori* in an additional 80 to 90% of patients. Resistance of *H. pylori* to metronidazole varies between 10 and 80% throughout the world. Clarithromycin resistance is increasing and is now estimated to be 5 to 10% in the United States because of the widespread use of macrolides to treat upper respiratory infections. Resistance to amoxicillin and tetracycline is rare and is not usually relevant in clinical practice. Sequential therapy may be superior to standard triple therapy and is a good alternative for both first- and second-line treatment.

Continuation of acid suppressive therapy after antibiotic treatment is needed only when symptoms persist[5] or in cases of complicated ulcer disease until eradication of *H. pylori* has been confirmed. Ascertainment of therapeutic efficacy must be delayed at least 1 month after the end of treatment to prevent false-negative results related to the organism's temporary suppression but not eradication. When repeat endoscopy is needed (e.g., a gastric ulcer requires repeated histologic examination to exclude underlying malignancy), repeat screening for *H. pylori* can be performed using the gastric biopsy specimens for histologic examination, culture, or urease testing. If no clinical indication exists for repeat endoscopy, *H. pylori* status can be determined by a carbon-13 urea breath test, stool *H. pylori* antigen, or repeated serology. Serologic determination is based on a more than 40 to 50% decrease in immunoglobulin G antibody levels in the first 6 months after treatment compared with pretreatment levels in that patient.

After successful *H. pylori* eradication, the risk of recurrent infection in most populations is small. In a minority of patients, ulcers recur either owing to re-infection or in the presence of another ulcerogenic factor, particularly NSAID use.

Disease Related to Nonsteroidal Anti-inflammatory Drug Use

In patients who are diagnosed with acid peptic disease while they are taking NSAIDs or aspirin, the first step is to stop such therapy. Acid suppression with a proton pump inhibitor (in doses similar to those used for *H. pylori*) leads to healing of 85% of NSAID-induced gastric ulcers and more than 90% of duodenal ulcers within 8 weeks of therapy, whereas acid suppression with an H_2-blocker, equivalent to ranitidine 300 mg twice daily, heals approximately 70% of ulcers within 8 weeks. The mucosal protective drug misoprostol (200 mg four times daily) has a similar effect. Treatment must be continued for at least 8 weeks, and maintenance therapy is needed in patients who continue to take NSAIDs. Gastric ulcers, larger lesions, and recurrent lesions heal more slowly.

Ulcer occurrence during NSAID therapy suggests a causative relationship, but patients should also be tested for *H. pylori*. In patients who are *H. pylori* positive, eradication therapy should be considered because there are no clear clinical parameters distinguishing between these etiologic factors. In patients who continue to take NSAIDs, maintenance therapy with a proton pump inhibitor is superior to *H. pylori* eradication for the prevention of recurrent ulcer,[6] except in patients who use aspirin, for whom *H. pylori* eradication alone may be curative.

Idiopathic Ulcer Disease

Patients with idiopathic ulcer disease despite a thorough assessment for underlying causes are treated primarily with an acid suppressant, usually a proton pump inhibitor, because they are at considerable risk for recurrent ulcer disease. After the underlying cause is identified and adequately treated, acid suppressive therapy can be withdrawn if there are no additional risk factors for ulcer disease, such as NSAID therapy or *H. pylori* infection.

PREVENTION

Primary Prevention

A test-and-treat strategy for *H. pylori* colonization may be considered for patients with dyspeptic symptoms, but there is no specific way to prevent *H. pylori*–associated ulcer disease. In contrast, primary prevention of NSAID-associated ulcer disease is widely advocated for patients at high risk because of a prior ulcer, severe concomitant disease, use of warfarin or high-dose corticosteroids, or older age (>65 years). H_2-blockers (at a dose equivalent to ranitidine 300 mg twice daily) partially prevents duodenal ulcer disease during NSAID therapy but has no effect on preventing gastric ulcers unless a higher dose (equivalent to famotidine 40 mg twice daily) is given. Proton

TABLE 141-4 OVERVIEW OF ANTIBIOTICS USED FOR *HELICOBACTER PYLORI* ERADICATION

DRUG CLASS	DRUG	TRIPLE THERAPY* DOSE	QUADRUPLE THERAPY† DOSE	SEQUENTIAL THERAPY‡ DOSE
Acid suppression	Proton pump inhibitor	20-40 mg bid§	20-40 mg bid§	20-40 mg bid§
Standard antimicrobials	Bismuth compound‖	2 tablets bid	2 tablets bid	
	Amoxicillin	1 g bid		1 g bid
	Metronidazole¶	500 mg bid	500 mg tid	500 mg bid
	Clarithromycin	500 mg bid		500 mg bid
	Tetracycline		500 mg qid	
Salvage antimicrobials	Levofloxacin	300 mg bid	300 mg bid	
	Rifabutin	150 mg bid		
	Furazolidone	100 mg bid		
	Doxycycline		100 mg bid	
	Nitazoxanide		1 g bid	

*Triple therapy consists of a proton pump inhibitor or bismuth compound, together with two of the listed antibiotics, usually given for 7-14 days.
†Quadruple therapy consists of a proton pump inhibitor plus either the combination of a bismuth compound, metronidazole, and tetracycline given for 4-10 days, or the combination of levofloxacin, doxycycline, and nitazoxanide for 10 days.
‡Sequential therapy consists of 10 days of proton pump inhibitor treatment, plus amoxicillin during days 1-5 and a combination of clarithromycin and an imidazole (when available, tinidazole; otherwise, metronidazole) during days 6-10.
§Proton pump inhibitor dose equivalent to omeprazole 20 mg bid.
‖Bismuth subsalicylate or subcitrate.
¶An alternative is tinidazole 500 mg bid.

pump inhibitors (at a dose equivalent to omeprazole 20 mg once daily) and misoprostol (in doses varying between 400 and 800 mg/day) partially protect against both gastric and duodenal ulcers during NSAID use. Misoprostol and proton pump inhibitors are equally effective,[7] but adherence with therapy is lower with misoprostol owing to its side effects. Patients should be advised of the importance of adherence because less than 80% adherence to gastroprotection is associated with a more than two-fold increased risk for ulcer disease compared with those who are fully adherent. During low-dose aspirin therapy, primary prevention of ulcers is advocated for the same risk groups, using a proton pump inhibitor or an H_2-receptor antagonist.[8]

Secondary Prevention

Secondary prevention of *H. pylori*–associated ulcer disease is mandatory and consists of successful bacterial eradication. Testing to ascertain *H. pylori* status after eradication therapy is indicated in patients with prior complicated ulcer disease or with persistent or recurrent symptoms after therapy, as well as in patients who fail to complete the therapeutic course.

Secondary prevention of NSAID-related ulcer disease is preferentially achieved by the withdrawal of NSAIDs. In patients who must continue taking NSAIDs, a change to a selective COX2 inhibitor in combination with a proton pump inhibitor at a dose equivalent to esomeprazole 20 mg twice daily is advocated, especially for patients with complicated ulcer disease.[9] This combination is associated with a lower risk of secondary peptic ulcer complications than treatment with a COX2 inhibitor alone.

Secondary prevention of recurrent ulcers in patients who use aspirin may depend on *H. pylori* status. In *H. pylori*–positive patients, *H. pylori* eradication is as effective as a proton pump inhibitor for the prevention of recurrent ulcers.[6] In *H. pylori*–negative patients, additional acid suppressive therapy at a dose equivalent to esomeprazole 20 mg twice daily should be prescribed. Secondary prevention of idiopathic ulcer disease consists primarily of maintenance therapy with a proton pump inhibitor and treatment of the underlying condition.

PROGNOSIS

The majority of peptic ulcers heal spontaneously within weeks to months. However, if the underlying condition is not adequately treated, a large proportion of ulcers recur. Both initial and recurrent ulcers can give rise to complications. The four major complications are intractability, perforation, hemorrhage, and stenosis. Each distinct situation requires specific management approaches. Patients with complicated ulcer disease are at particular risk for recurrent complications and need careful assessment for secondary prevention.

Hemorrhage

Hemorrhage (Chapter 137), which is the most common complication of peptic ulcer disease, occurs in about one in six patients with ulcers over the course of their ulcer activity. Ulcers caused by NSAIDs account for a larger proportion of these hemorrhages. Peptic ulcer is thus the most common cause of nonvariceal upper gastrointestinal bleeding, accounting for 40 to 60% of cases in most populations. Bleeding is associated with a 5 to 15% risk of rebleeding and up to a 10% risk of mortality. Hemorrhage may occur along a continuum from a serious acute event associated with hemodynamic shock and high mortality to slow or intermittent blood loss leading to chronic anemia. Approximately 80% of patients with bleeding ulcers describe a prior history of symptomatic disease, and about 20 to 30% have suffered a previous hemorrhage. Assessment of the magnitude of bleeding is of paramount importance in determining the need for transfusion and subsequent management (Table 141-5). Initial hematocrit levels may be misleading and are likely to fall because of hemodilution. Rapid bleeding is usually apparent on the basis of clinical signs (pallor, systolic blood pressure ≤100 mm Hg, pulse ≥100/minute); immediate fluid resuscitation and transfusions are indicated to prevent circulatory collapse. Mortality is particularly related to complications of the bleed, such as aspiration, and exacerbation of underlying disease, such as pulmonary, cardiovascular, renal, and hepatic disease. On rare occasions, patients may actually bleed to death, especially when a larger artery is affected, such as when an ulcer in the posterior wall of the duodenal bulb perforates the gastroduodenal artery.

Initial treatment aims at hemodynamic stabilization. Endoscopy is the mainstay of therapy and should be performed within 24 hours of presentation in high-risk cases, especially patients who are hemodynamically unstable, require transfusion, or have more severe comorbidities. Endoscopy can be performed to ascertain the origin of the bleeding, and, if necessary, provide therapy to stop the bleed and reduce the risk of rebleeding.

The appearance of the ulcer determines the need for endoscopic treatment and the risk of rebleeding (Table 141-6) and mortality. "Clean base" ulcers and those with flat pigmented spots carry a low risk of rebleeding and do not require endoscopic treatment. In contrast, ulcers with active bleeding or stigmata of recent bleeding, in particular a visible vessel or adherent clot, require treatment to stop the bleed and reduce the otherwise high risk of recurrence.

Endoscopic therapy may lead to a three-fold reduction in episodes of recurrent bleeding and in the need for surgical intervention, as well as a 40% reduction in mortality.[10] Treatment modalities include injection therapy with epinephrine or a sclerosant, thermocoagulation, and mechanical pressure by means of clips. Thermocoagulation can be performed by direct contact, such as with a heater probe, or by a noncontact method, such as argon plasma coagulation. The efficacy of these methods is generally comparable, except that epinephrine injection alone is inferior to the other modalities but can be useful when combined with any of the others.[10,11] If an adherent clot is found, an attempt should be made to remove it by water flushing or snaring to allow an assessment of the underlying ulcer base and the treatment of any underlying visible vessels to reduce the risk of rebleeding.[12]

The pre-endoscopy administration of intravenous proton pump inhibitor therapy (at a dose equivalent to a bolus of 80 mg esomeprazole, followed by a continuous infusion of 8 mg/hour until endoscopy) reduces bleeding and the need for emergent endoscopic treatment, but it has no effect on the need

TABLE 141-5 BLATCHFORD SCORING SYSTEM TO DETERMINE THE NEED FOR INTERVENTION IN PEPTIC ULCER BLEEDING

VARIABLE	VALUE AT ADMISSION	SCORE COMPONENT VALUE
Blood urea (mmol/L)	6.5-7.9	2
	8.0-9.9	3
	10.0-24.9	4
	≥25.0	6
Hemoglobin (g/L)		
Men	120-129	1
	100-119	2
	<100	6
Women	100-119	1
	<100	6
Systolic blood pressure (mm Hg)	100-109	1
	90-99	2
	<90	3
Other markers	Pulse ≥100/min	1
	Presentation with melena	1
	Presentation with syncope	2
	Hepatic disease	2
	Cardiac failure	2

Data from Stanley AJ, Ashley D, Dalton HR, et al. Outpatient management of patients with low-risk upper gastrointestinal haemorrhage: multicentre validation and prospective evaluation. *Lancet.* 2009;373:42-47. Intervention (endoscopic hemostasis, surgery, transfusion) is rarely needed for patients with an admission score ≤2 but is required in more than 40% of patients with a score ≥6.

TABLE 141-6 ENDOSCOPY RESULTS IN PATIENTS WITH BLEEDING ULCERS

ENDOSCOPY RESULT	ULCER CHARACTERISTICS*	RISK OF RECURRENT BLEEDING (%)
Active bleeding	Arterial bleeding	80-90
	Oozing bleeding	10-30
Stigmata of recent bleeding	Nonbleeding visible vessel	50-60
	Adherent clot	25-35
	Flat pigmented spot	0-8
No signs of bleeding	Clean ulcer base	0-12

*The ulcer characteristics determine the risk of recurrent bleeding during follow-up.

TABLE 141-7 ROCKALL SCORING SYSTEM FOR THE RISK OF MORTALITY FOLLOWING PEPTIC ULCER BLEEDING

	Score			
VARIABLE	**0**	**1**	**2**	**3**
Age (yr)	<60	60-79	80	—
Shock	Not present	Pulse >100	Systolic BP <100 mm Hg	—
Comorbidity	None		Cardiac failure Coronary insufficiency Other serious illness	Renal insufficiency Liver failure Metastatic malignancy
Diagnosis	Mallory-Weiss syndrome or no identifiable cause	Ulcer Varices	Malignancy of proximal digestive tract	—
Endoscopy	No signs of recent bleeding		Bleeding, clot, or visible vessel	—

BP = blood pressure.
Data from Rockall TA, Logan RFA, Devlin HB, et al. Risk assessment after acute upper gastrointestinal haemorrhage. *Gut.* 1996;38:316-321.

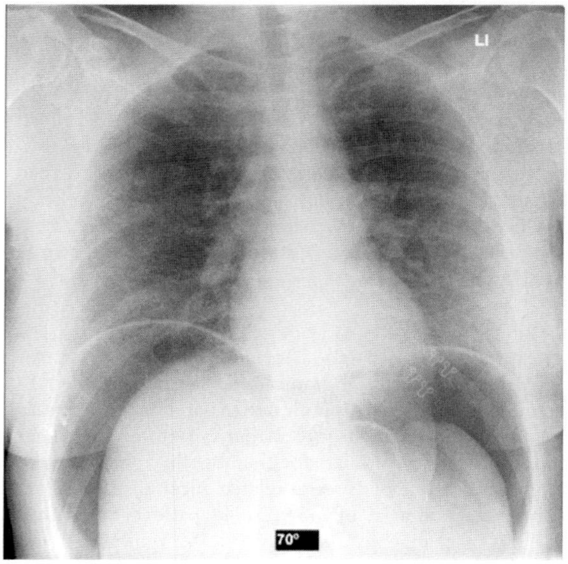

FIGURE 141-5. **Plain chest radiograph in an upright patient with a perforated ulcer.** The radiograph shows free air under the diaphragm.

for transfusion or the occurrence of rebleeding or death. For patients with active bleeding or stigmata of recent bleeding, endoscopic treatment should be followed by an intravenous proton pump inhibitor given as a bolus at a dose equivalent to 80 mg esomeprazole over 30 minutes, followed by a continuous infusion at a dose equivalent to esomeprazole 8 mg/hour for 72 hours, to reduce rebleeding and the need for further intervention.[13] Other therapies, including tranexamic acid, vasopressin, somatostatin, and octreotide, should be considered experimental (Chapter 137). Second-look endoscopy is not routinely indicated but can be considered in very high-risk cases, particularly when there is doubt about the adequacy of initial visualization or treatment.

About 70 to 80% of rebleeds occur within the first 3 days and generally should be managed by repeat endoscopy. If endoscopy fails to stop the bleed or prevent further rebleeding, surgery and interventional radiology are equivalent options. Surgery includes stitching of the ulcer and occlusion of the feeding artery, usually the gastroduodenal artery. Interventional radiology uses angiography to insert a coil in the culprit vessel at the site of the bleed. Single-center observational experience suggests that each of these methods is equally effective in the hands of experienced clinicians, and the choice depends on local availability and expertise.

The risk for a fatal outcome of an upper gastrointestinal hemorrhage can be estimated based on five clinical and endoscopic parameters (Table 141-7). In several studies, mortality in patients with a bleeding peptic ulcer was less than 2% among those with a score of 2 points or less, 10% in those with 3 to 5 points, and up to 46% in those with 6 points or more. Management of patients who recover after a peptic ulcer hemorrhage is similar to the treatment of patients with uncomplicated ulcers. Eradication of *H. pylori* provides excellent protection against both recurrence and rebleeding of *H. pylori*–related ulcers. NSAID-induced ulcers are preferentially managed by the withdrawal of NSAIDs or, if this is not feasible, by the combination of a COX2 inhibitor and a proton pump inhibitor at a dose equivalent to esomeprazole 20 mg twice daily. In patients with a history of ulcer bleeding and concomitant cardiovascular disease requiring antiplatelet therapy, the combination of low-dose aspirin and a proton pump inhibitor at a dose equivalent to esomeprazole 20 mg twice daily is associated with a lower risk of complicated ulcer than is clopidogrel monotherapy.[14] If a patient who requires antiplatelet therapy presents with a bleeding ulcer, antiplatelet therapy should be continued or restarted as soon as possible if the risk of a cardiovascular event outweighs the risk of recurrent bleeding.[15]

Perforation

Perforation may manifest as an acute event, whereby gastric contents spill into the peritoneal cavity, or more insidiously as the ulcer slowly penetrates into surrounding tissues. Acute free perforation typically causes abrupt and severe abdominal pain associated with abdominal muscular spasm that produces board-like rigidity of the abdomen and other manifestations of peritoneal irritation. Secondary hemodynamic shock is common. The clinical diagnosis can be confirmed in approximately 80% of patients by a plain chest radiograph with the patient standing (Fig. 141-5); a CT scan can be obtained if doubt persists. Leukocytosis and elevated C-reactive protein levels develop rapidly, and mild hyperamylasemia may occur. Treatment begins by correcting hemodynamic, fluid, and electrolyte imbalances. Nasogastric suction is helpful, and prophylactic antibiotics (e.g., amoxicillin-clavulanic acid 1 g every 8 hours intravenously) are usually administered. Unless a specific contraindication exists, emergency surgery is usually indicated, although more conservative approaches are sometimes appropriate. Given the success in achieving the long-term cure of ulcer disease through the eradication of *H. pylori* and the withdrawal of NSAIDs, suturing of the perforated ulcer may be adequate, permitting the patient to avoid a more radical vagotomy with or without gastric resection.

Intractability

Intractability is a term strictly applied to an ulcer that persists even after intensive and prolonged proton pump inhibitor therapy. Symptoms may or may not be present. These rare cases may result from poor compliance with recommended treatment, surreptitious use of ulcerogenic drugs, or other diseases (e.g., Crohn's disease, ischemia, infection with bacteria other than *H. pylori*, viral infection). If these issues are recognized and these diagnoses are pursued, further complications and interventions such as surgical vagotomy and pyloroplasty can almost always be avoided.

Acid peptic disease related to alcohol or bisphosphonates should be addressed by discontinuing the precipitating agent. Treatment of Zollinger-Ellison syndrome requires high-dose proton pump inhibitors and/or surgery (Chapter 201). Those rare ulcers caused by Crohn's disease (Chapter 143), vasculitis (Chapter 278), sarcoidosis (Chapter 95), polycythemia vera (Chapter 169), amyloidosis (Chapter 194), and other rare disorders should be addressed by treating the underlying condition. Stress ulcers and Cameron's ulcers are treated by potent acid suppression therapy (e.g., omeprazole 20 mg twice daily).

Stenosis

Gastric outlet obstruction is now a rare complication of ulcer disease because of the early detection and treatment of most ulcers. Most patients who develop clinically relevant gastric outlet obstruction have had an ulcer in the duodenal bulb and/or pyloric channel. Edema and inflammation play an important role, and occasionally a patient with active disease presents with symptoms of outlet obstruction as manifested by nausea, vomiting, and gastric stasis without a tight, chronic stenosis. Management therefore involves three key steps. This first is nasogastric tube aspiration and gastric lavage to clean the stomach of retained debris, followed by early endoscopy.

This step facilitates an accurate diagnosis. Nasogastric suction may need to be maintained for several days if vomiting resumes when the tube is clamped. The second step consists of intense antisecretory therapy using intravenous proton pump inhibitors in a dose equivalent to a bolus of 80 mg esomeprazole over 30 minutes, followed by a continuous infusion of 8 mg/hour. Finally, the cause of the ulcer needs to be addressed, usually by eradicating *H. pylori* and withdrawing NSAIDs. If the initial treatment resolves the clinical situation and the patient can resume eating, it is often not necessary to undertake further treatment of the outlet stenosis; however, tight, fibrous scarring may require endoscopic balloon dilation or surgery.

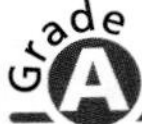

1. Moayyedi P, Soo S, Deeks J, et al. Eradication of *Helicobacter pylori* for non-ulcer dyspepsia. *Cochrane Database Syst Rev*. 2006;2:CD002096.
2. Ford AC, Delaney BC, Forman D, et al. Eradication therapy for peptic ulcer disease in *Helicobacter pylori*-positive patients. *Cochrane Database Syst Rev*. 2006;2:CD003840.
3. Fuccio L, Minardi ME, Zagari RM, et al. Meta-analysis: duration of first-line proton-pump inhibitor based triple therapy for the *Helicobacter pylori* eradication. *Ann Intern Med*. 2007;147:553-562.
4. Malfertheiner P, Bazzoli F, Delchier JC, et al. *Helicobacter pylori* eradication with a capsule containing bismuth subcitrate potassium, metronidazole, and tetracycline given with omeprazole versus clarithromycin-based triple therapy: a randomised, open-label, non-inferiority, phase 3 trial. *Lancet*. 2011;377:905-913.
5. Gisbert JP, Pajares JM. Systematic review and meta-analysis: is 1-week proton pump inhibitor-based triple therapy sufficient to heal peptic ulcer? *Aliment Pharmacol Ther*. 2005;21:795-804.
6. Chan FK, Chung SC, Suen BY, et al. Preventing recurrent upper gastrointestinal bleeding in patients with *Helicobacter pylori* infection who are taking low-dose aspirin or naproxen. *N Engl J Med*. 2001;344:967-973.
7. Graham DY, Agrawal NM, Campbell DR, et al. NSAID-Associated Gastric Ulcer Prevention Study Group. Ulcer prevention in long-term users of non-steroidal anti-inflammatory drugs: results of a double blind, randomized, multicenter, active- and placebo-controlled study of misoprostol versus lansoprazole. *Arch Intern Med*. 2002;162:169-175.
8. Taha AS, McCloskey C, Prasad R, et al. Famotidine for the prevention of peptic ulcers and oesophagitis in patients taking low-dose aspirin (FAMOUS): a phase III, randomised, double-blind, placebo-controlled trial. *Lancet*. 2009;374:119-125.
9. Barkun A, Bardou M, Kuipers EJ, et al. International consensus recommendations on the management of patients with non-variceal upper gastrointestinal bleeding. *Ann Intern Med*. 2010;152:101-113.
10. Barkun AN, Martel M, Toubouti Y, et al. Endoscopic hemostasis in peptic ulcer bleeding for patients with high-risk lesions: a series of meta-analyses. *Gastrointest Endosc*. 2009;69:786-799.
11. Laine L, McQuaid KR. Endoscopic therapy for bleeding ulcers: an evidence-based approach based on meta-analyses of randomized controlled trials. *Clin Gastroenterol Hepatol*. 2009;7:33-47.
12. Kahi CJ, Jansen DM, Sung JJ, et al. Endoscopic therapy versus medical therapy for bleeding peptic ulcer with adherent clot: a meta-analysis. *Gastroenterology*. 2005;129:855-862.
13. Sung JJ, Barkun A, Kuipers EJ, et al. Intravenous esomeprazole for prevention of recurrent peptic ulcer bleeding: a randomized trial. *Ann Intern Med*. 2009:150;455-464.
14. Chan FK, Ching JY, Hung LC, et al. Clopidogrel versus aspirin and esomeprazole to prevent recurrent ulcer bleeding. *N Engl J Med*. 2005;352:238-244.
15. Sung JJ, Lau YW, Ching JYL, et al. Continuation of low-dose aspirin in peptic ulcer bleeding: a randomized, controlled trial. *Ann Intern Med*. 2010;152:1-9.

SUGGESTED READINGS

Lanza FL, Chan FL, Quigley EM, et al. Guidelines for prevention of NSAID-related ulcer complications. *Am J Gastroenterol*. 2009;104:728-738. *International consensus guidelines on the prevention of NSAID-related ulcer disease.*

Madanick RD. Proton pump inhibitor side effects and drug interactions: much ado about nothing? *Cleve Clin J Med*. 2011;78:39-49. *Review.*

Malfertheiner P, Chan FK, McColl KE. Peptic ulcer disease. *Lancet*. 2009;374:1449-1461. *Review.*

McColl KE. *Helicobacter pylori* infection. *N Engl J Med*. 2010;362;1597-1604. *Review.*

142 APPROACH TO THE PATIENT WITH DIARRHEA AND MALABSORPTION

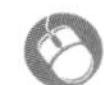

CAROL E. SEMRAD

DEFINITIONS

Normal stool frequency ranges from three times a week to three times a day. As a symptom, diarrhea can be described as a decrease in stool consistency (increased fluidity), stools that cause urgency or abdominal discomfort, or an increase in the frequency of stool. Consistency is defined as the ratio of fecal water to the water-holding capacity of fecal insoluble solids, which are composed of bacterial mass and dietary fiber. Because it is difficult to measure stool consistency and because stool is predominantly (60 to 85%) water, stool weight becomes a reasonable surrogate of consistency.

As a sign, diarrhea is defined by the weight or volume of stool measured over a 24- to 72-hour period. Daily stool weights of children and adults are less than 200 g, and greater stool weights are an objective definition of diarrhea; however, this definition misses 20% of diarrheal symptoms in patients who have loose stools that are less than this daily weight.

Acute diarrheas persist for less than 2 to 3 weeks or, rarely, 6 to 8 weeks. The most common cause of acute diarrhea is infection. Chronic diarrheal conditions persist for at least 4 weeks and, more typically, 6 to 8 weeks or longer. There are four mechanisms of diarrhea: osmotic, secretory, exudative, and altered motility. Because many diarrheal diseases are due to more than one of these mechanisms, it is clinically useful to categorize diarrhea as malabsorptive (fatty), watery, and inflammatory.

EPIDEMIOLOGY

Diarrhea is the second leading cause of mortality worldwide and is particularly problematic for elderly people and for children younger than 5 years of age in developing nations. Infectious diarrheal conditions cause 1.8 million childhood deaths annually, despite the improved use of oral rehydration solutions, zinc, and vitamin A supplements. About one third of these deaths have been due to rotavirus infection (Chapter 388), but the recently introduced oral monovalent rotavirus vaccination has diminished its incidence and mortality in developing and developed nations.

In the United States, about 48 million people suffer from food-borne illness each year, with 128,000 hospitalizations and 3000 deaths, most in elderly people. The complaint of diarrhea accounts for more than 7 million outpatient visits per year. Total costs for diarrheal diseases are about $1.2 billion in direct (health care) costs and $5.4 billion in indirect costs (days lost from work).

PATHOBIOLOGY

Abnormalities of Fluid and Electrolyte Transport

To understand the osmotic, secretory, and inflammatory mechanisms of diarrhea, it is necessary to understand how the normal intestine handles fluid and solutes in health and disease. Whether a hypotonic meal, such as a steak and water, or a hypertonic meal, such as milk and a doughnut, is consumed, the volume of the meal is augmented by gastric, pancreatic, biliary, and duodenal secretions. The permeable duodenum then renders the meal approximately isotonic with an electrolyte content similar to that of plasma by the time it reaches the proximal jejunum. As the intestinal slurry moves toward the colon, the Na^+ concentration in the luminal fluid remains constant, but Cl^- is reduced to 60 to 70 mmol/L, and bicarbonate (HCO_3^-) is increased to a similar concentration as the result of Cl^- and HCO_3^- transport mechanisms in the enterocyte and HCO_3^- secretion in the ileum (Fig. 142-1B and C). In the colon, K^{++} is secreted, and the Na^+ transport mechanism of the colonocyte, together with the low epithelial permeability, extracts Na^+ and fluid from the stool. As a result, the Na^+ content of stool decreases to 30 to 40 mmol/L; K^{++} increases from 5 to 10 mmol/L in the small bowel to 75 to 90 mmol/L; and poorly absorbed divalent cations, such as Mg^{2++} and Ca^{2++}, are concentrated in stool to values of 5 to 100 mmol/L. The anion concentrations in the colon change drastically because bacterial degradation of carbohydrate (i.e., unabsorbed starches, sugars, and fiber) creates short-chain fatty acids that attain concentrations of 80 to 180 mmol/L; at colonic pH, organic anions, such as acetate, propionate, and butyrate, are present. In the setting of carbohydrate malabsorption, the generation of high concentrations of these short-chain fatty acids may decrease stool pH to 4 or lower. The osmolality of the stool is approximately that of plasma (280 to 300 mOsm/kg H_2O) when it is passed.

At the cellular level Na^{++} transport by the epithelium from lumen to blood (by Na^{++}-coupled sugar and amino acid transport in the small intestine, by Na^{++}/H^{++} exchange proteins in the small intestine and proximal colon, and by aldosterone-regulated $^+$ Na^{++} channels in the distal colon) creates a favorable osmotic gradient for absorption (see Fig. 142-1A and B). Chloride transport by the epithelium from blood to lumen (by cystic fibrosis transmembrane conductance regulator [CFTR] and the calcium-activated chloride channel in the small intestine and colon) creates an osmotic gradient for secretion (see Fig. 142-1C). Normally, the intestine is in a net absorptive state, regulated by extrinsic adrenergic nerves and proabsorptive neuropeptides and hormones (see Fig. 142-1D). Stimulation of secretion by neurotransmitters, hormones, and inflammatory mediators (Table 142-1; see Fig. 142-1D) can offset this balance.

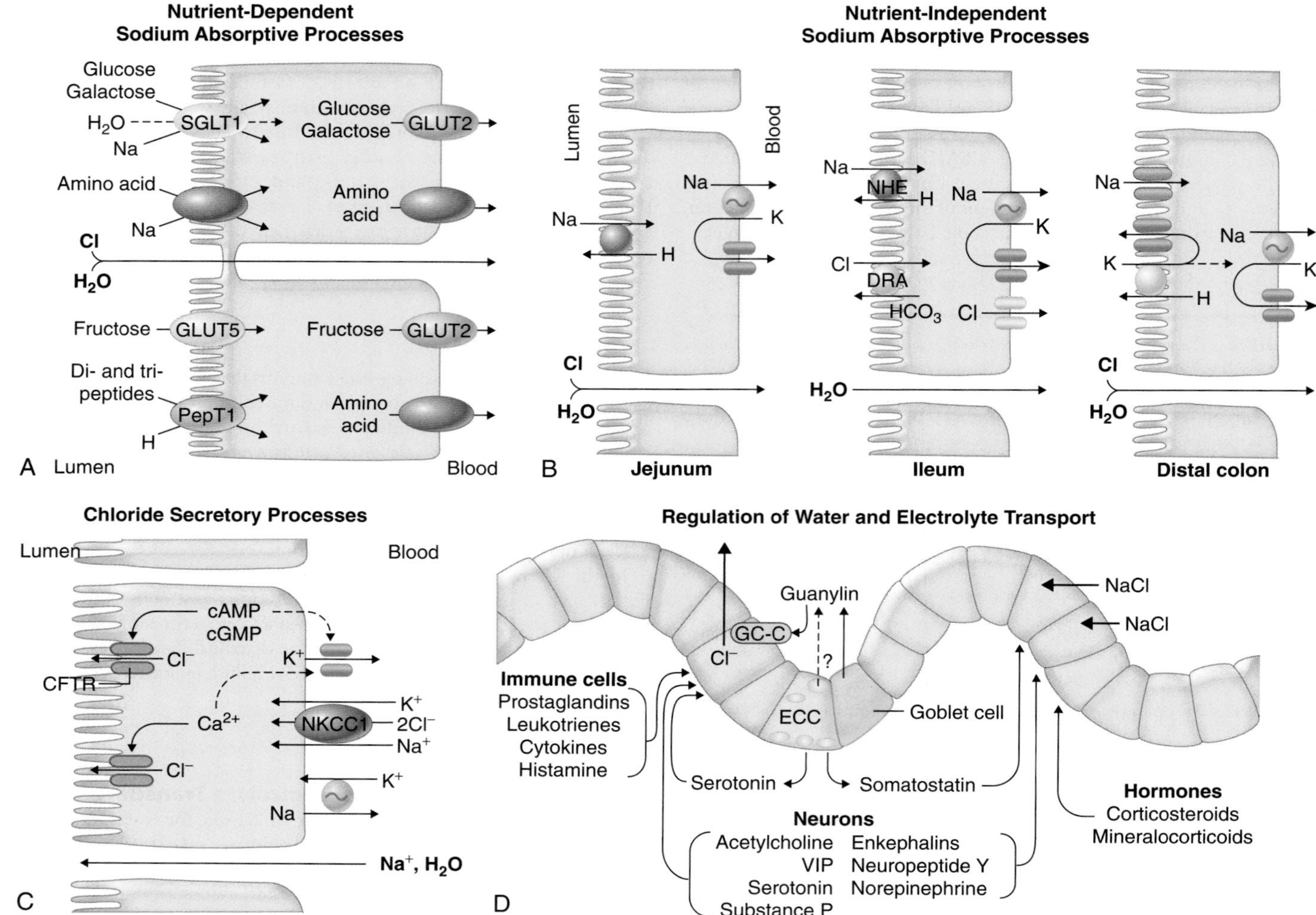

FIGURE 142-1. **Mechanisms of intestinal transport of water and electrolytes. A,** Intestinal sodium absorption. Sodium is actively absorbed in villus cells of the small intestine and surface cells of the colon. The sodium-potassium adenosine triphosphatase (Na^{++},K^{++}-ATPase) present on the cell basolateral membrane maintains a low intracellular Na^{+++} concentration and an electronegative cell interior favoring Na^{+++} movement across the apical membrane from lumen into cell. In the small intestine, glucose and galactose are taken up with sodium and water at the apical membrane by the sodium-glucose ligand transporter (SGLT1). Several different sodium-dependent amino acid carriers, some with overlapping substrate specificities, transport cationic, anionic, and neutral amino acids into villus cells. Dipeptides and tripeptides are transported by a hydrogen-coupled oligopeptide carrier, PepT1, that is driven by luminal hydrogen ions generated by the epithelial Na^+/H^{++} exchanger. Fructose is taken up by the facilitative glucose transporter (GLUT5). **B,** Sodium also is absorbed by nutrient-independent transport processes in the small intestine and colon. The Na^{++}/H^{++} (NHE) and Cl^-/HCO_3^- (DRA) exchangers are inhibited by agents that elevate intracellular cyclic adenosine monophosphate (cAMP), cyclic guanosine monophosphate (cGMP), or calcium. **C,** Chloride secretion by intestinal crypt cells. Chloride can be secreted actively throughout the small intestine and colon. Intracellular mediators of secretion (cAMP, cGMP, Ca^{2++}) open apical Cl^- channels (cystic fibrosis transmembrane conductance regulator [CFTR], calcium-activated chloride channel [TMEM16]) and basolateral K^{++} channels. Chloride moves from crypt cells into the intestinal lumen, favoring movement of Cl^- from the blood into cells by the Na^{++}/K^{++}/$2Cl^-$ cotransporter (NKCC1). Bicarbonate (HCO_3^-) also may be secreted via the CFTR channel. **D,** Regulation of intestinal water and electrolyte transport. Normally, the intestine is in a net absorptive state under the control of extrinsic adrenergic nerves from the sympathetic nervous system. Guanylin, the natural ligand for the *Escherichia coli* stable-toxin receptor (membrane-bound guanylyl cyclase [GC-C]), may be important in regulating local chloride secretion. The normal tone of the intestine is modified by the enteric nervous system, endocrine and inflammatory cells in the intestinal mucosa, and circulating hormones. The enteric nervous system releases a variety of neurotransmitters, some that stimulate chloride secretion (e.g., vasoactive intestinal peptide [VIP], acetylcholine) and others that promote sodium absorption (e.g., enkephalins, neuropeptide Y). Hormones produced locally from enterochromaffin cells (ECC) in the intestinal epithelium and inflammatory mediators released from immune cells directly affect enterocytes and nearby nerves. Circulating hormones (e.g., aldosterone, glucocorticoids) enhance sodium absorption in the intestine. Glucocorticoids also inhibit release of arachidonic acid and production of prostaglandin by inflammatory cells.

Diarrhea is due primarily to alterations of intestinal fluid and electrolyte transport and less to smooth muscle function. Each 24 hours, 8 to 10 L of fluid enters the duodenum. The diet supplies 2 L of this fluid; the remainder comes from salivary, gastric, hepatic, pancreatic, and intestinal secretions. The small intestine normally absorbs 8 to 9 L (80%) of this fluid and presents 1.5 L to the colon for absorption. Of the remaining fluid, the colon absorbs all but approximately 100 mL. Diarrhea can result from increased secretion by the small intestine or the colon if the maximal daily absorptive capacity of the colon (4 L) is exceeded. Alternatively, if the colon is diseased so that it cannot absorb even the 1.5 L normally presented to it by the small intestine, diarrhea results.

Watery diarrheas may be due to osmotic, secretory, or inflammatory mechanisms. With ingestion of a poorly absorbed (e.g., Mg^{2++}) or unabsorbable (polyethylene glycol, lactulose or, in lactase-deficient individuals, lactose) solute, the osmotic force of the solute pulls water and secondarily sodium and chloride ions into the intestinal lumen. A considerable proportion of the osmolality of stool results from the nonabsorbed solute. This gap between stool osmolality and the sum of the electrolytes in the stool causes osmotic diarrhea.

Active chloride secretion or inhibited sodium absorption, which also create an osmotic gradient favorable for the movement of fluids from blood to lumen, explains the pathophysiology of the secretory diarrheas. Agents that increase enterocyte cyclic adenosine monophosphate (cAMP) (e.g., cholera toxin, prostaglandins), cyclic guanosine monophosphate (cGMP) (e.g., *Escherichia coli* stable toxin), or intracellular ionized calcium (Ca^{2++}) (e.g., acetylcholine) (see Table 142-1) inhibit non-nutrient Na^{++} absorption and stimulate Cl^- secretion (see Table 142-1 and Fig. 142-1C and D).

Inflammatory diarrheas, which may be watery or bloody, are characterized by enterocyte damage, villus atrophy, and crypt hyperplasia. The damaged enterocyte membrane of the small intestine has decreased disaccharidase and peptide hydrolase activity, reduced or absent Na^{++}-coupled sugar or amino acid transport mechanisms, and reduced or absent sodium chloride absorptive transporters. Conversely, the hyperplastic crypt cells maintain their ability to secrete $^-$ Cl^- (and perhaps HCO_3^-). If the inflammation is severe, immune-mediated vascular damage or ulceration allows blood, pus, and protein to leak (exudate) from capillaries and lymphatics and contribute to the diarrhea. Activation of lymphocytes, phagocytes, and fibroblasts releases various inflammatory mediators that induce intestinal chloride secretion (see Fig. 142-1D). Interleukin-1 (IL-1) and tumor necrosis factor, which also are released into the blood, cause fever, anorexia, and malaise.

TABLE 142-1 STIMULI OF INTESTINAL SECRETION

AGENT	INTRACELLULAR MEDIATOR	RELATED DIARRHEAL ILLNESS
Enterotoxins		
Cholera, *E. coli* heat labile toxin, *Salmonella, Yersinia*	cAMP	Travelers, endemic
E. coli heat stable toxin	cGMP	
Rotatoxin (NSP4)	?	Viral gastroenteritis
Serotonin, PAF	Ca	Inflammatory, allergic
PG, leukotrienes	cAMP, Ca	Invasive enteric bacteria*
PG	cAMP	Villous adenoma
Histamine	Ca	Intestinal allergies, mastocytosis, scombroid poisoning
VIP	cAMP	VIPoma, ganglioneuromas
5-HT, substance P, bradykinin	Ca	Malignant carcinoid
Calcitonin	?	Medullary carcinoma thyroid
Acetylcholine	Ca	Insecticides, nerve gas poisoning, cholinergic drugs
Ricinoleic acid	cAMP, Ca	Laxative abuse†
Caffeine	cAMP	Coffee, sodas, tea

**Shigella* species, *Clostridium difficile*, enteroinvasive *E. coli, Vibrio parahaemolyticus, Clostridium perfringens.*
†Also phenolphthalein, anthraquinones, bisacodyl, dioctyl sodium sulfosuccinate, and senna.
5-HT = 5-hydroxytryptamine; Ca = calcium; cAMP = cyclic adenosine monophosphate; cGMP = cyclic guanosine monophosphate; PAF - platelet-activating factor; PG = prostaglandin; VIP = vasoactive intestinal peptide.

ACUTE DIARRHEA

CLINICAL MANIFESTATIONS

Approximately 80% of acute diarrheas are due to infections with viruses, bacteria, and parasites. The remainder is due to medications that have an osmotic force, stimulate intestinal fluid secretion, or contain poorly or nonabsorbable sugars (e.g., sorbitol), or less commonly to fecal impaction, pelvic inflammation (e.g., acute appendicitis [Chapter 144]), or intestinal ischemia (Chapter 145).

Food-Borne and Water-Borne Infectious Diarrhea

Most infectious diarrheas are acquired through fecal-oral transmission from water, food, or person-to-person contact (Table 142-2). Patients with infectious diarrhea often complain of nausea, vomiting, and abdominal cramps that are associated with watery, malabsorptive, or bloody diarrhea and fever (dysentery) (Chapters 310 through 320, 344, 345, 358 to 360, 364, 365, 387, and 388). As documented using polymerase chain reaction methods of diagnosis, most outbreaks of nonbacterial acute gastroenteritis in the United States and other countries are caused by noroviruses (Norwalk agent; Chapter 388). Rotavirus (Chapter 388) predominantly causes diarrhea in infants, usually in the winter months, but also may cause nonseasonal acute diarrhea in adults, particularly in elderly people. Mechanisms for diarrhea include decreased fluid absorption due to destruction of villus enterocytes and stimulation of fluid secretion by NSP4 rotatoxin and viral activation of the enteric nervous system.

Food-borne bacterial diseases in the United States are primarily due to *Salmonella* (Chapter 316), *Campylobacter jejuni* (Chapter 311), and *E. coli* O157:H7 (Chapter 312), and less commonly *Shigella* (Chapter 317). Outbreaks of *E. coli* O157:H7 have been associated with petting zoos, uncooked ground beef, and green leafy vegetables. These bacteria most often invade the distal small bowel and colon, where they multiply intracellularly and damage the epithelium. Diarrhea is due to the stimulation of intestinal secretion by inflammatory mediators, decreased absorption across the damaged epithelium, and exudation of protein into the lumen. *Shigella* species and enterohemorrhagic *E. coli* produce a similar toxin, the "Shiga toxin," which is cytotoxic to intestinal epithelial cells and causes inflammation, cell damage, and diarrhea with blood and pus.

Outbreaks of *Cryptosporidium* (Chapter 358) have been reported in water parks. This parasite causes diarrhea by adhering and fusing to the epithelial cell membrane in the small bowel, thereby causing cell damage. Organisms that are specific for seafood include *Vibrio parahaemolyticus* (Chapter 310),

TABLE 142-2 EPIDEMIOLOGY OF ACUTE INFECTIOUS DIARRHEA AND INFECTIOUS FOOD-BORNE ILLNESS

VEHICLE	CLASSIC PATHOGENS
Water (including foods washed in such water)	*Vibrio cholerae*, caliciviruses (Norwalk agent), *Giardia, Cryptosporidium*
Food	
Poultry	*Salmonella, Campylobacter, Shigella* species
Beef, unpasteurized fruit juice	Enterohemorrhagic *Escherichia coli*
Pork	Tapeworm
Seafood and shellfish (including raw sushi and gefilte fish)	*V. cholerae, Vibrio parahaemolyticus,* and *Vibrio vulnificus; Salmonella* and *Shigella* species; hepatitis A and B viruses; tapeworm; anisakiasis
Cheese, milk	*Listeria* species
Eggs	*Salmonella* species
Mayonnaise-containing foods and cream pies	Staphylococcal and clostridial food poisonings
Fried rice	*Bacillus cereus*
Fresh berries	*Cyclospora* species
Canned vegetables or fruits	*Clostridium* species
Sprouts	Enterohemorrhagic *E. coli, Salmonella* species
Animal-to-person (pets and livestock) contact	*Salmonella, Campylobacter, Cryptosporidium,* enterohemorrhagic *E. coli,* and *Giardia* species
Person-to-person (including sexual) contact	All enteric bacteria, viruses, and parasites
Daycare center	*Shigella, Campylobacter, Cryptosporidium,* and *Giardia* species; viruses; *Clostridium difficile*
Hospitalization, antibiotics, or chemotherapy	*C. difficile*
Swimming pool	*Giardia* and *Cryptosporidium* species
Foreign travel	*E. coli* of various types; *Salmonella, Shigella, Campylobacter, Giardia,* and *Cryptosporidium* species; *Entamoeba histolytica*

Adapted from Powell DW. Approach to the patient with diarrhea. In: Yamada T, Alpers DH, Owyang C, et al, eds. *Textbook of Gastroenterology*, 3rd ed. Philadelphia: Lippincott-Raven; 1999.

which causes either watery or bloody diarrhea, and *Vibrio vulnificus,* which causes watery diarrhea and, especially in patients with liver disease, a fatal septicemia. Ingestion of meat contaminated by anthrax (Chapter 302) causes fever, diffuse abdominal pain, and bloody stool or vomitus. Anthrax invades the intestinal mucosa; the organism, or anthrax toxin, causes inflammation, ulceration, and necrosis.

In addition to enteric infections, certain systemic infections (e.g., viral hepatitis [Chapter 150], listeriosis [Chapter 301], legionellosis [Chapter 322]) and emerging infections (e.g., Hanta virus [Chapter 389], severe acute respiratory syndrome [SARS, Chapter 374], avian influenza [Chapter 372]) may cause or manifest with substantial diarrhea.

Environmental and Food Poisonings

Food poisoning refers to the accumulation of toxin in food owing to the growth of toxin-producing organisms, most commonly *Staphylococcus aureus* (Chapter 296), *Bacillus cereus, Clostridium perfringens* (Chapter 304), and *Clostridium botulinum* (Chapter 304). Diarrhea is usually of rapid onset, as early as 4 hours after ingestion, and is often associated with vomiting. Natural toxins also are responsible for mushroom *(Amanita)* poisoning (Chapter 110), which can also cause acute liver and kidney failure.

Environmental poisonings may be caused by heavy metals (arsenic from rat poison, gold, lead, mercury) that impair cell energy production. Arsenic (Chapter 21) also induces cardiovascular collapse at high doses. Insecticide (organophosphates and carbamates) poisoning occurs most commonly in field workers or from the ingestion of contaminated herbs or teas (Chapter 110); diarrhea, excessive saliva, and pulmonary secretions are caused by acetylcholine-stimulated chloride secretion in intestine and other epithelia. Patients often have associated vomiting and abdominal cramps.

Seafood is a common source of food poisoning, particularly fin fish and bivalve shellfish. Most of these toxins cause varying combinations of gastrointestinal (nausea, vomiting, diarrhea) and neurologic symptoms (tingling and burning around the mouth, facial flushing, sweating, headache, palpitations, and dizziness) within hours of seafood ingestion (Chapter 114). Similar symptoms are reported in patients with scombroid poisoning, which is caused by ingestion of decaying flesh of blood fish (tuna, mahi-mahi, marlin, or mackerel) that release large amounts of histamine (Chapter 114).

Marine dinoflagellates (algae) produce toxins that can cause paralytic shellfish poisoning, diarrhetic shellfish poisoning, and ciguatera (Chapter 114). Sporadic outbreaks of diarrhetic shellfish poisoning "red tides" occur when bivalve mollusks ingest dinoflagellates that produce saxitoxins (voltage-sensitive sodium-channel blocker) and okadaic acid (a lipid-soluble toxin that inhibits serine and threonine protein phosphatases 1 and 2A). Ingestion of contaminated mollusks by humans results in diarrhea and neurologic symptoms. Saxitoxins cause predominantly neurologic symptoms (paralytic, neurotoxic, or amnestic shellfish poisonings) and okadaic acid gastrointestinal symptoms (diarrhetic shellfish poisoning).

Food-chain passage of another dinoflagellate species (*Gambierdiscus toxicus*) to fin fish (mackerel, amberjack, snapper, grouper, or barracuda) results in the accumulation of ciguatoxin (Chapter 114) that causes a seafood poisoning called ciguatera. Ciguatoxin activates voltage-sensitive sodium channels and causes neurologic and gastrointestinal symptoms. Fish from the Albemarle-Pamlico estuary (eastern United States) ingest toxic dinoflagellates that cause *Pfiesteria piscicida* poisoning. The dinoflagellate toxins cause nausea, vomiting, abdominal pain, diarrhea, and neurologic symptoms such as fatigue, myalgias, pruritus, circumoral paresthesias, reversal of hot and cold sensation, psychiatric abnormalities, and memory loss. The neurologic symptoms may persist for months to years. Puffer fish poisoning by tetrodotoxin, a voltage-sensitive sodium-channel blocker produced by the fish, causes neurologic symptoms, respiratory paralysis, and death.

Traveler's Diarrhea

North American travelers to developing countries and travelers on airplanes and cruise ships are at high risk for acute infectious diarrhea. Most traveler's diarrhea (85%) is due to enterotoxic *E. coli. E. coli* heat-stable toxin binds to guanylate cyclase in the enterocyte brush-border membrane, where it results in elevation of intracellular cGMP. *E. coli* heat-labile toxin, similar to cholera toxin, binds to the monosialoganglioside GM_1 in the brush-border membrane, thereby resulting in the activation of adenylate cyclase and the elevation of intracellular cAMP. Cyclic AMP and cGMP stimulate intestinal chloride secretion (see Fig. 142-1C) and inhibit the nutrient-independent absorption of sodium and chloride (see Fig. 142-1B). Sodium-glucose absorption is not affected, hence the basis for oral rehydration therapy. Cholera toxin permanently binds to adenylate cyclase until the natural turnover of the intestinal epithelium in 5 to 7 days, thereby resulting in persistent secretion and severe diarrhea. Of the 10 to 15 cases of cholera reported in the United States each year, about 60% are travel associated.

Antibiotic-Associated Diarrheas

Antibiotics are a common cause of hospital-acquired diarrheas that occur in about 20% of patients receiving broad-spectrum antibiotics; about 30% of these diarrheas are due to *Clostridium difficile* (Chapter 304). Hypervirulent, fluoroquinolone-resistant strains that produce increased levels of toxins A and B and a binary toxin have emerged. These strains are associated with an increase in the incidence and severity of *C. difficile* infections, including fulminant *C. difficile* colitis that can lead to colectomy or even death. The A and B toxins produced by *C. difficile* can cause diarrhea. In animal models, IL-8, substance P, and leukotriene B_4 were found to mediate toxin A–stimulated intestinal fluid secretion. *C. difficile* can cause severe diarrhea, pseudomembranous colitis, or toxic megacolon. Patients may have a relapsing course after seemingly successful therapy with metronidazole or vancomycin.

Nosocomial Hospital Diarrhea

Diarrhea is the most common nosocomial illness among hospitalized patients and residents in long-term care facilities. Common causes include antibiotic-associated diarrhea, *C. difficile* infection, medications, fecal impaction, tube feeding, and underlying illness. Magnesium-containing laxatives, antacids, and lactulose cause osmotic diarrheas. Bisacodyl laxatives cause secretory diarrhea. Colchicine, neomycin, methotrexate, and para-aminosalicylic acid damage the enterocyte membrane. Cholestyramine, colestipol, and colesevelam bind bile salts and can result in malabsorption. Gold therapy causes intestinal inflammation and diarrhea. Liquid formulations of medications cause diarrhea (elixir diarrhea) because of the high content of sorbitol or other nonabsorbable sugars (e.g., mannitol) used to sweeten the elixir; patients prescribed liquid medications through feeding tubes may receive more than 20 g of sorbitol daily. An important but poorly understood cause of diarrhea is enteral (tube) feeding (Chapter 223), particularly in critically ill patients, who often develop diarrhea. Dysmotility, increased intestinal permeability, and low sodium content in enteral formulas may be contributing factors.

Patients in mental health institutions and nursing homes have a high incidence of nosocomial infectious diarrhea (e.g., *C. difficile* and less commonly *Shigella, Salmonella,* hemorrhagic *E. coli, Giardia, Entamoeba histolytica*). Infectious diarrhea, 50% or more of which is caused by *C. difficile,* is also common in acute-care hospitals. Severe *C. difficile* infection has also been reported among peripartum women. If outside foods are not brought to hospitalized patients, the likelihood of a nosocomial infection caused by *Salmonella* or *Shigella* is extremely rare. Immunosuppressed patients are also susceptible to nosocomial viral infections (rotavirus, norovirus, adenovirus, and coxsackievirus).

Cancer Treatment–Related Diarrhea

Abdominal or whole body radiation virtually always causes an increased frequency of bowel movements that are often watery. Cancer chemotherapy with amsacrine, azacitidine, cytarabine, dactinomycin, daunorubicin, doxorubicin, floxuridine, 5-fluorouracil, 6-mercaptopurine, methotrexate, plicamycin, IL-2, and resveratrol may cause mild to moderate diarrhea. Irinotecan (CPT-11) and the combination of 5-fluorouracil plus leucovorin are frequent causes of severe watery diarrhea.

Daycare Diarrhea

More than 7 million children in the United States attend daycare, where diarrhea is extremely common, and secondary infection of family members occurs in 10 to 20% of cases. Most outbreaks of diarrhea are due to rotavirus or norovirus; less common causes are *Shigella* (Chapter 317), *Giardia* (Chapter 359), and *Cryptosporidium* (Chapter 358).

Runner's Diarrhea

Diarrhea occurs in 10 to 25% of individuals who exercise vigorously, especially women marathon runners and triathletes. Some athletes have associated abdominal cramps, urgency, nausea, or vomiting. The pathophysiology of runner's diarrhea is unknown. Release of intestinal secretogogues, especially prostaglandins, hormones, or ischemia, may be involved.

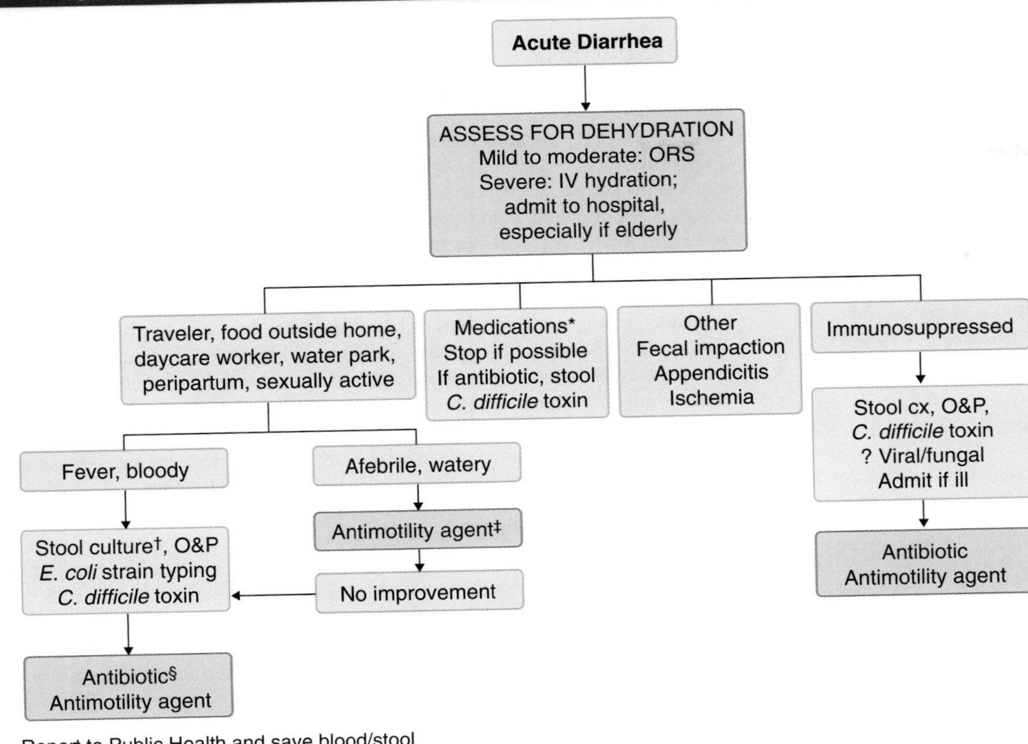

FIGURE 142-2. Approach to the diagnosis of acute diarrhea. *More than 700 medications cause diarrhea, including furosemide, caffeine, protease inhibitors, thyroid preparations, metformin, mycophenolate mofetil, sirolimus, cholinergic drugs, colchicine, theophylline, selective serotonin reuptake inhibitors, proton pump inhibitors, histamine-2 blockers, 5-ASA derivatives, angiotensin-converting enzyme inhibitors, bisacodyl, senna, aloe, anthraquinones, and magnesium- or phosphorus-containing medications. †Specifically request culture for *Yersinia, Plesiomonas,* enterohemorrhagic *Escherichia coli* serotype O157:H7, and *Aeromonas* if suspected. ‡If high suspicion for *Clostridium difficile* or invasive bacterial infection, wait for stool culture and toxin studies before starting. Racecadotril has antisecretory effects without paralyzing intestinal motility and can be used if available. §Not recommended for patients with bloody diarrhea due to *E. coli* O157:H7. CX = culture; IV therapy = intravenous rehydration; O&P = ova and parasites; ORS = oral rehydration solution.

DIAGNOSIS

Acute watery diarrhea may be due to infections, food toxins, or medications, or the acute diarrhea may signal the onset of a chronic disease (Fig. 142-2; see Tables 142-1 and 142-2) (Chapters 310 through 320, 344, 345, 359, 360, 364, 365, 387, and 388). The diagnostic approach in patients with fever and watery or bloody diarrhea should focus on stool cultures for *Campylobacter, Salmonella,* and *Shigella* species. Routine stool culture is not indicated when diarrhea occurs after 3 to 5 days of hospitalization, except in patients with neutropenia, human immunodeficiency virus infection, or signs of enteric infection. In patients with a history of recent antibiotic use, hospitalization, or peripartum, stools for *C. difficile* toxin should be obtained. Organisms that cause diarrhea but are not routinely tested by clinical microbiology laboratories include *Yersinia, Plesiomonas,* enterohemorrhagic *E. coli* serotype O157:H7, *Aeromonas, Cyclospora,* microsporidia, and noncholera *Vibrio.* Parasites such as *Giardia, Cryptosporidium,* and *Strongyloides* can be difficult to detect in stool but may be diagnosed by stool antigen testing or intestinal biopsy. Despite all testing techniques available, 20 to 40% of acute infectious diarrheas remain undiagnosed.

TREATMENT Rx

Goals for the treatment of diarrhea include fluid replacement, antidiarrheal agents, nutritional support, and antimicrobial therapy when indicated. Because death in patients with acute diarrhea is caused by dehydration, the first task is to assess the degree of dehydration and to replace fluid and electrolyte deficits.

Fluid Replacement

Severely dehydrated patients should be treated with intravenous Ringer's lactate or saline solution, with additional potassium and bicarbonate as needed. Oral rehydration solutions, which are used extensively to replace diarrheal fluid and electrolyte losses, are effective because they contain sodium, sugars, and, often, amino acids that use nutrient-dependent sodium uptake transporters. In alert patients with mild to moderate dehydration, oral rehydration solution is equally effective as intravenous hydration in repairing fluid and electrolyte losses. Oral rehydration solutions can be given to infants and children in volumes of 50 to 100 mL/kg over 4 to 6 hours; adults may need to drink 1000 mL/hr. Reduced-osmolarity solutions (Na^{++} 75 mmol/L, osmolarity 245 mmol/L versus Na^{++} 90 mmol/L, osmolarity 311 mmol/L in standard solutions) are better tolerated and effective in noncholera diarrhea but may cause hyponatremia in patients with high-volume diarrhea, particularly children. Glucose-based solutions, although effective in rehydrating the patient, may worsen the diarrhea. In contrast to glucose-based solutions, polymeric rice-based solutions decrease diarrhea in cholera victims; rice is digested to many glucose monomers that aid in the absorption of intestinal secretions. These solutions may not decrease stool output in acute diarrhea, but they will effectively rehydrate the patient despite continued diarrhea. After rehydration has been accomplished, oral rehydration solutions are given at rates equaling stool loss plus insensible losses until the diarrhea ceases.

Reducing Diarrhea

Bismuth subsalicylate (Pepto-Bismol, 525 mg orally every 30 minutes to 1 hour for five doses, may repeat on day 2) is safe and efficacious in bacterial infectious diarrheas. Opiates and anticholinergic drugs are not recommended for invasive bacterial infectious diarrheas because these drugs paralyze intestinal motility and predispose to increased colonization, invasion, and prolonged excretion of infectious organisms. The opiate loperamide is safe in acute or traveler's diarrhea, provided that it is not given to patients with dysentery (high fever, with blood or pus in the stool), and especially when administered concomitantly with effective antibiotics. A combination of loperamide (2 mg orally four times a day) plus simethicone (125 mg orally four times a day) may reduce the abdominal cramps and duration of traveler's diarrhea. Racecadotril (100 mg orally three times a day in adults, 1.5 mg/kg of body weight orally three times a day in children), an intestinal enkephalinase inhibitor that is antisecretory but does not paralyze intestinal motility, is effective in the treatment of acute diarrhea in children and adults. The diarrhea associated with enteral nutrition (Chapter 223) often can be managed with pectin (4 g/kg body weight daily) or, if there are no contraindications, with loperamide (2 mg orally four times a day for 3 to 7 days, maximal dose 16 mg daily), and diarrhea is not a reason to stop tube feeding unless stool volumes exceed 1 L/day.

Anxiolytics (e.g., diazepam 2 mg orally two to four times daily) and antiemetics (e.g., promethazine 12.5 to 25 mg orally once or twice daily) that decrease sensory perception may make symptoms more tolerable and are safe. Some foods or food-derived substances (green bananas, pectins [amylase-resistant starch], zinc) lessen the amount or duration of diarrhea in children. Unabsorbed amylase-resistant starches are metabolized in the colon to short-chain fatty acids that enhance fluid absorption. Zinc supplementation (20 mg of elemental zinc orally once a day) is effective in preventing recurrences of diarrhea in malnourished children; copper deficiency is a potential complication of prolonged zinc therapy.

Probiotics may be of benefit in children with acute diarrhea, predominantly that due to rotavirus infection. *Lactobacillus* GG (10^{10} colony-forming units [CFU]/250 mL daily until diarrhea stops) added to an oral rehydration solution decreases the duration of diarrhea.

Antibiotics

While the clinician is awaiting stool culture results to guide specific therapy (Chapter 295), the fluoroquinolones (e.g., ciprofloxacin, 500 mg orally twice a day for 1 to 3 days, or levofloxacin, 500 mg orally daily for 1 to 3 days) are the treatment of choice when antibiotics are indicated (see Fig. 142-2). Trimethoprim-sulfamethoxazole (one double-strength tablet orally twice a day for 5 days or two single-strength tablets orally twice a day for 5 days) is second-line therapy. If the symptom complex suggests *Campylobacter* infection, azithromycin (500 mg orally once a day for 3 days) should be added. Regardless of the cause of infectious diarrhea, patients should be treated with antibiotics if they are immunosuppressed; have valvular, vascular, or orthopedic prostheses; have congenital hemolytic anemias (especially if salmonellosis is involved); or are extremely young or old.

Certain infectious diarrheas should be treated with antibiotics, including those associated with shigellosis (Chapter 317), cholera (Chapter 310), pseudomembranous enterocolitis (Chapter 304), parasitic infestations (Chapters 358 to 360 and 365), and sexually transmitted diseases (Chapter 293). Treatment of *E. coli* serotype O157:H7 infection is not recommended at present because current antibiotics do not appear to be helpful and the incidence of complications (hemolytic-uremic syndrome) may be greater after antibiotic therapy. Antibiotics are not effective for viral diarrhea or cryptosporidiosis.

For traveler's diarrhea, ciprofloxacin (500 mg orally two times a day for 3 days) is an effective treatment. The nonabsorbable antibiotic rifaximin (200 mg taken orally three times a day or 400 mg two times a day for 3 days) is safe and effective for treatment of traveler's diarrhea in Mexico, but it may not be effective against *Campylobacter* and *Shigella* infections.

Fluoroquinolone-resistant and trimethoprim-sulfamethoxazole-resistant strains of *Shigella, E. coli, Salmonella, Campylobacter,* and *C. difficile* have emerged. Azithromycin, 500 mg orally on day 1 and 250 mg orally once a day for 4 days, may be an effective alternative treatment for resistant strains of *Shigella* and *Campylobacter* and for traveler's diarrhea acquired in Mexico.

If *C. difficile* is suspected on an epidemiologic basis, metronidazole (250 mg orally four times a day or 500 mg orally three times a day for 10 days) or oral vancomycin (125 to 250 mg orally four times a day for 10 days) should be prescribed. In patients with recurrent *C. difficile* infection that is associated with low serum antibody titers to toxin A, immunotherapy with monoclonal antibodies against toxin A and B[1] or fecal bacteriotherapy may decrease recurrence rates. Non–*C. difficile* antibiotic-induced diarrhea is generally mild and self-limited, and it usually clears spontaneously or in response to cholestyramine therapy (4 g orally four times a day for 2 weeks).

Treatment for chemotherapy-induced and radiation-induced mild to moderate diarrhea includes loperamide (2 mg orally four times a day) and nonsteroidal anti-inflammatory drugs (NSAIDs) (e.g., naproxen, 250 to 500 mg orally twice daily). Octreotide may be an effective treatment in those with severe diarrhea in doses up to 700 μg administered subcutaneously daily.

PREVENTION

Rotavirus vaccination (Chapter 388) reduces the risk of infection and generally results in milder symptoms among those infected.[2,3] Travelers to high-risk countries (Central America and parts of Latin America, Africa, Asia, the Middle East) should avoid ingestion of tap water and ice and of raw meat, raw seafood, and raw vegetables. An oral cholera vaccine against recombinant toxin B subunit and killed whole-cell (rBS-WC) is effective in preventing infection from the O1 El Tor strain and partially effective against enterotoxigenic *E. coli* strains.[4] Cholera vaccination is recommended for relief workers and health professionals who work in endemic countries and for individuals who are immunocompromised or have chronic illnesses or hypochlorhydria. Rifaximin (200 mg orally per day for 2 weeks) is safe and effective for preventing traveler's diarrhea in Mexico,[5] and the combination of rifaximin plus loperamide is better than either one alone. Bismuth subsalicylate (525 mg orally four times a day for up to 3 weeks) is also effective. Loperamide and NSAIDs are taken prophylactically by many runners who are susceptible to runner's diarrhea, but it is not clear whether they are effective.

CHRONIC DIARRHEA

An estimated 5% of the U.S. population suffers from chronic diarrhea, and about 40% of these individuals are older than 60 years of age. In 25 to 50% of cases, expert history and physical examination may be sufficient to make a definitive diagnosis (Fig. 142-3). The addition of stool culture and examination for ova and parasites, determination of stool fat, and flexible sigmoidoscopy or colonoscopy with biopsy raises the diagnostic rate to about 75%. The remaining 25% of patients with chronic diarrhea may need extensive testing and perhaps hospitalization to make a diagnosis.

Prolonged, Persistent Infectious Diarrheas

Prolonged infectious diarrheas (>2 weeks) may be due to persistent or recurrent infections. These diarrheas occur most commonly in children exposed to unsafe drinking water in developing countries, patients who have acquired immunodeficiency syndrome (AIDS) or are immunosuppressed for other reasons, and recent travelers. The most common causes in children in developing countries are enteropathogenic and enteroadherent *E. coli* infections (Chapter 312). Other common organisms include *Giardia* (Chapter 359), *Cryptosporidium* (Chapter 358), *Entamoeba* (Chapter 360), *Isospora* (Chapter 361), and microsporidia (Chapter 358). Recurrent or prolonged infectious diarrhea may lead to severe malnutrition and death (mortality rate, 50%). Treatment includes nutrition support with supplemental vitamin A (200,000

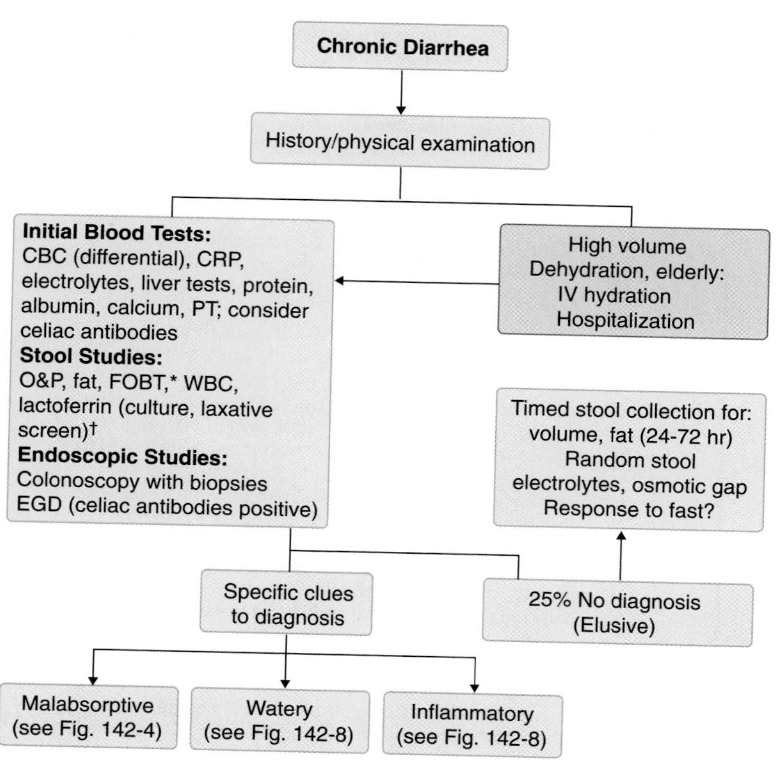

FIGURE 142-3. Initial approach to chronic diarrhea. *Fecal occult blood testing (FOBT) is a sensitive test for underlying bowel inflammation. †Perform stool culture in those who are immunosuppressed; perform laxative screen if laxative abuse is suspected. CBC = complete blood count; CRP = C-reactive protein; EGD = esophagogastroduodenoscopy; IV = intravenous; O&P = ova and parasites; PT = prothrombin time; WBC = white blood cells.

IU twice yearly) and zinc (20 mg elemental daily for 14 days). Severe disease may require total parenteral nutrition.

In AIDS patients, protracted diarrhea may be caused by treatable agents such as *Entamoeba histolytica, Giardia,* or *Strongyloides* or by organisms such as *Cryptosporidium, Isospora belli,* and microsporidia that are difficult to treat or untreatable. The most effective treatment is retroviral therapy to improve the immune system (Chapter 396).

Up to 10% of travelers returning from developing countries have infectious diarrhea that persists for longer than 3 to 4 weeks. Stool should be examined for culture and for ova and parasites; in patients with a recent history of antibiotic use, stool should also be sent for *C. difficile* toxin. Any specific organisms that are identified should be treated. If treatment with trimethoprim-sulfamethoxazole or a fluoroquinolone has been unsuccessful, tetracycline (250 mg orally four times a day for 7 to 10 days) or metronidazole (250 mg orally three times a day for 7 to 10 days) can be tried. After documented infectious diarrhea, 25% of patients experience pain, bloating, urgency, a sense of incomplete evacuation, and loose stools for 6 months or longer; some of these patients have celiac disease, so screening (see later) is warranted in this setting. When no other cause is found, these patients are deemed to have postinfectious irritable bowel syndrome (Chapter 139).

Sporadic outbreaks of severe, prolonged diarrhea, often greater than 1 year in duration, occasionally have been reported. This form of prolonged diarrhea is called *Brainerd's diarrhea.* The organism has yet to be identified. The diarrhea is difficult to treat; cholestyramine (4 g orally three times a day) may be helpful.

Malabsorptive Syndromes

Malabsorption is caused by many different diseases, drugs (e.g., the lipase inhibitor orlistat; Chapter 227), and nutritional products (the nonabsorbable fat olestra) that impair intraluminal digestion, mucosal absorption, or delivery of the nutrient to the systemic circulation (Fig. 142-5; Table 142-3). Dietary fat is the nutrient most difficult to absorb. Fatty stools (steatorrhea) are the hallmark of malabsorption; a stool test for fat is the best screening test. Malabsorption does not always cause diarrhea. Clinical signs of vitamin or mineral deficiencies may occur in the absence of diarrhea. A careful history is crucial in guiding further testing to confirm the suspicion of malabsorption and to make a specific diagnosis (see Fig. 142-4). The goals of treatment are to correct or treat the underlying disease and to replenish losses of water, electrolytes, and nutrients.

Conditions That Impair Intraluminal Digestion

Most digestion and absorption of nutrients occur in the small intestine (Fig. 142-5). Carbohydrates and most dietary proteins are water soluble and readily digested by pancreatic enzymes. Pancreatic proteases (trypsinogen, chymotrypsinogen, procarboxypeptidases) are secreted from acinar cells in inactive forms. The cleavage of trypsinogen to trypsin by the duodenal brush-border peptidase enteropeptidase (enterokinase) allows trypsin to cleave the remaining trypsinogen and other proteases to their active form.

Most dietary lipids (long-chain triglycerides, cholesterol, and fat-soluble vitamins) are water insoluble and must undergo lipolysis and incorporation into mixed micelles before they can be absorbed across the intestinal mucosa. Pancreatic lipase, in the presence of its cofactor, colipase, cleaves long-chain triglycerides into fatty acids and monoglycerides. The products of lipolysis interact with bile salts and phospholipids to form mixed micelles, which also incorporate cholesterol and fat-soluble vitamins (D, A, K, and E) in their hydrophobic centers. Bicarbonate secreted from pancreatic duct cells is physiologically important because pancreatic enzyme activity and bile salt micelle formation are optimum at a luminal pH of 6 to 8.

IMPAIRED MIXING

Surgical alterations, such as partial gastrectomy with gastrojejunostomy (Billroth II anastomosis) or gastrointestinal bypass surgeries for obesity, result in the release of biliary and pancreatic secretions into the intestine at a site remote from the site of entry of gastric contents. This imbalance can result in impaired lipolysis and impaired micelle formation, with subsequent fat malabsorption. Bypass of the duodenum also impairs absorption of iron, folate, and calcium. Rapid transit through the jejunum contributes to the malabsorption of nutrients. Individuals with these conditions also have surgical anastomoses that predispose to bacterial overgrowth.

DUMPING SYNDROME

After esophageal (distal esophagectomy, myomectomy for achalasia), gastric (Nissan wrap, hiatal hernia repair, gastrojejunostomy), and bariatric (Roux-en-Y and duodenal switch gastric bypass) surgeries, the unregulated delivery of concentrated sugars and food into the duodenum and jejunum results in altered insulin regulation, maldigestion, osmotic movement of fluid into the intestinal lumen, and rapid transit such that intestinal contact time is insufficient for absorption of nutrients.

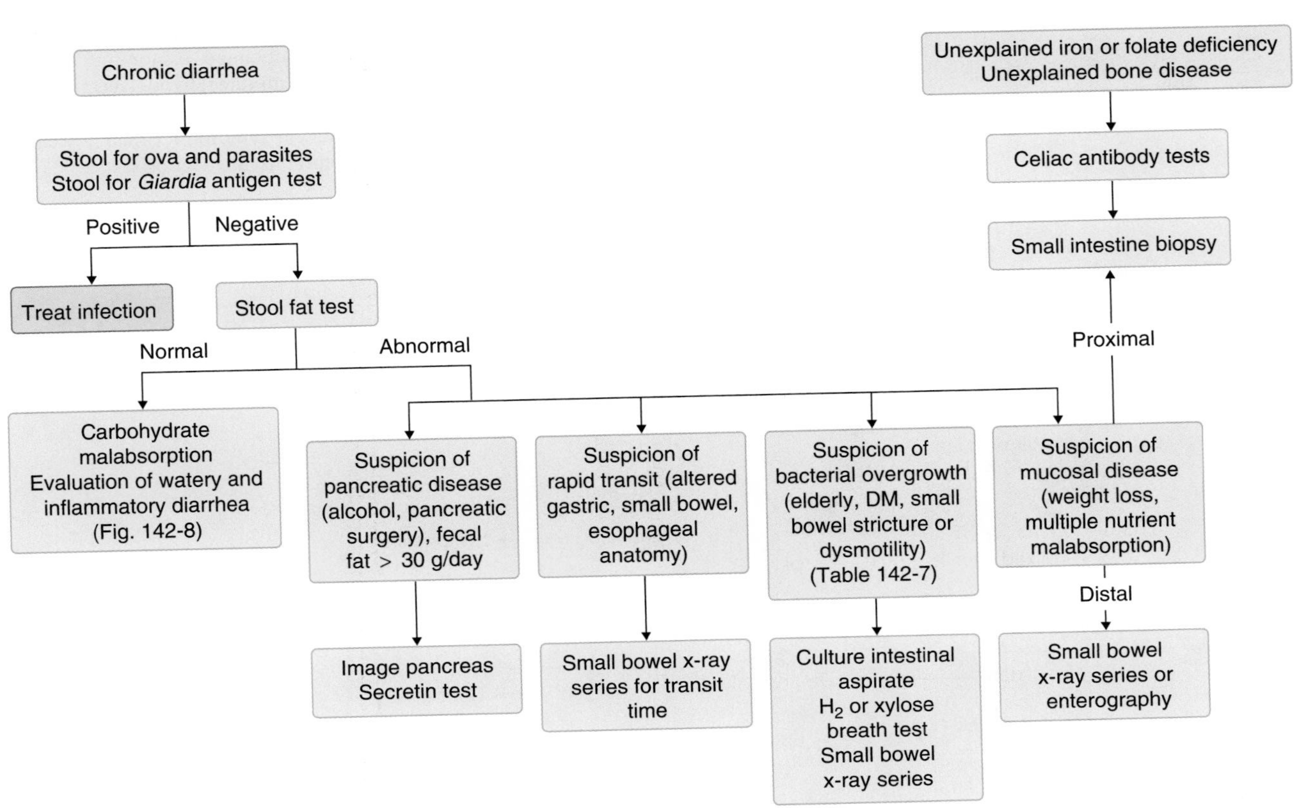

FIGURE 142-4. **Approach to the diagnosis of malabsorption.** DM = diabetes mellitus.

TABLE 142-3 CAUSES OF MALABSORPTION

MECHANISM OF MALABSORPTION	CONDITIONS
Impaired mixing	Partial/total gastrectomy Gastric bypass surgery
Impaired lipolysis	Chronic pancreatitis Pancreatic cancer Congenital pancreatic insufficiency Congenital colipase deficiency Gastrinoma
Impaired micelle formation	Severe chronic liver disease Cholestatic liver disease Bacterial overgrowth Crohn's disease Ileal resection Gastrinoma
Impaired mucosal absorption	Lactase deficiency Congenital enterokinase deficiency Abetalipoproteinemia Giardiasis Celiac disease Tropical sprue Agammaglobulinemia Amyloidosis AIDS-related (infections, enteropathy) Radiation enteritis Graft-versus-host disease Whipple's disease Eosinophilic gastroenteritis Megaloblastic gut Collagenous sprue Ulcerative jejunitis Lymphoma Bacterial overgrowth Short-bowel syndrome Mastocytosis
Impaired nutrient delivery	Congenital lymphangiectasia Lymphoma Tuberculosis Constrictive pericarditis Severe congestive heart failure
Unknown	Hypoparathyroidism Adrenal insufficiency Hyperthyroidism Carcinoid syndrome

AIDS = acquired immunodeficiency syndrome.

IMPAIRED LIPOLYSIS

A deficiency in pancreatic lipase may be caused by the congenital absence of pancreatic lipase or by destruction of the pancreatic gland due to alcohol-related pancreatitis, cystic fibrosis, or pancreatic cancer. Pancreatic lipase also can be denatured by excess secretion of gastric acid (e.g., Zollinger-Ellison syndrome; Chapter 201).

CHRONIC PANCREATITIS

Chronic pancreatitis (Chapter 146) is the most common cause of pancreatic insufficiency and impaired lipolysis. In the United States, chronic pancreatitis most commonly results from alcohol abuse; in contrast, tropical (nutritional) pancreatitis is most common worldwide. Malabsorption of fat does not occur until more than 90% of the pancreas is destroyed.

CLINICAL MANIFESTATIONS

Individuals with pancreatic causes of malabsorption typically present with bulky, fat-laden stools (usually >30 g of fat per day), abdominal pain, and diabetes, although some present with diabetes in the absence of gastrointestinal symptoms. Stools usually are not watery because undigested triglycerides form large emulsion droplets with little osmotic force and, in contrast to fatty acids, do not stimulate water and electrolyte secretion in the colon. Deficiency of fat-soluble vitamins is seen only rarely, presumably because gastric and residual pancreatic lipase generates enough fatty acids for some micelle formation. In severe disease, subclinical protein malabsorption, manifested by the presence of undigested meat fibers in the stool, and subclinical carbohydrate malabsorption, manifested by gas-filled, floating stools, can occur. Weight loss, when it occurs, is most often caused by decreased oral intake to avoid abdominal pain or diarrhea and less commonly by malabsorption.

In the dumping syndrome, patients may present with severe diarrhea, malabsorption, abdominal cramping, gas, and weight loss. Some have associated sweatiness, dizziness, and altered cognition due to postprandial hypoglycemia.

DIAGNOSIS

Between 30 and 40% of individuals with alcohol-related chronic pancreatitis have calcifications on abdominal radiographs. A qualitative or quantitative test for fecal fat is positive in individuals whose pancreas is more than 90% destroyed. Noninvasive tests of pancreatic function are not sensitive enough to detect mild to moderate insufficiency, so the secretin stimulation test is preferred (Table 142-4) if it can be obtained. A modified oral glucose tolerance test that shows late (120 to 180 minutes) hypoglycemia and an early (30 minutes) rise in hematocrit with an increased pulse rate suggests the dumping syndrome in patients with consistent symptoms. Small bowel barium study to assess transit time may be helpful in the diagnosis.

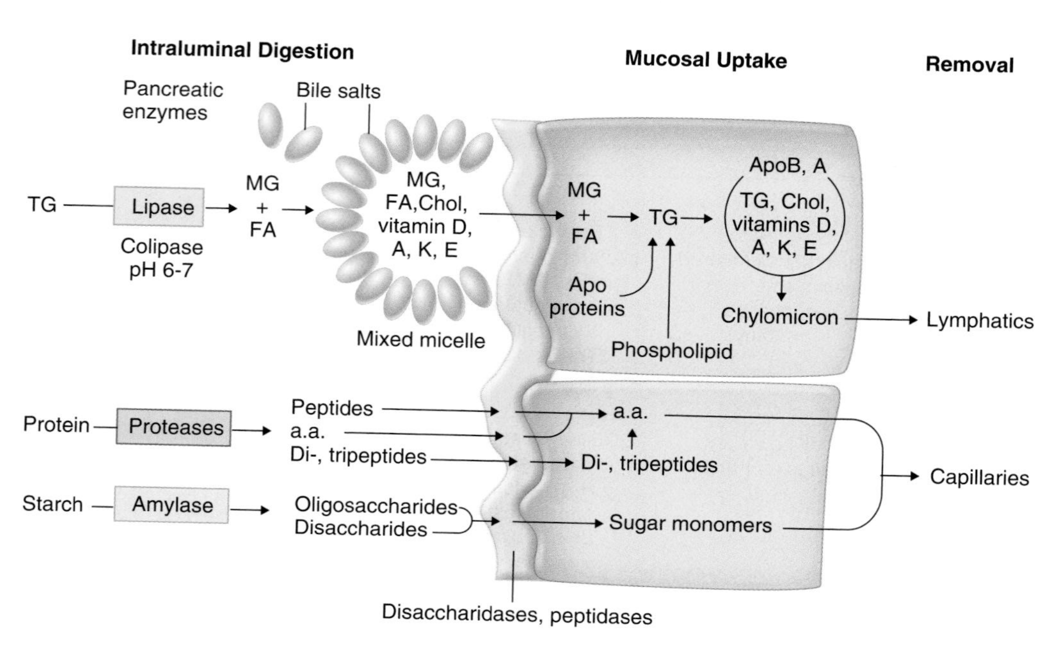

FIGURE 142-5. **Phases of intestinal digestion and absorption of dietary fat, protein, and carbohydrate.** a.a. = Amino acids; ApoB, A = apolipoproteins B and A; Chol = cholesterol; FA = fatty acids; MG = monoglycerides; TG = triglycerides.

TABLE 142-4 TESTS FOR THE EVALUATION OF MALABSORPTION*

TEST	COMMENTS
GENERAL TESTS OF ABSORPTION	
Quantitative stool fat test	Gold standard test of fat malabsorption, with which all other tests are compared. Requires ingestion of a high-fat diet (100 g) for 2 days before and during the collection. Stool is collected for 3 days. Normally, <7 g/24 hr is excreted on a high-fat diet. Borderline abnormalities of 8-14 g/24 hr may be seen in secretory or osmotic diarrheas that are not caused by malabsorption. There are false-negative findings if fat intake is inadequate. False-positive results can occur if mineral oil laxatives or rectal suppositories (e.g., cocoa butter) are given to the patient before stool collection.
Qualitative stool fat test	Sudan stain of a stool sample for fat. Many fat droplets per medium-power field (×40) constitute a positive test result. The nuclear magnetic resonance method determines the percentage of fat in the stool (normal, <20%). The test depends on an adequate fat intake (100 g/day). There is high sensitivity (90%) and specificity (90%) with fat malabsorption of >10 g/24 hr. Sensitivity drops with stool fat in the range of 6-10 g/24 hr.
D-Xylose test	A test of small intestinal mucosal absorption, used to distinguish mucosal malabsorption from malabsorption due to pancreatic insufficiency. An oral dose of D-xylose (25 g/500 mL water) is administered, and D-xylose excretion is measured in a 5-hr urine collection. Normally, >4 g of D-xylose is excreted in the urine over 5 hr. The test also may be positive in bacterial overgrowth owing to metabolism of D-xylose by bacteria in the intestinal lumen. False-positive test results occur with renal failure, ascites, and an incomplete urine collection. Blood levels at 1 and 3 hr improve sensitivity. May be normal with mild or limited mucosal disease.
Hydrogen breath test	Most useful in the diagnosis of lactase deficiency. An oral dose of lactose (1 g/kg body weight) is administered after measurement of basal breath H_2 levels. The sole source of H_2 in the mammal is bacterial fermentation; unabsorbed lactose makes its way to colonic bacteria, resulting in excess breath H_2. A *late peak* (within 3-6 hr) of >20 ppm of exhaled H_2 after lactose ingestion suggests lactose malabsorption. Absorption of other carbohydrates (e.g., sucrose, glucose, fructose) also can be tested.
SPECIFIC TESTS FOR MALABSORPTION	
Tests for Pancreatic Function	
Secretin stimulation test	The gold standard test of pancreatic function. Requires duodenal test intubation with a double-lumen tube and collection of pancreatic juice in response to IV secretin. Allows measurement of bicarbonate (HCO_3^-) and pancreatic enzymes. A sensitive test of pancreatic function, but labor intensive and invasive.
Fecal elastase-1 test	Stool test for pancreatic function. Equal sensitivity to the secretin stimulation test for the diagnosis of moderate-to-severe pancreatic insufficiency. More specific than the fecal chymotrypsin test. Unreliable with mild insufficiency. False-positive results occur with increased stool volume and intestinal mucosal diseases.
Tests for Bacterial Overgrowth	
Quantitative culture of small intestinal aspirate	Gold standard test for bacterial overgrowth. Greater than 10^5 colony-forming units (CFU)/mL in the jejunum suggests bacterial overgrowth. Requires special anaerobic sample collection, rapid anaerobic and aerobic plating, and care to avoid oropharyngeal contamination. False-negative results occur with focal jejunal diverticula and when overgrowth is distal to the site aspirated.
Hydrogen breath test	The 50-g glucose breath test has a sensitivity of 90% for growth of 10^5 colonic-type bacteria in the small intestine. If bacterial overgrowth is present, increased H_2 is excreted in the breath. A hydrogen level (within 2 hr) of >20 ppm suggests bacterial overgrowth. False-negative results occur with non-hydrogen-producing organisms.
^{14}C-D-xylose breath test	This test uses 1 g of carbon 14–labeled D-xylose. It has a sensitivity and specificity >90% for growth of 10^5 test colonic-type bacteria in the small intestine. Bacteria metabolize D-xylose with release of $^{14}CO_2$, which is absorbed and exhaled. Non-degraded D-xylose is absorbed in the small bowel and does not reach the colon, yielding a greater specificity than the lactulose H_2 breath test. A nonradioactive ^{13}C-D-xylose breath test is suitable for children and pregnant women.
Tests for Mucosal Disease	
Small bowel biopsy	Obtained for a specific diagnosis when there is a high index of suspicion for small intestinal disease. Several biopsy specimens (4-5) must be obtained to maximize the diagnostic yield. Distal duodenal biopsy specimens are usually adequate for diagnosis, but occasionally enteroscopy with jejunal biopsy specimens is necessary. Small intestinal biopsy provides a specific diagnosis in some diseases (e.g., intestinal infection, Whipple's disease, abetalipoproteinemia, agammaglobulinemia, lymphangiectasia, lymphoma, amyloidosis). In other conditions, such as celiac disease and tropical sprue, the biopsy specimens show characteristic findings, but the diagnosis is made on improvement after treatment.
Tests of Ileal Function	
Schilling test	A test of vitamin B_{12} absorption (see Table 167-1 in Chapter 167).
^{75}SeHCAT test	This is a test of bile acid absorption. Seven days after ingestion of radiolabeled synthetic selenium-homocholic acid conjugated with taurine (^{75}SeHCAT), whole body retention is measured by a gamma-counting device. The result is expressed as a fraction of baseline ingestion. Retention values of less than 10% are abnormal and indicate bile acid malabsorption with a sensitivity of 80-90% and specificity of 70-100%. The radiation dose is equivalent to a plain chest x-ray. Liver disease and bacterial overgrowth may give false results. Not approved for use in the United States.

*Not all these tests are readily available. A strong suspicion for any disease may warrant foregoing an extensive work-up and obtaining the test with highest diagnostic yield. In some cases, empirical treatment, such as removing lactose from the diet of an otherwise healthy individual with lactose intolerance, is warranted without any testing.

TREATMENT Rx

Pancreatic enzyme replacement and analgesics are the mainstays of treatment for chronic pancreatitis (Chapter 146). It is difficult to correct fat malabsorption completely with exogenous pancreatic enzymes because of their inactivation by acid and pepsin in the stomach. Normally, 28,000 U of lipase is present in the duodenal lumen with each meal. A high lipase-containing pancreatic enzyme preparation (25,000 to 40,000 U of lipase in the form of uncoated enzymes or enteric-coated, pH-sensitive microspheres) should be prescribed with each meal. Mini-microsphere preparations (e.g., 20,000 U of lipase taken orally with each meal) may be best tolerated owing to their small capsule size. Pancreatic proteases present in enzyme preparations may reduce abdominal pain by inactivating cholecystokinin-releasing factor in the duodenum. Uncoated preparations may be more effective in pain relief because coated preparations release enzymes predominantly distal to the duodenum.

A histamine-2 receptor antagonist (e.g., ranitidine, 150 mg orally taken two times a day) or a proton pump inhibitor (e.g., lansoprazole, 15 to 30 mg orally once a day) should be added to uncoated pancreatic enzyme replacement therapy in patients with a poor response.

In the dumping syndrome, treatment is with a diet that is low in concentrated sugars divided into six small meals. Administration of pectin (15 g with each meal) may slow gastric emptying. In patients who are refractory to dietary measures, a short-acting somatostatin analogue (e.g., octreotide, 25 to 200 μg subcutaneously three times a day) or the better tolerated long-acting octreotide preparation (10 to 20 mg subcutaneously monthly) improves dumping symptoms. In patients with predominant reactive hypoglycemia 1 to 3 hours after a meal (late dumping), an α-glycosidase hydrolase inhibitor (e.g., acarbose, 50 to 100 mg orally three times daily) that blocks carbohydrate absorption in the small bowel may be beneficial. Continuous tube feeding is also effective.

IMPAIRED MICELLE FORMATION

PATHOBIOLOGY

Bile salt concentrations in the intestinal lumen can fall to less than the critical concentration (2 to 3 mmol/L) needed for micelle formation because of decreased bile salt synthesis (severe liver disease), decreased bile salt delivery (cholestasis), or removal of luminal bile salts (bacterial overgrowth, terminal ileal disease or resection, cholestyramine therapy, acid hypersecretion). Fat malabsorption resulting from impaired micelle formation is generally not as severe as malabsorption resulting from pancreatic lipase deficiency, presumably because fatty acids and monoglycerides can form lamellar structures, which to a certain extent can be absorbed. Malabsorption of fat-soluble vitamins (D, A, K, and E) may be marked, however, because micelle formation is required for their absorption.

Decreased Bile Salt Synthesis and Delivery

Malabsorption can occur in individuals with cholestatic liver disease or bile duct obstruction. The clinical consequences of malabsorption are seen most often in women with primary biliary cirrhosis because of the prolonged nature of the illness. Although these individuals can present with steatorrhea, osteoporosis or, less commonly, osteomalacia is the most common presentation. The cause of bone disease in these patients is poorly understood and often is not related to vitamin D deficiency. Bone disease is treated with calcium supplements (and vitamin D if a deficiency is documented), weight-bearing exercise, and a bisphosphonate (e.g., alendronate, 10 mg orally once daily or 70 mg orally once weekly).

Intestinal Bacterial Overgrowth

In health, only small numbers of lactobacilli, enterococci, gram-positive aerobes, or facultative anaerobes can be cultured from the upper small bowel lumen. Motility and acid are the most important factors in keeping the number of bacteria in the upper small bowel low. Any condition that produces local stasis or recirculation of colonic luminal contents allows development of a predominantly "colonic" flora (coliforms and anaerobes, such as *Bacteroides* and *Clostridium*) in the small intestine (see Table 142-4). Anaerobic bacteria cause impaired micelle formation by releasing cholylamidases, which deconjugate bile salts. The unconjugated bile salts, with their higher pK_a, are more likely to be in the protonated form at the normal upper small intestinal pH of 6 to 7 and can be absorbed passively. As a result, the concentration of bile salts decreases in the intestinal lumen and can fall to less than the critical micellar concentration, causing malabsorption of fats and fat-soluble vitamins. Vitamin B_{12} deficiency and carbohydrate malabsorption also can occur with generalized bacterial overgrowth. Anaerobic bacteria ingest vitamin B_{12} and release proteases that degrade brush-border disaccharidases. Although anaerobic bacteria use vitamin B_{12}, they synthesize folate. Individuals with bacterial overgrowth usually have low serum vitamin B_{12} levels but normal or high folate levels; this helps distinguish bacterial overgrowth from tropical sprue, in which vitamin B_{12} and folate levels are usually low because of decreased mucosal uptake.

CLINICAL MANIFESTATIONS

Individuals with bacterial overgrowth can present with diarrhea, abdominal cramps, gas and bloating, weight loss, and signs and symptoms of vitamin B_{12} and fat-soluble vitamin deficiency. Watery diarrhea occurs because of the osmotic load of unabsorbed carbohydrates and stimulation of colonic secretion by unabsorbed fatty acids.

DIAGNOSIS

The diagnosis of bacterial overgrowth should be considered in elderly people and in individuals with predisposing underlying disorders (see Table 142-4). Bacterial overgrowth may be associated with the irritable bowel syndrome (Chapter 139). The identification of greater than 10^5 CFU/mL in a culture of small intestinal aspirate is the "gold standard" in diagnosis but is not readily available. The noninvasive tests with a sensitivity and specificity comparable to intestinal culture are the glucose hydrogen breath test and the ^{14}C- or ^{13}C-D-xylose breath test; in individuals with low vitamin B_{12} levels, a Schilling test before and after antibiotic therapy can be diagnostic (Chapter 167).

TREATMENT — Rx

The goals of treatment are to correct the structural or motility defect, if possible; to eradicate offending bacteria; and to provide nutritional support. Acid-reducing agents should be stopped, if possible. Treatment with antibiotics should be based on culture results whenever possible; otherwise, empirical treatment is given. Rifaximin (400 mg orally three times a day) is effective,[6] but less so in individuals with an excluded (blind) intestinal loop. Tetracycline (250 to 500 mg orally four times a day) or a broad-spectrum antibiotic against aerobes and enteric anaerobes (ciprofloxacin, 500 mg orally twice a day; amoxicillin–clavulanic acid, 250 to 500 mg orally three times a day; cephalexin, 250 mg orally four times a day with metronidazole, 250 mg three times a day) should be given for 14 days. Prokinetic agents such as metoclopramide (10 mg orally four times a day) or erythromycin (250 to 500 mg orally four times a day) can be tried to treat small bowel motility disorders, but often they are not efficacious. Octreotide (50 μg subcutaneously every day) may improve motility and reduce bacterial overgrowth in individuals with scleroderma. If the structural abnormality or motility disturbance cannot be corrected, the patient is at risk for malnutrition and deficiencies of vitamin B_{12} and fat-soluble vitamins. Cyclic treatment (1 to 3 weeks out of every 4 to 6 weeks) with rotating antibiotics may be required in these patients to prevent recurrent bouts of bacterial overgrowth. If supplemental calories are needed, medium-chain triglycerides should be given because they are not dependent on micelle formation for their absorption. Monthly treatment with vitamin B_{12} should be considered, along with supplemental vitamins D, A, K, and E and calcium.

ILEAL DISEASE OR RESECTION

Disease of the terminal ileum is most commonly due to Crohn's disease (Chapter 143), which also may lead to ileal resection, but it also can be caused by radiation enteritis, tropical sprue, tuberculosis, *Yersinia* infection, or idiopathic bile salt malabsorption. These diseases cause bile salt wasting in the colon.

The clinical consequences of bile salt malabsorption are related directly to the length of the diseased or resected terminal ileum. In an adult, if less than 100 cm of ileum is diseased or resected, watery diarrhea results because of stimulation of colonic fluid secretion by unabsorbed bile salts. Bile acid diarrhea responds to cholestyramine (2 to 4 g taken at breakfast, lunch, and dinner). If more than 100 cm of ileum is diseased or resected, bile salt losses (>3 g/day) in the colon exceed the capacity for increased bile salt synthesis in the liver, the bile salt pool shrinks, and micelle formation is impaired. As a result, steatorrhea ensues, and fatty acid–induced intestinal secretion synergizes with the bile acid–induced secretion to cause diarrhea. Treatment is with a low-fat diet, vitamin B_{12} (300 to 1000 μg subcutaneously once every month or 2 mg orally once a day), dietary supplements of calcium (500 mg orally two to three times a day, monitor 24-hour urine calcium for adequacy of dose), and a multiple vitamin and mineral supplement. An antimotility agent should be given for diarrhea. Bile salt binders may worsen diarrhea. Screening for fat-soluble vitamin deficiencies (vitamins A and E, 25-OH vitamin D, and prothrombin time) and bone disease (bone densitometry, serum calcium, intact parathyroid hormone, 24-hour urine for calcium) should be done.

Three long-term complications of chronic bile salt wasting and fat malabsorption are renal stones, bone disease (osteoporosis and osteomalacia), and gallstones. Oxalate renal stones occur as a consequence of excess free oxalate absorption in the colon. Free oxalate is generated when unabsorbed fatty acids bind luminal calcium, which is then unavailable for binding oxalate. Renal oxalate stones sometimes can be avoided with a low-fat, low-oxalate diet and calcium supplements. Bone disease is caused by impaired micelle formation with a resulting decrease in absorption of vitamin D; year-round sun exposure reduces this complication. Vitamin D (50,000 U orally one to three times a week) and calcium supplements (500 mg orally two to three times a day) should be given to susceptible individuals, but vitamin D levels and serum and urinary calcium must be monitored for response to treatment because excess vitamin D can be toxic. The mechanism of gallstone formation in these individuals is unclear; pigmented gallstones are most common.

Conditions that Impair Mucosal Absorption

PATHOBIOLOGY

Nutrients are absorbed along the entire length of the small intestine, with the exception of iron and folate, which are absorbed in the duodenum and proximal jejunum, and bile salts and cobalamin, which are absorbed in the distal ileum. The efficiency of nutrient uptake at the mucosa is influenced by the number of villus absorptive cells, the presence of functional hydrolases and specific nutrient transport proteins on the brush-border membrane, and transit time. Transit time determines the contact time of luminal contents with the brush-border membrane and influences the efficiency of nutrient uptake across the mucosa.

Mucosal malabsorption can be caused by specific (usually congenital) brush-border enzyme or nutrient transporter deficiencies or by generalized diseases that damage the small intestinal mucosa or result in surgical resection or bypass of small intestine. The nutrients malabsorbed in these general malabsorptive diseases depend on the site of intestinal injury (proximal, distal, or diffuse) and the severity of damage. The main mechanism of malabsorption in these conditions is a decrease in surface area available for absorption. Some conditions (infection, celiac disease, tropical sprue, food allergies, and graft-versus-host disease) are characterized by intestinal inflammation and villus flattening; others are characterized by ulceration (ulcerative jejunitis, NSAIDs, Crohn's disease), infiltration (amyloidosis), or ischemia (radiation enteritis, mesenteric ischemia).

Long-chain fatty acids are transported across the microvillus membrane of villus epithelial cells by the fatty acid transport protein FATP4. The bile salts from mixed micelles remain in the intestinal lumen and are absorbed in the distal ileum by sodium-dependent cotransport. Oligosaccharides and larger oligopeptides (products of pancreatic enzyme digestion), sucrose, and lactose are hydrolyzed further by enzymes present in the brush-border membrane of villus epithelial cells before they are absorbed. Although only sugar monomers (glucose, galactose, fructose) can be taken up at the apical epithelial cell membrane, dipeptides and tripeptides are readily taken into the cell.

Water-soluble vitamins are readily absorbed throughout the small intestine. Fat-soluble vitamins, minerals, and cobalamin are more difficult to absorb because of the requirement for micelle formation (vitamins D, A, K, and E), a divalent charge (magnesium, calcium, iron), or selected sites of uptake in the intestine (iron, cobalamin). Calcium is absorbed best in the proximal small intestine by a vitamin D–dependent calcium channel. Magnesium is absorbed by the small intestine (throughout its length) by a poorly understood mechanism. Ferrous iron is transported into intestinal epithelial cells by a proton-coupled metal-ion transporter (Nramp2) that has specificity for Fe^{2++} and other divalent cations (Zn^{2++}, Mn^{2++}, Co^{2++}, Cd^{2++}, Cu^{2++}, Ni^{2++}, and Pb^{2++}). The absorption of calcium and nonheme iron is enhanced by solubilization with hydrochloric acid. Intraluminal compounds such as oxalate, phytate, and long-chain fatty acids bind to calcium and magnesium, decreasing their absorption. Individuals with severe mucosal disease or short-bowel syndrome with high fecal fluid outputs lose magnesium and zinc from endogenous secretions.

Folates (Chapters 167 and 225) are both taken in the diet and produced by bacteria in the colon. Dietary folates are absorbed in the proximal small intestine through a reduced folate carrier (RFC1). Deficiency can be caused by poor intake or malabsorption secondary to intestinal disease or drugs. The cobalamins (Chapters 167 and 225) are abundant in foods containing animal proteins (e.g., meat, seafood, eggs, milk). Cobalamin deficiency in industrialized countries is rarely due to poor dietary intake but rather reflects the inability to absorb cobalamin. This inability may be caused by a lack of intrinsic factor, consumption of cobalamin by overgrowth of anaerobic bacteria in the small bowel lumen, ileal disease or resection, or defective transcobalamin II. Large amounts of cobalamin are present in the liver (2 to 5 mg), and cobalamin is reabsorbed from bile through the enterohepatic circulation, thereby limiting daily losses to less than 1 μg. It usually takes 10 to 12 years for cobalamin deficiency to develop after it is eliminated from the diet, but deficiency can occur more rapidly (2 to 5 years) with malabsorptive syndromes. If lack of gastric acid causes food-cobalamin malabsorption, treatment with oral cyanocobalamin supplementation (Chapter 167) is curative.

LACTASE DEFICIENCY

EPIDEMIOLOGY

Acquired lactase deficiency is the most common cause of selective carbohydrate malabsorption. Most individuals, except those of northern European descent, begin to lose lactase activity by the age of 2 years. The prevalence of lactase deficiency is highest (85 to 100%) in persons of Asian, African, and Native-American descent.

PATHOBIOLOGY

The persistence or nonpersistence of lactase activity is associated with a single nucleotide polymorphism C/T_{-13910} that is found upstream of the lactase gene on chromosome 2q21-22. Hypolactasia is associated with the C/C_{-13910} genotype in diverse ethnic groups. The mechanism by which this variant downregulates the lactase gene is not known, but functional studies suggest genotype-dependent alterations in levels of messenger RNA.

CLINICAL MANIFESTATIONS

Adults with lactase deficiency typically complain of gas, bloating, and diarrhea after the ingestion of milk or dairy products but do not lose weight. Unabsorbed lactose is osmotically active, drawing water followed by ions into the intestinal lumen. On reaching the colon, bacteria metabolize lactose to short-chain fatty acids, carbon dioxide, and hydrogen gas. Short-chain fatty acids are transported with sodium into colonic epithelial cells, facilitating the reabsorption of fluid in the colon. If the colonic capacity for the reabsorption of short-chain fatty acids is exceeded, an osmotic diarrhea results (see later discussion of carbohydrate malabsorption in watery diarrheas).

DIAGNOSIS

The diagnosis of acquired lactase deficiency can be made by empirical treatment with a lactose-free diet, which results in resolution of symptoms; by the hydrogen breath test after oral administration of lactose; or by genetic testing. Many intestinal diseases cause secondary reversible lactase deficiency, including viral gastroenteritis, celiac disease, giardiasis, and bacterial overgrowth.

Congenital Enteropeptidase (Enterokinase) Deficiency

Enteropeptidase is a brush-border protease that cleaves trypsinogen to trypsin, triggering the cascade of pancreatic protease activation in the intestinal lumen. The rare congenital deficiency of enteropeptidase results in inability to activate all pancreatic proteases and leads to severe protein malabsorption. It manifests in infancy as diarrhea, growth retardation, and hypoproteinemic edema.

Abetalipoproteinemia

Formation and exocytosis of chylomicrons at the basolateral membrane of intestinal epithelial cells are necessary for the delivery of lipids to the systemic circulation. One of the proteins required for assembly and secretion of chylomicrons is the microsomal triglyceride transfer protein, which is mutated in individuals with abetalipoproteinemia. Children with this disorder have fat malabsorption and the consequences of vitamin E deficiency (retinopathy and spinocerebellar degeneration). Biochemical tests show low plasma levels of apoprotein B, triglyceride, and cholesterol. Membrane lipid abnormalities result in red blood cell acanthosis (burr cells). Intestinal biopsy is diagnostic; the tissue is characterized by engorgement of epithelial cells with lipid droplets. Calories are provided by treatment with a low-fat diet containing medium-chain triglycerides. Poor absorption of long-chain fatty acids sometimes can result in essential fatty acid deficiency. High doses of fat-soluble vitamins, especially vitamin E, often are needed. Mutations in the apolipoprotein B gene (hypobetalipoproteinemia) and intracellular retention of chylomicrons (Anderson's disease) cause a similar although less severe clinical syndrome.

CELIAC DISEASE

DEFINITION AND EPIDEMIOLOGY

Celiac disease is an inflammatory condition of the small intestine precipitated by the ingestion of wheat, rye, and barley in individuals with certain genetic predispositions. Screening studies for the antiendomysial (EMA) and anti–tissue transglutaminase (anti-tTG) antibodies that are associated with celiac disease suggest a prevalence in white populations of about 1%. High-risk groups for celiac disease include first-degree relatives and individuals with type 1 diabetes mellitus, autoimmune thyroid disease, primary biliary cirrhosis, Turner's syndrome, or Down syndrome. About 20% of patients diagnosed with irritable bowel syndrome or with microscopic (lymphocytic) colitis have celiac disease.

PATHOBIOLOGY

Environmental and genetic factors are important in the development of celiac disease. The alcohol-soluble protein fraction of wheat gluten, the gliadins, and similar prolamins in rye and barley trigger intestinal inflammation in susceptible individuals. Oat grains, which have prolamins rich in glutamine but not proline, are rarely toxic. Gliadins and similar prolamins with high proline content are relatively resistant to digestion by human proteases. A 33-mer peptide that is a natural digestion product of α_2-gliadin may be important in the pathogenesis of celiac disease. This peptide resists terminal digestion by intestinal brush-border proteases and contains three previously identified antigenic epitopes. It also reacts with tissue transglutaminase and stimulates human leukocyte antigen (HLA)-DQ2-restricted intestinal T-cell clones from individuals with celiac disease.

Approximately 15% of first-degree relatives of affected individuals are found to have celiac disease. Predisposition has been mapped to the HLA-D region on chromosome 6. More than 90% of northern Europeans with celiac disease have the DQ2 heterodimer encoded by alleles *DQA1*0501* and *DQB1*0201*, compared with 20 to 30% of controls. A smaller celiac group carries HLA DQ8. The strongest candidate non-HLA alleles identified in genome-wide association studies are 4q27 and 3q28. The DQ2 protein expressed on antigen-presenting cells has positively charged binding pockets; tTG (the autoantigen recognized by EMA) may enhance intestinal inflammation by deamidation of select glutamine residues in gliadin to negatively charged glutamic acid. In the deamidated form, most gliadin peptides have a higher binding affinity for DQ2 and are more potent stimulants of gluten-sensitized T cells. Villous atrophy may be caused by inflammation that is triggered by γ-interferon released from DQ2- or DQ8-restricted CD4 T cells in the lamina propria. Alternatively, intraepithelial lymphocytes may directly kill intestinal epithelial cells under the influence of IL-15 released from stressed enterocytes.

CLINICAL MANIFESTATIONS

Celiac disease usually manifests early in life, at about 2 years of age (after wheat has been introduced into the diet), or later in the second to fourth decades of life, but it can occur at any age. It may first manifest clinically after abdominal surgery or an episode of infectious diarrhea.

Breast-feeding and the time of introduction of wheat in the diet may lessen the risk or delay the onset of celiac disease in children at risk. Adults with celiac disease in the United States often present with anemia or osteoporosis without diarrhea or other gastrointestinal symptoms. These individuals most likely have proximal disease that impairs iron, folate, and calcium absorption but an adequate surface area in the remaining intestine for absorption of other nutrients. Other extraintestinal manifestations of celiac disease include rash (dermatitis herpetiformis), neurologic disorders (peripheral neuropathy, ataxia, epilepsy), psychiatric disorders (depression, paranoia), reproductive disorders (infertility, spontaneous abortion), short stature, dental enamel hypoplasia, chronic hepatitis, or cardiomyopathy.

Individuals with significant mucosal involvement present with watery diarrhea, weight loss or growth retardation, and the clinical manifestations of vitamin and mineral deficiencies. Cobalamin deficiency is more common (10% of patients) than previously thought and usually corrects itself on a gluten-free diet. Symptomatic individuals require supplementation of vitamin B_{12}. Diarrhea is caused by many mechanisms, including a decreased surface area for water and electrolyte absorption, the osmotic effect of unabsorbed luminal nutrients, an increased surface area for chloride secretion (crypt hyperplasia), and the stimulation of intestinal fluid secretion by inflammatory mediators and unabsorbed fatty acids. Some individuals have impaired pancreatic enzyme secretion caused by decreased mucosal cholecystokinin release or bacterial overgrowth that may contribute to diarrhea.

DIAGNOSIS

The diagnosis of celiac disease is made by characteristic changes found on a small intestinal biopsy specimen and improvement when a gluten-free diet is instituted (Figs. 142-6 and 142-7). Mucosal flattening may be observed endoscopically as scalloped or reduced duodenal folds. Characteristic features found on intestinal biopsy include blunted or absent villi, crypt hyperplasia, increased intraepithelial lymphocytes, and infiltration of the lamina propria with plasma cells and lymphocytes. In some individuals, the only abnormal biopsy finding is increased intraepithelial lymphocytes. A hypoplastic mucosa indicates irreversible (end-stage) intestinal disease.

Serologic markers for celiac disease are useful in supporting the diagnosis, in screening first-degree relatives, and in monitoring the response to a gluten-free diet. EMA immunoglobulin A (IgA) antibodies, detected by indirect immunofluorescence, are highly sensitive (90%) and specific (90 to 100%) for active celiac disease in skilled laboratory testing. An enzyme-linked immunosorbent assay (ELISA) test to detect antibodies against tTG has equal sensitivity to the EMA test but is less specific. The newer anti-deamidated gliadin (a biotinylated synthetic γ-gliadin peptide with glutamic acid substituted for glutamine) IgA and IgG antibody immunofluorometric assay has a sensitivity and specificity that approaches that of EMA.

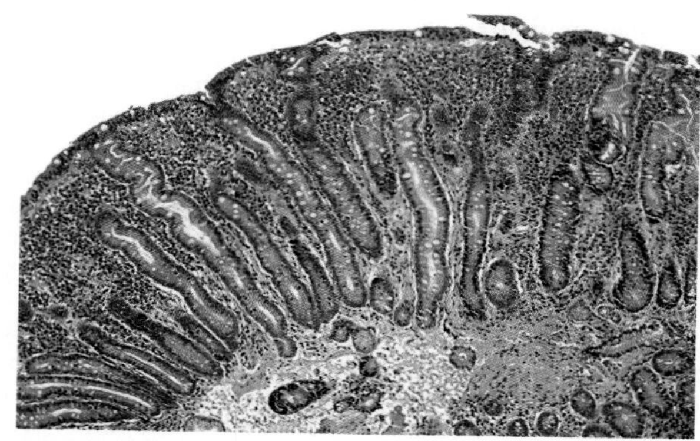

FIGURE 142-6. **Intestinal biopsy appearance of flattened villi, hyperplastic crypts, and increased intraepithelial lymphocytes.** (Courtesy of John Hart, MD.)

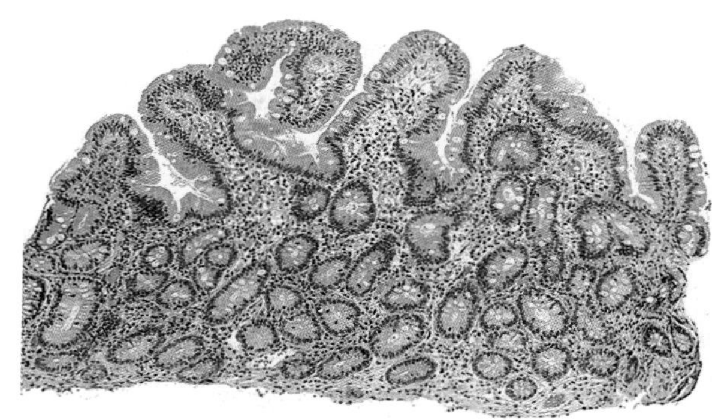

FIGURE 142-7. **Regeneration of villi after initiation of a gluten-free diet.** (Courtesy of John Hart, MD.)

The anti-tTG IgA antibody test, when obtained with a serum IgA level, is a cost-effective strategy for screening high-risk groups; very high titers of the anti-tTG IgA and EMA antibodies are virtually diagnostic of celiac disease. Patients with mild disease may have negative antibody studies. Anti-tTG, gliadin peptide, and EMA IgA antibodies tests are negative in individuals with selective IgA deficiency (present in up to 2.6% of individuals with celiac disease). In these patients, anti-tTG or gliadin peptide IgG antibodies may be helpful in diagnosis. In equivocal cases (negative serology and equivocal biopsy or positive serology and normal biopsy), HLA genotyping is useful to exclude the diagnosis of celiac disease in persons who lack the DQ2 or DQ8 gene.

TREATMENT Rx

Treatment consists of a lifelong gluten-free diet. Wheat, rye, and barley grains should be excluded from the diet. Rice and corn grains are tolerated. Oats (if not contaminated by wheat grain) are tolerated by most. Early referral to a reputable celiac support group or website is often helpful in maintaining dietary compliance. Owing to secondary lactase deficiency, a lactose-free diet should be recommended until symptoms improve. Bone densitometry should be performed on all individuals with celiac disease because up to 70% have osteopenia or osteoporosis. Patients with diarrhea and weight loss should be screened for vitamin and mineral deficiencies. Documented deficiencies of vitamins and minerals should be replenished (see Table 142-4), and women of childbearing age should take folic acid supplements. Bone mass often improves on a gluten-free diet alone. Patients with vitamin D or calcium deficiency should receive supplements (Chapter 225), with the dose monitored by 25-OH vitamin D levels and a 24-hour urine test for calcium.

PROGNOSIS

Of patients with celiac disease treated with a gluten-free diet, 90% experience symptomatic improvement within 2 weeks. The most common cause of a poor dietary response is continued ingestion of gluten. Other possibilities include a missed intestinal infection (see later), an alternative diagnosis (e.g., agammaglobulinemia [diagnosed by hypogammaglobulinemia and lack of plasma cells on small bowel biopsy], autoimmune enteritis [diagnosed by a positive antienterocyte antibody and crypt apoptosis or loss of goblet cells on small bowel biopsy]), bacterial overgrowth, pancreatic insufficiency, microscopic colitis, or other food allergies (cow's milk, soy protein).

In a small percentage of patients, symptoms and enteropathy persist despite a strict gluten-free diet. In such patients, repeat intestinal biopsy is indicated. Some patients will have collagen deposition beneath the surface epithelium (collagenous sprue). Others will have ulcerative jejunitis or a monoclonal population of intraepithelial T cells with an aberrant phenotype or clonal T-cell receptor-γ gene rearrangements, which are predictive of enteropathy-associated T-cell lymphoma (Chapter 191) that portends a poor prognosis. Video capsule endoscopy and balloon-assisted enteroscopy may be helpful in establishing these diagnoses. Patients with collagenous sprue, autoimmune enteritis, or refractory sprue with a polyclonal population of intraepithelial T lymphocytes often respond to prednisone (20 to 40 mg orally daily) or budesonide (3 mg orally three times a day).

Individuals with celiac disease are at increased risk for B-cell lymphoma (Chapter 191), gastrointestinal tract carcinomas (esophageal, small bowel, and colonic adenocarcinomas), and increased mortality; a strict gluten-free diet for life may lessen these risks. Intestinal T-cell lymphoma is rare and should be suspected in individuals who have abdominal pain, recurrence of symptoms after initial response to a gluten-free diet, or refractory celiac disease.

TROPICAL SPRUE

Tropical sprue is an inflammatory disease of the small intestine associated with the overgrowth of predominantly coliform bacteria. It occurs in residents or travelers to the tropics, especially India and Southeast Asia. Individuals classically present with diarrhea and megaloblastic anemia secondary to vitamin B_{12} and folate deficiency, but some have anemia only. Intestinal biopsy characteristically shows subtotal and patchy villous atrophy in the proximal and distal small intestine, which may be caused by the effect of bacterial toxins on gut structure or by the secondary effects of vitamin B_{12} deficiency on the gut (megaloblastic gut). Diagnosis is based on history, documentation of vitamin B_{12} or folate deficiency, and the presence of an abnormal small intestinal biopsy report. Treatment is a prolonged course of broad-spectrum antibiotics, oral folate, and vitamin B_{12} injections until symptoms resolve. Relapses occur mainly in natives of the tropics.

Infection

GIARDIA LAMBLIA

Giardia lamblia (Chapter 359) infection, the most common protozoal infection in the United States, can cause malabsorption in individuals infected with many trophozoites, especially the immunocompromised or IgA-deficient hosts. Malabsorption occurs when many organisms cover the epithelium and cause mucosal inflammation, which results in villous flattening and a decrease in absorptive surface area. Stool for ova and parasites at this stage of infection is often negative because of the attachment of organisms in the proximal small intestine. Diagnosis can be made by a stool antigen-capture ELISA test but may require duodenal aspiration and biopsies.

HUMAN IMMUNODEFICIENCY VIRUS

Diarrhea, malabsorption, and wasting are common in individuals with AIDS but are seen less frequently with improved antiretroviral therapy (Chapter 397). In patients who are receiving highly active antiretroviral therapy, diarrhea is more likely to be due to protease inhibitors than to enteric infection.

Malabsorption is usually due to infection with cryptosporidia, *Mycobacterium avium-intracellulare* complex, *I. belli*, or microsporidia. An organism can be identified by stool examination or intestinal biopsy about 50% of the time. *AIDS enteropathy* (a term used if no organism is identified) also can cause malabsorption. Mechanisms of malabsorption and diarrhea include villous atrophy, increased intestinal permeability, rapid small bowel transit (in patients with protozoal infection), and ultrastructural damage of enterocytes (in AIDS enteropathy). Among individuals with AIDS and diarrhea, results of fecal fat and D-xylose absorption are frequently abnormal. Serum albumin, vitamin B_{12}, and zinc levels are often low. Vitamin B_{12} deficiency is caused mainly by ileal disease, but low intrinsic factor and decreased transcobalamin II may be contributing factors. Management of malabsorption should focus on restoring the immune system by treating the underlying HIV infection with antiviral therapy. If possible, the offending organism should be treated with antibiotics. If the organism cannot be eradicated, chronic diarrhea and malabsorption result; treatment in these cases consists of antimotility agents and a lactose-free, low-fat diet. Pancreatic enzyme replacement therapy can be tried in HIV-infected individuals who are taking highly active antiretroviral therapy or nucleoside analogues and who have fat malabsorption of obscure origin. If supplemental calories are needed, liquid oral supplements that are predigested and high in medium-chain triglycerides (semi-elemental) are tolerated best. Vitamin and mineral deficiencies should be screened for and treated.

WHIPPLE'S DISEASE

Whipple's disease (Chapters 144 and 283), a rare cause of malabsorption, manifests with gastrointestinal complaints in association with systemic symptoms, such as fever, joint pain, or neurologic manifestations. About one third of patients have cardiac involvement, most commonly culture-negative endocarditis. Occasionally, individuals present with ocular or neurologic disease without gastrointestinal symptoms. Men are affected more commonly than women, particularly white men. The organism responsible for causing Whipple's disease is a gram-positive actinomycete, *Tropheryma whippelii.* The epidemiology and pathogenesis of Whipple's disease are poorly understood. The prevalence of the disease is higher in farmers compared with other workers, which suggests that the organism lives in the soil. Using the polymerase chain reaction, *T. whippelii* has been detected in sewage and in duodenal biopsy specimens, gastric juice, saliva, and stool of individuals without clinical disease. Whether the latter represents a carrier state or the presence of nonpathogenic organisms is not known. Immunologic defects and an association with the HLA-B27 gene may be disease factors. Small intestinal biopsy shows villous blunting and infiltration of the lamina propria with large macrophages that stain positive with the periodic acid–Schiff method and are filled with the organism. It is important to distinguish these macrophages from macrophages infected with *M. avium-intracellulare* complex, which stain positive on acid-fast staining and are found in individuals with AIDS. Treatment is with a prolonged course of broad-spectrum antibiotics (e.g., 10 to 14 days of parenteral penicillin G, 1.2 million U every day and streptomycin, 1 g every day; ceftriaxone, 2 g intravenously daily, or meropenem, 1 g intravenously three times daily; then, 160 mg of trimethoprim and 800 mg of sulfamethoxazole orally two times a day for 1 year or 160 mg of trimethoprim and 800 mg of sulfamethoxazole orally two times a day for 1 year). Relapses occur, but initial treatment with parenteral ceftriaxone or meropenem appears to be associated with a low relapse rate.

GRAFT-VERSUS-HOST DISEASE

Diarrhea occurs frequently after allogeneic bone marrow or stem cell transplantation (Chapter 181). Immediately after transplantation, diarrhea is caused by the toxic effects of cytoreductive therapy on the intestinal epithelium. Twenty to 100 days after transplantation, diarrhea is usually due to graft-versus-host disease (GVHD) or infection. Patients with GVHD present clinically with a skin rash, hepatic cholestasis, buccal mucositis, anorexia, nausea, vomiting, abdominal cramps, and diarrhea. The diagnosis of GVHD in the gastrointestinal tract can be made on biopsy of the stomach, small intestine, or colon. In mild cases, the mucosa appears normal on inspection at endoscopy, but apoptosis of gastric gland or crypt cells can be found on biopsy. In severe cases, denudation of the intestinal epithelium results in diarrhea and malabsorption and often requires parenteral nutritional support. Octreotide (50 to 250 μg subcutaneously three times a day) may be helpful in controlling voluminous diarrhea. Treatment of GVHD is with steroids and antithymocyte globulin combined with parenteral nutritional support until intestinal function returns.

SHORT-BOWEL SYNDROME

Malabsorption caused by small bowel resection or surgical bypass is called the short-bowel syndrome. The most common causes in the United States are massive resection due to adhesions, volvulus, ischemia (mesenteric or after intra-abdominal surgery), and gastric bypass surgery. Short-bowel syndrome due to Crohn's disease and radiation enteritis now is less common because of improved medical and radiation therapies. The severity of malabsorption depends on the site and extent of resection; the capacity for hyperplasia, dilation, and elongation; and the function of the residual bowel. Mechanisms of malabsorption after small bowel resection include a decreased absorptive surface area, decreased luminal bile salt concentration, rapid transit, and bacterial overgrowth. Limited jejunal resection usually is tolerated best because bile salt and vitamin B_{12} absorption remain normal. Ileal resection is less well tolerated because of the consequences of bile salt wasting and the limited capacity of the jejunum to undergo adaptive hyperplasia.

When less than 100 cm of jejunum remains, the colon takes on an important role in caloric salvage and fluid reabsorption. Malabsorbed carbohydrates are digested by colonic bacteria to short-chain fatty acids, which are absorbed in the colon.

TREATMENT

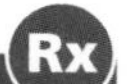

Parenteral nutrition may be avoided by a diet rich in complex carbohydrates, oral rehydration solutions, and an antimotility agent. In comparison, individuals with fewer than 100 cm of jejunum and no colon have high jejunostomy outputs and often require intravenous fluids or parenteral nutrition to survive. These individuals waste sodium, chloride, bicarbonate, magnesium, zinc, and water in their ostomy effluent. Dietary modifications should include a high-salt, nutrient-rich diet given in small meals. An oral rehydration solution with a sodium concentration greater than 90 mmol/L is absorbed best. Oral vitamin and mineral doses higher than the usual U.S. recommended daily allowances are required (Table 142-5). Vitamin B_{12} should be given parenterally (500 to 1000 μg subcutaneously every month). Magnesium deficiencies are often difficult to replenish with oral magnesium because of its osmotic effect in the intestinal lumen. A liquid magnesium preparation added to an oral rehydration solution and sipped throughout the day may minimize magnesium-induced fluid losses. Potent antimotility agents, such as tincture of opium (0.5 to 1 mL orally four times a day), often are needed to slow transit and maximize contact time for nutrient absorption. High-volume jejunostomy outputs can be lessened by inhibiting endogenous secretions with a proton pump inhibitor (e.g., omeprazole, 40 mg orally one to two times a day, or lansoprazole, 30 mg orally one to two times a day) and, in severe cases, octreotide (100 to 250 μg subcutaneously three times a day; if effective, convert to an equivalent long-acting monthly dosage). The benefit of octreotide may be offset by its potential to inhibit intestinal adaptation and impair pancreatic enzyme secretion with doses greater than 300 μg/day.

In the most severe cases, supplemental calories must be provided by nocturnal tube feeding or parenteral nutrition. Treatment with growth hormone (0.1 mg/kg/day subcutaneously) with or without glutamine (30 g once a day orally) for 4 weeks may reduce parenteral nutrition requirements in patients who have had massive intestinal resections.[7] Teduglutide (0.05 mg/kg/day subcutaneously), a glucagon-like peptide-2 analogue that stimulates adaptive hyperplasia in remnant intestine after resection, reduces parenteral nutrition requirements.[8]

TABLE 142-5 VITAMIN AND MINERAL DOSES USED IN THE TREATMENT OF MALABSORPTION

VITAMIN	ORAL DOSE	PARENTERAL DOSE
Vitamin A[*]	Water-soluble A, 25,000 U/day[†]	
Vitamin E	Water-soluble E, 400-800 U/day[†]	
Vitamin D[‡]	25,000-50,000 U/day	
Vitamin K	5 mg/day	
Folic acid	1 mg/day	
Calcium[§]	1500-2000 mg elemental calcium/day Calcium citrate, 500 mg calcium/tablet[†] Calcium carbonate, 500 mg calcium/tablet[†]	
Magnesium	Liquid magnesium gluconate[†] 1-3 tbsp (12-36 mEq magnesium) in 1-2 L of ORS or sports drink sipped throughout the day Magnesium chloride hexahydrate[†] 100-600 mg elemental magnesium/day	2 mL of a 50% solution (8 mEq) both buttocks IM
Zinc	Zinc gluconate[†] 20-50 mg elemental zinc/day[‖]	
Iron	150-300 mg elemental iron/day Polysaccharide-iron complex[†] Iron sulfate or gluconate	Iron sucrose[¶] Sodium ferric gluconate complex[¶] Iron dextran (as calculated for anemia) (IV or IM[¶]; Chapter 162)
B-complex vitamins	1 megadose tablet/day	
Vitamin B_{12}	2 mg/day	1 mg IM or SC/mo[**]

[*]Monitor serum vitamin A level to avoid toxicity, especially in patients with hypertriglyceridemia.
[†]Form best absorbed or with least side effects.
[‡]Monitor serum calcium and 25-OH vitamin D levels to avoid toxicity.
[§]Monitor 24-hr urine calcium to assess adequacy of dose.
[‖]If intestinal output is high, additional zinc should be given. Monitor for copper deficiency with high doses.
[¶]Parenteral therapy should be given in a supervised outpatient setting because of the risk of fatal reactions. Decreased risk of fatal reactions when compared with iron dextran.
[**]For vitamin B_{12} deficiency, 1 mg IM or SC twice a week for 4 wk, then once a month.
ORS = oral rehydration solution.

PROGNOSIS

Long-term complications include bone disease, renal stones (oxalate stones if the colon is present, urate stones with a jejunostomy), gallstones, bacterial overgrowth, fat-soluble vitamin deficiencies, essential fatty acid deficiency, and D-lactic acidosis. Small bowel transplantation should be considered for individuals who require parenteral nutrition to survive and then develop liver disease or venous access problems.

Conditions That Impair Nutrient Delivery to the Systemic Circulation

Insoluble lipids (present in chylomicrons) are exocytosed across the basolateral membrane of epithelial cells into the intestinal lymphatics. From there, they enter the mesenteric lymphatics and the general circulation through the thoracic duct. Sugar monomers, amino acids, and medium-chain fatty acids are transported across the basolateral membrane of intestinal epithelial cells into capillaries and into the portal circulation. Sugar monomers are transported across the basolateral membrane by the facilitative glucose transporter isoform (GLUT2) and amino acids by facilitative amino acid carriers (see Fig. 142-1A).

IMPAIRED LYMPHATIC DRAINAGE

Diseases that cause intestinal lymphatic obstruction, such as primary congenital lymphangiectasia (malunion of intestinal lymphatics), and diseases that result in secondary lymphangiectasia (lymphoma, tuberculosis, Kaposi's sarcoma, retroperitoneal fibrosis, constrictive pericarditis, severe heart failure) result in fat malabsorption. The increased pressure in the intestinal lymphatics leads to leakage and sometimes rupture of lymph into the intestinal lumen, with the loss of lipids, γ-globulins, albumin, and lymphocytes. The diagnosis of lymphangiectasia can be made by intestinal biopsy, but the specific cause may be more difficult to identify. Individuals with lymphangiectasia malabsorb fat and fat-soluble vitamins and have protein loss into the intestinal lumen. The most common presentation is hypoproteinemic edema. Nutritional management includes a low-fat diet and supplementation with medium-chain triglycerides, which are absorbed directly into the portal circulation. Fat-soluble vitamins should be given if deficiencies develop.

WATERY DIARRHEA

Watery diarrhea may be due to osmotic, secretory, inflammatory, or often combined mechanisms (Fig. 142-8).

Ingestion of Nonabsorbable or Poorly Absorbable Solutes

MAGNESIUM AND SODIUM PHOSPHATE AND SULFATE DIARRHEAS

Magnesium, phosphate, and sulfate are poorly absorbed minerals. Individuals who ingest significant amounts of magnesium-based antacids or high-potency multimineral and multivitamin supplements or those who surreptitiously ingest magnesium-containing laxatives or nonabsorbable anion laxatives, such as Na_2PO_4 (neutral phosphate) or Na_2SO_4 (Glauber's or Carlsbad salt) may develop osmotically induced, watery diarrhea that may be high volume.

SORBITOL AND FRUCTOSE DIARRHEA

Dietetic food, chewing gum, candies, and medication elixirs that are sweetened with sorbitol, which is an unabsorbable carbohydrate, can cause diarrhea. Excessive consumption of pears, prunes, peaches, and apple juice, which also contain sorbitol and fructose, a poorly absorbable sugar, can result in diarrhea. Most soft drinks are now sweetened with fructose-containing corn syrup and may be a cause of diarrhea when ingested in high concentrations.

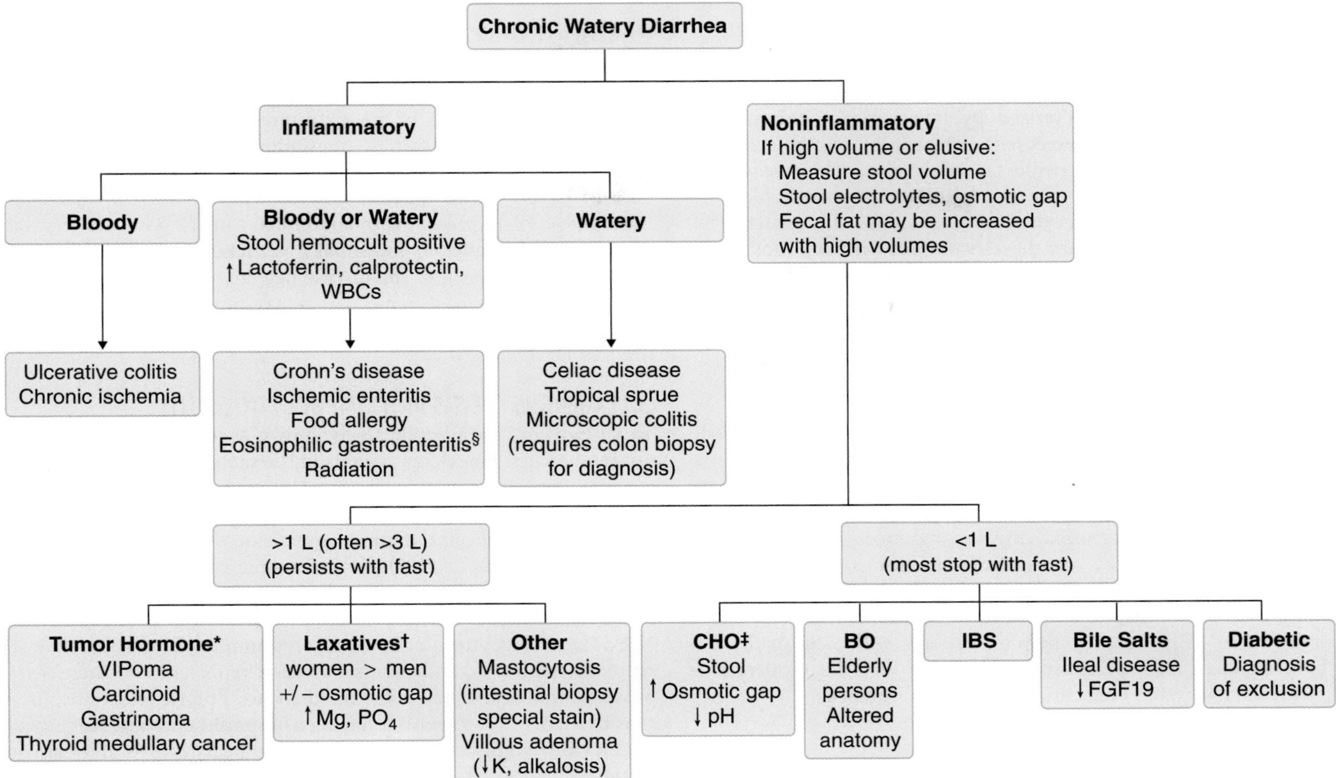

FIGURE 142-8. Approach to the evaluation of watery diarrheas. Many diarrheas have more than one mechanism (i.e., osmotic, secretory, inflammatory). Other causes include medications, postsurgical (vagotomy, Nissan wrap, cholecystectomy), hyperthyroidism, and alcohol. *VIPoma: >3 L output daily "pancreatic cholera," elevated VIP level. Carcinoid: elevated urine 5-hydroxyindole acetic acid, positive OctreoScan. Gastrinoma (Zollinger-Ellison syndrome): elevated gastrin level, positive secretin stimulation test, diarrhea due to high volume of acid secretion. Thyroid medullary cancer: elevated calcitonin level. †May be high or low volume depending on dose ingested, may respond to fast. ‡Carbohydrate malabsorption (CHO) may be due to lactase deficiency, dietary fructose, sorbitol in diabetic candies or liquid medications. §Full-thickness biopsy may be needed for diagnosis. BO = bacterial overgrowth; FGF = fibroblast growth factor; IBS = irritable bowel syndrome; WBCs = white blood cells.

GLUCOSE-GALACTOSE MALABSORPTION AND DISACCHARIDASE DEFICIENCIES

Primary and secondary lactase deficiency is the most common cause of disaccharidase deficiency (see malabsorption). Congenital lactase deficiency causes diarrhea at birth with the first breast feed. Congenital sucrose-isomaltose deficiency presents in infancy when table sugar is introduced into the diet. Glucose-galactose malabsorption is due to mutations in the *SGLT1* gene and causes diarrhea at birth. The mechanism of diarrhea in these disorders is osmotic. Stools are acidic owing to conversion of unabsorbed sugars to short-chain fatty acids in the colon. Treatment is the substitution of fructose for other sugars in the diet. Patients who develop gas, bloating, or diarrhea after the ingestion of mushrooms may have a deficiency in the disaccharidase trehalase.

RAPID INTESTINAL TRANSIT

A small amount of carbohydrate in the diet is unabsorbed by the normal small intestine. Diets that are high in carbohydrate and low in fat may allow rapid gastric emptying and rapid small intestinal motility, thereby leading to carbohydrate malabsorption and osmotic diarrhea. Rapid transit time also occurs in thyrotoxicosis (Chapter 233). Because of the production of H_2 and CO_2 gas by colonic bacteria, abdominal gas and cramping may be the predominant symptoms.

BILE ACID MALABSORPTION

Ileal malabsorption of bile salts results in the stimulation of colonic fluid secretion and watery diarrhea. Three types of bile acid malabsorption induce diarrhea. Type 1 results when severe disease (e.g., Crohn's disease), resection, or bypass of the distal ileum allows bile salts to escape absorption (see earlier). Type 2 may rarely be congenital, owing to a defect in the apical sodium bile acid transporter, or may more commonly be idiopathic. The idiopathic type has been associated with decreased levels of FGF19, an intestinal fibroblast growth factor that normally downregulates bile salt synthesis in the liver. The result is increased bile salt production that overwhelms reabsorption in the ileum. Type 3 is caused by various conditions, including prior cholecystectomy, celiac disease, pancreatic insufficiency, microscopic colitis, bacterial overgrowth, gastric surgery, or vagotomy. Postulated mechanisms include a bile salt storage problem, increased production, decreased recycling, or saturation of absorption.

TREATMENT Rx

Diarrhea due to types 1 and 2 often responds to cholestyramine, 2 to 4 g given orally two to four times daily, or the more potent and better tolerated bile salt binder, colesevelam, 625 mg tablet orally two to six times daily. Fat-soluble vitamin deficiency is a potential risk with chronic use of bile salt binders.

Although many patients with type 3 respond to cholestyramine, some do not. In these patients, motility-altering drugs such as opiates (e.g., loperamide, 2 to 4 mg orally two to four times daily) and anticholinergics (e.g., hyoscyamine sulfate, 0.125 to 0.250 mg orally two to four times daily) may be of benefit.

Functional Watery Diarrhea (Irritable Bowel Syndrome)

See Chapter 139.

TRUE SECRETORY DIARRHEAS

Endocrine diseases that can cause secretory diarrheas (see Fig. 142-8) include carcinoid tumors (Chapter 240), gastrinomas (Chapter 201), VIPomas of the pancreas (Chapter 201), and medullary carcinoma of the thyroid (Chapter 254). Diarrhea is also seen in 60 to 80% of patients with systemic mastocytosis (Chapter 263). Diarrhea due to gastrinoma is distinct in that it is caused by high volumes of hydrochloric acid secretion that overwhelm the reabsorptive capacity of the colon and by maldigestion of fat owing to pH inactivation of pancreatic lipase and precipitation of bile salts.

Villous Adenomas

Large (4 to 18 cm) villous adenomas (Chapter 199), particularly in the rectum or occasionally the sigmoid colon, may cause secretory diarrhea of 500 to 3000 mL/24 hours characterized by hypokalemia, chloride-rich stool, and metabolic alkalosis. Increased numbers of goblet cells and increased prostaglandin E_2 are responsible for the diarrhea. Chloride wasting in the stool and metabolic alkalosis are also found in congenital chloridorrhea, which is caused by a defect in the intestinal Cl^-/HCO_3^- transporter. The metabolic alkalosis distinguishes these two diarrheas from most other diarrheas that cause metabolic acidosis. A villous adenoma is usually diagnosed by colonoscopy. The prostaglandin antagonist indomethacin (25 to 100 mg orally daily) reduces the diarrhea in some patients; resection is curative.

Diabetes Mellitus–Related Diarrhea

Constipation is more common than diarrhea in patients with diabetes. High-volume, watery diarrhea, often with nocturnal incontinence, occurs in 20% of poorly controlled type 1 diabetic patients. These patients usually have concomitant neuropathy, nephropathy, and retinopathy. The diarrhea may be due to several causes, including celiac disease, anal incontinence, bacterial overgrowth related to dysmotility, medications (metformin, acarbose), and autonomic neuropathy. If no specific cause is found, clonidine (initial dose 0.1 mg orally twice daily and titrated slowly to a maximal dose of 0.5 to 0.6 mg orally twice daily) may be helpful. Patients with neuropathy frequently have impaired anal sphincter function, and high-dose loperamide (4 mg orally four times a day) may improve the incontinence.

Alcoholic Diarrhea

Diarrhea related to alcohol ingestion (Chapter 32) may be due to rapid intestinal transit, decreased bile and pancreatic secretion, nutritional deficiencies such as folate or vitamin B_{12}, or alcohol-related enteric neuropathy. Diarrhea may be acute with binge drinking, or it may be chronic and watery and persist for days or weeks. The diarrhea slowly resolves with abstinence from alcohol, proper nutrition, and the repletion of vitamin deficiencies.

Factitious Diarrhea

Approximately 30% of patients referred to tertiary centers have chronic diarrhea due to laxative abuse. The diarrhea is usually severe and watery, often with nocturnal symptoms. Some patients may have abdominal pain, weight loss, nausea, vomiting, hypokalemic myopathy, and acidosis. Stool volumes range from 300 to 3000 mL a day depending on the dose of laxative ingested. In the United States, bisacodyl is the most common cause. Other culprits include anthraquinone (senna, cascara, aloe, rhubarb) or osmotic laxatives (neutral phosphate, Epsom salts, and magnesium citrate). Some patients abuse other agents that cause diarrhea, such as the diuretics furosemide and ethacrynic acid.

More than 90% of laxative abusers are women who have underlying eating disorders such as anorexia nervosa or bulimia (Chapter 226) or middle-aged women who have complicated medical histories and who often work in health care. In patients with unexplained diarrhea, laxative screening of stool and urine (see later) should be performed to exclude this syndrome before an extensive medical evaluation is performed for other causes of chronic diarrhea.

Chronic Idiopathic Secretory Diarrhea

In a small subset of patients with secretory diarrhea, no cause is found despite an extensive evaluation. These cases are labeled as chronic idiopathic secretory diarrhea. In most patients, the diarrhea resolves within 6 to 24 months, which suggests a possible postinfectious or Brainerd's diarrhea. If no diagnosis is found after thorough testing and a search for surreptitious laxative abuse, a therapeutic trial with bile salt–binding drugs (e.g., cholestyramine, 4 g orally before meals three times a day, or the more potent colesevelam, 625-mg tablet two to six times daily) or opiates (e.g., loperamide, 2 mg orally four times a day, maximal dose 16 mg a day) is warranted.

INFLAMMATORY DIARRHEAS

Diarrhea due to inflammation is characterized by watery or bloody stools, fecal leukocytes, and loss of protein in the stool (see Fig. 142-8).

Inflammatory Bowel Disease

See Chapter 143.

Eosinophilic Gastroenteritis

Eosinophilic gastroenteritis is an increasingly recognized condition of unknown etiology characterized by infiltration of eosinophils in the mucosa, muscle, or serosal layers of the gastrointestinal tract. Approximately 50% of patients have atopic histories. Infestation with nematodes (Chapter 365) must be excluded before this diagnosis is made. Diarrhea occurs in 30 to 60% of patients with mucosal disease. Patients with involvement of the muscle layer often present with abdominal pain, nausea, and vomiting indicative of gastric outlet or intestinal obstruction. Peripheral eosinophilia is present in most patients. The disease may involve the entire gastrointestinal tract from esophagus to anus, or it may be isolated to a segment. With diffuse involvement, patients may have steatorrhea, protein-losing enteropathy, and blood loss.

COLLAGENOUS COLITIS AND LYMPHOCYTIC COLITIS

These two conditions, collectively known as *microscopic colitis*, may or may not be the same disease or variants of the same disease. Lymphocytic colitis is equally prevalent in men and women, whereas collagenous colitis occurs ten times more often in middle-aged or elderly women. These conditions may be associated with autoimmune disease or with NSAID use. There is an increased prevalence (15%) of microscopic colitis among individuals with celiac sprue. These diseases may be categorized as either inflammatory or secretory diarrheas. An epidemiologic relationship to medications such as NSAIDs, H_2-receptor blockers, proton pump inhibitors, selective serotonin reuptake inhibitors, and others has been reported, and increased luminal prostaglandin levels may cause the diarrhea. Enteric infections, food hypersensitivity, or intraluminal bile has been proposed as a trigger for prostaglandin release from lymphocytes. The disease disappears with fecal stream diversion. Antidiarrheal agents such as loperamide (2 mg orally four times a day) are the mainstay of therapy. Budesonide (9 mg orally once a day),[9,10] bismuth subsalicylate therapy (eight chewable 262-mg tablets orally once a day), and 5-aminosalicylates (e.g., mesalamine, 400 to 800 mg orally three times daily) may be useful. Those with refractory disease may require corticosteroids (e.g., prednisone, 40 mg orally once a day).

FOOD ALLERGY

Food allergies or sensitivities, especially to cow's milk and soy protein, are a well established cause of enterocolitis in children, with an estimated frequency of 5%. Symptoms of abdominal cramps, diarrhea, and sometimes vomiting occur shortly after ingestion of the allergen (Chapter 261). The role of food allergy in causing diarrhea in adults is less clear owing to the lack of a reliable diagnostic test. Allergy testing correlates poorly with intestinal allergy. The most common food allergens are milk, soy, eggs, seafood, nuts, and wheat. Sequential elimination diets can be diagnostic and therapeutic.

Protein-Losing Enteropathy

Severe protein loss through the gastrointestinal tract can be caused by mucosal diseases such as lymphangiectasia, lymphatic obstruction, bacterial or parasitic infection, gastritis (Chapter 141), gastric cancer, collagenous colitis, inflammatory bowel disease (Chapter 143), celiac disease, sarcoidosis (Chapter 95), lymphoma (Chapter 191), tuberculosis (Chapter 332), Ménétrier's disease (Chapter 198), eosinophilic gastroenteritis, and food allergies. A variety of extraintestinal diseases, including systemic lupus erythematosus (Chapter 274), heart failure (Chapter 58), and constrictive pericarditis (Chapter 77), also can be causative. Patients with systemic lupus erythematosus (Chapter 274) may present with protein-losing enteropathy as the only manifestation of their disease. Treatment focuses on the underlying disease.

Radiation Enteritis

Patients who receive pelvic radiation for malignancies of the female urogenital tract or the male prostate may develop chronic radiation enterocolitis 6 to 12 months after total doses of radiation greater than 40 to 60 Gy (Chapters 19 and 144). Symptoms can develop 20 years after treatment, however. Early abnormalities include an increase in inflammatory mediators, an increase in cholinergic stimulation of intestinal tissue, and endothelial cell apoptosis that precedes epithelial cell apoptosis. The last finding suggests that vascular injury is the primary event. Vascular endothelial growth factor, basic fibroblast growth factor, and IL-11 protect animal intestine from experimental radiation damage. Diarrhea may be caused by bile acid malabsorption if the ileum is damaged, by bacterial overgrowth if radiation causes small intestinal strictures or bypass, or by radiation-induced chronic inflammation of the small intestine and colon. Rapid transit also may contribute to malabsorption and diarrhea.

TREATMENT 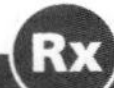

Treatment is often unsatisfactory. Anti-inflammatory drugs (sulfasalazine, corticosteroids) and antibiotics have been tried with little success. Cholestyramine (4 g orally three times a day) and NSAIDs (e.g., naproxen, 250 to 500 mg orally twice daily) may help, as may opiates (loperamide, 2 mg orally four times a day, or loperamide-*N*-oxide, 3 mg orally two times a day).

Miscellaneous Diseases

Although acute mesenteric arterial or venous thrombosis manifests as an acute bloody diarrhea, chronic mesenteric vascular ischemia (Chapter 145) may manifest as watery diarrhea. Gastrointestinal tuberculosis (Chapter 332) and histoplasmosis (Chapter 340) manifest as diarrhea that may be either bloody or watery, as do certain immunologic diseases, such as Behçet's syndrome or Churg-Strauss syndrome. All of these diseases may be misdiagnosed as inflammatory bowel disease (Chapter 143). Neutropenic enterocolitis, an ileocolitis that occurs in neutropenic leukemic patients, sometimes is caused by *C. difficile* infection.

CLINICAL MANIFESTATIONS OF CHRONIC DIARRHEA

Patients with malabsorption can present with a variety of gastrointestinal or extraintestinal manifestations (Table 142-6). Significant malabsorption of fat and carbohydrate usually causes chronic diarrhea, abdominal cramps, gas, bloating, and weight loss. Steatorrhea (fat in the stool) manifests as oily, foul-smelling stools that are difficult to flush down the toilet. Stools may be large and bulky (e.g., pancreatic insufficiency) or watery (e.g., bacterial overgrowth, mucosal diseases). Individuals with malabsorption also can present with manifestations of vitamin and mineral deficiencies. Dyspnea can be caused by anemia from iron, folate, or vitamin B_{12} deficiency. Manifestations of calcium, magnesium, or vitamin D malabsorption include paresthesias and tetany due to hypocalcemia or hypomagnesemia and bone pain due to osteomalacia or osteoporosis-related fractures. Paresthesias and ataxia are manifestations of cobalamin and vitamin E deficiency. Dermatitis herpetiformis is a blistering, burning, itchy rash on the extensor surfaces and buttocks that is associated with celiac disease.

Inflammatory diarrheas may present with fever and abdominal pain or with edema to suggest chronic protein loss. Patients may have multiple, low-volume, bloody stools with tenesmus to suggest proctitis, or have severe diarrhea due to GVHD or celiac disease. Systemic manifestations of inflammatory bowel disease include polymigratory arthritis, sacroiliitis, erythema nodosum, pyoderma gangrenosum, leukocytoclastic angiitis, uveitis, and oral aphthous ulcers.

TABLE 142-6 CLINICAL CONSEQUENCES OF MALABSORPTION OF NUTRIENTS, WATER, AND ELECTROLYTES

NUTRIENT MALABSORBED	CLINICAL MANIFESTATION
Protein	Wasting, edema
Carbohydrate and fat	Diarrhea, abdominal cramps and bloating, weight loss and growth retardation
Fluid and electrolytes	Diarrhea, dehydration
Iron	Anemia, cheilosis, angular stomatitis
Calcium and vitamin D	Bone pain, fractures, tetany
Magnesium	Paresthesias, tetany
Vitamin B_{12} and folate	Anemia, glossitis, cheilosis, paresthesias, ataxia (vitamin B_{12} only)
Vitamin E	Paresthesias, ataxia, retinopathy
Vitamin A	Night blindness, xerophthalmia, hyperkeratosis, diarrhea
Vitamin K	Ecchymoses
Riboflavin	Angular stomatitis, cheilosis
Zinc	Dermatitis, hypogeusia, diarrhea
Selenium	Cardiomyopathy
Essential fatty acids	Dermatitis

DIAGNOSIS OF CHRONIC DIARRHEA

A detailed history, physical examination, and certain screening tests lead to a diagnosis in 75 to 80% of patients with chronic diarrheas (see Table 142-1 and Fig. 142-3). A history of 10 to 20 daily bowel movements that do not respond to fasting suggests secretory diarrhea (see Fig. 142-8). A history of peptic ulcer should suggest gastrinoma (Chapter 201) or systemic mastocytosis (Chapter 263). Physical examination is helpful only if the thyromegaly of medullary carcinoma (Chapter 254), the cutaneous flushing of the neuroendocrine tumors and systemic mastocytosis, the dermatographism of systemic mastocytosis, or the migratory necrolytic erythema of glucagonoma (Chapter 201) is evident. Autonomic dysfunction (e.g., postural hypotension, impotence, gustatory sweating) is almost invariably present in diabetic diarrhea.

Evaluation for malabsorption begins with a careful elicitation of bowel habits, a description of the stool, weight loss, travel, food or milk tolerance, underlying gastrointestinal or liver diseases, abdominal surgery, radiation or chemotherapy treatments, family history, and drug and alcohol use.

Blood Tests

Blood measurements (see Fig. 142-3) of iron, folate, vitamin B_{12}, vitamin D, or prothrombin time (vitamin K) help evaluate malabsorption. Peripheral blood findings of leukocytosis, eosinophilia, elevated erythrocyte sedimentation rate, hypoalbuminemia, or low total serum protein suggests an inflammatory diarrhea, whose hallmark is the presence of blood, either gross or occult, and leukocytes in the stool. There are no bedside screening tests to establish the diagnosis in watery diarrheas.

Imaging

Malabsorption may be suggested if a flat plate radiograph of the abdomen shows pancreatic calcification (Chapter 135). Some diseases (e.g., previous gastric surgery, gastrocolic fistulas, blind loops from previous intestinal anastomoses, small intestine strictures, multiple jejunal diverticula, abnormal intestinal motility that could lead to bacterial overgrowth) may be shown by computed tomography or magnetic resonance imaging of the abdomen after administration of oral contrast agents or by a traditional upper gastrointestinal radiographic series with small intestine follow-through. A small bowel barium study may show thickening of the intestinal folds (e.g., amyloidosis, lymphoma or Whipple's disease), uniform or patchy abnormalities (e.g., lymphoma or lymphangiectasia), or flocculation of barium and ilealization of jejunum to suggest celiac disease. Routine contrast radiographs of the gastrointestinal tract usually are not helpful in the diagnosis of watery diarrheas, unless they show extensive small bowel resection, the presence of a tumor (carcinoid or villous adenoma), or a bowel filled with fluid (endocrine tumor). Abdominal contrast imaging may show diagnostic evidence of advanced inflammatory bowel disease or changes suggestive of eosinophilic gastroenteritis or radiation enterocolitis. Somatostatin receptor scintigraphy with indium-111-labeled octreotide can be useful in localizing gastrinomas, pancreatic endocrine tumors, and carcinoid tumors.

Endoscopy and Biopsy

Upper endoscopy with distal duodenal biopsy should be undertaken if serologic tests for celiac disease are positive or diagnostic clues suggest small bowel mucosal malabsorption (Chapter 136). Small bowel biopsy is virtually always abnormal when the tTG IgA antibody level is very high (more than five-fold the normal range), and EMA is positive. A biopsy may be avoided in this setting. Some patients may have patchy mucosal disease and require enteroscopy with jejunal biopsies for diagnosis. Wireless video capsule endoscopy (Chapter 136) and balloon-assisted enteroscopy are increasingly used to diagnose diseases that reside deep in the small bowel. Patients with severe watery or elusive diarrhea should have a colonoscopy to assess for villous adenomas, microscopic colitis, mastocytosis, or early inflammatory bowel disease. Colonoscopy may also show brown pigmentation suggestive of melanosis coli due to chronic use of anthracene laxatives. Terminal ileal biopsy may indicate infectious or inflammatory bowel disease.

Other Laboratory Tests

Malabsorption

If chronic diarrhea is the presenting symptom, a stool examination for ova and parasites and a stool antigen-capture ELISA test for *Giardia* should be

TABLE 142-7 ABNORMALITIES CONDUCIVE TO BACTERIAL OVERGROWTH

STRUCTURAL
Afferent loop syndrome after gastrojejunostomy
Ileocecal valve resection
End-to-side intestinal anastomoses
Duodenal and jejunal diverticula
Strictures (Crohn's disease, radiation enteritis)
Adhesions (postsurgical)
Gastrojejunocolic fistulas
MOTOR
Scleroderma
Diabetes mellitus
Idiopathic pseudo-obstruction
HYPOCHLORHYDRIA
Atrophic gastritis
Proton pump inhibitors
Acquired immunodeficiency syndrome
Acid-reducing surgery for peptic ulcer disease
MISCELLANEOUS
Immunodeficiency states
Pancreatitis
Cirrhosis
Chronic renal failure

obtained. A stool test for fat on a high-fat diet (70 to 100 g/day) is the best available screening test for malabsorption (see Table 142-6). If the fecal fat test result is negative, selective carbohydrate malabsorption or other causes of watery diarrhea should be considered. If the fecal fat test result is positive, further testing should be based on clinical suspicion for particular diseases. If pancreatic insufficiency is suspected, imaging studies of the pancreas should be performed. If proximal mucosal damage is suspected, multiple small intestinal biopsy specimens should be obtained. If there are no clues to the cause of malabsorption, a D-xylose test may help to distinguish mucosal disease from pancreatic insufficiency. However, the D-xylose test result also can be abnormal in individuals with bacterial overgrowth; if this condition is suspected, culture of an intestinal aspirate or a breath test should be obtained (see Table 142-6). Small bowel contrast imaging is useful in detecting ileal disease and structural abnormalities that predispose to bacterial overgrowth (Table 142-7). Some individuals with celiac disease present with selective nutrient deficiencies without diarrhea. In these cases, tTG antibody tests and intestinal biopsy should be performed. In patients hospitalized for severe diarrhea or malnutrition, a more streamlined evaluation usually includes a stool for culture, ova and parasites, and fat; an abdominal imaging study; and a biopsy of the small intestine and colon.

Watery Diarrhea

Breath tests to measure the respiratory excretion of labeled CO_2 after oral administration and metabolism of radioactive carbon-labeled substrates, or of H_2 after administration of carbohydrates, can assess carbohydrate and bile salt malabsorption or bacterial overgrowth (see Table 142-6).

The diagnosis of endocrine tumors, such as carcinoids, gastrinoma, VIPoma, medullary carcinoma of the thyroid, glucagonoma, somatostatinoma, and systemic mastocytosis, is made by showing elevated blood levels of serotonin or urinary 5-hydroxyindoleacetic acid and serum levels for gastrin, vasoactive intestinal peptide, calcitonin, glucagon, somatostatin, histamine, or prostaglandins (Chapter 201). Somatostatin receptor scintigraphy has proved to be sensitive and useful in the diagnosis and evaluation of Zollinger-Ellison syndrome (Chapter 201).

Inflammatory Diarrhea

Stool occult blood, white blood cells, or lactoferrin and calprotectin (components of leukocytes) are helpful tests for bowel inflammation. Video capsule endoscopy (Chapter 136) of the small bowel may detect ulcerations deep in the small bowel not reachable by standard upper or lower endoscopy and not detected with conventional barium contrast radiography. However, the risk of capsule retention in the small bowel is high in patients with Crohn's disease or NSAID use, particularly when there is a history of obstructive symptoms. The most sensitive test for protein-losing enteropathy is measurement of intestinal protein loss by 24-hour stool excretion or clearance of α_1-antitrypsin.

Stool Examination in Elusive Diarrhea

An important adjunct to diagnosing the cause of diarrhea is to examine the stool. The greasy, bulky stool of steatorrhea and the bloody stool of gut inflammation are distinctive. Stool collections (see Table 142-6) can be analyzed for weight, volume, fat, electrolytes ($^{+}Na^{++}$, K^{++}, Cl^{-}), osmolality, pH, and a laxative screen (SO_4^{2-}, PO_4^{2-}, Mg^{2+}). Stool or urine can be analyzed for emetine (a component of ipecac), bisacodyl, castor oil, or anthraquinone.

Carbohydrate malabsorption lowers stool pH because of colonic fermentation of carbohydrate to short-chain fatty acids. Stool pH less than 5.3 usually means pure carbohydrate malabsorption, whereas in the generalized malabsorptive diseases, stool pH is greater than 5.6 and usually greater than 6.0.

The normal stool osmotic gap, which is the difference between stool osmolality (or 290 mOsm) and twice the stool Na^{++} and K^{++} concentrations, is 50 to 125. In secretory diarrheas, the colon's capacity for adjusting electrolyte concentrations is overwhelmed, the stool osmotic gap is less than 50, and stool electrolytes more nearly resemble plasma electrolytes ($^{+}Na^{++}$ concentrations are usually >90 mmol/L, K^{+} concentrations usually <10 mmol/L), except for higher HCO_3^{-} concentrations (usually >50 mmol/L). In osmotic diarrhea, the presence of uncharged solute or unmeasured cation in the colonic lumen draws in water, depresses stool Na^{++} (usually <60 mmol/L) and K^{+} concentrations, and results in a stool osmotic gap >125. Stools with Na^{++} concentrations between 60 and 90 mmol/L and calculated osmotic gaps between 50 and 100 can result from either secretory or malabsorptive abnormalities. Patients with Mg^{2++}-induced diarrhea may be diagnosed by fecal Mg^{2+} values of more than 50 mmol/L. Sodium anion–induced diarrheas (Na_2SO_4, Na_2PO_4) mimic secretory diarrhea because the stool Na^{++} content is high (>90 mmol/L), and there is no osmotic gap; this diarrhea may be diagnosed by determining stool Cl^{-} concentration because these anions displace stool Cl^{-} resulting in a depressed stool Cl^{-} value (usually <20 mmol/L).

TREATMENT OF CHRONIC DIARRHEA Rx

Antidiarrheal Therapy

Antidiarrheal agents are of two types: those used for mild to moderate diarrheas and those used for severe secretory diarrheas. A major shortcoming of opiates, the most commonly prescribed antidiarrheal agents, is that they have no antisecretory effect. Rather, they act by decreasing intestinal motility, thereby allowing longer contact time with the mucosa for improved fluid absorption. The exception is racecadotril, an enkephalinase inhibitor, that blocks intestinal fluid secretion without affecting motility.

Bulk-forming agents (psyllium [7 g in 8 ounces water orally up to five times a day] and methylcellulose [three to six tablets twice a day with 300 mL of water]) act by binding water and increasing the consistency of stool. Pectin has been shown to have proabsorptive activity. These agents may be useful in patients with fecal incontinence. Bismuth subsalicylates (524 mg orally every hour up to eight doses a day) have mild antisecretory and antimotility effects and are effective and safe in mild diarrheas. Agents that bind bile salts (e.g., cholestyramine, 2 to 4 g orally two to four times a day) are effective in the treatment of bile acid diarrheas but may worsen diarrhea in patients with ileal resection or disease of more than 100 cm of ileum.

The opiates may be symptomatically useful in mild to moderate diarrheas. Paregoric, deodorized tincture of opium, codeine, and diphenoxylate with atropine largely have been supplanted by loperamide. Loperamide does not pass the blood-brain barrier and has a high first-pass metabolism in the liver; it has a high therapeutic-to-toxic ratio and is essentially devoid of addiction potential. It is safe in adults, even in total doses of 24 mg/day. The usual dose is 2 to 4 mg two to four times daily. Opiates may be harmful in patients with severe diarrheas because large volumes of fluid may pool in the intestinal lumen (third space), and stool output is no longer a reliable gauge for replacing fluid losses. The antimotility effects are a problem in infectious diarrheas because stasis may enhance bacterial invasion and delay clearance of microorganisms from the bowel. Opiates and anticholinergics also are dangerous in severe inflammatory bowel disease or severe *C. difficile* infection, where they may precipitate megacolon.

Antidiarrhea agents that are used for the treatment of severe secretory and inflammatory diarrheas generally have profiles with more serious side effects. The somatostatin analogue octreotide (initial dose, 100 to 600 μg subcutaneously in two to four divided doses daily; maximal dose, 1500 μg daily) lessens diarrhea in the carcinoid syndrome and in neuroendocrine tumors because it inhibits hormone secretion by the tumor. It is also effective in the treatment of dumping syndrome and chemotherapy-related diarrheas. Long-acting subcutaneous octreotide preparations (20 to 30 mg intramuscularly intragluteally every month) are now available for once-a-month dosing. Octreotide can suppress pancreatic enzyme secretion and make diarrhea worse; it also may be of only limited usefulness in short-bowel syndrome and AIDS diarrhea. Agents such as phenothiazine and calcium-channel blockers have mild antisecretory effects, but side effects limit their use. Clonidine (initial dose, 0.1 mg orally twice daily, titrated slowly to a maximal dose of 0.5 to 0.6 mg twice daily) is most useful in opiate withdrawal diarrhea and is sometimes useful in diabetic diarrhea; postural hypotension may limit its use, particularly in patients with diabetes. Alosetron (0.5 mg orally twice daily for four weeks, maximal dose 1 mg orally twice daily) may be justified for severe diarrhea-predominant irritable bowel syndrome; associations with ischemic colitis and severe constipation have limited its use. Indomethacin (250 to 500 mg orally twice daily), a cyclooxygenase blocker that inhibits prostaglandin production, is useful in the treatment of diarrheas caused by acute radiation, AIDS, or villous adenomas of the rectum or colon; occasionally, it may be useful in neuroendocrine tumors and food allergy. For eosinophilic gastroenteritis, corticosteroids (prednisone, 20 to 40 mg orally once a day for 7 to 10 days) are the mainstay of therapy, but disodium cromoglycate (200 mg orally four times daily) also may be useful; food elimination diets are not usually effective. Treatment of inflammatory bowel disease is described in Chapter 143.

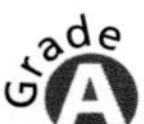

1. Lowy I, Molrine DC, Leav BA, et al. Treatment with monoclonal antibodies against *Clostridium difficile* toxins. *N Engl J Med.* 2010;362:197-205.
2. Richardson V, Hernandez-Pichardo J, Quintanar-Solares M, et al. Effect of rotavirus vaccination on death from childhood diarrhea in Mexico. *N Engl J Med.* 2010;362:299-305.
3. Madhi SA, Cunliffe NA, Steele D, et al. Effect of human rotavirus vaccine on severe diarrhea in African infants. *N Engl J Med.* 2010;362:289-298.
4. Sur D, Lopez AL, Kanungo S, et al. Efficacy and safety of modified killed-whole-cell oral cholera vaccine in India: an interim analysis of a cluster-randomised, double-blind, placebo-controlled trial. *Lancet.* 2009;374:1694-1702.
5. Dupont HL, Jiang ZD, Okhuysen PC, et al. A randomized, double-blind, placebo-controlled trial of rifaximin to prevent travelers' diarrhea. *Ann Intern Med.* 2005;142:805-812.
6. Lauritano EC, Gabrielli M, Scarpellini E, et al. Antibiotic therapy in small intestinal bacterial overgrowth: rifaximin versus metronidazole. *Eur Rev Med Pharmacol Sci.* 2009;13:111-116.
7. Byrne TA, Wilmore DW, Iyer K, et al. Growth hormone, glutamine, and an optimal diet reduces parenteral nutrition in patients with short bowel syndrome: a prospective, randomized, placebo-controlled, double-blind clinical trial. *Ann Surg.* 2005;242:655-661.
8. Jeppesen PB, Gilroy R, Pertkiewicz M, et al. Randomized placebo-controlled trial of teduglutide in reducing parenteral nutrition and/or intravenous fluid requirements in patients with short bowel syndrome. *Gut.* 2011. [Epub ahead of print.]
9. Miehlke S, Madisch A, Bethke B, et al. Oral budesonide for maintenance treatment of collagenous colitis: a randomized, double-blind, placebo-controlled trial. *Gastroenterology.* 2008;135:1510-1516.
10. Miehlke S, Madisch A, Karimi D, et al. Budesonide is effective in treating lymphocytic colitis: a randomized double-blind placebo-controlled study. *Gastroenterology.* 2009;136:2092-2100.

SUGGESTED READINGS

Feurle GE, Junga NS, Marth T. Efficacy of ceftriaxone or meropenem as initial therapies in Whipple's disease. *Gastroenterology.* 2010;138:478-486. *Either antibiotic is an effective initial therapy.*

Lopman BA, Hall AJ, Curns AT, et al. Increasing rates of gastroenteritis hospital discharges in U.S. adults and the contribution of norovirus, 1996-2007. *Clin Infect Dis.* 2011;52:466-474. *Norovirus, which causes 10% of cause-unspecified and 7% of all-cause admissions for gastroenteritis, should be routinely considered in hospitalized patients.*

van der Windt DA, Jellema P, Mulder CJ, et al. Diagnostic testing for celiac disease among patients with abdominal symptoms: a systematic review. *JAMA.* 2010;303:1738-1746. *IgA anti-tissue transglutaminase antibodies and IgA antiendomysial antibodies have a high sensitivity and specificity for diagnosing celiac disease among patients with abdominal symptoms.*

Williams JJ, Beck PL, Andrews CN, et al. Microscopic colitis: a common cause of diarrhea in older adults. *Age Aging.* 2010;39:162-168. *About 10 to 30% of older patients with diarrhea and normal colonoscopy have microscopic colitis.*

143

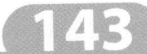

INFLAMMATORY BOWEL DISEASE

GARY R. LICHTENSTEIN

DEFINITION

Inflammatory bowel disease refers to two chronic idiopathic inflammatory disorders, ulcerative colitis and Crohn's disease. These disorders are diagnosed by characteristic clinical, endoscopic, and histologic features, but no single individual finding is absolutely diagnostic for one disease or the other. Ulceration from Crohn's disease may be transmural and may occur anywhere in the gastrointestinal tract, most commonly in the distal ileum and proximal colon. The hallmark of ulcerative colitis is continuous ulceration starting in the rectum and limited to the colon. Approximately 10% of patients with inflammatory bowel disease have indeterminant colitis, a term used when Crohn's colitis cannot be differentiated from ulcerative colitis.

EPIDEMIOLOGY

Inflammatory bowel disease occurs worldwide, but the highest incidence is found in North America, the United Kingdom, and northern Europe. The incidence of Crohn's disease has risen slowly over time, although ulcerative colitis remains slightly more prevalent than Crohn's disease. The incidence of ulcerative colitis in North America is estimated to be 2.2 to 14.3 per 100,000 person years, with a prevalence of 37 to 246 per 100,000. The incidence of Crohn's disease in North America is estimated to be 3.1 to 14.6 per 100,000 person years, with a prevalence of 26 to 199 per 100,000.

Crohn's disease and ulcerative colitis may occur at any age. The peak incidence of Crohn's disease occurs between age 15 and 30 years of age, with a second peak in the seventh decade. There is a 1.2 : 1 female-to-male ratio. Ulcerative colitis also has a bimodal peak age distribution, with an initial peak between 20 and 40 years of age and second smaller peak beyond the seventh decade. There is an equal gender distribution in ulcerative colitis.

Crohn's disease and ulcerative colitis are polygenic disorders, for which family history is a risk factor. Crohn's disease and ulcerative colitis occur in all ethnic groups and races, but their incidence is highest in whites and Jewish people of Eastern European (Ashkenazi Jews) descent. In North America and the United Kingdom, however, the incidence of Crohn's disease in African Americans and African Caribbeans appears to be approaching that of whites. Studies of migrants from underdeveloped countries in South Asia to the United Kingdom suggest an increased prevalence of inflammatory bowel disease in subsequent generations, presumably as a result of environmental influences.

Cigarette smoking is associated with a worse prognosis in patients with Crohn's disease but an improved course in ulcerative colitis. Nonsteroidal anti-inflammatory drugs (NSAIDs) appear to be associated with exacerbations of disease, although evidence for this is less definitive. Appendectomy has been suggested as protective against the development of ulcerative colitis. Diet does not clearly affect the course of inflammatory bowel disease.

PATHOBIOLOGY

Although the trigger for inflammatory bowel disease is not known, three major pathways likely activate the disease: a genetic predisposition, immune dysregulation, and an environmental antigen. A possible explanation is that the inability of the innate immune system to clear microbial antigens, combined with increased intestinal epithelial permeability to antigens, eventually leads to an overactive adaptive immune response.

Genetics

Of patients with inflammatory bowel disease, 5 to 20% have a positive family history. First-degree relatives have a 10- to 15-fold increased risk for developing inflammatory bowel disease. The concordance rate of developing Crohn's disease in identical twins, siblings, and first-degree relatives is 50%, 0 to 3%, and 5 to 10%, respectively. Ulcerative colitis follows similar genetic patterns but with slightly lower risk rates. Twenty percent of patients with a positive family history of inflammatory bowel disease will have discordant disease type: one family member with Crohn's disease and another with ulcerative colitis.

The initial gene associated with Crohn's disease is *NOD2/CARD15*, located on chromosome 16 (16q12), and is expressed in intestinal epithelial Paneth cells, macrophages, and dendritic cells. This gene is involved in the expression of an intracellular receptor that senses muramyl dipeptide, a peptidoglycan component of gram-positive bacteria. Activation of *NOD2* leads to activation of NF-κB, which mediates transcription of numerous proinflammatory cytokines. A mutation in the leucine-rich domain of the NOD2 protein, which interacts with bacterial lipopolysaccharide, leads to failure in activation of NF-κB and is associated with the development of Crohn's disease.

Toll-like receptor-4 gene polymorphisms are associated with both Crohn's disease and ulcerative colitis. Polymorphisms of the interleukin-23 (IL-23) receptor gene are associated with ulcerative colitis and a varied risk of Crohn's disease. Human leukocyte antigen (HLA) class II polymorphisms, especially in HLA-DR molecules, may confer increased risk for ulcerative colitis and possibly Crohn's as well. The *OCTN1* gene, located on chromosome 5, and the *DLG5* gene, located on chromosome 10, have also been associated with

Crohn's disease. *DLG5*, which encodes a scaffolding protein that is important for maintaining epithelial integrity in various organs, may interact with the *NOD2/CARD15* gene to increase susceptibility to Crohn's disease. Gene *OCTN1*, located on chromosome 5q31, codes for an ion channel and also increases the risk of Crohn's disease; mutations in this gene may disrupt ion channels through altered function of cation transporters and cell-to-cell signaling in the intestinal epithelium.

PATHOPHYSIOLOGY

Microbes likely play a part in the development of inflammatory bowel disease. In several animal models of colitis, colitis does not develop in a sterile environment but can be induced after the introduction of commensal bacteria. Diverting the fecal stream away from active mucosal inflammation, such as in an ileostomy, also helps alleviate inflammation in Crohn's disease. Antibiotics, particularly antibiotics with broad-spectrum anaerobic coverage, are helpful in the treatment of Crohn's disease. More recently, several genetic polymorphisms associated with sensing the intestinal microbial environment and triggering an immune response have been linked to inflammatory bowel disease.

Both Crohn's disease and ulcerative colitis are products of a dysregulated innate immune system that triggers T cells and a humoral response. T_H17 cells, which are activated in Crohn's disease and ulcerative colitis, are stimulated by IL-23, which is produced by antigen-presenting cells. Variations in single-nucleotide polymorphisms of the gene encoding the receptor for IL-23 are associated with Crohn's disease.

Pathology

Crohn's Disease

As a result of a dysregulated immune system, patients with Crohn's disease develop aphthous ulcers, which are superficial mucosal ulcers. As the disease progresses, the ulceration becomes deeper, transmural, and discrete; it may form a serpiginous pattern and may occur anywhere from the esophagus to the anus in a noncontinuous pattern. The most common location for ulceration is the ileocecal region. In some patients, chronic disease leads to the formation of fibrotic strictures, and approximately 30% of patients may develop fistulas.

In early Crohn's disease, the histopathology is characterized by an acute inflammatory infiltrate in the lamina propria, with cryptitis, and crypt abscesses. Later in the disease process, the crypt architecture becomes distorted, with a lymphocytic infiltrate and a resulting branching and shortening of the crypts. Noncaseating granulomas, which are present in up to 15% of endoscopic biopsy specimens and as many as 70% of surgical specimens, are not unique to Crohn's disease but help confirm the diagnosis when other classic features are present.

Surgical specimens also may show transmural intestinal wall inflammation and fat creeping on the serosal surface.

Ulcerative Colitis

In mild ulcerative colitis, the mucosa is granular, hyperemic, and edematous in appearance. As the disease becomes more severe, the mucosa ulcerates, and the ulcers may extend into the lamina propria. Ulcerative colitis starts in the rectum and may extend proximally in a continuous pattern, but it affects only the colon. Pseudopolyps may form owing to epithelial regeneration after recurrent acute attacks. With chronic disease, the colonic mucosa may lose the normal fold pattern, the colon may shorten, and the colon may appear narrowed.

In early ulcerative colitis, the histopathology is characterized by epithelial necrosis, an acute inflammatory infiltrate in the lamina propria, cryptitis, and crypt abscesses. In chronic disease, a predominant lymphocytic infiltrate and distortion of crypt architecture are seen.

CLINICAL MANIFESTATIONS

Symptoms of inflammatory bowel disease are varied and may be a consequence of the location of the disease, the duration of disease, and any anatomic complications of the disease, such as strictures and fistulas in Crohn's disease (Table 143-1).

TABLE 143-1 CLINICAL CHARACTERISTICS OF CROHN'S DISEASE AND ULCERATIVE COLITIS

	CROHN'S DISEASE	ULCERATIVE COLITIS
Peak age of onset (years of age)	15-30, 2nd peak in the 7th decade	20-40, 2nd smaller peak beyond the 7th decade
Sex distribution (F/M)	1.2/1	1/1
Potential sites of gastrointestinal involvement	Esophagus to anus	colon
Skipped areas of involvement	+	–
Transmural inflammation	+	–
Type of ulceration	Usually discrete	Continuous
Fistula	+	–
Stricture	–	–
Perianal disease (fissure, skin tags)	+	–

Symptoms

Crohn's Disease

The terminal ileum is affected in about 70% of patients with Crohn's disease. Primary ileal disease occurs in 30% of patients, whereas ileocolonic disease occurs in 40%. Symptoms may include abdominal pain, typically in the right lower quadrant, diarrhea, hematochezia, and fatigue. With more severe disease, fever and weight loss may be present. Some patients may present with obstructive symptoms, such as abdominal pain, abdominal distention, and nausea.

Only approximately 5% of patients develop Crohn's disease in the upper gastrointestinal tract, and esophageal Crohn's disease occurs in less than 2% of patients. Subjects with upper gastrointestinal Crohn's disease may present with dysphagia, odynophagia, chest pain, or heartburn. Gastroduodenal disease occurs in 0.5 to 4% of patients and commonly occurs along with distal disease. Symptoms may include upper abdominal pain. Isolated jejunal disease is rare; if the jejunum is involved, there is also distal small bowel involvement. Up to 30% of patients have perianal disease (Chapter 147) that may include the development of fistulas, abscesses, fissures, and skin tags. Symptoms of perianal disease include pain and discharge. Fever may be present if there is an abscess.

Fistulas, which are internal tracks that can occur anywhere in the gastrointestinal tract and connect to various sites, occur in 20 to 40% of Crohn's patients. Penetrating Crohn's disease may also cause intra-abdominal and perianal abscesses owing to a fistula with a blind end or intestinal perforation. External fistulas, which present with symptoms of fluid discharge from the cutaneous opening, can be enterocutaneous, or perianal. Internal fistulas can be enteroenteric, rectovaginal, or enterocolonic. Patients may present with persistent abdominal pain and fever with an abscess in this location.

Ulcerative Colitis

As with Crohn's disease, symptoms and signs of ulcerative colitis depend on the extent and severity of disease. At the time of diagnosis, 14 to 37% of patients have pancolitis, 36 to 41% have disease extending beyond the rectum, and 44 to 49% have proctosigmoiditis. Symptoms include hematochezia, diarrhea, tenesmus, passage of mucus, urgency to defecate, and abdominal pain. In the setting of proctitis or proctosigmoiditis, patients may have constipation with difficulty defecating. With more extensive and severe colonic involvement, patients may also have weight loss and fever. Patients may also have nausea and vomiting because of abdominal pain, fatigue because of anemia, and peripheral edema because of hypoalbuminemia.

Physical Examination

Signs on physical examination are representative of the type of disease as well as its location and severity. Oral ulcers may be present in Crohn's disease. The location of abdominal tenderness usually reflects the location of intestinal involvement. In Crohn's disease, abdominal tenderness is classically in the right lower quadrant and may include fullness or a mass depending on the severity of inflammation. Peritoneal signs may occur when penetrating Crohn's disease causes intestinal perforation. Rectal examination may reveal skin tags, hemorrhoids, fissure, and fistulas.

Extraintestinal Manifestations

Arthropathy, the most common extraintestinal manifestation (Table 143-2), affects up to 10 to 20% of subjects. Peripheral arthralgias, arthritis, ankylosing spondylitis (Chapter 273), and sacroiliitis may exacerbate with

TABLE 143-2 EXTRAINTESTINAL COMPLICATIONS OF INFLAMMATORY BOWEL DISEASE

	CROHN'S DISEASE	ULCERATIVE COLITIS
Ocular disorders (uveitis, episcleritis)	+	+
Arthropathy	+	+
Oral ulcers	+	–
Skin disorders (pyoderma gangrenosum, erythema nodosum)	+	+
Nephrolithiasis	+	+
Primary sclerosing cholangitis	+	+
Bone disorders (osteoporosis, osteomalacia)	+	–
Thromboembolic disease	+	+
B_{12} deficiency	+	–

TABLE 143-3 DIFFERENTIAL DIAGNOSIS OF ILEITIS AND COLITIS

INFECTIONS	MEDICATIONS/TOXINS
Bacterial *Aeromonas* *Campylobacter jejuni* *Chlamydia* (proctitis) *Clostridium difficile* *Mycobacterium tuberculosis* *Salmonella* *Shigella* Enterohemorrhagic *Escherichia coli* *Yersinia*	Nonsteroidal anti-inflammatory drugs Pancreatic enzyme supplements—"fibrosing colopathy" Phosphosoda bowel preparations Radiation
Viral Cytomegalovirus Herpes simplex virus (proctitis) Human immunodeficiency virus	
Fungal *Histoplasma capsulatum*	
Parasitic *Entamoeba histolytica* Helminths	
VASCULAR	**INFLAMMATORY**
Collagen vascular disease Behçet's disease Churg-Strauss syndrome Henoch-Schönlein purpura Systemic lupus erythematosus Polyarteritis nodosa	Appendicitis Diverticular disease Eosinophilic gastroenteritis Nongranulomatous ulcerative jejunoileitis (celiac disease)
Ischemia	
NEOPLASIA	**MISCELLANEOUS**
Carcinoid Carcinoma primary or metastatic Lymphoma Mycosis fungoides Malignant histiocytosis	Amyloidosis Sarcoidosis Endometriosis Tubo-ovarian abscesses

Adapted from Aberra FN, Lichtenstein GR. Crohn disease. In Talley NJ, Kane SV, Wallace MD, eds. *Practical Gastroenterology and Hepatology: Small and Large Intestine.* Wiley-Blackwell, 2010:225-235.

gastrointestinal symptoms. Dermatologic disorders, such as erythema nodosum (10 to 15%; see Fig. 448-23 in Chapter 448) and pyoderma gangrenosum (1 to 2%; Chapter 269), develop in up to 15% of patients. Eye disorders, especially uveitis and episcleritis (Chapter 431), may occur in 5 to 15%. Patients with inflammatory bowel disease also have up to a 10% risk of renal calculi, especially calcium oxalate stones (Chapter 128), in the setting of fat malabsorption with Crohn's disease in the small bowel. Uric acid stones can occur in the setting of severe volume depletion. Inflammatory bowel disease patients, especially patients with ulcerative colitis, are at increased risk for primary sclerosing cholangitis (Chapter 158).

Extraintestinal Complications

Patients with inflammatory bowel disease are susceptible to extraintestinal complications from the disease itself or medications used to treat disease. These complications include osteoporosis, osteomalacia, arthritic complications, thromboembolic events, pulmonary disease, and renal, dermatologic, and neurologic complications. Osteoporosis occurs in about 15% of patients, and steroid therapy (Chapter 34) is the major risk factor; avascular necrosis of the hip and septic arthritis are unusual complications of steroids or other immunosuppressive therapies. Cheilitis may be a result of iron deficiency anemia (Chapter 162). Patients with inflammatory bowel disease are at an increased risk for thromboembolic disease, especially in the setting of active intestinal disease, even when compared with other autoimmune diseases such as rheumatoid arthritis and celiac disease. Renal amyloidosis can be a consequence of chronic inflammation. Asthma is the most common pulmonary disorder in Crohn's disease. Patients also are at risk for multiple sclerosis (Chapter 419) and for peripheral neuropathy (Chapter 428) from vitamin B_{12} deficiency, which may occur as a result of poor absorption owing to active small bowel disease or surgical resection.

DIAGNOSIS

When diarrhea (Chapter 142) is the predominant symptom, the initial evaluation should include a thorough medical history, testing for infectious colitis (Chapter 142), and screening for endocrine-metabolic disorders such as hyperthyroidism (Chapter 233) and hypocalcemia (Chapter 253). Infections with organisms such as *Shigella* (Chapter 317), *Amoeba* (Chapter 360), *Giardia* (Chapter 359), *Escherichia coli* O157:H7 (Chapter 312), and *Campylobacter* (Chapter 311) can be accompanied by bloody diarrhea, abdominal cramps, and an endoscopic picture identical to ulcerative colitis. Stool studies are needed to diagnose or exclude these infections. If hematochezia or abdominal pain are the predominant symptom, the differential diagnosis is broad (Table 143-3).

Diagnostic Evaluation

Endoscopic Evaluation

In a patient with symptoms suggestive of inflammatory bowel disease and no evidence for an infection to explain their symptoms, endoscopic evaluation is essential. Colonoscopy is the initial endoscopic test for patients who present with lower gastrointestinal symptoms such as diarrhea and hematochezia, except in the presence of acute severe peritoneal symptoms. Colonoscopy to the terminal ileum is important if there is a potential diagnosis of inflammatory bowel disease. Small bowel imaging (such as small bowel follow-through or computed tomography [CT] enterography) may also be needed to determine whether there is small bowel disease or to determine the distribution of disease. Capsule endoscopy is useful if all other endoscopic and radiologic testing is nondiagnostic, but Crohn's disease of the small bowel is still suspected. Findings on capsule endoscopy should be followed by endoscopy to obtain biopsies. Capsule endoscopy should not be performed if Crohn's disease is complicated by a known small bowel stricture.

Crohn's Disease

Early endoscopic findings in Crohn's disease include superficial small mucosal ulcers, also called aphthous ulcers. As the severity of Crohn's disease progresses, the ulceration becomes deeper and may become round, linear, or serpiginous. A cobblestone appearance of the mucosa is caused by intersecting longitudinal and transverse ulcers, with "stone" areas representing normal mucosa (Fig. 143-1). Areas of ulceration, which are typically interspersed with normal "skip" areas, may occur anywhere from the esophagus to anus but are most common in the ileocecal region. Isolated colonic disease occurs in 25% of patients, and 60% will have rectal involvement, thereby making it at times difficult to differentiate from ulcerative colitis.

The diagnosis of inflammatory bowel disease is contingent on accurate histopathology, so biopsy of the affected area is key. Findings of an inflammatory infiltrate in the lamina propria and distortion of the crypt architecture support the diagnosis (Fig. 143-2). The diagnosis of Crohn's disease may be made by histopathology alone if noncaseating granulomas are seen, but

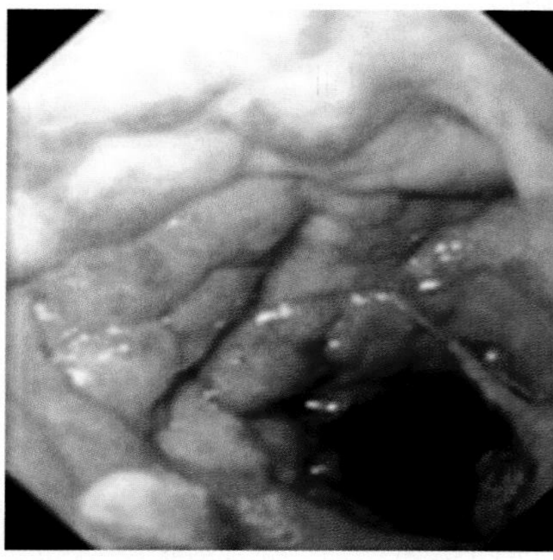

FIGURE 143-1. Endoscopic appearance of Crohn's disease with cobblestoning.

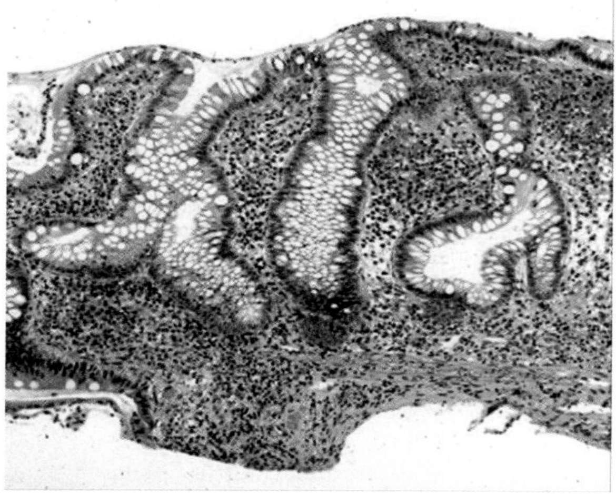

FIGURE 143-2. Colonic biopsy histopathology showing features of inflammatory bowel disease with crypt distortion and lymphocytic infiltration in the mucosa. (Adapted from AGA Institute GastroSlides 2010.)

granulomas are rarely found on endoscopic biopsies. The diagnosis of Crohn's disease is usually based on a combination of information gleaned from histopathology, colonoscopy, and small bowel imaging. A skipped pattern of ulceration, ulceration in the small bowel or upper gastrointestinal tract or the presence of fistulas supports the diagnosis of Crohn's disease. Colonic and small bowel ulceration occur in several other disorders, including infections that may not be detected by routine stool studies (such as enterohemorrhagic *Escherichia coli*), vascular disorders, immune-related enterocolitis, neoplasia, diverticulitis, radiation, and medications such as NSAIDs (see Table 143-3).

Ulcerative Colitis

The diagnosis of ulcerative colitis is based on endoscopic findings and histopathology. Early in the disease process, patients develop diffuse mucosal erythema with loss of the normal mucosal vascular pattern. In mild disease, the mucosa may have a granular and edematous appearance. As the disease becomes more severe, the mucosa becomes more friable, bleeds easily when the mucosa is touched, and may eventually ulcerate (Fig. 143-3). Endoscopic findings, which start in the rectum and may extend proximally in a continuous pattern, affect only the colon. Pseudopolyps may form owing to epithelial regeneration after recurrent attacks in patients with long-standing disease. With chronic disease, the colonic mucosa may lose its normal fold pattern, and the colon may shorten and appear narrowed.

Features such as crypt distortion, continuous mucosal inflammation starting from the rectum, absence of granulomas, and absence of small bowel disease are all consistent with ulcerative colitis. Early in the disease process, chronic inflammatory findings, such as crypt distortion, may not be present, and the diagnosis may be more difficult to confirm.

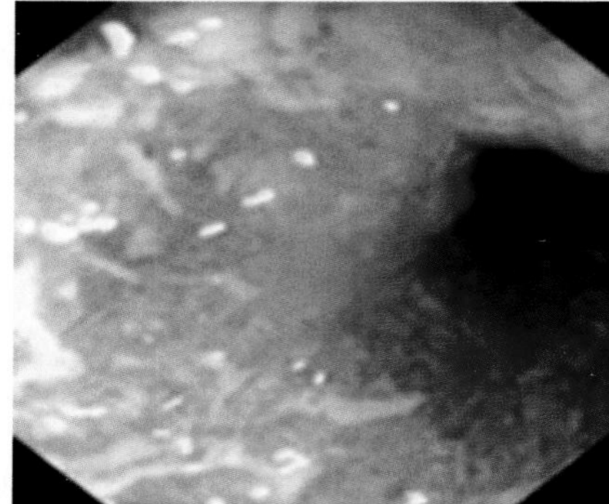

FIGURE 143-3. Endoscopic appearance of ulcerative colitis.

Radiology

Radiologic imaging is vital and should almost always be obtained when inflammatory bowel disease, particularly Crohn's disease, is suspected. Barium studies such as an upper gastrointestinal series, small bowel follow-through, and barium enema are usually necessary to diagnose fistulas and strictures in Crohn's disease. If Crohn's disease is suspected by colonoscopic examination, a small bowel follow-through is generally obtained to assess the extent, severity, and type of disease (strictures and fistulas) in the small intestine. CT enterography and magnetic resonance imaging (MRI) enterography are alternatives to a small bowel follow-through. CT enterography may be preferred for the detection of abdominal abscesses, whereas MRI may be preferred for the detection of perineal abscesses and strictures.

Laboratory Findings

Anemia may result from chronic disease, blood loss or nutritional deficiencies of iron, folate, or vitamin B_{12}. A modestly elevated leukocyte count is indicative of active disease, but a marked elevation suggests an abscess or another suppurative complication. The erythrocyte sedimentation rate and C-reactive protein are nonspecific serum inflammatory markers that are sometimes used to monitor the activity of disease. Hypoalbuminemia is an indication of malnutrition. Ileal disease or resection of more than 100 cm of distal ileum results in a diminished serum vitamin B_{12} level because of malabsorption.

Serologic Markers

Serologic markers are supportive but may not be used independently to diagnose inflammatory bowel disease. Anti-*Saccharomyces cerevisiae* antibodies (ASCA), which are antibodies to yeast, are present in 40 to 70% of patients with Crohn's disease and in less than 15% of patients with ulcerative colitis. The combination of elevated ASCA immunoglobulin A (IgA) and IgG titers is highly specific for Crohn's disease, ranging from 89 to 100%. Perinuclear antineutrophil cytoplasmic antibodies (pANCA) are present in 20% of Crohn's patients, primarily in colon-predominant disease, and in 55% of patients with ulcerative colitis. ASCA-positive and pANCA-negative disease is associated with a sensitivity of 55% and specificity of 93% for Crohn's disease. The antimicrobial antibodies anti-I2 (Crohn's disease–related protein from *Pseudomonas fluorescens*), anti-Cbir1 (flagellin-like antigen), and anti-OmpC (*E. coli* outer membrane porin C) are also associated with Crohn's disease, but the utility of these additional markers has yet to be determined.

TREATMENT

The aim of medical therapy is to reduce inflammation and subsequently induce and maintain clinical remission. Medications used to treat inflammatory bowel disease include the categories of 5-aminosalicylate (5-ASA), antibiotics, corticosteroids, immunomodulators, and biologics (infliximab, adalimumab, certolizumab pegol, and natalizumab) (Table 143-4). The specific medical therapy selected is based on the location, extent (nonpenetrating and nonstricturing, stricturing, and penetrating and fistulizing disease), and severity of disease (Fig. 143-4; see Fig. 143-3). Supportive medical therapy, such as antidiarrheal and antispasmodic medications, may also be used.

Categories of Medical Therapy

5-Aminosalicylate

5-ASA, which acts as a topical anti-inflammatory within the lumen of the intestine, is used to treat mild to moderate ulcerative colitis and also has a

TABLE 143-4 MEDICAL THERAPIES FOR INFLAMMATORY BOWEL DISEASE

DRUG	DOSE	RELEASE SITE
5-AMINOSALICYLATES		
Sulfasalazine (Azulfidine)	2-6 g/day	Colon
Mesalamine (Asacol, Lialda, Apriso)	2.4-4.8 g/day	Distal ileum, colon
Olsalazine (Dipentum)	1-3 g/day	Colon
Balsalazide (Colazal)	6.25 g/day	Colon
Mesalamine (Pentasa)	2-4 g/day	Duodenum, jejunum, ileum, colon
Mesalamine (Rowasa), enema, suppository	4 g/day (enema) 1 g/day (suppository)	Rectum/sigmoid Rectum
Mesalamine (Canasa), suppository	1 g/day (suppository)	Rectum
CORTICOSTEROIDS		
Budesonide (Entocort)	Induction: 9 mg PO qd Maintenance: 6 mg PO qd	Small intestine
Prednisone	0.25-0.75 mg/kg PO qd	Systemic
Methylprednisolone	40-60 mg IV qd	Systemic
IMMUNOMODULATORS		
6-Mercaptopurine	1.5 mg/kg/day	Systemic
Azathioprine	2.5 mg/kg/day	Systemic
Methotrexate	Induction: 25 mg SC q wk × 4 mo Maintenance: 15 mg SC q wk	Systemic
Cyclosporine	2-4 mg/kg/day	Systemic
BIOLOGICS		
Infliximab	Induction: 5 mg/kg IV weeks 0, 2, 6 Maintenance: 5 mg/kg IV q 8 wk	Systemic
Adalimumab	Induction: 160 mg SC week 0, 80 mg week 2 Maintenance: 40 mg SC every other week	Systemic
Certolizumab pegol	Induction: 400 mg SC weeks 0, 2, 4 Maintenance: 400 mg SC q 4 wk	Systemic
Natalizumab	300 mg IV q 4 wk	Systemic

IV = intravenously; PO = orally; SC = subcutaneously.

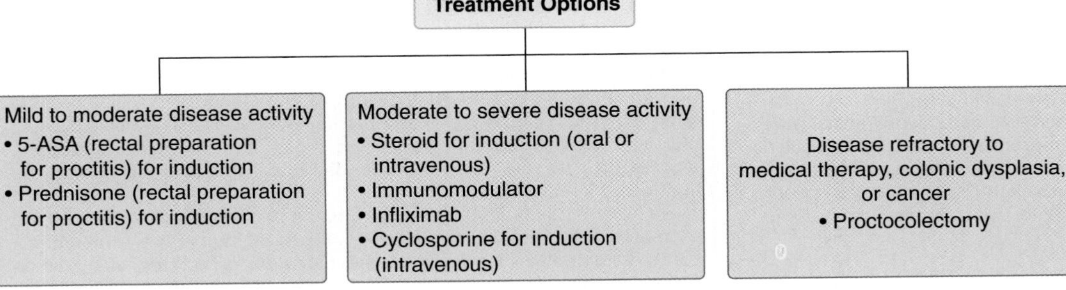

Treatment Options
Mild to moderate disease activity
• 5-ASA (rectal preparation for proctitis) for induction
• Prednisone (rectal preparation for proctitis) for induction
Moderate to severe disease activity
• Steroid for induction (oral or intravenous)
• Immunomodulator
• Infliximab
• Cyclosporine for induction (intravenous)
Disease refractory to medical therapy, colonic dysplasia, or cancer
• Proctocolectomy

FIGURE 143-4. Ulcerative colitis treatment algorithm.

limited role in Crohn's disease. Sulfasalazine is the combination of a sulfapyridine with 5-ASA; 5-ASA is responsible for the anti-inflammatory property of this drug, whereas sulfapyridine is the carrier that allows 5-ASA to be delivered into the colon. Other oral formulations of 5-ASA allow it to be delivered to the intestine by different mechanisms. Mesalamine is released in the intestine based on a pH delivery model, whereas sulfasalazine, olsalazine, and balsalazide are released in the intestine by bacterial cleavage of a covalent bond between 5-ASA and a prodrug. For rectal and sigmoid disease, 5-ASA suppository and enema preparations are also available. Adverse events associated with 5-ASAs are rare and may include nausea, dyspepsia, hair loss, headache, worsening diarrhea, and hypersensitivity reactions.

Corticosteroids

Corticosteroids are primarily used to treat flares of ulcerative colitis and Crohn's disease. Oral formulations may be used for mild to moderate disease, whereas systemic corticosteroids are used for moderate to severe disease.

Enteric coated budesonide, a pH-dependent ileal release formulation, is an oral corticosteroid with high topical activity and low systemic bioavailability (10%). Enteric coated budesonide is indicated for treatment of active mild to moderate Crohn's disease. Oral corticosteroids such as prednisone and methylprednisolone are used for moderate to severe disease, starting at doses ranging from 40 to 60 mg once a day. Intravenous methylprednisolone is used for severe disease, with dosing ranging from 40 to 60 mg once a day. Maintenance with systemic corticosteroids is not recommended because of their substantial side effects (Chapter 34).

Immune Modulators

In patients who remain symptomatic despite 5-ASA therapy or who have moderate to severe Crohn's disease or ulcerative colitis, the thiopurine analogues (6-mercaptopurine and azathioprine) may be used; methotrexate also may be used for moderate to severe Crohn's disease. Azathioprine, the prodrug of 6-mercaptopurine, typically is prescribed at a dose of 2 to 3 mg/kg/day; the equivalent dose of 6-mercaptopurine is 1.5 mg/kg/day. A disadvantage of the thiopurine analogs is the slow clinical response that may not be evident for as long as 12 weeks. Their side effects include allergic reactions, pancreatitis, myelosuppression, nausea, infections, hepatotoxicity, and malignancy, especially lymphoma. The white blood cell count and liver chemistries must be monitored routinely. Methotrexate, which is a folic acid antagonist, is given as 25 mg intramuscularly or subcutaneously once per week for 16 weeks for active Crohn's disease and, 15 mg to 25 mg intramuscularly or subcutaneously once per week for maintaining remission.

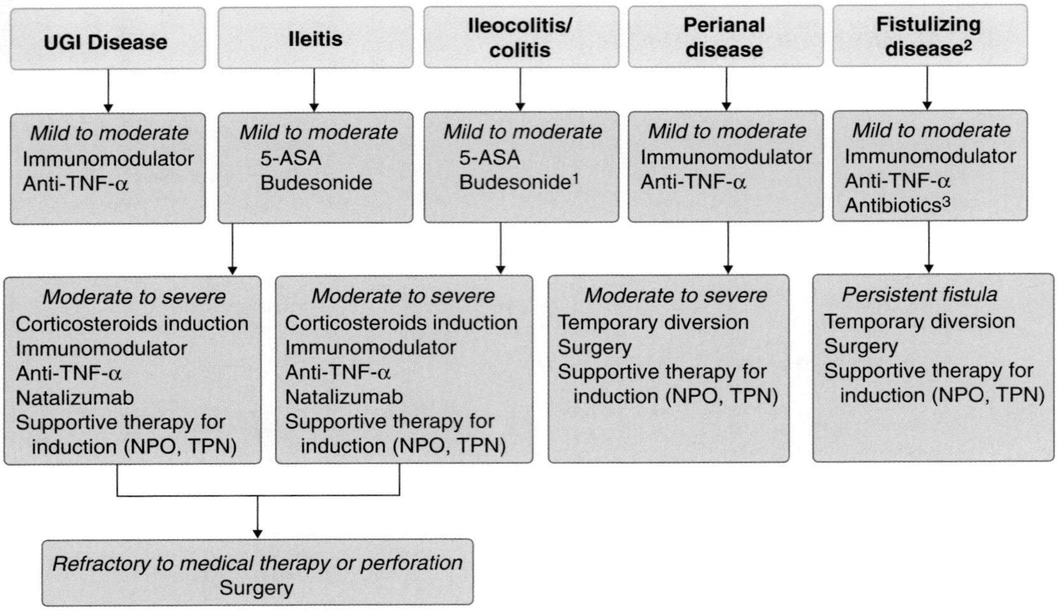

FIGURE 143-5. Crohn's disease treatment algorithm. NPO = nothing by mouth; TNF-α = tumor necrosis factor-α; TPN = total parenteral nutrition; UGI = upper gastrointestinal.

Antibiotics

The exact mechanism for the beneficial effect of broad-spectrum antibiotics in the treatment of inflammatory bowel disease is not known. Potential mechanisms include eliminating bacterial overgrowth, eradicating a bacterially mediated antigenic trigger, and potential immunosuppressive properties (e.g., metronidazole). The primary role of antibiotics is in Crohn's disease, where metronidazole (10 to 20 mg/kg daily for 4 to 8 weeks), ciprofloxacin (500 mg orally twice daily for 4 to 8 weeks), or both are primary inductive therapies for perianal fistulas and fissures. Metronidazole may also be a helpful adjunctive treatment for colonic Crohn's disease.

Biologicals

Anti–Tumor Necrosis Factor-α Agents

Antibodies to tumor necrosis factor-α (anti-TNF-α) include infliximab, which is a chimeric mouse-human IgG1 monoclonal antibody that is approved to treat moderate to severe Crohn's disease, fistulizing Crohn's disease, and moderate to severe ulcerative colitis that has failed to respond to conventional therapy. Adalimumab (Humira) and certolizumab pegol (Cimzia) have been approved to treat moderate to severe Crohn's disease that has failed to respond to conventional therapy. Adalimumab is a fully humanized IgG1 antibody that is self-administered subcutaneously. Certolizumab pegol, which is a chimeric pegylated Fab fragment to TNF-α, also is administered subcutaneously.

Antiadhesion molecules

Natalizumab, a humanized IgG4 monoclonal antibody, binds to the α_4 subunit of $\alpha_4\beta_1$ and $\alpha_4\beta_7$ integrins expressed on all leukocytes except neutrophils. Natalizumab inhibits the interactions between α_4 integrins on the surface of leukocytes and adhesion molecules on vascular endothelial cells in the gastrointestinal tract, thereby preventing adhesion and recruitment of leukocytes. Natalizumab is approved for the treatment of moderate to severe Crohn's disease that is refractory to conventional therapy, but there are strict guidelines for prescribing natalizumab because of its associated risk of progressive multifocal leukoencephalopathy (Chapter 378).

Crohn's Disease Medical Therapy

Mild to Moderate Crohn's Disease

Sulfasalazine, 3 to 6 g/day, is superior to placebo for treating active ileocolonic and colonic Crohn's disease, with response rates ranging from 45 to 55% for mild to moderate disease, but is not clearly effective for small bowel disease alone (Fig. 143-5). Mesalamine also has a modest benefit compared with placebo for mild to moderate disease.[1] However, the 5-ASAs are not effective for maintaining remission.

For mild to moderate Crohn's disease involving the distal small intestine or proximal colon budesonide (9 mg by mouth once a day) provides about a 70% response rate after 8 weeks and is significantly more effective than mesalamine, 4 g once a day, for distal ileal and right colonic disease.[2] As a maintenance agent at 3 or 6 mg, the effects of budesonide wane and disappear within 1 year.

Upper gastrointestinal Crohn's disease (jejunal, duodenal, gastric, and esophageal) is uncommon, so few clinical trials are available to assess therapies for this location. Because local therapies such as 5-ASAs and budesonide are not released in these locations, systemic immunosuppressants (azathioprine, mercaptopurine, infliximab, adalimumab, and certolizumab pegol) are the mainstays of therapy.

Moderate to Severe Crohn's Disease

Patients with moderate to severe disease are initially treated with systemic corticosteroids, but corticosteroids should not be used as maintenance therapy. Options to induce a remission or maintain a steroid-induced remission include 6-mercaptopurine, azathioprine, methotrexate, infliximab, adalimumab, and certolizumab.[3-5] After 1 year, approximately 20% more patients treated with combined therapy (corticosteroids, daily azathioprine, and infliximab, 5 mg/kg at weeks 1, 2, and 6) will be in remission compared with conventional treatment (corticosteroids plus azathioprine and then infliximab as needed according to current guidelines).[6] In a randomized trial, infliximab (5 mg/kg at 0, 2, and 6 weeks and then every 8 weeks) alone or infliximab plus azathioprine (2.5 mg/kg/day) was more effective than azathioprine alone.[7] Patients who have not responded to conventional therapy may be considered for natalizumab.

For severe Crohn's disease, patients should be hospitalized, given nothing by mouth, rehydrated with intravenous fluids, and administered parenteral corticosteroids. Patients who respond to parenteral corticosteroids should be switched to high-dose oral corticosteroids (prednisone, 40 to 60 mg/day), with the dose of prednisone gradually reduced. Patients who have severe Crohn's disease and who do not respond to parenteral corticosteroids within a week should be considered for either infliximab or surgery. A course of total parenteral nutrition (Chapter 224) may be useful as adjunctive therapy.

Fistulizing Crohn's disease

Fistulas occur in one third of patients with Crohn's disease, and perianal fistulas represent the most common location. Asymptomatic internal fistulas rarely require therapy. A concomitant abscess, which may occur in the setting of a fistula, must be excluded before initiating immunosuppressive therapy. Surgery may be required. Medical treatment depends on the location and associated complications.

High-output enterocutaneous fistulas in the setting of proximal small bowel involvement can lead to outputs of more than 500 mL/day and can cause severe volume depletion. Initial management requires volume repletion. In the postoperative setting, a fistulous opening is usually in the area of a wound, and it is imperative to protect the healing skin from infection caused by the drainage from either an ostomy bag or a catheter used for a high-output fistula. High-output fistulas will rarely close spontaneously and typically will require surgical closure. Low-output fistulas may be treated initially with azathioprine (or 6-mercaptopurine), methotrexate, or anti-TNF-α therapy (infliximab, adalimumab, or certolizumab).[8]

Perianal fistulas are classified into simple and complex fistulas. A simple fistula is located below most of the anal sphincter and has one track. A complex fistula passes through the intersphincteric (high location), transsphincteric, or suprasphincteric region and may have multiple tracks. Simple fistulas respond well to medical therapy, initially with metronidazole (10 to 20 mg/kg orally daily for 4 to 8 weeks) and ciprofloxacin (500 mg orally twice daily for 4 to 8 weeks) for the fistula and treatment of concurrent mucosal disease. Treatment with immunomodulators or anti-TNF-α agents is also beneficial.[8] Patients with fistulas without rectal mucosal Crohn's disease may respond well to fistulotomy, whereas patients with mucosal involvement may benefit from seton placement rather than fistulotomy. Complex fistulas usually require a combination of surgical and medical therapy. In the setting of intractable disease, colonic or ileal diversion may allow for rectal and perianal healing; in severe cases, proctocolectomy may be necessary.

For Crohn's disease–related rectovaginal fistulas, medical therapy with antimetabolite therapy, or anti-TNF-α agents is usually considered before surgery. Surgical therapy such as fistulotomy and mucosal flap may be considered.

Enterovesicular or colovesicular fistulas may be treated with antimetabolite therapy or anti- TNF-α agents, or both, but recurrent urinary tract infection is an indication for surgery. Surgery usually involves resection of involved bowel and closure of the bladder defect.

Asymptomatic internal fistulas, such as enteroenteric fistulas, do not require surgical intervention, but treatment with an immunomodulator may be considered. Internal fistulas, such as cologastric and coloduodenal, may cause substantial symptoms because of bypass of part of the intestine. If medical management fails or if an abscess forms, surgery is recommended.

Medical Management of Ulcerative Colitis

The anatomic distribution of ulcerative colitis guides therapy. Options include suppositories, retention enemas, topical foam, oral therapy, and parenteral therapy. Suppositories are effective to treat proctitis in the distal 20 cm of the colon. Topical foam and enemas are effective for distal and left-sided colitis. Oral therapy and parenteral therapy are effective for all locations of disease.

Proctitis

For active ulcerative proctitis, topical 5-ASA (enema and suppository) in combination with oral treatment is superior to oral treatment alone.[9] Topical 5-ASA is superior to topical corticosteroids for treatment of active ulcerative proctitis, rectal 5-ASA therapy produces a faster response when given with oral 5-ASA. Corticosteroid enemas, suppositories, or foam can also be used if 5-ASA fails. 5-ASA or corticosteroid retention enemas can be used for active disease up to the splenic flexure (i.e., the rectum, sigmoid colon, and descending colon). Another approach to proctitis or distal colitis is an oral aminosalicylate, although a response may not be evident for 3 to 4 weeks.

Extensive Colitis

In patients with ulcerative colitis of mild to moderate activity and extension of disease proximal to the splenic flexure, the initial drug of choice is an oral 5-ASA; efficacy increases with increasing doses.[10] Even with more extensive disease, supplementation of oral 5-ASA with 5-ASA enemas or suppositories may help reduce the symptoms of urgency that result from rectal involvement. In patients with more than five or six bowel movements per day, in patients in whom a more rapid response is desired, or in patients who have not responded to 3 to 4 weeks of 5-ASA, the treatment of choice is oral prednisone. Patients with severe diarrhea, systemic symptoms, or significant amounts of blood in stool should be started on 40 mg/day; most patients respond to oral corticosteroids within a few days. After the symptoms are controlled, prednisone can be tapered gradually by 5 mg every 1 to 2 weeks. Patients who respond to oral prednisone and can be fully withdrawn from it should be maintained on 5-ASA.

If patients with severe ulcerative colitis do not begin to respond to corticosteroids at the equivalent dose of 60 mg of intravenous methylprednisolone within 5 days or do not completely respond within 7 to 10 days, options include colectomy, infliximab, or cyclosporine. For patients whose disease flares whenever the corticosteroids are withdrawn or their corticosteroid dose is lowered, the continuation of high-dose corticosteroid therapy is the most common management error. If the patient requires a substantial dose (>15 mg/day of prednisone) for more than 6 months, a trial of an immunomodulator, infliximab, or colectomy should be given serious consideration.

The most common indication for hospitalization in patients with ulcerative colitis is intractable diarrhea, although blood loss is also common. Patients with severely active ulcerative colitis should be evaluated for toxic megacolon by abdominal radiography or CT. Antidiarrheal medications and anticholinergic medications are contraindicated in patients with severe ulcerative colitis because of the risk for precipitating toxic megacolon. The mainstays of therapy for severe ulcerative colitis are rehydration with intravenous fluids and intravenous corticosteroids (hydrocortisone, 300 mg/day; prednisolone, 60 to 80 mg/day; or methylprednisolone, 40 to 60 mg/day). Total parenteral nutrition (Chapter 224) may be necessary in patients with malnutrition. Patients with peritoneal signs or signs of systemic infection should be treated with parenteral antibiotics (Chapter 144). Patients who do not improve in 7 to 10 days should be considered for either colectomy, a trial of intravenous cyclosporine,[11] or a trial of infliximab.

Maintenance Therapy

Aminosalicylates reduce recurrent disease in patients with ulcerative colitis, and essentially all patients should receive maintenance therapy[12] with original or newer 5-ASA preparations. Corticosteroids are not effective as maintenance therapy and should not be used. Azathioprine, 6-mercaptopurine, and infliximab are effective for maintenance therapy in patients whose ulcerative colitis has not responded to 5-ASA.

Surgical Therapy

Crohn's Disease

Surgical resection does not cure Crohn's disease, and recurrences are likely after resection, so the approach should be conservative in terms of the amount of tissue removed. Nevertheless, about 40% of patients with Crohn's disease undergo surgery within 10 years of their diagnosis. Failure of medical management is a common cause for resection in patients with Crohn's disease, but complications (e.g., obstruction, fistula, abscess) are often the indications for resection. For Crohn's disease of the small bowel, the most common surgical procedure is segmental resection for obstruction or fistula; the incidence of a recurrence severe enough to require repeat surgery after ileal or ileocolic resection is about 25% after 10 years and 35% after 15 years. For patients with extensive colonic disease that includes the rectum, the procedure of choice is total proctocolectomy with a Brooke (end) ileostomy. Total colectomy with ileal pouch anal anastomosis is not appropriate in Crohn's colitis because recurrence of Crohn's disease in the ileal segment of the new pouch would require a repeat operation and loss of a long segment of ileum.

Ulcerative Colitis

For ulcerative colitis, colectomy is a curative procedure. Approximately 40% of patients with extensive ulcerative colitis eventually undergo colectomy, usually because their disease has not responded adequately to medical therapy. Emergency colectomy may be required in patients with toxic megacolon or a severe fulminant attack without toxic megacolon. The standard operation for ulcerative colitis is proctocolectomy and a Brooke ileostomy. The most popular alternative operation is total proctocolectomy with an ileal pouch anal anastomosis; in this procedure, a pouch is constructed from the terminal 30 cm of ileum, and the distal end of the pouch is pulled through the anal canal. Ileoanal anastomosis is sometimes complicated by inflammation in the ileal pouch (termed *pouchitis*), which can be treated with antibiotics (typically, metronidazole, 500 mg three times daily or 20 mg/kg daily, or ciprofloxacin, 500 mg twice daily for a duration of 2 weeks). The decision for or against colectomy and among types of surgery is influenced by the patient's age, social circumstances, and duration of disease, and this decision requires expert consultation. When other indications are equivocal, the risk of malignancy (see later) may be an indication for colectomy.

Complications

Crohn's Disease

Abscesses

Abscesses, which are common complications in Crohn's disease, result from extension of a mucosal fissure or ulcer through the intestinal wall and into extraintestinal tissue. Leakage of intestinal contents through a fissure into the peritoneal cavity results in an abscess. Abscesses occur in 15 to 20% of patients with Crohn's disease, especially in the terminal ileum. The typical clinical manifestation of an intra-abdominal abscess is fever, abdominal pain, abdominal tenderness, and leukocytosis. Abdominal abscess is most often diagnosed by a CT scan. Broad-spectrum antibiotic therapy, including anaerobic coverage, is indicated. Percutaneous drainage of abscesses in patients with Crohn's disease may improve the clinical picture but does not provide adequate therapy because of persistent communication between the abscess cavity and the intestinal lumen. Resection of the involved intestine is usually required for definitive therapy.

Obstruction

Obstruction is a common complication of Crohn's disease, particularly in the small intestine, and is a leading indication for surgery. Small bowel obstruction in Crohn's disease may be caused by mucosal thickening from acute inflammation, by muscular hyperplasia and scarring as a result of previous inflammation, or by adhesions. Obstruction may also occur because of impaction of a bolus of fibrous food in a stable, long-standing stricture. Obstruction is marked by cramping abdominal pain and diarrhea that worsen after meals and resolve with fasting. Strictures may be evaluated by CT enterography, MRI enterography, oral contrast studies, barium enema, or colonoscopy, depending on the anatomic location. Corticosteroids (e.g., intravenous methylprednisolone, 40 to 60 mg once a day, or intravenous hydrocortisone, 200 to 300 mg once a day, for 5 to 14 days) are useful if acute inflammation is an important component of the obstructive process, but not if the obstruction is caused by fibrosis. A common error in the management of Crohn's disease is inappropriate treatment with long courses of corticosteroids in patients who have obstructive symptoms from fixed anatomic lesions. If the obstruction does not resolve with nasogastric suction and corticosteroids, surgery is necessary.

Perianal Disease

Perianal disease is a potentially disabling complication of Crohn's disease. Ulcerations in the anal canal may coalesce and result in fistula formation. The fistulous openings are most commonly found in the perianal skin but can occur in the groin, the vulva, or the scrotum. Fistulas are accompanied by drainage of serous or purulent material. If the fistula does not drain freely, there is local accumulation of pus (perianal abscess) with redness, pain, and induration. The pain of a perianal abscess is exacerbated by local pressure that may result from defecation, sitting, or walking. The typical physical manifestation of an abscess is redness with tenderness on digital examination; fluctuance also may be present. Adequate evaluation of perianal disease generally requires proctoscopic examination under anesthesia. Cross-sectional CT or MRI can define the presence and extent of perianal abscesses. The goals of therapy for perianal disease are relief of local symptoms and preservation of the sphincter. Limited disease can be approached with sitz baths and metronidazole, but most cases also require adequate external drainage. Azathioprine, infliximab, adalimumab, or certolizumab pegol may be useful in healing perianal disease, but the disease may reactivate when the drug is stopped. Persistent severe perianal Crohn's disease can result in destruction of the anal sphincter and subsequent fecal incontinence.

Ulcerative Colitis

One of the most significant complications of ulcerative colitis is toxic megacolon, which is dilation of the colon to a diameter greater than 6 cm associated with worsening of the patient's clinical condition and the development of fever, tachycardia, and leukocytosis. Physical examination may reveal postural hypotension, abdominal tenderness over the distribution of the colon, and absent or hypoactive bowel sounds. Agents that reduce gastrointestinal motility, such as antispasmodics and antidiarrheal agents, are likely to initiate or exacerbate toxic megacolon. Medical therapy is designed to reduce the likelihood of perforation and return the colon to normal motor activity as rapidly as possible. The patient is given nothing by mouth, and nasogastric suction is begun. Intravenous fluids should be administered to replete water and electrolyte abnormalities, broad-spectrum antibiotics (e.g., ampicillin-sulbactam, given as 1 g ampicillin plus 0.5 g sulbactam, 1.5 to 3 g every 6 hours for 5 to 14 days; levofloxacin, 500 mg intravenously once daily plus metronidazole, 500 mg intravenously or orally twice daily; cefazolin, 500 mg intravenously three times daily plus metronidazole, 500 mg intravenously or orally twice daily; or trimethoprim-sulfamethoxazole, 8 to 10 mg/kg/day intravenously or orally in two to four divided doses plus metronidazole, 500 mg intravenously or orally twice daily for approximately 7 days or until symptomatic improvement) are given in anticipation of possible peritonitis as a result of perforation, and parenteral corticosteroids are administered at a dose equivalent to more than 40 to 60 mg of prednisone per day. Signs of improvement include a decrease in abdominal girth and the return of bowel sounds. Deterioration is marked by the development of rebound tenderness, increasing abdominal girth, and cardiovascular collapse. If the patient does not begin to show signs of clinical improvement during the first 24 to 48 hours of medical therapy, the risk for perforation increases markedly, and surgical intervention colectomy is indicated.

Follow-Up

Colon Cancer, Dysplasia, and Colonoscopic Surveillance

The risk of colorectal cancer is increased beginning after 8 years of disease and continues to increase in subsequent years. Patients with extensive ulcerative colitis have a markedly increased risk for colon cancer, patients with left-sided disease have an intermediate risk, and patients with long-standing ulcerative colitis are at risk for colorectal cancer even if their symptoms have been relatively mild or even quiescent for 10 to 15 years.

Colon cancers are commonly submucosal and may be missed at colonoscopy. Colon cancer in patients with ulcerative colitis is most commonly associated with dysplastic changes in the mucosa, often at multiple sites in the colon. Dysplasia cannot be always be identified by visual inspection, so microscopic examination of biopsy specimens is required.

Current practice guidelines recommend colonoscopy with random biopsies in patients with long-standing ulcerative colitis beginning 8 years after the onset of disease and repeated every 1 to 2 years. If the specimens show dysplasia, colectomy is recommended.

The risk for colon cancer in patients with Crohn's colitis is similar to the risk in patients with a similar extent of ulcerative colitis. Surveillance colonoscopy is also recommended in patients with Crohn's colitis.

Pregnancy

Fertility in women with inflammatory bowel disease usually is normal or only minimally impaired, and the incidence of prematurity, stillbirth, and developmental defects in the offspring of women with inflammatory bowel disease, except fetal complications may be somewhat more likely when the mother's disease is clinically active, regardless of drug therapy. Previous proctocolectomy or the presence of an ileostomy is not an impediment to successful completion of a pregnancy, but women who have had ileal pouch anal anastomosis surgery with a total proctocolectomy have markedly reduced fertility.

If a woman's disease is inactive at the time of conception, it is likely that it will remain inactive during the course of the pregnancy. Ulcerative colitis that is active at the time of conception tends to worsen. In patients with active Crohn's disease at the time of conception, the degree of activity remains the same in two thirds of women; of the other one third, some improve clinically, and others deteriorate.

Sulfasalazine does not harm the fetus, but pregnant women have an increased requirement for folic acid, and sulfasalazine interferes with folate absorption. Therefore, women who are taking sulfasalazine and who are pregnant or considering pregnancy should receive folate supplementation (1 mg twice daily) to ensure that the fetus receives adequate amounts for normal development. The use of corticosteroids by pregnant women with inflammatory bowel disease is associated with an increased rate of premature rupture of the membranes and a higher rate of cleft lip. In general, it appears that the risk to the pregnancy of treatment with sulfasalazine or corticosteroids is less than the risk of allowing disease activity to go untreated.

Most of the data on the teratogenicity of azathioprine and 6-mercaptopurine in pregnancy are derived from the transplant literature and involve higher doses than are commonly used for inflammatory bowel disease. Reported fetal effects in the transplant population include congenital malformations, immunosuppression, prematurity, and growth retardation. The risks of these medications in the inflammatory bowel disease population are not completely known, given that only small a number of such patients have been formally studied.

PROGNOSIS

Ulcerative Colitis

The prognosis of patients with ulcerative colitis is usually characterized by repeated flares and remissions. A rapidly progressive initial attack results in serious complications in about 10% of patients. Complete recovery after a single attack may occur in another 10% of patients, some of whom may actually have had an acute undetected infection rather than true ulcerative colitis. The probability that a patient with clinically inactive disease will remain in remission the following year is 80 to 90%. By comparison, patients with clinically active disease have a 70% probability of relapse during the following year.

Patients who present with ulcerative proctitis have the best overall prognosis, and only about 5% of patients with proctitis will require colectomy over a lifetime. Severe complications are very uncommon, but the disease will spread more proximally in the colon in approximately 10% to 30% of patients. Ulcerative colitis–related mortality has decreased substantially since the introduction of corticosteroids, and recent studies suggest that long-term survival rates for patients with ulcerative colitis are similar to those of the general population.

Crohn's Disease

Crohn's disease classically waxes and wanes. A patient with clinically active Crohn's disease has a 70 to 80% chance of having active disease in the subsequent year, whereas 80% of patients in remission will remain so over the following year. Over the course of a 4-year period, about 25% of patients will have persistently active disease after diagnosis, about 25% will remain in remission, and 50% will have a fluctuating course with years of remission and years with clinically active disease. Approximately 75 to 80% of all patients with luminal and fistulizing Crohn's disease will require surgical intervention for their disease, with approximately 50% of them requiring surgery within 6 months of diagnosis. The rate for a second surgery for luminal Crohn's disease ranges from 25 to 38% within 5 years, and 40 to 70% will need reoperation by 15 years.

Patients with Crohn's disease have an increased mortality rate, about 1.3 to 1.5 times higher than the general population, unrelated to whether they have small intestine or large intestine involvement, or both. This excess mortality, which is most notable in the first few years after diagnosis, is most commonly related to complications of Crohn's disease (e.g., colorectal cancer, shock, volume depletion, protein-calorie malnutrition, and anemia). Whether aggressive use of immunomodulators and biologic therapy will alter the natural course of disease is unknown.

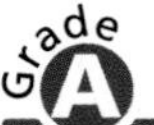

1. Hanauer SB, Stromberg U. Oral Pentasa in the treatment of Crohn's disease: a meta-analysis of double-blind, placebo-controlled trials. *Clin Gastroenterol Hepatol.* 2004;2:379-388.
2. Seow CH, Benchimol EI, Griffiths AM, et al. Budesonide for induction of remission in Crohn's disease. *Cochrane Database Syst Rev.* 2008;16:CD000296.

3. Prefontaine E, Macdonald JK, Sutherland LR. Azathioprine or 6-mercaptopurine for induction of remission in Crohn's disease. *Cochrane Database Syst Rev.* 2009;7:CD000545.
4. Patel V, Macdonald JD, McDonald JW, et al. Methotrexate for maintenance of remission in Crohn's disease. *Cochrane Database Syst Rev.* 2009;7:CD006884.
5. Behm BW, Bickston SJ. Tumor necrosis factor-alpha antibody for maintenance of remission in Crohn's disease. *Cochrane Database Syst Rev.* 2008;23:CD006893.
6. D'Haens G, Baert F, van Assche G, et al. Early combined immunosuppression or conventional management in patients with newly diagnosed Crohn's disease: an open randomised trial. *Lancet.* 2008;371:660-667.
7. Colombel JF, Sandborn WJ, Reinisch W, et al. Infliximab, azathioprine, or combination therapy for Crohn's disease. *N Engl J Med.* 2010;362:1383-1395.
8. Sands BE, Anderson FH, Bernstein CN, et al. Infliximab maintenance therapy for fistulizing Crohn's disease. *N Engl J Med.* 2004;350:876-885.
9. Marshall JK, Thabane M, Steinhart AH, et al. Rectal 5-aminosalicylic acid for induction of remission in ulcerative colitis. *Cochrane Database Syst Rev.* 2010;20:CD004115.
10. Sutherland L, Macdonald JK. Oral 5-aminosalicylic acid for induction of remission in ulcerative colitis. *Cochrane Database Syst Rev.* 2006;19:CD000543.
11. Van Assche G, D'Haens G, Noman M, et al. Randomized double-blind comparison of 4mg/kg versus 2 mg/kg IV cyclosporine in severe ulcerative colitis. *Gastroenterology.* 2003;125:1025-1031.
12. Sutherland L, Macdonald JK. Oral 5-aminosalicylic acid for maintenance of remission in ulcerative colitis. *Cochrane Database Syst Rev.* 2002;4:CD000544.

SUGGESTED READINGS

Abraham C, Cho JH. Inflammatory bowel disease. *N Engl J Med.* 2009;361:2066-2078. *Review.*

Kornbluth A, Sachar DB. Ulcerative colitis practice guidelines in adults: American College of Gastroenterology, Practice Parameters Committee. *Am J Gastroenterol.* 2010;105:501-523. *Comprehensive guidelines.*

Lichtenstein GR, Hanauer SB, Sandborn WJ, for the Practice Parameters Committee of American College of Gastroenterology. Management of Crohn's disease in adults. *Am J Gastroenterol.* 2009; 104:465-483; quiz 464, 484. *Comprehensive review.*

Nielsen OH, Seidelin JB, Munck LK, et al. Use of biological molecules in the treatment of inflammatory bowel disease. *J Intern Med.* 2011. [Epub ahead of print.] *Review.*

144

INFLAMMATORY AND ANATOMIC DISEASES OF THE INTESTINE, PERITONEUM, MESENTERY, AND OMENTUM

CHARLENE PRATHER

APPENDICITIS

DEFINITION AND EPIDEMIOLOGY

Acute appendicitis refers to inflammation of the appendix. Appendicitis is the most common acute surgical emergency involving the abdomen. Although appendicitis occurs most commonly in young adults, it can develop at any age. The lifetime prevalence of acute appendicitis is approximately 7%.

PATHOBIOLOGY

Obstruction of the appendix by a fecalith, which is thought to be the usual inciting event, is found in less than 30% of patients. Other causes of obstruction include ulceration of the appendiceal orifice, lymphoid hyperplasia, tumor (e.g., carcinoid; Chapter 240), inspissation of barium, and ascariasis (Chapter 365). Obstruction blocks the ongoing production of mucus by the appendix, thereby resulting in distention and subsequent mucosal ischemia. This process allows invasion by intraluminal bacteria, infection, and inflammation. Continued obstruction and inflammation can result in perforation, peritonitis, diarrhea, and abscess formation.

CLINICAL MANIFESTATIONS

More than 95% of patients with appendicitis have abdominal pain, but only 50 to 60% have the classic symptoms of appendicitis: an acute onset of periumbilical pain, often with nausea and vomiting and later localizing to the right lower quadrant. The position of the appendix has important implications for the location of pain, with pain from appendicitis occurring in the suprapubic region or the right upper quadrant. Anorexia is nearly universal, nausea is frequent, but vomiting is uncommon. Acute appendicitis occurs with nonspecific abdominal symptoms and signs in elderly patients and in patients who are immunosuppressed, as from corticosteroid use, organ transplantation, or diabetes mellitus. In elderly patients, the diagnosis is unsuspected 25% of the time.

Adults older than 50 years have a perforation rate of greater than 50%, with an intra-abdominal abscess in one third. Signs of perforation include the presence of peritoneal irritation, fever, and increasing abdominal pain.

DIAGNOSIS

A broad differential diagnosis (Table 144-1) may be narrowed by diagnostic testing, which usually includes a complete blood count, serum electrolytes, and tests of renal function, with the addition of amylase and lipase levels when pancreatitis (Chapter 146) is suspected and liver enzymes (aminotransferase levels and alkaline phosphatase) and a bilirubin level when gallbladder (Chapter 158) or bile duct conditions are suspected. An elevated white blood cell count, usually in the 12,000 to 18,000/mm^3 range, is common in acute appendicitis but may not be seen early in the course; the presence and degree of elevation are not helpful in identifying complicated appendicitis.

Computed tomography (CT), which is the preferred test [1] to confirm the diagnosis or suggest other causes (Fig. 144-1), has a sensitivity ranging from 88 to 100%, a specificity of 91 to 99%, a positive predictive value of 92 to 98%, and a negative predictive value of 95 to 100%. With a reported overall diagnostic accuracy of 94 to 98% and the ability to detect abscess formation (Fig. 144-2), CT has become the imaging diagnostic modality of choice. A disadvantage, which is more significant in children and young adults, is the need for ionizing radiation. Intravenous contrast may be used, but CT with rectal contrast is an alternative to avoid the risk of nephrotoxicity. [2] Ultrasound is useful when gynecologic causes, especially an ectopic pregnancy, are also in the differential diagnosis. Plain abdominal radiographs are not useful.

TABLE 144-1 DIFFERENTIAL DIAGNOSIS IN SUSPECTED APPENDICITIS

Crohn's ileitis
Mesenteric adenitis
Right-sided colonic diverticulitis
Yersinia, Campylobacter enterocolitis
Meckel's diverticulitis
Tuberculous colitis
Perforated right colon adenocarcinoma
Nephrolithiasis (right sided)
Foreign body perforation (e.g., toothpick bowel perforation)
Right tubo-ovarian abscess
Tubal pregnancy
Ovarian cyst rupture or torsion

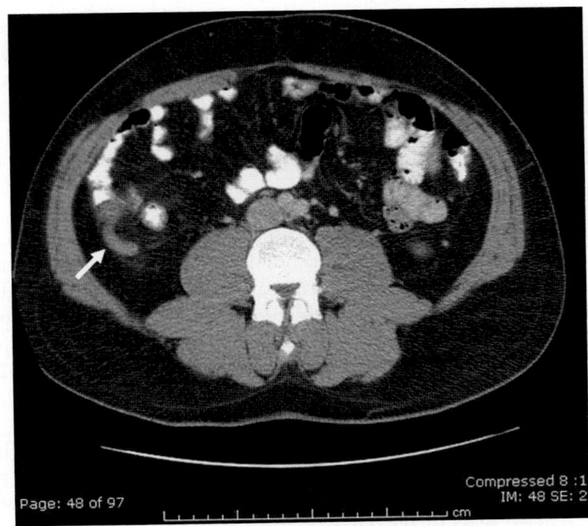

FIGURE 144-1. Appendicitis. A computed tomography scan shows an edematous appendix with a diameter greater than 1 cm *(arrow)*, consistent with acute, uncomplicated appendicitis.

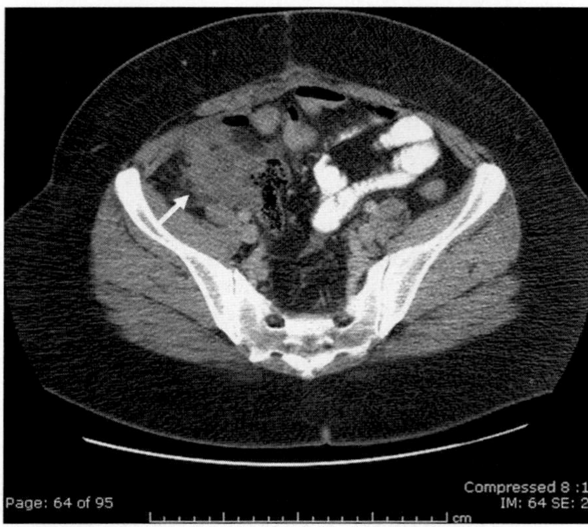

FIGURE 144-2. **Appendicitis.** A computed tomography scan shows appendicitis complicated by perforation with abscess formation *(arrow)*.

TREATMENT

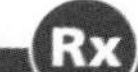

When appendicitis is suspected, emergent surgical consultation is indicated. Treatment of appendicitis is appendectomy, which is increasingly being performed laparoscopically. Two days of intravenous antibiotics followed by 10 days of oral antibiotics is a reasonable short-term alternative in the absence of evidence of perforation when surgery cannot be performed safely in the interim, but about one third of patients will require appendectomy.[3] Laparoscopic appendectomy generally takes longer than the open operation but results in faster recovery and a lower rate of wound infection.[4] Preoperative antibiotics (e.g., cefotetan, 2 g intravenously, or cefoxitin, 2 g intravenously, followed by three postoperative doses, or ticarcillin–clavulanic acid) reduce infectious complications in otherwise uncomplicated appendicitis.

In the presence of a perforated appendix with an appendicular abscess, immediate appendectomy yields similar results to a strategy of percutaneous ultrasound- or CT-guided drainage, intravenous antibiotics, and laparoscopic appendectomy about 10 weeks later.[5] In the setting of perforation, once-daily dosing with ceftriaxone and metronidazole for 7 to 10 days is as good as triple-dose therapy.[6]

PROGNOSIS

The frequency of complications associated with perforated appendicitis is greater than 18%, as opposed to a 10% frequency of complications in nonperforated appendicitis. Overall mortality in patients with perforated appendicitis is 3%, but it can be as high as 15% in elderly patients. Most patients who are operated on for suspected appendicitis, but who do not have it, have benign self-limited disease. In adults, however, appendiceal diverticulitis, granulomatous appendicitis, carcinoid tumors (Chapter 240), and occasionally other tumors may be found.

DIVERTICULITIS OF THE COLON

DEFINITION

Colonic diverticulosis refers to uncomplicated herniations of the colonic mucosa and submucosa through the muscular layer of the colon. Technically, these lesions are actually pseudodiverticula because all layers of the colon are not involved. Diverticular disease encompasses a spectrum of problems occurring in the setting of diverticulosis, including diverticulitis, painful diverticular disease, and complicated diverticular disease (Table 144-2).

EPIDEMIOLOGY

Although colonic diverticulosis is quite common and affects up to 10% of middle-aged adults and 50 to 80% of those older than 80 years, few people are aware that they have them. Diverticulosis is uncommon in individuals younger than 40 years of age. Diverticulosis is predominantly a disorder of industrialized or Western populations, where it correlates with low intake of dietary fiber. Obesity appears to be a risk factor for diverticulosis in young males.

TABLE 144-2 TERMINOLOGY IN DIVERTICULAR DISEASE

Diverticular disease	The entire spectrum of diverticulosis and its complications
Diverticulosis	The presence of one or more diverticula
Diverticulitis	Inflammation or infection of one or more colonic diverticula
Complicated diverticulitis	Diverticulitis with abscess, fistula formation, free perforation, or obstruction
Painful diverticular disease	Abdominal pain and altered bowel habit in the setting of diverticulosis without another explanation (may be a manifestation of irritable bowel syndrome)
Diverticular bleeding	Acute lower gastrointestinal bleeding from a colonic diverticulum

PATHOBIOLOGY

Colonic diverticulosis most commonly occurs at the location where the vasa recta (nutrient artery) penetrates through the muscularis propria. In Western populations, diverticulosis occurs more commonly in the left colon, with the sigmoid colon most frequently involved, perhaps because of the relatively higher pressure present in the lumen of the sigmoid colon. However, in Asian populations, a right-sided distribution is more common.

Diverticulitis, which is infection and inflammation of a diverticulum, develops in 10 to 25% of persons with diverticulosis during their lifetimes. Diverticulitis results from inflammation of a colonic diverticulum with subsequent microperforation, which is thought to occur when particulate debris within the diverticular sac compresses or erodes the blood vessel and thereby leads to perforation. Diverticulitis occurs most commonly in the sigmoid colon. Complications of diverticulitis, which include abscess formation, free perforation, colonic obstruction, and fistula formation, are more common in middle-aged and elderly patients but can also occur in young patients.

CLINICAL MANIFESTATIONS

Patients with diverticulitis most commonly have anorexia, left lower quadrant pain, and fever. The pain in diverticulitis may radiate to the flank, back, or suprapubic region. Patients may report loose stools or constipation. Additional associated symptoms include nausea, vomiting, altered bowel pattern, and urinary symptoms. On physical examination, left lower quadrant tenderness can usually be demonstrated. The examination may also identify localized guarding and, occasionally, a tender painful mass. The presence of peritoneal signs (e.g., rebound) suggests a free perforation.

Diverticular bleeding is manifested as painless rectal bleeding, with massive bleeding occurring in 5% of patients with diverticulosis (Chapter 137). Diverticular bleeding is rare in the setting of acute diverticulitis.

DIAGNOSIS

Leukocytosis is present in 70 to 80% of patients. When the diverticulitis is adjacent to the bladder, pyuria may occur. Conditions with findings similar to those of diverticulitis include gastroenteritis, appendicitis, inflammatory bowel disease (Chapter 143), and a perforating colon cancer (Chapter 199).

CT radiography, which reliably identifies the presence and location of inflammation, may show the colonic diverticula, inflammation involving the pericolic fat, and a colonic wall thicker than 4 mm (Fig. 144-3). Barium radiography, which can demonstrate diverticula (Fig. 144-4), will also identify whether the colon connects with the fluid collection in the setting of perforation and abscess formation; it is not recommended in the acute setting because of a higher risk for colonic perforation from contrast or air insufflation. After the acute syndrome has resolved and the patient has become stable, colonoscopy can also show diverticula (Fig. 144-5) and is essential to exclude malignancy, even in younger patients.

TREATMENT

Uncomplicated diverticulitis may be treated in the outpatient setting with broad-spectrum antibiotics such as ciprofloxacin and metronidazole for 7 to 10 days (Table 144-3). Oral antibiotics are as effective as the intravenous route,[7] and 4 days of treatment are as effective as 7 to 10 days for uncomplicated patients.[8] Patients are started on a clear liquid diet that can be advanced

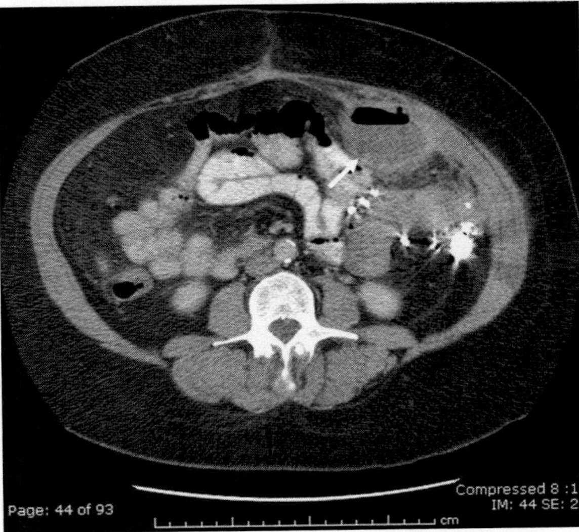

FIGURE 144-3. Diverticulitis. A computed tomography scan shows perforated diverticulitis with abscess formation *(arrow)*. The abscess is identified as the air-filled collection. Residual contrast remains in the diverticulum.

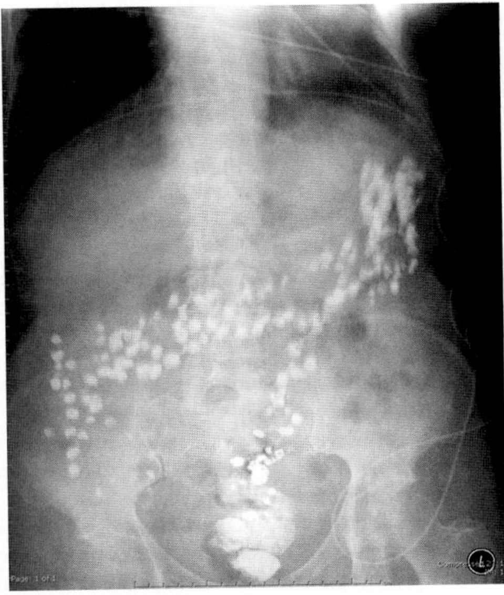

FIGURE 144-4. Colonic diverticula. An abdominal flat plate shows residual barium in diverticula scattered throughout the colon.

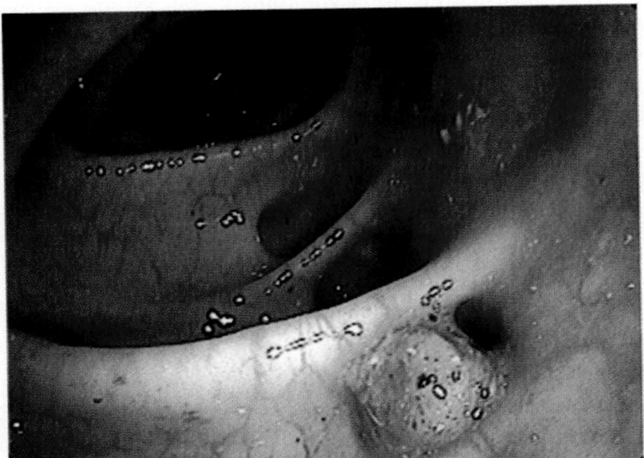

FIGURE 144-5. Sigmoid diverticula. A colonoscopic photograph shows sigmoid diverticula.

TABLE 144-3 ANTIBIOTIC OPTIONS FOR ACUTE DIVERTICULITIS*

Ciprofloxacin, 750 mg bid, and metronidazole, 500 mg q6h
Levofloxacin, 750 mg IV q24h, and metronidazole, 500 mg q6h
Trimethoprim-sulfamethoxazole-DS, bid
Piperacillin-tazobactam, 3.375 g q6h
Ampicillin-sulbactam, 3.0 g q6h
Imipenem–cilastatin sodium, 500 mg q6h (reserved for life-threatening infection)

*Four days in uncomplicated patients; 7 to 10 days in others.

as symptoms resolve. Patients unable to maintain oral intake require hospitalization for hydration and intravenous antibiotics.

Elective resection carries a mortality rate of 1 to 4%, and expectant management rather than operative treatment is probably associated with less mortality and fewer colostomies, and it is also less expensive.

However, patients younger than 40 years may experience a more aggressive form of the disease, so surgical resection is sometimes recommended after the first episode of diverticulitis. Patients with conditions resulting in immune system compromise may benefit from earlier (after a first episode) surgery because of their reduced ability to ward off infection and their increased risk for emergency surgery. For sigmoid diverticulitis, laparoscopic resection is preferred over open resection. 9

Patients with diverticular abscesses are treated by CT-guided drainage and subsequent surgery, usually 6 weeks after successful abscess drainage. Laparoscopic resection, which is increasingly being performed for diverticular disease, results in shorter hospitalization and an early return to full function. Patients with complicated diverticulitis have a mortality of 6.5% and morbidity of 41%; when perforated diverticulitis is excluded, the mortality is less than 2%. Older age, immunosuppressive medications, preexisting medical problems (especially preexisting cardiac and pulmonary disease), and perforated diverticulitis increase postoperative morbidity.

PREVENTION

Randomized trials show that the combination of fiber and rifaximin (400 mg twice daily for 7 days every month), a poorly absorbable antibiotic, decreases symptoms over a 12-month period. 10 Other medications used to reduce recurrent diverticular symptoms included mesalazine and calcium-channel blockers, although the evidence to support their use is inconclusive. The use of nonsteroidal anti-inflammatory drugs (NSAIDs) increases the risk for diverticular perforation.

PROGNOSIS

Most patients with diverticulitis improve quickly over a period of 2 to 3 days, and the risk for a second attack of diverticulitis is less than 25%. After a second attack of diverticulitis, the risk for subsequent episodes of diverticulitis exceeds 50%, and the risk increases with each subsequent episode. Surgical therapy to remove the segment of colon involved with diverticulosis is often recommended after a second episode of diverticulitis. After elective resection, 25% of patients have persistent symptoms, including altered bowel habits and pain that probably reflect a coexistent irritable bowel syndrome (Chapter 139), and 10% have recurrent diverticulitis.

OTHER INFLAMMATORY CONDITIONS

Neutropenic Enterocolitis

Neutropenic enterocolitis is also referred to as typhlitis. Although originally described in children after induction chemotherapy for acute leukemia, it is an increasingly recognized clinical syndrome in adults as well.

CLINICAL MANIFESTATIONS AND DIAGNOSIS

The syndrome occurs in neutropenic patients (absolute neutrophil count <500/μL) and consists of right lower quadrant abdominal pain, distention, fever, nausea, vomiting, and diarrhea, which may be bloody. Symptoms typically occur 10 to 14 days after high-dose chemotherapy. The clinical findings are nonspecific and overlap with symptoms seen in *Clostridium difficile* colitis (Chapter 304), ischemic colitis (Chapter 145), and colonic pseudo-obstruction (Chapter 138). CT findings include a thickened colonic wall (>4 mm), dilated cecum, and pericecal inflammatory changes (Fig. 144-6).

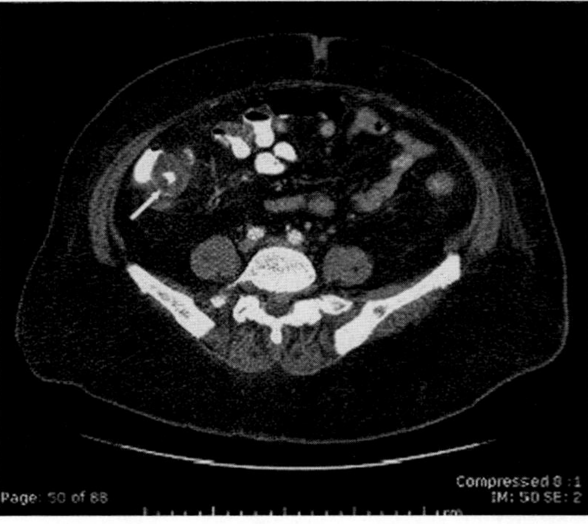
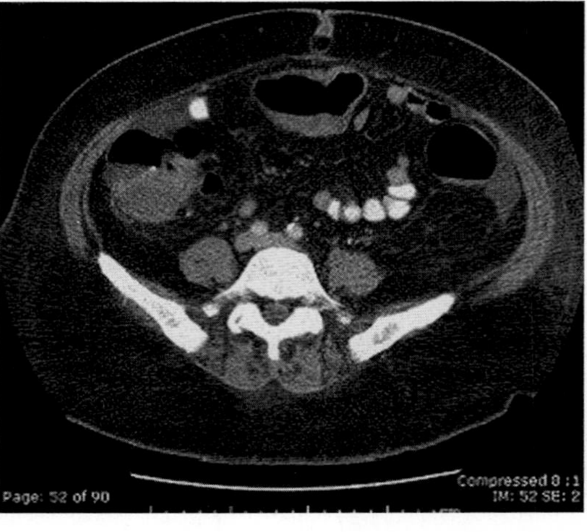

FIGURE 144-6. Computed tomography scans showing neutropenic colitis. The *left scan* shows a thickened cecal wall *(arrow)*. Eight days latter a follow-up scan showed resolution *(right scan)*.

TREATMENT

Conservative management includes bowel rest, nasogastric suction when bowel dilation is present, and broad-spectrum antibiotics to cover gram-positive and enteric gram-negative organisms, as well as anaerobes. Recombinant granulocyte colony-stimulating factor has been recommended to correct neutropenia. Lower gastrointestinal bleeding resulting from the colitis with a coexisting coagulopathy necessitates correction of the coagulopathy and blood transfusions. Surgery is indicated in the setting of impending or free perforation, when bleeding cannot be stopped, and for otherwise unexplained clinical deterioration. Symptoms improve rapidly as the neutropenia resolves.

Visceral Angioedema

Visceral angioedema is seen with hereditary and acquired C1 esterase inhibitor deficiency (Chapter 260), hypocomplementemia, drugs (especially angiotensin-converting enzyme inhibitors), or foods or may be idiopathic. Acquired C1 esterase inhibitor deficiency may occur as a paraneoplastic syndrome and is occasionally seen in autoimmune disorders. Angioedema of the gastrointestinal tract is commonly manifested as abdominal pain and distention, nausea, vomiting, and diarrhea. The symptoms may be accompanied by swelling of the mucous membrane, hives, wheezing, or dyspnea. CT findings include thickened, fluid-filled loops of small bowel. Ascites may also be present. The symptoms last 1 to 3 days and may recur periodically. The diagnosis is established by identifying suspect drugs, low serum levels of C4, low C1 esterase quantitative levels, or reduced C1 esterase functional activity. Hereditary and acquired C1 esterase inhibitor deficiency can be treated with C1 inhibitor therapy (Chapter 260).

Radiation Enterocolitis

Patients who receive radiation therapy for intra-abdominal and pelvic neoplasms are at risk for radiation-induced injury.

EPIDEMIOLOGY

The risk for injury varies according to the size of the radiation field and the dose received. Chronic radiation enterocolitis occurs approximately a year after completion of radiation therapy but may develop up to 20 years later. Doses greater than 50 Gy increase the risk for chronic changes, such as the development of obliterative arteritis, intestinal wall fibrosis, and serosal thickening. Other risk factors include older age, previous abdominal surgery, and a larger field of radiation. The quantity of small bowel in the radiation field is a strong predictor of subsequent complications.

CLINICAL MANIFESTATIONS AND DIAGNOSIS

Symptoms of acute radiation enterocolitis commonly include diarrhea, intestinal bleeding, and fecal incontinence. These symptoms are typically self-limited and resolve within a few months after the completion of radiation treatment.

Symptoms of chronic radiation enterocolitis commonly include abdominal pain and diarrhea. Gastrointestinal bleeding results from vascular ectasia. The bleeding is typically chronic and occult, with the development of iron deficiency anemia, but occasionally it is overt. Complete or partial bowel obstruction from adhesions or strictures, fistulas, small bowel bacterial overgrowth, and malabsorption can also occur.

Diagnostic imaging includes CT radiography or colonoscopy. The finding of a stricture necessitates an evaluation to exclude malignancy.

PREVENTION AND TREATMENT

Prevention of radiation enteritis includes minimizing the volume of small bowel and colon in the radiation field. Treatment is predominantly supportive. Management of bleeding includes endoscopic ablation of telangiectatic lesions and chronic iron therapy. Sucralfate enemas (2 g twice daily) may improve symptoms, but the data are not conclusive.

For acute obstruction, bowel rest and nasogastric suction may allow resolution; surgery is reserved for complete bowel obstruction that does not improve or perforation. Poor wound healing, anastomotic leaks, and fistulas may complicate surgical operations. Patients with diarrhea should be evaluated for small bowel bacterial overgrowth. Cholestyramine, loperamide, and diphenoxylate-atropine provide first-line options for treating diarrhea (Chapter 142), but stronger opiates such as codeine, morphine, or tincture of opium are sometimes required. Caution is necessary when using these agents because of the risk for development of bowel dilation and obstipation.

Nonsteroidal Anti-inflammatory Drugs

Small intestinal ulcerations are increasingly being recognized with the advent of small bowel capsule endoscopy (Chapter 136). The most common cause of small intestinal ulcers is the use of NSAIDs (Chapter 36). Small bowel and colonic erosions and ulcerations occur in 60 to 70% of long-term users of NSAIDs. Diaphragm-type strictures of the small bowel and, less frequently, the colon also result from chronic NSAID use.

CLINICAL MANIFESTATIONS AND DIAGNOSIS

Most NSAID-related lesions are asymptomatic, but symptoms suggesting NSAID enteropathy include gastrointestinal bleeding, abdominal pain, iron deficiency anemia, diarrhea, hypoalbuminemia, and obstructive symptoms. Ulceration can be detected by small bowel enteroscopy, small bowel capsule endoscopy, and colonoscopy.

TREATMENT

Treatment consists of discontinuing NSAIDs. When obstruction is present and conservative treatment fails, surgical resection may be required.

Systemic Inflammatory Conditions

Ulcerative jejunitis is an uncommon manifestation of celiac disease (Chapter 142). This diagnosis is suspected in patients with persistent symptoms despite a gluten-free diet.

Mycobacterium tuberculosis (Chapter 332) involvement of the small intestine and occasionally of the colon, especially in the cecum, most commonly manifests as abdominal pain, vomiting, and diarrhea. The disease may be subacute with waxing and waning symptoms or be marked by more fulminant sepsis. The intestinal lesions include nodularity, ulcerations, skip lesions, and strictures, features similar to those found in small bowel Crohn's disease. The diagnosis is made by biopsy, stains, and culture. When the small bowel is not accessible endoscopically, exploratory laparotomy for full-thickness biopsy may be required to make the diagnosis. Treatment with conventional antituberculous therapy results in symptomatic improvement.

Histoplasma capsulatum (Chapter 340) typically involves the gastrointestinal tract in the setting of disseminated disease in immunocompromised patients, predominately in patients with acquired immunodeficiency syndrome. Gastrointestinal involvement is accompanied by bleeding, obstruction, diarrhea, and malabsorption. Small bowel lesions include ulcerations, polypoid lesions, and masses that simulate carcinoma. The granulomatous changes present on biopsy must be differentiated from Crohn's disease, tuberculosis, and less commonly, sarcoidosis. Treatment is directed at the underlying disseminated infection.

Sarcoidosis (Chapter 95) of the gastrointestinal tract is relatively uncommon. Small bowel and colonic involvement has manifestations similar to those of Crohn's disease, with ulceration and non-necrotizing granulomas. Gastrointestinal involvement typically occurs in the setting of other systemic symptoms of sarcoidosis. Patients have abdominal pain, vomiting, diarrhea, or protein-losing enteropathy, or any combination of these findings. Treatment is aimed at the systemic disease.

Systemic lupus erythematosus (Chapter 274) frequently affects the gastrointestinal tract. Abdominal pain may be due to serositis, mesenteric ischemia, vasculitis, intestinal dysmotility, angioedema, or pancreatitis. Clinical manifestations include abdominal pain, nausea, vomiting, abdominal bloating, distention, diarrhea, and malabsorption. Small bowel bacterial overgrowth also occurs, presumably secondary to the underlying dysmotility. Treatment consists of management of the underlying systemic disease.

Ulceration of any part of the gastrointestinal tract may occur in *Behçet's disease* (Chapter 278). Symptoms include abdominal pain, diarrhea, and gastrointestinal bleeding. Most patients with gastrointestinal involvement have ileocecal involvement with a single or few ulcers. In the absence of obvious systemic symptoms, Behçet's disease can be difficult to differentiate from Crohn's disease.

Patients with *polyarteritis nodosa* (Chapter 278) may have intermittent or persistent abdominal complications. Gastrointestinal involvement occurs in half or more of patients with polyarteritis nodosa. Most have abdominal pain, nausea, vomiting, melena, hematochezia, diarrhea, and occasionally, constipation; however, severe abdominal pain can also develop as a result of mesenteric vasculitis with gastrointestinal infarction and perforation. These gastrointestinal complications of polyarteritis nodosa result in considerable morbidity and mortality, with a mortality rate of 23% to greater than 60% when the symptoms include an acute abdomen. The diagnosis is typically made by CT radiography and magnetic resonance or CT angiography; less frequently, angiography is required. Although colonoscopy can identify ischemia, its role is limited in the acute setting because of the risk for perforation. Treatment is directed at the systemic disease (Chapter 278).

Henoch-Schönlein purpura (Chapter 278) is an immunoglobulin A (IgA)-mediated vasculitis with skin, abdominal, and renal manifestations. Abdominal symptoms include pain, nausea, vomiting, diarrhea, and gastrointestinal bleeding. Small bowel thickening and intussusception can be seen on CT radiography. Upper endoscopy and colonoscopy are not usually necessary diagnostically but can show submucosal hemorrhage, erythema, swelling, and ulcerations. Similar changes are also present in the small intestine as imaged by capsule endoscopy. The disease is often self-limited but may require systemic therapy (Chapter 278).

PERITONEAL DISORDERS

Peritonitis

DEFINITION

The peritoneum is the smooth serous membrane that lines the abdominal and pelvic cavities. The most common clinical disorders of the peritoneum are ascites (Chapter 156) and peritonitis. Peritonitis may be acute or chronic, septic or aseptic, primary or secondary, and localized or diffuse.

EPIDEMIOLOGY AND PATHOBIOLOGY

Acute peritonitis results from acute disruption of the peritoneal cavity with infectious or inflammatory materials. In the setting of perforation of the bowel or an intra-abdominal viscus, the contents themselves may be inflammatory, such as with bile spillage, or may be infectious, such as with contamination from intraluminal contents (e.g., bacteria and fecal material). Aseptic peritonitis results from the introduction of sterile bile, digestive juices, or extrinsic materials (e.g., chemotherapeutic medications) into the peritoneal cavity. Aseptic peritonitis rarely remains that way, with infection typically following in due course. Primary peritonitis refers to spontaneous bacterial peritonitis without an identifiable cause, typically in the setting of chronic liver disease (Chapter 148). Secondary peritonitis results most commonly from a perforated viscus such as the appendix, a diverticulum, peptic ulcer disease, or trauma with secondary spillage of luminal contents into the peritoneum. The most common bacteriology in secondary peritonitis is a mixed flora with *Escherichia coli, Streptococcus faecalis, Pseudomonas aeruginosa, Klebsiella mirabilis, Bacteroides fragilis, Clostridium* species, and anaerobic streptococci.

CLINICAL MANIFESTATIONS

Clinical manifestations of acute diffuse peritonitis typically include the sudden onset of abdominal pain that is usually constant. The pain may be diffuse or referred to the umbilicus or the portion of the abdomen where the inciting event originated. The peritoneal inflammation may subside or localize, thereby resulting in a reduction in pain and improved localization. Additional symptoms include nausea, vomiting, and fever. The development of progressive tachycardia and a falling temperature are grave signs of impending peritoneal shock from bacterial toxemia and septicemia (Chapter 108) (Fig. 144-7).

Additional physical signs (Chapter 134) include a very still patient. Bowel sounds are typically diminished or absent in the setting of peritonitis. Percussion often reveals tympany from the resultant ileus. On palpation, tenderness and rigidity are present. Rebound tenderness, with increasing pain when the examining hand is lifted from the abdomen, is usually present. Increased pain may also be elicited in the affected area on examination of an uninvolved portion of the abdomen. The abdominal muscles may become boardlike with rigidity, although this sign is frequently absent in elderly patients and in immunosuppressed patients.

DIAGNOSIS

Identifying the cause of the peritonitis depends on the age and sex of the patient. In younger patients, appendicitis and a perforated duodenal ulcer (Chapter 141) are most common. In older patients, perforated diverticula and cancer (Chapter 199) are more common. The use of NSAIDs or aspirin increases the likelihood of a perforated ulcer or diverticula. In young females, tubal pregnancy and a ruptured tubo-ovarian abscess must be considered (Chapters 293 and 308). CT imaging identifies the presence of free air and often is the cause of the intra-abdominal calamity (see Fig. 144-3).

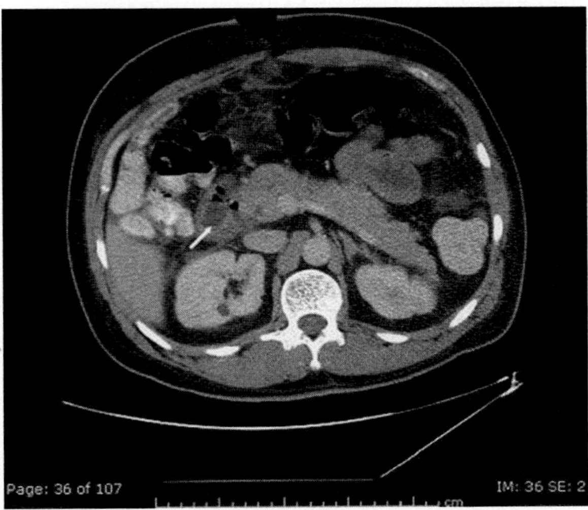

FIGURE 144-7. Computed tomography scan in a patient with peritonitis. Thickening of the duodenal wall *(arrow)* was identified at surgery as a perforated duodenal ulcer.

TREATMENT Rx

Treatment focuses on resuscitation, control of infection, and laparoscopy. The presence of suspected acute peritonitis necessitates surgical consultation. Correction of volume depletion and electrolyte disturbances with intravenous fluids is the cornerstone of initial management. Blood should be obtained for culture and broad-spectrum antibiotics administered prophylactically to cover gram-negative and anaerobic bacteria (Table 144-4).

PROGNOSIS

Peritonitis is a life-threatening disorder whose outcome depends on its cause as well as the rapidity of treatment. Mortality rates can be as low as 15% in patients who have correctable causes, such as a perforated appendix, and who do not develop multiorgan failure before treatment, but mortality rates can be as high as 50% for postoperative peritonitis.

Peritoneal Carcinomatosis and Malignant Ascites

Less than 10% of cases of ascites are malignant. Peritoneal carcinomatosis results from the metastatic spread of intra-abdominal malignancy (Table 144-5), usually in the setting of endometrial, colonic, gastric, and pancreatic carcinoma. The manifestation is similar to ascites of other causes (Chapter 148), although the ascites typically occurs rather suddenly in the absence of known portal hypertension, tuberculosis, or right heart failure.

DIAGNOSIS

In the setting of new-onset ascites, diagnostic paracentesis should be performed. Aspirated fluid should be sent for cell count and differential, Gram stain and culture, and measurement of albumin with simultaneous serum albumin measurement. A serum minus ascites albumin value of less than 1.1 g/mL (Chapter 156) supports the diagnosis of malignant ascites but is also seen in pancreatitis, nephrotic syndrome, and peritoneal tuberculosis. In the setting of hepatic metastases, the serum-ascites albumin gradient may be greater than 1.1. Ascitic fluid cytology will identify malignant cells 50 to 60% of the time.

Abnormal ultrasound findings can confirm the presence of ascites, but CT is preferred to help identify the underlying cause (Fig. 144-8). Malignant ascites is frequently loculated, sometimes from previous surgically related adhesions.

TABLE 144-4 ANTIBIOTIC OPTIONS FOR INTRA-ABDOMINAL SECONDARY PERITONITIS

Piperacillin-tazobactam, 3.375 g q6h
Ampicillin-sulbactam, 3.0 g q6h
Ciprofloxacin, 400 mg q12h, and metronidazole, 1 g q12h
Levofloxacin, 750 mg q24h
Cefepime, 2 g q12h, and metronidazole, 1 g q12h
Imipenem–cilastatin sodium, 500 mg q6h

TABLE 144-5 CAUSES OF PERITONEAL CARCINOMATOSIS

PRIMARY
Mesothelioma
Sarcoma
SECONDARY INTRA-ABDOMINAL MALIGNANCIES
Gastric adenocarcinoma
Colon adenocarcinoma
Pancreatic adenocarcinoma
Ovarian carcinoma
Neuroendocrine tumors, including carcinoid
Lymphoma
EXTRA-ABDOMINAL MALIGNANCIES
Breast
Melanoma
Lung

TREATMENT Rx

Treatment of malignant ascites is symptomatic and quite challenging. In general, malignant ascites does not respond to diuretic therapy, except that patients with malignant ascites in the setting of hepatic metastases may respond to spironolactone. Therapeutic paracentesis in the setting of tense ascites improves symptoms, including shortness of breath and abdominal discomfort. Unfortunately, malignant ascites rapidly reaccumulates. The use of intracavitary radioisotopes or chemotherapy has been advocated in some cases for palliation with variable success.

PROGNOSIS

The development of malignant ascites is usually a poor prognostic indicator, with few patients surviving beyond 4 months. An exception is the better prognosis with malignant ascites from ovarian (Chapter 205) or breast cancer (Chapter 204).

Peritoneal Tuberculosis

In the United States, tuberculosis (Chapter 332) is relatively uncommon, although it is increasingly being identified in immigrants. Tuberculous ascites also occurs in cirrhosis and in patients with chronic renal disease who are maintained on peritoneal dialysis.

Peritoneal tuberculosis is accompanied by abdominal swelling, fever, anorexia, and weight loss. The diagnosis should be considered in the setting of refractory ascites. Analysis of ascitic fluid reveals an exudative ascites. The fluid protein is typically greater than 2.5 g/100 mL, with a serum-ascites gradient of less than 1.1 g/mL.

TREATMENT AND PROGNOSIS 

Treatment involves conventional antituberculous therapy (Chapter 332). Prognosis is dependent on whether tuberculosis is systemic or restricted to the peritoneum. It is important to document clearance of the tuberculosis with repeat paracentesis.

Peritonitis Associated with Continuous Ambulatory Peritoneal Dialysis

Patients in whom peritonitis develops while undergoing continuous ambulatory peritoneal dialysis (Chapter 133) have abdominal pain and cloudy peritoneal fluid. Approximately 50% of patients have fever. Nausea and diarrhea may also occur. On physical examination, abdominal pain is usually present.

Diagnosis is based on the peritoneal fluid cell count and differential. Although Gram stain is rarely positive, any organisms that are seen are predictive of subsequent culture results. Peritoneal cultures are positive 90% of

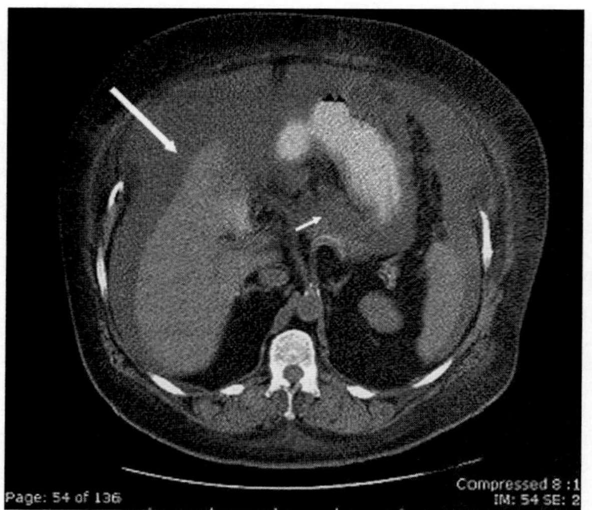

FIGURE 144-8. Malignant ascites. A computed tomography scan shows ascites *(large arrow)* and a gastric mass *(small arrow)*.

the time. Gram-positive organisms predominant, with coagulase-negative staphylococci and *Staphylococcus aureus* most commonly identified. Gram-negative organisms are present about 20% of the time, and 10% of patients have polymicrobial infections. Fungal peritonitis is infrequent and usually due to *Candida* species.

Antibiotic choices for empirical therapy include intraperitoneal cefazolin, cephalothin, and ceftazidime. Aminoglycosides should be used only when residual urine volume is less than 100 mL/day. Once culture results are available, antibiotics are adjusted according to the sensitivity of the organisms.

MISCELLANEOUS DISEASE OF THE MESENTERY AND OMENTUM

Mesenteric disorders are uncommon. Patients with mesenteric cysts complain of abdominal pain, fever, and emesis. Symptomatic cysts are treated surgically.

Mesenteric panniculitis refers to an inflammatory process of the adipose tissue of the mesentery. A variety of other terms are used, including lipodystrophy, sclerosing lipogranulomatosis, lipogranuloma of the mesentery, and mesenteritis. The disease is manifested as thickening or nodularity of the mesentery with fat necrosis. Mesenteric panniculitis is characterized by a variety of nonspecific abdominal symptoms, including fever, abdominal pain, anorexia, weight loss, and altered bowel habits. The diagnosis is made at laparoscopy. Laboratory studies are rarely helpful, although an elevated erythrocyte sedimentation rate may be seen. Surgical resection is required only when obstruction is present.

ANATOMIC AND MECHANICAL DISORDERS

Groin Hernias

In addition to hiatal hernias (Chapter 140), hernias may occur in the groin as inguinal or femoral hernias or as a result of weakness or abnormalities of other abdominal and pelvic muscles.

EPIDEMIOLOGY

About 3 to 4% of men have groin hernias, and the incidence increases with age. Indirect inguinal hernias, caused by a defect in the abdominal wall, account for about two thirds of hernias. Direct inguinal hernias, which protrude through an area bounded by the rectus abdominis muscle, the inferior upper gastric artery, and the inguinal ligament, account for about 30% of hernias in men and about 2% of hernias in women. Femoral hernias, which pass through an opening associated with the femoral artery and vein, represent about 30% of hernias in women and about 2% in men.

CLINICAL MANIFESTATIONS AND DIAGNOSIS

Groin hernias may be asymptomatic or be perceived as a mass that enlarges with standing or with increases in intra-abdominal pressure. If a hernia is not readily reducible (i.e., incarcerated), it may be associated with constant discomfort. With strangulation, ischemia or bowel obstruction may occur. The diagnosis is usually readily apparent by palpation of a soft groin mass that becomes larger with standing or with increases in intra-abdominal pressure.

TREATMENT Rx

Although femoral hernias should be repaired when first diagnosed because of the risk for strangulation, watchful waiting is an acceptable option for men with minimally symptomatic inguinal hernias.[11] Surgical options for both the initial operation and for recurrent hernias include laparoscopic repair and open mesh repair.[12,13]

Other Hernias

Incisional hernias develop after 1 to 4% of laparotomy incisions. These hernias may cause chronic abdominal discomfort, especially with maneuvers that increase intra-abdominal pressure. Repair is usually performed with prosthetic mesh.

Colonic Volvulus

Most cases of colonic volvulus involve the sigmoid colon (>90%), but volvulus can also involve the cecum and transverse colon. Elderly persons are at greatest risk. Volvulus results in colonic obstruction when the colon twists on its mesentery. Patients with volvulus frequently report a history of chronic constipation or laxative use or have previously been noted to have a dilated colon. A history of psychiatric illness or institutionalization is also associated with an increased risk for the development of volvulus.

CLINICAL MANIFESTATIONS

Symptoms of volvulus include the acute development of abdominal distention, nausea, and vomiting, with abdominal pain present initially in about one third of patients. Progressive or severe pain and tenderness suggest developing colonic ischemia and perforation. Much less commonly, patients have an intermittent history of obstructive symptoms and distention suggesting chronic volvulus.

DIAGNOSIS

The diagnosis of volvulus is made by abdominal radiographs, which show a dilated colon that may lack haustral folds and has a "bent inner tube" appearance, with the apex pointing to the right upper quadrant. Cecal volvulus is suspected radiographically when a dilated cecum is located in the epigastrium or left upper quadrant. Small bowel dilation may also be present. Water-soluble contrast enema will also confirm the presence and site of obstruction with the classic finding of a "bird's beak" configuration at the obstructed site.

TREATMENT Rx

Patients who have suspected colonic volvulus and who exhibit peritoneal signs or have complete obstruction on abdominal radiographs require fluid emergency exploratory laparotomy. In the absence of signs of complete obstruction or impending ischemia and when sigmoid volvulus is suspected, endoscopic sigmoidoscopic examination will document the site of obstruction and endoscopic reduction is the emergent treatment of choice for colonic decompression. Endoscopic procedures are generally avoided in patients with suspected cecal volvulus, however, and surgical resection is required emergently when endoscopic treatment is not appropriate or is unsuccessful or later after endoscopic treatment because of the risk of recurrence.

Intussusception

Intussusception results when a segment of intestine is drawn distally into another segment of intestine, thereby resulting in obstruction. Intussusception may occur in the small intestine itself, or the small intestine may intussuscept into the colon. Intussusception occurs most commonly in children, in whom it is seen in the setting of recent viral enteritis (e.g., rotavirus; Chapter 388), cystic fibrosis (Chapter 89), or Meckel's diverticulum. In adults, intussusception is more likely to occur in the setting of small bowel neoplasia (Chapter 199).

CLINICAL MANIFESTATIONS

Most patients have symptoms of partial small bowel obstruction—crampy abdominal pain, nausea, vomiting, and occasionally, diarrhea. An abdominal mass may be palpable on examination, and patients may have evidence of occult or overt gastrointestinal bleeding (the passage of "currant jelly" mucus-like stool is described in infants and children).

DIAGNOSIS AND MANAGEMENT

The diagnosis is most commonly confirmed by CT radiography, which classically shows a "target" lesion of the small bowel that represents the layers of the small bowel and intussuscepted segment. The finding of intussusception in an adult necessitates abdominal exploration and resection of the intussuscepted segment.

Adhesions

Peritoneal adhesions cause most cases of small bowel obstruction. Adhesions can result from previous laparotomy, with an increased risk for adhesions occurring in patients with intra-abdominal infections, ischemia, and foreign bodies. Symptomatic adhesive bowel obstruction will subsequently develop in 5 to 10% of patients undergoing laparotomy. Adhesive disease may also result in reduced fertility in females. After laparotomy, adhesive-related obstruction can occur at any time from the early postoperative period to many years later.

CLINICAL MANIFESTATIONS

Patients have crampy abdominal pain, nausea, vomiting, and increasing abdominal distention. In the setting of complete bowel obstruction, patients no longer pass stool or flatus.

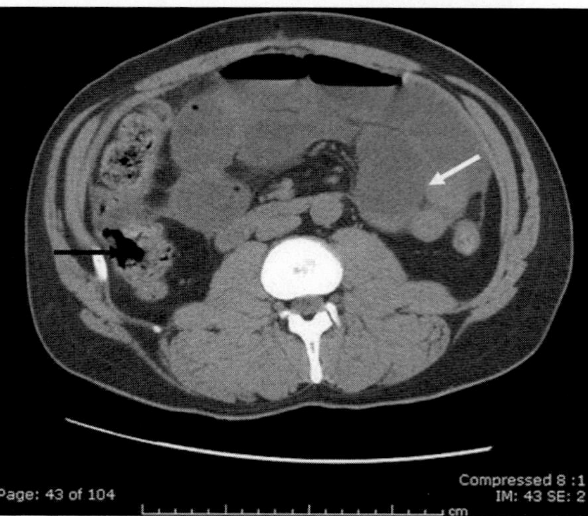

FIGURE 144-9. Adhesion-related small bowel obstruction. A computed tomography scan shows dilated, fluid-filled small bowel *(white arrow)* and a nondilated colon *(black arrow)*. At laparotomy, an obstruction secondary to adhesions was found in the midileum.

DIAGNOSIS AND TREATMENT

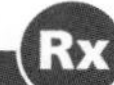

On an upright abdominal radiograph, findings of adhesive-related bowel obstruction include dilated loops of bowel (>6 cm of small bowel) and air-fluid levels, with reduced air distal to the obstruction. Similar findings are present on CT radiography (Fig. 144-9). Limitations of radiographic examination include subtle findings when the obstruction is very proximal in the bowel or the obstruction is only partial. In these settings, small bowel radiographs with water-soluble or barium contrast may be necessary to make the diagnosis.

Treatment of complete small bowel obstruction is fluid resuscitation and urgent laparotomy. Nasogastric tube decompression reduces nausea, vomiting, and distention. Nonoperative management may be tried in the setting of partial small bowel obstruction, with surgery reserved for patients whose obstruction fails to resolve. Patients with recurrent small bowel obstruction may benefit from a low-roughage diet to reduce the risk for obstruction from nondigestible food residue in a narrowed lumen.

The presence of chronic or recurrent abdominal pain in the absence of bowel obstruction has often been blamed on adhesions. Unless a clearly identified obstruction is present radiographically, surgical intervention for adhesiolysis is not warranted and does not reliably reduce abdominal pain symptoms. The search continues for intraoperative techniques or substances to reduce the development of adhesions.

Grade A

1. Terasawa T, Blackmore C, Bent S, et al. Systematic review: computed tomography and ultrasonography to detect acute appendicitis in adults and adolescents. *Ann Intern Med.* 2004;141:537-546.
2. Hershko DD, Awad N, Fischer D, et al. Focused helical CT using rectal contrast material only as the preferred technique for the diagnosis of suspected acute appendicitis: a prospective, randomized, controlled study comparing three different techniques. *Dis Colon Rectum.* 2007;50:1223-1229.
3. Varadhan KK, Humes DJ, Neal KR, et al. Antibiotic therapy versus appendectomy for acute appendicitis: a meta-analysis. *World J Surg.* 2010;34:199-209.
4. Sauerland S, Lefering R, Neugebauer EAM. Laparoscopic versus open surgery for suspected appendicitis. *Cochrane Database Syst Rev.* 2004;4:CD001546.
5. St. Peter SD, Aguayo P, Fraser JD, et al. Initial laparoscopic appendectomy versus initial nonoperative management and interval appendectomy for perforated appendicitis with abscess: a prospective, randomized trial. *J Pediatr Surg.* 2010;45:236-240.
6. St. Peter SD, Tsao K, Spilde TL, et al. Single daily dosing ceftriaxone and metronidazole vs standard triple antibiotic regimen for perforated appendix in children: a prospective randomized trial. *J Pediatr Surg.* 2008;43:981-985.
7. Ridgway PF, Latif A, Shabbir J, et al. Randomized controlled trial of oral vs intravenous therapy for the clinically diagnosed acute uncomplicated diverticulitis. *Colorectal Dis.* 2009;11:941-946.
8. Schug-Pass C, Geers P, Hugel O, et al. Prospective randomized trial comparing short-term antibiotic therapy versus standard therapy for acute uncomplicated sigmoid diverticulitis. *Int J Colorectal Dis.* 2010;25:751-759.
9. Klarenbeek BR, Veenhof AA, Bergamaschi R, et al. Laparoscopic sigmoid resection for diverticulitis decreases major morbidity rates: a randomized control trial: short-term results of the Sigma Trial. *Ann Surg.* 2009;249:39-44.
10. Latella G, Pimpo MT, Sottili S, et al. Rifaximin improves symptoms of acquired uncomplicated diverticular disease of the colon. *Int J Colorectal Dis.* 2003;18:55-62.
11. Fitzgibbons RJ Jr, Giobbie-Hurder A, Gibbs JO, et al. Watchful waiting vs repair of inguinal hernia in minimally symptomatic men: a randomized clinical trial. *JAMA.* 2006;295:285-292.
12. Amato B, Moja L, Panico S, et al. Shouldice technique versus other open techniques for inguinal hernia repair. *Cochrane Database Syst Rev.* 2009;4:CD001543.
13. Karthikesalingam A, Markar SR, Holt PJ, et al. Meta-analysis of randomized controlled trials comparing laparoscopic with open mesh repair of recurrent inguinal hernia. *Br J Surg.* 2010;97:4-11.

SUGGESTED READINGS

Eglinton T, Nguyen T, Raniga S, et al. Patterns of recurrence in patients with acute diverticulitis. *Br J Surg.* 2010;97:952-957. *Elective surgery to prevent recurrence and the development of complications should be used sparingly.*

Gupta RK, Agrawal CS, Yadav R, et al. Intussusception in adults: institutional review. *Int J Surg.* 2011;9:91-95. *Review of 38 cases, including causes (about 50% malignant) and rates of successful reduction (58% for ileocolic, 30% for colocolic).*

Merlin MA, Shah CN, Shiroff AM. Evidence-based appendicitis: the initial workup. *Postgrad Med.* 2010;122:189-195. *Review emphasizing CT diagnosis.*

Tan KK, Chong CS, Sim R. Management of acute sigmoid volvulus: an institution's experience over 9 years. *World J Surg.* 2010;34:1943-1948. *Elective definitive surgery is suggested in view of the high recurrence rate (>60%) and the considerable risks of emergency surgery.*

Zielinski MD, Elken PW, Bannon MP, et al. Small bowel obstruction—who needs an operation? A multivariate prediction model. *World J Surg.* 2010;34:910-919. *Intraperitoneal free fluid, mesenteric edema, lack of the "small bowel feces sign," and history of vomiting predict the need for surgery.*

145

VASCULAR DISEASES OF THE GASTROINTESTINAL TRACT

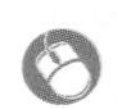

STEPHEN CRANE HAUSER

INTESTINAL ISCHEMIA

Intestinal ischemia can occur as a result of a variety of conditions that decrease intestinal blood flow. Both diminished arterial blood flow to the gut and compromised venous circulation from the intestine can cause intestinal or mesenteric ischemia. Several conditions, such as adhesions and malignancy (Chapter 199), may predispose to mesenteric ischemia by secondarily diminishing blood flow through extrinsic compression of otherwise normal intestinal arteries or veins (Table 145-1). These disorders and esophageal varices (Chapters 137 and 156) are discussed elsewhere.

EPIDEMIOLOGY

Intestinal ischemia is responsible for about 1 per 1000 hospital admissions. When considering the diagnosis of intestinal ischemia, it is important to distinguish *primary* (occlusive or nonocclusive) from *secondary* (extrinsic to the blood vessel) mesenteric ischemia, *acute* manifestations from *chronic, arterial* versus *venous,* and *small bowel* versus *colonic* ischemia. Risk factors for intestinal ischemia include older age (all the disorders discussed) and conditions that predispose to arterial embolism (e.g., cardiac arrhythmias, heart failure, cardiomegaly, dyskinesia, valvular heart disease, recent myocardial infarction, cardiac catheterization, intracardiac thrombus, atheromatous cholesterol embolism), occlusion of arteries (atherosclerosis, fibromuscular dysplasia, abdominal aortic aneurysm, trauma, vasculitis), low-flow states (sepsis, dialysis, reduced cardiac output, vasoconstrictive drugs), and pathologic thromboses (largely venous; hypercoagulable and hyperviscosity states, trauma, malignancy, inflammation).

TABLE 145-1 CONDITIONS PREDISPOSING TO SECONDARY MESENTERIC ISCHEMIA
Adhesions
Herniation
Volvulus
Intussusception
Mesenteric fibrosis
Retroperitoneal fibrosis
Carcinoid syndrome
Malignancy (peritoneal, mesenteric, colonic)
Neurofibromatosis
Amyloidosis
Trauma

PATHOBIOLOGY

Arterial or venous disease of the esophagus, stomach, duodenum, and rectum is very unusual for anatomic reasons. The esophagus receives its main blood supply segmentally through multiple small vessels from the aorta, right intercostal artery, bronchial arteries, inferior thyroid artery, left gastric artery, short gastric artery, and left phrenic artery. Likewise, the stomach, duodenum, and rectum have numerous arterial inputs with rich collateralization. Patients who have undergone extensive surgical resection of the esophagus, stomach, or duodenum are at increased risk for ischemia. Vasculitic disorders, which can involve small or large arteries or veins, may affect the esophagus, stomach, duodenum, or rectum.

The arterial supply of blood to the small and large intestine is from the *celiac artery, superior mesenteric artery* (SMA), and *inferior mesenteric artery* (IMA). Collateral vessels, which vary from person to person, may include the meandering mesenteric artery or arc of Riolan at the base of the mesentery (connecting the SMA and IMA), the marginal artery of Drummond along the mesenteric border (connecting the SMA and IMA), the pancreaticoduodenal arcade (connecting the celiac artery and SMA), the arc of Barkow (connecting the celiac artery and SMA), and the arc of Buhler (connecting the celiac artery and SMA). These collaterals can rapidly enlarge in response to localized mesenteric ischemia. During states of low arterial flow, such as in patients with low systemic arterial blood pressure, "watershed" areas such as the splenic flexure, which is farthest away from arterial flow, are more likely to be involved. In contrast, when a major arterial vessel such as the IMA is suddenly occluded, the splenic flexure is less likely to be involved because of collaterals from the SMA circulation.

Intestinal blood flow, which accounts for approximately 10% of cardiac output, increases to as much as 25% of cardiac output after eating a meal. Blood flow to the intestine is regulated by the sympathetic nervous system and a variety of systemic (angiotensin II, vasopressin) and local (prostaglandins, leukotrienes) humoral factors.

Mesenteric ischemia can occur as a result of decreased *arterial* blood flow, which can be *occlusive* (arterial embolus, arterial thrombus, and vasculitis) or *nonocclusive* (low-flow states). *Venous* obstruction (thrombosis, vasculitis) can also result in mesenteric ischemia.

Whatever the cause of mesenteric ischemia, the gut is able to adapt to as much as a 75% reduction in normal blood flow for as long as 12 hours. Increased flow through available and newly opened collateral vessels and increased oxygen extraction help compensate. However, with a more prolonged and more severe reduction in blood flow, generalized mesenteric arterial vasoconstriction often develops and can become irreversible, even with correction of the original underlying condition (i.e., relief of focal arterial obstruction or resolution of a low-flow state). Hypoxia and reperfusion injury by oxygen radicals, reduced endothelial synthesis of nitric oxide, and an enhanced cellular inflammatory response cause microvascular and end-organ damage. Initially, the end-organ damage is primarily mucosal, but damage can rapidly progress to transmural necrosis (gangrene). Some ischemic segments of bowel will heal with fibrosis (strictures).

CLINICAL MANIFESTATIONS

Symptoms of intestinal ischemia at initial evaluation may be acute (sudden, lasting hours), subacute (days), or chronic (intermittent, occurring over a period of weeks to months). With acute and many subacute manifestations, abdominal pain is often the cardinal symptom. Usually the pain is severe, persistent, and poorly localized. Initially, the pain is typically more severe than the findings on abdominal palpation (i.e., pain out of proportion to tenderness). With or without pain, other initial features may include fever, altered mental status, abdominal distention, difficulty eating, nausea, vomiting, and diarrhea. With small bowel ischemia, overt gastrointestinal bleeding (Chapter 137) is a late and ominous finding that often suggests small bowel infarction.

Findings on physical examination can include hypotension, tachycardia, abdominal distention, initially increased and later decreased bowel sounds, and nonspecific diffuse abdominal tenderness, often mild at first. Over time, peritoneal signs with localized to generalized abdominal tenderness, rebound, and rigidity may become manifest. Occult gastrointestinal bleeding can be an early finding.

DIAGNOSIS

Even as the diagnostic evaluation is begun, appropriate attention must be directed to emergency therapy, including fluid resuscitation, antibiotics, and invasive therapy (Fig. 145-1).

Initial Diagnostic Evaluation

The initial laboratory findings in patients with an acute onset of bowel ischemia can be entirely normal. Nonspecific abnormalities such as leukocytosis with a predominance of neutrophils and hemoconcentration may be observed. Elevated serum levels of amylase, lactate, aminotransferases, lactate dehydrogenase, creatine kinase, and phosphate often portend more advanced (necrotic) small bowel ischemia, but these findings lack sensitivity as well as specificity.

Noninvasive Imaging

The presence or absence of radiographic features suggestive of ischemia in patients with acute-onset mesenteric ischemia varies and depends on the duration and extent of ischemia. Plain abdominal radiographs are useful in helping exclude secondary causes of mesenteric ischemia, as well as other causes of acute abdominal pain, nausea, vomiting, or distention, such as obstruction and perforation. Radiographic findings such as "thumbprinting" (caused by submucosal hemorrhage), an ileus pattern, or formless loops of small bowel, or with more advanced disease, pneumatosis intestinalis or portal venous gas (often a sign of transmural necrosis or gangrene) may on occasion be seen. Contrast-enhanced abdominal-pelvic computed tomography (CT) is also helpful to exclude alternative diagnoses. CT may demonstrate entirely normal findings in acute mesenteric ischemia, or findings such as segmental bowel wall thickening, submucosal hemorrhage, mesenteric stranding, mesenteric venous thrombosis, pneumatosis, and portal venous gas may be present (Fig. 145-2). Multidetector CT angiography (MDCTA) has a greater sensitivity and specificity (each up to 95%) than traditional CT (about 65%). Magnetic resonance angiography (MRA) is less sensitive for more peripheral emboli. Subacute manifestations of bowel ischemia may be due to a wide variety of causes, including mesenteric venous thrombosis, which is best diagnosed by CT scan. However, the time needed to obtain a CT scan should not delay resuscitation or arteriography in very ill patients with suspected acute-onset ischemia.

TREATMENT Rx

Acutely ill patients require prompt, definitive diagnosis and treatment, which often requires selective mesenteric angiography (Fig. 145-3). If transmural intestinal necrosis (gangrene) is suspected from peritoneal signs, pneumatosis, or portal venous gas on imaging procedures, emergency laparotomy is indicated. The presence of predisposing conditions (e.g., arrhythmias, systemic hypotension) and their extraintestinal manifestations (e.g., heart failure, sepsis, respiratory insufficiency, acute renal failure, anemia) dictate the initial therapy: volume replacement, optimization of cardiac output, management of respiratory function, avoidance of splanchnic vasoconstrictors such as digoxin, and administration of broad-spectrum antibiotics (e.g., meropenem, imipenem/cilastatin, metronidazole and a third-generation cephalosporin, ciprofloxacin and metronidazole, or piperacillin until symptoms resolve to cover aerobic gram-negative and anaerobic organisms and to prevent sepsis secondary to translocation of bacteria across ischemic gut mucosa.

PROGNOSIS

Acute primary arterial mesenteric ischemia involving the small bowel is an urgent condition, which, if unidentified or untreated, can result in death within hours. Mortality rates may be as high as 70% but are much lower with early diagnosis and prompt therapy. Overall, colonic ischemia has a much better prognosis than does small bowel ischemia. Mesenteric venous thrombosis also has a much better prognosis than acute primary arterial mesenteric ischemia of the small intestine.

Specific Ischemic Bowel Syndromes

SUPERIOR MESENTERIC EMBOLISM

Embolization to the intestine through the SMA (*SMA embolus*) accounts for 5% of peripheral emboli and nearly 50% of cases of primary noncolonic mesenteric ischemia. Emboli originate most commonly from the heart, with an aortic origin being less common (Table 145-2), and tend to obstruct beyond the origin of the SMA.

CLINICAL MANIFESTATIONS AND DIAGNOSIS

Patients who are evaluated early in the course of their illness may have entirely normal CT scans, or the CT findings may be consistent with mesenteric

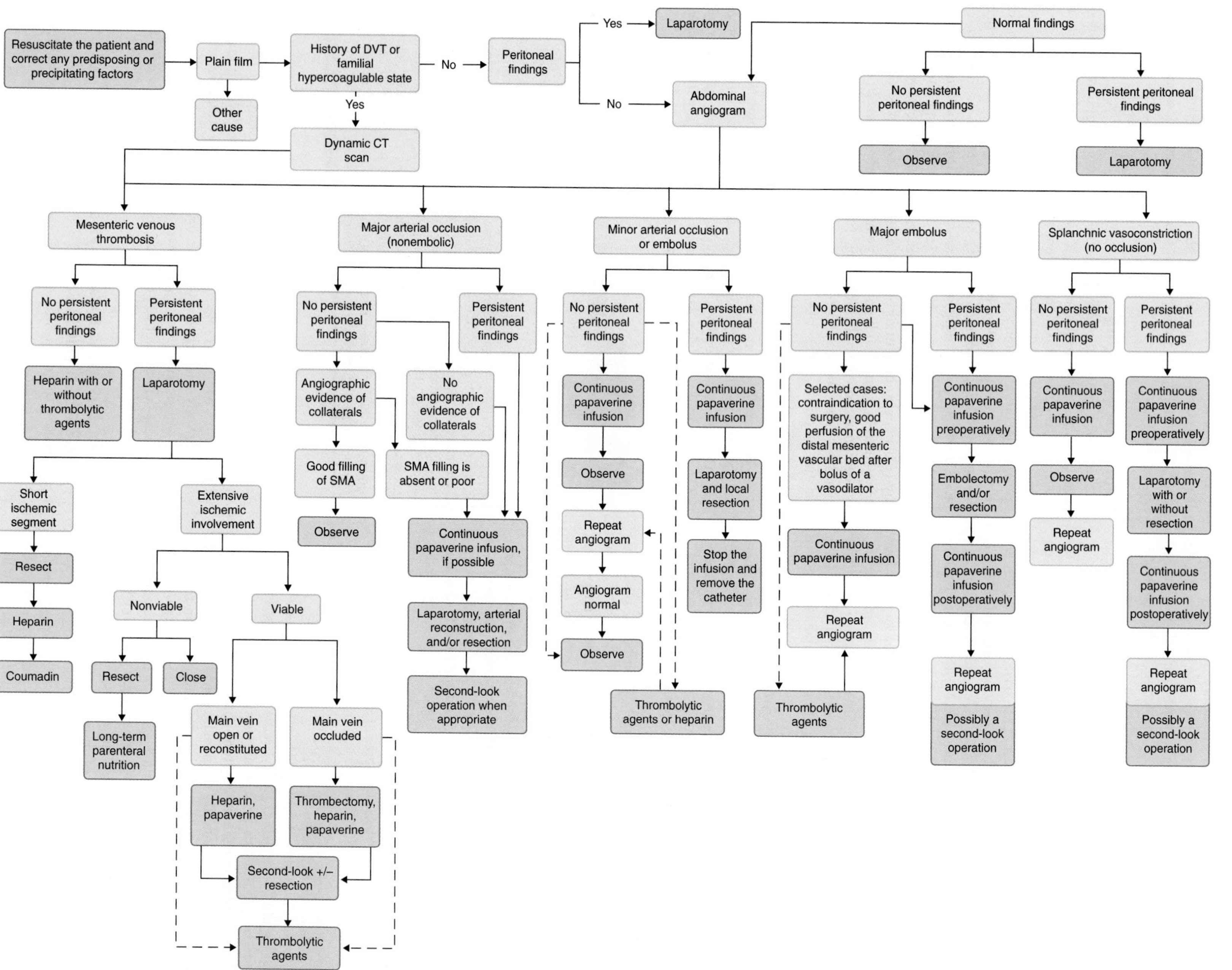

FIGURE 145-1. Algorithm for managing patients with suspected acute mesenteric ischemia: diagnosis and management. *Solid lines* indicate an accepted management plan; *dashed lines* indicate an alternative management plan. CT = computed tomography; DVT = deep venous thrombosis; SMA = superior mesenteric artery. (From American Gastroenterological Association Medical Position Statement: guidelines on intestinal ischemia. *Gastroenterology*. 2000;118:951-953 [corrected algorithm in *Gastroenterology*. 2000;119:281].)

ischemia without features that would suggest alternative diagnoses (e.g., perforation, obstruction). MDCTA is much more likely than standard CT to diagnose embolic disease reliably in the mesenteric arterial vasculature. Selective mesenteric angiography offers the possibility of therapy as well as diagnosis.

TREATMENT Rx

Select patients with acute onset of a partial or small SMA branch occlusion may be candidates for thrombolytic therapy (e.g., streptokinase, urokinase, tissue plasminogen activator) infused through an arterial catheter directly into the vicinity of the embolus; this therapy can lyse the embolus and resolve symptoms such as abdominal pain. Because segmental arterial embolic occlusion of a small portion of the SMA vascular bed results in widespread splanchnic visceral arterial vasoconstriction, which may persist even after the original inciting event (i.e., an embolus) is rectified, infusion of a vasodilator such as papaverine (often given as a 60-mg bolus, followed by a continuous infusion of 30 to 60 mg/hour for 12 to 48 hours) through an arterial catheter reverses this reflex vasoconstriction and improves the outcome, including mortality rates. The same scenario occurs with other arterial occlusive lesions (SMA thrombi), arterial nonocclusive disease (nonocclusive mesenteric ischemia), and disorders associated with mesenteric venous occlusion.

Patients evaluated in the course of their acute embolic illness with peritoneal signs require laparotomy, with or without resection and with or without embolectomy, which is usually performed during surgical exploration. A "second-look" operation 24 hours after embolectomy to make sure that all necrotic tissue has been resected may be necessary.

Any patient in whom SMA embolization is diagnosed requires preoperative systemic anticoagulation (e.g., intravenous heparin) to prevent propagation of clot around the embolus and to guard against further embolization to the intestine or other organs (i.e., brain, coronary arteries, kidneys, extremities). Anticoagulation is usually discontinued before surgery and is often resumed 24 to 48 hours postoperatively, depending on the operative findings. Mortality can be as high as 70%.

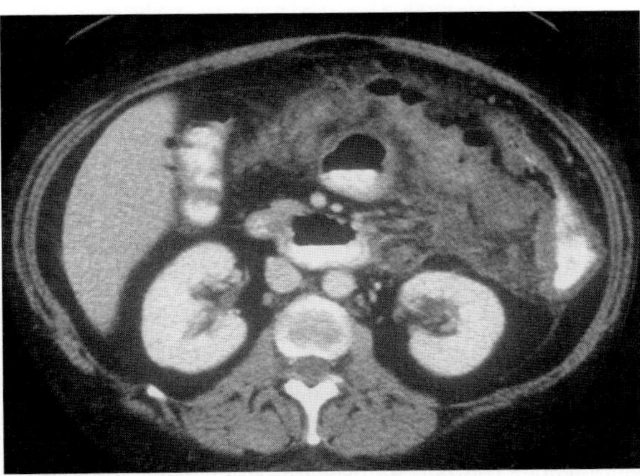

FIGURE 145-2. Computed tomography of the abdomen in a patient with ischemic colitis as a result of superior mesenteric vein thrombosis. A segmental area of the transverse colon demonstrates a thick wall, as well as considerable fluid and soft tissue stranding in the adjacent mesentery. (From Johnson CL, Schmit GD, eds. *Mayo Clinic Gastrointestinal Imaging Review*. Boca Raton, Fla: Mayo Clinic Scientific Press, Taylor and Francis Group; 2005. By permission of the Mayo Foundation for Medical Education and Research. All rights reserved).

SUPERIOR MESENTERIC THROMBOSIS

Thrombosis of the SMA *(SMA thrombus)* accounts for nearly 15% of cases of primary noncolonic mesenteric ischemia. Risk factors include older age, atherosclerosis (e.g., hypertension, diabetes mellitus, hyperlipidemia, smoking history), low-flow states, hypercoagulable states, and less often, vasculitis and aortic or mesenteric aneurysms.

CLINICAL MANIFESTATIONS AND DIAGNOSIS

Nearly one third of these patients have a history of symptomatic chronic mesenteric ischemia (see later) antedating their acute manifestation of SMA thrombosis. Proximal mesenteric arterial occlusions are well recognized by MDCTA, MRA, and Doppler ultrasound, but similar abnormalities are common in asymptomatic elderly persons. Similar to acute SMA embolism, the diagnosis is confirmed by selective mesenteric angiography, with intra-arterial infusion of a vasodilator used to reverse reflex-generalized vasoconstriction.

TREATMENT 

Although thrombolytic therapy has been helpful in a limited number of case reports, surgical thrombectomy or bypass grafting, with or without bowel resection, is the most common therapeutic approach. Because many thrombi occur near the SMA origin, angioplasty may be therapeutic in very select cases, but the risk for reocclusion is high. Similar to acute SMA embolism, anticoagulation (intravenous heparin) is important preoperatively and at some point postoperatively in the acute state, as is administration of broad-spectrum antibiotics (see earlier).

TABLE 145-2 CONDITIONS ASSOCIATED WITH EMBOLIZATION TO THE GASTROINTESTINAL TRACT

Cardiac arrhythmias
Valvular heart disease
Heart failure
Myocardial infarction
Intracardiac thrombus
Cardiac catheterization
Cardioversion
Atherosclerosis of the aorta

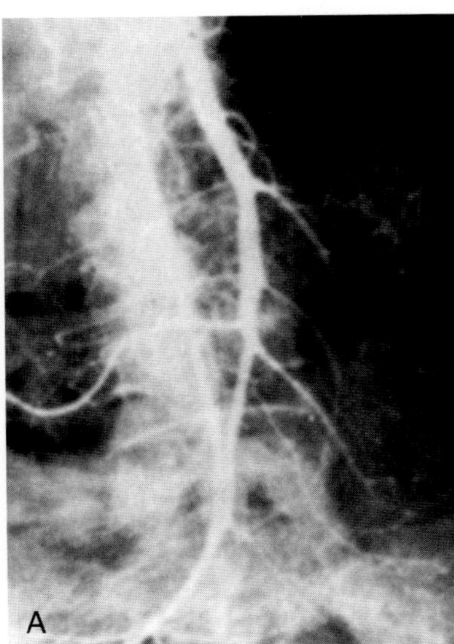

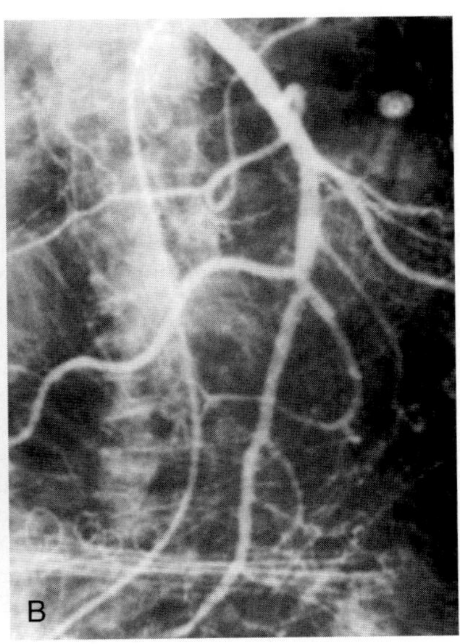

FIGURE 145-3. Selected films from superior mesenteric angiography. **A,** Diffuse vasoconstriction characteristic of nonocclusive mesenteric ischemia. **B,** Intra-arterial infusion of papaverine (30 to 60 mg/hour) resulted in vasodilation.

ACUTE NONOCCLUSIVE, NONCOLONIC PRIMARY ARTERIAL ISCHEMIA

Nonocclusive mesenteric ischemia, which accounts for about 20% of primary noncolonic mesenteric ischemia cases, is caused by low arterial blood flow to the intestine. Risk factors include advanced age, decreased systolic blood pressure (e.g., cardiac arrhythmia, heart failure, myocardial infarction, shock, sepsis, burns, pancreatitis, hemorrhage, multiple organ failure, dialysis, perioperative states), vasospasm (e.g., digoxin, vasopressin, amphetamines, cocaine), and atherosclerotic disease.

CLINICAL MANIFESTATIONS AND DIAGNOSIS

The clinical findings are generally indistinguishable from those of embolic or thrombotic vascular disease, except that symptoms may be less acute. As a result, patients initially may be seen without acute abdominal pain but rather with more nonspecific symptoms such as distention, nausea, fever, altered mental status, and borderline or low systolic blood pressure. Selected mesenteric angiography establishes the diagnosis (lack of embolus or thrombus, alternating areas of vessel spasm and dilation, vascular pruning and spasm).

TREATMENT Rx

The best specific treatment is prolonged intra-arterial instillation of a vasodilator (e.g., papaverine, often given as a 60-mg bolus, followed by a continuous infusion of 30 to 60 mg/hour) to reverse the vasospasm. Avoidance of vasospastic medications and optimization of cardiac output, blood volume, and blood pressure are crucial. Anticoagulation is generally not necessary, but broad-spectrum antibiotics (similar to those recommended earlier) should be administered to cover aerobic gram-negative and anaerobic organisms. Although many of these patients have serious conditions that predispose them to low-flow states and their ultimate prognosis is dependent on the outcomes of these serious conditions, diagnosis and treatment of acute nonocclusive mesenteric ischemia with therapeutic angiography can be life-saving.

MESENTERIC VENOUS THROMBOSIS

Occlusive disease of the mesenteric venous circulation *(mesenteric venous thrombosis)* usually involves the superior mesenteric vein (SMV) and may be accompanied by symptoms that are acute (hours to days) or subacute (weeks to months) in onset.

EPIDEMIOLOGY AND PATHOBIOLOGY

Thrombosis of the SMV accounts for about 10% of cases of primary noncolonic mesenteric ischemia. Colonic involvement with ischemic colitis is much less common. In contrast to arterial occlusive disease, risk factors and causes for SMV thrombosis are more numerous and diverse. Individuals with a personal or family history of a hypercoagulable state or deep venous thrombosis are at increased risk for SMV thrombosis. Hypercoagulable states, hyperviscosity syndromes, portal hypertension, intra-abdominal infections (e.g., pyelophlebitis, diverticulitis, appendicitis) or inflammation (e.g., Crohn's disease, pancreatitis), malignancy, vasculitis, and trauma may all cause thrombosis of the SMV (Table 145-3).

CLINICAL MANIFESTATIONS

Symptoms in acute-onset cases are similar to those observed in acute occlusive and nonocclusive arterial mesenteric ischemia—abdominal pain, anorexia, nausea, vomiting, abdominal fullness, diarrhea, and constipation—but tend to persist over a longer time period. Some patients may have bacteremia, especially infection with *Bacteroides.* Gastrointestinal hemorrhage, if present, is often indicative of infarction. However, many patients with SMV thrombosis experience more vague symptomatic abdominal pain, nausea, distention, or diarrhea over a period of weeks to months (subacute).

DIAGNOSIS

Abdominal-pelvic contrast-enhanced CT, which is the preferred diagnostic test, usually (>90% sensitivity) demonstrates SMV thrombosis with or without portal vein or splenic vein thrombosis. By definition, chronic mesenteric venous thrombosis is asymptomatic and usually detected as an incidental CT finding in patients with portal hypertension, pancreatitis (acute or chronic), or malignancy. The presence of abundant collateral vessels suggests chronic or sometimes subacute mesenteric venous obstruction.

TABLE 145-3 RISK FACTORS FOR MESENTERIC VENOUS THROMBOSIS

Hypercoagulable and hyperviscosity states
Protein S deficiency
Protein C deficiency
Antithrombin III deficiency
Factor V Leiden mutation
Hyperfibrinogenemia
Antiphospholipid syndrome
Primary myeloproliferative syndrome
Sickle cell disease
Estrogen or progesterone
Intra-abdominal infections and inflammation
Appendicitis
Diverticulitis
Crohn's disease
Abscess
Pancreatitis
Cholecystitis
Pyelophlebitis
Neonatal omphalitis
Portal hypertension
Variceal sclerotherapy
Malignancy
Trauma
Vasculitis

Small bowel radiography may demonstrate segmental bowel wall thickening and separation of bowel loops. Selective mesenteric angiography is not generally necessary.

TREATMENT

Therapy for acute-onset cases may include laparotomy with or without bowel resection when infarction is suspected, fluid resuscitation, broad-spectrum antibiotics (similar to those recommended earlier to cover aerobic gram-negative and anaerobic organisms), avoidance of vasoconstrictors, and anticoagulation (e.g., intravenous heparin) in the absence of gastrointestinal bleeding. Selected patients may be candidates for thrombolytic therapy (e.g., streptokinase, urokinase, tissue plasminogen activator), followed by anticoagulation. Underlying conditions such as hypercoagulable states, portal hypertension, intra-abdominal infections, intra-abdominal inflammation, and malignancy require concomitant diagnosis and therapy. The indications for anticoagulation in the chronic setting are uncertain, and it is generally avoided in patients who have portal hypertension but do not have symptoms related to their mesenteric venous thrombosis.

CHRONIC MESENTERIC ISCHEMIA

Chronic atherosclerotic stenosis of the visceral arteries is the cause of most cases of chronic mesenteric ischemia, sometimes called *intestinal angina.*

EPIDEMIOLOGY AND PATHOBIOLOGY

Risk factors for chronic mesenteric ischemia are principally older age and the risk factors for atherosclerosis. Rarely, vasculitis or an aortic aneurysm can be manifested as chronic mesenteric ischemia. Atherosclerotic stenoses usually involve the origins of two or all of the three major visceral arteries supplying the intestine. However, many age-matched patients also harbor atherosclerotic lesions and do not have symptoms of chronic mesenteric ischemia.

CLINICAL MANIFESTATIONS

Patients typically complain of episodic ischemic abdominal pain. The pain is usually upper or midabdominal, typically begins 15 to 30 minutes after a meal, lasts 1 to 3 hours, and progresses in severity over time, as well as occurs after smaller meals and more frequently after meals. Patients may lose weight as a result of fear of eating (sitophobia). Nausea, vomiting, bloating, diarrhea, and constipation can also occur. Malabsorption with steatorrhea, otherwise unexplained gastroduodenal ulcerations, and small bowel biopsy findings of villous atrophy, nonspecific surface cell flattening, and chronic inflammation may be seen in some patients. More than one half of patients have a bruit on abdominal examination. In some patients with episodic symptoms, acute thrombotic mesenteric ischemia develops suddenly.

DIAGNOSIS AND TREATMENT

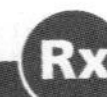

Atherosclerotic lesions usually can be identified by Doppler ultrasound because they are proximal in these vessels and demonstrate increased flow velocity through areas of marked stenosis. MDCTA and MRA are also useful to screen for arterial stenoses consistent with chronic mesenteric ischemia in symptomatic patients, but neither technique is adequately sensitive to exclude the diagnosis of chronic mesenteric ischemia when the pretest probability is high. Thus, selective mesenteric angiography is important to ensure that the anatomic findings are consistent with the diagnosis. Patients must be evaluated thoroughly to exclude other causes of abdominal pain (i.e., gastric cancer, gastroparesis, gastric volvulus, partial small bowel obstruction, small bowel bacterial overgrowth states, pancreatic cancer, biliary disease, paraesophageal hernias). For symptomatic patients with appropriate findings on angiography and no other causes of symptoms, surgical reconstruction provides better long-term outcomes than angioplasty and stenting.

ISCHEMIC COLITIS

EPIDEMIOLOGY AND PATHOBIOLOGY

Ischemic colitis, which is the single most common cause of mesenteric ischemia, accounts for nearly 50% of all cases and for almost 1 in 2000 hospital admissions. Many cases are acute and self-limited and occur in persons older than 60 years without any apparent cause; these cases are probably due to transient nonocclusive hypoperfusion involving a segment of the colon. It is controversial whether subtle hypercoagulable states contribute to the pathogenesis of idiopathic cases. Atherosclerotic or thrombotic occlusion of the IMA or its branches and low-flow states are recognizable causes of ischemic colitis. Less common causes include hypercoagulable states (especially in younger persons), iatrogenic ligation of the IMA (e.g., with aortic surgery), embolism, vasculitis, and any cause of colonic obstruction, including malignancy, stricture, and fecalith, that can produce localized compression of the vasculature with an upstream segment of ischemia. Other unusual associations include long-distance running (dehydration, mechanical trauma to the vasculature, generally involving the cecum), pit viper bite, scuba diving, and intra-abdominal infections or inflammatory disease. A variety of medications, illicit drugs, and chemicals also can result in a chemical picture identical or similar to ischemic colitis (Table 145-4), sometimes probably secondary to vasoconstriction that can affect other parts of the gastrointestinal tract, liver, and other organ systems (e.g., cocaine, amphetamines, pseudoephedrine), sometimes due to constipation (e.g., alosetron), sometimes due to a hypercoagulable effect (e.g., estrogens), and sometimes as a result of a chemical effect (e.g., sodium polystyrene with sorbitol enemas).

CLINICAL MANIFESTATIONS

The clinical presentation of ischemic colitis is acute and, in most patients, includes abdominal pain (mostly left lower quadrant), often with urgency, diarrhea, and passage of bright red blood per rectum. Anorexia, nausea, vomiting, abdominal distention, and passage of maroon material per rectum may also occur. Although the blood loss is not usually enough to require transfusion, some patients may be orthostatic because of loss of blood and fluid. Fever, tachycardia, abdominal tenderness over the affected portion of the colon, and distention may be found on physical examination.

TABLE 145-4 MEDICATIONS AND DRUGS ASSOCIATED WITH ISCHEMIC COLITIS

Digitalis
Vasopressin
Pseudoephedrine
Amphetamines
Cocaine
Ergot
Sumatriptan
Gold
Danazol
Estrogens
Progestins
Alosetron
Psychotropics
Nonsteroidal anti-inflammatory drugs
Various enemas
Tegaserod
Interferon/ribavirin

DIAGNOSIS

Laboratory findings range from normal to nonspecific findings such as leukocytosis and hemoconcentration to those observed in persons with bowel necrosis (see earlier). Evaluation of patients younger than 50 years should include tests for thrombophilic disorders (Chapter 179).

Plain radiographs of the abdomen may reveal "thumbprinting" or may be normal. Similar to small bowel ischemia, CT scanning can be useful to help exclude other disorders, especially in more symptomatic and ill patients; the findings may be consistent with segmental colonic edema and inflammation, with or without adjacent pericolonic inflammatory stranding. These radiographic features are consistent with ischemic colitis in an appropriate clinical setting but are nonspecific and may be seen in patients with other disorders such as acute diverticulitis (Chapter 144), infectious colitis (Chapter 142), and inflammatory bowel disease (Chapter 143). The diagnosis is best made by colonoscopy, which should provide endoscopic and histologic findings consistent with acute ischemic colitis: segmental patchy ulceration, edema, erythema, single stripe sign, and submucosal bluish purple hemorrhagic nodules (Fig. 145-4).

Typically, visceral angiography is not required because most patients with ischemic colitis have self-limited involvement of the left colon or distal transverse colon–splenic flexure with sparing of the rectum, and findings on urgent angiography in these patients are usually normal. However, about 10% of patients with acute ischemic colitis have predominantly right-sided involvement of the cecum, ascending colon, hepatic flexure, and proximal transverse colon. Because the arterial supply to the right colon is through the ileocolic branch of the SMA, there may be concomitant distal ileal ischemia, often owing to low-flow states (especially hemodialysis patients) or embolization. These patients have more pain, less bleeding, and a much worse outcome and are at risk for small bowel necrosis.

Differential Diagnosis

Gastrointestinal infections, such as with *Escherichia coli* O157:H7, *Clostridium difficile, Klebsiella oxytoca,* and cytomegalovirus, can mimic ischemic colitis clinically and even histologically. Acute-onset inflammatory bowel disease involving the colon can also be difficult to distinguish from ischemic colitis. However, patients with subacute or chronic pain, diarrhea, obstructive symptoms, weight loss, or bleeding may be thought to have complicated

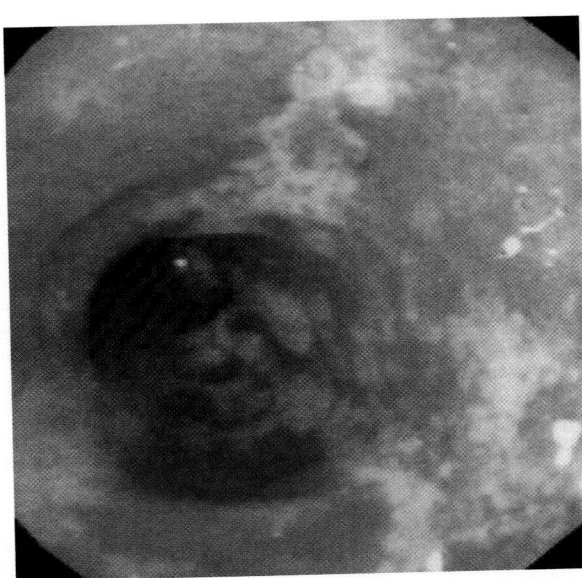

FIGURE 145-4. Endoscopy of the splenic flexure of the colon in a patient with ischemic colitis. Note the shallow, irregular, exudative ulceration with interspersed erythema. (From Emory TS, Carpenter HA, Gostout CJ, et al, eds. *Atlas of Gastrointestinal Endoscopy and Endoscopic Biopsies.* Washington, DC: Armed Forces Institute of Pathology, American Registry of Pathology; 2000.)

diverticular disease, Crohn's disease, or malignancy with stricture, and chronic ischemic stricture of the colon may not be correctly diagnosed until after surgery is performed.

Stool culture can exclude infection, especially with *E. coli* O157:H7, *C. difficile,* and parasites. In immunocompromised patients, colonic biopsy can be performed to diagnose cytomegalovirus infection.

TREATMENT Rx

Patients with right-sided ischemic colitis require visceral angiography not only for diagnosis but also for intra-arterial administration of vasodilators (e.g., papaverine as a 60-mg intravenous bolus followed by an infusion of 30 to 60 mg/hour). Some patients may require urgent surgery. The clinical course in patients with right-sided ischemic colitis may be subacute, with a mortality rate as high as 50% or greater.

By contrast, left-sided acute ischemic colitis, which accounts for most cases, tends to resolve within hours to a few days with supportive therapy, including volume replacement, correction of any low-flow state, broad-spectrum antibiotics (similar to those recommended earlier for patients with small bowel ischemia), avoidance of vasoconstrictive medications, and rarely, blood transfusion; surgery is required only in patients with signs and symptoms of transmural necrosis, perforation, or massive bleeding. Occasional patients with acute-onset left-sided ischemic colitis have persistent or recurrent symptoms of pain, diarrhea, bleeding, sepsis, or stricture formation that develop over a period of weeks to months and may require segmental surgical resection.

VASCULITIS

Many vasculitic syndromes can involve the gastrointestinal tract. Usually, but not always, other organ systems are also involved.

Large and Medium Vessel Vasculitis

Takayasu's arteritis (Chapters 78 and 278) and *giant cell arteritis* (Chapter 279), which affect large to medium-sized muscular arteries, rarely involve the gastrointestinal tract. Takayasu's arteritis has been associated rarely with inflammatory bowel disease.

Medium to Small Vessel Vasculitis

Polyarteritis nodosa (Chapter 278) is characterized by segmental microaneurysms typically involving small and medium-sized arteries. The small bowel is involved more commonly than the large bowel. Many patients will have abdominal pain, fever, hypertension, and multiple organ involvement. Gastrointestinal bleeding or perforation will develop in some patients. The gallbladder, spleen, pancreas, and liver may also be involved. Nearly half of patients with polyarteritis nodosa are infected with hepatitis B virus.

Both *Wegener's granulomatosis* (Chapter 278) and *Churg-Strauss syndrome* (Chapter 278) affect small and medium-sized arteries. Although gastrointestinal involvement is not common in Wegener's granulomatosis with granulomatous inflammation, in up to one third of patients with Churg-Strauss syndrome, abdominal pain or gastrointestinal bleeding may develop as a result of ischemia. Mesenteric venous involvement can also occur with Churg-Strauss syndrome.

Thromboangiitis obliterans (Buerger's disease; Chapter 80) involves small and medium-sized arteries and can cause multiple distal occlusions of the mesenteric arterial circulation. Patients with *Behçet's disease* (Chapter 278) often have lymphocytic inflammation of small and medium-sized arteries, as well as veins. Like Crohn's disease, the ileocecal region is frequently involved with ulceration. Abdominal pain, diarrhea, gastrointestinal bleeding, and perforation may occur.

Small Vessel Vasculitis

Small vessel involvement with immunoglobulin A immune complex deposition in blood vessel walls is typical in *Henoch-Schönlein purpura* (Chapter 278). These patients usually have palpable purpura, arthritis, and abdominal pain, as well as gastrointestinal bleeding. *Hypersensitivity vasculitis* (Chapter 278), which affects small arterioles, venules, and capillaries, is related to a variety of drugs, infections, and chemicals; on occasion there may be gastrointestinal involvement. *Cryoglobulinemia* (Chapter 193) with immune complex involvement of small blood vessels can sometimes involve the gastrointestinal tract. These patients are often infected with hepatitis C virus.

HEMORRHAGIC VASCULAR DISORDERS

Angiodysplasia

DEFINITION AND EPIDEMIOLOGY

Angiodysplasia or vascular ectasia is a thin-walled, dilated, punctate red vascular structure in the mucosa or submucosa of the bowel; it typically involves adjacent venules, capillaries, and arterioles. Angiodysplasia is found in the colon, especially the right colon, in up to 1% of persons and is found also in the stomach and small bowel but rarely in the esophagus. Angiodysplastic lesions may be single or multiple, and they increase in frequency with age. Some data suggest associations with chronic renal failure (Chapter 132), von Willebrand's disease (Chapter 176), and aortic stenosis (Chapter 75); whether correction of these associated disorders diminishes future gastrointestinal hemorrhage (Chapter 137) from angiodysplasia is uncertain.

CLINICAL MANIFESTATIONS

Clinically, these lesions can produce painless bleeding, which may be occult and manifest only by guaiac-positive stools or iron deficiency anemia, or the bleeding may be overt, with hematochezia, maroon stools, melena, and hematemesis.

DIAGNOSIS

Endoscopic procedures most often make the diagnosis of bleeding secondary to angiodysplasia (Fig. 145-5). In some patients, endoscopic procedures may need to be repeated, especially in volume-depleted patients and after the administration of narcotics. Small bowel angiodysplasia, beyond the reach of both a colonoscope from below and an extended-length endoscope from above, may be the cause of major bleeding (Chapter 137) and require video capsule endoscopy (Chapter 136) or small bowel enteroscopy for diagnosis.

TREATMENT Rx

Electrocoagulation laser therapy or argon plasma coagulation can be accomplished during endoscopy. When very active bleeding makes urgent colonoscopy technically difficult, visceral angiography can be diagnostic and also permit embolization of bleeding lesions or intra-arterial infusion of a vasoconstrictor. Rarely, bowel resection is required.

PROGNOSIS

More than 90% of gastrointestinal angiodysplasias never bleed. If found incidentally in patients without a history of bleeding, they should not be treated.

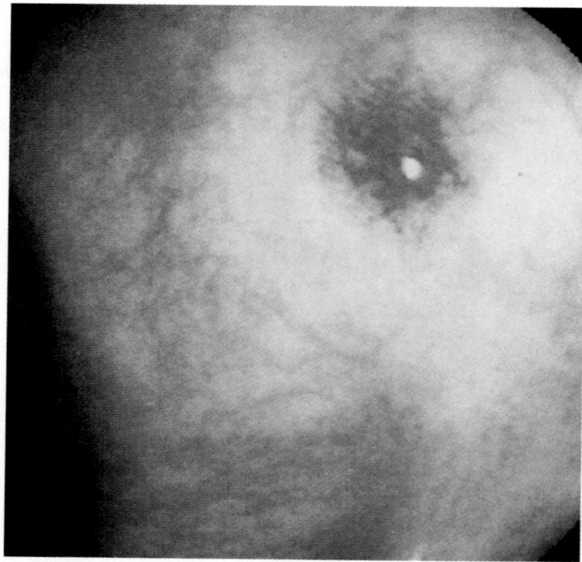

FIGURE 145-5. Endoscopy of the sigmoid colon in a patient with angiectasia. The lesion is discrete and contains a tight, radiating cluster of ectatic mucosal vessels. (From Emory TS, Carpenter HA, Gostout CJ, et al, eds. *Atlas of Gastrointestinal Endoscopy and Endoscopic Biopsies*. Washington, DC: Armed Forces Institute of Pathology, American Registry of Pathology; 2000.)

Dieulafoy's Lesion

Dieulafoy's lesion is an unusually large submucosal artery typically found in the proximal portion of the stomach within 6 cm of the gastroesophageal junction. Similar lesions may also occur in the rectum, colon, small bowel, and far less often, the esophagus. Dieulafoy's lesion is manifested clinically as sudden, massive bleeding, which may be recurrent.

DIAGNOSIS AND TREATMENT (Rx)

Urgent endoscopy is required to identify what is usually a very small vascular protuberance (Fig. 145-6) but can rapidly become inapparent once the acute bleeding stops. Ulceration is not seen, and repeat endoscopic procedures during active bleeding may be required to make the diagnosis. Sometimes the diagnosis requires angiography during a bleeding episode. Endoscopic injection and electrocoagulation therapy are generally effective, but endoscopic band therapy and hemoclips may also be used, and surgery is sometimes required.

PROGNOSIS

Endoscopic therapy is successful long-term in nearly 90% of patients.

Other Ectasias

Telangiectases are similar to angiodysplasias but occur in all the layers of the bowel wall, are usually congenital, and often occur in other organ systems. *Hereditary hemorrhagic telangiectasia* (Osler-Weber-Rendu disease; Chapter 176) is an autosomal dominant disorder with telangiectases involving the lips; mucous membranes, especially in the mouth and nose; gastrointestinal tract, especially the stomach and small bowel; liver; lung; retina; and central nervous system. Patients with *Turner's syndrome* (Chapter 243), *scleroderma* (Chapter 275), and the *CREST syndrome* (Chapter 275) (calcinosis, Raynaud's phenomenon, esophageal dysmotility, sclerodactyly, telangiectasia) may also have gastrointestinal tract telangiectases.

Vascular ectasias involving venules and capillaries can also be seen in the small bowel *(congestive enteropathy),* in the colon *(congestive colopathy),* and more commonly, in the stomach *(congestive gastropathy)* in patients with portal hypertension (Chapter 156). In contrast to angiodysplasias, these lesions tend to be more diffuse, appear as multiple, fine punctate red spots or as a mosaic pattern similar to the gastritis of *Helicobacter pylori,* and are more often found in the proximal than the distal part of the stomach. Therapies that decrease portal hypertension can reduce or eliminate these lesions and bleeding from them.

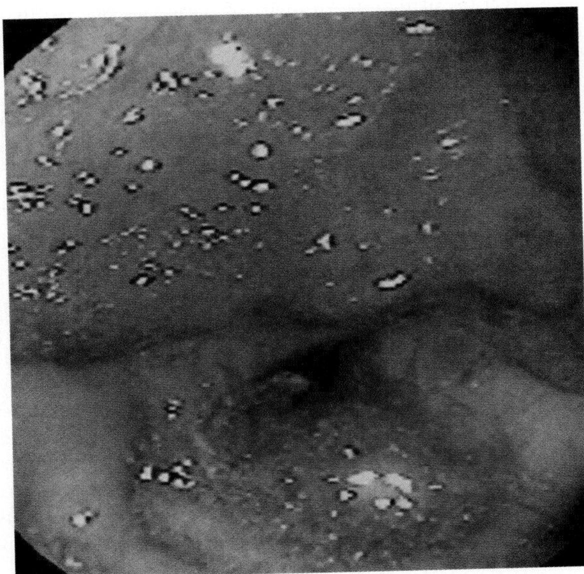

FIGURE 145-6. Endoscopy of the stomach in a patient with Dieulafoy's lesion. Note the visible vessel manifested as a pale protuberance surrounded by a clot with adjacent normal-appearing mucosa. (From Emory TS, Carpenter HA, Gostout CJ, et al, eds. *Atlas of Gastrointestinal Endoscopy and Endoscopic Biopsies*. Washington, DC: Armed Forces Institute of Pathology, American Registry of Pathology; 2000.)

Gastric antral vascular ectasia (GAVE), or watermelon stomach, also involves venules and capillaries with thrombosis as well as ectasia. Erythematous streaks similar to the stripes on a watermelon are typically seen in the antrum radiating toward the pylorus. Patients usually have occult bleeding and less often melena. GAVE is associated with connective tissue diseases (e.g., systemic lupus erythematosus [Chapter 274], mixed connective tissue disease [Chapter 275], scleroderma [Chapter 275]), pernicious anemia (Chapter 167), and portal hypertension (Chapter 156). However, unlike congestive gastropathy, treatment of portal hypertension does not eliminate GAVE or bleeding from it. Argon plasma coagulation is the usual therapy if iron replacement alone is not effective. Antrectomy is rarely needed.

Neoplastic Vascular Lesions

Hemangiomas are uncommon, usually benign vascular tumors that can be found throughout the gastrointestinal tract, often in the rectum or colon. They may be single or multiple, bluish purple, and sessile or polypoid. In some persons, these lesions are multiple and associated with skin lesions, such as the *blue rubber bleb nevus syndrome* with purple-blue cutaneous hemangiomas or the *Klippel-Trenaunay* syndrome with port-wine-colored cutaneous hemangiomas, hemihypertrophy, and varicose veins. Rare vascular malignant neoplasms of the gastrointestinal tract include *angiosarcomas* and *hemangioendotheliomas.*

Miscellaneous Vascular Disorders

Aortoenteric fistulas, which most commonly occur after surgery for an aortic aneurysm (Chapter 78), may be related to infection of the graft and can result in torrential gastrointestinal bleeding. Many of these fistulas communicate with the duodenum. Evaluation of bleeding in persons who have previously undergone abdominal aortic surgery should include urgent extended-length upper endoscopy to document a fistula or diagnose another definitive source of the bleeding. Angiography and radiographic tests (CT, magnetic resonance imaging [MRI]) are helpful only if the findings are abnormal (i.e., there is evidence of a fistula) because of their poor sensitivity for the presence of aortoenteric fistulas. If no clear alternative source for the bleeding can readily be found, explorative surgery is indicated.

Celiac artery compression syndrome (median arcuate ligament syndrome) is a very rare pseudo-ischemic syndrome. Patients are often young and healthy and have postprandial upper abdominal pain, most likely caused by extrinsic compression of the celiac axis by the median arcuate ligament of the diaphragm. Sitophobia can result in considerable weight loss, and there may be a loud systolic bruit in the epigastric region on physical examination. Visceral angiography supports the diagnosis, but bruits and celiac axis compression may occur without symptoms. Surgical therapy is indicated after other possible causes of the patient's symptoms have been excluded.

Bowel as well as large vessel rupture can occur as a complication of *Ehlers-Danlos syndrome type IV* (Chapter 268). Similar vascular catastrophes with gastrointestinal or intraperitoneal hemorrhage can occur in patients with *pseudoxanthoma elasticum type I* (Chapter 268) or with *visceral artery aneurysms* (secondary to atherosclerosis, fibrodysplasia, portal hypertension, pregnancy, pancreatitis, vasculitis, or trauma).

HEPATIC AND SPLENIC VASCULAR DISEASE

Budd-Chiari Syndrome

Budd-Chiari syndrome can occur as a result of any process that interferes with the normal flow of blood out of the liver, including constrictive pericarditis (Chapter 77) and veno-occlusive disease (Chapter 152). Hepatic vein thrombosis, which is the main cause of Budd-Chiari syndrome, may involve one, two, or all three of the major hepatic veins, with or without partial or complete occlusion of the inferior vena cava. Often, Budd-Chiari syndrome is due to a hypercoagulable state (Chapter 179), such as a chronic myeloproliferative disorder (e.g., polycythemia vera [Chapter 169], essential thrombocythemia [Chapter 169], myeloid metaplasia [Chapter 169]), paroxysmal nocturnal hemoglobinuria, or other hypercoagulable conditions (Chapter 179), such as factor V (Leiden) gene mutation, antiphospholipid antibody syndrome, protein C deficiency, protein S deficiency, or antithrombin III deficiency. A high percentage of these patients harbor *JAK2* V617F mutations. Nearly 50% of patients with Budd-Chiari syndrome have more than one risk factor. Malignancies (direct compression or invasion of hepatic veins, hypercoagulable state), infections (liver abscess), pregnancy, inflammatory disorders (e.g., Behçet's syndrome, inflammatory bowel disease, connective tissue disease, sarcoidosis), and membranous

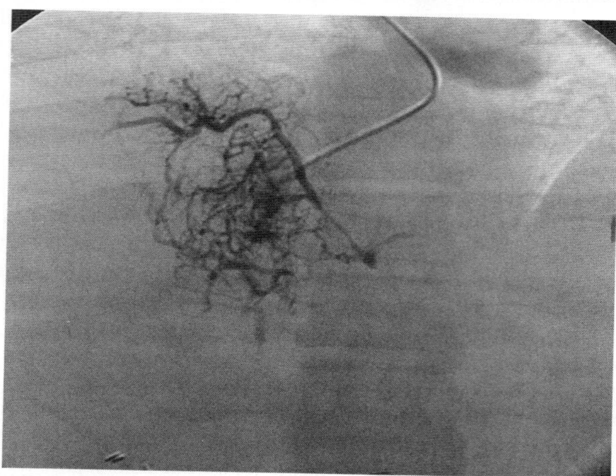

FIGURE 145-7. Budd-Chiari syndrome. A hepatic vein contrast study depicts the "spider web" pattern of venovenous collaterals attempting to bypass a thrombosed hepatic vein. (Courtesy of Patrick Kamath.)

obstruction (webs) of the inferior vena cava are also associated with Budd-Chiari syndrome.

CLINICAL MANIFESTATIONS

The syndrome is usually subacute or chronic, occurs over a period of weeks to months, and is characterized by the insidious onset of upper abdominal pain, hepatomegaly, and ascites. Fulminant or acute presentations, including encephalopathy, jaundice, ascites, and liver failure, are rare.

DIAGNOSIS

Liver function testing usually reveals normal or mild to moderate nonspecific elevations in serum aspartate and alanine aminotransferase levels. Doppler ultrasound of the liver is the initial diagnostic test of choice, but the absence of hepatic venous flow or venous thrombosis (or both) is also readily apparent with contrast-enhanced CT scanning or MRA. Hepatic venography can confirm the diagnosis (Fig. 145-7) and, with imaging of the inferior vena cava, as well as selective venous pressure measurements, can help guide therapy.

TREATMENT

Rx

Therapy includes diagnosis and treatment of underlying conditions, anticoagulation (intravenous heparin; see Table 81-4 in Chapter 81) to prevent the propagation of thrombi, and treatment of the ascites (e.g., diuretics; Chapter 156). To decompress the congested liver, most patients require interventional radiologic procedures, such as angioplasty, stenting, or transjugular intrahepatic portosystemic shunts, to restore hepatic venous flow. Surgical procedures such as surgical shunts to drain the portal or mesenteric venous system into the inferior vena cava can also decompress the liver. Liver transplantation (Chapter 157) should be considered for patients with fulminant liver failure or cirrhosis, or both. Most patients with Budd-Chiari syndrome require lifelong warfarin anticoagulation (Chapter 37), even after liver transplantation. Selective JAK2 inhibitors (Chapter 169) are being tested in preclinical and clinical studies.

PROGNOSIS

Overall, the 5-year survival rate of patients with the Budd-Chiari syndrome is more than 80%. Indices such as levels of serum albumin and bilirubin, the international normalized ratio, ascites, and encephalopathy, as well as the Child-Pugh score (see Table 156-2 in Chapter 156), can be useful in determining prognosis.

Portal Vein Thrombosis

In adults, cirrhosis, hypercoagulable states, intra-abdominal malignancy, inflammatory disorders (e.g., pancreatitis, Crohn's disease), and medical procedures (e.g., splenectomy, cholecystectomy, gastrectomy, liver transplantation, transjugular intrahepatic portosystemic shunt) are most often the cause of acute portal vein thrombosis. Similar to Budd-Chiari syndrome, a substantial number of these patients harbor JAK2 V617F mutations.

CLINICAL MANIFESTATIONS AND DIAGNOSIS

Clinical manifestations include portal hypertension with variceal bleeding and ascites. Abdominal pain and diarrhea may indicate extension of the thrombus into the SMV with intestinal ischemia. The diagnosis of acute portal vein thrombosis is confirmed by Doppler ultrasound, MDCTA, or MRA. CT imaging may reveal multiple small liver abscesses.

TREATMENT

Rx

Anticoagulation (see Table 81-4 in Chapter 81) therapy for at least 3 months is recommended for patients with acute portal vein thrombosis and should be continued long term in those persons with permanent thrombotic risk factors not otherwise correctable, as well as in patients with extension of thrombus into the mesenteric veins.

High fever, chills, a tender liver, and sepsis suggest pylephlebitis, which usually requires treatment with parenteral antibiotics such as piperacillin/tazobactam, ticarcillin/clavulanate, carbapenem, or a third-generation cephalosporin plus metronidazole for at least 6 weeks. Blood cultures can help to guide the choice and course of antibiotics, which should be administered intravenously for at least 2 weeks.

Treatment is less clear in cirrhotic patients with acute or chronic portal vein thrombosis. Endoscopy for the diagnosis and treatment of varices (Chapter 136), with or without pharmacologic treatment of the portal hypertension (e.g., β-blockade with propranolol; Chapter 156), is often beneficial, and surgical shunts are rarely necessary. Antibiotics, such as those recommended previously for pylephlebitis, should be administered in patients with any sign of infection.

Chronic portal vein thrombosis is defined as an obstructed portal vein replaced by collateral veins. Doppler ultrasound, MDCTA, or MRA will confirm the diagnosis. Patients may be asymptomatic but often have hypersplenism and portal hypertension (e.g., subclinical encephalopathy, rare ascites). Some patients may develop jaundice owing to biliary cholangiopathy and will require endoscopic placement of biliary stents. Endoscopic screening and treatment of varices (Chapter 136), with or without pharmacologic treatment of portal hypertension (Chapter 156), is recommended. After treatment of the varices, long-term anticoagulation therapy (see Table 81-4 in Chapter 81) should be considered in noncirrhotic patients whose permanent thrombotic risk factors are not otherwise correctable, unless there is a contraindication.

PROGNOSIS

Mortality rates after treatment of acute portal vein thrombosis are less than 10%, and the prognosis for patients with chronic portal vein thrombosis over 5 years is similar.

Splenic Vein Thrombosis

Splenic vein thrombosis is usually secondary to malignancy (e.g., pancreatic cancer), pancreatitis, or trauma. In many of these patients, isolated gastric varices develop and are difficult to treat by therapeutic endoscopy. Liver function and portal pressure are normal. Most patients with splenic vein thrombosis have splenomegaly (Chapter 171). Doppler ultrasound, MRI, and CT assist in making the diagnosis. Patients with symptomatic isolated splenic vein thrombosis (e.g., gastric variceal bleeding, hypersplenism) are best treated by splenectomy.

Hepatic and Splenic Arterial Disease

Hepatic arterial disease may be nonocclusive or occlusive. Nonocclusive disease, termed *ischemic hepatitis,* occurs when arterial blood flow to the liver is insufficient, usually because of cardiogenic hypotension, volume depletion, or sepsis. Typically, serum aminotransferase rises acutely to levels greater than 1000 U/L. With restoration of adequate hepatic arterial blood flow, serum aminotransferase levels eventually fall back to their baseline by about 40 to 60% per day. Hepatic artery thrombosis is extremely rare except in a post–liver transplantation (Chapter 157) patient, in whom it may be manifested as mild abnormalities in liver function test results, bile duct injury (e.g., biliary stricture, cholangitis, liver abscess), or liver failure. Doppler ultrasound and angiography will confirm the diagnosis, and these patients often require biliary stents, drainage of abscesses, surgical reconstruction of the hepatic artery, or retransplantation of the liver.

The splenic artery or hepatic artery may be predisposed to the development of aneurysmal dilation, usually secondary to atherosclerosis, trauma, portal hypertension, pancreatitis, pregnancy, infection, or vasculitis. Common clinical manifestations include abdominal pain and intra-abdominal hemorrhage. Hemobilia may occur with hepatic artery aneurysms.

Angiography is usually required to make the diagnosis. Symptomatic as well as sizable (variably defined, usually 1 cm or greater for a hepatic aneurysm and 2 cm or greater for a splenic artery aneurysm) aneurysms require surgery. Splenic artery aneurysms discovered during pregnancy are more likely to bleed and should be treated, usually by interventional radiology.

Fistulas from the hepatic artery to the portal vein can occur as a result of trauma, malignancy, or the inherited disorder hereditary hemorrhagic telangiectasia. The resultant portal hypertension may cause abdominal pain, ascites, and gastrointestinal bleeding, and involvement of the hepatic artery may result in biliary strictures and hepatobiliary infection. Radiographic embolization of these fistulas, surgery, or liver transplantation may be required.

SUGGESTED READINGS

Arthurs ZM, Titus J, Bannazadeh M, et al. A comparison of endovascular revascularization with traditional therapy for the treatment of acute mesenteric ischemia. *J Vasc Surg*. 2011;53:687-704. *Endovascular treatment was successful in 87% of patients with thrombotic or embolic arterial occlusions.*

DeLeve LD, Valla DC, Garcia-Tsao G. AASLD practice guidelines: vascular disorders of the liver. *Hepatology*. 2009;47:1729-1764. *Data-supported recommendations for diagnosis and treatment of vascular diseases of the liver.*

Feuerstadt P, Brandt LJ. Colon ischemia: recent insights and advances. *Curr Gastroenterol Rep*. 2010;12:383-390. *Review emphasizing that most patients respond to supportive therapy.*

Reissfelder C, Sweiti H, Antolovic D, et al. Ischemic colitis: who will survive? *Surgery*. 2011;149:585-592. *Nonocclusive ischemic colitis, acute renal failure, extent of bowel ischemia, serum lactate, and duration of catecholamine therapy predict survival.*

146

PANCREATITIS

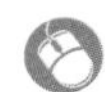

CHRIS E. FORSMARK

TABLE 146-1 CAUSES OF ACUTE PANCREATITIS

ETIOLOGY	EXAMPLES
Gallstones	Gallstones Microlithiasis
Drugs and toxins	Ethyl and methyl alcohol Tobacco Azathioprine, 6-mercaptopurine, pentamidine, didanosine, sulfonamides, thiazides, aminosalicylates, valproic acid, and others Scorpion venom Insecticides
Metabolic	Hyperlipidemia Hypercalcemia
Trauma	After endoscopic retrograde cholangiopancreatography Blunt or penetrating trauma Postoperative
Obstruction of the pancreatic duct	Benign pancreatic duct stricture Benign ampullary stricture (e.g., celiac disease, diverticulum) Ampullary adenoma or adenocarcinoma Pancreatic ductal adenocarcinoma Intraductal papillary mucinous neoplasm Pancreas divisum Sphincter of Oddi dysfunction
Infections	Cytomegalovirus, mumps, rubella, coxsackie B virus *Candida*, histoplasmosis *Ascaris*
Genetics	*PRSS1* mutations *CFTR* mutation *SPINK1* mutation
Autoimmune pancreatitis	
Idiopathic pancreatitis	

ACUTE PANCREATITIS

DEFINITION

Acute pancreatitis is defined as a discrete episode of cellular injury and inflammation in the pancreas, usually with symptoms of abdominal pain, nausea, and vomiting, and typically accompanied by elevations in serum levels of amylase or lipase and by radiographic evidence of pancreatic inflammation, edema, or necrosis. Although pancreatic morphology and function may appear to recover promptly after the attack, recovery may not be complete if the damage is substantial. With repeated episodes, there is a shift from acute inflammation, necrosis, and apoptosis to the chronic inflammation and fibrosis that is characteristic of chronic pancreatitis. In some patients, it may be difficult to distinguish acute pancreatitis from a flare of chronic pancreatitis.

EPIDEMIOLOGY

The incidence of acute pancreatitis in the United States is estimated to be between 5 and 30 cases per 100,000 population, thereby resulting in about 250,000 hospital admissions annually and making acute pancreatitis the second most common gastrointestinal discharge diagnosis in U.S. hospitals. The cost of caring for these patients is about $4 to $6 billion annually. The incidence of acute pancreatitis is increasing in the United States and many other developed countries, perhaps because of better diagnostic tests but also perhaps owing to an increasing prevalence of gallstones (Chapter 158) in the setting of the obesity epidemic.

PATHOBIOLOGY

Acute pancreatitis is characterized by premature activation of digestive enzymes within the pancreas. In particular, the activation of trypsinogen to trypsin appears to be a critical initial step, with trypsin then activating other proteases within the gland. These activated enzymes produce cellular injury and death, which is a mixture of necrosis, apoptosis, and autophagy. Necrosis may involve not only the pancreas but also the surrounding fat and structures, thereby leading to fluid extravasation into the retroperitoneal spaces ("third space" losses). Although necrosis may be present in many cases, necrosis visible on a contrast-enhanced computed tomography (CT) scan is usually termed *acute necrotizing pancreatitis* and distinguished from the milder interstitial pancreatitis, in which necrosis is not visible on a CT scan. In addition to the local damage, the release of proinflammatory cytokines and activated digestive enzymes into the systemic circulation can produce a systemic inflammatory response syndrome (SIRS; Chapter 108) with hypotension, renal failure, and respiratory failure. Gallstones and alcohol account for about 70 to 80% of all cases of acute pancreatitis, but the cause is unknown in about 10% (Table 146-1).

Gallstones

Passage of a gallstone (Chapter 158) through the ampulla of Vater with transient obstruction of the pancreatic duct is the initiating event for gallstone pancreatitis. Only about 5% of all patients with gallstones develop pancreatitis, and patients with smaller gallstones (≤5 mm), which can pass the cystic duct and reach the ampulla, are at highest risk. Patients with microlithiasis, defined as tiny gallstones or biliary sludge, may account for up to 75% of patients initially labeled as having acute idiopathic pancreatitis.

Alcohol

More than 5 years of alcohol intake averaging more than 5 to 8 drinks daily is usually required before pancreatitis develops, but most people with this level of intake do not develop pancreatitis. A variety of cofactors have been proposed, including a high-fat diet, genetic variability in detoxifying enzymes, and cigarette smoking. By the time patients present with a first episode of acute pancreatitis, most already have evidence of underlying chronic pancreatitis. The mechanism of alcoholic pancreatic injury likely involves a mixture of direct toxicity, oxidative stress, and alterations in pancreatic enzyme secretion.

Drugs, Toxins, and Metabolic Factors

Drug-induced pancreatitis is a rare and generally idiosyncratic event. Implicated drugs include 6-mercaptopurine and azathioprine (up to a 4% attack rate), didanosine, pentamidine, valproic acid, furosemide, sulfonamides, and aminosalicylates. Toxins that may cause acute pancreatitis include methyl alcohol, organophosphate insecticides, and venom from certain scorpions.

Levels of serum triglycerides above 500 mg/dL, and usually more than 1000 mg/dL, can cause acute pancreatitis, but the mechanism is not known. Hyperlipidemic pancreatitis can be caused by the administration of estrogens, which can worsen underlying hypertriglyceridemia. Hypercalcemia is an exceedingly rare cause of acute pancreatitis.

Trauma

Iatrogenic trauma to the pancreas and pancreatic duct during performance of an endoscopic retrograde cholangiopancreatography (ERCP; Chapter 136) is a common cause of pancreatitis, with the risk ranging from less than 5% for those with simple common bile duct stones or malignancy, to as high as 20% for those with suspected sphincter of Oddi dysfunction. The risk of post-ERCP pancreatitis is markedly reduced with the placement of small-caliber temporary pancreatic duct stents.

Penetrating and blunt trauma ranging from a contusion to severe crush injury and even transection of the gland can cause pancreatitis. Acute presentation is the rule, but some patients with milder injury may present in a subacute or chronic fashion. Ischemic injury to the gland can occur after surgical procedures, especially cardiopulmonary bypass, and can be quite severe.

Obstruction of the Pancreatic Duct

In addition to gallstones and microlithiasis, obstruction of the pancreatic duct by a pancreatic ductal adenocarcinoma, ampullary adenoma or carcinoma, or an intraductal papillary mucinous neoplasm can cause acute pancreatitis. The diagnosis is usually established with endoscopic ultrasound (EUS). Benign strictures of the pancreatic duct or ampulla of Vater may be caused by celiac disease and periampullary diverticula. Sphincter of Oddi dysfunction, which is defined by abnormal manometry of the sphincter at the time of ERCP, and pancreas divisum, in which the larger dorsal pancreas drains through the smaller minor papilla, may also cause pancreatitis by obstruction of the pancreatic duct and should be considered in patients with repeated episodes of otherwise unexplained acute pancreatitis.

Infections and Autoimmune Pancreatitis

Ascaris lumbricoides (Chapter 365) may cause pancreatitis by obstructing the pancreatic duct as the worms migrate through the ampulla. Viruses that may infect the pancreatic acinar cells directly include cytomegalovirus (Chapter 384), Coxsackie B virus (Chapter 387), and mumps virus (Chapter 377). Fungal infections of the pancreas are exceedingly rare but may be seen in the setting of immunosuppression. Autoimmune pancreatitis, which can be systemic, affects the salivary glands, retroperitoneum, biliary ducts, and kidneys.

Genetics

Mutations in the cationic trypsinogen gene (*PRSS1*), which have been identified in families with hereditary pancreatitis, are more commonly seen in association with chronic pancreatitis but can be observed rarely in acute pancreatitis. Mutations in the cystic fibrosis conductance regulator (*CFTR*; Chapter 89) and the serine protease inhibitor Kazal type 1 (*SPINK1*) predispose to pancreatitis but do not cause pancreatitis in the absence of other provocations.

Idiopathic Acute Pancreatitis

Of the 25% of patients who do not have an identified cause after a basic initial evaluation, surreptitious alcohol use and microlithiasis are probably the most common underlying explanations. With additional evaluation and testing, only about 10% of patients are ultimately labeled as having idiopathic pancreatitis.

CLINICAL MANIFESTATIONS

Abdominal pain, nausea, and vomiting are the hallmark symptoms of acute pancreatitis. The abdominal pain is usually maximum in the epigastric region and often radiates to the back. The pain is steady, reaches its maximal intensity over 30 to 60 minutes, and persists for days. These characteristic symptoms may be masked in patients who present with delirium, multiple-organ system failure, or coma.

The physical examination usually reveals tachycardia. Hypotension, tachypnea, dyspnea, and fever are seen in more severe cases. Confusion, delirium, and even coma may be present. The abdomen is often distended with diminished bowel sounds. Tenderness to palpation of the abdomen, which may be epigastric or more diffuse, is typical, and rebound and guarding are seen in more severe cases. Dullness to percussion in the lower lung fields may be noted owing to a pleural effusion. Rare physical findings include ecchymoses of the flank (Grey-Turner sign) or umbilicus (Cullen sign), which occur when fluid and blood tracks into these spaces from the retroperitoneum. Jaundice may be present if there is biliary obstruction by a stone.

The presence of tachycardia, dyspnea, tachypnea, orthostatic hypotension, pleural effusion, oxygen desaturation, or shock signal more substantial third space losses, a higher likelihood of a variety of complications (Table 146-2), and a worse prognosis. More severe pancreatitis is characterized by more substantial pancreatic and peripancreatic necrosis, more peripancreatic fluid collections, and more dysfunction of extrapancreatic organs.

TABLE 146-2 SCORING SYSTEMS TO ASSESS SEVERITY OF ACUTE PANCREATITIS

SYSTEM	CRITERIA	DEFINITION OF SEVERE PANCREATITIS
Ranson	At admission Age > 55 years WBC > 16,000/μL Glucose > 200 mg/dL LDH > 350 IU/L AST > 250 IU/L Within next 48 hours Decrease in hematocrit by > 10% Estimated fluid sequestration of > 6 L Serum calcium < 8.0 mg/dL Pao_2 < 60 mm Hg BUN increase > 5 mg/dL after hydration Base deficit > 4 mmol/L	Total score ≥ 3
APACHE-II	Multiple clinical and laboratory factors. Calculator available at *www.mdcalc.com/apache-ii-score-for-icu-mortality*	Total score ≥ 8
BISAP	BUN > 25 mg/dL Impaired mental status Presence of SIRS Age > 60 years Pleural effusion	Total score > 2
CT	A: Normal pancreas B: Focal or diffuse enlargement of pancreas C: Grade B plus pancreatic and/or peripancreatic inflammation D: Grade C plus a single fluid collection E: Grade C plus two or more fluid collections or gas in pancreas	Grade > C
CT severity index	CT grade A = 0 B = 1 C = 2 D = 3 E = 4 Plus necrosis grade No necrosis = 0 <30% necrosis = 2 30-50% necrosis = 4 >50% necrosis = 6	Score > 5

AST = aspartate aminotransferase; BUN = blood urea nitrogen; CT = computed tomography; LDH = lactate dehydrogenase; SIRS = systemic inflammatory response syndrome; WBC = white blood count.

DIAGNOSIS

The diagnosis of acute pancreatitis is suggested by the clinical features and confirmed by laboratory and imaging studies that exclude other serious intra-abdominal conditions, establish the presence of acute pancreatitis, and, hopefully, define the severity and most likely cause of the pancreatitis.

Laboratory Tests

Amylase and Lipase

Most patients with acute pancreatitis have elevations in serum levels of amylase or lipase within a few hours of the onset of symptoms. Lipase tends to remain elevated for longer than amylase, but both decline gradually over several days. Elevations more than three times the upper limit of normal are most specific for acute pancreatitis. Amylase and lipase levels may be normal in patients with acute pancreatitis, particularly if the measurement is delayed for several days after the onset of symptoms. Marked hypertriglyceridemia also can interfere with their accurate measurement. Both enzymes are cleared by the kidney, and renal failure can falsely raise the level of these enzymes up to five times the upper limit of normal in the absence of pancreatitis. Amylase and lipase also can be elevated in a variety of other conditions that may mimic acute pancreatitis, including intestinal ischemia and infarction (Chapter 145), bowel obstruction (Chapter 144), cholecystitis (Chapter 158), and choledocholithiasis (Chapter 158). In addition, amylase may be elevated from ectopic pregnancy, acute salpingitis, and a variety of extra-abdominal conditions such as parotitis, lung cancer, and head trauma. In some patients, only amylase or lipase may be elevated. Given its improved specificity, equal cost, and equal sensitivity, lipase is preferred over amylase as a single diagnostic test. Serial measurements of amylase or lipase in patients with established acute pancreatitis are not helpful in clinical decision making.

Other Laboratory Tests

In severe pancreatitis, leukocytosis and hemoconcentration may be seen. Failure of the blood urea nitrogen (BUN) level or hematocrit to normalize with fluid resuscitation is associated with a worse prognosis. Hyperglycemia, hypocalcemia, and mild hypertriglyceridemia can develop in more severe cases. Elevations in alanine aminotransferase levels more than three times the upper limit of normal are most suggestive of gallstones, although any significant elevation in liver chemistries should raise the possibility of gallstones (Chapter 158).

Imaging Studies

Imaging studies are used not only in establishing the diagnosis but also in determining etiology and prognosis. In most patients, both ultrasound and CT are used in a complementary fashion.

Abdominal ultrasound can confirm the presence of acute pancreatitis by documenting pancreatic enlargement, edema, or associated peripancreatic fluid collections. Visualization of the pancreas may be limited owing to body habitus or overlying intestinal gas. Importantly, ultrasound is most accurate in identifying gallstones in the gallbladder or a dilated common bile duct.

CT is more accurate than ultrasound in confirming the diagnosis of acute pancreatitis and in documenting the presence of pancreatic necrosis and peripancreatic fluid collections, but it is less accurate in identifying gallstones. CT is also particularly helpful in excluding intra-abdominal conditions that can mimic acute pancreatitis. On contrast-enhanced CT, pancreatic parenchyma that opacifies with intravenous contrast is considered still viable, whereas parenchyma that does not opacify is necrotic (Fig. 146-1). The extent of pancreatic necrosis, which is best seen about 3 days after presentation and may be missed in an early CT, has prognostic importance. CT scans are not routinely required in patients with acute pancreatitis but should be performed in patients with a first attack, with severe disease, with systemic complications, or when disease is slow to improve or the diagnosis is not clear.

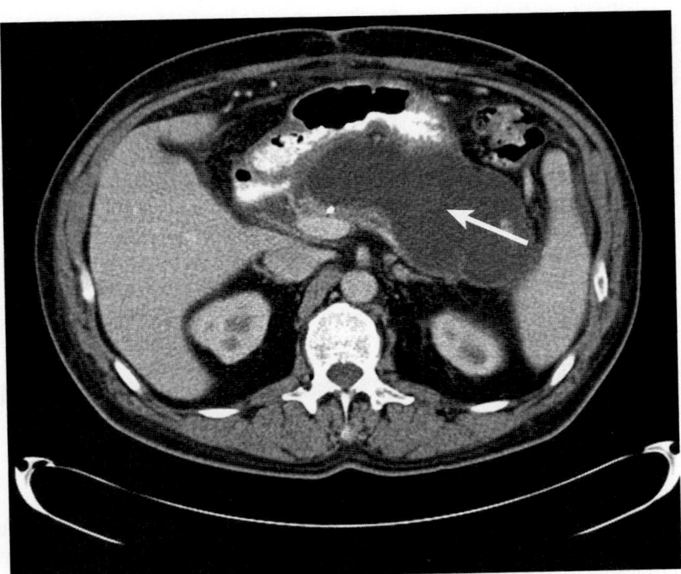

FIGURE 146-1. A computed tomographic scan demonstrating a large area of pancreas that does not enhance with intravenous contrast *(arrow)*, consistent with pancreatic necrosis.

Magnetic resonance imaging (MRI) is equivalent to CT in its ability to document acute pancreatitis, identify necrosis, and diagnose or exclude other diseases that could mimic acute pancreatitis. In addition, MRI with *magnetic resonance cholangiopancreatography* (MRCP) is much better than CT in identifying gallstones. MRI is more difficult than CT to perform in critically ill patients.

ERCP and EUS are important in both diagnosis and therapy of acute pancreatitis. EUS, which is primarily used to establish the cause when the initial evaluation is unrevealing, is particularly accurate in identifying underlying malignancy, premalignant lesions such as ampullary adenoma, and small gallstones or microlithiasis. ERCP is used primarily for therapeutic reasons, but it also may diagnose rare causes of pancreatitis such as pancreas divisum or sphincter of Oddi dysfunction.

Determining Etiology

To identify the cause of acute pancreatitis, the history should focus on alcohol and tobacco use, previous biliary colic, drug history, family history, and recent trauma. Alcohol use may need to be corroborated with family members. Gallstone pancreatitis should be suspected if stones are seen on imaging studies or if liver chemistries are abnormal and then improve over a few days. If these initial studies are unrevealing, EUS can detect small gallstones, microlithiasis, or underlying malignancy, particularly in patients older than 40 years. More specialized investigations like ERCP, sphincter of Oddi manometry, or genetic testing are usually reserved for patients seen in referral centers after multiple attacks of pancreatitis.

Determining Severity

Severe pancreatitis is characterized by organ system failure and by local pancreatic complications such as necrosis, fluid collections, or pseudocysts. Organ failure can be single or multiple, early or late onset, and progressive and persistent or transient. In severe acute pancreatitis, renal failure, pulmonary failure, and circulatory failure most commonly occur as part of the SIRS response. Severe pancreatitis also can be defined by local pancreatic and peripancreatic complications. Necrotizing pancreatitis as defined by CT is associated with a worse outcome, and the degree or amount of necrosis generally correlates with outcome, particularly if infection develops in the devitalized necrotic tissue.

During the acute attack, poorly demarcated fluid collections around the pancreas track into various retroperitoneal and peritoneal spaces. Much of this inflammatory fluid will resolve, but some will form into a more rounded and circumscribed fluid collection, called a *pseudocyst.* This process, which takes weeks, should be distinguished from early areas of pancreatic necrosis that may appear on CT as fluid collections and may be termed *pseudocysts* but in reality are collections of both liquid and solid necrotic material and are better described as *walled-off pancreatic necrosis.* Necrosis on CT, which can be seen in up to 25% of patients with acute pancreatitis and portends a worse outcome and particularly more substantial necrosis, is associated with higher rates of serious pancreatic infections. Organ system failure is quite rare in the absence of pancreatic necrosis.

Clinical features may help identify patients at higher risk, including patients who are older, are obese, or have more serious or more numerous comorbid conditions. In addition, a number of scoring systems can help guide clinicians in gauging prognosis.

The best known multiple-factor scoring systems are the Ranson criteria and Acute Physiology and Chronic Health Evaluation (APACHE) II score (see Table 146-2). Practice guidelines suggest a cutoff of more than 8 APACHE II points or more than 3 Ranson points as the definition of severe disease. Each approach has a high false-positive rate, in that many patients with high scores do not develop organ failure or die. An elevated admission BUN that does not return to normal with fluid therapy is associated with increased mortality, and a C-reactive protein level higher than 150 mg/L at 48 hours may be as accurate as multiple-factor scoring systems at predicting poor outcome. A simpler system is the "BISAP" score (*B*UN > 25 mg/dL, *I*mpaired mental status, *S*IRS, *A*ge > 60, and *P*leural effusion), in which mortality ranges from <1% for patients with none or only one of those risk factors (BISAP score of 0 or 1) to 27% for a BISAP score of 5. Each scoring system should be considered as a guide but not a replacement for clinical judgment.

TREATMENT

Rx

General Supportive Care

Most patients recover within several days, but it is usually not possible to identify these patients at the time of admission. All patients should be made NPO. Pain control usually requires parenteral narcotics, and hydromorphone (in divided doses of 1 to 2 mg given intravenously every 4 to 6 hours initially, with titration as needed, or more commonly as patient-controlled analgesia) is generally preferred. Patients with significant third space loss, often augmented by fluid losses through vomiting, will have evidence of intravascular fluid depletion. Even in mild pancreatitis, fluid losses may be substantial. Appropriate fluid resuscitation, which is one of the few medical interventions that appears to affect outcome, should be accomplished within the first 24 hours of admission to correct the blood pressure and pulse, to reduce the hematocrit and blood urea nitrogen levels to normal, and to ensure a urine output of at least 0.5 mL/kg/hour. Crystalloid, either normal or half-normal saline or lactated Ringer's solution, is preferred. If nausea and vomiting require treatment, promethazine (12.5 to 25 mg intravenously three times daily) is usually successful, although some patients may be more effectively treated with 5-HT3 antagonists (e.g., ondansetron, 8 mg orally or 4 or 8 mg intravenously up to every 8 hours). Nasogastric suction is needed for those with intractable nausea and vomiting. Patients can be fed, preferably with a full solid diet,[1] when bowel sounds and appetite have returned, nausea has resolved, enzyme levels are normalized, and pain is controlled.

In patients with more severe pancreatitis, based on the severity of their comorbid conditions, early organ system failure, or substantial third space fluid losses, admission to an intensive care unit (ICU) is appropriate. Vigorous fluid replacement, as outlined previously, which may reach 5 to 10 L/day, is required. Appropriate fluid resuscitation can be gauged by serial measurements of BUN and hematocrit as well as by urine output. Careful monitoring for progressive organ system failure and metabolic complications is critical in these patients.

Patients who appear to have sufficiently severe disease that they might not be able to eat for 5 to 7 days should be started on nutritional therapy. Trials suggest that enteral nutrition, using an elemental or semi-elemental formula, is associated with fewer complications, including hyperglycemia and line infections, compared with total parenteral nutrition.[2] Nasogastric feeding is easier and may be as good as nasojejunal feeding.[3]

Treatment of Complications

Most patients who develop acute gallstone pancreatitis have already passed the offending stone into the duodenum, but patients with a persistent stone or multiple stones are at higher risk of developing cholangitis and more severe pancreatitis. Data support current practice guidelines that recommend early ERCP in patients who have gallstone pancreatitis and evidence of concomitant cholangitis (e.g., fever, jaundice, right upper quadrant pain) or of a persistent bile duct stone (e.g., visible persistent stone on imaging study, jaundice, persistently dilated bile duct, worsening liver chemistries at 48 hours after admission).[4] Early ERCP is occasionally considered for patients who have severe pancreatitis, as evidenced by early and progressive organ system failure, but who do not have cholangitis or strong evidence of a stone; however, data do not support benefit from this intervention.[5] There is no other role for early endoscopic intervention in patients with acute pancreatitis.

The systemic complications (Table 146-3) that develop from multiple-organ system failure in patients with severe acute pancreatitis include some that are similar to those commonly encountered in other ICU patients as well as specific metabolic complications of severe pancreatitis. Hyperglycemia is commonly a result of the pancreatitis and may be seen with enteral nutrition; hyperglycemia may contribute to higher rates of infections. In severe acute pancreatitis, ionized calcium levels are usually normal, but hypocalcemia is common owing to a diminished serum albumin level; treatment (Chapter 253) is not needed in the absence of signs of hypocalcemia, such as tetany or a Chvostek's sign. Mild hypertriglyceridemia is common, but underlying hypertriglyceridemia is often the cause of acute pancreatitis when levels of triglycerides surpass 1000 mg/dL; triglyceride levels usually drop promptly when the patient is made NPO, but plasmapheresis may be required.

Any hospital-acquired infection dramatically worsens prognosis. Infections in patients with acute pancreatitis include urinary tract infections, pulmonary infections, line infections, and *Clostridium difficile* infection. High-quality nursing care, antibiotic stewardship, and careful attention to catheters and lines can minimize these infections.

For necrotizing pancreatitis, a step-up approach of percutaneous drainage followed, if necessary, by minimally invasive retroperitoneal necrosectomy reduces the risk of multiple-organ failure by more than two thirds and new diabetes by more than 50% with no change in in-hospital mortality compared with routine open necrosectomy.[6] Patients with necrotizing pancreatitis may develop infected pancreatic necrosis, which increases mortality to nearly 30%. Infection of preexisting necrosis typically occurs 2 to 3 weeks into the illness and is heralded by fever, leukocytosis, and worsening abdominal pain. The responsible organisms are usually gram-negative rods and other gut flora, but *Staphylococcus aureus* (Chapter 296) is an important agent as well. If infected necrosis is suspected, a CT scan should be obtained, followed by CT-directed fine-needle aspiration of the necrotic area for culture and Gram stain. If infection is documented, antibiotics tailored to the organism should be promptly initiated. Conservative therapy is continued, often for weeks, to allow the necrotic material to demarcate, begin to liquefy, and become encapsulated. When this walled-off necrosis is sufficiently liquefied to allow less invasive approaches, therapy can include percutaneous, endoscopic, or minimally invasive surgical therapy. Open surgical drainage is reserved for patients with progressive clinical deterioration and sepsis.

Given that infected necrosis has such substantial impact on prognosis, numerous studies have assessed the ability of prophylactic antibiotics to prevent infection in patients with preexisting sterile pancreatic necrosis. Data are unconvincing,[7] and current practice guidelines do not endorse prophylactic antibiotics in sterile pancreatic necrosis.

Fluid collections around the pancreas are common in acute pancreatitis and do not require any specific therapy. Most will resolve spontaneously, whereas some will mature into an encapsulated pseudocyst. It is important to distinguish a pseudocyst (usually outside the confines of the pancreas and filled with fluid) from an area of necrosis (usually inside the confines of the pancreas and a mixture of solid and liquid material). Therapy is not needed for asymptomatic pseudocysts, even if they are large, but therapy is indicated for pseudocysts that cause abdominal pain, obstruct a surrounding hollow viscus, or are associated with infection or bleeding. Bleeding may be limited to within the pseudocyst itself or may reach the intestine through the pancreatic duct if the pseudocyst is in communication with the duct. In some patients, bleeding into the pseudocyst may be caused by a pseudoaneurysm of a nearby visceral artery; this type of bleeding may be massive. Unexplained gastrointestinal bleeding or a sudden, unexplained drop in the hematocrit in a patient with pancreatitis or a pseudocyst should prompt an emergent CT scan, followed by embolization if a pseudoaneurysm is identified. A pseudocyst can be treated successfully using endoscopic, percutaneous or surgical techniques, and the choice among these approaches can be determined by local expertise.

Prevention of Relapse

Preventing relapse requires a clear knowledge of the precipitating causes. Abstinence from alcohol (Chapter 32) and tobacco (Chapter 31) should be strongly encouraged, including referral to appropriate resources. Cholecystectomy (Chapter 158) prevents subsequent attacks of gallstone pancreatitis and should be accomplished within a few weeks of discharge, if not sooner, if gallstones are the cause. In patients who have gallstone pancreatitis but who are not surgical candidates, endoscopic sphincterotomy provides reasonable protection from subsequent attacks. Control of serum lipids (Chapter 213) prevents subsequent attacks of hyperlipidemic pancreatitis. Therapy of lesions that obstruct the pancreatic duct, such as strictures, ampullary adenomas, and possibly sphincter of Oddi dysfunction and pancreas divisum, may also prevent relapse.

TABLE 146-3 COMPLICATIONS OF ACUTE PANCREATITIS

COMPLICATION	EXAMPLES
Systemic complications	Hypotension and shock Adult respiratory distress syndrome Acute renal failure Disseminated intravascular coagulation Hypocalcemia Hypertriglyceridemia Hyperglycemia Encephalopathy and coma
Gastrointestinal bleeding	Stress ulceration Pseudoaneurysm
Local (pancreatic) complications	Acute fluid collection Pseudocyst Pancreatic necrosis (infected and sterile) Duodenal and biliary obstruction

PROGNOSIS

More than 80% of all patients with acute pancreatitis recover promptly without developing severe pancreatitis. Mortality is usually from progressive multiple-organ system failure, either from the acute pancreatitis itself or from hospital-acquired infections, including infection of pancreatic fluid collections and pancreatic necrosis. The presence of early organ failure (within 24 hours of admission), multiple-organ system failure, and persistent or progressive (present beyond 48 hours after admission) organ failure are associated with prolonged hospitalization, ICU admission, need for surgery, and death. Overall mortality is about 2% but can be as high as 20% in patients referred to tertiary hospitals. Mortality can approach 30% in patients with more severe comorbid conditions and in patients who develop pancreatic necrosis, infection, or organ system failure. Although high-quality ICU care minimizes mortality, no specific therapy is currently available to affect these risks.

CHRONIC PANCREATITIS

DEFINITION

Chronic pancreatitis, which is a complex process rather than an isolated event, implies the presence of irreversible and permanent fibrosis, often with chronic mononuclear cell inflammation, damage to nerves, and loss of ducts, acini, and islets. Chronic pancreatitis evolves after episodes of acute pancreatitis, which may be subclinical, but the transition between acute and chronic pancreatitis may be difficult to identify.

EPIDEMIOLOGY

The prevalence of symptomatic chronic pancreatitis in Western countries is about 25 to 30 per 100,000 population, with an estimated incidence of 3 to 9 cases per 100,000. In the United States, chronic pancreatitis accounts for about 125,000 outpatient visits and 25,000 hospitalizations yearly. Interestingly, the prevalence of histologic evidence of chronic pancreatitis in autopsy studies approaches 5%, indicating that many people apparently develop chronic pancreatic damage as a consequence of normal aging, other diseases, or exposure to toxins, such as consumption of alcohol, but do not develop any symptoms or signs of chronic pancreatitis during life.

PATHOBIOLOGY

Multiple episodes of acute inflammation, whether clinical or subclinical, eventually change the inflammatory milieu of the pancreas, with a shift to chronic inflammation, the activation of pancreatic stellate cells, and the production of fibrosis. This process is self-sustaining and produces the characteristic histologic damage noted previously. Genetic mutations predispose to chronic pancreatitis, but the genetic predisposition is superimposed on exposure to various toxins, which precipitate acute pancreatitis, with cellular necrosis or apoptosis, that progresses in some individuals, particularly those with multiple episodes, to a chronic and fibrotic process. In Western countries, alcohol and tobacco abuse are the dominant causes of chronic pancreatitis.

One important contributor to the pain in chronic pancreatitis is damage to pancreatic nociceptive nerves and the complex neuroimmune interaction driven by the chronic inflammatory state. Chronic pain produces visceral, spinal cord, and central hyperalgesia, and the pain may become self-perpetuating even if therapy on the pancreas is successful. In addition to this neural mechanism, increased pressure within the gland, associated ischemia, obstruction of the pancreatic duct, and a pseudocyst can cause pain.

Alcohol and Tobacco

Alcohol (Chapter 32) causes about 70 to 80% of all cases of chronic pancreatitis in the United States and other major industrial countries. Substantial and prolonged ingestion of alcohol is usually required, on the order of 5 to 8 drinks daily over more than 5 years. Most people who consume this much alcohol do not develop chronic pancreatitis, pointing to important cofactors such as genetic background and cigarette smoking. There is evidence that tobacco alone (Chapter 31) can cause chronic pancreatitis, and the combination of alcohol and tobacco may be synergistic. Most patients will present initially with an episode of acute pancreatitis but will shortly thereafter develop evidence of chronic pancreatitis, but others will have obvious chronic pancreatitis at their first presentation.

Genetic

Hereditary pancreatitis is an autosomal dominant disease characterized by early onset of acute and chronic pancreatitis, the development of exocrine and endocrine pancreatic insufficiency, and a high risk of pancreatic adenocarcinoma. Mutations in the trypsinogen (*PRSS1*) gene in these families appear to cause a gain in function in which the mutant trypsinogen, once activated to trypsin, is difficult to inactivate. This trypsin, if present in an amount that overwhelms normal protective mechanisms, can activate other pancreatic enzymes and lead to pancreatic damage and eventually to chronic pancreatitis. One of the protective mechanisms is a trypsin inhibitor called *SPINK1*. Loss of function mutations in *SPINK1* may predispose to chronic pancreatitis, but unlike *PRSS1* mutations, are not sufficient to cause chronic pancreatitis. Major mutations in *CFTR* lead to cystic fibrosis (Chapter 89), which is associated with chronic pancreatitis and pancreatic atrophy. Milder mutations in *CFTR*, which predispose to chronic pancreatitis without causing the sinopulmonary features of cystic fibrosis, are encountered in patients with idiopathic chronic pancreatitis.

Other Causes

Autoimmune pancreatitis is a disease that most often presents as a masslike lesion with obstructive jaundice, mimicking cancer, but it also may present as chronic pancreatitis and rarely as acute pancreatitis. Characteristic features of the disease include a diffuse swelling of the pancreas, elevations in serum immunoglobulin G4 (IgG4), and involvement of other organs, especially biliary strictures, salivary gland inflammation, retroperitoneal fibrosis, and renal lesions. Histologically, these organs are infiltrated by chronic inflammatory cells, especially plasma cells bearing IgG4 on their surface.

Tropical pancreatitis is seen primarily in southern India. Characteristic features include childhood onset, exocrine insufficiency, diffuse pancreatic calcifications, and inevitable diabetes. There may be a genetic component (*SPINK1*), but cofactors such as malnutrition and dietary toxins have been suggested. In southern India, this disease is becoming uncommon and is being replaced by alcohol as the most common cause of idiopathic chronic pancreatitis.

Although most chronic pancreatitis evolves from multiple episodes of acute pancreatitis, a single severe acute attack that causes substantial pancreatic necrosis can destroy enough gland to produce exocrine and endocrine insufficiency. In addition, diseases that cause repeated attacks of pancreatitis can lead to chronic pancreatitis. For example, *hypertriglyceridemia* causes acute pancreatitis but commonly leads to chronic pancreatitis.

In about 20% of patients, no clear cause of chronic pancreatitis is found. Some patients may have underlying genetic mutations, and others may be surreptitiously using alcohol or tobacco. Two general forms of idiopathic chronic pancreatitis are seen. In the first, pain is the predominant feature, and the onset of disease is in young adulthood. In the second, the onset is in middle age, and exocrine and endocrine insufficiency, rather than abdominal pain, are the major clinical manifestations.

CLINICAL MANIFESTATIONS

The most common symptom of chronic pancreatitis is abdominal pain. The pain may be episodic or constant, and it is generally felt in the epigastrium with radiation to the back. If pain is episodic, the patient may be labeled as having acute pancreatitis or an acute flare of chronic pancreatitis. When pain is severe, nausea and vomiting may occur. Pain may worsen, improve, or remain stable over time. Up to 5% of patients do not have pain and instead present with exocrine (steatorrhea, weight loss) or endocrine (diabetes) pancreatic insufficiency. The disease tends to be progressive over time, even if the original cause (e.g., alcohol) is removed. The pathophysiology of pain is complex.

DIAGNOSIS

The diagnosis may be suspected based on the clinical features but should be confirmed by tests that identify structural damage to the pancreas or derangements in pancreatic function (Table 146-4). Chronic pancreatitis is a slowly

TABLE 146-4 DIAGNOSTIC TESTS FOR CHRONIC PANCREATITIS

STRUCTURAL	FUNCTIONAL
Biopsy	Hormonal (secretin) test
Endoscopic ultrasound	Fecal elastase
Endoscopic retrograde cholangiopancreatography	Serum trypsin
Magnetic resonance imaging with magnetic resonance cholangiopancreatography	Fecal fat
Computed tomography	Blood glucose
Ultrasonography	
Plain x-ray	

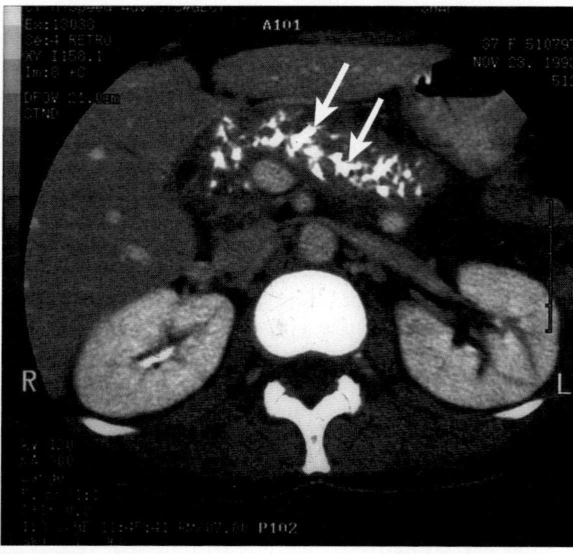

FIGURE 146-2. A computed tomography scan demonstrating diffuse pancreatic calcification in a patient with long-standing chronic pancreatitis *(arrows)*.

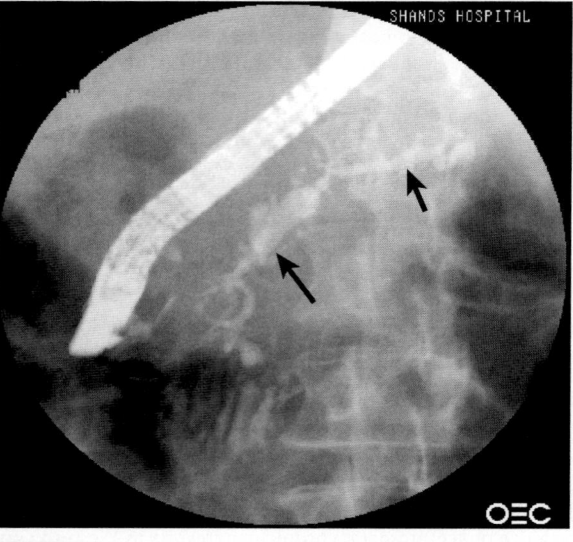

FIGURE 146-3. Endoscopic retrograde cholangiopancreatography demonstrating a very irregular pancreatic duct with areas of dilation and structuring in a patient with chronic pancreatitis *(arrows)*.

progressive disease in which visible damage to the gland (e.g., on a CT scan) and functional failure (e.g., steatorrhea or diabetes) may not be apparent for years. All diagnostic tests are most accurate when the disease is far advanced, and all are far less accurate in the early stages of disease.

Tests of Pancreatic Structure

Plain abdominal radiographs may demonstrate diffuse or focal pancreatic calcification in patients with advanced chronic pancreatitis. Although specific for chronic pancreatitis, these findings are quite insensitive.

Abdominal ultrasound is of limited utility because overlying gas often limits the ability to visualize the pancreas. An abnormal pancreatic duct, pancreatic calcifications, gland atrophy, or changes in echotexture are seen in about 60% of patients.

CT is the most widely used diagnostic test for chronic pancreatitis, and high-quality images can be obtained of the pancreas and pancreatic duct. Characteristic findings include a dilated pancreatic duct, ductal or parenchymal calcifications, and atrophy (Fig. 146-2). These structural changes take years to develop, so CT is not as accurate in early or less advanced disease. Like CT, MRI allows detailed images of the pancreas, and the addition of MRCP allows even better assessment of pancreatic duct morphology. At some centers, secretin is administered at the time of MRCP to allow better visualization of the pancreatic duct.

ERCP provides the most detailed images of the pancreatic duct. Changes in the duct, including dilation, irregularity, ductal stones, and strictures, can be appreciated (Fig. 146-3). These findings are not completely specific for chronic pancreatitis and can be seen in other situations, including with pancreatic cancer and in very elderly individuals. ERCP carries risk but has the advantage of providing both diagnostic and therapeutic impact.

EUS allows very detailed images of pancreatic parenchyma and duct (Fig. 146-4). A normal EUS essentially excludes chronic pancreatitis, whereas a very abnormal EUS is highly consistent with chronic pancreatitis.

Tests of Pancreatic Function

Serum trypsinogen (also called *trypsin*) is abnormally low in patients with far advanced chronic pancreatitis but is often normal in patients with less advanced disease. Levels lower than 20 ng/mL are seen in patients with chronic pancreatitis that is sufficient to cause functional failure (e.g., steatorrhea). Serum levels of amylase or lipase are not useful for chronic pancreatitis. Serum glucose levels will be elevated in those with endocrine insufficiency.

Quantification of fat in stool during a 72-hour collection while on a high-fat diet can be used to document steatorrhea (Chapter 142) but is rarely performed. Qualitative analysis of fat with Sudan staining of a stool specimen has poor sensitivity and specificity. Fecal levels of pancreatic elastase are diminished to less than 100 μg/g in patients with advanced chronic pancreatitis and steatorrhea. The test can be performed while patients are taking pancreatic enzyme therapy.

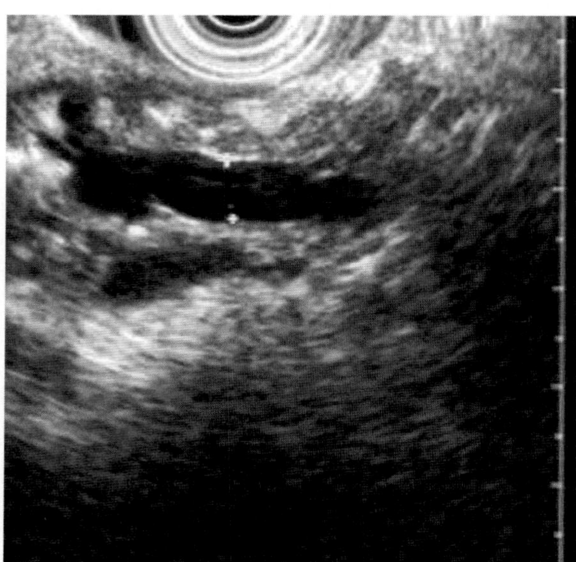

FIGURE 146-4. Endoscopic ultrasound in a patient with chronic pancreatitis, demonstrating a dilated pancreatic duct (*marks* on margin of main duct).

For a pancreatic function test, a tube is passed into the duodenum, where pancreatic secretions are collected over the course of 1 hour in 15-minute aliquots and analyzed for bicarbonate concentration after a supraphysiologic dose of secretin is administered. A normal study is defined by at least one of the samples having a bicarbonate concentration of more than 80 mEq/L. The test becomes abnormal earlier in the disease process than any other test, so it is well suited to diagnose chronic pancreatitis earlier in its clinical course; however, it is not widely available. An alternative, using endoscopy instead of a tube, is possible but somewhat less sensitive.

Diagnostic Approach

As the disease advances over years, structural and functional damage accumulate to the point that essentially all diagnostic tests are positive. In most patients, the diagnosis is established by routine tests such as CT or MRI; EUS and ERCP are rarely needed for diagnostic purposes in patients with long-standing chronic pancreatitis. The diagnostic challenge lies with patients who present with a severe pain syndrome suggestive of chronic pancreatitis but who have a normal CT or MRI. In these patients, EUS is the best choice unless the physician has access to a secretin-based pancreatic function test. ERCP should not be used for purely diagnostic purposes because patients with a normal-appearing pancreas are particularly prone to complications, especially post-ERCP pancreatitis.

TREATMENT

Rx

Abdominal Pain

A search for specifically treatable complications should be undertaken before initiating therapy for pain. Causes include a pseudocyst, obstruction of a surrounding hollow organ (e.g., duodenum or bile duct), or superimposed carcinoma. A good-quality CT or MRI image is usually sufficient to exclude these possibilities. These imaging tests also help in choosing appropriate therapy. Patients with a dilated pancreatic duct (generally >5 mm) are candidates for endoscopic and surgical therapy, which involves decompression of the dilated duct. Patients without duct dilation are generally not appropriate for endoscopic and surgical therapy and must rely instead on medical therapy (Table 146-5).

Medical therapy starts with vigorous attempts to assist patients in stopping alcohol and tobacco, if applicable. Most patients will require analgesics. It is appropriate to start with the less potent agents first, such as tramadol (50 mg, usually starting at one dose given every 6 hours). In patients who require more potent narcotics, it may be helpful to add an adjunctive antidepressant (e.g., amitriptyline, starting at 50 mg at night), selective serotonin reuptake inhibitors (see Table 404-5 in Chapter 404), gabapentin (starting at 100 mg at night), or pregabalin (starting at 50 mg three times daily). Antioxidants (mixtures of selenium, vitamins E and C, β-carotene, and methionine) may also have some beneficial effect on pain. [8] Finally, pancreatic enzyme therapy may have some beneficial effect on pain. Non-enteric-coated (tablet) pancreatic enzymes can reduce pancreatic stimulation and reduce pain by digesting a releasing factor present in the duodenum and providing negative feedback on the pancreas; conversely enteric-coated preparations, which are not active in the duodenum, have no proven effect on pain. These nonenteric preparations are not currently approved for clinical use but must be given with an agent to reduce gastric acid because acid will denature the proteases in these tablets. Autoimmune pancreatitis responds promptly to steroid therapy (usually 40 mg of prednisone daily for 4 weeks, with a taper of 5 mg/week over the next 7 weeks), but relapse may occur, particularly in the biliary tree.

Nerve Block and Neurolysis

EUS-guided celiac plexus block, using a local anesthetic and a steroid, or neurolysis, using absolute alcohol, can be performed relatively easily and safely, but substantial relief of pain is achieved for only weeks or months. [9] This therapy generally is considered only as a temporizing measure to provide relief from debilitating pain.

TABLE 146-5 TREATMENT FOR PAIN

TREATMENT	EXAMPLES
Medical therapy	Alcohol and tobacco cessation Analgesics and adjunctive agents Tramadol, 50 mg, one to three times daily Amitriptyline, starting at 50 mg at night Selective serotonin reuptake inhibitors (citalopram, fluoxetine, sertraline, paroxetine, and others) at recommended starting dose (see Table 404-5 in Chapter 404) Gabapentin, starting at 100 mg at night Pregabalin, starting at 50 mg three times daily Antioxidants Typical mixture containing vitamin C (1000 mg), vitamin E (300 IU), selenium (500 μg, methionine 2 g, and β-carotene 10,000 IU) total daily dose Non-enteric-coated enzymes (see Table 146-6)
Neurolysis	Endoscopic ultrasound–guided celiac plexus block or neurolysis Thoracoscopic splanchnicectomy
Endoscopic therapy	Stent Stone removal, lithotripsy
Surgical therapy	Pancreaticojejunostomy (modified Puestow operation) Partial pancreatic resection (Whipple operation, duodenum-preserving pancreatic head resection, others) Total pancreatectomy with islet cell autotransplantation

Endoscopic Therapy and Lithotripsy

At the time of ERCP, strictures can be dilated, and stents can be placed across the stricture. Ductal stones, if they are not too large and are not affected, may also be removed. Lithotripsy of larger stones is usually required to reduce the stone to fragments that are manageable. Only a subset of patients with chronic pancreatitis has ductal anatomy that is amenable to this type of therapy. In large case series from expert centers, therapy is technically successful in more than 80% of carefully selected patients, and pain relief may be seen in 70 to 80% of patients who undergo therapy. In patients with large stones, intraductal or extracorporeal lithotripsy is needed.

Surgical Therapy

Surgery for chronic pancreatitis is more effective and more durable than endoscopic therapy. [10,11] Surgery can involve decompression of the pancreatic duct, resection of the pancreas, or a combination of the two. The most commonly performed procedure, the modified Puestow procedure, involves a longitudinal incision of the pancreatic duct from the body of the pancreas to as close to the duodenum as possible, and this filleted duct is overlaid with a defunctionalized Roux limb. At the time of surgery, ductal strictures can be incised, and ductal stones can be removed. The procedure is relatively simple in patients with a dilated pancreatic duct (>5 mm). Pain relief in the short term is good (>80%), with about 50% obtaining long-term relief of pain. Alternative surgical procedures for pain include some resection of the pancreas, typically the head of the gland, in patients who have an inflammatory mass that causes biliary or duodenal obstruction. These operations, which include the classic pancreaticoduodenectomy (Whipple operation), provide equal short-term pain relief and better long-term pain relief than a modified Puestow, but with a higher morbidity. Total pancreatectomy, usually coupled with autotransplantation of harvested islet cells, is performed at a small number of centers but is generally considered a therapy of last resort, given the fact that diabetes mellitus is common after the procedure and pain relief is inconsistent.

Exocrine Insufficiency

Steatorrhea and maldigestion do not occur until approximately 90% of pancreatic enzyme secretion is lost, usually after 5 to 10 years of disease or even longer. Patients may note weight loss and oily stools, but often do not complain of diarrhea. Patients with chronic pancreatitis and exocrine insufficiency maldigest fat, protein, and carbohydrates, but fat maldigestion is usually most severe. In addition to weight loss, malabsorption of fat-soluble vitamins, particularly vitamin D, may occur. The diagnosis of exocrine insufficiency is usually suggested by symptoms of oily or floating stools and weight loss. A formal 72 stool fat analysis (Chapter 142) is the most accurate method to document steatorrhea and to gauge effectiveness of therapy but is rarely done. Instead, the clinical features and a fecal elastase of less than 100 μg/g stool, coupled with an appropriate response to enzyme replacement therapy, is the best substitute for 72-hour fecal fat testing.

Enzyme therapy (Table 146-6), which significantly reduces fecal fat levels and may reduce weight loss, [12] is divided into enteric-coated capsules and non-enteric-coated tablets. Non-enteric-coated preparations, as noted previously, are not clinically available but theoretically are the agents of choice if the goal is to treat pain. However, the enteric-coated preparations are used more frequently for exocrine insufficiency because they are more potent and require fewer pills. Enzymes are identified by the lipase content of the pill or capsule, although they all contain proteases and amylase as well. The goal of enzyme therapy, which is to administer at least 10% of normal pancreatic output with each meal, translates to approximately 30,000 IU of lipase with each meal. Most current products are measured in U.S. Pharmacopeia (USP) units, which are one third the amount of an international unit (IU) (e.g., up to 90,000 USP units of lipase with each meal). Because most patients are still producing some enzymes (including gastric lipase), it is usually not necessary to use the full dosage of 90,000 USP units with each meal.

Enzymes should be split during the meal (e.g., equally split before, during, and immediately after the meal). Supplementation with vitamin D (400 to 1000 IU daily) and calcium (1.0 to 1.5 g daily) is appropriate because osteoporosis (Chapter 251) and osteopenia are common. Success of enzyme therapy is generally defined as weight gain and reduction or absence of visible oil in the stool. Failure of enzyme therapy is most often due to inadequate dose. Increasing the dose up to the full 90,000 USP units with meals and encouraging compliance are appropriate as a first step. Some enteric-coated preparations may not release sufficient enzymes in the small bowel unless they are used with an agent to reduce gastric acid. Some patients may not respond owing to the presence of a second disease that also causes malabsorption, such as small intestinal bacterial overgrowth.

Endocrine Insufficiency

Like exocrine insufficiency, diabetes mellitus (Chapter 236) is a very late complication of chronic pancreatitis, occurring years or decades after disease onset. Unlike type 1 diabetes mellitus, there is destruction of the entire islet, which reduces secretion of both insulin and glucagon. As a result, overly aggressive therapy may lead to hypoglycemia, which cannot be reversed by

TABLE 146-6 ENZYME THERAPY FOR EXOCRINE INSUFFICIENCY*

AGENT[†]	DOSAGE
Creon 6000	10-15 with meals
Creon 12,000	5-8 with meals
Creon 24,000	3-4 with meals
Zenpep 5,000	12-18 with meals
Zenpep 10,000	6-10 with meals
Zenpep 15,000	4-6 with meals
Zenpep 20,000	3-5 with meals
Pancreaze 4200	15-18 with meals
Pancreaze 10,000	6-10 with meals
Pancreaze 16,800	4-5 with meals
Pancreaze 21,000	3-5 with meals

*Brand names. All contain pancrealipase.
[†]As more manufacturers receive U.S. Food and Drug Administration approval, this list may change.

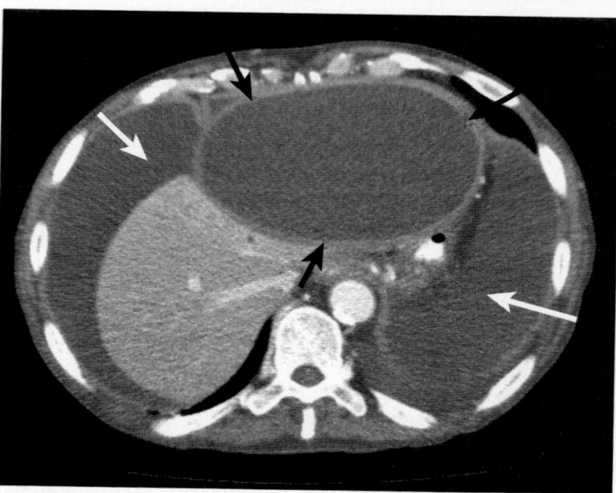

FIGURE 146-5. On computed tomography, a large pseudocyst is seen *(black arrows)*. In addition, ascites surrounding the liver *(white arrow)* is due to a leak from the pseudocyst (pancreatic ascites).

the usual natural glucagon surge. In most patients, therefore, insulin treatment is not aimed at exceedingly tight glucose control. Unfortunately, these patients are at similar risk for microvascular complications, as are all other patients with diabetes.

Complications

Pancreatic Pseudocyst

Pseudocysts, when they are discovered in patients with chronic pancreatitis, are generally mature and have a visible capsule surrounding them. As in acute pancreatitis, benign pseudocysts in chronic pancreatitis do not require therapy if they are not producing symptoms and are not rapidly enlarging. However, some cystic structures in and around the pancreas are cystic neoplasms, not pseudocysts. Symptomatic pseudocysts require drainage, whereas neoplasms require resection. Features that suggest a cystic neoplasm include a cyst with a thick or nodular wall, a cyst with multiple internal septations, or a cyst occurring in a patient who does not have a history of pancreatitis. Any combination of these features should lead to further investigation, generally with EUS and cyst aspiration.

Symptomatic pseudocysts can be treated with endoscopic, percutaneous, or surgical therapy with equal efficacy. In many centers, EUS-guided drainage is becoming first-line therapy. Both short-term and long-term results are excellent. Complications of pseudocysts include infection, bleeding, and rupture. A visceral artery pseudoaneurysm, which may develop as a consequence of a pseudocyst, can bleed torrentially, sometimes preceded by a brief self-limited bleed that stops when the blood is tamponaded within the pseudocyst. If the pseudocyst is in continuity with the pancreatic duct, blood may traverse the duct and enter the duodenum to cause melena; this release of pressure can produce exsanguinating bleeding. Any evidence of gastrointestinal bleeding or unexplained anemia in a patient with known pseudocyst or pancreatitis should raise the possibility of pseudoaneurysm. Embolization of the pseudoaneurysm is highly effective.

Pseudocysts may leak into the peritoneal compartment (pancreatic ascites) or track into the chest (pancreatic pleural effusion). Patients usually present with abdominal distention or dyspnea, rather than abdominal pain. Amylase level in the fluid is usually higher than 4000 U/L. Endoscopic therapy with stent placement across the connection between pseudocyst and pancreatic duct is highly effective in this situation (Fig. 146-5).

Malignancy

Chronic pancreatitis is a strong risk factor for pancreatic ductal adenocarcinoma (Chapter 200), with a lifetime risk of about 4%. The risk of cancer is much greater in patients with hereditary pancreatitis, in whom the risk may range as high as 40 to 70%. Equally importantly, it may be difficult to distinguish cancer from benign disease, particularly in patients with autoimmune pancreatitis.

PREVENTION

Currently, there are no reliable methods to prevent chronic pancreatitis. Patients at risk for chronic pancreatitis, such as members of families with hereditary pancreatitis and patients with established chronic pancreatitis, should avoid alcohol and tobacco and should probably be placed on a low-fat diet.

PROGNOSIS

With prolonged follow-up of 10 to 20 years, most patients will develop exocrine or endocrine insufficiency. The overall mortality is increased 3.6-fold compared with age-matched controls. Patients who are older, smoke, or have alcohol as the cause are at highest risk of mortality. Overall, 10-year survival approximates 70%, and 20-year survival is about 45%. Death is usually not due to pancreatitis itself, but rather to malignancy, postoperative complications, and complications of alcohol or tobacco.

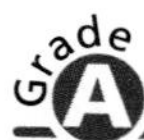

1. Moraes JM, Felga GE, Chebli LA, et al. A full solid diet as the initial meal in mild acute pancreatitis is safe and results in a shorter length of hospitalization: results from a prospective, randomized, controlled, double-blind clinical trial. *J Clin Gastroenterol.* 2010;44:517-522.
2. Petrov MS, van Santvoort HC, Besselink MG, et al. Enteral nutrition and the risk of mortality and infectious complications in patients with severe acute pancreatitis: a meta-analysis of randomized trials. *Arch Surg.* 2008;143:1111-1117.
3. Eatock FC, Chong P, Menezes N, et al. A randomized study of early nasogastric versus nasojejunal feeding in severe acute pancreatitis. *Am J Gastroenterol.* 2005;100:432-439.
4. Ayub K, Slavin J, Imada R. Endoscopic retrograde cholangiopancreatography in gallstone-associated acute pancreatitis. *Cochrane Database Syst Rev.* 2004;4:CD003630.
5. Petrov MS, van Santvoort HC, Besselink MG, et al. Early endoscopic retrograde cholangiopancreatography versus conservative management in acute biliary pancreatitis without cholangitis: a meta-analysis of randomized trials. *Ann Surg.* 2008;247:250-257.
6. van Santvoort HC, Besselink MG, Bakker OJ, et al. A step-up approach or open necrosectomy for necrotizing pancreatitis. *N Engl J Med.* 2010;362:1491-1502.
7. Segarra-Newnham M, Hough A. Antibiotic prophylaxis in acute necrotizing pancreatitis revisited. *Ann Pharmacother.* 2009;43:1486-1495.
8. Bhardwaj P, Garg PK, Maulik SK, et al. A randomized controlled trial of antioxidant supplementation for pain relief in patients with chronic pancreatitis. *Gastroenterology.* 2009;136:149-159.
9. Santosh D, Lakhtakia S, Gupta R, et al. Clinical trial: a randomized trial comparing fluoroscopy guided percutaneous technique vs. endoscopic ultrasound guided technique of celiac plexus block for treatment of pain in chronic pancreatitis. *Aliment Pharmacol Ther.* 2009;29:979-984.
10. Dite P, Ruzicka M, Zboril V, et al. A prospective, randomized trial comparing endoscopic with surgical therapy for chronic pancreatitis. *Endoscopy.* 2003;35:553-558.
11. Cahen DL, Gouma DJ, Nio Y, et al. Endoscopic versus surgical drainage of the pancreatic duct in chronic pancreatitis. *N Engl J Med.* 2007;356:676-684.
12. Shafiq N, Rana S, Bhasin D, et al. Pancreatic enzymes for chronic pancreatitis. *Cochrane Database Syst Rev.* 2009;7:CD006302.

SUGGESTED READINGS

Braganza JM, Lee SH, McCloy RF, et al. Chronic pancreatitis. *Lancet.* 2011;377:1184-1197. *Review.*

Chari ST, Kloeppel G, Zhang L, et al. Histopathologic and clinical subtypes of autoimmune pancreatitis: the Honolulu consensus document. *Pancreatology.* 2011;10:664-672. *Consensus definitions.*

Ksiadzyna D. Drug-induced acute pancreatitis related to medications commonly used in gastroenterology. *Eur J Intern Med.* 2011;22:20-25. *Review emphasizing importance of a high index of suspicion.*

147

DISEASES OF THE RECTUM AND ANUS

ROBERT D. MADOFF

DEFINITIONS

The rectum is best defined anatomically as the level of the large intestine where the taeniae coli splay to form a continuous longitudinal muscle layer. As a practical matter, the rectum begins about 15 cm proximal to the anal margin or verge, where the anus meets the perianal skin. The junction of the colon and rectum bears a variable relationship to the peritoneal reflection, which lies obliquely and at a variable distance from the anal margin.

The anus can be defined both anatomically and histologically. As a practical matter, it is best defined as the distal-most segment of the large bowel that extends from the pelvic floor muscles (levator ani) to the skin. The anorectal junction can be recognized as the point where the rectum angulates posteriorly from the axis of the anal canal. This junction, easily appreciated on digital rectal examination, is caused by the anterior pull of the puborectalis, a U-shaped muscle that loops behind the anorectal junction and pulls it forward. The puborectalis plays an important role in continence, and it is in continuity with the proximal external anal sphincter.

The dentate line lies about 2 cm proximal to the anal margin and roughly corresponds to the level where the distal squamous mucosa meets the more proximal columnar mucosa. Approximately 6 to 12 anal glands located around the perimeter of the dentate line can become infected and become the source of perianal abscesses and fistulas. The anal transition zone, which extends 1 to 2 cm proximal to the dentate line, is the site where many anal cancers develop and marks the proximal boundary for anal cancer surveillance. Hemorrhoids are classified based on their relationship to the dentate line: those proximal are deemed internal, and those distal are external. Anal papillae, the small triangular points of the dentate line, can become hypertrophied and may be mistaken for polyps. Finally, somatic sensation ceases 1 to 2 cm above the dentate line, which explains why hemorrhoid ligation can be performed without anesthesia.

The anal sphincter complex has three major components: the puborectalis, the external anal sphincter, and the internal anal sphincter. The external anal sphincter is composed of skeletal muscle and is under voluntary control. The internal anal sphincter is composed of smooth muscle and represents a continuous though thickened extension of the circular muscle coat of the rectum. The internal anal sphincter is responsible for about 70% of resting anal tone; augmentation of anal sphincter pressure occurs when the individual contracts the external anal sphincter.

SPECIFIC ANORECTAL CONDITIONS

Hemorrhoids

EPIDEMIOLOGY AND PATHOBIOLOGY

The prevalence of hemorrhoids in the United States has been estimated to be 4.4%. However, because many "hemorrhoidal" symptoms are in fact due to other causes, the true incidence and prevalence are unknown.

Despite the commonly held notion that hemorrhoids are always pathologic, hemorrhoids are normal structures, identifiable even in the fetus. Hemorrhoids are vascular cushions that consist of both arterioles and veins. The arteriolar component explains why hemorrhoidal bleeding is typically bright red in color and can be copious in quantity. Hemorrhoids are *not* rectal varices, which are a distinct entity caused by portal hypertension. Many causative factors have been proposed, including constipation, diarrhea, pregnancy, and prolonged straining at stool. Although none of these precipitating factors has been rigorously proved, each can cause either increased abdominal pressure or obstruction of venous return, leading to engorgement and enlargement of the vascular cushions.

CLINICAL MANIFESTATIONS AND DIAGNOSIS

The most common symptom of internal hemorrhoids is bright red rectal bleeding. This bleeding is typically painless and is most often seen on the toilet tissue or in the toilet bowl. The quantity of blood is variable, but some patients complain of blood dripping or squirting into the toilet bowl. Passage of dark blood or blood mixed in the stool suggests a more proximal source. Internal hemorrhoids are classified based on the symptoms they cause. As internal hemorrhoids enlarge, they become associated with redundant rectal mucosa that protrudes from the anus with defecation. Grade 1 hemorrhoids bleed but do not prolapse. Early protrusion reduces spontaneously (grade 2); more advanced protrusion requires digital reduction (grade 3) and, at its most advanced, becomes irreducible (grade 4). Internal hemorrhoids are insensate and are not itchy themselves, but they can cause itching due to associated perianal soiling or mucus deposition caused by mucosal prolapse.

Individuals with anorectal symptoms frequently present complaining of "hemorrhoids." It is always incorrect—and sometimes dangerous—for the physician to apply this diagnosis without completing an adequate evaluation. Fortunately, the initial evaluation is simple, and the correct diagnosis is often suspected based on history alone and confirmed by a limited endoscopic examination. For example, rectal bleeding should never be attributed to hemorrhoids alone, even if hemorrhoids are visible; at a minimum, sigmoidoscopy is required to exclude more proximal pathology. Internal hemorrhoids are best visualized with a slotted anoscope.

External hemorrhoids are usually asymptomatic and should be differentiated from perianal skin tags, which occasionally cause difficulties with hygiene. External hemorrhoids become symptomatic when they thrombose to cause acute-onset pain and swelling (Fig. 147-1). Thrombosed external hemorrhoids are diagnosed by simple inspection.

TREATMENT

Rx

Grade 1 hemorrhoids often respond to dietary manipulation: increased dietary fiber, addition of a fiber supplement,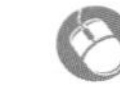 and increased water intake (Table 147-1). The goal, which may not be readily achievable, is approximately 25 g of fiber and 8 glasses of water daily. More advanced hemorrhoids require specific therapy, which is almost always office based. The most popular and simplest technique is rubber band ligation, whereby a tiny rubber band (internal diameter approximately 1 mm) is placed around a quantity of redundant rectal mucosa above the prolapsing hemorrhoid. The banded tissue sloughs in 7 to 14 days, an event sometimes heralded by rectal bleeding. Banding can be repeated at 3- to 4-week intervals until bleeding and protrusion are controlled. Bands placed too close to the dentate line cause immediate severe pain and must be removed promptly. Alternative therapies for moderate internal hemorrhoids include injection sclerotherapy and infrared coagulation, which can be performed in the office.

Operative hemorrhoidectomy is needed in only a small minority of patients. Indications for hemorrhoidectomy include irreducible prolapse, a substantial external component, and failure of more conservative therapies. The most common approach is an excisional hemorrhoidectomy, which is generally performed on an outpatient basis. A more recent approach is the stapled hemorrhoidopexy, which entails resecting a ring of rectal mucosa proximal to the internal hemorrhoids using a circular stapling device. This technique is quicker than conventional hemorrhoidectomy and is associated with less postoperative pain and a shorter period of disability; its drawbacks include a higher recurrence rate than conventional surgery and a small but worrisome risk of significant complications. Another alternative approach is Doppler-guided transanal devascularization of internal hemorrhoids, which is directed at obliterating the feeding arterioles. Although early results are promising, the experience to date is limited, and follow-up is short.

External hemorrhoids are usually treated by excision in the office under local anesthesia. However, because the pain associated with thrombosis generally abates within 7 to 10 days, patients who present with resolving symptoms are often best managed conservatively with standard doses of over-the-counter analgesics, sitz baths, and 25 g/day fiber supplementation.

Perianal Abscess

EPIDEMIOLOGY AND PATHOBIOLOGY

Although perianal abscess is a common condition, its exact incidence is not well documented. Most perianal abscesses are caused by infection of the anal glands that track toward the skin. Other causes include simple skin infections, trauma, anorectal surgery, and malignancy.

CLINICAL MANIFESTATIONS AND DIAGNOSIS

Patients most commonly present with complaints of perianal pain and swelling. In most cases, a local area of erythema, tenderness, and fluctuance can be appreciated. However, local swelling, erythema, and fluctuance are often absent in an intersphincteric abscess, which is a small abscess in the plane

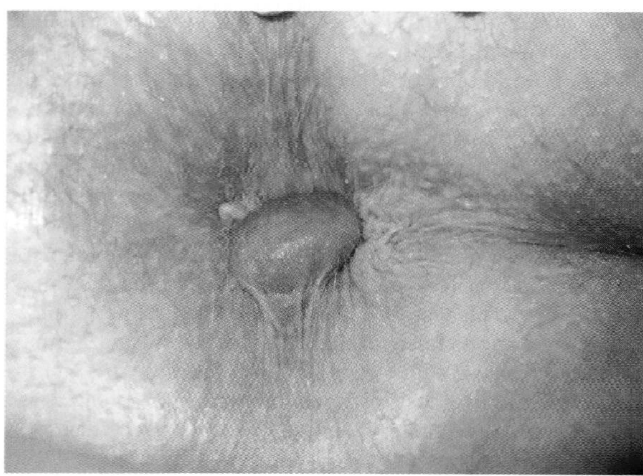

FIGURE 147-1. Thrombosed external hemorrhoids.

TABLE 147-1 INTERNAL HEMORRHOIDS: GRADING AND MANAGEMENT

GRADE	SYMPTOMS AND SIGNS	MANAGEMENT
1	Bleeding No prolapse	Dietary modifications* Rubber band ligation Infrared coagulation Injection sclerotherapy
2	Prolapse with spontaneous reduction Bleeding, seepage	Rubber band ligation Infrared coagulation Dietary modifications Injection sclerotherapy
3	Prolapse requiring digital reduction Bleeding, seepage	Surgical hemorrhoidectomy Rubber band ligation Dietary modifications
4	Prolapsed, cannot be reduced Strangulated	Surgical hemorrhoidectomy Urgent hemorrhoidectomy

*Dietary modifications include increasing the consumption of fiber, bran, or psyllium and water. Dietary modifications are always appropriate for the management of hemorrhoids and to prevent recurrence after banding or surgery (or both).
Adapted from Nelson H, Dozois RR. Anus. In: Townsend CM, ed. *Sabiston Textbook of Surgery*, 16th ed. Philadelphia: Saunders; 2001:979.

between the internal and external sphincter muscles; these abscesses are suspected based on the history of increasing pain and the physical finding of focal perianal tenderness.

As with all acutely painful anal conditions, digital examination should be avoided. Likewise, office instrumentation with an anoscope or proctoscope is contraindicated because these examinations cause substantial pain and yield little if any diagnostic information. When the cause of the acute pain cannot be determined in the office, prompt examination under anesthesia should be performed.

TREATMENT Rx

Treatment for perianal abscess is prompt incision and drainage, which can usually be performed in the office. Antibiotics do not adequately penetrate abscess cavities, and extension of a local infection can lead to severe local sepsis and complex long-term problems. Therefore, antibiotic therapy is inadequate and should never be given in an attempt to avoid or delay incision and drainage. Antibiotics usually are not indicated after incision and drainage; exceptions include immunocompromised patients (those with AIDS, transplant recipients, patients undergoing chemotherapy, diabetics) and those at high risk for endovascular infection (e.g., patients with cardiac shunts, prosthetic valves).

Anal Fistula

EPIDEMIOLOGY

An anal fistula represents the chronic form of a perianal abscess. The incidence of anal fistula is about 8.6 per 100,000. Fistulas are two to three times more common in men than in women.

PATHOBIOLOGY

After a perianal abscess is drained, there is about a 50% chance that the internal opening—the site at the dentate line where the infected gland originated—will remain patent, thereby leaving a source for recurrent infection. Multiple or atypical anal fistulas should always raise the diagnostic suspicion of Crohn's disease, which is isolated to the perianal area in approximately 10% of cases.

Anal fistulas are characterized by their relationship to the sphincter complex. The simplest fistula is intersphincteric—located in the plane between the internal and external sphincter muscles. Transsphincteric fistulas, which traverse both the internal and external sphincter muscles, are classified as low fistulas, which traverse only the distal external sphincter, or high fistulas, which traverse the more proximal portions of the external sphincter. Suprasphincteric fistulas loop over the entire sphincter complex. Extrasphincteric fistulas have internal openings remote from the dentate line; most originate from a pelvic abscess caused by a ruptured appendix (Chapter 144), diverticulitis (Chapter 144), or Crohn's disease (Chapter 143). A horseshoe fistula is one with external openings on both sides of the midsagittal plane; these most commonly have a single internal opening in the posterior midline.

CLINICAL MANIFESTATIONS AND DIAGNOSIS

Anal fistulas sometimes present as recurrent abscesses in the same location as the original one, and they sometimes present as persistent purulent drainage from an abscess site that has failed to heal completely. In either case, a persistent track between the external and internal openings remains.

The diagnosis of an anal fistula is established by history and by visualization of an external opening in the perianal skin. A fibrous fistula track can sometimes be palpated along the course of the fistula from the skin toward the anal canal. An internal opening is occasionally visible on anoscopy, but it is not necessary to identify one to make a presumptive diagnosis.

TREATMENT 

Treatment of anal fistulas is surgical. Most fistulas are cured by being laid open to eliminate the original source of infection at the internal opening. The fistula track heals by secondary intention. However, this approach divides sphincter muscle and puts the patient at risk for impaired fecal continence in proportion to the quantity of muscle involved. In general, intersphincteric and low transsphincteric fistulas can be safely laid open if the patient has normal baseline continence and no underlying predisposing factors for diarrhea (e.g., colitis) or recurrent fistulas (e.g., Crohn's disease). Because the anterior sphincter mechanism is relatively short and because the anterior sphincter is subject to injury following vaginal delivery, fistulotomy for anterior fistulas in women must be undertaken only after careful consideration.

Treatment of high fistulas is a challenge. When a high fistula is identified, the first step is often placement of a seton, a suture, or other material (now commonly a Silastic vessel loop) that is passed though the fistula track, out the anus, and secured to itself. The seton guarantees that the external fistula opening will not heal over, so a recurrent abscess cannot supervene. Once the track has "matured"—scarred around the seton and become fibrotic—treatment options to eliminate the internal opening include endorectal advancement flap repair and obliteration of the track using fibrin glue or a collagen fistula plug. For individuals with known or suspected Crohn's disease, fistulotomy is avoided, except for the most superficial fistulas. In general, patients with Crohn's disease are best served by placement of long-term draining setons and medical therapy for their underlying disease.

Anal Fissure

EPIDEMIOLOGY

Anal fissures can occur at any age but most frequently affect young adults. Men and women are equally affected.

PATHOBIOLOGY

An anal fissure is a longitudinal tear in the anoderm that occurs just inside the anal margin (Fig. 147-2). The underlying pathophysiology of anal fissures is hypertonia of the internal anal sphincter. Typical anal fissures occur at the midline; most commonly they occur posteriorly, but about 15% are found anteriorly or both anteriorly and posteriorly. "Off-the-midline" fissures should raise the question of other pathology such as anal cancer, Crohn's disease (Chapter 143), syphilis (Chapter 327), HIV, leukemia (Chapter 190), or tuberculosis (Chapter 332). Fissures may occur acutely owing to trauma but are more commonly a subacute condition.

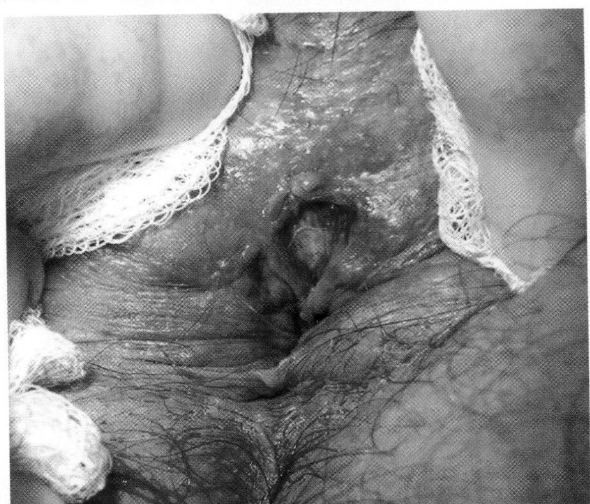

FIGURE 147-2. Anal fissure.

CLINICAL MANIFESTATIONS AND DIAGNOSIS

Patients with anal fissures generally have a typical presentation, and in most cases the correct diagnosis is suspected based on history alone. Following bowel movements, patients describe severe anal pain that may persist for hours or even continue until exacerbation by the next bowel movement. There is sometimes an association with minor red rectal bleeding, most commonly seen in small quantities on the toilet tissue. Anal fissures are frequently associated with a diagnostic triad: the fissure itself, a "sentinel" skin tag (so called because its presence should suggest the presence of an underlying fissure), and a hypertrophied anal papilla located just proximal to the fissure at the dentate line. Well-established fissures may have fibrotic margins and visible internal anal sphincter fibers at their base.

Most fissures can be readily seen on physical examination by applying opposing traction to the buttocks. Once a fissure is identified, no further examination is performed. Digital and endoscopic examination should generally be delayed until the patient has healed to avoid causing pain. However, patients should be advised that they will require subsequent sigmoidoscopy to exclude proximal pathology.

TREATMENT Rx

All therapies are directed at the underlying hypertonia of the internal anal sphincter. Approximately 40% of fissures heal with fiber supplementation and increased fluid intake. Patients are also advised to take warm sitz baths for symptomatic relief, especially following bowel movements.

Two pharmacologic approaches can augment diet and sitz baths: topical sphincter relaxants and botulinum toxin injection. Topical nitroglycerine ointment (0.2 to 0.5%) or diltiazem gel (2%) applied to the anal orifice two to three times daily reduces sphincter tone and usually leads to healing.[3] Both drugs have similar efficacy, but nitroglycerine has the significant disadvantage of causing headaches, lightheadedness, or syncope owing to systemic vasodilation in a substantial minority of patients; commercial 2% nitroglycerine ointment for cardiac use is too potent for perianal use. Botulinum toxin injection is another treatment option, but its usefulness is variable, and the risk of fissure relapse is significant.

For patients who fail medical therapy or who are simply too miserable to pursue it, lateral internal sphincterotomy is an appropriate and generally safe approach.[4] This simple operation is easily performed under monitored local anesthesia in an outpatient setting; recovery is rapid, and fissure healing is expected in more than 90% of cases. Sphincterotomy as first-line therapy provides higher healing rates, fewer relapses, and fewer side effects than topical nitroglycerine,[5] with fewer symptoms, greater satisfaction, and no difference in continence at long-term follow-up.[6] However, a small percentage of patients who undergo sphincterotomy develop minor seepage or actual incontinence, so sphincterotomy should be avoided in individuals who have underlying impaired continence, known sphincter injuries, or diarrheal disorders. When such patients have refractory fissures, a trial of botulinum toxin injection is often a good alternative.

Pruritus Ani

Pruritus ani, or perianal itching, is a very common complaint. It is a symptom and not a disease. The most common cause is inadequate perianal hygiene, often exacerbated by scratching, which leads to excoriation of the skin and further inflammation. Other causes include prolapsing hemorrhoids, anal fistulas, anal incontinence, and specific dermatologic conditions such as contact dermatitis (Chapter 446), psoriasis (Chapter 446), lichen sclerosus (Chapter 448), squamous intra-epithelial neoplasia (Bowen's disease), and perianal Paget's disease (intra-epidermal adenocarcinoma).

TREATMENT Rx

Most cases respond to treatment of the underlying pathology, improved hygiene, avoidance of potential contact allergens, and use of either talc to absorb excess moisture or a barrier cream such as zinc oxide. Some patients benefit from the avoidance of certain foods, including caffeinated beverages, alcohol, milk, chocolate, and tomatoes. Mild topical steroids such as 1% hydrocortisone are sometimes helpful, but stronger steroid preparations are frequently counterproductive and should be avoided when they are not indicated for a specific dermatologic diagnosis. Skin biopsies should be obtained when a primary dermatologic condition is suspected or when the perianal irritation fails to heal with conservative therapy.

Fecal Incontinence

EPIDEMIOLOGY AND PATHOBIOLOGY

Involuntary loss of stool or flatus is a relatively common problem that, when severe, can be socially isolating and debilitating. About 2% of individuals in the United States report incontinence symptoms, but the prevalence is substantially higher in patients visiting primary care providers and gastroenterologists. Almost half of U.S. nursing home patients suffer from fecal incontinence.

CLINICAL MANIFESTATIONS AND DIAGNOSIS

Fecal incontinence can be caused by many disorders. Sphincter disruption related to vaginal delivery is a common cause that often affects young women; many incontinent women who present later in life have an underlying sphincter injury for which they can no longer compensate. Other causes of incontinence include fecal impaction, surgical or traumatic sphincter injury, rectal prolapse, neurologic disorders (e.g., diabetic neuropathy, stroke, multiple sclerosis, brain or spinal cord injury), chronic diarrheal states, dementia, and impaired mobility.

Because incontinence is a symptom and not a disease, the diagnosis is based on history alone. Specific evaluation of the incontinent patient can include anal manometry, anal ultrasound, pudendal nerve testing, and defecography. Anal ultrasound, which is generally the most helpful test, accurately depicts sphincter anatomy and reliably identifies sphincter defects.

TREATMENT Rx

Mild incontinence is often treated successfully with dietary management, addition of a fiber supplement, and use of an antimotility agent such as loperamide 2 to 4 mg up to four times daily (Fig. 147-3). Biofeedback is successful in many patients. For individuals with sphincter disruption, surgical repair leads to substantial improvement in most patients. Sacral nerve stimulation is highly effective for fecal incontinence, although the implantable device has not yet been approved for this indication in the United States. In a randomized trial, transanal submucosal injections of dextranomer in stabilized hyaluronic acid reduced fecal incontinence by at least 50% with minimal adverse effects.[7] For patients with severe refractory incontinence, creation of a colostomy should be strongly considered. Initial reluctance notwithstanding, most patients regain control of their bowel function and report a substantially improved quality of life.

Rectal Prolapse

EPIDEMIOLOGY AND PATHOBIOLOGY

Rectal prolapse is a full-thickness protrusion of the rectum beyond the anal sphincter. The disorder can occur at any age, but prolapse is most frequently seen in older patients, and approximately 90% of adult patients are women. Prolapse is caused by an internal rectal intussusception that, as it becomes more severe, protrudes externally. Uncorrected prolapse frequently leads to

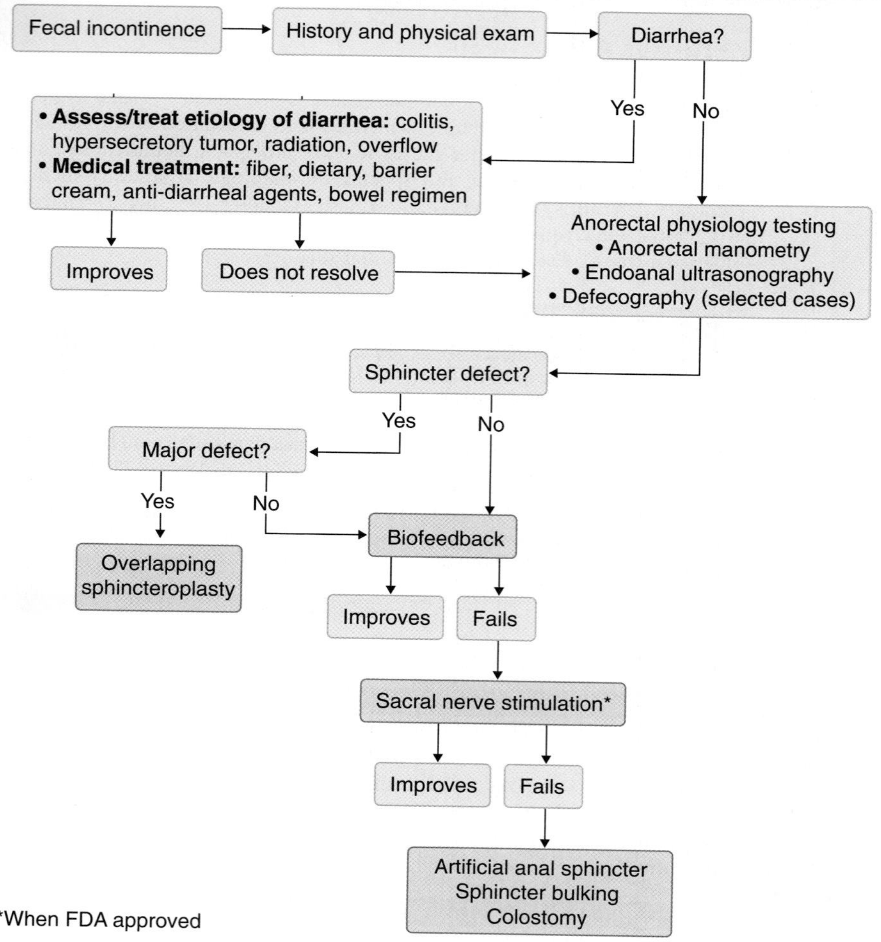

FIGURE 147-3. **Algorithm for fecal incontinence.** FDA = Food and Drug Administration. (Adapted from Madoff RD, Parker SC, Varma MG, Lowry AC. Faecal incontinence in adults. Lancet. 2004;364:621-632.)

fecal incontinence by mechanically stretching the sphincter complex and causing a stretch injury to the pudendal nerves.

CLINICAL MANIFESTATIONS AND DIAGNOSIS

The main clinical manifestation of rectal prolapse is the protruding rectal mass (Fig. 147-4). Most commonly the protrusion occurs with bowel movements, but with time it may occur with coughing or sneezing, and eventually it can occur spontaneously. Some patients present with complaints of fecal incontinence, and many also complain of "constipation," which may be caused by unsuccessful attempts to evacuate the intussuscepting rectum. The protruded rectum may cause minor bleeding and mucus discharge. Occasional patients present with an incarcerated or strangulated prolapse.

The diagnosis of rectal prolapse is confirmed on physical examination. Full-thickness prolapse, which is characterized by concentric mucosal folds, must be differentiated from circumferential mucosal prolapse, which is characterized by radial folds. The prolapse is often best demonstrated by having the patient strain on a commode. Defecography is sometimes helpful to diagnose internal rectal intussusception and associated pelvic floor abnormalities, such as rectocele and enterocele.

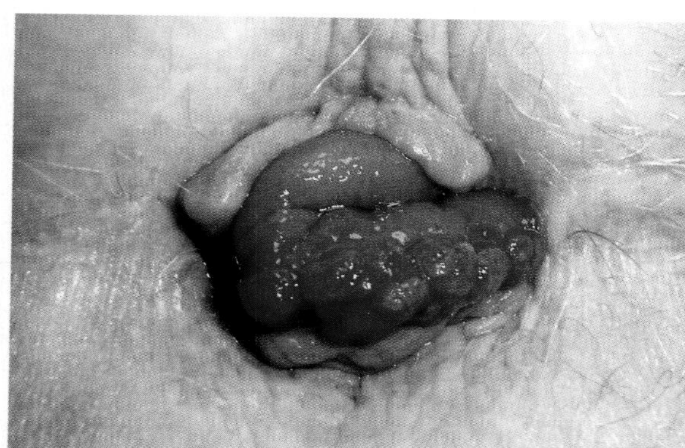

FIGURE 147-4. **Rectal mucosal prolapse.**

TREATMENT Rx

Rectal prolapse is treated by surgical correction. Both transabdominal and transperineal approaches are commonly used.

Human Papillomavirus

EPIDEMIOLOGY AND PATHOBIOLOGY

Human papillomavirus (HPV, Chapter 381), which is the most common sexually transmitted infection, is a cause of anal dysplasia and cancer. The approximately 40 HPV subtypes that can cause anogenital infections are divided into low-risk types (e.g., types 6 and 11) that cause anal warts (condyloma acuminata) and high-risk types (e.g., types 16, 18, and 33) that can cause anal dysplasia and cancer. HPV infection is associated with cervical, vulvar, vaginal, and penile cancers, and some patients have HPV-related dysplasia or cancer in multiple sites. Approximately 90% of anal cancers are attributable to HPV infection.

The incidence of anal cancer has been steadily increasing, from 0.6 per 100,000 in 1973 to 1.0 per 100,000 in 2001; the female-male ratio decreased from 1.6 : 1 to 1.2 : 1 over the same period. These epidemiologic trends have been attributed to a particularly rapid increase in anal cancers among men who have sex with men, especially men infected with HIV. Anal HPV, including the high-risk types, is highly prevalent in at-risk populations (sex workers, intravenous drug users, transplant recipients, men who have sex with men, and HIV-positive men and women). Furthermore, anal dysplasia is common in at-risk populations; indeed, the prevalence rates of high-grade anal dysplasia are reportedly 40 to 60% among HIV-positive men who have sex with men seen in specialty clinics in New York and San Francisco.

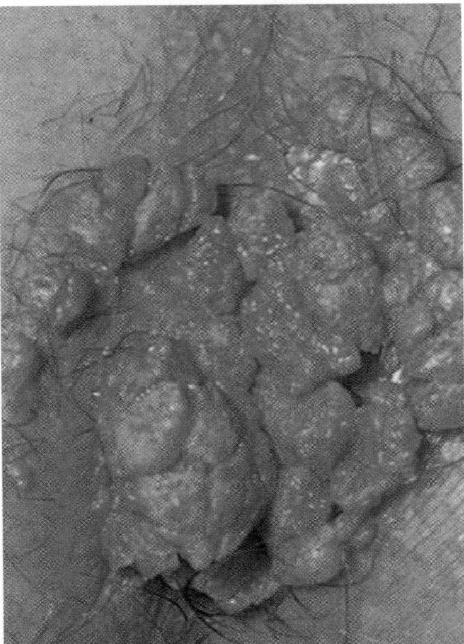

FIGURE 147-5. Perianal condylomata resulting from human papillomavirus infection.

TREATMENT Rx

Management of the patient with anal dysplasia is controversial. Many authorities advocate a screening and treatment approach based on that used for cervical cancer, another HPV-associated disease. High-risk individuals are screened with anal Papanicolaou smears, and high-definition anal microscopy (analogous to colposcopy of the cervix) is performed when abnormal cytology is detected. Using this technique, dysplastic lesions can be identified and focally ablated or treated with topical imiquimod. More extensive dysplasia requires microscopy-directed targeted ablation in the operating room. Although this overall approach is rational and provides good control of most dysplasia, it is also time-consuming and requires multiple follow-up visits. Cost, recurrence, compliance, and provider manpower all remain significant issues. However, even advocates of less aggressive surveillance report significant rates of anal cancer among patients with dysplasia, especially those who are immunocompromised.

Chemoradiotherapy is now standard first-line treatment for squamous cell cancer of the anal canal. Current radiation protocols most frequently use 45-Gy external beam radiation therapy in 25 fractions, with a boost to the primary tumor and involved inguinal nodes to a total dose of 54 to 59 Gy. Standard chemotherapy utilizes 5-fluorouracil (1000 mg/m^2 per 24 hours continuous infusion for 96 hours, starting on days 1 and 29) in combination with mitomycin C (most commonly 10 mg/m^2 intravenous bolus on days 1 and 29). Abdominoperineal resection with permanent colostomy is reserved for tumors that fail to respond to chemoradiation and those that recur. Similarly, groin dissection is performed only when involved inguinal nodes fail chemoradiation.

Early squamous cell cancers of the anal margin can be locally excised if a satisfactory margin can be obtained without injuring the anal sphincter and if there is no evidence of nodal spread. More advanced anal margin tumors are treated with chemoradiotherapy as described for anal canal tumors.

ANAL WARTS

CLINICAL MANIFESTATION AND DIAGNOSIS

Anal warts can occur in the perianal skin and within the anal canal. The lesions are raised, epithelialized (when external), and narrow based. They can appear as scattered individual warts or as a confluent mass (Fig. 147-5).

TREATMENT Rx

External warts can be treated with topical podophyllin or imiquimod, but extensive warts usually require surgical excision or fulguration. Untreated warts can rarely progress to form Bushke-Löwenstein tumors—giant, locally invasive condyloma acuminata that frequently contain in situ or invasive cancer.

ANAL CANCER

CLINICAL MANIFESTATIONS AND DIAGNOSIS

The most common symptoms of anal cancer are bleeding, pain, and a palpable mass. The cancer may be seen externally as an ulcerated mass or may be palpated within the anal canal. Anal dysplastic lesions may appear as anal warts or as flat, pigmented lesions, or they may be invisible to the naked eye. They are best visualized using anal microscopy after topical application of 3 to 5% acetic acid (see later). Biopsy is necessary to make the diagnosis.

The terminology of anal cancer is complex, but the great majority of tumors (including epidermoid, cloacogenic, and basaloid carcinomas) are variants of squamous cell carcinoma. The terminology of preinvasive squamous anal lesions is even more confusing because several terms exist for histologically identical pathology. The terms *anal dysplasia, anal intra-epithelial neoplasia* (AIN), and *squamous intra-epithelial lesion* (SIL) are used interchangeably. SILs are divided into low-grade and high-grade groups; AIN is similarly divided into AIN 1, 2, and 3, with AIN 2 and 3 being classified as high-grade lesions. Squamous cell carcinoma in situ corresponds to high-grade SIL and AIN 3; these terms are preferable to *Bowen's disease*, which has historically been applied to this lesion. Other significant but less common anal cancers include adenocarcinoma, melanoma, and Paget's disease.

Squamous cell carcinoma of the anus is divided into two groups based on tumor location: cancers of the anal margin (extending from the anal orifice for a distance up to 5 cm) and cancers of the anal canal. Tumors visible externally but extending into the anal canal are considered anal canal lesions.

Other Sexually Transmitted Anorectal Diseases

A number of sexually transmitted diseases (Chapter 293) of the anorectum occur most frequently in individuals who practice anoreceptive intercourse. Common causative agents include *Treponema pallidum* (Chapter 327), *Neisseria gonorrhoeae* (Chapter 307), *Chlamydia trachomatis* (Chapter 326), herpes simplex (Chapter 382), and HIV (Chapter 392). Other sexually transmitted pathogens are *Shigella* (Chapter 317), *Campylobacter jejuni* (Chapter 311), *Haemophilus ducreyi* (Chapter 309), *Calymmatobacterium granulomatis* (Chapter 324), *Entamoeba histolytica* (Chapter 360), *Giardia lamblia* (Chapter 359), and *Isospora belli* (Chapter 361).

The widely variable presentations range from asymptomatic to anal pain, pruritus, discharge, fever, cramps, and bloody diarrhea. Clinical suspicion followed by appropriate and specific testing is necessary to make the correct diagnosis, and clinicians should consider the possibility of simultaneous infections. Treatment addresses the specific infection.

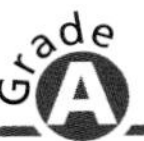

1. Alonso-Coello P, Mills E, Heels-Ansdell D, et al. Fiber for the treatment of hemorrhoids complications: a systematic review and meta-analysis. *Am J Gastroenterol*. 2006;101:181-188.
2. Jayaraman S, Colquhoun PH, Malthaner RA. Stapled versus conventional surgery for hemorrhoids. *Cochrane Database Syst Rev*. 2006.4.CD005393.
3. Nelson R. Nonsurgical therapy for anal fissure. *Cochrane Database Syst Rev*. 2006.4.CD003431.
4. Nelson RL. Operative procedures for fissure in ano. *Cochrane Database Syst Rev*. 2010.20.CD002199.
5. Richard CS, Gregoire R, Plewes EA, et al. Internal sphincterotomy is superior to topical nitroglycerin in the treatment of chronic anal fissure: results of a randomized, controlled trial by the Canadian Colorectal Surgical Trials Group. *Dis Colon Rectum*. 2000;43:1048-1057.
6. Brown CJ, Dubreuil D, Santoro L, et al. Lateral internal sphincterotomy is superior to topical nitroglycerin for healing chronic anal fissure and does not compromise long-term fecal continence: six-year follow-up of a multicenter, randomized, controlled trial. *Dis Colon Rectum*. 2007;50:442-448.
7. Graf W, Mellgren A, Matzel KE, et al. Efficacy of dextranomer in stabilised hyaluronic acid for treatment of faecal incontinence: a randomised, sham-controlled trial. *Lancet*. 2011;377:997-1003.

SUGGESTED READINGS

Balik SH, Gincherman M, Mutch MG, et al. Laparoscopic vs open resection for patients with rectal cancer: comparison of perioperative outcomes at long-term survival. *Dis Colon Rectum*. 2011;54:6-14. *Laparoscopic resection appears to be as good as open resection.*

Herzig DO, Lu KC. Anal fissure. *Surg Clin North Am*. 2010;90:33-44. *Review.*

Rao SS. Advances in diagnostic assessment of fecal incontinence and dyssynergic defecation. *Clin Gastroenterol Hepatol*. 2010;8:910-919. *Review.*

XIII

DISEASES OF THE LIVER, GALLBLADDER, AND BILE DUCTS

148

APPROACH TO THE PATIENT WITH LIVER DISEASE

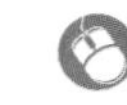

PAUL MARTIN

The liver has a variety of key functions, including metabolism of the products of ingested food, production of amino acids to form proteins, detoxification of ingested drugs, conversion of nitrogenous substances from the gut into urea for subsequent renal excretion, formation of clotting factors, metabolism of bilirubin, processing of lipids absorbed from the intestine, and excretion of its products as bile. The liver also stores glycogen, which is a source of glucose, and it has a role in containing bacterial infections by removing bacteria from the blood stream. These various functions are achieved by several types of liver cells, including hepatocytes, bile duct cells, and Kupffer cells.

The liver has a dual blood supply: 70% of its blood is delivered by the portal vein, which drains the intestine, and the remainder is from the hepatic artery. After delivery to the liver by the portal vein, nutrient-rich blood passes along the hepatic sinusoids in close contact with the hepatocytes that line them before draining into the hepatic vein. The hepatocytes detoxify, metabolize, and synthesize the products of digestion delivered to them. Bilirubin, the product of the breakdown of red cells and other hemoproteins, is produced by reticuloendothelial cells predominantly in the liver and spleen. Bilirubin is transported to the hepatocytes while bound to albumin; it is then solubilized by the hepatocytes for excretion into the bile ducts.

Clinical consequences of liver disease may reflect the loss of hepatocellular activity, with diminished detoxification, excretory, and synthetic functions. Interruption of bile flow may be caused by ineffective biliary excretion by diseased hepatocytes or by portal hypertension owing to disruption of portal blood flow through a diseased liver. Hepatocyte dysfunction results in diminished production of clotting factors, albumin, and other proteins, as well as the reduced endogenous formation of lipids. Hepatocyte injury from a variety of causes, including viruses, alcohol, autoimmune disorders, and drug hepatotoxicity, is accompanied by leakage of cellular enzymes into the systemic circulation (Chapter 149). Coagulopathy, decreased serum albumin, and hyperbilirubinemia are typical in more profound hepatocellular injury. Portal hypertension occurs because of disruption of the low-pressure intrahepatic blood flow from the portal to the systemic venous circulation, typically owing to fibrosis within the hepatic parenchyma. Consequences of portal hypertension include the accumulation of abdominal ascites and the development of portal-systemic venous collaterals with portal-systemic shunting, thereby resulting in the formation of varices and ultimately in hepatic encephalopathy. Vascular disorders, including portal vein thrombosis, can also result in portal hypertension.

Because of the diverse functions of the liver, its complicated blood supply, and its intimate relationship with the biliary tree, liver disease can present in a variety of ways. The presenting complaint often reflects whether the cause is diffuse, such as when acute viral hepatitis with widespread hepatocyte injury presents as malaise or fatigue, or discrete, such as when biliary obstruction from a gallstone in the common bile duct presents as severe abdominal pain. Patients with liver disease may present with multiple complaints, such as nausea and anorexia owing to hepatocellular disease accompanied by right upper quadrant discomfort due to stretching of the hepatic capsule by parenchymal cell edema and inflammation. Patients with more advanced liver disease, such as decompensated cirrhosis (Chapter 156), may have marked hepatocellular dysfunction with jaundice and coagulopathy in addition to portal hypertension with ascites and bleeding esophageal varices. Many patients who present with hepatic symptoms or signs may have extrahepatic disease; for example, a tender, swollen liver may be caused by a systemic disorder, such as heart failure with hepatic congestion, rather than a primary hepatic disorder. In cirrhotic patients, the initial presentation of previously undiagnosed liver disease may be a major complication such as variceal hemorrhage, which in turn can precipitate hepatic encephalopathy and other features of frank hepatic decompensation.

HISTORY

Patients with liver disorders come to medical attention for a number of reasons, ranging from the incidental discovery of abnormal liver chemistries to advanced cirrhosis. For patients with possible liver disease, however, a thorough history guides the appropriate diagnostic evaluation. Many complaints related to liver disease, such as fatigue, are nonspecific; unless liver disease is considered in the differential diagnosis, recognition of the hepatic origin of these complaints may be delayed.

In clinical practice, a frequent presentation of liver disease is an asymptomatic patient who is found to have abnormal liver biochemistries (Chapter 149) during a life insurance application, yearly physical examination, or attempt to donate blood. Such patients often have no prior history of liver disease, but it is important to inquire about past occasions when liver biochemistries may have been obtained to determine whether hepatic dysfunction is long-standing or more recent. In a patient with hepatic dysfunction, specific inquiries should be made about the presence of malaise, anorexia, fatigue, and weight change. Jaundice (Chapter 149) is the most typical manifestation of liver disease but is not specific. A patient may first notice lighter-colored stools or dark urine rather than scleral icterus. The absence of these changes suggests that unconjugated hyperbilirubinemia due to hemolysis may be the cause of jaundice rather than intrinsic liver disease. Not infrequently, a patient may be unaware of jaundice until it is noted by a family member or colleague.

Abdominal pain (Chapter 134) related to liver disease can have a variety of causes. Symptomatic gallstones (Chapter 158) can present with the abrupt onset of severe epigastric or right upper quadrant discomfort, often after a large meal and frequently associated with nausea and vomiting. The pain is often steady rather than colicky, and it can radiate widely, including to the chest and back. Patients may not be able to achieve a position that lessens the pain, which may last several hours. More persistent pain, particularly if associated with weight loss and jaundice, raises concern about malignant bile duct obstruction. Pain is also common in parenchymal liver disease in the absence of biliary tract disease. Many patients with chronic hepatocellular disorders, such as chronic hepatitis C (Chapter 151) or nonalcoholic fatty liver disease (Chapter 155), complain of vague right upper quadrant discomfort that has no particular relieving or aggravating factors. Abdominal pain, which can be severe, is also frequent in acute viral hepatitis (Chapter 150), as well as with the hepatic congestion that results from back pressure in heart failure or hepatic vein occlusion, as seen in Budd-Chiari syndrome (Chapter 145).

Fatigue, anorexia, and malaise can be present in both acute and chronic liver disease. In acute liver disorders such as acute viral hepatitis (Chapter 150), drug-induced liver disease (Chapter 152), or an acute presentation of autoimmune hepatitis (Chapter 151), patients may report profound fatigue, nausea, and malaise with decreased appetite and substantial associated weight loss. Distaste for cigarettes is said to be characteristic of acute viral hepatitis. Fatigue is also prominent in chronic liver disease such as chronic hepatitis C (Chapter 151). Pruritus is a prominent feature of cholestatic disorders, such as primary biliary cirrhosis, sclerosing cholangitis, or cholestatic drug reactions, particularly when patients are frankly icteric; however, pruritus also occurs in chronic parenchymal liver disease, most notably chronic hepatitis C, and in acute viral hepatitis. Easy bruisability in those with liver disease reflects coagulopathy and thrombocytopenia.

Fever in a patient with hepatic dysfunction is seen in the prodrome of acute hepatitis A, as well as in alcoholic hepatitis and drug-induced liver disease. In a patient with suspected biliary obstruction, fever suggests complicating bacterial cholangitis or acute cholecystitis.

Ascites is most frequently evidence of cirrhosis and portal hypertension in a patient with liver disease. Patients report increasing abdominal girth, which may be preceded by ankle edema. Weight gain owing to fluid retention may be masked by concomitant loss of muscle mass, and vice versa. The onset of ascites in the absence of a history of liver disease suggests a vascular event, such as hepatic vein occlusion (Chapter 145), or a nonhepatic cause of ascites, such as nephrotic syndrome or heart failure. Accumulation of ascites in a patient with liver disease may be subtle, with a slowly increasing waist circumference, or it may be more rapid, such as in a cirrhotic patient who receives fluid resuscitation following gastrointestinal bleeding. Although ascites in a patient with liver disease implies the presence of cirrhosis, ascites can also complicate severe acute liver disease, including alcoholic hepatitis and viral hepatitis, in which it suggests a poor prognosis.

Hepatic encephalopathy (Chapter 157), which is a neuropsychiatric disorder in patients with liver disease, can range from subtle cognitive impairment to deep coma. Early symptoms include a disturbed sleep pattern with nocturnal insomnia and daytime somnolence. More advanced encephalopathy can result in impairment of memory, confusion, and difficulty completing routine tasks. However, new-onset confusion or coma in a patient with liver disease should not be presumed to reflect hepatic encephalopathy unless other explanations, such as sedative overdose or subdural hematoma, have been ruled out. Important precipitants of hepatic encephalopathy in a cirrhotic patient include gastrointestinal bleeding, bacterial infection, and electrolyte imbalance, all of which need to be excluded during the initial clinical evaluation. In a patient with acute liver failure, coma owing to cerebral edema may be impossible to distinguish from advanced hepatic encephalopathy unless the increased intracranial pressure results in papilledema.

Gastrointestinal hemorrhage due to bleeding varices is usually profuse and often abrupt in onset. It classically presents with hematemesis or melena (Chapter 137), and coexisting postural hypotension and presyncope can reflect profound blood loss. The increased protein load in the gut can cause hepatic encephalopathy. Nonvariceal causes of gastrointestinal bleeding in a patient with liver disease include portal gastropathy (Chapter 137).

RISK FACTORS FOR LIVER DISEASE

An important aspect of the history is the identification of possible risk factors for liver disease. The history should include directed questioning about alcohol consumption, including frequency and pattern (Chapter 32). The age of initial alcohol use and whether its consumption has increased with age should be ascertained. Family members, if present, should also be asked about their perception of the patient's alcohol use and whether it has resulted in difficulties in personal relationships or work performance. Other clues to alcohol abuse are a history of convictions for driving under the influence of alcohol, motor vehicle accidents, and physical symptoms of alcohol dependence (Chapter 32). More circumspect questioning may be required to elicit a history of recreational drug use, especially given societal disapproval of this activity. Not infrequently, a patient with suspected viral hepatitis admits to smoking marijuana or snorting cocaine but does not acknowledge intravenous drug use. With the increasing frequency of nonalcoholic fatty liver disease as a cause of hepatic dysfunction (Chapter 155), the history should assess comorbid conditions such as diabetes mellitus, hyperlipidemia, or weight gain. Ingestion of medications, whether obtained by prescription or over the counter, must be assessed because drug-induced liver disease is an important cause of apparently cryptogenic hepatic dysfunction and is not limited to therapeutic drugs (Chapter 152). Increasingly, herbal and "natural" products (Chapter 38) are ingested for a variety of maladies, and patients may fail to disclose their use because they do not perceive these agents to have side effects or may sense that the physician does not endorse their use. As with alcohol, it is important to quantify the amount of medication ingested and over what period. The social history should also include details about recent travel and contact with individuals with viral hepatitis through intimate, household, or occupational contact. It is also important to ask about vigorous physical activity that can result in elevated aminotransferase levels of nonhepatic origin.

ASSESSING DURATION OF LIVER DISEASE

The differential diagnosis in a patient with liver disease is determined to a large extent by the presenting symptoms, such jaundice or ascites. In many patients, however, the timing of more subtle findings such as elevated aminotransferases is more difficult to determine. Prior blood test results should be retrieved to determine whether hepatic dysfunction is long-standing or more recent. Hepatic dysfunction of less than 6 months' duration is regarded as acute and is frequently self-limited, whereas abnormalities that persist for more than 6 months are chronic and unlikely to resolve spontaneously. If the patient has had a cholecystectomy, it is important to determine the indication; incidental gallstones are sometimes assumed to be the cause of hepatic abnormality in a patient with parenchymal liver disease, leading to unnecessary removal of the gallbladder. Thrombocytopenia owing to portal hypertension in a patient with unrecognized cirrhosis may have been investigated in the past without a firm conclusion being reached.

REVIEW OF OTHER ORGAN SYSTEMS

Despite the appropriate focus on liver-related symptoms, it is important not to overlook other clues, associated disorders, and complications. Sicca symptoms, including dry eyes and mouth, are common in primary biliary cirrhosis (Chapter 158); florid features of scleroderma and the CREST syndrome (Chapter 275) are also seen in association with this liver disease. Dyspnea in a patient with hepatic dysfunction may reflect cardiac failure with hepatic congestion (Chapter 58). Other explanations include the hepatopulmonary syndrome (Chapter 156), with the characteristic complaint of platypnea–dyspnea (often with chest tightness) that is worse in the upright position owing to aggravation of the ventilation-perfusion mismatch because of intrapulmonary shunting. The hepatopulmonary syndrome can also occur in association with cirrhosis (Chapter 156). A hydrothorax in decompensated cirrhosis can cause dyspnea, as can emphysema in patients with liver disease caused by α_1-antitrypsin deficiency (Chapter 153). A history of premature menopause is common in middle-aged women with cirrhosis, as is decreased libido and sexual potency in male cirrhotic patients. Arthralgias are often reported in viral hepatitis, and hemochromatosis (Chapter 219) may present with involvement of the proximal interphalangeal joints or chondrocalcinosis of the knees; increased skin pigmentation and diabetes mellitus are among other features of this disorder. Accelerated osteopenia occurs in many liver diseases, including primary cirrhosis, primary sclerosing cholangitis, and alcoholic cirrhosis; osteopenia may be aggravated by corticosteroid use in autoimmune chronic active hepatitis. Alcoholic peripheral neuropathy (Chapter 428) can present with pain as well as paresthesia. Tremor and inattentiveness in a younger patient with hepatic dysfunction suggests Wilson disease (Chapter 218). Diarrhea and rectal bleeding in a patient with cholestatic liver disease suggests associated inflammatory bowel disease (Chapter 143).

FAMILY HISTORY

The family history should inquire not only about relatives with liver disease but also about extrahepatic conditions associated with liver disease. Hereditary hepatic conditions, such as Wilson disease and hemochromatosis, may occur in several members of a sibship (Chapter 153). In α_1-antitrypsin deficiency, some family members may experience predominantly emphysema or cirrhosis of unclear cause (Chapter 153). Similarly, renal failure in a family member of a patient with hepatic cysts suggests adult polycystic disease (Chapter 129). A family history of inflammatory bowel disease may be a clue to primary sclerosing cholangitis in a patient with cholestatic liver chemistries. The family history in patients with suspected alcoholic liver disease may reveal other family members with alcoholism.

PHYSICAL EXAMINATION

General Condition

In a patient with suspected liver disease, it is crucial to resist the temptation to palpate the abdomen immediately and ignore other important clues to liver disease as a result. Apart from noting icterus, the initial observation should determine whether muscle wasting, cutaneous stigmata of liver disease, abdominal distention, and peripheral edema are present. The vital signs may reflect the hyperdynamic circulation characteristic of cirrhosis, with a resting tachycardia, wide pulse pressure, and low blood pressure due to peripheral vasodilation. Fetor hepaticus, which is described as a musty smell, may be detected when a cirrhotic patient exhales and must be distinguished from the more frequent halitosis due to poor dental hygiene.

Mucocutaneous Findings

Icterus (Fig. 148-1) is best confirmed by examination of the sclera or, if necessary, under the tongue, where elastin tissue retains bilirubin. Grayish skin discoloration in hemochromatosis may be most evident in the skin folds in

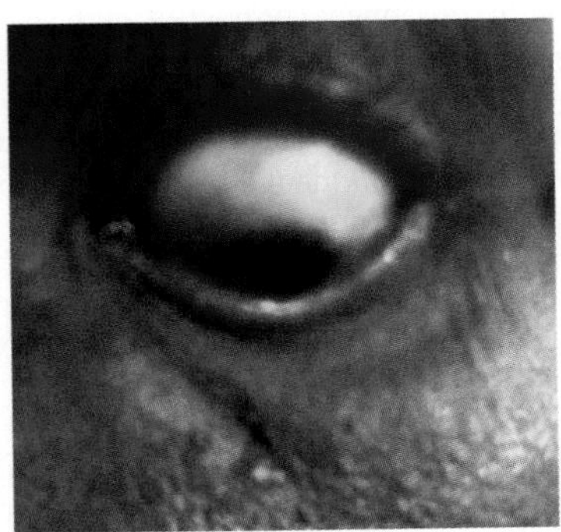

FIGURE 148-1. Scleral icterus.

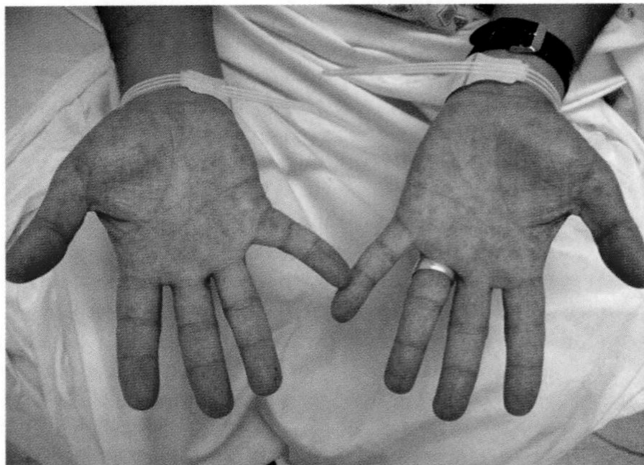

FIGURE 148-2. Palmar erythema.

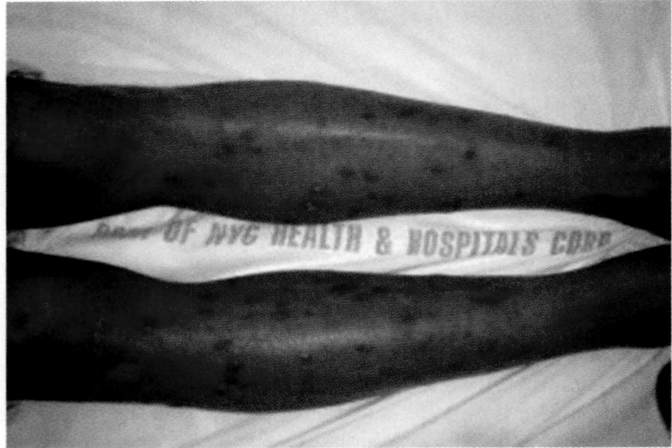

FIGURE 148-3. Prurigo nodularis.

the groin or axilla. A Kayser-Fleischer ring (see Fig. 218-1 in Chapter 218), caused by the deposition of copper in Descemet's membrane, is a brownish circle around the periphery of the iris and may require slit lamp examination to detect; it should always be sought in a patient with suspected Wilson disease (Chapter 218). Poor dentition is characteristic in alcoholic or drug-abusing individuals, and excessive dental caries may result from decreased saliva production in the sicca syndrome. Parotid gland swelling is occasionally observed in alcoholic patients. Central cyanosis and clubbing are found in the hepatopulmonary syndrome. Temporal muscle wasting and "paper money" facial skin, owing to atrophy with telangiectasia, are signs of advanced liver disease. Xanthelasma from lipid deposits may be observed on the eyelids and skin around the orbits in patients with cholestatic liver disease. Spider nevi on the face and thorax are not pathognomonic of liver disease, especially in women, but they are suggestive if more than a few are present. Palmar erythema (Fig. 148-2) may be normal in women but suggests liver disease in men. Dupuytren's contracture (see Fig. 155-1 in Chapter 155), the retraction of the palmar fascia with subsequent contracture of the palms and fingers, can be a sign of alcoholic liver disease, although it is also described in persons with epilepsy or diabetes mellitus. Petechiae and ecchymoses reflect impaired production of clotting factors and hypersplenism in advanced liver disease. Patches of white discoloration on the nails may be present in advanced liver disease. Scratch marks from pruritus may be observed on the trunk and extremities of patients with cholestatic liver disease (Fig. 148-3); sparing of the center of the back can lead to a less pigmented butterfly-shaped area, presumably because patients cannot reach that area with their fingernails.

Examination of the Abdomen

Abdominal distention and dilation of collateral veins are the most florid visible signs of advanced liver disease with ascites and portal hypertension. Caput medusae (Fig. 148-4) in the periumbilical area implies recanalization of the umbilical vein due to portal hypertension.

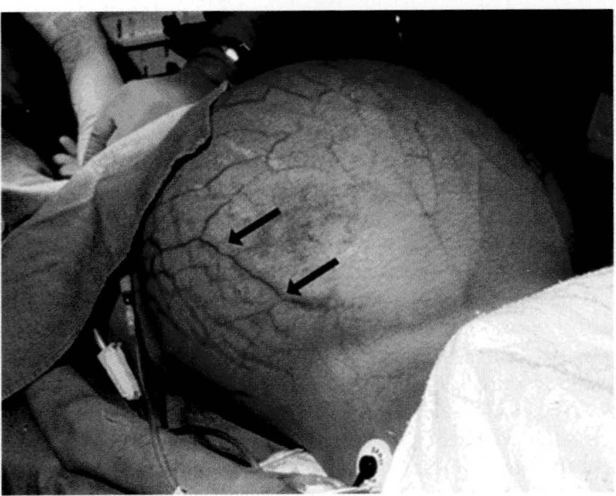

FIGURE 148-4. Caput medusae. Photograph shows a caput medusae accentuated by a large amount of ascites in a patient being prepared for liver transplantation. An extensive plexus of veins is seen emanating from the umbilical region and radiating across the anterior abdominal wall. Note the large vein coursing inferiorly along the right flank *(arrows)*. This is the superficial epigastric vein, which drains into the external iliac vein. (From Henseler KP, Pozniak MA, Le FT, et al. Three dimensional CT angiography of spontaneous portosystemic shunts. *Radiographics.* 2001;21:691-704.)

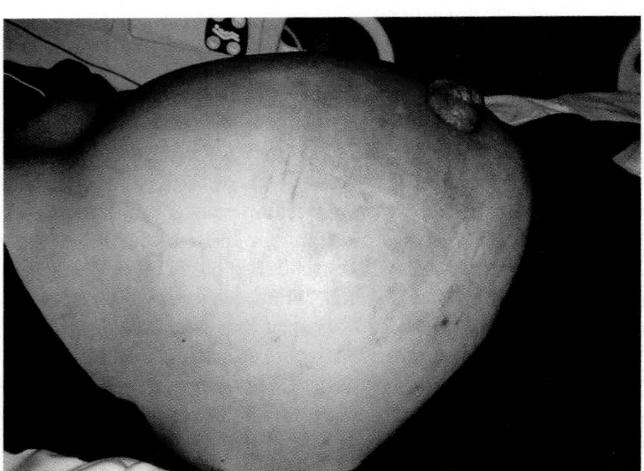

FIGURE 148-5. Ascites.

The presence of ascites (Fig. 148-5) can be assessed by percussion of the abdomen and the detection of shifting dullness or a fluid wave. Shifting dullness results from movement of the fluid to the most dependent portion of the abdomen. The subject should be examined in the supine position, and the abdomen should be percussed from the midline toward the right or left flank. A change from a tympanic sound to a dull sound signifies a change from air to fluid, and the location of that change identifies the surface of the fluid pool. Next, the examiner should percuss below the point at which dullness is elicited and ask the subject to turn toward the examiner. With the subject on his or her side, the examiner percusses again at the same point where tympany converted to dullness. If that spot is now tympanic, shifting dullness has been detected as a result of movement of the air-fluid boundary; this finding supports the presence of ascites. This maneuver should be performed sequentially on each side for confirmation. A fluid wave can be felt by placing the medial border of one hand on the abdomen and tapping the right or left lateral abdominal walls; the resulting wave is felt by the first hand. Scrotal edema and abdominal wall hernias are often present in patients with long-standing ascites. Abdominal tenderness in a patient with ascites suggests peritonitis (e.g., spontaneous bacterial peritonitis or due to a perforated viscus). However, it is important to note that abdominal tenderness is frequently absent, even with spontaneous bacterial peritonitis.

The liver is dull to percussion. Percussion of the right upper quadrant can assess the liver span, which is normally 6 to 12 cm in the midclavicular line. The liver span may be diminished in a patient with cirrhosis, whereas hepatomegaly (Fig. 148-6) is detected in hepatic congestion due to heart failure,

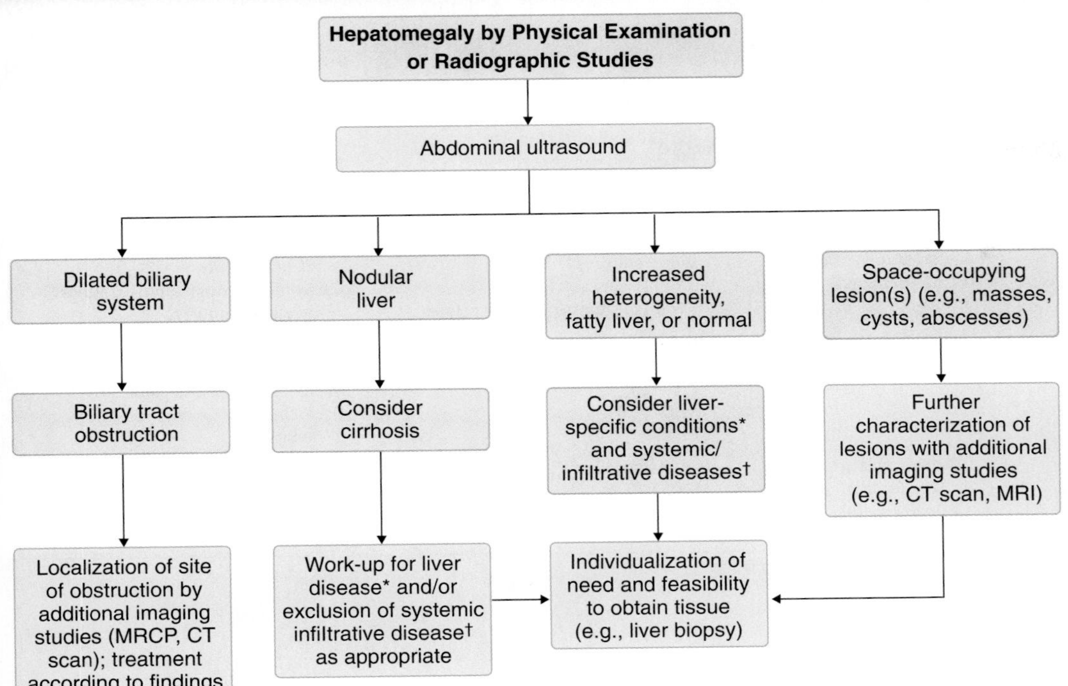

FIGURE 148-6. Diagnostic approach to hepatomegaly. *Conditions to be excluded include viral hepatitis, alcohol- and drug-induced liver disease, steatohepatitis, autoimmune liver diseases, and metabolic disorders, including hemochromatosis, Wilson disease, and α_1-antitrypsin deficiency. †Systemic and infiltrative diseases include amyloidosis, lymphoma, sarcoidosis, and infectious processes such as disseminated tuberculosis and fungemia. CT = computed tomography; MRCP = magnetic resonance cholangiopancreatography; MRI = magnetic resonance imaging.

nonalcoholic fatty liver disease, and cholestatic forms of cirrhosis. The liver is best examined with the patient in the supine position, arms parallel to the sides of the body, and knees bent to relax the abdominal muscles. To assess the liver, palpation should begin in the right lower quadrant of the abdomen and move upward toward the rib cage so that the liver edge is felt on the way up. A normal liver edge is smooth and sometimes slightly tender when palpated. In general, a liver edge that is felt up to 2 cm below the right costal margin is considered normal, but a normal-sized liver can be displaced downward by other abnormalities, such as emphysema. In thin subjects, the liver edge may be felt on deep inspiration, even if it is normal in size.

The liver can feel hard and irregular, as in cirrhosis, or slightly tender, enlarged, and smooth, as in acute viral hepatitis or hepatic congestion. The liver can extend across the midline, and the left lobe can be felt in the epigastrium. When the location of the edge of the liver is uncertain, the scratch test may be helpful. It is performed by placing the bell of the stethoscope on the right upper quadrant over the rib cage and scratching the surface of the abdominal wall from the midabdomen toward the liver; the sound of the scratch is amplified in an area under which the liver lies. In the presence of ascites, the liver edge may be detected by exerting quick pressure with the fingertips below the rib cage.

A palpable gallbladder suggests obstruction of the biliary system, whereas tenderness elicited by palpation during inspiration (Murphy's sign) suggests acute cholecystitis. Marked hepatic tenderness with hepatomegaly is observed in patients with a hepatic abscess (Chapter 154).

Splenomegaly may be suggested by dullness to percussion between the 9th and 11th ribs in the left midaxillary line. A palpable spleen tip is highly suggestive of portal hypertension in a patient with chronic liver disease, although an enlarged spleen can also be detected in acute viral hepatitis and infiltrative disorders that involve both the liver and the spleen (see Table 171-7 in Chapter 171). Rectal examination is obligatory if gastrointestinal bleeding is suspected because of melena, anemia, or unexplained hepatic encephalopathy.

Complete Physical Examination

The presence of rales and elevation of the jugular venous pressure suggest heart failure or pericardial disease as a cause of hepatic congestion. Loss of secondary sexual characteristics in liver disease is reflected by a loss of axillary and pubic hair, as well as feminization of body habitus in a male patient. Testicular atrophy may also be present. Peripheral edema is common in decompensated cirrhosis and may occur before ascites is obvious.

Neuropsychiatric alterations can include subtle changes in personality or more overt hepatic encephalopathy. Constructional apraxia (e.g., inability to draw a five-pointed star or to write legibly) in a fully conscious patient is a typical finding of hepatic encephalopathy. Asterixis, which is characterized by a series of extensor and flexor wrist movements, can be elicited by having the patient extend the arms, with dorsiflexion of the wrists, while separating the fingers for at least 15 seconds. Tremors (Chapter 417) are nonspecific but are also common in advanced cirrhosis.

DIAGNOSTIC STUDIES (TABLE 148-1)

Laboratory Studies

The initial evaluation for suspected liver disease involves a battery of blood tests that reflect hepatic necroinflammation (serum aminotransferases), cholestatic biliary tract dysfunction (alkaline phosphatase, γ-glutamyl transpeptidase), excretory function (bilirubin), and synthetic function (coagulation factors, albumin) (Chapter 149). In hepatocellular dysfunction caused by viral hepatitis (Chapter 150), the aminotransferase levels are elevated, with the serum alanine aminotransferase (ALT) level higher than the aspartate aminotransferase (AST) level. In alcoholic hepatitis (Chapter 155), AST elevation exceeds ALT elevation. In patients with biliary obstruction or cholestatic liver diseases (Chapter 158), such as primary biliary cirrhosis or a cholestatic drug reaction, the bilirubin and generally the alkaline phosphatase levels are elevated. Impairment of synthetic function, such as from cirrhosis or severe acute viral hepatitis, can lead to a low serum albumin level over days to weeks. The prothrombin time, expressed as the international normalized ratio (INR), is a more sensitive test of hepatic synthetic function and becomes prolonged within several hours after a major hepatic insult. Portal hypertension owing to advanced hepatic fibrosis or cirrhosis results in a decreased platelet count due to hypersplenism. Although these general patterns of liver dysfunction are helpful in the initial evaluation of liver disease, they are nonspecific. For example, a patient with a predominantly hepatocellular process commonly has elevated bilirubin and alkaline phosphatase levels and a low serum albumin level if the injury is severe. Nevertheless, these blood tests should identify the predominant pattern of abnormality and help focus further diagnostic evaluation with serologies and abdominal imaging.

Abdominal Imaging

Plain abdominal radiographs generally do not have a major role in the evaluation of suspected liver disease. An exception is a patient with severe abdominal pain in whom it is important to exclude a perforated viscus with free air under the diaphragm.

Ultrasonography should be the initial investigation in patients with obstructive jaundice. It can confirm dilated bile ducts in patients with biliary obstruction and can often identify the cause, such as a pancreatic mass or a

TABLE 148-1 APPROACH TO COMMON HEPATIC COMPLAINTS

PRESENTATION	COMMON SYMPTOMS	COMMON PHYSICAL SIGNS	DIAGNOSTIC STUDIES	COMMON DIAGNOSES
Ascites	Abdominal distention and pain, ankle edema	Flank dullness Shifting dullness Fluid wave	Ultrasound with Doppler Diagnostic paracentesis Urinalysis	Cirrhosis Budd-Chiari syndrome Heart failure Nephrotic syndrome
Hepatic encephalopathy	Sleep disorientation, confusion, coma	Asterixis Altered mentation Fetor hepaticus	Serum ammonia Blood cultures Stool Hemoccult Serum creatinine and electrolytes	Decompensated cirrhosis Acute liver failure Other metabolic encephalopathies (renal, respiratory)
Hepatic mass	None or abdominal pain	Hepatic bruit or rub	α-Fetoprotein Ultrasound CT scan MRI Biopsy	Benign lesions: hemangioma, adenoma, focal nodular hyperplasia Malignant lesions: hepatocellular carcinoma, cholangiocarcinoma, metastases
Abdominal pain	Nausea, vomiting, fever	Right upper quadrant tenderness Palpable gallbladder Murphy's sign	Ultrasound HIDA scan Paracentesis for ascites if present	Biliary colic Acute cholecystitis Hepatic congestion Hepatic metastases

CT = computed tomography; HIDA = hepatobiliary iminodiacetic acid; MRI = magnetic resonance imaging.

gallstone lodged in the common bile duct. Ultrasonography can also determine whether the hepatic parenchyma is diffusely abnormal, such as in a patient with acute viral hepatitis; it can identify bright hepatic echo texture in a patient with nonalcoholic fatty liver disease; or it can show a coarsened echo texture in cirrhosis. In addition to confirming the presence of ascites, ultrasonography can identify other signs of portal hypertension, such as splenomegaly or intra-abdominal varices. Blood flow through the portal and hepatic vessels can be assessed by adding a Doppler flow study. An ultrasound study can identify hepatic masses and distinguish a cystic mass from a solid lesion. Computed tomography (CT) and magnetic resonance imaging (MRI) add greater detail to the assessment of the hepatic vasculature, hepatic masses, and hepatic vascular structures. MRI can also obtain a very detailed cholangiogram (see Fig. 202-3 in Chapter 202), thereby avoiding the more invasive endoscopic retrograde cholangiopancreatography in many patients with suspected bile duct obstruction or disease (Chapters 135 and 136).

Liver biopsy remains the definitive test to assess the severity of hepatic inflammation and the extent of fibrosis in diffuse hepatocellular disease. In addition, it can confirm diagnoses suspected by noninvasive testing, such as autoimmune hepatitis, or it can suggest diagnoses, such as drug hepatotoxicity. Because of its potential complications, such as intra-abdominal bleeding, biopsy is recommended only when less invasive testing has not yielded a definitive diagnosis or prognosis or when additional information, such as quantitative determination of hepatic copper in Wilson disease or hepatic iron in hemochromatosis, is necessary for definitive diagnosis.

Transjugular pressure measurements are indicated in patients with atypical presentations of portal hypertension (e.g., when it is unclear whether liver disease is the cause) or to titrate medications to reduce portal pressure. A catheter is advanced under fluoroscopy into the hepatic vein, and the free hepatic venous pressure is measured. The catheter is then advanced farther until it becomes "wedged" in a small hepatic vein venule. The venule is occluded by a small balloon, and the wedged hepatic vein pressure, which reflects hepatic sinusoidal pressure, is obtained. The portal pressure gradient, which is derived by subtracting the free pressure measurement from the wedged pressure measurement, is normally less than 5 mm Hg. Varices form at a gradient above 10 mm Hg, whereas ascites and variceal hemorrhage occur only when the gradient exceeds 12 mm Hg. A transjugular approach also increases the safety of liver biopsy in the presence of ascites, coagulopathy, or thrombocytopenia when standard percutaneous liver biopsy is hazardous. Endoscopy is indicated to screen for varices in any patient suspected of having cirrhosis to determine the need for prophylaxis against hemorrhage.

SUGGESTED READING

Mutter D, Soler L, Marescaux J. Recent advances in liver imaging. *Expert Rev Gastroenterol Hepatol.* 2010;4:613-621. *Review.*

149

APPROACH TO THE PATIENT WITH JAUNDICE OR ABNORMAL LIVER TESTS

PAUL BERK AND KEVIN KORENBLAT

JAUNDICE

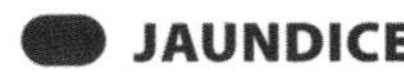

DEFINITION

Jaundice, from the French *jaune* (yellow), is the yellow-orange discoloration of the skin, conjunctivae, and mucous membranes that results from elevated concentrations of bilirubin in plasma. Mild hyperbilirubinemia may be clinically undetectable, but jaundice becomes evident at plasma bilirubin concentrations of 3 to 4 mg/dL, depending on the patient's normal pigmentation, the conditions of observation, and the bilirubin fraction that is elevated. Optimal interpretation of an elevated plasma bilirubin concentration is based on an appreciation of its sources and disposition.

Bilirubin Metabolism

Bilirubin Production

Bilirubin is the degradation product of the heme moiety of hemoproteins, a class of proteins involved in the transport or metabolism of oxygen (Fig. 149-1). Normal adults produce about 4 mg of bilirubin per kilogram of body weight per day. Between 70 and 90% of bilirubin is derived from the hemoglobin of erythrocytes, which in turn are sequestered and destroyed by the mononuclear phagocytic cells of the reticuloendothelial system, principally in the spleen, liver, and bone marrow. A minor fraction reflects ineffective erythropoiesis, the premature destruction of newly formed erythrocytes within the bone marrow. The remainder results primarily from the turnover of nonhemoglobin hemoproteins such as myoglobin, the P-450 cytochromes, catalase, and peroxidase. Although this occurs principally in the liver, bilirubin has proved to have antioxidant properties, and recent studies suggest that a limited, regulated production of bilirubin from heme may occur in many cell types and contribute to regulating the intracellular antioxidant environment.

The two-step conversion of heme to bilirubin commences with the opening of the heme molecule at its α bridge carbon by the microsomal enzyme *heme oxygenase*, a process that results in the formation of equimolar quantities of carbon monoxide and the green tetrapyrrole biliverdin, the main excretory product of heme in birds, reptiles, and amphibians. Because biliverdin cannot

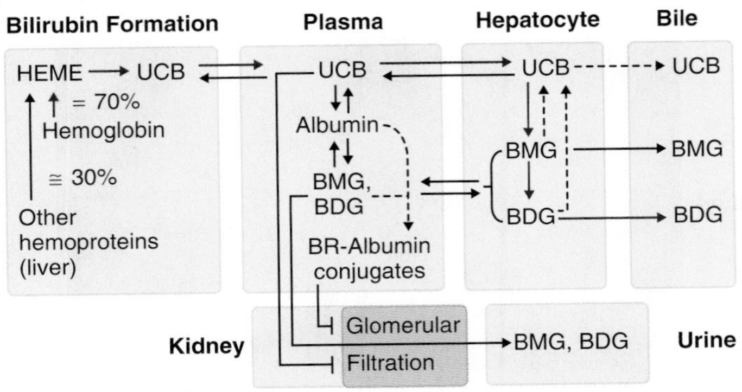

FIGURE 149-1. Overview of bilirubin metabolism. Unconjugated bilirubin (UCB) formed from the breakdown of heme from hemoglobin and other hemoproteins is transported in plasma reversibly bound to albumin and is converted in the liver to bilirubin monoglucuronide (BMG) and diglucuronide (BDG), the latter being the predominant form secreted in bile. BMG and BDG together normally account for less than 5% of normal serum bilirubin. In patients with hepatobiliary disease, BMG and BDG accumulate in plasma and appear in urine. Bilirubin glucuronides in plasma also react nonenzymatically with albumin and possibly other serum proteins to form protein conjugates, which do not appear in urine and have a plasma half-life similar to that of albumin. BR = bilirubin.

cross the placenta, its reduction to bilirubin in mammals by a second enzyme, *biliverdin reductase*, allows its transplacental removal from the fetus into the maternal circulation. The unconjugated bilirubin produced in the periphery is transported to the liver in plasma. Because of its insolubility in aqueous media, it is kept in solution by tight but reversible binding to albumin. A number of compounds, including sulfonamides, furosemide, and radiographic contrast agents, competitively displace bilirubin from its binding sites on albumin, a phenomenon of little clinical significance except in neonates, in whom the resulting increased concentration of unbound bilirubin raises the risk of kernicterus.

Disposition of Bilirubin by the Liver

Bilirubin excretion from the body is a major function of the liver (see Fig. 149-1), wherein specialized microanatomy enhances extraction of tightly protein-bound compounds from the circulation. Hepatic translocation of bilirubin from blood to bile involves four distinct steps: (1) uptake of unconjugated bilirubin, by both an incompletely characterized facilitated transport process and by diffusion; (2) intracellular binding, mainly to various cytosolic proteins of the glutathione-*S*-transferase family; (3) conversion of unconjugated bilirubin to bilirubin monoglucuronides and diglucuronides by a specific uridine diphosphate (UDP)-glucuronosyltransferase isoform designated UGT1A1; and (4) transfer of bilirubin monoglucuronides and diglucuronides into bile by a canalicular membrane adenosine triphosphate (ATP)-dependent transporter designated multidrug resistance–associated protein 2 (MRP2) or canalicular multispecific organic anion transporter (cMOAT). MRP2/cMOAT is a member of the *MRP* gene family, other members of which pump certain drug conjugates, as well as unmodified anticancer drugs, out of cells.

Conjugation to bilirubin monoglucuronides and diglucuronides greatly increases the aqueous solubility of bilirubin and thereby enhances its elimination from the body while simultaneously reducing its ability to diffuse across biologic membranes, including the blood-brain barrier. In newborns, a decreased capacity to conjugate bilirubin leads to unconjugated hyperbilirubinemia (physiologic jaundice of the newborn). If severe, this hyperbilirubinemia may lead to irreversible central nervous system toxicity. Phototherapy by exposure to blue light converts bilirubin to water-soluble photoisomers that are readily excreted in bile, protecting the central nervous system from bilirubin toxicity. Gilbert's syndrome and Crigler-Najjar syndrome types 1 and 2, which result from genetic defects in bilirubin conjugation, are characterized by unconjugated hyperbilirubinemia; in contrast, Dubin-Johnson syndrome, which results from inheritable defects in MRP2/cMOAT (see later), is characterized by conjugated or mixed hyperbilirubinemia.

Enterohepatic Circulation and Excretion of Bilirubin

Bilirubin in Bile

Normal bile contains an average of less than 5% unconjugated bilirubin, 7% bilirubin monoconjugates, and 90% bilirubin diconjugates. The proportion of monoconjugates increases with an increased bilirubin load (hemolysis) or defective conjugation (e.g., Gilbert's and Crigler-Najjar type 2 syndromes). After canalicular secretion, conjugated bilirubin passes down the gastrointestinal tract without reabsorption by either the gallbladder or intestinal mucosa.

Urobilinogen and the Enterohepatic Circulation

Although some bilirubin reaches the feces, most is converted to urobilinogen and related compounds by bacteria within the ileum and colon, where the urobilinogen is reabsorbed, returns to the liver through the portal circulation, and is re-excreted into bile in a process of enterohepatic recirculation. Any urobilinogen not taken up by the liver reaches the systemic circulation and is cleared by the kidneys. Normal urine urobilinogen excretion is 4 mg/day or less. With hemolysis, which increases the load of bilirubin entering the gut and therefore the amount of urobilinogen formed and reabsorbed, or with liver disease, which decreases its hepatic extraction, plasma urobilinogen levels rise, and more urobilinogen is excreted in the urine. Severe cholestasis, bile duct obstruction, or broad-spectrum antibiotics that reduce or eliminate bacterial conversion of bilirubin to urobilinogen markedly decrease the formation and urinary excretion of urobilinogen.

Unconjugated bilirubin ordinarily does not reach the gut except in neonates or by ill-defined alternative pathways in the presence of severe unconjugated hyperbilirubinemia (e.g., Crigler-Najjar type 1). In these circumstances, unconjugated bilirubin is reabsorbed from the gut, thereby amplifying the hyperbilirubinemia.

Measurement of Bilirubin in Plasma

The total plasma bilirubin concentration in normal adults is less than 1 to 1.5 mg/dL, depending on the measurement method used. Modern analytic techniques show that normal plasma contains principally unconjugated bilirubin, with only traces of conjugates. Clinical laboratories typically quantify plasma bilirubin by a reaction in which bilirubin is cleaved by a diazo reagent, such as diazotized sulfanilic acid, to azodipyrroles that are quantitated spectrophotometrically. Bilirubin conjugates react rapidly ("prompt" or "direct"-reacting bilirubin). Unconjugated bilirubin reacts slowly because the site of attack by the diazo reagent is protected by internal hydrogen bonding. Accordingly, accurate measurement of the total plasma bilirubin concentration requires addition of an accelerator, such as ethanol or urea, to disrupt this internal bonding and to ensure complete reaction of any unconjugated bilirubin. The "indirect"-reacting bilirubin is calculated by subtracting the direct-reacting bilirubin from the total. Although physicians traditionally equate the direct-reacting fraction of bilirubin in plasma with conjugated bilirubin and the indirect fraction with unconjugated bilirubin, this approach is, at best, a rough approximation, and the unqualified interpretation of direct and indirect fractions as reflecting conjugated and unconjugated bilirubin, respectively, may lead to diagnostic errors, particularly in the diagnosis of hereditary hyperbilirubinemias. In practice, 10 to 20% of bilirubin in normal plasma gives a prompt (direct) diazo reaction even though more than 95% of total bilirubin in normal plasma is unconjugated. Thus, at virtually any total bilirubin concentration, a direct-reacting fraction of less than 15% of the total can be considered as essentially all unconjugated. When the direct-reacting fraction is greater than 15%, a simple dipstick test for bilirubinuria may clarify the situation. Unconjugated bilirubin is not excreted in urine regardless of the height of its plasma concentration because its binding to albumin is too tight for effective glomerular filtration and it is not secreted by the tubules. The canalicular transport mechanism for excretion of bilirubin conjugates is especially sensitive to injury. Accordingly, in parenchymal liver disease or mechanical bile duct obstruction, bilirubin conjugates within the hepatocyte or biliary tract may reflux into the blood stream, resulting in a mixed or, less often, a purely conjugated hyperbilirubinemia. Conjugated bilirubin, which is normally loosely bound to albumin, is readily filtered at the glomerulus; even modest degrees of conjugated hyperbilirubinemia result in bilirubinuria, which is *always* a pathologic finding. With prolonged conjugated hyperbilirubinemia, some of the conjugated bilirubin binds *covalently* to albumin and produces what is designated the delta (δ) bilirubin fraction. Although δ -bilirubin gives a direct diazo reaction, it is not filterable by the glomerulus and does not appear in the urine; it disappears slowly from the plasma, with the 14- to 21-day half-life of the albumin to which it is bound. δ-Bilirubin accounts for the sometimes slow rate at which conjugated (direct) hyperbilirubinemia resolves as hepatitis improves or biliary obstruction is relieved. Although δ-bilirubin is not easily measured, its presence can be inferred when an elevated direct-reacting bilirubin persists after bilirubinuria resolves.

Bilirubin Kinetics

The plasma disappearance kinetics of radiolabeled bilirubin indicate that the plasma unconjugated bilirubin concentration ([UCB]) reflects a balance between the bilirubin production rate (BRP) and hepatic bilirubin clearance (C_{BR}) according to the relationship:

$$[UCB] \approx BRP/C_{BR}$$

C_{BR} is analogous to the creatinine clearance in the test of kidney function; it is a measure of the rate at which bilirubin is extracted from plasma, and is a true quantitative test of liver function. Whereas BRP and C_{BR} are not easily quantified in clinical settings, investigative measurements have yielded useful pathophysiologic insights. This equation indicates that [UCB] increases linearly with an increase in BRP or hyperbolically with a decrease in C_{BR}, thereby providing a basis for classifying unconjugated hyperbilirubinemias according to their pathogenesis.

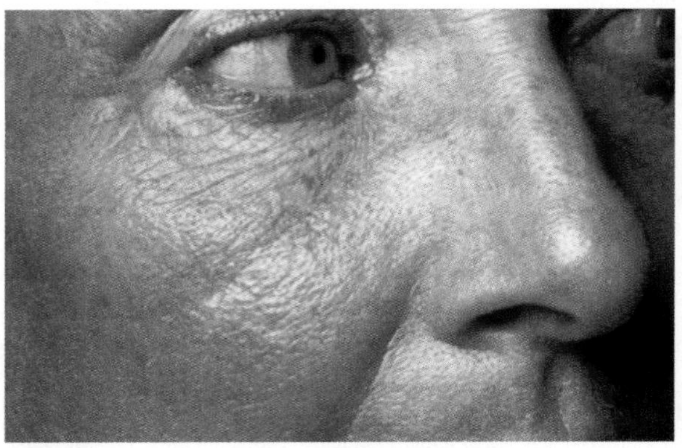

FIGURE 149-2. **Severe cholestatic jaundice in a patient with primary biliary cirrhosis.** The high level of conjugated bilirubin, maintained over a long period, gives a characteristic dark brown-orange pigmentation to the skin and sclerae. Patients with primary biliary cirrhosis usually develop large xanthelasmas and corneal arcus as a consequence of disordered lipid metabolism. (From Forbes CD, Jackson WF. *Color Atlas and Text of Clinical Medicine*, 3rd ed. London: Mosby; 2003.)

APPROACH TO THE PATIENT WITH HYPERBILIRUBINEMIA

Hyperbilirubinemia and jaundice (Fig. 149-2) may result from isolated disorders of bilirubin metabolism, liver disease, or obstruction of the biliary tract. Jaundice represents the most visible sign of hepatobiliary disease of many causes (Table 149-1).

TABLE 149-1 DIFFERENTIAL DIAGNOSIS OF HYPERBILIRUBINEMIA AND JAUNDICE

ISOLATED DISORDERS OF BILIRUBIN METABOLISM
Unconjugated hyperbilirubinemia
Increased bilirubin production
Examples: hemolysis, ineffective erythropoiesis, blood transfusion, resorption of hematomas
Decreased hepatocellular uptake
Examples: drugs (e.g., rifampin)
Decreased conjugation
Examples: Gilbert's and Crigler-Najjar syndromes, physiologic jaundice of the newborn, breast milk jaundice, HIV protease inhibitors
Conjugated or mixed hyperbilirubinemia
Decreased canalicular transport: Dubin-Johnson syndrome
Mechanism uncertain: Rotor's syndrome
LIVER DISEASE
Acute or chronic hepatocellular dysfunction
Acute or subacute hepatocellular injury
Examples: viral hepatitis A, B, and C, hepatotoxins (e.g., ethanol, acetaminophen, mushroom [*Amanita phalloides*] poisoning), drugs (e.g., isoniazid, α-methyldopa), metabolic diseases (e.g., Wilson's disease, Reye's syndrome), pregnancy-related (e.g., acute fatty liver of pregnancy, preeclampsia), hepatic ischemia (e.g., hypotension, postoperative, hepatic artery thrombosis)
Chronic hepatocellular disease
Examples: hepatitis B and C, hepatotoxins (e.g., vinyl chloride, vitamin A), nonalcoholic and alcoholic fatty liver disease, autoimmune hepatitis, metabolic disease (Wilson's disease, hemochromatosis, α_1-antitrypsin deficiency)
Hepatic disorders with prominent cholestasis
Familial cholestatic disorders
Single-gene disorders
Examples: benign recurrent intrahepatic cholestasis types 1-3; progressive familial intrahepatic cholestasis types 1-3
Familial cholestatic disorders of unknown pathogenesis
Examples: Aagenaes syndrome, Navajo neurohepatopathy, North American Indian cholestasis
Diffuse infiltrative disorders
Examples: granulomatous diseases (e.g., mycobacterial and fungal infections, sarcoidosis, lymphoma, drugs, Wegener's granulomatosis), amyloidosis, infiltrative malignancies
Inflammation of intrahepatic bile ductules and/or portal tracts
Examples: primary biliary cirrhosis, liver allograft rejection, graft-versus-host disease, drugs (e.g., chlorpromazine, erythromycin)
Miscellaneous conditions
Examples: uncommon presentations of viral or alcoholic hepatitis, intrahepatic cholestasis of pregnancy, contraceptive jaundice, estrogens, anabolic steroids, postoperative cholestasis, cholestasis of sepsis, total parenteral nutrition, bacterial infections, drugs
OBSTRUCTION OF THE BILE DUCTS
Choledocholithiasis
Examples: cholesterol gallstones, pigment gallstones
Diseases of the bile ducts
Inflammation/infection
Examples: primary sclerosing cholangitis, AIDS cholangiopathy, hepatic arterial chemotherapy, postsurgical strictures
Neoplasms (e.g., cholangiocarcinoma)
Extrinsic compression of the biliary tree
Neoplasms
Examples: pancreatic carcinoma, metastatic lymphadenopathy, hepatoma
Pancreatitis with or without pseudocyst formation
Vascular enlargement (e.g., aneurysm, cavernous transformation of portal vein)

AIDS = acquired immunodeficiency syndrome; HIV = human immunodeficiency syndrome.

DISORDERS OF BILIRUBIN METABOLISM

Hyperbilirubinemia in the absence of hepatocellular dysfunction (pure hyperbilirubinemia) may result from either increased bilirubin production or inherited or acquired defects in specific aspects of hepatic bilirubin disposition.

Increased Bilirubin Production

Increased bilirubin production and consequent unconjugated hyperbilirubinemia can be caused by hemolysis, accelerated destruction of transfused erythrocytes, resorption of hematomas, or ineffective erythropoiesis (e.g., lead poisoning, megaloblastic anemias related to deficiency of either folic acid or vitamin B_{12}, sideroblastic anemia, congenital erythropoietic porphyria, or myeloproliferative or myelodysplastic diseases). In these settings, other liver tests are typically normal and the hyperbilirubinemia is modest, rarely exceeding 4 mg/dL; higher values imply concomitant hepatic dysfunction. However, following brisk blood transfusion or resorption of massive hematomas, the increased bilirubin load may be transiently sufficient to lead to frank jaundice. The causes of hemolysis are numerous (Chapters 163 to 166). Besides specific blood disorders, mild hemolysis accompanies many acquired diseases. In the setting of systemic disease, which may include a degree of hepatic dysfunction, hemolysis may produce a component of conjugated hyperbilirubinemia in addition to an elevated unconjugated bilirubin concentration. Prolonged hemolysis may lead to the formation of bilirubin gallstones, which may cause cholecystitis, obstruction, or any other biliary tract consequence of calculous disease.

Decreased Hepatic Bilirubin Clearance

DECREASED BILIRUBIN UPTAKE

Several drugs (e.g., rifampin, flavaspidic acid, novobiocin, and various cholecystographic contrast agents) competitively inhibit the hepatocellular uptake of bilirubin. The resulting unconjugated hyperbilirubinemia resolves with cessation of the medication. Decreased hepatic bilirubin uptake is also believed to contribute to the unconjugated hyperbilirubinemia of Gilbert's syndrome, although the principal molecular basis for this syndrome is reduction of bilirubin conjugation.

IMPAIRED BILIRUBIN CONJUGATION

The most frequent cause of decreased bilirubin clearance is decreased bilirubin conjugating activity. Bilirubin conjugation with glucuronic acid is catalyzed by a specific UDP-glucuronosyltransferase, designated UGT1A1, encoded by the *UGT1* gene complex. The *UGT1A1* gene is assembled by alternative splicing of a bilirubin-specific variant of exon 1, designated exon A_1, with four common exons (exons 2 to 5) that encode the shared carboxyl terminal end of all *UGT1*-encoded proteins. Its promoter region normally contains an $A(TA)_6TAA$ TATA boxlike construct.

Genetic Disorders of Bilirubin Conjugation

The hereditary hyperbilirubinemias (Table 149-2) are a group of five syndromes in which hyperbilirubinemia occurs as an isolated biochemical abnormality, without evidence of either hepatocellular necrosis or cholestasis. The molecular defects have been identified in all but Rotor's syndrome.

CRIGLER-NAJJAR SYNDROME TYPES 1 AND 2 AND GILBERT'S SYNDROME

These are hereditary unconjugated hyperbilirubinemias that result from mutations in *UGT1A1*. In Crigler-Najjar type 1, essentially no functional enzyme activity is present, whereas patients with Crigler-Najjar type 2 have up to 10% of normal and patients with Gilbert's syndrome have 10 to 33% of normal, leading to bilirubin concentrations of 18 to 45, 6 to 25, and 1.5 to 4 mg/dL, respectively (see Table 149-2). Because total UGT1A1 enzymatic activity must be reduced to less than 50% of normal to produce unconjugated hyperbilirubinemia, phenotypic expression of mutations in this enzyme requires either homozygosity or double heterozygosity. Each of these disorders is inherited as an autosomal recessive trait. Patients with Crigler-Najjar types 1 and 2 are either homozygotes or double heterozygotes for structural mutations within the coding region. In Western countries, patients with Gilbert's syndrome are typically homozygous for an $A(TA)_7TAA$ promoter mutation. Structural mutations in exon 1 of *UGT1A1* causing modest reductions in UGT1A1 enzymatic activity have been reported in some Japanese patients with Gilbert's syndrome.

Crigler-Najjar type 1 is characterized by striking unconjugated hyperbilirubinemia that appears in the neonatal period, persists for life, and is unresponsive to phenobarbital. The majority of patients (type 1A) exhibit defects in the glucuronide conjugation of a spectrum of substrates in addition to bilirubin as the result of mutations in one of the common exons (2 to 5) of the *UGT1* complex. In a smaller subset (type 1B), a mutation in the bilirubin-specific exon A1 limits the defect to bilirubin conjugation. More than 85 structurally diverse *UGT1A1* mutations can cause Crigler-Najjar type 1; their common feature is that they all encode proteins with absent or, at most, traces of enzymatic activity. Before the availability of phototherapy, most patients with Crigler-Najjar type 1 died of bilirubin encephalopathy (kernicterus) in infancy or early childhood. Optimal treatment for a neurologically intact patient includes (1) about 12 hours/day of phototherapy from birth throughout childhood, perhaps supplemented by exchange transfusion in the neonatal period; (2) use of tin-protoporphyrin to blunt transient episodes of increased hyperbilirubinemia; and (3) early liver transplantation, before the onset of brain damage. Transplantation with isolated allogeneic hepatocytes continues to be evaluated as an experimental therapeutic approach.

Bilirubin concentrations are typically lower in Crigler-Najjar type 2, and plasma bilirubin levels can be reduced to 3 to 5 mg/dL by phenobarbital. At least 20 different mutations of *UGT1A1* have been associated with Crigler-Najjar type 2; all encode a bilirubin-UDP-glucuronosyl transferase with markedly reduced but detectable enzymatic activity. Although uncommon in Crigler-Najjar type 2, kernicterus has occurred at all ages, typically associated with factors that temporarily raise the plasma bilirubin concentration above baseline (e.g., fasting, intercurrent illness). For this reason, phenobarbital therapy is often recommended; a single bedtime dose usually maintains clinically safe plasma bilirubin concentrations.

Gilbert's syndrome is the most common hereditary hyperbilirubinemia, with a genotypic prevalence of 12% or less and a phenotypic prevalence of 7% or less. Its high prevalence may explain the frequency of mild unconjugated hyperbilirubinemia in liver transplant recipients. Plasma bilirubin concentrations are most often less than 3 mg/dL, although both higher and lower values are frequent, with increases of two- to three-fold commonly occurring with fasting and intercurrent illness. The phenotypic distinction between mild Gilbert's syndrome and a normal state is often blurred. Phenobarbital normalizes both the bilirubin concentration and C_{BR}. Oxidative drug metabolism and the disposition of most xenobiotics that are metabolized by glucuronidation appear to be normal in Gilbert's syndrome. A critical exception is the antitumor agent irinotecan (CPT-11), whose active metabolite (SN-38) is glucuronidated specifically by UGT1A1. In patients with Gilbert's syndrome, CPT-11 can cause intractable diarrhea, myelosuppression, and other serious toxicities. Life expectancy in Gilbert's syndrome is normal, and the denial of life insurance or employment to these patients is not medically justified.

UNCONJUGATED HYPERBILIRUBINEMIA RELATED TO SELECTIVE INHIBITION OF UGT1A1

This occurs with several human immunodeficiency virus (HIV) protease inhibitors (e.g., indinavir, atazanavir). Abnormal disposition of menthol, estradiol benzoate, acetaminophen, tolbutamide, rifamycin SV, and other agents has not been associated with significant complications, but prudence should be exercised in prescribing agents metabolized by glucuronidation to patients with Gilbert's syndrome.

UNCONJUGATED HYPERBILIRUBIN IN THE NEWBORN PERIOD

Most neonates develop mild unconjugated hyperbilirubinemia between days 2 and 5 after birth because of hepatic immaturity and low levels of UGT1A1. Peak bilirubin levels are typically less than 5 to 10 mg/dL, and levels return to normal within 2 weeks as mechanisms of bilirubin disposition mature. Prematurity, with hemolysis or hepatic immaturity, is associated with higher bilirubin levels that may require phototherapy. The progestational steroid $3\alpha,20\beta$-pregnanediol and certain fatty acids that are found in breast milk (but not serum) of some mothers inhibit bilirubin conjugation and can cause excessive neonatal hyperbilirubinemia (*breast milk jaundice*). By comparison, *transient familial neonatal hyperbilirubinemia* (Lucey-Driscoll syndrome) is caused by a UGT1A1 inhibitor found in maternal serum.

Acquired Conjugation Defects

A modest reduction in bilirubin conjugating capacity occurs in advanced hepatitis or cirrhosis (Chapter 156). However, in this setting, conjugation is better preserved than other aspects of bilirubin disposition, such as

TABLE 149-2 PRINCIPAL FEATURES OF THE HEREDITARY DISORDERS OF BILIRUBIN METABOLISM

FEATURE	Crigler-Najjar Syndrome TYPE I	Crigler-Najjar Syndrome TYPE II	GILBERT'S SYNDROME	DUBIN-JOHNSON SYNDROME	ROTOR'S SYNDROME
Incidence	Very rare	Uncommon	Up to 12% of population	Uncommon	Rare
Total serum bilirubin (mg/dL)	18-45 (usually >20), unconjugated	6-25 (usually ≤20), unconjugated	Typically ≤4 in absence of fasting or hemolysis; mostly unconjugated	Typically 2-5, less often ≤25; about 60% direct reacting	Usually 3-7, occasionally ≤20; about 60% direct reacting
Defect(s) in bilirubin metabolism*	Bilirubin UGT1A1 conjugating activity markedly reduced: trace to absent	Bilirubin UGT1A1 conjugating activity reduced: ≤10% of normal	Bilirubin UGT1A1 conjugating activity typically reduced to 10-33% of normal; reduced bilirubin uptake in some cases; mild hemolysis in up to 50% of patients	Impaired canalicular secretion of conjugated bilirubin due to MRP2/cMOAT mutation	Impaired hepatic secretion or storage of conjugated bilirubin; molecular defect not known
Routine liver tests	Normal	Normal	Normal	Normal	Normal
Serum bile acids	Normal	Normal	Normal	Usually normal	Normal
Plasma sulfobromophthalein removal (% retention of 5 mg/kg dose at 45 min)[†]	Normal	Normal	Usually normal (<5%); mild 45-min (<15%) retention in some patients	Slow initial decline in plasma concentration (retention ≤20% at 45 min) with secondary rise at 90-120 min	Very slow initial decline in plasma concentration (45-min retention = 30-45%) without secondary rise
Oral cholecystography	Normal	Normal	Normal	Faint or no visualization of gallbladder	Usually normal
Pharmacologic responses/special features	No response to phenobarbital	Phenobarbital reduces bilirubin by ≤75%	Phenobarbital reduces bilirubin, often to normal	Increased bilirubin concentration with estrogens; diagnostic urine coproporphyrin isomer pattern (total is normal, with isomer I increased to ≥80% of total)	Characteristic urine coproporphyrin excretion pattern (total is increased ≥2.5-fold in ~65% of cases, but isomer I always <80% of total)
Major clinical features	Kernicterus in infancy if untreated; may occur later despite therapy	Rare late-onset kernicterus with fasting	None	Occasional hepatosplenomegaly	None
Hepatic morphology/histology	Normal	Normal	Normal; occasionally increased lipofuscin pigment	Liver grossly black; coarse, dark centrilobular pigment	Normal
Bile bilirubin fractions[‡]	>90% unconjugated	Largest fraction (mean, 57%) monoconjugates	Mainly diconjugates but monoconjugates are increased (mean, 23%)	Mixed conjugates, reported increase in diconjugates	Increased conjugates
Inheritance (all autosomal)	Recessive	Recessive	Promoter mutation is recessive; missense mutation often dominant	Recessive; rare kindred appears dominant	Recessive
Diagnosis	Clinical and laboratory findings: lack of response to phenobarbital	Clinical and laboratory findings: response to phenobarbital	Clinical and laboratory findings: promoter genotyping; liver biopsy rarely necessary	Clinical and laboratory findings: liver biopsy unnecessary if coproporphyrin studies available; BSP disappearance	Clinical and laboratory findings: urine coproporphyrin analysis; BSP disappearance
Treatment	Phototherapy or tin protoporphyrin as short-term therapy; liver transplantation definitive	Consider phenobarbital if baseline bilirubin ≥8 mg/dL	None necessary	Avoid estrogens; no other therapy necessary	No treatment necessary

*UGT1A1 is the bilirubin specific isoform of the UGT1 family of uridine diphosphate glucuronosyl transferases.
[†]Sulfobromophthalein (BSP) studies: previously used to help distinguish Dubin-Johnson and Rotor's syndromes if coproporphyrin isomer studies not available. However, BSP is no longer approved for clinical use in the United States.
[‡]Bilirubin in normal bile: <5% unconjugated bilirubin, with an average of 7% bilirubin monoconjugates and 90% bilirubin diconjugates.
BSP = sulfobromophthalein; cMOAT = canalicular multispecific organic anion transporter; MRP2 = multidrug resistance–associated protein 2.

canalicular excretion. Pharmacologic and metabolic perturbations may also lead to acquired reductions in bilirubin conjugation. Various drugs (e.g., pregnanediol, novobiocin, chloramphenicol, gentamicin, and several HIV protease inhibitors) may cause unconjugated hyperbilirubinemia by inhibiting UGT1A1. In all settings in which UGT1A1 inhibitors cause unconjugated hyperbilirubinemia, the hyperbilirubinemia is greater in patients with underlying Gilbert's syndrome.

Conjugated or Mixed Hyperbilirubinemia

Two phenotypically similar but mechanistically distinct inherited disorders, *Dubin-Johnson syndrome* and *Rotor's syndrome*, are characterized by conjugated or mixed hyperbilirubinemia with normal values for other standard liver tests (see Table 149-2). Dubin-Johnson syndrome results from any of several mutations in the gene encoding the ATP-dependent canalicular organic anion transporter MPR2/cMOAT (see Fig. 149-1). The molecular defect in Rotor's syndrome remains unknown. Despite the conjugated hyperbilirubinemia, patients with these syndromes are not cholestatic and can be distinguished noninvasively by analysis of urine coproporphyrins (see Table 149-2), so liver biopsy is not required. Both syndromes carry a benign prognosis without specific therapy.

LIVER AND BILIARY TRACT DISEASE

Jaundice is a common sign of generalized hepatobiliary dysfunction, both acute and chronic. Icteric hepatobiliary disease is readily distinguished from the isolated disorders of bilirubin metabolism because the increase in plasma bilirubin concentration occurs in association with other markers of hepatobiliary injury. Liver diseases can be categorized as those in which the primary injury results from inflammation and hepatocellular necrosis, inhibition of bile flow (cholestasis), or a combination of the two. The cholestatic disorders can be further subdivided into those due to mechanical obstruction of the bile duct flow (Chapter 158) and those resulting from intrahepatic cholestasis, which may be the consequence of a multitude of conditions that include familial cholestatic syndromes and infiltrative disorders (Chapters 151 to 156), particularly those involving the intrahepatic biliary tree; sepsis (Chapter 108), and certain other inflammatory or neoplastic conditions; and drug reactions (see Table 149-1). It is important to note that chronic cholestasis from any cause may result in the intrahepatic accumulation of compounds such as bile acids, which may themselves be toxic, causing hepatocellular injury.

Familial Cholestasis Syndromes

Benign recurrent intrahepatic cholestasis (BRIC) is a rare disorder characterized by recurrent attacks of cholestatic jaundice beginning either in childhood or in adulthood and varying in duration from weeks to months. Intervals between attacks may vary from months to years. This benign disorder does not progress to chronic liver disease or cirrhosis. There is complete resolution between episodes; treatment during the cholestatic episodes is symptomatic. Three subtypes result from mutations in different canalicular transporters: *BRIC type 1* from a partial deficiency of the familial intrahepatic cholestasis 1 (FIC1) gene product, also designated ATP8B1; *BRIC type 2* from mutations in the bile salt export pump (BSEP, or ABCB11); and *BRIC type 3* from mutations in multidrug resistance–associated protein 3 (MDR3, ABCB4).

Progressive familial intrahepatic cholestasis (PFIC) is a heterogeneous group of cholestatic disorders of childhood that, by contrast, typically lead to hepatic fibrosis and end-stage liver disease before adulthood. The three best-characterized *PFIC* subtypes are type 1 (Byler's disease) and type 2, resulting from functionally more severe mutations in ATP8B1 and BSEP, respectively; and type 3, due to MDR3 deficiency. All forms of *BRIC* and *PFIC* are inherited as autosomal recessive disorders. Diagnostically, γ-glutamyl transpeptidase (GGT) levels are low despite elevations in alkaline phosphatase in types 1 and 2, whereas GGT and alkaline phosphatase are elevated in parallel in PFIC type 3, as in most other forms of cholestatic liver disease. In contrast to the selective bilirubin transport defect in Dubin-Johnson syndrome, the conjugated hyperbilirubinemia in these syndromes reflects generalized bile secretory failure.

Postoperative Jaundice

This multifactorial syndrome can be caused by increased bilirubin production (e.g., breakdown of transfused erythrocytes, resorption of hematomas) or decreased hepatic clearance (e.g., from bacteremia, endotoxemia, parenteral nutrition, perioperative hypoxia). Hyperbilirubinemia, the main biochemical feature, is often accompanied by a several-fold increase in alkaline phosphatase or GGT levels, or both. Aminotransferases are, at most, minimally elevated, and synthetic function is typically normal. The differential diagnosis includes biliary obstruction or hepatocellular injury related to shock, anesthetic injury (Chapter 152), or viral hepatitis (Chapter 150). Postoperative jaundice per se (Chapter 441) is not a threat to the patient, and it usually resolves in parallel with the patient's overall condition.

Jaundice in Pregnancy

Jaundice in pregnancy (Chapter 247) may result from any liver disease that also affects nonpregnant women or from conditions unique to pregnancy. The unique conditions include a generally modest, self-limited elevation of aminotransferase and bilirubin levels during the first trimester, often in patients with hyperemesis gravidarum; intrahepatic cholestasis of pregnancy (ICP), which occurs during the second and third trimesters and usually resolves spontaneously after delivery; or acute fatty liver or the HELLP (*h*emolysis, *e*levated *l*iver enzymes, and *l*ow *p*latelets) syndrome, in association with preeclampsia in the third trimester (Chapters 153, 178, and 247). ICP, as well as cholestasis occurring recurrently in some women taking oral contraceptives, is increasingly being linked to polymorphisms in the same genes responsible for BRIC and PFIC. Acute fatty liver may resemble fulminant hepatic failure, with early delivery a prerequisite to maternal recovery; a defect in the oxidation of long-chain fatty acids is found in some infants born after these pregnancies.

DIAGNOSTIC TOOLS FOR THE EVALUATION OF LIVER DISEASE

Accurate diagnosis and the distinction between acute and chronic disease are often dependent on appropriate selection and interpretation of a spectrum of laboratory and imaging studies.

Tests used in initial evaluation of liver disease fall into two categories: (1) tests that indicate injury, such as release of intracellular enzymes; and (2) tests that measure, or at least reflect, actual function. Tests that reflect injury usually do not measure liver function and should not be called liver function tests.

The important functions of the liver include clearance, biotransformation and detoxification of potentially toxic metabolites and exogenous compounds, synthesis and export of various plasma proteins, and a critical integrative role in the intermediary metabolism of carbohydrates, amino acids, and lipids. In specific diseases, some of these functions may be markedly compromised, whereas others are little affected. Liver tests must be chosen with care and interpreted within the total clinical context. In specific situations, serial determinations are often helpful to assess the course of disease or effects of therapy.

Serum Enzyme Tests

The levels of hepatic enzymes found in plasma are a measure of hepatocyte turnover or injury. Enzymes released during normal hepatocyte turnover are believed to be the principal basis for normal circulating levels. Cell injury and cell death activate phospholipases that create holes in the plasma membrane, thereby increasing the release of intracellular contents.

Aminotransferases

The aminotransferases (formerly called transaminases) catalyze transfer of the α-amino group of aspartate (aspartate aminotransferase, AST) or alanine (alanine aminotransferase, ALT) to the α-keto group of ketoglutarate, with pyridoxal phosphate (vitamin B_6) as a cofactor. Laboratory methods that assay aminotransferase activity require supplementation with vitamin B_6 to avoid falsely decreased activity in vitamin B_6-deficient subjects.

Normal ranges for serum aminotransferases are usually reported to be up to approximately 40 IU/L (see Appendix), but when particular care is taken to exclude obese patients and others with known fatty liver disease from the sampled population, results suggest that less than 30 IU/L is normal for men and less than 19 IU/L for women. Values can exceed 1000 IU/L in acute hepatocyte injury, for example, from viral infection (Chapter 150) or toxins (Chapter 152). ALT is a purely cytosolic enzyme. Distinct isoforms of AST are present in cytosol and mitochondria. Expression of the mitochondrial isoform and its physiologic export from the hepatocyte are upregulated by ethanol. Circulating levels of AST or ALT (or both) are elevated in most hepatic diseases, and the degree of aminotransferase activity found in plasma roughly reflects the current activity of the disease process. There are, however, critical exceptions, and the sensitivity of aminotransferases as markers of hepatocellular injury varies with the disease in question. A subset of patients with proven chronic hepatitis C have normal aminotransferase levels, approximately 25% of morbidly obese patients with biopsy-proven nonalcoholic steatohepatitis may have normal ALT levels, and aminotransferase levels greater than or equal to 200 to 300 IU/L are uncommon in even the most severe cases of alcoholic hepatitis (Chapter 155). By contrast, aminotransferases of 1000 IU/L or greater are often present in even mild acute viral hepatitis (Chapter 150) or shortly after acute biliary obstruction, for example, during passage of a gallstone (Chapter 158). Conversely, aminotransferase levels may decline during the course of massive hepatic necrosis because liver injury is so extensive that little enzyme activity remains (Chapter 157). In rare circumstances, autoantibodies to AST result in autoantibody-enzyme complexes called macroenzymes that have a delayed clearance, detected as an increase in enzyme concentrations in the absence of cellular turnover.

Aminotransferase levels are useful in several distinct ways. First, they provide a relatively specific screening test for hepatobiliary disease. Although AST levels may be increased with disease of other organs (notably myocardial and skeletal muscle), values ten times the upper limit of normal or greater almost invariably indicate hepatobiliary pathology. Moreover, in the total clinical context, the source of increased aminotransferase activity is usually obvious. Aminotransferase levels are also used to monitor the activity of an acute or chronic parenchymal liver disease and its response to therapy. However, levels in a given patient may correlate poorly with the severity of the disease as assessed by liver biopsy, particularly in chronic hepatitis C

(Chapter 151). Aminotransferases are also often normal in advanced cirrhosis (Chapter 156), in which they are of limited prognostic value. Finally, aminotransferase levels may provide diagnostic clues. AST levels 15 or more times normal are unusual in *chronic* bile duct obstruction unless there is concomitant cholangitis, and AST levels 6 or more times normal are uncommon in alcoholic liver disease in the absence of other causes. In most liver diseases, the ratio of AST to ALT is usually less than or equal to 1. However, ratios are typically 2 or higher in alcoholic fatty liver and alcoholic hepatitis (Chapter 155), reflecting increased mitochondrial AST synthesis and secretion into plasma and selective loss of ALT activity because of the pyridoxine deficiency commonly seen in alcoholism. An elevated AST/ALT ratio also occurs in fulminant hepatitis related to Wilson disease (Chapters 153 and 218).

Alkaline Phosphatase

Alkaline phosphatases are widely distributed enzymes (e.g., liver, bile ducts, intestine, bone, kidney, placenta, and leukocytes) that catalyze the release of orthophosphate from ester substrates at an alkaline pH. The normal activity level in adult serum is highly dependent on the measurement method, age, and sex. Two methods in current use have upper limits of normal in adults of 85 and 110 IU/L (see Appendix). Higher levels are normal in children and in pregnancy. Results must always be compared with the appropriate normal range. In bone, alkaline phosphatase participates in the deposition of hydroxyapatite in osteoid. In other sites, including liver, alkaline phosphatase activity may facilitate movement of molecules across cell membranes. Serum alkaline phosphatase activity usually reflects principally the hepatic and bone isozymes; the intestinal form may account for 20 to 60% of the total after a fatty meal. There is a substantial placental contribution to the alkaline phosphatase level late in pregnancy; the *Regan isozyme,* a variant that appears identical to the placental form, is associated with hepatomas (Chapter 202), lung cancer (Chapter 197), and other tumors.

Elevations in serum alkaline phosphatase activity in cholestatic hepatobiliary disease result from two distinct mechanisms: increased synthesis and secretion of the enzyme and solubilization from the apical (canalicular) surface of hepatocytes and the luminal surface of biliary epithelial cells by the increased local concentrations of bile acids that occur with cholestasis. Serum alkaline phosphatase activity may also be increased in bone disorders (e.g., Paget's disease [Chapter 255], osteomalacia [Chapter 252], bone metastases [Chapter 208]), during rapid bone growth in children, in the later stages of pregnancy, with chronic renal failure (Chapter 132), and, occasionally, in the presence of malignancy not involving bones or liver. The source is often obvious, but when it is not, methods such as heat stability and electrophoretic separation can distinguish hepatobiliary alkaline phosphatase from other forms. A simpler alternative is to measure serum levels of GGT or 5′-nucleotidase (5′-NT), which tend to parallel levels of alkaline phosphatase in hepatobiliary disease but are usually not increased in bone disease. With a serum half-life of approximately 1 week, serum alkaline phosphatase may remain elevated for days to weeks after resolution of biliary obstruction. This delay may be especially misleading when it is accompanied by prolonged direct-reacting hyperbilirubinemia owing to delayed clearance of δ-bilirubin.

Modest increases in serum alkaline phosphatase (three times normal or less) occur in many hepatic parenchymal disorders, including hepatitis and cirrhosis. In the absence of bone disease, larger increases (three to ten times normal) usually indicate obstruction of bile flow. Although the highest levels usually reflect obstruction of the common bile duct, elevations can also occur with obstruction of intrahepatic bile ducts from infiltrative conditions that arise from granulomatous processes (sarcoidosis, *Mycobacterium avium-intracellulare, Mycobacterium tuberculosis*), malignancy (lymphoma, cholangiocarcinoma, or metastatic cancer) or amyloidosis.

Other Hepatic Enzymes

5′-NT is a plasma membrane enzyme that cleaves orthophosphate from the 5′ position on the pentose sugar of adenosine or inosine phosphate. *Leucine aminopeptidase (LAP)* is a ubiquitous cellular peptidase. The serum levels of both usually increase in cholestasis. Accordingly, their major use is to confirm whether an elevated serum alkaline phosphatase is hepatic in origin. Both enzymes may be increased in the later stages of a healthy pregnancy.

γ-Glutamyl transpeptidase (GGT) is present in many tissues. Its serum activity increases in hepatobiliary disease but also after myocardial infarction; in neuromuscular diseases, pancreatic disease (even in the absence of biliary obstruction), pulmonary disease, and diabetes; and during the ingestion of ethanol and other inducers of microsomal enzymes. Nevertheless, because serum GGT levels are usually normal in bone disease, the enzyme may be helpful in confirming the hepatic origin of an elevated alkaline phosphatase. Measurement of GGT has been proposed as a sensitive screening test for hepatobiliary disease and for monitoring abstinence from ethanol. Because of its low specificity, many persons who test positive have no identifiable liver disease on further study. GGT offers no clear advantage over LAP or 5′-NT for identifying the source of increased serum alkaline phosphatase activity except in pregnancy. Serum GGT levels may be normal despite elevated hepatobiliary alkaline phosphatase levels in certain rare disorders, including benign recurrent intrahepatic cholestasis and progressive familial intrahepatic cholestasis types 1 and 2 (see earlier and Chapter 158).

Lactate dehydrogenase (LDH) levels are often elevated in hepatic ischemia; otherwise, the enzyme is too ubiquitous in other body tissues to be diagnostically useful.

Tests Based on Clearance of Metabolites and Drugs

A major liver function is to remove various metabolites and toxins from the blood (Chapter 152). In liver disease, clearance of such molecules may be impaired because of loss of parenchymal cells, diminished bile secretion, biliary obstruction, decreased cellular uptake or metabolism, or reduced or heterogeneous hepatic blood flow. When a metabolite is produced at a relatively constant rate (e.g., bilirubin), its serum level can be a sensitive indicator of liver function. The removal rate from plasma of certain exogenous drugs and dyes can be similarly interpreted.

Bilirubin

The differential diagnosis of hyperbilirubinemia (see earlier) includes generalized liver disease, inherited disorders of bilirubin metabolism (e.g., Gilbert's and Crigler-Najjar syndromes), and nonhepatic conditions (e.g., hemolysis). Higher bilirubin levels correlate with a poorer prognosis in acute alcoholic hepatitis (Chapter 155), fulminant hepatic failure (Chapter 157), primary biliary cirrhosis (Chapter 156), and most forms of chronic liver disease.

Ammonia

Ammonia, a byproduct of amino acid metabolism, is removed from blood by the liver, converted to urea in the Krebs-Henseleit cycle, and excreted by the kidneys (Chapter 117). In the setting of portosystemic shunting, severe hepatic dysfunction (e.g., fulminant hepatic failure), or defects in urea cycle metabolism, ammonia levels rise. Measurements of blood ammonia are sometimes used to confirm a diagnosis of hepatic encephalopathy and to monitor the success of therapy, but the correlation of ammonia levels with the degree of encephalopathy is only approximate (Chapter 157). Correlations may be somewhat better if the measurement is made rapidly on an iced arterial blood sample. Elevated ammonia levels also occur when ammonia production is increased by intestinal flora (e.g., after a high-protein meal or gastrointestinal bleeding), by the kidney (in response to metabolic alkalosis or hypokalemia), or in rare genetic diseases that affect the pathway of urea synthesis (Chapter 212).

Drug Clearance

The rate of hepatic clearance of compounds such as sulfobromophthalein, lidocaine, and aminopyrine from the circulation can be measured chemically or with radiolabeled tracers. Although such tests can quantify hepatic function, they are rarely used in clinical practice.

Tests Reflecting Hepatic Synthetic Function

Coagulation Tests

See also Chapters 37 and 174.

Prothrombin Time

The prothrombin time (PT) reflects the plasma concentrations of both extrinsic and common pathway factors, that is, factors VII, X, and V, prothrombin, and fibrinogen. A prolonged PT most often results from vitamin K deficiency, liver disease, or both. Vitamin K, a fat-soluble vitamin found in many foods, is also synthesized by gut bacteria (Chapter 177). Vitamin K deficiency can be caused by poor dietary intake and malabsorptive states, including fat malabsorption resulting from cholestasis, and also occurs with antibiotic suppression of gut flora, particularly in patients receiving inadequate vitamin K replacement.

The half-lives of clotting factors are typically less than 1 day. Factor VII, which has the shortest half-life, is usually the earliest and most severely depressed during periods of defective hepatic synthesis. Because the PT is dependent on the level of factor VII, it responds rapidly with changes in hepatic synthetic function; it is useful for following the course of acute liver diseases, in which a significant or growing prolongation of the PT may indicate a poor prognosis. An abnormal PT that is due solely to vitamin K deficiency usually becomes normal within 24 to 48 hours after parenteral repletion. However, if decreased synthesis of clotting factors reflects hepatocyte dysfunction, there may be little or no response to vitamin K. Finally, prolongation of the PT may also reflect disseminated intravascular coagulation (Chapter 178), which should always be considered in the context of both acute liver failure and end-stage chronic liver disease.

Partial Thromboplastin Time

This test reflects both intrinsic and common pathway factors, that is, all classical clotting factors except factor VII, and is, therefore, complementary to the PT. It is especially useful in detecting circulating anticoagulants (Chapter 178) but adds little to the PT in evaluating hepatic synthetic function.

Albumin

Albumin is produced solely by the liver. Its plasma concentration reflects a balance between its synthetic rate (100 to 200 mg/kg/day) and its plasma half-life of about 21 days. The synthetic rate is affected by the patient's nutritional state, thyroid and glucocorticoid hormone levels, plasma colloid osmotic pressure, exposure to hepatotoxins (e.g., alcohol), and presence of systemic disorders or liver disease. Many conditions increase albumin losses and shorten its plasma half-life, including nephrotic syndrome (Chapter 123), protein-losing enteropathy (Chapter 142), severe burns (Chapter 112), exfoliative dermatitis, and major gastrointestinal bleeding (Chapter 137). In cirrhosis with ascites (Chapters 156 and 157), hypoalbuminemia indicates diminished synthesis or redistribution into ascitic fluid. Thus, a reduced serum albumin concentration can confidently be considered an indicator of decreased hepatic synthetic function only when these other factors are not involved.

Examinations of Urine and Stool

Bilirubinuria always indicates a pathologic increase in plasma conjugated bilirubin levels. It is frequently seen with plasma conjugated bilirubin concentrations of 2 to 3 mg/dL, often appearing before the onset of clinical jaundice and persisting after jaundice has resolved. The quantification of urobilinogen in urine or feces is of limited clinical value. By contrast, stool culture or examination for ova and parasites may provide important information in selected patients. Testing of stool for occult blood may lead to discovery of a gastrointestinal lesion related to hepatobiliary disease (e.g., tumors metastatic to liver, ulcerative colitis associated with sclerosing cholangitis) or may explain the onset or worsening of hepatic encephalopathy.

Hematologic Tests in Liver Disease

In moderate to severe acute liver diseases, varying degrees of cytopenia occur in all three cell lineages. The most common finding is of thrombocytopenia from hypersplenism, which can be a surrogate marker of portal hypertension. Anemia may reflect low-grade hemolysis or marrow depression. Bone marrow suppression may be caused by ethanol or drugs, and aplastic anemia may sometimes complicate acute viral hepatitis (Chapters 150 and 168). Zieve's syndrome (hemolytic anemia and hypertriglyceridemia) is a rare but well-characterized complication of severe alcoholic liver disease (Chapters 155 and 156). Modest leukopenia, often with atypical lymphocytes, may also be present. Coagulopathy frequently complicates both acute and chronic liver failure owing to depressed hepatic synthesis of clotting factors or disseminated intravascular coagulation, or both (Chapters 177 and 178).

A modest increase in erythrocyte mean corpuscular volume occurs with alcohol consumption, hemolysis, or on occasion, liver disease per se. Chronic liver disease, especially if cholestatic, may be accompanied by target cells in the peripheral blood smear. Target cells are erythrocytes with an expanded cell membrane that reflects abnormalities in serum lipids. Spur cells (acanthocytes), most often found in advanced alcoholic cirrhosis, reflect a still greater increase in membrane cholesterol.

Tests for Specific Liver Diseases

Patients who present with a picture of acute or chronic parenchymal liver disease are most likely to fall into one of three categories: viral or toxic hepatitis, including alcoholic and nonalcoholic fatty liver disease; autoimmune liver disease; or an inherited metabolic disorder Specific tests for viral antigens, nucleic acids, and antibodies are available for the conventional hepatitis viruses (Chapters 150 and 151) as well as Epstein-Barr virus (Chapter 385), cytomegalovirus (Chapter 384), and herpesviruses (Chapters 382 and 383), which are well-established but less common causes of liver disease. The major hepatic autoimmune diseases include primary biliary cirrhosis (Chapter 158), autoimmune hepatitis (Chapter 151), and various overlap syndromes. The starting point for establishing a specific diagnosis within this category is the search for specific serum autoantibodies, including antimitochondrial antibodies against epitopes of the pyruvate dehydrogenase complex, which are virtually diagnostic of primary biliary cirrhosis (Chapter 158), and antinuclear, anti–smooth muscle, and anti–liver microsomal antibodies, which suggest one of the subtypes of autoimmune hepatitis (Chapter 148). The most prevalent of the hereditary metabolic disorders affecting the liver (Chapter 153) include hemochromatosis (Chapter 219), α_1-antitrypsin deficiency (Chapter 153), and Wilson disease (Chapter 218).

Liver Biopsy

Liver biopsy can be of great help in the diagnosis of diffuse or localized parenchymal diseases, including chronic hepatitis, cirrhosis, and primary or metastatic malignancy in the liver. The value of liver biopsy in acute hepatitis or acute cholestatic jaundice may be primarily prognostic because the histologic changes in these settings, although sometimes suggesting a specific diagnosis, are often nonspecific. However, toxic hepatitis (Chapter 152) related to certain medications may display diagnostic features. Liver biopsy for assessment of diffuse disease can be performed percutaneously after localization of the liver by physical examination or ultrasonographic visualization. When specific lesions, such as tumors, must be sampled, the biopsy can be guided by ultrasonographic or radiographic imaging or performed under direct visualization during laparoscopy or laparotomy. Relative or absolute contraindications include coagulopathy, high-grade biliary obstruction, biliary sepsis, ascites, and right pleural disease. Although liver biopsy remains the standard for assessment of hepatic histology in diffuse disease (Chapter 148), its invasiveness and concern for sampling error have generated interest in noninvasive measures of hepatic diseases. Transient elastography uses ultrasound to assess tissue stiffness as a measure of hepatic fibrosis. Commercially available biomarker panels have also been developed to provide a noninvasive assessment of hepatic fibrosis by blood testing alone. These panels typically include standard laboratory measures of hepatic injury (GGT, total bilirubin) and other serum markers (e.g., haptoglobin, hyaluronic acid, apolipoprotein A1). However, the ability of currently available noninvasive markers to assess the extent of hepatic fibrosis across the clinically relevant histologic spectrum remains to be established. Magnetic resonance elastography is another, emerging technique to characterize liver tissue elasticity, and hence fibrosis, noninvasively.

APPROACH TO THE PATIENT WITH JAUNDICE OR ABNORMAL LIVER TESTS

History, Physical Examination, and Initial Laboratory Studies

Patients with liver disease may present with jaundice or other signs or symptoms, or the disease may be detected in the asymptomatic patient by the finding of abnormal liver tests during a routine evaluation. Regardless of how the patient comes to medical attention, the diagnostic approach (Fig. 149-3) begins with a careful history and physical examination (Chapter 148), as well as screening laboratory studies (complete blood cell count, measurement of plasma bilirubin concentration, assay of ALT, AST, and alkaline phosphatase levels, and PT) to formulate an initial differential diagnosis. The ability to distinguish expeditiously between liver disease and extrahepatic biliary tract obstruction is the major goal of the initial evaluation, in part because the latter may require prompt surgical intervention. Appropriate choice of second-level laboratory tests and imaging studies leads to a definitive diagnosis in most patients. Care in selecting tests, particularly imaging studies, both maximizes the likelihood of making a correct diagnosis and protects the patient from unnecessary discomfort, risk, and expense.

If the patient is asymptomatic and hepatic tests other than bilirubin are normal, hemolysis or an isolated disorder of bilirubin metabolism should be considered. If signs, symptoms, or laboratory abnormalities indicate hepatobiliary disease, certain patterns of findings help to distinguish intrinsic liver disease from biliary obstruction (Table 149-3). Pain in the right upper quadrant accompanied by a predominant increase in serum alkaline phosphatase activity suggests biliary obstruction (Chapter 158), as does a history of prior biliary surgery, right upper quadrant scars, or an abdominal mass. Fever and

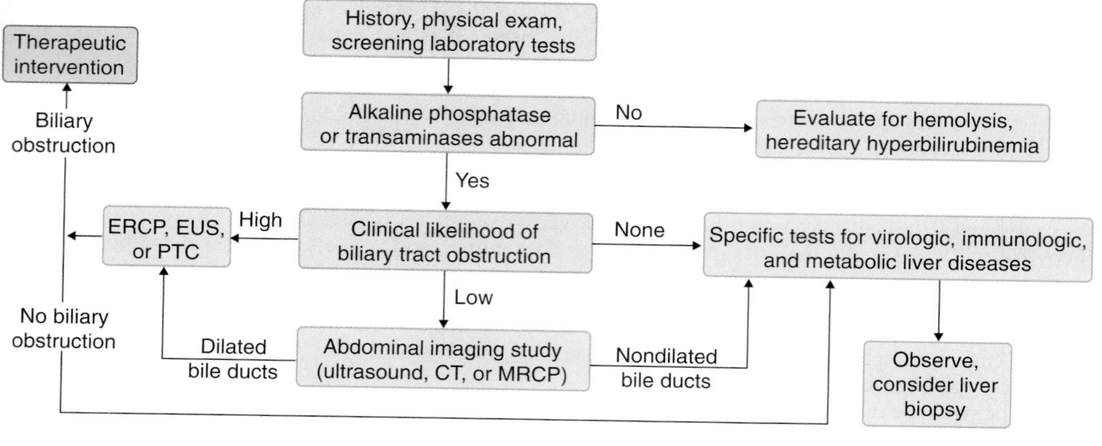

FIGURE 149-3. Diagnostic algorithm for the evaluation of hyperbilirubinemia and other liver test abnormalities and/or signs and symptoms suggestive of liver disease. CT = computed tomography; ERCP = endoscopic retrograde cholangiopancreatography; EUS = endoscopic ultrasound; PTC = percutaneous cholangiogram; MRCP = magnetic resonance cholangiopancreatography. (Modified from Lidofsky SD, Scharschmidt BF. Jaundice. In: Feldman M, Scharschmidt BF, Sleisenger MH, eds. *Gastrointestinal and Liver Disease*. 6th ed. Philadelphia: WB Saunders; 1998:227.)

TABLE 149-3 OBSTRUCTIVE JAUNDICE VERSUS CHOLESTATIC LIVER DISEASE

FEATURE	SUGGESTS OBSTRUCTIVE JAUNDICE	SUGGESTS PARENCHYMAL LIVER DISEASE
History	Abdominal pain Fever, rigors Previous biliary surgery Older age Acholic stools	Anorexia, malaise, myalgias, suggestive of a viral prodrome Known infectious exposure Receipt of blood products, use of intravenous drugs Exposure to a known hepatotoxin Family history of jaundice
Physical examination	High fever Abdominal tenderness Palpable abdominal mass Abdominal scar	Ascites Other stigmata of liver disease (e.g., prominent abdominal veins, gynecomastia, spider angiomas, asterixis, encephalopathy, Kayser-Fleischer rings)
Laboratory studies	Predominant elevation of serum bilirubin and alkaline phosphatase Prothrombin time that is normal or normalizes with vitamin K administration Elevated serum amylase	Predominant elevation of serum aminotransferases Prolonged prothrombin time that does not correct with vitamin K administration Blood tests indicative of specific liver disease

rigors, indicative of cholangitis, strengthen this conclusion. The incidences of gallstone disease and malignant neoplasm increase with age, although risk factors such as obesity or recent extensive diet-induced weight loss increase the risk of gallstones. Other risk factors (e.g., hepatitis exposure, transfusions, intravenous drug use, alcohol use, certain medications, and family history of genetic diseases) and a predominant elevation in serum aminotransferase levels favor a diagnosis of parenchymal liver disease. Physical evidence of cirrhosis (e.g., spider angiomas, gynecomastia, ascites, splenomegaly) supports the diagnosis of chronic parenchymal disease.

Despite the general validity of these patterns, many exceptions exist. In particular, parenchymal disorders with prominent cholestasis may mimic biliary obstruction. Both alkaline phosphatase and GGT are usually elevated in patients with cholestasis; the combination of an elevated alkaline phosphatase and normal GGT suggests that the alkaline phosphatase is from bone. Conversely, an isolated elevation of GGT may result from certain drugs (e.g., diphenylhydantoin) or alcohol even in the absence of liver disease. Because of the risk of life-threatening infection in the setting of unrelieved biliary tract obstruction, this possibility must always be considered and excluded if an alternative diagnosis is not definitely established.

Imaging Studies

If extrahepatic obstruction is suspected, it should be possible to determine its site and nature in virtually all patients (see Fig. 149-3). A reasonable initial step is the use of a noninvasive study such as ultrasonography or computed tomography (CT) to determine whether the intrahepatic or extrahepatic biliary system is dilated, implying mechanical obstruction. Because of its lesser expense, lack of radiation exposure, portability, and convenience, ultrasonography is often the procedure of choice and is substantially better than CT for detecting gallstones. CT may be preferred when better anatomic definition and information about the general level of obstruction are desired. Still more precise resolution may be obtained with magnetic resonance imaging cholangiopancreatography (MRCP). However, all of these techniques can fail to identify dilated ducts, particularly in patients with cirrhosis or primary sclerosing cholangitis. Conversely, a modest degree of ductal dilation is common in a patient with a previous cholecystectomy and does not necessarily signify current obstruction. Ultrasonography has the disadvantage of being highly operator dependent, whereas optimal CT imaging requires the use of intravenous contrast agents that may be nephrotoxic.

If dilated ducts are found, the biliary tree should be examined by endoscopic retrograde cholangiopancreatography (ERCP) or percutaneous transhepatic cholangiography (PTC) (Chapter 136). ERCP involves positioning an endoscope in the duodenum, inserting a catheter through the ampulla of Vater, and injecting contrast medium into the distal common bile duct or pancreatic duct, or both. PTC involves percutaneous passage of a needle through the hepatic parenchyma into a peripheral bile duct, followed by injection of contrast medium into the biliary tree through the peripheral duct. The choice of procedure is based on the suspected site of obstruction (proximal vs. distal); the presence of coagulopathy or a history of prior gastroduodenal surgery that might preclude PTC or ERCP, respectively; the likely need for a therapeutic procedure (e.g., stent placement or endoscopic sphincterotomy); and the skills of available staff. Endoscopic ultrasound (EUS) is a complementary approach that permits internal ultrasonographic analysis of the pancreas, extrahepatic bile ducts, and regional lymph nodes and blood vessels. EUS combined with fine-needle aspiration permits tissue sampling of abnormalities in areas such as the bile ducts and pancreas that typically have been difficult to sample percutaneously.

Selection of Imaging Tests

Liver ultrasound is an ideal screening test to evaluate the liver architecture, assess for surface nodularity and parenchymal mass lesions, and exclude biliary obstruction. Ultrasound is relatively inexpensive in comparison to other imaging modalities, is widely available, and avoids ionizing radiation. The identification of mass lesions on ultrasound commonly prompts further cross-sectional imaging with either CT or magnetic resonance imaging. If there is evidence of biliary obstruction on imaging, or if obstruction is still considered likely despite imaging findings, direct cholangiography by ERCP or PTC, which offer therapeutic as well as diagnostic capabilities, may be an appropriate choice. If obstruction is considered possible but not highly likely, noninvasive imaging with MRCP is a reasonable study. Individual radiology suites have different levels of expertise for these procedures, and the local radiology staff may be quite helpful in recommending the best procedure for a given patient.

APPROACH TO THE ASYMPTOMATIC PATIENT WITH ABNORMAL LIVER TESTS

The apparently healthy patient with an isolated abnormality of aminotransferase or alkaline phosphatase levels requires careful evaluation to identify any underlying disease while avoiding unneeded testing. Often, no significant disease is found despite extensive evaluation. Common causes of abnormal

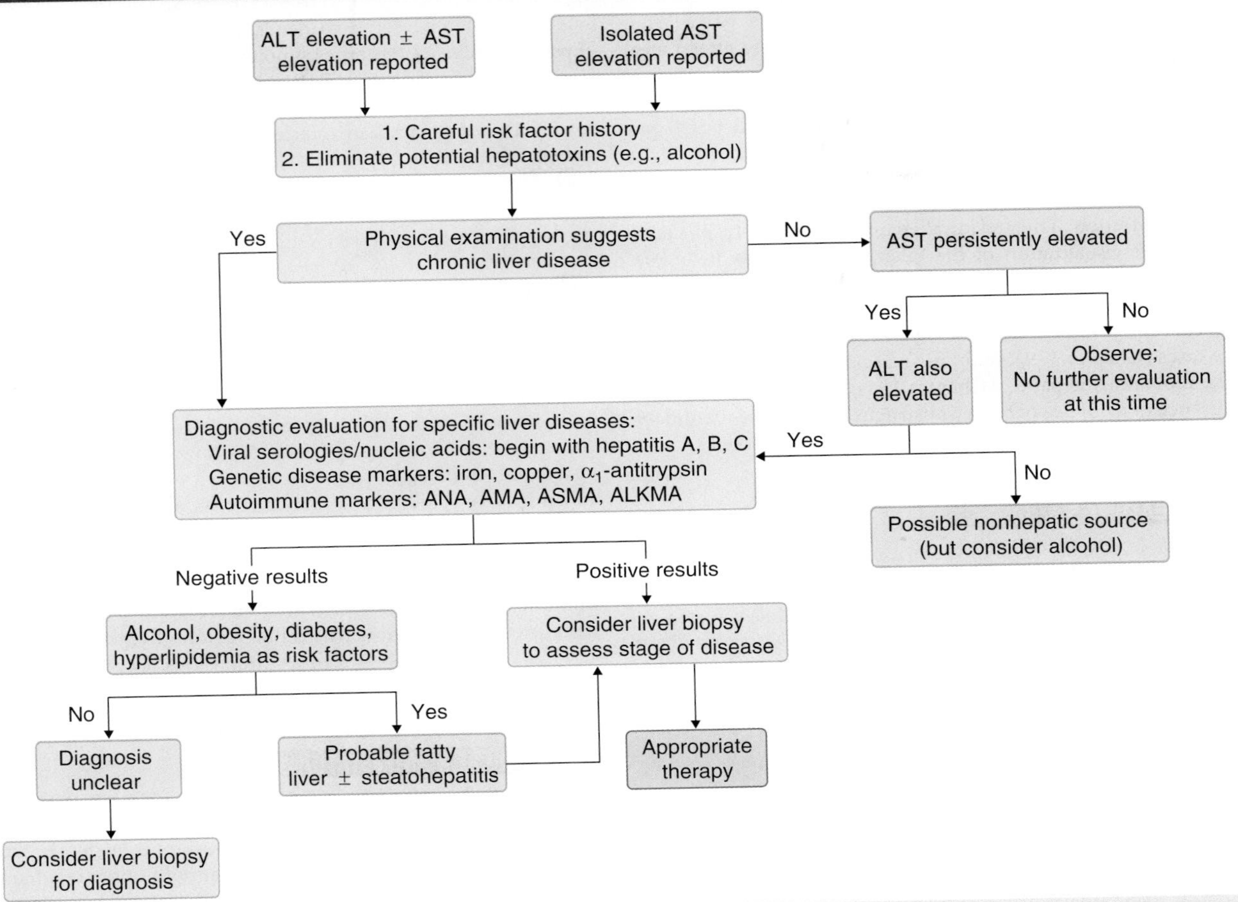

FIGURE 149-4. Approach to the evaluation of isolated elevated levels of serum alanine aminotransferase (ALT) and/or aspartate aminotransferase (AST) in the asymptomatic patient. ALKMA = anti-liver/kidney microsomal antibody; AMA = antimitochondrial antibody; ANA = antinuclear antibody; ASMA = anti–smooth muscle antibody.

enzyme tests include obesity, alcohol consumption, chronic hepatitis C, steatohepatitis, bone disease, and muscle injury.

Asymptomatic Aminotransferase Elevation

Epidemiologic data suggest that up to 25% of asymptomatic adult Americans have a mild to moderate elevation of aminotransferase levels. The incidental discovery of such abnormalities is currently the most frequent means by which liver disease is first recognized. Whereas up to one third of such patients have no elevation on subsequent testing, many others prove to have hepatic steatosis or steatohepatitis (Chapter 155) or chronic hepatitis C (Chapter 151) (Fig. 149-4). Further evaluation is generally indicated only in patients with persistent abnormalities. Initial screening should include a careful history of exposure to hepatotoxins (alcohol, prescription drugs, over-the-counter medications, herbs, chemicals, and occupational exposures). If the abnormal test was an AST, a hepatic origin for the enzyme elevation should be confirmed with an ALT determination. If the ALT is normal, a muscle source is likely, or the elevation may reflect the presence of a macroenzyme. If the ALT level is abnormal, the patient should be screened serologically for hepatitis B and C; young women in particular should also be screened for markers of autoimmune liver disease. Older persons should be screened for hemochromatosis with an iron and transferrin level (Chapter 219), whereas younger persons should be screened with ceruloplasmin and urine copper for Wilson disease (Chapter 218). If these tests are negative, screening for α_1-antitrypsin deficiency is indicated (Chapter 153). Malaria (Chapter 353), schistosomiasis (Chapter 363), and other parasitic diseases should be considered in appropriate settings. A substantial fraction of patients prove to have fatty liver, with or without nonalcoholic steatohepatitis (NASH; Chapter 155). AST abnormalities caused by alcohol-induced steatosis should become normal with several weeks of abstinence. If the abnormalities persist for 6 to 12 months without an apparent cause, liver biopsy should be considered.

Asymptomatic Alkaline Phosphatase Elevation

Many patients with isolated elevation of the alkaline phosphatase level have nonhepatic causes, such as pregnancy or bone disease (Fig. 149-5). The

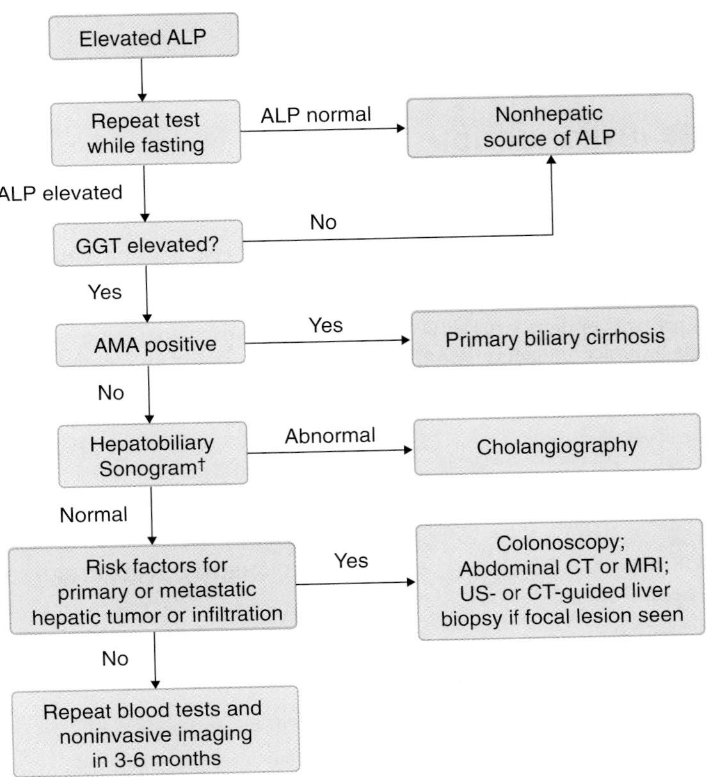

FIGURE 149-5. Approach to the asymptomatic patient with isolated elevated levels of serum alkaline phosphatase (ALP). †In cases with a high index of suspicion of biliary tract disease, such as sclerosing cholangitis, cholangiography may be warranted even in the face of normal ultrasound imaging. AMA = antimitochondrial antibody; CT = computed tomography; GGT = γ-glutamyl transpeptidase; MRI = magnetic resonance imaging; US = ultrasonography.

origin of an elevated alkaline phosphatase should be confirmed with a fasting sample because intestinal alkaline phosphatase may be elevated after a meal. A hepatic source is highly likely if the serum GGT is also abnormal. Women should be screened with an antimitochondrial antibody test; a positive result suggests primary biliary cirrhosis (Chapter 158). A careful history (Chapter 148) identifies patients at risk for intrahepatic cholestasis related to drugs or toxins. Essentially all other patients with persistently abnormal alkaline phosphatase should receive a hepatobiliary sonogram or other noninvasive imaging test. Demonstration of dilated intrahepatic or extrahepatic bile ducts should prompt direct visualization of the biliary tract by ERCP or PTC (Chapters 136 and 158). Evidence of an intrahepatic mass should prompt thorough evaluation for possible malignancy (Chapters 158 and 202). Because colon cancer often metastasizes to liver, colonoscopy may be useful in appropriate cases (Chapter 199). Infiltrative diseases, including schistosomiasis and granulomatous hepatitis (Chapter 154), should also be considered. In the absence of evidence of biliary obstruction or a cause identifiable by noninvasive means, liver biopsy should be strongly considered to complete the evaluation of cholestatic liver test abnormalities.

SUGGESTED READINGS

Castera L, Bedossa P. How to assess liver fibrosis in chronic hepatitis C: serum markers or transient elastography vs. liver biopsy? *Liver Int.* 2011;Suppl 1:13-17. *Discusses the advantages and limitations of liver biopsy and new, noninvasive diagnostic methods in clinical practice.*

Stapelbroek JM, van Erpecum KJ, Klomp LW, et al. Liver disease associated with canalicular transport defects: current and future therapies. *J Hepatol.* 2010;52:258-271. *Review of molecular transporters and their role in inherited and acquired cholestatic disease.*

Strassburg CP. Hyperbilirubinemia syndromes (Gilbert-Meulengracht, Criggler-Najjar, Dubin-Johnson, Rotor syndrome). *Best Pract Res Clin Gastroenterol.* 2010;24:555-571. *Summary of current knowledge.*

150

ACUTE VIRAL HEPATITIS

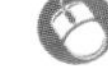

HEINER WEDEMEYER AND JEAN-MICHEL PAWLOTSKY

INTRODUCTION

Infection with a hepatotropic virus causes an acute episode of liver inflammation, referred to as *acute hepatitis,* which can lead to either spontaneous clearance of the infectious agent or its persistence, which in turn leads to chronic infection for a subset of these viruses. Five hepatitis viruses are responsible for the vast majority of acute hepatitis cases (Table 150-1): hepatitis A virus (HAV); hepatitis B virus (HBV); hepatitis C virus (HCV); hepatitis D or delta virus (HDV), which is a defective viroid using the hepatitis B surface antigen (HBsAg) as its envelope; and hepatitis E virus (HEV). Other viruses may also cause acute inflammatory liver disease, including members of the Herpesviridae family such as human cytomegalovirus, Epstein-Barr virus, or herpes simplex virus. It is unclear to what extent other viruses, such as parvovirus B19 or human herpesvirus 6, can also cause acute hepatitis. Patients who present with an acute viral hepatitis syndrome but negative virologic tests are referred to as having non A to E hepatitis, perhaps owing to unknown hepatotropic viruses. The worldwide incidence of acute viral hepatitis is decreasing because of global improvement in hygiene and the development and use of efficient vaccines against HAV and HBV, and perhaps in the future, HEV.

TABLE 150-1 VIRUSES RESPONSIBLE FOR ACUTE VIRAL HEPATITIS AND LIKELIHOOD OF CHRONIC EVOLUTION

VIRUS	EVOLUTION TO CHRONIC VIRAL HEPATITIS
Hepatitis A	Never
Hepatitis B	>90% (perinatal acquisition) to <1% (adult infection)
Hepatitis C	50-80%
Hepatitis D or delta	2% (coinfection) to 90% (superinfection)
Hepatitis E	Occasionally in immunosuppressed patients
Other viruses Human cytomegalovirus Epstein-Barr Herpes simplex Human herpesvirus 6 Parvovirus B19	May establish chronic infection, not associated with chronic hepatitis

GENERAL FEATURES OF ACUTE VIRAL HEPATITIS

PATHOBIOLOGY

Acute viral hepatitis is characterized by acute necroinflammation of the liver. Because none of the hepatotropic viruses is cytopathic, liver injury is thought to be mediated by a strong cytotoxic T-cell-mediated reaction against infected hepatocytes that express viral antigens at their surface. Proinflammatory cytokines, natural killer cells, and antibody-dependent cellular cytotoxicity also appear to play a role in liver necroinflammation. Successful immune elimination may lead to viral clearance, which may or may not be associated with lifelong immunity, depending on the infecting agent. The immune reaction is sometimes so potent that the patient develops subfulminant or even fulminant hepatitis that requires liver transplantation (Chapter 157). In some patients—the proportion varies, according to the virus responsible for acute hepatitis—the immune response fails and chronic infection is established (Chapter 151).

CLINICAL MANIFESTATIONS

After infection, there is an incubation period of a few days to a few weeks, depending on the causative agent (Fig. 150-1). This incubation period is generally characterized by nonspecific symptoms, including fatigue, nausea, loss of appetite, flu-like symptoms, and/or right upper quadrant pain (Table 150-2). The incubation period is often characterized by leukopenia and relative lymphocytosis. Immune-mediated symptoms, including rash, hives, arthralgias, angioneurotic edema, and fever, are observed in 10 to 20% of patients during the preicteric phase.

During the acute stage of the disease, symptoms may vary widely, from asymptomatic to subicteric, icteric or severe, and fulminant. The icteric form, which is not frequent, is characterized by fatigue, anorexia, nausea, dysgeusia, jaundice, dark urine, light colored stool, and weight loss. Physical

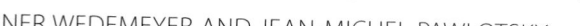

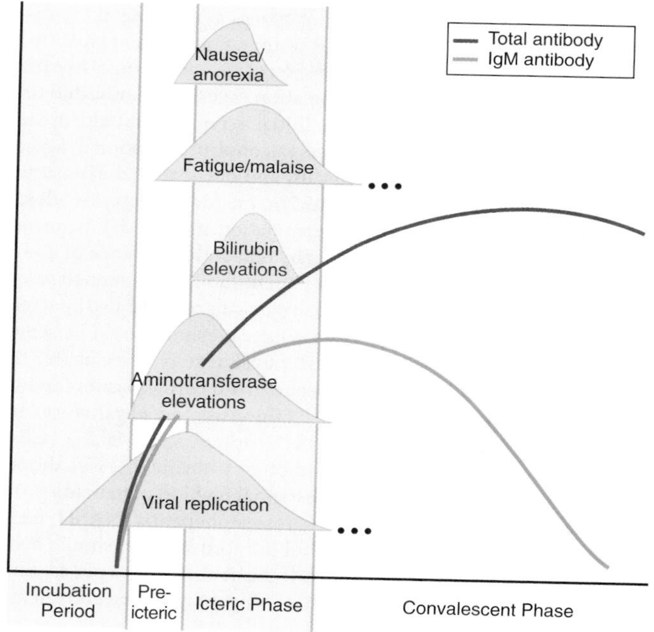

FIGURE 150-1. Typical course of acute viral hepatitis.

TABLE 150-2 CLINICAL MANIFESTATIONS OF VIRAL HEPATITIS

PHASES OF INFECTION	DURATION*	MANIFESTATIONS*
Inoculation	2-20 wk	Virus detectable in blood Aminotransferase and bilirubin levels normal No antibody detectable
Preicteric	3-10 days	Nonspecific symptoms: fatigue, anorexia, nausea, vague right upper quadrant pain Viral titers peak Aminotransferase levels begin to rise Serum sickness–like reaction (≈10-20% of cases) with rash, hives, arthralgias, fever
Icteric	1-3 wk	Jaundice appears; dark urine and light stools seen Nonspecific symptoms worsen Weight loss, dysgeusia, pruritus may occur Hepatosplenomegaly may develop Aminotransferase levels typically >10 times normal Antibodies appear Viral titers decline Rare extrahepatic manifestations (aseptic meningitis, encephalitis, seizures, ascending flaccid paralysis, nephrotic syndrome, seronegative arthritis)
Recovery	Up to 6 mo	Symptoms resolve gradually Antibody levels rise Aminotransferase and bilirubin levels normalize
Chronic	After 6 mo	See Chapter 151

*Varies by virus.

TABLE 150-3 LABORATORY TESTING FOR SUSPECTED ACUTE VIRAL HEPATITIS

GENERAL EVALUATION
Alanine aminotransferase Aspartate aminotransferase Alkaline phosphatase International normalized ratio
FIRST-LINE DIAGNOSTIC TESTS
Anti-HAV IgM HBsAg, anti-HBc IgM Anti-HCV antibodies HCV RNA
SECOND-LINE DIAGNOSTIC TESTS
Anti-HAV IgM present: none HBsAg present: HBeAg, anti-HBeAg, HBV DNA, HDV antigen, anti-HDV antibodies HCV RNA present with or without anti-HCV antibodies: none No virologic marker: see Figure 149-4

HAV = hepatitis A virus; HBc = hepatitis B core; HBeAg = hepatitis B e antigen; HBsAg = hepatitis B surface antigen; HBV = hepatitis B virus; HCV = hepatitis C virus; HDV = hepatitis D virus; IgM = immunoglobulin M.

examination reveals jaundice and hepatic tenderness. Hepatomegaly and splenomegaly may be present. On laboratory testing, acute viral hepatitis is characterized by elevated total and direct serum bilirubin levels and aminotransferase levels that are often more than 10 times the upper limit of normal. Cholestatic acute hepatitis is frequently associated with prolonged and fluctuating jaundice and pruritus. After 1 to 3 weeks, on average, both clinical and laboratory signs progressively improve and return to normal. Some patients, however, may experience a relapse before definitive resolution.

Fulminant forms of acute viral hepatitis are characterized by signs of hepatic failure, including changes in personality, aggressive behavior, sleeping disorders, and hepatic encephalopathy (Chapter 157). Coma can supervene rapidly, and widespread hemorrhage may develop.

DIAGNOSIS

The diagnosis of acute hepatitis is suspected based on elevated serum aminotransferase levels, which are generally more than 10 times the upper limit of normal (Table 150-3). Total and direct bilirubin levels are elevated if the acute hepatitis is subicteric or icteric. Alkaline phosphatase levels may be elevated in cases of cholestatic hepatitis.

Serologic and eventually molecular testing identifies the causal agent. Liver biopsy is generally not required. All cases of acute hepatitis should be reported to the local, state, or national health department as soon as possible after diagnosis.

TREATMENT Rx

In addition to virus-specific therapy for HBV and HCV, patients with acute viral hepatitis should avoid alcohol consumption. Sexual contact should be avoided if the partner is not protected. Patients with subfulminant or fulminant hepatitis should be evaluated for possible liver transplantation and supported in an intensive care unit setting (Chapter 157).

PROGNOSIS

Prognosis depends on the degree of prolongation of the prothrombin time, as well as how high the bilirubin and lactate levels are. A factor V level below 40% or any signs of encephalopathy are indications for hospitalization. Death is extremely rare and occurs only in fulminant cases. Other signs of poor prognosis are persistently worsening jaundice, ascites, and an acute decrease in the size of the liver. Serum aminotransferase levels and viral genome levels have no prognostic value.

HEPATITIS A

The Pathogen

HAV is a member of the Picornaviridae family, genus *Hepatovirus*. The hepatitis A viral particle is a 27-nm nonenveloped icosahedral nucleocapsid that expresses the hepatitis A antigen and contains a positive-stranded RNA genome approximately 7.5 kb long. At least four different HAV genotypes have been described in humans (genotypes I, II, III, and VII), with genotype I predominating worldwide. Other genotypes have been isolated in nonhuman primates. It is currently unclear to what extent different genotypes are associated with distinct clinical courses of infection.

EPIDEMIOLOGY

HAV infection has a worldwide distribution, and infections can be sporadic or occur in epidemic outbreaks. The incidence of acute cases and the seroprevalence vary according to the hygiene, sanitation, housing, and socioeconomic standards of the region, with seroprevalences as low as about 13% in Sweden but up to 100% in many developing countries. In developing countries, infection generally occurs at a young age, and most of the population has been exposed and is protected after age 10 years. In developed countries, however, infection can occur at any age, and the prevalence of exposed, immune subjects slowly increases with age. In the United States, the incidence of acute hepatitis A has declined from 12.0 cases per 100,000 individuals in 1995 to 1.0 case per 100,000 individuals in 2007.

HAV is generally transmitted via the oral-fecal route, most often directly from person to person or through the ingestion of fecally contaminated food or water. Transmission by blood transfusion has been reported, and isolated cases of apparent perinatal transmission have been described. High-risk groups for acute hepatitis A include travelers to developing countries, children in daycare centers and their parents, men who have sex with men, injection drug users, hemophiliacs who receive plasma products, and persons in institutions.

PATHOBIOLOGY

The genome serves as a messenger RNA and contains a single open reading frame that encodes both structural and nonstructural viral proteins. After attachment to a specific receptor at the surface of hepatocytes, the virus penetrates into cells and is uncoated. Subsequent events occurring exclusively in the cytoplasm include translation of the single open reading frame into a polyprotein that is later processed to generate the mature viral proteins; replication in a membrane-bound replication complex that generates new viral genomes, which are subsequently used for viral protein production and viral particle assembly; and packaging of newly formed genomes into new particles that are exported out of the cells. The virus is secreted into bile and, to a lesser extent, serum.

CLINICAL MANIFESTATIONS

Typically, the incubation period is 15 to 45 days (see Table 150-2). In most cases, acute infection takes a mild, often unrecognized course. The incidence of symptomatic, icteric cases increases with the age at infection. Acute hepatitis A in adults may require hospitalization in up to 13% of cases; prolonged courses of 6 to 9 months have been reported in 10% of adult patients with a diagnosis of acute hepatitis A. Hepatitis A is the most common cause of relapsing cholestatic hepatitis.

DIAGNOSIS

The diagnosis of acute hepatitis A is based on the detection of anti-HAV immunoglobulin (Ig) M in serum by enzyme immunoassay. IgM serum levels peak during the second month of infection (Fig. 150-2). HAV RNA can be transiently detected in stool and other body fluids by polymerase chain reaction (PCR) 3 to 10 days before the onset of illness and for 1 to 2 weeks thereafter; however, HAV RNA testing is generally not necessary. When the infection resolves, anti-HAV IgM disappears after 4 to 12 months, but anti-HAV IgG persists for life and confers definitive protection against infection.

TREATMENT Rx

Because HAV infection is self-limited, no specific antiviral treatment is required. In severe cases, patients may need to be hospitalized. If liver function is deteriorating, patients may need to be assessed for liver transplantation, which is the only therapeutic option for acute liver failure (Chapter 157).

PREVENTION

HAV vaccines consist of inactivated hepatitis A antigen purified from cell culture. Two doses of the vaccine at a 6- to 18-month interval are recommended. All vaccines are highly immunogenic, and virtually all healthy persons who are vaccinated develop protective anti-HAV antibodies. Patients with chronic liver disease also respond to vaccination but may display lower anti-HAV titers. An accelerated vaccine schedule, with vaccination on days 0, 7, and 21, is also effective and may be recommended for those planning to travel to endemic areas. HAV vaccines are well tolerated, and no serious adverse events have been linked with their administration; they can be safely administered with other vaccines or immune globulins without compromising the development of protective antibodies. A combination HAV and HBV vaccine is also available. Seroconversion rates are lower in patients with human immunodeficiency virus (HIV) infection and in other immunocompromised individuals.

HAV vaccination is recommended for nonimmune individuals who plan to travel to endemic countries, medical health professionals, men who have sex with men, persons who are in contact with hepatitis A patients, and individuals with chronic liver diseases. A childhood vaccination program leads to a significant decline in HAV infection, justifying its use as part of control efforts in endemic countries. Serologic testing for anti-HAV IgG can be performed before vaccination in adults born in endemic countries and in individuals older than 50 years born in industrialized areas; persons with detectable IgG are protected and should not be vaccinated. For postexposure prophylaxis, both HAV vaccination and immune globulin are effective; although immune globulin confers a slightly lower rate of infection, they should be used together.

Long-term follow-up studies after complete HAV vaccination show that anti-HAV titers sharply decline during the first year after vaccination but remain detectable in almost all individuals for at least 10 years. Protective anti-HAV antibody titers persist for at least 27 years after the successful vaccination of children and young adults.

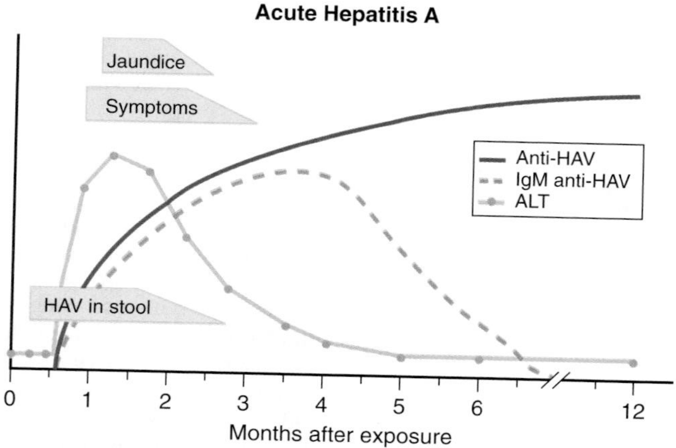

FIGURE 150-2. **Serologic course of acute hepatitis A.** ALT = alanine aminotransferase; HAV = hepatitis A virus; IgM = immunoglobulin M.

PROGNOSIS

Acute hepatitis A infection generally resolves without complications in 3 to 4 weeks and never evolves to chronic infection. Prolonged elevations of serum aminotransferase levels have been reported. Relapses a few weeks after the acute case have also been observed. Prolonged courses may occur in children and immunosuppressed individuals.

Cholestatic hepatitis A is unusual and has a good prognosis, with full recovery within a few weeks. Fulminant hepatitis A is rare, occurring in less than 0.1% of cases, but its incidence and mortality increase with the patient's age at acquisition. In the United States, 4% of all cases of fulminant hepatitis are caused by HAV infection. Overall, mortality of acute hepatitis A is 1.8% in patients older than 50 years. In patients with chronic hepatitis B, superinfection with HAV is associated with a 6- to 23-fold higher morbidity and mortality.

ACUTE HEPATITIS B

The Pathogen

HBV is a member of the Hepadnaviridae family, genus *Hepadnavirus*. The infectious virion, the Dane particle, is 42 to 47 nm in diameter. It possesses an envelope and a capsid or core that contains the partially double-stranded, circular DNA genome. The HBV genome is the smallest known human virus genome, with approximately 3000 nucleotides.

EPIDEMIOLOGY

Two billion individuals—that is, one third of the human population—have been in contact with HBV, and more than 350 million individuals have chronic infection. In the United States, approximately 0.5% of the population is chronically infected. HBV virions are produced and circulate in very high amounts in HBV-infected individuals, who are highly contagious. Four principal routes of transmission are responsible for acute HBV infections: (1) sexual transmission, which is the principal route in industrialized areas; (2) perinatal mother-to-infant transmission, which is associated with a very high (>90%) rate of chronic infection and is the principal cause of HBV transmission in Asia; (3) horizontal transmission through nonsexual interindividual contact, which is frequent at a young age in Africa and is associated with evolution to chronicity in approximately 15% of cases; and (4) percutaneous transmission by blood and blood products, unsafe medical or surgical materials, or injection drug use.

In industrialized countries, groups at high risk for HBV infection include individuals born in areas where HBV is endemic, including immigrants and adopted children; individuals who were not vaccinated as infants and whose parents were born in regions where HBV is endemic; household and sexual contacts of HBsAg-positive individuals; persons who have ever injected drugs; persons with multiple sexual partners or a history of sexually transmitted disease; men who have sex with men; inmates of correctional facilities; patients infected with HCV or HIV; patients undergoing renal dialysis; recipients of blood or blood products before 1987; and health care workers.

PATHOBIOLOGY

The HBV genome contains at least four overlapping open reading frames that encode a number of structural and nonstructural viral proteins. The pre-S/S gene encodes the three surface proteins—small (S), middle (M), and large (L)—which express HBsAg. The pre-C/C gene encodes the core protein that expresses the hepatitis B core (HBc) antigen and the hepatitis B e (HBe) protein, a nonstructural protein that plays a role in immune tolerance to HBV replication. The P gene encodes the HBV polymerase, whose two motifs—a reverse transcriptase motif and an RNAse H motif—code for two enzymes involved in HBV replication. Finally, the X gene encodes the X protein, which is a transactivator involved in HBV replication that bears oncogenic properties. The blood of infected patients contains not only infectious viruses but also a large excess of empty, noninfectious HBV envelopes.

The complex HBV life cycle involves multiple steps: fixation to an as yet unidentified receptor complex at the surface of hepatocytes; internalization; fusion and release of the nucleocapsid containing the HBV DNA genome and the associated HBV polymerase molecule in the cell cytoplasm; transport into the nucleus, where decapsidation occurs and the DNA genome molecule is released; transformation of the viral genome by the viral polymerase into a covalently closed circular DNA, which is the episomal form responsible for persistence of the HBV genome in the nucleus of infected hepatocytes; generation of messenger RNAs and viral protein synthesis; generation of a pregenomic RNA, which serves as a template for reverse transcription that generates the long DNA strand; degradation of the pregenomic RNA by the RNAse H activity of the viral polymerase; DNA-dependent DNA polymerase activity of the reverse transcriptase motif, which synthesizes the short complementary DNA strand in newly formed nucleocapsids; and, finally, budding into the endoplasmic reticulum, maturation, and export of newly formed virions.

Eight HBV genotypes (A through H), which differ by approximately 8% of their genomic nucleotide sequence, have different geographic distributions and may be associated with different clinical outcomes. Genotype A predominates in northern and western Europe, whereas genotype D is the most frequent genotype in the Mediterranean area and in eastern Europe. In non-Asian populations in the United States, genotype A predominates in men who have sex with men, whereas genotype D is the most frequent in intravenous drug users. In Asia and in Asian immigrants living in industrialized countries, genotypes B and C predominate. Genotype C has been associated with a higher incidence of severe liver disease and hepatocellular carcinoma compared with genotype B in Asia, perhaps because this genotype spread earlier than the others.

CLINICAL MANIFESTATIONS

Typically, the incubation period is 30 to 150 days. Jaundice has been reported in up to one third of adult patients with acute hepatitis B, but most cases are unrecognized. Among symptomatic patients (see Table 150-2), the manifestations are similar to those of other causes of acute viral hepatitis.

DIAGNOSIS

Four markers should be sought for the diagnosis of acute hepatitis B: HBsAg, total anti-HBc antibodies, anti-HBc IgM, and anti-HBs antibodies (Table 150-4). Acute hepatitis B is characterized by the simultaneous presence of both HBsAg and anti-HBc IgM (Fig. 150-3). Total anti-HBc antibodies are also present, whereas anti-HBs antibodies are not. During the convalescence phase, patients lose HBsAg before the appearance of anti-HBs antibodies; they have isolated anti-HBc antibodies, and the diagnosis is based on the presence of anti-HBc IgM. Recovery is characterized by the appearance of anti-HBs antibodies. The presence of both total anti-HBc and anti-HBs antibodies characterizes recovery from acute hepatitis B. Anti-HBc IgG remains at high levels for the patient's lifetime, whereas anti-HBs antibody titers may fluctuate and become undetectable after several years. Quantitative HBsAg assessment may be useful during the course of acute hepatitis B because if the HBsAg level does not rapidly decrease, the patient is at risk for chronic evolution. Patients who remain HBV DNA– and/or HBeAg-positive 6 weeks after the onset of symptoms are likely to develop chronic infection.

TABLE 150-4 SEROLOGIC PROFILES OBSERVED IN DIFFERENT PHASES OF ACUTE, SELF-RESOLVING HEPATITIS B

PHASE OF INFECTION	HBsAg	ANTI-HBc IgM	TOTAL ANTI-HBc ANTIBODIES	ANTI-HBs ANTIBODIES
Incubation	+	+/–	+/–	–
Acute hepatitis	+	+	+	–
Convalescence	–	+	+	–
Recovery	–	–	+	+

HBc = hepatitis B core; HBs = hepatitis B surface; HBsAg = hepatitis B surface antigen; IgM = immunoglobulin M.

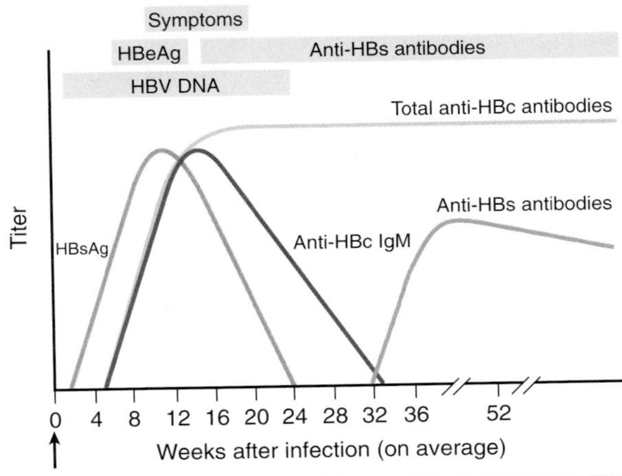

FIGURE 150-3. Kinetics of hepatitis B virus (HBV) markers during acute self-resolving hepatitis B. The arrow indicates infection. HBc = hepatitis B core; HBeAg = hepatitis B e antigen; HBs = hepatitis B surface; HBsAg = hepatitis B surface antigen; IgM = immunoglobulin M.

TREATMENT Rx

Acute HBV infection usually does not require antiviral therapy, and most patients spontaneously clear the infection. Antiviral therapy with lamivudine can decrease HBV DNA levels more rapidly but does not result in better clinical or biochemical improvement and may be associated with lower levels of protective anti-HBs at 1 year.[2] However, nonrandomized data in patients with severe acute or fulminant hepatitis B suggest that early antiviral therapy (lamivudine 100 mg daily) is safe and may reduce the need for liver transplantation.

PREVENTION

Because not everyone has been vaccinated, individuals who are aware that they are infected with HBV should take steps to avoid transmitting the infection to others. This is accomplished by ensuring that their sexual contacts and household members are vaccinated; using barrier protection during sexual intercourse; not sharing instruments such as toothbrushes, razors, and combs; cleaning blood spills with detergent or bleach; and not donating blood, organs, or sperm.

Prevention of HBV infection is based on vaccination. Universal infant vaccination programs have been initiated in many countries. High-risk individuals (e.g., health care workers, dialysis patients, family members and sexual partners of HBV carriers, pregnant women, and men who have sex with men) should be screened for HBV infection by HBsAg and anti-HBs antibody testing, and seronegative persons should be vaccinated.

Vaccination consists of the administration of recombinant HBsAg in three injections at 0, 1, and 6 months in adults. A lower dose is given at the same time points in newborns, children, and adolescents. Adults on dialysis require four injections at months 0, 1, 2, and 6. HBV vaccination elicits a potent neutralizing response, characterized by the presence of anti-HBs antibodies at titers greater than 10 U/L (protective titer). The seroconversion rate is higher than 90% in healthy individuals. HBV vaccines are well tolerated. Injection site reactions within 1 to 3 days, as well as mild general reactions, are common and transient. Postvaccination testing for anti-HBs antibodies to document seroconversion is not routinely recommended. However, persons who remain at risk for HBV infection, such as infants of HBsAg-positive mothers, health care workers, dialysis patients, and sexual partners of HBV carriers, should be tested to determine their response to vaccination.

Three percent to 10% of vaccinated subjects respond poorly or do not respond, especially smokers, obese patients, and elderly individuals. Nonresponders should receive another full course of vaccination, often with an increased dose. Other options include intradermal application and the coadministration of adjuvants and cytokines. One to two thirds of vaccinated individuals lose their anti-HBs antibodies after 10 to 15 years. It is unclear whether these subjects are still protected. Thus, persons at risk should receive booster immunization if anti-HBs antibodies have been lost.

When nonimmune persons or vaccinated individuals with an anti-HBs titer below 10 IU/L have contact with HBV-contaminated materials (e.g., needles) or have sexual intercourse with an HBV-infected person, active-passive immunization (i.e., infusion of hepatitis B immune globulin) plus active immunization (vaccination) is recommended within 48 hours after exposure. Vaccination alone is sufficient in persons with anti-HBs antibody titers between 10 and 100 IU/L, and no action is required if the anti-HBs titer is above 100 IU/L.

Infants born to HBsAg-positive mothers must receive hepatitis B immune globulin and be vaccinated within 12 hours of birth; this regimen reduces the rate of vertical HBV transmission from 95% to less than 5%. Mothers with HBV DNA levels above 5×10^7 IU/mL should also be treated during pregnancy with a potent nucleoside/nucleotide analogue with no teratogenic risk; the safest drugs in this setting are lamivudine and tenofovir, with the latter being more potent and having a higher barrier to resistance. Cesarean section is not needed if active-passive immunization is to be performed. Mothers of vaccinated infants can breast-feed, unless oral antiviral medications are present in the breast milk.

PROGNOSIS

Fulminant hepatitis is more frequent in acute HBV infection than in other types of acute viral hepatitis, with an incidence of about 0.1%. Factors associated with adverse outcomes of acute hepatitis B include advanced age, female sex, and perhaps some strains of virus. Whether infection with a precore mutant strain is associated with more severe or fulminant disease is still debated.

Among patients infected at birth, the rate of spontaneous recovery after an acute HBV infection is less than 5%, whereas adult infections spontaneously resolve in 95 to 99% of cases. Spontaneous resolution confers lifelong immunity, which is usually characterized by the presence of anti-HBs antibodies. Anti-HBs antibodies may become undetectable several years after resolution, but patients rapidly produce protective antibodies if they are re-exposed to HBV.

ACUTE HEPATITIS C

The Pathogen

HCV is a member of the Flaviviridae family, genus *Hepacivirus*. The genome is a single-stranded, positive, linear RNA molecule whose 5′ end contains an internal ribosome entry site involved in polyprotein translation; the genome also includes one single open reading frame and a short 3′ noncoding region involved in replication. The genome is contained in a protein capsid or core, which itself is surrounded by a lipid bilayer envelope into which two inserted viral glycoproteins mediate attachment of the viral particle to receptor molecules at the surface of target cells.

EPIDEMIOLOGY

HCV is present in all continents, and an estimated 120 to 130 million individuals, or 3% of the world population, are chronically infected. In industrialized countries, the incidence of HCV infection has declined considerably owing to blood screening and measures to prevent viral infections in intravenous drug users. However, about 35,000 new cases of acute hepatitis C still occur annually in the United States. In Germany, approximately 8 new infections per 100,000 inhabitants occur each year. HCV prevalence is higher in developing areas of the world, where the main route of HCV infection is unsafe medical or surgical procedures; only about 50% of blood products are screened for anti-HCV antibodies in these countries, and about 40% of all injections are given via reused equipment. Egypt's estimated 9% prevalence is the highest worldwide, owing to unsafe injection campaigns for the treatment of schistosomiasis. Although the incidence of acute hepatitis C has declined in Egypt during the past 15 years, up to 10% of cases of acute hepatitis are still caused by HCV.

HCV is transmitted almost exclusively by infected blood. Preventive screening with highly sensitive enzyme immunoassays and, more recently, nucleic acid testing has virtually eliminated the risk of post-transfusional HCV infection (theoretical risk: 1 in 2 million donations in the United States, 1 in 8 million donations in France). As a result, the principal route of HCV transmission in industrialized countries is now intravenous drug use, which is responsible for 60 to 80% of new cases. The incidence of HCV infection in this high-risk group is as high as 39 per 100 person years. In this context, imprisonment is an important risk factor for acquiring HCV infection in industrialized countries.

Nosocomial transmission through the use of improperly decontaminated materials or the contaminated hands or gloves of health care workers is responsible for a substantial number of new infections worldwide. HCV can also be transmitted by tattooing, piercing, or acupuncture if standard precautions are not implemented. Although HCV can be acquired after accidental needlestick exposure, the risk of infection is low (<1%), and health care workers have only a slightly higher prevalence of HCV than the general population. HCV can be transmitted to household members who share instruments such as scissors, razors, and combs. Sexual transmission is unusual, but outbreaks of acute hepatitis have been reported in HIV-positive communities of men who have sex with men. The risk of mother-to-infant transmission of HCV is less than 5% and is generally related to exposure to the mother's blood in the perinatal period. Cesarean sections are not recommended, and breast-feeding is not contraindicated. The risk of perinatal transmission is higher when the mother is coinfected with HIV. Other factors possibly associated with high transmission rates include the level of HCV viremia and maternal intravenous drug abuse. In 10 to 30% of cases, no apparent risk factor for HCV infection is identifiable, suggesting other potential sources of "community-acquired" hepatitis C.

PATHOBIOLOGY

Entry of HCV into cells is pH dependent through clathrin-mediated endocytosis and is followed by fusion. Decapsidation of viral nucleocapsids liberates free genomic RNAs into the cell cytoplasm, where they serve, together with newly synthesized RNAs, as messenger RNAs for synthesis of the HCV polyprotein. The post-translational processing of the HCV polyprotein results in the generation of at least 10 proteins, including 3 structural proteins (the core protein and the two envelope glycoproteins) and 7 nonstructural proteins. Infection with HCV leads to rearrangements of intracellular membranes, a prerequisite to the formation of the replication complex that associates viral proteins, cellular components, and nascent RNA strands in close proximity. HCV replication is catalyzed by a virally encoded RNA-dependent RNA polymerase within the replication complex. The positive-strand genome RNA serves as a template for the synthesis of a negative-strand intermediate of replication. Then, negative-strand RNA serves as a template to produce numerous strands that have a positive polarity and will subsequently be used for polyprotein translation, synthesis of new intermediates of replication, or packaging into new virus particles. Viral particle formation is initiated by the interaction of the core protein with genomic RNA. Budding of newly formed virions in the endoplasmic reticulum lumen leads to the formation of coated particles. Newly produced virus particles leave the host cell via constitutive secretory pathways.

Phylogenetic analyses of HCV strains isolated in various regions of the world have identified six main HCV genotypes, designated 1 through 6. These HCV types comprise a large number of subtypes, identified by lowercase letters (1a, 1b, etc.). The genotypes' nucleotide sequences differ by between 31 and 34%, and their amino acid sequences differ by approximately 30%; in contrast, the subtypes' nucleotide sequences differ by between 20 and 23%, with marked differences in particular genomic regions. The high prevalence and diversity of HCV genotype 3 and 6 strains in Asia and of genotype 1, 2, and 4 strains in Africa suggest that these types and subtypes emerged and diversified in these regions. In industrialized countries, a small number of HCV genotypes, including 1a, 1b, 2a, 2b, 2c, 3a, and 4a, have been introduced and spread rapidly among exposed populations. Subtypes 1a and 1b predominate all over the world. The most common genotypes in the United States are 1a and 1b (approximately 75%), 2a and 2b (approximately 15%), and 3a (approximately 7%). Genotype 3a is more prevalent in western Europe, where it accounts for up to 35% of cases, especially among intravenous drug users. Genotype 4 is highly prevalent in the Middle East and Africa. Its incidence and prevalence are increasing in intravenous drug users in industrialized countries. Genotype 5 is rare outside South Africa, and genotype 6 is rare outside Southeast Asia. Infections with different genotypes do not differ in terms of the clinical manifestations, progression, or disease severity (although this is debated), but the HCV genotype is a major determinant of the response to interferon-α–based therapies.

CLINICAL MANIFESTATIONS

HCV RNA becomes detectable in the serum 3 to 7 days after exposure. HCV RNA levels rise rapidly during the first weeks, followed by serum aminotransferase levels 2 to 8 weeks after exposure. Anti-HCV antibodies arise late in the course of acute hepatitis C and may not be present at the onset of symptoms and serum aminotransferase elevation.

TABLE 150-5 PATTERNS OF HEPATITIS C VIRUS (HCV) MARKERS AND THEIR SIGNIFICANCE DURING ACUTE HEPATITIS C

ANTI-HCV ANTIBODIES	HCV RNA	DIAGNOSIS
–	–	Not acute hepatitis C
–	+	Acute hepatitis C
+	–	Probably not acute hepatitis C (retest in a few weeks)
+	+	Difficult to differentiate acute from chronic hepatitis C

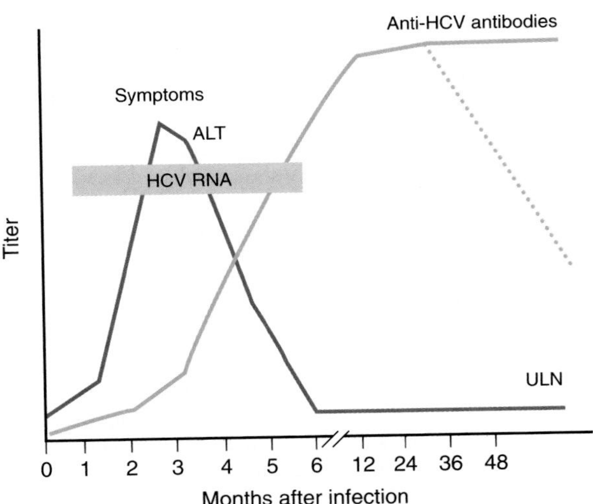

FIGURE 150-4. Kinetics of hepatitis C virus (HCV) markers during acute self-resolving hepatitis C. ALT = alanine aminotransferase; ULN = upper limit of normal.

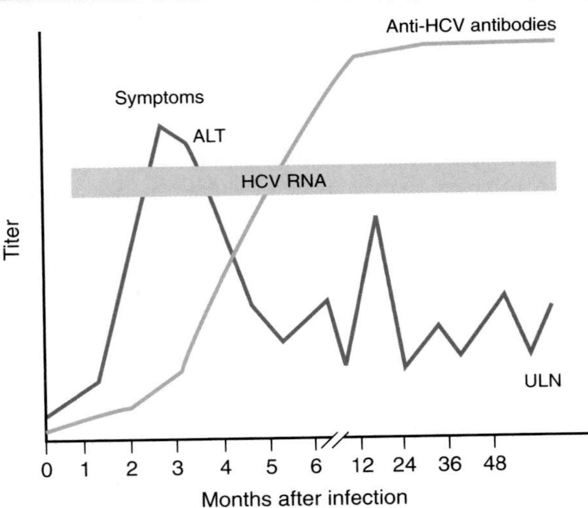

FIGURE 150-5. Kinetics of hepatitis C virus (HCV) markers during acute hepatitis C that evolves toward chronic infection. ALT = alanine aminotransferase; ULN = upper limit of normal.

After an incubation period that ranges from 15 to 120 days, acute hepatitis C usually remains asymptomatic and is undiagnosed. Nonspecific symptoms such as fatigue, low-grade fever, myalgias, nausea, vomiting, or itching may be present. Jaundice occurs in only 20 to 30% of patients, usually 2 to 12 weeks after infection. Serum aminotransferase levels commonly exceed 10 times the upper limit of normal in the acute stage, even in the absence of symptoms. Fulminant hepatitis C has been reported but appears to be exceptional in the absence of another chronic underlying liver disease.

DIAGNOSIS

When acute hepatitis C is suspected, patients should be tested for both anti-HCV antibodies by enzyme immunoassay and HCV RNA with a sensitive molecular biology technique (i.e., an HCV RNA assay with a lower limit of detection of ≤50 IU/mL). Four marker profiles can be observed, based on the presence or absence of either marker (Table 150-5). The presence of HCV RNA in the absence of anti-HCV antibodies is strongly indicative of acute HCV infection, which will be confirmed by seroconversion (i.e., the appearance of anti-HCV antibodies) a few days to weeks later. Acutely infected patients can have both HCV RNA and anti-HCV antibodies at the time of diagnosis; in this case, it is difficult to distinguish acute hepatitis C from an acute exacerbation of chronic hepatitis C or acute hepatitis of another cause in a patient with chronic hepatitis C.

Acute hepatitis C is very unlikely if both anti-HCV antibodies and HCV RNA are absent or if anti-HCV antibodies are present without HCV RNA (Fig. 150-4). Patients in the latter group should be retested in a few weeks, however, because HCV RNA may be temporarily undetectable owing to transient, partial control of viral replication before the infection becomes chronic (Fig. 150-5). Apart from such cases, the presence of anti-HCV antibodies in the absence of HCV RNA is generally seen in patients who have recovered from a past HCV infection. Nevertheless, this pattern cannot be differentiated from a false-positive enzyme immunoassay result, the exact prevalence of which is unknown.

TREATMENT Rx

Treatment of acute hepatitis C should be considered not only because it prevents chronic HCV infection, which can lead to serious clinical sequelae, but also because HCV viremia, which is associated with a risk of transmitting HCV to other persons, may have social, legal, and economic consequences, especially for infected health care workers. Treatment can be delayed for up to 3 months in patients with symptomatic acute hepatitis C, whereas immediate therapy is recommended if patients are infected with genotype 1 and have asymptomatic disease. Treatment of acute hepatitis C is based on the use of pegylated interferon-α2a or -α2b at doses of 180 μg/week or 1.5 μg/kg/week, respectively. Treatment should be administered for 24 weeks, but a shorter duration may be sufficient in patients with baseline parameters that predict a rapid viral clearance, such as symptomatic disease, high alanine aminotransferase levels, and low HCV RNA levels. Ribavirin should be added in patients who have a delayed or slow HCV RNA decrease with treatment, genotype 1 infection, and/or low or normal baseline alanine aminotransferase levels. With this treatment, 70% to more than 90% of patients have sustained viral clearance.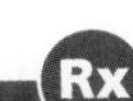 If treatment fails to clear the virus, patients can be retreated with a combination of pegylated interferon-α2a (180 μg/week) or -α2b (1.5 μg/kg/week) and ribavirin (0.8 g/day) for 48 weeks.

After accidental needlestick exposure, neither immune globulin nor preemptive therapy with pegylated interferon-α is recommended. Patients should be monitored with HCV RNA and aminotransferase level testing at baseline, week 2, and 4 and 6 months after exposure. Patients who have documented infection should be treated as above.

PREVENTION

Prevention of HCV transmission is based on standard precautions such as screening of blood and blood products, application of standard medical and surgical hygiene procedures, and safe use of syringes and materials for drug preparation in drug users. Needle exchange programs and education regarding the risks of drug use (including intranasal cocaine) and the risk of transmission from shared injection equipment are important.

No prophylactic vaccine is available against HCV. Phase I vaccine studies using HCV peptides, HCV proteins, or recombinant vectors expressing HCV proteins have induced HCV-specific T-cell responses or antibodies in healthy individuals, but full protection against infection by heterologous strains appears unlikely.

PROGNOSIS

About 50 to 80% of patients are unable to clear HCV spontaneously and develop chronic infection. Spontaneous recovery is more frequent if infection is acquired at birth (approximately 50%) and if acute hepatitis is symptomatic. It is unclear whether the genotype influences recovery rates. Other factors associated with better rates of spontaneous recovery include female sex, early decline of HCV RNA levels, and high aminotransferase or bilirubin levels. Patients who spontaneously recover may retain detectable anti-HCV antibodies for years to decades, but they are not protected against HCV reinfection.

ACUTE HEPATITIS D OR DELTA

The Pathogen

HDV, which is a satellite of HBV, can be transmitted only to patients who are acutely or chronically infected with HBV. Its single, negative-strand, circular RNA genome of approximately 1700 nucleotides folds in native conditions into a nearly complementary rod-like structure that contains a ribozyme. The HDV genome encodes one single structural protein, the hepatitis D (HD) protein, which expresses HDAg. The 36-nm infectious HDV virion comprises the HD protein and the genome, both enclosed within an HBsAg coat derived from empty HBV envelopes.

EPIDEMIOLOGY

Five percent of chronic HBV carriers, or 15 million to 20 million individuals worldwide, are also infected with HDV. The prevalence of HDV infection in HBV-infected patients varies according to the geographic area because it is transmitted primarily through parenteral exposure. As a result, its prevalence is relatively higher in HBsAg-positive intravenous drug users in Western countries, where approximately 8 to 12% of HBsAg-positive patients are infected with HDV. By comparison, the prevalence of HDV has decreased substantially in southern Europe, probably owing to universal HBV vaccination programs, improvement in hygiene and living conditions, and implementation of standard precautions to prevent HIV infection. The incidence of HDV is increasing in Russia, eastern Europe, Japan, and India.

PATHOBIOLOGY

HDV uses host RNA polymerase II for its replication, following the rolling circle model. Within cells, HDV RNA is associated with multiple copies of the HD protein to form a ribonucleoprotein complex. This complex is exported by the HBV envelope, which contains the three HBV envelope proteins, into the Golgi apparatus before being secreted.

HDV has at least eight genotypes, which differ from one another by at least 15% of their nucleotide sequences. Genotype I is the most prevalent HDV worldwide. Additional genotypes have recently been identified in Africa.

CLINICAL MANIFESTATIONS

HDV can be acquired at the same time as HBV (coinfection) or by a chronic HBsAg carrier (superinfection). Coinfection is characterized by one or two episodes of acute hepatitis, depending on the respective amounts of HBV and HDV present in the inoculum; acute hepatitis can range from mild to fulminant. In contrast, when chronic HBV carriers are superinfected by HDV, acute hepatitis D is generally severe, often fulminant, and chronic.

DIAGNOSIS

Three markers of HDV infection are total anti-HD antibodies, anti-HD IgM, and HDV RNA; each can be detected and quantified by real-time PCR. All HBsAg-positive patients should be tested.

In patients with an HBV-HDV coinfection, HDV RNA is only transiently present and is often missed. Anti-HBc IgM indicates concomitant acute HBV infection.

In HDV superinfection of a chronic HBsAg carrier, no anti-HBc IgM is present. HDV RNA is found in serum or plasma before and during the acute episode, whereas both total anti-HD antibodies and anti-HD IgM are present during the acute phase. Both serologic markers remain at high levels if the disease becomes chronic.

TREATMENT

Rx

No treatment of acute hepatitis D has been evaluated so far.

PREVENTION

The most effective means of preventing HDV infection is HBV vaccination, because individuals who are protected against HBV cannot be infected with HDV. In chronic HBsAg carriers, standard hygiene and behavioral precautions should be practiced to avoid superinfection with HDV.

PROGNOSIS

In patients who are acutely coinfected with HBV and HDV, only about 2% become chronic HDV carriers. In contrast, when HDV infection is acquired by chronic HBV carriers, about 90% also become chronic carriers of HDV.

ACUTE HEPATITIS E

The Pathogen

HEV is the sole known member of the genus *Hepevirus* in the Hepeviridae family. HEV is a small, nonenveloped virus. Its genome is a positive sense, single-stranded RNA molecule. Five HEV genotypes have been described: genotypes 1 and 2 appear to be strictly human, whereas genotypes 3 and 4 appear to be of swine origin but can also infect humans.

PATHOBIOLOGY AND EPIDEMIOLOGY

HEV transmission is principally oral-fecal. HEV is endemic in most developing areas of the world, where acute infections are sporadic or occur during large epidemics related to the contamination of drinking water. Genotype 1 has been found principally in Asia and North Africa, whereas genotype 2 has been isolated in cases from Central America and western Africa. No animal reservoir is known for these genotypes, and transmission appears to be linked to the contamination of food or drinking water. In industrialized countries, HEV genotypes 1 and 2 are not present. HEV genotypes 3 and 4 are endemic in swine, and zoonotic transmission appears to be the main route of transmission in Europe, the United States, and Asia. Diagnosed cases of acute hepatitis E have increased constantly in western Europe and North America in recent years, and high HEV seroprevalences have been described in special at-risk populations, such as butchers or farmers. Transmission may be favored by the consumption of uncooked meat and direct contact with infected animals.

CLINICAL MANIFESTATIONS

The incubation period is 15 to 60 days. HEV infection causes only mild, nonspecific symptoms in the majority of cases, especially if the infection is acquired early in life. Immunocompetent individuals clear the virus spontaneously. The peak of viremia occurs early during infection, whereas the peak of aminotransferase activity is reached approximately 6 weeks after infection. Severe disease is more frequent in pregnant women and in patients with underlying chronic liver disease, who may rarely progress to fulminant hepatic failure.

DIAGNOSIS

Diagnosis of acute hepatitis E is based on the detection of anti-HEV IgM antibodies, but current assays lack sensitivity and specificity. HEV RNA can also be detected in feces, serum, or plasma, where its presence is transient. Anti-HEV IgG generally persists for life after acute infection.

TREATMENT

Rx

Treatment of acute hepatitis E is not recommended because the vast majority of patients recover spontaneously. Severe and fulminant cases should be referred to specialized units.

PREVENTION

Improved public hygiene is the best defense against hepatitis E in developing countries. Travelers to areas of the world where HEV is endemic, particularly pregnant women, should be cautioned about drinking the water and eating uncooked food. An efficient prophylactic vaccine based on recombinant HEV proteins was 100% effective in a phase 3 trial.[4] However, the duration of protection is uncertain, so the vaccine's efficacy in preventing the spread of HEV has yet to be determined.

PROGNOSIS

Acute cases can be severe in elderly patients, and fulminant cases are frequent among pregnant women who are infected during large-scale water-borne epidemics. HEV genotypes 3 and 4 are less virulent than genotypes 1 and 2. Sporadic cases in industrialized areas are generally benign. HEV does not commonly evolve into chronic infection, but immunosuppressed patients and HIV-positive individuals can become chronic carriers.

OTHER TYPES OF ACUTE VIRAL HEPATITIS

Infection by members of the Herpesviridae family, such as cytomegalovirus (Chapter 384), Epstein-Barr virus (Chapter 385), and herpes simplex virus (Chapter 382), should be considered in the differential diagnosis of unclear episodes of elevated liver enzymes in the absence of markers of acute hepatitis virus infection, especially in immunocompromised individuals. For instance, cytomegalovirus infection can be associated with graft loss after liver transplantation (Chapter 157). Parvovirus B19 (Chapter 379) may persist in the liver and worsen liver disease in patients with chronic hepatitis B and perhaps in patients with chronic HCV infection. Human herpesvirus 6 variant A has been linked with syncytial giant-cell hepatitis.

Non A to E Hepatitis

Rare patients develop acute hepatitis of presumed viral cause but have no markers of known hepatitis viruses. Some of these cases may be due to variants of known hepatitis viruses, in particular HBV, that are not detected by the usual serologic and molecular methods. However, the existence of other, unknown hepatotropic viruses cannot be excluded.

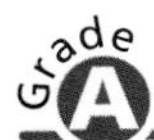

1. Victor JC, Monto AS, Surdina TY, et al. Hepatitis A vaccine versus immune globulin for postexposure prophylaxis. *N Engl J Med.* 2007;357:1685-1694.
2. Kumar M, Satapathy S, Monga R, et al. A randomized controlled trial of lamivudine to treat acute hepatitis B. *Hepatology.* 2007;45:97-101.
3. Jeckel E, Cornberg M, Wedemeyer H, et al. Treatment of acute hepatitis C with interferon alfa-2b. *N Engl J Med.* 2001;345:1452-1457.
4. Zhu FC, Zhang J, Zhang XF, et al. Efficacy and safety of a recombinant hepatitis E vaccine in healthy adults: a large-scale, randomised, double-blind placebo-controlled, phase 3 trial. *Lancet.* 2010;376:895-902.

SUGGESTED READINGS

Fitzsimmons D, Hendrickx G, Vorsters A, et al. Hepatitis A and E: update on prevention and epidemiology. *Vaccine.* 2010;28:583-588. *Review.*

Hadziyannis SJ. Milestones and perspectives in viral hepatitis B. *Liver Int.* 2011;1:129-134. *Review.*

Loomba R, Rivera MM, McBurney R, et al. The natural history of acute hepatitis C: clinical presentation, laboratory findings and treatment outcomes. *Aliment Pharmacol Ther.* 2011;33:559-565. *Review.*

Stramer SL, Wend U, Candotti D, et al. Nucleic acid testing to detect HBV infection in blood donors. *N Engl J Med.* 2011;364:236-247. *Triplex nucleic acid testing successfully detected HBV, HIV, and HCV during the window period before seroconversion.*

Wedemeyer H, Manns MP. Epidemiology, pathogenesis and management of hepatitis D: update and challenges ahead. *Nat Rev Gastroenterol Hepatol.* 2010;7:31-40. *Review.*

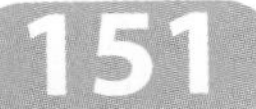

151 CHRONIC VIRAL AND AUTOIMMUNE HEPATITIS

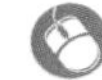

JEAN-MICHEL PAWLOTSKY AND JOHN MCHUTCHISON

DEFINITION

Chronic hepatitis is defined by chronic necroinflammation of the liver and may be due to various causes, including hepatotropic viruses, autoimmunity, alcohol (Chapter 155), and metabolic disorders (Chapter 153). Chronic infection by hepatitis viruses is by far the main cause of chronic hepatitis worldwide, with more than 500 million individuals chronically infected with hepatitis B virus (HBV) or hepatitis C virus (HCV). Chronic viral hepatitis B and C are the leading cause of cirrhosis (Chapter 156) and hepatocellular carcinoma (Chapter 202) worldwide and account for more than 1 million deaths per year. Chronic HBV infection can be associated with infection by hepatitis D virus (HDV). Hepatitis A virus does not cause chronic hepatitis. Hepatitis E virus (HEV) does not cause chronic hepatitis, except rarely in patients who undergo liver transplantation.

CLINICAL MANIFESTATIONS

The clinical symptoms of chronic viral and autoimmune hepatitis are typically nonspecific, and many patients have no symptoms. Fatigue, sleep disorders, and right upper quadrant pain may be present. Often the diagnosis is made when liver test abnormalities are identified by blood testing during a routine health evaluation or assessment for an unrelated problem or at the time of voluntary blood donation. More advanced symptoms include poor appetite, nausea, weight loss, muscle weakness, itching, dark urine, and jaundice. Patients can progress to full-blown cirrhosis (Chapter 156), with its typical clinical manifestations. If cirrhosis is present, weakness, weight loss, abdominal swelling, edema, bruisability, gastrointestinal bleeding, and hepatic encephalopathy with mental confusion may arise. Other findings may include spider angiomas, palmar erythema (see Fig. 148-2 in Chapter 148), ascites (see Fig. 148-5 in Chapter 148), edema, and skin excoriations (see Fig. 148-3 in Chapter 148).

TABLE 151-1 DIAGNOSIS OF CHRONIC HEPATITIS

DIAGNOSIS	SCREENING TESTS	CONFIRMATORY TESTS
Chronic hepatitis B	HBsAg	HBV DNA, HBeAg
Chronic hepatitis C	Anti-HCV antibodies	HCV RNA
Chronic hepatitis D	Anti-HDV antibodies	HDV RNA
Autoimmune hepatitis	ANA (anti-LKM1)	Exclusion of other causes and patterns of clinical disease
Drug-induced liver disease	History	Rechallenge, if necessary, is considered safe
Wilson disease	Ceruloplasmin	Urine copper concentration
Cryptogenic hepatitis	Exclusion of other causes	

ANA = antinuclear antibody; anti-LKM1 = anti–liver-kidney microsomal 1 antibody; HBeAg = hepatitis B e antigen; HBsAg = hepatitis B surface antigen; HBV = hepatitis B virus; HCV = hepatitis C virus; HDV = hepatitis D virus.

DIAGNOSIS

Levels of alanine aminotransferase (ALT) and aspartate aminotransferase (AST) are usually two to five times the upper limit of normal. The ALT level is generally higher than the AST level, but both can be normal in mild or inactive disease or 10 to 25 times the upper limit of normal during acute exacerbations. Biologic tests can establish the specific diagnosis (Table 151-1).

Alkaline phosphatase and γ-glutamyl transpeptidase levels are usually minimally elevated unless cirrhosis is present. Serum bilirubin and albumin levels and the prothrombin time are normal unless the disease is severe or advanced. Serum immunoglobulin levels are mildly elevated or normal in chronic viral hepatitis but may be very elevated in autoimmune hepatitis. Results that suggest the presence of advanced fibrosis are a platelet count below 160,000, AST levels higher than ALT levels, elevation in serum bilirubin, decrease in serum albumin, prolongation of the prothrombin time, elevation in α-fetoprotein levels, and presence of rheumatoid factor or high globulin levels.

Hepatic ultrasound can determine the texture and size of the liver and spleen, exclude hepatic masses, and assess the gallbladder, intrahepatic bile ducts, and portal venous flow. Computed tomography and magnetic resonance imaging of the liver are helpful if a mass or other abnormality is found by ultrasound. Hepatic elastography can assess liver stiffness as a marker of fibrosis.

Liver biopsy is usually critical for diagnosis and to determine the severity of disease. Hepatocellular necrosis is typically eosinophilic degeneration or ballooning degeneration throughout the parenchyma, greater in the periportal area, spotty, or piecemeal. Fibrosis also typically begins in the periportal regions and can link adjacent portal areas or portal and central areas (bridging fibrosis), distort the hepatic architecture, and lead to cirrhosis and portal hypertension. The histologic grade of chronic hepatitis can be determined by combining scores for periportal necrosis and inflammation, lobular necrosis and inflammation, and portal inflammation. Recently, ultrasound-based methods or serologic markers have proved accurate for the assessment of mild disease and cirrhosis, but they are less accurate for identifying moderate to severe inflammation, except in patients with chronic hepatitis C. Patients with suspected chronic viral or autoimmune hepatitis should be evaluated carefully for fatty liver, alcohol- (Chapter 155) or drug-induced (Chapter 152) liver disease, and metabolic liver diseases (Chapter 153), each of which can coexist with hepatitis. Liver biopsy can exclude other diagnoses that mimic chronic hepatitis, including fatty liver, alcoholic liver disease, steatohepatitis (Chapter 155), drug-induced liver disease (Chapter 152), sclerosing cholangitis (Chapter 158), iron overload (Chapter 219), and veno-occlusive disease (Chapter 145).

TREATMENT AND PROGNOSIS

Chronic HBV infection is not curable, but it can usually be controlled by appropriate antiviral drugs. HCV infection is curable, but less than 50% of patients who have access to therapy are cured. Autoimmune hepatitis responds to immunosuppression with corticosteroids and azathioprine.

CHRONIC HEPATITIS B

EPIDEMIOLOGY

More than 350 million individuals, or 8.5% of the world's population, are chronic HBV carriers. Two billion individuals, or one human being out of three, have been in contact with the virus. In North America, western and northern Europe, and Australia, less than 2% of the population are chronic hepatitis B surface antigen (HBsAg) carriers. In the United States, the prevalence is approximately 0.4%; that is, about 1.25 million Americans are infected. In eastern Europe, South America, the Mediterranean basin, and the Indian subcontinent, the prevalence of chronic HBsAg carriage is between 2 and 8%. Highly endemic areas, with a rate of chronic HBsAg carriage exceeding 8%, include China, Southeast Asia, sub-Saharan Africa, and the native populations of the Far North of America.

HBV is the main cause of primary liver cancer (hepatocellular carcinoma, Chapter 202) worldwide, with about 350,000 new cases attributable to HBV every year. Hepatocellular carcinoma is more likely in the presence of underlying cirrhosis, but HBV has oncogenic properties of its own, and hepatocellular carcinoma can occur in noncirrhotic HBV patients.

PATHOBIOLOGY

HBV is not a cytopathic virus. Rather, liver injury in chronic hepatitis B is a consequence of the local immune response at the immune elimination phase. In particular, liver injury is related to cytotoxic T cells that recognize and kill infected hepatocytes that express HBV antigens at their surface and to the local production of cytokines. Chronic inflammation triggers fibrogenesis through the activation of hepatic stellate cells. The hepatitis B X protein may also directly activate fibrogenesis. As a result, many patients with chronic hepatitis B have progressive fibrosis, which may evolve into cirrhosis.

The rate of chronicity after an acute HBV infection is more than 95% among patients infected at birth. This risk diminishes as the age at acquisition increases, and it is less than 5% in those infected as adults. Chronic HBV infection is defined by HBsAg carriage that persists for more than 6 months after the acute episode. Chronic HBsAg carriage typically evolves through three phases: immune tolerant, immune elimination, and inactive.

The immune tolerant phase is generally short if the infection occurred during adulthood, but it persists for years to decades in patients infected at birth or during early childhood. At the immune tolerant stage, the immune response of the host "tolerates" HBV infection and does not cause liver inflammation or hepatocyte destruction. The immune tolerant phase is characterized by the presence of hepatitis B e antigen (HBeAg), very high levels of HBV DNA in blood, normal serum or plasma aminotransferase levels, and no or minimal inflammatory activity on liver biopsy.

The immune elimination phase is characterized by an active immune response that causes necroinflammatory lesions and triggers hepatic fibrogenesis and progressive fibrosis. ALT and AST levels are increased, but HBV DNA levels are lower than during the immune tolerant phase and frequently fluctuate. The immune elimination phase has a variable duration, ranging from a few weeks to several decades. HBeAg, when present, defines HBeAg-positive chronic hepatitis B; it can be cleared and replaced by anti-HBe antibodies, defined as HBe seroconversion; or it can be absent while anti-HBe antibodies are present and to define HBeAg-negative chronic hepatitis B. Patients with HBeAg-positive chronic hepatitis B are infected with a wild-type virus and are able to secrete the HBe protein. Patients with HBeAg-negative chronic hepatitis B are infected with so-called precore mutant viruses, which cannot produce the HBe protein because they have a stop codon in the pre-C gene, and/or with core promoter mutant viruses, which produce considerably lower amounts of HBe protein.

The inactive HBsAg carriage phase is the result of successful immune elimination leading to HBe seroconversion. ALT and AST levels are normal, HBV DNA is undetectable or at very low levels, and patients without preexisting cirrhosis have normal liver histology.

CLINICAL MANIFESTATIONS

Chronic hepatitis B is usually asymptomatic. The most common symptom is fatigue, but sleep disorders, difficulty concentrating, and upper right quadrant pain are often observed. Chronic hepatitis B is characterized biologically by elevated aminotransferase levels, and ALT levels can fluctuate substantially during the immune elimination phase. Moderate cholestasis, with mildly elevated alkaline phosphatase and γ-glutamyl transpeptidase levels, can also be present, especially in patients with cirrhosis.

HBeAg-negative chronic hepatitis B is generally more severe than the HBeAg-positive variety. The incidence of spontaneous HBe seroconversion among HBeAg-positive patients is 8 to 12% per year when they are in the immune elimination phase; HBe seroconversion often follows a transient ALT flare. Some of these patients evolve toward inactive HBsAg carriage, whereas others switch into an HBeAg-negative form of chronic hepatitis B, with elevated ALT levels and an HBV DNA level greater than 2000 IU/mL.

The annual incidence of cirrhosis varies from 2 to 10% in patients with chronic HBV infection, with a cumulative incidence of approximately 20% at 5 years. The risk of cirrhosis is two- to four-fold higher in HBeAg-negative patients compared with HBeAg-positive ones, probably because they are older and have more severe disease at the time of diagnosis. The annual incidence of hepatocellular carcinoma in patients with chronic hepatitis B varies from 1% in patients without cirrhosis to 2 to 8% in cirrhotic patients, with the higher rates occurring in older patients. Patients with cirrhosis (Chapter 156) and/or hepatocellular carcinoma (Chapter 202) have the typical signs associated with these conditions. Rarely, chronic HBV infection is associated with extrahepatic manifestations, including glomerulonephritis (Chapter 123), most often in children, and polyarteritis nodosa (Chapter 278), mostly in adults.

DIAGNOSIS

Serologic markers used to diagnose chronic hepatitis B (Table 151-2) include HBsAg, anti-HBs antibodies, total anti–hepatitis B core (HBc) antibodies and anti-HBc immunoglobulin M (IgM), HBeAg, and anti-HBe antibodies. Molecular markers include HBV DNA and HBV resistance substitutions; real-time polymerase chain reaction (PCR)–based assays are the best way to detect and quantify HBV DNA

Chronic HBV infection is defined by the persistence of HBsAg in the serum for more than 6 months after the acute episode. The majority of subjects with isolated anti-HBc antibodies are not viremic. However, some individuals who test positive for anti-HBc antibodies, but not for HBsAg or anti-HBs antibodies, may be viremic; in these cases, the virus's amino acid

TABLE 151-2 VIROLOGIC MARKER PROFILES IN PATIENTS WITH CHRONIC HEPATITIS B VIRUS (HBV) INFECTION

					Anti-HBc Ab		
	HBsAg	ANTI-HBs Ab	HBeAg	ANTI-HBe Ab	IgM	TOTAL	HBV DNA
Chronic hepatitis							
HBeAg-positive	+	−	+	−	−*	+	>2 × 10^4 IU/mL
HBeAg-negative	+	−	−	+	−*	+	>2 × 10^3 IU/mL
Inactive carrier	+	−	−	+	−	+	<2 × 10^3 IU/mL
Reactivation	+	−	+/−	+/−	+/−	+	>2 × 10^3 IU/mL

*Anti-HBc IgM can be detected at low titers.
Ab = antibodies; Ag = antigen; HBc = hepatitis B core; HBe = hepatitis B e; HBs = hepatitis B surface; IgM = immunoglobulin M.

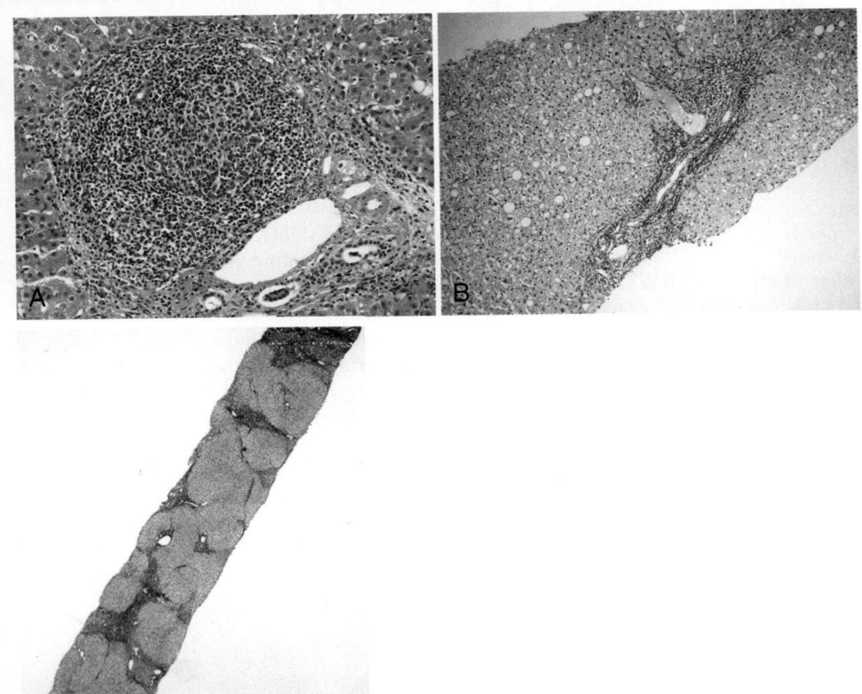

FIGURE 151-1. **Liver biopsies in patients with chronic hepatitis C. A,** Lymphoid nodule with germinal center; minimal interface hepatitis (hematein-eosin, magnification ×200). **B,** Mild fibrosis, Metavir score F1 (picrosirius-hemalun, magnification ×100). C, Extensive fibrosis, Metavir score F3 (picrosirius-hemalun, magnification ×20). (Courtesy of Prof. Elie-Serge Zafrani, Department of Pathology, Henri Mondor Hospital, Créteil, France.)

substitutions in the HBsAg sequence make HBsAg undetectable with current enzyme immunoassays. Other individuals may have such low-level HBV replication in their livers that HBV DNA is not detectable in blood ("occult" hepatitis B).

Serum or plasma ALT and HBV DNA levels are important markers of severity and prognosis. The assessment of severity, including the grade of necroinflammation and the stage of fibrosis, is based on the liver biopsy (Fig. 151-1). Noninvasive assessment using serologic markers or transient elastography can discriminate cirrhosis from mild hepatitis and fibrosis; although they are not accurate enough for intermediate stages, these methods will likely replace liver biopsy in the pretreatment assessment of the severity of chronic hepatitis B in many patients in the future.

PREVENTION AND TREATMENT

Rx

Patients with chronic hepatitis B should be vaccinated against hepatitis A virus, abstain from alcohol, and avoid immunosuppressive therapies unless absolutely necessary. HBV-infected patients who require corticosteroids or chemotherapy for other conditions should receive lamivudine 100 mg daily as prophylaxis against reactivation of hepatitis B.[1]

The goals of therapy are to suppress HBV replication, reduce the histologic activity of chronic hepatitis, and lessen the risk of cirrhosis and hepatocellular carcinoma. HBV infection cannot be completely eradicated because of the persistence of covalently closed circular DNA in the nucleus of infected hepatocytes. As a result, therapy attempts to reduce HBV DNA levels as much as possible—ideally, below the limit of detection of real-time PCR assays (10 to 15 IU/mL)—to ensure a degree of viral suppression that will lead to biochemical remission, histologic improvement, and prevention of complications.

Two different types of drugs for the treatment of chronic hepatitis B are pegylated interferon-α (IFN-α) and nucleoside/nucleotide analogues. Pegylated IFN-α2a, administered subcutaneously at a dose of 180 μg once a week for 48 weeks, improves various markers of HBV infection in both HBeAg-positive (Table 151-3) and HBeAg-negative (Table 151-4) patients.[2] Pegylated IFN-α2b (1.5 μg/kg) is very similar to IFN-α2a and is used by many liver experts, although it is not currently approved for HBV. The most frequent side effects of IFN-α are flu-like symptoms after the injections, fatigue, anorexia, weight loss, and alopecia. The most concerning side effects are neutropenia, thrombocytopenia, anxiety, irritability, depression, and even suicidal ideation.

Nucleoside analogues (lamivudine, telbivudine, and entecavir) require triple phosphorylation to be active, whereas nucleotide analogues (adefovir and tenofovir) need only two phosphorylations to be active. These drugs are given orally once a day at the following dosages: 100 mg for lamivudine, 600 mg for telbivudine, 0.5 mg for entecavir, 10 mg for adefovir (administered as the pro-drug adefovir dipivoxil), and 300 mg for tenofovir (administered as the pro-drug tenofovir disoproxil fumarate). All have short-term benefits on various markers of HBV infection in HBeAg-positive (see Table 151-3) and HBeAg-negative (see Table 151-4) patients. Entecavir and tenofovir are two of the most potent inhibitors of HBV replication,[3-5] and they are less likely to select for resistant HBV variants. These drugs are generally well tolerated. However, adefovir is nephrotoxic at doses higher than those used for HBV therapy, renal impairment and decreases in mineral bone density are rarely seen with tenofovir, myopathy is a rare complication of telbivudine, and peripheral neuropathy has been observed when telbivudine is combined with pegylated IFN-α.

Patients should be considered for treatment when their HBV DNA levels are greater than 2000 IU/mL and/or their serum ALT levels are abnormal if the liver biopsy shows moderate to severe active necroinflammation and/or fibrosis. Indications for treatment must also take into account the patient's age and health status and the availability of antiviral agents in individual countries. Patients in the immune tolerant phase and those with mild hepatitis on liver biopsy should not be treated, but follow-up ALT levels and HBV DNA assays are mandatory. Patients with compensated cirrhosis and detectable HBV DNA may be considered for treatment even if their ALT levels are normal and/or their HBV DNA levels are below 2000 IU/mL. Patients with decompensated cirrhosis require urgent antiviral treatment.

Two treatment strategies can be considered: a 48-week course of pegylated IFN-α or long-term oral treatment with nucleoside/nucleotide analogues. Whether their combined use improves the rate of sustained virologic response after treatment is currently under study. Pegylated IFN-α can provide a sustained virologic response, defined as a sustained HBe seroconversion (clearance of HBeAg, which is replaced by anti-HBe antibodies) and an HBV DNA level that remains below 2000 IU/mL after a 48-week course of treatment; however, an ALT flare can be observed at the time of HBeAg loss in patients in whom treatment is successful. Pegylated IFN-α treatment should be reserved for patients with the best chance of a sustained virologic response off treatment—HBeAg-positive patients with high baseline ALT levels (more than three times the upper limit of normal) and HBV DNA levels below 2.10^6 IU/mL. Pegylated IFN-α therapy is contraindicated in patients with advanced cirrhosis and in immunosuppressed patients. Patients infected with HBV genotypes A and B generally respond better to IFN-α therapy than do patients infected with genotypes C and D, but the predictive value of the HBV genotype for an individual patient is weak. Patients who fail to achieve a sustained virologic response after a single course of pegylated IFN-α are candidates for nucleoside/nucleotide analogue therapy.

Long-term treatment with nucleoside/nucleotide analogues is indicated in the majority of patients with chronic hepatitis B. Tenofovir or entecavir, which are the most potent drugs with an optimal resistance profile, are recommended as first-line monotherapies. HBV DNA should be suppressed to undetectable levels (<10 to 15 IU/mL) with a sensitive real-time PCR-based assay. If the HBV DNA level is reduced but still detectable in a compliant patient, the other agent may be added; however, the long-term safety of combined tenofovir and entecavir is unknown. When HBeAg-positive patients seroconvert to negative or HBeAg-negative patients lose their HBsAg, treatment should be continued for an additional 6 to 12 months. In all other cases, treatment should be continued for life, and adherence is particularly important.

Virologic breakthroughs—defined by a subsequent increase of the HBV DNA level of 1 log or more above the nadir level—in adherent patients are due to HBV resistance to the administered antiviral drug or drugs. HBV DNA levels most often increase back to baseline levels, and the virologic breakthrough is generally followed a few weeks later by a biochemical breakthrough in which a previously normal ALT level rises above normal. The cumulative rates of resistance in newly treated patients are 70% at 5 years for lamivudine, 17% at 2 years for telbivudine, 1.2% at 6 years for entecavir, 29% at 5 years for adefovir, and 0% at 2 years for tenofovir. These figures illustrate the high genetic barrier against resistance of entecavir and tenofovir. In a patient who develops resistance to any of the available nucleoside/nucleotide analogues, adding a second drug without cross-resistance is the only efficient strategy, although the long-term safety of some of these combinations is not known. In patients with lamivudine, telbivudine, or entecavir resistance, tenofovir should be added. Patients who have resistance to adefovir should be switched to tenofovir and also given lamivudine, telbivudine, or entecavir. In patients with tenofovir resistance, any of these three drugs should be added. The combination of tenofovir and emtricitabine, a nucleoside analogue similar to lamivudine, in a single tablet (approved for HIV but not for HBV therapy) is also a valid option in cases of resistance to any of these drugs.

In patients with cirrhosis, nucleoside/nucleotide analogue therapy is the only option because pegylated IFN-α is contraindicated if cirrhosis is decompensated. Because resistance in this population can be life threatening, some experts recommend de novo treatment with two potent drugs without cross-resistance. In those with decompensated disease, efficient antiviral treatment most often stabilizes the patient's condition and can also delay or obviate the need for liver transplantation. If transplantation is needed, post-transplant administration of anti-HBV immune globulins in combination with a potent nucleoside/nucleotide analogue prevents recurrent HBV in the vast majority of cases.

PROGNOSIS

Every year, approximately 0.5% of inactive HBsAg carriers spontaneously lose HBsAg, and most of them acquire anti-HBs antibodies. Reactivations are possible in inactive HBV carriers, especially if they become immunosuppressed, such as during chemotherapy or corticosteroid administration. HBV reactivations often evolve into a subfulminant or fulminant form.

The risk of cirrhosis in chronic hepatitis B is 2 to 10% per year, and it is significantly associated with a higher HBV DNA level, older age, alcohol consumption, coinfection with other hepatotropic viruses, and coinfection with HIV. The cumulative incidence of liver decompensation is about 15 to 20% at 5 years in patients with compensated cirrhosis. The complications of cirrhosis, including hepatocellular cancer, are among the main causes of mortality in HBV-infected patients, and the annual incidence of death is about 3 to 4%.

The likelihood of developing hepatocellular carcinoma is about 1% per year in patients without cirrhosis and 2 to 8% per year in those with cirrhosis, and it is significantly associated with a higher HBV DNA level, male sex, old age, reversion from anti-HBe-positive to HBeAg-positive, and coinfection with other hepatotropic viruses. HBV carriers at risk for hepatocellular cancer should be screened every 6 to 12 months, ideally with an ultrasound examination and an α-fetoprotein level.

CHRONIC HEPATITIS C

EPIDEMIOLOGY

HCV, which is present on all continents, is estimated to cause chronic infection in approximately 170 million individuals, or 3% of the world's population. The prevalence of chronic HCV infection, which varies geographically, is estimated to be about 1.3% in the United States (affecting 3.2 million individuals), 3.5% in Asia, 1.9% in the Americas overall, 5.2% in Africa, 1.7% in Europe, and 1.8% in Oceania. The highest prevalence is in Egypt (9% overall, but up to 40% in certain rural areas), where infection was initially spread by intramuscular injections for schistosomiasis during treatment campaigns several decades ago.

TABLE 151-3 SHORT-TERM (1-YEAR) RESPONSES TO APPROVED ANTIVIRAL THERAPIES AMONG TREATMENT-NAÏVE PATIENTS WITH HBeAg-POSITIVE CHRONIC HEPATITIS B

	PLACEBO/ CONTROL GROUPS	PEGYLATED IFN-α2A (48 WK)	LAMIVUDINE (48-52 WK)	TELBIVUDINE (52 WK)	ENTECAVIR (48 WK)	ADEFOVIR (48 WK)	TENOFOVIR (48 WK)
Loss of serum HBV DNA (%)*	0-17	25	40-44	60	67	21	76
HBeAg loss (%)	6-12	30/34†	17-32	26	22	24	NA
HBe seroconversion (%)	4-6	27/32†	16-21	22	21	12	21
HBsAg loss (%)	0-1	3	1	0	2	0	3
ALT normalization (%)	7-24	39	41-75	77	68	48	68
Histologic improvement (%)	NA	38‡	49-56	65	72	53	74
Durability of response (%)§	NA	NA	50-80	≈80	69	≈90	NA

*HBV DNA levels were assessed with various molecular assays, with different lower limits of detection.
†Responses at week 48/week 72 (24 weeks after stopping treatment).
‡Post-treatment biopsies at week 72 (24 weeks after stopping treatment).
§No or short duration of consolidation treatment for lamivudine and entecavir; most patients had consolidation treatment for adefovir and telbivudine.
Ag = antigen; ALT = alanine aminotransferase; HBe = hepatitis B e; HBs = hepatitis B surface; HBV = hepatitis B virus; IFN = interferon; NA = not available.
Adapted from Lok AS, McMahon BJ. American Association for the Study of Liver Diseases practice guidelines—chronic hepatitis B: update 2009, www.aasld.org.

TABLE 151-4 SHORT-TERM (1-YEAR) RESPONSES TO APPROVED ANTIVIRAL THERAPIES AMONG TREATMENT-NAÏVE PATIENTS WITH HBeAg-NEGATIVE CHRONIC HEPATITIS B

	PLACEBO/ CONTROL GROUPS	PEGYLATED IFN-α2A (48 WK)	LAMIVUDINE (48-52 WK)	TELBIVUDINE (52 WK)	ENTECAVIR (48 WK)	ADEFOVIR (48 WK)	TENOFOVIR (48 WK)
Loss of serum HBV DNA (%)*	0-20	63	60-73	88	90	51	93
ALT normalization (%)	10-29	38	60-79	74	78	72	76
Histologic improvement (%)	33	48	60-66	67	70	64	72
Durability of response (%)	NA	≈20	<10	NA	3	≈5	NA

*HBV DNA levels were assessed with various molecular assays, with different lower limits of detection. ALT = alanine aminotransferase; HBeAg = hepatitis B e antigen; HBV = hepatitis B virus; IFN = interferon; NA = not available.
Adapted from Lok AS, McMahon BJ. American Association for the Study of Liver Diseases practice guidelines—chronic hepatitis B: update 2009, www.aasld.org.

PATHOBIOLOGY

Acute HCV infection evolves into chronic infection in 50 to 80% of cases. Even patients who spontaneously recover and maintain detectable anti-HCV antibodies are not protected against reinfection. Persistence of infection is related to a qualitatively and quantitatively altered $CD4^+$ T-helper cell and cytotoxic T lymphocyte response that fails to eradicate infection. The plasticity of the viral genomes is responsible for the coexistence of closely related but genetically different viral populations in equilibrium in the patient's replicative environment. This genetic diversity allows continuously generated variant viral populations to be selected by timely changes in the replicative environment.

Chronic HCV infection is responsible for necroinflammatory lesions of varying severity, sometimes associated with steatosis, which is the accumulation of triglycerides in hepatocytes. HCV is not a cytopathic virus. Liver injury in chronic hepatitis C is related to the action of immune effectors that recognize and kill infected hepatocytes that express HCV antigens at their surface. Chronic inflammation triggers fibrogenesis through the activation of hepatic stellate cells. Fibrosis progresses at nonlinear rates that are generally faster in older patients, in males, and in the presence of chronic alcohol intake, viral coinfections, or immunosuppression. The severity of chronic hepatitis is independent of the HCV RNA level and of the HCV genotype. This chronic inflammation and progression of fibrosis predispose patients to cirrhosis (Chapter 156) and hepatocellular carcinoma (Chapter 202).

CLINICAL MANIFESTATIONS

Acute hepatitis C (Chapter 150) is most often asymptomatic and therefore undiagnosed. The most common symptom associated with chronic HCV infection is fatigue, but it may remain unapparent for years. ALT levels are usually moderately elevated and fluctuate, but they can remain normal for weeks to months despite active hepatitis on liver biopsy. Moderate cholestasis can be present in patients with cirrhosis. Patients with cirrhosis (Chapter 156) and/or hepatocellular carcinoma (Chapter 202) have the typical signs associated with these conditions.

HCV is the main cause of type II and type III mixed cryoglobulinemia (Chapter 193). Low levels of circulating cryoglobulins, which contain HCV RNA, anti-HCV antibodies, rheumatoid factor, and low levels of complement, can be found in 50 to 70% of cases, whereas elevated rheumatoid factor (Chapter 272) is found in 70% of cases. Less than 1% of HCV-infected patients develop symptoms of cryoglobulinemic vasculitis, including fatigue, myalgias, arthralgias, rash (purpura, hives, and leukocytoclastic vasculitis), neuropathy, and membranoproliferative glomerulonephritis. Cryoglobulinemia can be severe and lead to end-stage renal disease or severe neuropathies, and long-term cryoglobulinemia has been linked to non-Hodgkin's B-cell lymphomas (Chapter 191).

Low titers of antinuclear and anti–smooth muscle antibodies can be found in HCV-infected patients, but they do not have any clinical significance. HCV has been reported to trigger the symptoms of porphyria cutanea tarda (Chapter 217), and an association with lichen planus (Chapter 446) has been suggested.

DIAGNOSIS

Chronic HCV infection is defined by the persistence of HCV RNA for more than 6 months. In patients with clinical and/or biologic signs of chronic liver disease, chronic hepatitis C is diagnosed by the simultaneous presence of anti-HCV antibodies and HCV RNA. Detectable HCV replication in the absence of anti-HCV antibodies is observed almost exclusively in patients who are profoundly immunosuppressed, on hemodialysis, or agammaglobulinemic. The level of HCV replication does not correlate with the severity of liver disease or with the risk of progression to cirrhosis or hepatocellular carcinoma.

The HCV genotype, which has important therapeutic implications, should be determined. Anti-HCV IgM, which is found in about 50% of patients with chronic hepatitis, is of no significance. Laboratory testing often reveals high levels of monoclonal rheumatoid factor and cryoglobulins.

TREATMENT

Rx

Chronic HCV infection is curable. The goal of therapy is to achieve a sustained virologic response, defined by undetectable HCV RNA 24 weeks after the end of therapy using a sensitive HCV RNA assay with a lower limit of detection of 50 IU/mL or less.

The decision to treat chronic hepatitis C depends on a precise assessment of the severity of liver disease, the presence of absolute or relative contraindications to therapy, and the patient's willingness to be treated. Treatment typically requires a liver biopsy, but serologic markers of liver fibrosis and/or fibrogenesis and transient elastography have been validated in large series of patients with chronic hepatitis C.

In patients with no indication for therapy or with contraindications to therapy, repeated assessments of aminotransferase levels are recommended on a yearly basis. Assessment of liver inflammation and fibrosis by liver biopsy or noninvasive serologic or ultrasound-based testing is indicated for patients with persistent or intermittently elevated aminotransferase levels.

The current standard treatment for chronic hepatitis C is the combination of ribavirin (0.8 to 1.4 g/day orally) with either pegylated IFN-α2a (180 μg subcutaneously once weekly) or pegylated IFN-α2b (1.5 μg/kg subcutaneously once weekly). 6 The most common side effects of IFN-α are influenza-like symptoms (which can be prevented by acetaminophen), neutropenia, thrombocytopenia, irritability, difficulty concentrating, memory disturbances, thyroiditis, hair loss, sleep disorders, and weight loss. The principal side effect of ribavirin is hemolytic anemia. As a result of these side effects, dose modification is frequently required during therapy. Ribavirin should be decreased in 200-mg increments in patients with severe anemia. For IFN-induced side effects, the pegylated IFN-α dose should be decreased stepwise, from 180 to 135 to 90 μg/week for pegylated IFN-α2a, and from 1.5 to 1.0 to 0.5 μg/kg/week for pegylated IFN-α2b.

The main contraindications to therapy with pegylated IFN-α and ribavirin are decompensated liver disease, renal failure, severe immunosuppression, solid organ transplantation, cytopenias, severe psychiatric disease, and active substance abuse. Ribavirin is also contraindicated in patients with anemia, significant coronary or cerebrovascular disease, or renal insufficiency. Because ribavirin is teratogenic, it is essential that adequate contraception be practiced during therapy and for at least 6 months thereafter in both men and women.

In patients for whom therapy is deemed appropriate, the HCV genotype guides treatment and its duration (Fig. 151-2). Patients infected with HCV genotype 1 require 48 weeks of treatment and a higher, body-weight-based dose of ribavirin (1.0 to 1.4 g/day). Treatment should be tailored to the actual virologic response using a sensitive assay, such as a real-time PCR. The HCV RNA level should be measured before therapy and 4 and 12 weeks after its initiation. The lack of a virologic response (no change or an HCV RNA level that decreases by less than a factor of 100 [2 $\log_{10}$]) at 12 weeks indicates that the patient has virtually no chance of achieving a sustained virologic response and should stop treatment. In contrast, treatment must be continued if such a decline in HCV RNA level is observed at week 12. Patients who achieve a rapid virologic response (undetectable HCV RNA at week 4) can stop therapy after 24 weeks if their baseline HCV RNA level is below 400,000 IU/mL. Patients who do not achieve a complete virologic response (i.e., HCV RNA is still detectable) at week 4 but do so at week 12 should be treated for 48 weeks; then they can stop therapy. It is now generally accepted that patients with a slow virologic response (HCV RNA has decreased by more than 2 $\log_{10}$ but is still detectable at week 12) should be treated for 72 weeks because prolonged therapy significantly reduces the incidence of post-treatment relapse.

Patients infected with HCV genotypes 2 and 3 require 24 weeks of treatment, but at a lower ribavirin dose of 0.8 g/day. In patients who respond to treatment with an undetectable HCV RNA but relapse after the end of therapy, another 48 weeks of treatment with a higher, weight-based dose of ribavirin (1.0 to 1.4 g/day) is recommended.

Patients infected with HCV genotypes 4, 5, and 6 require 48 weeks of treatment and a higher, body-weight-based dose of ribavirin (1.0 to 1.4 g/day). The same approaches to monitoring and dose adjustment used for genotype 1 probably apply to these genotypes, but they have not been validated in sufficiently large cohorts of patients.

Currently, about 40 to 50% of patients infected with HCV genotypes 1 and 4 and 80% of patients infected with genotypes 2 and 3 achieve a sustained virologic response with the standard combination of pegylated IFN-α and ribavirin; rates for genotypes 5 and 6 are unknown. Predictors of a sustained virologic response include a baseline HCV RNA level less than 800,000 IU/mL, lack of extensive fibrosis or cirrhosis, young age, female sex, nonblack race, and single nucleotide polymorphisms in the host genome. However, none of these negative predictive factors should be used to deny treatment. Long-term maintenance therapy with a low dose of pegylated IFN-α is not beneficial, except perhaps in a small proportion of patients whose HCV RNA levels remain very low or undetectable on treatment.

The results of pegylated IFN-α and ribavirin therapy can be improved by reducing body weight and insulin resistance. Erythropoietin can control ribavirin-induced anemia and minimize ribavirin dose reductions. Granulocyte colony-stimulating factor can be used to reverse severe IFN-induced neutropenia. Careful management of anxiety, sleeping disorders, and depression is also important. Retreatment of patients who do not achieve a sustained virologic response with the same dose of pegylated IFN-α and ribavirin yields sustained virologic response rates of about 10 to 15%; retreatment with higher doses can be tried with careful monitoring and attention to side effects.

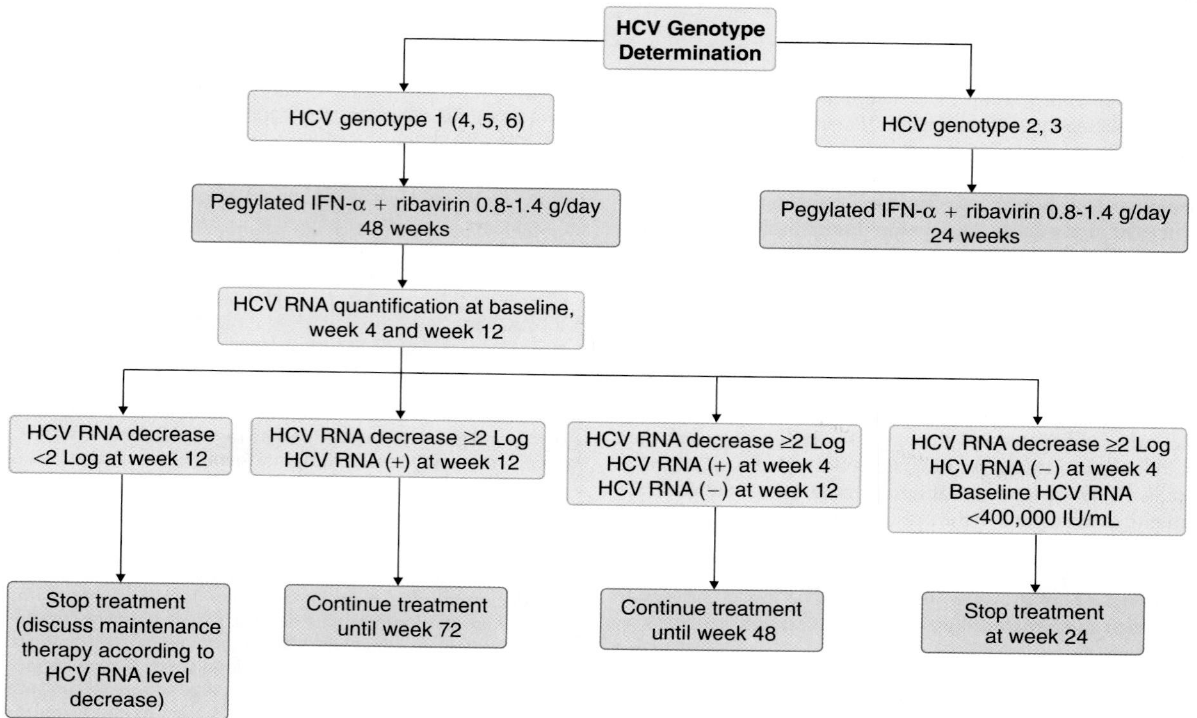

FIGURE 151-2. Pegylated interferon-α (IFN-α) and ribavirin treatment algorithm in patients with chronic hepatitis C, according to the hepatitis C virus (HCV) genotype.

New HCV drugs in trials include novel IFNs, alternatives to ribavirin, and direct-acting antiviral drugs that target various functions of the HCV life cycle. Telaprevir 750 mg three times daily or boceprevir 800 mg three times daily, in combination with the standard doses of pegylated IFN-α and ribavirin, has resulted in sustained virologic response rates of 70% in never-treated patients infected with HCV genotype 1 and in about 50% of patients who did not respond to a first course of standard two-drug therapy.[7,8] However, telaprevir frequently causes rashes and pruritus, and boceprevir can aggravate ribavirin-related anemia; furthermore, these drugs have little or no efficacy for genotypes 3 and 4. Similarly, the addition of boceprevir to standard therapy increases viral response in both never-treated[9] and previously treated[10] patients with genotype 1.

In patients with end-stage liver disease, liver transplantation (Chapter 157) is the only option. However, the graft becomes infected in 100% of patients who are viremic at the time of transplantation. Treatment with pegylated IFN-α and ribavirin is difficult in the post-transplant setting and yields disappointing results.

PROGNOSIS

Spontaneous HCV clearance in patients with chronic hepatitis C is exceptional. The HCV RNA level has no prognostic value in chronic hepatitis C.

It is estimated that 20% of patients with chronic hepatitis C develop cirrhosis; this occurs, on average, after 20 years of progression. Cirrhosis remains compensated for many years in the vast majority of patients, but decompensation occurs at an annual rate of 2 to 5% in cirrhotic patients. After a first decompensation, the mortality rate related to portal hypertension, hepatocellular insufficiency, and hepatocellular carcinoma is 10% per year, with a 50% survival rate at 5 years. The risk of death increases with advancing age, male gender, and the severity of cirrhosis.

Hepatocellular carcinoma is rare in patients with chronic hepatitis C without cirrhosis. In patients with cirrhosis, the incidence of hepatocellular carcinoma is 2 to 4% per year, most often in patients with compensated cirrhosis. HCV has become the most common cause of hepatocellular carcinoma in most industrialized countries.

Long-term follow-up shows that HCV does not recur in greater than 99% of patients who achieve a sustained virologic response, even in those who are immunosuppressed or receive chemotherapy. However, the liver disease may continue to evolve even after the infection has been eradicated. In addition, patients with chronic hepatitis C should abstain from alcohol and, unless there are other contraindications, should be vaccinated for hepatitis A and B (Chapter 17).

CHRONIC HEPATITIS D

EPIDEMIOLOGY

HDV infection occurs only in HBsAg carriers. Only approximately 2% of patients acutely coinfected with HDV and HBV develop chronic hepatitis D. In chronic HBV carriers superinfected by HDV, however, 90% of patients become chronic HDV carriers.

CLINICAL MANIFESTATIONS

Chronic hepatitis D is generally severe, with more than 80% of patients developing cirrhosis. Compared with patients who have chronic hepatitis B alone, patients with chronic infection with both HBV and HDV are three times as likely to develop hepatocellular carcinoma and twice as likely to die.

DIAGNOSIS

Markers of HDV infection should be sought at least once in every chronic HBsAg carrier. Both total anti-HD antibodies and anti-HD IgM remain at high levels in chronic HDV infection, and HDV RNA is present. Although all chronic HDV carriers also are chronic HBsAg carriers, chronic HDV carriers generally have low or undetectable HBV DNA levels because HDV inhibits HBV replication.

TREATMENT

Rx

High doses (9 million units three times/week for 1 year) of standard, non-pegylated IFN-α result in sustained normalization of ALT levels 24 weeks after the end of therapy in approximately 50% of cases, sometimes for as long as 20 years. Some patients clear HDV RNA and, eventually, HBsAg.

Pegylated IFN-α2b, 1.5 μg/kg once weekly for 12 months, provides a sustained virologic response in 20 to 40% of cases.[11] Although there is no clear consensus, most experts now recommend 1 year of pegylated IFN-α as first-line treatment of chronic HDV infection.

PREVENTION

Chronic HDV infection is best prevented by preventing primary HBV infection, because individuals who are protected against HBV cannot be infected with HDV. In chronic HBsAg carriers, standard hygiene and behavioral precautions should be practiced to avoid superinfection with HDV. Once acute HDV infection occurs, no secondary prevention strategy is successful.

CHRONIC HEPATITIS E

Although HEV infection was long thought to be self-limited, it can persist and cause liver inflammation in solid organ transplant recipients who harbor HEV RNA in their blood and liver tissues, either from a latent virus reactivated by immunosuppression or from a virus transmitted at the time of transplantation. All cases of chronic infection have been in immunosuppressed patients.

CLINICAL MANIFESTATIONS AND DIAGNOSIS

Chronic hepatitis E occurs after transplantation. Diagnosis is based on the detection of anti-HEV IgM antibodies, but current assays lack sensitivity and specificity. HEV RNA can also be detected in blood or feces, where its presence is transient. Solid organ transplant recipients with chronic hepatitis E harbor repeatedly positive anti-HEV antibodies and HEV RNA in blood.

TREATMENT AND PREVENTION

There is no validated treatment of chronic HEV infection. Whether candidates for transplantation or immunosuppressive therapies should be vaccinated to prevent chronic HEV infection remains to be determined.

AUTOIMMUNE HEPATITIS

Autoimmune hepatitis is a chronic inflammatory liver disorder characterized by the presence of autoantibodies in serum, high levels of serum immunoglobulins, and a frequent association with other autoimmune diseases.

EPIDEMIOLOGY AND PATHOBIOLOGY

Autoimmune hepatitis typically presents between the ages of 15 and 25 years or between the ages of 45 and 60 years, and it is more common in women. Along with primary biliary cirrhosis (Chapter 158) and primary sclerosing cholangitis (Chapter 158), autoimmune hepatitis is one of the three major autoimmune liver diseases.

Autoimmune hepatitis is believed to be caused by autoimmune reactions against normal hepatocytes in genetically predisposed persons or persons exposed to unidentified triggers of an autoimmune process against liver antigens. Associations are seen with the human leukocyte antigen (HLA) class I B8 and class II DR3 and DR52a loci. In Asians, autoimmune hepatitis is associated with HLA DR4.

CLINICAL MANIFESTATIONS AND DIAGNOSIS

Autoimmune hepatitis tends to be more severe at its onset than chronic hepatitis B or C, and it progresses to end-stage liver disease if not treated with immunosuppression. Although it is occasionally detected by elevated serum aminotransferase levels on a routine health evaluation, most patients present with fatigue and jaundice. Elevations of bilirubin or alkaline phosphatase indicate more severe or advanced disease. Patients typically have marked elevations in serum gamma globulin, specifically immunoglobulin G, as well as autoantibodies directed at non-organ-specific cellular constituents.

Type 1 (classic) autoimmune hepatitis is characterized by the presence of titers of 1:80 or higher (>1:20 in children) of antinuclear, anti–smooth muscle, antiactin, and anti-asialoglycoprotein receptor antibodies. Type 2 autoimmune hepatitis is characterized by similar elevations of anti–liver-kidney microsomal 1 antibodies and anti–liver cytosol 1 antibodies, without antinuclear or anti–smooth muscle antibodies. Liver biopsy shows features that are typical of all chronic types of hepatitis, except plasma cell infiltrates.

TREATMENT

The clinical symptoms and liver test abnormalities of autoimmune hepatitis generally respond promptly to prednisone, usually at a dose of 20 to 30 mg/day, with a decrease in serum aminotransferase levels to the normal or near-normal range within 1 to 3 months; higher doses may be required in patients with more severe disease. Lack of a biochemical or clinical response should lead to reevaluation of the diagnosis. Azathioprine 50 to 100 mg can be combined with prednisone or added later to reduce long-term steroid side effects. Maintenance doses, which are typically required indefinitely, are often 5 to 10 mg/day of prednisone combined with 50 to 150 mg/day of azathioprine. Sometimes patients can be maintained on azathioprine (2 mg/kg/day) alone. After 3 years or more of remission, therapy can be carefully withdrawn, but severe and even fatal flares can occur weeks to months later.

PROGNOSIS

The prognosis is generally related to the histologic stage of the disease. Patients who initially respond to therapy may do well for many years. Patients who progress to end-stage liver disease require liver transplantation (Chapter 157).

CRYPTOGENIC CHRONIC LIVER DISEASE

Cryptogenic chronic liver disease refers to chronic hepatitis or cirrhosis of unknown cause after excluding hepatitis B, C, D, and E; autoimmune hepatitis; steatohepatitis (Chapter 155); alcoholic liver disease (Chapter 155); drug-induced hepatitis (Chapter 152); and inherited and metabolic liver diseases (Chapter 153). Tests to exclude these conditions include serum levels of α_1-antitrypsin, iron, and ceruloplasmin and, if necessary, urine and liver copper concentrations. In its later stages, nonalcoholic steatohepatitis may be associated with little or no fat.

Grade A

1. Loomba R, Rowley A, Wesley R, et al. Systematic review: the effect of preventive lamivudine on hepatitis B reactivation during chemotherapy. *Ann Intern Med.* 2008;148:519-528.
2. Lau GK, Piravisuth T, Luo KX, et al. Peginterferon alfa-2a, lamivudine and the combination for HBeAg-positive chronic hepatitis B. *N Engl J Med.* 2005;352:2682-2695.
3. Chang TT, Gish RG, de Man R, et al. A comparison of entecavir and lamivudine for HBeAg-positive chronic hepatitis B. *N Engl J Med.* 2006;354:1001-1010.
4. Lai CL, Shouval D, Lok AS, et al. Entecavir versus lamivudine for patients with HBeAg-negative chronic hepatitis B. *N Engl J Med.* 2006;354:1011-1020.
5. Heathcote EJ, Marcellin P, Buti M, et al. Three-year efficacy and safety of tenofovir disoproxil fumarate treatment for chronic hepatitis B. *Gastroenterology.* 2011;140:132-143.
6. Fried MW, Shiffman ML, Reddy KR, et al. Peginterferon alfa-2a plus ribavirin for chronic hepatitis C virus infection. *N Engl J Med.* 2002;347:975-982.
7. McHutchison JG, Everson GT, Gordon SC, et al. Telaprevir with peginterferon and ribavirin for chronic HCV genotype 1 infection. *N Engl J Med.* 2009;360:1827-1838.
8. Hézode C, Forestier N, Dusheiko G, et al. Telaprevir and peginterferon with or without ribavirin for chronic HCV infection. *N Engl J Med.* 2009;360:1839-1850.
9. Poordad F, McCone J Jr, Bacon BR, et al. Boceprevir for untreated chronic HCV genotype 1 infection. *N Engl J Med.* 2011;364:1195-1206.
10. Bacon BR, Gordon SC, Lawitz E, et al. Boceprevir for previously treated chronic HCV genotype 1 infection. *N Engl J Med.* 2011;364:1207-1217.
11. Wedemeyer H, Yurdaydin C, Dalekos GN, et al. Peginterferon plus adefovir versus either drug alone for hepatitis delta. *N Engl J Med.* 2011;364:322-331.

SUGGESTED READINGS

Alberti A, Caporaso N. HBV therapy: guidelines and open issues. *Dig Liver Dis.* 2011;43:57-63. *Review of guidelines.*

Ghany MG, Strader DB, Thomas DL. Diagnosis, management and treatment of hepatitis C: an update. *Hepatology.* 2009;49:1335-1374. *Clinical practice guidelines of the American Association for the Study of Liver Diseases.*

Vergani D, Mieli-Vergani G. Pharmacological management of autoimmune hepatitis. *Expert Opin Pharmacother.* 2011;12:607-613. *Most patients respond rapidly to prednisolone and azathioprine.*

Woo G, Tomlinson G, Nishikawa Y, et al. Tenofovir and entecavir are most effective antiviral agents for chronic hepatitis B: a systematic review and Bayesian meta-analyses. *Gastroenterology.* 2010;139:1218-1229. *Conclusions based on meta-analysis.*

152

TOXIN- AND DRUG-INDUCED LIVER DISEASE

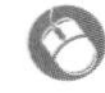

WILLIAM M. LEE

DEFINITION

Toxin-induced and drug-induced hepatotoxicity, defined as any degree of liver injury caused by a drug or a toxic substance, is a frequent cause of acute liver injury and accounts for more than 50% of all cases of acute liver failure with hepatic encephalopathy in the United States. Hepatotoxicity has been described with many drugs, although the number of cases is low, given the number of prescriptions written.

EPIDEMIOLOGY

Few data are available on the epidemiology of toxin- and drug-induced liver disease. The precise number of drug-induced liver injuries in the United States is unknown, but European data on adverse drug reactions indicate about 22 cases of drug-induced liver disease per 1 million people per year. In developing parts of the world, drug-induced liver disease is much less common and is related to fewer drugs. It is estimated that less than 10% of actual cases are reported, so the true incidence of toxin- and drug-induced liver disease may be impossible to determine.

PATHOBIOLOGY

The liver is central to the metabolism of exogenous substances. Most drugs and xenobiotics cross the intestinal brush border because they are lipophilic. *Biotransformation* is the process by which lipophilic therapeutic agents are rendered more hydrophilic by the liver, resulting in drug excretion in urine or bile. In most instances, biotransformation changes a nonpolar to a polar compound through several steps. Foremost are oxidative pathways (e.g., hydroxylation) mediated by the cytochromes (CYPs) P-450 (Chapter 28). The next step is typically esterification to form sulfates and glucuronides, a process that results in the addition of highly polar groups to the hydroxyl group. These two enzymatic steps are referred to as *phase I* (CYP oxidation) and *phase II* (esterification). Other important metabolic pathways involve glutathione-*S*-transferase, acetylating enzymes, and alcohol dehydrogenase, but the principal metabolic pathways for most pharmacologic agents involve CYPs and subsequent esterification.

Pathogenesis

The exact details of the pathogenesis of liver injury are unclear for most drugs. A single drug may cause toxic effects in several ways. One overarching approach suggests that high-energy unstable metabolites of the parent drug, the result of CYP activation, bind to cell proteins or DNA and disrupt cell function. Perhaps the best example is acetaminophen. Although used universally for non-narcotic pain relief, acetaminophen, when taken in large quantities, causes profound centrilobular necrosis. The metabolic pathway of acetaminophen involves phase I and phase II reactions, glutathione detoxification, and the formation of reactive intermediates (E-Fig. 152-1). The presence of alcohol, which competes for CYP P-450 2E1, not only inhibits the formation of *N*-aminoparaquinoneamine (NAPQI) but also induces the enzyme so that its half-life is slowed and more enzyme is present. After the cessation of alcohol ingestion, NAPQI formation is enhanced by the presence of the induced enzyme and the lack of competition from alcohol. Toxicity is a dynamic process and may be most pronounced in the 24 hours after the cessation of alcohol. Glucuronidation and sulfation occur as the initial detoxifying step because the parent compound contains a hydroxyl group. Glucuronidation and sulfation capacity greatly exceeds daily needs, so even patients with very advanced liver disease continue to have adequate glucuronidation capacity, which explains why no obvious enhancement of toxicity is observed when cirrhotic patients take acetaminophen.

Genetics

Enzyme Polymorphism

Although acetaminophen is a dose-related toxin, the rarity of idiosyncratic drug toxicity (1 in 10,000 patients) suggests the importance of environmental and host factors (Table 152-1). Genetically variant CYP isoenzymes may partially explain the observed individual variation in response to drugs. An example is debrisoquine, an antihypertensive drug marketed in Europe that is hydroxylated by CYP2D6, an isoform that is totally absent in 5% of normal individuals. Lack of CYP2D6 greatly prolongs the half-life of the parent compound in affected individuals. Another example is the phenomenon of fast versus slow acetylation, which affects different ethnic groups and has been implicated in the differential metabolism of isoniazid. Most of the known genetic variants that occur relatively frequently, however, cannot explain the formation of a toxic intermediate in only a rare individual.

Most drugs are small organic compounds, unlikely to evoke an immune response. Although some toxic drug reactions are associated with an obvious allergic response, most are not. Nevertheless, immune mechanisms not associated with systemic allergic immunoglobulin E (IgE) reactions or skin hypersensitivity might be involved. Studies suggest that the products of CYP P-450 metabolism, the highly reactive intermediates formed within the microsomes, covalently bind to the enzyme itself to form a drug-hapten adduct that disables the enzyme and injures the cell. Haptenization then evokes an immune response directed against the newly formed antigen or neoantigen. P-450s have been shown to traffic to the plasma membrane, thereby allowing the drug–P-450 adduct to become the target of a subsequent cytolytic attack. It is unclear whether the targets are these adducts or the smaller peptides processed and presented by the major histocompatibility complex class I and class II schemes. The association among neoantigens, autoantibodies, and hepatotoxic drugs implicates an immunologic mechanism.

Regardless of whether an individual drug causes significant cell necrosis, the drug–P-450 adducts can evoke an immune response. Any subsequent drug–P-450 adduct present on the hepatocyte surface would evoke a further response. Responses may be antibody mediated or occur as a result of direct cytolytic attack by primed T cells. Specific genetically determined components of the immune response may be important. A specific human leukocyte antigen (HLA) haplotype has been associated with amoxicillin-clavulanate–induced hepatitis, and polymorphisms have been identified for the interleukin-10 promoter and for tumor necrosis factor-α. For every patient with a severe injury caused by drugs, there are often many more individuals with asymptomatic aminotransferase elevations that subsided despite continuing the drug—sometimes referred to as an adaptive response.

Other Mechanisms

In drug-induced cholestasis, disruption of specific transport proteins or processes in hepatocytes or cholangiocytes may be the key event. Estrogen may cause multiple canalicular membrane transport changes that affect, among others, the canalicular bile salt pump. Uncoupling or inhibition of mitochondrial respiration may lead to microvesicular steatosis.

Hepatotoxic Agents

Although there are a few dose-related toxins, most drugs involved in liver disease cause idiosyncratic, unpredictable toxicity.

TABLE 152-1 FACTORS THAT MAY INFLUENCE THE METABOLIC FATE OF DRUGS

AGE
The elderly seem to be affected more often; adults are more susceptible than children to some drugs (acetaminophen, halothane, isoniazid) and less susceptible to others (aspirin, valproic acid)
ALCOHOL, ACUTE AND CHRONIC INGESTION
Induction of CYP2E1 affects drugs metabolized by this pathway, including acetaminophen and isoniazid
GENDER
Females are affected more often, but the reason is unknown
PREGNANCY
Effects of drugs in pregnancy have been poorly studied
PREEXISTING LIVER DISEASE
Hepatic disease may *protect* against idiosyncratic reactions and may *enhance* the toxicity of dose-dependent hepatotoxins (e.g., acetaminophen)
RENAL DISEASE
Slowed disappearance of the parent compound yields higher concentrations and affects P-450 (e.g., enhancement of tetracycline toxicity in renal disease)
CERTAIN FOODS
Grapefruit has an unknown substance that interferes with the metabolism of some drugs
CONCOMITANT DRUGS
Drug-drug interactions are common causes of adverse effects (e.g., valproate and chlorpromazine together lead to enhanced cholestasis)
GENETIC FACTORS
Enzyme polymorphisms (e.g., enhanced phenytoin liver disease in patients with defective epoxide hydrolase activity), HLA phenotypes (e.g., nitrofurantoin susceptibility)

TABLE 152-2 DRUGS AND TOXINS IN WHICH A DOSE-RESPONSE EFFECT IS OBSERVED

DRUG OR TOXIN	RESPONSE
Acetaminophen	Total dose, single vs. multiple time points
Amiodarone	Total dose over time
Bromfenac	Toxicity occurs only after extended use
Cocaine	Dose-related vascular collapse
Cyclophosphamide	Dose related, worse with previous ALT elevations
Cyclosporine	Cholestasis with toxic blood levels, CYP3A phenotype
Methotrexate	Aminotransferase, fibrosis; single dose/total dose
Niacin	Large doses cause vascular collapse
Oral contraceptives	Prolonged use causes hepatic adenomas
Tetracycline	Total dose, renal dysfunction
Toxins (yellow phosphorus, carbon tetrachloride, *Amanita* toxin, bacterial toxins)	Total dose

ALT = alanine aminotransferase.

TABLE 152-3 TYPES OF TOXIN AND DRUG REACTIONS

REACTION TYPE	IMPLICATED DRUGS OR TOXINS
Autoimmune (attack on cell surface markers)	Lovastatin, methyldopa, nitrofurantoin
Cholestatic (attack on bile ducts)	Anabolic steroids, carbamazepine, chlorpromazine, estrogen, erythromycin
Fibrosis (activation of stellate cells leads to fibrosis)	Methotrexate, vitamin A excess
Granulomatous (macrophage stimulation)	Allopurinol, diltiazem, nitrofurantoin, quinidine, sulfa drugs
Hepatocellular (damage to smooth endoplasmic reticulum and immune cell surface)	Acetaminophen, *Amanita* poisoning, diclofenac, isoniazid, lovastatin, nefazodone, trazodone, venlafaxine
Immunoallergic (cytotoxic cell attack on surface determinants)	Halothane, phenytoin, sulfamethoxazole
Mixed (see above)	Amoxicillin-clavulanate, carbamazepine, cyclosporine, herbs, methimazole
Oncogenic (hepatic adenoma formation)	Oral contraceptives, androgenic agents
Steatohepatitis (mitochondrial dysfunction: β-oxidation and respiratory chain)	Amiodarone, perhexiline maleate, tamoxifen
Vascular collapse (ischemic damage)	Cocaine, ecstasy, nicotinic acid
Veno-occlusive disease (endotheliitis of sinusoidal endothelial cells)	Busulfan, cytoxan

Intrinsic (Dose-Dependent) Agents

Acetaminophen (see later) and a few other agents seem to have a clear dose-response effect, although idiosyncrasy usually plays a role as well (Table 152-2). Some toxins, such as α-amanitine produced by *Amanita* mushrooms, cause dose-related injury. *Amanita* poisoning may occur after ingestion of the mushrooms *Amanita phalloides* (death cap) or *Amanita virosa* (deadly agaric). The dose-dependent toxic effect on the liver is attributed to amatoxin, an ingredient of the mushrooms that enhances the toxic effect by its enterohepatic recirculation characteristics; the toxic effect is exerted on each cycle of the recirculation through the liver.

Idiosyncratic Reactions

Drug reactions occur in 1 in 1000 to 1 in 200,000 patients. Characteristics of these idiosyncratic reactions include their infrequent occurrence, varying time intervals between the initial exposure and the reaction, and varying severity of reactions in affected individuals. There are also similarities such as "class effects" (similar drugs exhibit similar features; see Table 152-3), a consistent pattern for each drug, and the fact that rechallenge with a responsible agent usually leads to a more severe reaction with a shorter latency than seen after the initial exposure.

Antibiotics, anticonvulsants, and nonsteroidal anti-inflammatory drugs (NSAIDs) are associated more frequently with drug-induced liver disease, whereas hormones, antihypertensive drugs, digoxin, and antiarrhythmic drugs are implicated rarely. In some cases, idiosyncratic reactions are so infrequent that a drug continues to be used if its effectiveness or uniqueness makes the risk acceptable. An example is isoniazid, which is among the few drugs implicated in drug-induced liver injury in developing countries. In individuals receiving isoniazid as a single agent for tuberculosis prophylaxis, increased aminotransferase levels may develop in 15 to 20%, but severe hepatic necrosis develops in only 0.1 to 1% (Chapter 332)—a rate that is high in comparison to idiosyncratic drug reactions, yet low enough for isoniazid, because of its effectiveness, to remain a key drug.

CLINICAL MANIFESTATIONS

Patients may have few or nonspecific complaints despite elevated aminotransferase levels. Clinical features include nausea, fatigue, occasional right upper quadrant pain, and nonspecific symptoms similar to those seen in other forms of acute hepatitis (Chapter 150). Fever or pharyngitis (typically seen in phenytoin reactions) may be present. No specific physical findings to raise suspicion of drug toxicity are noted, except possibly a rash. Any patient in whom jaundice develops is at risk for having a severe or fatal outcome, and patients who continue taking the drug despite jaundice are at highest risk.

DIAGNOSIS

Abnormal aminotransferase levels with the use of a new drug should raise the suspicion of a drug-induced reaction and prompt immediate discontinuation of the drug rather than awaiting diagnostic tests to confirm or exclude the diagnosis. Immediate discontinuation of medication at the first sign of liver disease can prevent most fatal liver injuries.

Evaluation of a patient with a suspected drug reaction is directed toward establishing the timeline for all drugs or herbs the patient may have taken. Responsible drugs have usually been started between 5 and 90 days before the onset of symptoms. Evidence of viral hepatitis (Chapters 150), gallstones (Chapter 158), alcoholic liver disease (Chapter 155), pregnancy (Chapter 247), severe right heart failure (Chapter 58), or a period of hypotension (Chapter 106) points to these specific causes. Less commonly, cytomegalovirus (Chapter 384), Epstein-Barr virus (Chapter 385), or herpesviruses (Chapter 383) can cause hepatic injury, primarily in immunosuppressed individuals. If all these causes can be excluded, the temporal relationship fits, and the patient begins to improve after withdrawal of the drug, the diagnosis is more secure. Liver biopsy is of limited value because the histologic picture in most cases of drug-induced liver injury is no different from that of viral hepatitis (Chapter 150). Nevertheless, an occasional liver biopsy specimen in an enigmatic case might reveal eosinophils or granulomas, consistent with a drug reaction.

Types of Drug Reactions

Although most liver injury involves direct hepatocyte necrosis or apoptosis (hepatocellular injury), some drugs injure primarily the bile ducts or canaliculi and cause cholestasis without significant damage to hepatocytes. Other drugs affect sinusoidal cells or present a particular pattern of liver injury affecting multiple cell types (mixed type). Another approach to drug reactions emphasizes the histologic changes involved and the cell type (Table 152-3 and Fig. 152-1).

Hepatocellular Reactions

Hepatocellular reactions are the most common type of drug-induced liver disease and account for 90% of cases (Table 152-4). They are characterized by a pattern of serum liver test results that reflect hepatocellular injury. Usually, improvement is quick after discontinuation of the drug (1 to 2 months), and fulminant, acute liver failure with hepatic encephalopathy develops in only a few patients.

Histologic findings include necrosis and cellular infiltration. The necrosis may be zonal (e.g., induced by acetaminophen or carbon tetrachloride) or diffuse (e.g., induced by halothane), and the inflammatory response consists of lymphocytes or eosinophils. Massive necrosis may cause acute liver failure and death.

Acetaminophen toxicity is the most common form of acute liver failure in the United States and is the best understood example of direct hepatocyte toxicity. The incidence of acetaminophen poisoning varies widely throughout

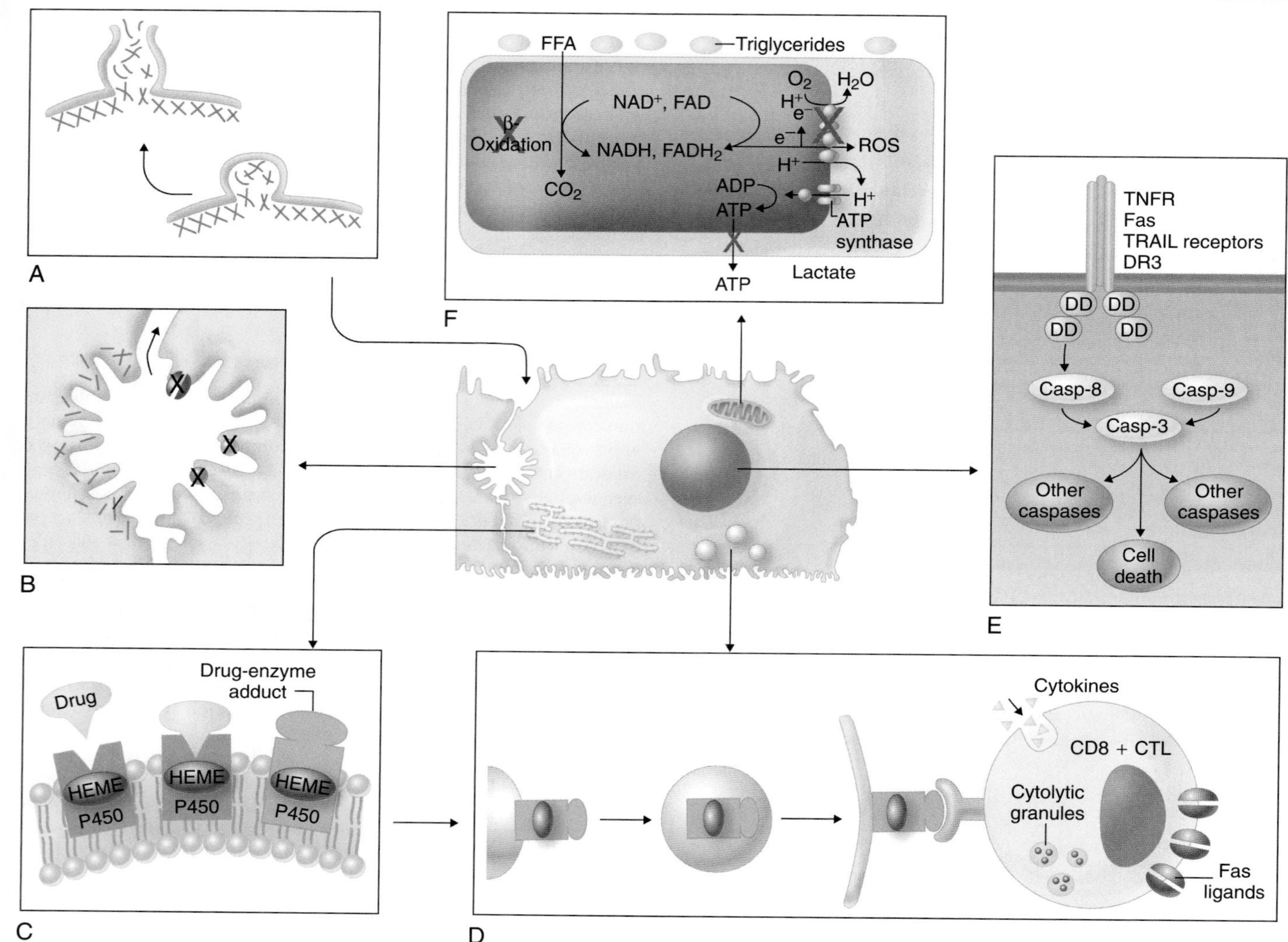

FIGURE 152-1. Mechanisms of liver injury. Each form of liver injury targets specific organelles, although multiple organelles may be affected. The hepatocyte in the center may be affected in at least six ways. **A,** Disruption of intracellular calcium leads to actin fibril disassembly at the hepatocyte surface, which results in blebbing of the cell membrane and subsequent rupture and cell lysis. **B,** In cholestatic diseases, disruption of actin filaments may occur with the loss of villous processes. Interference with ion pumps limits the excretion of bilirubin and other organic compounds. **C,** Most hepatocellular reactions involve the cytochrome P-450 system. The high-energy reaction involved may lead to binding of drug to enzyme and create a new adduct. **D,** Enzyme-drug adducts may traffic to the cell surface and serve as target immunogens for cytolytic attack by T cells. **E,** Activation of apoptotic pathways results in cell death. **F,** Inhibition of β-oxidation or respiration in mitochondria results in microvesicular fat accumulation and lactic acidosis, a pattern characteristic of a variety of agents, including nucleoside analogues, tetracycline, and aspirin. ATP = adenosine triphosphate; FAD = flavin adenine dinucleotide; FFA = free fatty acid; NAD = nicotinamide adenine dinucleotide; ROS = reactive oxygen species; TNFR = tumor necrosis factor receptor. (**A,** Adapted from Farrell GC. *Drug-Induced Liver Disease*. Edinburgh: Churchill Livingstone; 1994: 44; **B,** Adapted from Trauner M, Meier PJ, Boyer J. Mechanisms of disease: molecular pathogenesis of cholestasis. *N Engl J Med.* 1998;339:1217-1227; **C,** Adapted from Watkins Zimmerman HJ. *Hepatotoxicity*, 2nd ed. Philadelphia: Lippincott Williams & Wilkins; 2000; **D,** From Robin M-A, Le Roy M, Descatoire V, Pessayre D. Plasma membrane cytochromes P450 as neoantigens and autoimmune targets in drug-induced hepatitis. *J Hepatol.* 1997;26(Suppl 1):23-30; **E,** From Reed JC. Apoptosis-regulating proteins as targets for drug discovery. *Trends Mol Med.* 2001;7:314-319; **F,** Adapted from Pessayre D, personal communication.)

the world, but it is becoming more frequent and widespread. Liver injury occurs predictably after an intentional suicidal overdose (Chapter 110); it also occurs when acetaminophen is used in excessive doses or sometimes even in therapeutic doses for pain relief. Enhanced toxicity occurs when patients are fasting or are chronic alcohol users because of enzyme induction and depletion of glutathione by alcohol and fasting; by comparison, acute alcohol intake may protect against acetaminophen toxicity during the period of alcohol ingestion. Thereafter, a rebound increase in available CYP2E1 results in increased toxicity in the 12 hours after ingestion because of enzyme induction (see E-Fig. 152-1). Patients with an unintentional acetaminophen overdose may fare worse than suicidal patients because the former seek treatment later in their course, even though suicidal patients take larger doses. The better outcome after an acute overdose may be explained by earlier medical attention and the use of *N*-acetylcysteine, an effective antidote. Nevertheless, one fifth of suicide attempts using acetaminophen are associated with severe liver injury and the potential for a fatal outcome.

The extremely elevated aminotransferase values (often >6000 IU/L, and sometimes as high as 30,000 IU/L) observed in suicidal and unintentional acetaminophen ingestion help distinguish these cases from viral hepatitis or other drug injury. The antidote *N*-acetylcysteine (Chapter 110) may be given by nasogastric tube on admission and for the next 72 hours to provide glutathione substrate. The standard treatment is intravenous *N*-acetylcysteine beginning at a dose of 140 mg/kg in 300 mL of 5% dextrose given over 1 hour, followed by a dose of 70 mg/kg in 5% dextrose given over a 1-hour period every 4 hours for 48 hours. A loading dose of 140 mg/kg can be given orally, followed by 70 mg/kg every 4 hours for 17 doses (72 hours). Expected survival rates are greater than 80%, although liver transplantation is occasionally required.

Cholestatic Reactions

Cholestatic reactions have been described for many drugs. Cholestasis is best defined as failure of bile to reach the duodenum, and common symptoms are jaundice and pruritus. *Pure cholestasis,* with no signs of hepatocellular necrosis, is seen almost exclusively in patients taking oral contraceptives, anabolic steroids, or sex hormone antagonists such as tamoxifen. Acute *cholestatic hepatitis* is characterized histologically by cholestasis (dilated canaliculi, brown granules in the cytoplasm of hepatocytes), some degree of liver cell necrosis and bile duct injury, and inflammatory infiltration by polymorphonuclear leukocytes. Drugs that cause this type of reaction include carbamazepine, trimethoprim-sulfamethoxazole, and captopril.

TABLE 152-4 SCORING SYSTEM TO ASSESS CAUSALITY OF HEPATOCELLULAR REACTIONS

FACTOR	SCORE*
TEMPORAL RELATIONSHIP OF START OF DRUG TO START OF ILLNESS	
Initial treatment: 5-90 days; subsequent treatment course: 1-15 days	+2
Initial treatment: <5 or >90 days; subsequent treatment course: >15 days	+1
From cessation of drug: ≤15 days[†]	+1
COURSE	
ALT decreases ≥50% from peak within 8 days	+3
ALT decreases ≥50% from peak within 30 days	+2
If the drug is continued, inconclusive	0
RISK FACTORS	
Alcohol[‡]	+1
No alcohol[‡]	0
Age ≥ 55 yr	+1
Age < 55 yr	0
CONCOMITANT DRUG	
Concomitant drug with suggestive time of onset	−1
Concomitant drug known to be a hepatotoxin with suggestive time of onset	−2
Concomitant drug with further evidence of involvement (rechallenge)	−3
NUMBER OF NONDRUG CAUSES	
Hepatitis A, B, or C; biliary obstruction; alcoholism (AST ≥ 2 × ALT); recent hypotension; and CMV, EBV, and HSV infection all excluded	+2
4-5 causes excluded	+1
<4 causes excluded	−2
Nondrug cause highly probable	−3
PREVIOUS INFORMATION ON HEPATOTOXICITY OF DRUG IN QUESTION	
Package insert mentions	+2
Published case reports but not on package label	+1
Reaction unknown	0
RECHALLENGE	
Positive (ALT doubles with drug alone)[§]	+2
Compatible (ALT doubles, compounding features)[§]	+1
Negative (increase in ALT but ≤ 2 × ULN)[§]	−2
Not done	0

*Causality is highly probable (score >8), probable (score 6-8), possible (score 3-5), unlikely (score 1-2), or excluded (score ≤0).
[†]For cholestatic reactions, ≤30 days.
[‡]For cholestatic reactions, alcohol, or pregnancy.
[§]For cholestatic reactions, substitute alkaline phosphatase (or total bilirubin) for ALT.
ALT = alanine aminotransferase; AST = aspartate aminotransferase; CMV = cytomegalovirus; EBV = Epstein-Barr virus; HSV = herpes simplex virus; ULN = upper limit of normal.
Adapted from Danan G, Benichou C. Causality assessment of adverse reactions to drugs. I. A novel method based on the conclusions of international consensus meetings: application to drug-induced liver injuries. *J Clin Epidemiol.* 1993;46:1323-1330; Benichou C, Danan G, Flahault A. Causality assessment of adverse reactions to drugs. II. An original model for validation of drug causality assessment methods: case reports with positive rechallenge. *J Clin Epidemiol.* 1993;46:1331-1336.

Generally, drug-induced cholestasis takes longer to resolve than drug-induced hepatotoxicity. In some cases, segments of the intrahepatic biliary tree may be destroyed progressively, the so-called vanishing bile duct syndrome that occurs after a protracted course (>6 months) of drug-induced cholestasis. The result is a state of chronic cholestasis that resembles primary biliary cirrhosis (Chapter 158). Approximately 30 drugs have been implicated in the vanishing bile duct syndrome, including chlorpromazine and ajmaline. A sclerosing cholangitis–like syndrome with jaundice caused by intrahepatic and extrahepatic strictures in the bile ducts is sometimes observed in patients receiving intra-arterial floxuridine chemotherapy for hepatic metastases of colorectal cancer.

Immunoallergic Reactions

Drugs also may be associated with definite allergic reactions. A combined toxic-immunologic mechanism is involved in liver injury caused by halothane, a fluorinated hydrocarbon anesthetic that causes severe, often fatal liver injury after multiple exposures (Chapter 440). Other fluorinated hydrocarbons, including isoflurane and desflurane, occasionally result in the same response. Although halothane has never been withdrawn, its use has been limited by the advent of safer agents. Hypersensitivity reactions, such as fever, eosinophilia, and rash, are common. Halothane may induce fever, eosinophilia, and antimitochondrial antibodies. Direct cytotoxicity and immune-mediated toxicity are observed, consistent with the clinical observation that severe halothane toxicity occurs with repeated exposure. Although evidence of injury can usually be identified within 1 week of the first exposure, the interval to toxicity is shortened and the damage is more severe with each successive exposure, as befits an immune reaction.

Phenytoin (Chapter 410) induces the simultaneous onset of fever, rash, lymphadenopathy, and eosinophilia. The mechanisms responsible for the combined allergic and hepatotoxic reaction are unknown, but the slow resolution of the illness suggests that the allergen remains on the surface of the hepatocyte for weeks or months. A concurrent mononucleosis-like picture is frequently confused with a viral illness or streptococcal pharyngitis. If phenytoin is not discontinued promptly despite signs of hepatitis, a severe Stevens-Johnson drug eruption (Chapters 447 and 448) and prolonged fever may result. As with any therapeutic agent, rapid recognition of the presence of a toxic drug reaction and immediate discontinuation of the compound are key to limiting hepatic damage. Systemic features of an allergic reaction may not be obvious, even when eosinophilia or granulomas are present on liver biopsy.

Steatohepatitis

Steatosis in the liver (Chapter 155) can be present in a microvesicular or macrovesicular pattern. Macrovesicular steatosis, the most common form, is characterized histologically by a single vacuole of fat filling up the hepatocyte and displacing the nucleus to the cell's periphery. Macrovesicular steatosis is typically caused by alcohol, diabetes, or obesity. Sometimes drugs such as corticosteroids or methotrexate may cause these hepatic changes. Amiodarone (Chapters 64 and 65) has been associated with a picture resembling alcoholic hepatitis, occasionally with progression to cirrhosis. The pathophysiology involves accumulation of phospholipids in the liver, eyes, thyroid, and skin. Treatment is primarily withdrawal of the drug and observation, although the half-life of amiodarone is prolonged. Tamoxifen, which has been used in long-term regimens for the prevention of recurrent breast cancer (Chapter 204), has also been associated with steatohepatitis evolving to cirrhosis.

In microvesicular steatosis, hepatocytes contain numerous small fat vesicles that do not displace the nucleus. Valproic acid, an anticonvulsant (Chapter 410), causes hepatotoxicity, either as a result of microvesicular fat deposition, resembling Reye's syndrome, or in a more chronic, indolent fashion associated with macrovesicular fat accumulation. Toxicity is more severe and frequent in children. These lesions are associated with disruption of mitochondrial DNA, resulting in anaerobic metabolism that leads to lactic acidosis in the most severe cases. Macrovesicular and microvesicular lesions may be observed concomitantly in some patients, and microvesicular lesions are more often associated with a poor prognosis. Hepatocellular necrosis may also be present. Acute fatty liver of pregnancy (Chapter 153) and Reye's syndrome are two examples of severe liver diseases caused by microvesicular steatosis.

Drugs involved in microvesicular steatosis include valproate, tetracycline, and fialuridine. Aspirin use in children has been associated with Reye's syndrome, but the incidence of Reye's syndrome has decreased dramatically since warnings were issued concerning aspirin use in children.

Effects of Sex Steroids

Anabolic steroids, such as methyltestosterone, may cause cholestasis. Androgens may cause peliosis hepatis and benign or malignant tumors. Oral contraceptives (Chapter 246) may cause cholestasis, hepatic adenomas, or Budd-Chiari syndrome (hepatic vein thrombosis). Antiandrogens used to treat prostate cancer (Chapter 207), such as flutamide and nilutamide, and antipituitary drugs, such as cyproterone acetate, have also been associated with severe hepatocellular injury.

Other Drug Reactions

Other less severe drug reactions involving the liver include granulomatous reactions, fibrosis, ischemic injury, and chronic autoimmune liver injury (see Table 152-3). The type of reaction observed can be helpful in determining the probable agent because most drugs have a specific injury profile.

A pattern of veno-occlusive disease with obliteration of small intrahepatic veins, sinusoidal congestion, and necrosis is observed frequently in bone marrow transplant patients (Chapter 181) who receive chemotherapy with cyclophosphamide (Cytoxan) or busulfan. Symptoms, including rapidly accumulating ascites, painful hepatomegaly, and jaundice, develop soon after the chemotherapeutic regimen has begun. Rarely, herbal medicines (Chapter 38) such as pyrrolizidine alkaloids (*Crotalaria* and *Senecio* found in Jamaican bush tea) may cause veno-occlusive disease.

Toxins are associated with direct injury to hepatocytes in a dose-dependent fashion. Organic solvents such as carbon tetrachloride and trichloroethylene (Chapter 110) cause centrilobular injury. Yellow phosphorus, found in firecrackers and rat poisons, is a rare cause of liver injury from either accidental or intentional exposure. Symptoms of poisoning are similar to those of any other type of hepatitis.

Mushroom poisoning (Chapter 110), which follows the ingestion of *A. phalloides* and related species, typically occurs in amateur mushroom fanciers in a dose-related fashion. The associated muscarinic effects, including severe diarrhea, vomiting, and profuse sweating, predominate in the first hours after ingestion. Hepatic failure follows if antidotes (see later) are not given. The overall prognosis for spontaneous recovery is poor; liver transplantation may be life-saving.

Differential Diagnosis

The differential diagnosis of toxin- and drug-induced liver injury includes almost the entire spectrum of liver diseases. Because the clinical picture of drug-induced liver injury ranges from pure hepatocellular to pure cholestatic variants, a high index of suspicion must be maintained, even when toxin- or drug-induced liver injury is not obvious initially.

For dose-dependent hepatotoxins, the diagnosis may be easier to establish than for idiosyncratic drug reactions. Serum levels of acetaminophen, a thorough history, and characteristic biochemical abnormalities (high aminotransferase levels) usually reveal an acetaminophen overdose, whereas a diagnosis of *Amanita* poisoning depends on the history, symptoms of gastroenteritis (muscarinic reaction), and positive mushroom identification.

For idiosyncratic drug reactions, the diagnosis is sometimes more difficult to establish. A standardized reporting form called the RUCAM (Roussel-Uclaf causality assessment method; see Table 152-4), developed by an international panel, provides a worthwhile scoring system. These guidelines outline the steps an experienced clinician might use to assess the likelihood of a drug reaction. Causality assessment factors typically include the temporal relationship, course after cessation of the drug, risk factors, concomitant drugs, a search for nondrug causes (viral hepatitis), previous information concerning the drug, and response to rechallenge, which is typically not required.

TREATMENT Rx

Prompt discontinuation of a suspected drug is mandatory. Available antidotes should be used for acetaminophen (*N*-acetylcysteine) and *Amanita* poisoning (penicillin 300,000 to 1 million U/kg/day intravenously and thioctic acid 5 to 100 mg every 6 hours intravenously have been recommended, but there are no controlled trials). General supportive therapy ranges from intravenous fluid replacement to intensive monitoring and treatment of patients with hepatic encephalopathy secondary to acute liver failure (Chapter 157). Liver transplantation (Chapter 157) is performed in more than 50% of patients with idiosyncratic drug-induced acute liver failure because the survival rate in this setting without transplantation is less than 20%.

FUTURE DIRECTIONS

Research in pharmacogenomics may allow the patient's own genetic information to guide individualized drug therapy and monitoring of idiosyncratic drug reactions. The genetic information would probably concentrate initially on enzymes with variant alleles associated with poor metabolism, such as CYP1A2 or CYP2C19 for isoniazid, CYP2C9 for piroxicam, or CYP2D6 for nortriptyline. Better postmarketing surveillance of all drugs to identify those with previously unappreciated hepatotoxicity should be a high priority.

PREVENTION

It is reasonable to consider a drug reaction whenever an episode of apparent hepatitis is unexplained, particularly if a new agent has been introduced in the previous 3 months. It is prudent to defer embracing new drugs during their first year of introduction, particularly if they show no unique advantages over accepted formulations. Physicians must strive to instill in their patients a healthy level of alertness with regard to drug-induced liver injury, particularly for agents with known hepatotoxicity. Monitoring of aminotransferase levels on a monthly basis is suggested for known hepatotoxins such as isoniazid or diclofenac, but it is unlikely to be cost-effective when adverse reactions occur less frequently, such as in only 1 in 50,000 patients. Because many drug reactions develop within days, monitoring provides no guarantee. Most fatal drug reactions could have been prevented if the offending agent were withdrawn immediately, at the first sign of illness.

SUGGESTED READINGS

Bjornsson E. Review article: drug-induced liver injury in clinical practice. *Aliment Pharmacol Ther.* 2010;32:3-13. *Practical information for clinicians.*

Chalasani N, Björnsson E. Risk factors for idiosyncratic drug-induced liver injury. *Gastroenterology.* 2010;138:2246-2259. *Review of genetic and non-genetic risk factors.*

Khandelwal N, James LP, Sanders C, et al. Unrecognized acetaminophen toxicity as a cause of indeterminate acute liver failure. *Hepatology.* 2011;53:567-576. *Suggests that many indeterminate cases are unrecognized acetaminophen cases.*

Rockey DC, Seeff LB, Rochon J, et al. Causality assessment in drug-induced liver injury using a structured expert opinion process: comparison to the Roussel-Uclaf causality assessment method. *Hepatology.* 2010;51:2117-2126. *Review of the process of assessing causality.*

153 INHERITED AND METABOLIC DISORDERS OF THE LIVER

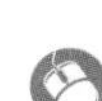

BRUCE R. BACON

DEFINITION

Inherited liver diseases (Table 153-1) include hereditary hemochromatosis, (Chapter 219), Wilson disease (Chapter 218), α_1-antitrypsin deficiency (Chapter 88), and cystic fibrosis. Metabolic liver diseases include nonalcoholic fatty liver disease (NAFLD), which is the most common cause of abnormal liver enzymes in Western societies; in addition, 3 to 5% of overweight or obese individuals in the United States may have nonalcoholic steatohepatitis (NASH) (Chapter 155), which has the potential to progress to advanced fibrosis. A variety of systemic metabolic abnormalities are less common causes of liver dysfunction or abnormal liver tests (Chapter 149).

INHERITED LIVER DISEASES

Hereditary Hemochromatosis

EPIDEMIOLOGY AND PATHOBIOLOGY

Hereditary hemochromatosis (Chapter 219) is the most common inherited disorder of the liver. The responsible gene for this inherited disorder of iron metabolism is *HFE,* which encodes for a major histocompatibility complex type 1 protein. Genetic testing is available for the two major mutations (C282Y, H63D) responsible for *HFE*-linked hereditary hemochromatosis. Large-scale population studies demonstrate that C282Y homozygosity is found in about 1 in 250 individuals of northern European descent, about 60% of whom have phenotypic expression of the disease. About 10% of the population are asymptomatic heterozygotes.

CLINICAL MANIFESTATIONS

Most individuals with hereditary hemochromatosis have no symptoms and are identified by screening laboratory tests or family studies. When

TABLE 153-1 INHERITED AND METABOLIC DISORDERS OF THE LIVER

INHERITED LIVER DISEASES
Hereditary hemochromatosis
α_1-Antitrypsin deficiency
Wilson disease
Cystic fibrosis
METABOLIC LIVER DISEASES
Nonalcoholic fatty liver disease
Porphyrias
Lipid storage diseases
Amyloidosis

symptoms are present, they are frequently nonspecific and include lethargy, fatigue, weight loss, and weakness. More organ-specific symptoms include right upper quadrant abdominal pain or arthralgias of the hands, hips, and knees. Occasionally, patients present with signs of advanced liver disease.

DIAGNOSIS

When symptoms and signs suggestive of hereditary hemochromatosis are present, it is reasonable to consider this diagnosis and order appropriate laboratory studies. Conversely, when abnormal iron studies (Chapter 162) are identified by routine screening or in patients being evaluated for anemia, hereditary hemochromatosis should be considered even in the absence of signs or symptoms.

Definitive diagnosis is relatively straightforward. Transferrin saturation (iron ÷ transferrin or total iron binding capacity × 100%) and ferritin levels are typically elevated in symptomatic patients in both the fasting and nonfasting states. Ferritin, which is an acute phase reactant, can be elevated without increased iron stores in acute illnesses, cancer, inflammatory arthritides, chronic viral hepatitis, and alcoholic and nonalcoholic fatty liver disease.

In patients with elevated transferrin saturation or ferritin levels, genetic testing should be performed. Detection of a C282Y homozygote or a compound heterozygote (C282Y/H63D) confirms the diagnosis of hereditary hemochromatosis. If the ferritin level is greater than 1000 μg/L, the patient should be considered for liver biopsy (Fig. 153-1) to determine whether fibrosis is present. Sensitive magnetic resonance imaging techniques can help determine hepatic iron concentrations when liver biopsy cannot be performed. On liver biopsy, iron deposition is found in periportal hepatocytes, with a periportal to pericentral gradient, and Kupffer cells are spared.

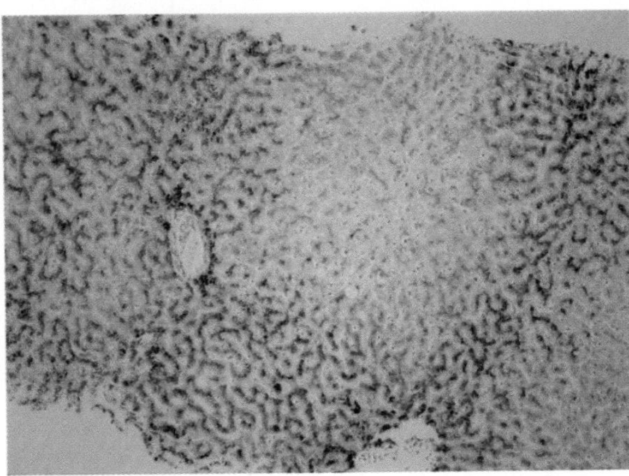

FIGURE 153-1. **Liver biopsy in hemochromatosis (Perls Prussian blue stain for iron).** Iron deposition is found in a periportal distribution, predominantly in parenchymal cells (hepatocytes).

TREATMENT AND PROGNOSIS (Rx)

Treatment of hereditary hemochromatosis is simple, safe, effective, and inexpensive. It consists of weekly phlebotomy of 1 unit of blood, which contains about 200 to 250 mg of iron, and is designed to reduce total body iron stores with a goal of reducing ferritin levels to 50 to 100 μg/L. Most patients require maintenance phlebotomy of 1 unit of blood every 2 to 3 months. Screening with iron studies and genetic testing should be offered to all first-degree relatives of identified probands. Complications of the disease can be avoided if patients are diagnosed and treated before they develop fibrosis.

α_1-Antitrypsin Deficiency

EPIDEMIOLOGY AND PATHOBIOLOGY

α_1-Antitrypsin deficiency has been identified in all populations, but the disorder is most common in individuals of northern European descent. In North America, about 1 in 1500 to 2000 individuals is affected by the disorder.

α_1-Antitrypsin is a 52-kD glycoprotein produced in hepatocytes, epithelial cells of the lungs, and phagocytes. It inhibits serine proteases, primarily neutrophil elastase. When patients are deficient in α_1-antitrypsin, increased amounts of neutrophil elastase degrade elastin and can lead to progressive lung injury and premature emphysema (Chapter 88). α_1-Antitrypsin deficiency causes liver disease in infancy, early childhood, adolescence, and adulthood.

More than 75 variants have been identified in the proteinase inhibitor (Pi) gene located on chromosome 14. Some alter protein structure, thereby interfering with hepatocellular export. As a result, deformed polymers of α_1-antitrypsin aggregate and accumulate in the endoplasmic reticulum of the hepatocyte. Conventional nomenclature identifies normal variants as PiMM; individuals with these variants have normal blood levels of α_1-antitrypsin. The most common abnormal variants of functional significance are identified as S and Z. Individuals who are homozygous for the Z mutation (PiZZ) have α_1-antitrypsin levels that are only about 15% of normal; these patients are susceptible to liver and/or lung disease, but only about 25% of PiZZ patients develop end-organ disease. Individuals with PiSZ are at risk for developing liver disease and cirrhosis. Null variants have undetectable α_1-antitrypsin and are susceptible to premature lung disease but not liver disease.

CLINICAL MANIFESTATIONS AND DIAGNOSIS

In adults, symptoms of liver disease may be absent, or patients may complain of symptoms ranging from fatigue to complications of chronic decompensated liver disease (Chapter 148). The diagnosis is most frequently considered in patients who present with abnormal liver enzymes (Chapter 149) or as part of an evaluation for the cause of cirrhosis (Chapter 156). Coexistent lung disease at a relatively young age or a family history of liver and/or lung disease can provide clues to the diagnosis. Lung disease is not necessarily present.

The diagnosis is confirmed by a reduced serum level of α_1-antitrypsin, which can be measured specifically or assumed based on a low level of α_1-protein on serum protein electrophoresis, accompanied by Pi determinations. Most patients with liver disease have either the PiZZ or the PiSZ variant; some patients with PiMZ have reduced α_1-antitrypsin levels, but they are usually not low enough to cause disease. Liver biopsy, which is performed to determine the degree of hepatic fibrosis, shows characteristic periodic acid–Schiff–positive, diastase-resistant globules in the periphery of the hepatic lobule (Fig. 153-2).

TREATMENT AND PROGNOSIS (Rx)

Unfortunately, there is no specific therapy for α_1-antitrypsin deficiency, so treatment is supportive. Other causes of liver injury, such as excessive alcohol ingestion, should be avoided. Evidence of other liver diseases (e.g., viral hepatitis B and C, hemochromatosis, NAFLD) should be sought, and such diseases should be treated if possible. Smoking, which can worsen the progression of lung disease but not liver disease in patients with α_1-antitrypsin deficiency, should be discontinued. In patients with lung disease, weekly infusions of α_1-antitrypsin given indefinitely can halt further lung damage.

The natural history of α_1-antitrypsin deficiency is variable because many individuals with the PiZZ variant never develop disease, whereas others develop cirrhosis in childhood, ultimately leading to liver transplantation. The risk of hepatocellular cancer is increased in patients with cirrhosis. If decompensated liver disease develops, liver transplantation (Chapter 157) should be curative. Following the transplant, patients express the Pi phenotype of the donor.

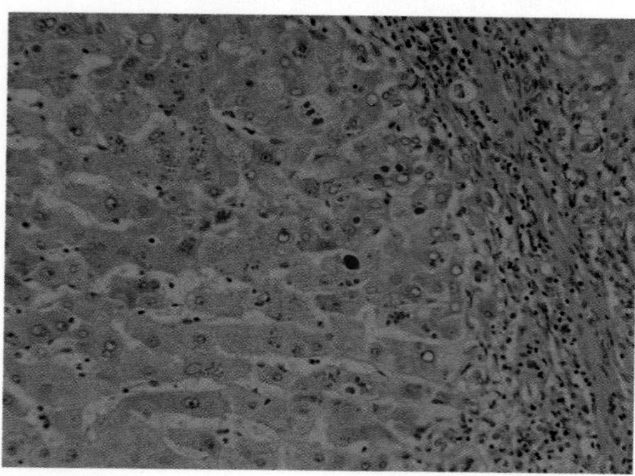

FIGURE 153-2. Liver biopsy in α_1-antitrypsin deficiency. On a periodic acid–Schiff, diastase-resistant stain, α_1-antitrypsin globules, with a characteristic magenta color, are found at the periphery of the lobule.

Wilson Disease

Wilson disease (Chapter 218), which is an inherited disorder of copper metabolism, leads to a progressive accumulation of copper in the liver and in various other tissues, ultimately causing toxicity and organ damage. The Wilson disease gene (*ATP7B*) encodes for a P-type ATPase that is involved in copper transport and is required for the removal of copper from hepatocytes into hepatic bile.

CLINICAL MANIFESTATIONS AND DIAGNOSIS

Wilson disease usually presents before age 35 years, but it can present in middle age or later. The clinical presentation is quite variable, and hepatic manifestations include chronic hepatitis, hepatic steatosis, and cirrhosis in adolescents and young adults. Patients who present with neurologic manifestations such as dysarthria or choreic or athetoid movement disorders always have concomitant liver disease. On physical examination, patients classically have Kayser-Fleischer rings (see Fig. 218-1 in Chapter 218) owing to copper deposition in Descemet's membrane in the cornea.

Diagnosis includes demonstration of a reduced ceruloplasmin level and an increased 24-hour urine copper excretion. In the presence of neurologic findings and clinical evidence of liver disease, a liver biopsy is not required. If a liver biopsy is obtained, however, the classic findings include an elevated hepatic copper level, hepatic steatosis, chronic hepatitis, and cirrhosis. The genetic diagnosis of Wilson disease is difficult because there are more than 200 mutations in *ATP7B*, with different degrees of frequency and penetration in certain populations.

TREATMENT AND PROGNOSIS Rx

Treatment consists of copper chelation using medications such as D-penicillamine (1 to 1.5 g/day indefinitely) and trientine. Zinc acetate (75 to 250 mg/day) has been used as maintenance therapy. Medical treatment should be lifelong because discontinuation of therapy has been associated with severe relapses, liver failure, and death. Liver transplantation (Chapter 157), which is indicated for either decompensated cirrhosis or fulminant liver failure, cures the underlying metabolic defect and restores normal copper homeostasis.

Cystic Fibrosis

Cystic fibrosis (Chapter 89) can cause chronic liver disease in adults, although its principal manifestations are chronic lung disease and pancreatic insufficiency. Some adult patients with cystic fibrosis develop biliary cirrhosis with portal hypertension. Combined lung-liver transplantation is recommended for these patients. Ursodeoxycholic acid (13 to 15 mg/kg/day) improves symptoms and liver test abnormalities but is not curative.

METABOLIC LIVER DISEASES

Nonalcoholic Fatty Liver Disease

NAFLD (Chapter 155), which is seen most commonly in obese, diabetic, and hyperlipidemic nonalcoholic patients, has a prevalence ranging from 15 to 30% in the United States. Not all obese patients have fatty liver disease, but NASH occurs in about 3 to 5% of the overweight and obese population, and liver fibrosis is increased in up to 40% of these individuals. Most patients with hepatic steatosis have stable, nonprogressive disease, but NASH can progress to cirrhosis. Many patients who were previously described as having cryptogenic cirrhosis are now thought to have NASH, especially because catabolic cirrhosis reduces macrovesicular steatosis, so late biopsy may show just a bland cirrhosis.

Symptoms usually include fatigue and/or vague right upper quadrant discomfort, most likely due to a distended hepatic capsule. However, most patients come to medical attention as a result of incidentally identified elevated liver enzymes or the finding of a fatty liver on imaging studies for other purposes.

Critical to the diagnosis of NAFLD is a careful history to be sure that alcohol ingestion is less than 20 g/day. Routine laboratory testing for other common liver diseases (e.g., hepatitis B and C, hemochromatosis), as well as less common ones (e.g., Wilson disease, α_1-antitrypsin deficiency, autoimmune liver diseases), should be performed. Imaging studies can confirm characteristic features of a fatty liver (e.g., bright liver on ultrasound). These findings are nonspecific, however, and the ultimate diagnosis of NAFLD or NASH requires liver biopsy.

The principal treatments are dietary changes and weight loss, but some medications can also be helpful in selected patients (Chapter 155).

Porphyrias

The porphyrias (Chapter 217) are characterized by defects in the synthesis of heme, which is necessary for incorporation into numerous hemoproteins such as hemoglobin, myoglobin, catalase, and cytochromes. The porphyrias can present both acutely and chronically, with the acute disorders causing recurring bouts of abdominal pain, and the chronic disorders being characterized by skin lesions.

The most commonly encountered porphyria is porphyria cutanea tarda, which is characterized by vesicular-type lesions that appear on sun-exposed areas of the skin, such as the backs of the hands (see Fig. 447-11 in Chapter 447), tips of the ears, or over the cheekbones. About 40% of patients with porphyria cutanea tarda have mutations in *HFE* (Chapter 219), and about 50% have chronic hepatitis C (Chapter 151).

Liver disease associated with the porphyrias typically presents as an asymptomatic elevation of liver enzymes. After appropriate testing to confirm porphyria (Chapter 217), *HFE* mutation analysis, iron studies, and hepatitis C testing should be performed in all patients who present with porphyria cutanea tarda. Excess alcohol use is also associated with porphyria cutanea tarda, so patients should be counseled to decrease or eliminate alcohol use. Iron reduction therapy, using therapeutic phlebotomy, is the cornerstone of treatment for porphyria cutanea tarda, even in the absence of iron overload (Chapter 219). Concomitant chronic hepatitis C should be treated as well (Chapter 151). Skin lesions reverse in the majority of patients. Acute intermittent porphyria (Chapter 217), which is much less common, presents with abdominal pain in the absence of typical findings on physical examination. Intravenous hematin is the treatment of choice.

Lipid Storage Diseases

Lipid storage diseases that involve the liver include Gaucher's disease (Chapter 215) and Niemann-Pick disease (Chapter 215). Other rare disorders include abetalipoproteinemia, Fabry's disease (Chapter 215), Tangier disease (Chapter 213), and types 1 and 5 hyperlipoproteinemia (Chapter 213). On physical examination, the liver is enlarged owing to both fat deposition and increased hepatic glycogen deposition. Liver enzymes may be elevated and diagnosis requires liver biopsy in the appropriate clinical setting. Treatment is supportive, with enzyme infusions as indicated.

Amyloidosis

In patients with systemic amyloidosis (Chapter 194), the liver is commonly involved, but this involvement is sometimes identified only in the premorbid state or documented at autopsy. Characteristic pathologic findings include positive staining with Congo red histochemical stain, where an apple-green birefringence is noted under polarizing light. Liver enzymes may be mildly elevated, but this finding is nonspecific. Treatment is as for the systemic disease.

LIVER DISEASE IN PREGNANCY

In a pregnant patient with liver enzyme abnormalities, it is important to distinguish between liver diseases that are unique to pregnancy and those

TABLE 153-2 LIVER DISEASES UNIQUE TO PREGNANCY

DISEASE	TRIMESTER OF ONSET	SYMPTOMS	LABORATORY ABNORMALITIES	RECURRENCE WITH FUTURE PREGNANCIES
Hyperemesis gravidarum	1	Nausea, vomiting	Mild to moderate elevation in ALT/AST, occasionally hyperbilirubinemia	
Cholestasis	2, 3	Pruritus, jaundice	Bile acids >8 μM, elevated ALT/AST and bilirubin in more severe cases	Common
Acute fatty liver	3	Nausea, vomiting, abdominal pain	Elevated ALT/AST (100-1000 U/L), bilirubin >5 mg/dL, prolonged prothrombin time*	Rare
HELLP syndrome	2, 3, or postpartum	Abdominal pain, nausea, vomiting	Elevated ALT/AST (60-1500 U/L), platelets <100,000/mm^3, LDH >600 U/L, hemolytic anemia	3-25%

*Useful diagnostic distinction from HELLP syndrome, in which the prothrombin time, partial thromboplastin time, and fibrinogen are usually normal.
ALT = alanine aminotransferase; AST = aspartate aminotransferase; HELLP = hemolysis, elevated liver enzymes, and low platelet count; LDH = lactate dehydrogenase.

that occur commonly in pregnancy (Table 153-2). In normal pregnancy, levels of alkaline phosphatase, bile acids, globulins, fibrinogen, and triglycerides may be increased, whereas levels of albumin, antithrombin 3, protein S, and γ-glutamyltransferase may be reduced.

Hyperemesis Gravidarum

Hyperemesis gravidarum is a syndrome of unknown cause in which patients have fairly intractable nausea and vomiting. It generally occurs in the first trimester, usually before 10 weeks of pregnancy. Risk factors include young age, obesity, and nulliparity. Aminotransferases levels may be increased up to 200 U/L, and bilirubin may be elevated up to 4 mg/dL. No specific abnormalities are found on liver biopsy, but some patients have mild steatosis or mild cholestasis. Treatment is symptomatic with antiemetics.

Intrahepatic Cholestasis of Pregnancy

Intrahepatic cholestasis of pregnancy presents with generalized pruritus. Most cases are associated with a mutation in the multiple drug resistance-3 gene. Ten percent to 25% of patients have visible jaundice, and laboratory abnormalities generally include hyperbilirubinemia less than 6 mg/dL. The alkaline phosphatase level may be elevated, and aminotransferase levels may be 2 to 10 times the upper limit of normal. Serum bile acids are also markedly increased at 2 to 100 times the upper limit of normal. If liver biopsy is performed, a bland cholestasis is identified. Ultrasonography is normal.

Treatment includes ursodeoxycholic acid or cholestyramine to bind bile salts. Phenobarbital has also been used. The syndrome resolves after delivery but is likely to recur with subsequent pregnancies.

Preeclampsia and HELLP Syndrome

Preeclampsia (Chapter 247), seen in as many as 7 to 10% of pregnancies, usually occurs in the third trimester or late in the second trimester. The triad of findings consists of hypertension, proteinuria, and edema. Some patients have severe hypertension, profound proteinuria, and seizures. Liver enzymes can be markedly elevated, and levels of lactate dehydrogenase and bilirubin can be increased by hemolysis. The prothrombin time is usually normal, but some patients may have thrombocytopenia. The *HELLP* syndrome (hemolysis, elevated liver enzymes, and low platelet count) is seen in about 10% of patients with preeclampsia and is considered a severe manifestation of eclampsia. Hepatic infarction is rare, but hepatic rupture can be catastrophic.

The diagnosis is generally made clinically, and a liver biopsy is usually not necessary. Treatment is by delivery.

Acute Fatty Liver Disease in Pregnancy

Acute fatty liver disease occurs in about 1 in 900 to 6000 pregnancies. Abnormalities in mitochondrial function and adenosine triphosphate (ATP) synthesis have been described, and about 20% of cases have a deficiency in long-chain 3-hydroxyacyl-CoA dehydrogenase, with an abnormality in the beta oxidation of fatty acids. Acute fatty liver is characteristically seen in the third trimester. Patients can have profound hepatic dysfunction, but liver enzymes are usually not markedly elevated and are characteristically less than 10 times the upper limit of normal. The prothrombin time may be prolonged, and the bilirubin level is elevated. Some patients have disseminated intravascular coagulation, and some may have hypoglycemia.

Clinical features are nonspecific, and the clinical course ranges from mild complications to more severe problems. Diagnosis is by ultrasound showing steatosis and liver biopsy showing microvesicular steatosis. Treatment requires urgent delivery.

Other Hepatobiliary Conditions in Pregnancy

Other hepatic conditions that can occur in pregnancy including gallstones (Chapter 158) and Budd-Chiari syndrome (Chapter 145). Acute herpes hepatitis, caused by herpesvirus type 2, occurs in the second and third trimesters and is associated with fever, chills, malaise, and nausea. Liver enzymes may be markedly elevated, and the prothrombin time may be prolonged. Liver biopsy shows typical viral inclusions. Treatment is with antiviral therapy (Chapter 368).

TOTAL PARENTERAL NUTRITION–INDUCED LIVER DISEASE

As many as 30 to 40% of patients who receive total parenteral nutrition (Chapter 224) develop abnormal liver enzyme levels. These abnormalities range from mild elevations of aminotransferase levels, owing to hepatic steatosis, to cholestatic liver disease with elevated alkaline phosphatase levels. Minor adjustments in the formula usually resolve the abnormalities. Some patients with cholestatic abnormalities may benefit from ursodeoxycholic acid.

SUGGESTED READINGS

Bacon BR, Adams PC, Kowdley KV, et al. AASLD Practice Guidelines. Diagnosis and management of hemochromatosis. *Hepatology.* 2011 (in press). *Practice guidelines.*
Huster D. Wilson disease. *Best Pract Res Clin Gastroenterol.* 2010;24:531-539. *Review.*
Joshi D, James A, Quaglia A, et al. Liver disease in pregnancy. *Lancet.* 2010;375:594-605. *Review.*

154 BACTERIAL, PARASITIC, FUNGAL, AND GRANULOMATOUS LIVER DISEASES

K. RAJENDER REDDY

INFECTIONS OF THE LIVER

Infections of the liver can be due to a variety of pathogens, including bacteria, fungi, amebae, protozoa, helminthes, spirochetes, and rickettsial infections. The manifestations of these infections are protean; some are generic to all infections, whereas others are specific to particular infections. The epidemiology can vary and depend on the geographic region of the world. In endemic areas, *Entamoeba histolytica* is a key consideration in the differential diagnosis of a liver abscess (Table 154-1).

TABLE 154-1 FEATURES OF BACTERIAL AND AMEBIC ABSCESSES

	DEMOGRAPHICS	RISK FACTORS	SYMPTOMS	LABORATORY FINDINGS	RADIOGRAPHIC FEATURES	DIAGNOSIS	TREATMENT
Bacterial liver abscess	50-70 years old Male = female	Recent bacterial infection, biliary obstruction, diabetes mellitus	Fevers, chills, malaise, anorexia, diarrhea, cough, pleuritic chest pain, RUQ pain	Leukocytosis, anemia, elevated alkaline phosphatase and bilirubin, low albumin, positive blood cultures (50%)	Multifocal (50%), usually right lobe, irregular margins	Aspirate (70-80% positive)	Percutaneous drainage and antibiotics
Amebic liver abscess	18-50 years old Male > female	Alcohol intake, HLA-DR3, oral and anal sex, contaminated enema apparatus, travel to or living in an endemic area	Fever, RUQ pain, hepatic tenderness, anorexia, weight loss, uncommon to have colitis	Leukocytosis, no eosinophilia, mild anemia, elevated alkaline phosphatase, elevated ESR, positive serology	Single abscess (80%), usually right lobe, wall enhancement seen on CT scan with IV contrast	Aspirate (trophozoites rarely seen) can rule out super-imposed bacterial infection, positive serology and risk factors	Metronidazole and iodoquinol

CT = computed tomography; ESR = erythrocyte sedimentation rate; IV = intravenous; RUQ = right upper quadrant.

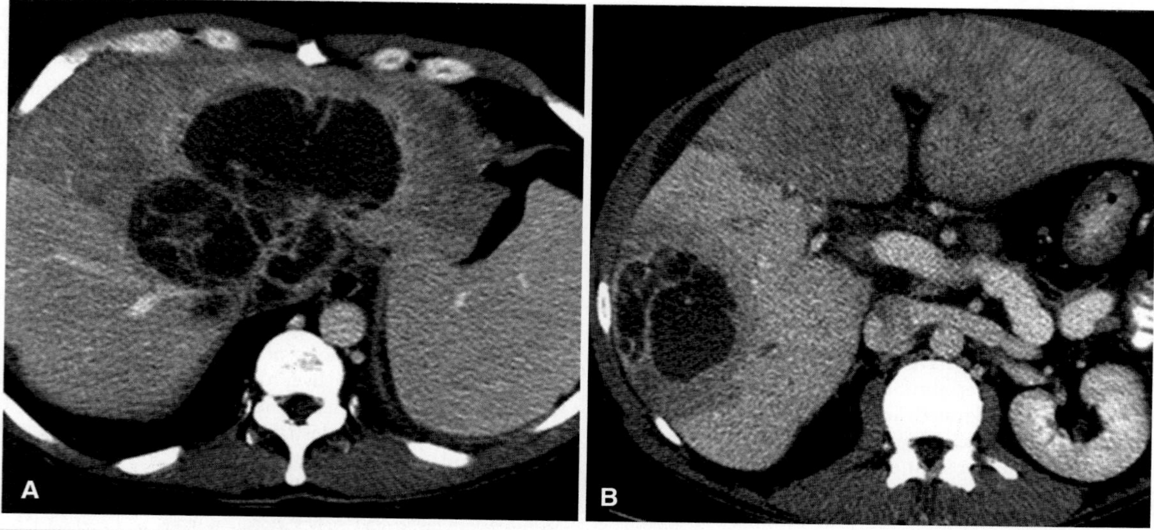

FIGURE 154-1. **A and B, Computed tomographic scans of a pyogenic liver abscess.** (Courtesy Dr. Chalermrat Bunchorntavakul, Bangkok, Thailand.)

Pyogenic Liver Abscess

DEFINITION

Pyogenic liver abscess is a focal collection of purulent bacterial material and necroinflammatory debris. It can be solitary or multiple and can be caused by one or more aerobic and anaerobic bacteria (Fig. 154-1).

EPIDEMIOLOGY

Pyogenic liver abscess has an estimated global incidence of approximately 1.1 to 2.3 per 100,000 person-years, whereas in the United States the incidence is reported to be approximately 3.6 per 100,000 and has been rising. Biliary obstruction, caused by a malignancy or benign disease, accounts for 50 to 60% of pyogenic liver abscesses, whereas portal pyemia, owing to appendicitis or other intra-abdominal infections, accounts for about 20% of cases.

PATHOBIOLOGY

Bacteria can enter the liver through the portal system from infections in areas drained by the mesenteric system into the portal system, such as appendicitis (Chapter 144). Other mechanisms for pyogenic liver abscess include bacterial cholangitis owing to benign or malignant obstruction, and infection of the liver from a systemic bacteremia, such as an infection of the oral cavity. Pyogenic liver abscess can also be caused by blunt or penetrating trauma, including such unusual causes as the ingestion of a toothpick or fish bone that can cause an intestinal perforation, fistula to the liver, and subsequent abscess formation. Liver abscesses can occur in a transplanted graft owing to vascular compromise caused by hepatic artery thrombosis and ischemic bile duct strictures.

Multiple organisms can cause pyogenic liver abscess. The most common organism, *Klebsiella pneumoniae,* often is associated with biliary tract disease. Other aerobes include *Escherichia coli,* group D streptococci, β-hemolytic streptococci, and *Staphylococcus aureus.* Anaerobic infection is often seen with colonic disease. Less common causes of liver abscesses include actinomyces, *Nocardia asteroides, Yersinia pseudotuberculosis* and *Yersinia enterocolitica, Listeria monocytogenes, Campylobacter jejuni, Legionella pneumophila, Mycobacterium tuberculosis, Salmonella typhi* or *Salmonella paratyphi, Candida albicans,* and *Bartonella henselae.* Most often the organism recovered from an abscess cavity is single, but multiple organisms can be isolated in as many as one third of patients. No bacteria may be isolated from the abscess because of prior antibiotic therapy or the failure to perform proper anaerobic cultures.

CLINICAL MANIFESTATIONS

The signs and symptoms associated with a liver abscess typically include fever, right upper quadrant abdominal pain, chills, nausea, vomiting, weight loss, and jaundice. The presentation can be acute or indolent. An associated bacteremia is seen in approximately 50% of the patients, but frank sepsis is rare.

DIAGNOSIS

Appropriate diagnosis requires a high degree of clinical suspicion, and diagnosis is sometimes delayed. Usually, however, the diagnosis is made promptly with the wide availability of the various radiologic modalities. The two common causes of liver abscesses are pyogenic and amebic abscess, and it is important to make a distinction because the prognosis and management differ. Amebic abscess can become secondarily infected with bacteria.

The diagnosis of an abscess is based on a constellation of clinical, bacteriologic, and radiologic features. Ultrasonography and computed tomography (CT) are the most common radiologic modalities to diagnose an abscess cavity reliably, as either single or multiple lesions, but CT is the preferred test, with sensitivity above 90%. Any concurrent biliary obstruction also can be diagnosed by these imaging studies. Approximately 50% of patients have multiple abscesses. On CT, the lesion is seen as a fluid collection with irregular borders and wall edema. One drawback to this imaging modality is that no specific features differentiate a pyogenic abscess from other infectious causes (i.e., amebic or fungal). Another drawback is that a very early stage abscess may not be well formed and may have characteristics more suggestive of a solid mass. Distinguishing an abscess from a tumor (Chapter 202) or a simple cyst can be difficult on noninvasive imaging if there is bleeding into a cyst, calcification, necrosis, or bleeding into a tumor. The presence of smaller (<2 cm) peripheral lesions that surround a central lesion argues strongly against a hepatic neoplasm. Calcification suggests bleeding into a tumor, but it also can be seen in the wall of an echinococcal cyst. Nonspecific radiologic features, including elevation of the right hemidiaphragm, right lower lung lobe atelectasis, and right pleural effusion, are seen in up to 30% of patients with pyogenic liver abscesses. Magnetic resonance imaging (MRI) and tagged white blood cell scans add little to the diagnosis of a liver abscess.

Microbial cultures are essential. In addition to blood cultures, the abscess cavity should be aspirated percutaneously, with either ultrasound or CT guidance, and the aspirate should be cultured for aerobic and anaerobic organisms as well as for amebae if there is any suspicion of an amebic abscess. Blood cultures are positive in only approximately 50% of cases. In approximately 15 to 20% of cases, multiple organisms are identified in the abscess cavity, but 20 to 30% of cases may have negative cultures despite appropriate culture techniques.

TREATMENT

Rx

Immediate broad-spectrum antibiotic coverage, as well as the prompt identification and treatment of the source of the infection, are essential for successful outcomes. Once the etiologic bacteria is identified, the antibiotic regimen can be tailored appropriately based on prevailing bacterial resistance patterns. Monotherapy with a β-lactam or β-lactamase inhibitor such as ampicillin-sulbactam (3 g intravenously every 6 hours), piperacillin-tazobactam (4.5 g intravenously every 6 hours), or ticarcillin-clavulanate (3.1 g intravenously every 6 hours) can be used, or a third-generation cephalosporin such as ceftriaxone (1 to 2 g intravenously daily) *plus* metronidazole (500 mg intravenously every 8 to 12 hours) can be used. Other potential regimens include a fluoroquinolone (e.g., ciprofloxacin, 400 mg intravenously every 12 hours, or levofloxacin, 500 or 750 mg intravenously daily) *plus* metronidazole (500 mg intravenously every 8 to 12 hours), or monotherapy with a carbapenem such as imipenem (500 mg intravenously every 6 hours), meropenem (1 g intravenously every 8 hours), or ertapenem (1 g intravenously daily).

The duration of therapy is partly based on the response to therapy. On an average, 4 to 6 weeks of antibiotic therapy appears reasonable, and the last 2 to 4 weeks of the antibiotic regimen can be administered orally. Abscesses that are hard to drain or are slow to demonstrate radiographic resolution require longer courses of therapy. Importantly, radiologic abnormalities resolve more slowly than clinical and biochemical features, so the latter should be used as an indicator for tailoring the therapeutic regimen.

Although antibiotics alone can sometimes successfully resolve small, multiple pyogenic abscesses, it also is critical to address the source of infection. Any underlying biliary source must be resolved, and any biliary obstruction must be relieved. More often, most patients will require drainage of the abscesses. The standard approach is placement of a drain for about 7 days. Alternatively, needle aspiration, repeated as needed when the abscess is large enough to drain percutaneously, provides equivalent results,[1] except in abscesses larger than 10 cm in diameter.[2] Surgical drainage seldom is the first option, except in patients who also have a surgically correctable precipitating lesion, such as appendicitis or biliary obstruction. More often, a biliary obstruction is treated with endoscopic retrograde cholangiopancreatography (ERCP) or transhepatic cholangiography with biliary drainage. For pyogenic abscesses in transplanted livers, management and proper biliary drainage may be difficult to achieve because of the diffuse nature of the biliary strictures.

PROGNOSIS

Abscesses smaller than 10 cm can take up to 16 weeks to resolve, whereas abscesses larger than 10 cm may take, on an average, another 6 weeks to resolve. Mortality from pyogenic liver abscess is associated with older age and with comorbidities such as cirrhosis, diabetes, chronic renal failure, and malignancy. Jaundice is an ominous sign. In developed countries, the mortality rate ranges from 2 to 12%. Patients with bacteremia have a four-fold higher risk for death.

Nonabscess Hepatic Bacterial Infections

Bacterial infections of the liver can also cause more diffuse infections without frank abscess formation. Implicated organisms include *L. monocytogenes* (Chapter 301), *Y. enterocolitica* (Chapter 320), *S. typhi* and *S. paratyphi* (Chapter 316), legionella (Chapter 322), ehrlichia (Chapter 335), and gonococci (Chapter 307). There are no specific features associated with these infections, and these organisms do not necessarily cause abscesses. Patients with chronic liver disease are especially at risk for listerial infection. Patients with active enteric yersinia infection can have secondary liver involvement with or without liver abscesses. Disseminated gonococcal infections (Chapter 307) can cause a perihepatitis (Fitz-Hugh-Curtis syndrome), which can present with right upper quadrant pain and tenderness.

Systemic bacteremia can cause a variety of hepatobiliary abnormalities, which may range from elevated aminotransferase and alkaline phosphatase levels (Chapter 149) to the cholestasis of sepsis with the development of jaundice. Common organisms that can disrupt normal liver function after entering the blood stream include *E. coli*, *Klebsiella* species, *Streptococcus pneumoniae*, and *S. aureus*, especially from pneumonias, urinary tract infections, or soft tissue infections. The hepatic biochemical abnormalities associated with bacteremia may be related to factors such as hemodynamic instability and liver hypoperfusion, as well as to the infection per se. Associated renal failure, a blood transfusion–derived bilirubin load, and drugs may complicate the picture. The course of cholestasis may be prolonged for several days to a few weeks, but it typically resolves with resolution of the systemic infection. There is no specific treatment for the cholestasis related to a systemic infection, but it is important to rule out drug-induced cholestasis that may evolve as a consequence of one or more of the antibiotics.

Fungal Diseases of the Liver

Except for hepatosplenic candidiasis with granuloma formation, clinically significant fungal diseases of the liver are unusual. Other fungal infections also commonly manifest as hepatic granulomas but usually are not accompanied by the high fever that is characteristic of hepatosplenic candidiasis.

HEPATOSPLENIC CANDIDIASIS

EPIDEMIOLOGY AND PATHOBIOLOGY

Hepatosplenic candidiasis typically is caused by *C. albicans*, but other *Candida* species, including *C. tropicalis*, *C. parapsilosis*, *C. glabrata*, and *C. krusei*, have occasionally been reported. It occurs as part of disseminated candidiasis (Chapter 346), almost exclusively in patients with acute leukemia, but rarely in patients with lymphoma, aplastic anemia, and sarcoma. Up to 7% of patients with acute leukemia may develop hepatosplenic candidiasis, and it is more common with acute lymphoblastic leukemia than acute myeloid leukemia. Recently, however, the incidence of hepatosplenic candidiasis has decreased by a factor of four owing to the widespread use of prophylactic antifungal agents early in the disease. Hepatosplenic candidiasis presumably results from translocation of *Candida* species from the gastrointestinal tract into the blood stream as a result of prolonged neutropenia and a breach in mucosal integrity.

CLINICAL MANIFESTATIONS AND DIAGNOSIS

Hepatosplenic candidiasis presents with persistent and high spiking fevers in a patient who was previously neutropenic and has now returned to a normal neutrophil count. The fever may be accompanied by right upper quadrant pain, nausea, vomiting, and anorexia.

Patients typically have elevated levels of alkaline phosphatase and less commonly of aminotransferases, bilirubin, and leukocytes. CT, which is the imaging modality of choice, classically shows multiple areas of lucency representing microabscesses in the liver, spleen, and kidneys. If the CT scan is nondiagnostic but clinical suspicion remains high, an MRI should be performed.

TREATMENT AND PROGNOSIS

Rx

The mainstay of therapy is with antifungal therapy for a long duration of treatment. In clinically stable patients, oral fluconazole can be used. In acutely ill patients, a lipid formulation of amphotericin B (3 to 5 mg/kg intravenously daily) is recommended. If the lipid formulation of amphotericin B is not used, other options are caspofungin (70 mg loading dose, then 50 mg intravenously daily), anidulafungin (200 mg loading dose, then 100 mg intravenously daily), or micafungin (100 mg intravenously daily). After 1 to 2 weeks, oral fluconazole (400 mg daily) should be started. Treatment should continue until lesions resolve on follow-up CT scans, typically within 6 months of treatment. In patients who are receiving chemotherapy or stem cell transplantation, however, the high risk for recurrent hepatosplenic candidiasis typically warrants continued prophylactic fluconazole (400 mg orally, daily) to prevent relapse until native immunity is restored.

A definitive diagnosis is usually made on liver biopsy specimens that show multiple granulomas, and, with special stains, yeast and hyphal forms. However, biopsy often will not show evidence of infection, especially in patients who have received prior antifungal therapy. Although biopsy is the only means to establish a definitive diagnosis, it is not often required because other clinical, laboratory, and radiographic manifestations are almost always sufficient for diagnosis.

PROGNOSIS

With prolonged treatment with antifungals, there has been good success at treating hepatosplenic candidiasis.

Other Fungal Diseases

Other fungal infections of the liver are quite rare. Fungal cultures are always necessary to establish a definitive diagnosis.

Coccidioides immitis (Chapter 341) is often asymptomatic but may lead to fungal hepatitis characterized by an increased alkaline phosphatase level and the development of hepatic granulomas. Hepatic *Cryptococcus neoformans* infections (Chapter 344) are rare but are seen in patients with AIDS, who typically develop hepatomegaly. In the much more rare non-HIV-infected patient, disseminated cryptococcosis can result in focal granulomatous hepatitis, which may clinically mimic viral hepatitis, or can present as obstructive jaundice secondary to sclerosing cholangitis. *Histoplasma capsulatum* (Chapter 340) infects individuals who inhale the fungus, but most cases are subclinical. In symptomatic hepatic histoplasmosis, two thirds of patients present with hepatomegaly, with some showing splenic enlargement as well. Histologically, histoplasmosis can cause multiple granulomas diffusely distributed throughout the liver, although a more common finding is portal lymphohistiocytic infiltrate. *Paracoccidioides brasiliensis* (Chapter 343) most commonly infects adult males, and autopsy series have shown hepatic involvement in up to 50% of patients who die from this infection. Some individuals may present with hepatomegaly or jaundice, although the latter is found in less than 6% of patients. Aminotransferase levels are often elevated in the early stages of the disease, with changes in alkaline phosphatase or bilirubin levels tending to occur in the later stages. Biopsy may reveal lesions ranging from small granulomas to diffuse fibrosis and infiltration of yeast forms, often with bile duct involvement.

PARASITIC, PROTOZOAL, AND HELMINTHIC INFECTIONS OF THE LIVER

Amebic Liver Abscess

EPIDEMIOLOGY

Entamoeba histolytica (Chapter 360) is found throughout the world where the barriers between human feces and food and water are inadequate. After malaria, it is the second leading cause of death from parasitic diseases worldwide, accounting for an estimated 40,000 to 100,000 deaths annually. In the United States, most cases of amebiasis arise in immigrants from endemic areas and people living in states that border Mexico. Travelers to endemic areas are also at risk; ingestion of amebic cysts and colonization of the gastrointestinal tract can occur years before the development of a liver abscess. Amebic liver abscesses mainly affect men between the ages of 18 and 50 years but are also more common in postmenopausal women, thereby suggesting a hormonal protective effect. Other risk factors include alcohol intake, HLA-DR3, oral and anal sex, and contaminated enema apparatuses.

TABLE 154-2 PARASITIC INFECTIONS INVOLVING THE LIVER

	CHARACTERISTICS	ENDEMIC AREAS	RISK FACTORS AND ENDEMIC AREAS	MAJOR HEPATIC MANIFESTATIONS
MAJOR PROTOZOA				
Entamoeba histolytica	Ingested cysts develop into invasive trophozoites that colonize the colon and occasionally spread to the liver by the portal blood	Mexico, regions of Central and South America, India, and regions of Africa	Male gender, alcohol intake, HLA-DR3, oral and anal sex, and contaminated enema apparatuses	Amebic liver abscesses develop as a tissue response to trophozoite invasion with acute and chronic manifestations (see text)
OTHER PROTOZOA				
Cryptosporidium species and microsporidia	Ingested cysts develop into trophozoites in intestinal mucosa	Worldwide distribution	AIDS	Biliary tract infection with obstruction and cholangitis
Toxoplasma gondii	Ingestion of oocysts in contaminated soil or water or in infected meat; systemic spread of tachyzoites in the circulation	Worldwide distribution	Consumption of undercooked meat, contact with soil, and travel outside the United States, Europe, or Canada	Immunocompetent: asymptomatic or hepatomegaly and mild LFT elevations Immunocompromised: occasional overt hepatitis
Leishmania species	Sand fly bite transmits promastigotes; proliferation in the reticuloendothelial system	Worldwide distribution	Children <10 yr and immunocompromised adults Contact with sand flies	Hepatosplenomegaly months to years after infection
Plasmodium species	Mosquito (*Anopheles*) bite transmits sporozoites	Multiple regions throughout the world	Exposure to anopheline mosquito bites	Proliferation in hepatocytes causes hepatomegaly, enzyme elevations, and jaundice
Babesia microti	Tick bite transmits the agent, which parasitizes erythrocytes	Europe	Asplenia is a risk for fatal hepatic failure, especially bovine babesiosis	Mild liver enzyme elevations

PATHOBIOLOGY

E. histolytica has a simple life cycle consisting of the cyst (infectious form) and trophozoite (the motile stage associated with disease); it infects only humans and some nonhuman primates. Cysts are ingested and mature into trophozoites in the intestinal lumen. The development of amebic colitis is not essential for liver abscess formation. *E. histolytica* trophozoites penetrate through the mucosa and submucosal tissues and enter the portal circulation. *E. histolytica* blocks intrahepatic portal venules. When the trophozoites reach the liver, they create their unique abscesses, which are well-circumscribed regions of dead hepatocytes, liquefied cells, and cellular debris that are surrounded by a rim of connective tissue, a few inflammatory cells, and amebic trophozoites. The adjacent liver parenchyma is unaffected. Given the small numbers of amebae relative to the size of the abscess, it is suggested that *E. histolytica* can cause hepatocyte death without direct contact.

CLINICAL MANIFESTATIONS

Patients can present with amebic liver abscesses months to years after traveling to an endemic area, so a detailed travel history is essential for the diagnosis. The disease should be suspected in patients with an appropriate travel history, fever, right upper quadrant pain, and substantial hepatic tenderness. Jaundice is extremely uncommon. Symptoms are usually acute (<10 days in duration) but can be chronic, with anorexia and weight loss. Patients with acute disease tend to have multifocal disease, whereas patients with a more indolent course tend to have a solitary lesion. Laboratory data tend to demonstrate a leukocytosis without eosinophilia, mild anemia, an elevated alkaline phosphatase level, and high erythrocyte sedimentation rate.

DIAGNOSIS

Although some individuals with amebic liver abscesses have concurrent amebic colitis, most have no bowel symptoms; hence, stool microscopy for *E. histolytica* trophozoites and cysts are usually negative. The diagnosis relies on identification of a space-occupying lesion in the liver and a positive amebic serology. Both ultrasound and CT scan are very sensitive (Fig. 154-2), but neither provides absolute specificity for amebic liver abscesses. Serologic testing is highly sensitive (>94%) and specific (>95%). False-negative testing can be obtained within the first 7 to 10 days of infection, but repeat testing will usually be positive. Aspiration of the lesion may be necessary to exclude a primary or secondary bacterial infection.

TREATMENT AND PROGNOSIS

Metronidazole (500 to 750 mg orally three times daily or a 15-mg/kg loading dose followed by 7.5 mg/kg every 6 hours intravenously) usually provides evidence of clinical improvement within 72 to 96 hours but should be continued for 5 to 10 days. Nitroimidazole tinidazole at 2 g daily for 3 days is also effective. Drainage is not necessary,[3] except in patients who do not respond within 5 days. For cysts larger than 10 cm, catheter drainage is preferred over repeated needle aspiration.[2] The abscess usually shrinks by about 50% within a week, but the mean time to complete radiologic resolution is 3 to 9 months. Repeated imaging in a clinically improving patient may lead to unwarranted concern and unnecessary treatment.

Treatment must also address the removal of all of the cysts from the intestinal lumen in patients with evidence of intraluminal infection. A recommended treatment is iodoquinol (650 mg orally three times a day for 20 days) to prevent continued colonization and possible recurrence of the liver abscess. With prompt diagnosis and adequate medical treatment, the mortality rate from amebic abscess is 1 to 3%.

Other Protozoal Liver Diseases

In addition to *E. histolytica*, other protozoal diseases that affect the liver include *Cryptosporidium* species, *Toxoplasma gondii, Leishmania* species, *Plasmodium* species, and *Babesia microti* (Table 154-2).

HELMINTH INFECTIONS

Echinococcosis and Hydatid Cyst Disease

EPIDEMIOLOGY AND PATHOBIOLOGY

Human cystic echinococcosis is a zoonosis caused by the larval cestode *E. granulosus*. It is often referred to as hydatid cyst disease because of the watery cysts that characterize the infection.

SYMPTOMS AND SIGNS	LABORATORY FINDINGS	RADIOGRAPHIC FEATURES	DIAGNOSIS	TREATMENT
Fever, RUQ pain, and substantial hepatic tenderness	Leukocytosis without eosinophilia, mild anemia, elevated serum AP, and high ESR	US, CT, and MRI can detect abscess but cannot always differentiate amebic from pyogenic. On CT or MRI, amebic abscess sometimes appears "cold" with bright rim.	Imaging, serology, stool antigen test (microscopic evaluation of stool has a poor yield)	Metronidazole, 500-750 mg PO tid × 5-10 days, or tinidazole, 2 g daily × 3 days; iodoquinol, 650 mg tid × 20 days, also needed to eradicate intestinal colonization
See Chapter 358	See Chapter 358	See Chapter 358	See Chapter 358	See Chapter 358
See Chapter 357	See Chapter 357	See Chapter 357	See Chapter 357	See Chapter 357
See Chapter 356	See Chapter 356	See Chapter 356	See Chapter 356	See Chapter 356
See Chapter 353	See Chapter 353	See Chapter 353	See Chapter 353	See Chapter 353
See Chapter 361	See Chapter 361	See Chapter 361	See Chapter 361	See Chapter 361

TABLE 154-2 PARASITIC INFECTIONS INVOLVING THE LIVER—cont'd

	CHARACTERISTICS	ENDEMIC AREAS	RISK FACTORS AND ENDEMIC AREAS	MAJOR HEPATIC MANIFESTATIONS
MAJOR HELMINTHS				
Schistosoma species	Cercaria in fresh water penetrate the skin, travel by the circulation to portal vein radicals	*S. mansoni* found in South America, Africa, and Middle East. *S. japonicum* found in Far East (mostly China and Philippines).	Contact with fresh water containing cercaria of schistosomes	Progressive presinusoidal blood flow obstruction, periportal fibrosis, portal hypertension, varices, ascites, splenomegaly
Echinococcus granulosus	Eggs of small (3-7 mm) tapeworms in stool of canid hosts; ingested eggs produce larval oncospheres that migrate to the liver and form cysts in sheep, humans, and other intermediate hosts	Worldwide distribution, found especially in sheep-raising areas (Africa, the Mediterranean region of Europe, the Middle East, Asia, South America, Australia, and New Zealand)	Ingestion of food or water fecally contaminated with eggs and human contact with sheepdogs	Initial infection asymptomatic; liver cysts increase in diameter by 1-5 cm yearly and cause variable abdominal pain, hepatomegaly, and variable eosinophilia; occasional cyst rupture, secondary bacterial infection
Echinococcus multilocularis	Eggs of small tapeworms in stool of foxes; ingested eggs produce oncospheres in the liver of rodents, humans, and other intermediate hosts	Endemic in Northern hemisphere	Human exposure increasing with growing fox populations	Metacestodes colonize the liver as a tumor-like mass of small vesicles
Fasciola species	Leaf-shaped flukes up to 13 × 30 mm derived from ingested cysts; the fluke excysts in the duodenum, migrates directly across the bowel wall into the peritoneal cavity, and burrows directly into the liver (or occasionally out to the skin)	Worldwide distribution	Consumption of freshwater or aquatic plants contaminated by colonized livestock	Adult flukes live in the common and hepatic bile ducts causing obstruction and leading to thickening of the ducts, dilation, and fibrosis of the proximal biliary tree
Opisthorchis species and *Clonorchis sinensis*	Flukes of 8-25 mm derived from ingested cysts; the fluke excysts in the duodenum and migrates into the bile ducts	*Opisthorchis* sp: Southeast Asia, Central and Eastern Europe (particularly Siberia) *C. sinensis:* China, Japan, Vietnam, Korea	Consumption of raw, pickled, dried, smoked, or salted freshwater fish or crayfish originating from East Asia or, in the case of *Opisthorchis felineus,* Russia and Eastern Europe	*Acute:* typically asymptomatic *Chronic:* abdominal pain, fever, anorexia, tender hepatomegaly, sometimes eosinophilia *Late sequelae:* intermittent biliary obstruction, cholelithiasis, cholecystitis, cholangitis, secondary bacterial abscesses, cholangiocarcinoma
Toxocara species	Nematode infection disseminates to cause visceral larva migrans after ingestion of soil contaminated with dog or cat feces	Highest prevalence in southeastern United States	Consumption of food contaminated with soil containing eggs; distributed throughout the United States	Often an asymptomatic cause of eosinophilia (exclude *Trichinella* sp, *Strongyloides* sp, filaria, hookworm, schistosomiasis); hepatomegaly is common, but nonhepatic manifestations dominate the clinical picture
OTHER HELMINTHS				
Ascaris lumbricoides	Ingested eggs develop into larvae that migrate to the lungs and are coughed and swallowed; develop into roundworms 15-30 mm long in the small intestine	Global distribution with higher prevalence in Africa, South America, India, and the Far East; 20% of the world's population is colonized	Consumption of fecally contaminated food or water, particularly in young children	Colonization is typically asymptomatic with eosinophilia; biliary migration of worms can cause symptomatic biliary obstruction, cholangitis, cholecystitis, and secondary bacterial liver abscess
Capillaria hepatica	Ingested eggs develop into larvae in the intestinal mucosa; larvae migrate to the liver by portal blood flow and develop into short-lived roundworms	Human infection is rare	Consumption of food contaminated with rodent feces	Fever, eosinophilia, and hepatomegaly; subsequent foci of liver fibrosis, granulomas, and calcification in involved areas
Strongyloides stercoralis	Ingested eggs develop into 1.5- to 2.5-mm nematodes that invade the hepatic vasculature, lymphatics, and biliary tract	Tropical and subtropical areas, including southeastern United States and Southern and Eastern Europe	Consumption of food contaminated with soil containing eggs, infection with HTLV-1, and immunocompromised individuals	Hepatic disease in the setting of immunosuppression: jaundice, abdominal pain; eosinophilia is uncommon

AP = alkaline phosphatase; CT = computed tomography; ELISA = enzyme-linked immunosorbent assay; ERCP = endoscopic retrograde cholangiopancreatography; ESR = erythrocyte sedimentation rate; HTLV = human T-cell lymphotrophic virus; LFT = liver function test; MRI = magnetic resonance imaging; RUQ = right upper quadrant; US = ultrasonography.

SYMPTOMS AND SIGNS	LABORATORY FINDINGS	RADIOGRAPHIC FEATURES	DIAGNOSIS	TREATMENT
Initial infection presents as itching. Later presentations include fever, diarrhea, chills, headaches, or hives. Hematemesis from ruptured gastroesophageal varices	Eosinophilia and splenomegaly; seroconversion occurs within 4 to 6 weeks	Extensive calcification with typical turtle-back appearance along portal tracts	Rectal biopsy, liver biopsy, microscopic examination of stool	Praziquantel (single dose, 40 mg/kg) with a second dose 6-12 weeks later if necessary
Enlarged hydatid cyst can cause abdominal pain, nausea, hepatomegaly, or a palpable mass. Mild RUQ pain, urticaria, and episodes of pruritus	Positive Weinberg reaction (false negative in 38% of cases) or ELISA analysis; eosinophilia seen in ruptured cysts	On US or CT, cysts appear flaky, sometimes showing daughter cysts or peripheral focal calcification. Fluid is of variable density.	Imaging, Weinberg reaction, or ELISA	Albendazole, 400 mg 2× daily for 3-6 monthly cycles with 10-14 day intervals. Drainage of the cyst is essential. Surgical resection if the cyst communicates with the biliary tree.
See Chapter 362	See Chapter 362	See Chapter 362	See Chapter 362	See Chapter 362
Acute: fever, abdominal pain, eosinophilia *Chronic:* symptomatic biliary obstruction, variable eosinophilia	Serologic tests include hemagglutination, complement fixation, ELISA, and counterimmunoelectrophoresis. Anemia, leukocytosis, eosinophilia, elevated AP, and hypergammaglobulinemia are often seen.	CT is most useful: liver shows hypodense nodules or tortuous tracks; thickening of the liver capsule, subcapsular hematoma, and parenchymal calcification may also be seen	Serology, stool examination	Triclabendazole, 10 mg/kg once or twice
Chronic infection presents as dyspepsia, abdominal pain, diarrhea, nausea, vomiting, anorexia, weight loss, fevers, hepatomegaly, and urticaria. Acute presentation includes serum sickness, intrahepatic pigment stones, and facial edema. Other rare complications are cholangitis, pancreatitis, and obstructive jaundice.	Anemia, leukocytosis, eosinophilia, elevated AP, and hypergammaglobulinemia	US may detect flukes in biliary tree. CT shows small hypodense nodules.	Serology and stool examination	Praziquantel, 25 mg/kg q8h × 3 doses
See Chapter 365	See Chapter 365	See Chapter 365	See Chapter 365	See Chapter 365
Sensitized patients during pulmonary phase present with asthma-like symptoms, hemoptysis, chest pain, and cyanosis. Urticaria and other allergic reactions are sometimes seen. Patients in intestinal phase show cognitive and nutritional impairment with abdominal pain, hepatomegaly, cholangitis, and obstructive jaundice.	Leukocytosis with eosinophilia; hyperbilirubinemia occasionally seen	Movement of the worms within the biliary tree can sometimes be observed. A bull's-eye appearance can be seen on cross-sectional imaging.	Stool examination, imaging, and ERCP	Albendazole, 400 mg once
Persistent fever, eosinophilia, and hepatomegaly are most common. Splenomegaly, anorexia, nausea, vomiting, night sweats, and altered bowel habits are also seen.	Anemia, eosinophilia, moderately elevated liver enzymes, increased ESR, and hypergammaglobulinemia	US shows nonspecific hyperechoic areas in the portal spaces.	Stool and liver biopsy	Mebendazole, 200 mg bid × 20 days
Recurrent urticaria, abdominal pain, diarrhea, and cough; mild jaundice and hepatomegaly in the absence of splenomegaly	Eosinophilia and hypoalbuminemia Patients may have elevated liver enzymes.	Imaging studies not used in diagnosis	Serology and stool examination	Ivermectin, 200 µg/kg/day × 2 days, or albendazole, 400 mg/day × 7 days

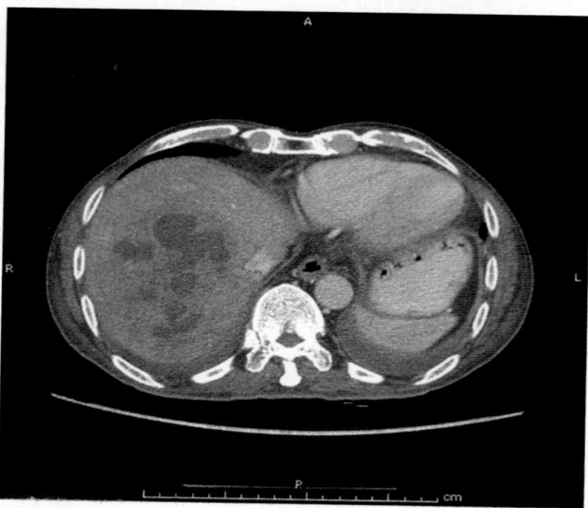

FIGURE 154-2. Computed tomographic scan of an amebic liver abscess. (Courtesy Dr. Chalermrat Bunchorntavakul, Bangkok, Thailand.)

The disease remains endemic in sheep-raising areas of the world, including Africa, the Mediterranean region of Europe, the Middle East, Asia, South America, Australia, and New Zealand. Dogs are the definitive hosts for *E. granulosus*, and sheep are the major intermediate hosts, although yaks, goats, and camels are other relevant intermediate hosts. Humans are only accidental hosts when they ingest food or water that is fecally contaminated with eggs. Human contact with sheepdogs that are in frequent contact with livestock is a major risk for infection.

The disease cycle begins when an adult tapeworm infects the intestinal tract of the definitive host (dogs usually). The adult tapeworm then produces eggs, which are expelled in the host's feces. Intermediate hosts become infected by ingesting the eggs of the parasite in fecally contaminated food. Inside the intermediate host, the eggs hatch and release tiny hooked embryos (called oncospheres), which travel in the blood stream and eventually lodge in the liver, lungs, or kidneys, where they develop into hydatid cysts. Inside these cysts grow thousands of tapeworm larvae, the next stage in the life cycle of the parasite.

CLINICAL MANIFESTATIONS

The initial infection is asymptomatic, but an enlarging hydatid liver cyst can cause abdominal pain, nausea, hepatomegaly, or a palpable mass. Patients may describe symptoms of mild upper right quadrant pain, urticarial skin rash, and episodes of pruritus. If the cyst ruptures, serious complications can develop. Cysts that perforate into the peritoneum can lead to the development of extrahepatic cysts and may induce an allergic reaction with eosinophilia, pruritic urticaria, and systemic anaphylaxis. In most cases, however, cysts rupture into bile ducts, where they cause cholestatic jaundice, cholangitis, or biliary pain.

DIAGNOSIS

On ultrasound or CT scans (Fig. 154-3), the hydatid cysts are often large with a flaky appearance that is referred to as *hydatid sand*. CT imaging also may show multiple daughter cysts or a fluid density cyst with peripheral focal areas of calcification. Fluid is of variable density depending on the amount of proteinaceous debris.

Hydatid cysts of liver can be diagnosed by a serologic assay, the Weinberg reaction, but this test can have false-negative results in up to 38% of cases. An enzyme-linked immunosorbent assay (ELISA) may be more sensitive. Eosinophilia is not a feature unless the cyst ruptures; in fact, usually there are no changes in blood chemistries.

TREATMENT AND PROGNOSIS

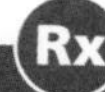

Drug therapy includes albendazole, 400 mg twice a day for 3 to 6 monthly cycles separated by 10 to 14 day intervals, but treatment with albendazole alone is not effective, so drainage is essential to the effective treatment of hydatid cysts. In a randomized trial, percutaneous drainage consisting of puncture, aspiration, injection, and reaspiration of scolicidal solutions resulted in a similar rate of cyst disappearance as open surgical drainage but with fewer side effects, provided that patients received preprocedure and postprocedure albendazole therapy.[4] Chlorhexidine, H_2O_2, 80% alcohol, and 0.5% cetrimide are the preferred scolicidal agents. If the cyst communicates with the biliary tree, however, injection of scolicidal agents carries an almost universal risk of secondary sclerosing cholangitis, and so it is contraindicated. In such cases, the cyst must be treated surgically, by either cystectomy or hepatic resection.

The prognosis is generally good, with complete cure expected after successful percutaneous or surgical treatment. However, spillage occurs in 2 to 25% of cases, depending on the location of the cyst and surgeon's experience, and the operative mortality rate varies from 0.5 to 4% for the same reasons.

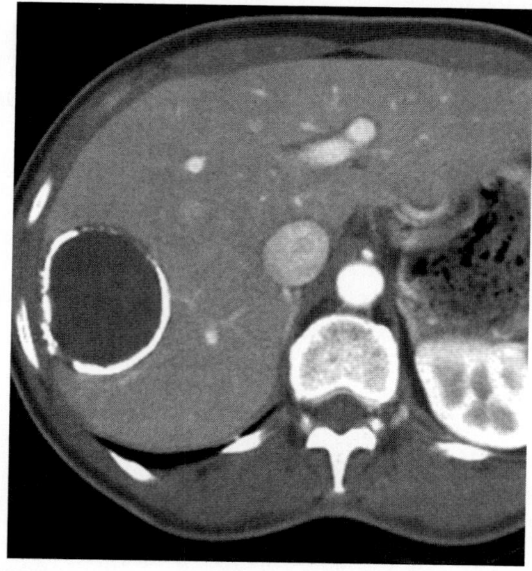

FIGURE 154-3. Computed tomographic scan of a hepatic echinococcal cyst.

Schistosomiasis

EPIDEMIOLOGY AND PATHOBIOLOGY

Schistosomiasis is an infection of trematodes. *Schistosoma* species (Chapter 363) cause periportal fibrosis and liver cirrhosis owing to deposition of eggs in the small portal venules. *Schistosoma mansoni* and *Schistosoma japonicum* lead to liver disease. Infection with *S. mansoni* is found in parts of South America, Africa, and the Middle East. Infection with *S. japonicum* is found in the Far East, mostly China and the Philippines. Although primary infection does not occur in the United States, 5% of the world's population may be infected, thereby making it a major international health concern and highly prevalent in immigrants.

Humans become infected after contact with water that contains the infective stage (cercaria) of schistosomes. After penetration of the skin, the larvae migrate to the lungs and then to the venules of the mesentery, urinary bladder, or ureters. They release eggs in the venules of the mesentery, and the eggs enter the liver through the portal vein, where they become lodged in the terminal branches of the portal venules. The lodged eggs cause a granulomatous inflammation, and the lesions heal by periportal fibrosis. *S. japonicum* is more virulent than *S. mansoni* because its infections produce ten times more eggs.

CLINICAL MANIFESTATIONS

Initial infection presents as itching that is caused by skin penetration by larvae. Several weeks later, patients may complain of fever, diarrhea, chills, headaches, or hives. At this time, patients will have eosinophilia. Over the next 5 to 15 years, periportal liver fibrosis develops and leads to presinusoidal portal hypertension, splenomegaly (Chapter 171), and gastroesophageal varices (Chapter 140). With *S. japonicum*, however, the progression can be much more rapid, with little interval between the acute and chronic disease. Hepatic function is generally well preserved, and patients usually present with hematemesis from ruptured gastroesophageal varices.

DIAGNOSIS

Schistosomal eggs typically have lateral or terminal spines and are easy to detect on microscopic examination of feces or on a rectal biopsy. Seroconversion occurs within 4 to 8 weeks of infection but cannot distinguish active infection from a history of exposure. Imaging may show extensive calcification with the typical turtle-back appearance along the portal tracts reflecting the clustered, calcified eggs along the portal triads.

TREATMENT AND PROGNOSIS Rx

Praziquantel (a single dose of 40 mg/kg) is effective in 70 to 100% of cases, but a second dose can be given 6 to 12 weeks later, particularly in patients with eosinophilia, high antibody titers, or persistent symptoms. Treatment of portal hypertension may be necessary (Chapter 156). The mortality rate is 0.05% for severe *S. mansoni* infection and 1.8% for severe *S. japonicum* infection. Bleeding from esophageal varices is the most serious complication. Chronic infection can lead to hepatocellular carcinoma.

GRANULOMATOUS DISEASES OF THE LIVER

Granulomas, which are found in up to 15% of liver biopsies, can be an incidental finding or may represent a wide array of liver diseases (Table 154-3). A granuloma is an accumulation of epithelioid cells, including transformed macrophages, mononuclear cells, and other inflammatory cells. Granulomas may have associated necrosis (caseating) as in tuberculosis (Chapter 332) or may be non-necrotizing (noncaseating) as in sarcoidosis (Chapter 95). In Q fever (Chapter 335), fibrin-ring granulomas are characterized by a vacuole encircled by a ring of fibrinoid necrosis and surrounded by lymphocytes and histiocytes.

An incidental granuloma requires minimal further evaluation. Tuberculosis should be excluded (Chapter 332). Sarcoidosis also should be considered because it is the most common cause of granulomas in the United States. An antimitochondrial antibody should be drawn to rule out primary biliary cirrhosis. The use of potentially causative drugs should be stopped (see Table 154-3).

Sarcoidosis

Sarcoidosis, which is the most frequently identified cause of hepatic granuloma in the United States, affects all racial and ethnic groups and occurs at all ages. In patients with sarcoidosis, the liver is the third most commonly involved organ, after the lymph nodes and lung; about 50 to 80% of patients with sarcoidosis have granulomas in their livers. The classic granuloma is found mainly in the portal triads, with a cluster of large epithelioid cells and often with multinucleated giant cells.

CLINICAL MANIFESTATIONS AND DIAGNOSIS

Hepatic involvement of sarcoidosis is often subclinical, and only a minority of patients present with pruritus, fever, abdominal pain, hepatomegaly, cholestatic jaundice, or portal hypertension. In some patients, the granulomatous injury and destruction of the interlobular bile ducts eventually causes ductopenia and a histologic picture similar to primary biliary cirrhosis (Chapter 158). In other patients, damage to the large bile ducts may lead to a syndrome that mimics primary sclerosing cholangitis (Chapter 158). Other patients may present with focal liver lesions suggestive of malignant neoplasm.

Patients typically have a marked elevation of the serum alkaline phosphatase level. Angiotensin-converting enzyme (ACE) levels also are characteristically elevated but may not be helpful in differentiating sarcoidosis from other chronic liver diseases, such as primary biliary cirrhosis, in which it also may be elevated. The presence of noncaseating granulomas in a patient with clinically suspected sarcoidosis generally establishes the diagnosis. However, granulomas do not correlate with liver function tests or duration of disease.

TREATMENT AND PROGNOSIS Rx

In general, hepatic sarcoidosis does not need to be treated except in patients with other indications for treatment (Chapter 95). Corticosteroids improve liver function tests but do not alleviate portal hypertension, and serial biopsies often show little improvement. Sarcoidosis that leads to portal hypertension and fibrosis may ultimately require liver transplantation (Chapter 157), and sarcoidosis may recur in the new organ.

Other Granulomatous Liver Diseases

In addition to sarcoidosis, another major cause of granulomatous liver disease is tuberculosis (Chapter 332). Military tuberculosis, caused by *Mycobacterium tuberculosis*, commonly results in hepatic granulomas, and patients present with hepatomegaly or abnormal liver function tests, or both. A biopsy revealing caseating granulomas along with a positive purified protein derivative test and active pulmonary tuberculosis can help in establishing a diagnosis. Other mycobacteria known to cause granulomatous liver disease include *M. avium-intracellulare*, *M. gevanese*, and *M. scrofulaceum* (Chapter 333).

Other causes of granulomatous liver disease include zoonotic infections such as cat-scratch disease (Chapter 323), Q fever (Chapter 335), and brucellosis (Chapter 318). Cat-scratch disease is caused by *B. henselae*, with cats serving as the main reservoir for the organism. The disease primarily affects children. Patients typically present with lymphadenopathy associated with persistent pyrexia of unknown origin, abdominal pain, and weight loss. *B. henselae* can be identified by a Warthin-Starry stain, or an imaging study may demonstrate scattered defects in the liver. Q fever is caused by the intracellular gram-negative rickettsial organism *Coxiella burnetii*. Most infections are

TABLE 154-3 CAUSES OF GRANULOMATOUS LIVER DISEASE

DIAGNOSIS	SPECIAL AND UNIQUE FEATURES
Sarcoidosis	Evidence of pulmonary sarcoidosis, granulomas found on biopsy specimens from other organs, elevated ACE level
Bacterial infections	
Mycobacteria tuberculosis	Caseating granulomas on biopsy, + PPD, active pulmonary tuberculosis
Other mycobacteria (*M. avium-intracellulare, M. lepra, M. mucogenicum, M. bovis*)	HIV, exposure history
Other bacteria (brucellosis, listeriosis, melioidosis, tularemia, yersiniosis, bartonellosis, Q fever, syphilis, psittacosis)	Fever, exposure history
Viral infections (cytomegalovirus, Epstein-Barr virus, hepatitis C, hepatitis B, hepatitis A)	Serology for acute or recent exposure
Fungal infections (histoplasmosis, coccidioidomycosis, blastomycosis, nocardiosis, candidiasis)	Fever, immunocompromised
Parasitic infections (schistosomiasis, *Ascaris lumbricoides* infection, toxoplasmosis, visceral leishmaniasis)	Travel to endemic regions, positive serologic testing
Primary biliary cirrhosis	Female sex, positive AMA, elevated IgM
Malignancies (Hodgkin's disease, non-Hodgkin's lymphoma, renal cell carcinoma)	Evidence of malignancy in kidney, lymph node, or bone marrow
Drug reactions (allopurinol, chlorpropamide, phenylbutazone, sulfonamides, carbamazepine, glyburide, quinidine, quinine, diltiazem, hydralazine, rosiglitazone, phenytoin, methyldopa, procainamide, amoxicillin–clavulanic acid, mebendazole, mesalamine, acetaminophen, pyrazinamide, halothane, isoniazid, norfloxacin)	Exposure history
Toxins (beryllium, copper sulfate, Thorotrast)	Previous exposure history
Miscellaneous (talc, Crohn's disease, Wegener's granulomatosis, after jejunoileal bypass, mineral oil lipogranulomas, hepatic allograft rejection, chronic granulomatous disease)	History of IV drug use, history of liver transplantation, diarrhea

ACE = angiotensin-converting enzyme; AMA = antimitochondrial antibody; HIV = human immunodeficiency virus; IV = intravenous; PPD = purified protein derivative.

asymptomatic, but patients may have self-limited influenza-like symptoms, pneumonia, and hepatitis. A liver biopsy may demonstrate fibrin-ring granulomas (doughnut shaped) in the background of nonspecific reactive hepatitis and steatosis. Brucellosis, which is not common in the United States, is caused by at least four species of Brucella: *B. abortus*, *B. suis*, *B. melitensis*, and *B. canis*. The disease presents as recurrent high fevers, drenching sweats, malaise, arthralgia, fatigue, abdominal pain, anorexia, and headaches. Patients often have hepatomegaly and increases in serum levels of aminotransferases and alkaline phosphatase. The granulomas formed by this infection are typically smaller than those caused by sarcoidosis or tuberculosis, and a definitive diagnosis can be established through serologic testing.

It is important to keep in mind that hepatic granulomas are formed naturally as a consequence of the immune response, so they may be seen in many infections with hepatic involvement (see Table 154-3). Examples of infections that can manifest as granulomatous liver disease include listeriosis, yersiniosis, candidiasis, histoplasmosis, coccidioidomycosis, and schistosomiasis. Viral infections (e.g., cytomegalovirus and hepatitis A, B, and C), primary biliary cirrhosis, malignancies, and certain drug reactions have all been etiologically linked to granulomatous liver disease.

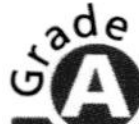

1. Yu SC, Ho SS, Lau WY, et al. Treatment of pyogenic liver abscess: prospective randomized comparison of catheter drainage and needle aspiration. *Hepatology*. 2004;39:932-938.
2. Singh O, Gupta S, Moses S, et al. Comparative study of catheter drainage and needle aspiration in management of large liver abscesses. *Indian J Gastroenterol*. 2009;28:88-92.
3. Chavez-Tapia NC, Hernandez Calleros J, Tellez-Avila FL, et al. Image-guided percutaneous procedure plus metronidazole versus metronidazole alone for uncomplicated amoebic liver abscess. *Cochrane Database Syst Rev*. 2009;21:CD004886.
4. Nasseri Moghaddam S, Abrishami A, Malekzade R. Percutaneous needle aspiration, injection, and reaspiration with or without benzimidazole coverage for uncomplicated hepatic hydatid cysts. *Cochrane Database Syst Rev*. 2006;19:CD003623.

SUGGESTED READINGS

Meddings L, Myers RP, Hubbard J, et al. A population-based study of pyogenic liver abscesses in the United States: incidence, mortality, and temporal trends. *Am J Gastroenterol*. 2010;105:117-124. *The most common causes were streptococci (30%) and Escherichia coli (18%).*

O'Farrell N, Collins CG, McEntee GP. Pyogenic liver abscesses: diminished role for operative treatment. *Surgeon*. 2010;8:192-196. *Emphasizes interventional radiology and antimicrobial therapy.*

Reid-Lombardo KM, Khan S, Sclabas G. Hepatic cysts and liver abscesses. *Surg Clin North Am*. 2010;90:679-697. *Review.*

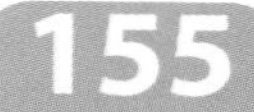

ALCOHOLIC AND NONALCOHOLIC STEATOHEPATITIS

NAGA P. CHALASANI

Alcoholic liver disease and nonalcoholic fatty liver disease (NAFLD), which represent two of the most common forms of liver disease, can lead to cirrhosis, liver failure, and death. Although these two conditions have different risk factors and natural histories, in both conditions (Table 155-1) the hepatocytes are characterized by macrovesicular steatosis, which is the accumulation of triglycerides as one large cytoplasmic globule that displaces the nucleus. In microvesicular steatosis, cytoplasmic accumulation of fat occurs as multiple small globules with a central nucleus.

ALCOHOLIC LIVER DISEASE

DEFINITION

Excessive alcoholic consumption (Chapter 32) causes alcoholic liver disease and can significantly worsen other liver disorders such as viral hepatitis (Chapter 151) and hemochromatosis (Chapter 219). Although most individuals who consume alcohol do not consume it excessively and do not develop any physical or social consequences, some alcoholics consume sufficient alcohol and, presumably owing to other predisposing factors, develop alcoholic liver disease. Alcoholic liver disease is a spectrum of chronic liver diseases, ranging from alcoholic fatty liver to alcoholic hepatitis and cirrhosis.

Alcoholic fatty liver disease will develop in nearly 90% of individuals who consume alcohol heavily (on average, >6 drinks per day), and some individuals develop the more severe conditions of alcoholic hepatitis and alcoholic cirrhosis. Nearly 50% of the patients with alcoholic hepatitis have preexisting cirrhosis (Chapter 156), and individuals who do not yet have cirrhosis are at high risk for developing it, especially if they continue to consume alcohol.

EPIDEMIOLOGY

The true prevalence of alcoholic liver disease is not known, but nearly 1% of North American adults are believed to have alcoholic liver disease. Even this figure is considered an underestimation because milder forms of alcoholic liver disease are asymptomatic and often unrecognized. It has been estimated that alcoholic liver disease accounts for 40% of deaths from cirrhosis and 28% of all deaths from liver disease. It is the second most common indication for liver transplantation in the United States once abstinence from alcohol has been established.

PATHOBIOLOGY

The mechanisms underlying alcoholic liver injury can be broadly categorized into those caused by the effects of alcohol directly on hepatocytes and those caused by the effects mediated by Kupffer cells. The hepatocyte mechanisms include the altered redox state induced by alcohol and aldehyde dehydrogenase reactions, the oxidative stress and lipid peroxidation caused by the induction of CYP2E1 enzymes and the mitochondrial electron transfer system, and the effects of alcohol on the nuclear transcription factors (AMP kinase and SREBP-1c), protein adduct formation, and altered methionine and folate metabolism with resulting endoplasmic reticulum stress. Chronic alcohol consumption increases gut permeability, and the resulting portal endotoxemia activates Kupffer cells. Activated Kupffer cells release a number of proinflammatory mediators, including tumor necrosis factor-α (TNF-α), transforming growth factor-β1 (TGF-β1), interleukins 1, 6, 8, and 10, and platelet-derived growth factor (PDGF). TNF-α has plethora of biologic effects and causes hepatocyte apoptosis, whereas TGF-β1 and PDGF play important roles in stellate cell activation, collagen production, and hepatic fibrosis.

Among the known risk factors for developing alcoholic liver disease (Table 155-2), the amount of alcohol consumed is the single most important. For

TABLE 155-1 COMMON CAUSES OF MACROVESICULAR AND MICROVESICULAR STEATOSIS

MACROVESICULAR STEATOSIS	MICROVESICULAR STEATOSIS
Obesity, type 2 diabetes, metabolic syndrome, and dyslipidemia (nonalcoholic fatty liver disease)	Reye's syndrome
Excessive alcohol consumption	Medications (valproate, antiretroviral medicines, intravenous tetracycline)
Hepatitis C (genotype 3)	Heat stroke
Wilson's disease	Acute fatty liver of pregnancy
Lipodystrophy	HELLP syndrome
Starvation	Inborn errors of metabolism (lecithin-cholesterol acyltransferase deficiency, cholesterol ester storage disease, Wolman's disease)
Jejunoileal bypass	
Parenteral nutrition	
Abetalipoproteinemia	
Medications (amiodarone, methotrexate, tamoxifen, corticosteroids, antipsychotics)	

HELLP = *h*emolysis, *e*levated *l*iver enzymes, and *l*ow *p*latelets.

TABLE 155-2 RISK FACTORS FOR ALCOHOLIC LIVER DISEASE AND NONALCOHOLIC FATTY LIVER DISEASE (NAFLD)

ALCOHOLIC LIVER DISEASE	NAFLD
MAJOR	**MAJOR**
Amount and duration of alcohol consumption	Obesity
Female gender	Type 2 diabetes
Genetic factors	Dyslipidemia
Protein-calorie malnutrition	Metabolic syndrome
MINOR	**MINOR**
Type of beverage	Polycystic ovary syndrome
Binge drinking	Hypothyroidism
Obesity	Sleep apnea
African-American and Hispanic ethnicity	Hypopituitarism

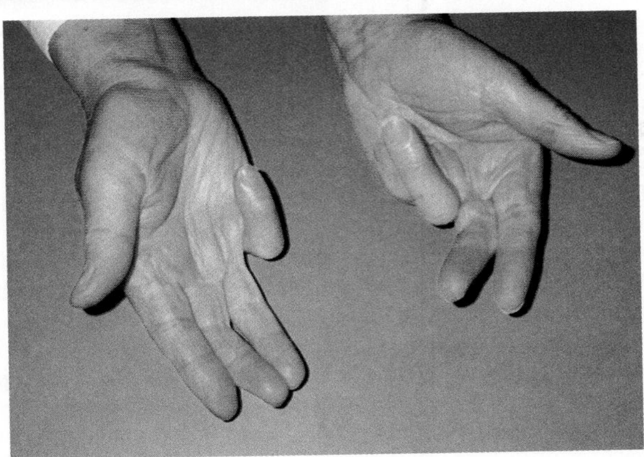

FIGURE 155-1. Dupuytren's contracture. (From Gudmundsson KG, Jonsson T, Arngrimsson R. Guillame Dupuytren and finger contractures. Lancet. 2003;362:165-168.)

unclear reasons, only 30 to 35% of individuals with heavy and long-term drinking develop alcoholic hepatitis, and less than 20% develop cirrhosis. Women are at higher risk; for example, the risk of alcoholic cirrhosis increases after 10 years of alcohol consumption at quantities of more than 60 to 80 g/day in men, whereas in women, it can develop at quantities of only more than 20 g/day. Moreover, the peak incidence of alcoholic liver disease in women is approximately a decade earlier than in men. The type of alcoholic beverage consumed may not be as critical, but "spirits" and beer may be more hepatotoxic than wine. African-American and Hispanic ethnic groups may be predisposed to more significant alcoholic liver injury. Both obesity and protein-calorie malnutrition, in which micronutrients and antioxidant capacity are diminished, also are important predispositions.

Polymorphisms in genes associated with alcohol metabolism (alcohol and aldehyde dehydrogenases and cytochrome P-450 enzymes) and dysregulated cytokine production (e.g., TNF-α) may also influence genetic susceptibility. In patients with other forms of chronic liver disease (e.g., viral hepatitis B or C), concomitant alcohol consumption significantly aggravates liver injury.

CLINICAL MANIFESTATIONS

Patients with alcoholic liver disease may have signs and symptoms from underlying alcoholism as well as those caused by liver disease. Stigmata of chronic alcoholism include palmar erythema (see Fig. 148-2 in Chapter 148), spider nevi, bilateral gynecomastia, testicular atrophy, bilateral parotid enlargement, and Dupuytren's contractures (Fig. 155-1). The clinical features of liver disease will depend on the stage of alcoholic liver disease, that is, whether a patient has alcoholic fatty liver or more advanced liver disease such as alcoholic hepatitis and cirrhosis.

Patients with alcoholic fatty liver disease are generally asymptomatic, but some patients may have anorexia, fatigue, right upper quadrant discomfort, and tender hepatomegaly. These patients may also have biochemical evidence of alcoholism and alcoholic liver disease with macrocytosis as well as elevated levels of aspartate aminotransferase (AST) and γ-glutamyl transpeptidase (GGT). Patients with alcoholic fatty liver typically do not have jaundice, ascites, or splenomegaly.

Patients with alcoholic hepatitis may have a more dramatic presentation with severe malaise, fatigue, anorexia, fever, evidence of protein-calorie malnutrition, and features of decompensated liver disease, including jaundice, coagulopathy, ascites, and encephalopathy. Physical examination invariably shows at least some features of chronic alcoholism, and jaundice (see Fig. 148-1 in Chapter 148), ascites (see Fig. 148-5 in Chapter 148), and splenomegaly are common. The laboratory examination is typically abnormal. Common hematologic abnormalities include leukocytosis with neutrophil predominance, macrocytic anemia (Chapter 167), thrombocytopenia (Chapter 175), and a prolonged prothrombin time. Liver biochemistries (Chapter 149) are abnormal with an elevated AST and ratio of AST to alanine transferase (ALT), alkaline phosphatase, GGT, and total bilirubin, but decreased levels of serum albumin. The AST rarely exceeds 300 IU/L. Serum electrolyte abnormalities including hypokalemia (Chapter 119), hypomagnesemia (Chapter 121), hypocalcemia (Chapter 253), and hypophosphatemia (Chapter 121) are frequent. Patients with alcoholic cirrhosis have the same clinical features that are common to other types of cirrhosis (Chapter 156), but also with striking features of underlying chronic alcoholism.

DIAGNOSIS

The diagnosis of alcoholic liver disease strongly depends on the history of excessive alcohol consumption and the presence of liver disease. Although laboratory abnormalities are not specific for alcoholic liver disease, they can be quite suggestive in the context of excessive alcohol consumption. An AST/ALT ratio of more than 2 is typical in alcoholic liver disease, and ALT values greater than 150 to 200 IU/L are very rare in alcoholic liver disease. Serology testing for co-existing chronic viral hepatitis (Chapter 151) is critical. Diagnostic dilemmas arise when a patient denies excessive alcohol consumption in the face of clinical features that are suggestive of alcoholic liver disease. Interviewing family members regarding specific alcohol consumption may be helpful in the accurate ascertainment of alcohol consumption. Elevated blood levels of carbohydrate-deficient transferrin, which is a form of transferrin with fewer than the four sialic acid chains present in normal transferrin, can identify recent heavy alcohol consumption. Hepatic imaging by ultrasound, computed tomography (CT), or magnetic resonance imaging (MRI) will show changes consistent with hepatic steatosis or more advanced forms of liver disease, such as alcoholic hepatitis and cirrhosis. Imaging is also important to exclude other forms of liver disease, including malignancy and biliary obstruction. Imaging findings specific for alcoholic liver disease include an enlarged caudate lobe, greater visualization of the right posterior hepatic notch, and focal fat sparing or geographic fat distribution.

Because specific treatment for alcoholic hepatitis may be harmful in patients with other liver diseases, it is very important to exclude other predominant or coexisting liver diseases, including chronic viral hepatitis (Chapter 151) and drug-induced liver injury, especially from acetaminophen (Chapter 152), by history, blood tests, and biopsy if needed. Hyperferritinemia generally reflects an acute phase reactant, rather than an iron overload disorder, so it usually will return to normal when the acute liver injury resolves.

Liver biopsy is the key to precisely characterizing the nature of alcoholic liver disease and determining whether a patient has fatty liver or more advanced alcoholic hepatitis. Histologic features of alcoholic fatty liver include macrovesicular steatosis that is predominantly zone 3 in nature. In alcoholic hepatitis, the biopsy is more striking and reveals macrovesicular steatosis, lobular neutrophilic infiltration, Mallory's hyaline, balloon degeneration of the hepatocytes, and perivenular fibrosis. In general, patients with alcoholic hepatitis also have histologic evidence of chronic liver injury in the form of more advanced fibrosis (periportal or bridging fibrosis, or cirrhosis).

TREATMENT Rx

Total abstinence, which is the most important treatment measure, is mandatory for the improvement of the clinical and histologic features of alcoholic liver disease. Its benefits are unequivocal, even in patients with severe decompensation. However, long-term abstinence is difficult to achieve, so a multidisciplinary approach with counseling and medications that promote abstinence should be considered. Disulfiram is not commonly used owing to its poor tolerability and hepatotoxicity. Opioid antagonists, such as naltrexone (50 mg/day for up to 6 months or even longer), nalmefene (20 mg/day as maintenance), and acamprosate (333 mg tablets, 2 tablets three times each day for 1 year) can help promote abstinence when used as part of a multidisciplinary approach (Chapter 32).

Alcoholic fatty liver disease requires no specific treatment other than abstinence. Patients with alcoholic hepatitis, however, have increased short- and long-term mortality and should be considered for therapeutic interventions in addition to mandatory abstinence. If a patient's liver biopsy is consistent with alcoholic hepatitis and there is no evidence of other inflammatory liver diseases, such as hepatitis C (Chapter 151), corticosteroids and pentoxifylline (400 mg three times daily for 28 days) are of some benefit. [1,2] Prednisolone (40 mg per day for 4 weeks) should be given to carefully selected patients who have a score of greater than 32 on Maddrey's discriminant function (4.6 × [patient's prothrombin time—control prothrombin time] + total bilirubin level) and encephalopathy, but do not have gastrointestinal bleeding or systemic infection. Recent studies suggested that a Model for End-Stage Liver Disease (MELD) score (see Table 156-2 in Chapter 156) higher than 21 can substitute for Maddrey's score for guiding the use of prednisolone. Two other anti-TNF-α agents, infliximab and etanercept, are not effective and have significant side effects. All patients with alcoholic hepatitis and alcoholic cirrhosis should be assessed and treated for protein-calorie malnutrition and micronutrient deficiency. Hospitalized patients with severe decompensation should be considered for enteral nutrition (Chapter 223).

Complications such as ascites, spontaneous bacterial peritonitis, encephalopathy, variceal bleeding, hepatorenal syndrome, osteoporosis, and hepatopulmonary syndrome may occur in patients with decompensated alcoholic cirrhosis and must be managed carefully (Chapter 156). Liver transplantation is a reasonable option in patients with decompensated alcoholic cirrhosis, but 6 months of abstinence and strong social support are generally required for eligibility (Chapter 157). Patients with alcoholic cirrhosis are at risk for hepatocellular carcinoma (Chapter 202) and should be screened with semiannual liver imaging and serum α-fetoprotein levels. They are also at risk for extrahepatic malignancy, notably head and neck, lung, and esophageal cancer. For Dupuytren's contracture, injection of collagenase clostridium histolyticum can reduce the severity and improve the range of motion significantly. 3

PROGNOSIS

Alcoholic fatty liver is generally reversible with total abstinence for a few months. Alcoholic hepatitis carries high mortality, with nearly 40% of patients dying within 6 months after its presentation.

NONALCOHOLIC FATTY LIVER DISEASE

DEFINITIONS

Histologically, NAFLD resembles alcoholic liver disease, but it occurs in individuals without significant alcohol consumption. Average alcohol consumption greater than two drinks per day in men and greater than one drink per day in women generally is not consistent with a diagnosis of NAFLD. In addition, the definition of NAFLD excludes patients with a history of exposure to steatogenic medications such as amiodarone, methotrexate, and tamoxifen.

NAFLD encompasses a spectrum of abnormal liver histology, ranging from simple steatosis to nonalcoholic steatohepatitis (NASH) and cirrhosis. In simple steatosis, liver histology reveals macrovesicular steatosis without ballooning degeneration of hepatocytes or liver fibrosis. NASH, which is a more advanced form of NAFLD, is histologically characterized by macrovesicular steatosis, ballooning degeneration of the hepatocytes, and sinusoidal fibrosis.

EPIDEMIOLOGY

NAFLD is one of the most common causes of elevated liver enzymes and chronic liver disease in the Western world. Its incidence in adults and children is rising rapidly owing to the ongoing epidemics of obesity (Chapter 227), type 2 diabetes mellitus (Chapter 237), and metabolic syndrome. Its prevalence is quite high in certain patient populations; for example, nearly 80% of type 2 diabetic patients and 90% of morbidly obese individuals have imaging evidence of NAFLD. Nearly one third of U.S. adults are estimated to have NAFLD, and up to 5% of U.S. adults may have NASH. These percentages compare reasonably well with other data suggesting that the prevalence of cirrhosis from NAFLD is about 2%. Hispanics and whites are at higher risk for NAFLD, whereas its prevalence is intriguingly quite low in African Americans.

PATHOBIOLOGY

The major risk factors for NAFLD include obesity, type 2 diabetes mellitus, metabolic syndrome, and dyslipidemia (see Table 155-2). Other comorbidities associated with NAFLD include polycystic ovary syndrome (Chapter 243), hypothyroidism (Chapter 233), hypopituitarism (Chapter 231), and sleep apnea (Chapter 100).

Two fundamental defects in NAFLD are insulin resistance/hyperinsulinemia and excessive levels of nonesterified fatty liver within the hepatocytes. An excessive influx of nonesterified fatty acids into the hepatocytes results in macrovesicular steatosis, which is predominantly centrilobular in location.

Additionally, patients with NAFLD have increased de novo intrahepatic lipogenesis. Although patients with NAFLD robustly esterify free fatty acids in neutral triglycerides, free fatty acids within the hepatocytes are considered the primary mediators of cell injury (lipotoxicity). In the background of hepatic steatosis, factors that promote cell injury, inflammation, and fibrosis include oxidative stress, endoplasmic reticulum stress, apoptosis, adipocytokines, and stellate cell activation. The sources of oxidative stress include mitochondria and microsomes. Adipocytokines that play an important role in the pathogenesis of NAFLD include adiponectin and TNF-α. It is unclear why some patients with NAFLD exhibit NASH, whereas other patients with a comparable risk factor profile have only simple steatosis. There is a consistent and significant relationship of *PNPLA3* genetic polymorphisms with the severity of steatosis and other histologic features of NAFLD. However, the genetic factors that play a role in NASH and NAFLD have not been fully elucidated.

CLINICAL MANIFESTATIONS

NAFLD is often asymptomatic but may rarely cause fatigue and right upper quadrant pain. Physical examination may reveal hepatomegaly, palmar erythema (see Fig. 148-2 in Chapter 148), and spider nevi. If liver disease is advanced, the features of liver failure, such as ascites, encephalopathy, and abdominal collateral vessels, are present. Simple steatosis is benign with a minimal risk of cirrhosis, whereas NASH is progressive and can lead to cirrhosis (Chapter 156) and liver failure (Chapter 157). In up to 20% of patients with NASH, liver histology will worsen and cirrhosis will develop over a 10- to 15-year period. Severe obesity, advancing age, and diabetes are believed to be risk factors for disease progression. Disease progression during the early phase can be identified only with a repeat liver biopsy, but in later stages, the signs and symptoms of portal hypertension (e.g., abdominal collateral vessels and low platelet count) indicate the development of cirrhosis. Patients with NASH-induced cirrhosis are at risk of developing hepatocellular carcinoma (Chapter 202). Patients with NAFLD have several metabolic risks that predispose them to atherosclerosis, and coronary artery disease is the single most common cause of death in patients with NAFLD.

DIAGNOSIS

NAFLD is generally suspected when aminotransferase levels are asymptomatically elevated in an individual with metabolic risk factors (obesity and diabetes) or when liver imaging (ultrasound, CT, or MRI) obtained for another reason shows fatty infiltration (Fig. 155-2). The diagnosis of NAFLD requires that there is no history of previous or ongoing significant alcohol consumption, no exposure to steatogenic medications, and no evidence of other causes of liver disease, such as viral hepatitis B or C. Elevated levels of aminotransferases, although common, are not required for the diagnosis of NAFLD. In contrast to alcoholic liver disease, ALT levels are higher than AST levels, but they rarely exceed 250 IU/L. In general, AST and ALT levels do not have diagnostic or prognostic significance. Mild hyperferritinemia is common and should not be confused with hereditary hemochromatosis (Chapter 219). Similarly, low-grade autoantibody (antinuclear antibody, anti–smooth muscle antibody) positivity is not uncommon and should not be confused with autoimmune liver disease (Chapter 151). Because steatosis is common in patients with Wilson's disease (Chapter 218), serum ceruloplasmin should be obtained as part of the diagnostic evaluation.

Fatty liver on ultrasonogram has a positive predictive value of only 77% and a negative predictive value of only 67% when compared with liver biopsy. Abdominal MRI is more accurate, but its high cost limits its usefulness in routine practice. Because none of these three tests can differentiate simple steatosis from NASH nor identify cirrhosis until hepatic fibrosis has caused overt portal hypertension, liver biopsy is required to establish the presence of NASH or cirrhosis. Common indications for a percutaneous liver biopsy

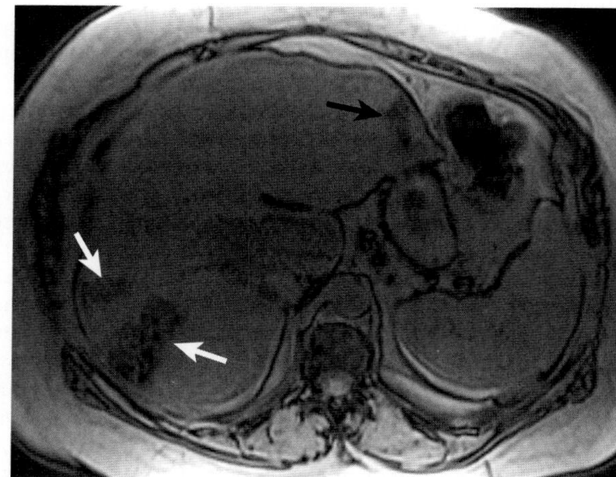

FIGURE 155-2. Magnetic resonance image of chronic liver disease due to nonalcoholic fatty liver disease. Out-of-phase T1-weighted images show focal fat infiltration of varying shapes in right lobe *(white arrows)* and left lobe *(black arrow)*. (Courtesy of Professor Kumar Sandrasegaran, Indiana University School of Medicine, Indianapolis, Ind.)

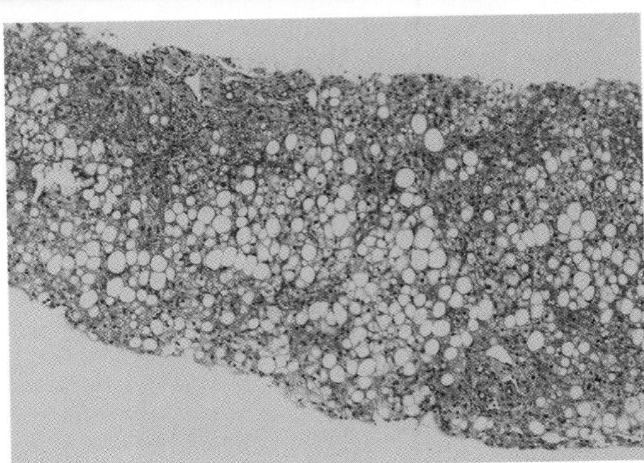

FIGURE 155-3. Liver biopsy showing nonalcoholic steatohepatitis, with increased fat and with early cirrhosis. (Courtesy of the NASH Clinical Research Network.)

in patients with NAFLD include persistently high aminotransferase levels, inability to exclude a competing or a coexisting cause (e.g., iron overload or autoimmune liver disease), or clinical suspicion of severe liver disease. In patients with NASH, liver histology shows steatosis, inflammation, ballooning, and fibrosis (Fig. 155-3).

TREATMENT

Rx

Lifestyle modification with dietary restriction and regular exercise is the first choice of treatment for NAFLD. It is generally recommended that patients with NAFLD lose 10% of their body weight in a gradual fashion, but this goal is difficult to achieve. If resources are available, a multidisciplinary approach with behavioral therapy, dietary advice, and monitoring by a professional nutritionist and an exercise expert is more successful than a prescriptive approach.[4]

Statins (e.g., atorvastatin 20 mg daily) with or without vitamins C and E can improve liver test results and reduce subsequent NAFLD.[5,6] In a large trial, 800 IU of vitamin E administered daily for 2 years significantly improved liver histology.[7] Thiazolidinedione insulin sensitizers (pioglitazone and rosiglitazone) improve steatosis, inflammation, and ballooning, but may not improve fibrosis.[8] Unfortunately, the weight gain that is common with thiazolidinediones may offset the histologic benefits that they offer. In morbidly obese individuals with NASH and other significant metabolic comorbidities, foregut bariatric surgery can lead to significant improvement in hepatic histology, but the physician must exclude the presence of portal hypertension before offering this type of surgery.[9] Patients with NAFLD often have dyslipidemia that puts them at excessive risk for coronary artery disease; their dyslipidemia (Chapter 213) should be treated aggressively with statins and other lipid-lowering agents, which can be safely administered to patients with NAFLD and NASH. Carefully selected patients with decompensated cirrhosis owing to NASH can be treated with liver transplantation (Chapter 157), but recurrence during the post-transplantation period is common.

PREVENTION

The measures to prevent NAFLD include maintaining optimal body weight, exercising regularly, and treating any associated metabolic comorbidities such as diabetes and dyslipidemia. Avoidance of saturated fat, high fructose intake, and alcohol consumption may reduce the development of NAFLD.

PROGNOSIS

Steatosis alone is generally benign, whereas steatohepatitis is often progressive. Otherwise, however, data are sparse regarding the risk and risk factors for the progression of NAFLD and NASH to cirrhosis and liver failure.

Because NAFLD often coexists with one or more components of the metabolic syndrome, its presence reflects guarded long-term overall prognosis. The long-term complications in patients with simple steatosis generally result from cardiovascular disease and atherosclerosis, not from liver failure.

Patients with NASH also are at risk for liver failure and liver cancer, in addition to their significantly increased risk of cardiovascular disease. For example, among patients with NASH on their initial biopsy, one third or more develop progressive fibrosis over a mean follow-up interval of about 5 years. Older age, diabetes, and ballooning and fibrosis on liver biopsy are important predictors of progression.

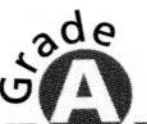

Grade A

1. Whitfield K, Rambaldi A, Wetterslev J, et al. Pentoxifylline for alcoholic hepatitis. *Cochrane Database Syst Rev.* 2009;4:CD007339.
2. De BK, Gangopadhyay S, Dutta D, et al. Pentoxifylline versus prednisolone for severe alcoholic hepatitis: a randomized controlled trial. *World J Gastroenterol.* 2009;15:1613-1619.
3. Hurst LC, Badalamente MA, Hentz VR, et al. Injectable collagenase clostridium histolyticum for Dupuytren's contracture. *N Engl J Med.* 2009;361:968-979.
4. Promrat K, Kleiner DE, Niemeier HM, et al. Randomized controlled trial testing the effects of weight loss on nonalcoholic steatohepatitis (NASH). *Hepatology.* 2010;51:121-129.
5. Athyros VG, Tziomalos K, Gossios TD, et al. Safety and efficacy of long-term statin treatment for cardiovascular events in patients with coronary heart disease and abnormal liver tests in the Greek Atorvastatin and Coronary Heart Disease Evaluation (GREACE) study: a post-hoc analysis. *Lancet.* 2010;376:1916-1922.
6. Foster T, Budoff MJ, Saab S, et al. Atorvastatin and antioxidants for the treatment of nonalcoholic fatty liver disease: the St. Francis Heart Study randomized clinical trial. *Am J Gastroenterol.* 2011;106:71-77.
7. Sanyal AJ, Chalasani N, Kowdley KV, et al. Pioglitazone, vitamin E, or placebo for nonalcoholic steatohepatitis. *N Engl J Med.* 2010;362:1675-1685.
8. Musso G, Gambino R, Cassader M, et al. A meta-analysis of randomized trials for the treatment of nonalcoholic fatty liver disease. *Hepatology.* 2010;52:79-104.
9. Mummadi RR, Kasturi KS, Chennareddygari S, et al. Effect of bariatric surgery on nonalcoholic fatty liver disease: systematic review and meta-analysis. *Clin Gastroenterol Hepatol.* 2008;6:1396-1402.

SUGGESTED READINGS

Beier JI, Arteel GE, McClain CJ. Advances in alcoholic liver disease. *Curr Gastroenterol Rep.* 2011;13:56-64. *Review.*

Dowman JK, Tomlinson JW, Newsome PN. Systematic review: the diagnosis and staging of non-alcoholic fatty liver disease and non-alcoholic steatohepatitis. *Aliment Pharmacol Ther.* 2011;33:525-540. *Review.*

Lucey MR, Mathurin P, Morgan TR. Alcoholic hepatitis. *N Engl J Med.* 2009;360:2758-2769. *A state-of-the-art review of pathogenesis, clinical features, and treatment of the alcoholic hepatitis.*

O'Shea RS, Dasarathy S, McCullough AJ, for the Practice Guideline Committee of the American Association for the Study of Liver Diseases and the Practice Parameters Committee of the American College of Gastroenterology. Alcoholic liver disease. *Hepatology.* 2010;51:307-328. *Comprehensive guidelines for the practicing physician.*

156

CIRRHOSIS AND ITS SEQUELAE

GUADALUPE GARCIA-TSAO

DEFINITION

Cirrhosis, which can be the final stage of any chronic liver disease, is a diffuse process characterized by fibrosis and conversion of normal architecture to structurally abnormal nodules (Fig. 156-1). These "regenerative" nodules lack normal lobular organization and are surrounded by fibrous tissue. The process involves the whole liver and is essentially irreversible. Although cirrhosis is histologically an "all or nothing" diagnosis, clinically it can be classified by its status as compensated or decompensated. Decompensated cirrhosis is defined by the presence of ascites, variceal bleeding, encephalopathy, or jaundice, which are complications that result from the main consequences of cirrhosis: portal hypertension and liver insufficiency.

EPIDEMIOLOGY

Because many patients with cirrhosis are asymptomatic until decompensation occurs, it is very difficult to assess the real prevalence and incidence of cirrhosis in the general population. The prevalence of chronic liver disease or cirrhosis worldwide is estimated to be 100 (range, 25 to 400) per 100,000 subjects, but it varies widely by country and by region.

Cirrhosis is an important cause of morbidity and mortality worldwide and in the United States. According to the World Health Organization, about 800,000 people die of cirrhosis annually. In the United States, cirrhosis accounts for about 27,500 deaths each year, or a death rate of 9.3 per 100,000, making it the 12th leading cause of death overall. Importantly, chronic liver disease and cirrhosis are the seventh leading cause of death in the United States in individuals between 25 and 64 years of age. Because chronic liver disease affects people in their most productive years of life, it has a significant impact on the economy as a result of premature death, illness, and disability.

Any chronic liver disease can lead to cirrhosis (Table 156-1). Chronic viral hepatitis C and alcoholic liver disease are the most common causes of

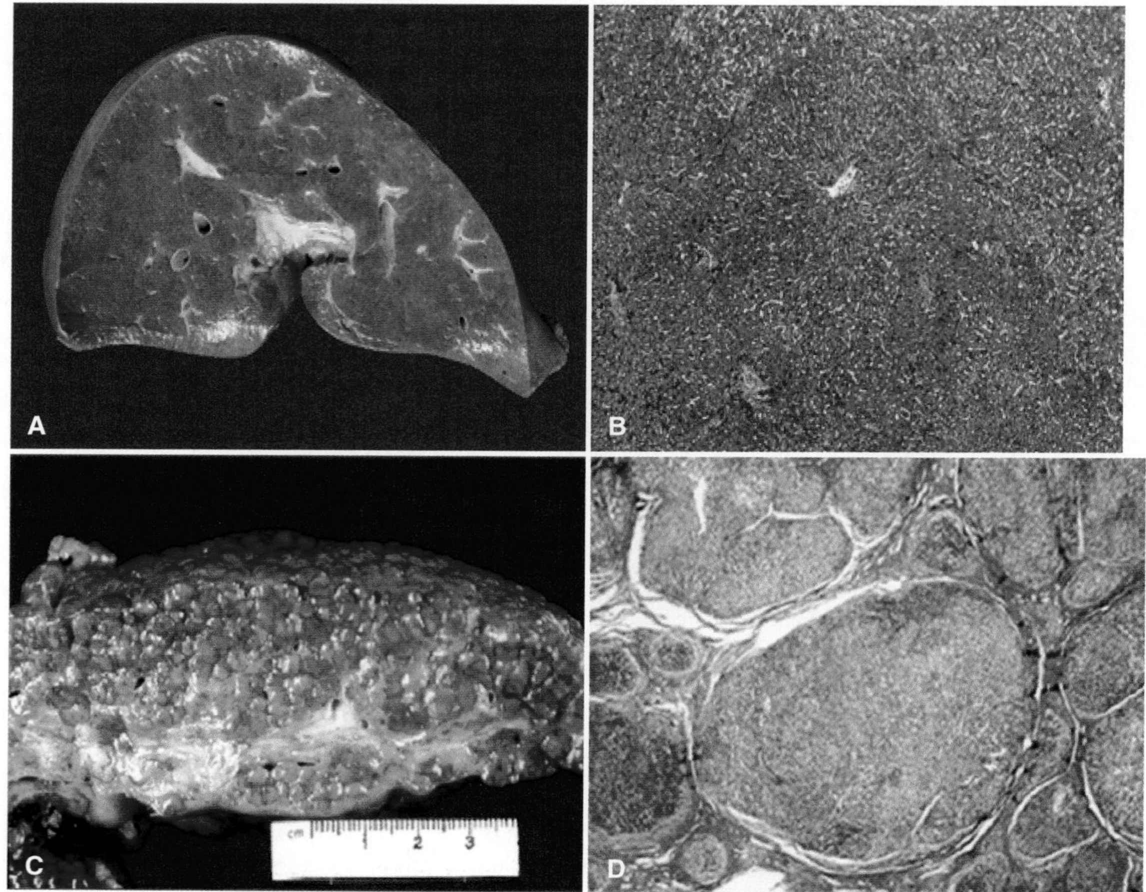

FIGURE 156-1. Gross and microscopic images of a normal and cirrhotic liver. A, Gross image of a normal liver with a smooth surface and homogeneous texture. **B,** Microscopically, liver sinusoids are organized, and vascular structures are normally distributed. **C,** Gross image of a cirrhotic liver. The liver has an orange-tawny color with an irregular surface and a nodular texture. **D,** Microscopically, the architecture is disorganized, and there are regenerative nodules surrounded by fibrous tissue.

TABLE 156-1 CAUSES OF CIRRHOSIS

MAIN FACTORS CAUSING CIRRHOSIS
Chronic hepatitis C
Alcoholic liver disease
Nonalcoholic fatty liver disease
Chronic hepatitis B
OTHER CAUSES OF CIRRHOSIS (<2% OF ALL CASES)
Cholestatic and autoimmune liver diseases
Primary biliary cirrhosis
Primary sclerosing cholangitis
Autoimmune hepatitis
Intrahepatic or extrahepatic biliary obstruction
Mechanical obstruction
Biliary atresia
Cystic fibrosis
Metabolic disorders
Hemochromatosis
Wilson's disease
α_1-Antitrypsin deficiency
Glycogen storage diseases
Abetalipoproteinemia
Porphyria
Hepatic venous outflow obstruction
Budd-Chiari syndrome
Veno-occlusive disease
Right-sided heart failure
Drugs and toxins
Intestinal bypass
Indian childhood cirrhosis

cirrhosis, followed by nonalcoholic fatty liver disease and chronic hepatitis B (Chapters 151 and 155). However, the many other causes of cirrhosis include cholestatic and autoimmune liver diseases such as primary biliary cirrhosis, primary sclerosing cholangitis (Chapter 158), autoimmune hepatitis (Chapter 151), and metabolic diseases such as hemochromatosis, Wilson's disease, and α_1-antitrypsin deficiency (Chapter 153). When all the causes have been investigated and excluded, cirrhosis is considered "cryptogenic." Many cases of cryptogenic cirrhosis are now thought to be due to nonalcoholic fatty liver disease (Chapter 155).

It is important to mention that although the entity termed *primary biliary cirrhosis* assumes the presence of cirrhosis, this term is actually misleading. Primary biliary cirrhosis (Chapter 158) is an immune-mediated cholestatic chronic liver disease that is characterized by progressive destruction of intrahepatic bile ducts and progresses over time from an initial stage in which fibrosis is minimal (stage 1) to a final stage in which there is well-established cirrhosis (stage 4).

PATHOBIOLOGY

Liver Fibrosis/Cirrhosis

The key pathogenic feature underlying liver fibrosis and cirrhosis is activation of hepatic stellate cells. Hepatic stellate cells, which are known as *Ito cells* or *perisinusoidal cells,* are located in the space of Disse between hepatocytes and sinusoidal endothelial cells. Normally, hepatic stellate cells are quiescent and serve as the main storage site for retinoids (vitamin A). In response to injury, hepatic stellate cells become activated, as a result of which they lose their vitamin A deposits, proliferate, develop a prominent rough endoplasmic reticulum, and secrete extracellular matrix (collagen types I and III, sulfated proteoglycans, and glycoproteins). Additionally, they become contractile hepatic myofibroblasts.

Unlike other capillaries, normal hepatic sinusoids lack a basement membrane. The sinusoidal endothelial cells themselves contain large fenestrae (100 to 200 nm in diameter) that allow the passage of large molecules with molecular weights up to 250,000. Collagen deposition in the space of Disse,

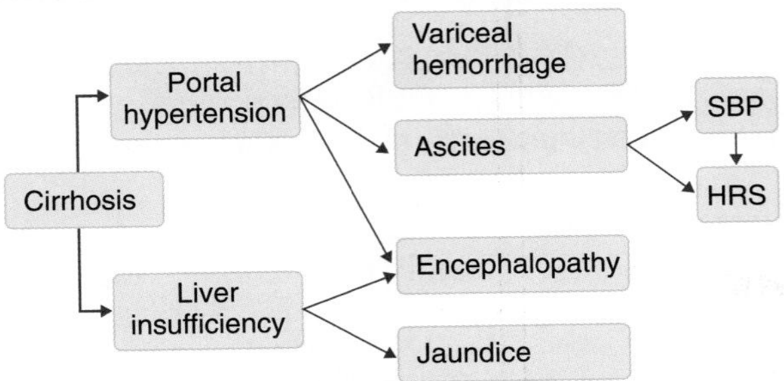

FIGURE 156-2. Complications of cirrhosis result from portal hypertension or liver insufficiency. Varices and variceal hemorrhage are a direct consequence of portal hypertension. Ascites results from sinusoidal portal hypertension and can be complicated by infection (spontaneous bacterial peritonitis [SBP]) or renal dysfunction (hepatorenal syndrome [HRS]). Hepatic encephalopathy results from portosystemic shunting (i.e., portal hypertension) and liver insufficiency. Jaundice results solely from liver insufficiency.

as occurs in cirrhosis, leads to defenestration of the sinusoidal endothelial cells ("capillarization" of the sinusoids), thereby altering exchange between plasma and hepatocytes and resulting in a decreased sinusoidal diameter that is further exacerbated by the contraction of stellate cells.

Complications of Cirrhosis

The two main consequences of cirrhosis are portal hypertension, with the accompanying hyperdynamic circulatory state, and liver insufficiency (Fig. 156-2). The development of varices and ascites is a direct consequence of portal hypertension and the hyperdynamic circulatory state, whereas jaundice occurs as a result of an inability of the liver to excrete bilirubin (i.e., liver insufficiency). Encephalopathy is the result of both portal hypertension and liver insufficiency. Ascites, in turn, can become complicated by infection, which is called *spontaneous bacterial peritonitis,* and by functional renal failure, which is called *hepatorenal syndrome.*

Portal Hypertension and the Hyperdynamic Circulatory State

In cirrhosis, portal hypertension results from both an increase in resistance to portal flow and an increase in portal venous inflow. The initial mechanism is increased sinusoidal vascular resistance secondary to (1) deposition of fibrous tissue and subsequent compression by regenerative nodules (fixed component) and (2) active vasoconstriction (functional component), which is amenable to the action of vasodilators such as nitroprusside and is caused by a deficiency in intrahepatic nitric oxide (NO), as well as enhanced activity of vasoconstrictors.

Early in the portal hypertensive process, the spleen grows and sequesters platelets and other formed blood cells, thereby leading to hypersplenism. In addition, vessels that normally drain into the portal system, such as the coronary vein, reverse their flow and shunt blood away from the portal system to the systemic circulation. These portosystemic collaterals are insufficient to decompress the portal venous system and offer additional resistance to portal flow. As collaterals develop, an increase in portal blood inflow maintains the portal hypertensive state as a result of splanchnic vasodilation, which in turn is secondary to increased production of NO. Thus, the paradox in portal hypertension is that a deficiency of NO in the intrahepatic vasculature leads to vasoconstriction and increased resistance, whereas overproduction of NO in the extrahepatic circulation leads to vasodilation and increased flow.

In addition to splanchnic vasodilation, there is systemic vasodilation, which by causing a decreased *effective* arterial blood volume, leads to activation of neurohumoral systems (renin-angiotensin-aldosterone system), retention of sodium, expansion of plasma volume, and development of a hyperdynamic circulatory state. This hyperdynamic circulatory state maintains portal hypertension, thereby leading to the formation and growth of varices, and plays an important role in the development of all other complications of cirrhosis.

Varices and Variceal Hemorrhage

The complication of cirrhosis that results most directly from portal hypertension is the development of portal-systemic collaterals, the most relevant of which are those that form through dilation of the coronary and gastric veins and constitute gastroesophageal varices. The initial formation of esophageal collaterals depends on a threshold portal pressure, clinically established by a hepatic venous pressure gradient of 10 to 12 mm Hg, below which varices do not develop.

Development of a hyperdynamic circulatory state leads to further dilation and growth of varices and eventually to their rupture and variceal hemorrhage, one of the most dreaded complications of portal hypertension. Tension in a varix determines variceal rupture and is directly proportional to variceal diameter and intravariceal pressure and inversely proportional to variceal wall thickness.

Ascites and Hepatorenal Syndrome

Ascites in cirrhosis is secondary to sinusoidal hypertension and retention of sodium. Cirrhosis leads to sinusoidal hypertension by blocking hepatic venous outflow both anatomically by fibrosis and regenerative nodules and functionally by increased postsinusoidal vascular tone. Similar to the formation of esophageal varices, a threshold hepatic venous pressure gradient of 12 mm Hg is needed for the formation of ascites. In addition, retention of sodium replenishes the intravascular volume and allows the continuous formation of ascites. Retention of sodium results from vasodilation that is mostly due to an increase in NO production because NO inhibition in experimental animals increases urinary sodium excretion, lowers plasma aldosterone levels, and reduces ascites. With progression of cirrhosis and portal hypertension, vasodilation is more pronounced, thereby leading to further activation of the renin-angiotensin-aldosterone and sympathetic nervous systems and resulting in further sodium retention (refractory ascites), water retention (hyponatremia), and renal vasoconstriction (hepatorenal syndrome).

Spontaneous Bacterial Peritonitis

Spontaneous bacterial peritonitis, an infection of ascitic fluid, occurs in the absence of perforation of a hollow viscus or an intra-abdominal inflammatory focus such as an abscess, acute pancreatitis, or cholecystitis. Bacterial translocation, or the migration of bacteria from the intestinal lumen to mesenteric lymph nodes and other extraintestinal sites, is the main mechanism implicated in spontaneous bacterial peritonitis. Impaired local and systemic immune defenses are a major element in promoting bacterial translocation and, together with shunting of blood away from the hepatic Kupffer cells through portosystemic collaterals, allow a transient bacteremia to become more prolonged, thereby colonizing ascitic fluid. Spontaneous bacterial peritonitis occurs in patients with reduced ascites defense mechanisms, such as a low complement level in ascitic fluid. Another factor that promotes bacterial translocation in cirrhosis is bacterial overgrowth attributed to a decrease in small bowel motility and intestinal transit time. Infections, particularly from gram-negative bacteria, can precipitate renal dysfunction through worsening of the hyperdynamic circulatory state.

Encephalopathy

Ammonia, a toxin normally removed by the liver, plays a key role in the pathogenesis of hepatic encephalopathy. In cirrhosis, ammonia accumulates in the systemic circulation because of shunting of blood through portosystemic collaterals and decreased liver metabolism (i.e., liver insufficiency). The presence of large amounts of ammonia in the brain damages supporting brain cells or astrocytes and leads to structural changes characteristic of hepatic encephalopathy (Alzheimer's type II astrocytosis). Ammonia results in upregulation of astrocytic peripheral-type benzodiazepine receptors, the most potent stimulants of neurosteroid production. Neurosteroids are the major modulators of γ-aminobutyric acid, which results in cortical depression and hepatic encephalopathy. Other toxins, such as manganese, also accumulate in the brain, particularly the globus pallidus, where they lead to impaired motor function. Other yet-to-be-elucidated toxins may also be involved in the pathogenesis of encephalopathy.

Jaundice

Jaundice (Chapter 149) in cirrhosis is a reflection of the inability of the liver to excrete bilirubin and is therefore the result of liver insufficiency. However, in cholestatic diseases leading to cirrhosis (e.g., primary biliary cirrhosis, primary sclerosing cholangitis, vanishing bile duct syndrome), jaundice is more likely due to biliary damage than liver insufficiency. Other indicators of liver insufficiency, such as the prothrombin time or the presence of encephalopathy, help determine the most likely contributor to hyperbilirubinemia (Chapter 149).

Cardiopulmonary Complications

The hyperdynamic circulatory state eventually results in high-output heart failure with decreased peripheral utilization of oxygen, a complication that

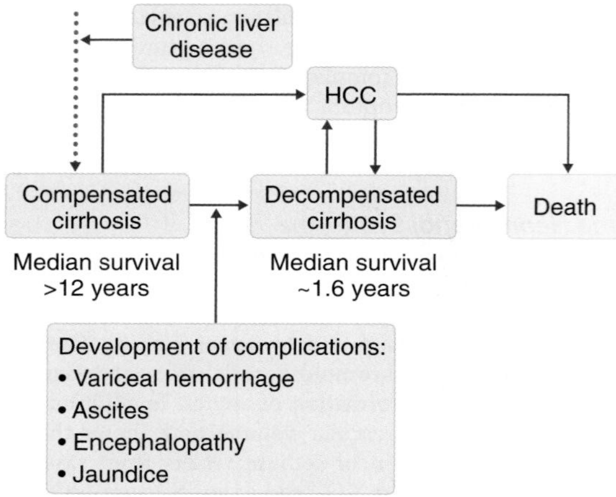

FIGURE 156-3. **Natural history of cirrhosis.** Any chronic liver disease will lead to cirrhosis. Initially, cirrhosis will be compensated (median survival, >12 years), but once complications (ascites, variceal hemorrhage, encephalopathy, jaundice) develop, it becomes decompensated (median survival, 1.6 years). Hepatocellular carcinoma (HCC) can develop at any stage and precipitate decompensation and death.

TABLE 156-2 THE TWO MOST COMMONLY USED SCORING SYSTEMS IN CIRRHOSIS

1. CHILD-TURCOTTE-PUGH (CTP) SCORE (RANGE, 5-15)

	Points Ascribed		
PARAMETERS	**1**	**2**	**3**
Ascites	None	Grade 1-2 (or easy to treat)	Grade 3-4 (or refractory)
Hepatic encephalopathy	None	Grade 1-2 (or induced by a precipitant)	Grade 3-4 (or spontaneous)
Bilirubin (mg/dL)	<2	2-3	>3
Albumin (g/dL)	>3.5	2.8-3.5	<2.8
Prothrombin time (seconds > control) or INR	<4 <1.7	4-6 1.7-2.3	>6 >2.3

CTP classification: Child A: score of 5-6; Child B: score of 7-9; Child C: score of 10-15

2. MODEL OF END-STAGE LIVER DISEASE (MELD) SCORE (RANGE, 6-40)

[0.957 × LN (creatinine in mg/dL) + 0.378 × LN (bilirubin in mg/dL) + 1.12 × LN (INR) + 0.643] × 10

INR = international normalized ratio; LN = natural logarithm.

has been referred to as *cirrhotic cardiomyopathy.* Vasodilation at the level of the pulmonary circulation leads to arterial hypoxemia, the hallmark of hepatopulmonary syndrome. Normal pulmonary capillaries are 8 μm in diameter, and red blood cells (slightly less than 8 μm) pass through them one cell at a time, thereby facilitating oxygenation. In hepatopulmonary syndrome, the pulmonary capillaries are dilated up to 500 μm, so passage of red cells through the pulmonary capillaries may be many cells thick. As a result, a large number of red cells are not oxygenated, which causes the equivalent of a right-to-left shunt.

Conversely, portopulmonary hypertension occurs when the pulmonary bed is exposed to vasoconstrictive substances that may be produced in the splanchnic circulation and bypass metabolism by the liver; the initial result is reversible pulmonary hypertension. However, because these factors result in endothelial proliferation, vasoconstriction, in situ thrombosis, and obliteration of vessels, irreversible pulmonary hypertension ensues.

CLINICAL MANIFESTATIONS

The clinical manifestations of cirrhosis range widely, depending on the stage of cirrhosis, from an asymptomatic patient with no signs of chronic liver disease to a patient who is confused and jaundiced and has severe muscle wasting and ascites. The natural history of cirrhosis is characterized by an initial phase, termed *compensated* cirrhosis, followed by a rapidly progressive phase marked by the development of complications of portal hypertension or liver dysfunction (or both), termed *decompensated* cirrhosis (Fig. 156-3). In the compensated phase, portal pressure may be normal or below the threshold level identified for the development of varices or ascites. As the disease progresses, portal pressure increases and liver function decreases, thereby resulting in the development of ascites, portal hypertensive gastrointestinal (GI) bleeding, encephalopathy, and jaundice. The development of any of these complications marks the transition from a compensated to a decompensated phase. Progression to death may be accelerated by the development of other complications such as recurrent GI bleeding, renal impairment (refractory ascites, hepatorenal syndrome), hepatopulmonary syndrome, and sepsis (spontaneous bacterial peritonitis). The development of hepatocellular carcinoma (Chapter 202) may accelerate the course of the disease at any stage (see Fig. 156-3). Transition from a compensated to a decompensated stage occurs at a rate of approximately 5 to 7% per year. The median time to decompensation, or the time at which half the patients with compensated cirrhosis will become decompensated, is about 6 years.

Compensated Cirrhosis

In this stage, cirrhosis is mostly asymptomatic and is diagnosed either during the evaluation of chronic liver disease or fortuitously during routine physical examination, biochemical testing, imaging for other reasons, endoscopy showing gastroesophageal varices, or abdominal surgery in which a nodular liver is detected. Nonspecific fatigue, decreased libido, or sleep disturbances may be the only complaints. About 40% of patients with compensated cirrhosis have esophageal varices. Nonbleeding gastroesophageal varices are asymptomatic, and their presence (without bleeding) does not denote decompensation.

Decompensated Cirrhosis

At this stage, there are signs of decompensation: ascites, variceal hemorrhage, jaundice, hepatic encephalopathy, or any combination of these findings. Ascites, which is the most frequent sign of decompensation, is present in 80% of patients with decompensated cirrhosis.

Variceal Hemorrhage

Gastroesophageal varices are present in approximately 50% of patients with newly diagnosed cirrhosis. The prevalence of varices correlates with the severity of liver disease and ranges from 40% in Child A cirrhotic patients (Table 156-2) to 85% in Child C cirrhotic patients.

Both the development of varices and the growth of small varices occur at a rate of 7 to 8% per year. The incidence of a first variceal hemorrhage in patients with small varices is about 5% per year, whereas medium and large varices bleed at a rate of approximately 15% per year. Large varices, severe liver disease, and red wale markings on varices are independent predictors of variceal hemorrhage. Bleeding from gastroesophageal varices can be manifested as overt hematemesis or melena, or both (Chapter 137).

Ascites and Hepatorenal Syndrome

Ascites is the most common cause of decompensation in cirrhosis and occurs at a rate of 7 to 10% per year. The most frequent symptoms associated with ascites are increased abdominal girth, which is often described by the patient as tightness of the belt or garments around the waist, and recent weight gain. When present in small to moderate amounts, ascites can be identified on examination by bulging flanks, flank dullness, and shifting dullness (Chapter 148).

Hepatorenal syndrome is a type of prerenal kidney injury that occurs in patients with cirrhosis and ascites. It is divided into two types based on clinical characteristics and prognosis. Type 1 hepatorenal syndrome is rapidly progressive *acute* kidney injury in which the rise in serum creatinine occurs within a 2-week period. Type 2 hepatorenal syndrome is more slowly progressive and associated with ascites that is refractory to diuretics. Patients with hepatorenal syndrome usually have tense ascites that responds poorly to diuretics, but no specific symptoms or signs typify this entity.

Spontaneous Bacterial Peritonitis

About one third of cirrhotic patients are admitted for or acquire bacterial infections during hospitalization, the most common being spontaneous bacterial peritonitis. The two most important predictors of the development of bacterial infection are the severity of liver disease and admission for GI hemorrhage. The most frequent clinical manifestations of spontaneous bacterial peritonitis are fever, jaundice, and abdominal pain. On physical examination, there is typically abdominal tenderness, with or without rebound tenderness, or ileus (or both). However, patients with spontaneous bacterial peritonitis may have just encephalopathy, acute kidney injury or evidence of shock. Up to one third of patients may be entirely asymptomatic.

Hepatic Encephalopathy

Hepatic encephalopathy, which is the neuropsychiatric manifestation of cirrhosis, occurs at a rate of approximately 2 to 3% per year. Hepatic encephalopathy associated with cirrhosis is of gradual onset and rarely fatal. Clinically, it is characterized by alterations in consciousness and behavior ranging from inversion of the sleep-wake pattern and forgetfulness (stage 1); to confusion, bizarre behavior, and disorientation (stage 2); to lethargy and profound disorientation (stage 3); to coma (stage 4). On physical examination, early stages may demonstrate only a distal tremor, but the hallmark of hepatic encephalopathy is the presence of asterixis (Chapter 157). Additionally, patients with hepatic encephalopathy may have sweet-smelling breath, a characteristic termed *fetor hepaticus.*

Pulmonary Complications

Hepatopulmonary syndrome is associated with exertional dyspnea, which can lead to extreme debilitation. Clubbing of the fingers, cyanosis, and vascular spiders may be seen on physical examination. Hepatopulmonary syndrome is present in approximately 5 to 10% of patients awaiting liver transplantation.

Portopulmonary hypertension is manifested as exertional dyspnea, syncope, and chest pain. On examination, an accentuated second sound and right ventricular heave are prominent (Chapter 68).

DIAGNOSIS

The diagnosis of cirrhosis should be considered in any patient with chronic liver disease. In asymptomatic patients with *compensated cirrhosis,* typical signs of cirrhosis may not be present, and the diagnosis may often require histologic confirmation by liver biopsy, which is the "gold standard" for the diagnosis of cirrhosis. In patients with symptoms or signs of chronic liver disease, however, the presence of cirrhosis can frequently be confirmed noninvasively by imaging studies without the need for liver biopsy.

Physical Examination

On physical examination, stigmata of cirrhosis consist of muscle atrophy, mainly involving the bitemporal muscle regions and the thenar and hypothenar eminences; spider angiomas, mostly on the trunk, face, and upper limbs; and palmar erythema involving the thenar and the hypothenar eminences and the tips of the fingers. Although muscular atrophy is a marker of liver insufficiency, spider angiomas and palmar erythema are markers of vasodilation and a hyperdynamic circulation. Males may have hair loss on the chest and abdomen, gynecomastia, and testicular atrophy. Petechiae and ecchymoses may be present as a result of thrombocytopenia or a prolonged prothrombin time. Dupuytren's contracture, which is a thickening of the palmar fascia, occurs mostly in alcoholic cirrhosis. A pathognomonic feature of cirrhosis is the finding on abdominal examination of a small right liver lobe, with a span of less than 7 cm on percussion, and a palpable left lobe that is nodular with increased consistency. Splenomegaly may also be present and is indicative of portal hypertension. Collateral circulation on the abdominal wall (caput medusae) may also develop as a consequence of portal hypertension. Absence of any of the aforementioned physical findings does not exclude cirrhosis.

Laboratory Tests

Laboratory test results suggestive of cirrhosis include even subtle abnormalities in serum levels of albumin or bilirubin or elevation of the international normalized ratio. The most sensitive and specific laboratory finding suggestive of cirrhosis in the setting of chronic liver disease is a low platelet count ($<150,000/mm^3$), which occurs as a result of portal hypertension and hypersplenism. Other serum markers that are often abnormal include levels of aspartate aminotransferase, γ-glutamyl transpeptidase, hyaluronic acid, α_2-macroglobulin, haptoglobin, tissue metalloproteinase inhibitor I, and apolipoprotein A. Although attempts have been made to use combinations of such markers to predict the presence of cirrhosis, none has sufficient sensitivity and specificity to be useful clinically.

Imaging Studies

Confirmatory imaging tests include computed tomography, ultrasound, and magnetic resonance imaging. Findings consistent with cirrhosis include a nodular contour of the liver, a small liver with or without hypertrophy of the left or caudate lobe, splenomegaly, and in particular, identification of intra-abdominal collateral vessels indicative of portal hypertension (Fig. 156-4). Transient elastography, a new noninvasive technique based on ultrasound wave propagation, measures liver stiffness and appears to be useful in the diagnosis of cirrhosis. Typical findings on any of these imaging studies, together with a compatible clinical picture, are indicative of the presence of cirrhosis. A liver biopsy then would not be required unless the degree of inflammation or other features require investigation.

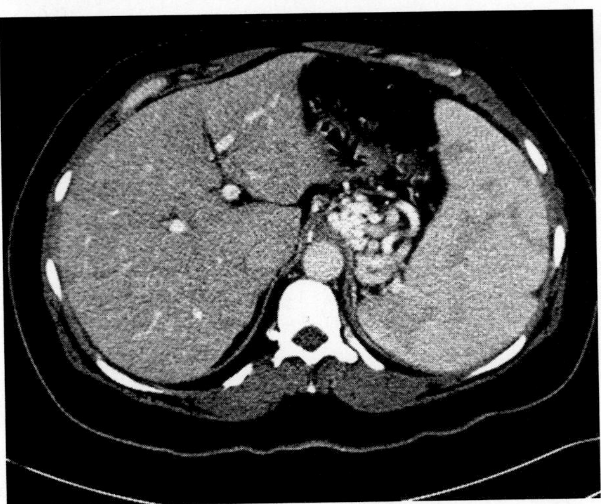

FIGURE 156-4. Computed tomography in a patient with compensated cirrhosis. The liver parenchyma is heterogeneous, there is splenomegaly, and, importantly, there are portosystemic collaterals.

In *decompensated cirrhosis,* detection of ascites, variceal bleeding, or encephalopathy in the setting of chronic liver disease essentially establishes the diagnosis of cirrhosis, so a liver biopsy is not necessary to establish the diagnosis. Patients with decompensated cirrhosis often exhibit malnutrition, more severe muscle wasting, more numerous vascular spiders, and hypotension and tachycardia as a result of the hyperdynamic circulatory state.

Portal Pressure Measurements

Direct measurements of portal pressure involve catheterization of the portal vein, are cumbersome, and may be associated with complications. Hepatic vein catheterization with measurement of wedged and free pressure is the simplest, safest, most reproducible, and most widely used method to indirectly measure portal pressure. Portal pressure measurements are expressed as the hepatic venous pressure gradient: the gradient between wedged hepatic venous pressure, which is a measure of sinusoidal pressure, and free hepatic or inferior vena cava pressure, which is used as an internal zero reference point. In a patient with clinical evidence of portal hypertension (e.g., varices), the hepatic venous pressure gradient is useful in the differential diagnosis of the cause of portal hypertension: it will be normal (3 to 5 mm Hg) in prehepatic causes of portal hypertension, such as portal vein thrombosis (Chapter 145), and in intrahepatic but presinusoidal causes, such as schistosomiasis (Chapter 363), but will be abnormal (≥6 mm Hg) in sinusoidal causes of portal hypertension, such as cirrhosis, and in postsinusoidal causes, such as veno-occlusive disease. A hepatic venous pressure gradient of 10 mm Hg or greater ("clinically significant" portal hypertension) predicts the development of complications of portal hypertension, and its reduction on pharmacologic therapy predicts a favorable outcome in patients with cirrhosis.

Complications of Cirrhosis

Varices and Variceal Hemorrhage

Upper GI endoscopy (Chapters 136) remains the main method for diagnosing varices and variceal hemorrhage. Varices are classified as small (straight, minimally elevated veins above the esophageal mucosal surface), medium (tortuous veins occupying less than one third of the esophageal lumen), or large (occupying more than one third of the esophageal lumen). The diagnosis of variceal hemorrhage is made when diagnostic esophagogastroduodenoscopy shows one of the following: active bleeding from a varix, a "white nipple" overlying a varix, clots overlying a varix, or varices with no other potential source of bleeding.

TABLE 156-3 USING THE SERUM-ASCITES ALBUMIN GRADIENT AND THE ASCITES TOTAL PROTEIN LEVEL TO DIAGNOSE THE CAUSE OF ASCITES

CONDITION	SERUM-ASCITES ALBUMIN GRADIENT*	ASCITES TOTAL PROTEIN LEVEL†
Cirrhosis	High	Low
Malignant ascites	Low	High
Cardiac ascites	High	High

*High is greater than 1.1 g/dL; low is less than 1.1 g/dL.
†High is greater than 2.5 g/dL; low is less than 2.5 g/dL.

Ascites

The most common cause of ascites is cirrhosis, which accounts for 80% of cases. Peritoneal malignancy (e.g., peritoneal metastases from GI tumors or ovarian cancer), heart failure (Chapter 58), and peritoneal tuberculosis (Chapter 332) together account for another 15% of cases. The initial, most cost-effective, and least invasive method to confirm the presence of ascites is abdominal ultrasonography.

Diagnostic paracentesis is a safe procedure that should be performed in every patient with new-onset ascites, even in those with coagulopathy. Ultrasound guidance should be used in patients in whom percussion cannot locate the ascites or in whom a first paracentesis attempt does not yield fluid. The fluid in a patient with new-onset ascites should always be evaluated for albumin (with simultaneous estimation of serum albumin), total protein, polymorphonuclear (PMN) blood cell count, bacteriologic cultures, and cytology. The PMN cell count and bacteriologic culture are useful to exclude infection (either spontaneous or secondary bacterial peritonitis), and cytologic evaluation is needed if peritoneal carcinomatosis is suspected. Depending on the clinical setting, additional tests can be performed on the fluid: glucose and lactate dehydrogenase levels (if secondary bacterial peritonitis is suspected), smear and culture for acid-fast bacilli (if peritoneal tuberculosis is suspected), and an amylase level (if pancreatic ascites is suspected).

The serum-ascites albumin gradient and ascites protein levels are useful in the differential diagnosis of ascites (Table 156-3). The serum-ascites albumin gradient correlates with sinusoidal pressure and will therefore be elevated (>1.1 g/dL) in patients in whom the source of ascites is the hepatic sinusoid (e.g., cirrhosis or cardiac ascites). Protein levels in ascitic fluid are an indirect marker of the integrity of the hepatic sinusoids: normal sinusoids are permeable structures that "leak" protein, whereas sinusoids in cirrhosis are "capillarized" and do not leak as much protein. The three main causes of ascites—cirrhosis, peritoneal malignancy or tuberculosis, and heart failure—can easily be distinguished by combining the results of both the serum-ascites albumin gradient and ascites total protein content. Cirrhotic ascites typically has a high serum-ascites albumin gradient and low protein, cardiac ascites has a high serum-ascites albumin gradient and high protein, and ascites secondary to peritoneal malignancy typically has a low serum-ascites albumin gradient and high protein.

Hepatorenal Syndrome

Hepatorenal syndrome represents the extreme of the spectrum of abnormalities that lead to cirrhotic ascites and is characterized by maximal peripheral vasodilation as well as maximal activation of hormones that cause the retention of sodium and water and intense vasoconstriction of renal arteries. Ascites unresponsive to diuretics is universal, and dilutional hyponatremia is almost always present.

Hepatorenal syndrome, which is a diagnosis of exclusion, should be made only after discontinuing diuretics, expanding intravascular volume with albumin, and excluding or treating any condition that leads to worsening of the hemodynamic status of the cirrhotic patient. The differential diagnosis includes conditions that worsen vasodilation, such as sepsis, the use of vasodilators, and large-volume paracentesis not accompanied by albumin infusion; conditions that decrease effective arterial blood volume, such as gastrointestinal hemorrhage, overdiuresis or diarrhea (often induced by overdoses of lactulose); conditions that induce renal vasoconstriction, such as nonsteroidal anti-inflammatory drugs; and nephrotoxic insults, such as from aminoglycosides.

Spontaneous Bacterial Peritonitis

A high index of suspicion and early diagnosis are key in the management of spontaneous bacterial peritonitis. Diagnostic paracentesis should be performed in any patient with symptoms or signs of spontaneous bacterial peritonitis, including unexplained encephalopathy and renal dysfunction. Because spontaneous bacterial peritonitis is often asymptomatic and frequently community acquired, diagnostic paracentesis should be performed when any cirrhotic patient is admitted to the hospital, regardless of the cause for admission.

The diagnosis of spontaneous bacterial peritonitis is established by an ascitic fluid PMN count greater than $250/mm^3$. Bacteria can be isolated from ascitic fluid in only 40 to 50% of cases, even with sensitive methods such as inoculation directly into a blood culture bottle. Spontaneous bacterial peritonitis is mostly a monobacterial infection, usually with gram-negative enteric organisms. Anaerobes and fungi very rarely cause spontaneous bacterial peritonitis; their presence, as well as a polymicrobial infection, should raise suspicion of secondary bacterial peritonitis.

Hepatic Encephalopathy

The diagnosis of hepatic encephalopathy is clinical and based on the history and physical examination showing alterations in consciousness and behavior, as well as the presence of asterixis. Ammonia levels are unreliable, and there is poor correlation between the stage of hepatic encephalopathy and ammonia blood levels. Therefore, measurements of ammonia are not useful. Psychometric tests and an electroencephalogram are typically used in research but are not useful for clinical diagnosis. Minimal hepatic encephalopathy, formerly called *subclinical* hepatic encephalopathy, which occurs in about 30 to 70% of patients who have cirrhosis without overt hepatic encephalopathy, is detected by psychometric and neuropsychological testing of attention (e.g., number connection test, digit symbol test) and psychomotor function (e.g., grooved pegboard) alone. However, screening of cirrhotic patients for asymptomatic hepatic encephalopathy is not recommended because diagnostic tests are not standardized and the benefits of treatment are unknown.

Hepatopulmonary Syndrome and Portopulmonary Hypertension

The diagnostic criteria for hepatopulmonary syndrome are arterial hypoxemia with a Pa_{O_2} of less than 80 mm Hg or an alveolar arterial oxygen gradient of greater than 15 mm Hg, along with evidence of pulmonary vascular shunting on contrast echocardiography (Chapter 55) or a ^{99m}Tc-labeled macroaggregated albumin scan demonstrating abnormal shunting of radioactivity to the brain. Portopulmonary hypertension is diagnosed by the presence of mean pulmonary arterial pressure higher than 25 mm Hg on right heart catheterization, provided that pulmonary capillary wedge pressure is less than 15 mm Hg.

TREATMENT Rx

Treatment of cirrhosis should ideally be aimed at interrupting or reversing fibrosis. However, antifibrotic drugs have not been shown to reverse fibrosis consistently or improve outcomes in cirrhotic patients. Treatment of compensated cirrhosis is currently directed at preventing the development of decompensation by (1) treating the underlying liver disease (e.g., antiviral therapy for hepatitis C or B) to reduce fibrosis and prevent decompensation; (2) avoiding factors that could worsen liver disease, such as alcohol and hepatotoxic drugs; and (3) screening for varices (to prevent variceal hemorrhage) and for hepatocellular carcinoma (to treat at an early stage) (Fig. 156-5). Treatment of decompensated cirrhosis focuses on specific decompensating events and the option of liver transplantation.

Varices and Variceal Bleeding

Reducing portal pressure decreases the risk for the development of varices and variceal hemorrhage, as well as the risk for ascites and death. Nonselective β-adrenergic blockers (propranolol, nadolol) reduce portal pressure by producing splanchnic vasoconstriction and decreasing portal venous inflow. In patients with cirrhosis and medium or large varices that have never bled, nonselective β-blockers significantly reduce the risk for first variceal hemorrhage.[1] Propranolol is initiated at a dose of 20 mg orally twice a day, whereas nadolol is initiated at a dose of 20 mg orally every day. The dose should be titrated to produce a resting heart rate of about 50 to 55 beats per minute. Endoscopic variceal ligation (Fig. 136-3 in Chapter 136), a therapy that aims to obliterate varices by placing rubber rings on variceal columns, is as useful as nonselective β-blockers to prevent a first variceal hemorrhage.[2] Because ligation is a local therapy that has no effect on portal pressure and that can lead to hemorrhage from ligation-induced ulcers, a rational approach is to start therapy with β-blockers and to use ligation in patients who cannot tolerate or have contraindications to β-blockers.

In patients with no varices, nonselective β-blockers do not prevent the development of varices and are associated with more side effects.[3] In

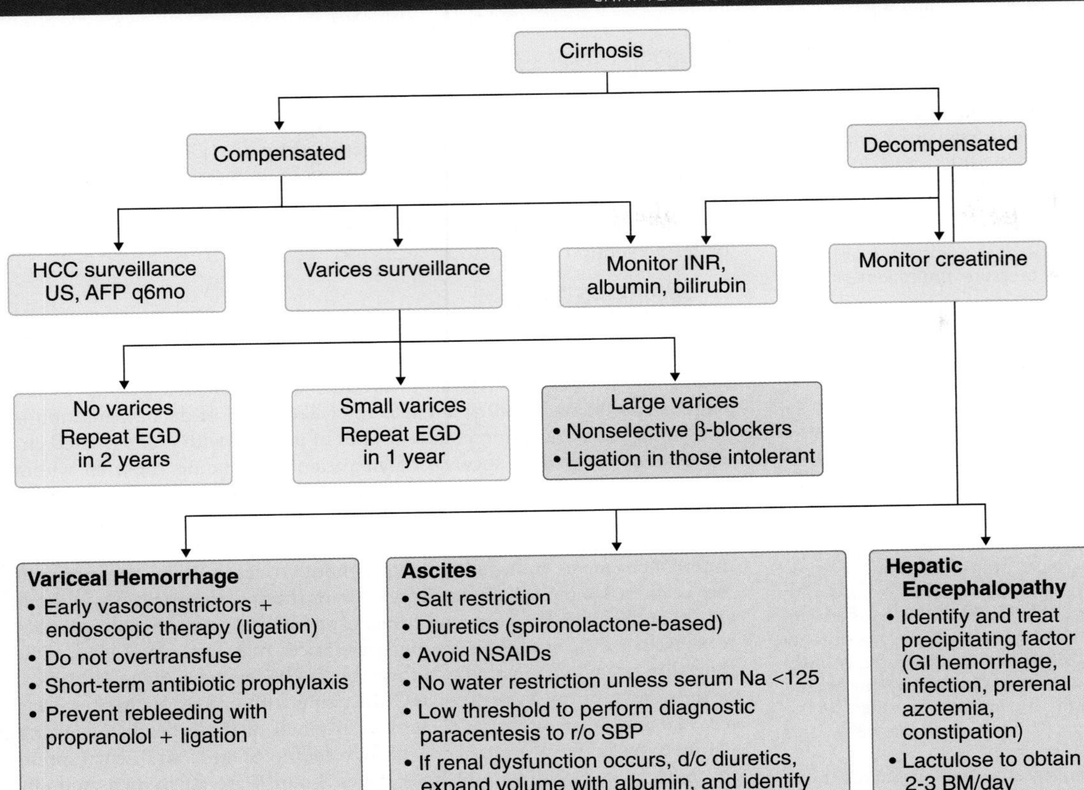

FIGURE 156-5. **Summary of the management of compensated and decompensated cirrhosis.** AFP = α-fetoprotein; BM = bowel movement; d/c = discontinue; EGD = esophagogastroduodenoscopy; GI = gastrointestinal; HCC = hepatocellular carcinoma; INR = international normalized ratio; Na = sodium; NSAIDs = nonsteroidal anti-inflammatory drugs; r/o = rule out; SBP = spontaneous bacterial peritonitis; US = ultrasound.

patients with small varices, data are insufficient to recommend therapy with nonselective β-blockers. Endoscopy should be repeated every 2 to 3 years in patients with no varices, every 1 to 2 years in patients with small varices, and sooner in patients with decompensated disease so that effective therapy can be instituted before the varices grow in size and bleed.

Patients with cirrhosis and variceal hemorrhage require resuscitation in an intensive care unit. However, overtransfusion should be avoided because it can precipitate rebleeding. Hemoglobin values should be maintained at about 7-8 g/dL. Prophylactic antibiotics should be used in this setting not only to prevent bacterial infections but also to decrease rebleeding[4] and death. The recommended antibiotic is oral norfloxacin at a dose of 400 mg twice daily for 5 to 7 days, although intravenous ceftriaxone at a dose of 1 g/day for 5 to 7 days is preferable in patients with advanced liver disease (malnutrition, ascites, encephalopathy, and jaundice) or in those already on norfloxacin prophylaxis.[5]

The most effective specific therapy for the control of active variceal hemorrhage is the combination of a vasoconstrictor with endoscopic therapy.[6] Safe vasoconstrictors include terlipressin, somatostatin, and the somatostatin analogues octreotide and vapreotide; they can be initiated at admission to the hospital and continued for 2 to 5 days. The vasoconstrictor currently available in the United States is octreotide, which is used as a 50-µg intravenous bolus followed by an infusion at 50 µg/hour.

After control of hemorrhage, the 1-year recurrence of hemorrhage without treatment is very high at about 60%. Therefore, therapy to prevent rebleeding should be instituted before the patient is discharged. The lowest rebleeding rates (about 10%) are observed in patients who achieve a significant reduction in the hepatic venous pressure gradient with pharmacologic therapy (β-blockers, at the same dose recommended for prevention of first hemorrhage, with or without isosorbide mononitrate at stepwise dosing starting at 20 mg/day orally and increased as tolerated up to 40 mg twice a day); however, because hepatic venous pressure gradient measurements are not widely used, the next best results (rebleeding rates of about 22%) are obtained with the combination of nonselective β-blockers (propranolol or nadolol), with or without isosorbide mononitrate, and endoscopic variceal ligation.[7] The dose of β-blockers should be the maximal dose tolerated, and endoscopic variceal ligation should be repeated every 2 to 4 weeks until the varices are obliterated.

Shunt therapy, either surgical or through radiologic placement of a transjugular intrahepatic portosystemic shunt (TIPS), should be used in patients whose variceal bleeding has persisted or recurred despite combined pharmacologic and endoscopic therapy. Both types of shunts are equally effective,[8] and the choice will depend on local expertise. Although uncovered TIPS stents frequently occlude, newer polytetrafluoroethylene-covered stents are associated with lower occlusion rates and lower rates of hepatic encephalopathy.[9]

Ascites

Salt restriction and diuretics constitute the mainstay of management of ascites. Dietary sodium intake should be restricted to 2 g/day. A more restrictive diet is not recommended and may compromise nutritional status. Fluid restriction is not required unless the serum sodium concentration is below 130 mEq/L.

Spironolactone, which is more effective than loop diuretics, should be started at a dose of 100 mg/day (once a day in the morning). The dose should be adjusted every 3 to 4 days to a maximal effective dose of 400 mg/day. Furosemide, at an escalated dose from 40 to 160 mg/day, can be started concurrently with spironolactone if weight loss is inadequate or if hyperkalemia develops on spironolactone alone. The goal is weight loss of 1 kg in the first week and 2 kg/week subsequently. However, diuretics should be reduced if the rate of weight loss is greater than 0.5 kg/day in patients without peripheral edema or more than 1 kg/day in patients with peripheral edema. Side effects of diuretic therapy include electrolyte abnormalities, renal dysfunction, encephalopathy, and painful gynecomastia (with spironolactone).

In the 10 to 20% of patients with ascites who are refractory to diuretics, large-volume paracentesis, aimed at removing all or most of the fluid, plus albumin at a dose of 6 to 8 g intravenously per liter of ascites removed, particularly when more than 5 L is removed at once, is a reasonable approach. The frequency of large-volume paracentesis is dictated by the rapidity at which the ascites reaccumulates. TIPS with uncovered stents is more effective than large-volume paracentesis plus albumin in preventing recurrent ascites but is associated with a higher rate of encephalopathy without a significant improvement in survival.[10] In patients requiring frequent large-volume paracentesis (more than twice per month), polytetrafluoroethylene-covered TIPS stents should be considered. A peritoneovenous shunt, using a subcutaneously placed silicone tube that transfers ascites from the peritoneal cavity to the systemic circulation, can be used in patients who are not candidates for TIPS or liver transplantation.

Hepatorenal Syndrome

Because hepatorenal syndrome is a functional kidney injury that results from hemodynamic abnormalities secondary to end-stage liver disease and severe portal hypertension, the mainstay of therapy is liver transplantation (Chapter 157). Therapies that have been used to "bridge" a patient to transplantation include vasoconstrictors (terlipressin, noradrenaline, octreotide plus midodrine) plus albumin, TIPS, and extracorporeal albumin dialysis, which is an experimental hemofiltration dialysis method that uses an albumin dialysate. The largest experience is with the use of terlipressin, which at a dose 0.5 to 2.0 mg intravenously every 4 to 6 hours leads to a higher reversal rate of hepatorenal syndrome compared with placebo.[11] Because terlipressin is not yet available in the United States, the most used combination is octreotide (100 to 200 μg subcutaneously three times a day) plus midodrine (7.5 to 12.5 mg orally three times a day), with the dose adjusted to obtain an increase of at least 15 mm Hg in mean arterial pressure. Improvements may become clinically noticeable at day 7.

Spontaneous Bacterial Peritonitis

Empirical antibiotic therapy with an intravenous third-generation cephalosporin (e.g., cefotaxime, 2 g intravenously every 12 hours, or ceftriaxone, 1 to 2 g intravenously every 24 hours) or amoxicillin-clavulanic acid (1 g/0.5 g intravenously every 8 hours) should be initiated as soon as the diagnosis is established and before culture results are available; the minimal duration of therapy should be 5 days. Aminoglycosides should be avoided because of the high incidence of renal toxicity in cirrhotic patients. Repeat diagnostic paracentesis should be performed 2 days after starting antibiotics, by which time the number of PMN neutrophils in ascitic fluid should have decreased by more than 25% from baseline. Lack of response should prompt further investigations to exclude secondary peritonitis. The renal dysfunction associated with spontaneous bacterial peritonitis can be prevented by the intravenous administration of albumin, particularly in patients who have any evidence of renal dysfunction (blood urea nitrogen >30 mg/dL or creatinine >1 mg/dL, or both) or serum bilirubin greater than 4 mg/dL at the time of diagnosis. Albumin has been used at a dose of 1.5 g/kg of body weight at diagnosis, repeated on the third day at an intravenous dose of 1 g/kg of body weight. However, this dosing is empirical and should not exceed 100 g per dose.

The administration of nonabsorbable (or poorly absorbable) antibiotics can prevent the development of spontaneous bacterial peritonitis and other infections in cirrhosis by selectively eliminating gram-negative organisms in the gut. However, the widespread use of prophylactic norfloxacin is associated with a higher rate of infections by antibiotic-resistant organisms. Long-term antibiotic prophylaxis with oral norfloxacin at a dose of 400 mg/day is justified only in two groups: patients who have recovered from a previous episode of spontaneous bacterial peritonitis, and patients who have an ascites protein level of less than 1 g/L with advanced liver and circulatory dysfunction as evidenced by the presence of jaundice, hyponatremia, or renal dysfunction.[12,13]

Hepatic Encephalopathy

Treatment of hepatic encephalopathy involves identifying and treating the precipitating factor and reducing the ammonia level. Precipitating factors include infections, overdiuresis, GI bleeding, a high oral protein load, and constipation. Narcotics and sedatives contribute to hepatic encephalopathy by directly depressing brain function. TIPS is a common precipitant of hepatic encephalopathy, and shunt reduction or occlusion may be required. Agents aimed at decreasing ammonia production in the gut are lactulose (15 to 30 mL orally twice daily adjusted to obtain two to three soft bowel movements per day) or orally administered nonabsorbable antibiotics such as neomycin (500 mg to 1 g three times per day), metronidazole (250 mg two to four times per day), or rifaximin (550 mg two times per day).[14] L-Ornithine, L-aspartate, and benzoate may increase ammonia fixation in the liver. Switching dietary protein from an animal source to a vegetable source may be beneficial, but protein restriction is not necessary and should not be used long term.[15]

Pulmonary Complications

Hepatopulmonary syndrome rarely resolves spontaneously, and medical therapy is disappointing. TIPS is not generally recommended. The only viable treatment is liver transplantation (Chapter 157).

By comparison, portopulmonary hypertension is not an indication for liver transplantation. In fact, a mean pulmonary arterial pressure higher than 50 mm Hg is an absolute contraindication to liver transplantation.

Surgical Therapy

Liver Transplantation

Orthotopic liver transplantation (Chapter 157), which is the definitive therapy for cirrhosis, is indicated when the risk for dying from liver disease is greater than the risk for dying from transplantation, as determined by a Child-Pugh score of 7 or higher (see Table 156-2) or a Model for End-Stage Liver Disease (MELD) score of 15 or higher. MELD (see Table 157-4 in Chapter 157), which is a mathematical model that estimates the risk for 3-month mortality, is used to determine the priority for liver transplantation. The number of available deceased donor organs is lower than the number of patients awaiting liver transplantation; as a result, 15 to 20% of patients awaiting liver transplantation in the United States die before an organ becomes available.

PRIMARY PREVENTION

Treatment of the underlying liver disease, before the development of cirrhosis, is a primary prevention strategy. Because the major causes of cirrhosis are related to lifestyle choices such as injection drug use (Chapter 33), alcohol consumption (Chapter 32), and unprotected sex, primary prevention programs that focus on encouraging alcohol abstinence, reducing high-risk behavior for hepatitis virus infection, and vaccinating for hepatitis B are even better prevention strategies.

PROGNOSIS

The outcome of cirrhosis depends on the patient's stage. Patients with compensated cirrhosis die of liver disease only after transition to a decompensated stage. The 10-year survival rate of patients who remain in a compensated stage is approximately 90%, whereas their likelihood of decompensation is 50% at 10 years. Inception cohort studies of patients with compensated cirrhosis show a median survival of all patients, including those in whom decompensation develops over time, of about 10 years, whereas the median survival after decompensation is about 2 years.

Four clinical stages of cirrhosis have recently been identified, each with a different prognosis. In stage 1 patients without varices or ascites, the mortality rate is about 1% per year. Stage 2 patients, or those with varices but without ascites or bleeding, have a mortality rate of about 4% per year. Stage 3 patients have ascites with or without esophageal varices that have never bled; their mortality rate while remaining in this stage is 20% per year. Stage 4 patients, or those with portal hypertensive GI bleeding with or without ascites, have a 1-year mortality rate of 57%, with nearly half of these deaths occurring within 6 weeks after the initial episode of bleeding. Stages 1 and 2 correspond to compensated cirrhosis, whereas stages 3 and 4 are decompensated cirrhosis. Hepatocellular carcinoma develops at a fairly constant rate of 3% per year and is associated with a worse outcome at whatever stage it develops.

Predictors of survival are different in compensated and decompensated patients, with parameters of portal hypertension (varices, splenomegaly, platelet count, γ-globulin) assuming greater importance in compensated patients, whereas renal dysfunction, hemorrhage, and hepatocellular carcinoma are important predictive factors in patients with decompensated cirrhosis. In clinical practice, the Child-Pugh score is applicable to all cirrhotic patients, and the MELD score is used in decompensated patients to determine priority for liver transplantation.

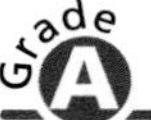

1. D'Amico G, Pagliaro L, Bosch J. Pharmacological treatment of portal hypertension: an evidence-based approach. *Semin Liver Dis.* 1999;19:475-505.
2. Gluud LL, Klingenberg S, Nikolova D, et al. Banding ligation versus beta-blockers as primary prophylaxis in esophageal varices: systematic review of randomized trials. *Am J Gastroenterol.* 2007;102:2842-2848.
3. Groszmann RJ, Garcia-Tsao G, Bosch J, et al. Beta-blockers to prevent gastroesophageal varices in patients with cirrhosis. *N Engl J Med.* 2005;353:2254-2261.
4. Hou MC, Lin HC, Liu TT, et al. Antibiotic prophylaxis after endoscopic therapy prevents rebleeding in acute variceal hemorrhage: a randomized trial. *Hepatology.* 2004;39:746-753.
5. Fernandez J, Ruiz del Arbol L, Gomez C, et al. Norfloxacin vs ceftriaxone in the prophylaxis of infections in patients with advanced cirrhosis and hemorrhage. *Gastroenterology.* 2006;131:1049-1056.
6. Banares R, Albillos A, Rincon D, et al. Endoscopic treatment versus endoscopic plus pharmacologic treatment for acute variceal bleeding: a meta-analysis. *Hepatology.* 2002;35:609-615.
7. Gonzalez R, Zamora J, Gomez-Camarero J, et al. Meta-analysis: combination endoscopic and drug therapy to prevent variceal rebleeding in cirrhosis. *Ann Intern Med.* 2008;149:109-122.
8. Henderson JM, Boyer TD, Kutner MH, et al. Distal splenorenal shunt versus transjugular intrahepatic portal systematic shunt for variceal bleeding: a randomized trial. *Gastroenterology.* 2006;130:1643-1651.
9. Bureau C, Garcia-Pagan JC, Otal P, et al. Improved clinical outcome using polytetrafluoroethylene-coated stents for TIPS: results of a randomized study. *Gastroenterology.* 2004;126:469-475.
10. D'Amico G, Luca A, Morabito A, et al. Uncovered transjugular intrahepatic portosystemic shunt for refractory ascites: a meta-analysis. *Gastroenterology.* 2005;129:1282-1293.
11. Sanyal AJ, Boyer T, Garcia-Tsao G, et al. A randomized, prospective, double-blind, placebo-controlled trial of terlipressin for type 1 hepatorenal syndrome. *Gastroenterology.* 2008;134:1360-1368.
12. Fernandez J, Navasa M, Planas R, et al. Primary prophylaxis of spontaneous bacterial peritonitis delays hepatorenal syndrome and improves survival in cirrhosis. *Gastroenterology.* 2007;133:818-824.
13. Loomba R, Wesley R, Bain A, et al. Role of fluoroquinolones in the primary prophylaxis of spontaneous bacterial peritonitis: meta-analysis. *Clin Gastroenterol Hepatol.* 2009;7:487-493.
14. Bass NM, Mullen KD, Sanyal A, et al. Rifaximin treatment in hepatic encephalopathy. *N Engl J Med.* 2010;362:1071-1081.
15. Cordoba J, Lopez-Hellin J, Planas M, et al. Normal protein diet for episodic hepatic encephalopathy: results of a randomized study. *J Hepatol.* 2004;41:38-43.

SUGGESTED READINGS

Beier JI, Arteel GE, McClain CJ. Advances in alcoholic liver disease. *Curr Gastroenterol Rep.* 2010;13:56-64. *Review of biology and treatment.*

Kremer AE, Oude Elferink RP, Beuers U. Pathophysiology and current management of pruritus in liver disease. *Gastroenterol Clin Biol.* 2011. [Epub ahead of print.] *Review emphasizing potential role of lysophosphatidic acid, a potent neuronal activator.*

Thabut D, Moreau R, Lebrec D. Noninvasive assessment of portal hypertension in patients with cirrhosis. *Hepatology.* 2011;53:683-694. *Noninvasive methods effectively identify severe portal hypertension but not less severe disease.*

Thalheimer U, Triantos C, Goulis J, et al. Management o f varices in cirrhosis. *Expert Opin Pharmacother.* 2011;12:721-735. *Review.*

157

HEPATIC FAILURE AND LIVER TRANSPLANTATION

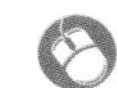

EMMET B. KEEFFE

Liver transplantation is the treatment of choice for patients with severe liver failure, end-stage liver disease, and certain metabolic liver diseases for which no alternative therapies are available. More than 6000 liver transplantations are performed in the United States annually, with a waiting list that has grown to approximately 16,000 patients. With modern immunosuppressive drug regimens, technical advances, and improved perioperative care, the current 1-year survival rate after liver transplantation is 85 to 90% (Table 157-1). Many studies show that liver transplantation significantly improves the physical, cognitive, and psychological functioning of the recipient. In recent years, the disparity between a limited supply of cadaver donor organs and much greater need for liver transplantation has resulted in an unacceptable number of deaths of patients listed for transplantation and created a mandate to optimize the selection of patients and timing of transplantation.

INDICATIONS AND SELECTION CRITERIA FOR LIVER TRANSPLANTATION

The indications and contraindications for liver transplantation, the most appropriate candidates to receive a transplant, and the organ allocation scheme continue to evolve. The diseases for which liver transplantation is performed in adults include cirrhosis with end-stage liver disease (Chapter 156), acute liver failure, hepatic malignancies (particularly hepatocellular carcinoma; Chapter 202), and metabolic diseases in which the inborn error of metabolism resides in the hepatocytes (e.g., hemochromatosis, α_1-antitrypsin deficiency, Wilson's disease; Chapter 153). The most common indications for liver transplantation are chronic hepatitis C and alcoholic liver disease in adults (together accounting for approximately 50% of transplantations) and biliary atresia and α_1-antitrypsin deficiency in children.

General selection criteria that should be considered in the referral of patients for liver transplantation include the following: (1) the absence of alternative forms of therapy that may reverse liver failure and defer the need for liver transplantation, (2) the absence of any absolute contraindication to transplantation (discussed later), (3) expected compliance with longitudinal follow-up care, and (4) the ability to provide for the financial costs of liver transplantation and follow-up care, including medications that may be expensive. Insurance coverage for transplantation is typically determined before referral by a financial counselor at the transplantation center.

TABLE 157-1 KAPLAN-MEIER PATIENT SURVIVAL RATES FOR LIVER TRANSPLANTATION PERFORMED FROM 1997 TO 2004

	Kaplan-Meier Survival Rate (%)		
DIAGNOSIS	**1-YEAR**	**3-YEAR**	**5-YEAR**
Acute hepatic necrosis	81	72	69
Cholestatic cirrhosis	90	85	80
Noncholestatic cirrhosis	86	77	70
Other liver disease	81	72	63
Metabolic disease	89	84	81
Malignant neoplasm	86	68	54
Benign neoplasm	86	81	68

From The Organ Procurement and Transplantation Network. http://www.unos.org → Data → View data reports → National Data → Survival/Liver/Patient → Survival by recipient diagnosis category. Accessed Nov. 25, 2009.

TABLE 157-2 BIOCHEMICAL AND CLINICAL INDICATIONS FOR LIVER TRANSPLANTATION IN CHRONIC LIVER DISEASE

CHOLESTATIC LIVER DISEASE

Bilirubin >10 mg/dL
Intractable pruritus
Progressive cholestatic bone disease
Recurrent bacterial cholangitis

HEPATOCELLULAR LIVER DISEASE

Serum albumin <3 g/dL
Prothrombin time >3 seconds above control

BOTH CHOLESTATIC AND HEPATOCELLULAR LIVER DISEASES

Recurrent or severe hepatic encephalopathy
Refractory ascites
Spontaneous bacterial peritonitis
Recurrent portal hypertensive bleeding
Severe chronic fatigue and weakness
Progressive malnutrition
Development of hepatorenal syndrome
Detection of small hepatocellular carcinoma

INR = International Normalized Ratio.
From Keeffe EB. Selection of patients for liver transplantation. In Maddrey WC, Sorrell MF, Schiff ER, eds. *Transplantation of the Liver*, 3rd ed. Philadelphia: Lippincott Williams & Wilkins; 2001:5-34.

TABLE 157-3 KING'S COLLEGE CRITERIA FOR LIVER TRANSPLANTATION IN FULMINANT HEPATIC FAILURE

PATIENTS TAKING ACETAMINOPHEN

pH <7.3, or prothrombin time >6.5 (INR) and serum creatinine >3.4 mg/dL

PATIENTS NOT TAKING ACETAMINOPHEN

Prothrombin time >6.5 (INR) *or* any three of the following:
1. Age <10 or >40 yr
2. Etiology: non-A, non-B hepatitis; halothane hepatitis; idiosyncratic drug reaction
3. Duration of jaundice before encephalopathy >7 days
4. Prothrombin time >3.5 (INR)
5. Serum bilirubin >17.6 mg/dL

INR = International Normalized Ratio.
Adapted from O'Grady JG, Alexander GJ, Hayllar KM, et al. Early indicators of prognosis in fulminant hepatic failure. *Gastroenterology.* 1989;97:439-445.

Referral for Liver Transplantation

Patients with chronic (Table 157-2) or acute (Table 157-3) liver disease should be referred when hepatic decompensation first develops or the presence of hepatocellular carcinoma is first detected. The greatest likelihood of survival and return to an excellent quality of life occurs in patients who undergo liver transplantation before the onset of multiorgan failure. Meticulous attention to medical management of the complications of cirrhosis, such as avoidance of excessive diuretic therapy or aminoglycosides to preserve renal function in patients with ascites or spontaneous bacterial peritonitis, is critical. Blood loss in patients with gastrointestinal bleeding should be replaced judiciously with blood products to avoid fluid overload and pulmonary edema.

For long-term management in patients with chronic liver disease who may ultimately become candidates for transplantation, nonsurgical interventions, such as transjugular intrahepatic portosystemic shunt (TIPS) for refractory portal hypertensive bleeding and endoscopic or radiologic approaches to dominant biliary strictures in patients with primary sclerosing cholangitis, are preferable to abdominal procedures that can cause adhesions. Patients with cirrhosis (Chapter 156) should undergo surveillance for hepatocellular carcinoma with ultrasound or computed tomography and α-fetoprotein testing every 6 months to facilitate early diagnosis of lesions, when they are small and amenable to treatment with modalities such as resection or liver transplantation.

Chronic Liver Disease

Although the survival of patients with compensated cirrhosis is excellent (approximately 90% at 5 years), the development of decompensation with ascites, portal hypertensive bleeding, or encephalopathy implies a lower 5-year survival rate of about 20%. A patient with a Child-Turcotte-Pugh (see Table 156-2 in Chapter 156) score of 5 or 6 (Child's class A cirrhosis) without a history of portal hypertensive bleeding or spontaneous bacterial peritonitis is likely to remain stable for a considerable period of time and does not require listing for transplantation. Suggested criteria for listing should be clinical decompensation or biochemical deterioration of synthetic function that results in a Child's class B or C status, any complication of portal hypertension, or the development of a small hepatocellular carcinoma, although one randomized trial showed no benefit to listing patients with Child's class B alcoholic cirrhosis compared with standard care.[1] Many centers are also using a Model for End-Stage Liver Disease (MELD; see Table 156-2 in Chapter 156) score of 10 to assist in the timing of evaluation for liver transplantation.

Liver transplantation for hepatocellular carcinoma (Chapter 202) is reserved for selected patients who have advanced cirrhosis, who do not have the hepatic reserve to undergo resection, and who have no evidence of extrahepatic tumor after thorough evaluation. Risks for recurrent hepatocellular carcinoma after transplantation include advanced disease (stage 3 or greater) as defined by lymph node involvement, gross vascular invasion by imaging studies, tumor burden (single lesion <5 cm, or two or more lesions >3 cm), or involvement of more than one lobe. In low-risk patients with stage 1 or 2 disease (single lesion of 5 cm, or two or three lesions of ≤3 cm), the actuarial survival rate is about 75% at 4 years, whereas the survival in patients with higher risk is about 50% at 4 years. Evolving data support expanding liver transplantation to patients with early stage 3 hepatocellular carcinoma, but use of these expanded criteria remains experimental.

Acute Liver Failure

Liver transplantation is a major advance in the management of severe acute liver failure. *Fulminant hepatic failure* refers to the presence of acute liver failure with superimposed hepatic encephalopathy developing within 2 to 8 weeks after the onset of illness in a patient without preexisting liver disease. *Subfulminant hepatic failure* (or *late-onset hepatic failure*) is applied to a syndrome that develops more slowly, after 2 to 8 weeks up to 3 to 6 months. The selection of patients with acute liver failure who are likely to die and therefore would benefit from liver transplantation is challenging but can be predicted by certain biochemical and clinical features, the most popular of which was established at King's College Hospital in London (see Table 157-3).

Aggressive supportive care is necessary in patients with fulminant hepatic failure to prevent and treat bleeding, infection, cerebral edema, renal failure, and respiratory failure. These complications are the main reasons that transplantation may not be possible and may also contribute to postoperative morbidity and mortality.

Potential alternative treatment strategies for fulminant hepatic failure include extracorporeal liver assist devices, hepatocyte transplantation, and heterotopic auxiliary liver transplantation, although all of these currently must be viewed as investigational. The goals of these therapies are to prevent irreversible brain damage, provide time for possible hepatic regeneration and recovery of acceptable function, and stabilize patients who do not recover until liver transplantation can be performed. Clinical experience with hepatic support devices, primarily using either porcine or human hepatocytes, is encouraging but limited to ongoing trials. Hepatocyte transplantation and heterotopic liver transplantation have a number of technical problems that limit their application.

Patients with fulminant hepatic failure should be treated in an intensive care unit, with the patient's head elevated at 20 to 30 degrees. Although lactulose is the cornerstone of treatment of chronic hepatic encephalopathy, it is less effective in patients with acute encephalopathy, and the role of antibiotics such as neomycin is unknown. However, a trial of lactulose, 30 mL two to four times daily, adjusted to achieve two to three loose bowel movements daily, is worthwhile, and the drug may need to be administrated by nasogastric tube or by rectal enema. Factors precipitating hepatic encephalopathy, such as gastrointestinal bleeding, hypokalemia, or sepsis, should be identified and treated.

Cerebral edema is manifest frequently by hypertension, bradycardia, and neurologic findings such as decerebrate posturing or abnormal pupillary reflexes. These findings may occur late; therefore, monitoring of intracranial pressure (ICP) with institution of therapy to maintain ICP at less than 20 mm Hg is preferred. ICP may be monitored with either a subdural or an epidural transducer, and the risk for hemorrhage as a complication of placement is outweighed by the benefit of monitoring and early intervention.

Initial treatment of increased ICP is with mannitol (0.5 to 1 g/kg by intravenous infusion over 5 minutes). Repeated doses of mannitol may be required to treat recurrent increases in ICP. Mannitol can be given only if the serum osmolality is less than 320 mOsm/L. Caution is advised in patients with renal failure, and mannitol may need to be administered in combination with hemodialysis or continuous arteriovenous hemofiltration. Other useful therapies include disturbing the patient as little as possible, controlling agitation, and administering moderate hyperventilation to a partial carbon dioxide pressure of 25 to 30 mm Hg. A persistent ICP greater than 40 mm Hg that is refractory to treatment precludes liver transplantation.

Listing for Liver Transplantation

Before final selection and listing for liver transplantation, prospective candidates with acute or chronic liver disease undergo a pretransplantation evaluation to define the current status of systemic diseases and to determine whether any absolute or relative contraindications are present. Routine evaluation includes blood bank and hematologic studies, complete liver and kidney chemistry profiles, viral serology assays (hepatitis A, B, and C viruses; human immunodeficiency virus [HIV]; cytomegalovirus [CMV]), chest radiography, and abdominal computed tomography or Doppler ultrasound studies of the hepatic vasculature. Additional routine tests include skin testing for tuberculosis, creatinine clearance, electrocardiogram, and, in the presence of lung disease, pulmonary function testing. Patients who are at risk for coronary artery disease undergo cardiology consultation and, if indicated, stress testing, cardiac catheterization, or both. Cancer screening, depending on age and gender, includes Papanicolaou smear, mammography, and colonoscopy. Consultations with a social worker, financial counselor, and psychiatrist are routinely performed at the transplantation center.

Patients are generally assigned to one of four categories by the liver transplantation center selection committee: (1) suitable and ready, with listing for transplantation; (2) suitable but too well, with placement on inactive status and continued follow-up with the referring physician; (3) potentially reversible relative contraindication, with treatment and recategorization at a later date; and (4) absolute contraindication, with denial of transplantation. Patients who are approved for liver transplantation are then listed for a donor organ with the United Network for Organ Sharing (UNOS), and final approval by the insurance carrier or third party payer is sought.

Allocation of Donor Organs

In the current UNOS system, patients with fulminant liver failure receive the first priority for available organs. The MELD score (see Table 156-2 in Chapter 156) was adopted by UNOS in 2002 as the severity measure to determine priority for transplantation and allocation of organs to patients with end-stage liver disease (Table 157-4). Recent data indicate that lower serum sodium levels also independently predict higher mortality over and beyond MELD scores alone, but serum sodium has not been included in the formula used to allocate organs.

Contraindications to Liver Transplantation

Absolute Contraindications

The list of absolute contraindications to transplantation is short: advanced cardiopulmonary disease, active untreated sepsis, extrahepatic malignancy, anatomic abnormality precluding transplantation, active alcohol or substance abuse, and documented poor compliance with medical care. In addition, patients should not undergo liver transplantation if they have compensated cirrhosis (Child's class A; Chapter 156) and no history of portal hypertensive bleeding. Patients are not candidates for liver transplantation if they have poor ventricular function or severe valvular heart disease. Coronary artery disease, if anatomically reversible by angioplasty or bypass surgery, is not a contraindication to listing if left ventricular function is adequate.

Nearly 50% of liver transplantation candidates have abnormal arterial oxygenation, but only patients with advanced chronic obstructive pulmonary disease or pulmonary fibrosis are precluded from liver transplantation. Previous tuberculosis is not a contraindication to liver transplantation. The

TABLE 157-4 RELATIONSHIP BETWEEN MELD SCORE AND 3-MONTH MORTALITY IN HOSPITALIZED CIRRHOTIC PATIENTS

MELD SCORE	NO. DEATHS/TOTAL NO. OF PATIENTS	MORTALITY RATE (%)
≤9	6/148	4
10-19	28/103	27
20-29	16/21	76
30-39	5/6	83
≥40	4/4	100

MELD = Model for End-Stage Liver Disease.
Adapted from Wiesner RH, McDiarmid SV, Kamath PS, et al. MELD and PELD: application of survival models to liver allocation. *Liver Transpl.* 2001;7:567-580.

benefits of treating latent tuberculosis before liver transplantation appear to outweigh the risks, providing justification for the strategy of performing a skin test and treating with isoniazid if positive. Active tuberculosis should be treated for at least 2 to 3 weeks and preferably for several months before liver transplantation and for up to 1 year afterward. Hepatopulmonary syndrome (Chapter 156), which is diagnosed on the basis of the triad of chronic liver disease with portal hypertension, intrapulmonary vascular dilation with right-to-left shunting, and arterial hypoxemia, may be reversed by liver transplantation. By contrast, portopulmonary hypertension is associated with high operative mortality; for example, patients with a mean pulmonary artery pressure of 50 mm Hg or greater have a postoperative mortality rate that approaches 100%. Conversely, patients with mean pulmonary artery pressures lower than 35 mm Hg do not have increased perioperative mortality.

Active untreated infection should be controlled before proceeding with liver transplantation. In the setting of spontaneous bacterial peritonitis, most programs defer transplantation until antibiotic treatment has been administered for 48 hours and resolution of infection is documented on repeat paracentesis. Sepsis and pneumonia remain absolute contraindications to liver transplantation. Serious chronic infections such as osteomyelitis, chronic fungal diseases, and abscesses preclude transplantation unless they can be treated effectively. Selected HIV-positive patients are currently undergoing liver transplantation in a few centers in the United States to determine whether the benefits outweigh the risks.

Liver transplantation is not performed in the presence of extrahepatic malignancy, except perhaps for patients with isolated liver metastases from slow-growing neuroendocrine tumors (Chapter 201), such as gastrinoma, insulinomas, glucagonomas, somatostatinomas, and carcinoid tumors. The results of liver transplantation are so poor with cholangiocarcinoma (Chapter 158) that most centers consider this diagnosis to be an absolute contraindication, although a few centers have demonstrated acceptable tumor-free survival rates when liver transplantation is combined with adjuvant chemotherapy and radiation in highly selected patients.

Most programs accept patients with alcoholic liver disease as candidates for liver transplantation only after proven alcohol abstinence for at least 6 months and completion of an inpatient or outpatient rehabilitation program. Isolated portal vein thrombosis, previously considered an absolute contraindication, is only a relative problem in light of novel reconstructive innovations, including thrombectomy or jump grafts.

Relative Contraindications

Patient selection should be based on an assessment of biologic age and absence of major systemic illnesses rather than an arbitrary chronologic age cutoff. Patients undergoing evaluation for liver transplantation may have hepatorenal syndrome, chronic renal failure, or reversible acute renal failure that may be related to intercurrent events such as spontaneous bacterial peritonitis, gastrointestinal bleeding, or excessive diuresis; however, these conditions are not contraindications to transplantation. Chronic renal failure secondary to intrinsic kidney disease is not a contraindication to liver transplantation but necessitates consideration for combined liver and kidney transplantation. Transient deterioration in renal function due to an acute injury usually is not a problem unless it is complicated by the development of hepatorenal syndrome, which is reversible only if urgent liver transplantation can be performed.

THE TRANSPLANTATION PROCEDURE

Donors and recipients are matched according to blood type and body size. In general, organs are transplanted into recipients in keeping with standard ABO compatibility rules. Most surgeons believe that a satisfactory size match exists if the donor's and recipient's body weights are within 20% of one another. The donor organ is harvested according to standard protocols to ensure that the physiologic condition of the donor is close to normal when the organ is removed and to limit warm ischemia time. The cold ischemia time while the organ is in a preservation solution is also kept as short as possible—the usual goal is less than 12 hours—to minimize the risk for delayed graft function or nonfunction.

The recipient undergoes bilateral subcostal incision with upper midline extension. The standard hepatectomy includes removal of both the vena cava and the liver, often with use of a pump-driven venovenous bypass to return the inferior vena cava and portal venous flow to the heart through the axillary vein. A popular alternative method is to preserve the retrohepatic vena cava during hepatectomy. After hepatectomy, the donor liver is put in place, with repair of the inferior vena cava if it was interrupted, portal reperfusion, hepatic arterial reconstruction, and, finally, duct-to-duct reconstruction of the common bile duct. A Roux-en-Y choledochojejunostomy is used when a duct-to-duct anastomosis is not suitable, such as in patients who have primary sclerosing cholangitis, in whom the diseased common bile duct is removed in its entirety.

Evolving Approaches to Liver Transplantation

The growing discrepancy between the number of available organs and the need for transplantation has led to increasing application of novel approaches to liver replacement, including deceased donor split-liver transplantation and adult living donor liver transplantation. Xenotransplantation and hepatocyte transplantation are investigational.

Split-liver transplantation allows two liver transplants from a single deceased donor liver, usually a right lobe implanted into an adult recipient and left lobe or left lateral segment implanted into a pediatric recipient. This technique has the potential to provide grafts to most listed pediatric patients and to decrease substantially the waiting time for adult patients.

Living donor liver transplantation uses the left lateral segment for adult-to-child donation, with a very low risk to the adult donor, who usually is a parent. Good results also have been achieved in recent years with elective adult-to-adult living donor liver transplantation grafting the right lobe (segments 5 to 8), which represents 60 to 65% of the liver, into the recipient. Advantages of living donor liver transplantation include thorough donor screening, optimization of the timing of transplantation, and minimal cold ischemia time. This operation has also been applied to urgent cases with good outcomes. Patients with small hepatocellular carcinomas and those with primary sclerosing cholangitis at risk for cholangiocarcinoma are excellent candidates for a timely living donor liver transplantation. Unfortunately, adult-to-adult living donor liver transplantation is just a partial solution to the donor shortage for adult liver transplantation because only about 15% of potential donors are satisfactory candidates after complete evaluation, and most liver transplantation centers do not routinely pursue this option. The morbidity and mortality rates for the donor average 15 to 30% and 0.3 to 0.5%, respectively, making the operation formidable and necessitating careful informed consent from the donor.

POST-TRANSPLANTATION MANAGEMENT

Allograft dysfunction is the most important complication after liver transplantation. Liver biopsy is critical in differentiating the various causes of dysfunction because many of them share similar but nonspecific clinical and biochemical presentations. Diagnostic evaluations may also include a cholangiogram and duplex ultrasound of the vessels supplying the liver.

Standard Medical Therapies

In general, all patients receive corticosteroids in large intravenous doses during the operation. Steroid doses are rapidly reduced over 5 days and can be discontinued by 3 to 12 months after transplantation in many patients, depending on the underlying disease and the presence or absence of rejection. Either cyclosporine or tacrolimus is initiated at the time of liver transplantation and is used long-term in most patients to prevent acute and chronic allograft rejection. Immunosuppression can be prednisone and a calcineurin agent (cyclosporine or tacrolimus) with early withdrawal of corticosteroids (from 14 days to 3 months after transplantation) followed by use of a calcineurin agent alone. Alternatively, a three-drug regimen (daclizumab, mycophenolate mofetil, and tacrolimus) may reduce rejection and avoid steroid side effects.[2] In patients with renal dysfunction, calcineurin-sparing regimens using mycophenolate mofetil with lower doses of a calcineurin agent or sirolimus alone are used. Calcineurin-sparing regimens reduce the incidence of late renal failure, which approaches 15 to 20% by 20 years after transplantation. Immunosuppressive drugs are typically titrated to therapeutic or slightly subtherapeutic blood levels, but different drug strategies are used in different centers. Other routine medications after liver transplantation include those used for preemptive prevention of viral and fungal infection (see later discussion).

Early Complications after Liver Transplantation

Problems that may occur in the first few days after liver transplantation include hepatic artery thrombosis, portal vein thrombosis, primary graft nonfunction, and hyperacute rejection. Hepatic artery thrombosis, which occurs in about 2 to 8% of adults and in 3 to 20% of children who undergo liver transplantation, is more common among patients who receive sirolimus. Hepatic artery thrombosis typically manifests early after transplantation as fulminant liver failure; occasionally, it occurs 1 to 2 months after transplantation and manifests with stenosis or intimal hyperplasia with eventual rearterialization from collaterals. Early hepatic artery thrombosis is first treated by immediate revascularization through thrombectomy or use of a surgical conduit, but it often requires urgent retransplantation. Hepatic artery stenosis without thrombosis is usually associated with multiple ischemic biliary strictures and manifests somewhat later. Retransplantation is indicated if biliary sepsis or graft failure develops.

Portal vein thrombosis complicates only 1 to 3% of liver transplantation cases. Early acute portal vein thrombosis leads to fulminant liver failure and requires immediate revascularization or urgent retransplantation. Conversely, late portal vein thrombosis manifests as portal hypertension.

Primary graft nonfunction, or delayed ischemia-reperfusion injury, is the most common cause of graft loss within the early postoperative period after a technically successful liver transplantation. The clinical presentation resembles that of fulminant liver failure, with persistent or new hepatic encephalopathy and elevated serum aminotransferase levels (>2500 IU/L).

Initial poor graft function is characteristic of a marginally functioning graft that typically recovers adequate function days to weeks after transplantation. This syndrome has a milder clinical presentation than primary nonfunction, and serum aminotransferases are usually less than 2500 IU/L. Treatment is largely supportive, and most grafts eventually recover.

Acute and Chronic Allograft Rejection

The most common cause of allograft dysfunction after the first postoperative week is acute cellular rejection, which occurs overall in one half to two thirds of cases and is seen within 5 to 30 days of transplantation. The incidence of acute rejection with the use of low-dose prednisone, tacrolimus, and mycophenolate mofetil is 25 to 30%. An acute rejection episode occurring beyond 6 weeks after transplantation should raise suspicion for a subtherapeutic immunosuppressive regimen or for noncompliance with the medical regimen. The patient is usually asymptomatic and presents with increases in serum bilirubin, alkaline phosphatase, and γ-glutamyltransferase in the early post-transplantation course and with predominant elevations in the serum aminotransferases if acute rejection occurs several weeks after transplantation. However, recipients may also present with fever, malaise, abdominal pain, or portal hypertensive changes such as ascites. Histologic examination reveals a mixed portal or periportal inflammatory infiltrate (with neutrophils, eosinophils, plasma cells, and lymphocytes) leading to destructive suppurative cholangitis and endotheliitis. Treatment, which reverses 65 to 85% of episodes, consists of high-dose intravenous corticosteroids, usually 1 g of methylprednisolone, followed by oral prednisone with a rapid taper over 7 days.

Chronic ductopenic rejection now occurs in 2 to 3% of patients, most commonly between 6 weeks and 6 months after transplantation. Cholestatic enzymes, such as alkaline phosphatase and γ-glutamyltransferase, gradually increase for weeks to months before the onset of jaundice that signals the late stage of chronic ductopenic rejection. Histologic evaluation reveals sparse lymphocytic portal inflammation but progressive loss of interlobular and septal bile ducts in at least half of the portal tracts—a condition known as vanishing bile duct syndrome. Approximately 10 to 20% of retransplantations are done because of chronic ductopenic rejection.

Biliary Complications after Liver Transplantation

The biliary tree has very poor regenerative and reparative capacity when damaged and is the most common site for technical complications after transplantation. Biliary complications occur in 10 to 25% of all recipients, with more than two thirds of cases diagnosed within 1 month and 80% within 6 months after transplantation. Causes of biliary complications include technical factors, preservation injury, hepatic artery thrombosis, immunologic factors, and infection, particularly with CMV. Bile leaks and strictures are the most common presentations of biliary complications in the first 3 months after surgery.

Choledochocholedochostomy and choledochojejunostomy are the two methods of primary biliary reconstruction in liver transplantation. The more commonly performed choledochocholedochostomy, or duct-to-duct anastomosis, preserves the sphincter of Oddi and endoscopic access to the biliary tree after transplantation. Choledochojejunostomy, or Roux-en-Y anastomosis, is used for retransplantation, for transplantation of small liver grafts, and in patients with intrinsic disease of the extrahepatic bile ducts, such as primary sclerosing cholangitis.

Bile leakage occurs in up to 25% of all recipients and can be diagnosed by cholangiogram or biliary scintigraphy if the leak is sufficiently large. Patients may present with fever, abdominal pain, peritonitis, hypotension, or sepsis with biloma. For patients who suffer from bile leak after T-tube removal, endoscopic placement of a nasobiliary drain or internal plastic stent allows the leakage to heal as the bile flows preferentially through the ampulla. Surgical creation or revision of choledochojejunostomy should be performed only after failure of endoscopic or radiologic interventions.

Anastomotic biliary stricture, which affects 4 to 10% of all recipients, occurs within the first 6 months after transplantation. Clinical presentation is typical of cholangitis but may be asymptomatic, with only elevation of cholestatic enzymes (predominantly alkaline phosphatase and γ-glutamyltransferase). Balloon dilation or stenting endoscopically or radiologically should be attempted before resorting to surgery. Nonanastomotic biliary strictures, affecting up to 20% of all recipients, occur within the first 4 months after transplantation. The biliary strictures are usually multiple and may be associated with extrahepatic and intrahepatic bile leaks. Management of these strictures depends on their number, location, and severity, as well as liver function. Diffuse strictures in the setting of bile leakage and biloma indicate the need for retransplantation. Focal intrahepatic strictures may benefit from repeated sessions of balloon dilation and stenting performed endoscopically or radiologically.

Infections

Most infections occur within the first 2 months after transplantation, whereas recipients are receiving a high-dose induction immunosuppressive regimen. Bacteria and fungi cause more than 90% of infections during this period. Pneumonia, urinary infection, intra-abdominal and hepatic abscesses, peritonitis, wound infection, and line sepsis are the most common infections. *Candida albicans* is the most common infecting fungal agent in the immediate post-transplantation period. Other frequently seen fungi include *Aspergillus fumigatus* and non-*albicans Candida* species. Despite its nephrotoxicity, amphotericin B is the treatment of choice for invasive fungal infections. Oral fluconazole, 100 mg daily, prevents most fungal infections and is the standard antifungal prophylaxis used for the first 6 weeks after transplantation.

The routine use of trimethoprim-sulfamethoxazole prophylaxis, one single-strength tablet (80/400) daily or one double-strength tablet three times weekly for 3 to 12 months, has made infection with *Pneumocystis jirovecii* (formerly *P. carinii*) rare in liver transplant recipients. Inhalational pentamidine, 300 mg every 4 weeks, and oral dapsone, 50 to 100 mg daily, are alternative prophylactic regimens for patients who are allergic to sulfa. Prophylaxis is administered for 3 months to 1 year after transplantation but should be extended for an extra year if the patient received additional high-dose immunosuppressants (e.g., steroid boluses, muromonab-CD3, increased tacrolimus) during the first year after transplantation.

CMV infection and disease are less common than in the past but remain a risk after liver transplantation. Prophylaxis with acyclovir, ganciclovir, or valganciclovir is effective and reduces mortality[3]; oral valganciclovir (900 mg daily) is most commonly used for the first 3 months after transplantation. Prophylaxis with oral acyclovir (200 mg daily) or valganciclovir is also a useful preventive strategy against the reactivation of oral or genital herpes simplex virus in the first 3 months after transplantation. Reactivation of varicella-zoster virus may manifest as localized dermatomal vesicles or, in patients who were seronegative before transplantation, as cutaneous and visceral dissemination; treatment is with high-dose acyclovir (800 mg four to five times daily for 5 to 7 days).

By 6 months after liver transplantation, recipients who have normal allograft function and are receiving standard doses of immunosuppressive drugs share the same risks as immunocompetent hosts for community-acquired infections and are not at increased risk for opportunistic infections. Conversely, recipients who have been receiving high-dose immunosuppressive drug regimens for antirejection therapy continue to be at high risk for life-threatening opportunistic infections.

Long-Term Follow-up

Long-term management after liver transplantation requires continuing communication and cooperation between the transplantation center and the primary care physician. Patients require careful routine medical management, screening for malignancy, and immunization updates and boosters.

Hypertension

Hypertension (Chapter 67) occurs in two thirds of all liver transplant recipients and is related to cyclosporine and tacrolimus, which cause vasoconstriction in the systemic and renal vasculature, and corticosteroids, which result in sodium retention, increased plasma volume, and weight gain. Management of hypertension in these patients follows a stepwise approach. Dietary sodium restriction, resumption of physical activity, and weight reduction are the first steps. Because of the pathophysiology of vasoconstriction, calcium-channel blockers are the drugs of first choice. The preferred calcium-channel blockers belong to the dihydropyridine class, such as nifedipine. Verapamil, diltiazem, and nicardipine are also effective, but they increase the drug levels of cyclosporine and tacrolimus. Second-line antihypertensive agents include diuretics, β-blockers, and α-adrenergic blockers. Angiotensin-converting enzyme inhibitors should be used with caution because they can aggravate hyperkalemia and, in rare instances, exacerbate leukopenia. Hypertension may improve with time as corticosteroids are discontinued and the dose of cyclosporine or tacrolimus is lowered.

Diabetes Mellitus

Diabetes mellitus (Chapter 237) develops in up to one third of liver recipients after transplantation, with most cases being insulin dependent. The pathogenesis is multifactorial, including genetic predisposition and use of tacrolimus, cyclosporine, and corticosteroids. Steroid tapering is the key to management of early post-transplantation hyperglycemia. Management is otherwise similar to that for the nontransplanted population.

Hyperlipidemia

Hyperlipidemia (Chapter 213) develops in approximately one fourth of all liver transplant recipients. The management of hyperlipidemia includes appropriate dietary restrictions of fat and carbohydrate, weight reduction, regular exercise, and smoking cessation. The preferred medication for patients with resistant hyperlipidemia is 3-hydroxy-3-methylglutaryl coenzyme A (HMG-CoA) reductase inhibitors.

Bone Mineral Density

Bone mineral density decreases during the first few months after transplantation but eventually regains its preoperative level. Fractures most frequently involve trabecular bones such as the vertebrae and the ribs. *Osteonecrosis* or *avascular necrosis* of the hips and, less often, the knees and the humerus bones, may occur. Contributing risk factors to bone disease include preexisting osteopenia, prolonged bed rest, malnutrition, corticosteroids, cyclosporine, tacrolimus, furosemide, and the original diagnosis of primary biliary cirrhosis or primary sclerosing cholangitis with associated metabolic osteodystrophy. Management includes regular exercise and pharmacologic therapies such as calcium supplementation, vitamin D derivatives, and bisphosphonates (Chapter 251).

Cancer

Skin cancer (Chapter 210) is the most common malignancy occurring in the setting of solid-organ transplantation and immunosuppression. Squamous cell carcinoma is more common than basal cell carcinoma or malignant melanoma in this population, and some recipients develop hundreds of squamous cell carcinomas. Patients should seek medical attention if they have a skin growth that bleeds or crusts, increases in size or thickness, or changes in color or texture. Sunscreen with a sun protection factor of at least 15 is recommended. Patients should undergo at least annual skin examinations depending on their previous history of skin cancers.

Colon cancer (Chapter 199) is a common de novo neoplasia after transplantation. Colonoscopic surveillance with multiple biopsies every 6 months for the first 2 years after transplantation, followed by annual examinations, has been recommended for high-risk patients with ulcerative colitis.

If not given before liver transplantation, hepatitis A, hepatitis B, and pneumococcal vaccines (Chapter 17) should be given. Other immunizations include influenza vaccine annually and tetanus toxoid booster every 5 years. Vaccines based on live or attenuated microorganisms should be avoided, including those for measles, mumps, rubella, chickenpox, polio, and bacille Calmette-Guérin (BCG).

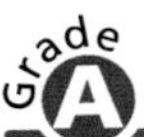

1. Vanlemmens C, Di Martino V, Milan C, et al. Immediate listing for liver transplantation versus standard care for Child-Pugh stage B alcoholic cirrhosis: a randomized trial. *Ann Intern Med.* 2009;150:153-161.
2. Otero A, Varo E, de Urbina JO, et al. A prospective randomized open study in liver transplant recipients: daclizumab, mycophenolate mofetil, and tacrolimus versus tacrolimus and steroids. *Liver Transpl.* 2009;15:1542-1552.
3. Hodson EM, Jones CA, Webster AC, et al. Antiviral medications to prevent cytomegalovirus disease and early death in recipients of solid-organ transplants: a systematic review of randomised controlled trials. *Lancet.* 2005;365:2105-2115.

SUGGESTED READINGS

Bernal W, Auzinger G, Dhawan A, et al. Acute liver failure. *Lancet.* 2010;376:190-201. *Review.*

Dutkowski P, De Rougemont O, Clavien PA, et al. Current and future trends in liver transplantation in Europe. *Gastroenterology.* 2010;138:802-809. *Overview of liver transplantation in Europe.*

Gali B, Rosen CB, Plevak DJ. Living donor liver transplantation: selection, perioperative care, and outcome. *J Intensive Care Med.* 2011. [Epub ahead of print.] *Review of surgical methods and donor risks.*

158

DISEASES OF THE GALLBLADDER AND BILE DUCTS

NEZAM H. AFDHAL

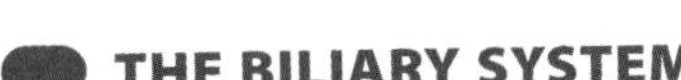

THE BILIARY SYSTEM

Definition

The biliary tract consists of the intrahepatic biliary canaliculus; the small, medium, and large intrahepatic bile ducts; the common bile duct; the gallbladder; the cystic duct; and the ampulla of Vater. The primary functions of the biliary system are secretion and storage of bile salts that solubilize intestinal lipids, excretion of cholesterol to maintain cholesterol homeostasis, excretion of excess bilirubin, and excretion of organic ions, including drug metabolites.

CHOLESTASIS

PATHOBIOLOGY

Cholestasis is the systemic retention of biliary constituents as a result of failure of formation and flow of bile (Table 158-1). In the liver, hepatocytes are organized into cribriform, anastomosing plates along the sinusoids. At the apical pole, between adjacent hepatocytes, is the 1- to 2-μM biliary canaliculus or space. Each hepatocyte can have multiple canaliculi (up to three), which are characterized by microvilli that protrude into the canalicular lumen. Bile consists of water, electrolytes, and organic solutes (Table 158-2). It is continuously modified both by the cholangiocytes that line the bile ducts and by the gallbladder mucosa; therefore, gallbladder bile is markedly different from hepatic bile. The gallbladder mucosa absorbs water and concentrates bile, so the total lipid content of gallbladder bile is much higher than that of hepatic bile (10 vs. 3 g/dL, respectively).

TABLE 158-1 CAUSES OF CHOLESTASIS

EXTRAHEPATIC	INTRAHEPATIC
Choledocholithiasis	Viral hepatitis
Bile duct stricture	Alcoholic hepatitis
Cholangiocarcinoma	Drug induced
Pancreatic carcinoma	Ductopenia syndromes
Chronic pancreatitis	Primary biliary cirrhosis
Papillary stenosis	Benign recurrent intrahepatic cholestasis
Ampullary cancer	Byler's disease
Primary sclerosing cholangitis	Primary sclerosing cholangitis
Choledochal cysts	Alagille's syndrome
Parasites (e.g., *Ascaris, Clonorchis*)	Sarcoid
Acquired immunodeficiency syndrome (AIDS) cholangiopathy	Lymphoma
Biliary atresia	Postoperative
Portal lymphadenopathy	Total parenteral nutrition
Mirrizzi's syndrome	α_1-Antitrypsin deficiency

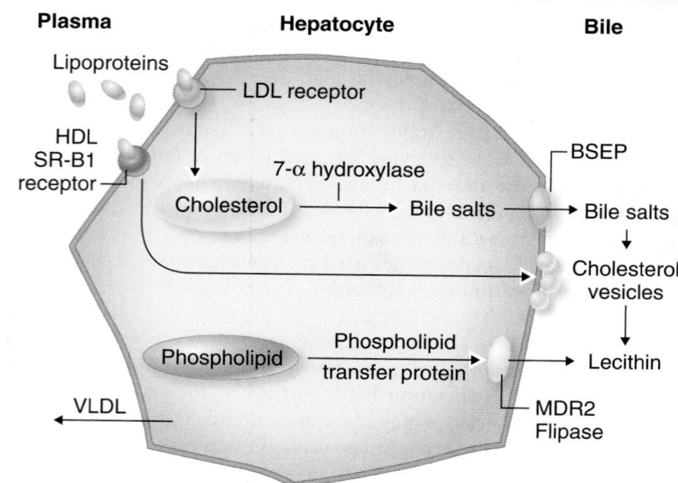

FIGURE 158-1. **Schematic diagram of the metabolism of phospholipid and cholesterol by the hepatocyte.** BSEP = bile salt export pump; HDL = high-density lipoprotein; LDL = low-density lipoprotein; MDR2 = multidrug resistant receptor 2 (a phospholipid lipase highly selective for phosphatidylcholine or lecithin); VLDL = very low density lipoprotein.

TABLE 158-2 CONSTITUENTS OF HUMAN CANALICULAR BILE

Bile salts, 12 g/L Glycine conjugates, 75% Taurine conjugates, 24.8% Free bile acids, 0.2%	Cholates, 35% Chenodeoxycholates, 35% Deoxycholates, 25% Lithocholates, 1% Miscellaneous, 40%
Phospholipids, 5 g/L	Phosphatidylcholine, 96% Phosphatidylethanolamine, 3%
Cholesterol, 1 g/L	Free, unesterified, 99%
Bilirubin, 0.2 g/L	Diglucuronide, 80% Monoglucuronide, 18% Unconjugated, 2%
Proteins, 2 g/L	Albumin, 50% Immunoglobulins, 23% Calcium binding protein/anionic peptide fraction, 17% Serum proteins, 9% Canalicular proteins, 1%
Electrolytes	Sodium, 150 mEq/L Magnesium, 2 mEq/L Calcium, 3 mEq/L Potassium, 5 mEq/L Chloride, 110 mEq/L Bicarbonate, 30 mEq/L

TABLE 158-3 CANALICULAR ATP-BINDING CASSETTE TRANSPORTERS FOR PRIMARY BILIARY CONSTITUENTS

TRANSPORTER NAME	GENE CODE	SUBSTRATE	ASSOCIATED HEREDITARY DISEASE
FIC1	*ATP8B1*	?	PFIC type 1 (Byler's disease)
BSEP	*ABCB11*	Bile salts	PFIC type 2
MDR3	*ABCB4*	Phosphatidylcholine	PFIC type 3
MDR1	*ABCB1*	Amphipathic drugs	
MRP2 (cMOAT)	*ABCC2*	Anionic neutral drugs	Dubin-Johnson syndrome
ABCG5/ABCG8	*ABCG5/8*	Cholesterol	Sitosterolemia

ATP = adenosine triphosphate; BSEP = bile salt export pump; cMOAT = canalicular multispecific organic anion transporter; MDR = multidrug-resistant receptor; MRP2 = multidrug resistance-associated protein 2; PFIC = progressive familial intrahepatic cholestasis.

The major primary bile acids are cholic and chenodeoxycholic acid. The secondary bile acids, lithocholic and deoxycholic acids, which are derived from the intestinal breakdown of primary bile acids, are more hydrophobic, increase in cholestasis, and can be toxic to hepatocytes. Amidation with glycine or taurine results in the formation of bile salts that are preferentially secreted into bile. Bile salts are amphophilic detergent-like molecules synthesized from cholesterol via a pathway dependent on either 7α-hydroxylase or sterol 27-hydroxylase. Bile salt synthesis accounts for approximately 50% of the liver metabolism of cholesterol. Bile salts are secreted into the canalicular space by an energy-dependent bile salt export pump (Fig. 158-1). In the canalicular membrane, bile salts exist as simple (bile salt only) or mixed (with phosphatidylcholine and cholesterol) micelles and are transported into the gallbladder. A fatty meal results in contraction of the gallbladder, with expulsion of bile salts into the duodenum, where they form micelles with intraluminal fat. About 95% of bile acids are absorbed by a sodium-dependent bile acid transporter in the terminal ileum. The total bile acid pool is circulated four to six times per day, and the volume of biliary secretion is approximately 1 L/day. The major phospholipid in bile is phosphatidylcholine, also called lecithin. Phosphatidylcholine in bile is derived from newly synthesized hepatic phosphatidylcholine, which is then transported through the hepatocyte by a phosphatidylcholine transfer protein and delivered to the multidrug resistance receptor 3 (MDR3), a phosphatidylcholine-specific transporter for final secretion into bile (see Fig. 158-1). All biliary lipids, including cholesterol, are secreted in a controlled manner by adenosine triphosphate (ATP)–binding cassette transporters (Table 158-3).

CLINICAL MANIFESTATIONS

The clinical manifestations depend on the location and cause of the obstructive process and the degree to which an associated increase in pro-inflammatory cytokines decreases bile salt synthesis and secretion. Intrahepatic cholestasis is usually the result of either hepatocellular dysfunction or injury to the small and medium bile ducts secondary to viruses, alcohol, or drugs.

Bile salt retention can lead to an excess of hydrophobic bile salts, such as deoxycholate, which are hepatotoxic. These retained bile salts can overflow out of the liver and lead to increased levels of bile salts in the serum and skin; the clinical manifestation is pruritus. Excess cholesterol is deposited in all tissues, particularly as tendinous xanthomas and periorbital xanthelasmas, but clinically significant atherosclerosis is uncommon.

In cholestasis, concentrations of intestinal bile salts are inadequate to solubilize dietary lipids; the result is the excretion of excess nonabsorbed fat. Long-chain dietary fats also irritate the colonic mucosa. Steatorrhea is suggested by the presence of stainable fat in stool and confirmed by quantitative analysis of a stool collection.

Because malabsorption of the fat-soluble vitamins A, D, E, and K can result in deficiency syndromes, fat-soluble vitamins and essential fatty acids should be given as dietary supplements. The combination of osteomalacia and osteoporosis is a serious consequence of cholestasis and chronic liver disease.

DIAGNOSIS

In pure cholestasis, alkaline phosphatase and γ-glutamyltransferase levels are elevated significantly, whereas aminotransferase levels are normal or only mildly increased (Chapter 149). Bilirubin may be elevated but can be normal even in severe intrahepatic cholestasis until the very late stages of disease. Dilation of the intrahepatic ducts on ultrasonography (US) suggests extrahepatic obstructive cholestasis.

TREATMENT (Rx)

Therapy should attempt to remove the cause of cholestasis, such as bypassing an obstructing pancreatic cancer (Chapter 200) with surgery or a stent. In the progressive cholestasis of intrahepatic biliary disease (e.g., primary biliary cirrhosis [PBC]), liver transplantation (Chapter 157) may be the only recourse.

Bile acid binders or sequestrants, such as cholestyramine, can lower the bile acid concentration but are associated with bloating and constipation (Table 158-4). Replacement of hydrophobic bile salts with hydrophilic bile salts, such as ursodeoxycholic acid (UDCA), treats all forms of intrahepatic cholestasis and the associated pruritus. The sensorineural pathway can also be blocked by using opioid antagonists such as naloxone and naltrexone, but care must be taken to avoid the risk for opioid withdrawal syndrome. Hepatic enzyme inducers such as phenobarbital and rifampicin have also been used successfully to treat pruritus. Rifampicin may induce drug-metabolizing transporters, resulting in increased excretion of pruritogens, but with a risk of hepatotoxicity. In some cases of intractable pruritus, marijuana or its synthetic form dronabinol (Marinol) has been useful in controlling symptoms. Finally, for situations such as the intractable pruritus of biliary cirrhosis, liver transplantation is the only option.

Supplementation with calcium, 1500 mg/day, plus vitamin D is essential. If bone density scans show osteopenia, therapy with bisphosphonates should be instituted (Chapter 251).

BILIARY TRACT DISEASES

Lesions of the intrahepatic and extrahepatic biliary tree, including the ampulla of Vater, are rare.

Biliary Atresia

Biliary atresia is a fibro-obliterative process that affects the perinatal bile ducts from the hilar bifurcation to the duodenum in 1 in every 13,000 live births in the United States. Associated genetic abnormalities in 25% of cases include polysplenia, anomalies of the portal vein and hepatic artery, abdominal situs inversus, intestinal malrotation, and cardiovascular and urinary tract anomalies. The clinical findings consist of jaundice with acholic stools persisting for 2 weeks after birth. The diagnosis can be suspected by endoscopic retrograde cholangiopancreatography (ERCP) or magnetic resonance cholangiopancreatography (MRCP) but is usually confirmed by laparotomy. Surgical correction by portoenterostomy should be performed within the first 60 days of life. About 80% of children grow normally through the first years of life, but subsequent stenosis of the anastomosis, with progressive biliary cirrhosis and liver failure, is common and is an indication for liver transplantation.

TABLE 158-4 CLINICAL FEATURES OF AND THERAPY FOR CHOLESTASIS

CLINICAL SYNDROME	TREATMENT
Pruritus	Bile salt binders (e.g., cholestyramine), ursodeoxycholic acid, rifampicin, naltrexone, carbinoids, phenobarbital
Hypercholesterolemia	Bile salt binders (e.g., cholestyramine) Statins—poor effect
Malabsorption	Medium-chain triglycerides, fat-soluble vitamins (A, D, E, K), essential fatty acids
Osteopenia	Calcium, vitamin D, bisphosphonates

Choledochal Cysts

Choledochal cysts are congenital ductal ectasias involving either a segment of the biliary tree or its entirety. The incidence is 1 per 13,000 live births in the United States, but it is 13 times higher in Japan and other parts of Asia. There is a four-fold greater prevalence in females, and choledochal cysts are associated with an abnormal pancreatic ductal junction and congenital hepatic fibrosis. The usual clinical manifestation is a right upper quadrant mass, jaundice, and pain. Acute pancreatitis, cholangitis, variceal hemorrhage, and cyst rupture are alternative findings. The diagnosis is usually made by imaging studies, including US, computed tomography (CT), MRCP, and ERCP. Therapy is generally surgical excision of the cyst with a Roux-en-Y hepaticojejunostomy because of the high (3 to 26%) incidence of malignant transformation of the cysts into cholangiocarcinoma. When there is extensive intrahepatic ductal dilation (Caroli's disease), recurrent cholangitis and intrahepatic stones are common, and liver transplantation is the optimal therapy.

Oriental Cholangiohepatitis

Recurrent cholangitis with hepatolithiasis is endemic in East Asia, especially in Taiwan, where the incidence is as high as 13% in areas where infection with *Ascaris lumbricoides* (Chapter 365) and *Clonorchis sinensis* (Chapter 364) is common. These worms cause local strictures and dilation of the intrahepatic biliary tree. Biliary stasis ensues, and the bile becomes infected with bacteria that are able to deconjugate bilirubin and cause brown stones to form. Recurrent cholangitis is the usual finding, but malignant transformation to cholangiocarcinoma can also occur. The diagnosis is made by US or CT. Treatment includes intravenous fluids and antibiotics. Endoscopic stone removal plus clearance of infected biliary segments is a primary option, but surgical resection of localized segments of the liver may be necessary.

Primary Sclerosing Cholangitis

Primary sclerosing cholangitis is a chronic cholestatic condition characterized by segmental fibrosing inflammation of the intrahepatic and extrahepatic bile ducts.

EPIDEMIOLOGY

The prevalence of primary sclerosing cholangitis is 1 to 6 cases per 100,000 in the U.S. population, with a male-to-female ratio of 2.3 : 1. The mean age at diagnosis is 32 to 40 years, but children can be affected.

PATHOBIOLOGY

The cause remains unknown, but primary sclerosing cholangitis is thought to be a primary autoimmune disease. Genome-wide association studies implicate loci near human leukocyte antigen (HLA)-B on chromosome 6p21 and loci not related to HLA on chromosomes 13q31, 2q35, and 3p21. Even more sophisticated technologies will likely identify specific genes and molecular pathways in the future. The disease is progressive, with the obliteration of small, medium, and large bile ducts leading to three distinct clinical syndromes: (1) cholestasis with eventual biliary cirrhosis, (2) recurrent cholangitis and large duct strictures, and (3) cholangiocarcinoma. The multiple causes of secondary sclerosing cholangitis can be accompanied by symptoms and signs indistinguishable from those of the primary form (Table 158-5).

Primary sclerosing cholangitis is associated with both ulcerative colitis and Crohn's disease of the colon (Chapter 143). Between 70 and 90% of patients with primary sclerosing cholangitis have clinical or microscopic colitis, and between 1.3 and 13% of patients with colitis have primary sclerosing cholangitis. Inflammatory bowel disease usually precedes primary sclerosing cholangitis, but in some cases the colitis is asymptomatic and is discovered by subsequent colonoscopy and biopsy. There is also a crossover syndrome between primary sclerosing cholangitis and primary autoimmune hepatitis (Chapter 151).

CLINICAL MANIFESTATIONS

The most common laboratory finding is an elevated alkaline phosphatase level, which is present in 90% of patients, and mildly elevated aminotransferase levels. The bilirubin level is initially normal in 60% of patients but increases over time and is an important prognostic factor. Autoantibodies, including antinuclear antibodies and anti–smooth muscle antibodies, are seen in 22% of patients, but a positive antimitochondrial antibody (AMA) is rare and suggests PBC. Perinuclear antineutrophilic cytoplasmic antibody (pANCA) is positive in 90% of patients with primary sclerosing cholangitis

TABLE 158-5 DISEASES ASSOCIATED WITH SCLEROSING CHOLANGITIS

PRIMARY SCLEROSING CHOLANGITIS	SECONDARY SCLEROSING CHOLANGITIS
Ulcerative colitis	Choledocholithiasis
Crohn's colitis or ileocolitis	Infections in immunocompromised patients (*Cryptosporidium, Trichosporon*, cytomegalovirus, *Cryptococcus*, visceral protothecosis)
Type 1 autoimmune hepatitis	HTLV-1-associated myelopathy Ischemic injury to the hepatic artery or arterioles Trauma Neoplasia Toxic injury Floxuridine (hepatic artery injection) Formalin injection of echinococcal cysts Congenital abnormalities Celiac sprue

HTLV = human T-lymphotropic virus.

and colitis, but pANCA is nonspecific and is also found in ulcerative colitis and in autoimmune hepatitis without primary sclerosing cholangitis.

DIAGNOSIS

The diagnosis is based on pathologic and radiologic findings, and all patients should undergo both liver biopsy and cholangiography. Large duct disease, which is diagnosed most frequently by ERCP or MRCP, includes strictures, beading, and dilation (Fig. 158-2). Liver biopsy shows an obliterative cholangitis with inflammation and characteristic periductular "onion ring" fibrosis (Fig. 158-3). As the disease progresses, ductopenia and secondary biliary cirrhosis predominate. In stage I, inflammation is confined to the portal tracts; in stage II, there is hepatitis and portal fibrosis; in stage III, bridging fibrosis appears; and stage IV is characterized by biliary cirrhosis and regenerative nodules. Associated conditions include pancreatitis (15% of patients), perihepatic lymphadenopathy, and cholangiocarcinoma (27 to 41% of patients at autopsy or transplantation).

TREATMENT Rx

No treatment slows disease progression. Medical therapy includes treatment of cholangitis and endoscopic therapy for large strictures via balloon dilation and stent insertion. Surgery is avoided, if possible, because it increases the risk for recurrent cholangitis. Immunosuppressive therapy is not effective. In randomized trials, UDCA (15 mg/kg/day) improved bilirubin, alkaline phosphatase, and albumin levels, but it provided no definite benefit in terms of survival or time to liver decompensation. Higher doses (>20 mg/kg) have often been used, but a randomized trial suggested that doses of 28 to 30 mg/kg are not beneficial and may actually increase morbidity when compared with placebo.[1]

Liver transplantation (Chapter 157), which is the only potentially curative therapy, provides an actuarial survival rate of 83% at 1 year and 73% at 5 years. All patients with primary sclerosing cholangitis who undergo transplantation should be screened periodically for colon carcinoma because they have chronic colitis (Chapter 143). Recurrent primary sclerosing cholangitis after transplantation is rare and difficult to distinguish from other causes of bile duct injury. If small (<1 cm), incidental cholangiocarcinomas are found at transplantation, survival is not affected, but larger cholangiocarcinomas (>2 cm) detected during the pretransplant evaluation by CT or magnetic resonance imaging are a contraindication to liver transplantation.

Patients with primary sclerosing cholangitis should be screened for possible cholangiocarcinoma by cholangiography of strictures every 6 to 12 months, with brushings and biopsies. If cholangiocarcinoma is detected, patients should be offered surgical resection or radiation therapy (Chapter 202).

PROGNOSIS

The natural history is variable. Some patients have severe recurrent cholangitis, whereas others progress to biliary cirrhosis. The median survival until death or transplantation is approximately 12 years, with a range of up to 21 years. Actuarial survival is greater for asymptomatic patients than for symptomatic ones (10-year survival rate of 80% vs. 50%).

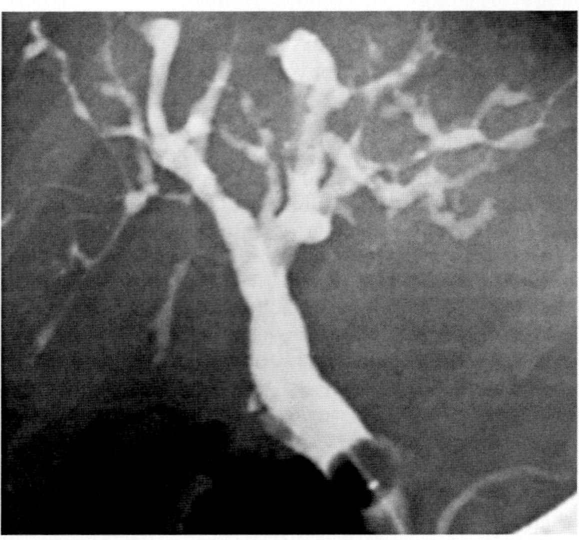

FIGURE 158-2. Endoscopic retrograde cholangiopancreatography for primary sclerosing cholangitis with contrast injected through a balloon catheter (seen in the lower common duct). The intrahepatic ducts are mainly affected and show diminished arborization (pruning); diffuse segmental strictures alternating with normal-caliber or mildly dilated duct segments (cholangiectases) have resulted in a beaded appearance. (From Mahadevan U, Bass NM. Sclerosing cholangitis and recurrent pyogenic cholangitis. In: Feldman M, Friedman LS, Sleisenger MH, eds. *Gastrointestinal and Liver Disease: Pathophysiology/Diagnosis/Management,* 7th ed. Philadelphia: Saunders; 2002:1137.)

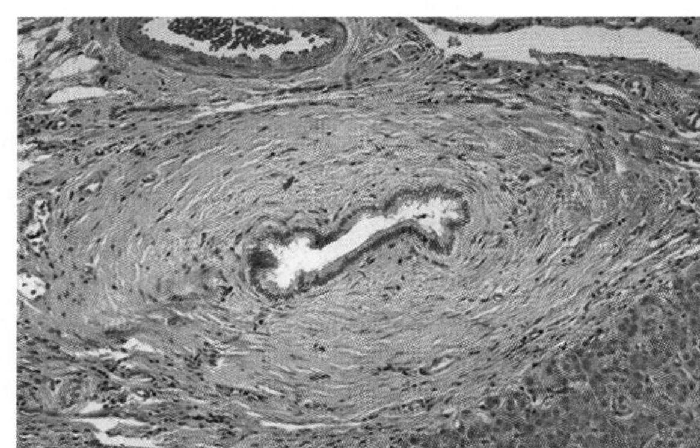

FIGURE 158-3. Microscopically, this bile duct in a case of sclerosing cholangitis is surrounded by marked collagenous connective tissue deposition. (Reproduced from http://library.med.utah.edu/WebPath/GUIDE/INTRO.html with permission.)

Primary Biliary Cirrhosis

DEFINITION

PBC is a slowly progressive, obliterative autoimmune cholangiopathy involving the small and medium-sized bile ducts. It leads to ductopenia, progressive fibrosis, cholestasis, and liver failure.

EPIDEMIOLOGY

PBC is predominantly a disease of women (95% of cases) between the ages of 20 and 60 years. The age- and gender-adjusted prevalence has been estimated at 65 and 12 per 100,000 persons, respectively, for women and men. The incidence of the disease may be increasing, and a U.S. study estimated it at 2.7 per 100,000 person years, or 4.5 and 0.7 for women and men, respectively.

PATHOBIOLOGY

PBC is thought to be an autoimmune disorder, but the mechanism of progressive destruction of the small interlobular ducts is unknown. Genome-wide studies show an association with HLA, interleukin (IL) 12A, and IL-12RB2 variants, suggesting that IL-12 signaling might be important. Mouse models have pointed to the potential roles of IL-12Rα and transforming growth factor-βII receptor. The human disease is slowly progressive and can eventually lead to biliary cirrhosis with portal hypertension and liver failure. The classic histologic finding is the presence of noncaseating granulomas associated with small bile ducts and an overall paucity of bile ducts in the portal tracts. The presence of significant bridging fibrosis or cirrhosis carries a worse prognosis.

CLINICAL MANIFESTATIONS

Almost 60% of patients with PBC are asymptomatic at diagnosis. The most common symptoms are fatigue (50%) and pruritus (30%). Fatigue is unrelated to the degree of underlying liver injury or cholestasis and can be extremely debilitating. Pruritus is often first noticed in pregnancy but persists after delivery, and many patients are initially referred for dermatologic evaluation.

In addition to the features of cholestasis, multiple clinical syndromes are associated with PBC and are suggestive of an autoimmune origin. Autoimmune thyroid dysfunction (Chapter 233), sicca syndrome (Chapter 276), Raynaud's phenomenon (Chapter 275), and celiac disease (Chapter 142) have all been associated with PBC. Metabolic bone disease can be particularly troublesome because of the long duration of cholestasis; bone density studies are mandatory every 2 years to guide and monitor therapy.

DIAGNOSIS

The most common biochemical abnormality is an elevation in serum alkaline phosphatase, which should be confirmed by an elevated γ-glutamyl transpeptidase and indicates cholestasis. The bilirubin level is not elevated until late in the course of the disease, and most of the elevation usually consists of conjugated bilirubin. US should be performed to image the biliary tree and confirm the absence of extrahepatic disease. AMA, which has a sensitivity and specificity higher than 95% when the titer is greater than 1:40, can be positive before there is any clinical or biochemical evidence of PBC. Total immunoglobulins are generally normal, but the immunoglobulin M fraction can be elevated. Liver biopsy is performed to stage the disease and occasionally to confirm the diagnosis, particularly in AMA-negative patients.

TREATMENT Rx

UDCA therapy reduces intracellular hydrophobic bile acids and may have a cytoprotective effect on cell membranes. Although initial randomized trials showed a significant increase in survival after up to 4 years of UDCA therapy (12 to 15 mg/kg), as judged by the time to liver transplantation, a more recent meta-analysis of 16 trials showed no benefit in terms of reducing mortality or delaying liver transplantation.[2] Serum bilirubin, alkaline phosphatase, and cholesterol levels improve with UDCA therapy, but treatment does not relieve the fatigue and has a variable effect on pruritus. Side effects are rare, the most common being diarrhea.

There is no definite benefit from steroids, colchicine, or azathioprine. Low-dose methotrexate (2.5 mg three times/week) has been tried, but data are insufficient to support its routine use at this time. PBC is a common indication for liver transplantation (Chapter 157), but there is considerable debate regarding the timing of transplantation.

PROGNOSIS

PBC is a progressive disease, with up to two thirds of asymptomatic patients becoming symptomatic in 2 to 4 years. Median survival is 9.3 years from diagnosis, and the most reliable determinants of prognosis are the serum bilirubin level and the Mayo risk score, a composite score that predicts clinical outcomes and is calculated as follows: $R = 0.871 \log(e)$ (bilirubin in mg/dL) + 2.53 log(e) (albumin in g/dL) + 0.039 (age in years) + 2.38 log(e) (prothrombin time in seconds) + 0.859 (edema score of 0, 0.5, or 1). Liver failure develops in 26% of patients by 10 years after diagnosis.

Vanishing Bile Duct Syndromes

Vanishing bile duct syndromes are characterized by a paucity of intrahepatic bile ducts and by eventual cholestasis and biliary cirrhosis. Causes include PBC, primary sclerosing cholangitis, autoimmune hepatitis (Chapter 151), graft-versus-host disease, chronic liver allograft rejection (Chapter 157), ischemia, intrahepatic chemotherapy, drug toxicity (e.g., ampicillin, amoxicillin, flucloxacillin, erythromycin, tetracycline, doxycycline, cotrimoxazole), human immunodeficiency virus (HIV) infection (Chapter 397), sarcoidosis (Chapter 95), idiopathic or paraneoplastic bile duct paucity, and histiocytosis. Almost all these conditions are accompanied by chronic cholestasis and elevated alkaline phosphatase levels. Treatment is for the complications of cholestasis, and UDCA (15 mg/kg) is given to increase bile flow. Most of these conditions are slowly progressive and result in biliary cirrhosis, which ultimately requires liver transplantation.

TABLE 158-6 RISK FACTORS FOR GALLSTONE DISEASE

Age
Female gender
Parity
Obesity
Rapid weight loss
Hypertriglyceridemia
Genetic (e.g., Pima Indians, Chileans)
Medications: estrogen, clofibrate, ceftriaxone, octreotide acetate (Sandostatin)
Terminal ileal resection
Gallbladder hypomotility: pregnancy, diabetes, after vagotomy
Somatostatinoma
Total parenteral nutrition
Spinal cord injury

GALLSTONE DISEASE

DEFINITION

There are three different types of gallstones: cholesterol gallstones, mixed gallstones, and pigment stones, which can be further divided into black and brown stones. Cholesterol and mixed stones account for 80% of gallstone disease in the United States. Cholesterol stones contain more than 70% cholesterol, whereas mixed stones also contain significant amounts of pigments such as bilirubin. Black pigment stones, which are generally associated with hemolytic diseases, contain calcium salts, bilirubin, and proteins. Brown pigment stones are more common in Asia, where they are associated with intrahepatic cholangitis and infection; in the United States, brown stones are seen after cholecystectomy, especially when they manifest as choledocholithiasis.

EPIDEMIOLOGY

Approximately 30 million people in the United States have gallstones, and the estimated annual cost of gallstone disease is $15 billion. In Europe, large ultrasound studies in subjects between 30 and 65 years of age have shown gallstones in 18.8% of women and 9.5% of men. In a study in which 1930 subjects were monitored for 10 years, the cumulative incidence of new stones was 4.6%.

Age is a major risk factor for gallstone disease (Table 158-6); less than 2% of cholecystectomies for gallstones are performed in children, usually because of hemolytic diseases. However, the increased prevalence of obesity in children may result in an earlier incidence of gallstone disease.

The age-adjusted female-to-male ratio for gallstone disease is 2.9:1 between the ages of 30 and 39 years, but it decreases to 1.2:1 between the ages of 50 and 59 years. Women with gallstone disease also appear to be more likely than men to undergo cholecystectomy. Pregnancy appears to be the major risk factor for gallstones in younger women, with a prevalence of 1.3% in nulliparous women versus 13% in multiparous women. Estrogen use is also associated with a higher risk for symptomatic gallstones and cholecystectomy: a relative risk of 2.1 to 3.7 versus no estrogen use. The mechanisms of increased risk include activation of estrogen α-receptor-mediated hepatic cholesterol secretion, a progesterone-induced reduction in gallbladder contraction, and a pregnancy-induced alteration in hydrophobic-hydrophilic bile salt balance.

Obesity increases the risk for gallstones as a result of enhanced cholesterol absorption, synthesis, and secretion. The risk is higher in women and in the morbidly obese, but rapid weight reduction by very low-calorie diets is also associated with gallstones. Diets high in polyunsaturated and monounsaturated fats may reduce the risk for gallstone disease.

PATHOBIOLOGY

Gallstone disease is predominantly an inability to maintain free cholesterol in solution in bile. As canalicular bile passes down the bile duct system, cholangiocytes maintain bile flow and volume by secreting chloride, bicarbonate, and water into bile. In cystic fibrosis (Chapter 89), defects in the cystic fibrosis transmembrane conductance regulator, which in the liver is found only on cholangiocytes, reduces choleresis and results in the formation of mucous plugs, with subsequent focal biliary cirrhosis and gallstone disease.

The gallbladder, which acts as the final storage reservoir for bile, concentrates bile by removing water and thereby increasing the lipid concentration from 3 g/dL in hepatic bile to 10 g/dL in gallbladder bile. Bile salt concentrations can be as high as 300 mM and would digest the biliary epithelium if the gallbladder did not secrete mucin for protection. The gallbladder mucosa also secretes hydrogen ions to prevent calcium salt deposition and maintain a bile pH of about 6.5. A normal gallbladder ejects 10 to 20% of its contents in response to duodenal-gallbladder enteric nervous stimulation. Postprandially, duodenal lipids cause an approximately 70% contraction of the gallbladder, mediated by both the enteric nervous system and cholecystokinin. Impaired contractility is one of the critical steps in the pathogenesis of gallstones.

Genetics

Family history studies have shown that gallstones are twice as common in first-degree relatives of gallstone patients as in age- and sex-matched control subjects. In the United States, descendants of the original Amerindians have a markedly increased prevalence of gallstones, with the highest rates in female Pima Indians older than 25 years, who have a 75% prevalence of cholesterol gallstones. Amerindians in South America and Mexico also have a very high prevalence of gallstones, and these populations have the highest rate of complications of gallstone disease, such as gallbladder cancer, in the world. South Americans of Hispanic origin have much lower rates of gallstone disease.

No specific gallstone genes have been found in humans, but lithogenic genes, including the bile salt export pump gene, have been described in gallstone-susceptible mice. Human gallstone disease is probably a combination of complex multigene susceptibility and environmental factors.

Cholesterol Gallstones

Cholesterol gallstones contain 50 to 90% cholesterol and are the most common form of stones in countries where people consume a Western diet high in protein and fat. Cholesterol is an intensely hydrophobic molecule that can remain soluble in aqueous solution only as saturated micelles and vesicles in conjunction with bile salts and lecithin. Cholesterol in gallbladder bile is found in multiple phases; in the presence of cholesterol supersaturation, unstable cholesterol vesicles nucleate to form cholesterol crystals (Fig. 158-4). Nucleation is promoted by a variety of factors, including proteins and lipids.

Increased biliary secretion of cholesterol results in cholesterol supersaturation of bile. The result is excess secretion of mucus into the gallbladder, formation of a gel layer, and stasis, which causes cholesterol to nucleate and cholesterol crystals to be deposited.

Cholesterol monohydrate crystals are only several hundred micrometers in size and should easily be expelled through the cystic duct. However, the mucous sludge containing calcium salts, bilirubin, mucin, and crystals is not easily expelled by contraction of the gallbladder. Biliary sludge, also known as microlithiasis, can be seen as an echogenic, freely mobile mass in the gallbladder on US. Biliary sludge can cause the symptoms of gallstone disease, including cholecystitis, cholangitis, and pancreatitis.

Biliary sludge can resolve, persist, or progress to stones when its crystals grow to form plates, in part because of an impairment in gallbladder contractility. Cholesterol supersaturation of bile is associated with increased absorption of cholesterol by the gallbladder smooth muscle, a process that impairs smooth muscle contractility and reduces the gallbladder's response to cholecystokinin.

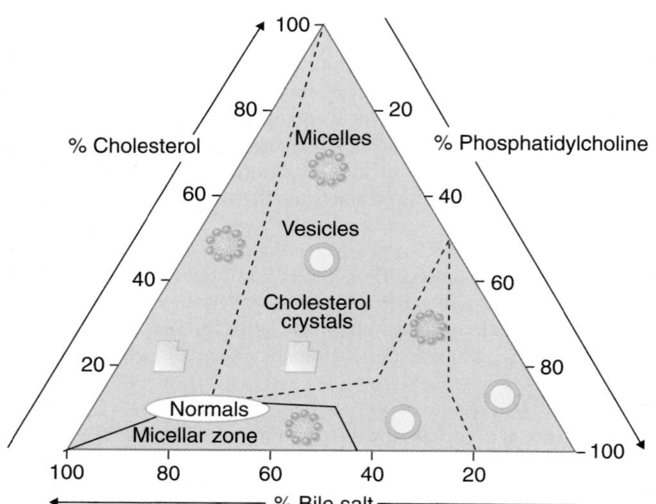

FIGURE 158-4. Equilibrium phase diagram for a lithogenic model bile system with a total lipid content of 10 g/dL.

Pigment Gallstones

Black pigment stones contain 10 to 90% calcium bilirubinate in combination with a variety of other calcium salts, such as hydroxyapatite and carbonate. These stones are common in India (40%) but rare in Minnesota (5%). Older age is associated with a higher incidence of pigment stones, as are total parenteral nutrition and hemolytic diseases.

Brown pigment stones represent 30% of gallstones in Japan and up to 90% of gallstones in rural China. They are related to low-calorie, high-vegetable diets; occur in both the biliary tract and the liver; and have a strong association with recurrent pyogenic cholangitis and cholangiohepatitis. In the United States, these stones are seen as postcholecystectomy cholelithiasis, presumably secondary to stasis and infection. Bacterial enzymes deconjugate bilirubin from its glucuronide and hydrolyze phospholipids, leading to precipitation of calcium, bilirubin, and free fatty acids. These stones, which are often soft and easy to crush endoscopically, are commonly treated by endoscopic extraction.

CLINICAL MANIFESTATIONS

The symptoms caused by gallstones are often nonspecific and include nausea, bloating, and right upper quadrant pain. Biliary pain, which is described as an intermittent right upper quadrant or epigastric pain occurring 15 to 30 minutes after a meal, often with radiation to the back, is unpredictable, severe, and usually constant rather than a true colic. The pain persists for 3 to 4 hours and may be associated with nausea and vomiting. In uncomplicated cholecystitis, fever and leukocytosis are absent, the pain can usually be adequately treated with a single dose of narcotic analgesics or nonsteroidal anti-inflammatory drugs (NSAIDs), and the pain generally subsides within 6 hours. Attacks of colic may be separated by days or months.

DIAGNOSIS

Asymptomatic Gallstones

Asymptomatic gallstones, which are frequently diagnosed by US performed for other indications, account for about 85% of gallstones. Patients with asymptomatic stones have a similar incidence of nonspecific symptoms of nausea and bloating as the general population, and complications of gallstone disease rarely develop. Biliary colic, however, is more predictive of gallstones, and it is an indicator of increased risk for cholecystitis or other complications. Because the current standard of care is to treat only symptomatic stones, it is critical to determine whether any symptoms are related to gallbladder stones.

Among patients with asymptomatic stones, biliary colic develops in about 2 to 3% annually. In the absence of antecedent symptoms, complications of gallstone disease (e.g., acute cholecystitis) develop at a rate of less than 1% per year. As a result, the recommendation is to delay cholecystectomy until after biliary colic develops, with prophylactic or incidental cholecystectomy recommended only for Amerindians, transplant recipients, or patients with sickle cell anemia, morbid obesity, an anomalous pancreatic ductal junction, porcelain gallbladder, or gallbladder polyps larger than 1 cm (see Cholecystectomy under Treatment).

Acute Calculous Cholecystitis

Acute cholecystitis, which is the most common serious complication of gallstone disease, can lead to perforation of the gallbladder, peritonitis, fistula into the intestine or duodenum with gallstone ileus or obstruction, and abscesses in the liver or abdominal cavity. Acute cholecystitis is caused by obstruction of the cystic duct, and the ensuing increased intraluminal pressure can lead to vascular compromise of the gallbladder. *Salmonella* and other less common microorganisms such as *Vibrio cholerae*, *Leptospira*, and *Listeria* can cause primary cholecystitis. Clinical differentiation of biliary colic from acute cholecystitis is difficult but can usually be made from clinical and radiologic findings (Table 158-7).

TABLE 158-7 CLINICAL FEATURES OF BILIARY COLIC COMPARED WITH ACUTE CHOLECYSTITIS

CLINICAL FINDINGS	BILIARY COLIC	ACUTE CHOLECYSTITIS
Right upper quadrant pain	Present	Present
Abdominal tenderness	Absent or mild	Moderate to severe, especially over the liver and/or gallbladder (Murphy's sign)
Fever	Absent	Usually present
Leukocytosis	Absent	Usually >11,000/μL
Duration of symptoms	<4 hr	>6 hr
Ultrasound	Gallstones	Gallstones, thickening of gallbladder wall
HIDA scan	Gallbladder visualized within 4 hr	No filling of gallbladder

HIDA = hepatobiliary iminodiacetic acid.

Blood Tests

In uncomplicated acute cholecystitis, laboratory testing usually shows leukocytosis but otherwise is not very helpful. Elevated liver enzyme levels, hyperbilirubinemia, and elevated amylase or lipase levels are not common in cholecystitis and suggest other complications of gallstone disease, such as cholangitis or pancreatitis. When acute cholecystitis is accompanied by an inflammatory mass, the gallbladder can compress the common duct and lead to bile duct obstruction (Mirrizzi's syndrome).

Imaging Studies

Right upper quadrant US noninvasively diagnoses gallstones in 95% of patients with cholecystitis (Fig. 158-5). US can also exclude common bile duct obstruction and may occasionally show bile duct stones. In cholecystitis, the gallbladder wall may be thickened, and free pericholecystic fluid may be present. Murphy's sign is also useful and can be elicited by the ultrasonographer or on physical examination. Gentle pressure is placed by the probe or hand at the border of the rectus sheath in the right upper quadrant, and the patient is asked to inspire. The gallbladder moves down with inspiration onto the examiner's hand or ultrasound probe, and the patient complains of pain when the inflamed gallbladder comes into contact with the examining hand. US can also exclude gangrenous cholecystitis with free air in the gallbladder wall, perforation, and abscess. The most specific test for acute cholecystitis is a technetium-labeled hepatobiliary iminodiacetic acid (HIDA) scan. Intravenously, HIDA is normally taken up by the liver, excreted into the biliary tract, and concentrated in the gallbladder. When a stone obstructs the cystic duct, the gallbladder fails to fill with HIDA; the sensitivity of HIDA scanning is 95%, but the specificity varies markedly and can be as poor as 50% in critically ill or jaundiced patients.

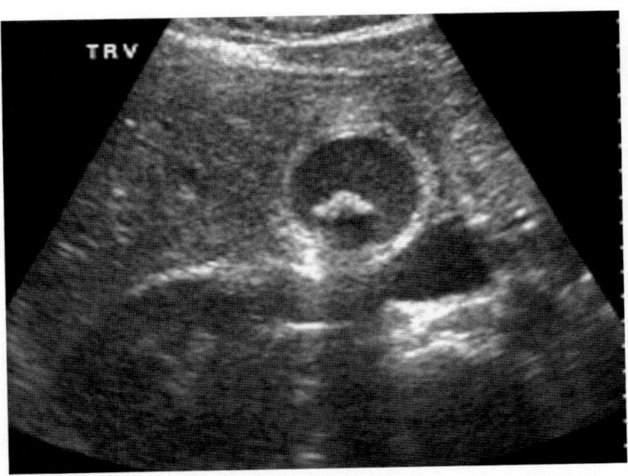

FIGURE 158-5. Ultrasound showing a gallstone.

TREATMENT

Medical Stabilization of Acute Cholecystitis

Treatment of uncomplicated acute cholecystitis is intravenous fluids, antibiotics for 7 to 10 days, and bowel rest. Antibiotic choices include ampicillin (2 g intravenously every 6 hours) and an aminoglycoside (gentamicin 5.1 mg/kg every 24 hours), but cephalosporins (ceftriaxone 1 to 2 g once daily) and ampicillin-sulbactam (1.5 to 3 g every 6 hours) can also be used. Broader coverage should be used in immunosuppressed patients, including the addition of metronidazole (500 mg every 8 hours), piperacillin-tazobactam (3.375 g every 6 hours), and levofloxacin (500 mg to 1 g once daily). Early cholecystectomy during the first hospital admission is generally recommended because it is safe and reduces total hospital stays.[3]

Cholecystectomy

Indications for cholecystectomy include biliary colic, acute and chronic cholecystitis, and acalculous cholecystitis. Diabetic patients may have fewer symptoms because of their neuropathy. As a result, their cholecystitis may be complicated more often by gangrene and perforation; however, prophylactic cholecystectomy is not recommended in patients with diabetes.

Laparoscopic cholecystectomy and small-incision cholecystectomy provide equivalent results for the treatment of gallstones,[4] with some data suggesting that small-incision cholecystectomy reduces operating time and complexity.[5,6] Most patients can be discharged a day after the procedure. A planned laparoscopic approach is changed to open cholecystectomy in only 3% of cases, usually because of difficulty identifying critical anatomic structures such as the cystic or common bile ducts.

Operative cholangiography can be performed during laparoscopic cholecystectomy, and bile duct stones can be removed concurrently or subsequently by ERCP. The incidence of unsuspected, retained common bile duct stones after laparoscopic cholecystectomy is about 2.3%.

The most serious complication of cholecystectomy is bile duct injury, which now occurs in 0.25% of cases. It is more common when the indication for surgery is acute cholecystitis, and it is less common after a surgeon has performed more than 25 laparoscopic surgeries. Bile duct injuries include cystic duct leak, laceration of the duct, complete transection of the duct, and thermal injuries to the duct. Early recognition permits primary open bile duct repair. Leakage from the cystic duct is usually recognized by jaundice, fever, and abdominal pain several days after the procedure; it can be treated successfully by ERCP, with insertion of an endoscopic stent, or by sphincterotomy.

Gallstone Dissolution Therapies

In patients who have relative or absolute contraindications to laparoscopic cholecystectomy, such as concomitant advanced cardiopulmonary or liver disease, a combination of chenodeoxycholic acid (10 mg/kg/day) and UDCA (7 to 15 mg/kg/day) or UDCA alone (15 mg/kg/day) can dissolve multiple small (<5 mm) stones in up to 60% of patients with functioning gallbladders. If CT shows the stones to be calcified, the efficacy is lower, and complete dissolution occurs in only about 10% of patients. Gallstones generally dissolve at a rate of 1 mm/month. After dissolution, gallstones recur at a rate of 10% per year for 5 years, but recurrence is unusual after that time. Continuous therapy may be necessary, thereby making this treatment unattractive except in selected patients in whom cholecystectomy cannot be performed safely.

Extracorporeal shock wave lithotripsy, which uses a focused ultrasound beam, can fragment larger stones. The fragmented stones can then be passed through the cystic duct and expelled into the common bile duct. The fragments that remain behind in the gallbladder should be treated with UDCA for dissolution. Gallstones disappear in more than 50% of patients, but they recur in 50% of successfully treated patients, particularly those with multiple stones and poorly functioning gallbladders.

Topical dissolution therapy involves the insertion of a catheter into the gallbladder under ultrasound guidance; stones are dissolved with methyl tert-butyl ether or ethyl propionate. The technique is still experimental but may soon be ready for widespread testing.

Choledocholithiasis

Common bile duct stones can descend from the gallbladder or arise de novo in a tortuous, dilated common bile duct as a result of infection and biliary stasis (usually cholesterol stones), or they can occur in a postcholecystectomy patient (usually brown stones), in whom they are frequently missed at surgery (2% of cholecystectomies). The clinical findings are cholangitis, pancreatitis, or biliary obstruction; large, obstructing stones can cause jaundice.

Acute bacterial cholangitis, which is most frequently caused by common duct stones that obstruct the common bile duct and raise intrabiliary pressure, is a medical emergency (Fig. 158-6). The bile in these patients is generally infected with *Escherichia coli*, *Bacteroides*, *Klebsiella*, or *Clostridium* species, and the increase in pressure results in transient bacteremia.

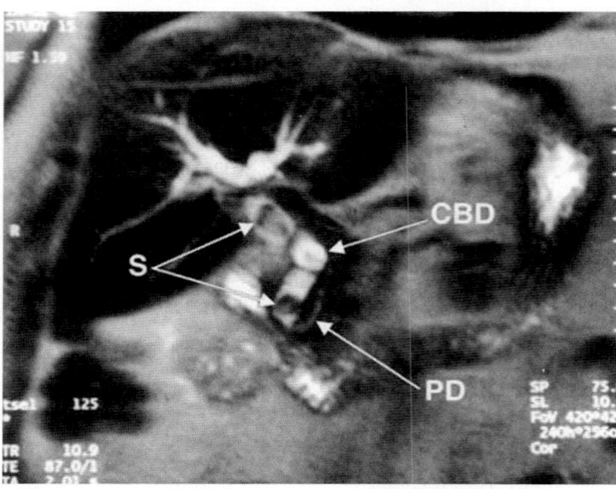

FIGURE 158-6. **Magnetic resonance cholangiopancreatogram of a dilated biliary tract.** The common bile duct (CBD), pancreatic duct (PD), and two large common duct stones (S) are shown.

DIAGNOSIS

Patients with bacterial cholangitis have Charcot's triad of jaundice, abdominal pain, and fever with rigors. Severe renal dysfunction and disseminated intravascular coagulation can complicate severe cholangitis. Aminotransferase, bilirubin, and alkaline phosphatase levels are usually increased. The diagnosis of common bile duct stones can be made with US, which generally shows dilated bile ducts and occasionally identifies a stone. MRCP can identify 95% of stones larger than 1 cm (see Fig. 158-6). ERCP remains the "gold standard" for the diagnosis and treatment of common bile duct stones. If cholangitis is suspected, ERCP should be performed.

TREATMENT Rx

In patients with concomitant stones in both the gallbladder and the common bile duct, laparoscopic cholecystectomy and bile duct exploration are preferable to a two-stage procedure (ERCP extraction of the common duct stone followed by laparoscopic cholecystectomy).[7,8] For isolated common duct stones, endoscopic therapy includes sphincterotomy and stone extraction with a balloon or basket. Small (<2 cm) stones can be removed easily, whereas larger stones may be crushed with mechanical or ultrasound lithotriptors before removal. Fluids and antibiotics with broad gram-negative coverage (e.g., ceftriaxone 1 to 2 g once daily, ampicillin-sulbactam 1.5 to 3 g every 6 hours, piperacillin-tazobactam 3.375 g every 6 hours, levofloxacin 500 mg to 1 g once daily) are recommended for bacterial cholangitis. In an acutely ill patient, initial decompression of a pus-filled common bile duct with a stent may be the first-line treatment, followed by definitive endoscopic or surgical therapy. After successful endoscopic therapy, laparoscopic cholecystectomy should be performed routinely because of the high risk for recurrent biliary events.[9]

In certain situations, such as after Roux-en-Y choledochojejunostomy, ERCP may not be possible. Alternative approaches include radiologic percutaneous transhepatic cholangiography (PTC) or open exploration of the common bile duct. During PTC, the radiologist can decompress the bile ducts with catheters or stents, and the stones can be removed through the fistula tract by direct cholangiography.

Unusual Complications of Gallstone Disease

Gallstone pancreatitis (Chapter 146) is more common in patients with multiple small stones; it has also been associated with microlithiasis and biliary sludge. Patients have acute epigastric pain radiating into the back, hyperamylasemia, and an imaging study that demonstrates an edematous or necrotic pancreas. Rarely, concomitant cholangitis or jaundice can be seen if the stone is obstructive. Clinical features that suggest gallstone pancreatitis include elevated aspartate aminotransferase and alkaline phosphatase levels. Early ERCP with sphincterotomy plus stone extraction within 24 hours of suspected acute gallstone pancreatitis reduces morbidity and mortality, but in 50% of cases, the stones are not visible or have passed by the time of ERCP. After the successful treatment of common duct stones, any patient who still has a gallbladder should have it removed electively.

Vascular compromise to the gallbladder and the presence of gas-forming bacteria, which are more common in patients who have diabetes or are immunocompromised, can cause gangrenous or emphysematous cholecystitis. Clinically, patients are usually very ill with a high temperature, features of systemic sepsis, and obtundation. US may show air in the gallbladder or gallbladder wall; perforation of the gallbladder with peritonitis may then occur. Emergency cholecystectomy is required.

If a fistula develops from the gallbladder to the duodenum, stomach, or colon, a large gallstone can pass through the fistula and into the bowel. If obstruction occurs at the duodenum or the ileocecal valve, gallstone ileus occurs, with symptoms and signs of intestinal obstruction. A plain abdominal radiograph shows bowel obstruction with free air in the gallbladder or biliary tract. Treatment is generally cholecystectomy and removal of the obstructing gallstone.

PREVENTION

UDCA, 600 mg at night, markedly reduces gallstone formation in patients on low-fat, low-calorie diets. Primary prevention of cholesterol gallstones is based on dietary alteration to avoid cholesterol supersaturation (i.e., a diet rich in whole grains and roughage and low in cholesterol and saturated fats). Secondary prevention includes using bile acid therapy with UDCA to reduce cholesterol supersaturation, improving gallbladder motility with cholecystokinin analogues, and reducing mucin secretion with aspirin and NSAIDs. All these strategies have been used effectively in high-risk groups, such as patients on low-calorie diets or those maintained on total parenteral nutrition.

PROGNOSIS

Overall, the prognosis of gallstone disease is excellent for younger and otherwise healthy patients. However, with the aging population, there is a higher prevalence of complicated gallstone disease with common duct stones, cholangitis, and pancreatitis, each of which is associated with substantial morbidity and mortality.

ACUTE ACALCULOUS CHOLECYSTITIS

EPIDEMIOLOGY AND PATHOBIOLOGY

Acalculous cholecystitis is inflammation of the gallbladder or the presence of gallbladder-related symptoms in the absence of stones. Acute acalculous cholecystitis accounts for 2 to 17% of all cholecystectomies. Ischemia, infection, chemical injury by biliary contents, and obstruction of the cystic duct have all been implicated as causes (Table 158-8).

TABLE 158-8 RISK FACTORS AND ORGANISMS ASSOCIATED WITH ACALCULOUS CHOLECYSTITIS

RISK FACTORS
Fasting
Total parenteral nutrition
Septicemia, biliary infections
Major trauma
Burns
Major nonbiliary surgery
Childbirth
Multiple blood transfusions
Mechanical ventilation
Opiates
Immunosuppression—chemotherapy, HIV infection, transplantation
Diabetes
Ischemic heart disease
Malignancy
ORGANISMS IMPLICATED AS A PRIMARY CAUSE
Salmonella typhi
Vibrio cholerae
Staphylococcus
Leptospira
Listeria
Pneumocystis carinii
Mycobacterium spp
Cytomegalovirus
Candida
Ascaris
Echinococcus

CLINICAL MANIFESTATIONS

Primary infection may manifest as acute cholecystitis with unexplained fever, right upper quadrant pain, or clinical deterioration postoperatively or after transplantation, trauma to the abdomen, chemotherapy, or total parenteral nutrition. Pain, fever, leukocytosis, and abnormal liver enzyme test results are common.

DIAGNOSIS

The diagnosis is confirmed by US showing a distended gallbladder, often with a thin wall, pericholecystic fluid, or a positive Murphy's sign (see earlier) in the absence of gallstones. Sludge may be present. Intraluminal gas or bubbles, the so-called champagne sign, indicates emphysematous cholecystitis.

TREATMENT

Rx

Treatment includes intravenous fluids, antibiotics as for gallstone disease, and general supportive measures. Because gangrene and perforation are more common in acalculous than calculous cholecystitis, urgent cholecystectomy is recommended. Postcholecystectomy complications such as leak, abscess, and wound infection are also more common and reflect the underlying multisystemic problems. In severely ill patients in whom cholecystectomy is contraindicated, radiologic decompression of the gallbladder via percutaneous cholecystostomy can be performed. The overall mortality associated with acute acalculous cholecystitis is 5 to 20%.

CHRONIC ACALCULOUS CHOLECYSTITIS

Chronic acalculous cholecystitis is a poorly understood clinical syndrome in which patients have symptoms of biliary colic in the absence of gallstones. The gallbladder may be normal or show changes of chronic inflammation. Cholesterolosis may also be present, with deposits of cholesterol in the mucosa and muscle layers of the gallbladder. Affected patients, who are often young and female, have abdominal pain and nonspecific symptoms such as nausea and intolerance of fatty food. Biliary dyskinesia may be diagnosed by food-cholecystokinin-stimulated US or a HIDA scan. In 80 to 90% of patients with abnormal stimulated motility, symptoms are relieved by cholecystectomy.

GALLBLADDER CANCER

Gallbladder cancer constitutes 0.76 to 1.2% of all cancers and is the most common biliary cancer, with about 7200 new cases reported in the United States each year. The highest incidence occurs in Amerindians, particularly in Chile, Mexico, and Colombia. Its incidence is also high in India, perhaps owing to the higher prevalence of pigmented gallstones. Gallbladder cancer is a disease of the elderly and is more common in women than in men. There is a strong association with cholelithiasis, chronic cholecystitis, and inflammation; 90% of patients with gallbladder cancer have concomitant stones. Patients who have a porcelain gallbladder, defined as calcification of the gallbladder wall, have a 25% risk for the development of gallbladder cancer, and patients with an anomalous pancreatic ductal junction in which the pancreatic duct drains into the lower common bile duct instead of the ampulla have an increased risk for gallbladder cancer. Both these lesions are indications for prophylactic cholecystectomy.

About 90% of gallbladder cancers are adenocarcinomas; the remainder are squamous cell or other cancers. Gallbladder cancer spreads locally, with invasion of the liver and to the local lymph nodes and peritoneal cavity. About 90% of patients have symptoms and signs suggestive of cholecystitis. Surgery, which is the only therapeutic option, can be curative when the tumor is confined to the gallbladder. Adjuvant radiation therapy and chemotherapy are not effective. The median survival for all patients with gallbladder cancer is 3 months, with a 1-year survival rate of 14% and a 5-year survival rate of 5%.

DISORDERS OF THE AMPULLA OF VATER

The ampulla of Vater is the final sphincter that controls entry of bile into the duodenum. Hormonal control of the sphincter is mediated by cholecystokinin, which causes the gallbladder to contract and the ampulla to relax. The most common disorder of the ampulla is stenosis or dysfunction after cholecystectomy, the so-called sphincter of Oddi dysfunction.

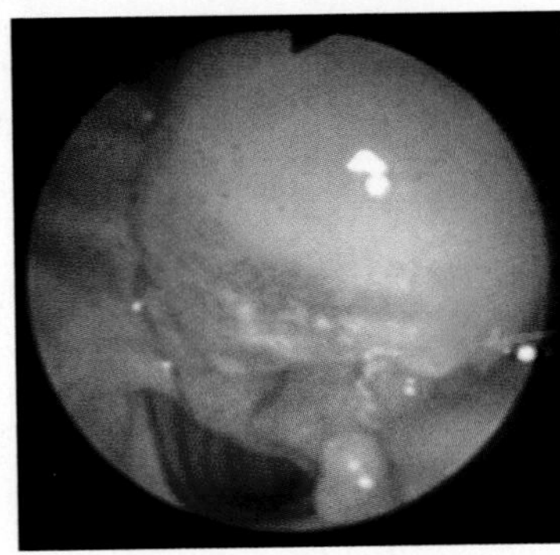

FIGURE 158-7. Carcinoma of the ampulla of Vater. The carcinoma can be seen toward the bottom of the picture. The bulging swelling above is the grossly dilated common bile duct, which is obstructed by the carcinoma. (From Forbes CD, Jackson WF. *Color Atlas and Text of Clinical Medicine*, 3rd ed. London: Mosby; 2003.)

Sphincter of Oddi Dysfunction or Biliary Dyskinesia

In true sphincter stenosis, the sphincter is narrowed by inflammation and fibrosis secondary to pancreatitis, passage of a gallstone through the papilla, intraoperative trauma, infection, or adenoma. Sphincter stenosis can manifest as abdominal pain and pancreatitis. The common bile duct is often dilated above the stenosis, and treatment is a large sphincterotomy performed at ERCP.

In sphincter of Oddi dyskinesia, a functional disorder of the sphincter leads to intermittent biliary obstruction. Most patients have undergone cholecystectomy and are being evaluated for recurrent biliary pain or, less frequently, pancreatitis. The diagnosis is usually made by ERCP, which can demonstrate delayed excretion of contrast material. In patients who have pain associated with abnormal aminotransferase levels on two or more occasions, a dilated common bile duct, and delayed drainage of contrast material, sphincterotomy is recommended. Patients without all three of these criteria are usually given a trial of relaxants, such as nitrates or calcium-channel blockers.

Ampullary Tumors

Adenocarcinoma of the ampulla has an incidence of 3 per million. Adenomas appear as protruding ampullary lesions, may grow either inside the ampulla or into the duodenum, and can transform into adenocarcinomas (Fig. 158-7). The cancer tends to be locally invasive. Ampullary adenomas are associated with familial adenomatous polyposis (Chapter 199) and the *APC* gene: almost 80% of patients with the *APC* gene have adenomas of the ampulla, and their risk for ampullary cancer is significantly higher than that of the normal population.

The average age at diagnosis is 50 years, with a peak at 70 years; there is no gender predilection. About 80% of patients have jaundice, which is usually progressive and associated with abdominal pain and weight loss. Liver enzymes are generally abnormal, and the diagnosis is suggested by US or CT findings of dilated biliary and pancreatic ducts all the way to the ampulla. Confirmation is by endoscopy, with biopsy and brushings. Staging of the tumor, particularly for lesions growing into the ampulla, is best performed by endoscopic US. Adenomas and small cancers can be removed by endoscopic ampullectomy. The standard, recommended curative operation is pancreaticoduodenectomy (the Whipple procedure), which provides a 25 to 55% 5-year survival rate, depending on the extent of the tumor. Adjuvant chemotherapy and radiation therapy have no proven benefit in the treatment of ampullary lesions.

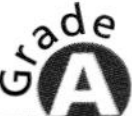

1. Poropat G, Giljaca V, Stimac D, et al. Bile acids for primary sclerosing cholangitis. *Cochrane Database Syst Rev*. 2011;1:CD003626.
2. Gong Y, Huang ZB, Christensen E, et al. Ursodeoxycholic acid for primary biliary cirrhosis. *Cochrane Database Syst Rev*. 2008;3:CD000551.
3. Gurusamy K, Samraj K, Gluud C, et al. Meta-analysis of randomized controlled trials on the safety and effectiveness of early versus delayed laparoscopic cholecystectomy for acute cholecystitis. *Br J Surg*. 2010;97:141-150.
4. Keus F, Gooszen HG, van Laarhoven CJ. Systematic review: open, small-incision or laparoscopic cholecystectomy for symptomatic cholecystolithiasis. *Aliment Pharmacol Ther*. 2009;29:359-378.
5. Keus F, Werner JE, Gooszen HG, et al. Randomized clinical trial of small-incision and laparoscopic cholecystectomy in patients with symptomatic cholecystolithiasis: primary and clinical outcomes. *Arch Surg*. 2008;143:371-377.

6. Keus F, Gooszen HG, van Laarhoven CJ. Open, small-incision, or laparoscopic cholecystectomy for patients with symptomatic cholecystolithiasis. An overview of Cochrane Hepato-Biliary Group reviews. *Cochrane Database Syst Rev* 2010;1:CD008318.
7. Rogers SJ, Cello JP, Horn JK, et al. Prospective randomized trial of LC+LCBDE vs ERCP/S+LC for common bile duct stone disease. *Arch Surg.* 2010;145:28-33.
8. Bansal VK, Misra MC, Garg P, et al. A prospective randomized trial comparing two-stage versus single-stage management of patients with gallstone disease and common bile duct stones. *Surg Endosc.* 2010;24:1986-1989.
9. Boerma D, Rauws EA, Keulemans YC, et al. Wait-and-see policy or laparoscopic cholecystectomy after endoscopic sphincterotomy for bile-duct stones: a randomised trial. *Lancet.* 2002;360: 761-765.

SUGGESTED READINGS

Barie PS, Eachempati SR. Acute acalculous cholecystitis. *Gastroenterol Clin North Am.* 2010;39:343-357. *Ultrasound of the gallbladder is most accurate for diagnosis.*

Ishibashi H, Komori A, Shimoda S, et al. Risk factors and prediction of long-term outcome in primary biliary cirrhosis. *Intern Med.* 2011;50:1-10. *Review emphasizing sustained serologic presence of anti-gp 210 antibodies as a risk factor.*

Shakespear JS, Shaaban AM, Rezvani M. CT findings of acute cholecystitis and its complications. *AJR Am J Roentgenol.* 2010;194:1523-1529. *Acute cholecystitis is unlikely with a normal CT scan, but an abnormal CT scan requires follow-up with abdominal ultrasound.*

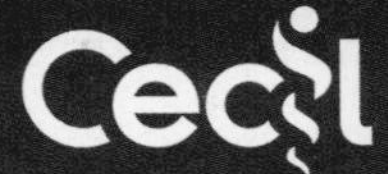

XIV

HEMATOLOGIC DISEASES

159

HEMATOPOIESIS AND HEMATOPOIETIC GROWTH FACTORS

KENNETH KAUSHANSKY

Hematopoiesis is the process by which bone marrow stem cells develop all of the cell types present in the blood (erythrocytes, neutrophils, eosinophils, basophils, monocytes, platelets, T lymphocytes, B lymphocytes, and natural killer cells) (Fig. 159-1). The regulation of the numbers of each cell type is carefully controlled by paracrine and endocrine hematopoietic growth factors, which exert antiapoptotic, proliferative, and differentiating effects on hematopoietic stem, progenitor, and maturing blood cells. Many of these glycoproteins are produced by recombinant DNA technology and have been among the most successful therapeutics in modern medicine.

HEMATOPOIETIC STEM AND PROGENITOR CELLS

Hematopoietic stem cells represent one in 10^5 to 10^6 bone marrow cells, are not morphologically distinguishable from other progenitors or small lymphocytes, but can be purified to homogeneity using physical characteristics and combinations of monoclonal antibodies to cell surface proteins. The two critical characteristics of a hematopoietic stem cell are its abilities to differentiate into all blood cell types and to self-renew. The decision to self-renew or differentiate is a stochastic process, at the stem cell stage and at the subsequent multipotent or unipotent stages of differentiation, that can be influenced by a number of cell extrinsic (growth factors and stromal proteins) and cell intrinsic (transcription factors) molecules.

HEMATOPOIETIC CELL EXPANSION—HEMATOPOIETIC GROWTH FACTORS

A large number of transcription factors regulate stem cell number and differentiation state. Several molecular switches have been identified that determine hematopoietic cell fate.

Equally important to hematopoiesis as the transcription factors is a group of hematopoietic growth factors, which share structural homology and bind to nonredundant type I transmembrane proteins belonging to the cytokine receptor family. Many of these proteins are the physiologic regulators of a specific lineage of blood cells; others appear to represent redundant hematopoietic growth-promoting activities of molecules essential for other biologic functions. Erythropoietin, granulocyte colony-stimulating factor (G-CSF), and thrombopoietin serve as examples of the former; interleukin-3 (IL-3), granulocyte-macrophage colony-stimulating factor (GM-CSF), and IL-11 serve as examples of the latter class of hematopoietic growth factors.

Erythropoietin is produced predominantly by the kidneys, and to a lesser extent in the liver, and acts on marrow erythroid progenitors to enhance their survival, proliferation, and differentiation. Levels of erythropoietin are inversely related to hemoglobin concentrations in the blood, as reflected in renal oxygen tension. In the presence of tissue (renal) hypoxia, the transcription factor hypoxia-induced factor (HIF)1α is stabilized against proteasome-mediated destruction and drives erythropoietin transcription by binding to a critical hypoxia-responsive element located in the 3′ untranslated region of the gene. Genetic elimination of erythropoietin or its receptor results in embryonic lethality, establishing that although other cytokines can influence erythropoiesis, red cell production is absolutely dependent on the hormone.

G-CSF stimulates the production of neutrophils from their marrow progenitors (Fig. 159-2). Levels of the hormone are also inversely related to neutrophil numbers but are regulated primarily by inflammatory stimuli, including tumor necrosis factor-α and IL-1α, acting on endothelial cells, fibroblasts and macrophages. Like the action of erythropoietin on erythroid progenitors, G-CSF acts to enhance the survival, proliferation, and differentiation of neutrophil progenitors. In addition, the cytokine acts to functionally activate the mature cells it helps to produce. Genetic elimination of G-CSF or its receptor in mice reduces neutrophil levels to 25% of normal, the only hormone known to exert this great an impact on granulopoiesis.

Thrombopoietin, the primary regulator of platelet production, is produced in the liver and kidney and by marrow stromal cells and is regulated by both platelet receptor–mediated uptake and destruction and by transcription feedback inhibition of the thrombopoietin gene in marrow stromal cells b platelet granule proteins. Like G-CSF, thrombopoietin stimulates the survival, proliferation, and differentiation of its corresponding lineage and megakaryocytes and their precursors, and also prime mature platelets to respon to platelet activation agonists. Genetic elimination of thrombopoietin or its receptor in mice and congenital non-sense or missense mutations in the thrombopoietin receptor in humans result in platelet levels approximate 10% of normal at birth, and in humans leads to aplastic anemia by 1 to 2 yea of age.

Other cytokine-receptor systems related to erythropoietin, G-CSF, an thrombopoietin essential for one or more aspects of hematopoiesis includ IL-7, critical for all types of lymphocyte production; IL-5, the primary regulator of eosinophil production; IL-4, responsible for immunoglobulin cla switching in B lymphocytes; IL-15, essential for normal natural killer ce differentiation; and IL-2, a lymphocyte activation cytokine. They displa modest effects on blood cell growth, but their genetic elimination fails t affect basal or stimulated production of those cells.

A second class of cytokines and receptors that influences hematopoiesis exemplified by the c-kit receptor, a member of the receptor tyrosine kinas family of surface proteins, and its cognate ligand, stem cell factor (also terme *steel* factor or *kit-ligand*). Although the c-kit receptor is structurally distin from members of the hematopoietic cytokine receptor family, possessing a intrinsic tyrosine kinase motif in its cytoplasmic domain, stem cell factor structurally related to the cytokines that bind to members of the hematopoietic growth factor family. Genetic elimination of stem cell factor or the c-k receptor results in the near elimination of hematopoietic stem cells, erythroi precursors, and basophils and mast cells. Two other hematopoietic membe of this family of cytokines and receptors are Flt3 ligand and its receptor Flt- and monocyte colony-stimulating factor and its receptor, c-Fms. Like ster cell factor, both Flt3 ligand and monocyte colony-stimulating factor pla nonredundant roles in hematopoiesis, inducing the formation of dendrit cells and monocytes, respectively.

The molecular mechanisms by which the hematopoietic growth facto affect blood cell survival, proliferation, and differentiation are becomin increasingly well understood. Binding of cognate ligand to each of the hema topoietic cytokine receptors results in activation of one or more tyrosin kinases, either tethered cytoplasmic kinases of the Janus (JAK) family for th hematopoietic cytokine receptor family, or the intrinsic kinase of the cyto kines that employ the receptor tyrosine kinase class of receptors (stem ce factor, Flt3 ligand, and monocyte colony-stimulating factor). Once activate these kinases phosphorylate tyrosine residues within the cytoplasmi domains of each receptor, providing docking sites for cytoplasmic signalin intermediates possessing Src homology (SH)2 domains. Among the bes characterized SH2 domain–containing proteins that bind to hematopoieti receptors are nascent transcription factors, such as the signal transducers an activators of transcription (STAT) proteins, adapter proteins, includin Grb2, Gab1, tensin2 and SHC, phosphatases (e.g., SHP1 and SHP2), and th regulatory subunit (p85) of phosphoinositol-3-kinase (PI3K). Once boun to one or more of the newly induced phosphotyrosine residues of the cyto kine receptor or receptor tyrosine kinase, these secondary molecules ar phosphorylated, either by the JAK kinase or by other kinases, making ther competent to bind additional molecules (e.g., the adapters that ultimatel activate Ras, and p85 PI3K that binds its kinase [p110] subunit) or are acti vated as transcription factors (e.g., STATs). The downstream effector mole cules then activated include a number kinases, transporter molecules, an transcription factors, ultimately leading to hematopoietic cell survival, proli eration, and differentiation.

CLINICAL USES OF HEMATOPOIETIC CELLS AND GROWTH FACTORS

The clinical development of erythropoietin, G-CSF, and thrombopoieti mimetics represents some of the very best examples of harnessing recombi nant DNA technology for therapeutic benefit. Patients with renal failure widespread inflammation, or marrow replacement and those undergoing che motherapy for cancer all suffer from variable degrees of anemia, often ver debilitating. Clinical trials have demonstrated the efficacy of recombinan erythropoietin in patients with renal failure and with cancer and inflamma tion. Administration of the drug almost invariably results in a rapid reticulo cyte response and correction of the anemia. The only patients who regularl demonstrate a poor response are individuals with severe inflammation. Mos

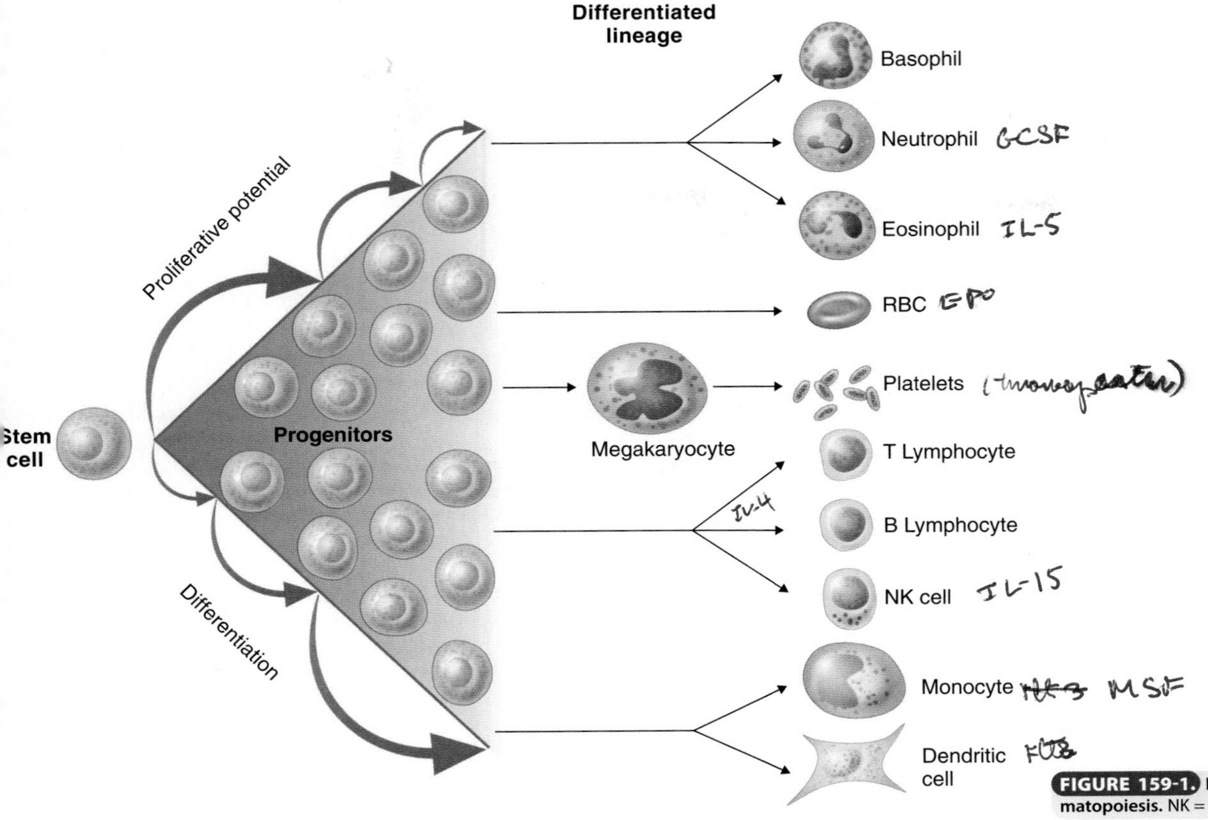

Differentiated lineage
Proliferative potential
Stem cell
Progenitors
Differentiation
Basophil
Neutrophil
Eosinophil
RBC
Megakaryocyte
Platelets
T Lymphocyte
B Lymphocyte
NK cell
Monocyte
Dendritic cell

FIGURE 159-1. Hierarchical model of lymphohematopoiesis. NK = natural killer; RBC = red blood cell.

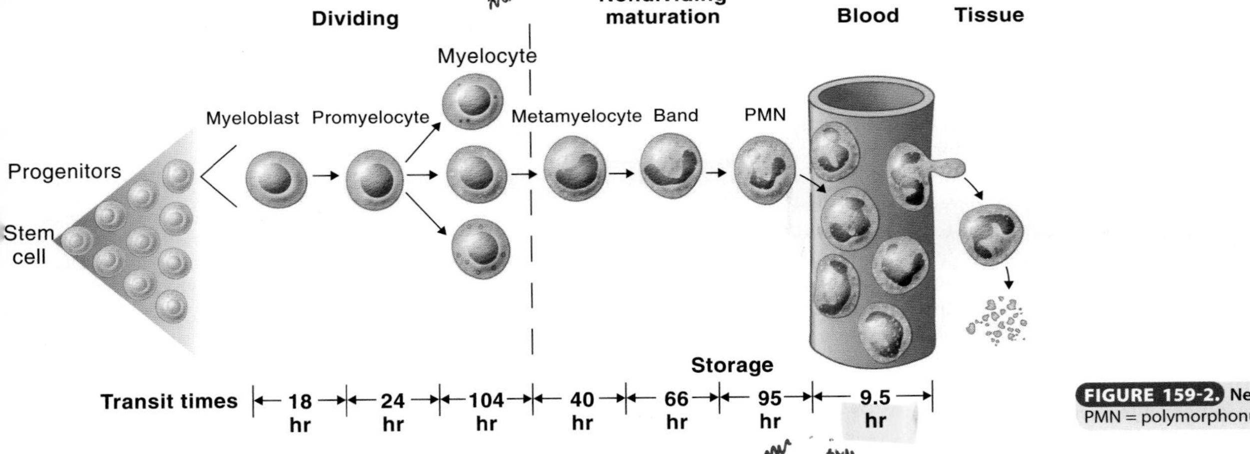

FIGURE 159-2. Neutrophil production system. PMN = polymorphonuclear leukocyte.

patients undergo an enhanced sense of well-being as the blood hemoglobin concentration rises to 10 g/dL. However, quality-of-life studies of doses of erythropoietin higher than those needed to result in a hemoglobin level of 10 g/dL failed to further enhance patient well-being and surprisingly resulted in a number of adverse effects. For example, patients receiving the drug for anemia secondary to kidney failure progressed to requiring dialysis more frequently and experienced greater cardiovascular events, such as myocardial infarction and stroke, than patients on low levels of the hormone sufficient to maintain their blood hemoglobin at 10 g/dL. Patients receiving erythropoietin for cancer also experienced greater relapses of their tumors than individuals not receiving the hormone. Overall, erythropoietin is a safe and effective drug for anemia due to a wide range of conditions, but its use and dose must be carefully considered.

Many patients undergoing cytotoxic therapy for cancer experience severe neutropenia and are thus at substantial risk for life-threatening infection. Clinical trials of recombinant G-CSF in patients undergoing aggressive chemotherapy for leukemia and solid tumors resulted in the U.S. Food and Drug Administration (FDA) approval of the drug for use in patients undergoing chemotherapy of intensity sufficient to produce severe neutropenia. The use of the drug is associated with the more rapid return of neutrophils to safe levels if administered soon after the inciting chemotherapy is completed, but not at the nadir of neutrophil production, and results in lower numbers of severe infections. However, the use of G-CSF has not enhanced survival in patients with any tumor type. Like the use of erythropoietin in patients with cancer, the administration of G-CSF to some patients receiving cytotoxic chemotherapy for cancer (e.g., breast cancer) has been associated with a statistically significant increase in cancer recurrence, although this finding is controversial.

Thrombopoietin was cloned and characterized in 1994 and was quickly advanced to clinical trials following the model of G-CSF use in patients undergoing cancer chemotherapy. Initial results with the intact hormone and a truncated version that included only the receptor-binding domain were mixed, and use of the truncated form of the drug, administration to healthy volunteer donors to improve platelet apheresis yields, resulted in a significant number of subjects developing antidrug antibodies, which cross-reacted with their native thrombopoietin, resulting in severe thrombocytopenia. This

experience caused both manufacturers of thrombopoietin to cease clinical trials. Instead, a series of small molecule mimics have been developed that bind to the thrombopoietin receptor and stimulate thrombopoiesis. Two such drugs are approved by the FDA for use in patients with severe immune thrombocytopenia, one a peptibody, which contains four thrombopoietin receptor–binding peptides grafted onto an immunoglobulin scaffold, and one a small organic molecule that is orally bioavailable and binds to a spatially distinct site on the thrombopoietin receptor. The use of each drug results in a high rate of platelet responses into the normal range in patients with severe immune thrombocytopenia (Chapter 175) who were refractory to conventional therapies. However, because thrombopoietin mimics do not affect the underlying immune destruction of platelets and megakaryocytes in patients with this disease, discontinuation of each drug results in rapid relapse to thrombocytopenia. Current clinical trials in other settings of transient myelosuppression are expected to improve platelet recovery but not be associated with rapid relapse.

Visit expertconsult.com for e-expanded chapter

SUGGESTED READINGS

Kaushansky K. Lineage specific hematopoietic growth factors. *N Engl J Med.* 2006;354:2034-2045. *Overview of the biochemistry, cell biology, clinical use, and potential side effects of these products of recombinant DNA technology.*

Laiosa CV, Stadfeld M, Graf T. Determinants of lymphoid-myeloid lineage diversification. *Ann Rev Immunol.* 2006;24:705-738. *Review of the cell intrinsic (transcription factors) and cell extrinsic (cytokines) factors that determine cell phenotypes.*

Yannaki E, Stamatoyannopoulos G. Hematopoietic stem cell mobilization strategies for gene therapy of beta thalassemia and sickle cell disease. *Ann N Y Acad Sci.* 2010;1202:59-63. *Overview of approaches for gene-engineered stem cell therapy.*

160 THE PERIPHERAL BLOOD SMEAR

BARBARA J. BAIN

With the development of sophisticated automated instruments to count and characterize blood cells, Romanowsky (Wright-Giemsa or May-Grünwald-Giemsa)-stained peripheral blood smears are now performed on only a minority of blood specimens received in a hematology laboratory. Nevertheless, the blood smear remains important for a number of reasons: it can (1) verify the result of an automated instrument, (2) provide an immediate specific diagnosis, or (3) indicate a narrow range of diagnostic possibilities, permitting a focused rather than indiscriminate investigation. A blood film can provide a rapid diagnosis in cases in which speed is crucial, such as in acute promyelocytic leukemia, thrombotic thrombocytopenic purpura, or Burkitt's lymphoma. Sometimes a smear provides unexpected information that is of value in patient management.

Usually, blood smears are initially interpreted by a laboratory scientist. In some countries it is customary for clinicians to examine the blood smears of their own patients because the clinician has the final responsibility for integrating all information and making a diagnosis. However, the interpretation of a blood smear can be difficult, and a trained laboratory hematologist or hematopathologist has a major role in interpreting smears that may have been initially examined by a laboratory scientist. It is crucial that, when requesting a blood count, the clinician provide all the essential information needed to interpret the count and any associated smear. Regardless of whether the clinician examines the blood film, he or she must be able to interpret the written report issued by the laboratory. To do so, the clinician must be familiar with the terms generally used by laboratory staff and the possible significance of the abnormalities described. The most important of these terms are illustrated in Figures 160-1 through 160-20.

REASONS FOR PERFORMING A BLOOD SMEAR

A blood smear may be requested by a clinician or initiated by a laboratory scientist or a laboratory hematologist. Clinical findings that should lead a clinician to request a blood smear are summarized in Table 160-1.

Laboratory scientists and physicians may initiate a blood smear that has not been requested by the clinician if the clinical details indicate the possibility of a significant hematologic abnormality. However, they are

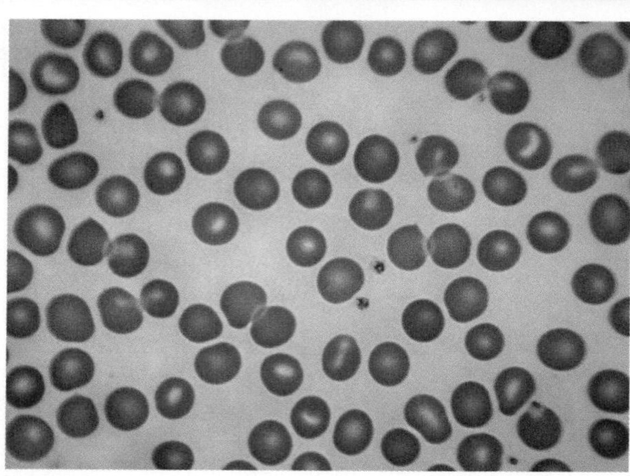

FIGURE 160-1. Normal peripheral blood smear. These normal red cells are described as *normocytic* (i.e., of normal size) and *normochromic* (i.e., their staining characteristics are normal). Normal erythrocytes are biconcave discs, causing them to have an area of central pallor that does not exceed one third the diameter of the cell. There are also scattered normal platelets (×1000).

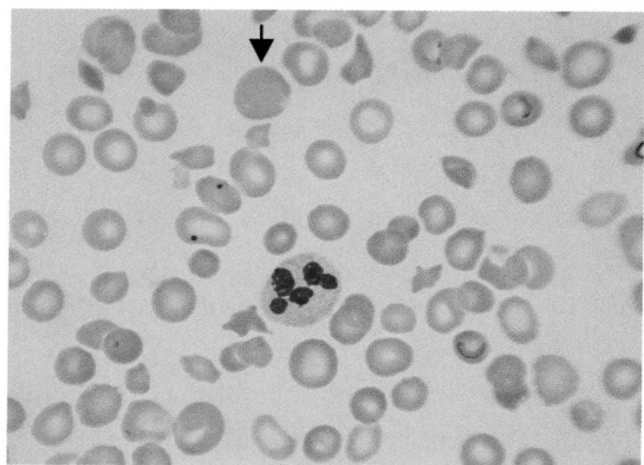

FIGURE 160-2. Smear showing multiple abnormalities. There is *anisocytosis,* defined as an increased variation in cell size; *poikilocytosis,* defined as an increased variation in cell shape; and *polychromasia,* defined as the presence of erythrocytes with a blue tinge to their cytoplasm—indicating a young cell recently released from the bone marrow in which the polychromasia is due to the presence of RNA. *Polychromatic cells* are erythrocytes with a blue tinge; because polychromatic cells are larger than normal mature erythrocytes, they are known as *polychromatic macrocytes (arrow).* The film also shows two cells containing bluish purple *Howell-Jolly bodies;* these inclusions are nuclear remnants (×1000).

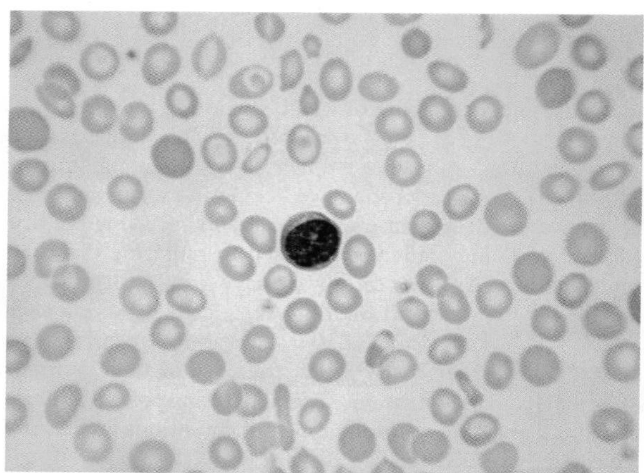

FIGURE 160-3. Microcytic red cells from a case of thalassemia minor. In a blood smear, a *microcyte* can be defined as a cell with a diameter less than that of the nucleus of a normal small lymphocyte. There are also some cells showing *hypochromia,* an area of central pallor that is larger than one third of the diameter of the red cell. In addition, there are two *target cells,* with a hemoglobinized area in the center of the area of pallor (×1000).

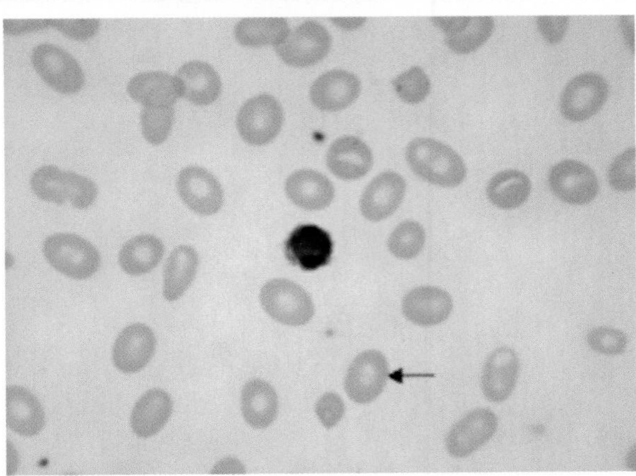

FIGURE 160-4. Macrocytic anemia. A *macrocyte* is recognized on a blood film as a cell with a diameter that is considerably greater than that of the nucleus of a small lymphocyte. In addition, this smear shows *oval macrocytes* (also known as *macro-ovalocytes*), defined as cells that are larger than normal and oval in shape *(arrow)*. They are of considerable diagnostic importance, being characteristic of megaloblastic anemia; they can also be seen in dyserythropoiesis (×1000).

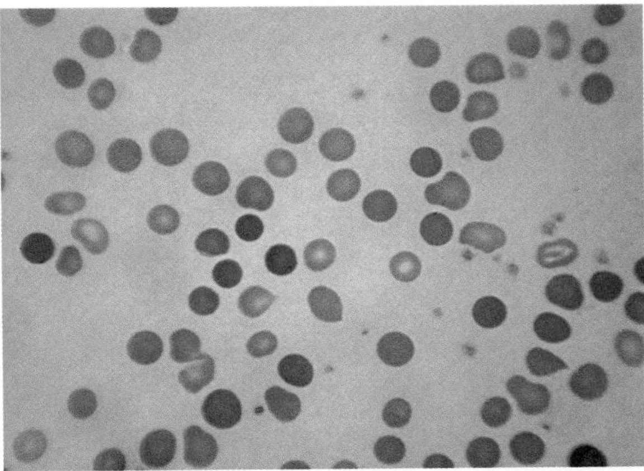

FIGURE 160-5. Hereditary spherocytosis. A *spherocyte* is a red cell that lacks central pallor because of its spherical shape. In hereditary spherocytosis, there are usually cells in which the central pallor is reduced rather than absent, and they are intermediate in shape between a spherocyte and a *discocyte*, which is an erythrocyte with the normal shape of a biconcave disc (×1000).

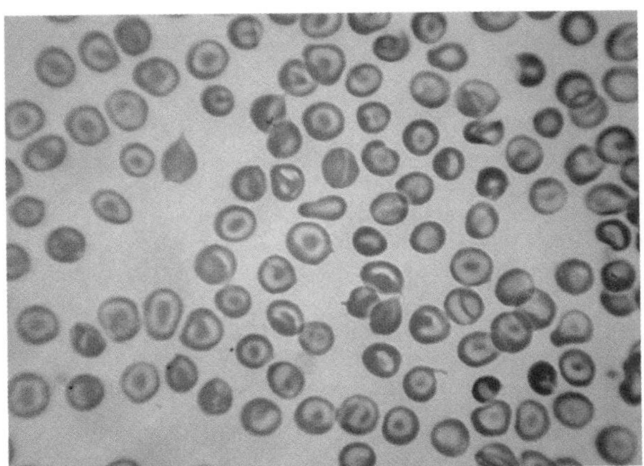

FIGURE 160-6. Target cells. A *target cell* is an erythrocyte with a hemoglobinized area in the middle of the normal area of central pallor (×1000).

also likely to evaluate a blood smear in response to abnormalities revealed by an automated instrument. These abnormalities may be quantitative or qualitative. Quantitative abnormalities that require evaluation include anemia, polycythemia, macrocytosis, microcytosis, neutrophilia, lymphocytosis, eosinophilia, thrombocytopenia, and thrombocytosis.

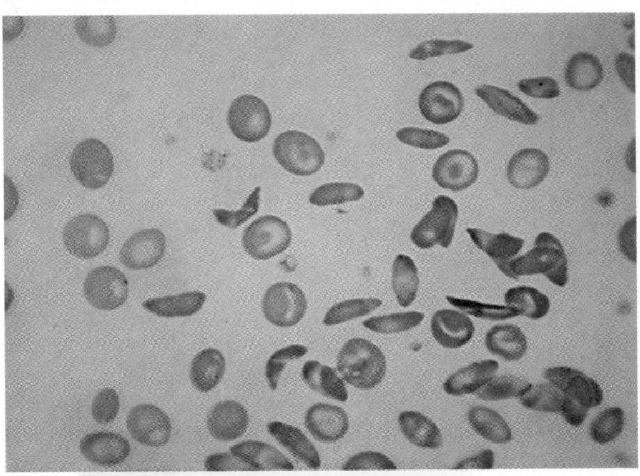

FIGURE 160-7. Sickle cells. A *sickle cell* is a cell with a sickle or crescent shape resulting from the polymerization of hemoglobin S. These cells are seen not only in sickle cell anemia (homozygosity for hemoglobin S) but also in compound heterozygous states such as sickle cell/hemoglobin C disease and sickle cell/β-thalassemia, which also lead to sickle cell disease. This smear also shows target cells and boat-shaped cells with a lesser degree of polymerization of hemoglobin S than in a classic sickle cell (×1000).

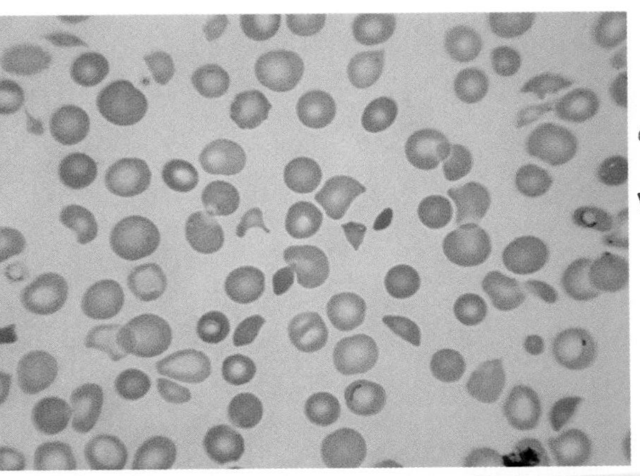

FIGURE 160-8. Red cell fragmentation. *Red cell fragments* or *schistocytes* are defined as fragments of erythrocytes. In addition to small angular fragments, there may be *microspherocytes,* cells of reduced size and spherical in form (also known as *spheroschistocytes*), and *keratocytes,* cells with two horn-like projections. Schistocytes are seen in microangiopathic hemolytic anemias and in mechanical hemolysis (×1000).

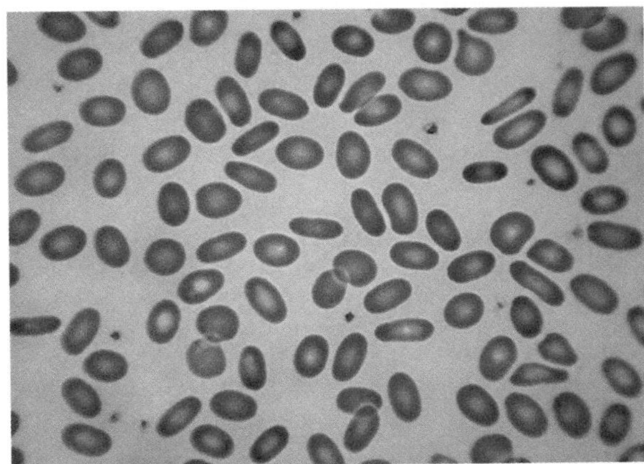

FIGURE 160-9. Hereditary elliptocytosis. An *elliptocyte* is an elliptical red cell. When seen in the numbers present in this smear, they are indicative of hereditary elliptocytosis; smaller numbers are seen in other conditions such as iron deficiency anemia, in which they are sometimes referred to as *pencil cells* (×1000).

Modern automated instruments are able to "flag" the presence of qualitative abnormalities that require a blood film to be examined for confirmation of the abnormality or for further elucidation. "Flags" are generated in response to the electrical impedance or the light scattering characteristics of individual cells. Some instruments are dependent on cytochemical

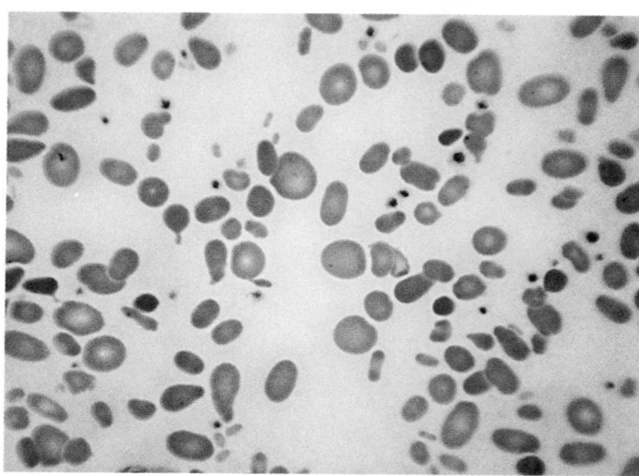

FIGURE 160-10. Hereditary pyropoikilocytosis. This smear shows striking poikilocytosis, including elliptocytes, microspherocytes and other fragments, and teardrop cells. This congenital condition, which is related to hereditary elliptocytosis, usually results from the inheritance of two different mutated genes from the two parents and is characterized by a severe hemolytic anemia (×1000).

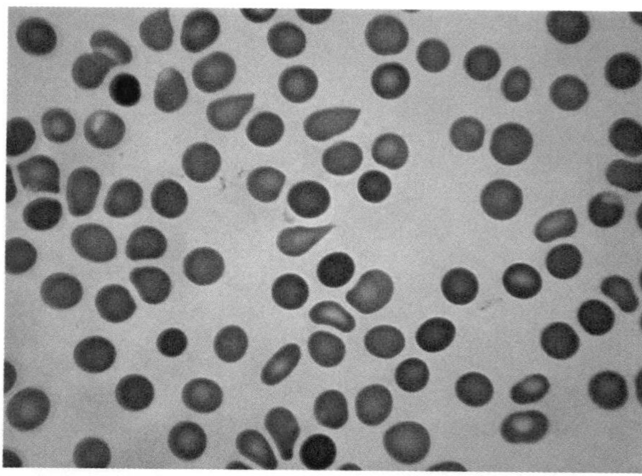

FIGURE 160-11. Teardrop poikilocytes. *Teardrop poikilocytes,* or *dacrocytes,* are teardrop-shaped red cells; they are characteristic of primary myelofibrosis but are also seen in megaloblastic anemia (×1000).

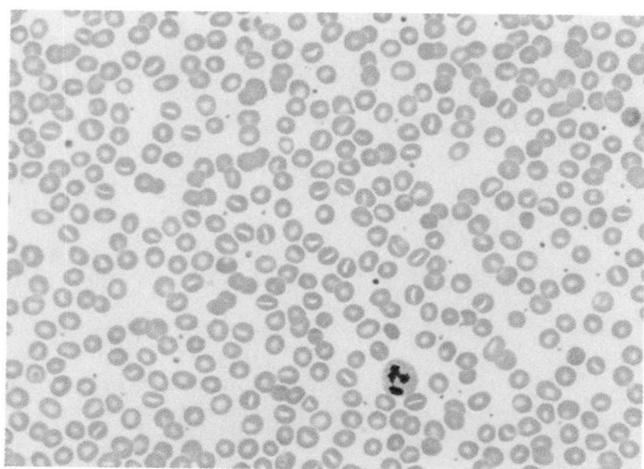

FIGURE 160-12. Stomatocytosis. A *stomatocyte* is a cell that appears to have a central mouth-shaped or slit-like stoma. Among the less common causes is hereditary stomatocytosis. Alcohol and hydroxycarbamide therapy are more common causes (×400).

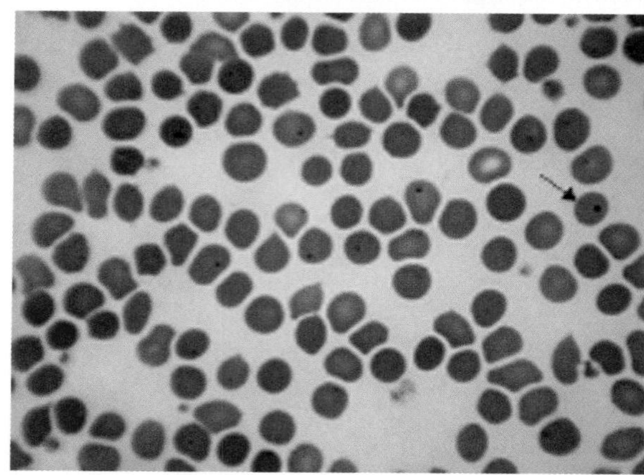

FIGURE 160-13. Numerous Pappenheimer bodies. A *Pappenheimer body* is an iron-containing red cell inclusion *(arrow)*. It is smaller and more angular than a Howell-Jolly body and stains navy blue rather than purple. Pappenheimer bodies are seen following splenectomy and in sideroblastic anemias (×1000).

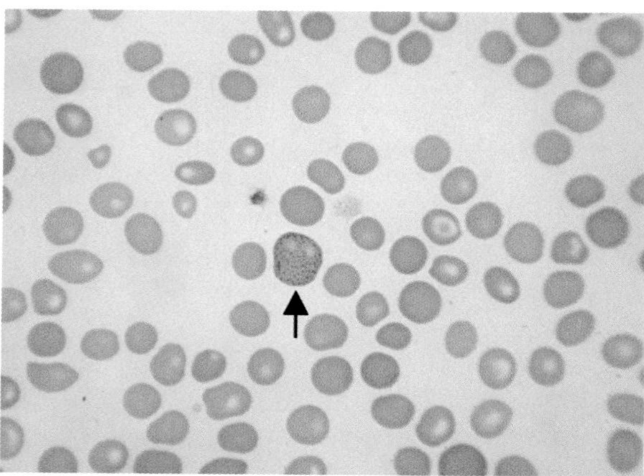

FIGURE 160-14. Basophilic stippling. *Basophilic stippling* means that there are fine (as in this case) or coarse purplish blue dots dispersed through the red cell *(arrow)*. They are a very nonspecific feature occurring in thalassemia trait, lead poisoning, 5′-nucleotidase deficiency, and dyserythropoiesis in general (×1000).

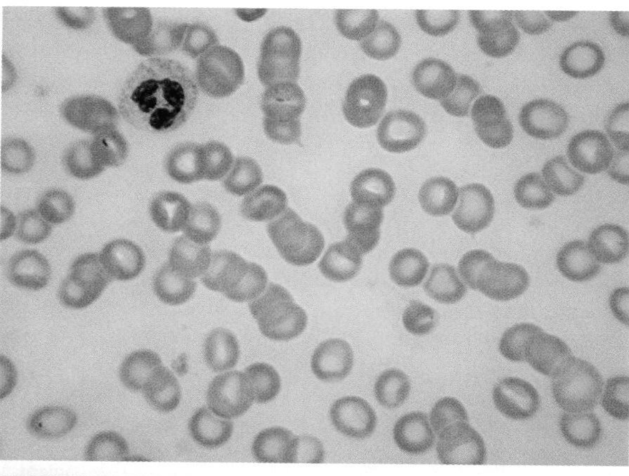

FIGURE 160-15. Rouleau formation. *Rouleaux* are stacks of red cells, often compared to stacks of coins. They result from an increase of high-molecular-weight globulins in the plasma, either as a reactive change or as a result of secretion of a paraprotein in a plasma cell neoplasm (×1000).

reactions of cells or on the cells' ability to polarize light. Most instruments can indicate the possibility of the presence of blast cells, reactive or other atypical lymphocytes, granulocyte precursors, or nucleated red blood cells. Instruments using a cytochemical reaction for peroxidase to help identify neutrophils, eosinophils, and monocytes may flag the appearance of large, unstained (i.e., peroxidase-negative) cells; such cells may indicate a harmless inherited peroxidase deficiency, but sometimes such cells are lymphoma cells, reactive lymphocytes, or leukemic blast cells. Instruments often flag the possibility of an erroneous platelet count, such as when there is an overlap in size between platelets and red cells or when light scattering characteristics suggest the presence of platelet aggregates (a potential cause of pseudothrombocytopenia).

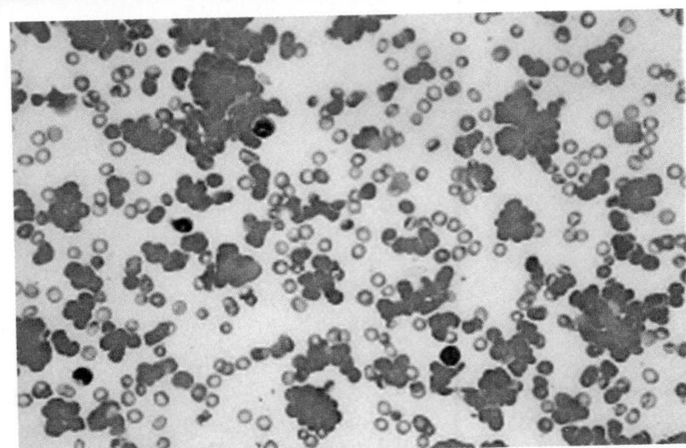

FIGURE 160-16. **Red cell agglutination.** *Red cell agglutinates* are irregular aggregates of red cells, as seen in *Mycoplasma pneumoniae* infection. They are also seen in other infections, such as infectious mononucleosis, and in chronic cold hemagglutinin disease (×100). (Courtesy of Jean Schafer.)

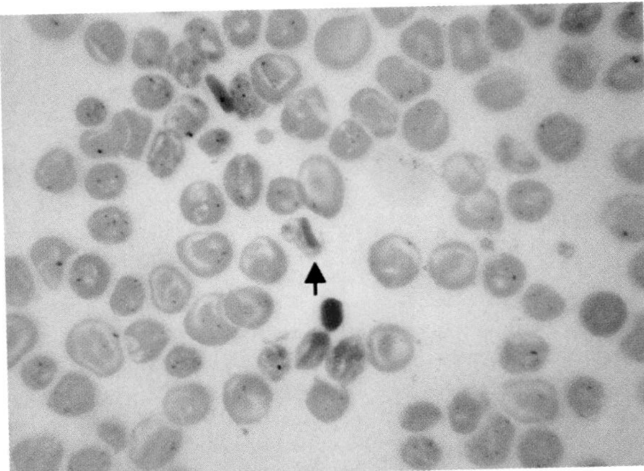

FIGURE 160-17. **Homozygous hemoglobin C.** Three *hemoglobin C crystals* are present, one indicated by an arrow. Hemoglobin C crystals are usually six-sided, with a long axis having parallel edges (×1000).

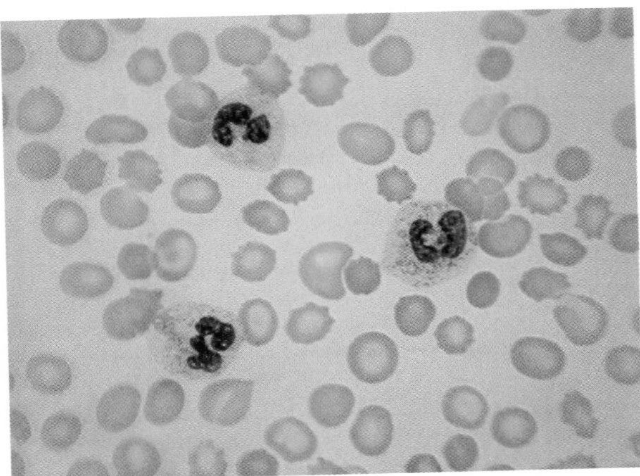

FIGURE 160-18. **Toxic granulation.** *Toxic granulation* refers to heavy staining of azurophilic granules of neutrophils. When accompanied by neutrophil vacuolation, it is often indicative of infection, but it can also result from inflammation, tissue damage, and normal pregnancy (×1000).

International consensus guidelines indicate which automated instrument results require blood smear review. Whether a review is needed is determined in part by whether that specimen is the first one obtained from that patient and whether there has been a significant change from a previously validated result (referred to as a delta check). Laboratory computers can be programmed to indicate when a result meets the criteria for smear review.

Automated red cell measurements can, to some extent, replace examination of the blood film. An increased red cell distribution width indicates the

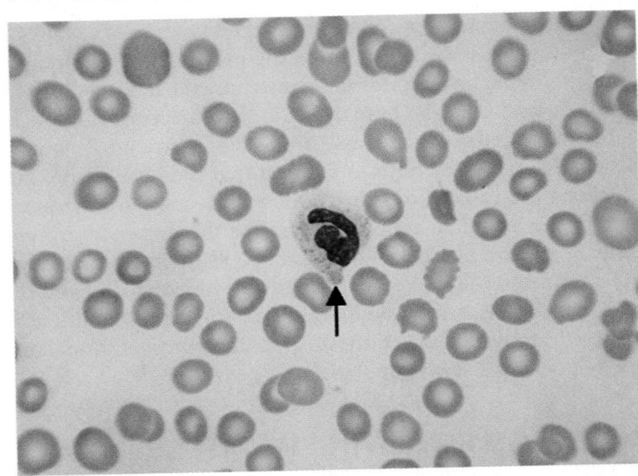

FIGURE 160-19. **Döhle's body.** A *Döhle's body* (arrow) is a pale blue-gray amorphous inclusion near the cell membrane of a neutrophil. Döhle's bodies can result from infection and inflammation. Similar but different inclusions (larger and more angular) are seen in the May-Hegglin anomaly (×1000).

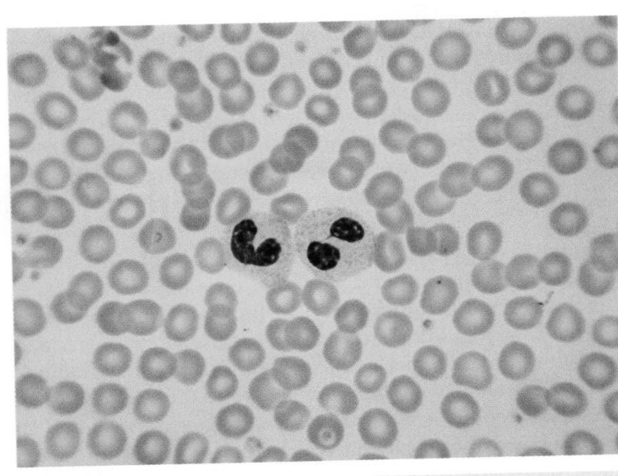

FIGURE 160-20. **Pelger-Huët anomaly.** A *Pelger-Huët anomaly* is a cytologic abnormality of neutrophils in which there is hypolobulation of nuclei and increased chromatin clumping. Nuclei may have a shape resembling a peanut or a pince-nez, as in the examples shown. The Pelger-Huët anomaly is inherited, but similar Pelger neutrophils are seen in myelodysplastic syndromes, in which the neutrophils may also be hypogranular (×1000).

TABLE 160-1 CLINICAL FEATURES SUGGESTING THE NEED FOR A BLOOD SMEAR

CLINICAL FEATURE	REASON TO PERFORM A BLOOD SMEAR
Lymphadenopathy or splenomegaly	May be indicative of infectious mononucleosis or another reactive condition, or of leukemia or lymphoma
Clinically evident anemia	Helps in the differential diagnosis
Bruising or bleeding tendency, including unexplained retinal hemorrhages	May confirm thrombocytopenia or show morphologically abnormal platelets (which may have defective function); sometimes owing to acute leukemia or other condition causing bone marrow failure
Acute renal failure	Hemolytic-uremic syndrome and thrombotic thrombocytopenic purpura should be confirmed or excluded
Jaundice and hypertension in a pregnant woman	May show schistocytes, supporting a diagnosis of HELLP syndrome
Bone pain	May indicate multiple myeloma, bone marrow infiltration, or sickle cell disease
Unexplained chest or abdominal pain or acute splenic enlargement in a child	Possible sickle cell disease
Unexplained hyperbilirubinemia	Assessment of possible hemolysis

HELLP = hemolysis, elevated liver enzymes, low platelets.

presence of anisocytosis. A decreased mean cell volume is usually a reliable indicator of microcytosis. A reduction in the mean cell hemoglobin concentration indicates hypochromia (for most instruments, however, this measurement is less sensitive than the human eye in the detection of hypochromia). An increased mean cell volume usually indicates macrocytosis, but examination of a smear is necessary both to confirm that the result is not artifactual and to elucidate the cause. Some instruments can measure the hemoglobin concentration in individual cells and thus flag the presence of hyperdense cells; however, a blood film is still necessary to distinguish spherocytes from irregularly contracted cells. Most instruments produce a histogram of the size distribution of red cells, and some do the same for the distribution of hemoglobin concentration; either of these graphic representations may show dimorphic red cells (i.e., two populations of cells).

THE BLOOD SMEAR IN THE DIFFERENTIAL DIAGNOSIS OF ANEMIA

Microcytic Anemias (Chapter 162)

In microcytic anemias, the automated count is of considerable importance and may permit a distinction between iron deficiency and thalassemia heterozygosity. In iron deficiency, there is initially a normocytic normochromic anemia; only when the deficiency becomes more severe is there microcytosis. Conversely, in β-thalassemia heterozygosity, there is usually a normal or near-normal hemoglobin concentration, but the red blood cell count is increased and there is marked microcytosis (low mean cell volume) together with a parallel reduction in mean cell hemoglobin. The blood film provides supplementary information that can favor one diagnosis or the other. Iron deficiency is more likely to be associated with hypochromia and elliptocytes ("pencil cells"), whereas in β-thalassemia heterozygosity there is microcytosis, hypochromia is less marked, and there are more likely to be target cells and basophilic stippling. Individuals with α-thalassemia involving the deletion of two α genes (−α/−α) or (– –/α α) have red cell indices similar to those of β-thalassemia heterozygosity; in this case, the blood film usually does not provide any additional diagnostically useful information, although individuals with nondeletional α-thalassemia due to hemoglobin Constant Spring have prominent basophilic stippling. When there is deletion of a single α gene, the blood count is either less abnormal or normal, and the blood smear does not provide any extra diagnostically useful information. The blood smear is, however, a useful supplement to the blood count in suggesting a diagnosis of hemoglobin H disease (Chapter 165). The count shows anemia, marked microcytosis (low mean cell volume and mean cell hemoglobin), and sometimes a reduction in the mean cell hemoglobin concentration. The smear usually shows marked poikilocytosis in addition to microcytosis, and there may be polychromasia, correlating with an elevated reticulocyte count. Iron deficiency anemia also needs to be distinguished from anemia of chronic disease. The blood counts may be quite similar, but in anemia of chronic disease, the smear often shows features of inflammation, such as increased rouleau formation, background staining (as a result of increased plasma proteins), and sometimes neutrophilia. Other rare microcytic anemias that must be distinguished from iron deficiency include congenital sideroblastic anemia and lead poisoning. In congenital sideroblastic anemia, the film is dimorphic, with one population of hypochromic microcytes and another of normochromic normocytic cells. In lead poisoning, the presence of basophilic stippling and polychromasia in a patient with microcytosis can suggest the diagnosis.

Macrocytic Anemias

A blood film can be important in distinguishing true macrocytosis from factitious macrocytosis as a result of the presence of red cell agglutinates (see Fig. 160-16). Diagnostic features that can suggest the cause of macrocytosis are shown in Table 160-2.

A smear is particularly important in evaluating the possibility of a megaloblastic anemia (Chapter 167) (Figs. 160-4 and 160-21). Sometimes assays of vitamin B_{12} and folate are normal despite a deficiency, and only the blood film features suggest the true diagnosis and indicate the need for further investigation.

Normocytic Normochromic Anemia (Chapter 161)

A blood smear is only occasionally useful in determining the cause of a normocytic normochromic anemia. Signs of inflammation may be present in anemia of chronic disease. Increased rouleau formation and background staining can also indicate multiple myeloma. Polychromasia suggests the possibility of young red cells as a result of recent blood loss or hemolysis. Small numbers of acanthocytes may indicate hypothyroidism or anorexia nervosa. Dysplastic features, such as in neutrophils, suggest a myelodysplastic syndrome.

TABLE 160-2 USEFUL FEATURES FOR DETERMINING THE CAUSE OF MACROCYTIC ANEMIA

CAUSE	SMEAR FEATURES
Megaloblastic anemia (vitamin B_{12} or folic acid deficiency)	Oval macrocytes, teardrop poikilocytes, hypersegmented neutrophils; when severe, marked anisocytosis and poikilocytosis, which may include red cell fragments
Ethanol excess	Target cells and stomatocytes; anisocytosis and poikilocytosis less than in megaloblastic anemia
Liver disease	Target cells, stomatocytes
Myelodysplastic syndromes, including sideroblastic anemias	Other dysplastic features such as hypogranular and hypolobulated neutrophils; if erythropoiesis is sideroblastic, a population of hypochromic microcytic cells and Pappenheimer bodies
Chronic hemolytic anemia	Polychromasia; characteristic poikilocytes sometimes present (e.g., irregularly contracted cells if there is an unstable hemoglobin)

TABLE 160-3 BLOOD SMEAR FEATURES SUGGESTING A SPECIFIC CAUSE OF INHERITED OR ACQUIRED HEMOLYTIC ANEMIA

BLOOD SMEAR FEATURES	CONDITIONS SUGGESTED
Spherocytes	Hereditary spherocytosis, autoimmune hemolytic anemia, alloimmune hemolytic anemia (e.g., hemolytic disease of the newborn, delayed hemolytic transfusion reaction), drug-induced immune hemolytic anemia, *Clostridium perfringens* sepsis
Irregularly contracted cells	Glucose-6-phosphate dehydrogenase deficiency, oxidant damage from chemicals or drugs in individuals with normal red cell enzymes (e.g., dapsone administration), liver failure due to Wilson disease (release of copper from liver), unstable hemoglobin, hemoglobin C homozygosity
Sickle cells and boat-shaped cells	Sickle cell disease (e.g., sickle cell anemia or compound heterozygous states such as S/C, S/D-Punjab, S/O-Arab, S/β-thalassemia)
Target cells	Hemoglobin C homozygosity, other hemoglobinopathies, hereditary xerocytosis
Stomatocytes	Hereditary stomatocytosis
Acanthocytes	Liver failure (spur cell hemolytic anemia)
Basophilic stippling	Lead poisoning, pyrimidine 5′-nucleotidase deficiency
Red cell fragments (schistocytes)	Microangiopathic hemolytic anemia (including hemolytic-uremic syndrome, thrombotic thrombocytopenic purpura, HELLP syndrome, and hemolysis associated with disseminated intravascular coagulation), mechanical hemolytic anemia (e.g., defective cardiac prosthetic valve, march hemoglobinuria)

HELLP = hemolysis, elevated liver enzymes, low platelets.

Hemolytic Anemias

The possibility of hemolysis is suggested by the presence of polychromasia and macrocytosis. Specific causes of hemolysis are suggested by the presence of various poikilocytes, as shown in Table 160-3.

The distinction between spherocytes and irregularly contracted cells is important; both are dense cells with absent central pallor, but the differential diagnosis is quite different. Recognition of the features of oxidant damage is important in diagnosing glucose-6-phosphate dehydrogenase (G6PD) deficiency, because sometimes an assay for G6PD performed during an acute hemolytic episode is normal (Chapter 164). In addition to irregularly contracted cells, there may be ghost cells, hemi-ghost cells ("blister cells"), and even Heinz bodies protruding from the red cells and confirmed on a Heinz body preparation. The observation of these features is an indication to repeat the assay when the acute hemolytic episode is over.

ASSESSMENT OF THROMBOCYTOPENIA, THROMBOCYTOSIS, AND PLATELET MORPHOLOGY

A blood smear is essential to validate the cell count whenever an automated count shows thrombocytopenia (e.g., a count <60 × 10^9/l). This should be done quickly before patient management is altered, such as by postponing surgery or initiating further diagnostic work-up. A platelet transfusion should never be given for an unexpected thrombocytopenia without microscopic confirmation of the count. A factitiously low platelet count is often the result of in vitro platelet aggregation and is occasionally the result of platelet satellitism (Chapter 174). To detect aggregates reliably, the edges and the tail of the smear should be examined for aggregates. The presence of fibrin strands also suggests the activation of coagulation and an erroneous count.

If a low platelet count is confirmed, the film may give clues to the cause (Chapter 175). Giant platelets (Figs. 160-22 and 160-23) occur in a number of inherited thrombocytopenias, including Bernard-Soulier syndrome and the May-Hegglin anomaly. Small platelets are less common but are a feature of Wiskott-Aldrich syndrome. Agranular platelets occur in the gray platelet syndrome, and platelets with a reduced number of larger-than-normal granules are seen in Jacobsen/Paris-Trousseau syndrome. The presence of May-Hegglin inclusions (Döhle-like bodies; see Fig. 160-19) in neutrophils indicates that this anomaly is the cause of the thrombocytopenia. In acquired thrombocytopenias, increased platelet turnover is often accompanied by the presence of large platelets, whereas bone marrow failure is associated with platelets of normal size. It is important to look for red cell fragments to confirm or exclude a diagnosis of thrombotic thrombocytopenic purpura in any patient with the apparent recent onset of thrombocytopenia; because platelet transfusions are usually contraindicated in this condition, the smear should be examined before platelet transfusion is contemplated. The smear of any patient with the apparent recent onset of severe thrombocytopenia should be examined carefully for evidence of acute promyelocytic leukemia; the leukemic cells may be infrequent in the circulating blood. Hemorrhagic manifestations and a low platelet count can also be indicative of meningococcal septicemia; in some patients, organisms are seen in the blood smear and the diagnosis is confirmed; in other patients, only marked toxic changes in neutrophils are detected.

Thrombocytosis should also be confirmed on a smear. Factitiously elevated counts may be the result of the presence of red cell fragments (in microangiopathic or mechanical hemolytic anemia, burns, or accidental in vitro heating of the blood sample), white cell fragments (in acute leukemia and, less often, in lymphoma), cryoglobulin precipitates, or microorganisms (particularly *Candida* species). If the count is confirmed, the blood smear may be useful to indicate a likely cause (e.g., features of hyposplenism or the presence of basophilia in a myeloproliferative disorder).

It is sometimes necessary to examine a smear to confirm that an apparently normal platelet count is valid. This should always be done in patients with acute leukemia and an elevated white cell count; the presence of white cell fragments of a similar size to platelets can suggest that the platelet count is at a safe level when it is in fact dangerously low. Counting the ratio of platelets to other particles of similar size permits the count to be corrected. Any unexpectedly normal count should be confirmed; for example, the sudden rise of the automated platelet count in a patient being treated for a hematologic neoplasm may be the result of fungi that have colonized an indwelling intravenous line and are being shed into the blood stream.

LEUKOCYTOSIS AND LEUKOPENIA (CHAPTER 170)

The finding of leukocytosis is not necessarily an indication for a blood smear. For example, this finding would be expected in a patient with infection or following surgery or trauma, in which case smear confirmation is not required. However, unexpected leukocytosis requires a smear. Artifactual elevation is unusual but can occur as a result of cryoglobulinemia, hyperlipidemia, or the presence of *Candida* species. Distinguishing reactive changes from leukemia on the basis of morphology is usually straightforward. In reactive leukocytosis, there is usually toxic granulation, and Döhle's bodies may be present (see Figs. 160-18 and 160-19). Vacuolation is particularly characteristic of bacterial infection, and there may be some degranulation of neutrophils. The hematologist should be aware of the changes induced by granulocyte colony-stimulating factor so that they are not confused with a response to infection;

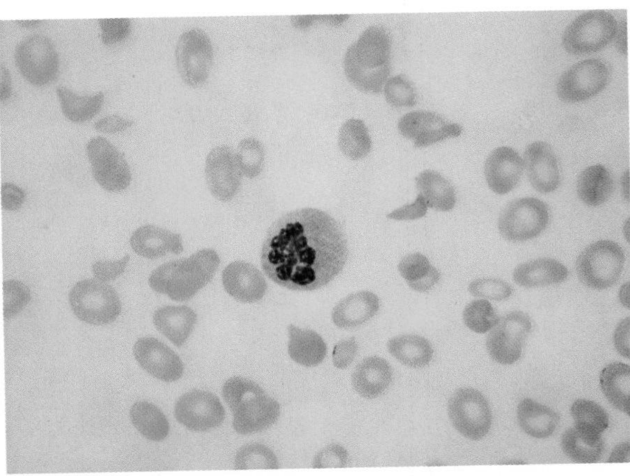

FIGURE 160-21. Hypersegmented neutrophils. A *hypersegmented neutrophil* is a neutrophil with more than five nuclear segments or lobes, as in this example from a patient with megaloblastic anemia. Neutrophil hypersegmentation is also said to be present if there are increased numbers of neutrophils with five lobes or if the median lobe count is increased (×1000).

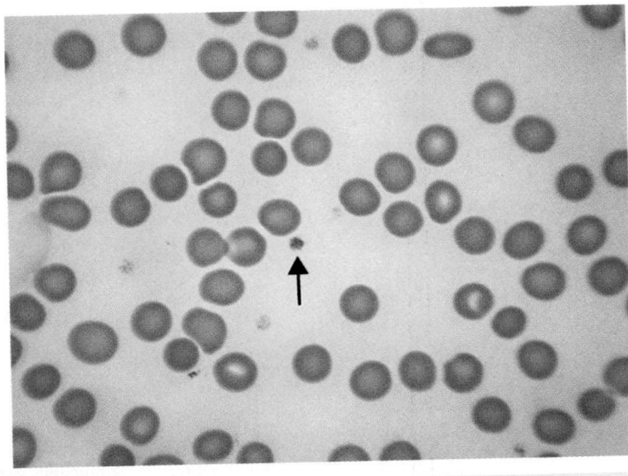

FIGURE 160-22. Normal-sized platelet (arrow). Platelets have central granules, although this is not apparent in this photomicrograph (×1000).

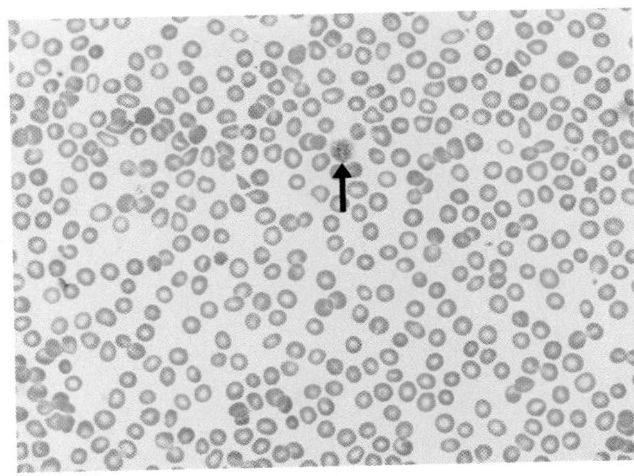

FIGURE 160-23. Giant platelet (arrow). Giant platelets are as large as or larger than normal red cells. Giant platelets can indicate increased platelet turnover or an inherited or acquired defect in thrombopoiesis (×1000).

this cytokine can cause toxic granulation, Döhle's bodies, vacuolation, and the presence of macropolycytes (giant neutrophils) and circulating neutrophil precursors. The changes typical of leukemia are discussed later.

Leukopenia usually requires a film for confirmation and elucidation. The exception is when it is expected in a given clinical context, such as when a patient has had recent chemotherapy. Rarely, an apparent leukopenia is artifactual, owing to the aggregation of neutrophils mediated by an autoantibody or resulting from infection-induced changes in adhesion molecules of the leukocyte surface membrane.

With some automated instruments, it is necessary to confirm that neutropenia is real. If the automated count is based on peroxidase cytochemistry, the presence of an inherited deficiency will lead to an apparent neutropenia associated with an increase of large, unstained (i.e., peroxidase-negative) cells. The scatter plot is characteristic, but because the same features could be due to acute leukemia with neutropenia and circulating blast cells, a smear is needed for confirmation.

LEUKEMIAS AND LYMPHOMAS

The blood smear is critical in the diagnosis of leukemias and lymphomas. The lymphoblasts of acute lymphoblastic leukemia are usually medium-sized agranular cells with relatively scanty cytoplasm (Fig. 160-24), whereas in acute myeloid leukemia, blast cells are generally larger, with more plentiful cytoplasm that may contain granules or Auer rods (Fig. 160-25). Myeloid blast cells vary in appearance according to whether they are myeloblasts or monoblasts. Myeloblasts are usually medium sized and may have plentiful granules, scanty granules, or no visible granules; they may contain Auer rods. Monoblasts are much larger cells with plentiful cytoplasm containing few granules and, very rarely, Auer rods. Megakaryoblasts are present in some patients and are sometimes cytologically distinctive because of their tendency to form cytoplasmic blebs or develop platelet-type granules.

Chronic myelogenous leukemia has a very characteristic blood smear (Fig. 160-26) in which the most numerous cells are myelocytes and mature neutrophils. Eosinophils and basophils are also present. Dysplastic features are generally absent. In atypical Philadelphia chromosome–negative chronic myeloid leukemia, monocytosis is more frequent and dysplastic features are present. Chronic myelomonocytic leukemia is characterized by increased monocytes, some of them immature, with inconspicuous dysplastic features and infrequent granulocyte precursors.

Chronic lymphocytic leukemia also has a very characteristic blood film, with an increase of small, mature lymphocytes of rather uniform appearance. The chromatin is often irregularly clumped, creating a mosaic effect (Fig. 160-27). Smear cells are almost always increased in number but are not pathognomonic.

Lymphoma in leukemic phase often has cytologic features that aid in the diagnosis. Follicular lymphoma, Burkitt's lymphoma, and splenic marginal zone lymphoma can all be distinctive.

THE INCIDENTAL DETECTION OF CLINICALLY SIGNIFICANT ABNORMALITIES

Sometimes the examination of a blood film reveals unexpected but clinically significant information. Examples are given in Table 160-4. Detection of microorganisms is particularly likely in patients with acquired immunodeficiency syndrome (AIDS), hyposplenic patients, and patients with overwhelming sepsis, but sometimes they are detected in immunologically normal patients with only trivial symptoms. It should be noted that microorganisms in blood smears sometimes represent contaminants, particularly if

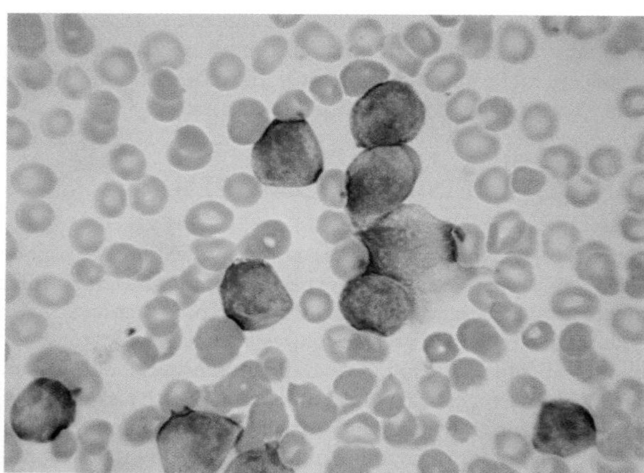

FIGURE 160-24. **Acute lymphoblastic leukemia.** Numerous agranular blast cells with a high nuclear-to-cytoplasmic ratio are present. Platelets are decreased in number (×1000).

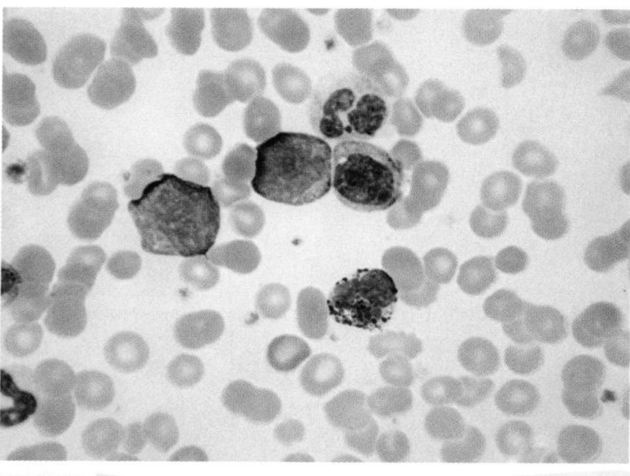

FIGURE 160-26. **Chronic myelogenous leukemia.** In this view there are myeloblasts, a myelocyte, a basophil, and a segmented neutrophil (×1000).

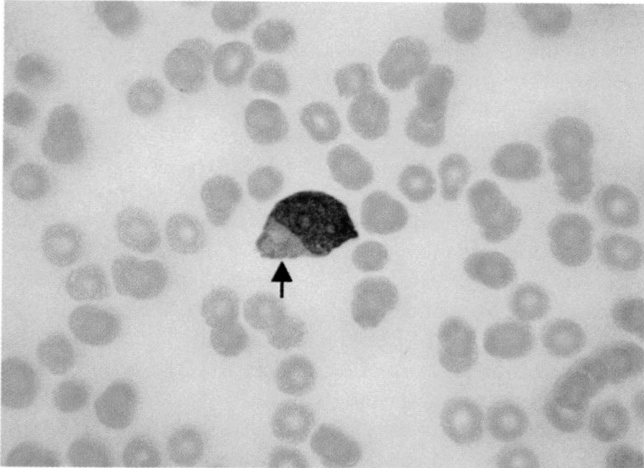

FIGURE 160-25. **Auer rod.** An Auer rod (arrow) is a rod-shaped inclusion in the cytoplasm of cells of myeloid lineage formed by the crystallization of azurophilic granule constituents. Auer rods are seen only in acute myeloid leukemia and high-grade myelodysplastic syndromes. They are usually seen in blast cells but are occasionally found in maturing cells (×1000).

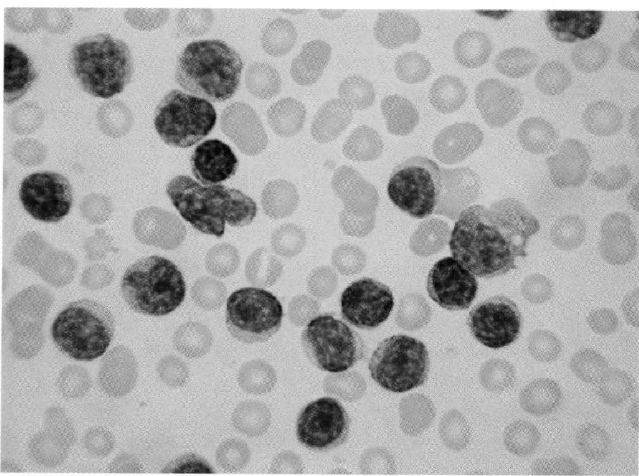

FIGURE 160-27. **Chronic lymphocytic leukemia.** There are large numbers of rather monotonous, mature small lymphocytes with chromatin clumping. Smear cells, reflecting the mechanical fragility of the cells, are characteristic but are not seen in this photomicrograph (×1000).

TABLE 160-4 INCIDENTAL BUT CLINICALLY RELEVANT BLOOD SMEAR OBSERVATIONS

OBSERVATION	POSSIBLE SIGNIFICANCE
Acanthocytes	Abetalipoproteinemia, neuroacanthocytosis, McLeod phenotype
Howell-Jolly bodies, target cells, and acanthocytes	Hyposplenism (congenital, previous splenectomy, celiac disease, amyloidosis)
Cryoglobulin	Hepatitis C, multiple myeloma
Vacuolated lymphocytes	Inherited metabolic disorders
Parasites (e.g., malaria parasites, *Babesia*, microfilaria, trypanosomes, *Leishmania*)	Parasitic infection
Fungi (*Candida* spp, *Histoplasma capsulatum*, *Penicillium marneffei*, *Cryptococcus neoformans*, *Malassezia furfur*)	Disseminated fungal infection or, in the case of *Candida*, colonization of an indwelling intravenous line
Bacteria (e.g., pneumococcus, meningococcus, *Capnocytophaga canimorsus*, *Borrelia*, *Ehrlichia*, *Anaplasma*, *Yersinia pestis*)	Bacterial infection
Leukoerythroblastic blood film	Bone marrow infiltration (e.g., metastatic malignancy)

specimens have been obtained by skin prick or from the umbilical cord and if there has been a delay in making the film.

CONCLUSION

Despite major advances in other diagnostic methods, the blood smear remains very useful in hematologic diagnosis. Sometimes it is critical either because it yields a diagnosis very quickly or because it provides information that is not available in any other way.

SUGGESTED READINGS

Bain BJ. Diagnosis from the blood smear. *N Engl J Med.* 2005;353:498-507. *More examples of how examining a blood smear contributes to diagnosis.*

Barnes PW, McFadden S, Machin SJ, et al. The International Consensus Group for Hematology Review. http://www.islh.org/web/index.php/2009/index.php?page=consensus_preface. Accessed Jan. 1, 2010. *Discussion of how abnormalities in the automated blood count may indicate that a blood film should be examined.*

Froom P, Havis R, Barak M. The rate of manual peripheral blood smear reviews in outpatients. *Clin Chem Lab Med.* 2009;47:1401-1405. *Fewer than 3% of automated peripheral blood smears in outpatients may require manual review.*

Prokocimer M, Potasman I. The added value of peripheral blood cell morphology in the diagnosis and management of infectious diseases—part 1: basic concepts. *Postgrad Med J.* 2008;84:579-585.

Prokocimer M, Potasman I. The added value of peripheral blood cell morphology in the diagnosis and management of infectious diseases—part 2: illustrative cases. *Postgrad Med J.* 2008;84:586-589. *Two articles that show the potential contribution of the blood smear examination to the diagnosis of infectious diseases.*

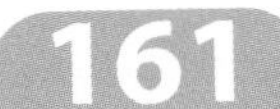

APPROACH TO THE ANEMIAS

H. FRANKLIN BUNN

Anemia is defined as a significant reduction in the mass of circulating red blood cells. As a result, the oxygen binding capacity of the blood is diminished. Because blood volume is normally maintained at a nearly constant level, anemic patients have a decrease in the concentration of red cells or hemoglobin in peripheral blood. As shown in Table 161-1, hemoglobin and hematocrit levels vary with the age of the individual and, in adults, with gender. The values in women of childbearing age are 10% lower than those in men. At altitude, higher values are found, roughly in proportion to the elevation above sea level. Anemic patients' values are more than one standard deviation below the mean values for their gender. However, because of the wide range in normal hemoglobin and hematocrit levels, it is often difficult to document mild anemia.

Sometimes the diagnosis of anemia is confounded by a concomitant change in the plasma volume. For example, if a patient with a low red cell mass sustains a loss of plasma volume from dehydration, diarrhea, vomiting, or severe burns, the blood hemoglobin and hematocrit levels will be increased and may even be in the normal range. Another important example, discussed in detail later in this chapter, is acute hemorrhage, in which the loss of both red blood cells and plasma results in a false elevation of hemoglobin and hematocrit. In contrast, hemoglobin and hematocrit values may be falsely low in patients with an expanded plasma volume, such as in pregnancy or congestive heart failure.

TABLE 161-1 NORMAL VALUES FOR RED BLOOD CELL MEASUREMENTS

MEASUREMENT	UNIT	NORMAL RANGE (APPROXIMATE)*
Hemoglobin	g/dL	Males: 13.5-17.5 Females: 12-16
Hematocrit	%	Males: 40-52 Females: 36-48
Red blood cell (RBC) count	$\times 10^6/\mu L$ of blood	Males: 4.5-6.0 Females: 4.0-5.4
Mean cell volume (MCV)	fL	81-99
Mean cell hemoglobin (MCH)	pg	30-34
Mean cell hemoglobin concentration (MCHC)	g/dL	30-36
RBC size distribution width		
RDW-CV	%	12-14
RDW-SD	fL	37-47
Reticulocyte count (absolute number)	No./μL of blood	20,000-100,000
Reticulocyte percentage	% of RBCs	0.5-1.5

*Actual normal ranges for many of these values may vary slightly, depending on factors such as the location and type of laboratory instruments used, altitude above sea level, and patient age.

O_2 Delivery = Blood Flow × Hb Concentration × (Asat − Vsat)

In anemia: ↑ Cardiac output, Altered flow distribution | ↑↑ Plasma Erythropoietin | ↓ RBC 2,3-DPG, RBC O_2 affinity

FIGURE 161-1. The Fick equation expresses the three independent variables that determine the transport of oxygen to a given organ or tissue. The impact of anemia on each of these variables is shown beneath the equation. Asat = oxygen saturation of arterial blood (oxyhemoglobin/oxyhemoglobin + deoxyhemoglobin); 2,3-DPG = 2,3-diphosphoglycerate (2,3-bisphosphoglycerate); Hb = hemoglobin; RBC = red blood cell; Vsat = oxygen saturation of venous blood.

PATHOBIOLOGY

Impact of Anemia on Oxygen Transport

In any organ or region of the body, the transport of oxygen is a product of three independent variables expressed in the Fick equation (Fig. 161-1). The middle variable—the oxygen carrying capacity of the blood—is, by definition, low in anemic patients. The two other variables in the Fick equation undergo compensatory changes that, as explained later, greatly enhance oxygen transport.

Blood Flow

Anemia has a marked impact on blood flow, the left-hand variable in the Fick equation. In all anemic individuals, there is enhanced flow to vital organs, including the heart, brain, liver, and kidneys, at the expense of nonvital organs. Anemic patients are pale because blood is diverted away from the skin and mucous membranes to preserve oxygen supply to the critical organs. Resting cardiac output is normal in patients with mild or moderate anemia, but with exercise, it increases more than that of a normal individual. In severe anemia, resting cardiac output is increased, putting patients at risk of developing high-output cardiac failure, particularly those with coronary artery insufficiency or other types of preexisting cardiac disease.

Oxygen Binding to Hemoglobin

The variable on the right side of the Fick equation is the difference in fractional oxygenation between the arterial and venous blood. This difference in

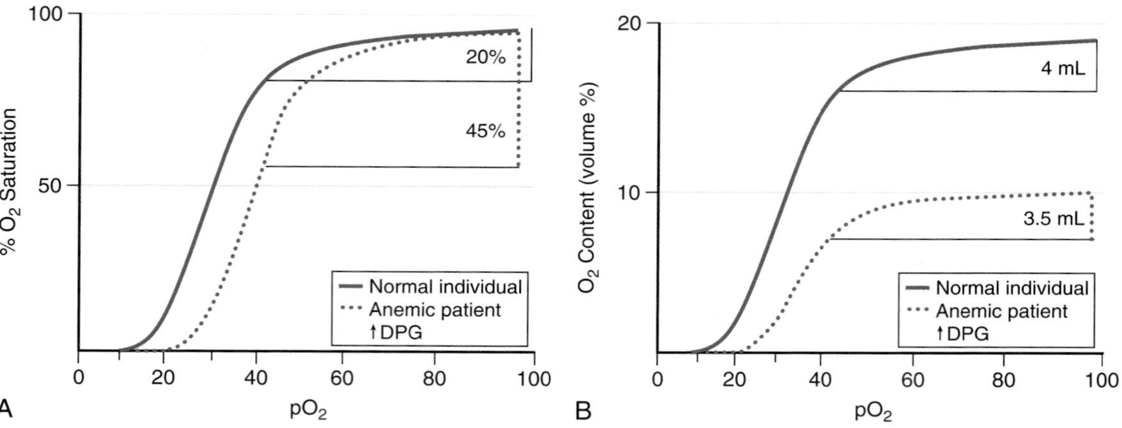

FIGURE 161-2. **Oxygen binding curves for hemoglobin of a normal individual and a patient with anemia. A,** Conventional plot of percent of oxygen (O_2) saturation versus oxygen tension (pO_2). **B,** The Y-axis shows the volume of oxygen in milliliters per 100 mL of blood. DPG = diphosphoglycerate.

oxygen saturation is determined by the hemoglobin oxygen binding curve. A comparison between a normal individual and an anemic patient is shown in Figure 161-2. As shown in part A, the curve is shifted to the right in an anemic patient. At any given oxygen tension (Po_2), the oxygen saturation of hemoglobin is lower. Thus, red cells of anemic patients have decreased oxygen affinity. This change is due entirely to elevated levels of red cell 2,3-diphosphoglycerate (2,3-DPG) in red cells. This glycolytic intermediate is the principal determinant of oxygen affinity in human red cells. The Po_2 in arterial blood is normally approximately 95 mm Hg, resulting in nearly 100% oxygen saturation. During the transit of red cells from an artery through its capillary bed to its vein, oxygen is released to respiring cells. In normal individuals, at a normal venous Po_2 of about 40 mm Hg, the oxygen saturation is approximately 80%. Thus, as shown in Figure 161-2A, 20% of the oxygen in the blood is unloaded. In contrast, in patients with anemia and elevated red cell 2,3-DPG levels, the lower oxygen affinity of their red cells enables a much higher fraction of the oxygen (about 45%) to be unloaded. In Figure 161-2B, the oxygen binding curves are depicted with the volume fraction of oxygen plotted on the Y-axis. One gram of hemoglobin binds up to 1.34 mL of oxygen under standard conditions of temperature and pressure. Thus, in a normal individual having a hemoglobin of 15 g/dL, the oxygen carrying capacity of the blood is 15 × 1.34, or 20 mL O_2/dL. As mentioned earlier, 20% of this oxygen will be unloaded—that is, 4 mL O_2/100 mL blood during arterial-venous transit. In contrast, an anemic patient with a hemoglobin of 7.5 g/dL has an oxygen binding capacity that is half normal, or 10 mL O_2/dL. If this patient had red cells with normal oxygen affinity, 20%, or only 2 mL of oxygen, would be unloaded per 100 mL of blood. However, because the patient's red cells have a lower affinity for oxygen, 3.5 mL is unloaded, nearly as much as normal. Thus, the decrease in oxygen affinity is an important mechanism by which anemic patients compensate for the deficit in red cell mass.

Methemoglobinemia

In order for hemoglobin to reversibly bind oxygen, the iron atom in the heme must be in the reduced (Fe^{2+}) valence state. As red cells circulate, the heme iron slowly auto-oxidizes to Fe^{3+}, forming methemoglobin, which is incapable of binding oxygen. Normal red cells are endowed with a very efficient enzymatic pathway composed of cytochrome b_5, cytochrome b_5 reductase, and NADH that rapidly reduces the iron in methemoglobin back to its functional Fe^{2+} form. Thus, normal red cells contain less than 0.5% methemoglobin. However, either an inherited deficiency in cytochrome b_5 reductase or exposure to an oxidant drug or toxin can result in methemoglobinemia. Laboratory samples of blood containing methemoglobin are dark brown, whereas patients with greater than 10% methemoglobinemia have cyanosis, a blue discoloration of the skin indistinguishable from that commonly seen in patients having normal hemoglobin but low oxygen saturation owing to pulmonary or cardiac disease. In many hospitals and large clinical laboratories, the instrument that measures oxygen saturation in blood samples also provides an accurate determination of methemoglobin.

Patients with congenital methemoglobinemia inherit an autosomal recessive deficiency in cytochrome b_5 reductase. Heterozygote relatives have low or undetectable methemoglobin levels, whereas affected individuals (homozygotes and compound heterozygotes) generally have 10 to 35% methemoglobin. These individuals are generally asymptomatic owing to the fact that the methemoglobin is distributed primarily in the older population of red cells. Nevertheless, many affected individuals have cosmetic concerns. Treatment with oral ascorbic acid or riboflavin is effective in lowering the level of methemoglobin below the threshold of detectable cyanosis.

A variety of drugs can cause methemoglobinemia, including acetaminophen (Tylenol), dapsone, nitroprusside, amyl nitrate, and procaine congeners used for local anesthesia. It is not clear why only a very small fraction of those using these drugs develop this complication, but some affected individuals have been shown to be heterozygous for cytochrome b_5 reductase deficiency. When these drugs are taken in prescribed doses, methemoglobinemia seldom reaches levels high enough to cause clinical concern.

In contrast, individuals exposed to industrial toxins such as nitrite, nitrate, or aniline may develop life-threatening levels of methemoglobin. The threshold at which symptoms occur is highly variable. Acute induction of 20% methemoglobin may cause fatigue; at 30%, individuals often develop tachycardia. When methemoglobin exceeds 50%, patients experience weakness, breathlessness, and confusion. At 70 to 80%, coma and death may occur. The toxicity of methemoglobinemia is not just because of the oxidized hemes' inability to bind oxygen; the remaining functional (Fe^{2+}) hemes in the hemoglobin tetramer have increased oxygen affinity and therefore, as suggested in Figure 161-2, are much less effective in releasing oxygen to tissues. Patients with toxic methemoglobinemia can be effectively treated with intravenous infusion of methylene blue (1 to 2 mg/kg).

Regulation of Erythropoiesis by Erythropoietin

Anemia also impacts the middle component of the Fick equation (see Fig. 161-1). As mentioned earlier, hemoglobin levels are, by definition, low in anemic patients. The resultant decrease in the oxygen carrying capacity of the blood causes cellular hypoxia. In all cells of the body, a molecular sensor detects even modest degrees of low oxygen tension and induces a hypoxia-inducible transcription factor called HIF. HIF upregulates expression of the hormone erythropoietin in the kidney and, to a lesser extent, in the liver. Erythropoietin (Chapter 159) binds to a specific receptor abundantly expressed on erythroid progenitor cells in the bone marrow and salvages these cells from apoptosis, thereby enhancing red blood cell production. Normal individuals maintain nearly constant levels of circulating red cells by finely tuned regulation of erythropoietin production. In anemic patients, the hypoxic signal in the kidneys and, to a lesser extent, in the liver results in a robust induction of erythropoietin expression. As the hematocrit falls, the plasma erythropoietin level rises markedly; in severely anemic patients, it may be 1000-fold higher than normal (Fig. 161-3). In patients with anemia due to impaired red cell production, their erythroid progenitors are unresponsive to such high levels of plasma erythropoietin. In contrast, in patients whose anemia is due to hemolysis or blood loss, elevated erythropoietin levels maximize red cell production.

CLINICAL MANIFESTATIONS

Figure 161-4 is a 17th-century painting of a pale young woman clutching her chest, apparently complaining of palpitations. Her physician is feeling her

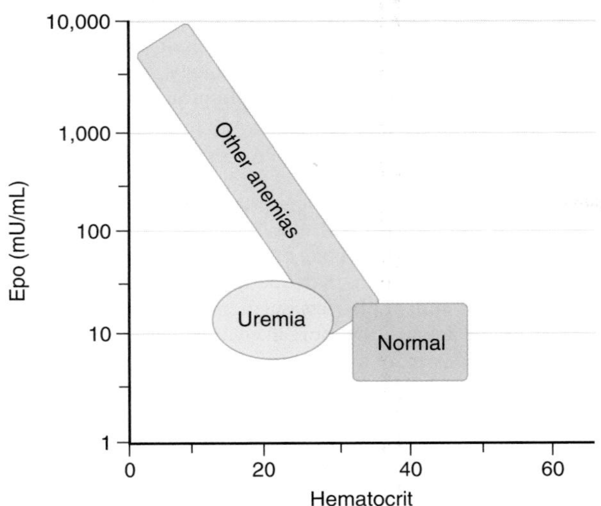

FIGURE 161-3. Plasma erythropoietin (Epo) levels in patients with different degrees of anemia. The subset of anemia patients with chronic renal disease (labeled "Uremia") have much lower plasma erythropoietin levels than those with other types of anemia. Values for normal individuals are also shown.

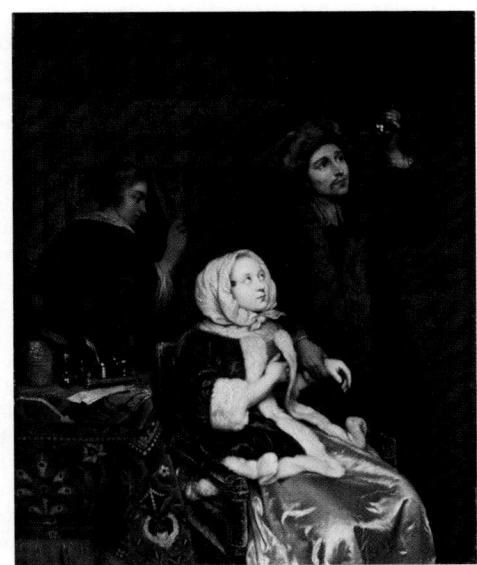

FIGURE 161-4. **"The Sick Lady," a 17th-century painting attributed to Caspar Netscher, from the Royal Collection, Buckingham Palace.**

pulse, documenting her rapid, forceful heartbeat. These signs and symptoms, common in patients with very low hemoglobin levels, can be readily explained by the cardiovascular adjustments discussed in the preceding section. These clinical findings pertain to anemia per se, irrespective of cause, and are dependent on its severity and chronicity. The history and physical examination may reveal additional findings peculiar to specific causes of anemia or to other comorbid conditions. The degree to which symptoms occur in an anemic patient depends on several contributing factors. If the anemia has developed rapidly, there may not have been adequate time for compensatory adjustments to take place, and the patient may have more marked symptoms than if an anemia of equivalent severity had developed insidiously. Furthermore, the patient's complaints may depend on the presence of local vascular disease. For example, symptoms owing to ischemia in patients with angina pectoris, intermittent claudication, or transient cerebral episodes may be triggered by the development of anemia.

Symptoms

Many individuals with mild anemia have no complaints and are unaware that they have "tired blood." Others may complain of fatigue as well as dyspnea and palpitations, particularly following exercise. Patients with severe anemia are often symptomatic at rest and are unable to tolerate significant exertion.

TABLE 161-2 INITIAL ASSESSMENT OF ANEMIA

Decreased red cell production
Usually acquired
Onset is insidious
Reticulocyte count is inappropriately low
Red cell indices (MCV, MCHC) are informative
Bone marrow examination is often required for diagnosis
Increased red cell destruction (hemolysis)
Often inherited
Onset may be abrupt or insidious
Reticulocyte count is increased
Red cell morphology is usually informative
Bone marrow examination is usually not indicated
Blood loss—must be ruled out in any patient with anemia

MCHC = mean cell hemoglobin concentration; MCV = mean cell volume.

If the hemoglobin concentration falls below 7.5 g/dL, resting cardiac output is likely to rise, with an increase in both stroke volume and heart rate. The patient may be aware of this hyperdynamic state and complain of a rapid, pounding sensation in the precordium. Patients with compromised myocardial reserve may develop complaints due to cardiac failure.

The symptoms of severe anemia often extend beyond the cardiac or circulatory system. Patients sometimes experience dizziness and headache and, less often, syncope, tinnitus, or vertigo. Many are irritable and have difficulty sleeping or concentrating. Because blood flow is shunted away from the skin, patients may complain of increased sensitivity to cold. In like manner, gastrointestinal symptoms such as indigestion, anorexia, or even nausea are attributable to the shunting of blood away from the splanchnic bed. Females commonly develop abnormal menstruation, either amenorrhea or increased bleeding. Males may experience impotence or loss of libido.

Physical Findings

Pallor is the most commonly encountered physical finding in patients with anemia. As mentioned earlier, this sign is due to the shunting of blood away from the skin and other peripheral tissues, permitting enhanced blood flow to vital organs. The usefulness of pallor as a physical finding is limited by other factors that affect the appearance of the skin. Blood flow to the skin may undergo wide fluctuations. Moreover, the skin's thickness and texture vary widely among individuals. Those with a fair complexion may appear pale even though they are not anemic, while pallor is difficult to detect in deeply pigmented individuals. The amount of melanin in the epidermis is an important determinant of skin color. Pallor may be difficult to detect in patients who have increased melanin pigmentation due to Addison's disease or hemochromatosis. Nevertheless, even in blacks, the presence of anemia may be suspected by the color of the palms or of noncutaneous tissues such as oral mucous membranes, nail beds, and palpebral conjunctivas. When the creases of the palm are as pale as the surrounding skin, the patient usually has a hemoglobin of less than 7 g/dL.

In addition to tachycardia, wide pulse pressure, and hyperdynamic precordium, a systolic ejection murmur is often heard over the precordium, particularly at the pulmonic area. In addition, a venous hum may be detected over the neck vessels. These findings disappear when the anemia is corrected.

DIAGNOSIS

Laboratory Evaluation of the Patient with Anemia

In the clinical assessment of the anemic patient, it is important to proceed in a systematic way so that the diagnosis can be established with a minimum of laboratory tests and procedures. A thorough history and careful physical examination are critical in the initial evaluation of the anemic patient. For example, a family history that reveals a dominant inheritance pattern would reinforce the tentative diagnosis of hereditary spherocytosis. The presence of fever, a new heart murmur, and splenomegaly is an anemic patient suggests subacute bacterial endocarditis.

In evaluating the anemic patient, the clinician must first ask whether the anemia is caused by decreased production of red cells or by loss of blood cells as a result of hemorrhage or hemolysis (Table 161-2). Blood loss may be either the sole cause of the anemia or a significant contributor. Therefore, examination of the stool for occult blood is an indispensable part of the evaluation of all anemic patients.

The laboratory work-up of anemia includes a complete blood count, red cell indices, reticulocyte count, and microscopic examination of the blood smear. In addition, in many cases a bone marrow examination is a critical component of the initial laboratory assessment.

Complete Blood Count

Most hospitals and clinical laboratories use equipment that provides high-throughput analyses of red cell, platelet, and white cell counts and white cell differential, along with measurements of cell size. The mean red cell volume (MCV) is normally 81 to 99 fL. These instruments also provide accurate determinations of hemoglobin concentration. The hematocrit, or fraction of packed red cells over total blood volume, is determined indirectly from the red cell count and the MCV. The mean concentration of hemoglobin within the red cell population (MCHC) is the quotient of hemoglobin divided by hematocrit. The MCV is particularly useful in classifying the anemias caused by decreased red cell production. Microcytic anemias have low MCV values and often low MCHC. Microscopic examination reveals small and often pale red cells. The MCV in the macrocytic anemias is increased, and large, oval cells (macro-ovalocytes) are seen. In contrast to the anemias of underproduction, the hemolytic anemias are either normocytic or slightly macrocytic owing to the preponderance of young red cells that are relatively large. Severe forms of thalassemia (Chapter 165) are an exception; there, microcytic red cells may be accompanied by brisk hemolysis.

Reticulocyte Count

This simple and cost-effective test is extremely useful for distinguishing anemias secondary to decreased red cell production from those caused by hemolysis. With the application of an appropriate supravital stain, the 1- to 2-day-old red cells in the peripheral blood reveal a network of purple strands, which are aggregates of ribosomes. The reticulocyte count in normal individuals is about 1%, consistent with a red cell lifespan of approximately 120 days. An elevated reticulocyte count reflects the release of an increased number of young cells from the bone marrow. The rate of red cell production can be assessed more quantitatively by determining the absolute reticulocyte count, the product of the percentage of reticulocytes and the red cell count. Thus, normal blood contains about 50,000 reticulocytes/mm^3. In interpreting this test, one should consider the distribution of reticulocytes between the bone marrow and the peripheral blood. When erythropoiesis is robust, marrow reticulocytes enter the circulation prematurely. These "shift reticulocytes" appear larger than average on a routine (Wright-stained) blood smear and have a lavender hue, called polychromatophilia. Because the circulation of shift reticulocytes in the peripheral blood is prolonged, the reticulocyte count should be divided by two. This correction should always be made if normoblasts are encountered in the peripheral blood because this finding indicates the premature release of newborn red cells into the circulation.

A failure to produce red cells is reflected in an inappropriately low reticulocyte count. In contrast, a significant elevation of reticulocytes is suggestive of hemolysis. Exceptions include the following:

- The brisk reticulocyte response seen in patients with hemorrhage
- Reticulocytosis encountered in patients recovering from impaired erythropoiesis (e.g., an individual with pernicious anemia who received an injection of cobalamin 1 week earlier)
- Mild to moderate elevations in reticulocytes (3 to 7%) encountered in myelophthisic anemia (Chapter 160), in which the orderly release of cells is affected by alterations of the marrow stroma owing to tumor, fibrosis, or granuloma

These exceptions are generally appreciated in the initial evaluation of the patient.

A number of ancillary laboratory tests described later under Hemolytic Anemias are useful in determining both the extent and the cause of hemolysis.

Examination of the Blood Smear

In the evaluation of any patient with unexplained anemia, the physician should take the time to examine a well-stained peripheral blood film (Chapter 160). Many subtleties escape the attention of the technologist, whose primary aim is to confirm or refine the white cell differential count provided by automated cell counters. The clinician approaches the specimen with a prepared mind and can scrutinize it for specific abnormalities. Examination of the blood film can confirm the size and color of red cells estimated by red blood cell indices. In contrast to the mean statistical values provided by automated cell counters, microscopic examination can reveal variations in red cell size (anisocytosis) or shape (poikilocytosis), abnormalities that are helpful in diagnosing specific anemias. Examination of the blood smear is particularly important in a patient with hemolysis. Many types of hemolytic anemia have characteristic abnormalities in red cell morphology. The presence of abnormal white cells may be the first clue to a lymphoproliferative or primary bone marrow disorder.

Bone Marrow Examination

A microscopic examination of the bone marrow (aspirate with or without a core biopsy) is often useful and may be critical in the work-up of any *unexplained* anemia. Study of the bone marrow is informative in the diagnosis of anemias of underproduction, particularly those accompanied by abnormalities in white cells and/or platelets, suggesting disordered hematopoiesis. The more severe the anemia, the more likely it is that the procedure will be informative. An assessment of the quantity and quality of red cell precursors may identify a defect in cell production due to either hypoplasia or ineffective erythropoiesis. A marrow biopsy is required for estimating overall cellularity. The ratio of myeloid (M) to erythroid (E) precursors is normally about 2 : 1, but it may be artifactually increased by the inclusion of circulating leukocytes. The ratio is increased in patients with infection, a leukemoid reaction, or neoplastic proliferation of myeloid cells. Rarely, a high M/E ratio is due to selective aplasia of the red cell precursors. A decreased M/E ratio indicates erythroid hyperplasia. Erythroid maturation is normal in hemolysis and hemorrhage, but it is disordered when erythropoiesis is ineffective, such as in megaloblastic and sideroblastic anemias and in β-thalassemia major or intermedia. The bone marrow examination is also important in demonstrating the presence of cellular infiltrates such as those found in leukemia, lymphoma, or multiple myeloma. The demonstration of tumor, fibrosis, or granuloma usually requires a bone marrow biopsy, not just a bone marrow aspiration. A portion of the marrow specimen should be stained with Prussian blue. In addition to providing an assessment of iron stores, this iron stain is required for the identification of erythroid sideroblasts.

ANEMIA DUE TO BLOOD LOSS

The clinical presentation of anemia resulting from blood loss varies considerably, depending on the site, severity, and rapidity of the hemorrhage. At opposite extremes are acute fulminant bleeding producing hypovolemic shock and chronic occult blood loss leading to iron deficiency anemia.

Acute Blood Loss

Patients who have had a sudden hemorrhage present with clinical findings secondary to hypovolemia and hypoxia. Symptoms and signs depend on the severity of the process. The patient may experience weakness, fatigue, lightheadedness, or stupor and may appear pale, diaphoretic, and irritable. The vital signs reflect cardiovascular compensation for the acute blood loss. The degree of hypotension and tachycardia depends on the extent of the hemorrhage. Elicitation of postural signs is useful in the initial evaluation of a patient with acute blood loss. When a patient is lifted from a supine to a sitting position, an increase in the pulse of 25% or more or a fall in the systolic blood pressure of 20 mm Hg or more signifies significant hypovolemia (blood loss >1000 mL). Acute blood loss in excess of 1500 mL usually leads to cardiovascular collapse.

Following acute hemorrhage, the red cell mass and plasma volume are contracted in parallel; accordingly, there is often not a significant decrease in the hemoglobin or hematocrit level initially. This stress induces a moderate leukocytosis and a "shift to the left" in the white cell differential count. In both acute and chronic blood loss, the platelet count is often increased, particularly if the patient is already iron deficient. During the first few days after acute blood loss, there is usually an increase in reticulocytes. Severe hypoxia may trigger the release of nucleated red cells from the bone marrow into the peripheral blood. Because young red cells are larger than old ones, the MCV generally rises slightly. If significant blood loss continues, reticulocytosis will persist until iron stores have been exhausted. Internal bleeding is often accompanied by an increase in unconjugated bilirubin, reflecting an increase in the catabolism of heme from extravasated red cells. Patients with acute gastrointestinal blood loss sometimes have an elevation of blood urea nitrogen owing to impaired renal blood flow and perhaps to the absorption of digested blood protein.

These patients must be assessed promptly, and treatment must be initiated without delay. Patients with severe acute blood loss require transfusion of packed red cells, with central monitoring of the appropriate amount of volume replacement. The site or sites of bleeding should be emergently identified and controlled. In addition, an emergency coagulation profile should be obtained. The approach to the patient with shock is discussed in detail in Chapter 106.

Chronic Blood Loss

Chronic blood loss is usually due to lesions in the gastrointestinal tract or the uterus. Testing of stool specimens for occult blood is an essential but frequently overlooked part of the evaluation of anemia. It is sometimes necessary to examine serial specimens over a prolonged period because gastrointestinal bleeding may be intermittent. The hematologic manifestations of chronic blood loss are those of iron deficiency anemia, discussed in detail in Chapter 162.

ANEMIAS DUE TO DECREASED RED CELL PRODUCTION

As shown in Table 161-3, anemias caused by the underproduction of red cells can be conveniently classified according to red cell size: microcytic, macrocytic, and normocytic.

Microcytic Anemias

The presence of small red cells (MCV <77 fL) indicates a defect in the production of hemoglobin. As shown in Figure 161-5, hemoglobin is composed of globin subunits into which heme is inserted. Heme is produced by the insertion of an iron atom into porphyrin (protoporphyrin IX). A defect in any of these three key components can cause microcytic anemia. Most individuals with microcytosis have either iron deficiency anemia (Chapter 162) or thalassemia (Chapter 165). A congenital or, more often, acquired impairment in porphyrin synthesis can lead to a buildup of excess iron in erythroid cells, resulting in the morphologic entity of ringed sideroblasts, which are identified in red cell precursors in the bone marrow (Chapter 162). Most patients with acquired sideroblastic anemia actually have a normal or somewhat elevated MCV but a broad distribution of red cell size, including a population of microcytes (because of this ambiguity, sideroblastic anemia appears in parentheses in Table 161-3). Iron deficiency anemia, the thalassemias, and sideroblastic anemia all involve some degree of ineffective erythropoiesis.

The anemias of chronic inflammation and malignancy, described in detail later, may be slightly microcytic owing to a defect in the availability of iron. However, these disorders are more often normocytic. Measurement of serum iron and iron binding capacity (Fig. 161-6A) and evaluation of marrow iron stores are particularly useful in distinguishing between iron deficiency and the anemia of chronic inflammation.

Macrocytic Anemias

A modest increase in red cell size is encountered in a variety of conditions, including liver disease, hypothyroidism, acute blood loss, hemolytic anemia, aplastic anemia, and alcoholism. The macrocytes in liver disease and hypothyroidism may be related to an increased deposition of lipid in the red cell membrane. If the MCV exceeds approximately 105 fL, the patient is likely to be deficient in either cobalamin (vitamin B_{12}) or folic acid. The bone marrow reveals megaloblastic morphology, reflecting impaired replication of DNA. Because nuclear maturation lags behind cytoplasmic development, large red cells tend to be produced in the bone marrow. Megaloblastic anemias are discussed in detail in Chapter 167. Like the microcytic anemias, these disorders are maturation defects associated with ineffective erythropoiesis.

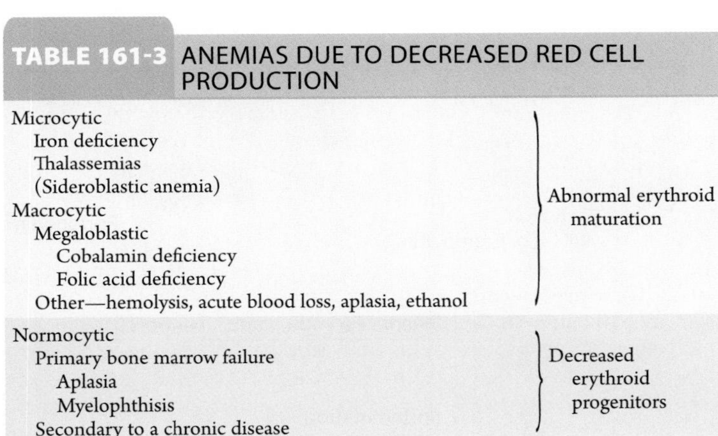

TABLE 161-3 ANEMIAS DUE TO DECREASED RED CELL PRODUCTION

Microcytic Iron deficiency Thalassemias (Sideroblastic anemia) Macrocytic Megaloblastic Cobalamin deficiency Folic acid deficiency Other—hemolysis, acute blood loss, aplasia, ethanol	Abnormal erythroid maturation
Normocytic Primary bone marrow failure Aplasia Myelophthisis Secondary to a chronic disease	Decreased erythroid progenitors

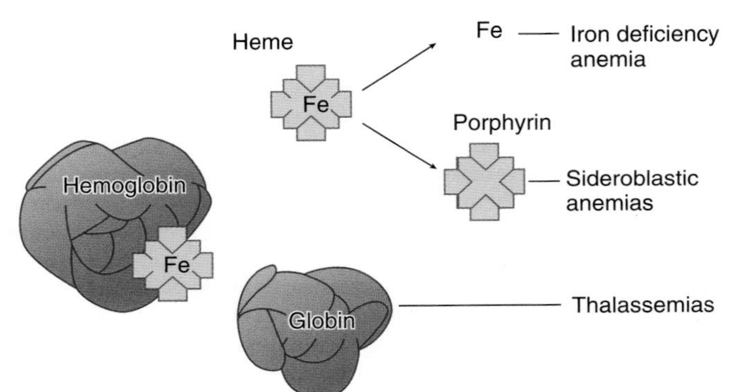

FIGURE 161-5. Components of hemoglobin that are deficient in the microcytic anemias.

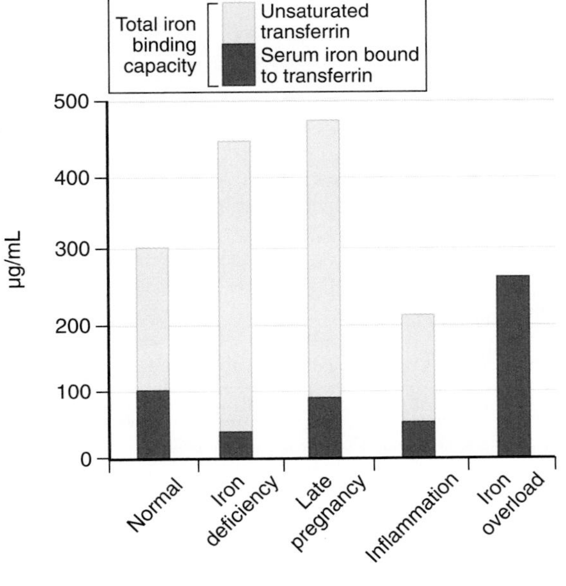

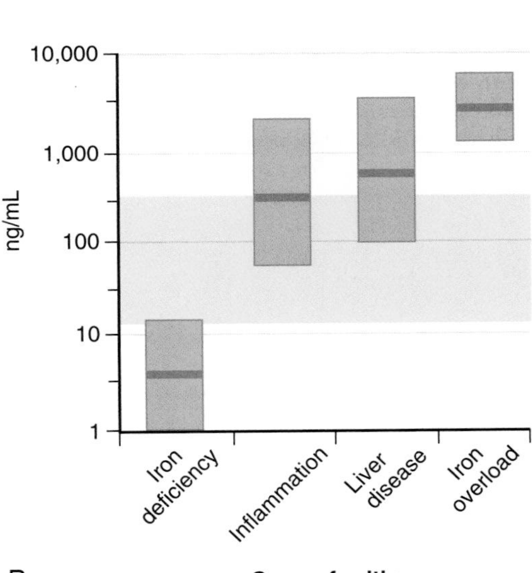

FIGURE 161-6. **A,** Serum iron and transferrin saturation in different conditions. **B,** Serum ferritin in different conditions. Note that the Y-axis in this panel is on a log scale. The normal range (10 to 200 ng/mL) is shown by the beige shaded area.

Normocytic Anemias

The normocytic anemias of underproduction are a diverse group of disorders. They can be conveniently divided into two categories: those due to intrinsic pathology within the bone marrow, and those secondary to some other underlying disease.

Primary Bone Marrow Disorders

The primary disorders of the bone marrow, such as the leukemias (Chapters 189 and 190), myelodysplasia (Chapter 188), aplastic anemia (Chapter 168), and myelophthisis, are best approached by microscopic examination of a marrow aspirate and biopsy. This group of anemias is often accompanied by leukopenia and thrombocytopenia. A lesser degree of pancytopenia can also occur in hypersplenism and in the megaloblastic anemias.

Anemias of Chronic Disease

Among the most common anemias and the ones most prevalent in patients hospitalized on a medical service are those secondary to an underlying chronic disease. The diagnosis is usually quite straightforward. However, in some patients the predisposing illness may not be apparent. Thus, the presence of an unexplained normocytic anemia should prompt the search for the disorders listed in Table 161-4. Even if the presence of an underlying illness is established, the physician should investigate whether other factors such as blood loss or a nutritional deficiency are contributing to the patient's anemia. Generally, the anemias due to chronic inflammation, an endocrinopathy, or liver disease are of only moderate severity. In contrast, the anemia of uremia is often severe.

ANEMIA OF CHRONIC INFLAMMATION

If a systemic inflammatory disorder persists for more than a few weeks, it is nearly always accompanied by anemia. As shown in Table 161-4, the most common causes of chronic inflammation are infection, tumor, or a connective tissue disorder. Many chronic infections can be responsible, including tuberculosis, lung abscess, subacute bacterial endocarditis, pyelonephritis, and osteomyelitis. The pathogenesis is more complex in some types of chronic infections. For example, in AIDS, the human immunodeficiency virus can directly attack hematopoietic cells and suppress erythropoiesis. In malaria and babesiosis, the parasite enters circulating red cells and triggers their destruction.

There is considerable variability in tumors' ability to evoke an inflammatory response. Many tumors express inflammatory cytokines as part of their profile of abnormal gene expression. In some cases, impaired supply of oxygen or nutrients to the interior of the tumor mass can lead to necrosis and an inflammatory response. Red cell production may be further compromised by encroachment of the bone marrow with leukemia, lymphoma, or metastatic tumor.

Anemia is also a feature of a broad range of inflammatory conditions that are not associated with either infection or cancer. In some of these disorders, the autoimmune attack on the patient's cells and tissues is met with a robust inflammatory response. Rheumatoid arthritis (Chapter 272) is the most commonly encountered connective tissue disorder and gives rise to the prototypical anemia of chronic inflammation. Even more intense inflammation and, accordingly, more severe anemia are seen in polymyalgia rheumatica and temporal arteritis (Chapter 279). In patients with systemic lupus erythematosus (Chapter 274), the anemia of chronic inflammation is often compounded by either immune hemolysis (Chapter 163) or renal insufficiency (discussed later).

TABLE 161-4 ANEMIAS SECONDARY TO CHRONIC DISEASE

Inflammation
Chronic infections
Cancer
Connective tissue disorders
Renal insufficiency
Endocrine disorders
Hypothyroidism
Hypoadrenalism
Hypopituitarism
Hypogonadism—males
Liver disease
Aging

PATHOBIOLOGY

Recently, the mechanism underlying the anemia of chronic inflammation has been elucidated by the discovery that plasma hepcidin levels are markedly increased as a result of induction by inflammatory cytokines. As shown in Figure 161-7, hepcidin blocks both iron absorption from the gut and the exit of iron from macrophages, thus explaining both reduced levels of serum iron and increased iron stores.

DIAGNOSIS

The anemia of chronic inflammation is associated with disordered iron homeostasis. Increased storage of iron in macrophages within the bone marrow, liver, and spleen results in elevated levels of serum ferritin (Fig. 161-6B). However, because of a block in the transfer of this excess iron into the plasma, serum iron is low (see Fig. 161-6A). The level of total transferrin in the serum is also low for unclear reasons. With the recent development of a reliable assay for hepcidin, elevated serum levels of this "master regulator" of iron homeostasis should become useful in the diagnosis of the anemia of chronic inflammation. Because of the impairment in iron availability, erythropoiesis is somewhat "iron deficient." The amount of cytoplasmic iron is

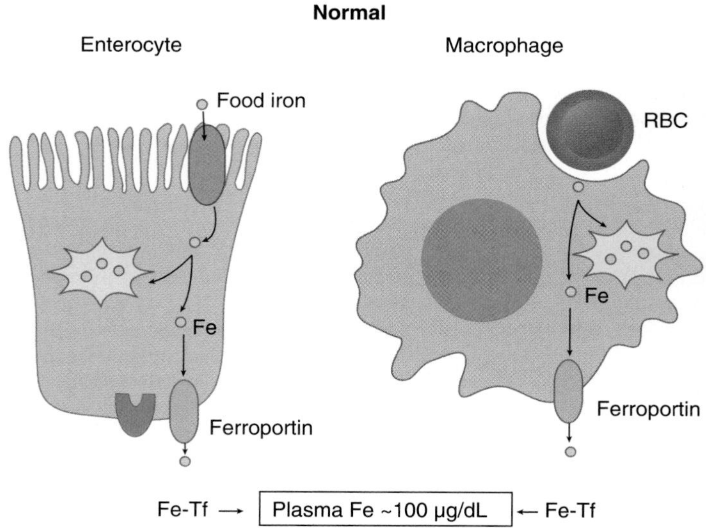

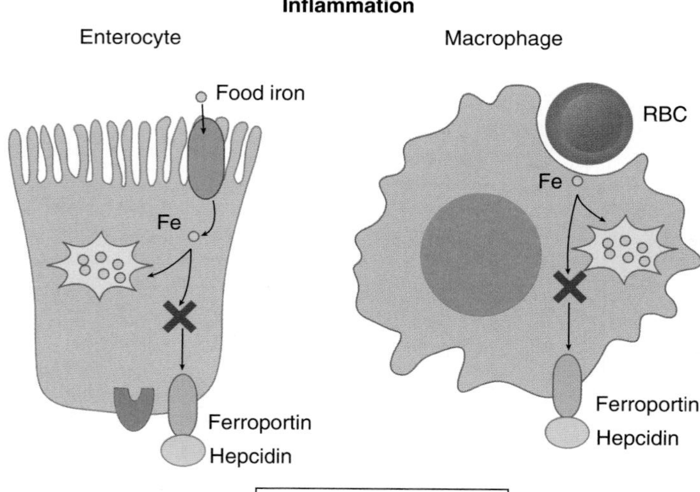

FIGURE 161-7. Pathogenesis of the block in iron availability in the anemia of chronic inflammation. The primary sources of iron in the plasma are from the breakdown of senescent red blood cells (RBCs) within macrophages and from duodenal absorption. **A,** In the presence of physiologically low levels of hepcidin in the plasma, there is efficient release of iron from the duodenal enterocyte and from macrophages via ferroportin. **B,** In patients with inflammation, the induction of plasma hepcidin by interleukin-6 and other cytokines results in the inactivation of ferroportin and the loss of iron egress from the duodenal enterocyte and from the macrophage.

decreased in erythroid precursors in the bone marrow, and the red cells that enter the circulation are slightly microcytic. This suppression of red cell production is earmarked by a low reticulocyte index. Because this block in iron utilization is subtle, the degree of anemia is seldom severe in patients with inflammatory disorders. If the hemoglobin is less than 8 g/dL, it is necessary to look for additional contributors such as hemolysis or bleeding.

TREATMENT Rx

Because the anemia of chronic inflammation is not severe, patients seldom require red cell transfusions. Some patients may benefit from recombinant erythropoietin therapy. However, the anemia is not fully corrected unless the underlying disease is effectively treated.

ANEMIA OF RENAL INSUFFICIENCY

A normocytic anemia almost always accompanies uremia (Chapter 132). Although the hemoglobin level is highly variable, the severity of the anemia is roughly proportional to the degree of impaired renal function. The cause of the kidney failure usually has little bearing on the extent of anemia. However, for any level of serum creatinine, patients with polycystic disease tend to be less anemic than those with other types of renal disease. In contrast to the anemias associated with other chronic disorders, the anemia of uremia can be very severe, with hemoglobin levels as low as 4 g/dL.

Examination of the bone marrow seldom reveals any abnormalities. Red cell morphology is usually normal. In a minority of patients, the peripheral blood smear reveals so-called burr cells characterized by an evenly scalloped border. Neither the degree of anemia nor the red blood cell lifespan is influenced by the presence of burr cells. In most patients, the corrected reticulocyte count is low, and the red blood cell survival is only modestly decreased. Thus, the low red blood cell mass is due to decreased red blood cell production.

PATHOBIOLOGY

The primary basis for the anemia is the diseased kidneys' inability to secrete adequate amounts of erythropoietin. Plasma erythropoietin levels are lower than those of nonuremic patients with a comparable degree of anemia (see Fig. 161-3). Erythropoiesis is further impaired but not abolished in patients who have undergone bilateral nephrectomy. In addition, red blood cell production may be suppressed by the accumulation of substances that are normally cleared by the kidneys.

Other factors may aggravate the anemia of renal disease. Uremic patients have a propensity to hemorrhage, owing to a qualitative defect in platelet function. As in other patients, chronic gastrointestinal blood loss leads to iron deficiency. Folic acid deficiency may also occur, owing to the poor nutrition of many patients or to the loss of this vitamin during dialysis. Patients whose renal failure is due to thrombotic thrombocytopenic purpura or hemolytic-uremic syndrome (Chapter 175) have a severe form of microangiopathic hemolytic anemia, with characteristic abnormalities of red blood cell morphology (Chapter 160).

TREATMENT Rx

Treatment of the anemia of uremia first focuses on reversing the renal failure. A prompt and dramatic correction of the anemia follows successful renal transplantation. Occasionally, polycythemia may be encountered following renal engraftment and may be a harbinger of impending rejection.

In patients who are not candidates for renal transplantation, the treatment of anemia of uremia has been revolutionized by the administration of recombinant human erythropoietin (rHuEPO). The rapid and complete responses that occur underscore the importance of erythropoietin in the pathogenesis of anemia. Figure 161-8 shows the hematologic response of one of the first patients treated with rHuEPO. Within a few days of initiating rHuEPO therapy, the hematocrit approached normal, necessitating a reduction in dose. Before rHuEPO treatment, this patient was overloaded with iron, as documented by increased serum ferritin and nearly full saturation of serum transferrin. As the red cell mass increased rapidly following treatment, the robust utilization of iron stores resulted in a decline in serum ferritin and transferrin saturation. In contrast to this patient with iron overload, many uremic patients on dialysis therapy have normal or low iron stores before rHuEPO therapy and need the concomitant administration of iron to maximize the erythropoietic response.

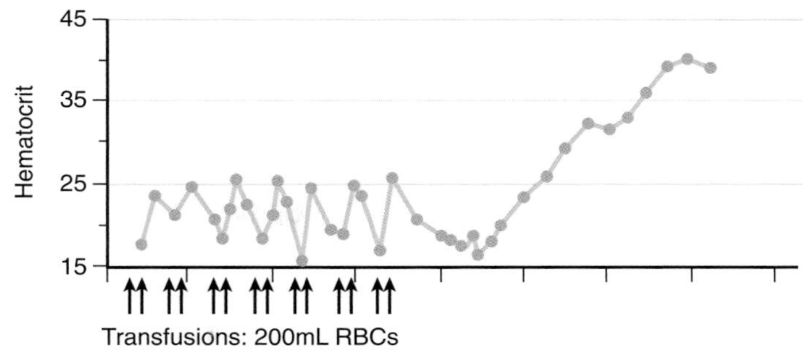

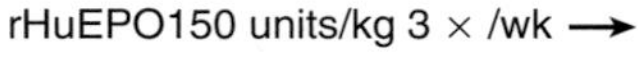

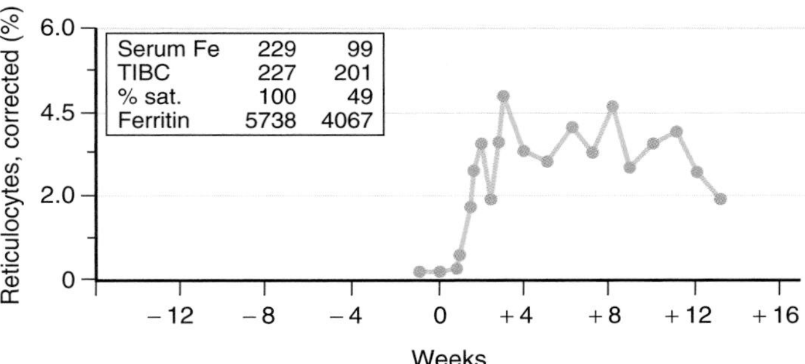

FIGURE 161-8. Response of a uremic patient to recombinant human erythropoietin (rHuEPO) therapy. Before therapy, the patient was severely anemic and transfusion dependent. Treatment with rHuEPO resulted in a reticulocytosis, followed by a progressive increase in hemoglobin. The dose of rHuEPO had to be lowered to prevent the hemoglobin from rising too high. Before rHuEPO therapy the patient was severely iron overloaded. The marked increase in red cell mass following therapy was accompanied by a significant reduction in iron stores. RBC = red blood cell; TIBC = total iron binding capacity. (From Eschbach JW, Egrie JC, Downing MR, et al. Correction of the anemia of end-stage renal disease with recombinant human erythropoietin: results of a combined phase I and II clinical trial. *N Engl J Med.* 1987;316:73-78.)

ANEMIA OF ENDOCRINE HYPOFUNCTION

The in vitro proliferation of erythroid cells is stimulated by a number of hormones, including thyroxine, glucocorticoids, testosterone, and growth hormone. Therefore, it is not surprising that a mild to moderate normocytic anemia generally accompanies endocrine deficiency states, including hypothyroidism, Addison's disease, hypogonadism, and panhypopituitarism.

In the anemia of hypothyroidism, erythropoiesis is suppressed, and the red blood cell lifespan is normal. A minority of patients have macrocytic red blood cells, often owing to cobalamin deficiency. Patients with hypothyroidism have an increased incidence of pernicious anemia. Some patients, particularly females with menorrhagia, develop iron deficiency and a microcytic anemia. The anemia of hypothyroidism may be masked because of a reduction in plasma volume. Because the signs and symptoms of hypothyroidism are sometimes elusive (Chapter 233), this diagnosis should be considered in any patient with unexplained anemia.

The anemia of adrenal insufficiency, including Addison's disease, may also be masked by a decrease in plasma volume. Untreated patients have an average hemoglobin level of about 13 g/dL. Upon hormone replacement, the plasma volume is rapidly reconstituted, and the hemoglobin level falls to 80% of its pretreatment value. With continued therapy, the red blood cell mass returns to normal.

Testosterone influences erythropoiesis in a physiologic manner. In males, the mean hemoglobin level increases from 13 to 15 g/dL during the transition from puberty to adulthood. Eunuchoid males usually have a mild anemia (hemoglobin ≈ 13 g/dL). Pituitary dysfunction or ablation is also associated with a mild anemia.

The anemias secondary to endocrine failure are all readily corrected when adequate hormone replacement is given.

ANEMIA OF CHRONIC LIVER DISEASE

Chronic liver disease, regardless of cause (Chapter 148), is usually accompanied by mild or moderate anemia that is normocytic or slightly macrocytic. An increased plasma volume may artificially lower the hematocrit, making the anemia seem worse than it is. Red cell morphology is normal, except for the presence of target cells and occasional stomatocytes that have a slitlike rather than a circular area of central pallor. These morphologic features reflect an increased red cell membrane surface area due to increased deposits of cholesterol and phospholipid. The bone marrow is usually normal. Erythropoiesis fails to compensate for a modest shortening of the red cell lifespan. The mechanism underlying the anemia of chronic liver disease is not understood. The anemia is usually corrected if the patient regains normal hepatic function.

In patients with alcoholic liver disease (Chapters 155 and 156), the situation is much more complex. Many factors can contribute to the development of anemia. Alcohol in high doses suppresses not only erythropoiesis but also neutrophil and platelet production. In alcoholics who continue to drink up to the time of clinical evaluation, the bone marrow often reveals vacuoles in the cytoplasm of red and white blood cell precursors. In addition, ringed sideroblasts may be observed, especially if there is concurrent malnutrition. Folic acid deficiency is common in alcoholics because of both a suboptimal diet and an impairment of folate utilization. Moreover, the anemia in alcoholics is often compounded by gastrointestinal hemorrhage as a result of gastric erosions, duodenal ulcers, or esophageal varices. The risk of blood loss is further increased by the presence of thrombocytopenia and/or deficiencies in soluble clotting factors. Although alcoholics usually have increased iron stores, they may become iron deficient after prolonged gastrointestinal bleeding. Rarely, patients with alcoholic cirrhosis develop a severe hemolytic anemia accompanied by the appearance of rigid blood cells with irregular borders called acanthocytes or "spur" cells.

ANEMIA OF THE ELDERLY

As individuals age there is a slight and gradual fall in hemoglobin and hematocrit levels. Elderly individuals whose values fall below two standard deviations of normal have significantly enhanced morbidity and mortality. As people age, there is also an increased incidence of cancer, myelodysplasia, renal insufficiency, and chronic inflammatory disorders, all of which can suppress red cell production. Because of the high likelihood of comorbid conditions among the elderly, it is not possible to affirm with any certainty whether aging per se is a cause of anemia. Nevertheless, a fall in hemoglobin in any patient, old or young, should prompt an investigation into the possible presence of one of these underlying disorders.

HEMOLYTIC ANEMIAS

With the exception of sickle cell disease (Chapter 166), hemolytic anemias are encountered much less frequently than those caused by decreased red cell production. Although they are a diverse group, the hemolytic anemias share a number of clinical and laboratory features. Patients with moderate or severe hemolysis may have icterus owing to an elevation in nonconjugated (indirect) bilirubin. In addition, individuals with various types of hemolytic anemia often have splenomegaly, signifying the primary site of enhanced red cell destruction.

PATHOBIOLOGY

The presence of hemolysis is established by the laboratory tests outlined in Table 161-6. Further evaluation is required to establish the specific diagnosis. The clinician saves both time and money by using the available tests in a rational and orderly manner. Diagnosis of hemolytic anemias is greatly facilitated by the use of a logical and pathophysiologically based classification scheme. Table 161-5 groups these disorders going from the outside of the red cell into the cytoplasm, as well as by whether the defect is inherited or acquired. Hemolytic anemias due to environmental factors such as immune destruction or traumatic rupture (Chapter 163) are acquired. Abnormalities of red cell membrane proteins can also cause hemolysis. Mutations in proteins of the red cell cytoskeleton may cause hemolysis of varying severity. The most commonly encountered is hereditary spherocytosis (Chapter 164). Acquired red cell membrane defects are rare. Paroxysmal nocturnal hemoglobinuria is discussed in Chapter 163, and spur cell anemia was mentioned earlier in the section on anemias secondary to chronic liver disease. The proteins in the cytosol of the red cell include hemoglobin and enzymes. Mutations in these proteins can result in inherited hemolytic anemias. Sickle cell disease (Chapter 166) and the thalassemias (Chapter 165) are the most commonly encountered hemoglobinopathies. Homozygous SS disease and the compound heterozygous states SC disease and S/β-thalassemia are pure hemolytic anemias. In contrast, anemia in the clinically significant forms of β-thalassemia is primarily due to ineffective erythropoiesis. By far the most

TABLE 161-5 CLASSIFICATION OF THE HEMOLYTIC ANEMIAS*

Environmental factors Antibody: immunohemolytic anemias Mechanical trauma: TTP, HUS, heart valve Toxins, infectious agents: malaria, etc. Membrane defects Paroxysmal nocturnal hemoglobinuria Spur cell anemia	Acquired
Hereditary spherocytosis, etc. Defects of cell interior Hemoglobinopathies: sickle cell, thalassemia Enzymopathies: G6PD deficiency, etc.	Congenital

*A more detailed differential diagnosis of the hemolytic anemias is presented in Table 163-2 in Chapter 163.
G6PD = glucose-6-phosphate dehydrogenase; HUS = hemolytic-uremic syndrome; TTP = thrombotic thrombocytopenic purpura.

TABLE 161-6 LABORATORY FEATURES COMMON TO HEMOLYTIC ANEMIAS

Peripheral blood
- Increased reticulocyte count
- Polychromasia

Bone marrow—erythroid hyperplasia

Serum
- Increased nonconjugated (indirect) bilirubin
- Elevated lactate dehydrogenase (isoenzymes 1, 2, and 3)
- Decreased or absent haptoglobin
- Plasma hemoglobin:
  - Extravascular hemolysis: moderately increased
  - Intravascular hemolysis: markedly increased

Urine
- Hemoglobinuria — In intravascular hemolysis
- Hemosiderin in urine sediment — In intravascular hemolysis

common red cell enzyme defect is glucose-6-phosphate dehydrogenase deficiency (Chapter 164).

DIAGNOSIS

A number of laboratory tests are used to establish the presence of accelerated breakdown of red cells (Table 161-6). As mentioned in the section Laboratory Evaluation of the Patient with Anemia, the reticulocyte count is the simplest and most cost-effective way to distinguish between hemolytic anemias and those due to decreased red cell production. In this test, a supervital stain or a probe for RNA reveals strands of polyribosomes that are present for only 24 to 48 hours after red cells exit the bone marrow. On a routine Wright or Romanowsky stain, these cells often appear relatively large, with a blue-gray hue (so-called polychromasia). The reticulocyte count is nearly always elevated in patients with hemolysis (unless there is concomitant marrow suppression, such as by folic acid or iron deficiency). This test is a reliable index of red cell production. Thus, in patients with hemolytic anemia, the bone marrow nearly always exhibits erythroid hyperplasia. Because this result is predictable, a bone marrow examination is seldom helpful in patients with hemolytic anemia, unless there is suspicion that the hemolysis is due to an underlying lymphoma.

A number of serum and urine tests are available to confirm the presence of hemolysis and assess its magnitude. As mentioned earlier, serum nonconjugated bilirubin is elevated in proportion to the severity of the hemolysis. Lactate dehydrogenase (LDH) isoforms type 1 through 3 are released from red cells during hemolysis, resulting in increased serum LDH. Most kinds of hemolytic anemia are extravascular, with red cell destruction mediated by macrophages in the spleen, liver, and bone marrow. In these patients, a relatively small amount of hemoglobin is released from engulfed red cells into the plasma, where it binds specifically to haptoglobin. The hemoglobin-haptoglobin complex is rapidly cleared from the circulation. Measurement of serum haptoglobin is a useful test of hemolysis. The great majority of patients with clinically significant hemolysis have very low or absent levels. Less often, patients have intravascular hemolysis with much higher levels of free hemoglobin in the plasma, sufficient to traverse renal glomeruli and exceed the tubular reabsorption capacity. These patients have red or brown urine that, after centrifugation, tests positive with a "dipstick" that detects heme protein. Hemoglobinuria can be readily distinguished from myoglobinuria. In the former, both the plasma and the urine are pigmented. In the latter, the plasma remains colorless because the smaller myoglobin molecule rapidly traverses the glomeruli. Hemoglobinuria is often transient. For a week or so after the episode has abated, the urine sediment will contain hemosiderin, which can be readily detected with the Prussian blue iron stain.

Once these general laboratory tests confirm the presence of hemolysis, an array of specific tests is available to establish the specific cause (Chapters 163 through 165).

APPROACH TO THE TREATMENT OF ANEMIA

As in other disorders, the effective treatment of anemia is based on a thorough diagnostic evaluation. Hematinics such as iron, cobalamin, or folic acid should not be administered unless a specific deficiency has been demonstrated or is anticipated. Although indiscriminate treatment with cobalamin is not harmful per se, it lulls both the patient and the physician into a false sense of security. In contrast, the inappropriate use of iron preparations over a prolonged period can be directly harmful, leading to a state of iron overload.

Many kinds of anemias can be corrected if a precipitating cause can be uncovered and reversed. If a drug or toxin is responsible, its withdrawal may allow full recovery. Correction of anemia secondary to a chronic disease usually depends on whether the underlying condition can be reversed. One of the most dramatic dividends of successful renal transplantation is the rapid correction of the anemia of uremia.

Erythropoietin Therapy

The administration of rHuEPO is remarkably effective in certain circumstances. In addition to those with the anemia of chronic renal failure, selected patients with other types of anemia may benefit from rHuEPO. Treatment can lower transfusion requirements in patients with cancer or HIV infection in whom anemia has been aggravated by chemotherapy. In comparison to patients with renal failure, higher doses are required for those with cancer or AIDS to achieve the same increase in red cell mass. Treatment with rHuEPO has also been effective in some patients with primary bone marrow disorders, particularly myelodysplasia (Chapter 188). Transfusion requirements in surgical patients, both perioperatively and postoperatively, may be reduced by prior short-term administration of rHuEPO. Treatment may also benefit rare patients who are unable to receive blood transfusions because of either antigen incompatibility or religious convictions.

A note of caution has emerged from a number of large studies suggesting that high doses of rHuEPO that drive the hemoglobin level above 12 g/dL are associated with a slight but significant increase in the risk of thrombosis and cardiovascular mortality. A meta-analysis of randomized controlled clinical trials of chronic kidney disease patients treated with rHuEPO showed that targeting higher levels of hemoglobin was associated with an increased risk of all-cause mortality and arteriovenous access thrombosis.[1] Administration of the erythropoiesis-stimulating agents erythropoietin and darbepoetin to patients with cancer has been associated with an increased risk of venous thromboembolism and mortality.[2] The possibility of increasing the risk of tumor progression may be mediated by erythropoietin receptors on malignant cells.

Primary bone marrow disorders pose a formidable therapeutic challenge when considering rHuEPO therapy. Aplastic anemia (Chapter 168) can be cured by both immunosuppressive therapy and stem cell transplantation. Long-lasting remissions can be achieved in an increasing fraction of patients with acute leukemias by chemotherapy, often coupled with stem cell transplantation (Chapter 181). Other primary bone marrow disorders that are unresponsive to these interventions are treated with supportive measures such as transfusions of red cells and platelets.

Red Cell Transfusion

The decision whether to transfuse an anemic patient is often challenging. The risks and complications of the administration of blood products are discussed in Chapter 180. Patients with chronic or long-standing anemia are able to compensate in several ways, discussed earlier in this chapter. A considerable reduction in red cell mass can be surprisingly well tolerated, especially if the patient is young or sedentary. Transfusion is seldom indicated in a patient with chronic anemia whose hemoglobin is 9 g/dL or greater. Those who are expected to respond to the administration of a specific agent such as iron, folic acid, or vitamin B_{12} can usually be spared transfusions. However, if the anemia is severe and accompanied by myocardial or cerebral ischemia or by congestive heart failure, prompt but slow administration of packed red cells is indicated. Whole blood should be given only if the patient is hypovolemic.

Splenectomy

Splenectomy is indicated in the treatment of certain hemolytic anemias. The efficacy of splenectomy correlates with the degree to which the abnormal or defective red cells are destroyed or sequestered in the spleen. Splenectomy is curative in nearly all patients with hereditary spherocytosis (Chapter 164). The operation may be also beneficial in selected patients with immunohemolytic anemia, congestive splenomegaly, spur cell anemia, and certain hemoglobinopathies and enzymopathies. The operative morbidity and mortality from elective splenectomy are very low. The procedure can often be done via mini-laparotomy. Occasional patients develop postoperative left subphrenic abscess. Following splenectomy, young children are at risk of developing overwhelming septicemia. This complication can be partially circumvented by vaccination against pneumococcus and meningococcus. Post-splenectomy sepsis occurs rarely in adults. The risk of sepsis can be circumvented by partial splenectomy. Thrombocytosis generally develops promptly following splenectomy. However, in most cases it is transient. In patients with continued hemolysis or with a myeloproliferative disorder (Chapter 169), the thrombocytosis usually persists and may occasionally be associated with thromboembolic complications.

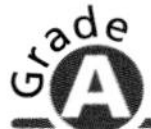

1. Phrommintikul A, Haas SJ, Elsik M, et al. Mortality and target haemoglobin concentrations in anaemic patients with chronic kidney disease treated with erythropoietin: a meta-analysis. *Lancet.* 2007;369:381-388.
2. Bennett CL, Silver SM, Djulbegovic B, et al. Venous thromboembolism and mortality associated with recombinant erythropoietin and darbepoetin administration for the treatment of cancer-associated anemia. *JAMA.* 2008;299:914-924.

SUGGESTED READINGS

Bunn HF, Aster JA. Pathophysiology of Blood Disorders. New York: McGraw Hill; 2010. *Overview of the anemias, with an emphasis on pathobiology.*
Hussein M, Haddad RY. Approach to anemia. *Dis Mon.* 2010;56:449-455. *Review.*
Price EA, Mehra R, Holmes TH, et al. Anemia in older persons: etiology and evaluation. *Blood Cells Mol Dis.* 2011;46:159-165. *Twelve percent had iron deficiency, 35% had unexplained anemia, and 16% had findings suspicious for myelodysplastic syndrome.*
Theurl I, Aigner E, Theurl M, et al. Regulation of iron homeostasis in anemia of chronic disease and iron deficiency: diagnostic and therapeutic implications. *Blood.* 2009;113:5277-5286. *Thorough and up-to-date review of clinically relevant aspects of iron homeostasis.*

162

MICROCYTIC AND HYPOCHROMIC ANEMIAS

GORDON D. GINDER

The oxygen-carrying hemoglobin molecule executes the principal function of the mature erythrocyte. The hemoglobin content of erythrocytes is determined by the coordinated production of globin protein, the heme porphyrin ring, and the availability of iron. A deficiency in any of these three critical components of hemoglobin results in hypochromic and/or microcytic anemia (see Fig. 161-5 in Chapter 161). Microcytic anemia is typically reported initially by automated red blood cell (RBC) indices. Hypochromic microcytic anemia can be confirmed on the peripheral blood smear (Fig. 162-1). Disorders of globin protein production typically produce microcytosis but not hypochromia and are discussed elsewhere (Chapter 165).

IRON DEFICIENCY ANEMIA

EPIDEMIOLOGY

Iron deficiency is by far the most common cause of anemia worldwide and is among the most frequently encountered medical problems seen by primary

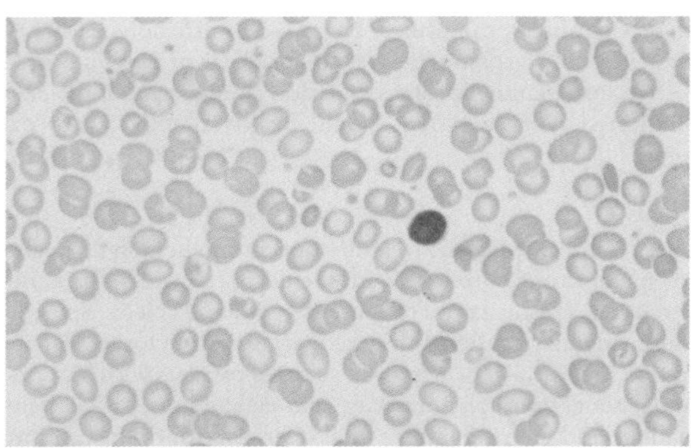

FIGURE 162-1. Iron deficiency anemia. Many of these red blood cells are microcytic (smaller than the nucleus of the normal lymphocyte near the center of the field) and hypochromic (with central areas of pallor that exceed half the diameter of the cells).

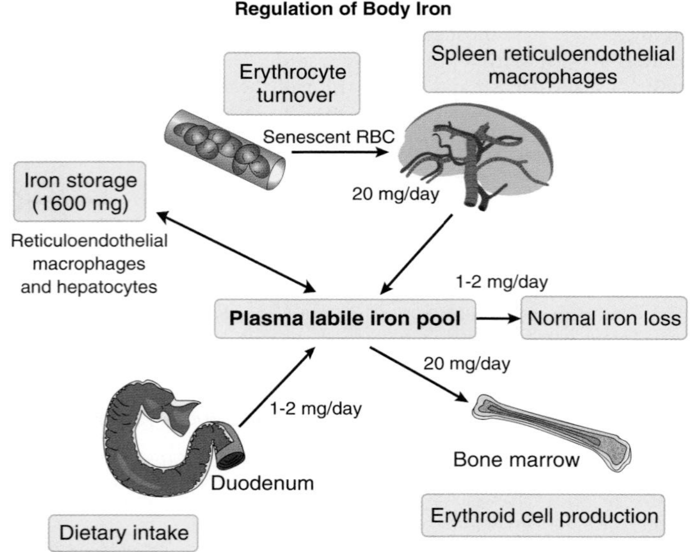

FIGURE 162-2. Iron homeostasis in normal humans. RBC = red blood cell.

care physicians in the United States. It is estimated that between 2 and 5% of adolescent females in the United States have iron deficiency sufficient to cause anemia. Elsewhere, the prevalence of iron deficiency–induced anemia is much higher, with estimates that up to 10% of the world population, or more than 500 million people, are affected. The prevalence rates are especially high in developing countries where dietary insufficiency and intestinal parasites are prevalent.

PATHOBIOLOGY

The majority of the approximately 4 g of iron in the adult human body is incorporated into hemoglobin (approximately 2100 mg) in erythrocytes or myoglobin (approximately 300 mg) in muscle. The remainder is chiefly present as storage iron in the liver (1000 mg) and in the reticuloendothelial macrophages of the bone marrow and spleen (600 mg) (Fig. 162-2). Only a small amount of iron (3 to 7 mg) is freely circulating in plasma bound to transferrin, but this pool is kinetically very active, turning over every 3 to 4 hours. Because of the potent conservation mechanisms of iron recycling through the reticuloendothelial macrophage system, only an average of about 1 to 2 mg of iron is normally lost per day, largely through mucosal sloughing, desquamation, and, in females of reproductive age, menstruation.

The ability of iron to donate or accept electrons readily through conversion between the ferrous (Fe^{2+}) and ferric (Fe^{3+}) states makes it a critical component of the hemoglobin and myoglobin porphyrin rings that transport oxygen as well as cytochromes and various other vital enzymes. Free iron is extremely toxic owing to its capacity to catalyze the formation of free radicals, which lead to cellular damage. Therefore, the majority of body iron that is not stably incorporated into porphyrin rings is associated with proteins. Transferrin is the major protein associated with circulating plasma iron, and ferritin is the major protein associated with stored intracellular iron both in the cytoplasm and in mitochondria. Because the normal rate of iron loss is low, only about 1 to 2 mg/day of dietary iron is needed to maintain homeostasis. The average Western diet contains about 20 mg/day, and the efficiency of iron absorption in the duodenum is usually sufficient to maintain the amount of iron required for homeostatic balance.

Control of iron absorption by the duodenal crypt cells is critical because of the lack of any regulated physiologic mechanism for iron excretion. As a result, excessive iron intake can lead to deleterious iron overload, with concomitant organ damage (Chapter 219). Nonheme dietary iron is dissolved in part by the low pH of the stomach effluent. After reduction to the ferrous state by ferroreductase, iron is transferred across the apical crypt cell membrane by divalent metal transporter-1 (DMT-1). Several levels of regulation are involved in iron absorption by the intestine. One of these is modulated by dietary intake; thus, after a large influx of dietary iron, the duodenal absorptive capacity is diminished. A second regulatory mechanism modulates the iron absorption capacity based on total body iron stores. Finally, the so-called erythropoietic regulator modulates the capacity for enterocyte absorption based on the iron needed for erythropoiesis. A paradoxical increase in iron absorption through this mechanism occurs in certain types of anemia characterized by intravascular and intramedullary destruction of erythroid cells: sideroblastic anemia, the thalassemias (Chapter 165), and congenital dyserythropoietic anemias.

Once inside the intestinal absorbing cell, iron is stored in complex with ferritin. Circulating plasma iron is complexed with the iron transport protein transferrin. The transferrin-iron complex is then taken up by erythroid precursors via the transferrin receptor. The high density of transferrin receptors on erythroid precursors ensures the preferential uptake of iron by these cells and explains why erythropoiesis proceeds normally until a critical deficiency of transferrin-bound iron, reflecting a depletion of total body iron, is present. The levels of transferrin, transferrin receptor, ferritin, and other proteins important in iron metabolism are regulated by the iron regulatory proteins IRP-1 and IRP-2.

Hepcidin, a 25–amino acid peptide, is the central regulator of iron homeostasis through its effects on intestinal absorption, macrophage recycling of iron from senescent RBCs, and iron mobilization from hepatic stores. Thus, hepcidin affects all major sites of iron uptake and storage. Hepcidin is produced in the liver and acts as a negative regulator of iron absorption by the intestine and of iron release from storage in the macrophages and hepatocytes (see Fig. 161-7 in Chapter 161). It is believed that hepcidin binds to ferroportin, the major iron transporter in the membranes of the enterocyte, macrophage, and hepatocyte, causing the internalization and degradation of ferroportin. This process blocks the transport of iron across the membrane of the basolateral crypt cell, preventing its incorporation into transferrin-bound plasma iron. Likewise, loss of ferroportin function blocks the major export pathway of iron stores from macrophages and hepatocytes. Hepcidin production is upregulated by iron and downregulated by hypoxia, consistent with its homeostatic role. Because hepcidin is also upregulated by inflammatory cytokines, it is believed to play an important role in the paradoxical lack of transferrin-bound iron available for erythropoiesis in the face of adequate or even excess iron stores found in the anemia of chronic inflammation (see later and Chapter 161).

Blood Loss

Iron deficiency anemia results from an imbalance between available body iron for hemoglobin production and the minimal amount needed to sustain normal hemoglobin production during erythropoiesis (see Fig. 162-2). Because of the combined effectiveness of dietary absorption and retention of iron under normal circumstances, this mismatch is most often due to blood loss, with the gastrointestinal (GI) tract being the most common site (Chapter 137). In developed countries, the blood loss is usually secondary to benign or neoplastic lesions of the GI tract (Chapters 198 and 199) or chronic ingestion of drugs that cause GI mucosal damage (Chapter 141). The most common offending agents are alcohol and salicylates or other nonsteroidal anti-inflammatory agents. In developing countries, helminthic infections, including hookworm (Chapter 365) and schistosomiasis (Chapter 363), are among the most common causes of GI blood loss.

Genitourinary tract blood loss resulting in iron deficiency is most common in menstruating women. Less common are urinary tract malignancies (Chapter 203) and hemoglobinuria due to intravascular hemolysis (Chapter

TABLE 162-1 LABORATORY FINDINGS FOR IRON STUDIES IN MICROCYTIC AND HYPOCHROMIC ANEMIAS

ANEMIA	SERUM IRON	TIBC	TRANSFERRIN SATURATION (%)	SERUM FERRITIN	SERUM TRANSFERRIN RECEPTOR	MARROW RE IRON	MARROW RINGED SIDEROBLASTS
Iron deficiency anemia	Low	High	0-15	Low (<30 μg/L)	High	Absent	Absent
Anemia of chronic disease	Low	Normal or low	5-15	Normal or high	Normal	Normal or high	Absent
Sideroblastic anemia	High	Normal	60-90	High	Normal or high	High	Present

RE = reticuloendothelial; TIBC = total iron binding capacity.

163). Respiratory tract blood loss is far less common as a cause of iron deficiency.

Reproduction and Growth

In most cases, an increased iron requirement is due to blood loss; other causes include rapid growth in infancy and adolescence and pregnancy and lactation in adulthood. It is estimated that failure to satisfy the increased iron requirements during pregnancy with supplemental iron may result in a deficiency equivalent to a cumulative blood loss of up to 1500 mL.

Inadequate Iron Intake

The other major cause of iron deficiency is inadequate iron intake. Only diets that lack 1 to 2 mg/day fail to provide adequate iron. The average Western meal contains about 6 mg of iron, so dietary insufficiency is not a common cause of iron deficiency. Certain diets that lack iron or contain large quantities of phytates from cereals or tannate from tea, both of which inhibit intestinal iron absorption, may result in iron deficiency. Although iron is usually readily absorbed, primarily in the duodenum, pathologic states that can impair the process include generalized intestinal malabsorption (Chapter 142), atrophic gastritis (Chapter 141) with achlorhydria, and extensive gastric surgery. In contrast, chronic use of H_2-receptor blockers or proton pump inhibitors does not appear to cause iron deficiency. In the United States, celiac disease (Chapter 142) is an increasingly common cause of iron deficiency, with resulting anemia.

CLINICAL MANIFESTATIONS

Because of compensatory physiologic mechanisms, patients with mild iron deficiency anemia may be asymptomatic. Iron deficiency in these patients may be recognized during the evaluation of an underlying disease process or as part of routine laboratory studies. The findings of microcytosis and hypochromia occur only after the hematocrit has fallen to approximately 30%, so neither finding may be present in early stages.

The anemia of iron deficiency, like other anemias, manifests with nonspecific symptoms such as weakness, pallor, dizziness, decreased exercise tolerance, or irritability. Because iron is a critical component of the porphyrin complex in muscle as well as many essential metabolic enzymes, its deficiency affects other organ systems besides the erythron, often resulting in a degree of fatigue, exercise intolerance, and weakness out of proportion to the hemoglobin level. Repletion of iron in iron-deficient individuals may improve cognitive and exercise performance. In addition, intravenous iron treatment in patients with heart failure and coexisting iron deficiency (to which heart failure patients are prone) can improve symptoms, functional capacity, and quality of life, irrespective of the presence or absence of anemia.[1]

Rare patients, most frequently elderly women, may have dysphagia due to an esophageal stricture or web (Plummer-Vinson syndrome). A clinical manifestation unique to iron deficiency is pica, which is an unusual craving for certain non-nutritional substances. Pica may manifest as a craving for ice (pagophagia) or, less commonly, for clay (geophagia) or starch (amylophagia); pagophagia is believed to be the most specific for iron deficiency.

Physical findings that may be associated with the iron-deficient state include glossitis and angular stomatitis. Other less common but highly specific findings are spooning of the fingernails (koilonychia) and blue-tinged sclerae.

DIAGNOSIS

The diagnosis of iron deficiency anemia is made by laboratory testing. Because microcytic hypochromic RBCs are a sine qua non of this type of anemia, initial screening consists of a determination of hemoglobin levels, mean corpuscular volume, erythrocyte hemoglobin content, and reticulocyte count. In experienced hands, the peripheral blood smear (Chapter 160) is an excellent indicator of iron deficiency anemia. In iron deficiency anemia, most erythrocytes are smaller in diameter than the nucleus of a typical lymphocyte, and the area of central pallor is greater than 50% of the total diameter of the erythrocyte (see Fig. 162-1). Variability of erythrocyte size distinguishes iron deficiency anemia from other conditions that give rise to microcytosis; the calculated variability in RBC volume (the so-called RBC volume distribution width, or RDW) is elevated early in iron deficiency anemia.

The definitive diagnosis of iron deficiency anemia is made by tests that measure total body iron stores: the absence of iron stores that can be mobilized is unique to this microcytic hypochromic anemia. Transferrin and transferrin-bound iron levels may not be reliable indicators of iron deficiency because they are also abnormal in the anemia of chronic disease, despite adequate total body iron stores (see Fig. 161-6 in Chapter 161).

The serum ferritin level is the most reliable, noninvasive, and cost-effective indicator that is routinely available in most clinical laboratories (Table 162-1). In a large study of 259 anemic patients, a serum ferritin level less than 18 μg/L was diagnostic of iron deficiency with greater than 95% specificity and a 55% sensitivity. At a serum ferritin level of 45 μg/L, the sensitivity rose to approximately 70%, and a level higher than 100 μg/L in populations with a less than 40% prevalence of iron deficiency excluded a diagnosis of iron deficiency with more than 90% sensitivity. Although some recent studies have questioned the accuracy of the routine determination of stainable marrow iron, this test is still generally considered to be the "gold standard" for tests of iron deficiency. However, determination of total bone marrow iron stores is rarely necessary to diagnose iron deficiency anemia, except when there is some other complicating process.

One setting in which serum ferritin levels can be spuriously elevated is chronic inflammation or chronic disease. The soluble serum transferrin receptor (StFR) level is an excellent measure of total erythroid precursor mass. The StFR is aberrantly elevated in the presence of iron deficiency, so it is considered a useful test for this condition. A number of studies have demonstrated the utility of the StFR/ferritin ratio in distinguishing iron deficiency from the anemia of chronic disease. However, the lack of reliable standards has prevented this assay from becoming routinely available in clinical practice.

TREATMENT Rx

The treatment of iron deficiency anemia is replenishment of body iron stores. However, the underlying cause should always be investigated before treatment is begun, because in many cases it is a correctable and potentially fatal GI lesion (Chapter 137).

Oral Administration

The preferred route of iron administration is oral. Oral iron is most readily absorbed in the absence of food, especially in the setting of decreased stomach acid production owing to atrophic gastritis, gastric surgery, or chronic suppression of gastric acid with an H_2 antagonist or proton pump inhibitor. The major obstacle to oral iron replacement is unacceptable side effects, chiefly epigastric discomfort or nausea; diarrhea or constipation also occurs in some patients. Reducing the dose often eliminates nausea and epigastric discomfort. Despite the development of a number of orally effective iron-containing compounds, the original salt, ferrous sulfate (325 mg three times daily), remains the most useful. Although some newer oral iron preparations, such as ferrous gluconate (300 mg two or three times daily) or ferrous fumarate (325 mg two or three times daily), may induce fewer GI side effects per milligram of iron, they are also less well absorbed, so there is no net advantage to these costlier formulations except for patients who cannot tolerate ferrous sulfate. Given both the low toxicity and the low cost of oral iron replacement, a therapeutic trial is an alternative means of confirming a diagnosis of iron deficiency anemia.

Parenteral Administration

In situations in which primary blood loss is uncontrollable, iron cannot be absorbed owing to severe malabsorption, or oral iron is not tolerated despite concerted efforts to minimize side effects, parenteral iron is an effective alternative treatment.[1] Intramuscular dosing is limited to 100 mg/injection, so intravenous administration is recommended. Sodium ferric gluconate (given intravenously at a dose of 125 mg over 10 minutes) is the preferred form of parenteral iron owing to the low incidence of adverse reactions. A multi-institutional, double-blind, randomized, placebo-controlled trial of more than 2500 patients showed similar adverse events in patients receiving sodium ferric gluconate versus those receiving placebo, and only one life-threatening complication occurred; in comparison, there were 23 such events among 3768 patients treated with iron dextran in a historical control arm.[2] One limitation of sodium ferric gluconate is that the maximum dose deliverable in a single injection is approximately 125 mg, and a total dose of 500 to 2000 mg is usually required for adequate repletion. Although large doses of iron dextran can be delivered in a single intravenous injection, this is currently reserved for situations in which rapid iron replacement is required because of the life-threatening anaphylactic and delayed adverse reactions that occur in 0.6 and 2.5% of cases, respectively. If iron dextran is to be given intravenously, premedication with diphenhydramine and a slow test-dose injection of 30 to 40 mg diluted in normal saline are recommended.

The response to iron repletion therapy is usually quite rapid, with elimination of symptoms within a few days. Increased reticulocytosis usually begins within 4 to 5 days, and the hemoglobin level often rises within 1 week and reaches a normal level after 6 weeks of therapy if adequate iron replacement is achieved. The goal of therapy, which is to reach a serum ferritin level of greater than 50 mg/L, usually takes 4 to 6 months. Therapy must be continued after adequate replacement is achieved if the underlying cause of iron deficiency is not reversible. Because of the avidity of transferrin receptor–rich erythroid precursors for transferrin-bound iron, the serum ferritin level usually does not rise until hemoglobin levels reach normal.

Failure to Respond to Iron Therapy

An incomplete or lack of response to oral iron therapy, as determined by failure to normalize the hemoglobin level, usually means either that iron replacement has not been adequate (most commonly due to noncompliance with oral iron because of its side effects) or that iron deficiency is not the primary cause of the anemia (e.g., coexisting anemia of chronic disease). Less common causes of failure to respond to oral iron include iron malabsorption (e.g., celiac disease, atrophic gastritis) or blood loss in excess of iron replacement.

TMPRSS6, also called matriptase-2, is a type II transmembrane serine protease that suppresses hepcidin production. Several types of mutations in *TMPRSS6* that are either sporadic or familial (usually autosomal recessive) have recently been described as causes of iron-refractory iron deficiency anemia (IRIDA). Associated with inappropriately increased levels of urinary hepcidin, the defect causes impaired iron absorption and recycling, leading to IRIDA. Characteristically, these patients exhibit no hematologic improvement in response to oral iron intake and are only partially responsive to parenteral iron because of abnormal iron utilization.

PROGNOSIS

In most cases, iron deficiency anemia can be corrected rapidly by either oral or parenteral replacement, but the long-term prognosis ultimately depends on the clinical course of the underlying cause. It is critical that the patient undergo a full evaluation to determine the underlying cause of the iron deficiency, especially because an occult gastrointestinal lesion, often malignant, may be present, particularly in patients older than 50 years (Chapters 198 and 199).

ANEMIA OF CHRONIC DISEASE AND INFLAMMATION

DEFINITION

Anemia of chronic disease refers to anemia that occurs in the setting of a chronic disease state, usually one associated with elevated levels of inflammatory cytokines. Because of this association, the condition is also referred to as anemia of inflammation. Although anemia of chronic inflammation usually manifests as a normochromic normocytic process (Chapter 161), between 20 and 50% of cases are associated with microcytic RBC indices. The anemia is usually mild to moderate, and it may not be symptomatic.

EPIDEMIOLOGY

Anemia of chronic inflammation is believed to be the second most common cause of anemia, after iron deficiency. It is the most common type of anemia encountered among hospitalized patients. The wide spectrum of underlying diseases includes acute and chronic infections, inflammatory and autoimmune diseases, cancers, and chronic kidney diseases.

PATHOBIOLOGY

There are three major mechanisms of anemia of chronic inflammation, and all are believed to result from the effects of abnormal levels of inflammatory cytokines. The first is dysregulated iron homeostasis, manifested by low serum iron (hypoferremia) in the presence of normal or elevated serum ferritin levels and abundant reticuloendothelial macrophage iron stores. The functional consequence is a limited availability of iron for erythroid progenitor cells and resultant restriction of erythropoiesis. Pro-inflammatory stimuli, including lipopolysaccharides, interferon-γ, and tumor necrosis factor-α (TNF-α), upregulate DMT-1, which increases iron uptake by the reticuloendothelial cells. At the same time, these stimuli cause the downregulation of ferroportin expression; ferroportin is the protein required for the release of ferrous iron from storage cells and for the transport of dietary iron from duodenal enterocytes into the circulation.

Because hepcidin is an iron-regulated, acute phase reactant peptide that blocks both iron uptake in the gut and iron release from hepatocytes and macrophage stores, its upregulation by lipopolysaccharides, interleukin (IL)-6, and possibly IL-1 (indirectly, through induction of IL-6) results in another mechanism of anemia. Also, patients with hepatic adenomas that secrete high levels of hepcidin have iron-refractory anemia in the presence of normal or elevated ferritin and macrophage iron stores, despite the absence of elevated inflammatory cytokine levels. Elevated urinary hepcidin concentrations correlate with ferritin levels in patients with anemia of inflammation, iron overload, and iron deficiency. These relationships are depicted in Figure 161-7 in Chapter 161.

A third pathophysiologic feature of anemia of chronic inflammation is the inhibition of erythroid progenitor expansion. Interferon-γ is the most potent inhibitory factor of erythropoiesis, but similar inhibition is believed to be mediated by IL-1, TNF-α, and interferon-β. These mediators of inflammation act to increase erythroid progenitor apoptosis, downregulate erythropoietin receptors, and antagonize pro-hematopoietic factors. The action of erythropoietin appears to be directly antagonized by these pro-inflammatory cytokines, which would explain why responsiveness to erythropoietin seems to be inversely related to the severity of the underlying chronic inflammation and the levels of interferon-γ and TNF-α. Finally, increased erythrophagocytosis in the presence of inflammation results in a modest shortening of RBC half-life.

CLINICAL MANIFESTATIONS

The clinical manifestations in patients with anemia of chronic inflammation are usually dominated by the underlying disease process. The anemia in this condition is usually mild, with hemoglobin levels in the range of 8 to 10 g/dL. However, supervening blood loss, absolute iron deficiency, or other aggravating factors can produce life-threatening anemia. Even mild to moderate anemia contributes to the debilitating effects of the underlying disease, adversely impacting performance status and quality of life. Moreover, the presence of anemia is associated with a poorer overall prognosis in many of the underlying chronic diseases, although correction of anemia has not been directly demonstrated to improve survival.

DIAGNOSIS

The clinical diagnosis of anemia of chronic disease presenting with microcytic hypochromic RBC indices is one of exclusion, based on low serum iron in the presence of normal or increased total body iron stores (see Table 162-1). Serum ferritin is the best single laboratory marker for assessing iron storage, and it is almost invariably normal or elevated in anemia of chronic disease. If both the serum iron and the transferrin saturation are reduced, reflecting dysregulation of iron homeostasis, the diagnosis of anemia of chronic disease can be made in the appropriate clinical setting after the exclusion of other causes of anemia, such as coexistent blood loss, thalassemia (Chapter 165), and drug-induced suppression of erythropoiesis. In the presence of inflammation, however, up to 30% of patients with true iron deficiency have serum ferritin levels greater than 100 μg/L, potentially obscuring the diagnosis of iron deficiency. Assays for StfR are useful to diagnose iron deficiency in the presence of the inflammation associated with anemia of chronic disease, but problems with standardization have limited this test's availability in clinical practice. Examination of the bone marrow for reticuloendothelial macrophage iron stores (hemosiderin) and erythroblasts containing iron granules (sideroblasts) can provide definitive evidence of absent iron stores in the setting of anemia of chronic inflammation. A low serum erythropoietin level is also useful in supporting a diagnosis of anemia of chronic inflammation, but only when the hemoglobin level is less than 10 g/dL.

TREATMENT Rx

Treatment of the Underlying Disease

The most effective treatment for anemia of chronic disease is successful treatment of the underlying inflammatory disease process, whether it is an acute or chronic infection, treatable cancer, renal failure, or rheumatoid arthritis. Even if definitive treatment is not possible, quality of life and perhaps prognosis can improve if symptomatic anemia is treated directly. Unfortunately, anemia of chronic inflammation remains undertreated, even in developed countries.

Blood Transfusion

Blood transfusion (Chapter 180) offers the immediate resolution of anemia, but it is indicated chiefly when the anemia is life threatening or seriously limits the patient's functioning. These situations almost always involve supervening blood loss or some other acute process that compounds the anemia of chronic disease. Transfusion is not recommended for the long-term treatment of mild or moderate anemia of chronic inflammation because of the secondary risks, which include transfusional iron overload, human leukocyte antigen (HLA) sensitization in the case of potential renal transplantation, and other side effects of transfusion.

Intravenous Iron and Erythropoietin Therapy

If iron replacement is needed for anemia of chronic inflammation, parenteral iron administration is usually required to replenish stores because of the block in intestinal absorption. In hemodialysis patients receiving erythropoietin therapy, intravenous iron therapy improves anemia; however, when intravenous iron replacement raises the transferrin saturation to greater than 20%, there appears to be an increased risk of developing bacteremia, underscoring the complex relationship between iron homeostasis and immunity.

Erythropoietin therapy is currently approved for use in patients with chronic kidney disease, those with HIV infection, and cancer patients who are undergoing myelosuppressive treatment. Patients with demonstrated iron deficiency should receive supplemental iron with intravenous iron gluconate (see the earlier discussion) while being treated with erythropoietin.

In patients undergoing chemotherapy for cancer whose hemoglobin is less than 10 g/dL, erythropoietin therapy improves quality of life and performance status.[3] However, erythropoietin therapy may be associated with cancer progression in some settings. Because of the decreased survival and increased thromboembolic complications that have been reported in cancer patients receiving erythropoiesis-stimulating agents, current recommendations are for cautious use during chemotherapy and against routine use in inpatients not receiving chemotherapy.[3,4]

PROGNOSIS

The overall prognosis of anemia of chronic inflammation is determined almost exclusively by the course of the underlying disease. It is well established that the degree of anemia correlates well with the severity of the underlying disease process and therefore with levels of inflammatory cytokines. In the absence of a supervening process, anemia of chronic inflammation is not life threatening, and treatment of the anemia per se has not been proved to affect overall survival.

SIDEROBLASTIC ANEMIAS

DEFINITION

This heterogeneous group of anemias is distinguished by the characteristic finding of excessive mitochondrial iron in erythroblasts, as manifested by iron-laden, ringed sideroblasts in the bone marrow in the presence of moderate to severe anemia. These disorders result from mitochondrial defects either in the biosynthesis of the heme porphyrin ring or in the metabolism of iron. Both hereditary and acquired types of sideroblastic anemia have been described. Although often characterized by microcytic and sometimes hypochromic anemia, these disorders can manifest with normochromic normocytic RBCs; if the anemia is associated with myelodysplasia (Chapter 188), macrocytic RBC indices may be present.

EPIDEMIOLOGY

Although acquired sideroblastic anemias are relatively rare, they are much more prevalent than hereditary forms. The true incidence of acquired

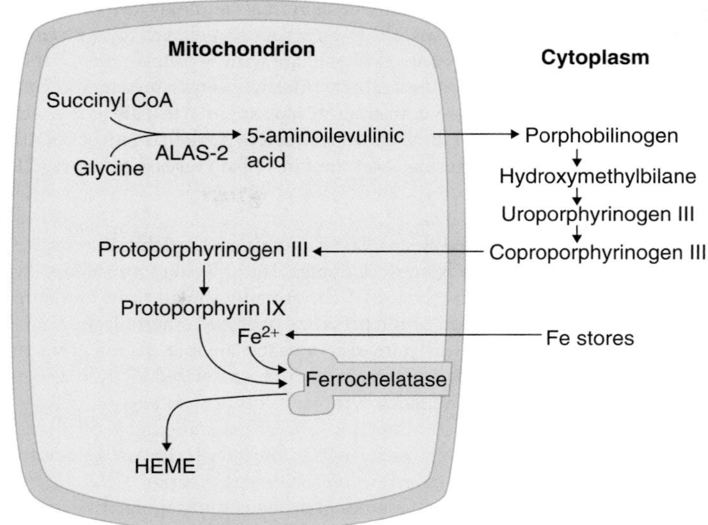

FIGURE 162-3. The heme synthesis pathway. ALAS-2 = δ-aminolevulinic acid synthase; CoA = coenzyme A.

sideroblastic anemia is not well established, in part owing to the heterogeneity of causes and clinical presentations. Hereditary X-linked sideroblastic anemias usually manifest in childhood or early adulthood.

PATHOBIOLOGY

Genetics

The pathophysiologic mechanisms of hereditary sideroblastic anemias are much better understood than those of the more common idiopathic, acquired variety associated with myelodysplasia. Two main forms of X-linked hereditary sideroblastic anemia have been characterized, and both result from defects in the heme synthesis pathway (Fig. 162-3). The first type is caused by mutations in the gene coding for erythroid-specific δ-aminolevulinic acid synthase, known as ALAS-2, on the X chromosome. These mutations may affect the affinity of the enzyme for pyridoxal phosphate or its structural stability, catalytic site, or susceptibility to mitochondrial proteases. In those cases in which the affinity of ALAS-2 for pyridoxal phosphate is altered, pyridoxine supplementation can ameliorate the associated anemia. The other major group of X-linked sideroblastic anemias results from defects in the adenosine triphosphate binding cassette (ABC) protein known as hABC7. The hABC7 protein is believed to be involved in iron-sulfur [FeS] cluster formation. Because [FeS] cluster–associated proteins include ferrochelatase and the cytosolic IRP-1, defects in hABC7 are believed to result in defective iron metabolism or inadequate incorporation of iron into the heme porphyrin ring by ferrochelatase. This type of X-linked sideroblastic anemia is associated with ataxia.

In addition to the two X-linked causes, both autosomal dominant and recessive forms of hereditary sideroblastic anemia have been described. However, the exact mechanisms involved in these disorders are not known.

Other types of hereditary sideroblastic anemia are believed to result from mutations in the mitochondrial genome rather than in nuclear genes. The inheritance of these disorders is complex, owing to the exclusively maternal inheritance pattern of mitochondria; the ovum is the only source of embryonic mitochondria.

Exposure to Drugs or Toxins

The most common form of acquired sideroblastic anemia results from nutritional deficiency or exposure to exogenous drugs or toxins, especially alcohol. Although sideroblastic anemia is not a common finding in alcoholism, the high incidence of alcohol abuse in Western cultures accounts for its frequency as a cause. Alcohol directly inhibits erythropoiesis, but sideroblastic anemia is usually seen only in the setting of concurrent alcoholism and nutritional deficiencies. Other well-documented drug exposures associated with sideroblastic anemia include isoniazid, chloramphenicol, and cycloserine. Sideroblastic anemia has also been attributed to lead exposure (Chapter 21), but there are limited primary data to support this association. Deficiency of pyridoxine causes sideroblastic anemia in animals and may also occur in the setting of alcoholism in humans, although ethanol is believed to be an antagonist of the interaction of pyridoxal phosphate with 5-aminolevulinic acid as a cofactor in the first step of heme biosynthesis. Copper deficiency, though rare, has also been associated with sideroblastic anemia, usually in the setting of an overdose of bivalent cation chelators such as penicillamine or trientine, used to treat the copper overloading found in Wilson disease (Chapter 218).

Idiopathic Forms

The major cause of acquired sideroblastic anemia is idiopathic, in association with myelodysplastic syndromes (Chapter 188). Refractory anemia with ringed sideroblasts is characterized by abnormalities in all three hematopoietic cell lineages, in addition to the presence of ringed sideroblasts.

A second form, known as pure sideroblastic anemia, is less frequently associated with cytogenetic abnormalities, is characterized by dysplasia only in erythroid progenitors, and lacks cytopenias other than anemia. The prognosis in this type of acquired idiopathic sideroblastic anemia is much better than that in refractory anemia with ringed sideroblasts, in part because of a very low incidence (≈10%) of evolution to acute leukemia.

Because of the important differences in prognosis, it is imperative to evaluate cytogenetics and marrow morphology at the time of diagnosis. Recent evidence suggests that mitochondrial DNA mutations and attendant mitochondrial cytopathies account for many, if not all, cases.

CLINICAL MANIFESTATIONS

Because of the heterogeneous nature of the sideroblastic anemias, many of the clinical manifestations vary according to the underlying pathophysiologic cause. The anemia is usually moderate to severe, with hemoglobin levels in the range of 4 to 10 g/dL. The peripheral blood smear frequently reveals hypochromia, often with basophilic stippling. Microcytosis is often seen in hereditary forms, but normochromic, normocytic, or even macrocytic RBCs may be seen, especially in the setting of myelodysplasia or in a rare X-linked hereditary form known as Pearson's syndrome.

DIAGNOSIS

The most useful diagnostic laboratory test for sideroblastic anemia is bone marrow morphology with Prussian blue iron staining, which reveals abnormally large and numerous bluish green siderosomes within at least 15% of erythroblasts, giving the characteristic appearance of ringed sideroblasts (Fig. 162-4). These ringed sideroblasts distinguish this disorder from iron deficiency anemia and anemia of chronic inflammation. Bone marrow findings in idiopathic acquired sideroblastic anemias include dyspoietic features of erythroid and/or myeloid and megakaryotic cell lineages.

Iron studies usually reveal normal iron stores or evidence of iron overload, which is caused by the ineffective erythropoiesis found in sideroblastic anemia as well as by the transfusion therapy often required for its treatment. Iron deficiency can occur coincident with sideroblastic anemia, complicating the diagnosis owing to the lack of characteristic ringed sideroblasts, particularly in myelodysplastic syndromes in which thrombocytopenia leads to GI blood loss. If coexisting iron deficiency is suspected, a repeat bone marrow examination after iron repletion has failed to correct the anemia reveals the diagnostic ringed sideroblasts.

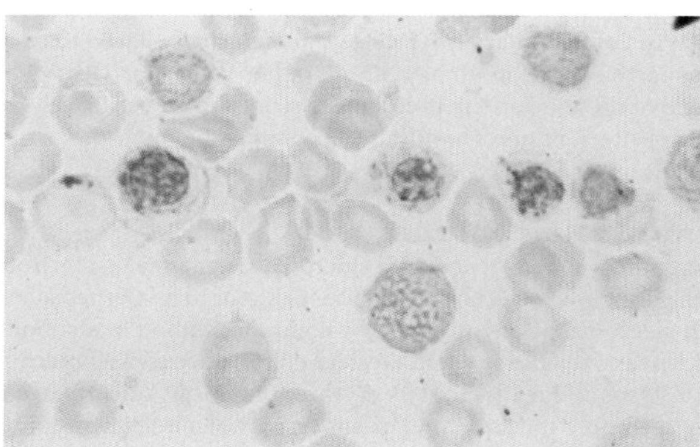

FIGURE 162-4. Sideroblastic anemia. Prussian blue iron stain of the bone marrow shows ringed sideroblasts, which are nucleated red blood cell precursors with perinuclear rings of iron-laden mitochondria.

TREATMENT Rx

Treatment of Underlying Disease

Most forms of sideroblastic anemia lack a specific therapy aimed at the underlying mechanism. Exceptions are those types caused by alcohol or drugs, for which removal of the offending agent usually results in resolution, or at least improvement, of the anemia. Abstinence from alcohol usually reverses the abnormalities in heme biosynthesis in 1 to 2 weeks, as evidenced by the disappearance of ringed sideroblasts in the marrow.

Pyridoxine markedly improves the relatively rare cases of nutritional deficiency, which are usually associated with alcoholism, and some forms of X-linked hereditary sideroblastic anemias in which the binding of pyridoxine by ALAS-2 is defective. Because of its low toxicity in moderate doses, a trial of pyridoxine, 100 to 200 mg/day orally for up to 3 months, is worthwhile in all patients. In responsive cases, reticulocytosis occurs within 2 to 3 weeks, and the hemoglobin level improves over several months. High-dose pyridoxine has been shown to overcome the defect in ALAS-2 activity in some patients with X-linked sideroblastic anemia, but prolonged high-dose therapy can be associated with peripheral neuropathy.

Transfusion

The mainstay of therapy for most severe sideroblastic anemias remains RBC transfusions. Because of the risks of long-term transfusion therapy, treatment should be aimed at achieving a normal performance status rather than a specific target hemoglobin level. Iron stores should be monitored regularly, and iron chelation therapy should be used in the setting of iron overload.

Erythropoietin

Therapy with erythropoietin, with or without granulocyte colony-stimulating factor (G-CSF), benefits a small percentage of patients with acquired sideroblastic anemia due to myelodysplasia. A meta-analysis of 17 studies in which 205 patients were treated with erythropoietin showed an overall response rate of only 16%. However, patients with a diagnosis other than refractory anemia with ringed sideroblasts who were not transfusion dependent had response rates greater than 50%, whereas none of the patients who had refractory anemia with ringed sideroblasts and a serum erythropoietin level greater than 200 U/L responded. Studies using a combination of erythropoietin and G-CSF showed somewhat higher response rates, although none of these studies were large or randomized. Allogeneic bone marrow transplantation (Chapter 181) benefits eligible patients whose myelodysplasia (Chapter 188) has a high risk of evolving into acute leukemia.

PROGNOSIS

As with the underlying pathophysiology, the prognosis in sideroblastic anemias is highly variable. Secondary acquired forms of the disease due to alcohol or toxins respond well to withdrawal of the offending agent, with rapid and often complete normalization of erythropoiesis. The pure sideroblastic anemia variant of myelodysplasia-associated sideroblastic anemia can usually be managed well for many years with transfusions and, if necessary, concordant iron chelation therapy. Other myelodysplasia-related sideroblastic anemias generally have a poor prognosis because of the frequent coexistence of pancytopenia and the relatively high incidence of progression to acute leukemia.

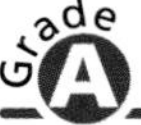

1. Anker SD, Colet JC, Filippatos G, et al. Ferric carboxymaltose in patients with heart failure and iron deficiency. *N Engl J Med.* 2009;361:2436-2448.
2. Michael B, Coyne DW, Fishbane S, et al. Sodium ferric gluconate complex in hemodialysis patients: adverse reactions compared to placebo and iron dextran. *Kidney Int.* 2002;61:1830-1839.
3. Ludwig H, Crawford J, Osterborg A, et al. Pooled analysis of individual patient-level data from all randomized, double-blind, placebo-controlled trials of darbepoetin alfa in the treatment of patients with chemotherapy-induced anemia. *J Clin Oncol.* 2009;27:2838-2847.
4. Bohlius J, Schmidlin K, Brillant C, et al. Recombinant human erythropoiesis-stimulating agents and mortality in patients with cancer: a meta-analysis of randomised trials. *Lancet.* 2009;373:1532-1542.

SUGGESTED READINGS

Camaschella C. Hereditary sideroblastic anemias: pathophysiology, diagnosis, and treatment. *Semin Hematol.* 2009;46:371-377. *Basic mechanisms and clinical approach to this heterogeneous group of rare anemias.*

Goodnough LT, Nemeth E, Ganz T. Detection, evaluation, and management of iron restricted erythropoiesis. *Blood.* 2010;116:4754-4761. *Comprehensive review of iron restricted anemias.*

Pietrangelo A. Hepcidin in human iron disorders: therapeutic implications. *J Hepatol.* 2011;54:173-181. *Review emphasizing the potential for therapeutic interventions.*

Zhu A, Kaneshiro M, Kaunitz JD. Evaluation and treatment of iron deficiency anemia: a gastroenterological perspective. *Dig Dis Sci.* 2010;55:548-559. *Approach to the evaluation of iron-deficient patients for a source of GI blood loss, including the frequent problem of nondiagnostic findings on upper and lower endoscopy.*

163

AUTOIMMUNE AND INTRAVASCULAR HEMOLYTIC ANEMIAS

ROBERT S. SCHWARTZ

DEFINITION

The immune-mediated hemolytic anemias are a group of disorders in which antibodies, complement, and macrophages, usually acting in concert, cause the patient's red blood cells to die prematurely. In the most common type, the antibodies bind to native constituents of the membrane of the patient's own red blood cells. For this reason, the antibodies qualify as autoantibodies, and the diseases they cause fall under the rubric of autoimmune hemolytic anemia.

There are also less common types of immune-mediated hemolytic anemia. Some drugs elicit antidrug antibodies that can cause hemolytic anemia if the drug plants itself in the erythrocyte membrane, thereby making the red cell a target of the antibodies. A high titer of immunoglobulin (Ig) M antierythrocyte autoantibodies that bind to red blood cells at cold temperatures is the distinguishing serologic feature of cold agglutinin disease. In paroxysmal cold hemoglobinuria, an IgG antibody binds to the erythrocyte at cold temperatures, setting the stage for complement-mediated hemolysis at warm temperatures. Paroxysmal nocturnal hemoglobinuria (PNH), another disease in which complement mediates hemolysis, arises from a somatic mutation in a hematopoietic stem cell that renders erythrocytes susceptible to complement-mediated lysis in the absence of antibody. The hemolytic transfusion reaction (Chapter 180) is another disorder in which complement-mediated destruction of erythrocytes occurs, but in such cases, the recipient's alloantibodies against the donor's red cell antigens trigger lysis of the transfused cells.

AUTOIMMUNE HEMOLYTIC ANEMIAS

Autoimmune Hemolytic Anemia with IgG Autoantibodies

EPIDEMIOLOGY

Autoimmune hemolytic anemia associated with IgG autoantibodies (generally referred to simply as autoimmune hemolytic anemia) accounts for about 75% of all autoimmune hemolytic anemias. It has also been called warm antibody autoimmune hemolytic anemia because the IgG autoantibodies in this disorder react best with red cells at 37° C. Autoimmune hemolytic anemia can be primary (idiopathic), or it can develop in association with another disease (secondary).

Autoimmune hemolytic anemia is uncommon. The estimated overall (not age-adjusted) annual incidence is about 1 case per 100,000 population; after age 60 years, the annual incidence reaches 10 per 100,000. The disorder can occur at any age, but most patients are older than 40 years. About 65% of patients with primary autoimmune hemolytic anemia are women, and almost all cases that complicate systemic lupus erythematosus (Chapter 274) occur in women.

PATHOBIOLOGY

Red Cell Antibodies

IgG anti–red cell autoantibodies mediate the destruction of red blood cells outside the circulating blood in a process called *extravascular hemolysis*. By contrast, when lytic components of the complement system participate in the process, the destruction of red cells usually occurs directly within the circulation (intravascular hemolysis). The participation of lytic complement components in IgG-mediated autoimmune hemolytic anemia is rare.

Structure of IgG Anti–Red Cell Autoantibodies

Chapter 44 reviews the structure and function of immunoglobulins. To understand how autoantibodies cause the destruction of red cells, recall that IgG antibodies consist of two identical heavy chains and two identical light chains (Fig. 163-1A); each kind of chain contains variable and constant

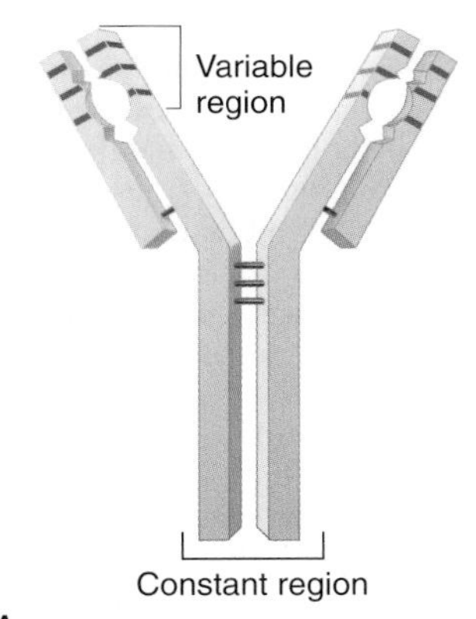

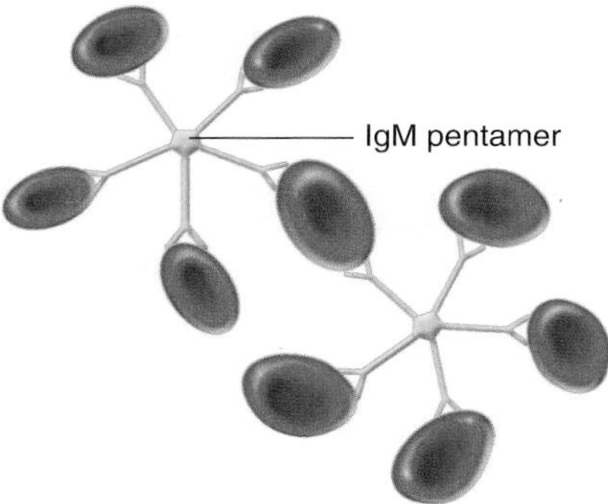

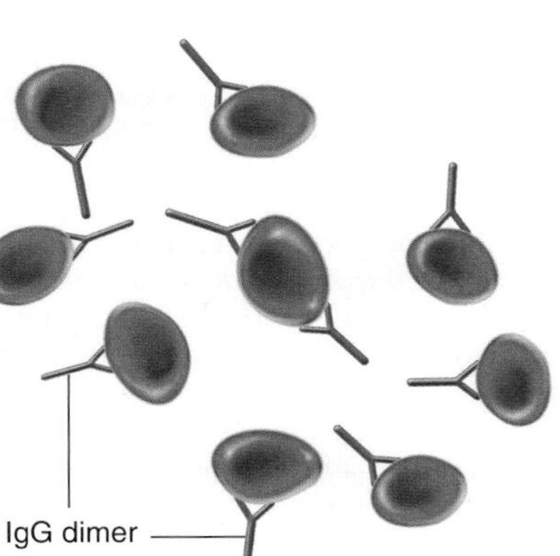

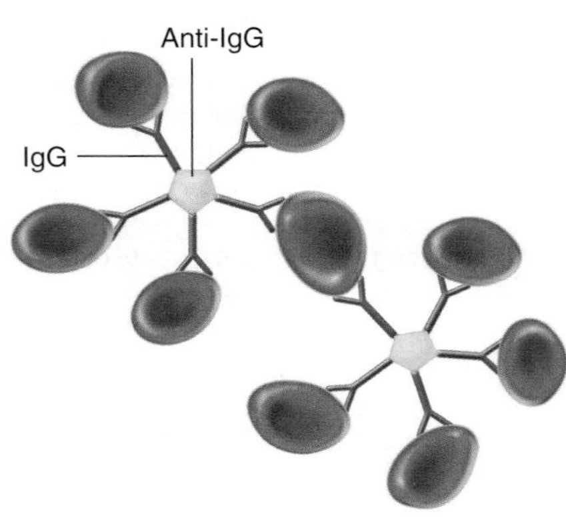

FIGURE 163-1. **IgG anti–red cell autoantibodies. A,** Structure of an IgG molecule demonstrating its variable and constant regions and the heavy and light chains. **B,** Agglutination of red cells by pentameric IgM antibodies, which can join the cells into a lattice. **C,** Coating of red cells by IgG antibodies. The antibodies are unable to agglutinate the cells. **D,** Agglutination of IgG-coated red cells by an anti-IgG antibody.

regions. The four variable regions of IgG form two identical antigen-binding pockets in the molecule. Disulfide bonds hold the constant regions of the heavy and light chains together and give the molecule its characteristic Y shape. An individual B cell produces a monoclonal antibody, a single kind of antibody with a structurally unique antigen-binding pocket, whereas polyclonal antibodies arise from a mixed population of B cells. The constant region (Fc) of the antibody consists of the constant regions of the two heavy chains.

There are two variants of the constant region of light chains: κ and λ. By contrast, the nine heavy chain constant region genes allow nine types of heavy chains: μ (IgM), δ (IgD), γ3 (IgG3), γ1 (IgG1), α1 (IgA1), γ2 (IgG2), γ4 (IgG4), ε1 (IgE1), and α2 (IgA2). These various constant regions determine the isotype of the antibody.

During the immune response, B cells produce IgM antibodies at first; later, under the influence of antigen-activated helper T cells ($CD4^+$), they switch to the production of an IgG, IgA, or IgE isotype. In autoimmune hemolytic anemia, the autoantibodies are a mixture of IgG κ and IgG λ molecules. Such a polyclonal population of antibodies marks the participation of activated $CD4^+$ T cells.

TABLE 163-1 CAUSES OF BLACK OR DARK BROWN URINE

Hemoglobinuria
Intravascular hemolysis
Myoglobinuria (from rhabdomyolysis, Chapter 115)
Ischemic muscle damage
Crush injury
March myoglobinuria
Drugs
Porphyria cutanea tarda (Chapter 217)
Melanin (metastatic malignant melanoma)
Alkaptonuria
Methemoglobinuria

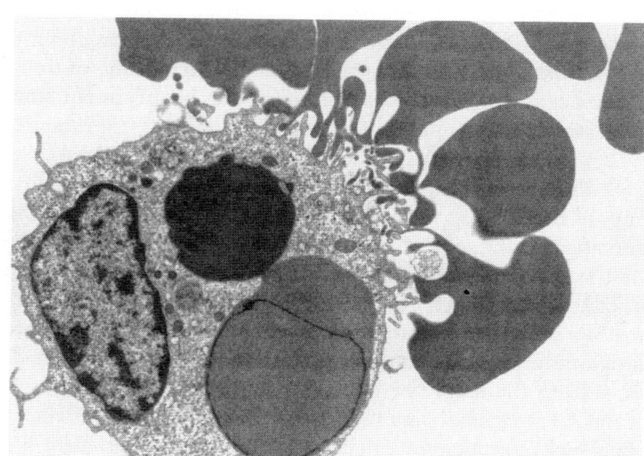

FIGURE 163-2. Electron micrograph of a macrophage that has ingested two spherocytes (dark circular structures within the cytoplasm) and is pinching off bits of membrane from antibody-coated red cells in contact with the surface of the macrophage. (From Jandl JH. Blood. In: *Textbook of Hematology,* 2nd ed. Boston: Little, Brown; 1996:432.)

Red Cell Destruction

Birth and Death of a Normal Erythrocyte

The blood of a normal adult contains about 2000 mL of erythrocytes, which arise in the bone marrow from hematopoietic precursors with a commitment to the red cell lineage. Under the primary influence of erythropoietin, these precursors differentiate, synthesize hemoglobin, and emerge from the marrow 3 days after they become proerythroblasts (Chapter 159). The earliest red cells in the blood are reticulocytes. They lose the blue-staining remnants of cytoplasmic RNA and ribosomes in a little more than a day to become mature oxygen-transporting erythrocytes. Its biconcave shape, the lack of a nucleus, and the lipid bilayer arrangement of its membrane give the red cell the flexibility it needs for the 100-mile journey it makes through the circulatory system during its lifespan of 4 months.

Normally, production and destruction of erythrocytes are matched. To maintain the steady state, the marrow of a 70-kg adult produces about 25 mL of red blood cells (2×10^{11} erythrocytes) daily. About 1% of the circulating red cells die every day, mainly because worn-out water pumps of the aged erythrocyte can no longer prevent intracellular water overload. The excessive water transforms red cell discs into spheres. These spherocytes constitute 1% of the erythrocytes in blood, a figure equal to the percentage of reticulocytes in blood. In sinusoids of the spleen, lymph nodes, and liver, where blood flow is sluggish, macrophages ingest spherocytes and break down their hemoglobin into bilirubin and amino acids.

In an adult, dead erythrocytes release 6 to 7 g of hemoglobin daily, mostly within macrophages. About 10% of dying spherocytes empty hemoglobin directly into the blood stream, where it binds with high affinity to haptoglobin. The haptoglobin-hemoglobin complexes turn plasma red (whereas in myoglobinuria—the result of massive muscle destruction—the plasma is pale amber because myoglobin does not bind to haptoglobin). Macrophages rapidly engulf the hemoglobin-haptoglobin complexes through the macrophage scavenger receptor (CD163), then catabolize the protein constituents of the complex and deliver the heme iron to transferrin. If massive intravascular hemolysis overwhelms the haptoglobin disposal mechanism, the kidneys excrete unbound (free) hemoglobin into the urine. Renal tubular cells take up and convert urinary hemoglobin into bile pigments and retain most of the heme iron. These tubular cells stain with Prussian blue; the blue cells and the cola-colored urine (hemoglobinuria) are diagnostic of chronic (or massive) intravascular hemolysis. Table 163-1 lists the causes of black or brown urine.

Mechanism of Antibody-Mediated Red Cell Destruction

IgG anti–red cell autoantibodies are opsonins; when bound to autoantigens on red cell membranes, they instigate phagocytosis of the cells by macrophages. Using its Fcγ receptors, the macrophage can ingest the entire IgG-coated erythrocyte or transform it into a spherocyte by nibbling away its surface (Fig. 163-2). Antibody-coated spherocytes cannot resist osmotic forces and ultimately surrender to macrophages, especially in the splenic sinusoids, where blood flows sluggishly.

Macrophages bind to structures in the constant regions of all four subclasses of IgG by means of Fcγ receptors. When IgG or IgM antibodies bind to an antigen, their Fc regions expose a binding site for C1q, the first component of the complement system (Chapter 49). The bound C1q, which resembles a bouquet of polypeptides, initiates activation of the classical complement pathway to its final step—formation of the lytic membrane attack complex. Macrophages display receptors for the later-acting C3b and C4b components of complement (CR1 receptors), and these components cooperate with the corresponding Fcγ receptors to hasten destruction of the red cell by acting as opsonins. In autoimmune hemolytic anemia, the complement system rarely proceeds to the late lytic components because molecules on the red cell surface can block generation of the membrane attack complex. The density and mobility of target antigens on the erythrocyte membrane are important because binding of C1q to the constant region of the anti–red cell antibody requires two closely adjacent Fcγ structures on the red cell membrane.

The Hemolytic Rate

The rate of hemolysis in autoimmune hemolytic anemia depends on the amount of autoantibody on the red cell surface, the affinity and avidity of autoantibodies for the red cell autoantigen, and the number of macrophages in the environment of the antibody-coated erythrocyte. Populations of autoantibodies with high avidity cause a higher rate of red cell destruction than populations with low avidity. Free (monomeric) IgG competes with the interaction of antibody-coated red cells with the Fc receptors of macrophages, but the IgG in plasma has only a minor influence on the hemolytic rate. The importance of the subclasses of IgG is unclear, but IgG3 antibodies seem more potent than IgG1 antibodies in promoting phagocytosis.

The degree of anemia in autoimmune hemolytic anemia depends not only on the rate of red cell destruction but also on the ability of marrow to generate a compensatory increase in erythrocyte production. With an adequate supply of nutrients and growth factors, the marrow can increase red cell production by six to eight times the normal rate. In such cases, there is erythroid hyperplasia in the marrow, and reticulocytes leave the marrow at an accelerated pace and in increased numbers; in some severe cases, even nucleated red cells enter the blood. Anemia does not appear until the half-life of the circulating red cell population drops to about 10 days (the half-life of a population of normal red cells is about 30 days). A half-life of 5 or 6 days is not unusual in autoimmune hemolytic anemia.

Causes of Autoimmune Hemolytic Anemia

The cause of autoimmune hemolytic anemia is unknown. In about a third of cases, the autoantibodies have specificity for an antigen in the Rh system. In another third, the antibodies target proteins in membrane glycoproteins (glycophorins) of the red cell; in other cases, the antibodies have specificity for antigens in the Kell or Duffy blood group system (very rarely for ABO antigens) or for structures in the membrane that are not blood group antigens (e.g., band 3). In all these cases, the patient's own erythrocytes display the relevant antigen.

During fetal life, the thymus deletes lymphocytes with receptors that can bind to autoantigen. This effect, one of the mechanisms of immunologic tolerance of endogenous ("self") antigens, prevents the development of autoantibodies against blood group antigens. The extreme rarity of autoimmune hemolytic anemia secondary to anti-A or anti-B antibodies indicates that the deletion occurs early in ontogeny, because the embryo begins to synthesize A and B substances at 5 weeks of gestation.

A population of $CD4^+/CD25^+$ T cells that express the transcription factor Foxp3 restrains immune responses against autoantigens. There is evidence that a deficiency of these regulatory T cells plays a role in the pathogenesis of autoimmune hemolytic anemia, but how this deficiency arises is unknown.

The anti–red cell autoantibodies in autoimmune hemolytic anemia constitute a polyclonal population of IgG antibodies—a typical feature of an antigen-driven immune response. Evidence that cultured T cells from patients with autoimmune hemolytic anemia proliferate in the presence of certain synthetic Rh peptides supports the idea that the patient's own Rh antigens, or exogenous cross-reactive antigens, drive the autoimmune response. These peptides are cryptic—they reside in regions of the Rh protein that are not normally exposed on the red cell surface. By contrast, T cells from Rh-negative persons who were alloimmunized by transfusion of Rh-positive blood respond to peptides in exposed regions of the Rh protein. The weak response of T cells from normal subjects to allogeneic Rh peptides suggests that cross-reactive environmental antigens may prime T cells for an anti-Rh response.

T cells from patients with chronic lymphocytic leukemia (Chapter 190) complicated by autoimmune hemolytic anemia also respond in vitro to self-Rh proteins. Notably, the leukemic B cells are highly effective in presenting Rh protein to T cells. In some cases of chronic lymphocytic leukemia with autoimmune hemolytic anemia, the leukemic cells display surface immunoglobulins with light chain isotypes that differ from those of the patient's anti–red cell autoantibodies, indicating that the source of the autoantibodies in these patients is not the leukemic clone.

Drug-Induced Immune Hemolytic Anemia

Many drugs or drug metabolites have the potential to elicit antidrug antibodies. Drugs that form covalent bonds with proteins in the red cell membrane can bind antidrug antibodies to the red cell surface, causing a positive direct antiglobulin test (see later) and, in some cases, initiating antibody-mediated destruction of red cells. Other drugs, such as the cephalosporins, can bind to red cell membranes and take up IgG nonspecifically from plasma. In these cases, there is no antidrug antibody. The diagnosis of drug-induced immune-mediated hemolytic anemia should be considered if the patient has a history of taking a suspected medication, there is acute complement-mediated hemolysis, only complement components are detectable on the red cell surface, or the patient's serum reacts with red cells in the presence of the suspected drug.

Some drugs can induce true autoantibodies against red cells. Fludarabine, a purine nucleoside analogue used in the treatment of chronic lymphocytic leukemia, and monoclonal antibodies against tumor necrosis factor-α (infliximab and adalimumab), T cells (alemtuzumab), α4 integrin (natalizumab), and interleukin-2 receptor (daclizumab) also have this property, the cause of which is unknown. Notably, there is no sure way of distinguishing drug-induced autoimmune hemolytic anemia from primary autoimmune hemolytic anemia.

CLINICAL MANIFESTATIONS

Autoimmune hemolytic anemia usually unfolds insidiously, but in some cases it begins abruptly with overt symptoms of severe anemia. When the disease is secondary to chronic lymphocytic leukemia (Chapter 190), systemic lupus erythematosus (Chapter 274), or some other disorder, the primary condition generally brings the patient to the physician.

The symptoms are nonspecific and varied. They depend on the age of the patient; the presence of comorbid conditions, especially cardiovascular disease; whether the autoimmune process is primary or a complication of another disorder; and the degree of anemia. In primary autoimmune hemolytic anemia, symptoms of anemia predominate; asthenia and easy fatigue are typical. Dyspnea suggests coexisting heart disease; angina or myocardial infarction can occur in patients with severe anemia and coronary artery disease.

DIAGNOSIS

History

The history can provide clues that help in the differential diagnosis of hemolytic anemia (Table 163-2). The patient's medical history is the key to the diagnosis of drug-induced hemolytic anemia. It is essential to question the patient about both prescribed and over-the-counter medications, because drug-induced hemolytic anemia can be confused with autoimmune hemolytic anemia, and management of the two conditions differs. It is also important to inquire about comorbid conditions; for example, symptoms of cardiovascular disease will influence management.

Autoimmune hemolytic anemia is a well-known complication of chronic lymphocytic leukemia (Chapter 190) and non-Hodgkin's B-cell lymphomas (Chapter 191). It can also occur occasionally in ulcerative colitis (Chapter 143), rheumatoid arthritis (Chapter 272), and various carcinomas. Autoimmune hemolytic anemia occurs in about 10% of cases of systemic lupus erythematosus (Chapter 274); it may be the initial clinical manifestation of the disease or occur later. It may also complicate the antiphospholipid antibody syndrome; such cases constitute a subset of systemic lupus erythematosus. In most diseases with autoimmune hemolytic anemia as a secondary feature, the primary disorder is at the center of the clinical problem.

Physical Examination

There are no diagnostic findings on physical examination. The combination of pallor, jaundice, and a palpable spleen (Chapter 171) points strongly to hemolytic anemia, but not necessarily to autoimmune hemolytic anemia. Pallor is often difficult to gauge; examination of the palmar creases, buccal mucosa, and subconjunctival membranes, as well as side-by side comparison of the examiner's nail beds with the patient's, can be revealing. More than half of patients have a palpable spleen. The tip of the spleen rarely descends more than 6 cm below the costal margin, except in the presence of lymphoma or chronic lymphocytic leukemia. Hepatomegaly is also frequent; a firm, nontender edge is easily palpable in about 50% of patients.

The examiner should search for an underlying disease because the differences between primary and secondary autoimmune hemolytic anemia influence management and prognosis. The malar rash of systemic lupus erythematosus and the enlarged lymph nodes of lymphoma or chronic lymphocytic leukemia should not be overlooked. A very large spleen also raises the possibility of coexisting lymphoma or chronic lymphocytic leukemia.

Laboratory Findings

The blood smear reflects the marrow's attempt to compensate for accelerated hemolysis and the effects of the interaction between antibody-coated red cells and macrophages. Two populations are evident: large, blue-tinged red cells, which correspond to reticulocytes, and small, dark red spherocytes (microspherocytes) (Fig. 163-3). Such a dimorphic population is characteristic of hemolytic anemia but is not diagnostic of any particular type of hemolytic anemia.

The white blood cell count is often moderately elevated, a reflection of a bone marrow stressed by severe hemolytic anemia. In uncomplicated cases, platelet counts are normal or occasionally increased slightly. Platelet counts may be low in systemic lupus erythematosus or in Evans syndrome, a rare combination of autoimmune hemolytic anemia and immune thrombocytopenia (Chapter 175).

The characteristic finding in bone marrow is erythroid hyperplasia. However, examination of marrow is necessary only if there are unexpected findings or suspicion of lymphoma.

Elevated serum levels of prehepatic (indirect) bilirubin and lactate dehydrogenase (LDH) and a reduced serum haptoglobin concentration are signs of hemolytic anemia. The indirect bilirubin in hemolytic anemia usually does not exceed 4.0 mg/dL unless there is coexisting liver disease. Serum LDH can be useful, especially in cases with intravascular hemolysis, but neither LDH nor the haptoglobin level is specific for hemolytic anemia. Moreover, the presence of inflammation negates the value of measuring haptoglobin, which is an acute phase protein. Oral contraceptives, estrogen replacement therapy, and tamoxifen all increase haptoglobin levels. Laboratory signs of intravascular destruction of red blood cells (hemoglobinemia, hemoglobinuria, and hemosiderinuria; see later) are unusual in autoimmune hemolytic anemia.

The Antiglobulin (Coombs) Test

The antiglobulin test is central to the diagnosis of autoimmune hemolytic anemia and to an understanding of the antibody-mediated mechanism of red blood cell destruction in this disorder (Fig. 163-1B to D).

The terms *complete* and *incomplete antibodies* refer to the ability (or inability) of antibodies to cross-link adjacent red cells, thereby building the lattice needed for the macroscopic clumping of red cells. The strong negative charge of red blood cells suspended in saline keeps them apart, even if they have a coating of antibodies—the average distance between cells is 24 nm. IgM antibodies, being pentamers, are efficient agglutinins; with five antigen-binding sites, they can bridge this distance. In contrast, bivalent IgG antibodies usually cannot cause the clumping of saline-suspended erythrocytes.

The test that reveals antibody-coated red blood cells is the direct Coombs (antiglobulin) test. The indirect Coombs test was devised to seek the presence of incomplete antibodies in the patient's serum. As presently used, the standard antiglobulin reagent contains antibodies against all four classes of IgG and components of complement (usually C3 and C4).

A positive Coombs test requires cautious interpretation when there are no other features of autoimmune hemolytic anemia. False-positive test results are not unusual. The reported incidence of positive antiglobulin tests in normal blood donors and general populations of hospitalized patients varies widely—from 1 in 100 to 1 in 15,000. Differences in the technique used to perform the test account for this variation. The usual reason for a false-positive direct antiglobulin test is nonspecific, low-avidity adherence of IgG to red cells. In rare cases, however, the result is not a false-positive but a harbinger of the development of autoimmune hemolytic anemia. False-negative direct antiglobulin tests are usually due to low-affinity autoantibodies that spontaneously elute from the red cell in vitro or to amounts of erythrocyte-coating antibodies that are below the limit of detection by the antiglobulin test. The distinction between a true-positive and a false-positive direct antiglobulin test can be made by eluting the antibody from the red cells and testing its ability to bind to normal red cells. In a false-positive reaction, the eluted antibody does not bind to normal red cells, whereas binding does occur in a true-positive test.

TREATMENT Rx

There are no controlled trials of the treatment of autoimmune hemolytic anemia. A corticosteroid, usually prednisone, is the standard initial treatment. Splenectomy is indicated in patients who fail to attain or sustain a remission. If splenectomy does not result in improvement, one or more immunosuppressive agents can be tried. The physician should not withhold red cell transfusions from symptomatic patients.

TABLE 163-2 DIFFERENTIAL DIAGNOSIS OF HEMOLYTIC ANEMIA

HEREDITARY HEMOLYTIC ANEMIA
The thalassemias
β-Thalassemia
α-Thalassemia
Combined thalassemia and hemoglobinopathy
The hemoglobinopathies
Sickle cell disease (hemoglobin S)
Hemoglobin C disease
Hemoglobin E disease
Combined hemoglobinopathies (hemoglobin SC disease)
Defects of the red cell membrane
Hereditary spherocytosis
Hereditary elliptocytosis
Acanthocytosis
Deficiencies in red cell enzymes
Glucose-6-phosphate dehydrogenase deficiency
Pyruvate kinase deficiency
Defects of the Embden-Meyerhof pathway
ACQUIRED HEMOLYTIC ANEMIA
Immune-mediated hemolytic anemia
Autoimmune hemolytic anemia
Cold agglutinin disease
Paroxysmal nocturnal hemoglobinuria
Paroxysmal cold hemoglobinuria
Drug-induced immune hemolytic anemia
Hemolytic transfusion reaction
Hemolytic disease of the newborn secondary to maternal alloantibodies
Systemic lupus erythematosus
Microangiopathic hemolytic anemia (Fig. 163-4)
Disseminated intravascular coagulation
Thrombotic thrombocytopenic purpura
Hemolytic-uremic syndrome
Infections (e.g., *Clostridium*, malaria, babesiosis, *Bartonella*)
Deficiency of factor H
Giant hemangioma
Disseminated carcinomatosis
Chemotherapy (e.g., mitomycin C)
Solid organ transplantation
Bone marrow transplantation
Malignant hypertension
Scleroderma
Eclampsia, preeclampsia, HELLP syndrome (hemolysis, elevated liver enzymes, low platelet count)
Prosthetic materials
Heart valves
Ventricular or atrial septal patches
Left ventricular assist devices
Vascular grafts
Transjugular intrahepatic portosystemic shunts
Physical or chemical injuries
Trauma to small vessels (e.g., exercise related)
Burn related
Venoms
Bacterial infection (e.g., *Clostridium*)
Copper
Freshwater near-drowning

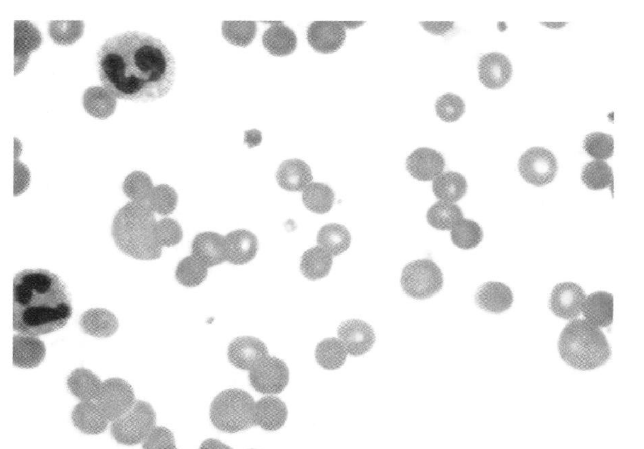

FIGURE 163-3. Representative peripheral blood smear in a patient with autoimmune hemolytic anemia. (Courtesy Thomas K. Chacko.)

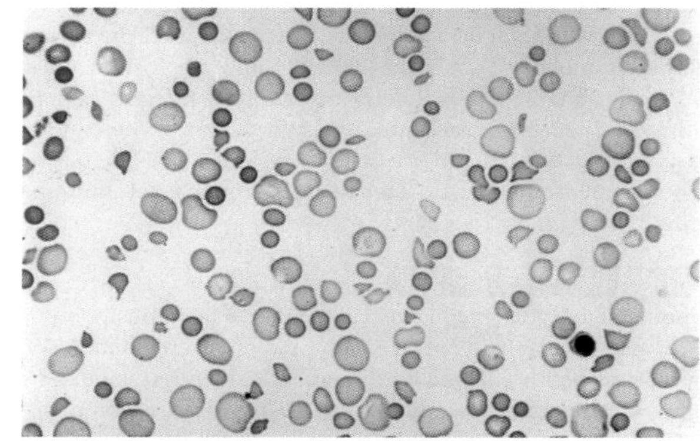

FIGURE 163-4. Microangiopathic hemolytic anemia. A peripheral smear shows fragmental red blood cells or schistocytes in a variety of shapes and sizes.

Initial Therapy

Corticosteroids

In the initial management of the disease, the standard of practice is to administer prednisone at a dose of 1.0 to 1.5 mg/kg/day. The duration of treatment at this dose is an unsettled question, but a response—manifested by a rise in the hematocrit and a fall in the reticulocyte count—is usually evident within 3 to 4 weeks. A patient who fails to improve within this time is unlikely to respond to further treatment with prednisone. In a patient who does respond, slow reduction of the dose of prednisone is essential to avoid a relapse. The usual tapering schedule is a weekly reduction of the initial dose by 10 mg/day to a dose of 30 mg/day, followed by a weekly reduction of 5 mg/day to 15 mg/day. Thereafter, slow, cautious tapering over at least 4 months is the rule. A rise in the reticulocyte count or a fall in the hematocrit should prompt an increase in the dose, usually to the previous level.

About 25% of patients treated with corticosteroids in this manner enter a stable, complete remission; half of patients require continuous, low-dose prednisone; and the remaining 25% respond only transiently or not at all or are unable to tolerate continuous corticosteroid treatment. There is no reliable evidence that alternate-day maintenance treatment is superior to daily treatment, but some patients tolerate this schedule better than daily prednisone. Very high doses of intravenous methylprednisolone have been advocated for stubborn cases, but such treatment is risky and should be considered experimental.

Transfusion

Red blood cell transfusions (Chapter 180) are indicated in patients with disabling symptoms of anemia: marked fatigue, reduced exercise tolerance, or an inability to work. These symptoms often develop when the hemoglobin concentration falls below 10 g/dL, but the decision to administer red cell transfusions should not depend primarily on laboratory tests—the patient's clinical status is the dominant factor. Some patients can tolerate a stable hemoglobin level as low as 8 g/dL; however, symptoms of coronary artery disease or heart failure may force the decision to transfuse before the hemoglobin level falls below 10 g/dL. Regardless of the patient's clinical status, rapid transfusion of large volumes of red cells can have serious adverse consequences. The blood should be administered at a rate that does not exceed 1 mL/kg/hour.

The risk of reactions to blood transfusions (Chapter 180) in patients with autoimmune hemolytic anemia is always present because of the destruction of transfused blood by the patient's autoantibodies. This hazard is increased if the patient also has alloantibodies that were induced by pregnancy or previous transfusions. For these reasons, the blood bank should be alerted to the diagnosis and should be informed if the patient was ever pregnant or has ever had transfusions.

It is important for the managing physician to understand that no patient with symptomatic autoimmune hemolytic anemia should be denied blood transfusions because of an "incompatible crossmatch." The patient's positive antiglobulin test always interferes with compatibility testing. Communication and cooperation between the patient's physician and specialists in transfusion medicine (Chapter 180) are essential in reducing the risks associated with transfusion in patients with autoimmune hemolytic anemia.

Splenectomy

Because the spleen is the major site of red cell destruction in autoimmune hemolytic anemia, splenectomy should be considered for patients who have not responded to corticosteroids or who have maintained a stable but corticosteroid-dependent remission. A complete, durable remission follows splenectomy in one half to two thirds of cases. Attempts to predict responsiveness to splenectomy by measuring the splenic sequestration of ^{51}Cr-labeled erythrocytes have not been reliable. The only way of determining the effectiveness of splenectomy in a given patient is to perform the procedure. Laparoscopic splenectomy, a safe method of removing the organ, is now the preferred surgical technique.

A major risk is post-splenectomy sepsis secondary to encapsulated bacteria, particularly pneumococci and especially in children. Splenectomy also increases susceptibility to babesiosis, ehrlichiosis, and malaria. Preoperative immunization with polyvalent pneumococcal and *Haemophilus influenzae* vaccines reduces the risk of post-splenectomy sepsis. In children, a prophylactic antibiotic, generally penicillin or amoxicillin, is essential after splenectomy. Evidence for the effectiveness of (or need for) prophylactic antibiotics in splenectomized adults is inconclusive. Education of the patient concerning the risk for serious infection after splenectomy is also important.

A rise in the platelet count occurs in almost all patients after splenectomy. The increase rarely exceeds 500,000/mL and usually subsides within 3 to 5 months. The low risk for thromboembolism related to post-splenectomy thrombocytosis argues against the need for routine antithrombotic prophylaxis.

Therapy in Refractory Patients

Rituximab

Rituximab is a chimeric monoclonal antibody with a high affinity for the CD20 antigen on the surface of normal and malignant B lymphocytes (Chapter 35). The antibody consists of murine variable region sequences and human constant region sequences. The usual dose is 375 mg/m^2 by intravenous infusion once a week for four or eight doses, but it may be continued weekly or biweekly if necessary. Rituximab rapidly depletes the circulation and lymphoid tissue of B cells; it can cause allergic reactions and increase the risk for infection.

Other Monoclonal Antibodies

Monoclonal antibodies against components of the immune system or cytokines have been used in the treatment of autoimmune hemolytic anemia, but most of the literature on this topic consists of small, uncontrolled series. Among the monoclonal antibodies that have been used are alemtuzumab (anti-CD52, a T-cell marker) and natalizumab (α4 integrin). These and similar monoclonal antibodies should be reserved for experimental use in refractory, transfusion-dependent cases.

Immunosuppressive Drugs and Other Modalities

Immunosuppressive drugs other than corticosteroids can be useful in stubborn cases of autoimmune hemolytic anemia, but no head-to-head trials have compared the efficacy of these drugs. The choice usually depends on safety and familiarity with the agent. Azathioprine has the least toxicity; cyclosporine is nephrotoxic; and cyclophosphamide damages the bone marrow, ovaries, and bladder and impairs spermatogenesis. Mycophenolate has also been tried, with some success in refractory cases. In general, these drugs should be administered only by specialists and should be reserved for patients who have failed to respond to splenectomy or who, because of comorbidities, are not suitable candidates for splenectomy.

A variety of other treatments have been used in refractory cases of autoimmune hemolytic anemia, including plasma exchange, vinca alkaloids, danazol (a synthetic androgen), and intravenous IgG. None of these forms of therapy is reliably effective, and none of them has been tested for efficacy in a randomized trial.

Cold Agglutinin Disease

DEFINITION AND EPIDEMIOLOGY

Of the two types of cold agglutinin disease, the acute form is a complication of infection, usually by *Mycoplasma pneumoniae* (Chapter 325) or Epstein-Barr virus (infectious mononucleosis [Chapter 385]). The onset in these cases is abrupt and generally appears during recovery from the infection. The acute disease, which almost always affects young adults, is rare, is self-limited, and seldom requires treatment. The usual type of cold agglutinin disease is a chronic disorder of older patients, many of whom have a B-cell lymphoma (Chapter 191), chronic lymphocytic leukemia (Chapter 190), or Waldenström's macroglobulinemia (Chapter 193). In these cases, the cold agglutinin is a monoclonal IgM antibody, in contrast to the polyclonal IgM cold agglutinins of postinfectious cold agglutinin disease.

PATHOBIOLOGY

Cold Agglutinins

Cold agglutinins are IgM autoantibodies that react with erythrocytes at temperatures below 37° C. Normal serum contains low titers of cold agglutinins, which are usually not detectable in a dilution higher than 1 : 10; in chronic cold agglutinin disease, however, the titer can exceed 1 : 10^5. The temperature at which cold agglutinins react with red cells in vitro—the thermal amplitude of the antibodies—varies considerably, but in almost all cases, red cells agglutinate readily at 4° C and quickly disaggregate at 37° C. The temperature-dependent reversibility of the reaction reflects the weak affinity of cold agglutinins for red cell antigens.

Most cold agglutinins react with polysaccharides on the red cell surface. The principal targets are the i antigen (a straight-chain paragloboside) and the I antigen (a branched paragloboside with the same composition as the i antigen). Less common are the Pr glycoproteins and sialylated polysaccharides. The erythrocytes of almost all adults are I$^+$ and lack the i antigen. The i antigen is characteristic of newborns, because the enzyme that converts i to I becomes active only after birth. Cold agglutinins associated with *M. pneumoniae* infection have anti-I specificity, whereas cold agglutinins related to infectious mononucleosis have anti-i specificity. In chronic cold agglutinin disease, the cold agglutinins are almost always monoclonal IgM, anti-I antibodies with a VH4-34 heavy chain; the shape of the antigen-binding surface of this heavy chain favors attachment to polysaccharides. About 10% of B cells from normal subjects display the VH-34 heavy chain; these cells are probably the source of the cold agglutinins in normal serum. Anti-Pr cold agglutinins tend to have a similar κ light chain variable region; presumably, the binding surface of this light chain promotes attachment of the agglutinins to red cell glycoproteins.

Erythrocyte Destruction in Cold Agglutinin Disease

The basis of red cell destruction in cold agglutinin disease is the ability of IgM antibodies to fix complement. Unlike IgG antibodies, each IgM molecule has two binding sites for C1q. An inhibitor on the red cell surface (the membrane inhibitor of reactive lysis) stops the complement cascade before lytic components can be activated, leaving behind C3b and C4b fragments. This step prepares the erythrocyte for engulfment by phagocytic cells with receptors for C3b and C4b. If such coated cells escape into the circulation, enzymes degrade the C3b and C4b fragments to harmless peptides (C3dg and C4d).

Blood cools sufficiently in the hands and feet to allow cold agglutinins to bind red cells. The adherent IgM attracts C1q, which initiates the generation of C3b and C4b on the erythrocyte's surface. On entering the warmer visceral circulation, the red cell releases the cold agglutinin, but the C3 fragments remain engaged to the CR1 of macrophages, thereby enabling phagocytosis of the red cell. The efficiency of this process depends on the amount of cold agglutinin on the red cell surface and the thermal amplitude of the cold agglutinin. An antibody that binds only at very low temperatures causes little harm, whereas an antibody that binds at a temperature close to 37° C can cause severe hemolytic anemia. These variables account for the widely different degrees of severity of cold agglutinin disease.

CLINICAL MANIFESTATIONS

Most cases of chronic cold agglutinin disease occur between the ages of 50 and 70 years. Anemia causes the main symptoms, which can worsen in cold weather. The degree of anemia, which is usually not severe, can remain static without treatment for many months because of the action of an inhibitor of C3b in serum.

In a patient with high-affinity cold agglutinins, exposure to cold can precipitate an attack of acrocyanosis by inducing massive agglutination of red cells in the capillary circulation of the hands, feet, or both. In such a case, intravascular hemolysis with hemoglobinuria and, rarely, acute renal failure can also occur. The acrocyanosis is neither Raynaud's phenomenon (white, blue, and red digits caused by vasospasm [Chapter 80]) nor the vasculitis of cryoglobulinemia (Chapter 193). Enlargement of the spleen is uncommon unless there is an associated B-cell neoplasm.

DIAGNOSIS

Agglutination of the patient's red cells at room temperature or, more often, on chilling of the blood, followed by disaggregation on warming the blood to 37° C, is typical. Hemagglutination causes red cell clumping in the blood smear and may interfere with automated blood counts. Spherocytosis is not prominent; the reticulocyte count is proportional to the degree of anemia.

The titer of cold agglutinins is often $1:10^5$ or higher, and the direct antiglobulin test is positive if the cold agglutinin has a high thermal amplitude. A monoclonal cold agglutinin indicates the presence of a B-cell lymphoma.

TREATMENT Rx

Cold agglutinin disease, whether postinfectious or chronic, often requires no treatment. Postinfectious cold agglutinin disease is self-limited and generally mild. When chronic cold agglutinin disease is stable, its management requires mainly avoidance of the cold. Safe transfusion is possible; there is no agreement concerning the need for transfusion with warmed blood.

In chronic cold agglutinin disease, prednisone, usually at a dose of 1.0 to 1.5 mg/kg/day for 3 to 6 weeks, can be tried, but it is rarely effective. The use of immunosuppressive drugs such as azathioprine or cyclophosphamide is not recommended. Splenectomy generally fails to induce a remission because the liver is a major site of destruction of C3b-coated red cells. Rituximab (375 mg/m^2 by intravenous infusion once a week for four or eight doses) has been used successfully in some cases. In patients with chronic cold agglutinin disease and a B-cell neoplasm, treatment should be directed against the tumor.

Paroxysmal Cold Hemoglobinuria

Paroxysmal cold hemoglobinuria is a rare form of immune-mediated hemolytic anemia in which C1q bound to an IgG autoantibody attaches to red cells at low temperatures. The target antigens are globoside and a glycosphingolipid. The antibody dissociates from red cells at 37° C, but C1q remains on the membrane; at the warmer temperature it triggers progression of the complement cascade to its lytic components. The result is intravascular hemolysis.

An unsolved problem is how the lytic components of complement are generated on the red cell surface in paroxysmal cold hemoglobinuria but not in cold agglutinin disease. With the waning of late syphilis in modern times, the so-called Donath-Landsteiner antibody of paroxysmal cold hemoglobinuria is encountered most often during convalescence from a viral infection, usually a childhood exanthem.

The Donath-Landsteiner autoantibody has no clinical effects unless the patient is exposed to cold temperatures. With cold exposure, even of just an arm or a leg, intravascular hemolysis begins soon after the return to a warm temperature. Chills, fever, back pain, abdominal cramps, and hemoglobinuria are typical. Urticaria is common, acute renal failure is rare, and anemia is an inevitable consequence of severe intravascular hemolysis. The attack is self-limited, lasting only 1 or 2 days.

A positive Donath-Landsteiner test is diagnostic, but the test is relatively insensitive. The procedure should demonstrate hemolysis in the test tube when the patient's blood is chilled and then warmed to 37° C. Addition of normal serum as a source of complement is often necessary to bring out the hemolytic phase of the reaction.

Treatment is generally unnecessary, and spontaneous recovery can be expected within weeks or a few months.

Paroxysmal Nocturnal Hemoglobinuria

DEFINITION

PNH is an acquired form of hemolytic anemia in which a somatic mutation in a hematopoietic stem cell renders erythrocytes susceptible to the lytic components of complement, thereby causing intravascular hemolysis in the absence of an anti–red blood cell antibody.

EPIDEMIOLOGY

PNH can occur at any age but is most common between 10 and 50 years. The median age at diagnosis is about 40 years; median survival after diagnosis is approximately 20 years. It is a rare disorder with an estimated prevalence in the population of 1 in 10^5 to 1 in 10^6. There is no sex preference, and a family history of PNH is unusual.

PATHOBIOLOGY

Genetics

PNH is due to a somatic mutation that causes a defect in the red cell membrane. The disease begins in a single hematopoietic stem cell when the *PIGA* gene on the short arm of the active X chromosome acquires a mutation. The *PIGA* gene encodes PIG-A, an enzyme that is essential for the synthesis of glycosylphosphatidylinositol (GPI). The location of *PIGA* on the X chromosome allows a single mutation in the gene to affect GPI synthesis. This lipid forms a peptide link with the C-terminal amino acid of numerous proteins, anchoring them to the red cell membrane. Molecular genetic studies indicate that the PNH clone upregulates genes that make the PNH clone resistant to apoptosis and immune attack.

The mutation in a hematopoietic stem cell affects PIG-A in blood cells of all lineages. Almost 150 different mutations of *PIGA* have been identified. Most of them inactivate PIG-A and cause total loss of GPI in the descendents of the carrier stem cell. Red cells with complete deficiency of GPI are termed PNH III erythrocytes, and those with partial deficiency are called PNH II erythrocytes. The coexistence of PNH III and PNH II red cells in the same patient indicates the presence of two mutant clones.

A small number of hematopoietic stem cells in normal people bear the *PIGA* mutation; they have no proliferative advantage and persist in small numbers. In normal blood, the frequency of PIG-A–deficient cells is about 1 : 50,000 red cells. In contrast to those with PNH, however, the deficient cells in normal subjects arise from committed hematopoietic cells. The presence of PIG-A–deficient cells in normal subjects suggest that PNH involves not only the *PIGA* mutation but also a second step, perhaps a mutation, that allows expansion of the mutated clone.

Functional Consequences of Deficiency of GPI

The membrane inhibitor of reactive hemolysis (CD59, or protectin) and CD55, an inhibitor of C3 convertase, are two of the many proteins that GPI anchors to the red cell. They prevent polymerization of C9, the final step in assembly of the membrane attack complex that begins with cleavage of C5 to C5b. The deficiencies of CD59 and CD55 allow unimpeded assembly of the membrane attack complex on the erythrocyte surface, thereby initiating intravascular hemolysis. A variety of nonspecific factors, such as a reduction in the pH of blood, can activate complement. The morning hemoglobinuria of PNH is probably the result of subtle acidification of blood during sleep.

CLINICAL MANIFESTATIONS

Classically, a patient with PNH arises in the morning and passes urine the color of a cola beverage. During the ensuing hours, the color of the urine gradually returns to yellow. The typical paroxysms of hemoglobinuria occur on a background of chronic, low-grade intravascular hemolysis, the cause of constant hemosiderinuria in PNH. About a third of cases evolve into aplastic anemia (Chapter 168). Transformation to acute myelogenous leukemia is a rare event. Abdominal pain, dysphagia, and erectile dysfunction are additional clinical features. The basis of these symptoms is probably scavenging by free plasma hemoglobin of nitric oxide, a regulator of vasomotor and smooth muscle tone. In about a third of cases, venous thrombosis occurs and can cause Budd-Chiari syndrome (Chapter 145) by obstructing the hepatic veins. Splenomegaly is uncommon; hepatomegaly and ascites point to the complication of hepatic vein thrombosis. Petechiae and susceptibility to infection are indications of bone marrow failure. Hemosiderinuria is the result of chronic intravascular hemolysis. Subtle or overt signs of bone marrow damage (leukopenia and thrombocytopenia) are frequent.

The extent of red cell destruction in PNH depends on the number of PNH red cells in blood, the level of GPI on the red cell membrane (PNH III cells are devoid of GPI), and the activation of complement. The anemia is often aggravated by iron deficiency caused by chronic urinary iron loss in the form of hemosiderinuria. The basis of the tendency to develop venous thrombosis is unclear; hypercoagulability caused by the release of prothrombotic materials in red cell and platelet membranes (which are also abnormal in PNH) and impaired fibrinolysis have been implicated. Nitric oxide scavenging by free plasma hemoglobin may also damage endothelial cells and cause aggregation of platelets.

DIAGNOSIS

Often, the clinical picture is virtually diagnostic. The diagnosis can be established by demonstrating, by flow cytometry, a deficiency of CD59 on erythrocytes. Another reagent with utility in flow cytometry is aerolysin, a bacterial protein that binds to the GPI anchor. Flow cytometry can also measure the proportions of PNH III and PNH II red cells in blood, providing information on the severity of the disease. Laboratory tests that depend on the sensitivity of PNH red cells to complement, such as the Ham acidification test, are insensitive and have largely been abandoned.

TREATMENT Rx

Eculizumab, a humanized monoclonal antibody against C5, which is essential for formation of the membrane attack complex, can reduce the signs of intravascular hemolysis, the requirement for transfusions, and the tendency to thrombosis. In a randomized trial,[1] the dose of the antibody was 600 mg every week for 4 weeks, followed 1 week later by a 900-mg dose, and then by 900 mg every other week through week 26. A thrombotic event is a strong indication for eculizumab treatment. Warfarin can also be used in patients with a history of a thrombotic event. Oral iron can correct the iron deficiency; treatment with iron does not exacerbate the hemolysis. Transfusions are helpful in supportive care. Aplastic anemia has been treated successfully with immunosuppressive agents (antithymocyte globulin, usually at a dose of 1.5 mg/kg/day for 7 to 14 days) or cyclosporine (3 to 5 mg/kg for at least 3 months). Bone marrow transplantation is risky but can be curative.

Hemolytic Transfusion Reactions

The cause of hemolytic transfusion reactions (Chapter 180) is intravascular lysis of the donor's red cells by antibodies (alloantibodies or isoantibodies) in the recipient that bind to one or more blood group antigens on the transfused cells. The recipient's isoantibodies can be natural anti-A or anti-B antibodies, or they can be induced by previous transfusions or pregnancy. Whether IgM or IgG, the isoantibodies trigger the assembly of lytic complement components on the surface of the donor's red cell. The rapid formation of large amounts of C3a and C5a fragments causes hypotension and bronchial and smooth muscle spasm. Renal failure is a consequence of severe, prolonged hypotension; the main renal lesion is renal cortical ischemia secondary to shunting of blood away from the kidneys. Hemoglobin itself is not nephrotoxic.

The signs and symptoms of a hemolytic transfusion reaction are nonspecific and include fever, back pain, urticaria, dyspnea, hypotension, and

TABLE 163-3 CAUSES OF EXTRAVASCULAR AND INTRAVASCULAR HEMOLYSIS

CONDITION	DIAGNOSTIC FINDING	RED CELL MORPHOLOGY	OTHER FINDINGS	TREATMENT
Autoimmune hemolytic anemia	Positive antiglobulin test	Spherocytosis	Splenomegaly	See text
Drug-induced hemolytic anemia	Drug-dependent antibody	Spherocytosis	History of drug ingestion	See text
Cold agglutinin disease	Cold agglutinins	Normal	Acrocyanosis	See text
Paroxysmal nocturnal hemoglobinuria	Lack of CD59	Normal	Hemoglobinuria, hemosiderinuria	See text
Paroxysmal cold hemoglobinuria	Donath-Landsteiner antibody	Normal	Cold-dependent hemoglobinuria	See text
Prosthetic heart valve	Heart murmur	Schistocytosis	Hemosiderinuria	Iron, folic acid, vitamin B_{12}; valve replacement for severe hemolysis (Chapter 75)
Thrombotic thrombocytopenic purpura	Intravascular hemolysis + thrombocytopenia	Schistocytosis	Renal failure, autoantibody against ADAMTS-13	Chapter 175
Hemolytic-uremic syndrome	Intravascular hemolysis + thrombocytopenia	Schistocytosis	Renal failure, *Shigella* toxin	Chapter 175
HELLP syndrome	Pregnancy	Schistocytosis	Thrombocytopenia, abnormal liver function tests	Chapter 175
Arteriovenous malformations (Kasabach-Merritt syndrome)	Large cavernous hemangioma	Schistocytosis	Thrombocytopenia, DIC	Chapter 175
Postperfusion syndrome	Cardiopulmonary bypass surgery	Ghost erythrocytes	Complement activation	Chapter 74
March hemoglobinuria	History of jogging	No consistent abnormality	Hematuria, hemoglobinuria	Symptomatic
Oxidative hemolysis	Drugs	Heinz bodies	G6PD deficiency	Avoid responsible drug (Chapter 164)
Chemical-induced hemolysis	Strong oxidizing chemicals (e.g., sodium chlorate)	Microspherocytes	Hemoglobinuria, methemoglobinemia, renal failure	Plasma exchange, dialysis
Burns	Severe burn	Spherocytes, schistocytes	Hemoglobinuria	Treatment of burn (Chapter 112)
Malaria	*Plasmodium falciparum* infection	Red cell sporozoites	Hemoglobinuria	Chapter 353
Babesiosis	Tick bite	Intracellular protozoa	Splenectomy scar	Chapter 361
Clostridium perfringens	*C. perfringens* bacteremia	Spherocytosis	Intravascular hemolysis	Chapter 304

DIC = disseminated intravascular coagulation; G6PD = glucose-6-phosphate dehydrogenase; HELLP = hemolysis, elevated liver enzymes, low platelet count.

evidence of disseminated intravascular coagulation. These nonspecific signs appear and worsen during administration of the transfusion. Immediate steps must be taken to stop the transfusion, submit the transfused blood and a sample of the patient's blood to the blood bank, and order tests of plasma and urine for free hemoglobin. Hydration is necessary to ward off renal failure; intravenous fluid, usually normal saline, should be started at once, together with a diuretic (usually furosemide) in amounts to keep urine flow at a rate of at least 100 mL/hour.

OTHER CAUSES OF INTRAVASCULAR HEMOLYSIS

Conditions in which vascular abnormalities, toxins, infections, or drugs damage red blood cells and cause them to lose pieces of membrane and ultimately fragment into hemoglobin-containing bits should be considered in the differential diagnosis of intravascular hemolysis (Table 163-3; see also Table 163-2). Most of these conditions are readily apparent from the history and physical examination. Treatment focuses on the underlying cause of the hemolysis (see Table 163-3).

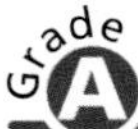

1. Brodsky RA, Young NS, Antonioli E, et al. Multicenter phase 3 trial of the complement inhibitor eculizumab for the treatment of paroxysmal hemoglobinuria. *Blood.* 2008;111:1840-1847.

SUGGESTED READINGS

Garratty G. Immune hemolytic anemia associated with drug therapy. *Blood Rev.* 2010;24:143-150. *Of about 125 implicated drugs, the most common are antimicrobials (e.g., cefotetan, ceftriaxone, and piperacillin).*

Gómez-Almaguer D, Solano-Genesta M, Tarin-Arzaga L, et al. Low-dose rituximab and alemtuzumab combination therapy for patients with steroid-refractory autoimmune cytopenias. *Blood.* 2010; 116:4783-4785. *Alemtuzumab 10 mg subcutaneously on days 1 and 3 plus rituximab 100 mg intravenously weekly in 4 doses provided an encouraging response rate.*

Kelly RJ, Hill A, Arnold LM, et al. Long-term treatment with eculizumab in paroxysmal nocturnal hemoglobinuria: sustained efficacy and improved survival. *Blood.* 2011. [Epub ahead of print.] *Survival in treated patients was similar to an age-matched control population and significantly better than historical controls with PNH.*

Rachidi S, Musallam KM, Taher AT. A closer look at paroxysmal nocturnal hemoglobinuria. *Eur J Intern Med.* 2010;21:260-267. *Practical clinical review.*

164 HEMOLYTIC ANEMIAS: RED CELL MEMBRANE AND METABOLIC DEFECTS

PATRICK G. GALLAGHER

The mature erythrocyte differs from all other cells in the body. Lacking a nucleus, DNA, RNA, and ribosomes, it cannot synthesize RNA, DNA, or protein. It does not divide, it has no mitochondria, it cannot perform the Krebs cycle, and it lacks an electron transport system for oxidative phosphorylation. After enucleation, the reticulocyte, the precursor of the mature erythrocyte, leaves the marrow and enters the circulation equipped with a full complement of enzymes, transporters, signaling molecules, and all other proteins necessary to perform the essential functions of the red cell during its life span.

The erythrocyte membrane accounts for only about 1% of the total weight of a red cell, yet it plays a critical role in the maintenance of normal red cell homeostasis through a number of mechanisms. These include retention of vital compounds and removal of metabolic waste, regulation of erythrocyte metabolism and pH, and import of iron required for hemoglobin synthesis during erythropoiesis. The membrane maintains a slippery exterior so that erythrocytes do not aggregate or adhere to endothelial cells. The membrane skeleton, a network of proteins on the inner surface of the red cell, provides the strength and flexibility needed to maintain the normal shape and deformability of the erythrocyte.

The principle functions of erythrocyte metabolism in the mature erythrocyte include maintenance of adequate supplies of adenosine triphosphate (ATP), production of reducing substances to act as antioxidants, and control of oxygen affinity of hemoglobin by production of adequate amounts of 2,3-diphosphoglycerate (2,3-DPG). Because the mature erythrocyte has lost its ability to perform oxidative phosphorylation, its energy is supplied by anaerobic glycolysis though the Embden-Meyerhof pathway, by oxidative glycolysis through the hexose monophosphate (HMP) shunt, and through nucleotide salvage pathways.

THE ERYTHROCYTE MEMBRANE

Composed of a lipid bilayer and an underlying cortical membrane skeleton (Fig. 164-1), the membrane provides the erythrocyte the deformability and stability required to withstand its travels through the circulation. In one circulatory cycle throughout the body, the erythrocyte is subjected to high sheer stress in the arterial system, dramatic size and shape changes in the microcirculation with capillary diameters as small as 7.5 μm, and marked fluctuations in tonicity, pH, and Po_2.

Membrane Lipids

Red cell membrane lipids are asymmetrically distributed across the bilayer membrane, reflecting a steady state involving a constant exchange of phospholipids between the two bilayer hemileaflets. Glycolipids and cholesterol are intercalated between the phospholipids in the bilayer with their long axes perpendicular to the bilayer plane. Glycolipids, located in the external half of the bilayer with their carbohydrate moieties extending into the aqueous phase, carry several important red cell antigens and serve other important functions. Phospholipids are asymmetrically organized, with the choline phospholipids, phosphatidylcholine and sphingomyelin, primarily in the outer half of the bilayer, and the amino phospholipids, phosphatidylethanolamine and phosphatidylserine (PS), in the inner half of the bilayer. In pathologic states, such as thalassemia, sickle cell disease, and diabetes, loss of phospholipid asymmetry with externalization of PS leads to activation of blood clotting through conversion of prothrombin to thrombin and facilitates macrophage attachment to erythrocytes, marking them for destruction. Mature erythrocytes are unable to synthesize fatty acids, phospholipids, or cholesterol de novo and depend on lipid exchange and fatty acid acylation as mechanisms for phospholipid repair and renewal.

Membrane Proteins

Membrane proteins are classified as *integral,* penetrating or crossing the lipid bilayer and interacting with the hydrophobic lipid core, or *peripheral,* interacting with integral proteins or lipids at the membrane surface but not penetrating into the bilayer core. Integral membrane proteins include the glycophorins, the Rh proteins, Kell and Duffy antigens, and transport proteins such as band 3 (AE1, anion exchanger 1, SLC4A1), Na^+,K^+-ATPase, Ca^{2+}-ATPase, and Mg^{2+}-ATPase. Numerous membrane receptors and antigens are present on integral membrane proteins. Peripheral membrane proteins are on the cytoplasmic membrane face and include enzymes such as glyceraldehyde 3-phosphate dehydrogenase and the structural proteins of the spectrin-actin–based membrane skeleton.

Integral Membrane Proteins

Band 3, the major integral protein of the red cell, has two primary functions: ion transport and maintenance of protein-protein interactions. Band 3 mediates chloride-bicarbonate exchange and provides a binding site for glycolytic enzymes, hemoglobin, and the skeletal proteins ankyrin, protein 4.1, and protein 4.2. A single *N*-glycan chain attached to an Asn in the membrane spanning domain of band 3 is composed of *N*-acetyl-D-lactosamine units arranged in an unbranched, linear fashion in fetal erythrocytes (i antigen) and in a branched fashion in adult cells (I antigen).

The glycophorins are the next most abundant family of integral membrane proteins. They provide most of the negative surface charge required by red cells to avoid sticking to each other and to the vascular wall. They are involved in transmembrane signaling and carry receptors for *Plasmodium falciparum,* a number of viruses and bacteria, and several blood group antigens.

Peripheral Membrane Proteins

Spectrin is the major component of the membrane skeleton. It is composed of two subunits, α and β spectrin, that are structurally related but functionally distinct. Spectrin is highly flexible and assumes a variety of conformations, an unusual property that may be critical for normal membrane pliancy. The spectrin-based membrane skeleton is linked to the plasma membrane through the actin-protein 4.1 junctional complex, through spectrin-ankyrin interactions, and through binding of a multiprotein complex containing Rh proteins, Rh-associated glycoproteins, CD47, LW, glycophorin B, and protein 4.2 to ankyrin. Protein 4.1, a protein necessary for normal membrane stability,

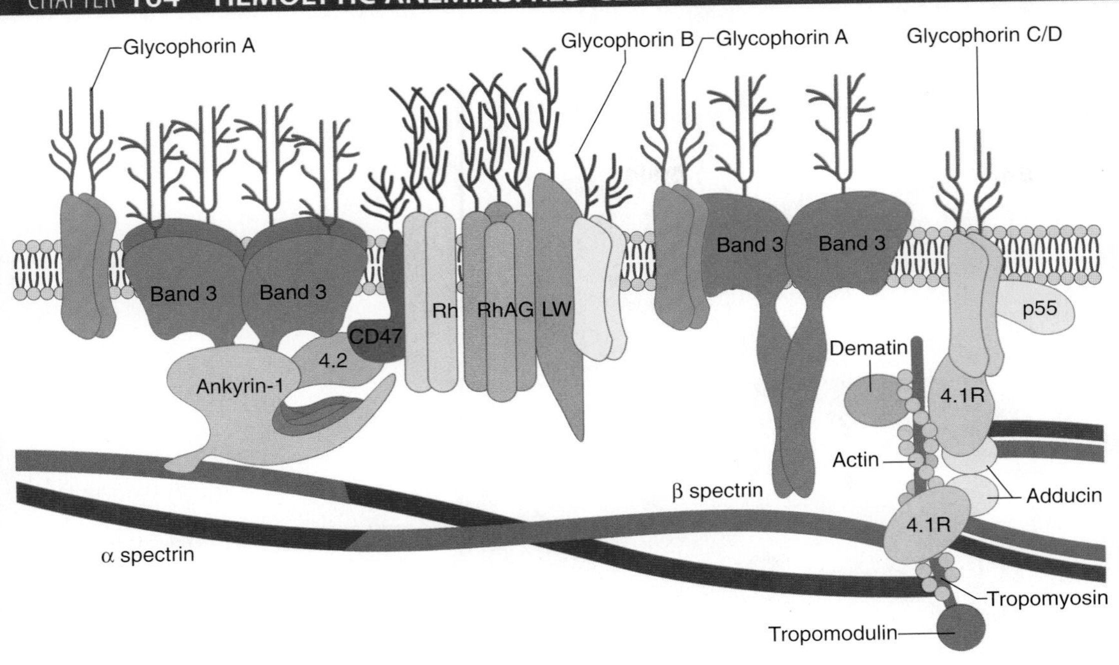

FIGURE 164-1. The erythrocyte membrane. A model of the major proteins of the erythrocyte membrane is shown: α and β spectrin, ankyrin, band 3 (the anion exchanger), 4.1 (protein 4.1) and 4.2 (protein 4.2), actin, and glycophorin. (From Perrotta S, Gallagher PG, Mohandas N. Hereditary spherocytosis. *Lancet.* 2008; 372:1411-1426.)

interacts with spectrin, actin, and other proteins of the red cell membrane. Ankyrin serves as the primary linkage protein for the high-affinity binding of spectrin to the inner membrane through interactions with the cytoplasmic domain of band 3. Protein 4.2 is a peripheral membrane protein that helps link the skeleton to the lipid bilayer through interactions with ankyrin and band 3.

Erythrocyte membrane disorders result from alterations in the quantity or quality (or both) of individual proteins and their dynamic interactions with each other. Disruption of the vertical protein-protein interactions of the membrane, that is, the spectrin-ankyrin–band 3 linkage or the band 3–protein 4.2 interaction, leads to uncoupling of the membrane skeleton from the lipid bilayer. This leads to membrane instability with loss of lipids and some integral membrane proteins, resulting in loss of membrane surface area and the phenotype of spherocytosis. Disruption of the horizontal interactions of membrane skeleton proteins, including perturbation of spectrin self-association or junctional complex protein-protein interactions, leads to membrane instability, altered membrane deformability and mechanical properties, and the phenotype of elliptocytosis.

DISORDERS OF THE ERYTHROCYTE MEMBRANE

Hemolytic anemias due to defects in the erythrocyte membrane comprise an important group of hereditary anemias. Hereditary spherocytosis (HS), hereditary elliptocytosis (HE), and hereditary pyropoikilocytosis (HPP) are the most common disorders among this group. Detailed clinical studies carried out years ago have now been complemented by biochemical and genetic studies, providing both a better understanding of the pathogenesis of these disorders and a better understanding of the normal biology of the erythrocyte membrane.

Hereditary Spherocytosis

DEFINITION

HS refers to a group of disorders characterized by spherical erythrocytes on the peripheral blood smear. Clinical, laboratory, and genetic heterogeneity characterize this group of disorders.

EPIDEMIOLOGY

HS affects approximately 1 in 2000 to 3000 individuals of northern European ancestry. Found worldwide, it is much more common in whites than individuals of African ancestry.

PATHOBIOLOGY

The primary defect in HS is the loss of erythrocyte membrane surface area due to defects in erythrocyte membrane proteins including α spectrin, β spectrin, ankyrin, band 3, and protein 4.2. Qualitative or quantitative defects of one or more of these membrane proteins lead to membrane instability, which, in turn, leads to membrane loss. In approximately two thirds of HS patients, inheritance is autosomal dominant. In the remaining patients, inheritance is nondominant owing to a de novo mutation or autosomal recessive inheritance. Cases with autosomal recessive inheritance are due to defects in either α spectrin or protein 4.2. Rare cases of homozygous HS have been reported, resulting in fetal death or severe hemolytic anemia. In most cases, HS mutations are "private," that is, each individual has a unique mutation, implying that there is no selective advantage to HS.

The spleen plays a critical, albeit secondary, role in the pathophysiology of HS. Splenic destruction of poorly deformable spherocytes is the primary cause of hemolysis experienced by HS patients. Abnormal erythrocytes are trapped in the splenic microcirculation and ingested by phagocytes. Moreover, the splenic environment is hostile to erythrocytes, with low pH, low glucose, and low ATP concentrations and high local concentrations of toxic free radicals produced by adjacent phagocytes, all contributing to membrane damage.

CLINICAL MANIFESTATIONS

The clinical manifestations of the spherocytosis syndromes vary widely. The classic triad of HS is anemia, jaundice, and splenomegaly. Rarely, patients may suffer from severe hemolytic anemia presenting in utero or shortly after birth, continuing through the first year of life. These patients may require multiple blood transfusions, and in some cases, splenectomy in the first year of life. Many HS patients escape detection throughout childhood. In these patients, the diagnosis of HS may not be made until they are being evaluated for unrelated disorders later in life or when complications related to anemia or chronic hemolysis occur. Although the life span of the erythrocyte in these patients may be shortened to only 20 to 30 days, they adequately compensate for their hemolysis with increased marrow erythropoiesis.

Chronic hemolysis leads to the formation of bilirubinate gallstones, the most frequently reported complication in HS patients. Although gallstones have been observed in early childhood, most appear in adolescents and young adults. Routine interval ultrasonography to detect gallstones should be performed, even if patients are asymptomatic.

Other complications of HS include aplastic, hemolytic, and megaloblastic crises. Aplastic crises occur after virally induced bone marrow suppression and present with anemia, jaundice, fever, and vomiting. The most common etiologic agent in these cases is parvovirus B19 (Chapter 379). Hemolytic crises, usually associated with viral illnesses and occurring before 6 years of age, are generally mild and present with jaundice, increased spleen size, and a decrease in hematocrit. Megaloblastic crises occur in HS patients with increased folate demands, such as the pregnant patient, growing children, or patients recovering from an aplastic crisis.

Uncommon manifestations of HS include skin ulceration, gout, chronic leg dermatitis, cardiomyopathy, spinal cord dysfunction, movement

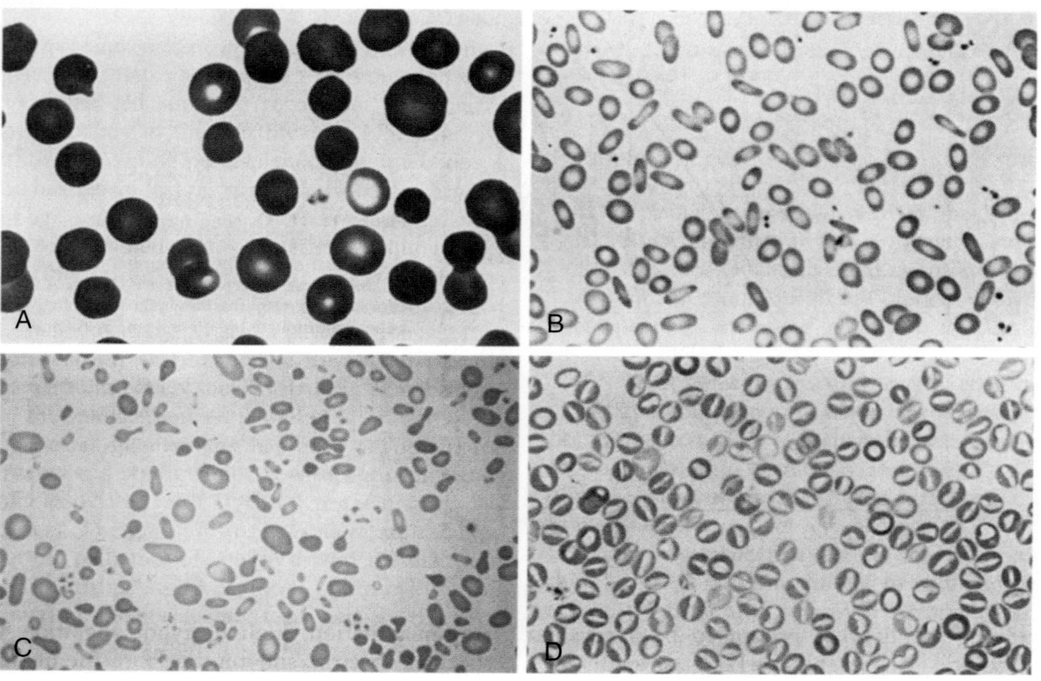

FIGURE 164-2. **Peripheral blood smears in disorders of erythrocyte shape. A,** Hereditary spherocytosis. Characteristic spherocytes lacking central pallor are seen. **B,** Hereditary elliptocytosis. Smooth, cigar-shaped elliptocytes are seen. **C,** Hereditary pyropoikilocytosis. Pronounced microcytosis, poikilocytosis, fragmentation of erythrocytes and elliptocytes are seen. **D,** Hereditary stomatocytosis.

disorders, and extramedullary erythropoiesis. In patients with untreated severe HS, poor growth and findings attributable to extramedullary hematopoiesis, such as hand and skull deformities, may be found.

DIAGNOSIS

Patients with HS may present at any age, usually with anemia, hyperbilirubinemia, or an abnormal blood smear. In evaluating a patient with suspected HS, particular attention should be paid to the family history, including questions about anemia, jaundice, gallstones, and splenectomy. Initial laboratory investigation should include a complete blood count with a peripheral smear, reticulocyte count, direct antiglobulin test (Coombs' test), and serum bilirubin. When the peripheral smear or family history is suggestive of hereditary spherocytosis, an incubated osmotic fragility test (discussed later) should be obtained. Rarely, additional, specialized testing is required to confirm the diagnosis.

Overall, laboratory findings in HS are heterogeneous. Erythrocyte morphology is distinctive but not diagnostic (Fig. 164-2A). Typical HS patients have blood smears with easily identifiable spherocytes lacking central pallor. Some patients present with only a few spherocytes on peripheral smear, whereas others present with numerous small, dense spherocytes and bizarre erythrocyte morphology. Specific morphologic findings have been identified in patients with certain membrane protein defects such as pincered erythrocytes (band 3) or spherocytic acanthocytes (β spectrin). When examining a smear in a case of suspected spherocytosis, it is important to have a high-quality smear with the erythrocytes well separated and some cells with central pallor in the field of examination because spherocytes are a common artifact on peripheral blood smears. The presence of spherocytosis on peripheral blood smear is not diagnostic of HS. Other disorders with spherocytes on peripheral blood smear are listed in Table 164-1.

The mean corpuscular hemoglobin concentration (MCHC) is increased (between 34.5 and 38) owing to relative cellular dehydration. The mean corpuscular volume (MCV) is usually normal or slightly decreased. Technicon and Advia (Siemens Diagnostics, Deerfield, Ill) blood counters provide a histogram of MCHCs claimed to be accurate enough to identify nearly all HS patients.

In the normal erythrocyte, a redundancy of cell membrane gives the cell its characteristic discoid shape and provides it with abundant surface area. In spherocytes, there is a decrease in surface area relative to cell volume, resulting in their abnormal shape. This change is reflected in the increased osmotic fragility found in these cells. Osmotic fragility is tested by adding increasingly hypotonic concentrations of saline to red cells. Normal erythrocytes are able to increase their volume by swelling, but spherocytes, which are already at maximal volume for surface area, burst at higher saline concentrations than normal. Approximately one fourth of HS individuals will have a normal

TABLE 164-1 DISORDERS WITH SPHEROCYTES ON PERIPHERAL BLOOD FILM

Hereditary spherocytosis
Autoimmune hemolytic anemia
Thermal injuries
Microangiopathic and macroangiopathic hemolytic anemias
Hepatic disease
Clostridial septicemia
Transfusion reactions with hemolysis
Poisoning with certain snake, spider, and Hymenoptera venoms
Severe hypophosphatemia
Heinz body anemias
ABO incompatibility (in neonates)

osmotic fragility on freshly drawn red blood cells, with the osmotic fragility curve approximating the number of spherocytes seen on peripheral smear. However, after incubation at 37° C for 24 hours, HS red cells lose membrane surface area more readily than normal because their membranes have become leaky and unstable. Thus, incubation accentuates the defect in HS erythrocytes and brings out the defect on osmotic fragility, making incubated osmotic fragility the standard test in diagnosing HS. When the spleen is present, a subpopulation of very fragile erythrocytes that have been conditioned by the spleen form the tail of the osmotic fragility curve. This tail disappears after splenectomy. The osmotic fragility test suffers from poor sensitivity, with as many as 20% of mild cases of HS missed after incubation. It is unreliable in patients who have small numbers of spherocytes and in patients who have been recently transfused. It is abnormal in other conditions in which spherocytes are present.

Specialized testing is available for studying difficult cases or cases in which additional information is desired. Useful tests for these purposes include structural and functional studies of erythrocyte membrane proteins, such as protein quantitation, limited tryptic digestion of spectrin, spectrin, and ion transport. Membrane frigidity and fragility may be examined using an ektacytometer. Complementary DNA and genomic DNA analyses are available when a molecular diagnosis is desired.

Other laboratory manifestations in HS are manifestations of ongoing hemolysis. Increased serum bilirubin, increased lactate dehydrogenase, increased urinary and fecal urobilinogen, and decreased serum haptoglobin reflect increased erythrocyte destruction.

After diagnosing a patient with HS, family members should be examined for the presence of HS. This can be of great epidemiologic importance, particularly for very old and very young patients. Prenatal diagnosis of HS has been made in a few cases, but this is rarely necessary.

TREATMENT AND OUTCOME Rx

Splenic sequestration and destruction is the primary determinant of erythrocyte survival in HS patients. Splenectomy cures or alleviates the anemia in most patients, reducing or eliminating the need for transfusions. The risk for cholelithiasis is also decreased to nearly background levels. After splenectomy, spherocytes remain in the peripheral blood, but their life span becomes near normal.

In the past, splenectomy was routinely performed in all HS patients. However, the risk of overwhelming postsplenectomy infection, the emergence of penicillin-resistant pneumococci, and the growing recognition of the increased risk of postsplenectomy cardiovascular disease, particularly thrombosis and pulmonary hypertension, have led to reevaluation of the role of splenectomy in the treatment of HS. In addition, with growing globalization, the important role of the spleen in protection of individuals living in or traveling to geographic regions where parasitic diseases such as malaria or babesiosis occur has re-emerged. When splenectomy is considered, health care providers, the patient, and family members must review and weigh the benefits of splenectomy against the immediate and long-term risks of the procedure. Considering the risks and benefits, a reasonable approach is to splenectomize all patients with severe spherocytosis and all patients suffering from significant signs or symptoms of anemia, including growth failure, skeletal changes, leg ulcers, and extramedullary hematopoietic tumors. Other candidates for splenectomy are older HS patients suffering from vascular compromise of vital organs. Whether patients with moderate HS and compensated, asymptomatic anemia should undergo splenectomy is controversial.

When splenectomy is indicated, laparoscopic splenectomy has become the method of choice. This technique results in less postoperative discomfort, a quicker return to preoperative diet and activities, shorter hospitalization, decreased costs, and smaller scars. Even massive spleens can be removed laparoscopically because the spleen is placed in a large bag, diced intraoperatively, and eliminated through suction catheters. Partial splenectomy, initially advocated for infants and young children with significant anemia associated with erythrocyte membrane disorders to allow for palliation of hemolysis and anemia while maintaining some residual splenic immune function, is now being suggested by some for most HS patients.

Before splenectomy, patients should be immunized with vaccines against pneumococcus, *Haemophilus influenzae* type B, and meningococcus. Postsplenectomy care includes counseling of patients or parents to seek prompt medical care in case of febrile illness. Use of routine antibiotics after splenectomy for prevention of pneumococcal sepsis is controversial. Data are lacking to indicate or refute their prescription. Before splenectomy and, in severe cases, after splenectomy, HS patients should take folic acid (1 mg/day orally) to prevent folate deficiency.

Hereditary Elliptocytosis and Related Disorders

DEFINITION

HE is characterized by the presence of elliptical or oval cigar-shaped erythrocytes on peripheral blood smears of affected individuals (see Fig. 164-2B).

EPIDEMIOLOGY

HE has been estimated to occur in approximately 1 in 2000 to 4000 individuals. The true incidence of HE is unknown because its clinical severity is heterogeneous and many patients are asymptomatic. It is common in African Americans and people of Mediterranean ancestry, presumably because elliptocytes confer some resistance to malaria. In parts of Africa, the incidence of HE approaches 1 in 100.

PATHOBIOLOGY

The principal defect in HE is mechanical weakness or fragility of the erythrocyte membrane skeleton. Qualitative and quantitative defects in a number of red cell membrane proteins have been described in HE, including α spectrin, β spectrin, protein 4.1, and glycophorin C. Most defects occur in spectrin, the principal structural protein of the erythrocyte membrane skeleton. αβ Spectrin heterodimers self-associate into tetramers and higher-order oligomers that are critical for erythrocyte membrane stability as well as erythrocyte shape and function. Most spectrin defects in HE impair the ability of spectrin dimers to self associate into tetramers and oligomers, thereby disrupting the membrane skeleton. Structural and functional defects of protein 4.1 appear to disrupt the spectrin-actin contact in the membrane skeleton. Glycophorin C variants are also deficient in protein 4.1. The precise pathobiology of how elliptocytes are formed in these syndromes is unclear.

Genetically, HE is heterogeneous with multiple genetic loci. A wide variety of mutations have been described in the α spectrin, β spectrin, protein 4.1, and glycophorin C genes, including point mutations, gene deletions and insertions, and messenger RNA processing defects. Several mutations have been identified in a number of individuals on the same genetic background, suggesting a "founder effect" for these mutants, which supports the hypothesis that there has been genetic selection for elliptocytosis because these red cells confer some resistance to malaria. Most cases of HE are inherited in an autosomal dominant pattern, with rare cases of de novo mutations.

CLINICAL MANIFESTATIONS

The clinical presentation of HE is heterogeneous, ranging from asymptomatic carriers to patients with severe, life-threatening anemia. Most HE patients are asymptomatic and are diagnosed incidentally during testing for unrelated conditions. Asymptomatic carriers have been identified who posses the same molecular defect as an affected HE relative but who have normal peripheral blood smears. The erythrocyte life span, normal in most patients, is decreased in only about 10% of patients. It is this subset of HE patients with decreased erythrocyte life span who experience hemolysis, anemia, splenomegaly, and intermittent jaundice. Many of these patients have parents with typical HE and thus are homozygotes or compound heterozygotes for defects inherited from each of the parents. Symptoms may vary among members of the same family, indeed, they may vary in the same individual at different times.

Hereditary Pyropoikilocytosis

HPP is a rare cause of anemia with distinctive erythrocyte morphology on peripheral blood smear (see Fig. 164-2C) and has a picture similar to that seen in patients suffering severe burns. Patients typically present in infancy with severe anemia and peripheral blood smear findings of elliptocytosis, poikilocytosis, pyknocytosis, and fragmentation. Microspherocytosis is common, and the MCV is usually very low (50 to 70 fL). The incubated osmotic fragility is increased. Most patients are of African ancestry, and at least one third of HPP patients have a parent or sibling with typical HE. Patients with HPP tend to experience severe hemolysis and anemia in infancy that gradually improves, evolving toward typical HE later in life.

DIAGNOSIS

Cigar-shaped elliptocytes on peripheral blood smear are the hallmark of HE (see Fig. 164-2B). These normochromic, normocytic elliptocytes vary in number from a few to 100%, with the likelihood of hemolysis not correlating with the number of elliptocytes present. Ovalocytes, spherocytes, stomatocytes, and fragmented cells may also be seen. In some cases, pyknocytes may be prominent. Elliptocytes may be seen in association with other disorders, including megaloblastic anemias, hypochromic microcytic anemias (iron deficiency anemia and thalassemia), myelodysplastic syndromes, and myelofibrosis; however, elliptocytes generally make up less than one third of red cells in these conditions. History and additional laboratory testing usually clarify the diagnosis of these disorders. In typical cases, the incubated osmotic fragility is normal, whereas in severe HE and HPP, osmotic fragility is increased.

Other laboratory findings in HE are similar to those found in other hemolytic anemias and are nonspecific markers of increased erythrocyte production and destruction. The reticulocyte count generally is less than 5% but may be higher when hemolysis is severe.

Like HS, specialized laboratory procedures are available to study the erythrocyte membranes of HE and HPP patients. These studies are not routinely required to make the diagnosis of HE or HPP, but they may be helpful in studying problematic cases and in elucidating the underlying molecular defects.

TREATMENT Rx

Therapy is rarely needed in patients with HE. In rare cases, occasional red blood cell transfusions may be required. In cases of severe HE and HPP, splenectomy has been palliative because the spleen is the site of erythrocyte sequestration and destruction. Many practitioners think that the same indications for splenectomy in HS should be applied to patients with symptomatic HE or HPP. Postsplenectomy patients with HE or HPP experience increased hematocrits, decreased reticulocyte counts, and improvement in clinical symptoms.

Patients should be followed for signs of decompensation during acute illnesses. Interval ultrasonography to detect gallstones should be performed. In patients with significant hemolysis, folate should be administered daily.

Hereditary Stomatocytosis Syndromes

Red cell hydration is primarily determined by the intracellular concentration of monovalent cations. A net increase in sodium and potassium ions causes water to enter, forming *stomatocytes* (see Fig. 164-2D) or *hydrocytes,* whereas a net loss of sodium and potassium produces dehydrated red cells, or *xerocytes*. Numerous descriptions of congenital or familial hemolytic anemias associated with abnormal cation permeability and, in some cases, disturbed red cell hydration have been reported. These span the range from severe hydrocytosis to severe xerocytosis. In most cases, the molecular bases of this group of disorders are unknown. An unusual characteristic of the stomatocytosis syndromes is a predisposition to thrombosis after splenectomy. Acquired stomatocytosis has been associated with acute alcoholism and hepatobiliary disease, vinca alkaloid administration, neoplasms, and cardiovascular disease. Stomatocytosis is also sometimes observed as a processing artifact.

OVERHYDRATED HEREDITARY STOMATOCYTOSIS (HYDROCYTOSIS)

This group of disorders is characterized by stomatocytes, erythrocytes with a mouth-shaped (stoma) area of central pallor on peripheral blood smear (see Fig. 164-2D), severe hemolysis, macrocytosis (110 to 150 fL), elevated erythrocyte sodium concentration, reduced potassium concentration, and increased total Na^+ and K^+ content. The excess cations elevate cell water, producing large, osmotically fragile cells with a low MCHC (24 to 30%). The clinical severity of overhydrated hereditary stomatocytosis is variable; some patients experience hemolysis and anemia, whereas others are asymptomatic.

DEHYDRATED HEREDITARY STOMATOCYTOSIS (XEROCYTOSIS)

Blood smears from patients with dehydrated hereditary stomatocytosis exhibit contracted and spiculated red cells, dessicytes, a variable number of stomatocytes, and target cells. Most patients have nearly normal erythrocyte morphology, with only a few target cells and an occasional echinocyte or stomatocyte. The MCHC and MCV (95 to 115 fL) are increased, and the osmotic fragility is decreased (i.e., resistance to osmotic lysis). The characteristic biochemical abnormality is a reduced potassium concentration and total monovalent cation content.

INTERMEDIATE SYNDROMES AND HEREDITARY STOMATOCYTOSIS VARIANTS

Hydrocytosis and xerocytosis represent the extremes of a spectrum of red cell permeability defects. A number of families with features of both conditions have been reported. Some patients with severe permeability defects have little or no hemolysis. The proportion of stomatocytes and the degree of sodium influx do not correlate with each other, and neither correlates with the amount of hemolysis or anemia.

ERYTHROCYTE METABOLISM

The primary functions of the erythrocyte, gas transport and exchange, are maintained without a net change in energy state. However, several critical functions of the erythrocyte depend on the production and expenditure of energy. As erythrocytes age, glucose utilization and ATP levels fall, leading to decreased membrane deformability and, ultimately, shortened life span. Lower potassium levels, higher sodium levels, and decreased membrane lipids are also seen in ATP-deficient, aging erythrocytes.

Erythrocytes do not undergo oxidative phosphorylation and do not store glycogen, thus they must constantly catabolize glucose from the blood stream through the Embden-Myerhof pathway and the hexose monophosphate shunt as a source of energy (Fig. 164-3). Erythrocytes incorporate glucose from the plasma through facilitated transfer, with erythrocyte glucose levels rapidly equilibrating with changes in blood glucose levels. Glucose is the preferred carbohydrate of the red cell, but fructose and mannose are metabolized almost as readily. Inside the erythrocyte, glucose is converted to glucose-6-phosphate or to fructose by sorbitol. Glucose-6-phosphate follows one of three pathways: (1) most (~90%) enters the Embden-Meyerhof pathway,

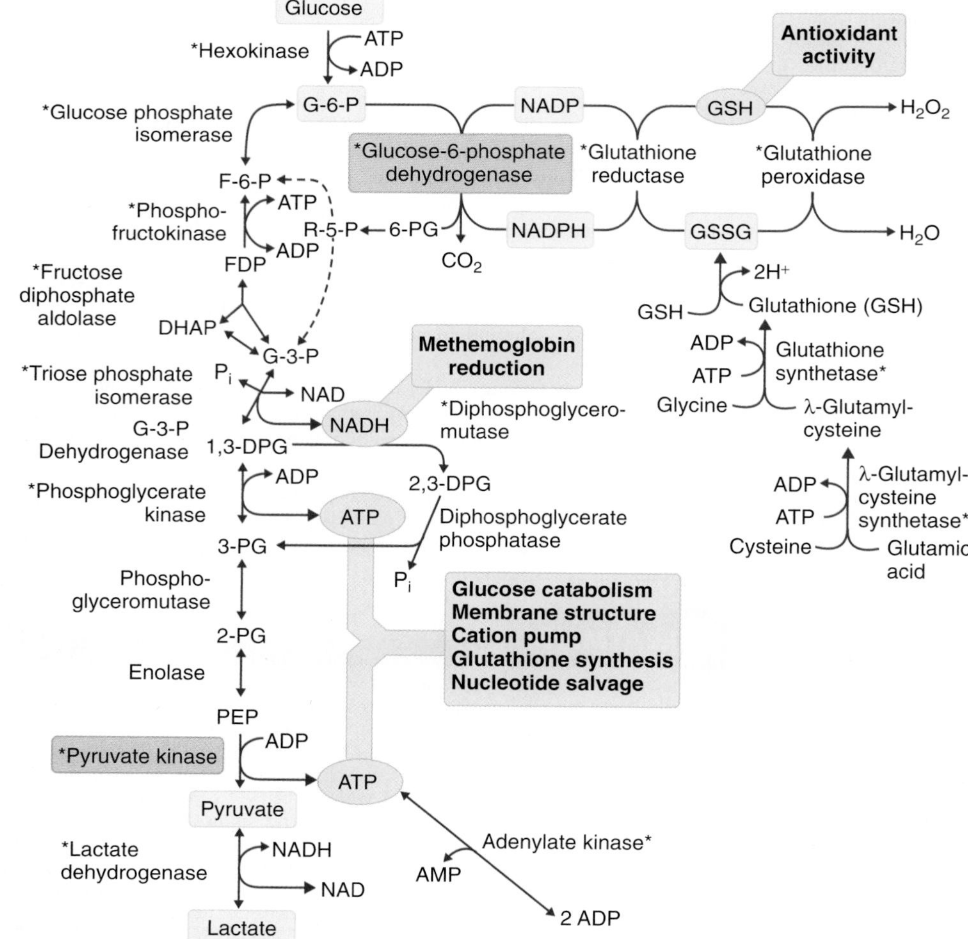

FIGURE 164-3. Pathways of energy metabolism in the erythrocyte. Glucose 6-phosphate may be degraded anaerobically to lactate through the Embden-Meyerhof pathway, or oxidatively through the hexose monophosphate shunt. Pentose phosphates (R-5-P) can reenter anaerobic glycolysis as fructose 6-phosphate (F-6-P) and glyceraldehyde 3-phosphate (G-3-P) after conversion by enzymes of the terminal pentose phosphate pathway or as a product of adenosine or inosine degradation. 2,3-Diphosphoglycerate (2,3-DPG) may be generated instead of adenosine triphosphate (ATP) through diversion of triose through the Rapoport-Luebering shunt. Glutathione may be synthesized directly from constituent amino acids; its cycling from oxidized (GSSG) to reduced forms (GSH) depends on reduced pyridine cofactor (NADPH) generation. ADP = adenosine diphosphate; DHAP = dihydroxyacetone phosphate; FDP = fructose 1,6-diphosphate; NAD = nicotinamide adenine dinucleotide; NADP = nicotinamide adenine dinucleotide phosphate; NADPH = nicotinamide adenine dinucleotide phosphate, reduced form; PEP = polyestradiol phosphate.

where it is converted into lactate, pyruvate, and ATP; (2) some (~5 to 10%) enters the hexose monophosphate shunt to produce reduced intermediates and ribulose 5-phosphate, the latter of which eventually enters the Embden-Meyerhof pathway; and (3) a tiny fraction (<1%) is converted to glucose-1-phosphate and then to glycogen.

Embden-Meyerhof Pathway

The Embden-Meyerhof Pathway of glycolysis is the primary source of ATP, 2,3-DPG and nicotinamide adenine dinucleotide, reduced form (NADH) in the erythrocyte (see Fig. 164-3). Most of the energy generated by erythrocytes is through the Embden-Meyerhof pathway, followed by storage as high-energy phosphates such as ATP or as reducing energy in the form of glutathione or pyridine nucleotides (NADH and nicotinamide adenine dinucleotide phosphate, reduced form [NADPH]). This pathway metabolizes about 90% of erythrocyte glucose with the catabolism of 1 mole of glucose yielding 2 moles of ATP and 2 moles of lactate. Two moles of ATP per mole of metabolized glucose seems insignificant compared with the Krebs cycle of intermediary metabolism, in which 1 mole of glucose metabolized produces 38 moles of ATP. However, this ATP production is adequate to renew 150 to 200% of the total red cell ATP every hour.

The Embden-Meyerhof pathway is also the primary source of NADH, a necessary cofactor for NADH methemoglobin reductase, which maintains heme iron in the reduced state. Without this reaction, heme iron would be oxidized to methemoglobin, which is not a functional oxygen transporter.

Finally, the Rapoport-Luebering shunt of the Embden-Meyerhof pathway (see Fig. 164-3) produces 2,3-DPG, a compound found in high concentrations in erythrocytes, but in low concentrations in other cells. Once formed, under physiologic conditions of pH and solute concentrations, 2,3-DPG binds reversibly to tetramers of deoxyhemoglobin with greater affinity than it does to oxyhemoglobin. By binding to deoxyhemoglobin, it allosterically upregulates the release of the remaining oxygen bound to the hemoglobin, enhancing the ability of erythrocytes to release oxygen near tissues that need it most.

Hexose Monophosphate Shunt (Pentose Phosphate Pathway)

In the HMP shunt (see Fig. 164-3), glucose-6-phosphate undergoes oxidation followed by a series of reactions to yield fructose-6-phosphate and glyceraldehyde-3-phosphate, intermediates in the glycolytic pathway. The HMP shunt is the primary source of erythrocyte NADPH, with 2 moles of NADPH produced for each mole of glucose metabolized. NADPH is required for the reduction of oxidized glutathione and some protein sulfhydryl groups.

Mature erythrocytes synthesize large amounts of reduced glutathione (GSH). GSH protects erythrocytes from oxidants, including hydrogen peroxide (H_2O_2), superoxide anions (O_2^-), and hydroxyl radicals (OH), which are produced as byproducts of the oxidation of heme by oxygen. Oxidants are also produced by activated phagocytes (e.g., during infection) and by erythrocytes after exposure to certain agents. When oxidants accumulate, they damage cellular proteins and lipids. Detoxification of H_2O_2 is significantly enhanced by glutathione peroxidase. GSH is converted to oxidized glutathione (GSSG) and to mixed disulfides with protein thiols. GSH levels are restored by glutathione reductase. In this process, NADPH is oxidized to nicotinamide adenine dinucleotide phosphate (NADP), which stimulates the HMP shunt to regenerate NADPH. After oxidant stress, hypoxia, or acidosis, erythrocytes can increase the amount of glucose metabolized through the HMP shunt up to 10- to 20-fold to generate increased amounts of reduced glutathione. The tight coupling of glutathione metabolism with the HMP shunt protects the mature erythrocyte from oxidative stress.

DISORDERS OF ERYTHROCYTE METABOLISM

Congenital nonspherocytic hemolytic anemia (CNSHA) traditionally includes erythrocyte disorders not due to defects of the red cell membrane or hemoglobin, immune-mediated disease, or other diseases such as paroxysmal nocturnal hemoglobinuria. CNSHA is a heterogeneous group of disorders associated with various metabolic abnormalities of the erythrocyte, including enzymopathies of glucose, glutathione, and nucleotide metabolism. Like the membrane disorders, clinical, biochemical, and genetic heterogeneity are typical within the enzymopathies. Hemolysis may develop as a result of either enzyme or antioxidant deficiency or dysfunction (e.g., abnormal substrate or cofactor binding), altered activation or inhibition characteristics, or decreased stability or specific activity.

Peripheral blood smears in CNSHA, with the exception of pyrimidine 5′-nucleotidase deficiency, are unremarkable. Osmotic fragility of fresh erythrocytes is normal. Response to splenectomy is variable. Inheritance is heterogeneous. A thorough family history is important and may be of assistance in determining the diagnosis. Manifestations of the metabolic defect are usually confined to the erythrocyte but may occasionally involve nonerythroid cells.

Definitive diagnosis of metabolic abnormalities of the red cell depend on qualitative or quantitative assays of specific enzyme activity or identification of the specific genetic mutation by DNA analysis. Results of enzyme assays should be interpreted with caution because (1) they only sample surviving red cells in the peripheral blood, and the metabolic milieu of these cells is not necessarily comparable to cells already hemolyzed; (2) in vitro enzyme assay conditions may not accurately reflect the in vivo environment; (3) transfusions before the assay may obscure the underlying metabolic defect, and (4) leukocyte contamination may lead to spurious results. Finally, average enzyme activity may not accurately reflect activity in subpopulations of erythrocytes. This is particularly true when there is reticulocytosis, which may yield artificially elevated mean enzyme activity owing to higher enzyme levels found in reticulocytes.

Disorders of the Embden-Meyerhof Pathway

Defects of the Embden-Meyerhof pathway are inherited in an autosomal recessive fashion, and usually hemolysis is seen only in homozygotes or compound heterozygotes. Heterozygotes, whose erythrocytes contain less than normal amounts of mutant enzyme, are clinically normal.

An exception is phosphoglycerate kinase deficiency, an X-linked disorder with hemolysis found only in males. In this group of disorders, hemolysis is chronic, is not typically influenced by drugs or other inciting agents, and is attributed to insufficient levels of erythrocyte ATP. Splenomegaly from trapping of mutant erythrocytes is common. The hostile splenic environment contributes to the shortened erythrocyte life span. When performing specific diagnostic enzyme assays, measurement of glycolytic intermediates may assist in diagnosis because concentrations of intermediates is increased upstream of a defect and decreased downstream of a defect.

PYRUVATE KINASE DEFICIENCY

Pyruvate kinase (PK) deficiency accounts for approximately 90% of inherited defects of the Embden-Meyerhof pathway and is the second most common inherited erythrocyte enzymopathy associated with anemia after glucose-6-phosphate dehydrogenase (G6PD) deficiency (see later). PK deficiency is found worldwide, but it is most common in individuals of northern European descent.

PATHOBIOLOGY

PK catalyzes the conversion of phosphoenolpyruvate (PEP) to pyruvate, generating ATP. Deficient or defective PK leads to decreased levels of erythrocyte ATP, disturbing many cellular processes such as signaling and maintenance of water and ion content, leading to energy failure and dehydration. Upstream catabolites accumulate in the erythrocyte, including 2,3-DPG, which shifts the oxygen dissociation curve to the right, enhancing tissue oxygenation and ameliorating some of the physiologic effects of anemia. Early PK-deficient reticulocytes retain the ability to utilize oxidative phosphorylation to produce ATP, bypassing their defect. This ability is lost as reticulocytes mature and is markedly dampened in the hypoxic environment of the spleen.

PK deficiency is inherited in an autosomal recessive manner. Affected individuals are homozygous or compound heterozygotes for PK defects. Heterozygotes are clinically normal or exhibit very minimal hemolysis.

CLINICAL MANIFESTATIONS

Clinical manifestations in PK deficiency are heterogeneous, ranging from asymptomatic to transfusion-dependent hemolytic anemia. More severely affected patients present in infancy or early childhood with anemia, jaundice, and splenomegaly. Occasionally, patients may escape detection until later in life when complications related to anemia and chronic hemolysis occur such as cholelithiasis or aplastic crisis or when the diagnosis is made during evaluation of the patient for another condition.

DIAGNOSIS

Peripheral blood smear demonstrates normocytic, normochromic erythrocytes, sometimes with spiculations (Fig. 164-4A). Poikilocytes and acanthocytes may also be seen. Reticulocytosis is common. Osmotic fragility of fresh erythrocytes is usually normal. Occasional patients exhibit a population of osmotically fragile cells after incubation.

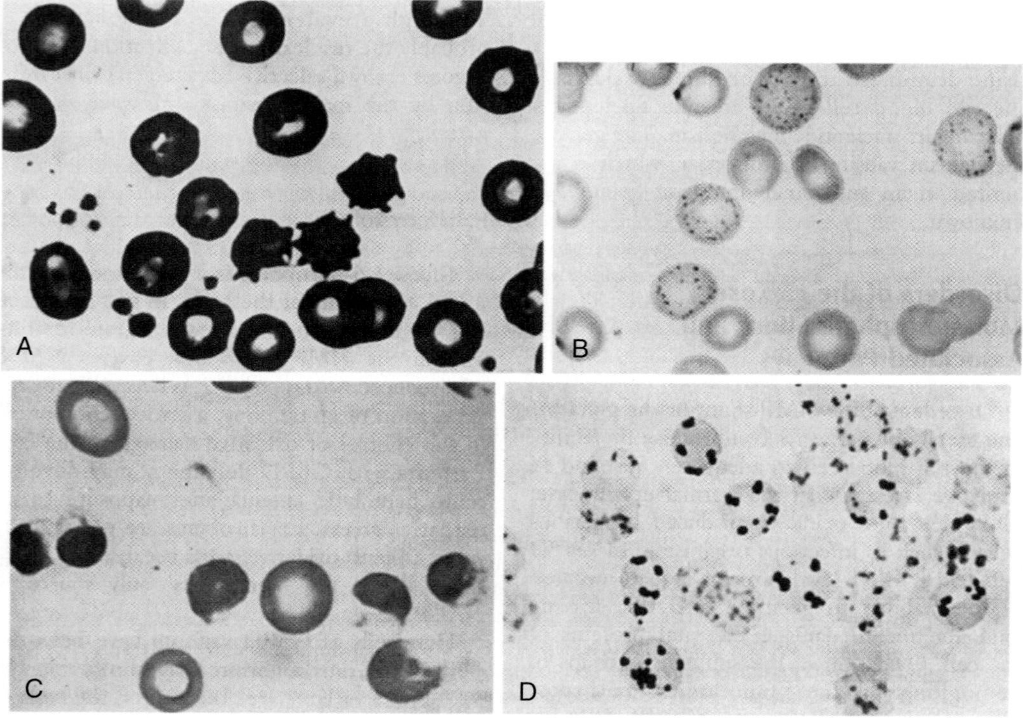

FIGURE 164-4. Peripheral blood smears in erythrocyte enzymopathies. **A,** Pyruvate kinase deficiency. **B,** Pyrimidine 5′-nucleotidase deficiency; **C,** Glucose-6-phosphate dehydrogenase (G6PD) deficiency. **D,** Heinz bodies in G6PD deficiency. (B from Paglia DE. Disorders of erythrocyte glycolysis and nucleotide metabolism. In: Handin RI, Lux SE, Stossel TP, eds. *Blood: Principles and Practice of Hematology.* Philadelphia: JB Lippincott; 1995:1877-1896.)

NADH fluorescence under ultraviolet light is a commonly used screening test for PK deficiency. PEP and NADH are mixed with the patient's blood, incubated, and spotted on filter paper, and fluorescence is measured. Direct enzyme assay, which uses PEP as substrate for PK, can be performed on leukocyte-free hemolysate to confirm abnormal fluorescence tests. Leukocytes must be carefully depleted from the samples because they contain over 300 times the PK activity of erythrocytes.

TREATMENT Rx

Most patients require only expectant management, with only rare transfusions, such as during an aplastic episode. In severe cases, patients may be transfusion dependent. In these cases, splenectomy typically lessens hemolysis and ameliorates the anemia. After splenectomy, some patients develop marked reticulocytosis, up to 50 to 70%. This paradoxical reticulocytosis is attributed to increased reticulocyte survival after removal of the hostile splenic environment.

OTHER DISORDERS OF THE EMBDEN-MEYERHOF PATHWAY

Other abnormalities of the Embden-Meyerhof pathway have been described. Hexokinase deficiency is quite uncommon, with great phenotypic variability in reported cases. Severely affected patients have suffered from anemia beginning in infancy and may require blood transfusion. Glucose phosphate isomerase (GPI) deficiency is the third most common hemolytic enzymopathy. GPI deficiency usually presents in infancy or early childhood with moderate to severe hemolytic anemia. Phosphofructokinase deficiency may involve erythrocytes, muscle, or both. Presentation is usually in adolescence with exertional myopathy. Hemolytic anemia has been described in isolated cases of 2,3-bisphosphoglycerate mutase deficiency and phosphoglycerate kinase deficiency.

Disorders of Nucleotide Metabolism

Mature erythrocytes lack the ability to synthesize purine and pyrimidine nucleotides de novo. However, they are able to form some nucleotides through salvage pathways.

PYRIMIDINE 5′-NUCLEOTIDASE DEFICIENCY

Pyrimidine 5′-nucleotidase (P5N) degrades the pyrimidine nucleotides of RNA to cytidine and uridine, which can diffuse out of the cell. When P5N is deficient, nondiffusible, partially degraded RNAs accumulate, leading to the marked basophilic stippling characteristic of P5N-deficient erythrocytes (see Fig. 164-4B). These accumulated pyrimidine nucleotides inhibit the transport of GSSG out of red cells, leading to high levels of erythrocyte glutathione. Clinically, there is mild to moderate hemolytic anemia and splenomegaly. The etiology of the hemolysis remains cryptic. Typically, splenectomy does not ameliorate the hemolysis and anemia.

Disorders of the Hexose Monophosphate Shunt (Pentose Phosphate Pathway) and Associated Pathways

Disorders of the HMP shunt or of the glutathione metabolic pathways (see Fig. 164-3) compromise the ability of the red cell to respond adequately to oxidative stress. In the normal erythrocyte, GSH detoxifies oxidants produced by various agents and infection. In G6PD-deficient erythrocytes, because of the inability to generate NADPH, GSH levels are inadequate, leaving the cell susceptible to oxidant stress. Oxidation of hemoglobin sulfhydryl groups leads to the production of methemoglobin and intracellular hemoglobin precipitates called Heinz bodies. Heinz bodies (see Fig. 164-4D), usually visualized on peripheral blood smears with supravital stains such as methyl violet, attach to and damage the erythrocyte membrane. They induce clustering of immunoglobulins and band 3 protein, marking the erythrocyte for opsonization by phagocytes and eventual removal from the circulation. Heinz bodies are "pitted" from circulating cells by the spleen and are commonly seen on smears of patients after splenectomy. "Bite cells," erythrocytes with localized invaginations, possibly at the site of Heinz body injury or removal, are seen during acute hemolytic episodes. In addition to damage from Heinz body formation, GSH-deficient erythrocytes also undergo peroxidation of membrane phospholipids and oxidative cross-linking of spectrin, decreasing membrane deformability and further promoting splenic trapping.

GLUCOSE-6-PHOSPHATE DEHYDROGENASE DEFICIENCY

G6PD deficiency is the most common inherited disorder of erythrocyte metabolism, affecting more than 400 million people worldwide. The high prevalence of G6PD deficiency is thought to be due to genetic selection because G6PD-deficient erythrocytes have a selective advantage against invasion by the malaria parasite *Plasmodium falciparum*.

EPIDEMIOLOGY AND PATHOBIOLOGY

G6PD is the initial and rate-limiting step in the HMP shunt (see Fig. 164-3), which converts NADP into NADPH. NADPH is required for the generation of glutathione, a critical constituent in the prevention of oxidative damage to the cell. G6PD-deficient patients may develop acute hemolytic anemia after exposure to oxidative stress. Although G6PD is a ubiquitous enzyme, erythroid cells are particularly susceptible to oxidative stress because the HMP shunt is their only source of NADPH.

Hundreds of G6PD variants have been described, but only a few are common. Variants are classified on the basis of biochemical characteristics, electrophoretic mobility, ability to use substrate analogue, Km for NADP and G6PD, pH activity profile, and thermal stability. The normal enzyme, Gd^{B}, is present in 99% of white Americans and 70% of African Americans. A normal variant, Gd^{A+}, found in 20% of African Americans, has a faster electrophoretic mobility than Gd^{B}. Gd^{A-}, the most common variant associated with hemolysis, is found in about 10% of African Americans and in many Africans. Gd^{A-} has decreased catalytic ability compared with Gd^{A+}. Gd^{Med}, the second most common variant associated with hemolysis, is common in the Mediterranean area, in India, and in southeast Asia, with a prevalence of up to 5 to 50%. Gd^{Med} exhibits markedly decreased catalytic activity. Gd^{Canton}, a variant common in Asian populations, produces a clinical syndrome similar to Gd^{A-}.

Gd^{B} activity decreases as normal cells age, with a half-life of approximately 60 days. Despite very low levels of or no active G6PD, older erythrocytes maintain the ability to produce NADPH and maintain a GSH response to oxidative stress. Gd^{A-} variant has a half-life of only 13 days, so young cells have a normal amount of enzyme activity whereas older red cells are grossly deficient. Because of this heterogeneity in G6PD levels, individuals with the Gd^{A-} variant experience only limited hemolysis after oxidant exposure.

More than 100 mutations in the *G6PD* gene, localized to Xq28, have been described. Most mutations are amino acid substitutions that influence enzyme kinetics, stability, or both, with a few rare deletions and splicing mutations described. Because it is X-linked, G6PD deficiency primarily affects males. Males have only one G6PD allele and express only one G6PD type. Females can express one or two G6PD types. The Lyon hypothesis specifies that only one X chromosome is active in any given cell; thus, any given cell in a heterozygous female is either normal or deficient. In females who are heterozygous for G6PD deficiency, average G6PD activity may be normal or mildly, moderately, or severely reduced, depending on the degree of lyonization. G6PD-deficient erythrocytes in heterozygous females are susceptible to the same oxidant stress as G6PD-deficient cells in males, but, typically, the overall degree of hemolysis is less because there is a smaller population of vulnerable cells.

CLINICAL MANIFESTATIONS

G6PD deficiency is divided into five classes based on clinical severity and degree of enzyme deficiency. Class I is characterized by CNSHA without precipitating cause and severe G6PD deficiency. Class II is characterized by intermittent hemolysis and severe G6PD deficiency. Class III is characterized by hemolysis after oxidant stress and mild G6PD deficiency. Class II and III together represent more than 90% of G6PD variants. Classes IV and V are clinically asymptomatic. The most clinically significant syndromes of G6PD deficiency are acute hemolytic anemia (AHA), neonatal jaundice (NNJ), and rarely, CNSHA.

AHA is the most dramatic clinical presentation of G6PD deficiency with acute intravascular hemolysis after exposure to an oxidative stress. Oxidative stresses include ingestion of certain drugs such as primaquine or sulfa-containing compounds, exposure to naphthalene (mothballs), ingestion of fava beans, or infection, the latter being the most common cause of hemolysis. Table 164-2 lists drugs that should be avoided in G6PD-deficient patients. Presenting symptoms include irritability, fever, nausea, abdominal pain, and diarrhea within 48 hours of oxidant exposure. Hemoglobinuria, jaundice, and anemia ensue. The spleen and liver may be enlarged and tender. Cases with severe anemia may precipitate congestive heart failure. Laboratory findings include a normochromic, normocytic anemia with anisocytosis and reticulocytosis. Poikilocytes and bite cells may be seen. Heinz bodies, a classic finding in G6PD deficiency, may be seen but are an inconsistent finding because these damaged cells are rapidly cleared from the circulation in the spleen. Additional laboratory findings include hemoglobinuria and the presence of free hemoglobin in the blood.

Another clinically significant syndrome of G6PD deficiency is NNJ. Jaundice is seldom present at birth, with the peak incidence of onset between days 2 and 3 of life. The severity of hyperbilirubinemia is variable. It may be severe, resulting in kernicterus or even death. In most cases, however, hyperbilirubinemia is adequately treated with phototherapy. In NNJ, it is important to note that the anemia is very rarely severe. The etiology of NNJ remains controversial. NNJ is increased in G6PD-deficient infants who also carry a polymorphism of the uridine diphosphoglucuronyl transferase (*UDPGT1*) gene associated with Gilbert syndrome.

Chronic nonspherocytic hemolytic anemia is associated with uncommon variants of G6PD deficiency, usually mutant enzymes unable to maintain basal NADPH production. Presentation may be in the neonatal period when NNJ is accompanied by anemia in a male. The degree of chronic anemia in CNSHA due to G6PD deficiency has been variable. Some patients have compensated hemolysis, whereas others require intermittent transfusions. Transfusion dependence occurs in the most severe cases.

TABLE 164-2 AGENTS TO BE AVOIDED BY GLUCOSE-6-PHOSPHATE DEHYDROGENASE–DEFICIENT PATIENTS*

ANTIMALARIALS
Primaquine (people with the African A^{-} variant may take it at reduced dosage, under surveillance)
Pamaquine
Chloroquine (may be used under surveillance when required for prophylaxis or treatment of malaria)
SULFONAMIDES AND SULFONES
Sulfanilamide
Sulfapyridine
Sulfadimidine
Sulfacetamide (Albucid)
Acetyl sulfisoxazole (Gantrisin)
Salicylazosulfapyridine (Salazopyrin)
Dapsone
Sulfoxone
Glucosulfone sodium (Promin)
Sulfamethoxazole-trimethoprim (Septrin)
OTHER ANTIBACTERIAL COMPOUNDS
Nitrofurans—nitrofurantoin, furazolidone, nitrofurazone
[Nalidixic acid]
Chloramphenicol
p-Aminosalicylic acid
ANALGESICS
Acetylsalicylic acid (aspirin): moderate doses can be used
Acetophenetidin (Phenacetin)
Safe alternative: Paracetamol
ANTHELMINTICS
β-Naphthol
Stibophen
Niridazole
MISCELLANEOUS
Vitamin K analogues (1 mg of menaphthone can be given to babies)
Naphthalene (moth balls)
Probenecid
Dimercaprol (BAL)
Methylene blue
Arsine†
Phenylhydrazine†
Acetylphenylhydrazine†
Toluidine blue
Mepacrine

*Drugs in bold print should be avoided by people with all forms of glucose-6-phosphate dehydrogenase (G6PD) deficiency. Drugs in normal print should be avoided, in addition, by G6PD-deficient people of Mediterranean, Middle Eastern, and Asian origin. Items in normal print and within square brackets apply only to people with the African A^{-} variant.
†These drugs or chemicals may cause hemolysis in normal people if given in large doses. Many other drugs may produce hemolysis in certain individuals.

DIAGNOSIS

The G6PD reaction (glucose-6-phosphate + $NADP^{+} \rightarrow$ 6-phosphoglucono-lactone + NADPH + H^{+}) reduces $NADP^{+}$ to NADPH. Formation of NADPH and NADH can be observed directly because they fluoresce in the visible spectrum when illuminated with long-wave ultraviolet light. Based on this observation, several simple screening tests performed using inexpensive long-wave ultraviolet light have been devised. These tests are semiquantitative, categorizing a sample as normal or deficient. They are unreliable after an acute hemolytic episode and do not typically detect female heterozygotes. Positive screening tests should be confirmed by spectrophotometric assay or DNA studies.

Definitive assay of the enzyme depends on direct spectrophotometric measurement of NADPH production. Although more sensitive than screening tests, this still requires 20 to 30% G6PD-deficient cells to obtain an abnormal result. Sensitivity can be increased by comparing the level of G6PD deficiency to levels of other age-dependent erythrocyte enzymes, especially when testing is temporally in close proximity to an acute hemolytic episode. The cyanide-ascorbate test measures the ability of erythrocytes to prevent the oxidation of hemoglobin by ascorbate. Employing intact erythrocytes, as few as 10 to 15% deficient cells can be detected, making this test useful for detecting female heterozygotes and males following a hemolytic episode. This test also detects other perturbations of the HMP shunt or glutathione metabolism.

TREATMENT

The best treatment for the individual with AHA is careful prescription of medications and avoidance of inciting agents (see Table 164-2). Outside of acute hemolytic episodes, these patients do not require any special therapy. AHA episodes are managed with particular attention to hematologic, cardiopulmonary, and renal complications of hemolysis. Management of NNJ does not differ from that recommended for other causes of neonatal hyperbilirubinemia. In CNSHA, management is expectant. Exposure to oxidant stresses should be avoided. Blood transfusions may be necessary during acute hemolytic episodes. In severe cases of CNSHA, splenectomy may ameliorate the anemia.

Disorders of Glutathione Metabolism

Defects of glutathione metabolism may be associated with hemolysis. Erythrocytes from patients lacking glutathione synthetase or γ-glutamylcysteine synthetase, enzymes involved in glutathione synthesis, have very low levels of GSH. Clinically, these disorders resemble G6PD deficiency. There is mild to moderate chronic hemolytic anemia with increased susceptibility to oxidant stress.

Visit expertconsult.com for e-expanded chapter

SUGGESTED READINGS

Bruce LJ. Hereditary stomatocytosis and cation leaky red cells—recent developments. *Blood Cells Mol Dis.* 2009;42:216-222. *Review of the molecular basis of hereditary stomatocytosis.*

Cappellini MD, Fiorelli G. Glucose-6-phosphate dehydrogenase deficiency. *Lancet.* 2008;371:64-74. *Comprehensive clinical review of the most common human enzyme defect worldwide.*

Iolascon A, Avvisati RA, Piscopo C. Hereditary spherocytosis. *Transfus Clin Biol.* 2010;17:138-142. *Review of the various forms of a condition with a prevalence of about 1 in 2000 among northern Europeans.*

Mohandas N, Gallagher PG. Red cell membrane: past, present and future. *Blood.* 2008;112:3939-3948. *Current concepts of red cell membrane structure and function in health and disease.*

165 THE THALASSEMIAS

MARIA DOMENICA CAPPELLINI

DEFINITION

The thalassemias—or, more comprehensively, the thalassemia syndromes—are a heterogeneous group of inherited hemolytic anemias characterized by deficient or absent production of one of the globin chains of hemoglobin. This leads to imbalanced globin chain synthesis, which is the hallmark of all the thalassemia syndromes.

EPIDEMIOLOGY

Taken together, the thalassemias are the most common single gene disorder in the world population. The estimated number of carriers exceeds 270 million, and more than 300,000 children are born each year with one of the thalassemia syndromes or one of the structural hemoglobin variants. The extremely high frequency of hemoglobin disorders compared with other monogenic diseases reflects natural selection mediated by the relative resistance of carriers against *Plasmodium falciparum* malaria. Other factors that may be involved include the widespread practice of consanguineous marriage and increased maternal age in poorer countries, and gene drift and founder effects. For these reasons, the thalassemias are most frequent in southeastern and southern Asia, the Middle East, the Mediterranean countries, and northern and central Africa. However, as a result of the mass migration of African populations from high-prevalence areas, thalassemias are now encountered worldwide.

PATHOBIOLOGY

The normal adult red cells contain 97% adult hemoglobin (HbA: $\alpha_2\beta_2$), with approximately 2.5% of the minor component HbA_2 ($\alpha_2\delta_2$) and a small amount of fetal hemoglobin (HbF: $\alpha_2\gamma_2$). Because the stable tetramer $\alpha_2\beta_2$ is the major component of hemoglobin after birth, there are two main forms of thalassemia: α-thalassemia and β-thalassemia. Because β-chain synthesis is fully activated only after birth, it follows that the β-thalassemias are not expressed as diseases in intrauterine life; they manifest as γ-chain synthesis declines during the first year of life. In contrast, because α chains are shared by both fetal and adult hemoglobin, α-thalassemias manifest in both fetal and adult life.

As knowledge about their genetic basis and pathophysiologic mechanisms has evolved, the thalassemia syndromes can now be classified at genetic and clinical levels (Table 165-1).

Genetics

Six different types of globin chains (α, β, γ, δ, ε, ζ) are found in normal human hemoglobin at different stages of development. In the very early embryo, hemoglobin synthesis is restricted to the yolk sac and to the production of Hb Gower 1 ($\zeta_2\varepsilon_2$), Gower 2 ($\alpha_2\varepsilon_2$), and Portland ($\zeta_2\gamma_2$). Subsequently, at about 8 weeks of gestation, the fetal liver takes over, synthesizing predominantly HbF ($\alpha_2\gamma_2$) and a small amount (<10%) of HbA. Between about 18 weeks and birth, the liver is progressively replaced by bone marrow as the major site of red cell production. This is accompanied in the later stages of gestation with a reciprocal switch in the production of HbF and HbA; this continues until, by the end of the first year of life, HbF production has dropped to less than 2%. The globin genes are encoded in separate gene clusters. The α cluster (ζ, α_2, α_1) lies at the telomere of chromosome 16, and the β cluster (ε, $^G\gamma$ and $^A\gamma$, δ, β) lies at chromosome 11p15.5. In both clusters the genes are aligned 5′ to 3′ in the order in which they are expressed during development. Both sets of genes are under the regulation of enhancer-like elements (hypersensitive site [HS]-40 for α cluster, and locus control region [LCR] for β cluster) that lie some distance away at the 5′ end of the cluster. Deletion of these enhancer elements results in inactivation of any related globin gene. There are two α genes/alleles (α_2 and α_1) that differ by a few nucleotides in intron 2 and the 3′ untranslated region but produce identical protein products. The output of the α_2 gene exceeds that of the α_1 gene by two- to three-fold. The α cluster also contains pseudo-ζ and pseudo-α genes that are not translated into protein products. The region around a DNase I

TABLE 165-1 GENETIC AND CLINICAL CLASSIFICATIONS OF THE THALASSEMIAS

	GENETIC	CLINICAL
α-Thalassemias	α^0 α^+ Deletion (−α) Nondeletion (α^T)	α-Minor HbH disease Hydrops fetalis
β-Thalassemias	β^0 β^+ Variant with high HbA_2 Normal HbA_2 Silent Dominant Unlinked to β-gene cluster	β-Minor Thalassemia intermedia Thalassemia major
δβ-Thalassemia	$(\delta\beta)^0$ $(\delta\beta)^+$ $(^A\gamma\delta\beta)^0$	δβ-Minor Thalassemia intermedia
HPFH	Deletion Nondeletion Unlinked to β-gene cluster	Silent increase in HbF

HbA = adult hemoglobin; HbF = fetal hemoglobin; HbH = hemoglobin H; HPFH = hereditary persistence of fetal hemoglobin.

HS at 40 kb upstream of the ζ-globin gene (HS-40) is the major regulator of α-globin gene expression. The β cluster contains a single pseudo-β gene; the β-cluster "enhancer" consists of five elements marked by erythroid-specific DNase I HSs lying 6 to 20 kb upstream of the ε-globin gene, each of which contains several binding sites for erythroid-specific and other transcription factors. All together, these elements are known as the LCR, and each element contributes to the overall LCR activity. In addition, there is an erythroid-specific HS approximately 20 kb downstream of the β-globin gene; when the cluster is activated, the upstream and downstream HSs are brought into close proximity with the gene promoters to activate their transcription. The individual globin genes share many general features: they consist of three coding sequence exons separated by two introns in identical positions but of variable length, for a total length of approximately 1500 nucleotides. This structure has been highly conserved throughout evolution. The upstream regions flanking the first exon contain a number of sequence motifs that are necessary for specifying correct transcriptional initiation. A TATA box is found at 30 base pairs upstream of the initiation site, together with one or more CCAAT sites at 70 base pairs upstream. The gene promoters also contain a CACCC or CCGCCC box that binds erythroid Krüppel-like factor (EKLF)-1, and some have binding sites for erythroid transcription factor GATA-1. In model systems, mutations introduced into such sequences lead to a reduction in the level of transcription.

All the thalassemias have a similar pattern of inheritance: in most cases, the gene defects are transmitted in a mendelian autosomal fashion. Thus the severe, symptomatic varieties usually result from the interaction of more than one genetic determinant. The inheritance of α-thalassemia is more complicated because it involves the products of the linked pairs of α genes (αα) (see Clinical Manifestations).

Molecular Basis

The α- and β-thalassemias are divided into disorders in which no chains are produced from the affected chromosomes (α^0 and β^0) and those in which the chain output is reduced (α^+ and β^+).

For the α-thalassemias, the most common molecular defects are deletions of one or both α genes, which are designated –α and – –, respectively. The single α gene is believed to have arisen by crossover between two misaligned α genes on the homologous chromosome, which can give rise to chromosomes with either single (–α) or triplicated (ααα) α-globin genes. Depending on the point of crossover, deletions may remove between 2.5 and 5.3 kb of sequence, with the loss of 3.7 ($-\alpha^{3.7}$) or 4.2 ($-\alpha^{4.2}$) kb being most prevalent. Full duplication of the α-globin gene locus, including the upstream regulatory element, has also been reported in subjects of different ancestries, suggesting that this type of homologous genetic recombination occurs relatively frequently in globin loci. To date, more than 20 different deletions that involve both α genes, resulting from illegitimate or nonhomologous recombination, have been reported. The lengths of deletion vary from 5.2 to more than 40 kb, with the most common being those from Southeast Asia, the Mediterranean, and the Philippines, designated $--^{SEA}$, $--^{MED}$, and $--^{FIL}$, respectively. Nondeletion types of α-thalassemia (α^T) are much less common than the deletion forms, and in most cases they result from single oligonucleotide mutations at regions of the α gene sequence that are critical for normal expression. Because expression of the α_2 gene is two to three times greater than that of the α_1 gene, it is not surprising that most of the nondeletion mutants affect predominantly expression of the α_2 gene. The mutations may affect the initiation codon or splicing signals, cause frameshifts, or introduce premature stop codons. At least five single-nucleotide variants affect the natural termination codon (TAA) of the α_2-globin gene. Among these, Hb Constant Spring ($\alpha^{CS}\alpha$) is the most common and extensively studied. Finally, there are several α-globin variants that are so unstable that they undergo very rapid, postsynthetic degradation. In such situations, β chains remain in excess within the red cell, and patient carriers of these α-chain variants, by definition, have α-thalassemia. To date, 17 unstable α variants have been shown to produce the phenotype of α-thalassemia to a greater or lesser extent.

As for the α-thalassemias, the β-thalassemias are classified as β^0 thalassemia (in which no β globin is produced) and β^+ thalassemia (in which some β globin is produced, but less than normal). In some cases the defects in β-chain production are so mild that they are designated β^{++}. So far, more than 200 different thalassemic mutations of the β-globin gene have been reported; the vast majority are point mutations within the gene or its immediate flanking sequence. A few β-thalassemia mutations that segregate independently of the β-globin gene cluster have been described, presumably involving transacting regulatory factors. The distribution of alleles is highly variable from one population to another, but within each population, only a few alleles are common. The nondeletion forms of β-thalassemia account for the vast majority of β-thalassemia alleles. An updated list of these mutations is accessible at the Globin Gene Server website: *http://globin.cse.psu.edu*. They include transcriptional mutations, RNA processing mutations, and mutations affecting translation.

Simple deletions of the β-globin gene are rare, ranging in size from 290 base pairs to more than 60 kb. The 619–base pair deletion at the 3′ end of the β gene is relatively common among Sind and Punjabi populations in India and Pakistan. The remaining deletions are restricted to single families and are necessarily β^0 thalassemias; interestingly, they are associated with an unusually high level of HbA_2 in heterozygotes. Large deletions that affect the entire β-globin gene cluster $(\varepsilon\gamma\gamma\delta\beta)^0$ are rare and restricted to single families. Finally, some highly unstable β-chain variants may manifest as a dominant form of β-thalassemia.

The δβ-thalassemias and the hereditary persistence of fetal hemoglobin (HPFH) are the result of deletions affecting various parts of the β-globin locus. These deletions are partially compensated by an increased expression of the γ genes, which raises the level of HbF. The length of deletion accounts for different forms of δβ-thalassemia, including both $^G\gamma$ and $^A\gamma$ genes or only $^A\gamma$, and this length varies from 9 to 100 kb. Hb Lepore is a hybrid of δ and β chains resulting from a crossover between the two misaligned genes; this hemoglobin is synthesized inefficiently and gives rise to a form of δβ-thalassemia. Deletions of δ and β genes are also the molecular basis for many forms of HPFH that usually have higher levels of compensatory HbF production than the δβ-thalassemias. Other forms of HPFH are due to point mutations in the promoter region upstream from the transcription start site in either the $^G\gamma$ or $^A\gamma$ genes that alter the binding of one or more transcription factors; they are known as nondeletion HPFH. Genetic studies have identified three major quantitative trait loci that account for 20 to 50% of the common variation in HbF levels in patients with β-thalassemia and sickle cell disease, as well as in healthy adults.

CLINICAL MANIFESTATIONS

The clinical manifestations (phenotype expression) of the thalassemia syndromes are extremely variable and depend on the degree of globin chain imbalance.

α-Thalassemias

As previously mentioned, there are two major classes of α-thalassemias: α^0, in which both α genes are inactivated (– –/), and α^+, in which only one of the pair is defective owing to either an α deletion or a mutation (–α or $\alpha\alpha^T$). The clinical spectrum of α-thalassemias correlates well with the number of affected α genes—that is, from normal to the loss of all four genes. The inheritance of a normal allele (αα) with one of the α^+ or α^0 alleles results, most frequently, in α-thalassemia minor (– –/αα, –α/αα, $-\alpha^T/\alpha\alpha$, $\alpha^T\alpha/-\alpha$, –α/–α). In general, carriers of such genotypes have lower levels of total hemoglobin, mean corpuscular volume, and mean cell hemoglobin but a higher than normal red blood cell count. The greatest differences are seen in mean cell hemoglobin, which is usually less than 26 pg. The peripheral blood smear is quite variable, showing different degrees of hypochromia, with some target cells and occasional poikilocytes (Chapter 160). In carriers of α^0-thalassemia (– –/αα), it is possible to generate a few red cell HbH inclusions (β_4). The carriers of nondeletional forms ($\alpha\alpha^T/\alpha\alpha$) show slightly more marked hematologic changes than carriers of deletional forms. The hemoglobin constitution of adults carriers of α^+- or α^0-thalassemia is indistinguishable from normal but has slightly lower levels of HbA_2. Traces of Hb Bart's (γ_4) in the neonatal period are detectable in a large proportion of neonates with α-thalassemia, and the levels decline during the first 6 months after birth. The α-thalassemias are common in areas where β-thalassemias are also found at a high frequency. Thus, the coinheritance of α- and β-thalassemia traits may occur and even ameliorate the hematologic parameters. For families in which both α- and β-thalassemias are present, genotype determination is essential to provide genetic counseling. The unstable mutant Hb^{CT} causes a severe reduction in α_2-globin expression from the affected chromosome; therefore, carriers and particularly homozygotes have a more severe phenotype than α-thalassemia minor but not as severe as most cases of HbH disease.

HbH disease most frequently results from the interaction of α^+ and α^0 thalassemia, and not surprisingly, most patients originate from southeastern Asia, the Mediterranean, and the Middle East. HbH disease is a diagnosis attributed to subjects older than 6 months with a sufficient globin imbalance to produce detectable levels of HbH (>1 to 2%) in their peripheral blood, together with inclusion bodies (β_4 tetramers) in their red cells. The clinical phenotypes encompass a wide spectrum, from mild clinical manifestations to thalassemia intermedia. The predominant features are a hypochromic microcytic anemia, with jaundice and hepatosplenomegaly. Because the main mechanism of the anemia is hemolysis rather than dyserythropoiesis, only a few patients have clinical evidence of an expanded erythron. The most common complication is the development of hypersplenism due to severe splenomegaly. Other complications include gallstones, leg ulcers, increased risk of infection, folic acid deficiency, and increased risk of venous thrombosis, mainly following splenectomy. Hemoglobin levels range from 3 to 12 g/dL in different series, and fluctuations may occur after exposure to an oxidant drug, infection, or transient aplasia possibly owing to intercurrent viral infection. Rarely, patients with HbH disease require regular blood transfusions. The anemia is associated with reticulocytosis and typical thalassemic changes of the red cell indices. The relative amount of HbH varies from 1 to 40%. HbA_2 values are always reduced. The peripheral blood film shows hypochromia with variable anisopoikilocytosis, target cells, and basophilic stippling. The characteristic feature of HbH disease is that it is always possible to generate multiple inclusions in the red cells after incubation with brilliant cresyl blue. The bone marrow shows marked erythroid hyperplasia.

The most severe form of α-thalassemia is hydrops fetalis, in which all four α-globin genes are deleted (genotype —/—). It is incompatible with life. In fact, because α-globin chains are absent during gestation, Hb Bart's (γ_4) becomes the dominant hemoglobin. Because of its very high oxygen affinity, Hb Bart's is unable to deliver oxygen to tissues, and the intrauterine consequences are progressive severe anemia, severe ineffective erythropoiesis with marked extramedullary erythropoiesis, massive organomegaly, heart failure, severe albuminemia, and edema. Infants with hydrops fetalis syndrome die either in utero (30 to 40 weeks' gestation) or soon after birth. The hemoglobin levels range from 3 to 20 g/dL; the peripheral blood film is characterized by marked anisopoikilocytosis, large hypochromic macrocytes, and many nucleated red cells. The hemoglobin consists almost entirely of Hb Bart's (80 to 90%), with some remaining HbH and Portland. Mothers of these infants often have a history of previous neonatal deaths. Without medical care, women carrying these fetuses may have delivery and postpartum complications (e.g., retained placenta, eclampsia, sepsis).

There are several reports describing α-thalassemia associated with mental retardation (so-called ATR-16 syndrome). These conditions are mainly owing to large deletions (1 to 2 megabases) of the tip of chromosome 16, including the α-globin gene cluster. However, several cases have no deletions or other apparent abnormalities of the α-globin gene cluster. It has been shown that these patients, with a peculiar phenotype characterized by severe mental retardation, dysmorphic facies, genital abnormalities, and α-thalassemia, have a disorder that maps to the X chromosome (ATR-X syndrome).

β-Thalassemias

The β-thalassemias include a heterogeneous group of disorders of hemoglobin synthesis, all of which are characterized by reduced output of the β chains of adult hemoglobin. The clinical classification includes thalassemia major (TM; transfusion dependent), thalassemia intermedia (TI; intermediate severity), and thalassemia minor (asymptomatic) (Fig. 165-1; see Table 165-1). The severity of the clinical manifestations correlates quite well with the degree of imbalance of the globin chains: depending on the β-globin gene defects and their interaction, the production of β-globin chains is quantitatively reduced to different degrees, whereas the synthesis of α-globin continues as normal, resulting in the accumulation of excess unmatched α-globin chains in the erythroid precursors. The free α-globin chains are unable to form stable tetramers; they therefore precipitate in the erythroid precursors, forming inclusion bodies that damage the red cell membrane, thereby causing premature destruction of erythroid precursors in the bone marrow (ineffective erythropoiesis). Ineffective erythropoiesis leads to a sequence of events

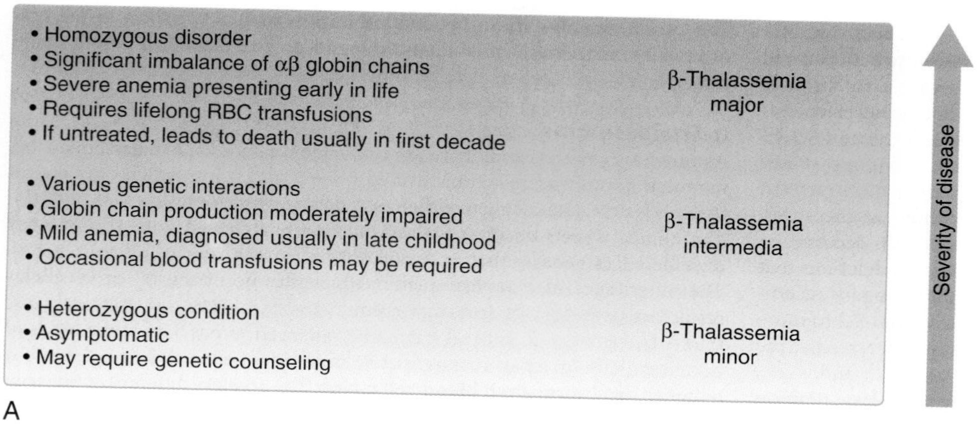

β-Thalassemia major
- Homozygous disorder
- Significant imbalance of αβ globin chains
- Severe anemia presenting early in life
- Requires lifelong RBC transfusions
- If untreated, leads to death usually in first decade

β-Thalassemia intermedia
- Various genetic interactions
- Globin chain production moderately impaired
- Mild anemia, diagnosed usually in late childhood
- Occasional blood transfusions may be required

β-Thalassemia minor
- Heterozygous condition
- Asymptomatic
- May require genetic counseling

Severity of disease

A

	Thalassemia major more likely	Thalassemia intermedia more likely
Clinical		
Presentation (years)	<2	>2
Hb levels (g/dL)	<7	7-10
Liver/spleen enlargement	Severe	Moderate to severe
Hematologic		
HbF (%)	>50	10-50 (may be up to 100%)
HbA_2 (%)	>3.5	<4-4.5
Genetic		
Parents	Both carriers of high HbA_2 β-thalassemia	One or both carriers: high HbF β-thalassemia, borderline HbA_2
Molecular		
Type of β-chain mutation	Severe	Mild/silent
Coinheritance of α-thalassemia	No/rare	Yes
Hereditary persistence of fetal hemoglobin	No	Yes
δβ-thalassemia	No	Yes
Gy XmnI polymorphism	No	Yes

B

FIGURE 165-1. **A,** Clinical classification of β-thalassemias. **B,** Tentative criteria to differentiate thalassemia major from thalassemia intermedia at presentation. HbA = adult hemoglobin; HbF = fetal hemoglobin; RBC = red blood cell.

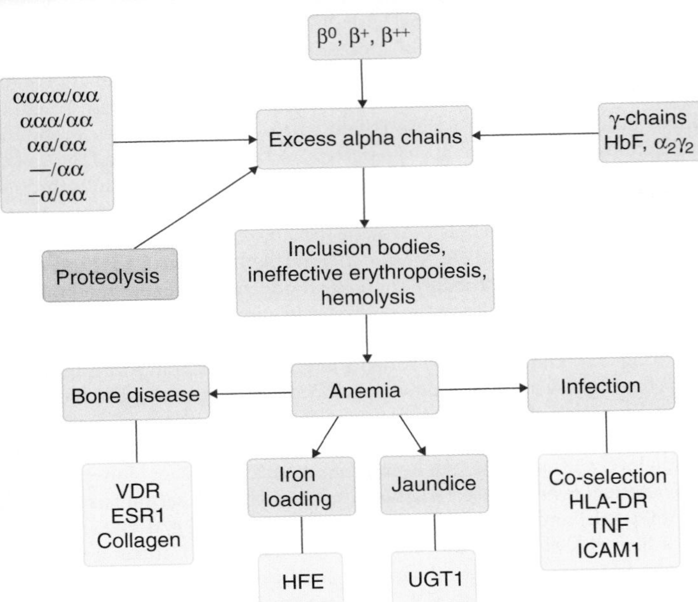

FIGURE 165-2. Pathophysiology of β-thalassemias and modifiers of globin chain imbalance. The severity of ineffective erythropoiesis is dependent on the degree of excess free α chains that result primarily from three different mechanisms: (1) inheritance of severe, mild, or silent β-chain mutations; (2) coinheritance of determinants associated with increased γ-chain production; and (3) coinheritance of α-thalassemia. A phenotype of thalassemia intermedia may result from the increased production of α-globin chains by a triplicated (ααα) or quadruplicated (αααα) α genotype associated with β heterozygosity. Inheritance of polymorphisms or mutations of genes involved in bone, iron, and bilirubin metabolism, as well as in infection, may contribute to modify the clinical course of the disease. ESR1 = estrogen receptor 1; HbF = fetal hemoglobin; HFE = hereditary hemochromatosis gene; HLA = human leukocyte antigen; ICAM1 = intercellular adhesion molecule-1; TNF = tumor necrosis factor; UGT1 = UDPglucose: glycoprotein glucosyltransferase 1; VDR = vitamin D receptor.

responsible for bone marrow expansion, anemia, hemolysis, splenomegaly, and increased iron absorption. Any factor that reduces the degree of chain imbalance and the magnitude of α-chain excess, such as coinheritance of α-thalassemia or an innate ability to increase HbF, will ameliorate the clinical expression of the disease (Fig. 165-2).

The major forms of β-thalassemia (still sometimes called Cooley's anemia) are disorders in which life can be sustained only by regular blood transfusions. This condition usually results from the homozygous state or from the compound heterozygous state for severe β gene mutations (β^0). The typical forms of TM manifest during the first year of life, during which γ chains are switched off but not replaced by β-chain synthesis. These infants, left untreated, are incapable of maintaining a hemoglobin level above 5 g/dL and show marked bone deformities and growth retardation. They develop thalassemic facies due to frontal bossing of the skull and protrusion of the jaws and cheekbones. The magnitude of the increase in erythropoiesis may result in extramedullary masses usually arising from the sternum and ribs. Progessive hepatosplenomegaly is a constant finding, leading to pancytopenia. The early childhood of untreated or inadequately treated TM patients includes various complications, such as recurrent infections, spontaneous fractures, gallstones, and leg ulcers. The mortality rate in such patients was once very high around puberty. Fortunately, this is no longer the case in children with well-treated TM. Children who are transfused to maintain a hemoglobin level above 9 g/dL have relatively normal growth and development, and their future course depends on whether they receive adequate iron chelation (see Treatment). Many children who are adequately transfused and are fully compliant with iron chelation therapy develop normally, enter puberty, and become sexually mature. At present, we are dealing with an adult population of TM patients who may suffer from the side effects of long-term treatment—namely, transfusion-associated infections (particularly hepatitis B and C and, in some populations, HIV) and organ damage (liver, heart, endocrine glands) due to unsatisfactory long-term iron chelation. The main causes of death in adult TM patients is still cardiac complications. Heart failure in these patients is multifactorial, involving chronic anemia, remaining iron overload, myocarditis, pericarditis, and probably many other mechanisms. Furthermore, in addition to the degree of globin chain imbalance, which is dependent on genetic factors linked to the globin genes (coinheritance of α-thalassemia, innate increased synthesis of HbF), there are many other genetic modifiers that may secondarily impact the outcome of complications. For example, the presence of a polymorphic variant in the UGT1A1 promoter responsible for Gilbert's syndrome (Chapter 149) may increase the predisposition to cholelithiasis, which is already a common complication in thalassemia. Likewise, polymorphisms in genes involved in iron homeostasis or bone metabolism may negatively or positively influence the degree of iron overload or osteopenia and osteoporosis, respectively (see Fig. 165-2). Environmental factors, including social conditions, nutrition, and the availability of medical care, have also been implicated in the variable severity of the clinical manifestations of TM.

TI is a clinical term used to describe patients with anemia and splenomegaly but without the full clinical spectrum of TM. The clinical phenotypes of TI lie between those of thalassemia minor and major, encompassing a wide spectrum. Mildly affected patients are almost completely asymptomatic until adult life, experiencing only mild anemia and spontaneously maintaining hemoglobin levels between 7 and 10 g/dL. Patients with more severe TI generally present between 2 and 6 years of age; although they are able to survive without regular transfusion therapy, growth and development may be retarded. Most TI patients are homozygotes or compound heterozygotes for mild to moderate β gene mutations (β^+/β^+, β^0/β^+); less commonly, only a single β-globin gene is affected. Because the clinical severity of the disease is dictated by the extent of globin chain imbalance, at least three different mechanisms can promote the mild clinical characteristics of TI versus those of TM: inheritance of mild or silent β gene mutations; coinheritance of determinants associated with increased γ-chain production, which contributes to neutralizing the large proportion of unbound α chains; and coinheritance of α-thalassemia, which reduces the synthesis of α chains, thereby reducing the α/non-α chain imbalance.

Three main factors are responsible for the clinical sequelae in TI patients: ineffective erythropoiesis, chronic anemia, and iron overload. The degree of ineffective erythropoiesis depends primarily on the underlying molecular defects (as already mentioned) and is due to the precipitation of free α chains into erythroid precursors in the bone marrow, causing membrane damage and premature cell death in the marrow. The degree of ineffective erythropoiesis is the primary determinant of the anemia of TI; the peripheral hemolysis of mature, circulating red cells and an overall reduction in hemoglobin synthesis are secondary. Hemolysis per se and damaged red cells that expose negatively charged membrane phosphatidyl-serine residues have been linked to the development of the hypercoagulable state and the increased risk of pulmonary hypertension found in the TI population. Chronic anemia and chronic ineffective erythropoiesis lead to an inappropriate increase in gastrointestinal iron absorption, resulting in iron overload. In contrast, in TM, iron loading results mainly from transfusional iron infusion. It has been shown that chronic anemia and ineffective erythropoiesis, which are characteristic of TI, are associated with the reduced expression of hepcidin, a hepatic peptide that plays a central role in iron homeostasis. Moreover, growth and differentiation factor 15 (GDF15), secreted by erythroid precursors and overexpressed in the presence of ineffective erythropoiesis, may suppress hepcidin synthesis. Taken together, ineffective erythropoiesis (leading to increased GDF15) and chronic anemia and hypoxia result in hepcidin suppression, increased dietary iron absorption from the gut, and increased release of recycled iron from the reticuloendothelial system, leading to an iron overload situation that is very similar to that observed in patients with hereditary hemochromatosis syndromes (which are characterized by impaired hepcidin production; Chapter 219). As a consequence of these pathophysiologic processes, several complications have been identified as unique in TI patients, especially in splenectomized naïve patients. Cholelithiasis is much more common in TI than in TM because of ineffective erythropoiesis and peripheral hemolysis. Extramedullary hematopoiesis, as a compensatory mechanism, leads to the formation of erythropoietic tissue masses that primarily affect the spleen, liver, lymph nodes, and vertebrae. These masses may cause neurologic problems such as spinal cord compression and paraplegia and intrathoracic masses. Leg ulcers are rare in well-transfused TM patients but are quite common in adult TI patients; it remains unclear why, at the same hemoglobin and HbF levels, some patients develop leg ulcers and others do not. Thrombotic risk is definitely increased in TI patients. Several studies have collectively shown that the incidence of thromboembolic events is higher in splenectomized TI patients. Although stroke is rare in TI, asymptomatic brain damage, including ischemia, has been documented by magnetic resonance imaging (MRI) and computed tomography in TI patients. Pulmonary hypertension (Chapter 68) is prevalent in TI patients (approximately 60%) and is thought to be the primary cause of heart failure in this population. Liver disease due to viral infection is less frequent than in TM; however, abnormal liver enzymes are frequently observed in TI patients, primarily owing to hepatocyte damage resulting from iron overload. In some of the oldest patients with TI (>40 years), hepatocellular carcinoma (Chapter 202) has been detected owing to long-term untreated iron accumulation with resultant cirrhosis, as found in genetic hemochromatosis (Chapter 219). Hypogonadism, hypothyroidism, and diabetes mellitus are quite rare. Although patients with TI generally experience puberty late, they have normal sexual development and are usually fertile. Women with TI may have spontaneous successful pregnancies, although complications may occur.

Thalassemia minor is the heterozygous state of β-thalassemia. Subjects with thalassemia minor are "carriers" of a single β-globin gene defect and are usually asymptomatic, except for a mild anemia of pregnancy. The carriers are usually identified as part of a family study, incidentally during an intercurrent illness, or as part of a population survey. The anemia is mild, microcytic, and hypochromic and is associated with an elevated level of HbA_2. The blood smear shows characteristic microcytosis and hypochromia, with some variation in size and shape of the red cells. The presence of target cells is very variable. The hematologic features are remarkably similar among different ethnic groups. Carriers of β-thalassemia with normal HbA_2 have been observed in settings in which an individual with mild TI was found to have one parent with typical β-thalassemia minor with elevated HbA_2 while the other showed either minimal or no hematologic abnormalities and normal HbA_2. Subjects with normal HbA_2 are usually carriers of silent β mutations (β^{++}).

δβ-Thalassemia and Hereditary Persistence of Fetal Hemoglobin

The clinical manifestations of $(\delta\beta)^0$-thalassemias are similar to those of TI, whereas the heterozygotes are distinguished from β-thalassemia heterozygotes by normal levels of HbA_2 and increased HbF levels of 5 to 20%. Homozygotes for Hb Lepore may have phenotypes similar to either TM or TI. Subjects affected by deletion or nondeletion forms of HPFH are usually asymptomatic.

Any of the β-thalassemia defects may be coinherited with β-chain variants (e.g., HbS, HbC, HbE) and cause a clinically relevant β-thalassemia phenotype of differing severity. These variants illustrate that β-thalassemia syndromes have a wide clinical spectrum and that specific therapeutic approaches may completely change the clinical course and natural history of these disorders.

DIAGNOSIS

The diagnosis of thalassemia may be required in a patient with a suspicious clinical picture or to identify a heterozygote subject as part of a family study or population screening program. The general diagnostic approach is common to any form of thalassemia, regardless of presentation. The primary evaluation is based on hematologic changes: the red cell indices obtained by electronic cell counter and the red cell morphology examined on a well-stained blood film are sufficient to direct further investigations. Individuals with a mean corpuscular volume below 80 fL and mean corpuscular hemoglobin below 27 pg with normal iron parameters need further investigation. The number of red blood cells is usually higher than normal. In the presence of anemia with thalassemic red cell changes, the next step is the evaluation of hemoglobin fractions (HbA, HbA_2, HbF, or Hb variants) by electrophoresis on cellulose acetate at alkaline pH or, even better, by high-performance liquid chromatography, which enables the precise measurement of HbA_2, HbF, and HbA and the provisional identification of a large number of Hb variants. An HbA_2 level greater than 3.5% associated with hypochromic microcytic red cells is diagnostic of β-thalassemia minor. HbA_2 values between 3.2 and 3.5% (borderline) should be interpreted with care because they could be due to the interaction of more than one thalassemic defect (α and β), a silent β mutation, or concomitant iron deficiency. If iron deficiency is present, it should be corrected and the HbA_2 estimation repeated. The majority of individuals with thalassemic red cell indices and normal or low HbA_2 and normal HbF are α^0-thalassemia carriers or α^+-thalassemia homozygotes. Carriers of α^0-thalassemia may have a few red cells with HbH inclusions. Microcytosis with low or normal HbA_2 levels and elevated HbF (2 to 20%) indicates heterozygosity for δβ-thalassemia. Patients with HPFH usually have normal red blood cell indices but increased levels of HbF with a different intercellular distribution (homogeneous or pancellular, with the exception of heterocellular HPFH) compared with δβ-thalassemia (uneven or heterocellular). A radioactive method for measuring the α/β-globin synthesis ratio was introduced in the mid to late 1960s and was largely directed at prenatal diagnosis in the pre-DNA era. Although it gives a quantitative assessment of globin production, today its use is limited to difficult cases caused by the interaction of different globin chain defects. Definitive diagnosis of the thalassemia syndromes involves identification of the underlying mutations through DNA analysis. There are several methods available for the diagnosis of any particular mutation, such as polymerase chain reaction (PCR) restriction-enzyme analysis, PCR allele-specific-oligonucleotides, gap PCR, and direct sequencing, which is probably the easiest and most reliable method. For deletion forms of α-thalassemia, multiplex ligation-dependent probe amplification is a useful, recently introduced method.

During their clinical course, patients affected by different forms of thalassemia develop several complications mainly due to iron overload, which must be monitored to direct iron chelation therapy. The principal methods of determining body iron levels (Chapter 219) are measurements of the serum ferritin level and assessment of liver iron concentration from biopsy tissue or, as an alternative noninvasive method, by R2 MRI. High serum ferritin levels (>2500 μg/L) and a high liver iron concentration (>15 g/dry weight) indicate a high risk of significant morbidity and mortality. Cardiac iron can be measured by a recently introduced T2* MRI procedure that allows estimation of the cardiac iron load. MRI T2* less than 10 msec is always associated with severe iron load and a high risk of heart failure within 1 year. MRI T2* greater than 20 msec is considered normal, meaning there is no iron in the heart. Echocardiography may also be useful to evaluate functional changes. For other complications, including endocrinopathies, liver disease, lung disease, thrombophilia, and bone disease, the diagnostic approaches are similar to those used in clinical practice, taking into consideration test cost, performance characteristics, and patient preferences.

TREATMENT

Rx

Conventional Treatment

No specific treatment is required for α- or β-thalassemia heterozygotes (carriers, thalassemia minor), but they should receive appropriate genetic counseling. During pregnancy, particularly during the second and third trimesters, thalassemia-carrying women may become more anemic, so they should be followed carefully and supported with folic acid. When real iron deficiency is associated with thalassemia traits, iron supplementation should be provided, while monitoring transferrin saturation and ferritin. Very few cases of in utero blood transfusions have been reported with Hb Bart's hydrops fetalis syndrome; most of these babies have been delivered prematurely by cesarean section, subsequent development has been abnormal, and survivors required regular blood transfusions after birth. HbH patients in general have rather high hemoglobin levels (8 to 9 g/dL) and do not need regular blood transfusion. Supplementation with folic acid (2 to 5 mg/day) is generally recommended, especially in pediatric patients. The major complications in HbH disease are hemolytic crises that may occur during or after acute infections; in such cases, immediate intervention, including blood transfusions and treatment for infection, should be promptly administered.

The clinical management of TM and TI remains the major issue. The lifespan and quality of life of TM and TI patients have been transformed over the last 10 years, with life expectancy increasing well into the third and fourth decades. Nevertheless, prolongation of life is accompanied by several complications, partly due to the underlying disorder and partly as a consequence of treatment with blood transfusions and iron overload. Moreover, we have to deal with aging-related complications in the context of a multiorgan disease that requires management by a team of clinicians with specific knowledge of thalassemias, working together with different specialists and well-trained nurses. The conventional treatment for TM patients includes regular transfusion therapy and iron chelation. Definition of the optimal transfusion and iron chelation regimen has been the most important advance in the management of TM patients, with the primary objective being to control the ineffective erythropoiesis, its consequences, and the iron burden. The optimal regimen involves regular blood transfusions, usually administered every 2 to 5 weeks, to maintain pretransfusion hemoglobin levels above 9 to 10.5 g/dL. The decision to initiate lifelong transfusion therapy should be based on a definitive diagnosis of severe thalassemia, taking into account the molecular defects, the severity of anemia on repeated measurements, the level of ineffective erythropoiesis, and clinical criteria such as failure to thrive or bone changes. It is advisable for TM patients to receive leukoreduced packed red cells to reduce transfusion reactions and pathogen transmission. Adverse reactions to red blood cell transfusions may occur during or after the transfusion, and they can be hemolytic or nonhemolytic. Transfusion-related acute lung injury (TRALI) is a very rare but severe complication and must be managed immediately

(Chapter 180). Many patients with TM require splenectomy because of hypersplenism. However, with optimal clinical management, the need for splenectomy may be delayed or even obviated. Splenectomy should be considered for patients whose annual blood consumption increases progressively and is responsible for significant increases in iron stores, despite good chelation therapy, and in those experiencing symptoms due to spleen enlargement. Clinical problems related to leukopenia or thrombocytopenia due to hypersplenism are other reasons to consider splenectomy. The major complication of splenectomy is severe and sometimes overwhelming infection. Because removal of the spleen may reduce the primary immune response to encapsulated organisms, it is advisable to delay splenectomy until patients are at least 5 years old. The mortality rate for overwhelming post-splenectomy infection in thalassemia patients is approximately 50%, despite intensive supportive care; therefore, preventive measures are mandatory, including immunoprophylaxis (vaccination against *Streptococcus pneumoniae*, pneumococcus, and meningococcus), chemoprophylaxis, and parent and patient education to recognize and report febrile illnesses.

Iron overload is an inevitable and serious complication of long-term blood transfusion therapy and hyperabsorption of dietary iron, and it requires adequate treatment to prevent early death from iron-induced cardiac disease. Optimal chelation therapy extends complication-free survival (Fig. 165-3). For more than 40 years, the standard chelation therapy has been deferoxamine (DFO), given for 10 to 24 hours a day as a continuous subcutaneous infusion 5 to 7 days per week. The long-term efficacy of DFO has been extensively documented in large cohorts of patients in Italy and elsewhere. Unfortunately, compliance with the rigorous daily regimen is a serious limiting factor, and in noncompliant patients, life expectancy is no different from that in the pre-DFO era. This has been the rationale behind the intensive effort to identify alternative, orally effective iron chelators. At present, two oral iron chelators are in the market: deferiprone (DFP) and deferasirox (DFX). DFP is registered in Europe but is not yet available in the United States. Based on the guidelines of the EMEA countries (Europe, Middle East, and Africa), treatment with DFP at doses of 75 to 100 mg/kg/day is restricted to patients unable to use DFO or those with an unsatisfactory response to DFO as judged by serum ferritin levels and liver iron concentrations. Recent studies indicate that DFP may be more effective than DFO in protecting the heart from the accumulation of iron.[1] A potential benefit of combined DFO/DFP therapy has been observed,[2,3] and according to the Thalassemia International Federation, combination DFO/DFP treatment should be considered for patients with very high levels of heart iron or cardiac dysfunction. The new orally effective iron chelator DFX is safe and effective for removing excess iron from different organs, including the heart. DFX is now available in most countries throughout the world as first-line treatment. Iron chelation therapy must be individualized according age, compliance history, and other factors. Monitoring and adjusting iron chelation based on repeated measurements of ferritin, calculation of iron intake by transfusions, and, whenever possible, measuring cardiac and liver iron by MRI (at least once) are mandatory.

The management of TI patients is more complicated owing to the wide heterogeneity of TI phenotypes. A number of options are currently available to treat TI patients, including transfusion therapy, splenectomy, modulation of HbF production, and hematopoietic stem cell transplantation. However, increasing evidence is delineating the benefit of transfusion therapy in decreasing the incidence of complications. Thus, although common practice in the past was to initiate transfusion when complications ensued, it may be worthwhile to start transfusion therapy earlier, as a preventive approach and to help alleviate the increased risk of alloimmunization with the delayed initiation of transfusion. The initiation of iron chelation therapy in patients with TI depends not only on the amount of excess iron but also on the rate of iron accumulation, the duration of exposure to excess iron, and various other factors in individual patients.

Bone Marrow Transplantation and Experimental Therapies

Allogeneic hematopoietic stem cell transplantation (HSCT) in thalassemia syndromes has been increasingly successful during the last 2 decades, mainly in β-thalassemia major. Predictors of poor transplant outcome are hepatomegaly, a history of irregular chelation, and hepatic fibrosis. Patients are categorized into three risk classes. Class 1 patients have none of these adverse risk factors, class 2 patients have one or two adverse risk factors, and class 3 patients have all three. In the most recent update of the Pesaro group's experience, the probability of thalassemia-free survival for patients younger than 17 years at the time of HSCT, receiving the allograft from a human leukocyte antigen (HLA)–identical relative, was 87% in class 1 patients, 85% in class 2 patients, and much lower in young class 3 patients. The progressive adjustment of conditioning therapy in class 3 patients and in adults (older than 17 years) has significantly reduced the incidence of transplant-related mortality. Only 25 to 30% of patients with diseases potentially curable by HSCT have suitable HLA-compatible siblings however, and bone marrow transplantation from unrelated donors significantly increases the incidence of acute and chronic graft-versus-host disease, particularly in thalassemia. A study from the Eurocord cooperative group reported the outcome of 33 class 1 and 2 patients with thalassemia who received cord blood HSCT from HLA-identical siblings: no patient died of transplant-related complications, suggesting that this is a safe procedure for thalassemia patients.

An alternative treatment of β-thalassemia consists of the pharmacologic stimulation of HbF synthesis. In humans, the hemoglobin switch from HbF to

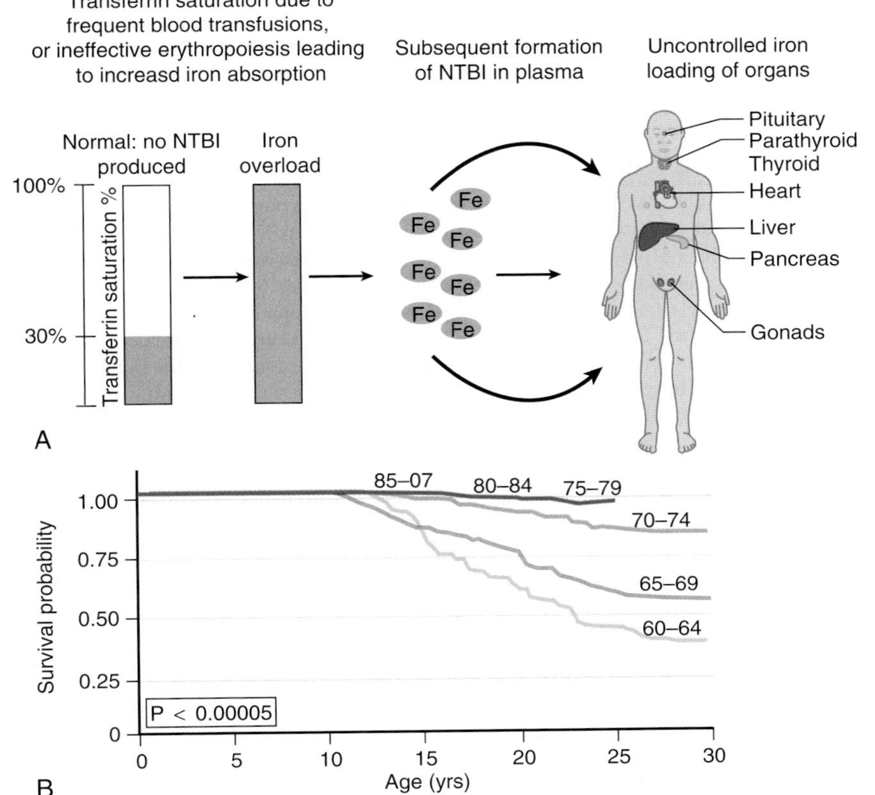

FIGURE 165-3. **A,** Transfusional iron overload and specific organ iron loading. **B,** Survival of Italian thalassemia major patients by cohort of birth: 1960 to 1964, 1965 to 1969, 1970 to 1974, 1975 to 1979, 1980 to 1984, and 1985 to 1997. NTBI = non–transferrin-bound iron. (From Borgna-Pignatti C, Rugolotto S, De Stefano P, et al. Survival and complications in patients with thalassemia major treated with transfusion and deferoxamine. *Haematologica.* 2004;89:1187-1193.)

HbA occurs in the period around birth as a result of γ- to β-globin gene switching. A number of pharmacologic agents with the ability to reactivate HbF synthesis have been identified, including hypomethylating agents, histone deacetylase inhibitors, and hydroxyurea. Although the effect of these treatments (particularly hydroxyurea) in sickle cell disease is clear (Chapter 166), their benefit on the clinical course of β-thalassemia is presently limited. This discrepancy in the response to HbF inducers may be related mainly to the higher level of HbF required to achieve clinical results in β-thalassemia compared to sickle cell disease. The limited clinical response to γ-globin inducers observed in the majority of β-thalassemia patients may also be a reflection of the unfavorable effects of these agents on the other globin genes (i.e., increased α-globin synthesis).

Gene therapy is an attractive approach for thalassemia syndromes; however, this strategy poses major challenges in terms of controlling transgene expression, which should be erythroid specific and sustained over time. Treatment of ß-thalassemia, sickle cell disease, and other disorders through lentivirus-mediated gene transfer has been reported in murine and primate models, but few human patients have been treated.

UNSTABLE HEMOGLOBINOPATHIES

More than 80 rare mutant hemoglobins have been reported to cause hemolytic anemia owing to amino acid replacements or deletions that significantly lower solubility. These mutant hemoglobins form intracellular precipitates that can be detected as so-called Heinz bodies when the blood smear is exposed to a supravital stain. Structural abnormalities include mutations that weaken the linkage between heme and globin, disrupt secondary (α-helical) structures, or introduce a charged or polar side group into the hydrophobic interior of the globin subunit.

This disorder, sometimes called congenital Heinz body hemolytic anemia, is inherited in an autosomal dominant manner. Severely affected individuals have jaundice, splenomegaly, and, on occasion, dark brown urine owing to the release of heme and aberrant conversion to dipyroles. The instability of a few of these globin mutants is so extreme that they cannot be detected by routine laboratory methods. This results in a thalassemia phenotype with microcytosis and ineffective erythropoiesis. Like individuals with glucose-6-phosphate dehydrogenase deficiency (Chapter 164), those with unstable hemoglobin mutants often lack clinical symptoms and signs of hemolysis until or unless they develop an infection or are exposed to an oxidant drug.

The diagnosis can be established by the combination of a positive Heinz body preparation and either abnormal hemoglobin electrophoresis or demonstration of a precipitate following exposure of a hemolysate to heat or isopropanol. Some clinics have access to a reference laboratory that can identify the specific mutation by α- and β-globin DNA sequencing.

Most individuals with this disorder do not require treatment. However, some are symptomatic from severe anemia. Splenectomy generally results in a significant increase in red cell mass, but the fraction of Heinz body–positive red cells increases markedly after splenectomy, putting these patients at significant risk of developing pulmonary hypertension and cor pulmonale.

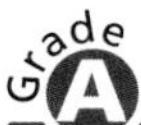

1. Pennell DJ, Berdoukas V, Karagiorga M, et al. Randomized controlled trial of deferiprone or deferoxamine in beta-thalassemia major patients with asymptomatic myocardial siderosis. *Blood.* 2006;107:3738-3744.
2. Tanner MA, Galanello R, Dessi C, et al. A randomized, placebo-controlled, double-blind trial of the effect of combined therapy with deferoxamine and deferiprone on myocardial iron in thalassemia major using cardiovascular magnetic resonance. *Circulation.* 2007;115:1876-1884.
3. Maggio A, Vitrano A, Capra M, et al. Long-term sequential deferiprone-deferoxamine versus deferiprone alone for thalassemia major patients: a randomized clinical trial. *Br J Haematol.* 2009;145:245-254.

SUGGESTED READINGS

Cao A, Galanello R. Beta thalassemia. *Genet Med.* 2010;12:61-74. *Review.*

Pennell DJ, Porter JB, Cappellini MD, et al. Continued improvement in myocardial T2* over two years of deferasirox therapy in β-thalassemia major patients with cardiac iron overload. *Haematologica.* 2011;96:48-54. *Continuous treatment with deferasirox (40 mg/kg/d) continued to remove iron from the heart.*

Pennell DJ, Porter JB, Cappellini MD, et al. Efficacy of deferasirox in reducing and preventing cardiac iron overload in beta-thalassemia. *Blood.* 2010;115:2364-2371. *Deferasirox is effective in removing and preventing myocardial iron accumulation.*

Serjeant GR, Serjeant BE, Fraser RA, et al. Hb S-β-thalassemia: molecular, hematological and clinical comparisons. *Hemoglobin.* 2011;35:1-12. *Clinically, Hb S-β(0)-thal and Hb S-β(+)-thal type I were generally severe.*

Smiers FJ, Krishnamurti L, Lucarelli G. Hematopoietic stem cell transplantation for hemoglobinopathies: current practice and emerging trends. *Pediatr Clin North Am.* 2010;57:181-205. *Improved results are possible with new conditioning regimens and expanded donor pools.*

Taher AT, Musallam KM, Karimi M, et al. Overview on practices in thalassemia intermedia management aiming for lowering complication-rates across a region of endemicity: the OPTIMAL CARE study. *Blood.* 2010;115:1886-1892. *Study of 584 thalassemia intermedia patients, searching for associations among disease characteristics, treatment received, and rate of complications.*

Testa U. Fetal hemoglobin chemical inducers for treatment of hemoglobinopathies. Review. *Ann Hematol.* 2009;88:505-528. *The increase in HbF in response to these drugs varies among patients with thalassemia and sickle cell disease owing to individual genetic determinants.*

Weatherall DJ. The inherited diseases of hemoglobin are an emerging global health burden. *Blood.* 2010;115:4331-4336. *Strong argument for recognition of inherited hemoglobinopathies as a major, growing global health burden.*

166

SICKLE CELL DISEASE AND OTHER HEMOGLOBINOPATHIES

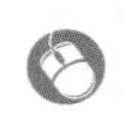

MARTIN H. STEINBERG

SICKLE CELL DISEASE

DEFINITION

Sickle cell disease, caused by a mutation in the β-globin gene (*HBB*), consists of a group of chronic hemolytic anemias, all characterized by vaso-occlusive events, hemolytic anemia, vasculopathy, widespread acute and chronic organ damage, and premature mortality.

EPIDEMIOLOGY

The prevalences of the various forms of sickle cell disease and of the sickle cell trait, which is not truly a form of sickle cell disease, vary in the United States and worldwide (Table 166-1; Fig. 166-1). The sickle hemoglobin mutation became prominent in equatorial Africa, the Middle East, and India several thousand years ago, when deforestation, the rise of agriculture, and stagnant pooling of water permitted *Plasmodium falciparum* infection to become endemic. Carriers of the sickle cell trait were more likely to survive to reproductive age and had a selective advantage where falciparum malaria was present. At least five distinct origins of this identical mutation can be distinguished by the accompanying haplotype of the β-globin gene–like cluster. Slave trading and war spread this mutation to the Americas, throughout the Mediterranean basin, and eastward to the Indian subcontinent. In some sites in Africa, half the population carries the sickle hemoglobin gene.

PATHOBIOLOGY

Globin, the protein portion of hemoglobin, harbors the porphyrin heme ring and permits the molecule to operate efficiently in oxygen transport and its other physiologic functions (Fig. 166-2). Mutations can alter the primary amino acid sequence of the globin polypeptide, sometimes resulting in clinically significant diseases called hemoglobinopathies, including sickle cell disease. Sickle hemoglobin (HbS; $\alpha_2\beta_2^S$) is caused by an adenine (A) to thymidine (T) substitution (GAG → GTG) in codon 6 of the β-globin gene, resulting in replacement of the normal glutamic acid residue by a valine (Glu6Val). HbS polymerizes when it is deoxygenated, a property only of hemoglobin variants that have the *HBB* Glu6Val substitution. Critical amounts of HbS polymer within sickle erythrocytes cause cellular injury and lead to the phenotype of sickle cell disease, which is recognized by hemolytic anemia and vaso-occlusion. Other hemoglobin variants, such as HbE and HbC, are also common. More than 1000 hemoglobin mutations are known, and occasionally they can affect the stability and function of hemoglobin and cause hemolytic anemia (Chapter 161), disordered oxygen transport (Chapter 169), or methemoglobinemia (Chapter 161). However, most globin mutations are clinically insignificant. Thalassemias (Chapter 165) are also caused by mutations in globin genes, but these mutations affect globin gene expression so that synthesis of a globin chain is reduced or absent, although the structure of any globin produced is usually normal.

In sickle cell disease, erythrocytes are heterogeneous as a result of membrane damage and the cellular distribution of fetal hemoglobin (HbF). HbF

TABLE 166-1 GENETIC AND LABORATORY FEATURES OF COMMON SICKLE HEMOGLOBINOPATHIES*

GENOTYPE	GENETICS	PREVALENCE AMONG AFRICAN AMERICANS†	HEMATOCRIT (%)	MCV (FL)	HBS (%)	HBA$_2$ (%)	HBF (%)	SEVERITY‡
Sickle cell anemia (HbSS)	Homozygous HbS	1 : 600	18-28	85-95	>85	2-3	2-15	4
HbSS-α-thalassemia	Homozygous HbS α$^+$-thalassemia	30% of HbSS patients	25-33	70-85	>85	4-6	2-15	4
HbSC disease (HbSC)	Compound heterozygous HbS, HbC	1 : 800	28-40	70-85	50	2-3	1-8	2
HbS-β^0-thalassemia (HbS-β^0-Thal)	Compound heterozygous HbS, β^0-thalassemia	1 : 1600	20-30	65-75	>85	4-6	5-15	4
HbS-β$^+$-thalassemia (HbS-β$^+$-Thal)	Compound heterozygous HbS, β$^+$-thalassemia	1 : 1600	30-40	60-70	70-95	4-6	2-10	1-3
HbSE disease (HbSE)	Compound heterozygous HbS, HbE	Rare§	30-45	70-80	60	2-3	1	1-2
HbS-HPFH	Compound heterozygous HbS and gene deletion HPFH	Rare	38-45	70-80	70	2	20-30	0
Sickle cell trait (HbAS)¶	Heterozygous HbS	1 : 12	38-50	80-90	35-40	2-3	<1	0
Normal (HbAA)	Homozygous HbA	—	38-50	80-90	0	2-3	<1	—

*Many other abnormal globin genes can be found as compound heterozygotes with the HbS gene. The most common of these are α-thalassemia, HbD, HbO (Arabia), HbG (Philadelphia), HPFH, Hb Hope, and Hb Lepore. Average ranges of laboratory values are shown, but these can vary according to patient age.

†These figures differ depending on the prevalence of the involved genes in the population studied. In West and Central Africa, where the disease is most common, approximately 2% of all newborns have sickle cell disease. The prevalence of the HbC trait in African Americans is 3%, and that of the β-thalassemia trait is 1%. About 30% of African Americans carry an α-thalassemia gene, which can alter the phenotype of sickle cell disease by causing microcytosis, reduced cell density, and less hemolysis.

‡Severity of disease compared with sickle cell anemia, clinically the most severe genotype. This is a qualitative ranking of the clinical severity of each genotype; within each genotype, there is great clinical heterogeneity.

§Although this combination is still a rare genotype, the rising Asian population in the United States (HbE is a Southeastern Asian gene) will make it more frequent with time. With few cases reported compared with the other genotypes, the phenotype of HbSE disease is not totally defined. It may resemble HbS-β$^+$ thalassemia with symptoms appearing mainly in adults.

¶Sickle cell trait should not be classified as a form of sickle cell disease. About 8% of African Americans are carriers of HbS. Carriers are hematologically normal with a normal life expectancy. The few abnormalities traceable to the presence of HbS besides the renal lesions (see Table 166-3) include a four-fold increased risk of pulmonary embolism, an increased risk of splenic infarction at high altitude, and a higher risk of dying during the course of exertional heat illness.

Hb = hemoglobin; HPFH = hereditary persistence of HbF; MCV = mean corpuscular volume.

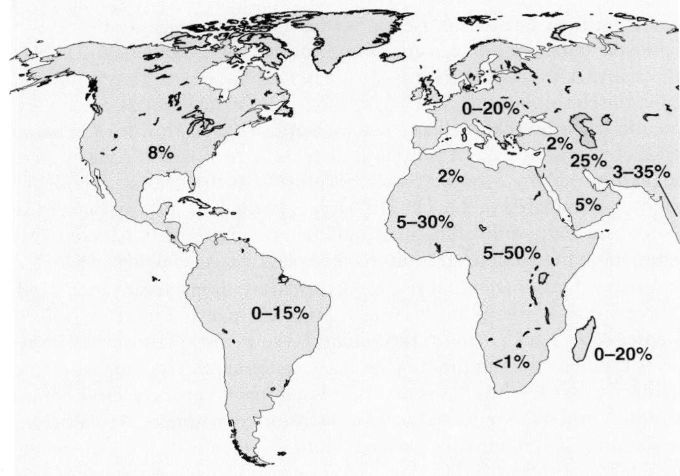

FIGURE 166-1. Worldwide prevalence of the sickle cell trait. Shown are the percentages of individuals with sickle cell trait in regions of the world where the hemoglobin S (HbS) gene is often present. In each geographic area, the prevalence of sickle cell trait can vary markedly according to racial or ethnic group, historical migration patterns, and even from village to village. Not shown is the high concentration of the HbS gene in areas of Europe such as London, Manchester, and Paris, where migrants from Africa or Afro-Caribbean populations have settled.

concentrations vary among patients with sickle cell anemia (homozygosity for HbS) and among erythrocytes of each individual. Because HbF inhibits HbS polymerization (see later discussion), its concentration within each cell and its distribution among all cells influence cell heterogeneity.

Sickle cell anemia is noteworthy for its clinical heterogeneity. Any patient can have almost all known disease complications; some have almost none but die suddenly; some skip one or more phases of the disease but suffer intensely from others. Thus, this prototypical single-gene, mendelian disorder behaves clinically as a multigenic trait with exceptional phenotypic variability. Understanding the vascular and inflammatory components of the disease provides many loci where the disease phenotype can be influenced by modifying genes. These genes potentially affect the pathogenesis of sickle cell anemia by modulating HbF concentration, inflammation, oxidant injury, nitric oxide (NO) biology, vasoregulation, cell-cell interaction, blood coagulation, and hemostasis. Polymorphisms have been noted in candidate genes that affect these functions, and some may be prognostically useful. The sickle mutation is found on several different haplotypes of the β-globin gene–like cluster, reflecting different origins of the mutation in Africa and the Middle East. The Senegal haplotype is often associated with higher HbF levels than other haplotypes and with a more benign clinical course. Conversely, the Bantu haplotype may be associated with more disease complications; however, there is phenotypic heterogeneity even within a particular haplotype group.

Cation homeostasis is impaired in some sickle cells. A reduced capacity of sickle cells to maintain normal potassium (K^+) gradients is mediated by activation of the Gardos and K^+/Cl^- cotransport channels. As a result, sickle erythrocytes vary in their density and deformability. Irreversibly sickled cells (ISCs; Fig. 166-3) always appear deformed because of permanent membrane damage, even though they may not contain HbS polymer. In some dense cells, the mean corpuscular hemoglobin concentration reaches 50 g/dL (normal, 27 to 38 g/dL), and HbS polymer is always present. Individuals with the highest numbers of ISCs and dense cells have the most hemolysis and anemia but not necessarily the highest incidence of acute vaso-occlusive events like painful episodes.

Hemolysis is mainly extravascular owing to erythrophagocytosis by reticuloendothelial cells that recognize the damaged sickle erythrocyte. In most patients, intravascular destruction of sickle erythrocytes liberates excessive amounts of hemoglobin into the circulation, thereby depleting haptoglobin and scavenging NO. This process promotes a vasoconstrictive, proinflammatory phenotype (Fig. 166-4). Certain complications of sickle disease, such as pulmonary hypertension, priapism, leg ulcer, and stroke, are epidemiologically linked to the intensity of hemolysis, whereas other complications, such as painful episodes, acute chest syndrome, and osteonecrosis, are linked to high blood viscosity and the interactions among sickle cells, leukocytes, and the endothelium.

Vaso-occlusive events probably depend on features intrinsic to the sickle erythrocyte, such as polymer content and the degree of cellular damage, interacting with factors in the cell's environment, such as endothelial injury, vascular tone, and other blood cells. In the first hours of a painful episode, the number of dense cells falls; it rises again as pain resolves. These observations suggest the possibility that more deformable, more adherent cells might

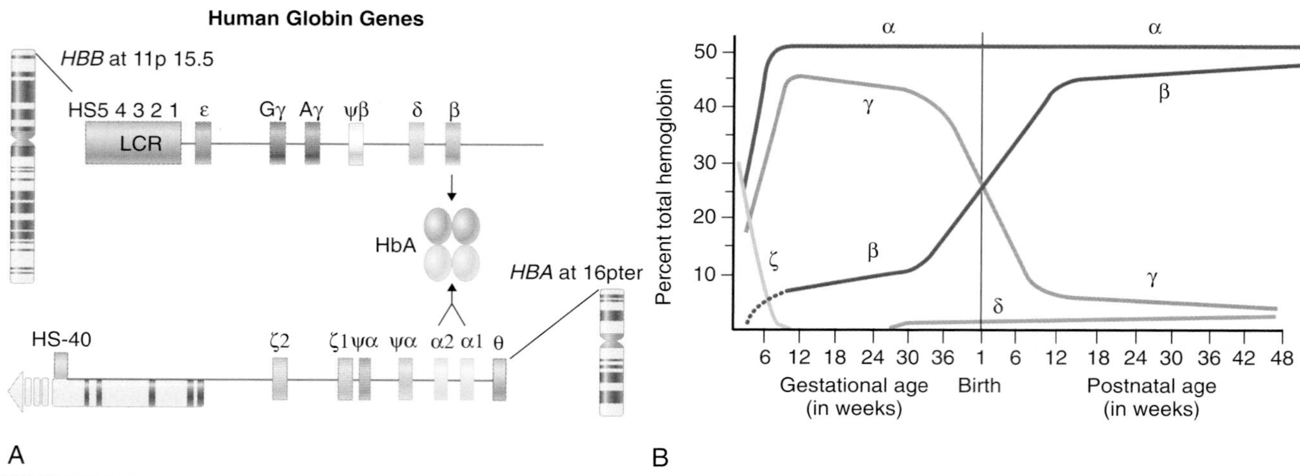

FIGURE 166-2. **Human globin genes. A,** The β-like globin gene cluster on chromosome 11 is shown above, and the α-like globin gene cluster below. Two β-globin chains and two α-globin chains combine to form the normal hemoglobin A (HbA) tetramer, represented between the globin genes. Each globin chain contains one heme group, and oxygen transport takes place sequentially at the four iron-containing heme groups. Fetal hemoglobin (HbF) is composed of two α- and two γ-globin chains; the minor hemoglobin of adults, HbA_2, contains two α- and two δ-globin chains. Normally present at a level of only 2 to 3%, HbA_2 concentration is increased to 4 to 6% in most carriers of β-thalassemia. The ζ *(HBZ)* and ε *(HBE1)* genes are normally expressed only in the embryo. The 5′ ψα gene has recently been found to be expressed at a very low level and is now called the μ-globin gene *(HBM)*. The θ-globin gene *(HBQ1)* is also expressed at low levels. Neither the θ nor the μ gene has been found in a functional hemoglobin. Any of the globin chains participating in hemoglobin formation may have a mutation altering its amino acid sequence. HbS, HbE, and HbC mutations affect the β-globin gene *(HBB)*. Other mutations can affect the α- *(HBA1, HBA2)*, γ- *(HBG1, HBG2)*, and δ-globin *(HBD)* genes. LCR = locus control region. **B,** Expression of globin genes during development. α-Chains are expressed throughout gestation and adult life, fetal γ-globin chains are expressed predominantly in utero, and the β- and δ-globin genes are expressed mainly postnatally. This switching of gene expression patterns accounts for the different hemoglobins present in the embryo, fetus, and adult. It also accounts for the observation that disorders of α-globin can affect both fetus and adult, whereas β-globin chain diseases usually are not clinically apparent in the first months of life, when HbF levels are still high.

initiate vaso-occlusion, whereas dense cells become sequestered or destroyed in the microvasculature. Endothelial cells are responsive to many biologic modifiers that can be generated during sickle vaso-occlusive episodes and infection. Their activation and damage may be provoked by adherent sickle cells and shear stresses that cause release of oxidant radicals, expression of endothelin, and disturbed NO balance. Cellular damage enables adhesive interactions among sickle cells, endothelial cells, and leukocytes. Reperfusion injury can also induce endothelial activation. The association of sickle and endothelial cells by a variety of adhesion molecules and their ligands may sufficiently delay cellular passage so that HbS polymerization, cell sickling, and vaso-occlusion happen before transit through the microvasculature is complete. Reticulocytes that are prematurely released from bone marrow display adhesive ligands that facilitate erythrocyte-endothelial interactions. Individuals with the greatest amount of hemolysis have the highest reticulocyte counts, and these adherent cells provide another link of hemolysis with vaso-occlusion. Neutrophils, which are modulators of inflammation and tissue damage, are increased in patients who have the acute chest syndrome, priapism, or stroke, and their numbers at baseline are a risk factor for survival.

CLINICAL MANIFESTATIONS

The clinical phenotype of sickle cell disease can be a result of many different genotypes, but most patients have either sickle cell anemia, HbSC disease, or HbS-β-thalassemia (see Table 166-1). Although hemolytic anemia and vaso-occlusive events are found in all genotypes, genotypes with higher cellular concentration of HbS are clinically more severe. Within milliseconds to seconds after HbS deoxygenation, depending on the intracellular concentration of HbS, HbS polymer appears in the sickle erythrocyte. In sickle cell trait (i.e., the simple heterozygote carriage of the HbS mutation), each cell contains only 30 to 40% HbS, so polymer is not found under most conditions (see Fig. 166-3). Therefore, carriers have few complications and a normal life expectancy.

The features of sickle cell anemia change as life advances (Table 166-2). The switch from HbF to HbS underlies the clinical shift in life's first decade. This time is typified by acute problems: high risks of severe life-threatening infection, acute chest syndrome, splenic sequestration, and stroke. Chronic organ damage (renal failure, pulmonary hypertension, and late effects of previous cerebrovascular disease) becomes paramount in adults.

Most patients with sickle cell anemia have moderate anemia with a hematocrit between 25 and 30%. Some patients appear to have more severe hemolysis, with hematocrit less than 20%, marked reticulocytosis, and extreme elevation of serum lactic dehydrogenase (LDH). Patients with the most profound hemolysis appear more likely to have stroke, pulmonary hypertension, priapism, and leg ulcers. Many patients with HbSC disease, especially adult men, have almost normal hematocrits and may have a higher incidence of sickle retinopathy, perhaps owing to their increased blood viscosity. Symptoms of anemia, such as weakness and dyspnea, are not the hallmarks of sickle cell disease, yet hemoglobin concentration can be a prognostic indicator for certain complications (see Table 166-2). Plasma volume in sickle cell anemia may be greatly expanded, making it difficult to predict the red blood cell (RBC) mass based on the hematocrit. Serum erythropoietin levels in sickle cell anemia are inappropriately low for the hematocrit. A consequence of hemolysis is increased turnover of bile pigments, regulated in part by promoter polymorphisms in the uridine diphosphate-glucuronosyltransferase 1A (*UGT1A*) gene, which is also associated with unconjugated hyperbilirubinemia and Gilbert's syndrome (Chapter 149). As a result, more than half of all adults have cholelithiasis (Chapter 158). Hemolytic anemia places patients at risk for acutely developing severe anemia when erythropoiesis is temporarily interrupted by parvovirus B19 infection (Chapter 379), which is the predominant cause of the aplastic crisis. Aplastic crisis is typified by a plummeting hematocrit, reticulocytopenia, and a bone marrow without erythroid precursors. It is a transient process, most common in children, and often requires blood transfusion to maintain circulatory competence until a spontaneous recovery follows. Rarely, if a patient's diet is inadequate, hemolysis-induced accelerated turnover of erythrocytes causes folic acid deficiency and megaloblastic anemia (Chapter 167).

First 20 Years

Although any complication can occur at any age, certain events tend to predominate in different age groups. In life's first decades, the most common sickle cell disease–related clinical events are painful episodes, acute chest syndrome, and stroke. Delayed growth and sexual development, more severe in patients with sickle cell anemia than in those with HbSC disease, become major issues of concern to the adolescent, but sexual maturation is eventually achieved.

Psychosocial problems are common in adolescents with sickle cell disease. Difficulties with medical staff often begin in adolescence and frequently center on issues of pain management and inpatient stay.

The Painful Episode

Pain, presumed to be caused by sickle vaso-occlusion, often starts in young children as the hand-foot syndrome: painful swelling of the hands and feet caused by inflammation of the metacarpal and metatarsal periosteum. Acute painful episodes are the most commonly encountered vaso-occlusive events in patients of all ages, but what triggers an acute painful episode is usually

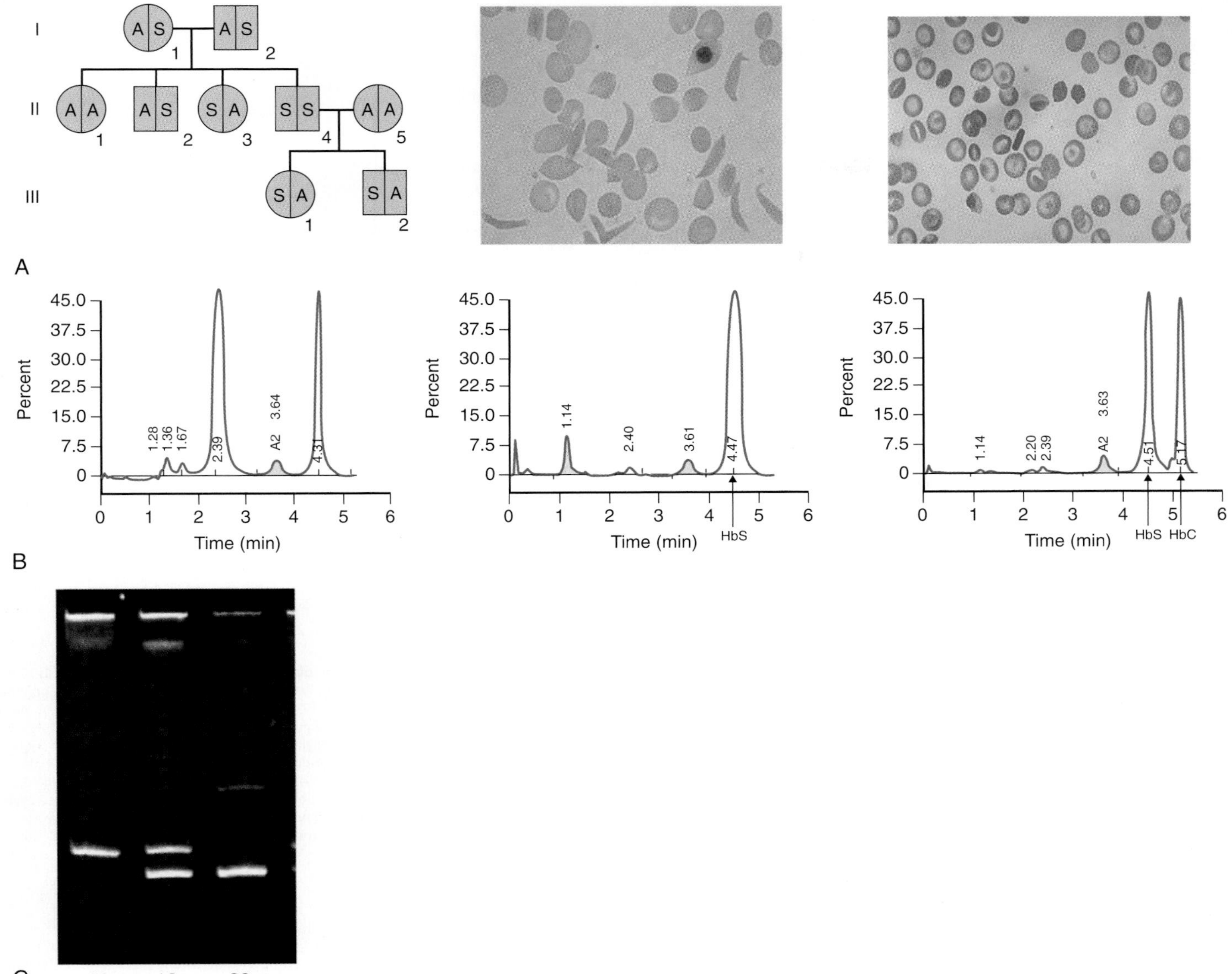

FIGURE 166-3. Diagnosis of sickle cell disease. A, A prototypical family structure in which both parents (I) have sickle cell trait and each offspring (II) has a 25% chance of having sickle cell anemia (SS). Each child of an affected parent (III) will have sickle cell trait (SA) if the other parent has a normal hemoglobin (AA) genotype. The center and right blood films are from patients with sickle cell anemia and HbSC disease, respectively. Note the irreversibly sickled cells (ISCs) in the former and the hemoglobin C (HbC) crystal and target cells in the latter. **B,** High-performance liquid chromatography (HPLC) profiles from patients with sickle cell trait (*left*), sickle cell anemia (*center*), and HbSC disease (*right*). **C,** Amplification refractory mutation system (ARMS)-based separation of the β-globin genes from a normal subject (AA), a carrier of sickle cell trait (AS), and a patient with sickle cell anemia (SS).

unknown. Commonly, painful episodes begin with little warning; some patients, however, may sense one in the offing. These episodes, which last from hours to many days, may wax and wane in intensity and migrate from site to site. No useful laboratory test can tell whether a vaso-occlusive pain episode is occurring, and the history remains the best clue. Sickle cell pain is described as worse than postoperative or traumatic pain. Some women describe the pain of childbirth as paling in comparison with the pain experienced during painful episodes. These agonizing attacks of acute pain must be separated from chronic pain perhaps caused by osteoporosis of the spine, pain associated with osteonecrosis of the hips and shoulders, neuropathic pain, iatrogenic pain, and the milder aches, pains, and soreness that are frequently present between severe episodes.

Patients vary greatly in the number, severity, and frequency of their painful episodes. Painful episodes are often stereotypical, affecting individuals in the same manner from episode to episode. Patients usually know whether the pain they are experiencing is different from their typical painful episode, and the wise physician should heed a patient's advice about the need for hospitalization or the likelihood that the pain has an alternative explanation.

About 40% of patients do not have pain requiring a hospital visit in a given year, whereas 3% have more than six painful episodes per year. Having more than three pain episodes requiring hospitalization per year is associated with increased mortality among patients 20 years and older. Recent studies suggest that pain is present on about half of all days; most episodes are managed at home and not in a medical setting, so hospital visits underestimate the frequency of pain.

HbF levels are inversely related to the frequency of painful episodes. Concurrent α-thalassemia may increase the pain rate because of its effect on the hematocrit. The day-to-day management of sickle cell disease often equates with the management of acute and chronic pain.

The pain accompanying acute chest syndrome, acute cholecystitis, splenic sequestration crisis, splenic infarction, or right upper quadrant syndrome may sometimes be mistaken for uncomplicated pain episodes. Acute painful episodes often herald the acute chest syndrome, and occasionally pain episodes end with multiorgan failure. Unexplained death can occur during acute painful episodes, perhaps as a result of an arrhythmia secondary to unrecognizable myocardial damage or perhaps as a sequela of pulmonary hypertension. Currently, it is not possible to foretell whether a "usual" pain episode will have an unexpected mortal outcome or presage acute chest syndrome, but the presence of atypically severe pain or an uncommonly high leukocyte count or low hematocrit should be cause for extra scrutiny.

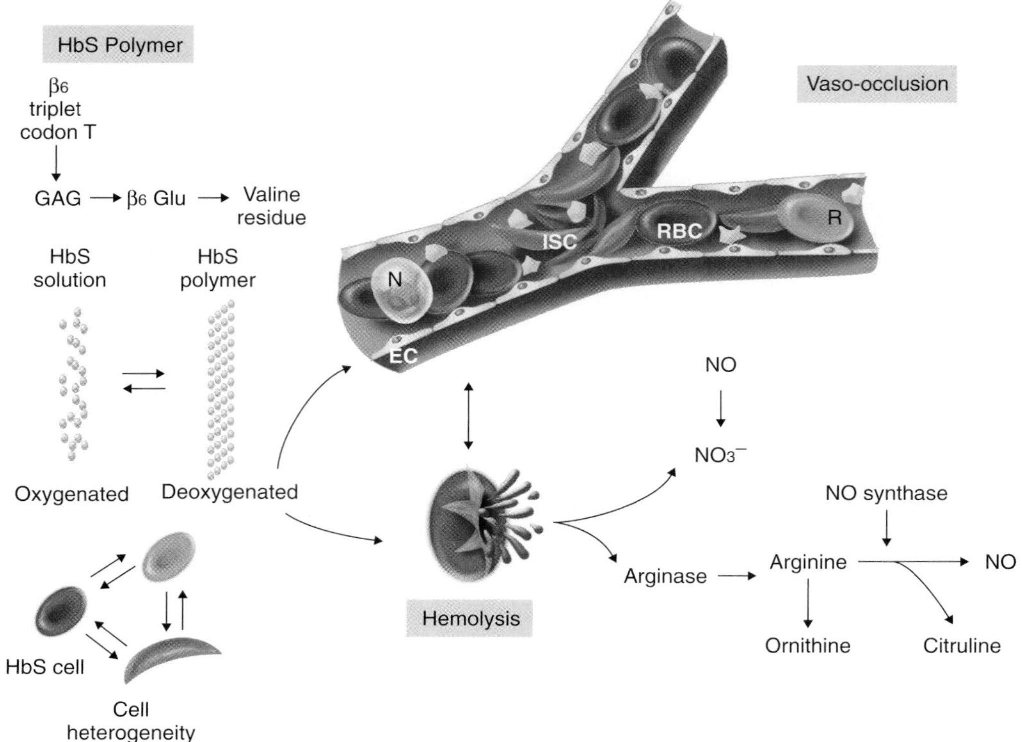

FIGURE 166-4. Pathophysiology of sickle cell disease. An adenine (A) to thymidine (T) transversion (A6T) at codon 6 in the β-hemoglobin gene on chromosome 11 *(HBB)* leads to the substitution of a glutamic acid codon by a valine codon. β^6 valine endows the hemoglobin S (HbS) molecule ($\alpha_2\beta_2^S$) with the property of polymerization when deoxygenated. HbS polymer injures the erythrocyte and leads to a heterogenous population of sickle cells with damaged membrane cytoskeleton, reduced cation and water content, and altered distribution of membrane lipids. In the vasculature, sickle cells interact with endothelium and other blood cells to cause vaso-occlusion. Some damaged erythrocytes hemolyze intravascularly, thereby releasing heme into the plasma to scavenge nitric oxide (NO) and to reduce hemoglobin to methemoglobin and nitrate. NO, by binding soluble guanylate cyclase, converts cyclic guanosine triphosphate (cGTP) to guanosine monophosphate (GMP), thereby relaxing vascular smooth muscle and causing vasodilation. A state of reduced endothelial NO bioavailability in sickle cell disease impairs the homeostatic vascular functions of NO, such as inhibition of platelet activation and aggregation and transcriptional repression of genes transcribing cell adhesion molecules. Hemoglobin, heme, and heme iron catalyze the production of oxygen radicals and protein nitration, potentially further limiting NO bioavailability and activating endothelium. Lysed erythrocytes also liberate arginase, which destroys L-arginine, the substrate for NO production, providing another mechanism for endothelial NO deficiency. The normal balance of vasoconstriction versus vasodilation is therefore skewed toward vasoconstriction as well as endothelial activation and proliferation. EC = epithelial cell; ISC = irreversibly sickled cell; N = neutrophil; R = reticulocyte; RBC = red blood cell.

TABLE 166-2 FEATURES OF SICKLE CELL ANEMIA

Painful episodes: associated with higher hemoglobin
Acute chest syndrome: associated with higher hemoglobin
Stroke: associated with lower hemoglobin
Osteonecrosis: associated with higher hemoglobin
Priapism: associated with lower hemoglobin
Proliferative retinopathy: associated with higher hemoglobin
Splenic infarction and sequestration
Leg ulcers: associated with lower hemoglobin
Gallstones
Aplastic crisis
Osteopenia—bone marrow hyperplasia
Nutritional deficiencies—folic acid, zinc, calories
Pneumococcal disease and sepsis
Placental insufficiency
Some complications are associated with hemoglobin concentration

Stroke

A major complication of sickle cell anemia in early life is stroke caused by stenosis and occlusion of large vessels (Chapter 414). Sickle erythrocytes and anemia-related high blood flow velocity lead to vascular damage. Hemorrhagic stroke is often caused by rupture of aneurysms. Moyamoya disease, a proliferation of small vessels found in sickle cell patients with stenotic lesions, may also cause hemorrhage in adults (Chapter 414). Hemorrhagic stroke is associated with a mortality rate of more than 20%. Stroke is most common among patients with sickle cell anemia, with much lower rates among those with HbSC disease or HbS-β^+-thalassemia. Beyond age 1 year, the incidence of stroke in sickle cell anemia is approximately 0.5 events per 100 patient years until age 40 years. The risk of having a first stroke is 11% by age 20 years, 15% by age 30 years, and 24% by age 45 years. Severe anemia, acute chest syndrome, and elevated systolic blood pressure are associated with ischemic strokes, whereas an elevated leukocyte count is a risk factor for hemorrhagic stroke. α-Thalassemia may protect patients with sickle cell anemia from stroke, perhaps because these patients have less hemolysis and a higher hematocrit. Subclinical neurologic events and silent cerebral infarction are even more common than stroke. The aberrant behavior of some sickle cell patients is most likely a result of otherwise silent cerebral infarction with deteriorating neurocognitive function.

Acute Chest Syndrome

Acute chest syndrome, characterized by fever, chest pain, wheezing, cough, hypoxia, and a new lung infiltrate, is a sometimes lethal complication that affects more than half of all patients with sickle cell anemia. It is the second most common reason for hospitalization and is a frequent cause of death in adults. The syndrome is more frequent in children, in whom its course is often mild, than in adults, in whom it tends to be more severe.

Commonly, acute chest syndrome develops after several days in individuals hospitalized for an acute painful episode (see earlier discussion). Acute chest syndrome also often occurs postoperatively, even when patients are properly prepared with blood transfusion. Other causes include rib infarction with atelectasis and regional hypoxia; fat emboli from the bone marrow (Chapter 98); infection with chlamydia, parvovirus B19, or other viral agents; microvascular or large vessel in situ thrombosis; thromboembolic disease; and vascular injury and inflammation. Fat embolism can be identified by finding lipid within pulmonary macrophages obtained by bronchopulmonary lavage, but this nonstandardized test is not recommended.

In most cases of acute chest syndrome, a cause cannot be found early enough to guide treatment. Elevated concentrations of phospholipase A_2

have been found in patients with sickle cell disease in association with acute chest syndrome and may predict its occurrence, but this test is not used widely.

Acute Anemia

Acute anemia can result from sequestration of blood in the spleen or liver, an aplastic crisis caused by parvovirus B19 infection (Chapter 379), or a severe vaso-occlusive event, such as acute chest syndrome or multiorgan failure. Transfusion may be needed. Megaloblastic arrest of erythropoiesis is uncommon if the diet is adequate in folic acid.

Infection

Because patients with sickle cell anemia are functionally asplenic early in life and hyposplenic later, they are susceptible to infection with encapsulated bacteria. Persistent gross splenomegaly but not normal splenic function is common in patients with sickle cell disease in Africa and is related to endemic malaria. Splenomegaly and splenic function often persist in patients with HbSC disease—hence the reduced incidence of infection but risk of splenic sequestration and infarction in adults. Prevention of mortality from pneumococcal infection is the basis for screening of newborns for sickle cell disease and the use of prophylactic oral penicillin in affected individuals. Pneumococcal vaccines (Chapter 17) are also recommended.

Age 20 to 40 Years

Pregnancy

There is no absolute contraindication to pregnancy for patients with sickle cell anemia, and fertility is probably normal. All approved methods of contraception can be used satisfactorily.

Modern medical management generally achieves good results of pregnancy, but the rates of pyelonephritis, pregnancy-induced hypertension (Chapter 247), and cesarean section are increased, and babies are more likely to have low birthweight. Some obstetricians believe that blood transfusions should be used routinely, but limited data suggest that, with good prenatal care, transfusions do not improve the outcome.

Osteonecrosis and Bone Diseases

Osteonecrosis of the hip and shoulder joints (Chapter 256) affects about half of all patients with sickle cell anemia or HbSC disease. Its onset is insidious but progressive, and most patients with early-stage disease progress to collapse of the femoral head within 2 years. Osteonecrosis of the hip usually manifests with pain in and around the affected joint, or at times with spasm of the surrounding muscles. Patients with higher hematocrits and with sickle cell anemia α-thalassemia have the highest prevalence of osteonecrosis. Osteonecrosis can be detected very early by magnetic resonance imaging, but only more advanced disease is visible on plain radiographs.

Osteomyelitis (Chapter 280) is often difficult to distinguish from bone infarction. Osteomyelitis is usually caused by staphylococcal infection, but salmonella infection is a particular cause of sickle cell osteomyelitis.

Leg Ulcers

About 5 to 10% of patients with sickle cell anemia older than 10 years of age develop leg ulcers, but leg ulcers are rare in HbSC disease or HbS-β^+-thalassemia and in children before age 10 years. In the tropics, leg ulcers are more common. Small and superficial leg ulcers heal spontaneously with rest and careful local hygiene. Control of local inflammation and infection remains the mainstay of treatment. Dressing the ulcer with an Unna boot protects the involved area and is a reasonable method of conservative management. Deep, large, painful ulcers may require large doses of narcotic analgesics, prolonged bed rest, and even surgery.

Priapism

Priapism, a prolonged undesirable painful erection, may be seen in 40% of men with sickle cell anemia. Priapism in sickle cell anemia is usually bicorporeal, with only the corpora cavernosa affected. Venous outflow is obstructed rather than arterial flow increased. In bicorporeal priapism, the glans remains soft, and urination is normal. Recurrent, self-limited attacks of priapism can last for several hours with tolerable discomfort. These episodes have been termed stuttering priapism and usually have a nocturnal onset. Erectile function is usually preserved between attacks. Major episodes of priapism often, but not always, follow a history of stuttering attacks, last for days, and can be excruciatingly painful; they often end in impotency. Affected patients have a higher incidence of stroke, pulmonary hypertension, renal failure, leg ulcers, and premature death than individuals without priapism, perhaps reflecting the severity of vasculopathy.

Digestive Diseases

Sickle hepatopathy, hepatic crisis, and right upper quadrant syndrome are terms applied to sickle cell–associated liver disease. Liver disease may be related to intrahepatic and extrahepatic cholestasis, viral hepatitis (Chapter 150), cirrhosis, hypoxia, infarction, erythrocyte sequestration, iron overload (Chapter 153), or drug reactions (Chapter 152). Differentiation among these potential causes can be difficult. Increased bilirubin levels (Chapter 149) are often the result of unconjugated bilirubinemia and are a manifestation of hemolytic anemia.

Gallstones

Cholelithiasis (Chapter 158), a consequence of the accelerated bile pigment turnover typical of hemolytic anemia, can appear in the first decade of life, and more than half of all adults are affected. Depending on the degree of calcification, pigmented gallstones may be either radiopaque or radiolucent. Ultrasonography is the preferred means of detection, and laparoscopic cholecystectomy is the preferred method of dealing with symptomatic stones. Documented episodes of acute cholecystitis and typical obstructive jaundice are much less frequent than the presence of stones. If stones are asymptomatic or symptoms and laboratory findings suggesting cholecystitis are equivocal, careful observation may be the best course.

Beyond the Fifth Decade

Pulmonary Hypertension

Echocardiographic studies show that 30 to 43% of adults with sickle cell anemia have a tricuspid regurgitant velocity (TRV) of more than 2.5 m/second (Chapter 55), suggestive of pulmonary hypertension (Chapter 68). This is associated with a six- to ten-fold increased risk in mortality. Although it is assumed that many patients with elevated TRV have pulmonary hypertension, pulmonary artery catheterization data in this population are limited, and it is likely that in many instances, an elevated TRV is not synonymous with true pulmonary hypertension. Pulmonary arterial hypertension is present in about half of catheterized patients, but with milder hemodynamics and symptoms compared with idiopathic pulmonary hypertension, particularly early in the course of disease. Increased TRV and the coexistence of relative systemic hypertension, renal disease, and intimal and smooth muscle proliferative changes in conduit vessels suggest the presence of a more widespread vasculopathy, which may be responsible for the observed mortality risk. Increased TRV is also seen in children and in patients with HbSC disease.

Nephropathy

Hyposthenuria is present in almost all patients with sickle cell anemia and even in most carriers of sickle cell trait (Table 166-3). Clinically, the loss of urine concentrating ability is not important unless access to fluid is restricted. Isosthenuria, distal renal tubular acidosis, and impaired potassium excretion are signs of medullary dysfunction.

Glomerular hyperfiltration, increased creatinine secretion, and a very low serum creatinine are characteristic of young patients with sickle cell anemia, so renal dysfunction can be present even with normal serum creatinine values. Glomerulopathy begins very early in life, but an increasing prevalence of renal failure is a hallmark of an aging population of sickle cell anemia patients. About 4% of patients with sickle cell anemia and 2% of those with HbSC develop renal failure, at median ages of 23 and 50 years, respectively. Among sickle cell patients, 60% of those older than 40 years of age have proteinuria, and 30% have renal insufficiency. Nephrotic syndrome is found in 40% of adults with creatinine levels greater than 1.5 mg/dL. Survival time for patients with sickle cell anemia after the diagnosis of sickle renal failure is 4 years, even with dialysis.

Eye Disease

Proliferative sickle retinopathy is present in fewer than 20% of patients with sickle cell anemia but in more than 40% of those with HbSC disease by the third decade of life. Vitreal hemorrhage and retinal detachment can occasionally lead to visual loss, but proliferative lesions may regress spontaneously. Screening for proliferative retinopathy using fluorescence angiography is recommended in patients with HbSC disease to guide possible laser photocoagulation.

TABLE 166-3 RENAL ABNORMALITIES IN SICKLE CELL DISEASE*

DISTAL NEPHRON
Impaired urine concentrating ability Impaired urine acidification—incomplete renal tubular acidosis Impaired K^+ excretion
HEMATURIA
PAPILLARY NECROSIS
PROXIMAL TUBULE
Increased phosphate reabsorption Increased β_2-microglobulin reabsorption Increased uric acid secretion Increased creatinine secretion
HEMODYNAMIC CHANGES
Increased glomerular filtration rate Increased renal plasma flow Decreased filtration fraction
GLOMERULAR ABNORMALITIES
Proteinuria Nephrotic syndrome with focal glomerular sclerosis Chronic renal failure

*In carriers of sickle cell trait, because of its hypertonicity and oxygen content, HbS can polymerize in the renal medulla and lead to hyposthenuria, a possible increased risk of urinary tract infection during pregnancy, papillary necrosis, and hematuria. A rare tumor, medullary carcinoma, arises from distal nephrons and is associated with sickle cell trait.

Cardiovascular Complications

The heart is usually enlarged, with a hyperactive precordium and systolic ejection murmurs. Myocardial infarction is rare and when present suggests small vessel disease. Sudden unexpected and unexplained death is common in adults and may be due to arrhythmias and pulmonary hypertension.

Patients with sickle cell anemia usually have blood pressures that are in the normal range yet inappropriately high compared with controls who have similar levels of anemia. "Relative" hypertension in sickle cell anemia may reflect endothelial cell damage and NO scavenging. Survival is decreased and the risk of stroke is increased as blood pressure rises. Treatment goals of 120/80 mm Hg or less are generally the same as for other patients (Chapter 67).

DIAGNOSIS

Normocytic, microcytic, or macrocytic hemolytic anemia with reticulocytosis, increased levels of lactate dehydrogenase and aspartate aminotransferase, and a compatible clinical history should suggest the presence of sickle cell disease. Nevertheless, because of the multiple genotypes and considerable clinical heterogeneity of each genotype, milder cases may not be diagnosed for many years.

The Blood

In sickle cell anemia, the erythrocytes are normocytic or macrocytic depending on the reticulocyte count. Microcytosis in a suspected case of sickle cell disease can be seen very early in life, when iron deficiency has developed, or when β-thalassemia or α-thalassemia is present. Sickled cells are usually present in the peripheral blood smear in sickle cell anemia and in HbS-β^0-thalassemia (see Fig. 166-3A) but are less common in other forms of sickle cell disease. In HbSC disease, target cells are prominent, and HbC crystalizes in some cells (see Fig. 166-3A). ISC numbers remain relatively constant over time, although their percentage may rise early during a painful episode. Finding ISCs has no value for establishing whether a patient is experiencing a vaso-occlusive episode.

Hemoglobin Composition of the Blood

After 1 year of age, hemoglobin fractions are sufficiently stable to be relied on for diagnosis, but the high HbF concentrations of early infancy often make the results of hemoglobin analysis at that time difficult to interpret. In patients with sickle cell anemia, except in infancy, HbS almost always forms more than 80% of the hemolysate. HbS is best detected by high-performance liquid chromatography (HPLC), which is also the method of choice for quantitation of the hemoglobin fractions in newborns and adults (see Fig. 166-3B), or by isoelectric focusing that provides qualitative information. HPLC provides excellent resolution of hemoglobin fractions, gives quantitative results, and is automated. HbF levels in adults average about 6% but can vary between 1 and 20%. DNA-based methods of detecting HbS are specific but usually are not needed for uncomplicated cases. Nevertheless, they are necessary for antenatal diagnosis and, sometimes, for genetic counseling (see Fig. 166-3C).

Family Studies

The *HBB* gene on chromosome 11 (see Fig. 166-2) is inherited as a codominant trait, implying that both normal and mutant alleles are expressed and are easily detectable. However, the sickle cell phenotype (see Table 166-1) is present only in homozygotes for HbS and in certain compound heterozygotes. Family studies (see Fig. 166-3) can suggest a patient's hemoglobin genotype.

PREVENTION AND TREATMENT Rx

Primary Prevention

In populations with a high prevalence of the HbS gene, heterozygote detection is simple, but there is little proven benefit of a broad screening effort to detect carriers. A preferred approach consists of educational programs about sickle cell disease and sickle cell trait, followed by counseling for couples who are planning families. These couples are offered the choice of testing, after which the risks of having affected fetuses can be discussed and the availability of antenatal diagnosis by chorionic villus sampling or amniocentesis presented.

General Measures

Sickle cell disease is a chronic disorder, for which good nutrition and timely immunizations are critical. Work should be encouraged.

Older children do not routinely need continued antibiotic prophylaxis. Neonatal screening to detect newborns with sickle cell disease allows early administration of prophylactic penicillin[1] and antipneumococcal immunization. These measures reduce the incidence of and mortality from pneumococcal bacteremia in children younger than 5 years of age who have sickle cell anemia.

Because of increased rates of RBC production and inadequate nutrition, folic acid, 1 mg daily, is generally recommended but may not be necessary with a good dietary intake. There is no evidence that high concentrations of inhaled oxygen are of preventive value.

Hydroxyurea

Hydroxyurea, the sole drug approved by the U.S. Food and Drug Administration for treatment of sickle cell anemia, increases HbF in these patients because its cytotoxicity causes erythroid regeneration and perhaps because its metabolism leads to NO-related increases in soluble guanylate cyclase, with a subsequent increase in cyclic guanosine monophosphate (cGMP) that augments γ-globin gene expression. In a multicenter trial in adults with sickle cell anemia, hydroxyurea reduced the incidence of pain and acute chest syndrome by almost 50%,[2] with little risk during more than 17.5 years of observation.[3,4] In follow-up studies, cumulative mortality was reduced almost 40%, and the favorable result was related to the ability of the drug to increase HbF and reduce painful episodes and the acute chest syndrome. Children have a more robust HbF response to hydroxyurea than adults. Cancer and leukemia have been reported in patients with sickle cell disease treated with hydroxyurea, but whether the incidence is higher than in the general population is not known. Hydroxyurea should be used in nearly all adults with sickle cell anemia and HbS-β^0 thalassemia (Table 166-4). However, not all patients who might benefit from this treatment receive it. The clinical benefits of hydroxyurea in HbSC disease are just beginning to be studied.

Red Blood Cell Transfusion

Acute transfusions of packed RBCs can be life-saving, and chronic transfusions reduce the incidence and severity of most complications of sickle cell disease. However, repeated transfusions produce iron overload, alloimmunization, loss of venous access, and viral infection. Whether exchange transfusion is preferable to simple transfusion in the acute chest syndrome, stroke, or other acute complications has not been tested in clinical trials. For severe symptomatic anemia or stroke prophylaxis, simple transfusions are preferred.

Treatment of Common Complications

Painful Episodes

A decision as to whether hospitalization is needed can be made after an assessment of the duration and severity of the pain and the response to treatment. Associated factors such as excessive tachycardia, hypotension, body temperature higher than 38.3° C (101° F), marked leukocytosis, a fall in the hematocrit and platelet count, hypoxia, or a new infiltrate on chest radiography should prompt admission.

TABLE 166-4 HYDROXYUREA TREATMENT IN SICKLE CELL ANEMIA*

BASELINE EVALUATION

Blood counts, RBC indices, HbF level, serum chemistries, pregnancy test, willingness to adhere to all recommendations for treatment, not receiving chronic RBC transfusions

INITIATION OF TREATMENT

Hydroxyurea 10-15 mg/kg/day or, for adults, 500 mg every morning for 6-8 wk

CONTINUATION OF TREATMENT

If counts are acceptable by CBC every 2 wk (granulocytes, ≥2000/mm^3; platelets, ≥80,000/mm^3), escalate dose in increments of 200 to 500 mg every 6-8 wk. When a stable nontoxic dose of hydroxyurea is reached, CBC may be done at 4- to 8-wk intervals. Most good responses require 1000 to 2000 mg/day and a final dose more than 30 mg/kg/day should be the top.

GOALS OF TREATMENT

Less pain, increase in HbF (usually measured every 6-8 wk) or MCV, increased hematocrit if severely anemic, acceptable toxicity. Failure of HbF to increase may be due to biologic inability to respond to treatment or, more often, to poor compliance with treatment. If compliance is documented, the dose can be increased cautiously to 2000-2500 mg/day (maximum dose, 30 mg/kg).

*Special caution should be exercised in patients with compromised renal or hepatic function and in those who are habituated to narcotics. Contraception should be practiced by both men and women. Without chronic RBC transfusions or an intercurrent illness suppressing erythropoiesis, a trial period of 6 to 12 months is probably adequate.
CBC = complete blood count; HbF = fetal hemoglobin; MCV = mean corpuscular volume; RBC = red blood cell.

TABLE 166-5 PULMONARY COMPLICATIONS OF SICKLE CELL DISEASE

ACUTE CHEST SYNDROME

Diagnosis: Chest pain, fever, cough wheezing, new infiltrate on chest radiograph, hypoxemia

Management: simple or exchange transfusions, pain relief, oxygen if hypoxemic, bronchodilators, incentive spirometry, antibiotics (broad coverage)

PULMONARY HYPERTENSION

Diagnosis: Tricuspid regurgitant velocity (TRV) ≥ 2.5 m/sec by echocardiography. May also have an elevated N-terminal pro–brain natriuretic peptide (NT-pro-BNP) (≥160 pg/mL) and a reduced 6-min walk distance (≤350 m).

Management: Screen by echocardiography beginning at age 18 yr, repeat echocardiogram periodically according to symptoms. If TRV > 3.0 m/sec, refer for right heart catheterization. Consider anticoagulation, treatment of iron overload and nocturnal hypoxemia. Optimize hydroxyurea, consider chronic transfusions and pulmonary vasodilator therapy.

ASTHMA

ABNORMAL PULMONARY FUNCTION

Physical examination is usually not helpful, but sometimes there is localized swelling and pain over an involved bone. Low-grade fever and a mild increase in leukocytosis can accompany uncomplicated painful episodes, but higher temperature elevations may point to infection or extensive tissue damage.

The cornerstones of pain management (Chapter 29) are fluid replacement and opioid analgesics. Because almost every patient is hyposthenuric, urinary output in patients with sickle cell anemia may exceed 2 L/day, making them susceptible to dehydration. Pain is often accompanied by reduced fluid intake and increased water losses, so increased fluid intake is essential. Administration of 5% dextrose in water and 0.25 to 0.5 normal saline should be used for initial fluid replacement. Although needs vary and hydration should be monitored closely to avoid iatrogenic heart failure or electrolyte imbalance, the daily fluid intake should be approximately 3 to 5 L for adults and 100 to 150 mL/kg for children. Oxygen should be reserved for patients who are hypoxic or have acute respiratory distress. Infection should always be considered and treated early if present, although bacterial infections are uncommon.

Analgesic management presupposes that other treatments, such as hydration, oxygen, and antimicrobial agents, are used if needed. The key to successful pain management is individualized treatment and dosing, taking into account prior pain management and prior use of opioids. Patient-controlled analgesia and a scheduled regimen of drug dosing are preferable, and PRN analgesics should be avoided. Frequent reassessment of the effects of treatment is paramount so that opioid doses can be titrated for pain relief and tapered when relief is obtained. Meperidine should be avoided because its metabolites (e.g., normeperidine) can cause central nervous system excitation. Pain management (Chapter 29) is complicated by the influence of learned pain behavior, pain memories, and pain therapy–induced pain. Management proves extremely difficult in perhaps 10% of all patients, and often enormous doses of opioids are required for relief.

Stroke

For new strokes, after initial stabilization and transfusion, chronic RBC transfusion reduces the chance of recurrent ischemic stroke. However, it is not known how long chronic transfusions should continue. In practice, transfusions are often stopped after children make the transition from pediatric to adult care. Long-term management of hemorrhagic stroke is unclear, and whether transfusion reduces their recurrence is unknown. Increased intracranial flow velocity, measurable only in children, increases the risk of stroke, but its sensitivity is only 10%, with a far from perfect specificity. Children found to be at risk for stroke by transcranial Doppler flow velocities should be started on chronic transfusions,[5] but it is unclear whether or when such transfusions may be discontinued.

Acute Chest Syndrome

Routine treatments for acute chest syndrome initially include bronchodilators (e.g., albuterol nebulizer 0.25 mL in 2.5 mL normal saline; or albuterol metered-dose inhaler during the acute episode), incentive spirometry, empirical antimicrobial agents as used for community-acquired pneumonia (e.g., ceftriaxone or azithromycin or levofloxacin for 5 to 7 days [Chapter 97]), and supplemental oxygen when hypoxia is noted by continuous or frequent monitoring of blood oxygen saturation. Opioid analgesics (e.g., morphine) are often needed, but their dose should be titrated carefully to avoid respiratory depression and worsening of hypoxia.

Blood transfusion is the cornerstone of treatment when a patient becomes hypoxic, develops respiratory distress, has a clinically significant fall in the hematocrit and platelet count or increase in leukocyte count, or shows any sign of multiorgan failure, such as impaired mentation, rhabdomyolysis, renal failure, or liver failure. Both simple transfusion and exchange transfusions appear to reverse many adverse findings of the acute chest syndrome, but controlled studies have never tested the superiority of either method. Although the death rate in acute chest syndrome is less than 10%, a few patients have a rapidly deteriorating course with sudden development of the acute respiratory distress syndrome (ARDS; Chapter 104), as manifested by increased oxygen requirements, extensive pulmonary opacification, and multiorgan failure. Excessive hydration and fat emboli are potential contributing causes. Successful management of severe acute chest syndrome and ARDS requires close coordination among physicians and nurses. Some patients have repeated episodes of severe acute chest syndrome, and chronic transfusion can reduce the recurrence rate. Hydroxyurea also reduces the rate of acute chest syndrome by about 50%.

Osteonecrosis and Bone Disease

Treatment with reduced weight bearing, nonsteroidal anti-inflammatory drugs (NSAIDs), and physical therapy is the mainstay of conservative management but does not retard progression of osteonecrosis and bone disease. Total hip arthroplasty can be very successful, but about one third of prostheses fail within 4 to 5 years.

Diffuse osteoporosis (Chapter 251) is usually present, and osteomalacia (Chapter 252) due to vitamin D deficiency is common in both children and adults. If vitamin D deficiency is present, treatment with calcium (1000 mg PO daily) and vitamin D (50,000 IU PO every week for 2 months, then 50,000 IU PO every other week) is reasonable.

Priapism

Conservative treatment of priapism includes analgesics, hydration, and transfusions. Aspiration and irrigation of the corporeal bodies should be performed within a 12-hour window from the onset of erection if the episode differs from prior episodes of stuttering priapism. Operative treatment, which should be considered after 24 to 48 hours of priapism, includes the creation of shunts between the corpora cavernosa and spongiosum. For a typical episode of low-flow priapism, a Winter shunt between the glans penis and corpora cavernosa should be performed within 24 to 48 hours. Oral or intracavernous administration of α-adrenergic agonists such as pseudoephedrine and sildenafil treatment are being studied.

Pulmonary Hypertension

Patients with sickle cell anemia should be screened by echocardiography for the presence of pulmonary hypertension because of the prognostic importance of an elevated TRV, although management of patients with few symptoms and minimally elevated TRV is ill defined. For symptomatic individuals, optimization of hydroxyurea, transfusions, sildenafil, bosentan, and epoprostenol have all been used, but controlled trials reporting their effectiveness in sickle cell patients have not been (Table 166-5) reported.

Renal Disease

In a small randomized trial, 6 months' treatment with 25 mg/day of captopril caused a 37% reduction in microalbuminuria, compared with a 17% increase in placebo-treated patients; such treatment would be reasonable in patients with known microalbuminuria, but whether screening or long-term treatment is worthwhile is unknown. NSAIDs reduce the glomerular filtration rate in sickle cell anemia and should be avoided in older individuals with creatinine levels of 1.2 mg/dL or higher. Dialysis and renal transplantation are used in end-stage sickle cell nephropathy, but with outcomes less favorable than in other types of renal failure.

Surgery and Anesthesia

Preoperative blood transfusion should be used for all surgeries requiring general anesthesia and selected other surgeries. Simple transfusion to a hematocrit of about 30% before surgery is as effective in preventing postoperative complications as exchange transfusion and causes fewer transfusion-related complications.[6] In some minor surgeries, it is likely that preoperative transfusion is unnecessary.

Implantable infusion ports and catheters have higher risks of complications in sickle cell anemia, including thrombosis of large veins and bacteremia. Low-dose warfarin may retard thrombosis of these devices.

Red Blood Cell Transfusion and Iron Chelation Therapy

The customary level of chronic stable anemia alone is seldom an indication for transfusion. With aging and the onset of renal failure, anemia worsens and can become symptomatic. Transfusion may become necessary, although judicious use of erythropoietin (e.g., darbepoetin, 0.45 μg/kg every 2 weeks, increased as needed) can often restore the hematocrit to prerenal failure levels and should not be higher because of the potential adverse effects of hyperviscosity.

It is advised that patients undergo erythrocyte phenotyping to determine their RBC antigens before embarking on a transfusion program. Otherwise, alloimmunization occurs in about one fourth of frequently transfused patients. In the presence of multiple alloantibodies, it may be difficult to find compatible blood.

With repeated transfusion, iron overload inevitably develops and can result in heart and liver failure and many other complications (Chapter 219). Serum ferritin is an inaccurate means of estimating the iron burden. Liver biopsy might be the most accurate means of determining tissue iron concentration and the response to chelation, but magnetic resonance imaging (FerriScan) correlates very well with this measurement and is noninvasive.

Chelation of excessive iron can be achieved using deferasirox (20 mg/kg orally daily).[7] Increases in serum creatinine and proteinuria occur in about 40% of patients. Desferrioxamine is a parenteral chelator and is usually started with 25 to 30 mg/kg given subcutaneously five times per week in 8- to 12-hour infusions (Chapter 219). Side effects include skin reactions, ototoxicity, retinal toxicity, bone and growth abnormalities, and *Yersinia* infection resulting from the sudden mobilization of iron. Another oral chelator, deferiprone, is less potent than deferasirox or desferrioxamine but is useful instead of or in addition to these drugs; at present, it is approved for use in more than 40 countries but not the United States. Side effects requiring discontinuation of deferiprone, seen in 5 to 10% of patients, include agranulocytosis, neutropenia, arthropathy, and gastrointestinal symptoms.

Stem Cell Transplantation

Successful stem cell transplantation (Chapter 181) can cure sickle cell anemia, but only about 10% of patients have suitable donors. Myeloablative stem cell transplantation carries a 5 to 10% mortality rate and is poorly tolerated in adults. A nonmyeloablative regimen that used total-body irradiation and treatment with alemtuzumab and sirolimus led to stable mixed chimerism in 10 adults transplanted with an HLA-identical family donor, with no graft versus host disease observed. If extended to a larger group of patients and to haploidentical transplants, this approach would be a major advance in treating the most severely ill patients.

FUTURE DIRECTIONS

Experimental treatments to induce higher levels of HbF more consistently and to reduce HbS polymer with drugs that may remodel chromosomal structure (e.g., short-chain fatty acids and their derivatives) or affect hypomethylation of the HbF gene promoters (e.g., decitabine) are undergoing clinical trials. Where malaria is endemic, antimalaria prophylaxis reduces episodes of malaria and increases mean hemoglobin levels. Gene therapy trials are slowly progressing.

PROGNOSIS

Average life expectancy for patients with sickle cell anemia in the United States is between 50 and 60 years; patients with HbSC disease typically live 60 to 70 years. Patients with HbS-β^0-thalassemia are likely to have a life expectancy similar to those with sickle cell anemia, and the lifespan for patients with the HbS-β^+ form may resemble that of patients with HbSC disease. Death is often caused by infection, and another 20% of deaths are related to organ failure. However, death in adults often is unexpected, happening in the midst of an acute event such as an acute painful episode, and occurring within the first 24 hours of hospitalization. In areas of the developing world without access to modern medical care, death in childhood is still common.

OTHER HEMOGLOBINOPATHIES

Hemoglobinopathies other than those associated with HbS, HbE, and HbC rarely cause clinically recognizable disorders. HbC (*HBB* Glu6Lys) and HbE (*HBB* Glu26Lys) are common β-globin variants. As with HbS, their high gene frequencies are a result of the positive selective pressure of endemic falciparum malaria. HbC is present in about 2% of African Americans, and HbE is seen in Southeast Asia, where, in some areas, the gene frequency may reach 50%. Heterozygotes with either mutation are asymptomatic, although the blood of HbC trait carriers contains target cells, and HbE carriers may have very mild anemia and microcytosis. Even homozygotes for HbC and HbE have virtually no clinical disease, only mild hematologic abnormalities such as microcytosis, target cells, and mild anemia. Compound heterozygotes for HbE and β-thalassemia usually have the phenotype of transfusion-dependent β-thalassemia, although genotype-phenotype correlations are difficult to make because of the likelihood that other genes affect the expression of disease.

Rare hemoglobinopathies may change the affinity of hemoglobin for oxygen, render it susceptible to oxidation, or cause molecular instability. Amino acid substitutions involving heme-binding residues may lead to irreversible iron oxidation, methemoglobinemia, and cyanosis (Chapter 161). Patients with these conditions have congenital pseudocyanosis but are usually asymptomatic and need no treatment.

Substitutions at contacts between globin subunits may alter the affinity of hemoglobin for oxygen. When hemoglobin-oxygen affinity is increased, less oxygen is available in tissues, erythropoietin production is enhanced, and erythrocytosis results (Chapter 169). Usually, no treatment is required because the erythrocytosis is mild. Hemoglobin-oxygen affinity may also be reduced by some mutations, resulting in anemia or cyanosis. Hemoglobin instability, produced by several molecular mechanisms (including introduction of proline residues into the α-helix, substitutions near the heme ring, and deletion or addition of amino acids) often causes loss of heme from the molecule and hemolytic anemia. Hb Koln is the most common example of this class of hemoglobinopathy, but more than 200 unstable variants have been described. Sometimes, oxidant drugs provoke increased hemolysis. Splenectomy is sometimes effective treatment when the anemia is severe.

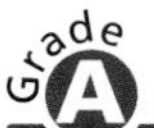

1. Gaston MH, Verter J, Woods G, et al. Prophylaxis with oral penicillin in children with sickle cell anemia. *N Engl J Med.* 1986;314:1593-1599.
2. Charache S, Terrin ML, Moore RD, et al. Effect of hydroxyurea on the frequency of painful crises in sickle cell anemia. *N Engl J Med.* 1995;332:1317-1322.
3. Lanzkron S, Strouse JJ, Wilson R, et al. Systematic review: hydroxyurea for the treatment of adults with sickle cell disease. *Ann Intern Med.* 2008;148:939-955.
4. Steinberg MH, McCarthy WF, Castro O, et al. The risks and benefits of long-term use of hydroxyurea in sickle cell anemia: a 17.5 year follow-up. *Am J Hematol.* 2010;85:403-408.
5. Adams RJ, McKie VC, Hsu L, et al. Prevention of a first stroke by transfusions in children with sickle cell anemia and abnormal results on transcranial Doppler ultrasonography [see comments]. *N Engl J Med.* 1998;339:5-11.
6. Vichinsky EP, Haberkern CM, Neumayr L, et al. A comparison of conservative and aggressive transfusion regimens in the perioperative management of sickle cell disease. *N Engl J Med.* 1995;333:206-213.
7. Meerpohl JJ, Antes G, Rücker G, et al. Deferasirox for managing transfusional iron overload in people with sickle cell disease. *Cochrane Database Syst Rev.* 2010;8:CD007477.

SUGGESTED READINGS

Bauer DE, Orkin SH. Update on fetal hemoglobin gene regulation in hemoglobinopathies. *Curr Opin Pediatr.* 2011;23:1-8. *Review.*

Brousseau DC, Owens PL, Mosso AL, et al. Acute care utilization and rehospitalizations for sickle cell disease. *JAMA.* 2010;303:1288-1294. *Acute care encounters and hospitalizations are very common.*

Hsieh MM, Kang EM, Fitzhugh CD, et al. Allogeneic hematopoietic stem-cell transplantation for sickle cell disease. *N Engl J Med.* 2009;361:2309-2317. *Stem cell transplantation with an HLA-identical donor can "cure" sickle cell anemia in adults.*

Rees DC, Williams TN, Gladwin MT. Sickle-cell disease. *Lancet.* 2010;376:2018-2031. *Review.*

Tsaras G, Owusu-Ansah A, Boateng FO, et al. Complications associated with sickle cell trait: a brief narrative review. *Am J Med.* 2009;122:507-512. *Sickle cell trait is "benign" but can be associated with certain complications.*

Wolfson JA, Schrager SM, Coates TD, et al. Sickle-cell disease in California: a population-based description of emergency department utilization. *Pediatr Blood Cancer.* 2011;56:413-419. *Nearly two thirds visited an emergency department each year, and almost 50% were on Medicaid.*

167

MEGALOBLASTIC ANEMIAS

AŚOK C. ANTONY

DEFINITION

Megaloblastic anemias, a group of disorders characterized by a distinct morphologic pattern in hematopoietic cells, are commonly due to a deficiency of vitamin B_{12} (cobalamin) or folates. These anemias are globally prevalent and carry a significant burden of morbidity. Folate and cobalamin are both required to sustain one-carbon metabolism, which involves the transfer of one-carbon groups such as methyl-, formyl-, methylene-, methenyl-, and formimino- in enzyme reactions essential for pyrimidine and purine biosynthesis, including the synthesis of three of the four nucleotides of DNA. Thus, a deficiency in cobalamin or folate results in the common biochemical feature of a defect in DNA synthesis, along with lesser alterations in RNA and protein synthesis, leading to a state of unbalanced cell growth and impaired cell division. The majority of megaloblastic cells have DNA values between 2 and 4 N because of delayed cell division. This is morphologically expressed as larger-than-normal "immature" nuclei with finely particulate chromatin, whereas the relatively unimpaired RNA and protein synthesis results in large cells with greater "mature" cytoplasm and cell volume. The microscopic appearance of this nuclear-cytoplasmic asynchrony (or dissociation) is morphologically described as *megaloblastic*. Megaloblastic hematopoiesis commonly presents with anemia, the most easily recognized manifestation of a global defect in DNA synthesis in all proliferating cells (especially of the gastrointestinal and reproductive tracts). Because vitamin replacement is curative, precise identification of the deficient vitamin is essential. In the case of cobalamin, the cause of the deficiency (Table 167-1) dictates the dose and duration of replacement therapy.

EPIDEMIOLOGY

Cobalamin

Nutrition

Cobalamin is a red, water-soluble vitamin with a complex structure that generally resembles the heme molecule, but with cobalt replacing iron in the center of the pyrrole ring. The recommended daily allowance of cobalamin is 2.4 μg for men and nonpregnant women, 2.6 μg for pregnant women, 2.8 μg for lactating women, and between 1.5 and 2 μg for children 9 to 18 years old. Cobalamin is produced in nature only by microorganisms, and humans receive cobalamin solely from the diet. Meat from parenchymal organs is richest in cobalamin (>10 μg/100 g wet weight); fish and animal muscle, milk products, and egg yolks have 1 to 10 μg/100 g wet weight. An average nonvegetarian Western diet with abundant meat, milk and other dairy products, and eggs contains 5 to 7 μg/day of cobalamin, which is adequate to sustain normal cobalamin equilibrium. For vegetarians, the consumption of eggs, milk, and dairy products generally provides less than 0.5 μg/day of cobalamin and cannot sustain cobalamin balance. Other foods, including *nori* (dried seaweed) and *tempeh* (fermented soybean cake), are not reliable sources of cobalamin. Near-vegetarians who consume meat infrequently (usually because of poverty) have a cobalamin status that is only marginally better than that of lacto-ovovegetarians.

Cobalamin is stored exceptionally well in tissues. Of the total body content of 2 to 5 mg in adults, half is in the liver. With a daily loss of 1 μg, dietary cobalamin deficiency can take 5 to 10 years to become apparent. However, it takes about 3 to 4 years to deplete cobalamin stores if dietary cobalamin is abruptly malabsorbed (e.g., ileal resection), thereby interfering with an efficient enterohepatic circulation, which accounts for the turnover of 5 to 10 μg of cobalamin per day and the reabsorption of 75% of cobalamin secreted into bile. Although cobalamin resists high-temperature cooking processes, it is unstable with light exposure and can be converted to inactive analogues.

Folates

Nutrition

Folates are synthesized by microorganisms and plants. Rich food sources include green leafy vegetables (spinach, lettuce, broccoli), beans, fruit (bananas, melons, lemons), yeast, mushrooms, and animal protein (liver, kidney). The recommended daily allowance of folate is 400 μg for adult men and nonpregnant women, 600 μg for pregnant women, 500 μg for lactating women, and 300 to 400 μg for children 9 to 18 years of age. A balanced Western diet can prevent folate deficiency, but the net dietary intake of folate in many developing countries may be insufficient to sustain folate balance and is often less than half of optimum. Folates are susceptible to breakdown during prolonged cooking (>15 minutes), which can destroy 50 to 95% of folate.

PATHOBIOLOGY

Cobalamin

Normal Physiology

Absorption and Transport

Cobalamin in food is usually in coenzyme form (as deoxyadenosylcobalamin and methylcobalamin) and bound to proteins (Fig. 167-1). In the stomach, peptic digestion at low pH is a prerequisite for the release of cobalamin from food protein. Once it is released by proteolysis, cobalamin preferentially binds to a high-affinity cobalamin-binding protein called R protein, which is secreted in salivary and gastric juice. These cobalamin–R protein complexes, along with unbound intrinsic factor, which is produced by gastric parietal cells, pass into the second part of the duodenum, where pancreatic proteases degrade R proteins. This allows the transfer of cobalamin to intrinsic factor.

The stable intrinsic factor–cobalamin complexes then pass through the jejunum to the ileum, where they bind to membrane-associated intrinsic factor–cobalamin receptors (also called *cubam* receptors because they are composed of a complex of two proteins, cubulin and amnionless) on the microvilli of ileal mucosal cells. Within enterocytes, cobalamin is transferred to transcobalamin II, which efficiently binds and delivers cobalamin ultimately to transcobalamin II receptors found on cell surfaces. Another protein, transcobalamin I, which binds approximately 75% of serum cobalamin but does not participate in transport, appears to be a storage protein for cobalamin in blood. A third quantitatively minor protein, transcobalamin III, binds a wide spectrum of cobalamin analogues that are rapidly cleared by the liver into bile for efficient fecal excretion.

Cellular Processing

More than 95% of intracellular cobalamin is bound to two intracellular enzymes: methylmalonyl-coenzyme A (CoA) mutase and methionine synthase. In mitochondria, deoxyadenosylcobalamin is a coenzyme for methylmalonyl-CoA mutase, which converts the product of propionate metabolism, methylmalonyl-CoA, to succinyl-CoA, a form that is easily metabolized. In the cytoplasm, methylcobalamin is a coenzyme for methionine synthase, which catalyzes the transfer of methyl groups from methylcobalamin to homocysteine to form methionine. The methyl group of 5-methyltetrahydrofolate (methyl-THF) is donated to regenerate methylcobalamin, thereby forming the THF that is essential to sustain one-carbon metabolism. The methionine so formed can be adenylated to S-adenosylmethionine, which donates its methyl group in a critical series of biologic methylation reactions involving more than 80 proteins, phospholipids, neurotransmitters, RNA, and DNA. An elevation of methylmalonic acid and homocysteine in the blood can point to cobalamin deficiency.

Pathogenesis of Cobalamin Deficiency

Nutritional Cobalamin Deficiency

Vegetarianism and poverty-imposed near-vegetarianism are the most common causes of nutritional cobalamin insufficiency worldwide in all age groups. In such patient populations, low maternal cobalamin status is associated with adverse pregnancy outcomes (preterm birth, intrauterine growth retardation, very early recurrent miscarriage), neural tube defects, reduced neurocognitive performance in children, accelerated bone turnover, and low bone mineral density with fractures.

Inadequate Dissociation of Cobalamin from Food Protein

Failure to release dietary cobalamin from food protein can lead to cobalamin deficiency despite the presence of intrinsic factor. This is a common cause of

TABLE 167-1 ETIOPATHOPHYSIOLOGIC CLASSIFICATION OF COBALAMIN AND FOLATE DEFICIENCIES

I. Cobalamin deficiency
  A. Nutritional cobalamin deficiency (insufficient cobalamin intake)—vegetarians, poverty-imposed near-vegetarians, breast-fed infants of mothers with pernicious anemia
  B. Abnormal intragastric events (inadequate proteolysis of food cobalamin)—atrophic gastritis, hypochlorhydria, proton pump inhibitors, H_2-blockers
  C. Loss/atrophy of gastric oxyntic mucosa (deficient intrinsic factor molecules)—total or partial gastrectomy, adult and juvenile pernicious anemia, caustic destruction (lye)
  D. Abnormal events in the small bowel lumen
    1. Inadequate pancreatic protease (R factor–cobalamin not degraded, cobalamin not transferred to intrinsic factor)
      a. Insufficient pancreatic protease—pancreatic insufficiency
      b. Inactivation of pancreatic protease—Zollinger-Ellison syndrome
    2. Usurping of luminal cobalamin (inadequate binding of cobalamin to intrinsic factor)
      a. By bacteria—stasis syndromes (blind loops, pouches of diverticulosis, strictures, fistulas, anastomosis), impaired bowel motility (scleroderma), hypogammaglobulinemia
      b. By *Diphyllobothrium latum* (fish tapeworm)
  E. Disorders of ileal mucosa/intrinsic factor–cobalamin receptors (intrinsic factor–cobalamin not bound to intrinsic factor–cobalamin receptors [a.k.a. cubam receptors])
    1. Diminished or absent cubam receptors—ileal bypass, resection, fistula
    2. Abnormal mucosal architecture or function—tropical/nontropical sprue, Crohn's disease, tuberculous ileitis, amyloidosis
    3. Cubam receptor defects—Imerslund-Gräsbeck syndrome, hereditary megaloblastic anemia
    4. Drug effects—metformin, cholestyramine, colchicine, neomycin
  F. Disorders of plasma cobalamin transport (TCII-cobalamin not delivered to TCII receptors)—congenital TCII deficiency, defective binding of TCII-cobalamin to TCII receptors (rare)
  G. Metabolic disorders (cobalamin not used by cells)
    1. Inborn enzyme errors (rare)
    2. Acquired disorders (cobalamin functionally inactivated by irreversible oxidation)—nitrous oxide inhalation

II. Folate deficiency
  A. Nutritional causes
    1. Decreased dietary intake—poverty and famine, institutionalization (psychiatric facilities, nursing homes), chronic debilitating disease, prolonged feeding of infants with goat's milk, special slimming diets or fad foods (folate-rich foods not consumed), cultural or ethnic cooking techniques (food folate destroyed)
    2. Decreased dietary intake and increased requirements
      a. Physiologic—pregnancy and lactation, prematurity, hyperemesis gravidarum, infancy
      b. Pathologic
        (1) Intrinsic hematologic diseases involving hemolysis with compensatory erythropoiesis, abnormal hematopoiesis, or bone marrow infiltration by malignant disease
        (2) Dermatologic disease—psoriasis
  B. Folate malabsorption
    1. With normal intestinal mucosa
      a. Drugs—sulfasalazine, pyrimethamine, proton pump inhibitors (via inhibition of proton-coupled folate transporters)
      b. Hereditary folate malabsorption (mutations in proton-coupled folate transporters) (rare)
    2. With mucosal abnormalities—tropical/nontropical sprue, regional enteritis
  C. Defective CSF folate transport—cerebral folate deficiency (autoantibodies to folate receptors) (rare)
  D. Inadequate cellular utilization
    1. Folate antagonists (methotrexate)
    2. Hereditary enzyme deficiencies involving folate
  E. Drugs (multiple effects on folate metabolism)—alcohol, sulfasalazine, triamterene, pyrimethamine, trimethoprim-sulfamethoxazole, phenytoin, barbiturates

III. Miscellaneous megaloblastic anemias not caused by cobalamin or folate deficiency
  A. Congenital disorders of DNA synthesis
    1. Orotic aciduria
    2. Lesch-Nyhan syndrome
    3. Congenital dyserythropoietic anemia
  B. Acquired disorders of DNA synthesis
    1. Deficiency—thiamine-responsive megaloblastic anemia (thiamine transporter 1 mutation)
    2. Erythroleukemia; refractory sideroblastic anemias (pyridoxine responsive?)

CSF = cerebrospinal fluid; HIV = human immunodeficiency virus; TCII = transcobalamin II.

cobalamin deficiency in affluent countries and occurs among 30 to 50% of elderly individuals with low cobalamin status. It is about 10-fold more common than pernicious anemia or loss of functional cubam receptors.

Absent Secretion of Acid and Intrinsic Factor

Deficiency of intrinsic factor as a result of gastric parietal cell atrophy is associated with insufficient hydrochloric acid secretion and can be caused by total or partial gastrectomy; autoimmune destruction (chronic atrophic gastritis), as found in classic pernicious anemia; or destruction of gastric mucosa by caustic (lye) ingestion.

Total gastrectomy invariably leads to cobalamin deficiency in 2 to 10 years, thus warranting prophylactic cobalamin (and iron) replacement. After partial gastrectomy, up to a third of patients may have multifactorial cobalamin deficiency from decreased secretion of intrinsic factor, hypochlorhydria, or intestinal bacterial overgrowth of cobalamin-consuming organisms. Morbidly obese patients following bariatric gastric bypass surgery (Chapter 227) also have food-cobalamin malabsorption, as do those on long-term H_2-blockers or proton pump inhibitors.

In pernicious anemia, the primary event is autoimmune destruction and atrophy of the gastric parietal cell mucosa, leading to the absence of intrinsic factor and hydrochloric acid, which causes severe cobalamin malabsorption and deficiency. The autoimmune gastritis that eventually leads to chronic atrophic gastritis involves the gastric fundus and body. Intrinsic factor antibodies are found in the serum of 60% and in the gastric juice of 75% of patients with pernicious anemia. The incidence of pernicious anemia is approximately 25 new cases per year per 100,000 persons older than 40 years. The average age at onset is about 60 years. Nearly 2% of free-living individuals older than 60 years in Southern California had undiagnosed pernicious anemia, with minimal clinical manifestations of cobalamin deficiency; significantly, in this cohort, 4% of white and African American women had pernicious anemia. Nonetheless, pernicious anemia can be found in persons of all ages, races, and ethnic origins. About 30% of patients have a positive family history, and there is an association with other autoimmune diseases (polyglandular autoimmune syndrome, Graves' disease, Hashimoto's thyroiditis, vitiligo, Addison's disease, idiopathic hypoparathyroidism, primary ovarian failure, myasthenia gravis, type 1 diabetes, adult hypogammaglobulinemia).

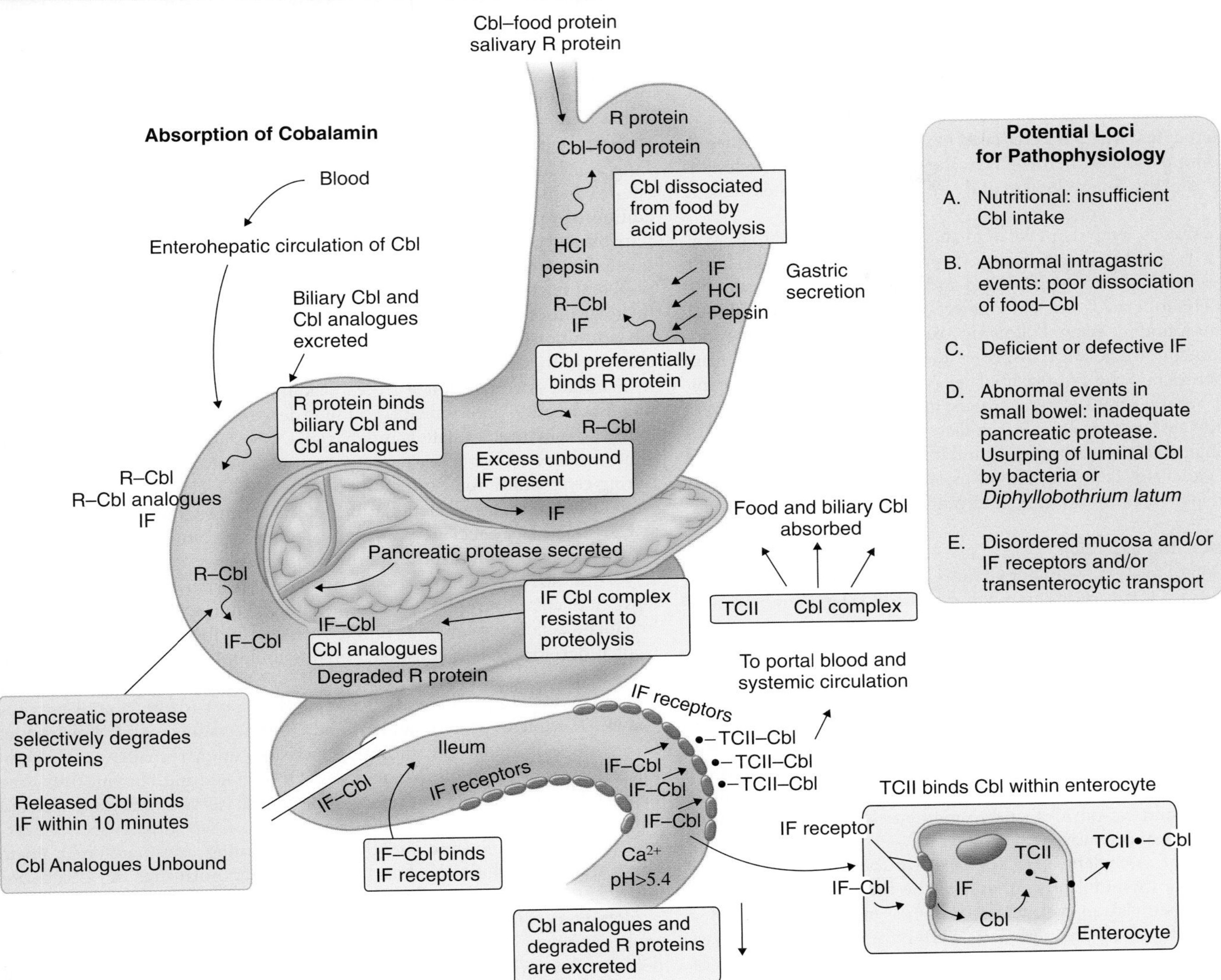

FIGURE 167-1. Components and mechanism of cobalamin absorption, with an indication of the locus for malabsorption. Cbl = cobalamin; IF = intrinsic factor; TCII = transcobalamin II. (From Antony AC. Megaloblastic anemias. In: Hoffman R, Benz EJ Jr, Shattil SJ, et al, eds. *Hematology: Basic Principles and Practice,* 4th ed. Philadelphia: Churchill Livingstone; 2005:519-556.)

Abnormal Events Precluding Absorption of Cobalamin

In pancreatic insufficiency (Chapter 142) with a deficiency of pancreatic protease, there is a failure to break down the R proteins to which cobalamin is preferentially bound in the stomach; this precludes the transfer of cobalamin to intrinsic factor. However, with the widespread early use of pancreatic protease replacement, frank cobalamin deficiency is uncommon. Endogenous pancreatic protease can be inactivated by massive gastric hypersecretion arising from a gastrinoma in Zollinger-Ellison syndrome (Chapter 201). Further, if the pH of the luminal contents in the ileum is less than 5.4, the binding of the intrinsic factor–cobalamin complex to cubam receptors will be precluded.

Bacterial overgrowth in the small bowel (arising from stasis, impaired motility, and hypogammaglobulinemia; Chapter 144) favors colonization by bacteria, which can usurp free cobalamin before it can bind to intrinsic factor. This problem can be reversed by a short course of antibiotic therapy. Individuals heavily infested with the fish tapeworm *Diphyllobothrium latum* (acquired by consuming raw or partially cooked freshwater fish from lakes in Russia, Japan, Switzerland, Germany, and the United States) can become cobalamin deficient when these long (10 m) adult worms in the jejunum avidly usurp cobalamin. After the worms have been expelled (with a single oral dose of praziquantel 10 to 20 mg/kg), cobalamin replenishment is curative.

Disorders of the Intrinsic Factor Receptors or Mucosa

Because the distal ileum has the greatest density of cubam receptors, the removal, bypass, or dysfunction of only 1 to 2 feet of terminal ileum can result in cobalamin malabsorption. Among drugs, the biguanides (e.g., metformin) decrease intrinsic factor and acid secretion and can inhibit the transenterocytic transport of cobalamin in up to a third of patients. This can be avoided by taking calcium (1.2 g/day). Other drugs (extended-release potassium chloride, cholestyramine, colchicine, neomycin) can also impair the transepithelial transport of cobalamin.

Acquired Cobalamin Deficiency

Nitrous oxide (N_2O) irreversibly inactivates cobalamin and results in a state of functional intracellular cobalamin deficiency, which can be bypassed by the administration of 5-formyl-THF (leucovorin). Although N_2O exposure during prolonged surgery can induce megaloblastosis, especially in those with marginal or low cobalamin stores, chronic intermittent (surreptitious, accidental, or occupational) exposure more frequently leads to neuromyelopathic manifestations, in which magnetic resonance imaging shows T2-weighted hyperintensity in affected areas of the spinal cord. Capsules used for making whipped cream are a cheap and easy source of N_2O in the community, and at one college, about 3% of students inhaled it monthly in an on-campus "nitrous club."

Folates

Normal Physiology

Absorption and Transport

In general, only half the folate in food, which is mainly in polyglutamylated form, is nutritionally available (bioavailable), whereas 85% of folic acid added to food or ingested as a supplement is bioavailable. The small intestine can absorb folic acid unchanged, but food folate polyglutamates must be hydrolyzed to monoglutamate by folate polyglutamate hydrolase at the brush border before transport into enterocytes. A luminal surface, proton-coupled, folate transporter protein, which has a low pH optimum in the acid microclimate of the duodenum and jejunum, facilitates the efficient transport of folates into enterocytes, where it is reduced to THF and methylated before being released into plasma as methyl-THF. The normal serum folate level is maintained by dietary folate intake and by an efficient enterohepatic circulation.

From plasma, there is a rapid uptake of folate (methyl-THF and folic acid) into tissues by two physiologic transport processes for cellular entry. Membrane-associated folate receptors bind and take up physiologically relevant methyl-THF, folic acid, and some newer antifolates with high affinity at concentrations found in serum. Following folate receptor–mediated endocytosis, a proton-coupled folate transporter then helps export folate from acidified endosomes into the cytoplasm of cells and also into the cerebrospinal fluid (CSF). Another transporter (reduced folate carrier) is a low-affinity but high-capacity system that can also mediate the uptake of methyl-THF and pharmacologic folates (methotrexate and folinic acid well, but folic acid poorly) into a variety of cells. Passive diffusion also operates to transport folate across biologic membranes at supraphysiologic folate concentrations.

Cellular Retention and Excretion

Polyglutamylation of folate is the major factor in intracellular retention. After glomerular filtration, folate receptors on the brush border membranes of proximal renal tubular cells bind luminal folate and transport it back into blood.

Intracellular Metabolism and Cobalamin-Folate Interactions

After cellular uptake, methyl-THF must first be converted to THF via methionine synthase. Only then can the THF be polyglutamylated by folate polyglutamate synthase, which allows it to play a central role in one-carbon metabolism. THF can be converted to 10-formyl-THF, which can be used for de novo biosynthesis of purines, and to methylene-THF, which can be used for the synthesis of thymidylate.

The central role of methylene-THF is that it can be used either in the thymidylate cycle via thymidylate synthase for the synthesis of thymidine and DNA or in the methylation cycle via methionine synthase, but only after its conversion to methyl-THF by methylene-THF reductase. Inactivation of methionine synthase during cobalamin deficiency results in accumulation of the substrate methyl-THF, which cannot be polyglutamylated and thus leaks out of the cell, resulting in an intracellular THF deficiency and the reduction of one-carbon metabolism. This process explains why cobalamin deficiency responds to replacement with folic acid, which can be converted to THF via dihydrofolate reductase, or to replacement with 5-formyl-THF (folinic acid), which bypasses methionine synthase and can be converted to methylene-THF or 10-formyl-THF via intermediates.

Pathogenesis of Folate Deficiency

Folate deficiency can arise from decreased supply (reduced intake, absorption, transport, or utilization) or increased requirements (from metabolic consumption, destruction, or excretion). One individual may have multiple causes of folate deficiency, but specific tests to define each mechanism are not available clinically. Folate deficiency varies among different populations, and nutritional folate insufficiency is the most common cause worldwide in all age groups, with women and children in developing countries at highest risk. Although food folate fortification has dramatically reduced the prevalence of folate deficiency in the United States, it can still be found among some elderly, infirm, or socially isolated individuals with poor diets.

Nutritional Causes (Decreased Intake or Increased Requirements)

With an abrupt reduction in folate consumption, body stores of folate are adequate for approximately 4 months. However, these stores are depleted faster in individuals who chronically have a negative folate balance and often have multiple nutritional deficiencies (and diseases) that tip them into frank folate deficiency. A seasonal reduction in folate-rich foods, poverty, cultural or ethnic diets that are intrinsically low in folates, cooking techniques that destroy folate, and the anorexia that accompanies chronic illnesses are among the many reasons for folate deficiency, especially in developing countries.

Patients with hematologic diseases involving increased intrinsic cell proliferation or with increased compensatory erythropoiesis in response to chronic peripheral red blood cell destruction are at risk. Folate deficiency in the face of chronic hemolysis can lead to an acute reticulocytopenic (aplastic) crisis, an unexpected increase in transfusion requirements, or a fall in platelets. Exfoliative skin diseases (Chapter 446) also cause folate deficiency when there is an increased demand from excess loss of skin cells.

Pregnancy and Infancy

Poor folate intake during pregnancy is a very common cause of megaloblastic anemia in developing countries because pregnancy and lactation require additional folate for growth of the fetus and maternal tissues. Physiologic transplacental folate transport, which relies on the continued intake of adequate dietary folate by the mother, involves the capture of maternal folate by placental folate receptors, followed by displacement of this pool by dietary folates, a process that leads to transfer to the fetal circulation along a downhill concentration gradient. However, mothers with short intervals between pregnancies, with twin pregnancies, or with hyperemesis gravidarum are unable to maintain adequate folate stores, leading to premature, low-birthweight infants and other predominantly midline developmental abnormalities in the fetus. Low maternal folate status has also been associated with behavioral abnormalities (hyperactivity-inattention and peer problems) in offspring during early childhood. Autoantibodies to folate receptors in mothers have been linked to recurrent neural tube defects among some populations.

Cerebral folate deficiency can be caused by a mutation in folate receptors that perturbs folate transport into the CSF, leading to severe developmental regression in early childhood associated with movement disturbances, epilepsy, and leukodystrophy that is reversed by folinic acid. Alternatively, cerebral folate deficiency can be acquired when autoantibodies to folate receptors (which develop against consumed bovine milk folate-binding proteins that share epitopes with human folate receptors) bind to folate receptors on the choroid plexus and thereby reduce folate transport to the central nervous system. The folate receptor autoantibody titer decreases with the restriction of bovine milk intake but promptly increases upon rechallenge. Cerebral folate deficiency responds to high doses of folinic acid and a bovine milk–free diet. Reduction of folate transport to the central nervous system associated with folate receptor autoantibodies also occurs in two autism spectrum disorders: Rett syndrome and infantile low-functioning autism with neurologic abnormalities. High doses of oral folinic acid can normalize the CSF folate and lead to partial or complete clinical recovery in 12 months.

Hereditary folate malabsorption, an autosomal recessive syndrome, is due to a mutation in the proton-coupled folate transporter that results in the defective transport of folates across the small intestine and across the choroid plexus into the CSF. The proton-coupled folate transporter functions distal to folate receptors in the choroid plexus to facilitate folate transfer to the CSF, and a loss-of-function mutation of the proton-coupled folate transporter can independently interrupt physiologic folate delivery to the brain, despite intact folate receptors. The CSF/blood folate ratio in healthy humans is 3 : 1, but in those with hereditary folate malabsorption, CSF folate is very low or undetectable. Patients present with folate deficiency anemia, hypoimmunoglobulinemia with recurrent infections, chronic diarrhea, and neurologic abnormalities (seizures or mental retardation) that are irreversible if left untreated. High parenteral doses of folinic acid can ensure passive diffusion into the CSF and lead to significant clinical improvement in these children.

Tropical and Nontropical (Celiac) Sprue

With the development of intestinal mucosal abnormalities, patients are at increased risk for folate malabsorption. In tropical sprue (Chapter 142), a dramatic response to a 4- to 6-month course of oral folic acid (5 mg/day) plus tetracycline (250 mg four times a day) can effect a cure in 60% or more of patients. In the short term, malabsorption leads to folate deficiency, but later in the chronic phase of the disease (>3 years), malabsorption of cobalamin also develops. In addition, iron deficiency (Chapter 162), pellagra, and beriberi (Chapter 225) may coexist in these patients.

Drugs

Excess alcohol consumption at the expense of a balanced diet may be the most common cause of folate deficiency in the United States. Inhibition of dihydrofolate reductase by trimethoprim and pyrimethamine or methotrexate can be acutely reversed by the administration of 5-formyl-THF (folinic acid). Sulfasalazine induces megaloblastosis in two thirds of subjects taking full doses (>2 g/day) by decreasing the breakdown of folate polyglutamates to monoglutamates before absorption or by inducing Heinz body hemolytic anemia, which leads to increased requirements. Sulfasalazine, pyrimethamine, and proton pump inhibitors also inhibit the human proton-coupled folate transporter, reducing folate absorption. Oral contraceptives may increase folate catabolism, whereas anticonvulsants can reduce absorption and induce microsomal liver enzymes. Antineoplastics and antiretroviral antinucleosides (azidothymidine) induce megaloblastosis by perturbing DNA synthesis.

CLINICAL MANIFESTATIONS

The finding of macrocytosis (increased mean corpuscular volume [MCV]) on a routine complete blood count may be the first clinical manifestation. In other patients, the findings may be dominated by the condition causing the deficiency of cobalamin or folate, such as malabsorption, alcoholism, or malnutrition (see Table 167-1).

The clinical manifestations of folate deficiency may include hematologic (pancytopenia with megaloblastic bone marrow), cardiopulmonary (secondary to anemia), gastrointestinal (megaloblastosis with or without malabsorption), dermatologic (hyperpigmentation of the skin, premature graying), genital (megaloblastosis of the cervical epithelium), infertility (sterility), and psychiatric (primarily a flat affect) symptoms. If patients have additional neurologic findings, other diseases that predispose to folate deficiency (e.g., alcoholism with thiamine deficiency) or associated cobalamin deficiency must be considered. Because megaloblastosis secondary to either folate or cobalamin deficiency results in functional folate deficiency, the hematologic manifestations of both deficiencies, including pancytopenia with megaloblastic bone marrow, are indistinguishable (see later). However, only cobalamin deficiency results in a patchy demyelinating process, which is expressed clinically as cerebral abnormalities and subacute combined degeneration of the spinal cord (Chapter 425). This widespread demyelination begins in the dorsal columns in the thoracic segments of the spinal cord and then spreads contiguously to involve the corticospinal tracts and later the spinothalamic and spinocerebellar tracts. Hematologic manifestations, neurologic manifestations, or both may dominate the clinical picture.

With chronic hyperhomocysteinemia associated with cobalamin or folate deficiency (or both), there may be additional clinical manifestations that stem from the fact that homocysteine is a risk factor for occlusive vascular diseases such as coronary artery disease, stroke, and peripheral arterial disease (Chapter 51), as well as arterial and venous thromboembolism (Chapters 81 and 179). Hyperhomocysteinemia is also associated with significant complications of pregnancy (preeclampsia, placental abruption or infarction, recurrent miscarriage) and poor pregnancy outcomes (preterm delivery, neural tube defects, congenital heart defects, intrauterine growth retardation). In addition, there is reduced bone mineral density, with an increased fracture risk, and a greater chance of small-vessel cerebrovascular disease–related stroke. Despite the failure of homocysteine-lowering therapy for the secondary prevention of atherosclerotic disease, this does not negate the risk. Several clinical conditions are benefited by folate supplementation or homocysteine-lowering therapy with combined folic acid, cobalamin, and pyridoxine.[1-7] By inference, patients can present clinically with any of these additional conditions when they have long-standing untreated hyperhomocysteinemia.

DIAGNOSIS

Diagnostic Approach to the Patient

The general approach to a patient with megaloblastic anemia is first to *recognize* that megaloblastic anemia is present; then to *distinguish* whether folate, cobalamin, or combined folate and cobalamin deficiencies have led to the anemia; and finally to diagnose the *underlying disease* and *mechanism* causing the deficiency (see Table 167-1).

Although deficiencies of cobalamin and folate are only two of the causes of macrocytosis, they become increasingly more likely as the MCV increases (see Fig. 167-2). Because perturbed DNA synthesis from any cause (including folate and cobalamin deficiency) results in megaloblastosis of bone marrow precursor cells, the red cells released into the circulation have an MCV that is often greater than 110 fL; on the peripheral blood smear, these large cells appear oval in shape (macro-ovalocytes). When compared with mature red cells, which normally have a central area of pallor that occupies about one third of the cell diameter, the central pallor of macro-ovalocytes is significantly reduced. Assessment of the corrected reticulocyte count is a good starting point to distinguish conditions in which macrocytes are not accompanied by megaloblastosis in the bone marrow (Fig. 167-2). On the hematoxylin-eosin–stained peripheral blood smear, reticulocytes, which are normally 20% larger than mature red cells, are recognized by their polychromatophilic staining; when they are prematurely released from the bone marrow during the stress of acute blood loss or hemolysis, these so-called shift reticulocytes are even larger. In liver disease, an altered lipid composition of the erythrocyte membrane results in an increased cell surface without a proportionate increase in volume; these so-called thin macrocytes are recognized on the peripheral blood smear by their larger area of central pallor (much greater than one third the cell diameter). Thin macrocytes are also found in the post-splenectomy state (because reticulocytes, which normally undergo a form of "remodeling" with a loss of membrane lipids during their maturation in the spleen, escape this process in splenectomized individuals).

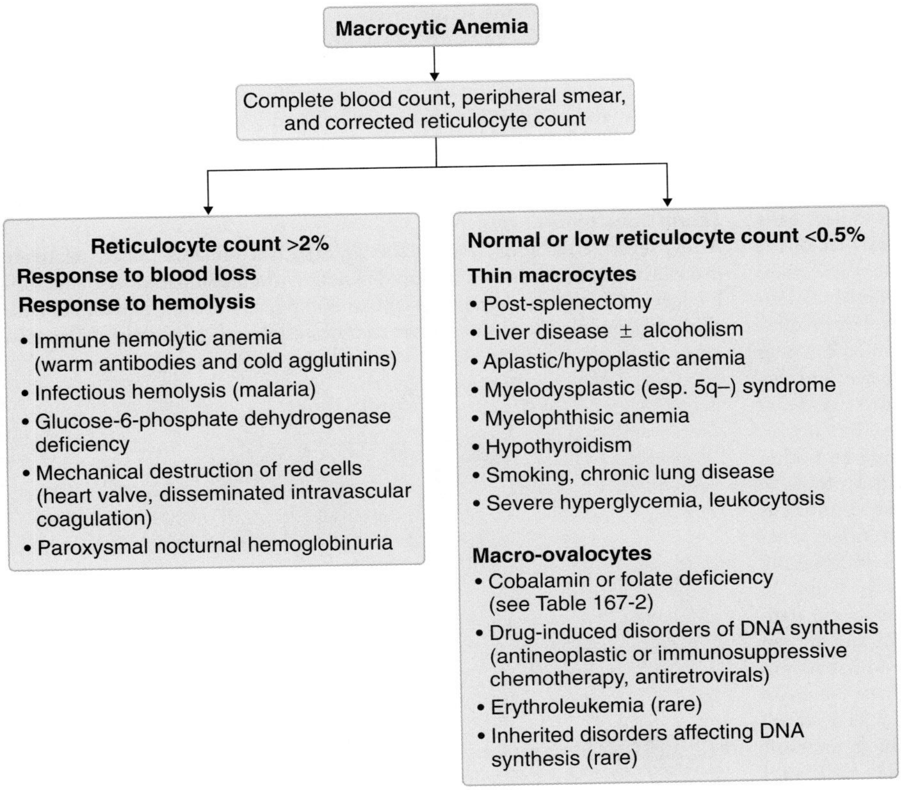

Macrocytic Anemia

↓

Complete blood count, peripheral smear, and corrected reticulocyte count

↓

Reticulocyte count >2%

Response to blood loss

Response to hemolysis

- Immune hemolytic anemia (warm antibodies and cold agglutinins)
- Infectious hemolysis (malaria)
- Glucose-6-phosphate dehydrogenase deficiency
- Mechanical destruction of red cells (heart valve, disseminated intravascular coagulation)
- Paroxysmal nocturnal hemoglobinuria

Normal or low reticulocyte count <0.5%

Thin macrocytes

- Post-splenectomy
- Liver disease ± alcoholism
- Aplastic/hypoplastic anemia
- Myelodysplastic (esp. 5q–) syndrome
- Myelophthisic anemia
- Hypothyroidism
- Smoking, chronic lung disease
- Severe hyperglycemia, leukocytosis

Macro-ovalocytes

- Cobalamin or folate deficiency (see Table 167-2)
- Drug-induced disorders of DNA synthesis (antineoplastic or immunosuppressive chemotherapy, antiretrovirals)
- Erythroleukemia (rare)
- Inherited disorders affecting DNA synthesis (rare)

FIGURE 167-2. Algorithm for the evaluation of patients with macrocytosis.

The frequency with which a high MCV is found depends on the patient population studied. Thus, in a U.S. hospital, up to two thirds of cases of macrocytosis (MCV ≥100) can be due to drug therapy (chemotherapy, antiretroviral therapy) or alcoholism and liver disease. But in a developing country where a substantial percentage of the population is vegetarian or near-vegetarian, insufficient intake of cobalamin, folate, or both, with an associated iron deficiency resulting in a dimorphic anemia (with a large red cell distribution width from a mix of macrocytic and microcytic cells), would be common.

The underlying condition predisposing to the development of folate deficiency usually began within the previous 6 months and often dominates the overall clinical picture. Alcoholism can be identified as the basis for folate deficiency from the history and physical examination, but associated thiamine deficiency may result in a more complex manifestation, such as heart failure from cardiovascular disease ("wet beriberi") and peripheral neuropathy ("dry beriberi") with Wernicke-Korsakoff syndrome (Chapters 225 and 425). By contrast, cobalamin deficiency takes several years to manifest clinically. Therefore, the underlying condition is more chronic, symptoms develop more insidiously, and defining the cause is a clinical challenge.

History and Physical Examination

The dietary history may be revealing (food faddism, vegetarianism), whereas the medical or family history may uncover blood diseases, gluten sensitivity, autoimmune diseases, epilepsy treated with an anticonvulsant, use of offending drugs, previous hemolytic anemia, past surgery (e.g., gastrectomy, fistula, bowel resection), inhalation of N_2O, or a travel history predictive for tropical sprue.

Physical examination of cobalamin-deficient vegetarians or those with pernicious anemia may reveal well-nourished individuals. By contrast, patients with folate deficiency are poorly nourished and may have other stigmata of multiple deficiencies from malabsorption (Chapter 142). Associated deficiency of vitamins A, D, and K or protein-calorie malnutrition, or both, may give rise to angular cheilosis, bleeding mucous membranes, dermatitis, osteomalacia, and chronic infections. Varying degrees of pallor with lemon-tint icterus (a combination of pallor and icterus best observed in fair-skinned individuals) are common features of megaloblastosis. The skin may reveal either a diffuse brownish pigmentation or abnormal blotchy tanning. Premature graying is observed in both light- and dark-haired individuals.

Examination of the mouth may reveal glossitis, with a smooth (depapillated), beefy-red tongue and occasional ulceration of the lateral surface. Thyromegaly may be observed with pernicious anemia and associated autoimmune thyroid disease, but it also raises suspicion for (nonmegaloblastic) macrocytosis related to hypothyroidism. The characteristic findings of heart failure from severe anemia may be accompanied by mild splenomegaly and extramedullary hematopoiesis.

In prolonged cobalamin deficiency, neurologic examination reveals evidence of involvement of the posterior columns as well as the pyramidal, spinocerebellar, and spinothalamic tracts. Posterior column dysfunction results in loss of position sense in the index toes (before great toe involvement) (Chapter 425) and loss of the ability to discern vibration of a high-pitched (256 cycles/second) tuning fork. Diminished vibratory sensation and proprioception of the lower extremities are the most common early objective signs. Neuropathic involvement of the legs precedes that of the arms. Upper motor neuron signs may be modulated by the subsequent involvement of peripheral nerves. A positive Romberg's sign and a Lhermitte's sign may be elicited. Loss of sphincter and bowel control or involvement of cranial nerves, such as optic neuritis, may be accompanied by other dysfunction of the cerebral cortex, including dementia, psychoses, and disturbances of mood. Folate deficiency in adults does not give rise to significant neurologic findings. Thus, the coexistence of folate deficiency with neurologic disease should prompt investigations to exclude cobalamin and other nutrient deficiencies arising from dietary insufficiency or malabsorption.

Nutritional cobalamin deficiency in developing countries can manifest as florid pancytopenia, mild hepatosplenomegaly, fever, and thrombocytopenia, with the neuropsychiatric syndrome developing as a later manifestation. However, cobalamin-related neurologic disease has also been found in patients with only mild to moderate anemia secondary to cobalamin deficiency in both developing and developed countries. Between 25 and 50% of patients who have neuropsychiatric abnormalities attributable to cobalamin deficiency may have a normal hematocrit and MCV if they have adequate folate stores to protect them from hematologic abnormalities. In fact, in the United States, there is often an inverse correlation between the hematocrit and neurologic disease in cobalamin deficiency—most subjects have mild neurologic deficits, and 25% have only moderate deficits, with paresthesias or ataxia as the initial symptoms.

Laboratory Tests

Megaloblastosis

To establish the diagnosis of megaloblastosis, the evaluation begins with a complete blood count, MCV (which often reveals a steady increase over a period of several months or years), peripheral smear, and reticulocyte count; a low reticulocyte count with macro-ovalocytes suggests an underlying megaloblastic anemia (see Fig. 167-2). Classic megaloblastosis from cobalamin or folate deficiency may be accompanied by a hemoglobin level of less than 5 g/dL. Neutropenia and thrombocytopenia occur less commonly than anemia and are usually not severe. Occasionally, however, neutrophil counts less than 1000/μL and platelet counts less than 50,000/μL can be seen. Additional abnormalities supporting intramedullary hemolysis include elevated levels of serum lactate dehydrogenase and bilirubin, as well as decreased serum haptoglobin levels.

Peripheral Smear

In peripheral blood, the earliest manifestation of megaloblastosis is an increase in MCV with macro-ovalocytes (up to 14 μm). Nuclear hypersegmentation of neutrophils, diagnosed if more than 5% of polymorphonuclear leukocytes have five lobes or if more than 1% have six lobes on the smear (Fig. 167-3), strongly suggests megaloblastosis, especially when associated with macro-ovalocytosis. However, neutrophil hypersegmentation is not sensitive for the diagnosis of *mild* cobalamin deficiency, and macrocytosis is absent in nearly 50% of cases. There may be associated teardrop-shaped erythrocytes and anisocytosis with mild leukopenia and thrombocytopenia.

Megaloblastic anemia can be masked when there is a coexisting condition that neutralizes the tendency to generate large cells, such as iron deficiency (Chapter 162) or thalassemia (Chapter 165). In these situations, giant myelocytes and metamyelocytes in bone marrow and hypersegmented neutrophils in bone marrow and peripheral blood (see Fig. 167-3) are important clues to a masked megaloblastosis. This problem is clinically relevant because appropriate replacement with cobalamin or folate elicits a maximal hematologic response only when any associated iron deficiency is corrected. Conversely, if a combined iron and cobalamin deficiency (after gastrectomy) or iron and folate deficiency (with pregnancy) is treated with iron alone, megaloblastosis will be unmasked.

Cobalamin and Folate Levels

Laboratory evaluation of suspected cobalamin or folate deficiency begins with measurement of the serum levels of these vitamins and then progresses to confirmatory tests (Table 167-2). Use of clinical information can improve the pretest probability of serum cobalamin and folate levels. Moreover, without detailed clinical information, the combined results of serum cobalamin, folate, and metabolite tests are not sufficiently unambiguous to diagnose and distinguish cobalamin deficiency from combined cobalamin plus folate deficiency.

Serum Cobalamin Levels

A low serum cobalamin level (<200 pg/mL) is a valuable (albeit relatively insensitive) indicator of cobalamin deficiency when compared with metabolite levels. Serum cobalamin is less than 300 pg/mL in 99% of patients with clinical hematologic or neurologic manifestations of cobalamin deficiency,

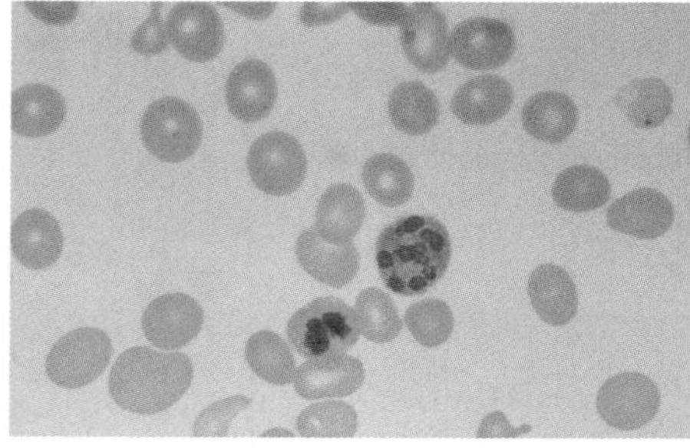

FIGURE 167-3. Megaloblastic anemia. The peripheral blood has oval macrocytes (large red blood cells) and marked neutrophil hypersegmentation.

TABLE 167-2 STEPWISE APPROACH TO THE DIAGNOSIS OF COBALAMIN AND FOLATE DEFICIENCY

MEGALOBLASTIC ANEMIA *OR* NEUROLOGIC-PSYCHIATRIC MANIFESTATIONS CONSISTENT WITH COBALAMIN DEFICIENCY *PLUS* TEST RESULTS ON SERUM COBALAMIN AND SERUM FOLATE

*Cobalamin** *(pg/mL)*	*Folate*† *(ng/mL)*	*Provisional Diagnosis*	*Proceed with Metabolites?*‡
>300	>4	Cobalamin/folate deficiency unlikely	No
<200	>4	Consistent with cobalamin deficiency	No
200-300	>4	Rule out cobalamin deficiency	Yes
>300	<2	Consistent with folate deficiency	No
<200	<2	Consistent with combined cobalamin plus folate deficiency or with isolated folate deficiency	Yes
>300	2-4	Consistent with folate deficiency or with anemia unrelated to vitamin deficiency	Yes

TEST RESULTS ON METABOLITES: SERUM METHYLMALONIC ACID AND TOTAL HOMOCYSTEINE

Methylmalonic Acid (Normal = 70-270 nM)	*Total Homocysteine (Normal = 5-14 μM)*	*Diagnosis*
Increased	Increased	Cobalamin deficiency confirmed; folate deficiency still possible (i.e., combined cobalamin plus folate deficiency possible)
Normal	Increased	Folate deficiency likely; <5% may have cobalamin deficiency
Normal	Normal	Cobalamin and folate deficiencies excluded

*Serum cobalamin levels: abnormally low = <200 pg/mL; clinically relevant low-normal range = 200-300 pg/mL.
†Serum folate levels: abnormally low = <2 ng/mL; clinically relevant low-normal range = 2-4 ng/mL.
‡Any frozen-over sample from the serum folate or cobalamin determination can be subjected to metabolite tests.

whereas a cobalamin level greater than 300 pg/mL suggests folate deficiency or another cause of macrocytosis or neurologic disease.

About 90% of older patients with serum cobalamin levels less than 200 pg/mL show evidence of true tissue cobalamin deficiency, but individuals with neuropsychiatric disorders attributed to cobalamin deficiency may not have anemia and may have normal or only minimally depressed cobalamin levels. The serum cobalamin concentration is falsely low in the absence of true cobalamin deficiency in patients with folate deficiency (one third of patients), pregnancy, multiple myeloma, transcobalamin I deficiency, megadose or vitamin C therapy, or when the serum contains other radioisotopes (e.g., ^{99m}Tc, ^{67}Ga, ^{125}I) from organ scanning.

A falsely raised cobalamin level in the presence of a true cobalamin deficiency leads to clinical manifestations if uncorrected. Examples include an artificial increase in transcobalamin I and II, which can occur with myeloproliferative disorders, hepatomas, and fibrolamellar hepatic tumors; when transcobalamin II–producing macrophages are activated in autoimmune diseases, monoblastic leukemias, and lymphomas; and on the release of cobalamin from hepatocytes during active liver disease in cobalamin-deficient patients. Studies suggest that approximately 10% of the U.S. population, especially the elderly, have true cobalamin deficiency manifested by low or low-normal serum cobalamin levels, as well as elevated levels of serum methylmalonic acid (MMA) and homocysteine that fall to normal with cobalamin therapy.

Serum Folate Levels

When combined with a clinical picture of megaloblastic anemia and the measurement of cobalamin levels, serum folate is the cheapest and best initial biochemical test to diagnose folate deficiency. Although red blood cell folate levels by microbiologic assay correlate well with hepatic folate stores, they are not widely available, and the newer radioisotopic or colorimetric assays are too unreliable for routine clinical use.

The serum folate level is highly sensitive to the intake of a single folate-rich meal. Nutritional folate deficiency first leads to a decline in the serum folate level below normal (<2 ng/mL) in about 3 weeks; thus, it is a sensitive indicator of negative folate balance. Isolated reduction of serum folate in the absence of megaloblastosis (i.e., a false-positive result) occurs in one third of hospitalized patients with anorexia and acute alcohol consumption, in normal pregnancy, and in those using anticonvulsants; because these groups are also at high risk for folate deficiency, additional testing with metabolites or an empirical therapeutic trial may be required. Conversely, in 25 to 50% of alcohol abusers (Chapter 32) with folate deficiency, serum folate levels may be low normal or borderline low.

Metabolite Levels—Homocysteine and Methylmalonic Acid

The serum homocysteine and MMA values rise in proportion to the severity of deficiency (see Table 167-2). Although serum MMA and homocysteine tests are the "gold standard" for confirming the diagnosis of cobalamin deficiency, they are too expensive to use for screening. Serum MMA levels are elevated in more than 95% of patients with clinically confirmed cobalamin deficiency (with median values of 3500 nM). Serum homocysteine concentrations are elevated in both cobalamin deficiency (median values of 70 μM) and folate deficiency (median values of 50 μM). Both homocysteine and MMA rise with dehydration or renal failure. Propionic acid, derived from anaerobic fecal bacterial metabolism, can also contribute to MMA values, which can be lowered by a course of metronidazole. Thus, although these metabolites can help distinguish between isolated cobalamin and folate deficiency, an increase in both metabolites cannot differentiate between isolated cobalamin deficiency and combined cobalamin plus folate deficiency. The abnormally high metabolites return to normal in a week when replaced with the appropriate (deficient) vitamin.

Clinicians can use serum MMA and homocysteine to assist in the diagnosis in patients with (1) borderline cobalamin and folate levels; (2) existing conditions known to perturb folate and cobalamin tests, leading to difficulties in interpreting the results; (3) low levels of both cobalamin and folate, in which case a high MMA level is useful to confirm cobalamin deficiency (rather than attributing the condition to folate deficiency alone); and (4) low serum cobalamin levels when there is an alternative explanation for the syndrome that led to the test (e.g., a diabetic or alcoholic patient with peripheral neuropathy or an alcoholic patient with a high MCV and low cobalamin level without anemia). In the context of diagnosing a subclinical deficiency of cobalamin (or folate) based on increased serum MMA or homocysteine (or both) despite normal serum cobalamin (or folate) levels, a positive diagnosis can be made only after reversal of laboratory values following treatment with cobalamin (and/or folate) has been demonstrated.

Bone Marrow Examination

In florid hematologic disease with or without neurologic disease suggestive of cobalamin or folate deficiency, the identification of nucleated red cells with megaloblastic changes in the peripheral smear—which reflects the morphology in the bone marrow—can clinch the diagnosis of megaloblastosis. If not found, a bone marrow aspirate can be invaluable in making the rapid diagnosis of megaloblastosis. However, in the outpatient setting, when there is less urgency because the anemia is mild to moderate and the patient has a suggestive peripheral smear, or when the manifestation is primarily neuropsychiatric, a good case can be made to initiate the sequence of diagnostic tests without bone marrow aspiration and proceed with the measurement of serum levels of vitamins or metabolites (see Table 167-2 and Fig. 167-2).

In a bone marrow aspirate (Fig. 167-4), which is better than biopsy for observing megaloblastosis, the cells are actually proliferating very slowly despite what looks like exuberant cell proliferation with numerous mitotic figures. In early cobalamin or folate deficiency, normoblasts may dominate the marrow, with only a few megaloblasts seen, but the full spectrum of megaloblastic hematopoiesis is observed in florid deficiency and is accompanied by varying degrees of pancytopenia. In contrast to the normally dense chromatin of comparable normoblasts, megaloblastic erythroid precursors have an open, finely stippled, reticular, sieve-like pattern. The orthochromatic megaloblast, with its hemoglobinized cytoplasm, continues to retain its large, sieve-like immature nucleus, in sharp contrast to the clumped chromatin of orthochromatic normoblasts. The majority of megaloblastic cells (80 to 90%) die in the bone marrow and are scavenged by macrophages in a process called *ineffective erythropoiesis* or *intramedullary hemolysis*. There is an

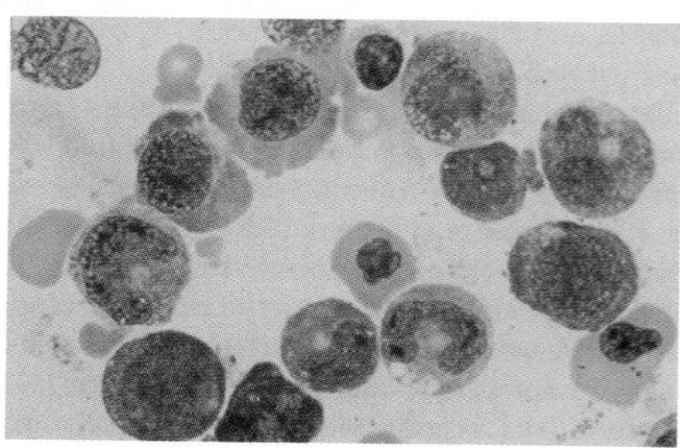

FIGURE 167-4. Megaloblastic anemia. A bone marrow aspirate shows red blood cell precursors that are giant megaloblasts with nuclear-cytoplasmic dissociation (nuclear maturation lagging behind cytoplasmic maturation). Megaloblastic changes in the leukocyte series are shown by the "giant metamyelocyte."

absolute increase in leukopoiesis, with megaloblastic cells also having a sieve-like chromatin. Giant (20 to 30 μm) metamyelocytes and "band" forms are pathognomonic for megaloblastosis. Hypersegmented polymorphonuclear leukocytes may be seen in the marrow and peripheral blood. Megakaryocytes may be normal or increased in number and can exhibit complex hypersegmentation, with liberation of fragments of cytoplasm and giant platelets into the circulation. The net output of platelets is decreased in severe megaloblastosis.

Determining the Cause of the Vitamin Deficiency

By the time the megaloblastic state is established, the cause of the folate deficiency is usually clear from the history, physical examination, and clinical setting. With rare exceptions, adults with cobalamin deficiency have either cobalamin malabsorption or dietary cobalamin insufficiency. All these conditions can be treated similarly with either monthly parenteral cobalamin or daily oral cobalamin. However, identifying the likely basis for malabsorption can point to the need for additional diagnostic tests (e.g., intestinal biopsy, examination of stool for malabsorption or *D. latum* infestation) and specific therapy (e.g., gluten-free diet, folate, antibiotics, anthelmintics). This evaluation, in turn, indicates whether cobalamin replacement should be lifelong. At this juncture in the diagnostic evaluation, the Schilling test, which was discontinued in 2003, once provided invaluable information on the locus and mechanism of cobalamin malabsorption. Now, only 60% of patients with pernicious anemia can be confidently identified through the measurement of serum anti–intrinsic factor antibodies. However, because most of the conditions predisposing to cobalamin deficiency (see Table 167-1) should be clinically evident by the time cobalamin deficiency is apparent, it is possible to identify several conditions through a detailed dietary history or past medical history that suggests esophagogastroduodenal disease, pancreatic insufficiency, impaired bowel motility, or other autoimmune diseases. The physical examination can provide additional clues and suggest focused testing for rarer conditions (stool for ova, anti–tissue transglutaminase antibodies, lipase, gastrin, intestinal biopsy, or radiographic contrast studies for stasis, strictures, or fistulas). For the younger patient with megaloblastic anemia, juvenile pernicious anemia and congenital intrinsic factor deficiency warrant the measurement of gastric juice for intrinsic factor and achlorhydria and DNA for mutations in cubam receptor (amnionless, cubulin genes) for hereditary megaloblastic anemia and Immerslund-Gräsbeck syndrome.

Measurement of a rise in blood holo-transcobalamin (cobalamin-bound transcobalamin II) levels after the administration of oral cobalamin can indicate the absorption of orally administered doses of cobalamin in otherwise healthy individuals or vegetarians; however, this test must still be clinically validated among various cohorts of patients with cobalamin malabsorption (see Table 167-1).

TREATMENT Rx

First, blood is drawn for a determination of serum folate and cobalamin levels (and enough for the measurement of metabolite levels later, if indicated), and bone marrow aspiration is performed, if necessary, to confirm megaloblastosis. If the patient is decompensated or decompensation is imminent, the patient is then transfused slowly with 1 U of packed red cells; diuretics are administered, if necessary; and both cobalamin and folate are started at full doses. If the patient is moderately symptomatic, transfusions should be avoided because a dramatic improvement in well-being is likely to occur within 2 to 3 days of starting appropriate vitamin replacement, even before hematologic improvement. If the patient is well compensated or is in the ambulatory setting, diagnostic testing should proceed in an orderly sequence (see Fig. 167-2 and Table 167-2) before initiating therapy.

Drug Dosage

Therapy with full doses of parenteral cobalamin (1 mg/day) and oral folate (folic acid 1 to 5 mg) before the type of vitamin deficiency has been established should be reserved for severely ill patients. An aggressive scheme to replace cobalamin rapidly is 1 mg/day of intramuscular or subcutaneous cyanocobalamin (week 1), 1 mg twice weekly (week 2), 1 mg/week for 4 weeks, and then 1 mg/month for life. Because 1 to 2% of an oral dose is absorbed by passive diffusion, even in patients with malabsorption of physiologic cobalamin for any reason, an equally effective alternative to maintenance therapy with monthly cobalamin injections is the daily administration of 2-mg cobalamin tablets orally after rapidly replenishing cobalamin parenterally. In patients with malabsorption of food-bound cobalamin, cobalamin doses of 1 mg/day are required. For patients with nutritional cobalamin deficiency (vegetarians) without absorptive problems, after cobalamin stores are replenished with 2 mg/day of oral cobalamin for at least 3 months, smaller oral cobalamin doses of 5 to 10 μg, using tablets or equivalent cobalamin-fortified foods, taken for life, are sufficient.

Subclinical cobalamin deficiency does not inexorably progress to clinical cobalamin deficiency; indeed, mild or borderline abnormal biochemical results tend to remain unchanged, fluctuate above or below normal values, or even spontaneously resolve. Some physicians follow these patients and treat them with cobalamin only when they exhibit symptoms or signs of frank cobalamin deficiency. Others err on the side of caution, preferring to preemptively replenish depleted cobalamin stores; these patients are treated for 6 months with high-dose daily oral cobalamin (1 mg), and then serum cobalamin levels are followed.

Oral folate (folic acid) at doses of 1 to 5 mg/day results in adequate absorption despite intestinal malabsorption of physiologic food folate. Therapy should be continued until complete hematologic recovery is documented; the subsequent duration of therapy is dictated by the cause. Folinic acid bypasses any block in one-carbon metabolism induced by methotrexate, trimethoprim-sulfamethoxazole, or N_2O.

Prophylaxis with Cobalamin or Folate

Cobalamin must be given to infants of cobalamin-deficient mothers, as well as to patients who have undergone total gastrectomy. For vegetarians, cobalamin-fortified foods (soy or rice beverages, fortified cereals, nutritional yeast) or oral cobalamin tablets 5 to 10 μg/day should suffice. For those with malabsorption of cobalamin from any other mechanism (see Table 167-1), cobalamin replacement is achieved with 1- to 2-mg tablets taken orally each day.

Periconceptional folate supplementation for all normal women (400 μg/day of folic acid) and for women who have previously delivered a baby with a neural tube defect (4 mg/day of folic acid) is now standard and prevents nearly three quarters of neural tube defects. Women of childbearing age who are taking anticonvulsant medications (phenytoin, phenobarbital, carbamazepine) are also at increased risk for delivering babies with neural tube defects and should routinely take 1 mg of folic acid daily. Folate supplementation throughout pregnancy also helps prevent premature delivery of low-birthweight infants and is recommended for premature infants and lactating mothers. Folic acid supplements (1 mg/day orally) are taken by patients with hemolysis or myeloproliferative diseases and to reduce the toxicity of methotrexate in patients with rheumatoid arthritis and psoriasis. Individuals in whom cobalamin deficiency develops while undergoing long-term folate replacement have a pure neurologic syndrome.

The mandatory fortification of food (flour, enriched pasta, cornmeal, cereal foods) with 140 and 150 μg of folic acid per 100 g in the United States and Canada, respectively, has led to several beneficial effects (Table 167-3). Indeed, 94% of U.S. adults who do not consume supplements or consume less than 400 μg/day of folic acid from supplements do not exceed the upper intake limit for folic acid (>1 mg/day), which has potential to mask cobalamin deficiency.

PROGNOSIS

The general response to cobalamin replacement is a dramatic improvement in well-being, with alertness, a good appetite, and resolution of a sore tongue. Megaloblastic hematopoiesis reverts to normal within 12 hours and resolves by 48 hours; the only persistent findings may be giant metamyelocytes in the bone marrow and hypersegmented neutrophils in the blood for up to 14 days. The reticulocyte count peaks by days 5 to 8, followed by a rise in the red cell count, hemoglobin level, and hematocrit. By the end of the first week, the white blood cell count rises, sometimes with a transient left shift, as does the platelet count; both normalize by approximately 2 months.

TABLE 167-3 BENEFICIAL EFFECTS OF HOMOCYSTEINE-LOWERING THERAPY ON NONHEMATOPOIETIC SYSTEMS

FOLIC ACID, COBALAMIN, PYRIDOXINE SUPPLEMENTATION
Reduction in hip fracture 1
Reduction in progression of carotid intima media thickness (surrogate marker of early subclinical arteriosclerosis) 2
Reduction in age-related macular degeneration 3
FOLIC ACID SUPPLEMENTATION
Reduction in stroke 4
Reduction in rate of cognitive decline among healthy elderly 5
Reduction in age-related (sensorineural) hearing loss 6
Reduction in recurrence of neural tube defects 7
FOLIC ACID FORTIFICATION OF FOOD (POPULATION-BASED STUDIES)
Reduction in neural tube defects (anencephaly, spina bifida, encephalocele, meningocele, iniencephaly)
Reduction in cleft lip with or without cleft palate
Reduction in severe congenital heart disease (endocardial cushion defects, conotruncal defects)
Reduction in congenital pyloric stenosis, stenosis of the pelvicoureteric junction, limb reduction defects, omphalocele
Reduction in stroke mortality
Decreased risk of low-birthweight and small-for-gestational-age babies

With cobalamin replacement, the degree of reversal of neurologic damage is generally inversely related to the extent of disease and the duration of signs and symptoms. Most neurologic abnormalities improve in up to 90% of patients with documented subacute combined degeneration, and most signs and symptoms of less than 3 months' duration are reversible. With signs and symptoms of longer duration, there is invariably some residual neurologic dysfunction. The maximal response often takes up to 6 months, but recovery beyond 12 months is unusual.

Incorrect treatment of cobalamin deficiency with folate does not improve the neuropsychiatric abnormalities, which will continue to progress; hematologic improvements often occur, however. Alternatively, there may be associated iron deficiency or hypothyroidism that needs treatment or another hemoglobinopathy (e.g., sickle cell disease, thalassemia) that limits the normalization of hemoglobin values.

In patients with pernicious anemia, subsequent iron deficiency anemia (Chapter 162), osteoporosis (Chapter 251) with fractures of the proximal end of the femur and vertebrae, gastric cancer (Chapter 198), and cancer of the buccal cavity and pharynx can develop. Some experts recommend periodic endoscopic surveillance.

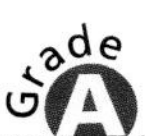

1. Sato Y, Honda Y, Iwamoto J, et al. Effect of folate and mecobalamin on hip fractures in patients with stroke: a randomized controlled trial. *JAMA.* 2005;293:1082-1088.
2. Hodis HN, Mack WJ, Dustin L, et al. High-dose B vitamin supplementation and progression of subclinical atherosclerosis: a randomized controlled trial. *Stroke.* 2009;40:730-736.
3. Christen WG, Glynn RJ, Chew EY, et al. Folic acid, pyridoxine, and cyanocobalamin combination treatment and age-related macular degeneration in women: the Women's Antioxidant and Folic Acid Cardiovascular Study. *Arch Intern Med.* 2009;169:335-341.
4. Wang X, Qin X, Demirtas H, et al. Efficacy of folic acid supplementation in stroke prevention: a meta-analysis. *Lancet.* 2007;369:1876-1882.
5. Durga J, van Boxtel MP, Schouten EG, et al. Effect of 3-year folic acid supplementation on cognitive function in older adults in the FACIT trial: a randomised, double blind, controlled trial. *Lancet.* 2007;369:208-216.
6. Durga J, Verhoef P, Anteunis LJ, et al. Effects of folic acid supplementation on hearing in older adults: a randomized, controlled trial. *Ann Intern Med.* 2007;146:1-9.
7. Grosse SD, Collins JS. Folic acid supplementation and neural tube defect recurrence prevention. *Birth Defects Res A Clin Mol Teratol.* 2007;79:737-742.

SUGGESTED READINGS

Andrès E, Fothergill H, Mecili M. Efficacy of oral cobalamin (vitamin B_{12}) therapy. *Expert Opin Pharmacother.* 2010;11:249-256. *Support for the routine use of oral cobalamin therapy in clinical practice.*

Bukowski R, Malone FD, Porter FT, et al. Preconceptional folate supplementation and the risk of spontaneous preterm birth: a cohort study. *PLoS Med.* 2009;6:e1000061. *This recent paper suggests a role for folate supplements in preventing spontaneous preterm births in developed countries.*

Carmel R. Mandatory fortification of the food supply with cobalamin: an idea whose time has not yet come. *J Inherit Metab Dis.* 2011;34:67-73. *Argues for randomized clinical trials before this potentially beneficial public health intervention is undertaken.*

Clarke R, Halsey J, Lewington S, et al. Effects of lowering homocysteine levels with B vitamins on cardiovascular disease, cancer, and cause-specific mortality: meta-analysis of 8 randomized trials involving 37,485 individuals. *Arch Intern Med.* 2010;170:1622-1631. *No benefit for incident or fatal cancer or cardiovascular disease, or for overall mortality.*

Schlotz W, Jones A, Phillips DI, et al. Lower maternal folate status in early pregnancy is associated with childhood hyperactivity and peer problems in offspring. *J Child Psychol Psychiatry.* 2010;51:594-602. *Maternal nutrition during early pregnancy contributes to an individual's neurodevelopment, with potential consequences for behavior later in life, similar to experimental studies in mice.*

168 APLASTIC ANEMIA AND RELATED BONE MARROW FAILURE STATES

GROVER C. BAGBY

DEFINITION

Aplastic anemia is a life-threatening syndrome characterized by failure of the bone marrow to produce peripheral blood cells and their progenitors. Diverse diseases and environmental factors can cause this syndrome, but its hallmark is bone marrow hypocellularity and hypoplasia of the erythroid, myeloid, and megakaryocyte lines (Fig. 168-1).

EPIDEMIOLOGY

In Europe and North America, the annual incidence is 2 per 1 million persons, and in Asia, 4 to 7 per 1 million. No age group is exempt, and although the syndrome occurs most often in young adults, the age distribution of newly diagnosed patients is bimodal, with peaks at 15 to 25 years and at 60 to 65 years.

PATHOBIOLOGY

Pathology

Peripheral blood pancytopenia is universally present in patients with aplastic anemia, but bone marrow biopsy is required to establish the diagnosis. The diagnosis will be clear-cut if the biopsy specimen is of sufficient size and has been obtained from an anatomic site that has never been exposed to extensive trauma or radiation. As shown in Figure 168-1B, some residual lymphoid cell populations can be found in marrow specimens. Although these lymphoid cells may be of pathophysiologic importance, it is the absence of *nonlymphoid* hematopoietic cells that is important in establishing the diagnosis of this syndrome. However, if the hematopoietic marrow has been suppressed (or "replaced") by the infiltration of neoplastic cells or fibroblasts, the diagnosis of aplastic anemia cannot be made. Therefore, the diagnosis requires not only a dearth of hematopoietic cells in the marrow but also an empty bone marrow.

Some bone marrow failure syndromes affect only one lineage. In those cases, only the marrow precursors of that lineage are missing. In patients with agranulocytosis, for example, there are rare neutrophils and neutrophil precursors present, and the ratio of erythroid to myeloid cells is very high. Likewise, in patients with the disorder known as pure red cell aplasia, few erythroid cells are detectable in the marrow, but the other lineages are well represented and functional. These two disorders are examples of bone marrow failure syndromes but are not examples of aplastic anemia, which involves global suppression of all hematopoietic lineages.

Pathophysiology

Marrow aplasia in a few patients (10%) can be attributed to an inherited bone marrow failure syndrome, but most cases are acquired and caused by factors other than an inherited gene mutation. In all cases, it is clear that the causative factors, genetic or environmental, injure pluripotent hematopoietic stem cells. This is in contrast to the case of the lineage-restricted disorders ,wherein the causative agents and factors suppress the growth and development of unipotent progenitor cells committed to that particular lineage. Radiation, viral diseases, cytotoxic drugs, and chemicals are known causes of aplastic anemia, but the most common form of acquired aplastic anemia is immunologically mediated, and evidence is emerging that some marrow failure states attributed to viral infection or to idiosyncratic drug reactions may also result

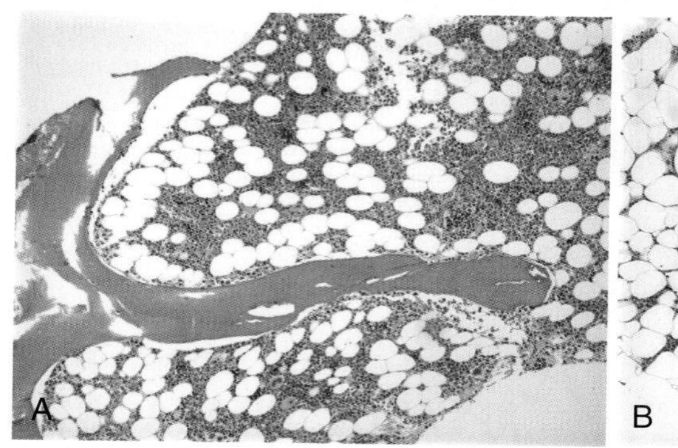

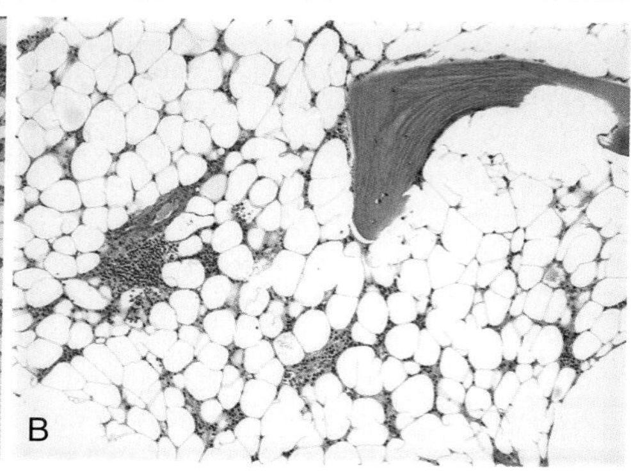

FIGURE 168-1. Two bone marrow biopsy samples from different patients. A. This specimen, from a normal individual, shows an abundance of hematopoietic cells, including myeloid and erythroid precursors and normal-appearing megakaryocytes. **B,** A specimen from a patient with severe aplastic anemia shows few detectable hematopoietic cells, and those that can be seen (one small nest) are largely lymphocytes. Lymphoid cells are often detectable and probably play an important pathophysiologic role in many cases of acquired idiopathic aplastic anemia, a disorder that is most often immunologically mediated. (Courtesy of Dr. Ken Gatter, Oregon Health and Science University.)

TABLE 168-1 MAJOR CAUSES OF APLASTIC ANEMIA AND RELATED BONE MARROW FAILURE STATES

1. Autoimmune aplastic anemia
   a. Acquired
   b. Drug induced
   c. Infections
      i. Hepatitis
      ii. Epstein-Barr virus
2. Autoimmune-mediated failure of single hematopoietic lineages
   a. Agranulocytosis
   b. Pure red cell aplasia
3. Direct stem cell toxicity
   a. Radiation
   b. Chemicals
   c. Drugs
4. Other aplastic states
   a. Pregnancy
   b. Paroxysmal nocturnal hemoglobinuria
   c. Inherited bone marrow failure syndromes

from immune suppression of hematopoiesis. The pathogenesis of the major causes of aplastic anemia and related bone marrow failure states is outlined in Table 168-1.

Pathogenesis

Autoimmune Aplastic Anemia

Acquired Aplastic Anemia

In patients with the most common form of acquired aplastic anemia, autologous lymphocytes suppress the replicative activity and induce the death of hematopoietic stem and progenitor cells. Evidence supporting this model are to be found in studies demonstrating that: (1) removal of T lymphocytes from cultured bone marrow cells enhances hematopoiesis in vitro; (2) patients with aplastic anemia can be effectively treated with immunosuppressive therapy alone; (3) oligoclonal T cells in the marrow and blood of aplastic anemia patients contain high intracellular levels of the myelosuppressive cytokines interferon-γ (IFN-γ) and tumor necrosis factor-α (TNF-α); (4) the IFN-γ/TNF-α-positive T-cell populations are suppressed in patients who respond to immunosuppressive therapy but are not suppressed in patients who do not respond; and (5) the syndrome can be modeled in mice by infusing alloreactive lymphocytes that induce marrow failure.

Drug Induced

Although a wide variety of drugs have been associated with aplastic anemia, the association is loose. Much of the evidence is circumstantial and, apart from drugs that are known to be directly toxic to the marrow (e.g., chemotherapeutic agents; Table 168-2), the cases are not related to total dose of the suspect agent. These "idiosyncratic" reactions are likely autoimmune. Some agents, chloramphenicol being the classic paradigm, are capable of inducing dose-related myelosuppression in all treated patients (which abates after discontinuation of the drug) and rare idiosyncratic aplastic responses as well (which do not remit after discontinuation of the agent). Drugs that have been repeatedly associated with aplastic anemia are listed in Table 168-2.

Infections

HEPATITIS. About 2 to 5% of patients with severe aplastic anemia have had viral hepatitis (Chapters 150 and 151). Some cases were associated with hepatitis A or B, but most patients with the hepatitis-aplasia syndrome have had hepatitis of unclear type (non-A, -B, -C, -E, or -G). Most patients with this syndrome are younger than 20 years. The natural course is rapid, with a 1-year mortality rate of more than 90%. The immune system is likely involved in the pathophysiology of this syndrome because immunosuppressive therapy has been reported to induce meaningful remissions.

EPSTEIN-BARR VIRUS. In rare patients with aplastic anemia, evidence of active Epstein-Barr virus (EBV) infection has been discovered (Chapter 385). Because the virus does not infect progenitor cells or stem cells, it is most likely that the virus induces an aberrant immune response that generates either immunoglobulin- or T-lymphocyte–mediated hematopoietic suppression. Because only a minority of EBV-infected aplastic patients describe a history of typical infectious mononucleosis, it is equally likely that the aplastic state came first and that EBV was later reactivated.

Autoimmune-Mediated Failure of Single Hematopoietic Lineages

Agranulocytosis

Agranulocytosis is characterized by severe neutropenia and suppression of granulopoiesis. This disorder can be an idiosyncratic reaction to certain drugs and most likely involves immune suppression of granulopoietic progenitor cells. The disease almost always abates when the offending drug is discontinued. Agranulocytosis also occurs in patients with established autoimmune diseases, including systemic lupus erythematosus, Sjögren's syndrome, and rheumatoid arthritis. In some cases, the disorder is caused by myelosuppressive antibodies, and in others, by T lymphocytes that suppress granulopoiesis. Immunosuppressive therapy is often effective in such patients and should be used in patients whose agranulocytosis is severe and associated with recurrent infections.

Pure Red Cell Aplasia

Severe normochromic, normocytic anemia with a marked decrease in reticulocyte number is sometimes associated with selective hypoplasia of the erythroid marrow without loss of megakaryocytes and myeloid precursor cells. In immunocompromised hosts and patients with chronic hemolytic diseases, this disorder, known as pure red cell aplasia, can be caused by parvovirus B19 infection (Chapter 379), an agent that infects erythroid precursor cells and likely generates an erythroid suppressive immune response. This disease can also be mediated by T lymphocytes or natural killer cells that suppress cells of the erythroid lineage and in more uncommon cases by antibody-dependent

TABLE 168-2 DRUGS AND TOXINS ASSOCIATED WITH APLASTIC ANEMIA

DOSE DEPENDENT
Antineoplastic Agents
Antimetabolites: fluorouracil, mercaptopurine, 6-thioguanine, methotrexate, cytosine arabinoside, gemcitabine, fludarabine, cladribine, pentostatin, hydroxyurea
Alkylating and cross-linking agents: busulfan, cyclophosphamide, chlorambucil, nitrogen mustard, melphalan, cisplatin, carboplatin, ifosfamide, nitrosoureas (BCNU and CCNU), mitomycin C
Cytotoxic antibiotics: daunorubicin, doxorubicin, mitoxantrone
Plant alkaloids: vinblastine, paclitaxel
Topoisomerase inhibitors: etoposide
Antimicrobial Agents
Chloramphenicol, dapsone, fluorocytosine
Anti-Inflammatory and Antirheumatic Agents
Colchicine
Insecticides
Chlordane, chlorophenothane (DDT), lindane, parathion
Other Chemicals
Benzene
Benzene-containing chemicals: kerosene, chlorophenols, carbon tetrachloride
DOSE INDEPENDENT
Idiosyncratic, likely immune mediated
(*Note:* Most agents on this list should be considered to be possibly associated with aplastic anemia.)
Antimicrobial Agents
Chloramphenicol, dapsone, sulfonamides, tetracycline, methicillin, amphotericin, quinacrine, chloroquine, pyrimethamine
Anticonvulsants
Hydantoins, carbamazepine, phenacemide, primidone, ethosuximide
Anti-Inflammatory Agents
Phenylbutazone, indomethacin, ibuprofen, oxyphenylbutazone, sulindac, naproxen
Antiarrhythmic Drugs
Quinidine, tocainide, procainamide
Metals
Gold, arsenic, mercury, bismuth
Antihistamines
Cimetidine, ranitidine, chlorpheniramine, pyrilamine, tripelennamine
Diuretics
Acetazolamide, furosemide, chlorothiazide, methazolamide
Hypoglycemic Agents
Chlorpropamide, tolbutamide
Antithyroid Drugs
Propylthiouracil, potassium perchlorate, methylthiouracil, methimazole, carbimazole
Antihypertensive Agents
Methyldopa, enalapril, captopril
Sedatives
Chlordiazepoxide, chlorpromazine, meprobamate, prochlorperazine

suppression of erythropoiesis. Pure red cell aplasia can also develop as a complication of thymoma (Chapters 99 and 430) and in these circumstances is likewise caused by oligoclonal T-cell expansion that specifically suppresses erythroid progenitor cells. This disorder can also be associated with drug exposure (e.g., isoniazid, chlorpropamide, and phenytoin), lymphoid neoplasms (chronic lymphocytic leukemia; Chapter 190), and myelodysplasia (Chapter 188). Rarely, adults with Diamond-Blackfan anemia present with isolated erythroid suppression, but the degree to which the erythroid marrow is suppressed rarely matches the profound suppression seen in acquired cases of immune-mediated pure red cell aplasia.

Direct Stem Cell Toxicity

Radiation

The severity of myelosuppression induced by radiation and the degree to which the marrow can recover from that injury depend on the radiation dose, the timing of exposure, and the fraction of hematopoietic tissues exposed. Low-dose total body radiation causes transient marrow suppression. High doses of total body radiation (700 to 1000 cGy) induce severe injury to the stem cell pool with persistent and life-threatening marrow failure. When limited bone marrow sites are radiated to very high doses (4000 cGy or more), the relatively radioresistant bone marrow stromal cells are eradicated, and thereafter that marrow space can never support hematopoietic activity.

Chemicals

Benzene suppresses the bone marrow in a dose-dependent manner, and chronic exposure to it has been linked with aplastic anemia and myeloid leukemogenesis. Benzene and many of its catabolites are directly toxic to stem cells, damage DNA, suppress the supportive function of the bone marrow microenvironment, and accentuate the responsiveness of hematopoietic progenitor cells to intramedullary apoptotic cues that arise during the inflammatory response. Kerosene, carbon-tetrachloride, and chlorophenols contain benzene, as do many other like products used for paint stripping, refinishing, and degreasing (see Table 168-2).

Drugs

Many agents in use for the treatment of malignant diseases are predictably myelosuppressive and can induce aplastic anemia because they are directly toxic to stem and progenitor cells in the marrow (see Table 168-2). These myelosuppressive responses are completely predictable and dose dependent. In practical terms, unless the patient receives a drug overdose or has an undiagnosed genetic disorder that predisposes the patient to respond to the agent in an exaggerated way (e.g., Fanconi anemia [FA]), most patients treated for neoplastic diseases develop reversible bone marrow aplasia or hypoplasia and recover bone marrow function within a matter of days.

Other Aplastic States

Pregnancy

Aplastic anemia can be diagnosed in pregnancy. In addition, some patients with aplastic anemia have become pregnant after the diagnosis. The prognosis in both instances is poor, and most fatal outcomes are due to bleeding complications. Some women, who have been fortunate enough to recover bone marrow function postpartum, develop aplastic anemia with a subsequent pregnancy. The pathogenesis and causal relationship between pregnancy and aplastic anemia remain unknown but may reflect immunologic activation during pregnancy.

Paroxysmal Nocturnal Hemoglobinuria

Paroxysmal nocturnal hemoglobinuria (PNH) is an acquired disorder that results from the expansion of a clone of hematopoietic stem cells whose progeny are incapable of anchoring essential proteins to their membranes (Chapter 163). The defect is caused by an inactivating somatic mutation of *PIGA*, an X-linked gene that encodes a protein essential for synthesis of the membrane anchor glycosyl phosphatidylinositol (GPI). Some of the GPI-anchored proteins (e.g., CD55 and CD59) are important in normal red cells to protect them from activated complement. Their loss results in chronic intravascular hemolysis. Two less clearly defined features of PNH are thromboembolism, of which there is a very high relative risk in the PNH patient population (Chapter 179), and aplastic anemia. The emergence of "PNH clones" is not uncommon in patients with acquired aplastic anemia, and experimental evidence supports the idea that the evolution of *PIGA*-deficient stem cells is an adaptive response to the immune attack. How the *PIGA*-deficient cells fend off cytotoxic T cells is less clear, but it is likely that their pool expands because they accomplish that task somehow. In effect, in the setting of an immune attack, *PIGA*-deficient stem cells are more fit than normal stem cells, but the complement-sensitive red cells to which they give rise have a short lifespan.

Inherited Bone Marrow Failure Syndromes

Some inherited bone marrow failure syndromes can present in adolescence and adulthood. They include dyskeratosis congenita, Fanconi anemia (FA), and Diamond-Blackfan anemia. The molecular pathogenesis of the bone marrow failure seen in these diseases is unclear. Although the genetic basis of these disorders has been well defined in the past decade, the canonical functions of the proteins encoded by these genes is distinct (Table 168-3) for each disease. For example, in dyskeratosis, the mutations occur in genes that encode proteins and RNAs involved in telomere maintenance. In FA, the mutations involve proteins involved in the DNA-damage response, and in

TABLE 168-3 DISTINGUISHING CLINICAL FEATURES OF THE INHERITED BONE MARROW FAILURE SYNDROMES THAT MAY BE INITIALLY DIAGNOSED IN ADULTHOOD

DISTINGUISHING FEATURES	*Diseases*		
	FANCONI ANEMIA	**DYSKERATOSIS CONGENITA**	**DIAMOND-BLACKFAN ANEMIA**
History	Skeletal and renal malformations, low birthweight, pancytopenia, family member with bone marrow failure, myelodysplasia (MDS), acute myelogenous leukemia (AML), or squamous cell carcinoma at an early age. Family member with Fanconi anemia	Intrauterine growth retardation, developmental delay, and short stature. Family history of MDS, AML, marrow failure, abnormal fingernails or toenails, leukoplakia, head and neck cancer, or pulmonary fibrosis	Low birthweight, arm and thumb deformities at birth
Physical findings	Thumb and radial malformations, hyperpigmented skin lesions (cafe au lait spots), short stature, MDS, AML, squamous cell carcinoma at young age, renal and cardiac malformations, microcephaly, hypogonadism	Lacy reticular pigmentation of skin, dystrophic fingernails and toenails, premature graying of hair, hair loss, short stature, oral leukoplakia, squamous cell cancer of head and neck, pulmonary fibrosis, osteopenia, hypogonadism	Triphalangeal thumbs, short stature, arm anomalies
Genes inactivated	*FANCA, FANCB, FANCC, FANCD1* (aka *BRCA2*), *FANCD2, FANCE, FANCF, FANCG* (aka *XRCC9*), *FANCI, FANCJ* (aka *BACH1* and *BRIP1*), *FANCL* (aka *PHF9* and *POG*), *FANCM* (aka *Hef*), and *FANCN* (aka *PALB2*) These genes encode proteins known to protect the genome from excessive damage induced by chemical crosslinking agents. These genes account for most cases of Fanconi anemia.	*DKC1, TERC, TERT, TINF2, NOLA2,* and *NOLA3* These genes encode proteins known to participate in maintenance of telomeres. They account for only half of dyskeratosis cases, so there are additional genes to be discovered.	*RPS17, RPS19, RPS24, RPL5, RPL11,* and *RPL35A* These genes encode ribosomal proteins. They account for only half of cases, so there are additional genes to be discovered.
Screening and diagnostic tests	1. Chromosomal breakage test (in response to mitomycin C or diepoxybutane) 2. Complementation analysis (flow cytometric analysis of G_2 arrest in melphalan-exposed cells after transduction with retroviral vectors expressing normal Fanconi anemia genes) 3. Gene sequencing	1. Quantitative analysis of telomere length ("flow FISH") 2. Gene sequencing	*Note:* Isolated erythroid failure is more common than full blown aplastic anemia. 1. There are no screening tests, although serum ADA is often elevated. 2. Gene sequencing

ADA = adenosine deaminase; FISH = fluorescent in situ hybridization.

Diamond-Blackfan anemia, inactivating mutations involve ribosomal proteins known to be involved in ribosome biogenesis. Whether loss of these canonical functions is linked with the pathogenesis of marrow failure is unclear. In fact, studies on hematopoietic cells have revealed noncanonical functions of some of these proteins. Some of the FA proteins, for example, not only function to protect the genome, but also participate directly in survival signaling pathways for hematopoietic cells. Interestingly, some of the pathways disrupted in mutant cells result in hyperactivation of precisely those same cytokine signaling pathways involved in the pathogenesis of acquired autoimmune aplastic anemia.

Genetics

The genetic basis of inherited bone marrow failure syndromes is being rapidly solved. Some of these syndromes (e.g., Shwachman-Diamond syndrome, amegakaryocytic thrombocytopenia, and severe congenital neutropenia) are almost always diagnosed in early life. However, some may be first diagnosed in adulthood (e.g., dyskeratosis congenita, FA, and Diamond-Blackfan anemia). It is critically important to consider these three disorders early in the evaluation of adults with aplastic anemia because the treatment of such patients with conventional stem cell transplantation regimens is associated with high mortality rates (especially in dyskeratosis congenita and FA). Furthermore, immunosuppressive therapy plays no role in these diseases. The clinical and laboratory manifestations of these three diseases and the findings that should prompt genetic testing in such patients are reviewed in Table 168-3. Importantly, adults who present with these diseases were not born with aplastic anemia. Instead, aplasia develops over time and gives rise to symptoms in adulthood. Prospective studies of children and adults who present with bone marrow failure have indicated that nearly 10% will have previously unsuspected FA.■ Diagnostic consideration of a hereditary form of aplastic anemia should not be limited to children.

CLINICAL MANIFESTATIONS

The natural course of aplastic anemia is influenced by its severity. Patients with hypoplastic bone marrow have severe aplastic anemia if they meet two of the following laboratory criteria: (1) absolute neutrophil count less than 0.5×10^9/L, (2) platelet count less than 20×10^9/L, or (3) reticulocytes less than 20×10^9/L. Patients who do not have severe aplastic anemia often progress to severe aplasia, but the pace is slow (about 40% will have progressed in 5 years). Severe aplastic anemia is a life-threatening condition that, untreated, is associated with a mortality rate of 80% in the 24 months after diagnosis. Treatment of any cohort of patients with severe aplastic anemia will prolong life, and many patients, particularly those who have received stem cell transplants, will be cured.

History

Symptoms of this syndrome, cause notwithstanding, are almost always reflective of low blood counts. The most common presenting symptoms are those associated with thrombocytopenia and anemia. Low platelet counts are associated with bleeding, often epistaxis and bleeding gums, bruising with minor or no trauma, and menorrhagia. Anemia accounts for the nearly universal symptoms of fatigue and dyspnea on mild exertion. Some aplastic patients may present with intercurrent bacterial or fungal infection (because of severe neutropenia), but these cases are less common. Family histories that include any of the features listed in Table 168-3 should raise suspicion of an inherited bone marrow failure syndrome.

Physical Examination

Pallor and tachycardia at rest are common signs of anemia but can be absent or unnoticeable in younger patients and in patients whose aplasia is of very recent onset. Often hemorrhagic manifestations classic for thrombocytopenia are found: petechiae (cutaneous or palatal), ecchymoses, and epistaxis. The most common form of aplastic anemia, autoimmune, is rarely associated with lymphadenopathy or hepatosplenomegaly, and when such findings are present, alternative diagnoses should be considered and painstakingly ruled out. Likewise, short stature, endocrinopathies, osteopenia, findings of developmental anomalies of the skin, nails, hands, or arms, or malformations of the heart, liver, or genitourinary tract should trigger concerns of an inherited bone marrow failure disease (see Table 168-3).

Initial Laboratory Findings

Pancytopenia (anemia, leukopenia, and thrombocytopenia) is a universal presenting finding. The morphology of neutrophils, platelets, and red cells on peripheral blood smear is usually normal unless there is concurrent iron deficiency due to bleeding.

DIAGNOSIS

Diagnostic Evaluation

The evaluation of pancytopenic patients first requires examination of the peripheral blood smear. If there are morphologic or clinical signs of vitamin B_{12} or folic acid deficiency (e.g., hypersegmented neutrophils and oval macrocytes), those disorders should be ruled out because a bone marrow aspiration and biopsy would not be required in those conditions. In severe aplastic anemia, the peripheral blood smear will not show nucleated red blood cells or other signs that the marrow might be infiltrated with abnormal cells. All patients in whom B_{12} and folate deficiency have been ruled out require a bone marrow aspiration and biopsy. Obtaining both types of samples is important. The biopsy best assesses overall bone marrow cellularity and provides the most sensitive evidence for some infiltrative processes. The aspirated sample can be examined microscopically for the presence of abnormal cells but also provides cells for cytogenetic analyses (which can provide evidence supporting hypoplastic myelodysplasia and acute leukemia). Rarely in the early stages of aplasia, the biopsy can be somewhat cellular. A repeat biopsy in 1 to 2 weeks might be required to establish the diagnosis clearly. As summarized in Figure 168-2, once the diagnosis of aplastic anemia has been made, a series of additional tests must be obtained. In light of the life-threatening nature of this disease, the tests must be obtained simultaneously, but they serve three distinct purposes.

Ruling Out Aplastic Anemia Variants that Are Treated Differently

The best therapeutic option for many different aplastic states is often matched sibling donor stem cell transplantation, but there are some aplastic states that are managed differently. For example, a child with an inherited marrow failure syndrome might have a human leukocyte antigen (HLA)-identical sibling who also has the same genetic defect. If such a diagnosis has been overlooked, the recipient will likely die from complications of the conditioning regimen (e.g., patients with FA are highly intolerant of radiation and crosslinking agents used in conventional conditioning regiments, and patients with dyskeratosis suffer excessive post-transplantation morbidity and mortality) or possibly because the transplanted stem cells (from the undiagnosed affected sibling donor) are equally unfit. Patients with dyskeratosis congenita and children with the Shwachman-Diamond syndrome are also intolerant of conventional transplantation regimens and often suffer severe pulmonary and hepatic toxicity. Although patients with Diamond-Blackfan anemia are more tolerant of standard conditioning regimens, they are more apt to respond to glucocorticosteroid therapy, and if they are transplanted with stem cells from an undiagnosed affected sibling, they too will do poorly. Finally, patients with PNH should be identified using flow cytometric quantification of CD55- and CD59-deficient red cells because more than half of patients with severe aplastic anemia will have PNH clones; when treated with immunosuppressive therapy, the PNH clone often expands and causes clinically significant signs of PNH (hemolysis and thrombosis).

Tests Helpful in Supportive Care

At some point during the course of the disease, red cell and platelet transfusions will be necessary. Radiated and filtered blood products are used to prevent transfusion-associated graft-versus-host disease (GVHD), reduce alloimmunization, and reduce the complication of cytomegalovirus (CMV) infection. ABO and HLA typing are required. Infections can be of bacterial, viral, or fungal origin and must be quickly diagnosed and treated not only because the patients are often neutropenic but also because, once definitive therapy begins, it is likely they will be receiving immunosuppressive therapy (either through primary immunosuppression or through stem cell transplantation). In the acutely infected, severely neutropenic patient, once cultures and biopsies are obtained, empirical antibiotic therapy should be prescribed even before the culture results are available. Post-transplantation CMV infection is best avoided in CMV-seronegative recipients by using CMV-negative blood products (Chapter 180). Many centers routinely infuse radiated and filtered ("CMV-safe") blood products and therefore no longer routinely screen for CMV seronegativity.

Evaluating the Patient as a Candidate for Stem Cell Transplantation

Timing of treatment depends on the severity of the aplastic anemia and the age of the patient (Table 168-4). Patients with mild marrow hypoplasia and mild bone marrow suppression can be followed closely to determine what the pace of hypoplasia might be. In patients up to 40 years of age with either severe acquired aplastic anemia or transfusion dependence, steps should be taken to evaluate them promptly for stem cell transplantation therapy by seeking HLA-identical siblings and, in appropriate cases, searching for matched unrelated donors.

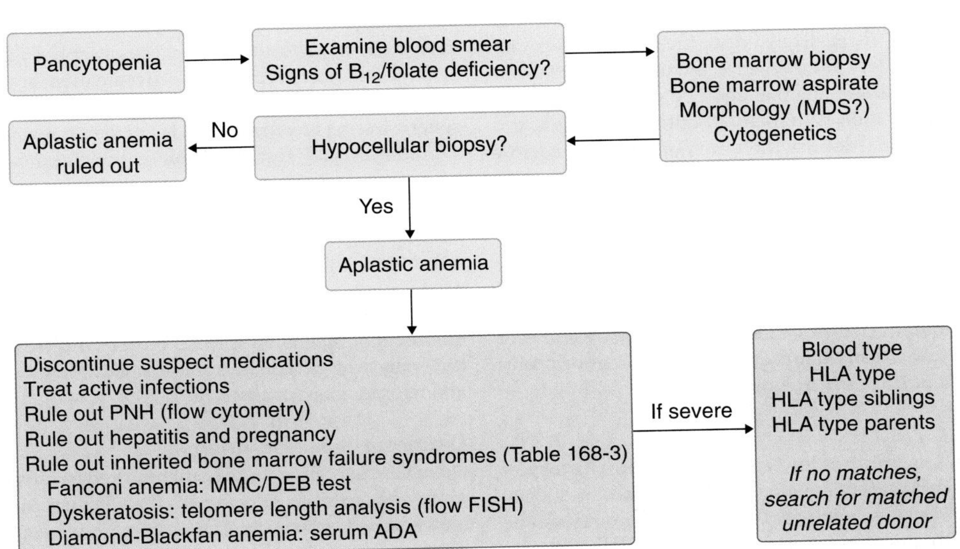

FIGURE 168-2. A pathway for the diagnostic management of patients with aplastic anemia. Patients who present with pancytopenia will require bone marrow biopsy and aspiration unless there are signs of vitamin B_{12} or folate deficiency. If the bone marrow is as cellular as that shown in Fig. 168-1A, the diagnosis of aplastic anemia has been effectively ruled out because the diagnosis requires bone marrow hypocellularity (see Fig. 168-1B). In all patients, regardless of severity, suspect medications should be discontinued, active infections should be treated without delay, and paroxysmal nocturnal hemoglobinuria (PNH) should be excluded, as should pregnancy and hepatitis. For patients with positive family histories or any one of the findings listed in Table 168-3, and all patients younger than 40 years, inherited marrow failure syndromes should be ruled out with screening tests. Patients with severe aplastic anemia are those who have at least two of the following: absolute neutrophil count of less than 0.5×10^9/L, platelet count of less than 20×10^9/L, or reticulocyte count of less than 20×10^9/L. These patients must be treated with definitive therapy and should be evaluated for stem cell transplantation with human leukocyte antigen (HLA) typing (patient and family members) and, if necessary, a search for matched unrelated donors. ADA = adenosine deaminase; DEB = diepoxybutane; FISH = fluorescent in situ hybridization; MDS = myelodysplasia; MMC = mitomycin C.

TABLE 168-4 TREATMENT RECOMMENDATIONS FOR PATIENTS WITH SEVERE ACQUIRED IDIOPATHIC APLASTIC ANEMIA*

	AGE < 20 YR		AGE 20-40 YR		AGE > 40 YR	
HLA-identical sibling?	Yes	No	Yes	No	Yes	No
First-line treatment	MSBMT	IST	MSBMT	IST	IST	IST
Second-line treatment	IST or second MSBMT	IST or MUDT or CBT	IST	IST or MUDT	MSBMT	IST. For failures, consider MUDT.

*This general set of recommendations cannot be applied to patients with inherited bone marrow failure syndromes because they do not respond to immunosuppressive therapy (IST).
CBT = umbilical cord blood transplantation; IST = immunosuppressive therapy; MSBMT = matched sibling bone marrow transplant; MUDT = matched unrelated donor transplant.
Adapted from Bacigalupo A, Passweg J. Diagnosis and treatment of acquired aplastic anemia. *Hematol Oncol Clin North Am.* 2009;23:159-170.

Differential Diagnosis

Most classic aplastic anemia patients have immunologically mediated disease. Notwithstanding strong evidence in support of this mechanism from some research laboratories over the past 30 years, there exists no validated screening tool that can either rule in or rule out immune-mediated disease, a fact that is complicated by the evidence that some cases of drug- and virus-induced disease are also immunologically mediated. Therefore, idiopathic autoimmune aplastic anemia remains a diagnosis of exclusion. For this reason, the obligation of the diagnostician is to consider disease induced by chemical or viral agents and radiation and disease associated with pregnancy. It is also most important to rule out PNH and inherited bone marrow failure syndromes (see Fig. 168-2).

Cytotoxic Drugs, Chemicals, and Radiation

A fastidiously obtained medication history is important. Any drug with the potential of inducing aplastic anemia should be discontinued. It is equally important to ask patients about alternative therapies that they might not consider being "medicines." Some herbal remedies are known to contain molecules (e.g., phenylbutazone) not listed on the label but associated with aplasia (see Table 168-2). A history of exposure to radiation or to chemicals with myelosuppressive capacities (see Table 168-2) should likewise be obtained. Tests for benzene metabolites detect only acute exposure and are not reliable indicators of cumulative exposure in individual patients. Although it is intuitively obvious and prudent to discontinue the use of agents that might have inflicted severe stem cell injury, by the time the injury has progressed to the point of severe aplastic anemia, most of these patients are in need of the same types of therapy prescribed for patients with autoimmune aplastic anemia.

Idiosyncratic Drug Responses

If a medication history unearths an exposure to an agent known to be associated with idiosyncratic (not related to dose) responses, the agent must likewise be discontinued. Because it is likely that these responses are immunologically mediated, the patient should be treated no differently from patients with severe idiopathic aplastic anemia, and the patient should be evaluated as a stem cell transplantation candidate. If, during the diagnostic evaluation of the patient and potential donors, there are signs that the marrow is recovering on its own, a more conservative approach can be taken.

Paroxysmal Nocturnal Hemoglobinuria

PNH can be ruled out by screening for CD55 and CD59 on the surface of granulocytes, monocytes, and red cells using flow cytometry. The proper diagnosis of PNH requires the absence of these or other GPI-anchored proteins on at least two hematopoietic cell types. Other characteristic features of this syndrome can be a high low-density lipoprotein level, high indirect bilirubin, low haptoglobin, and a positive urine hemosiderin test.

Fanconi Anemia

FA should be considered in any adult of any age with a family history of aplastic anemia, acute myelogenous leukemia or myelodysplasia, or a squamous cell carcinoma at an unusually young age. This disease should also be considered in any patient with any physical finding listed in Table 168-3 or in patients with a family member who has any of these findings. Unfortunately, some patients with FA meet none of these standards, so some hematologists advocate testing for it in all patients with aplastic anemia patients who are younger than 40 years. This disease can be ruled out by obtaining a chromosomal breakage test (see Table 168-3). Here, either lymphocytes or skin fibroblasts are exposed to mitomycin C or diepoxybutane for a period of 2 to 3 days, after which metaphase chromosomes are examined for chromosomal breaks and quadriradial forms (in FA cells, these four-armed interchromosomal forms involve at least two chromosomal breaks). If the clinical context is suggestive (see Table 168-3), but results of the lymphocyte chromosomal breakage test are negative or equivocal, testing of skin fibroblasts is required to rule out the diagnosis. Once the diagnosis is made, history, physical examination, blood counts, and chromosomal breakage tests should be performed on all immediate family members.

There are at least 13 different FA genes (see Table 168-3), and sequencing them all using cells from every patient is not practical at this time. Fortunately, the involved gene can be first identified by a variety of more affordable complementation analyses. In this type of test, normal FA genes are introduced into primary cells of the patient in vitro, and the one gene that corrects the defect (i.e. ,reduces hypersensitivity to cross-linking agents [melphalan, mitomycin C, or diepoxybutane]) represents the gene of interest. That gene can then be fully sequenced to identify the precise mutation, information that will be of value to family members for family planning purposes. In rare instances, it can also aid in applying preimplantation genetic diagnosis and in vitro fertilization, a process that has successfully resulted in unaffected offspring and ideal cord-blood stem cell donors for transplantation of an affected sibling.

Dyskeratosis Congenita

Dyskeratosis congenita should be considered in any aplastic adult of any age with a family member who has had aplastic anemia. It should be likewise considered if either the patient or a family member has had acute myelogenous leukemia, myelodysplasia, nail dystrophy, lacy skin pigmentation, pulmonary fibrosis, oral leukoplakia, squamous cell carcinoma at an unusually young age, or any other physical finding listed in Table 168-3. This disease can be frequently ruled out by quantifying the length of telomeres in circulating white cells using a flow cytometric method. Because some of the physical findings overlap, FA should be ruled out in all patients being evaluated for dyskeratosis congenita. The dyskeratosis test quantifies telomere length using fluorescence in situ hybridization. Lymphocytes from dyskeratosis patients have extremely short telomeres (i.e., at or less than the 1st percentile). If two or three leukocyte types from a given patient are above the 1st percentile, the diagnosis of dyskeratosis is unlikely. If telomeres are in the diagnostic range, genetic testing is warranted. It is not yet known whether this test will become a "gold-standard" test as reliable as the chromosomal breakage test is for FA because some investigators report that very short telomeres can be found in patients who have other causes of bone marrow failure. Unlike the genetic strategy employed with FA (at least today), complementation analyses are not routinely performed in dyskeratosis. The molecular diagnosis is based on gene sequencing. Once the diagnosis is made and even before the establishment of a molecular genetic diagnosis (see Table 168-3), all immediate family members of the patient should be seen individually, their history taken, and their physical examination performed along with peripheral blood counts and telomere length analysis.

Diamond-Blackfan Anemia

Diamond-Blackfan anemia is an inherited bone marrow failure syndrome that more often exhibits selective erythroid failure and is an unusual cause of full-blown severe aplastic anemia. Although some patients can present in adulthood, most are discovered within the first year of life and present with anemia but less commonly neutropenia and thrombocytopenia. Phenotypic abnormalities like short stature and skeletal defects are the exception in this disease. There are no screening tests as reliable as those used for FA and dyskeratosis congenita. However, in patients with unexplained erythroid failure, the finding of an elevated adenosine deaminase level in the serum, although unexplained, is strongly suggestive of this disease. Because no helpful screening test exists, there are no reliable or standardized complementation tests.

Consequently, genetic diagnosis requires the application of gene sequencing methods (see Table 168-3).

Other Diagnostic Considerations

Aplastic anemia has been reported in recipients of organ allografts (in which mismatched T cells [either from the donated graft or from blood products that had not been irradiated] induce severe aplasia), patients with myelodysplasia (Chapter 188), patients with congenital and acquired immunodeficiency states (Chapter 258), and patients with established autoimmune diseases including systemic lupus erythematosus (Chapter 274) and eosinophilic fasciitis (Chapter 448), a disease characterized by painful swelling of the skin and subcutaneous tissue.

TREATMENT

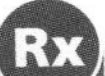

For patients with more mild forms of aplastic anemia, aggressive therapy may not be indicated. A passive approach is more problematic in patients with FA and dyskeratosis congenita because transplantation early in life is better tolerated, immunosuppressive therapy is ineffective, and stem cell transplantation provides the only hope for cure of bone marrow failure. If there is evidence of an underlying autoimmune-mediated disease (e.g., isolated granulopoietic or erythroid failure in patients with rheumatic diseases or thymoma), immunosuppressive therapy alone is often highly effective.

Hematopoietic Stem Cell Transplantation: Matched Sibling Donor

For patients with severe aplastic anemia, stem cell transplantation offers the advantages of immunosuppression, an infusion of new "healthy" stem cells, and the expectation that the lymphoid cells that suppressed the marrow in the first place will be replaced by more normal cells that have no myelosuppressive capacity. This expectation is borne out by large retrospective studies indicating the superiority of stem cell transplantation over immunosuppressive therapy alone in the treatment of severe aplastic anemia. Naturally, this approach is relevant to a minority of patients because only 25 to 30% will have an HLA-matched sibling.

Stem cells derived from the bone marrow, not the peripheral blood, should be the source of donor cells. Studies testing the comparative effectiveness of peripheral blood as a source of stem cells demonstrated that the peripheral blood source was associated with excess mortality stemming from an increased incidence of chronic GVHD. The recipient (in whom congenital marrow failure syndromes have been ruled out) initially receives high-dose cyclophosphamide with antithymocyte globulin (ATG) as the preparative regimen. Immunosuppressive therapy begins 2 to 4 days before infusion of stem cells. Common post-transplantation immunosuppression combines cyclosporine and methotrexate. The complication of graft failure with this approach is infrequently seen (<5%), grades II to IV acute GVHD is seen in 30 to 50% of recipients, 25% have chronic GVHD, and short-term (2-year) survival after transplantation is nearly 90%. Ten-year survival rates are highly age dependent: 83%, 73%, and 68% for recipients in the first, second, and third decades of life, respectively. In patients 40 years of age or older, the 10-year survival rate is only 51%. Treatment choices adjusted for patient age are presented in Table 168-4.

Hematopoietic Stem Cell Transplantation: Matched Unrelated Donor

The use of bone marrow from an HLA-matched unrelated donor should be considered for patients who have no HLA-identical siblings, have failed immunosuppressive therapy, and are refractory to transfused platelets. Results have not been as favorable as those associated with the use of marrow from HLA-identical siblings, but this strategy has improved in the past decade in part because of more accurate selection of HLA-matched donors and in part because of adjustments made with pretransplantation conditioning regimens. In fact, in some pediatric populations, some centers are now reporting identical outcomes in children transplanted with marrow cells from HLA-matched related and matched unrelated donors. Conditioning regimens without ATG are associated with inferior outcomes, and less toxic conditioning regimens appear to have improved survival (65% for patients older than 16 years and 75% for those 16 years of age or younger). The improvements have been encouraging enough to recommend strongly that unrelated donor searches be initiated at the time of diagnosis for any patient younger than 30 years. Adults older than 30 years should be considered candidates for alternative donor stem cell transplantation if they have failed two attempts at immunosuppressive therapy because newer fludarabine-based conditioning regimens have improved outcomes of matched unrelated donor transplants remarkably.

Immunosuppressive Therapy

Treatment with ATG alone prolongs survival when compared with supportive care alone, and for patients with mild aplastic anemia (not severe), either no treatment or ATG alone is sufficient. In patients with severe aplastic anemia, however, the combination of ATG and cyclosporine is superior to treatment with ATG alone.[1] The combination reduces mortality and induces more rapid and higher overall response rates than does ATG as a single agent. Doses vary from center to center, but ATG is given at doses of 12 to 40 mg/kg/day for 4 to 5 days, and cyclosporine doses of 5 to 10 mg/kg/day (targeting blood levels of 150 to 250 ng/mL) are prescribed for 6 months, after which cyclosporine is slowly tapered over a period of 1 year or more. The median time to response is 120 days. Complete responses are defined as the resolution of pancytopenia and the development of normal blood counts. Relapses are uncommon in complete responders (10%). Partial responders are those whose counts do not normalize but who no longer require transfusion support. Forty to 60% of these patients will relapse in 5 years, but most will respond to a repeat course of immunosuppressive therapy. Some will require chronic immunosuppressive therapy with cyclosporine to remain transfusion independent. Those with unresponsive relapses have a poor prognosis.

All age groups can benefit from immunosuppressive therapy. Long-term survival rates do vary with the age of the treated population. In patients younger than 20 years, 10-year survival rates are 80%, but these rates progressively decline to 25% in patients older than 70 years. However, when adjusted for the survival of an age-matched population using the standardized mortality ratio, the corrected risk for death is highest in young patients and declines as age increases. Advanced age is not a contraindication for the prescription of immunosuppressive therapy.

There are some caveats of importance related to the use of immunosuppressive therapy in aplastic anemia patients. First, patients may experience allergic reactions during infusions of ATG. This should not necessarily dissuade one from continuing this agent. Slowing the infusion after premedication with glucocorticosteroids and antihistamines often solves this problem. Fever and rigor can be signs of cytokine release from the targeted T-cell pool, so they likewise should not be used as a reason to stop treatment. Second, if a responsive patient later relapses, a second course of ATG is frequently effective and should be used. Third, it seems clear that a long interval between diagnosis of aplastic anemia and the initiation of immunosuppressive therapy is a negative predictor of response. Treatment should begin as soon as possible; certainly within 3 weeks of initial diagnosis. Fourth, the inclusion of hematopoietic growth factors during immunosuppressive therapy provides no benefit.[2]

Diamond-Blackfan Anemia and Pure Red Cell Aplasia

Although the mechanism by which glucocorticosteroids induce remissions in patients with Diamond-Blackfan anemia is unknown, nearly 80% of patients initially respond. Prednisone treatment is started at 2 mg/kg/day and is tapered after the hemoglobin increases to 10 g/dL. Most patients require a low every-other-day dose, but 15% remain in remission off steroids altogether. In those cases, survival to age 40 years is nearly universal. Of patients who require ongoing steroid support, 75% reach age 40 years. Only half of the patients with steroid-resistant severe anemia survive to age 40 years. Pure red cell aplasia may respond to a synthetic erythropoietin receptor agonist.

Supportive Care

Platelet Transfusions

In the absence of bleeding or infection, platelet transfusions are commonly administered only when the platelet count declines to 10,000/mL or less, but in the presence of active infection or bleeding, transfusion thresholds are often set at 20,000/mL or higher. If bleeding and infection coexist, it is prudent to rule out disseminated intravascular coagulation because fresh-frozen plasma or cryoprecipitate may be required along with platelet transfusions. Drugs (e.g., aspirin) that inhibit platelet function must be avoided, as should activities that might result in trauma. Menstrual activity should be suppressed with oral contraceptives or other agents.

Red Cell Transfusions

Filtered packed red blood cells should be provided to meet the needs of the patient's daily activities. There is no established hemoglobin target number for this purpose, but as a general rule, the number is higher in elderly patients than in young patients. Children with hemoglobin levels of as low as 6 g/dL can compensate reasonably. Adults with underlying cardiopulmonary disease may have symptomatic anemia at 8 g/dL. If chronic transfusion therapy is required, the development of iron overload may require chelation therapy.

Management of Infections

The major infectious challenges result from the immunosuppression used (either as primary therapy or as a component of a stem cell transplantation regimen) more than the neutropenia. For that reason, antibacterial, antiviral, and antifungal prophylaxis is routinely used in transplant recipients. In many centers, patients treated with immunosuppressive therapy alone are treated similarly for a 2- to 3-month period following ATG administration. Importantly, the onset of fever requires prompt clinical evaluation and antibiotic therapy as described in Chapter 289.

PREVENTION

Apart from public health measures controlling exposures to benzene, aromatic hydrocarbons, and radiation, little can be done to prevent acquired aplastic anemia. In the inherited bone marrow failure syndromes, prevention is quite achievable. Once the proband is identified, other affected family members, carriers, and siblings with no mutant allele can be identified, and genetic results can be applied in family planning even to the extent of preimplantation genetic diagnosis followed by in vitro fertilization. Because all somatic cells of children and adults with FA are hypersensitive to alkylating agents and oxidative stress, they must not receive standard doses of radiation or alkylating agents either for transplant conditioning or for treatment of squamous cell carcinoma.

Clonal evolution (e.g., to myelodysplasia and acute leukemia) occurs in 10 to 20% of patients with acquired aplastic anemia survivors and up to 40% of children and adults with dyskeratosis congenita and FA. This complication likely evolves through a process of clonal selection and adaptation and for that reason is seen less commonly in completely responsive patients than in those with less than complete responses (who therefore have ongoing suppression of hematopoiesis). This suggests that more effective strategies of immunosuppressive therapy may better control ongoing marrow damage and decrease the incidence of clonal evolution.

PROGNOSIS

Acquired Idiopathic Aplastic Anemia

The severity of aplastic anemia and age are key determinants of long-term survival. Both these factors influence the choice of therapy (see Table 168-4). Early intervention is associated with a better prognosis, which should inform the pace of diagnostic evaluation. Matched sibling donor transplants are associated with higher response rates, lower relapse rates, long-term survival rates approximating 80%, and a lower incidence of clonal evolution. Immunosuppressive therapy is associated with long-term (10-year) survival rates of 70 to 75% in responders. Infection represents the most common cause of death in patients of any age treated with either immunosuppression alone or stem cell transplantation.

Inherited Bone Marrow Failure Syndromes

Patients with dyskeratosis congenita and FA will not respond to immunosuppressive therapy. Stem cell transplantation with nonmyeloablative approaches has the potential of curing the marrow failure component of these diseases. There are good theoretical reasons for anticipating that successful transplantation will reduce the likelihood of clonal evolution to myelodysplasia and acute leukemia. Unfortunately, the decision to transplant is influenced by other key factors, as described earlier. In light of these complexities, no clear-cut when-to-transplant rule can be applied to all patients with these diseases. Taking these difficult issues into account, all patients should be evaluated early in an experienced transplantation center, and family members should be screened by hematologists, geneticists, and genetic counselors using specialty laboratories.

In patients with dyskeratosis, small case series report good outcomes after fludarabine-containing nonmyeloablative conditioning regimens, but studies of sufficient size are not available to permit concrete recommendations except that patients should be referred to an experienced center. In patients with FA, with proper conditioning regimens, matched sibling donor transplant recipients have expected 3-year survival rates of about 85% and matched unrelated recipients (when fludarabine containing nonmyeloablative approaches are used) have 3-year survival rates of 50%. In patients with Diamond-Blackfan anemia, sibling donor transplant recipients have 3-year survival rates of about 80%, but disease-free survival rates after matched unrelated donor transplants have been poor (20 to 30%).

Future Treatments

For patients with acquired aplastic anemia, studies designed to selectively target the T-cell clones responsible for hematopoietic suppression may provide more effective and less toxic strategies for immunosuppressive therapy. For all patients with aplastic anemia, further improvements in matched unrelated transplantation should make this modality more widely available for patients who are not now considered optimal candidates. GVHD control will continue to improve. For children with nonsevere aplastic anemia, the 10-year progression-free survival rate is only about 25%, suggesting that prospective trials of early intervention are warranted. For patients with inherited bone marrow failure syndromes, the genes for which have been largely identified, the possibility of stem cell gene therapy holds enormous theoretical promise.

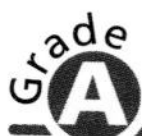

1. Gafter-Gvili A, Ram R, Gurion R, et al. ATG plus cyclosporine reduces all-cause mortality in patients with severe aplastic anemia: systematic review and meta-analysis. *Acta Haematol.* 2008;120:237-243.
2. Gurion R, Gafter-Gvili A, Vial PM, et al. Hematopoietic growth factors in aplastic anemia patients treated with immunosuppressive therapy: systematic review and meta-analysis. *Haematologica.* 2009;94:712-719.

SUGGESTED READINGS

Auerbach AD. Fanconi anemia and its diagnosis. *Mutat Res.* 2009;668:4-10. *A comprehensive, thoughtful up-to-date review of this disease by one of the founders of modern Fanconi anemia research.*

Gafter-Gvili A, Ram R, Raanani P, et al. Management of aplastic anemia: the role of systematic reviews and meta-analyses. *Acta Haematol.* 2011;125:47-54. *Review of hematopoietic cell transplantation, immunosuppressive therapy, hematopoietic growth factors, and supportive care.*

Kwon JH, Kim I, Lee YG, et al. Clinical course of non-severe aplastic anemia in adults. *Int J Hematol.* 2010;91:770-775. *About 20% of patients progress to severe disease, especially those with more severe initial abnormalities.*

Leguit RJ, van den Tweel JG. The pathology of bone marrow failure. *Histopathology.* 2010;57:655-670. *Review.*

Macdougall IC, Rossert J, Casadevall N, et al. A peptide-based erythropoietin-receptor agonist for pure red-cell aplasia. *N Engl J Med.* 2009;361:1848-1855. *A synthetic peptide-based erythropoietin-receptor agonist was effective for the treatment of anemia in pure red-cell aplasia, with 13 of 14 patients no longer requiring regular transfusions.*

Risitano AM. Immunosuppressive therapies in the management of immune-mediated marrow failure in adults: where we stand and where we are going. *Br J Haematol.* 2011;152:127-140. *Review of the pathophysiology and treatment of immune-mediated bone marrow failure states, with a comprehensive list of new immunosuppressive agents in various stages of clinical trial development.*

169 POLYCYTHEMIAS, ESSENTIAL THROMBOCYTHEMIA, AND PRIMARY MYELOFIBROSIS

AYALEW TEFFERI

DEFINITION

Polycythemia vera (PV), essential thrombocythemia (ET), and primary myelofibrosis (PMF) are categorized as myeloproliferative neoplasms (MPNs) in the 2008 World Health Organization (WHO) classification system for hematologic malignancies (Table 169-1). These disorders represent hematopoietic bone marrow stem cell–derived clonal myeloproliferations with a propensity to evolve into acute myeloid leukemia (also called blast-phase MPN). These three clinicopathologic entities, together with

TABLE 169-1 2008 WORLD HEALTH ORGANIZATION CLASSIFICATION OF MYELOID NEOPLASMS

1. Myeloproliferative neoplasms (MPNs)
   - 1.1. Chronic myelogenous leukemia, *BCR-ABL1* positive (CML)
   - 1.2. Polycythemia vera (PV)
   - 1.3. Essential thrombocythemia (ET)
   - 1.4. Primary myelofibrosis (PMF)
   - 1.5. Chronic neutrophilic leukemia (CNL)
   - 1.6. Chronic eosinophilic leukemia, not otherwise specified (CEL-NOS) (Chapter 173)
   - 1.7. Mast cell disease (MCD) (Chapter 263)
   - 1.8. MPN, unclassifiable (MPN-U)
2. Myeloid and lymphoid neoplasms with eosinophilia and abnormalities of *PDGFRA, PDGFRB*, or *FGFR1* (Chapter 173)
3. Myelodysplastic syndromes (MDS)/MPN
   - 3.1. Chronic myelomonocytic leukemia (CMML) (Chapter 190)
   - 3.2. Juvenile myelomonocytic leukemia (JMML)
   - 3.3. Atypical chronic myeloid leukemia, *BCR-ABL1* negative (aCML) (Chapter 190)
   - 3.4. MDS/MPN, unclassifiable
4. Myelodysplastic syndromes (MDS) (Chapter 188)
5. Acute myeloid leukemia (AML) and related neoplasms (Chapter 189)

chronic myelogenous leukemia (Chapter 190), used to be referred to as *myeloproliferative disorders*. Because chronic myelogenous leukemia is invariably linked to the Philadelphia translocation (i.e., *BCR-ABL1*), PV, ET, and PMF are operationally labeled *BCR-ABL1–negative MPNs*.

EPIDEMIOLOGY

Incidence figures for *BCR-ABL1*–negative MPNs are estimated at 0.2 to 2.5 per 100,000 for ET, 0.4 to 1.5 per 100,000 for PMF, and 0.8 to 2.6 per 100,000 for PV. The median age at diagnosis for all three MPNs is usually reported as 60 years, but population-based studies report a substantially older age. Family studies suggest a five- to seven-fold increased risk of MPN among first-degree relatives of patients with *BCR-ABL1*–negative MPN; the possibility of there being a hereditary component to disease susceptibility has been further supported by *JAK2* haplotype studies. ET appears to be more common in young women, but this gender imbalance is not as clear in other age groups. PMF has been associated with exposure to ionizing radiation (e.g., in Hiroshima survivors), heavy exposure to petroleum derivatives, and thorium dioxide (Thorotrast) contrast medium, but in the vast majority of cases there is no such exposure history.

PATHOBIOLOGY

The clonal nature of PV, ET, and PMF was established between 1976 and 1981 using glucose-6-phosphate dehydrogenase isoenzyme analysis. These diseases are now believed to derive from a genetically transformed bone marrow stem cell resulting in either monoclonal or oligoclonal myeloproliferation. In 2005, a *JAK2* gain-of-function mutation (*JAK2*V617F) was reported in *BCR-ABL1*–negative MPN, and subsequent studies using sensitive assays have revealed the presence of this mutation in approximately 95% of patients with PV and 60% of those with ET or PMF. Most of the remaining 5% of patients with PV carry another *JAK2* mutation (*JAK2* exon 12), whereas approximately 5 to 15% of *JAK2*V617F-negative patients with ET or PMF carry a *MPL*W515 mutation. All these mutations relate to the JAK-STAT intracellular signaling pathway in hematopoietic cells. The JAK-STAT pathway is normally activated by the occupancy of hematopoietic growth factor receptors (the receptor and the thrombopoietin receptor, also known as MPL) by their respective ligands (erythropoietin [Epo], thrombopoietin). Both *JAK2* and *MPL* mutations are also seen, albeit much less frequently, in other myeloid neoplasms. More recently, additional mutations have been described in PV, ET, and PMF and involve *TET2, ASXL1, CBL, IDH, IKZF1*, and *LNK* (Table 169-2). Most of these mutations originate at the progenitor cell level, but they do not necessarily represent the primary clonogenic event, are not mutually exclusive, and do not follow a predictable hierarchy.

The aforementioned molecular alterations in *BCR-ABL1*–negative MPN induce biologic changes that are demonstrated in animal models or ex vivo. For example, *JAK2* or *MPL* mutations induce PV-, ET-, or PMF-like diseases in mice by experimental manipulation of the mutant allele burden. These mutations are also believed to contribute to the growth factor independence or hypersensitivity of erythroid or megakaryocyte colony-forming progenitor cells and the accumulation of anti-apoptotic proteins such as Bcl-X_L. Bone marrow fibrosis, osteosclerosis, and angiogenesis in PMF are currently believed to be reactive and mediated by cytokines; that is, fibroblast proliferation in the bone marrow of patients with PMF is not a primary part of the clonal process.

TABLE 169-2 NOVEL MUTATIONS IN POLYCYTHEMIA VERA, ESSENTIAL THROMBOCYTHEMIA, PRIMARY MYELOFIBROSIS, AND BLAST-PHASE MYELOPROLIFERATIVE NEOPLASM

MUTATION	CHROMOSOME LOCATION	APPROXIMATE MUTATIONAL FREQUENCY (%)	PATHOGENETIC RELEVANCE
*JAK2*V617F exon 14 (Janus kinase 2)	9p24	PV: 96 ET: 55 PMF: 65 Blast-phase MPN: 50	Believed to contribute to myeloproliferation and progenitor cell growth factor hypersensitivity
JAK2 exon 12	9p24	PV: 3 ET: rare PMF: rare Blast-phase MPN: ?	Believed to contribute to primarily erythroid myeloproliferation
MPL exon 10 (myeloproliferative leukemia virus oncogene; encodes for thrombopoietin receptor)	1p34	PV: rare ET: 3 PMF: 10 Blast-phase MPN: ?	Believed to contribute to primarily megakaryocytic myeloproliferation
TET2 (mutations occur across several of the gene's 12 exons; TET oncogene family member 2)	4q24	PV: 16 ET: 5 PMF: 17 Blast-phase MPN: 17	Might contribute to epigenetic modulation of transcription (TET1 catalyzes conversion of 5-methylcytosine to 5-hydroxymethylcytosine)
ASXL1 exon 12 (Additional Sex Combs-Like 1)	20q11.1	PV: ? ET: ? PMF: ? Blast-phase MPN: 19	Believed to affect regulation of transcription and RAR-mediated signaling
CBL exons 8 and 9 (Casitas B-lineage lymphoma proto-oncogene)	11q23.3	PV: rare ET: rare PMF: 6 Blast-phase MPN: ?	Believed to alter the regulatory function of wild-type CBL against kinase signaling because of defective ubiquitylation of oncoproteins
IDH1/IDH2 exon 4/exon 4 (isocitrate dehydrogenase)	2q33.3/15q26.1	PV: rare ET: rare PMF: 4 Blast-phase MPN: 20	Induces accumulation of 2-hydroxyglutarate, a possible oncoprotein
IKZF1 (mostly deletions, including intragenic; IKAROS family zinc finger 1)	7p12	PV: rare ET: rare PMF: rare Blast-phase MPN: 19	Not clear at this point
LNK exon 2 (encodes a membrane-bound adaptor protein)	12q24.12	PV: rare ET: rare PMF: rare Blast-phase MPN: 10	Wild-type is a negative regulator of JAK2 signaling

ET = essential thrombocythemia; MPN = myeloproliferative neoplasm; PMF = primary myelofibrosis; PV = polycythemia vera; RAR = retinoic acid receptor.

TABLE 169-3 CLINICAL AND LABORATORY FEATURES OF POLYCYTHEMIA VERA

Persistent leukocytosis
Persistent thrombocytosis
Microcytosis secondary to iron deficiency
Increased leukocyte alkaline phosphatase
Splenomegaly
Generalized pruritus (usually after bathing)
Unusual thrombosis (e.g., Budd-Chiari syndrome)
Erythromelalgia (acral dysesthesia and erythema; see Fig. 169-1)

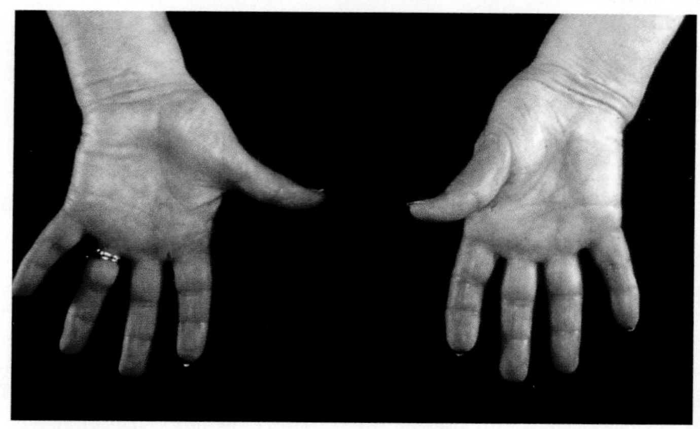

FIGURE 169-1. Erythromelalgia—a painful red discoloration of the hands or toes.

CLINICAL MANIFESTATIONS

Polycythemia Vera

Table 169-3 lists the typical clinical and laboratory features of PV. Increased red cell mass in PV might result in blood hyperviscosity, which leads to a plethora of symptoms and signs. Headaches are frequent, but blurry vision, altered hearing, mucous membrane bleeding, shortness of breath, and malaise are also observed. At least two thirds of PV patients have splenomegaly. Thrombosis occurs in about 40% of patients, most commonly arterial thrombosis. As in ET, venous thrombosis can occur in unusual sites, such as mesenteric or hepatic vessels, and hepatic vein thrombosis (Budd-Chiari syndrome) or portal vein thrombosis (Chapter 145) may be the presenting manifestation before the full hematologic picture of PV has emerged. Bleeding, especially gastrointestinal, is seen in PV, but it is less common than thrombosis. Pruritus is common in PV and may be provoked by warm water ("aquagenic"). Erythromelalgia (described later under Essential Thrombocythemia) may trouble some patients with PV, as do other vasomotor symptoms such as paresthesias and headaches.

Essential Thrombocythemia

At presentation, microvascular and vasomotor symptoms are found in 25 to 50% of ET patients. Major thrombosis is seen in 11 to 25% of patients at diagnosis and in 10 to 22% during follow-up; major hemorrhage is observed in 2 to 5% at diagnosis and in 1 to 7% during follow-up. Vasomotor disturbances (e.g., headaches, lightheadedness, visual symptoms such as blurring and scotomata, palpitations, chest pain, erythromelalgia, distal paresthesias) are not infrequent in ET and might be the result of abnormal platelet-endothelium interactions. Erythromelalgia (Fig. 169-1) is the most dramatic vasomotor symptom, characterized by erythema, warmth, and pain in the distal extremities; this symptom is rare but not entirely specific for ET. Splenomegaly is found in about 40% of patients with ET, but it is usually not prominent. Life-threatening complications of ET include large-vessel thrombosis (both arterial and venous), hemorrhage, and transformation of the disease into either a fibrotic phase resembling PMF or acute myeloid leukemia. Venous thrombosis in ET occurs both in sites common to other thrombotic diatheses (e.g., pulmonary embolism, lower extremity deep vein thrombosis) and in more unusual sites (e.g., cerebral sinus thrombosis, retinal vein thrombosis, hepatic and portal vein thrombosis).

Major hemorrhage in ET is most common in the gastrointestinal tract and may be precipitated by aspirin or other nonsteroidal anti-inflammatory drugs. Hemorrhage also occurs in the central nervous system and the retina, but such events are, fortunately, uncommon. Paradoxically, patients with extreme thrombocytosis may be at special risk for bleeding, in part related to the development of an acquired von Willebrand syndrome (Chapter 176) that is thought to be related to the adsorption of large multimers of von Willebrand protein from plasma onto the large number of abnormal circulating platelets. Fibrotic and leukemic transformations of ET are rare events (<5% of patients) during the first 10 years after diagnosis, but the risk increases with time.

Primary Myelofibrosis

Most patients with PMF present with anemia and marked splenomegaly. The anemia of PMF is multifactorial. Contributing factors include ineffective hematopoiesis and hypersplenism. Spleen and liver enlargement in PMF is secondary to extramedullary hematopoiesis (EMH) and may be associated with hypercatabolic symptoms including profound fatigue, weight loss, night sweats, and low-grade fever. Patients also experience peripheral edema, diarrhea, early satiety, and, occasionally, complications of portal hypertension, including variceal bleeding and ascites.

Splenomegaly in PMF may be complicated by splenic infarction that manifests with left upper quadrant abdominal pain and referred left shoulder pain. Computed tomography in such cases may be unremarkable, or it may show wedge-shaped or rounded low-attenuation lesions in the spleen. EMH occurs in many sites throughout the body. Besides the spleen and liver, common sites include the lymph nodes, skin, pleura, peritoneum, lung, and paraspinal and epidural spaces, where lesions may be found incidentally on imaging or may produce mass effects. The latter may result in spinal cord and/or nerve root compression, which is a medical emergency requiring corticosteroids to reduce edema and immediate radiation therapy.

DIAGNOSIS

At present, the 2008 WHO criteria are used for the diagnosis of ET, PV, and PMF (Table 169-4). These criteria are based on morphology and cytogenetic or molecular studies (Fig. 169-2). Almost all patients with PV carry a *JAK2* mutation (*JAK2*V617F or *JAK2* exon 12 mutation). Therefore, the absence of a *JAK2* mutation makes a diagnosis of PV unlikely. *JAK2*V617F is not specific to PV, however; it is also found in ET (≈55% of cases), PMF (≈65% of cases), and other myeloid neoplasms (usually <5% of cases). *JAK2* exon 12 mutations are relatively specific to *JAK2*V617F-negative PV and occur in approximately 3% of all patients with PV. Thus, the presence of a *JAK2* mutation excludes secondary myeloproliferation (e.g., secondary polycythemia or reactive thrombocytosis; see later), and its absence makes a diagnosis of PV very unlikely. The value of *MPL* and other MPN-associated mutations as diagnostic markers is undermined by their low prevalence in ET and PMF.

At present, neither red cell mass measurement nor bone marrow examination is essential for the diagnosis of PV (see Fig. 169-2). However, bone marrow examination with cytogenetic studies is often necessary for the accurate diagnosis of ET and PMF and is especially useful in distinguishing ET from prefibrotic PMF. Bone marrow fibrosis associated with *JAK2*V617F, trisomy 9, or del(13q) is highly suggestive of PMF. Figure 169-3 shows the typical peripheral blood smear seen in PMF, and the corresponding bone marrow histology is illustrated in Figure 169-4. Bone marrow morphology in ET also provides additional clues for distinguishing clonal from reactive thrombocytosis (Fig. 169-5).

Erythrocytosis (Polycythemias)

Polycythemia refers to either a real (true polycythemia) or a spurious (apparent polycythemia) perception of an increase in red blood cell mass. True polycythemia may represent either a clonal myeloproliferative disorder (PV) or a nonclonal increase in red blood cell mass that is often mediated by Epo (secondary polycythemia). Apparent polycythemia results from a decrease in plasma volume without an actual increase in red cell mass (relative polycythemia). Occasionally, a true increase in red blood cell mass may be masked by a normal-appearing hematocrit because of a concomitant increase in plasma volume, often accompanied by marked splenomegaly (inapparent polycythemia).

Most conditions that cause an acute depletion of plasma volume (i.e., relative polycythemia) are clinically obvious (e.g., severe dehydration, diarrhea, vomiting, use of diuretics, capillary leak syndrome, severe burns) and do not require specialized tests to confirm the diagnosis. Conversely, the existence

TABLE 169-4 2008 WORLD HEALTH ORGANIZATION DIAGNOSTIC CRITERIA FOR POLYCYTHEMIA VERA, ESSENTIAL THROMBOCYTHEMIA, AND PRIMARY MYELOFIBROSIS

CRITERIA	POLYCYTHEMIA VERA*	ESSENTIAL THROMBOCYTHEMIA*	PRIMARY MYELOFIBROSIS*
Major criteria	1 Hb >18.5 g/dL (men), >16.5 g/dL (women) or Hb/Hct >99th percentile of reference range or Hb >17 g/dL (men) or >15 g/dL (women) if associated with sustained increase of ≥2 g/dL from baseline, not otherwise explained or Elevated red cell mass >25% above mean normal predicted value	1 Platelet count ≥450 × 10^9/L	1 Megakaryocyte proliferation and atypia† accompanied by either reticulin or collagen fibrosis or In the absence of fibrosis, megakaryocyte changes accompanied by increased marrow cellularity and granulocytic proliferation
	2 Presence of *JAK2*V617F or similar mutation	2 Megakaryocyte proliferation with large and mature morphology; no or little granulocyte or erythroid proliferation	2 Not meeting WHO criteria for CML, PV, MDS, or other myeloid neoplasm
		3 Not meeting WHO criteria for CML, PV, PMF, MDS, or other myeloid neoplasm	3 Demonstration of *JAK2*V617F or other clonal marker or No evidence of reactive marrow fibrosis
		4 Demonstration of *JAK2*V617F or other clonal marker or No evidence of reactive thrombocytosis	
Minor criteria	1 Bone marrow trilineage myeloproliferation 2 Subnormal serum Epo level 3 EEC growth		1 Leukoerythroblastosis 2 Increased serum LDH 3 Anemia 4 Palpable splenomegaly

*Diagnosis of PV requires meeting either both major criteria and one minor criterion or the first major criterion and two minor criteria. Diagnosis of essential thrombocythemia requires meeting all four major criteria. Diagnosis of PMF requires meeting all three major criteria and two minor criteria.

†Small to large megakaryocytes with an aberrant nuclear-to-cytoplasmic ratio and hyperchromatic and irregularly folded nuclei and dense clustering.

CML = chronic myelogenous leukemia; EEC = endogenous erythroid colony; Epo = erythropoietin; Hct = hematocrit; Hb = hemoglobin; LDH = lactate dehydrogenase; MDS = myelodysplastic syndrome; PMF = primary myelofibrosis; PV = polycythemia vera; WHO = World Health Organization.

From Tefferi A, Vardiman JW. Classification and diagnosis of myeloproliferative neoplasms: the 2008 World Health Organization criteria and point-of-care diagnostic algorithms. *Leukemia.* 2008;22:14-22.

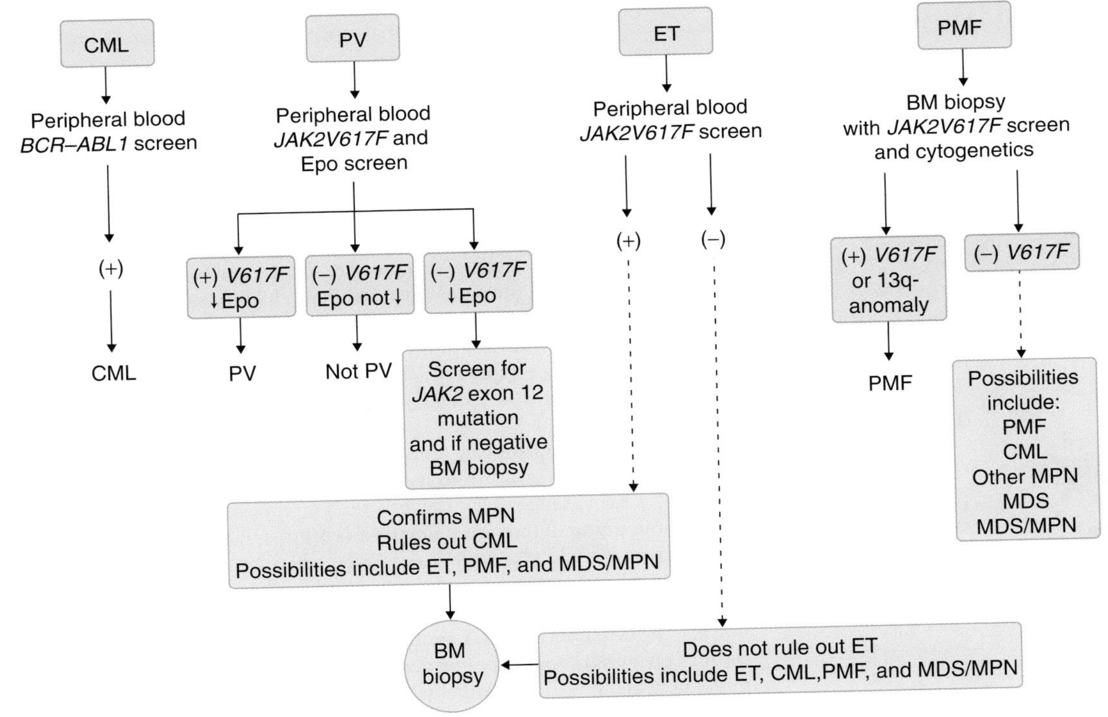

FIGURE 169-2. Diagnostic algorithm for the myeloproliferative neoplasms (MPNs). BM = bone marrow; CML = chronic myelogenous leukemia; Epo = erythropoietin; ET = essential thrombocythemia; MDS = myelodysplastic syndrome; PMF = primary myelofibrosis; PV = polycythemia vera. (From Tefferi A, Skoda R, Vardiman JW. Myeloproliferative neoplasms: contemporary diagnosis using histology and genetics. *Nat Rev Clin Oncol.* 2009;6:627-637.)

of chronic contraction of the plasma volume, such as that postulated to occur in Gaisböck's syndrome or stress polycythemia, is controversial. Accurate reference to the race- and sex-adjusted normal laboratory values should minimize the inappropriate use of the term *apparent polycythemia* in physiologically normal persons with hematocrit values in the upper percentiles of the normal range. In such instances, the performance of costly diagnostic tests, including the measurement of red blood cell mass, is unwarranted.

Table 169-5 provides a comprehensive list of causes of erythrocytosis (polycythemia), including acquired forms (both clonal and secondary) and congenital forms. In each of these, the serum Epo level is helpful in

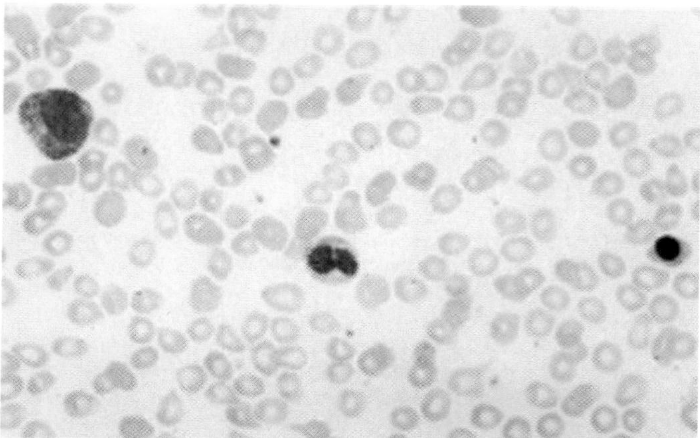

FIGURE 169-3. **Myeloproliferative disorder.** A peripheral blood smear from a patient with agnogenic myeloid metaplasia shows a leukoerythroblastic picture. The characteristic findings are teardrop-shaped red blood cells (dacryocytes), nucleated red blood cells (erythroblasts), and immature granulocyte precursors.

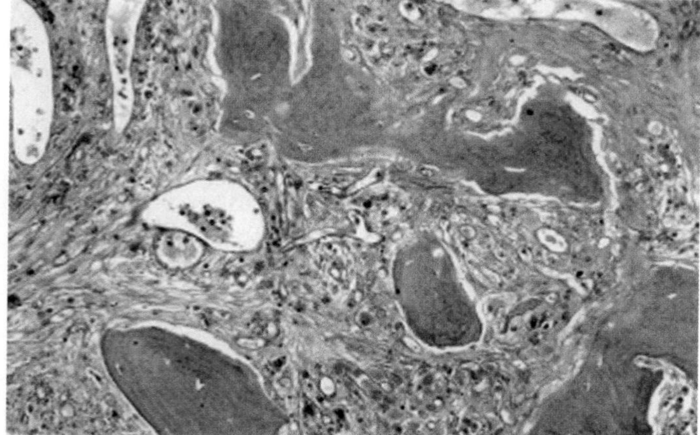

FIGURE 169-4. Bone marrow biopsy specimen from a patient with primary myelofibrosis shows reticulin fibrosis, osteosclerosis, and intrasinusoidal hematopoiesis.

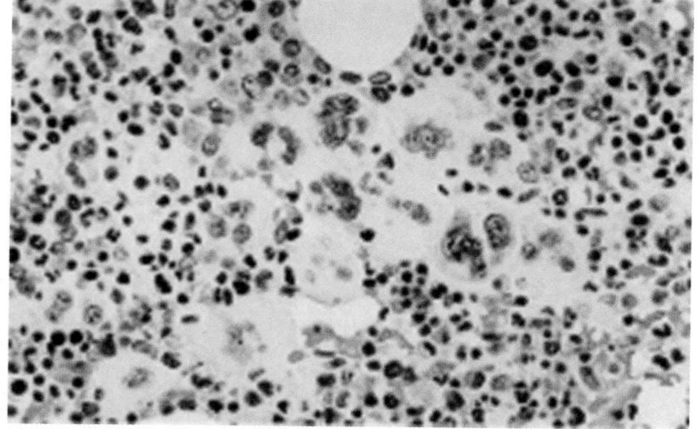

FIGURE 169-5. **Myeloproliferative disorder.** Bone marrow shows megakaryocytic clusters, seen in essential thrombocythemia and other conditions associated with clonal thrombocytosis.

establishing the differential diagnosis. Epo is a 35-kD glycosylated protein synthesized in response to tissue hypoxia, mainly by the peritubular capillary endothelial cells of the renal cortex by means of an intricate oxygen-sensing mechanism. Acquired secondary polycythemia is usually associated with increased Epo production that is either hypoxia driven or hypoxia independent. In the former instance, the hypoxic stimulus is usually central,

TABLE 169-5 CLASSIFICATION OF ERYTHROCYTOSIS

I. Acquired erythrocytosis
   A. Clonal (polycythemia vera)
   B. Secondary
      1. Hypoxia driven
         a. Chronic lung disease
         b. Right-to-left cardiopulmonary shunts
         c. High-altitude habitat
         d. Tobacco use, carbon monoxide poisoning
         e. Sleep apnea–hypoventilation syndrome
         f. Renal artery stenosis
      2. Hypoxia independent
         a. Use of androgen preparations, erythropoietin injection
         b. Post renal transplant
         c. Cerebellar hemangioblastoma, meningioma
         d. Pheochromocytoma, uterine leiomyoma, renal cysts, parathyroid adenoma
         e. Hepatocellular carcinoma, renal cell carcinoma

II. Congenital erythrocytosis
   A. Associated with reduced p50 (partial pressure of oxygen at which 50% of hemoglobin is saturated with oxygen)
      1. High-oxygen-affinity hemoglobinopathy (usually autosomal dominant)
      2. 2,3-bisphosphoglycerate deficiency (usually autosomal recessive)
      3. Methemoglobinemia (Chapter 161)
   B. Associated with normal p50
      1. *VHL* mutations, including Chuvash polycythemia (usually autosomal recessive)
      2. *PHD2* mutations
      3. *HIF2α* mutations
      4. *EPOR* mutations (usually autosomal dominant)

From Patnaik MM, Tefferi A. The complete evaluation of erythrocytosis: congenital and acquired. *Leukemia.* 2009;23:834-849.

with cardiopulmonary conditions most commonly responsible. Other causes of central hypoxia include high-altitude habitat and carbon monoxide poisoning. Hypoxia in peripheral tissues is exemplified by the acquired polycythemia associated with renal artery stenosis. In both central and peripheral hypoxia-driven secondary polycythemia, the serum Epo level is initially elevated but may fall to within the normal range after the hemoglobin level has stabilized at a higher level. In contrast, in Epo-mediated, hypoxia-independent secondary polycythemia, the serum Epo level often remains elevated despite the rise in hemoglobin. Hypoxia-independent elevation of Epo with an elevated hemoglobin level is associated with malignant or benign tumors of the liver, kidney, uterus, and cerebellum (see Table 169-5). Exogenous administration of drugs such as androgen preparations or Epo itself also causes acquired secondary polycythemia.

Congenital polycythemia can be associated with increased, normal, or decreased serum Epo levels. For example, the serum Epo level is usually increased or normal in the autosomal dominant, high-oxygen-affinity hemoglobinopathies (e.g., 2,3-diphosphoglycerate mutase deficiency) and the autosomal recessive Chuvash polycythemia that is endemic in Russia and is associated with a von Hippel-Lindau (*VHL*) gene mutation. Conversely, the serum Epo level is low in patients with an activating mutation of the Epo receptor gene.

The diagnostic approach to congenital polycythemia should start with measurement of the serum Epo level. The presence of a subnormal serum Epo level in the absence of PV suggests the presence of a germline mutation of the Epo receptor. If the serum Epo level is normal or elevated, the next step is to measure the p50 (the oxygen tension at which hemoglobin is 50% saturated). Decreased p50 suggests the presence of either a high-oxygen-affinity hemoglobinopathy or 2,3-bisphosphoglycerate deficiency. If the p50 is normal, the possibility of *VHL* mutations (usually associated with increased serum Epo levels) should be considered first because they constitute the most frequent mutations in congenital polycythemia.

Thrombocytosis

Table 169-6 outlines the different causes of thrombocytosis, and Figure 169-6 provides an algorithmic approach to the differential diagnosis. By far, the most common cause of thrombocytosis in general medical populations is a reactive or secondary process. Also, the degree of elevation in the platelet count does not clearly differentiate clonal from reactive thrombocytosis. Figure 169-7 illustrates the value of examining the peripheral blood smear in cases of thrombocytosis; the finding of Howell-Jolly bodies indicates a post-splenectomy or asplenic state as the cause of secondary (reactive) thrombocytosis.

Bone Marrow Fibrosis (Myelofibrosis)

Other causes of bone marrow fibrosis (myelofibrosis) are outlined in Table 169-7. The diagnosis of post-PV or post-ET myelofibrosis requires full documentation of a previous morphologic diagnosis of PV or ET, respectively.

TREATMENT Rx

Polycythemia Vera and Essential Thrombocythemia

Drug therapy in PV or ET does not improve survival or prevent disease transformation into post-ET or post-PV myelofibrosis or blast-phase MPN. Instead, the main objective of specific therapy is to prevent thrombosis in high-risk patients (i.e., those older than 60 years or with a history of thrombosis) or to alleviate non-life-threatening symptoms, including microvascular disturbances (e.g., headaches, acral paresthesia, erythromelalgia), pruritus, or symptomatic splenomegaly. Microvascular symptoms are usually effectively treated with low-dose aspirin (81 mg/day). The cause of MPN-associated

TABLE 169-6 CAUSES OF THROMBOCYTOSIS IN UNSELECTED COHORTS OF CONSECUTIVE PATIENTS

	Platelet Count (Approximate % of Patients)	
CONDITION	**ADULTS, >500,000/μL**	**>1 MILLION/μL**
Infection	22	31
Rebound thrombocytosis	19	3
Tissue damage (surgery)	18	14
Chronic inflammation	13	9
Malignancy	6	14
Renal disorders	5	<1
Hemolytic anemia	4	<1
Post-splenectomy status	2	19
Blood loss	NS	6
Primary thrombocythemia	3	14

NS = not stated.
From Tefferi A, Gilliland DG. Classification of chronic myeloid disorders: from Dameshek towards a semi-molecular system. *Best Pract Res Clin Haematol.* 2006;19:365-385.

TABLE 169-7 CAUSES OF BONE MARROW FIBROSIS

MYELOID DISORDERS

- Primary myelofibrosis
- Metastatic cancer
- Chronic myeloid leukemia
- Myelodysplastic syndrome
- Atypical myeloid disorder
- Acute megakaryocytic leukemia
- Other acute myeloid leukemias
- Gray platelet syndrome

LYMPHOID DISORDERS

- Hairy cell leukemia
- Multiple myeloma
- Lymphoma

NONHEMATOLOGIC DISORDERS

- Connective tissue disorder
- Infections (tuberculosis, kala-azar)
- Vitamin D deficiency rickets
- Renal osteodystrophy

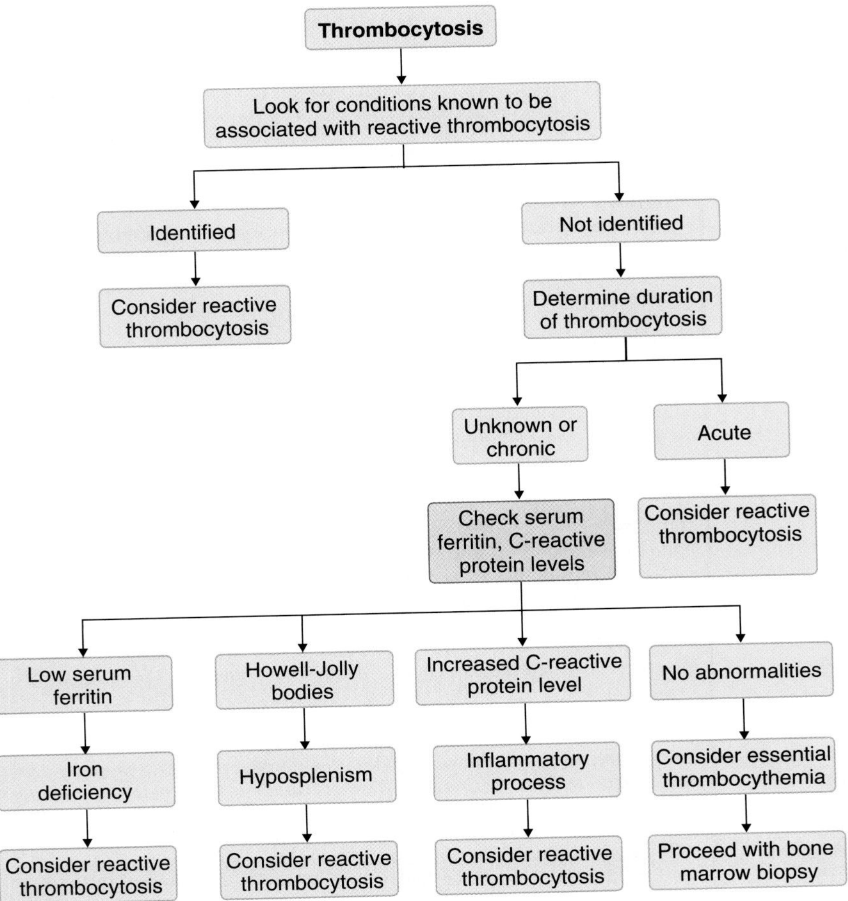

FIGURE 169-6. Diagnostic evaluation of thrombocytosis in routine clinical practice.

TABLE 169-8 RISK STRATIFICATION AND RISK-ADAPTED THERAPY IN ESSENTIAL THROMBOCYTHEMIA, POLYCYTHEMIA VERA, AND PRIMARY MYELOFIBROSIS

	Management			
RISK GROUPS FOR PV AND ET	**ET**	**PV**	**PMF**	**IPSS RISK GROUPS FOR PMF**
Low risk (age <60 yr and no thrombosis history)	Low-dose aspirin	Low-dose aspirin + phlebotomy*	Observation	Low risk (no risk factors†)
Low risk with extreme thrombocytosis‡	Low-dose aspirin§	Low-dose aspirin§ + phlebotomy	Conventional management‖	Intermediate-1 risk (1 risk factor†)
High risk (age ≥60 yr or thrombosis history)	Low-dose aspirin + hydroxyurea¶	Low-dose aspirin + phlebotomy + hydroxyurea¶	Allo-SCT if age <65 yr, or experimental therapy	Intermediate-1 risk with transfusions or unfavorable karyotype
			Allo-SCT if age <65 yr, or experimental therapy	Intermediate-2 risk (2 risk factors†)
			Allo-SCT if age <65 yr, or experimental therapy	High-risk (≥3 risk factors†)

*In the presence of aspirin therapy, the hematocrit target can range between 38 and 50% and is set at a level that maintains best performance status.
†The IPSS uses five risk factors for inferior survival: age >65 years, hemoglobin <10 g/dL, leukocyte count >25 × 10⁹/L, circulating blasts ≥1%, and presence of constitutional symptoms.
‡Extreme thrombocytosis is defined as a platelet count >1000 × 10⁹/L.
§Clinically significant acquired von Willebrand syndrome (ristocetin cofactor activity <30%) should be excluded before using aspirin in patients with extreme thrombocytosis.
‖Androgen preparations or thalidomide with prednisone for anemia; hydroxyurea for symptomatic splenomegaly.
¶In hydroxyurea-intolerant or -resistant cases, interferon-α (age <60 years) or busulfan or pipobroman (age >60 years) can be used.
Allo-SCT = allogeneic stem cell transplantation; ET = essential thrombocythemia; IPSS = International Prognostic Scoring System; PMF = primary myelofibrosis; PV = polycythemia vera.
From Tefferi A, Vainchenker W. Myeloproliferative neoplasms: molecular pathophysiology, essential clinical understanding, and treatment strategies. *J Clin Oncol.* 2011;29:573-582.

pruritus is poorly understood, but its dramatic response to JAK inhibitor therapy suggests a causal relationship with cytokines that use JAK-STAT signaling. Other therapies for MPN-associated pruritus include antihistamines, selective serotonin re-uptake inhibitors, interferon-α (IFN-α), and phototherapy. Symptomatic splenomegaly is usually managed with hydroxyurea (starting dose 500 mg orally twice a day).

Preventive cytoreductive therapy for thrombosis is indicated only in the presence of high-risk disease (see Prognosis later; Table 169-8). In this regard, randomized studies have demonstrated the value of low-dose aspirin (40 to 100 mg/day) in PV[1,2] and hydroxyurea (starting dose 500 mg orally twice a day) in high-risk ET. Hydroxyurea is a nonalkylating DNA synthesis inhibitor and a myelosuppressive agent. Based on noncontrolled but prospective evidence, most experts agree that low-dose aspirin therapy (81 mg/day) should also be considered for ET and hydroxyurea therapy for high-risk PV (see Table 169-8). In addition, phlebotomy is required for all patients with PV, and the target hematocrit in aspirin-treated individuals should be less than 50%—preferably around 45%. In high-risk patients with ET in whom cytoreductive therapy is indicated, a platelet target of less than 400 × 10⁹/L is reasonable and supported by data from retrospective studies.

High-risk PV or ET patients (see Prognosis) who cannot tolerate or are resistant to hydroxyurea are effectively managed by IFN-α or busulfan. IFN-α is the preferred second-line drug, at least for younger patients. Two recent studies of pegylated IFN-α (≈90 µg by weekly subcutaneous injection) in PV and ET patients reported hematologic remissions of approximately 80%, accompanied by decreases in the *JAK2*V617F allele burden (complete molecular remission rate of 5 to 10%). A controlled study is needed before IFN-α is recommended as first-line therapy in either PV or ET. For older patients, busulfan is started at 4 mg/day; it is withheld in the presence of platelets less than 100 × 10⁹/L or a white blood cell count less than 3 × 10⁹/L, and the dose is reduced to 2 mg/day if the corresponding levels are less than 150 × 10⁹/L and 5 × 10⁹/L.

There is unsubstantiated fear among primary caregivers regarding the leukemogenicity of hydroxyurea and busulfan; no controlled studies in either PV or ET have shown this to be the case. The most recent randomized study in this regard found no difference in leukemia risk among patients receiving either hydroxyurea or anagrelide. Similarly, the two largest noncontrolled studies in ET and PV, as well as long-term studies of patients receiving hydroxyurea for sickle cell disease, do not support the concern that leukemia might be caused by the use of hydroxyurea. The evidence for busulfan's leukemogenicity in the context of treatment for PV or ET is equally weak and inappropriately extrapolated from older patients with advanced disease who were exposed to multiple cytoreductive drugs. Similarly, the safety and efficacy of busulfan treatment in ET were underlined by a more recent long-term study of 36 patients older than 60 years in whom no instances of acute myeloid leukemia or other malignancies were documented after a median follow-up of 72 months.

Anagrelide is a cyclic adenosine monophosphate phosphodiesterase III inhibitor that relatively selectively reduces the platelet count by acting on platelet production in the bone marrow. A large randomized study compared anagrelide with hydroxyurea, both in combination with aspirin, in high-risk patients with ET and demonstrated hydroxyurea's overall superiority.[3] Hydroxyurea was better tolerated and was associated with significantly less risk of arterial thrombosis, major hemorrhage, and fibrotic transformation. In contrast, anagrelide displayed better activity against venous thrombosis. A more recent but smaller randomized study found no difference between hydroxyurea and anagrelide in terms of the incidence of ET-related events, but the treatment discontinuation rate was higher in the anagrelide arm. Other treatment options in PV and ET include pipobroman (not available in the United States) and radiophosphorus. The latter has been associated with a delayed risk of leukemic transformation in patients with PV, and its use is currently limited to patients older than 65 years.

ET is associated with an increased risk (approximately 35% vs. 15% in the control population) of spontaneous abortion in the first trimester of pregnancy. There is no association between the increased risk of spontaneous abortion and the degree of thrombocytosis. Low-risk pregnant patients with ET or PV are managed the same way as their nonpregnant counterparts, and the use of low-dose aspirin has been associated with a decreased prevalence of first trimester miscarriages in retrospective studies. High-risk pregnant women with ET (i.e., those with previous thrombosis) require cytoreductive therapy, just like other high-risk patients. In such patients, there is anecdotal evidence of the safety of using IFN-α and the potential teratogenicity of hydroxyurea.

Major bleeding occurs in less than 10% of ET patients. Extreme thrombocytosis (i.e., platelet count >1 million/µL) appears to be a risk factor for bleeding, in part because of the acquired von Willebrand syndrome (Chapter 176). One approach is to measure ristocetin cofactor activity in patients with extreme thrombocytosis and withhold aspirin therapy if the value is less than 30%.

Primary Myelofibrosis

Drug therapy does not modify the natural history of PMF, although survival has improved in recent years. Patients with PMF who are considered low risk, as determined by the International Prognostic Scoring System (IPSS), can be observed without any therapeutic intervention. IPSS high-risk or intermediate-2-risk patients should be considered for investigational drug therapy or allogeneic stem cell transplantation (Chapter 181). Intermediate-1-risk patients who are transfusion dependent or have an unfavorable karyotype are managed as high-risk patients.

Conventional therapy for PMF is largely palliative and does not improve survival. Anemia and symptomatic splenomegaly are the main indications for treatment. Conventional drugs used to treat PMF-associated anemia include androgen preparations (e.g., oral fluoxymesterone 10 mg twice daily), danazol (400 to 600 mg/day), prednisone (30 to 40 mg/day), and erythropoiesis-stimulating agents. Prostate cancer screening is required in men treated with androgen preparations. Response rates to prednisone, androgen preparations, or danazol are about 20%, and response durations average about 1 to 2 years. Erythropoiesis-stimulating agents may exacerbate PMF-associated splenomegaly and are usually ineffective in transfusion-dependent patients.

Thalidomide and thalidomide-like drugs such as lenalidomide may be effective in the treatment of anemia in PMF. Thalidomide as a single agent (50 to 200 mg/day) is not as effective as its combination with prednisone (30 mg/day), with reported response rates ranging from 20 to 62% for anemia, 25 to 80% for thrombocytopenia, and 7 to 30% for splenomegaly. Response rates with lenalidomide are similar, but the drug works best in the presence of a del(5q) cytogenetic abnormality. The occurrence of peripheral neuropathy with thalidomide and severe pancytopenia with lenalidomide therapy has limited their use in most patients.

The drug of choice for symptomatic splenomegaly in PMF is hydroxyurea (starting dose 500 mg twice daily). Hydroxyurea-refractory cases are often managed by splenectomy because the value of other conventional drugs in this regard is limited. Indications for splenectomy in PMF include mechanical discomfort, symptomatic portal hypertension (i.e., associated with ascites or variceal bleeding), and frequent red blood cell transfusions. The perioperative mortality of splenectomy in PMF is between 5 and 10%. Post-splenectomy complications occur in approximately 50% of patients and include bleeding, thrombosis, hepatomegaly, extreme thrombocytosis, leukocytosis, and an increase in circulating blasts. Prophylactic therapy with hydroxyurea is advised to prevent post-splenectomy thrombocytosis. A transjugular intrahepatic portosystemic shunt might be considered to alleviate symptoms of portal hypertension.

EMH is the main cause of hepatosplenomegaly in PMF and post-PV or post-ET myelofibrosis. Nonhepatosplenic EMH also occurs in PMF and might involve the vertebral column (causing cord compression), lymph nodes, lung (causing pulmonary hypertension), pleura (causing effusion), small bowel, peritoneum (causing ascites), urogenital tract, skin, and heart. Diagnosis is usually tissue based, but imaging studies are sometimes used; myelofibrosis-associated pulmonary hypertension is confirmed by technetium-99m sulfur colloid scintigraphy, which shows diffuse pulmonary uptake.

Radiation therapy is an attractive treatment option in both hepatosplenic and nonhepatosplenic EMH. Splenic irradiation (100 to 500 cGy in 5 to 10 fractions) induces a transient reduction in spleen size but might be associated with life-threatening pancytopenia. More recent studies suggest the relative safety and value of lower-dose treatment (100 cGy total dose in four daily fractions of 25 cGy). Radiation therapy works best for nonhepatosplenic EMH. Single-fraction (100 to 400 cGy) involved-field therapy has also been shown to benefit patients with myelofibrosis-associated pulmonary hypertension or extremity pain.

Symptoms in myelofibrosis that affect quality of life include profound fatigue, night sweats, weight loss, pruritus, bone pain, and nonproductive cough. In an international survey of 1179 patients, standardized fatigue metrics of the Functional Assessment of Cancer Therapy–Anemia (FACT-AN) and Brief Fatigue Inventory (BFI) were used to demonstrate that patients with PV, ET, and PMF suffer from anemia-independent fatigue exceeding that expected in age-matched controls. In a subset analysis of 458 patients with myelofibrosis, more than 50% suffered from moderate to severe fatigue, night sweats, pruritus, and symptomatic splenomegaly, whereas a smaller proportion listed bone pain, weight loss, and fever as additional symptoms. The study also documented the inadequacy of conventional therapy in the management of these symptoms. Recent studies of JAK inhibitor therapy in PMF or post-PV or post-ET myelofibrosis suggest major benefits in terms of constitutional symptoms and cachexia (see later).

Experimental Drug Therapy in Myeloproliferative Neoplasms

Because of the association between MPN and JAK-STAT–relevant mutations (e.g., *JAK2* and *MPL* mutations), several anti-JAK2 small-molecule drugs are currently undergoing clinical trials. One or more of these drugs have demonstrated remarkable activity against splenomegaly and constitutional symptoms, including pruritus, and resolution of leukocytosis and thrombocytosis, as well as reduction in the *JAK2*V617F allele burden. Side effects so far have included gastrointestinal symptoms; anemia; thrombocytopenia; reversible increases in transaminases, amylase, or lipase; and the phenomenon of "cytokine rebound." This phenomenon is seen in some patients receiving JAK2 inhibitors with particularly strong activity in suppressing pro-inflammatory cytokines and consists of the acute and immediate reappearance of symptoms on drug discontinuation.

Allogeneic Stem Cell Transplantation

The largest study of allogeneic stem cell transplantation in PMF was conducted by the Center for International Bone Marrow Transplant Research (CIBMTR) and included 289 subject with a variety of donor types and conditioning regimens. Five-year disease-free survival and treatment-related mortality were 33 and 35% for matched related transplants and 27 and 50% for unrelated transplants, respectively. Outcome was not favorably affected by reduced-intensity conditioning (Chapter 181). In another reduced-intensity conditioning transplant study from the Chronic Leukemia Working Party of the European Group for Blood and Marrow Transplantation, 103 patients (median age, 55 years) with PMF or post-PV or post-ET myelofibrosis were prospectively studied, and 5-year disease-free survival was estimated at 51%.[4] Chronic graft-versus-host disease (Chapter 181) occurred in 49% of these patients, and relapse (29%) was predicted by high-risk disease and prior splenectomy. The chronic graft-versus-host disease and relapse rates for matched related transplants in the CIBMTR study were 40 and 32%, respectively, and a history of splenectomy did not affect outcome.

Considering the lack of effective drug therapy for PMF, the risk of transplant-related complications might be justified in patients whose median survival is expected to be less than 5 years and whose leukemia risk is greater than 20%. Using the age-adjusted dynamic prognostic model, this group includes high- or intermediate-2-risk patients, as well as those with either red cell transfusion dependence or an unfavorable karyotype (see Prognosis). In general, post-transplant outcome is poor in the presence of high-risk disease, advanced age, unrelated donor, or human leukocyte antigen (HLA) mismatch. More studies are needed to clarify the impact of pretransplant *JAK2*V617F presence or allele burden on transplant outcome, but the persistent presence of the mutation after transplantation predicts clinical relapse.

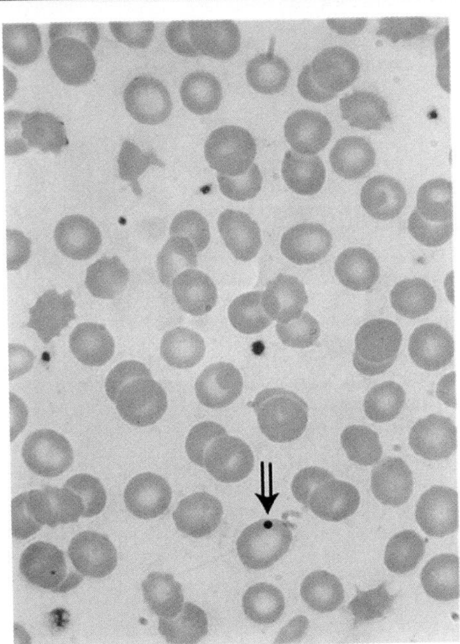

FIGURE 169-7. Peripheral smear showing Howell-Jolly bodies (arrow) in red blood cells. This finding is typical of surgical or functional hyposplenism.

PROGNOSIS

Essential Thrombocythemia and Polycythemia Vera

Neither ET nor PV is presently a curable disease, and current therapy has not been rigorously shown to prolong survival. Fortunately, a normal life expectancy is possible in most patients. Recent studies suggest a median survival that approaches 20 years in both diseases. Fibrotic or leukemic transformation in ET or PV is relatively infrequent (a combined rate of <10% in the first 15 years of disease).

Current risk stratification in PV and ET is designed to estimate the risk of thrombosis (see Table 169-8). Age 60 years or older and history of thrombosis are the two risk factors used to classify patients with PV or ET into low-risk (no risk factors) and high-risk (one or two risk factors) groups. In addition, because of the potential risk for bleeding, low-risk patients with extreme thrombocytosis (platelet count $>1000 \times 10^9/L$) are considered separately. The presence of cardiovascular risk factors is currently not taken into consideration during formal risk stratification.

Primary Myelofibrosis

The prognosis of PMF is worse than that of ET or PV. Median survival is approximately 6 years and appears to have improved in recent years. The IPSS uses five independent predictors of inferior survival: age older than 65 years, hemoglobin less than 10 g/dL, leukocyte count greater than $25 \times 10^9/L$, circulating blasts 1% or higher, and constitutional symptoms. The presence of zero, one, two, or three or more adverse risk factors defines low-, intermediate-1-, intermediate-2-, and high-risk disease, respectively, with corresponding median survivals of approximately 11.3, 7.9, 4, and 2.3 years. A dynamic prognostic model that uses the same variables but can be applied at any time during the disease course was recently published. In addition, red cell transfusion dependency, a platelet count less than $100 \times 10^9/L$, and an unfavorable karyotype carry an IPSS-independent prognostic value, and their presence warrants assignment to the high-risk category regardless of IPSS score.

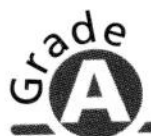

1. Landolfi R, Marchioli R, Kutti J, et al. Efficacy and safety of low-dose aspirin in polycythemia vera. *N Engl J Med*. 2004;350:114-124.

2. Squizzato A, Romualdi E, Middeldorp S. Antiplatelet drugs for polycythaemia vera and essential thrombocythaemia. *Cochrane Database Syst Rev.* 2008;16:CD006503.
3. Harrison CN, Campbell PJ, Buck G, et al. Hydroxyurea compared with anagrelide in high-risk essential thrombocythemia. *N Engl J Med.* 2005;353:33-45.
4. Kroger N, Holler E, Kobbe G, et al. Allogeneic stem cell transplantation after reduced-intensity conditioning in patients with myelofibrosis: a prospective, multicenter study of the Chronic Leukemia Working Party of the European Group for Blood and Marrow Transplantation. *Blood.* 2009;114:5264-5270.

SUGGESTED READINGS

Chen AT, Prchal JT. JAK2 kinase inhibitors and myeloproliferative disorders. *Curr Opin Hematol.* 2010;17:110-116. *Update on the status of early-phase clinical trials of molecularly targeted therapy.*

Harrison CN, Bareford D, Butt N, et al. Guideline for investigation and management of adults and children presenting with a thrombocytosis. *Br J Haematol.* 2010;149:352-375. *Guidelines from U.K. groups on the clinical approach to patients with thrombocytosis.*

Passamonti F, Cervantes F, Vannucchi AM, et al. A dynamic prognostic model to predict survival in primary myelofibrosis: a study by the IWG-MRT (International Working Group for Myeloproliferative Neoplasms Research and Treatment). *Blood.* 2010;115:1703-1708. *A novel model for assessing the prognosis of patients with primary myelofibrosis any time during their clinical course, which is useful for treatment decision making.*

Tefferi A, Vainchenker W. Myeloproliferative neoplasms: molecular pathophysiology, essential clinical understanding, and treatment strategies. *J Clin Oncol.* 2011;29:573-582. *Review.*

Vaidya R, Siragusa S, Huang J, et al. Mature survival data for 176 patients younger than 60 years with primary myelofibrosis diagnosed between 1976 and 2005: evidence for survival gains in recent years. *Mayo Clin Proc.* 2009;84:1114-1119. *Retrospective study of 176 consecutive patients at a single institution showing encouraging survival trends.*

170

LEUKOCYTOSIS AND LEUKOPENIA

NANCY BERLINER

The normal peripheral white blood cell count (WBC) ranges between 4500/μL and 10,000/μL, with a mean of 7500/μL and is composed of neutrophils, lymphocytes, monocytes, basophils, and eosinophils. Because neutrophils usually represent about 60% of the peripheral WBC, derangement in the WBC usually reflects elevation or reduction in the absolute neutrophil count. Leukocytosis, an elevated WBC, and leukopenia, a depressed WBC, may be secondary to an underlying disease or exposure, or they may be manifestations of a primary hematologic disorder. This chapter outlines both the primary and secondary causes of leukocytosis and leukopenia, focusing particularly on neutrophilia and neutropenia.

NORMAL NEUTROPHIL DYNAMICS

To understand the pathogenesis of a high or low WBC, one must understand normal neutrophil dynamics. Neutrophils arise from multipotent progenitor cells in the bone marrow that also give rise to erythrocytes, megakaryocytes, eosinophils, basophils, and monocytes. Neutrophil precursors in the marrow mature over 6 to 10 days to form a storage pool of mature neutrophils (Fig. 170-1). Together the marrow populations make up about 95% of the body's total granulocyte mass (20% neutrophil precursors, 75% mature bands and neutrophils). The circulating neutrophil pool thus represents only the remaining approximately 5% of the body's total neutrophils, just over half of which at any given time are adherent to the vascular endothelium and the spleen, a phenomenon termed *margination*. These marginated neutrophils are poised for immediate release into the circulation during times of stress. The remaining neutrophils circulate freely in the blood, where they can survive for 6 to 12 hours, or migrate into tissues, where they can survive for 1 to 4 days. In general, then, neutrophilia can occur as the result of increased marrow production, increased release of neutrophils from the storage pool, or mobilization of neutrophils from the marginated pool. Neutropenia, on the other hand, may be due to decreased marrow production, increased margination with or without sequestration by the spleen, or increased destruction of peripheral cells.

NEUTROPHILIA

Most cases of neutrophilia are reactive or secondary to an underlying inflammatory process. This includes neutrophilia due to infection, chronic inflammation, stress, drugs, nonhematologic malignancy, marrow stimulation (as in hemolysis or idiopathic thrombocytopenic purpura), or splenectomy. Primary causes of neutrophilia may be congenital, including hereditary neutrophilia, Down syndrome, and leukocyte adhesion deficiency (LAD), or acquired as in the case of chronic myelogenous leukemia and other myeloproliferative neoplasms (Table 170-1).

Secondary Causes of Neutrophilia

Infection

Many acute bacterial infections can present with a modest leukocytosis with a "left shift," referring to the circulation of more immature myeloid cells. This left shift most commonly is restricted to release of an increased number of band forms; however, in severe stress, one may see circulating metamyelocytes and even earlier cells (see Fig. 170-1) in the peripheral blood. Leukocytosis occurs within hours of infection owing to release of neutrophils from both the marrow and marginated pools. Examination of these neutrophils on peripheral smear may reveal evidence of toxic granulation (see Fig. 160-18 in Chapter 160), Döhle bodies (see Fig. 160-19 in Chapter 160), and cytoplasmic vacuoles. Certain infections (e.g., *Clostridium difficile* or tuberculosis in particular) are known to cause elevations in the WBC to greater than 30,000/μL in about one fourth of infected patients and may result in a *leukemoid reaction*, defined as a WBC of greater than 50,000/μL with a pronounced left shift (Fig. 170-2).

Chronic Inflammation

Leukocytosis due to chronic inflammation results from increased leukocyte (specifically neutrophil and monocyte) production as opposed to altered neutrophil distribution. Mature neutrophil pools become depleted with ongoing inflammation, and the myeloid compartment of the marrow expands to increase neutrophil production. A myriad of cytokines, including tumor necrosis factor-α (TNF-α), granulocyte colony-stimulating factor (G-CSF),

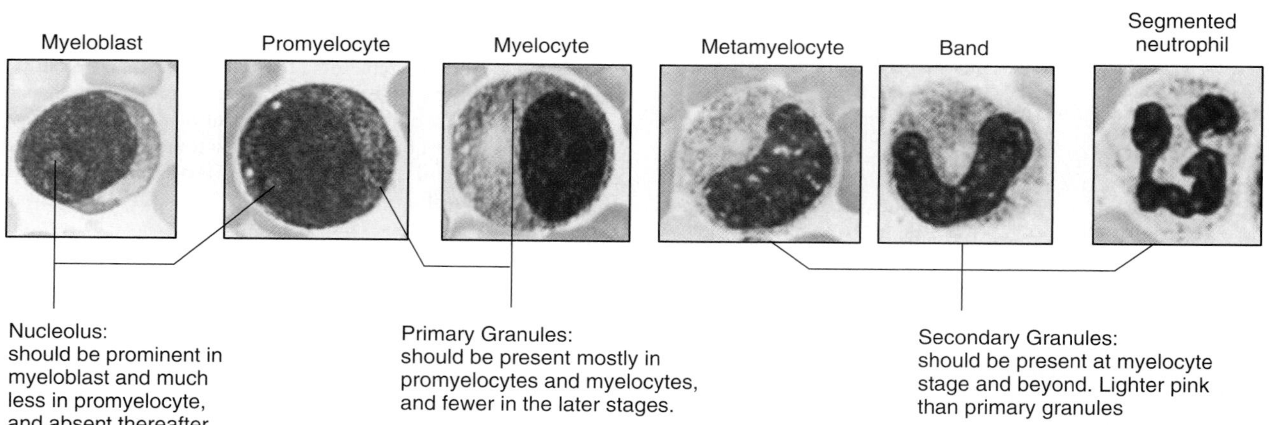

Myeloblast
Promyelocyte
Myelocyte
Metamyelocyte
Band
Segmented neutrophil
Nucleolus: should be prominent in myeloblast and much less in promyelocyte, and absent thereafter
Primary Granules: should be present mostly in promyelocytes and myelocytes, and fewer in the later stages.
Secondary Granules: should be present at myelocyte stage and beyond. Lighter pink than primary granules

FIGURE 170-1. Myeloid maturation in the bone marrow. Nucleoli are prominent in myeloblasts, much less frequent in promyelocytes, and absent in more mature forms. Primary granules are present in the cytoplasm of promyelocytes and myelocytes, and secondary granules predominate beyond the myelocyte stage.

TABLE 170-1 DIFFERENTIAL DIAGNOSIS OF NEUTROPHILIA

I. Primary hematologic etiologies
  a. Congenital neutrophilia
    i. Hereditary neutrophilia
    ii. Chronic idiopathic neutrophilia
    iii. Down syndrome
    iv. Leukocyte adhesion deficiency (LAD)
      1. LAD I
      2. LAD II
  b. Acquired hematologic neoplasms
    i. Myeloproliferative disease
      1. Chronic myelogenous leukemia
      2. Polycythemia vera
II. Secondary to other disease entities
  a. Infection
    i. Acute via release from marginated and storage pools
    ii. Chronic via increased myelopoiesis (e.g., tuberculosis, fungal infection, chronic abscess, other chronic infections)
  b. Chronic inflammation
    i. Rheumatic disease: juvenile rheumatoid arthritis, rheumatoid arthritis, Still's disease, and others
    ii. Inflammatory bowel disease
    iii. Granulomatous disease
    iv. Chronic hepatitis
  c. Cigarette smoking
  d. Stress
  e. Drug induced
    i. Corticosteroids
    ii. β-agonists
    iii. Lithium
    iv. Recombinant cytokine administration
  f. Nonhematologic malignancy
    i. Cytokine-secreting tumors (lung, tongue, kidney, urothelial tumors)
    ii. Marrow metastasis (myelophthisis)
  g. Marrow stimulation
    i. Hemolytic anemia, immune thrombocytopenia
    ii. Recovery from marrow suppression
    iii. Recombinant cytokine administration
  h. Postsplenectomy

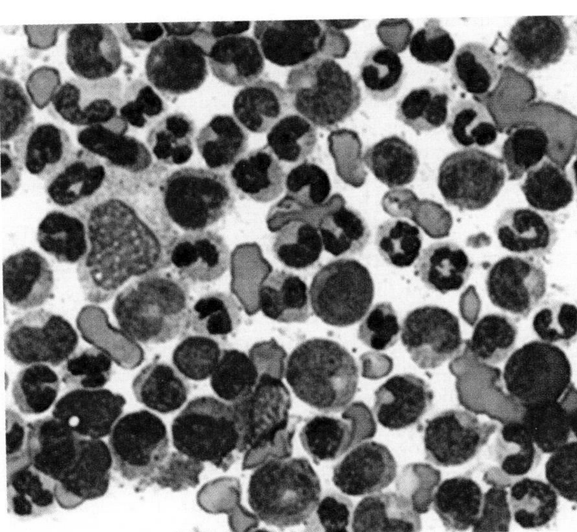

FIGURE 170-2. Peripheral blood from a patient with leukemoid reaction. From this smear, it would be impossible to distinguish this from chronic-phase chronic myelogenous leukemia (Chapter 190). Distinction would depend on determination of presence or absence of *BCR-ABL* fusion.

granulocyte-macrophage colony-stimulating factor (GM-CSF), macrophage inflammatory protein-1 (MIP-1), interleukin-1 (IL-1), IL-6, and IL-8, have been implicated in this marrow stimulation (Chapter 159). Chronic inflammatory conditions that are particularly associated with leukocytosis and neutrophilia include juvenile rheumatoid arthritis, rheumatoid arthritis, Still's disease, Crohn's disease, ulcerative colitis, granulomatous infection, and chronic hepatitis. The WBC and neutrophil elevation in these cases is typically more modest than that seen in acute infection or inflammation.

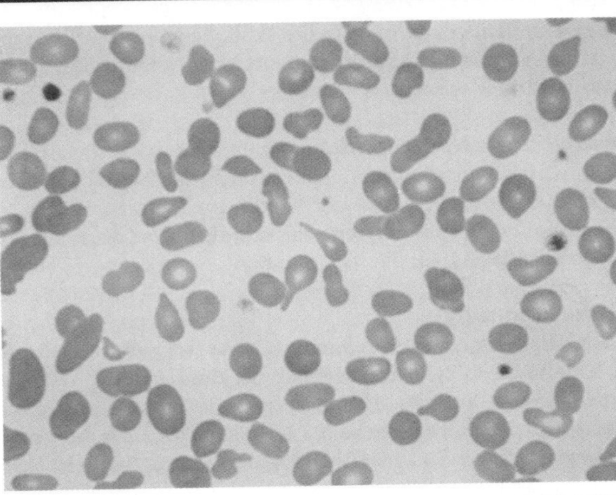

FIGURE 170-3. Myelophthisic changes in erythrocyte morphology. Note prominent teardrop forms. (From Rose M, Berliner N. Disorders of red blood cells. In Andreoli TE, Benjamin IJ, Griggs RC, et al, eds. *Andreoli and Carpenter's Cecil Essentials of Medicine,* 8th ed. Philadelphia: Saunders, 2010:522, Fig. 49-2.)

Cigarette Smoking

Cigarette smoking can cause a leukocytosis and neutrophilia in about 25 to 50% of chronic smokers that can persist for even up to 5 years after quitting smoking. The mechanism by which this occurs is unknown.

Stress

Within minutes of exercise, surgery, or stress, one can see an elevation in circulating neutrophils. This is presumed to be due to the effects of catecholamines on marginated neutrophils, with release of neutrophils into the circulation. Some cases of stress-induced neutrophilia can be prevented by pretreatment with β-adrenergic antagonists (e.g., propranolol), supporting the role of catecholamines in the process. Exercise-induced neutrophilia, however, is not blocked by propranolol, suggesting that it may instead be due to flow and mechanical perturbation of neutrophils in the lungs. An elevated WBC has also been noted in the setting of acute myocardial infarction, but whether this is a risk factor for cardiac ischemia or a result of inflammation is unclear.

Drug Induced

Probably the most well-known and widely used drugs associated with leukocytosis are corticosteroids. Other drugs that are associated with elevations in WBC and neutrophil count in particular include β-agonists and lithium. Lithium causes neutrophilia by increasing the production of endogenous colony-stimulating factors (CSFs).G-CSF or GM-CSF treatment likewise may result in neutrophilia, and although this is the desired effect, the neutrophilia can be quite pronounced if not appropriately monitored.

Nonhematologic Malignancy

Leukocytosis can be seen in a number of nonhematologic malignancies. Some tumors (lung, tongue, kidney, bladder) are thought to secrete G-CSF themselves as an ectopic hematopoietic growth factor. Other tumors (lung, stomach, breast), when metastasized to the bone and bone marrow, can cause a *leukoerythroblastic reaction*, characterized by left-shifted leukocytosis, thrombocytosis, and red cell abnormalities including nucleated and teardrop-shaped red blood cells (Fig. 170-3). The presence of nonhematopoietic entities invading the bone marrow (metastatic cancer, fibrosis, granulomatous disease) is termed *myelophthisis*.

Marrow Stimulation

Peripheral destruction of red cells and platelets, as seen with hemolytic anemia and idiopathic thrombocytopenic purpura, can result in stimulation of the bone marrow and a "spillover" leukocytosis. Recovery of cell counts following marrow suppression, as in the case of chemotherapy, can result in a rebound leukocytosis that may last several weeks.

Primary Causes of Neutrophilia

Hereditary Neutrophilia

Hereditary neutrophilia is an autosomal dominant genetic disease that is characterized by an elevated WBC in the 20,000 to 100,000/μL range with splenomegaly and widened diploe of the skull. The neutrophils in this disorder appear to function normally, and patients have no increased risk for bacterial infection or other sequelae.

Chronic Idiopathic Neutrophilia

Chronic idiopathic neutrophilia is a condition marked by leukocytosis in the 11,000 to 40,000/μL range with a normal bone marrow biopsy. In one series with a 20-year follow-up, patients with this condition had no medical sequelae from this elevated WBC.

Pelger-Huet Anomaly

Patients with the Pelger-Huet anomaly (PHA) are often misdiagnosed as having a left-shifted WBC because many of their mature neutrophils are misinterpreted as band forms. Although these patients do not actually have leukocytosis, the anomaly often raises suspicion for an acute infection or inflammatory process because of this apparent left shift. PHA is due to a mutation in the lamin B receptor gene and manifests with mature neutrophils and condensed, clumped chromatin within a bilobed nucleus (see Fig. 160-20 in Chapter 160). These neutrophils, however, function normally. A number of drugs can reversibly induce pseudo-PHA, including colchicine, sulfonamides, ibuprofen, taxoids, and valproate. Pseudo-PHA is also seen in some patients with myelodysplasia (Chapter 188). Vitamin B_{12} or folate deficiency can cause increased nuclear lobation of neutrophils in patients with PHA, perhaps leading a missed diagnosis. With correction of the vitamin deficiency, however, the aberrant neutrophil nuclear morphology returns.

Down Syndrome

Up to 10% of patients with Down syndrome develop transient myeloproliferative disorder (TMD) related to peripheral blood leukocytosis with blasts in association with an accumulation of megakaryoblasts in the blood, liver, and marrow. Similar reactions have also been reported in patients with trisomy 21 mosaicism who are phenotypically normal. TMD resolves spontaneously in most patients but can progress to acute megakaryoblastic leukemia (AMKL) in 23 to 30% of affected patients. This fascinating disorder is attributable to acquisition of mutations in the *GATA1* gene, which encodes a key transcription factor for hematopoietic regulation, leading to loss of normal GATA-1 expression and expression of a truncated GATA-1 protein. Evidence supports that these mutations are acquired during fetal life, and patients present in early infancy with TMD. The pathogenesis of progression to AMKL presumably requires additional genetic events and is the focus of intense study.

Leukocyte Adhesion Deficiency

Patients with LAD have persistent leukocytosis, defects in stimulus-dependent activation of neutrophils, recurrent infections, and delayed separation of the umbilical cord. LAD is an abnormality of leukocyte adhesion reflecting the loss of surface adhesion molecules. LAD I is due to absence or marked reduction in the common β chain of β_2 integrins, resulting in loss of expression of leukocyte function-associated antigen 1 (LFA-1), the C3bi receptor, and GP150;95. This results in a failure to ingest and kill microbes opsonized by C3bi. In LAD II, neutrophils lack sialyl Lewis X, the ligand for L-selectin expressed on endothelial cells. Neutrophils appear morphologically normal but are defective in chemotaxis, adherence, and phagocytosis.

Familial Cold Urticaria

Familial cold urticaria is marked by episodic fevers, leukocytosis, urticaria, rash, conjunctivitis, and muscle and skin tenderness with cold exposure. The rash is composed of infiltrating neutrophils. The syndrome appears to be related to decreased levels of C1-esterase inhibitor and is associated with mutations in the *CIAS1* gene on chromosome 1q.

Chronic Myelogenous Leukemia and Other Myeloproliferative Disorders

Chronic myelogenous leukemia (CML) and the other myeloproliferative neoplasms (namely polycythemia vera [PV] and essential thrombocythemia [ET]) are discussed in detail in Chapters 190 and 169, respectively. They are the principal acquired primary hematologic disorders associated with neutrophilia. They are marked by clonal expansion of myeloid precursors and increased release of both immature and mature myeloid cells into the peripheral blood. CML on presentation often has to be distinguished from a leukemoid reaction. In contrast to a leukemoid reaction, CML is characterized by the presence of abnormalities of other blood cell lines ("panmyelosis") and by the presence of specific abnormalities. Therefore, the peripheral blood smear in CML (but not leukemoid reaction) demonstrates increased numbers in all cells of the neutrophilic series, classically with a greater proportion of myelocytes to metamyelocytes, and may display concomitant basophilia, eosinophilia, anemia, and thrombocytosis. CML is characterized by the diagnostic presence of the Philadelphia chromosome [t(9;22)], which can be identified in the peripheral blood by the detection of the *BCR-ABL* translocation by fluorescence in situ hybridization (FISH) or reverse transcriptase–polymerase chain reaction (RT-PCR). PV and ET, on the other hand, are notable for a marked increase in red cell mass and a marked thrombocytosis, respectively, which is often accompanied by leukocytosis. Both PV and ET are associated with activating mutations in the *JAK2* gene (95 to 97% and 23 to 75% for PV and ET, respectively).

The leukocyte alkaline phosphatase (LAP) score was historically used in the laboratory evaluation of granulocytosis as a diagnostic marker for myeloproliferative disease. The LAP score is very low (usually 0) in the setting of CML and elevated in PV. The LAP score has a very wide normal range and in practical terms was only definitively helpful in the setting of CML because "high" LAP scores can also be seen in infectious and inflammatory settings. With the availability of direct molecular genetic diagnosis of CML by assay for the *BCR-ABL* fusion gene, it can no longer be recommended as a diagnostic test.

Postsplenectomy

Patients develop leukocytosis following splenectomy, and this may be longstanding, reflecting the loss of a major site of neutrophil margination. This is of no clinical importance, except insofar as it leads to unnecessary evaluation for other pathology.

CLINICAL MANIFESTATIONS AND DIAGNOSIS

As outlined previously, acquired leukocytosis is most commonly the result of acute or chronic infection or inflammation. When it occurs in the absence of fever, aberrations in acute phase reactants, effusions and edema, or other signs and symptoms of inflammation, it still may be secondary to drugs or an underlying nonhematologic malignancy. As such, it should be seen as the sign of a healthy hematopoietic system responding to an outside stress. Bone marrow evaluation is therefore rarely indicated. However, persistence of leukocytosis in the absence of signs and symptoms of inflammation or infection, nonhematologic malignancy, and offending drugs should prompt an evaluation for a primary myeloproliferative disease or clonal hematologic neoplasm, particularly when there is evidence of a leukoerythroblastic reaction. CML and PV can be ruled out by molecular diagnosis on the peripheral blood as described previously. In this setting, bone marrow examination is indicated to evaluate for marrow infiltration by infection, tumor, or fibrosis and should include cultures for tuberculosis and fungal infection as well as cytogenetics and flow cytometry (Fig. 170-4).

Leukocytosis Due to Expansion of Other Cell Lines

Monocytosis and lymphocytosis can also lead to elevations of the WBC. Monocytosis is defined by an absolute monocyte count of greater than 500/μL and usually occurs in the setting of chronic inflammation resulting from infections like tuberculosis, syphilis, or subacute bacterial endocarditis, autoimmune or granulomatous disease, and sarcoidosis. It can also be seen in malignancies, such as preleukemic states, nonlymphocytic leukemia including acute myelomonocytic and monocytic leukemia, histiocytosis, Hodgkin's disease, non-Hodgkin's lymphoma, and various carcinomas. Finally, it can be seen in the setting of chronic neutropenia, after splenectomy, and in the setting of recovery from marrow suppression (Table 170-2).

Lymphocytosis is defined by an absolute lymphocyte count of more than 5000/μL. The most common causes of an elevated lymphocyte count are viral infections such as Epstein-Barr virus and the hepatitis viruses. Although most bacterial infections cause neutrophilia, pertussis and cat-scratch disease due to *Bartonella henselae* can cause an impressive lymphocytosis. Other infections that may cause a secondary lymphocytosis include toxoplasmosis and babesiosis. Hypersensitivity reactions due to drugs or serum sickness may also be associated with lymphocytosis. Primary disorders that cause a lymphocytosis include chronic lymphocytic leukemia (CLL) and monoclonal B-cell lymphocytosis (Table 170-3; see also Table 190-2 and Chapter 190).

Eosinophilia is defined by an absolute eosinophil count of more than 400/μL. Eosinophils proliferate under the influence of IL-5 and play a role in phagocytosis and modulating toxicity due to mast cell degranulation in

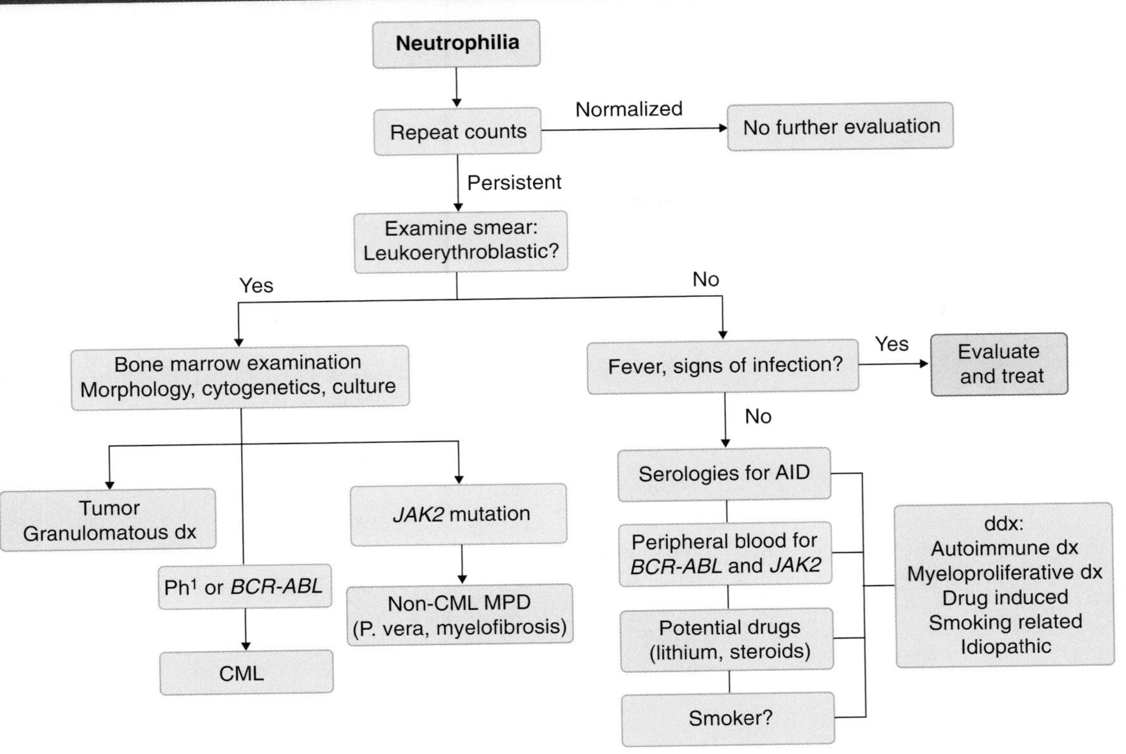

FIGURE 170-4. **Diagnostic approach to neutrophilia.** AID = autoimmune disease; CML = chronic myelogenous leukemia; ddx = differential diagnosis; dx = disease; MPD = myeloproliferative disorder; Ph[1] = Philadelphia chromosome; P. vera = polycythemia vera.

TABLE 170-2 DIFFERENTIAL DIAGNOSIS OF MONOCYTOSIS

- I. Infection
  - a. Granulomatous disease (tuberculosis, fungal disease)
  - b. Endocarditis
  - c. Syphilis
- II. Autoimmune diseases
  - a. Lupus, rheumatoid arthritis
  - b. Giant cell arteritis
  - c. Vasculitis
- III. Inflammatory bowel disease
- IV. Sarcoid
- V. Malignancy
  - a. Primary hematologic malignancy
    - i. Chronic myelomonocytic leukemia
    - ii. Acute myelomonocytic leukemia
    - iii. Lymphoma
  - b. Solid tumors
- VI. Neutropenia
  - a. Associated with chronic neutropenia
  - b. Recovery form marrow suppression
- VII. Postsplenectomy

TABLE 170-3 DIFFERENTIAL DIAGNOSIS OF LYMPHOCYTOSIS

- I. Infection
  - a. Viral infection
    - i. Epstein-Barr virus
    - ii. Cytomegalovirus
    - iii. Hepatitis
  - b. Bacterial infection
    - i. Pertussis
    - ii. Bartonella
    - iii. Tuberculosis
    - iv. Syphilis
    - v. Rickettsia
    - vi. Babesia
- II. Hypersensitivity reactions
  - a. Serum sickness
  - b. Drug hypersensitivity
- III. Primary hematologic disease
  - a. Chronic lymphocytic leukemia
  - b. Monoclonal B-cell lymphocytosis
  - c. Non-Hodgkin's lymphoma

hypersensitivity reactions. Eosinophilia is therefore most often seen in the setting of drug reactions, allergy, atopy, and asthma. A variety of infections, particularly parasitic infections and, to a lesser degree, fungal infections, can be associated with an increased number of circulating eosinophils. Eosinophilia can also be the result of autoimmune and inflammatory conditions, as in Churg-Strauss vasculitis. Atheroembolic disease and adrenal insufficiency may also cause eosinophilia. There are a number of cancers that have been associated with polytypic expansion of eosinophils, including lymphomas and solid tumors. There are also a number of clonal disorders of eosinophils that occur in the setting of some leukemias. Finally, there is a heterogeneous group of disorders termed *hypereosinophilic syndromes*. A *FIP1L1-PDGFRA* fusion gene has confirmed that some of these are primary clonal disorders of eosinophils; the clonality of other hypereosinophilic syndromes can be difficult to establish (see Table 173-1 in Chapter 173).

NEUTROPENIA

Neutropenia may reflect low numbers of circulating neutrophils with either low or normal neutrophil reserves. The risk for infection in the setting of neutropenia is therefore highly dependent on the size of the neutrophil storage pool. Although neutropenia is defined by an absolute neutrophil count of less than 1500/μL, patients with neutrophil counts below this number may have different risks and rates of infection depending on the cause of neutropenia. For instance, patients who are neutropenic owing to chemotherapy, marrow failure, or marrow exhaustion experience infection at much higher rates than those with chronic neutropenic syndromes and immune-mediated neutropenia. Neutropenia may be congenital or acquired. The following sections first discuss congenital neutropenic disorders, the study of which has provided critical insights into normal myelopoiesis, and then the secondary causes of neutropenia (Table 170-4).

Primary Causes of Neutropenia

Ethnic and Benign Familial (Constitutional) Neutropenia

The normal range of the neutrophil count is genetically determined and can be variable. A number of racial and ethnic groups have been observed to have a relatively large proportion of members who are neutropenic by comparison to the published normal range, usually based on young, largely white individuals. This is termed *constitutional neutropenia* and is seen among a variety of ethnic groups, including African Americans, Yemenite Jews, Falasha Jews, and African Bedouins. Single nucleotide polymorphisms in the gene for the Duffy antigen receptor for chemokine (DARC) have been shown to associate with race and are a postulated candidate to explain racial and ethnic differences in neutrophil counts. There is also an autosomal dominantly inherited

TABLE 170-4 DIFFERENTIAL DIAGNOSIS OF NEUTROPENIA

I. Congenital neutropenia
  a. Ethnic and benign familial (constitutional) neutropenia
  b. Severe congenital neutropenia
    i. Autosomal dominant (*ELANE* mutation)
    ii. Autosomal recessive (Kostmann's syndrome; *HAX2* mutation)
    iii. X-linked (*WASP* mutation)
    iv. Other rare defects (*G-CSFR* mutation, unknown)
  c. Cyclic neutropenia
  d. Shwachman-Diamond syndrome
  e. Fanconi anemia
  f. Dyskeratosis congenita
  g. Glycogen storage disease type Ib
  h. Myelokathexis
  i. Chédiak-Higashi syndrome
  j. Griscelli syndrome type II
  k. Hermansky-Pudlak syndrome II
II. Acquired neutropenia
  a. Infection
  b. Postinfection
  c. Drug induced
  d. Immune neutropenia
    i. Primary immune neutropenia
    ii. Secondary to autoimmune disease
      1. Rheumatoid arthritis
        (a) Felty's syndrome
        (b) Large granular lymphocyte disease
      2. Systemic lupus erythematosus
      3. Wegener's granulomatosis
      4. Hyperthyroidism
    iii. Pure white cell aplasia associated with thymoma
    iv. Large granular lymphocyte disease
  e. Primary bone marrow failure
    i. Aplastic anemia
    ii. Myelodysplastic syndrome
    iii. Acute leukemia
  f. Margination and hypersplenism
  g. Nutritional deficiency
  h. Chronic idiopathic neutropenia in adults (CINA)

ELANE = neutrophil elastase; G-CSFR: granulocyte colony-stimulating factor receptor; WASP = Wiskott-Aldrich syndrome protein.

TABLE 170-5 CONGENITAL NEUTROPENIA SYNDROMES

SYNDROME	INHERITANCE PATTERN	GENE
SCN	Autosomal dominant	ELANE (~60%)
	Autosomal recessive	HAX1 (~5%)
	X-linked	WASP (~5%)
	Autosomal recessive	G6PC3 (~2%)
	Autosomal dominant	Gfi1 (rare)
	Autosomal dominant	G-CSFR (rare)
Cyclic Neutropenia	Autosomal dominant	ELANE
Other Congenital Syndromes		
Shwachman-Diamond syndrome	X-Linked	SBDS
Fanconi anemia	Autosomal recessive	FANCA-FANCO
Dyskeratosis congenita	Variable	Telomerase and related genes
Glycogen storage disease type 1b	Autosomal recessive	G-6-PT
Myelokathexis	Autosomal dominant	CXCR4
Chédiak-Higashi Syndrome	Autosomal recessive	LYST
Griscelli syndrome type 2	Autosomal recessive	RAB27A
Hermansky-Pudlak syndrome type 2	Autosomal recessive	AP3B1

ELANE = neutrophil elastase; G6PC3 = glucose-6-phosphatase catalytic subunit 3; G-6-PT = glucose-6-phosphatase translocase; G-CSFR = granulocyte colony-stimulating factor receptor; LYST = lysosomal trafficking regulatory gene; SBDS = Shwachman-Bodian-Diamond syndrome; SCN = severe congenital neutropenia; WASP = Wiskott-Aldrich syndrome protein.

condition called *benign familial neutropenia* that is characterized by neutrophil counts in the 800 to 1400/μL range. Both ethnic and benign familial neutropenia have been shown to be associated with *no* increased risk for infection.

Severe Congenital Neutropenia

First described by Rolf Kostmann in 1956, severe congenital neutropenia (SCN) is a disorder of severe neutropenia with neutrophil counts of less than 500/μL, presenting in the neonatal period with recurrent bacterial infections. These infections can occur as early as the first months of life and often include omphalitis and perirectal abscesses. There is often an increase in other myeloid cell lines, including monocytes and eosinophils. Bone marrow biopsy in SCN patients reveals a "maturation arrest" with an absence of mature neutrophil elements. SCN can follow autosomal dominant and recessive and X-linked patterns of inheritance and has been shown to be associated with mutations in a variety of genes, as summarized in Table 170-5.

Neutrophil elastase (ELA2, now ELANE) is a serine protease that is synthesized at high levels in the promyelocyte stage of neutrophil maturation and is packaged in primary granules. It was originally hypothesized that mutations in ELANE led to its defective cellular trafficking and cytoplasmic accumulation, subsequently triggering neutrophil apoptosis. Newer evidence, however, supports a mechanism by which accumulation of the mutant neutrophil elastase in the endoplasmic reticulum activates the unfolded protein response, leading to apoptosis. SCN due to these mutations is inherited in an autosomal dominant fashion. Hax-1 is a mitochondrial protein with weak homology to bcl-2, and its absence results in mitochondrial-dependent apoptosis. It is the mutated protein implicated in the original autosomal recessive cases of SCN described by Kostmann. Although all SCN cases were originally referred to as *Kostmann's syndrome*, that term is now reserved for this subgroup of autosomal recessive SCN. Wiskott-Aldrich syndrome protein (WASP) regulates actin polymerization in hematopoietic cells, and deficiency in this protein results in the Wiskott-Aldrich syndrome, characterized by small platelets in low number, sinopulmonary infections, and eczema. Another phenotype of mutated WASP, however, is X-linked thrombocytopenia and neutropenia. Mutations in glucose-6-phosphatase catalytic subunit 3 (*G6PC3*) are the most recently discovered cause of a subset of SCN patients; homozygous loss of this metabolic enzyme also appears to lead to activation of the unfolded protein response and increased apoptosis of neutrophil precursors.

SCN was formerly a disease of infancy and early childhood because few, if any, patients survived to adulthood. However, the advent of the availability of recombinant G-CSF and the observation that G-CSF is able to raise neutrophil counts and prevent infection in most patients have allowed these children to survive. Some patients require very high doses of G-CSF, but responses are seen in 80 to 90% of individuals. Increased survival led to the emerging realization that SCN predisposes to the development of myelodysplasia and acute leukemia (MDS/AML), with the development of MDS/AML at a rate of approximately 2% per year, and a cumulative risk of about 30% over 10 years. Patients refractory to G-CSF appear to have a higher risk for leukemic transformation. As discussed later, development of MDS/AML is often associated with the acquisition of a mutation in the gene encoding for the G-CSF receptor. Considerable controversy exists concerning the potential contribution of G-CSF administration to the risk for malignant transformation in children with SCN who receive lifelong treatment with G-CSF (see later under Treatment).

Two classes of G-CSF receptor mutations have been associated with SCN and either hyper-responsiveness or hyporesponsiveness of the receptor. Initial studies aimed at demonstrating that SCN was caused by mutation of the G-CSF or G-CSF receptor gene did not implicate such mutations in the pathogenesis of a significant number of patients with SCN. However, a small number of patients have been shown to have mutations in the G-CSF receptor gene that block ligand binding and produce a G-CSF-resistant form of SCN. More important, however, the studies identified an acquired missense mutation that introduces a stop codon and leads to the deletion of the distal intracellular domain of the receptor known to be responsible for differentiation signaling. This has been hypothesized to cause proliferation of hematopoietic progenitors at the expense of maturation and to be associated with hypersensitivity to G-CSF, suggesting that this mutation may play an important role in the development of MDS/AML in the setting of SCN. However, whether this mutation is in fact of pathogenetic importance to the development of MDS/AML and whether G-CSF influences the risk of developing the mutation and influencing leukemic transformation remain subjects of significant controversy.

Cyclic Neutropenia

Cyclic neutropenia is defined as periods of neutropenia (≤200/µL) lasting 3 to 5 days and occurring at approximately 21-day intervals. These periods of neutropenia can be marked by recurrent fevers, mouth sores, and infections of the skin, upper respiratory tract, and ears. The disorder can be dominantly inherited or sporadic. Congenital cyclic neutropenia has also been shown to be associated with mutations in the gene for neutrophil elastase in all cases tested to date. The diagnosis formerly required demonstration of transient neutropenia through blood counts every 2 to 3 weeks over a course of 6 weeks but now can be established by sequencing of the neutrophil elastase gene. It is successfully treated with G-CSF and is not associated with an increased risk for leukemic transformation. Rare cases of cyclic neutropenia acquired in adulthood have been associated with systemic diseases such as large granular lymphocytosis or T-cell lymphoma.

Other Congenital Syndromes with Associated Neutropenia

A number of other congenital syndromes are associated with neutropenia as one of the constellation of disease-associated abnormalities. These include Shwachman-Diamond syndrome, Fanconi anemia, dyskeratosis congenita, glycogen storage disease Ib, myelokathexis, Chédiak-Higashi syndrome, Griscelli syndrome II, and Hermansky-Pudlak syndrome II.

Shwachman-Diamond syndrome usually begins as an isolated neutropenia but progresses to marrow failure and is also associated with pancreatic dysfunction and skeletal abnormalities. The responsible gene has been identified, the Shwachman-Bodian-Diamond syndrome gene (*SBDS*), and is involved in the regulation of ribosomal RNA. These patients carry an increased risk for leukemic transformation.

Fanconi anemia is due to mutations in genes involved in DNA repair, and as such, it takes more time for marrow failure to develop in these patients (median age, 7 years). Patients with Fanconi anemia often have, in addition to marrow failure, short stature with upper limb anomalies and hyperpigmented cafe au lait spots, although about one third have no physical abnormalities. Screening is done by chromosomal fragility testing following exposure to diepoxybutane or mitomycin C as well as direct assessment for known Fanconi gene mutations. Stem cell transplantation is curative but carries a high risk for morbidity and mortality.

Dyskeratosis congenita is a syndrome of nail dystrophy, leukoplakia, and skin pigmentation abnormalities with associated neutropenia or aplastic anemia, or both. It can be inherited in an autosomal dominant or recessive or X-linked fashion and has been shown to be associated with mutations in several genes that are implicated in telomere maintenance. It typically does not present until the second decade of life.

Glycogen storage disease Ib is inherited in an autosomal recessive fashion and characterized by intermittent neutropenia due to defects in the neutrophil respiratory burst with subsequent apoptosis of circulating neutrophils. Hepatomegaly and metabolic crises are also the hallmarks of this disease and are due to mutations in the gene for the glucose-6-phosphatase translocase enzyme.

The neutropenia of *myelokathexis* is due to retention of mature neutrophils in the bone marrow despite a low peripheral neutrophil count. During infection, however, patients with myelokathexis typically have a sudden rise in their neutrophil count, which makes their clinical course relatively more benign. There is an association between this condition and hypogammaglobulinemia and warts, the WHIM syndrome (*w*arts, *h*ypogammaglobulinemia, *i*mmunodeficiency, and *m*yelokathexis). It has been shown to be caused by heterozygous mutations in the gene encoding chemokine receptor CXCR4.

Chédiak-Higashi syndrome, Griscelli syndrome II, and *Hermansky-Pudlak syndrome II* are all syndromes of albinism and neutropenia due to defects in vesicular trafficking. Chédiak-Higashi syndrome is due to mutations in a lysosomal trafficking regulatory gene (*LYST*) and is characterized by oculocutaneous albinism, bleeding, progressive neurologic disease, and increased susceptibility to hemophagocytic syndrome. Patients with Griscelli syndrome II also have an increased susceptibility to hemophagocytic syndrome as well as albinism and periodic neutropenia; Griscelli syndrome II is caused by mutations in the gene encoding the small guanosine triphosphatase RAB27A, which is involved in the release of myeloperoxidase from the primary granules of neutrophils. Finally, Hermansky-Pudlak syndrome II is due to mutations in the *AP3B1* gene, which encodes a part of a protein transport complex that is involved in vesicular trafficking in many cell types and appears to be involved in the trafficking of neutrophil elastase. It is also marked by albinism, platelet abnormalities, and pulmonary fibrosis.

Secondary Causes of Neutropenia

Infection-Related Neutropenia

Several viral infections have been shown to cause a transient neutropenia that typically resolves as the viremia abates. These include varicella, measles, rubella, hepatitis A and B, Epstein-Barr virus, influenza, parvovirus, and cytomegalovirus. The mechanisms are diverse and can involve redistribution, decreased production, and immune destruction of neutrophils. Human immunodeficiency virus and acquired immunodeficiency syndrome can likewise cause leukopenia and neutropenia, perhaps through splenomegaly with increased sequestration as well as through immune-mediated destruction by antineutrophil antibodies. A myriad of atypical infections like *Mycobacterium tuberculosis*, ehrlichiosis, rickettsia, tularemia, brucellosis, and some staphylococcal infections can cause a moderate neutropenia. Any infection leading to overwhelming sepsis can cause neutropenia, but this is usually through consumption of the marrow neutrophil reserve and is typically seen in newborns and elderly patients and not in individuals with an otherwise healthy and mature marrow. There is also increased margination of neutrophils during sepsis due to systemic activation of complement, exacerbating the neutropenia.

Drug-Induced Neutropenia and Neutropenia Due to Marrow Injury

Drug-induced neutropenia is the most common cause of neutropenia. Multiple drugs have been implicated in neutropenia and agranulocytosis, in both predictable and idiosyncratic patterns. The mechanism of leukopenia is predominantly one that occurs within the marrow compartment, but certain drugs are also associated with increased destruction or clearance of peripheral neutrophils. Within the marrow compartment, many drugs cause direct dose-dependent marrow suppression, whereas others incite immune-mediated destruction. The typical pattern of drug-induced neutropenia is neutropenia that occurs after about 1 to 2 weeks of exposure to the drug with a recovery that begins within days of stopping the drug. However, atypical cases can present long after drug initiation, and others may be associated with a longer interval before recovery of the neutrophil count (Fig. 170-5). Patients with drug-induced agranulocytosis may present with acute sepsis, and it is associated with a significant risk for acute mortality. Recovery is often preceded by the appearance of monocytes and immature neutrophil forms. The more hypercellular the marrow is at diagnosis, the earlier marrow recovery may occur. Some common drugs known to cause neutropenia, in addition to antineoplastic, antiviral, and immunosuppressive agents, include clozapine, the thioamides, and sulfasalazine. Neutrophil recovery is speeded by G-CSF, although there are no definitive data that this improves survival.

Radiation can also result in marrow injury leading to an acute or chronic marrow failure state; in high doses, it is also a risk factor for the development of myelodysplasia and leukemia. These malignant hematopoietic diseases can themselves cause marrow failure because the malignant cells proliferate within the marrow-occupying space and can cause marrow fibrosis, both of which lead to cytopenias. These diseases are discussed in greater detail in Chapters 188 and 189, respectively. Likewise, metastatic carcinoma to the bone can also cause marrow failure because the marrow becomes increasingly occupied by the metastatic cells.

Immune Neutropenia

Infection and drugs cause immune-mediated neutrophil destruction. However, immune neutropenia can also occur as an isolated phenomenon (primary immune neutropenia) or as a manifestation of an underlying systemic autoimmune disease (secondary immune neutropenia). Primary autoimmune neutropenia is a disease of children younger than 4 years; median age of onset is 6 to 12 months. Although infectious risk is increased, treatment is restricted to prophylactic antibiotics, with G-CSF reserved for acute infectious episodes. Ninety-five percent of patients undergo spontaneous remissions within 2 years. Nearly all of these patients have antineutrophil antibodies directed against antigens derived from the FcγIIIb receptor; these antibodies mediate neutrophil destruction by either sequestration in the spleen or complement-mediated neutrophil lysis.

Secondary autoimmune neutropenia is a disease of adults and can be seen in association with hyperthyroidism, Wegener's granulomatosis, rheumatoid

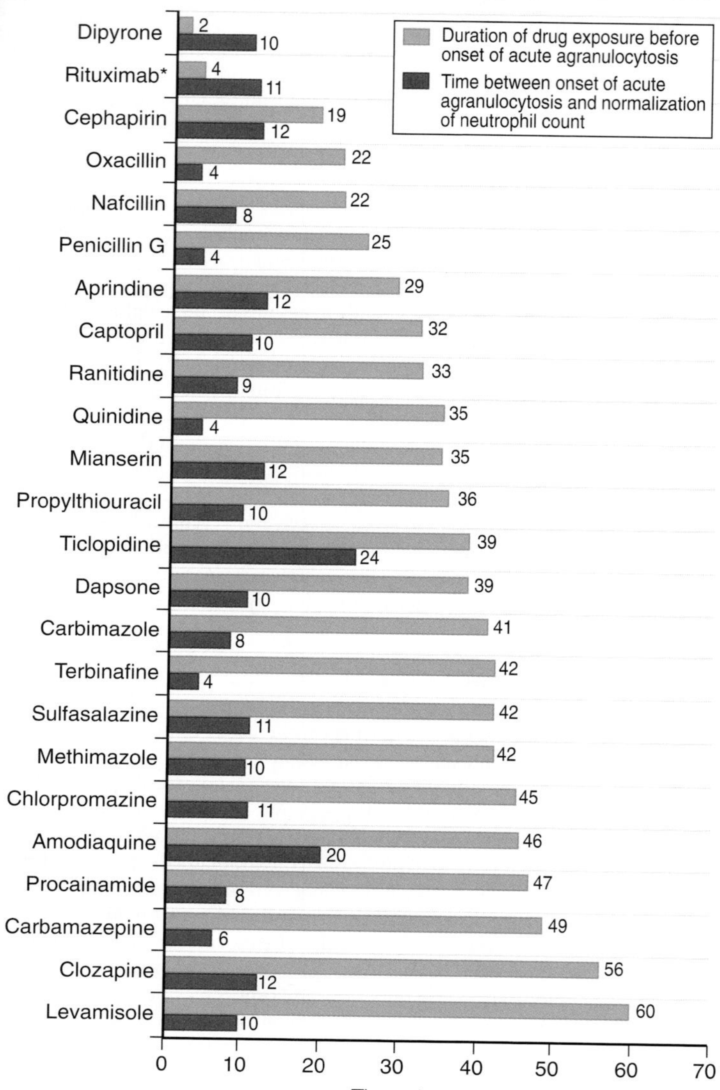

FIGURE 170-5. **Median duration of treatment and neutropenia.** Only drugs with more than three definite or probable reports of the time between onset of acute agranulocytosis and normalization of neutrophil count and the duration of treatment before onset of acute agranulocytosis were considered. (From Andersohn F, Konzen C, Garbe E. Systematic review: agranulocytosis induced by nonchemotherapy drugs. *Ann Intern Med.* 2007;146: 657-665.)

arthritis, and systemic lupus erythematosus (SLE). The role of antineutrophil antibodies in these patients is less clear. More than 50% of patients with SLE, for example, have antineutrophil antibodies, but many have normal neutrophil counts, and there is a poor correlation between the presence of the antibodies and neutrophil number.

Felty's syndrome and *large granular lymphocyte syndrome* deserve separate mention. Felty's syndrome occurs in association with long-standing rheumatoid arthritis (RA) (Chapter 272), and is characterized by splenomegaly and profound neutropenia. Large granular lymphocyte syndrome often occurs in the setting of RA but can also occur as an isolated phenomenon. Both Felty's syndrome and large granular lymphocyte syndrome are associated with a proliferation of large granular lymphocytes, with a characteristic surface phenotype ($CD3^+$, $CD8^+$, $CD16^+$, and $CD57^+$). In the setting of RA, these two syndromes were originally thought to be separate diseases, with Felty's syndrome being polyclonal and large granular lymphocyte syndrome representing a monoclonal proliferation of larger granular lymphocytes, but with increasing sensitivity of detection of monoclonal populations of lymphocytes, this distinction has become blurred. Finally, it has been observed that more than 90% of RA patients with either syndrome are human leukocyte antigen (HLA)-DR4-positive, leading to the postulate that the two entities represent the extremes of a single spectrum of disease. This HLA restriction is not found among non-RA patients with large granular lymphocytes. Both

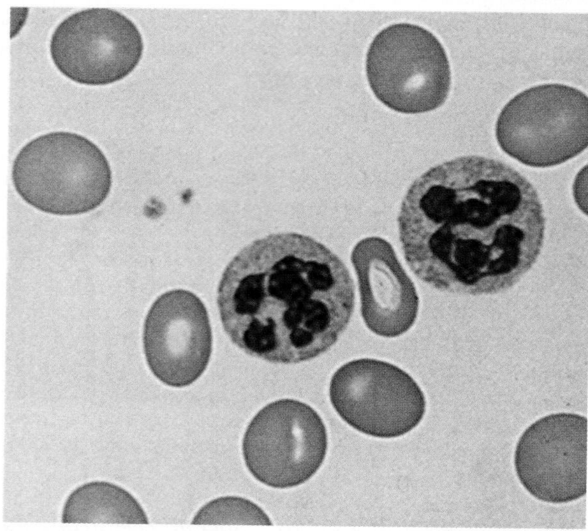

FIGURE 170-6. **Peripheral blood with macrocytosis and hypersegmented neutrophils in megaloblastic anemia.**

syndromes cause immune-mediated neutrophil destruction by a wide array of mechanisms, including antineutrophil antibodies and cell-mediated destruction. Some patients may also have G-CSF resistance mediated by inhibitory G-CSF antibodies.

There are other rare forms of immune neutropenia. Isoimmune neonatal neutropenia is a moderate to severe neutropenia of the newborn due to transplacental passage of maternal immunoglobulin G antibodies against alleles inherited from the father, resulting in neutropenia in a manner similar to the development of anemia in Rh hemolytic disease. Pure white cell aplasia is a rare disease associated with severe pyogenic infections, and also with thymoma in more than two thirds of cases. It has also occurred following ibuprofen therapy. There is a complete absence of myeloid precursors on bone marrow examination. It is immune-mediated, but removal of the thymoma in thymoma-associated cases may not be sufficient for remission. Adjuvant therapy with cyclophosphamide, corticosteroids, cyclosporine, and intravenous immunoglobulin may be needed.

Neutropenia Due to Increased Margination and Hypersplenism

Complement activation can result in both acute and chronic neutropenia as a result of increased margination of the circulating neutrophil pool. This is attributed to the fact that C5a renders neutrophils more adherent and thereby prone to aggregation within the pulmonary vasculature. This has been seen in patients suffering from burns and transfusion reactions. Complement activation may also lead to neutrophil destruction, as in paroxysmal nocturnal hemoglobinuria. The circulating neutrophil pool can also be diminished in association with hypersplenism, although this is typically less common and less pronounced than the anemia and thrombocytopenia seen in patients with an enlarged spleen.

Neutropenia Due to Nutritional Deficiency

Several vitamin and mineral deficiencies, particularly B_{12}, folate, and copper, are associated with neutropenia. Deficiencies in these vitamins and minerals result in ineffective myelopoiesis, maturation arrest, and megaloblastic changes with nuclear-cytoplasmic dyssynchrony. The characteristic finding in the setting of megaloblastic anemia is hypersegmentation of the neutrophil (Fig. 170-6).

Chronic Idiopathic Neutropenia

Chronic idiopathic neutropenia in adults (CINA) is perhaps the most puzzling form of neutropenia. Patients present with chronic neutropenia that is often an incidental finding on routine blood tests, making it impossible to know how long the neutropenia has been present. They have no evidence of autoimmune disease, nutritional deficiency, or myelodysplasia. The syndrome is heterogeneous, with a wide range of neutrophil counts. A group of these patients from Greece has been studied by Papadaki and colleagues, who reported increased production of transforming growth factor-β (TGF-β) and consequent marrow suppression, leading them to posit an undiagnosed underlying inflammatory disease. These patients, however, tend to have very mild neutropenia, with an absolute neutrophil count (ANC) that is rarely less than 800. It seems likely that these patients have an ethnic predisposition to neutropenia, and indeed the neutropenia has been demonstrated to be linked to a genetic polymorphism in the TGF-β locus. It seems likely, however, that these patients should be distinguished from other CINA patients, many of whom have an ANC below 200. The etiology of neutropenia in these patients is completely unknown. However, the natural history of CINA, even in the face of very low neutrophil counts, is generally benign. Most patients require no therapy, although those with very low counts must be treated with G-CSF when they develop fever in the setting of infections. Some patients with recurrent infections or troublesome aphthous ulcers require chronic G-CSF treatment. These patients typically respond to fairly low doses of G-CSF, and there is no reported increase in the development of MDS/AML.

CLINICAL MANIFESTATIONS AND DIAGNOSIS

Neutropenia by itself is not associated with many clinical signs and symptoms other than those of the condition that may be causing it. It becomes clinically evident, however, when it results in infection. Although patients with an ANC below 1000/μL do have a slightly increased risk for infection, the risk is substantially increased once the neutrophil count falls below 500/μL. Given the lack of neutrophils, the signs and symptoms of infection may be attenuated; as such, pneumonia may be present with minimal infiltrate on chest radiograph, or a urinary tract infection may yield only a very mild pyuria. Given this, fever in any neutropenic patient must be considered an emergency with prompt acquisition of cultures and administration of empirical antibiotic therapy.

When fever, infection or sepsis, and neutropenia present concomitantly for the first time, it can be difficult to determine whether the neutropenia predated the infection or, rather, is the result of the infection. Examination of the peripheral blood smear can be helpful in this regard because an elevation of band forms and evidence of toxic granulation suggest the latter.

Because drug-induced neutropenia is the most common cause of acquired neutropenia, a careful inventory of all drug and toxin exposures is warranted. Likewise, there should be a careful evaluation for underlying malignant and inflammatory conditions as the precipitant of neutropenia. The time course of the neutropenia and infections can provide clues to the etiology of the neutropenia (acute versus chronic, persistent versus cyclic, neonatal versus childhood versus adult onset). Attention should be paid to the skin, bones, appendages, and nails because abnormalities in these may point toward one of the congenital neutropenia syndromes. Evaluation of the complete blood count, peripheral blood smear, and vitamin B_{12} and folate levels should also be performed.

When the neutropenia is not severe and is associated with anemia and thrombocytopenia, one should consider the possibility of hypersplenism. In many cases, the diagnosis can be made by the finding of palpable splenomegaly. However, especially in obese patients, abdominal imaging should be used to evaluate spleen size. Abdominal ultrasound allows the assessment of portal venous flow with Doppler studies. If splenic enlargement is confirmed, the etiology of the splenomegaly (Chapter 171) should be determined. It may reflect congestive splenomegaly secondary to portal hypertension (as a result of cirrhosis, fatty liver, or congestive heart failure, among others) or infiltrative splenomegaly due to a benign or malignant process; Felty's syndrome should be considered in the setting of RA.

In patients with chronic neutropenia in the absence of a history of infection or drug or toxin exposure or an evident B_{12} or folate deficiency, bone marrow examination should be performed to rule out myelodysplasia, with assessment of morphology, flow cytometry for large granular lymphocyte syndrome, and cytogenetics. Once a normal marrow has been obtained, further bone marrow examination is not indicated in patients with CINA (Fig. 170-7).

TREATMENT AND MANAGEMENT Rx

The management of neutropenia (Chapter 289) is dependent on the etiology of the depressed neutrophil count as well as its severity and the presence or absence of fever or infection. Neutropenia with fever is a clinical emergency because these patients are at risk for hemodynamic collapse and septic shock. Therefore, these patients should be evaluated thoroughly and cultured promptly, and antibiotics should be administered within 30 to 60 minutes of presentation before obtaining the results of the cultures. The timely empirical administration of a combination of antipseudomonal antibiotics in patients with neutropenia at the onset of fever resulted in significant clinical benefit,

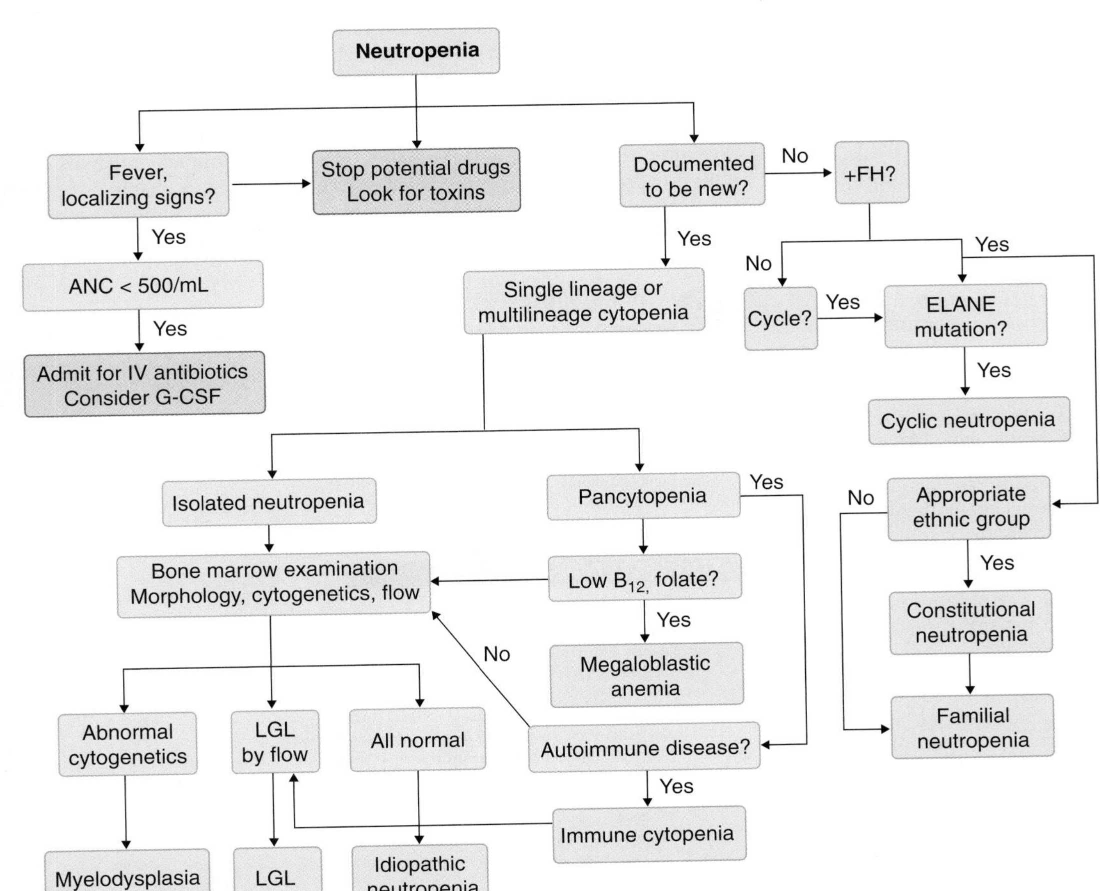

FIGURE 170-7. Diagnostic approach to neutropenia. ANC = absolute neutrophil count; ELANE = neutrophil elastase gene, FH = family history; G-CSF = granulocyte colony-stimulating factor; IV = intravenous; LGL = large granular lymphocyte syndrome.

both with respect to response and survival. With the advent of newer-generation cephalosporins, studies have shown that monotherapy with a third- or fourth-generation cephalosporin at the onset of fever may be sufficient. The addition of a second antipseudomonal agent, vancomycin, or antifungal agent is warranted in patients considered at risk for resistant pseudomonal infection, resistant gram-positive infection, or fungal infections, respectively, or in the face of a failure to defervesce within 3 to 5 days of antibiotic administration. These considerations are discussed in more detail in Chapter 289.

How to manage the uninfected and afebrile neutropenic patient is more nuanced and dependent on the etiology of the neutropenia. Patients with immune-mediated neutropenia are typically treated with immunosuppressive therapy, including steroids, antithymocyte globulin, or cyclosporine, or a combination of these, aimed primarily at treatment of the underlying autoimmune disease. Patients usually respond to G-CSF, although in the setting of RA, this may induce a flare of joint symptoms. Patients with large granular lymphocyte syndrome often respond to therapy with low-dose methotrexate, cyclosporine, or low-dose cyclophosphamide.

Patients with congenital neutropenia, including idiopathic, severe congenital, or cyclic neutropenia, are usually successfully managed with G-CSF for years. Before the use of G-CSF, the mean age of death for these patients was 2 to 3 years. Since the advent of G-CSF, however, life expectancy has been extended by decades into adulthood. Therapy is daily and chronic, with doses varying by the type of neutropenia and the individual responsiveness to therapy. It is usually well tolerated, although accelerated bone loss has been observed. Growth and development do not appear to be affected. Patients with SCN typically require the highest doses, whereas those with idiopathic neutropenia require the lowest, and patients with cyclic neutropenia fall somewhere in between. An increased rate of MDS/AML has been reported with the use of G-CSF in patients with SCN, but this has occurred coincidentally with improved survival. The increased incidence of MDS/AML may then be due to the fact that patients are living longer with a disease whose natural history includes a risk of developing MDS or AML. Certainly, the observation that acquired mutations in the G-CSF receptor are present in 65 to 80% of patients with SCN who develop MDS or AML suggests a potential mutagenic pathway towards leukemogenesis, but whether this is enhanced or accelerated by the administration of G-CSF has yet to be determined. Patients with idiopathic and cyclic neutropenia do not develop MDS or AML, despite therapy with G-CSF. However, recent evidence suggests that the risk for MDS/AML in SCN patients is much higher in those requiring high doses of G-CSF (>10 µg/kg/day), and patients with idiopathic and cyclic neutropenia are usually responsive to much lower G-CSF doses.

In patients with CINA, G-CSF should be reserved for acute febrile episodes unless the patient has recurrent infections. Patients with CINA treated with G-CSF may experience significant side effects, including fever, gastrointestinal symptoms, and splenomegaly. Consequently, in patients with CINA requiring chronic G-CSF administration, the cytokine should be administered at the lowest dose necessary to prevent infections; it is usually sufficient to treat to maintain the ANC higher than 500.

For patients with an inflammatory, infectious, or drug-induced neutropenia, the recommendation is to treat the underlying condition or stop the offending agent. This, however, is not always immediately possible, as in the cases of HIV-infected patients with opportunistic infections or on antiretroviral therapy, solid organ and bone marrow transplant recipients on immunosuppression and antiviral prophylaxis and treatment, and cancer patients undergoing chemotherapy. Prophylactic use of G-CSF in these patients has been shown to be effective in improving the ANC and decreasing rates of infection and febrile neutropenia, but has not been associated with a proven or consistent survival advantage.[1] In light of these findings, many oncologic professional society guidelines recommend the use of prophylactic G-CSF in patients receiving chemotherapy who have a 20% or greater risk of developing febrile neutropenia based on age, comorbid illness, disease characteristics, and myelotoxicity of the chemotherapy regimen. In addition, it is recommended for use during hematopoietic stem cell transplantation, for patients receiving chemotherapy for non-Hodgkin's lymphoma or dose-dense chemotherapy, and for patients with a history of febrile neutropenia receiving further chemotherapy.

The use of prophylactic antibiotics has also been investigated, predominantly in neutropenic patients receiving chemotherapy. Early studies in the 1980s and 1990s demonstrated an improvement in infection-related outcomes but not in infection-related or overall survival. Most recently, several randomized trials of prophylactic quinolones in patients receiving chemotherapy demonstrated an improvement in rates of infection and febrile neutropenia.[2-4] A meta-analysis of studies investigating the use of prophylactic quinolones in patients receiving chemotherapy was the first to document an overall survival benefit as well, although most of these patients had hematologic as opposed to solid tumor malignancies. The current Infectious Diseases Society of America guidelines do not recommend the use of prophylactic antibiotics in cancer patients undergoing myelosuppressive chemotherapy, with the exception of trimethoprim-sulfamethoxazole in patients at risk for *Pneumocystis jirovecii* pneumonia. Antibiotic prophylaxis is not generally used outside of the stem cell transplantation setting. The use of antibiotics to prevent infection in patients with neutropenia due to other causes has not been extensively studied but is typically not recommended and should be based on clinical context.

Stem cell transplantation (Chapter 181) can be curative for a number of the congenital neutropenia and bone marrow failure syndromes. It is, however, not without risk and should therefore be reserved for patients with severe neutropenia complicated by recurrent infection definitively shown to be due to marrow failure.

Leukopenia Due to Deficiency of Other Cell Lines

Lymphocyte production takes place in a variety of anatomic sites, and lymphocyte trafficking from those sites is bidirectional, making it difficult to understand lymphocyte dynamics in the same way that we do for neutrophils. Despite this, the peripheral lymphocyte count seems to be maintained in a narrow range at 2000 to 4000/µL, 20% of which are B cells and 70% of which are T cells. Lymphocytopenia, then, is a total lymphocyte count of less than 1500/µL. It can be the result of decreased production, defective trafficking, or increased loss or destruction. Decreased production can occur as a result of protein and calorie malnutrition; lymphocyte progenitor pool injury secondary to radiation, chemotherapy, or immunosuppressive agents; and congenital immunodeficiency states. Endogenous or exogenous glucocorticoid excess can cause lymphocytopenia by altering lymphocyte trafficking. This can also occur as the result of acute bacterial or fungal infections, certain viral infections, and granulomatous disease. Finally, many viruses can cause direct destruction of lymphocytes, as can antilymphocyte antibodies seen in patients with underlying autoimmune diseases. Lymphocytes can also be lost from intestinal lymphatics in cases of protein-losing enteropathy, primary disease of the gut or intestinal lymphatics, or gut edema secondary to severe heart failure. When lymphocytopenia is discovered, a comprehensive assessment of the immune system should be done, including lymphocyte subtyping, quantitative immunoglobulins, and skin testing to detect deficiencies of cell-mediated immunity. Treatment is typically aimed at the underlying disease, but intravenous immunoglobulin can be administered to patients who are hypogammaglobulinemic, and transplantation can be performed in patients with severe deficiencies of cell-mediated immunity due to impaired lymphocyte production and function.

Monocytopenia, eosinopenia, and basophilopenia can be seen in the setting of bone marrow failure syndromes or as a result of acute infection, malignancy, or severe injury. This is thought to be due to elevations in glucocorticoids, prostaglandins, and epinephrine. A rise in these humoral factors has the greatest impact on eosinophils such that a lack of eosinopenia in any of these settings should prompt suspicion for adrenal insufficiency, a primary myeloproliferative syndrome, parasitic infection, or primary hypereosinophilic syndrome. Monocytopenia is less frequently seen, probably owing to the diverse roles monocytes play in normal human physiology; prolonged and extreme monocytopenia may not be compatible with life.

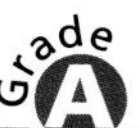

1. Sung L, Nathan PC, Alibhai SM, et al. Meta-analysis: effect of prophylactic hematopoietic colony-stimulating factors on mortality and outcomes of infection. *Ann Intern Med.* 2007;147:400-411.
2. Bucaneve G, Micozzi A, Menichetti F, et al. Levofloxacin to prevent bacterial infection in patients with cancer and neutropenia. *N Engl J Med.* 2005;353:977-987.
3. Cullen M, Steven N, Billingham L, et al. Antibacterial prophylaxis after chemotherapy for solid tumors and lymphomas. *N Engl J Med.* 2005;353:988-998.
4. Gafter-Gvili A, Fraser A, Paul M, et al. Meta-analysis: antibiotic prophylaxis reduces mortality in neutropenic patients. *Ann Intern Med.* 2005;142:979-995.

SUGGESTED READINGS

Aapro MS, Bohlius J, Cameron DA, et al. 2010 update of EORTC guidelines for the use of granulocyte-colony stimulating factor to reduce the incidence of chemotherapy-induced febrile neutropenia in adult patients with lymphoproliferative disorders and solid tumours. *Eur J Cancer.* 2011;47:8-32. *Consensus guidelines for targeted use.*

Apinantriyo B, Lekhakula A, Rujirojindakul P. Incidence, etiology and bone marrow characteristics of non-chemotherapy-induced agranulocytosis. *Hematology.* 2011;16:50-53. *Antimicrobial agents (63%) and antithyroid agents (14%) are the two most common causes.*

Berliner N. Lessons from congenital neutropenia: 50 years of progress in understanding myelopoiesis. *Blood.* 2008;111:5427-5432. *A review of congenital neutropenia in the context of our understanding of normal myeloid maturation.*

Dale DC, Welte K. Cyclic and chronic neutropenia. *Cancer Treat Res.* 2011;157:97-108. *Review of genetics, clinical manifestations, and the observation that most cyclic neutropenia responds well to G-CSF.*

Wilcox RA. Cancer-associated myeloproliferation: old association, new therapeutic target. *Mayo Clin Proc.* 2010;85:656-663. *New insights into the importance of cancer-associated paraneoplastic leukocytosis, the so-called leukemoid reaction.*

171

APPROACH TO THE PATIENT WITH LYMPHADENOPATHY AND SPLENOMEGALY

JAMES O. ARMITAGE

LYMPHADENOPATHY

Physiology and Anatomy

Lymph nodes are found throughout the body along the course of the lymphatics, strategically located to allow the filtering of lymphatic fluid and the interdiction of microorganisms and abnormal proteins. Lymphatic fluid enters the node in afferent lymphatic vessels that empty into the subcapsular sinus. The fluid then transverses the node and exits in a single efferent lymphatic vessel. In doing so, the lymph and its contents are exposed to immunologically active cells throughout the node. Lymph nodes are populated predominantly by macrophages, dendritic cells, B lymphocytes, and T lymphocytes. B lymphocytes are located primarily in the follicles and perifollicular areas, whereas T lymphocytes are found principally in the interfollicular or paracortical areas of the lymph node. These cells function together to provide antigen processing, antigen presentation, antigen recognition, and proliferation of effector B and T lymphocytes as part of the normal immune response to microorganisms or foreign proteins.

Because the normal immune response leads to the proliferation and expansion of one or more cellular components of lymph nodes, it often results in significant lymph node enlargement. In young children, who are continuously being exposed to new antigens, palpable lymphadenopathy is the rule. In fact, the absence of palpable lymphadenopathy would be considered abnormal. In adults, lymph nodes larger than 1 to 2 cm in diameter are generally considered abnormal. However, lymph nodes 1 to 2 cm in diameter in the groin are sufficiently common to be considered normal.

Lymphoid proliferation is a normal response to exposure to foreign antigens. The location of the enlarged lymph nodes often reflects the site of invasion. For example, cervical lymphadenopathy would be typical in a patient with pharyngitis. Generalized immune proliferation and lymphadenopathy can occur with a systemic disorder of the immune system, disseminated infection, or disseminated neoplasia. Malignancies of the immune system might manifest as localized or disseminated lymphadenopathy.

Differential Diagnosis

The differential diagnosis of lymphadenopathy (Table 171-1) is vast, and the underlying causes are responsible for either proliferation of immunologically active cells or infiltration of the lymph node by foreign cells or substances. In practice, the cause of enlarged lymph nodes is often uncertain even in retrospect; in such cases, unrecognized infectious processes are generally blamed.

Infections by bacteria, mycobacteria, fungi, chlamydiae, parasites, and viruses are the major causes of lymph node enlargement. Lymph nodes in the drainage area of essentially all pyogenic infections can enlarge. In certain infections, such as bubonic plague caused by *Yersinia pestis,* dramatic regional lymph node enlargement with fluctuant lymph nodes (i.e., buboes) can be a hallmark of the disease (Chapter 320). Other bacterial infections have lymph node enlargement as a prominent feature (e.g., cat-scratch disease, Chapter 323) and can mimic lymphoproliferative disorders. Mediastinal lymphadenopathy is seen in inhalational anthrax (Chapter 302). In some parts of the world, cervical lymphadenopathy is a sufficiently frequent manifestation of tuberculosis to lead to the institution of antituberculous therapy rather than biopsy. Disseminated lymphadenopathy can be seen in cases of infection by a variety of organisms such as *Toxoplasma,* Epstein-Barr virus (i.e., infectious mononucleosis), cytomegalovirus, and human immunodeficiency virus (HIV).

A variety of nonmalignant disorders of the immune system can lead to localized or disseminated lymphadenopathy. Autoimmune diseases such as rheumatoid arthritis (Chapter 272) and systemic lupus erythematosus (Chapter 274) often have accompanying lymphadenopathy, which can pose a diagnostic challenge because of the increased incidence of lymphoma in patients with these disorders. In the lymphadenopathy that occurs as a reaction to drugs such as phenytoin, lymph node biopsy findings can sometimes be confused with lymphoma. Benign proliferative diseases of the immune system that can also be confused with lymphoma include Castleman's disease (Chapters 191 and 400; angiofollicular lymph node hyperplasia), sinus histiocytosis with massive lymphadenopathy, and disorders seen more frequently in Asia, such as Kawasaki syndrome (Chapter 447) and Kimura's disease.

All the cells in the immune system can become malignant. Several of these malignancies typically manifest as lymphadenopathy, and it can be seen in all of them. Lymphadenopathy as the initial manifestation is the rule for Hodgkin's disease and non-Hodgkin's lymphoma, and it is common in Waldenström's macroglobulinemia and B-cell chronic lymphocytic leukemia; it is seen only occasionally in the myeloid leukemias (Chapters 189 through 192) and is rare in multiple myeloma. Malignancies of all organ systems can metastasize to the lymph nodes and cause lymphadenopathy, which is usually seen in the drainage area of the primary tumor—for example, axillary lymph nodes in patients with breast cancer, hilar and mediastinal lymph nodes in patients with lung cancer, and cervical lymph nodes in patients with head and neck cancer. However, widespread lymphadenopathy can also occur. Other disorders in which lymphadenopathy may be an initial finding include storage diseases such as Gaucher's disease (Chapter 215), endocrinopathies such as hyperthyroidism (Chapter 233), sarcoidosis (Chapter 95), and dermatopathic lymphadenitis. Amyloidosis (Chapter 194) can cause lymphadenopathy in patients with multiple myeloma, hereditary amyloidosis, or amyloidosis associated with chronic inflammatory states.

Among patients with lymphadenopathy actually seen in practices in the United States, diagnoses are not determined in a high proportion (Table 171-2). In such cases, the lymphadenopathy is usually blamed on infection. When the lymphadenopathy is in the drainage site of a known infection (e.g., cervical lymphadenopathy in a patient with pharyngitis) or the patient has a known infection associated with lymphadenopathy (e.g., infectious mononucleosis; Chapter 385), this infectious assumption is usually correct. Alternatively, if a patient has an immunologic disorder that is known to cause lymphadenopathy, such as rheumatoid arthritis, this disorder is usually an acceptable

TABLE 171-1 CAUSES OF LYMPHADENOPATHY

Infection
- Bacterial (e.g., all pyogenic bacteria, cat-scratch disease, syphilis, tularemia)
- Mycobacterial (e.g., tuberculosis, leprosy)
- Fungal (e.g., histoplasmosis, coccidioidomycosis)
- Chlamydial (e.g., lymphogranuloma venereum)
- Parasitic (e.g., toxoplasmosis, trypanosomiasis, filariasis)
- Viral (e.g., Epstein-Barr virus, cytomegalovirus, rubella, hepatitis, HIV)

Benign disorders of the immune system (e.g., rheumatoid arthritis, systemic lupus erythematosus, serum sickness, drug reactions such as to phenytoin, Castleman's disease, sinus histiocytosis with massive lymphadenopathy, Langerhans cell histiocytosis, Kawasaki syndrome, Kimura's disease)

Malignant disorders of the immune system (e.g., chronic and acute myeloid and lymphoid leukemia, non-Hodgkin's lymphoma, Hodgkin's disease, angioimmunoblastic-like T-cell lymphoma, Waldenström's macroglobulinemia, multiple myeloma with amyloidosis, malignant histiocytosis)

Other malignancies (e.g., breast carcinoma, lung carcinoma, melanoma, head and neck cancer, gastrointestinal malignancies, germ cell tumors, Kaposi's sarcoma)

Storage diseases (e.g., Gaucher's disease, Niemann-Pick disease)

Endocrinopathies (e.g., hyperthyroidism, adrenal insufficiency, thyroiditis)

Miscellaneous (e.g., sarcoidosis, amyloidosis, dermatopathic lymphadenitis)

TABLE 171-2 MOST FREQUENT CAUSES OF LYMPHADENOPATHY IN ADULTS IN THE UNITED STATES

Unexplained

Infection
- In drainage area of infection (e.g., cervical adenopathy with pharyngitis)
- Disseminated (e.g., mononucleosis, HIV infection)

Immune disorders (e.g., rheumatoid arthritis)

Neoplasms
- Immune system malignancies (e.g., leukemias, lymphomas)
- Metastatic carcinoma or sarcoma

TABLE 171-3 FACTORS TO CONSIDER IN THE DIAGNOSIS OF LYMPHADENOPATHY

Associated systemic symptoms
Patient's age
History of infection, trauma, medications, travel experience, previous malignancy
Location: cervical, supraclavicular, epitrochlear, axillary, intrathoracic (hilar vs. mediastinal), intra-abdominal (retroperitoneal vs. mesenteric vs. other), iliac, inguinal, femoral
Localized vs. disseminated
Presence of tenderness or inflammation
Size
Consistency

TABLE 171-4 METHODS OF LYMPH NODE EVALUATION

Physical examination
Imaging
- Chest radiography
- Ultrasonography
- Computed tomography
- Magnetic resonance imaging
- Positron emission tomography

Sampling
- Needle aspiration
- Cutting needle biopsy
- Excisional biopsy

explanation; however, progressive lymphadenopathy in such patients should trigger a biopsy because they are at increased risk for lymphoma. Localized, progressive lymphadenopathy, particularly when associated with fever, sweats, or weight loss, requires biopsy to exclude lymphoma.

Lymph Node Evaluation

Evaluation of a patient with lymphadenopathy includes a careful history, a thorough physical examination, laboratory tests, and sometimes imaging studies to determine the extent and character of the lymphadenopathy. The age of the patient and any associated systemic symptoms might be important clues (Table 171-3). Cervical lymphadenopathy in a child is much less worrisome than equally prominent lymphadenopathy in a 60-year-old adult. The occurrence of fever, sweats, or weight loss raises the possibility of a malignancy of the immune system. The explanation for the lymphadenopathy might become apparent with the identification of a site of infection, a particular medication, a travel history, or a previous malignancy.

Physical examination allows the identification of localized versus widespread lymphadenopathy. The particular sites of involvement can be important hints to the diagnosis because infection and carcinoma are likely to cause lymphadenopathy in the lymphatic drainage of the site of the disorder. In general, tender lymph nodes are more likely to be due to an infectious process, whereas painless adenopathy raises concern for malignancy. Lymph node consistency can also aid in the diagnosis: typically, lymph nodes containing metastatic carcinoma are rock hard, lymph nodes containing lymphoma are firm and rubbery, and lymph nodes enlarged in response to an infectious process are soft.

The larger the lymph node, the more likely it is that a serious underlying cause exists; lymph nodes greater than 3 to 4 cm in diameter in an adult are very worrisome. Physical examination to assess lymph node size is only marginally accurate and reproducible, although it is by far the most widely used method. More precise methods are available with various imaging techniques.

Imaging

Imaging studies, including routine radiographs, computed tomography (CT), ultrasonography, magnetic resonance imaging (MRI), and positron emission tomography (PET), can be used to assess the extent of lymphadenopathy in the chest and abdomen (Table 171-4). Chest radiographs are the most economical and easiest way to assess mediastinal and hilar lymphadenopathy but are not as accurate as CT of the chest. CT and ultrasonography are the most useful modalities for assessing abdominal and retroperitoneal lymphadenopathy. In most patients, CT is probably the most accurate approach, but ultrasonography has the advantage of being less expensive and not requiring radiation exposure. MRI and PET are not first-line studies for the assessment of lymphadenopathy. PET is frequently positive in patients with Hodgkin's disease and aggressive non-Hodgkin's lymphomas and can be used to assess the presence of active lymphoma in patients with lymphadenopathy and a proven diagnosis; it is especially useful for re-evaluating patients after therapy because lymph nodes do not always regress to normal size after treatment, particularly those in the mediastinum and retroperitoneum, even though the malignancy has been eradicated.

Interventional Evaluation

Lymph node aspiration or biopsy is often necessary for an accurate diagnosis of the cause of lymphadenopathy. Fine-needle aspiration is currently popular and is an accurate means of diagnosing infection or carcinoma involving a lymph node. Although lymphomas can occasionally be diagnosed with this approach, it is inappropriate as an initial diagnostic maneuver for lymphoma. Cutting needle biopsy occasionally provides sufficient material for an unequivocal diagnosis and subtyping of the lymphoma. However, excisional biopsy, which is most likely to provide the pathologist with adequate material to perform histologic, immunologic, and genetic studies, is also most likely to yield the correct diagnosis.

TABLE 171-5 APPROACH TO THE PATIENT WITH LYMPHADENOPATHY

Does the patient have a known illness that causes lymphadenopathy? Treat and monitor for resolution.
Is there an obvious infection to explain the lymphadenopathy (e.g., infectious mononucleosis)? Treat and monitor for resolution.
Are the nodes very large and/or very firm and thus suggestive of malignancy? Perform a biopsy.
Is the patient very concerned about malignancy and unable to be reassured that malignancy is unlikely? Perform a biopsy.
If none of the preceding are true, perform a complete blood cell count and, if unrevealing, monitor for a predetermined period (usually 2 to 8 weeks). If the nodes do not regress or if they increase in size, perform a biopsy.

An Approach to the Patient with Lymphadenopathy

Patients with lymphadenopathy (Table 171-5) come to medical attention in several ways. Perhaps most common is a patient who feels a lymph node in the neck, axilla, or groin and seeks a physician's opinion. Lymphadenopathy might also be an unexpected finding on a routine physical examination or as part of an evaluation for another complaint. Finally, patients might be found to have unexpected lymphadenopathy on imaging studies of the chest or abdomen. When the nodes are multiple or larger than 2 to 3 cm, biopsy via mediastinoscopy, a paramediastinal incision, laparoscopy, or laparotomy is often required for diagnosis.

The approach to a patient complaining of newly discovered lymphadenopathy in the neck, axilla, or groin depends on the size, consistency, and number of enlarged lymph nodes and the patient's general health. In most cases, very large or very firm lymph nodes in the presence of systemic symptoms such as unexplained fever, sweats, or weight loss should lead to lymph node biopsy. Patients who have enlarged lymph nodes in the drainage area of a previously treated malignancy (e.g., neck nodes in a patient with a history of head and neck cancer) might be best approached by lymph node aspiration. Carcinoma can often be diagnosed in this manner, although it is a poor approach for the diagnosis of lymphoid malignancies. For cervical lymph nodes, excisional biopsy should be delayed in a patient in whom head and neck cancer (Chapter 196) is a diagnostic consideration. These patients should initially undergo careful ear, nose, and throat examinations to avoid performing a biopsy that might complicate the patient's subsequent therapy. Some diagnostic possibilities for localized lymphadenopathy are presented in Table 171-6.

In the most common situation—that is, a lymph node is soft and is not larger than 2 to 3 cm and the patient has no obvious systemic illness—observation for a brief period is usually the best approach. Performance of a complete blood cell count and examination of a peripheral smear can be helpful in recognizing a systemic illness (e.g., infectious mononucleosis). These patients are often given antibiotics. If the lymph node does not regress over the course of a few weeks or if it gets bigger, a biopsy should be performed.

TABLE 171-6 SOME DIAGNOSTIC CONSIDERATIONS FOR LOCALIZED LYMPHADENOPATHY

SITE	INFECTIONS	NEOPLASMS	OTHER
Cervical	Pharyngitis, other head and neck infections, mononucleosis, toxoplasmosis, TB	Head and neck cancers, thyroid cancer, lymphoma	
Supraclavicular		Intra-abdominal cancer (particularly left-sided nodes), lung cancer, lymphoma	
Axillary	Cat-scratch disease, distal infections, plague	Breast cancer, melanoma, lymphoma	Silicone implants
Mediastinal	TB, fungal infection, anthrax	Lymphoma, lung cancer, germ cell tumor	Sarcoidosis
Retroperitoneal	TB	Lymphoma, testicular cancer, kidney cancer, upper GI malignancy	Sarcoidosis
Mesenteric	Appendicitis, cholecystitis, diverticulitis, Whipple's disease	Lymphoma, GI cancer	Inflammatory bowel disease, panniculitis
Inguinal	Distal or genital infection, plague, STDs	Lymphoma, melanoma, vulvar cancer	

GI = gastrointestinal; STD = sexually transmitted disease; TB = tuberculosis.

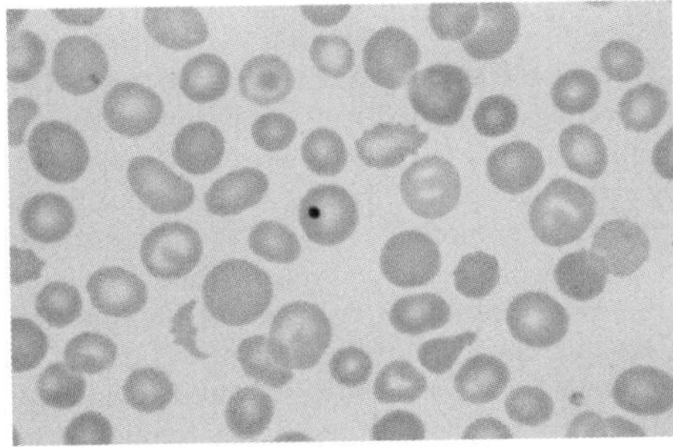

FIGURE 171-1. Howell-Jolly body in an erythrocyte. This is evidence of splenectomy or a nonfunctional spleen.

TABLE 171-7 CAUSES OF SPLENOMEGALY

Infection
- Bacterial (e.g., endocarditis, brucellosis, syphilis, typhoid, pyogenic abscess)
- Mycobacterial (e.g., tuberculosis)
- Fungal (e.g., histoplasmosis, toxoplasmosis)
- Parasitic (e.g., malaria, leishmaniasis)
- Rickettsial (e.g., Rocky Mountain spotted fever)
- Viral (e.g., Epstein-Barr virus, cytomegalovirus, HIV, hepatitis)

Benign disorders of the immune system (e.g., rheumatoid arthritis with Felty's syndrome, systemic lupus erythematosus, drug reactions such as to phenytoin, Langerhans cell histiocytosis, serum sickness)

Malignant disorders of the immune system (e.g., acute or chronic myeloid or lymphoid leukemia, non-Hodgkin's lymphoma, Hodgkin's disease, Waldenström's macroglobulinemia, malignant histiocytosis)

Other malignancies (e.g., melanoma, sarcoma)

Congestive splenomegaly (e.g., portal hypertension secondary to liver disease, splenic or portal vein thrombosis)

Hematologic disorders (e.g., autoimmune hemolytic anemia, hereditary spherocytosis, thalassemia major, hemoglobinopathies, elliptocytosis, extramedullary hematopoiesis)

Storage diseases (e.g., Gaucher's disease)

Endocrinopathies (e.g., hyperthyroidism)

Miscellaneous (e.g., sarcoidosis, amyloidosis, tropical splenomegaly, cysts)

Part of the care of such patients involves the art of medicine and being responsive to the patient's particular needs. For example, biopsy might be performed more quickly in a patient who is very anxious about malignancy or who needs a definitive diagnosis expeditiously.

SPLENOMEGALY

DEFINITION

The spleen is the largest lymphatic organ in the body and is sometimes approached clinically as though it were a very large lymph node. Although it participates in the primary immune response to invading microorganisms and foreign proteins, the spleen has many other functions. It functions as a filter for the blood and is responsible for removing senescent red blood cells from the circulation, as well as blood cells and other cells coated with immunoglobulins. Blood enters the spleen, filters through the splenic cords, and is exposed to immunologically active cells in the spleen.

The splenic red pulp occupies more than half the volume of the spleen and is the site where senescent red cells are identified and destroyed and red blood cell inclusions are removed by a process known as *pitting*. In the absence of splenic function, basophilic inclusions known as *Howell-Jolly bodies* are seen in circulating red blood cells. The presence of Howell-Jolly bodies (Fig. 171-1) in peripheral blood indicates that the patient has undergone splenectomy or has a process that has rendered the spleen nonfunctional (e.g., sickle cell disease with repeated splenic infarcts, chronic graft-versus-host disease).

The white pulp of the spleen contains macrophages, B lymphocytes, and T lymphocytes; participates in the recognition of microorganisms and foreign proteins; and is involved in the primary immune response. Absence of this splenic function makes individuals particularly susceptible to certain infections, including sepsis with encapsulated organisms such as *Streptococcus pneumoniae*. The risk for overwhelming sepsis is related to the age at the time of splenectomy or other cause of loss of splenic function. Children and young adults are at highest risk. If possible, all patients should undergo vaccination against *S. pneumoniae* and perhaps *Haemophilus influenzae* and *Neisseria meningitidis* before splenectomy. Some physicians have patients take oral penicillin (e.g., phenoxymethyl penicillin 250 mg twice daily) indefinitely if splenectomy has been performed in childhood or adolescence.

PATHOBIOLOGY

As with lymphadenopathy, numerous conditions are associated with splenomegaly (Table 171-7). Certain bacterial infections such as endocarditis (Chapter 76), brucellosis (Chapter 318), and typhoid fever (Chapter 316) have splenomegaly as a frequent manifestation. Disseminated tuberculosis (Chapter 332) is often associated with splenomegaly, and splenomegaly can also be seen in cases of disseminated histoplasmosis (Chapter 340) and toxoplasmosis (Chapter 357). Splenomegaly is an almost constant accompaniment of malaria (Chapter 353). Rickettsial disorders such as Rocky Mountain spotted fever are frequently associated with splenomegaly. A wide variety of viral infections typically cause splenomegaly, including infectious mononucleosis associated with Epstein-Barr virus (Chapter 385) and viral hepatitis (Chapters 150 and 151). Splenomegaly can accompany HIV infection. Splenic abscesses, which are usually the result of hematogenous spread of pyogenic organisms, represent an unusual and difficult to diagnose cause of splenomegaly.

Splenomegaly is also seen in a variety of benign disorders of the immune system, including rheumatoid arthritis (Chapter 272); some of these patients have Felty's syndrome and accompanying granulocytopenia. Splenomegaly can be detected in some patients with systemic lupus erythematosus (Chapter 274), certain drug reactions, and serum sickness.

Malignancies of the immune system and nonimmune organs can also lead to splenomegaly. Splenomegaly is usually seen in patients with chronic myeloid leukemia and is frequent in chronic lymphoid leukemia (Chapter 190). It can develop in patients with acute myeloid or lymphoid leukemia, non-Hodgkin's lymphoma, Hodgkin's disease, and Waldenström's macroglobulinemia but is rare in multiple myeloma (Chapter 193). Isolated splenomegaly (i.e., without any enlarged lymph nodes) is characteristic of certain immune system malignancies, including hairy cell leukemia (Chapter 190), the prolymphocytic variant of chronic lymphocytic leukemia (Chapter 190), and splenic marginal zone lymphoma (Chapter 191). Metastasis of carcinomas and sarcomas to the spleen is unusual except for malignant melanoma; even with melanoma, however, palpable splenomegaly is an unusual finding.

Splenomegaly can develop as a result of increased pressure in the splenic circulation, especially in patients with portal hypertension caused by a variety of hepatic disorders, including alcoholic cirrhosis (Chapter 155). However, it also can be due to splenic or portal vein thrombosis.

Hematologic disorders that can lead to palpable splenomegaly include autoimmune hemolytic anemia, hereditary spherocytosis, and a number of other anemias. In cases of idiopathic myelofibrosis, the spleen is frequently a site of extramedullary hematopoiesis (Chapter 169).

A variety of less common conditions can lead to splenomegaly. The storage disorder Gaucher's disease (Chapter 215) usually manifests as splenomegaly. Splenomegaly can be seen in endocrinopathies such as hyperthyroidism (Chapter 233). Sarcoidosis (Chapter 95) and amyloidosis (Chapter 194) can manifest as splenomegaly. *Tropical splenomegaly* is a term used to describe the palpable spleens found in patients who live in tropical areas, for which there may be numerous causes.

DIAGNOSIS

Evaluation of Spleen Size and Function

Physical Examination

The ability to perform an accurate physical examination and determine the presence of an enlarged spleen (Table 171-8) is an important skill, but it is not easily learned. Physical examination of the spleen can be performed with the patient supine or in the right lateral decubitus position. Inspection, percussion, auscultation, and palpation are all important parts of an accurate assessment. It is rare for a spleen to be so large that it is visible and can be seen to move with respiration. However, in patients with such a condition, it is possible to miss splenomegaly by failing to start palpation sufficiently low to find the edge. Occasionally, percussion of the left upper quadrant helps identify an area of dullness that moves with respiration and can lead to the identification of splenomegaly. Spleen size is generally recorded as the number of centimeters the spleen descends below the left costal margin in the midclavicular line on inspiration. Although auscultation is not usually a regular part of splenic examination, the existence of a splenic rub on inspiration can lead to the diagnosis of splenic infarction. The left kidney is sometimes confused with the spleen on physical examination, but its failure to move with respiration in the manner typical for the spleen usually allows its distinction.

Laboratory Evaluation

Laboratory studies are frequently valuable in assessing splenic function. In patients with an absent or nonfunctional spleen, Howell-Jolly bodies will be seen in circulating red blood cells (see Fig. 171-1). Splenic hyperfunction (a condition often referred to as *hypersplenism*) is associated with cytopenias: the spleen is the normal reservoir for a significant proportion of platelets, and this reservoir function can lead to thrombocytopenia in patients with splenomegaly. Patients with autoimmune hemolytic anemia usually have palpable splenomegaly, but patients with idiopathic (immune) thrombocytopenic purpura usually do not.

The spleen can be imaged with ultrasonography, CT, traditional radionuclide scans, and PET (Fig. 171-2). Ultrasonography can provide an accurate determination of spleen size and is easy to repeat. CT frequently gives a better view of the consistency of the spleen and can identify splenic tumors or abscesses that would otherwise be missed. PET can aid in evaluating focal lesions in the spleen. The technetium-labeled liver-spleen scan can be important in identifying liver disease as the cause of splenomegaly; in patients with cryptogenic cirrhosis who are found to have thrombocytopenia, a technetium liver-spleen scan that shows higher activity in the spleen than in the liver might be the first hint of liver disease.

Because of the spleen's location and its propensity to bleed, needle aspiration or cutting needle biopsy of the spleen is rarely performed. In general, splenic "biopsy" involves splenectomy, which can be performed at the time of laparotomy or via laparoscopy. However, performing splenectomy laparoscopically usually leads to maceration of the organ and can reduce the diagnostic information. In very young children, in whom splenectomy leads to a high risk for serious infections such as pneumococcal septicemia, partial splenectomy can sometimes be performed. Patients who undergo splenectomy at the time of splenic trauma and rupture may have seeding of splenic cells to other sites in the abdomen. Some patients have additional small or accessory spleens. Persistent, functional splenic tissue can be the explanation for recurrent immune thrombocytopenia after splenectomy and might be recognized by the absence of Howell-Jolly bodies in circulating red blood cells.

An Approach to the Patient with Splenomegaly

Patients with splenomegaly (Table 171-9) may come to medical attention for a variety of reasons. Patients may complain of left upper quadrant pain or fullness or early satiety. A splenic infarct, which typically manifests as left upper quadrant pain that sometimes radiates to the left shoulder, can be the first clue to the existence of an enlarged spleen. Rarely, splenomegaly initially manifests with the catastrophic symptoms of splenic rupture. Some patients are found to have splenomegaly as a result of evaluation for unexplained cytopenia. Splenomegaly can also be discovered incidentally on physical examination. In recent years, splenomegaly has frequently been discovered on imaging studies of the abdomen performed for other purposes.

The presence of a palpable spleen on physical examination is almost always abnormal. The one exception to this rule is a palpable spleen tip in a slender young woman. In general, the presence of a palpable spleen should be

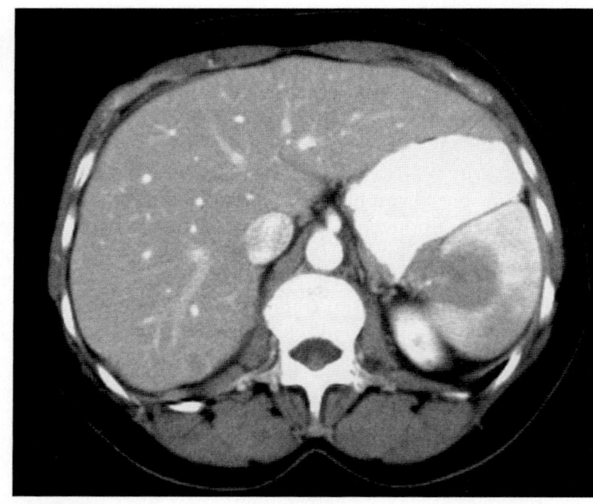

FIGURE 171-2. Enlarged spleen with metastatic adenocarcinoma.

TABLE 171-8 METHODS FOR EVALUATING THE SPLEEN

Physical examination
Imaging
Ultrasonography
Computed tomography
Liver-spleen scanning
Positron emission tomography
Biopsy
Needle aspiration
Splenectomy
Laparotomy (total or partial splenectomy)
Laparoscopy

TABLE 171-9 APPROACH TO THE PATIENT WITH SPLENOMEGALY

Does the patient have a known illness that causes splenomegaly (e.g., infectious mononucleosis)? Treat and monitor for resolution.
Search for an occult infection (e.g., infectious endocarditis), hematologic disorder (e.g., hereditary spherocytosis), occult liver disease (e.g., cryptogenic cirrhosis), autoimmune disease (e.g., systemic lupus erythematosus), or storage disease (e.g., Gaucher's disease). If found, manage appropriately.
If systemic symptoms are present and suggest malignancy, focal replacement of the spleen is seen on imaging studies, and no other site is available for biopsy, splenectomy is indicated.
If none of the above are true, monitor closely and repeat studies until the splenomegaly resolves or a diagnosis becomes apparent.

considered a serious finding, and an explanation should be sought. It is less clear whether the same rules apply to borderline splenomegaly discovered incidentally on routine imaging studies.

The approach to a patient with an enlarged spleen should focus initially on excluding a systemic illness that could explain the splenomegaly. Infectious mononucleosis, leukemia or lymphoma, rheumatoid arthritis, sarcoidosis, cirrhosis of the liver, malaria, and a host of other illnesses would be reasonable explanations for the splenomegaly. The systemic condition should be treated, and then the spleen should be re-evaluated. If the systemic illness can be treated successfully, the spleen should regress to normal size over time.

Patients with no obvious explanation for an enlarged spleen present a difficult diagnostic problem. Careful follow-up of these patients sometimes reveals occult liver disease or an autoimmune process that initially defied diagnosis. Concerns about malignancy, particularly in patients with systemic symptoms such as fever, sweats, or weight loss or in whom imaging studies show a focal abnormality, are sometimes indications for splenectomy. However, in the absence of such findings, it is generally preferable to monitor patients closely with repeated attempts to establish the diagnosis by approaches other than splenectomy. It is particularly important to avoid splenectomy in a patient with occult liver disease and portal hypertension.

Splenectomy was once performed routinely as part of the staging evaluation for Hodgkin's disease or other lymphomas. Today, this procedure is rarely needed to choose the correct therapy, and it should be avoided. Splenectomy can be an effective therapy for immune thrombocytopenic purpura (Chapter 175) and autoimmune hemolytic anemia (Chapter 163), and it is occasionally an appropriate therapy to relieve cytopenias in other conditions such as advanced myelofibrosis (Chapter 169).

SUGGESTED READINGS

Casaccia M, Torelli P, Cavaliere D, et al. Laparoscopic lymph node biopsy in intra-abdominal lymphoma: high diagnostic accuracy achieved with a minimally invasive procedure. *Surg Laparosc Endosc Percutan Tech.* 2007;17:175-178. *Laparoscopic procedures increase the number of patients who can have excisional biopsy.*

Casaccia M, Torelli P, Pasa A, et al. Putative predictive parameters for the outcome of laparoscopic splenectomy: a multicenter analysis performed on the Italian Registry of Laparoscopic Surgery of the Spleen. *Ann Surg.* 2010;251:287-291. *Only 6% of planned laparoscopic splenectomies were converted to open procedures, with an overall perioperative death rate of 0.4%.*

Feng K, Ma K, Liu Q, et al. Randomized clinical trial of splenic radiofrequency ablation versus splenectomy for severe hypersplenism. *Br J Surg.* 2011;98:354-361. *Ablation is an attractive alternative for hypersplenism induced by liver cirrhosis, particularly when more than 50% of the spleen is ablated.*

Harris A, Kamishima T, Hao HY, et al. Splenic volume measurements on computed tomography utilizing automatically contouring software and its relationship with age, gender, and anthropometric parameters. *Eur J Radiol.* 2010;75:e97-e101. *Normal spleen size correlates with age, body weight, body mass index, and body surface area.*

Yong M, Thomsen RW, Schoonen WM, et al. Mortality risk in splenectomised patients: a Danish population-based cohort study. *Eur J Intern Med.* 2010;21:12-16. *Most of the increased risk is due to the underlying indication for splenectomy, not to the splenectomy itself.*

172

DISORDERS OF PHAGOCYTE FUNCTION

MICHAEL GLOGAUER

Neutrophils and monocyte-macrophages are the key phagocytes of the innate immune system. Their principal innate immune role is to recognize and eliminate microorganisms that make their way past primary physical barriers, such as the epithelium and body secretions that protect the external and lining surfaces of the body. Phagocytes identify foreign invaders through a series of pattern recognition receptors, the majority of which belong to the Toll-like receptor family (Chapters 44 and 47). Whereas macrophages carry out sentinel duty looking for microbes in healthy tissue and act as a bridge between the innate and adaptive immune systems, neutrophils appear only in infected or damaged tissue after being recruited by inflammatory mediators released from activated macrophages and endothelial cells or by chemical signals released by invading microorganisms themselves (Table 172-1). After accumulation of these key immune cells at sites of infection, the microbes are eliminated through the process of phagocytosis, which is defined as the engulfment, internalization, and degradation of extracellular material.

NEUTROPHILS

Neutrophils develop in the bone marrow from myeloid precursors, migrate into the circulation, and, if required, make their way into infected or damaged tissue (Fig. 172-1). Their travels are essentially one-way trips because once they leave a compartment, they do not return. After release from the bone marrow compartment, a mature neutrophil has a blood half-life of about 10 hours and may survive up to an additional 48 hours within infected or damaged tissue.

TABLE 172-1 PRIMARY IMMUNE ROLES OF MONOCYTE-MACROPHAGES AND NEUTROPHILS

MONONUCLEAR PHAGOCYTE FUNCTIONS
Elimination of invading pathogens
Elimination of cellular debris from sites of tissue damage and the blood stream
Wound healing-remodeling of normal tissue
Amplification of the innate immune response: release of immune regulators
Bridge to the adaptive immune system: presentation of antigens to lymphocytes
NEUTROPHILS
Elimination of invading pathogens

The Bone Marrow Compartment: The Site of Granulopoiesis

Neutrophils are the most abundant white blood cell and account for up to 70% of circulating leukocytes. Neutrophil numbers can increase rapidly by as much as 5- to 10-fold during periods of acute infection. Because these cells have a very short half-life in blood, the bone marrow compartment provides a steady supply of mature neutrophils with the capability to upregulate cell production rapidly during times of infection. Neutrophils originate in the bone marrow from a common population of hematopoietic stem cells through a 10- to 14-day process of proliferation, differentiation, and maturation (Chapter 159).

Steps in Granulopoiesis

The stages of neutrophil granulopoiesis in the bone marrow (Fig. 172-2) are divided and identified by the major transitions from the pluripotent stem cell to the mature neutrophil. The *myeloblast* is the first recognizable progenitor cell committed to granulopoiesis. This proliferating cell is characterized by its large nucleus and agranular cytoplasm. The *promyelocyte* follows and displays the initial development of primary granules. *Myelocytes* occupy the next stage of neutrophil maturation and are characterized by development of the first specific or "secondary" (peroxidase-negative) granules. *Metamyelocytes,* which follow myelocytes, are incapable of further mitosis and are readily identifiable by their now numerous cytoplasmic granules. The functional maturation of metamyelocytes results in the development of *band* cells, which are usually slightly larger than mature neutrophils and have a 15-μm diameter, a horseshoe-shaped nucleus, and a moderate to abundant supply of specific granules. Band cells can be found in the circulation during periods of acute infection. The final mature *neutrophil,* which is released into the circulation, has a diameter of approximately 10 μm with a characteristic nucleus that is segmented and multilobed and occupies about 20% of the cell's volume; the remaining cytoplasm is taken up by granules.

Defects in granulopoiesis are manifested clinically as low circulating levels of neutrophils (neutropenia; Chapter 170). Verification of the stage at which neutrophil developmental arrest occurs can be determined by a bone marrow biopsy to assess the cellularity and characteristics of the neutrophil precursors present in the marrow space.

Regulation of Granulopoiesis

Granulopoiesis is driven by hematopoietic growth factors (Chapter 159). These factors, which are synthesized by a variety of cells, including fibroblasts and endothelial cells, are known to work together with other regulatory molecules, such as cytokines, to regulate hematopoiesis. Hematopoietic growth factors such as *interleukin-3* (IL-3), *granulocyte-macrophage colony-stimulating factor* (GM-CSF), and *granulocyte colony-stimulating factor* (G-CSF) bind to their target cells through specific receptors and are critical for the hematopoietic system to respond rapidly to infection or inflammation by dramatically increasing the production of leukocytes.

G-CSF is a potent cytokine that influences the proliferation, survival, maturation, and functional activation of cells from the neutrophil-granulocyte lineage. In normal individuals, circulating levels of G-CSF are very low (<100 pg/mL). However, in conditions of stress, G-CSF levels can rise to 20 times baseline levels, thereby resulting in a rapid increase in circulating neutrophils. G-CSF may regulate this increased granulopoiesis by increasing the

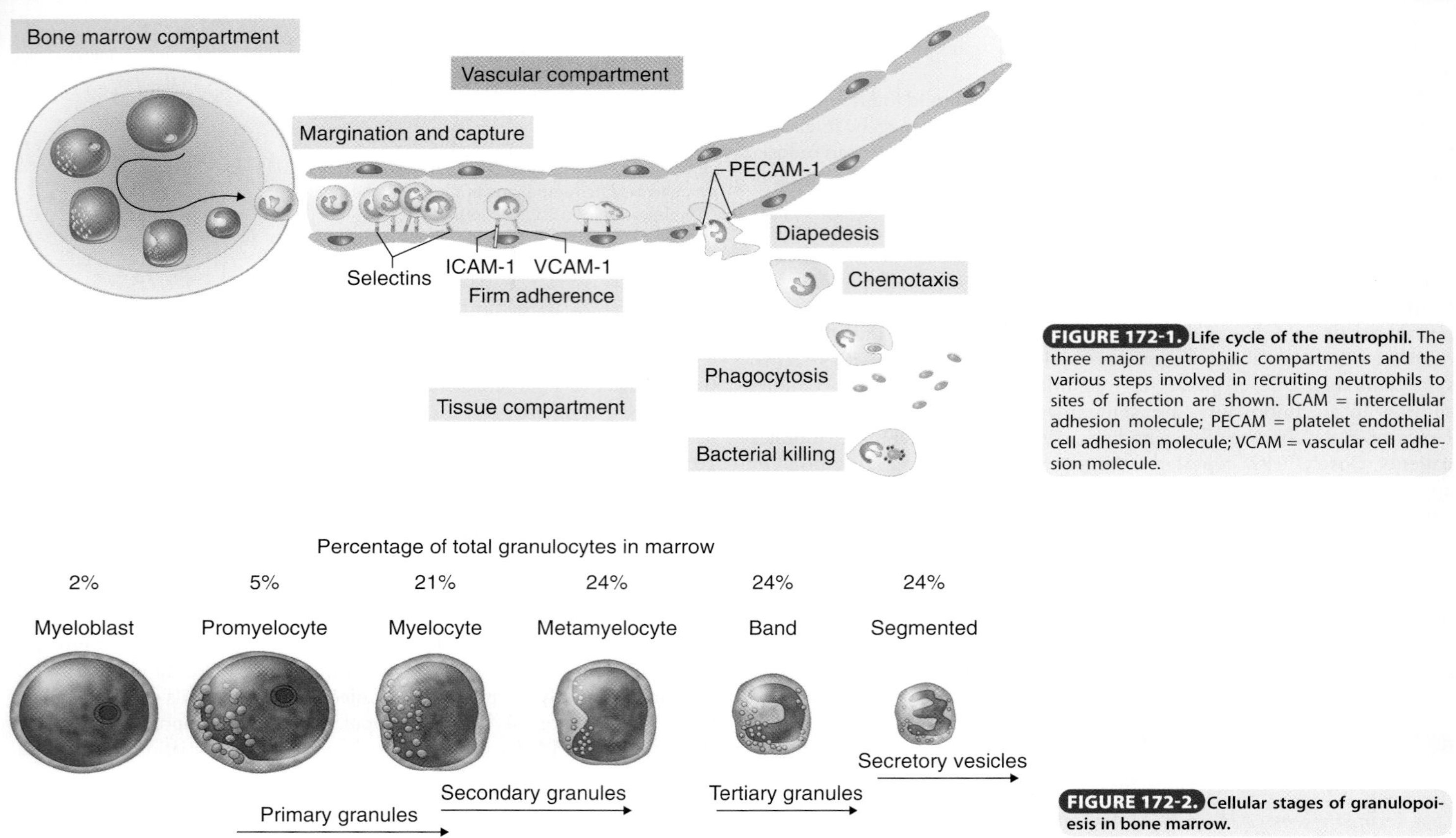

FIGURE 172-1. **Life cycle of the neutrophil.** The three major neutrophilic compartments and the various steps involved in recruiting neutrophils to sites of infection are shown. ICAM = intercellular adhesion molecule; PECAM = platelet endothelial cell adhesion molecule; VCAM = vascular cell adhesion molecule.

FIGURE 172-2. **Cellular stages of granulopoiesis in bone marrow.**

TABLE 172-2 MEMBRANE AND MATRIX COMPONENTS OF NEUTROPHILIC GRANULES

COMPONENT	AZUROPHIL GRANULES (PRIMARY; PEROXIDASE POSITIVE)	SPECIFIC GRANULES (SECONDARY; PEROXIDASE NEGATIVE)	GELATINASE GRANULES (TERTIARY; PEROXIDASE NEGATIVE)	SECRETORY VESICLES
Antimicrobial proteins	Defensins Lysozyme Elastase Myeloperoxidase Cathepsin G	Lysozyme Lactoferrin	Lysozyme	
Membrane proteins and receptors	CD63 CD68 Alkaline phosphatase	CD11b fMLP-R Cytochrome b_{558} CR3	CD11b fMLP-R Cytochrome b_{558} CR3 CD45	CD11b fMLP-R Cytochrome b_{558} CR1 CD14 CD16
Matrix proteins	β-Glucuronidase	Collagenase Gelatinase Laminin	Gelatinase	Albumin

Modified from Edwards SW. *Biochemistry and Physiology of the Neutrophil.* Cambridge, UK: Cambridge University Press; 2005:55.

mitotic pool at the promyelocyte and myelocyte stages and shortening neutrophil transit time in bone marrow.

Neutrophil Granules

One of the major mechanisms used by neutrophils to eliminate bacteria is a remarkable arsenal of antimicrobial proteins that are packed into cytoplasmic granules (Table 172-2). These antimicrobial proteins are securely contained within their respective granules and are released only when granules fuse with phagosomes or directly with the plasma membrane. Granulogenesis begins between the myeloblast and promyelocyte stages of neutrophil development and continues throughout the differentiation and maturation process of the cell. *Azurophilic* granules, which make up 30% of granules in a mature neutrophil, are the first to appear at the promyelocyte stage; they contain hydrolytic enzymes, microbicidal peptides, and myeloperoxidase. The *secondary,* or specific, granules appear later, beginning at the metamyelocyte stage; they are twice as abundant in the cytoplasm as azurophilic granules and contain proteins such as collagenase and lactoferrin. The *gelatinase-containing,* or *tertiary,* granules also appear at the metamyelocyte stage. A fourth category of granules, *secretory vesicles,* appear at the very final stages of neutrophil maturation, immediately before release of the cell into the circulation. All the granule types contain membrane proteins such as CR1, CR3, CD45, CD11c, and fMLP (*N*-formyl-methionyl-leucyl-phenylalanine) receptors, which are rapidly transported to the plasma membrane during activation to enhance neutrophil microbicidal activity.

A number of clinical conditions result from specific defects in granule development and formation. Initial assessment for granule defects can be made by microscopic evaluation of a peripheral blood smear (Chapter 160). Examples of obvious clinical diagnoses made with the peripheral smear include specific granule deficiency, which is characterized by bilobed nuclei in more than 80% of the neutrophils, and a significant decrease in cytoplasmic granularity. Abnormally large cytoplasmic granules are seen in individuals with Chédiak-Higashi syndrome.

The Vascular Compartment

Mature neutrophils are released from the postmitotic bone marrow compartment into the circulation, where they have an approximate lifespan of 8 to 12 hours and either circulate within the center of the blood vessel or attach to its endothelial lining, a process termed *margination*. Marginated neutrophils on the vessel walls are able to detach and reenter the circulation when required. For example, corticosteroids and epinephrine induce a rapid increase in circulating neutrophils by releasing neutrophils from the marginated pool. Neutrophils circulate until they are recruited to a site of infection. The initial phase of recruitment involves changes in the endothelial cell surface receptors lining the capillary beds closest to the site of infection or tissue damage. These critical changes in endothelial cells are mediated by immune regulators released by tissue macrophages, which initially detect the tissue damage or bacterial invasion. Emigration of circulating neutrophils from the vasculature to the site of infection or tissue damage requires three steps (see Fig. 172-1): capture and margination, firm adhesion to the endothelial wall, and diapedesis.

Margination and Capture

The marginated pool of neutrophils consists of neutrophils transiently retained against the walls of pulmonary capillaries and postcapillary venules. In the 20-μm diameter of a postcapillary venule, the smaller and faster circulating red blood cells displace the slower-moving and larger neutrophils, which move to the vessel margins, where a low-affinity molecular interaction occurs between surface adhesion molecules of the neutrophil and the endothelial cells. This interaction results in neutrophil rolling and capture along the vessel walls, an event that requires the specific neutrophil receptors *leukocyte selectin* (L-selectin) and the corresponding endothelial ligand, sLe. L-selectin is constitutively expressed in neutrophils, with highest expression in young circulating neutrophils and gradual decline with a cell's age, probably because previous margination events have depleted the receptor. The endothelial ligand for L-selectin, sLe, is a sialylated carbohydrate linked to a mucin-like molecule that can be upregulated by bacterial lipopolysaccharide or other mediators of inflammation. The selectin-ligand interactions are reversible and serve to promote and maintain accumulation of circulating neutrophils on inflamed endothelium.

Adherence to the Endothelial Wall

Low-affinity, selectin-mediated transient interactions must be replaced by high-affinity, adhesive contacts between neutrophils and endothelial cells. During an acute inflammatory event, mediators derived from bacteria, damaged host cells, complement activation, or other immune cells are released from the site of infection and diffuse to the capillary beds, where they induce an immediate and transient vascular response that results in vascular leakage, which further encourages neutrophil margination. Endothelial cells adjacent to the site of inflammation, as well as the activated neutrophils that are bound to them, express integrin receptors that lead to high-affinity attachments between the neutrophils and endothelial cells. These high-affinity connections occur between neutrophil β2 *integrins* and their endothelial counterparts, the intercellular adhesion molecules (ICAMs). Integrins, which are a receptor family of heterodimeric transmembrane glycoproteins made up of an α- and β-subunit, are integral for cell adhesion. Neutrophil β2 integrins consist of three different α-subunits (CD11a, CD11b, and CD11c) that bind to a common β-subunit (CD18). The cytoplasmic tails of these transmembrane receptors possess phosphorylation sites for attachment of signal transduction and cytoskeletal proteins. The neutrophil integrins that mediate this adhesion step are *macrophage antigen-1* (Mac-1; CD11b/CD18) and *lymphocyte-associated function antigen-1* (LFA-1; CD11a/CD18). The receptors are stored in the neutrophil granule compartments to facilitate quick transfer to the plasma membrane during cell stimulation. The integrins bind to endothelial ICAM-1 and ICAM-2 and *vascular cell adhesion molecule-1* (VCAM-1), which are upregulated on the endothelial cell membranes when a cell is exposed to inflammatory cytokines. L-selectin receptors on neutrophils are concentrated on microvillus projections of the cell membrane, whereas the integrins are restricted to the body of the neutrophil. As a result, soon after initial contact during rolling interactions, the projections retract, thereby allowing integrins to interact with their ligands.

Diapedesis

Firm adherence through the L-selectin and integrin receptors facilitates transendothelial migration, or diapedesis, which marks the "point of no return" in the process of neutrophil recruitment to the site of injury. Unlike rolling and firm adhesion, which require heterophilic interactions between one class of molecules on the neutrophil and another class of molecules on the endothelial cell, diapedesis involves homophilic interactions between the same class of molecules on both cells—the *platelet-endothelial cell adhesion molecule-1* (PECAM-1 or CD31). PECAM-1 is expressed evenly on the surface of neutrophils and concentrated at endothelial cell junctions. Once firmly bound to the endothelial cell surface, neutrophils migrate between the closest tricellular endothelial cell junctions through interactions with PECAM-1 receptors. The neutrophil has now entered the tissue compartment, where it is primed for its final critical role in the elimination of microorganisms and cellular debris.

Laboratory Evaluation of Margination and Firm Adhesion

A defect in neutrophil margination or adhesion to the endothelial lining of the vascular compartment results in neutrophilia (elevated circulating neutrophil levels). This condition is usually associated with leukocyte adhesion deficiency (LAD), which is the result of a lack of CD11/CD18 receptor surface expression in peripheral blood neutrophils. If LAD is suspected, surface expression of these receptors can be measured with a flow cytometer and specific antibodies to CD11, CD18, or CD15 receptors.

The Tissue Compartment

Chemotaxis

Chemotaxis is the directed movement of cells up a chemical concentration gradient of a *chemoattractant*. Chemoattractants are soluble proteins or peptides, including bacterial products, complement factors, and chemokines produced by both inflammatory and noninflammatory cells, that are released from damaged or infected tissue. A concentration difference of 1% at the opposite ends of the neutrophil is sufficient to activate neutrophil chemotaxis. Once a chemoattractant binds to its corresponding neutrophil membrane receptor, a series of cytoplasmic signaling pathways leads to activation of the neutrophil cytoskeleton. This activation results in the neutrophil assuming a polarized state characterized by an actin-rich leading lamella or pseudopod that drives cell motility.

Directional cell crawling, the intrinsic basis of chemotaxis, can be broken down into smaller processes, including extension of the cell membrane, adhesion to the tissue matrix, and contraction of the cell body in an organized and reversible manner. The actin-dependent protrusion of the leading edge, which is a sheetlike structure rich in actin filaments, is critical for normal neutrophil motility. The actin filaments within these lamellar regions are assembled into highly organized structures that push the membrane forward. These structures are formed by different collections of actin-binding proteins under the regulation of specific signal transduction cascades linking chemotactic receptors with cell movement. Defects in actin assembly also result in defects in chemotaxis and recurrent infections.

Actin Assembly Biology

Actin filaments are polar structures, with each end differing in its equilibrium-binding constant for actin monomers (Fig. 172-3). Filaments grow at the high-affinity or barbed end, whereas depolymerization occurs at the low-affinity or pointed end. This difference, generated by the ability of actin to bind and hydrolyze adenosine triphosphate, provides a physical polarity that regulatory proteins use to drive filament dynamics with high temporal and spatial precision. Three classes of proteins regulate the availability of high-affinity actin filament ends: filament-nucleating proteins (e.g., ARP2/3 de novo nucleation), filament-capping proteins (e.g., gelsolin), and filament-severing proteins (e.g., cofilin). Actin-nucleating factors bind actin monomers under conditions otherwise unfavorable for assembly and generate a new filament with a free high-affinity end available for assembly. Actin filament-capping proteins bind to the high-affinity filament end and regulate the addition of monomers by their presence or absence at the end of the filament. Actin-binding proteins are regulated by various second messengers, including calcium. On stimulation, localized changes in the intracellular Ca^{2+} concentration lead to the rapid initiation of actin assembly and disassembly. The changes in actin filament length and the extent of cross-linkage between the filaments may account for the directional extension of actin-rich lamellae and contraction of the tail-like uropod at the other end of the cell. Movement in the neutrophil is therefore the result of lamellar protrusions resulting from the growth of actin filaments. Actin-rich lamellae will continue to be maintained as long as the neutrophil detects the chemoattractant gradient.

Actin Assembly Regulation: Barbed End Regulation

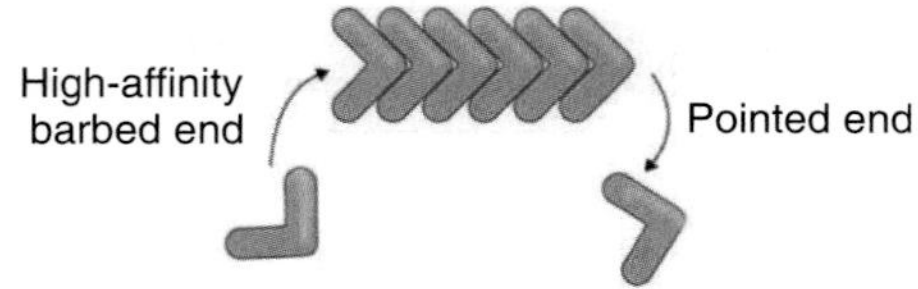

A. ARP 2/3 de novo nucleation

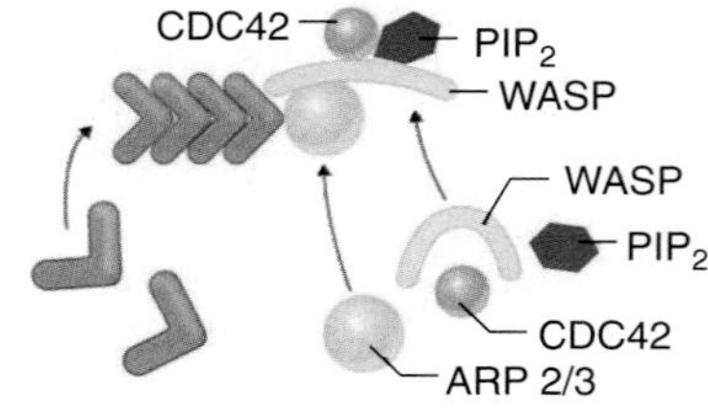

B. Capped barbed end

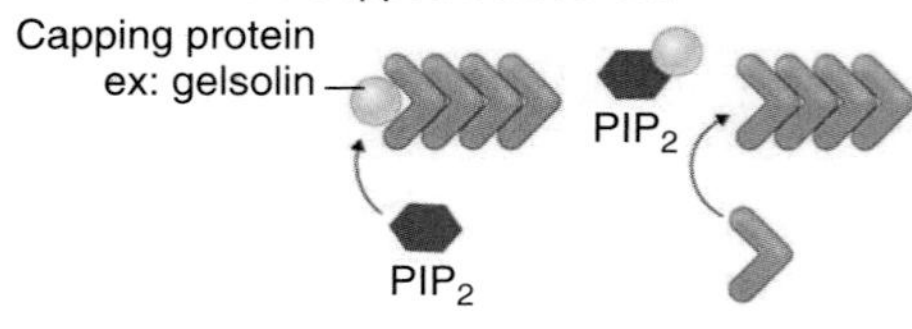

C. Cofilin-mediated severing

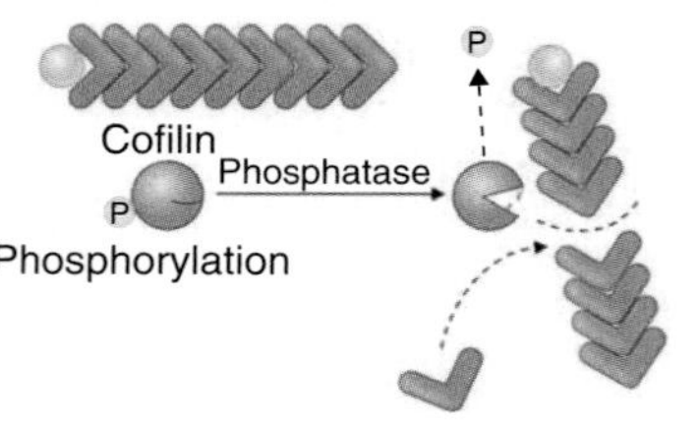

FIGURE 172-3. Regulation of actin assembly through the generation of free barbed ends by actin-binding proteins. A, The components below join together to form a nucleation complex (above). **B,** PIP_2 binds the capping protein, leading to its removal from the high-affinity end, allowing for addition and filament growth. **C,** A phosphatase removes the P from cofilin, thereby allowing it to sever the actin filament and leaving a free high affinity end. PIP_2 = phosphatidylinositol 4,5-biphosphate; WASP = Wiskott-Aldrich syndrome protein.

Laboratory Evaluation of Chemotaxis

A defect in neutrophil chemotaxis can be measured in the laboratory with a Boyden chamber, which uses a porous membrane to separate isolated neutrophils from a chemoattractant. A chemical gradient develops across the porous membrane and activates the neutrophils to crawl through the membrane toward the compartment containing the chemoattractant. Defects in chemotaxis can be determined by a lack of neutrophil transmigration through the membrane compared with control neutrophils from a healthy donor.

Phagocytosis

Phagocytosis is the process whereby neutrophils engulf and internalize invading pathogens into membrane compartments called *phagosomes.* Bacterial targets are "highlighted" or opsonized by antibodies (immunoglobulin G) or products from the classical complement pathway that coat the target and serve to mediate phagocytic adhesion. Neutrophilic phagocytosis involves two separate classes of receptors: *Fcγ receptors* (CD32 and CD16) for antibody-coated targets and *complement receptors* (CR1 and CR3) for complement-coated targets. CD32 and CR3 are functional receptors directly involved in neutrophilic phagocytosis, whereas CD16 and CR1 are coreceptors that assist their mate in completing binding and internalization. Activation of Fcγ receptors brings about phosphorylation of their cytoplasmic *immunoreceptor tyrosine-based activation motifs* (ITAMs) through activation of *Src family kinases;* the result is transduction of signals that induce extension of pseudopods, including signaling to the small Rho family of small guanosine triphosphatases (GTPases). These GTPases are responsible for the assembly of actin filaments, thereby leading to remodeling of the plasma membrane and the formation of actin-rich pseudopods, which are essential for the ingestion of particles and formation of phagosomes.

Laboratory Evaluation of Phagocytosis

Neutrophils can be incubated with fluorescently labeled bacteria after opsonization with serum from either the patient or a control. Phagocytosis is assessed by flow cytometry, which measures the increase in neutrophilic fluorescence after uptake of the fluorescently tagged bacteria.

Bacterial Killing

Phagocytes use two potent mechanisms for killing bacteria within the membrane-bound phagosome. The first involves fusion of the previously described storage granules with the phagosome to deliver microbicidal and lytic enzymes into the membrane compartment that contains the ingested microorganisms. The second mechanism uses a multiprotein enzyme complex to generate microbicidal oxidants through partial reduction of oxygen. The multiprotein enzyme complex known as reduced nicotinamide adenine dinucleotide phosphate (NADPH) oxidase generates oxidants by means of oxygen consumption, hence the term *respiratory burst.*

The NADPH enzyme system is made up of four essential polypeptide subunits that are denoted by their molecular weight (kD) and the superscript phox, which denotes phagocyte oxidase. Within the cytoplasmic membrane, the subunits $p22^{phox}$ and $gp91^{phox}$ bind the electron-carrying components of the oxidase (NADPH, a flavin adenine dinucleotide, and two nonidentical hemes) and form the cytochrome b_{558} redox center of the oxidase complex. Cellular activation by inflammatory mediators results in the addition of two cytosolic components, $p47^{phox}$ and $p67^{phox}$, to the complex along with the Rac small GTPase.

The membrane-bound electron transport chain NADPH oxidase catalyzes the reduction of molecular oxygen to superoxide (O_2^-). The superoxide generated by this process is in turn catalytically converted to hydrogen peroxide and serves as a cosubstrate for myeloperoxidase to oxidize halides and produce hypochlorous acid (HOCl), a very potent antimicrobial agent. These oxidants are able to kill bacteria within the phagosomes by oxidizing their cellular constituents.

Laboratory Evaluation of the Respiratory Burst and Bacterial Killing

Flow cytometry, a rapid and effective method for quantitatively assessing the respiratory burst, measures the fluorescence generated by cytoplasmic fluorescent probes such as dihydrorhodamine, which is converted to rhodamine by H_2O_2. The nitroblue tetrazolium (NBT) test is still used for rapid assessment of the respiratory burst when flow cytometry is not available.

Bacterial killing assays using a patient's neutrophils with either the patient's or control serum and bacteria such as *Staphylococcus aureus* or *Escherichia coli* are a definitive method to determine whether a given patient's neutrophils have an intracellular killing defect. Neutrophils from a healthy control subject phagocytose and kill approximately 95% of the bacteria within 2 hours. In assays in which an intracellular killing defect is present, neutrophils kill less than 10% of bacteria over a 2-hour period. It is necessary to confirm that there is no phagocytic defect before performing the bacterial killing assay to be sure that any defect in bacterial killing is not due to an internalization defect.

Neutrophil Extracellular Traps

It has recently been shown that neutrophils use a newly identified extracellular process to contain and kill bacteria. Neutrophil extracellular traps (NETs) are formed by the release of chromatin and antimicrobial proteins from the neutrophil cytoplasm and granules. The chromatin forms a netlike meshwork that traps the bacteria and brings them in closer proximity to the antimicrobial elements adhered to the chromatin. Activation of NET formation requires simultaneous activation by at least two different receptors and reactive oxygen species are essential to the process. IL-8 has been shown to be a potent activator of NET formation. The importance of NETs was highlighted by work showing that DNase expressing strains of GAS and *Streptococcus pneumoniae* are more virulent than their non-DNase-expressing counterparts because of their ability to escape NETs. The importance of this antibacterial function of neutrophils will become clearer in the years to come.

Clinical Manifestations of Phagocytic Defects

In addition to fever and recurrent infections, the most common findings in patients with phagocytic defects are oral infections resulting in gingival inflammation, periodontal bone loss, mobile or loose teeth, and premature

TABLE 172-3 SYMPTOMS SUGGESTIVE OF A PHAGOCYTIC DISORDER

Recurrent infections that fail to resolve with conventional treatment
Recurrent infections of unusual severity
Recurrent infections in the lung, liver, or bone
Normally nonpathogenic bacteria or fungi identified in cultures from the infection sites
Aphthous ulcers
Severe periodontal diseases, including gingivitis
Lymphadenopathy or hepatosplenomegaly
Severe recurrent cutaneous infections with *Staphylococcus aureus*
Recurrent mycobacterial infections

loss of teeth (Table 172-3). An oral examination should be performed at the initial evaluation, followed by a full dental examination, depending on the findings. The history and laboratory tests can differentiate among the various clinical causes of disordered phagocytosis (Table 172-4).

DEFECTS IN LEUKOCYTE ADHESION

A defect in neutrophil adhesion to the endothelial lining leads to neutrophilia—an accumulation of neutrophils in the circulation, with very few neutrophils at sites of infection. Defects in neutrophil adhesion can be induced by drugs or due to a genetic defect. Drugs such as corticosteroids and epinephrine result in a transient leukocyte adhesive defect that results in an apparent dramatic increase in circulating neutrophils because of release of the marginated neutrophil pool. The major genetic disease that results in an adhesion deficiency is termed *leukocyte adhesion deficiency.*

Leukocyte Adhesion Deficiency

LAD-I

LAD-I is an autosomal recessive inherited disorder in which patients have a mutation in the gene encoding CD18. The result is a deficiency of β2 integrin receptors, which are required for neutrophil migration from the vasculature into the tissues, thereby impairing the binding of neutrophils to C3bi and endothelial ICAM-1 and ICAM-2.

Patients have soft tissue bacterial and fungal infections, delayed wound healing, impaired pus formation, and severe destructive periodontitis with rapid tooth loss. This condition is also characterized by delayed separation of the umbilical cord. Patients usually die during childhood. Flow cytometry is used to measure CD11/CD18 surface expression levels on neutrophils.

Treatment is mainly supportive with prophylactic antibiotics in patients with recurrent infections. In severe cases, bone marrow transplantation is the treatment of choice.

LAD-II AND LAD-III

LAD-II, a variant of LAD-I, is associated with neutrophilia, the Bombay (hh) blood phenotype, dwarfism, and mental retardation. This disorder is due to a mutation in the guanosine diphosphate-fucose transporter gene, which results in impaired expression of CD15s and other selectin ligands. Symptoms are similar to those of LAD-I, and the diagnosis is confirmed by flow cytometry for CD15s. In the most recently described LAD-III, there is a primary activation defect in all three β integrins 1, 2, and 3, and mutations have been found in Kindlin 3, which binds the cytoplasmic tail of integrin.

DEFECTS IN NEUTROPHILIC CHEMOTAXIS

After phagocytes enter the tissue compartment from the vascular pool, they migrate up the concentration gradients of various chemoattractants to the site of focal infection. A number of chemotactic defects result in severe recurrent infections.

Hyperimmunoglobin E Syndrome

Hyperimmunoglobin E syndrome, or hyper-IgE syndrome, also referred to as Job's syndrome, is a group of genetically diverse, multisystem disorders of cytokine signaling. The most common form of the syndrome involves dominant mutations in the gene for signal transducer and activator of transcription 3 *(STAT3)*. The neutrophilic disorder is characterized by recurrent skin abscesses, pneumonia, and periodontal diseases. After birth, patients usually have moderate to severe dermatitis, eczematous skin eruptions, nonerythematous abscesses, pneumatoceles, and severe osteoporosis that can result in bone fractures. The organisms most commonly present at infected sites are *S. aureus, Haemophilus influenzae, E. coli,* and *Candida albicans.* Patients have elevated IgE levels and eosinophilia. The defect in neutrophilic chemotaxis is less severe than that in Chédiak-Higashi syndrome (see later). Treatment is prophylactic antibiotics and aggressive treatment of infections. In severe cases, bone marrow transplantation may be considered.

Familial Mediterranean Fever

Familial Mediterranean fever (Chapter 269), also known as recurrent polyserositis, is an autosomal recessive inflammatory disease that is widespread among people of Mediterranean descent, including Arabs, Armenians, and Sephardic Jews. The genetic defect is a missense mutation in the *MEFV* gene, which encodes the protein pyrin. Pyrin is believed to be a transcription factor involved in downregulating inflammation, possibly through an effect on chemotaxis in neutrophils and monocytes. The *MEFV* mutation results in a hyperinflammatory response characterized by abundant neutrophilic infiltration into the peritoneal, pleural, and joint spaces.

The most common findings include acute, self-limited attacks of fever accompanied by pleuritis, peritonitis, arthritis, pericarditis, and erythematous skin lesions. Although first attacks may be observed during infancy, clinical disease commonly occurs in childhood or adolescence.

Leukocytosis has been observed during attacks, but the leukocyte count is normal between episodes. Genetic testing is available for the most common mutations. This disease can be fatal if renal failure develops as a result of amyloidosis (Chapter 194), which occurs in up to 25% of those affected.

The hyperinflammatory attacks can be reduced significantly with 0.6 mg of prophylactic colchicine orally two or three times daily. The prognosis is generally good for most affected individuals maintained with colchicine.

DISORDERS OF NEUTROPHILIC DEGRANULATION

Granules supply key membrane proteins, including receptors required for phagocytosis. Granule-related defects result in profound defects in bacterial killing.

Chédiak-Higashi Syndrome

Chédiak-Higashi syndrome is a rare autosomal recessive disorder of the *LYST* gene, which encodes a protein responsible for lysosomal trafficking. Defective targeting of granules to the membrane results in large cytoplasmic granules that are unable to target to the plasma membrane in neutrophils, monocytes, and lymphocytes.

Symptoms are recurrent bacterial infections of the skin, mouth, and respiratory tract; partial albinism; peripheral neuropathy; and mild bleeding disorders as a result of a deficiency in serotonin- and adenosine phosphate–containing granules in platelets. Defects in myelopoiesis result in neutropenia. Death usually occurs by 7 years of age because of infection. Advanced disease is characterized by lymphocytic tissue infiltrates and pancytopenia.

Giant cytoplasmic granules are seen in the peripheral blood smear. Neutrophil function testing shows defects in chemotaxis and bacterial killing. Prophylactic antibiotics should be used to prevent infections. Bone marrow transplantation from an HLA-matched donor may be successful if performed before the disease becomes advanced.

Specific Granule Deficiency

Specific granule deficiency is an autosomal recessive disorder that manifests during infancy as the recurrent appearance of deep and superficial skin infections, respiratory infections, and abscesses. Azurophilic granules in neutrophils lack defensins, gelatinase, cytochrome *b,* and vitamin B_{12}. Neutrophils are morphologically altered and have a bilobed rather than a trilobed nucleus. This disorder is characterized by impaired neutrophil chemotaxis, reduced respiratory burst, and a defect in bacterial killing. Infections are commonly caused by *S. aureus, Pseudomonas aeruginosa,* and *C. albicans.* Aggressive treatment of infections is required.

DISORDERS OF OXYGEN-DEPENDENT BACTERIAL KILLING

A genetic defect in any component of the respiratory burst results in delayed or ineffective bacterial killing.

Chronic Granulomatous Disease

PATHOBIOLOGY

Chronic granulomatous disease (CGD) is a genetic disease that occurs in about 1 in 200,000 live births. Neutrophils and macrophages cannot generate

TABLE 172-4 DISORDERS OF PHAGOCYTIC FUNCTION

DISORDER	ETIOLOGY	IMPAIRED FUNCTION	CLINICAL CONSEQUENCE
DEGRANULATION ABNORMALITIES			
Chédiak-Higashi syndrome	Autosomal recessive; disordered coalescence of lysosomal granules Responsible gene found at 1q42-45. The encoded protein (LYST) has structural features homologous to a vacuolar sorting protein	Decreased neutrophilic chemotaxis, degranulation, and bactericidal activity; platelet storage pool defect; impaired NK function; failure to disperse melanosomes	Neutropenia, recurrent pyogenic infections, propensity for the development of marked hepatosplenomegaly in the accelerated phase, partial albinism
Specific granule deficiency	Autosomal recessive; abnormal regulation of various myeloid granule genes by a transacting factor	Impaired chemotaxis and bactericidal activity; bilobed nuclei in neutrophils; reduced content of neutrophil defensins, gelatinase, collagenase, vitamin B_{12}–binding protein, and lactoferrin	Recurrent infections, especially sinopulmonary and skin infections
ADHESION ABNORMALITIES			
Leukocyte adhesion deficiency type 1	Autosomal recessive; absence of CD11/CD18 surface adhesive glycoprotein (β2-integrins) on leukocyte membranes, most commonly arising from failure to express CD18 mRNA	Decreased binding of C3bi to neutrophils and impaired adhesion to ICAM-1 and ICAM-2	Neutrophilia, recurrent bacterial infection associated with lack of pus formation
Leukocyte adhesion deficiency type 2	Autosomal recessive; absence of neutrophil sialyl-Lewis^x	Decreased adhesion to activated endothelium expressing ELAM	Neutrophilia, recurrent bacterial infection without pus
Leukocyte adhesion deficiency type 3	Autosomal recessive; defects in activation of β1, β2, and β3 integrins	Severe leukocyte adhesion dysfunction; abnormal platelet aggregation	Neutrophilia, recurrent bacterial infection without pus, severe bleeding tendency
Neutrophil actin dysfunction	Altered polymerization of neutrophil cytoplasmic actin, perhaps arising from the presence of an inhibitor to F-actin formation	Impaired neutrophil adhesion, chemotaxis, and bacterial killing	Neutrophilia, recurrent bacterial infections without pus
DISORDERS OF CELL CHEMOTAXIS			
Hyperactive Chemotaxis			
Familial Mediterranean fever (FMF)	Autosomal recessive gene responsible for FMF on chromosome 16, which encodes for a protein called pyrin; pyrin may modify neutrophil activation	Excessive accumulation of neutrophils at inflamed sites	Recurrent fever, peritonitis, pleuritis, arthritis, amyloidosis
Depressed Chemotaxis			
Intrinsic defects of the neutrophil, e.g., leukocyte adhesion deficiency, Chédiak-Higashi syndrome, specific granule deficiency, neutrophil actin dysfunction, neonatal neutrophils	In the neonatal neutrophil, there is diminished ability to express β2 integrins and a qualitative impairment in β2 integrin function	Diminished chemotaxis	Propensity for the development of pyogenic infections
Direct inhibition of neutrophil mobility, e.g., drugs	Ethanol, glucocorticoids, cyclic AMP	Impaired locomotion and ingestion, impaired adherence	Possible causes of frequent infections; neutrophilia seen with epinephrine is the result of cyclic AMP release from the endothelium
Immune complexes	Bind to Fc receptors on neutrophils in patients with rheumatoid arthritis, systemic lupus erythematosus, and other inflammatory states	Impaired chemotaxis	Recurrent pyogenic infections
Hyperimmunoglobulin E syndrome	Disorders of cytokine signaling, most commonly due to autosomal dominant mutations in the *STAT3* gene	Impaired chemotaxis, impaired IgG opsonization of *Staphylococcus aureus*	Recurrent skin and sinopulmonary infections
DEFECTS OF MICROBICIDAL ACTIVITY			
Chronic granulomatous disease (CGD)	X-linked and autosomal recessive; failure to express functional gp91^{phox} (in the phagocyte membrane) and p22^{phox} (autosomal recessive). Other autosomal recessive forms of CGD arise from failure to express protein p47^{phox} or p67^{phox}	Failure to activate neutrophil respiratory burst leading to failure to kill catalase-positive microbes	Recurrent pyogenic infections with catalase-positive microorganisms
G6PD deficiency	Less than 5% of normal activity of G6PD	Failure to activate NADPH-dependent oxidase	Infections with catalase-positive microorganisms
Myeloperoxidase deficiency	Autosomal recessive; failure to process modified precursor protein arising from missense mutation	H_2O_2-dependent antimicrobial activity not potentiated by myeloperoxidase	None
Deficiencies of glutathione reductase and glutathione synthetase	Failure to detoxify H_2O_2	Excessive formation of H_2O_2	Minimal problems with recurrent pyogenic infections

TABLE 172-4 DISORDERS OF PHAGOCYTIC FUNCTION—cont'd

DISORDER	ETIOLOGY	IMPAIRED FUNCTION	CLINICAL CONSEQUENCE
IMPAIRED MACROPHAGE FUNCTION			
Defects in the interferon-γ–IL-12 axis	Interferon-γ receptor ligand-binding chain, interferon-γ receptor signaling chain, IL-12 receptor β1 chain, IL-12 p40 deficiency; the interferon-γ receptor abnormalities may be autosomal dominant or recessive; the IL-12 receptor and IL-12 abnormalities are autosomal recessive	Impaired killing of microorganisms. Fatal BCG infection secondary either to an inability to produce IL-12 by dendritic cells and macrophages or to depressed bactericidal activity of macrophages lacking normal function of the interferon receptor	Infection with atypical mycobacteria, *Salmonella*, and *Listeria*

AMP = adenosine monophosphate; BCG = bacille Calmette-Guérin; ELAM = endothelial leukocyte adhesion molecule; G6PD = glucose-6-phosphate dehydrogenase; ICAM = intracellular adhesion molecule; IL-12 = interleukin-12; NADPH = nicotinamide adenine dinucleotide phosphate; NK = natural killer; phox = phagocyte oxidase.
Modified from Boxer LA. Quantitative abnormalities of granulocytes. In: Beutler E, Lichtman MA, Coller BS, et al, eds. *Williams Hematology*, 6th ed. New York: McGraw-Hill; 2001:836.

superoxide and are therefore unable to kill catalase-positive organisms. This condition results from mutations in one of the four structural genes of the NADPH oxidase complex. The most common genetic defect occurs in the 91-kD component of cytochrome b_{558}, which is coded on the X chromosome. The other mutations are autosomal recessive and have been detected in the 22-, 47-, and 67-kD structural proteins.

CLINICAL MANIFESTATIONS AND DIAGNOSIS

Children are prone to infections or granulomatous lesions in the lungs, skin, and liver. *S. aureus* is the most common organism, but other organisms include *Serratia marcescens, Burkholderia cepacia, Aspergillus* species, and *Nocardia* species. Staphylococcal liver abscesses are pathognomonic of chronic granulomatous disease. Flow cytometry is used to measure the increase in fluorescence generated when dihydrorhodamine is converted to rhodamine by H_2O_2.

TREATMENT

Rx

Abscesses can be removed by surgery. Trimethoprim-sulfamethoxazole prophylaxis (5 mg/kg/day divided into two equal doses) and antifungal prophylaxis with itraconazole (100 mg/day for <50 kg, 200 mg/day for >50 kg) have been shown to reduce the frequency of infections in these patients. Interferon-γ (50 μg/m² subcutaneously three times per week) prophylaxis is now considered "standard of care" in many centers. Bone marrow transplantation can also be considered for patients with refractory infections. Gene therapy for CGD by gene-modified autologous hematopoietic stem cell transplantation has resulted in transient immune restoration but also genomic instability, monosomy 7, and clonal progression toward myelodysplasia.

Myeloperoxidase Deficiency

Myeloperoxidase deficiency is a relatively common disorder (1 in 4000) in which the enzyme for conversion of neutrophilic hydrogen peroxide to HOCl is absent. This deficiency is not associated with increased susceptibility to infections, probably because of the accumulation of hydrogen peroxide, which is also bactericidal. Myeloperoxidase deficiency is usually asymptomatic, although patients with diabetes mellitus may occasionally experience candidal infections. The diagnosis is made by observation of a negative peroxidase stain of the peripheral blood smear. Symptomatic patients may be treated with prophylactic antibiotics.

Glutathione Synthetase Deficiency

Glutathione, which is a potent antioxidant found in granulocytes, is required for a normal respiratory burst and bacterial killing. Patients with glutathione synthetase deficiency typically have recurrent otitis and hemolytic anemia. The diagnosis is confirmed by verifying low or no glutathione synthetase in red blood cells.

Severe Glucose-6-Phosphate Dehydrogenase Deficiency

Glucose-6-phosphate dehydrogenase (G6PD) deficiency is an X-linked disorder. White individuals with a severe reduction in G6PD activity are subject to recurrent infections, whereas Asians or blacks with similarly reduced G6PD levels are not. G6PD is crucial for regulating the availability of NADPH for the respiratory burst. G6PD deficiency results in recurrent bacterial infections, hemolytic anemia (Chapter 164), and jaundice. The diagnosis can be made with flow cytometry to assess the respiratory burst and to demonstrate the absence of G6PD in all blood cells.

MACROPHAGE-RELATED ABNORMALITIES

Accumulation of monocyte-macrophages at sites of infection occurs after the major influx of neutrophils. Macrophages have a critical role in antigen presentation to lymphocytes, thereby activating the adaptive arm of the immune system. A critical defect in macrophage signaling results in susceptibility to mycobacterial infection.

Interferon-γ Receptor 1 Defects

When macrophages phagocytose mycobacteria, they produce IL-12, which in turn stimulates T cells to produce interferon-γ (IFN-γ). IFN-γ is critical to the killing of mycobacteria and other intracellular bacteria. Patients with recurrent and severe mycobacterial infections who are not infected with human immunodeficiency virus should be assessed for abnormalities in pathways that lead to the generation and utilization of IFN-γ.

Patients with autosomal recessive mutations in the IFN-γ receptors typically have a complete loss of function of the IFN-γ receptors. Autosomal dominant mutations in the IFN-γ receptors result in normal ligand binding but defective intracellular signal transduction because of a cytoplasmically truncated form of the receptor.

Recessive mutations typically manifest as severe disseminated infections and poor formation of granulomas. Multifocal mycobacterial osteomyelitis is pathognomonic of an autosomal dominant mutation in the IFN-γ receptor. Flow cytometry confirms the absence of membrane expression of IFN-γ receptor 1 in the autosomal recessive form and up to ten-fold higher membrane expression levels of the cytoplasmically truncated receptor in the autosomal dominant form.

For patients with autosomal dominant mutations, subcutaneous IFN-γ is effective. For autosomal recessive patients completely lacking IFN-γ receptor function, bone marrow transplantation should be considered. Long-term antibiotic prophylaxis against mycobacterial infections with azithromycin or clarithromycin is recommended.

ASSESSING PHAGOCYTE FUNCTION: MAKING THE DIAGNOSIS

If a phagocyte functional disorder may be the underlying cause of recurrent infections in a patient, a complete blood count (CBC) and peripheral smear guide subsequent definitive testing (Fig. 172-4). Cultures from infected areas allow antimicrobial targeting and also provide critical diagnostic information. If the defect is a result of abnormal neutrophil development and maturation, the CBC will show neutropenia; a bone marrow biopsy might be required. Repeated CBC (twice per week for 6 weeks) is indicated if cyclic neutropenia is suspected because of a periodicity of the infections (Chapter 170).

If the CBC reveals neutrophilia, a defect in the recruitment of neutrophils into tissues is suggested. An assessment of the receptors required for transmigration by flow cytometry and specific antibodies to the surface receptors is indicated.

If circulating levels of phagocytes are normal yet the patient is experiencing recurrent infections, a phagocytic defect within the infected tissue is likely. Laboratory testing to evaluate chemotaxis, phagocytosis, and bacterial killing is indicated.

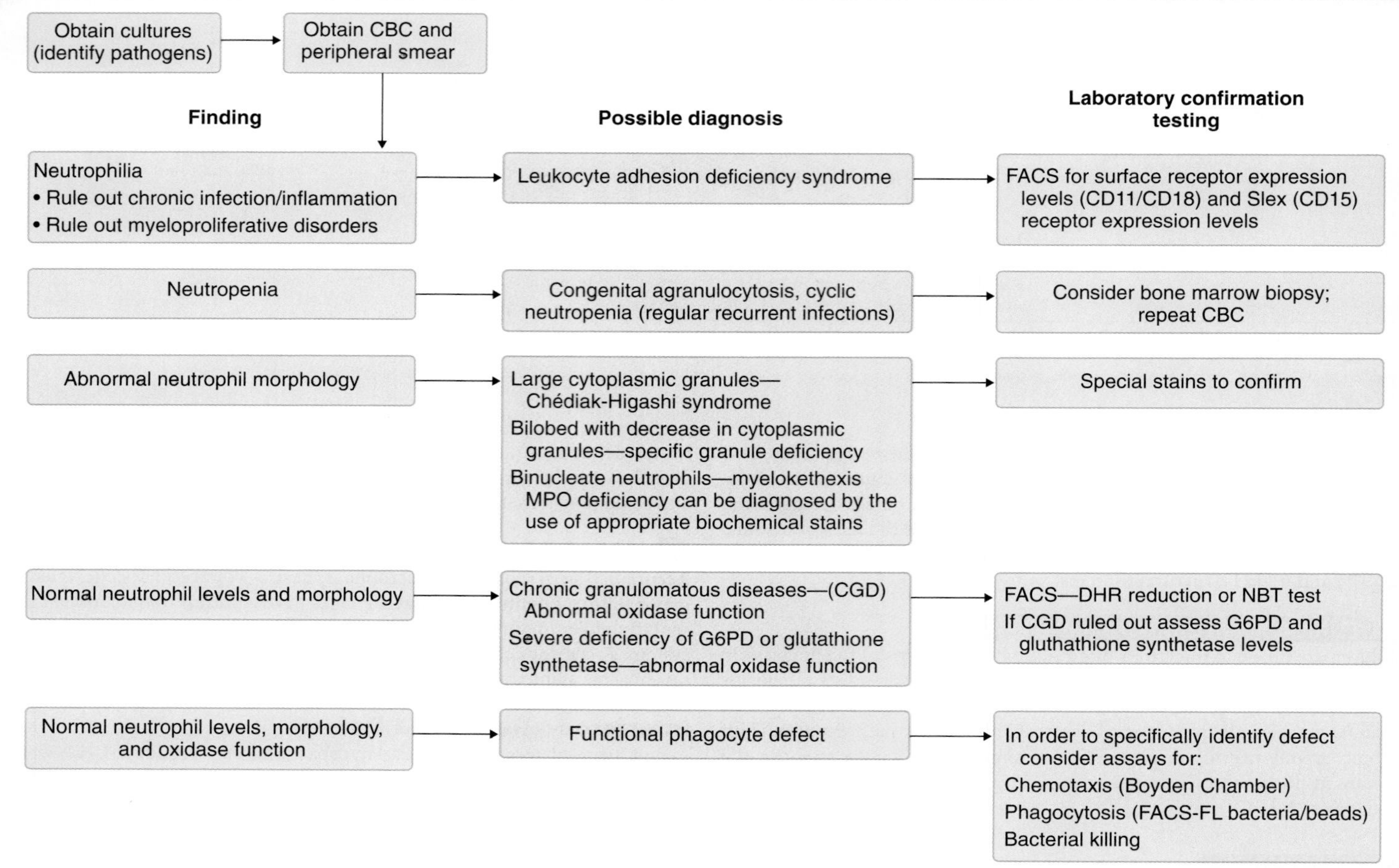

FIGURE 172-4. **Approach to diagnosing a suspected phagocytic defect.** CBC = complete blood count; DHR = dihydrorhodamine; FACS = flow cytometry; FL = fluorescent; G6PD = glucose-6-phosphate dehydrogenase; MPO = myeloperoxidase; NBT = nitroblue tetrazolium.

SUGGESTED READINGS

Bianchi M, Hakkim A, Brinkmann V, et al. Restoration of NET formation by gene therapy in CGD controls aspergillosis. *Blood.* 2009;114:2619-2622. *Positive effects of gene therapy on neutrophils in CGD.*

Bouma G, Ancliff PJ, Thrasher AJ, et al. Recent advances in the understanding of genetic defects of neutrophil number and function. *Br J Haematol.* 2010;151:312-326. *Review.*

Kuhns DB, Alvord WG, Heller T, et al. Residual NADPH oxidase and survival in chronic granulomatous disease. *N Engl J Med.* 2010;363:2600-2610. *Moderate residual production is associated with a significantly better survival.*

Lemos S, Jacob CM, Pastorino AC, et al. Neutropenia in antibody-deficient patients under IVIG replacement therapy. *Pediatr Allergy Immunol.* 2009;20:97-101 *Primary immunodeficient patients, even when treated with IVIg, require monitoring for neutropenia.*

Segal BH, Veys P, Malech H, et al. Chronic granulomatous disease: lessons from a rare disorder. *Biol Blood Marrow Transplant.* 2011;17:S123-S131. *Review.*

173 EOSINOPHILIC SYNDROMES

MARC E. ROTHENBERG

DEFINITION

Eosinophilic syndromes are a heterogeneous group of disorders that involve eosinophilia, which is defined as the accumulation of eosinophils in peripheral blood and/or tissues. Circulating eosinophils normally account for only 1 to 3% of peripheral blood leukocytes, and the upper limit of the normal range is 350 cells/mm^3 of blood. Eosinophilia occurs in a variety of disorders (Table 173-1) and is usually arbitrarily classified according to the degree of blood eosinophilia: mild (351 to 1500 cells/mm^3), moderate (>1500 to 5000 cells/mm^3), or severe (>5000 cells/mm^3). Tissue eosinophilic disorders, such as eosinophil-associated gastrointestinal disorders and eosinophilic fasciitis, are not necessarily associated with blood eosinophilia, so their

TABLE 173-1 CAUSES OF EOSINOPHILIA

REACTIVE EOSINOPHILIA
Allergic diseases—asthma, atopic dermatitis, allergic rhinitis
Drug reactions—including cytokine infusions
Infection—viral (human immunodeficiency virus) or fungal (allergic bronchopulmonary aspergillosis, coccidioidomycosis)
Parasitic infection—mostly helminths
EOSINOPHILIA ASSOCIATED WITH OTHER DISEASES
Eosinophil-associated gastrointestinal disorders—eosinophilic esophagitis, gastroenteritis
Skin—bullous pemphigoid, urticaria, eosinophilic cellulitis, episodic angioedema
Pulmonary—eosinophilic pneumonia, allergic bronchopulmonary aspergillosis
Neurologic—eosinophilic meningitis
Autoimmune—Churg-Strauss syndrome, eosinophilic fasciitis
Primary immunodeficiency—hyperimmunoglobulin E syndrome, Omenn's syndrome
Post-transplantation status—liver (in association with immunosuppression)
Transplant rejection—lung, kidney, liver
Malignancy—Hodgkin's disease, solid tumors
Hypoadrenalism—Addison's disease, adrenal hemorrhage
Renal—drug-induced interstitial nephritis, eosinophilic cystitis, dialysis
PRIMARY CLONAL EOSINOPHILIA
Chronic eosinophilic leukemia
Acute eosinophilic leukemia
Acute myelogenous leukemia with eosinophilia
Acute lymphoblastic leukemia with eosinophilia
Myeloblastic disorders with eosinophilia
Myeloproliferative disorders with eosinophilia
Systemic mastocytosis with eosinophilia
FIP1L1-PDGFRA fusion gene–positive disease
IDIOPATHIC HYPEREOSINOPHILIA

diagnosis is based on the microscopic identification of eosinophil-rich inflammatory infiltrates associated with tissue damage.

Historically, hypereosinophilic syndromes were generally classified as idiopathic and were defined by (1) the presence of eosinophilia (>1500 cells/mm^3 for at least 6 months) that remained unexplained despite a comprehensive evaluation for known causes of eosinophilia (such as drug reactions and infections) and (2) evidence of organ dysfunction directly attributable to the eosinophilia. Now, however, it is known that in some patients, a chromosome 4 microdeletion results in the generation of an activated tyrosine kinase (*FIP1L1*-platelet-derived growth factor receptor-α [*PDGFRA*]) that causes a clonal hematologic disorder now better classified as chronic eosinophilic leukemia. Identification of *FIP1L1-PDGFRA*-positive disease has important therapeutic implications because *PDGFRA*-associated disease can be treated with imatinib, a tyrosine kinase inhibitor.

EPIDEMIOLOGY

The most common cause of eosinophilia worldwide is helminth infections, which affect hundreds of millions of people. The most frequent cause in industrialized nations is atopic disease, which affects 10 to 30% of the population. Hypereosinophilic disorders such as *FIP1L1-PDGFRA*-associated disease and Churg-Strauss syndrome (Chapter 278) are very rare. For example, Churg-Strauss syndrome affects 4 to 6 cases per million per year, whereas true idiopathic hypereosinophilic syndromes may affect only 4000 to 5000 people worldwide. Other syndromes such as eosinophil-associated gastrointestinal disorders are more common, with a prevalence of approximately 1 in 10,000 individuals.

PATHOBIOLOGY

Eosinophils are produced in the bone marrow from pluripotential hematopoietic stem cells under regulation of the transcription factor GATA-1 and the cytokines interleukin-3 (IL-3), IL-5, and granulocyte-macrophage colony-stimulating factor (GM-CSF) (Fig. 173-1). Eosinophils are under the regulation of helper type 2 T cells (T_H2) that secrete IL-4, IL-5, and IL-13. Notably, IL-5 is a cytokine that specifically regulates the selective differentiation of eosinophils, their release from bone marrow into the peripheral circulation, and their survival. A humanized anti-IL-5 drug markedly lowers circulating eosinophilia and reduces tissue eosinophilia more modestly. Recent preliminary studies in patients with severe asthma have shown that anti-IL-5 therapy improves asthma control, including exacerbations, and allows steroid reduction. Similarly, anti-IL-5 has a steroid sparing effect in hypereosinophilic syndromes. Humanized anti-IL-5 therapy is currently in clinical testing for a variety of indications, including eosinophilic esophagitis, asthma, and hypereosinophilic syndromes. IL-4 and IL-13 induce eosinophil recruitment and survival, expression of critical adhesion molecules on the endothelium that bind to the β1 and β2 integrins on eosinophils (such as intercellular adhesion molecule 1 [ICAM-1] and vascular cell adhesion molecule 1 [VCAM-1]), and eosinophil-active chemokines such as the eotaxins. The eotaxins are three structurally related eosinophil chemoattractant and activating proteins that signal exclusively through the eosinophil-selective receptor CCR3. In addition to regulating the baseline homing of eosinophils into various tissues, such as the gastrointestinal tract, wherein most eosinophils reside, the eotaxins are induced by T_H2-associated inflammatory triggers (e.g., IL-13) and thereby promote tissue accumulation of eosinophils. Humanized antibodies against the eotaxins and small-molecule inhibitors against CCR3 are promising new approaches for treating eosinophilic disorders that are in clinical development.

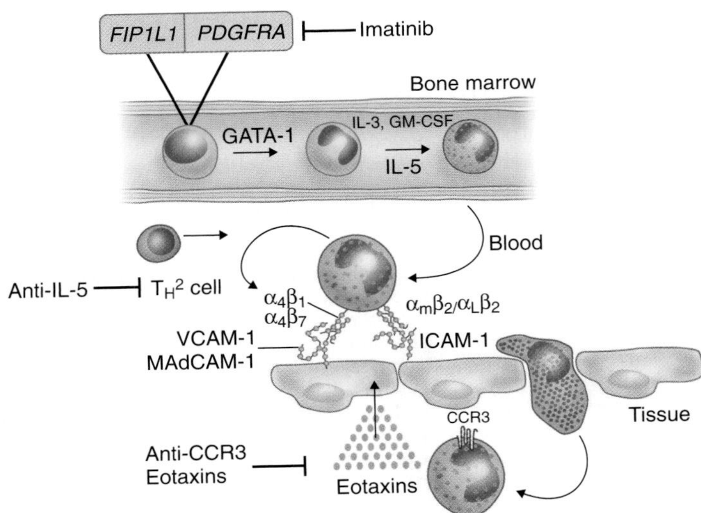

FIGURE 173-1. Schematic representation of eosinophil development, tissue recruitment, and therapeutic intervention. Eosinophil lineage development is specified by the GATA-1 transcription factor and promoted by the cytokines interleukin-3 (IL-3), IL-5, and granulocyte-macrophage colony-stimulating factor (GM-CSF). IL-5 is most selective to the eosinophil lineage and regulates eosinophil movement from the bone marrow into the peripheral blood. Eosinophil adhesion is mediated by β1, β2, and β7 integrins and their interaction with the endothelial adhesion molecules intercellular adhesion molecule 1 (ICAM-1), vascular cell adhesion molecule 1 (VCAM-1), and mucosal address in cell adhesion molecule 1 (MAdCAM-1). Recruitment of eosinophils into tissue is regulated by the eotaxin chemokines that stimulate eosinophilic chemoattraction and activation through their receptor CCR3. Hypereosinophilic syndromes can develop after an 800-kilobase microdeletion on chromosome 4 results in fusion of the *FIP1L1* and *PDGFRA* genes, thereby resulting in activation of an imatinib-sensitive tyrosine kinase. Targeted therapeutic intervention for eosinophilic syndromes includes anti-IL-5 and anti-CCR3/eotaxins, which are currently in clinical development.

Eosinophil granules contain a crystalloid core composed of major basic protein (MBP-1 and MBP-2), as well as a matrix composed of eosinophil cationic protein (ECP), eosinophil-derived neurotoxin (EDN), and eosinophil peroxidase (EPO). MBP, EPO, and ECP have cytotoxic effects on a variety of tissues in concentrations similar to those found in biologic fluids from patients with eosinophilia. Additionally, ECP and EDN belong to the ribonuclease A superfamily and possess antiviral and ribonuclease activity. ECP can insert voltage-insensitive, ion-nonselective toxic pores into the membranes of target cells, and these pores may facilitate the entry of other toxic molecules. MBP directly increases smooth muscle reactivity by causing dysfunction of vagal muscarinic M_2 receptors, and this process has been postulated to contribute to the airway hyperresponsiveness associated with asthma. MBP also triggers degranulation of mast cells and basophils. Triggering of eosinophils by engagement of receptors for cytokines, immunoglobulins, and complement can lead to the generation of a wide range of inflammatory cytokines, including IL-1, IL-3, IL-4, IL-5, IL-13, GM-CSF, transforming growth factor-α/β, tumor necrosis factor-α, RANTES, macrophage inflammatory protein 1α (MIP-1α), and the eotaxins, thus indicating that eosinophils have the potential to modulate multiple aspects of the immune response. Additionally, eosinophils can directly activate T cells by antigen presentation and help polarize dendritic cells to promote a T_H2 phenotype. Further eosinophil-mediated damage is caused by toxic hydrogen peroxide and halide acids generated by EPO and by superoxide generated by the respiratory burst oxidase enzyme pathway in eosinophils. Eosinophils also generate large amounts of cysteinyl leukotriene C_4 (LTC_4), which is metabolized to LTD_4 and LTE_4. These three lipid mediators increase vascular permeability and mucus secretion and are potent stimulators of smooth muscle contraction. Finally, bipyramidal Charcot-Leyden crystals are derived from a nongranule lysophospholipase in eosinophils and are frequently found in sputum, feces, and tissues infiltrated by eosinophils.

CLINICAL MANIFESTATIONS

Hypereosinophilia is often recognized on a routine blood count in a patient who is asymptomatic or being evaluated for unrelated or nonspecific signs or symptoms. On other occasions, the possibility of eosinophilia may be specifically investigated in a patient with gastrointestinal or respiratory symptoms because helminthic disease or allergic causes are suspected. The clinical signs and symptoms of hypereosinophilic syndromes are heterogeneous because of the diversity of the causes and potential organ involvement. Common signs and symptoms include dermatitis, heart failure, neuropathy, and abdominal pain. One of the most serious complications of hypereosinophilia is cardiac disease secondary to endomyocardial thrombus formation and restrictive fibrosis (Chapter 60). Mitral and tricuspid valve regurgitation may result from progressive fibrotic damage to the chordae tendineae, and resultant heart failure can develop from valvular insufficiency and endomyocardial fibrosis. Cardiac involvement can occur in association with eosinophilia from diverse causes, including parasitic infections. Hypereosinophilic syndromes can result in cerebral emboli from cardiac disease, diffuse encephalopathy, and peripheral neuropathy.

DIAGNOSIS

Differential Diagnosis

The differential diagnosis of eosinophilia includes reactive eosinophilia, eosinophilia associated with other primary disorders, and eosinophilia

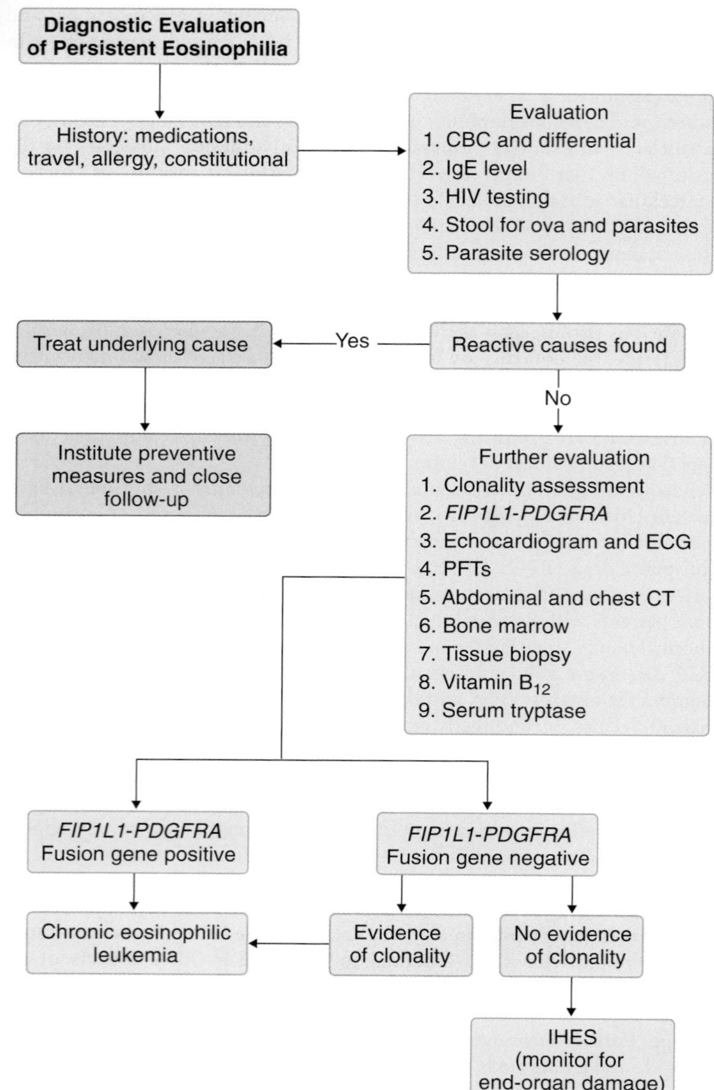

FIGURE 173-2. **Diagnostic evaluation of persistent eosinophilia.** CBC = complete blood count; CT = computed tomography; ECG = electrocardiogram; IgE = immunoglobulin E; IHES = idiopathic hypereosinophilic syndrome; HIV = human immunodeficiency virus; PDGFRA = platelet-derived growth factor-receptor α; PFTs = pulmonary function tests.

associated with clonal hematopoiesis (see Table 173-1). Evaluation of patients is based on their history and clinical characteristics (Fig. 173-2). The initial goal is to determine whether the eosinophilia is secondary to a reactive cause (i.e., in response to another primary trigger such as allergy, infection, solid tumor, vasculitis). If reactive causes are not identified, further evaluation should determine whether the eosinophilia is secondary to a clonal hematologic disorder. If no evidence of clonality is determined, the patient is considered to have an idiopathic hypereosinophilic syndrome.

The differential diagnosis of eosinophilia requires a review of the patient's history, which may reveal wheezing (Chapter 87), rhinitis (Chapter 259), or eczema (indicating atopic causes); travel to areas where helminth infections (e.g., schistosomiasis [Chapter 363]) are endemic; the presence of a pet dog (indicating possible infection with *Toxocara canis* [Chapter 365]); symptoms of cancer; or drug ingestion (indicating a possible hypersensitivity reaction [Chapter 262]). Eosinophilia caused by drugs (Chapter 262) is usually benign but can sometimes be accompanied by tissue damage, as in hypersensitivity pneumonitis (Chapter 97). In most cases, the eosinophilia resolves when use of the drug ceases, but in some cases, such as eosinophilia-myalgia syndrome secondary to the ingestion of contaminated L-tryptophan, the disease can persist despite withdrawal of the drug.

The presence of abnormal morphologic features of eosinophils, an increase in immature and dysplastic cells in the bone marrow or blood, elevated levels of vitamin B_{12}, and splenomegaly raises suspicion of a clonal hypereosinophilic syndrome. In such cases, evidence of clonality (e.g., by analysis of X chromosome inactivation patterns in female patients), an elevated level of mast cell tryptase (elevated in myelodysplastic variants of hypereosinophilic syndrome), the presence of aberrant lymphocyte phenotypes (elevated in lymphocytic variants of hypereosinophilic syndrome), abnormal cytogenetics, and the possible presence of specific fusion genes such as *FIP1L1-PDGFRA* should be investigated.

Other eosinophilic syndromes such as Churg-Strauss syndrome (Chapter 278) should be considered in patients with a history of worsening asthma, sinus disease, neuropathy, or blood eosinophilia and the presence of abnormal laboratory findings associated with autoimmunity, such as an elevated erythrocyte sedimentation rate, C-reactive protein, and antineutrophil cytoplasmic antibodies.

An accumulation of eosinophils that is limited to specific organs is characteristic of particular diseases, such as eosinophilic cellulitis (Wells' syndrome), eosinophilic esophagitis, eosinophilic pneumonias (e.g., Löffler's syndrome [Chapter 92]), and eosinophilic fasciitis (Shulman's syndrome).

Diagnostic Evaluation

Diagnostic studies that should be performed in patients with moderate to severe eosinophilia and considered in patients with persistent mild eosinophilia include morphologic examination of a blood smear, human immunodeficiency virus (HIV) screen, serial stool examinations for ova and parasites, parasite serology, and plasma immunoglobulin E (IgE) level. Parasitic infections that cause eosinophilia are usually limited to helminthic parasites, with the exception of two enteric protozoans, *Isospora belli* (Chapter 361) and *Dientamoeba fragilis* (Chapter 361). *Strongyloides stercoralis* (Chapter 366) infection is important to diagnose because it can cause disseminated fatal disease in immunosuppressed patients; detection of such infection often requires serologic testing. Other infections to consider include trichinosis (Chapter 366), *T. canis* infection (Chapter 365), and HIV infection (Chapter 400).

Patients with sustained hypereosinophilia should be monitored closely for the subsequent development of cardiac disease. A pathologically similar disease, Löffler's endomyocarditis (Chapter 60), has been noted in tropical regions, where antecedent parasite-elicited eosinophilia may be responsible for the cardiac damage.

TREATMENT

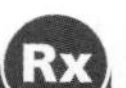

Reactive Hypereosinophilia and Hypereosinophilia Associated with Other Diseases

Treatment of reactive hypereosinophilia and hypereosinophilia associated with other diseases centers around identifying the cause and then treating the underlying disease process. For example, reactive eosinophilia typically responds by removal of the inciting triggers (e.g., allergens, parasites, and medications). Eosinophilia associated with other disease processes typically improves after treatment of the underlying disease, such as dietary manipulation in patients with allergic eosinophilic gastroenteritis.

FIP1L1-PDGFRA-Positive Disease

Imatinib should be considered as first-line therapy in patients in whom the *FIP1L1-PDGFRA* fusion gene has been demonstrated and in selected patients with the characteristic clinical and laboratory features of this myeloproliferative subtype of hypereosinophilic syndrome (e.g., male gender, tissue fibrosis, elevated serum vitamin B_{12} and tryptase levels). Clinical responses to imatinib in *FIP1L1-PDGFRA*-positive patients are rapid, with normalization of eosinophil counts generally occurring within 1 week of initiation of treatment and reversal of the signs and symptoms occurring within 1 month. Doses of imatinib as low as 100 mg daily appear to be effective in controlling symptoms and eosinophilia in most patients, but some recommend beginning imatinib treatment at 400 mg daily to achieve molecular remission and then decreasing the dose slowly while monitoring the patient closely for evidence of molecular relapse. In imatinib-resistant patients, sorafenib may be effective. The utility of imatinib therapy in hypereosinophilic patients without a demonstrable *FIP1L1-PDGFRA* mutation remains controversial, although some patients have responded. Nonmyeloablative allogeneic bone marrow transplantation (Chapter 181) has also been used successfully in several patients with hypereosinophilia.

Other Hypereosinophilic Syndromes

Corticosteroids, which have been used for decades in the treatment of idiopathic hypereosinophilic syndromes, remain the first-line treatment for most patients except those with *PDGFRA*-associated hypereosinophilia. The most appropriate initial corticosteroid dose and the duration of steroid therapy have not been subjected to randomized trials, but a general recommendation is to start with a moderate to high dose (≥40 mg prednisone equivalent) and taper very slowly while monitoring the eosinophil count closely. With this approach, most patients will respond initially, and some will be able to be maintained on low doses of corticosteroids for prolonged periods.

Monoclonal anti-IL-5 antibody therapy (e.g., mepolizumab or reslizumab) for hypereosinophilia and eosinophil-associated asthma[1,2] has a number of unique advantages related to the specificity of IL-5 for the eosinophil lineage. In patients treated with this agent, eosinophil counts are twice as likely to fall below 600/μL (95% vs. 45%, $P < .001$) with significantly lower prednisone doses.[3] Of the cytotoxic therapies that have been used for steroid-refractory hypereosinophilia, hydroxyurea has been the most extensively studied at doses of 1 to 3 g/day. Vincristine at a dose of 1 to 2 mg intravenously can rapidly lower eosinophilia in patients with extremely high eosinophil counts (>100,000/mm^3) and may be useful for the treatment of children whose aggressive disease is unresponsive to other therapies. In patients who have corticosteroid-refractory hypereosinophilic syndromes or who develop intolerable side effects of steroid treatment, immunomodulatory agents that are sometimes helpful include interferon-α, cyclosporine, and alemtuzumab. Responses can often be achieved with relatively low doses of interferon-α (1 to 2×10^6 U/day) and may persist for prolonged periods. Because the effects of interferon-α on eosinophil numbers in peripheral blood may not become evident for several weeks, escalation to an effective dose may require several months. Rarely, patients have remained in remission for extended periods after cessation of interferon-α therapy, suggesting that interferon-α may be curative in a small subset of individuals. Low-dose (500 mg daily) hydroxyurea appears to act synergistically with interferon-α to lower the eosinophil count without increasing side effects.

FUTURE DIRECTIONS

Treatments on the horizon for hypereosinophilic disorders include targeted therapy against the eotaxin chemokines and their receptor CCR3, as well as anti-IL-5 and anti-IL-5 receptor–based antibody therapy.

PROGNOSIS

The prognosis of hypereosinophilic syndromes depends on the primary cause. Whereas *FIP1L1-PDGFRA*-positive disease and other forms of clonal disorders have a poor prognosis (25 to 50% 5-year mortality rate if responsiveness to therapeutic intervention is not achieved), the prognosis of hypereosinophilia from reactive and other causes is usually better.

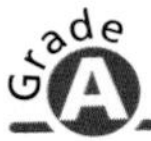

1. Nair P, Pizzichini MM, Kjarsgaard M, et al. Mepolizumab for prednisone-dependent asthma with sputum eosinophilia. *N Engl J Med*. 2009;360:985-993.
2. Haldar P, Brightling CE, Hargadon B, et al. Mepolizumab and exacerbations of refractory eosinophilic asthma. *N Engl J Med*. 2009;360:973-984.
3. Rothenberg ME, Klion AD, Roufosse FE, et al. Treatment of patients with the hypereosinophilic syndrome with mepolizumab. *N Engl J Med*. 2008;358:1215-1228.

SUGGESTED READINGS

Dulohery MM, Patel RR, Schneider F, et al. Lung involvement in hypereosinophilic syndromes. *Respir Med*. 2011;105:114-121. *About 25% of patients have pulmonary involvement with variable radiologic findings and oftentimes with asthma.*

Ogbogu PU, Bochner BS, Butterfield JH, et al. Hypereosinophilic syndromes: a multicenter, retrospective analysis of clinical characteristics and response to therapy. *J Allergy Clin Immunol*. 2009;124:1319-1325. *The 11% of patients who were F1P1L1-PDGFRA positive usually responded to imatinib, whereas the 17% with aberrant clonal T-cell populations usually responded to corticosteroids.*

Roufossue F, Weller PF. Practical approach to the patient with hypereosinophilia. *J Allergy Clin Immunol*. 2010;126:39-44. *Review.*

Sade K, Mysels A, Levo Y, et al. Eosinophilia: a study of 100 hospitalized patients. *Eur J Intern Med*. 2007;18:196-201. *Common causes were asthma or atopic disease (13%), eosinophilic pneumonia (10%), cancer (10%), infections (10%), and drug reactions (6%), but 34% were of unknown cause.*

Schwartz LB, Sheikh J, Singh A. Current strategies in the management of hypereosinophilic syndrome, including mepolizumab. *Curr Med Res Opin*. 2010;26:1933-1946. *Clinical review.*

Sheikh J, Weller PF. Advances in diagnosis and treatment of eosinophilia. *Curr Opin Hematol*. 2009;16:3-8. *Review of the lymphocytic (non-malignant T-cell expansion) and myeloproliferative (abnormal tyrosine kinase activity from a fusion product) variants.*

174

APPROACH TO THE PATIENT WITH BLEEDING AND THROMBOSIS

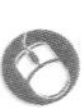

ANDREW I. SCHAFER

MECHANISMS OF HEMOSTASIS AND THROMBOSIS

The coagulation system is normally quiescent, and blood fluidity is maintained by the actions of a continuous monolayer of endothelial cells that line the intimal surface of the vasculature throughout the circulatory tree. At a site of vascular damage, the antithrombotic properties of endothelium are lost, and thrombogenic constituents of the subendothelial vessel wall become exposed to circulating blood. The result is rapid formation of a hemostatic clot that consists of platelets and fibrin and is localized to the area of vascular injury. Activation of platelets and formation of fibrin occur essentially simultaneously and interdependently to effect hemostasis. Subsequently, vascular repair is accomplished by thrombolysis and recanalization of the occluded site.

Platelet activation at a site of vascular injury begins with the adhesion of platelets to the locally de-endothelialized intimal surface (platelet–vessel wall interaction). Platelet adhesion is mediated by von Willebrand factor, which sticks circulating platelets to the area of damaged vessel wall by binding to its receptors located in platelet membrane glycoprotein Ib. The adherent platelets then undergo a "release reaction," during which they discharge constituents of their storage granules, including adenosine diphosphate (ADP), and simultaneously elaborate thromboxane A_2 from arachidonic acid through the aspirin-inhibitable cyclooxygenase reaction. ADP, thromboxane A_2, and other components of the release reaction act in concert to recruit and activate additional platelets from the circulation to the site of vascular injury. These activated platelets expose binding sites for fibrinogen by forming the surface membrane glycoprotein IIb/IIIa complex. In the process of platelet aggregation (platelet-platelet interactions), fibrinogen (or von Willebrand factor under conditions of high shear stress) mediates the final formation of an occlusive platelet plug.

Fibrin, which anchors the hemostatic platelet plug, is formed from soluble plasma fibrinogen by the action of the potent protease enzyme thrombin (Fig. 174-1). The fibrin mesh is stabilized by covalent cross-linking mediated by factor XIII. Thrombin is formed from its inactive (zymogen) plasma precursor, prothrombin, by the action of activated factor X (Xa) and its cofactor, factor Va. This sequence of reactions has classically been referred to as the *common pathway* of coagulation. Factor X can be activated by either the *tissue factor (extrinsic) pathway* or the *contact activation (intrinsic) pathway* of coagulation. The tissue factor pathway is now considered to be the major physiologic initiator of coagulation activation. It is triggered by the formation of the complex of tissue factor, which is exposed on the surfaces of activated vascular and blood cells, with activated factor VII (VIIa). The contact activation pathway involves a series (or cascade) of zymogen-protease reactions that are initiated by factor XII, high-molecular-weight kininogen, and prekallikrein. Activated factor XII (XIIa) converts factor XI to XIa, which in turn activates factor IX to IXa. Factor IXa is the enzyme that converts factor X to Xa, a reaction that requires factor VIIIa as a cofactor.

Intact, normal endothelium promotes blood fluidity by inhibiting platelet activation. It likewise plays a crucial role in preventing fibrin accumulation. Among the physiologic antithrombotic systems that produce this latter effect are (1) antithrombin III, (2) protein C and protein S, (3) tissue factor pathway inhibitor (TFPI), and (4) the fibrinolytic system. Antithrombin is the major protease inhibitor of the coagulation system: it inactivates thrombin and other activated coagulation factors. Heparin functions as an anticoagulant by binding to antithrombin and greatly accelerating these reactions. Heparin and heparin sulfate proteoglycans are naturally present on endothelial cells, so antithrombin inactivation of thrombin and other coagulation proteases most likely occurs physiologically on vascular surfaces rather than in fluid plasma. Activated protein C, with its cofactor protein S, functions as a natural anticoagulant by destroying factors Va and VIIIa, two essential cofactors of the coagulation cascade. Thrombin itself is the activator of protein C, and this reaction occurs rapidly only on the surfaces of intact vascular endothelial cells, where thrombin binds to the glycosaminoglycan thrombomodulin. TFPI is a plasma protease inhibitor that specifically quenches tissue factor–induced coagulation. Finally, what little fibrin can be produced, despite these potent physiologic antithrombotic mechanisms, is digested rapidly by the endogenous fibrinolytic system. Fibrinolysis is mediated by the protease plasmin, which is generated from plasminogen in plasma by the action of endothelium-derived plasminogen activators.

EVALUATION OF THE PATIENT WITH A POSSIBLE BLEEDING DISORDER

History and Physical Examination

A thorough history is paramount in evaluating a patient for a possible systemic bleeding disorder. In addition to asking the patient about spontaneous bleeding episodes in the past, responses to specific hemostatic challenges should be recorded. A bleeding tendency may be suspected if a patient previously experienced excessive hemorrhage after surgery or trauma, including common events such as circumcision, tonsillectomy, labor and delivery, menses, dental procedures, vaccinations, and injections. Conversely, a history of normal blood clotting after such specific challenges in the recent past is just as important to note. It may be a better test of the integrity of systemic hemostasis than any laboratory measurement can provide.

In a patient with a history of excessive or unexplained bleeding, the initial goal is to determine whether the cause is a systemic coagulopathy or an anatomic or mechanical problem with a blood vessel. This situation is encountered most frequently in patients with excessive postoperative bleeding, which could be due to either local surgical trauma or a coagulation abnormality. A history of prior bleeding suggests a coagulopathy, as does the finding of bleeding from multiple sites. However, this is not always the case. Even diffuse bleeding may arise from anatomic rather than hemostatic abnormalities. An example of this is recurrent mucosal hemorrhage in patients with hereditary hemorrhagic telangiectasia. Conversely, a single episode of bleeding from an isolated site may be the initial manifestation of a coagulopathy.

The history must include a survey of coexisting systemic diseases and drug ingestions that could affect hemostasis. Renal failure and the myeloproliferative disorders are associated with impaired platelet–vessel wall interactions and qualitative platelet abnormalities, connective tissue diseases and lymphomas are associated with thrombocytopenia, and liver disease causes a complex coagulopathy (Chapter 178). Ingestion of aspirin and other nonsteroidal anti-inflammatory drugs (NSAIDs) that cause nonselective inhibition of cyclooxygenase leads to platelet dysfunction; these drugs are often contained in over-the-counter preparations that patients may neglect to report without specific questioning. Other drugs, such as antibiotics, also may be associated with a bleeding tendency by causing abnormal platelet function or thrombocytopenia. Finally, it is important to elicit a family history of bleeding problems. Although a positive history provides an important clue to a possible inherited coagulopathy, a negative history does not exclude a familial cause; for example, 20% of patients with classic hemophilia have a completely negative family history of bleeding.

Patterns of clinical bleeding, as revealed by the history and physical examination, may be characteristic of certain types of coagulopathy (Table 174-1). In general, patients with thrombocytopenia or qualitative platelet or vascular disorders present with bleeding from superficial sites in the skin and mucous membranes. These may involve petechiae, which are pinpoint cutaneous hemorrhages that appear particularly over dependent extremities (characteristic of severe thrombocytopenia), ecchymoses (common bruises), purpura, gastrointestinal and genitourinary tract bleeding, epistaxis, and hemoptysis. In these types of disorders, bleeding tends to occur spontaneously or immediately after trauma. In contrast, patients with inherited or acquired coagulation factor deficiencies, such as hemophilia, or those on anticoagulant therapy tend to bleed from deeper tissue sites (e.g., hemarthroses, deep hematomas, retroperitoneal hemorrhage) and in a delayed manner after trauma.

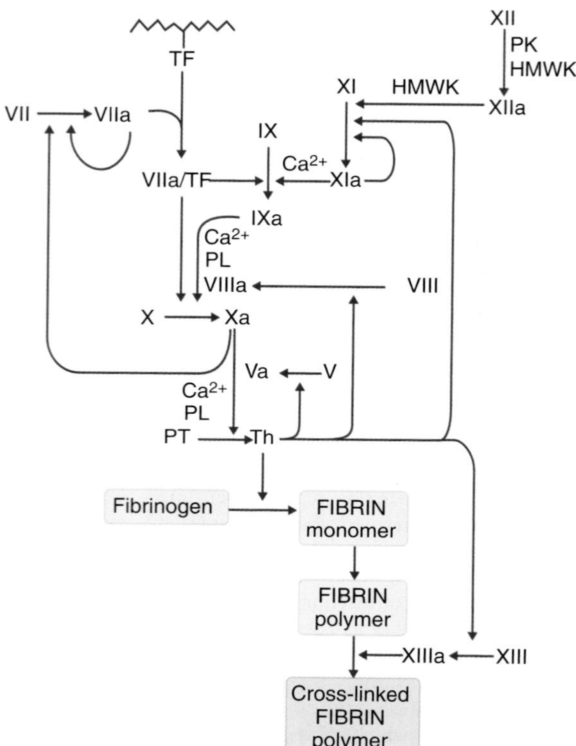

FIGURE 174-1. Coagulation cascade. This scheme emphasizes an understanding of (1) the importance of the tissue factor pathway in initiating clotting in vivo, (2) the interactions among pathways, and (3) the pivotal role of thrombin in sustaining the cascade by feedback activation of coagulation factors. HMWK = high-molecular-weight kininogen; PK = prekallikrein; PL = phospholipid; PT = prothrombin; TF = tissue factor; Th = thrombin. (From Schafer AI. Coagulation cascade: an overview. In: Loscalzo J, Schafer AI, eds. *Thrombosis and Hemorrhage.* Cambridge, MA: Blackwell Scientific Publications; 1994:3-12.)

Laboratory Testing

Four simple screening tests have traditionally been used in the initial evaluation of patients with a suspected coagulopathy: platelet count, bleeding time, prothrombin time (PT), and activated partial thromboplastin time (aPTT). Thrombocytopenia, reported by electronic particle counting, should be verified by examination of the peripheral smear. Pseudothrombocytopenia, a laboratory artifact of ex vivo platelet clumping, may be caused by the ethylenediaminetetraacetic acid (EDTA) anticoagulant used in tubes for blood cell counts, by other anticoagulants, or by nonphysiologic cold agglutinins acting at room temperature. It should be suspected whenever a very low platelet count is unexpectedly reported in a patient who does not exhibit any clinical bleeding. Pseudothrombocytopenia is indicated by the finding of platelet clumps on the peripheral smear, and the diagnosis is supported by the finding of simultaneously normal platelet counts in blood samples obtained by finger stick, in tubes containing other anticoagulants, or in a tube maintained at 37° C before platelet counting. Examination of the blood smear

TABLE 174-1 CHARACTERISTIC PATTERNS OF BLEEDING IN SYSTEMIC DISORDERS OF HEMOSTASIS

TYPE OF DISORDER	*Sites of Bleeding* GENERAL	SKIN	MUCOUS MEMBRANES	OTHER	ONSET OF BLEEDING	CLINICAL EXAMPLES
Platelet-vascular disorders	Superficial surfaces	Petechiae, ecchymoses	Common: oral, nasal, gastrointestinal, genitourinary	Rare	Spontaneous or immediately after trauma	Thrombocytopenia, functional platelet disorder, vascular fragility, disseminated intravascular coagulation, liver disease
Coagulation factor deficiency	Deep tissues	Hematomas	Rare	Common: joint, muscle, retroperitoneal	Delayed after trauma	Inherited coagulation factor deficiency, acquired inhibitor, anticoagulation, disseminated intravascular coagulation, liver disease

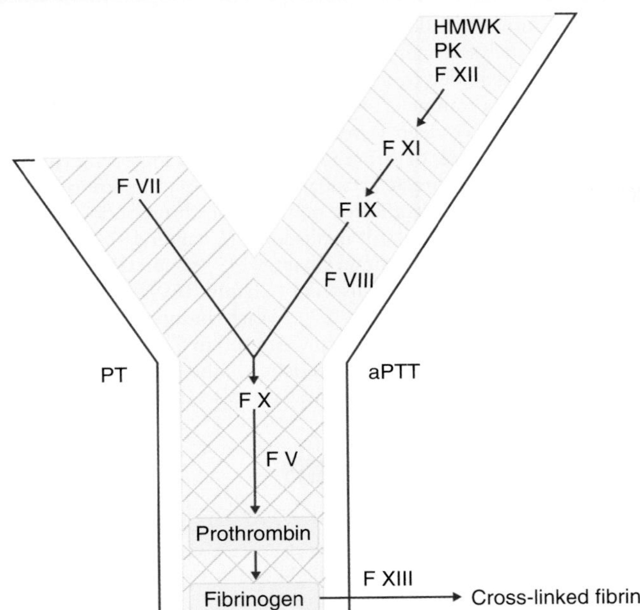

FIGURE 174-2. Classic coagulation cascade. The prothrombin time (PT) measures the integrity of the extrinsic and common pathways, whereas the activated partial thromboplastin time (aPTT) measures the integrity of the intrinsic and common pathways. Factor (F) XIII deficiency is not detected by PT or aPTT. HMWK = high-molecular-weight kininogen; PK = prekallikrein.

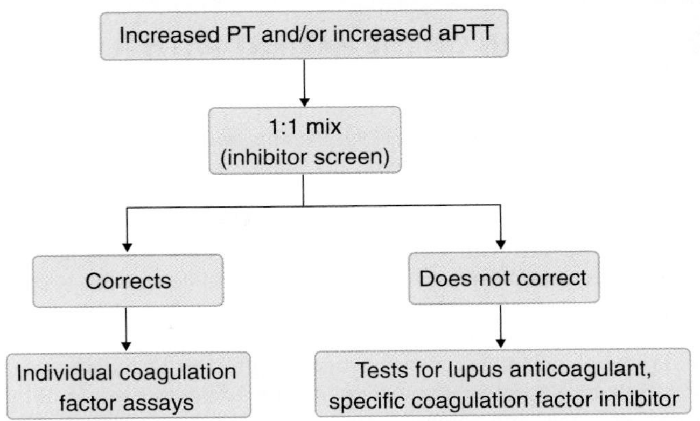

FIGURE 174-3. Approach to evaluating patients with prolonged prothrombin time (PT) or activated partial thromboplastin time (aPTT).

can also reveal clues to the cause of real thrombocytopenia, such as fragmented red blood cells in thrombotic thrombocytopenic purpura.

The bleeding time is a widely used clinical screening test for disorders of platelet–vessel wall interactions. It measures the time to cessation of bleeding after a standardized incision over the volar aspect of the forearm, now most commonly performed by disposable automated devices. The bleeding time is prolonged in thrombocytopenia, qualitative platelet abnormalities, defects in platelet–vessel wall interactions (e.g., von Willebrand disease), and primary vascular disorders. The bleeding time usually is not prolonged in patients with coagulation factor deficiencies. The test is prone to problems related to reproducibility, sensitivity, and specificity, however. Therefore, because von Willebrand disease is the most common genetic cause of abnormal platelet–vessel wall interactions, some experts now recommend replacing the bleeding time with specific tests for von Willebrand disease in the initial evaluation of patients with a suspected coagulopathy (Chapter 176).

The PT measures the integrity of the extrinsic and common pathways of coagulation (factors VII, X, and V; prothrombin; and fibrinogen) (Fig. 174-2). The aPTT measures the integrity of the intrinsic and common pathways of coagulation (high-molecular-weight kininogen; prekallikrein; factors XII, XI, IX, VIII, X, and V; prothrombin; and fibrinogen). The sensitivity of the PT and aPTT in detecting coagulation factor deficiencies may vary with the reagents used to perform these tests, and each laboratory must determine its own reference standards.

With a few notable exceptions, normal results for all these screening tests of hemostasis essentially exclude any clinically significant systemic coagulopathy. However, patients with factor XIII deficiency may have a serious bleeding diathesis but normal screening tests; specific tests for factor XIII deficiency should be performed if this disease is suspected. The PT and aPTT detect only the more severe deficiencies of coagulation factors, usually at levels less than 30% of normal; specific factor levels should be determined if a mild coagulation factor deficiency is suspected. Patients with von Willebrand disease sometimes have normal bleeding times and usually do not have sufficiently reduced levels of factor VIII to affect the aPTT, requiring specific testing for the disease. Rare disorders of fibrinolysis also may be associated with normal screening tests, necessitating more specialized tests when indicated. Abnormalities in the screening tests of hemostasis may be pursued by more specialized tests to establish a specific diagnosis.

The initial approach to a prolonged bleeding time in the absence of thrombocytopenia is to determine whether the patient is taking any drugs that might interfere with platelet function (e.g., aspirin, other NSAIDs) or has a coexisting disease that might explain the finding (e.g., renal failure). If these conditions are absent or if the bleeding time fails to correct after discontinuation of any potentially offending drugs, further specialized testing may include platelet aggregation studies to identify specific qualitative abnormalities of platelet function and specific assays to exclude one of the types of von Willebrand disease.

The finding of a prolonged PT and/or aPTT indicates either a deficiency of one or more coagulation factors or the presence of an inhibitor, usually an antibody, directed at one or more components of the coagulation system (Fig. 174-3). These two possibilities can be distinguished by performing a simple inhibitor screen, which involves a 1 : 1 mix of the patient's plasma and normal plasma. The premise of the test is that even if the patient's plasma is completely deficient (0% level) in a certain factor, mixing it 1 : 1 with normal plasma (100% level) should bring the concentration of that factor to 50% in the mixture; this is sufficient to correct the prolonged PT or aPTT. If correction occurs with the inhibitor screen, individual coagulation factor levels should be assayed for a specific deficiency state. If the 1 : 1 mix fails to correct the prolonged PT and/or aPTT, an inhibitor is likely to be present, and it is interfering with coagulation in vitro in both the patient's plasma and the normal plasma. Specific assays should then be performed to determine whether there is a true inhibitor against a coagulation factor (e.g., factor VIII antibody) or whether the inhibitor is a lupus anticoagulant.

EVALUATION OF THE ASYMPTOMATIC PATIENT WITH ABNORMAL COAGULATION TESTS

In asymptomatic individuals who are discovered incidentally to have abnormalities in screening laboratory tests of hemostasis, the first critical question is whether the findings are clinically relevant. Patients with inherited deficiencies of one of the contact activation coagulation factors (factor XII, high-molecular-weight kininogen, prekallikrein) characteristically have a markedly prolonged aPTT, yet they do not have a clinical bleeding tendency. Likewise, patients with lupus anticoagulants typically have prolongation of the aPTT and sometimes also the PT; they more often have thrombotic rather than bleeding complications. In patients with heparin-induced thrombocytopenia, a marked decrease in the platelet count is sometimes associated with arterial and venous thrombosis rather than bleeding. It is crucial to view the clinical setting, history, physical examination, and screening laboratory tests as complementary facets of the approach to patients with suspected coagulopathies.

EVALUATION OF THE PREOPERATIVE PATIENT

Routine screening of all preoperative patients with a platelet count, bleeding time, PT, and aPTT not only is uninformative but also may be counterproductive if follow-up testing causes unnecessary expense and delays in surgery (Chapter 439). Preoperative bleeding time, PT, and aPTT do not predict surgical bleeding risk in patients who are not found to be at increased risk on clinical grounds, so a thorough clinical assessment should guide the need for these preoperative screening tests. Laboratory testing and possibly further specialized tests of coagulation are indicated for patients whose bleeding histories are suspicious for a hemostatic abnormality. Preoperative screening tests of coagulation are probably warranted for patients who cannot cooperate with an adequate clinical assessment and for those who will be undergoing procedures in which even minimal postoperative hemorrhage could be hazardous.

EVALUATION OF THE PATIENT WITH A POSSIBLE HYPERCOAGULABLE STATE

Most patients with venous thromboembolism (VTE) have an inherited basis for hypercoagulability (Chapter 179). Patients with inherited hypercoagulable states (or thrombophilia) typically present with an initial episode of VTE in early adulthood, but thrombotic manifestations may begin at any time from early childhood to old age. Patients usually have deep vein thrombosis of the lower extremities or pulmonary embolism, but other uncommon sites of venous thrombosis may be involved. Arterial thrombosis is not characteristically associated with inherited hypercoagulable states. Arterial thrombosis that occurs prematurely or in the absence of apparent risk factors should trigger a different line of investigation, possibly including evaluation for vasculitis, myeloproliferative disorders, hyperhomocysteinemia, antiphospholipid syndrome, and potential sources of systemic embolization.

The primary or hereditary hypercoagulable states (see Table 179-1 in Chapter 179) result from specific mutations or polymorphisms that lead to decreased levels of physiologic antithrombotic proteins or increased levels of procoagulant proteins. In contrast, the secondary or acquired hypercoagulable states (see Fig. 179-2 in Chapter 179) are a heterogeneous group of disorders that predispose to thrombosis by complex mechanisms. VTE is often precipitated by the combination of an underlying hypercoagulable genotype and an acquired prothrombotic, hypercoagulable state such as pregnancy, immobilization, or the postoperative state. Certain clinical characteristics suggest the presence of an inherited hypercoagulable state (Table 174-2). Patients with recurrent thrombosis should be tested for these disorders and, in most cases, committed to lifelong prophylactic anticoagulation. It is not clear whether it is essential to order these tests after a single episode of VTE. Counterintuitively, it has been found that most of the common inherited hypercoagulable states—which, to varying extents, clearly increase the risk of a *first* episode of VTE—are at best only weak predictors of *recurrent* VTE. It has been argued, therefore, that making a specific thrombophilia diagnosis after an initial episode of VTE will not influence the decision about the duration of prophylactic anticoagulation. However, the increased risk of recurrent VTE with the more prothrombotic mutations (e.g., antithrombin III, protein C or S deficiency), combined inherited thrombophilias, or antiphospholipid syndrome may necessitate long-term anticoagulation, and their diagnosis after a first episode of VTE will in fact alter decisions about the duration of anticoagulation. Even if they are not maintained on long-term anticoagulation, patients with diagnosed primary hypercoagulable states should receive prophylactic anticoagulation during situations that pose a high risk for thrombosis, such as the peripartum period. There is no simple screening test for primary hypercoagulable states, and the timing of obtaining these tests is crucial to avoid erroneous diagnoses. Acute thrombosis itself can cause transient decreases in the levels of antithrombin, protein C, and protein S. Heparin therapy can cause a decrease in plasma antithrombin activity. Warfarin therapy lowers the functional levels of protein C and protein S. Inherited deficiency states can be diagnosed spuriously under these conditions.

Patients who present with VTE probably have an increased risk of harboring an occult malignancy (Chapter 187). This association is increased further in patients with recurrent and unprovoked thrombosis. There are conflicting opinions whether an evaluation for occult malignancy in these patients must be exhaustive. Some contend it can be limited to a thorough history, physical examination, routine complete blood cell count and chemistries, test of fecal occult blood, urinalysis, mammogram (in women), and chest radiograph, with further testing guided by any abnormalities found in this initial evaluation. Others argue for routine CT scanning of the chest, abdomen, and pelvis.

In addition to classic deep vein thrombosis and pulmonary embolism, certain characteristic types of thrombosis may provide important clues to the cause and trigger a more directed evaluation. Migratory, superficial thrombophlebitis (Trousseau's syndrome) or nonbacterial thrombotic endocarditis suggests the presence of an occult malignancy (Chapter 187). Hepatic vein thrombosis (Budd-Chiari syndrome; Chapter 145) or portal vein thrombosis may indicate a myeloproliferative disorder (Chapter 169) or paroxysmal nocturnal hemoglobinuria (Chapter 163). Warfarin-induced skin necrosis strongly suggests an underlying protein C or protein S deficiency. Recurrent, spontaneous miscarriages are characteristic of the antiphospholipid syndrome (Chapter 177), although they are also associated with other thrombophilias.

TABLE 174-2 CLINICAL CHARACTERISTICS OF PATIENTS WITH INHERITED HYPERCOAGULABLE STATES (THROMBOPHILIA)

- Venous thromboembolism (>90% of cases)
  - Deep vein thrombosis and/or pulmonary embolism most common
  - Mesenteric, cerebral vein thrombosis rare but characteristic
- Frequent family history of thrombosis
  - Typically autosomal dominant
- First episode of thrombosis typically in young adulthood (<40 yr)
- Often idiopathic (but an acquired thrombosis trigger is not infrequently identified with a careful history)
- More common thrombophilias (factor V Leiden, prothrombin 20210G→A) are associated with a lower thrombosis risk; rarer thrombophilias (antithrombin III, protein C, protein S deficiency) are associated with a higher thrombosis risk
- Warfarin-induced skin necrosis or neonatal purpura fulminans with protein C or protein S deficiency (very rare)

SUGGESTED READINGS

Favaloro EJ, Lippi G. Coagulation udate: what's new in hemostasis testing? *Thromb Res*. 2011;127:S13-S16. *Review of standard and newer tests.*

Favaloro EJ, McDonald D, Lippi G. Laboratory investigation of thrombophilia: the good, the bad, and the ugly. *Semin Thromb Hemostas*. 2009;35:695-710. *Review of the rationale for and current controversies over screening laboratory tests for thrombophilia.*

Kessler CM. The link between cancer and venous thromboembolism: a review. *Am J Clin Oncol*. 2009;32(4 Suppl):S3-S7. *Brief review of the relationship between cancer and venous thromboembolism (VTE) and the value of extensive screening for occult malignancy in patients with a first episode of idiopathic VTE.*

Tsoran I, Saharov G, Brenner B, et al. Prolonged travel and venous thromboembolism findings from the RIETE registry. *Thromb Res*. 2010;126:287-291. *Risk factors include high BMI, previous VTE, hormone use, and, in 16% of patients, a positive thrombophilia test.*

175

THROMBOCYTOPENIA

CHARLES S. ABRAMS

Thrombocytopenia is defined as a platelet count less than the normal range, typically below 150,000/μL. In the absence of qualitative platelet defects (Chapter 176), excessive bleeding does not occur in thrombocytopenic patients following trauma or surgery unless the platelet count is lower than 75,000/μL. In otherwise hemostatically normal patients, spontaneous hemorrhage typically does not occur with platelet counts above 30,000/μL. Patients with platelet counts less than 5000 to 10,000/μL are at high risk for spontaneous, life-threatening hemorrhage. However, there is no absolute threshold for spontaneous bleeding due to thrombocytopenia. It may occur at higher counts when fever, sepsis, severe anemia, and other hemostatic defects are present or when platelet function is impaired by medication. Notably, a prolonged cutaneous bleeding time test does not accurately predict the risk of clinical bleeding. Therefore, it is critical that the physician consider the gamut of possibilities when diagnosing and managing a patient with a low platelet count.

Typically, the first step in diagnosing a patient with a low platelet count is to determine whether the thrombocytopenia is attributable to one of the three broad mechanisms for developing thrombocytopenia: (1) increased destruction, such as that seen in immune-mediated causes; (2) decreased production, usually due to an underlying bone marrow disorder; or (3) sequestration of platelets within the spleen, as occurs in conditions that cause splenomegaly (hypersplenism).

Determining the cause of the patient's thrombocytopenia is essential to select the most appropriate therapy and to avoid unnecessary procedures. Because there is no easy test to differentiate among the three possibilities, clinical evaluation is critical. Therefore, a thorough history and physical examination, with attention to possible alternative explanations for thrombocytopenia, are mandatory. Particular attention should be paid to the duration of symptoms, which helps determine whether the patient has acute or chronic thrombocytopenia. Attention should also focus on the patient's recent exposure to new medications that might induce thrombocytopenia as a side effect.

Preliminary laboratory tests include a complete blood count (CBC) with a differential, along with an examination of the peripheral blood smear.

Abnormalities in the number or morphology of the leukocytes or erythrocytes may indicate a systemic inflammatory disorder or pathology within the bone marrow. Clumping of the platelets on the peripheral blood smear may indicate that the patient has pseudothrombocytopenia (Chapter 174). This anomaly is usually due to an antibody that binds to and thereby agglutinates platelets only in the presence of ethylenediaminetetraacetic acid (EDTA) or when the blood sample is allowed to cool to room temperature. Repeating the platelet count in a blood sample that has been anticoagulated with heparin and kept warm until it is analyzed can help exclude this spurious diagnosis. Any additional testing is based solely on the available clinical information; for example, human immunodeficiency virus (HIV) testing would be prudent in a patient with risk factors. A bone marrow aspirate and biopsy are typically not required for a patient with thrombocytopenia who has an otherwise normal CBC and peripheral blood smear count. However, a bone marrow aspirate and biopsy should be considered in older patients or in patients in whom standard therapy has not been effective.

GENERAL MECHANISMS OF THROMBOCYTOPENIAS

Increased Platelet Destruction

An acute drop in a patient's platelet count implies that a peripheral destructive process is the likely cause. For example, a patient who develops abrupt thrombocytopenia during hospitalization most likely has a low platelet count caused by an infection or a new medication. Both nonimmune and immune processes can lead to a shortened platelet lifespan. Nonimmune reasons for the accelerated destruction of platelets include sepsis, disseminated intravascular coagulation (DIC), thrombotic thrombocytopenic purpura (TTP), hemolytic-uremic syndrome (HUS), preeclampsia or eclampsia, cardiopulmonary bypass, and giant cavernous hemangioma. Thrombocytopenia that occurs in these circumstances usually resolves with treatment of the underlying disorder, and platelet transfusions are rarely necessary. Thrombocytopenia due to TTP, HUS, or heparin-induced thrombocytopenia (HIT) is associated with thrombosis rather than bleeding (Table 175-1), so platelet transfusions are rarely necessary. In addition, controversial reports have noted the clinical deterioration of patients with TTP or HIT following platelet transfusion, suggesting that platelets should not be given to most patients with these disorders.

Immune-mediated platelet destruction can occur owing to drugs, alloimmune sensitization, or autoimmunity. Medications should always be considered as a possible cause of acute thrombocytopenia. The list of potential offending agents is long, but drugs with strong evidence of antibody-mediated platelet destruction include quinine, quinidine, sulfonamides, and gold salts. In addition to stopping the offending medication, platelet transfusions might be required for severe thrombocytopenia.

Platelet Sequestration

Approximately 30% of the circulating platelet mass is normally sequestered within the spleen. Even more platelets may be sequestered when the spleen enlarges owing to portal hypertension or infiltrative diseases. This in turn can result in moderate thrombocytopenia. Because hypersplenism never causes a platelet count less than 40,000 to 50,000/μL, bleeding due to thrombocytopenia from hypersplenism alone is unusual.

Decreased Platelet Production

Decreased platelet production occurs in primary diseases of the bone marrow, such as acute leukemia and aplastic anemia; myelophthisic processes in which marrow is affected by metastatic carcinoma, fibrosis, or other clonal hematopoietic disorders; following chemotherapy and/or radiation therapy; with ethanol toxicity; and during infections with viruses such as HIV, cytomegalovirus (CMV), Epstein-Barr virus (EBV), and varicella. Thrombocytopenia also occurs when normal megakaryocyte proliferation is impaired by myelodysplasia.

TABLE 175-1 DISORDERS THAT CAUSE BOTH THROMBOCYTOPENIA AND THROMBOSIS

Thrombotic thrombocytopenic purpura (TTP)
Hemolytic-uremic syndrome (HUS)
Heparin-induced thrombocytopenia (HIT)
Disseminated intravascular coagulation (DIC)
Paroxysmal nocturnal hemoglobinuria (PNH)
Vasculitis (such as systemic lupus erythematosus)
Antiphospholipid antibody syndrome (APS)

PLATELET TRANSFUSIONS

Clinicians usually consider "wet" bleeding to be much more ominous than "dry" bleeding. Signs of wet bleeding include epistaxis, gingival bleeding, gastrointestinal or genitourinary bleeding, or bleeding around intravenous sites. Dry bleeding is defined as ecchymosis or petechiae. Overt wet bleeding that is clearly due to thrombocytopenia is usually treated with platelet transfusion. Prophylactic platelet transfusion for patients who are not bleeding is controversial. When making the decision whether to treat a nonbleeding patient with thrombocytopenia, the practitioner must consider the short lifespan of platelets (10 days), the 5-day shelf life of stored platelets, and the potential for the patient to develop transfusion-induced platelet alloantibodies. In patients undergoing treatment for acute leukemia, the outcome is unchanged when a platelet count as low as 5000 to 10,000/μL is used as the threshold for prophylactic platelet transfusion. In contrast, a higher platelet count is required when patients are bleeding or undergoing an invasive procedure or surgery. For patients experiencing the most extreme hemostatic challenges (e.g., neurosurgery, cardiopulmonary bypass, thyroid surgery, prostatectomy), a platelet count greater than 75,000 to 100,000/μL for the procedure and for the next several days is advisable. For minor invasive procedures, such as colonoscopy with biopsy, a platelet count of 30,000 to 50,000/μL is usually adequate.

A donated unit of blood contains approximately 50 billion platelets. Infusing this number of platelets into a patient should increase his or her platelet count by 20,000/μL divided by the patient's surface area in square meters. Therefore, transfusion into a typical patient should increase the recipient's platelet count by 10,000 to 12,000/μL. Bags of platelets used for transfusions are typically obtained by pooling platelets derived from four to eight blood donors. Therefore, a "unit" at one hospital may be derived from more donors than a "unit" obtained at another hospital.

Large quantities of platelets can be derived from a single donor by using apheresis technology (plateletpheresis). Because there is minimal loss of red blood cells with this technique, plateletpheresis allows one individual to donate very large numbers of platelets (equivalent to the number of platelets obtained from 6 to 10 units of donated blood). As discussed in the following section, the risk of platelet alloimmunization is partially dependent on the number of individuals donating platelets to a patient. Therefore, single-donor plateletpheresis platelets can prevent or at least minimize alloimmunization.

Several trials have addressed how many platelets should be transfused into thrombocytopenic patients to maintain hemostasis and minimize exposure to blood products. The largest of these trials was the multicenter Platelet Dose (PLADO) trial.[1] In this study, patients were randomized to receive transfusions of low-dose (110 billion), medium-dose (220 billion), or high-dose (440 billion) platelets per square meter for thrombocytopenia while recovering from hematopoietic stem cell transplantation. Patients who received the low-dose therapy required more frequent platelet transfusions, but overall, they received fewer transfused platelets over the course of the study. Importantly, bleeding complications were identical with all platelet transfusion strategies. This study demonstrates that low doses of platelets (110 billion/square meter of body surface area) are as safe as larger doses in patients with hypoproliferative thrombocytopenia receiving prophylactic platelet transfusion therapy.

Several complications of platelet transfusion therapy merit mention. First, some patients can become alloimmunized against platelet antigens and can become refractory to future platelet transfusion therapy (discussed in detail later). Second, bacterial contamination of stored platelets is a much more common complication than the infectious risk associated with red blood cell transfusions. Unlike red blood cells, which are stored frozen after being harvested from donated blood, platelets are sensitive to cool temperatures and therefore need to be stored at room temperature. This method of storage results in more bacterial overgrowth in the transfusion bags. Transfusion-associated bacterial sepsis is one of the most frequently reported causes of transfusion-induced mortality in the United States, and platelet transfusions are the most common blood products associated with sepsis. It should also be noted that room temperature storage of platelets contributes to their short shelf life of approximately 5 to 7 days. Consequently, unlike the blood-derived products that can be frozen (such as red blood cells and plasma), there is a constant need for platelet donations year-round. In contrast to the risk of bacterial infection, the risk of viral infection from platelet transfusions is no higher than it is for red blood cell transfusions. From a single unit of platelets, the risk of being exposed to HIV is less than 1 in 2.5 million, the risk of exposure to hepatitis B virus is less than 1 in 750,000, and the risk of exposure to hepatitis C virus is less than 1 in 1 million.

Platelet transfusions have been considered contraindicated for thrombocytopenia owing to TTP or HIT. This recommendation is driven entirely by case reports of thrombotic events occurring soon after platelet transfusions in such patients, not by randomized trials addressing this issue. Because thrombotic events are a known complication of both TTP and HIT, it is difficult to determine whether the thrombi were due to the platelet transfusions or merely the intrinsic prothrombotic risk of TTP and HIT. In any case, there is usually no indication for platelet transfusions in patients with TTP and HIT because thrombosis is a much greater risk than hemorrhage in these disorders.

The Transfusion-Refractory Patient

Many patients do not have an optimal increase in the platelet count following transfusion. Although there are various definitions of platelet refractoriness, it is simplest to base this definition on the timing of platelet loss following transfusion. A patient who does not have the predicted rise in platelet count (between 10,000 and 12,000/μL for every unit of donated platelets) should have the platelet count analyzed before the next platelet transfusion, 1 hour after that transfusion, and again 24 hours later. If the platelet count rises appropriately 1 hour after the transfusion but falls substantially 24 hours later, the patient has ongoing platelet consumption. This is often seen in patients with sepsis, DIC, or severe active hemorrhage or as a result of the drug-mediated immune destruction of platelets. In these situations, the best therapy is to treat the underlying cause and to continue to support the patient with platelet transfusions as clinically indicated. Alternatively, some patients fail to have a significant increase in platelets even 1 hour after a transfusion. These patients have (1) hypersplenism, (2) an autoantibody that eliminates not only endogenous platelets but also allogeneic platelets (as in patients with idiopathic thrombocytopenic purpura [ITP]), or (3) alloantibodies that react with antigens on the transfused platelets.

Alloantibodies develop in approximately 20% of patients who are repeatedly exposed to platelet transfusions, and these patients present some of the most challenging management issues in transfusion medicine (Chapter 180). The alloantibodies may be directed against human leukocyte antigen (HLA) class I antigens (HLA-A and HLA-B) or against platelet-specific antigens present on the surface of the platelets. Because it appears that HLA class II antigens present on the surface of leukocytes are essential for the development of antibodies directed against HLA class I antigens, efforts to remove the contamination of leukocytes in platelet transfusion preparations can minimize alloantibody formation. Therefore, the use of filters that trap leukocytes during transfusions are useful to prevent patients from becoming refractory to future platelet transfusions. Once a patient develops alloantibodies against transfused platelets, the clinician and the blood bank should attempt to identify whether the alloantibody is directed against an HLA or against a platelet-specific antigen. If the alloantibody can be identified, platelets derived from donors matched for HLA or the platelet-specific antigen can be used. Corticosteroids, intravenous immunoglobulin, splenectomy, and recombinant factor VIIa are probably of no value in maintaining hemostasis in platelet-refractory patients. Antifibrinolytic agents (e.g., ε-aminocaproic acid) might be helpful for patients with bleeding predominantly in the oral cavity or the genitourinary tract. However, antifibrinolytic agents are contraindicated in patients with DIC (Chapter 178) because these agents can precipitate thrombotic events.

SPECIFIC CAUSES OF THROMBOCYTOPENIA

Drug-Induced Thrombocytopenia

The abrupt onset of thrombocytopenia implies a high probability of the immune-mediated destruction of platelets. This is particularly likely if the thrombocytopenia is present in the absence of other abnormalities on the CBC. The clinician should first suspect either an infection (viral or bacterial) or a drug. A careful history and physical examination, along with a normal leukocyte count and differential, should help exclude an infectious cause of thrombocytopenia. Drug-induced thrombocytopenia is one of the most frequent causes of cytopenias evaluated by physicians.

The typical drug-induced thrombocytopenia is the result of an immune reaction elicited by either the drug or one of its metabolites. Sometimes the drug is simply deposited on the platelet surface, and antidrug antibodies lead to accelerated platelet clearance, primarily in the spleen. More frequently, the drug binds to a protein on the platelet surface and induces a neoantigen that is ultimately recognized by the immune system. In the absence of the drug or drug metabolites, this platelet neoantigen disappears, and the thrombocytopenia slowly resolves as new platelets are released from the bone marrow. This mechanism explains the vast majority of drug-induced thrombocytopenias, but there are some exceptions. For example, chemotherapy and other bone marrow toxins can decrease platelet production and thereby induce thrombocytopenia by a mechanism independent of the immune system.

Patients with drug-induced thrombocytopenia can have mild, moderate, or even severe forms. Almost all types of drug-induced thrombocytopenia predispose the patient to hemorrhagic but not thrombotic complications. The notable exception to this rule is HIT (discussed separately in the next section). The most difficult diagnostic dilemma is to discern drug-induced thrombocytopenia from ITP. For this distinction, the patient's medical history may be helpful. A gradually progressive thrombocytopenia is more consistent with ITP than with one induced by a medication. Conversely, the rapid onset of thrombocytopenia following the initiation of a new medication indicates that the drug is the most likely culprit. The time between initiation of the offending drug and development of thrombocytopenia has not been well documented for most medications. However, thrombocytopenia typically begins days to a few weeks after the administration of most medications with this type of toxicity. Presumably, this lag represents the period required for the patient to develop an immune response against the drug-platelet complex. Medications that have been taken safely for years before the onset of thrombocytopenia are unlikely to be the offending agents. In addition to an assessment of prescribed medications, a careful evaluation of over-the-counter medications is necessary. Agents that contain quinine lead the list of nonprescribed drugs that can induce life-threatening thrombocytopenia. Quinine is frequently contained in over-the-counter pills for leg cramps. Even the quinine in tonic water can induce severe thrombocytopenia ("gin and tonic purpura") when ingested by certain patients.

Some medications are much more likely to induce thrombocytopenia than others. Table 175-2 contains a partial list of drugs that frequently induce this type of toxicity. One particularly useful online database (*www.ouhsc.edu/platelets/ditp.html*) lists and periodically updates the level of evidence for specific drugs that may induce thrombocytopenia. With the exception of tests for HIT, laboratory tests for drug-induced thrombocytopenia do not have widespread applicability. Usually, drug-induced thrombocytopenia is proved only in retrospect, when the platelet count improves after discontinuation of the suspected medication. Even then, the diagnosis is not conclusive unless thrombocytopenia recurs after rechallenging the patient with the offending drug (a practice that is almost never recommended).

TABLE 175-2 DRUGS THAT ARE STRONGLY ASSOCIATED WITH THROMBOCYTOPENIA

ANTIBIOTICS AND ANTIVIRALS
Quinine/quinidine
Penicillins
Cephalosporins
Vancomycin
Trimethoprim/sulfamethoxazole
Sulfonamides/sulfonylureas
Linezolid
Valacyclovir
Ganciclovir
Indinavir
CARDIOVASCULAR MEDICATIONS
Abciximab
Tirofiban
Eptifibatide
Salicylates
Digoxin
Furosemide
MISCELLANEOUS
Cimetidine
Ranitidine
Famotidine
Valproate
Interferon

The most efficacious method of treating drug-induced thrombocytopenia is to stop all suspected offending medications. Usually, no additional therapy is indicated. The thrombocytopenia typically begins to resolve without further intervention within days to a week of stopping the drug. The notable exceptions involve drugs with particularly long half-lives. Sulfonamides, quinine, and quinidine are particularly notorious for inducing severe or even life-threatening thrombocytopenia. In patients with profound thrombocytopenia (<10,000 to 15,000/μL) or at high risk for bleeding, platelet transfusions are indicated. If ITP cannot be confidently excluded and the thrombocytopenia is life threatening, glucocorticoids can also be initiated (see the discussion of ITP treatment later).

Heparin-Induced Thrombocytopenia

A special case of drug-induced immune-mediated thrombocytopenia associated with arterial and venous thrombosis, rather than bleeding, is HIT. It is seen in 2 to 5% of patients exposed to unfractionated heparin and in 0.7% of patients given low-molecular-weight heparin; it almost never occurs in patients exposed only to fondaparinux. To understand this disease, one must know that platelets can secrete a protein, platelet factor 4 (PF4), that can bind to heparin. HIT is caused by an antibody that binds to this PF4-heparin complex (Fig. 175-1). Large complexes of antibodies directed against heparin-bound PF4 accumulate on the surface of platelets. At times, these anti-PF4 immunoglobulins bind to the Fc receptor that is also present on the platelet surface. The interaction of platelet Fc receptors and anti-PF4 antibodies causes activation of the platelet, release of more PF4, and a cycle of events that leads to the stimulation of even more platelets. Ultimately, it also leads to activation of the coagulation cascade. The activation of platelets and the clotting cascade leads to the formation of thrombi and thrombocytopenia.

When thrombocytopenia is detected in a hospitalized patient, HIT must always be considered. Patients with this syndrome often have multiple potential causes for thrombocytopenia (such as other medications or infections). Therefore, it is important to exclude these other causes. Large retrospective studies of HIT have suggested that the onset of thrombocytopenia relative to the initiation of heparin therapy is useful in establishing or excluding this diagnosis. HIT typically occurs 4 to 14 days after patients are given heparin by any route (even subcutaneously or in extremely low doses by heparin flush). This lag between heparin exposure and the appearance of HIT is due to the time it takes for the immune response to generate the requisite antibodies against the heparin-PF4 complex. Some patients who have been exposed to heparin within the past several months already have preexisting antibodies against the heparin-PF4 complex in their circulation. When these patients are re-exposed to heparin, they may develop an acute onset of HIT within the first day of reinitiating the drug.

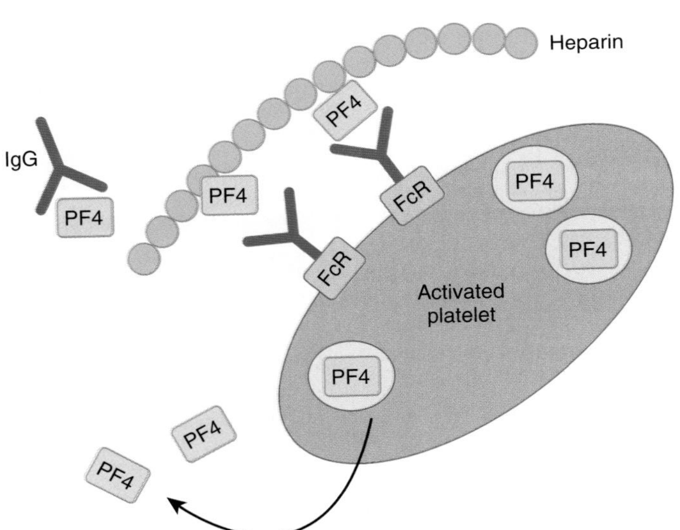

FIGURE 175-1. Pathophysiology of heparin-induced thrombocytopenia. Platelet factor 4 (PF4) is a protein stored in platelet granules and secreted from platelets upon their activation. Heparin can bind to PF4 and induce a conformational change within PF4 that in some patients produces an antibody-mediated immune response. Large complexes of immunoglobulin (Ig), heparin, and PF4 can accumulate on the platelet surface and stimulate the platelet when the Fc portion of the antibody interacts with the platelet's FcγRII receptor (FcR). Once activated, the platelets contribute to thrombosis. In addition, the activated platelets secrete more PF4, continuing the process.

The unique timing of acute-onset HIT within hours of heparin re-exposure and the more typical development of HIT within 4 to 14 days of initial heparin exposure emphasize the importance of a careful and critical history in establishing the diagnosis. HIT should be suspected in any patient who develops thrombocytopenia while on heparin therapy. It is important to note that the normal platelet count varies widely (150,000 to 450,000/μL), so some patients may have a substantial decrease in the platelet count but still remain within the normal range. Therefore, a greater than 50% decrease in the platelet count in a patient on heparin should raise suspicion for this syndrome. HIT should also be suspected in any patient who develops a thrombotic event while on heparin therapy.

Several antibody-based laboratory tests are available to confirm this diagnosis (Table 175-3). Although antibodies against the heparin-PF4 complex are almost always present in patients with HIT, these antibodies are also frequently present in heparin-treated patients who do not have this disorder (i.e., those with neither thrombocytopenia nor thrombosis). In addition, several days may elapse before the test results are available. Therefore, in practice, these laboratory assays provide only confirmatory information. Urgent clinical decisions should *not* be deferred until such test results are available. The timing of the thrombocytopenia with respect to the heparin exposure and the degree of platelet drop are the most important pieces of information needed by the physician evaluating a patient suspected of having HIT.

There are two general categories of laboratory assays for the diagnosis of HIT: functional assays and immunologic assays. Functional assays analyze whether the combination of heparin and the patient's plasma can induce normal platelets to aggregate or to secrete serotonin; these assays have very high specificity but relatively low sensitivity. Immunologic assays test the patient's plasma for antibodies that bind to the heparin-PF4 complex; they have very high sensitivity but lack specificity. Consequently, a *negative immunologic assay* is useful in excluding this diagnosis, and a *positive functional assay* is very useful in confirming the diagnosis of HIT.

Because platelets are consumed as they become activated, the clinical presentation of HIT is thrombocytopenia. However, it is unusual for the thrombocytopenia to actually cause bleeding. Instead, HIT is a highly prothrombotic disorder. Both venous and arterial thromboses are common in HIT. Patients with HIT who do not have thrombosis on initial presentation still have a 20 to 30% chance of developing a thrombus within the next month. Nevertheless, the incidence of HIT-related clinical events is greatest immediately after diagnosis. More importantly, clinical studies report that cessation of heparin frequently fails to prevent thromboses or the development of new thrombotic events.

If a patient has HIT, all heparin should be stopped immediately. This includes subcutaneous injections of "minidose" heparin, heparin flushes of intravenous lines, and low-molecular-weight heparin; even heparin-coated intravenous catheters should be withdrawn. Alternative anticoagulation, such as a direct thrombin inhibitor like recombinant hirudin or argatroban (Chapter 37), should be administered, at least until the platelet count normalizes. Warfarin should not be used in cases of acute HIT because of its delayed therapeutic effect and its association with venous limb gangrene. Because patients rarely become profoundly thrombocytopenic as a result of HIT alone, platelet transfusions are typically not required. In fact, some reports suggest that platelet transfusions can actually precipitate thrombotic complications, although this remains controversial.

TABLE 175-3 LABORATORY ASSAYS FOR HEPARIN-INDUCED THROMBOCYTOPENIA

ASSAY	SENSITIVITY (%)	SPECIFICITY (%)	POSITIVE PREDICTIVE VALUE (%)	NEGATIVE PREDICTIVE VALUE (%)
Functional assay (e.g., serotonin release assay)	88	≈100	≈100	81
PF4/heparin enzyme immunoassay (ELISA)	95-98	86	93	95

ELISA = enzyme-linked immunosorbent assay; PF4 = platelet factor 4.

Sepsis

Along with exposure to certain drugs, bacterial and viral infections are the most common cause of acute thrombocytopenia in hospitalized patients. Acute thrombocytopenia can be caused by the deposition of antibody-antigen complexes on the platelet surface via an "innocent bystander" phenomenon. These antibody-coated platelets are then cleared from the circulatory system by Fc receptor–expressing macrophages in the spleen. Thrombocytopenia associated with infections can also be due to DIC. The treatment of sepsis-induced thrombocytopenia is directed at the underlying cause, along with platelet transfusions as clinically indicated.

Idiopathic (Immune) Thrombocytopenic Purpura

DEFINITION

ITP is an autoimmune disorder caused by circulating antiplatelet autoantibodies. An ITP-like picture can also be found in patients with autoimmune diseases such as systemic lupus erythematosus (see later and Chapter 274), low-grade lymphoproliferative disorders such as chronic lymphocytic leukemia (Chapter 190), and HIV infection (Chapter 400).

CLINICAL MANIFESTATIONS

ITP was originally thought to be a disease of young women. Although this description is appropriate for many individuals with this disorder, more recent data indicate that ITP can occur in patients of either sex and at any age. ITP is a chronic, recurring disorder in the vast majority of adults with this disease. This is in stark contrast to pediatric patients, who usually suffer from acute ITP and rarely have the chronic variant of this disorder.

In contrast to patients with coagulation factor deficiencies who present with bleeding deep within tissues, individuals with ITP (or other disorders of platelets) typically have excessive mucocutaneous bleeding. Consequently, the clinician should inquire whether the patient has noticed epistaxis, gingival bleeding, easy bruising, hematuria, melena, or hematochezia. Female patients should also be asked about inappropriate or excessive vaginal bleeding. The physical examination should pay particular attention to signs of mucocutaneous bleeding. Consequently, the patient should be thoroughly examined for petechiae and ecchymosis, as well as for evidence of hemorrhage within the conjunctiva, retina, and central nervous system.

DIAGNOSIS

Except for the thrombocytopenia, the CBC is usually normal, and the peripheral blood smear is remarkable only for a decreased number of platelets, some of which may be larger than normal. Splenomegaly is absent unless the ITP is due to an underlying disorder, such as lymphoma, that is itself associated with splenomegaly. Bone marrow examination is usually not necessary in the absence of findings that suggest a different disease such as myelodysplasia. If performed, the bone marrow aspirate and biopsy typically show normal or increased numbers of megakaryocytes but are otherwise normal, characteristic of other forms of destructive thrombocytopenia.

TREATMENT Rx

Because platelet production is assumed to be increased in patients with ITP, traditional therapy has focused on moderating this immune response that ultimately leads to accelerated platelet destruction. For most of the latter half of the 20th century, splenectomy and corticosteroids were the sole therapies for ITP. Although they remain first-line therapeutic modalities, immunomodulating agents such as intravenous immunoglobulin (IVIG) and anti-D, as well as alternative immunosuppressives, have been introduced for the therapy of ITP. Corticosteroids in the form of high-dose dexamethasone (4-day pulses every 14 to 28 days for four to six cycles) are effective. For selected refractory patients, other immunosuppressives, such as cyclophosphamide, azathioprine, cyclosporine A, mycophenolate mofetil, dapsone, interferon, and etanercept, can be used.

For years, the basic mechanism of and rationale for ITP treatment revolved around altering the immune system through immunosuppressives, splenectomy, or immune modulators such as IVIG or anti-D. A more recent addition to the ITP treatment regimen is rituximab, a "humanized" murine monoclonal antibody against CD20, which is a B-cell antigen. Although rituximab has not been approved by the Food and Drug Administration (FDA) for the treatment of ITP, it is currently widely used in patients who are unresponsive to splenectomy and corticosteroids. Response rates vary significantly between studies, ranging from 28 to 44% in larger trials. The combination of high-dose dexamethasone and rituximab was recently shown to be more effective than dexamethasone alone.[2]

Although the vast majority of ITP patients have a compensatory increase in megakaryopoiesis in response to the rapid platelet destruction, plasma derived from some ITP patients was unexpectedly found to inhibit platelet production. This has prompted a re-evaluation of whether impaired megakaryopoiesis contributes to the development of thrombocytopenia in this disease. Thrombopoietin (TPO) is a potent megakaryocyte colony-stimulating factor and, along with other cytokines, increases the size and number of megakaryocytes (Chapter 159). TPO levels are not markedly elevated in ITP, suggesting that supplemental TPO could help increase platelet production and correct the thrombocytopenia.

Early experiments demonstrated that recombinant as well as truncated forms of TPO significantly increased the platelet count in some refractory ITP patients. However, this also induced autoimmune autoantibodies against endogenous TPO, which resulted in profound and persistent thrombocytopenia. Both recombinant TPO and its truncated form were therefore withdrawn from clinical trials. Subsequently, peptides were developed that bear no structural resemblance to TPO but still bind to and activate the TPO receptor; these agents are called *TPO receptor agonists*. Because these recombinant drugs bear little structural similarity to native TPO, they should not trigger autoimmune anti-TPO antibodies. The FDA has approved two of these drugs, and several more are being used in clinical trials. The first of these, called romiplostim, is composed of several copies of the TPO receptor–binding peptide spliced into a recombinant antibody. This peptide agonist competes with TPO for binding to the TPO receptor and activates the receptor in an identical fashion as endogenous TPO. The second FDA-approved TPO receptor agonist is eltrombopag (Promacta). It is an oral drug that activates the TPO receptor by binding to the receptor's transmembrane region.

Both subcutaneously administered romiplostim and orally administered eltrombopag are capable of increasing platelet counts in approximately 70% of patients with ITP. Remarkably, these drugs can also increase the platelet count in patients with ITP that is refractory to other treatment modalities, including splenectomy.[3-7] However, adverse events, including bone marrow fibrosis and thromboembolism, have been reported. It should be noted that the drugs' effects disappear soon after their discontinuation. Therefore, the TPO receptor agonists are not disease modifying and are probably most appropriate for short-term use when a temporary rise in platelet count is required.

General Principles of ITP Therapy

Management of ITP is guided by both symptoms and platelet count.[8] Asymptomatic patients with platelet counts greater than 30,000/µL can be followed without treatment. If the patient is bleeding and/or has a platelet count less than 30,000/µL, treatment with prednisone is recommended (Table 175-4). Refractory patients may require splenectomy, other immunosuppressive medications, or one of the new thrombopoiesis-stimulating agents (Table 175-5). Splenectomy has a long history of success in this disorder; durable complete response rates are approximately 66 to 70%. Approximately half the remaining patients who do not have normal platelet counts following splenectomy achieve a partial response that is clinically meaningful. Unfortunately, 10 to 15% of patients derive no benefit from splenectomy, and there is no test to predict whether a particular patient will respond to this treatment.

ITP patients with severe thrombocytopenia (<5000/µL) and/or internal bleeding should be promptly treated with high doses of pulse corticosteroids and IVIG. Platelet transfusion may be given concurrently with IVIG for critical bleeding. In Rh-positive patients who have not undergone splenectomy, anti-D immune globulin may be substituted for IVIG. However, some patients develop autoimmune hemolysis from this treatment.

TABLE 175-4 THERAPY FOR THE INITIAL MANAGEMENT OF IDIOPATHIC THROMBOCYTOPENIC PURPURA

ORAL PREDNISONE
Effect is dose dependent—approximately 80% of patients respond to 1 mg/kg/day. Toxicity also increases with dose and duration of treatment and includes glucose intolerance, immunosuppression, osteoporosis, and cataracts. Relapse is typical once therapy is discontinued.
INTRAVENOUS IMMUNOGLOBULIN (IVIG)
More rapid than daily prednisone. Administered at a dose of 1 g/kg/day for 2 consecutive days or 0.4 g/kg/day for 5 consecutive days. Response rates are approximately 80%, and effects typically last 2-4 wk. Toxicity includes headache, allergic reactions, and, rarely, thrombosis.
ANTI-D IMMUNOGLOBULIN
Administered at a dose of 50-75 µg/kg IV. Response rates are dose dependent but can approach 75-80%. Hemolysis is a common toxicity. Rarely, hemolysis can be life threatening and can be associated with disseminated intravascular coagulation, renal failure, and end-organ infarction.

Thrombotic Thrombocytopenic Purpura

DEFINITION

TTP is a consumptive thrombocytopenia associated with a mechanical hemolytic anemia. The classic pentad of symptoms—thrombocytopenia, anemia, fever, neurologic problems, and renal abnormalities—is fully present in only a minority of patients. Many patients today have only hemolytic anemia and thrombocytopenia. The poor specificity of the clinical features and laboratory abnormalities makes this disease difficult to diagnose. Historically, untreated TTP had a mortality of 90% within 3 months. With modern therapy, patients with TTP have a mortality of approximately 10 to 20%.

PATHOBIOLOGY

Some patients with recurrent TTP have very large multimers of von Willebrand factor (Chapter 176). Because larger multimers of von Willebrand factor are more efficient at binding and activating platelets than smaller ones, it was speculated that TTP could be due to a deficiency of a protease that cleaves large multimers of von Willebrand factor into smaller, less sticky ones. A genome-wide linkage analysis of patients with inherited recurrent TTP (Upshaw-Schulman syndrome) demonstrated a deficiency of a metalloproteinase that is now called ADAMTS13 (a disintegrin-like and metalloprotease with thrombospondin type 1 repeats). Many patients with adult-onset TTP have an antibody against ADAMTS13 that causes an acquired deficiency of the enzyme. Inherited or acquired ADAMTS13 deficiency causes the accumulation of ultra-large multimers of von Willebrand factor in plasma, which leads to platelet activation and the microvascular thrombosis characteristic of this disease (Fig. 175-2). Because many patients can have a partial deficiency of ADAMTS13 without having TTP, clinical assays of ADAMTS13 enzymatic activity have not been useful in diagnosing TTP. Levels of ADAMTS13 below 5% of normal are considered highly suggestive of TTP, but levels greater than this are not very helpful. This hypothesis still needs to be validated in large clinical trials. Consequently, analysis of ADAMTS13 enzymatic activity should not be used to diagnose TTP outside of a research setting.

Some patients reportedly developed TTP soon after taking an antiplatelet drug of the thienopyridine class. Approximately 1 of every 2000 patients taking ticlopidine will develop TTP. In several individuals with ticlopidine-induced TTP, an antibody against ADAMTS13 was identified. A few studies have also suggested that clopidogrel can induce TTP at an incidence of 1 in 15,000 to 1 in 250,000. Because the incidence of TTP in the general population is approximately 1 in 100,000, it is difficult to determine whether there is a significant risk of TTP in patients who are prescribed clopidogrel. It should be noted that some patients can also develop TTP after exposure to medications that directly injure the vascular endothelium. The majority of these patients do not have TTP but have the related disorder HUS (discussed later in this chapter).

TABLE 175-5 THERAPY FOR THE MANAGEMENT OF REFRACTORY IDIOPATHIC THROMBOCYTOPENIC PURPURA

ORAL PREDNISONE
Effect is dose dependent and rapidly dissipates after discontinuation of the medication. Some patients can be maintained on a very low and tolerable daily dose (e.g., 5 mg). Long-term use is associated with infections, diabetes, osteoporosis, avascular necrosis, weight gain, and cataracts.
ORAL DEXAMETHASONE
Administered at a dose of 40 mg/day for 4 consecutive days. Repeated every 2-4 wk for several months. Sustained response rates of 29-42% are possible. Toxicity is similar to that of oral prednisone.
SPLENECTOMY
Durable (often lifelong), significant responses are seen in 65-70% of patients who undergo this procedure. More modest benefits are seen in another 10-15% of patients. There is no useful way to predict who will respond. Splenectomy is associated with surgical morbidity and some mortality (≈1-2%). Produces lifelong immunosuppression to encapsulated and gram-positive organisms.
RITUXIMAB
Given at a dose of 375 mg/m^2/wk IV for a total of 4 wk. Significant responses are seen in 28-44% of patients and typically last for months. Toxicity includes reactivation of hepatitis B, immunosuppression, and, rarely, progressive multifocal leukoencephalopathy.
THROMBOPOIETIN RECEPTOR AGONISTS
Administered daily (eltrombopag) or weekly (romiplostim). An effect is typically seen in 2-3 wk and disappears a few weeks after discontinuation of the medication. Toxicity from long-term use is not well known but may include excessive thrombosis and bone marrow fibrosis.

CLINICAL MANIFESTATIONS AND DIAGNOSIS

Patients often present with symptoms of excessive mucocutaneous bleeding, but they might present with signs of a thrombotic event (including phlebitis, myocardial infarction, or stroke). Many patients complain of abdominal pain that is presumably due to intestinal ischemia. Signs of central nervous system disease, including somnolence and even frank coma, can also be seen on presentation.

The two major hallmarks of this disorder are microangiopathic hemolytic anemia and thrombocytopenia. Microangiopathic hemolytic anemia is a non-immune-mediated hemolytic anemia caused by red cell fragmentation. Patients with this disorder have typical laboratory findings of hemolytic anemia, including a decreasing hemoglobin concentration, high lactate dehydrogenase level, elevated indirect bilirubin, and increased reticulocyte count. Examination of the peripheral blood smear (Chapter 160) shows torn red blood cells (schistocytes) and, frequently, early red blood cell precursor cells (nucleated red blood cells). The thrombocytopenia may be mild if the disease is diagnosed at an early stage, but advanced cases of TTP can have platelet counts less than 10,000/μL. TTP should be considered in any patient who has evidence of hemolysis accompanied by thrombocytopenia.

Unlike most patients with typical thrombocytopenia, who tend to bleed excessively, patients with TTP have few hemorrhagic complications. Instead, they are markedly predisposed to thrombosis. In fact, a thrombotic complication in a thrombocytopenic patient is another clue that TTP might be the cause of the thrombocytopenia (see Table 175-1). Characteristically, the thrombotic occlusions are in the terminal arterioles and capillaries and are composed mainly of platelets within the damaged vascular lumen. In contrast to most blood clots, these occlusions contain very little fibrin and are referred to as hyaline thrombi. Before plasmapheresis was used, TTP typically progressed and caused renal disease, neurologic symptoms, and fever. These symptoms are believed to be due to ischemia and infarction of the affected

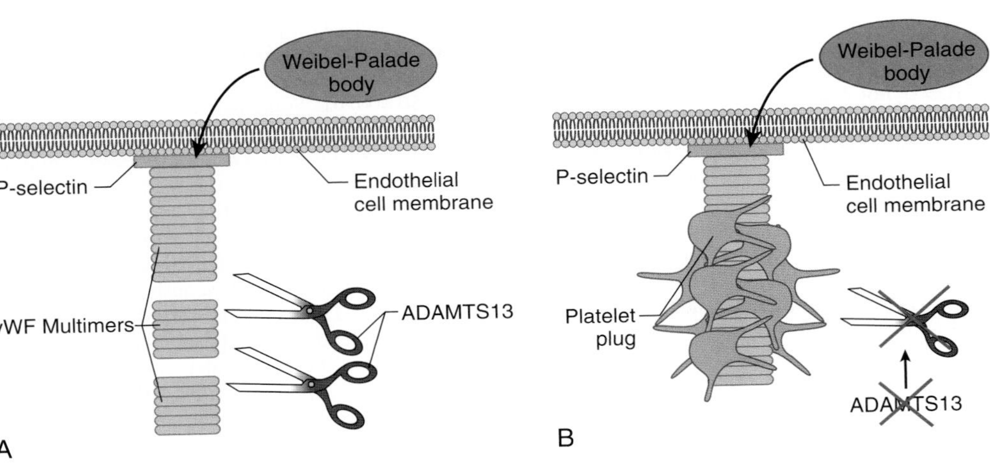

FIGURE 175-2. **Pathophysiology of thrombotic thrombocytopenia purpura (TTP). A,** Von Willebrand factor (vWF) is synthesized in endothelial cells and stored in Weibel-Palade bodies. The vWF is assembled into ultra-large multimers that are cleaved once they are released into the blood stream by the protease ADAMTS13. The resultant smaller multimers of vWF can bind to platelets to participate in normal hemostasis. **B,** Some patients with TTP have a deficiency of ADAMTS13. This results in the accumulation of ultra-large multimers of vWF within the circulation, promoting the excessive adhesion of platelets. This produces large hyaline plugs of vWF and platelets that cause vascular occlusions.

organs. Today, this disease is often diagnosed in its early stages, so patients may have only microangiopathic hemolytic anemia and thrombocytopenia.

TREATMENT[9]

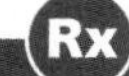

The prompt initiation of plasma exchange (plasmapheresis with plasma replacement) reduces the mortality of TTP from 90% to approximately 15%. The mechanism of this benefit is not entirely known. A randomized trial demonstrated that plasmapheresis is more beneficial than plasma infusion for the treatment of TTP, implying that some of the benefit of plasmapheresis is attributable to the removal of a pathologic substance from the patient's plasma. Assuming that the pathogenesis of most acquired forms of TTP is the antibody-mediated inhibition of ADAMTS13, plasmapheresis might have two benefits. First, it helps remove the pathogenic antibody from the plasma. Second, the normal plasma infused into the patient during plasmapheresis repletes the deficiency of ADAMTS13. Both these benefits probably play a role in the efficacy of plasma exchange in the treatment of this disease.

Because patients with TTP can develop sudden thrombotic events (including stroke and myocardial infarction) without warning and deteriorate quickly, it is prudent to initiate plasma exchange as rapidly as possible. Given the morbidity and mortality of untreated TTP and the relatively low risk of plasmapheresis, this therapy should be initiated even when the diagnosis is not certain. As discussed in the section on HUS, plasmapheresis is not beneficial in children with Shiga toxin–induced microangiopathic hemolytic anemia or in patients who develop HUS following exposure to endothelium-toxic drugs, such as chemotherapy.

Plasma exchange is administered to replace one entire plasma volume and is usually repeated once daily. An average-sized individual requires 20 to 30 units of fresh-frozen plasma for each plasmapheresis session. Therapy is usually administered daily, and the patient is monitored for signs of improvement in thrombocytopenia, hemolysis, neurologic symptoms, fever, and renal disease. Appropriate daily laboratory tests to monitor the patient are CBC, lactate dehydrogenase, reticulocyte count, and creatinine. Once the thrombocytopenia and hemolysis have been corrected for a few days, the daily plasmapheresis can be either discontinued or continued every other day for several more days. A typical duration of therapy is 1 to 2 weeks, although some patients require treatment far beyond this usual time course.

Approximately one third of patients relapse quickly after plasmapheresis is stopped. These patients require a reinitiation of plasma exchange and perhaps the addition of an immunosuppressive drug, such as a glucocorticoid. Some reports indicate that rituximab shows promise in reducing the incidence of relapse. However, given that this drug does not decrease antibody production for weeks to months after its administration, it is likely that if rituximab has any benefit in the treatment of TTP, it is probably only to minimize the incidence of late relapses.

Major complications of plasmapheresis do occur and are often attributable to the use of a central venous catheter. Hypotension, bacteremia, hemorrhage, and thrombosis are among the most common life-threatening complications of plasmapheresis therapy. Two specific complications deserve emphasis. First, patients on angiotensin-converting enzyme (ACE) inhibitor antihypertensives are susceptible to plasmapheresis-induced hypotension owing to these drugs' interference with bradykinin catabolism. Second, a patient who develops recurrent thrombocytopenia and fever several days to a week into treatment may not be having an exacerbation of TTP but may be developing central line–induced sepsis. Consequently, a vigorous investigation for infection should be initiated in patients who appear to be relapsing early.

Hemolytic-Uremic Syndrome

DEFINITION

HUS is another cause of microangiopathic hemolytic anemia, and it may be difficult to distinguish from TTP. When acute renal failure is predominant and there are no neurologic symptoms, many clinicians consider the syndrome to be HUS, not TTP. In contrast to TTP, HUS is not caused by a deficiency of ADAMTS13. However, at this point, it is not clear whether ADAMTS13 levels will be clinically useful to distinguish between HUS and TTP. Because there is such overlap between the signs and symptoms of TTP and those of HUS, the distinction and diagnosis may be impossible in some cases.

PATHOBIOLOGY AND CLINICAL MANIFESTATIONS

A toxin that directly damages endothelial cells can cause HUS. These direct endothelial toxins are either infectious or the result of a drug. Perhaps the best-characterized infectious agent that damages endothelial cells is Shiga toxin–producing enterohemorrhagic *Escherichia coli* (Chapter 312). In Shiga toxin–induced HUS, the renal disease and microangiopathic hemolytic anemia occur after an episode of diarrhea that is often bloody. *E. coli* O157:H7 is the cause of many cases in the United States. The toxin damages endothelial cells within the glomeruli and promotes the adhesion of platelets and the trapping of red blood cells.

Several drugs can induce HUS by directly damaging endothelial cells. These include calcineurin inhibitors such as tacrolimus and cyclosporine; sometimes, lowering the dose of these drugs can reverse the microangiopathic hemolytic anemia. Cytotoxic drugs such as mitomycin C, cisplatin, and bleomycin can also induce HUS by damaging endothelial cells.

Inherited forms of HUS have been described, and they usually involve dysregulation of the complement cascade (Chapter 49). The best-described genetic mutations cause the deficiency of factor H, a complement regulatory protease. HUS-inducing mutations in other components of complement regulation include those found in C3, CD46, and factor I.

TREATMENT AND PREVENTION

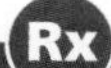

Reducing the spread of Shiga toxin–producing *E. coli* is vital, because antibiotics and antimotility drugs do not lower the risk of developing HUS symptoms. In contrast to TTP, there is little evidence that plasma exchange is beneficial.[9] The infusion of plasma or plasmapheresis is reportedly beneficial in the treatment of atypical forms of HUS caused by the dysregulation of complement.

Disseminated Intravascular Coagulation

DIC is a pathologic condition that depletes components of the coagulation system, including platelets. Therefore, in contrast to TTP and HUS, the thrombocytopenia of DIC is associated with the consumption of coagulation factors and increased fibrinolysis, often leading to prolongations of the prothrombin time and activated partial thromboplastin time, as well as increased levels of D-dimers. In its fully manifested state, DIC can be associated with arterial and venous thrombi, hemorrhage, microangiopathic hemolysis, thrombocytopenia, excessive fibrinolysis, and deficiency of coagulation factors such as fibrinogen. For a more complete review of DIC and related disorders, see Chapter 178.

Thrombocytopenia during Pregnancy

Thrombocytopenia occurs in approximately 5% of pregnant women. It may be due to a normal variant of pregnancy (gestational thrombocytopenia), a pregnancy-specific condition (preeclampsia and HELLP syndrome [hemolysis, elevated liver enzymes, and low platelets]), or a condition exacerbated by pregnancy (ITP, vasculitis, TTP). The prognosis and treatment vary tremendously based on the underlying cause.

Gestational thrombocytopenia (incidental thrombocytopenia of pregnancy) is a mild, asymptomatic thrombocytopenia that typically occurs late in pregnancy. There is no association with fetal thrombocytopenia, and this maternal thrombocytopenia resolves spontaneously after delivery. Other than thrombocytopenia during previous pregnancies, women with gestational thrombocytopenia have no prior history of a low platelet count. This lack of previous thrombocytopenia helps distinguish gestational thrombocytopenia from ITP. Additionally, in contrast to other causes of maternal thrombocytopenia, gestational thrombocytopenia does not produce a platelet count lower than 70,000/μL. Consequently, deviation from standard obstetric care is usually not required for a patient with gestational thrombocytopenia.

Preeclampsia is a syndrome that causes the gradual development of proteinuria and hypertension during the later stages of pregnancy (Chapter 247). A minority of women with preeclampsia progress to have seizures; when this occurs, the syndrome is called *eclampsia*. Approximately 15% of women with preeclampsia have thrombocytopenia, and 5% of patients with preeclampsia have platelet counts less than 50,000/μL. Some patients have a more severe form of preeclampsia associated with HELLP syndrome. Preeclampsia and HELLP syndrome are believed to be caused by a factor produced within the placenta, because these syndromes usually resolve rapidly and spontaneously after delivery. They can present post partum, but they still resolve within a few days of delivery. Consequently, immediate delivery of the child is recommended, if possible, because the microangiopathic process stops soon thereafter. If these syndromes do not resolve spontaneously within 3 days, alternative diagnoses such as ITP and TTP should be considered.

Most patients with ITP or vasculitis during pregnancy have a history of thrombocytopenia before pregnancy. The antiplatelet immunoglobulin G antibodies that cause this disease in the mother can cross the placenta and lead to thrombocytopenia in the fetus. However, the platelet count in the unborn child does not correlate well with the platelet count of the mother, and attempts to sample fetal blood to monitor platelet counts are associated with significant risk. Because the vast majority of children born to women with ITP have a platelet count high enough for a successful delivery, the management of ITP focuses on keeping the maternal platelet count acceptable for the mother's safety. In the early stages of pregnancy, a platelet count of 30,000 to 50,000/μL is considered safe. In preparation for delivery, a platelet count of 50,000 to 80,000/μL is more desirable. This can be managed by the use of oral glucocorticoids and, if necessary, by the administration of IVIG. The safety of rituximab and thrombopoiesis-stimulating agents during pregnancy is not known. Splenectomy performed during the first trimester has a risk of inducing miscarriage, and this operation is technically difficult during the later stages of pregnancy because of uterine enlargement. There is no evidence that a cesarean section is safer than vaginal delivery.

The diagnosis of TTP during pregnancy can be difficult because many of the symptoms are identical to those of preeclampsia. If the symptoms develop during the early stages of pregnancy, when preeclampsia is unlikely, the diagnosis of TTP is more certain. The presence of hyperuricemia, hypoproteinemia, elevated liver transaminases, and direct bilirubin is more consistent with preeclampsia. The development of microangiopathic hemolytic anemia and thrombocytopenia in the peripartum period is presumed to be attributable to preeclampsia, and immediate delivery of the fetus is desirable if it is safe to do so. Typically, the thrombocytopenia starts to resolve rapidly after delivery. If no improvement is seen by the third postpartum day, standard management for TTP, including plasma exchange, is recommended.

Post-Transfusion Purpura and Neonatal Alloimmune Thrombocytopenia

Alloimmune thrombocytopenia is due to sensitization to alloantigens such as Pl^{A1} (HPA-1a). These alloimmune antibodies can cause thrombocytopenia approximately a week after a blood transfusion (post-transfusion purpura, or PTP). A similar alloimmune antibody can cause thrombocytopenia in a fetus when it is produced by the mother (neonatal alloimmune thrombocytopenia, or NAIT). PTP causes profound thrombocytopenia 7 to 10 days after exposure to platelets that contaminate red blood cell transfusions. However, it can be treated with IVIG or plasma exchange. NAIT can cause severe thrombocytopenia and bleeding in neonates and is treated with the transfusion of platelets derived from a Pl^{A1}-negative donor (most conveniently the newborn's mother herself), corticosteroids, and IVIG.

Vasculitis

Autoimmune diseases such as systemic lupus erythematosus, rheumatoid arthritis, and other forms of vasculitis can also involve thrombocytopenia. This can be due to an ITP-like process that occurs in patients with a propensity for the development of autoantibodies. The treatment for these patients is immunosuppression, similar to the treatment for other patients with ITP. Some patients with active vasculitis and endothelial inflammation consume circulating platelets due to this damaged vessel wall, creating a clinical picture that is difficult to distinguish from that of TTP without a tissue diagnosis that documents vasculitis. Owing to the difficulty of discerning TTP from a flare-up of vasculitis, these patients are often treated with both plasma exchange and immunosuppression.

Dilutional Thrombocytopenia

Thrombocytopenia does not typically occur after blood loss, possibly due in part to the release of platelets from the splenic pool. Thrombocytopenia occasionally occurs after massive hemorrhage, but only when the hemorrhage is severe enough to necessitate replacement of 1.5 to 2 times the total blood volume, which usually requires transfusion of at least 15 to 20 units of packed red blood cells over a short period. Even in this circumstance, the thrombocytopenia is only mild to moderate. Therefore, the clinician should remain vigilant for another cause of the thrombocytopenia (such as DIC resulting from hemorrhage-induced hypotension and shock). There is no reason to routinely transfuse platelets in a fixed ratio to packed red blood cells unless thrombocytopenia is present and doing so is otherwise indicated. When indicated, dilutional thrombocytopenia can be corrected with platelet transfusions.

Congenital Thrombocytopenias

Lifelong thrombocytopenia can be due to an inherited defect that affects platelet production or survival. These disorders can be autosomal dominant (May-Hegglin anomaly, Alport's syndrome), autosomal recessive (Bernard-Soulier disease, Fanconi's anemia, gray platelet syndrome, thrombocytopenia with absent radius syndrome), or X-linked (Wiscott-Aldrich syndrome). Many of these disorders are associated with other abnormalities in addition to thrombocytopenia. A congenital cause of thrombocytopenia should be suspected in a patient who has long-standing moderate thrombocytopenia presumed to be treatment-refractory ITP.

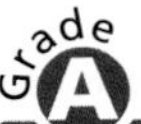

1. Slichter SJ, Kaufman RM, Assmann SF, et al. Dose of prophylactic platelet transfusions and prevention of hemorrhage. *N Engl J Med.* 2010;362:600-613.
2. Zaja F, Baccarani M, Mazza P, et al. Dexamethasone plus rituximab yields higher sustained response rates than dexamethasone monotherapy in adults with primary immune thrombocytopenia. *Blood.* 2010;115:2755-2762.
3. Kuter DJ, Bussel JB, Lyons RM, et al. Efficacy of romiplostim in patients with chronic immune thrombocytopenic purpura: a double-blind randomised controlled trial. *Lancet.* 2008;37:395-403.
4. Kuter DJ, Rummel M, Boccia R, et al. Romiplostim or standard of care in patients with immune thrombocytopenia. *N Engl J Med.* 2010;363:1889-1899.
5. George JN, Mathias SD, Go RS, et al. Improved quality of life for romiplostim-treated patients with chronic immune thrombocytopenic purpura: results from two randomized, placebo-controlled trials. *Br J Haematol.* 2009;144:409-415.
6. Bussel JB, Provan D, Shamsi T, et al. Effect of eltrombopag on platelet counts and bleeding during treatment of chronic idiopathic thrombocytopenic purpura: a randomised, double-blind, placebo-controlled trial. *Lancet.* 2009;373:641-648.
7. Cheng G, Saleh MN, Marcher C, et al. Eltrombopag for management of chronic immune thrombocytopenia (RAISE): a 6-month, randomised, phase 3 study. *Lancet.* 2011;377:393-402.
8. Provan D, Stasi R, Newland AC, et al. International consensus report on the investigation and management of primary immune thrombocytopenia. *Blood.* 2010;115:168-186.
9. Michael M, Elliott EJ, Ridley GF, et al. Interventions for haemolytic uraemic syndrome and thrombotic thrombocytopenic purpura. *Cochrane Database Syst Rev.* 2009;1:CD003595.

SUGGESTED READINGS

Arepally GM, Ortel TL. Heparin-induced thrombocytopenia. *Annu Rev Med.* 2010;61:77-90. *Review of current understanding of the pathogenesis, clinical features, diagnostic criteria, and management of this commonly encountered problem in inpatient medicine.*

Cines DB, Bussel JB, Liebman HA, et al. The ITP syndrome: pathogenic and clinical diversity. *Blood.* 2009;113:6511-6521. *Focus on the variety of underlying conditions associated with ITP.*

George JN, Aster RH. Drug-induced thrombocytopenia: pathogenesis, evaluation, and management. *Hematology Am Soc Hematol Program.* 2009;153-158. *Excellent review of an important consideration in determining the cause of thrombocytopenia.*

Kavanagh D, Goodship T. Haemolytic uraemic syndrome. *Nephron Clin Pract.* 2011;118:c37-c42. *Review.*

Provan D, Stasi R, Newland AC, et al. International consensus report on the investigation and management of primary immune thrombocytopenia. *Blood.* 2010;115:168-186. *Consensus guidelines.*

176 VON WILLEBRAND DISEASE AND HEMORRHAGIC ABNORMALITIES OF PLATELET AND VASCULAR FUNCTION

WILLIAM L. NICHOLS

VON WILLEBRAND DISEASE

DEFINITION AND EPIDEMIOLOGY

Von Willebrand disease (VWD), a usually autosomal dominantly inherited condition affecting both males and females of all ethnicities, is the most common hereditary bleeding disorder worldwide, with prevalence estimates dependent on case definition. It may also occur less frequently as an acquired disorder (acquired von Willebrand syndrome [AVWS]). Von Willebrand factor (VWF) plasma levels are variably decreased (minimally to substantially) in at least 2.5% of humans, whereas approximately 0.1% (1 in 1000) have definite VWD with medically significant bleeding symptoms related to low VWF, and approximately 0.01% (1 in 10,000) have more severe forms of VWD that often result in referral to tertiary care centers including hemophilia centers.

PATHOBIOLOGY

VWD reflects deficiency or dysfunction of VWF, a multimeric plasma glycoprotein that mediates platelet adhesion and aggregation at sites of vascular injury (Chapter 174), and that also carries and stabilizes blood coagulation factor VIII (FVIII) in the circulation. The *VWF* gene is located on chromosome 12, with a partial pseudogene on chromosome 22 that potentially complicates DNA-based mutation detection (which remains primarily a research application, with evolving clinical diagnostic potential). The protein is synthesized by vascular endothelium as ~270-kD subunits (protomers) that are dimerized, then processed and polymerized into very large (up to about 20,000 kD) hemostatically active VWF multimers, and finally secreted into the blood. Vascular endothelial cells additionally provide a storage reservoir of multimerized VWF (in intracellular Weibel-Palade bodies) from which it can be released by stress or drugs such as DDAVP (desmopressin). VWF is also synthesized and multimerized by bone marrow megakaryocytes and stored in circulating blood platelet α granules, from which it is secreted with platelet activation. Platelet-stored VWF represents about 10% of total blood VWF.

Multimerization of VWF is essential for its hemostatic activity that is mainly mediated by the higher-molecular-weight (larger) multimers. Circulating plasma VWF does not interact with platelets, but when VWF binds to injured (de-endothelialized) blood vessel walls, reflecting its collagen-binding activity, multimers can be stretched and unfolded by high intravascular shear forces, such as in the microvasculature, exposing and activating previously cryptic platelet-binding domains to promote platelet adhesion and aggregation to vessel-bound VWF. Simultaneously, activated (stretched) VWF multimers expose protomer cleavage sites for proteolysis by the circulating enzyme, ADAMTS13 (A Disintegrin And Metalloprotease domain with ThromboSpondin type 1 motifs, member 13), ultimately decreasing the size of VWF multimers and thereby downregulating VWF hemostatic function. Severe deficiency of ADAMTS13 is associated with the pathologic microangiopathy of thrombotic thrombocytopenic purpura (TTP) (Chapter 175), in which the microvascular thrombosis is mediated by ultralarge VWF multimers in the circulation.

VWD is classified into three major types that vary in severity and differ in clinical management, such that defining the VWD subtype is important. Type 1 VWD reflects partial quantitative deficiency of normally functioning VWF, of variable severity, and comprises 75 to 80% of individuals with symptomatic VWD. Type 2 VWD reflects qualitative VWF deficiency, with four subtypes (A, B, M, N), and comprises 20 to 25% of persons with VWD. Type 3 VWD reflects the virtual absence of VWF, with secondary near-absence of FVIII, and is rare (<1% of VWD). Inheritance of VWD is usually autosomal dominant, except that type 3 VWD is typically autosomal recessive in inheritance. Table 176-1 summarizes the classification of VWD subtypes and their basic pathophysiology.

The FVIII deficiency that often accompanies different types of VWD (see Table 176-1) is not genetically related to the disease; the gene that encodes FVIII is on the X chromosome, and its primary deficiency causes classic hemophilia (Chapter 177). FVIII deficiency in VWD is due to a primary deficiency or defect in the VWF molecule, which normally carries and stabilizes FVIII in the circulation. Therefore, FVIII is more rapidly cleared from the circulation, leading to its secondary deficiency in VWD.

TABLE 176-1 CLASSIFICATION OF VON WILLEBRAND DISEASE

TYPE	DESCRIPTION
1	Partial quantitative deficiency of VWF (~75-80% of VWD)
2	Qualitative VWF defect (~20-25% of VWD)
2A	Caused by VWF mutations that decrease the proportion of large functional VWF multimers, leading to decreased VWF-dependent platelet adhesion and aggregation
2B	Caused by VWF mutations that increase platelet-VWF binding, resulting in depletion of large, functional VWF multimers. Circulating platelets are coated with mutant VWF, which may impair platelet adhesion and aggregation at sites of injury. Thrombocytopenia, persistent or intermittent, is observed in most cases. Distinguishing type 2B VWD may require RIPA to detect increased (abnormal) platelet aggregation response to low-dose ristocetin; the latter may also reflect platelet-type (pseudo) VWD caused by rare mutations in the platelet VWF receptor.
2M	Caused by VWF mutations that decrease VWF-dependent platelet adhesion and aggregation, but do not deplete the large VWF multimers. Distinguishing between types 2A and 2M VWD requires VWF multimer gel electrophoretic analysis.
2N	Caused by VWF mutations that impair binding to FVIII, thereby shortening FVIII survival and lowering FVIII levels so that type 2N VWD can masquerade as an autosomal recessive form of hemophilia A. Discrimination from hemophilia A may require assays of VWF-FVIII binding.
3	Virtually complete VWF deficiency, associated with markedly decreased FVIII (<1% of VWD)

FVIII = factor VIII coagulant activity; RIPA = ristocetin-induced platelet aggregation/aggregometry; VWD = von Willebrand disease; VWF = von Willebrand factor.
Adapted and modified from National Heart, Lung, and Blood Institute. *The Diagnosis, Evaluation, and Management of von Willebrand Disease.* Bethesda, MD: National Institutes of Health Publication 08-5832. December 2007 (released Feb 29, 2008). Available at: http://www.nhlbi.nih.gov/guidelines/vwd; and Yawn BP, Nichols WL, Rick ME. Diagnosis and management of von Willebrand disease: guidelines for primary care. *Am Fam Physician.* 2009;80:1261-1268, 1269-1270.

CLINICAL MANIFESTATIONS

Individuals with VWD usually experience mucocutaneous bleeding symptoms such as easy bruising, prolonged or excessive bleeding from minor cuts or other injuries, nosebleeds or other mucosal bleeding such as gastrointestinal hemorrhage, or heavy menstrual bleeding (in women), and they may be at increased risk for bleeding following surgery or invasive procedures, dental extractions, traumatic injury, or childbirth. Symptoms can range from relatively mild or infrequent bleeding in type 1 VWD to severe, life-threatening bleeding in type 3 VWD. As a group, women with VWD may be more affected by bleeding symptoms than men because of hemostatic challenges of menstruation and childbirth.

DIAGNOSIS

Clinical Assessment

Diagnosis of VWD (or other bleeding disorders) begins with clinical assessment to evaluate for a personal and possible family history of abnormal bleeding, accompanied by focused physical examination to detect signs or symptoms of bleeding (e.g., petechiae, ecchymoses, hematomas, anemia), as well as findings that may suggest other causes of increased bleeding such as liver disease (e.g., hepatosplenomegaly, jaundice), joint or skin laxity (e.g., Ehlers-Danlos syndrome), telangiectasia (e.g., hereditary hemorrhagic telangiectasia), or anatomic lesions on gynecologic examination. Because bleeding symptoms are common in apparently normal individuals, with prevalence of certain symptoms as high as 25 to 50%, clinical assessment for VWD or other possible bleeding disorders can be challenging (Chapter 174).

The most important parts of the medical history include (1) family history of a known or suspected bleeding disorder; (2) review of personal surgical or other hemostatic challenges lifelong and recently, including dental extractions and traumatic injuries, and whether abnormal bleeding occurred and its severity; (3) mucocutaneous bleeding symptoms (e.g., bruising, nosebleeds, ecchymoses, gastrointestinal bleeding, menorrhagia), including frequency, severity and spontaneity of events; and (4) assessment for medical conditions that can increase risk for bleeding, such as use of certain drugs that can impede normal hemostasis, including aspirin or other nonsteroidal anti-inflammatory drugs (NSAIDs), clopidogrel, or warfarin or heparin anticoagulants; presence of liver or kidney disease (e.g., cirrhosis, uremia); and history of low or high platelet count and blood or bone marrow disorders.

Bleeding history scoring tools are being developed and applied for studying populations with VWD or other bleeding disorders but are not yet validated for routine clinical use. However, in general, an increasing number of positive or abnormal clinical bleeding history items increases the likelihood that an individual has a bleeding disorder, including VWD, and may merit undergoing appropriate laboratory evaluation (Chapter 174).

Laboratory Evaluation

Because no simple, single laboratory test is available to screen for VWD, the initial laboratory evaluation requires measurements of plasma: (1) VWF antigen (VWF:Ag); (2) ristocetin cofactor activity (VWF:RCo); and (3) factor VIII coagulant activity (FVIII). All three tests are recommended for initial evaluation, and the results may not only establish the diagnosis but also suggest the type and severity of VWD if it is present. These three tests are also used for monitoring therapy. Tests such as the bleeding time (BT) or platelet function analyzer (PFA-100, Siemens) assay lack sufficient sensitivity and specificity and are not recommended for routine screening.

If one or more of the three test results are abnormally low, or if the ratio of VWF:RCo to VWF:Ag is below 0.5 to 0.7, additional laboratory evaluation may include selecting one or more of the following tests, based on the pattern of initial results together with clinical assessment and experience: (1) repeating the three initial VWD tests with timing and procedures optimized for conditions of the patient, the blood sample, and laboratory testing (see later for additional information about these conditions); (2) VWF multimer analysis to help differentiate or exclude types 2A, 2B, or 2M VWD; (3) ristocetin-induced platelet aggregometry (RIPA), including low-dose ristocetin testing to evaluate for type 2B VWD or platelet-type (pseudo) VWD; (4) VWF-FVIII binding assay (or molecular DNA-based VWF testing) to evaluate for type 2N VWD; and (5) other tests such as VWF:CB (collagen-binding activity) to supplement VWF:RCo testing and the overall evaluation. Some of these tests have limited availability and are mainly performed in reference laboratories. Consultation with a hemostasis specialist can help guide test selection.

Multimer analysis visualizes the distribution of plasma VWF multimers, is technically complex, is qualitatively interpreted in conjunction with results of the initial three tests and available clinical information, and is used to help determine the VWD subtype. Therefore, VWF multimer analysis is not recommended for initial VWD screening and should only be performed if initial VWD testing identifies an abnormal result (e.g., abnormally low VWF:RCo or ratio of VWF:RCo to VWF:Ag) or clinical information suggests a high likelihood of abnormal VWF multimer analysis.

Table 176-2 provides prototypical laboratory values for VWD subtypes. Diagnosis, especially for individuals with mildly decreased VWF (30 to 50% or IU/dL), requires correlation of clinical assessment (personal and family history of bleeding) and results of laboratory testing, the latter preferably performed or repeated in the absence of conditions associated with elevation of baseline VWF and with careful attention to blood specimen collection, processing, transportation, and storage.

The laboratory evaluation of a person for possible VWD or AVWS is relatively complex, particularly because results of the laboratory tests can be influenced by certain conditions of the patient and by variables in the blood sample and laboratory testing methodology (Table 176-3). In interpreting test results, therefore, it is important to be aware of these variabilities and the status of the patient at the time of evaluation.

TABLE 176-2 PATTERNS OF LABORATORY TEST RESULTS FOR VON WILLEBRAND DISEASE DIAGNOSIS AND CLASSIFICATION*

CONDITION	VWF:RCo (IU/dL)	VWF:Ag (IU/dL)	FVIII (IU/dL)	VWF:RCo/VWF:Ag RATIO¶	RIPA	VWF MULTIMERS
Type 1 VWD	<30†	<30†‡	↓ or Normal	>0.5-0.7	Often normal	Normal
Type 2A VWD	<30†	<30-200†‡	↓ or Normal	<0.5-0.7	↓ or Normal	↓ HMW
Type 2B VWD	<30†	<30-200†‡	↓ or Normal	Usually <0.5-0.7	↑ (Low dose)	↓ HMW
Type 2M VWD	<30†	<30-200†‡	↓ or Normal	<0.5-0.7	↓ or Normal	No ↓ HMW
Type 2N VWD	30-200	30-200	↓↓	>0.5-0.7	Normal	Normal
Type 3 VWD	<3	<3	↓↓↓ (1-9)	NA	Absent	NA
"Low VWF"§	30-50§	30-50§	Normal	>0.5-0.7	Normal	Normal
Normal	50-200	50-200	Normal	>0.5-0.7	Normal	Normal

*Values in the table represent prototypical cases without additional VWF (or other disease) abnormalities. Exceptions occur, and repeat testing and clinical experience may be necessary for clarification and interpretation of laboratory test results.
†VWF values <30 IU/dL (or %) are designated as the level for definite diagnosis of VWD (especially type 1 VWD) because (1) there is a high frequency of blood type O that is associated with "low VWF" levels but not necessarily VWD; (2) bleeding symptoms are reported by a significant proportion of individuals with no disease; and (3) no abnormality in the VWF gene has been identified in many individuals who have only mildly to moderately decreased VWF levels. VWF values of 30-50 IU/dL include both apparently normal persons and those with mild VWD.
‡VWF:Ag is <50 IU/dL in most persons with types 2A, 2B, or 2M VWD.
§Diagnosis of VWD is not precluded for persons with VWF:RCo of 30-50 IU/dL if there is supporting clinical or family evidence for VWD, nor is the use of agents to increase VWF levels precluded in those who have VWF:RCo of 30-50 IU/dL and who may be at risk for bleeding.
¶Until more laboratories clearly define a reference range, the VWF:RCo/VWF:Ag ratio of <0.5-0.7 is recommended to distinguish type 1 vs. type 2 VWD variants (A, B, or M).
FVIII = factor VIII coagulant activity; HMW = high molecular weight VWF multimers; IU/dL = international units per deciliter (e.g., 100 IU/dL = 100% of mean normal level); NA = not applicable; RIPA = ristocetin-induced platelet aggregation/aggregometry; VWD, von Willebrand disease; VWF = von Willebrand factor; VWF:Ag = von Willebrand factor antigen; VWF:RCo = von Willebrand factor ristocetin cofactor activity; ↓, ↓↓, ↓↓↓, ↑, refer to varying degrees of decrease, or an increase, of the test result compared to the laboratory reference range.
Adapted and modified from National Heart, Lung, and Blood Institute. *The Diagnosis, Evaluation, and Management of von Willebrand Disease.* Bethesda, MD: National Institutes of Health Publication 08-5832. December 2007 (released Feb 29, 2008). Available at: http://www.nhlbi.nih.gov/guidelines/vwd; and Yawn BP, Nichols WL, Rick ME. Diagnosis and management of von Willebrand disease: guidelines for primary care. *Am Fam Physician.* 2009;80:1261-1268, 1269-1270.

TABLE 176-3 VARIABLE CONDITIONS OF THE PATIENT, BLOOD SAMPLING, AND LABORATORY TESTING AFFECTING LABORATORY EVALUATION FOR VON WILLEBRAND DISEASE

Phlebotomy conditions—An atraumatic blood draw limits the exposure of tissue factor from the site and the activation of clotting factors, minimizing falsely high or low values. Lipemia should be avoided because it may interfere with photo-optical testing methods, especially some used for VWF:RCo assay.

Patient stress level—Undue stress, such as struggling or crying in children or anxiety in adults, may falsely elevate VWF and FVIII levels. Very recent exercise can also elevate VWF levels.

Additional conditions in the individual—The presence of an acute or chronic inflammatory illness may elevate VWF and FVIII levels, as may pregnancy or administration of estrogen or oral contraceptives. Individuals with blood group O have VWF levels approximately 25% lower than those of other ABO blood groups. African Americans have higher VWF levels than whites.

Sample processing—To prevent cryoprecipitation of VWF and other proteins, blood samples for VWF assays should be transported to the laboratory at room temperature. Plasma should be separated from blood cells promptly at room temperature, and the plasma should be centrifuged thoroughly to remove platelets. If plasma samples will be assayed within 2 hours, they should be kept at room temperature. Frozen plasma samples should be carefully thawed at 37° C and kept at room temperature for <2 hours before assay.

Sample storage—Plasma samples that will be stored or transported to a reference laboratory must be frozen promptly at or below −40° C and remain frozen until assayed. A control sample that is drawn, processed, stored, and transported under the same conditions as the tested person's sample may be helpful in indicating problems in the handling of important test samples. Activity of FVIII typically is 10-20% lower in frozen-thawed plasma than in fresh (nonfrozen) plasma, and can be even lower if blood processing or storage conditions are suboptimal.

Laboratory testing—Calibrators for assays of VWF:Ag, VWF:RCo, and FVIII should be referenced to the World Health Organization (WHO) plasma standard. These three tests have relatively high coefficients of variation (CVs of 10-30%), especially the VWF:RCo assay. The quality of laboratory testing also varies considerably among laboratories (high interlaboratory CV). Test results can be reported as international units per deciliter (IU/dL), rather than as a percentage (%) of mean normal, if WHO-linked calibrators are used. Referencing VWF testing results to the population reference range, rather than to ABO-stratified reference ranges, may be clinically useful.

FVIII = coagulation factor VIII; VWF = von Willebrand factor; VWF:Ag = VWF antigen; VWF:RCo = VWF ristocetin cofactor activity.
Adapted and modified from National Heart, Lung, and Blood Institute. *The Diagnosis, Evaluation, and Management of von Willebrand Disease.* Bethesda, MD: National Institutes of Health Publication 08-5832. December 2007 (released Feb 29, 2008). Available at: http://www.nhlbi.nih.gov/guidelines/vwd; and Nichols WL, Rick ME, Ortel TL, et al. Clinical and laboratory diagnosis of von Willebrand disease: a synopsis of the 2008 NHLBI/NIH guidelines. *Am J Hematol.* 2009; 84: 366-370.

TABLE 176-4 SUGGESTED DURATIONS OF VON WILLEBRAND FACTOR REPLACEMENT FOR DIFFERENT TYPES OF SURGICAL PROCEDURES

MAJOR SURGERY 7-14 DAYS*	MINOR SURGERY 1-5 DAYS*	OTHER PROCEDURES: IF UNCOMPLICATED, SINGLE VWF TREATMENT
Cardiothoracic	Biopsy: breast, cervical	Cardiac catheterization
Cesarean section	Complicated dental extractions	Cataract surgery
Craniotomy	Gingival surgery	Endoscopy (without biopsy)
Hysterectomy	Central line placement	Liver biopsy
Open cholecystectomy	Laparoscopic procedures	Lacerations
Prostatectomy		Simple dental extractions

*Individual cases may need longer or shorter duration depending on the severity of VWD and the type of procedure.
VWF = von Willebrand factor.
Adapted and modified from National Heart, Lung, and Blood Institute. *The Diagnosis, Evaluation, and Management of von Willebrand Disease.* Bethesda, MD: National Institutes of Health Publication 08-5832. December 2007 (released Feb. 29, 2008). http://www.nhlbi.nih.gov/guidelines/vwd.

TABLE 176-5 INITIAL DOSING RECOMMENDATIONS FOR VON WILLEBRAND FACTOR CONCENTRATE REPLACEMENT FOR PREVENTION OR MANAGEMENT OF BLEEDING

MAJOR SURGERY/BLEEDING
Loading dose*: 40-60 U/kg
Maintenance dose[†]: 20-40 U/kg every 8 to 24 hours
Monitoring: VWF:RCo and FVIII trough and peak, at least daily
Therapeutic goal: trough VWF:RCo and FVIII >50 IU/dL for 7-14 days
Safety parameter: do not exceed VWF:RCo >200 IU/dL or FVIII >250-300 IU/dL
May alternate with desmopressin (DDAVP) for latter part of treatment
MINOR SURGERY/BLEEDING
Loading dose*: 30-60 U/kg
Maintenance dose[†]: 20-40 U/kg every 12 to 48 hours
Monitoring: VWF:RCo and FVIII trough and peak, at least once
Therapeutic goal: trough VWF:RCo and FVIII >50 IU/dL for 3-5 days
Safety parameter: do not exceed VWF:RCo >200 IU/dL or FVIII >250-300 IU/dL
May alternate with desmopressin (DDAVP) for latter part of treatment

*Loading dose is in VWF:RCo IU/dL.
[†]Dosing intervals reflect approximately 12-hour average half-lives of plasma VWF and FVIII, without conditions resulting in shortened survival or enhanced clearance such as bleeding or surgery.
FVIII = factor VIII; VWF = von Willebrand factor; VWF:RCo = VWF ristocetin cofactor activity.
Adapted and modified from National Heart, Lung, and Blood Institute. *The Diagnosis, Evaluation, and Management of von Willebrand Disease.* Bethesda, MD: National Institutes of Health Publication 08-5832. December 2007 (released Feb. 29, 2008). http://www.nhlbi.nih.gov/guidelines/vwd.

TREATMENT

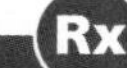

Management of patients with VWD is focused on treatment or prevention of bleeding episodes. There are three main approaches to treatment of VWD that are used individually or in combination: (1) increasing plasma concentration of VWF and FVIII by releasing endogenous VWF stores through stimulation of endothelial cells with DDAVP; (2) replacing or supplementing VWF and FVIII by using human plasma-derived, viral-inactivated concentrates; and (3) promoting hemostasis using hemostatic agents that work by mechanisms other than increasing VWF and FVIII. Regular prophylaxis is seldom required, and treatment is given primarily before and after planned invasive procedures or in response to episodes of bleeding. Table 176-4 outlines usual durations of treatment for a variety of surgical and other invasive procedures.

Desmopressin (DDAVP)

DDAVP (desmopressin: 1-desamino-8-D-arginine vasopressin) is a synthetic derivative of the antidiuretic hormone and causes release of preformed VWF from endothelial cells. It is mainly used in type 1 VWD, is contraindicated for type 2B VWD (because it can cause thrombocytopenia), has limited efficacy for types 2A, 2M, or 2N VWD, and has no efficacy for type 3 VWD. DDAVP is generally administered for short time periods (48 to 72 hours) and usually not more frequently than at 24- to 48-hour intervals, owing to tachyphylaxis and side effects. If it is required for longer periods or more frequently, the patient should be monitored for fluid and electrolyte problems because DDAVP may cause symptomatic hyponatremia. DDAVP therapy is potentially mildly thrombogenic, especially for persons who are at increased risk for atherosclerotic cardiovascular disorders such as stroke or myocardial infarction.

The hemostatic dose of DDAVP is 0.3 μg/kg body weight, infused intravenously over about 30 minutes, or administered subcutaneously; however, a concentrated formulation for the latter is not available in the United States. For outpatients, DDAVP can also be administered nasally, using a concentrated spray (Stimate, CSL Behring) that delivers 150 μg per nostril (300 μg total dose for persons ≥50 kg body weight). Peak increments of plasma VWF and FVIII occur about 1 to 2 hours after DDAVP, typically reaching two- to four-fold higher levels than at baseline, and decline toward baseline during the next 24 hours, reflecting VWF and FVIII plasma half-lives that are about 12 hours on average. However, plasma half-lives depend on the specific VWF subtype and phenotype and also vary considerably among individuals. Because of variability in response, before therapy with DDAVP, it is important to perform a treatment trial with pharmacokinetic monitoring of VWF and FVIII, measuring baseline (pre-DDAVP) and peak (~1 hour post-DDAVP) levels, supplemented with testing about 4 to 6 hours after DDAVP if shortened survival of endogenous VWF is a consideration. A DDAVP treatment trial with extended monitoring can also help diagnose VWD variants with intrinsically heightened VWF clearance. Because of the problem of rapid tachyphylaxis, the trial of DDAVP should be performed at least 1 to 2 weeks before an elective procedure.

Factor Replacement Therapy

Alphanate SD/HT (Grifols), Humate-P (CSL Behring), and Wilate (Octapharma) are U.S. Food and Drug Administration–approved plasma-derived VWF concentrates for treatment of VWD by intravenous infusions. They also contain FVIII but differ in VWF/FVIII ratios and in content of large (high-molecular-weight) VWF multimers. Other VWF-containing concentrates include Koate-DVI (Talecris) and Wilfactin (LFB, France), which lacks FVIII (endogenous levels of which rise secondarily within a few hours after infusion) and is not available in the United States. Cryoprecipitate is no longer recommended for VWF (or for FVIII) replacement, and its use should be limited to urgent situations when VWF concentrates are not available.

Table 176-5 outlines dosing and laboratory monitoring recommendations for treatment or prevention of bleeding in patients with VWD. Whenever possible, and particularly for individuals with more severe forms of VWD, major surgeries or bleeding events should be managed in hospitals with appropriate laboratory capability and clinical staff, including a hematologist and a surgeon skilled in the management of bleeding disorders.

Other Hemostatic Agents

Epsilon-aminocaproic acid and tranexamic acid are oral (or intravenous) antifibrinolytic agents that are useful for mucous membrane bleeding such as dental procedures. Antifibrinolytic therapy is potentially thrombogenic, particularly in patients who have coexisting disseminated intravascular coagulation (DIC) or advanced liver disease (Chapter 178), and caution should be applied for use. Topical agents such as bovine or human thrombin, or fibrin sealants, may be indicated for accessible bleeding sites.

Treatment with combined oral contraceptive pills can ameliorate menorrhagia in women with VWD, mediated partly by hormonal effects on uterine tissues as well as by elevating blood VWF and FVIII. Contraceptive hormonal skin patches have similar effects, and either type of therapy can also increase the risk for thromboembolic events. The levonorgestrel-releasing intrauterine device is an alternative to oral or skin-patch hormonal agents. For pregnancy and delivery in women with VWD, it is important to ensure that VWF and FVIII levels are normalized at the time of delivery, either spontaneously (which often occurs) or by therapy, including before administration of epidural anesthesia and postpartum.

ACQUIRED VON WILLEBRAND SYNDROME

AVWS refers to deficiencies or defects in VWF concentration, structure, or function that are not inherited but are consequences of other medical disorders. AVWS is less common than congenital (hereditary) VWD and is typically etiologically associated with several different mechanisms and medical conditions (Table 176-6).

Laboratory findings in AVWS are similar to those in congenital VWD (types 1, 2A, or 3). Although VWF:RCo values are typically decreased in AVWS (with variably decreased VWF:Ag or FVIII), sometimes only VWF multimer analysis is abnormal, with mild to moderate reduction or loss of the highest-molecular-weight (largest) multimers. This latter situation is more

TABLE 176-6 CAUSES OF ACQUIRED VON WILLEBRAND SYNDROME

PATHOPHYSIOLOGIC CATEGORY*	DISEASE OR ASSOCIATION
Antibodies to VWF	Monoclonal gammopathies, lymphoproliferative disorders, or autoimmune diseases such as systemic lupus erythematosus
Shear-induced VWF conformational changes leading to increased proteolysis of VWF	Aortic valvular stenosis, ventricular septal defect, hypertrophic obstructive cardiomyopathy, left ventricular assist device, or primary pulmonary hypertension
Markedly elevated blood platelet count	Essential thrombocythemia, polycythemia vera, myeloid metaplasia with myelofibrosis, or other myeloproliferative disorders
Removal of VWF from circulation by aberrant binding to tumor cells	Wilms' tumor and certain lymphoproliferative or plasma cell proliferative disorders
Decreased VWF synthesis	Hypothyroidism
Drugs associated with AVWS	Ciprofloxacin, valproic acid, hydroxyethyl starch or griseofulvin

*Pathophysiologic categories are listed in descending order of approximate prevalence.
AVWS = acquired von Willebrand syndrome; VWF, von Willebrand factor.
Adapted and modified from Nichols WL, Rick ME, Ortel TL, et al. Clinical and laboratory diagnosis of von Willebrand disease: a synopsis of the 2008 NHLBI/NIH guidelines. *Am J Hematol.* 2009;84:366-370.

likely for AVWS associated with enhanced VWF proteolysis reflecting shear-induced conformational changes in VWF leading to increased proteolysis of VWF by ADAMTS13, such as with severe aortic valvular stenosis and other conditions causing abnormally high shear forces somewhere in the circulation (see Table 176-6). Heyde's syndrome refers to AVWS caused by severe aortic stenosis and accompanied by gastrointestinal bleeding from arteriovenous malformations.

AVWS, and disorders causing it, should be considered in individuals found to have abnormal VWF test results and bleeding symptoms, without a personal or family history consistent with hereditary VWD. Conversely, when bleeding occurs in association with one of the known causative conditions, AVWS should be considered and initial VWD testing performed if indicated.

TREATMENT Rx

Treatment of AVWS should be focused first on elimination or amelioration of the associated causative disorder, if amenable to treatment (e.g., aortic valve replacement or repair for Heyde's syndrome). Survival of both endogenous and infused VWF is often shortened in AVWS, and replacement therapy should be monitored with measurement of plasma VWF (VWF:RCo and VWF:Ag) and FVIII. For AVWS due to immunoglobulin G MGUS (monoclonal gammopathy of undetermined significance), intravenous immunoglobulin infusion may temporarily normalize plasma VWF and FVIII and stop abnormal bleeding by abrogating heightened VWF clearance. However, such treatment reflects an off-label product use.

BLEEDING DUE TO QUALITATIVE PLATELET DISORDERS

Hereditary Platelet Bleeding Disorders

Hereditary defects in platelet function can occur at all stages of the linked sequence of events involved in hemostatic platelet activation at sites of vascular injury, as described in Chapter 174: (1) platelet adhesion (Bernard-Soulier syndrome [BSS]), (2) platelet release reaction (storage pool disorders), and (3) platelet aggregation (Glanzmann's thrombasthenia [GT]). They lead to varying levels of severity of bleeding.

BERNARD-SOULIER SYNDROME AND GLANZMANN THROMBASTHENIA

These rare, autosomally recessive platelet hypofunctional disorders typically manifest moderately severe (minimally provoked or spontaneous) mucocutaneous bleeding symptoms during childhood and beyond as well as abnormal bleeding with hemostatic challenges such as surgery. BSS results from deficiency or dysfunction of the platelet membrane glycoprotein (GP) Ib-IX-V complex that is the principal receptor for binding VWF, mediating platelet adhesion to injured blood vessels. (In some ways, therefore, BSS is the platelet counterpart of VWD as an adhesion defect, the latter being caused by an abnormality in the VWF rather than the platelets.) GT reflects deficiency or dysfunction of the platelet GPIIb-IIIa complex that is the principal receptor for binding plasma fibrinogen, mediating platelet aggregation. The platelet count and morphology are normal in GT, but BSS demonstrates moderate thrombocytopenia and enlarged (giant) platelets. BT or PFA-100 test results are typically markedly abnormal in both disorders, but nonspecific. Platelet aggregometry findings are usually diagnostic. BSS demonstrates absence of aggregation response to ristocetin, whereas responses to other agonists are relatively normal. GT demonstrates relatively normal response to ristocetin, contrasting with complete absence of aggregation response to other agonists, such as adenosine diphosphate, collagen, arachidonic acid, and epinephrine. Quantitative analysis of platelet membrane GPs by flow cytometry is evolving as a supplemental diagnostic tool for BSS and GT. Mutational DNA-based testing is primarily a research endeavor.

PLATELET STORAGE POOL DISORDERS

Platelet dense (δ) granule storage pool deficiency (DG-SPD) is more common than BSS and GT. Inheritance is typically autosomal recessive, or occasionally dominant, with evolving understanding of different mutational causes. Bleeding symptoms are usually mild but may be clinically significant. Hermansky-Pudlak syndrome (HPS) describes oculocutaneous albinism associated with platelet DG-SPD, with a propensity to develop pulmonary fibrosis or granulomatous colitis. DG-SPD can accompany some other hereditary disorders such as the X-linked Wiskott-Aldrich syndrome, in which it is associated with microthrombocytopenia, or Chédiak-Higashi syndrome with partial albinism and leukocyte inclusions. Isolated DG-SPD, including HPS, demonstrates normal blood platelet count and morphology by peripheral blood smear review. Results of BT, PFA-100, or platelet aggregometry testing may or may not be abnormal. Platelet content and secretion of adenosine triphosphate are decreased in DG-SPD, and platelet electron microscopy can diagnostically confirm absence or marked decrease of dense granules; however, these tests have limited availability.

Platelet α-granule deficiency manifests as the gray platelet syndrome, which is typically autosomal recessive in inheritance and may result in mild bleeding symptoms. Moderate thrombocytopenia is present, and peripheral blood smear review is usually diagnostic, demonstrating enlarged platelets that are "gray" (absence of granulomere staining, reflecting absence of α granules and their contents that include VWF). X-chromosome-linked mutations of *GATA1*, the gene encoding a transcription factor essential for erythropoiesis and megakaryocytopoiesis, can cause a gray platelet syndrome–like disorder affecting males.

OTHER HEREDITARY PLATELET HYPOFUNCTIONAL DISORDERS

Hereditary platelet secretion disorders (defective release of α- and δ-granule contents without granule deficiency) comprise a variety of abnormalities affecting various platelet receptors or mechanisms of signal transduction and platelet activation, including defective platelet procoagulant activity, with or without thrombocytopenia or other syndromic features, and with variable bleeding propensity and symptoms. Some of these disorders are reviewed in Chapter 175.

TREATMENT Rx

For treating or preventing major bleeding events (e.g., certain surgical challenges), judicious use of platelet transfusion may be indicated for patients with more severe hereditary platelet bleeding disorders such as BSS and GT. To reduce the risk for platelet alloimmunization, single-donor apheresis platelet concentrates are preferred when available, and HLA-matched transfusions may sometimes be indicated. DDAVP administration has been reported to improve hemostasis in DG-SPD, BSS, and some other hereditary platelet disorders. Treatment with recombinant activated coagulation factor VII (NovoSeven, NovoNordisk) has been reported as an alternative or salvage therapy for bleeding in GT and certain other platelet hypofunctional disorders. Antifibrinolytic therapy with epsilon-aminocaproic acid or tranexamic acid can be useful for dental extractions or for surgical procedures involving other tissues with high intrinsic fibrinolytic activity (e.g., nose, mouth and throat, extraocular tissues).

Acquired Platelet Bleeding Disorders

DRUGS

Drugs are a relatively common cause of platelet hypofunction that can result in mild bleeding symptoms, particularly if other bleeding propensities are present, such as thrombocytopenia. Aspirin, thienopyridines (e.g., clopidogrel, prasugrel, ticagrelor), dipyridamole, and inhibitors of platelet GPIIb/IIIa function are used therapeutically or prophylactically for atherosclerotic cardiovascular disorders such as coronary artery or cerebrovascular disease. In addition to aspirin, other NSAIDs can inhibit platelet arachidonic acid metabolism (Chapter 36) and contribute to bleeding. Other agents that may sometimes impair platelet function include certain selective serotonin reuptake inhibitors or antibiotics and some herbal or nutritional supplements. Laboratory testing for platelet hypofunction is not often indicated and may not yield diagnostic findings.

OTHER ACQUIRED PLATELET BLEEDING DISORDERS

Myelodysplastic or myeloproliferative disorders can sometimes manifest intrinsic platelet hypofunction, disproportionate to thrombocytopenia or thrombocytosis when they are present. Cirrhosis or liver failure can cause platelet hypofunction as well as thrombocytopenia. Uremia may induce platelet hypofunction that can be ameliorated by dialysis and erythropoietin therapy. Antibodies causing autoimmune thrombocytopenia (Chapter 175) can sometimes cause acquired platelet hypofunction (e.g., acquired GT or BSS) in addition to the low platelet count.

TREATMENT Rx

Review of patient medicaments and medical conditions, and modifications of them when feasible and indicated, can often suffice for recognition and management of acquired platelet hypofunctional disorders.

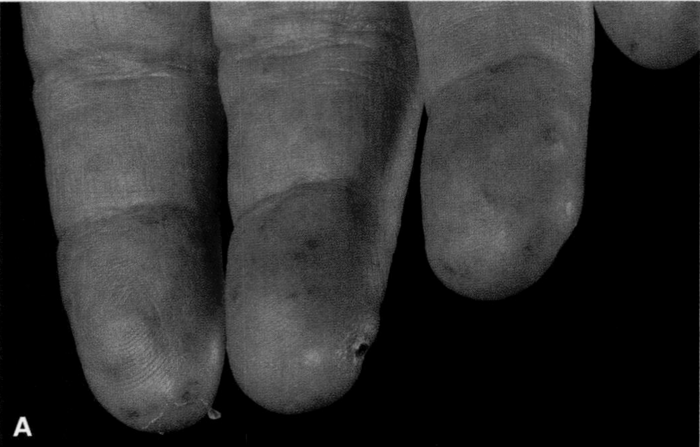

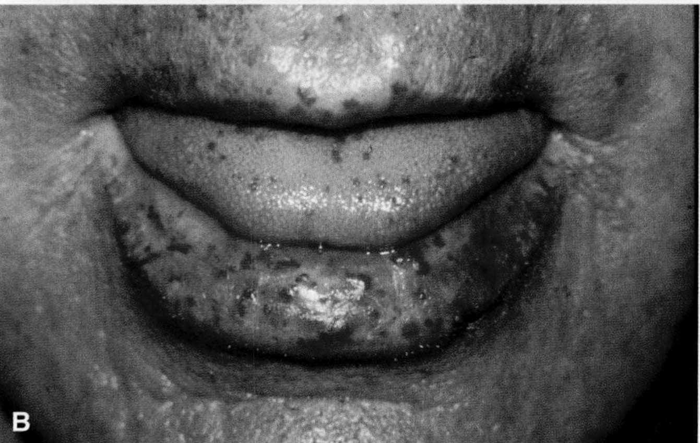

FIGURE 176-1. Hereditary hemorrhagic telangiectasia (HHT). Telangiectasias commonly occur on the face, lips, tongue, and fingers as well as in other areas, including nasal and gastrointestinal mucosa, and may develop in certain other internal organs. Skin or mucous membrane lesions typically blanch with pressure, in contrast to petechiae that do not. (**A**, Copyrighted and used with permission of the Mayo Foundation for Medical Education and Research, all rights reserved. **B**, Courtesy of Dr. Andrew Schafer.)

VASCULAR HEMORRHAGIC DISORDERS

Hereditary Vascular Hemorrhagic Disorders

Hereditary hemorrhagic telangiectasia (HHT), also called Osler-Weber-Rendu syndrome, is an autosomal dominant vascular disorder characterized by development of telangiectases and arteriovenous malformations in the skin, mucous membranes, and certain viscera (especially the central nervous system, lung, and liver), with a propensity for severe recurring nosebleeds and gastrointestinal bleeds resulting in chronic anemia and iron deficiency. Diagnosis primarily relies on physical examination (Fig. 176-1). Several mutations in two genes have been described: endoglin in HHT type 1 and activin receptor-like kinase-1 (ALK1) in HHT type 2. These genes encode proteins that modulate transforming growth factor-β signaling in vascular endothelial cells, and mutations in them in HHT lead to the development of fragile telangiectatic vessels and arteriovenous malformations. Molecular DNA-based testing has limited availability. Supportive treatment includes supplemental iron therapy for iron deficiency anemia. In a small randomized trial, tamoxifen (20 mg per day for 6 months) significantly reduced bleeding in patients with recurrent epistaxis caused by HHT.[1]

Ehlers-Danlos syndrome is caused by mutations in genes encoding fibrillar collagen or related genes and includes at least six subtypes that vary in clinical manifestations, severity, and prognosis. Inheritance is primarily autosomal dominant. Principal manifestations of Ehlers-Danlos syndrome include skin or joint hyperextensibility, with an associated bleeding tendency including easy bruisability (purpura), surgical bleeding, poor wound healing, and menorrhagia in women. Diagnosis depends mainly on physical examination, supplemented with molecular DNA-based testing that currently has limited availability.

Acquired Vascular Hemorrhagic Disorders

Systemic amyloidosis, Waldenström's macroglobulinemia, and cryoglobulinemia are dysproteinemic disorders reflecting monoclonal gammopathies or hyperglobulinemias (Chapters 193 and 194) that can manifest purpuric or other bleeding symptoms caused by either vascular deposition of immunoglobulin fragments (amyloidosis) or inhibition of platelet-vessel hemostatic functions by immunoglobulins. Henoch-Schönlein purpura is primarily a transient disease of children that typically presents with a palpable purpuric rash of the lower extremities, arthralgias, abdominal pain and renal symptoms (hematuria, proteinuria) in some cases, manifestations of a systemic vasculitis characterized by deposition of immunoglobulin A–containing immune complexes in the skin, gastrointestinal tract, and kidneys. Palpable purpura can also result from systemic sepsis or DIC. Scurvy is caused by the effects of vitamin C deficiency on collagen structure and often presents with bruising or petechiae, including tiny perifollicular hemorrhages. Senile purpura or purpura simplex is thought to reflect partly the age-related changes of skin vascular structure and is typified by easy bruisability of the dorsa of the hands, forearms, and lower legs. Psychogenic purpuras are controversial entities that include Gardner-Diamond syndrome, which is characterized by recurring focal pain preceding development of ecchymoses, believed to reflect poorly understood psychosomatic mechanisms. It can be difficult to differentiate this rare syndrome from factitious or self-induced purpura and bleeding.

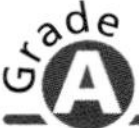

1. Yaniv E, Preis M, Hadar T, et al. Antiestrogen therapy for hereditary hemorrhagic telangiectasia: a double-blind placebo-controlled clinical trial. *Laryngoscope*. 2009;119:284-288.

SUGGESTED READINGS

Bowman M, Hopman WM, Rapson D, et al. A prospective evaluation of the prevalence of symptomatic von Willebrand disease (VWD) in a pediatric primary care population. *Pediatr Blood Cancer*. 2010;55:171-173. *Large prospective study using bleeding history scoring tool and laboratory testing, demonstrating about 5% prevalence of bleeding symptoms in children, with VWD prevalence of about 0.1%.*

Eby C. Pathogenesis and management of bleeding and thrombosis in plasma cell dyscrasias. *Br J Haematol*. 2009;145:151-163. *Review includes purpuric dysproteinemic disorders.*

Faughnan ME, Palda VA, Garcia-Tsao G, et al. International guidelines for the diagnosis and management of hereditary haemorrhagic telangiectasia. *J Med Genet*. 2011;48:73-87. *Consensus guidelines.*

Nichols WL, Rick ME, Ortel TL, et al. Clinical and laboratory diagnosis of von Willebrand disease: a synopsis of the 2008 NHLBI/NIH guidelines. *Am J Hematol*. 2009;84:366-370. *Updated synopsis of recommendations for clinical and laboratory diagnosis of VWD and AVWS, including algorithms.*

177

HEMORRHAGIC DISORDERS: COAGULATION FACTOR DEFICIENCIES

MARGARET V. RAGNI

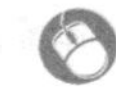

COAGULATION DEFICIENCIES

Severe coagulation deficiencies, or coagulopathies, are typically characterized by spontaneous or traumatic bleeding, such as during surgery or trauma, and may result in life- or limb-threatening complications. By contrast, moderate and mild coagulopathies may remain clinically silent until they are detected coincidentally on routine laboratory screening tests (e.g., prothrombin time [PT], activated partial thromboplastin time [aPTT]) or when these tests are ordered to evaluate the cause of abnormal bleeding or bruising. Much of the morbidity of coagulopathies can be minimized or avoided altogether by prophylactic replacement of the deficient clotting factor proteins. In contrast to the lifelong clinical manifestations of hereditary or congenital coagulopathies, acquired deficiencies usually appear acutely in previously asymptomatic individuals; they may not be suspected and often remit spontaneously or after eradication of an inciting disease state or withdrawal of an offending medication. Acquired coagulation disorders may be associated with more severe bleeding than congenital disorders, in part because of the delay in diagnosis. In general, coagulopathies may result from inadequate synthesis of coagulation factor proteins or from inhibition of activated clotting factor proteins by acquired antibodies or anticoagulant medications. Finally, qualitative defects, either congenital or acquired, may also result in bleeding.

Hereditary Hemophilias

DEFINITION

The hemophilias include hemophilia A and hemophilia B, caused by deficiencies or defects in clotting factor VIII (antihemophilic factor) and factor IX (antihemophilic factor B, or Christmas factor), respectively. A deficiency of either of these intrinsic coagulation pathway proteins results in inadequate formation of thrombin at sites of vascular injury.

EPIDEMIOLOGY

Hemophilia A and B are sex-linked recessive disorders estimated to occur in 1 in 5000 and 1 in 30,000 male births, respectively. The higher incidence of hemophilia A may be due to the greater amount of DNA "at risk" for mutation in the factor VIII gene (186,000 base pairs) compared with the factor IX gene (34,000 base pairs). Hemophilia A and B are observed in all racial and ethnic groups, and in the United States, more than 20,000 individuals are affected. Although carrier testing, genetic counseling, and prenatal diagnosis are widely available in the United States through the network of federally funded hemophilia treatment centers (HTCs), fecundity rates remain high, and few confirmed carriers elect to terminate their pregnancies, even if an affected fetus is detected in utero. These decisions are likely influenced by the wide availability of safe and effective coagulation factor replacement concentrates and by the prospect of an eventual cure for the hemophilias through gene transfer. A substantial proportion (30%) of hemophilia cases arise as new, spontaneous mutations. Overall, the hemophilias are much more common than the autosomal recessive coagulation disorders (see later), which often affect progeny from consanguineous relationships and require the inheritance of two defective alleles for the bleeding manifestations to become evident.

PATHOBIOLOGY

Genetics

As with other sex-linked recessive diseases, the genes for factor VIII and factor IX are located on the long arm of the X chromosome. Males with a defective allele on their single X chromosome transmit this gene to all their daughters, who are obligate carriers, but to none of their sons. Because the offspring of female carriers inherit one affected X chromosome, half of their sons develop the coagulation disorder, and half of their daughters are obligate carriers. Female carriers may manifest hemophilia-like symptoms if the alleles on the X chromosome are unequally inactivated (lyonization); the defective hemophilic allele is expressed in preference to the normal allele, plasma factor VIII levels are below 50%, and phenotypic hemophilia results. Female hemophilia may arise as a result of mating between a hemophilic male and a female carrier (homozygous for the defective factor VIII or IX gene) or in carrier females who have the 45 XO karyotype (Turner's syndrome) and are hemizygous for the defective hemophilia gene.

No single mutation is responsible for the hemophilias. Many missense and nonsense point mutations, deletions, and inversions have been described. Severe molecular defects predominate, with 40 to 50% of all cases of severe hemophilia A evolving from a unique inversion of intron 22 (the largest of the factor VIII introns). This inversion results from the recombination and translocation of DNA within intron 22 of the factor VIII gene, with areas of extragenic but homologous "nonfunctional" DNA located at a distance from intron 22. Other less common severe molecular defects include large gene deletions (5 to 10% of cases) and nonsense mutations (10 to 15% of cases). The encoded proteins resulting from these mutations are defective and do not express any factor VIII activity. Mild or moderate hemophilia A is commonly associated with point mutations and deletions. In contrast, factor IX mutations are more diverse, and severe hemophilia B is more likely caused by large deletions. Mutated clotting factor genes responsible for the hemophilias may also encode for the production of defective nonfunctional proteins that circulate in the plasma and are detected at normal quantitative levels by immunoassays but not by functional assays. A listing of the mutations that cause the hemophilias can be accessed via the Human Gene Mutation Database (*www.hgmd.org*).

CLINICAL MANIFESTATIONS

Hemophilia A and hemophilia B are said to be clinically indistinguishable, with clinical severity corresponding inversely to the circulating levels of plasma coagulant factor VIII or IX activity. Several studies have found a higher bleeding frequency, greater factor use, and more frequent hospitalizations in hemophilia A, suggesting a greater clinical severity than hemophilia B. Individuals with less than 1% of normal factor VIII or IX activity are classified as having "severe" disease, characterized by frequent spontaneous bleeding events in joints (hemarthrosis) and soft tissues and by profuse hemorrhage with trauma or surgery. Although spontaneous bleeding is uncommon in mild deficiencies (>5% normal activity), excess bleeding typically occurs with trauma or surgery. A moderate clinical course is associated with factor VIII or IX levels between 1 and 5%. Approximately 60% of all cases of hemophilia A are clinically severe, whereas only 20 to 45% of cases of hemophilia B are severe.

Severe hemophilia is typically suspected and diagnosed during infancy in the absence of a family history. Among newborns, intracranial hemorrhage is the leading cause of morbidity and mortality, with a cumulative incidence of 3.8%, according to data collected by the Centers for Disease Control and Prevention. Intracranial hemorrhage does not appear to be related to the mode of delivery, although half of such hemorrhages occur in the newborn period; whether prospective computed tomography screening should be instituted at birth remains unknown. Vacuum extraction may increase cephalohematoma formation and is discouraged. Circumcision within days after birth is accompanied by excessive bleeding in less than half of severely affected boys. The first spontaneous hemarthrosis in severely affected hemophiliacs usually occurs between 9 and 18 months of age, when ambulation begins; in moderately affected individuals, it generally does not occur until 2 to 5 years of age. The knees are the most prominent sites of spontaneous bleeds, followed by the elbows, ankles, shoulders, and hips; wrists are less commonly involved.

Acute hemarthroses (Fig. 177-1) originate from the subsynovial venous plexus underlying the joint capsule and produce a tingling or burning sensation, followed by the onset of intense pain and swelling. On physical examination, the joint is swollen, hot, and tender to palpation, with erythema of the overlying skin. Joint mobility is compromised by pain and stiffness, and the joint is usually maintained in a flexed position. Immediate or early replacement of the deficient clotting factor to normal hemostatic levels rapidly reverses the pain. Delayed treatment results in excess pain, morbidity, and joint damage. Optimal management includes rest, ice, (factor) concentrate, and elevation (RICE). Swelling and joint immobility improve as the intra-articular hematoma resolves. Intra-articular needle aspiration of fresh blood is not recommended because of the risk of introducing infection. Short courses of oral corticosteroids may be helpful to reduce the acute joint symptoms in children but are rarely used in adults.

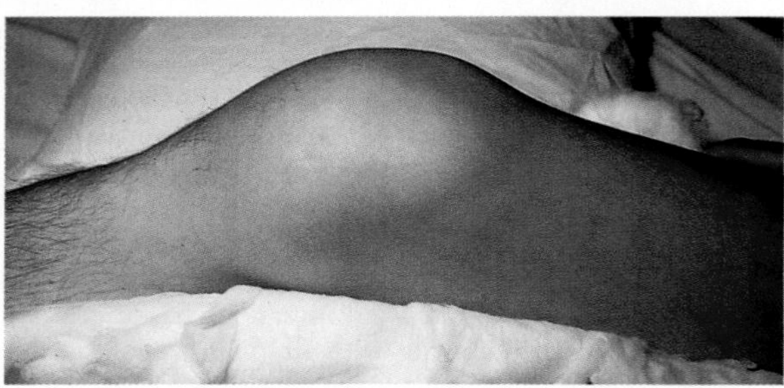

FIGURE 177-1. Acute hemarthrosis of the knee is a common complication of hemophilia. It may be confused with acute infection unless the patient's coagulation disorder is known, because the knee is hot, red, swollen, and painful. (From Forbes CD, Jackson WF. *Color Atlas and Text of Clinical Medicine*, 3rd ed. London: Mosby; 2003.)

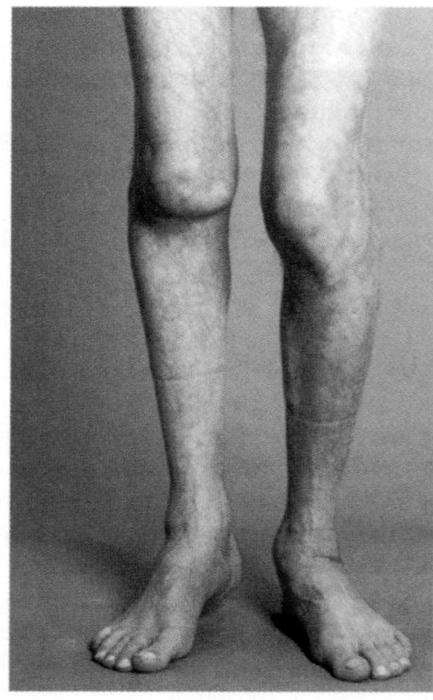

FIGURE 177-2. Severe chronic arthritis in hemophilia. The knee is the most commonly affected joint. Both knees are severely deranged in this patient. Note that he is unable to stand with both feet flat on the floor. (From Forbes CD, Jackson WF. *Color Atlas and Text of Clinical Medicine*, 3rd ed. London: Mosby; 2003.)

Recurrent or untreated bleeds result in chronic synovial hypertrophy and, eventually, damage to the underlying cartilage, with subsequent subchondral bone cyst formation, bony erosion, and flexion contractures. Abnormal mechanical forces from weight bearing can produce subluxation, misalignment, loss of mobility, and permanent deformities of the lower extremities (Fig. 177-2). These changes are accompanied by chronic pain, swelling, arthritis, and disability. Plain radiographs and clinical examination of chronic hemarthroses often underestimate the extent of bone and joint damage; serial magnetic resonance imaging is superior to radiography or computed tomography and is the most sensitive and specific means of detecting and monitoring early and progressive disease.

Intramuscular hematomas account for about 30% of hemophilia-related bleeding events and are rarely life threatening. They are usually precipitated by physical or iatrogenic trauma (e.g., after intramuscular injections) and may compromise sensory and motor function or arterial circulation if they entrap and compress vital structures in closed fascial compartments. The latter occurrence, termed *compartment syndrome*, presents with the rapid onset of swelling and severe pain in an extremity, unrelieved by factor infusion and standard analgesics. This is considered a medical emergency and may require fasciotomy to preserve tissue and provide pain relief. Retroperitoneal hematomas may be confused clinically with appendicitis or hip bleeds but should be suspected in a patient who is hunched over and unable to stand erect owing to the pain of muscle extension in the presence of hematoma. Unless these bleeding episodes are treated immediately and aggressively, permanent anatomic deformity, such as flexion contracture, nerve damage, or pseudotumor formation (expanding hematomas that erode and destroy adjacent skeletal structures), may occur. Bleeding from mucous membranes is very common and may be exaggerated by the degradation of fibrin clots by fibrinolytic enzymes contained in secretions. Bleeding involving the tongue or the retropharyngeal space may rapidly produce life-threatening compromise of the airway. Gastrointestinal hemorrhage typically originates from anatomic lesions proximal to the ligament of Treitz and may be exacerbated by esophageal varices secondary to cirrhosis and portal hypertension or by the use of nonsteroidal anti-inflammatory drugs (NSAIDs) for the treatment of hemarthroses. Spontaneous bleeding in the genitourinary tract secondary to hemophilia is a diagnosis of exclusion after ruling out renal stones and infection. Ureteral blood clots produce renal colic, which may be confused with nephrolithiasis and may be worsened by the use of antifibrinolytic agents. A short course of steroids may be helpful, especially in children, to hasten their resolution. Ninety percent of hemophiliacs experience at least one episode of gross hematuria or hemospermia.

Intracranial bleeds occur in 10% of patients, are usually induced by trauma, and may be fatal in 30% of cases. The risk of developing an intracranial hemorrhage is approximately 2% per year. Neuromuscular defects, seizure disorders, and intellectual deficits may ensue.

Individuals with hemophilia cared for at HTCs have lower mortality and reduced costs of care compared with those receiving treatment elsewhere. The chronic care model practiced at HTCs emphasizes prevention to reduce joint disease and complications, optimization of factor dosing, and counseling regarding safe sports and the avoidance of aspirin and other drugs that inhibit platelet function.

DIAGNOSIS

The diagnosis of hemophilia is suspected on the basis of a family and personal bleeding history and laboratory detection of prolongation of the aPTT (with normal PT). It is confirmed by significantly reduced plasma factor VIII or IX activity. As noted in Chapter 174, the aPTT is not a sufficiently sensitive screening test to be prolonged in mild hemophiliacs, in whom the factor VIII level is sometimes greater than 30% of normal. Severe hemophilia is usually recognized in infancy, with circumcision bleeding; by contrast, moderate or mild disease is recognized later in life after trauma or surgery. Hemophilia can be distinguished from von Willebrand disease (VWD; Chapter 176) by normal ristocetin cofactor and von Willebrand factor antigen levels. In type 2N VWD, factor VIII is significantly lower than ristocetin cofactor and von Willebrand factor antigen levels due to reduced factor VIII binding; this variant of VWD may require genotyping to distinguish it from hemophilia A. Other congenital intrinsic factor deficiencies (e.g., factor XI and XII) can be determined by coagulation factor–specific assays. Vitamin K deficiency (see later and Chapter 178) can be detected by the associated PT prolongation; deficiencies of factors II, VII, IX, and X; and resolution of the coagulation defect with vitamin K. The presence of heparin can be confirmed by correction of the aPTT after running the sample over a heparin absorption column. Failure of the aPTT to correct in a 1 : 1 mix with normal plasma suggests the presence of an inhibitor; specific inhibitors are associated with a single decreased factor level (usually factor VIII; see Alloantibody Inhibitors to Factors VIII and IX under Treatment), whereas blocking inhibitors cause nonspecific factor level changes associated with a positive hexagonal lipid assay (see Antiphospholipid Syndrome and Lupus Anticoagulant later).

TREATMENT

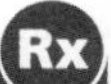

Treatment and prevention of acute bleeding events in hemophilia A and B are based on replacement of the missing or deficient clotting factor protein to restore adequate hemostasis (E-Table 177-1). The morbidity, mortality, and overall cost of care for individuals with hemophilia are reduced significantly if care is provided by comprehensive HTCs that have the multispecialty expertise and laboratory capabilities to coordinate and monitor specific patient needs.

The goal of replacement therapy (Table 177-1) is to achieve plasma factor VIII and IX activity levels of 25 to 30% for minor spontaneous or traumatic bleeds (e.g., hemarthroses, persistent hematuria), at least 50% clotting factor activity for the treatment or prevention of severe bleeds (e.g., major dental surgery, maintenance replacement therapy after major surgery or trauma), and 80 to 100% activity for any life-threatening or limb-threatening hemorrhagic event (e.g., major surgery, trauma). After major trauma or if visceral or intracranial bleeding is suspected, replacement therapy adequate to achieve 100% clotting factor activity should be administered *before* diagnostic procedures are initiated. To calculate the initial dose, plasma factor VIII activity generally increases about 2% (0.02 IU/mL) for each unit of factor VIII administered per kilogram of body weight, and factor IX activity increases about 1% (0.01 IU/mL) for each unit of factor IX administered per kilogram of body weight. Therefore, a 70-kg individual with severe hemophilia A or B (factor VIII or IX activity <1% of normal) who requires replacement to 100% activity for major

TABLE 177-1 FDA-APPROVED COAGULATION PROTEINS AND REPLACEMENT THERAPIES AVAILABLE IN THE UNITED STATES

COAGULATION PROTEIN DEFICIENCY	INHERITANCE PATTERN	PREVALENCE	MINIMUM HEMOSTATIC LEVEL	REPLACEMENT SOURCES
Factor I (fibrinogen)			50-100 mg/dL	Cryoprecipitate, FFP, fibrinogen concentrate
Afibrinogenemia	Autosomal recessive	Rare (<300 families)		
Dysfibrogenemia	Autosomal dominant or recessive	Rare (>300 variants)		
Factor II (prothrombin)	Autosomal dominant or recessive	Rare (25 kindreds)	30% of normal	FFP, factor IX complex concentrates
Factor V (labile factor)	Autosomal recessive	1 in 1 million births	25% of normal	FFP
Factor VII	Autosomal recessive	1 in 500,000 births	25% of normal	Recombinant factor VIIa (15-20 μg/kg), FFP, factor IX complex concentrates
Factor VIII (antihemophilic factor)	X-linked recessive	1 in 5000 male births	80-100% for surgery/ life-threatening bleeds, 50% for serious bleeds, 25-30% for minor bleeds	Factor VIII concentrates (see E-Table 177-1)
Von Willebrand disease			>50% VWF antigen and ristocetin cofactor activity	DDAVP for mild to moderate disease (except type 2B; variable response to 2A); cryoprecipitate and FFP (not preferred, except in emergencies); factor VIII/VWF concentrates, viral attenuated, intermediate purity (preferred for disease unresponsive to DDAVP and for type 3 (see E-Table 177-1)
Type 1 and 2 variants	Usually autosomal dominant	1% prevalence		
Type 3	Autosomal recessive	1 in 1 million births		
Factor IX (Christmas factor)	X-linked recessive	1 in 30,000 male births	25-50% of normal, depending on extent of bleeding, surgery	Factor IX concentrates; FFP not preferred except in dire emergencies (see E-Table 177-1)
Factor X (Stuart-Prower factor)	Autosomal recessive	1 in 500,000 births	10-25% of normal	FFP or factor IX complex concentrates
Factor XI (hemophilia C)	Autosomal dominant; severe type is recessive	4% of Ashkenazi Jews; 1 in 1 million general population	20-40% of normal	FFP or factor XI concentrate
Factor XII (Hageman factor), prekallikrein, high-molecular-weight kininogen	Autosomal recessive	Not available	No treatment necessary	—
Factor XIII (fibrin stabilizing factor)	Autosomal recessive	1 in 3 million births	5% of normal	FFP, cryoprecipitate, or viral-attenuated factor XIII concentrate

DDAVP = desmopressin; FDA = U.S. Food and Drug Administration; FFP = fresh-frozen plasma; VWF = von Willebrand factor.

surgery should initially receive 3500 IU of factor VIII or 7000 IU of factor IX concentrate. The circulating half-lives of factors VIII and IX require subsequent dosing at half the initial dose every 8 to 12 hours and every 18 to 24 hours, respectively. However, this empirical dosing (based on calculations) should be individualized according to the peak recovery increment within 10 to 15 minutes after bolus infusion, as well as trough activity levels. The frequency of repeat dosing is also determined by the rapidity of pain relief, recovery of joint function, and resolution of active bleeding. Replacement is usually maintained for 10 to 14 days after major surgery to allow proper wound healing. Bolus dosing typically results in wide fluctuations in clotting factor activity levels and requires frequent laboratory monitoring to avoid suboptimal troughs. A continuous infusion regimen, consisting of 1 to 2 IU of factor VIII or IX concentrate per kilogram per hour after a bolus dose, maintains a plateau level without the need for frequent laboratory testing. Continuous infusion also reduces total concentrate consumption by 30 to 75% in surgical settings. Long-acting recombinant factors VIII and IX, linked to the Fc domain of immunoglobulin G (IgG) or to liposomes, are currently in clinical trials. If these preparations prolong the circulation times of factors VIII and IX with similar efficacy and safety as standard recombinant products, they may allow simpler dosing schedules and fewer intravenous factor infusions.

Because of the potential thrombogenicity associated with the repeated administration of prothrombin complex concentrates to replace factor IX deficiency, high-purity, plasma-derived, or genetically engineered factor IX concentrates, which lack activated vitamin K–dependent clotting factors, are preferred in hemophilia B.

Cryoprecipitate (a cold precipitate of fresh-frozen plasma [FFP] after thawing at 4° C) and FFP contain factor VIII, but only FFP contains factor IX. However, neither cryoprecipitate nor FFP is an optimal replacement product for either hemophilia A or hemophilia B because these agents may transmit blood-borne pathogens. All clotting factor concentrates available in the United States (E-Table 177-1), whether plasma derived or genetically engineered, are equally efficacious and are considered extremely safe; none has ever been implicated in the transmission of blood-borne viral pathogens or prions. Newer second- and third-generation recombinant factor VIII and IX concentrates are manufactured free of added human or animal proteins in the culture medium or in the final formulation, eliminating the theoretical risks of transmission of prions or murine viruses.

Hemarthroses

The moderate or severe pain that accompanies acute hemarthroses responds to immediate analgesic relief, temporary immobilization, restraint from weight bearing, and clotting factor replacement. Narcotic analgesics, such as codeine or synthetic derivatives of codeine, should be prescribed alone or combined with doses of acetaminophen that are low enough to avoid hepatic toxicity in patients with chronic hepatitis. Although these medications do not possess significant anti-inflammatory activity, they are preferable to NSAIDs or aspirin, which can exacerbate bleeding complications through their inhibition of platelet aggregation.

Strategies intended to prevent end-stage joint destruction should be initiated at an early age. Although prophylaxis beginning soon after the first bleed is the optimal approach (see later), the majority of adults have not had the benefit of early prophylaxis and thus have advanced arthropathy with reduced motion, disability, and pain, for which surgery may be recommended. Synovectomy through open surgery or arthroscopy removes the inflamed tissue and should result in substantially decreased pain and less recurrent bleeding. Nonsurgical synovectomy (synoviorthosis), which involves the intra-articular administration of a radioisotope, is particularly useful for high-risk patients and for those with alloantibody inhibitors to factor VIII or IX (see later). The occurrence of leukemia in three hemophilic children receiving radioisotopic synoviorthosis has raised concerns about leukemogenesis, especially given the low background rate of cancers in individuals with hemophilia. Neither synovectomy nor synoviorthosis reverses joint damage, but both procedures may delay its progression. Non-weight-bearing exercises, such as swimming and isometrics, are important to periarticular muscle development and maintenance of joint stability for ambulation. Intractable pain and severe joint destruction secondary to repeated hemorrhage require prosthetic replacement. Chronic ankle pain responds best to open surgical or arthroscopic fixation and fusion (arthrodesis).

The ultimate strategy to minimize or eliminate progressive joint destruction by recurrent hemarthroses is predicated on the concept of prophylaxis—the scheduled administration of clotting factor concentrates several times weekly (twice a week for factor IX, three times a week for factor VIII) at doses to maintain trough factor activity levels greater than 1 to 2% of normal. In a prospective, randomized clinical trial, prophylaxis with factor VIII (25 IU/kg every other day) was superior to episodic therapy (on demand) in young children with severe hemophilia in reducing joint bleeding and joint damage as shown by magnetic resonance imaging and radiography.[1,2] Although prophylaxis uses more factor product at greater expense, the benefits of long-term prophylaxis to promote joint health and avert disability have led to the recommendation that it be initiated in young children with severe disease at the time of the first bleed. Compliance with this recommendation is not easy, given the invasiveness of intravenous factor administration, the requirement for central venous access devices, and the complication of access device infection. With the development of long-acting factor VIII and IX preparations, currently in clinical trials, bleeding management may become less invasive and simpler. Some unanswered questions include whether prophylaxis is necessary in adulthood and what the minimal effective dose is for prophylaxis or for acute bleeds. The risk of bleeding is thought to be related to the time spent at nadir factor levels less than 1% (0.01 IU/mL) between dosing. It is generally agreed that spontaneous bleeding may be averted by maintaining factor levels at 1% (0.01 U/mL) or greater, which is supported by animal studies of factor IX gene therapy.

Factor Concentrate–Transmitted Viral Infections

In contrast to other at-risk groups, individuals with hemophilia were exposed at a young age to transmissible agents through clotting factor concentrates. This included hepatitis C virus (HCV), leading to infection in 90% of those transfused from the late 1970s through the mid-1980s, and human immunodeficiency virus (HIV) infection in 80% of those transfused with factor VIII products and 50% of those transfused with factor IX products from 1978 through the mid-1980s. Overall, of those with HCV infection (Chapter 151), 40% have coinfection, and hepatitis C remains the leading cause of death in hemophilia. With the implementation of viral inactivation and recombinant technologies, new HCV and HIV infections have been virtually eliminated in hemophiliacs born since the 1990s. Nevertheless, among those exposed to HCV, a large multicenter biopsy study found that 25% have liver fibrosis, and those with HIV coinfection have a 1.4-fold greater fibrosis rate. Among the latter, those receiving highly active antiretroviral therapy (HAART) experience a significant slowing in the rate of HCV progression, to the rates observed in hemophilic men infected only with HCV.

Hepatitis G, observed in 15 to 25% of hemophiliacs, is susceptible to current viral attenuation procedures. Hepatitis B is now a rare problem for those with hemophilia because vaccination at an early age is the standard of care. Hepatitis A virus was transmitted to a small but significant number of patients through solvent detergent-treated factor VIII and factor IX concentrates in the past; hepatitis A vaccination now eliminates this risk. Parvovirus B19 seroprevalence approaches 80% in older adult hemophiliacs exposed to plasma-derived products. The long-term clinical consequences of hepatitis A and parvovirus B19 are unclear. Cadaver and living-donor liver transplantation (Chapter 157) has improved the survival of hemophilic men with chronic hepatitis-induced liver failure and has also resulted in the phenotypic cure of hemophilia, confirming that the liver is the predominant source of normal synthesis of factors VIII and IX. Liver transplantation can also be performed successfully in men coinfected with HIV and HCV with a good response to HAART therapy.

Ancillary and Other Therapies

Ancillary treatment strategies for the hemophilias include antifibrinolytic agents, such as ε-aminocaproic acid (50 mg/kg 3 to 4 times daily) or tranexamic acid (3 or 4 g PO daily in divided doses), to minimize mucous membrane bleeding and the application of fibrin glue to bleeding sites. Desmopressin (DDAVP) can be administered by nasal insufflation 2 hours before a scheduled surgical procedure (one spray per nostril, to provide a total dose of 300 μg; or, in patients weighing <50 kg, 150 μg administered as a single spray); alternatively, DDAVP can be administered intravenously (dissolved in 50 mL normal saline) over 30 minutes at a dose of 0.3 μg/kg. DDAVP is useful in patients with mild hemophilia A because an adequate incremental rise in factor VIII activity can circumvent the use of clotting factor concentrates. Repeated administration of DDAVP (intravenously or by intranasal spray) may be complicated by facial flushing, tachyphylaxis, hyponatremic seizures (primarily in children), and, rarely, angina.

Alloantibody Inhibitors to Factors VIII and IX

Alloantibodies—that is, antibodies to "foreign" infused factor VIII or, less frequently, factor IX—are usually detected in childhood after a median of 9 to 12 days of exposure to clotting factor. These inhibitors occur preferentially in those with a family history of inhibitors and those with large, multidomain factor VIII and factor IX gene deletions. The incidence of factor VIII alloantibodies among hemophilia A patients is 15 to 25%, with a higher frequency in blacks and Hispanics. Factor IX alloantibodies are observed in 1.5 to 3% of hemophilia B patients and predominate among Scandinavians. Patients with factor IX inhibitors seem to be susceptible to anaphylaxis and the development of nephrotic syndrome with subsequent exposure to sources of factor IX. Increasing evidence suggests that exposure to high-dose bolus treatment early in life increases the risk of inhibitor development, especially in those with a predisposition, such as a family history and an at-risk mutation (e.g., a large deletion mutation).

The development of an alloantibody inhibitor is suspected when replacement therapy is ineffective in controlling bleeding symptoms. These IgG antibodies, usually of the IgG4 subclass, completely neutralize clotting factor activity and prevent or reduce any increment in factor VIII or IX levels following bolus infusions of concentrate. Characterized as time and temperature dependent, inhibitors are quantitated in Bethesda units (BU): by definition, 1 BU is the amount of inhibitor that neutralizes 50% of the specific clotting factor activity in normal plasma. "High responders," or patients with high-titer inhibitors (>5 BU), mount an anamnestic antibody response to factor VIII clotting factor protein, usually within 5 to 7 days after subsequent exposure. "Low responders," or patients with low-titer inhibitors (≤5 BU), do not manifest anamnesis. Low-titer inhibitors can easily be overwhelmed by large amounts of human factor VIII or factor IX concentrate, usually three to four times the usual dose.

Treatment of patients with high-titer inhibitors against factor VIII or IX is difficult, and no single approach is uniformly successful. There are two components: first, assurance of hemostasis using "bypass therapy," and second, eradication of inhibitor formation. Hemostasis can be provided by "bypass" agents that are used to treat bleeding episodes (see E-Table 177-1); specifically, the activated prothrombin complex concentrate FEIBA VH (75 to 100 IU/kg initially, then 50 to 100 IU/kg every 6 to 8 hours) and recombinant factor VIIa (90 μ/kg every 2 to 3 hours) can be administered until bleeding is controlled. In studies of congenital hemophilia A patients with alloantibody inhibitors, one dose of FEIBA VH or two doses of recombinant factor VIIa controlled hemarthrosis episodes 81 and 79% of the time, respectively. The activated and unactivated prothrombin complex concentrates contain activated vitamin K–dependent clotting factors that "bypass" the intrinsic pathway (factor VIII or IX) inhibitor. As a result, repeated administration over a short time may be complicated by potential thrombogenicity: the aPTT and clotting factor assays are not helpful in monitoring hemostasis. In patients with high-titer inhibitors to factor VIII or IX, recombinant factor VIIa may achieve effective hemostasis, but its use is limited by the need for frequent intravenous dosing, usually every 2 hours to start. Although continuous dosing has been used in some patients, general experience dictates that for surgery or procedures in which significant bleeding is likely, bolus dosing is required to achieve optimal hemostasis—a "thrombin burst." The product has also been effective in patients who experience anaphylactic reactions or nephrotic syndrome after exposure to factor IX–containing replacement products or FFP. Eradication of inhibitor formation is usually attempted with "immune tolerance induction" regimens, which are generally effective if initiated within 12 months of the inhibitor's detection. Tolerance regimens consist of daily doses of factor concentrates to accomplish desensitization to infused factor, a process associated with a 68% success rate. Although factor dose is not critical in achieving tolerance, the higher the inhibitor titer, the greater the time required to achieve tolerance induction. After tolerance is achieved, maintenance prophylaxis with factor VIII or IX concentrate administered two or three times weekly (at 20 to 30 IU/kg) is necessary. Individuals with inhibitors since childhood who have not undergone immune tolerance induction before adulthood are unlikely to respond. An alternative approach involves treatment with single or combination immunosuppressive agents, including rituximab (currently in clinical trials), mycophenolate, or cyclosporine. Because only a minority respond, adults are typically managed with bypass agents alone.

PREVENTION

Carrier Detection and Prenatal Diagnosis

Carrier detection and prenatal diagnosis have become technically feasible, very sensitive, and widely available. The application of these diagnostic tools, however, is influenced by ethical, cultural, religious, economic, educational, and personal considerations. For instance, carrier detection is particularly useful in identifying women who may be at risk for hemorrhagic complications during the delivery process and male offspring who are particularly vulnerable to intracerebral bleeds at birth. Alternatively, these techniques can provide important information used to make difficult reproductive decisions.

PROGNOSIS

The life expectancy of individuals with severe hemophilia is approaching that of the normal population. The age-matched death rate in hemophilia is 2.7-fold greater than that in the general population, although ischemic heart disease mortality is 60% lower than in the general population. Life expectancy is related to the severity of hemophilia: the mortality rate of severely affected patients is 4- to 6-fold greater than that of patients with mild deficiency. Among those with alloantibody inhibitors, mortality rates are significantly higher than in noninhibitor patients. The three leading causes of death are hepatitis C, HIV/AIDS, and central nervous system bleeding. Hepatitis C has become the leading cause of death, accounting for over half; deaths from HIV have declined with the availability of HAART (Chapter 396). Among those with HIV/HCV coinfection, HAART also slows the progression of HCV-related liver disease. Predictors of hepatitis C disease progression in hemophilia include alcohol use, the use of acetaminophen for pain relief of hemophilic arthropathy, hepatitis B surface antigenemia, and HIV coinfection.

The lifetime risk of intracranial hemorrhage is 2 to 8%. It is the leading cause of morbidity and mortality in the newborn period, and prospective monitoring of central nervous system function is a priority as the population ages. Finally, with the essential elimination of disease transmission through blood products in this population, it is anticipated that the normal problems of aging will be increasingly recognized in those with hemophilia, including atherosclerosis, hypertension, hyperlipidemia, obesity, and diabetes. The impact of these conditions on the natural history of hemophilia, given the recognized lower mortality from ischemic heart disease, remains to be seen.

FUTURE DIRECTIONS

Gene Therapy for Hemophilia A and B

The hereditary hemophilias are model diseases for gene therapy because they are caused by specific, well-defined gene mutations; a small, incremental rise in clotting factor synthesis can lead to substantially improved treatment and quality of life; and inadvertent overexpression by successful gene transfer would not be detrimental. Although successful gene transfer techniques have been developed to provide long-term therapeutic benefits in hemophilic mice and dog models, sustained responses have not yet been achieved in patients with hemophilia—a problem at least in part related to immune responses directed against the vector that suppress long-term expression of clotting factor activity. Approaches under study to avert the immune response to vectors include short-term immunosuppression during the first weeks after vector-gene administration; use of modified, less immunogenic vectors; and use of innovative delivery systems, such as platelets.

Novel therapeutic approaches to enhance clotting factor replacement therapy include long-acting factor products pegylated with liposomes or linked to IgG molecules to prolong factor activity half-life, now in clinical trials; oral delivery systems using bioencapsulated proteins; and molecular modifications to enhance the desirable properties of clotting factor, so-called designer molecules.

Acquired Hemophilias

EPIDEMIOLOGY AND PATHOBIOLOGY

Autoantibody inhibitors occur spontaneously in individuals with previously normal hemostasis (nonhemophiliacs). In contrast to alloantibody inhibitors in hemophilic men, which are directed against foreign infused clotting factor, autoantibody inhibitors are directed against a "self" clotting factor, most commonly factor VIII. These autoantibodies typically arise in individuals with no past bleeding history; thus the diagnosis may be missed until a prolonged aPTT and aPTT mix tests are obtained (Chapter 174). Although half of those with autoantibody inhibitors have no obvious underlying cause, autoimmune diseases, lymphoproliferative disorders, idiosyncratic drug reactions, pregnancy, and advanced age are associated in the other half.

CLINICAL MANIFESTATIONS AND DIAGNOSIS

Massive hemorrhagic events, even more severe than in hemophilia patients with alloantibodies, may occur in those with autoantibodies because of a delay in diagnosis and treatment. The laboratory expression of autoantibodies is similar to that of alloantibodies, except that clotting factor activity is not completely neutralized. Residual clotting factor activities between 3 and 20% of normal are frequently observed in patients with autoantibodies.

TREATMENT

The same principles of replacement therapy for alloantibodies apply to these acquired autoantibody inhibitors. There are two goals of treatment: stop the bleeding and assure hemostasis, and eradicate the inhibitor. For hemostasis, recombinant factor VIIa or factor VIII bypass activity is commonly used, in similar doses used to achieve hemostasis with alloantibody. Porcine factor VIII concentrate is also useful in acquired hemophilia A because little cross-reactivity usually occurs, even with extremely high titers of anti–human factor VIII antibodies; however, its availability is limited. Clinical studies are under way to assess the utility of long-acting VIIa as well as genetically engineered forms of the porcine factor VIII protein. For eradication of the inhibitor, immunosuppressive therapy is generally more effective than in alloantibody patients; this includes corticosteroids (prednisone 1 mg/kg/day PO), cytotoxic agents (e.g., cyclophosphamide 150 mg/day PO or 500 to 750 mg/m^2 IV bolus every 3 to 4 weeks), or a combination, with dose titration based on inhibitor levels and complicating cytopenias. Anti-CD20 antibody (rituximab) 375 mg/m^2 intravenously weekly for 4 weeks is also effective. These agents are continued until the autoantibody inhibitor has disappeared; then they are tapered and discontinued. Whether these agents are also effective for the long-term eradication of autoantibody inhibitors is not known; the question has not been studied in randomized controlled trials. High-dose intravenous gamma globulin may be a useful adjunctive therapy. Immune tolerance induction regimens that combine alkylating agents, the daily administration of clotting factor concentrate, and high-dose corticosteroids have been successful in eradicating autoantibody inhibitors. Rarely, if inhibitor-related hemorrhage is refractory to bypassing agents, extracorporeal plasmapheresis over a staphylococcal protein A column may remove enough neutralizing IgG alloantibody or autoantibody to facilitate successful hemostasis after replacement therapy.

PROGNOSIS

Several large series of patients with acquired hemophilia reveal a substantial mortality rate of 15 to 25%, which is considerably higher than that observed with alloantibody factor VIII inhibitors. A large meta-analysis found that overall survival in acquired hemophilia was influenced primarily by the achievement of a complete remission, age younger than 65 years at diagnosis, and related diseases (malignancy vs. postpartum vs. others). As many as 17% of the deaths were associated with sepsis, and 71% of those arose as a complication of cyclophosphamide-induced neutropenia. Hemorrhagic complications were the primary cause of death, but these could be reduced if the inhibitor could be eradicated. Of note, complete remission was observed in 89% of cyclophosphamide-treated individuals, compared with 70% of those treated with corticosteroids alone and 41% of those who received no treatment.

Von Willebrand Disease

The most common congenital bleeding disorder is VWD. This disorder is inherited in an autosomal dominant fashion and affects both sexes, with a prevalence of 1 to 3% and no ethnic predominance. Homozygous patients are rare and carry a recessive mutant gene. Von Willebrand factor, the protein that is decreased or defective in VWD, is a large, multimeric glycoprotein encoded by the *VWF* gene, located on chromosome 12. Detailed discussion of VWD is provided in Chapter 176.

Factor XI Deficiency

EPIDEMIOLOGY

Factor XI deficiency has a prevalence of 1 in 1 million in the general population and 1 in 500 births in Ashkenazi Jewish families. Factor XI is the only component of the contact phase system (factor XII, prekallikrein, and high-molecular-weight kininogen) of the intrinsic pathway of coagulation that is associated with excessive bleeding complications when a deficiency exists.

PATHOBIOLOGY

Factor XI deficiency is predominantly an autosomal recessive trait, although some mutations may have a dominant transmission pattern. The factor XI gene (*FXI*) is located on chromosome 4, and the protein circulates as a homodimer, with each FXI monomer composed of 4 apple domains encoded by exons 3 through 10 and a protease domain encoded by exons 11 through 15. The Glu117 stop mutation in *FXI* is the most common cause of factor XI deficiency, secondary to poor secretion or stability of the truncated protein or decreased levels of messenger RNA. To date, more than 170 mutations of *FXI* have been identified in factor XI–deficient patients (see *www.factorxi.org*), but close correlation between hemorrhagic phenotype and genotype is lacking. Most are missense or nonsense mutations and are located across all 4 apple domains and the serine protease region. In Ashkenazi Jewish individuals, factor XI deficiency is common, with a heterozygote frequency of 8 to 10%; two predominant gene mutations occur with equal frequency and are designated type II (a stop codon in exon 5) and type III (a single base defect in exon 9). The most severe clinical disease is observed in patients homozygous for type II, who usually have less than 1% factor XI activity.

Homozygous type III individuals also manifest severe symptoms, but typically less severe than those of type II patients; they have slightly higher factor XI levels of about 10 to 20%. Compound heterozygotes, type II/III, make up the bulk of factor XI–deficient patients; they have clinically mild disease, with factor XI levels between 30 and 50%. In non-Jewish individuals, the mutations are more variable, although Cys128 stop has been described in several kindreds, and Cys38Arg has been found in several French Basque families. One third of those who develop inhibitors are homozygous for Glu117 stop, which results in an absent *FXI*. Genotypic identification of affected patients is determined by measuring factor XI levels rather than by defining the specific gene defect.

CLINICAL MANIFESTATIONS

The clinical bleeding tendencies in factor XI deficiency are less severe than those observed in severe hemophilia A or B and, in contrast to the hemophilias, do not correlate with the severity of the deficiency. Most individuals with less than 20% of normal factor XI activity experience excessive bleeding after trauma or surgery; however, a few do not bleed. In contrast, bleeding has been observed in approximately 35 to 50% of mildly affected patients with factor XI levels between 20 and 50% of normal. Spontaneous hemorrhagic episodes, hemarthroses, and intramuscular and intracerebral bleeds are unusual; traumatic and surgical bleeds typically involve the mucous membranes. Patients undergoing tonsillectomy, prostatectomy, or dental extraction are at highest risk for bleeding unless replacement therapy is administered. Women may experience significant menorrhagia, and it has been recommended that women with menorrhagia be screened for both VWD and factor XI deficiency. Patients with mild factor XI deficiency and coincident mild VWD have an increased risk of bleeding.

DIAGNOSIS

Factor XI deficiency is diagnosed in the laboratory by a prolonged aPTT, normal PT, and decreased factor XI activity ascertained in a specific quantitative clotting assay (normal range, 60 to 130%).

TREATMENT Rx

Not all individuals with factor XI deficiency bleed, so it may be reasonable to monitor with no treatment, especially if there is no family history of bleeding. For surgical or other major bleeding, FFP 15 to 20 mL/kg can be used, although potential complications include fluid overload and infection risk, which can be reduced with the use of pathogen-inactivated FFP, if available. Use of factor XI concentrate, which is available in Europe but not the United States, may be complicated by thrombosis, which occurs in approximately 10% of patients, particularly in older individuals with preexisting cardiovascular disease and malignancy. Replacement dosing levels should not exceed 70% of factor XI activity. Repeat dosing with FFP or factor XI concentrate should take into consideration the long (60- to 80-hour) biologic half-life of factor XI in vivo.

The decision to treat heterozygotes with factor XI at levels greater than 20% is empirical and should be based on the individual's prior history of bleeding after trauma or surgery. Alternatively, a family medical history of bleeding complications can be considered. There is no clear evidence of benefit with the use of DDAVP. Because hemorrhagic complications originate most commonly from mucous membrane surfaces, antifibrinolytic agents such as ε-aminocaproic acid or tranexamic acid are frequently helpful as adjunctive therapy. In women with menorrhagia or postpartum hemorrhage, testing for VWD is recommended because both diseases may be present.

Alloantibody inhibitors, which neutralize the hemostatic effects of exogenously administered factor XI replacement, can develop in patients with severe factor XI deficiency who have been exposed to plasma or factor XI concentrate. Recombinant factor VIIa can prevent bleeding during or after surgery in these patients.

Deficiencies of Contact Activation Factors

Although factor XI plays an important role in the activation of factor IX in the intrinsic pathway generation of thrombin, it is only one of the four components of the contact phase of coagulation. Deficiencies in any of the other three factors (factor XII, prekallikrein, and high-molecular-weight kininogen) produce in vitro laboratory abnormalities. Even among those with severe factor XII deficiency (<1% activity), there is no clinical bleeding; however, up to 8 to 10% with severe factor XII deficiency actually experience venous thromboembolic events, which are occasionally fatal. This finding has led to speculation that factor XII deficiency may lead to hypercoagulability through defective participation of the contact phase proteins in the activation of fibrinolysis.

DIAGNOSIS

Deficiencies of each of these factors prolong the aPTT, often markedly, which may normalize after prolonged incubation of the patient's plasma at 37° C with a negatively charged activator of the aPTT assay (i.e., kaolin or celite). Specific assays are also available to quantitate each of the contact factors.

TREATMENT Rx

Deficiencies of the contact activation factors, however severe they are and however prolonged the associated aPTT may be, do not cause clinical bleeding problems, even in response to surgery or trauma. Therefore, no therapy is indicated for factor XII deficiency, prekallikrein deficiency, or high-molecular-weight kininogen deficiency. Routine anticoagulation regimens are used to treat thrombogenic events.

Factor XIII (Fibrin-Stabilizing Factor) Deficiency

Factor XIII is a transglutaminase that is activated by thrombin and functions to cross-link fibrin to protect it from lysis by plasmin. It is also involved in wound healing and tissue repair and seems to be crucial for maintaining a viable pregnancy. Homozygous severe deficiency states are rare and are inherited in an autosomal recessive manner, with a prevalence of 1 per 3 million births. Consanguinity is common.

CLINICAL MANIFESTATIONS

Heterozygous carriers are usually asymptomatic, but homozygotes have lifelong bleeding that typically starts shortly after birth with persistent bleeding around the umbilical stump. Intracranial bleeding events, usually precipitated by minimal trauma, occur commonly enough in infants (25%) to justify the initiation of a primary prophylaxis regimen of replacement therapy. Delayed bleeding after surgery and trauma is the hallmark of the disease; however, easy bruising, poor wound healing with defective scar formation and dehiscence, and hemarthroses are characteristic. Spontaneous abortions are increased in severely affected women.

DIAGNOSIS

The diagnosis is usually suspected on clinical grounds, given that factor XIII deficiency is not detected by conventional screening coagulation assays (i.e., aPTT, PT). Most laboratories use a rapid screening assay that assesses the ability of a fibrin clot to remain intact with incubation in 5 mol/L of urea or 1% monochloroacetic acid. With factor XIII levels less than 1% of normal, the clot dissolves within 2 to 3 hours.

TREATMENT Rx

Replacement therapy for prophylaxis or the treatment of acute bleeds can be accomplished by administering cryoprecipitate, FFP, or, preferably, plasma-derived factor XIII concentrate (Fibrogammin P), which is pasteurized for viral safety. A clinical trial of Fibrogammin P for factor XIII deficiency is under way in the United States, and the product is available under compassionate investigational new drug use through ZLB-Behring Inc., Marburg, Germany, and CSL Behring Inc., King of Prussia, PA. Clinical studies are also in progress to evaluate a placentally derived product. Normal hemostasis is achieved with a factor XIII level of only 5% of normal. The dose of Fibrogammin P is 10 to 20 U/kg intravenously, and because it has a long half-life (10 days), prophylactic replacement can be given every 3 to 4 weeks. Acquired alloantibody inhibitors can develop in severely affected individuals. Autoantibodies also occur, usually in association with systemic lupus erythematosus.

Dysfibrinogenemia and Afibrinogenemia

Approximately 300 abnormal fibrinogens have been described, but few cause hemostatic symptoms. Abnormal fibrinogens are rare, autosomally inherited proteins. Quantitative fibrinogen deficiencies (afibrinogenemia and hypofibrinogenemia) may result from mutations affecting fibrinogen synthesis or processing, whereas qualitative defects (dysfibrinogenemia) are caused by mutations that lead to abnormal polymerization, defective cross-linking, or defective assembly of the fibrinolytic system.

CLINICAL MANIFESTATIONS

More than 50% of the dysfibrinogenemias are asymptomatic, 25% are associated with a mild hemorrhagic tendency (commonly caused by defective release of fibrinopeptide A), and 20% predispose individuals to thrombophilia (usually caused by impaired fibrinolysis) (Chapter 179). Concurrent bleeding and thrombosis also may occur. The prevalence of dysfibrinogenemia in patients with a history of thromboembolic episodes approaches 0.8%. A high prevalence of dysfibrinogenemia has been reported among patients with chronic thromboembolic hypertension, implicating changes in the molecular structure of fibrin in the development of this disorder. Women experience a high incidence of pregnancy-related complications, such as spontaneous abortion and postpartum thromboembolic events. Thrombin times and reptilase times (plasma-based clotting times with the substitution of reptilase snake venom for thrombin) are not helpful in predicting whether an abnormal fibrinogen will be prothrombotic, prohemorrhagic, or asymptomatic. However, clinical history, fibrinopeptide release studies, and fibrin polymerization studies may be useful. Clinically insignificant dysfibrinogenemias may be acquired in association with hepatocellular carcinoma (Chapter 202).

In contrast to the hepatic synthesis of a qualitatively abnormal protein in dysfibrinogenemia, congenital afibrinogenemia, an autosomal recessive disorder, represents the markedly deficient production of a normal protein. Severe life-threatening hemorrhagic complications can occur at any site, beginning at birth with umbilical bleeding. Intracranial hemorrhage is a frequent cause of death. Poor wound healing is characteristic. All coagulation-based assays that depend on the detection of a fibrin clot end point are markedly prolonged. Afibrinogenemia is usually detectable by specific functional or immunologic assays. Platelet dysfunction may accompany afibrinogenemia and exacerbate bleeding.

DIAGNOSIS

Abnormalities are usually detected incidentally when routine coagulation screening assays reveal decreased fibrinogen concentrations and prolonged thrombin clotting times. On further evaluation, discordance between functional and immunologic fibrinogen levels (>50 mg/dL more antigenic than functional) is observed; clotting times using snake venom (reptilase or ancrod) are variably prolonged.

TREATMENT Rx

Deficiencies of fibrinogen can be corrected by the administration of FFP or cryoprecipitate; however, viral safety remains an issue. A viral-attenuated (pasteurized), plasma-derived fibrinogen concentrate (Riastap, CSL Behring) was recently approved by the Food and Drug Administration (FDA) for use in congenital fibrinogen deficiency, with a target replacement goal of 100 mg/dL. With a circulating biologic half-life of at least 96 hours, treatment every 3 to 4 days is adequate. Primary prophylaxis regimens may be useful in afibrinogenemia, with on-demand or prophylactic replacement for trauma or surgery. Individuals with thrombophilic manifestations should receive anticoagulation long term, depending on risk-benefit assessment (Chapter 179). Riastap is not recommended for use in dysfibrinogenemia. Solvent detergent- or psoralen-treated FFP (when licensed by the FDA) may provide an alternative therapy.

Factor V Deficiency

Factor V is a component of the prothrombinase complex that assembles factors Va and Xa on the phospholipid membrane of the platelet for prothrombin (factor II) activation to thrombin (Chapter 174).

CONGENITAL FACTOR V DEFICIENCY

Deficiency of factor V is a rare, autosomal recessive disorder (1 in 1 million births). The factor V Leiden protein, which is responsible for resistance to activated protein C and thrombophilia, does not affect factor V coagulant activity (Chapter 179). The severity of plasma factor V deficiency correlates less well with the risk of clinical bleeding than does the factor V content in platelet α-granules. This observation illustrates the critical role of the platelet in promoting adequate hemostasis at bleeding sites and explains why transfusions of normal platelets may be preferred over FFP for the treatment of hemorrhagic episodes secondary to congenital or acquired factor V deficiency. Hemostasis can be maintained without correcting plasma factor V activity (>25% of normal).

COMBINED DEFICIENCIES OF FACTORS V AND VIII

Factors V and VIII are structurally homologous proteins, and combined deficiencies of these factors occur as an autosomal recessive disorder with a prevalence of 1 in 100,000 births among Jews of Sephardic origin. The severity of bleeding is determined by the levels of these factors, which usually range from 5 to 30% of normal. Replacement therapy should be aimed at normalizing both clotting protein activities.

ACQUIRED FACTOR V DEFICIENCY

Acquired factor V deficiency has been described in individuals exposed to bovine factor V, which contaminates the thrombin preparations used topically to control bleeding during cardiovascular surgery. This abnormality probably represents the development of anti–bovine factor V antibodies that cross-react with the human factor V protein. Profuse bleeding accompanies this complication.

Deficiencies of Vitamin K–Dependent Coagulation

DEFICIENCIES OF FACTORS II, VII, AND X

PATHOBIOLOGY AND CLINICAL MANIFESTATIONS

Congenital deficiencies of factors II (prothrombin), VII, and X are rare, autosomally inherited disorders. Heterozygotes (with factor levels approximately 20% of normal) are typically asymptomatic except in the immediate newborn period, when physiologic vitamin K deficiency exacerbates the underlying clotting factor deficiency. Homozygotes with clotting factor levels less than 10% of normal manifest variable symptoms. As with other coagulopathies, these deficiencies are usually suspected after neonatal umbilical stump bleeding. Thereafter, unless replacement or prophylactic therapy is provided, these patients are subject to mucosal bleeding from epistaxis, menorrhagia, and dental extractions; hemarthroses and intramuscular hematomas; and bleeding after surgery or trauma.

Acquired factor VII deficiency has been associated with Dubin-Johnson and Gilbert's syndromes (Chapter 149). Acquired factor IX deficiency has been associated with Gaucher's disease, because factor IX binds to glucocerebroside (Chapter 215). Acquired factor X deficiency and amyloidosis are discussed later.

DIAGNOSIS

In the coagulation laboratory, factor VII deficiency is associated with a prolonged PT and a normal aPTT. This pattern localizes the deficiency to the extrinsic pathway. In contrast, deficiencies of factors II (prothrombin) and X prolong both the PT and the aPTT, with the defects localized to the common pathway of coagulation. A Russell viper venom–based clotting assay can differentiate between these two deficiencies; as a direct activator of factor X, the assay is prolonged with factor X deficiency but not with factor II deficiency. Mixing patient plasma with normal plasma results in a correction of these assays, and specific clotting assays using plasma deficient in the coagulation protein to be studied can confirm the diagnosis.

TREATMENT Rx

Replacement therapy is indicated for acute symptomatic bleeds and for prophylaxis before surgery. In addition to FFP, which has the potential to transmit blood-borne viruses, factor IX complex concentrates can be administered to achieve hemostatic levels of any of these vitamin K–dependent factors (25 to 30% of normal).

Bleeding complications caused by acquired IgG autoantibodies directed against any coagulation factor protein can be reversed rapidly, albeit temporarily, by extracorporeal immunoadsorption over a Sepharose-bound polyclonal antihuman IgG or staphylococcal A column, with concomitant replacement therapy and initiation of immunosuppression. Recombinant factor VIIa is increasingly used for surgery in those with rare congenital coagulation deficiencies, but typically at lower doses than with hemophilia inhibitors—generally 10 to 15 μg/kg/day or less, for up to several days.

FACTOR DEFICIENCY IN AMYLOIDOSIS

Severe acquired deficiency of factor X, often accompanied by deficiencies of other vitamin K–dependent factors, occasionally occurs in individuals with systemic amyloidosis (Chapter 194). Because amyloid fibrils in the reticuloendothelial system bind endogenous and exogenous sources of factor X, replacement therapy with FFP or factor IX complex concentrates, even in large quantities, may not be sufficient. Recombinant factor VIIa concentrate has been used to reverse acute bleeding. Splenectomy may ameliorate recurrent bleeding complications.

Other Acquired Coagulation Abnormalities

ANTIPHOSPHOLIPID SYNDROME AND LUPUS ANTICOAGULANT

EPIDEMIOLOGY

The antiphospholipid antibody syndrome (APS) is associated with recurrent thrombosis or recurrent pregnancy loss with autoantibodies directed against phospholipids. Antiphospholipid antibodies (APAs) may include lupus anticoagulant (LA), anticardiolipin antibody (CL), or anti-β2-glycoprotein-I (anti-β2-GPI). Thrombocytopenia is also a common finding in this prothrombotic disorder. Rarely, multiorgan failure may arise from widespread thrombosis, termed *catastrophic APS.*

PATHOBIOLOGY

Our understanding of the role of individual antibodies in diagnosing APS continues to be enhanced with clinical studies, which may also contribute to the development of better diagnostic assays. It has been suggested that the prothrombotic effects of APAs may derive from their ability to complex with β2-GPI in vivo (thereby negating their modulatory phospholipid-binding function) or through APA inhibition of protein C activation, interference with antithrombin III activity, and/or disruption of the annexin V "shield," thereby preventing normal clot breakdown (fibrinolysis). Although complement and inflammation play a role in fetal loss in a murine model of APS, the pathogenic mechanism of APS-associated pregnancy loss remains unclear. Although non-β2-GPI antibodies detected by CL enzyme-linked immunosorbent assay (ELISA) may play a role in early obstetric APS, and anti-β2-GPI antibodies with LA activity play a role in late miscarriage, additional studies are needed to better classify, understand, and manage this syndrome.

CLINICAL MANIFESTATIONS

APAs prolong coagulation in in vitro assays but are not generally associated with clinical bleeding. Rarely, clinical bleeding may occur when APA interacts with factor II (prothrombin), producing an acquired prothrombin (factor II) deficiency associated with accelerated clearance of LA-prothrombin complexes from the circulation. Bleeding tendencies also may arise when LA targets platelet membranes and produces quantitative and/or qualitative platelet abnormalities. Other clinical findings in APS include livedo reticularis (Chapter 80), valvular heart lesions, and nephropathy. Clinically, although both arterial and venous thrombosis (Chapter 179) may occur in APS, the most relevant is venous thrombosis and stroke in young adults. A diagnostic work-up in those with arterial thrombosis should include transesophageal echocardiography to exclude a cardiac source for arterial clots. In obstetric patients, other causes of miscarriage should be excluded. Nonpregnant individuals with APS-associated thrombotic manifestations have a 50% risk of experiencing recurrent events over a 5-year period. Typically, recurrent hypercoagulable episodes occur in a pattern consistent with the initial findings (e.g., venous recurrence following an initial deep vein thrombosis).

DIAGNOSIS

By international consensus, a diagnosis of APS is based on both clinical and laboratory criteria. Clinical criteria include (1) arterial, venous, or small-vessel thrombosis in any tissue or organ and (2) pregnancy morbidity. The latter includes one or more pregnancy losses before 10 weeks' gestation; one or more pregnancy losses before 34 weeks due to eclampsia, preeclampsia, or placental insufficiency; or three or more spontaneous abortions before 10 weeks. APS may be suspected in the setting of recurrent spontaneous miscarriages or pregnancy-related thromboembolic events; with the detection of cerebral arterial thromboses in young adults; in those with systemic lupus erythematosus (20 to 40%; Chapter 274) or other autoimmune diseases or lymphoproliferative malignancies; in those receiving psychotropic medications (e.g., chlorpromazine); or when incidental coagulation assays reveal aPTT prolongation.

Laboratory criteria include one or more high-titer APAs (LA, CL, anti-β2-GPI) on at least two occasions at least 12 weeks apart. APAs can be detected by three assays: the LA assay, the CL ELISA assay, and the β2-GPI ELISA assay. The LA assay includes a screening test, based on a prolonged phospholipid-dependent clotting time; a mixing test that distinguishes the inhibitor (fails to correct in a 1 : 1 mix) from a deficiency state (corrects in a 1 : 1 mix); and a confirmatory test based on platelet neutralization to demonstrate that the inhibitor is phospholipid dependent (clotting time corrects) or a modified aPTT reagent based on the binding of hexagonal phase phospholipids to LA. The CL ELISA measures antibodies in dilute sera that bind to CL-coated plates, including those that bind to CL alone or bound to bovine β2-GPI and both IgG and IgM, but it may miss CL bound to human β2-GPI. The β2-GPI ELISA detects antibodies that bind to β2-GPI–coated irradiated plates, but it has reduced specificity owing to binding by nonpathogenic antibodies. Positivity in multiple assays is strongly associated with thrombosis and miscarriage. Of the three assays, the β2-GPI ELISA is most strongly associated with thrombosis and early recurrent miscarriage; the LA assay is associated with venous thrombosis, stroke, and late miscarriage. The greatest weight is given to a positive LA test. From a practical standpoint, testing for all three antibodies at diagnosis is recommended to guide follow-up, because oral anticoagulants may interfere with the LA test.

TREATMENT Rx

Because of the high risk of recurrent thromboembolism, patients with APS should receive antithrombotic therapy. The approach is based on achieving a balance between thrombosis risk and bleeding complications, especially in those with thrombocytopenia. Because of the limited information from randomized clinical trials, the recommendations for APS are similar to those for patients without APS—that is, to use unfractionated heparin or low-molecular-weight heparin (LMWH), with a 4- to 5-day overlap with warfarin, for acute venous thromboembolism (VTE), followed by long-term warfarin to a target international normalized ratio (INR) of 2.0 to 3.0. This recommendation is based on a randomized trial indicating no difference in bleeding rates with high-intensity (INR >3.0) versus low-intensity (INR 2.0 to 3.0) anticoagulation.[3] In individuals with thrombocytopenia, more frequent monitoring of the INR may be warranted to avoid bleeding complications. The duration of anticoagulation in those both with and without APS is based on a balance between VTE recurrence and bleeding.

For women with APS and pregnancy loss but no past thrombosis, the goal is to prevent recurrent pregnancy loss. Based on prospective studies indicating higher birth rates with aspirin plus heparin, recommendations include low-dose aspirin (81 mg) in combination with prophylactic heparin or LMWH in the antepartum period.

Among those with APS-associated thrombocytopenia and a platelet count below 20 to 30 × 10^9/L, in the setting of bleeding or when bleeding risk exceeds bleeding with VTE treatment, management is similar to that for idiopathic thrombocytopenic purpura (Chapter 175). This includes steroids, intravenous immunoglobulin, and immunosuppressive agents (e.g., cyclophosphamide, azathioprine, off-label rituximab). Case reports indicate that danazol, dapsone, aspirin, or chloroquine may be helpful adjuncts. In pregnant women with APS-associated thrombocytopenia, treatment is advised before epidural anesthesia or cesarean section. In the latter case, early delivery under cover of intravenous immunoglobulin is recommended.

Treatment of APS-associated bleeding is dependent on the site and severity of bleeding. For anticoagulation bleeding, the anticoagulant should be withheld and an antidote (e.g., protamine) given, if available. For thrombocytopenia bleeding, platelet transfusions should be given, along with red blood cell transfusions, if necessary. If both thrombosis and bleeding occur, treatment should be directed at the component that is most life threatening. In those with a high bleeding risk, anticoagulants should be withheld or given at a lower dosage; those with a high thrombotic risk, despite thrombocytopenia, should be anticoagulated and given agents to boost platelet count. For those who receive prolonged heparin, supplemental calcium and vitamin D should be administered to minimize the risks of osteoporosis.

Visit expertconsult.com for e-expanded chapter

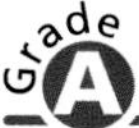

1. Manco-Johnson MJ, Abshire TC, Shapiro AD, et al. Prophylaxis versus episodic treatment to prevent joint disease in boys with severe hemophilia. *N Engl J Med.* 2007;357:535-544.
2. Gringeri A, Lundin B, von Mackensen SV, et al. A randomized clinical trial of prophylaxis in children with hemophilia A (the ESPRIR Study). *J Thromb Haemost.* 2011;9:700-710.
3. Crowther MA, Ginsberg JS, Julian J, et al. A comparison of two intensities of warfarin for the prevention of recurrent thrombosis in patients with the antiphospholipid antibody syndrome. *N Engl J Med.* 2003;349:1133-1138.

SUGGESTED READINGS

Baudo F, Caimi T, de Cataldo F. Diagnosis and treatment of acquired haemophilia. *Haemophilia.* 2010;16:102-106. *The diagnosis is associated with autoimmune diseases, solid tumors, lymphoproliferative diseases, and pregnancy, but 50% of causes are idiopathic.*

Berntorp E, de Moerloose P, Ljung RC. The role of prophylaxis in bleeding disorders. *Haemophilia.* 2010;16:189-193. *Review emphasizing benefits for joint- or life-threatening bleeds, arthropathy, and quality of life.*

Blancette VS. Prophylaxis in the haemophilia population. *Haemophilia.* 2010;16:181-188. *Review.*

Favaloro EJ, Wong RC. Laboratory testing for the antiphospholipid syndrome: making sense of antiphospholipid antibody assays. *Clin Chem Lab Med.* 2011;49:447-461. *Review.*

Giangrande PL, Escobar MA. Management of difficult-to-treat inhibitor patients. *Haemophilia.* 2010;16:52-57. *Case-based review.*

Iorio A, Matino D, D'Amico R, et al. Recombinant Factor VIIa concentrate versus plasma derived concentrates for the treatment of acute bleeding episodes in people with haemophilia and inhibitors. *Cochrane Database Syst Rev.* 2010;8:CD004449. *rFVIIa and aPCC have similar hemostatic effects without increasing thromboembolic risk.*

Kempton CL. Inhibitors in previously treated patients: a review of literature. *Haemophilia.* 2010;16:61-65. *Review.*

Pipe SW. Hemophilia: new protein therapeutics. *Hematology Am Soc Hematol Educ Program.* 2010;2010:203-209. *Review.*

Pengo V. APS—controversies in diagnosis and management, critical overview of current guidelines. *Thromb Res.* 2011;127(suppl 3):S51-S52. *Review.*

178

HEMORRHAGIC DISORDERS: DISSEMINATED INTRAVASCULAR COAGULATION, LIVER FAILURE, AND VITAMIN K DEFICIENCY

ANDREW I. SCHAFER

DISSEMINATED INTRAVASCULAR COAGULATION

DEFINITION

Disseminated intravascular coagulation (DIC), also referred to as *consumptive coagulopathy* or *defibrination*, is caused by a wide variety of serious disorders (Table 178-1). In most patients, the underlying process dominates the clinical picture, but in some cases (e.g., occult malignancy, envenomation), DIC may be the initial or predominant manifestation of the disorder. DIC never occurs in isolation, without an inciting cause.

PATHOBIOLOGY

DIC is primarily a thrombotic process, although its clinical manifestation may be widespread hemorrhage in acute, fulminant cases. The basic pathophysiology (Fig. 178-1), regardless of cause, is entry into the circulation of procoagulant substances that trigger systemic activation of the coagulation system and platelets with resultant disseminated deposition of fibrin-platelet

TABLE 178-1 MAJOR CAUSES OF DISSEMINATED INTRAVASCULAR COAGULATION

INFECTIONS
Gram-negative bacterial sepsis
Other bacteria, fungi, viruses, Rocky Mountain spotted fever, malaria
IMMUNOLOGIC REACTIONS
Transfusion reactions (ABO incompatibility)
Transplant rejection
OBSTETRIC COMPLICATIONS
Amniotic fluid embolism
Retained dead fetus
Abruptio placentae
Toxemia, preeclampsia
Septic abortion
MALIGNANCIES
Pancreatic carcinoma
Adenocarcinomas
Acute promyelocytic leukemia
Other neoplasms
LIVER FAILURE
ACUTE PANCREATITIS
ENVENOMATION
RESPIRATORY DISTRESS SYNDROME
TRAUMA, SHOCK
Brain injury
Crush injury
Burns
Hypothermia/hyperthermia
Fat embolism
Hypoxia, ischemia
Surgery
VASCULAR DISORDERS
Giant hemangioma (Kasabach-Merritt syndrome)
Aortic aneurysm
Vascular tumors

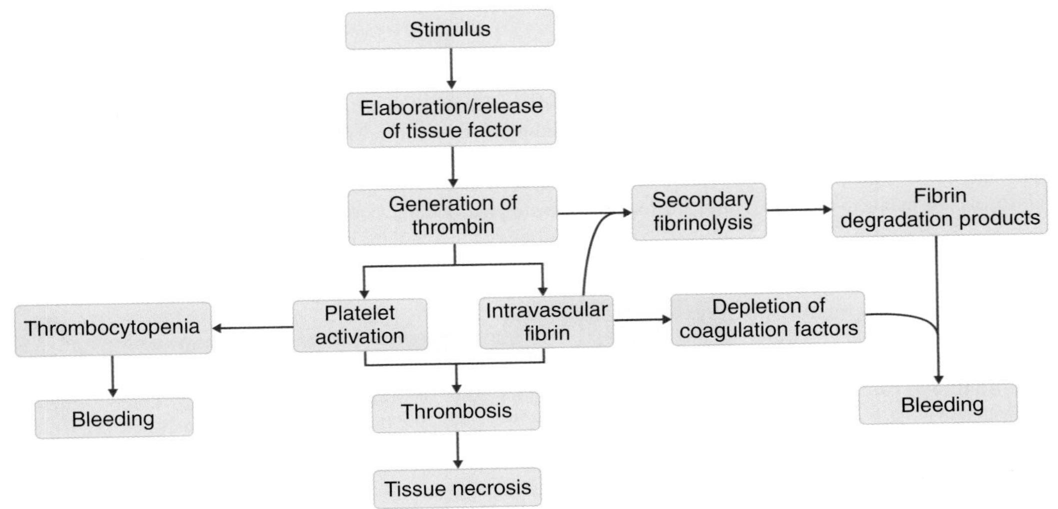

FIGURE 178-1. Pathophysiology of bleeding, thrombosis, and ischemic manifestations in patients with disseminated intravascular coagulation.

thrombi within the microvasculature. In most cases, the procoagulant stimulus is tissue factor, a lipoprotein that is not normally exposed to blood. In DIC, tissue factor gains access to blood by tissue injury, its elaboration by malignant cells, or its expression on the surface of monocytes and endothelial cells by inflammatory mediators. Components of the inflammatory response and the coagulation system are reciprocally activated in some forms of DIC, such as sepsis. Tissue factor triggers generation of the coagulation protease thrombin, which induces fibrin formation and platelet activation. In some specific cases of DIC, procoagulants other than tissue factor (e.g., a cysteine protease or mucin in certain malignancies) and proteases other than thrombin (e.g., trypsin in pancreatitis, exogenous enzymes in envenomation) provide the procoagulant stimulus.

In acute, uncompensated DIC, coagulation factors are consumed at a rate in excess of the capacity of the liver to synthesize them, and platelets are consumed in excess of the capacity of bone marrow megakaryocytes to release them. The resulting laboratory manifestations are a prolonged prothrombin time (PT) and activated partial thromboplastin time (aPTT) and thrombocytopenia. Increased fibrin formation in DIC stimulates the process of secondary fibrinolysis, in which plasminogen activators generate plasmin to digest fibrin (and fibrinogen) into fibrin(ogen) degradation products (FDPs). FDPs are potent circulating anticoagulants that further contribute to the bleeding manifestations of DIC. Intravascular fibrin deposition can cause fragmentation of red blood cells and lead to the appearance of schistocytes in blood smears; however, frank hemolytic anemia is unusual in DIC. Microvascular thrombosis in DIC can compromise the blood supply to some organs and lead to multiorgan failure, particularly when accompanied by systemic hemodynamic and metabolic derangements.

Underlying Causes

DIC always has an underlying cause that generally must be identified and eliminated if the coagulopathy is to be managed successfully. The development of DIC in many of these disorders is associated with an unfavorable outcome. Infection is the most common cause of DIC. The syndrome is particularly associated with gram-negative or gram-positive sepsis (Chapter 108), although it can be triggered by a variety of other bacterial, fungal, viral, rickettsial, and protozoal microorganisms. The placenta and uterine contents are rich sources of tissue factor and other procoagulants that are normally excluded from the maternal circulation; a spectrum of clinical manifestations of DIC may accompany obstetric complications when this barrier is breached, especially in the third trimester. These syndromes range from acute, fulminant, and often fatal DIC in amniotic fluid embolism to chronic or subacute DIC with a retained dead fetus. Other obstetric problems associated with DIC include abruptio placentae, toxemia, and septic abortion. Chronic forms of DIC are caused by a variety of malignancies, particularly pancreatic cancer (Chapter 200) and mucin-secreting adenocarcinomas of the gastrointestinal tract (Chapter 199), in which thrombotic rather than bleeding manifestations predominate. Treatment with all-*trans*-retinoic acid has greatly reduced the incidence of severe DIC in patients with acute promyelocytic leukemia (Chapter 189). It is not known whether liver failure (Chapter 157) can cause DIC or whether its coexistence merely exacerbates intravascular coagulation because of impaired clearance of activated clotting factors, plasmin, and FDPs. Snake venom contains a variety of substances that can affect coagulation and endothelial permeability. Bites from rattlesnakes and other vipers can induce profound DIC by introduction of these exogenous toxins and release of endogenous tissue factor via tissue necrosis. The likelihood and degree of DIC caused by trauma, surgery, and shock (Chapter 106) are related to the extent of tissue damage and the organs involved; the brain is a particularly rich source of tissue factor, so traumatic brain injury (Chapter 406) can precipitate acute DIC. Large aortic aneurysms (Chapter 78), giant hemangiomas, and other vascular malformations can cause subclinical or clinical DIC that is initiated locally within the abnormal vasculature but can "spill" into the systemic circulation.

CLINICAL MANIFESTATIONS

The clinical manifestations of DIC are determined by the nature, intensity, and duration of the underlying stimulus. The coexistence of liver disease exacerbates DIC of any etiology. Low-grade DIC is often asymptomatic and diagnosed only by laboratory abnormalities. Thrombotic complications of DIC occur most often with chronic underlying diseases, as exemplified by Trousseau's syndrome in cancer (Chapter 187). DIC can present as acrocyanosis and gangrene of the digits in critically ill, hemodynamically compromised patients on vasopressors. Hemorrhagic necrosis of the skin

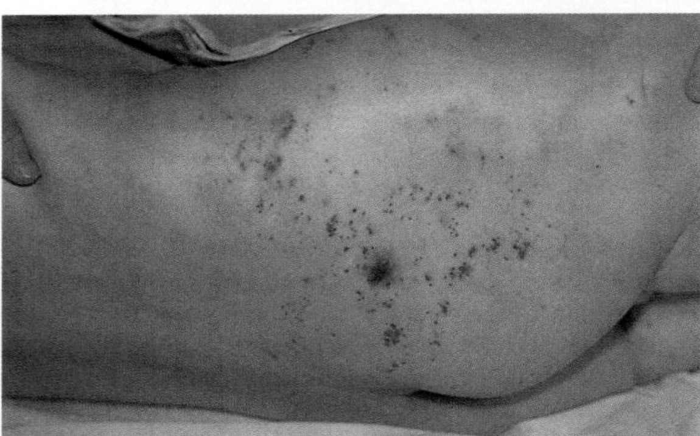

FIGURE 178-2. Disseminated intravascular coagulation resulting from staphylococcal septicemia. Note the characteristic skin hemorrhage ranging from small purpuric lesions to larger ecchymoses. (From Forbes CD, Jackson WF. *Color Atlas and Text of Clinical Medicine,* 3rd ed. London: Mosby; 2003.)

(Fig. 178-2) and purpura fulminans may also be manifestations of DIC. Bleeding is the most common clinical finding in acute, uncompensated DIC. Bleeding can be limited to sites of intervention or anatomic abnormalities, but it tends to be generalized in more severe cases, including widespread ecchymoses and diffuse oozing from mucosal surfaces and orifices.

DIAGNOSIS

The laboratory diagnosis of severe, acute DIC is not usually difficult. Consumption and inhibition of the function of clotting factors cause prolongation of the PT, aPTT, and thrombin time. Consumption of platelets causes thrombocytopenia. Secondary fibrinolysis generates increased titers of FDPs, which can be measured by latex agglutination or D-dimer assays. Some schistocytes may be seen in the peripheral blood smear, but this finding is neither sensitive nor specific for DIC. Chronic or compensated forms of DIC are more difficult to diagnose, with highly variable patterns of abnormalities in "DIC screen" coagulation tests. Increased D-dimers and a prolonged PT are generally more sensitive measures than are abnormalities of the aPTT and platelet count. Overcompensated synthesis of consumed clotting factors and platelets in some chronic forms of DIC may actually cause shortening of the PT and aPTT or thrombocytosis (or both), even though elevated levels of D-dimers indicate secondary fibrinolysis in such cases.

The most difficult differential diagnosis of DIC occurs in patients who have coexisting liver disease. The coagulopathy of liver failure is often indistinguishable from that of DIC, partly because advanced hepatic dysfunction is accompanied by a state of DIC. In liver failure, the combination of decreased synthesis of clotting factors, impaired clearance of activated clotting factors, secondary fibrinolysis, and thrombocytopenia from portal hypertension and hypersplenism may make the coagulopathy practically impossible to differentiate from DIC. In thrombotic microangiopathies, including thrombotic thrombocytopenic purpura and hemolytic-uremic syndrome, platelet consumption and thrombocytopenia are not accompanied by activation of clotting factors or secondary fibrinolysis; therefore the PT, aPTT, thrombin time, and D-dimers are generally normal in these disorders. Schistocytes, often with frank hemolysis, are much more prominent in the peripheral smear in thrombotic thrombocytopenic purpura and hemolytic-uremic syndrome (Chapter 175) than in DIC.

Primary fibrinolysis is disputed as a distinct entity. Some patients with a serious clinical bleeding diathesis, however, have laboratory evidence of predominantly fibrinolysis, including high levels of FDPs (D-dimers) and severe hypofibrinogenemia, with relatively little consumption of coagulation factors and normal or near-normal platelet counts. These unusual findings, which approximate the findings expected with fibrinolytic therapy, are encountered occasionally, particularly in patients with prostate cancer.

TREATMENT

Rx

Successful treatment of DIC (Table 178-2) requires that the underlying cause be identified and eliminated. All other therapies, including hemodynamic support, replacement of coagulation factors and platelets, and pharmacologic inhibitors of coagulation and fibrinolysis, are just temporizing measures. In many patients with asymptomatic, self-limited DIC who have only laboratory manifestations of the coagulopathy, no treatment may be necessary. In

TABLE 178-2 TREATMENT OF DISSEMINATED INTRAVASCULAR COAGULATION

Identify and eliminate the underlying cause
No treatment if mild, asymptomatic, and self-limited
Hemodynamic support, as indicated, in severe cases
Blood component therapy
- *Indications:* active bleeding or high risk for bleeding
  - Fresh-frozen plasma
  - Platelets
  - In some cases, consider cryoprecipitate, antithrombin III

Drug therapy
- *Indications:* heparin for DIC manifested by thrombosis or acrocyanosis; antifibrinolytic agents generally contraindicated except with life-threatening bleeding and failure of blood component therapy

DIC = disseminated intravascular coagulation.

patients with DIC who are actively bleeding or who are at high risk for bleeding, the blood component treatments of choice are transfusions of platelets to improve the thrombocytopenia and fresh-frozen plasma to replace all consumed coagulation factors and correct the prolonged PT and aPTT. Large volumes of plasma (e.g., >6 U/24 hours) may be required to ameliorate bleeding in severe cases. In some patients who have particularly profound hypofibrinogenemia, the additional transfusion of cryoprecipitate, a plasma concentrate that is enriched in fibrinogen, may be useful. The theoretical concern that these blood products could "fuel the fire" and exacerbate the DIC has not been supported by clinical experience.

The use of pharmacologic inhibitors of coagulation and fibrinolysis in DIC is controversial. Heparin is of theoretical benefit because it blocks thrombin activity and quenches intravascular coagulation and the resultant secondary fibrinolysis. In practice, heparin might exacerbate the bleeding tendency in acute DIC. Heparin is usually reserved for special forms of DIC, including those manifested by thrombosis or acrocyanosis and forms that accompany cancer, vascular malformations, retained dead fetus, and possibly acute promyelocytic leukemia. In cases of DIC in which thrombosis or acral ischemia predominates, unfractionated heparin should be used by continuous infusion owing to its short half-life and reversibility in the event of increased bleeding. Monitoring the aPTT in the presence of DIC may be problematic, so heparin infusion in this setting should be followed mainly by clinical response and improvement in other tests of coagulation (e.g., thrombocytopenia). Antifibrinolytic agents, including ε-aminocaproic acid and tranexamic acid, are generally contraindicated in DIC. By blocking the secondary fibrinolytic response to DIC, these drugs cause unopposed fibrin deposition and may precipitate thrombosis. Antifibrinolytic agents may be effective in decreasing life-threatening bleeding in DIC, however, particularly in extreme cases in which aggressive blood component replacement fails to control the hemorrhage; in such situations, simultaneous infusion of low doses of heparin may reduce the risk for thrombosis.

A 96-hour infusion of recombinant human activated protein C (rhAPC; drotrecogin alfa [activated]), which has both anticoagulant and anti-inflammatory properties, significantly reduces mortality in patients with severe sepsis and high risk of death; it should be urgently considered in such specific cases of DIC.[1] However, it does not benefit septic patients with a low risk of death, such as those with only single-organ failure or Acute Physiology and Chronic Health Evaluation (APACHE) II scores of less than 25; in fact, it is associated with increased serious bleeding complications in these patients.[2] Because of the increased risk for intracerebral hemorrhage with severe thrombocytopenia, rhAPC must be used cautiously in patients with DIC and in conjunction with platelet transfusion if the platelet count is less than 30,000/mm^3. Although recombinant tissue factor pathway inhibitor and antithrombin III concentrates may have some efficacy in improving laboratory parameters of DIC, the overall survival benefit with these agents in patients with DIC has not been demonstrated.

LIVER FAILURE

Bleeding complications in patients with advanced liver disease (Chapters 156 and 157) can be severe and even fatal and directly account for about 20% of the deaths associated with hepatic failure. The extent of the bleeding tendency depends on the severity and type of liver disease involved. About one third of deaths in patients undergoing liver transplantation are attributable to perioperative hemorrhage.

PATHOBIOLOGY

The pathophysiology of bleeding in liver failure is complex and multifactorial. Anatomic abnormalities resulting from portal hypertension are frequently the major cause of gastrointestinal bleeding in patients with liver disease.

TABLE 178-3 COAGULATION ABNORMALITIES IN LIVER DISEASE

ABNORMALITIES IN COAGULATION

Decreased synthesis of coagulation factors
Impaired vitamin K–dependent γ-carboxylation
Dysfibrinogenemia
Disseminated intravascular coagulation
Increased fibrinolytic activity

ABNORMALITIES IN PLATELETS

Thrombocytopenia (hypersplenism)
Abnormal platelet function

Upper gastrointestinal bleeding can be caused by esophageal varices or hemorrhagic gastritis (congestive gastropathy), whereas lower gastrointestinal bleeding, although seldom life-threatening, can be due to hemorrhoids.

The complexity of the systemic coagulopathy of liver failure is not surprising inasmuch as the liver is the principal organ site for the synthesis of coagulation and fibrinolytic factors as well as their protein inhibitors (Table 178-3). Hepatocytes produce all of the clotting factors except von Willebrand factor, and advanced parenchymal liver disease results in impaired synthesis of these proteins. Liver disease can also cause impairment in vitamin K–dependent γ-carboxylation of the procoagulant factors II, VII, IX, and X, as well as the anticoagulant proteins C and S. Functional abnormalities of fibrinogen, termed *dysfibrinogenemias,* are frequently found in various forms of liver disease, particularly in hepatocellular carcinoma. Most forms of advanced liver disease are accompanied by some degree of DIC caused by impaired synthesis of inhibitors of blood coagulation and defective hepatocellular clearance of activated coagulation factors. DIC is an especially important potential complication of LeVeen shunts used to treat intractable ascites because this procedure introduces procoagulant-rich ascitic fluid into the systemic circulation. In many of these cases, shunt ligation is required to terminate the DIC. DIC and bleeding risk are exacerbated by the enhanced fibrinolytic activity of liver disease caused by increased levels of tissue plasminogen activator accompanied by decreased synthesis of inhibitors of plasminogen activator and plasmin.

Quantitative and qualitative abnormalities of platelets also contribute to the bleeding diathesis of liver failure. Congestive splenomegaly secondary to portal hypertension causes increased pooling of platelets in the spleen (hypersplenism). The resultant thrombocytopenia, the degree of which generally correlates with spleen size, rarely causes a reduction in the platelet count to less than 50,000/mm^3. In alcoholic patients, suppression of bone marrow thrombopoiesis by the acute toxic effects of alcohol or folate deficiency may contribute to the thrombocytopenia. Qualitative platelet abnormalities have also been described in patients with liver disease.

Liver transplantation (Chapter 157) poses special problems to the coagulation system. During the anhepatic stage of surgery, which lasts about 2 hours, the complete cessation of synthesis of coagulation factors causes further prolongation of the PT and aPTT. Release of tissue plasminogen activator from the newly grafted liver leads to increased fibrinolysis and transient exacerbation of bleeding risk in the postoperative period.

CLINICAL MANIFESTATIONS

The most common hemorrhagic complication of liver disease is gastrointestinal bleeding, which is usually caused by anatomic abnormalities and exacerbated by the systemic coagulopathy of liver failure. Bleeding from other mucosal sites, extensive ecchymoses, or more serious hemorrhage into the retroperitoneum or central nervous system generally indicates more significant derangements of the coagulation system.

The severe coagulopathy in patients with liver disease makes liver biopsy a potentially hazardous procedure. The PT and platelet count are the best guides to bleeding risk. In general, liver biopsy can be performed safely if the PT and aPTT do not exceed 1.5 times control values and the platelet count is greater than 50,000/mm^3. Fresh-frozen plasma (see Treatment) can be infused to correct the prolonged PT and aPTT. Bleeding time is not a reliable predictor of bleeding risk after biopsy.

DIAGNOSIS

Although the PT and aPTT are often prolonged in patients with advanced liver disease, the former tends to be a more sensitive assay early in the course;

a disproportionate prolongation of the aPTT should raise suspicion of a coexisting coagulation abnormality, such as a lupus anticoagulant or clotting factor inhibitor. A prolonged PT is also a useful prognostic indicator of poor outcome in patients with cirrhosis, acute acetaminophen hepatotoxicity, and acute viral hepatitis; in the latter, it is a better index of prognosis than are serum albumin or transaminases. A disproportionate prolongation of the thrombin time should suggest the presence of dysfibrinogenemia. Hypersplenism (Chapter 171), possibly associated with nutritional folate deficiency or the acute toxic effects of alcohol on bone marrow, often causes mild to moderate thrombocytopenia in patients with liver disease; however, consideration should be given to other coexisting causes of thrombocytopenia if the platelet count is significantly less than 50,000/mm^3.

The coagulopathy of liver failure is often indistinguishable from that of DIC, in part because some degree of DIC is a necessary accompaniment of advanced liver disease. In general, patients with DIC have more marked decreases in levels of factor VIII and increases in D-dimer than patients with liver failure.

TREATMENT Rx

Therapy for the coagulopathy of liver disease may be directed at preventing the hemorrhagic complications of invasive procedures or treating active bleeding. The most effective treatment is blood component therapy with fresh-frozen plasma (which contains all the coagulation factors) and platelet transfusions (Chapter 180). Some patients require large volumes of fresh-frozen plasma (15 to 20 mL/kg) to lower the prolonged PT; rarely, plasmapheresis with plasma exchange is required to avoid fluid overload in these situations. Because of the short half-lives of some clotting factors, fresh-frozen plasma may have to be administered every 8 to 12 hours to maintain acceptable coagulation test parameters. In some patients, especially those with cholestasis, parenteral administration of vitamin K can at least partially reverse the coagulation abnormalities; however, in patients with advanced hepatocellular failure, vitamin K is largely ineffective. Prothrombin complex concentrates are relatively contraindicated in patients with liver failure, as in those with DIC, because of the risk of thrombotic complications. Because of immediate pooling of transfused platelets in the enlarged spleen of patients with hypersplenism, a higher than calculated dose of platelet concentrates is usually required to increase circulating platelet counts significantly.

A recent randomized, controlled trial failed to demonstrate a beneficial effect of recombinant activated factor VII (rhVIIa) for variceal bleeding in patients with advanced cirrhosis.[3] Routine use of rfVIIa for the coagulopathy of liver disease cannot be recommended at this time. Desmopressin (DDAVP), which can shorten the bleeding time of patients with cirrhosis, may be considered as ancillary therapy in patients undergoing invasive procedures.

VITAMIN K DEFICIENCY

Vitamin K is required for γ-carboxylation of glutamic acid residues of the procoagulant factors II (prothrombin), VII, IX, and X and the anticoagulant factors protein C and protein S. This post-translational modification normally renders these proteins functionally active in coagulation. The PT is more sensitive than the aPTT in detecting vitamin K deficiency states because factor VII, the only vitamin K–dependent factor that is in the extrinsic pathway of coagulation, is the most labile of these proteins.

The two major sources of vitamin K are dietary intake and synthesis by the bacterial flora of the intestine. In the absence of malabsorption, nutritional deficiency alone rarely causes clinically significant vitamin K deficiency. The condition can arise, however, when eradication of gut flora is combined with inadequate dietary intake. This situation typically occurs in critically ill patients in intensive care units who have no oral intake and are receiving broad-spectrum antibiotics for prolonged periods. Vitamin K deficiency can also develop in patients receiving total parenteral nutrition unless the infusions are supplemented with vitamin K.

Vitamin K is absorbed predominantly in the ileum and requires the presence of bile salts. Clinically significant vitamin K deficiency occurs with malabsorption of fat-soluble vitamins secondary to obstructive jaundice (Chapter 158) or with malabsorption caused by intrinsic small bowel diseases, including celiac sprue, short-bowel syndrome, and inflammatory bowel disease (Chapters 142 and 143).

Warfarin (Chapter 37) acts as an anticoagulant by competitive antagonism of vitamin K. Rare cases of hereditary deficiency of the vitamin K–dependent coagulation factors may cause a lifelong bleeding tendency.

Correction of vitamin K deficiency, when clinically significant, can be achieved with oral supplementation, unless malabsorption is present. In the latter case, parenteral vitamin K (10 mg subcutaneously daily) should be administered. Emergency treatment of bleeding caused by vitamin K deficiency is transfusion of fresh-frozen plasma.

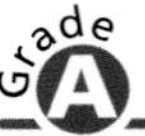

1. Bernard GR, Vincent JL, Laterre PF, et al. Efficacy and safety of recombinant human activated protein C for severe sepsis. *N Engl J Med.* 2001;344:699-709.
2. Abraham E, Laterre PF, Garg R. Drotrecogin alfa (activated) for adults with severe sepsis and a low risk of death. *N Engl J Med.* 2005;353:1332-1341.
3. Bosch J, Thabut D, Albillos A, et al. Recombinant factor VIIa for variceal bleeding in patients with advanced cirrhosis: a randomized, controlled trial. *Hepatology.* 2008;47:1604-1614.

SUGGESTED READINGS

Kitchens CS. Thrombocytopenia and thrombosis in disseminated intravascular coagulation (DIC). *Hematol Am Soc Hematol Educ Progr.* 2009;240-246. *Case-based discussion of contemporary issues in DIC.*

Levi M, Meijers JC. DIC: which laboratory tests are most useful. *Blood Rev.* 2011;25:33-37. *Review including more recently developed dynamic algorithms.*

Montagnana M, Franchi M, Danese E, et al. Disseminated intravascular coagulation in obstetric and gynecologic disorders. *Semin Thromb Hemost.* 2010;36:404-418. *Review.*

Munoz SJ, Stravitz RT, Gabriel DA. Coagulopathy of acute liver failure. *Clin Liver Dis.* 2009;13:95-107. *Review of the epidemiology, pathophysiology, presentation, evaluation, and management of coagulopathy in acute liver failure.*

Takemitsu T, Wada H, Hatada T, et al. Prospective evaluation of three different diagnostic criteria for disseminated intravascular coagulation. *Thromb Haemost.* 2011;115:40-44. *The platelet count, prothrombin time, fibrin and fibrinogen degradation products, and fibrinogen are the key diagnostic criteria.*

179 THROMBOTIC DISORDERS: HYPERCOAGULABLE STATES

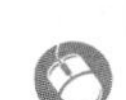

ANDREW I. SCHAFER

The *hypercoagulable states,* also referred to as *thrombophilias,* encompass a group of inherited or acquired conditions that cause a risk for thrombosis.

The primary hypercoagulable states are quantitative or qualitative abnormalities in specific coagulation proteins that induce a prothrombotic state. Most of these disorders involve inherited mutations and polymorphisms that lead to either (1) a deficiency of a physiologic antithrombotic factor or (2) an increased level of a prothrombotic factor (Table 179-1). Particularly when they are combined with other inherited prothrombotic mutations (multigene interactions), these primary hypercoagulable states are associated with a lifelong predisposition to thrombosis. The secondary hypercoagulable states, a diverse group of mostly acquired conditions, cause a thrombotic tendency by more complex, often multifactorial mechanisms. The trigger for a discrete, clinical thrombotic event is often the development of one of the acquired, secondary hypercoagulable states superimposed on an inherited state of hypercoagulability.

TABLE 179-1 PRIMARY HYPERCOAGULABLE STATES

DEFICIENCY OF ANTITHROMBOTIC FACTORS
Antithrombin (III) deficiency
Protein C deficiency
Protein S deficiency
INCREASED PROTHROMBOTIC FACTORS
Factor Va (activated protein C resistance; factor V Leiden)
Prothrombin (prothrombin G20210A mutation)
Factor IX Padua (factor IX R338L mutation)
Factors VII, XI, IX, VIII; von Willebrand's factor; fibrinogen (epidemiologic data; molecular mechanisms unknown)

PRIMARY HYPERCOAGULABLE STATES

Antithrombin III Deficiency

EPIDEMIOLOGY AND PATHOBIOLOGY

Inherited quantitative or qualitative deficiency of antithrombin III leads to increased fibrin accumulation and a lifelong propensity to thrombosis (Chapter 174). Antithrombin is the major physiologic inhibitor of thrombin and other activated coagulation factors; therefore, its deficiency leads to unregulated protease activity and fibrin formation.

The frequency of asymptomatic heterozygous antithrombin deficiency in the general population may be 1 in 350. Most of these individuals have clinically silent mutations and never have thrombotic manifestations. The frequency of symptomatic antithrombin deficiency in the general population has been estimated to be between 1 in 2000 and 1 in 5000. Among all patients seen with venous thromboembolism (VTE), antithrombin deficiency is detected in only about 1 to 2%, but it is found in approximately 2.5% of selected patients with recurrent thrombosis or onset of thrombosis at a younger age (<45 years old).

Patients with type I antithrombin deficiency have proportionately reduced plasma levels of antigenic and functional antithrombin that result from a quantitative deficiency of the normal protein. Impaired synthesis, defective secretion, or instability of antithrombin in type I antithrombin-deficient individuals is caused by major gene deletions, single nucleotide changes, or short insertions or deletions in the antithrombin gene. Patients with type II antithrombin deficiency have normal or nearly normal plasma antigen accompanied by low activity levels, characteristics indicative of a functionally defective molecule. Type II deficiency is usually caused by specific point mutations leading to single amino acid substitutions that produce a dysfunctional protein. More than 250 different mutations causing type I or type II antithrombin deficiency have been recognized to date.

The pattern of inheritance of antithrombin deficiency is autosomal dominant. Most affected individuals are heterozygotes whose antithrombin levels are typically about 40 to 60% of normal. These individuals may have the full clinical manifestations of lifelong hypercoagulability. Rare homozygous antithrombin-deficient patients generally have type II deficiency with reduced heparin affinity, a variant that is associated with a low risk for thrombosis in its heterozygous form; other forms of homozygous antithrombin deficiency are probably incompatible with life.

Protein C Deficiency

Protein C deficiency leads to unregulated fibrin generation because of impaired inactivation of factors VIIIa and Va, two essential cofactors in the coagulation cascade.

EPIDEMIOLOGY

The prevalence of heterozygous protein C deficiency in the general population is about 1 per 200 to 500. Protein C deficiency is found in 2 to 5% of all patients with VTE.

PATHOBIOLOGY

AS with antithrombin deficiency, two general forms of protein C deficiency are recognized: type I, in which quantitative deficiency of the protein is associated with a proportionate decrease in protein C antigen and activity, and type II, in which qualitative defects in protein C are associated with disproportionately reduced protein C activity relative to antigen. More than 160 mutations are known to cause protein C deficiency. In the more common type I deficiency, frameshift, nonsense, or missense mutations cause premature termination of synthesis or loss of protein C stability. In type II deficiency, different mutations can cause abnormalities in protein C activation or function. The mode of inheritance of protein C deficiency is autosomal dominant. As in antithrombin deficiency, most affected individuals are heterozygotes.

Protein S Deficiency

Protein S is the principal cofactor of activated protein C (APC), and its deficiency mimics that of protein C in causing loss of regulation of fibrin generation by impaired inactivation of factors VIIIa and Va.

EPIDEMIOLOGY

The exact prevalence of protein S deficiency in the general population is unknown but is estimated to be less than 0.5%. Its frequency in all patients evaluated for VTE (1 to 3%) is comparable to that of protein C deficiency.

PATHOBIOLOGY

Protein S circulates in plasma partly in complex with C4b binding protein; only free protein S, which normally constitutes about 35 to 40% of total protein S, can function as a cofactor of APC. As in antithrombin and protein C deficiencies, quantitative (type I) and qualitative (type II) forms of inherited protein S deficiency are known. In addition, type III protein S deficiency is characterized by normal plasma levels of total protein S but low levels of free protein S.

Relatively few specific mutations of the protein S gene have been described to date. Most involve frameshift, nonsense, or missense point mutations.

Activated Protein C Resistance (Factor V Leiden)

EPIDEMIOLOGY

The factor V Leiden mutation is remarkably frequent (3 to 7%) in healthy white populations but is far less prevalent in certain black and Asian populations. In various studies, APC resistance was found in a wide range of frequencies (10 to 64%) in patients with VTE.

PATHOBIOLOGY

Almost all subjects with functional APC resistance have a single, specific point mutation in the gene for factor V, which is a critical target of the physiologic anticoagulant action of APC. In this mutation, termed *factor V Leiden,* guanine is replaced with adenine at nucleotide 1691 (G1691A), which leads to the amino acid substitution of Arg504 by Gln and renders factor Va incapable of being inactivated by APC. Heterozygosity for the autosomally transmitted factor V Leiden mutation increases the risk for thrombosis by a factor of 5 to 10, whereas homozygosity increases the risk by a factor of 50 to 100.

Prothrombin Gene Mutation

The substitution of G for A at nucleotide 20210 of the prothrombin gene has been associated with elevated plasma levels of prothrombin and an increased risk for venous thrombosis. The allele frequency for this gain-of-function mutation is 1 to 6% in white populations, but it is much less prevalent in other racial groups. The prothrombin G20210A mutation is found in 3 to 8% of all patients with venous thromboembolism.

Other Primary Hypercoagulable States

The first X-linked thrombophilia was recently reported. A family with a gain-of-function mutation in the gene for coagulation factor IX (factor IX-R338L) had juvenile thrombophilia associated with a five- to ten-fold increase in factor IX clotting activity (with normal quantitative protein levels). Elevated levels of factor VIII coagulant activity are a significant risk factor for venous thrombosis, and family studies suggest that high factor VIII levels are often genetically determined. Increased levels of factors VII, IX, and XI, fibrinogen, von Willebrand factor, and thrombin-activatable fibrinolysis inhibitor, as well as very low levels of tissue factor pathway inhibitor, may also confer increased risk. Many other inherited abnormalities of specific physiologic antithrombotic systems may be associated with a thrombotic tendency. Most of these conditions are limited to case reports or family studies, their molecular genetic bases are less well defined, and their prevalence rates are unknown but are probably much lower than those of the disorders described earlier. The other primary hypercoagulable states include heparin cofactor II deficiency, dysfunctional thrombomodulin, and many fibrinolytic disorders that lead to impaired fibrin degradation, including hypoplasminogenemia, dysplasminogenemia, plasminogen activator deficiency, and certain dysfibrinogenemias that cause a thrombotic rather than a bleeding diathesis.

CLINICAL MANIFESTATIONS

The primary hypercoagulable states are associated with predominantly venous thromboembolic complications (see Table 174-2 in Chapter 174). Deep vein thrombosis of the lower extremities and pulmonary embolism are the most frequent clinical manifestations. Venous thromboses occurring in more unusual sites include superficial thrombophlebitis and mesenteric and cerebral venous thrombosis (see Table 174-2 in Chapter 174). Arterial thrombosis involving the coronary, cerebrovascular, and peripheral circulations is not linked to any of the primary hypercoagulable states, although some reports have described its occurrence with protein S deficiency and homozygous antithrombin deficiency. Venous thrombosis can also result in arterial occlusion by paradoxical embolism across a patent foramen ovale.

The initial episode of VTE can occur at any age in patients with primary hypercoagulable states, but it typically takes place in early adulthood. Positive family histories of thrombosis can frequently be elicited. The risk for thrombosis varies among the individual primary hypercoagulable states and is highest in patients with deficiencies of antithrombotic factors (Table 179-2); it is markedly increased with the coexistence of multiple prothrombotic mutations. Patients with homozygous deficiency states tend to have more severe thrombotic complications. A peculiar manifestation of homozygous protein C or protein S deficiency is neonatal purpura fulminans. This serious, sometimes fatal syndrome is caused by ischemic necrosis secondary to widespread thrombosis of small cutaneous and subcutaneous vessels. Fatal purpura fulminans associated with a bleeding diathesis has also been described in a patient with an acquired immunoglobulin G (IgG) inhibitor of protein C. Warfarin-induced skin necrosis (Fig. 179-1) very infrequently complicates the initiation of oral anticoagulant therapy in patients with heterozygous protein C or protein S deficiency. Because both these proteins depend on vitamin K for normal function, their plasma levels in patients with inherited deficiency states may drop to nearly zero within a few days of starting therapy with warfarin, a vitamin K antagonist, and lead to a transient prothrombotic imbalance and skin necrosis caused by dermal vascular thrombosis. Nevertheless, oral anticoagulation provides effective long-term antithrombotic prophylaxis in these individuals.

TABLE 179-2 INHERITED HYPERCOAGULABLE STATES (THROMBOPHILIAS): EPIDEMIOLOGY AND RISK OF VENOUS THROMBOEMBOLISM (VTE)

	Prevalence (%)		*Relative Risk*	
THROMBOPHILIA	**GENERAL POPULATION***	**UNSELECTED VTE**	**FIRST VTE**	**RECURRENT VTE**
Antithrombin deficiency	0.02-0.3	1-2	5-8	2.5
Protein C deficiency	0.2-0.5	2-5	5-8	2.5
Protein S deficiency	<0.5	1-3	1.7-8	2.5
Factor V Leiden	3-7	10-65	5-10†	1.3
Factor II G20210A	1-6	3-8	1.5-3.8	1.4
FV Leiden + FII G20210A	0.01	—	20-60	2.5

*Data refer to white populations. Prevalence of FV Leiden and FII G20210A is <0.1% in African, African American, and Asian populations.
†Relative risk of first VTE with homozygous FV Leiden is up to ten-fold higher (50-100).
Modified from Coppola A, Tufano A, Cerbone AM, et al. Inherited thrombophilia: implications for prevention and treatment of venous thromboembolism. *Semin Thromb Hemostas.* 2009; 35:683-694.

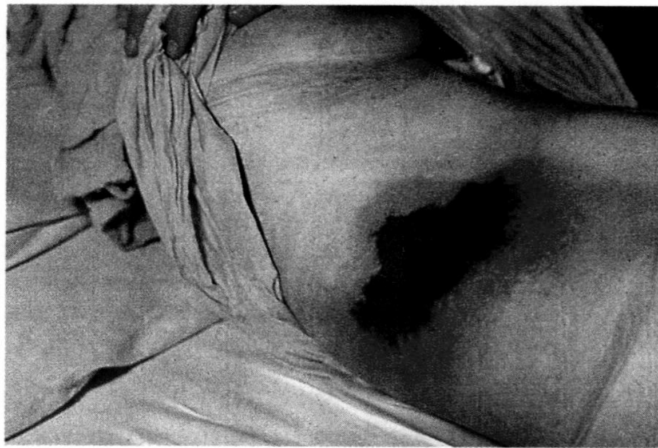

FIGURE 179-1. Acute skin necrosis in a patient with protein C deficiency who was treated with heparin and warfarin for deep vein thrombosis that occurred after elective hip surgery. Warfarin treatment was withdrawn and anticoagulation continued with heparin. Skin grafting of the affected area was required. (From Forbes CD, Jackson WF. *Color Atlas and Text of Clinical Medicine,* 3rd ed. London: Mosby; 2003.)

In most patients with primary hypercoagulable states, discrete clinical thrombotic complications appear to be precipitated by acquired prothrombotic events (e.g., pregnancy, use of oral contraceptives, surgery, trauma, immobilization), many of which are the secondary hypercoagulable states discussed subsequently. In particular, thrombosis complicates pregnancy, especially during the puerperium, in about 30 to 60% of women with antithrombin deficiency, 10 to 20% with protein C or protein S deficiency, and almost 30% with APC resistance (factor V Leiden), unless prophylactic anticoagulation is administered during this period.

DIAGNOSIS

Laboratory diagnosis (Chapter 174) of the primary hypercoagulable states requires testing for each of the disorders individually because no general screening test is available to determine whether a patient may have such a condition. Factor V Leiden can be diagnosed by a DNA-based assay or by a functional test for APC resistance: the former is required to distinguish between heterozygous and homozygous states. DNA-based assay is required to identify the prothrombin G20210A mutation. In contrast, many different mutations have been found in the genes for antithrombin, protein C, and protein S, so DNA-based tests are not practical for the diagnosis of these inherited deficiency states. Therefore, they are detected by functional and immunologic tests. Because type II ("qualitative") deficiencies of antithrombin, protein C, and protein S exhibit normal immunologic levels, functional assays for these proteins are better screening tests.

A reasonable diagnostic approach at this time is to screen at least all "strongly thrombophilic" patients after an initial episode of VTE: individuals with (1) a documented event before 50 years of age, (2) a positive family history, (3) massive or submassive pulmonary embolism, or (4) spontaneous thrombosis at an unusual site (e.g., intra-abdominal or cerebral). Analysis of results from a recent randomized trial showed that recurrent VTE was not increased in the presence of factor V Leiden, prothrombin G20210A mutation, antithrombin deficiency, or elevated levels of factor VIII, XI, or homocysteine.[1] However, there have been no controlled clinical trials to date that have assessed the benefit of testing for thrombophilia on the risk of recurrent VTE.[2] Although indefinite anticoagulation is recommended for patients who have had two or more VTE events, regardless of whether a primary hypercoagulable state is found, testing these individuals for thrombophilia may also be useful to guide family screening strategies. Individuals with arterial thrombosis generally should not be tested for any of these disorders because primary hypercoagulable states (see Table 179-1) are not clearly associated with an increased risk for arterial thrombosis. In contrast, some of the secondary hypercoagulable states, including hyperhomocysteinemia and the antiphospholipid syndrome (see later), are associated with an increased risk for arterial as well as venous thrombosis.

In general, testing for primary hypercoagulable states is not recommended immediately after a major thrombotic event, but rather in clinically stable patients at least 2 weeks after completing oral anticoagulation following a thrombotic episode. Active thrombosis may transiently consume and deplete some of the proteins in plasma and lead to the erroneous diagnosis of inherited antithrombin, protein C, or protein S deficiency. In addition to acute thrombosis, pregnancy, estrogen use, liver disease, and disseminated intravascular coagulation (DIC) may cause acquired deficiencies of antithrombin, protein C, or protein S. Anticoagulation may also interfere with some of the functional tests for primary hypercoagulable states. Heparin treatment can cause a decline in antithrombin levels to the deficiency range even in normal individuals. In contrast, warfarin can elevate antithrombin levels into the normal range in patients who do have an inherited deficiency state. Warfarin therapy also reduces the functional levels and, less prominently, the immunologic levels of protein C and protein S, thereby potentially leading to a misdiagnosis of inherited deficiency. When testing is indicated in patients in whom interruption of prophylactic oral anticoagulation is considered to be too risky, protein C and protein S levels can be determined after warfarin therapy has been discontinued under heparin coverage for at least 2 weeks.

As noted previously, functional assays are the best screening tests for antithrombin, protein C, and protein S deficiencies because they detect both quantitative and qualitative defects; antigenic (immunologic) assays detect only quantitative deficiencies of these proteins. Functional coagulation assays for protein C and protein S may yield spuriously low values, however, if APC resistance is present. APC resistance can be diagnosed by newer high-sensitivity and high-specificity coagulation assays or by DNA analysis of peripheral blood mononuclear cells for the factor V Leiden mutation.

TREATMENT Rx

The initial treatment of acute venous thrombosis or pulmonary embolism in patients with primary hypercoagulable states is not different from that in patients without genetic defects (Chapters 37 and 81). As in patients without known thrombophilia, thrombolytic therapy should be considered after massive venous thrombosis or pulmonary embolism. Acute management is initiated with at least 5 days of unfractionated or low-molecular-weight heparin. Oral anticoagulation with warfarin can be started on the first day of heparin use and continued for at least 6 months in patients with VTE in the absence of triggering factors (e.g., postoperative state), with regulation of the dose to maintain an international normalized ratio (INR) of the prothrombin time between 2.0 and 3.0.

Continuing oral anticoagulant prophylaxis beyond the initial 6 to 12 months after an acute episode of VTE must be weighed against continued exposure of the individual patient to the significant risk for bleeding complications. Patients with primary hypercoagulable states who have had two or more thrombotic events should receive indefinite or lifelong prophylactic anticoagulation with warfarin (Chapter 37). Indefinite or lifelong anticoagulation is probably indicated for individuals with recurrent thrombosis even in the absence of identifiable primary hypercoagulable states.

The decision to continue prophylactic oral anticoagulation beyond the initial period after the first episode of thrombosis is more difficult (Table 179-3). After a single episode of thrombosis, patients with inherited hypercoagulable states should probably receive indefinite or lifelong anticoagulation if their initial episodes were life-threatening or occurred in unusual sites (e.g., mesenteric, cerebral venous thrombosis) or if they have more than one prothrombotic genetic abnormality. Some authorities also recommend indefinite or lifelong anticoagulation after an initial venous thromboembolic event in patients whose risk of recurrence likewise appears to be increased: those with isolated heterozygous deficiencies of antithrombin, protein C, or protein S and patients with homozygous factor V Leiden. In the absence of these characteristics, particularly if the initial episode was precipitated by a transient acquired prothrombotic situation (e.g., pregnancy, postoperative state, immobilization), it is reasonable at this time to discontinue warfarin therapy after 6 to 12 months and administer subsequent prophylactic anticoagulation only during high-risk periods.

Asymptomatic individuals with known thrombophilia who have not had previous thrombotic complications do not require prophylactic anticoagulation except during periods of high risk for thrombosis. Because about half of the first-degree relatives of a patient with a primary hypercoagulable state should be affected, these individuals should be counseled about the implications of making a diagnosis.

Management of pregnancy in women with primary hypercoagulable states requires special consideration because of the high risk for thrombosis, particularly during the puerperium. Women with thrombophilia who have previously had thrombosis—and probably also asymptomatic women with thrombophilia—should receive prophylactic anticoagulation throughout pregnancy and for 4 to 6 weeks postpartum, a particularly high-risk period. Coumarin derivatives cross the placenta and have the potential to cause both bleeding and teratogenic effects in the fetus; therefore, oral anticoagulants should not be used during pregnancy. Heparin does not cross the placenta and does not cause these fetal complications. Therefore, either unfractionated heparin or fixed-dose, low-molecular-weight heparin is the anticoagulant of choice during pregnancy. Neither warfarin nor heparin induces an anticoagulant effect in a breast-fed infant when the drug is given to a nursing mother, so either can be given safely when indicated in the postpartum period.

Because warfarin-induced skin necrosis (see Fig. 179-1) is a rare problem, screening of all patients for inherited protein C or protein S deficiency, conditions that are known to predispose to this complication, is not indicated before starting warfarin therapy. Most cases can be avoided by not initiating warfarin therapy with high loading doses and by concomitant coverage with heparin. When the complication does occur, as manifested by painful red and subsequently dark, necrotic skin lesions within a few days of starting warfarin, such therapy must be discontinued immediately, vitamin K administered, and heparin started (Chapter 37). The use of fresh-frozen plasma or purified protein C concentrate to normalize protein C levels rapidly can improve results. Despite this rare complication, warfarin is an effective, long-term prophylactic anticoagulant in patients with inherited protein C or protein S deficiency.

Antithrombin III concentrate purified from normal human plasma may be a useful adjunct to anticoagulation in "heparin-resistant" patients, who represent unusual cases of type II antithrombin deficiency, and in antithrombin-deficient patients with recurrent thrombosis despite adequate anticoagulation. Infusion of antithrombin concentrate can also be considered in some perioperative or obstetric settings in which anticoagulation poses an unacceptable bleeding risk.

TABLE 179-3 LONG-TERM MANAGEMENT OF PATIENTS WITH PRIMARY HYPERCOAGULABLE STATES

RISK CLASSIFICATION	MANAGEMENT
High risk ≥2 spontaneous thromboses 1 spontaneous life-threatening thrombosis 1 spontaneous thrombosis at an unusual site (e.g., mesenteric, cerebral venous) 1 spontaneous thrombosis in the presence of antiphospholipid syndrome, antithrombin deficiency, or more than a single hypercoagulable state	Indefinite anticoagulation or lifelong chronic anticoagulation
Moderate risk 1 thrombosis with an acquired prothrombotic stimulus	Vigorous prophylaxis during high-risk situations
Asymptomatic	

Modified from Bauer K. Approach to thrombosis. In: Loscalzo J, Schafer AI, eds. *Thrombosis and Hemorrhage*, 3rd ed. Philadelphia: Lippincott Williams & Wilkins; 2003:330-342.

SECONDARY HYPERCOAGULABLE STATES

DEFINITION

The secondary hypercoagulable states (Fig. 179-2) are diverse, mostly acquired disorders that predispose patients to thrombosis by complex, multifactorial pathophysiologic mechanisms. Many of these conditions also represent the acquired precipitating stimuli for clinical thrombotic events in individuals with a genetic predisposition (primary hypercoagulable states). Although each disorder causes thrombosis primarily through abnormalities in blood flow (rheology), the composition of blood (coagulation factors and platelet function), or the vessel wall, multiple overlapping mechanisms are operative in many of them.

Hyperhomocysteinemia

Hyperhomocysteinemia is an elevated blood level of homocysteine, a sulfhydryl amino acid derived from methionine by a transmethylation pathway (E-Fig. 179-1). Homocysteine is remethylated to methionine or catabolized to cystathionine. The major remethylation pathway requires folate and cobalamin (vitamin B_{12}) and involves the action of methylenetetrahydrofolate reductase (MTHFR); a minor remethylation pathway is mediated by betaine-homocysteine methyltransferase. Alternatively, homocysteine is converted to cystathionine in a trans-sulfuration pathway catalyzed by cystathionine β-synthase (CBS), with pyridoxine used as a cofactor.

Homozygous CBS deficiency states that lead to severe hyperhomocysteinemia (homocystinuria) (Chapter 216) cause premature arterial atherosclerotic disease and VTE, as well as mental retardation, neurologic defects, lens ectopy, and skeletal abnormalities. By comparison, adults with heterozygous CBS deficiency, with resultant mild to moderate hyperhomocysteinemia, may have only venous or arterial thrombotic manifestations. Hyperhomocysteinemia resulting from inherited remethylation pathway defects usually involves reduced activity of MTHFR. In homozygous individuals with the autosomal recessive C677T mutation of the *MTHFR* gene, which occurs in 15% of certain populations, moderate hyperhomocysteinemia may occur and is correctable with folic acid, but it does not appear to be related to risk of venous thrombosis. Acquired causes of hyperhomocysteinemia in adults most commonly involve nutritional deficiencies of the cofactors required for homocysteine metabolism, including pyridoxine, cobalamin, and folate.

Acquired and inherited hyperhomocysteinemia is a probable risk factor for both arterial and venous thrombosis. The mechanism of homocysteine-induced thrombosis and atherogenesis involves complex, probably multifactorial effects on the vessel wall. Homocysteine can cause vascular endothelial injury, conversion of the endothelial surface of blood vessels from an antithrombotic to a prothrombotic state, and smooth muscle cell proliferation. These toxic effects of homocysteine on the vessel wall may be mediated by oxidant stress.

Vitamin supplementation with folate, pyridoxine, and cobalamin can normalize elevated blood levels of homocysteine. However, several prospective

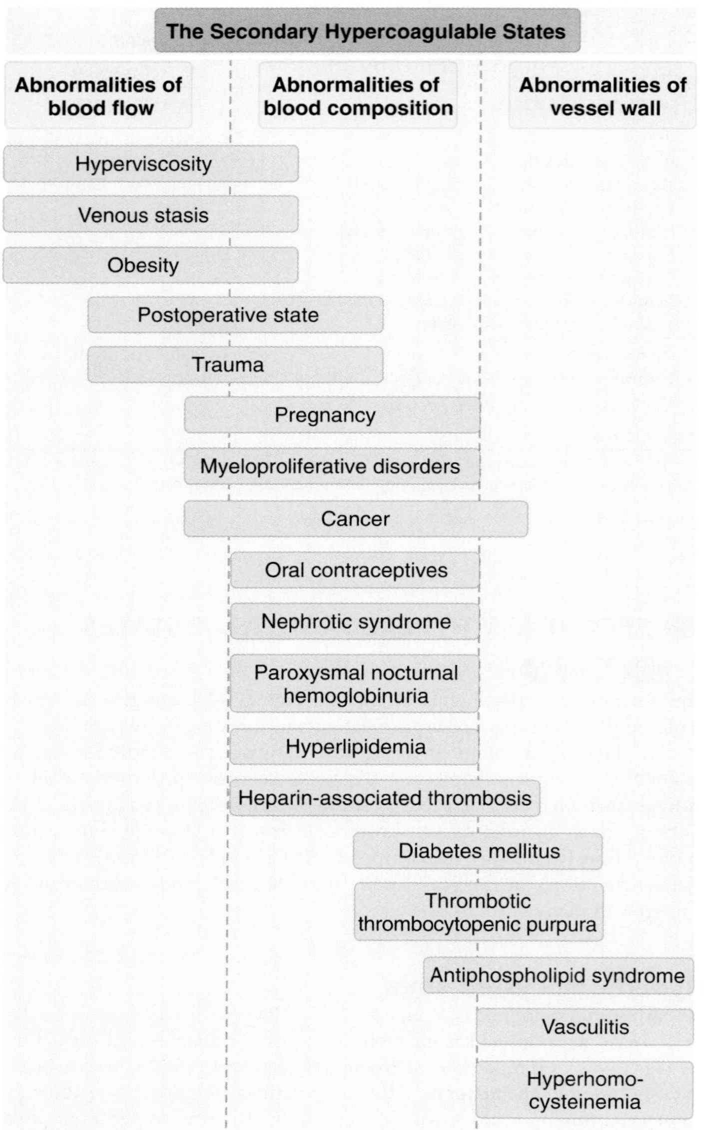

FIGURE 179-2. **Secondary hypercoagulable states.** The pathophysiologic basis of thrombotic risk in these diverse disorders is complex and multifactorial. Predominant mechanisms of thrombosis for the different secondary hypercoagulable states shown are based on Virchow's triad of thrombogenesis: abnormalities in blood flow, abnormalities in blood composition, and abnormalities of the vessel wall. (Modified from Schafer AI. The primary and secondary hypercoagulable states. In: Schafer AI, ed. *Molecular Mechanisms of Hypercoagulable States.* New York: Chapman & Hall; 1997:16.)

clinical trials of homocysteine-lowering therapy have failed to show reduced rates of vascular events in patients with established vascular disease. It remains to be determined whether this disappointing lack of clinical benefit with homocysteine-lowering vitamin therapy indicates that homocysteine is not a direct atherogenic factor, or that vitamin therapy in this setting might have other, offsetting deleterious effects, or that possibly other mechanisms are operative.

Malignancy

Multiple abnormalities of hemostasis are involved in the hypercoagulable state in cancer patients, many of which initiate a systemic process of chronic DIC (Chapter 178). The thrombotic tendency of patients with cancer may also be related to mechanical factors, such as immobility, indwelling central venous catheters, or a bulky tumor mass compressing vessels, and to comorbid conditions, such as sepsis, surgery, liver dysfunction secondary to metastases, and the prothrombotic effects of certain antineoplastic agents.

The incidence of thrombotic complications in cancer patients depends in part on the type of malignancy. Hypercoagulability is most prominent in patients with pancreatic cancer (Chapter 200), adenocarcinoma of the gastrointestinal tract (Chapters 198 and 199) or lung (Chapter 197), ovarian cancer (Chapter 205), and hematologic malignancies. The presence of underlying malignancy compounds the independent risk for thrombosis in the postoperative state. Thrombosis most commonly occurs in patients with established or concurrently diagnosed malignancy. In these patients, the risk of venous thrombosis has been found to be highest in the first few months after the diagnosis of malignancy, then decreases progressively over the subsequent 15 years. The same large case-control study showed that the risk of venous thrombosis in cancer patients is approximately 12- to 17-fold increased in those who also have the factor V Leiden or the prothrombin G20210A mutation.[3]

The most frequent thrombotic manifestations in patients with neoplasms are deep vein thrombosis and pulmonary embolism, but more unusual and distinctive thrombotic complications are also found. Trousseau's syndrome, characterized by migratory superficial thrombophlebitis of the upper or lower extremities, is strongly linked to cancer. Nonbacterial thrombotic endocarditis involves fibrin-platelet vegetations on heart valves, which produce clinical manifestations by systemic embolization (Chapter 60). Of patients with nonbacterial thrombotic endocarditis, 75% have underlying malignancies at autopsy. Trousseau's syndrome and nonbacterial thrombotic endocarditis are highly associated with adenocarcinomas. The occurrence of either syndrome in patients without known cancer demands a more vigorous search for occult malignancy than in patients with deep vein thrombosis or pulmonary embolism. Thrombotic microangiopathy (Chapter 175), characterized by hemolysis with red blood cell fragmentation, thrombocytopenia, and microvascular thrombosis with involvement of target organs, occurs in about 5% of patients with metastatic carcinomas, most commonly those with gastric (Chapter 198), lung (Chapter 197), and breast (Chapter 204) primary sites.

TREATMENT

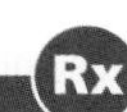

Treatment of acute VTE in cancer patients should be initiated as in other patients, but subsequent prophylactic anticoagulation should be continued while active malignancy is present. Anticoagulation can be difficult in many cancer patients; these patients may be resistant to warfarin prophylaxis. Anticoagulation can also be complicated by bleeding into tumors. Long-term treatment of cancer patients with low-molecular-weight heparin after VTE (Chapter 37) reduces recurrences and possibly decreases bleeding complications when compared with treatment with warfarin.[4]

Myeloproliferative Disorders and Paroxysmal Nocturnal Hemoglobinuria

Thrombosis and, apparently paradoxically, bleeding are major causes of morbidity and mortality in patients with myeloproliferative disorders (Chapter 169) and the related stem cell disorder paroxysmal nocturnal hemoglobinuria (Chapter 163). In uncontrolled polycythemia vera (Chapter 169), increased whole blood viscosity contributes to the thrombotic tendency. Thrombocytosis, abnormal platelet function, and other less well understood factors are also probably involved in the hemostatic defect of the myeloproliferative disorders and paroxysmal nocturnal hemoglobinuria.

In addition to deep vein thrombosis and pulmonary embolism, some distinctive thrombotic manifestations are seen. Hepatic vein thrombosis (Budd-Chiari syndrome) and portal and other intra-abdominal venous thromboses (Chapter 145) are associated with myeloproliferative disorders and paroxysmal nocturnal hemoglobinuria (Chapter 163) and may be the initial manifestations of the disease. Myeloproliferative disorders, particularly polycythemia vera (Chapter 169) and essential thrombocythemia (Chapter 169), may cause erythromelalgia, a syndrome of microvascular thrombosis manifested by intense pain accompanied by warmth, duskiness, and mottled erythema, sometimes resembling livedo reticularis, in a patchy distribution in the extremities, most prominently in the feet; digital microvascular ischemia progressing to vascular insufficiency and gangrene may ensue (Chapter 80). A wide spectrum of neurologic manifestations may be caused by cerebrovascular ischemia, especially in patients with essential thrombocythemia.

TREATMENT

Treatment of VTE in patients with the myeloproliferative disorders and paroxysmal nocturnal hemoglobinuria should be initiated as in patients without these hematologic disorders. In patients with thrombosis associated with polycythemia vera, the hematocrit should be maintained in the normal range with phlebotomies or chemotherapy, or with both (Chapter 169). Low-dose aspirin (100 mg daily) can prevent thrombotic complications without increasing the incidence of major bleeding in patients with polycythemia vera who have no contraindications to such treatment.[5] In patients with essential thrombocythemia, cytoreduction of the elevated platelet count should be achieved with chemotherapy (Chapter 169).

Antiphospholipid Syndrome

Antiphospholipid syndrome (Chapter 177) is characterized by venous and arterial thrombosis, recurrent spontaneous abortions (which may also be due to thrombosis), thrombocytopenia, and a variety of neuropsychiatric manifestations. The syndrome is associated with a heterogeneous group of autoantibodies that bind to anionic phospholipid-protein complexes, a protein cofactor of which is β_2-glycoprotein I. Patients with this syndrome have any combination of positive tests to detect different plasma antiphospholipid-protein antibodies (e.g., anticardiolipin antibodies) and phospholipid-based clotting tests (lupus anticoagulants) (Chapter 265). The predominant prothrombotic effects of these antibodies are probably directed to the vessel wall.

Deep vein thrombosis and pulmonary embolism are the most frequent venous thrombotic events in these patients. Cerebrovascular events are the most common arterial thrombotic complications and are manifested as stroke, transient ischemic attacks (Chapter 414), multi-infarct dementia (Chapter 409), or retinal artery occlusion. Peripheral and intra-abdominal vascular occlusion is encountered more rarely. About one third of these patients have nonbacterial heart valve vegetations (Libman-Sacks endocarditis). The most prominent obstetric complications are recurrent spontaneous abortions and fetal growth retardation, which are probably due to thrombosis of placental vessels. Patients are occasionally seen with "catastrophic" antiphospholipid syndrome involving a series of acute and sometimes fatal vascular occlusive events, or "thrombotic storm." Thrombotic complications are limited largely to patients with primary antiphospholipid syndrome and patients in whom the antibodies are associated with collagen vascular disease, not with drugs or infections.

TREATMENT Rx

Acute management of thrombosis in these patients is essentially the same as in other individuals. Monitoring of heparin anticoagulation is difficult in patients with a lupus anticoagulant because they already have a prolonged activated partial thromboplastin time at baseline; the use of low-molecular-weight heparin, which does not require monitoring, can circumvent this problem. Warfarin is effective in preventing recurrent thrombosis but usually requires prolonged or indefinite therapy with doses to achieve an INR of 2.0 to 3.0.[6] No established treatment of women with antiphospholipid syndrome has been shown to prevent recurrent fetal loss. Treatment with prednisone and aspirin during pregnancy is not effective in promoting live birth and may increase the risk for prematurity.

Pregnancy, Oral Contraceptives, and Hormone Replacement Therapy

The pathophysiology of hypercoagulability associated with pregnancy (Chapter 247) involves a progressive state of DIC throughout the course of pregnancy. Activation of the coagulation system is initiated locally in the uteroplacental circulation, where the placenta is the source of increased thrombin generation. Platelet activation and increased platelet turnover also occur during normal pregnancy, and about 8% of healthy women have mild thrombocytopenia at term. Simultaneously, the fibrinolytic system is progressively blunted throughout pregnancy because of the action of placental plasminogen activator inhibitor type 2. The net effect of these coagulation changes is creation of a state of hypercoagulability that makes pregnant women vulnerable to thrombosis, particularly in the puerperium. These systemic alterations are compounded by prothrombotic mechanical and rheologic factors in pregnancy, including venous stasis in the legs caused by the gravid uterus, pelvic vein injury during labor, and the trauma of cesarean section. Oral contraceptives induce a prothrombotic state by increasing procoagulant effects and decreasing physiologic anticoagulant effects. The use of oral contraceptives is associated with an increased risk for venous thrombosis, myocardial infarction, stroke, and peripheral arterial disease, particularly during the first year of use (Chapter 246). Unexpectedly, third-generation oral contraceptives, which contain less estrogen and a different progestin, double the risk for venous thromboembolism in comparison to second-generation preparations. Postmenopausal hormone replacement increases the risk for deep venous thromboembolism by a factor of 2 to 3.5, at least during the first year. Hormone replacement therapy has no beneficial and possibly even a detrimental effect on the risk for arterial disease (Chapter 248).

Deep vein thrombosis and pulmonary embolism are the most common thrombotic complications of pregnancy and the use of oral contraceptives or hormone replacement therapy. Coexisting primary hypercoagulable states are an additive risk factor in all these settings. In the absence of a clear family history of venous thromboembolism, there is little justification, however, to screen for prothrombotic mutations with pregnancy or before starting hormone replacement therapy or oral contraceptives. Increasing age, increasing parity, cesarean delivery, prolonged bedrest or immobilization, obesity, and previous thromboembolism are additional prothrombotic risk factors in pregnant women. Most thrombotic events associated with pregnancy occur in the peripartum period, especially after delivery. Special considerations for anticoagulation in the setting of pregnancy are noted in the section on treatment of primary hypercoagulable states.

Postoperative State, Immobilization, and Trauma

Postoperative thrombosis (Chapter 441) is caused by a combination of local mechanical factors, including decreased venous blood flow in the lower extremities, and systemic changes in coagulation (Chapter 81). The level of risk for postoperative thrombosis depends largely on the type of surgery performed. It is probably compounded by coexisting risk factors, such as an underlying inherited primary hypercoagulable state or malignancy, advanced age, and prolonged procedures. Postoperative deep vein thrombosis and pulmonary embolism, the most common thrombotic complications, are often asymptomatic but detectable by noninvasive studies. The incidence of deep vein thrombosis after general surgical procedures is about 20 to 25%, with almost 2% of these patients having clinically significant pulmonary embolism. The risk for deep vein thrombosis after hip surgery and knee reconstruction ranges from 45 to 70% without prophylaxis, and clinically significant pulmonary embolism occurs in 20% of patients undergoing hip surgery. Postoperative thrombosis risk after urologic and gynecologic surgery more closely approximates that found after general surgery. Although the process of thrombosis generally begins intraoperatively or within a few days of surgery, the risk for this complication can be protracted beyond the time of discharge from the hospital, particularly in hip replacement patients.

Patients who are bedridden or experiencing prolonged air travel are at increased risk for VTE. VTE is also one of the most common causes of morbidity and mortality in survivors of major trauma, and asymptomatic deep vein thrombosis of the lower extremities has been detected by venography in more than 50% of hospitalized trauma patients (Chapter 112). The risk for venous thrombosis after trauma is increased by advanced age, need for surgery or transfusions, and the presence of lower extremity fractures or spinal cord injury.

Mechanical methods of prophylaxis against VTE should be considered in high-risk postoperative patients and bedridden patients with medical conditions, either in combination with anticoagulant prophylaxis or instead of it in patients who have an unusually high risk for bleeding with anticoagulation. Such methods include graduated compression stockings, intermittent pneumatic compression devices, and venous foot pumps. For long-distance travelers with thrombophilia, either properly fitted below-knee graduated compression stockings or a single prophylactic dose of low-molecular-weight heparin injected before departure is recommended in addition to general measures such as avoidance of dehydration and frequent stretching of calf muscles.

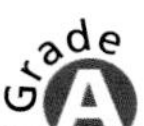

1. Kearon C, Julian JA, Kovacs MJ, et al. Influence of thrombophilia on risk of recurrent venous thromboembolism while on warfarin: results from a randomized trial. *Blood*. 2008;112:4432-4436.
2. Cohn D, Vansenne F, de Borgie C, et al. Thrombophilia testing for prevention of recurrent venous thromboembolism. *Cochrane Database Syst Rev*. 2009;1:CD007069.
3. Blom JW, Doggen CJ, Osanto S, et al. Malignancies, prothrombotic mutations, and the risk of venous thrombosis. *JAMA*. 2005;293:715-722.
4. Lee AY, Levine MN, Baker RI, et al. Low-molecular-weight heparin versus a coumarin for the prevention of recurrent venous thromboembolism in patients with cancer. *N Engl J Med*. 2003;349:146-153.
5. Landolfi R, Marchioli R, Kutti J, et al. Efficacy and safety of low-dose aspirin in polycythemia vera. *N Engl J Med*. 2004;350:114-124.

6. Crowther MA, Ginsberg JS, Julian J, et al. A comparison of two intensities of warfarin for the prevention of recurrent thrombosis in patients with the antiphospholipid antibody syndrome. *N Engl J Med.* 2003;349:1133-1138.

SUGGESTED READINGS

Coppola A, Tufano A, Cerbone AM, et al. Inherited thrombophilia: implications for prevention and treatment of venous thromboembolism. *Semin Thromb Hemostas.* 2009;35:683-694. *Review of approaches to prophylaxis and treatment of venous thromboembolism in patients with thrombophilia, based on epidemiology and risk assessment.*

Houbballah R, LaMuraglia GM. Clotting problems: diagnosis and management of underlying coagulopathies. *Semin Vasc Surg.* 2010;23:221-227. *A practical overview of diagnosis and treatment of hypercoagulable states, with a particular focus on patients with arterial thromboembolism seen by the vascular specialist.*

Lim W. Antiphospholipid antibody syndrome. *Hematol Am Soc Hematol Educ Progr.* 2009;233-239. *Concise review of the clinical approach to patients with antiphospholipid syndrome, with an emphasis on management.*

Luxembourg B, Delev D, Geisen C, et al. Molecular basis of antithrombin deficiency. *Thromb Haemost.* 2011;105:635-646. *Review citing nearly 90 different mutations.*

180

TRANSFUSION MEDICINE

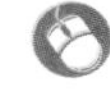

LAWRENCE T. GOODNOUGH

DEVELOPMENT OF TRANSFUSION MEDICINE

Issues in blood transfusion and blood conservation include the safety of blood, the formation of guidelines and consensus statements on the use of blood components and products, new strategies in blood conservation, emerging alternatives to blood transfusion, and informed consent for transfusion. The broad-based constituency of transfusion medicine includes blood collection facilities, hospital-based transfusion services, research laboratories, and the commercial sector.

THE TRANSFUSION MEDICINE SPECIALIST

Medical management of the blood bank involves issues related to blood inventory and safety, as well as the oversight of laboratory policies and procedures (Fig. 180-1). Management of the transfusion service includes coordinating blood transfusion and blood conservation activities and serving as a consultant to clinicians whose patients are undergoing massive transfusions, apheresis, or transplantation or who are having difficulty finding compatible blood products. Finally, the transfusion medicine specialist supervises quality assurance to satisfy regulatory and accreditation requirements.

TRANSFUSION

Worldwide, more than 75 million units of whole blood are estimated to be donated every year. In the United States, the yearly transfusion of more than 13 million units corresponds to the transfusion of 1 unit of blood every 0.39 second.

Blood Availability

Blood centers must be able to supply blood in response to acute crises. Sporadic shortages of blood and blood products (e.g., packed red cells, platelet products, albumin, intravenous immunoglobulin, and clotting factor concentrates) are potentially life threatening. Such shortages have been attributed to disruptions in production, increasingly strict criteria for accepting donors, product recalls, increased use (including off-label use), and stockpiling or other market issues.

In the United States, the Department of Health and Human Services monitors sentinel community blood services and hospital transfusion services to track blood collection and transfusion activity. Blood transfusion and collection activities peaked in 1986 and then declined until 1994. However, blood transfusion and collection subsequently increased 8.0% in 1997, 10.2% in 1999, and an estimated 4% to 5% annually thereafter.

Within the American Red Cross, which supplies about half of all blood products in the United States, a 3- to 4-day supply of red blood cell products is typical, but some independent centers have higher reserves. Use of frozen red cells as a hedge against inventory shortages has generally not been practical because the shelf life of thawed units is only 24 hours; however, an automated, functionally closed system for the glycerolization and deglycerolization processes allows a 2-week post-thaw shelf life. With such a system, many blood centers and transfusion services can expand their available red cell

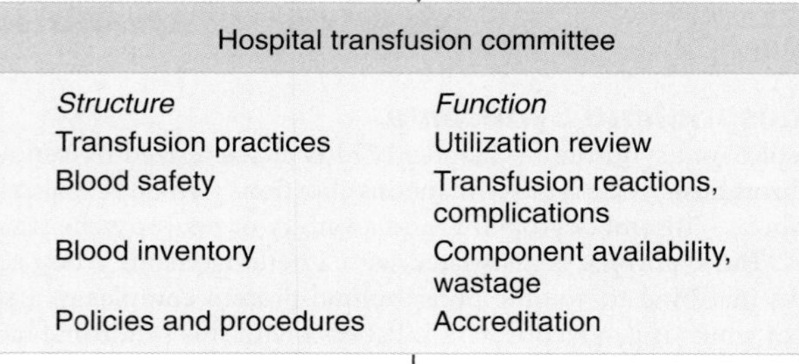

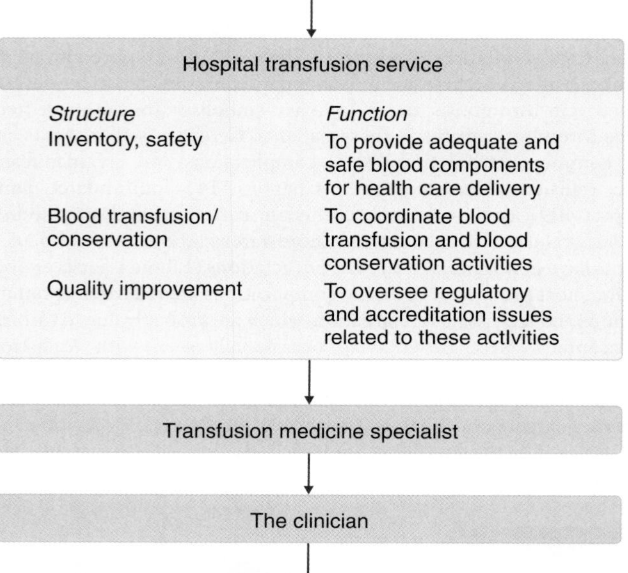

FIGURE 180-1. **A hospital's transfusion committee and transfusion service can help clinicians manage the availability, safety, and use of blood products.** (From Goodnough LT. What is a transfusion medicine specialist? *Transfusion.* 1999;39:1031-1033.)

inventories as reserves. After disasters—human or natural—on-hand blood supplies are adequate in the short term and can be rapidly mobilized over great distances. Because of the need to maintain reserves, blood collection must routinely surpass the anticipated need for blood transfusion.

Red Blood Cell Transfusion

Whole Blood

A unit of blood is collected as a donation of 450 mL ± 10% into a citrate anticoagulant that also contains phosphate and dextrose. The red cell and hemoglobin content is variable and dependent on the donor's hematocrit and the precise volume bled.

Whole blood is stored at 4 ± 2° C to diminish red cells' utilization of adenosine triphosphate and to preserve their viability, which should be at least 70% at the end of a shelf life of 35 days. After 10 days of storage, all predonation 2,3-diphosphoglycerate content in red cells is lost, but up to 50% is regenerated within 8 hours after transfusion.

In Western countries, whole blood is rarely used because within a few hours or days, some coagulation factors (especially factors V and VIII) and platelets decrease in quantity or lose viability. After a 7-day hold at 4° C, factor VIII levels fall to 0.32 ± 0.09 IU/mL, and factor V levels fall to 0.78 ± 0.15 IU/mL. At 4° C, platelets undergo a shape change from discoid to spherical that is irreversible after 8 hours, and their in vivo survival is reduced to 2 days.

Red Cell Components

Red cells are provided in various formats that differ with respect to the presence of additive solutions and the extent to which white cells are removed. Solutions that contain combinations of saline, adenine, phosphate, bicarbonate, glucose, and mannitol provide better red cell viability during storage and allow up to a 42-day shelf life. Red cells and red cells in additive solution can be used interchangeably, with the exception that red cells in additive solution are not recommended for exchange or massive transfusions in neonates.

Red cells should be refrigerated until the time of the transfusion because of the risk for bacterial proliferation within the pack at room temperature. Red cells that have been out of refrigeration for 30 minutes or longer cannot be returned to stock. A unit of red cells should be infused over a maximum period of 4 hours.

Irradiated Cellular Blood Components

Gamma-irradiated cellular blood components are used to prevent the occurrence of transfusion-associated graft-versus-host disease (see later).

Leukocyte-Reduced Blood Components

Blood components are depleted of leukocytes by means of filtration. A leukocyte-reduced component is defined as one with less than 5×10^6 residual white cells per liter, and 100% of tested units should meet this standard. Leukocyte removal should be performed while the cells are still intact by filtering the blood as soon as possible after collection.

Leukocyte reduction reduces the incidence of human leukocyte antigen (HLA) alloimmunization in multitransfused recipients, but immunization rates of 10 to 25% are still seen in women who have already been exposed to HLA alloantigens through previous pregnancy. Leukocyte reduction has less impact on refractoriness to random platelet donations because of the importance of nonimmune factors in the poor response to transfused platelets.

Leukocyte reduction also lowers the risk for nonhemolytic febrile reactions after the transfusion of red cells or platelets. Several, but not all, studies suggest that leukocyte reduction has a beneficial impact on the rate of postoperative infection. The impact of leukocyte reduction on the incidence of transfusion-associated graft-versus-host disease is unknown.

Preventing Transmission of Cytomegalovirus

A small number of studies of prestorage leukocyte reduction have suggested its efficacy in preventing transfusion-transmitted cytomegalovirus (CMV) infection (Chapter 384), which occurs in 4% of cases, even with seronegative components. Prestorage leukocyte depletion reduces the infection rate to less than 1%, suggesting that this technology may be at least equivalent to serologic testing for CMV antibodies for the prevention of CMV transmission; however, CMV testing of leukocyte-reduced components continues to be performed by most transfusion services. Indications for CMV-seronegative components include transfusion in pregnancy, intrauterine transfusion, transfusions to neonates less than 37 weeks' gestation, transfusions to CMV-seronegative patients who are potential or actual recipients of allogeneic bone marrow or peripheral blood progenitor transplants when the donor is also CMV seronegative, and patients infected with human immunodeficiency virus (HIV).

Immunomodulatory Effects

Previous transfusion has an immunomodulatory benefit for the survival of renal allografts, even with the use of potent immunosuppressive drugs, although the exact mechanism of this benefit remains unknown. Retrospective studies suggest an adverse effect of transfusion on the rate of perioperative infections or recurrent cancers.

Typing and Crossmatching

Blood and blood components for transfusion must be compatible with the same blood type as the patient. Obtaining an accurate ABO/Rh grouping for a patient is the most significant serologic test performed before transfusion. When type-specific blood and components are unavailable or emergency circumstances do not allow their identification or use, type O-negative red cells should be used. Group O is the only choice for group O recipients and is the alternative choice for groups A, B, and AB.

Red cell antigens other than ABO and D are not routinely considered when selecting *donor* blood products for transfusion; the exception is when unexpected, clinically significant red cell antibodies are present in the patient, as determined by an antibody screen or previous identification. Red cell alloantibodies are produced by exposure to foreign red cell antigens via previous transfusion, pregnancy, or both. For an antibody to be considered clinically significant, it must be associated with a hemolytic transfusion reaction or decreased survival of transfused incompatible red cells. Most of the clinically significant antibodies are optimally reactive at 37° C or are detected by the antiglobulin test. If an antibody screen is negative in the *recipient,* the probability is greater than 99% that an ABO and Rh crossmatch will also be compatible. If no unexpected, clinically significant antibodies are detected and there is no record of their previous detection, only serologic testing for ABO incompatibility is required (i.e., antiglobulin testing is not required when the crossmatch is performed).

Red Blood Cell Transfusion

If a transfusion is appropriate, a benefit should occur. In a large study of Jehovah's Witnesses (whose religious beliefs preclude the use of blood transfusion), the risk of death was higher in surgical patients with cardiovascular disease than in those without. A follow-up analysis of a subset of these patients reported that the odds of death in patients with a postoperative hemoglobin level less than 7 g/dL increased 2.5 times for each gram decrease in the hemoglobin level; although no deaths occurred in 98 patients with postoperative levels of 7.1 to 8.0 g/dL, 34.4% of 32 patients with postoperative levels of 4.1 to 5.0 g/dL died. These data suggest that in surgery-induced anemia, survival is improved if blood transfusion is administered to maintain the hemoglobin concentration at greater than 7 g/dL. In a large, retrospective study of elderly patients who underwent surgical repair of hip fractures, the use of perioperative transfusion in those with hemoglobin levels as low as 8 g/dL did not appear to influence 30- or 90-day mortality.

In a multi-institutional study, 418 critical care patients received red cell transfusions when their hemoglobin levels dropped below 7 g/dL and had their levels maintained between 7 and 9 g/dL, whereas another 420 patients received transfusions when their hemoglobin levels dropped below 10 g/dL and had their levels maintained between 10 and 12 g/dL. Thirty-day mortality rates were not significantly different in the two groups, suggesting that a transfusion threshold as low as 7 g/dL may be as safe as a higher threshold of 10 g/dL in critically ill patients.[1] A follow-up analysis found that the more restrictive strategy of red blood cell transfusion also appeared to be safe in most patients with cardiovascular disease.

A retrospective study analyzed the relationships among anemia, blood transfusion, and mortality in nearly 80,000 patients older than 65 years hospitalized for acute myocardial infarction. Anemia, defined as a hematocrit below 39%, was present on hospital admission in 44% of patients and was 33% or less in 10% of patients; blood transfusion in patients with hematocrit levels lower than 33% at admission was associated with a significantly lower 30-day mortality. On the basis of this study, transfusion to maintain hematocrit levels above 33% has been recommended in patients with acute myocardial infarction. In patients with heart failure, transfusion to maintain a hemoglobin level above 10 g/dL appears to improve outcomes. Among patients undergoing cardiac surgery, a restrictive perioperative transfusion strategy is as good as a more liberal strategy.[2]

Guidelines

Guidelines from several professional groups recommend that blood not be transfused prophylactically in patients without risk factors until the hemoglobin level is 6 to 8 g/dL; a threshold of 8 g/dL seems appropriate in surgical patients with no risk factors for ischemia, whereas a threshold of 10 to 11 g/dL can be justified for patients considered to be at risk: those with myocardial ischemia or infarction, heart failure, chronic lung disease, or chronic kidney disease. With substantial improvements in blood safety, now the concern is that some patients may be at risk for undertransfusion.

Platelet Transfusion

The use of intensive chemotherapy regimens and bone marrow or stem cell transplantation has increased the demand for platelet products, particularly in patients with severe thrombocytopenia or bleeding complications. The use of apheresis platelet transfusions (i.e., a platelet unit collected from a dedicated donor via an apheresis procedure) has increased substantially, driven by the need for platelet inventories to support cardiac surgery, oncology, and stem cell transplantation programs. Emerging issues in platelet transfusion therapy include re-evaluation of the platelet threshold for prophylactic transfusion and modification of the dose of platelet transfusions.

Threshold for Platelet Transfusion

The appropriate threshold for platelet transfusion depends on the clinical situation (Fig. 180-2). Prospective, randomized studies indicate that a platelet transfusion threshold of 10,000 cells/μL is as safe and effective as higher thresholds in patients undergoing chemotherapy or stem cell transplantation.[3]

For consumptive thrombocytopenias such as disseminated intravascular coagulation (Chapter 178), platelet therapy is supportive but not effective

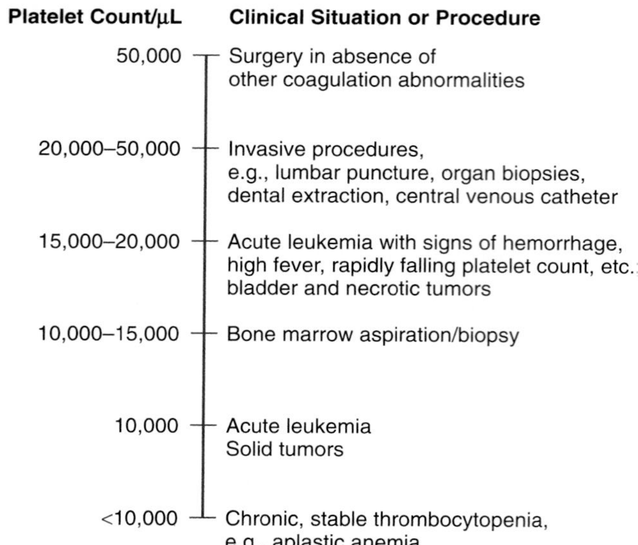

FIGURE 180-2. Threshold for providing platelet transfusions in thrombocytopenic patients.

until the underlying cause is treated. Platelet transfusions are generally not indicated in patients with idiopathic thrombocytopenic purpura or the thrombotic microangiopathies such as thrombotic thrombocytopenic purpura and hemolytic-uremic syndrome (Chapter 175).

Platelet Dose

American Association of Blood Bank (AABB) standards require that 75% of apheresis platelet products contain more than 3×10^{11} platelets; however, no consensus exists for a standardized platelet dose, and clinical trials have used a broad range of doses. In general, higher platelet doses result in greater incremental increases in the platelet count and prolonged time to the next transfusion; however, the estimated platelet half-life is similar, and there are no other differences in outcomes.

Low-dose platelet therapy (i.e., <1 platelet unit) may be more beneficial in thrombocytopenic patients who are receiving prophylactic platelet transfusions. The fixed platelet requirement for hemostasis is estimated to be $7100/\mu L^3$/day, and platelet needs above this threshold are mainly a result of platelet consumption. For patients who become thrombocytopenic as a result of myeloablative therapy, platelet survival decreases with increasing severity of thrombocytopenia. A trial of prophylactic platelet transfusions in patients with hypoproliferative thrombocytopenia found that low doses (1.1×10^{11} per square meter) of platelets led to a decreased number of transfusions but an increased number of platelets transfused (and donor exposures).[4] At doses between 1.1×10^{11} and 4.4×10^{4} platelets per square meter, no effect on the incidence of bleeding was demonstrated.

Plasma Transfusion

Plasma therapy provides a source of clotting factors for patients with inherited or acquired coagulation disorders. Patients with inherited disorders such as hemophilia (Chapter 177) or von Willebrand disease (Chapter 176) are now treated primarily with clotting factor concentrates, which are blood derivatives from processed and treated commercial lots from pooled donors. For patients with acquired coagulopathies, there is little systematically derived, evidence-based guidance to inform plasma transfusion decisions. For patients with mild prolongation of coagulation assays such as prothrombin time and partial thromboplastin time (Chapter 174), plasma therapy has little or no value in prophylaxis for invasive procedures. Plasma therapy is indicated in patients undergoing massive hemorrhage (trauma, postpartum hemorrhage, or gastrointestinal bleeding) or for emergent reversal of warfarin-associated coagulopathy (Chapter 37), such as in patients with intracranial hemorrhage. Recommended dosage in these settings is 15 to 30 mL/kg.

BLOOD SAFETY

Adverse reactions associated with transfusion are listed in Table 180-1.

TABLE 180-1 TRANSFUSION-ASSOCIATED ADVERSE REACTIONS

ADVERSE REACTION	RISK PER UNIT INFUSED
ABO-incompatible blood transfusions	1 in 30,000–60,000
Symptoms	40%
Fatalities	1 in 600,000
Delayed serologic reactions	1 in 1600
Delayed hemolytic reactions	1 in 6700
Transfusion-related acute lung injury	1 in 8000
Graft-versus-host disease	Rare
Fluid overload	Underestimated
Febrile, nonhemolytic transfusion reactions	
Red blood cells (non–leukocyte reduced/leukocyte reduced)	1 in 200/1 in 300
Platelets (non–leukocyte reduced/leukocyte reduced)	1 in 5–20/1 in 25–50
Allergic reactions	1 in 30–100
Anaphylactic reactions	1 in 150,000
Iron overload	After 80–100 U
Post-transfusion purpura	Rare
Immunosuppressive effects	Unknown

Modified from Goodnough LT. Current issues in transfusion medicine. *Clin Adv Hematol Oncol.* 2005;3:614-616.

Errors in Transfusion Medicine

The mistransfusion rate (blood transfused to other than the intended recipient) is about 1 in 14,000 to 28,000 units. About two thirds of the errors occur in the clinical arena (patient misidentification and/or specimen mislabeling at time of drawing blood for type and screen/crossmatch, incorrect identification of the recipient of the blood unit, and failure to recognize a transfusion reaction). About half of mistransfusions are ABO incompatible, and about 10% of these are fatal. The frequency of death as a result of ABO error can therefore be estimated at approximately 1 per 600,000 blood units, a risk that is higher than the risk of transmitting HIV or hepatitis C virus.

Transfusion Reactions

Acute Hemolytic Transfusion Reaction

An acute hemolytic transfusion reaction is most commonly defined as hemolysis of donor red cells within 25 hours of transfusion by preformed alloantibodies in the recipient's circulation. Life-threatening acute hemolytic transfusion reactions are most commonly due to ABO-incompatible blood being transfused to a recipient with naturally occurring ABO alloantibodies (anti-A, anti-B, anti-A, B). Clerical errors (mislabeling blood or misidentifying patients) account for 80% of such reactions.

Signs and symptoms of an acute intravascular hemolytic transfusion reaction may develop when as little as 10 to 15 mL of ABO-incompatible blood has been infused. Fever, which is the most common initial manifestation, is frequently accompanied by chills. The patient may complain of a general sense of anxiety or uneasiness or pain at the infusion site or in the back or chest (or both). The most serious sequela is acute renal failure. In an unconscious or anesthetized patient, diffuse bleeding at the surgical site may be the first indication of intravascular hemolysis and may be accompanied by hemoglobinuria and hypotension.

Treatment begins with immediate cessation of the transfusion. The risk for renal failure may be reduced by the administration of crystalloid fluids, including sodium bicarbonate (250 to 500 mg intravenously over a 1- to 4-hour period), to maintain urine pH at 7.0 and by diuresis with 20% mannitol (100 mL/m^2 in 30 to 60 minutes, followed by 30 mL/m^2/hour for 12 hours) or furosemide (40 to 120 mg intravenously).

Febrile Nonhemolytic Transfusion Reactions

Febrile nonhemolytic transfusion reactions are common and are estimated to occur in 0.5% of all red cell transfusions and up to 30% of platelet transfusions. A febrile transfusion reaction is defined as a rise in temperature greater than 1° C, which may be accompanied by chills, rigor, or both.

These reactions are thought to be due to a reaction of HLA or leukocyte-specific antigens (or both) on transfused lymphocytes, granulocytes, or platelets in the donor unit with antibodies in previously alloimmunized recipients. Multiply transfused individuals and multiparous women are most likely to experience this type of transfusion reaction. Febrile nonhemolytic transfusion reactions, especially those associated with platelet transfusions, may be caused by the infusion of biologic response modifiers, such as cytokines, that have accumulated in the platelet concentrate during storage.

Symptoms may occur during the transfusion or may not manifest until 1 to 2 hours after its completion. The diagnosis of a febrile nonhemolytic transfusion reaction is generally made by excluding other causes of fever (e.g., bacterial contamination of blood, acute hemolytic transfusion reaction).

Febrile nonhemolytic transfusion reactions in susceptible populations can often be prevented by administering antipyretics before the transfusion of blood components. Prestorage leukocyte reduction is recommended to prevent reactions resulting from the accumulation of cytokines during storage.

Allergic Reactions

Allergic reactions can be mild, moderate, or life threatening and are associated with the amount of plasma transfused. From 1 to 5% of all blood transfusion recipients experience mild allergic reactions.

Anaphylactic transfusion reactions are sometimes associated with antibodies to immunoglobulin (Ig) A, which are common and have an incidence of approximately 1 in 700 individuals. However, the incidence of anaphylactic transfusion reactions is much lower—1 in 20,000 to 50,000.

Urticarial reactions are not well understood but are believed to be an interaction between antibodies in the recipient's plasma and plasma proteins in the donor blood. There is usually no specific identifiable antigen to which the patient is reacting. Symptoms are generally mild and include localized urticaria, erythema, and itching.

Anaphylactic or anaphylactoid reactions, which can occur after the transfusion of only a few milliliters of blood or plasma, include skin flushing, nausea, abdominal cramps, vomiting, diarrhea, laryngeal edema, hypotension, shock, cardiac arrhythmia, cardiac arrest, and loss of consciousness. Fever is notably absent. In some cases, there may be symptoms indicative of airway involvement, such as hoarseness, wheezing, dyspnea, and substernal pain. Management begins with discontinuation of the transfusion. Treatment is diphenhydramine (25 to 50 mg intravenously), but more severe episodes may require aggressive therapy (Chapters 260 and 261).

Patients who experience recurrent allergic or urticarial reactions can be treated with antihistamines before transfusion. Washed red blood cells may be indicated for patients who experience repeated severe urticarial reactions.

Bacterial Contamination

Bacterial contamination may be introduced into a unit of blood through skin contaminants during venipuncture or from donors with asymptomatic bacteremia. Multiplication of bacteria can occur in blood and blood components stored at refrigerated temperatures but is more likely to occur in platelets stored at room temperature.

Bacterial contamination of red cells is most often due to *Yersinia enterocolitica,* followed by *Serratia liquefaciens,* whereas platelets are most often contaminated with *Staphylococcus* and Enterobacteriaceae. The incidence of bacterial contamination of red cells has been estimated to be 1 in 60,000, with an overall fatality rate of 1 in 1 million. The incidence of bacterial contamination of platelets was estimated to be 1 in 5000 before the initiation of bacterial detection systems in 2004, but it is now estimated to be 50% lower (1 in 10,000).

Recipients of units with low bacterial counts may have relatively mild symptoms such as fever and chills, but those receiving units with high bacterial counts may have severe or fatal reactions. Clinically, the patient may experience high fever, shock, hemoglobinuria, renal failure, and disseminated intravascular coagulation. The blood transfusion must be stopped immediately, the patient's blood and any untransfused blood must be cultured, and broad-spectrum antibiotics (Chapter 108) should be started.

Circulatory Overload

Acute pulmonary edema, caused by the circulatory system's inability to handle an increased fluid volume, can occur in any patient who is transfused too rapidly. Although the true frequency of this type of transfusion reaction is unknown, it is believed to be a common occurrence. Susceptible populations are primarily the very young, the elderly, and patients with a small total blood volume or cardiopulmonary disease. Treatment is the same as for heart failure (Chapter 59).

Delayed Reactions

A delayed hemolytic transfusion reaction generally occurs 3 to 7 days after transfusion of the implicated unit. Hemolysis is usually extravascular, and red cells are destroyed in the recipient's circulation by antibody produced as a result of an immune response to the transfusion. These reactions are most commonly due to an anamnestic response (secondary exposure to a red cell antigen) in a patient with a negative antibody screen despite a low level of antibody as a result of previous exposure to a foreign red cell antigen through either pregnancy or transfusion. Exposure to the same antigen a second time may cause IgG antibody to reappear within hours or days of the transfusion. This subsequent exposure to the antigen produces an anamnestic antibody response, resulting in increased production of IgG antibodies that are capable of reacting with any transfused cells present.

In most cases, anamnestic production of antibody does not result in acute hemolysis, but red cell destruction does occur between 3 days and 2 weeks after the transfusion. Patients are generally asymptomatic, and hemolysis may be noted only by a more rapid decline than usual in the patient's hemoglobin level or by an absence of the expected rise in hemoglobin. Fever, the most common initial symptom, is occasionally noted, along with jaundice; renal failure is rare. Prednisone (1 to 2 mg/kg/day) is indicated for more severe reactions.

Transfusion-Associated Graft-versus-Host Disease

Transfusion-associated graft-versus-host disease results from the transfusion of immunologically competent lymphocytes into an immunologically incompetent host. An individual's risk depends on whether the recipient is immunocompromised (and to what degree), the degree of HLA similarity between the transfusion donor and recipient, and the number of transfused T lymphocytes capable of multiplying and engrafting. The engrafted lymphocytes mount an immunologic response against the recipient's tissue, resulting in pancytopenia with bleeding and infectious complications. Symptoms usually appear within 12 days of transfusion. Transfusion-associated graft-versus-host disease is rare, but it is fatal in approximately 90% of affected patients.

Transfusion-Related Acute Lung Injury

Transfusion-related acute lung injury (TRALI; Chapter 94) is an acute respiratory distress syndrome (Chapter 104) that occurs within 6 hours after transfusion and is characterized by dyspnea and hypoxia secondary to noncardiogenic pulmonary edema. Although the actual incidence is almost certainly underreported, the estimated frequency is approximately 1 in 8000 transfusions. In a prospective nested case control study, 16 of 668 (2.4%) of cardiac surgery patients developed TRALI, suggesting that the incidence of TRALI is particularly high in this population. In approximately 50% of cases, blood donor antibodies with HLA or neutrophil antigenic specificity can be shown to react with the recipient's leukocytes, leading to increased permeability of the pulmonary microcirculation.

Most recently, reactive lipid products from donor blood cell membranes that arise during the storage of blood products have been implicated in the pathophysiology of TRALI. Such substances are capable of neutrophil priming, with subsequent damage to the pulmonary-capillary endothelium of the recipient, particularly in patients who receive massive transfusions during cardiac surgery or for trauma or in patients receiving chemotherapy for malignancy. In each of these settings, the true incidence of TRALI may be underreported because the findings may be blamed on the underlying disease process or the surgical procedure. Similar to other causes of acute respiratory distress syndrome, therapy is supportive, and 90% of patients recover. Ongoing initiatives to reduce TRALI risks include recruiting male plasma donors or female donors with no prior history of pregnancy, and screening female apheresis platelet donors for HLA antibodies and limiting donation to those who are HLA antibody negative.

Transmission of Viral Pathogens

Categories of transfusion-transmitted agents, as well as those currently screened, are listed in Table 180-2. The implementation of nucleic acid testing of multiple minipools (donation samples, test well) from blood donations has markedly reduced the transmission of HIV and hepatitis C virus during the infectious window period. Current estimates of the risk per unit of blood are 1 in 1.4 million to 2.4 million for HIV and 1 in 872,000 to 1.7 million for hepatitis C virus (Fig 180-3).

Only 43% of the World Health Organization's 191 member states test blood for HIV, hepatitis C virus, and hepatitis B virus, so at least 13 million units of blood donated every year are not tested for these transmissible viruses. In the poorest countries, the cost of testing ($40 to $50 per blood donation) is prohibitive. Every year, unsafe transfusions are estimated to account for 8 million to 16 million hepatitis B infections, 2.3 million to 4.7 million hepatitis C infections, and 80,000 to 160,000 HIV infections.

TABLE 180-2 CATEGORIES OF TRANSFUSION-TRANSMITTED AGENTS

AGENTS CAUSING TRANSFUSION-TRANSMITTED DISEASE FOR WHICH DONORS ARE ROUTINELY SCREENED
Hepatitis B virus
Human immunodeficiency virus
Hepatitis C virus
Human T-cell lymphotropic virus
West Nile virus
Bacteria
Trypanosoma cruzi
Cytomegalovirus
AGENTS THAT ARE TRANSFUSION TRANSMISSIBLE BUT HAVE NOT CAUSED ANY KNOWN DISEASE WHEN ACQUIRED THROUGH TRANSFUSION
Agents initially thought to cause hepatitis
Human herpesvirus 8
AGENTS CAUSING TRANSFUSION-TRANSMITTED DISEASE FOR WHICH DONORS ARE NOT ROUTINELY SCREENED
Hepatitis A virus
Parvovirus B19
Dengue fever virus
Babesia spp
Plasmodium spp
Leishmania spp
Brucella spp
Variant Creutzfeldt-Jakob disease prions
Other

Modified from Vamvakes EC, Blajchman MA. Transfusion-related mortality: the on-going risks of allogeneic blood transfusion and the available strategies for their prevention. *Blood.* 2009;113:3406-3417.

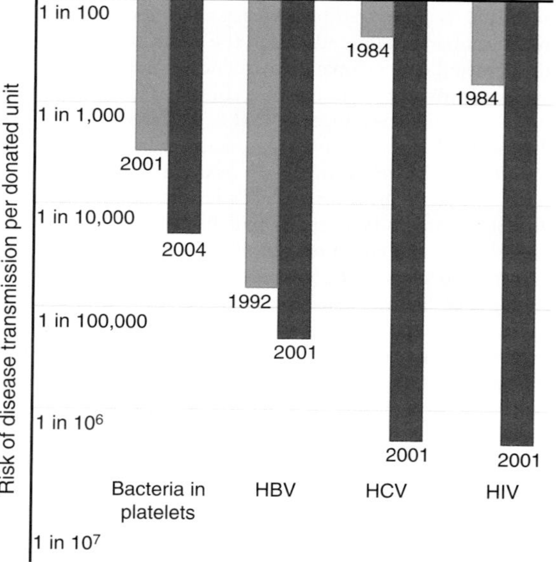

FIGURE 180-3. Risk of transmission of potentially fatal transfusion-acquired infections in the United States. The figures plotted pertain to risk reduction documented between 2001 and 2004 for bacteria in platelets, 1992 and 2001 for hepatitis B virus (HBV), and 1984 and 2001 for hepatitis C virus (HCV) and human immunodeficiency virus (HIV). The risk of bacteria in platelets today is considered to be the same as in 2004, and the risk of HBV, HCV, and HIV is considered to be the same as in 2001, because no further measures to protect the blood supply from these pathogens have been introduced. (From Vamvakas EC, Blajchman MA. Transfusion-related mortality: the on-going risks of allogeneic blood transfusion and the available strategies for their prevention. *Blood.* 2009;113:3406-3417.)

EMERGING ISSUES AND EVOLVING TECHNOLOGIES

Problems related to blood component storage have long been known, such as depletion of 2,3-diphosphoglycerate in red cell units during storage at 4° C for longer than 35 to 42 days. Recent evidence suggests that in patients undergoing cardiac surgery, transfusion of red cells stored for more than 14 days is associated with a significantly increased risk of postoperative complications, as well as reduced short-term and long-term survival. A prospective, randomized multicenter trial comparing the transfusion of blood less than 10 days old versus blood 21 days or older in adult patients undergoing cardiac surgery is currently under way in the United States. Erythropoiesis-stimulating agents, including recombinant human erythropoietin, modified erythropoietin molecules, and erythropoietin receptor agonists, along with artificial oxygen carriers, can potentially decrease the need for red cell transfusion. It is important that oversight of these biotechnology products and other specialized blood products (e.g., solvent- or detergent-treated plasma, leukoreduced blood products, irradiated blood components, CMV-negative blood components) be placed under the auspices of standing hospital medical committees, such as a transfusion medicine committee. Otherwise, promotion of such products by the commercial sector directly to consumers could undermine both institutional oversight and evidence-based rationales for their use.

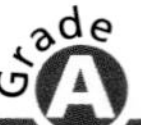

1. Herbert PC, Wells G, Blajchman MA, et al. A multicenter, randomized, controlled clinical trial of transfusion requirements in critical care. *N Engl J Med.* 1999;340:409-417.
2. Hajjar LA, Vincent JL, Galas FR, et al. Transfusion requirements after cardiac surgery: the TRACS randomized controlled trial. *JAMA.* 2010;304:1559-1567.
3. Diedrich B, Remberger M, Shanwell A, et al. A prospective randomized trial of a prophylactic platelet transfusion trigger of 10×10^9 per L versus 30×10^9 per L in allogeneic hematopoietic progenitor cell transplant recipients. *Transfusion.* 2005;45:1064-1072.
4. Slichter SJ, Kaufman RM, Assmann SF, et al. Dose of prophylactic platelet transfusion and prevention of hemorrhage. *N Engl J Med.* 2010;362:600-613.

SUGGESTED READINGS

Goodnough LT, Shander A. How we treat: management of warfarin-associated coagulopathy in patients with intracerebral hemorrhage. *Blood.* 2011, in press. *Review of management with personal perspective.*

Goodnough LT, Viele M, Fontaine MJ, et al. Implementation of a two specimen requirement for verification of ABO/Rh for blood transfusion. *Transfusion.* 2009;49:1321-1328. *The relevance of bedside errors in patient identification and specimen labeling.*

Koch CG, Li L, Sessler DI, et al. Duration of red-cell storage and complications after cardiac surgery. *N Engl J Med.* 2008;358:1229-1239. *Transfusion of red cells that had been stored for more than 2 weeks was associated with a significantly increased risk of postoperative complications and reduced survival.*

McCullough J. Overview of platelet transfusion. *Semin Hematol.* 2010;47:235-242. *Review.*

Shaz BH, Stowell SR, Hillyer CD. Transfusion-related acute lung injury: from bedside to bench and back. *Blood.* 2011;117:1463-1471. *Review.*

Vamakas EC, Blajchman MA. Transfusion-related mortality: the on-going risks of allogeneic blood transfusion and the available strategies for their prevention. *Blood.* 2009;113:3406-3417. *Review of blood risks.*

Vlaar AP, Hofstra JJ, Determann RM, et al. The incidence, risk factors and outcome of transfusion-related acute lung injury in a cohort of cardiac surgery patients: a prospective nested case control study. *Blood.* 2011;117:4218-4225. *Risk factors include age; time on bypass; larger transfusions of blood products, plasma, and RBCs stored for >14 days; and the presence of antibodies in donor blood.*

181 HEMATOPOIETIC STEM CELL TRANSPLANTATION

JULIE M. VOSE

Hematopoietic stem cell transplantation is the process of collecting and infusing hematopoietic stem cells obtained from bone marrow (bone marrow transplantation) or peripheral blood (peripheral blood stem cell transplantation). High-dose chemotherapy followed by bone marrow or peripheral blood stem cell transplantation is increasingly used for the treatment of many hematologic, immunologic, and neoplastic diseases. Hematopoietic stem cells can be obtained directly from bone marrow by multiple aspirations from the pelvic bones while the patient is under general anesthesia. Alternatively, hematopoietic stem cells can be obtained from peripheral blood, after stimulation with hematopoietic growth factors such as granulocyte colony-stimulating factor (G-CSF), followed by leukapheresis, or they can be obtained from cord blood sources. The availability of hematopoietic stem cell transplantation permits the administration of supralethal chemotherapy or combined chemotherapy and radiation therapy to patients with malignancies or, in selected cases, with nonmalignant diseases in an attempt to increase the destruction of the affected cells. Additionally, the healthy transplanted cells may reconstitute the patient's immune system to provide an antitumor effect or, in the case of bone marrow transplantation for congenital diseases, to provide cells that are no longer deficient in certain vital components.

ALLOGENEIC AND SYNGENEIC TRANSPLANTATION

Allogeneic bone marrow or peripheral blood stem cell transplantation involves the transfer of stem cells from a donor to another person. Syngeneic transplantation, which occurs in only about 1% of transplant procedures, is the special case of a donor and recipient who are genetically identical twins. Myeloablative allogeneic transplants are usually considered only for patients younger than 55 to 60 years; however, older patients are occasionally treated. Results tend to be poorer in older patients because of the increasing incidence of graft-versus-host disease (GVHD) with age. More recently, reduced-intensity nonmyeloablative allogeneic transplants have been used, especially in older patients and others who might not be good candidates for fully myeloablative transplants. In all cases, the decision whether to transplant must take into account all factors, including not only the patient's chronologic age but also his or her physiologic age.

The donor and recipient must be matched for human leukocyte antigens (HLAs); the most important gene pairs include HLA-A, HLA-B, HLA-C, HLA-DR, and HLA-DQ loci, all of which are closely linked on chromosome 6 and inherited in haplotypes. The chance of having an HLA match from a sibling is 25%; however, because of the relatively small size of families in the United States, only about 30% of patients have HLA-matched siblings. For patients who lack HLA-identical sibling donors, other possible solutions include identifying an unrelated but closely HLA-matched person through the National Marrow Donor Program (NMDP), using a partially matched related donor, or identifying one or more cord blood units from a cord blood bank. The genes encoding HLAs are numerous, and the odds that any two unrelated individuals are HLA identical for main loci are less than 1 in 10,000. About 10 million volunteer donors have been HLA-typed through the NMDP registry, however, and a donor can be found for about 50% of patients for whom a search is initiated. It usually takes about 4 months to locate an unrelated donor, which may be too long for some patients with rapidly progressive malignancies.

An allogeneic partially matched sibling or placental or umbilical cord blood is an alternative source of stem cells. Umbilical cord blood stem cells are already stored in cord blood banks, and no additional harvest procedures are needed. Because of the unique immature biology of umbilical cord blood stem cells, these transplants are associated with less GVHD; consequently, the HLA matching requirements are less strict. However, cord blood cells must be partially matched to the recipient, as well as to each other if more than 1 unit is given. The small volume of cord blood stem cells often makes these transplants unsuitable for adult recipients. The time to engraftment and immune reconstitution may also be different for this type of transplant, which sometimes causes late engraftment and an increased rate of post-transplant infection.

When an adequate donor has been identified, the patient is prepared for the allogeneic or syngeneic transplant with high doses of chemotherapy, alone or combined with radiation therapy. This treatment is designed to destroy any remaining malignant cells, provide sufficient immunosuppression to allow engraftment of the new cells, and clear the marrow space for engraftment of the new cells. The preparative agents must have few toxicities at high doses; for this reason, high doses of anthracyclines are often impractical because of their cardiac toxicities. Most regimens consist of total body irradiation combined with alkylating agents, etoposide, or cytarabine. With nonmyeloablative transplants, less intense chemotherapy and/or radiation is used, which is less damaging to the patient. However, acute and chronic GVHD is still a possibility, and in fact, the risk of chronic GVHD may be slightly higher.

An integral component of the regimens for allogeneic transplantation is immunosuppression to prevent GVHD and graft rejection (Chapter 48). Because the recipient's immune system is ablated with high-dose chemotherapy and radiation therapy, graft rejection is a rare event with related donors and a fully ablative transplant. However, reduced-intensity regimens can have a higher risk of nonengraftment. Drugs commonly used to prevent GVHD include tacrolimus, mycophenolate mofetil, rapamycin, and the combination of cyclosporine and methotrexate. For allogeneic hematopoietic stem cell transplantation, prophylactic immunosuppression is not lifelong; when immunologic tolerance is established, immunosuppressive agents can be slowly withdrawn and discontinued. Another strategy to prevent GVHD is to deplete the donor's T cells from the graft; the disadvantage of this approach is its association with increased rates of disease relapse and infection, and overall survival does not seem to be improved. To accelerate engraftment, hematopoietic growth factors such as G-CSF are administered after transplantation until the neutrophil count recovers. Allogeneic transplantation regimens also include prophylactic antiviral drugs (acyclovir, ganciclovir), antifungal drugs (fluconazole, voriconazole), broad-spectrum antibiotics (cephalosporins, fluoroquinolones), and anti-*Pneumocystis* drugs (trimethoprim-sulfamethoxazole, dapsone, pentamidine).

Leukemias and some indolent lymphomas that relapse after allogeneic stem cell transplantation can sometimes be controlled by further infusions of lymphocytes from the same allogeneic donor. The donor T lymphocytes destroy malignant cells by an immune mechanism called the *graft-versus-tumor effect*. For solid tumors, a graft-versus-tumor effect can sometimes be demonstrated. These observations led to the development of nonmyeloablative transplantation regimens, based on the concept that allogeneic stem cell transplantation is a form of immunotherapy by which the donor lymphocytes eradicate the malignant disease, with high-dose chemotherapy and irradiation not being necessary for success.

AUTOLOGOUS BONE MARROW TRANSPLANTATION

In autologous bone marrow transplantation, the patient's own hematopoietic cells are infused to reestablish bone marrow function after the administration of high-dose chemotherapy, with or without total body irradiation. These reinfused hematopoietic cells can come from the patient's bone marrow, peripheral blood, or both. Because a major limitation of allogeneic bone marrow transplantation is that only a few patients have HLA-matched sibling donors, the use of autologous hematopoietic cells greatly increases the number of patients eligible for transplantation (Table 181-1). Autologous transplantation can also be used safely in older patients because of the absence of GVHD, which is a major concern in this population. Disadvantages of autologous hematopoietic cell transplantation include the risk of contaminating the graft with viable tumor cells and the lack of graft-versus-tumor effects. Although patients undergoing autologous transplantation have higher relapse rates than those undergoing allogeneic transplantation, the lower rate of other complications seems to translate into similar long-term outcomes. A variety of methods have been developed to decrease the contamination of autologous grafts with tumor cells (graft "purging"), but no prospective data have yet confirmed that these interventions are beneficial because most relapses originate from incompletely eradicated disease in the host.

INDICATIONS FOR TRANSPLANTATION

For many diseases, hematopoietic stem cell transplantation is now part of standard therapy (Table 181-2). In the United States, more than 17,000 allogeneic and autologous transplants are performed each year for various diseases (Fig. 181-1).

Lymphoproliferative Malignancies

Non-Hodgkin's Lymphoma

As first-line treatment, autologous transplantation results in a higher rate of complete response but not better survival in patients with aggressive

TABLE 181-1 COMPARISON OF ALLOGENEIC AND AUTOLOGOUS TRANSPLANTATION

FEATURE	ALLOGENEIC	AUTOLOGOUS
Upper age limits	55–75 yr	Physiologic status limits
Availability	40–60% of patients	Only limitation may be the ability to collect enough stem cells
Main cause of failure	Graft-versus-host disease Infections	Disease relapse

TABLE 181-2 RESULTS OF STANDARD-OF-CARE ALLOGENEIC OR AUTOLOGOUS STEM CELL TRANSPLANTATION IN SPECIFIC DISEASES*

DISEASE	Three-Year Survival (%) ALLOGENEIC	AUTOLOGOUS
HEMATOLOGIC MALIGNANCIES		
Acute myelogenous leukemia	32–50	43–50
Chronic myelogenous leukemia	28–54	NU
Myelodysplastic syndrome	40–46	NU
Acute lymphocytic leukemia	25–51	NU
Chronic lymphocytic leukemia	35–45	66
Hodgkin's disease	NU	78
Follicular lymphoma	60	76
Diffuse large cell lymphoma	19–30	60
Multiple myeloma	12–40	66
Neuroblastoma	NU	60
NONMALIGNANT CONDITIONS		
Aplastic anemia	33–82	NA
Fanconi's anemia	16–81	NA
Thalassemia major	91 (1 yr)	NA
Sickle cell anemia	91	NA
Severe combined immunodeficiency	59.3	NA

*Information based on the Center for International Bone Marrow Transplant Research report for patients who underwent transplantation between 2000 and 2007. Results are typically better in patients younger than 20 years, patients in earlier stages of the disease, and recipients of HLA-identical sibling transplants.
NA = not applicable; NU = not routinely used.

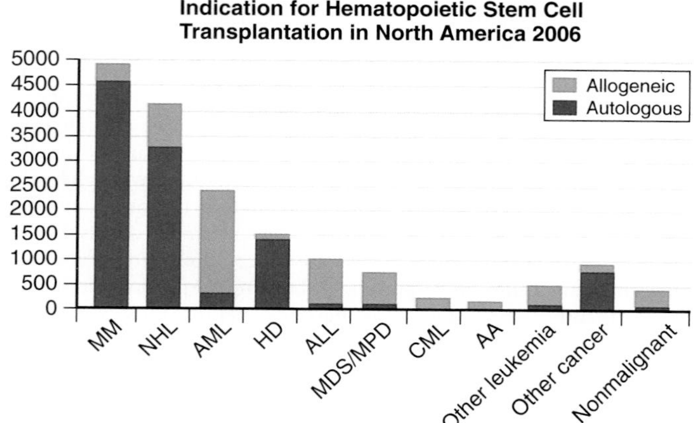

FIGURE 181-1. Indications for autologous and allogeneic blood and marrow transplantation in North America. AA = aplastic anemia; ALL = acute lymphocytic leukemia; AML = acute myelogenous leukemia; CML = chronic myelogenous leukemia; HD = Hodgkin's disease; MDS = myelodysplastic syndrome; MM = multiple myeloma; MPD = myeloproliferative disease; NHL = non-Hodgkin's lymphoma. (Information reprinted with permission from the Center for International Bone Marrow Transplant Research [CIBMTR], 2010.)

non-Hodgkin's lymphoma (Chapter 191).[1] Patients with relapsed disease seem to benefit most from this therapy if they undergo transplantation when they still have chemotherapy-sensitive disease. High-risk patients who undergo transplantation early in the course of the disease, during their first partial or complete response, may have a better outcome than similar patients treated with conventional therapy; however, this is considered controversial. The use of high-dose chemotherapy, radiation therapy, and autologous transplantation in patients with indolent disease is associated with a failure-free survival rate of 40 to 60% at a median follow-up of 3 years; because late relapses are common, much longer follow-up is necessary to assess the long-term results of this treatment. Allogeneic stem cell transplantation is typically used for patients who have relapsed after an autologous stem cell transplant or for some lymphomas in which an autologous transplant is not possible owing to circulating lymphoma cells.

Hodgkin's Disease

High-dose chemotherapy followed by autologous hematopoietic stem cell transplantation has been widely accepted for patients with relapsed Hodgkin's disease (Chapter 192). Allogeneic transplantation has not been used as extensively because of increased morbidity and mortality. The outcome is poorer in patients who have received multiple chemotherapy regimens than in those who have undergone less pretreatment. Autologous transplantation during the first remission is being evaluated in patients with "B" symptoms, disseminated disease with bone marrow or pulmonary involvement, and other high-risk features.

Multiple Myeloma

Autologous and allogeneic transplant procedures have been performed successfully in patients with multiple myeloma (Chapter 193). The major concern with conventional myeloablative allogeneic transplantation was its high mortality rate; however, with improvements in supportive care, the transplant-related mortality associated with autografts for multiple myeloma has been reduced to 1%, and randomized trials confirm better progression-free survival but not overall survival after autologous stem cell transplantation compared with conventional chemotherapy.[2] Autologous transplantation for multiple myeloma is more successful in patients who undergo less pretreatment and have a smaller tumor burden. Multiple myeloma is now the most common indication for autologous stem cell transplantation in North America. Studies using autologous tandem transplantation, or an autologous transplant followed by a nonmyeloablative transplant, have shown early promising results.

Lymphoid Leukemias

The results of conventional induction and consolidation chemotherapy for acute lymphoblastic leukemia (ALL) in children are excellent, except for ALL associated with the Philadelphia chromosome (Ph) (Chapter 189). Therefore, in children with ALL, transplantation is generally reserved for these high-risk patients and those who relapse after initial therapy. A much higher percentage of adults fail to respond to initial therapy and have higher-risk disease; therefore, allogeneic stem cell transplantation, which improves overall survival when performed in adults during a first complete remission,[3] should be considered in adult ALL patients, particularly those who are Ph positive.

Selected younger patients with B-cell chronic lymphocytic leukemia (B-CLL) that is refractory or who have relapsed more than once might benefit by transplantation from a related or unrelated donor; durable disease-free survival rates are 40 to 60% (Chapter 190). Because the allogeneic graft-versus-leukemia effect seems to be especially important against B-CLL, this disease is a common indication for nonmyeloablative allogeneic transplantation. Autologous transplantation also yields high rates of remission in pretreated B-CLL patients, but relapse rates are significant.

Myeloproliferative Malignancies

Myeloid Leukemias

Because patients with good-risk or average-risk acute myelogenous leukemia (AML) can be cured with conventional chemotherapy, most centers use transplantation only for relapsed AML in adults or as part of the initial therapy in patients with known poor prognostic characteristics, such as certain high-risk chromosomal abnormalities, including complex abnormalities or deletions (Chapter 189). In these intermediate- and high-risk patients, allogeneic transplantation improves progression-free survival and overall survival when performed during first complete remission.[4]

Most patients with chronic myelogenous leukemia (CML) are treated with tyrosine kinase inhibitors rather than allogeneic stem cell transplantation (Chapter 190). If the medications fail, allogeneic transplantation from an HLA-matched sibling donor produces long-term disease-free survival in 55 to 75% of patients with Ph-positive CML. The results seem to be better when younger patients undergo transplantation within the first year of diagnosis. When an HLA-matched related donor is not available, use of alternative donors can yield a cure in about 50% patients with chronic phase CML. However, the development of effective, nontoxic tyrosine kinase inhibitors for the treatment of *BCR-ABL*–positive CML is tempering enthusiasm for allogeneic transplantation in CML patients, so this procedure is rarely performed.

Myelodysplastic Syndromes

Myelodysplastic syndromes in young, otherwise healthy patients are best treated with an allogeneic transplant (Chapter 188). However, most patients with myelodysplastic syndromes are elderly, which often precludes the use of this therapy.

Solid Tumors

High-dose chemotherapy for the treatment of metastatic breast cancer can result in a higher complete response rate than conventional treatment (Chapter 204). The reported disease-free survival rate in chemotherapy-sensitive stage IV breast cancer is only 10 to 25%, however, and no overall survival benefit has been shown in several randomized trials. As a result, transplantation has lost favor in this condition.

High-dose chemotherapy plus transplantation has had success in the treatment of some chemotherapy-sensitive solid tumors, including testicular cancer (Chapter 206), ovarian carcinoma (Chapter 205), and childhood tumors such as neuroblastoma and Wilms' tumor. Other solid tumors that are refractory to chemotherapy, such as melanoma or many gastrointestinal malignancies, are poor targets for this therapy. Limited reports of a high rate of regression of metastatic renal carcinoma (Chapter 203) after nonmyeloablative allogeneic peripheral blood stem cell transplantation hold promise for its wider use.

Nonmalignant Conditions

Disorders such as Wiskott-Aldrich syndrome or severe combined immunodeficiency syndrome have been treated successfully with HLA-matched sibling transplants or transplants from alternative donors (Chapter 258).

Genetic disorders such as osteopetrosis (Chapter 256), Gaucher's disease (Chapter 215), and Hurler's syndrome (Chapter 268) can be treated successfully with an allogeneic transplant. Other indications for allogeneic transplantation include hemoglobinopathies such as sickle cell anemia (Chapter 166) and thalassemia (Chapter 165) and acquired blood disorders such as paroxysmal nocturnal hemoglobinuria (Chapter 163). The transplant must be performed before the onset of secondary organ failure.

Allogeneic transplantation can lead to long-term disease-free survival in more than 50% of patients with severe aplastic anemia (Chapter 168). When compared with standard immunosuppressive therapy, allogeneic transplantation is more likely to produce a complete and durable reversal of the hematologic abnormalities. Patients with aplastic anemia who are less heavily transfused have better outcomes with allogeneic transplantation. For patients with less severe aplastic anemia, patients older than 40 years, and those without a matched sibling donor, a trial of immunosuppression therapy is usually appropriate before consideration of allogeneic transplantation.

Autologous stem cell transplantation to engraft a tolerant immune system has had promising results in selected patients with systemic lupus erythematosus, rheumatoid arthritis, scleroderma, and multiple sclerosis. Randomized prospective trials comparing conventional treatments are currently under way.

Much attention has focused on the possible use of autologous bone marrow–derived or circulating peripheral blood stem cells to promote the recovery of myocardial function after acute myocardial infarction. To date, the infusion of such cells, usually directly into the relevant coronary artery after successful percutaneous coronary intervention, has shown promising results in improving regional but not necessarily global myocardial function. Further research is required to define the appropriate clinical role for such approaches.

COMPLICATIONS

Infections

Infections are a major cause of morbidity and mortality after hematopoietic stem cell transplantation, especially allogeneic transplantation, because of prolonged immunosuppression for the prevention or treatment of GVHD. Bacterial infections are frequently related to central venous catheters. Among fungal infections, *Aspergillus* infections typically occur in patients receiving prolonged high-dose steroids for the treatment of GVHD. Viral infections include reactivation cytomegalovirus (Chapter 384), human herpesvirus 6, and Epstein-Barr virus (Chapter 385) infections. These patients are also susceptible to seasonal respiratory viruses. Prophylactic use of G-CSF and granulocyte-macrophage colony-stimulating factor is helpful but does not improve survival.

At 1 year after allogeneic or autologous transplantation, patients should receive the following vaccinations: diphtheria, tetanus, *Haemophilus influenzae* type b, hepatitis A virus, hepatitis B virus, 23-valent pneumococcal polysaccharide, seasonal influenza virus, inactivated poliovirus, and, only in areas of outbreaks, meningococcal vaccine (Chapter 17). Live vaccines against measles, mumps, and rubella should not be administered until 2 years after transplantation, and only in the absence of chronic GVHD and immunosuppressive therapy. Family members can receive routine vaccines, including influenza virus vaccine, but patients should avoid contact with a child who has received oral poliovirus vaccine for about 1 month after vaccination. Despite these recommendations, vaccines may not always induce protective immunity in an immunodeficient patient who has chronic GVHD or is taking immunosuppressive drugs.

Cardiac Toxicity

Most transplant centers screen potential patients for underlying cardiac abnormalities that would place them at increased risk during the procedure. Nevertheless, a few patients experience cardiotoxicity, either acutely during the transplant procedure or later. Pericardial effusion can develop in patients who have disease near the pericardium or are receiving radiation therapy in that area (Chapter 77). An idiosyncratic cardiomyopathy can occur after high doses of cyclophosphamide. Viral cardiomyopathies can also develop.

Pulmonary Toxicity

Pulmonary toxicities include infections from bacterial, fungal, or viral sources during the transplant. In addition, in patients receiving certain chemotherapy agents, such as carmustine, chemotherapy-induced lung damage may develop, but this can usually be treated with steroids. Patients undergoing allogeneic transplantation are at increased risk for pneumonitis caused by cytomegalovirus and fungal infections, for adult respiratory distress syndrome, and for interstitial pneumonia of unknown cause. Chronic GVHD can also manifest in the lung as bronchiolitis obliterans, with or without obstructive pneumonia.

Liver Toxicity and Veno-occlusive Disease

The most frequent liver complication associated with transplantation is veno-occlusive disease of the liver (also called sinusoidal obstruction syndrome). The pathogenesis of this syndrome is damage to hepatic sinusoids, often with occlusion of hepatic venules, associated with chemotherapy drugs and total body irradiation used in conditioning regimens. Symptoms associated with this complication include jaundice, tender hepatomegaly, ascites, and weight gain. Total serum bilirubin is a sensitive but nonspecific test for veno-occlusive disease. Imaging studies may demonstrate hepatomegaly, ascites, periportal edema, and attenuated hepatic venous flow. The diagnosis can be made most definitively by transvenous liver biopsy and hepatic venous pressure measurements. Progressive hepatic failure and multiorgan system failure can develop, but at least 70% of patients recover spontaneously. Predisposing factors seem to be previous hepatic injury, the use of estrogens, and perhaps the use of HLA-mismatched donors.

Renal Toxicity

Acute renal failure requiring dialysis occurs infrequently during the transplant procedure. The judicious use of nephrotoxic agents can decrease the incidence of this complication. Idiopathic or cyclosporine-induced hemolytic-uremic syndrome (Chapter 175) can be a serious complication after allogeneic stem cell transplantation, with a high risk for end-stage renal disease or death.

Graft-versus-Host Disease

In the allogeneic transplant setting, acute GVHD manifests with symptoms in the skin, gastrointestinal tract, and liver within the first 100 days after transplantation. Skin involvement ranges from a maculopapular rash to generalized erythroderma or desquamation. The severity of liver disease is based on bilirubin levels, and the severity of the gastrointestinal disease is graded by the quantity of daily diarrhea. Patients who receive transplants from unrelated donors are at increased risk, and the incidence and severity of GVHD rise with the age of the patient. Other risk factors include a female donor (particularly a multiparous donor), advanced age, and cytomegalovirus seropositivity of the donor or patient. Prophylaxis with cyclosporine or tacrolimus, with or without methotrexate, corticosteroids, or mycophenolate mofetil, reduces the incidence and severity. Treatment of acute GVHD includes high-dose corticosteroids, antithymocyte globulin, or various monoclonal antibodies.

Chronic GVHD occurs more than 100 days after transplantation and is most likely to develop in older patients who also had acute GVHD. Symptoms include the sicca syndrome, chronic sinusitis, rashes, scleroderma-like skin thickening, diarrhea, wasting syndrome, and liver abnormalities. Patients are also at greatly increased risk for infectious complications resulting from either GVHD itself or treatment for it. Adverse prognostic factors for survival include thrombocytopenia, progressive clinical manifestations, involvement of more than 50% of the skin, poor performance status, and elevated bilirubin. Treatment of chronic GVHD includes corticosteroids, cyclosporine, tacrolimus, mycophenolate mofetil, ultraviolet light, and other immunosuppressive agents.

Graft Rejection

Graft rejection occurs when immunologically competent cells of host origin destroy the transplanted cells of donor origin. This complication is rare after fully matched, related donor transplants and occurs more commonly in patients who receive transplants from alternative donors or T-cell–depleted transplants. Graft rejection is less likely in nontransfused patients with aplastic anemia.

Late Complications

As the number of long-term post-transplant survivors increases, complications that develop years later are beginning to be recognized.

Secondary Malignancies

One complication of the chemotherapy or radiation therapy (or both) used to treat malignancy is the development of a secondary malignancy. There have been several reports of the development of secondary AML or myelodysplastic syndrome after autologous transplantation. Some studies have suggested that total body irradiation may increase the risk for these complications. After allogeneic transplantation, the overall incidence of secondary malignancies is 2.2% at 10 years and 6.7% at 15 years after transplantation. Within the first 1 to 2 years, the most common malignancies are Epstein-Barr virus–related lymphoproliferative disorders; solid tumors are more likely to occur more than 3 years after transplantation. Risk factors include the use of antithymocyte globulin to treat GVHD, the use of a T-cell–depleted graft, HLA incompatibility, and perhaps total body irradiation.

Infertility and Hypogonadism

The risk of gonadal failure is likely to be lower with nonmyeloablative preparative regimens. The use of total body irradiation is almost always associated with sterility, but successful pregnancies have occurred in some patients after other regimens. Gynecomastia (sometimes tender) occasionally occurs in males. To address all the complexities of functional castration from high-dose therapy, a reproductive endocrinologist should be consulted before transplantation in patients for whom future fertility is an issue.

Endocrine Dysfunction

Iatrogenic Cushing's syndrome is commonly due to long-term steroid therapy in patients with chronic GVHD (Chapter 34). Particularly disabling are steroid-induced myopathy, avascular necrosis of the hip, and osteoporosis. Because many patients take steroids for many months, tapering can be associated with malaise, nausea, hypotension, and musculoskeletal pains. In these situations, slower tapering over several months or reintroduction of physiologic replacement doses (e.g., 7.5 to 10 mg/day of prednisone) is appropriate. Hypothyroidism (Chapter 233) is typically related to the use of total body irradiation or local irradiation of the head and neck for lymphoma or other cancer. Osteoporosis (Chapter 251) occurs in 50 to 60% of patients after hematopoietic stem cell transplantation. The major contributing causes include hypogonadism, secondary hyperparathyroidism caused by low serum calcium, and post-transplant steroid therapy. Bone mineral density should be evaluated before and after transplantation; osteopenia should be treated as appropriate with bisphosphonates, calcium, vitamin D, estrogen, and testosterone.

Other Complications

The long-term incidence of cataracts is about 20 to 50%; the risk is related to the use of total body irradiation and corticosteroids (Chapter 431). About 50% of patients with cataracts require surgical therapy. Alopecia is typically reversible, but in rare cases it may be irreversible, especially after the use of busulfan-containing preparative regimens.

FUTURE DIRECTIONS

The safety and efficacy of transplantation may be improved by the use of hematopoietic cytokines to stimulate immunologic reconstitution, ex vivo expansion of progenitors, genetic modulation of cells, improved supportive care for transplant patients, better prophylaxis against GVHD, better HLA typing, and newer anticancer agents. Whether stem cells can be infused to improve the function of adult organs is an area of active investigation.

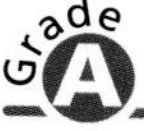

1. Greb A, Bohlius J, Schiefer D, et al. High-dose chemotherapy with autologous stem cell transplantation in the first line treatment of aggressive non-Hodgkin lymphoma (NHL) in adults. *Cochrane Database Syst Rev.* 2008;1:CD004024.
2. Koreth J, Cutler CS, Djulbegovic B, et al. High-dose therapy with single autologous transplantation versus chemotherapy for newly diagnosed multiple myeloma: a systematic review and meta-analysis of randomized controlled trials. *Biol Blood Marrow Transplant.* 2007;13:183-196.
3. Ram R, Gafter-Gvili A, Vidal L, et al. Management of adult patients with acute lymphoblastic leukemia in first complete remission: systematic review and meta-analysis. *Cancer.* 2010;116:3447-3457.
4. Koreth J, Schlenk R, Kopecky KJ, et al. Allogeneic stem cell transplantation for acute myeloid leukemia in first complete remission: systematic review and meta-analysis of prospective clinical trials. *JAMA.* 2009;301:2349-2361.

SUGGESTED READINGS

Choi SW, Levine JE, Ferrara JL. Pathogenesis and management of graft-versus-host disease. *Immunol Allergy Clin North Am.* 2010;30:75-101. *Review of the immunologic basis of GVHD, risk factors, and management.*

Gooley TA, Chien JW, Pergam SA, et al. Reduced mortality after allogeneic hematopoietic-cell transplantation. *N Engl J Med.* 2010;363:2091-2101. *Mortality from allogeneic hematopoietic stem cell transplantation decreased from 63% in 1993-1997 to 47% in 2003-2007, but the risk of relapse or progression of the underlying disease did not change.*

Wingard JR, Hsu J, Hiemenz JW. Hematopoietic stem cell transplantation: an overview of infection risks and epidemiology. *Hematol Oncol Clin North Am.* 2011;25:101-116. *Review.*

XV

ONCOLOGY

182

APPROACH TO THE PATIENT WITH CANCER

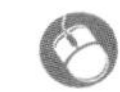

MICHAEL C. PERRY

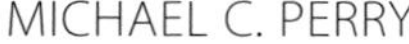

DIAGNOSIS

Few diagnoses produce such emotional responses as *cancer* or *leukemia,* and in the first few moments after those words are uttered, the patient often experiences a storm of feelings that limit useful discussion. When the time is right, however, the physician and the patient must discuss the diagnosis, its implications, and the therapeutic alternatives. It is often best for the patient if family members or close friends are present in the consulting room, both to provide emotional support and to be another "set of ears." It is often useful to ask, "What do you understand about your diagnosis?"

If the physician is not familiar with the latest treatments, consultation in advance with, for example, the National Cancer Institute's Physician Data Query will make the interview more meaningful. Prompt referral to a specialist, whether a surgical oncologist, radiation oncologist, or medical oncologist, is imperative. The generalist should not be a therapeutic nihilist unless he or she is intimately involved in the field and knows about all the current therapies and clinical trials.

The consulting medical oncologist, often advised by a local tumor board comprising medical, surgical, and radiation oncologists, usually outlines the prognosis and the alternatives: standard therapy, possible clinical trials, a second opinion, or no treatment. Many oncologists actively participate in clinical trials and may have investigational drugs available, or they may suggest referral to a tertiary cancer center as appropriate.

Diagnostic Procedures

In most settings, a lesion has been found on physical examination or by abnormal laboratory or radiographic studies, and a biopsy has confirmed the diagnosis. It is critical that the biopsy be representative of the entire tumor and that appropriate investigations (e.g., special stains, flow cytometry, cytogenetics, hormone assays) be performed before treatment is initiated. If there is a question whether the lesion is benign or malignant or about its proper classification, consideration should be given to additional biopsies, and consultation with a reference pathologist may be indicated. There is seldom a need for such rapid therapy that appropriate pretreatment evaluations cannot be performed. For many tumor sites, such as the colon (Chapter 199), there is one predominant histology; in others, such as the lung (Chapter 197), the distinction between small cell lung cancer and non–small cell lung cancer is critical for treatment. For breast cancer (Chapter 204), the treating physician is interested in a variety of factors, such as histology, tumor grade, the presence or absence of estrogen and progesterone receptors, and the presence of ERBB2 (HER2/neu) overexpression.

Staging and Work-up

After a diagnosis has been established, staging is next. The American Joint Committee on Cancer staging system is considered the standard in the United States and is based on the TNM (tumor, node, metastasis) system. The approach to staging depends on the type of cancer, but it commonly includes plain films such as chest radiographs, computed tomography (CT), magnetic resonance imaging (MRI), radionuclide scans, and, increasingly, positron emission tomography (PET). These studies are typically supplemented by routine hematologic and chemistry profiles, tumor markers, and, in some cases, bone marrow aspiration and biopsies.

The keys to the work-up are to identify sites of metastases and to establish an indicator lesion or lesions to monitor therapy. Thus, for most solid tumors, a CT scan and perhaps a bone scan can accomplish both goals, with brain CT or MRI reserved for cases in which central nervous system metastases are most likely (e.g., small cell lung cancer). PET scans supplement CT scans by establishing that a given lesion is likely to be malignant and by clarifying other sites of disease. In patients with known, established advanced disease, they are seldom needed.

TREATMENT

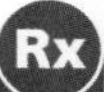

Development of a Treatment Plan

For cancers amenable to surgery, resection is usually the best alternative if the patient is a suitable candidate for anesthesia (Chapter 440) and is otherwise in acceptable condition in terms of concomitant or comorbid illnesses. A joint discussion among the internist, oncologist, surgeon, and anesthesiologist is often very useful in this regard. Determination of the patient's performance score (Table 182-1) is a simple means of assessing functional status. If life expectancy is limited or if the patient is not a good candidate for surgery, radiation therapy is usually considered the next best "local" therapy, with chemotherapy reserved for patients whose disease is extensive or metastatic. The increasing effectiveness of chemotherapy has resulted in its earlier incorporation into therapy, often as part of an "organ-sparing" approach. Ideally, the discussion of treatment with the patient should take a multidisciplinary approach, with clarification of the diagnosis, prognosis, treatment goals, alternatives, side effects, and risks and benefits.

Surgical Therapy

Surgery is used to biopsy a suspected lesion, to remove the primary tumor, to bypass obstructions, and to provide palliation. A preoperative discussion may determine the requirement for placement of a venous access device at the time of surgery, thus eliminating the need for a second anesthesia.

Surgery remains the most common method to cure localized cancers, such as breast cancer (Chapter 204), colorectal cancer (Chapter 199), and lung cancer (Chapter 197), but it is limited by the location of the tumor, its extension, and distant metastases. Even if a tumor cannot be removed, a biopsy provides confirmation of the diagnosis. Occasionally, an obstructing lesion can be bypassed to provide palliation.

Surgical staging also establishes the extent of the disease. For ovarian cancer (Chapter 205), surgical "debulking" aims to remove all visible disease, leaving minimal residual disease, to enhance chemotherapy.

In rare circumstances when the primary tumor is controlled, removal of a single metastasis (metastasectomy) can result in long-term survival; an example is resection of a single liver metastasis found at the time of colectomy for colorectal cancer. A variety of surgical techniques, such as radio frequency ablation or cryoablation, can treat hepatic metastases in carefully selected patients. Adjuvant chemotherapy is often given after surgery in this situation to treat microscopic metastases.

Reconstruction after a disfiguring procedure is critical to long-term physical and emotional functioning. Examples include post-mastectomy breast reconstruction (Chapter 204) and plastic surgery procedures to correct deformities after head and neck surgery (Chapter 196).

Radiation Therapy

Ionizing radiation (Chapter 19) can be delivered using high-energy rays, known as *teletherapy*, via a linear accelerator; by brachytherapy, through the application of radioactive implants, seeds, wires, or plaques; and intravenously by using radioisotopes. Radiation interacts with molecular oxygen, inducing the formation of superoxide, hydrogen peroxide, or hydroxyl radicals that damage DNA, leading to cell death. Like chemotherapy, radiation therapy is most effective against rapidly dividing cells.

As "local" therapies, both surgery and radiation therapy are limited in their effectiveness by the inapparent extension of disease, the location of tumors next to normal structures that must be preserved, and the presence of distant metastases. Normal tissue tolerance, which varies among the different organs and tissues, often prevents the use of radiation doses that could uniformly eradicate cancers. Radiation therapy is also limited by tumor hypoxia: large, bulky tumors are frequently relatively radioresistant, whereas well-oxygenated tumors can be more effectively treated at lower doses.

Radiation therapy can be used as the primary treatment, as part of multimodality therapy, in the adjuvant setting, and for palliation. As a single modality, radiation therapy can be curative for early-stage malignancies such as laryngeal cancer (Chapter 196), cervical cancer (Chapter 205), and prostate cancer (Chapter 207). Breast-conserving surgery (Chapter 204) requires the use of radiation to treat the remaining breast. Partial irradiation techniques using three-dimensional planning with external beam radiation or with a balloon catheter have recently been developed and used in selected patients with appropriately placed and sized breast cancers. For localized prostate cancer (Chapter 207), implanted radioactive seeds of gold or palladium offer an alternative to surgery or external beam radiation therapy, again in carefully selected patients.

It is important to note that the combination of chemotherapy and radiation therapy may result in synergistic toxicities, such as esophagitis (Chapter 140) in the treatment of lung cancer (Chapter 197) or mucositis in the treatment of head and neck cancer (Chapter 196).

Newer techniques, such as intensity-modulated radiation therapy, permit more exact tailoring of the dose to the target, thereby reducing damage to the surrounding normal tissues. Stereotactic radiation therapy or gamma knife techniques allow the treatment of primary or metastatic brain tumors (Chapter 195) measuring up to 3 cm with pinpoint accuracy, minimizing damage to normal brain. Proton therapy has only limited applicability at this time; it is

TABLE 182-1 KARNOFSKY AND ZUBROD PERFORMANCE SCALES

Karnofsky Performance Status Scale

VALUE	LEVEL OF FUNCTIONAL CAPACITY
100	Normal, no complaints, no evidence of disease
90	Able to carry on normal activity, minor signs or symptoms of disease
80	Normal activity with effort, some signs or symptoms of disease
70	Cares for self, unable to carry on normal activity or to do active work
60	Requires occasional assistance but is able to care for most needs
50	Requires considerable assistance and frequent medical care
40	Disabled, requires special care and assistance
30	Severely disabled, hospitalization is indicated although death is not imminent
20	Hospitalization is necessary, very sick, active supportive treatment necessary
10	Moribund, fatal processes progressing rapidly
0	Dead

Eastern Cooperative Oncology Group (Zubrod) Performance Scale

PERFORMANCE STATUS	DEFINITION
0	Asymptomatic
1	Symptomatic; fully ambulatory
2	Symptomatic; in bed <50% of day
3	Symptomatic; in bed >50% of day
4	Bedridden

used for some uveal melanomas, skull base tumors, and a few pediatric malignancies.

Low- to moderate-dose palliative radiation is used to ameliorate symptomatic cancer when cure is no longer the goal. For instance, radiation therapy can improve brain metastases (Chapter 195), relieve pain from bone lesions (Chapter 208), relieve obstructing lesions, and sometimes relieve hemoptysis caused by lung cancer (Chapter 197) or bleeding from a gynecologic malignancy (Chapter 205). Bone-seeking radioisotopes such as samarium or strontium may relieve pain from bone metastases in prostate cancer (Chapter 207) or breast cancer (Chapter 204).

Systemic Therapy

Chemotherapy

Pharmacogenomics, the study of inherited interindividual differences in drug disposition and effects, is becoming important in cancer therapy because genetic polymorphisms in drug-metabolizing enzymes are often responsible for the variations in efficacy and toxicity observed with many chemotherapeutic agents. Drugs potentially affected by polymorphisms identified to date include the thiopurines, 5-fluorouracil, irinotecan, and the platinum agents. In patients who are heterozygous or homozygous for deficiencies in metabolizing enzymes, toxicity can be dramatically enhanced.

Currently available tests cannot reliably assess the likelihood of response to therapy, so treatment is largely empirical and based on predictive factors from the tumor itself. Gene expression microarrays currently under development may reliably predict responses in the future. Gene profiles are increasingly used to determine the necessity of therapy, such as the adjuvant therapy of breast or lung cancer.

Assessing Treatment

Assessment of the response to therapy depends largely on tumor size, determined by either direct measurement or diagnostic imaging studies. The categories of response are complete response, with total absence of tumor and correction of tumor-associated changes; partial response, defined as greater than 50% reduction in tumor size; stable disease, defined as greater than 25% but less than 50% reduction in tumor size; and progressive disease, characterized by either tumor growth or the development of new tumors. Leukemias can be assessed by bone marrow aspirates, and multiple myeloma is typically assessed by the measurement of monoclonal proteins, peripheral blood counts, and percentages of malignant plasma cells in bone marrow samples, as well as radiographs of bone lesions.

Chemotherapy is now used in a variety of settings with or without and before, during, or after surgery and radiation therapy (Table 182-2). Considerable experimental evidence suggests that cancers are most sensitive to chemotherapy during the early stages of growth, as a result of the high growth fraction and shorter cell cycle times. Thus, a given dose of drug exerts a greater therapeutic effect against a rapidly growing tumor than against a larger, quiescent tumor.

TABLE 182-2 EXAMPLES OF TIMING OF CHEMOTHERAPY

ADJUVANT THERAPY	NEOADJUVANT THERAPY	ORGAN-SPARING THERAPY	COMBINATION CHEMOTHERAPY
Stage I and II breast cancer	Stage III breast cancer	Anal cancer	Metastatic solid tumors*
Stage III colorectal cancer		Laryngeal cancer	Hematologic malignancies
Stage III melanoma		Esophageal cancer	
Stage I–III lung cancer			

*Usually palliative.

Neoadjuvant Chemotherapy

Neoadjuvant therapy, also called *primary* or *induction chemotherapy*, is used before surgery or radiation therapy to decrease the size of locally advanced cancers, thereby permitting better surgical resection, and to eradicate undetectable metastases. It also affords an opportunity to evaluate the effectiveness of treatment by histologic analysis of resected tissue. This approach is most often used for locally advanced breast cancer (Chapter 204), although other primary tumors can be targeted. Disadvantages include the initially incomplete pathologic staging and the possibility that ineffective chemotherapy will permit the tumor to grow beyond the point of resection.

Organ-sparing therapy is the use of chemotherapy, radiation therapy, or both to salvage organs that would have been surgically removed if cure were the intended result. This technique is often effective in patients with cancers of the larynx (Chapter 196), esophagus (Chapter 198), bladder (Chapter 203), and anus (Chapter 199).

Adjuvant Chemotherapy

Adjuvant chemotherapy is used in patients whose primary tumor and all evidence of cancer (e.g., regional lymph nodes) have been surgically removed or treated definitively with radiation but in whom the risk of recurrence is high because of involved lymph nodes or certain morphologic or biologic characteristics of the cancer. Common examples include cancers of the breast (Chapter 204) and colon (Chapter 199). The typical end points of clinical chemotherapy, such as shrinkage of measurable tumor on serial radiographic studies, are not available in this situation; instead, relapse-free survival and overall survival are the principal measures of treatment effect. For an individual patient receiving adjuvant therapy, there is no way to determine whether such therapy is beneficial or necessary, so decisions are generally based on evidence from clinical trials.

Adjuvant therapy has been used in a wide variety of tumors, with variable success. In the case of breast cancer (Chapter 204) and colon cancer (Chapter 199), the number of lives saved by the use of adjuvant therapy is significant because of the large number of affected patients, despite the modest absolute differences between treated and control patients with current treatment programs. Resectable lung cancer (Chapter 197) has recently been added to this list.

Palliative Chemotherapy

Chemotherapy rarely cures cancers that remain after surgical or radiation treatment or that recur after such therapy. Pancreatic cancer (Chapter 200) is perhaps the best example of this scenario, because few patients are deemed eligible for surgery, and most have recurrent cancer after surgery. Most adult patients with recurrent or metastatic disease are considered for palliative therapy if there is no realistic chance of cure but the potential for prolongation of useful life and/or relief of tumor-related symptoms makes such therapy reasonable.

Combination Chemotherapy

Virtually all the curative chemotherapy regimens developed for hematologic malignancies or solid tumors use combinations of active agents. Combination chemotherapy is usually superior to the use of single agents in adjuvant and neoadjuvant therapy as well. The improved results achieved by combination chemotherapy can be explained in several ways. Resistance to any single agent is almost always present at diagnosis, even in clinically responsive tumors. Tumors that are initially "sensitive" to chemotherapy rapidly acquire resistance to single agents, either as a result of selection of a preexisting clone of resistant tumor cells or because of an increased rate of mutation leading to drug resistance. Combination chemotherapy theoretically addresses both phenomena by providing a broader range of coverage against initially resistant clones of cells and preventing or slowing the development of resistant clones.

Combination chemotherapy follows a set of principles. All drugs must be active against the tumor, and all drugs must be given at an optimal dose and on an optimal schedule. The drugs should have different mechanisms of antitumor activity as well as different toxicity profiles, and the drugs should be given at consistent intervals for the shortest possible treatment time.

Hormonal Therapy

Endocrine or hormonal therapy for cancer (Table 182-3), the earliest form of systemic therapy, is almost entirely limited to breast cancer (Chapter 204) and prostate cancer (Chapter 207). Many premenopausal breast cancers are thought to be under the influence of estrogens, and hormonal deprivation (ablation) may produce long-term responses in properly selected patients (those with estrogen and/or progesterone receptor positivity who have predominantly soft tissue or bone disease). This hormonal ablation may take the form of surgical removal of the ovaries, ablative radiation therapy, or the use of luteinizing hormone–releasing hormone antagonists. The antiestrogen tamoxifen is effective against breast cancer, and it may decrease the incidence of contralateral breast cancers in both premenopausal and postmenopausal women with breast cancer. It also has an estrogen-like activity that is responsible for an increased rate of endometrial cancers. Somewhat paradoxically, postmenopausal women who are candidates for hormonal therapy may also respond to tamoxifen.

Aromatase Inhibitors

Patients who have experienced a prolonged objective response or stable disease with hormonal therapy may be candidates for second-, third-, or fourth-line hormonal therapy. However, such responses tend to become less frequent and shorter, and many patients eventually need chemotherapy. Recently, aromatase inhibitors (e.g., anastrozole, letrozole, exemestane), which decrease the conversion of metabolites in fat and muscle into estrogen, have been found to be more effective than tamoxifen as first-line therapy in both the adjuvant and metastatic settings, although the optimal schedule for tamoxifen and the aromatase inhibitors in the adjuvant setting is still under study (Chapter 204).

Prostate cancer (Chapter 207) is androgen dependent, and androgen deprivation through castration or antiandrogens can produce meaningful responses. Estrogen therapy is now used infrequently because of its cardiovascular side effects and the availability of better alternatives. Once prostate cancer becomes androgen independent, second-line hormonal therapy rarely produces useful responses.

Corticosteroids

The corticosteroids (Chapter 34), typically prednisone or dexamethasone, are widely used in the treatment of hematologic and oncologic cancers. In Hodgkin's disease (Chapter 192), the non-Hodgkin's lymphomas (Chapter 191), and multiple myeloma (Chapter 193), corticosteroids have antitumor activity. In solid tumors, they are used as antiemetics and, rarely, for the treatment of hypercalcemia of cancer (Chapter 186), for symptomatic relief of cerebral edema in cases of central nervous system metastases (Chapter 195), or as an adjunct to radiation therapy for spinal cord metastases. Megestrol acetate (Megace) is often used in an attempt to relieve anorexia, which is common among cancer patients.

Immunotherapy

Two cancers characterized by often unpredictable clinical behavior, melanoma (Chapter 210) and renal cell carcinoma (Chapter 203), are treated with interferon, interleukin-2, or both (Table 182-4). Dramatic responses are uncommon, and immunotherapy is only a minor component of cancer therapy.

Molecularly Targeted Agents

Targeted agents (Table 182-5) are drugs directed at a specific molecular point, such as a protein tyrosine kinase, or at the presence of a specific antigen on a tumor cell. The first tyrosine kinase inhibitors were imatinib and erlotinib. The best example of the success of tyrosine kinase inhibitor therapy is the dramatic response of chronic myelogenous leukemia (Chapter 190) to imatinib (Gleevec). Imatinib also has activity against gastrointestinal stromal cell tumors.

Erlotinib, directed against the epidermal growth factor receptor (EGFR), has antitumor effects in patients whose non–small cell lung cancers (Chapter 197) have EGFR mutations. Current research aims to identify the specific types of mutations so that patients can be prospectively selected for therapy, analogous to the measurement of estrogen receptors to select breast cancer patients for hormonal therapy.

The vascular endothelial growth factor receptor (VEGFR) stimulates the formation of new blood vessels that are critical for tumor growth. Anti-VEGFR agents, such as the monoclonal antibody bevacizumab, prevent VEGF from transducing its signal in endothelial cells, thereby preventing their division. Bevacizumab has antitumor effects in metastatic colorectal cancer, non–small cell lung cancer, and breast cancer. Thalidomide inhibits angiogenesis through an unknown mechanism and is used against multiple myeloma (Chapter 193).

Bortezomib (Velcade), a unique drug, is a reversible inhibitor of the proteasome pathway that normally regulates the intracellular concentration of specific proteins, thus controlling homeostasis. It has been effective in the treatment of refractory multiple myeloma (Chapter 193) and non-Hodgkin's lymphomas (Chapter 191).

The development of monoclonal antibodies directed against antigens found on cancer cells represents an additional treatment modality, often complementary to conventional chemotherapy. Examples include alemtuzumab, cetuximab, rituximab, and trastuzumab. Trastuzumab has recently been shown to add significantly to disease-free survival time in patients positive for HER2/neu who receive adjuvant therapy for early-stage breast cancer (Chapter 204). These monoclonal antibodies can be used alone ("naked") or, in some cases,

TABLE 182-3 HORMONAL THERAPY

Corticosteroids
- Prednisone
- Dexamethasone (Decadron)

Androgens
- Fluoxymesterone (Halotestin)

Estrogens
- Diethylstilbestrol (DES)

Antiandrogens
- Bicalutamide (Casodex)
- Flutamide (Eulexin)
- Nilutamide (Nilandron)

Antiestrogens
- Tamoxifen (Nolvadex)
- Toremifene (Fareston)

Progestational agents
- Megestrol acetate (Megace)

Luteinizing hormone–releasing hormone analogues
- Leuprolide (Lupron)
- Goserelin (Zoladex)
- Degarelix

Aromatase inhibitors
- Anastrozole (Arimidex)
- Exemestane (Aromasin)
- Letrozole (Femara)

Estrogen receptor antagonist
- Fulvestrant (Faslodex)

TABLE 182-4 IMMUNOTHERAPY

Interferon-α (Intron A, Roferon)
Interleukin-2 (Proleukin)

TABLE 182-5 MOLECULARLY TARGETED AGENTS AND MONOCLONAL ANTIBODIES

MOLECULARLY TARGETED AGENTS

Imatinib (Gleevec)
Dasatinib (Sprycel)
Nilotinib (Tasigna)
Erlotinib (Tarceva)—EGFR TKI

Antiangiogenesis agents
- Bevacizumab (Avastin)—VEGF inhibitor
- Thalidomide (Thalomid)
- Lenalidomide (Revlimid)

Multikinase inhibitor
- Sorafenib (Nexavar)
- Sunitinib (Sutent)
- Temosirolimus (Torisel)
- Everloimus (Affinitor)
- Pazopanib (Votrient)
- Lapatinib (Tykerb)

Bortezomib (Velcade)—proteasome inhibitor

MONOCLONAL ANTIBODIES

Trastuzumab (Herceptin)
Rituximab (Rituxan)
Gemtuzumab ozogamicin (Mylotarg)
Alemtuzumab (Campath)
Cetuximab, C-225 (Erbitux)
Tositumomab iodine-131 (Bexxar)
Panitumumab (Vectibex)
Ofatumumab (Arzerra)
Ibritumomab tiuxetan Y 90 (Zevalin)

EGFR = epidermal growth factor receptor; TKI = tyrosine kinase inhibitor; VEGF = vascular endothelial growth factor.

labeled with a radioactive molecule to enhance cell killing. This radioimmunoconjugate approach has been most effective in the treatment of non-Hodgkin's lymphomas (Chapter 191) and chronic lymphocytic leukemia (Chapter 190). The effectiveness of monoclonal antibodies is limited by changes in the antigenic composition of neoplastic cells, called *antigenic drift*.

Individual Agents

A list of the most commonly used chemotherapeutic agents (Table 182-6) can help in understanding the key issues each one raises. In all cases, the most current information from the manufacturer should be sought before therapy is initiated. The number of new drugs continues to increase, and some older drugs included in previous editions of this textbook have been omitted.

The administration of chemotherapy is best done by specifically trained individuals because of the dual risks of hypersensitivity reactions and extravasation. No doses or schedules are suggested because these agents are often used in combination, and the doses must be reduced in many cases. End-organ function also affects dosing. The administration of chemotherapy during pregnancy is an especially difficult circumstance and requires a particularly high level of expertise.

Unless otherwise specified, all chemotherapeutic agents are capable of producing some degree of nausea and vomiting, myelosuppression, alopecia, mucositis, and/or diarrhea after treatment. Most agents are also teratogenic, mutagenic, and carcinogenic, so these toxicities are not repeated for each agent. Drugs used routinely to offset agent-specific toxicities are also included in Table 182-6.

Bone Marrow or Stem Cell Transplantation

Because the major dose-limiting toxicity of most chemotherapeutic agents is myelosuppression, approaches have been developed to harvest the pluripotent stem cells found in bone marrow, peripheral blood, or, less often, cord blood before marrow-damaging chemotherapy so that the stem cells can be reinfused later (Chapter 181). This technique is most effective for acute leukemias (Chapter 189), relapsed lymphomas (Chapter 191), and germ cell tumors (Chapter 206). The effectiveness of this approach is limited more by the inability to eradicate cancer cells than by the inability to achieve engraftment. Transplants may be syngeneic (from an identical twin), autologous (from oneself), allogeneic (from a matched donor, such as a sibling or parent), or from a matched unrelated donor. Nonablative hematopoietic transplants that do not completely abolish myelopoiesis reduce toxicity and allow the treatment of older and medically infirm patients.

Special Circumstances: Pregnant and Geriatric Patients

Pregnancy

Cancer during pregnancy is not uncommon, with breast, cervical, ovarian, melanoma, thyroid, and hematologic malignancies being most common. This is obviously an emotionally charged time, as the joy of a new birth is contrasted with the possible loss of the mother. Clinical decision making is complicated by ethical, moral, cultural, and religious issues. This is not an area for the inexperienced. If surgery can be safely accomplished, this may be the best course, even if it is only a temporizing measure. Radiation therapy carries the very real risk of radiation exposure to the fetus, and staging is almost always suboptimal and confined to ultrasound examinations. When the disease requires chemotherapy, changes in both the mother and the fetus must be taken into account; for instance, there are major changes is pharmacokinetics during pregnancy, along with changes in renal function and plasma volume, plasma protein levels, hepatic metabolism, gastrointestinal absorption, and placental transfer, not to mention fetal pharmacokinetics and placental excretion. Many of the commonly used chemotherapeutic drugs are classified by the Food and Drug Administration as category D (positive human fetal risk, but the benefits in pregnant women may be acceptable despite the risk) or category X (studies in humans and animal have shown fetal malformations or there is evidence of fetal risk based on human evidence). If the mother's condition permits, it is advisable to defer chemotherapy during the first and perhaps the second trimesters and to treat life-threatening situations during the third trimester after extensive counseling with the parents.

Geriatrics

The aging U.S. population has brought an increasing number of older patients with cancer to the attention of oncologists, and the field of geriatric oncology is a new area of specialization. An increasing proportion of cancers occurs in the older population. The changes that develop with age are covered in another chapter, but they can be briefly summarized here as decreased excretion of drugs and metabolites from the kidneys, decreased volume of distribution of water-soluble drugs, and increased susceptibility to myelosuppression, cardiomyopathy, and neuropathy. Many older adults also have comorbid illnesses that must be taken into account. As a general rule, the suitability of an older patient for therapy can be determined by a comprehensive geriatric assessment (CGA) that evaluates the patient's function, comorbidity, nutrition, medications, and resources. By itself, age is not a barrier to surgery; rather, the patient's performance status and the CGA should determine the likelihood of a good recovery. Tolerance of radiation therapy seems to remain largely intact with increasing age. Chemotherapy decisions are also based on the performance status and CGA, with the use of growth factors to increase the white blood cell count and to maintain a hemoglobin sufficient to minimize symptoms. Dosage adjustments are also made for individual glomerular filtration rates for patients aged 65 and older. The use of lower chemotherapy doses based on age alone is probably not advisable and may result in ineffective therapy.

Management of Complications

Supportive Care

Nutrition is always a concern for patients newly diagnosed with cancer, even if they have not experienced weight loss. In fact, significant weight loss is an adverse prognostic factor for several cancers, especially lung cancer. Patients are often concerned about whether their diet contributed to development of the cancer and whether diet can influence the results of therapy. In most settings, neither of these scenarios is the case. Malnourished patients should be evaluated by a dietitian to determine whether they are ingesting sufficient calories and whether dietary supplements might be needed. Some patients, such as those with head and neck cancers (Chapter 196) or esophageal cancers (Chapter 198), may require parenteral nutrition through a percutaneous endoscopic gastrostomy tube. Total parenteral nutrition (Chapter 224) is rarely indicated, is not particularly helpful, and is likely to produce an ethical dilemma when therapy fails and the decision to discontinue it must be discussed. Corticosteroids increase appetite but have many undesirable side effects. Megestrol acetate (Megace) at a dose of 800 mg/day improves appetite and allows weight gain in many patients; it is expensive, although the suspension is less costly than the tablets. The synthetic cannabinoid dronabinol (Marinol) stimulates appetite and reduces nausea in some patients, but it can produce dysphoria, particularly in older patients. A multiple vitamin with zinc may help with abnormal taste and provide trace minerals. Larger than recommended doses of vitamins are not helpful and may be toxic. It is always useful to inquire what over-the-counter and alternative medications (Chapter 38) are being contemplated or used by the patient.

Symptom Management

Symptom management is key to successful treatment and the patient's quality of life. Pain control (Chapter 29) can be accomplished with a variety of analgesics, both non-narcotic and narcotic. Oncologists use a 10-point scale for evaluating pain control (Fig. 182-1) and start with nonsteroidal anti-inflammatory drugs (NSAIDs) such as aspirin and acetaminophen, progress through ibuprofen and related drugs, and then through combinations of NSAIDs and narcotics to stronger narcotics.[1] Newer narcotics are available in both short-duration and long-duration forms; some patches last 72 hours, which are ideal for patients who have severe pain and are unable to take oral medications. Oral transmucosal fentanyl is more effective than standard-release morphine in this setting. Oral mucositis, a common complication of intensive therapy for hematologic malignancies, can be treated with local measures or with recombinant human keratinocyte growth factor.[2,3] Oral anti-*Candida* drugs that are absorbed or partially absorbed from the gastrointestinal tract can help prevent oral candidiasis.[4]

Many patients still fear chemotherapy because of the risk of nausea and vomiting. New antiemetics, used in combination, have made this side effect much less common. Chemotherapeutic drugs can be ranked according to their probability of causing nausea and vomiting, with prophylactic treatment given accordingly. The availability of the serotonin 5-hydroxytryptamine type 3 ($5\text{-}HT_3$) receptor antagonists (dolasetron, granisetron, ondansetron) has dramatically improved the ability to completely control nausea and vomiting. Although prochlorperazine may be adequate for mildly emetogenic chemotherapy, more emetogenic regimens require combination therapy with a corticosteroid (usually dexamethasone), a $5\text{-}HT_3$ antagonist, and a benzodiazepine (e.g., lorazepam). A newer antiemetic, aprepitant, is particularly useful for the treatment of delayed nausea and vomiting. Treating patients before the development of nausea and vomiting is much more effective and helps patients adhere to their treatment schedules.

Growth factors, such as granulocyte colony-stimulating factor (G-CSF) and granulocyte-macrophage colony-stimulating factor (GM-CSF), permit the more rapid recovery of white blood cell nadirs, thus permitting chemotherapy to be given on schedule, without reducing the dosage in many cases.[5] However, such therapy does not decrease hospitalizations or improve survival. It is possible to determine which individuals are at greatest risk for febrile neutropenia (Chapters 170 and 289) and treat them in advance, based on published guidelines.[6,7] Anemia induced by chemotherapy can be alleviated, the need for transfusions reduced, and quality of life improved by the use of either erythropoietin (Procrit) or darbepoetin (Aranesp).

The bisphosphonates pamidronate (Aredia) and zoledronate (Zometa) are very effective not only to treat tumor-induced hypercalcemia (Chapter 186) but also to reduce pathologic fractures in bones with metastatic lesions, particularly from breast cancer (Chapter 204), prostate cancer (Chapter 207), and myeloma (Chapter 193). They are also used to treat osteoporosis caused by chemotherapy-induced premature menopause in young women with breast cancer. Denosumab (Xgeva) is a human monoclonal antibody that binds to

Text continues on p. 1177

TABLE 182-6 CHEMOTHERAPEUTIC AGENTS

AGENT	CLASS	ACTION	EXCRETION	UNIQUE SIDE EFFECTS	DRUG INTERACTIONS	INDICATIONS
ALKYLATING AGENTS						
Bendamustine (Treanda)	Alkylating agent	Bifunctional with both alkylating and purine-like antimetabolite action	Biotransformation in liver	None	Synergistic with rituximab	CLL, myeloma, Hodgkin's and non-Hodgkin's lymphoma
Carboplatin (Paraplatin)	Platinum coordination compound	Produces interstrand DNA cross-links, similar to those with bifunctional alkylating agents; cell cycle nonspecific	Renal	Nephrotoxicity, ototoxicity, neuropathy, hypomagnesemia, hypersensitivity reactions, hepatotoxicity	Avoid other nephrotoxic or ototoxic drugs	Ovarian cancer, testicular cancer, lung cancer, head and neck cancer, breast cancer
Chlorambucil (Leukeran)	Bifunctional alkylating agent	Formation of interstrand DNA cross-links with resultant inactivation of DNA; cell cycle nonspecific	Hepatic biotransformation, renal excretion	Hepatotoxicity, pulmonary toxicity	None	CLL, Waldenström's macroglobulinemia, Hodgkin's and non-Hodgkin's lymphomas, myeloproliferative disorders, ovarian cancer
Cisplatin (Platinol)	Platinum coordination compound	Produces interstrand DNA cross-links similar to bifunctional alkylating agents; cell cycle nonspecific	Renal	Nephrotoxicity, ototoxicity, neuropathy, hypomagnesemia, hypersensitivity reactions, hemolytic anemia, SIADH	Avoid other nephrotoxic or ototoxic drugs	Testicular cancer, other germ cell tumors, ovarian cancer, bladder cancer, prostate cancer, lung cancer, sarcomas, cervical cancer, endometrial cancer, gastric cancer, breast cancer, adrenal cancer, head and neck cancer
Cyclophosphamide (Cytoxan, Neosar)	Alkylating agent of nitrogen mustard type	Cross-linking of DNA and RNA, inhibits protein synthesis; cell cycle nonspecific	Hepatic biotransformation, renal excretion	Hemorrhagic cystitis, SIADH	Phenobarbital increases rate of metabolism and leukopenia; cyclophosphamide potentiates effects of succinylcholine and may increase oral anticoagulant activity	Breast cancer, ovarian cancer, Hodgkin's and non-Hodgkin's lymphomas, leukemias, neuroblastoma, retinoblastoma, other sarcomas, bladder cancer, lung cancer, cervical cancer, endometrial cancer, prostate cancer, osteogenic sarcoma, Wilms' tumor
Dacarbazine (DTIC-Dome)	Nonclassic alkylating agent	Inhibits DNA and RNA synthesis via formation of carbonium ions; cell cycle nonspecific	Hepatic biotransformation, renal excretion	Pain on injection, flu-like syndrome, hepatic veno-occlusive disease, photosensitivity	Heparin, lidocaine, hydrocortisone, phenytoin, phenobarbital, interleukin-2	Melanoma, Hodgkin's disease, sarcomas
Ifosfamide (Ifex)	Alkylating agent of nitrogen mustard type	Alkylated metabolites interact with DNA; cell cycle nonspecific	Hepatic biotransformation, renal elimination	Hemorrhagic cystitis, nephrotoxicity, CNS toxicity	None	Germ cell tumors, sarcomas, non-Hodgkin's lymphomas, cervical cancer, Ewing's sarcoma, lung cancer
Mechlorethamine, nitrogen mustard (Mustargen)	Bifunctional alkylating agent	Cross-links strands of DNA and RNA, inhibits protein synthesis; cell cycle nonspecific	Rapidly deactivated in body fluids and tissues	Extravasation	None	Hodgkin's disease, intracavitary treatment of effusions; topically for mycosis fungoides
Melphalan (Alkeran)	Alkylating agent of nitrogen mustard type	Forms interstrand, intrastrand, or DNA protein cross-links; cell cycle nonspecific	Deactivated in body fluids and tissues, renal elimination 50%	Pulmonary toxicity	Cimetidine decreases oral bioavailability; cyclosporine enhances risk of renal toxicity	Multiple myeloma, breast cancer, ovarian cancer, rhabdomyosarcoma, bone marrow ablation for stem cell transplantation
Mitomycin (Mutamycin)	Antitumor antibiotic	Acts as bifunctional alkylating agent, inhibiting DNA synthesis; cell cycle nonspecific, but most active in G and S phases	Hepatic biotransformation, renal elimination	Cumulative myelosuppression, extravasation, renal toxicity, pulmonary toxicity, cardiac toxicity, hemolytic-uremic syndrome	Prior treatment with vinca alkaloids may predispose to pulmonary toxicity; if used with doxorubicin, may potentiate cardiotoxicity	Gastric cancer, pancreatic cancer, anal cancer, lung cancer, head and neck cancer, cervical cancer

Oxaliplatin (Eloxatin)	Platinum coordination compound	Produces interstrand DNA cross-links similar to bifunctional alkylating agents; cell cycle nonspecific	Renal	Nephrotoxicity, neurotoxicity (worse with cold), allergic reactions	Avoid other nephrotoxic drugs, incompatible with 5-fluorouracil	Colorectal cancer
Procarbazine (Matulane)	Nonclassic alkylating agent and MAO inhibitor	Unknown; metabolism produces highly active free radicals that may alkylate and methylate DNA; cell cycle specific, S phase	Renal 70% after hepatic biotransformation	Disulfiram (Antabuse)-like side effects with alcohol ingestion; patients should avoid foods containing tyramine due to the drug's MAO inhibitory effects; central and peripheral neurotoxicity, hepatotoxicity, pulmonary toxicity	>100, including alcohol, antihistamines, anticoagulants, anticonvulsants, hypoglycemics, certain antihypertensives, caffeine-containing preparations, narcotics, methyldopa, metrizamide, sympathomimetics, tyramine or other high pressor amine-containing foods	Hodgkin's disease, brain tumors
Streptozocin (Zanosar)	Nitrosourea	Inhibits DNA synthesis	Renal	Cumulative, dose-related renal toxicity, hepatotoxicity, glucose intolerance	None	Islet cell tumors of pancreas, carcinoid tumors
Temozolomide (Temodar)	Nonclassic alkylating agent	Inhibits DNA and RNA synthesis via formation of carbonium ions; cell cycle nonspecific	Hepatic biotransformation, renal excretion	Photosensitivity	None	Melanoma, brain tumors
DIFFERENTIATING AGENTS						
All-*trans*-retinoic acid (ATRA)	Retinoid	Induces differentiation and/or inhibition of clonogenicity	Conjugation to glucuronic acid with subsequent biliary excretion and enterohepatic circulation	Mucocutaneous toxicity, ocular toxicity, musculoskeletal toxicity, neurologic toxicity, hepatotoxicity, lipid toxicity	None	Acute progranulocytic leukemia
Arsenic trioxide (Trisenox)	Natural product	Induces differentiation of acute progranulocytic leukemia cells	Hepatic metabolism, excreted in urine	Prolonged QT interval, acute progranulocytic leukemia differentiation syndrome, leukocytosis, peripheral neuropathy	Medications that increase QT interval, such as antiarrhythmics and amphotericin	Acute progranulocytic leukemia
ENZYMES						
L-Asparaginase (Elspar)	Enzyme	Hydrolyzes 1-asparagine to aspartic acid and ammonia, resulting in cellular deficiency of 1-asparagine; sensitive tumor cells lack asparagine synthetase; interferes with protein, DNA, and RNA synthesis; cell cycle specific for G1 phase of cell division	Metabolized in liver	Hypersensitivity reactions, inhibitory effects on protein synthesis with resultant decreases in hepatic synthesis of coagulation factors, pancreatitis, hyperglycemia, CNS depression, hepatotoxicity	Abolishes effects of methotrexate on malignant cells; concurrent vincristine may enhance hyperglycemic effects of asparaginase and increase risk of neuropathy	Acute lymphoblastic leukemia
ANTIMETABOLITES						
5-Azacitidine (Vidaza)	Antimetabolite; pyrimidine nucleoside analogue of cytidine	Causes hypomethylation of DNA and direct cytotoxicity on abnormal hematopoietic cells	Hepatic metabolism, excreted in urine	Renal toxicity, low serum bicarbonate levels	None	Myelodysplasia
Capecitabine (Xeloda)	Antimetabolite of pyrimidine analogue type	Fluoropyrimidine carbamate prodrug form of 5-fluorouracil; given orally; inactive as itself; inhibits DNA and RNA synthesis; cell cycle specific, S phase	Hepatic catabolism	Hand and foot syndrome, angina	Warfarin potentiation, phenytoin, antacids, leucovorin, thymidine	Breast cancer, colorectal cancer

TABLE 182-6 CHEMOTHERAPEUTIC AGENTS—cont'd

AGENT	CLASS	ACTION	EXCRETION	UNIQUE SIDE EFFECTS	DRUG INTERACTIONS	INDICATIONS
Cladribine (Leustatin), 2-chloro-2-deoxy-D-adenosine	Antimetabolite	Purine nucleoside analogue, inhibits both DNA synthesis and repair	Uncertain	Bone marrow suppression, fever, paralysis, and/or acute renal failure when used at very high doses for BMT	None known	Hairy cell leukemia
Clofarabine (Clofar)	Purine nucleoside antimetabolite	Inhibits DNA synthesis and DNA repair	Excreted in urine and other?	Bone marrow suppression, hepatotoxicity	Other renal and hepatotoxic drugs	Relapsed acute lymphoblastic leukemia
Cytarabine (Cytosar-U, Tarabine PFS)	Antimetabolite	Activated to cytarabine triphosphate in tissues, inhibits DNA synthesis; cell cycle specific, S phase	Deaminated in blood and tissues	Pancreatitis; with high doses, cerebral dysfunction, GI damage, hepatotoxicity, pulmonary edema, corneal damage, "Ara-C syndrome"	With high-dose cyclophosphamide, may increase cardiotoxicity	Acute granulocytic leukemia and its variants, non-Hodgkin's lymphoma, myelodysplasia*
Fludarabine phosphate (Fludara)	Antimetabolite of purine type	2-Fluoro-ara-ATP inhibits DNA synthesis by inhibition of ribonucleotide reductase and the DNA polymerases; cell cycle specific, S phase	Renal	Neurologic, pulmonary toxicity	None	CLL
Fluorouracil (5-FU, Adrucil)	Antimetabolite of pyrimidine analogue type	Inhibits DNA and RNA synthesis; cell cycle specific, S phase	Respiratory, small renal elimination	Cerebellar ataxia, myocardial ischemia	None	Breast cancer, GI cancers, head and neck cancer, bladder cancer, ovarian cancer, endometrial cancer, effusions
Floxuridine (FUDR)	Antimetabolite of pyrimidine analogue type	Inhibits DNA and RNA synthesis; cell cycle specific, S phase	Respiratory, small renal elimination	Cerebellar ataxia, myocardial ischemia, hepatotoxicity	Leucovorin enhances activity and toxicity; thymidine rescues toxic effects	Intra-arterial therapy for hepatic malignancies
Hydroxyurea (Hydrea)	Antimetabolite	Inhibits ribonucleotide reductase, causing inhibition of DNA synthesis; cell cycle specific, S phase	Renal after hepatic biotransformation	Megaloblastosis	May enhance effects of anti-HIV drugs	Myeloproliferative neoplasms, ovarian cancer, head and neck cancer, cervical cancer (with radiation therapy)
Mercaptopurine (Purinethol, 6-MP)	Antimetabolite of purine analogue type	Inhibits DNA synthesis; cell cycle specific, S phase	Metabolic alteration by xanthine oxidase, renal excretion	Hepatotoxicity, skin rashes	Dose must be reduced when used with allopurinol; concomitant methotrexate enhances bioavailability of 6-MP; inhibits warfarin (Coumadin) effects	Acute lymphoblastic leukemia
Methotrexate (Folex, Mexate)	Antimetabolite of folic acid analogue type	Inhibits DNA, RNA, thymidylate, and protein synthesis as a result of binding to dihydrofolate reductase; cell cycle specific, S phase	Renal	Hepatotoxicity, lung disease; in high doses, acute renal failure, acute neurologic dysfunction; avoid use with ascites, pleural effusions	Salicylates, NSAIDs, folic acid–containing vitamins, oral nonabsorbable broad-spectrum antibiotics, trimethoprim/sulfamethoxazole, other nephrotoxic drugs	Breast cancer, head and neck cancer, choriocarcinoma, acute lymphoblastic leukemia, non-Hodgkin's lymphomas, osteosarcoma, intrathecal treatment of meningeal leukemia, bladder cancer, lung cancer
Pemetrexed (Alimta)	Antimetabolite of folic acid analogue type	Inhibits thymidylate synthetase, dihydrofolate reductase, and de novo purine synthesis; cell cycle specific, S phase	Renal, after hepatic metabolism	Must be given with folic acid and vitamin B_{12}; avoid use with ascites, pleural effusions	Salicylates, NSAIDs	Mesothelioma, breast cancer, lung cancer
Pentostatin (Nipent)	Purine antagonist	Inhibits adenosine deaminase; also inhibits RNA synthesis	Renal	Fever, fatigue, rash, pain, hepatotoxicity, chronic immunosuppression	Enhances effects of vidarabine, a purine nucleoside with antiviral activity; must not be given with fludarabine because of fatal pulmonary toxicity	Hairy cell leukemia, CLL
Pralatrexate (Fotolyn)	Antimetabolite type		Renal	Requires vitamin B_{12} and folate supplementation	Myelosuppression	Relapsed peripheral T-cell lymphomas

NONCOVALENT DNA-BINDING DRUGS						
Bleomycin (Blenoxane)	Antitumor antibiotic	Inhibition of DNA synthesis; most effective in G2 phase of cell division	Renal	Dose-related pulmonary fibrosis, hypersensitivity reactions, skin and mucocutaneous toxicity, including Raynaud's phenomenon (in combination with other agents), fever, chills; usually considered nonmyelosuppressive	Cisplatin may decrease renal clearance; high oxygen concentrations may enhance pulmonary toxicity, even after therapy	Testicular cancer and other germ cell tumors; Hodgkin's and non-Hodgkin's lymphomas; mycosis fungoides; squamous cell carcinomas of head and neck, cervix, and vulva; pleural effusions
Daunorubicin (Cerubidine)	Antitumor antibiotic	Binds to DNA by intercalation between base pairs and inhibits DNA and RNA synthesis by template disordering and steric obstruction; most active in S phase but not cell cycle phase specific	Hepatic biotransformation with 40% biliary excretion	Dose-related cardiotoxicity, extravasation, red urine	None	Acute granulocytic leukemia and its variants, acute lymphoblastic leukemia
Doxorubicin (Adriamycin, Rubex)	Antitumor antibiotic	Binds to DNA by intercalation between base pairs and inhibits DNA and RNA synthesis by template disordering and steric obstruction; cell cycle specific, S phase	Hepatic biotransformation with 50% biliary excretion	Dose-related cardiotoxicity, extravasation, red urine	None	Acute granulocytic leukemia and its variants, acute lymphoblastic leukemia, breast cancer, bladder cancer, ovarian cancer, thyroid cancer, lung cancer, Hodgkin's and non-Hodgkin's lymphomas, sarcomas, gastric cancer, multiple myeloma, endometrial cancer, bladder cancer, prostate cancer, Wilms' tumor, neuroblastoma
Doxorubicin liposomal (Doxil)	Anthracycline antibiotic	Topoisomerase inhibitor	Liver	Dose-related cardiotoxicity, extravasation, hand-foot syndrome	None	Ovarian cancer, myeloma, Kaposi's sarcoma
Epirubicin (Ellence)	Antitumor antibiotic	Intercalates with DNA	Liver	Dose-related cardiotoxicity	None	Breast cancer adjuvant therapy
Idarubicin (Idamycin)	Anthracycline glycoside	Intercalates DNA and inhibits DNA synthesis, interacts with RNA polymerases, and inhibits topoisomerase II	Hepatic biotransformation, biliary excretion	Dose-related cardiotoxicity, extravasation	None	Acute granulocytic leukemia and its variants
Mitoxantrone (Novantrone)	Antitumor antibiotic	Binds to DNA by intercalation between base pairs and nonintercalative electrostatic interaction, resulting in inhibition of DNA and RNA synthesis; not cell cycle specific, but most active in late S phase	Hepatic biotransformation, biliary/fecal excretion	Dose-related cardiotoxicity, extravasation, blue-green urine	None	Prostate cancer, acute myelogenous leukemia and its variants, breast cancer, non-Hodgkin's lymphomas
INHIBITORS OF CHROMATIN FUNCTION						
Docetaxel (Taxotere)	Mitotic spindle poison	Unique mitotic spindle inhibitor; cell cycle specific, M phase	Hepatic metabolism, biliary	Hypersensitivity reactions, fluid retention syndrome, nail discoloration, neuropathy, arthralgias	Inhibitors or activators of liver cytochrome P-450 CYP34A enzyme system may affect metabolism	Breast cancer, prostate cancer, lung cancer, ovarian cancer, esophageal cancer, gastric cancer, head and neck cancer, bladder cancer
Etoposide (VP-16, VePesid)	Epipodophyllo toxin	Inhibits DNA synthesis; cell cycle dependent and phase specific, with maximum effect in S and G2 phases	Hepatic biotransformation, renal elimination	Allergic reactions, hepatotoxicity, CNS toxicity, hypotension	None	Testicular cancer, lung cancer, Hodgkin's and non-Hodgkin's lymphomas, choriocarcinoma, Ewing's sarcoma, acute granulocytic leukemia
Irinotecan (Camptosar)	Topoisomerase I inhibitor	Binds to topoisomerase I–DNA complex and prevents relegation of these single-strand breaks	Metabolized in liver	Early and late diarrhea may be severe	None	Colorectal cancer, small cell lung cancer

TABLE 182-6 CHEMOTHERAPEUTIC AGENTS—cont'd

AGENT	CLASS	ACTION	EXCRETION	UNIQUE SIDE EFFECTS	DRUG INTERACTIONS	INDICATIONS
Paclitaxel (Taxol)	Mitotic spindle poison	Unique mitotic spindle inhibitor; cell cycle specific, M phase	Hepatic metabolism, biliary	Hypersensitivity reactions, neuropathy, arthralgias, cardiotoxicity	Enhanced myelosuppression with doxorubicin	Lung cancer, ovarian cancer, breast cancer, esophageal cancer, gastric cancer, head and neck cancer
Paclitaxel protein-bound particles (Abraxane)	Mitotic spindle poison	Unique mitotic spindle inhibitor; cell cycle specific, M phase	Hepatic metabolism, biliary	Hypersensitivity reactions, neuropathy, arthralgias/myalgias, cardiotoxicity	Enhanced myelosuppression with doxorubicin	Metastatic breast cancer
Topotecan (Hycamtin)	Topoisomerase I inhibitor	Binds to topoisomerase I–DNA complex and prevents relegation of these single-strand breaks	Excreted unchanged in urine	—	None	Relapsed ovarian cancer, small cell lung cancer
Vinblastine (Velban)	Vinca alkaloid	Blocks mitosis by arresting cells in metaphase; cell cycle specific, M phase	Biliary/fecal	Extravasation, neurotoxicity	None	Testicular cancer, breast cancer, choriocarcinoma, Hodgkin's and non-Hodgkin's lymphomas, Kaposi's sarcoma, bladder cancer, neuroblastoma, renal carcinoma
Vincristine (Oncovin)	Vinca alkaloid	Blocks mitosis by arresting cells in metaphase; cell cycle specific, M phase	Biliary/fecal	Extravasation, neurotoxicity, constipation, SIADH	Concurrent use with L-asparaginase may increase neurotoxicity	Acute lymphocytic leukemia, neuroblastoma, Wilms' tumor, Hodgkin's and non-Hodgkin's lymphomas, rhabdomyosarcoma, Ewing's sarcoma, breast cancer, small cell lung cancer, multiple myeloma
Vinorelbine (Navelbine)	Vinca alkaloid	Inhibits tubulin polymerization, disrupting formation of microtubule assembly during mitosis; cell cycle specific, M phase	Biliary/fecal	Extravasation, neurotoxicity, constipation, SIADH	Drugs metabolized by liver P-450 system, phenytoin	Non–small cell lung cancer, breast cancer, non- Hodgkin's lymphomas
HORMONAL AGENTS						
Anastrozole (Arimidex)	Nonsteroidal aromatase inhibitor	Inhibits synthesis of estrogens by inhibiting conversion of adrenal androgens to estrogens	Metabolized in liver	Hot flashes, arthralgias	None	Adjuvant and metastatic breast cancer in postmenopausal women
Bicalutamide (Casodex)	Nonsteroidal antiandrogen	Binds to androgen receptors in prostate	Hepatic metabolism	Worsening bone pain, gynecomastia, hot flashes	None	Prostate cancer (usually in conjunction with LHRH antagonist)
Degarelix (Firmagon)	GnRH receptor antagonist	Binds to GnRH receptors in pituitary		Injection site reactions, increased LFTs, QT interval prolongation	None	Prostate cancer
Dexamethasone (Decadron)	Corticosteroid	Multiple	Renal excretion of inactive metabolites	Cushingoid appearance, hyperglycemia, fluid retention, osteoporosis, muscular weakness, peptic ulcer disease, cataracts, psychosis, aseptic necrosis	Efficacy impaired by phenytoin	Acute lymphoblastic leukemia, Hodgkin's and non-Hodgkin's lymphomas, CLL, multiple myeloma, Waldenström's macroglobulinemia, cerebral edema, hypercalcemia, lymphangitic metastases, antiemetic
Diethylstilbestrol (DES)	Estrogen	Stimulation of autocrine growth factors	Renal	Feminization in men, fluid retention, thromboembolic phenomena, induction of endometrial cancer	None	Breast cancer, prostate cancer

Estradiol	Estrogen	Stimulation of autocrine growth factors	Renal	Feminization in men, fluid retention, thromboembolic phenomena, induction of endometrial cancer	None	Breast cancer, prostate cancer
Estramustine (Emcyt)	Phosphorylated combination of estradiol and nitrogen mustard	Inhibits microtubule structure and function; cell cycle specific, M-phase	Biliary/fecal	Feminization, fluid retention	None	Prostate cancer
Estrogens (conjugated or esterified)	Estrogen	Stimulation of autocrine growth factors, inhibition of pituitary secretion of LH, resulting in decreased serum testosterone concentration	Primarily renal	Feminization in men, fluid retention, thromboembolic phenomena, induction of endometrial cancer	None	Breast cancer, prostate cancer
Exemestane (Aromasin)	Steroidal aromatase inhibitor	Permanently binds to and irreversibly inhibits aromatase, inhibits synthesis of estrogens by inhibiting conversion of adrenal androgens to estrogens	Metabolized in liver	Hot flashes, arthralgias	None	Metastatic breast cancer in postmenopausal women
Fluoxymesterone (Halotestin)	Androgen	Suppresses GnRH, LH, and FSH through negative feedback mechanism involving hypothalamus and anterior pituitary	Renal	Masculinization in women, hepatotoxicity	May increase anticoagulant effects of warfarin (Coumadin); decreased blood glucose, resulting in potential for hypoglycemia in diabetics	Breast cancer
Flutamide (Eulexin)	Antiandrogen	Inhibition of androgen uptake and/or inhibition of nuclear binding of androgen in target tissues; its interference with testosterone at cellular level complements "medical castration" produced by LHRH analogues	Renal	Worsening bone pain, hot flashes, gynecomastia	None	Prostate cancer (usually in conjunction with LHRH antagonist)
Fulvestrant (Faslodex)	Estrogen receptor antagonist	Competitively binds to estrogen receptor and downregulates estrogen receptor protein in breast cancer cells	Cleared by hepatobiliary route	Arthralgias	None	Recurrent breast cancer in postmenopausal women
Goserelin (Zoladex)	Synthetic decapeptide analogue of LHRH	Suppresses pituitary gonadotropins, with fall of serum testosterone into castrate range	Metabolism	Worsening bone pain, hot flashes	None	Breast cancer, prostate cancer
Letrozole (Femara)	Nonsteroidal competitive inhibitor of aromatase	Inhibits synthesis of estrogens by inhibiting conversion of adrenal androgens to estrogens	Metabolized in liver	Hot flashes, arthralgias	None	Adjuvant and metastatic breast cancer in postmenopausal women
Leuprolide (Lupron, Lupron Depot)	Synthetic LHRH analogue	Suppresses secretion of GnRH, with resultant fall in testosterone secretion, producing "medical castration"	Metabolized in liver	Increased bone pain, hot flashes, thromboembolic phenomena	None	Prostate cancer, breast cancer
Medroxyprogesterone (Provera, Depo- Provera)	Progestational drug	Inhibition of pituitary gonadotropin production with resultant decrease in estrogen secretion	Renal	Weight gain, thromboembolic phenomena, fetal hazard	None	Breast cancer, endometrial cancer
Megestrol acetate (Megace)	Progestational drug	Inhibition of pituitary gonadotropin production, with resultant decrease in estrogen secretion	Renal	Weight gain, thromboembolic phenomena, fetal hazard	None	Breast cancer, endometrial cancer

TABLE 182-6 CHEMOTHERAPEUTIC AGENTS—cont'd

AGENT	CLASS	ACTION	EXCRETION	UNIQUE SIDE EFFECTS	DRUG INTERACTIONS	INDICATIONS
Nilutamide (Nilandron)	Nonsteroidal antiandrogen	Binds to androgen receptors in prostate, inhibiting androgen uptake and binding in nucleus	Hepatic metabolism	Worsening bone pain, gynecomastia, hot flashes, visual disturbances, interstitial pneumonitis	Increased warfarin effect; inhibits liver cytochrome P-450 system; increased risk of alcohol intolerance	Prostate cancer (usually in conjunction with LHRH antagonist)
Octreotide (Sandostatin)	Synthetic octapeptide analogue of somatostatin	Suppresses secretion of serotonin and GI peptides; blocks carcinoid flush, decreases serum 5-HIAA, and controls other symptoms associated with carcinoid syndrome	Renal	Hyper/hypoglycemia, hepatic dysfunction	None	Palliative treatment of carcinoid tumors and vasoactive intestinal peptide tumors (VIPomas)
Prednisone (Deltasone)	Corticosteroid	Multiple	Renal excretion of inactive metabolites	Cushingoid appearance, hyperglycemia, fluid retention, osteoporosis, muscular weakness, peptic ulcer disease, cataracts, psychosis, aseptic necrosis	Efficacy impaired by phenytoin	Acute lymphoblastic leukemia, Hodgkin's and non-Hodgkin's lymphomas, CLL, multiple myeloma, Waldenström's macroglobulinemia, cerebral edema, hypercalcemia, lymphangitic metastases, antiemetic
Tamoxifen (Nolvadex)	Nonsteroidal antiestrogen	Competes with estradiol for estrogen receptor protein	In feces, mainly as conjugates	Hot flashes, nausea/vomiting, vaginal bleeding or discharge, hypercalcemia, visual disturbances, thrombocytopenia, endometrial cancer, rare liver dysfunction	When used with coumarin anticoagulants, significant increase in anticoagulant effect may be seen	Adjuvant and metastatic breast cancer
BIOLOGIC RESPONSE MODIFIERS						
Aldesleukin (Human Recombinant IL-2, Proleukin)	Lymphokine	Supports T-cell proliferation, augments natural killer cytotoxicity, induces lymphokine-activated killer (LAK) cell development, and participates in activation of monocytes and B cells	Renal	Cardiovascular toxicity, nephrotoxicity, pulmonary toxicity, GI toxicity, endocrine toxicity, dermatologic complications, CNS toxicity, hematologic toxicity, fever and chills, infection, capillary leak syndrome	May potentiate effects of psychotropics, nephrotoxic drugs, and antihypertensive agents; corticosteroids may reduce effectiveness	Renal cancer, melanoma
Erythropoietin (Aranesp, Epogen, Procrit)[†]	Hematopoietic growth factor	Stimulates division and differentiation of committed erythroid progenitors in bone marrow	Metabolized in liver	Headache, hypertension, possible seizures, allergic reactions	None	Correction of anemia in chronic renal failure, azathioprine-treated HIV infection, myelodysplasia, multiple myeloma, chemotherapy-induced anemia
Filgrastim (G-CSF, Neupogen)	Class II hematopoietic growth factor (acts on progenitor cells capable of forming only one differentiated cell type, the neutrophil)	CSFs bind to specific cell surface receptors and stimulate proliferation and differentiation	Metabolized in liver	Pain at site of subcutaneous injection, allergic reactions, arthralgias, bone pain	None	Decreases incidence of infection after myelosuppressive chemotherapy, enhances myeloid engraftment after BMT, enhances peripheral progenitor cell yield
Interferon-α (Intron-A, Roferon)[†]	Interferon	Antiviral, antiproliferative, and immunomodulatory properties	Renal	Fever, flu-like symptoms, cardiotoxicity, neurotoxicity	None	Hairy cell leukemia, Kaposi's sarcoma, renal cancer, non-Hodgkin's lymphoma

Sargramostim (GM-CSF, Leukine, Prokine)	Class I hematopoietic growth factor (stimulates formation of granulocytes and macrophages and is not lineage specific)	CSFs bind to specific cell surface receptors and stimulate proliferation and differentiation	Metabolized in liver	Fever, capillary leak syndrome, pain at site of subcutaneous injection, allergic reactions, arthralgias, bone pain	None	Decreases incidence of infection after myelosuppressive chemotherapy, enhances myeloid engraftment after BMT, enhances peripheral progenitor cell yield
TARGETED AGENTS						
Alemtuzumab (Campath)	Humanized monoclonal antibody	Targets CD52 antigen present on surface of most normal lymphocytes and malignant B and T lymphocytes	Metabolism unclear	Hypersensitivity reactions, immunosuppressive	None	Relapsed B-cell CLL, T-cell prolymphocytic leukemia
Bevacizumab (Avastin)	Recombinant humanized monoclonal antibody to VEGF; inhibits angiogenesis	Binds to all human forms of VEGF, preventing it from binding to its receptors, reducing blood vessel formation	Metabolized	Hemorrhage, hypertension, proteinuria, thrombophlebitis	SN-38 metabolite of irinotecan is higher with concurrent use	Metastatic colorectal cancer, lung cancer, breast cancer
Bortezomib (Velcade)	Targeted agent	Reversible inhibitor of 26S proteasome; inhibits breakdown of ubiquitinated intracellular proteins and disrupts ubiquitin-proteasome pathway, eventually leading to apoptosis	Undergoes oxidative metabolism via cytochrome P-450 enzymes	Myelosuppression, peripheral neuropathy, asthenia, hypotension	Unknown	Relapsed multiple myeloma
Cetuximab (Erbitux)	Chimeric monoclonal antibody targeted against EGFR	Blocks growth factor from binding to EGFR, preventing cell signaling by tyrosine kinase phosphorylation	Metabolized	Hypersensitivity reactions, rash, diarrhea	None	Metastatic colorectal cancer
Dasatinib (Sprycel)	Multitargeted TKI	Inhibits multiple kinases	Metabolized by P-450 microenzyme CYP3A4	Myelosuppression	Multiple	Resistant/refractory CML
Erlotinib (Tarceva)	Targeted agent	Inhibits tyrosine kinase domain of EGFR	Metabolized	Rash, diarrhea, interstitial lung disease	CYP3A4 inducers and inhibitors may alter metabolism	Second- or third-line non–small cell lung cancer
Everolimus (Affinitor)	mTOR inhibitor	Inhibits mTOR	Metabolized by CYP3A4 in liver		CYP3A4 inhibitors/inducers, grapefruit juice	Renal cell carcinoma
Imatinib (Gleevec)	Targeted agent; signal transduction inhibitor	Inhibits BCR-ABL tyrosine kinase	Hepatic metabolism, excreted in feces	Myelosuppression, hypophosphatemia, fluid retention	Drugs inhibiting/stimulating liver microsomal CYP3A4 enzyme	CML, GISTs
Lapatinib (Tykerb)	Tyrosine kinase inhibitor	TKIs of EGFR and HER2/neu inhibitors/inducers	Metabolized by CYP3A4	Diarrhea, hand-foot syndrome	Capecitabine, CYP3A4	HER2/neu+ breast cancer
Lenalidomide[§] (Revlimid, CC-5013)	Targeted agent	Induces apoptosis	Renal excretion	Neutropenia, thrombocytopenia, diarrhea, pruritus, rash, fatigue, leg cramps	Other myelosuppressive agents	Myelodysplasia, myeloma
Nexavar (Sorafenib)	Targeted agent	Multikinase inhibitor, inhibits RAF kinase, VEGF, and PDGF receptors	Hepatic	Rash, hand-foot syndrome, fatigue, diarrhea, hair loss	CYP2C9 inducers, UGT1A1 pathway-excreted agents	Renal cell carcinoma
Nilotinib (Tasigna)	Tyrosine kinase inhibitor	Inhibits ATP site of ABL	Metabolized in liver	Prolonged QTc interval	CYP3A 4 inhibitors/inducers (irinotecan)	Resistant/intolerant CML
Ofatumumab (Arzerra)	Monoclonal antibody	Anti-CD20 antibody	Metabolized	Infusion reactions, infections	None	Resistant CLL
Pazopanib (Votrient)	Tyrosine kinase inhibitor	Inhibits multiple TKIs	Metabolized	Hepatotoxicity	CYP3A4 inducers/inhibitors	Renal cell cancer
Rituximab (Rituxan)	Chimeric anti- CD20 antibody	Targets CD20 antigen expressed on lymphocytes	Metabolized	Hypersensitivity reactions, lymphopenia	None	Relapsed low-grade non- Hodgkin's lymphomas

TABLE 182-6 CHEMOTHERAPEUTIC AGENTS—cont'd

AGENT	CLASS	ACTION	EXCRETION	UNIQUE SIDE EFFECTS	DRUG INTERACTIONS	INDICATIONS
Sunitinib (Sutent)	Multitargeted TKI	Inhibits TKIs and angiogenesis	Metabolized by P-450	Bleeding, CHF, prolonged QTc	CYP3A4 inhibitors/inducers	GIST, renal cell cancer
Temosirolimus (Torisel)	mTOR inhibitor	Inhibits mTOR kinase responsible for cell division	Metabolized in liver	Bowel perforation, interstitial lung disease	Affected by CYP3A4 inhibitors/inducers	Renal cell cancer
Thalidomide (Thalomid)	Immunomodulatory agent, antigenic agent	Inhibits TNF-α, may inhibit angiogenesis through inhibition of bFGF and VEGF	Nonenzymatic hydrolysis	Teratogenicity, sedation, constipation, peripheral neuropathy, rash	Sedation enhanced with alcohol, other sedatives	Multiple myeloma
Trastuzumab (Herceptin)	Recombinant humanized monoclonal antibody against HER2/neu	Downregulates expression of ERBB2 pathways	Metabolized	Hypersensitivity reactions	Increased risk of cardiotoxicity when used with anthracyclines or taxanes	Metastatic or adjuvant HER2/neu+ breast cancer
DRUGS TO OFFSET SIDE EFFECTS OF CHEMOTHERAPY						
Amifostine (Ethyol)	Cytoprotectant	Free thiol metabolites	Metabolized	Nausea/vomiting,	Hypertension	Reduces renal toxicity from cisplatin
Dexrazoxane (Zinecard)	Cardioprotector	Unclear	Excreted in urine	Myelosuppression		Reduces cardiotoxicity
Leucovorin (folinic acid, citrovorum factor, Wellcovorin)	Water-soluble folate vitamin	Increases general body pool of reduced folates	Metabolized in liver	None	In large amounts may counteract action of anticonvulsives	Prophylaxis and treatment of hematopoietic side effects of folic acid antagonists
Kepivance (Palifermin)	Keratinocyte growth factor	Stimulates growth of epithelial cells?		Rash	Heparin, myelotoxic chemotherapy	Decreases mucositis after BMT
Mesna (Mesnex)	Synthetic sulfhydryl compound	Only metabolite, mesna disulfide, reacts chemically with urotoxic ifosfamide metabolites, resulting in their detoxification	Renal	Bad taste, diarrhea	None	Prophylaxis of cyclophosphamide/ifosfamide-induced hemorrhagic cystitis

*An intrathecal formulation, DepoCyt, is used for the treatment of carcinomatous meningitis.
†Dosing differs among agents.
‡Dosages differ among brands.
§An analogue of thalidomide, which is a severe human teratogen; restricted prescribing.

ATP = adenosine triphosphate; bFGF, basic fibroblast growth factor; BMT = bone marrow transplantation; CHF = congestive heart failure; CLL = chronic lymphocytic leukemia; CML = chronic myelogenous leukemia; CNS = central nervous system; CSF = colony-stimulating factor; EGFR = epidermal growth factor receptor; ERBB2 = HER2/neu; FSH = follicle-stimulating hormone; G-CSF = granulocyte colony-stimulating factor; GM-CSF = granulocyte-macrophage colony-stimulating factor; GI = gastrointestinal; GIST = gastrointestinal stromal tumor; GnRH = gonadotropin-releasing hormone; 5-HIAA = 5-hydroxyindolacetic acid; HIV = human immunodeficiency virus; IL = interleukin; LFT = liver function test; LH = luteinizing hormone; LHRH = luteinizing hormone–releasing hormone; MAO = monoamine oxidase; mTOR = mammalian target of rapamycin; NSAID = nonsteroidal anti-inflammatory drug; PDGF = platelet-derived growth factor; SIADH = syndrome of inappropriate secretion of antidiuretic hormone; TKI = tyrosine kinase inhibitor; TNF = tumor necrosis factor; VEGF = vascular endothelial growth factor.

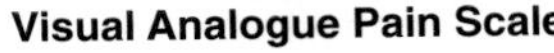

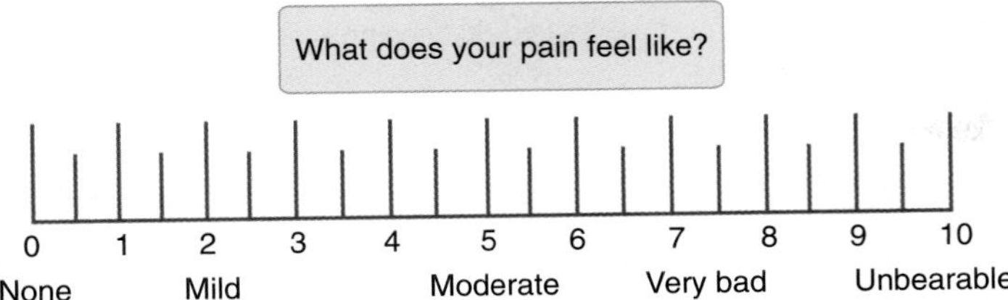

FIGURE 182-1. Grading pain in cancer patients.

RANK ligand, a protein found on osteoclasts and involved in bone breakdown. It is administered subcutaneously. Some clinical trials have found denosumab to be superior to zoledronic acid for the prevention of skeletal-related events in cancer patients with bone metastases.[8]

Hematologic malignancies and chemosensitive solid tumors should be treated with prophylactic allopurinol to prevent gout and renal colic from hyperuricemia. The acute tumor lysis syndrome can be defined by laboratory findings—elevated levels of uric acid, potassium, and phosphorus and decreased levels of calcium—or clinically—elevated creatinine, cardiac arrhythmias or sudden death, and seizures. The effects can be minimized by the use of allopurinol, vigorous hydration, and rasburicase and by the careful assessment of serum electrolytes, but anticipating the possibility of its occurrence is the best strategy.

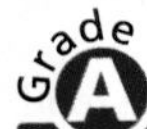

1. Zeppetella G, Ribeiro MD. Opioids for the management of breakthrough (episodic) pain in cancer patients. *Cochrane Database Syst Rev.* 2006;1:CD004311.
2. Worthington HV, Clarkson JE, Bryan G, et al. Interventions for preventing oral mucositis for patients with cancer receiving treatment. *Cochrane Database Syst Rev.* 2010;12:CD000978.
3. Clarkson JE, Worthington HV, Furness S, et al. Interventions for treating oral mucositis for patients with cancer receiving treatment. *Cochrane Database Syst Rev.* 2010;8:CD001973.
4. Worthington HV, Clarkson JE, Khalid T, et al. Interventions for treating oral candidiasis for patients with cancer receiving treatment. *Cochrane Database Syst Rev.* 2010;7:CD001972.
5. Sung L, Nathan PC, Alibhai SM, et al. Meta-analysis: effect of prophylactic hematopoietic colony-stimulating factors on mortality and outcomes of infection. *Ann Intern Med.* 2007;147:400-411.
6. Bucaneve G, Micozzi A, Menichetti F, et al. Levofloxacin to prevent bacterial infection in patients with cancer and neutropenia. *N Engl J Med.* 2005;353:977-987.
7. Cullen M, Steven N, Billingham L, et al. Antibacterial prophylaxis after chemotherapy for solid tumors and lymphomas. *N Engl J Med.* 2005;353:988-998.
8. Fizazi K, Carducci M, Smith M, et al. Denosumab versus zoledronic acid for treatment of bone metastases in men with castration-resistant prostate cancer: a randomized, double-blind study. *Lancet.* 2011;377:785-786.

SUGGESTED READINGS

Aapro MS, Bohlius J, Cameron DA, et al. 2010 update of EORTC guidelines for the use of granulocyte-colony stimulating factor to reduce the incidence of chemotherapy-induced febrile neutropenia in adult patients with lymphoproliferative disorders and solid tumours. *Eur J Cancer.* 2011;47:8-32. *Consensus guidelines recommending their use in patients with ≥20% chance of developing febrile neutropenia.*

Behl D, Hendrickson AW, Moynihan TJ. Oncologic emergencies. *Crit Care Clin.* 2010;26:181-205. *Review including metabolic, cardiac, neurologic, and infectious disorders.*

García Gómez J, Pérez López ME, García Mata J, et al. SEOM clinical guidelines for the treatment of antiemetic prophylaxis in cancer patients receiving chemotherapy. *Clin Transl Oncol.* 2010;12:770-774. *Consensus guidelines.*

Mitera G, Swaminath A, Wong S, et al. Radiotherapy for oncologic emergencies on weekends: examining reasons for treatment and patterns of practice at a Canadian cancer centre. *Curr Oncol.* 2009;16:55-60. *The top reasons for emergency weekend treatment included spinal cord compression (56%), brain metastases (15%), and superior vena cava obstruction (6%).*

National Cancer Institute's Patient Data Query (PDQ). Current version of therapy for cancers and hematologic malignancies, updated every three months. *www.cancer.gov.* Accessed March 9, 2011. *Addresses common management issues.*

Soussain C, Richard D, Fike JR, et al. CNS complications of radiotherapy and chemotherapy. *Lancet.* 2009;374:1639-1651. *Review.*

Swarm R, Abernethy AP, Anghelescu DL, et al. Adult cancer pain. *J Natl Compr Canc Netw.* 2010;8:1046-1086. *Comprehensive review.*

EPIDEMIOLOGY OF CANCER

MICHAEL J. THUN AND AHMEDIN JEMAL

EPIDEMIOLOGY

Overview

All cancers combined account for about 23% of deaths in the United States, placing cancer second only to heart disease as a cause of death. Cancer has also become the second leading cause of death worldwide after heart diseases, owing to increasing longevity, the global dispersion of tobacco use, and Western patterns of diet, physical inactivity, and reproduction. At current rates, nearly one in two men and more than one in three women in the United States will be diagnosed with cancer at some point in life. The National Institutes of Health estimates that the overall costs of cancer in 2008 equaled $228.1 billion.

Research has identified the causes of many types of cancer as well as basic mechanisms that drive carcinogenesis. Various control measures have reduced exposure to tobacco (Chapter 31) and occupational carcinogens (Chapter 18) in most industrialized countries. These advances in prevention, together with progress in early detection and treatment, have achieved a nearly 16% reduction in the death rate from all cancers combined in the United States from 1991 to 2006, and a 6% reduction in the incidence rate from 1999 to 2006.

Measures of Occurrence and Survival

Incidence and Death Rates

Cancer *incidence* and *death rates* are usually expressed per 100,000 people per year and are age-standardized to allow valid comparisons across populations of different sizes and age structures. Age-standardized rates must be standardized to the same age distribution in order for different time periods and geographic areas to be comparable. Conventionally, rates within the United States are standardized to the age distribution of the U.S. population (currently the year 2000 age standard), whereas international comparisons are based on the world population standard in 1960. Data on cancer incidence rates in the United States are collected by population-based tumor registries that now encompass 92% of the population. Temporal trends in cancer incidence have been monitored since 1973 in 10% of the population by the National Cancer Institute (NCI) Surveillance, Epidemiology, and End Results (SEER) program. Deaths from cancer have been tabulated nationally in U.S. vital statistics since 1930. Mortality rates are based on the underlying cause of death as coded from death certificates using systematic nosologic rules. Validation studies have documented that, despite the well-known limitations of death certificates, there is greater than 90% agreement between the clinical diagnosis and the underlying cause of death coded systematically from death certificates for the 17 cancer sites that represent more than two thirds of cancers in the United States.

Relative Survival

Survival in patients with cancer is usually expressed as *relative survival*, which compares the percentage of cancer patients alive after a designated period (often 5 years) with the corresponding percentage in a population without cancer but of similar age, race, and sex. A *relative survival* of 100% signifies that cancer patients have the same survival as people of the same age without cancer. *Relative survival* is different from *absolute survival* in that the latter reflects death from any condition, whether or not it relates to cancer. Trends in *relative survival* have been monitored by the NCI SEER program since 1975. Relative survival has improved substantially for many types of cancer (Table 183-1). Caution is advised, however, in interpreting trends in relative survival for cancer sites detected by screening because of the potential for lead-time bias (see Screening).

Cumulative Incidence

The terms *cumulative incidence* and *cumulative risk* describe the average probability of developing or dying from a specified condition (in this case all cancers or specific cancer sites) over a defined period. Annual incidence and death rates per 100,000 people per year (or alternatively per 1 million

TABLE 183-1 RELATIVE 5-YEAR SURVIVAL RATES* (%) FOR SELECTED CANCER SITES DURING THREE TIME PERIODS, UNITED STATES, SEER

SITE	1975-1977	1984-1986	1999-2005
All sites	50	53	67
Breast (female)	75	79	89
Colon	51	59	67
Leukemia	35	42	54
Lung and bronchus	13	13	16
Melanoma of the skin	82	86	93
Non-Hodgkin lymphoma	48	53	69
Ovary	37	40	46†
Pancreas	2	3	6
Prostate	69	76	100
Rectum	49	57	66
Urinary bladder	73	78	82

*Five-year relative survival rates based on follow-up of patients through 2005.
†Recent changes in the classification of ovarian cancer have affected 1996 to 2005 survival rates.
From Surveillance, Epidemiology and End Results Program (SEER), 1975-2006, Division of Cancer Control and Population Sciences, National Cancer Institute, 2009.

people per year for childhood cancers) correspond to 1-year cumulative risks. The cumulative risk of developing or dying from cancer increases with age. Lifetime cumulative incidence is strongly influenced by life expectancy; improvements in longevity increase the cumulative risk of developing cancer, even if the annual incidence and death rates at every age remain the same.

Geographic Variation

Cancer occurs in all countries of the world, although the predominant types of cancer vary widely (E-Table 183-1). In general, cancers caused by chronic infections (e.g., stomach, liver, cervix) predominate in economically developing countries, whereas those related to Western patterns of tobacco use and diet (lung, breast, prostate, and colon) are most common in high-resource countries. Some of the geographic variation reflects differences in diagnostic capabilities and data quality, yet much of the difference is real, reflecting geographic variation in causal factors. The regional cancer registries that provide these data are maintained by the International Agency for Research on Cancer (IARC), which makes special efforts to improve the completeness of registration. The international variation in cancer occurrence has historically provided important evidence that much of the disease burden from cancer is caused by exposures rather than inherited genetic susceptibility and could, in principle, be prevented.

Lung cancer (Chapter 197) is the most common cancer worldwide in terms of both new cases and deaths. The incidence rate varies from more than 70 per 100,000 among men in Eastern Europe to less than 5 per 100,000 among men in West Africa. The geography of lung cancer principally reflects the progression of populations through the stages of the tobacco epidemic. Within a country, the uptake of smoking manufactured cigarettes typically begins among middle-aged men and then spreads progressively to younger men and women. The resulting increase in lung cancer begins 25 to 30 years later and continues until publicity about the adverse effects of smoking and tobacco control measures cause a downturn in smoking, which is later followed by a downturn in lung cancer.

Breast cancer (Chapter 204) is the most common incident cancer in women worldwide. Incidence rates have increased, even in developing countries, but continue to be about five times higher in North America, Europe, and other Western industrial countries than among women in rural Asia. Increased longevity and the widespread use of screening contribute to the high lifetime risk (12.7%) of breast cancer among women in the United States, as does the prevalence of risk factors such as delayed childrearing, excess body weight, physical inactivity, and hormone use.

Prostate cancer (Chapter 207) is the second most commonly diagnosed cancer in men globally, with nearly three fourths of all cases diagnosed in economically developed countries. Incidence rates are especially high in the United States because of widespread screening with prostate-specific antigen (PSA), which finds tumors that might otherwise be missed. In contrast, the much higher incidence and death rates among men of African descent in Africa, the Caribbean, and the United States represents a true disparity that is currently unexplained.

Cancers of the colon and rectum (Chapter 199) are more common in economically developed than in developing countries. The incidence rate in the United States is 20 to 30 times higher than in rural India and Southeast Asia. Risk factors thought to contribute to the geographic variation include obesity, physical inactivity, high consumption of red and processed meat, cigarette smoking, and heavy alcohol consumption.

The geographic distribution of several cancers caused by infectious agents or behavioral practices closely parallels the prevalence of the causal agent. For example, the high incidence of liver cancer (Chapter 202) in parts of Asia and sub-Saharan Africa matches the geographic patterns of *hepatitis B virus* (HBV) infection in childhood, just as mortality from stomach (Chapter 198) and cervical (Chapter 205) cancer correlates closely with the prevalence of infection with pathogenic strains of *Helicobacter pylori* and *human papillomavirus* (HPV), respectively. The exceptionally high incidence of oropharyngeal (Chapter 196) cancer throughout much of the Indian subcontinent and Southeast Asia is caused by the practice of chewing betel quid and areca nut, often mixed with tobacco. In contrast, it is not fully understood why squamous cell carcinoma of the esophagus (Chapter 198) was extraordinarily common until the late 20th century in countries surrounding the Caspian Sea. This was attributed to a combination of severe nutritional deficiency corresponding to a seasonal lack of vegetables and the practice of swallowing the charred residue from opium pipes. The incidence of this cancer has decreased rapidly over the past 20 years following improvement of the food supply. Other incompletely understood geographic variations involve why ovarian cancer (Chapter 205) is more common in certain European countries than in others, or how dietary consumption of salted fish may interact with Epstein-Barr virus (EBV) infections and genetic susceptibility to cause nasopharyngeal cancer (Chapter 196) in southern China and in Eskimos in Alaska and Greenland.

Geographic and demographic variations in cancer risk are seen for all cancers combined as well as for individual sites. An extreme example is that the cumulative incidence of being diagnosed with any type of cancer is almost ten times higher among African American men than men of similar age in parts of India. These large variations in overall cancer risk indicate that geographic variability does not simply reflect substitution of one form of cancer for another, but affects disease occurrence overall.

Temporal Variation

Temporal variations in the incidence or death rates from certain cancers further illustrate the importance of potentially modifiable "environmental" factors on the burden of disease. For example, the large changes in mortality from stomach and lung cancer among men and women in the United States (Fig. 183-1A and B) reflect changes in external exposure rather than inherited genetic susceptibility. Cancer of the stomach was one of the most common fatal cancers in the United States in 1930, as was cancer of the uterus (principally uterine cervix) in women. Mortality from these cancers has decreased dramatically over the past 75 years. The global decrease in stomach cancer (Chapter 198) probably reflects an unintended benefit of changes in food preservation and reduced prevalence of *H. pylori* infection. The advent of refrigeration increased the availability of fresh vegetables and fruit and decreased reliance on salted, smoked, and pickled foods, whereas improvements in sanitation and housing and widespread antibiotic use decreased the prevalence of chronic infection with *H. pylori*. Progress in reducing the incidence and death rate from cervical cancer (Chapter 205) is largely attributable to the introduction of Papanicolaou testing and early removal of premalignant and cancerous lesions. The close relationship between global trends in lung cancer (Chapter 197) and cigarette smoking was discussed previously.

Screening

Trends in cancer incidence rates are more difficult to interpret than trends in mortality, especially for sites that are detectable by screening. The introduction of a new screening test can create the appearance of a sudden increase in cancer incidence, especially when the test detects prevalent but undiagnosed tumors that would otherwise be missed. For example, a sudden increase in the incidence rate of prostate cancer (Chapter 207) in the United States in the late 1980s (Fig. 183-2A) coincided with the introduction of PSA screening. The upward trend reversed after 1992 because of saturation of

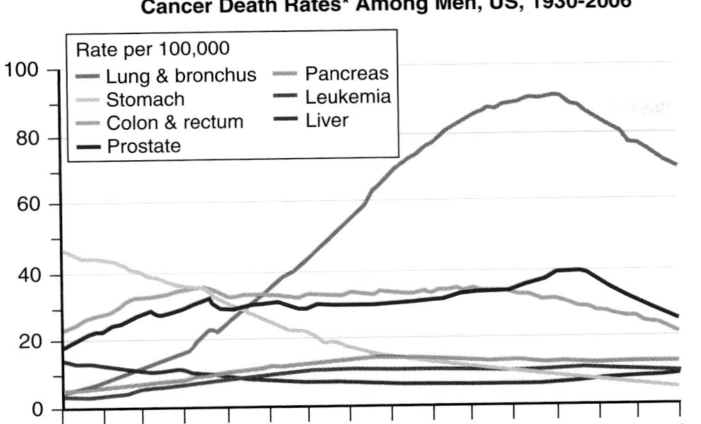

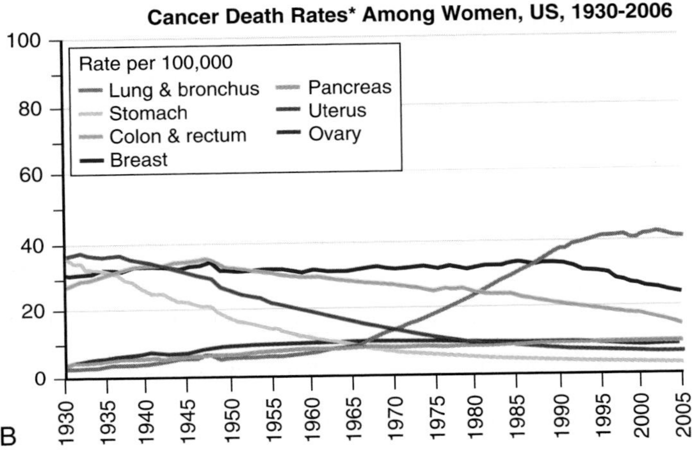

FIGURE 183-1. Cancer mortality rates. A, Temporal trends in cancer mortality rates, United States, 1930 to 2006, men. **B,** Temporal trends in cancer mortality rates, United States, 1930 to 2006, women. *Age-adjusted to the 2000 U.S. standard population. (Data from U.S. Mortality Data 1960-2005, U.S. Mortality Volumes 1930-1959, National Center for Health Statistics, Centers for Disease Control and Prevention, 2008.)

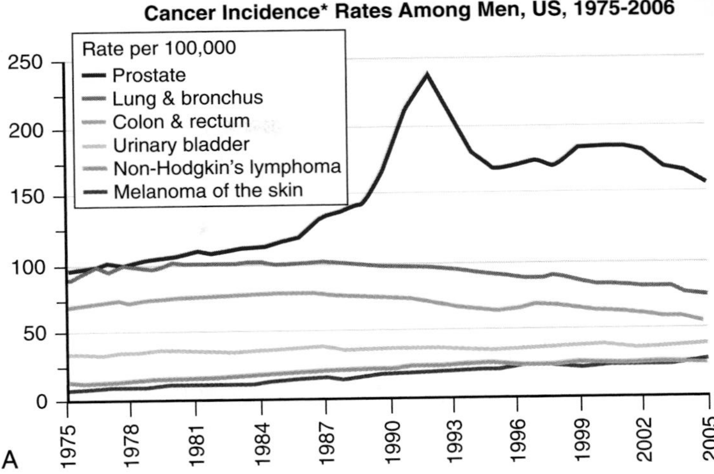

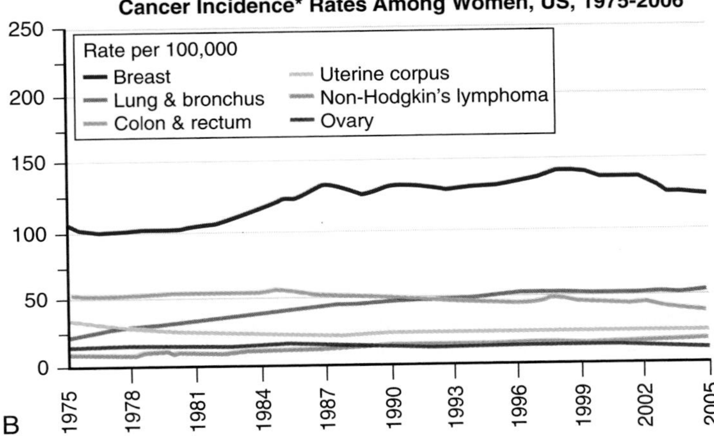

FIGURE 183-2. Cancer incidence rates. A, Temporal trends in cancer incidence rates adjusted for delayed reporting, Surveillance, Epidemiology, and End Results (SEER), 1975 to 2006, men. **B,** Temporal trends in cancer incidence rates adjusted for delayed reporting, SEER, 1975 to 2006, women. *Age-adjusted to the 2000 U.S. standard population and adjusted for delays in reporting. (Data from Surveillance, Epidemiology, and End Results Program, Delay-Adjusted Incidence Database: SEER Incidence Delay-Adjusted Rates, 9 Registries, 1975-2005, National Cancer Institute, 2008.)

screening among older men. The upward trend in reported incidence has since returned to the more gradual increase that prevailed before the introduction of PSA testing. Likewise, the introduction of mammography screening during the 1980s contributed to the increase in breast cancer incidence among women (see Fig. 183-2B), although the impact was considerably smaller than that of PSA screening on prostate cancer incidence (see Fig. 183-2A). The introduction of mammography had a much larger impact on the detection of ductal carcinoma in situ (DCIS), which is not included in the incidence rates, than invasive breast cancer.

The introduction of new screening tests also complicates the interpretation of temporal trends in *relative survival* among patients with cancer (see Table 183-1). Screening tests detect cancer earlier, before the tumor would otherwise have been diagnosed, thus creating an apparent lengthening of survival that exaggerates actual progress. This so-called lead-time bias can be difficult to separate completely from improvements in relative survival for sites that are commonly diagnosed by screening, such as breast and prostate cancer, even in analyses that stratify for stage at diagnosis. New screening tests can also alter the mix of cancers being diagnosed by increasing the detection of indolent tumors that may not be life-threatening. Advances in the molecular characterization of tumors may ultimately resolve this problem by providing more homogeneous groupings of tumors in which to measure relative survival.

Demographic Factors

Age

The incidence of most cancers increases exponentially with age from 10 to 84 years (Fig. 183-3). Age is a stronger predictor of cancer risk than any other factor. About three fourths (77%) of all cancers occur in the approximately 19% of the U.S. population 55 years or older. This age-related increase reflects the multistage nature of carcinogenesis and the time required for a single cell line to accumulate all the mutations and epigenetic events needed for malignant transformation (Chapter 185). The apparent decrease in the incidence of cancer after 85 years of age reflects incomplete diagnosis of cancer in elderly people as well as the fact that generations born before 1920 preceded the peak of cigarette smoking.

Age affects the types of cancer that occur as well as their frequency. In the United States, the five most common fatal cancers before age 20 are acute lymphocytic leukemia, cancer of the brain and other nervous system, bones and joints, endocrine system, and soft tissues. In women aged 20 to 59 years, breast cancer is the most common fatal cancer. At age 60 and older, the four most common cancers are lung and bronchus (Chapters 197), breast (Chapter 204), prostate (Chapter 207), and colon and rectum cancer (Chapter 199).

Sex

For most cancers that affect both sexes, the incidence rate is higher in men than women, the exceptions being cancers of the breast, thyroid, gallbladder, and anus. The incidence rate from all cancers combined is higher in men than women except in the age range of 30 to 54 years, when, because of breast cancer, women have higher incidence rates (see Fig. 183-3). The male excess for cancers of the oropharynx, esophagus, larynx, lung, pancreas, and kidney can be attributed to higher tobacco or alcohol use, or both. For other sites, such as brain, hematopoietic, and childhood cancers, however, the reasons for higher risk in men are unclear.

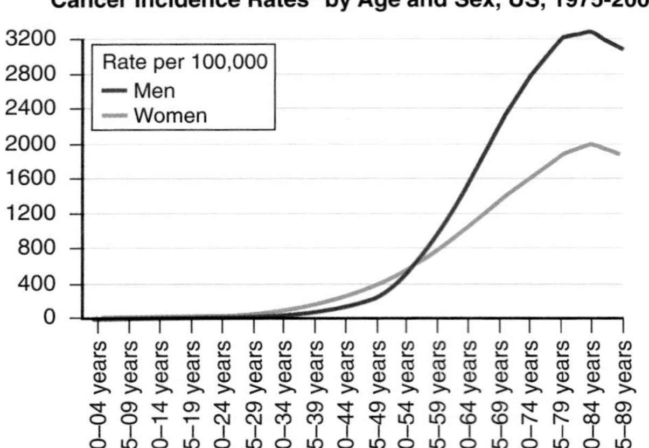

FIGURE 183-3. **Age- and sex-specific incidence rates for all cancer combined in the nine Surveillance, Epidemiology and End Results (SEER) areas.** *Age-adjusted to the 2000 U.S. standard population. (Data from U.S. Mortality Data, National Center for Health Statistics.)

Socioeconomic Status, Race, and Ethnicity

African Americans experience disproportionately high incidence and death rates from most cancers. Racial disparities in death rates are largest for cancers of the prostate, stomach, larynx (men), myeloma, and uterine cervix. Relatively few studies have attempted to separate the impact of biologic differences associated with race from factors related to poverty and its effects on education, risk factors, and access to high-quality care for prevention, early detection, and treatment. Accumulating data suggest that socioeconomic factors account for most of these disparities (Chapter 5). For example, black women have the highest death rate from breast cancer among all racial or ethnic groups in the United States. Although the incidence rate is higher in white than in black women, this paradox likely results from underdiagnosis of breast cancer in black women. Survival among women with breast cancer is lower in black than in white women in the general population, but it is similar in military hospitals where both races have equal access to care. Relative survival is lower in African Americans than in whites for many other cancers, including prostate, uterine cervix and corpus, colon, and rectum cancer.

Other ethnic groups in the United States also have distinctive cancer patterns. Relative to whites, age-adjusted incidence and mortality rates among Hispanics are higher for gallbladder, stomach, and cervical cancer; those among American Indians are higher for cancer of the gallbladder, stomach, and cervix; rates in Japanese Americans are higher for stomach and liver cancer; those in Chinese Americans are higher for nasopharynx, liver, and stomach cancer; Native Hawaiians have higher death rates from breast, esophagus, liver, pancreas, lung, and cervical cancer; and Filipino Americans have a lower risk of most cancers except for cancers of the stomach, liver, oral cavity, and esophagus. Many of these ethnic differences are known to reflect differences in the use of tobacco, dietary habits, infectious exposure, or medical care. Research is needed to identify practical interventions to reduce these disparities.

Causes of Cancer

Whereas infectious diseases are defined by exposure to a specific microorganism, chronic diseases such as cancer may have multiple causes, none of which need be necessary or sufficient for the disease to occur (Table 183-2). For instance, tobacco smoking is the major cause of lung cancer, but it is neither necessary nor sufficient for the disease to occur. Approximately 10 to 15% of lung cancers occur in people who have never smoked actively, and in only about 20% of long-term cigarette smokers does lung cancer develop.

Tobacco

Exposure to tobacco (Chapter 31) is the single largest cause of cancer in the United States. Tobacco smoke contains more than 4000 chemicals, at least 40 of which are known to be carcinogenic in humans or animals, or both. All forms of tobacco can cause cancer. Cigarette smoking causes cancer of the lip, oral cavity, nasal cavity, paranasal sinuses, pharynx (nasal, oral, and hypopharynx), larynx, lung, esophagus (squamous cell and adenocarcinoma), stomach, colorectum, pancreas, liver, kidney (adenocarcinoma and renal pelvis), urinary bladder, uterine cervix, and myeloid leukemia. Secondhand smoke, or environmental tobacco smoke, contains a similar mix of carcinogens as active smoking at varying concentrations. Each year in the United States, secondhand smoke causes an estimated 3000 deaths from lung cancer and 30,000 to 40,000 deaths from heart disease.

Diet, Obesity, Physical Inactivity

Other important modifiable determinants of cancer risk are dietary patterns, physical inactivity, and obesity. Approximately one third of cancer deaths in the United States are attributed to nutritional factors. Obesity, physical inactivity, and an excess of caloric intake over energy expenditure are known to increase the risk for several types of cancer. Obesity (Chapter 227) is causally related to cancer of the endometrium, kidney, breast (in postmenopausal but not premenopausal women), esophagus, colon (especially in men), and gallbladder (particularly in women). More limited evidence suggests that obesity may also increase the risk for cancer of the liver, pancreas, and stomach as well as some hematopoietic cancers. Excessive alcohol consumption (Chapter 32) is an established cause of cancer of the oropharynx, larynx, esophagus, and liver; even moderate drinking increases the risk for breast cancer. The importance of other specific components of diet to the risk for cancer in Western populations is more controversial. The strongest evidence pertains to increased risk for colon cancer in people who have inadequate intake of folic acid or excessive consumption of red or processed meat.

Infectious Agents

It is estimated that about 17% of cancer cases worldwide are attributable to infectious agents. This percentage is higher in economically developing (26%) than in developed (7.2%) countries. Viruses known to cause cancer in humans include *HPV* (Chapter 381), *hepatitis B virus (HBV)* (Chapter 151), *hepatitis C virus* (HCV) (Chapter 151), *EBV* (Chapter 385), *human immunodeficiency virus (HIV)* (Chapter 400), and *human herpesvirus-8* (Chapter 382). Viruses increase the risk for cancer through a variety of mechanisms, including direct effects on DNA, promotion of tumor development by means of chronic inflammation *(HPV, HBV, HCV)*, or suppression of specific elements of the immune system (e.g., *HIV*) (Chapter 185).

H. pylori, which is the only bacterial infection known to cause cancer, is a gram-negative, spiral bacteria that colonizes the mucous layer of the stomach. Chronic inflammation caused by strains of *H. pylori* that express the CagA (a 128-kD cytotoxin-associated gene–A positive) protein promotes the development of gastric ulcers, gastric carcinoma, and mucosa-associated lymphoid tissue (MALT) lymphoma of the stomach (Chapter 198). Parasitic infections known to increase the risk for cancer include *Schistosoma haematobium* (Chapter 363) (bladder cancer) and liver flukes such as *Clonorchis sinensis* (Chapter 364) and *Opisthorchis viverrini* (Chapter 364) (biliary tract cancer, Chapter 202).

Ionizing Radiation

Ionizing radiation (Chapter 19) from x-rays, gamma radiation, and other sources is one of the most extensively studied human carcinogens. Leukemia and cancer of the thyroid and female breast are most strongly associated with radiation, although cancer of the lung, esophagus, stomach, colon, brain, and bladder and myeloma are also causally related. The risk for development of cancer from ionizing radiation depends not only on cumulative exposure but also on the intensity, rate, and nature of the exposure as well as on the age at which it occurs. Childhood exposure from medical treatments or fallout from atomic bombs or nuclear accidents principally increases the risk for leukemia and thyroid cancer. Girls exposed to radiation during adolescence and young adulthood are more susceptible to breast cancer from this exposure than are women exposed later in life. Radioactive isotopes such as iodine-131, radium-224, -226, and -236, and phosphorus-32 concentrate in the thyroid, bone, and bone marrow, respectively, and deliver high localized doses to radiosensitive tissues. Radon-222, a naturally occurring radioactive decay product of uranium-238, was first discovered to cause lung cancer in occupational studies of highly exposed uranium miners. Radon gas is also a common contaminant of household basements and unventilated underground spaces, albeit at much lower concentrations. Exposure to ultraviolet radiation from sunlight and tanning booths is the principal cause of melanoma as well as squamous and basal cell skin cancer. Nonionizing radiation, such as the electromagnetic frequency emissions from cell phones, has not been thought to cause cancer because the energy that is imparted to tissues is too weak to

TABLE 183-2 SELECTED KNOWN CAUSES OF CANCER AND THE ASSOCIATED CANCER SITES*

Cause	Cancer Site
TOBACCO	
Active and passive smoking	Multiple sites: see text
Spit tobacco (snuff, chewing)	Oral cavity, pancreas
NUTRITION, OBESITY, PHYSICAL INACTIVITY, AND FOOD CONTAMINANTS	
Aflatoxins	Liver
Alcohol	Mouth, pharynx, larynx, esophagus, breast,[†] liver[†]
Chinese salted fish†	Nasopharynx
Obesity	Multiple sites: see text
Physical inactivity	Colon, breast
MEDICAL	
Chemotherapy	
Chlorambucil	Acute nonlymphocytic leukemia
Cyclophosphamide	Bladder, leukemia
Melphalan	Acute nonlymphocytic leukemia
Methyl-CCNU, Myleran, Thiotepa	Leukemia
Radiotherapy (see Ionizing Radiation)	
Hormones	
Diethylstilbestrol	Breast, endometrium, cervix, vagina, testicles
Estrogen, steroidal	Endometrium, breast
Tamoxifen	Endometrium (reduces breast cancer risk)
Other Drugs	
Analgesic mixtures containing phenacetin	Kidney, bladder
Azathioprine	Non-Hodgkin lymphoma, skin, liver, mesenchyma
Chlornaphazine†	Bladder
Cyclosporine	Lymphoma, skin
Methoxsalen with ultraviolet A therapy (PUVA)	Skin
INFECTIOUS AGENTS	
Viruses	
Epstein-Barr virus	Non-Hodgkin lymphoma (Burkitt lymphoma), Hodgkin lymphoma, nasopharynx
Hepatitis B and hepatitis C	Liver
Human immunodeficiency virus	Kaposi sarcoma, Hodgkin lymphoma, non-Hodgkin lymphoma
Human papillomavirus	Cervix, vulva, vagina, penis, anus, oral cavity, oropharynx, and tonsil
Human herpesvirus 8	Kaposi sarcoma, lymphoma
Human T-cell lymphotrophic virus	Leukemia
Bacteria	
Helicobacter pylori	Stomach
Parasites	
Liver flukes (*Clonorchis sinensis* and *Opisthorchis viverrini*)	Bile duct, liver
Schistosoma haematobium	Bladder
RADIATION	
Nonionizing Radiation	
Broad-spectrum solar ultraviolet radiation	Skin
Sun lamps or sun beds	Skin, eye
Ionizing Radiation	
X-radiation and gamma radiation	Leukemia, thyroid, breast, lung
Radium	Bone sarcoma
Radon	Lung
Thorium dioxide	Liver, leukemia, bone
Neutrons	Leukemia, thyroid, breast, lung
OCCUPATION AND ENVIRONMENTAL CHEMICALS	
4-Aminobiphenyl	Bladder
Arsenic compounds, inorganic	Skin, lung, digestive tract, liver, bladder, kidney, lymphatic and hematopoietic systems
Asbestos	Respiratory tract, pleural and peritoneal mesothelioma
Benzene	Acute myeloid leukemia
Benzidine and dyes	Bladder
Beryllium and beryllium compounds	Lung
1,3-Butadiene	Lymphatic, hematopoietic systems
Cadmium and cadmium compounds	Lung, prostate, kidney, bladder
Bis(chloromethyl) ether and technical-grade chloromethyl methyl ether	Lung
Chromium hexavalent compounds	Lung, sinonasal cavity
Coal tar and coal tar pitch	Skin, scrotum, lung, bladder, kidney, digestive tract, leukemia
Coke oven emissions	Skin, respiratory tract, kidney, bladder
Dioxin	Lung, non-Hodgkin lymphoma
Erionite	Mesothelioma, lung
Ethylene oxide	Leukemia, stomach
Formaldehyde†	Nasopharynx
Mineral oils (untreated and mildly treated)	Skin, gastrointestinal tract, sinonasal, scrotum, bladder
Mustard gas	Respiratory tract
2-Napthylamine	Bladder
Nickel compounds	Lung, nasal
Silica, crystalline	Lung
Soot	Scrotum, skin, lung, prostate, bladder, hematopoietic and lymphatic systems
Strong inorganic acid mists containing sulfuric acid	Larynx, lung
Vinyl chloride	Liver, brain, lung, lymphatic and hematopoietic systems
Wood dust	Nasal cavity, paranasal sinus

*Modified from lists compiled by the International Agency for Research on Cancer (IARC) and the National Toxicology Program (NTP).
†Classified as carcinogenic by the IARC but not by the NTP.

damage DNA. Because of the widespread use of cell phones, however, this remains an active area of research.

Iatrogenic Exposures

Many medical diagnostic and therapeutic interventions have been found to increase the risk for cancer, either directly as chemical or physical carcinogens or indirectly through suppression of immune responses. Alkylating drugs and other cytotoxic agents used to treat cancer increase the risk for development of a secondary malignancy, as does radiation therapy. Hormone replacement therapy increases the risk for breast cancer in postmenopausal women. Tamoxifen increases the risk for endometrial cancer, even though this risk is outweighed by the reduction in breast cancer in high-risk women. The practice of treating pregnant women with diethylstilbestrol was discontinued because of the increased incidence of clear cell vaginal cancer in the daughters of these women during adolescence. Immunosuppressive drugs used to prevent graft rejection in organ transplantation and other autoimmune conditions increase the risk for certain lymphomas (non-Hodgkin B-cell lymphomas), Kaposi sarcoma, malignant melanoma, and liver cancer. Repeated use of diagnostic procedures such as whole body computed tomography results in substantial radiation exposure, although the potential long-term consequences receive surprisingly little attention.

Occupational and Environmental Carcinogens

Occupationally exposed workers (Chapter 18) have unfortunately served as the sentinel for many of the recognized industrial carcinogens, especially in workplaces where prolonged, heavy exposure caused unusual clusters of rare cancers. For example, clusters of scrotal cancer in London chimney sweeps, osteosarcoma of the jaw in watch dial painters exposed to radium, mesothelioma in asbestos workers, and angiosarcoma of the liver in chemical workers exposed to vinyl chloride monomer attest to the carcinogenicity of coal tar, radium, asbestos, and vinyl chloride monomer. In other instances, increases in the risk for common cancers have been sufficiently large to be detected in epidemiologic studies of several thousand workers. Examples include arsenic, asbestos, beryllium, bis(chloromethyl) ether, cadmium, chromium (hexavalent), coal tar, coke oven emissions, nickel, polycyclic aromatic hydrocarbons, and radon.

What Constitutes "Proof" of Causation?

There has been vigorous philosophic and scientific debate over what constitutes "proof" of causation in scientific studies of chronic (i.e., noninfectious) diseases. When policy decisions relate to exposures judged to be harmful, epidemiologic evidence alone is often considered sufficient to justify protective intervention. It is unethical to propose randomized clinical trials to confirm that smoking causes lung cancer, that ionizing radiation causes leukemia, or that HPV causes cervical cancer. Moreover, in these examples, the observational evidence is so strong that the epidemiologic evidence itself is virtually incontrovertible. In other instances, especially when the exposure of interest is difficult to measure and the observed association is weaker, judgments about causality must be based on the weight of the evidence with consideration of all potentially relevant information from observational, clinical, experimental, and basic studies.

The inference that an association is causal is supported when a number of the following apply:

1. The association is strong (higher relative risk being more likely to indicate cause).
2. The risk increases or decreases with exposure in a dose-response gradient.
3. Consistent findings are seen in multiple studies with different investigators, study populations, and designs.
4. The exposure or cause precedes disease onset.
5. It is biologically plausible that the exposure could cause the disease.
6. The association is specific between the exposure and a single disease.
7. The epidemiologic findings fit coherently with information from other types of research and other epidemiologic studies.

Reviews and listings of substances known or suspected to cause cancer in humans are maintained by the National Toxicology Program (NTP) and by the IARC, a branch of the World Health Organization (see Table 183-2). The IARC evaluations classify exposures into one of four categories: (1) "sufficient evidence" of carcinogenicity in humans (in the working group's opinion, chance, bias, and confounding can be excluded with reasonable confidence); (2) "limited evidence" of carcinogenicity (a causal relationship between the agent and risk of cancer in humans is plausible, but chance, bias, and confounding cannot be ruled out with reasonable confidence); (3) "inadequate evidence" of carcinogenicity (available studies are of insufficient quality, consistency, or statistical power to permit a conclusion regarding the carcinogenicity of the agent, or no data on carcinogenicity in humans are available); and (4) "evidence suggesting lack of carcinogenic activity" (several adequate studies of use or exposure are mutually consistent in not showing an increased risk for specified cancer sites, conditions, and levels of exposure). The NTP uses only two categories, "known to be a human carcinogen" and "reasonably anticipated to be a human carcinogen."

FUTURE DIRECTIONS

An exciting frontier in cancer epidemiology involves efforts to integrate insights from molecular biology and genetics into large-scale population studies to examine how the interaction of inherited genetic susceptibility (nature) with exposure after conception (nurture) influences an individual's risk for the development of cancer. In some cases, information on inherited genetic polymorphisms is now being used clinically to tailor the selection and dose of certain drugs used for chemotherapy or treatment of other conditions. Until now it has been difficult to identify well-established examples of gene-environment interactions that affect cancer risk, mostly because the technology for rapidly genotyping tens of thousands of people has only recently become available and affordable. Advances in proteomics, metabolomics, and epigenetics may soon make it possible to identify early markers and intermediate factors that affect tumor development. These may provide therapeutic targets by which to influence the development or progression of cancer, just as cardiovascular research has identified lipid abnormalities and hypertension as modifiable intermediates of heart disease.

SUGGESTED READINGS

International Agency for Research on Cancer website. http://www.iarc.fr. Accessed Feb. 4, 2011. *Listing of numerous resources on cancer available through the branch of the World Health Organization.*

Jemal A, Siegel R, Ward E, et al. Cancer statistics, 2010. *CA Cancer J Clin.* 2010;60:277-300. *Documents an ongoing decline in cancer-related mortality in 2004, the second consecutive year.*

Garcia M, Jemal A, Ward EM, et al. Global cancer facts and figures 2010. Atlanta, GA: American Cancer Society; http://ntp.niehs.nih.gov. Accessed Feb. 4, 2011. *International cancer statistics.*

National Toxicology Program website. Department of Health and Human Services. http://ntp-server.niehs.nih.gov. Accessed Feb. 4, 2011. *Website lists substances that are known or "reasonably anticipated to be" human carcinogens.*

184

CANCER GENETICS

HENRY T. LYNCH AND C. RICHARD BOLAND

CANCER IS A GENETIC DISEASE

Cancer is caused by alterations in genes. Many genes are involved in the process, and there is a broad range of mechanisms by which the genes may be altered. The genetic alterations are tumor specific, but there are common features to the genes that cause cancer. Also, one must individually consider the differences between somatic mutations (found in the cancers, but not present throughout the rest of the body) and germline mutations (inherited, and present in every cell of the body).

Oncogenes are normal cellular genes that participate in the stimulation of growth pathways and become abnormally activated in cancer. There are several ways for activation to occur. Point mutations may make the protein product unresponsive to downregulating signals, as in the case of mutant *KRAS*. The transcription factor *MYC* is often activated by copy number amplification, or it may be put under the control of an inappropriate promoter, achieving the same result. In the case of the *BCR-ABL* mutation, which is ubiquitous in certain leukemias, a chromosomal translocation relocates a promoter that is active in myeloid cells to a position that drives the unregulated production of a proliferation-promoting tyrosine kinase.

Tumor suppressor genes normally suppress cellular growth or mediate cellular differentiation, and these are inactivated in cancers. Because humans are born with two copies of almost every gene (the X and Y chromosomes in males are the exceptions), it takes two lesions or "hits" to release the cell from the regulatory effects of these genes. Tumor suppressor genes provide the conceptual basis for many of the hereditary forms of predisposition to cancer. The affected person is born with a "germline" mutation in one allele, which is present in every cell of the body. The cancer occurs in a specific cell lineage after the other allele suffers an inactivating "somatic" mutation, which is the second hit. Examples of tumor suppressor genes include the *Rb* gene, *p53*, and *p16*, which are inactivated in some cancers.

DNA repair genes are important in cancer. There are multiple types of DNA repair, each specific to one or more types of DNA damage. When these genes are inactivated, a hypermutability ensues within that cell, and this leads to numerous somatic mutations in the target genes, which will include oncogenes or tumor suppressors, and then leads to cancer. Defective DNA repair states also provide an additional explanation for certain inherited diseases. DNA repair systems inactivated in cancer include the DNA mismatch repair (MMR) system (which is involved in Lynch syndrome [LS]), the base excision repair system (which leads to an autosomal recessive form of familial polyposis called *MYH*-associated polyposis), and nucleotide excision repair (which leads to the autosomal recessive disease xeroderma pigmentosa).

HEREDITARY CANCER SYNDROMES

The tumor suppressor gene concept provides an explanation for how a person could be born with a predisposition to cancer, which occurs when one allele of a gene is mutated in every cell, greatly increasing the likelihood that some cell would eventually lose both copies of the gene—a situation that would be statistically unlikely without the germline mutation. In fact, germline mutations in the previously mentioned tumor suppressors *Rb*, *p53*, and *p16* give rise to familial retinoblastoma, Li-Fraumeni syndrome, and the familial atypical multiple mole melanoma–pancreatic cancer (FAMMM-PC) syndromes, respectively.

Germline mutations in the DNA repair genes create more complex clinical scenarios. In case of hereditary nonpolyposis colon cancer, also known as LS, the most common hereditary CRC syndrome, accounting for approximately 3% of CRC incidence, a germline mutation occurs in one allele of a DNA MMR gene (including *MSH2, MLH1, MSH6*, or *PMS2*), and the loss of the other allele creates a cell without any DNA MMR activity. The affected cell becomes hypermutable, and mutations accumulate in growth-regulating target genes; this causes the cancer. (There are rare instances in which biallelic mutations in DNA MMR genes create constitutional MMR deficiency and a pediatric cancer diathesis.) More recently it has been discovered that a deletion in the *EPCAM* gene (previously called *TACSTD1*), upstream of *MSH2*, can silence *MSH2*, thereby causing LS without a mutation in the *MSH2* gene itself. Thus, LS is inherited in a classic dominant mendelian fashion, but the cancers occur only after the second hit occurs, meaning that the disease is recessive at the tissue level. Constitutional deficiency of base excision repair occurs when there are biallelic mutations in the *MUTHY* genes (called *MUTHY*-associated polyposis); these patients develop multiple colorectal adenomas and are highly prone to CRC. Similarly, constitutional deficiency of nucleotide excision repair causes xeroderma pigmentosa (Chapter 444), in which patients are unable to tolerate even minimal degrees of sunlight, because the enzyme complex required to repair ultraviolet light–induced DNA changes is defective. These two conditions are classic recessive diseases, and the monoallelic carrier state does not lead to a clinically substantial increase in risk for cancer.

DIAGNOSIS OF FAMILIAL CANCER SYNDROMES

The primary care physician is often the first to apply cancer genetics to clinical care when there is the suspicion of a familial cancer-prone syndrome. It would not be possible to predict which mutations cause what familial cancers based on knowledge of the gene function. The diagnoses depend on pattern recognition and linkage to the known mutations. The recognition of a familial pattern of disease may result in further investigation of potentially affected patients and families. The goal will be effective screening and management recommendations. Examples of the most common familial cancer syndromes include the following:

- Breast and ovarian cancers with *BRCA1/BRCA2* mutations (the hereditary breast and ovarian cancer, or HBOC, syndrome)
- CRC, endometrial, ovarian, stomach, pancreas, and other cancer types with DNA MMR mutations in LS
- Sarcomas, breast cancers, brain tumors, leukemia, lymphoma, and adrenal cortical cancers with *p53* mutations in the Li-Fraumeni syndrome
- Medullary thyroid carcinoma and pheochromocytoma with the *RET* proto-oncogene mutation in the multiple endocrine neoplasia syndromes MEN 2a and 2b
- Malignant melanoma and pancreatic cancer with *CDKN2A* (*p16*) mutation in familial multiple mole melanoma syndrome
- Diffuse gastric cancer and lobular breast cancer with *CDH1* mutation in the hereditary diffuse gastric cancer (HDGC) syndrome
- Multiple adenomatous colonic polyps and CRC with mutations of the *APC* gene in familial adenomatous polyposis (FAP), or biallelic mutations in the *MUTHY* gene in *MUTHY*-associated polyposis

The differential diagnosis is highly complex for common cancers, such as breast and CRC, as shown in Figures 184-1 and 184-2, respectively. Ideally, the family pedigree will cover a minimum of three generations. It must incorporate cancer of all anatomic sites with age of cancer onset and pathology documentation. Older individuals will often have passed through the cancer risk age and therefore will be more informative genetically. Pertinent noncancerous phenotypic features, such as perioral pigmentations in Peutz-Jeghers syndrome, multiple colonic adenomas in FAP, multiple atypical moles in the FAMMM syndrome, and the presence of sebaceous adenomas, sebaceous carcinomas, or multiple keratoacanthomas in the Muir-Torre syndrome variant of LS should also be included.

Referral to a medical geneticist or a hereditary cancer center can be made at any time, depending on the physician's individual expertise as well as resources he or she has available. When referral is made, key medical, genetic, and genealogic findings must be made available to the center with the patient's written permission. In every potential hereditary cancer syndrome, it is essential to determine who needs to be tested. Unfortunately, even when a patient has a very strong family history of cancer and would be a candidate for DNA testing for a cancer-causing mutation, rates of referral for such testing are low. Many physicians are intimidated by the profusion of genes linked to cancer and the complexities involved in ordering and interpreting the tests.

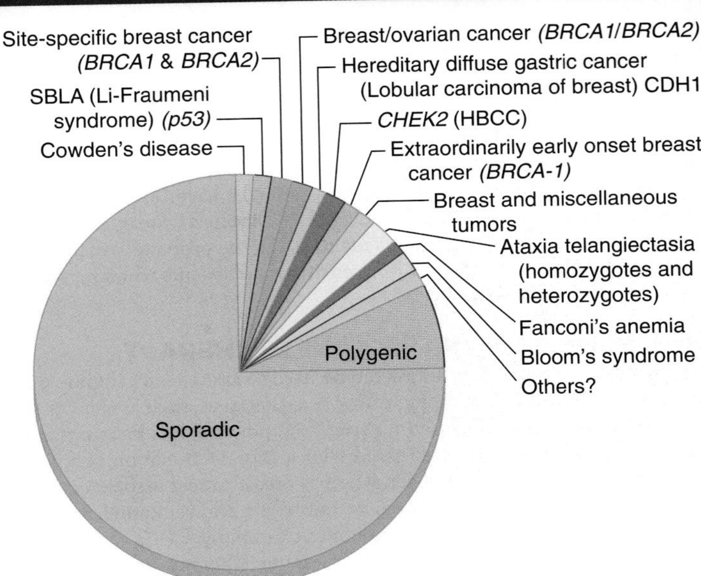

FIGURE 184-1. Schematic depicting heterogeneity in breast cancer. HBCC = hereditary breast and colorectal cancer; SBLA = sarcoma, breast and brain tumors, leukemia, laryngeal and lung cancer, and adrenal cortical carcinoma. (From Lynch HT, Fitzgibbons RJ Jr, Lynch JF. Heterogeneity and natural history of hereditary breast cancer. *Surg Clin North Am.* 1990;70:753.)

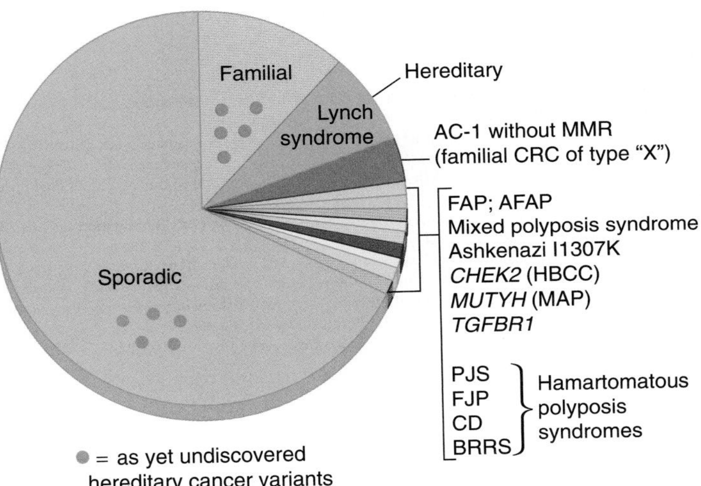

FIGURE 184-2. Circle graph depicting the marked genotypic and phenotypic heterogeneity in hereditary colorectal cancer syndromes. AC-1 = Amsterdam Criteria 1; AFAP = attenuated familial adenomatous polyposis; BRRS = Bannayan-Ruvalcaba-Riley syndrome; CD = Cowden's disease; FAP = familial adenomatous polyposis; FJP = familial juvenile polyposis; HBCC = hereditary breast and colorectal cancer; MAP = MUTYH-associated polyposis; MMR = mismatch repair; PJS = Peutz-Jeghers syndrome; TGFBR1 = transforming growth factor-β receptor type 1. (Revised from Lynch HT, Riley BD, Weissman SM, et al. Hereditary nonpolyposis colorectal carcinoma [HNPCC] and HNPCC-like families: problems in diagnosis, surveillance, and management. *Cancer.* 2004;100:53-64.)

Therefore, many patients are not receiving critical information that is available at this time.

The ideal candidate for initial genetic testing will be an individual with an early-onset syndrome cancer who is in the direct line of hereditary descent, and will be the most likely candidate to carry the family's pathogenic mutation. If that mutation can be identified in a likely syndrome carrier, it is then possible for other at-risk members of the family to have "mutation-specific testing." Although the initial genetic diagnosis is limited by technical considerations, once the index mutation is identified in the proband, confirmatory testing is cheaper and is nearly 100% sensitive and specific when performed by the same reference laboratory.

USE OF GENETICS IN CANCER THERAPY

Genetic tests of somatic mutations can be used to assist in developing prognostic estimates and in predicting response to therapies, such as using trastuzumab in breast cancer patients who are *HER2* positive. It is known that the phenotype of breast cancer associated with a *BRCA1* mutation is different from that of sporadic breast cancer, whereas breast cancer associated with a *BRCA2* mutation is similar to sporadic tumors; it is not yet known, however, how these differences should affect treatment. Similarly, CRCs showing MSI do not respond favorably to adjuvant 5-fluorouracil therapy. Imatinib is effective in the treatment of some cancers, including chronic myelogenous leukemia and gastric stromal tumors, which share activating mutations in a tyrosine kinase. Finally, genetic profiling and studies looking for single nucleotide polymorphisms are being investigated as a way to identify incremental forms of cancer predisposition. Genome-wide association studies (Chapter 42) are providing a wealth of new information about risk and are likely to provide clues to developing personalized treatments of cancer.

SUGGESTED READINGS

Boland CR, Goel A. Microsatellite instability in colorectal cancer. *Gastroenterology*. 2010;138:2073-2087. *Scholarly review.*

Leemans CR, Braakhuis BJ, Brakenhoff RH. The molecular biology of head and neck cancer. *Net Rev Cancer*. 2011;11:9-22. *Review of tumor heterogeneity, field cancerization, and molecular pathogenesis.*

McDermott U, Downing JR, Stratton MR. Genomics and the continuum of cancer care. *N Engl J Med*. 2011;364:340-350. *Review.*

Milne RL, Antoniou AC. Genetic modifiers of cancer risk for *BRCA1* and *BRCA2* mutation carriers. *Ann Oncol*. 2011;22:i11-i17. *Review based on GWAS.*

Park YJ, Claus R, Weichenhan D, et al. Genome-wide epigenetic modifications in cancer. *Prog Drug Res*. 2011;67:25-49. *Review of the potential use of DNA methylation for disease detection and prognosis.*

Plon SE, Cooper HP, Parks B, et al. Genetic testing and cancer risk management recommendations by physicians for at-risk relatives. *Genet Med*. 2011;13:148-154. *Review.*

Taylor BS, Ladanyi M. Clinical cancer genomics: how soon is now? *J Pathol*. 2011;223:318-326. *Review of germline and somatic alterations in DNA.*

185 BIOLOGY OF CANCER

JEFFREY A. MOSCOW AND KENNETH H. COWAN

GENETIC CANCER BIOLOGY

Cancer is an acquired genetic disease (Chapter 184). Spontaneous genetic changes overwhelm the mechanisms that maintain normal cellular homeostasis, disrupt the normal tight control of cell division and death, and result in the malignant phenotype.

The genetic damage that results in cancer can occur in several ways: translocations of genes can juxtapose two genes in ways that cause dysregulation of their function; mutations can activate cancer-causing genes or deactivate cancer-preventing genes; and epigenetic modifications of proteins that associate with DNA can alter the expression of critical genes (Chapter 184). Sometimes, the first step is the mutation of genes that normally prevent mutations in other genes—cells then quickly gain additional mutations that, through a morbid natural selection, ultimately produce the mutant clone that gives rise to a malignancy.

The very processes that generate malignant transformations also present obstacles to their treatment. The genetic plasticity that can manufacture cancer-causing mutations can also generate mutations that result in resistance to anticancer drugs.

Tumor formation after malignant transformation requires changes in cell biology that, in the processes of invasion and metastases, favor propagation of the malignant cells. Because individual cells, like organisms, are programmed to die, cancer cells must learn to evade the intricate systems of apoptosis that ensure cell death. Cancer cells must also enable the formation of new blood vessels to provide nutrition for the growing mass and develop strategies to escape the immune surveillance that suppresses tumor formation. These processes that give rise to malignant tumors can again raise barriers to successful therapies; for example, cells with impaired apoptosis may be resistant to anticancer drugs that kill cells through activation of apoptosis. However, the distinctive biology of malignancies can also provide opportunities for directed therapies.

Specific Mutations, Targeted Therapies

All cancer cells contain some genomic damage. In most cases, several abnormalities must occur, but sometimes even a single mutation appears sufficient to produce malignant transformation. The latter examples demonstrate clearly that cancer is a genetic disease of dysregulated growth, and they demonstrate that identification of a genetic cause can lead to a specific targeted therapy aimed at the product of the damaged gene.

In the case of acute promyelocytic leukemia (APL; Chapter 189), the characteristic t(15;17) translocation is the only identified genetic lesion. This genetic mishap splices the retinoic acid receptor *(RAR)* gene to another gene called *PML*, and the resulting hybrid RAR-PML protein does not function properly. The functional defect of the RAR-PML hybrid protein product can be overcome with pharmacologic doses of a vitamin A analogue, all-*trans*-retinoic acid (ATRA). The addition of ATRA to chemotherapy for APL doubles disease-free survival, from approximately 40% to approximately 80%. Similarly, the accidental genetic recombination that creates the BCR/ABL hybrid protein results in malignant transformation of myeloid cells (Chapter 190), and can be treated with specific inhibitors of the BCR/ABL kinase. Cancers driven by single mutations appear to be restricted to specific tissue types. Thus, genetic alterations that lead to malignant transformation are also dependent on the cellular context in which they occur.

Multistage Evolution of Malignancy

Most cancers do not have a single cause but rather are the products of a progression of genetic lesions that can be years in the making, as evidenced by their multiple and complex genetic alterations. The classical model of two stages of cancer development, initiation and promotion, has been replaced by a more dynamic and multistep model in which accumulated genetic damage leads to dysregulation of cell division and the disarming of the mechanisms of cell death.

Often the first step in the creation of a tumor is the development of genomic instability. During each cell division, some 3 billion nucleotide pairs must be faithfully copied to produce exact replicas in each daughter cell. The process of cancer can begin with alterations in any one of a number of factors that influence the accuracy of this process of genetic replication. Two major mechanisms create this acquired genetic damage: spontaneous mutations can disable the machinery that edits DNA replication and removes damaged genes, or, more frequently, cells are exposed to carcinogens that directly damage DNA, and the imprecise repair of damaged DNA results in an increase in spontaneous mutations.

Heritable conditions that impair the proteins that ensure genomic fidelity cause a predisposition to a variety of types of cancer. Examples of defects in genes that repair DNA damage, leading to increased hereditary cancer risk, are listed in Table 185-1.

Because cancer is a genetic disease, carcinogens are genomic toxins that damage DNA and create mutations. The DNA damage from cigarette smoke (Chapter 31) results from exposure to dangerous hydrocarbon products that bind DNA and disrupt faithful replication. Ultraviolet irradiation causes characteristic DNA damage in the skin that can lead to melanoma and other skin cancers (Chapter 210). Ionizing radiation (Chapter 19) from diagnostic and therapeutic radiation also cause genetic damage and cancer.

One key regulator of genomic integrity is the p53 protein, the product of a tumor suppressor gene that is commonly referred to as the "guardian of the

TABLE 185-1 GENOMIC INSTABILITY GENES ASSOCIATED WITH INCREASED HEREDITARY CANCER RISK

GENES	SYNDROME	HEREDITARY TUMOR TYPES
MUTYH	Attenuated polyposis	Colon
ATM	Ataxia-telangiectasia	Leukemias, lymphomas, brain
BLM	Bloom's	Leukemias, lymphomas, skin
BRCA1, BRCA2	Hereditary breast cancer	Breast, ovary
FANCA, FANCC, FANCD2, FANCE, FANCF, FANCG	Fanconi's anemia A, C, D2, E, F, and G	Leukemias
NBS1	Nijmegen breakage	Lymphomas, brain
MSH2, MLH1, MSH6, PMS2	Hereditary nonpolyposis colon cancer (Lynch syndrome)	Colon
XPA, XPC, ERCC2, ERCC3, ERCC4, ERCC5, DDB2	Xeroderma pigmentosum	Skin

TABLE 185-2 TUMOR SUPPRESSOR GENES ASSOCIATED WITH INCREASED HEREDITARY CANCER RISK

GENES	SYNDROME	HEREDITARY TUMOR TYPES
p53	Li-Fraumeni	Breast, sarcoma, adrenal, brain
APC	Familial adenomatous polyposis	Colon, thyroid, stomach, intestine
CDHI	Familial gastric carcinoma	Stomach
VHL	von Hippel-Lindau	Kidney
WT1	Familial Wilms' tumor	Wilms'
PTEN	Cowden's	Hamartoma, glioma, uterus
CDKN2A	Familial malignant melanoma	Melanoma, pancreas
CDK4	Familial malignant melanoma	Melanoma
RB1	Hereditary retinoblastoma	Eye
NF1	Neurofibromatosis	Neurofibroma, brain tumors
MEN1	Multiple endocrine neoplasia type 1	Parathyroid, pituitary, islet cell
NF2	Neurofibromatosis	Meningioma, acoustic neuromas

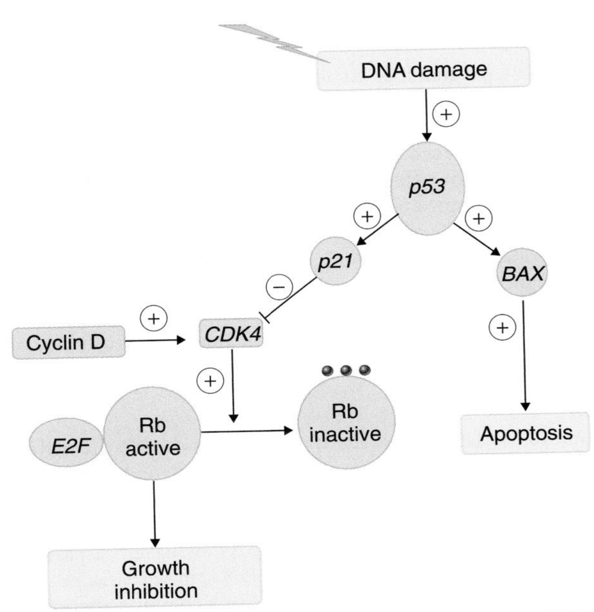

FIGURE 185-1. Response to p53 and DNA damage. After DNA damage, *p53* expression induces the cyclin kinase inhibitor p21, resulting in cell cycle arrest, and *BAX*, which induces apoptosis. Rb = retinoblastoma.

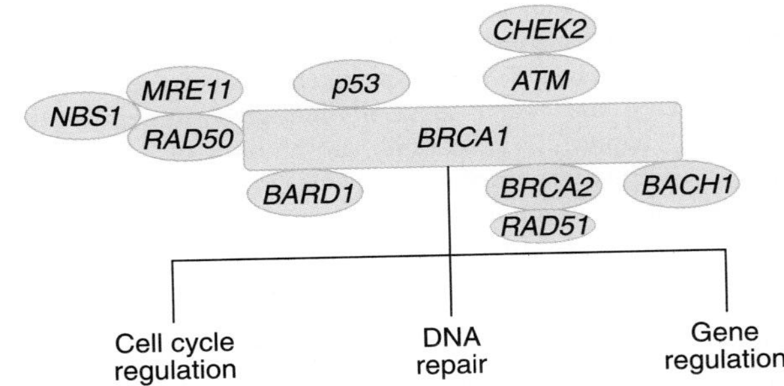

FIGURE 185-2. Protein interactions with *BRCA1* and *BRCA2*. *BRCA1* and *BRCA2* act as molecular scaffolds and promote assembly of protein complexes involved in cell cycle regulation in response to DNA damage as well as DNA repair. Signaling scaffolds, like *BRCA1*, bring together proteins belonging to interlinked pathways and orchestrate specific interactions among signaling proteins. Some of the more than 50 proteins that interact with *BRCA1* are shown.

genome." The p53 protein can sense DNA damage and direct the cell either to cell cycle arrest by increased expression of the cyclin kinase inhibitor p21 (Fig. 185-1), which provides the cell with the opportunity to repair genetic damage before cell division, or down the path of programmed cell death (apoptosis). Inactivating mutations in p53 are among the most common abnormalities observed in cancer, emphasizing the critical role of unrepaired genetic damage in the etiology of cancer. Individuals with inherited mutations of the *p53* gene have the Li-Fraumeni syndrome (Chapter 184), with increased susceptibility to specific types of cancer. The retinoblastoma (*RB*) gene is another tumor suppressor gene whose normal function is to regulate cell growth (see Fig. 185-1). Mutations in a number of other tumor suppressor genes are also associated with specific cancer syndromes (Table 185-2).

Similarly, the heritable breast cancer predisposition genes *BRCA1* and *BRCA2* encode proteins that associate with many intracellular proteins that are involved in DNA repair, including rad50, rad51, ATM, and p53 (Fig. 185-2). Cells defective in *BRCA1* or *BRCA2* display defects both in the response to DNA and in DNA repair. Mutations in the *BRCA1* and *BRCA2* (Chapter 204) are rare, so relatively few women inherit abnormal copies of these gene alleles from their parents, and only approximately 10% of breast cancers can be attributed to *BRCA1* and *BRCA2* mutations.

DNA damage, whether from heritable conditions, from somatic mutations in the DNA repair mechanisms themselves, or from carcinogen exposure, increases the rate of spontaneous mutations in cells and sets the stage for the natural selection of malignant clones. Although mutations of most of the approximately 25,000 genes in the genome do not result in malignancy, mutations or other disruptions of the right genes in the right cellular context can confer a selective proliferative or survival advantage, and set the stage for malignant progression.

Disease of the Messenger Proteins

In health, cells respond to external stimuli with complex and redundant protein networks that interact with external stimuli and transmit appropriate signals to the nucleus. The proteins involved in signal transduction include cell surface receptors, second messenger systems, and multiple transcription factors that directly regulate gene expression. Each of these elements of the signal transduction network is controlled by multiple proteins that tightly regulate the activation state of each element of the network. Disruption of any of the genes that encode the proteins involved in signal transduction—proteins that relay the external stimulus to the nucleus—occurs frequently in cancer.

Cell surface receptors for external stimuli involve families of receptor tyrosine kinases, proteins that become activated after binding to specific ligands. For example, the epidermal growth factor (ErbB) family receptor kinases are often amplified or found activated by mutations in breast, ovary, gastric, and lung cancers. Identification of such genetic abnormalities in cancer cells has

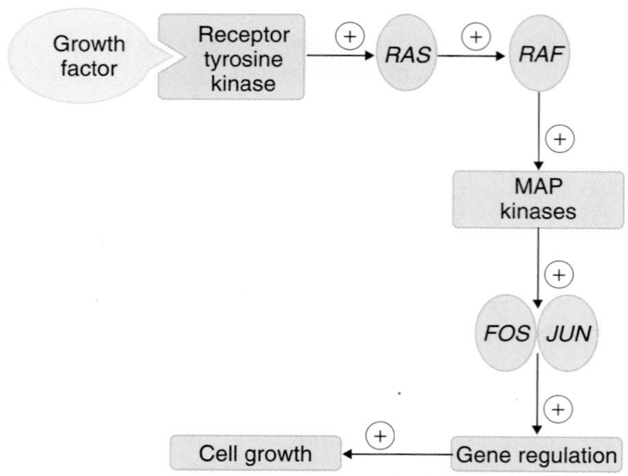

FIGURE 185-3. Growth factor–mediated signal transduction. Upon binding to specific receptor ligands, receptor tyrosine kinases activate downstream signal transduction cascades that result in changes in gene expression and enhanced cell growth. Alterations in various steps in the signal transduction cascade are frequently observed in cancer. MAP = mitogen-activated protein.

provided valuable targets for selective therapies. Thus, trastuzumab, a monoclonal antibody directed against the ErbB2/Her2neu protein, which is amplified and overexpressed in 25% of breast cancers, has been shown to improve disease-free survival and overall survival when given in combination with chemotherapy (Chapter 204). Erlotinib, an inhibitor of ErbB1 (epidermal growth factor [EGF]) receptor, may be effective in treatment of lung cancers that contain mutations in the ErbB1 (EGF) receptor (Chapter 197).

Unregulated growth can also result from mutations that affect downstream signal transduction networks (Fig. 185-3). Receptor tyrosine kinases transmit their signals through biochemical pathways and ultimately drive gene transcription. In some pathways, receptor tyrosine kinases activate Ras proteins, which act as second messengers that amplify and direct signals from receptor tyrosine kinases to other intracellular proteins, which then ultimately generate the cellular response to the stimulus. Ras mutations, which are frequently found in cancer, typically result in the Ras protein being stuck in the "on," or activated, position, which provides a constant, unregulated stimulus to downstream proteins, which in turn creates a cascading effect that stimulates cell growth. Although mutations in other genes are also commonly found in tumors that harbor Ras mutations, mutation of Ras alone has been shown to transform normal cells into malignant cells. Activating mutations of Ras family proteins can frequently be found in melanoma, myeloid leukemias, and cancers of the colon, pancreas, and lung. Genetic abnormalities are also frequently found in the other signaling pathways that transmit signals from receptor tyrosine kinases, including the PIP3/PDK1/Akt pathway, as well as in the nonreceptor tyrosine kinases signaling pathways, including the Jak/STAT and the c-Src pathways.

Disruption of the genes that encode the proteins that regulate gene transcription, which are the downstream targets of signal transduction cascades, can also create malignancy. For example, amplification of the Myc family of transcription factors is frequently observed in neuroblastoma and in cancers of the lung, bladder, breast, stomach, and colon. Certain acute leukemias (Chapter 189) arise when the normal gene recombination process that produces diverse immune responses goes awry and an immunoglobulin or T-cell receptor locus is accidentally spliced onto a gene encoding a transcription factor, resulting in loss of regulation of the transcription factor activity. Several pathognomonic oncogenic chromosomal translocations commonly found in sarcomas also involve genes for transcription factors; for example, the t(11;22) of Ewing's sarcoma (Chapter 209) creates the *EWSR1-FLI1* hybrid transcription factor, and the characteristic t(2;13) of alveolar rhabdomyosarcoma creates the hybrid *PAX3-FOXO1A* DNA binding protein.

Suppression of Tumor Suppressors

Normal cells contain proteins that prevent malignant transformation. Inactivation of the tumor suppressor genes that encode these proteins also leads to cancer. Because a loss of function is required for a malignant effect, both copies of the tumor suppressor gene must be affected. In almost all cases, patients have a physical loss of one copy of a gene and an acquired mutation of the other. The spontaneous deletion of genetic material, called loss of heterozygosity, is a frequently observed genetic abnormality in tumors.

Some familial cancer predisposition syndromes are based on the inheritance of one damaged copy of a tumor suppressor gene (Chapter 184). Hereditary retinoblastoma, which results from inheritance of a mutated *RB* gene, and the Li-Fraumeni syndrome (Chapter 184), which results from inheritance of a mutant *p53* gene, predispose affected individuals to cancers. Both the Rb and p53 proteins play critical roles in regulating the progression of proliferating cells through the cell cycle, and the loss of this checkpoint regulation can contribute to uncontrolled cell growth and cancer.

The importance of the p53 and Rb signaling pathways in tumor suppression is further revealed by the mechanism by which infection with the human papillomavirus (HPV; Chapter 381) in cervical epithelial cells leads to cervical cancer (Chapter 205). HPV proteins E6 and E7 inactivate p53 and Rb proteins, respectively, thereby creating a virally induced premalignant state in which the machinery that prevents damaged cells from proliferating has been turned off. For this reason, vaccination against certain HPV serotypes holds the promise of preventing most cases of cervical cancer.

DISTINCTIVE CANCER BIOLOGY

Cancer cells do not behave like normal cells. The alterations in the regulation of cell growth, differentiation, and death that give rise to cancer also produce common abnormal biologic characteristics, which are shared by tumors that arise from different cells of origin. These common features conspire to allow the transformed cell to grow into a tumor.

Telomerase

Normal cells are programmed to differentiate and ultimately to die, and this programming is regulated through enzymatic pathways that lead to terminal differentiation, senescence, or apoptosis. Cancer cells evade the mechanisms that are designed to steer cells toward terminal differentiation and senescence by altering the function of telomerase. As primitive cells divide and differentiate, the ends of chromosomes, called telomeres, progressively shorten and ultimately lead to a growth arrest that is termed replicative senescence. An enzyme called telomerase adds length back to the telomeres and reverses the process of replicative senescence. Telomerase is usually expressed at significant levels only in stem cells. However, telomerase is highly expressed in most malignant tissues, demonstrating a common alteration of cell biology that is necessary for creation and maintenance of the malignant phenotype.

Apoptosis

In addition to bypassing senescence, cancer cells disable the pathways that lead to apoptosis. Because apoptosis is literally a life-and-death decision for the cell, it must be tightly controlled by intricate pathways of regulatory proteins. Apoptosis can be triggered through either external or internal pathways that converge to activate a family of enzymes, called caspases, that systematically degrade cellular proteins and DNA in a characteristic pattern resulting in cell death. Cancer cells contain many common aberrations in the machinery that regulates apoptosis, including increased activity of antiapoptotic proteins, such as Bcl-2 and Mcl-1, or increased levels of inhibitors of apoptosis, such as the protein survivin, which inhibits caspase activity.

Cancer Epigenetics

Epigenetic changes in gene expression are also hallmarks of malignancy (Chapter 184). In normal cells, gene expression is controlled by epigenetic processes that limit the physical accessibility of genes to transcription factors. Gene expression can be silenced by processes that methylate specific DNA sequences on chromosomes, called CpG islands. In cancer, tumor suppressor genes are frequently found to be abnormally methylated, leading to a loss of their expression and function. The drugs 5-azacytidine and decitabine reverse methylation and have activity in the myelodysplastic syndrome (Chapter 188) and leukemia. Gene expression is also controlled by histone acetylases, which influence how tightly genomic DNA is spooled around large complex nuclear proteins called histones and alter the interaction of chromatin proteins with DNA. A novel group of drugs called histone deacetylase inhibitors are currently under development as anticancer agents.

Energy Metabolism

Cancer cells also demonstrate characteristic alterations in glucose metabolism, known as the Warburg effect. Malignant cells tend preferentially to shunt glucose into the glycolytic pathway, taking up excessive amounts of glucose and metabolizing glucose into lactate instead of channeling glucose into the typical aerobic pathway that more efficiently captures energy and creates the end products of carbon dioxide and water. This disruption of normal cellular energy metabolism is thought to be due to dysregulation of a gene that is also involved in the regulation of apoptosis, Akt, and its downstream effectors. This abnormal metabolism of glucose in cancer cells is also the principle behind the use of positron emission tomographic scans to image tumors. Inherited inactivating mutations of the phosphatase and tensin homologue *(PTEN)*, which inactivates Akt, are also responsible for Cowden's syndrome, in which the susceptibility to breast and thyroid cancers is increased.

Ubiquitinylation and Proteasomes

Normal cells have tightly regulated mechanisms to degrade and recycle proteins by attaching one or more ubiquitin molecules to a protein. Ubiquitinylation can serve as a signal that a protein should be trafficked to and degraded by lysosomes or the proteasome. Ubiquitinylation plays an important role in the regulation of receptor tyrosine kinases, in cell cycle progression, and in repair of DNA damage. This regulatory mechanism is altered in many types of cancer. The first anticancer drug targeted at this abnormality in cancer cells is bortezomib, which inhibits proteasome activity and is effective in the treatment of multiple myeloma (Chapter 193).

Angiogenesis

Because tumors must find mechanisms to feed themselves as they grow, the malignant transformation must include the ability to stimulate new blood vessel formation, or angiogenesis. Malignant cells have in common the ability to stimulate the formation of endothelial cells and the breakdown of extracellular membranes, often by secreting vasculature endothelial growth factor (VEGF). The resulting tumor vasculature, although functional, does not have the vessel architecture or endothelial wall characteristics of a normal vascular bed. The realization that tumor cells have unique angiogenesis has led to the novel therapeutic approach of targeting tumor vessel formation, and not the malignant cell itself, such as with the monoclonal anti-VEGF antibody bevacizumab in metastatic colorectal cancer (Chapter 199).

Tumor Immune Evasion

Tumors also develop strategies to evade immune surveillance. The T cells and natural killer cells of the immune system play a role in protecting the host against malignancy, just as they also protect against infectious agents. Tumors can grow unimpeded after malignant cells have been selected with properties that disarm the host's immune response to tumors; these mechanisms include downregulation of costimulatory and major histocompatibility complex molecules, as well as secretion of cytokines that inhibit the immune system, such as transforming growth factor-β. The development of therapies designed to harness the immune system for cancer treatment, including tumor antigen vaccines, has been hindered by properties that allow tumors to escape immune destruction.

Drug Resistance

The same genetic plasticity that leads to cancer also gives cancer cells access to the human genome repertoire, with the capability to express and mutate any of its genes—sometimes resulting in resistance to anticancer therapy. Cancer cells can specifically alter the chemotherapy target to become resistant. In the case of imatinib mesylate, the targeted therapy for chronic myeloid leukemia (Chapter 190), cells can become resistant by mutating the binding site of the drug to the already mutant BCR/ABL protein. Cancer cellular resistance to older targeted drugs such as methotrexate, which targets the enzyme dihydrofolate reductase, can be mediated by multiple steps in the folate metabolic pathway. Cancer cells can also reach into their genomes and call on more general mechanisms of protection from stress. Normal cells can upregulate genes to protect against environmental toxins. In cancer, malignant cells use the same proteins to evade chemotherapy, such as adenosine triphosphate–dependent efflux drug pumps MDR1 (for multidrug resistance) and the MRP (for multidrug resistance–related protein) family of transmembrane proteins. Cancer cells also use other detoxification pathways, such as those involving glutathione, for protection against chemotherapy. For every anticancer drug developed, a cancer cell has found a way to circumvent it.

Cancer Stem Cells

Tissues are composed of a vast majority of cells that are irreversibly committed toward terminal differentiation. Hidden within tissues are also a very small minority of primitive, seemingly nondescript cells that are capable of repopulating the tissue with new cells and have the potential for self-renewal, that is, the ability to divide without differentiating; these are called stem cells. The view of cancer as a homogeneous mass of clonally derived malignant cells has been replaced by a view that, in some tumors, cancer cell division is organized more like a tissue in that most of the cells of a tumor do not have unlimited capacity for self-renewal but rather are the progeny of a minute population of cancer-initiating (or stem) cells. In hematopoietic malignancies and other tumors, flow cytometric techniques have demonstrated small, unique populations of cancer cells within tumors that have the ability to re-form the tumor, whereas the vast majority of cells in a malignancy do not have this potential.

This concept of cancer has enormous consequences for the study and treatment of cancer. Most important, all previous studies that have examined the overall expression of genes in a malignancy may not reveal critical and unique characteristics of the cancer-initiating cells from which the tumor has arisen. The pattern of treatment response followed by treatment relapse may be due not only to the acquisition of drug resistance but also to a failure of the therapy to treat the distinctive biology of the cancer stem cell. Isolation and characterization of cancer stem cells may reveal new cancer stem cell–specific targets that distinguish them from both their malignant progeny and normal stem cells. Treatments aimed at cancer stem cells hold the potential for markedly improving cancer therapy.

SUGGESTED READINGS

Frezza C, Pollard PJ, Gottlieb E. Inborn and acquired metabolic defects in cancer. *J Mol Med.* 2011;89:213-220. *Review of pro-oncogenic signaling.*

Goh AM, Coffill CR, Lane DP. The role of mutant p53 in human cancer. *J Pathol.* 2011;223:116-126. *Review.*

Tsai HC, Baylin SB. Cancer epigenetics: linking basic biology to clinical medicine. *Cell Res.* 2011;21:502-517. *Review of molecular mechanisms and the possibilities for pharmacological targeting of cancer-specific epigenetic alterations.*

Vander Heiden MG, Cantley LC, Thompson CB. Understanding the Warburg effect: the metabolic requirements of cell proliferation. *Science.* 2009;324:1029-1033. *Review of molecular mechanisms underlying altered glucose metabolism in cancer.*

186

ENDOCRINE MANIFESTATIONS OF TUMORS: "ECTOPIC" HORMONE PRODUCTION

ROBERT F. GAGEL

It is now commonly accepted that genetic abnormalities, either activating or inactivating mutations, cause disordered cell growth leading to cellular transformation. A corollary of this fundamental tenet is that changes in a handful of important cellular genes can result in altered expression of other genes and thereby lead to the production of cellular proteins not normally expressed in the differentiated cell type. Among the more interesting and clinically relevant types of abnormal proteins are those associated with "ectopic" hormone syndromes, a small but clinically important group of disorders.

There are several patterns of "ectopic" hormone production. The most common is the production of small polypeptide hormones by tumors derived from a specific class of neuroendocrine cells. These neuroendocrine cells are widely dispersed throughout the lung, gastrointestinal tract, pancreas, thyroid gland, adrenal medulla, breast, prostate, and skin; they share several common cytologic and biochemical characteristics (amine precursor uptake and decarboxylation), are often derived from the neural crest, and normally produce both biogenic amines and small polypeptide hormones. The list of hormones produced by tumors derived from members of this group of neuroendocrine cells includes adrenocorticotropic hormone (corticotropin, ACTH), calcitonin, vasoactive intestinal peptide, growth hormone–releasing hormone, corticotropin-releasing hormone (CRH), somatostatin, and other small peptides. A second group of tumors, generally derived from squamous epithelium, produces parathyroid hormone–related protein (PTHrP) and vasopressin.

Current evidence suggests that aberrant hormone production is due to reversion to an earlier state of differentiation and an earlier developmental

TABLE 186-1 CLINICAL SYNDROMES OF ECTOPIC HORMONE PRODUCTION

HUMORAL HYPERCALCEMIA
Parathyroid hormone–related protein
Squamous cell carcinoma
Breast cancer
Neuroendocrine tumors
Renal cell cancer
Melanoma
Prostate cancer
Increased calcitriol
Lymphoma
Benign conditions: sarcoidosis, berylliosis, tuberculosis, fungal infection
CORTICOTROPIN
Proopiomelanocortin
Small cell lung cancer
Pulmonary carcinoid
Medullary thyroid cancer
Islet cell tumor
Pheochromocytoma
Ganglioneuroma
Corticotropin-releasing hormone
Medullary thyroid cancer
Paraganglioma
Prostate cancer
Islet cell tumor
HUMAN CHORIONIC GONADOTROPIN
Choriocarcinoma
Testicular embryonal cell carcinoma
Seminoma
HYPOGLYCEMIA
Insulinoma
Sarcomas or large retroperitoneal tumors
INAPPROPRIATE ANTIDIURETIC HORMONE SECRETION
Small cell lung cancer
Squamous cell head and neck cancer
ERYTHROPOIETIN
Renal cell cancer
Hepatoma
Pheochromocytoma
Benign conditions: cerebellar hemangioblastoma, uterine fibroid

pattern of transcription factor expression. In hypercalcemia caused by ectopic production of PTHrP, activation of the *ras*–mitogen-activated protein kinase signaling pathway, through mutation, appears to be responsible for PTHrP production by squamous epithelium. For example, normal fibroblasts can be stimulated to express PTHrP by combined expression of an activated *ras* gene and mutated tumor suppressor gene *p53*. In this example, a combinatorial effect of common genetic changes in human cancer results in abnormal expression of this hypercalcemic peptide.

The clinical syndromes associated with ectopic hormone production are important because they are often difficult diagnostic dilemmas, they are a major cause of morbidity and death in cancer patients, and their therapy can be challenging (Table 186-1). Management of these clinical syndromes is often difficult because of the necessity to treat both the cancer and the syndrome caused by excessive hormone production.

HUMORAL HYPERCALCEMIA OF MALIGNANCY

Hypercalcemia (Chapter 253) is one of the most common hormonal syndromes associated with cancer and is caused by several different pathophysiologic processes. To differentiate among these possibilities and initiate appropriate treatment, each patient must be approached in an organized manner.

PATHOBIOLOGY

Parathyroid Hormone–Related Protein

PTHrP is normally involved in chondrocytic and dermatologic differentiation. Eight of the first 16 amino acids of PTHrP are homologous with parathyroid hormone (PTH), and both peptides exert their various effects through interaction with the PTH receptor. Activation of this receptor in the osteoblast increases the expression of an osteoblast-specific cell surface protein called receptor activator of nuclear factor-kappa B ligand (RANKL). Interaction of RANKL with the RANK receptor on undifferentiated osteoclasts causes increased osteoclast differentiation and formation, bone resorption, and hypercalcemia. Ectopic production of PTHrP by a wide variety of tumors is one of the most common causes of hypercalcemia associated with malignancy; ectopic production of PTH itself is uncommon.

Increased Production of Calcitriol

Increased production of calcitriol occurs in a high percentage of patients with lymphoma (Chapters 191 and 192). There is compelling evidence for increased expression of 1α-hydroxylase by lymphomatous tissue. Other granulomatous conditions such as sarcoidosis (Chapter 95), berylliosis (Chapter 93), tuberculosis (Chapter 332), or fungal infection can also cause this clinical syndrome. Calcitriol-mediated hypercalcemia is caused by increased calcium absorption and is characterized by a suppression of serum immunoreactive PTH.

Bone Metastasis

Bone metastasis (Chapter 208) should always be considered in the differential diagnosis of hypercalcemia in a cancer patient. Bone metastases are frequently associated with local production of cytokines, PTHrP, or other substances that cause increased bone resorption. Indeed, the distinction between humoral hypercalcemia of malignancy and localized osteolysis has become blurred because of evidence that tumors such as breast cancer (Chapter 204) or myeloma (Chapter 193) cause localized osteolysis by the local production and secretion of PTHrP in addition to RANKL. In breast cancer there is considerable evidence of a local regulatory loop between transforming growth factor-β (TGF-β) and PTHrP production. TGF-β is a normal component of bone matrix. Local PTHrP production by breast cancer cells can stimulate osteoclastic bone resorption and the release of TGF-β. The release of TGF-β in turn stimulates breast cancer growth and greater PTHrP production, accelerating the osteolytic process. Other activators of bone resorption, including tumor necrosis factor, lymphotoxin, endothelin, interleukin (IL)-1, and IL-6, can be produced by other tumors that metastasize to (renal cell carcinoma) or reside in (myeloma) bone.

CLINICAL MANIFESTATIONS

The clinical syndrome associated with elevated levels of PTHrP is nearly identical to that observed with hyperparathyroidism and includes increased osteoclast-mediated bone resorption, as well as an increase in renal tubular calcium resorption and a decrease in renal phosphorus resorption. The only significant clinical difference between PTHrP- and PTH-mediated hypercalcemia is the finding of increased serum calcitriol (1,25-dihydroxycholecalciferol) levels in hyperparathyroidism and low or normal values in PTHrP-mediated hypercalcemia, presumably because of the inhibitory effects of cancer on 1α-hydroxylase, the enzyme that produces calcitriol. PTHrP production is most commonly associated with squamous cell carcinoma (Chapter 197), although production has been observed in other types of cancer as well, including breast (Chapter 204), neuroendocrine (Chapter 201), renal (Chapter 203), skin (Chapter 210), and prostate (Chapter 207) cancer. A notable trend over the past decade has been the reduction of hypercalcemia in patients with breast cancer. Routine bisphosphonate use and more effective therapies for breast cancer, particularly the widespread use of aromatase inhibitors, have led to decreased bone metastasis and hence a substantial reduction in hypercalcemia.

Clinical features that differentiate patients with increased production of calcitriol from those with PTHrP-mediated hypercalcemia include a suppressed intact serum PTH level (Fig. 186-1), an increased or normal serum phosphorus level, hypercalciuria, and no evidence of bone metastasis. An elevated serum calcitriol concentration is found in approximately half of patients with calcitriol-mediated hypercalcemia with a malignancy.

DIAGNOSIS

Measurement of intact PTH provides a useful starting point for diagnosis (see Fig. 186-1). An elevated PTH level in the context of hypercalcemia should prompt further evaluation for parathyroid disease (Chapter 253). However, in the majority of cancer patients with hypercalcemia, the intact PTH value is suppressed, indicating that the malignancy is causing the hypercalcemia. It should be kept in mind that hyperparathyroidism is not an uncommon disease, and a small percentage of patients with hypercalcemia and cancer may have both hyperparathyroidism and cancer-mediated hypercalcemia.

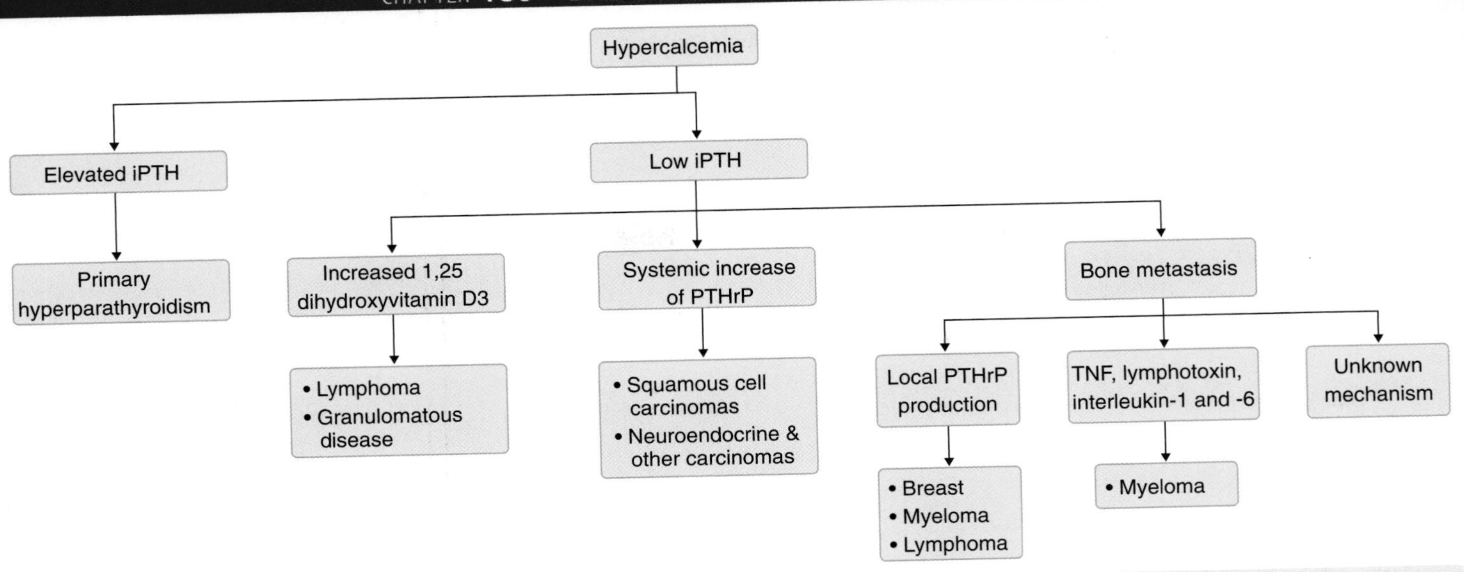

FIGURE 186-1. **Strategy for evaluation of hypercalcemia in the context of malignancy based on measurement of intact parathyroid hormone (iPTH).** PTHrP = parathyroid hormone–related protein; TNF = tumor necrosis factor.

TREATMENT Rx

The initial management of hypercalcemia should focus on reversing dehydration and increasing urine calcium excretion by the infusion of normal saline solution at rates of 100 to 300 mL/hour, depending on the patient's cardiac status. A patient with a serum calcium concentration greater than 13 mg/dL (3.25 mM/L), altered mental status, or renal dysfunction should also be treated with a bisphosphonate (intravenous pamidronate 60 to 90 mg over 4 hours, or intravenous zoledronate 4 mg over a 15-minute period), glucocorticoids (prednisone or methylprednisolone 40 to 60 mg/day), gallium nitrate (200 mg/m²/day, infused for 7 days), or salmon calcitonin (100 to 200 U intravenously or subcutaneously every 6 to 12 hours), alone or in combination. PTHrP-mediated or localized osteolysis is most responsive to bisphosphonates or gallium nitrate; vitamin D–mediated hypercalcemia is most responsive to glucocorticoid therapy (Chapter 253).

Use of high-dose intravenous bisphosphonates for extended periods has been associated with osteonecrosis of the jaw, a condition in which the mandibular or maxillary bone becomes devascularized, leading to loss of the overlying mucosa and exposed bone (Chapter 256). This condition developed in approximately 1 to 2% of patients with breast cancer and 2 to 3% with myeloma who received monthly intravenous pamidronate or zoledronate. Replacement of the devascularized and sclerotic bone occurs slowly—some patients have exposed bone for 3 to 5 years. Because many cases have been associated with dental procedures, such as removal of a tooth or tooth implantation, or with poorly fitting dentures, patients should have any dental issues addressed before the initiation of intravenous bisphosphonate therapy. The benefits of intravenous bisphosphonates in the context of bone metastasis or myeloma are substantial, and their continued use seems appropriate; however, trials are ongoing to determine whether the use of bone turnover markers to monitor suppression of bone resorption will permit use of less intensive bisphosphonate therapy.

Long-term management is focused on treatment of the underlying malignancy. Average survival in a patient with PTHrP-mediated hypercalcemia is less than 3 months, in part related to the underlying malignancy. Long-term therapy for PTHrP-mediated hypercalcemia, like that associated with parathyroid carcinoma, is difficult: patients tend to become less responsive to the effects of bisphosphonate or salmon calcitonin therapy over time and may experience renal toxicity when gallium nitrate therapy is used for extended periods.

Identification of the aforementioned RANKL/RANK receptor system has led to the development of a monoclonal antibody that binds to RANKL, thereby preventing activation of the RANK receptor. This agent, denosumab, is administered subcutaneously and recently approved for treatment of bone metastases; it is comparable to intravenous bisphosphonates in suppressing bone turnover and reducing the risk of skeletal events in patients with cancer-related bone metastases. 1 2

ECTOPIC ADRENOCORTICOTROPIC HORMONE SECRETION

PATHOBIOLOGY

Inappropriate secretion of ACTH is a rare but important cause of morbidity and mortality in cancer patients. It can be caused by two different mechanisms: expression of the proopiomelanocortin (POMC) gene by a tumor, or ectopic expression of CRH. In cell types that express the POMC gene, post-translational processing of this gene product can proceed down one of several mutually exclusive pathways and result in the expression of β-lipotropin, γ-lipotropin, and β-endorphin or the expression of big melanocyte-stimulating hormone and ACTH. Although POMC expression by malignant tumors is relatively common, expression of the enzymes necessary to cleave ACTH from the precursor is found less frequently outside the pituitary gland. ACTH production occurs in a broad spectrum of tumors, but it is most commonly associated with small cell carcinoma of the lung (Chapter 197) or classic neuroendocrine tumors such as pulmonary carcinoid (Chapter 240), medullary thyroid carcinoma (Chapter 233), islet cell adenoma or carcinoma (Chapter 238), pheochromocytoma (Chapter 235), and occasional neural tumors such as ganglioneuroma. Ectopic ACTH production causes adrenal cortical hyperplasia and excessive cortisol production (Chapter 234).

CLINICAL MANIFESTATIONS

Ectopic production of CRH causes a clinical syndrome characterized by pituitary corticotrope hyperplasia and laboratory results that mimic those of pituitary Cushing's disease (Chapter 231). Diagnosis requires a high index of suspicion combined with either measurement of CRH in blood or identification of a neoplasm outside the pituitary. Some neoplasms produce both ACTH and CRH. Tumors reported to produce CRH include medullary thyroid carcinoma, paraganglioma, prostate cancer, and islet cell neoplasms.

Hypercorticism associated with ectopic ACTH syndrome may manifest with classic features of Cushing's syndrome, such as easy bruisability, centripetal obesity, muscle wasting, hypertension, diabetes, and metabolic alkalosis. In other patients, particularly those with rapidly growing small cell carcinoma of the lung, the clinical picture may be dominated by profound hypokalemic metabolic alkalosis and hypertension, without the other clinical findings of Cushing's syndrome.

DIAGNOSIS

Evaluation of Cushing's syndrome (Chapter 234) is based on the plasma ACTH measurement in a patient with suggestive clinical and laboratory features (Fig. 186-2). The finding of a marked elevation in the plasma ACTH concentration (>100 pg/mL) should prompt a search for an ectopic source of ACTH. In a patient with a plasma ACTH value greater than 10 pg/mL but

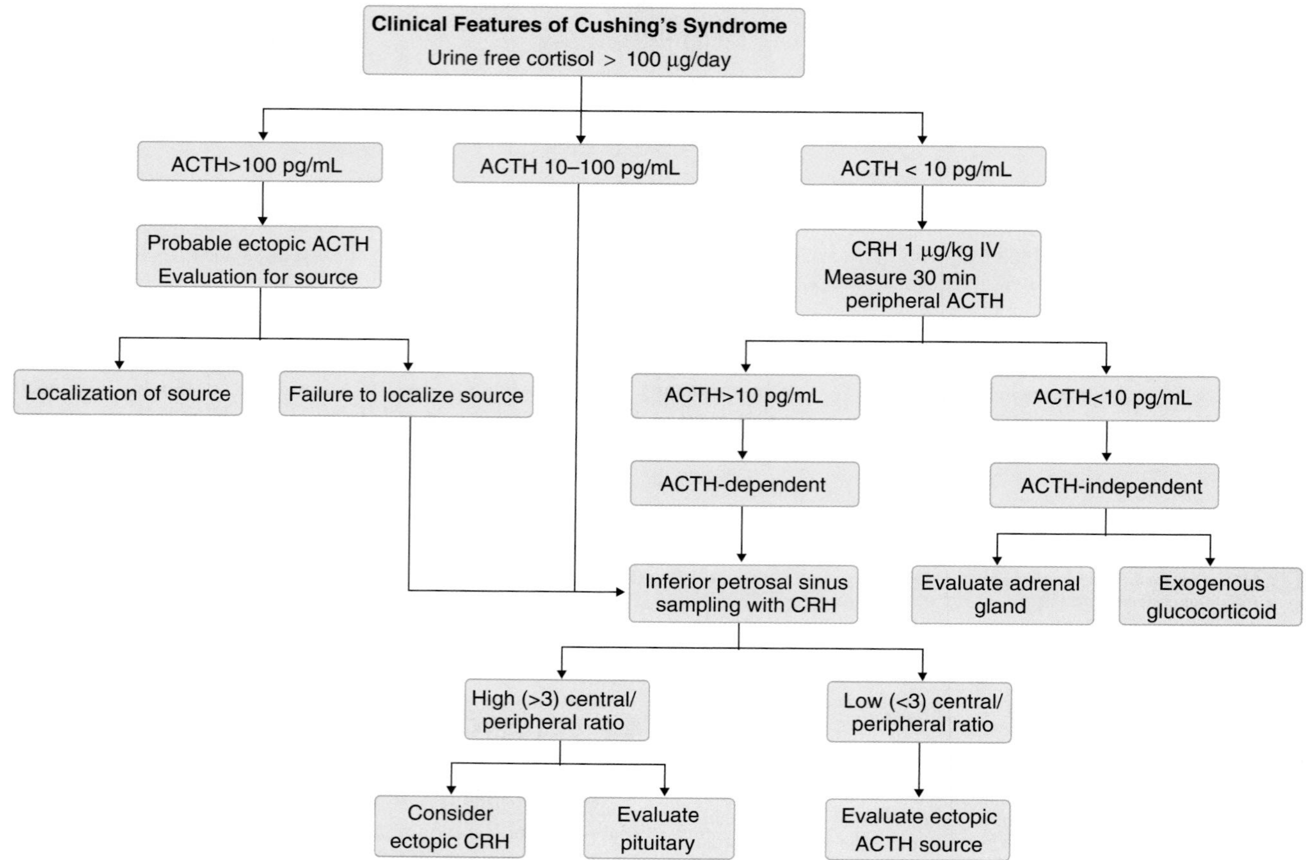

FIGURE 186-2. Evaluation strategy for a patient with Cushing's syndrome and suspected ectopic adrenocorticotropic hormone (ACTH) production. In patients with a plasma ACTH concentration greater than 100 pg/mL, an ectopic ACTH source should be considered, although some patients with pituitary Cushing's disease may have values in this range. In patients with a plasma ACTH concentration between 10 and 100 pg/mL, inferior petrosal sinus sampling for ACTH should be performed after peripheral corticotropin-releasing hormone (CRH) injection (Chapter 234) to separate a pituitary (high central-peripheral ACTH ratio) from an ectopic (low central-peripheral ACTH ratio) ACTH source. In patients with a low basal peripheral ACTH value (<10 pg/mL), a low-dose CRH test (1 μg/kg) should be performed, followed by inferior petrosal sinus sampling in individuals whose plasma ACTH concentration rises to greater than 10 pg/mL.

less than 100 pg/mL, a more detailed evaluation is appropriate. Differentiation between a pituitary and an ectopic source may require stimulation of ACTH secretion by CRH combined with measurement of ACTH in blood from the pituitary venous drainage (inferior petrosal sinus sampling). Lack of an increase in the inferior petrosal sinus ACTH concentration (less than three times the peripheral ACTH concentration) after peripheral CRH stimulation should prompt a search for an ectopic source. In patients with an increased (more than three times the peripheral level) inferior petrosal sinus ACTH level after CRH, a pituitary source is likely. Ectopic CRH can yield confusing results and may not be diagnosed unless the clinician considers the possibility and measures plasma CRH or looks for an ectopic source.

Other approaches have also been applied to the diagnosis of ectopic ACTH syndrome. For example, ACTH production from an ectopic source is not generally suppressed by high-dose dexamethasone. In a patient with an ACTH concentration greater than 10 pg/mL, administration of a single 8-mg oral dose of dexamethasone at 11:00 PM, followed by measurement of the serum cortisol level at 8:00 AM, can differentiate between a pituitary and an ectopic source. The serum cortisol level in pituitary Cushing's disease (caused by a pituitary tumor) is generally suppressed 50% after dexamethasone, whereas levels in ectopic ACTH are usually not suppressed. However, false-positive or false-negative results occur with each of these testing procedures, making the differential diagnosis of Cushing's syndrome one of the most challenging in medicine.

TREATMENT Rx

Hypercortisolism associated with ectopic ACTH can be managed by removal of the ACTH- or CRH-producing tumor or by inhibition of cortisol synthesis with metyrapone (1 to 4 g/day orally), aminoglutethimide (250 mg orally four times/day with upward titration), or ketoconazole (200 to 400 mg orally twice a day). Parenteral etomidate, used for sedation and induction of anesthesia, rapidly inhibits cortisol synthesis at subhypnotic concentrations. It is titrated from 0.3 to 4 mg/kg/hour to normalize serum cortisol measurements and has been used to rapidly reverse hypercorticism in a small number of patients. Replacement glucocorticoid therapy is needed to prevent adrenal insufficiency in patients receiving inhibitors of cortisol synthesis (Chapter 234). If surgical removal of an ACTH- or CRH-producing tumor is not possible and inhibition of cortisol synthesis is inadequate, bilateral adrenalectomy (with replacement glucocorticoid and mineralocorticoid therapy) may be required. In patients with a rapidly progressive small cell carcinoma of the lung and ectopic ACTH syndrome, the oncologic imperative to initiate immediate cytotoxic therapy must be counterbalanced by the desire to normalize cell-mediated immunity by normalizing cortisol secretion, hypokalemia, and metabolic alkalosis. Cytotoxic chemotherapy should generally be delayed, if possible, until the serum cortisol level is normalized because neutropenic patients with hypercortisolism have a high rate of infection that often causes death. If cancer treatment is initiated, prophylactic therapy for pulmonary *Pneumocystis carinii* (Chapter 349) and fungal infections should be considered.

HUMAN CHORIONIC GONADOTROPIN PRODUCTION

PATHOBIOLOGY

Two different genes encode the α- and β-subunits of human chorionic gonadotropin (HCG). The β-subunit is common to all the pituitary glycoprotein hormones (luteinizing hormone, follicle-stimulating hormone, thyroid-stimulating hormone [TSH], and HCG), whereas each of these hormones has a unique β-subunit gene. Inappropriate production of the α-subunit occurs in a variety of pituitary and nonpituitary tumors and does not cause any discernible clinical syndrome. The β-subunit confers biologic specificity. Production of intact HCG occurs commonly in trophoblastic tumors (choriocarcinoma, testicular embryonal carcinoma, and seminoma; Chapter 206) and less commonly in other tumors such as those of the lung and pancreas.

CLINICAL MANIFESTATIONS AND DIAGNOSIS

Clinical syndromes associated with the production of HCG include precocious puberty, gynecomastia, and hyperthyroidism. Hyperthyroidism results from the low-affinity interaction of HCG with the TSH receptor when β-HCG is present in high concentrations. β-HCG concentrations that are several orders of magnitude higher than normal interact with the TSH receptor and increase the production of thyroid hormone, thereby suppressing endogenous TSH production below normal.

TREATMENT Rx

Therapy for precocious puberty and gynecomastia is directed toward removal or treatment of the underlying tumor. Hyperthyroidism is treated by inhibiting thyroid hormone synthesis, usually with thionamide therapy, followed by therapy for the underlying tumor. Treatment of hyperthyroidism by surgical removal of the thyroid gland or ablation with radioactive iodine is rarely required because the hyperthyroidism resolves rapidly after treatment of the underlying tumor.

HYPOGLYCEMIA ASSOCIATED WITH CANCER

PATHOBIOLOGY

Tumor-associated hypoglycemia is a rare but important cause of morbidity in cancer patients. Three different clinical syndromes cause most cancer-related hypoglycemia. The first is production of insulin by an islet tumor. Although primary insulinomas are rare, dedifferentiation and bulky hepatic metastasis of an islet cell carcinoma may be associated with excessive insulin production (Chapter 238). A second cause of hypoglycemia, insufficient hepatic gluconeogenesis to maintain the plasma glucose concentration in the fasting state, is caused by nearly complete replacement of the liver by metastatic tumor. A third cause of hypoglycemia is increased concentrations of insulin-like growth factor type II (IGF-II), which activates the insulin receptor associated with large abdominal or retroperitoneal tumors such as fibrosarcoma, hemangiopericytoma, or hepatoma. This increased activity appears to be due to the failure to form a normal IGF binding protein 3 (IGFBP-3) and the acid-labile subunit (ALS) complex that normally binds IGF-II; the result is an increase in free IGF-II concentrations. It is usually possible to differentiate among the three causes by measuring serum insulin, C-peptide, proinsulin, IGF-I, IGF-II, and ALS levels during a controlled fast that causes hypoglycemia (Chapter 238).

CLINICAL MANIFESTATIONS, DIAGNOSIS, AND TREATMENT Rx

In all three types of hypoglycemia, the patient is at greatest risk for symptoms during periods of fasting, most commonly while sleeping. Therapy should focus on surgical excision, when possible, or antineoplastic therapy directed at the tumor. Initial therapy for hypoglycemia is focused on frequent meals, and patients occasionally remain symptom free if awakened for one or more snacks during sleeping hours. If the tumor progresses or the patient's caloric intake is inadequate, additional measures may be required. If hepatic replacement by tumor is evident, a continuous infusion of 20% dextrose through a central line may be required, especially during sleep. In patients with insulin-producing or large retroperitoneal tumors, glucagon infusion (0.5 to 2 mg/hour) stimulates hepatic gluconeogenesis and prevents hypoglycemia; however, in rare patients a rash associated with glucagonoma may develop. An increase in glucose concentration after a single injection of glucagon (1 mg) should be documented before initiating therapy. In patients with large retroperitoneal tumors, treatment with growth hormone (3 to 6 μg/kg subcutaneously) or glucocorticoids (20 to 40 mg/day) may reverse the hypoglycemia, possibly by facilitating IGFBP-3/ALS complex formation, thereby reducing free serum IGF-II levels. This condition has also been treated with growth hormone doses as high as 2600 μg/day; long-term treatment with this dose may cause acromegaly. Somatostatin analogues (octreotide or lanreotide) are not generally effective for normalizing the plasma glucose level in patients with islet cell tumors; diazoxide (3 to 8 mg/kg/day in two or three divided doses) may be effective, but problems with fluid retention frequently preclude its long-term use.

SYNDROME OF INAPPROPRIATE ANTIDIURETIC HORMONE SECRETION

PATHOBIOLOGY

Ectopic production of vasopressin by head and neck tumors (3%), small cell carcinoma of the lung (15%), and other lung carcinomas (1%) causes the clinical syndrome of inappropriate antidiuretic hormone (SIADH), which is characterized by hyponatremia, hypo-osmolality, excessive urine sodium excretion, an inappropriately high urine osmolality for the low serum osmolality, and normal function of the kidneys and adrenal and thyroid glands. Other malignant neoplasms (primary brain tumors; hematologic neoplasms; skin tumors; gastrointestinal, gynecologic, breast, and prostate cancers; and sarcomas) are rare causes of this clinical syndrome.

CLINICAL MANIFESTATIONS AND DIAGNOSIS

In most cases the hyponatremia is asymptomatic, although altered mental status and seizures may develop when the serum sodium concentration falls below 120 mEq/L. Hyponatremic women of reproductive age may experience profound cerebral degeneration.

TREATMENT Rx

Fluid restriction may be effective for short-term management, but it is difficult to maintain over long periods. Hypertonic fluids can be given with great caution to symptomatic patients (Chapter 118); the serum sodium concentration should be monitored to prevent an increase of more than 12 mEq/day. Treatment with 150 to 300 mg/day demeclocycline can block the effects of vasopressin on the kidney and is an effective long-term therapy in patients with cancer. Oral tolvaptan and intravenous conivaptan are vasopressin receptor type 2 antagonists that are effective treatments for hyponatremia.

RARE ECTOPIC HORMONE SYNDROMES

Tumor-Induced Osteomalacia

A clinical syndrome characterized by profound hypophosphatemia, muscle weakness, and osteomalacia (Chapter 252) can be produced by mesenchymal tumors (osteoblastoma, giant cell osteosarcoma, hemangiocytoma, and, rarely, prostate and lung carcinoma). Fibroblast growth factor 23 (FGF-23), mutated in autosomal dominant hypophosphatemic rickets (Chapter 252), is overexpressed in neoplasms causing this disorder. Therapy is directed toward correction of hypophosphatemia with either oral or intravenous supplementation and vitamin D treatment. Surgical removal of the tumor is curative. Identification of FGF-23 overexpression as a cause may lead to the development of specific antagonists.

Hematologic Syndromes

The kidney is the primary site of erythropoietin production; therefore, the relatively common erythropoietin production by benign or malignant renal tumors is not an "ectopic" hormone syndrome. Production of erythropoietin by cerebellar hemangioblastomas (Chapter 195), uterine fibroids, pheochromocytomas (Chapter 235), and ovarian (Chapter 205) and hepatic (Chapter 202) tumors is generally considered "ectopic." Patients with excessive erythropoietin production may or may not have polycythemia (Chapter 169). Other ectopic syndromes, less well defined, include production of thrombopoietin or colony-stimulating factor by some tumors. These conditions are treated by removal of the tumor or by appropriate chemotherapy.

Hypertension

Renal (Wilms' tumor, renal cell carcinoma, hemangiopericytoma), lung (small cell carcinoma of the lung, adenocarcinoma), hepatic, pancreatic, and ovarian carcinomas may produce renin. The clinical findings in these patients can include hypertension, hypokalemia, and evidence of increased aldosterone production. Therapy with aldosterone antagonists or angiotensin-converting enzyme inhibitors may be effective.

Growth Hormone and Prolactin Production

Rare examples of growth hormone production have been identified in lung and gastric adenocarcinoma. Ectopic production of growth hormone–releasing hormone has been documented for islet cell tumors (Chapter 238), bronchogenic carcinoids (Chapter 240), and small cell carcinoma of the lung (Chapter 197). Increased prolactin production is a rare phenomenon associated with lymphomas and cancer of the lung, colon, kidney, and oral cavity. Hyperprolactinemia produces galactorrhea and amenorrhea in women and hypogonadism and gynecomastia in men. Treatment with dopamine agonists (bromocriptine, quinagolide, or cabergoline), which is effective in pituitary prolactinoma (Chapter 231), should be tried, but it is most commonly ineffective.

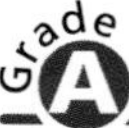

1. Lipton A, Steger GG, Figueroa J, et al. Randomized active-controlled phase II study of denosumab efficacy and safety in patients with breast cancer-related bone metastases. *J Clin Oncol.* 2007;25:4431-4437.
2. Body JJ, Lipton A, Gralow J, et al. Effects of denosumab in patients with bone metastases with and without previous bisphosphonate exposure. *J Bone Miner Res.* 2010:25:440-446.
3. Schrier RW, Gross P, Gheorghiade M, et al. SALT Investigators. Tolvaptan, a selective oral vasopressin V2-receptor antagonist, for hyponatremia. *N Engl J Med.* 2007;355:2099-2112.

SUGGESTED READINGS

Alexandraki KI, Grossman AB. The ectopic ACTH syndrome. *Rev Endocr Metab Disord.* 2010;11:117-126. *Review of pathogenesis and diagnosis.*

Kacprowicz RF, Lloyd JD. Electrolyte complications of malignancy. *Hematol Oncol Clin North Am.* 2010;24:553-565. *Concise review of the diagnosis and treatment of life-threatening electrolyte abnormalities in cancer patients, including hyponatremia, hypoglycemia, and hypercalcemia.*

Peri A, Pirozzi N, Parenti G, et al. Hyponatremia and the syndrome of inappropriate secretion of antidiuretic hormone (SIADH). *J Endocrinol Invest.* 2010;33:671-682. *Review.*

Santarpia L, Koch CA, Sarlis NJ. Hypercalcemia in cancer patients: pathobiology and management. *Horm Metab Res.* 2010;42:153-164. *Synthesis of peer-reviewed evidence regarding the pathophysiology and treatment of hypercalcemia in cancer.*

Verbalis JG. Managing hyponatremia in patients with syndrome of inappropriate antidiuretic hormone secretion. *Endocrinol Nutr.* 2010;57:30-40. *Review including the use of tolvaptan.*

187

PARANEOPLASTIC SYNDROMES AND OTHER NON-NEOPLASTIC EFFECTS OF CANCER

HOPE S. RUGO

DEFINITION

The direct clinical manifestations of cancer are usually due to local effects of tumor growth, either in the primary site or at a distant site, or are nonspecific such as anorexia, malaise, weight loss, night sweats, and fever. The term *paraneoplasia,* which means "alongside cancer," has been commonly used to denote remote effects of cancer that cannot be attributed either to direct invasion or to distant metastases.

EPIDEMIOLOGY

These syndromes may be the first sign of a malignancy and affect up to 15% of patients with cancer. However, if patients with cachexia are excluded, the incidence probably drops to only a few percent.

Paraneoplastic syndromes are important clinically for a number of reasons. First, they may be the initial presenting sign or symptom of an underlying malignancy. Up to two thirds of paraneoplastic syndromes arise before an associated malignancy is diagnosed. In some cases, the paraneoplastic syndrome may be associated with relatively small tumors; recognition of these associations may lead to earlier diagnosis and possibly more effective therapy. Second, one of the hallmarks in defining a paraneoplastic syndrome is that the course of the syndrome generally parallels the course of the tumor. Therefore, effective treatment of the underlying malignancy is often accompanied by improvement or resolution of the syndrome. Conversely, recurrence of the cancer may be heralded by return of systemic symptoms. One exception is the neurologic paraneoplastic syndromes, in which damage to structures within the nervous system may not be reversible. Third, the clinical manifestations of the paraneoplastic syndrome (or the toxic effects of electrolyte disturbances) may constitute a more urgent hazard to life or have a greater impact on quality of life than the underlying cancer.

PATHOBIOLOGY

Paraneoplastic syndromes may be caused by a variety of mechanisms; the endocrine (Chapter 186) and neurologic syndromes are the best understood. Possible etiologies include (1) secretion of proteins that are not associated with the normal tissue equivalent of the cancer (e.g., ectopic endocrine syndromes, local destruction of tissues by tumor-secreted cytokines), (2) antibodies that are directed against aberrantly expressed antigens on the tumor cell that cross-react with antigens that are normally expressed on other tissues (e.g., neurologic syndromes), and (3) effects related to unknown mechanisms, such as unidentified tumor products or circulating immune complexes stimulated by the tumor (e.g., osteoarthropathy associated with bronchogenic carcinoma; Chapter 197). Clinical findings may resemble those of primary metabolic, hematologic, dermatologic, or neuromuscular disorders or be specific to a cancer-related syndrome. Even such nonspecific symptoms as fever and weight loss are truly paraneoplastic and are due to the production of specific factors (e.g., tumor necrosis factor) by tumor cells or by normal cells in response to the tumor (see later).

DIAGNOSIS

In a patient who presents with symptoms or signs of a paraneoplastic syndrome, the screening evaluation (Table 187-1) should focus on the most common associated malignancies. If the initial evaluation is unrevealing, a repeated evaluation should be considered after several months. If the relationship between the syndrome and malignancy is less clear or less frequently observed, the evaluation should be focused on the patient's individual risks and symptoms.

The most common cancer associated with paraneoplastic syndromes is small cell cancer of the lung (Chapter 197), probably because of its neuroectodermal origin. Other neoplasms commonly associated with paraneoplastic syndrome include carcinomas of the breast (Chapter 204), ovary (Chapter 205), other adenocarcinomas, lymphoproliferative diseases (especially Hodgkin's disease; Chapter 192), and thymoma (Chapter 99).

NEUROLOGIC PARANEOPLASTIC SYNDROMES

PATHOBIOLOGY

Increasing evidence suggests that the underlying mechanisms of most neurologic syndromes associated with cancer are autoimmune in origin (Table 187-2). Tumors express antigens that are normally isolated to the nervous system and are found on neurons, referred to as onconeuronal antigens. Antineuronal antibodies that are produced against the new tumor cell antigen circulate in serum and spinal fluid and, at least in some patients, cause damage at the primary site of normal antigen expression. Pathologically, perivascular and interstitial lymphocytic infiltrates are found in the affected area of the brain. Indirect immunofluorescence of serum detects antibodies reactive with neurons. Disorders mediated by antibodies against neuronal cell surface or synaptic proteins may occur with or without tumor association; both may respond to immunotherapy.

It is unclear what susceptibility factors lead to development of a neurologic paraneoplastic syndrome. In addition to direct antibody-mediated damage, there is evidence that cell-mediated autoimmune mechanisms may

TABLE 187-1 EVALUATION AND DIAGNOSIS OF PARANEOPLASTIC SYNDROMES

Characterize abnormality; obtain laboratory studies and biopsy as necessary.
Carefully elicit any additional symptoms and signs.
Eliminate common causes.
If there is no obvious etiology, consider a paraneoplastic syndrome.
If findings are consistent with a known syndrome, screen for underlying malignancy.
If signs and symptoms are consistent with a known paraneoplastic syndrome, undertake a search for an unknown primary cancer or recurrence or progression of a known primary tumor.
Screening should include a careful physical examination with breast, gynecologic, and prostate evaluations; basic hematology, chemistry, and urine studies; chest radiograph; and mammogram.
Computed tomography (CT) of the abdomen and pelvis or positron emission tomography CT scan is indicated if there are any suspicious symptoms, signs, or laboratory abnormalities. Antibody testing for paraneoplastic neurologic syndromes and/or skin biopsy should be performed as indicated.
Consider treatment of cancer and/or appropriate palliative treatment, including immunosuppressive therapy for paraneoplastic symptoms when possible.

TABLE 187-2 PARANEOPLASTIC NEUROLOGIC SYNDROMES, ASSOCIATED ANTIBODIES, AND MALIGNANCIES

NEUROLOGIC SYNDROME	CLINICAL PRESENTATION	ANTIBODY	ASSOCIATED MALIGNANCY
Lambert-Eaton myasthenic syndrome	See text	Anti-VGCC Anti-SOX1	SCLC (>80%)
Paraneoplastic encephalomyelitis/ subacute sensory neuropathy	See text	Anti-Hu Anti-SOX1 Anti-amphiphysin Anti-Ma Anti-Trk (sensory)	SCLC (75-80%), neuroblastoma SCLC, breast Various carcinomas Lymphoma
	Acute psychosis	Anti-NMDA	Ovarian teratoma
Paraneoplastic cerebellar degeneration	See text	Anti-Yo Anti-SOX1 Anti-Ri Anti-Hu Anti-Tr, Anti-GluR Anti-Ma	Breast, ovarian, and other gynecologic malignancies Breast (50%) SCLC Hodgkin's lymphoma Various carcinomas
Limbic encephalopathy	Subacute amnestic syndrome, affective disorder, seizures DDX: herpes encephali*tis* Improvement common with treatment of underlying tumor; immunosuppression is of unclear benefit	Anti-Hu, Antiamphiphysin, Anti-SOX1, Anti-VGKC, Anti-AMPA Anti-Ta	SCLC Testicular, breast
Opsoclonus/myoclonus	Saccadic eye movements with ataxia and myoclonus Most occur in children with neuroblastomas Pathology reveals diffuse dropout of Purkinje cells Treatment of underlying tumor may improve symptoms; ACTH, steroids, and IVIG may also benefit	Anti-Ri Anti-Hu Antiamphiphysin Anti-Ta	Breast (70%), ovarian SCLC, neuroblastoma (50%) SCLC Testicular
Stiff-person syndrome	Progressive muscle stiffness and rigidity, with intermittent and painful muscle spasms. EMG: continuous firing of motor unit potentials Treat with muscle relaxants; may improve with cancer therapy	Antiamphiphysin Anti-GAD	Breast, SCLC Breast
Neuromyotonia	Diffuse muscle stiffness and cramps; may be associated with myasthenia gravis Responds to treatment of tumor and immunosuppression	Anti-VGCC	Thymoma
VISUAL SYNDROMES			
CAR	Gradual to acute and progressive visual loss	Antiretinal, antirecoverin	SCLC
MAR	Reports of response to immunosuppressive therapy and plasmapheresis	Antibipolar cell	Melanoma
Bilateral diffuse melanocytic proliferation (BDUMP)		?	Gynecologic malignancy Various adenocarcinomas
SYNDROMES WITH NO ASSOCIATED ANTIBODY IDENTIFIED			
Demyelinating neuropathies (including CDP, mononeuritis multiplex)	Sensory more common than motor or both May improve with treatment of paraprotein, plasmapheresis	IgM paraprotein may cross-react with MAG, cryoglobulins	Plasma cell and lymphoproliferative neoplasms, osteosclerotic myeloma, POEMS, amyloid, SCLC, other carcinomas
Necrotizing myelopathy	Symptoms associated with specific levels of spinal cord dysfunction Rapid deterioration and death		Variety of carcinomas and lymphomas
Motor neuron disease	Similar to ALS with progressive weakness; may improve with plasmapheresis and treatment of paraproteinemia		Plasma cell and lymphoproliferative neoplasms
Polymyositis/dermatomyositis	Unclear relationship to cancer, higher risk with dermatomyositis May improve with treatment of cancer, otherwise treat as idiopathic		Variety of carcinomas

ACTH = adrenocorticotropic hormone; AGNA = antiglial nuclear antibody; ALS = amyotrophic lateral sclerosis; AMPA = α-amino-3-hydroxy-5-methyl-4-isoxazolepropionic acid; amphiphysin = synaptic vesicle–associated protein; CAR = carcinoma-associated retinopathy; CDP = chronic demyelinating polyneuropathy; DDX = differential diagnosis; EMG = electromyogram; GAD = glutamic acid decarboxylase; GluR = glutamate receptor; IgM = immunoglobulin M; IVIG = intravenous immunoglobulin; MAG = myelin-associated glycoprotein; MAR = melanoma-associated retinopathy; NMDA = *N*-methyl-D-aspartate; POEMS = polyneuropathy, organomegaly, endocrinopathy, monoclonal protein, and skin changes associated with osteosclerotic myeloma; SCLC = small cell lung cancer; VGCC = voltage-gated calcium channel, VGKC = voltage-gated potassium channel.

contribute. The finding of $CD8^+$ T lymphocytes infiltrating neurologic tissue in postmortem studies of patients with neurologic paraneoplastic syndromes, combined with data that patients with antibodies (with or without neurologic paraneoplastic syndromes) may have longer survival rates than otherwise similar patients without circulating antibodies, suggests that $CD8^+$ T lymphocytes play a beneficial role in tumor-directed immune responses. This immune response may be mediated by aberrant expression of native antigens.

CLINICAL MANIFESTATIONS

Neurologic paraneoplastic syndromes may involve the brain, cranial nerves, spinal cord, dorsal root ganglia, peripheral nerves, neuromuscular junction, muscle, or multiple levels of the nervous system. Perhaps because of cross-reactivity of antibodies, it is not uncommon for patients to develop more than one paraneoplastic syndrome, making the diagnosis of a particular syndrome more difficult. Classic paraneoplastic disorders include those whose clinical manifestations are unique and are frequently associated with cancer;

TABLE 187-3 GENETIC SYNDROMES WITH CUTANEOUS MANIFESTATIONS ASSOCIATED WITH AN INCREASED RISK OF SYSTEMIC CANCERS

GENETIC SYNDROME	SKIN LESION	GENETIC MUTATION	ASSOCIATED CANCERS	RISK
Torre's (Muir-Torre)	Multiple sebaceous gland tumors, basal cell cancers	Mutations in DNA mismatch repair genes leading to microsatellite instability (*MSH2*, 2p22-p21)	GI and GU cancers	High
Gardner's	Multiple epidermal and sebaceous cysts of face and scalp, desmoid tumors of skin, osteomas of face and head, GI polyps	Adenomatous polyposis coli tumor suppressor gene (5q21-q22)	GI cancers	High
Cowden's	Multiple hamartomas of skin, mucous membranes (trichilemmomas), lipomas	*PTEN/MMAC1* tumor suppressor gene	Breast, thyroid cancers	High
MEN 2B	Multiple papular mucosal neuromas on lips, oropharynx, conjunctiva	Receptor tyrosine kinase (*RET*) protooncogene	Medullary carcinoma of thyroid, pheochromocytoma	High
Ataxia-telangiectasia	Telangiectasias over face, conjunctiva	*ATM* gene (11q22-23)	Lymphomas	Medium
Neurofibromatosis type 1	Cafe au lait spots, axillary freckles, neurofibromas	*NF1* gene (17q11.2)	Neurofibrosarcoma, pheochromocytoma, acoustic neuromas	Low
Peutz-Jeghers	Pigmented macules on the lips, oral mucosa, hands, feet; hamartomatous GI polyps	*STK11/LKB1* gene (19p13.3)	GI, pancreas, ovary, testes	Low
Basal cell carcinoma nevus (Gorlin's)	Multiple basal cell cancers	*PTCH1* gene (9q22) resulting in activation of hedgehog signaling	Basal cell cancers, medulloblastoma, fibrosarcoma	Low
Bloom's	Telangiectatic redness of skin in photo-exposed areas, stunted growth	DNA helicase gene (*RECQL3*)	Lymphomas, leukemias	Medium

GI = gastrointestinal; GU = genitourinary; MEN = multiple endocrine neoplasia.

nonclassic syndromes frequently occur without cancer and may be difficult to identify. The differential diagnosis of neurologic paraneoplastic syndromes includes idiopathic presentations of the same syndrome, side effects of chemotherapy (Chapter 182) and radiation therapy (Chapter 19; Table 187-2), infections (usually associated with lymphoproliferative diseases), vascular disease (including infarction and hemorrhage), and metabolic and nutritional abnormalities (including hormonal paraneoplastic syndromes). Therapy includes treatment of the underlying tumor as well as immunosuppressive therapy with or without plasmapheresis. Unfortunately, this approach usually results in only modest, if any, improvement of the neurologic deficit.

DIAGNOSIS

A patient presenting with neurologic complaints regardless of a prior diagnosis of malignancy should undergo a standard evaluation for diseases such as a primary central nervous system (CNS) malignancy, a metastatic malignancy, bleeding, vascular events, and infection. Generally, this evaluation includes a careful history regarding onset, associated symptoms, and other general medical conditions, as well as a careful physical and neurologic examination. Studies should include initial contrast-enhanced magnetic resonance imaging (MRI) and examination of the cerebrospinal fluid (CSF) for protein and cells if the MRI is normal or showed leptomeningeal enhancement. If the evaluation does not reveal evidence of primary CNS disease, a body positron emission tomography (PET) or computed tomography (CT) scan along with standard laboratory testing may be useful to screen for undetected malignancies.

If a neurologic paraneoplastic syndrome is suspected, serum and CSF should be tested for antineuronal antibodies targeted to either intracellular or cell surface proteins (see Table 187-2). However, a high degree of specificity of an antibody for a particular syndrome does not prove that the antibody is pathogenic. Finding a circulating antibody is useful but not diagnostic of any particular syndrome; patients can have circulating antibodies without the associated clinical syndrome, and most lung cancers as well as many breast and gynecologic malignancies express neuronal antigens, although the antibody titer is usually much lower than that seen with a neurologic paraneoplastic syndrome. High serum antibody levels and the presence of antibody in the CSF are more specific findings. Diagnosis of a neurologic paraneoplastic syndrome should instigate a reasonable search for the commonly associated malignancy (see Table 187-1). PET and CT scans have been shown to improve the detection of cancers when other screening tests are negative, particularly when patients are found to have antineuronal antibodies.

Lambert-Eaton Myasthenic Syndrome—Anti-VGCC and Anti-SOX1 Antibodies

DEFINITION AND EPIDEMIOLOGY

The Lambert-Eaton myasthenic syndrome (LEMS) is one of the first recognized and most common neurologic paraneoplastic syndromes, and it is one of the only syndromes with direct evidence to support the role of autoantibodies in producing clinical disease. This disorder affects 1 to 2% of patients with small cell cancer of the lung (SCLC), and up to two thirds of the cases are associated with an underlying malignancy.

PATHOBIOLOGY

LEMS is associated with a defect in the release of neurotransmitters (acetylcholine) from the presynaptic neurons at the neuromuscular junction and other sites. Acetylcholine release is mediated by P-type voltage-gated calcium channels (VGCCs); antibodies to VGCC are found in the serum of more than 85% of patients with Lambert-Eaton myasthenic syndrome. Paraneoplastic LEMS and idiopathic LEMS are clinically and immunologically similar, but a recently discovered antibody significantly associates with the presence of SCLC. Antiglial nuclear antibody (AGNA) binds to the SOX1 antigen, found in nuclei of specialized glia cells in the cerebellum. Anti-SOX1 antibodies have been identified in the sera of more than 60% of patients with paraneoplastic LEMS and appear to be a relatively specific marker of an associated underlying malignancy. SOX antibodies, as well as antibodies to the Zic protein, have been found in patients with a number of other paraneoplastic neurologic syndromes associated with SCLC as well as in the serum of patients with SCLC without neurologic symptoms.

CLINICAL MANIFESTATIONS AND DIAGNOSIS

Clinically, patients present with proximal lower limb weakness, with improvement in strength after several seconds of sustained voluntary contraction (Chapter 430). Autonomic symptoms, including dry mouth, ptosis, and impotence, are also common. Patients may also have associated CNS dysfunction, such as encephalomyelitis, cerebellar dysfunction, and peripheral neuropathy resulting from cross-reactivity or the presence of combinations of antibodies. The diagnosis is made by an electromyogram, which shows *increased* muscle action potential with repeated nerve stimulation greater than 10 Hz (the opposite of myasthenia gravis; Chapter 430). As noted previously, the finding of SOX1 antibodies significantly associates with the presence of SCLC.

TREATMENT 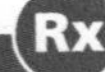

Treatment consists of a combination of plasmapheresis, intravenous immunoglobulin (IVIG) to bind circulating antibodies, and immunosuppression (to remove antibodies and suppress their production), as well as treatment of the underlying malignancy. Successful removal of the primary malignancy may result in resolution of symptoms. Pharmacologic facilitation of neuromuscular transmission with pyridostigmine, 3,4-diaminopyridine, and guanidine may be useful. 1

Paraneoplastic Encephalomyelitis and Subacute Sensory Neuropathy—Anti-Hu Antibodies

This heterogeneous group of disorders can affect the cerebral hemispheres, limbic system, cerebellum, brain stem, spinal cord, dorsal root, and autonomic ganglia.

PATHOBIOLOGY

About 75 to 80% of paraneoplastic encephalomyelitis and subacute sensory neuropathy (Chapter 428) is associated with SCLC (Chapter 197), with a variety of other neoplasms representing the remainder. Most patients have circulating antineuronal anti-Hu autoantibodies; a small number have either no antibodies or antibodies to other proteins. One report found evidence of impairment of the Trk-neurotrophin receptor by the serum of a patient with subacute sensory neuropathy, suggesting production of anti-Trk autoantibodies. Although neuronal loss is accompanied by perivascular and leptomeningeal infiltration of lymphocytes, the pathogenesis of this syndrome is unknown.

CLINICAL MANIFESTATIONS

The most common manifestations are related to subacute sensory neuropathy, including patchy or asymmetrical numbness, burning or aching paresthesias, and sensory ataxia with loss of proprioception and vibration sense. Patients may also present primarily with subacute cerebellar degeneration or brain stem encephalitis, and nearly all patients have evidence of multifocal involvement of the CNS and dorsal root ganglia.

DIAGNOSIS

The diagnosis is made on clinical grounds and is aided by finding circulating antibody in serum. MRIs are usually normal, and the CSF can show elevated protein levels with a lymphocytosis. The usual course is deterioration over weeks to months, with stabilization at a level of severe neurologic disability.

TREATMENT 

Treatment has been largely unsuccessful, but a small number of patients have improved with immunosuppressive therapy, including prednisone and IVIG.

Paraneoplastic Cerebellar Degeneration—Anti-Yo Antibodies

Paraneoplastic cerebellar degeneration is usually the initial manifestation of cancer. About 90% of patients have breast cancer, ovarian or other gynecologic tumors, SCLC, or Hodgkin's disease.

PATHOBIOLOGY

Patients with paraneoplastic cerebellar degeneration and carcinomas of the breast or ovary or other gynecologic cancers have been found to have high titers of an anti–Purkinje cell antibody, anti-Yo, in the serum and CSF, but other antibodies that react against Purkinje cell antigens can also be found (see Table 187-2). Autopsy reveals nearly complete loss of cerebellar Purkinje cells, with occasional inflammatory infiltrates.

CLINICAL MANIFESTATIONS AND DIAGNOSIS

Symptoms are often abrupt in onset and include dysarthria, ataxia, and oculomotor dysfunction. Syndromes such as paraneoplastic encephalomyelitis or LEMS may be superimposed. The diagnosis is based on clinical signs and may be aided by the presence of circulating antibody; however, anti-Yo antibodies are also found in patients who have a variety of cerebellar disorders but no evidence of cancer even on follow-up. CSF may reveal a pleocytosis and an elevated protein level or may be normal. MRI may show diffuse cerebellar atrophy but is often normal.

TREATMENT 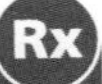

Treatment of the underlying malignancy occasionally results in significant improvement of cerebellar function. Rarely, responses have been seen to immunosuppressive therapy.

DERMATOLOGIC PARANEOPLASTIC SYNDROMES

CLINICAL MANIFESTATIONS AND DIAGNOSIS

Recognition of cutaneous manifestations of malignancy can be critical for the early diagnosis and successful treatment of malignancy, but some syndromes are seen only with advanced, incurable disease. Cutaneous manifestations include direct involvement of the skin with tumor as well as the remote effects of cancer.

Benign skin changes may be the only sign of genetic syndromes that predispose to an increased risk for malignancy over a lifetime (see Table 187-3). Recognition of these syndromes is critical for screening, early diagnosis, and genetic counseling of affected family members.

Associations between cutaneous syndromes and underlying malignancies may be difficult to confirm. Generally, and unlike the situation in neurologic paraneoplastic syndromes, the skin condition and cancer should follow a parallel course, and the two diagnoses should be made at about the same time (Table 187-4). Some skin lesions are almost always associated with malignancy. Others, however, are nonspecific and are most commonly seen with nonmalignant conditions, making it difficult or impossible to connect the skin disease with the underlying malignancy. In addition, biopsies of the skin lesion are usually nonspecific, showing features identical to those when the same lesion is seen with a nonmalignant condition. The formation of tumor-related autoantibodies has been rarely associated with dermatologic paraneoplastic syndromes, although inflammatory cell infiltration may be seen.

The finding of a new skin lesion that is almost always associated with an underlying malignancy (e.g., Bazex's syndrome, erythema gyratum repens) should prompt a directed evaluation for that tumor. In contrast, diagnosis of a common problem that is only occasionally associated with cancer (e.g., pruritus, dermatomyositis) should prompt a careful physical examination and routine cancer screening as well as continued awareness of this possible association over time. The etiology of most dermatologic paraneoplastic syndromes is not well understood. The diagnosis of a paraneoplastic dermatologic syndrome is based on characteristic clinical and pathologic findings, including deposition of immunoglobulin G (IgG) and C3 at the basement membrane of affected skin in a variety of syndromes and the finding of an underlying malignancy.

Selected Specific Syndromes

ACANTHOSIS NIGRICANS

One of the most well-known paraneoplastic syndromes is acanthosis nigricans, whose pathogenesis is unclear. The tumor may produce factors that activate insulin-like growth factors or the insulin receptor in skin. Many tumors are known to produce transforming growth factor-α (TGF-α), which might activate epidermal growth factor receptors in skin, causing hyperpigmentation and thickening.

CLINICAL MANIFESTATIONS AND DIAGNOSIS

The skin lesions (Fig. 187-1) arise as velvety, verrucous hyperpigmentation of the neck, axilla, groin, and mucosal membranes, including the lips,

TABLE 187-4 EXAMPLES OF CUTANEOUS AND RHEUMATOLOGIC LESIONS ASSOCIATED WITH MALIGNANT DISEASE

SYNDROME	CLINICAL PRESENTATION	ASSOCIATED MALIGNANCY	ASSOCIATION/RISK
CUTANEOUS			
Acanthosis nigricans	Velvety, verrucous, brown hyperpigmentation involving body folds and mucosal membranes	Gastric cancer (also endocrinopathies)	High
Acquired hypertrichosis lanuginosa (malignant down)	Long, fine, nonpigmented lanugo hairs on face, trunk, limbs, axillae	Carcinomas of the lung, colon, breast, uterus, bladder, and lymphoma (also seen with AIDS, anorexia, thyrotoxicosis, porphyria, medications)	Moderate to high
Acquired tylosis	Hyperkeratosis of palms	Lung cancer, esophageal cancer	Likely low
Bazex's syndrome	Acral hyperkeratotic papulosquamous lesions, onychodystrophy	Squamous cell carcinomas of the oropharynx, larynx, bronchi, esophagus	High
Extramammary Paget's	Nonhealing superficial dermatitis	Genitourinary and rectal cancers	Moderate to high
Sign of Leser-Trélat	Diffuse eruption of seborrheic keratoses	Gastrointestinal cancers (also seen with aging)	Likely moderate
Tripe palms	Thickened, velvety palms	Lung and gastric cancers (almost always seen with acanthosis nigricans)	High
Necrolytic migratory erythema	Circinate erosive erythematous rash, stomatitis	Glucagonoma	Likely moderate
Erythema gyratum repens	Concentric rings on trunk and proximal extremities; may have pruritus	Carcinomas of the lung, esophagus, and breast	High
Erythroderma	Diffuse erythema	Lymphoma	Low to moderate
Paraneoplastic pemphigus	Painful erythematous lesions with blistering; mucous membrane ulcerations	Lymphoma	High
Sweet's syndrome	Red nodules or plaques, fever, dermal neutrophilic infiltrates	Acute myelogenous leukemia (also seen with infection)	Moderate
Pruritus	Excoriations, pruritus occurs on extremities, upper trunk, extensor surfaces	Lymphoma and myeloproliferative neoplasms (especially polycythemia vera)	Low
CUTANEOUS WITH ARTHRITIS OR MYOPATHY			
Amyloidosis	Waxy papules and nodules, occasionally with associated symmetrical arthritis; renal insufficiency	Multiple myeloma	Moderate
Palmar fasciitis-polyarthritis	Thickening of the palmar fascia; inflammatory distal symmetrical arthritis	Ovarian cancer	Low
Panniculitis-arthritis	Erythematous subcutaneous tender nodules; inflammatory monoarticular or polyarticular arthritis	Cancer of the pancreas (also pancreatitis)	Low
Eosinophilic fasciitis	Edema, thickening of the dermis and fascia associated with joint contractures	Breast cancer, myeloproliferative neoplasm, lymphoproliferative disease	Low
Dermatomyositis/polymyositis	Heliotrope rash (erythema in periorbital area); Gottron's papules (erythematous papules over phalangeal joints); proximal myopathy	Various tumors, primarily adenocarcinomas	Low to moderate, more with dermatomyositis
ARTICULAR			
Digital clubbing	Loss of nail bed angle	Lung cancer (also seen with benign cardiopulmonary disorders)	Low
Hypertrophic pulmonary osteoarthropathy	Periostosis of long bones; pain and swelling in distal joints	Lung cancer	High
Carcinoma polyarthropathy	Sudden onset of seronegative arthritis at a late age	Cancers of the breast and lung	Low to moderate
Gout	Classic acute painful gouty arthritis	Acute leukemias, lymphomas associated with rapid tumor cell turnover and tumor lysis	Low
VASCULAR			
Leukocytoclastic vasculitis	Palpable purpura, urticaria, maculopapular rash with or without arthritis	Myeloproliferative and lymphoproliferative neoplasms, myelodysplasia; rarely with adenocarcinoma and melanoma	Low to moderate
Polyarteritis nodosa	Cutaneous and/or mesenteric vasculitis; fever, myalgia; arthritis; mononeuritis multiplex	Hairy cell leukemia	Low
Raynaud's syndrome	Classic Raynaud's with progression to digital necrosis or gangrene common	Lymphoma, leukemia, myeloma, and cancers of the lung, ovary, small bowel, breast, pancreas, kidney	Low to moderate in patients older than 50 years
Erythromelalgia	Painful, erythematous digits, relieved by aspirin	Myeloproliferative neoplasms (especially essential thrombocythemia)	Moderate to high

periocular area, and anus. Although acanthosis nigricans clearly occurs as a benign entity associated with obesity and endocrinopathy, its appearance in older adults, especially when it includes mucosal lesions, has been highly associated with malignancies of the gastrointestinal tract as well as other adenocarcinomas. The lesions often regress with successful treatment of the underlying tumor.

PARANEOPLASTIC PEMPHIGUS

This syndrome is manifested by ulcerative and blistering mucocutaneous lesions with acantholysis; it is primarily associated with lymphoma (Chapters 191 and 192), other lymphoproliferative diseases, and thymic cancers. Patients have high titers of autoantibodies to tumor antigens that cross-react with antigens at the epidermal cell junction, including the plakin family of

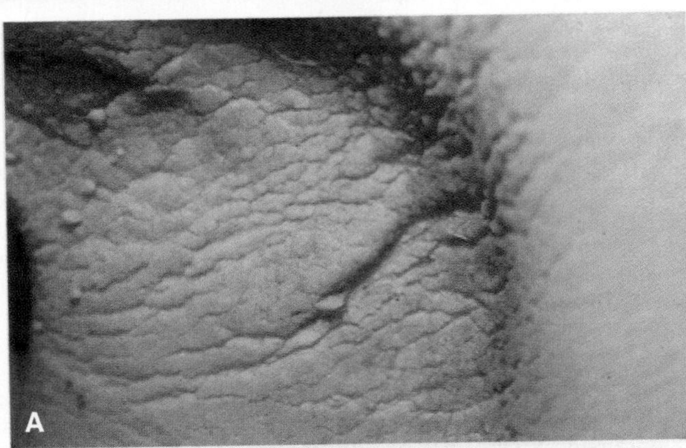

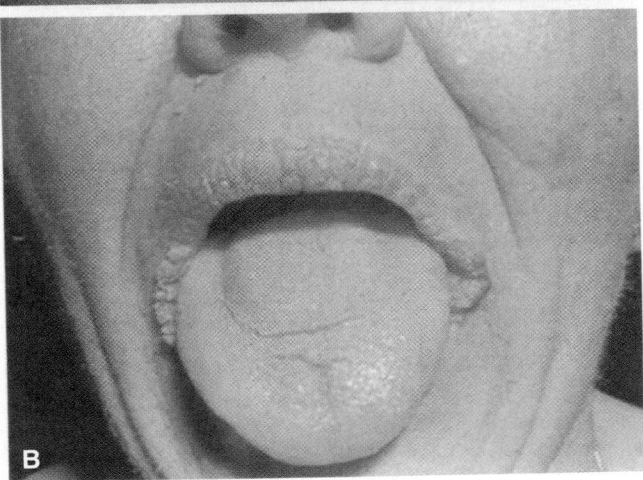

FIGURE 187-1. **Acanthosis nigricans. A,** Paraneoplastic acanthosis nigricans with a velvety hyperpigmented rash in the axilla in a patient with gastric cancer. **B,** Acanthosis nigricans of the oral mucosa. This pattern of involvement is almost always associated with cancer. (Courtesy of Dr. Timothy Berger.)

desmosomal proteins and desmogleins; indirect immunofluorescent staining shows IgG and C3 deposition on the surface of keratinocytes and on the basement membrane zone. Antibody titers may correlate with the severity of the skin disease and its response to therapy.

DIAGNOSIS

The diagnosis of paraneoplastic pemphigus should include finding specific major criteria including a polymorphic cutaneous eruption, concurrent internal neoplasia, and a specific immunoprecipitation pattern on testing of serum. Minor criteria include histologic evidence of acantholysis, intercellular and basement membrane staining with antibodies to IgG and C3 on direct immunofluorescence, and staining of rat urothelium with antibodies to desmoplakin on indirect immunofluorescence. The development of paraneoplastic pemphigus in patients with lymphoma (Chapters 191 and 192), chronic lymphocytic leukemia (Chapter 190), Castleman's disease (Chapter 191), and, less commonly, other malignancies is associated with a very poor prognosis and is often associated with pulmonary involvement.

BAZEX'S SYNDROME

Bazex's syndrome is a papulosquamous eruption that is also termed acrokeratosis paraneoplasia owing to the characteristic location of the hyperkeratotic lesions on the palms and soles. It is seen in association with squamous cell carcinoma of the head and neck (Chapter 196) as well as other malignancies involving the oropharynx or larynx. Bazex's syndrome has been postulated to be caused by antibodies that are directed against the tumor but that cross-react with keratinocyte or basement membrane antigens, similar to those in paraneoplastic pemphigus, or a T-cell-mediated immune response to epidermal tumor–like antigens.

CLINICAL MANIFESTATIONS AND DIAGNOSIS

The findings are similar in appearance to psoriatic plaques but are seen in unexpected locations including the ears, nails, nodes, fingers, palms, and soles. These lesions can predate the diagnosis of malignancy by as long as 1 year, and they may progress in parallel with the underlying tumor. The main differential diagnosis involves exclusion of benign acral variants of psoriasis.

RHEUMATOLOGIC PARANEOPLASTIC SYNDROMES

DEFINITION AND EPIDEMIOLOGY

A wide variety of rheumatologic paraneoplastic syndromes have been associated with underlying malignancies, but almost all of these syndromes are identical to their benign counterparts (see Table 187-4). The rheumatologic paraneoplastic syndromes can be classified as cutaneous with arthritis, articular, or vasculitic. Paraneoplastic rheumatologic syndromes may either coincide with the diagnosis of malignancy or precede it by several years, although the longer the interval between diagnoses, the less likely the association with cancer. Patients with a variety of rheumatologic diseases are known to have an increased risk of subsequent malignancy. For example, Sjögren's syndrome (Chapter 276) is associated with a slightly increased risk of lymphoproliferative disease, although the cause of this relationship remains unclear.

CLINICAL MANIFESTATIONS

In contrast to the nonparaneoplastic rheumatologic syndromes, rheumatologic paraneoplastic syndromes are associated with rapid onset, late age at onset (>50 years), negative serologies, and effusions characterized by the absence of inflammatory markers. Considerable overlap exists among the rheumatologic, dermatologic, and neurologic paraneoplastic syndromes.

DIAGNOSIS

In general, when a rheumatologic paraneoplastic syndrome is suspected, screening should include a physical examination, laboratory tests, and standard radiographic tests, such as a mammogram.

POEMS Syndrome

Osteosclerotic myeloma (Chapter 193) associated with the POEMS syndrome (*p*olyneuropathy, *o*rganomegaly, *e*ndocrinopathy, *m*onoclonal protein, and *s*kin changes suggestive of *s*cleroderma) is a rare condition that has features of neurologic, rheumatologic, and dermatologic paraneoplastic syndromes owing to the effects of a circulating paraprotein. It is likely that other factors also play a role in the pathogenesis of POEMS syndrome, including production of high levels of vascular endothelial growth factor and inflammatory cytokines.

Hypertrophic Osteoarthropathy

One of the more common and specific rheumatologic paraneoplastic syndromes is hypertrophic osteoarthropathy, which arises as an oligoarthritis or polyarthritis of the distal joints with clubbing, tender periostitis of the distal long bones, and noninflammatory synovial effusions. Hypertrophic osteoarthropathy may affect up to 10% of patients with adenocarcinoma of the lung. It is also seen with a variety of other pulmonary malignancies, including lung metastases from other primary sites. The etiology is unknown. Laboratory studies often reveal an elevation in the erythrocyte sedimentation rate; bone radiographs show linear ossification of the distal long bones separated by a radiolucent zone from the underlying cortex (Fig. 187-2). Treatment is symptomatic with anti-inflammatory agents; successful treatment of the underlying tumor may also improve the signs and symptoms of this syndrome.

Tumor-Induced Osteomalacia

Tumor-induced osteomalacia, a rare paraneoplastic syndrome associated with benign mesenchymal tumors and characterized by inappropriately low levels of serum 1,25-dihydroxyvitamin D and renal phosphate wasting thought to be due to tumor expression of fibroblast growth factor 23, is discussed in detail in Chapter 186.

Dermatomyositis and Polymyositis

Dermatomyositis or polymyositis has been reported to be associated with an underlying malignancy in less than 10% to as high as 60% of cases (Chapter 277). Dermatomyositis is more strongly and frequently associated with malignancy than is polymyositis. Studies of patients with dermatomyositis report a two- to four-fold increased risk of underlying malignancy, including cancer of the lung, ovaries, breast, gastrointestinal tract, and testes. The true incidence of malignancy in patients diagnosed with

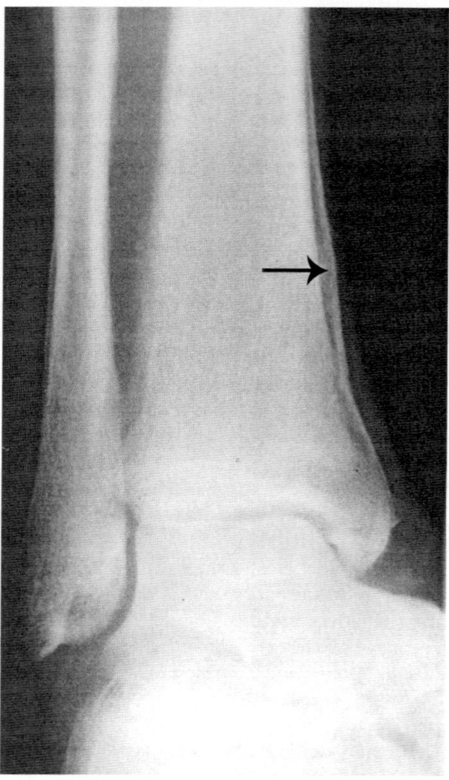

FIGURE 187-2. **Hypertrophic pulmonary osteoarthropathy characterized by periosteal elevation of the tibia (*arrow*).** (Courtesy of Dr. Lynne S. Steinbach.)

dermatomyositis is probably in the range 10 to 15%. Although the etiology is unknown, autoantibodies to muscle have been described. These autoantibodies are not well characterized and do not appear to be directed to known tumor antigens. The diagnosis of malignancy should be made within 1 year preceding or following the diagnosis of suspected paraneoplastic dermatomyositis; a longer duration of dermatomyositis without the development of cancer substantially decreases the risk of an associated malignancy.

Hematologic Paraneoplastic Syndromes

Routine blood testing may identify a hematologic paraneoplastic syndrome as well as the underlying malignancy. Hematologic paraneoplastic syndromes may involve all three cell lines.

RED CELLS

One of the most prevalent and commonly recognized paraneoplastic syndromes, seen with many cancers, is normochromic, normocytic anemia associated with a low reticulocyte count (Chapter 161). This hypoproductive anemia, generally termed *anemia of chronic disease,* or *anemia of chronic inflammation,* must be differentiated from anemia as a result of side effects of treatment or direct tumor infiltration of the bone marrow. It is associated with inappropriately low serum erythropoietin levels as well as the inability to reuse iron. Cytokines, including interleukin-1 (IL-1), tumor necrosis factor (TNF), and TGF-β, released by the tumor or local inflammatory cells mediate this disorder. Hypoproductive anemia may be effectively treated in patients with advanced malignancies with subcutaneous injections of erythropoietin or darbepoetin, although this treatment may possibly be associated with increased risk of thromboembolism (at high hemoglobin levels) and cancer progression (Chapter 161). Because of the potential risk of tumor stimulation, erythropoietic growth factors are not recommended for use in patients with early-stage or curable cancer. Pure red cell aplasia (Chapter 168) is a rare syndrome associated with cancer of the thymus gland (thymoma; Chapter 99) and is thought to be due to an autoimmune mechanism. Bone marrow examination shows absent red cell precursors.

Paraneoplastic anemia can also be caused by hemolysis (Chapter 163) related to warm- or cold-reacting antibodies in the setting of B-cell malignancies, especially chronic lymphocytic leukemia (Chapter 190) and lymphoma (Chapters 191 and 192). Treatment is directed toward the underlying lymphoproliferative disease but may also include IVIG, steroids, and possibly splenectomy for warm antibody hemolysis; cold-reacting hemolysis may require plasmapheresis. Microangiopathic hemolytic anemia (Chapter 163) with thrombocytopenia may occur with mucinous adenocarcinomas or after specific types of chemotherapy. Erythrocytosis is an uncommon paraneoplastic syndrome that is associated with tumors that produce erythropoietin, including renal cell cancer, hepatocellular carcinoma, and posterior fossa tumors (e.g., cerebellar hemangioblastoma) (Chapters 169 and 195).

WHITE CELLS

Leukocytosis (Chapter 170) is common in advanced cancer. Although infection and myeloproliferative disease must be excluded, the leukocytosis is generally caused by cytokines that are probably produced by the tumor itself, including granulocyte colony-stimulating factor and granulocyte-macrophage colony-stimulating factor. Although paraneoplastic leukocytosis requires no specific treatment, it may represent a poor prognostic sign. Eosinophilia (Chapter 173) can be seen with lymphoproliferative diseases.

PLATELETS

Paraneoplastic thrombocytosis, which is a relatively common laboratory finding, is caused by tumors that produce stimulatory cytokines (IL-6, thrombopoietin); platelet counts usually do not exceed 1 million. This type of secondary or reactive thrombocytosis, in contrast to the myeloproliferative neoplasm essential thrombocythemia (Chapter 169), is generally not associated with complications and does not require specific treatment. However, the underlying neoplasm may cause hypercoagulability by other mechanisms (see later). Iron deficiency, especially caused by gastrointestinal blood loss, should be excluded. Thrombocytopenia is uncommon except when it is associated with microangiopathic hemolytic anemia, disseminated intravascular coagulopathy (DIC), or marrow infiltration.

THROMBOSIS

EPIDEMIOLOGY

The best known and one of the first described hematologic paraneoplastic syndromes is Trousseau's syndrome, or the association of venous or arterial thrombosis with malignancy (Fig. 187-3). Although thrombosis frequently complicates progressive cancer, it may also be the first sign of cancer and predate diagnosis by a year or more. In approximately 10% of patients, deep vein thrombosis may herald an underlying malignancy, particularly in patients who present with an initial episode without other obvious risk factors, in the setting of recurrent thrombosis despite adequate doses of warfarin (warfarin resistance), or when the thrombosis occurs in unusual sites (e.g., subclavian vein, Budd-Chiari syndrome, portal vein thrombosis).

PATHOBIOLOGY

Paraneoplastic thrombosis is most commonly associated with adenocarcinomas, particularly of the stomach, breast, pancreas, and ovary. The etiology of thrombosis in patients with cancer is complex; tumor cells can activate coagulation through a number of mechanisms, including production of procoagulant mediators (e.g., sialic residues of tumor-secreted mucin), release of proangiogenic or inflammatory cytokines, direct interaction with host vasculature (endothelial damage) and blood cells through adhesion molecules, and tumor-mediated endothelial damage . Thrombosis may be associated with low-grade DIC (Chapter 178) and abnormal platelet activation. Risk factors for thrombosis in patients with known malignancy (Chapter 179) include the procoagulant effects of chemotherapy, indwelling catheters, immobility, surgery, older age, infection, obesity, prior thrombosis, and advanced stage of disease.

DIAGNOSIS

The evaluation of patients with a malignancy-associated thrombosis should include laboratory testing for DIC as well as a careful assessment of bleeding risk at sites of tumor, such as metastases to the nervous system, involvement of the gastrointestinal tract, or varices from portal hypertension in patients with liver involvement. It is important to exclude inherited clotting disorders, especially in younger patients who present with deep vein thrombosis without known underlying cause (Chapter 179) and in patients who develop a clot while taking tamoxifen.

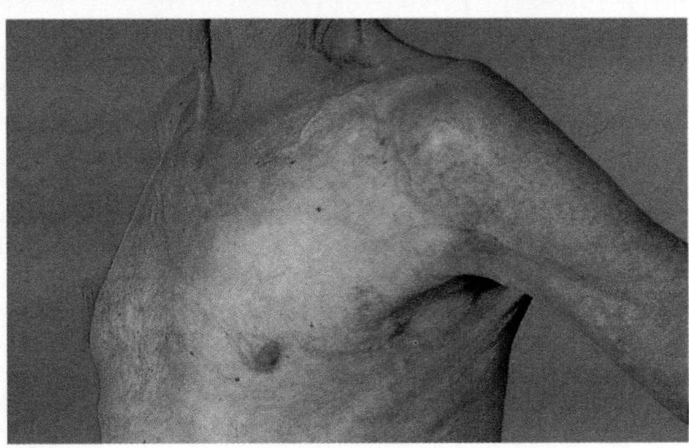

FIGURE 187-3. Thrombophlebitis in superficial or deep veins is relatively common in many forms of malignant disease, but it is particularly associated with carcinoma of the pancreas and sometimes is the presenting feature. In this patient, thrombosis in the veins of the upper arm is associated with an extensive collateral circulation in the superficial veins around the shoulder. Recurrent episodes of thrombophlebitis may precede the diagnosis of carcinoma by many months, and their occurrence in an otherwise apparently fit patient should lead to a search for underlying malignancy, especially in the pancreas. (From Forbes CD, Jackson WF. *Color Atlas and Text of Clinical Medicine*, 3rd ed. London: Mosby; 2003.)

TREATMENT Rx

Treatment for thrombosis without evidence of DIC should include initial standard anticoagulation with heparin. Long-term treatment with low-molecular-weight heparin has been demonstrated to be superior to warfarin for preventing recurrent thromboembolism without increasing the risk of bleeding.[2] Prophylactic low-dose or dose-adjusted subtherapeutic warfarin does not prevent or reduce catheter-related thromboses in patients with cancer.[3] Venous interruption (Chapters 81 and 98) is associated with significant complications and should be reserved for patients without other treatment options; temporary devices may be placed when anticoagulation must be delayed for surgery or other reasons. Successful treatment of the underlying malignancy is the most effective way to reduce the risk of thrombosis.

HEMORRHAGIC PARANEOPLASTIC SYNDROMES

DIC caused by activation of the hemostatic system with consumption of coagulation factors and platelets can result in both thrombosis and hemorrhage (Chapter 178). Acute DIC can be seen with a variety of malignancies. Essentially all patients with acute promyelocytic leukemia (Chapter 189) either present with acute DIC and associated hemorrhage or develop it during treatment. Procoagulant material released from the leukemia cells activates the fibrinolytic pathway; treatment with all-*trans*-retinoic acid and low-dose heparin has significantly reduced the complications of hemorrhage with this leukemia.

Other causes of malignancy-associated bleeding disorders include paraproteins that interfere with fibrin polymerization, amyloid deposits associated with monoclonal gammopathies such as multiple myeloma (Chapters 194), and, rarely, acquired von Willebrand's disease associated with lymphoproliferative and myeloproliferative disorders (Chapter 176). Increased fibrinolysis may be seen in patients with advanced prostate cancer (Chapter 207).

RENAL PARANEOPLASTIC SYNDROMES

Renal involvement in the setting of malignancy may be due to direct tumor infiltration of the renal parenchyma or, less commonly, to a paraneoplastic syndrome. Paraneoplastic syndromes involving the kidney may be caused by tumor-related hormone production, may directly involve the glomerulus or the microvasculature, may be related to proteins produced by the tumor (e.g., amyloid, paraproteins), or may be caused by electrolyte disorders (hyponatremia, hyperuricemia). Hyponatremia due to the syndrome of inappropriate antidiuretic hormone secretion (SIADH) is commonly associated with both limited and advanced-stage SCLC; some series have suggested a worse outcome in these patients (Chapter 186).

Glomerulonephritis

The renal paraneoplastic syndrome most clearly linked to malignancy is membranous glomerulonephritis, which is characterized by nephrotic range proteinuria, edema, hypoalbuminemia, microscopic hematuria, hypertension, and increased risk of thrombosis (Chapter 123). Associated cancers include adenocarcinomas of the lung (Chapter 197), breast (Chapter 204), and stomach (Chapter 198), as well as others. The pathology is related to thickening of the glomerular basement membrane from subepithelial deposition of tumor antigen that has reacted with circulating immunoglobulins (IgG) and complement. Other glomerular lesions include minimal change nephropathy complicating lymphoproliferative disorders, in particular Hodgkin's disease (Chapter 192); rapidly progressive glomerulonephritis associated with lymphoplasmacytic diseases; and other glomerulopathies (including nephrotic syndrome and minimal change disease) associated with a variety of malignant diseases.

It may be very difficult to differentiate a renal paraneoplastic syndrome from a benign disorder of the kidney; a biopsy demonstrating immune complex deposition, as well as a parallel course with an underlying malignancy, can help make the diagnosis.

Microvascular Disease

Renal microvascular involvement is uncommon and may be due to vasculitis or microangiopathy. Vasculitis may be caused by cryoglobulinemia in patients with hepatitis C–related hepatocellular carcinoma (Chapter 202) or rarely in patients with IgA monoclonal gammopathy in association with cancer of the lung. Thrombotic microangiopathy (hemolytic-uremic syndrome) or thrombotic thrombocytopenic microangiopathy (Chapter 175) is most commonly a complication of chemotherapy, including mitomycin C, cisplatin, and other drugs, but it may also be seen in association with a variety of advanced-stage adenocarcinomas as well as with promyelocytic leukemia. The etiology is unknown; the underlying malignancy should be treated, if possible, and plasma exchange may be helpful.

HEPATOPATHY

Paraneoplastic hepatopathy is an uncommon disorder characterized by hepatic dysfunction with elevated liver enzymes and abnormal synthetic function with fever and weight loss. This syndrome has been associated with nonmetastatic renal cell cancer (Chapter 203) and is probably due to either autoimmune effects or direct toxicity from tumor-related products. This unusual syndrome resolves with resection of the tumor.

FEVER AND CACHEXIA

Fever (Chapters 289), night sweats, and cachexia are nonspecific symptoms that, when seen in the absence of infection or a known disorder, suggest the diagnosis of an underlying malignancy. Cytokines clearly play a pathogenetic role in inducing both fever and cachexia. TNF-α (previously known as cachectin), interleukins (including IL-1 and IL-6), and interferon-γ are produced directly by the tumor or by tumor-associated host inflammatory cells, such as macrophages, which then results in a catabolic state. Cytokines may produce fever directly by acting at the hypothalamic thermoregulatory center (Chapters 289). In addition to the burden of tumor and the production of cytokines, cachexia may be caused or worsened by the side effects of cancer treatment, by intestinal blockage or malabsorption caused by tumor infiltration, and by depression.

Fever is generally cyclic and may be associated with drenching night sweats. Symptoms resolve with treatment of the underlying tumor, and return of fever usually heralds relapse. When treatment of the tumor is not possible or is ineffective, nonsteroidal anti-inflammatory agents or steroids given around the clock significantly improve quality of life. Although fever is most commonly seen in association with lymphoproliferative disease (Chapters 191 and 192), renal cell carcinoma (Chapter 203), and leukemias (Chapters 189 and 190), it may also occur with other cancers.

Cachexia, or the cancer wasting syndrome, is probably the single most common paraneoplastic syndrome, eventually affecting up to 80% of patients with cancer. This syndrome is characterized by anorexia, muscle wasting, loss of subcutaneous fat, and fatigue. It appears to be caused by a combination of protein wasting, malabsorption, immune dysregulation, and increased glucose turnover in the setting of tumor-induced increases in energy expenditure. Successful treatment of the underlying tumor reverses the process; most patients have advanced disease, for which treatment results in modest success at best. Megestrol acetate given in high concentrations in liquid form (400 to 800 mg/day) can significantly improve appetite and result in weight gain, as can dronabinol (Marinol; 2.5 to 5 mg three times a day). Corticosteroids may also help. Although agents that block TNF production are theoretically attractive to treat cancer-related cachexia, there is also concern that such agents may block cytokines that inhibit tumor growth. In addition, preclinical data suggest that antibodies to parathyroid hormone–related protein may block the production of inflammatory cytokines in cancer; whether this effect is of clinical value remains a research question.

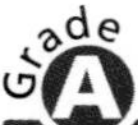

1. Wirtz PW, Verschuuren JJ, van Dijk JG, et al. Efficacy of 3,4-diaminopyridine and pyridostigmine in the treatment of Lambert-Eaton myasthenic syndrome: a randomized, double-blind, placebo-controlled, crossover study. *Clin Pharmacol Ther.* 2009;86:44-48.
2. Hull RD, Pineo GF, Brant RF, et al. Long-term low-molecular-weight heparin versus usual care in proximal-vein thrombosis patients with cancer. *Am J Med.* 2006;119:1062-1072.
3. Young AM, Billingham LJ, Begum G, et al. Warfarin thromboprophylaxis in cancer patients with central venous catheters (WARP): an open-label randomised trial. *Lancet.* 2009;373:567-574.

SUGGESTED READINGS

Blum D, Omlin A, Baracos VE, et al. Cancer cachexia: a systematic literature review of items and domains associated with involuntary weight loss in cancer. *Crit Rev Oncol Hematol.* 2011. [Epub ahead of print.] *Review of reduced nutritional intake and catabolic/hypermetabolic changes.*

Giometto B, Grisold W, Vitaliani R, et al. Paraneoplastic neurologic syndrome in the PNS Euronetwork database: a European study from 20 centers. *Arch Neurol.* 2010;67:330-335. *This large study of more than 900 patients suggests that patients with cancer and a PNS have a worse prognosis than those with the underlying malignancy alone.*

Noble S, Pasi J. Epidemiology and pathophysiology of cancer-associated thrombosis. *Br J Cancer.* 2010;102(Suppl 1):S2-S9. *The overall risk of venous thrombosis is increased seven-fold in patients with a malignancy, and thrombosis is associated with significant morbidity and mortality.*

Pelosof LC, Gerber DE. Paraneoplastic syndromes: an approach to diagnosis and treatment. *Mayo Clin Proc.* 2010;85:838-854. *Comprehensive review.*

Rosenfeld MR, Dalmau J. Update on paraneoplastic and autoimmune disorders of the central nervous system. *Semin Neurol.* 2010;30:320-331. *Excellent updated review with a discussion of differential diagnosis, antibodies, and specific syndromes.*

188

MYELODYSPLASTIC SYNDROME

ALAN F. LIST AND RAMI S. KOMROKJI

DEFINITION

Myelodysplastic syndrome (MDS) comprises a heterogeneous group of hematopoietic stem cell malignancies resulting in variable degrees of cytopenias with a tendency to progress to acute myeloid leukemia (AML). Pathologically, the disease is characterized by abnormal morphology and cytologic dysplasia.

EPIDEMIOLOGY

For many years, the incidence of MDS was not well characterized and was underestimated. In 2001, MDS became reportable to the Surveillance, Epidemiology, and End Results (SEER) cancer registry database; from these data, it is estimated that approximately 10,000 MDS cases are diagnosed annually in the United States. The overall incidence of MDS approaches 4 per 100,000, with a male predominance and a clear increase in incidence with age. In populations older than 60 years, the incidence of MDS approaches that for other hematologic malignancies like multiple myeloma and chronic lymphocytic leukemia (CLL), reaching approximately 50 per 100,000. Nonetheless, the complexities in diagnosis, nonspecific symptomatology, and underreporting make accurate estimates of incidence difficult.

Most cases of MDS are sporadic. There are few hereditary syndromes associated with MDS per se, but two ill-defined pediatric conditions, juvenile myelomonocytic leukemia (JMML) and the monosomy 7 syndrome, mimic MDS and show a familial tendency. Heterozygous germline mutations of the runt-related transcription factor 1 *(RUNX1)* gene are associated with an autosomal dominant familial predisposition to platelet abnormalities and MDS, with a median incidence of either MDS or AML among carriers of 35%. In the elderly population, other than senescence, the exact causes of MDS are not well recognized. Risk factors include benzene exposure, chemical or solvent exposure, tobacco smoke, and family history.

Therapy-related MDS (t-MDS) refers to a subset of MDS that is associated with prior exposure to mutagenic antineoplastic drugs or radiation. The increasing success in treatment of solid tumors is accompanied by a challenge whereby the incidence of t-MDS in survivors is on the rise. The risk of t-MDS varies from less than 1% (adjuvant breast cancer chemotherapy studies) to 15% (heavily treated lymphoma patients), depending on the age of the individual, class of antineoplastics, and duration of cytotoxic therapy.

PATHOBIOLOGY

The pathobiology of MDS is complex and remains under intense investigation. As opposed to other hematologic disorders like chronic myeloid leukemia (CML), there is unlikely to be a sentinel genetic event [i.e., t(9:22)]. The observed morphologic dysplasia is a common pathologic phenotype for the different underlying biology in various subsets of MDS patients. Ineffective erythropoiesis, genetic abnormalities, allelic haploinsufficiency, immune derangements, and microenvironment changes are examples of underlying disease biology.

Accelerated apoptosis is the hallmark of early MDS, which explains the paradoxical findings of normal or hypercellular bone marrow in most patients, accompanied by peripheral cytopenias. The malignant clone has an inherent susceptibility to premature apoptotic cell death. Other factors are recognized that amplify apoptotic sensitivity in MDS and include hematopoietic suppression from stromal production of inhibitory cytokines (e.g., tumor necrosis factor-α) and direct T-cell suppression akin to aplastic anemia. As the disease progresses, additional antiapoptotic signals are acquired, resulting sometimes in clonal evolution and transformation to higher-risk disease and, in some cases, to acute myeloid leukemia.

Cytogenetic Abnormalities

Cytogenetic abnormalities are observed in approximately 50% of MDS patients. The loss of genetic material is highly conserved among MDS and has led to a haploinsufficiency model of tumorigenesis. It is hypothesized that loss of even a single allele in the affected chromosomal regions may decrease the level and activity of critical gene products, presumably tumor suppressor genes. This may lead to dysplastic features, cytopenias, and the propensity to transform to AML. The most common cytogenetic abnormalities in MDS are deletions of the long arm of chromosomes 5, 7, and 20. Chromosome 5q deletion is present in approximately 15% of de novo MDS and 50% of t-MDS; abnormalities of 5q or 7, or both, are present in 70% of t-MDS. A potential validation of the haploinsufficiency model is illustrated in the analysis of a hematologic phenotype resulting from inactivation of genes encoded within the chromosome 5q common deleted region (CDR). Early growth response factor 1 *(EGR1)*, a member of the Wilms' tumor 1 (WT1) family of transcription factors, is one such gene located on 5q. It is a direct transcriptional activator of TP53, an important tumor suppressor, and is downstream of many signaling pathways. Ribosomal protein S14 *(RPS14)* is another candidate gene located more distally on 5q, and within the CDR linked to the 5q− syndrome (discussed later). This gene product is required in the 40s subunit of the ribosome and has tumor suppressor properties as well as direct action on erythropoiesis. Haploinsufficiency of the *RPS14* gene alone recapitulates the hematologic features of the 5q− syndrome, resulting in impaired erythroid differentiation and proliferation.

There are some chromosomal abnormalities that are associated with specific MDS subtypes. For example, the *MLL (HRX)* gene localized to chromosome 11q23 has been implicated in the pathogenesis of de novo AML and in t-MDS/AML. It is a translocation t(11;16)(q23;p13), which results in a fusion protein between *MLL* and the promoter of CBP (cyclic adenosine monophosphate response element binding protein [CREB] binding protein). The t(3;21)(q22;q22) translocation is also associated with t-MDS and results in fusion of *RUNX1* (formerly *AML1*) with one of several fusion partners on chromosome 3, including *EAP, EVI1,* and *MDS. RUNX1*'s product has been implicated in regulating the expression of important granulocyte elements such as myeloperoxidase and neutrophil elastase. Another translocation, t(5;12)(q33;p13), results in an activating mutation of *PDGFR*-β and is associated with chronic myelomonocytic leukemia (CMML). This is important because the *PDGFR* mutation renders the disease vulnerable to imatinib is some cases.

Epigenetics

Although loss of genetic material is common in MDS, 50% of patients with MDS have a normal karyotype. Therefore, undetectable translocations, point mutations, or epigenetic changes controlling gene expression may be responsible for the hypothesized loss of function. Because of the activity of hypomethylating agents in MDS, the role of epigenetic changes has emerged as a key contributor. DNA methyl transferase (DNMT) is responsible for methylating, and thus inactivating, gene promoters within CpG islands. Aberrant methylation of presumed tumor suppressor genes such as *p15* has been observed in MDS with adverse prognostic connotations, thereby providing an alternate mechanism by which tumor suppressors are inactivated in the pathogenesis of MDS.

Point Mutations

Point mutations represent another mechanism by which tumor suppressor function can be altered. Several activating mutations have been observed in a minority of MDS cases. Activating mutations in the *RAS* gene family occur in 5 to 15% of patients with MDS and are associated with progression to AML. Activating *FLT3* mutations have also been reported and are associated with progression to AML. Recent investigation has described multiple, novel, loss-of-function mutations in a presumed tumor suppressor protein known as TET2. It is hypothesized that these mutations may have a role in MDS progression and AML prognosis, and may be present in up to 15% of MDS cases. Also, previously cryptic mutations have been elucidated using single nucleotide polymorphism technology on c-Cbl, a known regulator of tyrosine kinase. The *c-Cbl* mutation has been seen most in CMML and, in vivo, confers a proliferative advantage.

CLINICAL MANIFESTATIONS

The hallmark clinical manifestation in MDS is persistent or progressive cytopenias. The cytopenia is usually insidious and, in retrospect, may have been present for months before diagnosis. Neutropenia has been reported in 24 to 39% of patients, anemia in 45 to 93%, and thrombocytopenia in 28 to 45%. Symptoms from MDS reflect the magnitude and lineage of cytopenias and their interactions with comorbidities. For example, a patient with coronary artery disease may present with mild anemia associated with an increase in the frequency and duration of angina. A patient on chronic anticoagulation may present with petechiae, bruising, or frank hemorrhage secondary to thrombocytopenia or platelet dysfunction. Or, a diabetic patient may present with signs and symptoms of poor wound healing and infection secondary to neutropenia or neutrophil dysfunction (i.e., impaired chemotaxis and microbial killing in those neutrophils that are produced despite adequate absolute number).

The clinical course of MDS can be subdivided in two broad categories. Approximately 70% of patients with MDS have a clinical course primarily involving progressive cytopenia. The rate of progression of these cytopenias is highly variable, as is their effect on morbidity and mortality. Approximately half of the theses patients die of causes unrelated to MDS, whereas the other half succumb to complications of marrow failure.

The remaining 30% of patients evolve into AML. The clinical course of these patients is grimmer because the transformed AML is notoriously refractory to conventional chemotherapy. If a complete remission is achieved, bone marrow transplantation remains the mainstay of therapy and the only chance for a durable remission.

DIAGNOSIS

The diagnosis of MDS requires the presence of dysplastic hematopoiesis along with the exclusion of disorders that may be a secondary cause of dysplasia. Dysplasia can first be recognized by inspection of the peripheral smear. Neutrophils may show degranulation in the cytoplasm and hyposegmentation of the nucleus (the pseudo-Pelger-Huët anomaly) (Fig. 188-1). The erythrocytes may be mildly macrocytic, a hallmark of MDS, or in cases of refractory anemia with ring sideroblasts, microcytic. The mean corpuscular volume (MCV) ranges between 100 and 110 mm^3, and the erythrocytes are usually hypochromic. Other changes can be seen in the erythrocyte morphology that reflects a hypercellular marrow or even splenomegaly seen in CMML, an MDS variant with myeloproliferative features. Some of these changes include tear drops (dacryocytes), red cell fragments, rouleaux formation, and helmet cells.

Bone marrow aspirate and biopsy are indispensable in the diagnosis of MDS. Dysplastic features may be seen in one or all three hematopoietic lineages. Dysgranulopoiesis, for example, can result in abnormal cytoplasmic granules and pleomorphic nuclear forms. Hyposegmentation of the nucleus and Auer rods (see Fig. 160-25 in Chapter 160) may be seen, with a greater proportion of immature forms including myeloblasts. Dyserythropoiesis is characterized by pleomorphic nuclear forms, ringed sideroblasts, megaloblastic changes, and nuclear-cytoplasmic dyssynchrony. Lastly, dysplasia affecting megakaryocytes can include bizarre nuclear figures, decreased ploidy, separated nuclei (so-called nuclear dispersion), and small micromegakaryocytes. The marrow cellularity is usually increased as a result of ineffective hematopoiesis. Myeloblasts may also be increased, and indeed the percent increase is important in the classification and prognosis of MDS.

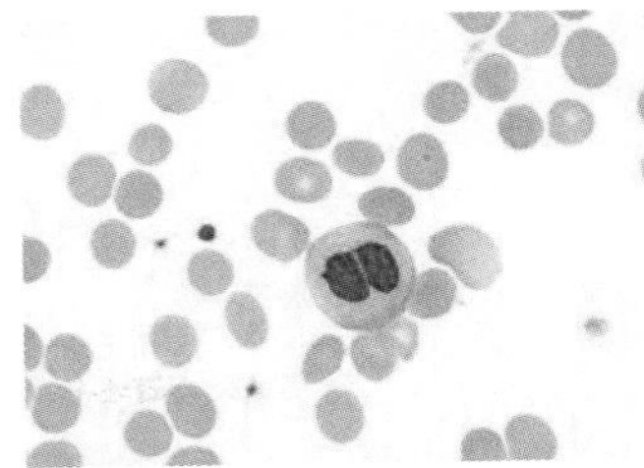

FIGURE 188-1. Pseudo-Pelger-Huët phenomenon. Abnormal, acquired, hyposegmented (usually bilobed) nucleus in neutrophil of a patient with MDS, resembling the familial Pelger-Huët anomaly (see Fig. 160-20 in Chapter 160).

TABLE 188-1 DIFFERENTIAL DIAGNOSIS OF MYELODYSPLASTIC SYNDROME

CONGENITAL DISORDERS
Hereditary sideroblastic anemia
Fanconi's anemia
Diamond-Blackfan syndrome
Kostmann's syndrome
Shwachman's syndrome
Down syndrome
VITAMIN DEFICIENCY
B_{12}, folate, or iron deficiency
DRUG TOXICITY
Marrow suppression from oral or parenteral medications
Toxins
Chemotherapy and/or radiation therapy
Alcohol
ANEMIA OF CHRONIC DISEASE
Renal failure
Chronic infection, including tuberculosis
Rheumatologic disorders
VIRAL MARROW SUPPRESSION
Including Epstein-Barr virus, parvovirus B19, human immunodeficiency virus, and others
MARROW INFILTRATION
Acute and chronic leukemias
Metastatic solid tumor infiltration
PAROXYSMAL NOCTURNAL HEMOGLOBINURIA
HYPERSPLENISM

Characteristic clonal cytogenetic abnormalities are another helpful clue in the diagnosis of MDS, although normal cytogenetics do not exclude the diagnosis. Most cytogenetic abnormalities in MDS are characterized by loss of genetic material through deletions. Nonrandom chromosomal abnormalities associated with MDS include isolated chromosome 5q deletion (5q−), which occurs in approximately 15% of de novo MDS and 50% of secondary MDS; monosomy 7; trisomy 8; 21q−; 17q−; and 20q−.

Differential Diagnosis

Although MDS should be considered in older adults with an insidious presentation of cytopenia, more common causes should be excluded (Table 188-1). Because this disease predominantly affects elderly people, polypharmacy and vitamin deficiencies (iron, folate, and B_{12} deficiency) should be strongly considered as a cause of cytopenia and corrected before proceeding in the diagnosis of MDS. Infectious causes should be considered to include parvovirus B19, human immunodeficiency virus (HIV), and viral hepatitis. Splenic sequestration should also be considered in the presence of splenomegaly on physical examination, potentially arising from portal hypertension from cirrhosis, myelofibrosis, and infiltrating splenic diseases such as lymphoma. Alcoholism can cause cytopenia secondary to direct myelosuppression, vitamin deficiency, and with intrinsic liver disease, sequestration by the spleen. Autoimmune disorders and hypogonadism in men rarely cause cytopenia. Lastly, a careful history should focus on a personal history of congenital disorders that may causes cytopenias. Once a thorough history and physical examination, review of peripheral smear, and exclusion of the above causes is complete, a bone marrow (BM) biopsy with cytogenetic analysis is warranted. The BM biopsy may then reveal hypercellularity with cytologic dysplasia (MDS), BM aplasia (aplastic anemia), or marrow infiltration with neoplastic cells (metastatic disease, leukemia).

Classification

In 1976, the French-American-British (FAB) classification was first reported and later revised in 1982 to include five MDS subtypes: refractory anemia (RA); refractory anemia with ring sideroblasts (RARS); refractory anemia with excess blasts (RAEB); CMML; and refractory anemia with excess blasts in transformation (RAEB-t). The FAB classification has since been revised by the World Health Organization (WHO) (Table 188-2) and expanded to more accurately classify patients into more homogeneous subgroups. The most important changes include lowering the threshold for AML diagnosis to 20% blasts instead of 30% and thereby omitting FAB RAEB-t subtype; recognizing CMML as a related but stand-alone MDS subtype included in the new category of myelodysplastic myeloproliferative neoplasms (MDS/MPN), and inclusion of the 5q− syndrome, a subtype of MDS that is characterized by this isolated cytogenetic abnormality, clinical distinctness, and unique response to lenalidomide.

TABLE 188-2 WORLD HEALTH ORGANIZATION CLASSIFICATION OF MYELODYSPLASTIC SYNDROME

CATEGORY	PERIPHERAL BLOOD	BONE MARROW
1a. RA without dysplasia	Blasts <1%; monocytes <1000/mm^3	Blasts <5%; ringed sideroblasts <15%
1b. RA with dysplasia	Same + dysgranulocytes and/or giant platelets	Same + dysgranulocytes and/or dysmegakaryocytes
2a. RARS without dysplasia	Blasts <1%; monocytes <1000/mm^3	Blasts <5%; ≥15% ringed sideroblasts
2b. RARS with dysplasia	Same + dysgranulocytes and/or giant platelets	Same + dysgranulocytes and/or dysmegakaryocytes
3a. RAEB-I	Blasts 1-4%; monocytes <1000/mm^3	Blasts 5-10%
3b. RAEB-II	Blasts 5-19%; monocytes <1000/mm^3	Blasts 11-19%

RA = refractory anemia; RAEB = refractory anemia with excess blasts; RARS = refractory anemia with ringed sideroblasts.

TABLE 188-3 INTERNATIONAL PROGNOSTIC SCORING SYSTEM (IPSS)

	Points				
PROGNOSTIC VARIABLE	0	0.5	1.0	1.5	2.0
Bone marrow blasts	<5%	6-10%	—	11-20%	21-30%
Karyotype*	Good	Intermediate	Poor	—	—
Cytopenias	0-1	2-3	—	—	—

*Good = normal, -Y, -5q, -20q; intermediate =other abnormal; poor = complex (>3) or monosomy 7. IPSS groups: (1) low = 0 points; (2) intermediate-1 = 0.5-1.0 points; (3) intermediate-2 = 1.5-2.0 points; (4) high = >2.5 points.

TREATMENT Rx

The International Prognostic Scoring System (IPSS) is currently the most widely used risk stratification tool to tailor treatment options (Table 188-3). In patients in the low and intermediate-1 risk groups, the goals of treatment are improve quality of life and improve cytopenias. In higher-risk MDS patients, (intermediate-2 or high-risk IPSS), the goal of treatment is to alter the natural history of the disease by approaches such as allogeneic stem cell transplantation or hypomethylating agents in order to extend survival and suppress leukemia potential.

Hematopoietic Growth Factors

About 15 to 30% of patients have an erythropoietic response to treatment with a recombinant erythropoietic stimulating agent (ESA), favoring those with low (<200 U/mL) serum endogenous erythropoietin (EPO) levels and low transfusion burden (<2 units/month). Addition of granulocyte-colony stimulating factor (G-CSF) can increase the erythroid response rate in some patients. Responders to ESA may derive a survival benefit with improvement in erythropoiesis.

Epigenetic Therapy

Aberrant hypermethylation of tumor suppressor genes has been implicated in the pathogenesis of MDS. Hypomethylating agents like 5-azacytidine (5-aza) and decitabine aim to reverse this aberrant hypermethylation and restore transcription of tumor suppressor genes. Several trials have explored the use of 5-aza in MDS. A randomized phase III trial compared 5-aza with best supportive care (BSC) in patients with all FAB subtypes and yielded improvements in cytopenias, transfusion dependency, quality of life, and time to AML progression.[1] A more recent phase III trial, Aza-001, compared 5-aza with conventional therapy that included low-dose and intensive chemotherapy in patients with higher risk (intermediate-2, high-risk) MDS. This trial demonstrated a significant improvement in median overall survival (24 months versus 15 months).[2] 5-aza likewise improved overall survival compared with conventional care regimens in the MDS subgroup of elderly patients with low BM blast count AML.[3] Romiplostim, which activates the thrombopoietin receptor, may provide incremental benefit during 5-aza therapy.[4] Decitabine has also been found in a phase III clinical trial to improve time to AML transformation and death compared with BSC; however, no survival advantage was observed compared with BSC.[5,6]

Immunomodulatory Drugs

Lenalidomide, a more potent and less toxic analogue of thalidomide, is approved for the treatment of transfusion-dependent anemia in patients with lower-risk MDS with a chromosomal 5q deletion. In the registration phase II study, 76% experienced a transfusion response, and 67% became transfusion independent that was sustained for a median duration greater than 2 years. Unlike treatment with ESAs, lenalidomide suppresses the del(5q) MDS clone to yield cytogenetic improvement in more 70% of patients. Neutropenia and thrombocytopenia are commonly seen, especially in the initial months of treatment, but are also predictive for hematologic and cytogenetic response. Activity also exists in those without a chromosome 5q deletion, albeit less robust. A multicenter trial in lower-risk patients without del(5q) reported 43% overall transfusion response, with 26% achieving transfusion independence.[7] The mechanism of action of lenalidomide is karyotype specific with clonal suppression in patients with deletion of 5q and erythropoiesis stimulation in non-5q-deletion patients.

Immunosuppressive Therapy

Based on clinical similarities between a subset of hypocellular MDS and aplastic anemia, antithymocyte globulin plus cyclosporine has been used with success in select patients with MDS. A phase III randomized trial has recently demonstrated that immunosuppressive therapy with antithymocyte globulin (15 mg/kg for 5 days) in combination with oral cyclosporine) for 180 days (average daily dose 290 mg) was associated with hematologic response in a subset of patients with MDS, compared with best supportive care, without apparent impact on transformation-free or overall survival.[8]

Hematopoietic Stem Cell Transplantation

Despite novel therapies, allogeneic hematopoietic stem cell transplantation (HSCT) remains the only curative option for MDS (Chapter 181). The overall 5-year survival rate approaches 40%. Based on decision analysis and limited data from randomized trials , the best timing for allogeneic HSCT is on a diagnosis of higher-risk MDS[9]; deferring HSCT until disease progression optimizes survival potential in patients with lower-risk disease with a compatible donor.

Conventional Chemotherapy

Response rates to conventional acute leukemia chemotherapy regimens for MDS patients are low, and mortality and morbidity can be substantial owing to comorbidities and age. Conventional chemotherapies are generally reserved for the setting of hypomethylating agent failure with disease progression.

Signal Transduction Inhibitors

Multiple signal transduction pathways have been implicated in the pathogenesis of MDS. In the rare MDS patient with *PDGFR*-activating mutations, imatinib is an effective agent. Several other agents are currently in clinical trials targeting different pathways implicated in the pathobiology of MDS.

Iron Chelation

An important consideration in lower-risk patients who are transfusion dependent is iron overload. Iron overload as measured by incremental rise in serum ferritin is an independent prognostic factor in lower-risk MDS, with increased cardiac comorbidity and decrease in survival. In practice, iron chelation therapy is considered in transfusion-dependent lower-risk MDS patients with persistent elevation in ferritin greater than 1000 ng/mL and in patients who have received more than 15 to 20 units of red blood cells. Newer oral iron-chelating agents (e.g., deferasirox) are more appealing and offer a higher expectation for patient compliance.

PROGNOSIS

Unfortunately, most MDS patients will ultimately succumb to complications from the disease or transformation to AML. The IPSS can be applied at the time of diagnosis to estimate the natural history of the disease and therefore guide treatment selection. The cumulative score is based on BM myeloblast percentage, karyotype, and number of cytopenias to risk-stratify patients into four distinct groups: low, intermediate-1, intermediate-2, and high-risk MDS (see Table 188-3). Newer risk models have been proposed to further enhance our ability to predict outcome but more importantly to tailor our therapy according to risk and disease behavior.

FUTURE DIRECTIONS

As our understanding of underlying disease biology improves, one can expect to individualize therapy based on biologic response signatures and enhanced risk stratification.

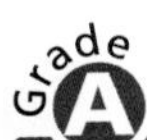

1. Kornblith AB, Herndon JE 2nd, Silverman LR, et al. Impact of azacytidine on the quality of life of patients with myelodysplastic syndrome treated in a randomized phase III trial: a Cancer and Leukemia Group B study. *J Clin Oncol.* 2002;20:2441-2452.
2. Fenaux P, Mufti GJ, Hellström-Lindberg E, et al. Efficacy of azacitidine compared with that of conventional care regimens in the treatment of higher-risk myelodysplastic syndromes: a randomised, open-label, phase III study. *Lancet Oncol.* 2009;10:223-232.
3. Fenaux P, Mufti GJ, Hellström-Lindberg E, et al. Azacitidine prolongs overall survival compared with conventional care regimens in elderly patients with low bone marrow blast count acute myeloid leukemia. *J Clin Oncol.* 2010;28:562-569.
4. Kantarjian HM, Giles FJ, Greenberg PL, et al. Phase 2 study of romiplostim in patients with low- or intermediate-risk myelodysplastic syndrome receiving azacitidine therapy. *Blood.* 2010;116:3163-3170.
5. Kantarjian H, Issa JP, Rosenfeld CS, et al. Decitabine improves patient outcomes in myelodysplastic syndromes: results of a phase III randomized study. *Cancer.* 2006;106:1794-1803.
6. Wijermans P, Suciu S, Baila L, et al. Low dose decitabine versus best supportive care in elderly patients with intermediate or high risk MDS not eligible for intensive chemotherapy: final results of the randomized phase III study (06011) of the EORTC Leukemia and German MDS Study Groups. *ASH Annual Meeting Abstracts.* 2008;112:226.
7. Raza A, Reeves JA, Feldman EJ, et al. Phase 2 study of lenalidomide in transfusion-dependent, low-risk, and intermediate-1 risk myelodysplastic syndromes with karyotypes other than deletion 5q. *Blood.* 2008;111:86-93.
8. Passweg JR, Glagounidis AA, Simcock M, et al. Immunosuppressive therapy for patients with myelodysplastic syndrome: a prospective randomized multicenter phase III trial comparing antithymocyte globulin plus cyclosporine with best supportive care—SAKK 33/99. *J Clin Oncol.* 2011;29:303-309.
9. de Witte T, Hagemeijer A, Suciu S, et al. Value of allogeneic versus autologous stem cell transplantation and chemotherapy in patients with myelodysplastic syndromes and secondary acute myeloid leukemia: final results of a prospective randomized European Intergroup Trial. *Haematologica.* 2010;95:1754-1761.

SUGGESTED READINGS

Epling-Burnette PK, List AF. Advancements in the molecular pathogenesis of myelodysplastic syndrome. *Curr Opin Hematol.* 2009;16:70-76. *Review of advances in our understanding of the molecular pathogenesis of myelodysplastic syndrome (MDS).*

Greenberg PL, Attar E, Bennett JM, et al. Myelodysplastic syndromes. *J Natl Compr Canc Netw.* 2011;9:30-56. *Review of five subtypes: refractory anemia with or without ringed sideroblasts or excess or blasts, RAEB in transformation, or chronic myelomonocytic leukemia.*

Komrokji RS, Zhang L, Bennett JM. Myelodysplastic syndromes classification and risk stratification. *Hematol Oncol Clin North Am.* 2010;24:443-457. *Comprehensive review of MDS classification and risk stratification.*

Leitch HA. Controversies surrounding iron chelation therapy for MDS. *Blood Rev.* 2011;25:17-31. *Review.*

Loaiza-Bonilla A, Gore SD, Carraway HE. Novel approaches for myelodysplastic syndromes: beyond hypomethylating agents. *Curr Opin Hematol.* 2010;17:104-109. *Review of recent advances in new strategies and targeted therapies for treatment of MDS.*

Tefferi A, Vardiman JW. Myelodysplastic syndromes. *N Engl J Med.* 2009;361:1872-1885. *Review.*

Tehranchi R, Woll PS, Anderson K, et al. Persistent malignant stem cells in del(5q) myelodysplasia in remission. *N Engl J Med.* 2010;363:1025-1037. *Rare treatment-resistant del(5q) myelodysplastic stem cells can be found in patients in remission and can serve as the presumed source of recurrence.*

189 THE ACUTE LEUKEMIAS

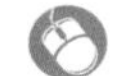

FREDERICK R. APPELBAUM

DEFINITION

Normal hematopoiesis (Chapter 159) requires tightly regulated proliferation and differentiation of pluripotent hematopoietic stem cells that become mature peripheral blood cells. Acute leukemia is the result of a malignant event or events occurring in an early hematopoietic precursor. Instead of proliferating and differentiating normally, the affected cell gives rise to progeny that fail to differentiate but continue to proliferate in an uncontrolled fashion. As a result, immature myeloid cells in acute myeloid leukemia (AML) or lymphoid cells in acute lymphoblastic leukemia (ALL)—often called blasts—rapidly accumulate and progressively replace the bone marrow, diminishing the production of normal red cells, white cells, and platelets. This loss of normal marrow function in turn gives rise to the common clinical complications of leukemia: anemia, infection, and bleeding. With time, the leukemic blasts pour out into the blood stream and eventually occupy the lymph nodes, spleen, and other vital organs. If untreated, acute leukemia is rapidly fatal; most patients die within several months after diagnosis. With appropriate therapy, however, the natural history of acute leukemia can be markedly altered, and many patients can be cured.

EPIDEMIOLOGY

Incidence

About 39,000 new cases of leukemia were diagnosed in the United States in 2009, at a rate of about 8.5 cases per 100,000 persons; this rate has remained relatively consistent for the past 3 decades. The leukemias account for about 3% of all cancers in the United States. The impact of leukemia is heightened because of the young age of some patients. For example, with a maximum incidence between ages 2 and 10 years, ALL is the most common cancer and the second leading cause of death in children younger than 15 years. In contrast, the incidence of AML gradually increases with age, without an early peak. The median age at diagnosis of AML is about 60 years.

Determinants

In most cases, acute leukemia develops for no known reason, but sometimes a possible cause can be identified.

Radiation

Ionizing radiation (Chapter 19) is leukemogenic. The incidence of ALL, AML, and chronic myeloid leukemia (CML) is increased in patients given radiation therapy for ankylosing spondylitis and among survivors of the atomic bomb blasts at Hiroshima and Nagasaki. The magnitude of the risk depends on the dose of radiation, its distribution in time, and the age of the individual. Greater risk results from higher doses of radiation delivered over shorter periods to younger patients. In areas of high natural background radiation (often from radon), chromosomal aberrations are reportedly more frequent, but an increase in acute leukemia has not been consistently found. Concern has been raised about the possible leukemogenic effects of extremely low-frequency nonionizing electromagnetic fields emitted by electrical installations. If such an effect exists at all, its magnitude is small.

Oncogenic Viruses

The search for a viral cause of leukemia has been pursued intensely, but only two clear associations have been found. Human T-cell lymphotropic virus type I (HTLV-I), an enveloped, single-stranded RNA virus, is considered the causative agent of adult T-cell leukemia (Chapter 386). This distinct form of leukemia is found within geographic clusters in southwestern Japan, the Caribbean basin, and Africa. Because HTLV-I seropositivity was found with increasing frequency among heavily transfused patients and intravenous drug users, screening of blood products for antibodies to HTLV-I is now routine practice in blood banks in the United States. Epstein-Barr virus (Chapter 385), the DNA virus that causes infectious mononucleosis, is associated with Burkitt's lymphoma (Chapter 191) and its leukemic counterpart, mature B-cell ALL.

Chemicals and Drugs

Heavy occupational exposure to benzene and benzene-containing compounds such as kerosene and carbon tetrachloride may lead to marrow damage, which can take the form of aplastic anemia, myelodysplasia, or AML. A link between leukemia and tobacco use has recently been reported.

With the increasing use of chemotherapy to treat other malignancies, the incidence of AML secondary to prior chemotherapy has increased and may represent 6 to 10% of all cases. Prior exposure to alkylating agents such as melphalan and the nitrosoureas is associated with an increased risk of secondary AML, which often manifests initially as a myelodysplastic syndrome (Chapter 188), frequently with abnormalities of chromosomes 5, 7, and 8 but with no distinct morphologic features. These secondary AMLs typically develop 4 to 6 years after exposure to alkylating agents, and their incidence may be increased with greater intensity and duration of drug exposure. Secondary AML associated with epipodophyllotoxin (teniposide or etoposide) exposure tends to have a shorter latency period (1 to 2 years), lacks a myelodysplastic phase, has a monocytic morphology, and involves abnormalities of the long arm of chromosome 11 (band q23) or chromosome 21 (band q22). Because patients frequently receive combination chemotherapy, it is often difficult to identify a single causative agent.

PATHOBIOLOGY

Genetics

If leukemia develops before 10 years of age in a patient with an identical twin, the unaffected twin has a 20% chance of developing leukemia. Several syndromes with somatic cell chromosome aneuploidy, including trisomy 21 (Down), trisomy 13 (Patau), and XXY (Klinefelter), are associated with an increased incidence of AML. Other inherited mutations, for example, a mutation at 21q22, have been associated with a high incidence of AML in rare families. Several autosomal recessive disorders associated with chromosomal instability are prone to terminate in acute leukemia, including Bloom's syndrome, Fanconi's anemia (Chapter 168), and ataxia-telangiectasia (Chapter 258).

Clonality and Cell of Origin

The acute leukemias are clonal disorders, and all leukemic cells in a given patient are descended from a common progenitor. The clonal nature of acute leukemia suggests that there are leukemic stem cells capable of both self-renewal and proliferation. Recent studies suggest that the leukemic stem cells in AML are rare among the leukemic mass, with a frequency of 0.2 to 10 per 10^6, and are within the primitive $CD34^{++}$ $CD38^{-}$ fraction. Less is known about the ALL stem cell.

Classification

The World Health Organization (WHO) classification of acute leukemias is based on clinical, morphologic, immunophenotypic, cytogenetic, and molecular features (Table 189-1).

TABLE 189-1 WORLD HEALTH ORGANIZATION CLASSIFICATION OF ACUTE LEUKEMIAS

CLASSIFICATION SUBTYPES (2008)
Acute Myeloid Leukemia (AML) and Related Neoplasms
AML with recurrent genetic abnormalities
AML with t(8;21)(q22;q22); *RUNX1-RUNX1T1*
AML with inv(16)(p13.1q22) or t(16;16)(p13.1;q22); *CBFB-MYH11*
Acute promyelocytic leukemia (APL) with t(15;17)(q22;q12); *PML-RARA*
AML with t(9;11)(p22;q23); *MLLT3-MLL*
AML with t(6;9)(p23;q34); *DEK-NUP214*
AML with inv(3)(q21q26.2) or t(3;3)(q21;q26.2); *RPN1-EVI1*
AML (megakaryoblastic) with t(1;22)(p13;q13); *RBM15-MKL1*
Provisional entity: AML with mutated *NPM1*
Provisional entity: AML with mutated *CEBPA*
AML with myelodysplasia-related changes
Therapy-related myeloid neoplasms
AML, not otherwise specified
AML with minimal differentiation
AML without maturation
AML with maturation
Acute myelomonocytic leukemia
Acute monoblastic/monocytic leukemia
Acute erythroid leukemia
Pure erythroid leukemia
Erythroleukemia, erythroid/myeloid
Acute megakaryoblastic leukemia
Acute basophilic leukemia
Acute panmyelosis with myelofibrosis
Myeloid sarcoma
Myeloid proliferations related to Down syndrome
Transient abnormal myelopoiesis
Myeloid leukemia associated with Down syndrome
Blastic plasmacytoid dendritic cell neoplasm
B Lymphoblastic Leukemia (ALL)/Lymphoma
B lymphoblastic leukemia/lymphoma, not otherwise specified
B lymphoblastic leukemia/lymphoma with recurrent genetic abnormalities
B lymphoblastic leukemia/lymphoma with t(9;22)(q34;q11.2); *BCR-ABL1* (Philadelphia chromosome–positive ALL)
B lymphoblastic leukemia/lymphoma with t(v;11q23); *MLL* rearranged
B lymphoblastic leukemia/lymphoma with t(12;21)(p13;q22); *TEL-AML1* (*ETV6-RUNX1*)
B lymphoblastic leukemia/lymphoma with hyperdiploidy
B lymphoblastic leukemia/lymphoma with hypodiploidy
B lymphoblastic leukemia/lymphoma with t(5;14)(q31;q32); *IL3-IGH*
B lymphoblastic leukemia/lymphoma with t(1;19)(q23;p13.3); *TCF3-PBX1*
T Lymphoblastic Leukemia (ALL)/Lymphoma

ALL = acute lymphoblastic leukemia.

Morphology

Leukemic cells in AML are typically 12 to 20 nm in diameter, with discrete nuclear chromatin, multiple nucleoli, and cytoplasm that usually contains azurophilic granules. Auer rods, which are slender, fusiform cytoplasmic inclusions that stain red with Wright-Giemsa stain, are virtually pathognomonic of AML. The French-American-British (FAB) morphologic system divides AML into eight subtypes: M0, M1, M2, and M3 reflect increasing degrees of differentiation of myeloid leukemic cells; M4 and M5 leukemias have features of the monocytic lineage; M6 has features of the erythroid cell lineage; and M7 is acute megakaryocytic leukemia. The WHO system also recognizes acute basophilic leukemia and acute leukemia with predominant myelofibrosis.

The leukemic cells in ALL tend to be smaller than AML blasts and relatively devoid of granules. ALL can be divided by FAB criteria into L1, L2, and L3 subgroups. L1 blasts are uniform in size, with homogeneous nuclear chromatin, indistinct nucleoli, and scanty cytoplasm with few, if any, granules. L2 blasts are larger and more variable in size and may have nucleoli. L3 blasts are distinct, with prominent nucleoli and deeply basophilic cytoplasm with vacuoles.

Immunophenotyping

Immunophenotyping by multiparameter flow cytometry is used to determine lineage involvement of newly diagnosed acute leukemias and to detect aberrant immunophenotypes, allowing the measurement of minimal residual disease after therapy. Antibodies that react with antigens found on normal immature myeloid cells, including CD13, CD14, CD33, and CD34, also react with blast cells from most patients with AML. Exceptions are the M6 and M7 variants, which have antigens restricted to the red cell and the platelet lineage, respectively. Myeloid leukemia blasts also express human leukocyte antigen (HLA)-DR antigens but usually lack T-cell, B-cell, and other lymphoid antigens. In 10 to 20% of patients, however, otherwise typical AML blasts also express antigens usually restricted to B- or T-cell lineage. Expression of lymphoid antigens by AML cells does not change either the natural history or the therapeutic response of these leukemias.

Approximately 75% of cases of ALL express B-lineage antigens and can be subdivided into four categories. The most immature group, pro-B ALL, expresses CD19 but not other B-lineage antigens and represents about 10% of cases of ALL. Approximately 50 to 60% of cases of ALL express the common ALL antigen (CALLA, or CD10), a glycoprotein that is also found occasionally on normal early lymphocytes and other nonhematopoietic tissues. CALLA-positive ALL is thought to represent an early pre-B-cell differentiation state. Approximately 10% of cases of ALL have intracytoplasmic immunoglobulin and are termed pre-B-cell ALL. B-cell ALL is signified by the presence of immunoglobulin on the cell surface and accounts for less than 5% of cases of ALL. In general, the best therapeutic outcomes among B-cell ALL types are with early pre-B-cell (CALLA positive) ALL. Among the 25% of cases of ALL that express T-lineage antigens, less than half are so-called pre-T-cell types that express CD3 with either CD4 and CD8 or neither CD4 nor CD8; the majority of cases, termed T-cell ALL, express CD3 and either CD4 or CD8. The prognosis for T-cell ALL is superior to that for pre-T-cell ALL. In about 25% of patients with ALL, the leukemic cells also express myeloid antigens. Historically, the presence of such antigens defined a group of patients with a somewhat worse prognosis; however, with current, more aggressive regimens, the impact of myeloid antigen expression has disappeared.

Acute leukemias of ambiguous lineage are rare cases with no evidence of lineage differentiation (i.e., acute undifferentiated leukemia [AUL]) or those with blasts that express markers of more than one lineage (i.e., mixed phenotype acute leukemia [MPAL]). MPAL can contain either distinct blast populations of different lineages (bilineal) or a single population expressing features of both lineages (biphenotypic). In general, the prognosis of patients with AUL or MPAL is poor when treated with standard chemotherapy.

Cytogenetics and Molecular Biology

In most cases of acute leukemia, an abnormality in chromosome number or structure is found. These abnormalities are clonal, involving all the malignant cells in a given patient; they are acquired and are not found in the normal cells of the patient; and they are referred to as "nonrandom," because specific abnormalities are found in multiple cases and are associated with distinct morphologic or clinical subtypes of the disease. These abnormalities may be simply the gain or loss of whole chromosomes, but more often they include chromosomal translocations, deletions, or inversions. When patients with acute leukemia and a chromosomal abnormality receive treatment and enter into complete remission, the chromosomal abnormality disappears; when relapse occurs, the abnormality reappears. In many cases, these abnormalities have provided clues into the pathobiology of acute leukemia.

The most common cytogenetic abnormalities seen in AML can be categorized according to their underlying biology and prognostic significance. The translocation t(8;21) and the inversion inv(16) result in abnormalities of a transcription factor made up of core binding factor-α (CBF-α) and CBF-β. The t(8;21) results in the fusion of CBF-α on chromosome 21 with the *MTG8* gene on chromosome 8, whereas inv(16) results in the fusion of CBF-β on the q arm of chromosome 16 with the *MYH11* gene on the p arm. Both of these "core binding factor" AMLs are characterized by a high complete response rate and relatively favorable long-term survival. An additional translocation with a favorable prognosis, t(15;17), involves two genes, *PML* and *RAR-α* (a gene encoding the α-retinoic acid receptor), and is invariably associated with acute promyelocytic leukemia (APL), the M3 subtype of AML. Translocations involving the *MLL* gene, located at chromosome band 11q23, carry an intermediate prognosis. *MLL* is perhaps the most promiscuous oncogene partner in oncology, with more than 30 fusion partners identified. Trisomy 8 is among the most common nonrandom cytogenetic abnormalities seen in AML; it accounts for 9% of cases and carries an intermediate prognosis. Trisomies of chromosome 21, chromosome 11, and other chromosomes are sometimes seen as well. Deletions of part or all of chromosome 5 or 7 each account for 6 to 8% of cases of AML. These abnormalities are seen with greater frequency in older patients and in patients with AML secondary to myelodysplasia or prior exposure to alkylating agents, and they are associated with an unfavorable prognosis.

In addition to the abnormalities detectable by routine cytogenetic analysis, other mutations exist in the malignant cells in a substantial proportion of AML cases. Many of these involve signal transduction pathways. Activating mutations in the FLT3 receptor have been found in 20 to 40% of cases of AML. These mutations may be internal tandem repeats (15 to 30%) or point mutations (5 to 10%) and are associated with a poorer overall response to therapy. Mutations in FMS, which, like FLT3, is a receptor tyrosine kinase, are seen in 10 to 20% of cases of AML, and mutations in HRAS, KRAS2, and NRAS1, which are cellular proteins involved with signal transduction, are seen in 15 to 20% of AML cases. Mutations in the nucleophosmin gene (*NPM1*) have been identified in 20 to 30% of AML cases and appear to be associated with a favorable clinical outcome. *CEBPA*, a gene encoding a leucine zipper transcription factor involved in myeloid differentiation, is mutated in 4 to 15% of cases of AML and may be associated with a more favorable outcome. All these mutations are of interest not only for their prognostic importance but also because they may serve as targets for new therapies.

The most common cytogenetic abnormality seen in adults with ALL is the Philadelphia (Ph) chromosome, or t(9;22). This translocation results in fusion of the *BCR* gene on chromosome 22 to the *ABL* tyrosine kinase gene on chromosome 9. This results in the constitutive activation of *ABL*, but the precise mechanism by which this activity leads to leukemia is unclear. The *BCR-ABL* fusion is associated with both ALL and CML (Chapter 190), with a difference in the breakpoint of *BCR* distinguishing the two. A slightly smaller 190-kD fusion protein is usually found in ALL, whereas a larger 210-kD protein is characteristic of CML. The frequency of t(9;22) in ALL increases with age: it is found in approximately 5% of childhood cases, 25% of adults, and 50% of adults older than age 50. Before the development of specific tyrosine kinase inhibitors, ALL with t(9;22) had a poor prognosis; newer regimens combining tyrosine kinase inhibitors with chemotherapy are providing improved outcomes. The most common translocation seen in childhood ALL is t(12;21), which involves the genes *TEL* and *AML1*. Like the AML-associated t(8;21) and inv(16), t(12;21) is thought to result in abnormal DNA transcription by interfering with the normal function of CBF. Although t(12;21) is difficult to diagnose by routine cytogenetics, by molecular studies it has been shown to account for 25% of childhood ALL and 4% of adult ALL and has a favorable prognosis. Partial deletions in 9p, seen in 5 to 7% of adult ALL, are also associated with a favorable outcome. Other abnormalities sometimes seen in B-cell ALL include t(8;14) and t(8;22), which result in translocation of the *MYC* gene on chromosome 8 and immunoglobulin enhancer response genes on chromosomes 14 or 22; they are associated with a poor therapeutic outcome. T-cell ALLs are frequently associated with abnormalities of chromosome 7 or 14 at the sites of T-cell receptor enhancer genes on these chromosomes. The leukemia cells in about 20% of patients with ALL have a propensity to gain chromosomes, sometimes reaching an average of 50 to 60 chromosomes per cell. Patients with such hyperdiploid leukemias tend to respond well to chemotherapy.

CLINICAL MANIFESTATIONS

The signs and symptoms of acute leukemia are usually rapid in onset, developing over a few weeks to a few months at most; they result from decreased normal marrow function and invasion of normal organs by leukemic blasts. Anemia is present at diagnosis in most patients and causes fatigue, pallor, headache, and, in predisposed patients, angina or heart failure. Thrombocytopenia is usually present, and approximately one third of patients have clinically evident bleeding at diagnosis, usually in the form of petechiae, ecchymoses, bleeding gums, epistaxis, or hemorrhage. Most patients with acute leukemia are significantly granulocytopenic at diagnosis. As a result, approximately one third of patients with AML and slightly fewer patients with ALL have significant or life-threatening infections when initially seen, most of which are bacterial in origin.

In addition to suppressing normal marrow function, leukemic cells can infiltrate normal organs. In general, ALL tends to infiltrate normal organs more often than AML does. Enlargement of lymph nodes, liver, and spleen is common at diagnosis. Bone pain, thought to result from leukemic infiltration of the periosteum or expansion of the medullary cavity, is a common complaint, particularly in children with ALL. Leukemic cells sometimes infiltrate the skin and result in a raised, nonpruritic rash, a condition termed *leukemia cutis*. Leukemic cells may infiltrate the leptomeninges and cause leukemic meningitis, typically manifested by headache and nausea. As the disease progresses, central nervous system (CNS) palsies and seizures may develop. Although less than 5% of patients with ALL have CNS involvement at diagnosis, the CNS is a frequent site of relapse; therefore, CNS prophylaxis is an essential component of ALL therapy. Because the incidence of CNS disease is low in AML, there is no proven benefit to CNS surveillance or prophylaxis. Testicular involvement is seen in ALL, and the testicles are a frequent site of relapse. In AML, collections of leukemic blast cells, often referred to as *chloromas* or *myeloblastomas*, can occur in virtually any soft tissue and appear as rubbery, fast-growing masses.

Certain clinical manifestations are unique to specific subtypes of leukemia. Patients with APL of the M3 type commonly have subclinical or clinically evident disseminated intravascular coagulation (DIC; Chapter 178) caused by tissue thromboplastins released by the leukemic cells. Acute monocytic or myelomonocytic leukemias are the forms of AML most likely to have extramedullary involvement. M6 leukemia often has a long prodromal phase. Patients with T-cell ALL frequently have mediastinal masses.

DIAGNOSIS

Abnormalities in peripheral blood counts are usually the initial laboratory evidence of acute leukemia. Anemia is present in most patients. Most are also at least mildly thrombocytopenic, and up to one fourth have severe thrombocytopenia (platelets <20,000/μL). Although most patients are granulocytopenic at diagnosis, the total peripheral white cell count is more variable; approximately 25% of patients have very high white cell counts (>50,000/μL), approximately 50% have white cell counts between 5000 and 50,000/μL, and about 25% have low white cell counts (<5000/μL). In most cases, blasts are present in the peripheral blood, although in some patients the percentage of blasts is quite low or absent.

The diagnosis of acute leukemia is typically established by marrow aspiration and biopsy, usually from the posterior iliac crest. Marrow aspirates and biopsy specimens are usually hypercellular and contain 20 to 100% blast cells, which largely replace the normal marrow (Figs. 189-1 and 189-2). Occasionally, in addition to the blast cell infiltrate, other findings are present, such as marrow fibrosis (especially with M7 AML) or bone marrow necrosis. Marrow

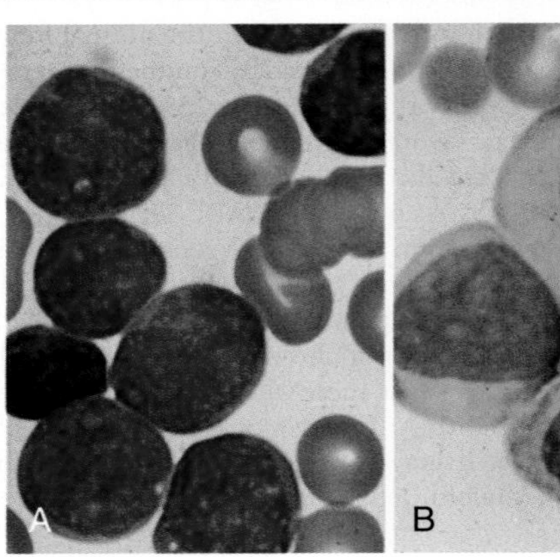

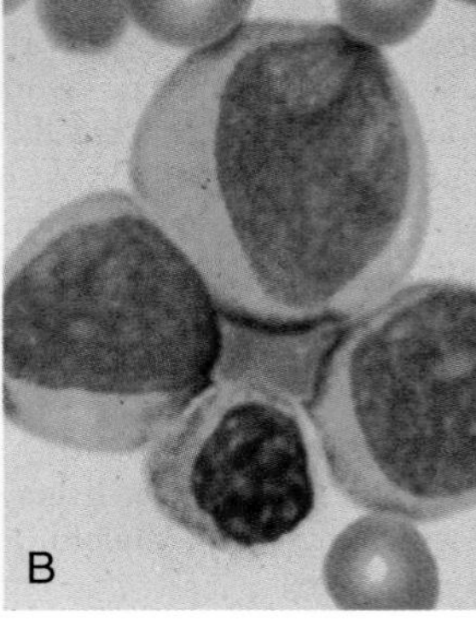

FIGURE 189-1. **Acute leukemia. A,** Acute lymphoblastic leukemia (ALL). **B,** Acute myeloid leukemia (AML). Lymphoblasts in ALL are smaller, with a higher ratio of nuclear to cytoplasmic material and less distinct nucleoli than in the myeloblasts in AML. The nucleoli in the myeloblasts are clear and "punched out."

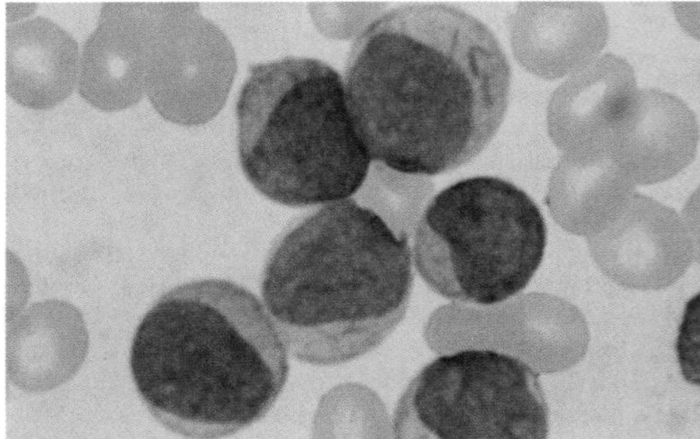

FIGURE 189-2. **Acute myeloid leukemia.** The myeloblasts in the smear show Auer rods as cytoplasmic inclusions.

samples should also be evaluated by immunophenotyping and cytogenetics. If AML is suspected, samples should be evaluated for the presence of mutations in *FLT3*, *NPM1*, and *CEBPA*. A diagnostic lumbar puncture is generally recommended in suspected cases of ALL, but not in asymptomatic cases of AML.

The prothrombin and partial thromboplastin times are sometimes elevated. In APL, reduced fibrinogen and evidence of DIC are often seen. Other laboratory abnormalities frequently present are hyperuricemia, especially in ALL, and increased serum lactate dehydrogenase. In cases of high cell turnover and cell death (e.g., L3 ALL), evidence of tumor lysis syndrome may be noted at diagnosis, including hypocalcemia, hyperkalemia, hyperphosphatemia, hyperuricemia, and renal insufficiency. This syndrome, which is more commonly seen shortly after therapy is begun, can be rapidly fatal if untreated.

Differential Diagnosis

The diagnosis of acute leukemia is usually straightforward but can occasionally be difficult. Both leukemia and aplastic anemia (Chapter 168) can manifest with peripheral pancytopenia, but the finding of a hypoplastic marrow without blasts usually distinguishes aplastic anemia. An occasional patient has hypocellular marrow and a clonal cytogenetic abnormality, which establishes the diagnosis of myelodysplasia or hypocellular leukemia. A number of processes other than leukemia can lead to the appearance of immature cells in the peripheral blood. Although other small round cell neoplasms can infiltrate the marrow and mimic leukemia, immunologic markers are effective in differentiating the two. Leukemoid reactions to infections such as tuberculosis can result in the outpouring of large numbers of young myeloid cells, but the proportion of blasts in marrow or peripheral blood almost never reaches 20% in a leukemoid reaction (Chapter 170). Infectious mononucleosis (Chapter 385) and other viral illnesses can sometimes resemble ALL, particularly if large numbers of atypical lymphocytes are present in the peripheral blood and the disease is accompanied by immune thrombocytopenia or hemolytic anemia.

TREATMENT Rx

With the development of effective programs of combination chemotherapy and advances in hematopoietic cell transplantation, many patients with acute leukemia can be cured. These therapeutic measures are complex and are best carried out at centers with appropriate support services and experience in treating leukemia. Because leukemia is a rapidly progressive disease, specific antileukemic therapy should be started as soon after diagnosis as possible, usually within 48 hours. The goal of initial chemotherapy is to induce a complete remission (CR) with restoration of normal marrow function. In general, induction chemotherapy is intensive and is accompanied by significant toxicities. Therefore, patients should be stabilized to the extent possible before specific antileukemic therapy is begun.

Preparing the Patient for Therapy

Severe bleeding usually results from thrombocytopenia, which can be reversed with platelet transfusions (Chapter 180). Once thrombocytopenic bleeding is stopped, continued prophylactic transfusions of platelets may be warranted to maintain the platelet count higher than 10,000 to 20,000/μL. Occasionally, patients also have evidence of DIC, usually associated with the diagnosis of M3 AML. If M3 AML is suspected as the cause, all-*trans*-retinoic acid (ATRA) should be started without waiting for molecular confirmation of the diagnosis; the drug can be discontinued if the diagnosis is not M3 AML. If active bleeding is due to DIC (Chapter 178), low doses of heparin (50 U/kg) given intravenously every 6 hours can be of benefit. Platelets and fresh-frozen plasma (or cryoprecipitate) should be transfused to maintain the platelet count higher than 50,000/μL and the fibrinogen level greater than 100 mg/dL until the DIC abates. Whether heparin should be given prophylactically to patients with laboratory evidence of DIC but no active bleeding is an often debated but unsettled question.

Blood cultures should be obtained in patients with fever and granulocytopenia; while awaiting culture results, infection should be assumed and broad-spectrum antibiotics begun empirically (Chapters 170 and 289). It is preferable to bring an infection under control before starting initial chemotherapy if the patient has an adequate granulocyte count. However, patients often have infection but essentially no granulocytes; in this situation, delaying chemotherapy is unlikely to be beneficial.

Patients with very high blast counts (>100,000/μL) may have symptoms attributable to the effect of masses of these immature cells on blood flow. The leukostasis may evolve into vascular injury and local hemorrhage. If this situation occurs in the CNS, the outcome can be fatal. Leukapheresis, immediate whole brain irradiation (600 cGy in one dose), and administration of hydroxyurea (3 g/m^2/day orally for 2 or 3 days) can usually prevent this complication.

Before treatment, management in all patients should be aimed at preventing the tumor lysis syndrome. Patients should be hydrated, have their urine alkalinized with acetazolamide 500 mg/day, and be given allopurinol 100 to 200 mg orally three times a day before chemotherapy is initiated. Patients with very high white cell counts may have uremia and anuria secondary to greatly increased serum uric acid levels, with subsequent intratubular crystallization, even before starting therapy. Hyperuricemia usually responds rapidly to rasburicase 0.20 mg/kg/day for up to 5 days intravenously, given over 30 minutes.

The diagnosis of leukemia usually comes as a profound psychological shock to the patient and family. Therefore, in addition to stabilizing the patient hematologically and metabolically, it is worthwhile to have at least one formal conference in which the patient and family are advised about the meaning of the diagnosis of leukemia and the consequences of therapy before treatment is initiated.

Treatment of Acute Lymphoblastic Leukemia

After the patient's condition has been stabilized, antileukemic therapy should be started as soon as possible. Treatment of newly diagnosed ALL can be divided into three phases: remission induction, postremission therapy, and CNS prophylaxis.

Remission Induction

The initial goal of treatment is to induce CR, defined as the reduction of leukemic blasts to undetectable levels and the restoration of normal marrow function. A number of different chemotherapeutic combinations can be used to induce remission; all include vincristine and prednisone, and most add L-asparaginase and daunorubicin, administered over a period of 3 to 4 weeks. With such regimens, CR is achieved in 90% of children and 80 to 90% of adults (Table 189-2). Because vincristine, prednisone, and L-asparaginase are relatively nontoxic to normal marrow precursors, the disease often enters CR after a relatively brief period of myelosuppression. Failure to achieve CR is usually due to either the leukemic cells' resistance to the drugs or progressive infection. These two complications occur with approximately equal frequency.

Postremission Chemotherapy

If no further therapy is given after induction of CR, relapse occurs in almost all cases, usually within several months. Chemotherapy after CR can be given in a variety of combinations, dosages, and schedules. The term *consolidation chemotherapy* refers to short courses of further chemotherapy given at doses

TABLE 189-2 COMMON REGIMENS FOR COMMON FORMS OF ACUTE LEUKEMIA

I. MANAGEMENT OF NEWLY DIAGNOSED ACUTE MYELOID LEUKEMIA

A. Induction—daunorubicin 60-90 mg/m^2/day for 3 days (or idarubicin 10-12 mg/m^2/day for 3 days) and cytarabine 200 mg/day for 7 days
B. Postremission
 1. Favorable risk—cytarabine 3 g/m^2 over 3 hr q12h on days 1, 3, and 5 every month for 4 mo
 2. Intermediate risk—as for favorable risk; or, if HLA-matched donor sibling exists, allogeneic hematopoietic cell transplantation
 3. Unfavorable risk—if HLA-matched donor is available, proceed to allogeneic transplantation; if not, treat as for intermediate risk

II. MANAGEMENT OF NEWLY DIAGNOSED ACUTE PROMYELOCYTIC LEUKEMIA

A. Induction—ATRA 45 mg/m^2/day until complete remission plus daunomycin 45-60 mg/m^2/day for 3 days and cytarabine 200 mg/m^2/day for 7 days
B. Consolidation #1—arsenic trioxide 0.15 mg/kg/day 5 days/wk for 5 wk; repeat course after 2-wk rest
 Consolidation #2—ATRA 45 mg/m^2/day for 7 days and daunomycin 50 mg/m^2/day for 3 days; repeat course 1 mo later
C. Maintenance—ATRA 45 mg/m^2/day for 15 days every 3 mo plus 6-MP 100 mg/m^2/day and MTX 10 mg/m^2/wk for 2 yr

III. MANAGEMENT OF NEWLY DIAGNOSED ADULT Ph-NEGATIVE ACUTE LYMPHOID LEUKEMIA

A. Induction (and courses 3, 5, 7)—cyclophosphamide 300 mg/m^2 over 3 hr q12h for 6 doses on days 1, 2, 3; doxorubicin 50 mg/m^2 on day 4; vincristine 2 mg/day on days 4 and 11; and dexamethasone 40 mg/day on days 1-4 and days 11-14
B. Consolidation (courses 2, 4, 6, 8)—MTX 200 mg/m^2 over 2 hr, followed by 800 mg/m^2 over 22 hr on day 1; high-dose cytarabine 3 g/m^2 over 2 hr q12h for 4 doses on days 2 and 3
C. Four intrathecal treatments of MTX 12 mg alternating with cytarabine 100 mg are given during the first four courses of systemic therapy

ATRA = all-*trans*-retinoic acid; HLA = human leukocyte antigen; 6-MP = 6-mercaptopurine; MTX = methotrexate; Ph = Philadelphia chromosome [t(9;22)].

similar to those used for initial induction (requiring rehospitalization). Usually, different drugs are selected for consolidation chemotherapy than were used to induce the initial remission. In the case of ALL, such drugs include high-dose methotrexate, cyclophosphamide, and cytarabine, among others. Maintenance involves the administration of low-dose chemotherapy on a daily or weekly outpatient basis for long periods. The most commonly used maintenance regimen in ALL combines daily 6-mercaptopurine and weekly or biweekly methotrexate. The optimal duration of maintenance chemotherapy is unknown, but it is usually given for 2 to 3 years. Optimal chemotherapy for ALL requires both consolidation and maintenance chemotherapy.

Central Nervous System Prophylaxis

Most chemotherapeutic agents that are given intravenously or orally do not penetrate the CNS well, and if no form of CNS prophylaxis is given, at least 35% of adults will develop CNS leukemia. With prophylaxis, relapse in the CNS as an isolated event occurs in less than 10% of patients. Systemic chemotherapy with high-dose methotrexate (e.g., 200 mg/m^2 intravenously over 2 hours, followed by 800 mg/m^2 over 22 hours) and cytarabine (e.g., 3 g/m^2 over 2 hours every 12 hours for 4 doses) can achieve therapeutic drug levels within the CNS. Alternatives are intrathecal methotrexate, intrathecal methotrexate combined with 2400 cGy radiation to the cranium, or 2400 cGy to the craniospinal axis.

Burkitt-Like ALL

Burkitt-like ALL (also called FAB L3 or mature B-cell ALL) is characterized by the presence of monoclonal surface immunoglobulin, cytogenetics showing t(8;14), and the constitutive expression of the *MYC* oncogene. Burkitt-like ALL, which accounts for 3 to 5% of adult cases of ALL, responds well to regimens that incorporate short, intensive courses of high-dose methotrexate (1.5 g/m^2 over 24 hours with leucovorin), cytarabine (3 g/m^2 over 2 hours every 12 hours for 4 doses), and cyclophosphamide (200 mg/m^2/day for 5 days); this regimen yields high rates of complete response and cures about 50% of patients. Recent results suggest that the addition of rituximab may further improve outcomes.

Philadelphia Chromosome–Positive ALL

Approximately 5% of pediatric cases and 25% of adult cases of ALL have cytogenetics showing t(9;22), the Ph chromosome. Historically, such patients had CR rates slightly lower than those seen in Ph-negative ALL and markedly reduced remission durations, averaging less than a year; few if any such patients were cured with conventional chemotherapy. Therefore, the general recommendation has been that such patients receive an allogeneic transplant from a matched sibling or a matched unrelated donor during the first remission, if possible. With this approach, approximately 50% of patients can be cured. More recently, the addition of the tyrosine kinase inhibitor imatinib mesylate to conventional chemotherapeutic regimens has increased complete response rates, equaling those seen in Ph-negative ALL, but the impact of the addition of imatinib mesylate on the duration of remission is not yet known. The general recommendation remains transplantation during the first remission for this high-risk group of patients.

Prognosis of ALL after Initial Chemotherapy

A number of factors are predictive of outcome in ALL, the most important of which are younger age, a lower white cell count at diagnosis, and favorable cytogenetics. With currently available treatment regimens, 80 to 85% of children and 35 to 40% of adults who initially achieve CR maintain that state for more than 5 years, and these patients are probably cured of their disease.

Treatment of Relapsed ALL

Most relapses occur within 2 years after diagnosis, and most occur in the marrow. Occasionally, relapse is initially found in an extramedullary site such as the CNS or testes. Extramedullary relapse is usually followed shortly by systemic (marrow) relapse and should be considered part of a systemic recurrence. With the use of chemotherapeutic regimens similar to those used for initial induction, 50 to 70% of patients achieve at least a short-lived second remission. A small percentage of patients for whom the initial remission was longer than 2 years may be cured with salvage chemotherapy. If the CNS or testes is the initial site of the relapse, specific therapy at that site is also required, along with systemic retreatment. Because the prognosis of relapsed leukemia treated with chemotherapy is so poor, marrow transplantation is usually recommended in this setting.

Hematopoietic Cell Transplantation

The use of high-dose chemoradiotherapy followed by hematopoietic cell transplantation (Chapter 181) from an HLA-identical sibling can cure 20 to 40% of patients with ALL who fail to achieve an initial remission or who have a relapse after an initial CR; it can cure 50 to 60% of patients who undergo transplantation during a first remission. Although there is still considerable debate, several recent studies have reported improved survival for adults with high-risk or standard-risk ALL who receive a stem cell transplant during a first remission rather than being treated with standard chemotherapy. 1,2 The major limitations of transplantation are graft-versus-host disease, interstitial pneumonia, and recurrence of disease. If an HLA-identical sibling is not available, transplantation from a matched unrelated donor or transplantation of cord blood from a partially matched unrelated donor can be conducted, with results that approach those seen with matched related donors.

Treatment of Acute Myeloid Leukemia

Remission Induction

Treatment with a combination of an anthracycline and cytarabine (100 to 200 mg/m^2/day for 7 days) leads to CR in 60 to 80% of patients with AML. Prospective randomized trials have demonstrated that idarubicin (10 to 12 mg/m^2/day for 3 days) or a higher dose of daunorubicin (60 to 90 mg/m^2/day for 3 days) is superior to the conventional daunorubicin dose of 45 mg/m^2/day for 3 days. 3-5 Profound myelosuppression always follows when these agents are used at doses capable of achieving CR. Failure to achieve CR is usually due to either drug resistance or fatal complications of myelosuppression.

Postremission Therapy

Intensive consolidation chemotherapy with repeated courses of daunorubicin and cytarabine at doses similar to those used for induction, high-dose cytarabine (1 to 3 g/m^2/day for 3 to 6 days), or other agents prolongs the average remission duration and improves the chances for long-term disease-free survival. The best results reported to date have generally been achieved with repeated cycles of high-dose cytarabine. Unlike the situation with ALL, low-dose maintenance therapy is of limited benefit after intensive consolidation treatment. In AML, leukemic recurrence occurs less often in the CNS (appropximately 10% of cases), most commonly in patients with the M4 or M5 variant. There is no evidence that CNS prophylaxis improves survival in AML.

Prognosis of AML after Initial Chemotherapy

Among patients in whom CR is achieved, 20 to 40% remain alive in continuous CR for more than 5 years, suggesting a probable cure. As with ALL, younger patients and those with a low white cell count at diagnosis have a more favorable outcome. Patients whose disease is characterized by certain chromosomal abnormalities, particularly t(8;21) and inv(16), or those with normal cytogenetics but mutated *CEBPA* and those with normal cytogenetics but mutated *NPM1* and wild-type *FLT3* do somewhat better, whereas those with 5q−, −7, 11q23, inv(3), or t(6;9) do worse. Patients who have a preleukemic phase before their condition evolves into acute leukemia and those whose leukemia is secondary to prior exposure to chemotherapy have a poorer prognosis. Increased expression of the multidrug resistance gene 1 *(MDR1)* is also associated with a worse outcome.

Treatment of Recurrent AML

Patients whose AML recurs after initial chemotherapy can achieve a second remission in about 50% of cases after retreatment with daunorubicin-cytarabine or high-dose cytarabine. The likelihood of achieving a second remission is predicted by the duration of the first remission: 70% in patients whose first remission persisted beyond 2 years, compared with less than 15% in those whose first remission lasted less than 6 months. Older patients may benefit from gemtuzumab ozogamicin (9 mg/m^2 on days 1 and 15), a form of antibody-targeted chemotherapy. Second remissions tend to be short-lived, however, and few patients in whom relapse occurs after first-line chemotherapy are cured by salvage chemotherapy.

Treatment of Acute Promyelocytic Leukemia

CR can be induced in at least 90% of patients with APL by using ATRA (45 mg/m^2/day until CR is achieved) in combination with an anthracycline. Patients treated with ATRA usually have their coagulation disorders corrected within several days. A unique toxicity of ATRA in the treatment of APL is the development of hyperleukocytosis accompanied by respiratory distress and pulmonary infiltrates. The syndrome responds to temporary discontinuation of ATRA and the addition of corticosteroids. By combining ATRA with anthracyclines for induction and consolidation and then using ATRA as maintenance therapy, approximately 70% of patients can be cured. Patients with higher white cell counts at diagnosis do worse. Arsenic trioxide (0.15 mg/kg/day until CR is achieved) is effective in patients with recurrent APL and appears to improve overall survival if used as part of consolidation therapy for patients in their first CR.

Hematopoietic Cell Transplantation

For patients with AML in whom an initial remission cannot be achieved or for those who have a relapse after chemotherapy, hematopoietic cell transplantation (Chapter 181) from an HLA-identical sibling offers the best chance for cure. Fifteen percent of patients with end-stage disease can be saved by this treatment. If the procedure is applied earlier, the outcome is better: approximately 30% of patients who undergo hematopoietic cell transplantation at first relapse or second remission are cured, and 50 to 60% of patients are cured if hematopoietic cell transplantation is performed during the first remission. A large number of studies have prospectively compared the outcome of allogeneic hematopoietic cell transplantation with that of chemotherapy in patients with AML in first remission. The trends in all these studies have been toward higher treatment-related mortality but improved disease-free and overall survival time with allogeneic transplantation. Meta-analyses conclude that survival is improved with allogeneic transplantation from a matched sibling in first remission when compared with continued chemotherapy.[6] This improvement is clearest in patients with high-risk or intermediate-risk cytogenetics and is not seen in those with good-risk cytogenetics. The major limitations of allogeneic hematopoietic cell transplantation are lack of a matched sibling donor, graft-versus-host disease, interstitial pneumonia, and disease recurrence. Because transplant-related toxicities increase with patient age, some centers limit hematopoietic cell transplantation to those 60 years of age or younger. However, recent studies of reduced-intensity or non-myeloablative allogeneic transplantation have shown encouraging results in patients with AML in remission at ages up to 70 years. The results of allogeneic transplantation using matched unrelated donors are not too dissimilar from those using matched siblings, although there is a higher incidence of complications. Autologous hematopoietic cell transplantation offers an alternative for patients without matched siblings to serve as donors. In randomized trials, the use of autologous bone marrow transplantation after consolidation chemotherapy significantly prolonged the duration of disease-free survival for patients with AML in first remission but did not alter overall survival.

Treatment of AML in Older Patients

The benefits of intensive consolidation chemotherapy in younger patients do not translate to patients older than 60 years, in part because older patients are less able to tolerate therapy, but also because AML in older patients is more often associated with unfavorable cytogenetics (particularly abnormalities of chromosomes 5 and 7) and more often overexpresses P-glycoprotein, resulting in the multidrug resistance phenotype. Accordingly, long-term survival rates of only 10 to 15% are seen with chemotherapy in patients older than 60 years. Otherwise healthy older patients can usually tolerate intensive chemotherapy and should be offered this treatment. However, intensive chemotherapy can cause more harm than good in older patients with poor performance status, and such patients may be candidates for supportive care only or for alternative therapies currently under study.

Management of Complications

Treatment of acute leukemia, especially AML, is accompanied by a number of complications, the two most serious and frequent being infection and bleeding. During the granulocytopenic period that follows induction and consolidation chemotherapy, the risk of bacterial infection is high. A Cochrane review examined results of antibiotic prophylaxis compared with placebo in afebrile neutropenic patients. Antibiotic prophylaxis significantly decreased infection-related deaths, with the best results seen with quinolones.[7] Invasive fungal infections are also common following chemotherapy for AML. A review of randomized trials found a significant reduction in death from fungal infection in patients given antifungal prophylaxis. Posaconazole may be more effective than fluconazole or itraconazole. Despite antibiotic and antifungal prophylaxis, many patients are febrile while neutropenic. The most commonly isolated organisms vary somewhat from medical center to medical center, but gram-positive organisms such as *Staphylococcus epidermidis* and gram-negative enteric organisms such as *Pseudomonas aeruginosa*, *Escherichia coli*, and *Klebsiella* (*Aerobacter*) are the most commonly isolated bacteria. Even if no cause for fever is found, bacterial infection should be assumed, and, in general, all patients with fever and neutropenia should begin receiving broad-spectrum antibiotics (Chapters 170 and 289). Commonly used antibiotic approaches include monotherapy with imipenem or a combination of an antipseudomonal penicillin and a third-generation cephalosporin. Once begun, antibiotics should be continued until patients recover their granulocyte counts, even if they become afebrile first. If documented bacterial infection persists despite appropriate antibiotics, the physician should consider removal of indwelling catheters.

In addition to being granulocytopenic, patients undergoing induction chemotherapy for leukemia have deficient cellular and humoral immunity, at least temporarily, and therefore are subject to infections common in other immunodeficiency states, including *Pneumocystis jirovecii* (formerly *Pneumocystis carinii*) infection and a variety of viral infections. *P. jirovecii* infection can be prevented by the prophylactic use of trimethoprim-sulfamethoxazole. Cytomegalovirus (CMV) infection can be prevented in a CMV-seronegative patient by the sole use of CMV-seronegative blood products (Chapter 384). Herpes simplex (Chapter 382) can often complicate existing mucositis and can be prevented with prophylactic acyclovir. Acyclovir is also useful for the treatment of disseminated varicella-zoster virus infection (Chapter 383).

Myeloid growth factors (granulocyte or granulocyte-macrophage colony-stimulating factor; Chapter 159), if given shortly after the completion of chemotherapy, shorten the period of severe myelosuppression by, on average, 4 days. In most studies, this accelerated recovery has resulted in fewer days with fever and less use of antibiotics, but it has not improved the complete response rate or altered survival.

The platelet count that signals a need for platelet transfusion has been the subject of debate. Traditionally, platelet transfusions from random donors were used to maintain platelet counts greater than 20,000/μL, but more recently it has been demonstrated that lowering this threshold to 10,000/μL is safe in patients with no active bleeding. In 30 to 50% of cases, patients eventually become alloimmunized and require the use of HLA-matched platelets (Chapter 180). Transfusion-induced graft-versus-host disease (Chapter 180), manifesting as a rash, low-grade fever, elevated values in liver function tests, and decreasing blood counts, can be prevented by irradiating all blood products before transfusion.

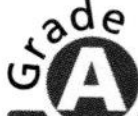

1. Goldstone AH, Richards SM, Lazarus HM, et al. In adults with standard-risk acute lymphoblastic leukemia, the greatest benefit is achieved from a matched sibling allogeneic transplantation in first complete remission, and an autologous transplantation is less effective than conventional consolidation/maintenance chemotherapy in all patients: final results of the International ALL Trial (MRC UKALL XII/ECOG E2993). *Blood*. 2008;111:1827-1833.
2. Ram R, Gafter-Gvili A, Vidal L, et al. Management of adult patients with acute lymphoblastic leukemia in first complete remission: systematic review and meta-analysis. *Cancer*. 2010;116:3447-3457.
3. Mandelli F, Vignetti M, Suciu S, et al. Daunorubicin versus mitoxantrone versus idarubicin as induction and consolidation chemotherapy for adults with acute myeloid leukemia: the EORTC and GIMEMA Groups Study AML-10. *J Clin Oncol*. 2009;27:5397-5403.
4. Fernandez HF, Sun Z, Yao X, et al. Anthracycline dose intensification in acute myeloid leukemia. *N Engl J Med*. 2009;361:1249-1259.
5. Lowenberg B, Ossenkoppele GJ, van Putten W, et al. High-dose daunorubicin in older patients with acute myeloid leukemia. *N Engl J Med*. 2009;361:1235-1248.
6. Koreth J, Schlenk R, Kopecky KJ, et al. Allogeneic stem cell transplantation for acute myeloid leukemia in first complete remission: a systematic review and meta-analysis of prospective clinical trials. *JAMA*. 2009;301:2349-2360.
7. Gafter-Gvili A, Fraser A, Paul M, et al. Meta-analysis: antibiotic prophylaxis reduces mortality in neutropenic patients. *Ann Intern Med*. 2005;142:979-995; erratum in *Ann Intern Med*. 2006;144:704.

SUGGESTED READINGS

Döhner H, Estey EH, Amadori S, et al. Diagnosis and management of acute myeloid leukemia in adults: recommendations from an international expert panel, on behalf of the European LeukemiaNet. *Blood*. 2010;115:453-474. *A comprehensive review of AML from an international group of experts.*

Marcucci G, Haferlach T, Döhner H. Molecular genetics of adult acute myeloid leukemia: prognostic and therapeutic implications. *J Clin Oncol.* 2011;29:475-486. *Review.*

Sanz MA, Lo-Coco F. Modern approaches to treating acute promyelocytic leukemia. *J Clin Oncol.* 2011;29:495-503. *Review including chemotherapy and the use of arsenic trioxide.*

Smith ML, Hills RK, Grimwade D. Independent prognostic variables in acute myeloid leukaemia. *Blood Rev.* 2011;25:39-51. *Review of clinical and molecular risk factors.*

190

THE CHRONIC LEUKEMIAS

HAGOP KANTARJIAN AND SUSAN O'BRIEN

CHRONIC MYELOGENOUS LEUKEMIA

DEFINITION

Chronic myelogenous leukemia (CML), also called chronic myeloid leukemia, chronic myelocytic leukemia, and chronic granulocytic leukemia, is a clonal myeloproliferative disorder of the primitive hematopoietic stem cell that is characterized by overproduction of cells of the myeloid series, which results in marked splenomegaly and leukocytosis. Basophilia and thrombocytosis are common. A characteristic cytogenetic abnormality, the Philadelphia (Ph) chromosome, is present in the bone marrow cells in more than 90% of cases. Most patients (85 to 90%) present in the chronic phase. Eventually, if poorly controlled, CML evolves into the accelerated and blastic phases.

EPIDEMIOLOGY

CML constitutes one fifth of all cases of leukemia in the United States. It is diagnosed in 1 or 2 persons per 100,000 per year and has a slight male preponderance. This incidence of 5000 to 6000 cases annually has not changed significantly in the past few decades. The incidence of CML increases with age; the median age at diagnosis is 50 to 55 years. Ph-positive CML is uncommon in children and adolescents. No familial association of CML has been noted; for example, the risk is not increased in monozygotic twins or in relatives of patients with CML. Because of the availability of effective therapy, the annual mortality has been reduced from 15 to 20% before 2000 to 1 to 2% at present. Thus, the prevalence of CML is predicted to increase gradually, from 15,000 to 20,000 cases before 2000 up to 250,000 cases by 2040 in the United States.

Often, no etiologic agent is incriminated in CML. Exposure to ionizing radiation (e.g., in survivors of the atomic bomb explosions in Japan in 1945, in those undergoing radiation treatment of ankylosing spondylitis or cervical cancer) increases the risk of CML; the peak incidence occurs 5 to 12 years after exposure and is dose related. No increase in the risk of CML has been demonstrated among individuals working in the nuclear industry. Radiologists working without adequate protection before 1940 were more likely to develop myeloid leukemia, but no such association has been found in recent studies. Benzene exposure increases the risk of acute myelogenous leukemia (AML) but not of CML. CML is not a frequent secondary leukemia after treatment of other cancers with radiation, alkylating agents, or both.

PATHOBIOLOGY

Molecular Pathogenesis

The Ph chromosome abnormality, present in more than 90% of patients with typical CML (Fig. 190-1), results from a balanced translocation of genetic material between the long arms of chromosomes 9 and 22: t(9;22)(q34;q11.2). The breakpoint at band q34 of chromosome 9 results in translocation of the cellular oncogene *ABL1* (previously *c-ABL*) to a region on chromosome 22 coding for the major breakpoint cluster region (BCR). *ABL1* is a homologue of *v-ABL*, the Abelson virus that causes leukemia in mice. This translocation allows juxtaposition of a 5′ portion of a BCR and 3′ position of ABL; the two genetic sequences produce a new hybrid oncogene (*BCR-ABL*), which codes for a novel BCR-ABL oncoprotein with a molecular weight of 210 kD ($p210^{BCR\text{-}ABL}$). The $p210^{BCR\text{-}ABL}$ oncoprotein results in uncontrolled kinase activity of BCR-ABL, which triggers the excessive proliferation and reduced apoptosis of CML cells, thereby giving CML cells a growth advantage over normal cells and suppressing normal hematopoiesis. Although in most cases 100% of the metaphases on cytogenetic analysis show BCR-ABL, some normal stem cells emerge on long-term bone marrow culture and after treatment with interferon-α (IFN-α), imatinib, high-dose chemotherapy, and autologous stem cell transplantation.

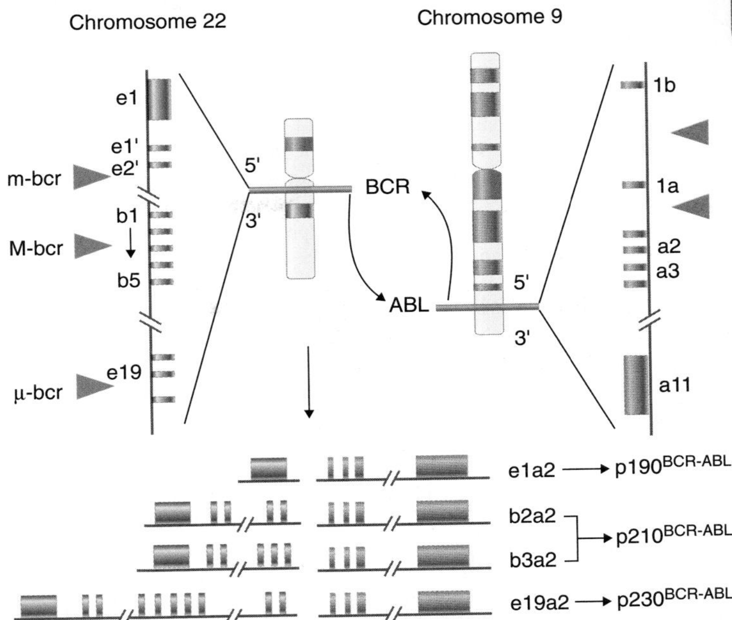

FIGURE 190-1. **The Philadelphia chromosome.** Originally described as a shortened long arm of chromosome 22, the Philadelphia chromosome (Ph) was later found to be the result of a balanced translocation of genetic material between the long arms of chromosomes 9 and 22: t(9;22)(q34;q11.2). This results in the juxtaposition of *ABL* to *BCR*, producing a hybrid *BCR-ABL* oncogene. Depending on the breakpoint on *BCR*, three oncoproteins may be produced: $p210^{BCR\text{-}ABL}$, which is associated with 98% or more of the cases of Ph-positive chronic myelogenous leukemia (CML); $p190^{BCR\text{-}ABL}$, which is associated with 60 to 80% of cases of Ph-positive acute lymphocytic leukemia (the other 20 to 40% of cases are $p210^{BCR\text{-}ABL}$); and $p230^{BCR\text{-}ABL}$, which is associated with rare cases of Ph-positive CML. The dysregulated expression of *BCR-ABL*, through phosphorylation of substrate proteins, triggers the abnormal signal transduction of multiple downstream events, some of them thought to cause excessive proliferation, reduced apoptosis, abnormal cytoskeletal regulation and cytoadhesion, and other events contributing to the growth advantage of CML cells.

The constitutive activation of BCR-ABL results in autophosphorylation and activation of multiple downstream pathways that affect gene transcription, apoptosis, cytoskeletal organization, cytoadhesions, and degradation of inhibitory proteins. The signal transduction pathways implicated involve RAS, mitogen-activated-protein (MAP) kinases, signal transducers and activators of transcription (STAT), phosphatidyl inositol 3-kinase (PI3K), MYC, and others. Many of these interactions are mediated through tyrosine phosphorylation and require binding of the BCR-ABL to adapter proteins such as GRB-2, CRK, CRK-like protein (CRKL), and SCR-homology containing proteins (SHC). Although imatinib has been extremely successful at targeting BCR-ABL, understanding of the pathophysiology of the downstream events of BCR-ABL is important for the future development of agents that may target these events.

In Ph-positive acute lymphocytic leukemia (ALL), the breakpoint in BCR is proximal, in the minor BCR, resulting in a smaller *BCR* gene apposing *ABL*; the resulting fusion gene, messenger RNA, and BCR-ABL oncoprotein ($p190^{BCR\text{-}ABL}$) are smaller. A third rare, mu (μ) BCR breakpoint distal to the major BCR produces a $p230^{BCR\text{-}ABL}$ hybrid oncoprotein, which is associated with a more indolent CML course.

What induces this molecular rearrangement is unknown. Molecular techniques that amplify detection of *BCR-ABL* have demonstrated its presence in the marrow cells of 25 to 30% of healthy volunteers and 5% of infants, but not in cord blood. Because clinical CML develops in only 1 to 2 of 100,000 individuals (i.e., 1 to 2 per 25,000 to 30,000 individuals who express *BCR-ABL* in their bone marrow), immune regulatory processes or additional molecular events presumably contribute to the development of CML.

BCR-ABL is found only in hematopoietic cells and has its origin close to the pluripotent stem cell. For example, the Ph chromosome occurs in erythroid, myeloid, monocytic, and megakaryocytic cells; less commonly in B lymphocytes; rarely in T lymphocytes; and not at all in marrow fibroblasts. The fusion *BCR-ABL* gene and the p210 protein can be found in cases of typical morphologic CML in which no cytogenetic abnormality occurs or in which changes other than the typical t(9;22) (q34;q11.2) are identified. These patients have a survival rate and a response to therapy similar to those of patients with Ph-positive CML. Patients with atypical CML (usually older and more frequently exhibiting anemia, thrombocytopenia, monocytosis, and dysplasia) who are Ph negative and *BCR-ABL* negative have a worse prognosis than those who are either Ph-positive or Ph-negative and *BCR-ABL*–positive; they more closely resemble patients with myelodysplastic syndrome (Chapter 188). Thus, three groups of patients with CML can be identified: (1) those who are positive for Ph and *BCR-ABL,* (2) those who are Ph negative but *BCR-ABL* positive, and (3) those who are negative for Ph and *BCR-ABL. PDGFB* (previously *SIS*), which codes for platelet-derived growth factor (PDGF) and is the homologue of the simian sarcoma virus, is also translocated from chromosome 22 to chromosome 9 in CML, but it is distant from the breakpoint and is not expressed.

CLINICAL MANIFESTATIONS

About 40 to 50% of patients diagnosed with CML are asymptomatic until the disease is found on routine physical examinations or blood tests. In these patients, the white blood cell (WBC) count may be relatively low at diagnosis. The degree of leukocytosis correlates with tumor burden, as defined by spleen size.

The symptoms of CML, when present, are due to anemia and splenomegaly; they include fatigue, weight loss, malaise, easy satiety, and left upper quadrant fullness or pain. Rarely, bleeding (associated with a low platelet count or platelet dysfunction) or thrombosis (associated with thrombocytosis or marked leukocytosis) occurs. Other rare presentations include gouty arthritis (from elevated uric acid levels), priapism (usually with marked leukocytosis or thrombocytosis), retinal hemorrhages, and upper gastrointestinal ulceration and bleeding (from elevated histamine levels due to basophilia). Headaches, bone pain, arthralgias, pain from splenic infarction, and fever are uncommon in the chronic phase but more frequent as CML progresses. Symptoms of leukostasis, such as dyspnea, drowsiness, loss of coordination, or confusion, which are due to leukocyte sludging in the pulmonary or cerebral vessels, are uncommon in the chronic phase despite WBC counts exceeding 50,000 cells/μL, but these symptoms appear more frequently in the accelerated or blastic phases.

Splenomegaly, the most consistent physical sign in CML, occurs in 50 to 60% of cases. Hepatomegaly is less common (10 to 20%) and usually minor (1 to 3 cm below the right costal margin). Lymphadenopathy is uncommon, as is infiltration of skin or other tissues. If present, these findings suggest Ph-negative CML or the accelerated or blastic phase of CML.

DIAGNOSIS

The diagnosis of typical CML is not difficult. Patients with untreated CML usually have leukocytosis ranging from 10,000 to 500,000/μL. The predominant cells are neutrophils, with a left shift extending to blast cells. Basophils and eosinophils are commonly increased. Monocytes may be slightly increased in some cases that overlap with chronic myelomonocytic leukemia (CMML; see later discussion). Thrombocytosis is common, whereas thrombocytopenia is rare and, if present, suggests a worse prognosis. A hemoglobin level of less than 11 g/dL is present in one third of patients. Biochemical abnormalities in CML include a low leukocyte alkaline phosphatase (LAP) score. A low LAP score also occurs in some patients with agnogenic myeloid metaplasia. Serum levels of vitamin B_{12}, lactate dehydrogenase, uric acid, and lysozyme are often increased. Some patients demonstrate a cyclic oscillation of the WBC count. The presence of unexplained myeloid leukocytosis (Fig. 190-2) with splenomegaly should lead to a bone marrow examination and cytogenetic analysis.

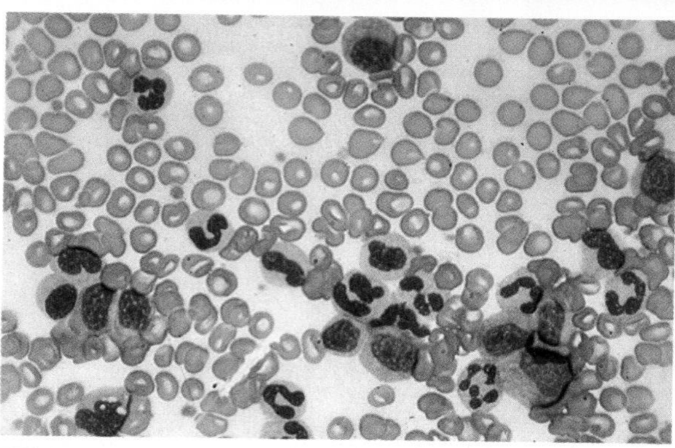

FIGURE 190-2. Chronic myelogenous leukemia, chronic phase. Peripheral smear shows leukocytosis, with representation by the entire spectrum of leukocyte differentiation, ranging from myeloblasts to mature neutrophils. (Courtesy of Andrew Schafer, MD.)

Bone Marrow

The bone marrow is hypercellular, with marked myeloid hyperplasia and, at times, evidence of increased reticulin or collagen fibrosis. The myeloid-erythroid ratio is 15 : 1 to 20 : 1. About 15% of patients have 5% or more blast cells in the peripheral blood or bone marrow at diagnosis.

Cytogenetics

The presence of the t(9;22)(q34;q11.2) abnormality establishes the diagnosis of CML. If the Ph chromosome is not found in a patient with suspected CML, molecular studies for the presence of the hybrid *BCR-ABL* gene should be performed. About 25 to 30% of patients with a typical morphologic picture of CML who are Ph negative have the *BCR-ABL* rearrangement. The Ph chromosome is usually present in 100% of metaphases, often as the sole abnormality. Between 10 and 15% of patients have additional chromosomal changes (loss of the Y chromosome, trisomy 8, an additional loss of material from 22q, or double Ph). Some patients have complex chromosomal changes involving chromosome 9 or chromosome 22 (Ph variants, three-way translocations).

Differential Diagnosis

CML must be differentiated from leukemoid reactions (Chapter 170), which usually produce WBC counts lower than 50,000/μL, toxic granulocytic vacuolation, Döhle's bodies in the granulocytes, absence of basophilia, and normal or increased LAP levels; the clinical history and physical examination generally suggest the origin of the leukemoid reaction. Corticosteroids can rarely cause extreme neutrophilia with a left shift, but this abnormality is self-limited and of short duration.

CML may be more difficult to differentiate from other myeloproliferative or myelodysplastic syndromes (Chapters 169 and 188). Patients with agnogenic myeloid metaplasia with or without myelofibrosis frequently have splenomegaly, neutrophilia, and thrombocytosis. Polycythemia vera with associated iron deficiency, which causes normal hemoglobin and hematocrit values, can manifest with leukocytosis and thrombocytosis. Such patients usually have a normal or increased LAP score, a WBC count less than 25,000/μL, and no Ph chromosome.

The greatest diagnostic difficulty lies with patients who have splenomegaly and leukocytosis but do not have the Ph chromosome. In some, the *BCR-ABL* hybrid gene can be demonstrated despite a normal or atypical cytogenetic pattern. Patients who are Ph negative and *BCR-ABL* negative are considered to have Ph-negative CML or CMML (see later discussion). Rarely, patients have myeloid hyperplasia, which involves almost exclusively the neutrophil, eosinophil, or basophil cell lineage. These patients are described as having chronic neutrophilic, eosinophilic, or basophilic leukemia and do not have evidence of the Ph chromosome or the *BCR-ABL* gene. Isolated megakaryocytic hyperplasia can be seen in essential thrombocythemia (Chapter 169), with marked thrombocytosis and splenomegaly. Some patients who present with clinical characteristics of essential thrombocythemia (with marked thrombocytosis but without leukocytosis) have CML; cytogenetic and molecular studies showing the Ph chromosome, the *BCR-ABL* rearrangement, or both lead to the appropriate diagnosis and treatment.

Clinical Course

Evolution to Accelerated and Blastic Phases

More than 90% of patients present with CML in the benign or chronic phase, which becomes asymptomatic once the disease is controlled. Death rarely occurs during the chronic phase of CML.

When poorly controlled, CML evolves into an accelerated phase, usually defined by the presence of 15% or more blasts, 30% or more blasts plus promyelocytes, 20% or more basophils, thrombocytopenia less than 100,000/μL unrelated to therapy, or cytogenetic clonal evolution. The accelerated phase is also characterized by worsening anemia; increasing splenomegaly or hepatomegaly; infiltration of nodes, skin, bones, or other tissues; and fever, malaise, and weight loss. In the accelerated phase, bone marrow studies may

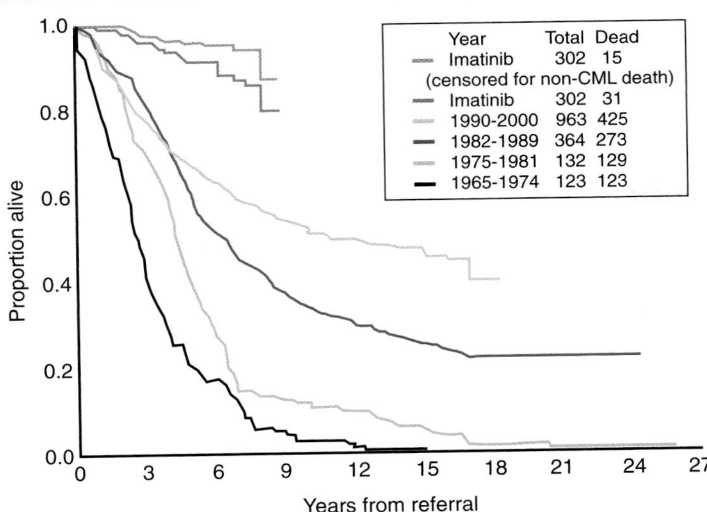

FIGURE 190-3. **Survival of patients with Ph-positive chronic myelogenous leukemia in chronic phase.** (M. D. Anderson data; 1884 patients from 1965 to 2008.)

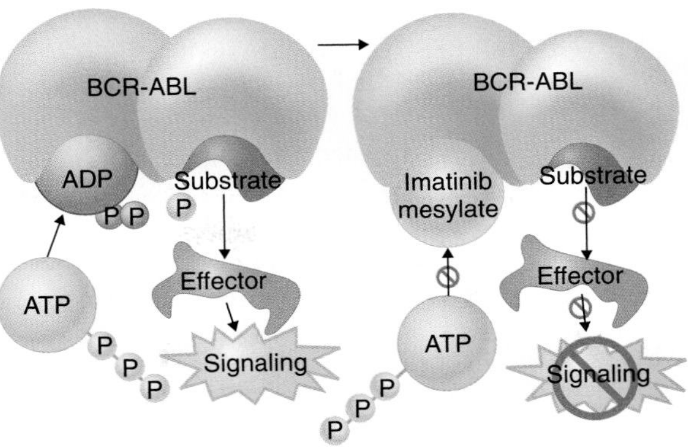

FIGURE 190-4. **Mechanism of action of imatinib.** By occupying the ATP binding pocket of the ABL kinase domain, imatinib prevents substrate phosphorylation and downstream activation of signals, thus inhibiting the leukemogenic effects of BCR-ABL on cells in chronic myelogenous leukemia. ADP = adenosine diphosphate; ATP = adenosine triphosphate; P = phosphate group.

show dysplastic changes, increased percentages of blasts and basophils, myelofibrosis, and chromosomal abnormalities in addition to the Ph chromosome (clonal evolution). About 5 to 10% of patients present in the accelerated phase.

Before the era of imatinib therapy, the risk of developing accelerated or blastic phase CML was 10% per year in the first 2 years after diagnosis and 15 to 20% per year thereafter, unless therapies such as IFN-α or allogeneic stem cell transplantation were used. With imatinib, the annual incidence of progression of CML from the chronic to the accelerated or blastic phase has been 2% in the first 10 years of observation (Fig. 190-3). Before imatinib therapy, the median survival of accelerated phase CML was 18 months or less, but survival has now increased to 4 years or more.

The blastic phase of CML is diagnosed when 30% or more blast cells are present in the bone marrow and/or peripheral blood or when extramedullary blastic disease is present. Most patients develop features of the accelerated phase before progressing to the blastic phase, but 20% of patients evolve quickly into a blastic phase without warning. Most patients in the accelerated or blastic phase have additional chromosomal abnormalities (clonal evolution) such as duplication of the Ph chromosome, trisomy of chromosome 8, or development of an isochromosome 17. The extramedullary blastic phase of CML can occur in the spleen, lymph nodes, skin, meninges (especially in the lymphoid blastic phase), bones, and other sites; extramedullary transformation is usually followed shortly by evidence of marrow involvement. Blastic phase CML is associated with a very poor median survival time of 5 months. About 25% of patients develop a lymphoid blastic phase; their response rate to anti-ALL–like chemotherapy and imatinib is about 60%, and their median survival time is about 1 year.

Ph-negative and *BCR-ABL*–negative CML often appear to overlap clinically with CMML in terms of behavior, progress, and response to therapy and seem to resemble the myelodysplastic syndromes (Chapter 188) more than Ph-positive CML. A male preponderance and older age are noted; splenomegaly is common (60 to 70%). The WBC count is usually in the range of 25,000 to 100,000/μL. Anemia, thrombocytopenia, and monocytosis are more common than in Ph-positive CML, whereas eosinophilia and basophilia are less common. The median survival time is 18 to 24 months; patients die of infection, bleeding, or transformation to acute leukemia.

TREATMENT Rx

Choice of Therapy in Chronic Myelogenous Leukemia

Treatment decisions in CML are based on the phase of CML, the patient's age, and the availability of a stem cell donor. For patients presenting in chronic phase CML (>90% of newly diagnosed patients), imatinib mesylate, a selective BCR-ABL tyrosine kinase inhibitor, is first-line therapy in the vast majority of patients. Allogeneic stem cell transplantation is considered effective second-line therapy in chronic phase CML after imatinib failure. Alternative second-line therapies are more potent second-generation tyrosine kinase inhibitors, including dasatinib (dual SRC-ABL kinase inhibitor) and nilotinib (selective and more potent BCR-ABL kinase inhibitor). Patients with CML in the accelerated or blastic phase should consider allogeneic stem cell transplantation as immediate, definitive therapy; in this situation, the use of tyrosine kinase inhibitors as an interim measure before stem cell transplantation may reduce the CML burden significantly and improve the results of allogeneic stem cell transplantation.

Imatinib Mesylate

Since its discovery in 1999, imatinib mesylate has become standard therapy for CML. Imatinib is a 2-phenylaminopyrimidine derivative that binds to the canonical adenosine triphosphate (ATP) lining the groove between the N and C lobes of the ABL kinase domain, thus blocking the phosphorylation of tyrosine residues on substrate protein. Blocking of ATP binding inactivates the ABL kinase, because it cannot transfer phosphate to its substrate. By inhibiting phosphorylation, imatinib prevents the activation of signal transduction pathways that induce the leukemic transformation processes that cause CML (Fig. 190-4). Imatinib inhibits several tyrosine kinases, including $p210^{BCR-ABL}$, $p190^{BCR-ABL}$, v-ABL, c-ABL, C-kit, and PDGF receptor.

In a randomized trial of 1106 patients with newly diagnosed CML, imatinib 400 mg/day orally provided significantly higher rates of major cytogenetic response (87% vs. 35%) and complete cytogenetic response (76% vs. 14%), as well as lower rates of progression (8% vs. 26%) and transformation (3% vs. 9%) after 12 months of therapy, compared with the prior standard nontransplantation therapy (a combination of IFN-α and cytosine arabinoside).[1,2] The longer-term follow-up results continue to demonstrate outstanding outcomes with imatinib therapy (Table 190-1; see Fig. 190-3): with a median follow-up of 7 years, the complete cytogenetic response rate (occurring at least once on therapy) is 87%, the estimated 5-year durable complete cytogenetic response rate is 65 to 70%, the annual rate of progression to accelerated or blastic phase is only 1 to 2%, and the estimated 7-year survival rate is above 86% (94% if non-CML deaths are censored).[3] Imatinib plus peginterferon alfa-2a is somewhat superior to imatinib alone for providing a persisting molecular response at 12 months,[4] but its precise role in routine treatment remains to be determined.

Most CML experts and physicians now consider imatinib frontline therapy for all patients with newly diagnosed Ph-positive CML in the chronic phase, regardless of age and donor availability. The only possible exceptions are the rare patients who present with $p190^{BCR-ABL}$ CML, who may have a worse prognosis on imatinib.

Imatinib has a 5% or lower rate of serious side effects, which include nausea, vomiting, diarrhea, skin rashes, muscle cramps, bone aches, periorbital or leg edema, weight gain, and, rarely, hepatic, renal, or cardiopulmonary dysfunction; most of these are manageable with dose reductions or treatment interruptions. Drug-related myelosuppression occurs in 10 to 20% of patients with newly diagnosed CML and is manageable with brief treatment interruptions, dose modifications, or both or with the administration of growth factors (erythropoietin for anemia, granulocyte colony-stimulating factor for neutropenia). Hypophosphatemia associated with altered bone metabolism can occur, and the serum phosphate level should be monitored. Chromosomal abnormalities may appear in the Ph-negative diploid cells in 5 to 10% of responding patients, probably due to unmasking of a fragile stem cell prone to the development of CML or to chromosomal instability; such changes disappear spontaneously in 70% of cases and rarely evolve into a myelodysplastic syndrome or acute myeloid leukemia, probably as part of the natural course of CML.

Allogeneic Stem Cell Transplantation

Allogeneic stem cell transplantation, a potentially curative therapy in selected patients with CML, is most effective during the chronic phase, when

TABLE 190-1 EARLY RESULTS OF IMATINIB MESYLATE THERAPY IN CHRONIC MYELOGENOUS LEUKEMIA

	% Cytogenetic Response		
PHASE	COMPLETE (Ph 0%)	MAJOR (Ph < 35%)	ESTIMATED SURVIVAL
Blastic	7	10-20	10-15% at 4 yr
Accelerated	20-40	40-60	40-50% at 4 yr
Chronic, after failure of IFN-α	55-63	60-80	80-85% at 4 yr
Chronic, newly diagnosed	65-85	80-90	86-94% at 7-8 yr

IFN-α = interferon-α; Ph = Philadelphia chromosome.

it is associated with a 20-year survival rate of 40 to 50%. Transplant-related mortality ranges from 5 to 50%, depending on the patient's age, whether the donor is related or unrelated, the degree of matching, and other, less important factors such as positivity for cytomegalovirus, preparative and post-transplantation regimens, and institutional expertise. Disease-free survival rates with related allogeneic stem cell transplantation are 40 to 80% in chronic phase, 15 to 40% in accelerated phase, and 5 to 20% in blastic phase. In chronic phase CML, patients younger than 30 to 40 years have disease-free survival rates of 60 to 80%, compared with only 30 to 40% for patients older than 50 years. A major limitation of allogeneic stem cell transplantation is the availability of related donors. Human leukocyte antigen (HLA)–compatible unrelated donors can be found for 50% of patients; the median time from initiation of the donor search to transplantation is 3 to 6 months.

Nonmyeloablative preparative regimens have expanded the indications for allogeneic stem cell transplantation to older patients and have reduced transplant-related mortality and complications (Chapter 181). Early results show acceptable degrees of engraftment, less mortality and organ damage, more persistent residual disease, and similar degrees of graft-versus-host disease. Patients whose CML recurs after allogeneic stem cell transplantation may respond to donor lymphocyte infusions, imatinib or second-generation tyrosine kinase inhibitors (dasatinib, nilotinib), IFN-α, or a second allogeneic transplant.

The advantage of allogeneic stem cell transplantation is its proven track record, with an estimated cure rate of 40% at 20 years. However, it is associated with a 1-year mortality rate of 5 to 40% and with morbidities such as cataracts, infertility, second cancers (5 to 10%), immune-mediated complications, and chronic graft-versus-host disease. Delaying allogeneic stem cell transplantation beyond 1 to 3 years after diagnosis may be associated with worse results and with occasional sudden blastic transformation, which may not be salvageable. The outcome of allogeneic stem cell transplantation may be even better after imatinib exposure.

Treatment of CML after Imatinib Failure

Imatinib failure is strictly defined as (1) lack of any cytogenetic response after 6 months of imatinib therapy, (2) no major cytogenetic response (Ph ≤35%) after 12 months, (3) no complete cytogenetic response (Ph 0%) beyond the first year of therapy (generally at 18 months or later), or (4) hematologic or cytogenetic relapse or CML transformation at any time. Patients with chronic phase CML on imatinib should be considered for allogeneic stem cell transplantation only if imatinib therapy fails. Alternatively, a more potent tyrosine kinase inhibitor may be tried if imatinib resistance is noted. These include nilotinib (AMN107), which is 20 to 50 times more potent than imatinib, and dasatinib (BMS-354825), which is 300 times more potent than imatinib. Both agents are now approved for the treatment of CML after imatinib failure (dasatinib for all CML phases; nilotinib for chronic and accelerated phases). Dasatinib and nilotinib have been associated with complete hematologic response rates of 70 to 80% and complete cytogenetic response rates of 40 to 50% in chronic phase CML, with estimated 2-year survival rates of 90% (compared with annual mortalities of 10 to 20% after imatinib failure before their availability). They have also shown encouraging results in accelerated or blastic phase CML after imatinib failure. 5,6 An important question is whether these second-generation tyrosine kinase inhibitors can be used as more definitive therapy, thus delaying the consideration of allogeneic stem cell transplantation until the failure of drug therapy. This depends on the patient's age (patients 70 years or older may decide to forgo the risks of allogeneic stem cell transplantation, even though it might be curative), the availability of an ideal donor (e.g., related vs. unrelated; matched vs. mismatched), the initial response to tyrosine kinase inhibitors (major cytogenetic response by 12 months predicts long-term favorable disease control), and the presence and specific type of mutations (e.g., *T315I* mutations are resistant to all currently approved tyrosine kinase inhibitors; mutations with a high IC_{50} in vitro [drug concentration that suppresses 50% of clonal growth] to a particular agent are associated with poor long-term disease control).

Treatment of Accelerated and Blastic Phase Chronic Myelogenous Leukemia

Patients with accelerated or blastic phase CML may receive initial imatinib therapy to reduce the CML burden, but they should be considered for early allogeneic stem cell transplantation. Response rates to combination chemotherapy are 20% in nonlymphoid blastic phase CML and 60% in lymphoid blastic phase CML. Median survival times are 3 to 6 months and 9 to 12 months, respectively. The addition of imatinib to chemotherapy has improved the response rates and prolonged the median survival time in blastic phase CML from 3 to 5 months to 6 to 12 months.

At present, allogeneic stem cell transplantation is the only curative therapy for accelerated and blastic phase CML: overall cure rates are in the range of 15 to 40% and 5 to 20%, respectively, and patients with cytogenetic clonal evolution as the only accelerated phase criterion have a long-term event-free survival rate of about 60%. Otherwise, imatinib provides hematologic responses in 80% of patients and an estimated 4-year survival rate of 40 to 55% in accelerated phase CML, but only a 40% response rate and a median survival of 7 months in blastic phase CML. Patients in the accelerated or blastic phase should be encouraged to participate in investigational strategies to improve their prognosis. Combinations of imatinib with chemotherapy may improve results in CML transformation, as may the new tyrosine kinase inhibitors.

Special Therapeutic Considerations

Patients with severe leukocytosis and manifestations of leukostasis may benefit from initial leukapheresis. Severe thrombocytosis uncontrolled with anti-CML measures may respond to anagrelide, thiotepa, IFN-α, 6-mercaptopurine, 6-thioguanine, and platelet pheresis. CML during pregnancy may be controlled with pheresis in the first trimester and then with hydroxyurea until delivery. Use of IFN-α during pregnancy has been reported anecdotally to be safe. There is little experience with the use of imatinib during pregnancy. Splenectomy can be useful as a palliative measure in patients with massive painful splenomegaly, hypersplenism, or thrombocytopenia.

Follow-up

Monitoring Response to Therapy in CML

With improved therapy, the incidences of complete cytogenetic response and minimal residual disease have increased. This has required the development of new techniques to measure these responses more accurately (rather than relying on only 20 metaphases by cytogenetic analysis), less tedious and less painful procedures (peripheral blood rather than marrow studies), and techniques that can measure minimal (molecular) disease below the level of detection by routine cytogenetic studies. Fluorescence in situ hybridization (FISH) studies with improved probes can measure 200 interphase cells using peripheral blood, and they have false-positive rates of less than 2 to 3%. Quantitative polymerase chain reaction (QPCR) studies usually measure the ratio of the abnormal message, BCR-ABL, to a normal message, such as ABL. A BCR-ABL/ABL ratio of 0.1% (International Standard) or less, about a 3-log reduction of disease, has been associated with a very low risk of CML relapse on imatinib therapy. This is now referred to as a *major molecular response*. A negative QPCR analysis (i.e., undetectable BCR-ABL levels, usually $<10^{-5}$ to 10^{-6}) may be dependent on the technique used and could be referred to as a *complete molecular response*.

In monitoring the response to imatinib-based therapies, patients require a bone marrow analysis before therapy (to determine the percentages of blasts and basophils and clonal evolution), at 6 and 12 months (to assess cytogenetic response and confirm complete cytogenetic response), and once every 1 to 3 years in those with stable, durable complete cytogenetic responses (to look for chromosomal abnormalities in both Ph-positive and Ph-negative cells). Monitoring in patients with confirmed, durable complete cytogenetic responses can be continued with either FISH or QPCR studies every 6 months (or more often, such as every 3 months, if there are concerns about significant and consistent increases in QPCR levels). The frequency of monitoring depends on the treatment plan; monitoring is more frequent in younger patients, less frequent in very old patients.

"Resistance" to imatinib therapy can be defined as persistent 100% Ph positivity after 6 months of therapy, Ph positivity of more than 35% after 12 months of therapy, or cytogenetic or hematologic relapse. A positive QPCR in a patient with a complete cytogenetic response does not, at present, indicate imatinib resistance or the need to change therapy. The rate of resistance to imatinib in chronic phase CML is less than 4% per year; for those who achieve a complete cytogenetic response, the rate of resistance beyond year 3 of imatinib therapy is 1% or less, suggesting the durable stability of a complete cytogenetic response on imatinib and the predictability of the CML course once such a response is obtained. Several mechanisms of resistance have been identified; the most common are mutations in the BCR-ABL kinase domain. More than 50 different mutations have been reported and can involve any of the important domains in the BCR-ABL structure, including the P-loop (the area where ATP binds), the activation loop, and the catalytic domain, as well as the amino acids where imatinib makes contact with BCR-ABL. The different mutations have considerable variability with respect to resistance to imatinib. Some mutations are overcome by slightly higher concentrations of imatinib than required to inhibit the wild-type form; others are completely insensitive to imatinib. Mutational analysis is useful in patients with imatinib resistance to identify those with the *T315I* mutation, who do not respond to imatinib or the second-generation tyrosine kinase inhibitors (dasatinib, nilotinib, bosutinib) and should be considered for immediate allogeneic stem cell transplantation or therapy with *T315I*-selective inhibitors. In addition, knowledge of the sensitivity of the different mutations, as determined by the IC_{50} for particular agents, can help select the tyrosine kinase inhibitor. Mutational studies may also be helpful in patients who develop cytogenetic or hematologic resistance or relapse on imatinib therapy.

FUTURE DIRECTIONS

Two second-generation tyrosine kinase inhibitors, dasatinib and nilotinib, are now approved for the treatment of CML after imatinib failure. Other tyrosine kinase inhibitors (bosutinib) are under investigation, with promising results. Three randomized studies of the more potent second-generation tyrosine kinase inhibitors nilotinib, dasatinib, and bosutinib against the standard of care, imatinib, are ongoing in patients with newly diagnosed CML. Maturing data suggest that they may significantly improve the complete cytogenetic and major molecular response rates, as well as reduce the transformation rate to the accelerated and blastic phases.[5,6] Equally important are the "third-generation" tyrosine kinase inhibitors such as AP24534, which are also active against CML with the *T315I* mutation. Other active anti-CML agents under development include omacetaxine (previously known as homoharringtonine), decitabine (a hypomethylating agent), and pegylated formulations of interferon. Immunotherapeutic strategies, including vaccines, may improve the eradication of minimal residual disease, potentially obviating the need for indefinite therapy with imatinib. Further understanding of the pathophysiology and events downstream of BCR-ABL may help in the development of new strategies to target these events. Such strategies may include inhibitors of pathways involving Raf, protein farnesylation, mTOR, JAK/STAT, proteasome, MEK/MAPK, PI3K/AKT, or others.

PROGNOSIS

Imatinib therapy has revolutionized the treatment of CML. In cases of newly diagnosed CML, imatinib therapy is associated with an estimated 7-year survival rate of 86% (94% if non-CML deaths are censored). If this favorable trend continues with longer follow-up, the median survival time in CML may exceed 25 years. During the first 7 years of follow-up, the annual mortality has been about 2%. Many well-established poor prognostic factors in CML (e.g., older age, splenomegaly, presence of marrow fibrosis, deletion of derivative 9q) have lost much of their importance since the advent of imatinib therapy. With allogeneic stem cell transplantation, cures can be expected in 40 to 80% of patients with chronic phase CML, 15 to 40% of those with accelerated phase CML, and 5 to 20% of those with blastic phase CML.

CHRONIC MYELOMONOCYTIC LEUKEMIA

DEFINITION AND EPIDEMIOLOGY

Although superficially resembling CML in its clinical and morphologic presentation, CMML should be considered a separate entity because of its particular clinical, therapeutic, and prognostic aspects. CMML is a hybrid entity manifesting as a proliferation of the myeloid monocytic series and dysplasia of the erythroid-megakaryocytic series. Patients with CMML are older (median age, 65 to 70 years) than most patients with CML.

PATHOBIOLOGY

The cytogenetic findings in patients with CMML are normal or involve an additional chromosome 8 or findings other than the Ph chromosome. Patients with CMML have *RAS* mutations in 40 to 60% of cases.

CLINICAL MANIFESTATIONS AND DIAGNOSIS

Patients often present with symptoms related to anemia and thrombocytopenia (fatigue, bleeding). Other typical features include splenomegaly, leukocytosis, and monocytosis. Organ infiltration (lymph nodes, skin, liver) is less common. Basophilia and thrombocytosis are not presenting features.

TREATMENT AND PROGNOSIS (Rx)

Allogeneic stem cell transplantation (Chapter 181), which is the only curative modality, should be considered frontline therapy in candidate patients. Other therapies include hydroxyurea to control leukocytosis, erythropoietin to improve anemia, azacitidine or decitabine (both approved by the U.S. Food and Drug Administration [FDA] for the treatment of CMML), topotecan and cytarabine or other intensive anti-AML (Chapter 189) regimens for CMML transformation, splenectomy for symptomatic splenomegaly and/or hypersplenism, and investigational agents.

Poor prognostic factors include the presence of anemia (hemoglobin <10 g/dL), thrombocytopenia, and more than 5% blasts. Median survival time is 12 to 18 months.

HAIRY CELL LEUKEMIA

DEFINITION AND EPIDEMIOLOGY

Hairy cell leukemia (HCL) is an uncommon and indolent B-cell leukemia (1 to 2% of all leukemias). The median age at diagnosis is 50 years, and there is a 4 : 1 male preponderance.

PATHOBIOLOGY

The cell of origin of HCL is the B lymphocyte, as documented by the demonstration of heavy and light chain immunoglobulin gene rearrangements. Hairy cells express CD19, CD20, CD11C, CD103, FMC7, and CD22, but not CD21, CD5, CD10, or CD23. The cells demonstrate a κ or γ light chain phenotype excess. The cells also express CD25 (TAC), the low-affinity interleukin-2 (IL-2) receptor, and CD103, a unique hairy cell antigen. High levels of soluble IL-2 receptor (>5 times normal) are present in the sera of almost all patients with HCL, with extremely high levels noted in many cases. A number of different cytogenetic abnormalities have been reported in HCL, but none appears to be consistently present, and all have been described in other hematologic malignancies. Immune dysfunction is wide ranging in HCL. Monocytopenia is universal; B and T lymphocytes are decreased in number; the CD4/CD8 (T helper/T suppressor) ratio is often inverted; and skin test reactivity to recall antigens is impaired, as is antibody-dependent cellular cytotoxicity. Humoral immunity is relatively preserved, with normal immunoglobulin levels. Marrow failure in HCL may be due in part to inhibitory factors (e.g., tumor necrosis factor) produced by the leukemic infiltrate; the pancytopenia is often more marked than would be anticipated from the degree of leukemic infiltration.

CLINICAL MANIFESTATIONS

The majority of patients present with pancytopenia and splenomegaly. Patients may also have fatigue, fever, weight loss, and infection secondary to granulocytopenia or monocytopenia. Leukocytosis is uncommon, and lymphadenopathy is rare. Anemia is present in up to 85% of patients, whereas leukopenia and thrombocytopenia are present in 60 to 75%. The cytopenias are caused by a combination of bone marrow failure due to leukemic infiltration and hypersplenism. Patients may experience repeated infections and, rarely, a systemic vasculitis resembling polyarteritis nodosa. Although bacterial infections occur, as would be expected with neutropenia, patients with HCL have a predilection to develop tuberculosis, atypical mycobacterial infections, and fungal infections, perhaps related to the severe monocytopenia that is characteristic of this disorder.

DIAGNOSIS

In conjunction with the clinical features, careful examination of the peripheral blood smear may demonstrate the occasional typical cells with cytoplasmic projections, giving rise to the name *hairy cell leukemia* (Fig. 190-5). The hairy cells are 10 to 15 mm in diameter, with pale blue cytoplasm, a nucleus with a loose chromatin structure, and one or two indistinct nucleoli. Bone marrow aspiration is often inadequate owing to increased deposition of reticulin, collagen, and fibrin; bone marrow biopsy is usually necessary. Bone marrow involvement is interstitial or patchy, and the infiltrate is characterized by widely spaced nuclei due to the abundant cytoplasm, giving rise to the commonly described "fried egg" appearance.

Hairy cells exhibit a strong acid phosphatase (isoenzyme 5) cytochemical reaction in 95% of cases, a reaction that is resistant to the inhibitory effect of tartaric acid (TRAP). Other lymphoproliferative diseases are rarely TRAP positive. Electron microscopy clearly demonstrates the microvillar

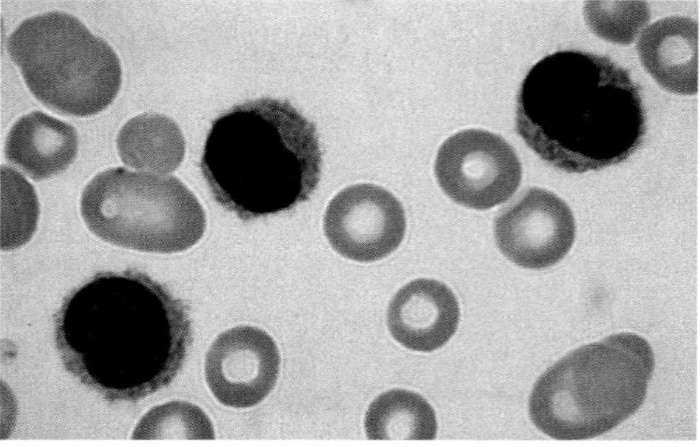

FIGURE 190-5. Hairy cell leukemia. Peripheral smear shows hairy cells with blue-gray cytoplasm; fine, hair-like projections (resembling ruffles); and oval or slightly indented nuclei with loose chromatin and indistinct nucleoli. (Courtesy of Andrew Schafer, MD.)

projections. Often, ribosomal-lamellar complexes, which are characteristic but not diagnostic of HCL, can be identified. The peroxidase stain is negative, and lysozyme activity is absent in hairy cells, thereby differentiating these cells from monocytes.

Differential Diagnosis

The differential diagnosis must distinguish HCL from lymphoma (Chapter 191) or chronic lymphocytic leukemia (CLL), which can manifest with predominant splenomegaly and minimal lymphadenopathy. Some patients with a myelodysplastic syndrome (Chapter 188) or a myeloproliferative syndrome (Chapter 169) have splenomegaly and pancytopenia with only a few atypical cells. Patients with other diseases, such as systemic lupus erythematosus (Chapter 274) and other autoimmune diseases, B-cell and T-cell prolymphocytic leukemias (see later), infiltrative splenomegaly (Chapter 171), or tuberculosis (Chapter 332), may have splenomegaly and cytopenia, but these diagnoses can usually be made by history, physical examination, and appropriate blood and bone marrow tests. Splenomegaly, cytopenia, and nonaspirable marrow in a middle-aged man should create a high index of suspicion for HCL. Splenectomy and lymph node biopsy are sometimes necessary to establish the diagnosis in difficult cases. Cases of HCL variant manifest with higher WBC counts, are TRAP negative, have prominent nucleoli, and are only occasionally positive for antibodies against CD25. HCL variant does not respond as well to the agents that are usually effective in the management of typical HCL.

TREATMENT Rx

A small proportion (<5%) of patients with HCL do not require therapy. These patients have mild cytopenias, are not transfusion dependent, have no history of infections, and have a low level of marrow infiltration by hairy cells.

2-Chlorodeoxyadenosine (cladribine), an adenosine analogue that is resistant to deamination by adenosine deaminase, produces complete remission in more than 80% of HCL patients after a single course of 0.1 mg/kg/day for 7 days given by continuous intravenous infusion, and it is now the recommended first-line therapy. Remissions are durable, and patients who relapse can often attain a second remission after retreatment with cladribine. The drug is well tolerated, with a low infection rate. Despite long-lasting suppression of $CD4^+$ lymphocyte counts, there does not appear to be an increase in late opportunistic infections or second malignancies.

Deoxycoformycin (pentostatin; 4 mg/m^2 weekly or every 2 weeks for up to 6 months), an adenosine deaminase inhibitor, produces complete remission in 70 to 80% of patients. The response to treatment is rapid, and the drug is active in patients previously treated with IFN. Toxicity includes nausea and vomiting, infection, renal and hepatic dysfunction, conjunctivitis, and photosensitivity, albeit mild in most cases.

Human leukocyte interferon (HuIFN), or r-IFN-α, rapidly improves granulocyte, platelet, and hemoglobin levels (1 to 3 months); reduces spleen size; and decreases marrow infiltration. Peripheral blood cell counts return to normal in 80% of cases, but complete remission is uncommon. In addition, when treatment is discontinued, relapse occurs within 1 to 2 years.

Rituximab, the monoclonal antibody targeting CD20, can also produce responses; 8 weekly infusions appear to be more effective than four.

Two immunotoxins can produce responses in refractory patients. LMB2 is composed of the Fc portion of the anti-TAC antibody linked to a *Pseudomonas* exotoxin. BL22 also contains *Pseudomonas* exotoxin linked to an antibody targeting CD22. Splenectomy is recommended mainly for patients with splenic infarcts or massive splenomegaly.

PROGNOSIS

More than 85 to 90% of patients treated with cladribine or pentostatin are expected to be alive at 10 years.

CHRONIC LYMPHOCYTIC LEUKEMIA

DEFINITION

CLL is a neoplasm characterized by the accumulation of monoclonal lymphocytes of B-cell origin. The cells accumulate in the bone marrow, lymph nodes, liver, spleen, and occasionally other organs.

EPIDEMIOLOGY

CLL is the most common leukemia (one third of all cases) in the Western world and is twice as common as CML. The disease occurs rarely in those younger than 30 years; most patients with CLL are older than 60 years. CLL increases in incidence exponentially with time; by age 80, the incidence rate is 20 cases per 100,000 persons per year. The male-female ratio is approximately 2 : 1. The incidence of CLL among Asians in Japan and China is only 10% of that in the United States and other Western countries. Intermediate incidence rates are seen in persons of Hispanic origin.

The cause of CLL is unknown. Ionizing radiation and viruses have not been associated with CLL, although hepatitis C infection has recently been associated with splenic lymphoma with villous lymphocytes (another indolent B-cell disorder). Familial clustering in CLL is more common than in other leukemias; first-degree relatives of patients have a two- to four-fold higher risk and develop CLL at a younger age compared with the general population (anticipation). Farmers have a higher incidence of CLL than do those in other occupations, raising the possibility of an etiologic role for herbicides or pesticides. Agent Orange, the defoliating agent used in Vietnam, has been associated with the development of CLL.

PATHOBIOLOGY

Leukemia cells in CLL are homogeneous and have the appearance of normal mature lymphocytes. However, clonality can be documented by the presence of immunoglobulin gene rearrangements and the restriction to either κ or γ light chains on the cell surface. The cells express low-intensity monoclonal surface immunoglobulin (SmIg; usually immunoglobulin [Ig] M ± IgD) and the pan-B-cell antigens CD19, CD20, CD23, and CD24 in almost all cases, as well as CD21 (which includes the receptor for the Epstein-Barr virus and the C3d component of complement) in more than 75% of cases. Almost all cells exhibit Ia antigen and receptors for the Fc fragment of IgG and spontaneously form rosettes with mouse erythrocytes. In addition to B-cell antigens, CLL cells express CD5 (Leu 1, T1, and T101), a pan-T-cell antigen. Other T-cell antigens are absent. CD25 (TAC, IL-2 receptor) antigen is positive in about 25% of cases. T cells are increased in number at diagnosis, and the CD4/CD8 ratio is often inverted, owing to a relatively greater increase in $CD8^+$ cells. The CD4/CD8 ratio declines as the disease progresses and after therapy. The T cells have a blunted response to T-cell mitogens and decreased delayed hypersensitivity reactions to recall antigens. However, these T-cell functions may be impaired by factors produced by the CLL cells, because purified T cells have a normal response to T-cell mitogens.

GENETICS

Standard cytogenetic analysis identifies abnormalities in 40 to 50% of cases of CLL, but CLL cells have low mitotic activity. By FISH, the likelihood of detecting abnormalities increases to 80%. A 13q deletion is the most common abnormality; other abnormalities include 11q deletion (15 to 20%), trisomy 12 (15 to 20%), and 17p deletion (5 to 10%). The 17p deletion increases in frequency as the disease progresses, recurs after therapy, and is associated with a very poor prognosis. The 11q deletion also is associated with a poorer prognosis, whereas the 13q deletion, if present as the sole abnormality, is associated with a favorable prognosis.

CLINICAL MANIFESTATIONS

Most patients with CLL are asymptomatic, and the disease is diagnosed when absolute lymphocytosis is noted in the peripheral blood (see Fig. 190-6) during evaluation for other illnesses or when the patient undergoes a routine physical examination. Symptoms such as fatigue, lethargy, loss of appetite, weight loss, and reduced exercise tolerance are nonspecific. Many patients have enlarged lymph nodes. B symptoms (fever, night sweats, weight loss) are rarely present initially, and their presence in later stages of the disease suggests transformation to large cell lymphoma. The most common infections are sinopulmonary. As the disease progresses, the frequency of neutropenia, T-cell deficiency, and hypogammaglobulinemia increases, resulting in infections with gram-negative bacteria, fungi, and viruses such as herpes zoster and herpes simplex.

The major physical findings relate to infiltration of the reticuloendothelial system. Lymphadenopathy with discrete, rubbery, mobile lymph nodes is present in two thirds of patients at diagnosis. Later, as the lymph nodes enlarge, they can become matted. Enlargement of the liver or spleen is less common at diagnosis (approximately 10% and 40% of cases, respectively) but occurs more frequently with progression. Organ failure resulting from infiltration with CLL is uncommon. Infiltration of the central nervous system in CLL is rare, and central nervous system symptoms are more likely to be caused by opportunistic infections such as cryptococcosis or listeriosis.

DIAGNOSIS

CLL is characterized by absolute lymphocyte counts that typically range from 5000 to 600,000/μL in the peripheral blood. Even with markedly elevated WBC counts, hyperviscosity symptoms rarely occur, probably because of the small size and pliability of the cells. Anemia (hemoglobin <11 g/dL) is present in 15 to 20% of patients at diagnosis, and thrombocytopenia (platelet count <100,000/μL) in 10%. However, bone marrow replacement and hypersplenism, which are seen with progressive disease, increase the frequency of anemia and thrombocytopenia. The anemia is usually normochromic and normocytic, and the reticulocyte count is normal unless the patient has autoimmune hemolytic anemia (Chapter 163), which usually results from the development of a warm-reacting IgG antibody. The diagnosis of autoimmune hemolytic anemia, which occurs in 10% of cases, is confirmed by a positive direct Coombs test (80 to 90% of cases), reticulocytosis, a low serum haptoglobulin concentration, and an elevated unconjugated serum bilirubin level. In such patients, reactive erythroid hyperplasia as a response to the hemolysis may be masked in the bone marrow by the marked lymphocytic infiltration. Cold agglutinin hemolysis occurs rarely in CLL. Autoimmune thrombocytopenia (immune thrombocytopenic purpura; Chapter 175) can be diagnosed in 10 to 15% of cases. The antibodies causing red cell and platelet destruction are not produced by the CLL cells, and the mechanisms for the associated autoimmune diseases are not known. Pure red cell aplasia (Chapter 168) is an additional, underappreciated cause of anemia in CLL.

The lymphocytes in CLL are indistinguishable on light or electron microscopy from normal small B lymphocytes (Fig. 190-6). On bone marrow aspiration, the proportion of lymphocytes is greater than 30% and may be up to 100%. Four patterns of lymphocyte infiltration on bone marrow biopsy occur: nodular (15%), interstitial (30%), mixed nodular and interstitial (30%), and diffuse (35%). Most early-stage cases have one of the first three patterns; diffuse histology is common in advanced-stage disease and becomes more prominent as the disease evolves. A diffuse histologic pattern confers a poor prognosis regardless of the stage of disease.

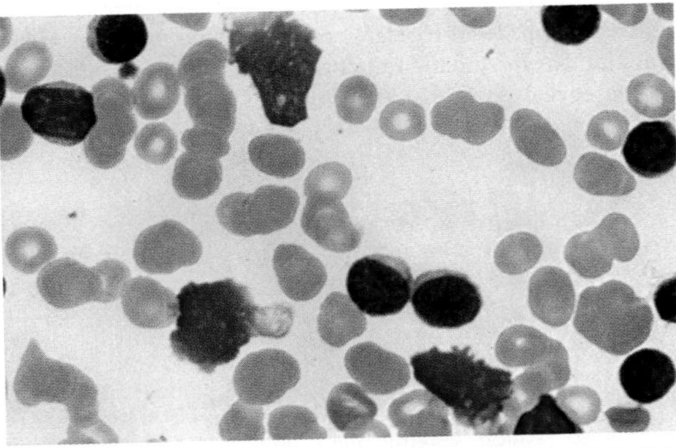

FIGURE 190-6. Chronic lymphocytic leukemia. Peripheral smear shows that the predominant leukocytes are "normal," mature-appearing lymphocytes, with occasional "smudge" cells. (Courtesy of Andrew Schafer, MD.)

Differential Diagnosis

There are many diseases that can cause lymphocytosis, including pertussis (Chapter 321), cytomegalovirus (Chapter 384), Epstein-Barr virus mononucleosis (Chapter 385), tuberculosis (Chapter 332), toxoplasmosis (Chapter 357), chronic inflammatory disorders, and autoimmune syndromes. These diseases are seldom confused with B-cell CLL, largely because the lymphocytosis in these conditions is usually less than 15,000/μL and is not sustained. If doubt persists, immunophenotypic or molecular studies can distinguish the monoclonal lymphocytosis in CLL from the T-cell or polyclonal B-cell proliferation in the other disorders.

In individuals 62 to 80 years old, monoclonal CLL-phenotype B cells are found in about 5% of individuals with normal blood counts. In patients with greater than 4000 lymphocytes/mL, about 45% have CLL, about 40% have reactive lymphocytosis, and about 15% have monoclonal CLL-phenotype B cells that confer a 1.1% per year risk of developing CLL. In patients ultimately diagnosed with CLL, B-cell clones were previously present in peripheral blood in 98% of patients, sometimes many years before diagnosis.

Other Chronic Lymphocytic Leukemias

The more difficult differential diagnosis is distinguishing CLL from other lymphoproliferative disorders such as prolymphocytic leukemia (PLL), splenic lymphoma with villous lymphocytes, HCL, the leukemic phase of mantle cell lymphoma, and Waldenström's macroglobulinemia. Although certain clinical features are more common in some of these disorders (e.g., marked splenomegaly with minimal or no lymphadenopathy in PLL, splenic lymphoma, and HCL vs. extensive lymphadenopathy with or without splenomegaly in CLL), none of these clinical features is specific. The differential diagnosis therefore depends largely on histopathologic and, more specifically, immunophenotypic features (Table 190-2).

Prolymphocytic Leukemia

PLL is an uncommon disease (incidence <5% that of CLL), and its characteristics of massive splenomegaly, minimal lymphadenopathy, and markedly elevated WBC count (often >100,000/μL), with 10 to 90% of the cells being prolymphocytes, distinguish this disease from typical B-cell CLL. Prolymphocytes are larger cells that have a distinct nucleolus and express FMC-7. The male-female ratio is 4 : 1, and the median age at diagnosis is 70 years. Survival is shorter than in CLL (median 3 years), and response to therapies usually applied in CLL is poor. A serum paraprotein, typically IgG or IgA, is present in one third of cases. The immunoglobulin on the surface of the cells is occasionally IgG or IgA, not IgM ± IgD, as in CLL. Several karyotypic abnormalities have been reported in PLL, including t(11;14)(q13;q32). Deletions of 11q3, 23, and 17p are more common in B-cell PLL than in CLL. Abnormalities in the *TP53* oncogene are found in 75% of cases of B-cell PLL. One fifth of PLL cases express a T-cell phenotype.

Small Lymphocytic Lymphoma

Small lymphocytic lymphoma (SLL) shares histopathologic and immunophenotypic features with CLL, differing only in the lack of lymphocytosis in the peripheral blood. The bone marrow in SLL may or may not have more than 30% lymphocytes. LFA-1 adhesion protein is much more commonly expressed on SLL cells than on CLL cells. Other lymphomas, such as follicular and mantle cell lymphomas (Chapter 191), occasionally manifest a leukemic phase on initial presentation. Follicular lymphoma cells are often cleaved on light microscopy, have bright staining for SmIg, and are positive for FMC-7 and CD10. Lymph node biopsy should be performed to identify these cases with greater precision. The presence of lymphoma cells in the blood in follicular lymphoma is more common with advanced disease. Follicular lymphoma can usually be identified by the presence of the translocation t(14;18) and consequent *BCL2* rearrangement, both of which are rare in CLL. The WBC count in Waldenström's macroglobulinemia (Chapter 193) is usually much lower than in CLL (<10,000/μL), and many patients are leukopenic. The cells have a plasmacytoid appearance, CD38 and PCA-1 positivity, and more SmIg and cytoplasmic Ig. A serum monoclonal IgM peak is present in almost all cases of Waldenström's macroglobulinemia but is uncommon in CLL.

TABLE 190-2 DIFFERENTIAL DIAGNOSIS OF INDOLENT LYMPHOPROLIFERATIVE DISORDERS

DISEASE	LYMPHADENOPATHY (%)	SPLENOMEGALY (%)	CELL OF ORIGIN (B/T)	Positive Markers* SmIg	CD5	CD19, CD20 (%)	OTHER
Chronic lymphocytic leukemia (CLL)	75	50	B (20:1)	Weak	>90%	≥90	Mouse red blood cell receptors
Prolymphocytic leukemia (PLL)	33	95	B (4:1)	Bright	T-cell PLL	75	FMC-7
Hairy cell leukemia	<10	80	B (T rare)	Bright	—	>90	CD25, CD11C, CD103
Lymphoma (leukemic phase)	90	90	B (T rare)	Bright	Some	>90	CD10
Splenic lymphoma with villous lymphocytes	10	80	B	Bright	20%	>90	FMC-7, CD22
Waldenström's macroglobulinemia	33	33	All B	Weak	Some	Many	CD38, PCA-1
Large granular lymphocytosis	10	10	All T	Absent	—	—	CD2, CD3, CD8

*CD2 = pan-T cell; CD3 = pan–mature T cell; CD5 = pan-T cell, B-cell CLL; CD8 = T cell (suppressor cytotoxic); CD10 = early B cell; CD11C = hairy cell, activated T cell, NK cell; CD19 = early pan-B cell; CD20 = pan-B cell; CD25 = low-affinity interleukin-2 receptor; CD38 = activated B cell, thymocyte, plasma cell; FMC-7 = PLL, hairy cell leukemia; PCA-1 = plasma cell; SmIg = monoclonal surface immunoglobulin.

TABLE 190-3 RAI AND BINET STAGING SYSTEMS IN CHRONIC LYMPHOCYTIC LEUKEMIA

STAGE	LYMPHOCYTOSIS	LYMPHADENOPATHY	HEPATOMEGALY OR SPLENOMEGALY	HEMOGLOBIN (G/DL)	PLATELETS ×10³/ML
RAI STAGING SYSTEM					
0	+	−	−	≥11	≥100
I	+	+	−	≥11	≥100
II	+	±	+	≥11	≥100
III	+	±	±	<11	≥100
IV	+	±	±	Any	<100
BINET STAGING SYSTEM					
A	+	±	± (<3 lymphatic groups* positive)	≥10	≥100
B	+	±	± (≥3 lymphatic groups* positive)	≥10	≥100
C	+	±	±	<10†	<100†

*The three lymphatic groups are (1) cervical, axillary, and inguinal nodes; (2) liver; and (3) spleen. Each group is considered one group whether unilateral or bilateral.
†The criterion is hemoglobin <10 g/dL and/or platelets <100 × 10³/mL.

T-Cell Leukemias

The predominant clinical manifestation of Sézary's syndrome (a $CD4^+$ T-cell malignant disorder related to mycosis fungoides) is chronic exfoliative erythroderma with a low number of circulating monoclonal T cells. The clinical and laboratory differentiation from CLL is not difficult. Other T-cell malignant disorders with peripheral blood involvement are adult T-cell leukemia-lymphoma and large granular lymphocytosis, also referred to as large granular lymphoproliferative disorder, T-cell lymphocytosis with neutropenia, or T-gamma lymphocytosis syndrome. Adult T-cell leukemia-lymphoma is associated with a retrovirus (human T-lymphotropic virus I) and is common in Japan and the Caribbean. It frequently manifests with lytic bone lesions and hypercalcemia. In T-cell large granular lymphoproliferative disorders, the absolute lymphocyte count is usually low (<5000/μL), with a $CD2^+$, $CD3^+$, $CD8^+$, and $CD16^+$ (T-suppressor) phenotype (T-gamma cells). These patients often have splenomegaly, neutropenia, and rheumatoid arthritis–like symptoms. A subset, called natural killer (NK) cell large granular lymphocytosis, has an NK cell phenotype ($CD16^-$) and no molecular evidence of T-cell receptor rearrangement. The lymphocytes have abundant cytoplasm with azurophilic granules. Most patients have a benign course, although repeated infections can occur.

Staging and Prognostic Factors

The natural history of CLL is heterogeneous, with survival times ranging from 2 to 20 years after diagnosis. Either of two validated clinical staging systems can be used. The Rai staging system (1975) defines five stages and is most frequently used in the United States, whereas the Binet system (1981) defines three stages and is most frequently used in Europe (Table 190-3). Patients with anemia and thrombocytopenia (Rai III and IV, Binet C) have the worst prognosis; patients with lymphocytosis alone (Rai 0, some Binet A patients) have an excellent prognosis. A group of patients with a lymphocyte count less than 30,000/μL, hemoglobin greater than 13 g/dL, platelet count greater than 100,000/μL, fewer than three involved node areas, and lymphocyte doubling time greater than 12 months has been described as having "smoldering" CLL, with survival equal to that of an age- and sex-matched control population. Patients tend to progress through stages, with many patients developing more sites of involvement over time and eventually experiencing marrow failure; however, anemia and thrombocytopenia can develop abruptly, even without antibody-mediated destruction or markedly increased tumor burden.

Other adverse factors include a diffuse pattern of lymphocytic infiltration observed on bone marrow biopsy; molecular abnormalities, including deletion of 11q or 17p; advanced age; male sex; elevated serum levels of thymidine kinase, β_2-microglobulin, and soluble CD23; rapid lymphocyte doubling time; an increased proportion of large or atypical lymphocytes in the peripheral blood; and lack of somatic mutation of the *VH* gene within the B-CLL cell or the presence of the ZAP-70 protein or CD38 on the CLL cell surface.

TREATMENT

The major therapeutic questions are when to treat and which therapeutic regimen to use. Patients with CLL are usually older, and the prognosis of the disease is variable (with some early-stage cases being stable for 10 to 20 years). Treatment of early-stage CLL (Rai 0, Binet A) is delayed until the disease progresses. In randomized trials, early treatment with alkylating agents did not prolong survival and was associated with a heightened risk of developing second malignant tumors. Two large clinical trials are currently investigating, in a randomized fashion, whether early treatment benefits asymptomatic patients with high-risk disease. Treatment of Rai stages III and IV (Binet stage C) is recommended at the time of diagnosis because of the morbidities associated with cytopenias and the poor survival time of these patients. Treatment of intermediate-stage disease (Rai I and II, Binet B) is recommended if symptomatic disease (fever, sweats, weight loss, severe fatigue) or massive lymphadenopathy, with or without hepatosplenomegaly, is present.

Medical Therapy

Chemotherapy

Fludarabine monophosphate (25 mg/m^2/day for 5 days every 4 weeks), an adenosine analogue, is approved by the FDA for treatment of relapsed CLL, with overall response rates of 50 to 60%. The dose-limiting toxicity is myelosuppression. When used in conjunction with steroids, the treatment may be complicated by infections with organisms usually associated with immunodeficiency syndromes involving T lymphocytes (e.g., those caused by *Pneumocystis jirovecii* or herpesviruses). In a large randomized trial of initial therapy for CLL, fludarabine resulted in higher overall and complete remission rates, longer duration of remission, and improved response rates on crossover, but there was no survival advantage compared with chlorambucil, the prior standard therapy.[7] However, 10-year follow-up has now shown a survival benefit in the fludarabine arm. Cladribine is used primarily in Europe, where it appears to have efficacy similar to fludarabine; pentostatin has not been as widely studied in CLL as in HCL.

Before the advent of fludarabine, combination regimens were based on alkylating agents and borrowed from regimens used to treat lymphoma. The COP regimen (cyclophosphamide 100 to 300 mg/m^2/day orally on days 1 through 5, vincristine [Oncovin] 2 mg intravenously on day 1, and prednisone 100 mg orally on days 1 through 5) does not have any advantage over chlorambucil alone, usually given at a dose of 0.1 to 0.2 mg/kg/day for 3 to 6 weeks until the desired effect is obtained or until thrombocytopenia or neutropenia develops; the dose is then adjusted for maintenance and is continued for 6 to 12 months. Regimens using cyclophosphamide, doxorubicin, and prednisone with vincristine (CHOP) or without vincristine (CAP) have produced response rates of 50 to 70% in those with Binet stage C disease.

The combination of fludarabine and cyclophosphamide (FC) was a logical attempt to improve on the efficacy of fludarabine alone by combining it with the other most active agent in this disease, an alkylating agent. The FC combination has been compared to fludarabine alone in three randomized trials.[8-10] All these trials consistently showed a higher complete response rate, higher overall response rate, and longer progression-free survival with the FC combination.

After therapy, many patients remain stable for months to years before progressive disease indicates the need for further treatment. The goal of treatment is to achieve complete response (Table 190-4).

Bendamustine is a potent alkylating agent that has some structural similarity to nucleoside analogues, but preclinical data suggest that it does not function as a nucleoside analogue. Bendamustine was recently approved by the FDA for the treatment of CLL based on a randomized trial comparing this agent to chlorambucil as initial therapy for patients with CLL.[11] Complete and overall response rates were higher with bendamustine, and progression-free survival was longer. The main side effect is myelosuppression.

Monoclonal Antibodies

Rituximab, a monoclonal antibody targeting the CD20 antigen, is associated with response rates of about 50% when given at the standard dose (375 mg/m^2/week for 4 weeks) as initial therapy for CLL and significantly lower rates when used in the salvage setting, but complete responses are rare in either setting. The major benefit of this antibody appears to be its use in combination with chemotherapy. Fludarabine combined with rituximab appears to produce better responses than those seen historically with fludarabine alone. In addition, progression-free and overall survival are better than that seen in the historical cohort. A three-drug regimen of fludarabine, cyclophosphamide, and rituximab (FCR) appears to produce the best and most durable complete remission rates when used as first-line therapy. A recent randomized trial compared the activity of FC to that of FCR. More than 800 patients were accrued, and the patient characteristics were balanced between the two arms. FCR produced slightly more neutropenia than FC, but there was no difference in grade 3 or 4 infections. The complete response rate and the overall response rate were significantly higher with FCR, and progression-free and overall survival were significantly longer than with chemotherapy alone.[12] Alemtuzumab (Campath-1H; 30 mg intravenously three times a week for 4 to 12 weeks), a monoclonal antibody that binds to the CD52 antigen, was originally approved for the treatment of fludarabine-refractory CLL. One third of such patients can achieve remission. Recently, alemtuzumab was compared with chlorambucil as initial therapy for symptomatic patients with CLL. Alemtuzumab produced higher complete and overall response rates and longer progression-free survival.[13]

Ofatumumab is a humanized monoclonal antibody that binds to CD20, but to a different epitope than rituximab. This drug was recently approved by the FDA for the treatment of fludarabine- and alemtuzumab-refractory CLL. In the pivotal trial, the drug was given intravenously for 8 weeks and then monthly for 4 months. The overall response rate in this highly refractory population was 58%; the median progression-free survival was 6 months, with a median overall survival of 13.7 months. As with other monoclonal antibodies, the predominant side effects are infusion reactions, which tend to be more common with the initial doses.

TABLE 190-4 DEFINITION OF REMISSION IN CHRONIC LYMPHOCYTIC LEUKEMIA: THE INTERNATIONAL WORKSHOP IN CHRONIC LYMPHOCYTIC LEUKEMIA–NATIONAL CANCER INSTITUTE WORKING GROUP CRITERIA

CRITERION	COMPLETE REMISSION	PARTIAL REMISSION
Physical examination		
Nodes	None ≥1.5 cm	≥50% decrease
Liver/spleen	Not palpable	≥50% decrease
Symptoms	None	N/A
Peripheral blood		
Neutrophils	≥1500/mL	≥1500/mL or ≥50% increase from baseline
Platelets	>100,000/μL	100,000/μL or ≥50% increase from baseline
Hemoglobin	>11 g/dL	>11 g/dL or >50% increase from baseline
Lymphocytes	≤4000/mL	>50% decrease
Bone marrow	<30%, no B-lymphoid nodules	50% reduction in infiltrate or B-lymphoid nodules

Stem Cell Transplantation

Autologous stem cell transplantation has no proven benefit in terms of survival or long-term disease control in CLL. Data on allogeneic stem cell transplantation are limited to young patients with refractory disease, in whom a long-term control rate of 40 to 55% has been reported. Nonmyeloablative stem cell transplantation, which works mainly by its graft-versus-leukemia effect, has been used in older patients with CLL, with some success.

Radiation Therapy

In CLL, radiation therapy is used palliatively to shrink unsightly or painfully enlarged nodal masses or an enlarged spleen.

Autoimmune and Infectious Manifestations

Autoimmune hemolytic anemia and immune-mediated thrombocytopenia do not correlate closely with the activity of CLL. Prednisone (60 to 100 mg/day) is indicated as treatment for autoimmune hemolytic anemia (Chapter 163) and for some cases of immune-mediated thrombocytopenia (Chapter 175) in CLL. If there is no response in 3 to 4 weeks, the treatment has failed, and the dose should be tapered over 1 to 2 weeks. If a response is obtained, the dose is reduced by 25% each week over 4 weeks. Patients for whom corticosteroids fail often respond to low-dose oral cyclosporin 100 mg three times a day. Other therapeutic options include splenectomy, intravenous immunoglobulin, rituximab, and alemtuzumab.

Intravenous immunoglobulin (400 mg/kg every 3 to 4 weeks) significantly decreases the incidence of infections in patients with recurrent infections and hypogammaglobulinemia. However, the cost of this therapy is substantial.

PROGNOSIS

Approximately one third of patients who present with early-stage CLL never require therapy and have the same survival of age-matched controls. Frequent characteristics of such patients include WBC less than 30,000/μL, hemoglobin greater than 13 g/dL, nondiffuse pattern on bone marrow biopsy, and slow lymphocyte doubling time.

A poor response to therapy is an adverse factor in all phases of the disease. As CLL progresses, the development of a prolymphocytic transformation (10% of cases) or transformation to large cell lymphoma portends a median survival time of less than 6 months. Other factors that may suggest transformation are the development of B symptoms, a markedly elevated lactate dehydrogenase level, or fludeoxyglucose-avid disease on positron emission tomography. A high incidence of second malignant tumors (10 to 20% of patients) either precedes or follows the diagnosis of CLL; the roles of therapy versus impaired immune surveillance as causative factors are unclear. Skin cancer, including melanoma, as well as colorectal and lung cancers are common. CLL tends to develop in older people; in indolent cases, death occurs from other intercurrent illnesses seen in this age group. Almost all patients younger than 60 years and those with progressive disease die as a result of CLL, primarily from infections. Gram-positive organisms usually cause nonfatal infections early in CLL, but most deaths due to infection are associated with gram-negative bacterial or fungal infections. Infection with other opportunistic organisms, such as *Mycobacterium tuberculosis,* herpesvirus, and *P. jiroveci,* may also be fatal.

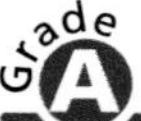

1. O'Brien SG, Guilhot F, Larson RA, et al. Imatinib compared with interferon and low-dose cytarabine for newly diagnosed chronic-phase chronic myeloid leukemia. *N Engl J Med.* 2003;348:994-1004.
2. Hughes T, Kaeda J, Branford S, et al. Frequency of major molecular responses to imatinib or interferon alfa plus cytarabine in newly diagnosed chronic myeloid leukemia. *N Engl J Med.* 2003;349:1423-1432.
3. Druker B, Guilhot F, O'Brien S, et al. Five-year follow-up of patients receiving imatinib for chronic myeloid leukemia. *N Engl J Med.* 2006;355:2408-2417.
4. Preudhomme C, Guilhot J, Nicolini FE, et al. Imatinib plus peginterferon alfa-2a in chronic myeloid leukemia. *N Engl J Med.* 2010;363:2511-2521.
5. Saglio G, Kim DW, Issaragrisil S, et al. Nilotinib versus imatinib for newly diagnosed chronic myeloid leukemia. *N Engl J Med.* 2010;362:2251-2259.
6. Kantarjian H, Shah N, Hochhaus N, et al. Dasatinib versus imatinib in newly diagnosed chronic-phase chronic myeloid leukemia. *N Engl J Med.* 2010;362:2260-2270.
7. Rai KR, Peterson BL, Appelbaum FR, et al. Fludarabine compared with chlorambucil as primary therapy for chronic lymphocytic leukemia. *N Engl J Med.* 2000;343:1750-1757.
8. Eichhorst BF, Busch R, Hopfinger G, et al. Fludarabine plus cyclophosphamide versus fludarabine alone in first-line therapy of younger patients with chronic lymphocytic leukemia. *Blood.* 2006;107:885-891.
9. Flinn IW, Neuberg DS, Grever MR, et al. Phase III trial of fludarabine plus cyclophosphamide compared with fludarabine for patients with previously untreated chronic lymphocytic leukemia: US Intergroup Trial E2997. *J Clin Oncol.* 2007;25:793-798.
10. Catovsky D, Richards S, Matutes E, et al. Assessment of fludarabine plus cyclophosphamide for patients with chronic lymphocytic leukaemia (the LRF CLL4 Trial): a randomized controlled trial. *Lancet.* 2007;370:230-239.
11. Knauf WU, Lissichkov T, Aldaoud A, et al. Phase III randomized study of bendamustine compared with chlorambucil in previously untreated patients with chronic lymphocytic leukemia. *J Clin Oncol.* 2009;27:4378-4384.
12. Hallek M, Fischer K, Fingerle-Rowson G, et al. Addition of rituximab to fludarabine and cyclophosphamide in patients with chronic lymphocytic leukaemia: a randomised, open-label, phase 3 trial. *Lancet.* 2010;376:1164-1174.
13. Hillmen P, Skotnicki AB, Robak T, et al. Alemtuzumab compared with chlorambucil as first-line therapy for chronic lymphocytic leukemia. *J Clin Oncol.* 2007;25:5616-5623.

SUGGESTED READINGS

Bixby D, Talpaz M. Seeking the causes and solutions to imatinib-resistance in chronic myeloid leukemia. *Leukemia.* 2011;25:7-22. *Review.*

Cramer P, Hallek M. Prognostic factors in chronic lymphocytic leukemia—what do we need to know? *Natl Rev Clin Oncol.* 2011;8:38-47. *Review.*

Hallek M. Therapy of chronic lymphocytic leukaemia. *Best Pract Res Clin Haematol.* 2010;23:85-96. *Review including fludarabine, bendamustine, alemtuzumab, and rituximab.*

Keating GM. Rituximab: a review of its use in chronic lymphocytic leukaemia, low-grade or follicular lymphoma and diffuse large B-cell lymphoma. *Drugs.* 2010;70:1445-1476. *Review.*

Okimoto RA, Van Etten RA. Navigating the road toward optimal initial therapy for chronic myeloid leukemia. *Curr Opin Hematol.* 2011;18:89-97. *Review including imatinib, nilotinib, and dasatinib.*

191 NON-HODGKIN'S LYMPHOMAS

PHILIP J. BIERMAN AND JAMES O. ARMITAGE

DEFINITION

Lymphomas are solid tumors of the immune system. Rapidly increasing knowledge of the biology of the immune system has led to a corresponding increase in the understanding of these malignancies. In addition to better systems of classification and clinical evaluation, this new knowledge has led to the development of new therapies. Beneficial treatment is available for essentially every patient with non-Hodgkin's lymphoma, and many patients can be cured.

EPIDEMIOLOGY

In the United States, about 66,000 new cases of non-Hodgkin's lymphoma are diagnosed annually, and about 20,000 people are estimated to die each year of this disease. Non-Hodgkin's lymphomas account for about 4% of new cancers in the United States and result in about 4% of cancer deaths. The U.S. lifetime risk of developing non-Hodgkin's lymphoma is 2.18% (1 in 46) for men and 1.80% (1 in 56) for women. In 2002 the U.S. age-adjusted incidence rate for non-Hodgkin's lymphoma was about 23.2 per 100,000 for men and 16.3 per 100,000 for women. The incidence rate increases dramatically with age and is higher in whites than in other ethnic groups.

Geographic differences in the incidence of non-Hodgkin's lymphomas vary as much as five-fold. The highest rates are seen in the United States, Europe, and Australia, whereas lower rates are seen in Asia. Even more striking are geographic differences in the incidence of certain types of non-Hodgkin's lymphoma, such as Burkitt's lymphoma, follicular lymphoma, extranodal natural killer (NK)/T-cell nasal lymphoma, and adult T-cell leukemia/lymphoma (see later).

Between 1950 and the early 1990s, the incidence rate for non-Hodgkin's lymphomas in the United States increased by about 3 to 4% yearly, but it has declined slightly since the mid-1990s. Increases have occurred among both men and women in all parts of the world. This increase in incidence is partially related to the aging population (Fig. 191-1) and to the acquired immunodeficiency syndrome (AIDS) epidemic (Chapter 400); occupational and environmental exposures (e.g., farm chemicals) may also explain some of the increase. Finally, some of the increase may be explained by improvements in the ability of pathologists to diagnose lymphoma and by improvements in imaging techniques.

PATHOBIOLOGY

For most cases of non-Hodgkin's lymphoma, the cause is unknown, although genetic, environmental, and infectious agents have been implicated (Table 191-1).

Genetic Factors

Familial clusters have been described, and there is a slightly higher risk of non-Hodgkin's lymphoma among siblings and first-degree relatives of patients with lymphoma or other hematologic malignancies. Tumor necrosis factor (308G→A), interleukin (IL)-10 (3575 T→A), and other polymorphisms are associated with the development of diffuse large B-cell lymphoma.

Immune System Abnormalities

Several inherited disorders increase the risk of developing non-Hodgkin's lymphoma as much as 250-fold (see Table 191-1). In some of these conditions, the lymphoma may be related to Epstein-Barr virus (EBV; Chapter 385). For example, patients with X-linked lymphoproliferative disorder have mutations in the *SH2D1A* gene, which encodes proteins that regulate the host immune response against EBV-infected cells; they may develop fatal infectious mononucleosis or non-Hodgkin's lymphoma after primary

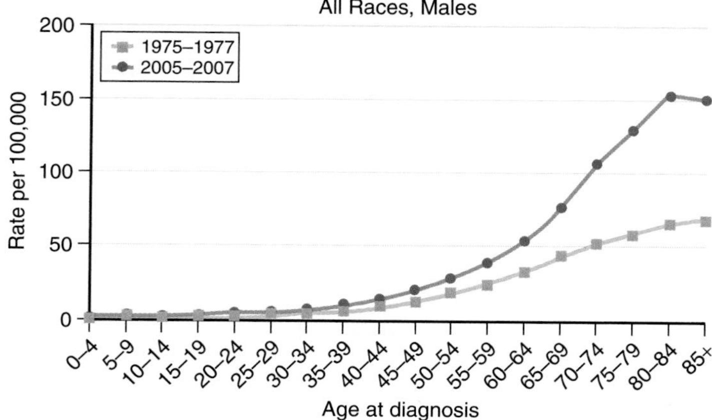

FIGURE 191-1. **Non-Hodgkin's lymphoma incidence by age in men, 1975-1977 versus 2005-2007.** (From the Surveillance, Epidemiology, and End Results [SEER] Program of the National Cancer Institute, http://seer.cancer.gov/csr/1975_2007/.)

exposure to EBV. Acquired immunodeficiency states are also associated with an increased risk of non-Hodgkin's lymphoma. For example, post-transplantation lymphoproliferative disorders occur in as many as 20% of solid organ transplant recipients, related to the proliferation of B lymphocytes that have been transformed during immunosuppressive therapy. The risk of non-Hodgkin's lymphoma is also increased more than 100-fold in patients infected with human immunodeficiency virus (HIV); almost all central nervous system (CNS) lymphomas and approximately 50% of other lymphomas in patients with AIDS are related to EBV. Some studies have shown a two-fold increase in the incidence of non-Hodgkin's lymphomas among patients with rheumatoid arthritis (Chapter 272), and the risk of marginal zone lymphomas is increased approximately 30- to 40-fold in patients with Sjögren's syndrome (Chapter 276). Increases in the incidence of thyroid lymphoma are seen in patients with Hashimoto's thyroiditis (Chapter 233). Enteropathy-type T-cell lymphomas are associated with celiac disease (Chapter 142).

TABLE 191-1 FACTORS ASSOCIATED WITH THE DEVELOPMENT OF NON-HODGKIN'S LYMPHOMA

Inherited immune disorders
- Severe combined immunodeficiency disease
- Common variable immunodeficiency disease
- Wiskott-Aldrich syndrome
- Ataxia-telangiectasia
- X-linked lymphoproliferative disorder

Acquired immune disorders
- Solid organ transplantation
- Acquired immunodeficiency syndrome (AIDS)
- Methotrexate therapy for autoimmune disorders
- Rheumatoid arthritis and systemic lupus erythematosus
- Sjögren's syndrome
- Hashimoto's thyroiditis

Infectious agents
- Epstein-Barr virus
- Human T- lymphotropic virus type 1
- Human herpesvirus 8
- Hepatitis C virus
- *Helicobacter pylori*
- *Borrelia burgdorferi*
- *Chlamydia psittaci*
- *Campylobacter jejuni*

Occupational and environmental exposure
- Herbicides
- Organic solvents
- Hair dyes
- Ultraviolet light
- Diet
- Smoking

Infectious Agents

EBV is associated with the majority of post-transplantation lymphoproliferative disorders and many AIDS-associated lymphomas. This viral genome is detectable in more than 95% of cases of endemic Burkitt's lymphoma and in approximately 40% of cases of sporadic Burkitt's lymphoma and AIDS-associated lymphomas.

The human T-lymphotropic virus type 1 (HTLV-1; Chapter 386) is detectable in virtually all cases of adult T-cell leukemia/lymphoma. The risk of lymphoma is approximately 3% in patients infected with HTLV-1; in endemic areas, up to 50% of all non-Hodgkin's lymphomas may be related to HTLV-1. Reports of an association between simian virus 40 and non-Hodgkin's lymphoma have not been supported by further research.

Human herpesvirus 8 (HHV-8, Kaposi's sarcoma–associated herpesvirus; Chapter 400), which is associated with expansion of the B-cell population, is also associated with primary effusion lymphoma (see later) in immunocompromised patients and with multicentric Castleman's disease. Patients with primary effusion lymphoma are often coinfected with EBV.

Epidemiologic evidence has linked hepatitis C virus (Chapter 151) to lymphoplasmacytic lymphoma and splenic marginal zone lymphoma. Chronic antigenic stimulation from this virus may lead to the emergence of malignant B-cell clones.

Helicobacter pylori is associated with gastric lymphoma (Chapter 198) of extranodal marginal zone/mucosa-associated lymphoid tissue (MALT). Colonized patients develop gastritis from chronic antigenic stimulation mediated by T cells, which respond to *H. pylori*–specific antigens; malignant B-cell clones emerge. *Borrelia burgdorferi* (Chapter 329) has been associated with marginal zone B-cell lymphoma of the skin. Evidence also links *Chlamydia psittaci* (Chapter 326) with ocular adnexal lymphomas and *Campylobacter jejuni* with immunoproliferative small intestinal disease (Chapter 311).

Environmental and Occupational Exposure

Agricultural chemicals have been associated with an increased risk of developing non-Hodgkin's lymphomas, and the strongest associations involve phenoxy herbicides such as 2,4-dichlorophenoxyacetic acid (2,4-D), which was also a component of Agent Orange (Chapter 18). An increased risk has also been associated with ionizing radiation (Chapter 19), organic solvents, hair dyes, and nitrates in drinking water, although contradictory results have been reported. Some studies have also linked non-Hodgkin's lymphomas to high-fat diets and ultraviolet radiation (Chapter 183). The risk of non-Hodgkin's lymphomas is increased approximately 20-fold after treatment for Hodgkin's disease (Chapter 192). Heavy smokers (Chapter 31) have an increased risk of developing follicular lymphoma.

Pathology

Non-Hodgkin's lymphomas are derived from cells of the immune system at varying stages of differentiation. In some cases, the cell of origin is directly linked to the morphology, immunophenotype, and clinical behavior of the lymphoma (Fig. 191-2 and Table 191-2).

TABLE 191-2 TYPICAL IMMUNOPHENOTYPES OF COMMON NON-HODGKIN'S LYMPHOMAS

LYMPHOMA	CD20	CD3	CD10	CD5	CD23	OTHER
Small lymphocytic	+	–	–	+	+	
Lymphoplasmacytic	+	–	–	–	–	Cytoplasmic Ig+
Extranodal marginal zone MALT	+	–	–	–	–	
Nodal marginal zone	+	–	–	–	–	
Follicular	+	–	+	–		
Mantle cell	+		–	+	–	Cyclin D1+
Diffuse large B cell	+	–				
Mediastinal large B cell	+	–				
Burkitt's	+	–	+	–		TdT–
Precursor T lymphoblastic	–	+/–				TdT+, CD1a +/–, CD7+
Anaplastic large T cell	–	+/–				CD30+, CD15–, EMA+, ALK+
Peripheral T cell	–	+/–				Other pan-T variable

ALK = anaplastic lymphoma kinase; EMA = epithelial membrane antigen; MALT = mucosa-associated lymphoid tissue; TdT = terminal deoxynucleotidyl transferase.

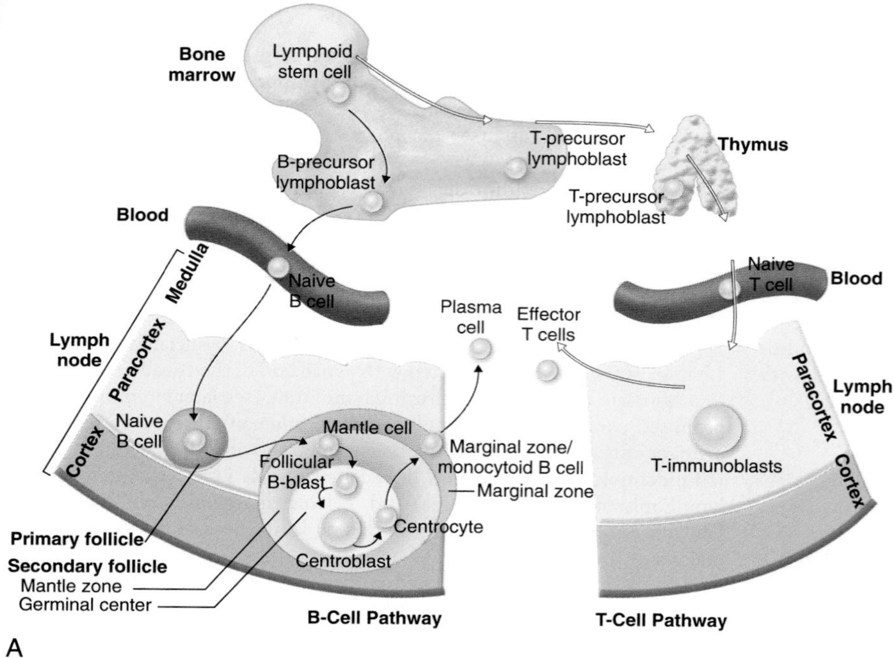

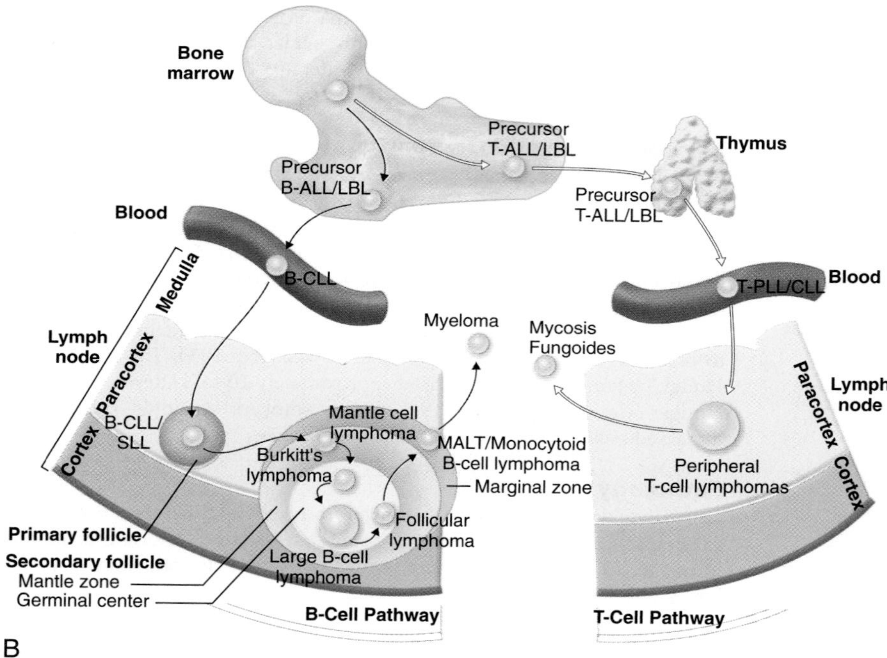

FIGURE 191-2. Postulated normal counterparts of currently recognized B- and T-cell malignancies. A, Schema of normal B- and T-cell differentiation. Bone marrow–derived lymphoid stem cells differentiate into committed B-cell precursors or into T-cell precursors that undergo further maturation in the thymus. These B- and T-cell precursors mature into naïve B or T cells that circulate to lymph nodes. After antigen exposure, normal B blasts proliferate and undergo further differentiation in the germinal center of the secondary follicle. The germinal center is surrounded by a mantle zone and a marginal zone. Antigen-specific B cells generated in the germinal center leave the follicle and reappear in the marginal zone. Thereafter, immunoglobulin-producing plasma cells accumulate in the lymph node medulla and subsequently exit to the periphery. Antigen-dependent T-cell proliferation occurs in the lymph node paracortex. After antigen exposure, mature T cells become immunoblasts and, subsequently, antigen-specific effector T cells that exit to the periphery. The postulated normal counterparts of many currently recognized T- and B-cell neoplasms are shown. **B,** T- and B-cell malignancies derived from the postulated normal counterparts shown in **A.** ALL = acute lymphoblastic leukemia; CLL = chronic lymphocytic leukemia; LBL = lymphoblastic lymphoma; MALT = mucosa-associated lymphoid tissue; SLL = small lymphocytic lymphoma.

The transformation of cells from the normal immune system into malignant lymphoma reflects the acquisition of specific genetic abnormalities. In many cases, cytogenetic studies can identify chromosomal translocations that underlie the development or progression of the lymphoma. In most cases of non-Hodgkin's lymphoma, the activation of proto-oncogenes is the major abnormality, but occasionally chromosomal translocations can lead to fusion genes that code for chimeric proteins. In addition, some cases are associated with deletion of tumor suppressor genes. Specific genetic abnormalities are associated with some specific subtypes of non-Hodgkin's lymphoma (Table 191-3). It is becoming clear that the tumor microenvironment (i.e., stromal cells associated with the lymphoma cells) is important in tumor cell survival and response to therapy.

Classification

Recognition of the Reed-Sternberg cell approximately 100 years ago made it possible to define Hodgkin's disease (Chapter 192) as a distinct entity, whereas other lymphomas were included under the heading "non-Hodgkin's lymphomas." In the 1990s a classification system incorporating morphologic, immunologic, genetic, and clinical information (the Revised European-American Lymphoma classification, or REAL) was developed to identify distinct clinicopathologic subgroups representing diseases that can be recognized by clinicians. This system was subsequently adopted as the World Health Organization (WHO) classification of lymphomas in 2008 (Table 191-4).

The WHO classification divides lymphomas on the basis of B-cell or T/NK-cell origin and whether they are derived from primitive precursor cells or from more mature "peripheral" cells. Specific clinical and pathologic entities are recognized within each of these groupings. In the United States and Europe, 85 to 90% of non-Hodgkin's lymphomas are B cell in origin.

The most frequent type is diffuse large B-cell lymphoma, which represents 31% of all non-Hodgkin's lymphomas worldwide. The next most frequent type is follicular lymphoma, which represents 22% of cases; follicular lymphoma is relatively more frequent in North America and western Europe and less frequent in Asia. Less common types, each representing between 5 and

TABLE 191-3 CHROMOSOMAL TRANSLOCATIONS CHARACTERISTIC OF NON-HODGKIN'S LYMPHOMA

LYMPHOMA SUBTYPE	TRANSLOCATION	GENES INVOLVED	FREQUENCY (%)
Diffuse large B cell	t(3q27) t(14;18)(q32;q21) t(18;14)(q24;q32)	*BCL6* *IgH, BCL2* *MYC (c-Myc), IgH*	35 15-20 <5
Burkitt's	t(8;14)(q24;q32) t(8;22)(q24;q11) t(2;8)(p12;q24)	*MYC, IgH* *MYC, IgL* *IgK, MYC*	100% have one of these, most commonly t(8;14)
Follicular	t(14;18)(q32;q21)	*IgH, BCL2*	~90
Mantle cell	t(11;14)(q13;q32)	*BCL1, IgH*	>90
ALCL	t(2;5)(p23;q35)	*ALK, NPM*	>80 of ALK+ ALCLs
MALT	t(11;18)(q21;q21) t(14;18)(q21;q32) t(1;14)(p22;q32)	*API2, MALT1* *IgH, MALT1* *BCL10, IgH*	35 20 10

ALCL = anaplastic large cell lymphoma; ALK = anaplastic lymphoma kinase; MALT = mucosa-associated lymphoid tissue.

TABLE 191-4 WORLD HEALTH ORGANIZATION CLASSIFICATION OF NON-HODGKIN'S LYMPHOMA (2008)

PRECURSOR LYMPHOID NEOPLASMS
B-lymphoblastic leukemia/lymphoma T-lymphoblastic leukemia/lymphoma
MATURE B-CELL NEOPLASMS
Chronic lymphocytic leukemia/small lymphocytic lymphoma Splenic marginal zone lymphoma Lymphoplasmacytic lymphoma Extranodal marginal zone lymphoma of MALT (MALT lymphoma) Nodal marginal zone lymphoma Follicular lymphoma Primary cutaneous follicle center lymphoma Mantle cell lymphoma Diffuse large B-cell lymphoma, NOS Burkitt's lymphoma
MATURE T-CELL NEOPLASMS
Adult T-cell leukemia/lymphoma Extranodal NK/T-cell lymphoma, nasal type Enteropathy-associated T-cell lymphoma Hepatosplenic T-cell lymphoma Subcutaneous panniculitis-like T-cell lymphoma Mycosis fungoides Sézary's syndrome Primary cutaneous $CD30^+$ T-cell lymphoproliferative disorders Peripheral T-cell lymphoma, NOS Angioimmunoblastic T-cell lymphoma Anaplastic large cell lymphoma, ALK positive Anaplastic large cell lymphoma, ALK negative

ALK = anaplastic lymphoma kinase; MALT = mucosa-associated lymphoid tissue; NK = natural killer; NOS = not otherwise specified.

10% of all non-Hodgkin's lymphomas, are extranodal marginal zone/MALT lymphomas, peripheral T-cell lymphomas, small lymphocytic lymphoma, and mantle cell lymphoma. Other types each represent less than 2% of non-Hodgkin's lymphomas seen in the United States.

The non-Hodgkin's lymphomas recognized in the WHO classification have clinically distinctive characteristics (Table 191-5), such that an experienced hematopathologist can accurately classify 85% or more of patients by WHO criteria when adequate material is available. Some diagnoses, such as follicular lymphoma, can be made with a high degree of accuracy without immunologic or genetic studies. The diagnosis of T-cell lymphomas cannot be made accurately without immunophenotyping. Cytogenetic studies and molecular genetic studies can help resolve difficult differential diagnoses. For example, the presence of a t(8;14) translocation supports the diagnosis of Burkitt's lymphoma, whereas a t(11;14) with cyclin D1 overexpression can confirm the diagnosis of mantle cell lymphoma (see Tables 191-2 and 191-3).

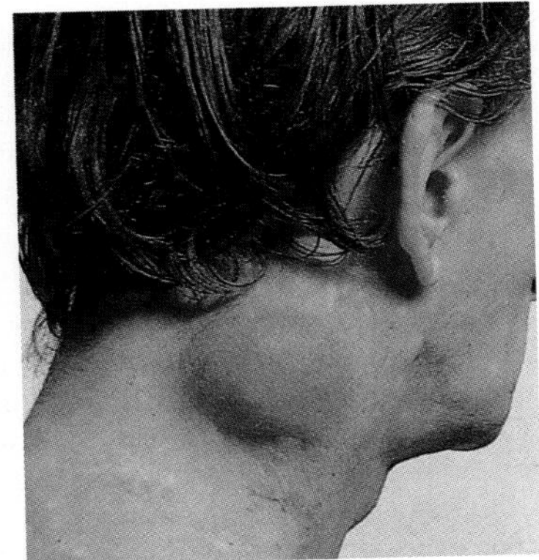

FIGURE 191-3. Non-Hodgkin's lymphoma. Despite the redness of the skin over the enlarged lymph node in this patient, the lesion was completely painless. (From Forbes CD, Jackson WF. *Color Atlas and Text of Clinical Medicine,* 3rd ed. London: Mosby; 2003.)

The use of complementary DNA microarrays has allowed the identification of distinct subsets of patients with diffuse large B-cell lymphoma. Patients with histologically identical lymphomas can be divided into those with tumor gene expression patterns resembling normal germinal center B cells, those whose tumors resemble activated post–germinal center B cells, or those with patterns resembling that seen in Hodgkin's lymphoma; the last pattern is most frequently found in young women who present with large mediastinal masses.

CLINICAL MANIFESTATIONS

The most common presentation of non-Hodgkin's lymphoma is lymphadenopathy (Fig. 191-3; Chapter 171). In many cases, patients notice cervical, axillary, or inguinal adenopathy and seek a physician's advice. In general, lymph nodes containing lymphoma are firm, nontender, and not associated with a regional infection. However, patients are frequently treated with a course of antibiotics before a biopsy is performed to confirm the diagnosis of lymphoma. In other patients, lymphadenopathy occurring in sites such as the mediastinum or retroperitoneum causes symptoms that bring the patient to the physician. Chest pain, cough, superior vena cava syndrome, abdominal pain, back pain, spinal cord compression, and symptoms of renal insufficiency associated with ureteral compression are characteristic.

Non-Hodgkin's lymphomas are often associated with systemic symptoms that may lead to the diagnosis. The most obvious symptoms are fevers, night sweats, and unexplained weight loss. Any of these symptoms without an obvious cause should lead a physician to consider the diagnosis of lymphoma. Other, less characteristic symptoms include fatigue, which is frequently present at the time of diagnosis if the patient is questioned carefully, and pruritus.

Non-Hodgkin's lymphomas can involve essentially any organ in the body, and malfunction of that organ can cause symptoms that lead to the diagnosis.

TABLE 191-5 PRESENTING CLINICAL CHARACTERISTICS OF COMMON NON-HODGKIN'S LYMPHOMA SUBTYPES

TYPE OF LYMPHOMA	MEDIAN AGE (YR)	% MALE	Stage (%) I	Stage (%) IV	B SYMPTOMS (%)	BONE MARROW INVOLVED (%)	5-YR SURVIVAL (%)
B-CELL LYMPHOMAS							
Small lymphocytic	65	53	4	83	33	72	51
Lymphoplasmacytic	63	53	7	73	13	73	59
Extranodal marginal zone MALT	60	48	39	31	19	14	74
Nodal marginal zone	58	42	13	40	37	32	57
Follicular	59	42	18	51	28	42	72
Mantle cell	63	74	13	71	28	64	27
Diffuse large B cell	64	55	25	33	33	16	46
Mediastinal large B cell	37	34	10	31	38	3	50
Burkitt's	31	89	37	38	22	33	44
PRECURSOR B/T-CELL LYMPHOMAS							
Precursor T-lymphoblastic	28	64	0	75	21	50	26
T-CELL LYMPHOMAS							
Anaplastic large T cell	34	69	19	39	53	13	77
Peripheral T cell	61	55	8	65	50	36	25

B symptoms = fevers, night sweats, and weight loss; MALT = mucosa-associated lymphoid tissue.
Adapted from Armitage JO, Weisenburger DD, for the Non-Hodgkin's Lymphoma Classification Project. New approach to classifying non-Hodgkin's lymphomas: clinical features of the major histologic subtypes. *J Clin Oncol.* 1998;16:2780-2795.

Examples include neurologic symptoms with primary brain lymphoma (Chapter 195), shortness of breath with MALT lymphomas in the lung, epigastric pain and vomiting with gastric MALT lymphomas or diffuse large B-cell lymphomas (Chapter 198), bowel obstruction with small bowel lymphomas (Chapter 199), testicular masses with diffuse large B-cell lymphoma (Chapter 206), and skin lesions with cutaneous lymphomas (Chapter 448). Many lymphomas involve the bone marrow and occasionally cause extensive myelophthisis (Chapter 168) and bone marrow failure; these patients may present with infections, bleeding, and anemia.

Non-Hodgkin's lymphomas can also manifest with a variety of immunologic abnormalities. For example, autoimmune hemolytic anemia (Chapter 163) and immune thrombocytopenia (Chapter 175) can be the presenting manifestations of non-Hodgkin's lymphoma, especially small lymphocytic lymphoma/chronic lymphocytic leukemia as well as other subtypes, including diffuse large B-cell lymphoma. Peripheral neuropathies (Chapter 428), often associated with overproduction of a monoclonal protein, can be seen in a variety of subtypes but are most characteristic of lymphoplasmacytic lymphoma; sometimes they are also seen with POEMS syndrome (polyneuropathy, organomegaly, endocrinopathy, M protein, skin changes; Chapter 193). Paraneoplastic neurologic complications of non-Hodgkin's lymphoma include demyelinating polyneuropathy, Guillain-Barré syndrome, autonomic dysfunction, and peripheral neuropathy. Paraneoplastic syndromes (Chapter 187) associated with non-Hodgkin's lymphoma can affect the skin (e.g., pemphigus), kidney (e.g., glomerulonephritis), and miscellaneous organ systems (e.g., vasculitis, dermatomyositis, cholestatic jaundice).

The differential diagnosis in patients with non-Hodgkin's lymphoma is broad. Any cause of lymphadenopathy or splenomegaly can potentially be confused with non-Hodgkin's lymphoma (Chapter 171). However, this confusion is resolved by an appropriate biopsy. It is extremely important to recognize that the diagnosis of non-Hodgkin's lymphoma must be considered in patients with compatible clinical presentations and then confirmed by an adequate biopsy read by an experienced hematopathologist. The diagnosis should never be inferred, and patients should not be treated until the diagnosis is confirmed by biopsy. This is also true for patients who achieve a complete remission with initial therapy; they should not be treated for presumed relapse on the basis of symptoms or abnormal images without a biopsy.

DIAGNOSIS

Each new patient with a non-Hodgkin's lymphoma should be thoroughly evaluated in a systematic manner (Table 191-6). Because subtle pathologic distinctions may alter therapy, the most important issue in managing non-Hodgkin's lymphoma is to establish an accurate diagnosis. Core needle biopsies can occasionally be used for a primary diagnosis if the specimen is handled properly. Fine-needle aspirates should not be used to diagnose lymphoma, and they preclude an accurate diagnosis of the specific subtype of non-Hodgkin's lymphoma. In most cases, an excisional biopsy is necessary (and is always preferred) for the initial diagnosis; another biopsy should be performed if sufficient material is not obtained. Review by an experienced hematopathologist is essential.

TABLE 191-6 TYPICAL EVALUATION OF A PATIENT NEWLY DIAGNOSED WITH NON-HODGKIN'S LYMPHOMA

1. Biopsy to establish diagnosis
2. Careful history and physical examination
3. Laboratory evaluation
   A. Complete blood count
   B. Chemistry screen, including lactate dehydrogenase
4. Imaging studies
   A. Computed tomography of chest, abdomen, and pelvis
   B. Positron emission tomography
5. Additional biopsies
   A. Bone marrow
   B. Any other suspicious site if results would change therapy

Staging and Prognostic Systems

After diagnosis, a meticulous staging evaluation is necessary to estimate prognosis and determine therapy. Staging requires a careful history and physical examination; complete blood count; renal and hepatic function tests; serum lactate dehydrogenase (LDH) level; computed tomography (CT) of the chest, abdomen, and pelvis; and bone marrow biopsy. Positron emission tomography (PET) can be helpful to identify initial sites of involvement and, after treatment, to distinguish persisting lymphoma from residual fibrosis in masses seen on CT. The most common staging system is the Ann Arbor classification, which separates patients into four stages based on anatomic sites of disease (Table 191-7). In addition, each stage is subdivided into A (no defined general symptoms) and B (unexplained weight loss >10% of body weight in the previous 6 months, unexplained temperature >38° C, or night sweats) categories. Known sites of disease can be reexamined later to evaluate the response to therapy.

Although a wide variety of patient factors (e.g., age, symptoms, LDH level) and tumor factors (e.g., bulk, gene expression pattern, proliferation rate) can affect treatment outcomes, two prognostic systems can help in choosing

TABLE 191-7 STAGING OF NON-HODGKIN'S LYMPHOMA

STAGE	DESCRIPTION
I	Involvement of a single lymph node region (I) or a single extralymphatic organ or site (I_E)
II	Involvement of ≥2 lymph node regions on the same side of the diaphragm (II) or localized involvement of an extralymphatic organ or site and ≥1 lymph node regions on the same side of the diaphragm (II_E)
III	Involvement of lymph node regions on both sides of the diaphragm (III), which may also be accompanied by localized involvement of an extralymphatic organ or site (III_E) or by involvement of the spleen (III_S) or both (III_{SE})
IV	Diffuse or disseminated involvement of ≥1 extralymphatic organ or tissues with or without associated lymph node enlargement
Subtypes	
A	No B symptoms
B	B symptoms: unexplained weight loss ≥10% of body weight in prior 6 months, unexplained fever >38° C, or night sweats

Adapted from Carbone PP, Kaplan HS, Musshoff K, et al. Report of the Committee on Hodgkin's Disease Staging Classification. *Cancer Res.* 1971;31:1860-1861.

TABLE 191-8 INTERNATIONAL PROGNOSTIC INDEX

CATEGORY	SCORE (NO. OF RISK FACTORS)
ALL PATIENTS*	
Low	0 or 1
Low intermediate	2
High intermediate	3
High	4 or 5
AGE-ADJUSTED INDEX, PATIENTS ≤60 YR†	
Low	0
Low intermediate	1
High intermediate	2
High	3

*Adverse factors for all patients: age >60 yr, ↑LDH, performance status 2–4, >1 extranodal site, Ann Arbor stage III or IV.
†Adverse factors for patients ≤60 yr: ↑LDH, performance status 2–4, Ann Arbor stage III or IV.
LDH = lactate dehydrogenase.
Adapted from Shipp M, Harrington D, Anderson J, et al. A predictive model for aggressive non-Hodgkin's lymphoma. *N Engl J Med.* 1993;329:987-994.

therapy and determining an accurate prognosis. The International Prognostic Index (IPI; Table 191-8) is the most widely used method to predict treatment outcome and survival. The IPI is based on five adverse factors (age older than 60 years, performance status ≤2, elevated serum LDH level, two or more extranodal sites of disease, Ann Arbor stage III or IV), which are summed to give the score. This index was developed for patients with diffuse aggressive lymphoma (predominantly diffuse large B-cell lymphoma), but it can be used to predict treatment outcome with any subtype. For young patients, an abbreviated index that uses only reduced performance status, elevated serum LDH level, and high stage can be applied. Because patients with follicular lymphoma rarely have a reduced performance status or a large number of extranodal sites, an alternative index termed the *Follicular Lymphoma International Prognostic Index* (FLIPI) was developed; it substitutes more than four nodal areas of involvement and a hemoglobin less than 12 g as staging criteria and does a somewhat better job of predicting treatment outcome in follicular lymphoma.

TREATMENT Rx

Lymphomas may behave in an indolent or an aggressive manner. The behavior of many of these neoplasms is distinctive, but within each category, behavior is frequently influenced by disease site, tumor bulk, and performance status of the patient. Some lymphomas can be managed, at least initially, with observation, whereas other situations are medical emergencies, such as spinal cord compression (Chapter 195). It is important to consider three questions before starting therapy: (1) Does treatment have curative potential? (2) Can treatment prolong survival? (3) Will treatment alleviate symptoms?

SPECIFIC TYPES OF NON-HODGKIN'S LYMPHOMAS

Precursor T-Cell and B-Cell Lymphomas

These tumors are nodal or other solid tissue infiltrates of cells that are morphologically and immunophenotypically identical to the immature cells seen in B-cell or T-cell acute lymphoblastic leukemia (Chapter 189). Patients who have predominantly nodal disease with minimal or no involvement of the bone marrow are frequently classified as having *lymphoblastic lymphoma,* whereas those with more than 25% neoplastic cells in the marrow are classified as having *lymphoblastic leukemia.* These distinctions are arbitrary and reflect the stage of disease rather than different diagnoses. These neoplasms are more common in children than in adults.

B-cell precursor lymphomas frequently manifest as solid tumors with involvement of the skin and bones, whereas T-cell neoplasms typically manifest as a mediastinal mass in a young male. Involvement of the CNS is common. Approximately 90% of patients who present with lymphoblastic lymphoma have a T-cell phenotype, whereas about 85% of patients who present with acute lymphoblastic leukemia have a B-cell phenotype. Adverse prognostic characteristics include CNS involvement, stage IV disease, and an elevated LDH level.

TREATMENT Rx

Patients with either T-cell lymphoblastic lymphoma or precursor B-cell lymphoblastic lymphoma are typically treated with regimens modeled after those used for acute lymphoblastic leukemia (Chapter 189). These regimens frequently contain cytarabine and high-dose methotrexate, and they often include maintenance therapy. CNS prophylaxis with intrathecal chemotherapy, high-dose methotrexate, or cranial irradiation is also a component of these regimens.

Mature B-Cell Lymphomas

SMALL LYMPHOCYTIC LYMPHOMA/CHRONIC LYMPHOCYTIC LEUKEMIA

Small lymphocytic lymphoma is defined as a lymph node or other tissue infiltrate that is morphologically and immunophenotypically identical to chronic lymphocytic leukemia (Chapter 190). Patients are frequently asymptomatic, and the diagnosis is often made when blood counts are performed for other reasons. Patients frequently have lymphadenopathy or splenomegaly. Fatigue is common. Hypogammaglobulinemia can occur and may lead to an increased susceptibility to infection.

A poor prognosis is associated with advanced stage and systemic symptoms, expression of high levels of CD38 and ZAP-70 on tumor cells, lack of rearranged immunoglobulin heavy chain genes, and genetic abnormalities such as del(17p) and del(11q). Approximately 10% of patients exhibit transformation to diffuse large B-cell lymphoma (Richter's syndrome), which is associated with a poor prognosis.

The median survival time is more than 10 years for patients without adverse characteristics, and these patients can often be managed with observation. Therapy is necessary for patients who have rapidly progressive or symptomatic lymphadenopathy and for those who develop cytopenias.

TREATMENT 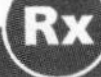

Management must be individualized because therapy is not curative, and patients are often elderly. A regimen consisting of fludarabine in combination with cyclophosphamide and rituximab (Table 191-9) is frequently used in the United States for relatively young, fit patients. Single-agent fludarabine plus rituximab is more commonly used in elderly patients. Fludarabine is more effective than chlorambucil, but because chlorambucil is administered orally

TABLE 191-9 COMBINATION CHEMOTHERAPY REGIMENS FOR NON-HODGKIN'S LYMPHOMA

REGIMEN	DOSE	DAYS OF ADMINISTRATION	FREQUENCY
CHOP-R			Every 21 days
Cyclophosphamide	750 mg/m^2 IV	1	
Doxorubicin	50 mg/m^2 IV	1	
Vincristine	1.4 mg/m^2 IV*	1	
Prednisone, fixed dose	100 PO	1-5	
Rituximab	375 mg/m^2 IV	1	
CVP-R			Every 21 days
Cyclophosphamide	1000 mg/m^2 IV	1	
Vincristine	1.4 mg/m^2 IV*	1	
Prednisone, fixed dose	100 mg PO	1-5	
Rituximab	375 mg/m^2 IV	1	
FCR			Every 28 days
Fludarabine	25 mg/m^2 IV	1-3	
Cyclophosphamide	250 mg/m^2 IV	1-3	
Rituximab	375 mg/m^2	1	

*Vincristine dose often capped at 2 mg total.

and has few side effects, it is sometimes used in older patients. Bendamustine is an active, newly available drug. Alemtuzumab, a monoclonal antibody directed against the CD52 antigen, is sometimes effective after other treatments have failed. Allogeneic hematopoietic stem cell transplantation may be curative, but few patients are candidates for this approach.

Patients may develop autoimmune thrombocytopenia (Chapter 175), autoimmune neutropenia (Chapter 170), and red blood cell aplasia (Chapter 168). These autoimmune disorders may respond to treatment with corticosteroids, intravenous immune globulin, or splenectomy, as used in patients without underlying lymphoma.

EXTRANODAL MARGINAL ZONE LYMPHOMA OF MUCOSA-ASSOCIATED LYMPHOID TISSUE (MALT LYMPHOMA)

MALT lymphomas are indolent tumors that originate in association with epithelial cells and are seen most commonly in the gastrointestinal tract, salivary glands, breast, thyroid, orbit, conjunctiva, skin, and lung. The majority of cases are stage I or II at diagnosis, although in some series as many as 30% disseminate to bone marrow or other sites. These lymphomas tend to remain localized for extended periods. Local treatment with surgery or radiation therapy cures a high proportion of localized neoplasms. Disseminated disease is treated similarly to follicular lymphoma (see later).

Gastric MALT lymphomas are usually associated with infection by *H. pylori.* Eradication of *H. pylori* with antibiotics leads to complete regression in more than 50% of gastric MALT lymphomas, although polymerase chain reaction analysis demonstrates minimal residual disease in many patients, and the long-term outcome of this approach is unknown. Response to antibiotic therapy is less likely if invasion is deeper, lymph node metastases are found, or the t(11;18) chromosomal translocation is present.

TREATMENT Rx

Patients may have tumors in more than one extranodal site, and these locations can sometimes be successfully treated with local therapy. Asymptomatic patients can be monitored closely without antilymphoma therapy until symptoms progress. Gastric MALT lymphoma that does not respond to antibiotics can be treated with radiation, rituximab as a single agent (similar to its use in follicular lymphoma), or several traditional combination chemotherapy regimens (see Table 191-9).

FOLLICULAR LYMPHOMA

Follicular lymphoma accounts for the majority of indolent or "low-grade" lymphomas in the United States. Follicular lymphoma is divided into three grades based on the proportion of large, transformed cells (centroblasts).

Patients with follicular lymphoma are frequently asymptomatic. The most common presenting complaint is painless lymphadenopathy. Some patients have cough or dyspnea related to pulmonary or mediastinal involvement or pleural effusions. Other patients have symptoms of abdominal pain or fullness related to subdiaphragmatic or splenic disease. A minority of patients have systemic symptoms of fevers, night sweats, or weight loss.

The clinical behavior and treatment of follicular lymphoma grades 1 and 2 are the same and are discussed in this section. Grade 3 follicular lymphoma may have a more aggressive clinical course and is frequently treated similarly to diffuse large B-cell lymphoma (see later).

TREATMENT

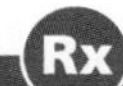

Localized Disease

Approximately 5 to 15% of patients have localized disease (stage I or minimal stage II disease) at diagnosis. These lymphomas are usually treated with involved-field radiation, and most series report 10-year disease-free survival rates of approximately 50% and overall survival rates of 60 to 70%. Some retrospective series have reported improved outcomes when chemotherapy is combined with radiation.

Advanced Disease

Most patients with follicular lymphoma have extensive disease at diagnosis. The median survival time of these patients is more than 10 years. Although spontaneous regression has been described, 30 to 50% of patients experience transformation to a more aggressive histology—usually diffuse large B-cell lymphoma. Transformation is frequently associated with new systemic symptoms and rapidly progressive lymphadenopathy, an aggressive clinical course, and a poor prognosis.

Asymptomatic patients, especially elderly patients and those with other medical illnesses, are frequently managed with a "watch and wait" approach. Prospective trials have demonstrated that this approach does not influence overall survival, and patients can sometimes be observed for long periods before treatment is required.

Most patients with follicular lymphoma eventually require treatment because of systemic symptoms, symptomatic or progressive lymphadenopathy, splenomegaly, effusions, or cytopenias. In elderly patients, those who are poor candidates for intensive chemotherapy regimens, and those who want to avoid the side effects (e.g., alopecia) of chemotherapy, single-agent rituximab (375 mg/m^2 intravenously, given weekly for 4 consecutive weeks) yields an objective response rate of well over 50%. The median duration of response is approximately 1 to 2 years for patients who receive no additional therapy, but the response can be extended with ongoing administration of rituximab once every 2 or 3 months or by repeating the initial four doses every 6 months. When rituximab is combined with standard chemotherapy regimens such as CVP (cyclophosphamide, vincristine, prednisone) or CHOP (cyclophosphamide, doxorubicin, vincristine, prednisone) (see Table 191-9), the response rate, duration of response, and survival are increased compared with the chemotherapy regimen alone, and maintenance rituximab further extends the duration of remission.[1] For aggressive lymphomas, high dose intensity doxorubicin can significantly improve survival.[2] Fludarabine, used alone or in combination with mitoxantrone, is also effective. In one study, ^{131}I-tositumomab radioimmunotherapy appeared to provide a prolonged benefit. Interferon-α may be beneficial in follicular lymphoma when combined with initial chemotherapy,[3] but it is rarely used as primary therapy in the United States because of its side effects. Some studies have shown an improvement in failure-free survival with the use of autologous bone marrow transplantation in patients who achieve an initial remission, but overall survival is not prolonged.

Salvage Therapy

Most patients respond to initial chemotherapy, and initial responses typically persist for 1 to 3 years. However, follicular lymphoma eventually progresses in most patients with advanced-stage disease. Patients who have a relapse usually respond to additional therapy, often with the same agents, although the duration of response becomes progressively shorter with repeated courses of therapy. Approximately 50 to 60% of patients with relapsed follicular lymphoma respond to rituximab, and maintenance therapy prolongs remission in responding patients; however, less than 10% attain a complete response. Some patients who do not respond to rituximab respond to the radiolabeled antibodies tositumomab or ibritumomab. Radiation therapy may also be useful for patients with a localized site of symptomatic disease.

Prolonged remissions have been observed after autologous hematopoietic stem cell transplantation. Allogeneic hematopoietic stem cell transplantation may cure some patients with relapsed follicular lymphoma.

MANTLE CELL LYMPHOMA

Mantle cell lymphoma is a B-cell neoplasm composed of small lymphoid cells that may resemble small lymphocytic lymphoma or follicular lymphoma. It is most common in elderly patients and is usually at an advanced stage at the time of diagnosis. Males are more frequently affected, and extranodal disease, especially involvement of the bone marrow, Waldeyer's ring, and the gastrointestinal tract, is common. Mantle cell lymphoma is the most common cause of multiple lymphomatous polyposis, and the gastrointestinal tract should be evaluated with endoscopy during the initial evaluation.

Some patients present with involvement of the peripheral blood as well as the bone marrow, a clinical picture that resembles chronic lymphocytic leukemia (Chapter 190). The lymphocytes in both disorders are $CD5^+$, but the t(11;14) and overexpression of cyclin D1 seen in mantle cell lymphoma usually allow an accurate diagnosis.

Mantle cell lymphoma usually has a poor prognosis, with a median survival of 3 to 4 years, although occasional patients may have an indolent course. There is some evidence that prognosis may be improved with aggressive chemotherapy, but mantle cell lymphoma is usually not curable with standard chemotherapy regimens. Autologous hematopoietic stem cell transplantation for patients in their first remission may improve survival, but randomized trials have not been performed. Allogeneic transplantation can be curative but is associated with considerable morbidity and mortality.

DIFFUSE LARGE B-CELL LYMPHOMA

These tumors are the most common type of non-Hodgkin's lymphoma, but their morphology and genetic features are heterogeneous. Signs and symptoms are similar to those of other subtypes, although patients are more likely to have B symptoms or symptoms from the local tumor than are patients with follicular lymphoma.

The WHO classification of non-Hodgkin's lymphomas has identified several variants and subtypes of diffuse large B-cell lymphoma (Table 191-10). Many of these are histologic or genetic subtypes or variants for which treatment is the same as the standard approach for diffuse large B-cell lymphoma. Other subtypes present unusual clinical syndromes or specific therapeutic problems.

TREATMENT Rx

Localized Disease

As many as 30% of patients with diffuse large B-cell lymphoma have stage I or minimal stage II disease. These patients are occasionally cured with radiation therapy alone, but initial treatment with chemotherapy is more effective. Although one study in France suggested that a very intensive chemotherapy regimen alone might be better than CHOP plus radiation, most patients in the United States receive CHOP plus rituximab (CHOP-R; see Table 191-9), followed by consolidative radiation therapy.[4] Although the necessity of radiation therapy after CHOP-R has not been tested, this combination is still widely used.

Advanced Disease

CHOP-R is generally considered the "gold standard" treatment for adults of all ages with advanced-stage diffuse large B-cell lymphoma. Among patients older than 60 years, 75% achieve a complete response, with a 5-year event-free survival rate of 47% and a 5-year overall survival rate of 58%. In younger patients the outcome is better.[5]

Salvage Therapy

A variety of chemotherapy regimens have been developed for patients who relapse after attaining a remission with initial chemotherapy. These regimens commonly contain agents such as cisplatin, cytarabine, etoposide, carboplatin, and ifosfamide. Response rates exceeding 50% can be observed with these combinations, although no more than 10% of patients achieve long-term disease-free survival. High-dose therapy followed by autologous hematopoietic stem cell transplantation has become accepted therapy for patients with relapsed diffuse large B-cell lymphoma; approximately 20 to 40% of these patients attain long-term disease-free survival with transplantation if they are still responsive to conventional salvage chemotherapy.

Subtypes of Diffuse Large B-Cell Lymphoma

Primary mediastinal large B-cell lymphoma originates in the thymus and is most common in young women. This entity is distinguished by the presence of a mediastinal mass, which usually causes symptoms of cough, chest pain, or superior vena cava syndrome. A very large mass (>10 cm) or the existence of a malignant pleural effusion is associated with a worse prognosis.

TABLE 191-10 DIFFUSE LARGE B-CELL LYMPHOMA, VARIANTS AND SUBTYPES

Diffuse large B-cell lymphoma, not otherwise specified (NOS)
Common morphologic variants
Centroblastic
Immunoblastic
Anaplastic
Immunohistochemical subgroups
$CD5^+$ DLBCL
Germinal center B-cell–like (GCB)
Non–germinal center B-cell–like (non-GCB)
Diffuse large B-cell lymphoma, subtypes
T-cell/histiocyte-rich large B-cell lymphoma
Primary DLBCL of the CNS
Primary cutaneous DLBCL, leg type
EBV-positive DLBCL of the elderly
Other large B-cell lymphomas
Primary mediastinal (thymic) large B-cell lymphoma
Intravascular large B-cell lymphoma
DLBCL associated with chronic inflammation
Lymphomatoid granulomatosis
ALK-positive large B-cell lymphoma
Plasmablastic lymphoma
Large B-cell lymphoma arising in HHV-8-associated multicentric Castleman's disease
Primary effusion lymphoma

ALK = anaplastic lymphoma kinase; CNS = central nervous system; DLBCL = diffuse large B-cell lymphoma; EBV = Epstein-Barr virus; HHV = human herpesvirus.

Mediastinal large B-cell lymphoma is treated with the same chemotherapy regimens used for diffuse large B-cell lymphoma, followed, in some cases, by consolidative radiation therapy. The prognosis is similar to that of other diffuse large B-cell lymphomas. Relapses often occur in extranodal sites such as the CNS, lungs, gastrointestinal tract, liver, ovaries, and kidneys.

Intravascular large B-cell lymphoma is an aggressive lymphoma caused by cells that infiltrate the lumens of small blood vessels. Widespread extranodal involvement is common. Focal neurologic deficits and mental status changes are frequent. Cases are often diagnosed at autopsy, although durable responses to combination chemotherapy have been described.

Primary effusion lymphoma is associated with HHV-8 and is seen in HIV-infected and other immunosuppressed patients. Effusions occur in serous body cavities; peripheral lymphadenopathy is not seen. Prognosis is poor despite chemotherapy.

Plasmablastic lymphoma is most often seen in patients with HIV infection and frequently presents with involvement of the head and neck. This tumor does not express CD20 and thus does not benefit from treatment with rituximab.

Primary cutaneous diffuse large B-cell lymphoma of the leg (leg type) is one of two presentations of B-cell lymphoma in the skin. This tumor occurs mostly in older patients and follows an aggressive course. This neoplasm must be distinguished from primary cutaneous follicle center lymphoma, which might also be diagnosed as a cutaneous diffuse large B-cell lymphoma but follows an indolent course and requires only local therapy.

BURKITT'S LYMPHOMA

Burkitt's lymphoma is a highly aggressive B-cell lymphoma that is more common in children and immunosuppressed individuals than in healthy adults (see later). Widespread extranodal involvement is common. The endemic form of Burkitt's lymphoma is seen most frequently in children who reside in equatorial Africa. Involvement of bones of the jaw is common in this form. The sporadic form of Burkitt's lymphoma is seen most commonly in children in the United States. Males are more frequently affected. Both children and adults frequently have bulky abdominal disease, sometimes with involvement of the kidneys, ovaries, and breasts. Bone marrow involvement is seen in about one third of cases.

TREATMENT Rx

Tumors may progress extremely rapidly, so therapy should be started as soon as possible. Tumor lysis syndrome may occur because of the frequent presence of bulky disease, the high rate of tumor proliferation, and the extreme sensitivity of the tumor to chemotherapy. Patients are usually treated with specialized high-intensity regimens, including rituximab, of relatively short duration. Treatment with the CHOP-R regimen used for diffuse large B-cell lymphoma has a poor outcome. CNS prophylaxis with intrathecal chemotherapy or high-dose methotrexate is required. Cure rates well in excess of 50% are typical with appropriate therapy.

RARE TYPES OF B-CELL LYMPHOMA

Several rare types of lymphoma have distinct clinical features.

Lymphoplasmacytic lymphoma is an indolent lymphoma that frequently involves the bone marrow, peripheral blood, and spleen. Patients frequently have an immunoglobulin M paraprotein (and therefore could be called Waldenström's macroglobulinemia) that may lead to symptoms of hyperviscosity, autoimmune phenomena, or neuropathies (Chapter 193). Plasmapheresis can reduce symptoms of hyperviscosity. Chemotherapy with alkylating agents, combination chemotherapy, or fludarabine may be used. Rituximab is also effective, as are new agents such as the proteosome inhibitor bortezomib.

Splenic marginal zone lymphoma is an indolent lymphoma that usually manifests with splenomegaly and lymphocytosis. A monoclonal gammopathy is frequently seen. Peripheral lymphadenopathy is unusual. Anemia and thrombocytopenia may respond to splenectomy. Chemotherapy with single agents or anthracycline-based combinations may be useful, and when the lymphoma is associated with hepatitis C, antiviral therapy may be effective. Responses to interferon have been described. This lymphoma appears to be particularly responsive to rituximab.

Nodal marginal zone B-cell lymphoma is an indolent disorder that is usually associated with generalized lymphadenopathy. The clinical course and prognosis are similar to those of follicular lymphoma, and it is usually treated in a similar manner.

Small intestinal immunoproliferative disease, a disorder seen most frequently in the Middle East, begins as a polyclonal process and can progress to a large B-cell lymphoma. The process is often associated with *Campylobacter jejuni* infection. Early in the disease, patients may respond to antibiotics, and frank lymphoma may respond to combination chemotherapy regimens.

Mature T-Cell Lymphomas (Peripheral T-Cell Lymphomas)

Peripheral (or mature) T-cell lymphomas are neoplasms of post-thymic T cells. These include relatively indolent disorders such as mycosis fungoides and CD30$^+$ cutaneous lymphoproliferative disorders, but most patients diagnosed with peripheral T-cell lymphoma have an aggressive neoplasm. Peripheral T-cell lymphomas represent only 10% of the non-Hodgkin's lymphomas occurring in the United States. Unfortunately, the treatment for these lymphomas has not progressed as rapidly as the treatments for B-cell lymphomas.

MYCOSIS FUNGOIDES

Mycosis fungoides (often referred to as *cutaneous T-cell lymphoma*) is an indolent malignancy that is most common in middle-aged and older adults. The clinical course is usually a slow progression from isolated patches or plaques to thickened, more widespread plaques and then to multiple cutaneous tumors that may ulcerate (Chapter 446). A subset of patients presents with generalized erythroderma and circulating tumor cells, called *Sézary's syndrome*. Lymph node and visceral involvement may occur late in the course of the disease.

TREATMENT Rx

Cutaneous radiation therapy may be curative for patients with limited patch or plaque disease. Patients with early-stage disease (<10% body surface area) are frequently treated with skin-directed therapy that may include ultraviolet radiation, topical steroids, or topical nitrogen mustard.

Patients with more advanced disease frequently benefit from total skin electron beam therapy or extracorporeal photopheresis. Medical treatments include interferon-α, retinoids, monoclonal antibodies, histone deacetylase inhibitors (vorinostat, depsipeptide), the fusion toxin denileukin diftitox, and traditional cytotoxic chemotherapeutic agents; however, these treatments are usually only palliative. Results with autologous hematopoietic stem cell transplantation are usually poor, although allogeneic stem cell transplantation has yielded promising results in some cases.

ADULT T-CELL LYMPHOMA/LEUKEMIA

Adult T-cell lymphoma/leukemia, which is associated with HTLV-1 infection (Chapter 386), is most commonly seen in southern Japan and the Caribbean. Most infected patients are asymptomatic, and the lifetime risk of developing adult T-cell lymphoma/leukemia is approximately 3%.

Patients may have acute leukemia, aggressive lymphoma, or an indolent lymphoproliferative disease. Patients with aggressive disease present with generalized lymphadenopathy, hepatosplenomegaly, cutaneous infiltration, and hypercalcemia. Many patients have characteristic circulating tumor cells with a "flower" or "cloverleaf" nucleus.

TREATMENT Rx

Patients with indolent disease can sometimes be monitored without therapy. Aggressive disease is usually treated with combination chemotherapy, but there is no consensus on the best regimen. Historically, the 5-year survival rate has been less than 10%, although recent trials have reported better outcomes.

CD30$^+$ CUTANEOUS LYMPHOPROLIFERATIVE DISORDERS

These disorders represent a spectrum of diseases that may have an identical histologic appearance and overlapping clinical manifestations. Treatment decisions are often based on the clinical behavior of the lesions. These lymphomas express CD30 but do not express the anaplastic lymphoma kinase (ALK) protein (see later).

Lymphomatoid papulosis is a "histologically malignant" clonal disorder consisting of erythematous or skin-colored papules that frequently undergo spontaneous ulceration and necrosis over a period of weeks. The prognosis is excellent, although patients may eventually develop lymphoma.

Primary cutaneous anaplastic large cell lymphoma occurs most commonly in older men and also undergoes frequent spontaneous regression. The 5-year survival rate is greater than 90%. Treatment usually consists of local measures (surgery or radiation), although chemotherapy may be required.

PRIMARY SYSTEMIC ANAPLASTIC LARGE CELL LYMPHOMA

Anaplastic large cell lymphoma (ALCL) is an aggressive, CD30$^+$, T-cell non-Hodgkin's lymphoma that is seen most frequently in young males. B-cell lymphomas with similar morphology can occur, but they have clinical features identical to other diffuse large B-cell lymphomas and are not considered part of this disease. A morphologically similar but biologically unrelated and clinically distinct neoplasm, primary cutaneous ALCL, occurs predominantly in older adults and represents part of the spectrum of cutaneous CD30$^+$ lymphoproliferative disorders (see earlier). Primary systemic ALCL frequently has a t(2;5) chromosomal translocation that leads to overexpression of ALK, a protein not normally detectable in lymphoid cells.

Patients usually have lymphadenopathy, and involvement of the skin, bone, and gastrointestinal tract may be observed.

TREATMENT Rx

Patients are usually treated with chemotherapy regimens such as CHOP. Patients whose tumors express ALK have an excellent outcome, and 5-year survival rates of 70 to 90% have been observed. ALK-negative ALCL is more common in older patients and is associated with an inferior response rate and shorter survival time. Autologous hematopoietic stem cell transplantation may be curative for patients who relapse.

PERIPHERAL T-CELL LYMPHOMAS, UNSPECIFIED

The largest group of patients with peripheral T-cell lymphomas are defined in the WHO classification as having "peripheral T-cell lymphoma, unspecified." These patients' signs and symptoms are similar to those of patients with aggressive B-cell lymphomas, although systemic symptoms (fevers, night sweats, and weight loss) and extranodal involvement are frequent. The diagnosis of peripheral T-cell lymphoma requires immunophenotyping to demonstrate the T-cell origin.

TREATMENT 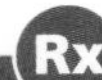

Patients are generally treated with the same regimens used for diffuse large B-cell lymphomas (e.g., CHOP), although the outcome is substantially worse (see Table 191-5). Patients who relapse after complete remission can sometimes be cured with hematopoietic stem cell transplantation.

UNUSUAL SUBTYPES OF T-CELL LYMPHOMA

Angioimmunoblastic T-cell lymphoma is associated with generalized lymphadenopathy, fever, weight loss, skin rash, and polyclonal hypergammaglobulinemia. Results of therapy are similar to those for peripheral T-cell lymphoma, unspecified.

Extranodal NK/T-cell lymphoma usually occurs in extranodal sites, especially the nose, palate, and nasopharynx. Involvement of the nose and face leads to the syndrome that was previously called lethal midline granuloma. This disorder is unusual in the United States, but it is frequent in Southeast Asia and Latin America. The prognosis is extremely poor, although patients with localized disease can sometimes be cured with aggressive combination radiation therapy and chemotherapy.

Hepatosplenic T-cell lymphoma is characterized by sinusoidal infiltration of the spleen, liver, and bone marrow, which leads to hepatosplenomegaly, systemic symptoms, and cytopenias. Lymphadenopathy is unusual. Patients are typically young males, and this disease can occur in allograft recipients and in the setting of immune dysfunction. The prognosis is poor, and remissions are rarely observed with chemotherapy.

Enteropathy-type T-cell lymphoma is usually seen in patients with gluten-sensitive enteropathy (Chapter 142). Patients typically present with abdominal pain and diarrhea and sometimes with bowel perforation. Treatment of celiac disease with a gluten-free diet appears to reduce the risk of lymphoma. The prognosis in these often undernourished patients is poor.

Subcutaneous panniculitis-like T-cell lymphoma manifests with multiple subcutaneous nodules and is often misdiagnosed as panniculitis. Patients with disseminated disease can have a syndrome consisting of fevers, weight loss, hepatosplenomegaly, pancytopenia, and phagocytosis of blood cells (hemophagocytic syndrome). Patients sometimes respond to combination chemotherapy regimens used for diffuse large B-cell lymphoma, interferon, and radiation therapy, but long-term disease-free survival is unusual.

SPECIAL CLINICAL SITUATIONS

The diagnosis and management of patients with the various types of non-Hodgkin's lymphoma can be profoundly influenced by the site of origin of the lymphoma and by certain clinical characteristics of the patients. Examples of the latter include pregnant patients with lymphoma, elderly patients with lymphoma, and lymphoma in patients who are severely immunosuppressed.

Specific Primary Sites of Diffuse Large B-Cell Lymphoma

Approximately 30% of diffuse large B-cell lymphomas originate in extranodal sites. Presentation in certain extranodal sites is associated with unique clinical behaviors that may necessitate diagnostic studies or additional therapy beyond that used for patients with nodal presentations.

Patients with primary CNS lymphoma (Chapter 195) commonly have ocular involvement, and all patients with this diagnosis should have a slit lamp examination. Surgical resection of primary CNS lymphoma is not beneficial, and the only role for surgery is in diagnosis. Primary lymphomas of the CNS are very sensitive to corticosteroids, but the best results have been observed with chemotherapy regimens that use high-dose methotrexate alone or in combination with other agents such as cytarabine. By comparison, conventional chemotherapy regimens, such as CHOP, are of little benefit. Whole brain irradiation is also effective therapy, although the incidence of leukoencephalopathy is extremely high, especially in elderly patients. Radiation therapy is frequently reserved for relapse rather than being used as adjunctive treatment with primary chemotherapy.

Treatment of primary testicular lymphoma, the most common testicular cancer in men older than 60 years (Chapter 206), usually consists of orchiectomy followed by combination chemotherapy. Relapse in the contralateral testicle is common, and most oncologists recommend adjuvant radiation to the scrotum. CNS involvement is common, and prophylactic intrathecal chemotherapy is usually recommended. Late relapses occur frequently.

Diffuse large B-cell lymphoma of the stomach and gastrointestinal tract is treated differently from gastric MALT lymphoma, even if there is a history of prior MALT lymphoma. Patients can be cured with surgery and adjunctive radiation or chemotherapy, although surgery is rarely performed for gastric lymphomas because of the morbidity associated with gastric resection. Patients should be treated with chemotherapy regimens used for other diffuse large B-cell lymphomas. Radiation therapy is sometimes used after chemotherapy, although the role of combined-modality treatment is not defined.

Lymphoma in AIDS and Post-Transplantation Lymphoproliferative Disorders

Non-Hodgkin's lymphoma is an AIDS-defining illness in HIV-infected individuals (Chapter 400), and the risk of developing a non-Hodgkin's lymphoma is increased more than 150-fold after the diagnosis of another AIDS-defining illness. Most cases are diffuse large B-cell lymphomas or Burkitt's lymphomas. AIDS-associated lymphomas behave aggressively and frequently involve the CNS and other unusual sites, such as the gastrointestinal tract, anus, rectum, skin, and soft tissue (Chapter 400). Factors associated with poor survival include low CD4 counts, poor performance status, older age, and advanced stage. The prognosis of these lymphomas is poor, with median survival times of approximately 6 months in the absence of concomitant aggressive therapy for HIV. If chemotherapy is given in association with highly active antiretroviral agents to patients with a good performance status, the likelihood of controlling the lymphoma is similar to that in patients without HIV infection. Intrathecal prophylaxis is generally recommended because of a higher risk of CNS involvement.

The risk of developing a non-Hodgkin's lymphoma is also markedly increased in patients who have received a solid organ transplant. The histologic appearance of these lymphomas is variable, but they frequently resemble aggressive lymphomas in nonimmunocompromised patients. Similar disorders can be seen in patients who are treated with methotrexate and other drugs for autoimmune disorders and in recipients of allogeneic hematopoietic stem cell transplants, especially if the transplants are T-cell depleted. These post-transplantation lymphoproliferative disorders, which may develop within weeks after surgery, are more common in patients who receive aggressive immunosuppression after transplantation. Involvement of extranodal sites is common, and lymphoma frequently involves the transplanted organ. Post-transplantation lymphoproliferative disorders may respond to reduction or withdrawal of immunosuppression. Some investigators have advocated the use of acyclovir or ganciclovir, because these lymphomas are usually related to EBV, but this practice is controversial. High response rates are also seen with rituximab. Other patients require treatment with combination chemotherapy regimens.

Non-Hodgkin's Lymphoma in Elderly Patients

More than 50% of patients who develop non-Hodgkin's lymphomas are older than 60 years, and the prognosis is generally worse for elderly patients. These poorer outcomes are related to increased toxicity of drug therapy, lower remission rates, increased rates of relapse, and higher death rates from cardiovascular disease and causes other than the lymphoma itself. Older patients are more likely to have other adverse prognostic characteristics (see Table 191-8), which also contribute to poorer outcomes. The practice of arbitrary dose reductions based solely on age should be discouraged if patients have a good performance status and no comorbid illnesses.[6]

Non-Hodgkin's Lymphoma and Pregnancy

Non-Hodgkin's lymphoma in pregnancy involves major clinical and ethical issues, and a multidisciplinary approach is needed (Chapter 247). Although chest radiographs are generally considered safe, ultrasound examination is usually used instead of CT for staging in the abdomen and pelvis.

Treatment can occasionally be delayed until after delivery; however, most women have a tumor that is potentially curable, and treatment delays may decrease the chance for cure. Other patients have conditions such as superior vena cava syndrome that require immediate treatment. After the first trimester, full-dose standard therapy such as CHOP-R may be used; several studies indicate high probabilities of cure without adverse long-term physical or intellectual deficits for the child. Although it is reasonable to offer therapeutic abortion for women in the first trimester, chemotherapy may also be successful in this situation. Regimens using methotrexate must be avoided.

DISEASES SOMETIMES CONFUSED WITH LYMPHOMA

The most common atypical lymphoid proliferations that can be confused with lymphoma are florid reactions to immune stimulation. Follicular hyperplasia with diffuse proliferation of B cells and T cells can be seen in a variety of autoimmune diseases (e.g., Sjögren's syndrome, systemic lupus erythematosus, rheumatoid arthritis) and infectious processes (e.g., EBV, cytomegalovirus, cat-scratch disease) (Chapter 171). If the definitive diagnosis of lymphoma cannot be made even after immunologic and molecular studies, the patient should be closely observed. The clinical course or subsequent biopsies can usually resolve the confusion.

Castleman's disease, or angiofollicular lymph node hyperplasia, usually appears with a hyaline vascular pattern of lymphoid proliferation, but a subset of patients has hyperplastic lymphoid follicles and sheets of plasma cells. Patients with Castleman's disease often present with a localized lymphoid mass, but some patients have a systemic illness with fevers, night sweats, weight loss, and fatigue. Frequently, the systemic symptoms of Castleman's disease are related to excessive production of interleukin-6 (IL-6). Castleman's disease in HIV-infected patients is frequently associated with HHV-8. Patients with disseminated and plasma cell–rich forms of Castleman's disease may occasionally progress to lymphoma. Patients with localized Castleman's disease can be treated with surgical removal or radiation therapy. Patients with systemic disease may respond to treatment with high-dose corticosteroids. Patients with overexpression of IL-6 frequently benefit from treatment with an anti–IL-6 antibody. If other treatments fail, patients sometimes benefit from combination chemotherapy regimens, autologous or allogeneic hematopoietic stem cell transplantation, or both.

Sinus histiocytosis with massive lymphadenopathy, also known as *Rosai-Dorfman disease,* manifests as bulky lymphadenopathy in children and young adults. Extranodal sites such as the skin, upper airways, gastrointestinal tract, and CNS can be involved. The disease is usually self-limited, but it has been associated with autoimmune hemolytic anemia.

Kikuchi's disease (histiocytic necrotizing lymphadenitis) is a disease of unknown origin that most commonly affects young women. Symptoms most commonly consist of painless cervical lymphadenopathy that is often accompanied by fever, flu-like symptoms, and rash. Treatment is symptomatic, and manifestations usually resolve within weeks or months.

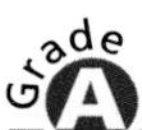

1. Salles G, Seymour JF, Offner F, et al. Rituximab maintenance for 2 years in patients with high tumour burden follicular lymphoma responding to rituximab plus chemotherapy (PRIMA): a phase 3, randomised controlled trial. *Lancet.* 2011;377:42-51.
2. Azim HA, Santoro L, Bociek RG, et al. High dose intensity doxorubicin in aggressive non-Hodgkin's lymphoma: a literature-based meta-analysis. *Ann Oncol.* 2010;21:1064-1071.
3. Baldo P, Rupolo M, Compagnoni A, et al. Interferon-alpha for maintenance of follicular lymphoma. *Cochrane Database Syst Rev.* 2010;1:CD004629.
4. Persky DO, Unger JM, Spier CM, et al. Phase II study of rituximab plus three cycles of CHOP and involved-field radiotherapy for patients with limited-stage aggressive B-cell lymphoma: Southwest Oncology Group study 0014. *J Clin Oncol.* 2008;26:2258-2263.
5. Pfreundschuh M, Trumper L, Osterborg A, et al. CHOP-like chemotherapy plus rituximab versus CHOP-like chemotherapy alone in young patients with good-prognosis diffuse large-B-cell lymphoma: a randomized controlled trial by the MabThera International Trial (MInT) Group. *Lancet Oncol.* 2006;7:379-391.
6. Pfreundschuh M, Schubert J, Ziepert M, et al. Six versus eight cycles of bi-weekly CHOP-14 with or without rituximab in elderly patients with aggressive $CD20^+$ B-cell lymphomas: a randomized controlled trial (RICOVER-60). *Lancet Oncol.* 2008;9:105-116.

SUGGESTED READINGS

Chan WC, Armitage JO. Genomic analysis of lymphoma: potential for clinical application. *J Natl Compr Canc Netw.* 2010;8:353-360. *Review of the application of gene expression profiling to the diagnosis and treatment of lymphomas.*

Lenz G, Staudt LM. Aggressive lymphomas. *N Engl J Med.* 2010;362:1417-1429. *Recent progress in the molecular genetics of aggressive lymphomas, focusing on the most common form of this disease: diffuse large B-cell lymphoma.*

Pirani M, Marcheselli R, Marcheselli L, et al. Risk for second malignancies in non-Hodgkin's lymphoma survivors: a meta-analysis. *Ann Oncol.* 2011. [Epub ahead of print.] *Review showing a 1.9-fold increased risk.*

Schultz CJ, Bovi J. Current management of primary central nervous system lymphoma. *Int J Radiat Oncol Biol Phys.* 2010;76:666-678. *Review of most effective whole brain radiation therapy and chemotherapy regimens and the limited role of surgery.*

Tay K, Dunleavy K, Wilson WH. Novel agents for B-cell non-Hodgkin lymphoma: science and the promise. *Blood Rev.* 2010;24:69-82. *Novel agents for lymphoma, including immunotherapy and small molecules.*

192

HODGKIN'S LYMPHOMA

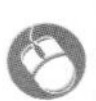

JOSEPH M. CONNORS

DEFINITION

Hodgkin's lymphoma, formerly called Hodgkin's disease, is one of the B-cell lymphomas. It has a characteristic neoplastic cell, the Hodgkin-Reed-Sternberg cell, a distinct natural history, and most important, an excellent response to treatment, with the large majority of patients being cured. Its management, which requires careful multidisciplinary cooperation, serves as a paradigm for the successful application of modern oncologic concepts. Highly effective chemotherapy is the cornerstone of treatment. Carefully selected patients may require the addition of radiation or, if the lymphoma recurs after primary treatment, high-dose chemoradiation therapy and autologous hematologic stem cell transplantation (HDC/HSCT). The current challenge to clinicians managing this neoplasm is to cure the disease while minimizing long-term toxicity.

EPIDEMIOLOGY

The incidence of Hodgkin's lymphoma varies substantially around the world. The highest rates occur in the United States, Canada, Switzerland, and northern Europe. Intermediate rates are seen in southern and eastern Europe and low rates in eastern Asia. No clear explanation for this variation in incidence has been found. Postulated reasons include differences in the age at onset or genotype of any associated Epstein-Barr virus (EBV) infection; crowding during childhood as a result of lower socioeconomic status, predisposing to passage of an as yet undiscovered infectious vector; and intrinsic genetic differences in susceptibility.

Approximately 20,000 new cases are seen annually in North America and Europe. The age-adjusted incidence of Hodgkin's lymphoma declined modestly over the 20 years before 1990 at a rate of approximately 0.9% per year but has leveled off since then and is now approximately 2.7 per 100,000. Age-adjusted annual mortality is 0.5 per 100,000. Hodgkin's lymphoma occurs slightly more often in men and is seen more frequently in whites than African Americans and much less frequently in Asian populations. Much of the difference in incidence between whites and blacks in North America can be attributed to the higher incidence seen in higher socioeconomic classes. The cumulative lifetime risk for development of Hodgkin's lymphoma is approximately 1 in 250 to 1 in 300 in North America.

The incidence of Hodgkin's lymphoma rises from a very low level in childhood to a plateau in early adulthood and then remains stable. In the Western world, only about 5% of cases occur in persons younger than 15 years and 5% in persons older than 70 years. In contrast, however, the age distribution in the Indian subcontinent is strongly shifted into childhood.

PATHOBIOLOGY

The cause of Hodgkin's lymphoma remains unclear. Hodgkin's lymphoma is not associated with exposure to radiation, chemicals, biocidal agents, working in health care–related professions, or previous tonsillectomy. The leading suspect remains EBV, based on much suggestive evidence but no definitive proof.

Epstein-Barr Virus

EBV is a large B-lymphocyte tropic herpesvirus (Chapter 385). Approximately 90% of the general population acquires infection with EBV by early adulthood. In the developing world, this infection usually occurs in childhood, but in developed countries, infection is often delayed into the teens, when it is associated with the syndrome of infectious mononucleosis in up to 30% of new cases. A history of infectious mononucleosis increases the likelihood for subsequent Hodgkin's lymphoma three-fold. Antibodies to the viral capsid antigen reach higher levels in patients with Hodgkin's lymphoma than in controls, and these higher levels appear several years before the neoplasm. In situ hybridization studies have demonstrated that the Hodgkin-Reed-Sternberg cells in approximately 50% of cases of Hodgkin's lymphoma contain EBV-encoded small RNA (EBER), and in these cases, virtually all the Hodgkin-Reed-Sternberg cells are positive for the virus. The EBV genome is amplified 50-fold or more in Hodgkin-Reed-Sternberg cells and is monoclonal in an individual patient's Hodgkin-Reed-Sternberg cells. In some populations, virtually all cases of Hodgkin's lymphoma occur in EBV-positive individuals, but up to 50% of patients in developed countries do not have EBV in their Hodgkin-Reed-Sternberg cells. Thus, although EBV may play an important role in the development of Hodgkin's lymphoma, that role is neither straightforward nor universal.

Genetic Factors

Circumstantial evidence for a genetic contribution to the etiology of Hodgkin's lymphoma comes from studies showing that Hodgkin's lymphoma is almost 100-fold more likely to develop in the monozygotic twin of an affected individual than in a dizygotic twin. First-degree relatives of individuals with the disease have up to a five-fold increased risk for development of the lymphoma. Perhaps genetically predisposed individuals react differently to EBV, thereby increasing the chance that a lymphoid neoplasm will develop.

Polymerase chain reaction–based genotypic analysis has demonstrated the clonal derivation of Hodgkin-Reed-Sternberg cells, including identical *p53* mutations from multiple Hodgkin-Reed-Sternberg cells extracted from a single biopsy specimen, thereby unequivocally establishing clonality. The presence of clonal immunoglobulin gene rearrangements from multiple cells in the same biopsy specimen also confirms a B-cell origin. Only a few rare cases with a T-cell genotype have been reported, but these are obviously exceptional. The presence of clonal somatic mutations provides proof of the germinal center origin of the neoplastic cells. Finally, identification of cells with identical immunoglobulin gene rearrangements both at diagnosis and at relapse verify that the B-cell clonality of the disease is preserved over time.

Despite their B-cell origin, the neoplastic cells of Hodgkin's lymphoma are incapable of making intact antibodies, perhaps because they lack the ability to make the transcription factors necessary to activate the immunoglobulin promoter. B cells that are incapable of manufacturing antibody should undergo apoptosis, but the Hodgkin-Reed-Sternberg cells avoid this self-destruction. The observation that the antiapoptotic nuclear transcription factor NFκB is constitutively activated in these cells may provide an explanation.

Classic cytogenetics has been unrevealing in Hodgkin's lymphoma. Aneuploidy and hyperploidy consistent with the multinucleated nature of Hodgkin-Reed-Sternberg cells are frequent, but no consistent translocations have been detected.

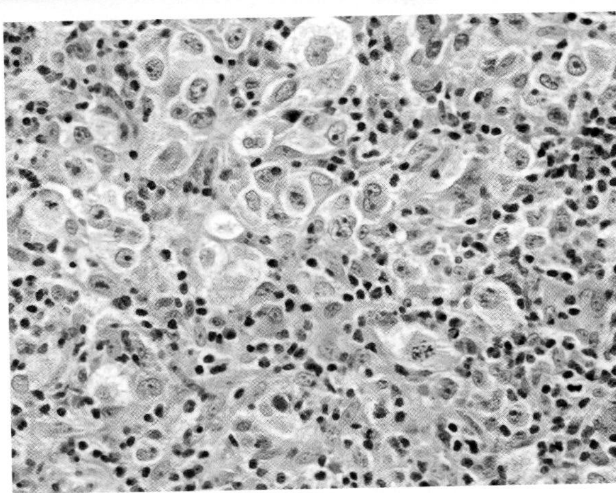

FIGURE 192-1. Nodular sclerosing Hodgkin's lymphoma. This figure shows a typical case of classic nodular sclerosing Hodgkin's lymphoma with many lacunar cells, occasional diagnostic Hodgkin-Reed-Sternberg cells, and the characteristic background of lymphocytes and eosinophils. (Photomicrograph courtesy of Randy D. Gascoyne, MD, British Columbia Cancer Agency.)

TABLE 192-1 WORLD HEALTH ORGANIZATION CLASSIFICATION OF HODGKIN'S LYMPHOMA SUBTYPES

SUBTYPE NAME	FREQUENCY (%)*
Classic Hodgkin's lymphoma	
Nodular sclerosis	70
Lymphocyte rich	3
Mixed cellularity	10
Lymphocyte depleted	1
Nodular lymphocyte-predominant Hodgkin's lymphoma	7
Hodgkin's lymphoma, not otherwise classifiable	9

*Frequency based on all new cases ($N = 1043$) seen in British Columbia since January 1998 when the category of lymphocyte-rich classic Hodgkin's lymphoma became well established.

CLINICAL MANIFESTATIONS

Hodgkin's lymphoma is usually manifested as lymphadenopathy (Chapter 171), typically in the cervical, axillary, or mediastinal areas, and only about 10% of the time as nodal disease below the diaphragm. Although peripherally located nodes seldom reach large size, very large mediastinal masses or, less often, retroperitoneal masses can develop with only modest symptoms. Lymph node involvement in Hodgkin's lymphoma is usually painless, but an occasional patient notes discomfort in involved nodal sites immediately after drinking alcohol.

Approximately 25% of patients with Hodgkin's lymphoma have constitutional symptoms. The classic B symptoms, significant weight loss (>10% of baseline), night sweats, and persistent fever, usually signal widespread or locally extensive disease and imply a need for systemic treatment. Generalized pruritus, occasionally severe, can antedate the diagnosis of Hodgkin's lymphoma by up to several years. Some patients have symptoms suggestive of a growing mass lesion, such as cough or stridor as a result of tracheobronchial compression from mediastinal disease or bone pain secondary to metastatic involvement. Because Hodgkin's lymphoma can involve the bone marrow extensively, an occasional patient has symptomatic anemia or incidentally noted pancytopenia. Paraneoplastic neurologic or endocrine syndromes have been reported with Hodgkin's lymphoma but are rare.

DIAGNOSIS

The diagnosis of Hodgkin's lymphoma is based on recognition of Hodgkin-Reed-Sternberg cells (Fig. 192-1) or Hodgkin's cells (or both) in an appropriate cellular background in tissue sections from a lymph node or extralymphatic organ, such as bone marrow, lung, or bone. Fine-needle aspiration biopsy is not adequate for the diagnosis of Hodgkin's lymphoma. Open biopsy and standard histochemical staining are required to establish the diagnosis unequivocally and to determine the histologic subtype. Immunohistochemical studies can prove helpful in difficult cases or to distinguish special subtypes such as lymphocyte-rich classic Hodgkin's lymphoma and the nodular lymphocyte-predominant type. In classic Hodgkin's lymphoma, scattered large Hodgkin-Reed-Sternberg cells either are multinucleated or have large polyploid nuclei. Variations include mononuclear cells that are similar to the usual polylobated or multinuclear cells but have only one large nucleus with a prominent nucleolus, as well as lacunar cells, which are Hodgkin-Reed-Sternberg variants with abundant cytoplasm that has retracted as an artifact of formalin fixation. The infrequent Hodgkin-Reed-Sternberg cells are usually present in a background mixture of polyclonal lymphocytes, eosinophils, neutrophils, plasma cells, fibroblasts, and histiocytes. Recently, a high number of associated macrophages have been demonstrated to be a strong predictor of treatment resistance. Occasionally, granulomas form with a prominent histiocytic component.

Hodgkin's lymphoma can typically be classified into one of five well-described subtypes (Table 192-1). Reproducibility of the distinctions among these subtypes has been confirmed in the current widely accepted World Health Organization classification of lymphoid neoplasms. With addition of the new category of lymphocyte-rich classic Hodgkin's lymphoma, this newest classification scheme permits confident identification of nodular lymphocyte-predominant Hodgkin's lymphoma as a separate entity. The most common subtype is nodular sclerosing, which has characteristic course bands of sclerosis surrounding nodules composed of typical Hodgkin-Reed-Sternberg cells in the usual background mixture of reactive and inflammatory cells.

The immunophenotype of the neoplastic cells in Hodgkin's lymphoma can help identify the specific subtype. Typically, the Hodgkin-Reed-Sternberg cells stain positively for CD30 (80 to 100% of cases), CD15 (75 to 85% of cases), and B-cell-specific activating protein (BSAP), which is the product of the *PAX5* gene (>90% of cases). However, often only a minority of the malignant cells stain positively for the CD15 and BSAP markers. CD20, a generally reliable marker of B-cell lineage, is positive in about 40% of cases of classic

Hodgkin's lymphoma, but usually only in a minority of cells, and the staining can be weak. In contrast, nodular lymphocyte-predominant Hodgkin's lymphoma almost always stains strongly positive for CD20 and for the specialized B-cell markers CD79a and CD45, but it is negative for CD30 and CD15. Finally, anaplastic large cell lymphoma (Chapter 191) is reliably negative for CD15, CD20, and CD79a but frequently positive for anaplastic lymphoma kinase (ALK).

Differential Diagnosis

Depending on the site of occurrence and associated symptoms, the differential diagnosis of Hodgkin's lymphoma includes non-Hodgkin's lymphoma (Chapter 191), germ cell tumors (Chapter 206), thymoma (Chapter 430), sarcoidosis (Chapter 95), and tuberculosis (Chapter 332). However, the specific diagnosis is readily determined by obtaining an adequate biopsy specimen for review by an experienced hematopathologist. Proceeding to such a biopsy early in the assessment of patients with lymphadenopathy (Chapter 171), especially of the mediastinum, often saves time and spares the patient needless testing and delay in diagnosis.

With computed tomography (CT) and appropriate biopsy procedures to investigate enlarged central thoracic or intra-abdominal lymph nodes, the diagnosis of Hodgkin's lymphoma seldom presents difficulty. The immunophenotype helps distinguish Hodgkin's lymphoma from other diseases. For example, T-cell-rich B-cell lymphoma (Chapter 191) is distinguished from classic Hodgkin's lymphoma by being CD30 and CD15 negative but positive for CD20 and CD45. However, T-cell-rich B-cell lymphoma (Chapter 191) can be very difficult to distinguish from nodular lymphocyte-predominant Hodgkin's lymphoma because both are negative for CD30 and CD15 but positive for CD45. This distinction is best made by focusing on the histologic pattern of the neoplastic cells. In fact, the combination of appropriate immunohistopathologic evaluation by an expert hematopathologist and clinical assessment has virtually eliminated difficulties with the differential diagnosis. Problems mostly arise when inadequate or improperly processed material is all that is available for diagnosis.

Staging

Physical Examination

Given its tendency to spread in an orderly fashion, usually from initially involved lymph nodes, the stage of Hodgkin's lymphoma can be established by using readily available imaging and laboratory tests (Fig. 192-2 and Table 192-2). The evaluation should start with a careful history to search for the presence of localizing signs, such as bone pain, or the constitutional symptoms of fever, weight loss, or night sweats. The history may also reveal comorbid conditions that may affect the safe delivery of planned treatment. The physical examination may identify lymphadenopathy or organomegaly.

Laboratory Testing

Laboratory testing should include blood cell counts and the erythrocyte sedimentation rate, assessment of liver and renal function, serum albumin level, serum protein electrophoresis, and serologic testing for hepatitis B. Also, the patient should be tested for hepatitis C if liver enzyme abnormalities are detected and human immunodeficiency virus (HIV) antibody if the history indicates an increased risk or if the sites of disease are unusual. Bone marrow aspiration and biopsy are only useful for the minority of patients with constitutional (B) symptoms or those with lower than normal peripheral blood counts at diagnosis.

Imaging

Imaging techniques to evaluate Hodgkin's lymphoma continue to evolve (Fig. 192-3). All patients should undergo contrast-enhanced CT scanning of the thorax, abdomen, and pelvis with slices at intervals of 1 cm or less. Magnetic resonance imaging is occasionally useful when the extent of bone or soft tissue involvement must be determined precisely or for a patient with an absolute contraindication to the use of intravenous contrast agents.

Positron Emission Tomography

Positron emission tomography (PET) is more sensitive and specific than CT or gallium scanning both for staging and for assessment of residual masses after treatment. However, it has not been proved that the addition of PET to standard staging imaging tests for Hodgkin's lymphoma will actually improve outcome, so whether PET could replace other studies is not clear. The greatest usefulness of PET presently appears to be the assessment of residual masses during or after planned treatment so that the minority of patients who should receive altered or additional therapy, especially radiotherapy, can be identified.

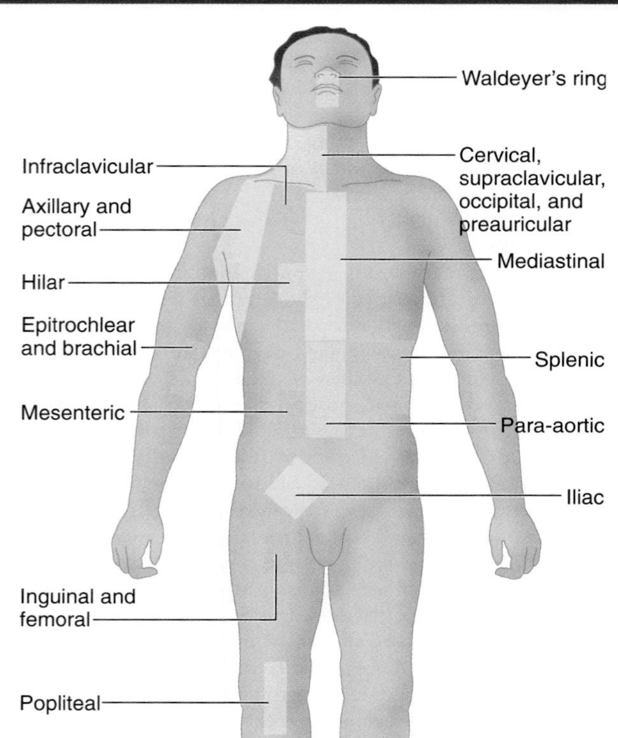

FIGURE 192-2. Anatomic definition of lymph node regions for staging of Hodgkin's disease. (From Kaplan HS, Rosenberg SA. The treatment of Hodgkin's disease. *Med Clin North Am.* 1966;50:1591-1610.)

TABLE 192-2 TESTS REQUIRED FOR STAGING OF HODGKIN'S LYMPHOMA

Complete history to search for B symptoms (fever, weight loss, night sweats) or other symptomatic problems suggesting more advanced disease
Physical examination for lymphadenopathy or organomegaly
Complete blood count
Serum creatinine, alkaline phosphatase, lactate dehydrogenase, bilirubin, and protein electrophoresis (including serum albumin level)
Chest radiograph, posteroanterior and lateral views
Computed tomography scan of the neck, thorax, abdomen, and pelvis
Certain tests are required only for specific manifestations

MANIFESTATION/CONDITION	TEST
B symptoms or WBC count <4.0 × 10^9/L, Hgb <120 g/L (women) or 130 g/L (men), or platelets <125 × 10^9/L	Bone marrow biopsy and aspiration
Stage IA or IIA disease with upper cervical lymph node involvement (suprahyoid)	ENT examination

ENT = ear, nose, and throat; Hgb = hemoglobin; WBC = white blood cell.

Staging System

The Ann Arbor staging system with the Cotswold modification (Table 192-3) categorizes patients into four stages. The first three indicate the expanding extent of lymph node disease (see Fig. 192-2): stage I, a single nodal area; stage II, two or more nodal areas but still on one side of the diaphragm; and stage III, nodal disease on both sides of the diaphragm. The spleen and the lymphoid tissue of Waldeyer's ring each count as nodal sites in this system. Stage IV is reserved for extranodal disease, which for all practical purposes is disease in the bone marrow, lung, bone, or liver. Hodgkin's lymphoma at any other extranodal site should prompt questioning of the diagnosis or a search for HIV infection.

Bulky disease is defined as the presence of any tumor mass with the largest diameter greater than 10 cm or a mediastinal mass with a transverse diameter exceeding one third of the largest transverse transthoracic diameter. With CT scanning, use of the mediastinal mass ratio is obsolete, and the term *bulky* is best assigned to tumors exceeding 10 cm in largest single diameter.

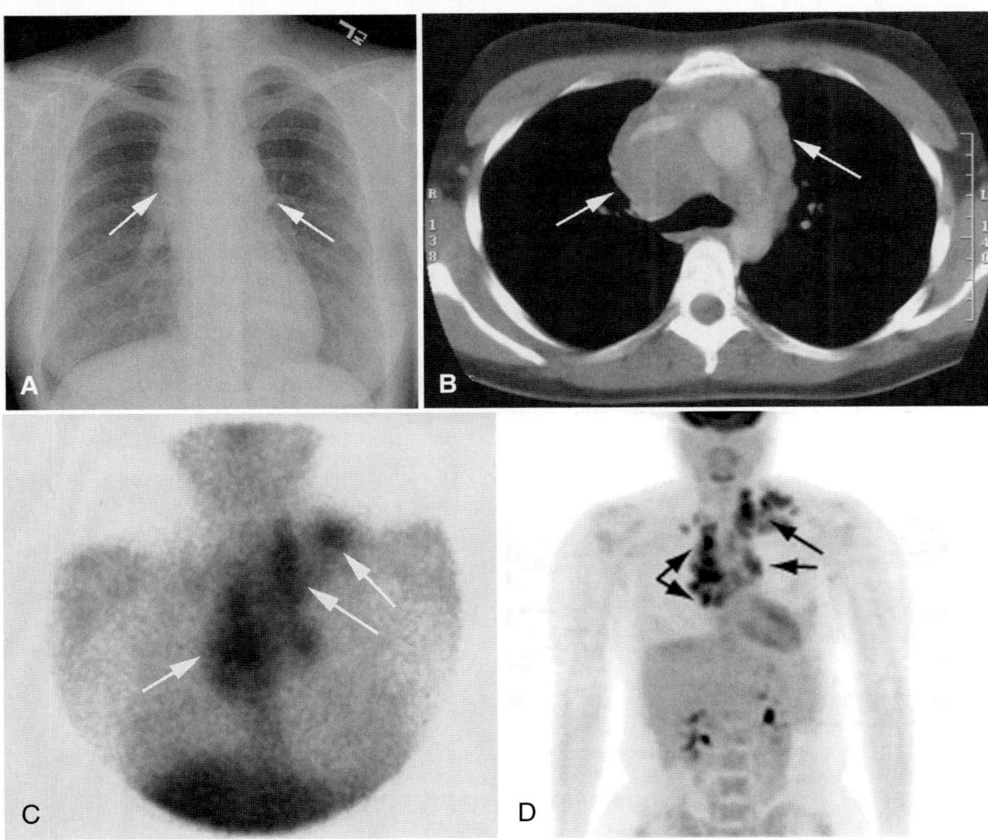

FIGURE 192-3. **Imaging of Hodgkin's lymphoma.** Bulky Hodgkin's disease as seen on chest radiograph (**A**), computed tomography (CT) of the chest (**B**), gallium scan (**C**), and positron emission tomography (PET) (**D**). The *arrows* indicate sites of disease. Note that the PET and CT scans provide more detailed information than the chest radiograph and gallium scan.

TABLE 192-3 MODIFIED ANN ARBOR STAGING SYSTEM FOR HODGKIN'S LYMPHOMA

STAGE	INVOLVEMENT
I	Single lymph node region (I) or one extralymphatic site (I_E)
II	Two or more lymph node regions, same side of the diaphragm (II), or local extralymphatic extension plus one or more lymph node regions, same side of the diaphragm (II_E)
III	Lymph node regions on both sides of the diaphragm (III); may be accompanied by local extralymphatic extension (III_E)
IV	Diffuse involvement of one or more extralymphatic organs or sites
A	No "B" symptoms
B	Presence of at least one of the following: Unexplained weight loss >10% of baseline during 6 mo before staging Recurrent unexplained fever >38° C Recurrent night sweats

TABLE 192-4 RATES OF PROGRESSION IN 5 YEARS IN PATIENTS WITH ADVANCED-STAGE HODGKIN'S LYMPHOMA

NO. OF FACTORS*	FREQUENCY (%)	PERCENTAGE WITH PROGRESSION-FREE SURVIVAL AT 5 YEARS
0-3	81	70
4-7	19	47

*Male sex, age older than 45 years, stage IV, hemoglobin level less than 10.5 g/dL, white blood cell count greater than 15,000/mL, lymphocyte count less than 600/mL or less than 8% of the white cell count, or serum albumin less than 4 g/dL.

The E lesion designation identifies patients whose limited extranodal extension of Hodgkin's lymphoma could be included in a reasonable involved field of irradiation. After staging, patients are further subdivided into those with or without fever, night sweats, or weight loss (B symptoms).

TREATMENT

Rx

Over the past 60 years, Hodgkin's lymphoma has been transformed from a nearly uniformly fatal illness to one that is usually cured. This remarkable success has provided a paradigm on which much of modern oncologic treatment is based. The principles underlying combined-modality treatment and multiagent chemotherapy, the mainstays of today's successful treatment of many malignancies, were first demonstrated to be effective with Hodgkin's lymphoma. The essential involvement of a multidisciplinary team, including pathologists, experts in diagnostic imaging, medical and radiation oncologists, nurses, and support staff, has served as a model for all cancer. The necessity to balance greater efficacy of initial treatment, which often requires an increase in intensity and therefore toxicity, against troublesome and occasionally fatal late complications has encouraged a long-term perspective.

From a practical therapeutic viewpoint, patients with stage III or IV disease, bulky disease, or B symptoms are defined as having advanced disease, whereas patients without these characteristics have limited-stage disease. In Europe, patients with limited disease are further subdivided into those with favorable and unfavorable outcomes, but cure rates exceed 90 to 95% for all patients with nonbulky stage IA or IIA (limited) disease. However, for patients with advanced-stage disease, independent predictors of progression include gender, age, stage, hemoglobin level, white blood cell count, lymphocyte count, and serum albumin level (Table 192-4). Based on results obtained in the 1980s, the 80% of patients with fewer than four factors had a progression-free survival of 70%, but for the 20% who had four or more factors, the progression-free survival rate fell to less than 50%. However, with better attention to dose delivery, more current results indicate a spread of only 80% to 60% between these two groups. A straightforward plan of treatment for the 90% of patients in whom Hodgkin's lymphoma is diagnosed between the ages of 16 and 70 years can be based on clinical stage, the presence of B symptoms, and bulk of the largest tumor mass (Table 192-5).

Treatment of Limited-Stage Hodgkin's Lymphoma

More than 95% of the one third of patients with Hodgkin's lymphoma initially found to have limited-stage disease can be cured regardless of the site

TABLE 192-5 TREATMENT PLAN FOR ADULT PATIENTS WITH HODGKIN'S LYMPHOMA

STAGE	PROGNOSTIC CATEGORY	TREATMENT
IA or IIA, no bulky disease*		ABVD‡ × 4 if CR after 2 cycles or ABVD × 2 + IRRT
IB, IIB, or any stage III or IV or bulky disease, any stage	≤3 adverse factors†	ABVD‡ until 2 cycles past CR (minimum 6, maximum 8)
	≥4 adverse factors†	Escalated BEACOPP‡

*Bulky refers to disease with the largest diameter of any single mass equal to or greater than 10 cm.
†See Table 192-4 note.
‡See text for drugs in each regimen. Optimal dosing must be individualized.
CR = complete response; IRRT = involved-region radiation therapy.

of occurrence, the presence of disease above or below the diaphragm, or the histologic subtype. The challenge is to achieve this goal with the least toxicity and cost.

Two cycles of ABVD (Adriamycin [doxorubicin], bleomycin, vinblastine, and dacarbazine) chemotherapy followed by involved-field irradiation cures nearly 95% of patients with limited-stage disease and nearly completely eliminates the risk for infertility, premature menopause, and leukemia and minimizes cardiopulmonary toxicity.[1-3] The chemotherapy in the combined-modality treatment of limited-stage Hodgkin's lymphoma eradicates subclinical disease and allows smaller fields of irradiation to be used. However, a substantial proportion of the excess, long-term mortality in patients with limited-stage Hodgkin's lymphoma is due to cardiovascular disease and second neoplasms that are closely related to the use of irradiation. In a randomized trial that compared four to six cycles of ABVD chemotherapy alone versus irradiation, either alone or augmented with two cycles of ABVD chemotherapy, the strategy of chemotherapy alone proved equivalent to irradiation-based treatment in terms of event-free and overall survival, although the irradiation-based approach did produce a modest improvement in progression-free survival.[4] Longer follow-up will be necessary to see whether the goal of a reduction in cardiovascular events and second neoplasms was accomplished. This trial suggests that more than 90% of patients with limited-stage Hodgkin's lymphoma can be treated with four to six cycles of ABVD alone; for the minority whose lymphoma does not completely regress after two cycles, probably best assessed by PET scanning, the addition of radiation may be optimum.

Treatment of Advanced-Stage Hodgkin's Lymphoma

In advanced-stage Hodgkin's lymphoma (stages IIIA, IIIB, IVA, and IVB), both ABVD and MOPP (mechlorethamine, Oncovin [vincristine], procarbazine, and prednisone)/ABVD are superior to MOPP alone in terms of progression-free survival. Today, ABVD is the most widely used regimen for patients with advanced-stage Hodgkin's lymphoma. The addition of radiation therapy significantly improves progression-free survival at 10 years in patients with advanced-stage Hodgkin's lymphoma, but it does not improve overall survival because it causes significantly more deaths unrelated to lymphoma. Even the addition of radiation therapy for patients in complete remission after chemotherapy for advanced-stage Hodgkin's lymphoma has no significant impact. The adverse long-term effects of radiation therapy and its lack of improvement in overall survival appear to outweigh any benefits for the usual patient with advanced-stage disease. The ability of PET scanning to distinguish between residual fibrosis and persistent lymphoma may provide a mechanism to identify selected patients who might benefit from localized radiation therapy.

Recently devised regimens for patients with advanced Hodgkin's lymphoma are the Stanford V regimen (doxorubicin, vinblastine, mechlorethamine, etoposide, vincristine, bleomycin, and prednisone) and escalated BEACOPP (bleomycin, etoposide, doxorubicin, cyclophosphamide, vincristine, prednisone, and procarbazine) (see Table 192-5). As originally described, both include postchemotherapy irradiation to sites of initial or residual tumor bulk (≥5 cm). Although initial results appeared quite promising, recent results indicate that the Stanford V regimen is no more effective than standard ABVD.[5] BEACOPP plus radiation therapy provides better progression-free and overall survival at a median follow-up of 6.9 years than COPP/ABVD plus radiation therapy despite a higher rate of hematologic toxicity and infertility.[6]

The overall approach to managing advanced-stage Hodgkin's lymphoma must factor in the fact that about 50% of patients who are not cured by primary chemotherapy can be effectively treated with HDC/HSCT (Chapter 181). Thus, for the 80% of patients with zero to three adverse prognostic factors at presentation, who have a 75% chance of cure with primary chemotherapy, the most widely used approach is to start with ABVD. For the 20% of these low-risk patients in whom progressive lymphoma develops despite primary treatment, HDC/HSCT (Chapter 181) should be offered. Such a strategy confines the high cost and toxicity of intensified treatment to the minority of patients whose disease demands it. Conversely, for the 20% of patients with high-risk disease who have four or more adverse factors and only a 60% likelihood of cure with primary chemotherapy, more intense initial treatment with the BEACOPP protocol is reasonable.

Management of Refractory or Relapsed Hodgkin's Lymphoma

HDC/HSCT has become the established treatment for most patients whose Hodgkin's lymphoma persists or recurs despite primary chemotherapy.[7] However, the treatment-related mortality, high levels of toxicity, and cost associated with HDC/HSCT demand that it be reserved for patients in whom it clearly increases the chance of cure over alternative treatments; such patients include those whose disease progresses during or within 3 months of initial multiagent chemotherapy (refractory Hodgkin's lymphoma) and those who relapse more than 3 months after multiagent chemotherapy (relapsed Hodgkin's lymphoma). For relapsed lymphoma, controversy remains, however, for two special subgroups: patients who relapse solely in originally involved but unirradiated lymph nodes and without B symptoms or extranodal disease, who may obtain up to a 40 to 50% cure rate with wide-field irradiation, and patients who relapse without B symptoms more than 1 year after completion of primary chemotherapy, who may achieve up to a 30 to 40% cure rate with additional chemotherapy with or without irradiation. However, even these two subgroups may achieve up to an 80% 10-year disease-free survival rate after HDC/HSCT. Thus, data suggest that standard treatment for patients with progressive Hodgkin's lymphoma after primary chemotherapy for advanced-stage disease should be HDC/HSCT regardless of the characteristics of the relapse.

HDC/HSCT should be reserved for patients who have progressive lymphoma after primary chemotherapy because randomized trials of HDC/HSCT for patients in complete or partial remission after primary chemotherapy for advanced Hodgkin's lymphoma failed to show a difference in outcome.[8]

Management of Complications

Follow-up and Late Complications of Treatment

Most adult patients with Hodgkin's lymphoma are cured and experience minimal long-term toxicity from their treatment. However, the risk for certain predictable and occasional rare and less predictable late effects warrants careful but not intrusive follow-up and selective intervention (Table 192-6). At the conclusion of treatment, a thorough reassessment of the initial sites of lymphoma should be completed to provide post-treatment baseline measurements. Patients should be seen by a specialist knowledgeable in the management of lymphoma, preferably about every 3 months for 2 years, then every 6 months for 3 years, then annually. Patients should be strongly encouraged to refrain from smoking, to perform careful breast and skin examinations on a regular basis, and to undergo regular immunizations for influenza annually, pneumococcus at diagnosis and 5 years after treatment, and diphtheria and tetanus every 10 years (Chapter 17). Patients who have received radiation to the head or neck area should follow a vigorous program of dental prophylaxis in anticipation of the deleterious effect of reduced saliva production and have their thyroid-stimulating hormone (TSH) level checked annually in recognition of the 50% risk for eventual hypothyroidism.

Special Problems in the Management of Hodgkin's Lymphoma

Hodgkin's Lymphoma during Pregnancy

Between 0.5 and 1.0% of cases of Hodgkin's lymphoma occur coincident with pregnancy (Chapter 247). When the lymphoma is discovered during pregnancy, it is almost always possible to keep it under control and allow the pregnancy to go to full term.

Standard staging tests (see Table 192-2) should be completed, except that imaging requiring radiation must be minimized. For example, abdominal ultrasonography can identify bulky retroperitoneal disease, and a single posteroanterior radiograph of the chest, with proper shielding, can identify bulky mediastinal disease.

More than 50% of patients can continue the pregnancy to term without any treatment of the lymphoma. If symptomatic or progressive disease develops, systemic chemotherapy can be given in the second and third trimester with very small risk of injuring the fetus. An attractive alternative is intermittent single-agent vinblastine, given in the lowest dose that can control symptoms until delivery, followed by a full course of six to eight cycles of multiagent chemotherapy after delivery.

Hodgkin's Lymphoma and Acquired Immunodeficiency Syndrome

In patients with HIV infection, the incidence of Hodgkin's lymphoma is increased as much as five- to ten-fold, and the lymphoma manifests differently and pursues a more aggressive natural history (Chapter 400). Hodgkin's lymphoma in HIV-positive individuals is almost always associated with EBV within Hodgkin-Reed-Sternberg cells. The histology is much more likely to be mixed cellularity or lymphocyte depleted. The disease most commonly develops in extranodal sites, especially the bone marrow. More than 80% of patients have advanced-stage disease, and most patients have B symptoms.

TABLE 192-6 MONITORING AFTER SUCCESSFUL PRIMARY TREATMENT OF HODGKIN'S LYMPHOMA

RISK/PROBLEM	INCIDENCE/RESPONSE
Relapse	Ten to 30% of patients experience relapse. Careful attention should be directed to lymph node sites, especially if previously involved with disease and not treated with radiation. New persistent focal symptoms such as bone pain should be investigated with appropriate laboratory and imaging studies.
Dental caries	Neck or oropharyngeal irradiation may cause decreased salivation. Patients should have regular dental care and should make their dentist aware of the previous irradiation.
Hypothyroidism	After external beam thyroid irradiation at doses sufficient to cure Hodgkin's lymphoma, at least 50% of patients eventually become hypothyroid. All patients who have been exposed to neck irradiation should have an annual TSH level determined. Patients whose TSH level becomes elevated should be treated with lifelong thyroxine replacement in doses sufficient to suppress TSH levels to low normal (Chapter 233).
Infertility	ABVD is not known to cause permanent gonadal toxicity, although temporary oligospermia or irregular menses may persist for 1 to 2 years after treatment. Direct or scatter radiation to gonadal tissue may cause infertility, amenorrhea, or premature menopause, but this adverse event seldom occurs with the current fields used for the treatment of Hodgkin's lymphoma. In general, women who continue menstruating are fertile, but men require semen analysis to provide a specific answer.
Secondary neoplasms	Although uncommon, certain secondary neoplasms occur with increased frequency in patients who have been treated for Hodgkin's lymphoma: acute myelogenous leukemia; thyroid, breast, lung, cervical, and upper gastrointestinal carcinoma; and melanoma. It is appropriate to "be vigilant" for these neoplasms for the remainder of the patient's life because they may have a lengthy induction period.

ABVD = doxorubicin (Adriamycin), bleomycin, vinblastine, and dacarbazine; TSH = thyroid-stimulating hormone.

Patients are prone to opportunistic infections, and the interaction of chemotherapeutic agents with other medications may compromise the patient's ability to tolerate treatment. The best approach is a combination of highly active antiretroviral agents (Chapter 396), vigorous supportive care with antiherpetic and antifungal agents and neutrophil-stimulating growth factors, and standard multiagent chemotherapy. With appropriate supportive care, regimens such as ABVD can be delivered. However, more severe than normal toxicity must be anticipated, and cure rates are much lower than in the non-HIV-infected population. Median survival is typically 3 to 4 years.

Hodgkin's Lymphoma in the Elderly Population

Elderly patients with Hodgkin's lymphoma have a worse outcome. For example, the 5-year overall survival rate falls from 80% in patients younger than 65 years to less than 50% in patients older than 65 years. Explanations include more advanced stage at diagnosis, comorbid diseases, delay in diagnosis, incomplete staging, inadequate adherence to treatment protocols, and failure to maintain full dose intensity.

Of note is that elderly patients achieve outcomes equivalent to those of younger patients when they receive similar doses of chemotherapy. The best approach for elderly patients is to attempt to treat them in a manner similar to younger patients, with vigorous supportive care and the addition of neutrophil growth factors if necessary to enable safe delivery of full doses. For patients with preexisting pulmonary or cardiac disease, it might be necessary to reduce or eliminate bleomycin or doxorubicin, respectively.

FUTURE DIRECTIONS

The ability to profile multigene expression patterns and identify genetic polymorphisms associated with specific malignancies may provide better insight into the molecular genesis of Hodgkin's and other lymphomas. Therapeutic agents more specifically targeted at the malignant Hodgkin-Reed-Sternberg cells, such as those coupling an antibody to the CD30 antigen with a cellular toxin, hold substantial promise to improve treatment outcome.

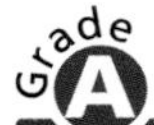

1. Engert A, Schiller P, Josting A, et al. Involved-field radiotherapy is equally effective and less toxic compared with extended-field radiotherapy after four cycles of chemotherapy in patients with early-stage unfavorable Hodgkin's lymphoma: results of the HD8 trials of the German Hodgkin's Lymphoma Study Group. *J Clin Oncol.* 2003;21:3601-3608.
2. Bonadonna G, Bonfante V, Viviani S, et al. ABVD plus subtotal nodal versus involved-field radiotherapy in early-stage Hodgkin's disease: long-term results. *J Clin Oncol.* 2004;22:2835-2841.
3. Engert A, Plütschow A, Eich HT, et al. Reduced treatment intensity in patients with early-stage Hodgkin's lymphoma. *N Engl J Med.* 2010;363:640-652.
4. Meyer RM, Gospodarowicz MK, Connors JM, et al. Randomized comparison of ABVD chemotherapy with a strategy that includes radiation therapy in patients with limited-stage Hodgkin's lymphoma: National Cancer Institute of Canada Clinical Trials Group and the Eastern Cooperative Oncology Group. *J Clin Oncol.* 2005;23:4634-4642.
5. Hoskin PJ, Lowry L, Horwich A, et al. Randomized comparison of the Stanford V regimen and ABVD in the treatment of advanced Hodgkin's Lymphoma: United Kingdom National Cancer Research Institute Lymphoma Group Study ISRCTN 64141244. *J Clin Oncol.* 2009;27:5390-5396.
6. Engert A, Diehl V, Franklin J, et al. Escalated-dose BEACOPP in the treatment of patients with advanced-stage Hodgkin's lymphoma: 10 years of follow-up of the GHSG HD9 study. *J Clin Oncol.* 2009;27:4548-4554.
7. Schmitz N, Pfistner B, Sextro M, et al. Aggressive conventional chemotherapy compared with high-dose chemotherapy with autologous haemopoietic stem-cell transplantation for relapsed chemosensitive Hodgkin's disease: a randomised trial. *Lancet.* 2002;359:2065-2071.
8. Federico M, Bellei M, Brice P, et al. High-dose therapy and autologous stem-cell transplantation versus conventional therapy for patients with advanced Hodgkin's lymphoma responding to front-line therapy. *J Clin Oncol.* 2003;21:2320-2325.

SUGGESTED READINGS

Armitage JO. Current concepts: early-stage Hodgkin's lymphoma. *N Engl J Med.* 2010;363:653-662. *Review.*

Farrell K, Jarrett RF. The molecular pathogenesis of Hodgkin lymphoma. *Histopathology.* 2011;58:15-25. *Review.*

Punnett A, Tsang RW, Hodgson DC. Hodgkin lymphoma across the age spectrum: epidemiology, therapy, and late effects. *Semin Radiat Oncol.* 2010;20:30-44. *Differences in epidemiology, disease biology, and new approaches to prognostic and therapeutic stratification in light of the strong age gradient that exists with respect to patient outcomes in Hodgkin's lymphoma.*

Steidl C, Lee T, Shah SP, et al. Tumor-associated macrophages and survival in classic Hodgkin's lymphoma. *N Engl J Med.* 2010;362:875-885. *Histochemical assessment of tumor-infiltrating macrophages strongly predicts outcome.*

193

PLASMA CELL DISORDERS

S. VINCENT RAJKUMAR

INTRODUCTION

Plasma cell disorders are neoplastic or potentially neoplastic diseases associated with the clonal proliferation of immunoglobulin-secreting plasma cells (Table 193-1). They are characterized by the secretion of electrophoretically and immunologically homogeneous (monoclonal) proteins that represent intact or incomplete immunoglobulin molecules. Monoclonal proteins are commonly referred to as M proteins, myeloma proteins, or paraproteins.

Syndromes associated with plasma cell disorders and monoclonal proteins include monoclonal gammopathy of undetermined significance, multiple myeloma, Waldenström's macroglobulinemia, cryoglobulinemia, and primary amyloidosis (see Table 193-1). Occasionally, free hemoglobin-haptoglobin complexes resulting from hemolysis, large amounts of transferrin in patients with iron deficiency anemia, or increased levels of fibrinogen may simulate the presence of a monoclonal protein in serum.

Serum Immunoglobulins

Intact immunoglobulins consist of two heavy (H) polypeptide chains of the same class and subclass and two light (L) polypeptide chains of the same type (Chapter 44). The heavy polypeptide chains are designated by Greek letters: γ in immunoglobulin G (IgG), α in immunoglobulin A (IgA), μ in immunoglobulin M (IgM), δ in immunoglobulin D (IgD), and ε in immunoglobulin E (IgE). The light chain types are kappa (κ) and lambda (λ). Both heavy

TABLE 193-1 PLASMA CELL PROLIFERATIVE DISORDERS

I. Premalignant monoclonal gammopathies
  A. Monoclonal gammopathy of undetermined significance (MGUS)
  B. MGUS in association with chronic lymphocytic leukemia and non-Hodgkin's lymphoma
  C. Biclonal and triclonal gammopathies of undetermined significance
  D. Idiopathic Bence Jones proteinuria and light chain MGUS
  E. Smoldering multiple myeloma
II. Malignant monoclonal gammopathies
  A. Multiple myeloma and related malignancies (IgG, IgA, IgD, IgE, and free light chains)
    1. Symptomatic multiple myeloma
    2. Plasma cell leukemia
    3. Osteosclerotic myeloma (including POEMS syndrome)
    4. Solitary plasmacytoma of bone
    5. Solitary extramedullary plasmacytoma
  B. Waldenström's macroglobulinemia (IgM)
III. Heavy chain diseases (HCDs)
  A. γ-HCD
  B. α-HCD
  C. μ-HCD
IV. Cryoglobulinemia (types I, II, and III)
V. Immunoglobulin light chain amyloidosis

Ig = immunoglobulin; POEMS = polyneuropathy, organomegaly, endocrinopathy, M protein, and skin changes.

chains and light chains have "constant" and "variable" regions with respect to the amino acid sequence. The class specificity of each immunoglobulin is defined by a series of antigenic determinants on the constant regions of the heavy chains (γ, α, μ, δ, and ε) and the two major classes of light chains (κ and λ). The amino acid sequence in the variable regions of the immunoglobulin molecule corresponds to the active antigen-combining site of the antibody.

In the majority of clonal plasma cell disorders, intact immunoglobulin molecules are secreted as monoclonal (M) proteins. In some patients, however, heavy chain expression is completely lost, and only monoclonal light chains (Bence Jones proteins) are secreted. Even less frequently, only heavy chains are secreted, resulting in heavy chain diseases (HCDs). Rare patients with multiple myeloma secrete no identifiable immunoglobulin ("nonsecretory myeloma").

Identification of Monoclonal Proteins

Protein electrophoresis of the serum and urine detects M protein as a narrow peak (like a church spire) on the densitometer tracing or as a dense, discrete band on agarose gel (Fig. 193-1). Electrophoresis also permits quantitation of M proteins. Monoclonal light chains (Bence Jones proteinemia) are rarely seen on serum electrophoresis but are easily detected on urine electrophoresis. Urine electrophoresis requires a 24-hour urine collection.

Immunofixation of the serum and urine is performed when a peak or band is first seen on protein electrophoresis to identify the heavy and light chain type of the M protein. Immunofixation is also a more sensitive test than protein electrophoresis, and it should always be performed in conjunction with electrophoresis when multiple myeloma or related disorders are first suspected in order to detect small, unmeasurable M proteins that may be missed on electrophoresis. This is particularly important in oligosecretory myeloma, primary amyloidosis, and solitary plasmacytoma and after successful treatment of multiple myeloma or macroglobulinemia. In these instances, a small M protein can be concealed in the normal β or γ areas of the electrophoresis gel and may be overlooked. In 5% of patients there is an additional M protein of a different immunoglobulin class; this condition is designated a biclonal gammopathy.

In some patients the M protein has specificity to one of the various antigens. Examples include actin, dextran, antistreptolysin O, antinuclear antibody, riboflavin, von Willebrand's factor, thyroglobulin, insulin, double-stranded DNA, and apolipoprotein. Binding of calcium by an M protein may produce hypercalcemia without symptomatic or pathologic consequences. M proteins have also been found to bind to copper and to phosphate.

Monoclonal proteins must be distinguished from an excess of polyclonal immunoglobulins (one or more heavy chain types and both κ and λ light chains, usually limited to the γ region), which produce a broad-based peak or broad band (Fig. 193-2). This finding is associated with chronic infectious or inflammatory states.

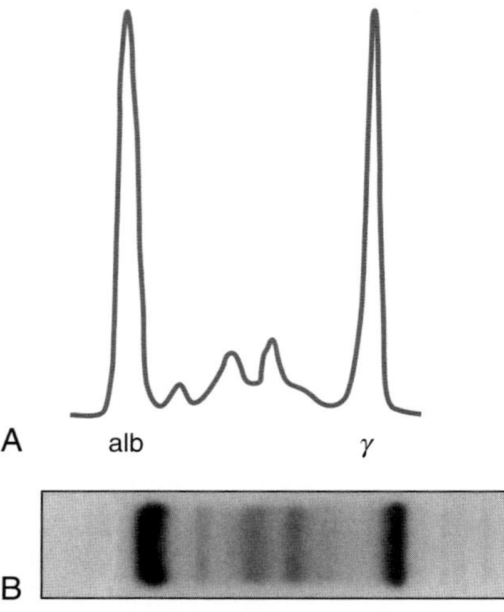

FIGURE 193-1. Serum protein electrophoresis showing a monoclonal (M) protein. A, Monoclonal pattern of serum protein as traced by a densitometer after electrophoresis on agarose gel: tall, narrow-based peak of γ mobility. **B,** Monoclonal pattern from electrophoresis of serum on agarose gel (anode on the left): dense, localized band representing monoclonal protein of γ mobility. (From Kyle RA, Katzmann JA. Immunochemical characterization of immunoglobulins. In: Rose NR, Conway de Macario E, Folds JD, et al, eds. *Manual of Clinical Laboratory Immunology,* 5th ed. Washington, DC: ASM Press; 1997:156, with permission of the American Society for Microbiology.)

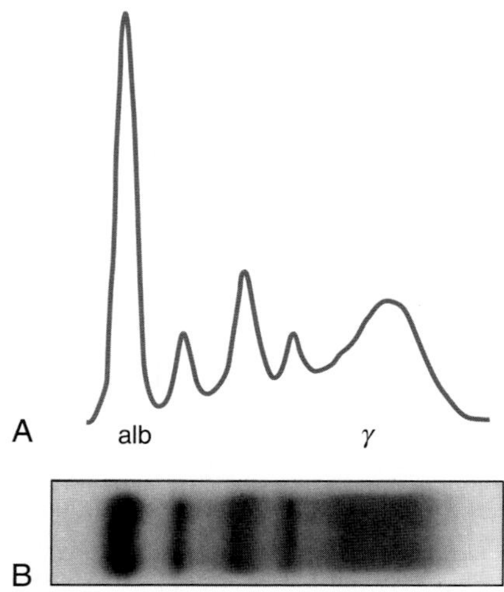

FIGURE 193-2. Serum protein electrophoresis showing increased polyclonal immunoglobulins. A, Polyclonal pattern from a densitometer tracing of agarose gel: broad-based peak of γ mobility. **B,** Polyclonal pattern from electrophoresis of agarose gel (anode on the left). The band at the right is broad and extends throughout the γ area. (From Kyle RA, Katzmann JA. Immunochemical characterization of immunoglobulins. In: Rose NR, Conway de Macario E, Folds JD, et al, eds. *Manual of Clinical Laboratory Immunology,* 5th ed. Washington, DC: ASM Press; 1997:156, with permission of the American Society for Microbiology.)

Detection of Serum Free Light Chains

The serum free light chain assay measures the level of free κ and λ immunoglobulin light chains (i.e., light chains that are not bound to intact immunoglobulin). An abnormal κ/λ free light chain ratio (normal range, 0.26 to 1.65) indicates an excess of one light chain type versus the other and is interpreted as representing a monoclonal elevation of the corresponding light chain type. The serum free light chain assay is more sensitive than electrophoresis or immunofixation in detecting free monoclonal light chains and is useful in the diagnostic evaluation of plasma cell disorders and in risk stratification.

MONOCLONAL GAMMOPATHY OF UNDETERMINED SIGNIFICANCE

DEFINITION

Monoclonal gammopathy of undetermined significance (MGUS; formerly called *benign monoclonal gammopathy*) is a premalignant clonal plasma cell

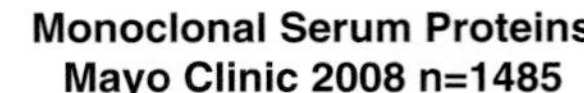

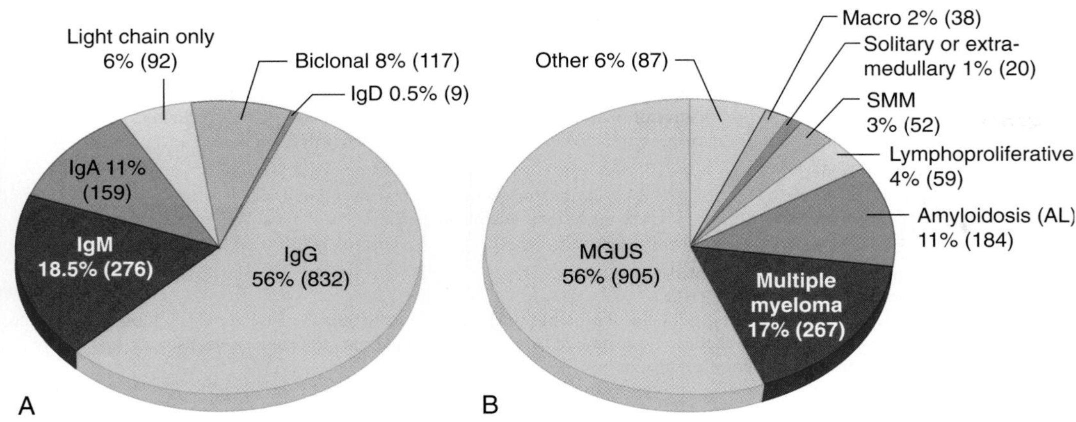

FIGURE 193-3. **Monoclonal gammopathy.** **A,** Distribution of serum monoclonal proteins in 1485 patients seen at the Mayo Clinic during 2008. **B,** Diagnoses in 1612 cases of monoclonal gammopathy seen at the Mayo Clinic during 2008. Ig = immunoglobulin; Macro = Waldenström's macroglobulinemia; MGUS = monoclonal gammopathy of undetermined significance; SMM = smoldering multiple myeloma.

disorder characterized by the presence of a serum M protein in persons who lack evidence of multiple myeloma, macroglobulinemia, amyloidosis, or other related diseases. MGUS is defined by a serum M protein concentration lower than 3 g/dL, less than 10% clonal plasma cells in the bone marrow, and absence of lytic bone lesions, anemia, hypercalcemia, and renal insufficiency that can be attributed to a plasma cell disorder. The main clinical significance of MGUS is its lifelong risk of transformation to myeloma or related malignancy at a fixed but unrelenting rate of 1% per year.

EPIDEMIOLOGY

More than 50% of patients in whom a serum M protein is detected have MGUS (Fig. 193-3). The prevalence of MGUS in the general population increases with age, from approximately 1% in persons 50 to 60 years old to greater than 5% in those older than 70 years. The age-adjusted prevalence is higher in males than in females and is twice as high in blacks compared with whites.

PATHOBIOLOGY

MGUS represents a limited, nonmalignant expansion of monoclonal plasma cells. The etiology of MGUS is unknown, but age, male gender, family history, immunosuppression, and exposure to certain pesticides are known risk factors. It is hypothesized that infection, inflammation, or other antigenic stimuli, acting in concert with the development of cytogenetic abnormalities in the plasma cells, are the initiating pathogenetic events in most patients. Approximately 50% of MGUS is associated with plasma cell translocations involving the immunoglobulin heavy chain (IgH) locus on chromosome 14q32 (IgH translocated MGUS). These primary IgH translocations commonly involve one of five recurrent partner chromosome loci: 11q13 (*CCND1* [cyclin D1 gene]), 4p16.3 (*FGFR-3* and *MMSET*), 6p21 (*CCND3* [cyclin D3 gene]), 16q23 (*c-maf*), and 20q11 (*mafB*). The remaining 50% lack IgH translocations but are usually associated with hyperdiploidy (hyperdiploid MGUS).

CLINICAL MANIFESTATIONS

MGUS is asymptomatic and is usually diagnosed incidentally on laboratory testing. Patients with MGUS progress to multiple myeloma or related malignancy at a rate of approximately 1% per year. The interval from the time of recognition of the M protein to the diagnosis of serious disease ranges from 1 to 32 years (median, 10.6 years), and the relative risk versus a control population is 25.0 for progression to multiple myeloma, 8.4 for primary amyloidosis, 46.0 for Waldenström's macroglobulinemia, 2.4 for the development of other forms of non-Hodgkin's lymphoma, and 8.5 for plasmacytoma. The relative risk for chronic lymphocytic leukemia (CLL) is not increased. In addition, in a small percentage of patients, the M protein level increases to greater than 3 g/dL and/or the percentage of plasma cells in bone marrow increases to more than 10% without progression to overt myeloma or a related disorder (smoldering multiple myeloma).

DIAGNOSIS

MGUS is differentiated from multiple myeloma and smoldering multiple myeloma by the size of the M protein, the bone marrow plasma cell percentage, and the presence or absence of anemia, renal failure, hypercalcemia, or lytic bone lesions (Table 193-2). Because anemia and renal insufficiency are relatively common in the elderly population with MGUS, the causes of these conditions should be carefully investigated with adequate laboratory studies. For example, in a patient with anemia, tests to exclude iron, vitamin B_{12}, or folate deficiency must be performed. In certain instances, such as unexplained renal failure, a renal biopsy may be needed. Only patients with strong evidence of end-organ damage thought to be directly related to a plasma cell disorder can be considered to have myeloma or a related malignancy.

Levels of the immunoglobulin classes other than M protein (i.e., the normal polyclonal or background immunoglobulins) are generally reduced in multiple myeloma or Waldenström's macroglobulinemia, but a reduction also occurs in almost 40% of patients with MGUS. The presence of osteolytic lesions strongly suggests multiple myeloma, but metastatic carcinoma may produce lytic lesions as well as polyclonal plasmacytosis and must be differentiated from MGUS.

Association of MGUS with Other Diseases

MGUS is associated with numerous diseases. However, because 3% of the general population older than 50 years has MGUS, it is often difficult to determine whether these reported associations are causal or coincidental. Some associations have been verified based on epidemiologic studies; these include peripheral neuropathy (Chapter 428), deep vein thrombosis (Chapter 81), osteoporosis (Chapter 251), and lymphoproliferative disorders (Chapter 191). A secondary form of MGUS also occurs with immunosuppression after organ transplantation (Chapter 48) and autologous or allogeneic stem cell transplantation (Chapter 181). M proteins also occur in the sera of some patients with CLL (Chapter 190) but have no recognizable effect on the clinical course.

Approximately 5% of patients with sensorimotor peripheral neuropathy of unknown cause (Chapter 428) have an associated monoclonal gammopathy (MGUS-associated neuropathy). In half of such patients, the M protein binds to myelin-associated glycoprotein. These patients have a slowly progressive sensory neuropathy more than motor neuropathy, beginning in the distal ends of the extremities and extending proximally. The clinical and electrodiagnostic manifestations of MGUS neuropathy resemble those of a chronic inflammatory demyelinating polyneuropathy. A causal relationship is usually assumed in younger patients and those without other conditions known to cause neuropathy in whom the neuropathy is severe and progressive. Therapeutic approaches include plasmapheresis and, occasionally, chemotherapy (similar to myeloma for IgG or IgA monoclonal proteins, and rituximab or chlorambucil for IgM monoclonal proteins; see the later section on the treatment of multiple myeloma).

TABLE 193-2 CRITERIA FOR THE DIAGNOSIS OF PLASMA CELL DISORDERS

DISORDER	DISEASE DEFINITION
Monoclonal gammopathy of undetermined significance (MGUS)	All 3 criteria must be met: 1. Serum monoclonal protein (IgG, IgA, or IgM) <3 g/dL 2. Clonal bone marrow plasma cells <10% 3. Absence of end-organ damage such as hypercalcemia, renal insufficiency, anemia, and bone lesions that can be attributed to the plasma cell proliferative disorder (or, in the case of IgM MGUS, no evidence of anemia, constitutional symptoms, hyperviscosity, lymphadenopathy, or hepatosplenomegaly)
Smoldering multiple myeloma (also referred to as *asymptomatic multiple myeloma*)	Both criteria must be met: 1. Serum monoclonal protein (IgG or IgA) ≥3 g/dL and/or clonal bone marrow plasma cells ≥10% 2. Absence of end-organ damage such as lytic bone lesions, anemia, hypercalcemia, or renal failure that can be attributed to a plasma cell proliferative disorder
Multiple myeloma	All 3 criteria must be met, except as noted: 1. Clonal bone marrow plasma cells ≥10% 2. Presence of serum and/or urinary monoclonal protein (except in patients with true nonsecretory multiple myeloma) 3. Evidence of end-organ damage that can be attributed to the underlying plasma cell proliferative disorder, specifically hypercalcemia, renal insufficiency, anemia, or bone lesions
Waldenström's macroglobulinemia	Both criteria must be met: 1. IgM monoclonal gammopathy (regardless of the size of the M protein) 2. >10% bone marrow lymphoplasmacytic infiltration (usually intertrabecular) by small lymphocytes that exhibit plasmacytoid or plasma cell differentiation and a typical immunophenotype (surface IgM$^+$, CD5$^{+/-}$, CD10$^-$, CD19$^+$, CD20$^+$, CD23$^-$) that satisfactorily excludes other lymphoproliferative disorders, including chronic lymphocytic leukemia and mantle cell lymphoma
Smoldering Waldenström's macroglobulinemia (also referred to as *indolent* or *asymptomatic Waldenström's macroglobulinemia*)	1. Serum IgM monoclonal protein ≥3 g/dL and/or bone marrow lymphoplasmacytic infiltration ≥10% 2. No evidence of end-organ damage such as anemia, constitutional symptoms, hyperviscosity, lymphadenopathy, or hepatosplenomegaly that can be attributed to a lymphoplasma cell proliferative disorder
Solitary plasmacytoma	All 4 criteria must be met: 1. Biopsy-proven solitary lesion of bone or soft tissue with evidence of clonal plasma cells 2. Normal bone marrow with no evidence of clonal plasma cells 3. Normal skeletal survey and MRI of spine and pelvis (except for the primary solitary lesion) 4. Absence of end-organ damage such as hypercalcemia, renal insufficiency, anemia, or bone lesions that can be attributed to a plasma cell proliferative disorder
POEMS syndrome	All 4 criteria must be met: 1. Presence of a monoclonal plasma cell disorder (almost always λ-type) 2. Peripheral neuropathy 3. Any one of the following 3 major features: sclerotic bone lesions, Castleman's disease, elevated levels of vascular endothelial growth factor (VEGF) 4. Any one of the following 6 minor features: organomegaly, edema, endocrinopathy (excluding diabetes mellitus or hypothyroidism), typical skin changes, papilledema, thrombocytosis, polycythemia The features should have a temporal relationship to one another, with no other attributable cause

Modified from Rajkumar SV, Dispenzieri A, Kyle RA. Monoclonal gammopathy of undetermined significance, Waldenstrom macroglobulinemia, AL amyloidosis, and related plasma cell disorders: diagnosis and treatment. *Mayo Clin Proc.* 2006;81:693-703; and Kyle RA, Rajkumar SV. Criteria for diagnosis, staging, risk stratification and response assessment of multiple myeloma. *Leukemia.* 2009;23:3-9.

Certain skin disorders are known to be associated with MGUS. Lichen myxedematosus (papular mucinosis, scleromyxedema) is associated with a cathodal IgG γ protein. Pyoderma gangrenosum and necrobiotic xanthogranuloma are other associated skin disorders.

PREVENTION AND TREATMENT

No treatment is necessary for MGUS. Low-risk patients (Table 193-3) can be evaluated when symptoms suggestive of myeloma or related disorders occur. In all other patients with MGUS, the M protein level in serum and urine should be measured serially, together with periodic reevaluation of clinical and other laboratory findings, to determine whether multiple myeloma or another related disorder is present. In general, electrophoresis, complete blood count, and creatinine and calcium levels should be repeated at 6 months and, if stable, yearly thereafter.

PROGNOSIS

Differentiating a patient with MGUS in whom the disorder will remain stable for life from one in whom multiple myeloma, macroglobulinemia, or a related disorder will eventually develop is difficult when the M protein is first recognized. The size and type of the M protein at diagnosis of MGUS and an abnormal serum free light chain ratio are prognostic factors for progression (see Table 193-3).

BICLONAL GAMMOPATHIES

Biclonal gammopathies occur in at least 5% of patients with clonal plasma cell disorders. A biclonal gammopathy of undetermined significance (analogous to MGUS) accounts for about two thirds of such patients. The remainder have multiple myeloma, macroglobulinemia, or other lymphoproliferative diseases. Rarely, triclonal gammopathies may occur.

LIGHT CHAIN MGUS AND IDIOPATHIC BENCE JONES PROTEINURIA

The diagnosis of typical MGUS requires expression of an intact heavy chain type. In some patients a premalignant clonal plasma cell disorder characterized by the presence of monoclonal immunoglobulin light chains without expression of heavy chains can occur (light chain MGUS). Some patients with light chain MGUS may secrete adequate amounts of monoclonal light chains in the urine, resulting in idiopathic Bence Jones proteinuria. Idiopathic Bence Jones proteinuria is analogous to MGUS, and the urinary excretion of monoclonal light chains can persist for many years without evidence of end-organ damage suggestive of multiple myeloma or related disorders. No therapy is indicated unless progression to malignancy occurs.

MULTIPLE MYELOMA

DEFINITION

Multiple myeloma is a malignancy of plasma cells characterized by bone marrow infiltration and extensive skeletal destruction resulting in anemia, bone pain, and fractures. Multiple myeloma (commonly referred to as *myeloma*) is defined by the presence of 10% or more clonal plasma cells on bone marrow examination, M protein in serum or urine (except in the case of nonsecretory myeloma), and evidence of hypercalcemia, renal insufficiency, anemia, or bone lesions thought to be related to the plasma cell proliferative disorder. Patients with multiple myeloma must be differentiated from those with MGUS and smoldering multiple myeloma (see Table 193-2).

TABLE 193-3 RISK OF PROGRESSION OF MONOCLONAL GAMMOPATHY OF UNDETERMINED SIGNIFICANCE TO MYELOMA OR RELATED DISORDERS

RISK GROUP	RELATIVE RISK	CUMULATIVE ABSOLUTE RISK OF PROGRESSION AT 20 YEARS (%)*	CUMULATIVE ABSOLUTE RISK OF PROGRESSION AT 20 YEARS ACCOUNTING FOR DEATH AS A COMPETING RISK (%)†
Low risk: serum M protein <1.5 g/dL, IgG subtype, normal free light chain ratio (0.26-1.65)	1	5	2
Low-intermediate risk: any 1 factor abnormal	5.4	21	10
High-intermediate risk: any 2 factors abnormal	10.1	37	18
High risk: all 3 factors abnormal	20.8	58	27

*Estimates in this column represent the risk of progression assuming that patients do not die of other causes during this period.
†Estimates in this column represent the risk of progression calculated by using a model that accounts for the fact that patients can die of unrelated causes during this time.
Ig = immunoglobulin.
Adapted from Rajkumar SV, Kyle RA, Therneau TM, et al. Serum free light chain ratio is an independent risk factor for progression in monoclonal gammopathy of undetermined significance (MGUS). *Blood.* 2005;106:812-817. © The American Society of Hematology.

EPIDEMIOLOGY

Multiple myeloma accounts for 1% of all malignant disease and slightly more than 10% of hematologic malignancies in the United States. The annual incidence of multiple myeloma is 4 per 100,000. Its incidence in blacks is almost twice that in whites. Multiple myeloma is slightly more common in men than in women. The median age of patients at the time of diagnosis is about 65 years; only 2% of patients are younger than 40.

PATHOBIOLOGY

The cause of multiple myeloma is unclear. Exposure to radiation, benzene, and other organic solvents, herbicides, and insecticides may play a role. Multiple myeloma has been reported in familial clusters of two or more first-degree relatives and in identical twins.

Almost all cases of myeloma evolve from a premalignant MGUS phase, although the MGUS is clinically recognized before the diagnosis of myeloma in only a small minority of patients. The progression of MGUS to myeloma suggests a simple, random, two-hit genetic model of malignancy in which the risk of progression is fixed (approximately 1% per year) regardless of the duration of MGUS. Unfortunately, the precise mechanisms of progression are unknown, although several potentially pathogenetic abnormalities have been described in the clonal plasma cells. These include *RAS* and *p53* mutations, p16 methylation, *MYC* abnormalities, and secondary translocations. Changes in the bone marrow microenvironment may also play a role in the pathogenesis, including induction of angiogenesis and abnormal paracrine loops involving cytokines such as interleukin-6 (IL-6), which serves as a major growth factor for plasma cells.

The lytic bone lesions, osteopenia, hypercalcemia, and pathologic fractures in patients with myeloma are a result of abnormal osteoclast activity induced by the neoplastic plasma cells, as well as inhibition of osteoblast differentiation. Osteoclasts are activated by stimulation of the transmembrane receptor RANK (receptor activator of nuclear factor κB), which belongs to the tumor necrosis factor (TNF) receptor superfamily. The ligand for this receptor (RANKL) also has a decoy receptor, osteoprotegerin (OPG). In myeloma, there is an increase in RANKL expression by osteoblasts (and possibly plasma cells), accompanied by a reduction in the level of OPG. The resultant increase in the RANKL/OPG ratio causes osteoclast activation and increased bone resorption and turnover (Chapter 250).

Cytogenetic Abnormalities

As discussed earlier (see Pathobiology of MGUS), primary translocations involving the immunoglobulin heavy chain loci (chromosome 14q32) are seen in up to 50% of patients with multiple myeloma (IgH-translocated or nonhyperdiploid myeloma). The remaining 50% of patients do not have IgH translocations but have evidence of hyperdiploidy (hyperdiploid myeloma). In a small percentage of patients the disease cannot be classified into either of these two types (unclassified). Besides these cytogenetic abnormalities, other secondary cytogenetic abnormalities occur as late events during the course of symptomatic myeloma; these include activating mutations of N- and K-*RAS*, inactivating mutations of *p53*, and dysregulation of c-*MYC*. Complete or partial deletions of chromosome 13 are well described in myeloma and have prognostic value, but they also occur at the MGUS stage.

TABLE 193-4 MAJOR CLINICAL MANIFESTATIONS OF MULTIPLE MYELOMA

CLINICAL FINDINGS	APPROXIMATE PERCENTAGE OF PATIENTS WITH ABNORMALITY AT DIAGNOSIS
Skeletal involvement: pain, reduced height, lytic bone lesions, pathologic fractures	80
Anemia (hemoglobin ≤12 g/dL): caused mainly by decreased erythropoiesis; produces weakness and fatigue	75
Renal insufficiency (serum creatinine ≥2 mg/dL): caused mainly by "myeloma kidney" from light chains or hypercalcemia, rarely from amyloidosis	20
Hypercalcemia (≥11 mg/dL)	15
Light chain amyloidosis	10
Evidence of monoclonal protein by immunofixation and serum free light chain assay	97
Evidence of clonal plasma cells ≥10% in bone marrow	96

CLINICAL MANIFESTATIONS

History

Bone pain, particularly in the back or chest and less often in the extremities, is present at the time of diagnosis in more than two thirds of patients (Table 193-4). The patient's height may be reduced by several inches because of vertebral collapse. Weakness and fatigue are common and are often associated with anemia. Fever is rare and, when present, is generally from an infection; in some patients the infection itself is the initial feature. Other symptoms may result from renal insufficiency, hypercalcemia, nephrotic syndrome, radiculopathy, or amyloidosis (Chapter 194).

Physical Examination

Pallor is the most frequent physical finding. The liver is palpable in about 5% of patients, and the spleen in 1%. Tenderness may be noted at sites of bone involvement. Radiculopathy may be caused by spinal compression fractures. Occasionally, extramedullary plasmacytomas are palpable.

DIAGNOSIS

Laboratory Findings

A normocytic, normochromic anemia (Chapter 161) is present initially in approximately 75% of patients, but it eventually occurs in nearly every patient with multiple myeloma. Serum protein electrophoresis shows an M protein in 80% of patients. With serum immunofixation, an M protein can be detected in 93% of patients. When these serum studies are combined with urine electrophoresis plus immunofixation, an M protein can be detected in 97% of patients with myeloma. The serum free light chain assay is more convenient and can be used in place of urine studies in the diagnostic evaluation. The

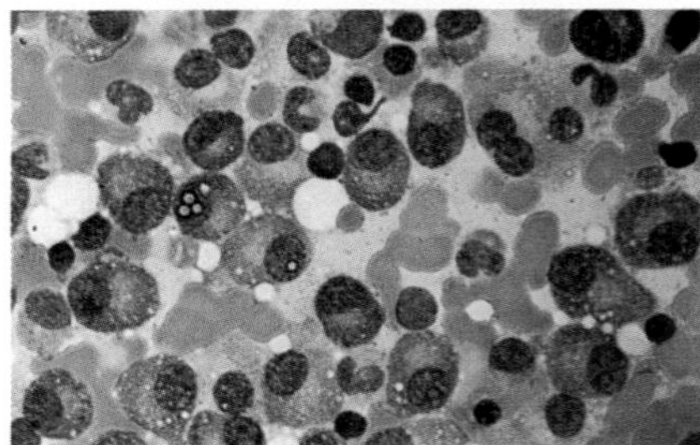

FIGURE 193-4. Multiple myeloma. A bone marrow aspirate shows a predominance of plasma cells.

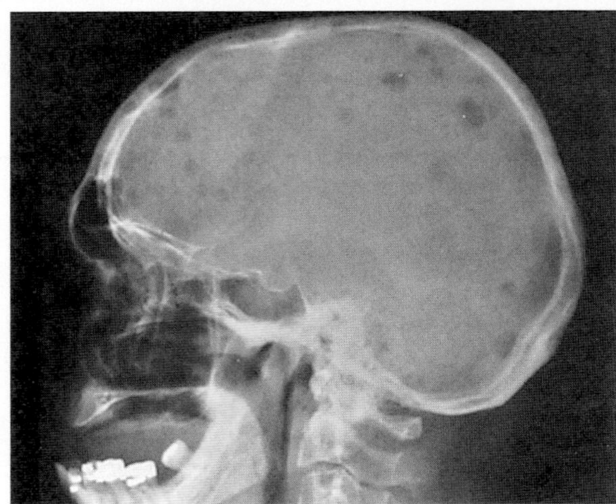

FIGURE 193-5. Skull radiograph showing multiple lytic lesions.

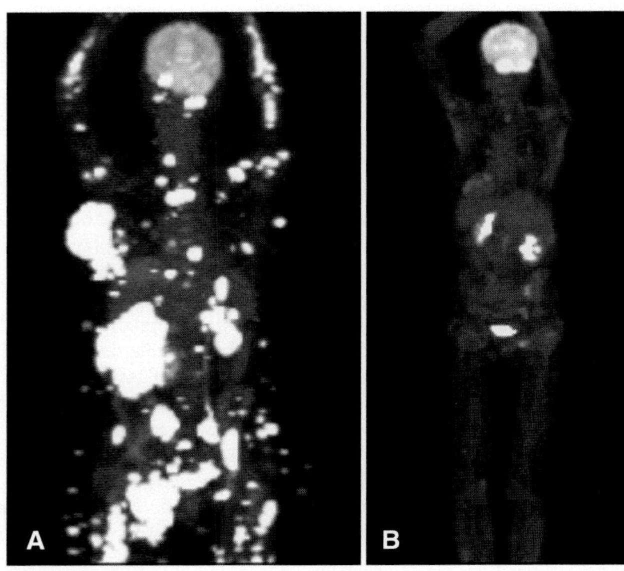

FIGURE 193-6. Positron emission tomography in multiple myeloma. A, Extensive bony and extramedullary disease. **B,** Significant improvement after systemic chemotherapy for myeloma.

type of M protein is IgG in 52%, IgA in 21%, light chain only (Bence Jones proteinemia) in 16%, IgD in 2%, and biclonal gammopathy in 2%; the light chain type is κ in 65% of cases and λ in 35%. In 3% of patients, no secreted M protein can be identified; these patients are considered to have nonsecretory myeloma.

In the bone marrow, plasma cells account for greater than 10% of all nucleated cells in 96% of patients (Fig. 193-4). In 4% of patients, bone marrow examination shows less than 10% plasma cells, even though the patient otherwise meets the criteria for myeloma; because bone marrow involvement in myeloma may be focal rather than diffuse, repeated bone marrow examinations or biopsy of a discrete bone or extramedullary lesion may be required. In most cases, the plasma cells in myeloma are cytoplasmic Ig^+, $CD38^+$, and $CD138^+$; only a minority express CD10 and human leukocyte antigen (HLA)-DR, and 20% express CD20. The clonality of the plasma cells is established using the κ/λ ratio, which is abnormal in myeloma (either >4 : 1, indicating a clonal κ population, or <1 : 2, indicating a clonal λ population). This is helpful for differentiating monoclonal plasma cell proliferation in multiple myeloma from reactive plasmacytosis related to connective tissue disease, metastatic carcinoma, liver disease, and infection.

Radiologic Findings

Conventional radiographs reveal abnormalities consisting of punched-out lytic lesions (Fig. 193-5), osteoporosis, or fractures in nearly 80% of patients. The vertebrae, skull, thoracic cage, pelvis, and proximal ends of the humerus and femur are the most frequent sites of involvement. Technetium-99m bone scanning is inferior to conventional radiography and should not be used. Positron emission tomography (PET; Fig. 193-6) and magnetic resonance imaging (MRI) are helpful in patients who have skeletal pain but no abnormality on radiographs and for monitoring the response to therapy.

Organ Involvement

Renal

At diagnosis, the serum creatinine value is increased initially in almost half of patients and is greater than 2 mg/dL in 20%.

The two major causes of renal insufficiency are light chain cast nephropathy *(myeloma kidney)* and hypercalcemia. Light chain cast nephropathy is characterized by the presence of large, waxy, laminated casts in the distal and collecting tubules. The casts are composed mainly of precipitated monoclonal light chains. The extent of cast formation correlates directly with the amount of free urinary light chain and with the severity of renal insufficiency. Dehydration may precipitate acute renal failure.

Hypercalcemia (Chapters 186 and 253), which is present in 15 to 20% of patients initially, is a major and treatable cause of renal insufficiency. It results from destruction of bone. Hyperuricemia may contribute to renal failure. Besides light chain cast nephropathy and hypercalcemia, there are other mechanisms by which renal dysfunction can occur in myeloma. For example, light chain amyloidosis occurs in nearly 10% of patients and may produce nephrotic syndrome, renal insufficiency, or both. Acquired Fanconi's syndrome (Chapter 124), characterized by proximal tubular dysfunction, results in glycosuria, phosphaturia, and aminoaciduria. Deposition of monoclonal light chains in the renal glomerulus (light chain deposition disease) may also produce renal insufficiency and nephrotic syndrome.

Neurologic

Radiculopathy (Chapter 407), the single most frequent neurologic complication, usually occurs in the thoracic or lumbosacral area and results from compression of the nerve by the vertebral lesion or by the collapsed bone itself. Compression of the spinal cord occurs in up to 10% of patients. Peripheral neuropathy (Chapter 428) is uncommon in multiple myeloma and, when present, is generally caused by amyloidosis. Rarely, myeloma cells diffusely infiltrate the meninges. Intracranial plasmacytomas almost always represent extensions of myelomatous lesions of the skull.

Other Systemic Involvement

Hepatomegaly from plasma cell infiltration is uncommon. Plasmacytomas of the ribs are common and arise either as expanding bone lesions or as soft tissue masses. The incidence of infections is increased in patients with multiple myeloma. Historically, *Streptococcus pneumoniae* and *Staphylococcus aureus* have been the most frequent pathogens, but gram-negative organisms now account for more than half of all infections. The propensity for infection results from impairment of the antibody response, deficiency of normal immunoglobulins, and neutropenia. Bleeding from coating of the platelets by M protein may occur. Myeloma patients have an increased risk of deep vein thrombosis.

PREVENTION AND TREATMENT Rx

Patients with MGUS or smoldering multiple myeloma should not be treated until evidence of multiple myeloma develops. The approach to treatment of multiple myeloma is illustrated in Figure 193-7.

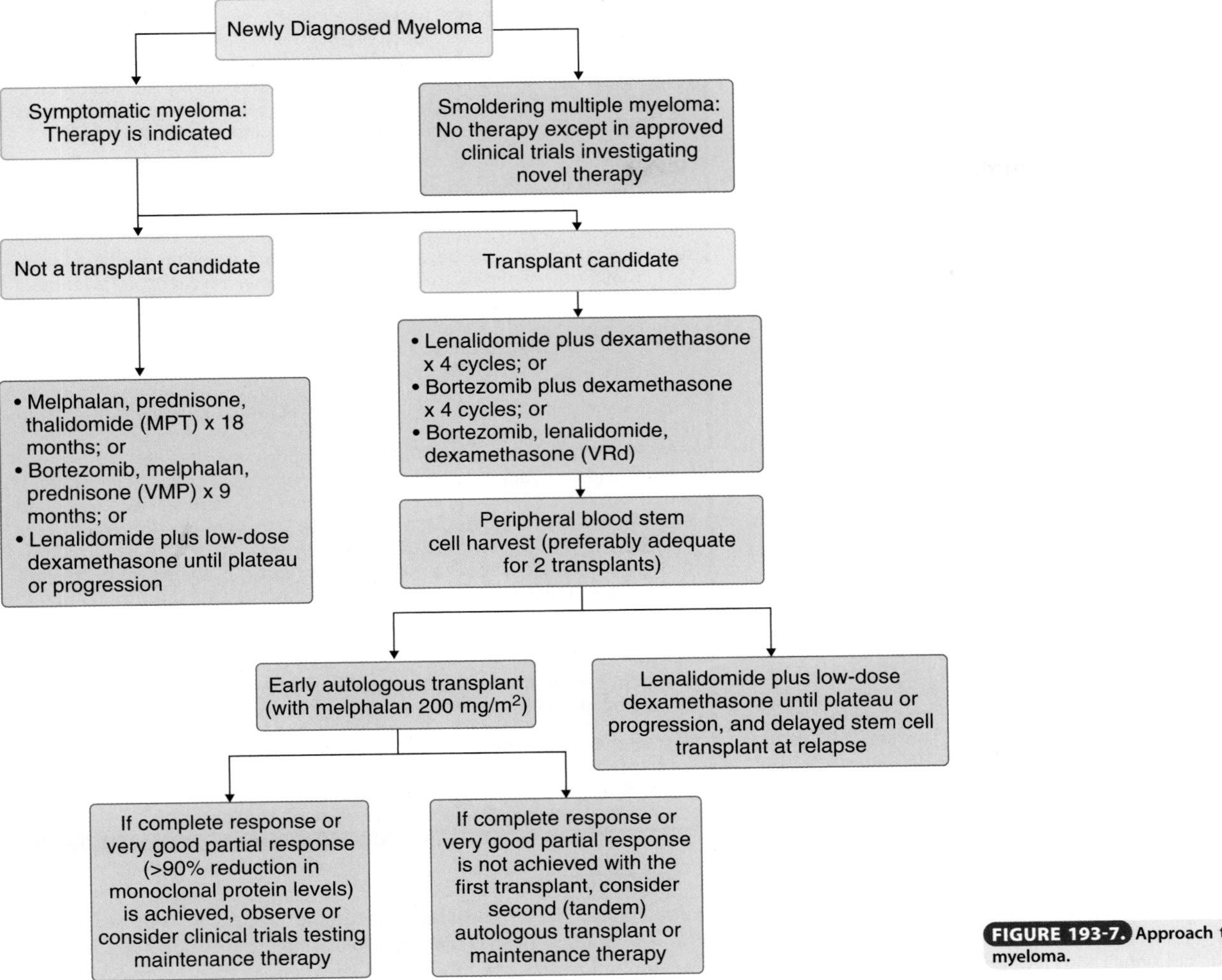

FIGURE 193-7. Approach to newly diagnosed multiple myeloma.

Initial Therapy of Patients Who Are Candidates for Stem Cell Transplantation

In the approximately 50% of patients with newly diagnosed multiple myeloma who are considered candidates for autologous stem cell transplantation based on good performance status, no or limited comorbid conditions, and younger physiologic age (<65 to 70 years), autologous peripheral blood stem cell transplantation (Chapter 181) with high-dose chemotherapy improves overall survival in comparison to conventional chemotherapy.[1] Currently, it is not possible to eradicate myeloma cells completely with conditioning regimens, and reinfused autologous stem cells are usually contaminated by myeloma cells or their precursors. As a result, autologous transplantation is not curative, but it prolongs event-free and overall survival.

Initial therapy typically consists of low-dose dexamethasone (40 mg once a week) plus lenalidomide (25 mg/day on days 1 to 21, every 28 days) and/or bortezomib (1.3 mg/m^2 on days 1, 4, 8, and 11, every 21 days) for approximately 4 months to reduce the number of tumor cells in the bone marrow and peripheral blood. As induction before stem cell transplantation in previously untreated myeloma, bortezomib plus dexamethasone has been found to be superior to vincristine plus doxorubicin plus dexamethasone (VAD).[2] Lenalidomide plus high-dose dexamethasone, compared with high-dose dexamethasone only, produced superior 1-year progression-free survival, overall and partial response rates, but not 1-year overall survival.[3] In a randomized trial, lenalidomide plus low-dose dexamethasone (40 mg once a week) was associated with superior overall survival compared with lenalidomide and high-dose dexamethasone (40 mg on days 1 to 4, 9 to 12, and 17 to 20).[4] As a result, high-dose pulse dexamethasone is no longer recommended in the context of initial therapy. Reducing the dose of bortezomib to once a week instead of days 1, 4, 8, and 11 decreases the risk of serious neuropathy and should be considered after the first 1 to 2 months if a bortezomib-based regimen is used.[5] Toxicities of lenalidomide plus dexamethasone include deep vein thrombosis, and all patients must be treated with prophylactic aspirin or an anticoagulant. After induction therapy, peripheral blood stem cells adequate for two stem cell transplants are collected with the use of granulocyte colony-stimulating factor with or without cyclophosphamide to aid in mobilization. Autologous stem cell transplantation (Chapter 181) is performed with melphalan 200 mg/m^2 as the conditioning regimen, followed by infusion of the peripheral blood stem cells. Patients who do not achieve a complete or very good partial response with the first autologous transplant are considered for a second autologous transplant.[6]

An alternative approach in patients with newly diagnosed disease is to cryopreserve stem cells for future use after initial therapy. Patients then continue initial therapy, such as lenalidomide plus low-dose dexamethasone, until progression or achievement of a plateau phase, reserving stem cell transplantation for the first relapse. Data from randomized trials comparing early versus delayed transplantation indicate no significant difference in survival between the two strategies. The choice is based on the patient's preferences and other clinical conditions, but early transplantation is often preferred because its mortality is low (<1%) and it avoids the inconvenience, cost, and potential side effects of prolonged chemotherapy.

Role of Allogeneic Bone Marrow Transplantation

Ninety to 95% of patients with multiple myeloma cannot undergo allogeneic bone marrow transplantation because of their age, lack of an HLA-matched sibling donor, or inadequate renal, pulmonary, or cardiac function (Chapter 181). Although a complete response occurs in 40% of patients, most have a relapse; in long-term follow-up there is no apparent survival plateau. The mortality rate from the procedure is approximately 25%, and conventional allogeneic bone marrow transplantation is rarely used in myeloma. An alternative is autologous stem cell transplantation followed by nonmyeloablative ("mini") allogeneic transplantation, but treatment-related mortality is still approximately 20%. Nonmyeloablative allogeneic transplantation for myeloma is best performed only in the context of clinical trials.

Initial Therapy of Patients Who Are Not Candidates for Transplantation

Approximately 50% of newly diagnosed patients are not considered candidates for stem cell transplantation. For decades, the oral administration of melphalan (8 to 10 mg/day for 7 days) and prednisone (20 mg three times a day for the same 7 days) repeated every 6 weeks has been the standard of care. When using melphalan, the leukocyte and platelet levels should be measured every 3 weeks, and the dosage of melphalan must be adjusted until midcycle cytopenia occurs. The addition of thalidomide to the standard regimen of melphalan plus prednisone improves event-free and overall survival compared with melphalan plus prednisone alone in patients with newly diagnosed myeloma who are not candidates for transplantation. [7-9] Similarly, in a randomized trial, the addition of bortezomib to melphalan plus prednisone prolonged event-free and overall survival compared with melphalan plus prednisone alone by 39% among patients not eligible for high-dose chemotherapy and stem cell transplantation. [10] Based on these data, melphalan and prednisone plus either thalidomide (MPT) or bortezomib (VMP) are two recommended treatments for this patient population. Lenalidomide plus low-dose dexamethasone is a third option based on its high efficacy and low toxicity in elderly patients.

MPT is typically administered for 18 months, whereas VMP is given for 9 months. Lenalidomide plus low-dose dexamethasone can be given for 1 year or until progression, based on tolerability. Maintenance therapy is not generally recommended following MPT or VMP. If relapse occurs during the plateau state 6 to 12 or more months after cessation of therapy, the initial chemotherapeutic regimen can be reinstituted. Most patients respond, but the duration and quality of the response are usually inferior to those of the initial response.

Treatment of Relapsed Refractory Myeloma

Almost all patients with multiple myeloma eventually relapse. Single-agent dexamethasone, alkylating agents, thalidomide, lenalidomide, and bortezomib, administered alone or in combination, are all options for the treatment of relapsed refractory myeloma. Methylprednisolone 2 g three times a week intravenously for a minimum of 4 weeks, then reduced to once or twice a week if there is a response, is helpful for patients with pancytopenia and may be associated with fewer side effects than dexamethasone.

Thalidomide (50 to 200 mg/day orally) produces an objective response, with a median duration of about 1 year, in about a third of patients with refractory myeloma. Side effects are sedation, constipation, peripheral neuropathy, rash, bradycardia, and thrombotic events. The addition of dexamethasone to thalidomide increases the response rate to approximately 50%, and combinations of thalidomide, dexamethasone, and alkylating agents produce response rates exceeding 70% in patients with relapsed refractory disease.

The thalidomide analogue lenalidomide is better tolerated and produces objective benefits in approximately 40% of patients with relapsed refractory myeloma as a single agent; in combination with dexamethasone, 60% of patients benefit. Lenalidomide plus dexamethasone significantly prolongs time to progression and overall survival compared with dexamethasone alone. [11,12] The starting dose of lenalidomide is 25 mg orally on days 1 to 21, every 28 days. Lenalidomide has significantly fewer nonhematologic toxicities than thalidomide does; myelosuppression is the most common adverse event.

Bortezomib, an inhibitor of the ubiquitin-proteasome pathway, acts through multiple mechanisms to arrest tumor growth, tumor spread, and angiogenesis. It produces objective responses in about a third of patients with refractory myeloma and is superior to single-agent dexamethasone. [13] Like thalidomide and lenalidomide, bortezomib can also be combined with dexamethasone and other active agents to increase response rates. [10] The starting dose is 1.3 mg/m^2 administered intravenously on days 1, 4, 8, and 11, every 21 days. The most common adverse events are gastrointestinal side effects, fatigue, and neuropathy.

Other novel agents that have shown promise but are not commercially available at this time include pomalidomide (a new analogue of thalidomide) and carfilzomib (a new proteasome inhibitor). Several other novel agents are in clinical trials.

Role of Radiation Therapy

Palliative radiation in a dose of 20 to 30 Gy should be limited to patients who have multiple myeloma with disabling pain and a well-defined focal process that has not responded to chemotherapy and to patients with spinal cord compression from a plasmacytoma. Analgesics in combination with chemotherapy can usually control the pain (Chapter 29).

Management of Complications

Hypercalcemia

Hypercalcemia, present in 15 to 20% of patients at diagnosis, should be suspected in those with anorexia, nausea, vomiting, polyuria, polydipsia, constipation, weakness, confusion, or stupor. If hypercalcemia is untreated, renal insufficiency may develop. Hydration, preferably with isotonic saline plus prednisone (25 mg four times/day), usually relieves the hypercalcemia. Bisphosphonates such as zoledronic acid or pamidronate are recommended and will correct hypercalcemia in almost all patients (Chapter 251).

Renal Insufficiency

The most common cause of acute renal failure is light chain cast nephropathy in patients who have excess excretion of monoclonal protein in urine (myeloma kidney). Aggressive treatment of acute renal failure due to light chain cast nephropathy is critical for long-term overall survival. If the patient is not oliguric, intravenous fluids and furosemide are needed to maintain a high urine flow rate (100 mL/hour). If the underlying cause is thought to be light chain cast nephropathy based on clinical findings (e.g., serum free light chains >150 mg/dL) or renal biopsy, plasmapheresis is recommended daily for 5 days to reduce the levels of circulating light chains. Hemodialysis is necessary for symptomatic azotemia. The mainstay of therapy is aggressive treatment of myeloma with a regimen such as bortezomib, thalidomide, and dexamethasone (VTD). Allopurinol is necessary if hyperuricemia is present.

Infection

Prompt, appropriate therapy for bacterial infections is necessary. Prophylactic antibiotics such as trimethoprim-sulfamethoxazole should be considered in patients taking high-dose corticosteroids, but trimethoprim-sulfamethoxazole should be avoided in patients receiving thalidomide or lenalidomide to minimize the risk of serious skin reactions. Intravenously administered gamma globulin is reserved for patients with hypogammaglobulinemia and recurrent severe infections. Pneumococcal and influenza immunizations (Chapter 17) should be given to all patients.

Skeletal Lesions

Patients should be encouraged to be as active as possible but to avoid trauma. Pamidronate (90 mg infused intravenously over a 4-hour period every 4 weeks) or zoledronic acid (4 mg intravenously over at least 15 minutes every 4 weeks) reduces the incidence of bone pain, pathologic fractures, and spinal cord compression; such prophylaxis is now routinely recommended for all patients with myeloma bone disease and may improve overall survival. [14] After 1 to 2 years the dosing can be reduced to once every 3 months in patients who are stable, to minimize the risk of osteonecrosis of the jaw, which is a complication of long-term bisphosphonate therapy.

Spinal cord compression from an extramedullary plasmacytoma (Chapter 407) should be suspected in patients who have severe back pain, weakness or paresthesias of the lower extremities, or bladder or bowel dysfunction. Initial treatment is with dexamethasone-based therapy and/or radiation therapy. If the neurologic deficit increases, surgical decompression is necessary.

Miscellaneous Complications

Symptomatic hyperviscosity (see later) is less common than in Waldenström's macroglobulinemia. Anemia that persists despite adequate treatment of underlying myeloma often responds to erythropoietin.

PROGNOSIS

Multiple myeloma is considered incurable at present, but survival has improved significantly in recent years following the arrival of new agents such as lenalidomide and bortezomib. The median survival is approximately 4 years, but it varies widely according to clinical stage and risk stratification factors (Table 193-5). In some patients an acute or aggressive terminal phase is characterized by rapid tumor growth, pancytopenia, soft tissue subcutaneous masses, decreased M protein levels, and fever; survival in this subset is generally only a few months.

FUTURE DIRECTIONS

Future efforts must be directed toward identifying new active agents and developing effective combinations of active drugs. Studies are under way to improve the conditioning regimen used in autologous stem cell transplantation and to better integrate novel therapies with stem cell transplantation.

TABLE 193-5 STAGING AND PROGNOSTIC FACTORS IN MULTIPLE MYELOMA

STAGE/RISK FACTOR	MEDIAN SURVIVAL (MO)
INTERNATIONAL STAGING SYSTEM	
Stage I (serum β_2-microglobulin <3.5 mg/L and serum albumin ≥3.5 g/dL)	62
Stage II (neither stage I nor stage III)	44
Stage III (serum β_2-microglobulin ≥5.5 mg/L)	29
RISK STRATIFICATION	
High-risk myeloma (any one of the following): Fluorescence in situ hybridization: t14;16, t14;20, deletion 17p	24-36
OTHER ADVERSE PROGNOSTIC FACTORS	
Elevated lactate dehydrogenase level	
Poor performance status	
Increased circulating plasma cells	
Plasmablastic morphology	
Increased plasma cell labeling index ≥1%	

VARIANT FORMS OF MULTIPLE MYELOMA

Smoldering Multiple Myeloma

Smoldering (asymptomatic) multiple myeloma is defined by the presence of an M protein level greater than 3 g/dL in serum or 10% or more plasma cells in bone marrow in the absence of anemia, renal insufficiency, hypercalcemia, or skeletal lesions. Biologically, patients with smoldering multiple myeloma are similar to those with MGUS but carry a much higher risk for progression to myeloma or related malignancy: 10% per year for the first 5 years, 5% per year for the next 5 years, and 1 to 2% per year thereafter. As a result, patients must be observed more closely (every 3 to 4 months), but they should not be treated unless progression to symptomatic multiple myeloma occurs.

Plasma Cell Leukemia

Patients with plasma cell leukemia have more than 20% plasma cells in the peripheral blood and an absolute plasma cell count of 2000/μL or greater. Plasma cell leukemia is classified as primary when it is diagnosed in the leukemic phase (60%) or as secondary when there is leukemic transformation of a previously recognized multiple myeloma (40%). Patients with primary plasma cell leukemia are younger and have a greater incidence of hepatosplenomegaly and lymphadenopathy, a higher platelet count, fewer bone lesions, a smaller serum M protein component, and longer survival (median, 6.8 vs. 1.3 months) than do patients with secondary plasma cell leukemia. Treatment of plasma cell leukemia is unsatisfactory. An aggressive initial treatment regimen that contains bortezomib, dexamethasone, and either thalidomide or lenalidomide for two or three cycles, followed by autologous stem cell transplantation and subsequent maintenance therapy with lenalidomide, is a reasonable strategy if the patient's clinical condition permits such an approach. Secondary plasma cell leukemia rarely responds to chemotherapy because the patients have already received chemotherapy and are resistant.

Nonsecretory Myeloma

Patients with nonsecretory myeloma have no M protein in either serum or urine and account for only 3% of cases of myeloma. To make the diagnosis, the clonal nature of bone marrow plasma cells should be established by immunoperoxidase, immunofluorescence, or flow cytometric methods. Treatment and survival are similar to those in patients with typical myeloma. The serum free light chain assay is abnormal in more than 60% of patients and can be used to monitor the response to therapy.

Osteosclerotic Myeloma (POEMS Syndrome)

This syndrome is characterized by polyneuropathy, organomegaly, endocrinopathy, M protein, and skin changes (POEMS). The diagnosis of POEMS syndrome requires the presence of a monoclonal plasma cell disorder, peripheral neuropathy, plus at least one of the following seven features: osteosclerotic bone lesions, Castleman's disease, organomegaly, endocrinopathy (excluding diabetes mellitus or hypothyroidism), edema, typical skin changes, and papilledema. However, not every patient meeting these criteria has POEMS syndrome; the features should have a temporal relationship to one another, with no other attributable cause. The absence of osteosclerotic lesions makes the diagnosis suspect. Elevations in plasma or serum levels of vascular endothelial growth factor and thrombocytosis are common features of the syndrome and are helpful when the diagnosis is difficult. The major clinical features are a chronic inflammatory-demyelinating polyneuropathy with predominantly motor disability and sclerotic skeletal lesions. The bone marrow usually contains less than 5% plasma cells, and hypercalcemia and renal insufficiency rarely occur. Almost all patients have a λ-type M protein. The diagnosis is confirmed by identification of monoclonal plasma cells obtained at biopsy of an osteosclerotic lesion.

If the lesions are in a limited area, radiation therapy substantially improves the neuropathy in more than 50% of patients. If the patient has widespread osteosclerotic lesions, treatment is with autologous stem cell transplantation or other systemic therapy similar to that used for myeloma.

Solitary Plasmacytoma (Solitary Myeloma) of Bone

The diagnosis of solitary bone plasmacytoma is based on histologic evidence of a solitary tumor consisting of monoclonal plasma cells identical to those in multiple myeloma. In addition, complete skeletal radiographs and MRI of the spine and pelvis must show no other lesions of myeloma, and the bone marrow aspirate must contain no evidence of clonal plasma cells. An M protein may be present in serum or urine at diagnosis, but persistence of the M protein after radiation therapy is associated with an increased risk for progression to multiple myeloma. Treatment consists of radiation in the range of 40 to 50 Gy. Almost 50% of patients who have a solitary plasmacytoma are alive at 10 years, and disease-free survival rates at 10 years range from 15 to 25%. Progression to myeloma, when it occurs, usually takes place within 3 years, but patients must be monitored indefinitely. There is no convincing evidence that adjuvant chemotherapy decreases the rate of conversion to multiple myeloma.

Extramedullary Plasmacytoma

Extramedullary plasmacytomas outside the bone marrow are most commonly found in the upper respiratory tract (80% of cases), especially in the nasal cavity and sinuses, nasopharynx, and larynx. Extramedullary plasmacytomas may also occur in the gastrointestinal tract, central nervous system, urinary bladder, thyroid, breast, testes, parotid gland, or lymph nodes. Extramedullary plasmacytomas may be solitary, or they may occur in the context of existing myeloma. The diagnosis of solitary extramedullary plasmacytoma is based on detection of a plasma cell tumor in an extramedullary site, absence of clonal plasma cells on bone marrow examination, and absence of other bony or extramedullary lesions on radiographic studies. Treatment of solitary extramedullary plasmacytoma consists of either complete surgical resection or tumoricidal irradiation. The plasmacytoma may recur locally, metastasize to regional nodes, or, rarely, develop into multiple myeloma.

WALDENSTRÖM'S MACROGLOBULINEMIA (PRIMARY MACROGLOBULINEMIA)

DEFINITION

Waldenström's macroglobulinemia is the result of the uncontrolled proliferation of lymphocytes and plasma cells in which an IgM M protein is produced. The cause is unknown; familial clusters have been reported. The median age of patients at the time of diagnosis is about 65 years, and approximately 60% are male. The diagnostic criteria are IgM monoclonal gammopathy (regardless of the size of the M protein), 10% or greater bone marrow infiltration (usually intertrabecular) by clonal lymphocytes that exhibit plasmacytoid or plasma cell differentiation, and a typical immunophenotype (e.g., surface IgM^+, $CD5^{+/-}$, $CD10^-$, $CD19^+$, $CD20^+$, $CD23^-$) that would satisfactorily exclude other lymphoproliferative disorders, including CLL (Chapter 190) and mantle cell lymphoma (Chapter 191).

CLINICAL MANIFESTATIONS

Weakness, fatigue, and bleeding (especially oozing from the oronasal area) are common initial symptoms. Blurred or impaired vision, dyspnea, weight loss, neurologic symptoms, recurrent infections, and heart failure may occur. In contrast to multiple myeloma, lytic bone lesions, renal insufficiency, and amyloidosis are rare. Physical findings include pallor, hepatosplenomegaly, and lymphadenopathy. Retinal hemorrhages, exudates, and venous congestion with vascular segmentation ("sausage" formation) may occur. Sensorimotor peripheral neuropathy is common. Pulmonary involvement is manifested by diffuse pulmonary infiltrates and isolated masses.

Laboratory Evaluation

Almost all patients have moderate to severe normocytic, normochromic anemia. The serum electrophoretic pattern is characterized by a tall, narrow peak or dense band that is of the IgM type on immunofixation. Quantitative IgM levels are high. A monoclonal light chain is detected in the urine of 80% of patients, but the amount of urinary protein is generally modest.

The bone marrow aspirate is often hypocellular, but the biopsy is hypercellular and extensively infiltrated with lymphoid cells and plasma cells. The number of mast cells is frequently increased. Rouleau formation is prominent (Chapter 160), and the sedimentation rate is markedly increased. About 10% of cases may have an associated type I cryoglobulinemia (see later).

DIAGNOSIS

Diagnosis requires the combination of typical symptoms and physical findings, the presence of an IgM M protein, and 10% or greater lymphoplasmacytic infiltration of the bone marrow. The lymphoplasmacytic cells express CD19, CD20, and CD22, whereas expression of CD5 and CD10 occurs in a minority. Asymptomatic patients with 10% or greater lymphoplasmacytic infiltration of the bone marrow are considered to have smoldering Waldenström's macroglobulinemia. Multiple myeloma, CLL, and MGUS of the IgM type must be excluded.

Patients meeting the diagnostic criteria for Waldenström's macroglobulinemia but who have less than 3 g/dL IgM protein at diagnosis have sometimes been classified as having "lymphoplasmacytic lymphoma with an IgM M protein" (Chapter 191). However, except for hyperviscosity, the clinical picture, therapy, and prognosis for these patients do not differ from those of patients with an IgM level of 3 g/dL or greater; thus, these patients are also considered to have Waldenström's macroglobulinemia by the current definition.

PREVENTION AND TREATMENT Rx

Patients should not be treated unless they have anemia; constitutional symptoms such as weakness, fatigue, night sweats, or weight loss; hyperviscosity; or significant hepatosplenomegaly or lymphadenopathy. Rituximab, a chimeric anti-CD20 monoclonal antibody (Chapter 35), produces a response in at least 50% of untreated patients. Alkylating agents such as cyclophosphamide and chlorambucil with or without corticosteroids are also effective. Another choice for therapy is a purine nucleoside analogue, either fludarabine or 2-chlorodeoxyadenosine. In general, for minimally symptomatic patients, rituximab as a single agent is an excellent choice for initial therapy. For patients with more advanced symptoms, including severe anemia or hyperviscosity, combination approaches are preferred. The combination of rituximab, cyclophosphamide, and dexamethasone is highly active and also preserves the ability to mobilize stem cells for transplantation, if necessary. An alternative is cladribine with or without rituximab.

For relapse, the agents used as initial therapy can be given alone or in combination. Autologous stem cell transplantation can be considered for eligible patients with relapsed disease.

Spuriously low hemoglobin and hematocrit levels may occur because of the increased plasma volume from the large amount of intravascular M protein. Consequently, transfusions should not be given solely on the basis of the hemoglobin or hematocrit value. Symptomatic hyperviscosity should be treated by plasmapheresis. The median survival of patients with macroglobulinemia is 5 years.

HYPERVISCOSITY SYNDROME

Hyperviscosity syndrome occurs in patients with Waldenström's macroglobulinemia who have high levels of serum IgM M protein (>5 g/dL) and occasionally in those with myeloma, especially of the IgA type. Hyperviscosity is disproportionately more common relative to the same serum concentration of IgM and IgA M proteins compared with IgG M proteins, owing to the inherent tendency of IgM and IgA molecules to polymerize. Typically, IgM forms pentamers, whereas IgA forms dimers or sometimes trimers, resulting in high-molecular-weight complexes. Chronic nasal bleeding and oozing from the gums are the most frequent symptoms of hyperviscosity, but postsurgical or gastrointestinal bleeding may also occur. Retinal hemorrhages are common, and venous congestion with sausage-like segmentation and papilledema may be seen (Fig. 193-8). The patient occasionally complains of blurring or loss of vision. Dizziness, headache, vertigo, nystagmus, decreased hearing, ataxia, paresthesias, diplopia, somnolence, and coma may occur. Hyperviscosity can precipitate or exacerbate heart failure. Most patients have symptoms when the relative viscosity is greater than 4 cP, but the relationship between serum viscosity and clinical manifestations is not precise. Patients with symptomatic hyperviscosity should be treated with plasmapheresis and with chemotherapy to treat the underlying malignancy. Plasma exchange of 3 to 4 L with albumin should be performed daily until the patient is asymptomatic. Plasma exchange is rapidly effective (two to three exchanges) in the case of IgM M proteins, which are primarily intravascular; with IgG M proteins, multiple attempts may be needed because a significant amount of IgG can exist in the extravascular space.

HEAVY CHAIN DISEASES

The HCDs are characterized by the presence of an M protein consisting of a portion of the immunoglobulin heavy chain in serum, urine, or both. These heavy chains are devoid of light chains and represent a lymphoplasma cell proliferative process. There are three major types: γ-HCD, α-HCD, and μ-HCD.

γ-HCD

Patients with γ-HCD often initially have a lymphoma-like illness, but the clinical findings are diverse and range from an aggressive lymphoproliferative process (Chapter 191) to an asymptomatic state. Hepatosplenomegaly and lymphadenopathy occur in about 60% of patients. Anemia is found in approximately 80% initially and in nearly all eventually. The electrophoretic pattern often shows a broad-based band more suggestive of a polyclonal increase than an M protein. The diagnosis depends on the identification of an isolated monoclonal γ heavy chain on serum immunofixation, without evidence of either monoclonal κ or λ light chain expression.

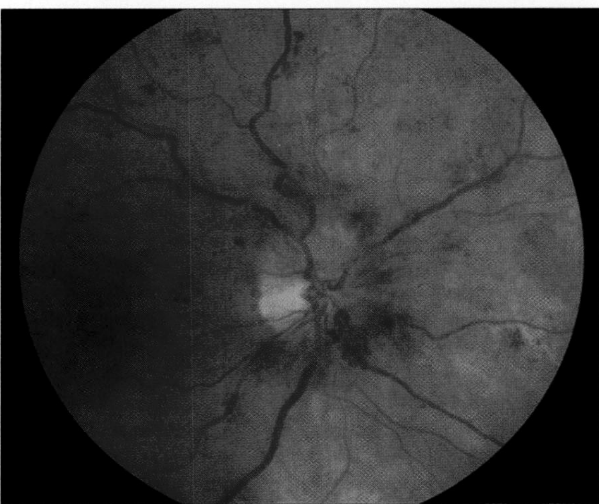

FIGURE 193-8. Hyperviscosity syndrome. Right eye retinal image in a patient with Waldenström's macroglobulinemia and hyperviscosity syndrome showing sausaging (focal venular dilations), intraretinal hemorrhages, microaneurysms, and peripapillary cotton-wool spots and disc swelling (papilledema).

Treatment is indicated only for symptomatic patients and consists of chemotherapy with melphalan plus prednisone or regimens used to treat non-Hodgkin's lymphoma (Chapter 191), such as cyclophosphamide, vincristine, and prednisone. The prognosis of γ-HCD is variable and ranges from a rapidly progressive downhill course of a few weeks' duration to the asymptomatic presence of a stable monoclonal heavy chain in serum or urine.

α-HCD

α-HCD is the most common form of HCD and occurs in patients from the Mediterranean region or the Middle East, generally in the second or third decade of life. About 60% are men. Most commonly the gastrointestinal tract is involved, and severe malabsorption with diarrhea, steatorrhea, and weight loss is noted (Chapter 142). Plasma cell infiltration of the jejunal mucosa is the most frequent pathologic feature. Immunoproliferative small intestinal disease is restricted to patients with small intestinal lesions who have the pathologic features of α-HCD but do not synthesize α heavy chains.

The serum protein electrophoretic pattern is normal in half the cases; in the remainder an unimpressive broad band may appear in the α2 or β region. The diagnosis depends on identification of an isolated monoclonal α heavy chain on serum immunofixation, without evidence of either monoclonal κ or λ light chain expression. The amount of α heavy chain in urine is small.

In the absence of therapy, α-HCD is typically progressive and fatal. The usual treatment consists of antibiotics, such as tetracyclines, and the eradication of any concurrent parasitic infection. Patients who do not respond adequately to antibiotics are given chemotherapy similar to that used to treat non-Hodgkin's lymphoma, for example, the cyclophosphamide, hydroxydaunomycin, vincristine (Oncovin), and prednisone (CHOP) regimen (Chapter 191).

μ-HCD

This disease is characterized by the demonstration of an isolated monoclonal μ chain fragment on serum immunofixation, without evidence of either monoclonal κ or λ light chain expression.

The serum protein electrophoretic pattern is usually normal, except for hypogammaglobulinemia. Bence Jones proteinuria has been found in two thirds of cases. Lymphocytes, plasma cells, and lymphoplasmacytoid cells are increased in the bone marrow. Vacuolization of the plasma cells is common and should suggest the possibility of HCD. The course of μ-HCD is variable, and survival ranges from a few months to many years. Treatment is with corticosteroids and alkylating agents.

CRYOGLOBULINEMIA

Cryoglobulins are plasma proteins that precipitate when cooled and dissolve when heated. They are designated as idiopathic or essential when they are not associated with any recognizable disease. Cryoglobulins are classified into

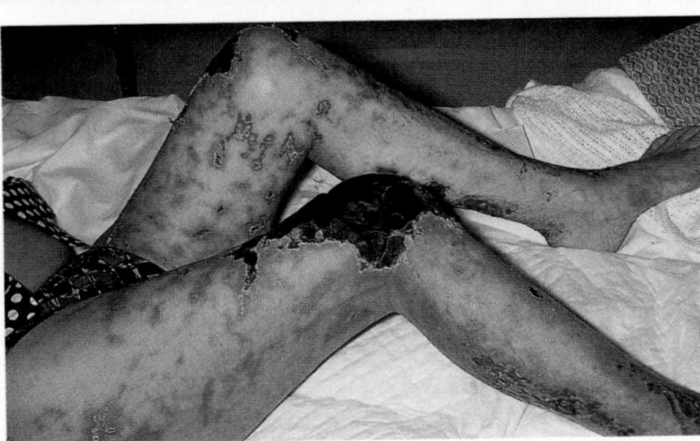

FIGURE 193-9. Skin infarction in cryoglobulinemia. The skin has a reticulated pattern as a result of leakage of red blood cells from damaged skin capillaries. Necrosis and ulceration have occurred in peripheral sites because of vessel blockage. This patient eventually required plastic surgery. (From Forbes CD, Jackson WF. *Color Atlas and Text of Clinical Medicine*, 3rd ed. London: Mosby; 2003.)

three types: type I (monoclonal), type II (mixed monoclonal plus polyclonal), and type III (polyclonal).

Type I Cryoglobulinemia

Type I (monoclonal) cryoglobulinemia is most commonly of the IgM or IgG class, but IgA and Bence Jones cryoglobulins have been reported. Most patients, even with large amounts of type I cryoglobulin, are completely asymptomatic from this source. Others with monoclonal cryoglobulins in the range of 1 to 2 g/dL may have evidence of vasculitis with pain, purpura, Raynaud's phenomenon, cyanosis, and even ulceration and sloughing of skin and subcutaneous tissue (Fig. 193-9) on exposure to cold because their cryoglobulins precipitate at relatively high temperatures. Type I cryoglobulins are associated with macroglobulinemia, multiple myeloma, or MGUS. Therapy for patients with symptomatic type I cryoglobulinemia and significant symptoms is similar to that for Waldenström's macroglobulinemia for the IgM type and multiple myeloma for the non-IgM type.

Type II Cryoglobulinemia

Type II (mixed) cryoglobulinemia typically consists of an immune complex of IgM M protein and polyclonal IgG, although monoclonal IgG or monoclonal IgA may also be seen with polyclonal IgM. Serum protein electrophoresis generally shows a normal pattern or a diffuse, polyclonal hypergammaglobulinemic pattern. The quantity of mixed cryoglobulin is usually less than 0.2 g/dL. Despite the monoclonal component, most patients do not have a clonal plasma cell disorder; rather, they have serologic evidence of infection with hepatitis C virus (Chapter 151). At present, hepatitis C is thought to be the cause of most cases of type II cryoglobulinemia.

Most clinical manifestations are related to the development of vasculitis and include palpable purpura, livedo reticularis, polyarthralgias, and neuropathy. Involvement of the joints is symmetrical, but joint deformities rarely develop. Raynaud's phenomenon, necrosis of the skin, and neurologic involvement may be present. In almost 80% of renal biopsy specimens, glomerular damage can be identified. Nephrotic syndrome may result, but severe renal insufficiency is uncommon.

Early administration of corticosteroids is the most frequent therapy. Treatment should also target underlying hepatitis C infection with interferon-α2 or ribavirin (Chapter 151). Agents to treat the monoclonal component, such as cyclophosphamide, chlorambucil, azathioprine, or rituximab, are used if there is no response. Plasmapheresis (with a warmed circuit) is helpful in the acute management of symptoms by removing circulating immune complexes.

Type III Cryoglobulinemia

Type III (polyclonal) cryoglobulinemia does not have a monoclonal component and is not associated with a clonal plasma cell proliferative disorder. Type III cryoglobulins are found in many patients with chronic infections or inflammatory diseases and are usually of no clinical significance unless associated with hepatitis C infection.

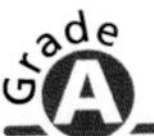

1. Child JA, Morgan GJ, Davies FE, et al. High-dose chemotherapy with hematopoietic stem-cell rescue for multiple myeloma. *N Engl J Med*. 2003;348:1875-1883.
2. Harousseau JL, Attal M, Avet-Loiseau H, et al. Bortezomib plus dexamethasone as induction treatment prior to autologous stem-cell transplantation in newly diagnosed multiple myeloma: results of the IFM 2005-01 phase III trial. *J Clin Oncol*. 2010;28:4621-4629.
3. Zonder JA, Crowley J, Hussein MA, et al. Lenalidomide and high-dose dexamethasone compared with dexamethasone as initial therapy for multiple myeloma: a randomized Southwest Oncology Group Trial (S0232). *Blood*. 2010;116:5838-5841.
4. Rajkumar SV, Jacobus S, Callander NS, et al. Lenalidomide plus high-dose dexamethasone versus lenalidomide plus low-dose dexamethasone as initial therapy for newly diagnosed multiple myeloma: an open-label randomised controlled trial. *Lancet Oncol*. 2010;11:29-37.
5. Mateos MV, Oriol A, Martinez-Lopez J, et al. Bortezomib, melphalan, and prednisone versus bortezomib, thalidomide, and prednisone as induction therapy followed by maintenance treatment with bortezomib and thalidomide versus bortezomib and prednisone in elderly patients with untreated multiple myeloma: a randomised trial. *Lancet Oncol*. 2010;11:934-941.
6. Attal M, Harousseau JL, Facon T, et al. Single versus double autologous stem-cell transplantation for multiple myeloma. *N Engl J Med*. 2003;349:2495-2502.
7. Facon T, Mary JY, Hulin C, et al. Melphalan and prednisone plus thalidomide versus melphalan and prednisone alone or reduced-intensity autologous stem cell transplantation in elderly patients with multiple myeloma (IFM 99-06): a randomised trial. *Lancet*. 2007;370:1209-1218.
8. Palumbo A, Bringhen S, Caravita T, et al. Oral melphalan and prednisone chemotherapy plus thalidomide compared with melphalan and prednisone alone in elderly patients with multiple myeloma: randomised controlled trial. *Lancet*. 2006;367:825-831.
9. Hulin C, Facon T, Rodon P, et al. Efficacy of melphalan and prednisone plus thalidomide in patients older than 75 years with newly diagnosed multiple myeloma: IFM 01/01 Trial. *J Clin Oncol*. 2009;27:3664-3670.
10. San Miguel JF, Schlag R, Khuageva NK, et al. Bortezomib plus melphalan and prednisone for initial treatment of multiple myeloma. *N Engl J Med*. 2008;359:906-917.
11. Dimopoulos M, Spencer A, Attal M, et al. Lenalidomide plus dexamethasone for relapsed or refractory multiple myeloma. *N Engl J Med*. 2007;357:2123-2132.
12. Weber DM, Chen C, Niesvizky R, et al. Lenalidomide plus dexamethasone for relapsed multiple myeloma in North America. *N Engl J Med*. 2007;357:2133-2142.
13. Richardson PG, Sonneveld P, Schuster MW, et al. Bortezomib or high-dose dexamethasone for relapsed multiple myeloma. *N Engl J Med*. 2005;352:2487-2498.
14. Morgan GJ, Davies FE, Gregory WM, et al. First-line treatment with zoledronic acid as compared with clodronic acid in multiple myeloma (MRC Myeloma IX): a randomised controlled trial. *Lancet*. 2010;376:1989-1999.

SUGGESTED READINGS

Landgren O, Waxman AJ. Multiple myeloma precursor disease. *JAMA*. 2010;304:2397-2404. *Review of monoclonal gammopathy of undetermined significance.*

Laubach J, Richardson P, Anderson K. Multiple myeloma. *Annu Rev Med*. 2011;62:249-264. *Review.*

Palumbo A, Anderson K. Multiple myeloma. *N Engl J Med*. 2011;364:1046-1060. *Review.*

Rajkumar SV. Multiple myeloma: 2011 update on diagnosis, risk-stratification and management. *Am J Hematol*. 2011;86:57-65. *Provides a detailed, risk-adapted approach to the treatment of myeloma.*

194

AMYLOIDOSIS

MORIE A. GERTZ

DEFINITION

Immunoglobulin light chain amyloidosis is characterized by a clonal population of bone marrow plasma cells that produces a monoclonal light chain of the κ or λ type, as either an intact molecule or a fragment. The light chain protein, instead of conforming to the α-helical configuration of most proteins, misfolds and forms a β-pleated sheet. This insoluble protein deposits in tissues and interferes with organ function. The β-pleated sheet configuration is responsible for the tinctorial properties; when the protein is stained with Congo red and viewed under polarized light, apple-green birefringence is demonstrated and is required for the diagnosis. Systemic light chain amyloidosis (AL) must be distinguished from the much less common amyloidosis associated with chronic infection and inflammatory arthropathies (secondary or AA) or with inherited amyloid cardiomyopathies and neuropathies (familial or AF).

CLINICAL MANIFESTATIONS

Amyloidosis is particularly difficult to diagnose and is a challenge for internists. The presenting symptoms can be very broad and are mimicked by far more common disorders (Table 194-1). The signs include tongue enlargement with dental indentations and "pinch" or periorbital purpura, a result of vascular fragility. The signs are specific but lack sensitivity, in that they are present in no more than 20% of patients. No single imaging procedure or

TABLE 194-1 SYMPTOMS, SIGNS, AND SYNDROMES IN AMYLOIDOSIS

SYMPTOMS AND SIGNS
Common symptoms: fatigue, edema, dyspnea, anorexia, paresthesias
Rare symptoms: claudication, joint pain and stiffness, sicca syndrome
Common signs: periorbital purpura, glossomegaly, hepatomegaly
Rare signs: waxy infiltration of eyelids, shoulder pad sign
SYNDROMES
Nondiabetic nephrotic syndrome
Nonischemic cardiomyopathy with an echocardiogram showing "hypertrophy"
Hepatomegaly or increased alkaline phosphatase with no imaging abnormality
Peripheral neuropathy with monoclonal gammopathy of undetermined significance or chronic inflammatory demyelinating polyneuropathy with autonomic features
Atypical myeloma with monoclonal light chains and modest marrow plasmacytosis

laboratory study is diagnostic for the disease. The clinician must therefore be aware of the possibility of amyloidosis, or it may be overlooked. The kidney is commonly involved in amyloidosis. The diagnosis should be suspected in any patient who presents with nondiabetic nephrotic-range proteinuria (Chapter 123). One third of patients with amyloidosis have nephrotic syndrome that presents with dramatic increases in the blood cholesterol level (median, 270 mg/dL), and urinalysis for proteinuria should be done in patients with a sudden increase in the serum cholesterol level. A patient with nondiabetic proteinuria may receive an empirical course of corticosteroids for possible minimal-change glomerulopathy. This treatment delays the diagnosis of amyloidosis and allows other organs to become involved. Ten percent of renal biopsy specimens in nondiabetic nephrotic syndrome are subsequently shown to be involved by amyloidosis. The incidence of bleeding after percutaneous renal biopsy is not increased in AL.

The heart is involved in approximately 50% of patients with amyloidosis, and the presentation is subtle because fatigue is often the only manifestation. Because amyloid heart disease (Chapter 60) is a disorder of diastolic failure, the typical findings of cardiomyopathy (enlarged cardiac silhouette on chest radiography, depressed ejection fraction by echocardiography, and pulmonary vascular redistribution) are absent. The effect of amyloidosis on the heart is poor filling during diastole. Patients have low end-diastolic volume and, as a consequence, poor stroke volume despite a completely normal ejection fraction. Electrocardiography frequently shows a pseudoinfarct pattern, which can be interpreted as demonstrating silent ischemic infarction; this finding leads to coronary angiography, which is invariably negative (unless there is coincidental coronary artery disease). Echocardiography, which shows thickening of the heart walls due to amyloid infiltration, is frequently interpreted as showing left ventricular hypertrophy, and the cause of heart failure can be ascribed to silent hypertension or, alternatively, hypertrophic cardiomyopathy. Echocardiography frequently shows valvular insufficiency of the mitral and tricuspid valves. Restrictive cardiomyopathy has been confused with pericardial disease, and patients have undergone unnecessary pericardiectomy, without clinical benefit. The classic granular sparkling appearance of the echocardiogram is not a useful diagnostic finding. Patients with amyloidosis rarely have symptoms of ischemic heart disease. Enhancement on magnetic resonance imaging with gadolinium is delayed in 69% of patients with cardiac amyloidosis. Myocardial enhancement is associated with increased ventricular mass and impaired left ventricular systolic function.

The liver is involved in 13% of patients (Chapter 153). The typical presentation is hepatomegaly and an increased serum alkaline phosphatase value. An increased transaminase value and hyperbilirubinemia are late signs. Imaging is not helpful, and liver uptake is homogeneous. Many patients undergo an evaluation for metastatic malignancy. Liver biopsy is not associated with an increased rate of bleeding and is not contraindicated in the presence of hepatic amyloidosis. Rare patients present with spontaneous splenic rupture. Acquired deficiency of coagulation factor X is specific to AL and can be associated with clinically severe hemorrhage. Levels improve with effective therapy because the cause is binding of the factor to the fibrils of amyloid.

The peripheral neuropathy (Chapter 428) associated with amyloidosis begins in the lower extremities, is symmetrical, and is generally sensory or mixed sensorimotor. When a monoclonal protein is recognized, frequent diagnoses are chronic inflammatory demyelinating polyneuropathy or neuropathy associated with monoclonal gammopathy of undetermined significance, because amyloidosis has not been considered in the differential diagnosis. Associated autonomic neuropathy occurs in approximately 4% of patients and can be characterized by orthostatic hypotension, which may be misattributed to the cardiac failure. Autonomic dysmotility of the bowel is a common associated finding (Chapter 138). It can be upper intestinal, leading to pseudo-obstruction and recurrent emesis, or lower intestinal, which is characterized by alternating obstipation and fecal incontinence. Diarrhea caused by autonomic failure has been misdiagnosed as collagenous colitis when eosinophilic deposits are found in the bowel mucosa on hematoxylin-eosin staining in the absence of Congo red staining. Carpal tunnel syndrome (Chapter 428) occurs in approximately 13% of patients; it is not clinically distinguishable from the syndrome associated with repetitive stress injury but frequently fails to improve after surgical release. Rarely, interstitial lung disease, pseudoclaudication, periarticular deposits, and unexplained weight loss are presenting symptoms.

Systemic amyloidosis can be confused with early multiple myeloma (Chapter 193). Patients who present with vague symptoms of fatigue and edema are found to have a monoclonal protein in the urine, and a bone marrow biopsy shows a clonal plasmacytosis with a median of 5% plasma cells in the bone marrow; however, a quarter of patients have more than 10% plasma cells in the bone marrow, a finding that qualifies as a diagnosis of multiple myeloma. These patients are often considered to have atypical multiple myeloma when the underlying amyloid syndrome goes undetected. In these patients, a misdiagnosis of myeloma kidney or demyelinating neuropathy is made when an adequate diagnostic evaluation to exclude amyloidosis has not been performed.

DIAGNOSIS

Screening for Amyloidosis

In a patient with nondiabetic proteinuria, cardiomyopathy without ischemic risk factors, unexplained hepatomegaly, peripheral or autonomic neuropathy, or carpal tunnel syndrome, amyloidosis is not the most likely cause. The disorder occurs in only 8 per million persons per year, and routine biopsy is not appropriate whenever consistent symptoms are found. The classic physical finding of periorbital purpura occurs in only 10% of patients, is often limited to petechial eruptions over the eyelids, and is easily overlooked. Enlargement of the tongue occurs in 10 to 15% of patients; therefore, although it is specific, it is not sensitive for the diagnosis. Patients with enlarged tongues may be unrecognized, or they may be evaluated for acromegaly or undergo unnecessary tongue biopsies because of the suspicion of squamous cell cancer. If biopsy is not an appropriate screening technique, what algorithm should be used to recognize light chain amyloidosis?

By definition, amyloidosis is a plasma cell dyscrasia (Chapter 193); therefore, virtually all patients have a detectable immunoglobulin abnormality by immunofixation of the serum or urine, or they have abnormal results on a serum immunoglobulin free light chain assay. When a patient presents with a compatible clinical syndrome, these diagnostic studies should be completed before performing invasive diagnostic studies (Fig. 194-1). Simple electrophoresis without immunofixation is inadequate because the monoclonal proteins are very small in most patients and will not cause a detectable peak on serum protein electrophoresis. When these three diagnostic studies are used in combination, the sensitivity is 100%. If a monoclonal protein is detected, further investigations for amyloid should proceed, as described later. If a monoclonal protein is not found, three possibilities exist: (1) the patient does not have amyloidosis; (2) if the patient is known to have amyloidosis, it may be localized rather than systemic; (3) if the patient is known to have systemic amyloidosis, it may be the senile systemic or familial type rather than the light chain type.

Confirming the Diagnosis of Amyloidosis

In view of the grave prognosis associated with light chain amyloidosis, the diagnosis must be confirmed by biopsy (with Congo red staining) in all cases. Although it is reasonable to biopsy the kidney when proteinuria is the presenting symptom, the heart when cardiomyopathy is recognized, the liver when there is hepatomegaly and increased alkaline phosphatase, or the nerve when there is a sensorimotor functional loss, these invasive and occasionally risky procedures are not required. Subcutaneous fat aspiration is an outpatient procedure that has a 24-hour turnaround time and recognizes amyloid deposits in 70% of patients. Bone marrow is a second convenient biopsy site, and this test is often required to exclude the possibility of associated multiple myeloma. Bone marrow biopsy is positive in 50% of patients. When both

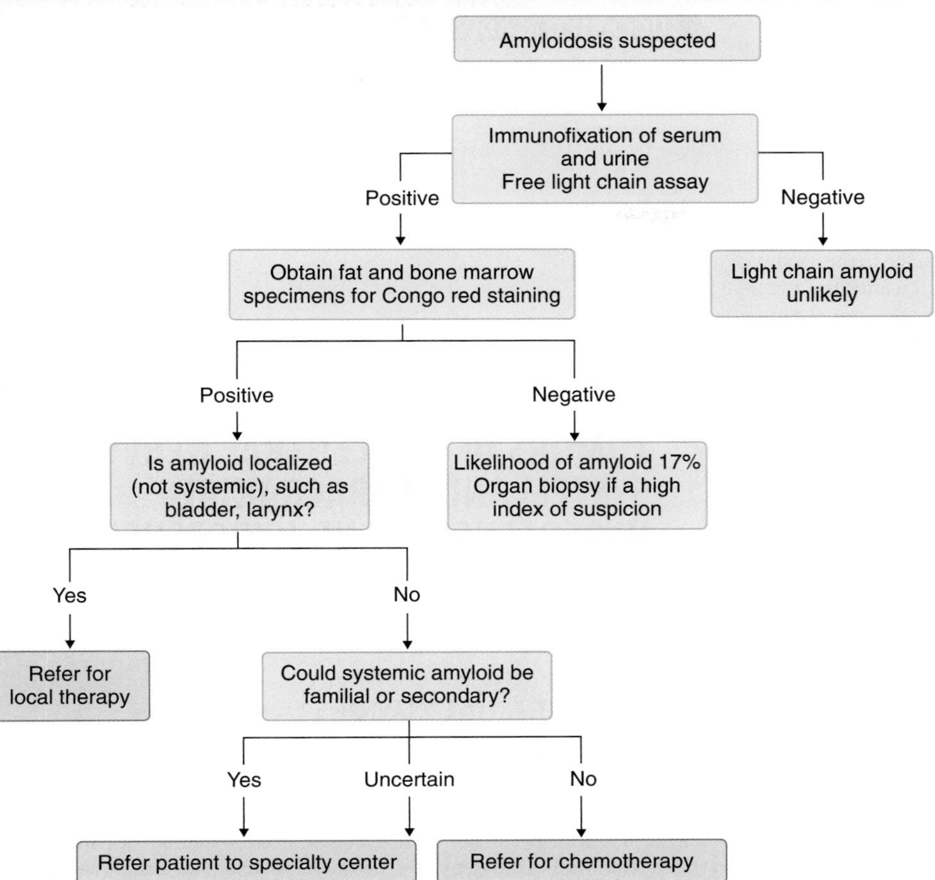

FIGURE 194-1. Algorithm for the cost-effective pursuit of a diagnosis of systemic light chain amyloidosis.

subcutaneous fat aspiration and bone marrow biopsy are done, amyloid is detected in 87% of patients. The remaining patients should have biopsy of the appropriate organ.

Once amyloid deposits are detected in tissues, further diagnostic evaluation is required. The presence of a monoclonal protein in the serum or urine and the presence of congophilic deposits in tissue do not verify that amyloidosis is light chain in origin. Further diagnostic studies are essential to classify the type of amyloid before therapy is initiated. Immunohistochemical studies on the tissue may be useful, but misfolding of the amyloid light chain often prevents epitopes from being recognized by commercial antisera; thus false-negative results are common. Mass spectroscopic analysis of the amyloid deposit can be done on paraffin-embedded tissue and validates the type of amyloid by direct amino acid sequencing, leaving no question about the origin of the amyloid protein as an immunoglobulin light chain. The incidence of monoclonal gammopathies in the elderly ranges from 3 to 5%. Therefore, that fraction of patients with senile systemic, localized, and familial amyloidosis could be expected to have an associated monoclonal gammopathy, which would be misleading. Mass spectroscopic analysis is feasible on subcutaneous fat tissue.

TREATMENT

Rx

Previously, amyloidosis was thought to be untreatable and invariably fatal. With current therapy, response rates of about 70% regularly occur, and the median duration of survival is reportedly upward of 5 years. Agents to reverse the misfolding of the protein and render it soluble would be ideal, but they are not available. The source of the immunoglobulin light chain is the clonal plasma cell population in the bone marrow. All known therapies are directed at destruction of the plasma cell clone. The two choices are generally traditional-dose chemotherapy or high-dose chemotherapy with autologous stem cell transplantation. Most patients are not candidates for high-dose therapy because of age, advanced cardiac dysfunction, or renal insufficiency. Current therapies include combinations of melphalan, dexamethasone, bortezomib, and lenalidomide. The role of high-dose therapy with stem cell transplantation in the management of amyloidosis remains controversial.[1,2] Effective therapy has been associated with resolution of nephrotic syndrome, cardiac failure, and hepatomegaly. Imaging has shown amyloid deposits to regress after the suppression of light chain synthesis.

Assessing the Effect of Therapy

The serum immunoglobulin free light chain assay has been cited as a useful screening test for patients with a compatible clinical syndrome. This assay is also used to measure the therapeutic effect of intervention because the light chain level is quantifiable and reproducible. Based on current hematologic response criteria, successful therapy is characterized by a 50% reduction in the abnormal free light chain level. Because the tissue toxicity associated with amyloid is related to the deposition of small amounts of light chain, it is unclear whether a successful outcome requires complete eradication of the light chain product. Studies have shown that patients achieving complete normalization of the free light chain have a better outcome, but it is uncertain whether patients who do not achieve this level of response should be subjected to more intensive treatment in an effort to remove this pathogenic amyloid serum precursor.

PROGNOSIS

The outcome of patients with light chain amyloidosis depends on the extent of cardiac involvement (Chapter 60). With the advent of routine hemodialysis for this population, death due to renal failure is uncommon. The greater the involvement of the heart, the shorter a patient's survival. Echocardiography provides useful information about the ejection fraction, the thickness of the ventricular septum and left ventricular free wall, and the strain percentage (the rate at which wall shortening occurs). Doppler echocardiography allows quantitative measurements of diastolic function and reflects the slowing of blood flow into the ventricular chamber as the noncompliant left ventricle fills. This "stiffness" measured by the deceleration time provides useful information and correlates well with survival.

Cardiac biomarkers are extremely sensitive measures of myocardial function, are reproducible, and can be used not only for prognosis but also to follow cardiac response after effective therapy. The serum troponin value is a powerful predictor of survival in patients with amyloidosis, and the N-terminal pro-brain natriuretic peptide value predicts survival after a diagnosis of amyloidosis. A staging system has been developed using these two cardiac biomarkers to accurately predict survival. In clinical trials of amyloidosis, half the patients with extreme increases in these markers have been incapable of completing 3 months of therapy.

Other Forms of Amyloidosis

Localized amyloidosis can be confused with systemic amyloidosis, but it has a much better prognosis. Patients with localized amyloidosis generally do not require systemic therapy; management can be supportive or localized to the deposition. The location of the amyloid deposits can be a clue to the localized nature. Typical sites for localized amyloid deposition include the ureter, bladder, urethra, and prostate. Therapy entails cystoscopic resection or intravesical instillation of dimethyl sulfoxide. Most forms of cutaneous amyloidosis are localized, although nodular cutaneous amyloidosis has occurred in systemic light chain AL. Tracheobronchial and laryngeal amyloidosis and nodular pulmonary amyloidosis are localized, are not associated with a plasma cell dyscrasia, and generally require only local therapy. Nodular pulmonary amyloidosis is often diagnosed after thoracotomy for a presumed malignant pulmonary nodule. Most cases of laryngeal amyloidosis are found when the patient presents to an otorhinolaryngologist with hoarseness and amyloid deposits are found on endoscopic biopsy. Patients with localized amyloidosis do not have a demonstrable monoclonal protein in the serum or urine and have a normal free light chain ratio. The localized amyloidosis found in Alzheimer's disease is chemically unrelated to light chain amyloidosis, and patients with light chain amyloidosis have no increased risk of dementia.

Senile systemic amyloidosis results from the deposition of a normal serum protein, transthyretin, in the myocardium. It has a much better prognosis than cardiac AL and generally necessitates endomyocardial biopsy for diagnosis; most patients are older than 70 years. When a monoclonal protein is present, it is incidental, and confirmation generally requires analysis of the amyloid-laden tissues. Therapy is supportive. The clinical presentation of senile systemic amyloidosis is not distinguishable from that of cardiac AL.

Familial amyloidosis is uncommon in the United States and represents only 3% of the cases of systemic amyloidosis. Patients present with the full clinical spectrum associated with amyloidosis, including cardiomyopathy, peripheral neuropathy, and proteinuria. Patients do not have a monoclonal protein because the deposited precursor is a mutant form of transthyretin, fibrinogen, lysozyme, or apolipoprotein A. Selected patients with familial amyloidosis have benefited from liver transplantation. One very important form of familial amyloidosis in the United States is associated with an allele of the normal serum protein transthyretin in which isoleucine is substituted for valine at position 122 (TTR Val-122-Ile). The prevalence of this mutation in blacks in the United States is as high as 3.9%. Heterozygous inheritance of this mutant TTR is associated with late-onset cardiomyopathy in this population. Wall thickening is found on echocardiography. The heart failure is often mild at onset. The prognosis is far better than that of cardiac AL, and its recognition has important implications for genetic counseling.

Secondary Amyloidosis

Secondary systemic amyloidosis is the rarest form in Western nations. Previously, it was a consequence of uncontrolled sustained inflammation, usually infectious, and causes included tuberculosis and osteomyelitis. Today it occurs primarily in patients with difficult-to-control inflammatory rheumatic syndromes, including juvenile arthritis and ankylosing spondylitis. These patients present with nephrotic syndrome, diarrhea related to intestinal involvement, and thyromegaly. Suppression of the inflammatory process results in regression of tissue amyloid deposits. There are familial forms of secondary amyloidosis associated with familial periodic fever syndromes, the most common being familial Mediterranean fever (Chapter 269) due to mutations in the tumor necrosis factor receptor.

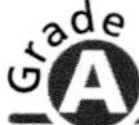

1. Mhaskar R, Kumar A, Behera M, et al. Role of high-dose chemotherapy and autologous hematopoietic cell transplantation in primary systemic amyloidosis: a systematic review. *Biol Blood Marrow Transplant.* 2009;15:893-902.
2. Jaccard A, Moreau P, Leblond V, et al. High-dose melphalan versus melphalan plus dexamethasone for AL amyloidosis. *N Engl J Med.* 2007;357:1083-1093.

SUGGESTED READINGS

Cohen AD, Comenzo RL. Systemic light-chain amyloidosis: advances in diagnosis, prognosis, and therapy. *Hematology Am Soc Hematol Educ Program.* 2010;2010:287-294. *Review.*
Gertz MA. Immunoglobulin light chain amyloidosis: 2011 update on diagnosis, risk-stratification, and management. *Am J Hematol.* 2011;86:180-186. *Review.*
Kumar SK, Gertz MA, Lacy MQ, et al. Recent improvements in survival in primary systemic amyloidosis and the importance of an early mortality risk score. *Mayo Clin Proc.* 2011;86:12-18. *Four-year survival has increased from 21% in 1977-1986 to 42% now.*
Stangou AJ, Banner NR, Hendry BM, et al. Hereditary fibrinogen A alpha-chain amyloidosis: phenotypic characterization of a systemic disease and the role of liver transplantation. *Blood.* 2010;115:2998-3007. *Liver-kidney transplant is curative.*

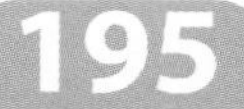

195 TUMORS OF THE CENTRAL NERVOUS SYSTEM AND INTRACRANIAL HYPERTENSION AND HYPOTENSION

LISA M. DEANGELIS

INTRACRANIAL TUMORS

General Approach to Brain Tumors

EPIDEMIOLOGY

About 17,000 new primary brain tumors and nervous system cancers are diagnosed annually in the United States, making central nervous system (CNS) tumors more than twice as common as Hodgkin's disease and approximately one third as common as melanoma. In contrast, intracranial metastases are five times more common than primary brain tumors. More than 120 types of primary brain tumors arise from the different cells that make up the CNS (Table 195-1). In addition to classifying tumors by their cell of origin, in clinical practice it is often useful to classify a tumor by its intracranial site as well, such as pineal region tumors or pituitary and suprasellar tumors.

PATHOBIOLOGY

In contrast to tumors arising elsewhere in the body, there is little distinction between benign and malignant tumors when they occur in the brain. The growth of brain tumors is restricted to the CNS; they rarely, if ever, metastasize to other organs. In the CNS, a malignant tumor is characterized by aggressive pathologic features, including local tissue invasion, neovascularity, regional necrosis, and cytologic atypia. These features confer a growth advantage to malignant cells and lead to rapid expansion and, frequently, to early regrowth after treatment. Tumors lacking these aggressive histologic features are preferably classified as low-grade rather than benign. Many low-grade tumors continue to grow within the CNS, causing progressive neurologic disability, and some may acquire a more malignant phenotype over time. The low-grade tumors that transform into high-grade neoplasms are primarily the intra-axial tumors that cannot be cured by resection because of their diffuse infiltration of brain. Almost all truly benign CNS tumors are extra-axial tumors, such as meningiomas and acoustic neuromas that can be cured with complete surgical resection.

CLINICAL MANIFESTATIONS

A patient with a brain tumor can present with one or both of two types of symptoms and signs. *Generalized symptoms,* which typically reflect the increased intracranial pressure (ICP) that often accompanies cerebral tumors, include headache, lethargy, personality change, nausea, and vomiting. *Lateralizing symptoms,* which reflect the specific location of the tumor, include hemiparesis, hemisensory deficits, aphasia, visual field impairment, and seizures (Table 195-2).

Most patients have symptoms that progress over a week to a few months. A sudden intensification of symptoms may precipitate the patient's initial visit to the physician; however, a careful history usually reveals symptoms that predated the acute deterioration and slowly worsened over time. Two exceptions are the new appearance of a seizure in a previously asymptomatic individual (Chapter 410) and sudden hemorrhage into a tumor.

TABLE 195-1 WORLD HEALTH ORGANIZATION CLASSIFICATION OF BRAIN TUMORS*

TUMORS OF NEUROEPITHELIAL TISSUE

Astrocytic tumors
- Astrocytoma
- Anaplastic (malignant) astrocytoma
- Glioblastoma multiforme
- Pilocytic astrocytoma
- Pleomorphic xanthoastrocytoma
- Subependymal giant cell astrocytoma

Oligodendroglial tumors
- Oligodendroglioma
- Anaplastic (malignant) oligodendroglioma

Ependymal tumors
- Ependymoma
- Anaplastic (malignant) ependymoma
- Myxopapillary ependymoma (spinal tumor)
- Subependymoma

Mixed gliomas
- Oligoastrocytoma
- Anaplastic (malignant) oligoastrocytoma

Choroid plexus
- Choroid plexus papilloma
- Choroid plexus carcinoma

Neuronal and mixed neuronal-glial tumors
- Gangliocytoma
- Dysembryoplastic neuroepithelial tumor
- Ganglioglioma
- Anaplastic (malignant) ganglioglioma
- Central neurocytoma

Pineal parenchymal tumors
- Pineocytoma
- Pineoblastoma

Embryonal tumors
- Medulloblastoma
- Primitive neuroectodermal tumor

TUMORS OF CRANIAL AND SPINAL NERVES

Schwannoma
Neurofibroma

TUMORS OF MENINGES

Meningioma
Hemangiopericytoma
Hemangioblastoma

PRIMARY CENTRAL NERVOUS SYSTEM LYMPHOMAS

GERM CELL TUMORS

Germinoma
Embryonal carcinoma
Yolk sac tumor (endodermal sinus tumor)
Choriocarcinoma
Teratoma
Mixed germ cell tumors

CYSTS AND TUMOR-LIKE LESIONS

Rathke cleft cyst
Epidermoid cyst
Dermoid cyst
Colloid cyst of the third ventricle

TUMORS OF THE SELLAR REGION

Pituitary adenoma
Pituitary carcinoma
Craniopharyngioma

METASTATIC TUMORS

*Abridged and modified from World Health Organization classification.

TABLE 195-2 FOCAL CLINICAL MANIFESTATIONS OF BRAIN TUMORS

Frontal lobe
- Generalized seizures
- Focal motor seizures (contralateral)
- Expressive aphasia (dominant side)
- Behavioral changes
- Dementia
- Gait disorders, incontinence
- Hemiparesis

Basal ganglia
- Hemiparesis (contralateral)
- Movement disorders (rare)

Parietal lobe
- Receptive aphasia (dominant side)
- Spatial disorientation (nondominant side)
- Cortical sensory dysfunction (contralateral)
- Hemianopia (contralateral)
- Agnosias

Occipital lobe
- Hemianopia (contralateral)
- Visual disturbances (unformed)

Temporal lobe
- Complex partial (psychomotor) seizures
- Generalized seizures
- Behavioral changes
- Olfactory and complex visual auras
- Language disorder (dominant side)
- Visual field defect

Corpus callosum
- Dementia (anterior)
- Memory loss (posterior)
- Behavioral changes
- Asymptomatic (middle)

Thalamus
- Sensory loss (contralateral)
- Behavioral changes
- Language disorder (dominant side)

Midbrain/pineal
- Paresis of vertical eye movement
- Pupillary abnormalities
- Precocious puberty (boys)

Sella/optic nerve/pituitary
- Endocrinopathy
- Bitemporal hemianopia
- Monocular visual defects
- Ophthalmoplegia (cavernous sinus)

Pons/medulla
- Cranial nerve dysfunction
- Ataxia, nystagmus
- Weakness, sensory loss
- Spasticity

Cerebellopontine angle
- Deafness (ipsilateral)
- Loss of facial sensation (ipsilateral)
- Facial weakness (ipsilateral)
- Ataxia

Cerebellum
- Ataxia (ipsilateral)
- Nystagmus

Symptoms of brain tumors can be produced by tumor invading brain parenchyma, tumor and edema compressing brain tissue, cerebrospinal fluid (CSF) obstruction caused directly by the tumor or by a shift of brain tissue, and herniation. Invasion and compression typically produce focal symptoms, many of which can be relieved if the compression is reduced. Obstruction of CSF flow and herniation are frequently a consequence of elevated ICP and typically produce generalized symptoms of headache, nausea, and vomiting, but they can also cause false localizing signs, such as an abducens nerve palsy, as a result of diffuse increased ICP.

Headache (Chapter 405) is a presenting symptom of approximately 35% of brain tumors. It is more common in younger than older patients and more common in patients who have rapidly growing tumors than in those whose tumors have evolved slowly (Fig. 195-1). Mental and cognitive abnormalities may be a reflection of local tumor (e.g., aphasia, alexia, agnosia) or of general impairment (e.g., lethargy, confusion, word finding difficulty, apathy). Seizures affect approximately one third of patients with brain tumors, and they are especially common as the presenting and only symptom of a low-grade tumor. The seizures, which are focal because they originate at the site of the tumor, may remain restricted (e.g., focal motor seizures), or they may generalize secondarily, producing loss of consciousness (Chapter 410), sometimes so quickly that the focal signature is missed by the patient or even an observant witness.

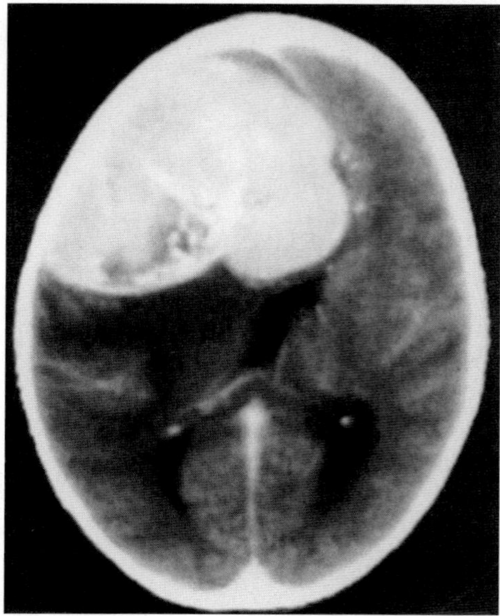

FIGURE 195-1. Meningioma. Computed tomography scan with contrast of a meningioma in a patient who presented with mild cognitive deficits, illustrative of the size a slow-growing tumor can attain in the brain. The tumor was completely resected.

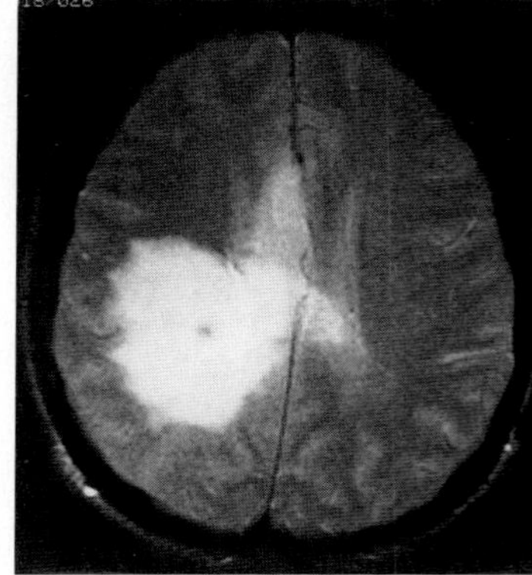
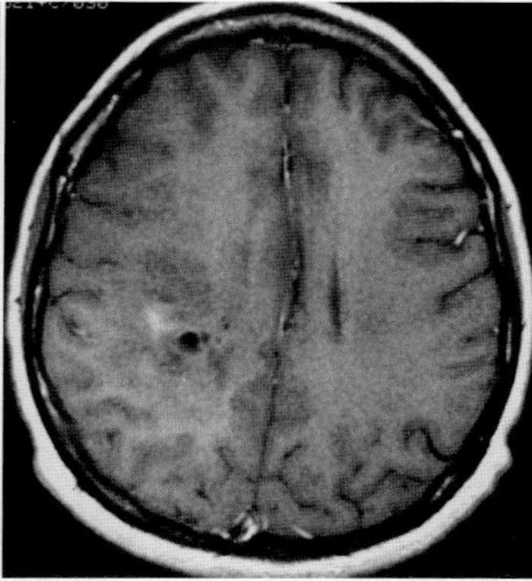

FIGURE 195-2. Glioma. Magnetic resonance imaging (MRI) view of a low-grade glioma. **Left,** T2-weighted image; **right,** T1-weighted image, gadolinium contrast with minimum enhancement. The images are typical of this tumor, which is being detected with increasing frequency by MRI in seizure patients. Many are invisible on computed tomographic scans.

TABLE 195-3 MAGNETIC RESONANCE IMAGING OF COMMON BRAIN TUMORS

TUMOR TYPE	NONCONTRAST T1	CONTRAST T1	T2
Malignant glioma	↓ density	+	↑ density
Low-grade glioma	↓ density	–	↑ density
Primary central nervous system lymphoma	↑ density	+	↑ density
Meningioma	Iso to ↑	+	Iso to ↓
Acoustic neuroma	↓ to Iso	+	Iso to ↑
Metastases	↑ to ↓	+	Variable, ↑ to ↓

DIAGNOSIS

Imaging

Magnetic resonance imaging (MRI) is far superior to computed tomography (CT) and should be used in all cases of suspected intracranial tumor. MRI should be performed both without and with intravenous gadolinium. A well-performed MRI scan identifies any intracranial tumor, and normal MRI results effectively exclude a neoplasm. The MRI of some extra-axial tumors (e.g., acoustic neuromas, meningiomas) is so characteristic that histologic confirmation is not required (Table 195-3). A non-contrast-enhancing infiltrative lesion that is visible primarily on T2 or fluid-attenuated inversion recovery (FLAIR) images is most consistent with a low-grade glioma (Fig. 195-2), whereas a contrast-enhancing lesion with an area of central necrosis and surrounding edema is most likely to be a glioblastoma or possibly a brain metastasis. Although these diagnoses must be confirmed histologically, the preoperative diagnostic possibilities affect the choice of surgical procedure and the surgical approach to the lesion.

Perfusion MRI after rapid infusion of gadolinium can measure the relative cerebral blood volume and neovascularity associated with a tumor; high perfusion is associated with higher grade of malignancy. This technique can help estimate the tumor grade preoperatively and guide the planning of treatment.

Magnetic resonance spectroscopy (MRS) noninvasively assesses tissue composition. High-grade primary brain tumors are associated with a decrease in *N*-acetylaspartate (NAA) and an increase in choline (Cho). More malignant tumors are associated with a greater Cho/NAA ratio and frequently contain areas with elevation of lactate and lipid.

Surgical resection is a major objective in the treatment of almost every kind of brain tumor, but resection must be balanced against possible damage to adjacent normal brain. The development of functional MRI (fMRI), which measures cerebral blood flow when areas of cortex are activated, has greatly enhanced the ability to localize critical neurologic functions and their relationship to the tumor preoperatively. When the fMRI is fused with the anatomic MRI, critical functions can be identified in relationship to the patient's tumor, and a safer and more complete resection may be planned.

On positron emission tomography (PET), high-grade tumors are usually hypermetabolic, whereas low-grade tumors are hypometabolic. New technologies using ^{11}C-methionine PET may differentiate low- from high-grade gliomas much more efficiently than deoxyglucose PET.

CT, without and with intravenous contrast, should be used only for patients who cannot undergo MRI. A CT scan, even with contrast, may miss low-grade tumors and tumors in the posterior fossa.

Currently, angiography has no role in the diagnosis of intracranial tumors. However, angiographic embolization is occasionally useful preoperatively to reduce the vascularity of some meningiomas, thereby making a complete resection safer and more feasible.

Other Tests

Electroencephalography (EEG) is rarely needed in the diagnosis or management of brain tumors. An EEG can occasionally be useful in a patient who has prolonged or unexplained stupor and in whom nonconvulsive status epilepticus is a consideration. Intraoperative monitoring is also frequently used to help guide resection of epileptogenic cortex adjacent to or within brain tumor tissue.

CSF analysis has little role in the diagnosis of most intracranial neoplasms. In primary CNS lymphoma (PCNSL), the diagnosis may be established on CSF cytologic examination in about 15% of patients. Rarely, a lumbar puncture is required to exclude inflammatory conditions or other processes that may be confused with a primary brain tumor. Lumbar puncture must be avoided in patients with cerebellar tumors because the release of pressure through the spinal needle may result in herniation of the cerebellar tonsils through the foramen magnum.

Differential Diagnosis

Patients who present with symptoms of raised ICP or the new onset of central neurologic symptoms such as hemiparesis or seizure should be hospitalized and evaluated rapidly. Prompt neuroimaging discloses a mass, and the radiographic features narrow the differential diagnosis (Table 195-4). Extra-axial tumors, such as a meningioma or acoustic neuroma, can be confused with a dural metastasis. Low-grade intra-axial tumors, which are nonenhancing on MRI, have been confused with infections such as herpes encephalitis when they involve the temporal lobe. Contrast-enhancing intra-axial tumors can be confused with a stroke, brain abscess, or focal plaque of demyelination. Subacute infarction can show brisk contrast enhancement, usually in a gyral pattern, unlike brain tumors, in which enhancement is primarily in the white matter; occasionally, however, the two are indistinguishable radiographically. Brain abscesses typically have a thinner enhancing wall than a malignant tumor, but they sometimes appear similar on MRI. Despite careful evaluation, patients thought to have a malignant glioma occasionally are found at surgery to have a brain abscess. A single large plaque of demyelination can

TABLE 195-4 DIFFERENTIAL DIAGNOSIS OF INTRACRANIAL TUMORS

Infection
- Brain abscess
  - Bacterial
  - Fungal
  - Parasitic (e.g., cysticercosis)
- Herpes encephalitis

Vascular disease
- Stroke
- Intracranial hemorrhage

Inflammatory conditions
- Granuloma (sarcoid)
- Multiple sclerosis: single large lesion

Vascular malformations
- Cavernous angiomas
- Venous angiomas

Congenital abnormalities
- Cortical dysplasia
- Heterotopia

also be confused radiographically with a brain tumor, and sometimes the diagnosis can be established only by biopsy.

When MRI suggests a primary brain tumor, there is no need for an extensive systemic search for a possible source of metastasis. Brain metastases are more common than primary brain tumors, but most occur in patients with known cancer, typically with active systemic disease. If an obvious systemic cancer is not revealed by a thorough general examination, chest radiograph, routine blood tests, and urinalysis, then the patient should proceed to craniotomy. Even if a brain metastasis is found at surgery, resection of a single brain metastasis is the appropriate treatment, and the pathology of the lesion guides the subsequent search for the primary tumor.

TREATMENT Rx

The treatment for all brain tumors can be divided into two main categories: symptomatic and definitive (Table 195-5). Symptomatic treatment addresses the associated problems, such as cerebral edema, seizures, and thromboembolic disease, which can contribute substantially to clinical symptoms. Definitive treatment addresses the tumor itself.

Symptomatic Treatment

Symptomatic management includes the use of corticosteroids, anticonvulsants, and prophylaxis for deep vein thrombosis (DVT) (Chapter 37). Corticosteroids decrease the vasogenic edema that surrounds primary and metastatic brain tumors. Blood vessels associated with tumor formation are leaky and do not share the normal morphologic and physiologic features that form the blood-brain barrier; corticosteroids effectively reconstitute the blood-brain barrier by decreasing the abnormal permeability of these neovessels. Clinical improvement may begin within minutes, and frequently patients are dramatically improved within 24 to 48 hours.

Dexamethasone is the most commonly used glucocorticoid because it has the least mineralocorticoid activity. The usual starting dose is 12 to 16 mg/day, but this can be adjusted to find the lowest possible dose that alleviates neurologic symptoms. After definitive treatment is instituted, many patients can be tapered off their corticosteroid completely. Chronic high-dose corticosteroid therapy is associated with substantial side effects (Chapter 34). Patients who will be taking glucocorticoids for 6 weeks or longer should receive prophylaxis against *Pneumocystis jiroveci* (formerly *Pneumocystis carinii;* Chapter 349).

Anticonvulsants are administered to any patient who has had a seizure, but prophylactic anticonvulsants should not be prescribed for patients who have never had a seizure, except they may be useful in the perioperative period.[1,2]

DVT, which occurs in about 25% of patients with brain tumors, can occur early in the illness or at any time during treatment. All patients undergoing neurosurgery should have pneumatic compression boots in the postoperative period to reduce the incidence of DVT. Prophylactic anticoagulants have also been used successfully in the immediate postoperative period without increasing postoperative hemorrhage. Appropriately regulated anticoagulation (Chapter 37) is the optimal therapy for DVT and is not associated with an increased risk of intracerebral hemorrhage in patients with intracranial tumors. Inferior vena cava filters can be used for patients who have DVTs or pulmonary emboli and who cannot be fully anticoagulated.

TABLE 195-5 TREATMENT FOR BRAIN TUMORS

SYMPTOMATIC

Glucocorticoids
Anticonvulsants
Deep vein thrombosis prophylaxis and treatment

DEFINITIVE

Surgery
- Goal is gross total excision

Radiotherapy
- Standard external beam
  - Fractionated
  - Usually focal
- Stereotactic radiosurgery

Chemotherapy
- Limited by intrinsic drug resistance and blood-brain barrier

Definitive Treatment

Surgery

Complete excision is the goal for a primary brain tumor. Surgical excision can often be accomplished for primary extra-axial tumors, such as meningiomas and acoustic neuromas. However, meningiomas often occur in intracranial locations that make resection impossible. Tumors of the skull base are particularly difficult to remove, and partial resection for decompression is often performed to preserve neurologic function. The safe boundaries for resecting cortical lesions while preserving function can often be elucidated by preoperative fMRI and intraoperative cortical mapping. However, lesions involving many critical structures, such as the brain stem or thalamus, cannot be excised safely.

Lesions that cannot be resected are still amenable to biopsy for diagnostic purposes. In particular, the use of stereotactic biopsy has made it feasible to reach lesions in almost any area of the brain with minimal morbidity. The risks of stereotactic biopsy include (1) inadequate tissue sample to make a diagnosis, (2) a tissue sample that does not accurately reflect the most malignant grade of the tumor, and (3) a procedure-related complication, such as hemorrhage. Hemorrhage that causes neurologic impairment occurs in only 2% of stereotactic biopsies, typically in patients with glioblastoma multiforme.

Complete excision can cure extra-axial primary brain tumor and is associated with prolonged survival and better neurologic outcome even in patients with primary intra-axial tumors. Gross total excision, as measured by postoperative neuroimaging, is associated with prolonged survival in patients with malignant gliomas and probably in those with low-grade gliomas as well. However, most low-grade gliomas are not amenable to gross total excision, and usually only partial excision is feasible. Macroscopic tumor can frequently be removed completely in patients with high-grade gliomas, but there is always remaining microscopic disease that infiltrates surrounding brain.

Some tumors, such as brain stem gliomas, are in such critical locations that biopsy is not attempted. Their characteristic radiographic appearance permits diagnosis and initiation of medical treatment.

Radiation Therapy

A course of external beam radiation therapy is delivered in small daily fractions to a total cumulative dose usually between 45 and 60 Gy. Dividing the treatment into small daily fractions permits sublethal repair in normal tissues and markedly reduces neurologic toxicity associated with cerebral radiation. External beam irradiation, which is the most effective nonsurgical treatment for brain tumors, doubles median survival time of patients with malignant primary brain tumors or metastatic lesions. It can also be useful for recurrent meningiomas and acoustic neuromas. However, it only rarely cures any of these lesions, and most patients develop recurrent disease despite maximal radiation therapy.

Stereotactic radiosurgery has been developed to deliver high fractions of focused radiation therapy that spare normal surrounding tissue. The technique is limited to tumors that are 3 cm in diameter or smaller and is less useful for malignant gliomas because of their infiltrative nature.

The neurologic complications of radiation therapy, which are usually observed in patients months to years after completion of treatment, include radionecrosis, dementia, and leukoencephalopathy. The incidence is reported as less than 5%, and most patients die of their brain tumor before the delayed consequences of treatment can be observed. However, in long-term survivors (e.g., patients with low-grade glioma or children with medulloblastoma), the late consequences of radiation therapy are important. Dementia accompanying radiation-induced leukoencephalopathy can progress and result in severe neurologic impairment. Radionecrosis can mimic recurrent tumor with a large contrast-enhancing lesion on MRI. Corticosteroids can reduce the edema and sometimes are sufficient to treat small areas of radionecrosis. However, if the lesion is sufficiently large, resection may be required to decompress the mass and reduce the steroid requirements.

Chemotherapy

Chemotherapy for brain tumors has usually been disappointing because of the intrinsic resistance of these tumors to most conventional agents. Carboplatin and cisplatin are active agents against medulloblastoma, even when the tumor is disseminated in the CSF. Temozolomide (150 to 200 mg/m^2 for 5 days every 4 weeks) is active in all gliomas, and high-dose methotrexate (3 to 8 g/m^2 for 3 to 12 months) is effective for PCNSL. For patients with glioblastoma, polymers impregnated with carmustine (BCNU) and placed in a resection cavity offer modest benefit when compared with no chemotherapy, but they are associated with local tissue injury and edema.

SPECIFIC TYPES OF BRAIN TUMORS

Primary Extra-axial Tumors

The most common primary extra-axial tumors are meningiomas, pituitary adenomas, and acoustic neuromas. These tumors arise within the intracranial cavity but are not tumors of brain tissue. Almost all are benign; because the brain is rarely invaded, complete excision often enables cure with full recovery of neurologic function. These tumors produce neurologic symptoms and signs by compressing the underlying brain; however, edema of the underlying brain is infrequent, so glucocorticoids have a limited role.

MENINGIOMAS

EPIDEMIOLOGY

Meningiomas are usually benign. Between 5 and 10% of meningiomas are atypical or malignant variants with a more aggressive course. Meningiomas are more common in women, may be multiple in about 10% of patients with sporadic meningioma, and are occasionally part of a familial syndrome. They occur with increased frequency in patients with neurofibromatosis type 2 (Chapter 426).

DIAGNOSIS

Meningiomas grow slowly and produce symptoms that are insidious in onset and typically slowly progressive. Tumors can reach a considerable size, but they grow so slowly that the brain accommodates to the progressive compression. Meningiomas typically occur in specific locations: over the convexity, along the falx and parasagittal area, the olfactory groove, base of the skull near the sphenoid bone, cavernous sinus, cerebellopontine angle, and foramen magnum. Cortical and parasagittal tumors typically manifest with seizures or progressive hemiparesis. Tumors in the anterior cranial fossa can cause slowly progressive changes in personality and cognition. Meningiomas at the base of the skull manifest with cranial neuropathies and gait difficulties when there is brain stem compression. Frequently, tumors are completely asymptomatic and are identified on neuroimaging done for another purpose, such as head trauma.

On MRI, meningiomas have a characteristic appearance consisting of a diffusely enhancing, dural-based lesion that is associated with a thin enhancing dural tail extending from the tumor. Often the radiographic features are so characteristic that surgery is performed for therapeutic purposes only. The radiographic differential diagnosis includes the less common hemangiopericytoma and dural metastasis. Most meningiomas are not accompanied by significant edema, but marked edema is seen with high-grade malignant lesions or the secretory variant.

If small meningiomas are discovered in the absence of clinical symptoms or the symptoms are minor, lesions may be monitored with serial images because growth can be so slow.

TREATMENT

If treatment is indicated, complete resection is often curative, but even completely resected benign tumors may recur (as many as 20% in some series), so radiologic follow-up is essential. Tumors at the base of the skull often cannot be resected completely and tend to recur despite successive attempts at surgical resection. Radiation therapy can sometimes slow progression and is essential for the treatment of malignant meningiomas. No effective chemotherapy has yet been identified.

Acoustic Neuromas

Acoustic neuromas (Chapter 436), better called vestibular schwannomas, are benign tumors that arise from the eighth cranial nerve. Acoustic neuromas are twice as common in women as in men; the peak age is between 40 and 60 years. Sporadic vestibular schwannomas are unilateral; bilateral acoustic neuromas are pathognomonic of neurofibromatosis type 2 (Chapter 426).

Acoustic neuromas usually arise from the vestibular portion of the nerve and typically manifest with unilateral hearing loss, sometimes preceded or accompanied by tinnitus and a sensation of dizziness or unsteadiness but not true vertigo. The slow, progressive enlargement of the tumor produces ipsilateral facial numbness or weakness by compressing the fifth or seventh cranial nerve, respectively. Tumors originate within the internal auditory meatus but grow out of the acoustic canal and into the cerebellopontine angle, where they can compress the brain stem and cause ataxia and ipsilateral cerebellar signs. Cranial MRI with gadolinium delineates even small acoustic neuromas with ease.

Treatment is often surgical; stereotactic radiosurgery may be an alternative for lesions smaller than 3 cm. It is preferable to treat the tumors when they are small, to preserve facial nerve function and hearing.

Pituitary Adenomas

Pituitary adenomas (Chapter 231) can be classified according to their size as microadenomas (<1 cm in diameter) or macroadenomas; by the presence or absence of endocrine function; and by the endocrinologic syndromes or neurologic syndromes caused by tumor compression. Microadenomas typically manifest with endocrine symptoms as described in Chapter 231. As pituitary tumors enlarge and become macroadenomas, they compress the surrounding neural structures, including the optic chiasm and optic nerves, typically causing bitemporal hemianopia and occasionally causing unilateral visual loss. Macroadenomas are frequently nonsecreting but destroy pituitary tissue, causing panhypopituitarism. Rarely, pituitary tumors manifest with the abrupt onset of headache, ophthalmoplegia, unilateral blindness, and even a depressed level of alertness or coma—a syndrome of *pituitary apoplexy* caused by hemorrhage or infarction.

Cranial MRI, particularly with coronal images and gadolinium administration, can completely outline the pituitary tumor and surrounding neural structures. All macroadenomas and some microadenomas can be treated with transsphenoidal pituitary surgery, which is associated with minimal morbidity. Occasionally, residual or recurrent tumor necessitates radiation therapy. Some hormone-secreting tumors, particularly prolactinomas or growth hormone–secreting tumors, can be treated medically with cabergoline or octreotide, respectively (Chapter 231). These medications not only correct the hormonal excess but also shrink the tumor; they must be taken for life.

Other tumors in the pituitary and suprasellar region include craniopharyngiomas, suprasellar epidermoid cysts, Rathke cleft cysts, germinomas (discussed later), and lymphocytic hypophysitis, which is a benign inflammatory condition that usually manifests with diabetes insipidus (Chapter 232). MRI frequently differentiates these conditions, which are usually suprasellar and erode into the pituitary fossa only secondarily. Some of these lesions also have characteristic radiographic features. These lesions are benign. Except for hypophysitis, which resolves completely with corticosteroid treatment (e.g., methylprednisolone, 120 mg daily for 2 weeks and then tapered for 1 additional week), complete surgical excision is the curative therapy.

Other Extra-axial Tumors

Pineal region tumors all have a characteristic clinical presentation that includes Parinaud's syndrome, which consists of paresis of upward gaze, poor pupillary reaction to light with brisk reaction on accommodation, impairment of convergence, and convergence-retraction nystagmus. Some of these lesions may also cause hydrocephalus and symptoms of increased ICP. Pineal region tumors include pineal parenchymal tumors, such as pineocytomas and the more aggressive pineoblastomas, and germ cell tumors, including germinomas and nongerminomatous germ cell tumors. Germinomas can be completely cured with focal radiation therapy, whereas nongerminomatous germ cell tumors are more aggressive and frequently relapse despite chemotherapy plus cranial irradiation.

Chordomas are rare tumors of residual notochordal tissue. They usually occur at the base of the skull, are locally invasive, and are characterized by multiple recurrences despite surgery and radiation therapy.

Lipomas are benign tumors that can occur in midline structures, particularly near the corpus callosum. They can be cured by complete removal.

Arachnoid cysts are not tumors per se but can manifest with headaches, seizures, or focal neurologic symptoms if they become large enough to compress underlying brain tissue. Many are completely asymptomatic and are found incidentally on neuroimaging. Only symptomatic cysts require removal.

Primary Intra-axial Tumors

Most primary intra-axial brain tumors are gliomas, including the astrocytomas, oligodendrogliomas, and ependymomas. Less common are medulloblastomas, other rare neuroectodermal tumors, and PCNSLs. All of these tumors have a tendency to invade brain tissue, and none can be completely excised surgically.

GLIOMAS

DEFINITION

Astrocytomas, which are the most common glioma, are classified into one of four World Health Organization (WHO) categories: grade I is the pilocytic astrocytoma, grade II is the fibrillary astrocytoma, grade III is the anaplastic astrocytoma, and grade IV is the glioblastoma multiforme. Pilocytic astrocytomas (grade I) are extremely low-grade focal tumors that are more common in children and may be associated with neurofibromatosis type 1; they are often cured by complete surgical excision. Astrocytomas, anaplastic astrocytomas, and glioblastomas are diffuse tumors that tend to infiltrate widely into brain; even grade II tumors progress over time, and most acquire the histologic features and growth patterns of grade III and IV tumors.

EPIDEMIOLOGY

Gliomas occur at any age, but the peak age is 20 to 30 years for an astrocytoma, 40 years for anaplastic astrocytoma, and 55 to 60 years for glioblastoma. Age is the single most important prognostic factor: younger patients live substantially longer than older patients. Histology is also critical: patients with glioblastoma do significantly worse than patients with lower-grade lesions. Performance status, duration of symptoms, and whether a complete resection has been achieved are also strong predictors of improved outcome and prolonged survival. For all grades of glioma, men are more frequently affected than women, and whites significantly more frequently than blacks. Gliomas are typically single lesions, but multifocal disease is seen in approximately 5% of patients with high-grade tumors. A variant of gliomas, called *gliomatosis cerebri,* causes widespread infiltration of the entire brain; most patients have relatively low-grade pathology on biopsy, but focal regions of high-grade transformation can exist.

PATHOBIOLOGY

At least 95% of gliomas are sporadic, and only 5% occur in patients with a family history of brain tumor. Furthermore, patients with a familial history of glioma usually do not fall into a well-recognized hereditary syndrome. However, neurofibromatosis 1 (von Recklinghausen's disease; Chapter 426) is associated with an increased incidence of gliomas, particularly in the optic pathway, hypothalamus, and brain stem. Gliomas also occur with increased frequency in Turcot's syndrome, in which colorectal neoplasms are seen in association with a variety of CNS tumors. Somatic mutations of the isocitrate dehydrogenase 1 and 2 genes (*IDH1* and *IDH2*) have been identified in most low-grade gliomas and secondary glioblastomas: these patients had a better outcome than those with wild-type *IDH* genes.

CLINICAL MANIFESTATIONS AND DIAGNOSIS

Patients with gliomas often present with seizures, headache, and lateralizing signs such as hemiparesis, aphasia, or a visual field deficit. On MRI, low-grade gliomas typically appear as diffuse, nonenhancing lesions with a propensity to occur in the frontal lobe and insular cortex. High-grade gliomas, which typically enhance with contrast, occur in the cortical white matter and are accompanied by significant surrounding edema. Glioblastomas frequently have regions of central necrosis (Fig. 195-3), and hemorrhage can occur in 5 to 8% of patients.

TREATMENT Rx

For all gliomas, treatment frequently involves surgery, radiation therapy, and chemotherapy. The surgical goal of complete removal of all visible disease is often impossible. The adequacy of resection is best assessed on a postoperative MRI study, without and with gadolinium, performed within 72 to 96 hours after surgery. Surgical removal usually improves neurologic function and reduces dependency on corticosteroids.

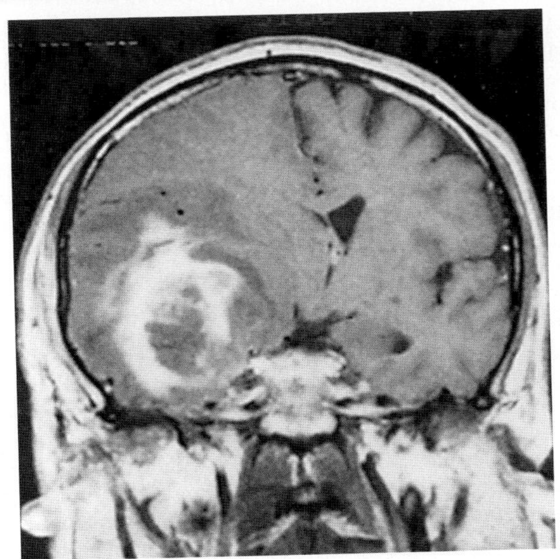

FIGURE 195-3. Temporal lobe glioblastoma. This T1-weighted gadolinium-enhanced magnetic resonance imaging view shows a typical ring configuration of contrast with central necrosis and marked mass effect.

ANAPLASTIC ASTROCYTOMAS AND GLIOBLASTOMAS

All anaplastic astrocytomas and glioblastomas should be treated with postoperative radiation therapy to a dose of approximately 60 Gy. In a randomized trial of patients with glioblastoma, the alkylating agent temozolomide (75 mg/m^2 daily), administered concurrently with radiation therapy and followed by adjuvant temozolomide (150 to 200 mg/m^2 for 5 consecutive days every 4 weeks for 6 cycles), significantly improved survival (median, 14.6 months) compared with radiation therapy alone (median, 12.1 months; $P <$ .001), and the 2-year survival rate more than doubled to 26.5%.[3] Patients whose tumors contained a methylated promoter of the O6-methylguanine-DNA methyltransferase (*MGMT*) DNA repair gene benefited most from the addition of temozolomide. Based on these data, combined treatment is the current standard of care for patients with glioblastoma. Chemotherapy is generally well tolerated and associated with minimal toxicity. Elderly patients often do poorly, but a randomized trial showed that radiotherapy (compared with supportive care only) results in a modest improvement in survival, without reducing quality of life or cognition, in elderly patients with glioblastoma.[4] Recurrences can be treated with re-resection, additional chemotherapy, or, occasionally, stereotactic radiosurgery, or a combination of these. Despite aggressive treatment, disease recurs in almost all patients, and the median survival time is 14 to 15 months for glioblastoma. Patients with anaplastic gliomas (including anaplastic oligodendrogliomas) had identical median survivals of about 7 years whether the initial treatment was radiotherapy or chemotherapy.[5] However, some young patients with anaplastic astrocytoma can survive many years before the tumor recurs.

OPTIC AND BRAIN STEM GLIOMAS

Optic gliomas, which can involve the optic nerve or optic chiasm, are usually associated with neurofibromatosis type 1. These gliomas are typically pilocytic tumors that can have an indolent course, including rare spontaneous regression. Often they are not amenable to surgical resection, and they can have a stuttering clinical course, with periods of visual loss punctuated by prolonged periods of visual stability. When necessary, radiation or even chemotherapy may be useful, but often no treatment is required. Brain stem gliomas usually involve the pons, less often the medulla or midbrain. Brain stem gliomas are most commonly seen in children in the first decade of life but can be found even in elderly people; they can have a low-grade or a high-grade histology, but outcome is primarily determined by the location of the tumor. In general, most brain stem gliomas have a dismal outcome with survival of 1 year or less, but relatively benign variants occasionally occur.

LOW-GRADE ASTROCYTOMAS

Low-grade astrocytomas have a variable course. In patients who present with isolated seizures that can be easily controlled with anticonvulsants, treatment with radiation therapy or chemotherapy immediately after surgery does not prolong survival, and patients can be monitored until there is clinical or radiographic evidence of tumor progression.[6] Patients with progressive neurologic symptoms or cognitive impairment require immediate treatment after diagnosis, and focal radiation therapy to a total of about 54 Gy is the optimal choice. An astrocytoma can progress as a low-grade tumor or transform to a higher-grade malignancy, a change that typically is associated with the appearance of contrast enhancement on MRI. Resection or a biopsy may be necessary in these patients, followed by radiation therapy if they have not received it previously; chemotherapy with temozolomide (150 to 200 mg/m^2 for 5 days every 4 weeks for anywhere from 6 to 24 cycles) is also used. Patients with astrocytomas have a median survival of about 5 years.

OLIGODENDROGLIOMAS

Oligodendrogliomas occur as low-grade tumors and, less commonly, as anaplastic lesions. Treatment of these tumors differs from that of their astrocytic counterparts because oligodendrogliomas are uniquely chemosensitive, owing to their characteristic loss of chromosomes 1p and 19q. As with the low-grade astrocytomas, treatment should be withheld in patients with low-grade oligodendrogliomas who have no symptoms other than well-controlled seizures. Patients with progressive neurologic symptoms require treatment, and initial therapy is often chemotherapy, usually with single-agent temozolomide (150 to 200 mg/m^2 for 5 days every 4 weeks for 6 to 24 cycles) or the combination of procarbazine, lomustine, and vincristine. Radiation therapy is withheld until chemotherapy fails.

By comparison, all anaplastic oligodendrogliomas require immediate treatment. The standard approach includes focal radiation therapy. Adjuvant chemotherapy significantly prolongs disease-free survival but not overall survival time.[7] However, there is a growing movement toward treating high-grade tumors with chemotherapy alone and, in some cases, using high-dose chemotherapy with autologous stem cell rescue (Chapter 181). Some success has been reported with this approach, but it should still be considered experimental. Tumor progression should be treated with re-resection, radiation therapy if not previously administered, and additional chemotherapy. Patients with low-grade oligodendrogliomas have a median survival time in excess of 15 years, and those who have anaplastic oligodendrogliomas survive a median of 4 to 5 years.

MEDULLOBLASTOMAS

Medulloblastomas usually occur in the vermis of the cerebellum and principally affect children and young adults. Boys outnumber girls by about 2 : 1, and peak onset is at age 7 years; medulloblastoma in adulthood is rare and usually affects the cerebellar hemisphere.

The most common chromosomal abnormality associated with medulloblastoma is isochromosome 17q, which is found in as many as 60% of tumors. Tumors with an identical histology but different genetics may arise in the cerebral hemispheres and are called *primitive neuroectodermal tumors* (PNETs). PNETs usually have an aggressive course, leading to rapid death despite vigorous treatment.

Medulloblastomas have a characteristic clinical presentation, with ataxia (due to cerebellar and brain stem involvement) and headache, nausea, and vomiting (due to increased ICP from obstructive hydrocephalus). Aggressive surgery with complete excision is strongly associated with improved outcome. Surgery is always followed by neuraxis radiation therapy. Chemotherapy with vincristine, etoposide, carboplatin, and cyclophosphamide significantly improves 5-year event-free survival from 60 to 74% but has not significantly prolonged overall survival, which is about 70 to 80% at 5 years. This vigorous therapy often results in significant delayed complications in survivors, including intellectual deficits, growth impairment, and endocrinologic dysfunction. Late relapses as well as secondary neoplasms compromise long-term outcome.

GANGLIOGLIOMAS

Gangliogliomas, as the name implies, possess both a glial component and a neoplastic neural component (ganglion cell). Some low-grade gangliogliomas are indolent and do not require additional treatment after surgical extirpation. Patients with anaplastic tumors may fare better than patients with malignant gliomas, but recurrence is the rule despite surgery and radiation therapy.

PRIMARY CENTRAL NERVOUS SYSTEM LYMPHOMAS

PCNSLs are associated with immunodeficiency states, particularly acquired immunodeficiency syndrome and organ transplantation, and are seen with increased frequency among the apparently immunocompetent population as well. Men are more frequently affected than women, and the median age at diagnosis is about 60 years. These tumors are usually large cell, B-cell non-Hodgkin's lymphomas identical to systemic lymphoma (Chapter 191). The tumor can involve the CSF, the eye, and the brain, where it is multifocal in about 40% of patients at presentation. In contrast to all other brain tumors, surgical resection is not associated with improved survival and can cause significant neurologic morbidity; therefore, biopsy, not resection, is the better surgical approach. Chemotherapy is the primary treatment, and high-dose methotrexate (3 to 8 g/m^2 on alternate weeks for 3 to 12 months) is the most important chemotherapeutic agent. In older patients, radiation therapy is avoided because the necessary whole brain irradiation causes significant cognitive impairment when combined with chemotherapy. Furthermore, radiation therapy alone produces a response but is followed by relapse within 1 year. Corticosteroids (e.g., dexamethasone 8 to 16 mg/day), which are frequently used as part of the chemotherapeutic regimen, not only help manage the associated cerebral edema but also can cause tumor regression. With the use of multiagent chemotherapy, with or without cranial irradiation, median survival times are now in the 3- to 5-year range.

OTHER INTRA-AXIAL TUMORS

Rare, intra-axial cerebral tumors include the *ependymoma,* which is optimally treated with surgical excision followed by radiation therapy. *Choroid plexus papillomas* and carcinomas may manifest with hydrocephalus or lateralizing signs. Resection may be sufficient for the benign papilloma, but carcinomas rapidly recur even when postoperative radiation therapy is also used. *Colloid cysts* of the third ventricle are benign tumors that can cause obstructive hydrocephalus; they may be treated with a ventricular peritoneal shunt or with resection using an intraventricular endoscope. *Hemangioblastomas* occur primarily in the cerebellum but can also occur in the spinal cord and the hemispheres. About 15% of patients with a hemangioblastoma have the autosomal dominant disorder, von Hippel-Lindau disease (Chapter 426), which is characterized by hemangioblastomas in the CNS and retina, renal cell carcinoma, pheochromocytoma, endolymphatic sac tumors, and cysts in a variety of visceral organs. Hemangioblastomas are treated by surgical excision and require radiation therapy only for recurrence. Complete removal usually results in cure.

Metastatic Tumors

BRAIN METASTASES

DEFINITION AND EPIDEMIOLOGY

Every systemic cancer is capable of metastasizing to the brain. Melanoma (Chapter 210) has the greatest propensity to spread to the CNS, but the most common causes of CNS metastases are cancers of the breast (Chapter 204) and lung (Chapter 197), followed by cancers of the colon (Chapter 199) and kidney (Chapter 203). CNS metastases are being seen with greater frequency as patients with systemic cancers have prolonged survival with better treatments. In most patients with brain metastases, CNS disease develops late in the course of their illness, but a brain metastasis may be the initial presentation of a systemic cancer. In most of the latter patients, lung cancer is the primary site; in some, however, a primary site is never identified (Chapter 211).

CLINICAL MANIFESTATIONS AND DIAGNOSIS

Patients with brain metastases present with progressive neurologic symptoms and signs that typically include headache, seizures, and lateralizing signs. Metastases are best diagnosed by a cranial MRI with gadolinium enhancement (Fig. 195-4). All lesions can be clearly seen by MRI, which is better than CT for visualizing the posterior fossa. Metastases, which are usually well-circumscribed lesions at the gray matter–white matter junction, are often associated with extensive edema. Hemorrhage into a metastasis occurs most frequently with metastases from melanoma, renal cancer, and thyroid cancer; however, because brain metastases from lung cancer are so common, they are the type most commonly associated with hemorrhage. Sometimes, hemorrhage into a brain metastasis is best visualized by noncontrast head CT.

TREATMENT Rx

Because brain metastases do not widely infiltrate into brain tissue and tend to have a pseudocapsule around them, they can be completely excised surgically. In randomized controlled studies, complete removal of a single brain metastasis substantially prolonged life and maintained neurologic function for

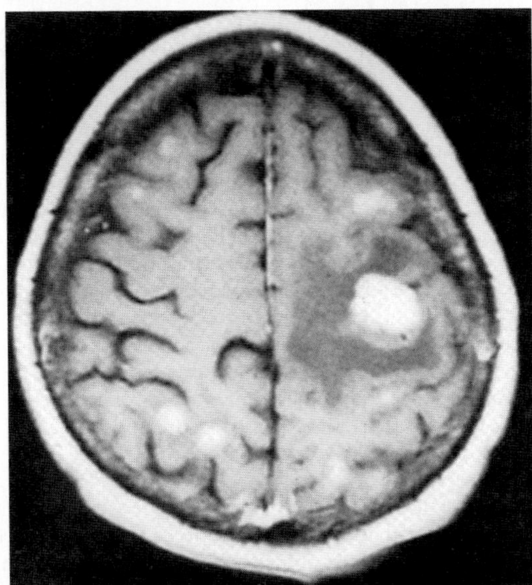

FIGURE 195-4. **Brain metastasis.** Multiple metastases from breast carcinoma are seen on this T1-weighted gadolinium-enhanced magnetic resonance imaging view. The multiple smaller tumors were not visible on computed tomography, even after a contrast agent was given.

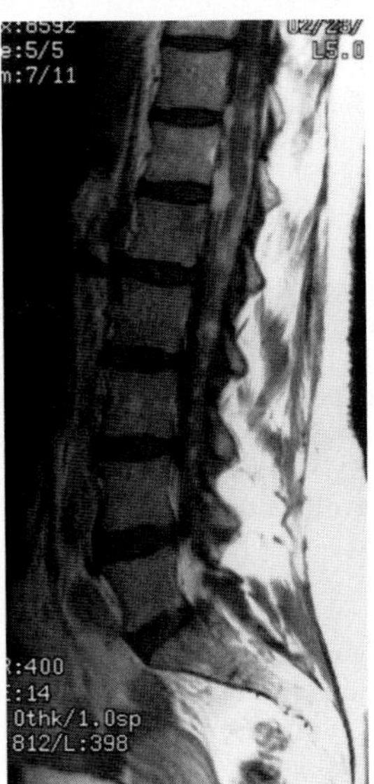

FIGURE 195-5. **Leptomeningeal metastases.** Gadolinium-enhanced magnetic resonance imaging of the lumbosacral spine in a patient with leptomeningeal metastases from melanoma. Multiple enhancing nodules are seen on the cauda equina, and the conus medullaris and lower spinal cord are encased by tumor.

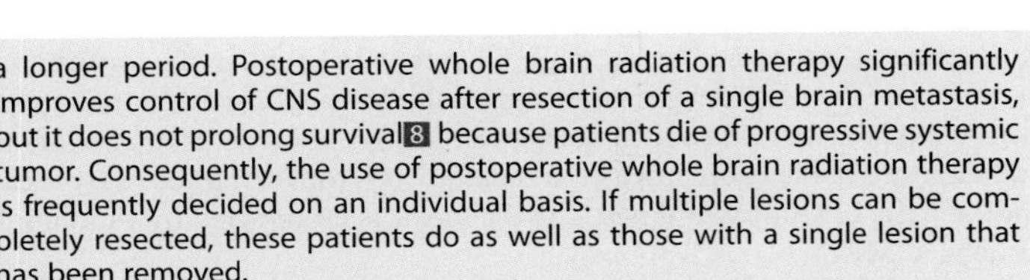

a longer period. Postoperative whole brain radiation therapy significantly improves control of CNS disease after resection of a single brain metastasis, but it does not prolong survival[8] because patients die of progressive systemic tumor. Consequently, the use of postoperative whole brain radiation therapy is frequently decided on an individual basis. If multiple lesions can be completely resected, these patients do as well as those with a single lesion that has been removed.

Most patients with multiple brain metastases are best treated with a course of whole brain radiation therapy, most commonly 3 Gy in 10 fractions for a total of 30 Gy. Some patients with single brain metastasis are also treated with whole brain irradiation if they are in poor general condition, have uncontrolled systemic disease, or are not good candidates for surgical treatment.

Stereotactic radiosurgery, using either a gamma knife that delivers gamma radiation from multiple cobalt sources or a linear accelerator that delivers x-rays to a highly focused area involving the tumor, has been quite effective for the treatment of one or a few brain metastases. Most patients tolerate radiosurgery without difficulty, but occasionally the procedure is complicated by seizures or acute swelling that causes more neurologic dysfunction. Approximately 20 to 30% of patients develop radionecrosis, which may be indistinguishable clinically and on MRI from recurrent tumor. One advantage of stereotactic radiosurgery is that most of the normal brain is not exposed to the radiation.

Chemotherapy is used to treat brain metastases from only a few chemosensitive primary cancers such as choriocarcinoma, small cell lung cancer, and, to a lesser extent, breast cancer. Because few patients have a significant response to chemotherapy, it is usually used as a last resort. The oral agent temozolomide (150 to 200 mg/m^2 for 5 days every 4 weeks) has shown some activity against brain metastases from lung cancer and is very well tolerated.

LEPTOMENINGEAL METASTASES

The brain is the most common intracranial site of metastases, but systemic cancer can spread to the dura and the leptomeninges as well. Dural metastases most commonly arise from breast or prostate cancer, frequently from a metastasis in the overlying calvaria. Metastasis to the leptomeninges often manifests as multifocal neurologic symptoms and signs. These metastases involve the cranial nerves to cause diplopia or bulbar palsy; the cervical and lumbar roots to cause limb pain or weakness; and the intracranial space to cause headache, nausea, vomiting, and elevated ICP. The diagnosis is established by the presence of tumor cells in the CSF or by neuroimaging that definitively outlines tumor in the subarachnoid space (Fig. 195-5). Treatment frequently involves radiation therapy to symptomatic sites; intrathecal chemotherapy, usually through an intraventricular cannula (Ommaya reservoir); or systemic chemotherapy with agents at doses that penetrate into the CSF.

TABLE 195-6 SPINAL TUMORS

Extradural
Metastasis
Primary bone tumors arising in the spine
Intradural extramedullary
Meningiomas
Neurofibromas
Schwannomas
Lipomas
Arachnoid cysts
Epidermoid cysts
Metastasis
Intramedullary
Ependymoma
Glioma
Hemangioblastoma
Lipoma
Metastasis

Spinal Tumors

Tumors involving the spine can be classified according to the anatomic area they involve: extradural, intradural extramedullary, and intramedullary tumors (Table 195-6). Extradural tumors typically arise from the bony elements of the spine and cause neurologic symptoms and signs by spinal cord compression. Intradural but extramedullary tumors arise from the pachymeninges or nerve roots (meningiomas or schwannomas) and can cause either radicular symptoms or spinal cord compression. Intramedullary spinal cord tumors arise from the spinal cord parenchyma and have a biology similar to brain tumors. Intramedullary tumors are rare.

EXTRADURAL TUMORS

EPIDEMIOLOGY AND CLINICAL MANIFESTATIONS

Most extradural tumors originate from a metastasis to the bony elements of the spine, typically the vertebral body and occasionally the vertebral lamina or spinous process. Less common are primary tumors of the spine, including chordoma, osteogenic sarcoma, plasmacytoma, and chondrosarcoma. Expansile growth of the bone tumor impinges on the spinal canal and, if untreated, compresses the spinal cord or the nerve roots as they exit the intervertebral foramina. Whereas most of these lesions arise from bony metastases, extradural tumors can also arise from paravertebral metastases that can grow through the intervertebral foramina and into the epidural space; very rarely, a direct metastasis to the epidural space is also seen. The most common primary cancers that cause extradural metastases are prostate (Chapter 207), breast (Chapter 204), and lung cancer (Chapter 197), as well as the lymphomas (Chapter 191). Hematologic malignancies may also be associated with paravertebral disease that grows through the intervertebral foramina.

Whether the mass is a primary bone tumor or a metastasis from a distant source, 98% of patients present with pain that is usually local at the site of the tumor. Because there are more thoracic than cervical or lumbar vertebrae, the tumor and pain are likely to be in the middle or high back, a less common site for benign pain (Chapter 407). Motor impairment and sensory symptoms are present in about 50% of patients, whereas sphincter disturbances are found in only about 25% of patients. Back pain often precedes the development of any other neurologic symptom or sign, frequently by weeks and occasionally by months.

DIAGNOSIS

Severe back pain in a patient with cancer should be evaluated by MRI, which does not require intravenous contrast. Plain films of the spine, bone scans, or even CT scans may show bony disease, but epidural tumor can be seen only on MRI. Furthermore, MRI is the only technique that can reveal paravertebral or direct epidural metastasis. Patients who cannot have an MRI should be imaged by CT myelography.

Differential Diagnosis

The differential diagnosis of extradural tumors includes epidural abscess (Chapter 421), acute or subacute epidural hematomas (Chapter 407), herniated intervertebral discs (Chapter 407), spondylosis (Chapter 407), epidural lipomatosis, and, rarely, extramedullary hematopoiesis. Occasionally, a percutaneous needle biopsy or decompressive laminectomy is required to make a definitive diagnosis.

TREATMENT Rx

Extradural metastases require immediate treatment because patients can develop acute and unpredictable neurologic deterioration resulting in paraplegia. Patients should be started on high-dose corticosteroids, usually 100 mg IV dexamethasone, which rapidly relieve pain and may contribute to neurologic recovery. Surgery followed by postoperative radiation therapy is superior to radiotherapy alone in preserving the ability to walk[9] and may prolong survival in a wide population of patients with metastatic spinal cord compression. It is much easier to preserve neurologic function than to reverse impairment, so clinically silent areas of extradural tumor that are detected on MRI should be treated before neurologic compromise develops. Patients whose primary tumor arises in the spine, such as an osteogenic sarcoma (Chapter 208), should undergo definitive surgery; the need for postoperative radiation therapy is determined on the basis of the tumor's histology. Patients with extradural metastases can have a good neurologic outcome if treated before the onset of severe neurologic compromise, but their overall survival is usually short because of the presence of widespread metastatic disease.

INTRADURAL EXTRAMEDULLARY TUMORS

Meningiomas

Most intradural extramedullary tumors are benign. Meningiomas are benign, slow-growing tumors that occur primarily in middle-aged women and are predominantly located in the thoracic region. Back pain is a common symptom, but about 25% of patients have no pain and present with slowly progressive neurologic dysfunction, typically a gait disorder that has been slowly progressing, frequently for years. Spinal MRI with gadolinium clearly delineates the lesion. Surgical resection is curative, and a complete resection can usually be accomplished easily.

Nerve Sheath Tumors

Nerve sheath tumors include schwannomas and neurofibromas. Both typically arise from the dorsal root, and the first symptom is often radicular pain that precedes symptoms of spinal cord compression by months or even years. Some patients with spinal neurofibroma or schwannoma have neurofibromatosis type 1 (Chapter 426), but most do not. The diagnosis is clearly established by gadolinium-enhanced MRI of the spine. The treatment is surgical, and complete removal results in cure.

Metastases

Metastasis to the spinal leptomeninges can manifest as an intradural extramedullary lesion. A single large tumor nodule can cause focal symptoms and signs referable to that spinal level, but in most patients, multiple levels of the neuraxis are involved, causing multifocal neurologic symptoms and signs. Cervical and lumbosacral radicular pain, as well as sensory and motor loss, is seen in more than half of patients. The diagnosis is established by gadolinium-enhanced MRI showing multifocal nodules or sometimes a layer of cells coating the spinal cord or nerve roots (see Fig. 195-5). If imaging is negative, the diagnosis can be established by demonstrating tumor cells in the CSF. Treatment is complicated and frequently requires radiation therapy to symptomatic sites of disease, intrathecal chemotherapy best administered through an intraventricular cannula (Ommaya device), and occasionally systemic chemotherapy. Radiation therapy can ameliorate neurologic symptoms, particularly pain, but the disease often has a relentless progressive course, resulting in death in 3 to 6 months despite aggressive therapy. Because of the diffuse nature of the disease, surgery is not an option.

INTRAMEDULLARY TUMORS

Intramedullary spinal cord tumors are similar to neoplasms that arise in brain parenchyma. The most common spinal cord tumors are ependymomas and astrocytomas; hemangioblastomas (particularly in association with von Hippel-Lindau disease; Chapter 426), lipomas, and, rarely, intramedullary metastases are also seen.

CLINICAL MANIFESTATIONS AND DIAGNOSIS

All intramedullary tumors have a similar clinical presentation, and pain is a common initial symptom. Signs of spinal cord dysfunction subsequently ensue and reflect the location of the lesion. In addition, some intramedullary tumors are accompanied by a syrinx (Chapter 426), which can contribute to symptoms. The classic signs of intramedullary spinal cord lesions, such as dissociated sensory loss, sacral sparing, and early sphincter problems, are not sufficiently reliable to distinguish intramedullary from extramedullary lesions on the basis of clinical findings. The diagnosis is established by gadolinium-enhanced MRI.

TREATMENT Rx

Surgery is the first therapeutic intervention, both to obtain a definitive diagnosis and to resect the lesion. Complete resection of spinal cord tumors is possible, particularly in the case of ependymomas and hemangioblastomas. However, spinal cord tumors are rare, and only neurosurgeons experienced in removal of this type of lesion should perform the procedure. High-grade gliomas and residual ependymomas should be treated with postoperative radiation therapy. Low-grade astrocytomas of the spinal cord can be treated with radiation therapy when the patient develops symptomatic neurologic impairment, but presymptomatic treatment does not prevent the development of impairment nor necessarily delay it. Intramedullary metastases do not require surgery because the diagnosis is usually straightforward; radiation therapy provides limited benefit because these patients typically have other CNS metastases.

INTRACRANIAL HYPERTENSION AND HYPOTENSION

CSF is made, in part, by the choroid plexus in the ventricular system; newly formed fluid circulates out the foramina of Luschka and Magendie, at the bottom of the fourth ventricle, to surround the entire spinal cord and cerebrum. It is reabsorbed back into the circulation through the arachnoid granulations over the convexities. Balance between CSF production and reabsorption keeps the volume relatively constant at about 150 mL in the normal healthy adult. CSF is produced at a rate of roughly 20 mL/hour, implying that the entire volume of CSF is replaced three to four times each day. CSF circulates nutrients to the nervous system and removes waste products from the only organ in the body that lacks a lymphatic system. In addition, CSF performs an important mechanical function by absorbing shock to the brain and spinal cord, cushioning them from the bony surroundings of the skull and spine.

A lumbar puncture provides the opportunity not only for sampling the CSF composition to detect disease processes but also for measuring ICP. CSF

TABLE 195-7 SYMPTOMS AND SIGNS OF INTRACRANIAL HYPERTENSION

COMMON
Headache
Tinnitus
Vomiting (with or without nausea)
Visual obscurations, visual loss, photopsias
Papilledema
Diplopia
Lethargy and increased sleep
Psychomotor retardation
Pain on eye movement
LESS COMMON
Hearing distortion or loss
Vertigo
Facial weakness
Shoulder or arm pain
Neck pain or rigidity
Ataxia
Paresthesias of extremities
Anosmia
Trigeminal neuralgia

pressure is normally maintained between 70 and 195 mm H_2O. ICP is maintained within this narrow window because significant fluctuations, either up or down, can cause marked neurologic dysfunction.

Intracranial Hypertension

Elevated ICP causes symptoms by compressing neural tissue, a process that causes ischemia and sometimes hemorrhage due to associated arterial and venous compression. ICP is partially maintained through the autoregulatory mechanisms of the cerebral blood vessels. Low ICP is caused by diminished CSF volume, and symptoms result from the loss of buoyancy of the brain as it floats within the CSF liquid. Pulling or stretching of the dura and cortical veins, which are the pain-sensitive structures in the cranial vault, causes headache; compensatory vasodilation may also contribute to headache.

The principal symptoms and signs associated with increased ICP are headache, nausea, vomiting, and lethargy; other symptoms are less frequent (Table 195-7). Focal mass lesions that cause a herniation syndrome may produce lateralizing signs such as hemiparesis; by comparison, diffuse elevation of ICP, as in communicating hydrocephalus, rarely does. Three main herniation syndromes are (1) herniation of the medial frontal gyrus under the falx; (2) transtentorial herniation of the uncus, pushing the diencephalon and the brain stem downward and laterally; and (3) herniation of the cerebellar tonsils through the foramen magnum. Generalized increased ICP may be due to obstruction of CSF, which may be caused by blockage of the ventricular system (obstructive or noncommunicating hydrocephalus) or by impairment of CSF reabsorption (nonobstructive or communicating hydrocephalus).

Increased ICP of any cause may produce pressure or plateau waves (episodic increases in ICP), leading to transient symptoms such as headache, vertigo, or diminished consciousness. Plateau waves occur normally and are associated with symptoms only when the baseline ICP is elevated. Plateau waves may be precipitated by a change in body position.

Hydrocephalus

Hydrocephalus refers to ventricular dilation caused by accumulated CSF. Hydrocephalus can be acute, resulting from sudden blockage of CSF outflow, or chronic, developing slowly over many months to years (Table 195-8). Patients with chronic hydrocephalus sometimes have normal CSF pressures, whereas those with acute hydrocephalus always have elevated CSF pressure.

CLINICAL MANIFESTATIONS

Acute hydrocephalus usually manifests with severe headache, lethargy, nausea, vomiting, papilledema, and diplopia from abducens palsy as well as signs from the causative lesion. Diffuse hyperreflexia and bilateral Babinski signs are common. Patients with chronic communicating hydrocephalus often have normal CSF pressure, so-called normal pressure hydrocephalus (NPH), and may present with progressive dementia characterized by memory loss and psychomotor retardation, an unsteady gait, and urgency incontinence (Chapter 409). Some patients have features of parkinsonism (Chapter 416) because of the bradykinesia and psychomotor retardation associated with hydrocephalus, but resting tremor is absent.

TABLE 195-8 CAUSES OF HYDROCEPHALUS

ACUTE
Cerebellar hemorrhage/infarction
Colloid cyst of the third ventricle
Exudative meningitis
Head trauma
Intracranial tumor or hematoma
Spontaneous subarachnoid hemorrhage
Viral encephalitis
CHRONIC
Aqueductal stenosis
Ectasia and elongation of the basilar artery (rare)
Granulomatous meningitis
Head trauma
Hindbrain malformations
Leptomeningeal metastasis
Brain and spinal cord tumors
Spontaneous subarachnoid hemorrhage

DIAGNOSIS

Ventriculomegaly is readily diagnosed by MRI or CT. In older patients, cerebral atrophy and the associated compensating increase in ventricular volume that accompanies normal aging (hydrocephalus ex vacuo) must be considered. Periventricular hyperintensity on T2-weighted or FLAIR MRI may help separate patients with NPH from those with hydrocephalus ex vacuo. MRI is the best test to identify a cause of hydrocephalus.

TREATMENT Rx

If the ICP approaches or exceeds the systolic blood pressure, the cerebral perfusion pressure decreases, and ischemia develops. Marked elevation of ICP is a neurologic emergency that requires immediate intervention (Table 195-9) to reduce the volume of the intracranial contents and to prevent permanent brain damage. Hyperventilation to lower the arterial partial pressure of carbon dioxide ($PaCO_2$) to 25 to 30 mm Hg causes immediate vasoconstriction, which reduces cerebral blood volume. Intravenous mannitol or hypertonic saline can cause a rapid diuresis, which reduces intravascular plasma volume and helps to withdraw water from the extracellular space in the brain. Glucocorticoids, typically as dexamethasone 50 to 100 mg by IV bolus, will require hours to reduce underlying edema; vasogenic edema from brain tumor or brain abscess responds rapidly to corticosteroids, but cytotoxic edema accompanying an acute ischemic stroke or hematoma seldom responds to corticosteroids.

Ultimately, however, definitive treatment of the specific cause is necessary. If such treatment is not immediately feasible, hydrocephalus often responds promptly to ventricular drainage. If temporary drainage is necessary, an external ventricular drain can be placed until the underlying obstruction is relieved. A ventriculoperitoneal shunt is the definitive treatment for chronic hydrocephalus, but it is not reliably effective for "idiopathic" NPH. The clinical response to several days of external lumbar CSF drainage has a high predictive value for determining which patients with NPH are likely to benefit from a shunt. Complications of shunting include subdural hematomas and infection.

Idiopathic Intracranial Hypertension

DEFINITION AND EPIDEMIOLOGY

Idiopathic intracranial hypertension, also called benign intracranial hypertension or pseudotumor cerebri, refers to elevated ICP that develops in an otherwise healthy individual without evidence of a structural CNS

TABLE 195-9 EMERGENCY TREATMENT OF ELEVATED INTRACRANIAL PRESSURE IN ACUTELY DECOMPENSATING PATIENTS

THERAPY	TREATMENT	ONSET (DURATION OF ACTION)	OTHER
Hyperventilation	Lower $Paco_2$ to 25-30 mm Hg	Seconds (minutes)	Usually requires intubation and mechanical ventilation
Osmotherapy	Mannitol 0.5-2 g/kg IV, repeat as necessary	Minutes (hours)	Brisk diuresis Requires Foley catheter Strict attention to electrolytes
Corticosteroids	Dexamethasone 50-100 mg IV, followed by 50-100 mg/day in divided doses	Hours (days)	Most effective on vasogenic edema (tumors, abscesses) Less effective on cytotoxic edema (stroke)

$Paco_2$ = arterial partial pressure of carbon dioxide.

TABLE 195-10 SYSTEMIC AND IATROGENIC CONDITIONS ASSOCIATED WITH BENIGN INTRACRANIAL HYPERTENSION

COMMONLY PRESCRIBED DRUGS

Nalidixic acid
Nitrofurantoin
Phenytoin
Sulfonamides
Tetracycline
Vitamin A
Retinoic acid (*cis* or *trans*)

ENDOCRINE AND METABOLIC DISORDERS

Addison's disease
Cushing's syndrome
Hypoparathyroidism
Menarche, pregnancy, oral contraceptives
Obesity (often associated with irregular menses)
Corticosteroid therapy or withdrawal

HEMATOLOGIC DISORDERS

Cryoglobulinemia
Iron deficiency anemia

MISCELLANEOUS DISORDERS

Dural venous sinus obstruction or thrombosis
Head trauma
Internal jugular vein ligation
Systemic lupus erythematosus
Middle ear disease

abnormality. Most patients are obese young women, but the disorder can also occur in men, thin patients, older adults, and children. Idiopathic intracranial hypertension can be associated with a variety of systemic disorders and medications (Table 195-10), but the direct cause of ICP elevation is usually unknown. Chronic elevations of ICP can lead to the "empty sella syndrome" (Chapter 231), which refers to enlargement of the sella turcica due to an incompetent diaphragma sellae, leading to CT or MRI evidence of CSF in the sella; the result is a compressed but functioning pituitary gland.

CLINICAL MANIFESTATIONS

Patients usually present with headache that may be accompanied by visual disturbances, including visual loss, nausea, vomiting, diplopia, tinnitus, and vertigo. Examination is notable for bilateral papilledema in an otherwise healthy patient. Loss of vision, which is the most feared complication, is uncommon. Visual fields typically reveal an enlarged blind spot owing to the papilledema, but no other visual impairment. Diplopia can occur from an abducens palsy as a false localizing sign.

DIAGNOSIS

The diagnosis is established by excluding any structural cause of elevated ICP by MRI. Magnetic resonance venography (MRV) also should be performed to exclude dural venous sinus thrombosis or stenosis. Lumbar puncture is performed after neuroimaging and is required to confirm the diagnosis by establishing an elevated opening pressure, frequently greater than 300 mm H_2O; however, the composition of the fluid is normal, and the protein concentration is typically in the low-normal range (<20 mg/dL).

TABLE 195-11 CAUSES OF INTRACRANIAL HYPOTENSION

Postlumbar puncture
CSF leak following CNS surgery or trauma
CSF fistula
Post-thoracotomy leak into pleural space
Spontaneous/idiopathic dural tear

CNS = central nervous system; CSF = cerebrospinal fluid.

TREATMENT Rx

The need to treat chronic intractable elevation of ICP is based on the patient's symptoms and serial visual field testing. Headache or new or progressive visual loss on eye examination or perimetry testing should trigger one or more of five treatments: (1) weight reduction (e.g., 20 lb) or correction of underlying endocrinologic or hematologic disorders, or both; (2) repeated lumbar punctures; (3) acute pharmacologic treatments, including corticosteroids, loop diuretics, and acetazolamide, although corticosteroids can contribute to weight gain and their tapering may exacerbate the syndrome; (4) ventriculoperitoneal or lumboperitoneal shunt; and (5) fenestration of the optic nerve sheath, especially for patients with persistently elevated ICP and deteriorating vision.

PROGNOSIS

Outcome is variable: spontaneous remissions may occur; clinical improvement is not always accompanied by a reduction in CSF pressure; and the CSF pressure may remain persistently elevated despite intervention. Furthermore, patients with chronically elevated ICP from idiopathic intracranial hypertension never develop hydrocephalus, so CSF pressure and ventriculomegaly are not linked.

Intracranial Hypotension

Intracranial hypotension occurs most commonly after lumbar puncture or after an idiopathic tear of the spinal dura. Evidence suggests that new "atraumatic" needles, as well as smaller-bore needles and few passes of the needle to perform the lumbar puncture, are associated with a lower incidence of postspinal headache.

CLINICAL MANIFESTATIONS AND DIAGNOSIS

Low CSF pressure (Table 195-11) can cause clinical symptoms that are usually mild but occasionally severe and debilitating. Postural headaches occur within 30 seconds after assuming the erect posture and subside completely when the patient lies flat (Chapter 405). The headaches, which are usually bifrontal or occipital, are typically severe, generalized, and throbbing. Headaches may be accompanied by nausea, dizziness, photophobia, neck stiffness, and, rarely, an abducens nerve palsy. All symptoms are relieved when the patient lies down.

TREATMENT AND PROGNOSIS Rx

In most patients, symptoms resolve spontaneously and can be treated with simple analgesics. Some patients develop persistent, symptomatic intracranial hypotension that does not respond to simple measures.

In patients whose symptoms are persistent or disabling, an epidural blood patch is performed by injecting approximately 10 mL of the patient's own blood into the epidural space to seal the presumed dural leak. Occasionally, CSF radioisotope studies must be performed to identify the site of the leak so that surgical repair of the dura can be performed.

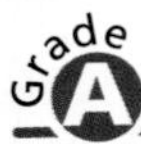

1. Forsyth PA, Weaver S, Fulton D, et al. Prophylactic anticonvulsants in patients with brain tumour. *Can J Neurol Sci*. 2003;30:106-112.
2. Mikkelsen T, Paleologos NA, Robinson PD, et al. The role of prophylactic anticonvulsants in the management of brain metastases: a systematic review and evidence-based clinical practice guideline. *J Neurooncol*. 2010;96:97-102.
3. Stupp R, Hegi ME, Mason WP, et al. Effects of radiotherapy with concomitant and adjuvant temozolomide versus radiotherapy alone on survival in glioblastoma in a randomised phase III study: 5-year analysis of the EORTC-NCIC trial. *Lancet Oncol*. 2009;10:459-466.
4. Keime-Guibert F, Chinot O, Taillandier L, et al. Radiotherapy for glioblastoma in the elderly. *N Engl J Med*. 2007;356:1527-1535.
5. Wick W, Hartmann C, Engel C, et al. NOA-04 randomized phase III trial of sequential radiochemotherapy of anaplastic glioma with procarbazine, lomustine, and vincristine or temozolomide. *J Clin Oncol*. 2009;27:5874-5880.
6. Karim AB, Afra D, Cornu P, et al. Randomized trial on the efficacy of radiotherapy for cerebral low grade glioma in the adult. *Int J Radiat Oncol Biol Phys*. 2002;52:316-324.
7. Cairncross G, Berkey B, Shaw E, et al. Phase III trial of chemotherapy plus radiotherapy compared with radiotherapy alone for pure and mixed anaplastic oligodendroglioma: Intergroup Radiation Therapy Oncology Group Trial 9402. *J Clin Oncol*. 2006;24:2707-2714.
8. Aoyama H, Shirato H, Tago M, et al. Stereotactic radiosurgery plus whole-brain radiation therapy vs stereotactic radiosurgery alone for treatment of brain metastases: a randomized controlled trial. *JAMA*. 2006;295:2483-2491.
9. Patchell RA, Tibbs, PA, Regine WF, et al. Direct decompressive surgical resection in the treatment of spinal cord compression caused by metastatic cancer: a randomised trial. *Lancet*. 2005; 366:643-648.

SUGGESTED READING

McPherson CM, Suki D, Feiz-Erfan I, et al. Adjuvant whole-brain radiation therapy after surgical resection of single brain metastases. *Neuro-Oncology*. 2010;12:711-719. *Role of adjuvant whole-brain radiation therapy in reducing local and distal recurrences in subsets of patients following surgical resection of single brain metastases.*

Robertson T, Koszyca B, Gonzales M. Overview and recent advances in neuropathology. Part 1: central nervous system tumours. *Pathology*. 2011;43:88-92. *Review.*

Ryken TC, McDermott M, Robinson PD, et al. The role of steroids in the management of brain metastases: a systematic review and evidence-based clinical practice guideline. *J Neurooncol*. 2010;96:103-114. *Limited data suggest a benefit with a preference toward dexamethasone 16 mg/day tapered slowly over a 2-week time period, or longer in symptomatic patients.*

Suh JH. Stereotactic radiosurgery for the management of brain metastases. *N Engl Med*. 2010;362:1119-1127. *Review.*

196 HEAD AND NECK CANCER

MARSHALL R. POSNER

DEFINITION

The principal cancers of the head and neck include squamous cell cancers arising from the mucosal surfaces of the upper aerodigestive tract and a diverse group of salivary gland neoplasms. Unique cancers of the region include nasopharyngeal carcinoma, thyroid malignancies (Chapter 233), esthesioneuroblastoma, and sinonasal undifferentiated carcinoma. A variety of other cancers arise from structures and tissues in the head and neck, including the more common skin cancers (Chapter 210), lymphomas (Chapters 191 and 192), and sarcomas (Chapter 209).

EPIDEMIOLOGY

Squamous cell carcinomas account for 95% of all malignancies of the head and neck, whereas salivary gland cancers represent nearly all of the remaining 5%. They represent 4% of all malignancies in the United States. Squamous cell cancers of the head and neck can be divided into two distinct groups based on pathogenesis, biology, and prognosis. Environmentally related cancers, caused principally by tobacco and alcohol, have been declining in incidence; however, they remain common. There has been an increasing incidence of human papillomavirus (HPV)-related oropharynx cancer (HPVOC). HPVOC now represents about 65% of oropharynx cancers seen in the United States and Europe. HPVOC affects a younger population (50 to 60 years) than environmental cancers (55 to 65 years). HPVOC patients are also generally healthier.

The mucosal surfaces of the head and neck are divided into six anatomic regions: the oral cavity, oropharynx, hypopharynx, larynx, nasopharynx, and paranasal sinuses. The site of anatomic origin for a squamous cell carcinoma of the head and neck has important, albeit imperfect implications for diagnosis, pathogenesis, spread, prognosis, and treatment because of intrinsic differences in the biology of the mucosal cells and subsequent cancers at the sites of origin, as well as differences in lymphatic drainage patterns and proximity to other structures in this compact region.

Oral Cavity

The oral cavity includes the floor of the mouth, anterior or oral aspect of the tongue, lips, buccal surfaces, hard palate, retromolar trigone, and gums. This region is easily appreciable by physical examination, and thus tumors in this area can frequently be detected early in their course. Tumors of the oral cavity, which are strongly related to the use of smokeless tobacco and other oral tobacco products (Chapter 31), appear on the buccal and gingival surfaces in the sites where tobacco products are held in contact with the mucosa for long periods. Anterior tongue cancers are more common in smokers. Lip cancers are particularly prevalent in transplant recipients and can be caused by DNA damage from solar ultraviolet light.

Oropharynx

The oropharynx consists of the tongue from the circumvallate papillae, posteriorly to the epiglottis, the tonsils, the associated pharyngeal walls, and the soft palate. The oropharynx has become the most common location for head and neck tumors in the United States and is a common site of origin in Europe. This is due to a high rate of HPVOC, which continues to increase in incidence. HPVOC is caused almost exclusively by HPV-16, a high-risk HPV type associated with cervical, anal, and vulvar cancers. HPVOC presents with lower primary T stage (T1 and T2) and higher nodal stage (N2 and N3) than environmental cancers and is frequently a cause of unknown primary cancer because of small and hard to identify primary tumors.

Hypopharynx

The hypopharynx comprises the piriform sinuses, the lateral and posterior pharyngeal walls, and the posterior surfaces of the larynx. These structures surround the larynx posteriorly and laterally. Tumors in this region can be difficult to detect because of the recesses and spaces surrounding the larynx. As a result, primary hypopharyngeal tumors may be asymptomatic and, like oropharyngeal tumors, may initially be recognized in an advanced state or diagnosed as an "unknown primary" (Chapter 211). These tumors are associated with tobacco (Chapter 31) and alcohol (Chapter 32) use.

Larynx

The larynx includes the vocal cords, the subglottis, and the supraglottic larynx, as well as the thyroid, cricoid, and arytenoid cartilages. Tumors arising in the true vocal cords are frequently symptomatic early and rarely spread beyond the confines of the larynx, whereas subglottic and supraglottic cancers can be relatively asymptomatic and have a much higher and earlier risk of spread to the lymphatics and regional sites. Laryngeal cancers are strongly associated with smoking (Chapter 31).

Nasopharynx

The nasopharynx includes the mucosal surfaces and structures of the cavity behind the nasal passages. Nasopharyngeal cancers are common in the Pacific Rim, northern Africa, and the Middle East. In some areas of China and Southeast Asia, nasopharyngeal cancers occur with a frequency that rivals lung cancer. In North America, there are about 2000 cases each year, but numbers are increasing as high-risk ethnic populations settle in North America. Nasopharyngeal cancers are frequently associated with the presence of latent infection of the epithelial tumor cells by Epstein-Barr virus (EBV), the etiologic agent of infectious mononucleosis (Chapter 385). Nasopharyngeal cancers are also associated with both environmental and genetic factors in susceptible populations that have migrated to North America and remain at high risk for this disease. Unlike other squamous cell carcinomas of the head and neck, nasopharyngeal cancers can occur at an early age, with a distinct peak in adolescence and young adulthood. Nasopharyngeal cancers are categorized into three histologic subtypes by the World Health Organization (WHO): the undifferentiated (WHO III) and nonkeratinizing forms (WHO II) are latently infected with EBV in 95% of cases and represent the majority of cases in North America and worldwide; the well-differentiated (WHO I) form is rarer and represents about 5% worldwide but about 15 to 25% of all nasopharyngeal cancers in North America, and it is usually associated with traditional risk factors such as smoking. Nasopharyngeal cancers have a high risk of early regional lymph node involvement, a prolonged natural history, and a very high risk of spread to distant sites.

Paranasal Sinuses

The paranasal sinuses comprise the maxillary, ethmoid, sphenoid, and frontal sinuses as well as the nasal cavity. These are relatively rare locations for tumors of the head and neck in North America, but there is an unexplained higher rate of malignant sinus disease among the Japanese. Squamous maxillary sinus cancers are more common in smokers. Up to 50% of cancers of the sinuses may be of salivary gland origin, often related to exposure to dust from woodworking, tanning, or leather working (Chapter 18). Occasionally, neuroendocrine tumors and the rare sinonasal undifferentiated carcinoma are found. Sinus cancers are frequently diagnosed late in their course at the time of symptomatic invasion of surrounding structures, including the orbit, nasal cavity, base of the skull, and cranial nerves.

Salivary Glands

Salivary glands occur in all the regions described, as well as in the trachea and esophagus. Tumors can develop in all of the major and minor salivary glands with an incidence that is roughly proportional to the quantity of glandular tissue. The most common single site is the parotid. Although tumors can develop at any age, including childhood, the peak incidence is between 55 and 65 years of age. Salivary gland cancers have diverse histologic findings and manifest different behavior based on their histologic classification. A substantial fraction of parotid salivary tumors can be benign. Risk factors for salivary gland cancers are poorly understood, but previous radiation therapy in adjacent areas increases the risk (Chapter 19).

PATHOBIOLOGY

Tobacco products and alcohol are major etiologic and risk factors for squamous cell carcinoma of the head and neck. Both show a clear dose response. Any irritating smoked product increases the risk for local cancer, but nicotine in tobacco, as well as in other tobacco leaf components, directly affects the oral mucosa and increases the risk for squamous cancer (Chapter 31). Alcohol is also a carcinogen, and alcohol consumption (Chapter 32), as well as its direct application in mouthwashes, is associated with an increased risk. Moreover, alcohol affects local and systemic detoxification enzymes and may increase the carcinogenic potential of other environmental carcinogens. Other environmental risk factors include radiation exposure and solar radiation; welding, metal refining, diesel exhaust, wood stove, and asbestos exposure; chronic irritants; vitamin A deficiency; and immunosuppression.

Carcinogenic viruses are responsible for the increasing incidence of head and neck cancer in the United States and Europe. Pathogenic HPV subtypes, specifically HPV-16, independently account for approximately 65% of oropharyngeal cancer cases. HPV is transmitted by epithelial contact, and there is increased risk of HPVOC associated with increasing numbers of individual sexual partners. HPV-16 DNA can be found in the tumor cells, and the oncogenic viral proteins E6 and E7 are responsible and necessary for the growth and survival of the cancer cells by effecting critical signaling pathways. HPVOC patients have a three-fold better prognosis than patients with environmentally related cancers. Nasopharyngeal cancer is predominantly associated with keratinocyte infection with EBV (Chapter 385). The classic nasopharyngeal cancer, which is also called *lymphoepithelioma,* is associated with a brisk lymphoid infiltrate that can be confused with a lymphoma. Careful examination reveals the malignant epithelial cells in the tumor. EBV is also rarely associated with epithelial tumors of the oropharynx, tonsil, and salivary gland.

Several inherited diseases and genetic abnormalities are associated with the development of head and neck cancer. Fanconi's anemia (Chapter 168), a rare disorder of a family of related gene products, has been linked to the development of tongue cancer, as has Cowden's syndrome (Chapter 184), which is associated with mutation of the *PTEN* gene. Finally, common inherited allelic variants of the alcohol dehydrogenase and P-450 genes may be associated with increased susceptibility to alcohol and other environmental carcinogens.

The development of squamous cell carcinoma of the head and neck is a multistep process in which early genetic changes evolve into frank malignancy. In environmentally related cancers, an abnormal premalignant clone of mucosal cells may be localized to a single site within the head and neck, or clones may occur independently in many sites. The pathogenesis of HPVOC is less well understood. Second cancers are rare with HPVOC in the short term, and long-term risk is unknown. In contrast, about 20% of patients with environmentally caused cancers will develop a second primary cancer, most commonly in the head and neck, lung, and esophagus; 5% of patients are initially seen with a synchronous second primary. In environmentally related cancers, the cell cycle is dysregulated by the early loss of p16, an inhibitor of cyclin D1, or by upregulation of cyclin D1; p53 is disabled through a number of mechanisms preventing programmed cell death; mitogenic signaling is enhanced by upregulation of epidermal growth factor (EGF) receptor function; cyclooxygenase-2 is overexpressed, thereby inhibiting apoptosis and promoting angiogenesis; and chromosomal instability with aneuploidy develops. Many of these early molecular and functional changes occur without obvious alteration in the physical appearance of the oral mucosa, although leukoplakia can occur. In HPVOC, the RB and p53 pathways are inactivated by the HPV oncogenic proteins E6 and E7. As a result, the p16 protein is upregulated as a biomarker of HPV tumor origin. As a consequence of RB and p53 inactivation, these patients have dysregulation of cell growth and DNA damage control/programmed cell death, respectively. The differences between the genetic and molecular determinants of cancer in HPVOC and environmentally related cancers can be differentially targeted for therapy.

In environmentally related cancers, high-risk early lesions can occasionally be identified as leukoplakia and erythroplakia. Leukoplakia (Fig. 196-1A) is diagnosed clinically as a white patch of mucosal tissue in the oral mucosa or larynx. It can unpredictably progresses to cancer over a period of several years in approximately 30% of patients. Erythroplakia (see Fig. 196-1B), a red hyperkeratotic change in the mucosa, is a more advanced premalignant lesion with an approximately 60% rate of progression to oral cancer. Surgical resection of leukoplakia or erythroplakia has no effect on the subsequent development of invasive cancer. There is no proven chemopreventive therapy for persons with oral premalignant lesions. Because continued smoking or alcohol consumption increases the risk for recurrence and second primaries dramatically, patients with prior cancers should stop alcohol and tobacco use.

CLINICAL MANIFESTATIONS

The symptoms and clinical manifestations of tumors in the head and neck can vary broadly and are related to the structures at the site of the primary tumor, as well as regional lymph node drainage. Small tumors of the oral cavity and larynx can be easily appreciated because of physical self-discovery

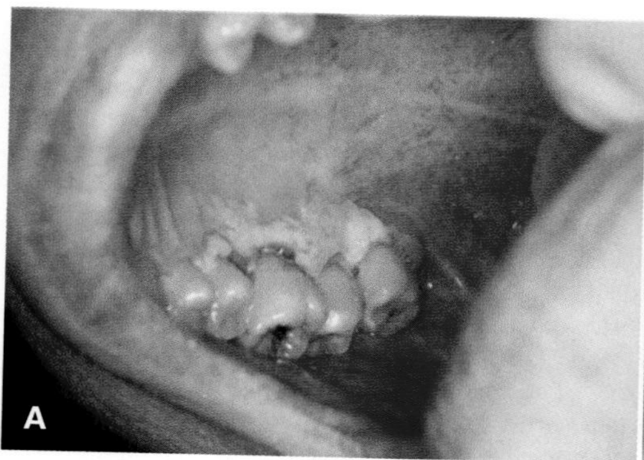

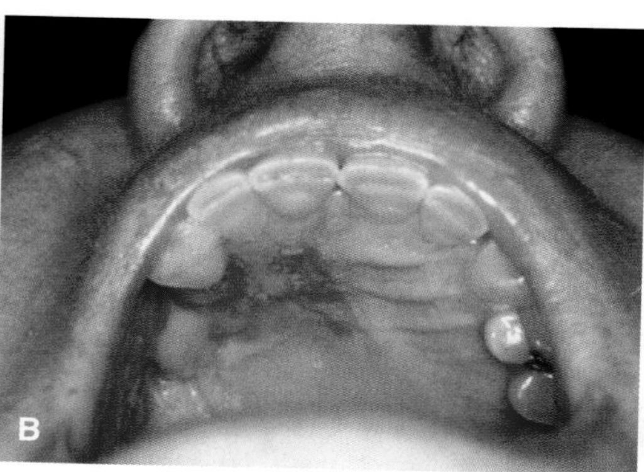

FIGURE 196-1. High-risk early mouth lesions. **A,** Oral leukoplakia. **B,** Oral erythroplakia.

or early compromise of the function of a critical structure. As a result of the propensity for squamous cell carcinoma of the head and neck to remain a local and regional disease, it is unusual for this cancer to be associated with abnormalities outside the head and neck. Salivary gland malignancies are less constrained and frequently spread distantly; however, because the primary tumors are also frequently accessible to direct physical examination and discovery, it is still uncommon to identify these tumors as a result of metastatic spread outside the region.

Clinical manifestations of *tumors in the oral cavity* include a painless lump, a painful mass or ulcer, or simple thickening of the mucosa. Small lesions in the lateral aspect of the tongue and the floor of the mouth can cause pain referred to the mandible, gums, and ear because of the shared sensory nerves supplying these areas. Antibiotics can relieve symptoms and even reduce the size of a tumor or lymph nodes when superficial infection and inflammation are contributing to the pain; however, recurrent or continued pain in an adult should trigger suspicion about more ominous disease. Speech may be affected late if the tumor causes restricted tongue motion or cranial nerve XII dysfunction. Gingival tumors can loosen teeth and invade the mandible along tooth sockets.

In true vocal cord cancer, hoarseness and other forms of voice change are common and expected early symptoms, but they may be later manifestations of *supraglottic and subglottic laryngeal tumors,* which become relatively large without affecting the voice. Tumors of the piriform sinus can affect the voice when they become large and impair the recurrent laryngeal nerve, or they are associated with deep local invasion; pain in the ear or pain on swallowing referred to the ear is also a common and important feature of these tumors. Adults with ear pain or persistent hoarseness should be referred to an otolaryngologist for evaluation. Because this posterior area is difficult to assess, primary tumors are frequently missed in routine office examinations. *Tumors of the supraglottic region, subglottic cancers, and cancers of the piriform sinus* can also be manifested as acute, emergency airway obstruction. Frequently, patients have a history of wheezing and mild upper airway distress in the period leading up to the emergency situation. Occasionally, such findings are confused with adult-onset asthma.

A middle ear infection or effusion in an adult should also prompt an ear, nose, and throat (ENT) evaluation. Nasopharyngeal cancer may be manifested as an ear infection in young adults. Hemoptysis or epistaxis may be the only clue to a nasopharyngeal cancer or a *paranasal sinus tumor.* Cranial nerve findings from deep invasion of the base of skull are late events and include lateral gaze abnormalities, diplopia, facial pain, or facial nerve paralysis. *Sinus tumors* can also be associated with these later findings, although nasal stuffiness occurs frequently and can be confused with sinusitis. New and persistent symptoms of sinusitis or facial pain should raise suspicion of sinus cancer and prompt an evaluation.

Tumors in the tonsil or base of the tongue can cause local pain and referred ear pain; however, they are frequently asymptomatic and can attain a large size before becoming evident as a result of changes in speech ("hot potato voice"), a sense of globus, or restriction of tongue movement. Manifestation as a painless lump in the neck is increasingly common with the increased incidence of HPVOC. Tumors of the tonsil or base of the tongue may also lose their mucosal component, not be seen or felt on direct inspection, and occur as a solid or cystic neck mass. Isolated neck masses can wax and wane with antibiotics. A mass, especially a cystic mass, in the neck in an adult is cancer and specifically HPVOC until proved otherwise and should prompt an ENT evaluation, before fine-needle aspiration (FNA) or excisional biopsy.

The staging of squamous cell carcinoma of the head and neck is based on the TNM (tumor, node, metastasis) staging system, and prognosis is related primarily to the N and T stages (Table 196-1). The risk of the cancer spreading to lymph nodes is directly related to the location of the primary and secondarily to the size of the primary. Tumors of the oropharynx have a high risk for nodal metastases, followed in risk by the supraglottic larynx and piriform sinus (hypopharynx), oral portion of the tongue, soft palate, oral cavity and floor of the mouth, and larynx. Nasopharyngeal cancer is highly associated with extensive nodal spread, whereas paranasal sinus cancers rarely spread to the lymph nodes. The location of lymph node spread is determined in part by site. Nasopharyngeal cancer spreads to the posterior cervical lymph nodes, as well as the high cervical nodes. Oropharynx, larynx, and piriform sinus tumors spread to the high cervical nodes. Nodal metastases from these locations can be bilateral. Oral cavity tumors spread to the submental nodes and submandibular nodes. Spread tends to be orderly from the submandibular nodes to the midcervical nodes. Oral cavity cancers can have as high as a 20% risk of clinically unappreciated contralateral spread.

DIAGNOSIS

The relative accessibility of the head and neck to direct inspection makes physical examination critical for diagnosis and staging. Patients with localized symptoms or a sign such as an ulcer or a small mass should have a thorough head and neck office examination performed by their primary physician and by a specialist, including inspection of the visible structures and palpation of the base of the tongue and tonsil areas, as well as the neck. Specialized office examination with fiberoptics should be included in the preliminary assessment. Regardless of whether cancer is suspected, excisional biopsies should be discouraged because margins are frequently violated and inadequate, thereby leading to larger re-excisions. A simple punch biopsy is sufficient for diagnosis, particularly in the oral portion of the tongue where tumors can spread readily though lymphatics.

When cancer is highly suspected and before definitive surgical intervention, a computed tomography (CT) scan from the base of the skull to the clavicles, preferably with the spiral technique, and a chest radiograph should be obtained. Magnetic resonance imaging (MRI) provides added information in evaluating soft tissue involvement, especially in the base of the tongue and the parapharyngeal spaces and for sinus tumors. MRI can distinguish between soft tissue masses and retained secretions, whereas CT is more helpful in assessing nodal spread in the neck and bone invasion. Positron emission tomography (PET) provides an adjunct to CT scanning and can identify occult disease. PET scanning should be performed when cancer is suspected and when the patient has an "unknown primary tumor," before biopsy, in order to guide the evaluation and reduce the risk of inadequate diagnostic and premature therapeutic procedures (Fig. 196-2).

When a biopsy indicates cancer or cancer is highly suspected, an examination under anesthesia with endoscopy should be performed to stage the primary tumor before definitive therapy is undertaken. This procedure, which provides information regarding the extent of disease, the appropriateness of the planned definitive procedure, and the presence of second primaries, is an absolute requirement before definitive therapy can be discussed with a patient. Endoscopy and palpation under anesthesia can identify unexpected local spread or a synchronous second primary (found in about 5% of patients with environmentally related cancers).

Approach to the Patient with an Unknown Primary Site

Patients frequently seek care from their primary physician because of an enlarged lymph node, a cystic mass, or a collection of lymph nodes in the

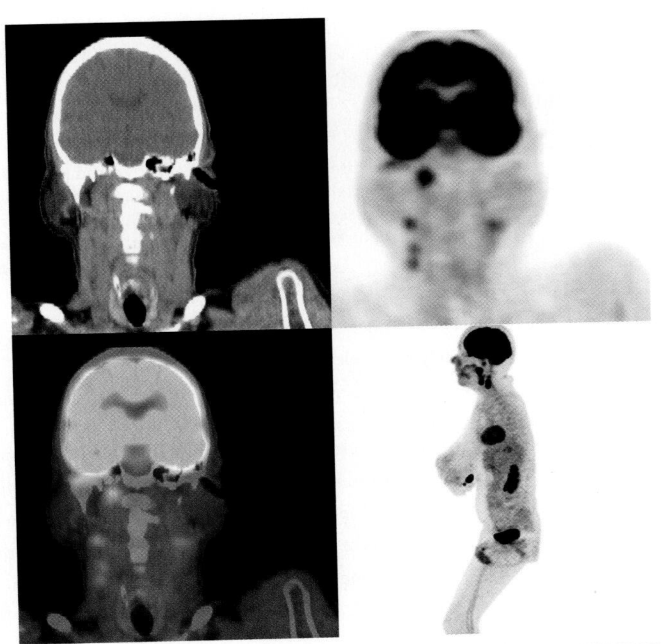

FIGURE 196-2. Positron emission tomography and computed tomography fused images. A primary human papillomavirus–positive base of tongue cancer and neck adenopathy is shown.

TABLE 196-1 AMERICAN JOINT COMMITTEE ON CANCER STAGING FOR HEAD AND NECK SQUAMOUS CELL CARCINOMA

TUMOR	LARYNX	LIP AND ORAL CAVITY	OROPHARYNX	HYPOPHARYNX
Tis	Carcinoma in situ	Carcinoma in situ	Carcinoma in situ	Carcinoma in situ
T1 T1a T1b	*Supraglottis:* Tumor limited to one subsite of supraglottis with normal vocal cord ability *Glottis:* Tumor limited to the vocal cord(s) (may involve anterior or posterior commissure) with normal mobility Tumor limited to one vocal cord Tumor involves both vocal cords *Subglottis:* Tumor limited to the subglottis	Tumor 2 cm or less in greatest dimension	Tumor 2 cm or less in greatest dimension	Tumor limited to one subsite of hypopharynx and/or 2 cm or less in greatest dimension
T2	*Supraglottis:* Tumor invades mucosa of more than one adjacent subsite of supraglottis or glottis or region outside the supraglottis (e.g., mucosa of base of tongue, vallecula, medial wall of pyriform sinus) without fixation of the larynx *Glottis:* Tumor extends to supraglottis and/or subglottis, and/or with impaired vocal cord mobility *Subglottis:* Tumor extends to vocal cord(s) with normal or impaired mobility	Tumor more than 2 cm but not more than 4 cm in greatest dimension	Tumor more than 2 cm but not more than 4 cm in greatest dimension	Tumor invades more than one subsite of hypopharynx or an adjacent site, or measures more than 2 cm but not more than 4 cm in greatest dimension without fixation of hemilarynx
T3	*Supraglottis:* Tumor limited to larynx with vocal cord fixation and/or invades any of the following: postcricoid area, pre-epiglottic space, paraglottic space, and/or inner cortex of thyroid cartilage *Glottis:* Tumor limited to the larynx with vocal cord fixation and/or invasion of paraglottic space, and/or inner cortex of the thyroid cartilage	Tumor more than 4 cm in greatest dimension	Tumor more than 4 cm in greatest dimension or extension to lingual surface of epiglottis	Tumor more than 4 cm in greatest dimension or with fixation of hemilarynx or extension to esophagus
T4a	Moderately advanced local disease Tumor invades through the thyroid cartilage and/or invades tissues beyond the larynx (e.g., trachea, soft tissues of neck including deep extrinsic muscle of the tongue, strap muscles, thyroid, or esophagus)	Moderately advanced local disease Lip: Tumor invades through cortical bone, inferior alveolar nerve, floor of mouth, or skin of face, i.e., chin or nose Oral cavity: Tumor invades adjacent structures only (e.g., through cortical bone [mandible or maxilla] into deep [extrinsic] muscle of tongue [genioglossus, hyoglossus, palatoglossus, and styloglossus], maxillary sinus, skin of face)	Moderately advanced local disease Tumor invades the larynx, extrinsic muscle of tongue, medial pterygoid, hard palate, or mandible (Note: Mucosal extension to lingual surface of epiglottis from primary tumors of the base of the tongue and vallecula does not constitute invasion of larynx)	Moderately advanced local disease Tumor invades thyroid/cricoid cartilage, hyoid bone, thyroid gland, or central compartment soft tissue (Note: Central compartment soft tissue includes prelaryngeal strap muscles and subcutaneous fat).
T4b	Very advanced local disease Tumor invades prevertebral space, encases carotid artery, or invades mediastinal structures	Very advanced local disease Tumor invades masticator space, pterygoid plates, or skull base and/or encases internal carotid artery	Very advanced local disease Tumor invades lateral pterygoid muscle, pterygoid plates, lateral nasopharynx, or skull base or encases carotid artery	Very advanced local disease Tumor invades prevertebral fascia, encases carotid artery, or involves mediastinal structures

NODE	DEFINITION
NX	Regional lymph nodes cannot be assessed
N0	No regional lymph node metastasis
N1*	Metastasis in a single ipsilateral lymph node, 3 cm or less in greatest dimension
N2*	Metastasis in a single ipsilateral lymph node, more than 3 cm but not more than 6 cm in greatest dimension; or in multiple ipsilateral lymph nodes, none more than 6 cm in greatest dimension; or in bilateral or contralateral lymph nodes, none more than 6 cm in greatest dimension
N2a*	Metastasis in single ipsilateral lymph node more than 3 cm but not more than 6 cm in greatest dimension
N2b*	Metastasis in multiple ipsilateral lymph nodes, none more than 6 cm in greatest dimension
N2c*	Metastasis in bilateral or contralateral lymph nodes, none more than 6 cm in greatest dimension
N3*	Metastasis in lymph node more than 6 cm in greatest dimension

METASTASIS	DEFINITION
M0	No distant metastasis
M1	Distant metastasis present

TABLE 196-1 AMERICAN JOINT COMMITTEE ON CANCER STAGING FOR HEAD AND NECK SQUAMOUS CELL CARCINOMA—cont'd

STAGE	T	N	M
0	Tis	N0	M0
I	T1	N0	M0
II	T2	N0	M0
III	T3	N0	M0
	T1	N1	M0
	T2	N1	M0
	T3	N1	M0
IVa	T4a	N0	M0
	T4a	N1	M0
	T1	N2	M0
	T2	N2	M0
	T3	N2	M0
	T4a	N2	M0
IVb	Any T	N3	M0
	T4b	Any N	M0
IVc	Any T	Any N	M1

*Distribution and prognostic impact of regional lymph node spread from nasopharynx cancer are different from those of other head and neck mucosal cancers and justify the use of a different N classification scheme.
From *AJCC Cancer Staging Manual*. 7th ed. New York: Springer-Verlag; 2010.

upper part of the neck (Fig. 196-3). Such masses in an adult should be considered cancer until proved otherwise. Unless there is an obvious symptom or sign that leads the clinician to the identification of a primary site in the head and neck, such patients are considered to have an unknown primary. Masses in the supraclavicular areas represent primary tumors below the clavicles, and masses in the midneck and cervical regions are almost always from the head and neck. Identification of a primary site is critical to focus therapy, reduce morbidity, and determine prognosis.

The most common primary sites for painless lumps are the oropharynx (base of the tongue and tonsil) and piriform sinus. Oropharynx cancers are frequently due to HPV and a positive HPV-16 polymerase chain reaction test of the biopsy or FNA is presumptive evidence of oropharynx origin. Salivary gland cancers, lymphomas, melanomas, and skin cancers can also be manifested in this manner. Bilateral nodal disease or nodal disease with systemic symptoms may suggest lymphoma. By comparison, pain, warmth, and erythema may suggest an infectious etiology. Intraparotid nodes most likely represent metastases from skin malignancies. Physical examination should include a careful investigation for primary skin cancers. CT, PET, and MRI should be part of the initial evaluation. FNA should be performed and repeated if initially negative. CT-guided biopsy may be indicated if the mass is difficult to approach. If squamous cells are identified, the tumor is most likely a squamous cell carcinoma of the head and neck. Next, endoscopy under anesthesia should be performed with bilateral tonsillectomy and directed biopsies of any abnormalities, areas of firmness, and the base of the tongue, nasopharynx, and ipsilateral piriform sinus, even if they appear normal. Core or excisional (single node <3 cm) biopsy of the lymph node should be performed if the pathology is equivocal and a primary site is not confirmed. Neck dissection can be accomplished if a primary site is not identified and the patient has an N1 or small N2a/b manifestation. Some unknown primaries with squamous histology are never identified. Currently, HPV-16 and EBV are the only molecular markers to distinguish head and neck cancer from skin or salivary gland squamous cancer. EBV positivity indicates a nasopharyngeal cancer, and HPV-16 is an oropharyngeal primary.

In contrast to squamous cell carcinoma of the head and neck, salivary gland cancers are heterogeneous in their natural history and treatment. The three most common histologic types are adenoid cystic carcinoma, mucoepidermoid cancer, and adenocarcinoma. Other histologic types include the aggressive salivary duct cancer and squamous cell cancers, whereas less aggressive histologic varieties include adenocarcinoma ex pleomorphic adenoma and acinic cell carcinoma. Because adenoid cystic carcinoma travels along nerves and can spread hematogenously, careful assessment of the cranial nerves and the chest by CT is indicated before major surgery is undertaken. Patients should also be evaluated for bone and liver metastases. Formal lymph node dissection is not indicated. Ethmoid and sphenoid sinus adenoid cystic carcinomas are locally and regionally aggressive and require specialized surgery and radiation therapy techniques for local and regional control. The behavior of mucoepidermoid carcinoma is determined by histology. Low- and intermediate-grade lesions rarely metastasize. Isolated high-grade tumors spread to local lymph nodes and by hematogenous routes and carry a high risk for the development of lung metastases. The work-up for high-grade lesions should be similar to that for adenoid cystic carcinoma. Local therapy should be directed at local and regional control with lymph node dissection. Radiation therapy is indicated for close microscopic margins or lymph node involvement. Adenocarcinoma, salivary duct cancers, and squamous cell carcinoma are also poor-prognosis lesions with aggressive local and distant behavior. These tumors should be evaluated in the same fashion as aggressive mucoepidermoid carcinomas. Acinic cell carcinoma and carcinoma ex pleomorphic adenoma are relatively rare. They have a propensity for local and regional recurrence if they are not removed in toto. Metastases are rare and tend to be slow growing.

Other Tumors of the Head and Neck

Lymphomas in the head and neck frequently manifest either as nodal disease in the neck or as tumor involving the lymphoid tissues of Waldeyer's ring (Chapters 191 and 192). A primary head and neck cancer may later develop in patients with lymphoma as a consequence of past exposure to tobacco, radiation therapy, or immunosuppression. The tonsil is a preferred site for mantle cell and undifferentiated lymphomas. Mucosa-associated lymphoid tissue (MALT) lymphomas can affect the salivary glands.

In the context of an isolated neck mass, a systematic evaluation (see Fig. 196-3) should be undertaken, even in young adults without a smoking history. The sinonasal T-cell and natural killer cell lymphomas, also known as *lethal midline granulomas*, represent a unique family of lymphomas of the head and neck. These lymphomas are associated with EBV infection (Chapter 385). Solitary, extramedullary plasmacytoma can also occur in the nasopharynx or paranasal sinuses (Chapter 193).

Sarcomas that arise in the head and neck include osteogenic sarcomas (Chapters 208 and 209) and nerve sheath tumors. Paragangliomas, which are rare malignant tumors of the chief cells of nerve paranglia, can be extensive, multicentric, and vascular. Rhabdomyosarcomas, which have a predilection for the orbit and sinuses, occur in younger persons; the prognosis tends to be better for tumors of the head and neck than for other locations. Olfactory

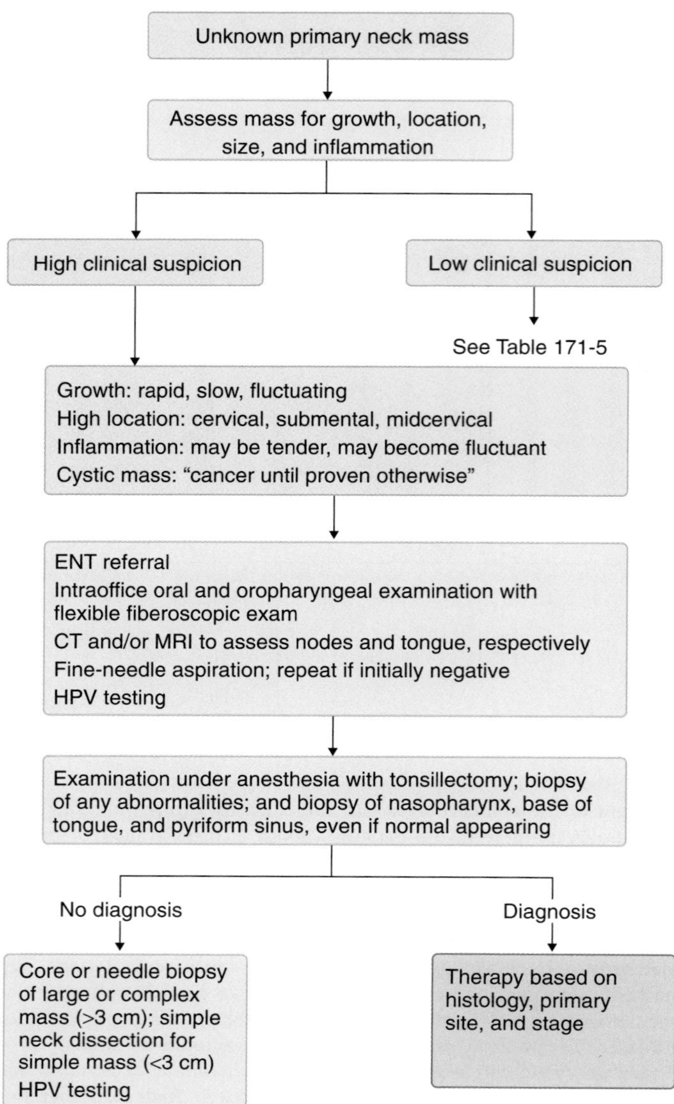
Unknown primary neck mass
Assess mass for growth, location, size, and inflammation
High clinical suspicion
Low clinical suspicion
See Table 171-5
Growth: rapid, slow, fluctuating
High location: cervical, submental, midcervical
Inflammation: may be tender, may become fluctuant
Cystic mass: "cancer until proven otherwise"
ENT referral
Intraoffice oral and oropharyngeal examination with flexible fiberoscopic exam
CT and/or MRI to assess nodes and tongue, respectively
Fine-needle aspiration; repeat if initially negative
HPV testing
Examination under anesthesia with tonsillectomy; biopsy of any abnormalities; and biopsy of nasopharynx, base of tongue, and pyriform sinus, even if normal appearing
No diagnosis
Diagnosis
Core or needle biopsy of large or complex mass (>3 cm); simple neck dissection for simple mass (<3 cm)
HPV testing
Therapy based on histology, primary site, and stage

FIGURE 196-3. **Evaluation of an unknown primary neck mass.** CT = computed tomography; ENT = ear, nose, and throat; HPV = human papillomavirus; MRI = magnetic resonance imaging.

neuroblastomas or esthesioneuroblastomas invade the nasal cavity and base of the skull.

Many skin tumors, including melanoma and squamous cell cancer, can be accompanied by adenopathy of the neck or parotid area (Chapter 210). An unusual skin appendage tumor, Merkel cell cancer, can be confused with other neuroendocrine epithelial tumors.

PREVENTION AND TREATMENT Rx

Selection of a treatment program for an individual patient is based on three factors: the primary site and stage of the tumor, the patient's comorbid conditions and preferences, and the biology of the tumor (Table 196-2). Early-stage lesions, T1N0 and T2N0, are defined by their size, and their prognosis is site specific. For example, early *larynx cancer* involving the true vocal cords has an excellent prognosis and can be treated by local excision. Voice-preserving larynx conservation surgery is effective for selected patients. Radiation therapy is equally effective for early cancer. When there is a risk of lymph node spread, radiation therapy must be given postoperatively, and the primary value of surgery is diminished. Intensity-modulated radiation therapy (IMRT) allows radiation to be delivered in a more conformal manner to the tumor and areas at risk while sparing critical structures such as the spinal cord and noncritical but important structures such as the salivary glands. IMRT is now a standard of care for patients with head and neck cancer.

Oral tongue, piriform sinus, and environmentally related oropharynx tumors have a worse prognosis and are difficult to stage accurately because of submucosal spread or lymphatic involvement. Stage I and II cancers are cured with local and regional surgery or radiation therapy in 70% to 90% of cases. Surgery may be preferred for oral cavity and anterior lesions. In surgically treated patients, those with a positive margin, two or more positive lymph nodes, or extracapsular spread have a poorer survival rate (<30%) at 5 years. Perineural invasion and lymphovascular invasion may also be associated with a poor prognosis. Postoperative cisplatin-based chemoradiotherapy improves local and regional control, as well as survival, and should be given to poor-prognosis patients if their condition permits.[1] At present, aside from HPV status and p16 immunohistochemistry, no molecular or immunohistochemical finding definitively adds to the information gleaned from pathology, staging, and performance status.

When organ preservation and function are issues for stage III or IV cancers or when radiation therapy is required regardless of surgical outcome, primary chemoradiotherapy or sequential therapy should be considered.[2,3] The curative treatment of intermediate (stage III, T1-3N1, T3N0) and locally advanced (stage IV, T1-3N2-3, T4) disease remains controversial. Long-term (3 years) survival rates in patients with stage III disease are generally between 50 and 75%, whereas only 15 to 50% of stage IV patients survive for 3 years. Intermediate-stage tumors are usually resectable, but organ preservation may be an important consideration. In many of these cases, a combined-modality approach that includes chemotherapy is the standard of care.

Patients with anterior lesions may do better with initial surgical treatment. The oral cavity is easy to assess and is relatively forgiving for surgery and reconstruction; postoperative radiation therapy or chemoradiotherapy can be moderated in the absence of bad prognostic features. For intermediate and advanced tumors, radiation therapy or chemoradiotherapy is a necessary adjunct to prevent recurrence. For example, a T3 or N1 lesion of the oropharyngeal tongue or hypopharynx is almost always more extensive than clinically appreciated and may be more suited to a nonsurgical regional and systemic approach. In addition, patients with rapidly growing tumors are more suitable for a combined-modality approach. Patients with extensive N2 or N3 nodal disease (stage IV) should be considered relatively unresectable because of a poor prognosis from regional recurrence and distant metastases. Certain locations such as the nasopharynx and posterior pharynx should also be considered for definitive radiation therapy, sequential therapy, or chemoradiotherapy.

Radiation therapy has been proved by randomized trials to yield better local control and disease-free survival if given in twice-daily fractionated treatments rather than as daily therapy. However, the absolute benefit of hyperfractionated radiation therapy at 5 years is only 3 to 4%, and it is unclear whether a twice-daily schedule is advantageous with chemotherapy.[4]

Induction chemotherapy is the delivery of chemotherapy before definitive local-regional treatment. Sequential therapy adds chemoradiotherapy (see later) to induction chemotherapy. Induction chemotherapy with docetaxel (75 mg/m^2), cisplatin (75 to 100 mg/m^2 by intravenous bolus), plus 5-fluorouracil (750 to 1000 mg/m^2/day for 4 to 5 days by intravenous infusion), repeated every 3 or 4 weeks (TPF) are effective, standard regimens. For patients with advanced oropharynx, larynx, and hypopharynx tumors, sequential chemotherapy with chemoradiotherapy using concomitant carboplatin and once-daily radiotherapy improves survival and preserves function compared with radiation, surgery, or cisplatin and 5-fluorouracil chemotherapy (PF).[5,6]

Chemoradiotherapy integrates chemotherapy and radiation therapy together and has led to significant improvements in overall survival in patients with advanced disease compared with radiation therapy alone. For example, patients with unresectable disease who received cisplatin (100 mg/m^2 by intravenous bolus) every 3 weeks during radiation therapy have significantly better survival than do those treated with radiation therapy alone.[7] In a trial of patients with oropharyngeal carcinoma, those treated with carboplatin and 5-fluorouracil plus simultaneous radiation therapy had significantly better survival than did those treated by radiation therapy alone.[8] Cetuximab plus radiotherapy has also proved effective in improving survival in patients with locally advanced head and neck cancer compared with radiotherapy alone.[9]

Patients with locally advanced or unresectable disease (or both) should receive chemotherapy as part of a combined-modality approach. Sequential therapy, induction chemotherapy, and chemoradiotherapy all prolong survival compared with surgery or radiotherapy, or both, and support an organ preservation approach. Organ preservation should be offered to patients who can tolerate the treatment and participate in the post-treatment rehabilitation.

Treatment of *tumors of the paranasal sinuses* is a special case. They rarely metastasize, and treatment should focus on surgical resection with postoperative radiation therapy for resectable stage III and IV disease and on chemoradiotherapy for local and regional control of unresectable disease. Proton beam irradiation may be more suited for tumors in and around the base of the skull and brain.

Follow-up

Patients need lifelong follow-up. A chest radiograph should be performed at least yearly, and surveillance examinations for second primaries and

TABLE 196-2 GENERAL APPROACH TO SQUAMOUS CELL HEAD AND NECK CANCER

STAGE	TNM	DISEASE-SPECIFIC SURVIVAL	TREATMENT APPROACH	SPECIAL CONDITIONS
I	T1N0	85-95%	Surgery or radiation therapy	Consider organ function and long-term toxicity
II	T2N0	75-90%	Surgery, radiation therapy, or chemoradiotherapy	Consider organ function Combined-modality treatment for high-volume tumor Postoperative chemoradiotherapy for poor prognostic findings on pathologic staging
III	T3N0 T1-3N1	50-75%	Combined-modality treatment	Primary chemoradiotherapy or TPF induction therapy or sequential therapy for organ function Postoperative chemoradiotherapy More aggressive approach (sequential therapy) for high-volume disease or hypopharynx tumors
IV	T1-3N2-3 T4N0-3 Any M1	20-60%	Combined-modality treatment	Combined-modality therapy Limited surgery Postoperative chemoradiotherapy Palliative therapy for M1 (curative therapy for isolated lung metastases)

recurrences should be performed monthly to bimonthly in the first year and then less frequently over time. Treatment failure after 3 years is uncommon, but second primaries may continue to be identified in environmentally related cancers. It is important to counsel these patients to avoid tobacco products and any exposure to alcohol.

During therapy and immediately after therapy, patients benefit from pain medications, local anesthetics, mucolytics, and saline mouthwash. Patients must avoid alcohol-containing preparations or irritants. Long-acting agents such as fentanyl or time-release narcotics should be added when needed (Chapter 29). A percutaneous endoscopic gastrostomy feeding tube is effective for maintaining weight, improving healing, and managing nutrition during radiation therapy. Because depression is a major problem, psychiatric support and antidepressants may be very helpful. Salivary function improves over more than 4 years after radiation therapy, but most improvement occurs in the first 2 years. Pilocarpine and cevimeline (Evoxac) are effective stimulants of salivary flow in about 20% of patients.

Long-term sequelae of radiation therapy include dependence on a feeding tube in patients treated with aggressive chemoradiotherapy or radiation therapy alone. Attention should be paid to preserving swallowing function by means of training in speech and swallowing, as well as dilation in selected patients. Hypothyroidism occurs in up to 50% of patients and as early as 3 months after treatment. Patients should be monitored by determining serum thyroid-stimulating hormone levels at regular intervals and then be treated as appropriate (Chapter 233). Dental failure is a common problem. Patients must be counseled to see their dentists regularly for cleanings and to obtain fluoride therapy daily for dental preservation. Patients are at substantial lifelong risk for complications from dental manipulations after radiation therapy. Bone necrosis is painful, can be confused with recurrent tumor, and requires vigorous antibiotic therapy, débridement, and possibly hyperbaric oxygen to promote healing.

Patients with recurrent disease, a second primary, or metastatic disease must be evaluated for potential curability. If patients have a recurrence or second primary, curative treatment options are defined by their current stage, their previous therapy, and the interval from their original therapy. Patients who have previously been treated with surgery but not radiation therapy can undergo surgery, radiation therapy, and chemotherapy as part of a curative treatment plan. Patients with a surgically treatable recurrence in an irradiated field should undergo surgery as appropriate. It is important to recognize that the surgery must encompass the entire recurrence. Symptomatically, persistent pain may be the most important indicator of a recurrence, and repeat biopsy should be considered when a suspicious lesion is observed. Surgical salvage may cure as many as 30% of patients with recurrent oral cavity, larynx, or hypopharyngeal tumors. A repeat course of radiation therapy is also acceptable in selected patients.

Patients who are incurable can be managed effectively with palliative therapy to improve quality of life and survival (e.g., tracheostomy for airway control, laryngectomy for pain and aspiration, percutaneous endoscopic gastrostomy tube for feeding). These maneuvers can improve comfort and care in appropriate patients.

Palliative chemotherapy can provide meaningful benefit to some patients. Response rates with single agents are generally poor, and combination therapy offers higher response rates (30 to 50%). The combination of a platinum (cisplatin or carboplatin) plus 5-fluorouracil with an anti-EGF receptor antibody, cetuximab, significantly improves survival, response rate, and progression-free survival compared with the same chemotherapy without cetuximab.

Salivary Gland Tumors

In contrast to squamous cell carcinoma of the head and neck, salivary gland cancers are heterogeneous in their natural history and treatment; however, the mainstays of therapy for these tumors are surgery and radiotherapy. Early symptoms of local-regional recurrence include cranial nerve dysfunction and progressive pain. A PET scan may be useful in distinguishing recurrence from the neuropathy that may result from radiation therapy.

There are no highly active agents or combinations for treatment of metastatic salivary gland tumors. Local therapy can include surgical removal of isolated metastases, radio frequency ablation, and radiation therapy. Response rates are generally in the 20 to 35% range, but prolonged responses are occasionally seen.

Future Directions

Antibodies that target the EGF receptor and other molecular targets may improve local and regional control, as well as survival, when delivered with radiation therapy. Vaccines against EBV and HPV may prevent malignancy in high-risk populations.

PROGNOSIS

The prognosis for patients with squamous cell carcinoma of the head and neck (see Table 196-2) is directly related to the presence of HPV, stage, and performance status. The risk for recurrence declines dramatically at 2 years after definitive treatment, and survival and possible cure can be defined after 3 years. HPV status and then N (nodal) stage are the most important prognostic indicators of potential recurrence, with T (tumor) stage and smoking history being next. Stage I patients (T1N0) have a 90% likelihood of tumor control, whereas stage II patients (T2N0) have greater than 70 to 85% tumor control. Tumor control in stage III patients (T1-2N1, T3N0-1) is site dependent and HPV status dependent and varies from 35 to 85%. Patients with stage IVa and IVb environmentally related disease (T1-3, N2-3, or T4NX) have a 20 to 50% tumor-specific 5-year survival rate compared with 60 to 90% 5-year survival for HPVOC. Bad prognostic signs in advanced-stage (IVb) patients are related to N3 nodal disease and invasion of basic structures (carotid artery encasement, base of the skull, pterygoid muscles). Patients with M1 disease are categorized as stage IVc. Isolated patients with single lung metastases can be cured, whether as a second primary or as an isolated recurrence. Patients with recurrent disease and no curative options have a median survival of 6 to 9 months. Death can occur as a result of compromise of local critical structures, including vessels, breathing, and swallowing.

Distant metastases occur in about 15 to 20% of patients, but this rate is increasing as better local and regional control prolongs survival in patients with locally advanced disease. Oropharyngeal, tonsil, and piriform sinus tumors have the highest risk for distant metastases. In approximately 5% of patients, a synchronous lung tumor or metastasis develops. A single lung metastasis in a patient at initial evaluation or at follow-up can be cured in about 20% of cases.

Salivary gland cancers vary in behavior, depending on their histology. Adenocarcinoma, salivary duct cancer, salivary squamous cell cancer, and high-grade mucoepidermoid cancer not only spread to lymph nodes but also spread rapidly hematogenously. The presence of lymph node metastases signals a high risk for distant metastases. Adenoid cystic carcinoma infrequently involves lymph nodes but spreads along nerves. Regional recurrences along cranial nerves are frequent and associated with "skip" lesions. Adenoid cystic carcinoma is also associated with the late development of lung metastases, but these patients can have a prolonged lifespan lasting more than 20 years. Low-grade mucoepidermoid cancer and acinic cell carcinoma have little risk of distant spread and are more notable for local recurrence if not completely removed.

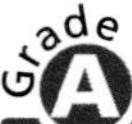

1. Bernier J, Domenge C, Ozsahin M, et al. Postoperative irradiation with or without concomitant chemotherapy for locally advanced head and neck cancer. *N Engl J Med.* 2004;350:1945-1952.
2. Forastiere AA, Goepfert H, Maor M, et al. Concurrent chemotherapy and radiotherapy for organ preservation in advanced larynx cancer. *N Engl J Med.* 2003;349:2091-2098.
3. Pointreau Y, Garaud P, Chapet S, et al. Randomized trial of induction chemotherapy with cisplatin and 5-fluorouracil with or without docetaxel for larynx preservation. *J Natl Cancer Inst.* 2009; 101:498-506.
4. Baujat B, Bourhis J, Blanchard P, et al. Hyperfractionated or accelerated radiotherapy for head and neck cancer. *Cochrane Database Syst Rev.* 2010;12:CD002026.
5. Vermorken JB, Remenar E, van Herpen C, et al. Cisplatin, fluorouracil, and docetaxel in unresectable head and neck cancer. *N Engl J Med.* 2007;357:1695-1704.
6. Lorch JH, Goloubeva O, Haddad RI, et al. Induction chemotherapy with cisplatin and fluorouracil alone or in combination with docetaxel in locally advanced squamous-cell cancer of the head and neck: long-term results of the TAX 324 randomised phase 3 trial. *Lancet Oncol.* 2011;12:153-159.
7. Adelstein D, Li Y, Adams G, et al. An Intergroup Phase III comparison of standard radiation therapy and two schedules of concurrent chemoradiotherapy in patients with unresectable squamous cell head and neck cancer. *J Clin Oncol.* 2003;21:92-98.
8. Denis F, Garaud P, Bardet E, et al. Final results of the 94-01 French Head and Neck Oncology and Radiotherapy Group randomized trial comparing radiotherapy alone with concomitant radiochemotherapy in advanced-stage oropharynx carcinoma. *J Clin Oncol.* 2004;22:69-76.
9. Bonner JA, Harari PM, Giralt J, et al. Radiotherapy plus cetuximab for squamous-cell carcinoma of the head and neck. *N Engl J Med.* 2006;354:567-578.

SUGGESTED READINGS

Ang KK, Harris J, Wheeler R, et al. Human papillomavirus and survival of patients with oropharyngeal cancer. *N Engl J Med.* 2010;363:24-25. *Patients with HPV positive tumors had a significantly better 3-year survival (82% vs 57%).*

Leemans CR, Braakhuis BJ, Brakenhoff RH. The molecular biology of head and neck cancer. *Nat Rev Cancer.* 2011;11:9-22. *Review of tumor heterogeneity and molecular pathogenesis.*

Tham IW, Lu JJ. Controversies and challenges in the current management of nasopharyngeal cancer. *Expert Rev Anticancer Ther.* 2010;10:1439-1450. *Review.*

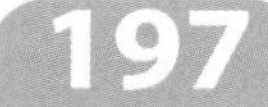

LUNG CANCER AND OTHER PULMONARY NEOPLASMS

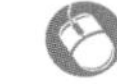

DAVID S. ETTINGER

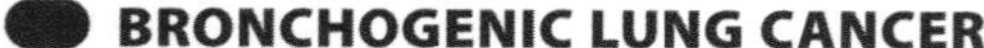

BRONCHOGENIC LUNG CANCER

DEFINITION

Lung cancer (e.g., bronchogenic carcinoma) arises from the respiratory epithelium. Lung cancer is divided into two major histologic groups: non–small cell lung cancer (NSCLC) and small cell lung cancer (SCLC). NSCLC accounts for approximately 85% of all lung cancer. Other less common pulmonary neoplasms include adenosquamous carcinoma, carcinoid tumors, bronchial gland tumors, soft tissue tumors (e.g., sarcomas), pulmonary blastomas, and lymphoma.

EPIDEMIOLOGY

Worldwide, lung cancer accounts for approximately 13% of all cancer; more than 1.1 million cases of lung cancer are diagnosed annually, and more than 1 million deaths are caused by the disease. In the United States, 28% of all annual cancer deaths (30% in men, 26% in women) are due to lung cancer; lung cancer is the leading cause of cancer death in both men and women.

The incidence and mortality of lung cancer in American men and women reflect their smoking habits (Chapter 31). Lung cancer deaths started rising in men in the 1950s and in women 10 to 15 years later. Cancer death rates from lung cancer decreased in men by 37% between 1990 and 2005; however, in women, the cancer death rate from lung cancer between 1991 and 2005 increased approximately 8%. Worldwide, increasing lung cancer rates are predicted to continue in less developed countries as a result of increasing endemic use of tobacco.

TABLE 197-1 LUNG CANCER INCIDENCE AND MORTALITY RATES BY RACE/ETHNICITY AND GENDER

	Incidence			Mortality		
	WHITE	AFRICAN AMERICAN	HISPANIC	WHITE	AFRICAN AMERICAN	HISPANIC
Male	77.6	104.3	43.2	69.9	90.1	33.9
Female	54.8	54.7	24.7	41.9	40.0	14.4

Incidence and death rates per 100,000 population, 2002 to 2006, from the Surveillance, Epidemiology and End Results (SEER) program in the United States.

The U.S. Surveillance, Epidemiology and End Results (SEER) program estimated that 1 in 14 men and women will be at risk for the development of lung cancer during their lifetime. Incidence and mortality rates vary by race/ethnicity (Table 197-1), with African American men having a higher incidence and mortality rate than other racial/ethnic groups. Incidence rates of lung cancer for men and women in the United States from the period 2002 to 2006 are 77.7 and 52.5 per 100,000 people, respectively. The median age at diagnosis in both sexes is 71 years.

Unfortunately, tobacco use in high-school students increased until the mid-1990s, but now it is slowly declining. Despite this decline, 38% of high-school seniors smoke. This smoking at an earlier age may in part explain the occurrence of lung cancer in younger patients.

Risk Factors

Tobacco

It is estimated that cigarette smoking is responsible for approximately 85 to 90% of all cases of lung cancer, including 90% of cases in men and 80% in women. More than 40 carcinogens have been identified in cigarette smoke (Chapter 31). The risk for development of lung cancer correlates with the number of cigarettes smoked per day, lifetime duration of smoking, age at onset of smoking, degree of inhalation, tar and nicotine content of the cigarettes, and use of unfiltered cigarettes. If a lifelong nonsmoker has a relative risk ratio of 1 for the development of lung cancer, cigarette smokers of less than ½ pack/day, ½ to 1 pack/day, 1 to 2 packs/day, and more than 2 packs/day have risk ratios of 15, 17, 42, and 64, respectively. The risk ratio in ex-smokers is dependent on the duration of abstinence of cigarette smoking; to reach a risk ratio of 1.5 to 2.0 requires abstinence of approximately 30 years.

Pipe and cigar smoking are also risk factors for lung cancer, but the risk is thought to be less than that associated with cigarette smoking, possibly because such tobacco products tend to be inhaled less deeply than cigarette smoke. Marijuana and cocaine smoking probably cause an increased risk for lung cancer, but the carcinogenicity of the two drugs is less well studied than that of cigarette smoking.

Environmental Tobacco Smoke

Exposure to environmental tobacco smoke (i.e., passive smoking) by nonsmokers, especially in the workplace, increases the risk for the development of lung cancer. The exposure levels of environmental tobacco smoke depend on the size of the enclosed space and the intensity of smoking.

Other Exposure

The International Agency for Research on Cancer classified the following as group 1 known carcinogens for lung cancer: radon, asbestos, arsenic, beryllium, bis(chloromethyl)ether, cadmium, chromium, nickel, vinyl chloride, and polycyclic aromatic hydrocarbons (PAHs) (Chapters 18 and 93). Group 2A probable carcinogens include acrylonitrile, formaldehyde, and diesel exhaust. Group 2B possible carcinogens include acetaldehyde, silica, and welding fumes. It is estimated that 9% of lung cancers in men and 2% in women are caused by occupational exposure.

Radon, a gaseous decay product of uranium-238 and radium-226, damages lung tissue by emitting alpha particles. Underground mining of uranium

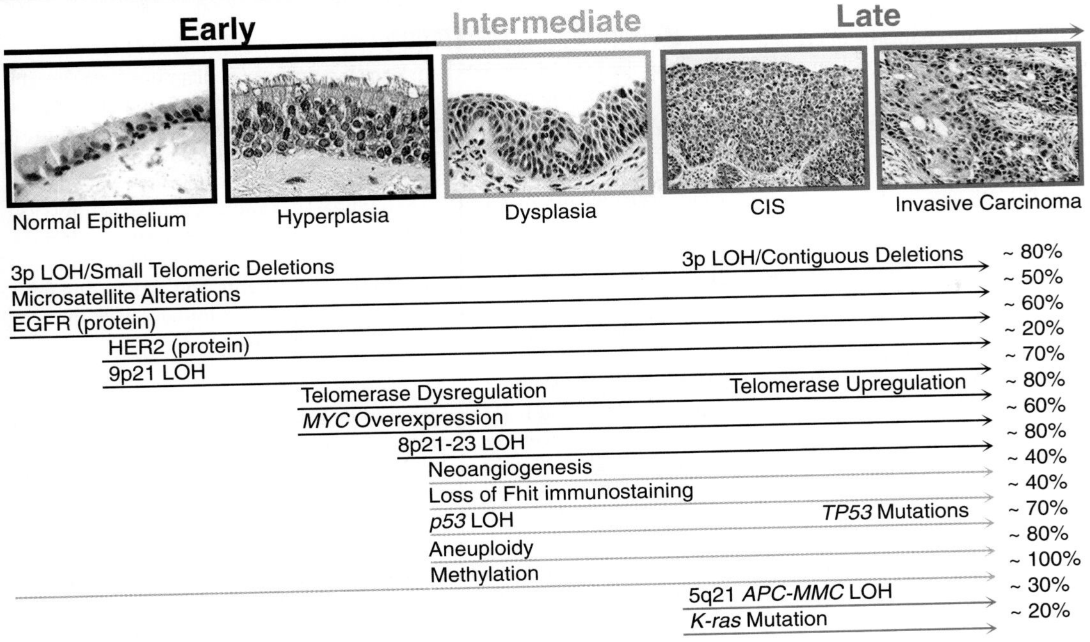

Early | Intermediate | Late

Normal Epithelium | Hyperplasia | Dysplasia | CIS | Invasive Carcinoma

3p LOH/Small Telomeric Deletions — 3p LOH/Contiguous Deletions ~ 80%
Microsatellite Alterations ~ 50%
EGFR (protein) ~ 60%
HER2 (protein) ~ 20%
9p21 LOH ~ 70%
Telomerase Dysregulation — Telomerase Upregulation ~ 80%
MYC Overexpression ~ 60%
8p21-23 LOH ~ 80%
Neoangiogenesis ~ 40%
Loss of Fhit immunostaining ~ 40%
p53 LOH — *TP53* Mutations ~ 70%
Aneuploidy ~ 80%
Methylation ~ 100%
5q21 *APC-MMC* LOH ~ 30%
K-ras Mutation ~ 20%

FIGURE 197-1. Sequential changes during the pathogenesis of lung cancer. CIS = carcinoma in situ; LOH = loss of heterozygosity. (From Hirsch FR, Franklin WA, Gazdar AF, et al. Early detection of lung cancer: clinical perspectives of recent advances in biology and radiology. *Clin Cancer Res.* 2001;7:5-22. Updated courtesy of Fred R. Hirsch, MD, PhD, Department of Medical Oncology, University of Colorado Health Sciences Center, and Adi F. Gazdar, MD, Department of Pathology, Southwestern Medical Center.)

exposes miners to radon and its decay products, thus increasing their risk for lung cancer. Radon may appear in homes, especially basements, because it is present in soil rock and ground water and enters the home through defects in pipes or the foundation. The indoor radon level depends on the soil concentration and ventilation rate. Data are conflicting about the risk for lung cancer with exposure to domestic radon, but the consensus is that the risk is increased.

Exposure to asbestos fibers (Chapter 93) occurs in automobile shops, shipyards, mines, and textile and cement plants and in construction and insulation workers. Workers with asbestosis, not just asbestos exposure, have an increased risk for lung cancer. Cigarette smokers with asbestos exposure have a risk of lung cancer that is multiplicative—a 50-fold relative risk compared with unexposed nonsmokers. The latency period for the development of lung cancer in workers exposed to asbestos is 25 to 40 years.

Arsenic, a naturally occurring metal, is a byproduct of copper, lead, zinc, and tin ore smelting. The metal is also present in agricultural pesticides and marine organisms. Exposure to arsenic occurs through air, soil, water, and foods. Cigarette smokers exposed to arsenic are at greater risk for the development of lung cancer than those not exposed to arsenic.

Beryllium, a metal used for alloys, is a pulmonary carcinogen. Exposure occurs in mining and in the manufacture of ceramics and electronic equipment. Bis(chloromethyl)ether is a product of chloromethylation processes used in the manufacture of ion exchange resins, polymers, and plastics. The relative risk for lung cancer in exposed workers is 10, especially for SCLC. Cadmium is a metal used for electroplating metals, batteries, plastics, and pigments. Exposure to cadmium causes an increased risk for lung cancer. Chromium is commonly used for metal alloys, paint pigments, electroplating, cement, rubber, photoengraving, and the composition of floor covering. Exposure to chromium increases the risk for lung cancer two- to three-fold. Nickel is used in electroplating, manufacturing of steel and other alloys, ceramics, storage batteries, electric circuits, and petroleum refining. Nickel exposure increases the risk for lung cancer 1.56-fold. Vinyl chloride is used to make plastics, packaging materials, propellant in cosmetic products, and vinyl floor tiles. Although the risk for development of lung cancer after exposure to vinyl chloride is increased, it is considered small. PAHs are formed from the incomplete combustion of organic material. Exposure to PAHs occurs with cigarette smoke; smelting of nickel-containing ores; aluminum, iron, steel, and coke production; coal tar; and diesel exhaust. PAHs carry a 1.5 to 2.5 relative risk for lung cancer.

Preexisting Lung Disease

Tobacco smoking causes chronic inflammation and destruction of lung tissue, which results in chronic obstructive pulmonary disease (COPD) (Chapter 88). Patients with COPD have an approximately four-fold increased risk for lung cancer. In addition, patients in whom idiopathic pulmonary fibrosis or pulmonary fibrosis from asbestosis or silica develops are at increased risk for the development of lung cancer.

Dietary Factors

Increased consumption of fruits and green and yellow vegetables is associated with a reduced risk for lung cancer, whereas low serum concentrations of antioxidant vitamins such as vitamins A and E are associated with the development of lung cancer. However, β-carotene supplementation increases the incidence of lung cancer.

Increased consumption of dietary fat is also associated with an increased incidence of lung cancer. High blood concentrations of selenium, a mineral involved in the protection of cellular membranes, has been associated with a lower risk for lung cancer.

Gender and Racial Differences

Women who smoke have a 1.2- to 1.7-fold higher risk ratio than men, especially for adenocarcinoma and SCLC. Possible explanations for this difference in lung cancer risk include (1) effects of hormones such as estrogen on the development of lung cancer, (2) gender differences in nicotine metabolism, and (3) gender variations in cytochrome P-450 enzymes involved in the bioactivation of toxic components in cigarette smoke condensate.

The high incidence and mortality of lung cancer in African American males may be due, in part, to (1) increased tobacco use, (2) differences in the metabolism of tobacco smoke, and (3) higher intake of dietary fat.

Human Immunodeficiency Virus Infection

Some studies suggest that the risk for lung cancer is increased in patients infected with human immunodeficiency virus (HIV) (Chapter 398), mostly as a result of cigarette smoking. Most patients are male (10 : 1) and young, in part reflecting the demographics of HIV infection.

Inheritance

First-degree relatives of patients with lung cancer have a two- to six-fold increase in the risk for lung cancer after adjusting for tobacco use. Second-degree relatives of lung cancer patients have a relative risk of 1.28, and third-degree relatives have a relative risk of 1.14. Nonsmokers with a family history of lung cancer have a two- to four-fold increased risk for lung cancer. The familial risk may be due to shared exposure, such as environmental tobacco smoke, or to shared genetic susceptibility to environmental carcinogens.

PATHOBIOLOGY

The development of lung cancer is the result of a multistep process from a premalignant lesion to frank cancer (Fig. 197-1) after a number of years.

Tobacco smoke or other carcinogens promote sequential genetic and epigenetic changes that result in the loss of normal control mechanisms of cellular growth. These changes affect (1) oncogenes, which are homologues of normal cellular genes and, when mutated, result in activation and gain of function; (2) tumor suppressor genes, which are "cancer" genes, in which loss of function by mutation removes inhibitions to control cell growth; and (3) growth factors (Chapter 185).

Oncogenes

The oncogenes that play a role in the pathogenesis of lung cancer include *ras,* the *myc* family, *HER-2/neu* (*ERBB2*), and *Bcl-2*. The *ras* family of oncogenes has three primary members (H-*ras,* K-*ras,* and N-*ras*), one of which, K-*ras,* is activated by point mutations in codon 12 of lung cancer cells. The mutation occurs in 30% of adenocarcinomas of the lung, most often in patients with a history of smoking, but it has not been found in SCLC. Patients who have the K-*ras* mutation have a poorer prognosis, stage for stage.

Amplification and overexpression of the *myc* family oncogenes (a-*myc,* L-*myc,* N-*myc*) are seen in 10 to 40% of SCLC and 10% of NSCLC. The most frequently altered gene, however, is c-*myc,* whose amplification in SCLC tumors that relapse is associated with shorter survival. However, overexpression of the *myc* oncogene is not present in most lung cancers, so its overexpression is probably not a primary event.

The *HER-2/neu* (*ERBB2*) gene, which encodes growth factor receptor or p185 neu (a tyrosine kinase glycoprotein), is activated in NSCLC but not SCLC. Overexpression of *HER-2/neu* in patients with adenocarcinoma of the lung portends a poor survival. *Bcl-2*, an oncogene that encodes a protein that inhibits programmed cell death (apoptosis), is also overexpressed in lung cancer, especially in SCLC.

Tumor Suppressor Genes

Tumor suppressor genes include *p53, Rb,* and *3p* (Chapter 185). The *p53* mutation correlates with cigarette smoking and has been detected in preneoplastic lesions of the lung. Mutations of *p53* are common in both NSCLC (~50%) and SCLC (~80%).

In SCLC, *Rb* is often mutated or deleted, so the Rb protein is not expressed in 90% of SCLC. In NSCLC, Rb is normally expressed, but when Rb is phosphorylated, uncontrolled cell division can occur in NSCLC.

One of the earliest genetic abnormalities in lung cancer occurs with the deletion of genetic material on the short arm of chromosome 3(3p) (p14-p23). The deletion occurs in approximately 50% of NSCLC and 90% of SCLC. The *FHIT* (fragile histidine triad) gene (3p14.2) is abnormal in many lung cancers and may function as a tumor suppressor gene by suppressing tumor growth and causing apoptosis.

Growth Factors

Growth factors secreted by lung cancer cells may reflect adjacent or regional cells (paracrine stimulation) or cause autonomous proliferation of the cells from which they were secreted (autocrine stimulation). Cells that are affected by this autocrine stimulation secrete a biologically active growth factor. Antibodies that bind to this growth factor will inhibit cell growth.

Autocrine (peptide) growth factors that are important in the growth of lung cancer cells, particularly SCLC, include gastrin-releasing peptide (GRP), insulin-like growth factor type I (IGF-I), and hepatocyte growth factor. GRP occurs in approximately 20 to 60% of SCLC and less frequently in NSCLC. Hepatocyte growth factor is expressed mainly in NSCLC.

The oncogene c-*erB*-1 encodes the epidermal growth factor receptor (EGFR), a 170-kD tyrosine kinase glycoprotein. Activation of EGFR initiates autophosphorylation of the receptor and eventually leads to cell cycle proliferation. Activating mutations in the *EGFR* gene have been found in 10 to 17% of patients with NSCLC; these patients have had an up to 75% response rate to the tyrosine kinase inhibitors, gefitinib or erlotinib.

Epigenetics

Epigenetics refers to a change in gene expression that is heritable but does not involve a change in DNA sequence. One of these epigenetic modifications involves changes in DNA methylation. These changes, which are very common in lung cancer, can include hypomethylation, dysregulation of DNA methyltransferase I, and hypermethylation. Genes that are methylated in NSCLC include *p16, RAR-β, RASSFIA,* methylguanine-methyltransferase, and death-associated protein kinase (DAP-kinase). This hypermethylation can silence tumor suppressor genes, thereby permitting unregulated cell growth.

CLINICAL MANIFESTATIONS

As many as 15% of patients in whom lung cancer is diagnosed are initially asymptomatic. The diagnosis is usually made incidentally on a chest radiograph obtained for other reasons (e.g., a preoperative study). However, most patients have symptoms and signs that are (1) caused by the pulmonary lesion itself—local tumor growth, invasion, or obstruction; (2) intrathoracic—regional tumor spreading to lymph nodes and adjacent structures; (3) extrathoracic—distant spread of disease; and (4) paraneoplastic syndromes. Nonspecific signs and symptoms of lung cancer include anorexia in about 30% of patients, weight loss, fatigue in third of patients, and anemia and fever in 10 to 20% of patients. More than 80% of patients initially have three or more symptoms or signs as a result of the lung cancer.

Pulmonary Lesion

Symptoms resulting from the primary lung cancer depend on the location and size of the cancer. Such symptoms can be secondary to endobronchial or peripheral growth of the primary tumor. The most common, cough, occurs in approximately 45% of cases, but it is nonspecific and also common in patients who smoke and have COPD. Hemoptysis occurs in more than 30% of patients, but the most common causes of hemoptysis are bronchitis and bronchiectasis. Dyspnea also occurs in 30 to 50% of patients. Wheezing is uncommon as an initial symptom in lung cancer and may signify major airway obstruction, which can cause a postobstructive pneumonia that may not initially be evident on chest radiographs and may be diagnosed only when the pneumonia fails to respond to standard therapy (Chapter 97). Lesions may be cavitary and may be associated with an abscess at the time of diagnosis of the lung cancer.

Peripheral lung tumors may be asymptomatic but are more frequently associated with symptoms of cough and pain from involvement of the pleura or chest wall. Chest pain, which occurs in more than 25% of patients, may be dull in nature, but chest pain that is severe and persists may be due to chest wall involvement.

Intrathoracic Spread

Symptoms associated with intrathoracic spread may be related to direct extension of the tumor or metastasis to regional lymph nodes. Dysphagia may occur secondary to esophageal compression. Although tracheoesophageal or bronchoesophageal fistulas are uncommon, coughing associated with swallowing or the development of aspiration pneumonitis (Chapter 97) should point to this possibility. Hoarseness, which is associated with recurrent laryngeal nerve paralysis, occurs in less than 20% of cases; it is more common with left-sided lung tumors because the nerve on this side has a longer intrathoracic course than the right-sided nerve. Phrenic nerve paralysis with hemidiaphragmatic elevation is associated with dyspnea and hiccups. Apical tumors, such as superior sulcus NSCLC (Pancoast's syndrome), may cause Horner's syndrome (Chapter 427), pain secondary to rib destruction, atrophy of hand muscles, and pain in the distribution of the C8, T1, and T2 nerve roots because of tumor invasion of the brachial plexus.

Blockage of the superior vena cava (SVC) (Chapter 99) as a result of compression or direct invasion by the tumor itself or by enlarged mediastinal lymph nodes may cause dyspnea. Signs of SVC syndrome include facial swelling, plethora, upper extremity swelling, dilated neck veins, and a prominent venous pattern on the anterior surface of the chest. Lung cancer accounts for most cases of SVC syndrome, with most cancer being SCLC and located on the right side.

Other manifestations of intrathoracic spread include pleural effusion (Chapter 99) causing dyspnea; pericardial effusion (Chapter 77) and cardiac extension of the tumor (Chapter 60) causing heart failure, arrhythmia, or tamponade; and lymphangitic spread through the lungs causing dyspnea and hypoxemia.

Extrathoracic Spread

At diagnosis, 30 to 40% of patients with NSCLC and approximately 60% of patients with SCLC have extrathoracic hematogenous spread of their tumor. Bone metastasis occurs in 30 to 40% of patients with lung cancer and commonly involves the vertebrae, ribs, and pelvic bones. Pain is the primary symptom. Liver metastases can produce right upper quadrant abdominal pain as well as nonspecific symptoms of fatigue and weight loss. Adrenal metastases can cause pain but most often cause no symptoms. One gland is usually involved, but bilateral metastases may occur. Brain metastasis, which occurs in 25 to 50% of SCLC and 25% of adenocarcinomas of the lung, may cause no symptoms but is more commonly associated with nausea, vomiting, headaches, seizures, confusion, personality changes, and focal neurologic signs and symptoms, depending on the site of metastatic disease. Epidural, intramedullary spinal cord metastasis and diffuse leptomeningeal involvement are less common than cerebral and cerebellar metastases.

Paraneoplastic Syndromes

Paraneoplastic syndromes (Chapter 187) occur in approximately 10 to 20% of patients with lung cancer. Endocrine syndromes include hypercalcemia, the syndrome of inappropriate antidiuretic hormone secretion, and ectopic adrenocorticotropic hormone secretion (Chapter 186). Other endocrine paraneoplastic syndromes of lesser clinical significance produce hormones such as the β-subunit of human chorionic gonadotropin, prolactin, gastrin, growth hormone, thyroid-stimulating factor, insulin-like substance, and calcitonin.

Neurologic syndromes are relatively rare, are most commonly associated with SCLC, and may have autoimmune mechanisms. Such syndromes include Eaton-Lambert syndrome, limbic encephalopathy, cerebellar degeneration, subacute sensory neuropathy, autonomic neuropathy, and optic neuritis (Chapter 187). Skeletal manifestations include digital clubbing (see Fig. 450-5 in Chapter 450) and hypertrophic pulmonary osteoarthropathy (Chapter 187).

Hematologic and vascular syndromes include hypercoagulable states, migratory thrombophlebitis (Trousseau's syndrome), and nonbacterial thrombotic endocarditis (Chapters 60 and 179). Cutaneous manifestations include dermatomyositis, acanthosis nigricans, erythema gyratum repens, and hyperkeratosis of the palms and soles of the feet (Chapter 187).

DIAGNOSIS

The diagnosis of lung cancer is made by cytologic examination of tissue biopsy specimens, sputum (Fig. 197-2), bronchial washings and brushings of suspicious lesions (Fig. 197-3), bronchoalveolar lavage fluid, and transbronchial and transthoracic needle aspirates (Fig. 197-4). The greater number of viable tumor cells in biopsy specimens from transthoracic, endobronchial, transbronchial, or open biopsy procedures increases the probability of accurate diagnosis. Sputum cytology may be only 20% sensitive for peripheral lung lesions, but it may be 80% sensitive for central lesions. In general, the sensitivity of a single sputum specimen is approximately 50%, whereas examination of three or more specimens increases the sensitivity to nearly 90%. The sensitivity of a single bronchial washing and brushing for detecting lung cancer is approximately 65%. For bronchoalveolar lavage fluid, the sensitivity is 60 to 65%. The sensitivity of fine-needle aspiration biopsy for detecting lung cancer exceeds 85%.

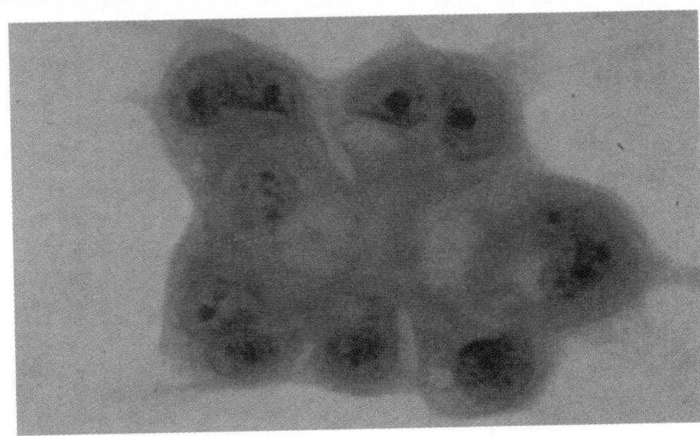

FIGURE 197-2. Adenocarcinoma cells in a sputum smear. (From Forbes CD, Jackson WF. *Color Atlas and Text of Clinical Medicine*, 3rd ed. London, Mosby, 2003.)

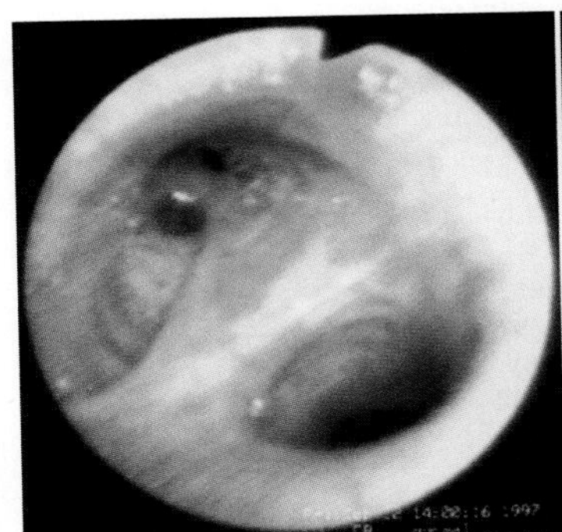
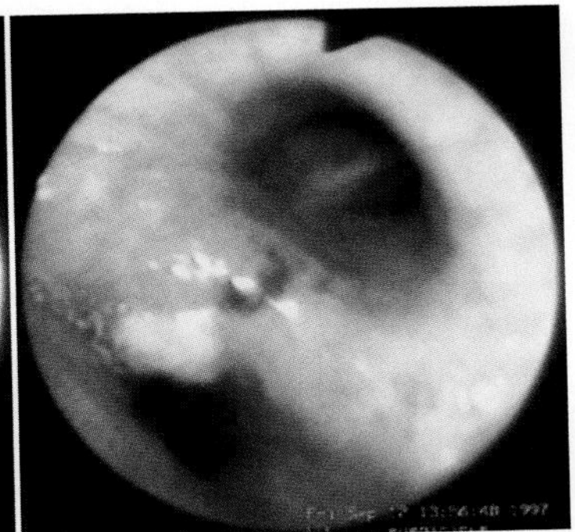

FIGURE 197-3. Squamous cell carcinoma. Left, Carina between the lingular and upper division bronchus of the left upper lobe. Note the well-defined, sharp features of the carina. **Right,** Carina between the left upper and lower lobes in the same patient. Note the swollen, red, infiltrated appearance of the mucosa and the white exophytic lesion. In addition, there is subepithelial hemorrhage. A biopsy specimen demonstrates squamous cell carcinoma. The patient had increased sputum production, positive sputum cytologic findings, and a nonlocalizing chest radiograph and computed tomography scan.

Solitary Pulmonary Nodule

A solitary pulmonary nodule is an asymptomatic lesion less than 3 cm in diameter surrounded by normal lung parenchyma that is incidentally found on a chest radiograph or computed tomography (CT) scan (Fig. 197-5). A solitary pulmonary nodule is found in up to 0.2% of all chest radiographs, and 10 to 70% are malignant. The chance of any solitary pulmonary nodule being cancerous correlates with the size and growth rate of the nodule, the age of the patient, any history of smoking, and a previous history of a malignancy. It is important to compare previous chest radiographs with the one demonstrating the nodule. A nodule that has not changed in size for at least 2 years is probably benign; a high-resolution CT scan with a resolution of 0.3 mm can best assess its size and growth characteristics. Solitary pulmonary nodules smaller than 4 mm have a 1% risk of malignancy, whereas a nodule larger than 8 mm has a 10 to 20% risk. In the latter situation, serial CT scans are indicated; positron emission tomography (PET) and biopsy should be considered. PET is 96.8% sensitive and 77.8% specific for identifying a malignancy, but because both false-negative and false-positive results can occur, tissue is needed for a definitive diagnosis. Transthoracic fine-needle aspiration biopsy, bronchoscopy, thoracotomy, and video-assisted thoracoscopic surgery (VATS) can establish a diagnosis.

Pathology

The histologic classification of lung cancer includes adenocarcinoma (about 40%), squamous cell (epidermoid) carcinoma (~30%), large cell carcinoma (~15%), and small cell carcinoma (~15%). These four histologic types represent more than 95% of all lung cancer.

Squamous cell carcinoma and adenocarcinoma are further classified by their differentiation: well differentiated, moderately differentiated, and poorly differentiated. The latter types of cells are more aggressive and may have a worse prognosis than well-differentiated tumors. Adenocarcinoma is the most frequent histologic type in women and nonsmokers. Bronchoalveolar carcinoma, a subtype of adenocarcinoma, is well differentiated, grows along intact alveolar septa, and can be localized, multinodular, multifocal, or diffuse.

From a practical perspective based on biologic differences, clinical features, growth properties, and treatment, bronchogenic lung cancer is divided into two main categories: NSCLC and SCLC. In general, all NSCLCs are generally treated the same way based on the stage of the disease. SCLC is usually characterized by more aggressive biology, and treatment is dependent on whether the SCLC is limited stage (i.e., locally advanced) or extensive stage (i.e., metastatic disease).

Staging

Staging of NSCLC involves classification according to T (tumor size), N (regional lymph node involvement), and M (presence or absence of distant metastases). In October 2009, the TNM staging for NSCLC changed (Table 197-2). For SCLC, TNM staging is not generally used; rather, SCLC is staged as limited disease, defined as disease that can be encompassed by a single radiation portal, or extensive disease, that extending beyond a single radiation portal (usually metastatic).

Staging Procedures

All patients with lung cancer should be clinically staged using a complete history with a focus on performance status and weight loss; physical examination; pathologic review of all biopsy material; complete blood cell and platelet counts; chemistry profile, including renal and liver function tests, electrolytes, glucose, calcium, and phosphorus; and chest radiograph and chest CT (including the upper part of the abdomen and adrenal glands). Magnetic resonance imaging (MRI) of the brain and radionuclide scan of

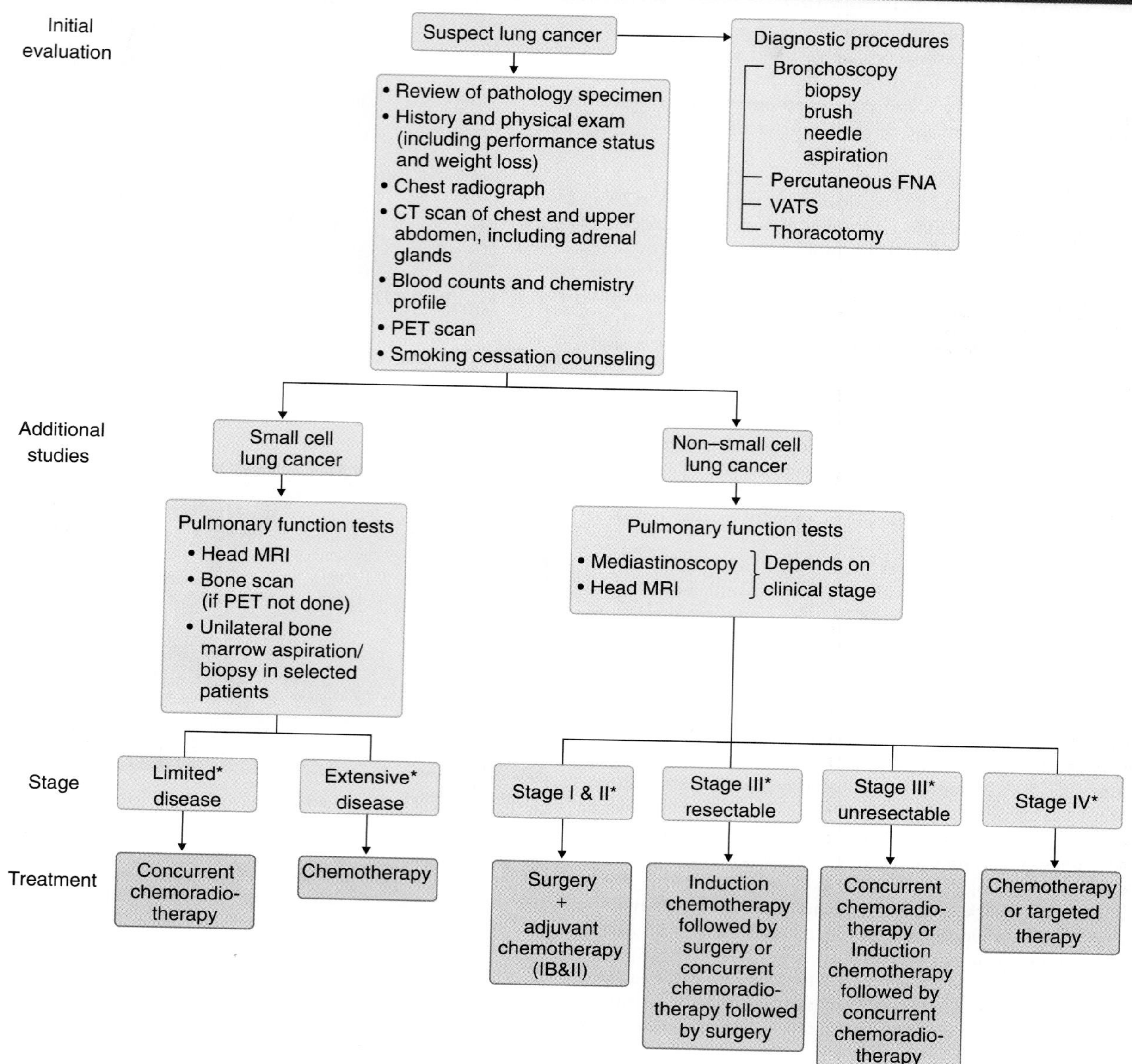

FIGURE 197-4. Schematic overview for diagnosing, staging, and treating non–small cell and small cell lung cancer. See text for details. (Consult practice guidelines in oncology, non–small cell lung cancer, and small cell lung cancer at www.nccn.org as well for specifics.) *See Tables 197-2 and 197-3. CT = computed tomography; FNA = fine-needle aspiration; MRI = magnetic resonance imaging; PET = positron emission tomography; VATS = video-assisted thoracic surgery.

bones should be performed if metastases to these organs are suspected. Radiographs or MRI should be obtained if bone lesions are suggested by radionuclide scanning. PET is used to assess both regional and metastatic spread of tumor. Pulmonary function tests and arterial blood gas determinations should be obtained only if needed for treatment purposes.

For patients with SCLC, the initial pretreatment staging evaluation is similar to that used for NSCLC patients. For patients with peripheral blood count abnormalities, bone marrow aspiration and biopsy are recommended. Twenty to 30% of patients with SCLC will have tumor in bone marrow at the time of diagnosis.

Imaging

Radiography

A standard posteroanterior and lateral chest radiograph, although inexpensive and easy to perform, has limited value in the staging of lung cancer. Although it can detect pulmonary nodules as small as 3 to 4 mm, it is not reliable in detecting hilar or mediastinal lymphadenopathy.

Computed Tomography

A CT scan is commonly used to evaluate whether lung cancer is present in the hilar and mediastinal lymph nodes, liver, and adrenal glands, but its accuracy in identifying mediastinal lymph node involvement is suboptimal (sensitivity of 40 to 65% and specificity of 45 to 90% versus either a PET scan or mediastinoscopy). Most importantly, CT will miss small metastatic foci that do not result in mediastinal lymph node enlargement. Mediastinal lymph nodes that are normal in size (≤1 cm) have an 8 to 15% probability of having metastatic disease, whereas mediastinal lymph nodes that are 1 to 1.5 cm, 1.5 to 2 cm, and greater than 2 cm in size will contain metastases 15 to 30%, approximately 50%, and about 90% of the time, respectively.

Positron Emission Tomography

PET, which uses 2-[^{18}F]fluoro-2-deoxy-D-glucose to identify areas of increased glucose metabolism in lung tumors, is more sensitive than CT in staging lung cancer (see Fig. 197-5); it has a sensitivity of 83%, specificity of 96%, and negative predictive value of 96%. However, increased glucose metabolism also occurs with inflammatory processes. Obtaining both PET and CT scans can enhance accuracy in the staging of lung cancer. 1 PET also enhances detection of bone, liver, and adrenal metastases. However, if treatment decisions are to be based on PET scan results, positive PET scan findings require pathologic or other radiologic confirmation.

Evaluation of Mediastinal Tissue

After initial clinical staging, if a patient with NSCLC has potentially surgically resectable disease, the regional lymph nodes (mediastinum) must be sampled

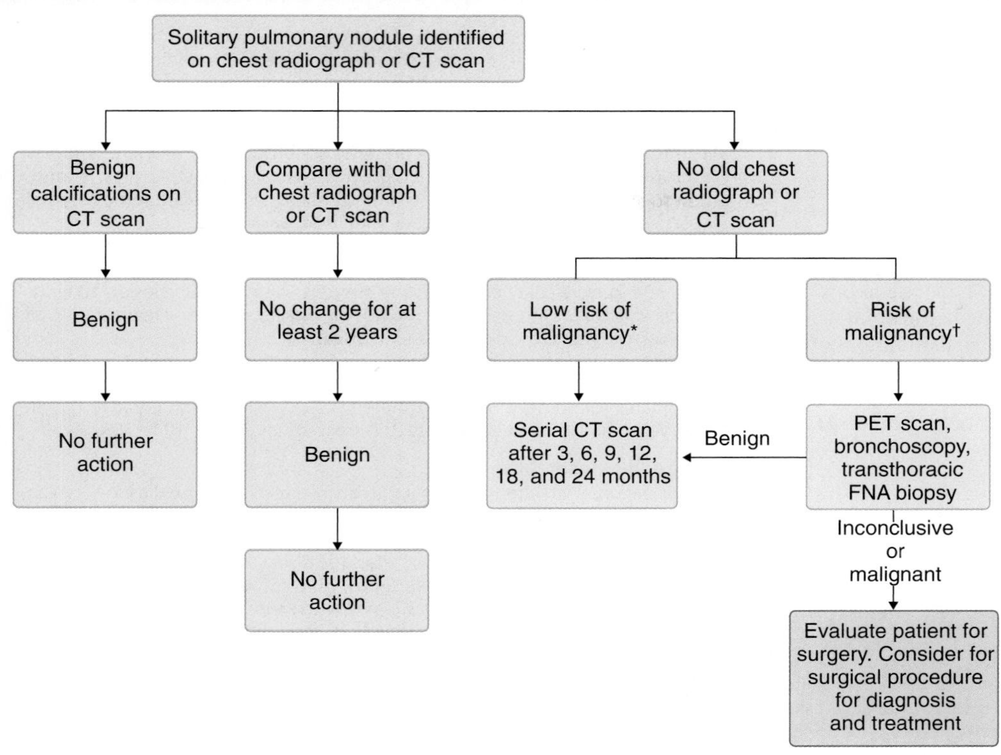

FIGURE 197-5. Evaluation of a patient with a solitary pulmonary nodule. *Patient with a minimal or absent history of smoking and other known risk factors for the development of lung cancer and a nodule 8 mm or smaller in size. †Patient with a history of smoking and other risk factors for the development of lung cancer and a nodule 8 mm or larger in size. CT = computed tomography; FNA = fine-needle aspiration; PET = positron emission tomography.

TABLE 197-2 STAGING OF LUNG CANCER

STAGE	TUMOR	NODE	METASTASIS	GENERAL DESCRIPTION
NON–SMALL CELL LUNG CANCER*				
Local				
IA	T1a,b	N0	M0	T1 tumor: ≤3 cm, surrounded by lung or visceral pleura, not more proximal than the lobar bronchus T1a ≤ 2, T1b > 2 but ≤3 cm
IB	T2a	N0	M0	T2 tumor: >3 cm, but ≤7 cm; or tumor with any of the following: invades visceral pleura; involves main bronchus ≥2 cm distal to the carina; associated with atelectasis/obstructive pneumonia extending to hilum but not involving the entire lung; T2a > 3 but ≤5 cm
IIA	T1a,b T2a T2b	N1 N1 N0	M0	T2b > 5 but ≤ 7 cm N1: involvement of the ipsilateral peribronchial or hilar nodes and intrapulmonary nodes including involvement by direct extension
Locally Advanced				
IIB	T2b T3	N1 N0	M0 M0	T3 tumor: tumor >7 cm or directly invading chest wall, diaphragm, mediastinal pleura, pericardium; or tumor in the main bronchus, <2 cm distal to the carina; or atelectasis or pneumonitis of the entire lung; or separate tumor nodules in the same lobe
IIIA	T1-3 T3 T4	N2 N1 N0,1	M0 M0 M0	N2: involvement of the ipsilateral mediastinal or subcarinal nodes T4 tumor: tumors of any size with invasion of the heart, great vessels, trachea, recurrent laryngeal nerve, esophagus, vertebral body, carina; or separate tumor nodules in a different ipsilateral lobe
Advanced				
IIIB	T4 T1-4	N2 N3	M0 M0	N3: involvement of the contralateral mediastinal or hilar nodes or any supraclavicular nodes
IV	Any T	Any N	M1a,b	M1a: separate tumor nodules in a contralateral lobe; or tumor with pleural nodules or malignant pleural dissemination M1b: distant metastasis
SMALL CELL LUNG CANCER†				
Limited disease				Evidence of tumor confined to the ipsilateral hemithorax; can be encompassed by a single radiation port
Extensive disease				All other diseases, including metastatic disease

The staging classification system was refined by the Union Internationale Contre le Cancer (UICC) and the American Joint Committee on Cancer (AJCC) with help from the International Association for the Study of Lung Cancer (IASLC). T = tumor, N = node, M = metastases. SCLC staging was developed by the Veterans Administration Lung Study Group.

*Detterbeck FC, Boffa DJ and Tanoue LT. The new lung cancer staging system. *Chest.* 2009;136:260-271.

†Stahel RA, Ginsberg R, Havermann K, et al. Staging and prognostic factors in small cell lung cancer: a consensus. *Lung Cancer.* 1989;5:119-126.

for possible metastases. Fiberoptic bronchoscopy to assess the bronchi and transbronchial needle aspirates to evaluate for mediastinal lymphadenopathy are recommended. Transbronchial needle aspirates are positive in 35 to 40% of patients when a CT scan demonstrates hilar or mediastinal lymphadenopathy. The larger the size of the lymph node on CT scan, the greater the chance for the aspirate to be positive.

The gold standard for evaluating the mediastinal lymph nodes for metastatic disease during life is transcervical mediastinoscopy. The subaortic and aortopulmonary window lymph nodes are inaccessible by routine mediastinoscopy, and the subcarinal lymph nodes may be difficult to access. The accuracy of the procedure ranges from 80 to 90%, with a false-negative rate of 10 to 12%. Other procedures used to evaluate the mediastinal lymph nodes include extended cervical mediastinoscopy, anterior mediastinotomy, thoracoscopy, and VATS. Endoscopic ultrasound (EUS) and endobronchial ultrasound (EBUS) biopsies of mediastinal lymph nodes can significantly reduce unnecessary thoracotomies when used in the staging of lung cancer.[2]

TREATMENT

Rx

Refer also to Table 197-3 and Figure 197-4.

Non–Small Cell Lung Cancer

Stage I and II Disease

For stage I and II NSCLC, surgery is the initial treatment of choice. Before surgical resection, a comprehensive preoperative medical evaluation is mandatory (Chapter 439). This evaluation must be supplemented by pulmonary function tests (forced expiratory volume at 1 second [FEV_1] and diffusing capacity of the lung for carbon monoxide [DLCO]), as well as blood gas analysis (Chapter 85). FEV_1 and DLCO will determine what surgical procedure can be performed safely—pneumonectomy, lobectomy, wedge resection, or segmentectomy. A preoperative FEV_1 less than 40% of predicted and a DLCO less than 40% of normal are associated with an increase in operative mortality. Threshold levels to define resectability include a preoperative FEV_1 greater than 2.0 L and DLCO greater than 60% for pneumonectomy and a preoperative FEV_1 greater than 1.5 L and DLCO greater than 50% for lobectomy. Other factors for determining resectability include exercise tolerance and comorbid disease. The curability of the patient is dependent on the stage of disease and completeness of the resection and not whether lobectomy or pneumonectomy is performed. By comparison, there is a significant risk of local recurrence in patients undergoing wedge resection or segmentectomy rather than more extensive resection of the tumor. Mortality rates for lobectomy and pneumonectomy are 3% and 9%, respectively. For patients older than 70 years, the mortality rate for pneumonectomy rises to 16 to 25%.

For patients with stage I NSCLC who either refuse surgery or have coexisting illnesses that preclude surgery, the use of stereotactic radiotherapy (SRT) shows high local control rates with minimal toxicity. Randomized trials of SRT and surgery for stage I NSCLC are ongoing.

At surgery, a tumor is considered to be unresectable if metastasis is found in the pleura or contralateral mediastinal lymph nodes or if there is tumor invasion of the mediastinum, heart, great vessels, or other structures. In addition to surgical resection of the tumor, sampling or complete removal of all accessible mediastinal lymph nodes should be performed.

Adjuvant cisplatin-based chemotherapy (e.g., cisplatin, 80 mg/m^2 every 3 weeks for four doses or 100 mg/m^2 every 4 weeks for four doses, plus vinorelbine 30 mg/m^2 weekly or vinblastine 4 mg/m^2 weekly or etoposide 100 mg/m^2 per day for 3 days per cycle) provides a small absolute increase in overall survival at 5 years for stage I, II, and III disease.[3]

Adjuvant radiation therapy for stage I and II disease is not indicated. However, in patients with stage I NSCLC who for medical reasons are not candidates for surgery, radiation therapy can be given with curative intent. Five-year survival rates in patients thus treated range from 10 to 30%.

Stage III—Resectable

For patients with stage III resectable disease (ipsilateral mediastinal spread of disease [N2], tumors [T3] involving the chest wall, diaphragm, or pleura; or superior sulcus tumors [Pancoast's]), surgery alone is suboptimal treatment because of the presence of occult metastatic disease. Neoadjuvant (i.e., induction) chemotherapy given in sequence with or concurrent with radiation therapy before surgery improves survival when compared with surgery alone or surgery plus postoperative radiation therapy.[4] However, concurrent chemoradiation therapy causes significant esophagitis when compared with the use of sequential chemotherapy and radiation therapy.

Stage III—Unresectable

Stage IIIA or IIIB disease may be unresectable. Thoracic radiation therapy (total dose, 60 Gy) relieves symptoms in the chest but has little effect on 5-year survival rates unless combined with induction chemotherapy (e.g., vinblastine plus cisplatin for two cycles), which improves median survival from 9.7 months to 13.8 months and the 5-year survival rate from 7 to 19% when compared with radiation therapy alone.

Concurrent chemotherapy and radiation therapy rather than sequential therapy can improve survival in patients with locally advanced NSCLC but increases side effects, particularly esophagitis, by five-fold. To improve the effectiveness of radiation therapy, different fractionation approaches are under evaluation. Three-dimensional treatment planning permits delivery of higher doses of radiation to the primary tumor and regional lymph nodes without increasing toxicity.

Stage IV—Disseminated Disease

For patients with disseminated NSCLC, treatment generally consists of cisplatin or carboplatin combined with paclitaxel, docetaxel, gemcitabine, vinorelbine, pemetrexed, irinotecan, or topotecan. The response rate to such

TABLE 197-3 GENERAL APPROACH TO THE TREATMENT OF LUNG CANCER ACCORDING TO STAGE*

STAGE	PRIMARY TREATMENT	ADJUVANT THERAPY	OUTCOME
NON–SMALL CELL LUNG CANCER			
I	Surgical resection	Chemotherapy (stage 1B)	5-yr survival rate >60-70%
II	Surgical resection	Chemotherapy	5-yr survival rate >40-50%
IIIA (resectable)	Preoperative chemotherapy followed by surgical resection (preferable) or chemotherapy followed by radiation therapy	Chemotherapy with or without radiation therapy	5-yr survival rate 15-30%
IIIA (unresectable) or IIIB (involvement of the contralateral or supraclavicular lymph nodes)	Chemotherapy plus concurrent radiation therapy (preferable) or chemotherapy followed by radiation therapy	None	5-yr survival rate, 10-20%
IV	Chemotherapy with 2 agents for 4-6 cycles Chemotherapy + bevacizumab (selected patients) EGFR-TKI (erlotinib, gefitinib) in patients with positive *EGFR* gene mutation Surgical resection of solitary brain metastasis and surgical resection of primary (T1) lesion	None	Median survival 8-10 mo 1-yr survival rate 30-35% >70% response rate; PFS-HR 0.48; median survival >20 mo 2-yr survival rate 10-15% 5-yr survival rate 10-15%
SMALL CELL LUNG CANCER			
Limited disease†	Chemotherapy plus concurrent radiation therapy	None	5-yr survival rate 15-25%
Extensive disease†	Chemotherapy	None	5-yr survival rate <5%

*All chemotherapy regimens include either cisplatin or carboplatin. The second drug used as part of the regimen may include etoposide, paclitaxel, docetaxel, vinorelbine, gemcitabine, or irinotecan.
†Prophylactic cranial irradiation is recommended for all patients with a complete response to initial therapy.
EGFR = epidermal growth factor receptor; PFS HR = progression-free survival hazard ratio.
Modified from Spira A, Ettinger DS. Multidisciplinary management of lung cancer. *N Engl J Med.* 2004;350:379-392.

therapy is 20 to 50%, with a median survival of 8 to 10 months, 1-year survival rate of 30 to 35%, and 2-year survival rate of 10 to 15%. Data suggest that two-drug combinations are better than single-agent therapy, but three-drug combinations are not more effective than two-drug combinations. The duration of therapy is four to six cycles, and patients older than 70 years who have good performance status respond to and tolerate chemotherapy as well as younger patients.

Over the past several years, the treatment of patients with disseminated NSCLC has changed. The era of "personalized therapy" has arrived, with treatment decisions being made based on histologic subtypes (nonsquamous vs. squamous cell carcinoma) and EGFR mutation analysis. Pemetrexed in combination with cisplatin has been approved for first-line treatment of patients with metastatic nonsquamous NSCLC.[5] The use of bevacizumab (an antiangiogenesis drug) in combination with paclitaxel plus carboplatin demonstrated a significant improvement in overall response rate, progression-free survival, and overall survival compared with chemotherapy alone in patients with non–squamous cell advanced NSCLC.[6] EGFR–tyrosine kinase inhibitors such as erlotinib or gefitinib in patients having tumors with activating mutations in the *EGFR* gene have significant clinical efficacy compared with standard chemotherapy when given as first-line treatment in patients with disseminated NSCLC.[7] Future therapies for patients with NSCLC will be based on genomic, pharmacogenomic, and proteomic strategies.

Patients with a solitary metastasis may occasionally benefit from resection of the isolated metastatic lesion. For example, resection of a solitary brain metastasis followed by whole brain irradiation can potentially be curative, with 5-year survival rates as high as 20%. Patients with metastatic NSCLC can benefit from palliative radiation therapy to specific lesions that cause bronchial obstruction, SVC syndrome, bone pain, brain masses, and spinal cord compression. Early palliative care promotes quality of life and mood as well as survival in patients with metastatic non–small cell lung cancer.[8]

Small Cell Lung Cancer

The mainstay of treatment of SCLC is chemotherapy because the disease is characterized by its propensity for a rapid growth rate and spread to distant sites. Unfortunately, management of SCLC has changed little in the past decade.

Limited Stage

Thirty to 40% of SCLC patients have limited-stage disease. Management usually consists of chemotherapy and radiation therapy, and surgery is indicated only in the approximately 5% of patients who have a solitary peripheral pulmonary nodule without evidence of mediastinal lymph node involvement with clinical staging. After surgical removal of the SCLC nodule, patients with negative mediastinal lymph nodes at surgery require only postoperative chemotherapy with etoposide and cisplatin. The 5-year survival rate in patients with no mediastinal lymph node involvement is 30 to 60%. If the nodes contain metastases, chest irradiation is recommended in addition to chemotherapy.

For most patients with limited-stage SCLC, concurrent chemotherapy and radiation therapy appear to be more effective than sequential therapy. In the United States, etoposide and cisplatin plus concurrent radiation therapy (i.e., twice-a-day irradiation—total dose of 45 Gy) is the treatment of choice and produces a 5-year survival rate of 26% compared with 16% when given with the same dose of radiation once a day.

In patients who achieve a complete response to therapy, prophylactic cranial irradiation (24 to 36 Gy) reduces the risk for brain metastases and provides about a 5% survival advantage, but its higher risk of precipitating cognitive abnormalities must be taken into consideration, especially in elderly patients.

Extensive Stage

For extensive-stage SCLC, chemotherapy is the treatment of choice. In the United States, etoposide plus cisplatin or carboplatin is commonly used. Carboplatin causes significantly less nausea, vomiting, and neurotoxicity. The chemotherapy is administered every 3 weeks for four to six cycles. At this time, there is no evidence that maintenance therapy with either chemotherapy or targeted molecular therapy increases survival rates.

SCREENING AND PREVENTION

Screening

Unfortunately, most patients with lung cancer are initially found to have advanced disease that is not curable. Screening chest radiographs have been unsuccessful in improving outcome. Spiral CT scanning is four- to five-fold more sensitive than chest radiography for detecting malignant nodules in high-risk patients, but spiral CT also detects seven to eight benign nodules for every malignant nodule found. A large trial is currently ongoing to determine whether current or former smokers benefit from screening with spiral CT.

Prevention

Primary prevention of lung cancer focuses on ways to prevent individuals from smoking and promotion of smoking cessation (Chapter 31). Trials of supplemental doses of β-carotene and vitamin E, stimulated by epidemiologic evidence of lower serum levels of these antioxidants in patients with lung cancer, have not only been unsuccessful but actually produced a higher risk of lung cancer in smokers who received either of these supplements. High concentrations of selenium in blood are associated with a lower risk of lung cancer, and an ongoing trial is comparing selenium with placebo in patients who have survived resection for stage I lung cancer.

PROGNOSIS

Most patients in whom lung cancer is diagnosed have incurable disease, with an overall 5-year survival rate of approximately 15%. What determines the chance for survival is the stage of disease in NSCLC and whether the disease is extensive or limited in the case of SCLC (Table 197-4).

OTHER PULMONARY NEOPLASMS

Neuroendocrine Lung Tumors

Neuroendocrine lung tumors are classified into four types: carcinoid tumors, atypical carcinoids, SCLC, and large cell neuroendocrine carcinomas. Carcinoid tumors are low-grade neuroendocrine tumors with a 10-year survival rate of greater than 90%. Atypical carcinoid tumors are intermediate-grade tumors, more aggressive than carcinoid, with survival ranging from 10 months to 3 years. Large cell neuroendocrine carcinoma is an aggressive neuroendocrine tumor that does not meet the criteria for either carcinoid, atypical carcinoid, or SCLC.

Bronchial Carcinoid Tumors

Carcinoid tumors (Chapter 240) of the lung account for 1 to 2% of all lung neoplasms. They are neuroendocrine tumors that trace their origin to the Kulchitsky cell present in bronchial epithelium. Typical and atypical carcinoids differ in the number of mitoses (<2 per 10 high-power fields [HPF] vs. 2 to 10 per 10 HPF, respectively), nuclear pleomorphism (absent vs. present), regional lymph node metastases (5 to 15% vs. 20 to 28%), and distant metastases at initial evaluation (rare vs. 20%). Patients with a typical carcinoid tumors rarely die, whereas patients with atypical carcinoid tumors have a 5-year mortality rate of 27 to 47%. Carcinoid tumors are not associated with cigarette smoking, are twice as common in women as in men, usually occur in patients younger than 40 years, and arise in the perihilar area of the lung. Treatment of bronchial carcinoid tumors is based on the stage of the disease. Usually, mediastinal staging is followed by surgical resection. With mediastinal lymph node involvement, radiation therapy is recommended for typical carcinoid tumors if surgery cannot be performed. For atypical carcinoid or metastatic disease, chemotherapy (etoposide plus cisplatin every 3 weeks for four cycles) plus radiation therapy is commonly used, but there is no evidence for the benefit of one therapy over another.

TABLE 197-4 FIVE-YEAR SURVIVAL RATE FOR NON–SMALL CELL LUNG CANCER BY THE CLINICAL AND SURGICAL TNM (TUMOR, NODE, METASTASIS) INTERNATIONAL STAGING SYSTEM FOR LUNG CANCER

		5-Year Survival Rate (%)	
STAGE	**TNM SUBGROUPS**	**CLINICAL STAGE**	**SURGICAL STAGE**
IA	T1a,b N0 M0	50	73
IB	T2a N0 M0	43	58
IIA	T1a,b N1 M0 T2a N1 M0 T2b N0 M0	36	46
IIB	T2b N1 M0 T3 N0 M0	25	36
IIIA	T3 N1 M0 T1-3 N2 M0 T4 N0 M0	19	24
IIIB	T4 Any N M0 Any T N3 M0	7	9
IV	Any T Any N M1a,b	2	13

Malignant Mesothelioma

Pleural mesotheliomas (Chapter 99) are related to asbestos exposure (Chapter 93), with a peak risk 30 to 35 years after the initial exposure to asbestos. Approximately 50% of patients in whom a mesothelioma develops give no history of direct asbestos exposure. Other possible risk factors for mesothelioma include radiation and SV40 virus. Mesothelioma is generally diagnosed in the fifth to seventh decade of life (median age, 60 years), with the neoplasm developing in men five times more frequently than in women. Common symptoms include shortness of breath (60%) and chest wall pain or discomfort (60%). Chest radiographs usually reveal the presence of a unilateral pleural effusion. When the tumor progresses, it is generally local; symptomatic distant metastases are a late occurrence, if at all. Cytologic evaluation of pleural fluid to establish the diagnosis is difficult and may be inaccurate. The diagnosis is usually made by a biopsy procedure—under CT guidance or thoracoscopically, including VATS if necessary. Several staging systems have been proposed, but none has achieved complete acceptance. Treatment, which depends on the extent of disease, includes surgery (thoracoscopy with sclerosis, pleurectomy, extrapleural pneumonectomy), radiation therapy, and, often, chemotherapy. These three modalities individually have not significantly improved survival rates, and chemotherapy also has not helped control symptoms.[9] Multimodality and molecularly targeted agents are being evaluated. Mesothelioma remains a fatal disease, with a median survival of 9 to 12 months from the time of diagnosis.

Other Lung Tumors

Carcinomas of the salivary gland type include mucoepidermoid carcinoma and adenoid cystic carcinoma. These tumors are slow-growing neoplasms that arise from the bronchial glands. They represent approximately 0.2% of lung cancers and are usually treated surgically.

Primary sarcomas of the lung are very rare and include malignant fibrous histiocytoma, fibrosarcoma, leiomyosarcoma, rhabdomyosarcoma, epithelioid hemangioendothelioma, angiosarcoma, and liposarcoma. Surgery is the primary treatment, but radiation therapy or chemotherapy, or both, may be necessary, depending on the size and grade of the tumor and whether the margins are clear (Chapter 209).

Primary lymphomas of the lung account for approximately 0.3% of all primary cancers of the lung. The most common type is a low-grade small lymphocytic lymphoma. Surgery and chemotherapy (Chapter 191) are the usual treatments.

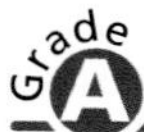

1. Maziak DE, Darling GE, Inculet RI, et al. Positron emission tomography in staging early lung cancer: a randomized trial. *Ann Intern Med.* 2009;151:221-228.
2. Annema JT, van Meerbeeck JP, Rintoul RC, et al. Mediastinoscopy vs endosonography for mediastinal nodal staging of lung cancer: a randomized trial. *JAMA.* 2010;304:2245-2252.
3. Winton T, Livingston R, Johnson D, et al. Vinorelbine plus cisplatin vs. observation in resected non-small-cell lung cancer. *N Engl J Med.* 2005;352:2589-2597.
4. Albain KS, Swann RS, Rusch VW, et al. Radiotherapy plus chemotherapy with or without surgical resection for stage III non-small cell lung cancer: a phase III randomized control trial. *Lancet.* 2009;374:379-386.
5. Scagliotti GV, Parikh P, von Pawel J, et al. Phase III study comparing cisplatin plus gemcitabine with cisplatin plus pemetrexed in chemotherapy naïve patients with advanced-stage non-small cell lung cancer. *J Clin Oncol.* 2008;26:3543-3551.
6. Sandler A, Gray R, Perry M, et al. Paclitaxel-carboplatin alone or with bevacizumab for non-small-cell lung cancer. *N Engl J Med.* 2006;355:2542-2550.
7. Mok TS, Wu YL, Thongprasert S, et al. Gefitinib or carboplatin-paclitaxel in pulmonary adenocarcinoma. *N Engl J Med.* 2009;361:1-10.
8. Temel JS, Green JA, Muzikansky A, et al. Early palliative care for patients with metastatic non–small-cell lung cancer. *N Engl J Med.* 2010;363:733-742.
9. Muers MF, Stephens RJ, Fisher P, et al. Symptom control with or without chemotherapy in the treatment of patients with malignant pleural mesothelioma (MS01): a multicentre randomized trial. *Lancet.* 2008;371:1685-1694.

SUGGESTED READINGS

Cataldo VD, Gibbons DL, Pérez-Soler R, et al. Treatment of non–small-cell lung cancer with erlotinib or gefitinib. *N Engl J Med.* 2011;364:947-955. *These epidermal growth factor receptor tyrosine kinase inhibitors have a role in advanced disease.*

Clinical Practice Guidelines in Oncology. Non-Small Cell Lung Cancer and Small Cell Lung Cancer. Version 3.2011 (NSCLC), version 1.2011 (SCLC). Available from the National Comprehensive Cancer Network at http://www.nccn.org. *Up-to-date approaches to the treatment of non–small cell and small cell lung cancer.*

NSCLC Meta-analyses Collaborative Group. Adjuvant chemotherapy, with or without postoperative radiotherapy, in operable non–small-cell lung cancer: two meta-analyses of individual patient data. *Lancet.* 2010;375:1267-1277. *In two meta-analyses, adjuvant chemotherapy improved survival of operable non–small cell lung cancer by 14%.*

Ray M, Kindler HL. Malignant pleural mesothelioma: an update on biomarkers and treatment. *Chest.* 2009;136:888-896. *A concise review of the present and future treatments in pleural mesothelioma.*

Tomaszek SC, Wigle DA. Pretreatment assessment for the optimal management of early-stage lung cancer. *Cancer. J* 2001;17:11-17. *Review.*

Travis WD, Brambilla E, Noguchi M, et al. International association for the study of lung cancer/American Thoracic Society/European Respiratory Society international multidisciplinary classification of lung adenocarcinoma. *J Thorac Oncol.* 2011;6:244-285. *Proposed new classification strategy.*

van Klaveren RJ, Oudkerk M, Prokop M, et al. Management of lung nodules detected by volume CT scanning. *N Engl J Med.* 2009;361:2221-2229. *After one negative screening CT scan, the risk of finding lung cancer on a subsequent screening CT scan was 1/1000 at 1 year and 3/1000 at 2 years.*

198

NEOPLASMS OF THE ESOPHAGUS AND STOMACH

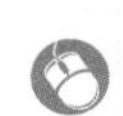

ANIL K. RUSTGI

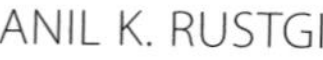

NEOPLASMS OF THE ESOPHAGUS

DEFINITION

The esophagus is a hollow tubular organ with primary physiologic functions related to contraction to permit propulsion of solid and liquid food contents into the stomach. Benign disorders of contraction are designated as esophageal motility disorders and discussed in Chapters 138 and 140. The mucosa is a stratified squamous epithelium that covers the submucosa and muscle; the latter is skeletal muscle in the proximal esophagus and smooth muscle in the mid-distal esophagus. Cancers of the esophagus may be classified broadly into epithelial versus nonepithelial. There are benign epithelial tumors referred to as *squamous cell papillomas.* Malignant epithelial tumors are classified into two main subtypes: esophageal squamous cell carcinoma (ESCC) and esophageal adenocarcinoma (EAC) (Table 198-1), which serves as the focus of this chapter's section. Apart from ESCC and EAC, other esophageal epithelially derived tumors include verrucous squamous cell carcinoma, adenosquamous carcinoma, adenoid cystic carcinoma, and mucoepidermoid carcinoma. Benign nonepithelial tumors include leiomyoma, granular cell tumors, fibrovascular polyp, hemangioma, lymphangioma, lipoma, and fibroma. Malignant nonepithelial tumors include leiomyosarcoma and other sarcomas, metastatic carcinoma (originating from breast, lung), and lymphoma.

Esophageal Squamous Cell Carcinoma

EPIDEMIOLOGY

ESCC is the more common type of esophageal cancer worldwide and represents a leading cause of cancer-related mortality in men. ESCC may have rates of up to 100 per 100,000 population in what is often termed the *central Asian belt*, including regions around the Caspian Sea, Iran, India, and China; other areas of high incidence include some Mediterranean countries and South Africa. In the United States, ESCC is more common among African American males than white males, with risks of 15.1 per 100,000 compared with 2.9 per 100,000, respectively. Overall, although the incidence of ESCC

TABLE 198-1 RISK FACTORS FOR ESOPHAGEAL CANCER

Esophageal squamous cell cancer
- Tylosis palmaris et plantaris
- Achalasia
- Plummer-Vinson syndrome
- Cigarette smoking
- Alcohol
- Chronic lye ingestion
- Human papilloma virus infection
- Radiation injury
- Celiac sprue

Esophageal adenocarcinoma
- Gastroesophageal acid reflux
- Bile reflux
- Obesity
- Barrett's esophagus

is low in males or females younger than 50 years, it does increase with advancing age.

Risk Factors

Cancers in general are viewed in the context of hereditary or inherited forms versus sporadic or seemingly random diseases that are related to age, environmental exposures, and genetic alterations (see Table 198-1). That being said, the hereditary basis for ESCC is exceedingly rare, consisting of a desquamating condition termed *tylosis palmaris et plantaris*. As implied, the desquamation most dramatically affects the hands and feet, but this extends to the esophagus as well. Another uncommon condition is called *Plummer-Vinson syndrome* or *Paterson-Brown Kelly syndrome*, which entails glossitis, cervical esophageal webs, and iron deficiency anemia. In both conditions, it is likely that chronic inflammation triggers the cascade of events that culminate in ESCC.

The vast preponderance of ESCC cases are attributable to cigarette smoking or alcohol, but especially so in combination because there appear to be synergistic deleterious effects of various chemical carcinogens in both, including *N*-nitroso compounds, polycyclic aromatic hydrocarbons, and aromatic amines. The relative risk for ESCC is 6.2 in those who smoke more than 25 cigarettes on a daily basis. Cessation of cigarette smoking is helpful in attenuating risk after 10 years of abstinence. Cigarette smokers who partake in beer and whiskey have a 10- to 25-fold enhanced risk of developing ESCC. Indeed, it is the type of alcohol and the manner of distillation that are most critical. In endemic areas of the world, deficiencies of vitamins A, B_{12}, C, and E, folic acid, and certain minerals (zinc, selenium, molybdenum) are important risk factors. All these vitamins and minerals exert direct or indirect antioxidant effects, and their deficiencies impair epithelial and tissue homeostasis and regeneration.

Other risk factors for ESCC include achalasia (Chapter 140), a disorder that involves agangliosis of Auerbach's plexus, resulting in dysphagia, chest pain, and weight loss, among other symptoms. The emergence of ESCC may be observed 10 to 20 years after the identification of achalasia in patients. Because head and neck squamous cell carcinoma (HNSCC) (Chapter 196) shares many of the environmental and lifestyle risk factors with ESCC, HNSCC and ESCC may occur synchronously or metachronously. In different parts of the world, ESCC is also associated with chronic esophageal stricture due to lye ingestion, consumption of maté (a hot herb-based beverage), celiac sprue, human papillomavirus infection, and radiation injury.

PATHOBIOLOGY

ESCC involves the transition over time from normal squamous epithelium to squamous dysplasia to cancer. ESCC initiation, progression, and metastasis are associated with a number of genetic alterations. Among the genetic alterations are overexpression of *epidermal growth factor receptor* and *cyclin D1* oncogenes, and inactivation of *TP53*, *p16INK4A*, and *E-cadherin* tumor suppressor genes. The frequency of these changes varies greatly based on the studies, but the oncogenic alterations appear to be generally early onset in dysplasia and early ESCC, whereas the inactivation of the tumor suppressor genes appear to be late events in established primary and metastatic ESCC. From a genomic viewpoint, the SOX-2 transcriptional factor, important in the pluripotent capacity of somatic cells, has been shown to be an important gene involved in ESCC pathogenesis and transformation by virtue of SOX-2 amplification. The ability to model ESCC in vitro and in vivo has witnessed great strides in recent years through the advent and characterization of three-dimensional organotypic culture models, xenograft transplantation mouse models, and genetically engineered mouse models.

CLINICAL MANIFESTATIONS

Symptoms and Signs

Although esophageal squamous dysplasia is typically not associated with symptoms, ESCC, which has a predilection for the proximal to mid esophagus, may be associated with dysphagia, odynophagia, atypical or typical chest pain, gastrointestinal bleeding, nausea, vomiting, weight loss, and malnutrition. ESCC may metastasize to local lymph nodes, lung, liver, and bone. Symptoms attributable to metastatic ESCC may involve bone-related pain, dyspnea, and evidence of jaundice and liver failure, depending on the extent of metastatic disease.

Physical Examination

The patient should be evaluated for changes in hair, skin integrity, and nail beds as a reflection of malnutrition. Weight loss may result in general cachexia and muscle wasting. There may be lymphadenopathy in the anterior cervical and superclavicular regions. Hepatomegaly and complications of liver disease may be present with metastatic disease to the liver.

Laboratory Studies

There may be progressive iron deficiency anemia due to chronic, indolent upper gastrointestinal bleeding. Additional abnormalities may be reflected in metabolic disturbances, such as metabolic alkalosis due to vomiting and hypernatremia due to dehydration. Liver enzyme abnormalities, both hepatocellular and cholestatic, may reflect metastasis to the liver. There are no specific markers for ESCC, but an elevated carcinoembryonic antigen (CEA) level may be used to aid in diagnosis or to monitor disease recurrence after therapy.

DIAGNOSIS

Barium swallow radiography is useful for the diagnosis of ESCC with depiction of a filling defect due to the mucosal lesion or impaired transit of barium due to luminal growth. However, definitive diagnosis involves direct visualization with upper endoscopy; once the mass is visualized, biopsies are necessary for confirmation by histopathology and possibly immunohistochemistry for cytokeratins associated with proliferation and differentiation. ESCC may involve local lymph nodes, which are best detected by endoscopic ultrasound; as needed, samples can be then analyzed for cytopathology by fine-needle aspiration. Evaluation of metastatic disease involves chest and abdominal/computed tomography (CT) scans. Bone scan might be useful in patients who are symptomatic with bone-related pain. Positron emission tomography (PET) has become increasingly used in some settings, although there are no guidelines for its routine use. In totality, these diagnostic modalities also allow for staging of ESCC (Table 198-2), which is important in guiding therapeutic options.

TREATMENT Rx

Surgical Therapy

Surgery is the cornerstone of therapy for curative intent. Technical advances have led to improvements in both operative mortality and postoperative morbidity. The different surgical techniques include transthoracic, transhiatal, and radical en bloc resections. Depending on the location of the ESCC, either total esophagectomy or subtotal esophagectomy is pursued. For the latter, jejunal or colonic interposition can be done.

Minimally invasive surgery may be done for esophagectomy in selected patients.

Medical Therapy

Depending on the stage, there is some variation in whether to proceed with preoperative (neoadjuvant) chemoradiation therapy or postoperative (adjuvant) chemoradiation therapy.

A study in which patients were randomized to receive surgery alone or surgery plus postoperative chemotherapy with 5-fluorouracil and leucovorin and concurrent radiation therapy revealed that the median survival was 36 months for patients in the adjuvant arm compared with 26 months for those in the surgery-only arm. The 3-year overall survival rates were 50% compared with 40%, respectively.

PROGNOSIS

The 5-year survival for treated ESCC is dependent on stage and types of therapies used as indicated previously. For stages T1 and T2 without lymphadenopathy, surgery alone may be curative in more than 60% of cases. For patients with metastatic disease, therapy is palliative involving endoscopically placed expandable prosthetic stents to open the nearly obstructed lumen for passage of food contents, percutaneous endoscopic gastrotomy tubes for delivery of nutrition to the stomach distal to the mass lesion, total parenteral nutrition, pain control, and systemic chemotherapy.

Esophageal Adenocarcinoma

EPIDEMIOLOGY

EAC affects whites more than African Americans and males much more than females (3 : 1 to 5.5 : 1) and increases in incidence after the age of 40 years. The age-adjusted incidence annually is 1.3 per 100,000. We will deal with EAC as a separate entity from gastroesophageal (GE) adenocarcinomas (so-called GE junctional cancer) and gastric cardia adenocarcinomas, although there has been a tendency by some to think of these in aggregate. That being stated, the incidence of EAC is increasing dramatically in developed

TABLE 198-2 TNM STAGING SYSTEM FOR CANCER OF THE ESOPHAGUS (AMERICAN JOINT COMMITTEE ON CANCER CRITERIA)

PRIMARY TUMOR (T)*	
TX	Primary tumor cannot be assessed
T0	No evidence of primary tumor
Tis	High-grade dysplasia†
T1	Tumor invades lamina propria, muscularis mucosae, or submucosa
T1a	Tumor invades lamina propria or muscularis mucosae
T1b	Tumor invades submucosa
T2	Tumor invades muscularis propria
T3	Tumor invades adventitia
T4	Tumor invades adjacent structures
T4a	Resectable tumor invading pleura, pericardium, or diaphragm
T4b	Unresectable tumor invading other adjacent structures, such as aorta, vertebral body, trachea, etc.

*(1) At least maximal dimension of the tumor must be recorded and (2) multiple tumors require the T(m) suffix.
†High-grade dysplasia includes all noninvasive neoplastic epithelia that was formerly called carcinoma in situ.

LYMPH NODE (N)*	
NX	Regional lymph nodes cannot be assessed
N0	No regional lymph node metastasis
N1	Metastasis in 1-2 regional lymph nodes
N2	Metastasis in 3-6 regional lymph nodes
N3	Metastasis in 7 or more regional lymph nodes

*Number must be recorded for total number of regional nodes sampled and total number of reported nodes with metastasis.

DISTANT METASTASIS (M)	
MX	Metastasis cannot be assessed
M0	No distant metastasis
M1	Distant metastasis

From *AJCC Cancer Staging Manual*, 7th ed. New York: Springer-Verlag; 2010.

countries, especially in the United States (by 4 to 10% annually) and western and northern Europe.

Etiology

Obesity (central) is an important risk factor for EAC. This may be related to either mechanical factors that foster greater gastroesophageal acid reflux disease (GERD) or the release of proinflammatory cytokines and adipokines that track to the esophagus, or both. The major recognized precursor of EAC is Barrett's esophagus (BE). BE is the replacement of the normal stratified squamous epithelium by an incomplete small intestinal type of epithelium (metaplasia) in the distal esophagus projecting from the GE junction in a distal-proximal gradient. In turn, it has been demonstrated that BE is fostered by GERD but also by an admixture of bile acids in the acid refluxate. Patients with scleroderma (Chapter 275) may be at increased risk for BE. A small subset of BE patients may progress to EAC through intermediate stages of low-grade and high-grade dysplasia. In BE, one case of EAC is estimated to arise in 55 to 441 patient years, which corresponds to an approximately 125-fold increased risk for EAC compared with that in the general population.

PATHOBIOLOGY

BE, or incomplete intestinal metaplasia, involves transdifferentiation from normal esophageal epithelium to an epithelium of the small intestine with columnar enterocytes and secretory goblet cells, but without Paneth cells and enteroendocrine cells—hence the designation of incomplete intestinal metaplasia. By itself, BE metaplasia cannot become EAC. However, if and when BE transitions to low-grade and high-grade dysplasia, there is the aforementioned risk for EAC. BE is associated with abnormal DNA ploidy based on flow cytometry analysis, and certain genetic alterations in epidermal growth factor receptor signaling, *TP53* and *p16INK4A*. Microsatellite instability may be noted as well. Whole genome approaches are revealing gains and losses of chromosomal regions that might lead to identification of known and previously unknown genes critical in the pathogenesis of EAC.

CLINICAL MANIFESTATIONS

Symptoms and Signs

It is estimated that 5 to 15% of GERD patients may develop BE, but such population-based studies are difficult to pursue because vast millions of people are affected with GERD, and most GERD patients do not undergo upper endoscopy. Patients with BE may or may not have symptoms related to GERD. Chronic GERD with BE may be associated with distal esophageal strictures. With EAC, patients may suffer from dysphagia, odynophagia, upper gastrointestinal bleeding, chest pain, nausea, vomiting, early satiety, weight loss, and malnutrition.

Physical Examination

Examination of the patient may reveal signs consistent with malnutrition and weight loss. Lymph adenopathy should be explored. There may be hepatomegaly. Paraneoplastic syndromes are unusual with EAC (as well as with ESCC) in contrast to non–small cell lung cancer (NSCLC) or pancreatic adenocarcinoma. Nevertheless, it is important to ensure that EAC is not mistaken for a benign entity such as a primary esophageal motility disorder.

Laboratory Studies

Patients with EAC may suffer from iron deficiency anemia, metabolic derangements, and abnormal liver enzyme tests due to metastatic disease. CEA may be elevated as a tumor serologic marker.

DIAGNOSIS

Barium swallow radiography may lead one to the suspicion of BE and can diagnose luminal mass lesions consistent with EAC in the distal esophagus. However, the mainstay of diagnosis is upper endoscopy. At that time, one will appreciate a salmon-colored mucosa from the GE junction with frondlike projections in a proximal direction. If the extent of BE is less than or equal to 3 cm, it is termed *short-segment BE;* if it is more than 3 cm, it is referred to as *long-segment BE*. This distinction is important in that the risk for EAC in long-segment BE is greater than in short-segment BE. Noting that the normal esophageal mucosa is more pink-white in hue, one can visually distinguish the two different types of epithelia, with the caveat that the gastric cardia mucosa at the GE junction should not be mistaken for BE. With that in mind, endoscopic mucosal biopsies from the BE region (with control biopsies from the normal esophagus and gastric cardia) are required for diagnosis histopathologically. Features of dysplasia are best appreciated in the absence of reflux-related esophagitis that can lead to nuclear architectural distortion; hence, suppression of acid production with proton pump inhibitor therapy for 6 to 8 weeks is needed, with a view to repeat biopsies.

If the patient has BE metaplasia, upper endoscopy should be repeated every 2 to 3 years. However, low-grade dysplasia requires surveillance endoscopy every 6 to 12 months. High-grade dysplasia, if properly evaluated by the pathologist, may require reconfirmation, but then leads to either medical (radiofrequency ablation, endoscopic mucosal resection) or surgical intervention due to the possibility of missed contiguous EAC. Endoscopic ultrasound may be helpful in discriminating between high-grade dysplasia and EAC.

TREATMENT

The principles are very similar to those applied to ESCC in terms of surgery. Data support adjuvant chemoradiation therapy for EAC, with median survival of 27 months for surgery alone versus 36 months for surgery plus chemoradiation therapy. Overall prognosis for EAC is not too dissimilar from that noted in ESCC. The treatment options of BE, the main precursor of EAC, have witnessed dramatic growth. Initially, photodynamic therapy was viewed with favor. However, for patients who are not surgical candidates because of comorbid illnesses, endoscopic mucosal resection (EMR) and radio frequency ablation[1] are credible options, especially for BE-related high-grade dysplasia or BE associated with intramucosal EAC.

NEOPLASMS OF THE STOMACH

DEFINITION

Gastric neoplasms are predominantly malignant, and nearly 90 to 95% of these tumors are adenocarcinomas. Less frequently observed malignant diseases include lymphomas, especially non-Hodgkin's lymphoma, and sarcomas, such as leiomyosarcoma. Benign gastric neoplasms include leiomyomas, carcinoid tumors, and lipomas.

Adenocarcinoma of the Stomach

EPIDEMIOLOGY

The great geographic variation in the incidence of gastric cancer worldwide strongly indicates that environmental factors influence the pathogenesis of gastric carcinogenesis. Further support for this notion comes from observations that groups emigrating from high-risk to low-risk areas, such as Japanese individuals moving to Hawaii and Brazil, acquire the low risk of the area into which they emigrate, presumably because of adoption of the endogenous lifestyle and exposure to different environmental factors.

Gastric adenocarcinoma was the most frequently observed malignant disease in the world until the mid-1980s, and it remains extremely common among men in certain regions, such as tropical South America, some parts of the Caribbean, and Eastern Europe. Regardless of gender, it remains one of the most common malignancies in Japan and China.

Whereas gastric cancer was the most common cancer in the United States in the 1930s, its annual incidence has steadily decreased. The annual incidence is now fewer than 20,000 new cases per year. However, although the incidence of gastric adenocarcinoma localized to the distal stomach has declined, the incidence of proximal gastric and gastroesophageal adenocarcinomas has been steadily increasing in the United States, a finding that perhaps reflects differences in pathogenic factors. Typically, gastric cancer occurs between the ages of 50 and 70 years and is uncommon before age 30 years. The rates are higher in men than in women by 2 to 1. Five-year survival is less than 20%.

Risk Factors

Risk factors for the development of gastric adenocarcinoma can be divided into environmental and genetic factors as well as precursor conditions (Table 198-3). For example, *Helicobacter pylori* infection is significantly more common in patients with gastric cancer than in matched control groups. Epidemiologic studies of high-risk populations have also suggested that genotoxic agents such as *N*-nitroso compounds may play a role in gastric tumorigenesis. *N*-nitroso compounds can be formed in the human stomach by nitrosation of ingested nitrates, which are common constituents of the diet. High nitrate concentrations in soil and drinking water have been observed in areas with high death rates from gastric cancer. Atrophic gastritis (Chapter 141), with or without intestinal metaplasia, is observed in association with gastric cancer, especially in endemic areas. Pernicious anemia (Chapter 167) is associated with a several-fold increase in gastric cancer. Atrophic gastritis and gastric cancer have certain environmental risk factors in common. It is likely that atrophic gastritis and intestinal metaplasia represent intermediary steps to gastric cancer. The achlorhydria associated with gastritis related to *H. pylori* infection, pernicious anemia, or other causes favors the growth of bacteria capable of converting nitrates to nitrites. The nitrosamine *N*-methyl-*N′*-nitro-*N*-nitrosoguanidine causes a high rate of induction of adenocarcinoma in the glandular stomach of rats. At the same time, most patients with atrophic gastritis do not develop gastric cancer, a finding suggesting that neither atrophic gastritis nor achlorhydria alone is responsible.

Benign gastric ulcers do not appear to predispose patients to gastric cancer. However, patients who have a gastric remnant after subtotal gastrectomy for benign disorders have an increased relative risk for gastric cancer of 1.5 to 3 by 15 to 20 years after surgery.

PATHOBIOLOGY

Gastric adenocarcinomas can be divided into two types based on the Lauren classification: intestinal and diffuse. The intestinal type is typically in the distal stomach with ulcerations, is often preceded by premalignant lesions, and is declining in incidence in the United States. By contrast, the diffuse type involves widespread thickening of the stomach, especially in the cardia, and it often affects younger patients; this form may present as linitis plastica, a nondistensible stomach with the absence of folds and narrowed lumen caused by infiltration of the stomach wall with tumor. Diffuse-type gastric cancers harbor mucin-producing cells. Other conditions may result in linitis plastica, such as lymphoma (Chapter 191), tuberculosis (Chapter 332), syphilis (Chapter 327), and amyloidosis (Chapter 194). The prognosis is generally worse in the diffuse type.

Key histopathologic features of gastric cancer include degree of differentiation, invasion through the gastric wall, lymph node involvement, and the presence or absence of signet ring cells within the tumor itself. Other pathologic manifestations include a polypoid mass, which may be difficult to distinguish from a benign polyp. Early gastric cancer, a condition that is not uncommon in Japan and that has a relatively favorable prognosis, consists of superficial lesions with or without lymph node involvement.

TABLE 198-3 CONDITIONS PREDISPOSING TO OR ASSOCIATED WITH GASTRIC CANCER

ENVIRONMENTAL
Helicobacter pylori infection
Dietary: excess of salt (salted pickled foods), nitrates/nitrites, carbohydrates; deficiency of fresh fruit, vegetables, vitamins A and C, refrigeration
Low socioeconomic status
Cigarette smoking
GENETIC
Familial gastric cancer (rare)
Associated with hereditary nonpolyposis colorectal cancer
Blood group A
PREDISPOSING CONDITIONS
Chronic gastritis, especially atrophic gastritis with or without intestinal metaplasia
Pernicious anemia
Intestinal metaplasia
Gastric adenomatous polyps (>2 cm)
Postgastrectomy stumps
Gastric epithelial dysplasia
Ménétrier's disease (hypertrophic gastropathy)
Chronic peptic ulcer

The leading hypothesis explaining the way in which *H. pylori* predisposes to gastric cancer risk is the induction of an inflammatory response, in which interleukin-1β may be pivotal. Chronic *H. pylori* infection also leads to chronic atrophic gastritis with resulting achlorhydria, which, in turn, favors bacterial growth that can convert nitrates (dietary components) to nitrites. These nitrites, in combination with genetic factors, promote abnormal cellular proliferation, genetic mutations, and eventually cancer. In a mouse model of gastric cancer, *H. pylori* infection may play a role in the recruitment of bone marrow–derived stem cells that facilitate gastric carcinogenesis. Animal models now recapitulate the cardinal features of gastric adenocarcinoma, either through the use of carcinogens or through genetic approaches.

GENETICS

It is clear that genetic factors play a role in gastric cancer. For example, blood group A is associated with a higher incidence rate of gastric cancer, even in nonendemic areas. A three-fold increase in gastric cancer has been reported among first-degree relatives of patients with the disease. Furthermore, albeit rare, germline or inherited mutations in the *E-cadherin* gene have been described in diffuse hereditary gastric cancer, which is seen in young patients. In addition, in hereditary nonpolyposis colorectal cancer type II (Chapter 199), patients have associated extracolonic cancers, including gastric cancer.

It now appears that several genetic mechanisms are important in gastric cancer: oncogene activation, tumor suppressor gene inactivation, and DNA microsatellite instability. For example, loss of heterozygosity of the *APC* (adenomatous polyposis coli) gene has been observed in gastric cancers. The p53 tumor suppressor gene product regulates the cell cycle at the G_1-S phase transition and probably also functions in DNA repair and apoptosis (programmed cell death). The *p53* gene is mutated not only in gastric cancer but also in gastric precancerous lesions, a finding suggesting that mutation of the *p53* gene is an early event in gastric carcinogenesis. Microsatellite DNA alterations or instability in dinucleotide repeats that were originally identified in hereditary nonpolyposis colorectal cancer also occur frequently in sporadic gastric carcinoma. Mutations in genes may accumulate as a result of DNA microsatellite instability.

CLINICAL MANIFESTATIONS

Symptoms and Signs

In its early stages, gastric cancer may often be asymptomatic or may produce only nonspecific symptoms that make early diagnosis difficult. Later symptoms include bloating, dysphagia, epigastric pain, or early satiety. Early satiety or vomiting may suggest partial gastric outlet obstruction, although gastric dysmotility may contribute to the vomiting in patients with nonobstructive cases. Epigastric pain, reminiscent of that associated with peptic ulcer (Chapter 141), occurs in about one fourth of patients, but in most patients with gastric cancer, the pain is not relieved by food or antacids. Pain that radiates to the back may indicate that the tumor has penetrated the pancreas.

When dysphagia is associated with gastric cancer, this symptom suggests a more proximal gastric tumor at the GE junction or in the fundus.

Signs of gastric cancer include bleeding, which can result in anemia that produces the symptoms of weakness, fatigue, and malaise, as well as more serious cardiovascular and cerebral consequences. Perforation related to gastric cancer is unusual. Gastric cancer metastatic to the liver can lead to right upper quadrant pain, jaundice, and fever. Lung metastases can cause cough, hiccups, and hemoptysis. Peritoneal carcinomatosis can lead to malignant ascites unresponsive to diuretics. Gastric cancer can also metastasize to bone.

Physical Examination

In the earliest stages of gastric cancer, the physical examination may be unremarkable. At later stages, patients become cachectic, and an epigastric mass may be palpated. If the tumor has metastasized to the liver, hepatomegaly with jaundice and ascites may be present. Portal or splenic vein invasion can cause splenomegaly. Lymph node involvement in the left supraclavicular area is termed *Virchow's node,* and periumbilical nodal involvement is called *Sister Mary Joseph's node.* The fecal occult blood test may be positive. Metastasis to the ovary is termed *Krukenberg's tumor.*

Paraneoplastic syndromes may precede or occur concurrently with gastric cancer. Examples include the following: Trousseau's syndrome (Chapter 187), which is recurrent migratory superficial thrombophlebitis indicating a possible hypercoagulable state (Chapter 179); acanthosis nigricans (see Fig. 187-1 in Chapter 187), which arises as raised and hyperpigmented skin lesions of flexor areas, neck, axilla, groin, and mucosal membranes; neuromyopathy with involvement of the sensory and motor pathways; and central nervous system syndromes with altered mental status and ataxia (Chapter 187).

Laboratory Studies

Laboratory studies may reveal iron deficiency anemia. Microangiopathic hemolytic anemia has been reported. Abnormalities in liver tests generally indicate metastatic disease. Hypoalbuminemia is a marker of malnutrition. Protein-losing enteropathy is rare but can be seen in Ménétrier's disease, another predisposing condition. Serologic test results, such as those for CEA and CA 72.4, may be abnormal. Although these tests are not recommended for initial diagnosis, they may be useful for monitoring disease after surgical resection.

DIAGNOSIS

The diagnostic accuracy of upper endoscopy with biopsy and cytologic examination approaches 95 to 99% for both types of gastric cancer. Cancer may arise as a small mucosal ulceration, a polyp, or a mass (Fig. 198-1). In some patients, gastric ulceration may first be noted in an upper gastrointestinal barium contrast study. A benign gastric ulcer is suggested by a smooth, regular base, whereas a malignant ulcer is manifested by a surrounding mass, irregular folds, and an irregular base. Although these and other radiographic characteristics historically helped to predict benign versus malignant disease, upper gastrointestinal endoscopy with biopsy and cytologic examination is mandatory whenever a gastric ulcer is found in the radiologic study, even if the ulcer has benign characteristics.

Staging of gastric cancer and, at times, diagnosis have been greatly enhanced by the advent of endoscopic ultrasonography (EUS) (Table 198-4). The extent of tumor, including gastric wall invasion and local lymph node involvement, can be assessed by EUS (Fig. 198-2), which provides information complementary to that obtained from CT scans. EUS can help guide aspiration biopsies of lymph nodes to determine their malignant features, if any.

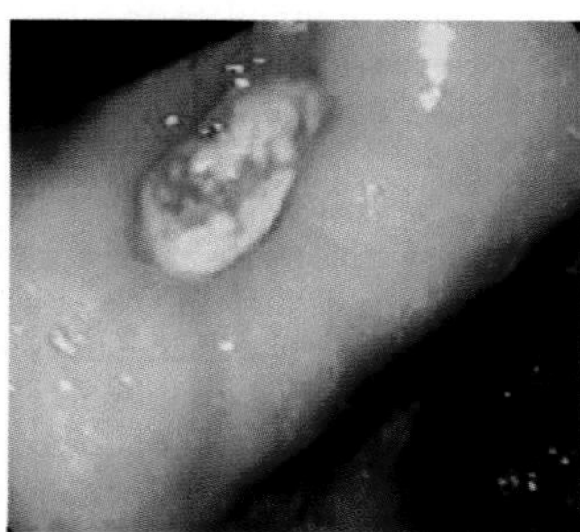
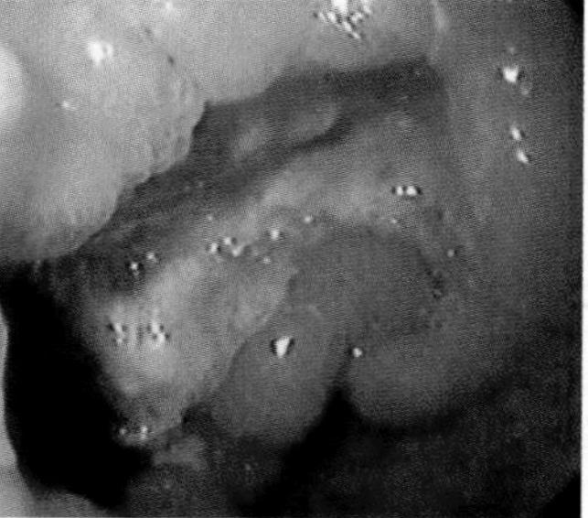

FIGURE 198-1. Benign *(left)* and malignant *(right)* gastric ulcer. Note the shaggy, thickened, and overhanging edges of the cancer. (Courtesy of Pankaj Jay Pasricha, MD.)

CT of the chest, abdomen, and pelvis should be performed to document lymphadenopathy and extragastric organ (especially lung and liver) involvement. In some centers, staging of gastric cancer entails bone scans because of the proclivity of gastric cancer to metastasize to bone.

TREATMENT Rx

Surgical Therapy

The only chance for cure of gastric cancer remains surgical resection, which is possible in only 25 to 30% of cases. If the tumor is confined to the distal stomach, subtotal gastrectomy is performed with resection of lymph nodes in the porta hepatis and in the pancreatic head. By contrast, tumors of the proximal stomach merit total gastrectomy to obtain an adequate margin and to remove lymph nodes; distal pancreatectomy and splenectomy are usually also performed as part of this procedure, which carries with it higher mortality and morbidity rates. The addition of para-aorta nodal dissection does not improve survival. Even if a curative procedure is not possible because of metastasis, limited gastric resection may be necessary for patients with excessive bleeding or obstruction. If cancer recurs in the gastric remnant, limited resection may again be necessary for palliation. Most recurrences in both types of gastric cancer are in the local or regional area of the original tumor.

Medical Therapy

Gastric cancer is one of the few gastrointestinal cancers that is somewhat responsive to chemotherapy.[2] In patients with gastric cancer who undergo gastrectomy and extended lymph node dissection with curative intent, S-1 (an oral fluoropyrimidine, 80 mg daily for 4 weeks followed by 2 weeks off, repeated in 6-week cycles for 1 year starting within 6 weeks after surgery) significantly improves 3-year survival from 70% to 80%.[3] Chemotherapy with the combination of epirubicin, cisplatin, and fluorouracil, given both

TABLE 198-4 TNM STAGING OF STOMACH CANCER

PRIMARY TUMOR (T)	
TX	Primary tumor cannot be assessed
T0	No evidence of primary tumor
Tis	Carcinoma in situ: intraepithelial tumor without invasion of the lamina propria
T1	Tumor invades lamina propria, muscularis mucosa, or submucosa
T1a	Tumor invades lamina propria or muscularis mucosa
T1b	Tumor invades submucosa
T2	Tumor invades muscularis propria*
T3	Tumor penetrates subserosal connective tissue without invasion of visceral peritoneum or adjacent structures[†,‡]
T4	Tumor invades serosa (visceral peritoneum) or adjacent structures[†,‡]
T4a	Tumor invades serosa (visceral peritoneum)
T4b	Tumor invades adjacent structures
REGIONAL LYMPH NODES (N)	
NX	Regional lymph nodes(s) cannot be assessed
N0	No regional lymph nodes metastasis[§]
N1	Metastasis in 1 to 2 regional lymph nodes
N2	Metastasis in 3 to 6 regional lymph nodes
N3	Metastasis in 7 or more regional lymph nodes
N3a	Metastasis in 7 to 15 regional lymph nodes
N3b	Metastasis in 16 or more regional lymph nodes
DISTANT METASTASIS (M)	
M0	No distant metastasis
M1	Distant metastasis

**Note:* A tumor may penetrate the muscularis propria with extension into the gastrocolic or gastrohepatic ligaments, or into the greater or lesser omentum, without perforation of the visceral peritoneum covering these structures. In this case, the tumor is classified T3. If there is perforation of the visceral peritoneum covering the gastric ligaments or the omentum, the tumor should be classified T4.

†The adjacent structures of the stomach include the spleen, transverse colon, liver, diaphragm, pancreas, abdominal wall, adrenal gland, kidney, small intestine, and retroperitoneum.

‡Intramural extension to the duodenum or esophagus is classified by the depth of the greatest invasion in any of these sites, including the stomach.

§*Note:* A designation of pN0 should be used if all examined lymph nodes are negative, regardless of the total number removed and examined.

From *AJCC Cancer Staging Manual,* 7th ed. New York: Springer-Verlag, 2010.

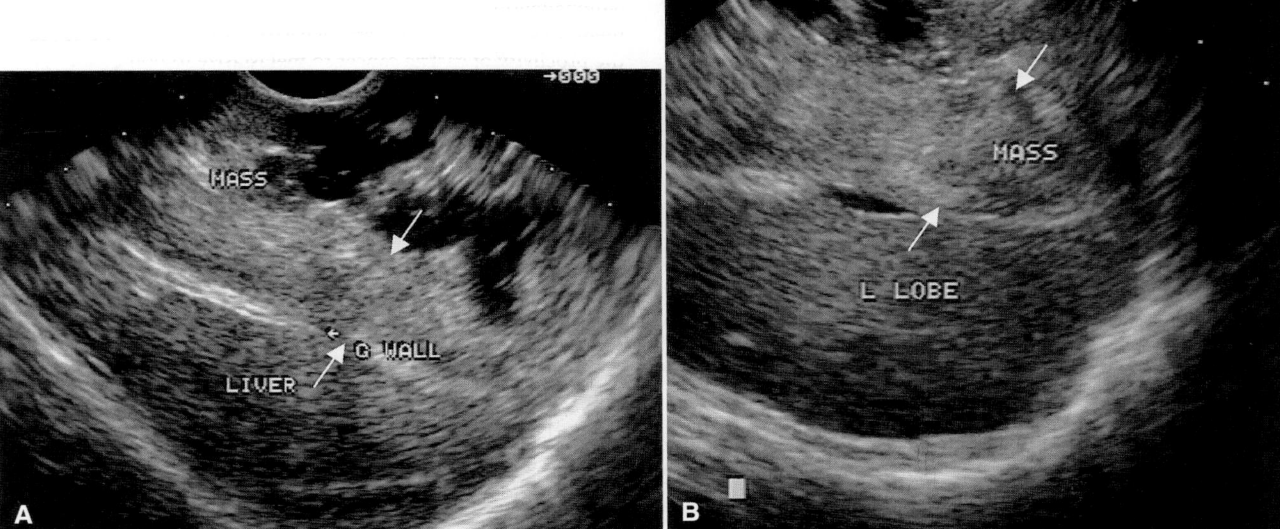

FIGURE 198-2. **Gastric mass.** Endoscopic ultrasonography depicting a large gastric mass that is compressing the liver and gallbladder wall (**A**) and, on a different view, the left lobe of the liver (**B**).

preoperatively and postoperatively, significantly improves 5-year survival from 23% to 36% in patients with resectable gastroesophageal cancer.[4] Similarly, the combination of chemotherapy (fluorouracil and leucovorin) with radiation therapy has been shown to improve median survival from 27 months to 36 months compared with surgery alone in patients with adenocarcinoma of the stomach or gastroesophageal junction.[5]

Single-agent chemotherapy treatment, which provides partial response rates of 20 to 30%, is reserved for patients with a poor performance status. Combination regimens that can yield partial response rates of 35 to 50% include the following: ECF, which is most popular in Europe (epirubicin, 50 mg/m^2 on day 1; cisplatin, 60 mg/m^2 on day 1; 5-fluorouracil, 200 mg/m^2/day as a continuous infusion through a central venous access device [CVAD] given throughout treatment, repeated every 21 days for a maximum of eight cycles); CF (5-fluorouracil infusion, 1000 mg/m^2/day for 4 days; cisplatin, 75 to 100 mg/m^2 on day 1, every 4 weeks); or TCF (docetaxel [Taxotere], 75 mg/m^2 on day 1; cisplatin, 75 mg/m^2 on day 1; and 5-fluorouracil, 750 mg/m^2/day for 5 days, every 3 weeks), or capecitabine plus cisplatin. A randomized trial of triple chemotherapy for advanced esophagogastric cancer showed that oral capecitabine is at least as effective as infused fluorouracil and that oxaliplatin (which does not require hydration) is at least as effective as cisplatin (which does require hydration) with respect to overall survival.[6] Trastuzumab (8 mg/kg intravenously once, then 6 mg/kg every 3 weeks) can increase survival of HER2-positive advanced gastric or gastro-esophageal junction cancer from 11.1 months to 13.8 months.[7] Radiation therapy alone is ineffective and is generally employed only for palliative purposes in the setting of bleeding, obstruction, or pain. Gene therapy and immune-based therapy are currently only investigational in animal models.

General Methods

Implicit in the management of the patient with gastric cancer is meticulous attention to nutrition (jejunal enteral feedings or total parenteral nutrition), correction of metabolic abnormalities that arise from vomiting or diarrhea, and treatment of infection from aspiration or spontaneous bacterial peritonitis. *H. pylori* eradication treatment reduces the risk for metachronous gastric carcinoma by about two thirds.[8] To maintain lumen patency, endoscopic laser treatment or prosthesis placement can be used in a palliative fashion.

PROGNOSIS

Approximately one third of patients who undergo a curative resection are alive after 5 years. In aggregate, the overall 5-year survival rate in patients with gastric cancer is less than 10%. Prognostic factors include anatomic location and nodal status. Distal gastric cancers without lymph node involvement have a better prognosis than proximal gastric cancers with or without lymph node involvement. Other prognostic factors include depth of penetration and tumor cell DNA aneuploidy. Linitis plastica and infiltrating lesions have a much worse prognosis than polypoid disease or exophytic masses. In the subset of mostly Japanese patients with early gastric cancer that is confined to the mucosa and submucosa, surgical resection may be curative and definitely improves the 5-year survival rate to more than 50%. In fact, when early gastric cancer is confined to the mucosa, endoscopic mucosal resection may be an alternative.

Lymphoma of the Stomach

EPIDEMIOLOGY

Gastric lymphoma represents about 5% of all malignant gastric tumors and is increasing in incidence. Most gastric lymphomas are non-Hodgkin's lymphomas (Chapter 191), and the stomach is the most common extranodal site for non-Hodgkin's lymphomas. Patients with gastric lymphoma are generally younger than those with gastric adenocarcinoma, but the male predominance remains.

CLINICAL MANIFESTATIONS

Patients commonly present with symptoms and signs similar to those of gastric adenocarcinoma. Lymphoma in the stomach can be a primary tumor, or it can be secondary to disseminated lymphoma.

B-cell lymphomas (Chapter 191) of the stomach are most commonly large cell with a high-grade type. Low-grade variants are noted in the setting of chronic gastritis and are termed *mucosa-associated lymphoid tissue* (MALT) lymphomas. MALT lesions are strongly associated with *H. pylori* infection.

DIAGNOSIS

Radiographically, gastric lymphomas usually arise as ulcers or exophytic masses; diffusely infiltrating lymphoma is more suggestive of secondary lymphoma. Thus, upper gastrointestinal barium studies usually show multiple nodules and ulcers for a primary gastric lymphoma and typically have the appearance of linitis plastica with secondary lymphoma. As with gastric adenocarcinoma, however, upper endoscopy with biopsy and cytologic examination are required for diagnosis and have an accuracy of nearly 90%. Apart from conventional histopathologic analysis, immunoperoxidase staining for lymphocyte markers is helpful in diagnosis. As with gastric adenocarcinoma, proper staging of gastric lymphoma involves EUS, chest and abdominal/pelvic CT scans, and bone marrow biopsy as needed.

TREATMENT Rx

Treatment of gastric diffuse large B-cell lymphoma is best pursued with combination chemotherapy with or without radiation therapy (Chapter 191). For MALT lesions, eradication of *H. pylori* infection with antibiotics should be attempted (Chapter 141), but patients with refractory lesions that are confined to the stomach can sometimes be cured with radiotherapy (Chapter 191).

Other Malignant Tumors of the Stomach

Leiomyosarcoma, which constitutes approximately 1% of all gastric cancers, usually occurs as an intramural mass with central ulceration. Symptoms may include bleeding accompanied by a palpable mass. Leiomyosarcomas are often relatively indolent; surgical resection yields a 5-year survival rate of about 50%. Metastasis can occur to lymph nodes and the liver. Other gastric sarcomas include liposarcomas, fibrosarcomas, myosarcomas, and neurogenic sarcomas.

Most gastrointestinal stromal tumors (GISTs) have been associated with activating mutations in the C-*kit* gene; a subset of such tumors are associated with mutations in the platelet-derived growth factor receptor *(PDGFR)* gene. C-*kit* mutations are also found in chronic and acute myelogenous leukemia (Chapters 189 and 190), and approximately 50% of GISTs respond to imatinib mesylate, which is also used in chronic myelogenous leukemia. If imatinib is not successful, sunitinib increases survival.[9] Carcinoid tumors (Chapter 240) may begin in the stomach and are curable by removal if they have not yet spread to the liver.

Primary tumors can also spread to the stomach. In addition to lymphomas, other tumors found in the stomach include primary lung (Chapter 197) and breast (Chapter 204) cancers as well as malignant melanoma (Chapter 210).

LEIOMYOMAS AND BENIGN TUMORS

Leiomyomas, which are smooth muscle tumors of benign origin, occur with equal frequency in men and women and are typically located in the middle and distal stomach. Leiomyomas can grow into the lumen, with secondary ulceration and consequent bleeding. Alternatively, they can expand to the serosa with extrinsic compression. Endoscopy may reveal a mass that has overlying mucosa or mucosa replaced by ulceration. On upper gastrointestinal series, leiomyomas are usually smooth with an intramural filling defect, with or without central ulceration. However, benign leiomyomas can be difficult to distinguish from their malignant counterparts radiographically or endoscopically; tissue diagnosis is imperative. Symptomatic leiomyomas should be removed, but those without associated symptoms do not require therapy.

Other benign gastric tumors include lipoma, neurofibroma, lymphangioma, ganglioneuroma, and hamartoma, the last associated with Peutz-Jeghers syndrome (Chapter 199) or juvenile polyposis (restricted to the stomach).

ADENOMAS

Gastric adenomas and hyperplastic polyps are unusual but may be found in middle-aged and elderly patients. Polyps may be sessile or pedunculated and are also found in nearly 50% of patients with familial adenomatosis polyposis (Chapter 199). Gastric adenocarcinoma arising in the antrum has been described in such patients. Although isolated gastric adenomatous polyps are generally asymptomatic, some patients may have dyspepsia, nausea, or bleeding. Gastric adenomas and hyperplastic polyps are smooth and regular on upper gastrointestinal series, but the diagnosis must be confirmed by upper endoscopy with biopsy. Pedunculated polyps that are larger than 2 cm or that have associated symptoms should be removed by endoscopic snare cautery polypectomy, whereas large sessile gastric adenomatous polyps may merit segmental surgical resection. If polyps progress to an intermediary stage of severe dysplasia or culminate in cancer, treatment is the same as for gastric adenocarcinoma.

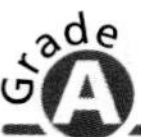

1. Shaheen NJ, Sharma P, Overholt BF, et al. Radiofrequency ablation in Barrett's esophagus with dysplasia. *N Engl J Med.* 2009;360:2277-2288.
2. GASTRIC (Global Advanced/Adjuvant Stomach Tumor Reasearch International Collaboration) Group. Benefit of adjuvant chemotherapy for resectable gastric cancer: a meta-analysis. *JAMA.* 2010;303:1729-1737.
3. Sakuramoto S, Sasako M, Yamaguchi T, et al. Adjuvant chemotherapy for gastric cancer with S-1, an oral fluoropyrimidine. *N Engl J Med.* 2007;357:1810-1820.
4. Cunningham D, Allum WH, Stenning SP, et al. Perioperative chemotherapy versus surgery alone for resectable gastro esophageal cancer. *N Engl J Med.* 2006;355:11-20.
5. Macdonald JS, Smalley SR, Benedetti J, et al. Chemoradiotherapy after surgery compared with surgery alone for adenocarcinoma of the stomach or gastroesophageal junction. *N Engl J Med.* 2001;345:725-730.
6. Cunningham D, Starling N, Rao S, et al. Capecitabine and oxaliplatin for advanced esophagogastric cancer. *N Engl J Med.* 2008;358:36-46.
7. Bang YJ, Van Cutsem E, Feyereislova A, et al. Trastuzumab in combination with chemotherapy versus chemotherapy alone for treatement of HER2-positive advanced gastric or gastro-oesophageal junction cancer (ToGA): a phase 3, open-label, randomised controlled trial. *Lancet.* 2010;376:687-697.
8. Fukase K, Kato M, Kikuchi S, et al. Effect of eradication of *Helicobacter pylori* on incidence of metachronous gastric carcinoma after endoscopic resection of early gastric cancer: an open-label, randomised controlled trial. *Lancet.* 2008;372:392-397.
9. Demetri GD, Oosterom AT, Garrett CR, et al. Efficacy and safety of sunitinib in patients with advanced gastrointestinal stromal tumour after failure of imatinib: a randomised controlled trial. *Lancet.* 2006;368:1329-1338.

SUGGESTED READINGS

Ng T, Vezeridis MP. Advances in the surgical treatment of esophageal cancer. *J Surg Oncol.* 2010;101:725-729. *Review of technical improvements in surgical resection of esophageal cancer.*

Paoletti X, Oba K, Burzykowski T, et al, for the GASTRIC (Global Advanced/Adjuvant Stomach Tumor Research International Collaboration) Group. Benefit of adjuvant chemotherapy for resectable gastric cancer: a meta-analysis. *JAMA.* 2010;303:1729-1737. *Meta-analysis showing superiority of fluorouracil-based adjuvant chemotherapy compared with surgery alone in reducing mortality.*

Polk DB, Peek RM Jr. *Helicobacter pylori*: gastric cancer and beyond. *Nat Rev Cancer.* 2010;10:403-414. *Review of mechanisms that regulate the biological interactions of* H. pylori *with its hosts and that promote carcinogenesis.*

Spechler SJ, Fitzgerald RC, Prasad GA, et al. History, molecular mechanisms, and endoscopic treatment of Barrett's esophagus. *Gastroenterology.* 2010;138:854-869. *An excellent review of the diagnosis and management of Barrett's esophagus.*

Wang J, Yu JC, Kang WM, et al. Treatment strategy for early gastric cancer. *Surg Oncol.* 2011. [Epub ahead of print.] *Review.*

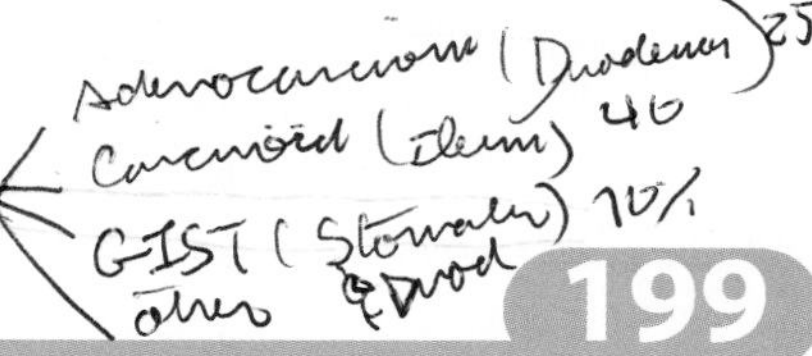

199 NEOPLASMS OF THE SMALL AND LARGE INTESTINE

CHARLES D. BLANKE AND DOUGLAS O. FAIGEL

NEOPLASMS OF THE SMALL INTESTINE

EPIDEMIOLOGY

The small intestine accounts for the majority of the length (≈75%) and surface (≈90%) of the gastrointestinal (GI) tract. Nonetheless, it is a rare site for the development of neoplastic disease, as only 1 to 2% of primary GI tumors originate in the duodenum, jejunum, or ileum. In fact, half of all small bowel neoplasms represent metastatic disease from other sites, particularly elsewhere in the GI tract. Small bowel malignancies constitute less than 0.5% of all cancers, although the incidence of small bowel tumors (especially carcinoids) seems to be increasing. Overall, the mean age at diagnosis of a small bowel tumor is about 67 years; neoplasms are more common in males, and they occur more commonly in African Americans than in whites.

PATHOBIOLOGY

Adenocarcinomas, arising from mucosal glands, were formerly the most frequent primary small bowel tumor. They now constitute 25% of small bowel neoplasms, including benign growths, and 40% of all malignant tumors. Adenocarcinomas most commonly arise in the duodenum (65% of all small intestinal adenocarcinomas), even though the duodenum represents only a tiny fraction of the length of the small bowel. They occur less commonly in the jejunum and least commonly in the ileum. The majority are well or moderately differentiated.

Small bowel carcinoids, which derive from enterochromaffin cells in the crypts of Lieberkühn, are now the most common small bowel tumors, accounting for approximately 30 to 40% of malignancies. They tend to be quite well differentiated. In contrast to glandular tumors, small intestinal carcinoids tend to arise in the distal ileum, and up to 30% are multifocal. Other small bowel neuroendocrine tumors are occasionally seen, including biochemically active neoplasms such as gastrinomas and somatostatinomas. Very rarely, high-grade true small cell carcinomas occur.

Malignant connective tissue tumors account for 10% of small bowel neoplasms. Gastrointestinal stromal tumors (GISTs), which derive from the interstitial cells of Cajal or a common precursor, account for approximately 85% of these neoplasms (Fig. 199-1). GISTs, like adenocarcinomas, disproportionately arise in the duodenum, and the small bowel itself is the second most common primary site for these mesenchymal neoplasms (33% derive from small bowel). Morphologically, GISTs often resemble leiomyosarcomas

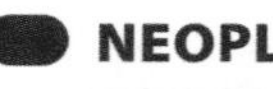

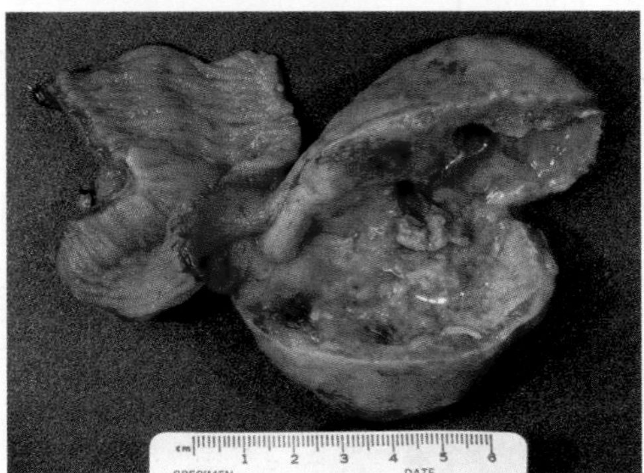

FIGURE 199-1. Small bowel gastrointestinal stromal tumor with ulceration.

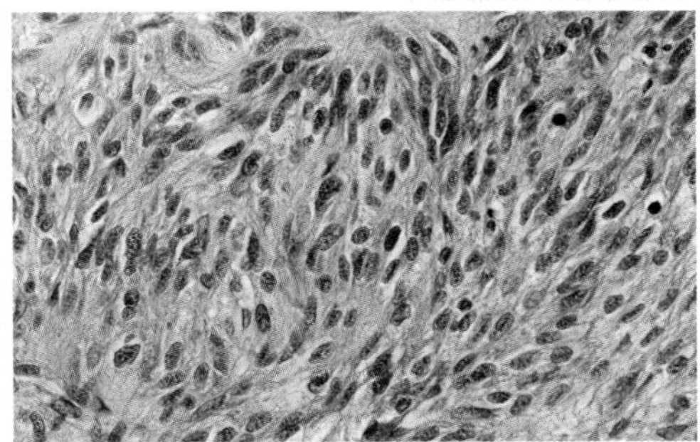

FIGURE 199-2. Histopathology of gastrointestinal stromal tumor.

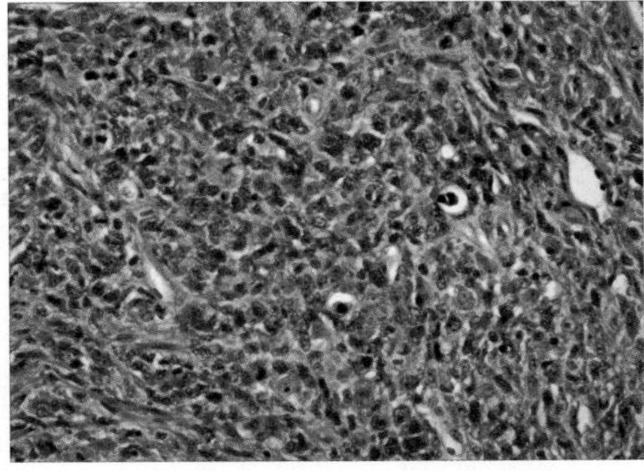

FIGURE 199-3. Histopathology of small bowel non-Hodgkin's lymphoma. (Courtesy Dr. M. K. Washington.)

(Fig. 199-2), but they can be differentiated by the expression of the Kit protein (CD117). Other small bowel sarcomas such as true leiomyosarcomas are seen more rarely (Chapter 209).

Primary GI lymphomas are the most common extranodal lymphomatous variation, and the small intestine is the second most common GI site for such tumors (Chapter 191). The ileum, rich in submucosal lymphoid follicles, is the most common small bowel site. Tumors may be low or higher grade and can arise from precursor B or T lymphocytes. The overwhelming majority are non-Hodgkin's tumors (Fig. 199-3). Lymphomas involving the small bowel may also be a manifestation of true systemic disease.

Malignant melanoma (Chapter 210) can develop as a primary mucosal small bowel tumor, probably arising from schwannian neuroblasts associated with GI innervation. In addition, the small bowel is the most common GI site for melanoma metastases.

Finally, a variety of common benign tumors may originate in the small bowel, including adenomas, leiomyomas, and lipomas. Desmoids, most often seen in patients with familial adenomatous polyposis (FAP); hamartomas; and hemangiomas are relatively rare. Benign growths are more common in the distal small intestine.

The small intestine can be involved by advanced cancers from other sites through direct invasion, extension of peritoneal metastases, or hematogenous spread. As noted, the small bowel is the most common GI site for melanoma metastases; in addition, involvement is fairly common with ovarian, breast, lung, and other GI neoplasms.

Predisposing Conditions

Inflammatory bowel disease (Chapter 143) predisposes to adenocarcinoma. Additionally, many of the polyposis syndromes are associated with small bowel neoplasms. Most notably, FAP (see later) is associated with adenomas and carcinomas of the duodenum and jejunum, but especially in the ampullary and periampullary region. At least 90% of FAP patients develop duodenal adenomas, and up to 10% develop cancer. The risk of cancer is related to the number of polyps, their size and histologic type, and the presence of high-grade dysplasia. Patients with FAP should undergo regular screening for duodenal neoplasia with both forward- and side-viewing endoscopes beginning around the time of colectomy and repeated at 1- to 5-year intervals, depending on the presence and degree of duodenal polyposis. Patients with MUTYH polyposis likewise develop duodenal neoplasia and should undergo screening. Patients with hereditary nonpolyposis colon cancer (HNPCC) are also at increased risk for small intestine adenocarcinoma, which may be the first manifestation of their disease. HNPCC-associated small bowel cancer may present at a young age (median, 39 years) and occurs with decreasing frequency from the duodenum to the ileum, with about 50% of occurrences in the duodenum. Screening may be considered beginning at age 30. Patients with sprue are at an increased risk for small bowel lymphomas.

CLINICAL MANIFESTATIONS

The most common presenting symptom of small bowel tumors is abdominal pain, especially for those that are true cancers. Less common are symptoms such as weight loss, nausea, GI bleeding, and symptoms related to perforation. Approximately 25% of patients have GI obstruction, and duodenal periampullary tumors can lead to obstructive jaundice. Only a minority of malignancies are asymptomatic, whereas benign tumors may cause no symptoms in up to half of patients. Carcinoid tumors in the small bowel are often asymptomatic, although in the setting of advanced disease they may secrete bioactive amines, leading to flushing, diarrhea, wheezing, and eventually symptoms of right heart failure (related to valvular fibrosis) (Chapter 240). This is more common with tumors originating in the jejunum and ileum. Benign tumors tend to be found incidentally, although intraluminal growth may eventually cause symptoms of obstruction, and some may grow large enough to ulcerate and bleed.

DIAGNOSIS

The physical examination in patients with small bowel tumors is often unremarkable, although there is occasionally a palpable mass and, in more advanced cases, ascites. As discussed earlier, patients with periampullary neoplasms may be jaundiced and/or icteric. Obstructive signs such as hyperperistalsis may be present, and those with lymphoma may also have splenomegaly or other signs of systemic involvement, such as lymphadenopathy. Laboratory findings may include iron deficiency anemia or increased hepatic enzymes (the latter is especially common in those with liver metastases or biliary obstruction). Serum levels of the carcinoembryonic antigen (CEA) tumor marker may be elevated in small bowel adenocarcinoma, especially in advanced cases, but it is neither sensitive nor specific enough for routine diagnostic use. Patients with neuroendocrine tumors may demonstrate elevated levels of serotonin, chromogranin A, tumor-specific bioactive amines (e.g., gastrin), or urinary 5-hydroxyindoleacetic acid. Variants of intestinal lymphomas may show heavy chain immunoglobulin A fragments in serum and urine.

Proper imaging is crucial for both diagnosis and staging of small bowel neoplasms, but no one method is clearly the best. Standard radiographic techniques of value include upper GI with small bowel follow-through (helpful in demonstrating both masses and potential mucosal defects), angiography (which may show a site of bleeding or tumor blush with specific neoplasms), and computed tomography (CT) or magnetic resonance imaging (MRI) enteroclysis (double-contrast studies are both sensitive and specific for small bowel masses). Transabdominal ultrasound and standard CT may indicate a primary mass as well as metastases; MRI appears to be superior to CT in detecting and characterizing liver metastases.

Primary neuroendocrine tumors and their metastases are often apparent on indium-111 octreotide scanning. A wide variety of histologies may have uptake on positron emission tomography (PET) scanning. However, PET does not yet have a well-defined role in the diagnosis of most small bowel malignancies, although PET scans are useful in those with GISTs to monitor response to systemic therapy (see later). Plain films rarely help make the diagnosis, but they may demonstrate intestinal obstruction.

Capsule endoscopy uses a wireless endoscopic device that allows minimally invasive imaging of the small intestine. The system consists of the capsule camera—a swallowable, self-contained battery-operated device that transmits two images per second—a receiver worn on the patient's belt, and a computerized work station for downloading and viewing the images. The primary indications for capsule endoscopy are the evaluation of obscure GI bleeding and Crohn's disease. Tumors are found in about 2 to 3% of patients undergoing capsule endoscopy for obscure GI bleeding, and they may be more common in younger patients. Tumors detected include lymphoma, adenocarcinoma, metastatic disease, carcinoid tumor, and GIST. Capsule endoscopy has also been used to assess the small intestines of patients with FAP and Peutz-Jeghers syndrome (PJS), although its clinical utility for the routine screening of these patients has not been established.

Surveillance

Patients with FAP, MUTYH polyposis, PJS, and probably HNPCC require regular surveillance of the small intestine, with specific recommendations as noted earlier. Patients with sporadic small intestine adenomas and possibly carcinoid tumors should undergo colonoscopy, because they are at increased risk for colonic neoplasia. No specific guidelines exist for following patients with resected small bowel adenocarcinomas.

Staging

The staging systems for small bowel tumors vary by histology. Adenocarcinomas and, more recently, neuroendocrine cancers and GISTs are staged using the American Joint Committee on Cancer's TNM classification of malignant tumors system. Intestinal non-Hodgkin's lymphomas, whether primary or part of a systemic process, are staged in accordance with a modified Ann Arbor system originally used in Hodgkin's disease (Chapter 191).

TREATMENT

Rx

In general, surgical excision is the treatment of choice for most localized small bowel tumors. The extent of excision necessary depends on the tumor's location and histology. Adenocarcinomas involving the first and second portions of the duodenum require pancreaticoduodenectomy, whereas those in the more distal small intestine may be treated with segmental or wide local resection, including regional lymph nodes. Low-grade neuroendocrine tumors should be managed with en bloc resection, again including regional nodes. GISTs, which very rarely spread to regional nodes, may be treated with excision without lymphadenectomy (except in cases with gross involvement of nodes). Primary surgery for lymphomas may be offered for low-stage malignancies and may also be required for complications of disease (e.g., intussusception). Local management of benign small bowel tumors varies from observation (incidentally discovered lipomas) to endoscopic polypectomy (small adenomas) to pancreaticoduodenectomy (periampullary villous adenomas).

The need for and types of adjuvant therapy vary as well. Fully resected benign tumors require no additional therapy. Adenocarcinomas are often treated according to the principles developed for colorectal cancer, with some experts advocating fluoropyrimidine-based systemic chemotherapy, at least for patients with nodal involvement. Chemoradiotherapy has also been recommended for those with more locally advanced duodenal adenocarcinomas. So far, no randomized trials have proved either strategy to be superior to surgery alone. Fully excised well- to moderately differentiated neuroendocrine cancers do not require adjuvant therapy. Postoperative imatinib mesylate treatment (see later) clearly postpones the recurrence of intermediate- and high-risk GISTs, but it is not yet known whether the cure rate is improved, and questions remain with regard to dose and duration of therapy. There is no defined role for the postoperative treatment of other mesenchymal tumors. Lymphomas treated with excision alone have high rates of recurrence, and systemic chemotherapy is advocated for high-grade variants; some experts also recommend chemotherapy for low-grade subtypes.

Patients with advanced small bowel adenocarcinomas are often treated with systemic chemotherapy regimens known to be effective against cancers of similar histology originating in the colon. However, the data supporting any specific regimen are scant and are not derived from randomized trials. Approximately 90% of patients with incurable GISTs have durable disease control when treated with the tyrosine kinase inhibitor imatinib mesylate, and the median survival for patients with metastatic disease has recently improved from approximately 18 months to 5 years.

Patients with small bowel lymphomas may be treated with chemotherapy that is effective in tumors of nodal origin.

PROGNOSIS

Patients with small bowel adenocarcinomas generally do worse than those with similarly staged colonic glandular tumors. Also, patients with duodenal primaries may have poorer outcomes than those with more distal small bowel cancers. In general, 5-year survival rates range from 4% for those with metastases to 80% for those with very early disease confined to the small bowel wall. Five-year survival in patients with small bowel carcinoids exceeds 50%. In the pre-imatinib era, patients with surgically resected small bowel GISTs had recurrence rates from 0 to 90% or higher, depending on the tumor's size, precise location, and mitotic rates, and those with more distal tumors had a worse prognosis than those with duodenal primaries. Patients with recurrences almost invariably died within 2 years because salvage surgery and systemic chemotherapy were ineffective. True life expectancy in this era of postoperative imatinib use is unknown, but the median survival of patients with advanced GISTs likely exceeds 5 years. Small intestinal lymphomas have 5-year survival rates surpassing 60%, although this is highly variable and depends on the histologic subtype.

NEOPLASMS OF THE LARGE INTESTINE

Colorectal cancer is the third most common cancer in the United States. Disease that has spread beyond regional lymph nodes is, for the most part, incurable, and colorectal cancer in general remains the second leading cause of neoplastic death. The lifetime risk of developing colorectal cancer for the average patient is about 1 in 18 to 20.

EPIDEMIOLOGY

Almost three quarters of large bowel cancers arise proximally (i.e., are of colonic origin). Although colorectal cancer is primarily a disease of the elderly (median age, ≈73 years), about 10% of cases occur in those 50 years of age or younger. Colorectal cancer incidence and mortality have decreased overall recently, although the incidence has been increasing in the young. Incidence rates for right-sided cancers have also been decreasing, possibly but not solely owing to effective distal large bowel screening with flexible sigmoidoscopy. Colorectal cancer is slightly more common in men than in women and in African Americans than in whites. Men develop colorectal cancer an average of 5 to 10 years earlier than women; similarly, large bowel cancers seem to arise an average of 5 to 10 years earlier in African Americans than in whites. There is much geographic variation in incidence that is probably based more on environmental factors than on genetic ones, as suggested by migration studies.

PATHOBIOLOGY

Between 96 and 98% of colorectal cancers are adenocarcinomas. Rarely seen histologies include neuroendocrine cancers, epidermoid carcinomas, lymphomas, and sarcomas (including GISTs). Additionally, composites, such as adenocarcinomas with neuroendocrine differentiation, are increasingly being described.

Adenocarcinomas derive from colonic columnar glandular epithelium in the colorectal mucosal lining. They are equally common in males and females and are most frequently reported in the sigmoid colon. Adenocarcinomas most commonly present at a localized or regional (nodal) stage. About two thirds are of moderate grade. The majority are nonmucinous, although the mucinous phenotype constitutes up to one fifth of all colorectal cancers. Another variant is the true signet ring carcinoma, identified by large quantities of single tumor cells with nuclear displacement by intracytoplasmic mucin. Mucinous tumors likely have a worse prognosis (data are controversial to date), whereas a signet ring histology almost always indicates a poorly differentiated or undifferentiated tumor and is clearly associated with a worse outcome.

Neuroendocrine cancers can have a variety of histologies, ranging from bland, well-differentiated carcinoids to high-grade small cell carcinomas. True carcinoids are the second most common histologic colorectal subtype. They are more common in nonwhites and make up the vast majority of non-adenocarcinoma epithelial cancers.

Distal bowel carcinoids are hormonally inactive. Noncarcinoid neuroendocrine cancers tend to be high grade and commonly present with hepatic and other distant metastases.

Epidermoid carcinomas are rare overall but still account for up to one fourth of colorectal cancers. Most are squamous cell subtypes. They are more common in women and Hispanics. Epidermoid carcinomas are located in the rectum more than 90% of the time, and they are usually moderately or poorly

TABLE 199-1 GENERAL FEATURES OF THE INHERITED COLORECTAL CANCER SYNDROMES

SYNDROME	POLYP HISTOLOGY	POLYP DISTRIBUTION	AGE OF ONSET	RISK OF COLON CANCER	GENETIC LESION	CLINICAL MANIFESTATIONS	ASSOCIATED LESIONS
Familial adenomatous polyposis	Adenoma	Large intestine, duodenum	16 yr (range, 8-34 yr)	100%	5q (*APC* gene)	Rectal bleeding, abdominal pain, bowel obstruction	Desmoids, CHRPE
Peutz-Jeghers syndrome	Hamartoma	Large and small intestine	First decade	Slightly above average	19p (*STK11*)	Possible rectal bleeding, abdominal pain, intussusception	Orocutaneous melanin pigment spots, other tumors
MUTYH-associated polyposis	Adenoma	Large intestine, duodenum	45-50 yr (range, 13-60 yr)	75% (range, 50-100%)	1p (*MYH* gene)	Rectal bleeding, abdominal pain, bowel obstruction	CHRPE, osteomas
Juvenile polyposis	Hamartoma (rarely adenoma)	Large and small intestine	First decade	≈9%	*PTEN, SMAD4, BMPR1*	Possible rectal bleeding, abdominal pain, intussusception	Pulmonary AVMs
Hereditary nonpolyposis colon cancer	Adenoma	Large intestine	40 yr (range, 18-65 yr)	30%	Mismatch repair genes*	Rectal bleeding, abdominal pain, bowel obstruction	Other tumors (e.g., ovary, uterus, pancreas, stomach)

*Including *hMSH2, hMSH3, hMSH6, hMLH1, hPMS1,* and *hPMS2.*
AVM = arteriovenous malformation; CHRPE = congenital hypertrophy of the retinal pigment epithelium.

differentiated. Interestingly, they commonly present as localized cancers, regardless of their degree of differentiation.

Primary colorectal lymphomas are fairly rare, constituting 10 to 20% of all GI lymphomas but less than 1% of colorectal cancers. They are much more common in males and in the elderly. The cecum is the most common site of origin. Tumors are usually of B-cell origin.

Sarcomas of the large bowel have no gender or racial predilections. More than 50% have been classified as leiomyosarcomas, most commonly found in the rectum. They are usually diagnosed at a localized stage, regardless of grade, although about 40% are actually poorly differentiated. Kaposi's sarcomas and GISTs are other sarcoma histologies found in the large bowel; many of the distal tumors called *leiomyosarcomas* in older registries were likely true GISTs.

Predisposing Conditions

Predisposing conditions for colonic neoplasia include age (discussed previously), gender, race, inflammatory bowel disease, family history, and defined inherited syndromes. Defined genetic cancer syndromes, however, account for only a small percentage of colorectal cancers (see later). Patients with first-degree relatives who also have colon neoplasia (adenomas or carcinomas) are commonly seen. Individuals with a first-degree relative with colorectal cancer face a two- to three-fold increased risk for malignancy, and this risk rises to five- or six-fold if two first-degree relatives are affected. Patients whose relatives have adenomas face a 1.8-fold increased risk for colorectal cancer, and this rises to 2.6 if the relative is younger than 60 years.

Patients with ulcerative colitis and Crohn's disease (Chapter 143) are at increased risk for colorectal cancer in proportion to the amount of bowel involved and the duration of illness. For example, adenocarcinoma of the colon is 10 to 20 times more common in persons with ulcerative colitis than in the general population. Between 2 and 4% of all patients with long-term ulcerative colitis develop this malignancy, and the cumulative incidence over a 25-year period is approximately 12%. Patients with both ulcerative colitis and primary sclerosing cholangitis seem to be at even greater risk. For those with Crohn's colitis, patients with extensive disease involving more than one third of the colon are at increased risk (six- to eight-fold), similar to those with ulcerative colitis. Isolated proctitis is not a risk factor. Patients with ulcerative colitis or extensive Crohn's disease should undergo screening colonoscopy every 1 to 2 years beginning 8 to 10 years after disease onset. At colonoscopy, multiple biopsies (at least 32 for pan-colitis) are obtained, and any suspicious lesions are sampled. The purpose of this is to identify the presence of dysplasia. The presence of high-grade dysplasia, any dysplasia in a mass or lesion that cannot be excised endoscopically, or multifocal low-grade dysplasia should prompt colectomy.

Patients who have had ureterocolostomy and those with acromegaly are also at increased risk. Case-control studies suggest that obesity, low physical activity, smoking, excessive alcohol, high-fat diet, and lack of dietary fiber increase the colorectal cancer risk. Patients with *Streptococcus bovis* bacteremia or endocarditis have increased rates of colorectal cancer and should undergo colonoscopy.

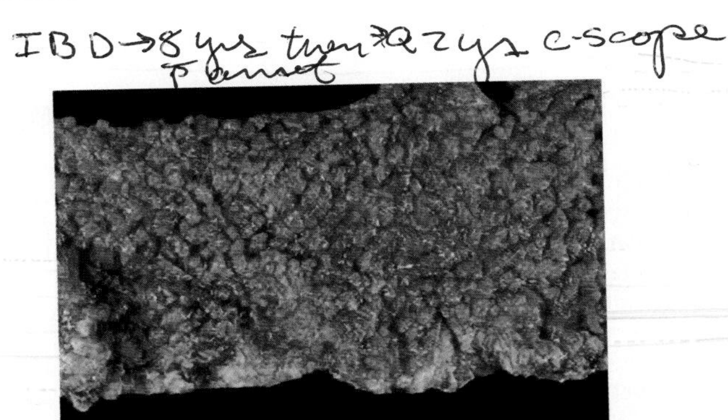

FIGURE 199-4. Resected colon lined with hundreds of adenomatous polyps in a patient with familial adenomatous polyposis.

Polyposis Syndromes

Several defined dominant and recessive genetic conditions have been identified that convey an increased risk of colorectal cancer (Table 199-1). These include FAP, HNPCC, MUTYH-associated polyposis, PJS, juvenile polyposis, PTEN hamartoma syndrome, and Cronkhite-Canada syndrome.

FAMILIAL ADENOMATOUS POLYPOSIS

FAP is an autosomal dominant condition characterized by the development of hundreds to thousands of adenomatous polyps and colorectal cancer by age 40 (Fig. 199-4). Estimates of disease prevalence are 1 in 8000 to 15,000 births.

PATHOBIOLOGY

FAP is inherited as an autosomal dominant disease with incomplete penetrance. It has been mapped to the adenomatous polyposis coli (*APC*) gene located on the long arm of chromosome 5 (5q21). *APC* is a tumor suppressor gene that is a critical regulator of intestinal epithelial cell growth. Inherited mutations generally result in a truncated gene product. Patients with the familial syndrome inherit one mutant copy of *APC*; when a loss-of-function mutation develops in the other *APC* allele, mucosal epithelial cell growth is no longer controlled normally, and polyps develop. Variable phenotypes can be partly attributed to differences in the location of the *APC* mutation, with attenuated FAP being seen in mutations at the 5′ and 3′ ends of the gene.

CLINICAL MANIFESTATIONS AND DIAGNOSIS

Adenomas begin to appear early in the second decade of life, and GI symptoms begin to appear in the third or fourth decade. Polyps are distributed relatively evenly throughout the colon, although a slight predominance has been noted in the distal colon. Almost all patients with FAP develop frank colorectal carcinoma by age 40 years if the condition is left untreated. Gastric polyps (mostly nonadenomatous) occur in 30 to 100% of patients, and duodenal adenomas are found in 45 to 90%. Periampullary duodenal cancer develops in approximately 10% of cases. Small bowel lesions that are distal to the duodenum rarely progress to malignancy. In attenuated FAP, fewer than 100 colonic adenomas develop, there is a right colon predominance, and cancer develops approximately 10 years later. Genetic testing may identify the mutation in up to 85% of affected individuals and is useful for family screening.

TREATMENT Rx

The primary treatment option in FAP patients is total proctocolectomy with conventional ileostomy or ileoanal (pouch) anastomosis. Individuals with *APC* mutations and those with no identified mutation but clinical FAP in their families should be screened with annual sigmoidoscopy beginning at age 10 to 12 years. In families with known *APC* mutations, individuals who test negative do not require heightened surveillance but should undergo routine risk screening. FAP patients should be screened for duodenal polyposis with upper endoscopy beginning at age 20 years, with subsequent surveillance depending on polyp burden and histology.

GARDNER'S SYNDROME

Gardner's syndrome is a phenotypic subtype of FAP that is also caused by mutations in the *APC* gene. It is distinguished by the presence of extraintestinal manifestations, including osteomas (particularly mandibular), soft tissue tumors (including lipomas, sebaceous cysts, and fibrosarcomas), supernumerary teeth, desmoid tumors, mesenteric fibromatosis, and congenital hypertrophy of the retinal pigment epithelium. The phenotypic differences between Gardner's syndrome and FAP appear to result from variations in the location of the *APC* mutation, the presence of modifying genes, and environmental factors. Adenomatous polyps in Gardner's syndrome have the same malignant potential as those found in FAP, and colorectal cancer screening and treatment recommendations are the same.

TURCOT'S SYNDROME

A hallmark of Turcot's syndrome is the combination of colorectal polyposis and malignant diseases of the central nervous system. Mutations in the *APC* gene account for two thirds of cases, and the remaining one third result from mutations in the DNA mismatch repair genes that are also mutated in HNPCC. Central nervous system manifestations include medulloblastomas, glioblastomas, and ependymomas.

HEREDITARY NONPOLYPOSIS COLON CANCER

HNPCC, also known as *Lynch syndrome*, is the most common hereditary colorectal cancer syndrome and accounts for approximately 2% of all cases of colorectal cancer (Chapter 184). It is an autosomal dominant trait and is highly penetrant. Clinically, HNPCC has been defined by the presence of all three of the following: (1) three or more relatives with histologically verified HNPCC-associated cancer (colorectal cancer or cancer of the endometrium, small bowel, ureter, or renal pelvis), one of whom is a first-degree relative of the other two, in the absence of FAP; (2) colorectal cancer involving at least two generations; and (3) one or more family members with cancer diagnosed before age 50 years.

PATHOBIOLOGY

HNPCC is caused by loss-of-function germline mutations in a set of genes involved in the repair of DNA base pair mismatches that occur during DNA replication (also known as the *mutation mismatch repair system*). The genetic basis of HNPCC (Lynch syndrome) is described in greater detail in Chapter 184.

CLINICAL MANIFESTATIONS AND DIAGNOSIS

The median age for diagnosis of HNPCC is the mid-40s. Although several adenomas may be present, the diffuse polyposis characteristic of FAP is not found. Colonic neoplasia has a right-sided predominance (proximal to the splenic flexure). Although the cancers tend to be poorly differentiated, they generally have a better prognosis than similar sporadic colorectal cancers. Synchronous and metachronous colorectal cancer is common. Patients with HNPCC are also at high risk for other malignant diseases, especially endometrial carcinoma, as well as cancers of the ovary, stomach, small bowel, hepatobiliary tract, ureter, and pancreas. The Muir-Torre syndrome variant is associated with cutaneous lesions and visceral malignancies. Screening for HNPCC may begin with testing of the tumor for microsatellite instability, performing immunohistochemical staining for products of mismatch repair genes (including *hMSH2, hMSH3, hMSH6, hMLH1, hPMS1,* and *hPMS2*), and/or *BRAF* gene mutation testing. A positive screen does not definitely indicate HNPCC because up to 15% of sporadic tumors may have these features; this should be followed with germline testing.

TREATMENT Rx

Persons potentially affected with HNPCC should undergo a colonoscopy every 2 years beginning at age 21 years and annually beginning at age 40. Patients with colorectal cancer or large adenomas should undergo subtotal colectomy. Women in HNPCC-affected families should have pelvic examinations every 1 to 3 years beginning at age 18 years; annual pelvic examinations, transvaginal ultrasonography, and endometrial biopsy have been recommended beginning at age 25 years. Prophylactic total abdominal hysterectomy with bilateral salpingo-oophorectomy may also be considered at the time of colectomy.

MUTYH-ASSOCIATED POLYPOSIS

MUTYH-associated polyposis is a recently described autosomal recessive syndrome caused by mutations in the *MYH* gene. It is characterized by colonic polyposis and a high rate of colorectal cancer. In a Finnish colon cancer registry, 0.4% of patients were homozygous for *MYH* mutations.

PATHOBIOLOGY

MUTYH-associated polyposis is caused by a biallelic inherited defect in the *MYH* gene located on chromosome 1p. Inherited as an autosomal recessive trait, this leads to defects in base excision repair and acquired mutations of the *APC* gene and other genes, such as *KRAS*. This results in adenoma formation and the subsequent development of adenocarcinoma.

CLINICAL MANIFESTATIONS AND DIAGNOSIS

Phenotypically, affected patients are similar to those with attenuated FAP. Patients have five to hundreds of adenomas. The onset is later than in classic FAP, with cancers more likely to be right sided and to occur at age 45 to 50 years. Associated extracolonic features include gastroduodenal polyps, duodenal carcinoma, breast and ovarian cancer in female carriers, bladder cancer, skin cancer, congenital hypertrophy of the retinal pigment epithelium, and osteoma. Monoallelic carriers do not appear to have an increased cancer risk.

The diagnosis is suggested by the presence of colonic polyposis in the absence of FAP, or when there appears to be recessive inheritance. In these cases, genetic testing for *MYH* gene mutations should be considered. Whether heterozygote carriers are at increased risk has not been established, but screening similar to that for individuals with first-degree relatives with colorectal cancer may be advisable (i.e., colonoscopy at age 40 and then every 5 years).

TREATMENT Rx

Patients with numerous polyps should undergo colectomy. Patients with mild disease and a relatively small number of polyps may be considered for colonoscopy with polypectomy and regular surveillance. Colonoscopy should be performed beginning at age 18 to 20 and repeated every 1 to 2 years. Regular endoscopic surveillance for duodenal polyps should also be performed beginning at age 25 to 30.

PEUTZ-JEGHERS SYNDROME

PJS is an intestinal hamartomatous polyposis of the upper and lower GI tract that is associated with characteristic mucocutaneous pigmentation. The

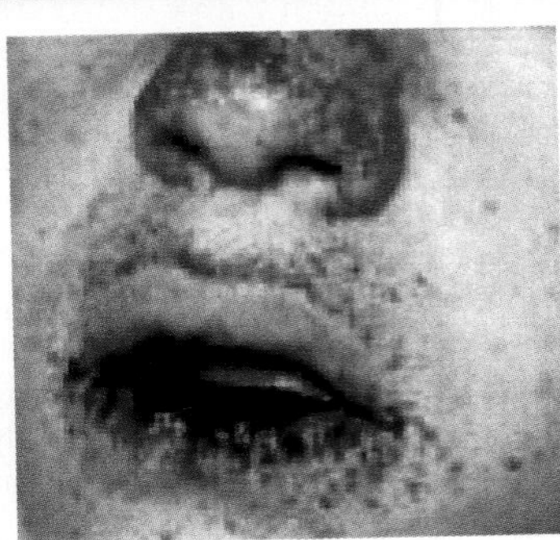

FIGURE 199-5. Mucosal pigmentation in a patient with Peutz-Jeghers syndrome.

average age at diagnosis is in the mid-20s. PHS predisposes to both intestinal and extraintestinal malignancies.

PATHOBIOLOGY

PJS is a rare autosomal dominant syndrome with high penetrance. The prevalence is between 1 in 8300 and 1 in 29,000. The gene responsible for the syndrome is the serine-threonine kinase *(STK11)* gene located on chromosome 19p; a mutation in *STK11* is found in approximately 60% of patients with this syndrome. The hamartomatous polyps in PJS are located predominantly in the small intestine (64 to 96%), stomach (24 to 49%), and colon (60%). Histologically, these polyps are benign; they are unique, in that a layer of muscle that extends into the submucosa or muscularis propria may surround the glandular tissue. Adenomatous and hyperplastic polyps may also be found.

CLINICAL MANIFESTATIONS AND DIAGNOSIS

The most common symptoms are small bowel intussusception, obstruction, and GI bleeding that may require surgery and may be recurrent. PJS is associated with an increased risk of cancer, with an estimated 47% of patients developing a malignancy by age 65. The most common cancers are those of the small intestine, stomach, colon, pancreas, testes, breast, ovary, cervix, and uterus. More than 95% of patients have a characteristic pattern of melanin spots on the lips, buccal mucosa, and skin (Fig. 199-5). Because genetic testing is not widely available, first-degree relatives should be screened beginning at birth with an annual history, physical examination, and evaluation for melanotic spots, precocious puberty, and testicular tumors.

TREATMENT Rx

Standard medical care for patients with PJS involves an annual physical examination that includes evaluation of the breasts, abdomen, pelvis, and testes, as well as a complete blood count. Surveillance for cancer includes small bowel radiography every 2 years, esophagogastroduodenoscopy and colonoscopy every 2 years, and endoscopic ultrasound of the pancreas every 1 to 2 years. For women, annual Pap smear, transvaginal ultrasound, CA125, and mammography are recommended. Polyps larger than 1 cm should be removed endoscopically. Laparotomy and resection are recommended for recurrent or persistent small intestinal intussusception, obstruction, or intestinal bleeding.

JUVENILE POLYPOSIS

Familial juvenile (non-neoplastic, hamartomatous) polyposis is a rare (<1 in 100,000 births) syndrome characterized by 10 or more non-neoplastic, hamartomatous polyps throughout the GI tract or any number of polyps in a patient with a family history of juvenile polyposis. The syndrome is inherited in an autosomal dominant manner with high penetrance and is caused by mutations in the *SMAD4, PTEN,* or *BMPR1A* gene. The hamartomas are histologically distinct from the polyps seen in PJS. Patients generally present with rectal bleeding, anemia, abdominal pain, or intestinal obstruction in childhood or early adolescence. Extraintestinal symptoms include pulmonary arteriovenous malformations in some probands. The risk of malignancy in juvenile polyposis is reportedly as high as 20% and occurs in adulthood (median age, 37 years). Affected individuals should undergo regular colonoscopic surveillance. Patients with numerous, large, or high-grade dysplastic polyps may be considered for subtotal colectomy. Family members should be screened with colonoscopy every 3 to 5 years beginning at age 12 until age 40.

PTEN HAMARTOMA SYNDROME

PTEN hamartoma syndrome is a rare, autosomal dominant syndrome consisting of multiple hamartomatous polyps of the skin and mucous membranes, including GI polyps, facial tricholemmomas, oral papillomas, and keratoses of the hands and feet. It was previously referred to as Cowden's syndrome and Bannayan-Riley-Ruvalcaba syndrome. The causative genetic lesion has been mapped to the *PTEN* tumor suppressor gene. The rate of associated malignancy is high, particularly in the thyroid, breast, and reproductive organs. The polyps in PTEN hamartoma syndrome are benign.

CRONKHITE-CANADA SYNDROME

Cronkhite-Canada syndrome is a rare, sporadic, acquired condition characterized by multiple hamartomatous polyps throughout the GI tract, along with alopecia, dermal pigmentation, and atrophy of the nail beds. Symptoms include diarrhea, protein-losing enteropathy, GI bleeding, intussusception, and rectal prolapse. It carries a poor prognosis, with 5-year mortality rates as high as 55%. Patients are at risk for gastric and colorectal cancer, and endoscopic surveillance has been recommended.

Polyps of the Colon

A *polyp* is defined as a grossly visible mass of epithelial cells that protrudes from the mucosal surface into the lumen of the intestine. A polyp may be sessile, flat, or pedunculated when it is attached by a stalk. Polyps are classified as either non-neoplastic or neoplastic (adenomatous). Polyps may rarely cause symptoms such as bleeding, prolapse, or obstruction. Neoplastic polyps have the potential to become malignant.

NONADENOMATOUS POLYPS

Nonadenomatous polyps, which account for approximately 90% of all mucosal polyps detected in the large bowel, can be found in more than 50% of people older than 60 years. These polyps, which are also termed *non-neoplastic polyps,* can be subcategorized into hyperplastic, inflammatory, lymphoid, and juvenile polyps. Most non-neoplastic polyps are hyperplastic polyps that arise as a result of abnormal maturation of the mucosal epithelial cells; these polyps are usually small in diameter and are found predominantly in the distal sigmoid colon and rectum. Hyperplastic polyps are not malignant and are not thought to be associated with any measurable increase in malignant potential. However, those with multiple, large right-sided hyperplastic polyps may be at increased risk. Patients with inflammatory bowel disease may develop inflammatory pseudopolyps, which may require biopsy or removal to distinguish them from neoplastic polyps. Lymphoid polyps are regions of the mucosa that contain exaggerated intramucosal lymphoid tissue. Juvenile polyps usually develop in the rectum of children younger than 5 years and are termed *hamartomatous* because they are focal malformations that resemble tumors but are caused by abnormal development of the lamina propria; these polyps require no therapy unless they cause symptoms, such as obstruction or severe bleeding, or are part of a genetic syndrome.

ADENOMATOUS POLYPS

DEFINITION

Adenomatous polyps (or adenomas) are neoplastic polyps with malignant potential. They are benign glandular tumors that exhibit either low- or high-grade dysplasia under microscopy. Their anatomic distribution parallels that of colorectal adenocarcinoma. Adenomatous polyps manifest in a range of sizes and may be sessile, flat, or pedunculated in morphology. They are believed to be the precursor lesion to colorectal adenocarcinoma, a process that occurs according to the adenoma-carcinoma sequence. Evidence supporting the adenoma-carcinoma sequence comes from several sources. Patients with genetic conditions that predispose to adenoma formation (e.g., FAP) develop cancer at high rates. Animal studies in which adenomas are induced by either carcinogens or genetic manipulation show carcinoma formation. Correlative evidence includes the observations that the epidemiology is similar for adenomas and carcinomas, that both lesions are more common in the same anatomic locations, and that adenomatous tissue can often be found in small adenocarcinomas. Intervention studies have shown that the removal of adenomatous polyps leads to a significant decrease in the risk for colorectal cancer.

EPIDEMIOLOGY

Adenomatous polyps are relatively common, particularly in elderly populations. Among healthy screening populations older than 50 years, adenomas are found in more than 15% of women and 25% of men. The prevalence of adenomas tends to be high in regions of the world where colorectal cancer is common. The importance of genetic risk factors is clear in the hereditary polyposis syndromes, and sporadic adenomas have a familial component; for example, individuals with a positive first-degree family history have a fourfold greater risk of developing adenomatous polyps. Blacks in the United States have an increased risk for developing adenomas and carcinomas relative to whites; the risk in Asians and Hispanics is similar to that in whites.

PATHOBIOLOGY

The layer of epithelial cells lining the surface of the normal large bowel undergoes continuous self-renewal, with a turnover period of 3 to 8 days. Undifferentiated stem cells located at the base of invaginated crypts give rise to cells that migrate toward the lumen as they differentiate further into specialized enterocytes; these cells are subsequently removed by apoptosis, by extrusion, or by phagocytes underlying the epithelial layer. The development of adenomatous polyps is associated with a sequence-specific accumulation of genetic lesions that cause an imbalance between epithelial cell proliferation and cell death. As a result, cells accumulate at the luminal surface, where they remain undifferentiated and continue to undergo cell division, eventually leading to the abnormal development of a mass of adenomatous tissue.

Adenomas are classified into three main histologic subtypes: tubular adenomas, villous adenomas (Fig. 199-6), and tubulovillous adenomas. Tubular adenomas, which are the most common type, account for 70 to 85% of all adenomas removed at colonoscopy. They are often small and pedunculated, and they consist of dysplastic tubular glands that divide and branch out from the mucosal surface; they rarely contain concomitant high-grade dysplasia or carcinoma. In contrast, villous adenomas are rarer (<5% of all adenomas), are generally large and sessile, and are composed of strands of dysplastic epithelium that project, finger-like, into the lumen of the gut; they have a much higher prevalence of high-grade dysplasia or carcinoma. Tubulovillous adenomas (10 to 25% of all adenomas) have a mixture of tubular and villous architecture. Advanced adenomas are defined as those that measure 1 cm or greater or have any villous histology or high-grade dysplasia. Patients with advanced adenomas or multiple adenomas (three or more) are at much greater risk for synchronous (developing simultaneously) or metachronous (developing after a time interval) colorectal cancer.

CLINICAL MANIFESTATIONS

Patients with adenomatous polyps generally remain asymptomatic, but they may present with an asymptomatic positive stool occult blood test or with evident hematochezia. The lifetime incidence of additional adenomas in a patient with one known adenoma is 30 to 50%. Less than 5% of all adenomas eventually develop into carcinomas. Two critical factors that determine the likelihood of an adenoma developing into an invasive lesion are the size of the polyp and the grade of dysplasia. For polyps less than 1 cm, the risk for carcinoma is 1 to 3%; polyps between 1 and 2 cm have a 10% risk of becoming cancerous; and more than 40% of polyps greater than 2 cm progress to an invasive lesion. All adenomatous polyps contain some degree of dysplasia, but they can be further categorized as low or high grade to indicate the degree of dysplasia and the corresponding risk for invasive carcinoma. High-grade dysplasia is associated with a 27% rate of eventual transformation into carcinoma.

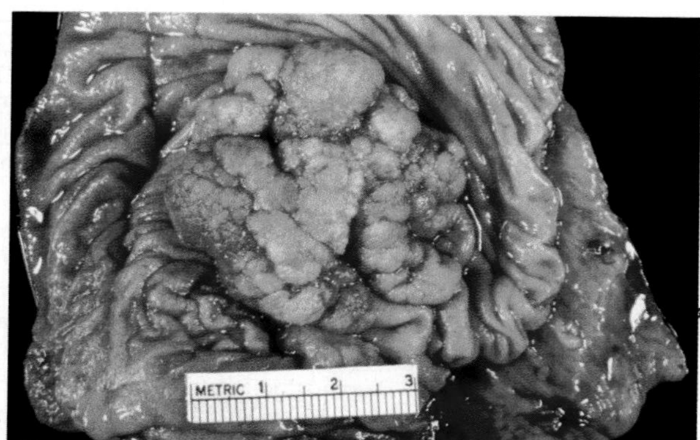

FIGURE 199-6. Villous adenoma. Large and sessile villous adenomas of the large bowel with finger-like projections into the gut lumen. (Courtesy Dr. M. K. Washington.)

DIAGNOSIS

Adenomatous polyps in the colon and rectum can be diagnosed by endoscopy, barium radiography, or CT scanning (CT colography or virtual colonoscopy). Colonoscopy is the preferred method for diagnosing adenomas because of its high accuracy and the ability to immediately biopsy and resection most polyps. Barium enema, as assessed in the National Polyp Study, missed 52% of polyps measuring 1 cm or more. CT colography has good sensitivity for detecting large (>1 cm) polyps (>85%) and for detecting cancers (96%), but it is less sensitive and specific for smaller polyps. CT colography requires bowel preparation, exposes the patient to ionizing radiation, and cannot remove polyps. Colonoscopy may miss 6 to 12% of large (≥1 cm) polyps and 5% of cancers. Of note is that nonpolypoid (flat and depressed) colorectal neoplasms are found in about 9% of asymptomatic and symptomatic adults on colonoscopy and are more likely to contain a carcinoma than are polypoid lesions; these lesions may not be visible on barium radiography or CT.

Flexible sigmoidoscopy, which is often used to screen asymptomatic persons at average risk for colorectal adenocarcinoma, detects 50 to 60% of all polyps and cancers. Generally, patients who have polyps detected by barium radiography, CT colography, or flexible sigmoidoscopy should undergo colonoscopy to remove the lesion and search for additional polyps. In one study in which patients with polyps discovered by flexible sigmoidoscopy underwent subsequent colonoscopy, there was an 80% reduction in the incidence of colorectal cancer.

TREATMENT Rx

The goal of treatment for adenomatous polyps is to remove or destroy the lesion during endoscopy. This recommendation is based on overwhelming evidence that endoscopic polypectomy reduces the subsequent incidence and mortality of colorectal cancer. Pedunculated adenomas are generally removed by snare polypectomy, with subsequent submission of the tissue for pathologic analysis. Piecemeal snare resection may be required to remove sessile polyps. Surgical resection of a polyp is indicated when endoscopic resection of an advanced adenoma is not possible. The biopsied polyp must be evaluated histologically to determine the presence or absence of carcinoma; if a malignant lesion is found, its histologic grade, vascular and lymphatic involvement, and proximity to the margin of resection should be determined. Unfavorable histopathologic factors that should prompt surgical resection include poorly differentiated histology, vascular invasion, lymphatic invasion, and incomplete endoscopic resection. Pedunculated polyps with cancer confined to the submucosa, with no evidence of unfavorable histologic features, can be definitively treated with endoscopic resection, without the need for surgical resection. Whether similar malignant sessile polyps can be managed nonoperatively is controversial. In these cases, the risk of surgery versus the risk of recurrence or lymphatic metastases needs to be balanced.

PROGNOSIS

Patients who have undergone resection of an adenomatous polyp are at increased risk for the subsequent development of adenoma and colorectal adenocarcinoma. This risk is influenced by the size, histology, and number of adenomas, and the surveillance intervals differ (Table 199-2). Low-risk patients—those with only one or two small tubular adenomas—should

TABLE 199-2 POST–ADENOMA RESECTION SURVEILLANCE INTERVALS

FINDINGS	INTERVAL
1-2 adenomas, <1 cm	5 yr
3-10 adenomas, adenoma with villous features, ≥1 cm, or with high-grade dysplasia	3 yr
>10 adenomas	<3 yr
Sessile adenoma ≥2 cm, piecemeal excision	2-6 mo

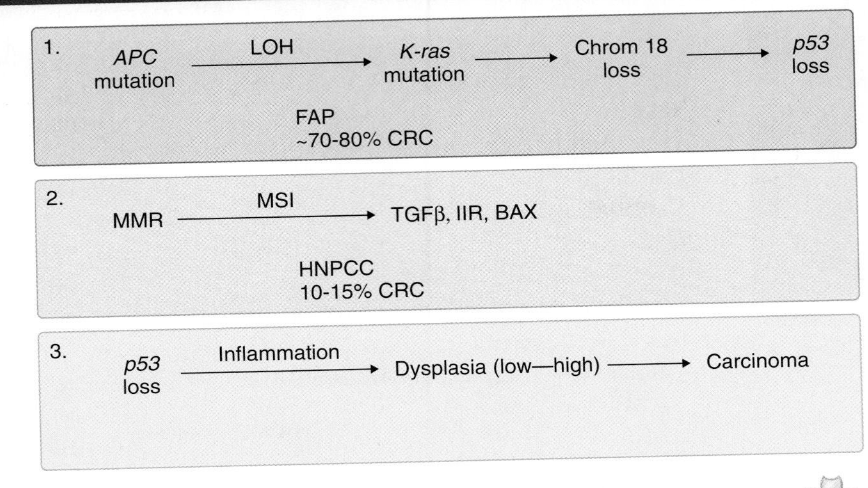

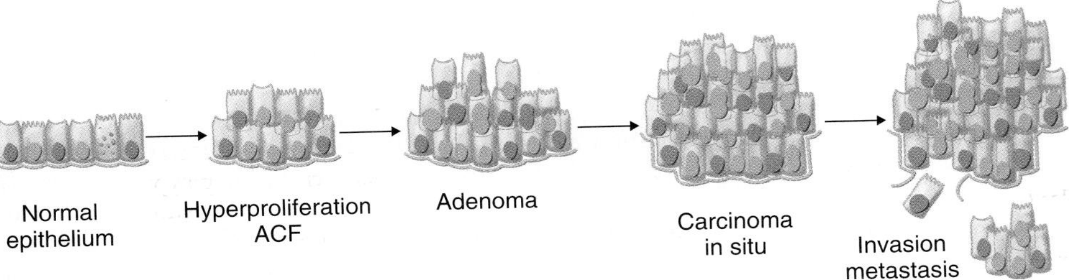

FIGURE 199-7. The molecular basis of colorectal cancer. Sequence-specific genetic lesions result in the transition from normal large bowel mucosa to invasive carcinoma. ACF = aberrant crypt foci; BAX = apoptosis-related protein; CRC = colorectal cancer; HNPCC = hereditary nonpolyposis colorectal cancer; IIR = type II receptor; LOH = loss of heterozygosity; MMR = mutation mismatch repair; MSI = microsatellite instability; TGFβ = transforming growth factor-β.

undergo colonoscopy in 5 years. Patients with multiple (more than two) adenomas, large (≥1 cm) adenomas, or adenomas with villous or high-grade histology should undergo colonoscopy in 3 years. Patients with numerous (>10) adenomas should undergo colonoscopy within 3 years. Patients who have had polypectomy of a large (≥2 cm) adenoma or an adenoma that had to be removed in pieces (piecemeal resection) should undergo colonoscopy within 6 months to evaluate the completeness of the resection.

Adenocarcinoma of the Colon and Rectum

PATHOBIOLOGY

Colorectal cancer is caused by the accumulation of multiple genetic lesions in sequence over time. Both the tissue architecture and the cellular genotype change as the disease progresses (Fig. 199-7). Early in the pathogenesis, mutations occur in either the *APC* gene (approximately 80% of sporadic colon cancers) or one of the mismatch repair genes (15% of sporadic colon cancers). The *APC* gene regulates cell growth and apoptosis, and mutations result in aberrant crypt foci, crypt dysplasia, and adenoma formation; 50% of sporadic adenomas have *APC* mutations. Mismatch repair gene mutations result in the failure to repair DNA transcription errors and the accumulation of additional mutations. Germline mutations in *APC* are the cause of FAP, and germline mutations of mismatch repair genes cause HNPCC (Lynch syndrome). Colorectal cancer pathogenesis requires additional mutations, including *DCC* ("deleted in colon cancer"), a tumor suppressor gene; *p53*, a regulator of the cell cycle; and *KRAS*, involved in the transduction of mitogenic signals across cell membranes. The accumulation of mutations leads to genetic instability and loss of heterozygosity where cells have only one allele of a gene owing to the loss of individual chromosomes during mitosis. DNA methylation can result in inactivation of tumor suppressor genes such as *p14* and *p16*. Other genetic and epigenetic alterations, including the expression of genes capable of cleaving extracellular matrix and a protein tyrosine phosphatase, lead to metastasis.

CLINICAL MANIFESTATIONS

The majority of patients with colorectal cancer present with symptoms that may be emergent. Common symptoms related to primary disease include rectal bleeding with or without manifestations of anemia, abdominal pain, and change in bowel function. Patients with systemic disease may exhibit anorexia, weight loss, and symptoms related to hepatic dysfunction, such as jaundice, icterus, and ascites (the last may also be seen with peritoneal metastases). Symptoms vary, depending on the primary site (Fig. 199-8):

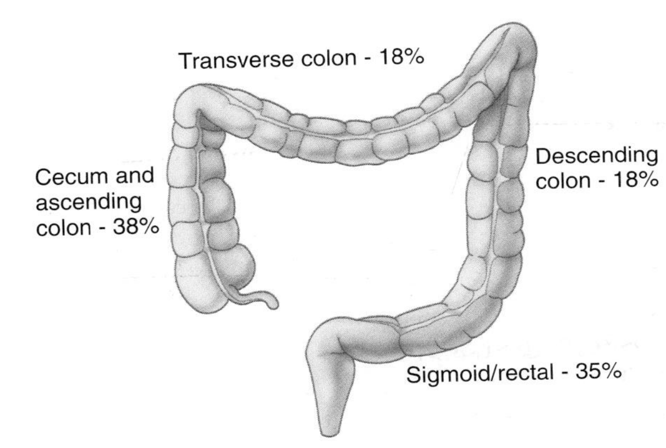

FIGURE 199-8. Sites of development of large bowel adenocarcinoma.

proximal lesions are more likely to present with bleeding and associated symptoms; more distal disease has a higher risk of obstruction and perforation. Rectal cancers can also manifest with tenesmus and changes in stool caliber. They involve sacral nerve plexi, causing significant neuropathic pain. Patients with PJS or Gardner's syndrome may exhibit extraintestinal manifestations.

DIAGNOSIS

The history, physical examination, and judicious use of both laboratory and radiologic tests are important in diagnosing colorectal cancer. The history should include prior colorectal cancer or adenomatous polyps, inflammatory bowel disease, and family history of colonic neoplasia. On physical examination, extraintestinal lesions characteristic of PJS or Gardner's syndrome may be noticed. Metastatic disease is suggested by enlargement, characteristically of the supraclavicular lymph nodes (Virchow's nodes) or the liver, or by the presence of an umbilical mass (Sister Mary Joseph's node) or ascites. The digital rectal examination may reveal a distal rectal cancer or spread of the tumor to the rectal shelf or pelvis (Blumer's shelf). The stool shows evidence of frank or occult blood in 40 to 80% of advanced cases. Iron deficiency anemia or an elevation in liver enzymes may aid in the diagnosis. The CEA level may be elevated, but it cannot be relied on for diagnosis owing to inadequate sensitivity.

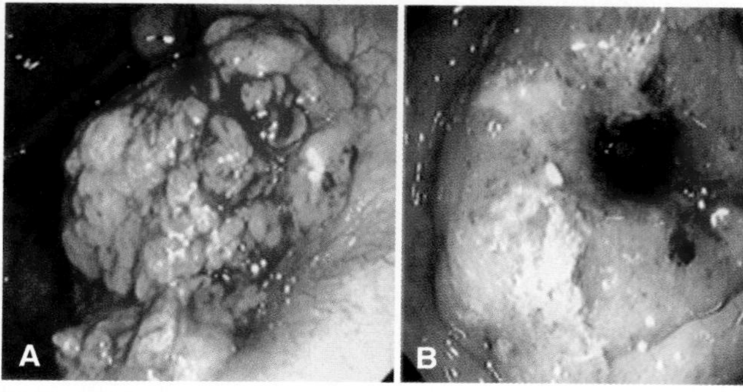

FIGURE 199-9. **Two manifestations of large bowel adenocarcinoma. A,** Exophytic growth within the lumen. **B,** Stricturing ("apple core") lesion.

TABLE 199-3 OPTIONS FOR COLORECTAL NEOPLASIA SCREENING*

TEST	INTERVAL
TESTS THAT DETECT ADENOMATOUS POLYPS OR CANCER	
Colonoscopy	Every 10 yr
Flexible sigmoidoscopy†	Every 5 yr
CT colography†	Every 5 yr
Double-contrast barium enema†	Every 5 yr
TESTS THAT DETECT PRIMARILY CANCER†	
Fecal occult blood tests	
High-sensitivity guaiac-based fecal occult blood test	Annually
Fecal immunochemical test	Annually
Stool DNA	Interval uncertain

*Beginning at age 50 for average-risk individuals.
†A positive test should prompt full colonoscopy.
CT = computed tomography.

Methods for diagnosing colorectal cancer are similar to those used to detect adenomatous polyps. Colonoscopy is the procedure of choice for all patients who have occult blood in their stools, unexplained iron deficiency anemia, or signs and symptoms suggestive of colorectal cancer (Fig. 199-9). Colonoscopy is more accurate than barium radiographic studies for the detection of colorectal neoplasms of all sizes and has the advantage of enabling the clinician to detect synchronous cancers and to obtain tissue for histologic analysis.

Additionally, accurate *local* staging of rectal cancers is paramount. Endoscopic ultrasound combines high-frequency ultrasonography with videoendoscopy. It is superior to CT and allows an accurate determination of the degree of invasion and detection and sampling of enlarged lymph nodes. Endoscopic ultrasound is also highly sensitive for the detection of rectal cancer recurrence after local resection or low anterior resection. MRI using either endorectal or phased array coils can also provide accurate local staging of rectal cancer. Local staging of nonrectal large bowel cancer is generally not performed preoperatively because this information is not used to guide therapy.

Many expert consensus guidelines now recommend CT scans of the abdomen and pelvis for colorectal cancer patients because liver metastases would preclude resection of an asymptomatic primary. Chest imaging with plain films or CT is recommended as well. PET scans have specific uses in defined cases of colorectal cancer, such as precluding additional systemic disease before resection of a solitary metastatic site. They may also be used to further describe abnormalities seen on CT. However, there is no role for PET in the routine work-up. Plain abdominal films are useful only in diagnosing obstruction.

Screening

The purpose of screening is to reduce colorectal cancer–related mortality by removing the precursor adenomas and detecting prevalent cancers at earlier, more curable stages. The long latency between adenoma development and subsequent cancer, on the order of 10 to 20 years, makes colorectal cancer a preventable disease through colonoscopy with polypectomy. It is an age-associated disease, and most patients should begin screening at age 50. There is a range of options for average-risk individuals (Table 199-3). These can be divided into two categories: stool tests, which include tests for occult blood and abnormal DNA, and structural tests, which include colonoscopy, flexible sigmoidoscopy, CT colography, and double-contrast barium enema. Stool tests are best suited for detecting prevalent cancers (and some advanced adenomas), whereas structural tests detect both cancers and adenomas. These tests may be used alone or in combination. Current multisociety guidelines recognize the multiple screening options but encourage the use of structural tests that have the ability to both detect and prevent colorectal cancer.

Tests for fecal occult blood detect hemoglobin in the stool from bleeding tumors. These tests are either guaiac based or immunochemical based. The guaiac tests detect blood in stool through the pseudoperoxidase activity of heme or hemoglobin. The immunochemical tests react with human globin and are therefore more specific. Guaiac testing consists of collecting two samples from three consecutive stools. To improve test accuracy, individuals undergoing guaiac testing are instructed to avoid aspirin, nonsteroidal anti-inflammatory drugs (NSAIDs), vitamin C, red meat, poultry, fish, and some vegetables. Three large, prospective randomized trials demonstrated that guaiac-based testing decreased colorectal cancer mortality by 15 to 33%, with one large U.S. study also showing a 20% decrease in colorectal cancer incidence, attributed to the relatively higher rates of colonoscopy in the study group. Guaiac-based tests have sensitivities for cancer from 35 to 80%. Immunochemical-based tests do not rely on a peroxidase reaction and therefore may have fewer false-positives and false-negatives. They do not require the dietary restrictions of guaiac-based tests. Despite these advantages, studies have not demonstrated a clear-cut benefit of immunochemical tests over highly sensitive guaiac-based tests. Fecal occult blood tests are repeated annually, and any positive test should prompt colonoscopy.

Stool DNA tests rely on the observation that both adenomas and carcinomas contain altered DNA, and this DNA is shed in the stool. Tests contain a multiple marker panel designed to detect mutations in *KRAS*, *APC*, and *p53*; a probe for BAT-26 (a marker of microsatellite instability); and a marker of DNA integrity analysis. Collection kits are designed to facilitate stool collection (at least 30 g) and mailing. In a screening population, stool DNA had better sensitivity for colorectal cancer (52%) than a relatively insensitive guaiac-based test (unrehydrated Hemoccult II; 13% sensitivity). Stool DNA did not have good sensitivity for advanced adenomas (defined as >1 cm, villous, or with high-grade dysplasia), detecting only 15%. Stool DNA testing is more expensive than fecal occult blood testing, and the optimal screening interval has not been defined.

Flexible sigmoidoscopy is capable of examining the distal 60 cm of the colon, or roughly the splenic flexure to the rectum. It can be done with minimal bowel preparation, does not require sedation, and can be performed by primary care providers, nurses, or physician's assistants. Flexible sigmoidoscopy can detect either left-sided cancers or polyps. The detection of an adenoma should prompt referral for full colonoscopy, owing to the high prevalence of synchronous neoplasia in the unexamined proximal colon. In case-control studies, flexible sigmoidoscopy is associated with 60 to 80% reduction in colorectal cancer mortality in the area of the examined colon—an effect that persists for up to 10 years. In one randomized trial, a single flexible sigmoidoscopy performed once between ages 55 to 64 years reduced colorectal cancer incidence by 23% and mortality by 31%.[1] Sigmoidoscopy should be repeated every 5 years and may be combined with yearly fecal occult blood testing.

Colonoscopy allows complete examination of the colon, as well as adenoma removal and thus cancer prevention. In the United States it is generally done under sedation, after an oral bowel preparation, and by physicians with specific training in colonoscopy and polypectomy. There are no direct randomized studies assessing the efficacy of colonoscopy for screening, although there is a large amount of indirect evidence. Colonoscopy is generally used as the "gold standard" in assessing other screening methods. In a large, randomized Minnesota study of fecal occult blood testing, a decrease in cancer incidence was observed that could be explained only by the use of colonoscopy and polypectomy at a higher rate in the screened population. Case-control studies of sigmoidoscopy demonstrate a colorectal cancer mortality benefit that should also apply to colonoscopy. The National Polyp Study, which followed patients after polypectomy, found that the incidence of colorectal cancer was reduced 76 to 90% compared to three reference populations. However, recent dietary and chemotherapeutic intervention trials found less of an effect, so the magnitude of the benefit is currently uncertain. If the initial screening colonoscopy is normal, further screening can be deferred for 10 years.

Double-contrast barium enema evaluates the entire colon by coating the mucosal surface with high-density barium and insufflating with air via a rectal tube. Multiple radiographs are obtained while varying the patient's position under fluoroscopy. It requires a colon preparation and exposes the patient to a small amount of ionizing radiation. There are no studies of double-contrast barium enema as a screening test. It is 85 to 97% sensitive for colon cancer, but its sensitivity for detecting large adenomas is only 48 to 73%. It should be repeated every 5 years. The finding of a polyp larger than 5 mm should prompt colonoscopy.

CT colography (also known as *virtual colonoscopy*) uses multidetector CT technology to obtain two- and three-dimensional images of the entire colon. It requires an adequate colon preparation and gaseous distention of the bowel using a rectal tube. Tagging of residual stool with barium or iodinated contrast material is frequently used. CT scanning is performed with the patient in the supine and prone positions. No studies have been done to evaluate the efficacy of CT colography in decreasing colorectal cancer incidence or mortality. CT colography has been compared with standard colonoscopy for the detection of neoplasia in screening populations.[2] The sensitivity of CT colography for large (≥10 mm) polyps is 85 to 93%, with a specificity of 97%. For polyps 6 to 9 mm, CT colography is 70 to 86% sensitive and 86 to 93% specific. Sensitivity for colorectal cancer (96%) is similar to that of colonoscopy. Although the optimal interval for testing has not been established, it is recommended that CT colography screening begin at age 50; if negative, it should be repeated at 5-year intervals. If a polyp greater than 5 mm is found, colonoscopy should be performed.

TABLE 199-4 STAGING FOR COLORECTAL ADENOCARCINOMAS

STAGE	TUMOR	NODE	METASTASIS
0	Tis	N0	M0
I	T1, T2	N0	M0
IIA	T3	N0	M0
IIB	T4a	N0	M0
IIC	T4b	N0	M0
IIIA	T1, T2 T1	N1 N2a	M0 M0
IIIB	T3, T4a T2, T3 T1, T2	N1 N2a N2b	M0 M0 M0
IIIC	T4a T3, T4a T4b	N2a N2b N1, N2	M0 M0 M0
IVA	Any T	Any N	M1a
IVB	Any T	Any N	M1b

Tis = in situ; T1 = submucosa; T2 = muscularis propria; T3 = subserosa, pericolorectal tissues; T4a = visceral peritoneum; T4b = other structures.
N1a = 1 regional node; N1b = 2-3 regional nodes; N1c = satellite(s) without regional nodes; N2a = 4-6 regional nodes; N2b = ≥7 regional nodes.
M1a = 1 organ; M1b = >1 organ, peritoneum.

Staging

Accurate staging of colorectal cancer is of the utmost importance in determining both prognosis and the most relevant and effective therapy. The versions of the TNM classification system for large bowel cancers used by the American Joint Committee on Cancer and the International Union Against Cancer are identical (Table 199-4). Differing from many solid tumors (although not those of other GI origin, except for anal cancer), colorectal cancers are not staged according to size. Stage I cancers penetrate into but not through the bowel wall (T1–2N0M0), while stage II cancers penetrate through the wall without spreading to regional lymph nodes. About 40% of patients present with stage I or II disease in the United States. Stage III cancers involve regional lymph nodes and constitute about 40% of presenting cases. Stage IV colorectal tumors commonly spread to liver, lung, distant nodes, and peritoneum, with about 20% of patients presenting with distant disease. Rectal primaries, because of early access to the systemic circulation, may involve the lungs without liver metastases; this pattern of spread is distinctly unusual in proximal large bowel cancers.

Surveillance

Surveillance should be undertaken in patients fit enough to undergo metastasectomy or systemic therapy for recurrent colorectal cancer. The American Society of Clinical Oncology recommends annual CT of the chest and abdomen for 3 years following resection of high-risk primary tumors, with pelvic CT added in cases of rectal origin. Colonoscopy should also be done at 3 years and then every 5 years, with flexible proctosigmoidoscopy offered to rectal cancer patients who have not received irradiation. Physical examinations should be performed every 3 to 6 months for 3 years, then biannually for at least 2 more years. CEA levels should be checked every 3 months for at least 3 years.

PROGNOSIS

The prognosis for patients with colorectal cancer depends primarily on stage. Five-year survival for patients with proximal (colonic) adenocarcinomas ranges from a low of 6 to 8% for those with metastatic disease to approximately 95% for those with stage I resected tumors. Corresponding rates for rectal cancers are similar to slightly inferior overall, ranging from 4 to 72%. Besides TNM stage, additional factors that are prognostic for poorer outcomes in patients undergoing potentially curative resection include signet ring histologic subtype (see the preceding discussion under Pathobiology), lymphovascular and perineural invasion, absence of host lymphoid response, presence of clinical obstruction preoperatively, high preoperative serum levels of the CEA tumor marker, positive margins, high tumor grade, and microsatellite-stable disease. Differing from many solid tumors originating outside the GI tract, colorectal cancers do not have different prognoses based on size.

Genetic factors are important as well, even in the metastatic setting. Patients with tumors harboring *BRAF* mutations appear to have a worse outcome. *KRAS* mutations were formerly thought to be prognostic but now appear to be only predictive for lack of benefit from certain types of systemic therapy.

TREATMENT

Rx

Chemoprevention

NSAIDs, including aspirin, are believed to reduce adenoma formation and inhibit colon cancer development by inhibiting cyclooxygenase and subsequent prostaglandin generation (Chapter 36). Prostaglandins (e.g., E_2) promote cell proliferation and tumor growth. The NSAID sulindac causes regression of existing adenomas and inhibits the formation of new adenomas in patients with FAP. Epidemiologic studies have shown decreased colorectal cancer rates in regular users of NSAIDs. Randomized trials of aspirin have shown 20 to 40% reductions in adenoma recurrence and a 70% reduction in the incidence of colorectal cancer when at least 75 mg of aspirin daily is continual for 5 or more years.[3] The selective cyclooxygenase 2 inhibitor celecoxib has shown similar decreases in adenoma recurrence, but its use is limited by concerns about cardiovascular risk. Calcium supplementation (1200 mg/day) was shown to decrease the rate of metachronous adenomas by 20%. However, the large Women's Health Trial, with 36,000 participants, found that calcium (1000 mg) plus vitamin D (400 IU) had no effect in reducing colorectal cancer incidence.[4] Currently, the routine use of aspirin and calcium for prevention is not recommended, but it may be considered on an individual basis.

Dietary Prevention

Epidemiologic studies have reported correlations between colorectal cancer and obesity, smoking, inactivity, excessive alcohol use, and diets high in fat and low in fruits, vegetables, and fiber. These observations suggest that lifestyle modifications may decrease colorectal cancer risk. Unfortunately, three randomized intervention trials of modest dietary changes (10% less fat, 25 to 75% more fiber, 50% more fruits and vegetables) found no significant reductions in adenomas or colorectal cancer over 3 to 8 years of follow-up.

Surgery

Resection is the primary treatment modality for patients with regionally confined colorectal cancer. Highly selected patients with metastatic disease may also undergo surgery with curative intent. The goal of curative surgery for colonic adenocarcinoma is margin-negative elimination of the tumor, plus en bloc removal of the primary feeding arterial vessel and corresponding lymphatics for that segment of bowel. A minimum of 12 lymph nodes should be retrieved for microscopic examination to assure staging accuracy. Synchronous colon cancers may be removed individually or with subtotal colectomy, and tumors adherent to adjacent structures should be resected en bloc. Prophylactic oophorectomy is no longer recommended, but women with one ovary grossly involved with cancer should undergo bilateral oophorectomy because of the relatively high risk of involvement of the other side. Laparoscopic resection is currently thought to be as effective as open resection and requires a modestly shorter recovery time. 5

In general, surgical considerations for rectal primaries are similar. Total mesorectal excision (en bloc removal of the lymphovascular and fatty envelope surrounding the rectum) is recommended for distal cancers, whereas tumor-specific mesorectal excision (en bloc removal of the mesorectum 5 cm distal to the tumor) should suffice for upper rectal tumors. Local transanal excision is acceptable for selected low rectal cancers thought to have minimal risk of nodal involvement. Selection criteria include the following: T1 disease, size less than 3 cm, low grade (well differentiated), location within 8 cm of the anal verge, no lymphovascular invasion, and less than one-third circumferential.

Until fairly recently, patients presenting with synchronous colorectal cancer primaries and unresectable metastases underwent resection of the primary tumor, regardless of whether they were symptomatic. This practice pattern could obviously delay systemic treatment in patients who are markedly more likely to die from their metastases before suffering significant complications from the intact large bowel tumor. Recent data suggest that stage IV patients with an asymptomatic primary tumor can safely begin systemic therapy without undergoing surgery, with only a small chance of developing serious complications requiring urgent operative interaction. Patients with rectal primaries may be at slightly higher risk for developing complications than those with tumors originating in the proximal large bowel.

Obstructing tumors that can be fully removed should be resected, with bowel anastomosis usually being acceptable in this setting. Proximal diversion alone, especially in the setting of very locally advanced unresectable cancer, may be necessary; if the primary tumor responds to the point where it can later be removed, resection followed by ostomy closure is reasonable. Endoscopic stenting may be useful to relieve acute obstruction. Perforated bowel is usually resected, with the choice of anastomosis, with or without diversion, depending on a number of factors, including degree of fecal contamination and general health of the patient.

Radiation Therapy

Radiation therapy may be used as curative or palliative treatment of large bowel cancers. In general, it plays a markedly larger role in treating rectal than colonic primaries. Single-institution trials have shown that irradiation improves local control following resection of high-risk proximal large bowel (colonic) cancers, but these findings were not confirmed in a randomized intergroup trial that closed early owing to slow accrual. Current recommendations for adjuvant radiation to the tumor bed following colon cancer resection include positive margins and localized perforation. Some authorities also advocate its use in colon cancers at particularly high risk of local recurrence (T4, T3N1–2 tumors in the ascending or descending colon), but that recommendation is not universally accepted. Irradiation may still play a role in treating colon cancer metastases to bone, brain, liver, and lung, as well as in cases of bleeding, obstruction, and locally advanced unresectable disease.

A major use for radiation in the definitive treatment of large bowel adenocarcinoma involves perioperative therapy for resectable rectal cancer. It is also commonly employed with chemotherapy for locally advanced invasive tumors, which occasionally become resectable after therapy. As with colon primaries, irradiation may be used to palliate bleeding, obstruction, or selected metastases from rectal cancers.

Systemic and Combination Therapies

The backbone of colorectal cancer treatment in both the adjuvant and metastatic settings is a fluorinated pyrimidine. The most commonly used drug is 5-fluorouracil (5-FU), although oral prodrugs are increasingly been utilized. 5FU targets the enzyme thymidylate synthase, inhibiting DNA synthesis and/or repair. It also may be incorporated into RNA, interfering with further processing. Although not particularly effective as a single agent (see later), 5-FU's efficacy can be enhanced by changing its means of administration (prolonging infusion) and by administering it with a variety of biochemical modulators, most commonly leucovorin. Other agents commonly used in treating colorectal cancer include irinotecan, a topoisomerase I inhibitor, and oxaliplatin, a later-generation platin that forms bulky DNA adducts that inhibit replication.

Patients with resected stage I colon cancers have a high cure rate, and this cannot easily be improved on with systemic therapy. Stage II patients have a higher chance of relapse (event-free survival ≈76% at 3 years), and systemic therapy with 5-FU and leucovorin improved that figure by about 3% for an unselected group of node-negative patients. Patients harboring highly microsatellite-unstable tumors have a better prognosis in general but may actually have worse outcomes with 5-FU treatment, although that is controversial. Treatment of stage II patients remains controversial in general: some experts suggest that the proportional benefit of systemic therapy is as great as it is in stage III disease, while others point out the low absolute magnitude of benefit and do not advocate its use. Some categories of stage II disease are believed to be at particularly high risk for recurrence (e.g., clinical obstruction). These patients usually receive postoperative chemotherapy, often with regimens commonly prescribed for patients with stage III cancer. Radiation has been tested in patients thought to be at higher than average risk of local relapse (T4 tumors), but its use is not standard. Finally, it is likely that gene studies will eventually be used to identify patients at higher risk of relapse or who have a greater chance of benefiting from systemic therapy, and treatment of carefully selected patients with stage II disease may become standard.

Five-year disease-free survival for patients with stage III colon cancer is only in the 40 to 45% range. Barring significant comorbidities or other confounding factors, all patients with node-positive disease receive adjuvant systemic therapy. Combinations of 5-FU and oxaliplatin (usually FOLFOX [fluorouracil, leucovorin, oxaliplatin]) clearly improve long-term survival rates and represent standard care. 6 Regimens containing irinotecan and biologics (bevacizumab, cetuximab) are highly effective in the treatment of advanced disease (see later), but oddly, they do not clearly benefit patients when they are given in the postoperative setting. Patients who are not candidates for combination chemotherapy are sometimes offered capecitabine, an oral prodrug activated to 5-FU in sequential enzymatic steps. Capecitabine has also been combined effectively and relatively safely with oxaliplatin for adjuvant use. Important outstanding questions regarding adjuvant chemotherapy is whether a shorter duration (3 months vs. the standard 6) might be equally effective, and whether elderly patients obtain greater benefit from newer combination regimens versus simple fluoropyrimidine use.

Rectal Adenocarcinoma

Radiation considerations are slightly different for patients with primary rectal adenocarcinomas, owing to the difficulty of achieving negative circumferential (radial) margins. Specifically, the risk of local recurrence is much more significant. In general, rectal cancer patients undergoing standard resection for stage I tumors do not receive additional treatment. However, higher-risk patients (T2 disease, T1 with poorly differentiated histology, perineural or lymphovascular invasion, or close margins) treated with local excision should receive postoperative pelvic irradiation with or without 5-FU chemotherapy, or they should return to the operating room for total mesorectal excision. Irradiation is standard for those with stage II and III rectal adenocarcinomas to decrease local relapse rates, increase the chance of sphincter preservation (when used in selected preoperative settings for low-lying cancers), and possibly improve survival. The major considerations are timing (pre- or postoperative use), course (short or long), and whether to combine it with fluoropyrimidine-based chemotherapy. Short-course (5-day) preoperative irradiation without chemotherapy may be considered and used if tumor downsizing is not necessary. When short-course radiation is used, patients still require postoperative systemic therapy, with either a fluoropyrimidine alone (stage II) or a fluoropyrimidine-oxaliplatin combination regimen (node-positive disease), to minimize the risk of distant metastases. Long-course irradiation (approximately 5.5 weeks) is particularly important when tumor response is necessary to make surgery easier or more feasible. It is usually combined with continuous-infusion 5-FU or capecitabine, and it can be given preoperatively or postoperatively (if the patient did not receive preoperative short-course radiation). Including oxaliplatin preoperatively does not improve results and is not recommended independent of a clinical trial, owing to its higher toxicity profile. Oxaliplatin may be used postoperatively if the pathology specimen demonstrates nodal involvement. With long-course irradiation, preoperative (compared with postoperative) treatment is less toxic and may offer improved local control. 7 However, it requires accurate preoperative staging (to avoid treating patients who might have stage I disease). Highly selected rectal cancer patients thought to be at low risk of local recurrence (T3N0 or T1–2N1) may receive total mesorectal excision plus best systemic therapy without irradiation, usually postoperatively.

Metastatic Colorectal Cancer

Metastatic disease is treated identically, regardless of the site of origin (colon vs. rectum). Patients with incurable metastatic colorectal cancer have a median survival of approximately 6 months with best supportive care alone; however, incremental gains made through the adoption of new systemic therapies have extended that time to almost 2 years. For example, treatment with single-agent fluoropyrimidines leads to median survival in the 10- to 13-month range; adding one more effective chemotherapy drug (either irinotecan or oxaliplatin) affords survival of about 15 to 20 months, and adding both drugs to 5-FU has been reported to extend life to 23 months. Interestingly, long-term results seem to be similar regardless of which drug (oxaliplatin or irinotecan) is added to 5-FU first (although the toxicity pattern varies, depending on which drug is given), or even regardless of whether 5-FU is used first and combination chemotherapy is used subsequently, as long as patients are eventually exposed to all active agents.

Additional improvements have arisen through the development of drugs that are more convenient and/or less toxic than standard agents, although they may not be more effective. Capecitabine, an oral prodrug activated to 5-FU in three sequential enzymatic steps, can be substituted for that agent alone and in combination with oxaliplatin (although patients still need intravenous access for the latter drug).

Recent breakthroughs have all been related to use of biological agents (Chapter 35). Successful drugs to date have all been monoclonal antibodies, whereas small molecule tyrosine kinase inhibitors generally appear to be ineffective. Bevacizumab is a humanized monoclonal antibody directed against vascular endothelial growth factor, an important mediator of angiogenesis. Bevacizumab has little single-agent activity against colorectal cancer, but it improves the interval without progression when added to irinotecan- or oxaliplatin-containing chemotherapy.[8,9] Bevacizumab with FOLFOX or FOLFIRI (fluorouracil, leucovorin, irinotecan) now represents first-line treatment for patients with advanced large bowel cancer in the United States.

The epidermal growth factor receptor (EGFR) is another important target in advanced colorectal cancer. Cetuximab and panitumumab are monoclonal antibodies (chimeric and human, respectively) directed against the EGFR. They have single-agent activity against colorectal cancers,[10] and both may be combined with chemotherapy to improve at least progression-free survival.[11] Although both agents appear effective in front-line or later use, efficacy is restricted to patients whose tumors harbor no mutations in *KRAS*.

Locally Directed Treatment of Metastatic Disease

Complete resection of hepatic or pulmonary metastases may result in long-term survival and is the standard of care for selected patients with colorectal cancer. The majority of data exist for hepatic metastasectomy. Actuarial 5-year survival rates from single-institution series have been in the 25 to 40% range. However, relapse after 5 years still occurs, suggesting that this percentage does not reflect the number actually *cured* with surgery. That figure, calculated from 10-year survival rates, is probably between 17 and 25%, which still compares quite favorably with the survival rate for patients with colorectal cancer metastatic to the liver who do not undergo surgery. The actual role of perioperative systemic therapy in those undergoing metastasectomy is not well defined, but most experts advocate 6 months of fluoropyrimidine-based chemotherapy, with or without oxaliplatin. Importantly, bevacizumab can affect wound healing and should not be used in the immediate perioperative period.

Small liver metastases that are not resectable because of anatomic location or in a frail patient unable to undergo hepatic resection may be treated with radio frequency ablation, which uses alternating electrical current to generate heat, destroying malignant cells through protein coagulation. Although it has never been directly compared with resection in a randomized trial, radio frequency ablation appears to offer inferior local control of disease. Some advocate the placement of a hepatic artery pump to infuse fluoropyrimidine-based chemotherapy to treat unresectable liver-predominant metastases. Other techniques useful in noncolorectal liver-based tumors (e.g., hepatocellular carcinoma), such as chemoembolization, have no proven role for large bowel liver metastases.

CONCLUSION

Colorectal cancer remains a significant problem, despite the fact that most cases can be prevented. Large gains have been made in terms of overall survival, but the vast majority of patients with advanced disease still succumb to their malignancy. Although minimal tailoring can be offered to patients (e.g., selecting a chemotherapeutic agent based on toxicity or not using an anti-EGFR antibody in those with *KRAS*-mutated tumors), the dream of truly individualized therapy remains elusive.

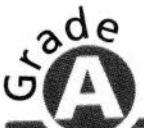

1. Atkin WS, Edwards R, Kralj-Hans I, et al. Once-only flexible sigmoidoscopy screening in prevention of colorectal cancer: a multicentre randomised controlled trial. *Lancet.* 2010;375:1624-1633.
2. Johnson CD, Chen MH, Toledano AY, et al. Accuracy of CT colonography for detection of large adenomas and cancers. *N Engl J Med.* 2008;359:1207-1217.
3. Rothwell PM, Wilson M, Elwin CE, et al. Long-term effect of aspirin on colorectal cancer incidence and mortality: 20-year follow-up of five randomised trials. *Lancet.* 2010;376:1741-1750.
4. Wactawski-Wende J, Kotchen JM, Anderson GL, et al. Calcium plus vitamin D supplementation and the risk of colorectal cancer. *N Engl J Med.* 2006;354:684-696.
5. Fleshman J, Sargent DJ, Green E, et al. Laparoscopic colectomy for cancer is not inferior to open surgery based on 5-year data from the COST study group trial. *Ann Surg.* 2007;246:655-664.
6. Andre T, Boni C, Navarro M, et al. Improved overall survival with oxaliplatin, fluorouracil, and leucovorin as adjuvant treatment in stage II or III colon cancer in the MOSAIC trial. *J Clin Oncol.* 2009;27:3109-3116.
7. Sauer R, Becker H, Hohenberger W, et al. Preoperative versus postoperative chemoradiotherapy for rectal cancer. *N Engl J Med.* 2004;351:1731-1740.
8. Hurwitz H, Fehrenbacher L, Novotny W, et al. Bevacizumab plus irinotecan, fluorouracil, and leucovorin for metastatic colorectal cancer. *N Engl J Med.* 2004;350:2335-2342.
9. Saltz LB, Clarke S, Diaz-Rubio E, et al. Bevacizumab in combination with oxaliplatin-based chemotherapy as first-line therapy in metastatic colorectal cancer: a randomized phase III study. *J Clin Oncol.* 2008;26:2013-2019.
10. Van Cutsem E, Siena S, Humblet Y, et al. An open-label randomized phase 3 clinical trial of panitumumab plus best supportive care versus best supportive care in patients with chemotherapy-refractory metastatic colorectal cancer. *J Clin Oncol.* 2007;25:1658-1664.
11. Van Cutsem E, Köhne C-H, Hitre E, et al. Cetuximab and chemotherapy as initial treatment for metastatic colorectal cancer. *N Engl J Med.* 2009;360:1408-1417.

SUGGESTED READINGS

Cunningham D, Atkin W, Lenz HJ, et al. Colorectal cancer. *Lancet.* 2010;375:1030-1047. *Review.*

Damjanaov N, Weiss J, Haller DG. Resection of the primary colorectal cancer is not necessary in non-obstructed patients with metastatic disease. *Oncologist.* 2009;14:963-969. *Modern literature review with recommendations for treatment (or not) of primary colorectal cancer in patients who also have metastatic disease.*

Gastrointestinal Stromal Tumor Meta-Analysis Group (MetaGIST). Comparison of two doses of imatinib for the treatment of unresectable or metastatic gastrointestinal stromal tumors: a meta-analysis of 1640 patients. *J Clin Oncol.* 2010;28:1247-1253. *Though not limited to intestinal GISTs, this meta-analysis provides results of imatinib therapy for advanced disease, including results for patients with tumors harboring exon 9 mutations (markedly more common in those with small bowel primaries).*

Holden DJ, Jonas DE, Porterfield DS, et al. Systematic review: enhancing the use and quality of colorectal cancer screening. *Ann Intern Med.* 2010;152:668-676. *Review.*

Hyslop T, Weinberg DS, Schulz S, et al. Occult tumor burden predicts disease recurrence in lymph node–negative colorectal cancer. *Clin Cancer Res.* 2011;17:3293-3303. *Molecular tumor burden in lymph nodes is independently associated with time to recurrence and disease-free survival in node-negative colorectal cancer.*

200

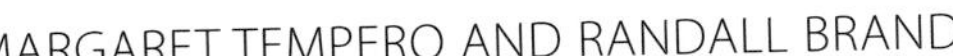

PANCREATIC CANCER

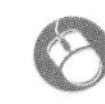

MARGARET TEMPERO AND RANDALL BRAND

DEFINITION

The term *pancreatic cancer* usually refers to ductal adenocarcinomas because more than 90% of pancreatic neoplasms are of ductal epithelial origin. Other pancreatic tumors include endocrine tumors (Chapter 201), carcinoid tumors (Chapter 240), lymphomas, cystic neoplasms, and the rare squamous cell carcinomas, giant cell carcinomas, carcinosarcomas, malignant fibrous histiocytomas, solid pseudopapillary neoplasms, sarcomas, and pancreaticoblastomas.

EPIDEMIOLOGY

Pancreatic cancer is the fourth most common cause of cancer death in the United States despite its low incidence: about 42,500 pancreatic neoplasms are diagnosed and 35,200 will die annually from cancer-related causes. Worldwide, pancreatic cancer accounts for 2% of all malignant diseases. Its incidence is higher in developed than in developing countries, but there is less than a two-fold variation in incidence worldwide. The 5-year survival rate for adenocarcinoma of the pancreas is less than 5%, and most patients die within the first 2 years. The risk for developing a pancreatic carcinoma increases with age, with a mean age of onset in the seventh and eighth decades of life. There is almost an equivalent risk in men and women.

Pancreatic cancer is more common in African Americans, Maori New Zealanders, and Polynesians. Cigarette smoking is the most reproducible environmental risk factor, causing a 1.5- to 5.5-fold increased rate of pancreatic cancer. Other risk factors include increased body mass index, chronic pancreatitis (Chapter 146), high intake of animal fat, and prolonged contact with petroleum products and wood pulp. A modest, less than two-fold increased risk for pancreatic cancer is associated with blood groups A, AB, and B relative to blood group O, and with selected polymorphisms that map to three loci on chromosomes *13q22.1*, *1q32.1*, and *5p15.33*.

The association between pancreatic cancer and diabetes is complex. Diabetes or impaired glucose tolerance is observed in up to 80% of patients at the time of diagnosis of their pancreatic cancer, and diabetes is often described as a risk factor. However, the diabetes is usually of recent onset and may improve or resolve after resection of the tumor. A population-based study suggests that about 1% of patients who develop diabetes after age 50 years will have a diagnosis of pancreatic cancer within 3 years before or after the onset of diabetes, and most of these individuals will be diagnosed with diabetes within 6 months of detection of the pancreatic cancer. Thus, diabetes may be a sign of underlying pancreatic cancer.

The greatest risk factor for developing pancreatic cancer is genetic predisposition. It is estimated that up to 10% of patients with pancreatic cancer have one or more first- or second-degree relatives with the disease. Recognized inherited syndromes include hereditary pancreatitis (Chapter 146), mutation of the *BRCA2* gene (Chapter 204), familial atypical multiple mole–melanoma syndrome and a *p16* germline mutation, hereditary nonpolyposis colorectal cancer (Chapter 199), Peutz-Jeghers polyposis (Chapter 199), and ataxia-telangiectasia (Chapter 258). In most families, the genetic factors responsible for the predisposition are unknown.

Pancreatic cysts are increasingly recognized with the widespread use of abdominal imaging and can be categorized as neoplastic or non-neoplastic. Neoplastic cystic lesions consist of those with malignant potential such as intraductal papillary mucinous neoplasms (IPMNs), mucinous cystic neoplasms, and the rare solid pseudopapillary tumors. Those without malignant potential include serous cystadenomas and lymphoepithelial cysts. IPMNs equally affect women and men and are usually located in the head of the pancreas. Other cystic neoplasms most commonly occur in young to middle-aged women and are located in the body or tail of the pancreas.

PATHOBIOLOGY

Three major precursors to invasive pancreatic adenocarcinoma have been identified: pancreatic intraepithelial neoplasia (PanIN), IPMN, and mucinous cystic neoplasm (MCN). The PanIN is the most prevalent type of precursor lesion, arising from the ductal epithelial cells. It is presumed that these lesions follow a pathway of progression from no dysplasia to moderate dysplasia (borderline) to high-grade dysplasia (carcinoma in situ) to invasive carcinoma. As the extent of ductal atypia rises, there is an increasing frequency of associated genetic alterations (Fig. 200-1). Unlike PanIN lesions, the IPMNs and MCNs are detectable by computed tomography (CT) or endoscopic ultrasound (EUS). Although only responsible for a minority of pancreatic cancers (less than 15%), IPMNs and MCNs do offer the opportunity to identify a premalignant lesion in the pancreas, especially with the increasing use of high-resolution noninvasive abdominal imaging procedures.

Ductal adenocarcinoma and its variants are characterized by a dense, desmoplastic reaction surrounding a compact mass of hard pancreatic tissue that can invade surrounding mesenteric vessels and can involve perineuronal tissue and lymphatic channels or nodes. Because approximately 75% of pancreatic carcinomas are located in the head of the pancreas, the usual clinical presentations are related to invasion or compression of the bile or pancreatic ducts. The duodenum, stomach, and colon may be invaded or compressed. Pancreatic cancers other than ductal adenocarcinoma, such as islet cell tumors or lymphomas, tend to be softer and less fibrotic and thus tend to cause distortion rather than encasement or compression of adjacent structures.

Tumor suppressor genes that are most frequently mutated in pancreatic adenocarcinoma are *p16* (95%), *p53* (50 to 75%), and *DPC4* (55%). *K-ras*, which is the most commonly activated oncogene, occurs in about 95% of advanced pancreatic cancers. An extensive genetic analysis of 24 pancreatic cancers, performed using state-of-the-art DNA sequencing of 20,735 genes, as well as both gene expression and gene copy number analysis, revealed on average a total of 63 altered genes per tumor. Although there was marked variability from tumor to tumor in the specific genes that were mutated, 12 cellular signaling pathways and processes that had at least one gene genetically altered in at least 70% of the tumors were identified. The six specific pathways that had alterations of at least one of the genes in all of the 24 pancreatic cancers were *K-ras* signaling, apoptosis, Wnt/Notch signaling, transforming growth factor-β (TGF-β) signaling, hedgehog signaling, and regulation of G_1 to S phase transition.

CLINICAL MANIFESTATIONS

Early symptoms include nonspecific abdominal discomfort, nausea, vomiting, sleeping difficulties, anorexia, and generalized malaise. Despite the historic perception that a mass in the head of the pancreas manifests initially with painless jaundice, the more common presenting symptoms are epigastric pain, obstructive jaundice, and weight loss. Although these symptoms prompt evaluation of the pancreas and biliary tree, they occur late in the disease and are usually associated with advanced tumor at the time of diagnosis. The finding of a palpably distended, nontender gallbladder as a result of obstruction of the distal common bile duct by pancreatic cancer has been called *Courvoisier's sign*. Patients may manifest superficial or deep vein thrombosis (Trousseau's syndrome; Chapter 187).

The most common laboratory abnormalities include anemia and elevation of serum levels of alkaline phosphatase, bilirubin, and aminotransferases. Approximately 80% of patients have jaundice related to biliary obstruction. Diabetes or hyperglycemia is seen in up to 80% of patients, and pancreatic cancer should be considered in the differential diagnosis of the cause of new-onset diabetes in patients who older than 50 years and who do not have a family history of diabetes.

Tumors of other histologic types arising in the pancreas may also cause nonspecific symptoms. Patients with functioning islet cell tumors can present with symptoms related to the overproduction of peptides manufactured in the islets (Chapter 201). Cystic neoplasms generally remain asymptomatic until they become quite large, at which point patients can present with a palpable mass, abdominal pain, nausea, emesis, and weight loss. Obstruction of the common bile duct is less common than with ductal adenocarcinoma. Intraductal papillary mucinous tumors may cause symptoms of acute pancreatitis or pancreatic insufficiency owing to obstruction of the pancreatic duct.

DIAGNOSIS

Differential Diagnosis

The differential diagnosis of pancreatic ductal cancer includes conditions that can manifest as a solid mass in the pancreas or especially acute or, more commonly, chronic pancreatitis (Chapter 146). Ampullary carcinomas and distal cholangiocarcinomas also manifest with biliary obstruction and jaundice (Chapters 158 and 202). It may be difficult to differentiate cystic pancreatic neoplasms from non-neoplastic pancreatic pseudocysts based on noninvasive imaging studies; a cystic neoplasm should always be considered in patients who present with isolated cystic lesions and have no prior history of acute or chronic pancreatitis.

Imaging

For all patients with suspected pancreatic tumors, the preferred imaging study is a multidetector CT scan using dynamic contrast with thin cuts

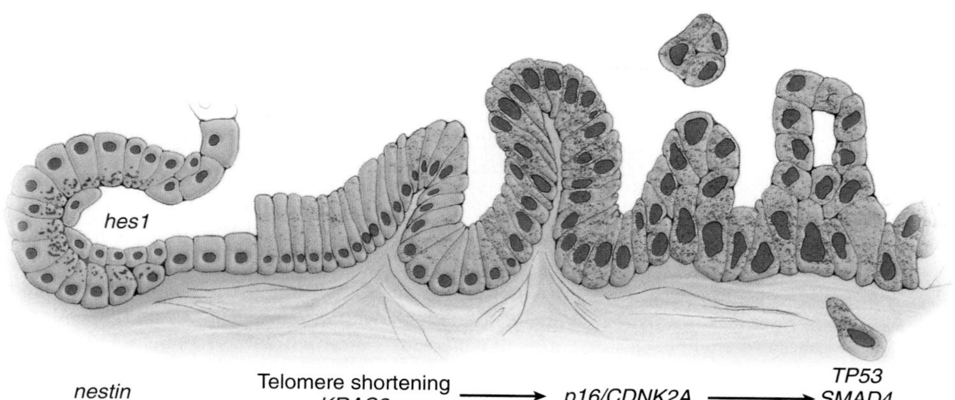

FIGURE 200-1. Molecular progression model of pancreatic cancer (PanINs). Molecular abnormalities in PanINs can usually be stratified into "early" changes (e.g., expression of *MUC5* and prostate stem antigen, or loss of *p16*), "intermediate" changes (e.g., expression of cyclin D1), and "late" changes (e.g., expression of *p53*, proliferation antigens, *MUC1*, mesothelin, and 14-3-3s, or loss of *SMAD4/DPC4*). (Adapted from Maitra A, Adsay NV, Argani P, et al. Multicomponent analysis of the pancreatic adenocarcinoma progression model using a pancreatic intraepithelial neoplasia tissue microarray. *Mod Pathol.* 2003;16:902-912).

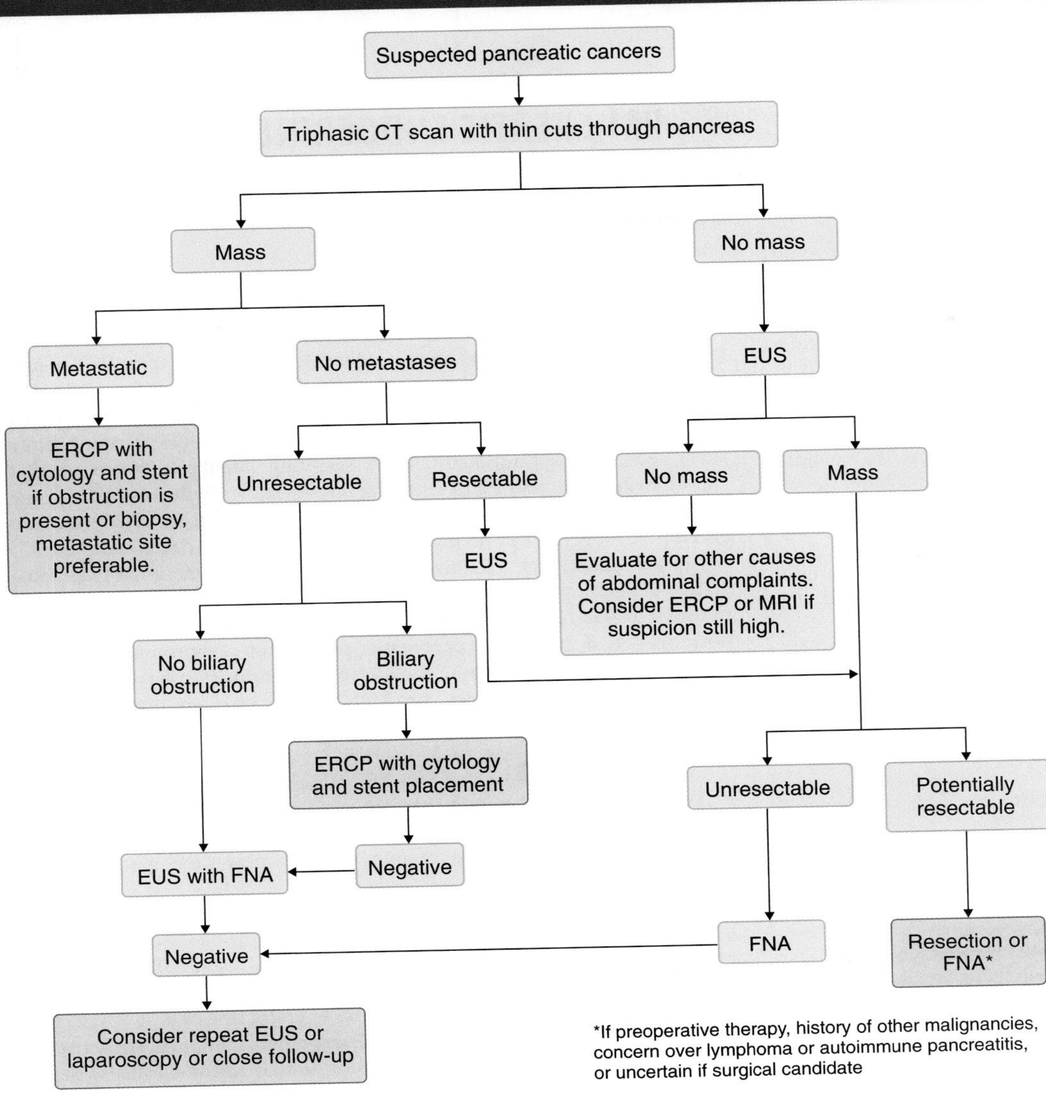

FIGURE 200-2. Diagnostic algorithm for pancreatic cancer. Intraoperative fine-needle aspiration (FNA) is used if the tumor is found to be inoperable during surgery. CT = computed tomography; ERCP = endoscopic retrograde cholangiopancreatography; EUS = endoscopic ultrasonography; MRI = magnetic resonance imaging.

through the pancreas (Fig. 200-2). The CT scan provides important information about vascular involvement and metastases, and it is approximately 90% accurate in assessing resectability. EUS may be useful in patients with equivocal findings on the CT scan. When a preoperative biopsy is needed, it is preferable to obtain a fine-needle aspiration under endoscopic guidance to minimize the chance of tumor seeding, but patients with potentially resectable disease can proceed directly to surgery. False-negative biopsy findings can result from the desmoplastic reaction characteristic of pancreatic ductal adenocarcinoma. Laparoscopy can identify patients who may have occult metastases in the peritoneum or the surface of the liver. Patients whose CT scans indicate an unresectable tumor based on local extension or the presence of metastases should have a definitive diagnosis established by a fine-needle aspiration biopsy of the primary or metastatic site.

Biomarkers

The clinical role for tumor markers is limited. CA-19-9, a sialylated Lewis[a] antigen associated with circulating mucins, is the most widely used marker for pancreatic disease. At the most commonly used cutoff level of 37 U/mL, its sensitivity ranges from 81 to 85%, and its specificity ranges from 81 to 90%; CA-19-9 levels higher than 1000 U/mL are associated with unresectable disease. Although this test is not a substitute for a histologic diagnosis, it is useful for monitoring the response to treatment.

The aforementioned radiographic studies also apply to other pancreatic tumors. EUS with fine-needle aspiration can be useful in the evaluation of cystic lesions, and it often provides additional detail not seen by CT and permits sampling of the cystic fluid for tumor marker levels, amylase content, viscosity, and cytologic examination. Carcinoembryonic antigen (CEA) levels of 192 mg/mL are approximately 80% accurate for identifying mucinous as compared with nonmucinous cystic lesions. For obvious reasons, it is important to clarify whether the lesion is a simple cyst, which would suggest a pseudocyst, or a cystic neoplasm.

TREATMENT AND PROGNOSIS Rx

In the absence of metastatic disease, surgical resection is the initial treatment of choice for all patients with pancreatic adenocarcinomas. The procedure should be performed in centers that have a high volume of pancreatectomies because surgical outcomes are improved with more volume and experience. Routine preoperative biliary drainage in patients with obstructive jaundice caused by pancreatic head tumor increases the rate of complications of surgery for the cancer.[1] For periampullary adenocarcinoma, pancreaticoduodenectomy is the standard of care, and distal gastrectomy and extended lymphadenectomy do not improve outcome.[2] Tumors are considered resectable if a clear fat plane is present around the celiac and superior mesenteric arteries and if the mesenteric and portal veins are patent. After successful resection, adjuvant therapy with intravenous 5-fluorouracil (425 mg/m^2) and folinic acid (20 mg/m^2) daily for 5 days and then monthly for 6 months or gemcitabine (1000 mg/m^2 over 30 minutes) weekly for 3 weeks out of 4 for 6 months improves survival compared with observation alone,[3,4] but the addition of gemcitabine to fluorouracil plus folinic acid does not provide incremental benefit.[5] Radiation therapy may not confer any added value beyond chemotherapy alone. In general, successful resection followed by adjuvant therapy results in a 5-year survival rate of approximately 20%.

Borderline resectable tumors include those with venous involvement of the superior mesenteric vein (SMV)–portal vein demonstrating tumor abutment with or without impingement and narrowing of the lumen, encasement of the SMV–portal vein but without encasement of the nearby arteries, short-segment venous occlusion secondary to either tumor thrombus, or encasement but with suitable vessel proximal and distal to the area of vessel involvement allowing for safe resection and reconstruction, gastroduodenal artery encasement up to the hepatic artery with either short-segment encasement or direct abutment of the hepatic artery without extension to the celiac axis, and tumor abutment of the superior mesenteric artery (SMA) not to exceed more than 180 degrees of the circumference of the vessel wall. Because there is a higher risk for positive margins with these tumors, some advocate preoperative chemotherapy and radiation, although this is controversial.

Surgery can also have an important palliative role. Patients who undergo surgical exploration but who are found not to have a resectable tumor may benefit from a biliary or gastric bypass procedure, depending on the clinical setting. However, there is now substantial experience in the placement of both biliary and luminal (duodenal) stents, so the more invasive operative procedure can be avoided in most instances. In addition, intraoperative, EUS-guided, or percutaneous chemical splanchnicectomy can provide protracted pain control.

Patients with locally unresectable disease are usually managed with a combination of chemotherapy and radiation therapy, followed by additional chemotherapy. The most commonly used drug is 5-fluorouracil, given by low-dose continuous infusion, combined with radiation therapy, but gemcitabine is also being studied. The median survival time for these patients is 10 to 12 months.

For patients with metastatic disease, single-agent gemcitabine (1000 mg/m^2 intravenously, weekly times 7 for 8 weeks and then weekly times 3 every 4 weeks) remains the standard of care and improves survival. A small improvement in survival has been observed with the addition of erlotinib (orally, 100 mg/day). [6]

For all patients with locally advanced and metastatic disease, optimal management of pain and of local complications is critical. Biliary obstruction can be managed surgically or with placement of a plastic or expandable metal stent. Narcotic analgesics (Chapter 29) and palliative care (Chapter 3) are cornerstones of therapy.

Most patients with a cystic neoplasm should be considered for surgical resection. The long-term survival rate following resection of malignant pancreatic cystic neoplasms exceeds 70%, and adjuvant therapy is currently not recommended.

FUTURE DIRECTIONS

Future research in pancreatic adenocarcinoma will focus on identifying individuals at high risk, developing strategies for early detection, and optimizing treatment. Drugs that interact with tyrosine kinase receptors, downstream signaling events, or tumor-supporting pathways in the microenvironment are under active investigation.

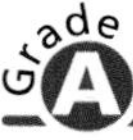

1. van der Gaag NA, Rauws EA, van Eijck CH, et al. Preoperative biliary drainage for cancer of the head of the pancreas. *N Engl J Med*. 2010;362:129-137.
2. Neoptolemos JP, Stocken DD, Friess H, et al. A randomized trial of chemoradiotherapy and chemotherapy after resection of pancreatic cancer. *N Engl J Med*. 2004;351:726.
3. Oettle H, Post S, Neuhaus P, et al. Adjuvant chemotherapy with gemcitabine vs observation in patients undergoing curative-intent resection of pancreatic cancer: a randomized controlled trial. *JAMA*. 2007;297:311-313.
4. Regine WF, Winter KA, Abrams RA, et al. Fluorouracil vs gemcitabine chemotherapy before and after fluorouracil-based chemoradiation following resection of pancreatic adenocarcinoma: a randomized controlled trial. *JAMA*. 2008;299:1019-1026.
5. Neoptolemos JP, Stocken DD, Bassi C, et al. Adjuvant chemotherapy with fluorouracil plus folinic acid vs gemcitabine following pancreatic cancer resection: a randomized controlled trial. *JAMA*. 2010;304:1073-1081.
6. Moore MJ, Goldstein D, Hamm J, et al. Erlotinib plus gemcitabine compared with gemcitabine alone in patients with advanced pancreatic cancer: a phase III trial of the National Cancer Institute of Canada Clinical Trials Group. *J Clin Oncol*. 2007;25:1960-1966.

SUGGESTED READINGS

Brand RE, Nolen BM, Zeh HJ, et al. Serum biomarker panels for the detection of pancreatic cancer. *Clin Cancer Res*. 2011;17:805-816. *Review of promising new approaches.*

Callery MP, Chang KJ, Fishman EK, et al. Pretreatment assessment of resectable and borderline resectable pancreas cancer: expert consensus statement. *Ann Surg Oncol*. 2009;16:1727-1733. *This is the first attempt to define criteria for high-risk resectable tumors.*

Greer JB, Brand RE. New developments in pancreatic cancer. *Curr Gastroenterol Rep*. 2011;13:131-139. *Review of etiology and diagnosis.*

Hidalgo M. Pancreatic cancer. *N Engl J Med*. 2010;362:1605-1617. *Review.*

Petersen GM, Amundadottir L, Fuchs CS, et al. A genome-wide association study identifies pancreatic cancer susceptibility loci on chromosomes 13q122.1, 1q32.1 and 5p15.33. *Nat Genet*. 2010;42:224-228. *Details results of extensive genome-wide association studies on germline DNA and identifies several new susceptibility loci.*

Thomas A, Dajani K, Neoptolemos JP, et al. Adjuvant therapy in pancreatic cancer. *Dig Dis*. 2010;28:684-692. *Review emphasizing 5-fluorouracil and gemcitabine.*

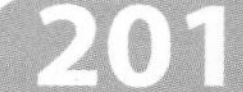

201 PANCREATIC ENDOCRINE TUMORS

ROBERT T. JENSEN

DEFINITION

Pancreatic endocrine tumors (PETs) are also called islet cell tumors; however, because the cell of origin of most is unknown, the general term PET is preferred. This term is also a misnomer because PETs can also occur outside the pancreas. Ten PETs are well established (Table 201-1). Other additional functional PET syndromes have been rarely reported: PETs secreting renin, PETs secreting erythropoietin, PETs secreting luteinizing hormone that causes virilization, and PETs secreting insulin-like growth factor II causing hypoglycemia. In addition, PETs synthesizing neurotensin, calcitonin, and ghrelin are reported, but no distinct syndrome has been described.

PETs frequently are classified as functional or nonfunctional (see Table 201-1) depending on whether a clinical syndrome resulting from the autonomously released hormone is present. Nonfunctional PETs frequently release hormones and peptides (pancreatic polypeptide, neurotensin, α- and β-subunits of human chorionic gonadotropin, neuron-specific enolase, chromogranin A and breakdown products) that cause no distinct clinical syndromes.

EPIDEMIOLOGY

PETs are uncommon, having a prevalence of less than ten cases per 1 million population. Insulinomas, gastrinomas, and nonfunctional PETs are the most common, with an incidence of one to three new cases per 1 million population.

PATHOBIOLOGY

All PETs share certain features. PETs are classified as APUDomas (amine precursor uptake and decarboxylation), which share cytochemical features with carcinoid tumors, melanomas, and other endocrine tumors (pheochromocytomas, medullary thyroid cancer). Except for insulinomas, these tumors are frequently malignant. All PETs appear similar histologically, with few mitotic figures. Ultrastructurally, they have dense granules containing peptides, amines, and products of neuroendocrine differentiation (neuron-specific enolase, chromogranins, synaptophysin). The presence of chromogranin immunoreactivity in the tumor is now widely used to identify these tumors as endocrine tumors.

Molecular studies show that PETs have a different pathogenesis than common gastrointestinal adenocarcinomas because they infrequently demonstrate alterations in common tumor suppressor genes (e.g., retinoblastoma gene, *p53*) or common oncogenes (*ras*, *c-Jun*, *c-Fos*). Alterations in p16^{INK4a}, the *MEN1* gene, and the expression of growth factors, as well as chromosomal losses (1q, 3p, 3q, 6p, X) and gains (17p, 17q, 20q), have been associated with a worse prognosis in numerous studies. A number of other factors have prognostic significance, the most important of which is the presence of liver metastases. Recently, a World Health Organization TNM grading and classification system has been proposed for PETs based on tumor size, presence of metastases, invasiveness, and proliferative indices and has been recently shown to have prognostic value in a number of studies.

Four autosomal dominant–inherited disorders are associated with an increased occurrence of PETs: multiple endocrine neoplasia type 1 (MEN 1; 80 to 100% develop PETs), von Hippel-Lindau disease (VHL; 10 to 17% have PETs), von Recklinghausen's disease (neurofibromatosis 1([NF-1]; 12% develop duodenal somatostatinomas), and tuberous sclerosis (<1% develop PETs).

FUNCTIONAL PANCREATIC ENDOCRINE TUMOR SYNDROMES

Zollinger-Ellison Syndrome (Gastrinomas)

DEFINITION AND EPIDEMIOLOGY

Zollinger-Ellison syndrome (ZES) is a clinical syndrome caused by a gastrin-releasing endocrine tumor usually located in the pancreas or duodenum and characterized by clinical symptoms and signs resulting from gastric acid

TABLE 201-1 PANCREATIC ENDOCRINE TUMORS

NAME OF TUMOR	NAME OF SYNDROME	MAIN SIGNS OR SYMPTOMS	LOCATION	MALIGNANCY (%)	HORMONE CAUSING SYNDROME
I. FUNCTIONAL PET					
Gastrinoma	Zollinger-Ellison syndrome	Abdominal pain, diarrhea, esophageal symptoms	Pancreas—30% Duodenum—60% Other—10%	60-90	Gastrin
Insulinoma	Insulinoma	Hypoglycemic symptoms	Pancreas—100%	5-15	Insulin
Glucagonoma	Glucagonoma	Dermatitis, diabetes/glucose intolerance, weight loss	Pancreas—100%	60	Glucagon
VIPoma	Verner-Morrison, pancreatic cholera, WDHA	Severe watery diarrhea, hypokalemia	Pancreas—90% Other—10% (neural, adrenal, periganglionic tissue)	80	Vasoactive intestinal peptide (VIP)
Somatostatinoma	Somatostatinoma	Diabetes mellitus, cholelithiasis, diarrhea	Pancreas—56% Duodenum/jejunum—44%	60	Somatostatin
GRFoma	GRFoma	Acromegaly	Pancreas—30% Lung—54% Jejunum—7% Other—13% (adrenal, foregut, retroperitoneum)	30	Growth hormone–releasing factor (GRF)
ACTHoma	ACTHoma	Cushing's syndrome	Pancreas—4-16% of all ectopic Cushing's cases	>95	Adrenocorticotropic hormone (ACTH)
PET causing carcinoid syndrome	PET causing carcinoid syndrome	Diarrhea, flushing	Pancreas—<1% of all carcinoids	60-90	Serotonin, tachykinins
PET causing hypercalcemia	PET causing hypercalcemia	Signs/symptoms of hypercalcemia	Pancreas (rare cause of hypercalcemia)	>85	PTHrP, other unknown
II. NONFUNCTIONAL PET					
Nonfunctioning PPoma	Nonfunctional PPoma	Weight loss, abdominal mass, hepatomegaly	Pancreas—100%	60-90	None: pancreatic polypeptide chromogranin released but no known symptoms due to hypersecretion

PET = pancreatic endocrine tumor; PP = pancreatic polypeptide; PTHrP = parathormone-related peptide; WDHA = watery diarrhea, hypokalemia, and achlorhydria.

hypersecretion (peptic ulcer disease, diarrhea, esophageal reflux disease). ZES occurs most frequently between the ages of 35 and 65 years and is slightly more common in men (60%).

PATHOBIOLOGY

In recent surgical series, gastrinomas occur two to five times more frequently in the duodenum than in the pancreas. Duodenal gastrinomas are generally small (<1cm), whereas pancreatic gastrinomas are generally larger. Occasionally ZES results from a gastrinoma in the splenic hilum, mesentery, stomach, or only in a lymph node or in the ovary. Extrapancreatic gastrinomas producing ZES have been reported in the heart and as a result of small cell lung cancer. As with other PETs, malignancy can be reliably determined only by demonstrating the presence of metastatic disease, and no light microscopic or ultrastructural finding can clearly establish malignant behavior.

Gastrin stimulates parietal cells to secrete acid and also has a growth effect on cells of the gastric mucosa. Chronic hypergastrinemia thus leads to increased gastric mucosal thickness, prominent gastric folds, and increased numbers of parietal cells and gastric enterochromaffin-like cells. Patients with gastrinomas have increased basal and maximal acid outputs. *Helicobacter pylori* appears not to be important in the pathogenesis of the ulcer disease in ZES, in contrast to that of routine peptic ulcers (Chapter 141). Diarrhea is common because the large-volume gastric acid output leads to structural damage to the small intestine (inflammation, blunted villi, edema), interference with fat transport, inactivation of pancreatic lipase, and precipitation of bile acids. These same mechanisms, if prolonged, can lead to steatorrhea. If acid hypersecretion is controlled, the diarrhea will stop.

CLINICAL MANIFESTATIONS

Abdominal pain resulting from a peptic ulcer is the most common symptom (>80%). Most ulcers occur in the duodenum (>85%), but they occasionally occur in the postbulbar area, jejunum, or stomach, or in multiple locations. Initially, the pain is usually similar to that of patients with typical peptic ulcers (Chapter 141). With time, the symptoms become persistent and, in general, respond poorly to treatments aimed at eliminating *H. pylori* and to conventional doses of histamine-2 receptor antagonists, as well as to the now rarely used surgical treatments for ulcer disease. By comparison, conventional doses of proton pump inhibitors (PPIs) (e.g., omeprazole, lansoprazole, pantoprazole, esomeprazole, rabeprazole) can mask the symptoms of most patients with ZES and can also cause hypergastrinemia as seen in ZES. The widespread use of PPIs has delayed the diagnosis of ZES.

Heartburn is also common (20%). Diarrhea (60 to 70%) occurs frequently and may be the first symptom (10 to 20%). Twenty to 25% of ZES patients have MEN 1 (Chapter 239). These patients have hyperplasia or tumors of multiple endocrine glands (parathyroid hyperplasia [>90%], pituitary tumors [60%], and PETs [80 to 100%]). In MEN 1, ZES is the most common functional PET syndrome (54%), although patients typically first develop renal stones related to hypercalcemia from hyperparathyroidism or have elevated prolactin levels resulting from pituitary tumors and only later develop ZES. However, studies show that 20 to 40% of patients with MEN and ZES initially present with ZES symptoms.

In ZES patients, almost all the symptoms result from the effects of gastric acid hypersecretion, but late in the disease, patients can have tumor-related symptoms. Approximately one third of patients have metastatic liver disease at presentation, but less than 20% of other patients develop metastatic disease to the liver during a 10-year follow-up period.

Up to 5% of patients with ZES develop Cushing's syndrome (Chapter 234) as a result of adrenocorticotropic hormone (ACTH) secretion by the gastrinoma. These patients usually have a metastatic gastrinoma in the liver, ZES without MEN 1, and a poor prognosis.

DIAGNOSIS

ZES should be suspected in any patient whose peptic ulcer disease is accompanied by diarrhea, is recurrent, does not heal with treatment, is not associated with *H. pylori* infection, is associated with a complication (bleeding, obstruction, esophageal stricture), is multiple or occurs in unusual locations, or is associated with a pancreatic tumor. ZES should also be suspected in patients with chronic secretory diarrhea (Chapter 142), peptic ulcer disease associated with large gastric folds, a family or personal history of renal stones or endocrinopathies, or the laboratory finding of hypercalcemia, hypergastrinemia, or gastric acid hypersecretion.

When suspected, the initial test is a fasting serum gastrin level, which is elevated in 99 to 100% of ZES patients. However, other causes of hypergastrinemia include renal failure, *H. pylori* infections, and a physiologic response to achlorhydria or hypochlorhydria because of pernicious anemia, atrophic gastritis, or the use of PPIs. If the serum gastrin level is elevated, the fasting gastric pH should be determined. If the serum gastrin is more than 1000 pg/mL (normal, <100) and the pH is less than 2.0, the patient almost certainly has ZES; approximately 40% of patients have this combination. If the gastrin is increased more than ten-fold and the pH is less than 2.0, basal acid output and a secretin test should be performed. Basal acid output is increased in patients with ZES, and more than 95% have a value greater than 15 mEq/hour if no previous gastric acid–reducing surgery has been performed. Because of their long duration of action, PPIs must be stopped for at least 1 week, if possible, to ensure that the cause of the hypergastrinemia is not the drug itself.

Differential Diagnosis

A secretin test can exclude *H. pylori* infection, retained gastric-antrum syndrome, antral G-cell hyperfunction or hyperplasia, chronic renal failure, and gastric outlet obstruction that may mimic ZES. Physiologically normal individuals show a less than 120 pg/mL increase in the gastrin level after intravenous secretin, whereas 94% of ZES patients with a fasting gastrin level that is elevated less than ten-fold above normal have a positive test. No false-positive results are reported, except in patients with achlorhydria. In all patients with ZES, evaluation must exclude MEN 1 syndrome by searching for other endocrinopathies and assessing family history.

Imaging and Endoscopy

All patients should have imaging studies to localize the tumor. Somatostatin receptor scintigraphy using single photon emission computed tomography after injection of indium-111–[diethylenetriamine pentaacetic acid-D-phenylalanine-1] octreotide is the localization method of choice; it identifies 60% of primary gastrinomas and more than 90% of patients with metastatic liver disease with a sensitivity equal to all conventional imaging studies (magnetic resonance imaging [MRI], computed tomography [CT], ultrasound, angiography) combined. For pancreatic gastrinomas, endoscopic ultrasound is particularly sensitive. Small duodenal gastrinomas (<1 cm) are frequently not detected by an imaging modality but can be found at surgery if routine duodenotomy is performed. Recent studies show that two new imaging techniques may be useful for small gastrinomas and other PETs: the use of hybrid scanning with CT or MRI and somatostatin receptor scintigraphy (SRS) and the use of positron emission tomographic scanning, especially with gallium-68-labeled somatostatin analogues.

TREATMENT Rx

Medical Therapy

Patients need medical therapy directed at controlling the gastric acid hypersecretion and, if possible, surgical therapy to remove the gastrinoma. PPIs are now the drugs of choice. Because of their long duration of action, acid hypersecretion can be controlled in all patients with once- or twice-daily doses. The recommended starting dose for omeprazole is 60 mg once a day. In 30% of patients, higher doses are needed, particularly in patients with MEN 1, previous gastric surgery, or a history of severe esophageal reflux. Patients must be treated indefinitely unless surgically cured. Long-term therapy is safe, and patients have been treated for up to 20 years with omeprazole without loss of efficacy, although reduced vitamin B_{12} levels may occur and require vitamin B_{12} supplementation (Chapter 167). Histamine-2 receptor antagonists are also effective, but frequent (every 4 to 6 hours) high doses are needed. Total gastrectomy, the historical treatment, is now performed only for patients who cannot or will not take oral antisecretory medications. Selective vagotomy reduces acid secretion, but many patients continue to require a low dose of drug. Parathyroidectomy should be performed in MEN 1 patients with hyperparathyroidism and ZES because it reduces acid secretion and increases the sensitivity to antisecretory drugs.

Surgical Therapy

Surgical exploration for cure is recommended in all patients without liver metastases, MEN 1, or complicating medical conditions that limit life expectancy. Tumors are found by experienced endocrine surgeons in 95% of patients at surgery. Surgical resection decreases the metastatic rate, increases survival, and results in a 5-year cure rate of 30%. Patients with metastatic gastrinoma in the liver have a poor prognosis, with a 5-year survival rate of 30%.

Metastatic Disease

If the metastatic disease is slowly increasing in size or is symptomatic, treatment with octreotide (100 to 450 μg two to three times daily) alone or in combination with interferon-α (1 to 5 million U 3 to 7 days/week) is effective in inhibiting further tumor growth in 50 to 60% of patients. If this treatment fails or if the tumor is rapidly growing, chemotherapeutic agents (streptozotocin, 5-fluorouracil, doxorubicin) are recommended. For patients with extensive metastatic disease, somatostatin receptor–directed radiation therapy using analogues labeled with yttrium-90, lutetium-177, or indium-111 is increasingly used. Newer treatments targeting PETs using radiolabeled somatostatin analogues or targeting PET growth factors or their receptors, intracellular signaling cascades (mTor), and a DTIC-related compound, temozolomide, show some promise in a small number of gastrinomas and other PET patients. Liver transplantation is occasionally performed in the rare patient with metastases limited to the liver.

PROGNOSIS

Approximately 25% of gastrinomas show aggressive growth. The most important prognostic predictor is the development of liver metastases. The presence of a large primary tumor, a pancreatic tumor, bone metastases, development of ectopic Cushing's syndrome, or a high fasting gastrin level is associated with aggressive growth.

Glucagonomas

DEFINITION

Glucagonomas are endocrine tumors of the pancreas that ectopically secrete glucagons, causing a specific syndrome (see Table 201-1).

PATHOBIOLOGY

Glucagon hypersecretion explains the glucose intolerance. The exact origin of the rash is unclear; some studies report that prolonged glucagon infusions can cause the characteristic skin lesions. A role for possible zinc deficiency has been proposed because of the similarity of the rash to that seen with zinc deficiency (acrodermatitis enteropathica) and because the rash improves in some patients who are given zinc. The hypoaminoacidemia is thought to be secondary to the effect of glucagon on amino acid metabolism by altering gluconeogenesis. The wasting and weight loss are intrinsic parts of the glucagonoma syndrome, and recent studies suggest that a novel anorectic substance distinct from glucagon is responsible.

CLINICAL MANIFESTATIONS

The cardinal clinical features are a distinct dermatitis (necrolytic migratory erythema, seen in 70 to 90%), diabetes mellitus and glucose intolerance (40 to 90%), weight loss (70 to 96%), anemia (30 to 85%), hypoaminoacidemia (80 to 90%) with deficiencies of essential fatty acids, thromboembolism (10 to 25%), diarrhea (15 to 30%), and psychiatric disturbances (0 to 20%). The characteristic skin rash is usually found at intertriginous and periorificial sites, especially in the groin and buttocks (Fig. 201-1). It is initially erythematous, becomes raised, and develops central bullae whose tops detach, with the eroded areas becoming crusty. Healing occurs with hyperpigmentation.

DIAGNOSIS

The diagnosis is established by demonstrating elevated plasma glucagon levels. Normal levels are 150 to 200 pg/mL; in patients with glucagonomas, levels usually (>90%) are higher than 1000 pg/mL. However, in some recent studies, up to 40% of patients had plasma glucagon values of 500 to 1000 pg/mL. Increased plasma glucagon levels also occur in renal insufficiency, acute pancreatitis, hypercorticism, hepatic diseases, celiac disease, severe stress and prolonged fasting, in patients treated with danazol, and in familial hyperglucagonemia. In these conditions, the level is usually less than 500 pg/mL except in patients with hepatic diseases or in those with familial hyperglucagonemia.

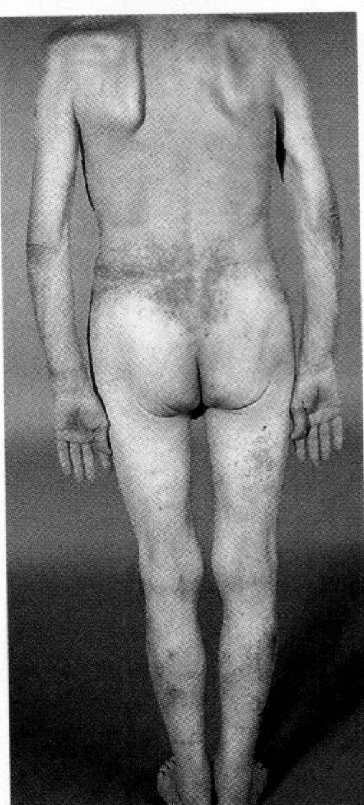

FIGURE 201-1. A patient with a glucagonoma with the characteristic rash (necrolytic migratory erythema). The rash is usually at intertriginous areas or periorificial sites and shows various stages of erythema, blistering, and crusting. (From Forbes CD, Jackson WF. *Color Atlas and Text of Clinical Medicine*, 3rd ed. London: Mosby; 2003.)

Glucagonomas are generally large when discovered (mean, 5 to 10 cm), and they most frequently occur in the pancreatic tail (>50%). Liver metastases are commonly present at the time of diagnosis (45 to 80%).

TREATMENT

Rx

Subcutaneous administration of the synthetic long-acting somatostatin analogue, octreotide (100 to 400 micrograms two to three times daily), controls the rash in 80% of patients and improves weight loss, diarrhea, and hypoaminoacidemia, but it usually does not improve the diabetes mellitus. Increasingly, long-acting depot formulations of octreotide (octreotide-LAR) or lanreotide autogel are being given by monthly injection. Zinc supplementation and infusions of amino acids or fatty acids, or both, can diminish the severity of the rash. After tumor localization, surgical resection is preferred; even debulking of metastatic tumor may be of benefit. For advanced disease, chemotherapy (with dacarbazine or streptozotocin and doxorubicin), hepatic embolization, or chemoembolization may control symptoms in refractory cases.

PROGNOSIS

The prognosis is now largely determined by the growth of the tumor per se because the symptoms of glucagon excess can be largely controlled by somatostatin analogues. This is particularly true with glucagonomas because in many series more than 50 to 80% are metastatic at presentation, and patients usually present late with large primary tumors. The mean 5-year survival rate is 50%; however, extended survivals (>15 years) are reported in some patients with treatment with somatostatin analogues and other tumor-directed therapies.

VIPomas

DEFINITION

The VIPoma syndrome, also called the Verner-Morrison syndrome, pancreatic cholera, and the WDHA syndrome (for watery diarrhea, hypokalemia, and achlorhydria), results from an endocrine tumor, usually in the pancreas that ectopically secretes vasoactive intestinal polypeptide (VIP).

EPIDEMIOLOGY AND PATHOBIOLOGY

VIPomas in adults are found in the pancreas in 80 to 90% of cases; rare cases result from intestinal carcinoids, ganglioneuromas, ganglioneuroblastomas, and pheochromocytomas. In children younger than 10 years and rarely in adults (<5%), the VIPoma syndrome is caused by ganglioneuromas or ganglioneuroblastomas at extrapancreatic sites. VIPomas are usually large and solitary; 50 to 75% of these tumors occur in the pancreatic tail, and 40 to 70% have metastasized at diagnosis. VIPomas frequently secrete both VIP and peptide histidine methionine, but VIP is responsible for the symptoms. VIP is a potent stimulant of secretion in the small and large intestine, which causes the cardinal clinical features of the VIPoma syndrome. VIP also causes relaxation of gastrointestinal smooth muscle, and this may contribute to the dilated loops of bowel that are common in this syndrome as well as a dilated, atonic gallbladder that is sometimes seen. Hypochlorhydria is thought to result from the inhibitory effect of VIP on acid secretion, the flushing is related to the vasodilatory effects of VIP, and the hyperglycemia is caused by the glycogenolytic effect of VIP. The mechanism of the hypercalcemia remains unclear.

CLINICAL MANIFESTATIONS

The cardinal clinical feature is severe, large-volume, watery diarrhea (>1 L/day) (100%), which is secretory and occurs during fasting. Hypokalemia (67 to 100%) and dehydration (83%) commonly occur because of the volume of the diarrhea. Achlorhydria is occasionally noted, but hypochlorhydria is usually found (34 to 72% of cases). Flushing occurs in 20% of patients, hyperglycemia in 25 to 50%, and hypercalcemia in 41 to 50%. Steatorrhea is uncommon (16%) despite the volume of diarrhea.

DIAGNOSIS

The diarrhea of VIPomas characteristically persists during fasting and is large in volume (>3 L/day in 70 to 80%); the diagnosis is excluded when fasting stool volume is less than 700 mL/day. To differentiate VIPomas from other causes of large-volume, fasting diarrhea, fasting plasma VIP levels should be determined. The normal value in most laboratories is less than 190 pg/mL, and elevated levels are present in 90 to 100% of patients in various series. The differential diagnosis of large-volume, fasting diarrhea (>700 mL/day) includes ZES, diffuse islet cell hyperplasia, surreptitious use of laxatives, the pseudopancreatic cholera syndrome, and, rarely, human immunodeficiency virus (HIV) infection (Chapter 397). Serum gastrin levels identify patients with ZES, and plasma VIP levels are normal in most patients who abuse laxatives, in 82% of patients with pancreatic islet cell hyperplasias, and in patients with HIV-induced secretory diarrhea.

TREATMENT

The symptoms caused by the VIP are controlled initially in more than 85% of patients by daily doses of octreotide (50 to 400 μg once to three times daily) or by monthly injections of the depot form, octreotide-LAR or lanreotide autogel, but increased doses may be needed over time. Before the availability of octreotide, small numbers of patients were reported to respond to a variety of agents, including high-dose prednisone (60 to 100 mg/day; 40 to 50%), clonidine, lithium carbonate, indomethacin, loperamide, metoclopramide, and phenothiazines. After tumor localization studies, surgical resection should be attempted if it is possible to remove all visible tumor; however, more than 50% of patients have generalized liver metastases at diagnosis, so complete resection may not be possible. For patients with advanced cases and refractory symptoms, chemotherapy with streptozotocin and doxorubicin, hepatic chemoembolization, and hepatic embolization have been beneficial.

PROGNOSIS

The prognosis is now largely determined by the growth of the tumor per se because the symptoms of VIP excess can be largely controlled by somatostatin analogues. This is particularly true in patients with VIPomas because they frequently (>50%) present with advanced metastatic disease. The mean 5-year survival is 50 to 70%.

Somatostatinomas

DEFINITION AND PATHOBIOLOGY

Somatostatinomas are endocrine tumors that occur in the pancreas or upper small intestine and ectopically secrete somatostatin. In the gastrointestinal tract, somatostatin inhibits basal and stimulated acid secretion, pancreatic secretion, intestinal absorption of amino acids, gallbladder contractility, and release of numerous hormones, including cholecystokinin and gastrin.

CLINICAL MANIFESTATIONS

Most reported somatostatinomas are diagnosed histologically as an endocrine tumor containing somatostatin-like immunoreactivity and are not associated with a distinct clinical syndrome (the somatostatinoma syndrome). The somatostatinoma syndrome includes diabetes mellitus, gallbladder disease, diarrhea, steatorrhea, and weight loss. Sixty percent of somatostatinomas occur in the pancreas, and 40% are found in the duodenum or jejunum. Pancreatic somatostatinomas occur in the pancreatic head in 60 to 80% of cases; 70 to 92% have metastasized at diagnosis, and they are usually large (mean, 5 cm) and solitary. In contrast, duodenal somatostatinomas are smaller (mean, 2.4 cm), frequently associated with psammoma bodies on histologic examination (11%), and less frequently have metastases at diagnosis (30 to 40%).

The somatostatinoma syndrome occurs much more commonly (80 to 95% of all cases) in patients with pancreatic than duodenal or intestinal somatostatinomas. Duodenal somatostatinomas occur in up to 10% of patients with von Recklinghausen's disease and are usually asymptomatic.

DIAGNOSIS

Somatostatinomas are usually found by accident, particularly during exploratory laparotomy for cholecystectomy, during endoscopy, or on imaging studies. The presence of psammoma bodies on histologic examination of a duodenal endocrine tumor or any duodenal lesions in patients with von Recklinghausen's disease should raise the suspicion of a duodenal somatostatinoma. The diagnosis of the somatostatinoma syndrome requires the demonstration of increased concentrations of somatostatin-like immunoreactivity in the plasma and the resected tumor. However, other tumors outside the pancreas or intestine, such as small cell lung cancer, medullary thyroid carcinoma, pheochromocytomas, and paragangliomas, may also have elevated concentrations of somatostatin-like immunoreactivity. Somatostatinomas can be imaged using somatostatin receptor scintigraphy or, if needed, other conventional imaging studies to assess the tumor's location.

TREATMENT 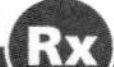

Treatment with octreotide or lanreotide can improve symptoms. Surgery, if possible, or chemotherapy, hepatic chemoembolization, or hepatic embolization may be of value.

PROGNOSIS

Patients with intestinal somatostatinomas, which uncommonly cause the somatostatinoma syndrome and are less malignant, have an excellent prognosis (5-year survival rate, >80%), whereas those with pancreatic somatostatinomas, which frequently cause the somatostatinoma syndrome and present with metastatic disease (>70%), have a much reduced 5-year survival rate (<50%).

GRFomas

DEFINITION

GRFomas are endocrine tumors that frequently originate in the pancreas but also occur in other extrapancreatic locations and ectopically release growth hormone–releasing factor (GRF). The GRF causes acromegaly that is clinically indistinguishable from that caused by a pituitary adenoma.

PATHOBIOLOGY

GRFomas most commonly occur in the lung (54%). Most of the remainder occur in the gastrointestinal tract, including 30% in the pancreas. Pancreatic GRFomas are usually large (mean, 6 cm), 39% are metastatic at diagnosis, 40% occur in combination with ZES, and 33% are in patients with MEN1.

DIAGNOSIS

GRFomas are an uncommon cause of acromegaly. These tumors occurred in none of 177 unselected patients with acromegaly in one study. However, any patient with acromegaly and abdominal complaints, with acromegaly but no pituitary tumor, or with acromegaly and hyperprolactinemia (which occurs in 70% of GRFomas) should be suspected of having a GRFoma. The intra-abdominal features of GRFomas result from its metastases and are typical of any malignant PET. The diagnosis is confirmed by performing a plasma assay for GRF and growth hormone.

TREATMENT 

The effects of the GRF can be controlled with octreotide or lanreotide in more than 90% of patients. Treatment should be directed at the GRFoma per se, as described for the other more common PETs.

Nonfunctional Pancreatic Endocrine Tumors

DEFINITION

Nonfunctional PETs are endocrine tumors that originate in the pancreas and either secrete no peptides or secrete products that do not cause clinical symptoms.

PATHOBIOLOGY

Frequently secreted, nonfunctional peptides include chromogranin A (100%), pancreatic polypeptide (60%), and the α-subunit (40%) and β-subunit of human chorionic gonadotrophin. Immunocytochemically, even higher percentages contain these peptides as well as insulin (50%), glucagons (30%), and somatostatin (13%).

CLINICAL MANIFESTATIONS

Nonfunctional PETs are frequently diagnosed only late in the course of disease after the patient presents with symptoms or signs of metastatic disease and a liver biopsy reveals metastatic PET. Any symptoms or signs result from the tumor per se and include abdominal pain (36 to 56%), abdominal mass or hepatosplenomegaly (8 to 40%), weight loss or cachexia (8 to 46%), and jaundice (27 to 40%). In 20% of asymptomatic patients, tumors are found incidentally at surgery.

DIAGNOSIS

Any patients with a long survival (>5 years) after a diagnosis of metastatic pancreatic adenocarcinoma should be suspected of having a nonfunctional PET. Most primary tumors are large (70% are >5 cm), and 70% occur in the pancreatic head. Liver metastases are frequent (38 to 62%) at presentation. An elevated plasma chromogranin A or pancreatic polypeptide level or a positive somatostatin receptor scintigraphic scan is strong evidence that a pancreatic mass is a PET. Malignancy correlates with vascular or perineural invasion, a proliferative index of more than 2%, a mitotic rate of 2 or higher, a size of at least 4 cm, capsular penetration, nuclear atypia, lack of progesterone receptors, and the presence of calcitonin immunoreactivity in the tumor.

TREATMENT 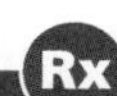

Tumor localization, surgical resection, and, for advanced cases, chemotherapy with streptozotocin and doxorubicin, hepatic embolization, or chemoembolization are useful. Survival is better in patients with smaller tumors, patients who are asymptomatic at presentation, patients with no metastases, and patients in whom surgical resection can be performed.

Two novel agents have been recently found to prolong progression-free and probably overall survival in patients with advanced pancreatic neuroendocrine tumors, major proportions of which were nonfunctional. The multitargeted tyrosine kinase inhibitor sunitinib was administered by a daily oral dose of 37.5 mg [1]; the oral inhibitor of mTOR, everolimus, was given at a dose of 10 mg once daily. [2]

PROGNOSIS

The overall 5-year survival rate varies in different series from 30 to 70%, but it is heavily dependent on the extent of the disease at diagnosis, with survival rates of 96% in patients without metastases at presentation, decreasing to 30 to 50% for those with metastatic disease.

ACTHomas and Other Uncommon Tumors

PETs that ectopically secrete ACTH cause 4 to 16% of the cases of ectopic Cushing's syndrome. Cushing's syndrome (Chapter 234) occurs in 5% of all cases of ZES, but in patients with sporadic ZES, it is a late feature, occurring with metastatic liver disease. Its development is associated with a poor prognosis, and the response to chemotherapy is generally poor; however, occasional patients benefit from the use of long-acting somatostatin analogues (octreotide, lanreotide).

Paraneoplastic hypercalcemia (Chapter 186) can result from a PET that releases parathormone-related peptide or an unknown hypercalcemic substance. Tumors are generally large with metastatic liver disease at diagnosis. Somatostatin analogues may help control the hypercalcemia, but surgery, chemotherapy, hepatic embolization, and chemoembolization are the mainstays of treatment.

PETs causing the carcinoid syndrome (Chapter 240) are usually large, and 68 to 88% are malignant. Octreotide may control the symptoms. Surgery, chemotherapy, or hepatic embolization or chemoembolization may be helpful.

A single case of a PET that secreted renin manifested with severe hypertension; the tumor was localized with somatostatin receptor scintigraphy, and the patient's symptoms improved significantly after tumor resection. A single case of an erythropoietin-secreting PET resulting in polycythemia and a single case of a PET secreting insulin-like growth factor II causing hypoglycemia have been described.

Two symptomatic cases of PETs that secreted luteinizing hormone have been described; virilization occurred in the female patient, whereas the male patient had increased acne and a skin rash. In both cases, the tumors were resectable, and symptoms improved postoperatively.

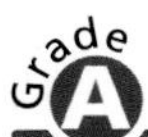

1. Raymond E, Dahan L, Raoul JL, et al. Sunitinib malate for the treatment of pancreatic neuroendocrine tumors. *N Engl J Med.* 2011;364:501-513.
2. Yao JC, Shah MH, Ito T, et al. Everolimus for advanced pancreatic neuroendocrine tumor. *N Engl J Med.* 2011;364:514-523.

SUGGESTED READINGS

Kuiper P, Verspaget HW, Overbeek LI, et al. An overview of the current diagnosis and recent developments in neuroendocrine tumors of the gastroenteropancreatic tract: the diagnostic approach. *Neth J Med.* 2011;69:14-20. *Review of epidemioloty, pathology, and diagnosis.*

Oberg K. Pancreatic endocrine tumors. *Semin Oncol.* 2010;37:594-618. *Review of diagnosis and treatment.*

Wilcox CM, Seay T, Arcury JT, et al. Zollinger-Ellison syndrome: presentation, response to therapy, and outcome. *Dig Liver Dis.* 2011. [Epub ahead of print.] *In a case series, symptoms preceded diagnosis by a median of 9 years and survival was principally related to underlying comorbidity.*

202 LIVER AND BILIARY TRACT TUMORS

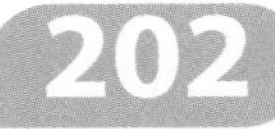

LEWIS R. ROBERTS

Liver and biliary tract tumors are a diverse group of benign and malignant tumors that arise from the different epithelial and stromal tissues of the liver. Various malignant diseases of other tissues metastasize to the liver or extend into or metastasize to the vicinity of the biliary tract, but not all mass lesions of the liver and biliary tract are malignant (Table 202-1).

TABLE 202-1 LIVER AND BILIARY TRACT TUMORS

TUMOR	CHARACTERISTICS ON IMAGING
BENIGN TUMORS USUALLY REQUIRING OBSERVATION ONLY	
Cavernous hemangioma	Peripheral enhancement filling into the center on delayed contrast imaging
Focal nodular hyperplasia	Rapid arterial enhancement with return to isointensity in venous phase; possible central scar with feeding vessel
Simple cyst	Hypoechoic on ultrasound
Focal fatty change	Best characterized by in- and out-of-phase sequences on magnetic resonance imaging
Angiolipoma	Arterial enhancement on contrast imaging
BENIGN TUMORS REQUIRING FURTHER EVALUATION AND TREATMENT	
Hepatic adenoma	Heterogeneous lesion with rapid arterial enhancement
Nodular regenerative hyperplasia	Nonspecific and variable
Cystadenoma	Cystic lesion on ultrasonography with solid components, enhancement of cyst wall; possible septations
Hepatic abscess (Chapter 154)	Cystic lesion on ultrasonography
Inflammatory pseudotumor	Atypical enhancing mass on contrast imaging
Echinococcal cyst (Chapter 154)	Cystic mass with septations, calcified rims, daughter cysts
MALIGNANT TUMORS REQUIRING APPROPRIATE MANAGEMENT	
Hepatocellular carcinoma	Arterial enhancement with portal venous "washout"
Cholangiocarcinoma	Late arterial enhancement that persists in portal phase
Mixed hepatocellular-cholangiocarcinoma	Early to late arterial enhancement
Liver metastases	Peripheral arterial enhancement, usually bilobar, multifocal disease
Cystadenocarcinoma	Solid enhancing mass in cystic lesion
Sarcoma	Solid mass with arterial enhancement
Mixed hepatic tumor	Solid mass with arterial enhancement; possible areas of calcification
Non-Hodgkin's lymphoma (Chapter 191)	Less intense arterial enhancement than hepatocellular carcinoma; possibly diffuse or mimicking hepatocellular carcinoma with venous invasion

EVALUATION OF MASS LESIONS OF THE LIVER

Diagnostic Approach

Mass lesions of the liver can be classified as benign lesions usually requiring observation only, benign lesions requiring further evaluation and treatment, or malignant lesions requiring appropriate management (see Table 202-1). The clinical approach to liver mass lesions requires careful history taking, physical examination, appropriate laboratory and imaging studies, judicious use of liver biopsy for histologic confirmation, and optimal management that considers the patient's age and comorbidities (Fig. 202-1).

History and Physical Examination

Because of the increasing use of imaging techniques for the evaluation of abdominal symptoms, many mass lesions of the liver are discovered incidentally as a result of imaging performed to evaluate nonhepatic diseases, such as abdominal pain or discomfort (Chapter 134). Right upper quadrant discomfort is frequently nonspecific and unhelpful in the evaluation of liver masses. Nevertheless, large liver masses may distend the liver capsule and cause pain, which is occasionally referred to the right shoulder. Patients also may present with episodes of acute, severe pain, which results from bleeding into a hepatic adenoma, a primary hepatocellular carcinoma, or the liver surrounding the lesion. Patients with advanced malignant disease and regional lymph metastases may present with epigastric pain.

Patients with malignant liver disease, whether primary or metastatic, frequently present with constitutional symptoms, which include night sweats, low-grade fever, unintended weight loss, anorexia, and diarrhea. In the United States, the most common malignant lesions in the liver are metastases from other primary cancers, including the esophagus, stomach, colon, pancreas, breast, lung, neuroendocrine, kidney, bladder, and skin cancer. Patients with hepatocellular carcinoma often have symptoms related to their underlying liver disease, such as fatigue from chronic hepatitis or ascites, spontaneous bacterial peritonitis, variceal bleeding, or hepatic encephalopathy resulting from cirrhosis with portal hypertension. Patients with cholangiocarcinoma may present with jaundice from a dominant stricture or with episodes of acute cholangitis in the setting of primary or secondary sclerosing cholangitis (Chapter 158).

When available, previous imaging studies of the liver can be helpful in determining whether a liver lesion is new or enlarging. The patient's characteristics, including age, sex, history of oral contraceptive use (associated with an increased incidence of hepatic adenomas), geographic residence, travel history (relevant in cases of amebic liver abscess and hydatid cysts), alcohol

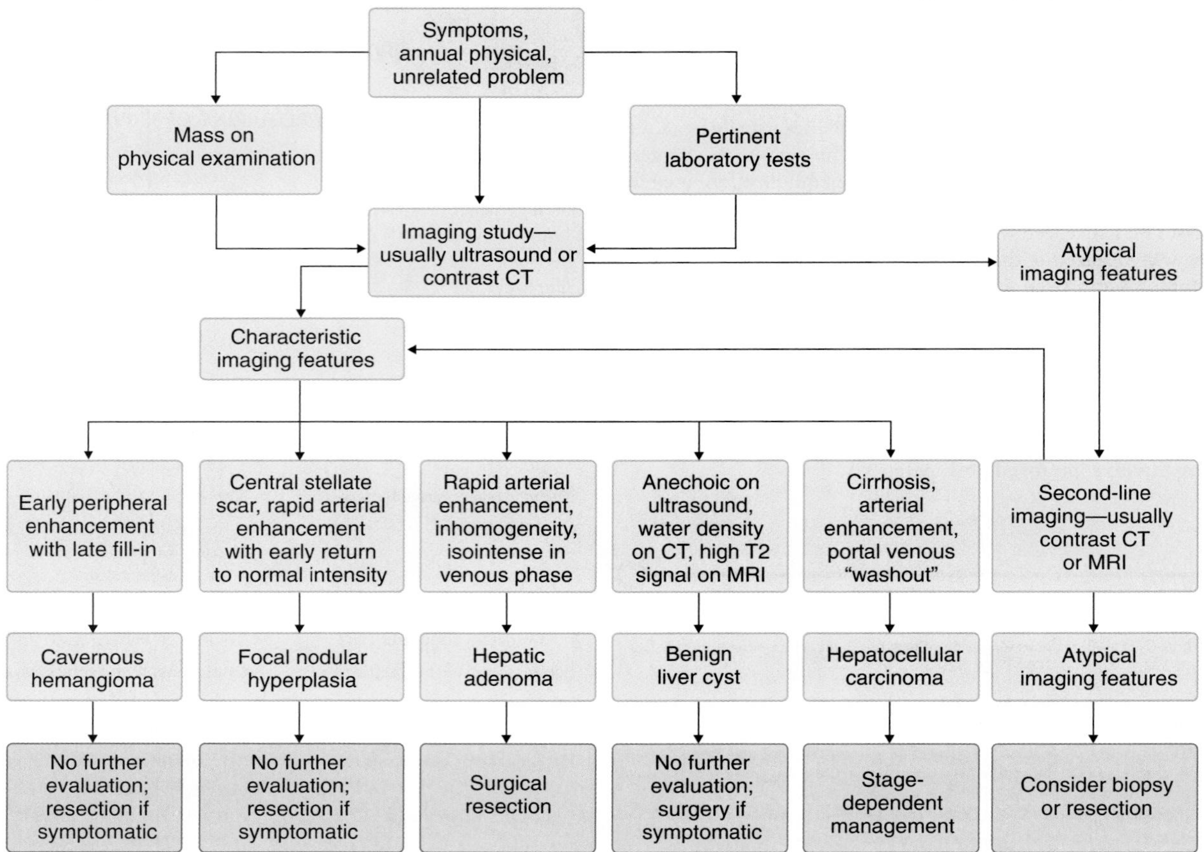

FIGURE 202-1. **Approach to evaluating the patient with a mass lesion in the liver.** Flow chart showing an algorithm for evaluating and managing common liver mass lesions. CT = computed tomography; MRI = magnetic resonance imaging.

consumption, and comorbid illnesses (e.g., association between chronic hepatitis or liver cirrhosis and hepatocellular carcinoma; association between ulcerative colitis or primary sclerosing cholangitis and cholangiocarcinoma) can also provide clues to the diagnosis.

On physical examination, patients with chronic liver disease typically have cutaneous stigmata (spider angiomas and palmar erythema), splenomegaly, and bilobar enlargement of the liver or caudate lobe hypertrophy. They may also have an abdominal bruit over a vascular hepatocellular carcinoma. Patients with metastatic disease may have peripheral or intra-abdominal lymphadenopathy or palpable peritoneal carcinomatosis. Jaundice, peripheral edema, and ascites are nonspecific features that may be related to benign or malignant liver disease.

Laboratory Findings

Laboratory studies are often useful in determining the nature of a liver mass or its underlying cause. Laboratory features of chronic liver disease include the following: thrombocytopenia; elevated levels of serum aminotransferase (elevated in active inflammatory liver disease or infiltrative neoplastic diseases), alkaline phosphatase, and bilirubin (markedly elevated in bile duct obstruction from biliary tumor or mass effect; Chapter 149); and low serum albumin levels and an elevated prothrombin time (abnormal in chronic liver disease). Viral markers (e.g., hepatitis B surface antigen and antibody, hepatitis B e antigen and antibody, hepatitis B virus DNA, and hepatitis C antibody and hepatitis C virus RNA), iron studies, and autoimmune markers (e.g., antimitochondrial antibody, antinuclear antibody, and anti–smooth muscle antibody) often help to determine the cause of chronic liver disease. Finally, tumor markers such as α-fetoprotein (AFP; hepatocellular carcinoma), CA-19-9 (cholangiocarcinoma), carcinoembryonic antigen (colorectal metastases or cholangiocarcinoma), and lactate dehydrogenase (lymphoma) have variable sensitivity and utility as screening tests but may be useful in confirming the diagnosis or in predicting prognosis.

COMMON BENIGN TUMORS OF THE LIVER

Cavernous Hemangioma

EPIDEMIOLOGY

Cavernous hemangioma, which is the most common benign tumor of the liver, is present in up to 7% of individuals in autopsy studies. There is a female predominance of 1.5 : 1 to 5 : 1, and hemangiomas are more common in multiparous women. Hemangiomas are multicentric in up to 30% of cases.

CLINICAL MANIFESTATIONS

Cavernous hemangiomas are usually asymptomatic, although large, subcapsular hemangiomas may cause abdominal pain or discomfort. Thrombosis of giant hemangiomas (>10 cm) may cause systemic features of inflammation such as fever, weight loss, and anemia.

Rarely, large hemangiomas are associated with the Kasabach-Merritt syndrome, which is local or disseminated intravascular coagulation with thrombocytopenia, hypofibrinogenemia, and increased fibrin degradation products, usually seen initially in infants (Chapter 178). Most cavernous hemangiomas remain stable over time, and malignant transformation does not occur. Rupture of cavernous hemangiomas is exceedingly rare, considering the high prevalence of hepatic hemangiomas.

DIAGNOSIS

Imaging

Hepatic cavernous hemangiomas have characteristic imaging features. On *ultrasound,* they appear as well-circumscribed, homogeneously hyperechoic lesions with smooth margins. Hemangiomas may also appear hypoechoic in fatty livers. Atypical features include hypoechoic lesions with a thin hyperechoic rim or a thick rind and scalloped borders.

On *dynamic contrast-enhanced multiphasic computed tomography* (CT), hemangiomas are hypoattenuating lesions on nonenhanced scans, with peripheral nodular enhancement during the arterial phase and later filling in toward the center of the lesion. On *contrast magnetic resonance imaging* (MRI) *with gadolinium,* hemangiomas appear as homogeneous, low-intensity lesions on T1-weighted images and as sharply demarcated, hyperintense lesions on T2-weighted images. In the arterial phase, peripheral enhancement occurs and fills in toward the center of the lesion on delayed images.

Technetium-99m-labeled red blood cell scintigraphy is very specific for hemangiomas. It shows low perfusion on early images and a high concentration of isotope that completely fills the lesion on late images. Larger hemangiomas that are complicated by fibrosis, thrombosis, or bleeding may have incomplete filling in on contrast or technetium-99m studies.

Because the imaging features are often characteristic, biopsy is seldom needed to confirm the diagnosis. Biopsy is occasionally useful for small indeterminate lesions and for large lesions with scarring and atypical imaging features. Histologic examination shows a network of vascular spaces lined by endothelial cells and separated by a thin, fibrous stroma. Large hemangiomas may have areas of thrombosis, scarring, and calcification.

TREATMENT **Rx**

Observation is the optimal management for most patients with asymptomatic hemangiomas. Surgical enucleation or anatomic resection is recommended for hemangiomas that cause significant pain, enlarge over time, are of uncertain diagnosis, or are associated with the Kasabach-Merritt syndrome. Rarely, liver transplantation has been used for massive unresectable hepatic hemangiomas, particularly in the presence of Kasabach-Merritt syndrome.

Focal Nodular Hyperplasia

DEFINITION

Focal nodular hyperplasia is a benign reaction to a congenital arterial malformation within the liver. The lesion typically consists of a vascular stellate scar with connective tissue, bile ductules surrounded by proliferated hepatocytes, and Kupffer cells separated by fibrous septa.

EPIDEMIOLOGY

Focal nodular hyperplasia occurs predominantly in women of childbearing age. The relationship with oral contraceptive use is controversial; some studies suggest an association of long-term oral contraceptive use with focal nodular hyperplasia and with complications such as hemorrhage or infarction. However, discontinuation of oral contraceptive use usually does not lead to resolution of focal nodular hyperplasia. There is a female predominance of 2 : 1 to 4 : 1, and the lesions are typically diagnosed in women aged 20 to 50 years. Focal nodular hyperplasias are occasionally multiple (10 to 20%) or are associated with cavernous hemangiomas (20%).

CLINICAL MANIFESTATIONS

Most focal nodular hyperplasias are asymptomatic. Patients with large or subcapsular lesions may present with abdominal discomfort or an abdominal mass. In contrast to hepatic adenoma, presentation with acute abdominal pain from tumor bleeding or necrosis is very rare.

DIAGNOSIS

On *ultrasound,* focal nodular hyperplasias are variably hypoechoic, hyperechoic, or isoechoic. The lesions are most commonly hypoechoic except for the central scar. Doppler evaluation frequently shows blood flow within the central stellate scar.

On *dynamic CT,* focal nodular hyperplasias are isoattenuating or slightly hypoattenuating on noncontrast CT. One sees rapid, intense contrast enhancement in the arterial phase and rapid loss of contrast from the lesion, so it becomes isointense in the venous phase. An avascular central scar is often seen, sometimes with a feeding artery coursing into the middle of the lesion.

On *contrast MRI,* the lesions are isointense on T1-weighted images and remain isointense or are slightly hyperintense on T2-weighted images. The central scar is hypointense on T1-weighted images but hyperintense on T2-weighted images. As with contrast CT, rapid, intense contrast enhancement in the arterial phase quickly dissipates. Typically, the central scar has a low signal on T1-weighted images and enhances with contrast.

Technetium-99m-sulfur colloid scintigraphy is occasionally used to characterize focal nodular hyperplasias. Hyperintense or isointense uptake occurs in 50 to 70% of focal nodular hyperplasias because of uptake by Kupffer cells. In contrast, most hepatic adenomas do not have Kupffer cells and so do not take up technetium-99m-sulfur colloid. *Kupffer cell–specific MRI agents* such as ferumoxide are taken up by Kupffer cells and lead to significant signal intensity loss on ferumoxide-enhanced T2-weighted images, which may help to distinguish focal nodular hyperplasia from hepatic adenoma and hepatocellular carcinoma.

Diagnosis is usually made by radiologic studies, and biopsy is rarely needed. When a histologic diagnosis of focal nodular hyperplasia is needed, a core needle biopsy should be performed because fine-needle aspirates may only show benign-appearing hepatocytes in both focal nodular hyperplasia and hepatic adenoma. Histopathologic examination shows a benign hepatic parenchyma with bile ductules in septal fibrosis.

TREATMENT **Rx**

The management of asymptomatic focal nodular hyperplasias with characteristic imaging or biopsy features is observation because lesions usually do not enlarge, bleed, or undergo malignant transformation. Patients do not need to discontinue oral contraceptive use because no convincing evidence indicates that discontinuation leads to reduction in size of the lesions. Surgical resection is recommended for indeterminate or symptomatic lesions.

Hepatic Adenoma

EPIDEMIOLOGY

Hepatic adenoma is a benign liver tumor that occurs predominantly in the third and fourth decades of life. There is a female predominance of 2 : 1 to 6 : 1 as well as a strong association with oral contraceptive use. The relative risk of developing a hepatic adenoma is 2.5 after 3 to 5 years of oral contraceptive use and 25 to 40 after 9 years of use, resulting in an incidence of 4 per 100,000 versus 1 per million in the general population.

PATHOBIOLOGY

Hepatic adenomas also occur in users of androgenic steroids, in a familial pattern associated with diabetes mellitus, in the syndrome of maturity-onset diabetes of the young, and in patients with glycogen storage disease types 1A and 3 (Chapter 214), hemochromatosis (Chapter 219), and acromegaly (Chapter 231). Adenomas are multiple in 20% of cases, particularly in patients with glycogen storage disease.

CLINICAL MANIFESTATIONS

Hepatic adenomas are usually asymptomatic and are discovered on imaging studies, but patients may present with intermittent pain or discomfort in the upper abdomen or right upper quadrant of the abdomen. Adenomas also have a propensity to rupture, with intrahepatic hemorrhage and pain or rarely with hemoperitoneum and shock. They may decrease in size after withdrawal of oral contraceptives, but typically they do not, and sometimes they even increase in size.

DIAGNOSIS

On *ultrasound,* hepatic adenomas are variably homogeneous or heterogeneous (because of hemorrhage or necrosis within the tumor). On *dynamic CT,* adenomas, like focal nodular hyperplasias, are isoattenuating on nonenhanced scans; with intravenous contrast, they show early enhancement and then become rapidly isoattenuating in the portal venous phase. Adenomas are often hyperattenuating in a fatty liver. Adenomas typically have well-defined borders and are not lobulated. Approximately 40% of adenomas have intralesional hemorrhage with heterogenous regions of high attenuation. Approximately 5% of adenomas show coarse calcifications within the lesion.

On *contrast MRI,* adenomas are hyperintense or isointense on T1-weighted images and are slightly hyperintense on T2-weighted images. They show early enhancement in the arterial phase and become isointense on delayed imaging.

Technetium-99m-sulfur colloid scintigraphy shows no uptake in 70% of adenomas because of the absence of Kupffer cells. Overall, the relatively nonspecific imaging features make adenomas difficult to differentiate from other lesions.

Biopsy is often required for diagnosis, but a significant risk of misdiagnosis exists in differentiating hepatic adenomas from focal nodular hyperplasias, as well as a potential risk of hemorrhage from core biopsies. Histologic examination shows sheets of well-differentiated hepatocytes without bile ductules, fibrous septa, portal tracts, or central veins. Most adenomas do not contain Kupffer cells.

TREATMENT AND PROGNOSIS

Management of hepatic adenoma is usually by surgical resection because of the risks of hemorrhage (≤30% for large adenomas) and malignant transformation (the exact risk is unknown). Radiofrequency ablation is used in patients who are high surgical risks. Oral contraceptives should be discontinued, and patients should avoid pregnancy until the adenoma is resected because these lesions often grow during pregnancy. The risk of malignant transformation is small but real.

Benign Liver Cysts

EPIDEMIOLOGY

Benign liver cysts occur in approximately 4% of individuals. There is a female predominance of 4 : 1, and the prevalence increases with age. Liver cysts are often multiple and coexist with other mass lesions in the liver. The inherited autosomal dominant and recessive polycystic kidney diseases (Chapter 129) are both associated with the development of multiple liver cysts. Liver cysts are lined by cuboidal bile duct epithelium and are filled with isotonic fluid. Cysts are typically asymptomatic, but large cysts can cause pressure symptoms or biliary obstruction. Hemorrhage, infection, or rupture of cysts is rare.

DIAGNOSIS

Ultrasound is the best imaging test to confirm the fluid-filled nature of cysts, which are anechoic and show no vascular flow on color flow or duplex Doppler. They demonstrate through-transmission and well-defined posterior walls. Simple cysts may have thin echogenic septa. On *dynamic CT,* cysts appear as water-density lesions. On *contrast MRI,* cysts are hyperintense on T2-weighted images. Small cysts may be difficult to differentiate from a cavernous hemangioma or other small hepatic lesions on CT or MRI because of the volume averaging from adjacent tissue. Biopsy is typically unnecessary because of the classical imaging findings.

Lesions with Focal Fat or Fat Sparing

PATHOBIOLOGY

Fatty infiltration of the liver (Chapter 155) is increasingly common as populations increase in weight across the world. Focal fatty infiltration can look like a mass on imaging studies, as can focal sparing in a liver that is diffusely infiltrated by fat. Associations with fatty change in the liver include obesity, diabetes mellitus, high alcohol consumption, and altered nutritional status as a result of chemotherapy.

CLINICAL MANIFESTATIONS

Patients with focal fatty infiltration are typically asymptomatic. The lesions are usually discovered incidentally and are sometimes mistaken for more sinister masses.

DIAGNOSIS

The characteristic imaging feature of focal fat is that it does not distort the contour of the liver, so normal vessels, especially veins, can be seen coursing through the lesion. Focal fat usually occurs in vascular watersheds such as the region around the falciform ligament. Fat sparing usually occurs adjacent to the gallbladder fossa, in subcapsular areas, and in the posterior aspect of segment IV. On ultrasound, fat is usually hyperechoic. On dynamic CT, fatty liver is hypodense compared with the spleen, but not as low in density as adipose tissue. Venous structures can be seen in the lesion on venous phase studies. On contrast MRI, fatty liver is occasionally hyperintense on T1-weighted and T2-weighted images. The decreased signal intensity on out-of-phase gradient imaging is diagnostic of focal fat.

Biopsy is occasionally useful to rule out other lesions. On histologic examination, areas of fatty infiltration show fat-laden cells.

PRIMARY MALIGNANT TUMORS OF THE LIVER AND BILIARY TRACT

Hepatocellular Carcinoma

EPIDEMIOLOGY

Hepatocellular carcinoma, the third most common cause of death from cancer worldwide, accounts for approximately 700,000 deaths annually. There is a male preponderance of 2 : 1 to 4 : 1. The major predisposing factor for the development of hepatocellular carcinoma is cirrhosis of the liver (Chapter 156). The risk factors for the development of hepatocellular carcinoma include chronic hepatitis B or C virus infection (Chapter 151), alcoholic cirrhosis, nonalcoholic steatohepatitis (Chapter 155), hereditary hemochromatosis (Chapter 219), α_1-antitrypsin deficiency (Chapter 153), primary biliary cirrhosis (Chapter 158), and autoimmune hepatitis (Chapter 151). The hepatitis B virus almost always integrates into the host genomic DNA and can lead to development of hepatocellular carcinoma in the absence of cirrhosis. The availability of an effective vaccine against hepatitis B has reduced the incidence of hepatitis B–related hepatocellular carcinomas in high-prevalence regions. Long-term exposure to fungal aflatoxins in the diet significantly increases the risk of hepatocellular carcinoma. The fungi are ubiquitous and invade and grow in grains, legumes, and peanuts when they are stored in conditions of high humidity and temperature. The aflatoxin-producing fungal species, *Aspergillus flavus* and *Aspergillus parasiticus,* produce at least 13 different types of aflatoxin, with aflatoxin B1 the most potent. In most parts of the world, the most rapidly increasing groups of patients with hepatocellular carcinoma includes those with chronic hepatitis C virus infection. More than 90% of individuals with hepatitis C virus infection develop chronic infection, and up to 20% of patients with chronic hepatitis C develop cirrhosis. Hepatocellular carcinoma then develops in up to 20% of individuals with cirrhosis from chronic hepatitis C virus, at a rate of 2 to 6% per year. More recently, there has been a progressive increase in obesity-related nonalcoholic fatty liver disease (Chapter 155), which can progress to steatohepatitis, cirrhosis (often previously considered to be of unknown origin or "cryptogenic"), and hepatocellular carcinoma. Diabetes, also obesity related, has recently been shown to be an independent risk factor for the development of hepatocellular carcinoma.

PATHOBIOLOGY

Like most other malignant diseases, hepatocellular carcinoma develops as a result of a combination of the activation of cellular oncogenic pathways and abrogation of tumor suppressor pathways. Chronic hepatic injury resulting from viruses, alcohol, and metabolic or autoimmune mechanisms leads to repeated cycles of liver cell death, regeneration, and repair that ultimately lead to premature senescence of the liver.

Cellular senescence is characterized by a progressive decrease in length of the telomeric regions that protect the ends of chromosomes, with resulting development of chromosomal and genetic instabilities that are recognized by cellular stress response pathways and that trigger the apoptosis of senescent cells in a process known as *telomeric crisis.* In some senescent cells, apoptosis is avoided, and the cells become immortal, either through activation of the cellular telomerase enzyme complex, which maintains telomere ends, or through non-telomerase-dependent mechanisms. These genetically unstable, immortal cells are then prone to the development of additional genetic and epigenetic alterations that result in the cancer phenotype of unconstrained cell proliferation, resistance to apoptosis, enhanced cell migration and invasion, and activation of new vessel formation (angiogenesis).

Many oncogenic pathways normally have intrinsic tumor suppressor activities that limit their growth-promoting procarcinogenic effects; during carcinogenesis, mutations or epigenetic alterations lead to loss of the intrinsic tumor suppressing activity of the oncogenic pathways and result in unconstrained cellular proliferation and the secondary development of the other characteristics of the tumor phenotype. This hypothesis is well illustrated by the phenomenon of aflatoxin-induced mutation of the p53 tumor suppressor. During metabolism of aflatoxin in the liver, an aflatoxin B1-8,9-exo-epoxide intermediate is formed, and it interacts with cellular DNA to mediate formation of specific mutations, most frequently leading to a G-to-T transversion in codon 249 of the *p53* tumor suppressor gene. This mutation leads to loss of the p53 tumor suppressor function. Oncogenic pathways that normally activate p53 and limit proliferation are left without their natural "brake" on proliferation and result in an increased tendency to carcinogenesis. It is well known that aflatoxin B1 has a synergistic effect with the hepatitis B virus in the development of hepatocellular carcinoma.

Another important concept in the pathogenesis of malignant liver diseases is that of the development of malignant diseases within the epithelial stem cell compartment. Progenitor oval cells from the canals of Hering in the liver are capable of differentiating into both the hepatic and biliary lineages during liver regeneration. The development of a neoplastic phenotype within this compartment can result in the formation of cells that subsequently mature partially into more differentiated tumor cells and lead to the formation of a cancer with a "parent" clone of more immature progenitor cells and "daughter" clones of more mature cells. The existence of a tumor stem cell compartment (Chapter 185) has important implications for the development of anticancer therapy because agents that are active against carcinogenic pathways in the daughter cells but not in the parent clones may be capable of suppressing or arresting tumor growth but will not be curative unless they also target the growth pathways within the tumor stem cell compartment.

Integration of hepatitis B virus into host hepatocyte genomic DNA can lead to the development of hepatocellular carcinoma in the absence of cirrhosis. The pathogenic mechanisms include activation of oncogenic pathways through the activity of hepatitis B virus enhancer sequences and mutational inactivation of tumor suppressor genes by insertional mutagenesis. Certain proteins encoded by the hepatitis viruses have been shown to have oncogenic effects; these include the hepatitis B virus X protein, a truncated carboxy terminal variant of the hepatitis B virus S protein, the hepatitis C virus core protein, and NS5A protein.

Specific tumor suppressor and oncogenic molecules and pathways that have been shown to be important in liver carcinogenesis include the p53/p21^{WAF1} pathway, the p16^{INK4a}/CDK4/RB1/E2F pathway, the Wnt/β catenin signaling pathway, transforming growth factor-α, c-myc, the transcription factor NFκB, insulin/insulin-like growth factor I, and the receptor tyrosine kinases (fibroblast growth factor, hepatocyte growth factor, and vascular endothelial growth factor) and their downstream activators.

CLINICAL MANIFESTATIONS

Most patients are asymptomatic except for symptoms of chronic liver disease at cancer diagnosis because ultrasound surveillance in high-risk patients detects cancer in asymptomatic patients. Symptomatic presentation such as abdominal pain often suggests advanced stage cancer. Mild decompensation of cirrhosis can be observed from the replacement of functioning liver tissue with tumor. The sudden onset of severe abdominal pain from hemorrhage within the tumor mass is a rare presentation. Signs on physical examination may include a palpable liver mass and a vascular bruit over the tumor. Hepatocellular carcinomas occasionally cause a variety of paraneoplastic syndromes, including hypoglycemia mediated by insulin-like growth factors, erythrocytosis from erythropoietin generation by the tumor, hypercalcemia related to production of a parathyroid-like hormone, and watery diarrhea from tumor production of vasoactive intestinal peptide and other neuroendocrine hormones (Chapters 186 and 187).

DIAGNOSIS

Approximately 80 to 90% of hepatocellular carcinomas occur in a cirrhotic liver, so the early diagnosis of most hepatocellular carcinomas depends on rigorous efforts of intermittent long-term surveillance for cancer in patients with cirrhosis. Surveillance is usually performed using liver ultrasound every 6 months in patients with any cause of cirrhosis. In patients with chronic hepatitis B who are at increased risk of hepatocellular carcinoma (family history of hepatocellular carcinoma; high viral load or transaminases; Africans older than 20 years; Asian males older than 40 years; Asian females older than 50 years), ultrasound surveillance is indicated even in patients without liver cirrhosis. Any suspicious nodules found by ultrasound are then examined with additional contrast imaging studies.

A serum AFP level is a specific tumor marker for hepatocellular carcinoma. A level greater than 200 ng/mL has a 95 to 100% specificity for hepatocellular carcinoma, and lesions larger than 2 cm with AFP greater than 200 ng/mL is diagnostic for hepatocellular carcinoma; but at the cutoff value of 200 ng/mL, the sensitivity of AFP is only about 20%. Therefore, use of AFP alone for hepatocellular carcinoma surveillance is not recommended.

Contrast imaging studies are diagnostic modalities of choice once suspected nodules are detected during surveillance. On contrast imaging studies, including contrast CT, MRI, ultrasound, and angiography, hepatocellular carcinomas are characterized by bright enhancement in the arterial phase, followed by a loss of enhancement as contrast washes out of the arterial circulation, and a characteristic decreased intensity below that of the surrounding liver during the portal phase, when the surrounding liver is perfused

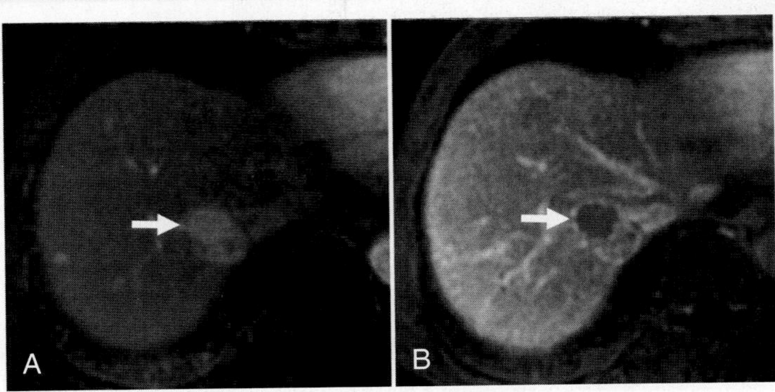

FIGURE 202-2. Hepatocellular carcinoma. A T1-weighted magnetic resonance image is shown during the arterial (**A**) and portal (**B**) phases after the administration of intravenous gadolinium contrast. The tumor *(arrows)* shows contrast enhancement in the arterial phase and washout in the portal phase.

by contrast to a higher intensity than that of the tumor nodule. This feature, referred to as *washout,* is highly specific for hepatocellular carcinomas occurring in a cirrhotic liver (Fig. 202-2). In patients with cirrhosis, almost all hepatocellular carcinomas 2 cm or larger can be confidently diagnosed using noninvasive imaging criteria. When lesions are between 1 and 2 cm in a cirrhotic liver, characteristic imaging findings should be present in two dynamic imaging studies to diagnose hepatocellular carcinoma.

Lesions smaller than 1 cm should be closely followed at an interval of 3 to 6 months for up to 2 years. Should a lesion not change, the patient can return to routine surveillance.

The diagnosis of small equivocal lesions in a noncirrhotic liver or any lesions in noncirrhotic liver can be established by needle biopsy of the lesion. However, because of the small but real risks of tumor seeding (0.5 to 2%), hemorrhage, and false-negative results from biopsy, many centers avoid biopsy, particularly in patients who may be candidates for liver transplantation and instead rely on imaging characteristics for the diagnosis of hepatocellular carcinoma.

PREVENTION

Universal vaccination against hepatitis B has been shown to reduce the incidence of hepatocellular carcinoma. 1 No vaccine is available against the hepatitis C virus. Individuals who have durable responses to treatment for hepatitis B and C appear to have a reduced risk of developing hepatocellular carcinoma.

TREATMENT Rx

Patients who have early-stage hepatocellular carcinoma and who do not have significant underlying liver dysfunction can be treated by surgical resection. Liver transplantation (Chapter 157) of patients who meet the Milan criteria (one tumor mass lesion ≤5 cm or two to three lesions each ≤3 cm, with no evidence of extrahepatic spread or vascular invasion) provides long-term survival results no different from those of patients receiving liver transplants for nonmalignant indications. In patients who are not candidates for liver transplantation, local ablation of small tumors up to 3 to 4 cm is performed with percutaneous ethanol injection or radiofrequency ablation, which uses probes with small tines that can be deployed through the tumor and energized with high-frequency electrical current to produce coagulation of the tumor and a surrounding rim of benign tissue. Although surgical resection and the local ablative therapies are effective treatments for small hepatocellular carcinomas, patients with cirrhosis still have a residual molecular defect in the remaining liver that makes them susceptible to recurrent tumor, at a rate of approximately 50% by 3 years after surgical resection or local ablation.

Patients with tumors that do not meet the criteria for surgical resection, liver transplantation, or local ablation but that are still limited to the liver are considered to have intermediate-stage disease. Intermediate-stage disease is currently treated using transarterial chemoembolization with chemotherapeutic agents, such as doxorubicin, mitomycin C, and cisplatin, as well as polyvinyl alcohol (Ivalon) or absorbable gelatin (Gelfoam) particles, sometimes combined with iodized poppy-seed oil (Lipiodol or Ethiodol). Randomized trials and meta-analyses have confirmed that transarterial chemoembolization improves survival of patients with intermediate-stage hepatocellular carcinoma. 2 Radioembolization with yttrium-90-impregnated glass microspheres, which is an alternative to transarterial chemoembolization, can be used for patients with portal vein thrombosis because, unlike the Ivalon or Gelfoam particles used for chemoembolization, the 20- to 30-μg glass microspheres used for radioembolization do not occlude the hepatic arterial vascular bed. However, radioembolization has not as yet been subjected to rigorous randomized trials.

Treatment using systemic chemotherapy is complicated by the presence of underlying chronic liver disease and a significantly increased risk of drug toxicity. Current efforts are focused on the use of targeted therapies directed against molecular pathways known to be involved in hepatocarcinogenesis, including receptor tyrosine kinases and the Wnt signaling pathway. Sorafenib, 400 mg twice daily, has been shown to increase median survival significantly in patients with advanced-stage hepatocellular carcinoma, typically by slowing progression but not by inducing remission.[3] Recently, sorafenib, 400 mg twice daily, combined with doxorubicin, 60 mg/m^2 intravenously every 21 days, was shown to be superior to doxorubicin alone in prolonging progression-free survival and overall survival among patients with advanced hepatocellular carcinoma.[4]

PROGNOSIS

Patients with early disease who undergo liver transplantation have an excellent outcome with a 5-year survival rate of 70 to 80% and 5-year recurrence rate of 10% or less. Patients who are ineligible for liver transplantation who undergo surgical resection or local treatment by radiofrequency ablation or percutaneous ethanol injection also have relatively high 5-year survival rates of 50 to 70%; however, because they still have a cirrhotic liver with a predisposition to cancer, these patients have a 3-year recurrence rate of approximately 50%. Patients with intermediate-stage disease who are treated with transarterial chemoembolization have a 1-year survival rate of 50 to 80% and a 2-year survival rate of 25 to 60%. Appropriate selection of individuals with preserved liver function is important for achieving the best outcomes with transarterial chemoembolization because it can decrease survival by inducing liver decompensation. Patients with advanced-stage disease who are currently candidates for treatment trials or symptomatic treatment have a median survival of only 6 to 8 months and a 1-year survival rate of 10 to 30%.

Cholangiocarcinoma

EPIDEMIOLOGY

Although the overall incidence of biliary cancers, or cholangiocarcinomas, is relatively low, these tumors are associated with perhaps the most rapidly rising incidence of any cancer in Western industrial nations. The reason for this trend is unknown. Most cholangiocarcinomas occur incidentally, but the known risk factors for cholangiocarcinoma include primary sclerosing cholangitis (Chapter 158), which is often associated with inflammatory bowel disease (Chapter 143); congenital choledochal cysts or other biliary tract abnormalities; Asian cholangiopathies secondary to liver fluke infections; and secondary chronic bacterial cholangitis, which frequently occurs in individuals who have had intrahepatic biliary stones or a prior biliary-enteric anastomosis. Chronic liver disease from viral or nonviral hepatitis is associated with cholangiocarcinoma, although the strength of association is weaker than with hepatocellular carcinoma.

PATHOBIOLOGY

The pathogenesis of cholangiocarcinoma is not well understood. Current concepts suggest that biliary inflammation results in impairment of DNA repair mechanisms, with the subsequent development of genomic instability and cancer. Genes in pathways shown to be involved in biliary carcinogenesis include *p53, K-ras, c-met, c-erbB2, mcl-1, Bcl-xl,* $p16^{INK4a}$, $p14^{ARF}$, *iNOS,* and *IL-6.*

CLINICAL MANIFESTATIONS

Patients with cholangiocarcinomas typically present with painless jaundice resulting from the presence of hilar or distal biliary strictures or with an intrahepatic mass causing abdominal pain, which may be referred to the shoulder. These patients often have associated pruritus, pale stools, and dark urine. Nonspecific symptoms such as weight loss and low-grade fever may also occur.

DIAGNOSIS

Cholangiocarcinomas are classified as intrahepatic or extrahepatic based on the location of the tumor within the biliary tree. The use of MRI with magnetic resonance cholangiography provides a noninvasive means of imaging the obstructed biliary tract before endoscopic retrograde cholangiopancreatography and allows the endoscopist and surgeon to plan an optimal approach for evaluation and therapy. Patients with unilateral biliary obstruction often have atrophy of the involved liver lobe and compensatory hypertrophy of the other lobe, referred to as the *atrophy-hypertrophy complex* (Fig. 202-3). Because of the presence of a dense fibrous stroma around a relatively sparse number of malignant glandular epithelial elements in many cholangiocarcinomas, cytologic examination from brushings of malignant strictures has a relatively low sensitivity, particularly in early cancers most amenable to successful therapy. However, the examination of biliary brush cytology specimens using advanced cytologic techniques such as DNA flow cytometry, digital image analysis, and fluorescence in situ hybridization with DNA probes for the detection of chromosomal polysomy has improved diagnostic accuracy (Fig. 202-4). These techniques can be applied in patients with primary sclerosing cholangitis who present with a new dominant stricture or clinical deterioration to improve the early detection of malignant transformation. Advanced endoscopic methods such as endoscopic ultrasound, intraductal ultrasound, and choledochoscopy also improve visualization and characterization of biliary strictures and associated metastatic lymphadenopathy.

The CA-19-9 marker is a commonly used tumor marker in cholangiocarcinoma. Although the sensitivity is modest and cholestasis and inflammation of the biliary tract can lead to false positive elevation, CA-19-9 is a tool for determining the effect of treatment or for monitoring recurrence after curative treatment.

TREATMENT (Rx)

The outcome after development of cholangiocarcinoma is generally poor because the tumor is relatively resistant to chemotherapy and also frequently results in biliary obstruction, which is complicated by episodes of bacterial cholangitis and cholestatic liver dysfunction. The treatment of biliary cancers depends on the extent of involvement of the biliary tree and on the presence of extrahepatic disease.

For disease limited to the liver and biliary tree, with malignant strictures that do not extend beyond the secondary branching of the right or left intrahepatic

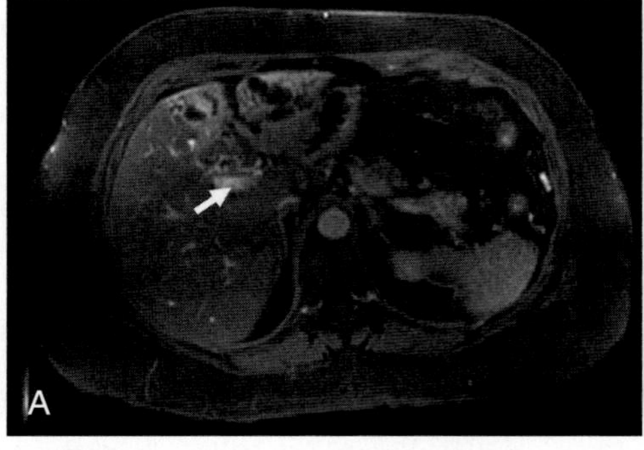

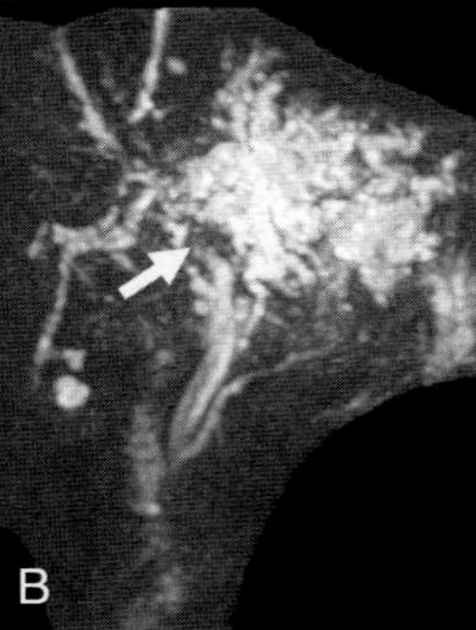

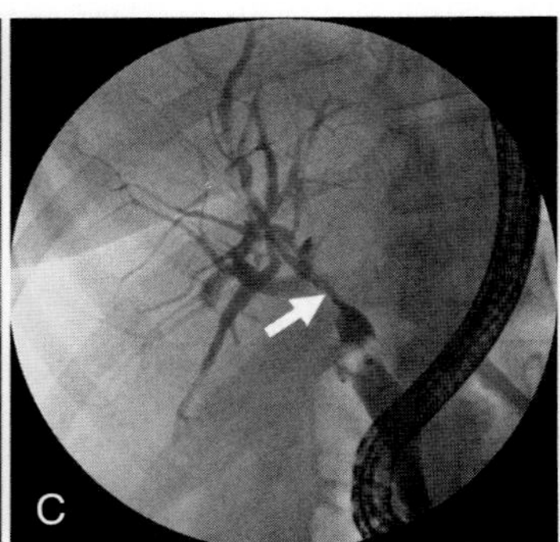

FIGURE 202-3. Cholangiocarcinoma. A, A T1-weighted magnetic resonance image during the arterial phase after the administration of intravenous gadolinium. The tumor *(arrow)* occludes the left hepatic duct, leading to marked dilation of the left biliary system and atrophy with enhanced contrast enhancement of the left lobe; the right lobe of the liver shows compensatory hypertrophy. This combination of features is called the *atrophy-hypertrophy complex.* **B,** Magnetic resonance cholangiopancreatography from the same patient showing narrowing of the common hepatic duct by the cholangiocarcinoma *(arrow)* and grossly dilated left biliary system. **C,** Endoscopic retrograde cholangiopancreatography showing filling of the right biliary system through the narrowed common hepatic duct *(arrow)*; the left biliary system is completely isolated and not filled during injection of contrast.

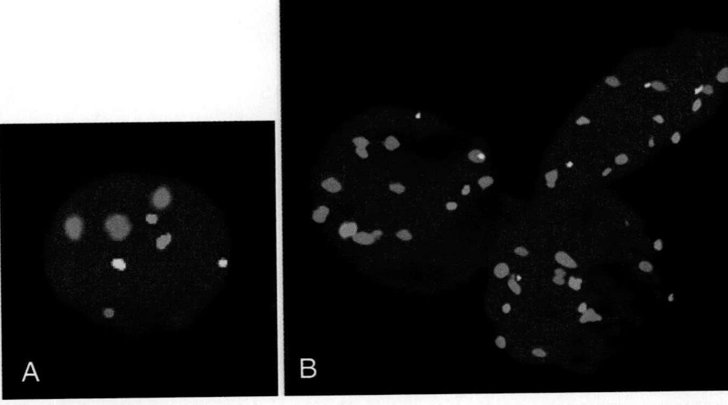

FIGURE 202-4. Fluorescence in situ hybridization for diagnosis of malignancy in biliary strictures. Fluorescent DNA probes for the centromeres of chromosomes 3 (red), 7 (green), 17 (aqua), and the p16 locus at chromosome 9p21 (yellow) are hybridized to brush cytology specimens obtained from biliary strictures at endoscopic retrograde cholangiopancreatography. The normal diploid cell (**A**) has two copies of each of the probes; the malignant polysomic cells (**B**) each have multiple copies of chromosomes 3, 7, and 17.

bile ducts, treatment by surgical resection results in a 5-year survival rate of approximately 20% after successful resection. Patients with distal biliary cancers without distant spread are usually treated by bile duct resection or by Whipple's pancreaticoduodenectomy.

Patients with unresectable disease are generally treated by palliative biliary stenting using plastic or metal stents. Effective stenting of approximately 25% of the total liver volume using the less affected lobe of the liver is usually sufficient to relieve cholestasis and is significantly less likely to result in repeated episodes of cholangitis.

Adjuvant chemotherapy and radiation, with staging laparotomy followed by liver transplantation for selected patients with early hilar cholangiocarcinomas, have resulted in a remarkable 5-year survival rate of 80% in patients who can successfully complete the treatment protocol. Photodynamic therapy with 630-nm laser light treatment administered using a fiber inserted across the biliary stricture after intravenous infusion of a photosensitizing porfimer, which is preferentially taken up by malignant cells, can preserve biliary patency and can improve survival in patients with unresectable malignant biliary strictures.5

In patients with locally advanced or metastatic cholangiocarcinoma, gallbladder cancer, or ampullary cancer, combination chemotherapy with cisplatin plus gemcitabine has been found to have survival advantage without the addition of substantial toxicity compared with gemcitabine alone.6

PROGNOSIS

Patients eligible for liver transplantation have the best prognosis with a 5-year rate survival of about 80%. Patients with curative resection have 5-year survival rate of about 20 to 40%. In patients with unresectable disease, biliary stenting, photodynamic therapy, and the use of chemotherapy regimens such as gemcitabine and cisplatin generally result in improvements in survival that are measured only in months.

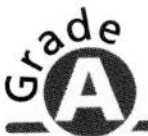

1. Chang MH, Shau WY, Chen CJ, et al. Hepatitis B vaccination and hepatocellular carcinoma rates in boys and girls. *JAMA*. 2000;284:3040-3042.
2. Llovet JM, Bruix J. Systematic review of randomized trials for unresectable hepatocellular carcinoma: chemoembolization improves survival. *Hepatology*. 2003;37:429-442.
3. Llovet JM, Ricci S, Mazzaferro V, et al. Sorafenib in advanced hepatocellular carcinoma. *N Engl J Med*. 2008;359:378-390.
4. Abou-Alfa GK, Johnson P, Knox JJ, et al. Doxorubicin plus sorafenib vs doxorubicin alone in patients with advanced hepatocellular carcinoma: a randomized trial. *JAMA*. 2010;304:2154-2160.
5. Ortner ME, Caca K, Berr F, et al. Successful photodynamic therapy for nonresectable cholangiocarcinoma: a randomized prospective study. *Gastroenterology*. 2003;125:1355-1363.
6. Valle J, Wasan H, Palmer DH, et al. Cisplatin plus gemcitabine versus gemcitabine for biliary tract cancer. *N Engl J Med*. 2010;362:1273-1281.

SUGGESTED READINGS

Alves RC, Alves D, Guz B, et al. Advanced hepatocellular carcinoma: review of targeted molecular drugs. *Ann Hepatol*. 2011;10:21-27. *Review emphasizing sorafenib.*

Burak KW, Kneteman NM. An evidence-based multidisciplinary approach to the management of hepatocellular carcinoma (HCC): the Alberta HCC algorithm. *Can J Gastroenterol*. 2010;24:643-650. *Recommendations regarding resection, ablative techniques, liver transplantation, transarterial chemoembolization, transarterial radioembolization, and sorafenib.*

Everhart JE, Ruhl CE. Burden of digestive diseases in the United States. Part III. Liver, biliary tract, and pancreas. *Gastroenterology*. 2009;136:1134-1144. *Documents the increasing incidence of hepatocellular carcinoma and cholangiocarcinoma in the United States over the past 25 years.*

Kim JH, Won HJ, Shin YM, et al. Radiofrequency ablation for the treatment of primary intrahepatic cholangiocarcinoma. *AJR Am J Roentgenol*. 2011;196:W205-W209. *An approach for local tumor control of primary intrahepatic cholangiocarcinomas <5 cm in diameter.*

Marrero JA, Feng Z, Wang Y, et al. Alpha-fetoprotein, des-gamma carboxyprothrombin, and lectin-bound alpha-fetoprotein in early hepatocellular carcinoma. *Gastroenterology*. 2009;137:110-118. *Overview of the diagnostic utility of these assays.*

Rahbari NN, Mehrabi A, Mollberg NM, et al. Hepatocellular carcinoma: current management and perspectives for the future. *Ann Surg*. 2011;253:453-459. *Review.*

Zografos GN, Farfaras A, Zagouri F, et al. Cholangiocarcinoma: principles and current trends. *Hepatobiliary Pancreat Dis Int*. 2011;10:10-20. *Review of surgical and medical treatments.*

203 TUMORS OF THE KIDNEY, BLADDER, URETERS, AND RENAL PELVIS

DEAN F. BAJORIN

RENAL CELL CARCINOMA

DEFINITION

Cancers of the kidney are a heterogeneous group of neoplasms, most of which are of epithelial origin and malignant. Renal cell carcinoma (RCC), classically referred to as clear cell carcinoma or hypernephroma, is not a single malignancy. Rather, RCC comprises a group of distinguishable entities, each with a strong relationship between its morphologic and genetic features. The World Health Organization recognizes these biologic and histologic differences in the classification system of kidney cancers (Table 203-1). The metastatic potential is dependent on the histologic subtype and ranges from the most virulent conventional clear cell carcinomas (75% of total tumors but accounting for 90% of the metastases), to the more indolent papillary and chromophobe carcinomas (20% of the total but only 10% of the metastases), to the benign oncocytomas (5% of all tumors).

EPIDEMIOLOGY

In the year 2009, it is estimated that there will be more than 49,000 new cases and approximately 11,000 deaths from kidney cancer in the United States. Since 1950, there has been a 126% increase in the incidence of renal cancer and a 36.5% increase in annual mortality. The increase in incidence of RCC may be in part related to early detection as a consequence of computed tomography (CT) and magnetic resonance imaging (MRI) of the abdomen for other medical conditions. The male-to-female ratio is approximately 2:1 to 3:1, and the increase in incidence is highest in African Americans and lowest in Asians and Pacific Islanders. The mean age at diagnosis is in the sixth to seventh decade of life. Aside from genetic predisposition, risk factors associated with RCC include cigarette smoking, obesity, hypertension, and the use of diuretics. Increased cigarette smoking has been associated with greater risk in both men and women. The risk may decrease after smoking cessation but requires about 20 years. Obese persons have an increased risk

TABLE 203-1 CLASSIFICATION OF RENAL CELL NEOPLASMS

BENIGN	MALIGNANT
Oncocytoma	Clear cell (conventional) renal cell carcinoma
Papillary (chromophil) adenoma	Papillary (chromophil) renal cell carcinoma
Metanephric adenoma	Chromophobe renal cell carcinoma
Nephrogenic adenofibroma	Collecting duct carcinoma
	Medullary carcinoma
	Mixed tubular and spindle cell carcinoma
	Renal cell carcinoma, unclassified

Modified from Storkel S, Eble JN, Adlakha K, et al. Classification of renal cell carcinoma: Workgroup No. 1. Union Internationale Contre le Cancer (UICC) and the American Joint Committee on Cancer (AJCC). *Cancer.* 1997;80:987-989.

TABLE 203-2 HISTOLOGIC SUBTYPES, GENETICS, AND SYNDROMES

HISTOLOGIC SUBTYPE	%	MAJOR GENETIC/ MOLECULAR DEFECTS	OTHER GENETIC/MOLECULAR DEFECTS	ASSOCIATED SYNDROMES
Conventional (clear cell)	75	LOH* 3p Mutation of 3p25 (VHL)	+5q, −8p, −9p, −14q *p53* mutation, c-*erB-1* oncogene expression	VHL Hereditary RCC
Papillary 1	5	c-*Met* gene mutation 7q31	Trisomy 7, 12, 16, and 17; −Y, +7, +17	Hereditary papillary RCC
Papillary 2	10	Fumarate hydratase 1q42	Trisomy 7, 12, 16, 17, 20; −1p, −3p, −9p, −Y, +5q	Hereditary leiomyomatosis RCC
Chromophobe	5	Birt-Hogg-Dubé 17p11	−1p, −2p, −6p, −13q, 21q, −Y *p53* mutation	Birt-Hogg-Dubé
Oncocytoma	5	Birt-Hogg-Dubé 17p11	−1, −Y, 11q rearrangement	Familial oncocytoma Birt-Hogg-Dubé
Collecting duct	0.4	−18, −Y	−1q, −6p, −8p, −11, −13q, −21q c-*erB-1* oncogene expression	Renal medullary carcinoma

LOH = loss of heterozygosity; RCC = renal cell carcinoma; VHL = von Hippel-Lindau disease.
Modified from Zambrano NR. Histopathology and molecular genetics of renal tumors *J Urol.* 1999;162:1246-1258; and Klatte T, Pantuck AJ, Said JW, et al. Cytogenetic and molecular tumor profiling for type 1 and type 2 papillary renal cell carcinoma. *Clin Cancer Res.* 2009;15:1162-1169.

of RCC, and the risk rises with increasing body mass index. Although there is an elevated risk associated with diuretic use, this association is hard to distinguish from the increased risk associated with hypertension. RCC is more prevalent in patients with preexisting renal conditions such as polycystic kidney disease, horseshoe kidney, and chronic renal failure requiring hemodialysis.

PATHOBIOLOGY

The new classification system for RCC permits a better understanding of the cell of origin for the various subtypes and their chromosomal abnormalities (Table 203-2). The classic clear cell carcinoma constitutes approximately 65% of tumors and is believed to be derived from the proximal convoluted tubule. It is generally solitary and well circumscribed with a golden yellow color because of abundant cytoplasmic lipid. Higher-grade tumors contain less lipid and glycogen. About half of the tumors exhibit either a solid or acinar growth pattern characterized by solid sheets of tumor cells and accompanied by a rich capillary vascular network. Papillary RCCs represent approximately 15% of primary epithelial renal neoplasms. Multifocality, either bilateral or multifocal lesions in the same kidney, is present in about 45% of cases. Most of these tumors exhibit a broad morphologic spectrum, including papillary, papillary-trabecular, and papillary-solid areas; associated necrosis is a common finding. The classic papillary pattern is characterized by discrete papillary fronds lined by neoplastic epithelial cells and containing a central fibrovascular core, easily recognized on low magnification. These tumors are divided into type 1 and type 2 lesions, based on cytologic features and genetic differences. Chromophobe renal cancers make up 5% of renal epithelial tumors. Characteristically, these tumors are solitary and discrete but not encapsulated. The typical histology consists of large round-to-polygonal cells with well-defined cell borders and pale basophilic cytoplasm admixed with a smaller population of polygonal cells with eosinophilic cytoplasm. These tumors may be quite large at diagnosis, with resectable tumors reported as big as 23 cm.

Clear cell carcinoma is characterized by the loss of genetic material of the short arm of chromosome 3 (3p) and mutations in the von Hippel-Lindau (*VHL*) gene. In patients with von Hippel-Lindau disease, these losses and mutations occur in virtually all cases. The more common sporadic tumors also have somatic mutations or hypermethylation in the same region in approximately 75 to 80% of cases. Conventional clear cell tumors have a mutation in the *VHL* gene, which is inactivated by a point mutation or by epigenetic gene silencing by promoter methylation. The loss of *VHL*, responsible for ubiquination and degradation of hypoxia-inducible factor (*HIF*) genes, leads to upregulation of HIF-responsive genes responsible for angiogenesis and cell growth. Two of these upregulated genes are platelet-derived growth factor (*PDGF*) and vascular endothelial growth factor (*VEGF*), which are angiogenic factors thought to induce the neovascularity seen in both primary and metastatic clear cell cancers. Patients with the VHL syndrome more commonly develop tumors at an earlier age and frequently have multiple tumors. Other tumors associated with the syndrome include central nervous system hemangioblastomas (Chapter 195), pancreatic neuroendocrine tumors (Chapter 201), pheochromocytomas, retinal angiomas, and epididymal cystadenomas.

Most sporadic papillary RCCs are characterized by trisomy of chromosomes 7 and 17 as well as loss of chromosome Y. Hereditary papillary renal cancer is a result of germline mutations and activation of the *MET* proto-oncogene, which is located on chromosome 7p. These cells have aberrant hepatocyte growth factor receptors that are unable to deactivate after binding by the growth factor. Somatic *MET* gene amplifications have also been observed in about 10% of sporadic papillary renal cancer. The syndrome of hereditary leiomyomatosis and papillary renal cancers is associated with the gene for fumarate hydratase. Birt-Hogg-Dubé syndrome is a rare disorder predominantly associated with the chromophobe renal cancers but in which clear cell tumors and chromophobe and oncocytic tumors can develop. The gene associated with the Birt-Hogg-Dubé syndrome has been mapped to 17p and expresses a novel protein, folliculin, whose function is not yet characterized. Chromophobe RCCs have genetic loss on chromosomes 1 and Y as well as combined chromosomal losses affecting chromosomes 1, 6, 10, 13, 17, and 21.

CLINICAL MANIFESTATIONS

Although RCC has a high propensity for metastases and has associated paraneoplastic syndromes, most patients are asymptomatic at presentation. Historically, RCC tumor was characterized by the presenting triad of hematuria, a palpable mass, and pain in as many as 10% of patients. However, there has been a migration to the detection of earlier-stage tumors with the increased use of abdominal imaging for unrelated medical conditions in modern series. Up to 48% of tumors may be discovered in this manner, and less than 5% of patients now have a palpable mass at presentation. The more common presenting symptoms are anemia, weight loss, malaise, and anorexia (Table 203-3). The presence of these symptoms has been associated with the disease-free survival after nephrectomy. Patients presenting with RCC frequently have associated paraneoplastic syndromes. Hypercalcemia (Chapter 186) has been observed in approximately 20% of patients and can be due to the secretion of parathyroid hormone, parathyroid hormone–like peptide, and interleukin-6, shown to stimulate osteoclastic bone resorption. Other associated syndromes include hypertension, erythrocytosis (from ectopic erythropoietin production) and the rare Stauffer's syndrome, which is the presence of liver dysfunction without the presence of hepatic metastases; the hepatic dysfunction resolves after surgical resection of the tumor.

DIAGNOSIS

The complete evaluation for patients with suspected RCC should include a complete blood count, chemistry profile, bone scan, and CT scan of the chest, abdomen, and pelvis. CT is the most reliable method for detecting and staging of RCC. The "ideal" CT scan for renal masses can be divided into four phases, including the precontrast images, the arterial phase (about 25 seconds after injection), the nephrographic phase (about 90 seconds into the injection), and the excretory phase. The most important phases for imaging renal tumors are the precontrast and nephrographic images because renal lesions appear low in density in contrast to the uniformly enhanced renal parenchyma. The arterial phase is helpful for identifying renal arteries and small hypervascular masses. The excretory phase aids in assessing the collecting system and the renal pelvis. The CT scan is also helpful in detecting regional

TABLE 203-3 PRESENTING SYMPTOMS AND SIGNS OF RENAL CELL CARCINOMA (BOTH LOCALIZED AND METASTATIC DISEASE)

Anemia	52%
Hepatic dysfunction	32%
Weight loss	23%
Hypoalbuminemia	20%
Malaise	19%
Hypercalcemia	13%
Anorexia	11%
Thrombocytosis	9%
Night sweats	8%
Fever	8%
Erythrocytosis	4%
Hypertension	3%
Chills	3%

Modified from Kim HI, Belldegrun AS, Freitas DG, et al. Paraneoplastic signs and symptoms of renal cell carcinoma: implications for prognosis. *J Urol.* 2003;170:1742-1746.

metastases, and three-dimensional CT imaging is now possible in cases in which "nephron-sparing surgery" or partial nephrectomy is planned. The additional use of ultrasonography and MRI can help distinguish benign from malignant lesions of the kidney and in treatment planning. Ultrasound is used when distinguishing cysts from solid lesions. MRI has the advantage of imaging tumors in patients with poor renal function in which intravenous contrast may be contraindicated. MRI is also helpful for delineating any thrombi that may be extending into the renal vein or inferior vena cava, and magnetic resonance angiography can be used to determine the number and location of renal arteries in patients who are candidates for partial nephrectomy. Once the evaluation is complete, the clinical stage is assessed using the TNM (tumor, node, metastasis) system (Table 203-4).

TREATMENT Rx

Localized Disease

The historical standard of care for patients with an RCC is a radical nephrectomy. Kidney cancers routinely selected for radical nephrectomy include large and centrally localized tumors that have effectively replaced most of the normal renal parenchyma, tumors associated with regional adenopathy (of benign or malignant etiology), those with inferior vena cava or right atrial extension, and even those in which metastatic disease is evident. Nephrectomy can be performed through a flank, transperitoneal, or a transthoracic incision. The ipsilateral adrenal gland is also removed, but a regional lymph node dissection is optional and controversial. The increasing percentage of small tumors has resulted in a corresponding decrease in patients undergoing radical nephrectomy. Partial nephrectomy for tumors of 7 cm or smaller offers rates of local tumor control and survival similar to radical nephrectomy but also reduces the risk of renal insufficiency over time. Partial nephrectomy is further supported by the fact that approximately 35% of renal cortical tumors are the indolent papillary or chromophobe carcinomas. Laparoscopic nephrectomy offers a minimally invasive alternative to the classical radical nephrectomy. Both open and laparoscopic approaches can be used for partial nephrectomy to control disease and preserve renal function.

RCCs are resistant to both radiation therapy and traditional chemotherapy. Neither are used in either the neoadjuvant or adjuvant surgical setting. Immunotherapy with interferon and interleukin-2, used in the treatment of metastatic disease, have shown no benefit in the adjuvant setting after nephrectomy.

Metastatic Disease

About 30% of patients with RCC present with metastatic disease, and an additional 20 to 30% of patients with surgically resected primary tumors relapse with metastases. Complications of metastatic disease include pain from either an unresectable primary tumor or from skeletal metastases. Radiation therapy is frequently used for palliation of bone metastases and in patients with multiple brain metastases. Palliative nephrectomy is sometimes used to provide symptomatic relief of pain. Surgical resection of the primary tumor is considered a mainstay of treatment even in patients with metastatic

TABLE 203-4 TNM STAGING OF RENAL CELL CARCINOMA

TUMOR, NODES, AND METASTASES CLINICAL CLASSIFICATION	
PRIMARY TUMOR (T)	
TX	Primary tumor cannot be assessed
T0	No evidence of primary tumor
T1	Tumor 7 cm or less in greatest dimension, limited to the kidney
T1a	Tumor 4 cm or less in greatest dimension, limited to the kidney
T1b	Tumor more than 4 cm but not more than 7 cm in greatest dimension, limited to kidney
T2	Tumor more than 7 cm in greatest dimension, limited to kidney
T2a	Tumor more than 7 cm but less than or equal to 10 cm in greatest dimension, limited to the kidney
T2b	Tumor more than 10 cm, limited to the kidney
T3	Tumor extends into major veins or the perinephric tissues but not into the ipsilateral adrenal gland but not beyond Gerota's fascia
T3a	Tumor grossly extends into renal vein or its segmental (muscle-containing) branches, or tumor invades perirenal and/or renal sinus fat but not beyond Gerota's fascia
T3b	Tumor grossly extends into the vena cava below the diaphragm
T3c	Tumor grossly extends into vena cava above the diaphragm or invades the wall of the vena cava
T4	Tumor invades beyond Gerota's fascia (including contiguous extension into the ipsilateral adrenal gland)
Regional Lymph Nodes (N)	
NX	Regional lymph nodes cannot be assessed
N0	No regional lymph node metastasis
N1	Metastasis in regional lymph node(s)
Distant Metastasis (M)	
MX	Distant metastasis cannot be assessed
M0	No distant metastasis
M1	Distant metastasis
STAGE GROUPING	
Stage I	T1, N0, M0
Stage II	T2, N0, M0
Stage III	T1 or T2, N1, M0
	T3, N0 or N1, M0
Stage IV	T4, Any N, M0
	Any T, Any N, M1

From *AJCC Cancer Staging Manual*, 7th ed. New York: Springer-Verlag; 2010.

disease and has been shown to extend survival in these patients.[1] Surgical resection of metastatic sites of disease (i.e., "metastectomy") may also extend survival and even cure a subset of patients. The patients most likely to benefit from surgical resection of metastatic disease are those with a disease-free interval of greater than 1 year, those with a solitary site of metastases, and those with lung metastases. Long-term survival has been observed when the solitary site of resection was the lung (up to 45%) and even the brain (up to 20%). RCC is resistant to most conventional chemotherapy agents, with responses seen in less than 10% of patients.

Immunotherapy with either interleukin-2 or interferon-α (Chapter 35) has been the historical treatment for patients with metastatic disease. High-dose intravenous interleukin-2, a potentially curative treatment, requires a dedicated inpatient setting because of the severe toxicities associated with this therapy, including hypotension, pulmonary edema, renal failure, and central nervous system toxicity. However, most toxicities are reversible, and complete or partial responses are seen in approximately 15 to 20%; approximately 4% of patients achieve long-term, disease-free survival. Interferon-α therapy is given as three to five subcutaneous injections per week, is less toxic than interleukin-2, and has an overall response rate of approximately 15%. However, the number of patients achieving a complete response and long-term survival is substantially less than seen with interleukin-2. Reversible toxicities of interferon-α treatment include influenza-like symptoms such as fever, chills, myalgias, mild myelosuppression, and mild hepatic dysfunction.

RCC has been an ideal candidate for the development of new "targeted" therapies, exploiting the downstream effects of *VHL* mutations. Randomized trials have shown the benefit of tyrosine kinase inhibitors (TKIs), such as sunitinib and sorafenib, that block the actions of *VEGF* and PDGF, and bevacizumab, an antibody that blocks the endothelial growth factor receptor. Sunitinib was found to be superior to interferon as initial therapy and is now a standard of care.[2] Common side effects include fatigue, diarrhea, hypertension, and hand-foot-syndrome, a condition in which blisters appear at areas of contact. The addition of bevacizumab to interferon is superior to interferon alone, and this combination has been approved for first-line treatment as well. Side effects include hypertension and an increased risk of bleeding.[3] Sorafenib was found to be superior to placebo in patients whose disease progressed after cytokine therapy. Side effects are similar to sunitinib. Two new drugs active in RCC target the mammalian target of rapamycin (mTOR) pathway and have also been approved for treatment. Temsirolimus, an intravenous mTOR inhibitor, improves survival of patients with untreated poor-risk disease (those with three or more risk factors; see later).[4] Everolimus, an oral mTOR inhibitor, improves the outcomes of patients who have been previously treated with sunitinib, sorafenib, or bevacizumab.[5] Common side effects include fatigue, skin rashes, and mouth sores.

PROGNOSIS

Survival rates for resected nonmetastatic renal cortical tumors range between 60 and 100% depending on the mode of presentation, tumor histology, tumor size, and pathologic stage (E-Fig. 203-1). The prognosis declines considerably for patients with more advanced disease, with long-term survival seen in only 20% of stage III patients and 5% or less of stage IV patients. Of the more common histologic subtypes of RCC, the prognosis of clear cell carcinoma is less favorable than papillary RCC; chromophobe RCC is the most favorable. For patients with metastatic disease, five clinical features associated with shorter survival are low performance status, high lactate dehydrogenase, low hemoglobin, high calcium, and absence of prior nephrectomy. Three groups have been defined using survival data from patients treated with immunotherapy: favorable (0 zero risk factors), with a median survival of 20 months; intermediate (one or two risk factors), with a median survival of 10 months; and poor (three or more risk factors), with a median survival of 4 months. Immunotherapy treatment of patients and surgical resection of metastases can result in long-term survival of a small percentage of RCC patients. New targeted drugs, a direct result of increased understanding of RCC biology, are now the standard of care for patients with metastatic disease.

BLADDER CANCER

DEFINITION

A spectrum of tumors arise from the urothelial lining of the bladder, renal pelvis, ureters, and urethra, of which transitional cell carcinoma is the most common. Most tumors arise from the bladder, with a minority arising from the upper tracts (renal pelvis and ureters) and even fewer from the proximal urethra. Although transitional cell cancers possess a variable natural history, they have a proclivity for multifocality, high recurrence rates, and progression to higher pathologic stages. These tumors are generally grouped into the three broad categories of superficial, muscle-invasive, and metastatic disease, each of which differs in clinical behavior, prognosis, and primary management. For superficial tumors, the aim is to prevent recurrences and progression to a more advanced stage. In muscle-invasive disease, the medical challenge is to integrate the modalities of surgery, chemotherapy, and radiation to optimize cure and minimize morbidity. For metastatic disease, chemotherapy is used to palliate the symptoms of most patients, but there is a subset of patients in whom combination chemotherapy may result in long-term cure. During the past 30 years, improvements in diagnosis, management, and therapies has resulted in a 5-year survival rate that has increased from 73% in the 1974 to 1976 time period to 82% for those patients diagnosed between 1998 and 2001.

EPIDEMIOLOGY

More than 68,000 estimated new cases of bladder cancer were diagnosed in 2008, of which 14,000 patients are expected to succumb to their disease. The male-to-female ratio of 3:1 is similar in all racial groups, making this disease the fourth most common cancer in men and the ninth in women. The combined bladder cancer incidence for men and women has remained stable from 1986 to 2001 after rising 0.7% per year from 1975 to 1986, whereas the death rate from bladder cancer continues to decline. Bladder cancer is twice as prevalent in whites as in African Americans and is less frequently observed in Asians. The median age at diagnosis is approximately 70 years, and the disease is rarely diagnosed before the age of 40 years.

Carcinogens or their metabolites implicated in the carcinogenesis of bladder cancer are believed to be excreted in the urine, where they can act directly on the urothelial lining. The latency period from initial exposure to the development of cancer is almost 20 years, making it difficult to establish a definitive cause-and-effect relationship between a putative carcinogen and the development of the disease. Cigarette smoking is the leading risk factor for bladder cancer, believed to contribute to 48% of the cancers in men and 28% of the cancers in women. A longer duration of exposure is associated with a higher risk than a more intense exposure (in cigarettes/day) over a shorter time period of time. Overall, smokers have a two- to four-fold higher relative risk of bladder cancer than nonsmokers. Smoking is associated with cellular atypia of the urothelium; individuals who never smoked show atypia in only 4% of cases, in contrast to a 50% incidence of atypia in smokers.

Polycyclic aromatic hydrocarbons such as 2-naphthylamine, 4-aminobiphenyl, and benzidine and benzene or exhausts from combustion gases are associated with an increased risk of bladder cancer. Occupations reported to be at higher risk include aluminum work, dry cleaning, manufacturing of preservatives and polychlorinated biphenyls, and pesticide application. Arylamines, also implicated in carcinogenesis, are metabolically activated to electrophilic compounds by *N*-hydroxylation in the liver by cytochrome P-450 IA2 and detoxified by *N*-acetylation; studies suggest that individuals with a fast oxidizer and slow acetylator phenotype are at highest risk. Patients with occupations associated with a higher exposure to arylamines, such as workers in the dye, rubber, or leather manufacturing industries, are believed to be at higher risk of bladder cancer. *Schistosoma haematobium* infection enhances formation of carcinogenic *N*-nitroso compounds and results in an increased risk of both squamous and transitional cell carcinomas of the bladder. An association has been observed between squamous cell carcinoma (but not transitional cell tumors) and the presence of chronic urinary tract infections seen in paraplegic patients and those with chronic bladder stones and indwelling Foley catheters. The chemotherapy agent cyclophosphamide can increase the risk of bladder cancer nine-fold, and phenacetin-containing compounds have been implicated in the development of renal pelvis and ureteral tumors.

PATHOBIOLOGY

Urothelial tumors can occur anywhere along the urinary tract, including the renal pelvis, ureters, bladder, and urethra. More than 90% of tumors originate in the bladder, 8% in the renal pelvis, and the remaining 2% in the ureter and urethra. Transitional cell carcinomas make up 90 to 95% of urothelial tumors; squamous cell (keratinizing) tumors (3%), adenocarcinomas (2%), and small cell tumors (1%) constitute the remainder. Mixed-histology tumors, consisting of predominantly transitional cell carcinoma with areas of squamous, adenocarcinomatous, or neuroendocrine elements, are frequently observed. Squamous cell tumors are more common in the distal urethra, and adenocarcinomas occur in the embryonal remnant of the urachus on the dome of the bladder and in periurethral tissues. In endemic areas of *S. haematobium* (Chapter 363) infections (such as Egypt), 40% of tumors are squamous cell carcinomas. Rare tumors of the bladder include lymphoma, sarcoma, and melanoma.

Most (70 to 80%) newly detected bladder cancers are classified as superficial tumors and include exophytic papillary tumors confined to the mucosa (Ta), tumors invading the lamina propria (T1), and carcinoma in situ (CIS, also called Tis). Superficial bladder tumors are typically graded according to the World Health Organization/International Society of Urologic Pathology (WHO/ISUP) grading system as low or high grade. If the grading system is not specified, a numerical system can be used: well differentiated (G1), moderately differentiated (G2), poorly differentiated (G3), and undifferentiated (G4). Grading is more important for noninvasive Ta tumors because almost all invasive bladder tumors (T1 or greater) are high grade. Primary CIS (or Tis) without a concurrent Ta or T1 tumor constitutes 1 to 2% of new bladder cancer cases. More frequently, CIS is found in the presence of multiple papillary tumors, either immediately adjacent to another lesion or involving remote mucosa in the bladder. CIS is, by definition, high-grade disease; it is regarded as a precursor to more invasive tumors because 60% of untreated tumors develop more invasive disease within 5 years. A T1 tumor is an aggressive, invasive malignancy. Virtually all T1 tumors are high grade, and 50% have associated CIS. Fifty percent of patients have disease recurrence by 1 year, and 90% within 5 years. A minority of primary tumors at diagnosis are found to invade the muscularis propria (T2), extend to perivesicular fat (T3), or extend into immediately adjacent organs (T4); all primary tumors stage T2 or higher are high grade.

The natural history of a urothelial tumor is to recur either at the same location or at a separate site in the urothelial tract and at the same or a more advanced stage. Several studies support the controversial concept that these recurrences are clonal in origin. Chromosome 9 deletions are the most commonly observed chromosomal changes in bladder cancer. Chromosomal deletions of 17p (the *TP53* locus), 18q (the *DCC* gene locus), and the *RB* gene locus are frequently observed in invasive tumors; deletions of 3p and 11p occur in both superficial and invasive tumors. Associations between specific gene deletions and prognosis have been attempted, particularly for the *TP53* and *RB* genes, but inconsistent findings among studies preclude their routine use in clinical management. The epidermal growth factor receptor is highly expressed (~80%) on bladder cancer tumors, and the Her-2/Neu growth factor receptor is less frequently expressed (~50%). Studies suggest that higher expression of these receptors on bladder cancers is associated with a more advanced and more aggressive phenotype of disease.

CLINICAL MANIFESTATIONS

Hematuria is the presenting symptom in 80 to 90% of bladder cancer cases, but others present with a urinary tract infection. Individuals older than 40 years who develop hematuria should have an evaluation for the presence of urothelial cancer that includes urinary cytology, cystoscopy, and imaging of the urinary tract by either an ultrasound or CT. Screening of asymptomatic subjects for hematuria increases the probability of diagnosing bladder cancer at an earlier stage but does not improve survival; thus, it is not routinely recommended. Urinary frequency and nocturia may be present as a consequence of either irritative symptoms or reduced bladder capacity. Pain, when present, typically reflects the location of the bladder tumor. Lower abdominal pain may occur as a result of a bladder mass, and rectal discomfort and perineal pain can result from tumors invading into the prostate or pelvis. Tumors of the renal pelvis, ureter, or bladder in which the ureteral orifice is obstructed can cause hydronephrosis, reduced renal function, and flank pain. Patients with more advanced disease can present with anorexia, fatigue, weight loss, or pain from a metastatic bone lesion. The physical examination is frequently unremarkable in patients presenting with bladder tumors because most patients have organ-confined tumors.

DIAGNOSIS

The mainstay of bladder cancer diagnosis and staging is the cystoscopic evaluation. The procedure includes the examination under anesthesia to determine whether a palpable mass (either mobile or not) is present. A nonmobile tumor mass is indicative of disease invading the pelvic sidewall, which is unlikely to be resectable. Urine is obtained to evaluate for the presence of malignant cells. A cystoscope is inserted to visually inspect the bladder and detail the size, number, location, and growth pattern (papillary or solid) of all lesions. All visible tumors undergo transurethral resection of the bladder tumor to determine the histologic subtype and depth of invasion. Adequate evaluation, particularly in large tumors that may be invasive, requires that muscle be identified in the pathologic specimen. Repeat biopsy of the resected area is occasionally required to ensure that no muscle invasion is present because invasion into muscle requires consideration of surgical removal of the bladder rather than just endoscopic resection of the tumor. Biopsies from any areas of erythema are performed to assess for CIS. The urethra is inspected during withdrawal of the cystoscope, and specimens are taken if clinically indicated. Patients with a positive cytology but no apparent tumor within the bladder undergo selective retrograde catheterization of the ureters up to the renal pelves to assess for upper tract disease.

The decision whether to image the abdomen and pelvis is based on the cystoscopy results and the pathology of the tumor. An intravenous pyelogram or CT urogram can evaluate the upper urinary tracts, and CT or MRI may distinguish whether a tumor extends to the perivesical fat (T3) or prostate or vagina (T4) and whether regional lymph nodes are involved. In the case of larger, invasive tumors, the presence or absence of distal metastases can be documented with physical examination, CT of the abdomen and pelvis, chest radiograph, and radionuclide bone scan.

All patients with carcinoma of the bladder or of related sites are staged using the TNM system advocated by the American Joint Committee on Cancer (AJCC) (Table 203-5). The TNM system categorizes the depth of invasion of the primary tumor, nodal metastases in the pelvis (or retroperitoneum for upper tract disease) on the basis of the number and size of regional nodes involved, other nonregional lymph node sites, and any visceral sites of disease.

TREATMENT Rx

Superficial Disease

The standard treatment for superficial tumors is a complete endoscopic resection. Most patients develop new tumors, 30% of which progress to a higher stage, mandating vigilant surveillance at 3-month intervals with cystoscopy, urine cytology, and repeat transurethral resection when indicated. Additional treatment in the form of adjuvant intravesical therapy is dependent on the number of lesions, the size, the depth of invasion, and the number of prior tumors in that individual. Prophylactic or adjuvant intravesical therapy is typically instituted in the setting when a patient has shown either a repeated tendency to develop new lesions in the bladder or is at high risk for recurrence or progression de novo. Intravesical therapy is not warranted for the first Ta tumor that is low grade. Instances of high recurrence and progression warranting intravesical therapy include multifocal or large lesions, high-grade papillary lesions, T1 tumors, CIS, or a combination. It is never advised for muscle-invasive tumors because agents instilled in the bladder do not penetrate beyond a few layers of cells. After allowing sufficient time for healing after the endoscopic resection, intravesical therapy is most frequently initiated with the immunologic agent bacillus Calmette-Guérin (BCG) weekly for 6 weeks. 6 Occasionally, other chemotherapy and cytokines are used when BCG is contraindicated. Treatment outcome is assessed at the 3- and 6-month evaluations following treatment to determine whether the bladder has been rendered tumor free. If disease persists, either a repeat course of BCG treatment or even an immediate cystectomy may be recommended. Bladder toxicity can result from urothelial irritation, including bladder irritability or spasms, hematuria, and pain on urination. A rare complication of BCG is development of a systemic tuberculosis infection requiring treatment with systemic antituberculosis agents. BCG is highly effective in eradicating CIS, with 70% of patients disease free at 1 year and 40% at 10 years. Selected tumors in the ureter or renal pelvis can be managed by ureteroscopic resection, in some cases by instillation of BCG through the renal pelvis, or nephroureterectomy. Tumors of the prostatic urethra are frequently managed by cystoprostatectomy, particularly if a complete resection cannot be accomplished.

Muscle-Invasive Tumors

For patients with tumors infiltrating the muscularis propria, the standard of care in the United States is a radical cystectomy and pelvic lymphadenectomy because of the high incidence of cancer extending into the perivesicular fat or into regional lymph nodes. A prostatectomy is also performed in men; in women, the urethra, uterus, fallopian tubes, ovaries, and anterior vaginal wall are removed. Urinary flow can be directed through either a conduit diversion or a continent reservoir. With a conduit diversion, urine is drained directly from the ureters to a loop of small bowel that is anastomosed to the skin surface with no internal reservoir. Urine is collected in an external appliance. Alternatively, a low-pressure continent reservoir can be created from a detubularized segment of bowel attached to the abdominal wall with a continent stoma that can be self-catheterized at regular intervals. Low-pressure reservoirs can also be anastomosed to the urethra, creating an internal orthotopic neobladder and permitting the patient to void through the normal urethra. The standard pelvic lymphadenectomy includes the distal common iliac, external iliac, obturator, and hypogastric nodes; improved survival and decreased local recurrence are associated with an increased number of lymph nodes removed. Complications of cystectomy include recurrent urinary infections, hyperchloremic acidosis (Chapter 120), oxalate stones (Chapter 128), incontinence, and impotence.

Neoadjuvant chemotherapy before cystectomy for muscle-invasive bladder cancer increases survival. 7 This survival benefit is achieved only with cisplatin-based combinations, which require the patient to have normal renal function and a good performance status. Some physicians prefer immediate cystectomy followed by adjuvant chemotherapy if the pathologic evaluation demonstrates a high risk of recurrence, such as disease extending to either the perivesicular fat or the lymph nodes. Radical cystectomy is effective in providing long-term disease control in 75 to 80% of patients with organ-confined disease, approximately 50% of those with tumors extending into the perivesical tissues, and nearly one third of patients with regional lymph node involvement. Some patients prefer a bladder-sparing approach using radiation treatment rather than a cystectomy. The best candidates for this approach are patients with a solitary early-stage lesion and no evidence of hydronephrosis. This trimodality treatment for bladder preservation first requires a successful, near-complete transurethral resection of tumor followed by concurrent chemotherapy and radiation. External beam treatments are delivered in five daily fractions a week, starting with the whole pelvis to a total dose of 40 to 45 Gy followed by 20 to 25 Gy reduced volume to the bladder tumor. Toxicities include inflammation of the skin, impotence, fatigue, and irritative symptoms from the bladder and bowel; persistent proctitis is rare. In this approach, cystectomy is reserved for patients failing to achieve complete response. The 5-year disease-free survival rate with this approach is 50%, with most patients retaining a normally functioning bladder.

TABLE 203-5 TNM DEFINITIONS FOR CANCERS OF THE BLADDER, URETER, AND RENAL PELVIS

PRIMARY TUMORS OF THE BLADDER (T)	
TX	Primary tumor cannot be assessed
T0	No evidence of primary tumor
Ta	Noninvasive papillary carcinoma
Tis	Carcinoma in situ ("flat tumor")
T1	Tumor invades subepithelial connective tissue
T2	Tumor invades muscularis propria
pT2a	Tumor invades superficial muscularis propria (inner half)
pT2b	Tumor invades deep muscularis propria (outer half)
T3	Tumor invades perivesical tissue
pT3a	Microscopically
pT3b	Macroscopically (extravesical mass)
T4	Tumor invades any of the following: prostatic stroma, seminal vesicles, uterus, vagina, pelvic wall, abdominal wall
T4a	Tumor invades the prostatic stroma, uterus, vagina
T4b	Tumor invades the pelvic wall, abdominal wall
REGIONAL LYMPH NODES FOR UROTHELIAL TUMORS OF THE BLADDER (N)	
Regional lymph nodes include both the primary and secondary drainage regions. All other nodes above the aortic bifurcation are considered distant lymph nodes.	
NX	Lymph nodes cannot be assessed
N0	No lymph node metastasis
N1	Single regional lymph node metastasis in the true pelvis (hypogastric, obturator, external iliac, or presacral node)
N2	Multiple regional lymph node metastases in the true pelvis (hypogastric, obturator, external iliac, or presacral node)
N3	Lymph node metastasis to the common iliac lymph nodes
PRIMARY TUMORS OF THE URETER AND RENAL PELVIS (T)	
TX	Primary tumor cannot be assessed
T0	No evidence of primary tumor
Ta	Papillary noninvasive carcinoma
Tis	Carcinoma in situ
T1	Tumor invades subepithelial connective tissue
T2	Tumor invades the muscularis
T3	(For renal pelvis only) Tumor invades beyond muscularis into peripelvic fat or the renal parenchyma
T3	(For ureter only) Tumor invades beyond muscularis into periureteric fat
T4	Tumor invades adjacent organs or through the kidney into perinephric fat
REGIONAL LYMPH NODES FOR UROTHELIAL TUMORS (N)* OF URETER AND RENAL PELVIS	
NX	Regional lymph nodes cannot be assessed
N0	No regional lymph node metastasis
N1	Metastasis in a single lymph node, 2 cm or less in greatest dimension
N2	Metastasis in a single lymph node, more than 2 cm but not more than 5 cm in greatest dimension; or multiple lymph nodes, none more than 5 cm in greatest dimension
N3	Metastasis in a lymph node, more than 5 cm in greatest dimension
*Note: Laterality does not affect the N classification.	
DISTANT METASTASIS FOR ALL UROTHELIAL TUMORS (M)	
MX	Distant metastasis cannot be assessed
M0	No distant metastasis
M1	Distant metastasis
AJCC STAGE GROUPINGS FOR BLADDER CANCER	
0a	Ta, N0, M0
0is	Tis, N0, M0
I	T1, N0, M0
II	T2a, N0, M0
	T2b, N0, M0
III	T3a, N0, M0
	T3b, N0, M0
	T4a, N0, M0
IV	T4b, N0, M0
	Any T, N1-3, M0
	Any T, Any, N M1
AJCC STAGE GROUPINGS FOR CANCER OF THE RENAL PELVIS AND URETER	
0a	Ta, N0, M0
0is	Tis, N0, M0
I	T1, N0, M0
II	T2, N0, M0
III	T3, N0, M0
IV	T4, N0, M0
	Any T, N1, M0
	Any T, N2, M0
	Any T, N3, M0
	Any T, Any, N M1

From *AJCC Cancer Staging Manual*, 7th ed. New York: Springer-Verlag; 2010.

Metastatic Disease

Patients with metastatic disease are treated predominantly with chemotherapy. Cisplatin-based chemotherapy is the standard of care. The two most commonly used regimens are gemcitabine plus cisplatin (GC) and the four-drug regimen of methotrexate, vinblastine, doxorubicin, and cisplatin (MVAC); six cycles of therapy are given are over a 6-month period. The most frequently observed toxicities include anemia, thrombocytopenia, neutropenic fever, mucositis, and fatigue. The GC regimen is better tolerated and has less severe toxicities than MVAC.[8] The median survival of patients treated with both regimens is approximately 14 months, and the 5-year survival rate is 15% or less. Patients with a good performance status and whose metastatic disease is limited to the lymph nodes (i.e., no visceral metastases) have the highest likelihood for response and a 20 to 33% chance of 5-year disease-free survival. Patients with impaired renal function are treated with carboplatin rather than cisplatin owing to less toxicity to the kidney with carboplatin.[9] Carboplatin is administered with either gemcitabine or paclitaxel, and toxicities include myelosuppression and fatigue.

PROGNOSIS

Urinary bladder cancer is a common but heterogeneous disease with a decreasing mortality rate because of improvements in therapy. Superficial Ta G1 lesions, easily treated with endoscopic resection alone, almost never progress. At the other end of the spectrum of superficial disease, aggressive transitional cell CIS requires intravesical immunotherapy therapy with BCG in addition to endoscopic resection. This intravesical treatment can substantially reduce recurrence and progression, with a 5-year disease-free survival rate of 60%. Muscle-invasive disease is most frequently cured with an integrated approach of systemic chemotherapy for micrometastases followed by cystectomy and pelvic lymphadenectomy; cure rates for T2 tumors can be as high as 80% with this multimodality approach. Bladder-sparing approaches associated with an improved quality of life are possible using external beam radiation. Metastatic urinary bladder cancer is a fast growing and often lethal malignancy; despite aggressive chemotherapy, only a small proportion (~15%) of patients are disease free at 5 years.

CANCERS OF THE RENAL PELVIS AND URETERS

Approximately 10% of transitional cell carcinomas occur in the ureters and the renal pelvis. These tumors can arise either de novo or in the setting of prior tumors. The risk of developing an upper tract tumor in patients with multifocal CIS of the bladder approaches 25% by 10 years. These tumors are morphologically similar to the tumors in the bladder and behave in a similar manner. Hematuria is the most common presenting symptom, although patients with large tumors or ureteral obstruction can present with flank pain. An intravenous pyelogram, CT, or MRI is used to stage the extent of primary disease and to detect regional metastases. Low-grade tumors can be treated endoscopically, but high-grade tumors are most commonly treated with a nephroureterectomy. In contrast to cystectomy, a regional lymphadenectomy is not routinely performed. In renal pelvis tumors, the ureter is removed in addition to a nephrectomy because of the high risk of multifocal tumors along the entire upper tract and the inability to monitor the ureteral stump with accuracy. Systemic chemotherapy is used for unresectable primary tumors, patients with regional adenopathy, or recurrent tumors. Upper tract transitional cell carcinomas are staged according to the TNM system (see Table 203-5). Treatment of advanced, nonsurgical disease is with chemotherapy, and these urothelial tumors have the same sensitivity to chemotherapy as bladder cancer, with similar response rates and 5-year survival rates. Cisplatin-based chemotherapy is used in patients with normal renal function. Carboplatin-based chemotherapy is considered if there is renal insufficiency either from obstruction, a prior nephroureterectomy, or medical comorbidity.

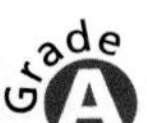

1. Flanigan RC, Salmon SE, Blumenstein BA, et al. Nephrectomy followed by interferon alfa-2b compared with interferon alfa-2b alone for metastatic renal-cell cancer. *N Engl J Med*. 2001;345:1655-1659.
2. Motzer RJ, Hutson TE, Tomczak P, et al. Sunitinib versus interferon alfa in metastatic renal-cell carcinoma. *N Engl J Med*. 2007;356:115-124.
3. Escudier B, Pluzanska A, Koralewski, et al, for the AVOREN Trial investigators. Bevacizumab plus interferon alfa-2a for treatment of metastatic renal cell carcinoma: a randomised, double-blind phase III trial. *Lancet*. 2007;370:2103-2111.
4. Hudes G, Carducci M, Tomczak P, et al. Global ARCC Trial. Temsirolimus, interferon alfa, or both for advanced renal-cell carcinoma. *N Engl J Med*. 2007;356:2271-2281.
5. Motzer RJ, Escudier B, Oudard S, et al, for the RECORD-1 Study Group. Efficacy of everolimus in advanced renal cell carcinoma: a double-blind, randomised, placebo-controlled phase III trial. *Lancet*. 2008;372:449-456.
6. Shelley MD, Mason MD, Kynaston H. Intravesical therapy for superficial bladder cancer: a systematic review of randomised trials and meta-analyses. *Cancer Treat Rev*. 2010;36:195-205.
7. Grossman HB, Natale RB, Tangen CM, et al. Neoadjuvant chemotherapy plus cystectomy compared with cystectomy alone for locally advanced bladder cancer. *N Engl J Med*. 2003;349:859-866.
8. von der Maase H, Hansen SW, Roberts JT, et al. Gemcitabine and cisplatin versus methotrexate, vinblastine, doxorubicin, and cisplatin in advanced or metastatic bladder cancer: results of a large, randomized, multinational, multicenter, phase III study. *J Clin Oncol*. 2000;18:3068-3077.
9. De Santis M, Bellmunt J, Mead G, et al. Randomized phase II/III trial assessing gemcitabine/carboplatin and methotrexate/carboplatin/vinblastine in patients with advanced urothelial cancer "unfit" for cisplatin-based chemotherapy: phase II—results of EORTC study 30986. *J Clin Oncol*. 2009;27:5634-5639.

SUGGESTED READINGS

Chou R, Dana T. Screening adults for bladder cancer: a review of the evidence for the U.S. preventive services task force. *Ann Intern Med*. 2010;153:461-468. *Clinical guidelines recommending against screening.*

Morgan TM, Keegan KA, Clark PE. Bladder cancer. *Curr Opin Oncol*. 2011;23:275-282. *Comprehensive review of epidemiology, diagnosis, and management.*

Rouprêt M, Zigeuner R, Palou J, et al. European guidelines for the diagnosis and management of upper urinary tract urothelial cell carcinomas: 2011 update. *Eur Urol*. 2011;59:584-594. *Consensus guidelines.*

Singer EA, Gupta GN, Srinivasan R. Update on targeted therapies for clear cell renal cell carcinoma. *Curr Opin Oncol*. 2011;23:283-289. *Review including rapamycin and new biologies.*

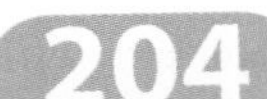

BREAST CANCER AND BENIGN BREAST DISORDERS

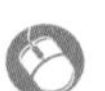

NANCY DAVIDSON

Invasive breast cancer, the most common nonskin cancer in women in the United States, will be diagnosed in about 180,000 women in 2010 and will result in approximately 40,000 deaths. Incidence and mortality from breast cancer appear to be dropping in the United States and parts of western Europe. This decline is believed to reflect early detection by screening mammography and widespread use of adjuvant systemic therapy as well as decreased use of hormone replacement therapy.

BREAST CANCER

EPIDEMIOLOGY AND PATHOBIOLOGY

Multiple risk factors for the development of breast cancer have been identified (Table 204-1). The principal risk factor is gender. Breast cancer is largely a disease of women, although it does occur in men at an incidence of about 1% that seen in women. A second critical risk factor is age. About 75% of breast cancer cases in the United States are diagnosed in women older than 50 years of age.

TABLE 204-1 RISK FACTORS FOR BREAST CANCER

RISK FACTOR	RELATIVE RISK
Any benign breast disease	1.5
Postmenopausal hormone replacement (estrogen with or without progestin)	1.5
Menarche at <12 yr	1.1-1.9
Moderate alcohol intake (two to three drinks/day)	1.1-1.9
Menopause at >55 yr	1.1-1.9
Increased bone density	1.1-1.9
Sedentary lifestyle and lack of exercise	1.1-1.9
Proliferative breast disease without atypia	2
Age at first birth >30 yr or nulliparous	2-4
First-degree relative with breast cancer	2-4
Postmenopausal obesity	2-4
Upper socioeconomic class	2-4
Personal history of endometrial or ovarian cancer	2-4
Significant radiation to chest	2-4
Increased breast density on mammogram	2-4
Older age	>4
Personal history of breast cancer (in situ or invasive)	>4
Proliferative breast disease with atypia	>4
Two first-degree relatives with breast cancer	5
Atypical hyperplasia and first-degree relative with breast cancer	10

Family history is a third critical risk factor. About 20% of breast cancer occurs in women with a family history of breast cancer; increased risk is associated with diagnosis of breast cancer in first-degree relatives younger than 50 years. Five to 8% of breast cancer cases occur in high-risk families. Several familial breast cancer syndromes with associated molecular abnormalities have been identified. Chief among them is the breast ovarian cancer syndrome, which is linked to germline mutations in the breast cancer susceptibility genes, *BRCA1* and *BRCA2*. These mutations are inherited in an autosomal dominant fashion and can therefore be transmitted through the maternal or paternal line. Extensive studies suggest that a germline mutation in either of these genes is associated with a 50 to 85% lifetime risk of developing breast cancer. Testing for *BRCA1* and *BRCA2* mutations is now viewed as a standard option for women with clinical features suggestive of a hereditary breast cancer syndrome; these include multiple family members with early-onset breast or ovarian cancer, bilateral breast cancer, or Ashkenazi Jewish heritage. Careful counseling about the implications of a positive or negative test and about the limitations of testing is a prerequisite for testing.

Other hereditary cancer syndromes (Chapter 184) include Li-Fraumeni syndrome, which is linked with germline mutations in the *p53* tumor suppressor gene, and Cowden's syndrome, which is associated with inherited mutations in the *PTEN* gene. Finally, in addition to these high-penetrance genetic susceptibility syndromes, recent results from genome-wide association studies have identified a number of low-penetrance genetic associations, including single nucleotide polymorphisms in a variety of genes. If or how to incorporate these low-penetrance traits into clinical practice remains to be established.

Reproductive risk factors include early menarche, late menopause, nulliparity, and late first pregnancy. In aggregate, these factors result in prolonged estrogen exposure of the breast. The emerging association between postmenopausal obesity and breast cancer likely reflects estrogen exposure as well. Certain types of breast pathology, including atypical hyperplasia and lobular carcinoma in situ, are also associated with increased risk. The possibility that increased breast density as assessed by mammography is a risk factor has also been raised. Finally, much interest has focused on the possibility that exogenous environmental factors predispose to breast cancer. Among the factors that appear to enhance breast cancer risk are ionizing radiation during adolescence, prolonged use of hormone replacement therapy, ongoing use of oral contraceptives, and alcohol consumption. Large studies have failed to show any convincing association between exposure to estrogenic pesticides or a high-fat diet and breast cancer.

CLINICAL MANIFESTATIONS

Breast cancer usually presents as a mammographic abnormality or a physical change in the breast including a mass or asymmetrical thickening, nipple discharge, or skin or nipple changes. Two unusual clinical presentations include Paget's disease of the nipple and inflammatory breast cancer. The former is a form of adenocarcinoma involving the skin and ducts and is manifested as nipple excoriation. The latter is recognized as a constellation of redness, warmth, and edema that often reflects tumor cell infiltration of dermal lymphatics of the breast; it should not be mistaken for a simple mastitis.

Nipple discharge may be associated with breast malignancy. Although milky discharge is seldom associated with a malignant diagnosis, patients with a clear or bloody nipple discharge require breast examination and mammography and often excisional biopsy of any suspicious area. Ductography and sometimes ductoscopy may be used to identify the inciting lesion. A bloody discharge is frequently caused by an intraductal papilloma.

Breast pain is common, especially as a premenstrual symptom in premenopausal women. But it may also be associated with an underlying malignancy. Patients with localized noncyclic breast pain should undergo breast examination and bilateral mammography. If these are normal, ultrasound or magnetic resonance imaging (MRI) may be used to exclude the small probability of a malignancy.

DIAGNOSIS

Diagnostic evaluation is generally triggered by suspicious findings on screening mammogram or detection of a palpable breast abnormality by the patient or health care provider. For both clinically occult and clinically apparent lesions, pathologic evaluation is mandatory to establish a diagnosis. Today, fine-needle aspiration and core needle biopsy have replaced incisional or excisional biopsy as the standard diagnostic measures. These procedures can be performed in the office in patients with suspicious palpable lesions. For women with nonpalpable lesions, biopsy guided by mammography, ultrasonography, or MRI is now standard. A recently published systematic review showed that stereotactic- or ultrasound-guided core needle biopsies are almost as accurate as and associated with lower complication rates than open surgical biopsy. These technologies permit an accurate diagnosis that can be followed by definitive treatment planning. It is axiomatic, however, that further evaluation must be undertaken for suspicious lesions that give an equivocal diagnosis after needle aspiration or core biopsy. Finally, bilateral breast imaging is always recommended to identify any unsuspected lesions in the contralateral breast that may also require evaluation.

Staging and Prognostic and Predictive Markers

Although staging originally reflected the clinical assessment of tumor size, nodal status, and evidence of metastatic disease, pathologic staging is the most accurate estimate of tumor involvement and prognosis. The staging system for breast cancer was revised in 2002 (Tables 204-2 and 204-3).

Most patients with breast cancer present with stage I or II disease in the absence of symptoms. In these patients, laboratory studies can be limited to blood counts, chemistry panel, and chest radiograph, and more extensive radiologic evaluation is not warranted because of low yield. In contrast, women with clinical evidence of stage III or IV disease should undergo more intensive evaluation of common sites for metastases, including lung, liver, and bone, through computed tomography and radionuclide scanning.

The two most important determinants of prognosis for early-stage breast cancer are pathological lymph node status and tumor size. Other factors that contribute to prognosis are the expression of the estrogen receptor-α (ER), progesterone receptor (PR), and HER2 proteins; these are conventionally measured by immunohistochemistry, although fluorescence in situ hybridization (FISH) for *HER2* gene amplification is also employed. Poor prognosis is associated with high lymph node burden, poor histologic grade, large tumor size, absence of ER and PR expression, and overexpression of HER2.

Recently, the focus has been on the development of predictive markers to guide selection of therapy. There are three established predictive markers for breast cancer—ER, PR, and HER2—and these should be routinely evaluated in every invasive cancer. Most tumors that express ER or PR, or both, are responsive to endocrine therapy, whereas those that lack ER and PR expression seldom respond to such therapy. Overexpression of the HER2 protein by immunohistochemistry or *HER2* gene amplification by FISH is associated with response to the HER2-targeted monoclonal antibody, trastuzumab, or the receptor tyrosine kinase inhibitor, lapatinib. Evidence that links expression of ER, PR, or HER2 to chemotherapy efficacy is equivocal.

Modern molecular techniques have provided further insight into molecular classification of breast cancer. Transcriptional profiling has suggested that breast cancers can be divided into at least five molecular subsets—normal mammary, luminal A and B, HER2, and basal. The luminal subtypes frequently express ER, but luminal A appears to be associated with a better

TABLE 204-2 STAGING OF BREAST CANCER: TNM SYSTEM

TUMOR SIZE: T (LARGEST DIAMETER)	
TX	Primary tumor cannot be assessed
T0	No evidence of primary tumor
Tis	Carcinoma in situ
Tis (DCIS)	Ductal carcinoma in situ
Tis (LCIS)	Lobular carcinoma in situ
Tis (Paget's)	Paget's disease of the nipple NOT associated with invasive carcinoma and/or carcinoma in situ (DCIS and/or LCIS) in the underlying breast parenchyma. Carcinomas in the breast parenchyma associated with Paget's disease are categorized based on the size and characteristics of the parenchymal disease, although the presence of Paget's disease should still be noted.
T1	Tumor ≤20 mm in greatest dimension
T1mi	Tumor ≤1 mm in greatest dimension
T1a	Tumor >1 mm but ≤5 mm in greatest dimension
T1b	Tumor >5 mm but ≤10 mm in greatest dimension
T1c	Tumor >10 mm but ≤20 mm in greatest dimension
T2	Tumor >20 mm but not ≤50 mm in greatest dimension
T3	Tumor >50 mm in greatest dimension
T4	Tumor of any size with direct extension to chest wall or skin (includes inflammatory carcinoma)
NODAL INVOLVEMENT: N (NODAL STATUS)	
NX	Regional lymph nodes cannot be assessed (e.g., previously removed, not removed)
N0	No regional lymph node metastases histologically
N1	Metastases to movable ipsilateral level I, II axillary lymph node(s)
N2	Metastases in ipsilateral level I, II axillary lymph nodes that are clinically fixed or matted; or in clinically detected* ipsilateral internal mammary nodes in the *absence* of clinically evident axillary lymph node metastases.
N3	Metastases in ipsilateral infraclavicular (level III axillary) lymph node(s) with or without level I, II axillary lymph node involvement; or in clinically detected* ipsilateral internal mammary lymph node(s) with clinically evident level I, II axillary lymph node metastases; or metastases in ipsilateral supraclavicular lymph node(s) with or without axillary or internal mammary lymph node involvement
N3a	Metastases in ipsilateral infraclavicular lymph node(s)
N3b	Metastases in ipsilateral internal mammary lymph node(s) and axillary lymph node(s)
N3c	Metastases in ipsilateral supraclavicular lymph node(s)
METASTASES: M	
M0	No clinical or radiographic evidence of distant metastases
cM0(i+)	No clinical or radiographic evidence of distant metastases, but deposits of molecularly or microscopically detected tumor cells in circulating blood, bone marrow, or other nonregional nodal tissue that are no larger than 0.2 mm in a patient without symptoms or signs of metastases
M1	Distant detectable metastases as determined by classic clinical and radiographic means and/or histologically proven larger than 0.2 mm

**Clinically detected* is defined as detected by imaging studies (excluding lymphoscintigraphy) or by clinical examination and having characteristics highly suspicious for malignancy or a presumed pathologic macrometastasis based on fine-needle biopsy with cytologic examination.
From *AJCC Cancer Staging Manual*, 7th ed. New York: Springer-Verlag; 2010.

TABLE 204-3 TNM STAGE AND SURVIVAL

STAGE	TNM CATEGORY*	RECURRENCE FREE AT 10 YEARS (NO SYSTEMIC ADJUVANT THERAPY)
0	TisN0M0	98%
I	T1N0M0	80% (all stage I patients)
	T < 1 cm	90%
	T > 1-2 cm	80-90%
IIA	T0N1M0; T2N0M0	60-80%
IIA	T1N1M0	50-60%
IIB	T2 N1M0	5-10% worse than IIA and based on node status
IIB	T3N0M0	30-50%
IIIA	T0 or T1 or T2N2M0; or T3N1 or N2M0	10-40%
IIIB	T4N0 or N1 or N2M0	5-30%
IIIC	Any T, N3M0	15-20%
IV	Any T, any NM1	<5%

*See Table 204-2 for TNM definitions.

TABLE 204-4 CARCINOMA IN SITU: DUCTAL VERSUS LOBULAR

FEATURE	LOBULAR CARCINOMA IN SITU	DUCTAL CARCINOMA IN SITU
Age	Younger	Older
Palpable mass	No	Uncommon
Mammographic appearance	Not detected on mammography	Microcalcifications, mass
Immunophenotype	E-cadherin negative	E-cadherin positive
Usual manifestation	Incidental finding on breast biopsy	Microcalcifications on mammography or breast mass
Bilateral involvement	Common	Uncertain
Risk and site of subsequent breast cancer	25% risk for invasive breast cancer in either breast over remaining lifespan	At site of initial lesion; 0.5% risk/yr of invasive breast cancer in opposite breast
Prevention	Consider tamoxifen or raloxifene	Consider tamoxifen or raloxifene if estrogen receptor positive
Treatment	Yearly mammography and breast examination	Lumpectomy ± radiation; mastectomy for large or multifocal lesions

prognosis and higher likelihood of response to endocrine therapy than luminal B. The basal subtype is dominated by tumors that lack expression of ER, PR, and HER2—the so-called triple-negative breast cancer that lacks a readily identified molecular target. Multigene assays that evaluate these gene expression patterns are under investigation, and several multigene assays are available in clinical practice. One such assay, Oncotype Dx, may assist in the identification of women with early-stage steroid receptor–positive breast cancer who would benefit from the addition of chemotherapy to tamoxifen. A second assay, Mammaprint, may be useful to identify young women with breast cancer with poor prognosis. A number of other assays are under development, and both the Oncotype Dx and Mammaprint assays are the subject of large randomized trials to refine the conditions for their optimal use.

TREATMENT Rx

Local Treatment of Early-Stage Breast Cancer

In Situ Carcinoma

Thanks to heightened breast cancer awareness and use of screening mammography, in situ carcinomas now account for 20 to 25% of newly diagnosed cases of breast cancer (Table 204-4). Most of these are ductal carcinoma in situ (DCIS). These lesions are associated with about a 30% risk for subsequent invasive breast cancer in the same breast. The risk for metastatic breast cancer with a diagnosis of DCIS is extremely small. As a consequence, management decisions are centered on the involved breast, and axillary lymph node evaluation is not routinely performed. Total mastectomy, the traditional therapy, has a high likelihood of cure, but studies suggest that breast conservation is appropriate for many women with DCIS. The major contraindications include poor cosmesis, extensive disease, or patient preference. Several models have suggested that size and grade of lesion and surgical margin status are important determinants of local outcome. Excision to obtain tumor-free margins is critical. Careful mammographic examination of the specimen and postexcision mammography of the breast are crucial to confirm that the DCIS has been adequately excised. A large randomized trial showed that radiotherapy plus lumpectomy decreased the likelihood of in situ or invasive recurrence when compared with lumpectomy alone. Other data sets suggest that some women with favorable histology who are willing to undergo close surveillance are candidates for local excision alone. In addition, the use of tamoxifen for 5 years can reduce ipsilateral breast cancer recurrence and contralateral breast cancer diagnosis by about 50%.

Controversy continues over whether lobular carcinoma in situ (LCIS) is truly a malignant lesion. LCIS is usually an incidental finding on a breast biopsy done for other indications, and it appears to be associated with a 25% risk for development of invasive breast cancer in either breast. Women with LCIS are generally managed expectantly with regular breast examination and mammography. Bilateral total mastectomy is sometimes considered for women with LCIS who have other risk factors or extreme anxiety. Finally, these women are candidates for tamoxifen or raloxifene as a risk-reduction strategy based on the results of several large breast cancer chemoprevention trials.

Invasive Breast Cancer

Surgery

Although radical mastectomy (removal of the breast, axillary contents, and underlying chest musculature) was the mainstay for breast cancer treatment for many years, it is seldom performed today. Multiple randomized trials have consistently shown that breast conservation therapy (BCT) with lumpectomy plus radiotherapy provides identical survival rates to modified radical mastectomy (removal of the breast and lymph nodes) for women with stages I and II breast cancer. Medical contraindications to BCT include multifocal disease, previous radiotherapy, ongoing pregnancy that precludes the timely use of radiotherapy, poor cosmesis, and patient preference. Although the number of patients who receive BCT has increased substantially, there are wide geographic differences within the United States. Patients who undergo mastectomy should be counseled about the availability of a number of autologous tissue and implant options for reconstruction, either at the time of surgery or anytime thereafter.

Because the likelihood of distant micrometastatic spread is highly correlated with the number of pathologically involved axillary lymph nodes, axillary dissection has traditionally been used to provide prognostic information. A drive toward limiting axillary surgery to minimize the incidence of postoperative lymphedema (see later) has led to the development of sentinel node techniques. Here a radioactive tracer or blue dye or both are injected into the area around the primary breast tumor. The injected substance tracks rapidly to the dominant axillary lymph node—the sentinel node—that can be located and removed by the surgeon. If the sentinel node is tumor free, the remaining nodes are likely to be tumor free as well, and no further axillary surgery is required. Currently, women with palpable axillary nodes and those with a histologically involved sentinel node are counseled to undergo axillary dissection. For women with small tumors and a clinically negative axilla, large randomized trials of sentinel node management and traditional axillary dissection suggest similar outcomes.

Adjuvant Radiotherapy

Radiotherapy has been a cornerstone in BCT because women who undergo lumpectomy alone have a breast cancer recurrence rate of up to 40%, whereas the rate of recurrence is less than 10% with whole-breast radiotherapy. 1 Attempts to identify women whose tumors are so favorable that radiotherapy can be withheld are ongoing. One large trial suggested that women older than 70 years with small ER-positive tumors who receive tamoxifen gain little with radiotherapy. Current research is also focused on the possibility that radiotherapy can be delivered safely and effectively to a smaller field (partial breast radiotherapy) or over a shorter period of time.

The role of postmastectomy radiotherapy continues to be a matter of debate. Based on the results of individual randomized trials as well as a meta-analysis suggesting a survival advantage, many radiation oncologists recommend postmastectomy radiation to women with more than three involved nodes and discuss its use for those with involvement of one to three nodes.

Adjuvant Systemic Therapy for Early Breast Cancer

Adjuvant systemic therapy is defined as the use of chemotherapy, endocrine therapy, or biological therapy, or a combination of these, after definitive local therapy for early breast cancer. Its goal is to suppress or eradicate clinically occult micrometastases. Because current testing does not permit the definitive identification of the patient with micrometastases, recommendations for adjuvant systemic therapy are based on menopausal status, lymph node status, tumor size, and the extent of expression of the ER, PR, and HER2 proteins in breast cancer cells. The treatment algorithms that are currently used are the result of more than 50 years of clinical trials[2]; the results of these trials have been compiled in sequential overview analyses that have evaluated the worldwide experience with use of endocrine therapy and chemotherapy. These analyses have shown that adjuvant therapy results in a proportional reduction in risk of recurrence across all patients regardless of risk of recurrence; this implies that the absolute benefit of adjuvant systemic therapy is greatest for individuals with the greatest risk of recurrence. Tools to assist the clinician and patient to make decisions about the use of adjuvant therapy include guidelines based on evidence and expert consensus such as the National Comprehensive Care Network (NCCN) and St. Gallen conference guidelines, as well as web-based algorithms like Adjuvant Online (Table 204-5).

Adjuvant Endocrine Therapy

Tamoxifen (20 mg/day for 5 years) has been the most widely used endocrine therapy. It improves outcomes in women of all ages with ER- or PR-positive breast cancer. Its side-effect profile includes an increased risk for thromboembolic events and uterine cancer, especially in postmenopausal women, because of its estrogen agonist properties. Potential benefits include promotion of bone density and lowering of cholesterol. The effects of altered activity of the tamoxifen metabolizing enzyme, CYP2D6, by coadministration of pharmacologic inhibitors or single-nucleotide polymorphism variants in the *CYP2D6* gene on outcome with tamoxifen is an area of active research.

In recent years, the role of estrogen deprivation has been the subject of intense scrutiny—ovarian suppression or ablation for premenopausal women and aromatase inhibition for postmenopausal women. Ovarian ablation through surgery or radiotherapy is the oldest form of systemic therapy for breast cancer. More recent work has focused on the use of luteinizing hormone-releasing hormone (LHRH) agonists as a means of effecting a temporary and reversible ovarian suppression. Two large meta-analyses have sought to define the role of these approaches. A meta-analysis of trials addressing the efficacy of LHRH agonists in women with early-stage ER-positive breast cancer suggested the following: (1) monotherapy with LHRH agonist has significant activity; (2) the efficacy of LHRH monotherapy is similar to that of certain chemotherapy regimens; and (3) LHRH agonists appear to add benefit to adjuvant chemotherapy, especially in women younger than 40 years, who are less likely than older women to become postmenopausal as a consequence of adjuvant chemotherapy. Unfortunately, these trials did not routinely include tamoxifen because its value in premenopausal breast cancer was recognized only after accrual for these ovarian suppression studies was completed. In sum, however, it appears that ovarian ablation or suppression is a viable strategy for premenopausal women with steroid receptor–positive breast cancer.

In postmenopausal women, the primary source of estrogen is the conversion of androgens synthesized by the adrenal glands to estrogen through the activity of CYP19 or aromatase in peripheral tissues such as the mammary and adipose tissues. The aromatase inhibitors (anastrozole, letrozole, and exemestane) specifically inhibit this conversion, leading to further estrogen deprivation in older women. Randomized trials have shown that efficacy of aromatase inhibitors is similar or superior to that of tamoxifen and that these drugs have an acceptable side-effect profile.[3] Multiple trials have compared monotherapy with tamoxifen or aromatase inhibitor or sequential therapy; in aggregate, they suggest that the use of an aromatase inhibitor at some point should be considered for most postmenopausal women with steroid receptor–positive invasive breast cancer. Side effects include postmenopausal symptoms, osteoporosis and fractures, and arthralgias. Aromatase inhibitors are not useful for receptor-negative breast cancer, nor should they be used as monotherapy in premenopausal women. The simultaneous administration of tamoxifen plus aromatase inhibitor does not improve outcome over aromatase inhibitor alone. In premenopausal women, the combination of LHRH agonist plus aromatase inhibitor is no better than LHRH agonist plus tamoxifen in initial studies.

Duration of endocrine therapy appears to be quite important. Direct evidence suggests that at least 5 years of adjuvant endocrine therapy is associated with better outcomes than shorter periods. Whether longer durations will be more useful remains uncertain.

Adjuvant Anti-HER2 Therapy

Increased understanding of growth and death pathways of breast cancer has led to the identification of critical nonendocrine pathways that are potential targets for therapy. The transmembrane HER2/neu protein is overexpressed in about 20% of breast cancers, generally because of gene amplification. The efficacy and safety of the monoclonal antibody, trastuzumab, in the treatment of women with HER-overexpressing metastatic breast cancer laid the foundation for several adjuvant trials that in aggregate showed that the addition of 1 year of trastuzumab to chemotherapy reduced the risk for recurrence by about 50% in women with high-risk early breast cancer. Thus, use of trastuzumab is considered for many women with HER2-positive tumors. Important questions remain regarding long-term risks and benefits, optimal duration of therapy, use of trastuzumab in the absence of chemotherapy, and role of other anti-HER2 agents such as lapatinib in addition to or in place of trastuzumab.

TABLE 204-5 ADJUVANT TREATMENT GUIDELINES FOR PATIENTS WITH EARLY-STAGE INVASIVE BREAST CANCER*

PATIENT GROUP*	TREATMENT
FAVORABLE HISTOLOGY (TUBULAR OR COLLOID)	
ER- and/or PR-Positive Breast Cancer	
<1 cm	No adjuvant therapy
1-2.9 cm	Consider adjuvant hormonal therapy†
≥3 cm or node-positive	Adjuvant hormonal therapy ± adjuvant chemotherapy†
ER- and PR-Negative Breast Cancer	
<1 cm	No adjuvant therapy
1-2.9 cm	Consider adjuvant chemotherapy
≥3 cm or node-positive	Adjuvant chemotherapy
HORMONE RECEPTOR–POSITIVE (ER- AND/OR PR-POSITIVE) BREAST CANCER	
Lymph Nodes Negative	
≤0.5 cm	No adjuvant therapy
0.6-1.0 cm well differentiated and no unfavorable features‡	Consider adjuvant hormonal therapy
0.6-1.0 cm moderate or poorly differentiated or unfavorable features	Adjuvant hormonal therapy ± adjuvant chemotherapy
>1 cm	Adjuvant hormonal therapy ± adjuvant chemotherapy
Lymph Nodes Positive	
	Adjuvant hormonal therapy + adjuvant chemotherapy
HORMONE RECEPTOR–NEGATIVE (ER- AND PR-NEGATIVE) BREAST CANCER	
≤0.5 cm	No adjuvant therapy
0.6-1.0 cm	Consider chemotherapy
>1 cm or lymph-node positive	Adjuvant chemotherapy
HER2 POSITIVE	
	Trastuzumab should be added to the suggested treatment above for all node-positive patients; trastuzumab not recommended for tumors ≤1 cm for most node-negative patients; for tumors >1 cm, trastuzumab should be considered for most patients

*Data are insufficient to make chemotherapy recommendations for patients 70 years and older. Treatment should be individualized for these patients based on life expectancy and comorbidity.
†In ER-positive or PR-positive patients, decisions regarding the added value of chemotherapy in addition to hormonal therapy alone can be aided by accurately assessing the added value of chemotherapy in individual patients using a web-based model: *www.adjuvantonline.com* or Oncotype Dx assay.
‡Unfavorable characteristics include high-grade tumor, blood vessel or lymphatic invasion by tumor, and high tumor proliferation rate (high S phase by flow cytometry or high Ki-67 value by immunohistochemistry) or HER2-positive status.
ER = estrogen receptor; PR = progesterone receptor.
Modified from National Comprehensive Cancer Network Guidelines. Available at www.nccn.org.

Adjuvant Chemotherapy

Individual trials and the Early Breast Cancer Trialists Collaborative Group meta-analysis have shown the benefit of adjuvant chemotherapy. Benefit varies by age and nodal status such that, in the meta-analysis, the absolute benefit is greatest in women younger than 50 years, in whom 15-year breast cancer mortality decreased from 42% to 32%, whereas it decreased from 50% to 47% for women aged 50 to 69 years.

These trials have established several principles that guide chemotherapy use. Combination therapy appears to be more effective than single-agent chemotherapy. Effective agents include anthracyclines, taxanes, antimetabolites, and cyclophosphamide.[4] Randomized trials have shown that 3 to 6 months of therapy is preferred over longer durations. Dose reduction below the standard level was associated with inferior outcome, but dose escalation through the use of colony-stimulating factors or autologous stem cell support led to excess toxicity without improved outcome. Regimens that use colony-stimulating factors to accelerate schedule of chemotherapy administration have been more successful.

Increased use of adjuvant chemotherapy and longer survival have led to concerns about toxicity. Acute side effects of therapy are nausea and vomiting, bone marrow suppression, and hair loss; all are reversible, and the first may be mitigated by the use of modern antiemetics. Careful use of colony-stimulating agents can minimize complications of neutropenia, but current evidence argues against the use of erythroid-stimulating agents for chemotherapy-induced anemia. Induction of menopause is a common concern for pre-menopausal women. Its likelihood is related to the type and duration of chemotherapy and the age of the patient; most women older than 40 years will suffer drug-induced menopause. Doxorubicin-related cardiomyopathy is noted in about 1% of women who received doxorubicin-containing adjuvant chemotherapy. Use of standard adjuvant chemotherapy regimens results in a very small incidence of acute leukemia, but there is no evidence of increased incidence of other second tumors. Concerns about cognitive impairment are under evaluation.

Sequencing of Adjuvant Therapy

Women frequently receive several adjuvant interventions, including chemotherapy, radiotherapy, endocrine therapy, or anti-HER2 therapy. A logical question is how best to sequence these therapies. A randomized trial showed no clear difference between the sequence of chemotherapy to radiotherapy and radiotherapy followed by chemotherapy. Concurrent chemoradiotherapy requires that certain drugs be omitted during the radiotherapy to limit toxicity. A common algorithm is surgery followed by chemotherapy followed by radiotherapy. Radiotherapy can be safely administered with endocrine or anti-HER2 therapy.

Because a large randomized trial showed that concurrent chemotherapy plus tamoxifen led to worse outcome than chemotherapy followed by tamoxifen, most practitioners delay the administration of endocrine therapy until after completion of chemotherapy. Conversely, the benefit of trastuzumab appears to be greater when it is coadministered with taxane chemotherapy rather than following completion of taxane.

A number of trials have tested the concept that administration of systemic therapy before primary surgery would improve outcome over the standard sequence of surgery followed by systemic therapy. Together they suggest that, compared with adjuvant therapy, preoperative (also termed *neoadjuvant*) systemic therapy improves the rate of breast conservation but does not enhance disease-free or overall survival. The possibility that preoperative therapy can provide an in vivo assessment of tumor response to therapy is suggested by the correlation between the finding of a pathologic complete response (absence of invasive cancer in the surgical specimen) and long-term disease-free survival in some studies.

Follow-up of Early Breast Cancer Survivors

A critical question is how longitudinal medical follow-up should be conducted in women who have received appropriate local and systemic therapy for early breast cancer. Randomized trials have addressed the question of the value of serial laboratory and radiology testing as well as the role of primary care versus oncology specialist follow-up. On the basis of these and other studies, the American Society of Clinical Oncology has published evidence-based guidelines for follow-up of asymptomatic survivors of early-stage breast cancer. These guidelines are summarized in Table 204-6.

TABLE 204-6 FOLLOW-UP GUIDELINES FOR PATIENTS WITH EARLY-STAGE BREAST CANCER: AMERICAN SOCIETY OF CLINICAL ONCOLOGY GUIDELINES*

PROCEDURE OR TEST	FREQUENCY
History and physical examination* (eliciting of symptoms of breast cancer)	Every 3-6 mo for first 3 yr, every 6-12 mo for next yr, then yearly
MAMMOGRAPHY	
Mastectomy patients	Yearly
Lumpectomy patients	Yearly
Pelvic examination	Yearly
Breast self-examination	Monthly
Complete blood cell counts and chemistry studies	The literature does not support the use of these tests
Chest radiography, bone scans, PET scans, breast MRI, liver imaging, and tumor marker studies	Not recommended for routine follow-up in asymptomatic patients
Patient education regarding signs and symptoms of recurrence	Each visit

*Limited evaluation: assess for pain, dyspnea, weight loss, and other major changes in function. The limited examination should include an assessment of nodes, axillae, lumpectomy or mastectomy site, chest, and abdomen. Patients should be instructed regarding symptoms of recurrence.

Modified from Khatcheressian JL, Wolff AC, Smith TJ, et al. American Society of Clinical Oncology 2006 update of the breast cancer follow-up and management guidelines in the adjuvant setting. *J Clin Oncol.* 2006;24:5091-5097.

Stage III Breast Cancer

Locally advanced or inoperable stage III breast cancer accounts for about 10% of breast cancers. It is characterized by large primary tumor or fixed tumor or lymph nodes or neoplastic invasion of the skin or chest wall. Inflammatory breast cancer falls into this category. It has a clinical presentation of breast swelling, warmth, and erythema and may or may not be associated with a mass. Because as many as one third of women with locally advanced breast cancer have distant metastases at the time of diagnosis, many oncologists perform an evaluation for distant disease even in asymptomatic patients. Diagnosis is usually established by fine-needle aspiration or core biopsy, and combined-modality therapy is used to maximize control of local disease and distant micrometastases. Several months of preoperative endocrine therapy or chemotherapy results in tumor regression in most patients, thereby allowing definitive breast surgery of some type to be performed. Postoperative radiotherapy is generally employed to enhance local control, and some studies suggest that administration of further chemotherapy, hormone therapy, anti-HER2 therapy, or a combination thereof (depending on the features of the cancer) is then desirable. Multimodality therapy results in a 5-year disease-free survival rate of about 50%.

Stage IV or Metastatic Breast Cancer

Although seldom curable, advanced breast cancer is a highly treatable illness. Palliation or prevention of symptoms without excess toxicity is the primary goal of treatment. The median survival after diagnosis of metastatic breast cancer is 2 to 3 years, although the range is great, and a small cadre of long-term survivors has been described. Several recent clinical trials have documented small improvements in survival with some of the newer therapies.

Most women with metastatic breast cancer present with symptoms or abnormalities on physical examination. Less than 10% of women present with metastatic disease; rather advanced disease is normally diagnosed in women with a previous diagnosis of early breast cancer for which they received treatment. Common sites for metastases include bone, soft tissues, lung, liver, and brain. If metastatic disease is suspected, relevant hematologic, biochemical, and radiographic evaluation is indicated to assess location and severity of involvement. Because of the import of the diagnosis, pathologic confirmation is preferred. This permits verification of recurrent disease, exclusion of other diagnoses, and reassessment of biologic features such ER, PR, and HER2. Elevation of tumor markers (e.g., CA-2729, carcinoembryonic antigen) or the presence of circulating tumor cells is not diagnostic of recurrent disease, although these markers may be useful adjuncts in the assessment of the effects of therapy.

The role of surgery in metastatic breast cancer is limited. It is useful in certain circumstances such as resection of a chest wall nodule or solitary brain metastasis or orthopedic stabilization to treat or prevent a long-bone fracture. Radiotherapy is a mainstay in the management of advanced disease. It may be used at any time during the patient's course to treat localized disease such as chest wall recurrence, brain metastases, or painful bony metastases. Systemic treatment is the primary mode for management of disseminated disease. Key principles for selection of therapy include maximal palliation of symptoms, minimization of treatment-related toxicity, and prevention of disease complications. An algorithm for treatment of stage IV breast cancer is shown in Figure 204-1.

Endocrine Therapy

Endocrine therapy is preferred as the first intervention for metastatic breast cancer whenever feasible because of its favorable therapeutic index. Factors that support the use of endocrine therapy include the expression of hormone receptors, a long disease-free interval, and absence of symptoms or visceral disease. More than half of the women who meet these criteria respond to an initial course of hormone therapy, with a median response duration of 9 to 12 months. Length of response is a good predictor for the likelihood of response to a second course of endocrine therapy when the first agent fails. A second course of endocrine therapy is less likely to be successful, and the duration of response is shorter; again, duration of response predicts for likelihood of success with third-line therapy. Successful application of this algorithm can result in good disease control with little toxicity for several years in some women.

A number of types of hormone therapy are now available. These include the selective estrogen receptor modulator (SERM) tamoxifen; the selective estrogen receptor–degrading agent, fulvestrant; the aromatase inhibitors; and ovarian suppression by oophorectomy or LHRH agonists. Selection is usually made on the basis of efficacy, toxicity, and menopausal status. Serial

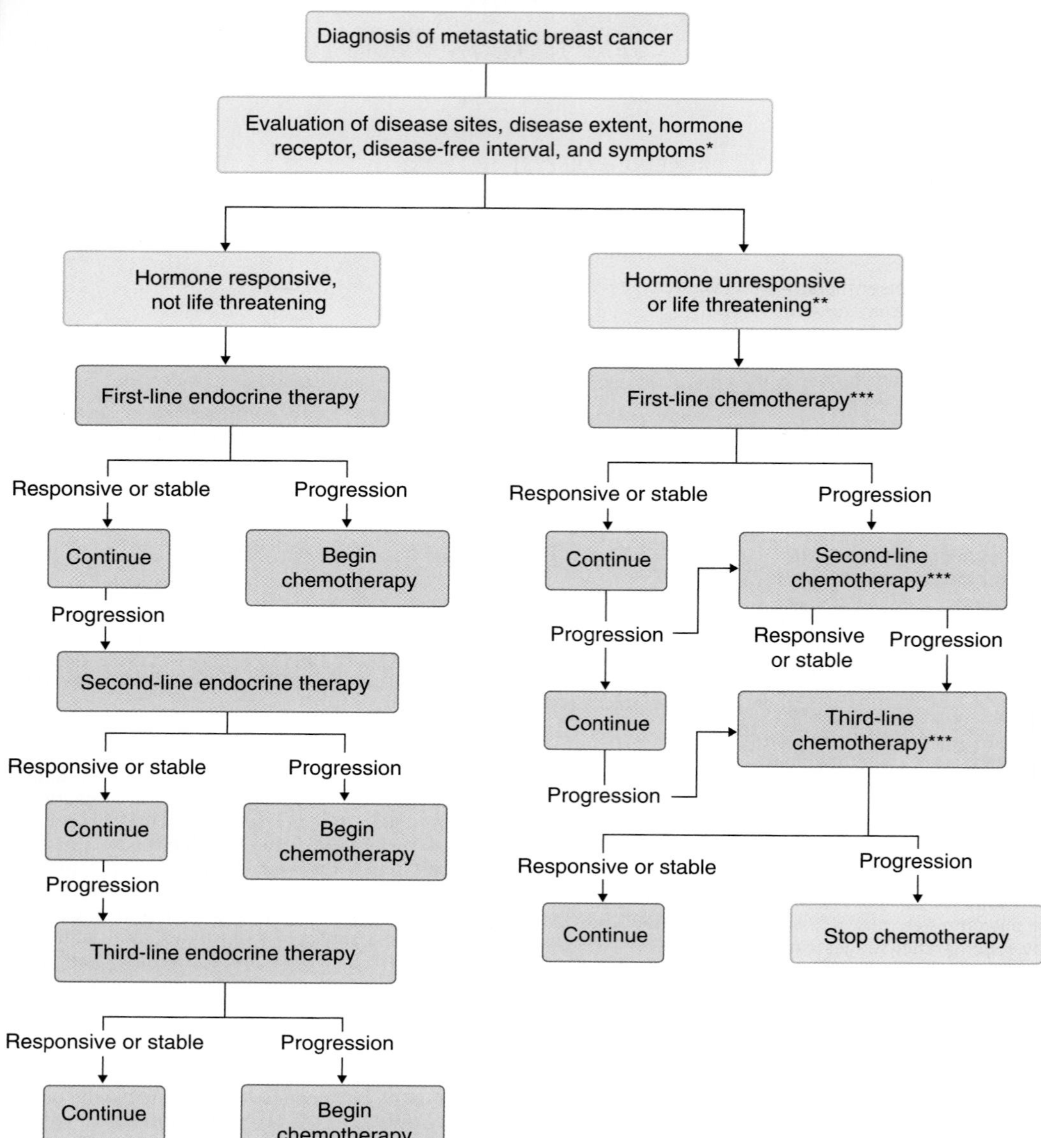

FIGURE 204-1. **An algorithm used for the systemic treatment of stage IV breast cancer.** *Consider role of bisphosphonate if bone involvement. **Consider integration of anti-HER2 therapy if tumor is HER2 overexpressing. ***Consider using bevacizumab.

administration of agents is the norm; combination therapy (with the possible exception of ovarian suppression plus tamoxifen) does not improve outcomes.

Several months of therapy are needed before the efficacy of a newly introduced endocrine therapy can be assessed. Patients and clinicians should be aware of the possibility of treatment-related tumor flare—a syndrome of worsening symptoms and increased circulating tumor markers—that can occur within the first few weeks of treatment. This response is usually of short duration and should not be confused with disease progression.

Chemotherapy

Most women with advanced breast cancer experience endocrine-unresponsive disease at some point and become candidates for palliative chemotherapy. Serial chemotherapy is the norm. Patients receive two to four cycles of therapy and then are evaluated for disease stabilization or improvement. Duration of therapy is variable for those who are responding to therapy. Several trials compared the approach of continuing therapy until time of disease progression with the approach of administering therapy, followed by a "drug holiday," with resumption of therapy at the time of disease progression. In sum, these studies suggest that survival is the same with these two approaches but that quality of life, as judged by the patients, is often better with continued therapy. Thus, decisions about continuation or cessation of a therapy are driven by perception of side effects and benefits by the patient and clinician.

Many active agents for breast cancer are now available. These include well-established drugs such as cyclophosphamide, doxorubicin, and methotrexate as well as newer agents like paclitaxel, docetaxel, vinorelbine, capecitabine, gemcitabine, carboplatin, ixabepilone, pegylated doxorubicin, and nano-albumin-bound paclitaxel. All these agents are active individually and in combination. There is considerable debate about the value of combination therapy compared with sequential single-agent therapy for metastatic breast cancer. In addition, much attention has been focused on schedule of administration. For example, weekly paclitaxel regimens appear to be more effective and better tolerated than every-3-week regimens for many women. As with endocrine therapy, response rates and duration diminish with each successive change in therapy. As with early breast cancer, high-dose chemotherapy combined with autologous stem cell or bone marrow support has not shown benefit. A difficult question for patient and doctor is when to stop chemotherapy. No fixed rules exist, but many patients and physicians move to a program of supportive care if two successive chemotherapy regimens fail to produce a tumor response or disease stabilization.

Biological Agents

Enhanced understanding of breast cancer biology has resulted in the identification of new targets for therapy beyond the estrogen receptor pathway. The first agent brought into clinical practice was the monoclonal antibody, trastuzumab (Herceptin), which is active against the transmembrane HER2/neu protein. Administration of trastuzumab monotherapy to women with metastatic HER2-overexpressing breast cancer led to partial or complete tumor regression in about 30% of untreated women. Concurrent trastuzumab with paclitaxel increased response rate and duration and survival compared with paclitaxel alone for women with newly diagnosed metastatic breast cancer. Similar results were seen with concurrent administration of trastuzumab and doxorubicin, but this combination was associated with a 20% incidence of congestive heart failure. This unexpected finding demonstrates the need for careful evaluation of new biological agents as they enter the clinic. Dose and schedule of trastuzumab have been studied, and it appears that every-3-week administration is active with less patient inconvenience. One unanswered question has been how long to continue trastuzumab in advanced breast cancer because discontinuation of a therapy at the time of progression has been the norm. A small provocative study suggests that patients who develop progressive disease while taking paclitaxel and trastuzumab fare better if they are changed to a regimen of trastuzumab and capecitabine rather than capecitabine alone.

Another molecular target of interest is the epidermal growth factor receptor (EGFR, or HER1). Small molecules that target the EGFR tyrosine kinase, gefitinib and erlotinib, or the monoclonal antibody against EGFR, cetuximab, have shown little activity as monotherapy in women with advanced breast cancer. But the dual HER1 and HER2 receptor inhibitor, lapatinib, has been shown to improve outcome for women with advanced HER2-overexpressing breast cancer when added to capecitabine. Further, clinical trials have suggested that addition of lapatinib to trastuzumab at the time of progression on trastuzumab gives superior results to lapatinib alone. Studies of both these agents suggest that their benefit is most marked in women whose tumors overexpress HER2 protein. Other agents that target the HER family members are in clinical testing.

Strategies to block tumor angiogenesis are also employed. One such agent is bevacizumab, a monoclonal antibody that targets the vascular endothelial growth factor. This agent has only modest activity as monotherapy in metastatic breast cancer, but its addition to taxane-based chemotherapy for women with newly diagnosed stage IV breast cancer appears to improve progression-free survival without a major impact on survival. Other studies suggest that it has similar effects when added to subsequent chemotherapy regimens as well. Its use in concert with standard adjuvant chemotherapies is under evaluation.

Multiple other targeted agents are also under development. Of recent interest are the poly-ADP-ribose polymerase (PARP) inhibitors. These small molecule inhibitors of DNA repair show particular activity in women with *BRCA* mutant breast cancer in early studies. In addition, early information suggests that coadministration of PARP inhibitor with chemotherapy improves outcomes over chemotherapy alone for women with stage IV triple-negative breast cancer. More definitive testing is in progress.

Supportive Care

Bone Health

Because palliation of symptoms and prevention of complications of metastatic disease are the primary goals of treatment for advanced breast cancer, careful attention to supportive care is vital. Bone is the most common site of metastasis in breast cancer, and bone disease can be a source of significant morbidity. Several studies have shown that regular administration of a bisphosphonate such as zoledronate or pamidronate in addition to endocrine therapy or chemotherapy can reduce pain and lower the incidence of skeletal complications of disease. Although such therapy is now the norm, several issues remain unaddressed, including the optimal treatment interval and duration of therapy.

Given the propensity of breast cancer therapy to lead to estrogen deprivation and osteopenia or osteoporosis (Chapter 251), the use of bisphosphonates in the adjuvant setting is under evaluation. Small trials have raised the possibility that bisphosphonates might prevent or delay the development of metastases in women with early-stage breast cancer, and the results of large randomized trials are awaited.

Postmenopausal Symptoms

Postmenopausal symptoms as a consequence of therapy or natural aging are common in breast cancer survivors. In general, hormone replacement therapy should be avoided in women with a history of breast cancer. A short course of treatment can be considered in patients with early-stage breast cancer who have truly disabling symptoms. Topical estrogens are considered for women with vaginal dryness that does not respond to lubricants. Vasomotor symptoms may be reduced with the use of certain antidepressants of the selective serotonin release inhibitor family. Multiple studies have failed to show consistent benefit from many alternative therapies.

Lymphedema

Lymphedema develops in the ipsilateral arm in up to 15% of women after treatment for early breast cancer. Its incidence is lower with sentinel lymph node procedures and meticulous radiotherapy planning. Prevention includes avoidance of trauma and possibly exercises. Early recognition of symptoms is key. Affected patients should be referred to specialists for consideration of treatment such as manual drainage or the use of compression stockings or pumps.

Special Circumstances

The risk for breast cancer is slightly increased during and just after pregnancy. Suspicious breast findings during pregnancy should be investigated vigorously. Surgical therapy for breast cancer can be safely performed after the first trimester of pregnancy, but radiotherapy should be delayed until after delivery. Current data suggest that certain adjuvant chemotherapy regimens can be safely administered in the second and third trimesters of pregnancy, and development is normal in children of mothers who receive this chemotherapy. Administration of antimetabolites should be avoided because of the potential for damage to the placenta. Initiation of endocrine therapy is generally delayed until after delivery. Pregnancy after a diagnosis of early breast cancer does not appear to increase the risk for metastatic disease in limited data sets. The major considerations for women contemplating pregnancy should be its timing with regard to endocrine therapy, which may require 5 or more years to complete, as well as the underlying risk for disease recurrence.

Men account for not more than 1% of breast cancer cases. Failure of the patient or health care provider to diagnose the disease means that it may be diagnosed at a later stage. Most breast cancers in men express ER, and treatment recommendations for these men are generally similar to those for postmenopausal women.

PREVENTION AND SCREENING

There is enormous interest in the development of breast cancer prevention strategies. Currently these include surgical, chemopreventive, and lifestyle modification approaches.

Prophylactic Mastectomy and Oophorectomy

Prophylactic mastectomy appears to reduce the risk of developing breast cancer by about 90% in individuals who are at high risk because of a strong family history or carriage of a germline *BRCA1* or *BRCA2* mutation. Prophylactic oophorectomy in *BRCA* mutation carriers has also been shown to decrease breast cancer incidence by about 50%, presumably because of reduction in ovarian steroids. It is critical that women who opt for prophylactic mastectomy be counseled about the possibility that cancer may develop in remnants of breast tissue that remain after prophylactic mastectomy.

Chemoprevention

The observation that adjuvant endocrine therapy with the SERM tamoxifen also decreased contralateral breast cancer led to evaluation of tamoxifen as a chemopreventive for well women who are at high risk for breast cancer. Meta-analysis of four randomized trials of tamoxifen versus placebo for high-risk women confirmed a 38% reduction in invasive breast cancer with tamoxifen. The largest trial, NSABP P01, randomized 13,388 high-risk women to receive either tamoxifen or placebo for 5 years. Risk factors used to determine eligibility were age ≥60 years, a diagnosis of LCIS, or age 35 to 59 years with a constellation of risk factors that, when combined, resulted in a 1.67% or greater risk for breast cancer within 5 years. This study showed a 50% decrease in the diagnosis of breast cancer across all age groups at a cost of increased risk for endometrial cancer and thromboembolic events in women older than 50 years. These data led to the approval of tamoxifen to reduce incidence of breast cancer in women at high risk as defined by the eligibility criteria for this prevention trial.

Other SERMs have been studied as chemopreventive agents. Two trials have documented the utility of raloxifene as a breast cancer risk-reduction strategy.[5] In one trial, raloxifene administration reduced the incidence of breast cancer in postmenopausal women of average breast cancer risk and elevated cardiovascular risk. A second trial showed that raloxifene was as effective as tamoxifen in preventing invasive breast cancer in postmenopausal women at high risk for breast cancer. Raloxifene use was associated with fewer uterine cancers than tamoxifen but carries the same risk for thromboembolic events. It is approved by the U.S. Food and Drug Administration (FDA) for risk reduction in high-risk postmenopausal women. A vitamin A derivative, fenretinide, showed some impact as a chemopreventive agent for secondary prevention in premenopausal breast cancer survivors but has not found a place in routine practice. Finally, large epidemiologic studies have raised the possibility that aspirin or certain statins might also decrease breast cancer risk, but these agents have not been prospectively tested.

Lifestyle Modification

Prevention strategies that involve lifestyle alterations have been suggested. The Women's Health Initiative did not show a clear role for a low-fat diet as a means of breast cancer prevention. Regular exercise, especially during adolescence, may be associated with reduced breast cancer risk. By extrapolation from the epidemiologic studies mentioned previously, abstinence from alcohol might slightly reduce the risk for breast cancer.

Screening

Screening strategies for breast cancer have traditionally included the triad of breast self-examination (BSE), clinical breast examination (CBE) by a health

TABLE 204-7 BREAST CANCER SCREENING

TEST	ACS	USPSTF
Mammography		
40-49 yr	Annual	Insufficient evidence to support
>49 yr	Annual if healthy	Every 2 yr, 50-75 yr
Clinical breast examination	Every 3 yr, 20-39 yr Annually, ≥40 yr	Insufficient evidence to support
Breast self-examination	Optional	Not recommended

ACS = American Cancer Society; USPSTF = U.S. Preventive Services Task Force.

care professional, and screening mammography in well women. Although widely promulgated as an important component of early detection, two large randomized trials of conventional BSE versus observation failed to show any clinical advantage with BSE. As a result, many experts now promote breast awareness rather than regular BSE. The independent value of CBEs has not been rigorously assessed. Rather, it has been studied in conjunction with screening mammography, in which case the two interventions appear to decrease mortality from breast cancer by 25 to 30% in women older than 50 years. Considerable controversy continues over the value of screening mammography in women 40 to 50 years of age and those over 70 years of age as well as the optimal interval between mammograms for women aged 50 to 70 years. Currently, the American Cancer Society and the National Cancer Institute recommend annual screening mammography for women older than 40 years of age who are at standard risk for breast cancer. In contrast, the U.S. Preventive Services Task Force, advising the Department of Health and Human Services, recommended in 2009 that women between 40 and 50 years of age be counseled about the risks and benefits of screening mammography and that screening mammography can be used at 2-year intervals for women aged 50 to 75 years (Table 204-7). A study of digital versus conventional film screen mammography failed to show an overall advantage for digital mammography but suggest that digital mammography may be more useful for women with dense breasts.

The knowledge that screening mammography fails to diagnose about 10 to 15% of breast cancers has led to the evaluation of other imaging modalities. Of these, MRI is the most mature. MRI has been promoted as a useful screening tool for women at high risk by virtue of the *BRCA* mutation; indeed, the American Cancer Society has recommended consideration of screening MRI for women whose predicted risk for breast cancer exceeds 20%. MRI has been shown to detect breast cancer in the contralateral breast in 3% of women with a newly diagnosed breast cancer whose contralateral mammogram showed no abnormality. Use of MRI in the general population is limited by the fact that it is highly sensitive but lacks specificity. Insufficient information exists about other breast imaging modalities such as ultrasound and radionuclide imaging to support their use in screening asymptomatic women.

BENIGN BREAST LESIONS

Benign breast disease includes *mastalgia* (pain and tenderness), mastitis (including infectious and noninfectious inflammatory conditions), trauma, and benign tumors. In addition, mastalgia can be caused by extramammary conditions, such as myocardial ischemia, pneumonia, pleural irritation, esophageal spasm, costochondritis, rib fracture, and varicella-zoster virus (preceding the skin eruption). After these conditions have been ruled out, mastalgia is considered to be a benign condition that is self-limited. It can be cyclical or noncyclical in timing (where it is thought to be related to hormonal activity), and it may occur in postmenopausal women, even in the absence of hormone replacement therapy.

Mastitis is due to breast inflammation or infection, and it can occur in either nonlactating or lactating women. The typical presentation in nonlactating women is occurrence in their 40s with the acute onset of severe breast pain and tenderness followed by erythema and swelling that tends to be localized in the nipple-areolar area. The cause in most cases is considered to be rupture of dilated subareolar ducts that leads to an inflammatory response to leakage of intraductal contents into periductal tissue. Infection is difficult to rule out, and, in practice, patients are often treated with empirical antibiotics; if symptoms do not resolve within 7 to 10 days on antibiotics, ultrasound is required to rule out abscess. If the latter is found, incision and drainage are required. The most important differential diagnosis with mastitis is inflammatory carcinoma, as noted previously. Therefore, failure to improve with antibiotics or to find an abscess should lead to evaluation by a breast surgeon. Mastitis in lactating women is often due to infection caused by a break in the skin of the nipple or milk stasis. *Staphylococcal aureus, Staphylococcus albus,* and sometimes *Escherichia coli* or streptococci are the most common pathogens. Treatment requires antibiotics and milk removal.

Nonproliferative and Proliferative Benign Breast Lesions

Nonproliferative benign breast lesions include (1) inflammatory fat necrosis, which follows surgical or blunt trauma, and generally resolves spontaneously; (2) lymphocytic mastitis, which may be seen in diabetic patients; and (3) granulomatous mastitis, associated with foreign body reactions (e.g., silicone and paraffin for breast augmentation and reconstruction after cancer surgery), sarcoid, or certain infections. Other nonproliferative benign breast lesions appear as tumor-like processes, including (4) fibroadenoma, a very common (about 25% of women), usually solitary, sharply demarcated, smooth lesion in younger age groups; (5) phyllodes tumor (previously known as cystosarcoma phyllodes); (6) intraductal papilloma, solitary lesions that may be accompanied by bloody nipple discharge; (7) fibrocystic breast disease, which is now more appropriately called “fibrocystic changes” because it is observed clinically in up to 50% and histologically in 90% of women, composed of varying amounts of fibrosis and cysts sometimes associated with calcifications and inflammation; and (8) simple or complex cysts, which should be aspirated with ultrasound guidance and, when the fluid is not clear, sent for cytologic analysis.

Proliferative benign breast lesions include ductal or lobular hyperplasia; atypical hyperplasias are associated with increased risk for breast cancer.

Breast Cancer Risk

The increasing use of mammography has increased the frequency of breast biopsies, which, in turn, has increased the finding of benign breast lesions, the most common findings on biopsy. The benign breast lesions listed in the previous section encompass the general histologic spectrum of (1) nonproliferative lesions, (2) proliferative lesions without atypia, and (3) atypical hyperplasia, listed in ascending order of risk for breast cancer. A large number of retrospective and prospective studies have shown an overall relative risk for breast cancer of 1.5 to 1.6 for women with biopsy-proven benign breast disease compared with women in the general population. A study of 9087 women with all types of benign histology, followed for a median of 15 years at the Mayo Clinic, found that 707 of them developed breast cancers. Increased risk for cancer persisted for at least 25 years after the original biopsy. Of the three broad histologic categories, the relative risk for cancer development was 4.24 associated with atypia, 1.88 with proliferative changes without atypia, and 1.27 with nonproliferative lesions. It is not known if the finding of a benign breast lesion with atypical histology represents an actual precursor lesion for cancer or if it is only a marker for a general tendency to develop breast cancer. The observations that about half of breast cancers in these patients arise in the contralateral breast suggests the latter hypothesis.

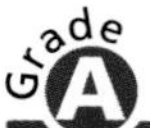

1. Clarke M, Collins R, Darby S, et al, for the Early Breast Cancer Trialists' Collaborative Group (EBCTCG). Effects of radiotherapy and of differences in the extent of surgery for early breast cancer on local recurrence and 15-year survival: an overview of the randomised trials. *Lancet.* 2005; 366:2087-2106.
2. Early Breast Cancer Trialists' Collaborative Group (EBCTCG). Effects of chemotherapy and hormonal therapy for early breast cancer on recurrence and 15-year survival: an overview of the randomised trials. *Lancet.* 2005;365:1687-1717.
3. Dowsett M, Cuzick J, Ingle J, et al. Meta-analysis of breast cancer outcomes in adjuvant trials of aromatase inhibitors versus tamoxifen. *J Clin Oncol.* 2010;28:509-518.
4. Swain SM, Jeong JH, Geyer CE Jr, et al. Longer therapy, iatrogenic amenorrhea, and survival in early breast cancer. *N Engl J Med.* 2010;362:2053-2065.
5. Vogel VG, Costantino JP, Wickerham DL, et al. Update of the National Surgical Adjuvant Breast and Bowel Project Study of Tamoxifen and Raloxifene (STAR) P-2 Trial: preventing breast cancer. *Cancer Prev Res.* 2010;3:696-706.

SUGGESTED READINGS

Bruening W, Fontanarosa J, Tipton K, et al. Systematic review: comparative effectiveness of core-needle and open surgical biopsy to diagnose breast lesions. *Ann Intern Med.* 2010;152:238-246. *Stereotactic and ultrasound-guided breast biopsies are nearly as accurate as open surgical biopsies.*

Burstein HJ, Prestrud AA, Seidenfeld J, et al. American Society of Clinical Oncology clinical practice guideline: update on adjuvant endocrine therapy for women with hormone receptor–positive breast cancer. *J Clin Oncol.* 2010;28:3784-3796. *Consensus guidelines.*

Carlson RW, Allred DC, Anderson BO, et al. Invasive breast cancer. *J Natl Comp Canc Netw*. 2011;9:136-222. *Comprehensive review.*

Henderson TO, Amsterdam A, Bhatia S, et al. Systematic review: surveillance for breast cancer in women treated with chest radiation for childhood, adolescent, or young adult cancer. *Ann Intern Med*. 2010;152:444-455; W144-154. *Women treated with chest radiation for childhood, adolescent, or young adult cancer have a higher risk of breast cancer at a young age and likely benefit from early cancer screening.*

Kabat GC, Jones JG, Olson N, et al. A multi-center prospective cohort study of benign breast disease and risk of subsequent breast cancer. *Cancer Causes Control*. 2010;21:821-882. *Women with proliferative disease without atypia have a modestly increased risk of breast cancer, whereas women with atypical hyperplasia have a substantially increased risk.*

Meissner HI, Klabunde CN, Han PK, et al. Breast cancer screening beliefs, recommendations and practices: primary care physicians in the United States. *Cancer*. 2011. [Epub ahead of print.] *Recommendations of primary care physicians generally followed national guidelines.*

205

GYNECOLOGIC CANCERS

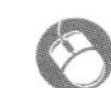

MAURIE MARKMAN

CERVICAL CANCER

Worldwide there are more than 450,000 cases of invasive cancer of the cervix each year, leading to 250,000 deaths. Overall, this malignancy is the second most common cancer (after breast cancer) in women and the third most common cancer overall.

However, owing to the availability of a highly effective screening strategy (Pap smear), the incidence of invasive cervical cancer and deaths from this illness have decreased substantially in the developed world over the past several decades, with the majority of cases (and deaths) found in the developing world. For example, in the United States it is anticipated that there will be approximately 11,000 new cases accounting for 4000 deaths each year, making cancer of the cervix the 12th most common malignancy in women in this country.

EPIDEMIOLOGY

It is well established that essentially all cases of cervical cancer result from persistent infection (transmitted through sexual exposure) by oncogenic types of human papillomavirus (HPV; Chapter 381). Risk factors for cancer include early age of first sexual encounter; history of other sexually transmitted illnesses (Chapter 293), such as herpes simplex, chlamydia, and human immunodeficiency virus (HIV); multiple sexual partners and pregnancies; extended duration of oral contraceptive use; history of cigarette smoking; and chronic immunosuppression (e.g., renal transplantation, HIV).

Epidemiologic surveys demonstrate that as many as 50% of women will be exposed to HPV within 4 years of their initial sexual encounters. However, the large majority of individuals can spontaneously clear the infection, with subsequent cervical cytologic abnormalities being observed in only 5 to 10% of women experiencing an HPV infection.

The strongest association with cervical cancer involves HPV types 16 and 18, which together are implicated in approximately 70% of cases of the malignancy worldwide. An additional 30 types of HPV have been documented to be oncogenic, and another 70 have been described that are not known to have the potential to lead to cancer of the cervix. Besides types 16 and 18, other relatively common oncogenic HPV types that are responsible for varying percentages of cases in different regions of the world are 45, 31, 33, 52, 58, and 35.

PATHOBIOLOGY

It is important to note that the current level of understanding of the pathogenesis of cervical cancer from the time of viral infection to the development of invasive disease is greater than for any other human malignancy. Evidence suggests that once an oncogenic HPV successfully incorporates into the host genome (becoming a "persistent infection"), viral proteins (E6, E7) are produced that bind to and inactivate essential tumor suppressor proteins (RB1, TP53), leading to a cascade effect that ultimately results in a malignancy.

CLINICAL MANIFESTATIONS

Most cancers of the cervix are of squamous cell histology, although adenocarcinomas currently account for as many as one quarter of all cases of this malignancy. Other less common histologies include neuroendocrine and carcinoid tumors, lymphomas, and sarcomas.

The most common symptoms of invasive cervical cancer are abnormal vaginal or postcoital bleeding and vaginal discharge. These complaints are certainly not specific for cancer, but if they persist or another obvious cause is not evident, the diagnosis of cancer should be considered. A negative Pap test should not preclude further examination of the cervix as a possible site of malignancy in the appropriate clinical setting, because one half of women with documented invasive cervical cancer have a negative test.

With more advanced disease, pelvic pain and difficulty with both defecation and urination may be noted. Finally, with locally advanced cancer or metastatic spread, the patient may complain of back pain, leg swelling (from direct interference with blood flow to the region or development of deep venous thrombosis), or neuropathic pain (from nerve involvement).

DIAGNOSIS

Common diagnostic testing for cervical cancer includes physical examination (which may reveal a mass lesion or friable or necrotic tissue), laboratory testing (revealing possible renal dysfunction due to urethral obstruction), and radiographic imaging. In general, magnetic resonance imaging (MRI) is more sensitive than computed tomography in defining tumor size and extent of disease. Recent data have revealed the superiority of positron emission tomography in determining the presence or absence of nodal involvement in cancer of the cervix.

Screening for Preinvasive Disease

It would not be hyperbole to state that the initial development and subsequent routine use of Pap smears constitute one of the most important public health advances of the past 50 years (Fig. 205-1). It has long been recognized that preinvasive cervical abnormalities precede the development of invasive cancer by many years, permitting highly effective (essentially 100%, if correctly applied) and relatively nonmorbid local interventions.

Liquid-based cytologic testing procedures and HPV testing have improved both the sensitivity and the specificity of screening. However, the basic principle of screening remains the same: early discovery and removal of preinvasive lesions that, if left untreated, would have a substantial risk of developing into invasive cancer. The magnitude of this risk is highlighted by data revealing that as many as one third of documented, untreated carcinoma in situ abnormalities may progress to frank invasive cancer of the cervix over a 10-year period.

Patients with a concerning Pap smear result should be referred to undergo colposcopy and directed biopsies. Subsequent treatment and follow-up are based on the findings from this evaluation.

Recently revised guidelines from the American College of Obstetricians and Gynecologists for routine screening for cervical cancer are as follows:

- Screening should begin at age 21.
- Screening is recommended every 2 years for women aged 21 to 29.
- Either conventional or liquid-based cytology is acceptable.

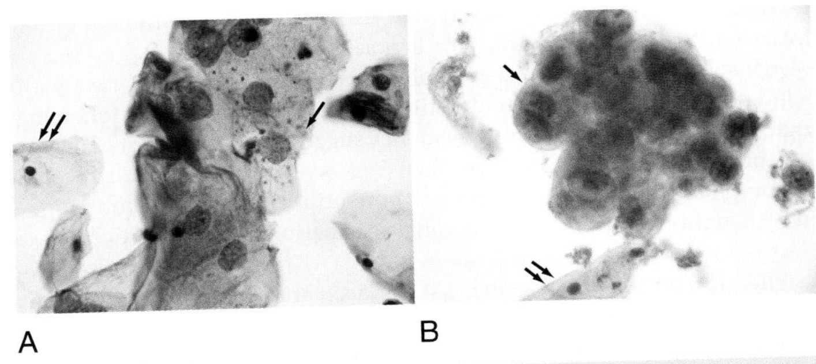

FIGURE 205-1. Cervical abnormalities on Pap smear. A, Low-grade squamous intraepithelial neoplasia. Note the group of mildly dysplastic cells with an increased nuclear-to-cytoplasmic ratio *(single arrow)* contrasted with a normal squamous epithelial cell *(double arrows)* (Papanicolaou stain, × 400). **B,** Cervical adenocarcinoma. Note the three-dimensional cluster of pleomorphic cells with a markedly increased nuclear-to-cytoplasmic ratio, dense nuclear chromatin, and macronucleoli *(single arrow)* contrasted with a normal squamous epithelial cell *(double arrows)* (Papanicolaou stain, × 400).

- Women 30 years of age and older with three consecutive negative results for intra-epithelial lesions can change to an every-3-year screening schedule.
- Women with any of the following risk factors may require more frequent screening: (1) HIV infection; (2) receiving immunosuppressive medication; (3) history of exposure to diethylstilbestrol in utero (see the section on vaginal cancer); (4) prior treatment for cervical intra-epithelial neoplasia (CIN) 2, CIN 3, or cancer.
- Women older than 65 to 70 years with three or more consecutive negative test results over the preceding 10 years can discontinue routine screening.
- Women who have had a total hysterectomy performed for a nonmalignant condition can discontinue routine screening.

TREATMENT

Rx

Localized Disease

Following evaluation for the extent of disease involvement, patients with localized cancer of the cervix can be managed with a variety of approaches, including (1) simple hysterectomy (if pretreatment clinical characteristics suggest the risk of lymph node involvement is very low), (2) radical hysterectomy (with removal of pelvic and para-aortic lymph nodes), (3) surgery plus external beam radiation, or (4) external beam radiation plus concurrent chemotherapy (so-called chemo-radiation).

Invasive Disease

Several randomized trials have revealed the superior outcome associated with radiation plus cisplatin-based chemotherapy, compared with radiation alone, in the management of locally advanced, invasive cervical cancer.[1] In patients with nonmetastatic, invasive cervical cancer, long-term disease-free survival is strongly influenced by a number of factors (most prominently, initial tumor stage) and ranges from as high as 95% (early-stage disease without lymphovascular space invasion) to less than 20% for stage IV cancer.

In the presence of metastatic cancer at diagnosis, or if the cancer has recurred following initial management, currently available treatment options provide quite modest palliative benefits. Cisplatin is the single most active antineoplastic agent in cancer of the cervix (20% objective response rate). Patients with an adequate baseline performance status that permits a more intensive approach may be treated with a cisplatin-based combination chemotherapy regimen.[1] Responses in this setting are generally limited in duration (3 to 4 months) and are more likely to occur in areas not previously radiated. In this difficult clinical setting, the limited potential for therapeutic benefit must be weighed against the risk of toxic effects that may negatively impact the quality of a patient's remaining life.

PREVENTION

Two recently licensed vaccines based on HPV types 16 and 18 are highly effective in reducing the risk of developing persistent HPV infection and type-specific cervical dysplasia *if administered before evidence of sexual exposure to the virus.*[2,3] In the large randomized trials conducted to obtain regulatory approval of these preparations, and in extensive post-marketing surveillance evaluations, few serious vaccine-related side effects (e.g., hypersensitivity reactions) have been documented.

There is no convincing evidence of the utility of HPV vaccination in an individual already infected with HPV. These data emphasize the importance of vaccination before an individual's first sexual contact.

Unanswered questions and unresolved issues regarding HPV vaccination include the following: (1) the duration of protective immunity following a single vaccination series (current evidence suggests that sufficient concentrations of antibody persist for more than 5 to 6 years in individuals receiving the complete vaccination regimen); (2) the utility of strategies consisting of fewer than three individual shots (initial vaccination followed by two booster injections) delivered over several months; (3) the benefit of approaches designed to increase the effectiveness of vaccination by adding other oncogenic types (in addition to 16 and 18); (4) the impact on cervical cancer prevention associated with the vaccination of males; and (5) cost, religious, and other societal objections to vaccine use (e.g., mandated vs. voluntary vaccination).

ENDOMETRIAL CANCER

Endometrial cancer is the most common female pelvic malignancy in the United States; approximately 40,000 new cases are diagnosed each year, resulting in almost 8000 deaths. Overall, endometrial cancer accounts for almost 50% of all female pelvic malignancies and is the fourth most common cancer type in women. The reported high incidence of endometrial cancer is likely due to several factors, including longer life expectancies, earlier diagnosis, and the reduced incidence of cervical cancer. Worldwide, endometrial cancer trails only cervical cancer as the leading cause of malignant disease in women.

EPIDEMIOLOGY

The major recognized risk factor for the development of endometrial cancer is estrogen exposure, either endogenous or exogenous. Case-control studies conducted more than 20 years ago demonstrated that women exposed to long-term unopposed estrogen have a 4- to 15-fold increased risk of developing this malignancy. In contrast to the impact of unopposed estrogens, the past use of oral contraceptives containing a progestin (either high or low potency) has been shown to reduce the risk for the development of endometrial cancer.

Other risk factors include obesity (an increased mass of fatty tissue is associated with greater aromatization of androstenedione to estrone), nulliparity, eating a "Western-type" (i.e., high-fat) diet, the documented presence of endometrial hyperplasia, a history of hereditary nonpolyposis colorectal cancer, and prior or current treatment with tamoxifen (used to treat or prevent breast cancer, leading to a 3- to 7-fold increased risk for this pelvic malignancy). There is also a documented greater risk of endometrial cancer in women with diabetes (3-fold higher) and in those with hypertension (1.5-fold higher), likely due to these conditions' association with obesity. This is the likely explanation for the "classic triad" frequently used to characterize the endometrial cancer patient: overweight, diabetic, and hypertensive.

For as many as 75% of all patients with endometrial cancer (type 1), it is possible to identify a clinical factor suggesting excessive estrogen exposure (e.g., replacement therapy, obesity). The malignancy in these individuals often begins as endometrial hyperplasia, is well differentiated (grade 1) and of low stage, and has a very favorable prognosis.

Conversely, 25% of patients with this cancer (type 2) have no evidence of excessive estrogen exposure. These women frequently have an atrophic endometrium, the malignancies are of higher grade (grade 3 or undifferentiated) and stage, and their overall survival is poorer.

CLINICAL MANIFESTATIONS

Endometrial cancer is seen predominantly in the postmenopausal population, although in some series as many as one quarter of patients were premenopausal. It is uncommon for endometrial cancer to be diagnosed in a woman younger than 40 years.

The most common presenting symptom is postmenopausal bleeding (80 to 90% of cases), which should lead to a formal gynecologic evaluation (with biopsy). In more advanced cases, pelvic pressure or pain may be noted.

Approximately 90 to 95% of all endometrial cancers are adenocarcinomas. Fortunately, most tumors are low grade and stage I (80%) at diagnosis. However, as previously noted, patients with type 2 endometrial cancer are more likely to present with both a higher-grade and higher-stage malignancy.

Endometrial sarcomas (e.g., uterine leiomyosarcomas) are far less common than adenocarcinomas and have a different natural history. Even in the setting of stage I cancer, as many as half of these patients experience subsequent disease progression.

Uterine carcinosarcomas (mixed müllerian tumors) are another uncommon subtype that frequently demonstrates rapid progression. Despite its name, this tumor is currently considered to be a poorly differentiated epithelial malignancy rather than a true sarcoma.

TREATMENT

Surgical resection is the standard initial treatment for the large majority of women with endometrial cancer, and it is generally considered sufficient therapy for patients with early-stage, low-grade disease. The role of routine postoperative adjuvant therapy is controversial. There is evidence that pelvic radiation decreases the risk of local recurrence, but the impact on overall survival is uncertain.

In patients with disease documented in the upper abdomen (stage III), phase III trial data have revealed the superiority of combination chemotherapy compared with whole abdominal radiotherapy.[4] Despite these data, many oncologists favor a multimodality strategy in the management of high-risk endometrial cancer patients (e.g., those with completely surgically resected disease in the upper abdomen or locally advanced grade 3 cancer), which might include several cycles of systemic chemotherapy followed by pelvic radiotherapy (to reduce the chance of relapse in this region). Unfortunately, phase III trial data are not available to definitively prove the benefits of this approach. Vaginal brachytherapy appears to be as good as external beam radiotherapy.5

A number of chemotherapeutic agents have demonstrated biologic activity (objective response rates >20%) in endometrial cancer, including doxorubicin, paclitaxel, cisplatin, and carboplatin. In metastatic disease or in the setting of recurrent cancer, such agents are frequently administered as a combination strategy (e.g., carboplatin plus paclitaxel, cisplatin plus doxorubicin plus paclitaxel), and response rates greater than 50% have been reported. An optimal treatment regimen in this setting has not been defined.6

It is also known that patients with low-grade advanced or metastatic endometrial cancer may exhibit clinically meaningful and prolonged responses to high doses of progestational agents (anticipated 15 to 30% response rate). There is no evidence of an added benefit obtained by combining chemotherapy with hormonal therapy in patients with endometrial cancer, and high-grade tumors rarely (if ever) respond to progestational drugs.

Overall 5-year survival in patients with endometrial cancer varies, based on tumor stage. It ranges from greater than 80% for stage I cancer to approximately 25% for individuals who present with metastatic disease. Other factors that influence survival include patient age, evidence of vascular invasion, hormone receptor status (the presence of which suggests a more indolent clinical course), tumor grade, and histologic subtype (papillary, serous, and clear cell morphology being associated with poorer outcomes).

Management of both endometrial sarcoma and carcinosarcoma includes surgical staging and frequently an attempt at maximal surgical cytoreduction. Owing to the substantial risk of recurrence, adjuvant radiation and/or chemotherapy may be employed, but the utility of such treatment is uncertain. Chemotherapy of metastatic disease may prolong survival and favorably impact cancer-related symptoms.

EPITHELIAL OVARIAN CANCER

Epithelial ovarian cancer is the sixth most common cancer in women in the United States, accounting for approximately one quarter of all female pelvic malignancies. However, far more significant than its incidence is the disturbing fact that the majority of women (>70%) initially present with advanced cancer, and overall survival is inferior to that observed in other female pelvic malignancies.

EPIDEMIOLOGY

In rather striking contrast to cancers of the endometrium and cervix, there is no unifying hypothesis or etiologic factor that defines either the epidemiology or the risk of developing this malignancy. Perhaps the most widely accepted theory is that carcinogenesis is initiated during the normal process of damage and repair associated with a woman's monthly ovulatory cycle. This hypothesis is supported by population-based data revealing a lower incidence of ovarian cancer in women with a history of multiple pregnancies, lactation, extended use of oral contraceptives, and late menarche or early menopause. Each of these clinical features is associated with fewer lifetime ovulatory cycles. Conversely, women with a history of infertility, early menarche, or late menopause have a statistically increased risk of experiencing this malignancy.

Overall, an individual woman has a 1 in 70 lifetime risk for the development of ovarian cancer. The single well-established risk factor for ovarian cancer is a family history of either ovarian or early-onset breast cancer, which appears to account for approximately 5 to 15% of all cases of the malignancy. Existing data reveal that the large majority of women with such a family history have either a *BRCA1* or *BRCA2* mutation, which results in a lifetime ovarian cancer risk of 40 to 50% or 10 to 20%, respectively.

CLINICAL MANIFESTATIONS

The large majority of epithelial ovarian cancers are adenocarcinomas. Until recently, the specific ovarian histologic subtypes were not thought to have major prognostic relevance beyond that identified by tumor grade, but it has become evident that both mucinous and clear cell cancers respond poorly to standard ovarian cancer chemotherapy and have a much worse prognosis (when found in an advanced stage) compared with the more common papillary, serous, or endometrioid types.

Unfortunately, symptoms of ovarian cancer are quite nonspecific (abdominal bloating, discomfort, and pain; loss of appetite; early satiety; fatigue) and in the large majority of cases are an indication of advanced disease. Many women present with abdominal fullness and early satiety due to ascites and omental tumor implants. Ascites is commonly observed in patients with advanced disease. There is no evidence that any particular symptom or symptom complex is more suggestive of ovarian cancer in contrast to other equally (or more) common conditions that may be the cause of the reported complaints.

TREATMENT Rx

Standard treatment of suspected or documented epithelial ovarian cancer includes surgical staging and a reasonably aggressive attempt to resect all macroscopic disease (including disease present in the upper abdomen) before the administration of cytotoxic chemotherapy. Extensive published retrospective experience supports the utility of this basic management approach, with superior outcomes anticipated for women who initiate chemotherapy with small-volume macroscopic or only microscopic cancer.

However, it is relevant to note the complete absence of evidence-based data from randomized, controlled trials documenting the superiority of surgery followed by chemotherapy compared with a primary chemotherapy approach (after histologic confirmation of malignant disease) in the treatment of stage III or IV epithelial ovarian cancer. A recently reported international phase III trial demonstrated equivalent survival and reduced morbidity for individuals managed by primary chemotherapy followed by an attempt at surgical resection compared with "standard" cytoreductive surgery followed by chemotherapy.7 This provides important support for the concept that in certain settings it may be most appropriate for initial treatment to focus on cytotoxic drug delivery.

Ovarian cancer is a highly chemotherapy-sensitive malignancy, with major objective response rates to combination platinum-taxane chemotherapy exceeding 70 to 80%.8 Prolonged disease-free survival (>5 years) is a realistic possibility for a minority of women who present with advanced (stage III and IV) disease. In women with small-volume residual intraperitoneal disease following surgical cytoreduction, direct delivery of cisplatin into the peritoneal cavity has been shown to improve survival in several randomized trials.

Unfortunately, the majority of responding patients ultimately experience a relapse of the malignancy. Although a number of second-line treatment approaches have been shown to favorably impact symptoms of recurrent disease and improve overall survival, there is no evidence that any such approach can cure the malignancy.

There may also be a role for secondary cytoreductive surgery at the time of documented recurrence of ovarian cancer. In general, patients who have experienced relatively long disease-free intervals (>12 months) following completion of the primary treatment program are the best candidates for surgery designed to remove all visible macroscopic cancer before the initiation of second-line chemotherapy.

It is important to note that carefully considered surgical procedures designed to palliate distressing cancer-related symptoms (e.g., colostomy for large bowel obstruction) may be reasonable therapeutic options, even in the setting of progressive cancer. External beam radiation may also play an important role in the palliation of painful masses in the setting of chemotherapy-resistant disease. Despite encouraging early results, the intraperitoneal administration of chemotherapy has not been incorporated into the mainstream management of advanced ovarian cancer.

PREVENTION

Currently, there is no indication that any screening strategy (e.g., tumor markers such as CA-125, radiographic imaging) can detect recurrent9 or "early-stage" ovarian cancer, although several such approaches have been proposed. Although it may be tempting to suggest that women at high risk (those with known genetic abnormalities) for the development of ovarian cancer may benefit from some form of routine screening (biomarker or imaging), it must be emphasized that no valid data support the utility of such an approach.

For women with a strong family history of ovarian cancer, particularly those documented to have a *BRCA1* or *BRCA2* genetic abnormality, available data support the conclusion that bilateral oophorectomies can reduce the risk of developing the malignancy by more than 80%. However, the actual extent of the absolute reduction in lifetime risk remains uncertain, because most series have followed individuals for less than 10 years following this cancer prevention surgery. For an individual woman with the appropriate genetic background who is considering undergoing such surgery, it is important to consider the negative aspects of this approach, including infertility, potentially distressing symptoms of early menopause, and the risk of accelerated bone loss.

NONEPITHELIAL OVARIAN MALIGNANCIES

Germ Cell Tumors of the Ovary

Ovarian germ cell cancers are uncommon malignancies observed in adolescent girls and young women. Like their male germ cell counterparts (Chapter 206), these malignances are extremely chemosensitive and have a high cure rate, even if discovered at an advanced stage. Both the diagnosis and the treatment of ovarian germ cell tumors are aided by the presence of two sensitive serum markers (human gonadotropin and α-fetoprotein).

Standard management of ovarian germ cell tumors includes surgical staging and an attempt to remove all gross macroscopic cancer (in the presence of metastatic spread). The majority of ovarian germ cell tumors are unilateral at presentation, permitting the performance of a salpingo-oophorectomy on the involved side and potentially preserving fertility in this young patient population.

Early-stage dysgerminomas can be managed with observation following surgical staging; less than 25% of such patients will experience a relapse. For more advanced disease, chemotherapy is indicated. However, the large majority of nondysgerminous germ cell tumors require chemotherapy because of the high recurrence rate (80% in stage I disease).

Stromal Ovarian Tumors

Granulosa cell and Sertoli-Leydig tumors are uncommon ovarian tumors characterized by being generally localized at presentation and exhibiting long natural histories, even when metastatic spread is documented. In contrast to epithelial ovarian cancer and germ cell tumors, this group of malignancies exhibits modest responsiveness to cytotoxic chemotherapy, which is usually employed only when disease progression has been documented.

VULVAR CANCER

Primary vulvar cancers account for less than 5% of cancers involving the female reproductive tract. As with cervical cancer, HPV has been strongly implicated in the pathogenesis of this malignancy (HPV DNA documented in 70 to 80% of cases).

The majority of patients are symptomatic at presentation (pain, local irritation, pruritus), and these complaints have commonly (>80% of cases) been present for more than 6 months before diagnosis. Most vulvar cancers are of squamous cell histology (Fig. 205-2), but malignant melanoma is also observed in this region.

Standard treatment is surgical excision of the primary tumor and dissection of inguinal lymph nodes. The risk of tumor recurrence is related to the size and extent of tumor involvement, the ability of the surgeon to achieve adequate surgical margins, and the documented presence of metastatic cancer in the inguinal nodes. With advanced local disease, concurrent external beam radiation and chemotherapy are generally employed. There is little evidence for the effectiveness of cytotoxic antineoplastic drugs in the setting of metastatic vulvar cancer.

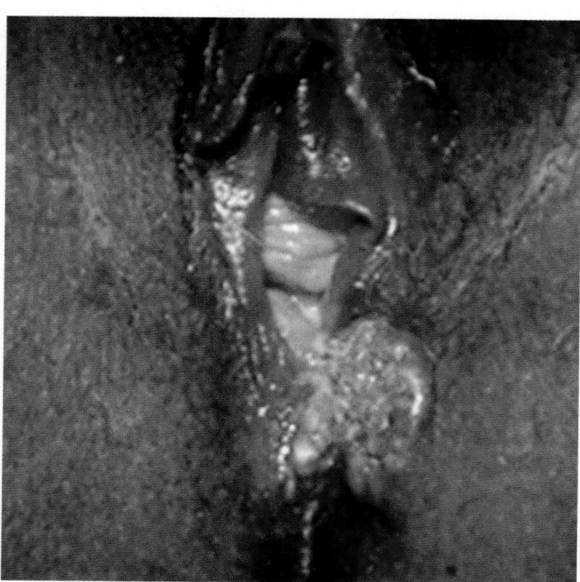

FIGURE 205-2. **Vulvar cancer.** Invasive squamous cell carcinoma of the vulva.

VAGINAL CANCER

Vaginal cancers are uncommon malignancies associated with prior persistent HPV infection, and they are generally seen in an elderly population (older than 60 years). The large majority of primary cancers in this region are of squamous cell histology (80 to 90% of cases). Melanomas and sarcomas can also originate at this site.

Women who have undergone successful treatment for cervical cancer have an increased risk for the development of vaginal cancer. Although mainly of historical interest, there is a well-recognized association between in utero exposure to diethylstilbestrol and the development of very rare clear cell vaginal cancer.

The major presenting symptom is vaginal bleeding. Dysuria and vaginal discharge are also noted. In patients with advanced disease, pelvic pain is frequently described.

Depending on the clinical circumstances, standard treatment of vaginal cancers may focus on either radiation or surgical resection. Combined chemo-radiation therapy may be employed in locally advanced disease, but the overall experience with this strategy is limited. In a patient whose performance status is adequate, systemic chemotherapy may provide a modest level of benefit in recurrent or metastatic disease.

UTERINE FIBROIDS

Though not a malignancy, it is appropriate to discuss the management of uterine fibroids in this chapter because this condition is the most common female pelvic tumor (70 to 80% incidence in the female population by age 50). During the reproductive years, the incidence of fibroids may be as high as 40%.

The majority of fibroids are asymptomatic. When present, symptoms can range from mild inconvenience to heavy bleeding and pelvic pressure and pain.

In the past, the most common treatment was surgical removal of the fibroid or of the uterus itself. This procedure can be performed during laparotomy or through less invasive laparoscopic surgery. Over the years, a variety of invasive strategies have been introduced into routine medical practice for the treatment of symptomatic uterine fibroids, including uterine artery embolization, transvaginal temporary uterine artery occlusion, and MRI-guided focused ultrasound.

Noninterventional, hormonally based approaches (e.g., antiprogestins such as mifepristone) have been examined in the management of uterine fibroids. Although they are effective in relieving symptoms, these strategies are potentially limited by long-term drug-related side effects. However, these agents are clinically helpful in reducing the size of fibroids, decreasing dysfunctional uterine bleeding and pain, and improving overall quality of life.

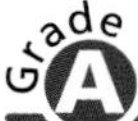

1. Monk BJ, Sill MW, McMeekin DS, et al. Phase III trial of four cisplatin-containing doublet combinations in stage IVB, recurrent, or persistent cervical carcinoma: a Gynecologic Oncology Group study. *J Clin Oncol.* 2009;27:4649-4655.
2. Muñoz N, Manalastas R Jr, Pitisuttithum P, et al. Safety, immunogenicity, and efficacy of quadrivalent human papillomavirus (types 6, 11, 16, 18) recombinant vaccine in women aged 24-45 years: a randomised, double-blind trial. *Lancet.* 2009;373:1949-1957.
3. Paavonen J, Naud P, Salmeron J, et al. Efficacy of human papillomavirus (HPV)-16/18 AS04-adjuvanted vaccine against cervical infection and precancer caused by oncogenic HPV types (PATRICIA): final analysis of a double-blind, randomised study in young women. *Lancet.* 2009;374:301-314.
4. Randall ME, Filiaci VL, Muss H, et al. Randomized phase III trial of whole-abdominal irradiation versus doxorubicin and cisplatin chemotherapy in advanced endometrial carcinoma: a Gynecologic Oncology Group study. *J Clin Oncol.* 2006;24:36-44.
5. Nout RA, Smit VT, Putter H, et al. Vaginal brachytherapy versus pelvic external beam radiotherapy for patients with endometrial cancer of high-intermediate risk (PORTEC-2): an open-label, non-inferiority, randomised trial. *Lancet.* 2010;375:816-823.
6. Humber CE, Tierney JF, Symonds RP, et al. Chemotherapy for advanced, recurrent or metastatic endometrial cancer: a systematic review of Cochrane collaboration. *Ann Oncol.* 2007;18:409-420.
7. Bookman MA, Brady MF, McGuire WP, et al. Evaluation of new platinum-based treatment regimens in advanced-stage ovarian cancer: a Phase III trial of the Gynecologic Cancer Intergroup. *J Clin Oncol.* 2009;27:1419-1425.
8. Vergote I, Tropé CG, Amant F, et al. Neoadjuvant chemotherapy or primary surgery in stage IIIC or IV ovarian cancer. *N Engl J Med.* 2010;363:943-953.
9. Rustin GJ, van der Burg ME, Griffin CL, et al. Early versus delayed treatment of relapsed ovarian cancer (MRC OV05/EORTC 55955): a randomised trial. *Lancet.* 2010;376:1155-1163.

SUGGESTED READINGS

Amant F, Coosemans A, Debiec-Rychter M, et al. Clinical management of uterine sarcomas. *Lancet Oncol.* 2009;10:1188-1198. *A comprehensive review of the management of uterine sarcomas.*

Cragun JM. Screening for ovarian cancer. *Cancer Control.* 2011;18:16-21. *Review concluding that neither CA-125 nor ultrasound has adequate sensitivity or specificity for routine screening.*

Hennessy BT, Coleman RL, Markman M. Ovarian cancer. *Lancet.* 2009;374:1371-1382. *A comprehensive review of the management of ovarian cancer.*

Ramirez I, Chon HS, Apte SM. The role of surgery in the management of epithelial ovarian cancer. *Cancer Control.* 2011;18:22-30. *Review emphasizing that optimal cytoreductive surgery positively impacts survival.*

Wiegand KC, Shah SP, Al-Agha OM, et al. ARID1A mutations in endometriosis-associated ovarian carcinomas. *N Engl J Med.* 2010;363:1532-1543. *ARID1A mutations may predispose to the transformation of endometriosis into cancer.*

Winter-Roach B, Kitchener H, Dickinson H. Adjuvant (post-surgery) chemotherapy for early stage epithelial ovarian cancer. Cochrane Database Syst Rev. 2009;3:CD004706. *Meta-analysis revealing the impact of chemotherapy on high-risk early-stage ovarian cancer.*

206 TESTICULAR CANCER

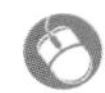

LAWRENCE H. EINHORN

EPIDEMIOLOGY

Testicular tumors are relatively uncommon and account for only 1% of male malignancies in the United States. The highest worldwide incidence occurs in Scandinavian countries; by contrast, testicular cancer is rare in African Americans and Asian Americans. The primary age group is 15 to 35 years for nonseminomatous tumors and a decade older for seminomas.

Male patients with a history of cryptorchidism have a 10- to 40-fold increased risk for the development of testicular cancer. The normally descended testis in these men is also at higher risk, suggesting a dysgenetic abnormality.

PATHOBIOLOGY

More than 95% of tumors of the testis originate from germ cells. Germ cell tumors can be seminomas or nonseminomatous germ cell tumors. Seminomas are more likely to be confined to the testis (stage I) and are exquisitely sensitive to radiation therapy. Pure seminomas never have elevated serum α-fetoprotein (AFP) levels. Nonseminomatous germ cell tumors consist of embryonal cell carcinomas, choriocarcinomas, yolk sac tumors, or teratomas, alone or mixed with other elements. Teratomas do not secrete human chorionic gonadotropin (HCG) or AFP and do not usually metastasize; they grow by local extension and are completely resistant to radiation therapy and chemotherapy.

Most germ cell testicular cancers in adults are associated with the cytogenetic abnormality i12p—an isochromosome of the short arm of chromosome 12—which is a highly specific finding in germ cell tumors. Sertoli cell tumors, Leydig cell tumors, and lymphomas are the most common non–germ cell tumors. In men older than 60 years, most tumors are non-Hodgkin's lymphoma (Chapter 191), with a predilection for bilateral involvement.

CLINICAL MANIFESTATIONS

Most patients with testicular cancer are initially evaluated because of testicular pain or because of a mass in or enlargement of one testis. Others are asymptomatic, and the cancer is first detected during a routine physical examination. Less commonly, the diagnosis is made during an evaluation for infertility, in part because testicular cancer can cause oligospermia.

Metastatic spread is either lymphatic or hematogenous. Lymphatic metastases usually go initially to the ipsilateral retroperitoneal lymph nodes, where they may be associated with flank pain. Lymphatic metastases may continue in a superior direction to the posterior mediastinum and eventually to the left supraclavicular lymph nodes. A large retroperitoneal mass or a supraclavicular lymph node may be palpable on physical examination. Hematogenous spread usually occurs first to the pulmonary parenchyma bilaterally. Pulmonary symptoms such as chest pain, shortness of breath, dyspnea on exertion, coughing, or hemoptysis are seen only with extensive pulmonary metastases. Other sites of hematogenous spread include the liver, bone, or brain. Significant elevation of the serum HCG level may produce gynecomastia.

DIAGNOSIS

Patients with a palpable mass in the testis should be suspected of having testicular cancer, especially if there is a history of cryptorchidism. Other causes of testicular and scrotal abnormalities may be included in the differential diagnosis. Acute pain in the testis suggests torsion. Painful enlargement may be due to a hydrocele, which may be caused by an underlying primary testicular malignancy. Pain and tenderness adjacent to the testis may be due to epididymitis or a varicocele. Tenderness of the testis itself on physical examination may reflect orchitis. However, an underlying neoplasm should always be considered.

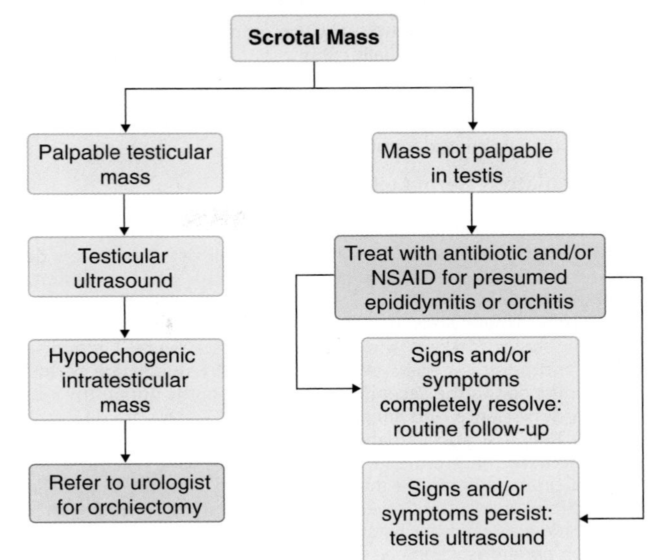

FIGURE 206-1. Management of a scrotal mass. NSAID = nonsteroidal anti-inflammatory drug.

Any testicular symptoms, including pain or a suspected mass, require evaluation. Testicular ultrasound is the test of choice in all suspicious cases. A hypoechogenic mass within the testis must be presumed to be testicular cancer and requires referral to a urologist (Fig. 206-1).

When orchiectomy reveals the diagnosis of testicular cancer, a staging evaluation is performed to determine the extent of disease and appropriate therapy. Clinical stage I disease is confined to the testis; stage II disease reflects spread to the retroperitoneal lymph nodes; and stage III is supradiaphragmatic disease, with either nodal metastases to the posterior mediastinum or supraclavicular region or hematogenous spread, especially to the lungs.

In addition to a full history and physical examination, serum HCG and AFP levels should be determined. Because the serum half-life is 1 day for HCG and 5 days for AFP, an AFP level of 1000 may take more than a month to normalize after orchiectomy, even if the tumor has been completely removed. Imaging studies to define the extent of disease include abdominal and pelvic computed tomography (CT) and a chest radiograph. If the chest radiograph does not show pulmonary metastases, a chest CT scan should be performed. Bone scans and head CT scans can be reserved for patients with symptoms suggestive of osseous and central nervous system metastases, respectively.

PREVENTION AND TREATMENT Rx

A careful testicular examination is a mandatory part of the physical examination in men, especially young men (Chapter 14), and is the key means of detecting tumors at an early stage. With the patient lying supine or standing up, the testis is gently palpated with the thumb and second and third fingers; the entire anterior, posterior, and lateral surfaces of the testis should be examined.

Local and Regional Disease

Seminomas

About 70% of seminomas are initially diagnosed at clinical stage I. Although the cure rate with orchiectomy alone is 80 to 95%, treatment can also include 2000 cGy para-aortic irradiation [1] or adjuvant carboplatin. [2]

Twenty percent of patients with seminoma are initially found to have stage II disease (positive abdominal CT scan). For these patients, radiation therapy has a 90% cure rate; in patients who are not cured by radiation therapy, subsequent combination chemotherapy (cisplatin combined with etoposide, with or without bleomycin) is usually curative. If the transverse diameter of the tumor is greater than 3 cm, if there are multiple anatomic levels of nodal metastases, or if stage III disease is present, the preferred initial treatment is cisplatin combination chemotherapy without irradiation; the cure rate is 70 to 100%, depending on the extent of the disease.

Nonseminomatous Germ Cell Tumors

Management of clinical stage I nonseminomatous germ cell tumors begins with orchiectomy, which has a 70% cure rate. This is followed by either retroperitoneal lymph node dissection or close surveillance (which can detect metastases early and guide curative chemotherapy), with or without one course of bleomycin, etoposide, and cisplatin. Most relapses occur in the first year, during which meticulous surveillance should include history and physical examination, serum markers, and chest radiograph every 2 months and abdominal and pelvic CT scans every 4 months. All studies are performed every 4 months during the second year, every 6 months during the third to fifth years of surveillance, and annually thereafter. CT scans are discontinued after 5 years. The physical examination should include palpation of the remaining testis, because these patients have a 1 to 2% chance of developing a contralateral primary tumor. The major complication of retroperitoneal lymph node dissection is inadvertent severing of the sympathetic plexus, with resultant retrograde ejaculation or failure of ejaculation. Nerve-sparing retroperitoneal lymph node dissection can retain antegrade ejaculation in more than 95% of patients. Some centers advocate primary chemotherapy for high-risk clinical stage I disease (embryonal predominant or vascular or lymphatic invasion) with cisplatin combination chemotherapy.[3] However, surveillance is still an option in this patient population.

For clinical stage II disease with persistently elevated serum markers or a transverse tumor diameter greater than 3 cm, chemotherapy is preferred. Other stage II patients are treated with retroperitoneal lymph node dissection, often followed by close surveillance (as described earlier, but without abdominal CT scans) or adjuvant chemotherapy. Testicular cancer has a higher cure rate with surgery alone, despite nodal metastases, than any other cancer.

Chemotherapy for Disseminated or Persistent Disease

The combination of bleomycin, etoposide, and cisplatin repeated every 3 weeks for three to four courses cures 70% of patients with metastatic disease and is the standard chemotherapy for disseminated testicular cancer. Poor-risk disease (Table 206-1) has a 50 to 60% cure rate with standard three-drug therapy, intermediate-risk disease (HCG 5000 to 50,000 IU/mL or AFP 1000 to 10,000 ng/mL) has a 70% cure rate, and all other forms of metastatic disease (good risk) have a 90 to 100% cure rate.

In the 30% of metastatic germ cell tumors that are not cured by initial combination chemotherapy, the use of standard-dose salvage therapy (ifosfamide, cisplatin, and either vinblastine or paclitaxel) or high-dose carboplatin and etoposide therapy, followed by peripheral blood stem cell transplantation, can cure 25 to 70% of refractory cases, depending on patient characteristics.

TABLE 206-1 DEFINITION OF POOR-RISK DISEASE (ALL NONSEMINOMATOUS TESTICULAR CANCER PATIENTS)

Presence of any of the following:
Lactate dehydrogenase >10 times the upper limit of normal, human chorionic gonadotropin >50,000 IU/mL, or α-fetoprotein >10,000 ng/mL
Any primary mediastinal nonseminomatous germ cell tumor
Nonpulmonary visceral metastases (e.g., bone, liver, brain)

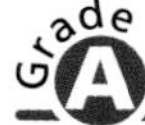

1. Jones WG, Fossa SD, Mead GM, et al. Randomized trial of 30 versus 20 Gy in the adjuvant treatment of stage I testicular seminoma. *J Clin Oncol.* 2005;23:1200-1208.
2. Oliver RTD, Mason MD, Mead GM, et al. Radiotherapy versus single-dose carboplatin in adjuvant treatment of stage I seminoma: a randomised trial. *Lancet.* 2005;366:293-300.
3. Alberts P, Siener R, Krege S, et al. Randomized phase III trial comparing retroperitoneal lymph node dissection with one course of bleomycin and etoposide plus cisplatin in the adjuvant treatment of clinical stage I non-seminomatous germ cell tumors. *J Clin Oncol.* 2008;26:2966-2972.

SUGGESTED READINGS

Fosså SD, Cvancarova M, Chen L, et al. Adverse prognostic factors for testicular cancer-specific survival: a population-based study of 27,948 patients. *J Clin Oncol.* 2011;29:963-970. *Age over 40 (RR = 2), non-seminomic histology (RR = 2), and metastatic disease (RR = 9) were predictive, but survival has improved significantly in the past 25 years.*

Hotte SJ, Mayhew LA, Jewett M, et al. Management of stage I non-seminomatous testicular cancer: a systematic review and meta-analysis. *Clin Oncol (R Coll Radiol).* 2010;22:17-26. *Review.*

Ilic D, Misso ML. Screening for testicular cancer. *Cochrane Database Syst Rev.* 2011;2:CD007853. *Review emphasizing importance of family history, undescended testis, and testicular atrophy.*

Nakamura T, Miki T. Recent strategy for the management of advanced testicular cancer. *Int J Urol.* 2010;17:148-157. *Comprehensive overview.*

U.S. Preventive Services Task Force. Screening for testicular cancer: U.S. Preventive Services Task Force reaffirmation recommendation statement. *Ann Intern Med.* 2011;154:483-486. *Guidelines recommending against routine screening.*

Winter C, Albers P. Testicular germ cell tumors: pathogenesis, diagnosis and treatment. *Nat Rev Endocrinol.* 2011;7:43-53. *Review.*

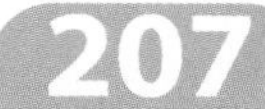

PROSTATE CANCER

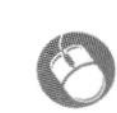

ERIC J. SMALL

DEFINITION

Prostate cancer is the most common noncutaneous malignant neoplasm in men in the United States, where it results in about 32,000 deaths each year, making it the second most common cause of cancer death in men. Prostate cancer is a single histologic disease with marked clinical heterogeneity ranging from indolent, clinically irrelevant disease to a virulent, rapidly lethal phenotype.

EPIDEMIOLOGY

The incidence of clinically diagnosed prostate cancer reflects the effects of screening by the prostate-specific antigen (PSA) assay. Before PSA testing was available, about 19,000 new cases of prostate cancer were reported each year in the United States; this number reached 84,000 by 1993 and peaked at about 300,000 new cases in 1996. Since 1996, the reported annual incidence of prostate cancer in the United States has declined to about 190,000, a number that may more closely estimate the true incidence of clinically detectable disease. The death rate due to prostate cancer has declined by about 1% per year since 1990. The age-specific decrease in mortality has been greatest in men younger than 75 years. Men older than 75 years still account for two thirds of all prostate cancer deaths. Whether this decline is due to early detection (screening) or to improved therapy has not been proved.

Risk factors for prostate cancer include increasing age, family history, African American race, and dietary factors. Epidemiologic studies have suggested that nutritional factors such as reduced fat intake and increased soy protein may have a protective effect against the development of prostate cancer. The incidence of prostate cancer among African Americans is nearly twice that observed among white Americans. Prostate cancer is diagnosed in African Americans at a more advanced stage, and disease-specific survival is lower in African Americans. The relative contributions of biologic, genetic, and environmental differences, as well as differences in health care access, are not well established. Prior vasectomy and benign prostatic hypertrophy (Chapter 131) do not increase the risk. Prostatic intraepithelial neoplasia, particularly when it is high grade, is recognized as a premalignant lesion, so its presence on biopsy increases the likelihood of subsequent malignancy.

PATHOBIOLOGY

Prostate cancer appears to be common among relatives of men with early-onset prostate cancer. At the molecular level, there appears to be a susceptibility locus for the development of prostate cancer at an early age on chromosome 1, band q24; however, an abnormality at this locus occurs in less than 10% of patients with prostate cancer. Although many genetic abnormalities with both loss and gain of function have been identified, consistent patterns of changes associated with an increased likelihood for the development of prostate cancer have not been identified. Approximately half of prostate cancers demonstrate genetic rearrangements, with fusion of promoters or enhancers of androgen-responsive genes such as *TMPRSS2* (transmembrane protease, serine 2) with oncogenic *ETS* (*E-twenty six*) transcription factors such as *ERG* (*ETS-related gene*). These fusions lead to overexpression of oncogenic transcription factors and appear to define a subset of tumors with more aggressive behavior.

Testosterone is required for maintenance of a normal, healthy prostatic epithelium, but it is also a prerequisite for the development of prostate cancer.

Prostate cancers express robust levels of androgen receptor, and signaling through the androgen receptor results in growth, progression, and invasion of prostate cancer. Inhibition of signaling, typically by the surgical or pharmacologic reduction of testosterone levels, results in prostate cancer apoptosis and involution. Ultimately, however, androgen-deprivation therapy loses clinical efficacy. The biologic events surrounding the clinical development of "androgen deprivation–resistant prostate cancer" are not well delineated, but amplification of the androgen receptor, which is a common event in these patients, presumably makes the cancer sensitive to minute levels of androgen or other ligands of the androgen receptor. The identification of androgen receptor splice variants that are constitutively active and ligand independent raises this as a potential mechanism by which true hormone resistance develops.

CLINICAL MANIFESTATIONS

Most patients with early-stage, organ-confined disease are asymptomatic. Obstructive voiding symptoms (hesitancy, intermittent urinary stream, decreased force of stream) generally reflect locally advanced disease with growth into the urethra or bladder neck, although these symptoms can be indistinguishable from benign prostatic hypertrophy (Chapter 131). Locally advanced tumors can also result in hematuria and hematospermia. Prostate cancer that has spread to the regional pelvic lymph nodes occasionally causes edema of the lower extremities or discomfort in the pelvic and perineal areas. Metastasis occurs most commonly to bone, where it is frequently asymptomatic, but it can also cause severe and unremitting pain. Bone metastasis can result in pathologic fractures or spinal cord compression. Although visceral metastases are rare as presenting features of prostate cancer, patients can have pulmonary, hepatic, pleural, peritoneal, and central nervous system metastases late in the natural history or after androgen-deprivation therapy fails.

DIAGNOSIS

More than 60% of patients with prostate cancer are asymptomatic, and the diagnosis is made solely because of an elevated screening PSA level. A palpable nodule on digital rectal examination, which is the next most common clinical presentation, generally prompts biopsy. Much less commonly, prostate cancer is diagnosed because of advanced disease that causes obstructive voiding symptoms, pelvic or perineal discomfort, lower extremity edema, or symptomatic bone lesions.

Although the digital rectal examination has a low sensitivity and specificity for the diagnosis of prostate cancer, biopsy of a nodule or area of induration reveals cancer 50% of the time, suggesting that prostate biopsy should be undertaken in all men with palpable nodules. The PSA level has a far better sensitivity but a low specificity because conditions such as benign prostatic hypertrophy and prostatitis can cause false-positive PSA elevations (Chapter 131). By use of a PSA threshold of 4 ng/mL, 70 to 80% of tumors are detected. Far greater accuracy is achieved with age-specific PSA thresholds. Thus, for men aged 40 to 49, a PSA greater than 2.5 is considered abnormal; for men 50 to 59, a PSA greater than 3.5 is abnormal; for men 60 to 69, a PSA greater than 4.5 should prompt further evaluation; and patients aged 70 to 79 should have a PSA of 6.5 or less. The positive predictive value for a single PSA level above 10 ng/mL is greater than 60% for cancer, but the positive predictive value for a PSA level between 4 and 10 ng/mL is only about 30%. Assays of the PSA fraction that circulates unbound (percentage of free PSA) may help distinguish prostate cancer from benign processes; in patients with PSA levels of 4 to 10 ng/mL, the percentage of free PSA appears to be an independent predictor of prostate cancer, and a cutoff value of free PSA less than 25% can detect 95% of cancers while avoiding 20% of unnecessary biopsies.

Transrectal ultrasonography with biopsies is indicated when the PSA level is elevated, when the percentage of free PSA is less than 25%, or when an abnormality is noted on digital rectal examination. Extended field specimens (preferably up to six biopsies on each side) are generally obtained. Seminal vesicles are sampled in high-risk patients. A bone scan is warranted only in patients with PSA levels above 10 ng/mL, and abdominal and pelvic computed tomography or magnetic resonance imaging is usually unrevealing in patients with a PSA level below 10 to 20 ng/mL.

The prognosis of prostate cancer correlates with histologic grade and extent (stage) of disease. More than 95% of prostate cancers are adenocarcinomas, and multifocality is common. The histologic (Gleason) grade ranges from 1 to 5, although in the modern era, Gleason grades of 1 and 2 are exceedingly rare; the Gleason score, which refers to the sum of the two most common histologic patterns seen on each tissue specimen, ranges from 4 (2+2) to 10 (5+5). In general, tumors are classified as well differentiated (Gleason score 2 to 6), of intermediate differentiation (Gleason score 7), or poorly differentiated (Gleason score 8 to 10).

Clinical stage is defined by the extent of disease based on the physical examination, imaging studies, and pathology. Stage T1 is nonpalpable prostate cancer detected only on pathologic examination, noted either incidentally after transurethral resection for benign hypertrophy (T1a and T1b) or on a biopsy specimen obtained because of an elevated PSA level (T1c, the most common clinical stage at diagnosis). Stage T2 is a palpable tumor that appears to be confined to the prostate gland (T2a in one lobe, T2b in two lobes), and stage T3 is tumor with extension through the prostatic capsule (T3a if it is focal, T3b if seminal vesicles are involved). T4 tumors are those with invasion of adjacent structures, such as the bladder neck, external urinary sphincter, rectum, levator muscles, or pelvic sidewall. Nodal metastases can be microscopic and detectable only by biopsy or lymphadenectomy, or they can be visible on imaging studies. Distant metastases are predominantly to bone, but occasional visceral metastases occur.

PREVENTION

The precise role for screening remains controversial. Currently, many organizations recommend screening with PSA, but the U.S. Preventive Services Task Force recommends against screening for men older than 70 years, and it is neither for nor against screening in younger men. Of two large randomized screening trials using PSA levels, one reported a reduction in prostate-cancer–specific mortality,[1] but neither found an overall reduction in mortality.[1,2] At best, an estimated 1410 men would need to be screened to prevent one prostate cancer death over a 10-year period. Randomized trials have shown that vitamins E and C and selenium are not effective at preventing prostate cancer. The use of 5a-reductase inhibitors (both finasteride and dutasteride) reduces the risk for development of prostate cancer.[3,4] However, this approach has not been widely adopted.

TREATMENT

Rx

Localized Prostate Cancer

Principles of Therapy

The principal therapeutic options for men with localized prostate cancer include the following: active surveillance; androgen deprivation; retropubic or perineal radical prostatectomy, with or without postoperative radiation therapy to the prostate margins and pelvis; external beam radiation therapy; and brachytherapy (either permanent or temporary radioactive seed implants), with or without external beam radiation therapy to the prostate margins and pelvis.

Treatment options require individualization, taking into account the patient's comorbidity, life expectancy, likelihood of cure, and personal preferences based on an understanding of the potential morbidity associated with each treatment. A multidisciplinary approach to integrate surgery, radiation therapy, and androgen deprivation is increasingly recommended. For higher-risk patients with a greater likelihood of nodal micrometastases, androgen deprivation is often combined with radiation therapy encompassing both the prostate and the pelvis. In patients at extremely high risk of micrometastatic disease or with comorbidities, systemic therapy alone without concurrent local therapy may be appropriate.

PSA screening has led to the early detection of a large number of nonpalpable tumors, for which conventional clinical means of staging are inadequate. Thus, less emphasis is being placed on clinical stage and more emphasis is being placed on PSA values and other predictors of outcome. Careful risk assessment is required to identify patients who are appropriate candidates for definitive local treatment.

Several studies have confirmed that serum PSA level, clinical stage, and biopsy Gleason score can be used to predict the final pathologic stage after prostatectomy, and that these are independent predictors of survival without PSA elevation after external beam radiation therapy or radical prostatectomy. For example, in a radiation therapy series, clinical stage T3 or higher, PSA level above 10 ng/mL, and biopsy Gleason score of 7 or higher were risk factors for poor outcome (death or PSA elevation); 5-year survival without PSA elevation was 85% for patients with none of these adverse features (good risk), 65% for patients with one adverse feature (intermediate risk), and 35% for patients with two or three adverse features (poor risk). Similar statistics are cited in radical prostatectomy series. The percentage of biopsy specimens that are positive and the rate of increase in the PSA value are each independent predictors of outcome after radical prostatectomy and can be used to counsel patients about their therapeutic options. A number of multivariable prognostic models have been developed and validated and have been used to develop simple nomograms or online risk calculators.

Low- to Intermediate-Risk Disease

In a randomized trial of patients younger than 75 years with clinical stage T1b, T1c, or T2 prostate cancer, radical prostatectomy compared with no therapy significantly reduced the relative risk of death due to prostate cancer by 50% (a 2% absolute risk reduction) and overall mortality by a similar absolute amount at 8.6 years.[5] Reductions in progressive disease and metastases were also significant. The adverse effects on quality of life differed between the two strategies—more sexual dysfunction and urinary leakage after radical prostatectomy, more urinary obstruction with active surveillance—but were of similar magnitude.[6] Nerve-sparing radical prostatectomy was not routinely performed in this study, and many patients already had palpable disease, so the implications for less advanced disease with newer surgical techniques are not known. Nonrandomized data suggest that active surveillance may be judiciously used in patients with low disease volume, Gleason score of 6 or lower, and slow PSA doubling times. Active surveillance is probably not appropriate for young, otherwise healthy men with high-risk features as described earlier (PSA >10 ng/mL, Gleason score of 7 or higher, clinical stage T3 or higher). Whether active surveillance is appropriate for men with intermediate-risk, nonpalpable tumors remains debated. Androgen deprivation has not been carefully studied as primary therapy for localized disease, but it is becoming a more common approach in men who wish to receive some therapy but are not suited for or decline to undergo prostatectomy or radiation therapy.

Men with T1 or T2 prostate cancer who otherwise have a life expectancy of more than 10 years and no significant comorbid illnesses usually should have definitive local therapy with either surgery or radiation therapy. Long-term survival is excellent. Men with T1 or T2 tumors with Gleason scores of 7 or less have 8-year survival rates of 85 to 95%. Patients with T1 or T2 tumors with Gleason scores of 8 to 10 have 8-year survival rates of about 70%.

Nerve-sparing procedures and careful dissection techniques have decreased the risk of postoperative urinary incontinence and impotence. Postoperative urinary incontinence is reported to occur in less than 10% of cases. Postoperative impotence is dependent on a variety of factors, including the patient's age, preoperative erectile function, extent of cancer, and whether a nerve-sparing procedure was performed. In general, impotence rates of 10 to 50% are cited. Robotic-assisted laparoscopic prostatectomies have gained popularity but have not been shown to result in better outcomes. After a radical prostatectomy, the PSA should become undetectable; a detectable PSA implies the presence of cancer cells, either locally or at a metastatic site. Immediate (adjuvant) postoperative radiation therapy improves biochemical progression-free survival and local control in patients with one or more pathologic risk factors (capsule penetration, positive surgical margins, invasion of a seminal vesicle) after radical prostatectomy.[6]

Conventional external beam radiation therapy is being replaced by three-dimensional conformal radiation therapy or intensity-modulated radiation therapy, which permits higher doses to the target tissue with less toxicity. Randomized trials suggest a benefit with higher doses of radiation. Brachytherapy, which is the placement of permanent or temporary radioactive seeds directly into the prostate, is adequate for intracapsular disease with no more than minimal transcapsular extension; otherwise, it should be combined with external beam radiation therapy.

High-Risk Disease

Patients with adverse risk features (Gleason score 8 to 10, PSA >10, stage T3) are at high risk of nodal and micrometastatic disease and are generally treated with aggressive local therapy in combination with androgen deprivation, which is synergistic with radiation therapy.[7] Taken in the aggregate, trials suggest that 4 months of androgen deprivation with radiation therapy can improve local control and prolong progression-free survival in patients with intermediate-risk features, whereas long-term androgen deprivation (up to 3 years) prolongs local control, progression-free survival, and overall survival in patients with high-risk features compared with radiation therapy alone.[8,9] Patients with stage T3 disease and Gleason scores of 7 have intermediate outcomes, with 8-year survival rates of about 70%; patients with stage T3 disease and Gleason scores of 8 to 10 have 8-year survival rates, after radiation therapy, of about 50%. Several randomized controlled trials suggest that patients with high-risk disease who are treated surgically and have capsule penetration, positive margins, or seminal vesicle involvement should receive immediate adjuvant radiation therapy.

Recurrent Disease

Between 30 and 50% of men treated with radiation therapy or prostatectomy have evidence of disease recurrence, as defined by a climbing PSA level. PSA doubling time is predictive of survival, and a short PSA doubling time (<3 to 6 months) is associated with a higher likelihood of systemic disease. For selected patients with clear local recurrences, low PSA levels, and prolonged PSA doubling times (generally), local salvage therapy (surgery for patients previously treated with radiation therapy, radiation therapy for patients previously treated with surgery,[10] and androgen deprivation) can be considered. Although androgen-deprivation therapy readily controls PSA levels, it is unknown whether it prolongs life in patients with PSA-only recurrent disease.

Advanced Disease

In patients whose radical prostatectomy surgery reveals microscopic involvement of lymph nodes, immediate androgen deprivation prolongs survival compared with deferment of androgen deprivation until osseous metastases are detected. Similarly, patients who are at high risk of nodal invasion and who undergo external beam radiation benefit from concurrent short-term hormonal therapy.[9]

In patients with newly diagnosed metastatic prostate cancer, androgen deprivation is the mainstay of treatment and results in symptomatic improvement and disease regression in approximately 80 to 90% of patients. Androgen deprivation can be achieved by orchiectomy or by medical castration with a luteinizing hormone–releasing hormone (LHRH) agonist (leuprolide acetate, goserelin acetate).

Some LHRH agonists cause a transient worsening of signs and symptoms during the first week of therapy as a result of a surge in luteinizing hormone and testosterone, which peaks within 72 hours; an antiandrogen (flutamide, bicalutamide, or nilutamide) should be given with the first LHRH injection to prevent a tumor flare. Medical castration occurs within 4 weeks. The duration of hormone sensitivity is 5 to 10 years for node-positive or high-risk localized (or recurrent) prostate cancer, but it is closer to 24 months in patients with overt metastatic disease. The most common side effects of androgen ablation are loss of libido, impotence, hot flashes, weight gain, fatigue, anemia, and osteoporosis. Bisphosphonates reduce bone mineral loss associated with androgen deprivation.

Castration-Resistant Prostate Cancer

Typically, the first manifestation of resistance to androgen deprivation is a climbing PSA level in the setting of anorchid levels of testosterone. In about 15% of patients, discontinuation of antiandrogen therapy (flutamide, bicalutamide, nilutamide) while continuing treatment with LHRH agonists results in a PSA decline that can be associated with symptomatic improvement and can persist for 4 months or more. If antiandrogen withdrawal fails, treatment with secondary hormonal manipulations, such as ketoconazole or estrogens, is appropriate. Sipuleucel-T is an autologous dendritic cell product that has been shown to prolong life[11] and is appropriate for patients with castration-resistant metastatic prostate cancer who do not have cancer-associated pain, visceral metastases, rapidly progressive disease, or the need for systemic steroids. Thereafter, treatment with chemotherapeutic regimens, such as docetaxel plus corticosteroids or mitoxantrone plus corticosteroids, may be effective. Randomized phase III trials have demonstrated a survival advantage of approximately 25% in patients receiving taxol-based therapy compared with mitoxantrone,[12,13] and docetaxol-prednisone is now considered a standard therapeutic approach in patients with metastatic, androgen deprivation–resistant prostate cancer. Following therapy with docetaxel, patients who remain candidates for further chemotherapy can be treated with cabazitaxel, an agent shown to prolong life in this group of patients. In general, serial PSA levels are the best (albeit imperfect) way to follow up patients, and a decline of 30 to 50% is associated with improved survival. Zoledronic acid or denosumab is indicated in castration-resistant prostate cancer patients with bone metastases, as each reduces the incidence of skeletal-related events.

Palliative Care

Many patients with advanced prostate cancer have bone pain or functional impairments that adversely affect quality of life, and the provision of appropriate palliative care is an integral component of their management. In addition to the usual analgesics, glucocorticoids serve as anti-inflammatory agents and can alleviate bone pain. For patients with widespread bone metastases and pain not easily controlled with analgesics or local irradiation, strontium-89 and samarium-153 can be administered intravenously; they are selectively concentrated in bone metastases and alleviate pain in 70% or more of treated patients.

The approach to the treatment of prostate cancer is detailed in Table 207-1.

PROGNOSIS

In general, the 10-year PSA progression-free survival is 70 to 80% with Gleason scores of 2 to 6, whether treatment is with radiation therapy or surgery; 50 to 70% for Gleason scores of 7; and 15 to 30% for Gleason scores of 8 to 10. For patients with a climbing PSA level after radical prostatectomy, time to detectable PSA, Gleason score at the time of prostatectomy, and PSA doubling time are important prognostic variables. The likelihood of bone metastases at 7 years ranges from 20% for good-prognosis patients to 80% for poor-prognosis patients.

For patients with microscopic nodal disease, 10-year survival approaches 80% in men treated with androgen deprivation. Median survival in men treated with androgen deprivation for established metastatic disease ranges

TABLE 207-1 APPROACH TO THE TREATMENT OF PROSTATE CANCER

EXTENT OF CANCER	THERAPEUTIC OPTIONS
Organ confined: low risk (usually T1 or T2, GS <7, PSA <10 ng/mL)	Surveillance Radical prostatectomy External beam radiation therapy to prostate Brachytherapy
Organ confined: intermediate risk (usually T2, GS = 7, PSA = 10-20 ng/mL)	Radical prostatectomy External beam radiation therapy to prostate, possibly to pelvis, with or without AD Brachytherapy
Organ confined: high risk (usually T3, GS >7, PSA >20 ng/mL)	Radical prostatectomy (with adjuvant radiation therapy, if needed) External beam radiation therapy to prostate and pelvis (usually with AD) Brachytherapy plus radiation therapy (usually with AD)
Climbing PSA level after local therapy	AD: antiandrogen monotherapy or combined AD Salvage radiation therapy (for patients with prior prostatectomy) Salvage radical prostatectomy (for patients with prior radiation therapy) Surveillance Investigational therapy
Node positive	Surveillance AD Pelvic or prostate radiation therapy + AD Investigational therapy
Metastatic: untreated hormone-refractory prostate cancer	AD Second-line hormones Sipuleucel-T immunotherapy Chemotherapy Investigational therapy

AD = androgen deprivation; GS = Gleason score; PSA = prostate-specific antigen.

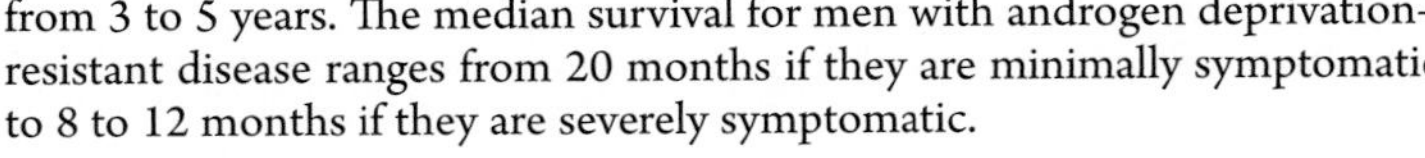

from 3 to 5 years. The median survival for men with androgen deprivation–resistant disease ranges from 20 months if they are minimally symptomatic to 8 to 12 months if they are severely symptomatic.

FUTURE DIRECTIONS

Molecular markers can not only identify patients at risk for the development of progressive disease but also act as therapeutic targets. In addition, the genomic characterization of prostate cancer subtypes will lead to risk-adapted therapy. Enhanced understanding of androgen receptor biology may permit the development of specific hormonal therapies and guide the more rational use of existing agents.

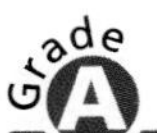

1. Schröder FH, Hugosson J, Roobol MJ, et al. Screening and prostate-cancer mortality in a randomized European study. *N Engl J Med.* 2009;360:1320-1328.
2. Andriole GL, Grubb RL 3rd, Buys SS, et al. Mortality results from a randomized prostate-cancer screening trial. *N Engl J Med.* 2009;360:1310-1319.
3. Thompson IM, Goodman PJ, Tangen CM, et al. The influence of finasteride on the development of prostate cancer. *N Engl J Med.* 2003;349:215-224.
4. Andriole GL, Bostwick DG, Brawley OW, et al. Effect of dutasteride on the risk of prostate cancer. *N Engl J Med.* 2010;362:1192-1202.
5. Bill-Axelson A, Holmberg L, Ruutu M, et al. Radical prostatectomy versus watchful waiting in early prostate cancer. *N Engl J Med.* 2005;352:1977-1984.
6. Steineck G, Helgesen F, Adolfsson J, et al. Quality of life after radical prostatectomy or watchful waiting. *N Engl J Med.* 2002;347:790-796.
7. D'Amico AV, Chen MH, Renshaw AA, et al. Androgen suppression and radiation vs radiation alone for prostate cancer: a randomized trial. *JAMA.* 2008;299:289-295.
8. Bolla M, van Poppel H, Collette L, et al. Postoperative radiotherapy after radical prostatectomy: a randomized controlled trial (EORTC trial 22911). *Lancet.* 2005;366:572-578.
9. Roach M 3rd, DeSilvio M, Lawton C, et al. Phase III trial comparing whole-pelvic versus prostate-only radiotherapy and neoadjuvant versus adjuvant combined androgen suppression: radiation Therapy Oncology Group 9413. *J Clin Oncol.* 2003;21:1904-1911.
10. Stephenson AJ, Shariat SF, Zelefsky MJ, et al. Salvage radiotherapy for recurrent prostate cancer after radical prostatectomy. *JAMA.* 2004;291:1325-1332.
11. Kantoff PW, Higano CS, Shore ND, et al. Sipuleucel-T immunotherapy for castration-resistant prostate cancer. *N Engl J Med.* 2010;363:411-422.
12. Tannock IF, de Wit R, Berry WR, et al. Docetaxel plus prednisone or mitoxantrone plus prednisone for advanced prostate cancer. *N Engl J Med.* 2004;351:1502-1512.
13. de Bono JS, Oudard S, Ozguroglu M, et al. Prednisone plus cabazitaxel or mitoxantrone for metastatic castration-resistant prostate cancer progressing after docetaxel treatment: a randomised open-label trial. *Lancet.* 2010;376:1147-1154.

SUGGESTED READINGS

Berger MF, Lawrence MS, Demichelis F, et al. The genomic complexity of primary human prostate cancer. *Nature.* 2011;470:214-220. *Review of multiple genomic abnormalities.*

Gaster B, Edwards K, Trinidad SB, et al. Patient-centered discussions about prostate cancer screening: a real-world approach. *Ann Intern Med.* 2010;153:661-665. *Practical suggestions for physicians.*

Hayes JH, Ollendorf DA, Pearson SD, et al. Active surveillance compared with initial treatment for men with low-risk prostate cancer: a decision analysis. *JAMA.* 2010;304:2373-2380. *Decision analysis suggests that active surveillance is as effective as initial treatment for men with low-risk prostate cancer.*

Heidenreich A, Bellmunt J, Bolla M, et al. EAU Guidelines on Prostate Cancer. Part I: Screening, Diagnosis, and Treatment of Clinically Localised Disease. *Eur Urol.* 2011;59:61-71. *Consensus guidelines.*

Mottet N, Bellmunt J, Bolla M, et al. EAU Guidelines on Prostate Cancer. Part II: Treatment of Advanced, Relapsing, and Castration-Resistant Prostate Cancer. *Eur Urol.* 2011;59:572-583. *Consensus guidelines.*

Whitson JM, Porten SP, Carroll PR. Prostate cancer: reducing overtreatment: active surveillance in low-risk disease. *Nat Rev Urol.* 2011;8:124-125. *Makes the case for "watchful waiting."*

Wu Y, Rosenberg JE, Taplin ME. Novel agents and new therapeutics in castration-resistant prostate cancer. *Curr Opin Oncol.* 2011;23:290-296. *Review including denosumab, abiraterone, cabazitaxel, and provenge.*

208 PRIMARY AND METASTATIC MALIGNANT BONE LESIONS

ADAM LERNER AND KAREN H. ANTMAN

PRIMARY BONE TUMORS

DEFINITION

Primary bone malignancies are relatively uncommon tumors (0.2% of all neoplasms in the Surveillance, Epidemiology, and End Results [SEER] database, 1.8 new cases/100,000 population/year) that arise from cells that are normal components of bone tissues and that have the potential to metastasize. Malignant tumors are to be distinguished from a variety of more common benign bone lesions, such as osteochondromas and enchondromas, which lack the ability to metastasize.

CLINICAL MANIFESTATIONS AND DIAGNOSIS

Patients with primary malignant and benign bone tumors present with pain, swelling and occasionally pathologic fracture of the involved bone. If radiologic studies suggest a malignant primary bone tumor (see characteristics of each subtype described later), an orthopedic oncologist should be consulted before carrying out a biopsy because improper biopsy technique may compromise subsequent surgical care, particularly limb-sparing surgery. Staging of patients with bone tumors generally requires computed tomography (CT) scans of the chest, abdomen, and pelvis to assess for metastatic disease. Characterization of the primary bone tumor may benefit from magnetic resonance imaging (MRI) assessment of soft tissue extension or CT scan assessment of cortical bone involvement, or both.

MAJOR PRIMARY MALIGNANT BONE TUMORS

Myeloma, the most common primary bone malignancy, is covered in Chapter 193.

Osteosarcoma

Osteosarcoma is the most common malignant sarcoma of bone, representing about 35% of cases. It has a bimodal age distribution, with highest incidence in patients younger than 20 years, most likely related to the normal rapid bone growth that occurs during adolescence. In this age group, most tumors arise in the metaphyseal areas of the long bones of the extremities, particularly around the knee. Males are affected more commonly than females at a ratio of 3:2. A second peak of incidence occurs in adults older than 60 years. The sites of origin in these older patients are somewhat more heterogeneous, with craniofacial and pelvic bones each accounting for 20% of tumors. Radiographically, osteosarcomas usually present as mixed osteoblastic and osteolytic lesions, although pure forms of either appearance can occur. Periosteal elevation (Codman's triangle), cortical destruction, and tumor extension into soft tissue are common on plain films or MRI.

The incidence of osteosarcoma is increased in families that carry germline deletion of retinoblastoma (*Rb*), *p53* (Li-Fraumeni), or *RecQ* DNA helicase (Rothman-Thompson, Werner, or Bloom syndrome) genes. Consistent with these observations, although most younger patients with osteosarcomas have no apparent predisposing factor or family history of bone tumors, alterations in the *p53* and *Rb* genes of such sporadic tumors occur in 40% and 60%, respectively. In older patients, a variety of conditions may predispose patients to osteosarcoma, most convincingly antecedent Paget's disease or prior radiation therapy.

TREATMENT Rx

Osteosarcoma is a highly proliferative neoplasm that metastasizes rapidly. As for most sarcomas, osteosarcoma spreads hematogenously, and the most common site of metastasis is the lung. Despite aggressive surgical resection of the primary bone tumor, the incidence of recurrence with metastatic disease is high in the absence of systemic treatment, consistent with the concept that most patients present with clinically inapparent micrometastatic disease. The development of effective systemic chemotherapy with doxorubicin (Adriamycin) and cisplatin, with or without methotrexate, has had a profoundly positive effect on treatment outcome, with 5-year disease-free survival rates exceeding 65% in patients younger than 40 years with nonmetastatic extremity tumors.[1] Most patients are managed with initial neoadjuvant chemotherapy, delayed resection of the primary tumor, and then further postoperative chemotherapy. Serum alkaline phosphatase levels, often elevated in osteosarcoma patients, can be used to monitor disease status.

Modern surgical techniques have allowed surgical resection of most extremity osteosarcomas without amputation. Although resection of lung metastases can be curative in about 20% of selected patients, detection of radiologically apparent metastatic disease at presentation significantly worsens prognosis. Long-term disease control in older adults with osteosarcoma is substantially lower than in younger patients, with a 5-year overall survival rate of 22% in one series of patients older than 65 years, most likely because of fundamental differences in the underlying molecular pathophysiology of tumors in older adults. Although osteosarcoma is generally considered to be relatively radiation resistant, radiation can play a palliative role in selected patients.

Chondrosarcoma

Chondrosarcoma, a malignant tumor characterized by hyaline cartilage differentiation, is the second most common sarcoma of bone, representing 25% of bone sarcomas. The peak incidence is in the fifth to seventh decades of life. The most common primary sites are in the pelvis, proximal femur, and proximal humerus. Patients present with long-standing complaints of swelling, pain, or both. Radiographically, chondrosarcoma is detected as an area of radiolucency with variable punctate mineralization, with frequent cortical bone erosion or thickening, sometimes with extension into adjacent soft tissue. Distinguishing low-grade chondrosarcomas from benign central enchondromas can be difficult: location in the axial skeleton and size greater than 5 cm favor malignancy.

Up to 15% of chondrosarcomas arise from preexisting peripheral osteochondromas and, like their benign counterparts, harbor mutations in the exostosin *(EXT)* genes. The remaining 85% of chondrosarcomas arise in a central location, some in preexisting enchondromas. Chondrosarcomas are divided into three grades, with higher-grade tumors characterized by greater cellularity and cellular atypia. In one series, 61% of patients had grade 1 tumors; only 4% of such patients developed metastases. In contrast, 36% of patients had grade 2 and 3% grade 3 tumors; among this combined group, 29% developed metastases.

TREATMENT 

Unlike osteosarcoma and Ewing's sarcoma, chondrosarcomas generally grow slowly, metastasize less commonly, and have an excellent prognosis after adequate surgical resection. Although chondrosarcomas are considered relatively radiation resistant, radiation therapy may provide palliation for patients with large or recurrent unresectable central chondrosarcomas.

Ewing's Sarcoma

Ewing's sarcoma and primitive neuroectodermal tumor (PNET) are a family of small round cell sarcomas that represent 16% of primary bone sarcomas. As with osteosarcoma, the peak incidence occurs during the second decade of life, but unlike osteosarcoma, the incidence of Ewing's is unimodal, being distinctly unusual in older adults and in nonwhites. Ewing's sarcoma tends to arise in the diaphyseal region of long bones, in the pelvis, or in ribs. Ewing's tumors are characterized radiologically by a permeative or "moth-eaten" appearance of the affected bone, with a multilayered "onion-skin" periosteal reaction. MRI studies frequently document a significant soft tissue mass associated with the bone lesion. Unlike other sarcomas of bone, Ewing's sarcoma may present with symptoms of an inflammatory systemic illness, with intermittent fevers, anemia, leukocytosis, and an increased sedimentation rate.

Eighty-five percent of patients with Ewing's family sarcomas contain a t(11;22)(9q24;q12) chromosomal translocation that juxtaposes the *EWS* gene on chromosome 22 with *FLI1*, an ETS family transcription factor. Another 15% contain a variant in which *EWS* is juxtaposed to *ERG*, another ETS family member on chromosome band 21q22. Because Ewing's sarcoma resembles other small round cell tumors microscopically, reverse transcription–polymerase chain reaction and fluorescent in situ hybridization studies that document such translocations play a critical role in confirming the diagnosis. Ewing's sarcoma/PNET cells characteristically express CD99/MIC2.

TREATMENT 

The development of effective systemic chemotherapy regimens has substantially improved long-term control of Ewing's sarcoma. After completion of staging procedures, patients are treated with neoadjuvant chemotherapy. One highly active regimen alternates cycles of vincristine, doxorubicin, and cyclophosphamide with ifosfamide and etoposide. After 3 months of chemotherapy, the primary tumor is resected, radiated, or both, depending on the location and extent of the primary tumor. Chemotherapy is then resumed for a total of up to 1 year of treatment. Using such an approach, the mean 5-year event-free survival rate for patients who present with nonmetastatic disease is 69%.[2] Insulin-like growth factor-1 receptor antagonists have demonstrated clinical activity in recent clinical trials for chemotherapy-refractory disease.

METASTATIC TUMORS TO BONE

Tumors metastatic to bone are important causes of cancer-related morbidity. Effective prevention and treatment of skeleton-related metastases are an important part of clinical care for many cancer patients. The most common tumors to metastasize to bone are breast in women and prostate in men, followed by lung, kidney, gastrointestinal tract, and thyroid.

Bone metastases typically present as localized or referred pain and less commonly as a fracture. Plain radiographs may demonstrate blastic or lytic lesions. Although prostate cancer is generally blastic and multiple myeloma usually lytic, most other tumors have a mixed appearance. In patients with one documented bone metastasis or in patients with widely metastatic disease and bone pain, a radiologic survey can identify bone metastases that may ultimately place the patient at risk for a pathologic fracture. Technetium diphosphonate bone scans are useful to delineate the extent of bony metastases and in following response to therapy. However, a negative study must be interpreted cautiously for tumors that are potentially purely lytic because these may be undetectable by bone scan. In such tumors (e.g., multiple myeloma), a skeletal survey is therefore preferable. Routine screening for bone metastases is not indicated for cancer patients with no symptoms or signs of bone involvement.

TREATMENT

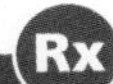

In the absence of fracture or impending fracture, painful bone metastases are treated with external beam radiation therapy. In patients with numerous bone metastases, systemic chemotherapy or endocrine therapy can play an important palliative role. Pathologic fractures or imminent fractures are generally managed by operative internal fixation.

PREVENTION

In breast cancer, prostate cancer, and multiple myeloma patients, bisphosphonate therapy increases the time to a first skeletal event. Bisphosphonate therapy also appears to prolong survival in patients with metastatic breast cancer. The optimal schedule and duration of administration of bisphosphonates to maximize benefit and minimize potential complications remain to be established.

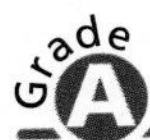

1. Grier HE, Krailo MD, Tarbell NJ, et al. Addition of ifosfamide and etoposide to standard chemotherapy for Ewing's sarcoma and primitive neuroectodermal tumor of bone. *N Engl J Med.* 2003;348:694-701.
2. Meyers PA, Schwartz CL, Krailo MD, et al. Osteosarcoma: the addition of muramyl tripeptide to chemotherapy improves overall survival—a report from the Children's Oncology Group. *J Clin Oncol.* 2008;26:633-638.

SUGGESTED READINGS

Balamuth NJ, Womer RB. Ewing's sarcoma. *Lancet Oncol.* 2010;11:184-192. *Opportunities for new treatment approaches in a sarcoma of children and adolescents, in which survival has improved from about 10% to about 75% with chemotherapy for localized tumors but patients with metastases still fare badly.*

Geller DS, Gorlick R. Osteosarcoma: a review of diagnosis, management, and treatment strategies. *Clin Adv Hematol Oncol.* 2010;8:705-718. *Review including multiagent chemotherapy.*

Jamil N, Howie S, Salter DM. Therapeutic molecular targets in human chondrosarcoma. *Int J Exp Pathol.* 2010;91:387-393. *Review.*

O'Day K, Gorlick R. Novel therapeutic agents for osteosarcoma. *Expert Rev Anticancer Ther.* 2009;9:511-523. *New therapeutic approaches, including targeted agents, inhibitors of tumor microenvironment, and immunomodulatory agents.*

Riedel RF, Larrier N, Dodd L, et al. The clinical management of chondrosarcoma. *Curr Treat Options Oncol.* 2009;10:94-106. *This review highlights the need for a coordinated multidisciplinary approach to management of these patients.*

209

SARCOMAS OF SOFT TISSUE AND BONE, AND OTHER NEOPLASMS OF CONNECTIVE TISSUES

GEORGE D. DEMETRI

DEFINITION

Sarcomas are a very heterogeneous group of malignant neoplasms of connective tissues, including bone and soft tissue. Sarcomas, as well as other putatively "nonmalignant" neoplasms that affect soft tissue and bone, share a mesenchymal cell of origin with aberrant differentiation and growth potential. Mesenchymal cells (derived from mesoderm), as well as neural crest cells (from ectoderm), are critical for the normal structure and function of humans because they give rise to the connective tissues that hold the organism together and also provide critical functions such as support and nourishment of neural tissues. When the growth, differentiation, or survival of these cells is aberrant, tumors arise, and this is the family of neoplasms to which sarcomas belong. Sarcomas include a vast array of tumor types related to muscle, stromal tissue, adipose tissue, blood and lymphatic vessels, nerves and nerve sheaths, cartilage, bone, and other fibrous tissues.

Sarcomas are tumors with distinct histopathologic abnormalities; other forms of connective tissue neoplasms may also cause significant disease without being classified as sarcomas per se. For example, because of the histopathologically bland appearance of desmoid tumors, pathologists do not classify these myofibroblastic neoplasms as sarcomas, even though they can cause significant morbidity and even death if they are recurrent and unresectable. Similarly, the sarcoma known as gastrointestinal stromal tumor (GIST) was not considered a true sarcoma before 2000, although many GISTs certainly exhibit all the characteristics of aggressive malignancy. In brief, sarcomas represent a broad group of different diseases that can affect any anatomic location, and for this reason, they have puzzled clinicians and intrigued developmental biologists and fundamental researchers.

EPIDEMIOLOGY

True sarcomas represent a very uncommon subset of human malignancies, accounting for less than 1% of cancers in adults but a disproportionately large number of cancers in the pediatric population (approximately 15% of pediatric cancers). The overall incidence of sarcomas of soft tissue and bone is approximately 15,000 cases per year in the United States. Given the fact that there are no sarcoma-specific disease diagnostic codes, however, such numbers must be viewed as rough approximations at best. Nonetheless, it is clear that sarcomas are uncommon compared with carcinomas. The prevalence of sarcomas significantly exceeds the incidence, because sarcomas can be cured with expert multidisciplinary care. This makes it critical that the initial evaluation and management of patients suspected of having sarcomas be performed by an experienced team with relevant expertise and interdisciplinary capabilities (including pathology diagnostic capabilities, surgical specialization, and radiotherapeutic experience and judgment, as well as access to the latest systemic therapy agents and data on their use). Certain patients are at high risk of developing sarcomas, most notably individuals in families with Li-Fraumeni syndrome and those with neurofibromatosis (at risk for malignant peripheral nerve sheath tumors and GISTs) or familial polyposis (at risk for intra-abdominal desmoid tumors). Other risk factors include exposure to radiation (including radiation therapy for other cancers, such as patients with prior irradiated breast cancer or survivors of retinoblastoma). Chemical carcinogens can also increase the risk of sarcoma development, such as the increased risk of sarcomas in Vietnam veterans exposed to Agent Orange or the greatly increased risk of hepatic angiosarcomas associated with occupational exposure to polyvinyl chloride. However, the vast majority of sarcomas appear to be sporadic, with no evident inciting risk factors.

PATHOBIOLOGY

Sarcomas and other connective tissue neoplasms are an overwhelmingly complex and heterogeneous mixture of diseases with a wide range of clinical behaviors and outcomes. Some soft tissue neoplasms, such as localized tenosynovial giant cell tumors, can be cured by expert resection, whereas more advanced tumors of this type (referred to as pigmented villonodular tenosynovitis) often lead to debilitating amputations or even death due to metastatic disease. The bewildering array of polysyllabic names used by pathologists has caused confusion among clinicians and basic science investigators alike. In brief, expert pathologists strive to develop concise, systematic, and reproducible criteria for the diagnosis of specific sarcoma subtypes, but interobserver variability can plague the application of elegant diagnostic categories such as those promulgated by the World Health Organization. Increasing knowledge of the molecular pathways that drive sarcomas has provided more objective diagnostic tools with novel immunohistochemical staining patterns and genetic markers (e.g., pathognomonic chromosomal translocations have defined diseases such as Ewing's sarcoma or synovial sarcoma more objectively than any histopathologic appearance determined by simple light microscopy). In general, sarcomas may exhibit differentiation patterns consistent with defined connective tissues (e.g., well-differentiated liposarcoma may appear as only slightly bizarre fat cells under the microscope), or they may be absolutely unclassifiable. In fact, the terminology used by pathologists for very poorly differentiated sarcomas has also evolved: the current diagnostic category is "unclassifiable pleomorphic sarcoma," whereas 20 years ago most pathologists grouped such poorly differentiated tumors under the misnomer "malignant fibrous histiocytoma." In any case, as diagnostic tools have evolved, it has become possible to place such poorly differentiated tumors more accurately into certain histopathologic categories based on the expression of lineage-related proteins (e.g., smooth muscle actin expression may help categorize tumors as leiomyosarcomas) or on the basis of genomic markers (e.g., overexpression of chromosome 12 material or the *mdm2* gene locus is most consistent with a dedifferentiated liposarcoma).

It may be necessary to refer patient material to expert reference pathologists to accurately define the type of connective tissue neoplasm, and such referral can make an enormous difference in patient care (e.g., differentiating between a benign process that may self-resolve and a truly malignant sarcoma). The complexity of sarcoma and connective tissue tumor diagnosis cannot be overstated, and that is a major reason why all international clinical practice guidelines emphasize the importance of experienced diagnosticians and a low threshold for referral to expert pathology review for patients with connective tissue tumors.

CLINICAL MANIFESTATIONS AND DIAGNOSIS

Given the broad range of sarcomas, it is understandable that the clinical course can range from rapidly evolving and immediately life-threatening cancers (such as most Ewing's sarcomas) to indolent lesions that can take decades to evolve (such as atypical lipomatous tumors, also known as well-differentiated liposarcomas). Most patients with sarcomas present with a mass, often nontender, with a history of abnormal growth over time. For extremity tumors of soft tissues, it is important to note that many benign tumors (e.g., lipomas) cannot be easily distinguished from more worrisome neoplasms or even from frankly malignant sarcomas. Therefore, it is important to include sarcoma in the differential diagnosis of any mass.

The initial biopsy or surgical approach to a sarcomatous lesion is often the most important, and a poorly oriented biopsy or a suboptimal surgical procedure can make the difference between cure with full limb function and disease recurrence with the need for amputation or mutilating surgical re-resection. This lesson was first learned by orthopedic specialists with regard to bone sarcoma (osteosarcoma), but it is true for soft tissue sarcomas as well. The National Comprehensive Cancer Network (NCCN) has developed expert consensus guidelines for clinical practice that emphasize the importance of expert management from the moment a suspected sarcoma presents. The initial diagnosis includes appropriate imaging studies of relevant anatomic areas, including plain radiographs, computed tomography, or magnetic resonance imaging to define the anatomic area of the mass and surrounding tissue, as well as systemic staging because sarcomas can spread in well-defined patterns to distal sites such as the lung or liver. The decision to proceed to diagnostic biopsy, with optimal orientation, is an important one, and for certain lesions, forgoing incisional biopsy and proceeding directly to expertly planned surgical excision may be justified. The most important consideration is to make the correct diagnosis, and there must be sufficient amounts of properly prepared and expertly oriented tissues for optimal diagnostic analysis. In certain tumors with pathognomonic molecular markers (such as the translocation between chromosomes X and 18 that characterizes synovial sarcoma, or the balanced translocation between chromosomes 12 and 16 that defines myxoid and round cell liposarcoma), molecular analyses such as fluorescence in situ hybridization (FISH) may help make the diagnosis. New molecular subtypes of sarcomas enter the pathology literature on an annual basis, and this supports the need for expert pathology review of tumors of soft tissue and bone. These new diagnostic categories may lead to new molecularly targeted therapies. Nowhere has this been more evident than in the rapid evolution of effective therapy against the major pathobiologic cause of GISTs[1] (see later, under Treatment).

The diagnosis of a soft tissue or bone tumor is made by evaluating biopsy material in the clinical context, which includes understanding the tumor's anatomic location and imaging characteristics. Such contextual diagnostics are key to understanding whether a lesion may represent a primary sarcoma or whether it may be the first presentation of metastases from an occult primary tumor located elsewhere. Given the broad spectrum of sarcomas, the diagnostic considerations are quite far-reaching, especially because many benign pathophysiologic conditions can mimic sarcomas. For example, it may be very difficult for an inexperienced pathologist to distinguish among normal fat, inflammatory infiltrates, and liposarcoma. Similarly, certain fibroblastic neoplasms might simulate inflammation or scar. Therefore, a broad differential diagnosis is needed when considering any neoplasm of soft tissue or bone.

TREATMENT

Rx

The most important element of treatment is expert multidisciplinary care. The range of options is too broad to categorize simply, and the specific details of each patient's anatomy, comorbidities, functional status, and personal preferences must be taken into account when defining treatment options and management plans. Therefore, the care of virtually all sarcoma patients should be managed by an expert multidisciplinary team with expertise in advanced surgical and/or orthopedic oncology techniques, radiation therapy, reconstructive surgery, physical therapy and rehabilitation medicine, systemic therapies such as conventional cytotoxic chemotherapy, hormonal therapy, and modern molecularly targeted therapy with agents such as kinase inhibitors, as well as psychosocial support and specialized nursing care. Sarcomas represent such a complex family of diseases that referral to academic centers makes good sense for patients as well as for the health care system overall. Therefore, appropriate referral to obtain expert opinion and to define the diagnostic and treatment options for patients with suspected sarcomas is exceedingly important.

For most primary localized masses in which sarcoma is in the differential diagnosis, the first step is to obtain the correct diagnosis in a manner that does not compromise patient outcome or function. The need for biopsy must be considered first, because some small, localized sarcomas are best approached through definitive surgical excision following careful staging and expert review of imaging studies. For suspected sarcomas in deeper locations, such as deep within muscle compartments, or for large visceral lesions, biopsy may be necessary to ascertain that the process is in fact a sarcoma, as well as to fully characterize the histopathologic subtype. This may make the difference between initial management with chemotherapy, as might be appropriate for a highly chemosensitive disease such as Ewing's sarcoma, versus surgery, which might be appropriate for a less chemosensitive disease such as dedifferentiated liposarcoma. Expert opinion varies regarding the utility and timing of adjuncts to surgical resection, such as radiation therapy or systemic cytotoxic chemotherapy. This variation can best be appreciated by noting the variety of management options for extremity sarcomas in the NCCN's consensus practice guidelines.

In general, expert surgical resection is first-line therapy for localized sarcomas. Preoperative systemic chemotherapy is standard for most common forms of osteosarcoma, as well as for Ewing's sarcoma and certain rhabdomyosarcomas. Many expert teams favor preoperative radiation therapy for certain sarcomas; irradiation of a large primary tumor can deliver smaller doses to surrounding normal tissues preoperatively compared with postoperatively, but this is a matter of personal preference. A reasonably sized randomized trial of preoperative versus postoperative radiation therapy for large sarcomas of the extremity was performed in Canada, and outcomes were similar, with subtle differences: patients who received preoperative radiation had a higher incidence of serious postoperative wound complications, but the long-term functional outcomes were slightly more favorable.[2] Because of such subtleties in results, sarcoma care is based largely on expert opinion and personal experience, and the vast range of sarcoma diagnoses and clinical presentations adds to this complexity.

Many sarcoma centers disagree about the relative value of cytotoxic chemotherapy, although there is no doubt that chemotherapy has greatly improved disease control rates and cure rates of certain subtypes of aggressive sarcomas such as intermediate- and high-grade osteosarcomas, Ewing's sarcomas, and rhabdomyosarcomas. For other forms of sarcomas originating in bone (e.g., chondrosarcoma) or soft tissue (e.g., leiomyosarcoma, synovial sarcoma), there is no strong evidence that systemic chemotherapy increases cure rates or long-term clinical outcomes, although there may be some improvement in local disease control and recurrence-free survival. This has led to discordant expert opinion: many experts believe that the risks and toxicities of aggressive chemotherapy justify the benefit of longer disease-free survival, whereas others feel that such toxicities are not reasonable without a major improvement in overall survival. Limited series of postoperative adjuvant therapy are often contradictory owing to the relatively small patient groups under study, as well as divergent patient selection factors, such as the inclusion of those with a lower risk of recurrence or death from metastatic disease. Inclusion of a sizable percentage of sarcoma patients with low-risk disease no doubt dilutes the results of even a reasonably effective therapy and runs the risk of making the study result negative; this possibility has remained an irreconcilable point of controversy among sarcoma centers across the United States and around the world.

It is also critical to recognize that treatment may differ radically depending on the histologic diagnosis. The best example of this is GIST, a form of sarcoma that, in more than 95% of cases, is driven by aberrant tyrosine kinase signaling. Routine systemic chemotherapy is completely ineffectual against this disease once it has metastasized or become unresectable owing to extensive local disease. By understanding the pathobiology of the disease and the "short-circuits" of intracellular kinase signaling, it is now possible to use targeted tyrosine kinase inhibitor drugs (e.g., imatinib mesylate, sunitinib malate) to block the abnormally activated tumor cell signaling, leading to dramatic tumor regression and tumor control in more than 85% of patients. Therefore, correctly diagnosing GIST is critical for choosing the proper therapy, and it can have life-or-death consequences for patients. Fortunately, pathologists are increasingly able to recognize this histopathologically and molecularly defined sarcoma. Immunohistochemistry to detect antigens such as CD117 (the Kit receptor tyrosine kinase) and DOG1 (a membrane antigen that is reasonably specific for GIST) and tumor genotyping via molecular genetics have significantly increased the accuracy of GIST diagnosis in the past decade. Tyrosine kinase inhibitor therapy with imatinib has been approved by the Food and

Drug Administration to decrease the risk of disease recurrence following resection of GISTs with significant potential for relapse. It is important to note that patients with a low risk of relapse have not derived substantive benefits from adjuvant imatinib because they have a very good chance of being cured by expert surgery alone.[3] GIST is therefore a paradigmatic example of a sarcoma in which critical therapy decisions must be made in the context of the proper diagnosis and with access to the latest evidence-based medical information.

For soft tissue sarcomas other than GIST, radiation therapy can play a meaningful role in preventing disease recurrence, especially for lesions that arise in the extremities. Radiation therapy can also provide significant palliation of unresectable disease, and it can be surprisingly effective in certain tumors such as desmoid tumor. However, radiation-associated sarcomas are increasingly common after therapeutic radiation therapy (e.g., in patients cured of breast cancer with radiation therapy), and an increasing incidence of poorly differentiated sarcomas or vascular sarcomas has been reported in patients following irradiation for other diseases.

As noted earlier, traditional cytotoxic chemotherapy is dramatically effective at increasing disease control and cure rates for certain sarcomas (especially those most prevalent in pediatric patients, such as osteosarcoma, Ewing's sarcoma, and rhabdomyosarcoma). It appears to be somewhat less effective in improving long-term cure rates for patients with most other forms of soft tissue and bone sarcomas, such as liposarcoma, leiomyosarcoma, synovial sarcoma, and other subtypes. Nonetheless, appropriate use of chemotherapy can lead to objective responses in certain patients and can palliate metastatic disease with disease control and prolongation of progression-free survival. Sarcoma experts often disagree about the relative value and toxicity of combination chemotherapy as opposed to sequential single-agent chemotherapy. In patients with very aggressive and highly symptomatic sarcomas, clinicians may wish to "hedge their bets" and choose a combination chemotherapy regimen, even if there is a greater risk of toxicity, to ensure some measure of rapid disease control or even a greater chance of disease regression. In contrast, in patients with asymptomatic metastatic disease (e.g., a sarcoma patient with indolent pulmonary metastases and no symptoms), the optimal choice might be single-agent chemotherapy to avoid toxicity and to maximize the choice of subsequent chemotherapeutic agents after the benefit of the first agent is fully realized. There is no single "best" choice for all patients, and each clinical situation requires individualization based on the specific details of the case and the patient's preferences. There are no definitive data from rigorously conducted and properly powered randomized trials that any chemotherapy for metastatic sarcoma of soft tissue (other than GIST) improves overall survival, yet there is no room for nihilism. All experts agree that owing to the complexity of the trials, the diseases, and the clinical settings, one must allow for variations in interpretations for individual patients. This explains the greatly discordant practice patterns observed across the country based on referrals, provider experience, and patient characteristics and preferences.

PROGNOSIS

As noted earlier, it is relatively meaningless to discuss prognosis for sarcomas overall because they represent such a variety of diseases with widely divergent natural histories. It is estimated that approximately 50% of patients with localized sarcomas can be cured, and the risk of recurrence is related to variables such as tumor grade (low-grade tumors have a lower risk of recurrence or metastasis compared with intermediate- or high-grade tumors), tumor size, and tumor location or depth. For patients with recurrent or metastatic sarcoma, outcome depends on many factors, including the time from initial diagnosis to the first appearance of metastatic disease: a longer disease-free interval is associated with longer survival, probably indicating a slower rate of tumor proliferation. Another factor that may determine outcome is the number of metastatic lesions: it is possible that oligoclonal metastases, with few lesions, can be surgically resected, which itself may be associated with improved survival. Advances in chemotherapy and targeted therapies may also affect survival, as documented by the dramatic improvements in survival and disease control for GIST and other kinase-driven sarcomas, such as dermatofibrosarcoma protuberans, as well as the more recent molecular therapeutic targeting of giant cell tumor of bone, perivascular epithelioid cell–oma (PEComa), and tenosynovial giant cell tumor. The natural history of these diseases will almost certainly be changed by a more complete and mechanistic understanding of the underlying neoplasia-promoting signals that cause the transformation and maintenance of the sarcoma.

The complexities of soft tissue and bone neoplasms and sarcomas are rivaled only by the spectrum of molecular pathways and aberrancies that are at the root of these diseases. Virtually every disease mechanism can be associated with some form of mesenchymal cell neoplasm. Better understanding of sarcoma biology is translating into improvements in sarcoma outcomes, and this is being extrapolated to improved understanding of the pathophysiology of other stromal-mediated diseases, such as pathologic conditions of fibrosis (e.g., interstitial pulmonary fibrosis and fibrocystic diseases such as lymphangioleiomatosis). Expert multidisciplinary management of sarcomas is critical to improving outcomes, and ongoing translational and therapeutic research will provide dividends far beyond the relatively low incidence and prevalence of these mesenchymal cell neoplastic disorders.

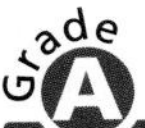

1. Gastrointestinal Stromal Tumor Meta-Analysis Group (MetaGIST). Comparison of two doses of imatinib for the treatment of unresectable or metastatic gastrointestinal stromal tumors: a meta-analysis of 1640 patients. *J Clin Oncol.* 2010;28:1247-1253.
2. Davis AM, O'Sullivan B, Turcotte R, et al. Canadian Sarcoma Group; NCI Canada Clinical Trial Group Randomized Trial. Late radiation morbidity following randomization to preoperative versus postoperative radiotherapy in extremity soft tissue sarcoma. *Radiother Oncol.* 2005;75:48-53.
3. DeMatteo RP, Ballman KV, Antonescu CR, et al. Placebo-controlled randomized trial of adjuvant imatinib mesylate following the resection of localized, primary gastrointestinal stromal tumor (GIST). *Lancet.* 2009;373:1097-1104.

SUGGESTED READINGS

Bannasch H, Eisenhardt SU, Grosu AL, et al. The diagnosis and treatment of soft tissue sarcomas of the limbs. *Dtsch Arztebl Int.* 2011;108:32-38. *Clinical review with a useful algorithm.*

Casali PG, Blay JY; ESMO/CONTICANET/EUROBONET Consensus Panel of experts. Soft tissue sarcomas: ESMO clinical practice guidelines for diagnosis, treatment and follow-up. *Ann Oncol.* 2010;21:v198-203. *Consensus guidelines.*

Le Cesne A, Ray-Coquard I, Bui BN, et al. Discontinuation of imatinib in patients with advanced gastrointestinal stromal tumours after 3 years of treatment: an open-label multicentre randomised phase 3 trial. *Lancet Oncol.* 2010;11:942-949. *Discontinuation led to high risk of rapid tumor progression.*

National Comprehensive Cancer Network Clinical Practice Guidelines for Soft Tissue Sarcoma and Gastrointestinal Stromal Tumor. http://www.nccn.org/professionals/physician_gls/f_guidelines.asp. *Definitive clinical practice guidelines that cover the complexities of sarcoma management and present algorithms ranging from initial presentation through diagnosis, primary disease management, surveillance, and care of metastatic or recurrent disease.*

Sarcoma on Cancer.Net from the American Society of Clinical Oncology: http://www.cancer.net/patient/Cancer+Types/Sarcoma. *Patient-focused information on sarcomas from the leading professional organization of oncologists.*

Verweij J, Baker LH. Future treatment of soft tissue sarcomas will be driven by histological subtype and molecular aberrations. *Eur J Cancer.* 2010;46:863-868. *Review emphasizing the need for a change in approach to soft tissue sarcomas, a highly heterogeneous group of diseases that have often been studied and treated as if they were all the same.*

210 MELANOMA AND NONMELANOMA SKIN CANCERS

LYNN SCHUCHTER

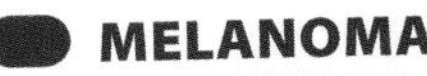

MELANOMA

EPIDEMIOLOGY

Current estimates are that 1 out of 39 men and 1 of out of 58 women will be diagnosed with melanoma during their lifetime. Each year in the United States, approximately 62,000 new cases of invasive melanoma are detected, and 8400 patients die of melanoma. The explanation for the rising incidence is thought to be increasing sun exposure, especially early in life. Melanoma is the leading cause of death from cutaneous malignant disease, and it accounts for 1 to 2% of all cancer deaths in the United States. Melanoma affects all age groups; the median age at diagnosis is 50 years. Melanoma is largely a disease of whites, with a very low incidence in African Americans, Asians, and Hispanics.

PATHOBIOLOGY

Exposure to sunlight, and especially ultraviolet (UV) radiation (Chapter 19), has been strongly implicated as a causative factor in the development of melanoma. Melanomas originate from melanocytes, which are located predominantly in the basal cell layer of the epidermis and use the enzyme tyrosinase to synthesize melanin pigment, which serves to protect against UV damage (Chapter 443). Worldwide, the incidence of melanoma in whites generally correlates inversely with latitude; that is, rates are generally higher closer to the equator and become progressively lower near the poles.

Risk Factors

Risk factors for melanoma include family history of melanoma, prior melanoma or nonmelanoma skin cancer, inherited genetic susceptibility, and sun exposure. Individuals with fair complexion, blond or red hair, blue eye color, and freckles, who have a tendency to burn rather than tan, have higher rates of melanoma. The pattern of sun exposure may also be important; intermittent intense exposure, rather than long-term exposure, may carry a higher risk of melanoma.

Individuals with an increased number of typical or benign moles or atypical moles or dysplastic nevi (Figs. 210-1 and 210-2) also have an increased risk for melanoma. Atypical moles or dysplastic nevi are important precursor lesions of melanoma and also serve as markers for increasing risk. For example, individuals with dysplastic nevi have a 6% lifetime chance of developing melanoma, and this risk increases to as high as 80% in individuals who have dysplastic nevi and a strong family history of melanoma.

Genetics

Approximately 10% of patients with melanoma have a family history of melanoma. Several chromosomal loci determine susceptibility to melanoma, the most important of which is *p16/CDKN2A,* a gene located on chromosome 9p21. This gene is a member of a class of molecules that play a central role in cell cycle regulation. Of the members of melanoma-prone families, 25 to 40% have mutations in this gene. The risk of developing cutaneous melanoma in an individual who is a CDKN2A carrier is between 30 and 90% by age 80 years and varies by geographic location. Testing for mutations in the *p16/CDKN2A* locus is commercially available, but its clinical utility is unclear at this time. Genetic variability in melancortin-1 receptor (MC1R) plays a key role in pigmentation of skin and hair and more recently has been implicated in melanoma predisposition.

Somatic mutations in primary and metastatic melanoma primarily involve the mitogen activated protein kinase pathway. Activating mutations in *B-RAF* can be found in approximately 40% of melanomas, and 10 to 15% of melanomas are associated with a mutation in *N-RAS.* Recent studies have found that melanoma on mucous membranes, acral skin (soles, palms), and skin with chronic sun damage (i.e., lentigo maligna melanoma) have frequent mutations in *c-kit.* Thus, distinct patterns of genetic alterations are found in primary melanomas based on anatomic location and extent of sun exposure. The discovery of somatic mutations in melanoma and associated aberrant signal transduction pathways has provided leads for the development of molecularly targeted therapy for patients with advanced melanoma.

CLINICAL MANIFESTATIONS

Early detection and recognition of melanoma are key to improving survival. The signs of early melanoma are based on the clinical appearance of the pigmented lesion and a change in the shape, color, or surface of an existing mole. Most patients report a preexisting mole at the site of the melanoma. Itching, burning, or pain in a pigmented lesion should increase suspicion, although melanomas often are not associated with local discomfort. Bleeding and ulceration are signs of a more advanced melanoma. Most melanomas are varying shades of brown, but they may be black, blue, or pink. The ABCDEs for the recognition of melanoma are asymmetry, border irregularity, color variation, diameter greater than 6 mm, and evolution or a change in a skin lesion.

Cutaneous melanoma has been divided into four subtypes. Superficial spreading melanoma, which accounts for 70% of all melanomas, can be located on any anatomic site (Fig. 210-3). Lentigo maligna melanoma, which represents 4 to 10% of all melanomas, tends to occur more commonly in chronically sun-exposed skin in older patients, frequently on the head and neck (Fig. 210-4); clinically, it appears as a macular (flat) lesion, arising in a lentigo maligna. Nodular melanoma (Fig. 210-5) accounts for 15 to 30% of melanomas and manifests as a rapidly enlarging elevated or polypoid lesion, often blue or black. The ABCDE rule does not always apply as well to nodular melanomas. Acral lentiginous melanoma manifests as a darkly pigmented, flat to nodular lesion on the palm, on the sole, and subungually; sunlight is not thought to play a causative role in this form of melanoma. Histologic subtype does not directly correlate with clinical behavior. However, recent data suggest that histologic subtype may correlate with specific genetic abnormalities.

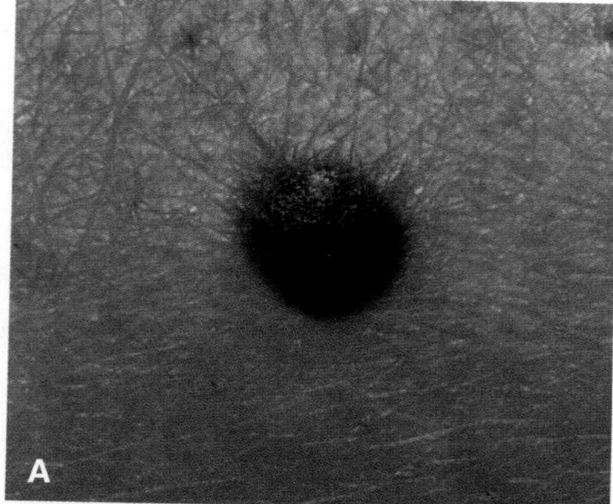

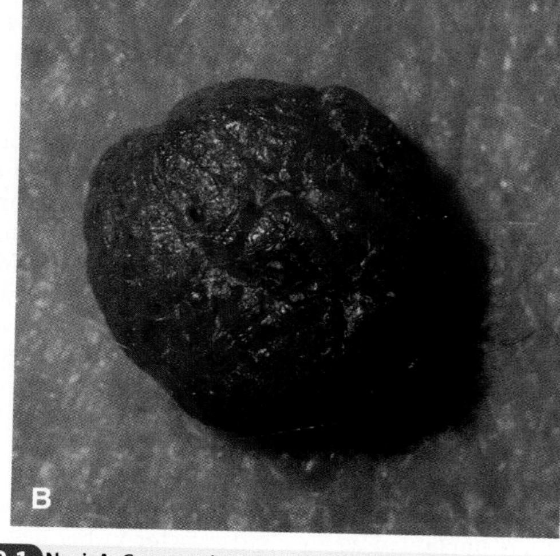

FIGURE 210-1. Nevi. **A,** Common benign nevus. **B,** Dermal nevus.

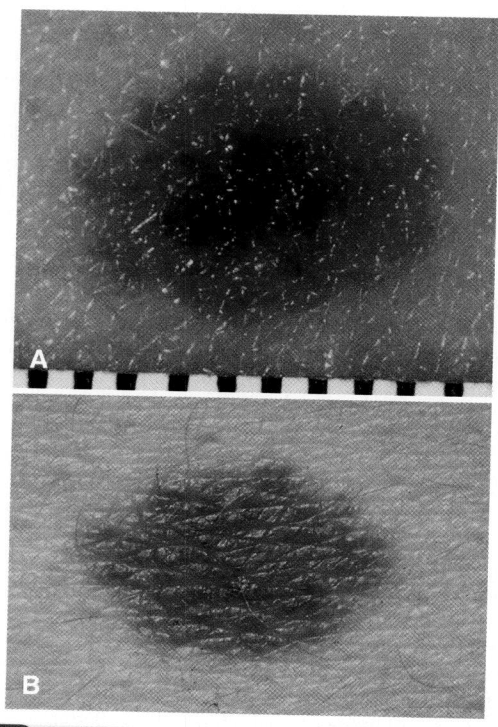

FIGURE 210-2. Dysplastic nevi. **A** and **B,** Examples of dysplastic nevi.

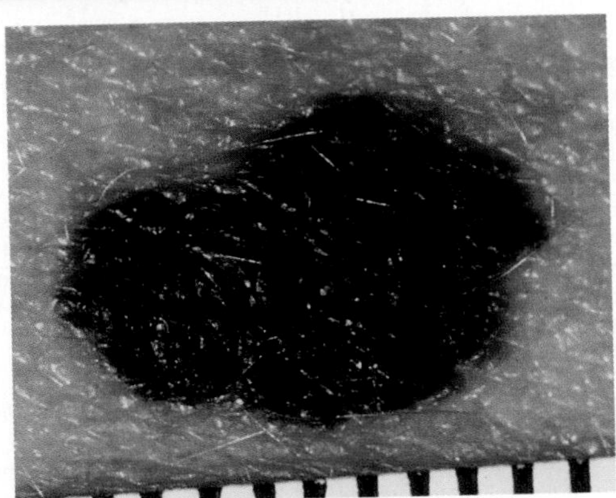

FIGURE 210-3. Superficial spreading melanoma.

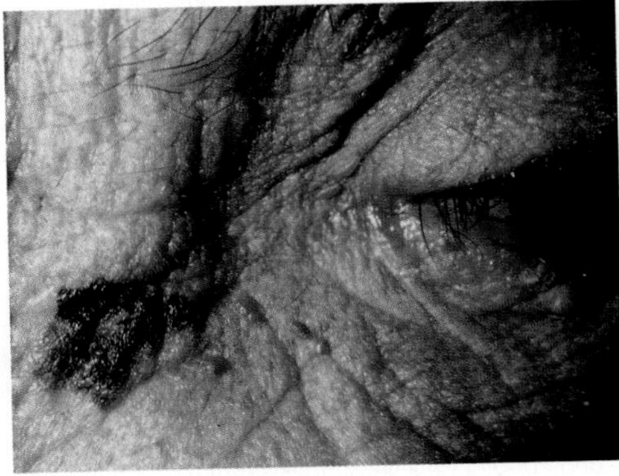

FIGURE 210-4. Lentigo maligna melanoma.

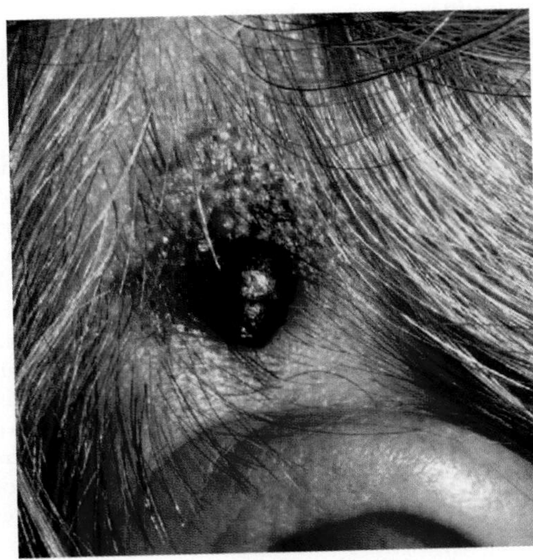

FIGURE 210-5. Nodular melanoma. (From Internal Medicine for Clerkship Students. American College of Physicians, 2006.)

Ocular melanomas arise from the pigmented layer of the eye. Uveal melanoma is the most common intraocular malignancy of adults. Melanomas can also arise from noncutaneous sites, including mucosal epithelium in the gastrointestinal tract, anorectal area, genitourinary tract, and nasal and nasopharyngeal mucosa. Melanomas of the vulva and vagina are relatively rare. In general, mucosal melanomas are diagnosed at a more advanced stage of disease. The mainstay of treatment is surgical.

DIAGNOSIS

Any skin lesion suggestive of melanoma should be sampled using biopsy with complete excision, including a 1- to 2-mm margin of normal skin and some subcutaneous fat. An incisional biopsy may be necessary for lesions too large for complete excision. Shallow shave biopsies, curettage, cryosurgery, laser, and electrodessication are contraindicated in lesions suggestive of melanoma. Other lesions that can be confused with melanoma include blue nevi, pigmented basal cell carcinoma, seborrheic keratosis, and hemangiomas (Table 210-1).

TABLE 210-1 CLINICAL FEATURES OF COMMON NEVI, DYSPLASTIC NEVI, AND MELANOMAS

DISEASE	CHARACTERISTICS
Common acquired nevi (moles)	These tend to be small, flat, and round; the border is regular, smooth, and well defined; the color is homogeneous, usually no more than two shades of brown; any site is affected; lesions are usually <6 mm.
Dysplastic nevi (atypical moles)	These occur predominantly on the trunk; they tend to be large, usually >5 mm, with a flat component; the border is characteristically fuzzy and ill defined. The shape can be round, oval, or misshapen. The color is usually brown but can be mottled with dark brown, pink, and tan. Some individuals have only 1 to 5 moles, others more than 100.
Melanoma	The border is more irregular; lesions tend to be larger, often >6 mm; substantial heterogeneity of color is noted, ranging from tan-brown, dark brown, black, pink, red, gray, blue, or white.

Prognostic Factors

As with most malignancies, the outcome of melanoma is dependent on the stage and extent of disease at presentation. For localized melanoma, the most important prognostic factor is involvement of regional lymph nodes. The most important prognostic factor related to the primary tumor is the depth of invasion (Breslow's thickness) of the melanoma, which is measured in millimeters from the top of the epidermis to the underlying dermis. Increasing thickness is associated with an increased risk for recurrence, regional lymph node involvement, and death from melanoma. Patients whose melanomas are less than 1 mm thick have about an 80 to 90% 10-year survival rate, whereas patients whose melanomas are greater than 4 mm thick have only a 40 to 50% 10-year survival rate. Other poor prognostic factors related to the primary melanoma include the presence of ulceration, an increasing level of invasion (Clark's level), a high mitotic rate, and the presence of microscopic satellites. Regional lymph node involvement (stage III) has a major impact on survival, with 5-year survival rates ranging from 20 to 70%, depending on the number of involved lymph nodes. Melanomas that arise on the extremity tend to have a better prognosis, and women tend to do better than men.

Staging System for Melanoma

Staging and prognosis for melanoma are based on the TNM system, in which T refers to tumor, N to nodes, and M to metastasis, which was updated in 2009 (E-Table 210-1). Stages I and II indicate clinically localized primary melanoma, stage III melanoma indicates regional involvement (lymph nodes or in-transit metastases), and stage IV is metastatic disease beyond the regional lymph nodes (i.e., lung, liver, brain).

Patient Evaluation

The initial evaluation of a patient with melanoma includes a personal history, a family history, a total skin examination, and palpation of regional (draining) lymph nodes. The focus is to identify risk factors, signs or symptoms of metastases, dysplastic nevi, and additional melanomas. A chest radiograph and liver enzyme tests may be performed at the discretion of the physician. Most patients who present with melanoma do not have distant metastatic disease at presentation; therefore, extensive evaluations with computed tomography (CT) to search for distant metastases have an extremely low yield and are not indicated in asymptomatic patients. More extensive staging evaluation with CT or positron emission tomography (PET) can be considered in patients with high-risk disease (primary melanoma >4 mm thick or node-positive disease), in whom the risk of distant metastatic disease is higher.

TREATMENT

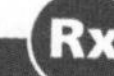

Primary Melanoma

Once melanoma is diagnosed, the standard treatment is surgical excision. Several prospective randomized trials have been conducted to define the optimal surgery for primary melanoma.[1] The extent of the surgery depends on the thickness of the primary melanoma. Large surgical excisions are no longer required, and most wide excisions can be performed with primary closure. For melanoma in situ, excision with a 0.5-cm border of clinically normal skin is sufficient. For melanomas less than 1 mm thick, a 1-cm margin is recommended. If the thickness is between 1 and 4 mm, a 1- to 2-cm margin is recommended. For melanomas thicker than 4 mm, at least a 2-cm margin should be taken. In cosmetically sensitive areas (face) or anatomically difficult areas (ear, hands), it may be difficult to achieve the desired margin, but at least a 1-cm margin should be obtained whenever possible.

Management of Regional Lymph Nodes

Clinically Normal Regional Lymph Nodes

In approximately 10 to 20% of patients who do not have clinically apparent lymph node involvement, lymph nodes contain occult micrometastases. The risk for occult lymph node involvement rises with increasing tumor thickness. Results from randomized trials fail to show a survival benefit from elective or prophylactic lymph node dissections in patients with clinically negative lymph nodes.

Sentinel lymph node biopsy (SLNB) is a technique that accurately evaluates whether microscopic melanoma cells involve regional lymph nodes. The technique relies on the concept that specific regions of the skin drain specifically to an initial lymph node within the regional nodal basin through an organized pathway of afferent lymphatic channels. This technique is performed by injecting the primary melanoma site with blue dye (isosulfan blue) or radiolabeled colloid, or both. When both modalities are used in combination, a sentinel node can be identified in 98% of patients; biopsy of the node accurately determines whether melanoma cells have metastasized to that specific lymph node basin. The sentinel node technique also promotes a more comprehensive histologic examination of lymph nodes because limited amounts of pathologic material are submitted.

SLNB allows earlier identification of metastases and earlier lymphadenectomy.[2] The likelihood of detecting melanoma in SLNB increases with thickness of the primary lesion providing the rationale for determining which patients may benefit from the procedure. SLNB is recommended to patients with melanoma 1 mm thick or thicker. The use of this technique for patients with thinner melanomas, that is, less than 1 mm thick, is controversial. The SLNB is generally performed at the same time as the wide excision of the primary tumor. If the SLNB is negative for melanoma, no further lymph node surgery is required. If melanoma is detected by the SLNB, complete lymph node dissection remains the standard of care. SLNB is a useful staging tool; however, its impact on the overall survival of patients is uncertain.

Clinically Apparent Regional Lymph Nodes

Surgical (therapeutic) lymphadenectomy is the preferred treatment of cytologically (fine-needle aspiration) positive or pathologically proven regional lymph node involvement with melanoma. The goal is to provide long-term, disease-free survival and reduce local morbidity of enlarged lymph nodes.

Adjuvant Therapy

Postsurgical adjuvant therapy can be considered for patients at high risk for recurrence (melanomas ≥4 mm thick or node-positive disease). These patients have at least a 25 to 75% chance of dying of melanoma. Adjuvant treatment options include interferon-α (IFN-α), enrollment in a clinical trial, or observation. High-dose IFN-α is the only U.S. Food and Drug Administration (FDA)-approved adjuvant therapy for patients with melanoma. Randomized clinical trials have shown that therapy with IFN-α can prolong disease-free survival but has not improved overall survival.[3] The treatment is given for 1 year and is associated with considerable side effects, which require close monitoring. Intermediate and low doses of IFN-α as well as pegylated IFN-α have also been evaluated in a series of clinical trials. These regimens are not considered standard in the United States but are offered in Europe. Numerous vaccine studies are ongoing but are considered experimental at present.

Treatment and Course of Advanced Melanoma (Stage IV)

The treatment of a patient with metastatic melanoma emphasizes palliation. No evidence indicates that treatment of metastatic melanoma has any impact on survival, which ranges from 5 to 11 months, with a median of 8.5 months. Treatment options include surgery for resection of solitary metastases, single-agent chemotherapy such as dacarbazine, temozolomide (an oral version of dacarbazine), combination chemotherapy, immunotherapy (vaccines, interleukin-2, interferon), or combined immunotherapy. Melanoma can metastasize to virtually any organ, especially the lung, skin, liver, and brain.

The discovery of somatic genetic mutations in melanoma has provided leads for the development of molecularly targeted therapies. The MAP kinase pathway, which is activated in most melanomas due to mutations in *BRAF*, *NRAS*, and *c-kit*, has been the focus of most clinical investigations of signal transduction (kinase) inhibitors. Recent results of a phase I study of PLX4032, a potent and specific BRAF inhibitor in patients with metastatic melanoma whose tumors harbor the V600E BRAF mutation demonstrated a response rate of almost 80% and an estimated median progression free survival of at least 7 months. Recent and preliminary results also show that imatinib can induce regression in patients whose melanoma is driven by *KIT* mutations.

New immunotherapy approaches are being tested in patients with advanced melanoma. Encouraging results have been reported with ipilimumab, which blocks cytotoxic T-lymphocyte antigen 4 (CTLA-4) in patients with metastatic melanoma.[4]

Surveillance and Follow-up

Patients should be educated on the clinical characteristics of melanoma, the importance of safe sun strategies, and the performance of monthly self-examinations of the skin. Patients should be followed regularly for evidence of local or regional recurrence, distant metastatic disease, and a second primary melanoma. The intensity of the surveillance and the extent of the investigation is influenced by risk for recurrence with more frequent follow-up visits in patients who have thicker tumors or node-positive disease because these patients are at greater risk for recurrence.

For patients with low-risk melanoma (≤1 mm), visits are recommended every 6 months for 2 years and then annually. The surveillance guidelines for patients with high-risk melanoma include evaluation every 3 to 4 months for 2 years, then every 6 months for 3 years. After 5 years, patients are seen once a year. Patients are generally followed for 10 years. However, lifelong dermatologic examination is recommended, particularly for patients with dysplastic nevi or a family history of melanoma. In general, a history and physical examination are performed at each visit. Periodic chest radiographs, laboratory studies, and other imaging studies are performed at the discretion of the treating physician. The physical examination should include a thorough skin examination, because at least 3% of patients develop an additional primary cutaneous melanoma within 3 years. Regional lymph nodes should be thoroughly examined, especially in patients without prior nodal surgery. For the remainder of the examination, one should keep in mind the frequency of metastases to lung, liver, and brain. Follow-up studies may include a complete blood cell count and chemistry studies, including liver enzyme tests. An elevated lactate dehydrogenase level suggests metastatic melanoma.

PREVENTION

The most important measures to prevent melanoma are to reduce excessive sun exposure, particularly to the midday sun, and to avoid sunburns. Sunscreen products with a sun protection factor of 15 or greater and protective clothing are recommended, and one randomized trial found that regular sunscreen use reduced incident melanoma by 50% and invasive melanoma by 75%.[5] Sunscreens block primarily UVB rays, which are considered to be the major causative agent of cutaneous cancers. Newer sunscreen products also block UVA rays, which may contribute to the risk of melanoma.

Screening for skin cancer, whether by self-examination or by a health care provider, is controversial (Chapter 14). Many public health experts do not recommend screening for adults in the general population, but some organizations do. On the basis of the type and number of nevi, family history of melanoma, prior melanoma, and history of severe sunburns, clinicians can identify patients who are at high risk for melanoma and who may benefit from screening programs. In several population studies, screening has detected melanomas at an earlier, curable stage. Physicians, other health care providers, and the public should be educated regarding the early signs of melanoma and the need for prompt biopsy of a suspicious pigmented lesion.

Patients with clinically atypical nevi (see Fig. 210-2), particularly if they have a family history of melanoma, require a regular dermatologic surveillance program. Regular skin examinations should be performed every 6 to 12 months, preferably assisted by the use of serial photography.

Recent studies have focused on the impact of vitamin D levels on the risk for melanoma, and results have been conflicting. The potential health benefits of vitamin D continue to be evaluated, both in terms of melanoma prevention and risk.

BASAL AND SQUAMOUS CELL SKIN CANCER

Nonmelanoma skin cancer (basal cell cancer [BCC] and squamous cell skin cancer [SCC]) is the most common malignant disease in the United States. Although national statistics are imprecise, an estimated 900,000 to 1,200,000 of nonmelanoma skin cancers are diagnosed annually in the United States. SCC accounts for 20%, and most of the remainder are BCC. SCC is associated with a higher absolute mortality rate; most of the 2300 annual deaths from nonmelanoma skin cancer in the United States arise from this tumor.

EPIDEMIOLOGY

Overall, skin cancer incidence rates are rising because of increased recreational sun exposure, longer life expectancy, and depletion of the ozone layer. More than 99% of nonmelanoma skin cancers occur in whites. These skin cancers are most commonly seen in elderly persons, especially those with fair skin and long-standing sun exposure. However, nonmelanoma skin cancers are increasingly being seen in people in their 30s and 40s. The lifetime risk of developing BCC is 30%.

PATHOBIOLOGY

BCC arises from a pluripotential stem cell within the skin. Acquired mutations in the patched gene 1 *(PTCH1),* a tumor suppressor gene in the hedgehog signaling pathway, have been identified in cases of sporadic BCC. Sporadic BCC are also associated with mutations in the genes encoding p53 and ras.

SCC of the skin is a malignant disease of epidermal keratinocytes. Many such carcinomas are derived from actinic keratoses, a precursor that appears as a rough, scaly, often erythematous papule, which often is more apparent on palpation than on visual examination. Estimates of the likelihood of progression of actinic keratoses to squamous cell carcinoma range from 0.025% to as high as 20%. Mutations in the gene encoding the p53 protein and in the *RAS* oncogene have been found in both actinic keratoses and squamous cell carcinomas. Mutations in *p16* have also been reported in squamous cell carcinomas.

Risk Factors

The most important risk factor is exposure to UV radiation from sunlight. The most clearly established association is with UVB radiation, but increasing evidence suggests that UVA is probably carcinogenic as well (Chapter 19). The timing and pattern of sun exposure are associated with different types of skin cancer. In general, SCC is associated with cumulative sun exposure and occurs most frequently in areas maximally exposed to the sun (e.g., the face, back of hands, and forearms). Intermittent, intense exposure to the sun, particularly in childhood, is associated with an increased risk for BCC. Individuals who have fair skin, light-colored eyes, red hair, a tendency to burn rather than tan, and a history of severe sunburns are at increased risk for nonmelanoma skin cancers. Other risk factors, primarily for SCC, include chronic arsenic exposure, therapeutic radiation, chronic inflammatory skin conditions, psoralen plus UVA (PUVA) treatment for psoriasis and other diseases, and immunosuppression. Most cases in African American patients are associated with scarring or burns rather than UV exposure. Human papillomavirus infection (Chapter 381) has also been implicated in some SCCs, particularly in the autosomal dominant disorder epidermodysplasia verruciformis.

BCC can be seen in association with several conditions, including the basal cell nevus syndrome (also called nevoid basal cell carcinoma syndrome or Gorlin's syndrome), albinism, and xeroderma pigmentosum. The basal cell nevus syndrome is a rare autosomal dominant disorder caused by germline mutations in the patched gene *(PTCH).*

CLINICAL MANIFESTATIONS

Basal Cell Carcinoma

Approximately 90% of BCCs occur on sun-exposed areas such as the face, neck, ears, scalp, and arms. The nose is the most common site. Typical BCC appears as slowly growing, shiny, skin-colored to pink translucent papules with telangiectasia and a "pearly" rolled border (Fig. 210-6). As the tumor grows, the center may become ulcerated and bleed, although there is usually no associated pain or tenderness. BCC rarely metastasizes and is usually curable with a variety of treatments. Although the mortality rate is low, these cancers may result in significant morbidity owing to invasive local growth with potential disfigurement and destruction of skin, bone, and cartilage. Clinical trials with inhibitors of the hedgehog pathway for patients with advanced BCC are under way, with very encouraging clinical activity demonstrated.

Squamous Cell Carcinoma

This type of skin cancer usually appears on areas of skin that are heavily damaged by sun exposure. The most common sites include the head or neck, back, forearms, and dorsum of the hand. Clinically, SCC occurs as a discrete scaly erythematous papule on an indurated base that can develop on normal-appearing skin or on an actinic keratosis (Fig. 210-7). The lesion may grow over time and may become ulcerated, itchy, painful, or bleeding. Keratoacanthoma is a variant that is characterized by rapid growth and a crateriform appearance with a central plug. Bowen's disease, or squamous cell carcinoma in situ, manifests as an erythematous, scaly, sharply defined plaque.

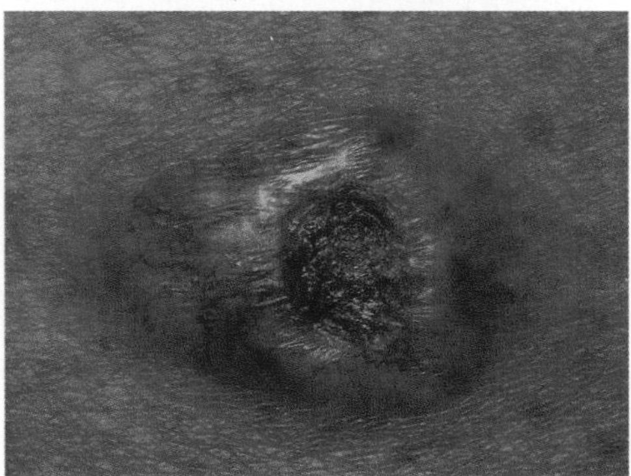

FIGURE 210-6. Basal cell carcinoma.

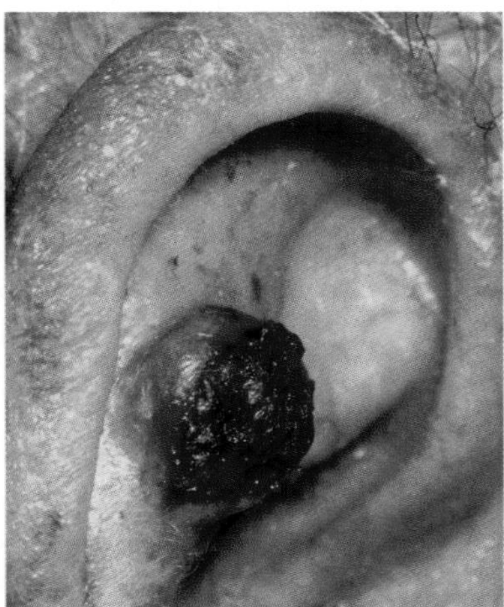

FIGURE 210-7. Squamous cell carcinoma of the skin.

Untreated SCC may cause significant local destruction. However, unlike BCC, SCC carries a 0.5 to 5% risk for metastasis. Higher-risk lesions are those that are larger than 2 cm, are moderately or poorly differentiated, have perineural involvement, or are located on the ear or the lip, arise in scars, or occur in immunosuppressed patients. Most metastases develop in regional lymph nodes, although metastases may also occur in lung, liver, brain, skin, or bone. For patients with lymph node metastases, the 5-year survival rate is less than 50%.

DIAGNOSIS

The diagnosis of BCC and SCC is frequently suspected by inspection alone, but histologic confirmation is usually indicated. Either a shave or a punch biopsy technique is acceptable (Chapter 444). Care should be taken to include the base of the lesion if a shave biopsy technique is used.

TREATMENT Rx

Basal Cell Carcinoma

BCCs are classified as low or high risk, based on their clinical features, location, and histology. Treatment options includes cryotherapy (liquid nitrogen), electrosurgery (i.e., curettage and electrodessication), topical treatment (i.e., 5-fluorouracil, photodynamic therapy, or imiquimod), surgical excision, Mohs' surgery, or radiation therapy. Mohs' microsurgery should be considered when treating recurrent cases; microscopically aggressive forms, such as the morpheaform subtype; lesions greater than 2 cm in greatest diameter; and tumors of the ears, eyelids, nose, nasolabial folds, and lips. Cure rates for BCC range between 90 and 99%.

Squamous Cell Carcinoma

As with BCC, SCC can also be cured by traditional surgical excision or Mohs' surgery, cryotherapy, topical therapies, and radiation therapy. Topical 5-fluorouracil, photodynamic therapy, or imiquimod have a role in the management of in situ squamous cell cancers. The optimal approach for a specific patient requires consideration of likelihood of the lesion recurring or metastatic potential, cosmetic factors, and the expertise of the treating physicians.

Mohs' micrographic surgery provides the lowest recurrence rate, with cure rates greater than 90%. Mohs' microsurgery is especially useful for recurrent tumors or lesions that have an increased risk of metastasis.

Follow-up

Patients with BCC and SCC require ongoing follow-up to detect local recurrences and to recognize new skin cancers. The likelihood of developing a second basal cell carcinoma or squamous cell carcinoma has been estimated to be 15% over 3 years. In addition, these patients have an increased risk of developing cutaneous melanoma. Patient education regarding modification of risk factors (i.e., sun exposure) is an important component of follow-up.

PREVENTION

Primary prevention strategies are aimed at reducing long-term sun exposure. Public education and patient education should encourage the regular use of sunscreens with a sun protection factor of 15 or greater, especially in childhood, and sun-protective clothing (e.g., a broad-brimmed hat). Avoidance of tanning parlors and minimizing of total sun exposure, especially to the midday sun, is recommended. The thinning of the ozone layer has been linked to increased UV radiation and increases in the incidence of nonmelanoma skin cancers. Currently, no evidence indicates that total body skin examination is effective at reducing mortality or morbidity from nonmelanoma skin cancer.

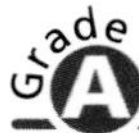

1. Thomas JM, Newton-Bishop J, A'Hern R, et al. Excision margins in high-risk malignant melanoma. *N Engl J Med.* 2004;350:757-766.
2. Morton DL, Thompson JF, Cochran AJ, et al. Sentinel-node biopsy or nodal observation in melanoma. *N Engl J Med.* 2006;355:1307-1317.
3. Eggermont AM, Suciu S, Santinami M, et al. Adjuvant therapy with pegylated interferon alfa-2b versus observation alone is resected stage III melanoma: final results of EORTC 18991, a randomised phase III trial. *Lancet.* 2008;372:117-126.
4. Hodi FS, O'Day SJ, McDermott DF, et al. Improved survival with ipilimumab in patients with metastatic melanoma. *N Engl J Med.* 2010;363:711-723.
5. Green AC, Williams GM, Logan V, et al. Reduced melanoma after regular sunscreen use: randomized trial follow-up. *J Clin Oncol.* 2011;29:257-263.

SUGGESTED READINGS

Bower MR, Scoggins CR, Martin RC 2nd, et al. Second primary melanomas: incidence and outcome. *Am Surg.* 2010;76:675-681. *About 2% of patients developed a second primary melanoma during a median follow-up of 5.5 years.*

Lin JS, Eder M, Weinmann S. Behavioral counseling to prevent skin cancer: a systematic review for the U.S. Preventive Services task force. *Ann Intern Med.* 2011;154:190-201. *Consensus guidelines recommending counseling to increase sun-protective behaviors.*

Madan V, Lear JT, Szeimies RM. Non-melanoma skin cancer. *Lancet.* 2010;375:673-685. *Concise review of recent advances.*

211 CANCER OF UNKNOWN PRIMARY ORIGIN

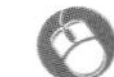

JOHN D. HAINSWORTH AND F. ANTHONY GRECO

DEFINITION

The first signs or symptoms of cancer are frequently the result of metastases to visceral or nodal sites. In most such patients, routine clinical evaluation with a comprehensive history, physical examination, complete blood cell count, screening chemistries, and directed radiologic studies based on specific symptoms or signs identifies the primary tumor. Patients who have no primary tumor located after this routine clinical evaluation are defined as having cancer of unknown primary origin. Further clinical and pathologic evaluation identifies the primary site in only a few patients, and approximately 80% never have a primary site identified during their subsequent clinical course.

EPIDEMIOLOGY

In patients whose primary site of cancer remains undetectable, the primary site has presumably remained small or, less likely, regressed spontaneously. Before the routine use of computed tomography (CT) or magnetic resonance imaging (MRI) for diagnosis, large autopsy series identified small primary sites of cancer in 85% of patients with previously unidentified primary tumors, usually in the pancreas, lung, and various other gastrointestinal sites; with the use of CT and MRI for diagnosis, however, primary sites are identified at autopsy in only 50 to 70% of patients.

Approximately 3% of all patients with cancer have metastatic disease without a known primary site; the annual incidence is approximately 50,000 to 60,000 cases in the United States. Cancer of unknown primary site occurs with approximately equal frequency in men and women, and it increases in incidence with advancing age.

DIAGNOSIS

The initial clinical and pathologic evaluation should focus on identifying a primary site, when possible, and on identifying patients for whom specific treatment is indicated. In most patients with cancer of unknown primary site, the diagnosis of advanced cancer is strongly suspected after the initial history and physical examination. A brief additional evaluation, including complete blood cell counts, chemistry profile, and CT of the chest and abdomen, should be performed. Any specific symptoms or signs should be evaluated with appropriate radiologic and endoscopic studies.

Biopsy

The diagnosis of metastatic cancer should be confirmed by biopsy of the most accessible metastatic lesion. Fine-needle aspiration may or may not provide sufficient material for optimal histologic examination and special pathologic procedures. If tissue is inadequate, a larger biopsy sample should be obtained so that all necessary stains and special studies can be performed.

The initial light microscopic evaluation identifies adenocarcinoma in approximately 60% of patients with cancer of unknown primary site. Other diagnoses obtained by initial light microscopy include poorly differentiated carcinoma (25%), squamous carcinoma (10%), and poorly differentiated neoplasm (inability to distinguish among carcinoma, lymphoma, melanoma, and sarcoma; 5%).

In patients with adenocarcinoma, it is seldom possible for the pathologist to determine a primary site by light microscopic characteristics or with additional pathologic techniques. Specific exceptions include immunoperoxidase staining for prostate-specific antigen (PSA), which is relatively specific for adenocarcinoma of the prostate (Chapter 207); for estrogen and progesterone receptors, which are suggestive of breast cancer (Chapter 204); and for leukocyte common antigen, which can identify non-Hodgkin's lymphoma (Chapter 191) as the primary tumor in up to 50% of patients with poorly differentiated neoplasms. Other diagnoses suggested by immunoperoxidase staining include neuroendocrine carcinomas, melanomas (Chapter 210), and sarcomas (Chapter 209). Electron microscopy should be considered when light microscopy and immunoperoxidase staining fail to identify the tumor, especially in young patients with anaplastic tumors; specific ultrastructural features may suggest neuroendocrine carcinoma (neurosecretory granules), melanoma (premelanosomes), and certain sarcomas.

Occasionally, detection of a tumor-specific chromosomal abnormality can provide a definitive diagnosis. Cancers with recognized specific chromosomal abnormalities include germ cell tumors (i12p; Chapter 206), peripheral neuroepithelioma and Ewing's tumor (t11;22; Chapter 208), and non-Hodgkin's lymphoma (Chapter 191). Chromosomal analysis should therefore be considered, especially in young men who have poorly differentiated mediastinal or retroperitoneal tumors and in whom other pathologic studies have been inconclusive.

Recently, specific gene expression profiles based on the tissue of origin have been identified for many tumor types. Several currently available multigene assays have 80 to 90% accuracy in determining the tissue of origin when performed on metastatic tissue in patients with tumors of known origin. The contribution of molecular profiling to the diagnosis and management of carcinoma of unknown primary site is still being defined; however, it is likely to

TABLE 211-1 RECOMMENDED EVALUATION FOLLOWING INITIAL LIGHT MICROSCOPIC DIAGNOSIS

DIAGNOSIS	CLINICAL EVALUATION*	SPECIAL PATHOLOGIC STUDIES
Adenocarcinoma (or poorly differentiated adenocarcinoma)	PET CT of chest, abdomen Men: serum PSA Women: mammogram Additional directed radiologic or endoscopic studies to evaluate abnormal symptoms, signs, laboratory values	Men: PSA stain Women: estrogen and progesterone receptor stains (if clinical features suggest metastatic breast cancer)
Poorly differentiated carcinoma	PET CT of chest, abdomen Serum hCG, AFP Additional directed radiologic or endoscopic studies to evaluate abnormal symptoms, signs, laboratory values	Immunoperoxidase staining Electron microscopy (if immunoperoxidase stains indeterminate)
Squamous carcinoma, cervical nodes	PET Direct laryngoscopy with visualization; biopsy of nasopharynx, pharynx, hypopharynx, larynx Fiberoptic bronchoscopy (if laryngoscopy is negative)	—
Squamous carcinoma, inguinal nodes	PET Complete examination of perineal area (including pelvic examination) Anoscopy Cystoscopy	—

*In addition to a history, physical examination, complete blood cell counts, chemistry profile, and chest radiograph.
AFP = α-fetoprotein; CT = computed tomography; hCG = human chorionic gonadotropin; PET = positron emission tomography; PSA = prostate-specific antigen.

have an important role in the future both in diagnosing the site of tumor origin and in allowing more site-specific therapy.

Search for the Primary Site

After completion of the brief, directed initial evaluation outlined previously, further diagnostic studies should be limited (Table 211-1). Positron emission tomography (PET) identifies a primary site and guides therapy in about one third of patients, so it should be obtained in all patients with an initially unknown primary tumor. By comparison, other routine radiologic and endoscopic evaluations of asymptomatic areas are not useful in identifying a primary site and therefore are not recommended. Levels of serum tumor markers, including carcinoembryonic antigen, CA-125, CA-19-9, and CA-15-3, are frequently increased in patients with carcinoma of unknown primary site; however, these elevations are nonspecific and should not be used to infer a primary site, even though they can be useful in monitoring response to treatment.

In all men with metastatic adenocarcinoma, serum PSA should be measured. Mammograms and breast MRI should be considered in women with metastatic adenocarcinoma, particularly if clinical features are consistent with metastatic breast cancer (e.g., axillary node involvement, pleural effusion, lytic or blastic bone metastases). In patients younger than 50 years with poorly differentiated carcinoma, serum human chorionic gonadotropin and α-fetoprotein levels should be measured. Patients with metastatic squamous carcinoma involving cervical lymph nodes should have a thorough endoscopic evaluation of the head and neck, including visualization of the structures from the nasopharynx to the larynx and biopsy of any suspicious areas (Chapter 196). Fiberoptic bronchoscopy should also be considered in patients who have low cervical adenopathy and in whom no head or neck primary site is established by endoscopic examination. In patients with metastatic squamous carcinoma involving inguinal lymph nodes, all perineal structures should be carefully inspected, including anoscopy, a urologic evaluation, and a pelvic examination in women.

TREATMENT Rx

Management of Specific Treatable Subsets

Because patients with cancer of unknown primary site have advanced disease, therapeutic nihilism has been common. However, several subsets of patients can benefit from specific treatment, and they can be identified on the basis of clinical and pathologic features (Table 211-2). These patients are important to recognize and treat appropriately, because some individuals in each group have the potential for long-term survival.

Adenocarcinoma

Women with Axillary Lymph Node Metastases

Metastatic breast cancer should be suspected in women who have axillary lymph node involvement with adenocarcinoma, particularly when other metastatic sites are not evident. In these patients, pathologic evaluation of the initial lymph node biopsy should include staining for estrogen and progesterone receptors and for HER-2 expression; elevated levels provide strong evidence for the diagnosis of breast cancer. When no other metastases are identified, these women should be treated as if they had stage II breast cancer, which is potentially curable with appropriate therapy (Chapter 204). Modified radical mastectomy identifies a breast primary site in 44 to 82% of women, even when the breast examination and mammographic findings are normal. Axillary lymph node dissection followed by radiation therapy to the breast appears to give results similar to those of mastectomy, although these two options for primary therapy have not been compared directly. Adjuvant systemic therapy should follow standard guidelines for the treatment of women with stage II breast cancer.

Women with Peritoneal Carcinomatosis

Adenocarcinoma involving the peritoneum in women usually originates from the ovary (Chapter 205), although carcinomas arising in the gastrointestinal tract or breast can occasionally produce this syndrome. However, diffuse peritoneal carcinomatosis occasionally occurs in women who have histologically normal ovaries or who have had previous bilateral oophorectomy. The peritoneum is frequently the only site of tumor involvement, and serum CA-125 levels are usually elevated. When histologic features suggest ovarian cancer, this syndrome has been called *peritoneal papillary serous carcinoma* or *primary extraovarian serous carcinoma.*

Even when the histologic features are not typical, women with adenocarcinoma of unknown primary site involving the peritoneum often have cancers with biologic characteristics similar to those of ovarian cancer (Chapter 205). Treatment of these patients should follow guidelines for stage III ovarian cancer. When feasible, a full laparotomy with maximal surgical cytoreduction should be performed, followed by combination chemotherapy with a taxane/platinum–containing regimen. Measurement of serial serum CA-125 levels provides an accurate assessment of the efficacy of treatment. A few of these patients may have complete responses and long-term survival, particularly when initial surgical cytoreduction leaves minimal residual disease. A similar syndrome of peritoneal carcinomatosis that is responsive to chemotherapy for ovarian cancer has occasionally been reported in men.

Men with Skeletal Metastases and/or Elevated Serum Prostate-Specific Antigen Levels

Metastatic prostate cancer (Chapter 207) should be suspected in men with adenocarcinoma predominantly involving bone, particularly if the metastases are blastic. An elevated serum PSA level or tumor immunostaining for PSA confirms the diagnosis of prostate cancer. Occasionally, men with adenocarcinoma of unknown primary site and patterns of metastasis unusual for prostate cancer (e.g., lung metastases, mediastinal lymph node metastases) are found to have elevated serum PSA levels. These patients should be treated according to guidelines for advanced prostate cancer. Androgen ablation produces excellent responses and substantial palliation in most patients.

Single Metastatic Lesion

Occasionally, a single metastatic lesion containing adenocarcinoma or poorly differentiated carcinoma is identified, and a complete evaluation reveals no other evidence of disease. Such presentations can include a single

TABLE 211-2 SPECIFIC PATIENT SUBSETS AND RECOMMENDED TREATMENT

Subset-Identifying Features		
HISTOLOGIC	**CLINICAL**	**TREATMENT RECOMMENDATIONS**
Adenocarcinoma	Women, isolated axillary adenopathy	Treat as stage II breast cancer
Adenocarcinoma	Women, peritoneal carcinomatosis (Occasionally men?)	Treat as stage III ovarian cancer
Adenocarcinoma	Men, elevated PSA and/or blastic bone metastases	Treat as advanced prostate cancer
Adenocarcinoma, poorly differentiated carcinoma	Single metastatic lesion	Definitive local therapy (resection and/or radiation therapy) with or without chemotherapy
Adenocarcinoma	Colon cancer profile	Treat as metastatic colorectal cancer
Squamous	Cervical adenopathy	Treat as locally advanced head or neck cancer
Squamous	Inguinal adenopathy	Definitive local therapy (node dissection with or without radiation therapy) with or without chemotherapy
Poorly differentiated carcinoma	Young men with midline tumor and/or elevated hCG, AFP	Treat as extragonadal germ cell tumor
Poorly differentiated carcinoma	Diverse clinical features	Empirical chemotherapy with paclitaxel, ,platinum, etoposide
Neuroendocrine carcinoma, poorly differentiated	Diverse clinical presentations	Treat with platinum, etoposide
Neuroendocrine carcinoma, well differentiated	Usually liver metastases	Treat as metastatic carcinoid tumor

AFP = α-fetoprotein; hCG = human chorionic gonadotropin; PSA = prostate-specific antigen.

lymph node or subcutaneous site or single lesions at various visceral sites, including bone, liver, lung, brain, and adrenal gland. The possibility of an unusual primary site mimicking a metastatic lesion should be considered (e.g., a subcutaneous nodule from a primary apocrine or sebaceous carcinoma rather than a metastasis), but this possibility can usually be excluded on the basis of clinical or pathologic features. PET is useful in excluding other metastatic lesions. For patients with only a single identifiable lesion, definitive local therapy is recommended, guided by the site of tumor involvement. Such therapy may include surgical resection, radiation therapy, or a combination of these modalities. Although most of these patients eventually develop other metastatic sites, a significant disease-free interval is often experienced, and local treatment provides substantial palliation. The role of systemic chemotherapy in addition to definitive local therapy is not well defined; younger patients with poorly differentiated carcinoma or poorly differentiated adenocarcinoma are often treated with a short course of a taxane/platinum–based regimen (see Empirical Chemotherapy).

Colon Cancer Profile

The accurate recognition of patients likely to respond to colon cancer regimens has become increasingly important as treatment for this cancer has improved substantially. A "colon cancer profile" has been defined and includes (1) metastases predominantly in the liver and/or peritoneum, (2) adenocarcinoma with histologic features typical of gastrointestinal origin, and (3) typical immunohistochemical staining that is CK20 positive, CK7 negative, and CDX-2 positive. Patients with this profile should be treated according to guidelines for metastatic colorectal cancer (Chapter 199).

Squamous Carcinoma

Cervical Adenopathy

Squamous carcinoma of unknown primary site is relatively uncommon. Most patients with this syndrome have involvement of cervical lymph nodes, usually in the upper or midcervical area. Often, patients with this syndrome are middle-aged or elderly and have a history of substantial tobacco or alcohol use or both. A primary site in the head and neck region should be suspected (Chapter 196); however, complete endoscopic evaluation fails to identify a primary site in approximately 15% of these patients. Even if other tests are negative, PET identifies a primary site in the head and neck region in approximately 25% of such patients and should be part of the initial evaluation.

Even when no primary site is identified, management of these patients should follow standard guidelines for the treatment of locally advanced squamous carcinoma arising in the head and neck. Many reports have documented long-term survival rates of 30 to 60% following definitive local treatment, which should include radiation therapy or combined radiation and cervical lymph node dissection. Outcome of treatment depends on the size and number of involved cervical lymph nodes. Concurrent chemotherapy and radiation therapy are now considered the standard treatment approach for patients with locally advanced head and neck cancers and should be considered in patients with multiple involved lymph nodes or nodes larger than 2 cm in diameter (Chapter 196).

Inguinal Adenopathy

Occasionally, metastatic squamous cancer is found in inguinal lymph nodes. In most of these patients, a primary site can be located in the perineal or anorectal area. For the occasional patient in whom no primary site is identified, long-term survival can result from local therapy with inguinal lymph node dissection, with or without radiation therapy. Recently, combined-modality treatment with concurrent chemotherapy and radiation therapy has improved cure rates in patients with several squamous cancers arising in this region (e.g., cervix, anus, bladder). Although data are incomplete, a reasonable approach is the addition of chemotherapy with a platinum/5-fluorouracil regimen, as described for locally advanced carcinoma of the cervix.

Poorly Differentiated Carcinoma

Extragonadal Germ Cell Cancer Syndrome

Young men with clinical features of extragonadal germ cell tumors, including tumors in the mediastinum or retroperitoneum or those associated with elevated serum levels of human chorionic gonadotropin or α-fetoprotein, should be treated according to guidelines for extragonadal germ cell tumors (Chapter 206). Some of these patients can be proved to have germ cell tumors by identifying an i12p chromosomal abnormality, even when the diagnosis is not possible with other standard pathologic techniques. Approximately 30 to 40% of these patients achieve complete responses and long-term survival following chemotherapy with cisplatin, etoposide, and bleomycin, as used for advanced germ cell tumors.

Anaplastic Lymphoma

An appropriate initial pathologic evaluation should identify most histologically atypical lymphomas. Occasionally, immunoperoxidase staining for leukocyte common antigen is negative or cannot be adequately performed in patients with anaplastic lymphoma. The disease in some of these patients can be recognized using other immunoperoxidase stains (e.g., Ki-1, CD-30) or molecular genetic analysis (detection of immunoglobulin gene rearrangements). All patients with lymphomas identified by special pathologic studies should be treated using standard guidelines for aggressive non-Hodgkin's lymphoma (Chapter 191).

Neuroendocrine Carcinoma

In approximately 10% of poorly differentiated carcinomas, neuroendocrine features are identified by either immunoperoxidase staining or electron microscopy. Treatment of these patients is discussed later (see Neuroendocrine Carcinoma).

Other Poorly Differentiated Carcinomas

In most patients with poorly differentiated carcinoma, there are no clinical or pathologic features that allow their assignment to one of the three preceding subsets. However, this heterogeneous group contains some patients whose carcinomas are highly sensitive to platinum-based chemotherapy. Clinical factors predictive of sensitivity to chemotherapy include site of tumor involvement (lymph nodes as compared with visceral metastases), fewer sites of metastatic disease, and younger age. In selected patients with one or more of these favorable clinical features, treatment with cisplatin-based chemotherapy can produce a greater than 60% response rate, and approximately 15% of patients remain free of disease more than 8 years after completing treatment. Therefore, a brief trial of empirical chemotherapy (see later) is recommended for all patients with poorly differentiated carcinoma, unless they are extremely debilitated at the time of diagnosis. Patients with highly sensitive tumors can be identified within the first 4 to 6 weeks of treatment, and ineffective treatment can be discontinued in the remainder.

Neuroendocrine Carcinoma

Poorly Differentiated Neuroendocrine Carcinoma or Small Cell Anaplastic Carcinoma

These high-grade neuroendocrine tumors are now reliably identified using widely available immunoperoxidase stains. Although the origin of these tumors remains unknown, they are often highly sensitive to combination chemotherapy; with platinum/etoposide chemotherapy, the overall response rate is about 75%, and 25% of patients have complete responses. In patients with locoregional disease, the addition of radiation therapy following chemotherapy is reasonable.

Low-Grade (Carcinoid-Type) Neuroendocrine Tumors

Occasionally, low-grade neuroendocrine tumors are found at a metastatic site. In almost all cases, the liver is the site of involvement, and the histologic features suggest a carcinoid (Chapter 240) or islet cell tumor of gastrointestinal origin (Chapter 201). Various clinical syndromes caused by the secretion of vasoactive peptides (e.g., serotonin, vasoactive intestinal peptide, gastrin) have been described. Like other carcinoid tumors, these tumors often have indolent biologic characteristics, and patients can frequently survive for several years despite multiple liver metastases. Unlike poorly differentiated neuroendocrine tumors, these tumors are relatively resistant to chemotherapy, and intensive combination regimens should usually be avoided. Management of these patients should follow guidelines for metastatic carcinoid tumors (Chapter 240) and may include the use of somatostatin analogues, local ablative procedures (e.g., surgical resection, radiofrequency ablation, chemoembolization), targeted agents (e.g., sunitinib, everolimus), or fluorouracil-based chemotherapy regimens.

Empirical Chemotherapy

Approximately 60 to 70% of patients with carcinoma of unknown primary site do not fit into any of these defined clinical subsets. In these patients, earlier reports of empirical chemotherapy were discouraging, with overall response rates of only 20 to 25% and short median survival times (5 to 7 months). The combination of paclitaxel (200 mg/m^2 IV on day 1) and carboplatin (AUC 6.0 IV on day 1), with or without etoposide (50 mg alternating with 100 mg PO on days 1 to 10), all repeated every 21 days for four courses, produces objective responses in 30 to 45% of patients, with median survival in the 9- to 12-month range. In addition, a few patients obtain a major benefit from treatment; the 2-year survival rate with taxane-containing regimens is 20 to 25%. Regimens containing gemcitabine and cisplatin have produced similar results. The most effective treatment is unknown because randomized comparisons are lacking in this area.

At present, patients with carcinoma of unknown primary site who have a reasonable performance status should be considered for an empirical trial of combination chemotherapy. Patients with responsive tumors can be identified after 4 to 6 weeks of treatment, and they should continue treatment for a standard 4- to 5-month course. Patients who do not respond to initial combination chemotherapy are unlikely to respond to further treatment; palliative care is appropriate in these patients (Chapter 3). For patients who have a poor performance status at the time of diagnosis, palliative care alone is an appropriate approach.

SUGGESTED READINGS

Cerezo L, Raboso E, Ballesteros AI. Unknown primary cancer of the head and neck: a multidisciplinary approach. *Clin Trans Oncol*. 2011;13:88-97. *Review*.

Greco FA, Spigel DR, Yardley DA, et al. Molecular profiling in unknown primary cancer: accuracy of tissue of origin prediction. *Oncologist*. 2010;15:500-506. *Molecular profiling correctly identified the primary site in 15 of 20 cases*.

Morris GJ, Greco FA, Hainsworth JD, et al. Cancer of unknown primary site. *Semin Oncol*. 2010;37:71-79. *Review*.

Pavlidis N, Briasoulis E, Pentheroudakis G; ESMO Guidelines Working Group. Cancers of unknown primary site: ESMO Clinical Practice Guidelines for diagnosis, treatment and follow-up. *Ann Oncol*. 2010;21:v228-v231. *Consensus guidelines*.

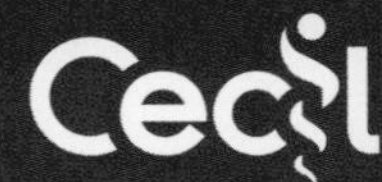

INDEX

Page numbers followed by "f" indicate figures, "t" indicate tables, and "b" indicate boxes. **Boldface** numbers refer to main discussions; **boldface** terms indicate supplemental online material.

B

E

F

G

J

K

O

U

V

W

X

Y

Z

GUIDE TO THE APPROACH TO COMMON SYMPTOMS, SIGNS, AND LABORATORY ABNORMALITIES

	CHAPTER	SPECIFIC TABLES OR FIGURES
MPTOMS		
nstitutional		
ver	288	Tables 288-1 to 288-8
igue	282	Table 282-3
or appetite	134	Table 134-1
ight loss	134, 226	Figure 134-4; Tables 134-4, 226-1, 226-2
esity	227	Figure 227-1
oring, sleep disturbances	100, 412	Tables 412-2, 412-4
ad, Eyes, Ears, Nose, Throat		
adache	405	Tables 405-1, 405-2
ual loss, transient	431, 432	Tables 431-1, 432-2
pain	434	Table 434-2
aring loss	436	Figure 436-1
ging in ears (tinnitus)	436	Figure 436-2
tigo	436	Figure 436-3
sal congestion, rhinitis or sneezing	259, 434	Figure 259-1, Table 259-2
ss of smell or taste	435	Table 435-1
y mouth	433	Table 433-7
e throat	437	Figure 437-2; Table 437-1
arseness	437	
rdiopulmonary		
est pain	50	Tables 50-2, 139-5, 139-6
nchitis	90	Table 90-1
rtness of breath	50	Figures 50-1, 83-3
pitations	50, 62	Figure 62-1; Tables 50-4, 62-2, 62-3
ziness	50, 62	Figure 62-1
cope	62	Figure 62-1; Tables 62-1, 62-2, 62-3
rdiac arrest	63	Figures 63-2, 63-3
ugh	83	Figure 83-1; Tables 83-1, 83-2
moptysis	83	Tables 83-4, 83-5
strointestinal		
usea and vomiting	134	Figure 134-5; Table 134-5
sphagia, odynophagia	134, 140	Table 134-1
matemesis	137, 156	Figure 137-3; Table 137-1
artburn/dyspepsia	134, 139, 140, 141	Figures 134-6, 139-3, 140-2; Table 141-1
dominal pain: Acute Chronic	 134, 144 134, 139	 Figure 134-1; Tables 134-2, 134-3, 144-1 Figure 134-2; Tables 134-2, 139-1
rrhea	139, 142	Figures 139-1, 142-2, 142-3, 142-4, 142-8
lena, blood in stool	137	Figures 137-3, 137-4, 137-6; Table 137-4
nstipation	138, 139	Figures 138-3, 138-5, 139-1; Table 138-2
al incontinence	147	Figure 147-3
al pain	147	
nitourinary		
suria	292, 293	Tables 292-4, 292-8, 293-2
quency	292	Tables 292-4
ontinence	25	Tables 25-1 to 25-3
nary obstruction	125	Tables 125-1 to 125-3
nal colic	128	Figure 128-3
ginal discharge	293	
nstrual irregularities	244	Figure 244-3; Tables 244-3, 244-4
nale infertility	244	Table 244-5
t flushes	248	Table 248-1
ctile dysfunction	242	
le infertility	242	Figures 242-8, 242-9; Table 242-7
otal mass	206	Figure 206-1

	CHAPTER	SPECIFIC TABLES OR FIGURES
Genital ulcers or warts	293	
Musculoskeletal		
Neck or back pain	407	Figures 407-4, 407-5; Tables 407-3 to 407-6
Painful joints	264	Table 264-2
Extremities		
Swollen feet, ankles, or legs		
Bilateral	50	Figure 50-8
Unilateral	81	Figure 81-2; Table 81-2
Claudication	79	Table 79-2
Acute limb ischemia	79	Figure 79-5; Table 79-3
Neurologic		
Weakness	403, 428, 429, 430	Tables 403-1, 428-2, 429-2, 429-4
Sensory loss	403, 428	Figure 428-1; Tables 428-1, 428-4 to 428-7
Memory loss	409	Figures 409-1, 409-2; Tables 409-1 to 409-6
Abnormal gait	403	Table 403-2
Seizures	410	Tables 410-1 to 410-6
Integumentary		
Abnormal bleeding	174	Table 174-1
Rash	444, 449	Figure 444-1; Tables 444-1 to 444-4, 449-4
Hives	261, 448	Figure 261-1; Tables 261-1, 448-1
Abnormal pigmentation	449	Table 449-2
Hirsutism and alopecia	450	Tables 261-1, 450-1, 450-2
Nail disorders	450	Table 450-3
SIGNS		
Vital Signs		
Fever	288, 289	Figure 289-1; Tables 288-1 to 288-8, 289-2
Hypothermia	7, 109	Table 109-4
Tachycardia/bradycardia	7, 62, 64, 65	Figures 62-2, 62-3; Tables 64-4, 65-2
Hypertension	67	Table 67-4
Hypotension/shock	7, 106	Figures 106-3, 108-3; Tables 106-1, 107-1, 107-2
Altered respiration	7, 86, 104	Tables 86-1, 86-2, 104-2
Head, Eyes, Ears, Nose, Throat		
Eye pain	431	Table 431-3
Red eye	431	Tables 431-4, 431-6
Dilated pupil	432	Figure 432-4
Nystagmus	432	Table 432-5
Papilledema	432	Table 432-2
Strabismus	432	Figure 432-6
Jaundice	149	Figure 149-3; Tables 149-1 to 149-3
Otitis	434	Table 434-2
Sinusitis	259, 434	Tables 259-3, 434-1
Oral ulcer	433	Tables 433-1 to 433-4
Salivary gland enlargement	433	Table 433-6
Neck		
Neck mass	196	Figure 196-3
Lymphadenopathy	171	Tables 171-1 to 171-6
Thyroid nodule	233	Figure 233-4
Thyromegaly/goiter	233	Figures 233-1, 233-3
Breast		
Breast mass	204	
Lungs		
Wheezes	83	Table 83-3
Cardiac		
Heart murmur or extra sounds	50	Figure 50-6; Tables 50-7, 50-8
Jugular venous distention	50	Table 50-6
Carotid pulse abnormalities	50	Figure 50-5